American Medical Association

Physicians dedicated to the health of America

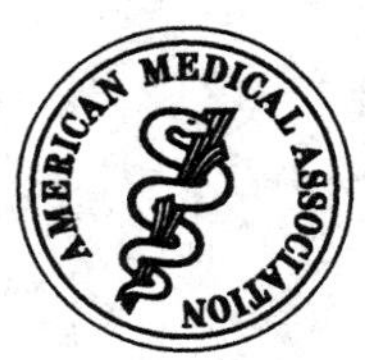

Drug Evaluations Annual 1995

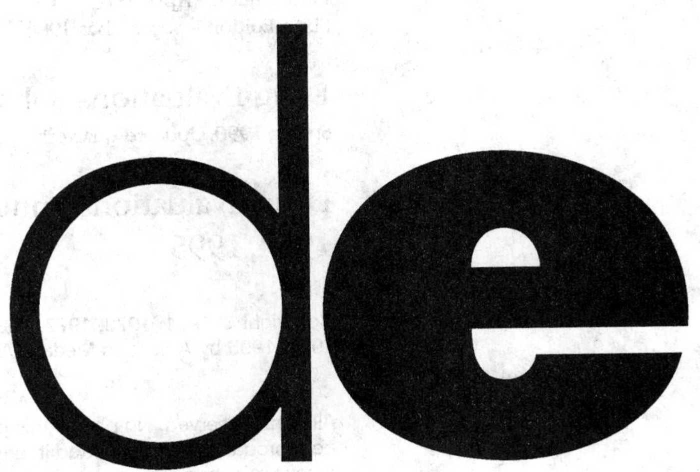

Prepared by the
Division of Drugs and Toxicology

AMA Drug Evaluations

First Edition - January 1971
Second Edition - September 1973
Third Edition - March 1977
Fourth Edition - February 1980
Fifth Edition - April 1983
Sixth Edition - September 1986

Drug Evaluations Subscription

Spring 1990. Updated quarterly.

Drug Evaluations Annual 1991, 1992, 1993, 1994, 1995

Printed in the United States of America.

Additional copies may be purchased from:
Order Dept. (OP 025595)
American Medical Association
For order information
call toll free 800 621-8335

ISBN 0-89970-677-0

FA16/5633:94-808:13M:12/94

Preface

DRUG EVALUATIONS (DE) is in its third decade of use. Its original goal is unaltered: To provide physicians and other health care professionals with up-to-date, unbiased, practical information—including comparative evaluations—on the clinical use of drugs.

DRUG EVALUATIONS has been available in several formats: (1) this hardbound version, which is published annually; (2) a CD-ROM format as part of the STAT!-Ref medical library (Teton Data Systems); and (3) a three-volume subscription product that contains updated chapters and a newsletter, *DE Monitor*, and is distributed four times yearly. The *DE Annual* and *DE Subscription* formats are now being discontinued with publication of this 1995 Annual edition, and the information in *DRUG EVALUATIONS* is to be merged with that in *United States Pharmacopeia Drug Information (USP DI)* to create one national drug and therapeutic database. The objective of this alliance is to provide a single authoritative, consistent, unbiased, and rapidly updated source of information for physicians and other healthcare professionals, as well as for caregivers and patients in private, institutional, managed care, and ambulatory settings. The integrated AMA DE/USP DI database will be maintained by the USP, and multiple print and electronic formats are being planned.

The following criteria for inclusion of therapeutic and individual drug information in *DE* remain applicable in this edition, and these objective criteria will continue to be employed in the AMA DE/USP DI database.

Evaluative Process: Chapters initially are prepared by the professional staff of the AMA Division of Drugs and Toxicology on the basis of the current scientific literature. Chapter drafts then are reviewed by distinguished expert consultants (more than 800 participate for the entire text) and by the medical staffs of the pharmaceutical manufacturers whose products are evaluated. Thus, the principles of therapeutics and comparative information contained in the introductions to the chapters and in the individual drug evaluations that follow represent a scientific contribution to the field of applied therapeutics that is based on a distillation of the current scientific literature plus the combined wisdom of many experienced clinicians.

Every effort has been made to include information on newly introduced drugs and dosage forms and on significant investigational drugs. In a project of this scope, however, the inadvertent omission of some products and the inclusion of others no longer marketed are inevitable.

The inclusion of a particular drug in *DE* does not imply endorsement by the American Medical Association. An evaluation may be favorable, unfavorable, or variable based on patient characteristics or other factors; it represents a statement of the expected value of the drug in all or selected subsets of patients but not its specific usefulness in a given patient. The limitations of use, adverse reactions, contraindications, precautions, or dosage should be considered for each patient.

The opinions expressed in this book, particularly on controversial matters, may differ from those in other sources. For other information, and even for varying points of view, the physician is encouraged to consult other sources of information on drugs.

Scope and Organization: *DE* is organized into sections and chapters that are based, insofar as possible, on therapeutic classifications. The five initial chapters contain general information on therapeutic principles, prescribing practices, adverse drug events, management of poisoning, and orphan drugs.

In most of the remaining chapters, the *introductory section* discusses basic pharmacologic information, principles of therapeutics, pathogenesis or diagnosis of disease to the extent deemed necessary to facilitate the use of drugs in patients, and comparative drug evaluations within a pharmacologic or therapeutic category. Drug selection is based principally on the nature and severity of the disease or disorder, the pharmacologic profile of each drug, and individual patient considerations. When possible, drugs of choice are recommended within the therapeutic or pharmacologic class. Discussions on the comparative merits of drugs are emphasized, and the utilization of tables for ready reference continues to increase. When appropriate, the relative merits of drug therapy and nondrug management are discussed.

The introductory section of each chapter is followed by *individual drug evaluations,* including selected mixtures. Occasionally, individual evaluations on newly approved drugs evaluated after the chapter was prepared appear at the end of the chapter. Information on investigational drugs and uses usually appears in the introductory section of the chapter; however, an individual evaluation of an investigational drug may appear if (1) approval is considered likely in the near future; (2) it is available under a Treatment IND protocol; or (3) it is of sufficient clinical importance to warrant such inclusion. Listings of evaluations on drugs marketed since the previous edition and on investigational drugs appear in the section on General Information.

Generally, titled headings in the evaluations include *Actions, Uses, Adverse Reactions and Precautions, Drug Interactions, Pharmacokinetics,* and *Dosage and Preparations.*

Discussion of diagnostic information and drug *action* generally is limited to that considered necessary to facilitate clinical drug use.

The indications cited in *official* labeling for a drug are limited to those that are approved by the FDA for purposes of marketing or advertising. The labeling does not constrain a physician's use of the drug for an unlabeled indication in individual patients so long as that use is based on rational scientific evidence or theory, expert medical judgment, or controlled clinical studies. Therefore, because indications approved for labeling by the FDA often lag behind both the world literature and medical practice or because the manufacturer has not submitted an application for a new use, both labeled and unlabeled (off-label) *uses* of drugs are evaluated in *DE*.

Information on *adverse reactions and precautions* and *drug interactions* usually represents that most essential for use of the drugs. Accordingly, rare, minor, or unconfirmed adverse reactions, precautions, or drug interactions are often omitted.

Pharmacokinetic information, especially that in the evaluations, continues to be emphasized. Information that is applicable to special patient populations (eg, pediatric, elderly, those with renal impairment) is included for many drugs. Therapeutic drug concentrations in blood, plasma, or serum are included when relevant.

The *dosage* information cited in *DE* falls within the ranges suggested by manufacturers and the FDA or that considered appropriate by other authorities. For many drugs, however, the correct dosage depends on the size, age, and condition of the patient; response to treatment; sensitivity or tolerance; and the possible synergistic or antagonistic effect of concomitant medication. If the clinical situation permits, establishment of the dose should be cautious and exploratory unless a wide margin of safety prevails. In either situation, the physician should remember that improper dosage of the proper drug is probably as common a cause of inadequate response or therapeutic failure as the use of an improper drug. Accordingly, many doses are stated as ranges, but even the limits of these ranges are not inviolable. The upper limits given for most ranges, however, do suggest that larger amounts either may increase the risks of toxicity beyond the degree ordinarily acceptable or may fail to provide a significant additional therapeutic effect. Similarly, the lower limits often indicate that smaller doses will not provide therapeutic effects for most patients. For a small number of drugs, no dosage is suggested.

The *preparations* listed for each drug, including those available generically, appear at the end of each evaluation. However, clinical experience often is limited to products of one or only a few manufacturers. Adequate clinical comparisons of all brands of the same drug are rarely available. For this reason, a valid comparison of brands usually is not possible or attempted. Although most drugs described in this volume are dispensed exclusively or principally by prescription, some are nonprescription and these are so indicated.

Considerable effort is made to provide up-to-date cited and selected *references* at the end of each chapter. Specific statements often are cited, but general references also may be included for additional information. Frequently, instead of listing all relevant primary references, secondary reviews in which original citations can be found are included.

The single comprehensive *index,* which includes drug names (both generic and trademark), indications, adverse reactions and interactions, and table and figure titles, continues to expand to improve access to the information.

We hope that *DRUG EVALUATIONS* has met the need for timely drug information for the medical profession and others who provide medical care. Suggestions for improving *DE*'s usefulness, particularly with the planned development of new product formats in the integration of information with USP DI, are welcome.

Contents

SYSTEMIC ANTI-INFECTIVES

TOPICAL ANTI-INFECTIVES

MISCELLANEOUS ANTI-INFECTIVES

ANTI-INFLAMMATORY, ANTIALLERGIC, AND IMMUNOLOGIC DRUGS

ONCOLYTIC DRUGS

OPHTHALMIC DRUGS

METABOLIC DRUGS

APPENDIX

Acknowledgments

Appreciation is expressed to the following members of the staff of the AMA Division of Drugs and Toxicology for their assistance in the preparation of *DRUG EVALUATIONS Annual 1995*:

STAFF AUTHORS:	John J. Ambre, M.D., Ph.D. Donald R. Bennett, M.D., Ph.D. Joseph W. Cranston, Jr., Ph.D. Barry D. Dickinson, Ph.D. Mary Ann McCann David C. Pang, Ph.D. Carol M. Proudfit, Ph.D., M.B.A. Norbert P. Rapoza, Ph.D. Jerome Seidenfeld, Ph.D. Steven J. Smith, Ph.D.

EDITORIAL AND TECHNICAL STAFF:

Editor-In-Chief:	Donald R. Bennett, M.D., Ph.D.
Project Manager:	Carol M. Proudfit, Ph.D., M.B.A.
Scientific Editor:	Barry D. Dickinson, Ph.D.
Managing Editor:	Beverly J. Rodgers
Associate Editors:	Sandra McVeigh Marsha Meyer
Assistant Editor:	Jerri M. Schwartz
Senior Research Associate:	Joaquin Chang
Consultant Coordinator:	Sandra Van Laan
Technical Associate:	Marilyn A. Mayo

REVIEWERS AND CONSULTANTS

The AMA Division of Drugs and Toxicology expresses its appreciation to the following individuals for their assistance in reviewing the content of *DRUG EVALUATIONS Annual 1995*:

Consultants

Walter H. Abelmann, M.D.
Charles F. Abildgaard, M.D.
Jonathan Abrams, M.D.
Steven B. Abramson, M.D.
Elias Abrutyn, M.D.
Lori J. Acuncius, M.D.
Rodney Adam, M.D.
Harold P. Adams, Jr., M.D.
David G. Addiss, M.D.
John Affronti, M.D.
Suhail Ahmad, M.D.
A. Leland Albright, M.D.
Louis M. Aledort, M.D.
James R. Allen, M.D.
Robert H. Allen, M.D.
Roy D. Altman, M.D.
Barbara M. Alving, M.D.
John C. Alverdy, M.D.
Raza Aly, Ph.D.
Richard D. Amelar, M.D.
Marvin Ament, M.D.
Elias Anaissie, M.D.
Betty Jane Anderson, J.D.
James W. Anderson, M.D.
Jeffrey L. Anderson, M.D.
Philip Anderson, M.D.
Richard J. Andrassy, M.D.
Thomas W. Andrews, M.D.
Vincent T. Andriole, M.D.
Jack E. Ansell, M.D.
Joseph H. Antin, M.D.
Lawrence J. Appel, M.D.
Frederick R. Appelbaum, M.D.
Allen I. Arieff, M.D.
Jenifer Aronoff
Wilbert S. Aronow, M.D.
Jeffrey Askanazi, M.D.
Martin Ast, M.D.
Arthur J. Atkinson, Jr., M.D.
William Atkinson, M.D.
Melissa A. Austin, Ph.D.
Michael J. Avram, Ph.D.
Bernard M. Babior, M.D., Ph.D.
David B. Badesch, M.D.
John D. Bagdade, M.D.
Laurence Baker, D.O.
Ross J. Baldessarini, M.D.
Edward D. Ball, M.D.
William Banner, Jr., M.D., Ph.D.
Robert Barbieri, M.D.
Adrian Barbul, M.D.
Ariel L. Barkan, M.D.
John G. Bartlett, M.D.
Doris G. Bartuska, M.D.
Michael Barza, M.D.
Robert C. Bast, Jr., M.D.
John H. Bauer, M.D.
Kenneth A. Bauer, M.D.
Jules Baum, M.D.
Harold E. Bays, M.D.
William T. Beaver, M.D.
William K. Becker, M.D.
Rodolfo Begue, M.D.
Robert B. Belshe, M.D.
Leslie Z. Benet, Ph.D.
Joel S. Bennett, M.D.
William M. Bennett, M.D.
Honorio Benzon, M.D.
Harold S. Berenson, M.D.
K. G. Berge, M.D.
Barbara J. Berger, M.D.
Nathan A. Berger, M.D.
Jonathan D. Berman, M.D., Ph.D.
I. Leonard Bernstein, M.D.
Jonathan A. Bernstein, M.D.
Richard E. Besinger, M.D.
Joseph Biederman, M.D.
Edwin L. Bierman, M.D.
David W. Bilheimer, M.D.
Henry J. Binder, M.D.
Alan L. Bisno, M.D.
Robert M. Black, M.D.
George L. Blackburn, M.D.
Paul A. Blake, M.D.
David H. Blankenhorn, M.D.
Martin J. Blaser, M.D.
Bruce R. Blazar, M.D.
Thomas P. Bleck, M.D.
E. Richard Blonsky, M.D.
Joseph R. Bloomer, M.D.
John Blundell, M.D.
Hooshang Bolooki, M.D.
Ruth A. Bolton, M.D.
Roger C. Bone, M.D.
Robert O. Bonow, M.D.
Ernest C. Borden, M.D.

Charles Bowden, M.D.
James Bowen, M.D.
Norman F. Boyd, M.D.
Samuel A. Bozzette, M.D.
Reagan H. Bradford, M.D.
Michael T. Brady, M.D.
William E. Brady, M.P.H.
Larry E. Bragg, M.D.
D. Craig Brater, M.D.
Glenn D. Braunstein, M.D.
George A. Bray, M.D.
Robert F. Breiman, M.D.
Kenneth R. Bridges, M.D.
David C. Brittain, M.D.
Claire V. Broome, M.D.
Ben H. Brouhard, M.D.
B. Greg Brown, M.D.
W. Virgil Brown, M.D.
Bruce H. Brundage, M.D.
Saul W. Brusilow, M.D.
Ralph T. Bryan, M.D.
Henry Buchwald, M.D., Ph.D.
Ronald M. Burde, M.D.
Julie E. Buring, ScD.
Gregory L. Burke, M.D.
William Busse, M.D.
John M. Butitta, M.D.
Terri M. Byrd, M.D.
John A. Cairns, M.D.
David H. Calhoun, Ph.D.
Robert M. Califf, M.D.
Paul L. Canner, Ph.D.
Louis R. Cantilena, Jr., M.D., Ph.D.
Louis R. Caplan, M.D.
Steve N. Caritis, M.D.
Ralph Carmel, M.D.
Paul C. Carpenter, M.D.
H. F. Carvajal, M.D.
William P. Castelli, M.D.
Peter Cassileth, M.D.
Kenneth Castro, M.D.
Dwight Cavanagh, M.D., Ph.D.
David R. Cave, M.D.
Frank B. Cerra, M.D.
Bruce A. Chabner, M.D.
Robert Chen, M.D.
Ronald A. Chez, M.D.
George C. Y. Chiou, Ph.D.
Anthony W. Chow, M.D.
Michael Cleman, M.D.
Mary Lou Clements, M.D.
Beverly Clevidence, M.D.
Ronald I. Clyman, M.D.
Margaret M. Cobb, M.D.
Yank D. Coble, Jr., M.D.
Stephen Cochi, M.D.
Jay D. Coffman, M.D.
Bruce E. Cohan, M.D.
Elizabeth Cohen, M.D.
Harvey J. Cohen, M.D., Ph.D.
Clair I. Colvin, Ph.D.
Michael Colvin, M.D.
Philip C. Comp, M.D., Ph.D.
Elizabeth B. Connell, M.D.
William E. Connor, M.D.
Alan J. Cooper, M.D.
Gerald R. Cooper, M.D., Ph.D.
Jacquelynne P. Corey, M.D.
Lawrence Corey, M.D.
Roger C. Cornell, M.D.
Michael L. Corrado, M.D.
Gregory H. Corsan, M.D.
Jean A. Courtner, M.D.
Diane D. Cousins
William A. Craig, M.D.
Michael H. Criqui, M.D.
William R. Crom, Pharm.D.
Philip E. Cryer, M.D.
Ronald G. Crystal, M.D.
Jeffrey Cummings, M.D.
Burke A. Cunha, M.D.
Leona Cuttler, M.D.
Adnan S. Dajani, M.D.
John M. Daly, M.D.
Gilbert H. Daniels, M.D.
David R. Dantzker, M.D.
William H. Daughaday, M.D.
Mayer B. Davidson, M.D.
Michael H. Davidson, M.D., M.P.H.
Gary L. Davis, M.D.
John Davis, M.D.
Leslie J. DeGroot, M.D.
Vincent A. DeLeo, M.D.
E. Patchen Dellinger, M.D.
Gregory J. Del Zoppo, M.D.
Robert H. Demling, M.D.
Robert J. Desnick, M.D., Ph.D.
Roz Dewart
Seymour Diamond, M.D.
Adrian M. DiBesceglie, M.D.
Gordon M. Dickinson, M.D.
Rodger L. Dierker, Pharm.D.
Jack A. DiPalma, M.D.
Joseph DiPiro, Pharm.D.
Richard L. Dobson, M.D.
W. Edwin Dodson, M.D.
Peter C. Donshik, M.D.
John M. Douglas, Jr., M.D.
R. Gordon Douglas, Jr., M.D.
David A. Drachman, M.D.
Darlene M. Dreon, M.S., M.P.H.
Robert C. Drews, M.D.
Thomas D. DuBose, Jr., M.D.
David K. Dueker, M.D.
Carlos A. Dujovne, M.D.
Brian O. L. Duke, M.D.
Herbert L. DuPont, M.D.
Anna Durbin, M.D.

Paul J. Edelson, M.D.
Randall S. Edson, M.D.
J. Edwards, M.D.
Merrill J. Egorin, M.D.
Lawrence H. Einhorn, M.D.
George W. Ellison, M.D.
Ivor A. Emanuel, M.D.
Mary G. Enig, Ph.D.
Robert H. K. Eng, M.D.
Andrew Engel, M.D.
Jay S. Epstein, M.D.
James O. Ertle, M.D.
Joseph W. Eschbach, M.D.
Bruce Ettinger, M.D.
David S. Ettinger, M.D.
Walter H. Ettinger, Jr., M.D.
Gary Euler, M.D.
Richard G. Fadal, M.D.
Gerald Faich, M.D.
Constantine J. Falliers, M.D.
Thomas A. Farrell, M.D.
Karim A. Fawaz, M.D.
David S. Fedson, M.D.
Laura Fehrs, M.D.
Judith Feinberg, M.D.
Arthur M. Feldman, M.D., Ph.D.
Robert L. Feldman, M.D.
Carlos M. Ferrario, M.D.
Sydney M. Finegold, M.D.
Mieczyslaw Finster, M.D.
Michael C. Fiore, M.D., M.P.H.
Josef E. Fischer, M.D.
Thomas J. Fischer, M.D.
Marvin A. Fishman, M.D.
John D. Folts, M.D.
John S. Fordtran, M.D.
C. Stephen Foster, M.D.
Charles W. Francis, M.D.
Gary S. Francis, M.D.
Elliot Francke, M.D.
Gary E. Fraser, Ph.D.
Joseph C. Fratantoni, M.D.
Michael D. Freed, M.D.
Ruta Freimanis, Pharm.D.
Ilona J. Frieden, M.D.
William Frishman, M.D.
Edward D. Frohlich, M.D.
Lawrence A. Frohman, M.D.
Donald E. Fry, M.D.
Valentin Fuster, M.D.
John N. Galgiani, M.D.
Abhimanyu Garg, M.D.
Irene Gavras, M.D.
Gerald Gebhart, Ph.D.
Layne O. Gentry, M.D.
Jeffrey S. Gerdes, M.D.
Anne A. Gershon, M.D.
Samuel Gershon, M.D.
Welton M. Gersony, M.D.
Mihai Gheorghiade, M.D.
Milo Gibaldi, Ph.D.
Samuel S. Gidding, M.D.
Ray W. Gifford, Jr., M.D.
Mark R. Gilbert, M.D.
J. Christian Gillin, M.D.
Henry N. Ginsberg, M.D.
Richard M. Glass, M.D.
David B. Glasser, M.D.
Alexander Glassman, M.D.
William M. Glazer, M.D.
Charles J. Glueck, M.D.
Christopher Goetz, M.D.
Anne Carol Goldberg, M.D.
M. R. Goldberg, M.D.
Stephen E. Goldfinger, M.D.
Steven Goldman, M.D.
Ellie J.C. Goldstein, M.D.
Michael Goldstein, M.D.
Robert A. Goldstein, M.D., Ph.D.
Robert E. Goldstein, M.D.
Sidney Goldstein, M.D.
Donald E. Goodkin, M.D.
John F. Goodwin, M.D.
Marshall P. Goren, M.D.
Glenn J. Gormley, M.D.
Stephen S. Gottlieb, M.D.
Antonio M. Gotto, M.D., DPhil
Steven A. Gould, M.D.
Mark Grabowsky, M.D.
Thomas B. Graboys, M.D.
David Y. Graham, M.D.
Thomas P. Graham, Jr., M.D.
David S. Gray, M.D.
David Green, M.D.
Peter L. Greenberg, M.D.
Richard N. Greenberg, M.D.
Paul A. Greenberger, M.D.
John H. Greist, M.D.
David A. Grimes, M.D.
Stephen C. Groft, Pharm.D.
Scott M. Grundy, M.D., Ph.D.
Duane J. Gubler, Sc.D.
Richard L. Guerrant, M.D.
Philip Gunby
Rolf M. Gunnar, M.D.
Andrzej Gutkowski
Stephen Hadler, M.D.
Marlene E. Haffner, M.D.
Jerome A. Halperin, M.P.H.
Robert N. Hamburger, M.D.
Margaret Hammerschlag, M.D.
Charles B. Hammond, M.D.
M. Hamosh, M.D.
Stephen B. Hanauer, M.D.
H. Hunter Handsfield, M.D.
Arthur F. Haney, M.D.
Laurence A. Harker, M.D.
Edward D. Harris, Jr., M.D.

Barry Jay Hartman, M.D.
Charles Haskell, M.D.
Paul J. Hesketh, M.D.
Herbert A. Haupt, M.D.
Richard J. Havel, M.D.
Robert H. Hayashi, M.D.
Frederick G. Hayden, M.D.
William R. Hazzard, M.D.
William C. Heird, M.D.
William M. Heller, Ph.D.
Richard A. Helms, Pharm.D.
David L. Hemsell, M.D.
Leslie Hendeles, Pharm.D.
Charles H. Hennekens, M.D.
Jack E. Henningfield, Ph.D.
Thomas K. Henthorn, M.D.
Paul E. Hermans, M.D.
Harry W. Herr, M.D.
Michael S. Hershfield, M.D.
Barbara L. Herwaldt, M.D.
Paul J. Hesketh, M.D.
Michael A. Heymann, M.D.
Steven B. Heymsfield, M.D.
William R. Hiatt, M.D.
Eve Juliet Higginbotham, M.D.
Jack Hirsh, M.D.
Basil I. Hirschowitz, M.D.
Ronald A. Hoffman, M.D.
Alan F. Hofmann, M.D.
Judith Hochman, M.D.
Marika J. Hohol, M.D.
Paul V. Holland, M.D.
Norman K. Hollenberg, M.D., Ph.D.
William J. Holloway, M.D.
Victoria Holt, Ph.D.
David C. Hooper, M.D.
Paul N. Hopkins, M.D.
P. Ann Hoppe
Benson J. Horowitz, M.D.
C. Robert Horsburgh, Jr., M.D.
Robert H. Howland, M.D.
Richard C. Hubbard, M.D.
Robin E. Huebner, M.D.
George R. Huggins, M.D.
John R. Hughes, M.D.
Walter T. Hughes, M.D.
Christine E. Huls, Pharm.D.
Donald B. Hunninghake, M.D.
Lawrence M. Hurvitz, M.D.
Richard S. Hurwitz, M.D.
J. Thomas Hutton, M.D.
D. Roger Illingworth, M.D., Ph.D.
John H. Ip, M.D.
Richard S. Irwin, M.D.
Jon I. Isenberg, M.D.
Douglas H. Israel, M.D.
David R. Jacobs, Jr., Ph.D.
Robert R. Jacobson, M.D., Ph.D.
Israeli A. Jaffe, M.D.
R. L. Jamison, M.D.
Henry D. Jampel, M.D.
Joseph Jankovic, M.D.
Michael Jastremski, M.D.
Manucher J. Javid, M.D.
Michael A. Jenike, M.D.
John W. Jenne, M.D.
G.L. Jensen, M.D.
Raphael Jewelewicz, M.D.
Cynda A. Johnson, M.D.
Greg Johnson, M.D.
Jonas T. Johnson, M.D.
Joyce Johnson, D.O., M.A.
Keith W. Johnson, R.Ph.
Judith K. Jones, M.D., Ph.D.
Franklyn N. Judson, M.D.
Stevo Julius, M.D.
Dennis D. Juranek, D.V.M.
Allen B. Kaiser, M.D.
Edward L. Kaplan, M.D.
Marshall M. Kaplan, M.D.
Norman M. Kaplan, M.D.
Selna Kaplan, M.D., Ph.D.
John E. Kasik, M.D., Ph.D.
Ralph E. Kauffman, M.D.
Todd B. Kaye, M.D.
Alan P. Kendal, M.D.
B. J. Kennedy, M.D.
Dianne Kennedy, R.Ph.
Paul A. Keown, M.D.
Craig M. Kessler, M.D.
Jay S. Keystone, M.D.
Janardan D. Khandekar, M.D.
Dr. Khin-Maung-U
Charles Kilo, M.D.
Charles H. King, M.D.
Spencer B. King III, M.D.
Joseph B. Kirsner, M.D., Ph.D.
Albert S. Klainer, M.D.
George G. Klee, M.D., Ph.D.
Michael Kleerekoper, M.D.
Harvey G. Klein, M.D.
Jerome O. Klein, M.D.
Lloyd W. Klein, M.D.
W. Peter Klinke, M.D.
Charles Kochakian, Ph.D.
Emre Kokmen, M.D.
William Koller, M.D.
Anthony L. Komaroff, M.D.
Winston Koo, M.D.
Burton Korelitz, M.D.
John B. Kostis, M.D.
Peter Kowey, M.D.
Harry B. Kram, M.D.
Margot S. Kruskall, M.D.
Howard E. Kulin, M.D.
Calvin M. Kunin, M.D.
Roger Kurlan, M.D.
Hau C. Kwaan, M.D.

Peter O. Kwiterovich, Jr., M.D.
Stephen LaFranchi, M.D.
Peter Lakatos, M.D.
Charles R. Lambert, M.D., Ph.D.
Anthony E. Lang, M.D.
Craig B. Langman, M.D.
Allan M. Lansing, M.D., Ph.D.
John C. LaRosa, M.D.
Elaine Larson, R.N., Ph.D.
Paul O. Larson, M.D.
Jonathan H. Lass, M.D.
Louisa Laue, M.D.
Carl J. Lavie, M.D.
Frank A. Lederle, M.D.
William J. Ledger, M.D.
Peter A. Lee, M.D., Ph.D.
William Lee, M.D.
Howard M. Leibowitz, M.D.
Ilo Leppik, M.D.
Robert L. Lesser, M.D.
Stuart Levin, M.D.
Donald P. Levine, M.D.
Joel S. Levine, M.D.
Steven R. Levine, M.D.
David C. Lewis, M.D.
Jeffrey Lieberman, M.D.
Shari Lieberman, Ph.D.
John J. Lima, Pharm.D.
Michael B. Limberg, M.D.
Mary Lou Lindegren, M.D.
John Lindenbaum, M.D.
Scott M. Lippman, M.D.
Larry I. Lipshultz, M.D.
John D. Lloyd-Still, M.D.
Charles L. Loprinzi, M.D.
Joseph Loscalzo, M.D., Ph.D.
Michael T. Lotze, M.D.
Richard R. Love, M.D.
Franklin C. Lowe, M.D.
David T. Lowenthal, M.D., Ph.D.
Tom F. Lue, M.D.
Jeanne M. Lusher, M.D.
Catherine M. MacLeod, M.D.
Anne-Marie Maddox, M.D.
Howard I. Maibach, M.D.
Mark A. Malangoni, M.D.
Laxmaiah Manchikanti, M.D.
Gerald L. Mandell, M.D.
Andrea Manni, M.D.
Lyndon E. Mansfield, M.D.
Michael J. Manyak, M.D.
Marsha Marcus, Ph.D.
Harold S. Margolis, M.D.
Stephen Marder, M.D.
Victor J. Marder, M.D.
Maurie Markman, M.D.
James Marsh, M.D.
John B. Marshall, M.D.
David H. Martin, M.D.
Henry Masur, M.D.
Barry J. Materson, M.D.
James B. McAuley, M.D.
Daniel J. McCarty, M.D.
H. Juhling McClung, M.D.
John A. McCulloch, M.D.
Edward J. McGuire, M.D.
Charles R. McKay, M.D.
M. M. Meguid, M.D.
David R. Meldrum, M.D.
Shlomo Melmed, M.D.
Victor D. Menashe, M.D.
Wallace B. Mendelson, M.D.
Jay E. Menitove, M.D.
John Merrill, M.D.
T. Allen Merritt, M.D.
Gregory J. Mertz, M.D.
Franz H. Messerli, M.D.
Boyd E. Metzger, M.D.
Francois Meyer, M.D., ScD.
Walter J. Meyer III, M.D.
Abbey S. Meyers
Burt R. Meyers, M.D.
Frederick J. Meyers, M.D.
Jay M. Meythaler, M.D.
Kenneth Miller, M.D.
Lucinda G. Miller, Pharm.D.
Myron Miller, M.D.
Richard A. Miller, M.D.
Sohrab Mobarhan, M.D.
Robert C. Moellering, Jr., M.D.
Kamran S. Moghissi, M.D.
Bartly J. Mondino, M.D.
Ernest E. Moore, M.D.
Neil C. Moran, M.D.
Gary R. Morrow, Ph.D.
Edward J. Mortimer, Jr., M.D.
Joanne E. Mortimer, M.D.
Marvin Moser, M.D.
Deane F. Mosher, M.D.
John Mullen
Gregory R. Mundy, M.D.
Michael B. Murphy, M.D.
Scott Murphy, M.D.
Thomas F. Myers, M.D.
Robert M. Naclerio, M.D.
Donald J. Nalebuff, M.D.
Neal Nathanson, M.D.
Paul A. Nausieda, M.D.
Kenneth H. Neldner, M.D.
John D. Nelson, M.D.
John Nemunaitis, M.D.
Paul M. Ness, M.D.
Harold C. Neu, M.D.
Eric D. Newman, M.D.
John H. Newman, M.D.
Ronald Lee Nichols, M.D.
Jennifer R. Niebyl, M.D.
Andrew A. Nierenberg, M.D.

Stuart L. Nightingale, M.D.
Carl W. Norden, M.D.
Russell Noyes, M.D.
John Gordon Nutt, M.D.
William Nyhan, M.D., Ph.D.
Richard J. O'Brien, M.D.
Susan O'Donoghue, M.D.
Edward J. O'Connell, M.D.
Peter J. O'Dwyer, M.D.
Maria-Teresa Olivari, M.D.
Elise Olsen, M.D.
Walter A. Orenstein, M.D.
Avrin M. Overbach, M.D.
Robert Ozols, M.D.
Harold I. Palevsky, M.D.
Stephen J. Pancoast, M.D.
Eugene Pantuck, M.D.
Vasilios Papademetriou, M.D.
Lawrence C. Parish, M.D.
Michael F. Parry, M.D.
Madhu A. Pathak, M.B., Ph.D.
Mary Elaine Patrinos, M.D.
Wolfgang Patsch, M.D.
Steven M. Paul, M.D.
Harold E. Paulus
Ronald G. Pearl, M.D.
Thomas A. Pearson, M.D., Ph.D.
John M. Pellock, M.D.
Richard Penn, M.D.
Mark Peppercorn, M.D.
Peter L. Perrine, M.D., M.P.H.
Ora Hirsch Pescovitz, M.D.
Georges Peter, M.D.
John C. Petricciani, M.D.
Thomas L. Petty, M.D.
Marc A. Pfeffer, M.D., Ph.D.
John P. Phair, M.D.
Larry K. Pickering, M.D.
Bertram Pitt, M.D.
Hiram C. Polk, M.D.
Ronald E. Polk, Ph.D.
George H. Pollock, M.D.
James L. Pool, M.D.
A. T. Porter, M.D.
Russell K. Portenoy, M.D.
Kathleen I. Pritchard, M.D.
Charles G. Prober, M.D.
Richard Quintiliani, M.D.
Ralph H. Raasch, Pharm.D.
Lawrence G. Raisz, M.D.
Salvatore Raiti, M.D.
Andres A. Ramos, M.D.
Samuel I. Rapaport, M.D.
Neil H. Raskin, M.D.
James E. Rasmussen, M.D.
Eddie Reed, M.D.
Jane M. Rees, M.S., R.D.
Theobald Reich, M.D.
Lee B. Reichman, M.D., M.P.H.
Richard C. Reichman, M.D.
Marcus M. Reidenberg, M.D.
John R. Reigart, M.D.
Michael F. Rein, M.D.
Neil Resnick, M.D.
Shereif Rezkalla, M.D.
Peter H. Rheinstein, M.D., J.D.
Stuart Rich, M.D.
Gail Richards, M.D.
Donald W. Richardson, M.D.
Joel E. Richter, M.D.
Matthew Riddle, Jr., M.D.
Paul M. Ridker, M.D.
Robert J. Roberts, M.D., Ph.D.
David Robertson, M.D.
Ralph G. Robinson, M.D.
Allan R. Ronald, M.D.
Allen W. Root, M.D.
Franz W. Rosa, M.D., M.P.H.
Leslie Rose, M.D.
Alan H. Rosenbaum, M.D.
Jerrold F. Rosenbaum, M.D.
Robert L. Rosenfield, M.D.
Douglas S. Ross, M.D.
Sanford H. Roth, M.D.
Thomas Roth, Ph.D.
Lewis P. Rowland, M.D.
Peter Roy-Byrne, M.D.
Lewis J. Rubin, M.D.
Ross N. Rubin, J.D.
Cheryl Ruble, M.D.
Stephen G. Ruby, M.D.
T. Donald Rucker, Ph.D.
Lorne A. Runge, M.D.
Allan J. Ryan, M.D.
Sheila M. Ryan, M.D.
R. Bradley Sack, M.D.
Gerald Salen, M.D.
Daniel R. Salomon, M.D.
Mary Samuels, M.D.
Peter Sand, M.D.
W. Eugene Sanders, M.D.
Wayne Sandler, M.D., Ph.D.
Jay P. Sanford, M.D.
Grannum R. Sant, M.D.
Joel R. Saper, M.D.
Felix A Sarubbi, M.D.
Richard J. Sassetti, M.D.
Seddon R. Savage, M.D.
Ernst J. Schaefer, M.D.
Saul Schaefer, M.D.
Anthony J. Schaeffer, M.D.
Gary L. Schaer, M.D.
Peter M. Schantz, V.M.D, Ph.D.
Martin B. Scharf, Ph.D.
Irwin J. Schatz, M.D.
Gisela F. Schecter, M.D., M.P.H.
Oliver Schein, M.D.
Charles Schiffer, M.D.

Joan H. Schiller, M.D.
Richard L. Schilsky, M.D.
Stephen C. Schimpff, M.D.
Barton D. Schmitt, M.D.
David E. Schteingart, M.D.
Harold Schulman, M.D.
H. Ralph Schumacher, Jr., M.D.
Bernard Schwartz, M.D.
Ira K. Schwartz, M.D.
Curtis L. Scribner, M.D.
Jack E. Sebben, M.D.
Demetrios S. Sgoutas, Ph.D.
Colin A. Shanks, M.D.
Samuel Shapiro, M.D.
Leslie R. Sheeler, M.D.
Ethan M. Shevach, M.D.
Andrew Shrake, Ph.D.
Eva P. Shronts, R.D.
Stanford T. Shulman, M.D.
Edward B. Silberstein, M.D.
David E. Silverstone, M.D.
Trevor Silverstone, M.D.
Tommy C. Sim, M.D.
Lee S. Simon, M.D.
Patricia Simone, M.D.
F. Estelle R. Simons, M.D.
Frederick R. Singer, M.D.
Michael D. Sitrin, M.D.
Arthur Skarin, M.D.
Boris Skurkovich, M.D.
Gregory L. Skuta, M.D.
Jay S. Skyler, M.D.
Richard Smiley, M.D., Ph.D.
Edgar B. Smith, M.D.
Laurie Smith, M.D.
Leon G. Smith, M.D.
O. Carter Snead III, M.D.
David R. Snydman, M.D.
Jack D. Sobel, M.D.
Glen D. Solomon, M.D.
Lawrence M. Solomon, M.D.
Seymour Solomon, M.D.
Edmund H. Sonnenblick, M.D.
George Sopko, M.D.
Nicholas A. Soter, M.D.
Sheldon L. Spector, M.D.
Harrison C. Spencer, M.D., M.P.H.
K. B. Sperling, M.D.
Leon Speroff, M.D.
Jerry L. Spivak, M.D.
Walter E. Stamm, M.D.
Meir J. Stampfer, M.D., Ph.D.
Harold C. Standiford, M.D.
Walter J. Stark, M.D.
Thomas E. Starzl, M.D., Ph.D.
Russell W. Steele, M.D.
Linda C. Stehling, M.D.
C. A. Stein, M.D., Ph.D.
Roger F. Steinert, M.D.
W. Jack Stelmach, M.D.
George A. Stern, M.D.
John J. Stern, M.D.
Robert S. Stern, M.D.
Paul Sternberg, Jr., M.D.
Irmin Sternlieb, M.D.
Richard H. Sterns, M.D.
John Stewart, M.D.
Gary L. Stiles, M.D.
Neil J. Stone, M.D.
D. E. Strandness, Jr., M.D.
Charles W. Stratton, M.D.
Michael B. Strauss, M.D.
Richard H. Strauss, M.D.
Peter Strebel, M.D.
Ray Strikas, M.D.
Alan M. Sugar, M.D.
Martin I. Surks, M.D.
Gordon L. Sussman, M.D.
Roland Sutter, M.D.
Wendy S. Swails, R.D.
Richard L. Sweet, M.D.
Debra J. Szeluga, Ph.D., R.D.
L. Ann Tanner, M.P.H., R.Ph.
David Taplin, M.D.
Ira N. Targoff, M.D.
Andrew L. Taylor, M.D.
Sam S. Thatcher, M.D., Ph.D.
Theoharid C. Theoharides, M.D.
Pierre Theroux, M.D.
Jess G. Thoene, M.D.
Angus W. Thomson, Ph.D.
Frank K. Thorp, M.D.
Douglas M. Tollefsen, M.D., Ph.D.
Gary D. Tollefson, M.D., Ph.D.
Eric J. Topol, M.D.
Philip P. Toskes, M.D.
William J. Tremaine, M.D.
Kenneth F. Trofatter, Jr., M.D., Ph.D.
B. Todd Troost, M.D.
Allan S. Troupin, M.D.
Donald L. Trump, M.D.
Paul Turner, M.D.
Wulf Utian, M.D., Ph.D.
Harry Uy, M.D.
Martin D. Valentine, M.D.
Robert E. Vestal, M.D.
Garry Vickar, M.D.
Donald G. Vidt, M.D.
Nicholas J. Vogelzang, M.D.
Kelly Vollmer, M.D.
Robert Volpe, M.D.
Robert Voy, M.D.
Thomas A. Wadden, M.D.
Scott Wadler, M.D.
Arnold Wald, M.D.
Randall C. Walker, M.D.
Wayne A. Wallace, M.D.
Edward E. Wallach, M.D.

Raymond P. Warrell, Jr., M.D.
Leonard Wartofsky, M.D.
John A. Washington, M.D.
Albert J. Wasserman, M.D.
Jay Watson, M.D.
Lawrence C. Weaver, Ph.D.
Alan J. Wein, M.D.
Myron H. Weinberger, M.D.
Howard L. Weiner, M.D.
Robert N. Weinreb, M.D.
Michael Weintraub, M.D.
Geoffrey R. Weiss, M.D.
Sigmund A. Weitzman, M.D.
Jay D. Wenger, M.D.
Anne Colston Wentz, M.D.
Melinda Wharton, M.D.
Andrew Whelton, M.D.
Randall W. Whitcomb, M.D.
William B. White, M.D.
Richard J. Whitley, M.D.
Jacob T. Wilensky, M.D.
William S. Wilke, M.D.
Jonathan K. Wilkin, M.D.
Grant Wilkinson, Ph.D.
Walter C. Willett, M.D., Ph.D.
David N. Williams, M.D.
Russell Williams, Jr., M.D.
Walter Williams, M.D.
Douglas W. Wilmore, M.D.
Mary Wilson, M.D.
Carey L. Winkler, M.D.
Brian Wispelwey, M.D.
Robert Wittes, M.D.
Robert Wolk, Pharm.D.
Charles D. Wood, Ph.D.
Elaine Wyllie, M.D.
Robert Yarchoan, M.D.
William Yates, M.D.
Charles Yesalis, M.P.H., Sc.D.
Jack Z. Yetiv, M.D., Ph.D.
Barbara A. Yetter, Pharm.D.
Norman N. Yoshimura, M.D.
Mei-Ying Yu, Ph.D.
Michael Zarski, J.D.
Steven H. Zeisel, M.D. Ph.D.
Jonathan M. Zenilman, M.D.
Irwin Ziment, M.D.
Thom J. Zimmerman, M.D.

New Drugs Evaluated in DRUG EVALUATIONS Annual *1995*

Drug	Indication/Classification
*†Acrivastine [Semprex-D]	Antihistamine
Aldesleukin (Interleukin 2) [Proleukin]	Antineoplastic (biological response modifier)
Antihemophilic Factor (Recombinant) [Bioclate, Helixate, Kogenate, Recombinate]	Hemostatic
Aprotinin [Trasylol]	Prophylaxis of perioperative blood loss during coronary artery bypass surgery
Budesonide [Rhinocort]	Rhinitis; asthma (bronchodilator)
Cisapride Monohydrate [Propulsid]	Upper gastrointestinal tract motility stimulator
Enoxaparin [Lovenox]	Anticoagulant
Famciclovir [Famvir]	Antiviral
Felbamate [Felbatol]	Antiepileptic
Fenofibrate [Lipidil]	Antilipidemic
Fluvastatin Sodium [Lescol]	Antilipidemic
Gabapentin [Neurontin]	Antiepileptic
Granisetron Hydrochloride [Kytril]	Antiemetic
*†Halofantrine Hydrochloride [Halfan]	Antiprotozoal (malaria)
Interferon Beta-1b [Betaseron]	Immunomodulator (multiple sclerosis); antiviral; antineoplastic (biological response modifier)
*Itraconazole [Sporanox]	Antifungal
†Levocabastine Hydrochloride [Livostin]	Antihistamine
†Loratadine [Claritin]	Antihistamine
Mesalamine (Oral) [Asacol, Pentasa]	Gastrointestinal anti-inflammatory
Pegaspargase [Oncaspar]	Antineoplastic (enzyme)
Piperacillin Sodium/Tazobactam Sodium [Zosyn]	Antibiotic
Rimantadine Hydrochloride [Flumadine]	Antiviral
Risperidone [Risperdal]	Antipsychotic
†Salmeterol Xinafoate [Serevent]	Bronchodilator
Strontium Chloride Sr 89 [Metastron]	Antineoplastic (palliation of bone pain caused by skeletal metastases)
Tacrine Hydrochloride [Cognex]	Mild to moderate Alzheimer's dementia
*Terbinafine Hydrochloride [Lamisil]	Antifungal (tinea)
†Torsemide [Demadex]	Antihypertensive
*Trimetrexate Glucuronate [NeuTrexin]	*Pneumocystis carinii* pneumonia; antineoplastic (antimetabolite)

* Evaluated as investigational drug; now approved but chapter not yet revised.
† Drug not evaluated separately.

Investigational Drugs Evaluated in DRUG EVALUATIONS Annual *1995*

Drug	Indication/Classification
Albendazole	Anthelmintic
Amonafide	Antineoplastic (synthetic intercalator)
Amsacrine	Antineoplastic (DNA binding)
Azacitidine	Antineoplastic (antimetabolite)
Bezafibrate	Antilipidemic
Brequinar Sodium	Antineoplastic (antimetabolite)
Buserelin Acetate	Antineoplastic (gonadotropin releasing hormone analogue)
Buthionine Sulfoximine	Antineoplastic (antimetabolite)
Caracemide	Antineoplastic (antimetabolite)
†Cetirizine Hydrochloride	Antihistamine
Dehydroemetine	Amebiasis
Deoxyspergualin	Antineoplastic (antibiotic)
Diaziquone	Antineoplastic (DNA binding)
Didemnin B	Antineoplastic (peptide antibiotic)
Diloxanide Furoate	Amebiasis
Domperidone	Antiemetic
Echinomycin	Antineoplastic (peptide antibiotic)
Epirubicin Hydrochloride	Antineoplastic (anthracycline)
Esorubicin Hydrochloride	Antineoplastic (anthracycline)
Fluocortin Butyl	Rhinitis
Fluticasone Propionate	Rhinitis
Heparins and heparinoids, low-molecular-weight	Anticoagulants
Hexamethylene-*bis*-acetamide	Antineoplastic (biological response modifier)
Homoharringtonine	Antineoplastic (alkaloid)
Interleukin 1 (IL-1)	Antineoplastic (biological response modifier)
Ivermectin	Anthelmintic
Lamotrigine	Antiepileptic
Meglumine Antimoniate	Leishmaniasis
Melarsoprol	Trypanosomiasis, African
Menogaril	Antineoplastic (anthracycline)
Merbarone	Antineoplastic (topoisomerase II inhibitor)
Metrifonate	Anthelmintic
Midodrine Hydrochloride	Orthostatic hypotension
Mitoguazone	Antineoplastic (polyamine synthesis inhibitor, DNA binding)
Moxisylyte Hydrochloride	Ophthalmic drug
Muramyl Dipeptide	Immunomodulator

Nifurtimox	Trypanosomiasis, South American
Nimustine Hydrochloride	Antineoplastic (DNA cross-linker)
N-Methylformamide	Antineoplastic (differentiation inducer)
N-(phosphonoacetyl)-L-aspartate	Antineoplastic (antimetabolite)
PCNU	Antineoplastic (DNA cross-linker)
Phenformin Hydrochloride	Antidiabetic agent
Piroxantrone Hydrochloride	Antineoplastic (anthrapyrazole)
Razoxane	Antineoplastic (actions unknown)
Semustine	Antineoplastic (DNA cross-linker)
Sodium Stibogluconate	Leishmaniasis
Suramin Sodium	Trypanosomiasis; antineoplastic (biological response modifier)
Tegafur	Antineoplastic (antimetabolite)
Teicoplanin	Antimicrobial (glycopeptide)
Thymic Hormones	Immunomodulators
Tiazofurin	Antineoplastic (antimetabolite)
Tumor Necrosis Factor	Antineoplastic (biological response modifier)
Vindesine Sulfate	Antineoplastic (alkaloid)

† Drug not evaluated separately.

Prescription Practices and Regulatory Agencies

1

GOOD PRESCRIPTION PRACTICES

The prescription of a drug represents the culmination of a deliberative process between physician and patient aimed at the prevention, amelioration, or elimination of a disease, disorder, or condition. This deliberation requires that the physician understand a broad spectrum of scientific and psychosocial issues germane to the success of treatment. Following is a discussion of ways in which good prescription practices enhance a drug's effectiveness and minimize misuse, abuse, and noncompliance.

The prescribing process encompasses selecting the appropriate drug, communicating the treatment program and information about the drug to the appropriate individuals (eg, patient, family, other health professionals), writing the prescription, and monitoring the treatment program to determine if changes are needed to optimize the effectiveness and safety of drug therapy.

Drug Selection Process

Nondrug therapy influences the extent of drug therapy required, and such therapy alone may be adequate. However, because some patients consider the prescription of a drug to be the most tangible evidence of a meaningful interaction with the physician, counseling and encouragement by the physician often will be necessary to gain patient acceptance of a treatment program that is limited to nondrug therapy.

Prior to writing a prescription, certain factors need to be assessed to maximize appropriate selection of therapy for an individual patient. The *status, severity, and duration of the disease, disorder, or condition* will be the initial determinants in identifying the drug(s) to be considered in the selection process. Rational drug selection demands that the efficacy and safety of all *potentially useful drug classes be considered* for their relevance to the medical problem being treated and that the most effective, least hazardous, and least costly drug(s) be chosen.

Anticipated individual variation in drug response also must be considered in the drug selection process, because it is usually the major obstacle to the rapid delivery of optimum therapy. The determinants of drug response variation are endogenous and exogenous. The former includes factors such as age, health status, genetic profile, and presence of other abnormal conditions (eg, diseases, disorders, trauma) and even normal conditions (eg, pregnancy). Significant exogenous factors are dietary intake including health store remedies, exposure to environmental chemicals, and all drugs being taken concurrently regardless of source (prescription or nonprescription [OTC]). For further discussion of variations in drug response, see index entry Drug Response Variation. It is especially important to *minimize adverse events (ie, adverse drug reactions, therapeutic failures) that may occur because of drug-drug, drug-food, and drug-environmental chemical interactions.*

Once the status of the patient's disease or disorder and the factors that will likely influence drug response have been identified, the pharmacologic profiles of drugs within a therapeutic class can be compared in order to select the most appropriate agent. *DRUG EVALUATIONS* is especially designed to provide comparative data for the drug selection process.

When the optimum drug(s) has been chosen for the patient, the *dosage schedule* and *form* are selected. These choices are often just as critical in optimizing drug therapy as the choice of the drug itself. They include: (1) dose (based not only on age, weight, and surface area of the patient but also on severity of disease, possible loading dose requirement, and presence of interacting drugs); (2) timing of administration (eg, bedtime dose to minimize undesirable daytime sedation); (3) route of administration (eg, parenteral administration to assure compliance and attainment of peak drug concentrations rapidly); and (4) dosage form (eg, tablets or suspension depending on age of the patient, lotion in preference to ointment in intertriginous areas, prolonged-release preparations to improve compliance).

The Prescription

After the drug selection process, a number of decisions are required to complete the written prescription properly. The following major issues should be considered.

WRITING THE PRESCRIPTION. Based on reports received through the USP Medication Errors Reporting Program, the following suggestions are offered to avoid misinterpretations in prescription writing: (1) use preprinted prescription blanks for physician identification or print in block lettering; (2) supply the complete drug name, strength, dosage, and form; (3) use metric not apothecary units of measure; (4) avoid use of "as directed" or "as needed" (knowing the desired dosing regimen helps nurses and pharmacists confirm the drug name and instructions); and (5) avoid use of abbreviations. To prevent dispensing errors due to look-alike (handwritten) or sound-alike (telephone order) drugs, physicians may consider including a general indication for use provided the patient agrees (ie, confidentiality is not breached).

PATIENT CONTAINER LABEL. The American Medical Association encourages physicians to include the direction, "label," on the prescription. Exceptions should be made only when such disclosures are inadvisable for psychological reasons or are otherwise detrimental to the welfare of the patient.

Numerous reasons exist for including the name and strength of a prescription drug on the container label. Patient container label information (1) fulfills the right of the patient to be informed about the medication(s) prescribed, (2) minimizes mistaken ingestion and may be lifesaving in accidental poisoning or overdose by providing immediate identification of the drug, (3) is of value when the patient has multiple attending physicians, takes multiple medications, or moves to another locality, (4) identifies the drug for patients who have allergies or who develop an allergic reaction while taking the medication, (5) enables the pharmacist and patient to validate the fact that the prescribed medication has been dispensed, and (6) alerts patients when a warning is subsequently issued for a specific drug.

PRESCRIBED AMOUNT OF DRUG. Generally, for nonchronic illnesses, the amount of drug prescribed should be sufficient to ameliorate or cure the illness or condition prior to the next patient visit. Initial prescribing of excessive amounts of a drug is costly, permits subsequent inappropriate self-treatment with the residual drug supply, enhances the potential for unsupervised use by other family members or friends, and contributes to the potential for accidental poisoning, willful overdose, or other misuse. Furthermore, patients cannot return the amount unused to pharmacies for credit. Conversely, if a drug must be taken for a prolonged period, the correct dose has been established, and the patient can be trusted to follow instructions properly, a prescription for a quantity to cover an extended time (eg, three months) is often more economical than repeated prescriptions or refills for small quantities. Therefore, judicious prescribing of the amount of drug, or the occasional use of drug samples initially, may obviate some of these problems and provide a considerable economic benefit for the patient.

REFILLS. Refills for certain drugs are regulated by federal and state controlled substances acts (see the section on Prescribing Controlled Psychotropic Drugs). Prescriptions for all other drugs remain valid indefinitely if marked "refill prn" unless state law directs otherwise. However, an open-ended authorization for refills usually is not advisable. Limiting the number of refills allows the physician to monitor the patient's course of illness periodically, which is particularly important during long-term therapy to detect intolerance, development of tolerance, drug interactions, and compliance. After individual response variation and appropriate dosage have been determined from experience, the number of refills may be increased for the patient's convenience.

CHILDPROOF PACKAGING. The Poison Prevention Packaging Act (PPPA) requires that prescription drugs be dispensed in containers that meet child protection packaging standards. The purpose of this law is to protect against accidental poisoning of children because of easy access to unattended drug products. The PPPA applies to drugs dispensed both by the pharmacist and physician. The law does allow conventional packaging at the consumer's request or direction of the prescribing physician. This does not exempt drugs dispensed by the physician from the provisions of the law, but rather it allows the physician to determine for a particular patient whether childproof packaging is necessary or detrimental (eg, for elderly patients with arthritis of the hands).

Communication of the Treatment Program

Because the prescription conveys only part of the treatment program, it is imperative that the complete treatment program and its rationale be documented in the patient's record for continuing review as well as for legal reasons. Verbal communication of the treatment program between the physician and patient (and/or family when indicated), followed by giving written drug information to the patient, will improve compliance and patient cooperation for the entire management plan (see the following sections on Compliance and AMA Patient Medication Information). In many situations, verbal and/or written communication with the pharmacist and/or other health professionals and caregivers can significantly increase the chances for success of the treatment program.

AMA PATIENT MEDICATION INSTRUCTIONS. The American Medical Association-Patient Medication Instruction (AMA-PMI) program, initiated in 1982, provides physicians with easily understood written information on approximately 100 widely used prescription and some nonprescription (eg, acetaminophen, salicylates, antihistamines) drugs or drug classes for distribution to their patients. These supplementary instructions present a balanced summary of the anticipated benefits and possible risks of the prescribed drug. The information is intended to augment, but not replace, the oral communication that should take place between the physician and the patient.

The Patient Medication Instruction (PMI) sheet describes the uses of the prescribed drug or drug class. It includes background information that the patient should be aware of and inform the physician of to facilitate selection of the optimal treatment regimen. Instructions for the proper use of the drug, as well as precautions that the patient should be aware of are also specified. The importance of drug compliance in chronic disease states (eg, hypertension, epilepsy, diabetes) is stressed. Finally, common documented side effects that may be anticipated are listed, as are more serious reactions that require notification of the physician and possibly discontinuation of the drug.

The PMI program is intended to reinforce the importance of informing patients about their medications and instructing them in proper use. These supplementary written instructions enhance the physician's capacity to accomplish these two goals, thereby improving the effectiveness of drug therapy; reducing the risk of adverse reactions, dispensing errors, or improper use of the drugs; and reinforcing the physician-patient relationship. A list of available AMA-PMI sheets with ordering information can be obtained from the United States Pharmacopeial Convention, Inc., 12601 Twinbrook Parkway, Rockville, MD, 20852 (telephone 1-800/227-8772 or 1-301/881-0666).

Monitoring the Treatment Program

Proper prescription practices do not end when the patient receives the prescription from the physician. Plans to monitor for drug efficacy and safety, compliance, and potential development of tolerance to relevant pharmacologic actions must be formulated at the time the prescription is given to the patient. It is especially important to monitor the dose of any medication for possible adjustment in patients with chronic disorders who require prolonged therapy or those in population groups who may not respond to a drug in the usual manner. Subjective symptoms can be used for monitoring, but preferably objective clinical signs (eg, body weight, pulse rate, temperature, blood pressure, concentration of drug in blood) can serve as early indications of therapeutic failure or unacceptable adverse drug reactions that will require alteration of therapy. Monitoring is especially critical when newer drugs for which less experience is available are prescribed. Requesting patients to keep logs of signs and symptoms gives them a sense of participation in their own treatment program and facilitates physician review of therapeutic progress and adverse events at the next scheduled visit. No treatment program should be left open-ended; termination of drug therapy is a desirable goal whenever possible to minimize drug exposure and reduce expense. Rational drug therapy demands that a drug not continue to be administered despite proven ineffectiveness or beyond the time required to achieve the desired therapeutic effect.

COMPLIANCE. Compliance is defined as strict adherence to a prescribed treatment plan. Once the drug selection process has been followed, much of the responsibility for success of treatment, particularly in the outpatient setting, falls on the patient. However, the physician can influence the extent of compliance. The patient's perception of the severity of the disorder and the importance of taking the prescribed treatment may be derived primarily from interaction with the physician (Solomon, 1980).

Compliance is reported to be approximately 75% for short-term therapy but only 50% for long-term treatment (Sackett, 1980). Therefore, the physician often overestimates the degree to which a patient is following the prescribed regimen (Roth and Caron, 1978), and prior awareness of the possibility of noncompliance, especially during prolonged treatment, can be a significant step toward improving compliance. Vials with caps containing a computerized chip that is unknown to the patient and that allows investigators to determine the time and frequency of opening of the vial have proven to be exceptionally helpful in determining compliance in clinical trials (Urquhart, 1990). Nevertheless, substantiation of a therapeutic blood drug concentration is probably the most conclusive proof of compliance. Lack of response to drug therapy and/or lack of side effects are only suggestive of noncompliance (Peck, 1980).

Simplification of the drug regimen, patient education and counseling by the physician and pharmacist, telephone calls to patients, home visits by nursing personnel, convenient packaging of medication, and monitoring of serum drug levels with positive feedback (eg, praise) are beneficial (Peck, 1980). Parenteral therapy administered by medical personnel may be necessary if compliance cannot be assured.

Rapidly metabolized or excreted drugs whose effects must be maintained steadily for long periods must be administered repeatedly at short intervals. Therefore, their use in a prolonged-release dosage form can simplify a drug regimen and thus improve compliance—*provided the medication is actually delivered in the measured manner that is intended.* The use of prolonged-release preparations of drugs with inherently long half-lives generally is not warranted. However, for patients who eliminate these drugs rapidly, prolonged-release preparation may be useful if an effective plasma concentration can be maintained.

Mixtures (drug combinations) also can simplify a drug regimen by decreasing the number of medications that must be ingested. When they represent the drugs of choice in appropriate amounts, mixtures, like prolonged-release preparations, would be expected to improve compliance.

Finally, the cost of a drug is a significant factor in compliance for some patients and may be one reason why 5% to 10% of prescriptions are never filled. "Drug expense" is preferred terminology to "drug cost," because expense is defined as value per unit cost. The add-on value of quality obtained from certain products (eg, an elegant dermatologic formulation, an enteric-coated preparation, convenient packaging, a skin patch that improves compliance) may be worth an additional cost to the individual patient. Expense is the final criterion of importance when more than one product can provide comparable efficacy and safety.

SPECIAL PRESCRIBING PRACTICES

Prescribing Controlled Substances

CONTROLLED SUBSTANCES ACT. The Controlled Substances Act (Title II of the Federal Comprehensive Drug Abuse Prevention and Control Act of 1970) is designed to improve regulation of the manufacturing, distribution, and dispensing of controlled substances by providing a "closed" system for legitimate handlers of these drugs. If not specifically exempted, every person who manufactures, distributes, prescribes, administers, or dispenses any controlled substance must register annually with the Drug Enforcement Administration. Accurate records of drugs purchased, distributed, and dispensed must be maintained and kept on file for two years by all persons who regularly dispense and administer controlled substances during the course of their practice.

Each drug or substance subject to control is assigned to one of five schedules depending on the potential for abuse, medical use, and degree of dependence if abused. The five schedules and the drugs included in them follow:

Schedule I: Drugs and other substances having a high potential for abuse and no current accepted medical use. Included are certain opium derivatives (eg, heroin), some synthetic opioids (eg, alpha-methylfentanyl), and hallucinogens (eg, LSD).

Schedule II: Drugs having a high potential for abuse and accepted medical use; abuse leads to severe psychological or physical dependence. In general, drugs in this schedule were previously controlled under the Narcotic Acts (eg, opium and derivatives, other opioids, cocaine). Stimulants, such as amphetamine and related compounds, and the short-acting barbiturates also are in this schedule.

Schedule III: Drugs having less abuse potential and accepted medical use; abuse leads to moderate dependence. Included in this schedule are certain stimulants and depressants (eg, barbiturates not included in other schedules), as well as preparations containing limited quantities of codeine.

Schedule IV: Drugs having a low abuse potential, accepted medical use, and limited dependence. Included in this schedule are certain depressants not in another schedule (eg, chloral hydrate, phenobarbital, benzodiazepines).

Schedule V: Drugs, including a few OTC preparations, having a lower abuse potential than a Schedule IV drug, accepted medical use, and limited likelihood of dependence. Antitussive, antidiarrheal, and other mixtures containing limited quantities of opioids are included in this schedule.

The Act also provides that no prescription order for drugs in Schedule II can be renewed. Emergency telephone prescriptions for drugs in this schedule may be dispensed if the practitioner limits the amount to that needed during the emergency period and furnishes a written, signed prescription order to the pharmacy within 72 hours. Prescription orders for drugs in Schedules III and IV may be redispensed up to five times within six months after the date of issue if authorized by the prescriber. Prescription orders for Schedule V drugs may be redispensed only as expressly authorized by the practitioner on the prescription.

Many states have controlled substances acts patterned after the federal law. Because there may be differences in the scheduling of drugs among states (some states are more restrictive for specific drugs, but none are less restrictive), physicians are urged to become acquainted with the provisions of the statutes and regulations in their local jurisdictions.

Precautions: The physician should take the following precautions to minimize the chances of controlled substances being procured illegally:

Keep prescription blanks where they cannot be stolen easily. Never sign them in advance and do not use them for writing notes. The prescriber's name, address, and Drug Enforcement Administration's (DEA) registration number; the full name and address of the patient; and the directions for use must be given when controlled substances are prescribed.

The DEA registration number should not be included on preprinted prescription blanks.

The written prescription order should be precise and legible to enhance communication between physician and pharmacist. It also must be dated.

The prescription order should indicate whether or not the prescription may be refilled and, if so, the number of times or duration of time a refill is authorized.

When prescribing a controlled substance, write out the actual amount in addition to giving an arabic number or roman numeral in order to discourage alterations in written prescription orders.

Use a separate prescription blank for each controlled substance prescribed. Avoid the use of prescription blanks that are preprinted with the name of a proprietary preparation.

Avoid writing prescription orders for large quantities of controlled drugs unless such amounts are absolutely necessary.

Maintain an accurate record of controlled drugs dispensed (preferably separate from the patient's record), as required by the Controlled Substances Act Amendments of 1984 and state law.

Store office supplies of controlled drugs in locked receptacles.

Maintain only a minimum stock of controlled drugs in the medical bag, which should not be left unattended.

Assist any pharmacist who telephones to verify information about a written prescription order.

Institutions should discourage the use of institutional prescription blanks for prescribing controlled substances; if institutional prescription blanks are used, the physician should print his/her name, address, and DEA registration number on each blank.

PRESCRIBING CONTROLLED PSYCHOTROPIC DRUGS. The following is a brief commentary on the prescribing of controlled narcotic and psychotropic drugs. Included are the opioids, the antianxiety and hypnotic agents, and the central nervous system stimulants. More detailed information on the benefits and risks associated with these drugs is presented in the chapters on these classes of drugs (see index entries).

Opioids: Morphine and morphine-like drugs, such as codeine, have legitimate clinical usefulness, and the physician should not hesitate to prescribe them when indicated for patients who require analgesia or symptomatic relief not provided by nonopioid analgesics.

Special attention should be given to patients with current dependence on opioids or other central nervous system depressants or a history of such dependence who also have other medical or surgical problems. If a genuine symptomatic need is confirmed by adequate diagnostic evaluation and if other analgesics or nondrug therapy for pain are ineffective or impractical, it is the physician's responsibility to prescribe opioid analgesics as for any other patient. The physician must, however, remain constantly alert to certain considerations: (1) the patient may be simulating a disease or condition in order to obtain a dependence-producing drug; (2) the effective dose level will vary, depending on the degree of tolerance; and (3) abrupt discontinuation can precipitate a withdrawal syndrome that increases morbidity or can even cause death if the patient with established dependence on a morphine-like drug undergoes major medical or surgical trauma. Drug dependence can be maintained until the patient begins to recover from the other illness. A regimen of gradual withdrawal then should be considered.

Antianxiety and Hypnotic Agents: Although the specific indications for the benzodiazepines, barbiturates, and other antianxiety and hypnotic agents vary, their principal use is to relieve anxiety and/or insomnia. Other indications for some drugs in these categories include preanesthetic medication and seizure disorders. Drugs that are neither benzodiazepines nor barbiturates but that possess hypnotic activity as well as abuse potential and dependence liability include chloral hydrate, ethchlorvynol, and glutethimide. Meprobamate is a nonbenzodiazepine, nonbarbiturate drug with antianxiety action, abuse potential, and dependence liability. All of the above drugs are scheduled under the Controlled Substances Act.

The shorter acting barbiturates are listed under Schedule II of the Controlled Substances Act, and the longer acting barbiturates are in Schedules III and IV. Because nonbarbiturate-nonbenzodiazepine hypnotics also have a high abuse potential, substituting one of these drugs for a barbiturate does not necessarily reduce the risk of drug dependence.

The physician must caution any patient for whom an antianxiety or hypnotic drug is prescribed about the potentiating effects of alcohol and should seldom prescribe these drugs for individuals with a history of alcohol abuse or alcoholism.

Amphetamines and Other Stimulants: Amphetamines and several chemically related drugs are central nervous system stimulants. Small doses give the user a feeling of increased mental alertness and a sense of well being. As doses are increased, apprehension, decreased appetite, volubility, tremor, and excitement occur. Because tolerance and psychological dependence can develop rather quickly with large doses, the physician should prescribe amphetamines and other stimulants only for an appropriate indication.

Abusers of stimulants usually prefer amphetamine or methamphetamine, but phenmetrazine or another stimulant is commonly substituted when the preferred drug is not readily available. The chosen route of administration may be oral or intravenous. Under the Controlled Substances Act, amphetamines, phenmetrazine, and methylphenidate are included in Schedule II; other stimulant-anorexiants are classed as Schedule III or IV drugs. In addition, numerous states have adopted legislation or regulations restricting the prescribing of amphetamines to specific indications—usually only narcolepsy and attention-deficit hyperactivity disorder.

The combined stimulant and euphoric effects of "crack" (free base) cocaine make it the fastest growing form of stimulant drug abuse today, but the medical use of pharmaceutical cocaine is limited to topical anesthesia of the eye, nose, and oropharynx. There is considerable evidence that tolerance, profound psychological dependence, and perhaps physical dependence develop with relatively short-term use of cocaine.

The administration of stimulants to alcohol- and sedative-dependent individuals is not appropriate, because such use can induce the patient to take increasing amounts of depressant drugs. Amphetamine-type drugs also are contraindicated in other individuals with a history of drug dependence.

The physician who prescribes stimulants for any indication must always be alert to their dependence liability and recognize that some patients may seek other sources of supply, either illegally or from another physician. There also is the danger that the efficacy of a stimulant in helping a person achieve a time-limited goal may predispose that person to regard amphetamine-type drugs as desirable rather than potentially dangerous substances and thus may encourage future abuse.

Stimulant abuse can cause three types of medical problems: (1) medical complications associated with drug effects (eg, exacerbation of hypertension, arrhythmias, stroke, retinal damage due to intense vasospasm); (2) emergency conditions, such as acute amphetamine psychosis, or hyperthermia and convulsions arising from use of toxic doses; and (3) signs and symptoms during the abstinence period following regular use that indicate drug dependence. Of course, any drug administered with shared or unclean needles poses the risk of septicemia, endocarditis, hepatitis, and HIV infection.

Prescribing Mixtures

Prescribing a combination drug product, ie, a single preparation containing two or more active ingredients in a fixed ratio in which each ingredient contributes to overall therapeutic effectiveness, is a means to enhance therapeutic effect, decrease the potential for adverse reactions, increase compliance, and reduce cost. The therapeutic effect may be enhanced by synergism (eg, trimethoprim/sulfamethoxazole [Bactrim, Septra]), by improved efficacy of the primary ingredient (eg, levodopa/carbidopa [Sinemet], imipenem/cilastatin [Primaxin]), or by improved patient compliance (ie, fewer medications). Cost should be reduced all along the manufacturer-to-consumer chain, since only one product must be handled. However, the selection of a mixture in preference to individual drugs is often controversial.

In its Combination Drug Policy, the Food and Drug Administration requires that each component of a mixture contribute to the claimed therapeutic effects or, alternatively, that the added component enhance the safety or efficacy of the principal component or minimize its potential for abuse (eg, naloxone added to pentazocine [Talwin Nx]). Criticisms of selected mixtures include inflexibility of dosage ratio, inclusion of a low-potency drug(s) that contributes only marginally if at all to the therapeutic effect, or inclusion of an ingredient(s) that actually impairs the effectiveness of the primary ingredient (MacCannell and Giraud, 1980).

It is critical that the physician be aware of all active ingredients in a mixture, their indications, and their amounts. Mixtures should be prescribed only if all of the active ingredients contribute significantly to the desired therapeutic effect and thus reduce patient discomfort, cost, and noncompliance.

Prescribing Drug Samples

A drug sample is defined as a unit of drug that is not intended to be sold but is intended to promote the sale of the drug. In addition to this marketing objective, drug samples allow a physician to begin therapy immediately. Samples also permit a physician to determine the patient's therapeutic response and tolerance, including potential allergic reactions, before prescribing larger amounts for a full course of treatment. This option may be important from the standpoint of drug efficacy, safety, and cost. Finally, physicians often use samples to supply drugs for low-income patients.

In order to minimize or eliminate any potential problems associated with drug samples (eg, uncontrolled storage, distribution of expired drugs, illicit drug diversion), the Prescription Drug Marketing Act was enacted by Congress in 1988. The law principally affects pharmaceutical manufacturers and their representatives who distribute drug samples to physicians. This law does not prevent physicians from receiving or dispensing drug samples; however, they are specifically prohibited from selling samples and they are required to sign a written request form supplied by the manufacturer verifying the identity of the drug sample and the quantity requested. Although the law does not require physicians to maintain these records, some manufacturers will seek physician help in assuring that the requested samples were received. The physician may continue to receive drug samples from the sales representatives as well as by mail or common carrier.

This law is designed to safeguard the integrity of the drug sampling process. Physicians also can improve the medical practice of drug sampling and assure its continued availability by documenting the prescribing of drug samples in the patient's record for reference and review at the next visit. Furthermore, providing medication information with drug samples is no less important than for drug products procured by prescription. Unneeded or expired samples should be destroyed; they must not be sold or traded to pharmacists, hospitals, nursing homes, or other physicians.

Prescribing Generic Drugs

A generic drug is one that is no longer the exclusive property of the pharmaceutical company that developed or first marketed it. The company that developed the drug may have marketed it exclusively and/or cross-licensed other companies to manufacture and market the drug under the same or a different trademark for the life of the patent. Following expiration of the patent, the prescription drug can be marketed generically by any pharmaceutical manufacturer that fulfills certain requirements of the Food, Drug and Cosmetic Act, including proper manufacture and interstate marketing.

The following definitions were adopted by the AMA House of Delegates to improve communication among physicians and their patients when discussing generic substitution.

Generic name is the established (official) United States Adopted Name (USAN) of a drug. It is a nonproprietary name.

Pioneer brand name is the name of a drug manufactured by its innovator, ie, the manufacturer who holds the patent on the drug and whose brand name often has become a synonym for the drug itself (eg, Valium, Darvon, Tagamet) or by a company who has an exclusive license from the innovator to sell the drug.

A drug's *brand* (or *trade*) *name* is a proprietary name that is registered to protect the name for the sole use of the company holding the trademark. It usually identifies a particular product or formulation sold by a pharmaceutical manufacturer. However, the law permits the manufacturer to change the inactive ingredients in single-entity preparations, and even the active ingredients of combination products, without loss of the trademark. Prior to a drug's patent expiration, a number of proprietary names may exist that include not only the pioneer's brand name but also brand names trademarked by manufacturers who have cross-licensing arrangements with the innovator.

A *generic drug product* contains a drug dispensed as an alternative to the pioneer's brand-name drug (or another manufacturer's cross-licensed brand-name drug) whose patent has expired or has been successfully challenged. The generic drug product has the identical biologically active drug(s) as its corresponding brand-name counterparts; however, excipients (ie, inactive ingredients included as fillers, binders, preservatives, and coloring agents), as well as manufacturing processes, may vary. After availability of the drug in the public domain, a generic drug product may be sold under the established (official) generic name (*generic-named product*) or under a brand name (*branded generic drug product*).

Examples of the above types of drug products are pioneer brand-named: *Elavil*; generic-named: *Amitriptyline*; branded generic: *Endep*.

The Drug Price Competition and Patent Term Restoration Act, enacted in 1984, has substantially shortened the approval process for generic drug products through the use of Abbreviated New Drug Applications (ANDAs) (see Drug Approval Process in the section on Official and Regulatory Agencies). In order for the FDA to regard a generic drug product for systemic use as therapeutically equivalent to an already approved brand-name drug product, the generic drug product must contain the same active ingredient(s); be identical in strength, dosage form, and route of administration; have at least one of the same indications and the same precautions, warnings, and other instructions on the labeling as the brand-name drug; and be bioequivalent (ie, following oral ingestion or application of a transdermal patch, the same amount of drug must be absorbed systemically at a similar rate with a predetermined statistical certainty as the brand-name drug product).

Inert ingredients, color, taste, tablet shape, and packaging may vary. Tablets, capsules, and suspensions are considered different dosage forms.

Some brand-name drugs may have one or more additional indications than their generic counterparts if approval for the indication has been obtained and its period of exclusivity has not expired. Under the Drug Price Competition and Patent Term Restoration Act of 1984, a manufacturer is granted three years of exclusivity for a new indication(s) for which clinical trials were required for FDA approval. This exclusivity provides that only that manufacturer can promote the new indication and list it in the product labeling. It does not restrict the physician's ability to prescribe or the pharmacist's ability to dispense that drug for another indication.

GENERIC EQUIVALENTS. The federal government and every state have enacted legislation that permits, encourages, or even mandates (Florida, Hawaii, Kentucky, Massachusetts, Michigan, Mississippi, New Jersey, New York, Pennsylvania, Rhode Island, Vermont, Washington, West Virginia) (Parker et al, 1991 A, 1991 B) the substitution of a less costly generic equivalent for a more expensive (brand-name) drug that may have been prescribed. Many states also have compiled lists of acceptable (positive formulary) and unacceptable (negative formulary) generic drug product substitutions. However, even in states with mandatory generic substitution laws, the physician can prohibit substitution. Each state has specific rules on how a physician should designate the fact that a generic product should *not* be substituted. Examples include two-line signature prescription blanks, a box that indicates "brand medically necessary," or a written indication by the physician (ie, "dispense as written").

The FDA's *Approved Drug Products With Therapeutic Equivalence Evaluations* (the "Orange Book" or "The List"), published annually, lists currently marketed drug products that have been approved for safety and effectiveness. The list includes both prescription and OTC products and both single and multisource products with approved New Drug Applications (NDAs), as well as approved blood and blood products. This annual publication is updated monthly by cumulative supplements. Therapeutic equivalence evaluations are provided for multisource products. The list is prepared as an *advisory* to purchasers of pharmaceuticals and is used by health professionals seeking to determine whether a given drug product can be expected to have the same therapeutic effect when administered to patients under conditions specified in the labeling compared with a reference drug product assigned by the FDA having the same active ingredient(s).

For every multiple source product, the "Orange Book" cites a letter code that indicates the agency's evaluation regarding the therapeutic equivalence of the product relative to the reference pioneer or a brand-name drug product. The major codes are Class A (not expected to have bioequivalence problems based on test data supplied by the manufacturer) and Class B (documented or potential bioequivalence problems exist). Class AB (drug originally designated as Class B, but applicant has subsequently provided data from studies in human subjects to assure bioavailability and bioequivalence to the reference standard) is a subset of Class A. An FDA rating of Class B usually means that the agency currently lacks sufficient evidence to establish equivalence. Class BD (products that have been found to be nonequivalent [Nightingale, 1988]) is a subset of Class B. The AMA House of Delegates has adopted a policy that recommends that no generic drug products with a B rating be dispensed (American Medical Association, 1993 A, 1993 B). Drugs that were marketed before the existence of the NDA procedures do not have to provide evidence of bioequivalence (eg, codeine phosphate tablets, phenobarbital tablets, many OTC tablets and capsules).

The annual publication, *Approved Drug Products With Therapeutic Equivalence Evaluations,* and cumulative supplements can be obtained from the Superintendent of Documents, US Government Printing Office, Washington, DC 20402-9371 (telephone 1-202/783-3238) at a cost of $91.00 ($113.75 for foreign subscriptions) or as *USP DI Volume III, Approved Drug Products and Legal Requirements,* from the United States Pharmacopeial Convention, Inc, Order Processing Department, 12601 Twinbrook Parkway, Rockville, MD, 20852 (telephone 1-800/227-8772 or 1-301/881-0666) at a cost of $97.00.

The practice of generic drug substitution for a pioneer drug product has grown since the Drug Price Competition and Patent Term Restoration Act of 1984 was enacted. Two questions continue to be debated: (1) Is the bioavailability of the generic drug product equivalent to that of its assigned reference standard (usually the pioneer drug product)? (2) If it is, will the patient benefit financially from use of the generic drug product?

Bioequivalence: The FDA procedure for approving generic drug products has been summarized for practicing physicians (Nightingale and Morrison, 1987). The agency believes its process for determining bioequivalence, and thus therapeutic equivalence, is accurate and reliable. Although the agency warns that prescribers and pharmacists should always be aware of the possibility of a generic or nongeneric drug product not being effective in every patient to whom it is administered, it encourages physicians to feel confident in substituting generic drug products that are designated therapeutically equivalent (Class A) when they are available.

Bio*in*equivalence is a concern only when drug efficacy or safety is altered. A bioinequivalent product is usually detected clinically when another product containing the same active ingredient is substituted. Altered response may be manifested as diminished efficacy (therapeutic failure), enhanced efficacy, or adverse drug reaction (toxicity). Failure to recognize the reason for the altered response may result in improper diagnosis and treatment following patient re-evaluation. For example, the physician usually considers a drug as potentially causal when an adverse event occurs or is enhanced. On the other hand, when a diminution or lack of efficacy is observed, the physician may consider inadequate dosage, development of tolerance, inaccurate diagnosis, or progression of the disease as being responsible and may not think of inadequate drug bioavailability as causal.

Bioequivalence based on equal bioavailability between a generic and reference solid drug product intended for oral or transdermal absorption can be resolved only in controlled cross-over studies in humans when the area under the curve (AUC), time to maximum effect (Tmax), and maximum concentration attained (Cmax) (for both the active parent drug and all other active metabolites) are determined from serum drug concentration-time curves and compared. Ideally, this test should be conducted in patients with the disease, disorder, or condition for which the drug is intended. However, the studies often are conducted in 18 to 24 healthy individuals (usually males 21 to 35 years of age); therefore, the data may not always be relevant for an individual patient. Furthermore, when data from an in vitro dissolution test can be shown to correlate with drug serum concentration-time data, the agency allows the in vitro test to be used to compare continuing production lots of reference (usually innovator) and generic drug products. These and other unresolved scientific, educational, regulatory, and epidemiologic issues regarding generic substitution have been discussed by various authors (Strom, 1987; Turner et al, 1987; Schwartz and Stanton, 1987; Weinberger, 1987).

The AMA is concerned that survey results indicate that only 12.9% of 245 responding physicians had knowledge of FDA procedures for testing generic products (Friedman et al, 1987). The AMA House of Delegates adopted reports on generic substitution in 1987 and 1989 that reviewed the current status and emphasized that the issue involves not only generic versus pioneer drug product substitution but drug product substitution in general (American Medical Association, 1993 A, 1993 B).

Until the methodology for determining bioequivalence for all drug products is resolved, the AMA recommends the following: (1) The dose of any medication should continue to be titrated for optimum efficacy and safety, especially in patients with chronic disorders who require prolonged therapy or in those in special population groups who may not respond to a drug in the usual manner. (2) When multiple refills for chronic diseases are anticipated, the physician should avoid substitution unless the products have been proven to be bioequivalent and, once a medication has been prescribed and begun (whether generic or nongeneric drug product), should stipulate that no further substitution be made without the attending physician's permission. (3) When serious or unusual problems develop that may be related to drug substitution, the findings should be documented. An FDA reporting form is included at the end of this publication. Physicians are urged to include the manufacturer's name and the lot number of the drug product on the reporting form. (4) Physicians should improve their awareness of the controversial issues regarding generic drug substitution. They also should become familiar with specific laws governing generic drug substitution in their state, and, where applicable, they should obtain a copy of the current generic drug substitution drug formulary in their state (provided in individual state supplements as part of the subscription to the aforementioned *USP DI Volume III*).

Savings: The intent of state legislatures in enacting generic drug substitution laws was to transfer to the patient any savings that might accrue to the pharmacy as a result of competitive pricing, less complex inventories, and price reduction on bulk purchasing. However, although patients can benefit financially from the prescription of a generic drug, the amount of money saved has varied from nothing to substantial sums.

The price of a particular drug product can vary greatly from pharmacy to pharmacy. If an expensive product or prolonged therapy is required, the physician should, if possible, suggest a pharmacy that dispenses the drug at a reasonable price while maintaining the quality of its service. The relative cost to consumers charged by pharmacies can be determined by comparing their prices for several commonly used drugs. Pharmacy and therapeutics committees of local hospitals—which often base their review of products for inclusion in the hospital's formulary on reports in the literature, experiences of local physicians, availability, and cost in their region—also may be valuable sources of information and guidance; however, many drug companies charge much lower prices to hospitals (especially teaching and nonprofit hospitals) so that a hospital price per se cannot be assumed to be typical of community pharmacy prices.

IMPROPER PRESCRIPTION PRACTICES

The avoidance of inappropriate drug selection, undermedication (underprescribing), overmedication (overprescribing), and drug abuse often are significant factors in drug selection. Some physicians prefer the general synonyms of drug misuse or drug misadventuring (Manasse, 1989) to include undermedication, overmedication, and inappropriate drug selection but to exclude drug abuse.

INAPPROPRIATE DRUG SELECTION. Selecting the most appropriate drug for a patient is dependent principally on correct diagnosis; knowledge of comparative drug therapy for the disease, disorder, or condition; coexisting conditions and therapy being administered for those conditions; anticipated individual variation; the probable effectiveness of nondrug therapy; and knowledge of comparative costs of the potentially useful drugs after medical factors have been considered (see the section on Drug Selection Process). Any deviations or exceptions from a rational program of drug selection for an individual, as well as a disregard for cost-effective prescribing, could be considered inappropriate drug selection. Obviously, inappropriate drug selection that results in a clinically significant unfavorable outcome is of most concern.

UNDERMEDICATION. *Undermedication* occurs when the patient fails to receive adequate drug therapy (Morgan, 1980). For example, the negative impact of excessive concern about psychological and/or physical dependence is revealed by reports that the severe chronic pain accompanying terminal cancer is often inadequately treated. Potent analgesics, particularly opioids, are indicated for the sometimes excruciating pain of terminal cancer, and physicians should not hesitate to use them in these patients.

Relief of suffering is a legitimate goal of medical practice. Failure to provide such relief may result from timidity ("pharmacophobia"), incorrect or downgraded diagnosis in the context of severity, or lack of knowledge or faith in the value of a controversial drug, even when its administration is indicated. Finally, patients may fail to comply or to convey the severity of their symptoms to the physician (Weintraub, 1981). Thus, the factors contributing to undermedication are diverse and span the fields of medicine, psychology, economics, and sociology.

OVERMEDICATION. *Overmedication* occurs when the dose and/or duration of drug use is excessive, when a mixture is used and only one of the components is indicated, or when more drugs are prescribed than are required (polypharmacy).

DRUG ABUSE. *Drug abuse* is the use of a drug, usually by self-administration, in a manner that deviates from approved medical, legal, and social standards (Jaffe, 1980). The issues of drug abuse and overmedication are often inextricably related. Acquisition of prescription drugs for purposes of abuse can occur by either illicit or licit means. The illicit mode has many variations, including prescription "kiting" (ie, alteration of written prescriptions to increase the amount prescribed) and counterfeiting; theft and forgery of prescription blanks; and theft of drugs from manufacturers, wholesalers, pharmacies, and physicians' offices. The smuggling of drugs into the United States and the clandestine manufacture of drugs within this country also are significant illegal sources of otherwise legal medication.

Prescription drug abuse may take any of the following forms (Council on Scientific Affairs, 1982):

1. The willful and conscious misprescribing of controlled substances by physicians for abuse purposes, usually for profit. These are the "script (or dishonest) doctors." Physicians responsible for this type of prescribing should be prosecuted to the full extent of the law.
2. Inappropriate prescribing by physicians who unwittingly acquiesce to insistent demands by patients for medication. These are "deceived doctors." In these instances, drugs are prescribed in excessive amounts or for longer periods than necessary, which may initiate or perpetuate drug abuse or dependence or permit diversion of the drug to other persons for abuse purposes.
3. Uninformed prescribing by physicians who have not kept abreast of new developments in pharmacology and drug therapy. These are the "dated doctors." In addition to prescribing drugs in excessive quantities or for excessive periods, these physicians prescribe drugs for conditions that do not warrant such therapy or that might be better treated with other drugs.
4. Self-prescribing and administration by physicians who abuse or are dependent on drugs. These are "disabled doctors" who need treatment. Rehabilitation and disciplinary programs exist in every state through medical societies and boards of medical examiners.

The major risk associated with a psychotropic drug is that a patient may feel compelled to continue to experience the drug's reinforcing effects after the medical indications for its use have disappeared. Such compulsive use constitutes *psychological dependence* on the drug. Tolerance characteristically develops, and larger doses are necessary to achieve the same desired effects. Chronic self-administration of increasing doses often alters the normal physiologic state to such an extent that the abuser becomes *physically dependent* on the continuous use of the drug to prevent withdrawal symptoms, which range in severity from unpleasant (eg, insomnia) to life-threatening (eg, seizures).

Iatrogenic drug abuse and dependence are adverse reactions that every physician should seek to avoid. To do so, practitioners must guard against injudicious prescribing practices and must avoid acquiescing to the demands of patients for instant chemical solutions to their problems. The physician should convey to patients through attitude and manner that drugs, no matter how helpful, are only one part of an overall plan of treatment and management. In essence, a preventive role can be played by the physician who exercises good judgment in administering and prescribing psychotropic drugs so that diversion to illicit use is averted and drug dependence is minimized or prevented.

DRUG UTILIZATION REVIEW

Problems associated with drug utilization by prescribers, dispensers, and consumers have been documented. These shortcomings provide the rationale for organized drug utilization review (DUR, drug use review) initiatives. DUR can be defined as a formal program for assessing data on drug use against explicit, prospective criteria and standards and, as necessary, introducing remedial strategies to achieve some desired end (eg, improve quality of care, control fraud and abuse, control costs).

DUR is a routine function in acute-care hospitals and long-term care facilities and is emerging rapidly in outpatient environments. For example, it is estimated that over 75% of health maintenance organizations (HMOs) have some form of DUR program. Furthermore, the US Congress passed Section 4401 of the Omnibus Budget Reconciliation Act (OBRA '90) that mandated DUR in every state Medicaid outpatient prescription drug program by January 1, 1993.

Two types of DUR are now required in Medicaid. *Prospective DUR* is a review conducted (currently most often by a pharmacist) before the prescription is dispensed, and it provides the potential to modify an individual patient's prescription. *Retrospective DUR* occurs after the prescription is dispensed and usually involves computerized screening of large batches of prescription claims data. Another element of DUR programs involves an *educational component* that is intended to educate physicians and pharmacists on common drug therapy problems with the aim of improving prescribing and dispensing practices.

The emergence and continuing development of DUR programs will dramatically influence the use of medications in coming years. Such influence should be targeted to assuring quality therapeutic outcomes that are both clinically appropriate and economically sound. Thus, it is essential that physicians accept the responsibility to participate in the development and operation of DUR programs to assure that quality of patient care is the primary objective.

In order to provide guidance in the development of appropriate DUR programs, the AMA House of Delegates adopted "Principles of Drug Utilization Review" in June 1991 (American Medical Association, 1993 C). These principles and associated characteristics also were adopted by the American Pharmaceutical Association (APhA) in June 1991 and by the Pharmaceutical Manufacturers Association (PMA) in July 1991 (see Table). They address the goals of a DUR program, its major elements, confidentiality between the physician and patient, and program operations. The four basic components of a DUR program are (1) explicit criteria (eg, appropriate indication, dose, drug interactions) and standards (ie, acceptable variation); (2) data processing and analysis; (3) intervention and education; and (4) feedback and update of criteria and standards. The AMA encourages careful consideration and adoption of these DUR principles by all those who are involved in the drug therapy process.

PRINCIPLES OF DRUG USE REVIEW

PRINCIPLE 1 • The primary emphasis of a DUR program must be to enhance quality of care for patients by assuring appropriate drug therapy.

Characteristics:

- While a desired therapeutic outcome should be cost-effective, the cost of drug therapy should be considered only after clinical and patient considerations are addressed.
- Sufficient professional prerogatives should exist for individualized patient drug therapy.

PRINCIPLE 2 • Criteria and standards for DUR must be clinically relevant.

Characteristics:

- The criteria and standards should be derived through an evaluation of the peer-reviewed clinical and scientific literature and compendia; relevant guidelines obtained from professional groups through consensus-derived processes; the experience of practitioners with expertise in drug therapy; drug therapy information supplied by pharmaceutical manufacturers; and data and experience obtained from DUR program operations.
- Criteria and standards should identify underutilization as well as overutilization and inappropriate utilization.
- Criteria and standards should be validated prior to use.

PRINCIPLE 3 • Criteria and standards for DUR must be nonproprietary and must be developed and revised through an open professional consensus process.

Characteristics:

- The criteria and standards development and revision process should allow for and consider public comment in a timely manner before the criteria and standards are adopted.
- The criteria and standards development and revision process should include broad-based involvement of physicians and pharmacists from a variety of practice settings.
- The criteria and standards should be reviewed and revised in a timely manner.
- If a nationally developed set of criteria and standards are to be used, there should be a provision at the state level for appropriate modification.

PRINCIPLE 4 • Interventions must focus on improving therapeutic outcomes.

Characteristics:

- Focused education to change professional or patient behavior should be the primary intervention strategy used to enhance drug therapy.
- The degree of intervention should match the severity of the problem.
- All retrospective DUR profiles/reports that are generated via computer screening should be subjected to subsequent review by a committee of peers prior to an intervention.

- If potential fraud is detected by the DUR system, the primary intervention should be a referral to appropriate bodies (eg, Surveillance Utilization Review systems).
- On-line prospective DUR programs should deny services only in cases of patient ineligibility, coverage limitations, or obvious fraud. In other instances, decisions regarding appropriate drug therapy should remain the prerogative of licensed practitioners.

PRINCIPLE 5 • Confidentiality of the relationship between patients and practitioners must be protected.

Characteristic:

- The DUR program must assure the security of its database.

PRINCIPLE 6 • Principles of DUR must apply to the full range of DUR activities, including prospective, concurrent, and retrospective drug use evaluation.

PRINCIPLE 7 • DUR program operations must be structured to achieve the principles of DUR.

Characteristics:

- DUR programs should maximize physician and pharmacist involvement in program development, operation, and evaluation.
- DUR programs should have an explicit process for system evaluation (eg, total program costs, validation).
- DUR programs should have a positive impact on improving therapeutic outcomes and controlling overall health care costs.
- DUR programs should minimize administrative burdens to patients and practitioners.

OFFICIAL AND REGULATORY AGENCIES

Several official governmental and quasi-official voluntary bodies are concerned with standards for the manufacturing, distribution, labeling, and advertising of drug products. To acquaint the reader with the functions of these agencies and their spheres of influence as they pertain to medicinal agents, brief descriptions of their organization and duties follow.

Food and Drug Administration

DRUG APPROVAL PROCESS. The Pure Food and Drugs Act of 1906 required only that drugs distributed in interstate commerce meet the official standards of strength, quality, and purity delineated in the United States Pharmacopeia (USP) and the National Formulary (NF). This Act was replaced by the Federal Food, Drug and Cosmetic (FDC) Act of 1938. Provisions regarding adherence to the USP-NF standards continued to be included; in addition, the FDC Act of 1938 required that drugs be proved safe prior to marketing. In 1962, Amendments to the Act added the requirement that drugs be proved effective for the labeled indications prior to marketing and that efficacy be established for those drugs marketed for the first time between 1938 and 1962. The Secretary of Health and Human Services is charged by the Act and its Amendments with assuring the safety and efficacy of prescription drugs, including biologic products, marketed in interstate commerce. This responsibility is delegated to the FDA.

Two additional Acts have had considerable influence on improving drug availability to benefit patients with rare diseases and to reduce drug costs: The Orphan Drug Act of 1983 fostered orphan drug development, and the Drug Price Competition and Patent Term Restoration Act of 1984 expanded the number of generic drugs suitable for an Abbreviated New Drug Application (ANDA). Although they do not involve changes in the law, four revisions of FDA's drug regulations have been made in an attempt to hasten and improve the process of new drug development: Revision of New Drug Application (NDA) Regulations (1985), Revision of Investigational New Drug Application Regulations—the "IND Rewrite" (1987), and Proposed Revision of Generic Drug Review Process and Regulations (1989). A fourth revision, Treatment Use of Investigational New Drugs (1987) expedites availability of experimental drugs for patients with serious or immediately life-threatening diseases. (See the following section on Premarket Drug Availability.)

The FDA's regulatory jurisdiction over drugs encompasses the standardization of nomenclature, the approval process for new drugs and new indications, official labeling, surveillance of adverse drug events, and methods of manufacture and distribution. The FDA regulates advertisements only for prescription drugs and biologics; OTC drug advertising is regulated by the Federal Trade Commission. The developmental history and current status of the regulatory authority for drugs and devices have been summarized (FDA, 1981; Hayes, 1981; Kessler et al, 1987; Kessler, 1989).

Official Drug Name: The Secretary of Health and Human Services is given the authority to designate an official (established) name for any drug if it is determined that such action is necessary or desirable in the interest of usefulness and simplicity. This name is to be used in any official compendium as the only official title for that drug. In practice, the official name will be one that has been adopted by the USAN Council (see the discussion on The United States Adopted Names Council). This official name is the only nonproprietary (generic) name, other than the chemical name or formula, that can appear on the label. The official name also must appear in conjunction with the brand name in other labeling (eg, package insert, patient information). The label for an OTC drug must disclose the official names of all active ingredient(s), but disclosure of the quantity(ies) or ratios of ingredients is not required for combination products.

Investigational New Drug (IND): Before an investigation of a new drug entity in humans can be initiated, the sponsor must submit to the FDA an Investigational New Drug application, more commonly referred to as an "IND." An IND sponsored by a clinical investigator usually is intended to permit use of the drug in early clinical trials in order to advance scientific knowledge. An IND sponsored by a pharmaceutical company is generated to supply information to support an application for the drug to be marketed for specific approved uses. The former is about three to four times more common than pharmaceutical company-sponsored INDs; however, the latter is much more comprehensive and includes the entire clinical program to develop the drug for marketing. It includes information about the chemical composition of the drug, results of all preclinical investigations (including animal safety studies), a protocol for the proposed clinical investigation, information on the experience of clinical investigators, arrangements and procedures for protecting the rights and safety of human subjects developed in accordance with the requirements of Human Subjects Protection Committees (Institutional Review Boards), and an agreement to submit annual progress reports. After the IND has been submitted to the FDA, the Agency legally has 30 days to review the proposed clinical study for safety issues; the sponsor of the IND may proceed with the planned studies in humans after notification of approval or absence of comment from the FDA within the 30-day review period.

The FDA has formulated IND regulations for the clinical study of a new drug's safety and efficacy and has divided this evaluation into three phases. Phase I is intended to determine the safety of the new drug in normal subjects and to identify the tolerable dosage range. Pharmacokinetic data on absorption, distribution, metabolism, and excretion also are obtained in this usually small group of healthy volunteers. In Phase II trials, controlled studies are performed in limited numbers of patients with the target disease or disorder to establish efficacy and appropriate dosage. Additional pharmacokinetic data may be obtained and compared with the data from normal subjects. If Phase I and II studies demonstrate that the drug is reasonably safe and potentially effective or may have benefits that outweigh any observed risks, more extensive clinical trials are initiated in Phase III.

Phase III trials verify that the acceptable benefit/risk ratio determined in Phase II studies persists under conditions of anticipated usage and in groups of patients large enough to identify statistically and clinically significant responses. Conferences between the sponsor and FDA, sometimes including outside medical experts, usually are held during all three phases of development.

While an IND is in effect, the sponsor must report in writing to the FDA and all participating investigators within 10 working days any serious and unexpected adverse events that may be drug related. Fatal or immediately life-threatening drug-related events require that the FDA be notified by telephone within three working days.

A Treatment IND is discussed in the section on Premarket Drug Availability below.

New Drug Application (NDA): To market a new drug for human use in interstate commerce, a manufacturer must have an NDA approved by the FDA. When the IND sponsor feels that data are sufficient to fulfill the requirements for approval of the drug by the FDA, a New Drug Application is filed. By statute, the FDA must review the NDA within 180 days. Usually, additional information and/or clarification is requested by the FDA and at least one to three years are needed for the manufacturer to complete any additional adequate and well-controlled trials necessary to support the claimed indications or supply further information regarding the drug's safety, efficacy, or manufacturing characteristics and for the Agency to review and approve an NDA (Commission on the Federal Drug Approval Process, 1982).

Accelerated Approval of an NDA: The timely availability of new drug approvals and the efficiency of the new drug development process remain the subject of considerable debate (Miller and Young, 1989; Lasagna, 1989; Advisory Committee on the Food and Drug Administration, 1991). In December 1992, in response to criticism that the FDA new drug approval processes are too protracted and deny patients access to needed medications, the Agency published new regulations to accelerate approval of certain new drug, antibiotic, and biologic products that provide meaningful therapeutic benefit to patients with serious or life-threatening illnesses compared with existing treatments (ie, treatment of patients unresponsive to or intolerant of available therapy, improvement in patient response over available therapy). These regulations allow the Agency to grant marketing approval for a new drug product (1) on the basis of adequate and well-controlled clinical trials establishing that the product has an effect on a clinical endpoint that, based on epidemiologic, therapeutic, pathophysiologic, or other evidence, is reasonably likely, to be predictive of clinical benefit, or (2) on the basis of an effect on a clinical endpoint other than survival or irreversible morbidity (surrogate endpoint). The applicant is required to conduct postmarketing studies with due diligence if there is uncertainty regarding the relation of the surrogate endpoint to the clinical benefit. NDA applicants are not mandated to use this accelerated approval mechanism.

Supplemental New Drug Application: After a drug product has been marketed, the FDA requires further clinical proof of safety and efficacy if new or additional indications or statements are to be added to the product's labeling. A supplemental NDA is required.

As a general rule, whether new claims are added to the official labeling depends on whether the pharmaceutical company has sufficient interest to initiate and follow the procedures necessary to obtain a supplemental NDA. The process of approval for a supplemental NDA, although less demanding than the initial NDA, still requires considerable time and monetary investment before the new claim can appear on the official labeling and exclusivity be granted to the manufacturer.

Abbreviated New Drug Application (ANDA): The Drug Price Competition and Patent Term Restoration Act of 1984 provides the opportunity to extend patents on drug products to encourage the development of new drugs, as well as amends the Federal Food, Drug and Cosmetic Act to expand the universe of drugs for which the FDA may accept ANDAs. Before enactment of this new law, ANDAs were permitted only for duplicates, ie, generic versions of drug products first approved between 1938 and 1962. Copies of pre-1938 drugs (eg, codeine, digoxin, phenobarbital) may be marketed without FDA approval provided there is no change in the product or its labeling that could cause the Agency to reclassify the drug as "new" and hence subject to NDA requirements. The law now provides for the submission of ANDAs for duplicates of any previously approved drug product, including post-1962 drug products. Therefore, use of the ANDA has been expanded by the increasing number of pharmaceutical companies desiring to market generic versions of post-1962 drugs and generic drug products become available more quickly. Since the NDA process has already been satisfactorily completed (either by the same or a different manufacturer), the clinical investigations for safety and efficacy need not be repeated.

However, the manufacturer must demonstrate that the proposed formulation meets USP standards for identity, strength, quality, and purity before approval. Bioequivalence testing is required for each active ingredient.

PREMARKET DRUG AVAILABILITY. Several compassionate-use procedures are available to enable a physician to have earlier access to a promising investigational drug for a patient who is not responding to conventional therapies. These include Treatment INDs, parallel track program, single patient compassionate use, and clinical trials.

Treatment Investigational New Drug Application (Treatment IND): The Treatment IND program is part of the FDA's efforts to facilitate the development and availability of significant new therapies. Under this program, treatment protocols for use of an investigational drug can be sought (usually by the sponsor) for life-threatening or serious conditions when there is no comparable or satisfactory alternative or other therapy to treat the disease or a particular stage of the disease in the intended population. To qualify for Treatment IND status, a drug also must be under investigation in a controlled clinical trial under an IND unless all clinical trials have been completed, and the sponsor must be actively pursuing marketing approval of the investigational drug. Furthermore, even when a life-threatening disease is involved, there must be a reasonable basis in the scientific evidence for concluding that the drug may be effective for the intended patient population and that it would not expose patients to unreasonable risk. Information on the availability of an investigational drug under the Treatment IND is published in the "From the Food and Drug Administration" column in *JAMA* and other vehicles (eg, press releases).

The most common way for a physician to obtain a Treatment IND drug is by direct contact with the sponsor (usually a pharmaceutical manufacturer) who already has obtained FDA approval of the treatment protocol. The sponsor will make the drug available to the physician, provide a brochure containing technical information about the drug, and describe the conditions of use allowed under the treatment protocol. In contrast to a regular IND, sponsors can charge for a Treatment IND drug, but experience to date indicates that most manufacturers do not charge for these drugs. For additional information, see *FDA Drug Bull,* 1988; Young et al, 1988.

Parallel Track Drug Availability Program: The FDA published regulations on a parallel track policy in April 1992. The program covers only drugs designed for AIDS patients, and it is an effort to make investigational drugs available more quickly without the restrictions inherent in well-controlled clinical trials. However, conducting controlled clinical trials concurrently for ultimate marketing approval is a condition that must be met by the drug sponsor to enable a drug to gain parallel track status.

The parallel track program is a more liberal mechanism of compassionate use than a Treatment IND for drug approval, because a parallel track drug may be approved without evidence of a drug's threshold of effectiveness that would be required for a Treatment IND. Concern exists that the parallel track drug program may interfere with the recruitment of subjects in concurrent controlled studies conducted in the normal drug approval process because patients who may be willing to try anything as quickly as possible will stop enrolling in controlled studies in sufficient numbers. The FDA may place a parallel track drug on clinical hold if it determines that this form of compassionate use is interfering with ongoing clinical trials as well as for other reasons (eg, an adequate and well-controlled study suggests that the drug is not effective; the drug sponsor is not pursuing market approval with due diligence; insufficient quantities of the drug exist to conduct the adequate, well-controlled studies as well as the uncontrolled concurrent parallel track studies).

In October 1992, stavudine [Bristol-Myers Squibb] became the first drug available under the FDA's parallel track program. Only patients with AIDS who are ineligible for both zidovudine [Retrovir] and didanosine [Videx] therapy due to intolerance, treatment failure, or contraindications are eligible to receive stavudine free of charge. In addition, patients must be over 13 years of age and have a CD4 cell count <300.

Single Patient Compassionate Use: The Code of Federal Regulations does not have a section on or define a "compassionate IND." This form of compassionate use describes an approval requested from the FDA by a physician to use a drug for a single patient, usually in a desperate situation and when there is no response to other therapies or in which no approved or generally recognized treatment is available. Approval for a compassionate use for a single patient might be sought in the following situations: (1) when an IND is in effect, but, unlike a Treatment IND or Parallel Track Drug Availability Program, the drug is still in the early stages of testing; (2) when an IND is in effect, but the physician needs the drug for purposes not described in the IND protocol; (3) when a drug has FDA approval, but it is not marketed; (4) when a drug had FDA approval but has been withdrawn from the market, usually because of questions regarding safety; or (5) when a drug is being investigated or marketed abroad but no IND is in effect in the United States. The physician must contact the review division of the FDA that is responsible for the drug or disease in question. In these situations, the FDA often will permit the proposed use under a commercial sponsor's IND or under a new IND filed by the patient's physician for an identified patient. In such cases, the FDA requires that the physician provide a report on the efficacy and any adverse reactions observed with the drug. This form of compassionate use is limited to one or a small number of patients per physician; however, the aggregate number of patients may be quite substantial.

The FDA has a drug import policy that permits patients with life-threatening disorders for which there is no treatment to acquire from any foreign country (including by mail) small quantities of unproved remedies for personal use. Because this policy potentially permits fraud that might result in exposure to unsafe medications, the FDA encourages such patients to notify their physician of this action so that they can be monitored for adverse drug reactions.

Clinical Trials: If the inclusion and exclusion criteria are met, entering a patient into an ongoing clinical trial of the desired investigational drug is a relatively common means of obtaining an investigational drug. Because scientific determination of efficacy and safety of the drug is the goal, a clinical trial generally is controlled and randomized; therefore, the patient may or may not receive the agent, at least initially, in most protocol designs. Open clinical trials are usually less restrictive regarding access to a desired drug.

A special program to facilitate access to investigational agents for cancer chemotherapy is available. Under its Cancer Therapy Evaluation, the Division of Cancer Treatment of the National Cancer Institute (NCI), in cooperation with the FDA, distributes certain drugs for use in clinical trials in patients with cancer. Unlike some drugs distributed by the NCI, drugs in one group, designated Group C drugs, are not limited to use in clinical trials for the purpose of testing their efficacy. Drugs are classified in Group C only if there is sufficient evidence demonstrating their efficacy for a tumor type and they can be administered safely. Although the drugs may be used for treatment outside of clinical trials, their most significant use is as part of combination chemotherapeutic regimens (not approved by the FDA) in clinical trials under NCI-sponsored protocols. Information about these drugs may be obtained from the Office of the Chief, Investigational Drug Branch, Division of Cancer Treatment, CTEP, Bldg 37, Room 6E20, National Cancer Institute, Bethesda, MD 20205.

POSTMARKETING DRUG ISSUES. Postmarketing Surveillance: Clinical experience with a new drug not approved in another country at the time of U.S. approval typically includes no more than 1,000 or 2,000 patients and often no more than a few hundred. The detection of adverse drug reactions (ADRs) occurring at frequencies of 1:1,000 or less is not reliable until hundreds of thousands of people have been exposed. "Phase IV" postmarketing surveillance studies may be conducted after NDA approval to obtain data to support additional safety and efficacy claims. The manufacturer (or a contract organization) may initiate such a study. Thus, postmarketing surveillance is designed to improve detection of ADRs. Orderly postmarketing surveillance also permits better estimation of the incidence and severity of known adverse drug reactions, which in turn permits physicians to make better judgments in drug use and patient counseling.

Manufacturers are required to submit to the FDA all reports of adverse effects, additional clinical experience, and other relevant data on marketed drugs. The following types of adverse drug reactions (ADRs) must be reported to the FDA by the manufacturer: Reports of ADRs (domestic, foreign, literature, or study) (1) that are serious and unexpected (ie, not already listed on the labeling) or (2) that are already labeled serious ADRs but that increase significantly in frequency. The agency can require label updating to keep precautionary information current. It also can take steps to have claims deleted that it considers no longer warranted or even to revoke an NDA and remove the drug from the market if there is evidence that it is not as safe and effective as originally believed. Legal remedies are available by which manufacturers may contest such actions if they disagree.

Official Labeling: The legal (Humphrey-Durham Amendment to the Food, Drug and Cosmetic Act, 1951) distinction between a prescription drug and an OTC drug is not founded on relative safety per se, but rather involves a regulatory decision on whether adequate directions for the proper (effective and safe) use of a particular drug can be written for the layman. If the FDA determines that adequate directions can be written, the manufacturer is not allowed to identify the drug with a prescription legend. Conversely, for a prescription drug, the manufacturer's directions or FDA-approved labeling (package insert) are intended for the physician, pharmacist, and nurse and provide a summary of information about the chemical and physical nature of the product, pharmacology, indications and contraindications, means of administration, appropriate dosages, side effects and adverse reactions, how the drug is supplied, and any other information pertinent to its safe and effective use. This summary, or official labeling, is developed by discussions between the FDA and the sponsor. Drug product information published in the *Physicians' Desk Reference* is usually a verbatim presentation of the FDA-approved labeling.

The FDA's jurisdiction over the uses of marketed drugs, dosage, and related matters extends only to what the manufacturer may recommend and must disclose in its labeling. It was not the intent of the Congress (under the 1962 amendment of the Food, Drug and Cosmetic Act) to charge the FDA with dictating how a physician should practice medicine (Erickson et al, 1980; Roth, 1982). Rather, the FDA is concerned with sanctioning the marketing and assuring the availability of drugs that have demonstrated substantial evidence of an acceptable benefit/risk ratio for labeled indications. The proper and successful therapeutic use of these drugs is the responsibility of the physician and requires a critical awareness and understanding of the present medical literature and careful monitoring of the patient's response.

Unlabeled (Off-Label) Use: The prescription of a drug for an unlabeled (off-label) indication is entirely proper if the proposed use is based on rational scientific theory, expert medical opinion, or controlled clinical studies. The FDA has made it eminently clear that it neither has nor wants the authority to compel physicians to adhere to officially labeled uses, because experience demonstrates that the official label lags behind scientific knowledge and publications. New uses for drugs already on the market are often first discovered through the serendipitous observations and therapeutic innovations of physicians (Hayes, 1981; *FDA Drug Bull*, 1982).

The physician is well advised to be *aware* of the content of a package insert and to give it due weight, especially the information on precautions, contraindications, and warnings. However, a decision on how to use a drug must be based on what is good medicine and best for the patient. This statement applies whether the physician's use of a drug conforms to official labeling or departs from it. In a professional liability suit, such drug labeling *may* have evidentiary weight for or against a physician, but drug labeling *per se* is not intended to set the standard for what is good medical practice.

In *DRUG EVALUATIONS,* the use of the term, investigational drug, means that the drug has not received FDA approval for marketing in this country. Uses of approved drugs for indications not included in the FDA-approved labeling (ie, off-label use, unlabeled use) also are included in *DE*. Such uses usually are referenced and may include discussion of their relative place in medical practice compared with other drug or nondrug therapy.

At present, many health care organizations are interested in the development of criteria that define degrees of acceptable and unacceptable medical practice; nevertheless, a widely accepted, consensus-derived mechanism(s) to define such criteria is not yet universally agreed upon. However, with regard to unlabeled uses, statutory language in the Omnibus Budget Reconciliation Act of 1990 names three compendia (*AMA DRUG EVALUATIONS;* Volume I of the United States Pharmacopeial Convention entitled *Drug Information for the Health Care Professional; and American Hospital Formulary Service-Drug Information*) and the peer-reviewed literature as the basis for defining a medically accepted indication for coverage and reimbursement purposes in state Medicaid prescription drug benefits programs.

The FDA does not have jurisdiction over drug formulations that the physician may devise for use in the normal course of his/her practice, provided the physician does not introduce these products into interstate commerce. Such formulations include those compounded from separate ingredients, certain readily available chemicals, or other nonpharmaceutical products that have therapeutic uses.

Advertising: The Federal Food, Drug and Cosmetic Act provides that the advertising of prescription drugs must conform to the labeling in specified ways. Any advertisement that describes or alludes to a drug's use in patients must contain the generic name and amount of the active ingredient(s), the name and address of the manufacturer, and a brief summary of prescribing information, including contraindications, warnings, and other pertinent information. A prescription drug advertisement that implies incorrectly that a drug is the treatment of choice or is useful for an unlabeled indication is unlawful. Manufacturers may voluntarily submit anticipated advertising to the FDA to ensure that the information conforms to legal requirements.

Regulation of advertising of nonprescription (OTC) drugs is the responsibility of the Federal Trade Commission.

Manufacturing and Distribution: Detailed manufacturing information to assure uniform purity and potency of drugs is an important part of the NDA and continuing FDA inspection program. The method of preparing the drug must be outlined, along with a complete description of how quality, purity, and strength are maintained. The manufacturing facilities, production methods, and quality control measures of a pharmaceutical company are subject to FDA inspection and review. The FDA conducts regular inspections of manufacturing plants for compliance with Good Manufacturing Practices (GMP) regulations. These are usually conducted at intervals not exceeding two years but may occur more frequently if manufacturers have many products and complex production processes. In addition, batch certification procedures for compliance with USP standards are conducted by the FDA for insulin preparations. Finally, the FDA is responsible for ensuring the safe distribution of drugs used in interstate commerce.

Other Official and Regulatory Agencies

FEDERAL TRADE COMMISSION (FTC). The Federal Trade Commission (FTC) is an independent agency of the federal government with five commissioners appointed by the President. The Commission administers several laws, the principal one being the Federal Trade Commission Act, which deals with the regulation of commercial trade practices.

The principal power of the FTC with respect to drugs is contained in the Federal Trade Commission Act (Chapter 2 of Title 15 of the U.S. Code): This Act gives the Commission broad power to prevent the dissemination of false or misleading advertising of foods, drugs, and cosmetics to the general public. For nonprescription (OTC) drugs, the FTC relies on FDA determinations of efficacy and safety and has taken action against advertising claims that are inconsistent with these criteria. Regulation of advertising for prescription drugs is the responsibility of the FDA.

DRUG ENFORCEMENT ADMINISTRATION (DEA). Responsibility for administration of the Controlled Substances Act is assigned to the Drug Enforcement Administration (DEA) in the Department of Justice. The DEA is charged with enforcing the provisions of the Act, which regulate the manufacture, purchase, prescribing, and dispensing of controlled substances and includes: (1) registration of physicians, pharmacists, and other handlers; (2) record-keeping and inspection requirements; (3) quotas on manufacturing; (4) restrictions on distribution; (5) restrictions on dispensing; (6) limitations on imports and exports; (7) conditions for storage of drugs; (8) reports of transactions to the government; and (9) criminal, civil, and administrative penalties for illegal acts. As a convenience, the *United States Pharmacopeia-National Formulary (USP-NF)* includes the latest DEA regulations that affect practicing physicians and pharmacists.

CONSUMER PRODUCT SAFETY COMMISSION (CPSC). The Consumer Product Safety Commission is responsible for administration of the Poison Prevention Packaging Act (PPPA). The Commission sets standards for childproof packaging, grants exemptions from these standards for certain products, and enforces the Act.

UNITED STATES PHARMACOPEIAL CONVENTION (USPC), INC. Through the General Committee of Revision, the United States Pharmacopeial Convention, Inc, issues the combined *United States Pharmacopeia (USP)-National Formulary (NF)* at five-year intervals with semiannual *Supplements* and *Interim Revisions* as needed. This is a private body incorporated in the District of Columbia and is composed of representatives from medical and pharmacy schools, state medical and pharmaceutical associations, the American Medical Association, the American Pharmaceutical Association, the American Chemical Society, many other scientific and trade associations, various interested federal agencies, and several foreign countries that recognize this volume as an official compendium.

Under authority of the Federal Food, Drug and Cosmetic Act, the standards of strength, quality, purity, packaging, and labeling for products described in *USP-NF* are official.

The Pharmacopeial Convention also publishes annually the text entitled *Drug Information for the Health Care Professional (USP DI)*. Volume I includes drug information for the health professional (an expansion of the information that formerly appeared in the official compendia); Volume II includes information designed expressly for the patient and is entitled *Ad-*

vice for the Patient; and Volume III consists of *Approved Drug Products* (the FDA's "Orange Book") and *Legal Requirements*. The latter include both state and federal requirements that are applicable to the prescribing-dispensing interface. These volumes are supplemented by a single monthly *USP DI Update*.

USAN and the USP Dictionary of Drug Names, a cumulation of United States Adopted Names and other designations for drugs, both current and retrospective, also is published annually by the United States Pharmacopeial Convention, Inc.

UNITED STATES ADOPTED NAMES (USAN) COUNCIL. The USAN Council adopts appropriate nonproprietary names for all new single-entity drugs marketed in the United States; it was organized in January 1964 and is sponsored by the American Medical Association, the American Pharmaceutical Association, and the United States Pharmacopeial Convention, Inc. The Council has five members: one member appointed by each sponsor, one member-at-large who must be approved by all three sponsors, and one liaison member from the FDA.

The primary functions of the USAN Council are: (1) to negotiate with pharmaceutical manufacturers in the selection of meaningful and distinctive nonproprietary names for new drug entities; (2) to publicize the adopted names, the guiding principles used in devising these names, and the procedures involved in their adoption; and (3) to cooperate with other national and international agencies, particularly the World Health Organization International Nonproprietary Names (INN) Committee, in standardizing the nonproprietary nomenclature for drugs.

Following adoption, new USAN designations are published in *Clinical Pharmacology and Therapeutics, USP DI Update, USP Pharmacopeial Forum, Hospital Pharmacy*, and *Unlisted Drugs*. The current version of The Guiding Principles for Coining United States Adopted Names for Drugs appears in the annual cumulative publication, *USAN and the USP Dictionary of Drug Names*, in each edition of the *USAN Handbook*, and in Remington's *Pharmaceutical Sciences*. The *USAN Handbook* is available on request from the AMA Department of Drugs. This booklet describes the process of establishing nonproprietary names and the information required to process an application for a U.S. Adopted Name.

Cited References

Use of approved drugs for unlabeled indications. *FDA Drug Bull* 12:4-5, (April) 1982.

Drugs available under Treatment IND. *FDA Drug Bull* 18:14-15, (Aug) 1988.

Advisory Committee on the Food and Drug Administration: *Final Report of the Advisory Committee on the Food and Drug Administration.* Washington, DC, US Department of Health and Human Services, (May) 1991.

Generic substitution, policy no. 125.994 (A-87), in: *Policy Compendium.* Chicago, Ill, American Medical Association, 1993 A, 94-95.

Generic substitution, policy no. 125.992 (A-90), in: *Policy Compendium.* Chicago, Ill, American Medical Association, 1993 B, 93-94.

Principles of drug utilization review, policy no. 120.978 (A-91), in: *Policy Compendium.* Chicago, Ill, American Medical Association, 1993 C, 90.

Commission on Federal Drug Approval Process: Final report. (March 31) 1982.

Council on Scientific Affairs: Drug abuse related to prescribing practices. *JAMA* 247:862-866, 1982.

Erickson SH, et al: Use of drugs for unlabeled indications. *JAMA* 243:1543-1546, 1980.

FDA: 75th Anniversary Issue. *FDA Consumer* 15:1-68, (June) 1981.

Friedman D, et al: Physicians attitudes toward and knowledge about generic drug substitution. *NY State J Med* 87:539-542, 1987.

Hayes AH Jr: Food and drug regulation after 75 years. *JAMA* 246:1223-1226, 1981.

Jaffe JH: Drug addiction and drug abuse, in Gilman AG, et al (eds): *The Pharmacological Basis of Therapeutics,* ed 6. New York, Macmillan, 1980, 535-584.

Kessler DA: Regulation of investigational drugs. *N Engl J Med* 320:281-288, 1989.

Kessler DA, et al: Federal regulation of medical devices. *N Engl J Med* 317:357-366, 1987.

Lasagna L: Congress, the FDA, and new drug development: Before and after 1962. *Perspect Biol Med* 32:322-343, 1989.

MacCannell KL, Giraud G: Fixed ratio drug combinations: Sense and nonsense, in Lasagna L (ed): *Controversies in Therapeutics.* Philadelphia, WB Saunders, 1980, 172-179.

Manasse HR Jr: *Medication Use in an Imperfect World: Drug Misadventuring as an Issue of Public Policy.* Bethesda, Md, American Society of Hospital Pharmacists Research and Education Foundation, 1989.

Miller HI, Young FE: Drug approval process at the Food and Drug Administration: New biotechnology as paradigm of science-based activist approach. *Arch Intern Med* 149:655-657, 1989.

Morgan JP: Politics of medication, in Lasagna L (ed): *Controversies in Therapeutics.* Philadelphia, WB Saunders, 1980, 16-22.

Nightingale SL: Generic drugs. *Am Fam Physician* 38:369-370, (Sept) 1988.

Nightingale SL, Morrison JC: Generic drugs and the prescribing physician. *JAMA* 258:1200-1204, 1987.

Parker RE, et al: Drug product selection—Part 1: History and legal overview. *Am Pharm* NS31:72-79, (July) 1991 A.

Parker RE, et al: Drug product selection—Part 3: The orange book. *Am Pharm* NS31:47-55, (Sept) 1991 B.

Peck CC: Should we improve patient compliance with therapeutic regimens and if so how? in Lasagna L (ed): *Controversies in Therapeutics.* Philadelphia, WB Saunders, 1980, 559-566.

Roth SH: Drug use, package insert, and practice of medicine, editorial. *Arch Intern Med* 142:871-872, 1982.

Roth HP, Caron HS: Accuracy of doctors' estimates and patients' statements on adherence to drug regimen. *Clin Pharm Ther* 23:361-370, 1978.

Sackett DL: Is there a patient compliance problem? If so, what do we do about it? in Lasagna L (ed): *Controversies in Therapeutics.* Philadelphia, WB Saunders, 1980, 552-558.

Schwartz LL, Stanton MA: Generic drugs, letter. *N Engl J Med* 317:1411-1412, 1987.

Solomon HS: How to improve patient compliance, in Lasagna L (ed): *Controversies in Therapeutics.* Philadelphia, WB Saunders, 1980, 567-571.

Strom BL: Generic drug substitution revisited. *N Engl J Med* 316:1456-1462, 1987.

Turner P, et al: Generic bioinequivalence, letter. *Lancet* 2:517, 1987.

Urquhart J: Real-time compliance monitoring in clinical trials: Methods, early results, prospects, in Hindmarch I, Stonier P (eds): *Human Psychopharmacology.* Chichester, United Kingdom, John Wiley, 1990, vol 3, 129-147.

Weinberger M: Generic drugs, letter. *N Engl J Med* 317:1412, 1987.

Weintraub M: Undertreatment: Who is to blame? *Drug Ther (Hosp)* 11:58-63, (Dec) 1981.

Young FE, et al: FDA's new procedures for use of investigational drugs in treatment. *JAMA* 259:2267-2270, 1988.

Drug Response Variation and Dosing Information 2

PROCESSES IN DRUG DISPOSITION

- **Absorption**
- **Distribution**
- **Biotransformation**
- **Excretion**

BASIC CONCEPTS OF CLINICAL PHARMACOKINETICS

- **Clearance**
- **Volume of Distribution**
- **Half-Life**
- **Steady State**
- **Designing a Dosage Regimen**
- **Nonlinear Elimination**
- **Therapeutic Drug Monitoring**

FACTORS AFFECTING PATIENT RESPONSE TO DRUGS

- **Influence of Disease**
  - **Renal Impairment**
  - **Hepatic Impairment**
  - **Other Disease States**
- **Influence of Age**
  - **Pediatric Patients**
  - **Geriatric Patients**
- **Influence of Other Conditions**
  - **Pregnancy**
  - **Obesity**
- **Influence of Pharmacogenetics**
- **Influence of Diet and Environmental Chemicals**
- **Influence of Biological Rhythms**

Patients vary widely in their response to the standard doses of many drugs. Such interpatient variation in response is especially relevant clinically for drugs with narrow therapeutic indexes. A drug's therapeutic index is the ratio of the dose (or plasma concentration) that is likely to produce toxic effects compared with the dose (or plasma concentration) required to produce therapeutic effects.

Differences in pharmacodynamic factors (ie, sensitivity or response of target tissues or organs to drug effects) exist within the population. These differences are more apparent in patients taking certain drugs (eg, beta blockers, central nervous system depressants, analgesics) and in the elderly. Superimposed on pharmacodynamic differences, individual pharmacokinetic factors, particularly genetic and developmentally related determinants of drug metabolism, contribute significantly to the patient variability in drug response to a particular dose. In addition, age, gender, body size and composition, diet, exposure to environmental chemicals, use of alcohol or tobacco, pregnancy, concurrent illness or disease states, and drug interactions also can modify drug disposition and/or response, thereby contributing to interpatient variability. Dosage forms that differ in bioequivalence may further complicate the relationship between the dose and the plasma concentration. Therefore, drug dosage must be individualized to obtain the desired therapeutic response with minimal side effects.

PROCESSES IN DRUG DISPOSITION

Pharmacokinetics refers to the quantitative analysis of the time course of drug (and metabolite) concentration in various tissues of the body. It includes analysis of the processes of drug disposition (ie, absorption; distribution, including storage; biotransformation; excretion).

Absorption

Most drugs are administered orally. This route is convenient, and linking drug ingestion to daily routines such as mealtime can improve compliance. Tablets and capsules must disintegrate and dissolve before the drug is available for absorption (see Figure 1). Once solubilized, a drug can diffuse through the gastrointestinal epithelium into the portal circulation. Drug absorption proceeds via passive diffusion, although there are exceptions (eg, levodopa). Absorption may be incomplete because of the physiochemical properties of the drug (eg, aqueous or lipid solubility, degree of ionization, stability, molecular size) or because the pharmaceutical preparation may disintegrate or deaggregate too slowly. This is a particular concern with some prolonged-release formulations.

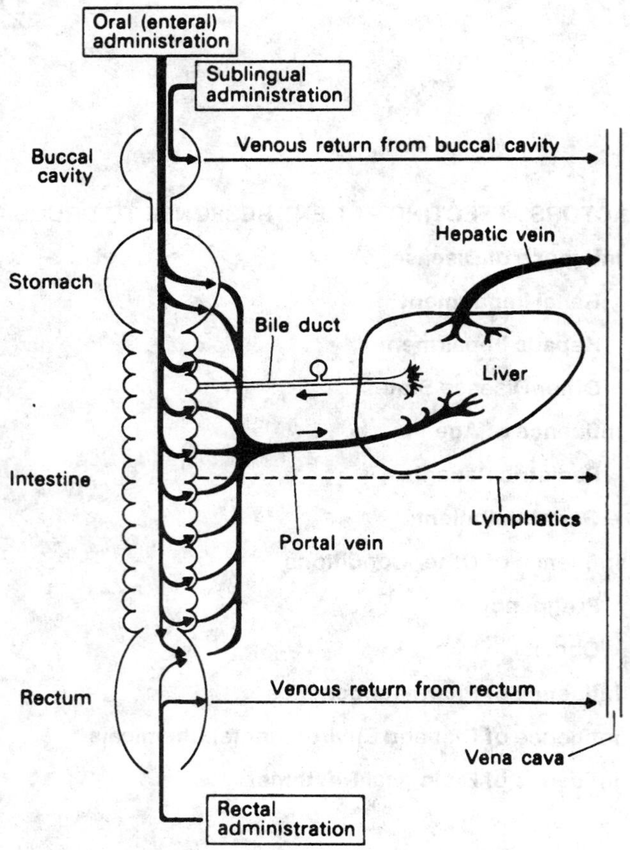

Figure 1. Absorptive processes following oral, sublingual, and rectal administration. From Bowman WC, Rand MJ: Textbook of Pharmacology, *ed 2. St. Louis, Blackwell Mosby, 1980. Reprinted with permission.*

Drug absorption generally occurs in the small intestine; few drugs are absorbed to an important degree from the stomach. The presence of food or other substances in the intestine, gastric emptying and intestinal transit times, and local pH can influence both the rate and extent of drug absorption. Some drugs (eg, ranitidine, levodopa) reduce the rate of gastric emptying and hence their own rate of absorption. Such factors can be important for drugs that must act promptly (eg, analgesics, sedatives). Food can reduce the absorption of some drugs (eg, acid-labile compounds) but may increase the bioavailability of others because of effects on solubility (eg, griseofulvin, quinidine gluconate) or presystemic clearance (eg, propranolol, phenytoin) (Winstanley and Orme, 1989). (See also the discussion in the section on Influence of Diet and Environmental Chemicals.)

Once absorbed into the portal circulation, the drug must pass through the liver to gain access to the systemic circulation. However, the intestinal wall and the liver are major sites of biotransformation. Biotransformation that takes place before the drug reaches the systemic circulation is called *first-pass* metabolism.

Rectally administered drugs may or may not bypass the liver, since the upper two-thirds of the rectum drains to the portal circulation. Use of the rectal route is clinically advantageous for certain medications and conditions (eg, opioids, antiemetics, diazepam for febrile seizures, preoperative medication) (van Hoogdalem et al, 1991).

Other routes of administration can avoid first-pass metabolism or provide a more rapid onset. Sublingual, buccal, nasal, and transdermal administration can result in greater systemic bioavailability of some drugs that, when administered orally, are degraded in the gastrointestinal tract or extensively metabolized by the liver.

The intramuscular and subcutaneous routes usually result in more rapid and complete absorption than with oral administration while minimizing the hazards of intravascular injection. The rate of absorption with these routes depends on drug solubility, concentration of the injected solution, site of administration, and area blood flow. Absorption is most rapid after intramuscular injection into the deltoid, followed by injection into the vastus lateralis, and is slowest after injection into gluteal muscle.

Drugs that are poorly absorbed after intramuscular injection because they are insoluble in water (eg, diazepam) must be given in an organic, water-miscible vehicle such as propylene glycol. After administration, the local concentration of the vehicle decreases and the drug precipitates into the tissue; the absorption rate then depends on the dissolution rate of precipitated drug. The result is slow systemic absorption following intramuscular injection.

Prolonged-release preparations are formulated to release a drug slowly, thereby extending plasma concentrations and duration of action. These products deserve special consideration because their bioavailability and duration of action are potentially variable. The general terms, "prolonged-release" or "delayed-release," used to describe preparations in this text are synonymous with the term, "controlled-release," used by the Food and Drug Administration, and include formulations variously referred to as "timed-release," "delayed-action," "extended-release," "prolonged-action," "slow-release," "sustained-release," or "sustained-action."

Data on which to base an evaluation of effectiveness are inadequate or unavailable for the prolonged-release forms of many drugs; however, when a drug has been tested for effectiveness in this form, the assessment of its value is indicated in the evaluations in appropriate chapters.

A number of factors stimulate interest in developing and marketing prolonged-release preparations. These dosage forms potentially increase patient compliance and minimize fluctuations in plasma drug concentrations. However, in some instances, a pharmaceutical manufacturer develops a prolonged-release product solely to permit extension and/or retention of a competitive position in the marketplace while providing no significant advantage to the patient (Gibaldi, 1984). Physicians should ensure that a prolonged-release preparation, which typically is more expensive than a standard preparation, is of significant benefit to a patient. Properties of a drug that are conducive to development of prolonged-release formulations are short half-life (eg, three to six hours) and strong relationship between plasma drug concentration and pharmacologic response; administration for a chronic condition without the need for immediate response is also advantageous for these formulations.

Most prolonged-release products are administered orally. A number of pharmaceutical techniques are used to produce *oral* prolonged-release preparations. These include ion-exchange resins that bind the drug, semipermeable membranes with small laser-drilled holes, slowly eroding coatings or matrixes, and slowly dissolving physical or chemical forms.

In *parenteral* preparations, prolonged release is achieved by using relatively insoluble salts or esters of the active drug or a special vehicle. When some latitude in the range of safe and effective blood levels is permissible, substitution of slowly released preparations for intermittent injections may provide a more uniform blood concentration, and this type of preparation is certainly more convenient. Examples of such preparations include benzathine penicillin G, depot antipsychotic agents, leuprolide, and various corticosteroids, androgens, estrogens, and progestins (eg, medroxyprogesterone).

The *topical* application of drugs for systemic activity has become more frequent since commercial development of transdermal patches. These prolonged-release products are easy to use, can be applied daily or even weekly, avoid large fluctuations in plasma drug concentrations, and avoid first-pass metabolism by the liver and in the intestinal wall. Transdermal formulations of scopolamine, nitroglycerin, clonidine, fentanyl, nicotine, and estradiol are now commercially available.

Transdermal patches employ various techniques to allow the diffusion of a relatively constant amount of drug over a period of time. The drug diffuses passively through the skin; four principal factors determine the rate of percutaneous absorption. The first is the thickness of the stratum corneum of the epidermis, which provides the main resistance to the transdermal absorption of drugs. The rate of absorption is inversely related to thickness of the skin and can influence the effectiveness of a drug. For example, if the site of application is rotated from an area where the skin is thin, such as the chest, to an area where the skin is thick, such as the inner arm, the amount of drug absorbed will decline and therapeutic activity may decrease. A second factor is the physicochemical properties of a drug. The drug must be both lipophilic and hydrophilic for optimal diffusion through the skin. A third factor is the quantity of drug on the skin surface; a greater amount increases the concentration gradient between the skin surface and the vascular bed and increases diffusion. The final principal factor is the patient's state of hydration. In hydrated patients, the epidermal packing is looser and more drug penetrates through the barrier.

A number of controlled-release systems that deliver a drug at a predetermined rate for a definite period of time have been developed recently. Externally worn or implantable pumps, polymeric subdermal reservoirs or materials placed in other body compartments, and injectable microspheres are but a few examples of novel drug delivery approaches that already have improved clinical treatment (Langer, 1990).

Distribution

After entering the systemic circulation, a drug distributes throughout the body in a characteristic fashion that depends on its physicochemical characteristics (molecular size, lipid solubility, degree of ionization). For a few drugs, an equilibrium between tissue and plasma (or serum) drug concentrations is reached very rapidly. However, for most drugs, there is a significant time lag before equilibrium is reached. The rate of drug distribution may be controlled by diffusion across capillary endothelium cell membranes (diffusion-rate limitation) or by tissue blood flow (perfusion-rate limitation).

Another factor affecting drug distribution is the binding of drugs to plasma and tissue proteins. Drugs that are weak acids (eg, warfarin, phenytoin, aspirin) generally bind to albumin. Drugs that are weak bases (eg, propranolol, imipramine, quinidine) also bind to lipoproteins and alpha$_1$-acid glycoprotein (AAG). In general, plasma protein binding is a reversible process governed by the protein and drug concentrations and the drug's affinity for the binding sites. With the exception of a few drugs (eg, ceftriaxone, disopyramide, prednisolone, valproate), the fraction of drug that is bound to plasma proteins remains relatively constant throughout the usual therapeutic range, even though the total plasma concentration changes.

The fraction of drug bound to plasma proteins may be altered by other drugs and endogenous substances that compete for protein binding sites. Displacement of a drug from plasma or tissue protein increases its unbound fraction and may alter the drug's pharmacokinetic behavior. The clinical sequelae depend on a variety of factors, but displacement per se seldom causes serious adverse drug reactions (see the discussion in the section on Therapeutic Drug Monitoring).

Biotransformation

In general, biotransformation converts lipophilic drugs into more polar, water-soluble metabolites that are more suitable for renal excretion. Usually, this is a detoxification process, but, for some drugs, metabolites are pharmacologically active and contribute important therapeutic or toxic effects. Drug metabolic reactions may be characterized as phase I or phase II. In phase I (nonsynthetic) reactions, the polarity of the drug molecule is increased via oxidation, hydrolysis, or reduction. Most lipophilic drugs are eliminated by oxidation in the liver. Hydrolytic reactions, which are important for drugs containing ester or amide groups, occur in the brain, blood, liver, and many other tissues. Gastrointestinal bacteria may contribute to reduction reactions. In phase II (synthetic) reactions, the parent compound is conjugated with an endogenous substrate (eg, glucuronic acid, acetate, glycine, sulfate). Phase II metabolites are generally inactive and are readily excreted in the urine, although hydrolysis of enterally secreted glucuronides by bacterial enzymes may restore the parent compound, which may be cycled enterohepatically.

Drug oxidations are predominantly catalyzed in the liver by cytochrome P450, which is a collective term for a group of microsomal enzymes characterized as mixed function oxidases. Other organs (eg, lungs, gastrointestinal tract, kidneys, placenta, skin) also contain significant amounts of cytochrome P450. Related enzymes in the mitochondria of various organs participate in the oxidation of steroid hormones.

Each enzyme shares a common component (heme group) but is encoded by a separate gene. The enzymes are grouped into families and subfamilies (Gonzalez, 1989). Considerable overlap in substrate specificity exists among the various isoforms, although a particular drug may have such a high affinity for one isoform that its relative rate of biotransformation in vivo is essentially dependent on that isoform. Mutations or deletions of a particular gene can lead to dramatic interpatient variations in the rate of drug oxidation for particular substrates (see the section on Influence of Pharmacogenetics).

Certain cytochrome P450 enzymes can be induced by a number of exogenous factors, including cigarette smoking (ie, polycyclic hydrocarbons), exposure to environmental chemicals, diet, ingestion of alcohol, and presence of certain drugs (eg, phenytoin, phenobarbital, rifampin, carbamazepine). This induction process may lead to increased metabolism for the specific agent (autoinduction) or to increased metabolism for a number of other drugs (heteroinduction). Also, the general catalytic activity of cytochrome P450 may be impaired (eg, cimetidine), selective isoform inhibition may occur (eg, erythromycin, quinidine, ketoconazole), or substrates may compete for oxidation.

Excretion

Drugs are eliminated from the body either unchanged or as metabolites. Quantitatively, the kidney is the most important organ for excretion of drugs and their metabolites. Many metabolites formed in the liver may be secreted into the bile for delivery to the intestinal tract, where they are excreted in the feces, or, more commonly, are reabsorbed for eventual urinary excretion. Pulmonary excretion is important for anesthetic gases and volatile compounds.

The excretion of drugs by the kidneys may involve glomerular filtration, tubular secretion, and tubular reabsorption. The kidneys receive about one-fourth of the total cardiac output, of which 10% is filtered by the glomerulus. The resulting glomerular filtration rate is approximately 120 ml/minute for the average young adult. Only unbound drugs are cleared by renal filtration. Thus, the fraction of drug that is bound to blood components affects the rate of renal elimination. The maximal rate of drug clearance by renal filtration is equal to the product of the glomerular filtration rate and the fraction of drug unbound in the blood.

Renal tubular secretion is an active process that occurs primarily in the proximal tubule. Two separate systems add certain organic anions (acids) and cations (bases) to the glomerular filtrate by carrier-mediated, tubular secretion. A wide variety of drugs and their metabolites, as well as numerous endogenous substances, are excreted in this manner (van Ginneken and Russel, 1989). Although protein binding decreases the extent of drug clearance by glomerular filtration, the tubular secretion of most organic anions seems to be relatively unaffected. Both carrier systems are relatively nonselective, and organic ions of similar charge compete for transport. Saturation of tubular secretion may lead to a decrease in drug clearance with increasing plasma concentration. In addition, drug interactions at the level of tubular secretion have been described (see the discussion on Drug Interactions, Mechanisms, in the following chapter).

Renal tubular reabsorption usually is a passive process that decreases drug clearance. It occurs all along the nephron and tends to follow the movement of free water. Because the tubular cell membrane is relatively impermeable to the ionized form of weak electrolytes, passive reabsorption is influenced by changes in urinary pH. When the tubular fluid is made more alkaline (eg, sodium bicarbonate), the ionization of weak acids (eg, salicylates, phenobarbital) is increased and they are excreted more rapidly. On the other hand, acidification of the urine (eg, ammonium chloride, ascorbic acid) increases the ionization and renal excretion of drugs that are weak bases (eg, quinidine). Occasionally, such manipulation may be useful adjunctively to hasten the renal elimination of certain drugs in the management of acute toxicity (see the chapter on Drugs Used in the Management of Poisoning).

BASIC CONCEPTS OF CLINICAL PHARMACOKINETICS

Drug disposition usually proceeds according to linear kinetics. In linear (first-order) kinetics, the rate of drug disposition is proportional to the drug concentration. Analysis of drug disposition can be facilitated by the use of mathematical models. Depending on the drug's pharmacokinetic and pharmacodynamic characteristics, a one-compartment model often is sufficient for clinical applications. This model, which depicts the body as a single homogeneous compartment, is useful for defining important variables and is broadly applicable to many clinical situations. For other drugs, a multicompartment model may be required. Occasionally, a Michaelis-Menten or nonlinear model is necessary.

For drugs that conform to linear kinetics, bioavailability, volume of distribution, and systemic clearance are useful parameters for the design and modification of therapeutic regimens.

Bioavailability is the rate and extent of absorption following nonvascular administration. A drug is completely available (ie, the total administered dose reaches the systemic circulation) when it is given intravenously. Administration by any other route may result in less than complete absorption or presystemic clearance, and the fraction of drug that reaches the systemic circulation (F) may be less than unity. One way of measuring the extent of absorption is by comparing the area under a serum drug concentration-time curve (AUC) following oral administration with the AUC following intravenous administration (Equation 1). Correction must be made for any difference between doses.

$$F = \frac{AUC_{oral}}{AUC_{iv}} \qquad \text{(Eq. 1)}$$

Although a drug may be absorbed completely, the absorption rate also is important, since it may be too slow to achieve a therapeutic blood level of the drug or so rapid that initial high concentrations produce adverse effects.

Differences in the bioavailability of various pharmaceutical formulations of a given drug (ie, lack of bioequivalence) may have clinical significance, since therapeutic or toxic effects usually depend on serum drug concentrations. Problems are more likely to be encountered during long-term therapy when a patient who is stabilized on one pharmaceutical product receives a nonequivalent substitute. (For a discussion on generic substitution, see index entry Prescription Practices.)

Clearance

Clearance is the most important parameter for individualizing a dosage regimen. It may be defined as the virtual volume of biological fluid (eg, blood, plasma, serum) from which a drug is removed over a period of time. Clearance is commonly adjusted for body weight or, occasionally, for body surface area and is expressed as ml/minute, ml/kg/minute, L/kg/hour, ml/M^2/minute, or L/M^2/hour. As will be discussed later, the clearance value is used to predict drug concentrations at steady state and to forecast the dosage regimen required to achieve a desired drug concentration (Gibaldi, 1986).

The total body clearance (CL) is a summation of clearances from the various drug-eliminating organs, including the liver, kidneys, lungs, and intestinal mucosa. Clearance of most drugs is constant over the range of plasma drug concentrations encountered clinically. For drugs with linear elimination kinetics, CL can be estimated from the following relationship:

$$CL = \frac{Dose_{iv}}{AUC}$$

(Eq. 2)

Hepatic Clearance: The rate of drug removal from the blood by the liver is the product of the hepatic blood flow and the fraction of drug removed from the portal circulation as the blood percolates through the liver (ie, the extraction ratio, E).

Factors that affect E include the degree of binding to blood proteins and components, the diffusion of unbound drug between blood and the hepatocyte, the rate of secretion of drug from the hepatocyte into the biliary tract, and the rate of hepatic biotransformation. The maximal ability of the liver to remove a drug by all pathways in the absence of blood flow limitations is termed intrinsic clearance (CL_{int}) (Wilkinson and Shand, 1975). Intrinsic clearance usually reflects the activity of hepatic drug metabolizing enzymes.

When the hepatic intrinsic clearance of a drug is efficient, the hepatic extraction is high ($E \geq 0.7$). The hepatic clearance of drugs in this category is dependent on the amount of drug (bound and unbound) delivered to the liver and therefore is dependent on blood flow. Conversely, when the hepatic intrinsic clearance of a drug is inefficient, the rate of metabolism of these poorly extracted drugs ($E \leq 0.3$) is independent of hepatic blood flow and is limited by the hepatic metabolizing capacity and the amount of drug available for metabolism. The hepatic clearance of many low extraction drugs is proportional to the concentration of free (unbound) drug in plasma. Clearance that is sensitive to changes in the unbound fraction is termed restrictive (Benet and Massoud, 1984). (See Table 1.)

TABLE 1.
DRUGS WITH HIGH AND LOW HEPATIC INTRINSIC CLEARANCE*

Category	Approximate Hepatic Extraction Ratio	% Bound
HIGH		
Propoxyphene	0.95	70
Pentazocine	0.80	60-70
Labetalol	0.70	50
Lidocaine	0.70	45-80
LOW RESTRICTIVE		
Quinidine	0.27	82-90
Clindamycin	0.23	93
Chlorpromazine	0.22	98
Phenytoin	0.03	90
Diazepam	0.03	98
Tolbutamide	0.02	95
Warfarin	0.003	99
Digitoxin	0.005	97
LOW NONRESTRICTIVE		
Thiopental	0.28	72-86
Chloramphenicol	0.28	60-80
Theophylline	0.09	50-60
Amobarbital	0.03	61

**Adapted from Blaschke, 1977.*

Intrinsic clearance explains why the systemic clearance of certain drugs is affected by changes in hepatic metabolic enzyme activity while the clearance of others is not. For drugs with a low extraction ratio, hepatic enzyme induction and inhibition result in a change in the rate-limiting factor of hepatic elimination. However, their systemic clearance is essentially unchanged by variations in hepatic blood flow. In contrast, for drugs with a high extraction ratio, intrinsic clearance is not a rate-limiting factor and systemic clearance is resistant to changes in hepatic enzyme activity. Systemic clearance is, however, susceptible to changes in hepatic blood flow. Importantly, changes in intrinsic clearance are proportionally reflected in a drug's oral clearance, regardless of the magnitude of the extraction ratio (Wilkinson, 1987).

Drugs such as quinidine, desipramine, and nortriptyline have an intermediate extraction ratio and are more equally affected by changes in hepatic enzyme activity and blood flow.

Renal Clearance: Renal clearance results in the appearance of drug in the urine as the net result of the three renal processes of glomerular filtration, tubular secretion, and tubular reabsorption. Consequently, renal clearance is quite sensitive to changes in renal function or in those variables that affect elimination by renal processes (ie, protein binding, renal blood flow, urinary pH). Renal clearance (CL_R) of a drug can be assessed directly from urinary data (Equation 3).

$$CL_R = \frac{V \cdot C_u}{C}$$

(Eq. 3)

V equals urine flow rate, C_u is the urinary drug concentration, and C is the blood or plasma drug concentration at the midpoint of the urine collection interval.

Changes in renal function are commonly assessed by estimating endogenous creatinine clearance. If creatinine clearance cannot be determined directly, it can be estimated from a serum creatinine value if age, sex, and body weight are known and renal function is stable. Nomograms that provide reasonable estimates of creatinine clearance have been published (eg, Siersbaek-Nielsen et al, 1971). An estimation for adult males may be calculated from the following equation (Cockcroft and Gault, 1976):

$$\text{Creatinine Clearance (men)} = \frac{(140 - \text{age}) \cdot (\text{body weight in kg})}{72 \cdot \text{serum creatinine}}$$

(Eq. 4)

For women, the creatinine clearance is 85% of the value calculated by this equation. Creatinine clearance calculated from Equation 4 may be higher than the actual creatinine clearance in certain patients (eg, pregnant women, elderly patients with muscle atrophy, patients with markedly reduced renal function [<10 ml/minute]). Formulas also have been developed for boys and girls (Schwartz et al, 1976; Schwartz and Gauthier, 1985).

Volume of Distribution

Conceptually, if the body is considered a single compartment, the (apparent) volume of distribution (Vd) represents the volume necessary to account for the total amount of drug in the body if it were present at the same concentration found in plasma, and C_o represents the estimated plasma concentration at time zero (see Figure 2). This can be expressed mathematically as:

$$Vd = \frac{Dose_{iv}}{C_o} = \frac{\text{Amount in body}}{C}$$

(Eq. 5)

For example, if 300 mg of theophylline is present in the body and the plasma theophylline concentration is equal to 10 mg/L, the apparent Vd for theophylline is 30 L. Vd is an important concept because it is a proportionality constant that relates the total amount of drug in the body to the plasma concentration. It also is a particularly useful parameter for designing regimens that involve loading doses. In addition, Vd and clearance (see Equation 6) determine the rate constant of elimination and hence the half-life of a drug.

For most drugs, Vd is constant over a wide dosage range. Factors affecting Vd include lipid solubility, degree of ionization, molecular size, and the degree of binding to plasma and tissue proteins. The Vd can be altered significantly by major illness. For example, severe renal failure markedly decreases the Vd for digoxin, probably because of decreased plasma protein binding.

Although Vd is based on the extent of drug distribution outside the plasma compartment, it usually has no obvious anatomic counterpart. Distribution volumes vary greatly. The smallest Vd corresponds to the extracellular fluid space (Atkinson et al, 1991), but is more than 20 L/kg for nortriptyline. The Vd defined in Equation 5 considers the body a single, homogeneous compartment. Utilizing this model for drug elimination that proceeds by first-order kinetics, a semilogarithmic plot of the drug's plasma concentration versus time following intravenous administration shows a linear decline (Figure 2). The slope of this line reflects the elimination rate constant, k. In a linear, one-compartment model:

$$k = \frac{CL}{Vd}$$

(Eq. 6)

Therefore, the effect of a given plasma clearance on the rate of removal of drug from the body depends on Vd.

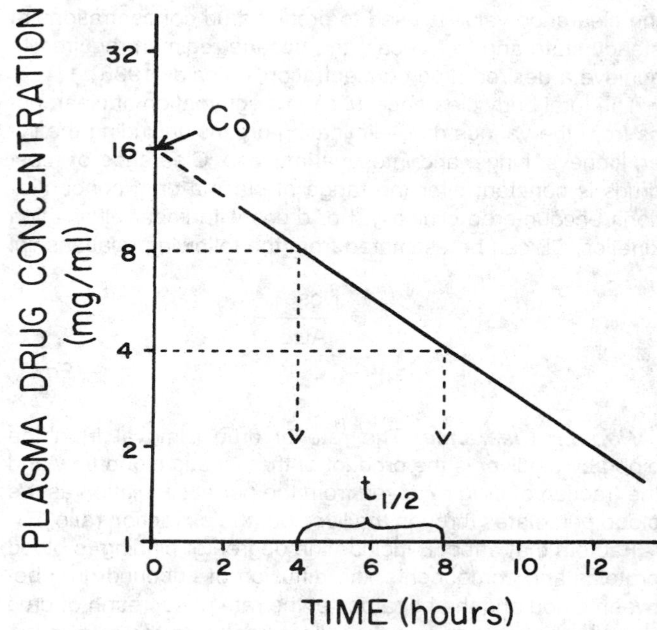

Figure 2. Plasma concentration-time curve following intravenous administration of a drug. The first sample is taken at two hours postadministration. Semilogarithmic plot appears to indicate a drug that follows linear, one-compartment kinetics. Extrapolation of the linear decline yields intercept C_o on the left ordinate that can be used for estimation of Vd according to equation 5 in text. Half-life ($t_{1/2}$) is four hours.

Alternatively, with earlier multiple samples, a semilogarithmic plot of plasma concentration versus time may yield an initial curve followed by a slower linear decline (Figure 3). This is characteristic of a drug with biexponential kinetics. Usually, the initial segment (α phase) *primarily* reflects the drug's distribution to highly perfused organs and readily accessible body fluids; the second segment (β phase) primarily reflects drug elimination. Even more exponential phases may be required to characterize the disposition of some drugs. However, the k and $t_{1/2}$ generally are determined from the terminal exponential phase. For some drugs with multiexponential kinetics, failure to identify or consider the distribution phase may lead to significant errors in the estimation of clearance (Equation 2).

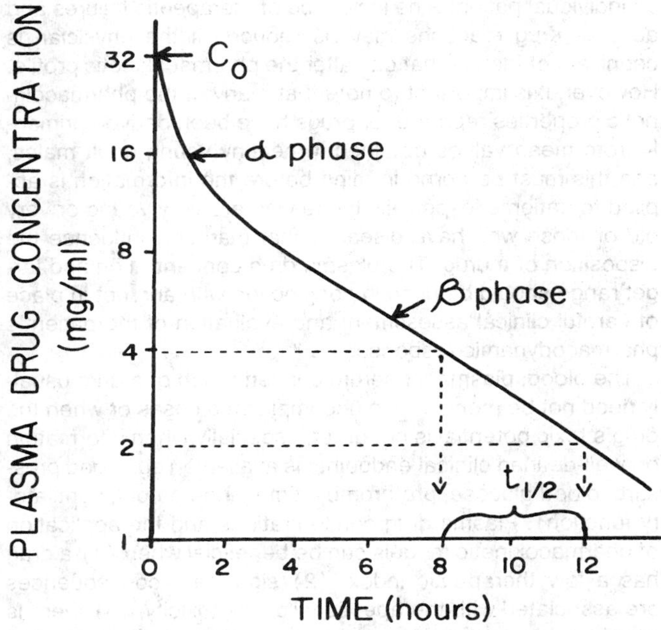

Figure 3. Semilogarithmic plot of plasma concentration-time curve following intravenous administration of a drug that follows multiexponential kinetics. Multiple sampling within the first two hours identifies an initial rapid decline (α phase) followed by slower linear decline (β phase) that can be used to estimate $t_{1/2}$.

Other volume terms may be used to describe the distribution of drugs with multiexponential kinetics. The term Vd_{SS} (volume of distribution at steady state) may be most useful, since it relates the total amount of drug in the body to the plasma concentration at steady state (Benet and Galeazzi, 1979).

Half-Life

The elimination rate constant is more conveniently expressed in terms of half-life ($t_{1/2}$). The $t_{1/2}$ is the time required for the plasma drug concentration to decline by one-half, and in a linear system its value is independent of the plasma drug concentration (Figure 2). The relationship of $t_{1/2}$ to k, Vd, and CL is provided by Equation 7.

$$t_{1/2} = \frac{0.693}{k} = \frac{0.693 \cdot Vd}{CL} \qquad (Eq.\ 7)$$

Neither the rate constant of elimination nor the $t_{1/2}$ are fundamental pharmacokinetic properties since they are derived from clearance and Vd. Therefore, it is not valid to make any assumptions about clearance (or Vd) from the $t_{1/2}$, because either clearance or Vd may change independently. However, the $t_{1/2}$ is quite useful for estimating the time course of drug elimination or drug accumulation to steady state. For practical purposes, a drug is considered to be eliminated in four half-lives (over 90% eliminated) as shown in Table 2. The half-life also can be used to determine the appropriate dosing interval for maintenance therapy after consideration of what constitutes acceptable fluctuations in the plasma drug concentration during the dosing interval.

TABLE 2.
DECLINE IN PLASMA DRUG CONCENTRATION FOLLOWING BOLUS INJECTION AND ACCUMULATION DURING CONTINUOUS INFUSION

Time (half-lives)	Single Bolus Intravenous Dose (% of initial plasma concentration)	Continuous Intravenous Infusion (% of steady-state plasma concentration)
0	100	0
1	50	50
2	25	75
3	12.5	87.5
4	6.25	93.8
5	3.12	96.9
6	1.56	98.4

Steady State

When a drug with first-order, monoexponential kinetics is administered by continuous intravenous infusion, the plasma concentration gradually increases to a steady state (C_{SS}) at a rate determined by the $t_{1/2}$. Technically, steady-state is established when the rate of drug elimination equals the rate at which the drug is delivered to the systemic circulation. Plasma concentrations will reach almost 94% of their eventual steady-state value after four half-lives have elapsed (Table 2). A comparable situation exists when a drug is administered intermittently at fixed intervals. The mean steady-state concentration ($\overline{C}_{SS}$) is the average plasma concentration obtained during each dosing interval.

Loading Dose: When the time required to attain steady-state is long relative to the temporal demands of the condition being treated, it may be desirable to administer a loading dose. The loading dose is one or a series of doses given at the onset of therapy to achieve therapeutic plasma concentrations rapidly. The loading dose may be estimated by:

$$LD = \frac{(C)\,(V_{SS})}{F} \qquad (Eq.\ 8)$$

in which C is the desired (or therapeutic) concentration to be produced. For intravenous loading, F equals 1.

Designing a Dosage Regimen

If values for systemic clearance (CL) and bioavailability are known, Equation 9 takes into account the calculation of the steady-state plasma concentration (C_{ss}) resulting from constant intravenous infusion (F = 1; Dose/τ = infusion rate) or mean steady-state concentration ($\overline{C}_{ss}$) from a fixed-rate, multiple-dose oral regimen (τ = dosing interval).

$$\overline{C}_{ss} = \frac{(F)\,(Dose)}{(\tau)\,(CL)} = \frac{\text{dosing rate} \cdot F}{(CL)} \qquad (Eq.\ 9)$$

Equation 9 emphasizes the fact that $\overline{C}_{ss}$ depends on the primary disposition parameter, which is clearance. Rearrangement (Equation 10) yields the dosing rate required to achieve a targeted steady-state concentration.

$$\frac{Dose}{\tau} = \frac{(\overline{C}_{ss})\,(CL)}{F} \qquad (Eq.\ 10)$$

Nonlinear Elimination

For a few drugs, therapeutic concentrations will exceed the linear range of metabolic and/or excretory processes. These drugs are generally described in the clinical literature as having *nonlinear kinetics*. Other drug disposition processes (eg, systemic drug input arising from drug absorption/first-pass metabolism and drug distribution/protein binding) also may display nonlinear features. For drugs that exhibit saturable or dose-dependent elimination, clearance will vary with the concentration of drug, often according to the Michaelis-Menten equation:

$$CL = \frac{V_{max}}{K_m + C} \qquad (Eq.\ 11)$$

in which K_m represents the plasma concentration at which one-half of the maximal rate of elimination is reached and V_{max} is equal to the maximal rate of elimination. The Michaelis-Menten equation is often used to describe enzyme kinetics.

Of particular significance is the fact that increases in the dosing rate may result in disproportionate increases in the plasma drug concentration and time required for elimination. Dosage modifications for these drugs, notably phenytoin, salicylates, heparin, and, in some patients, theophylline, are best determined by monitoring the clinical response or by measuring plasma concentrations. Nonlinear kinetics also are observed for drugs that bind to saturable sites in tissues or on plasma proteins (eg, disopyramide, valproate, prednisolone).

Therapeutic Drug Monitoring

Therapeutic drug monitoring (TDM) is the use of plasma drug concentrations, pharmacokinetic models, and clinical acumen to maximize the safety and efficacy of drug therapy in an individual patient. The incidence of therapeutic failures and adverse drug reactions may be reduced if the physician is cognizant of factors that can alter the pharmacokinetic profile. However, it is important to note that many of the pharmacokinetic properties reported for drugs have been derived primarily from mean values obtained in healthy young adult males, and this must be borne in mind before the information is applied to patients, especially those who are very young or very old or those who have diseases that markedly influence the disposition of a drug. The plasma drug concentration and target range should be used in conjunction with and not in place of careful clinical assessment and evaluation of the patient's pharmacodynamic response.

The blood, plasma, or serum concentration of a drug usually need not be monitored in uncomplicated cases or when the drug's toxic potential is not great, especially when information on well-defined clinical endpoints is available (eg, blood pressure, blood glucose, prothrombin time, urine output, ventilatory function). Plasma drug concentrations and the application of pharmacokinetic models can be beneficial when (1) a drug has a low therapeutic index, (2) significant consequences are associated with therapeutic failure or toxicity, (3) there is considerable interpatient variability in drug disposition, (4) there is a correlation between plasma concentration and therapeutic response (for many drugs, this criterion is poorly established or lacking), (5) an interacting drug is added to or removed from the regimen, and (6) therapeutic effects are not precisely quantifiable (eg, phenytoin to prevent seizures, procainamide to prevent arrhythmias). Numerous dosing methods have been developed in an attempt to improve the relationship between dosing, plasma concentration, and response (Perucca et al, 1985; Peck and Rodman, 1986).

TDM also is useful to monitor compliance or the treatment of overdose in selected patients. Nonlinear kinetics often are evident after overdosage and can be detected with multiple sampling. TDM may help to establish the severity of the toxicity, to provide an index to monitor the efficacy of management, and to estimate the duration of the excessive plasma level of the drug.

Sampling Time: One of the most common errors in therapeutic drug monitoring is obtaining blood samples at inappropriate (or unrecorded) times. Such measurements may mislead a physician into altering a dosage regimen based on faulty data and expose a patient to the risk of subtherapeutic response or toxicity.

When interpreting a plasma drug concentration, the drug, route of administration, and condition of the patient must be considered. An acutely ill patient requires closer monitoring than one who is stabilized. The plasma concentrations of a drug with a short half-life fluctuate markedly between doses, making the timing of the sample critical. If, however, a drug is administered by continuous intravenous infusion, a sample may be obtained any time after steady state is reached.

The time at which a blood sample is drawn for measuring the plasma concentration of a drug with a very long half-life or a prolonged-release preparation is less critical except when samples are drawn before steady state is reached in order to forecast whether the concentrations are likely to be subtherapeutic, therapeutic, or toxic at steady state. In this case, the relative rate of tissue distribution is very important. Once steady state is reached, the specimen usually can be obtained any time between the completion of the distribution phase and the next dose.

For orally administered drugs, the best time to draw a blood sample for determining drug concentrations is immediately before the next dose (trough concentration). Sampling at this time minimizes the variation in absorption rate and distribution.

Protein Binding: Routinely, drug plasma concentration assays measure total drug concentrations, which reflect both unbound and protein-bound drug. However, pharmacologic actions generally correlate better with the amount of unbound (free) drug in the plasma and, in some clinical situations, it is important to measure these concentrations. Factors that may alter the percentage of free drug are a change in the plasma protein concentration resulting in an alteration in the number of available binding sites; a change in the drug concentration because of an alteration in the number of molecules competing for the binding sites; and the presence of other chemicals (including other drugs) that compete for the same binding sites on the proteins, thereby displacing the bound drug.

Acidic and neutral drugs often bind to plasma albumin, and the plasma concentration of albumin decreases in a number of conditions (see Table 3). Basic drugs also frequently bind to alpha$_1$-acid glycoprotein (AAG), also known as orosomucoid. AAG is an acute phase-reactant protein, and its plasma concentration increases in the presence of inflammation or malignancy. Lowering the concentration of albumin would increase the free fraction of acidic drugs. Conversely, increasing the concentration of AAG would be expected to decrease the free fraction of basic drugs.

TABLE 3. CONDITIONS THAT ALTER THE PLASMA CONCENTRATIONS OF ALBUMIN AND ALPHA$_1$-ACID GLYCOPROTEIN

Conditions Decreasing Albumin Concentration	Conditions Increasing Alpha$_1$-Acid Glycoprotein Concentration
Advanced age	Advanced age
Burns	Burns
Cancer	Cancer
Cardiac failure	Chronic pain
Hepatic disease	Crohn's disease
Inflammatory disease	Inflammatory disease
Malnutrition	Myocardial infarction
Nephrotic syndrome	Obesity
Surgery (postoperative period)	Surgery (postoperative period)
Pregnancy	Trauma
Renal disease	

For drugs that are cleared by the liver, the clinical relevance of altering plasma protein concentrations or drug displacement that leads to an increase in free fraction depends on whether the intrinsic hepatic clearance of a drug is high or low (see Table 1). For drugs with low (restrictive) intrinsic clearance, the relationship between the rate of clearance and the fraction of unbound drug in blood is proportional. If the free fraction and total amount of unbound drug increases, hepatic extraction increases. Ultimately, the total plasma drug concentration will decrease, but the concentration of free drug will return to its original value. Therefore, the concentration of free drug remains unchanged and there is no long-term effect as a result of the displacement. The total plasma concentration that is routinely measured has declined, however, and this may lead to misinterpretation of plasma drug concentration data. The elimination of drugs with high intrinsic clearance is relatively unaffected by altered plasma protein concentrations. Consequently, a decrease in the unbound fraction results in a reduced steady-state concentration of unbound drug and an increase in the fraction results in an increased steady state concentration.

Drug protein binding also can be influenced by an alteration in the drug concentration relative to the number of available drug-protein binding sites. If the plasma drug concentration is high enough to saturate the protein binding sites, the free fraction of drug will increase as the plasma drug concentration increases. Drugs that display this type of concentration-dependent protein binding within the therapeutic range include disopyramide, valproate, ceftriaxone, prednisolone, and possibly salicylates at high dosages.

Active Metabolites: A number of drugs have active metabolites (Garattini, 1985), which should be considered when monitoring plasma concentrations because, unless specifically requested by a physician, their plasma concentration may not be determined routinely by clinical laboratories. Active metabolites occasionally have clinically relevant pharmacokinetic and pharmacodynamic characteristics that are quite different from those of the parent compound (eg, N-acetylprocainamide) and may accumulate to toxic levels, especially in patients with impaired renal function.

FACTORS AFFECTING PATIENT RESPONSE TO DRUGS

An important factor affecting patient response to a drug is variation in pharmacokinetic parameters. Some of this variation in the clearance of drugs can be explained by factors such as patient age, gender, or renal and hepatic function. However, the cause of much of the variability cannot be determined, and it is difficult to predict the extent of variation when developing a dosage regimen.

The pharmacodynamic response to a drug also may be affected by certain diseases that cause a reduction in the number of receptors (eg, myasthenia gravis, Parkinson's disease). Receptor activity also may be increased. Thus, one to two weeks after acute denervation (soft tissue trauma, major burns, cord transection), succinylcholine may liberate sufficient potassium from the affected muscle to induce cardiac arrest. Hyperthyroidism enhances the anticoagulant response to warfarin. The role of changing pharmacodynamic response is unknown for many disorders, but further studies may demonstrate that this is a major factor in drug response variation.

Influence of Disease

RENAL IMPAIRMENT. In addition to decreasing renal excretion, renal dysfunction can alter the bioavailability, distribution, protein binding, and hepatic metabolism of drugs (Gibson, 1986). Even for parent drugs that are not excreted renally, renal dysfunction may cause toxic metabolites to accumulate.

Distribution: Drug distribution may be affected by (1) changes in systemic pH, such as the acidosis of uremia or the alkalosis following severe potassium depletion; (2) alterations in protein binding that result from hypoalbuminemia produced by the nephrotic syndrome or pregnancy, by displacement of drugs by endogenous acids that accumulate in those with uremia, or by the altered configuration of albumin in that condition; and (3) alterations in the degree of hydration.

In end stage renal disease, digoxin's volume of distribution is reduced and a smaller than usual loading dose will produce the normal therapeutic range of plasma drug concentrations. In uremia or hypoalbuminemia, protein binding of a number of drugs (eg, valproate, morphine, furosemide, salicylates, phenytoin, warfarin, diazepam, triamterene, sulfonamides, certain penicillins and cephalosporins) is decreased. For highly protein bound drugs, the effect of renal disease on hepatic clearance depends on the mode (restrictive versus nonrestrictive) of hepatic elimination. For example, the therapeutic dose of phenytoin usually remains the same, but the total plasma concentration may be one-half to one-third that of patients with normal renal function.

Systemic acidosis increases the central nervous system distribution, and therefore the toxicity, of salicylates and phenobarbital but does not affect the plasma concentration of these agents. Whether increased sensitivity to other drugs is due to similar alterations in distribution has not been established.

Metabolism: The clinical significance of drug metabolism within the kidneys has not been widely evaluated, but it may be considerable (Anders, 1980). Renal disease sometimes affects hepatic clearance of drugs. Elimination of most drugs dependent on cytochrome P450 oxidation is normal, although some oxidations are accelerated (Reidenberg and Drayer, 1980). However, uremic patients often eliminate drugs dependent on hepatic acetylase or plasma esterase activity more slowly.

Dosage Alteration for Patients with Renal Impairment: Drugs that are excreted mostly unchanged by the kidney (eg, aminoglycosides, cephalosporins, some sulfonamides, digoxin, lithium, ethambutol, methotrexate) or those with pharmacologically active metabolites that are eliminated by renal excretion (eg, allopurinol, clofibrate, procainamide, meperidine, amobarbital, some oral sulfonylureas) may produce adverse effects in patients with impaired renal function if usual doses are administered. Guidelines for specific drugs have been published (Bennett, 1988), and some are included in the evaluations. See also Fillastre and Singlas, 1991; Singlas and Fillastre, 1991.

To prevent accumulation and toxic effects caused by increased plasma concentrations of such drugs or their metabolites, the dosage must be reduced. The goal is to modify the dosage so that the plasma concentration profile (eg, steady-state concentration, fluctuations) is similar to that expected in patients with normal renal function. This can be accomplished by reducing the size of the dose while maintaining the usual dosing interval or by increasing the interval while using the standard dose. Loading doses are unchanged unless the distribution is altered.

Dosage adjustment may be important if renal function is less than 50% of normal, if the percentage of drug excreted unchanged is greater than 50%, or if active metabolites are extensively excreted by the kidney. As the percentage of drug excreted by the kidney decreases with reduction in renal function, there is a corresponding increase in the importance of extrarenal routes (biliary and metabolic) of elimination. If extrarenal elimination also is compromised, further dose reduction must be considered *in addition* to the dosage adjustment made for the loss in renal function.

The dosage adjustment factor is dependent on the ratio of the drug's clearance (or rate of elimination) in renal failure to that in uncompromised individuals. Calculation of dosage based on clearance of the drug is most accurate. However, use of dosage adjustment factors or nomograms for calculating dosage in those with renal failure is often based on the assumption that a linear relationship exists between the drug clearance and glomerular filtration as determined by the endogenous creatinine clearance (CL_{cr}). Although it is seldom practical to determine creatinine clearance directly, the serum creatinine is often used to estimate this value (Equation 4). However, these estimates will be unreliable in patients with acute renal failure, severe uremia, rapidly changing renal function, or systemic muscular disease.

The dosage adjustment factor is the ratio of systemic drug clearance in the presence of renal insufficiency (CL_{ri}) to systemic clearance with normal renal function (CL), in which:

$$CL = CL_R + CL_{NR} \qquad \textit{(Eq. 12)}$$

and

$$CL_{ri} = CL_R \times \frac{\text{measured } CL_{cr}}{100 \text{ ml/min}} + CL_{NR} \qquad \textit{(Eq. 13)}$$

The dose in those with renal insufficiency is equal to:

$$\text{Normal dose} \times \frac{CL_{ri}}{CL} \qquad \textit{(Eq. 14)}$$

Alternatively, the normal dose is administered but the dosage interval is increased by dividing the normal dosage interval by the modification factor.

$$\text{Dosage Interval} = \frac{\text{Normal dosage interval}}{CL_{ri}/CL} \quad (Eq. 15)$$

The dosage adjustment factor is preferred when a relatively constant plasma concentration of the drug is desired.

Nomograms also are useful for dosage calculation in renal failure (Figure 4). The nomogram can be used to reduce the maintenance dose or prolong the dosage interval by determining the individual drug clearance fraction (P), which is similar to the dosage adjustment factor described above. The fraction of total systemic clearance attributable to nonrenal mechanisms (P_0) is plotted on the left ordinate and a line is drawn to the upper right hand corner. The patient's endogenous creatinine clearance is plotted on the lower abscissa and a vertical intersecting line is constructed. The point of intersection extended to the left ordinate represents P. The maintenance dose may be reduced by multiplying with P, or the dosage interval is extended by dividing with P. For some bactericidal antibiotics with an extremely low P_0 and a dosage interval longer than the normal $t_{1/2}$, the maintenance dose may be more appropriately determined by the decay fraction (d). The drug's $t_{1/2}$ in those with renal impairment is estimated from the normal $t_{1/2}$ by dividing with P. The dosage interval (T) is expressed as half-life in renal impairment and is termed the relative dosage interval (ϵ). The point of intersection between ϵ on the upper abscissa and the curved interrupted line extended to the right ordinate is the decay fraction (d). The appropriate maintenance dose (D^*) at the selected dosage interval is then:

$$D^* = D \times d \quad (Eq. 16)$$

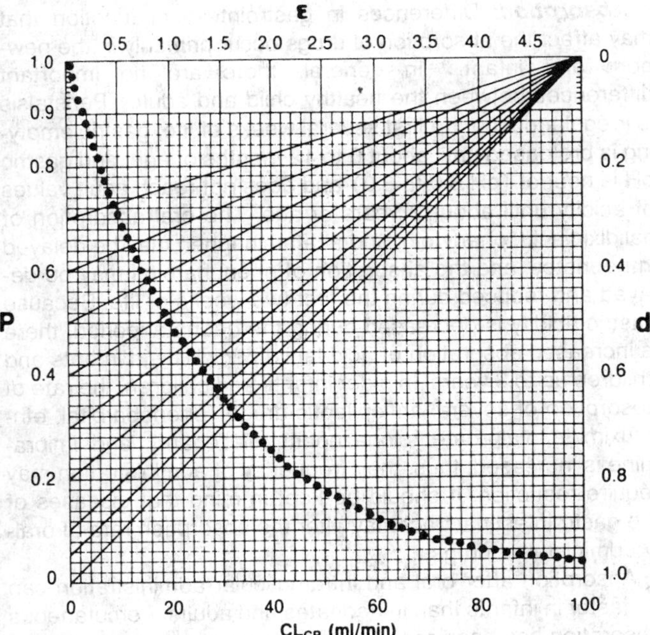

Figure 4. Nomogram for the determination of the individual drug clearance fraction (P) from creatinine clearance (CL_{cr}). See text for explanation and description of the relative dosage interval (ϵ), and the decay fraction (d). (From Spring, 1975; reprinted by permission.)

HEPATIC IMPAIRMENT. The importance of hepatic dysfunction as a determinant of pharmacokinetics depends, for the most part, on the extent that the liver and metabolic pathway (ie, oxidation versus conjugation) contribute to the drug's elimination. For many patients, intersubject variability in hepatic metabolism is greater than the variability caused by liver disease. The extraction ratio (see the discussion on Hepatic Clearance for definition) may be modified by changes in protein binding (presence of cirrhosis, ascites, renal disease). Changes in hepatic blood flow also may alter hepatic clearance. Total hepatic blood flow is somewhat decreased in patients with chronic liver disease but may be unchanged or even slightly elevated in those with acute viral hepatitis. In cirrhotic patients, the bioavailability of orally administered drugs with high extraction ratios may be enhanced.

The stage of disease also is an important determinant of hepatic drug elimination. Metabolizing capacity is reduced by hepatic necrosis. Oxidative metabolism generally is impaired in patients with cirrhosis and other types of liver disease, but the effect on clearance of individual drugs varies widely. Metabolism by glucuronidation tends to be well maintained for the majority of drugs that have been studied to date, but metabolism by other conjugative enzymes may be decreased (Pacifici et al, 1990).

Disorders of biliary excretion affect the clearance of drugs excreted primarily in the bile, which are mostly agents of high molecular weight (eg, rifampin).

General dosage guidelines for patients with hepatic disease have been developed (Bircher, 1983; Wedlund and Branch, 1983; Bass and Williams, 1988). Unfortunately, in contrast to renal disease, there is no specific quantitative method for adjusting dosage in patients with liver disease because of the variability of involvement and the lack of reliable indicators of hepatic function analogous to creatinine clearance (Bennett, 1981).

Factors to be considered when administering a drug to a patient with liver disease include the route of administration, the route of elimination (including enzyme-limited or flow-limited), the therapeutic index, and an approximation of the extent of liver disease. Doses should be reduced if the drug is administered orally, is metabolized extensively by the liver (and is flow-limited), and has a narrow therapeutic index and the function of the liver is significantly impaired.

OTHER DISEASE STATES. Most of the information about the effect of *congestive heart failure* on pharmacokinetics has been derived from studies of drugs used in the treatment of this disorder (Shammas and Dickstein, 1988). Gastrointestinal edema, delayed gastric emptying, decreased intestinal motility, and decreased splanchnic blood flow may reduce the rate of absorption and peak plasma concentration of orally administered drugs (eg, furosemide, bumetanide, digoxin, quinidine). Organ hypoperfusion may result in reduced renal (eg, furosemide, hydrochlorothiazide, captopril, procainamide) or hepatic (eg, prazosin, amrinone, quinidine, lidocaine) clearance. Reduced clearance may require a decrease in the maintenance dose. Congestion and peripheral vasoconstriction may alter the Vd of some drugs. A reduction in Vd (eg, quinidine, procainamide, lidocaine) may necessitate reduction of the loading dose. Changes in the elimination half-life depend on whether both clearance and Vd are altered and on the extent of that change. If the $t_{1/2}$ is prolonged, the time required to achieve steady state is lengthened. If, as is the case in cardiac failure, the Vd is reduced at the same time that clearance is reduced, there may be little change in the $t_{1/2}$ but the steady-state plasma concentration will increase. However, for most of the agents used to treat congestive heart failure, dosage alterations are dictated by hemodynamic or electrophysiologic endpoints in conjunction with therapeutic drug monitoring.

Pulmonary disease (cor pulmonale, acute hypoxia) may produce hemodynamic disturbances that are associated with decreases in renal and hepatic blood flow, thus reducing the clearance of drugs with flow-dependent elimination. The half-life of aminoglycosides is prolonged significantly in preterm neonates with hypoxia, and the clearance of theophylline is reduced up to 75% in patients with severe respiratory insufficiency. Hypoxia may affect a drug's metabolic pathways and extent of metabolism (eg, increased liberation of the nephrotoxic fluoride ion from halothane).

Hyperthyroidism affects many physiologic parameters that influence drug disposition (O'Connor and Feely, 1987). These alterations may be especially relevant for drugs used to treat symptoms or complications of this disorder. Gastrointestinal motility is increased; plasma binding proteins (eg, albumin, AAG) are reduced; cardiac output, hepatic blood flow, and enzymatic activity are elevated; and the glomerular filtration rate may be increased in some patients. Gastrointestinal absorption of some drugs may be increased (eg, acetaminophen, propranolol) or decreased (eg, riboflavin). Protein binding of propranolol and warfarin is decreased. The oxidative metabolism (eg, metoprolol, propranolol, tolbutamide, theophylline) and conjugation of certain drugs (eg, acetaminophen, oxazepam) are increased. The hepatic metabolism of other drugs (eg, diazepam, phenytoin) apparently is unchanged. Renal clearance of digoxin may be increased (Shenfield, 1981).

Less information is available on the effects of *hypothyroidism,* but, in general, the influences on drug disposition processes are the opposite of those observed in hyperthyroidism.

Influence of Age

The patient's age may be responsible for variations in drug response. Particular problems in dosage selection occur in the very young and the very old; the former are undergoing nonuniform organ maturation while the latter are experiencing nonuniform organ deterioration. Both of these age groups differ from young adults in the kinetics of absorption and elimination, volume of distribution, and receptor sensitivity. It must be emphasized that any method devised to calculate drug dosage for both children and adults provides an estimate only, to be verified or corrected by clinical experience and/or measurement of drug concentrations.

PEDIATRIC PATIENTS. There are many challenges in choosing the most appropriate drugs and determining the dosage in pediatric patients, who are typically assigned to one of the following age groups: premature infant (gestational age, less than 36 weeks); full-term infant (gestational age, 36 to 40 weeks); neonate (first month of life); infant (5 to 52 weeks); child (1 to 12 years); and adolescent (12 to 16 years). Whether children and infants will respond to a particular drug in the same manner as adults can be determined only through research and clinical experience. Indeed, their quantitative and/or qualitative responses to many drugs are known to be different. The age and size of the individual, as well as the disease state, affect dosage in these patients.

The pharmacokinetics of many drugs change with the continuing development of several physiologic functions. Many metabolic mechanisms in premature and newborn infants are not fully developed, and drugs may accumulate to toxic concentrations if dosage is based on traditional criteria. In fact, the infant's response to drugs during the first weeks of life probably varies more, overall, from that of a 1-year-old than the response of a 1-year-old varies from that of an adult.

Although an increasing number of studies are being conducted on the pharmacokinetics of drugs in pediatric patients, data on which to base dosage recommendations for specific drugs are limited. Consequently, many drugs do not have established doses for infants and children. Nevertheless, some generalizations can be made on the basis of the information available.

The basic pharmacokinetic functions (absorption, distribution, metabolism, and excretion) affect a drug's concentration at receptor sites and hence its actions; as for adults, these should be considered when treating pediatric patients.

Absorption: Differences in gastrointestinal function that may affect the absorption of drugs occur primarily in the newborn and infant. (In general, there are no important differences between the healthy child and adult.) Peristalsis is irregular during the first several weeks of life, gastric emptying is prolonged until about 6 to 12 months of age, and gastric pH is neutral (pH 6.0 to 8.0) and does not reach adult values of acidity until about 2 years of age. The oral absorption of nalidixic acid, phenytoin, and acetaminophen may be delayed in neonates, and the absorption of phenobarbital may be delayed and reduced during the first two weeks of life. Because gastric acidity is decreased during the neonatal period, there is increased absorption of acid-labile penicillins in infants and children up to 3 years. In older infants and children, the rate of absorption of several antiepileptic drugs (phenobarbital, ethosuximide, valproate, clonazepam, diazepam) and imipramine is increased; thus, their frequency of administration may require reduction. It should be kept in mind that diseases of the gastrointestinal tract may alter the absorption rate of orally administered drugs.

Absorption after oral and intramuscular administration can be faster in infants than in neonates and adults. Percutaneous absorption has been reported to be more rapid and complete in infants than in adults because of differences in skin thickness.

Distribution: The distribution of drugs in neonates and infants may differ from that in older children and adults because body composition varies markedly with age. The proportion of body water (total and extracellular) is greater in the premature and full-term infant but gradually decreases to adult values by about 12 months. The relative mass of subcutaneous tissue also varies; it is greatest at 9 months, decreases until about 6 years, and increases again in adolescence. Premature infants, however, have very little fatty tissue. These changes affect the distribution of lipid-soluble drugs.

Plasma protein binding capacity for several drugs is decreased in neonates and infants because the concentration of plasma protein is lower than in adults, and endogenous factors, including free fatty acids and bilirubin, compete with a drug for the existing binding sites. The adult values for protein binding typically are reached in about 10 to 12 months. Protein binding of salicylates, penicillins, sulfonamides, phenytoin, phenobarbital, and imipramine is decreased in infants. The protein binding of diazepam and digoxin is similar in infants and adults. In neonates with hyperbilirubinemia, drugs that are very highly bound to plasma proteins (eg, sulfonamides, salicylates, phenytoin) may compete with bilirubin protein binding.

Since cardiac output and blood flow are related to body surface area rather than to body weight, drug distribution and equilibration rates may be faster in children than in adults.

Metabolism: The capacity of the infant's liver to metabolize certain drugs may be reduced but increases rapidly during the first weeks to months after birth. It varies for different drugs depending on the enzymes involved, since the various enzyme systems do not mature at the same rate.

In general, hydroxylation rates are diminished most frequently. Drugs that depend on hepatic mixed function oxidase metabolism for elimination may have longer apparent plasma half-lives in neonates; for those drugs, the interval between doses should be increased (daily dose decreased). Esterase activity parallels the increase in plasma proteins during the first 12 months of life. Phase II reactions, especially conjugation with glucuronic acid, are variably reduced. However, methylation, glycine conjugation, and possibly sulfation appear to be similar in neonates and adults (Milsap and Szefler, 1986).

If drug metabolism is reduced in the neonate, the increases that occur after 2 to 4 weeks of age may exceed the rates in adults. Metabolic rates of hepatic drug oxidation may remain markedly elevated for the first 2 to 3 years and then gradually decrease with age until puberty, at which time adult values are reached (Morselli, 1989).

Certain drugs administered to the mother during pregnancy may affect metabolism in the newborn through induction of hepatic enzymes. For example, phenytoin and carbamazepine have shorter half-lives in neonates who were exposed to these drugs prenatally. Therefore, the possibility of previous exposure to an inducing agent might be considered when administering drugs to a newborn infant, although the clinical significance of prenatal enzyme induction has not been assessed.

Data on specific drugs are limited; the plasma half-lives of diazepam, digoxin, indomethacin, nalidixic acid, nortriptyline, phenylbutazone, phenobarbital, salicylates, and tolbutamide appear to be longer in *infants*. Conversely, theophylline, phenylbutazone, and most antiepileptic drugs can be metabolized faster in infants and *older children* than in adults. It should be kept in mind that hepatic disease may affect the metabolizing ability in children as well as in adults.

Excretion: Renal blood flow in relation to body surface area is reduced in neonates and infants but approaches adult values in about 5 to 12 months. Glomerular filtration approaches adult values by about 3 to 5 months of age (Kearns and Reed, 1989). Generally, maturation of glomerular and tubular function is complete at 6 to 8 months of age. Clearance values for some drugs (eg, aminoglycosides, digoxin, indomethacin) may be reduced during this period, particularly in infants who were born prematurely. Therefore, the dosage of these and other drugs that depend on renal excretion for elimination must be adjusted to avoid accumulation and toxic reactions.

Dosage schedules for several antibiotics that are eliminated by the kidney (eg, penicillins, gentamicin) have been developed (see the evaluations in the appropriate chapters in the section on Systemic Anti-Infectives). Other drugs that are excreted at reduced rates include indomethacin, salicylic acid, and sulfonamides. (See the section on Renal Impairment.)

Calculation of Doses for Children: Usually, dosages recommended for infants, children, and adolescents are based on body weight (in milligram per kilogram) or, less commonly, on body surface area; some drugs are given in higher dosages for younger children. The dose of many drugs is not a simple linear function of body weight, however, and calculation of the dose as so much per kilogram of body weight is often inaccurate, especially as children reach adult heights. Another common practice in determining a child's dose has been to give some fraction of an adult dose, using the age of the patient as a rough guide. Because of the great variation in size among children of the same age, this method is not acceptable.

For drugs eliminated by the liver, identification of the primary metabolic pathway may help to determine the best method of dosage calculation. Findings in one study suggest that calculation of dosage based on body surface area provides more uniform dosing in pediatric and adolescent age groups for drugs eliminated by oxidation; for drugs eliminated by conjugation, dosage calculated based on body weight may be appropriate (Crom et al, 1991). Surface area generally is not a satisfactory basis for dosage calculations in premature infants or neonates.

The pediatric doses cited for individual drugs in this publication follow the method of conversion developed for the particular drug. Some conversions are based on weight, some on body surface area, and some on age. If adequate dosage information based on actual pediatric use is either nonexistent or not readily available, suggested guidelines sometimes are furnished even when it is recognized that more data would be desirable. For some drugs, lack of information has been specifically acknowledged. When the dosage for children has been established, it is given in the text and should be used in preference to any calculated dose. When information is inadequate, it is suggested that the body surface area be taken as the criterion—*provided* there is no specific evidence that a child will react to the drug differently from an adult.

GERIATRIC PATIENTS. Elderly patients also should receive special consideration when determining the dosage of certain drugs. Two-thirds of all Americans over the age of 65 take at least one prescription drug, and of these, at least one-third take three or more. Because they use relatively more drugs than other age groups, the appropriate choice of drugs and dosage is of primary importance in their health care. This is emphasized by results of one study that found that 28% of hospital admissions for elderly patients were drug related (12% for noncompliance and 16% for adverse drug reactions) (Col et al, 1990).

Although a specific age cannot be applied to define this group, patients over 60 or 65 are usually included. There is some interest in further stratification of the over-65 age group. Two clinically important phenomena occur with aging: physiologic decline and an increase in the prevalence of disease. However, it should be kept in mind that chronological age is not necessarily closely related to physiologic age in the elderly. There is growing realization that characteristics once considered to be inevitable consequences of aging (eg, decline in cardiac output and in glomerular filtration rate, loss of lean body mass, glucose intolerance) often are not apparent in physically fit elderly patients (Bortz, 1989). Indeed, the differences between individuals of the same age are so great that *increased* biological variation is characteristic of this age group. This may be especially true of physiologic functions that affect drug disposition and response. Each patient must be evaluated individually.

Absorption: There is little evidence that the extent of absorption of passively absorbed drugs is diminished in the elderly. However, conditions such as decreased gastric acidity and gastrointestinal motility, which reduce gastric emptying, may delay or impair drug absorption. Drugs that affect these functions (eg, laxatives, antacids, H_2 antagonists, anticholinergic agents, levodopa) may affect the absorption of other agents. The active absorption of nutrients, vitamins, and minerals also may be impaired in the elderly. For example, it has been reported that iron, calcium, thiamine, and vitamin B_{12} absorption is decreased and, thus, larger doses may be necessary (Massoud, 1984).

Distribution: Alterations in circulation and changes in body composition may affect the distribution and equilibration rate of drugs. Total body weight may decrease, especially in the very elderly, but the ratio of fat to lean is usually greater. Adipose tissue increases from an average of 18% to 30% in men and from 35% to 48% in women (Greenblatt et al, 1982). The enlarged fat compartment may increase the weight-normalized distribution volume of lipid-soluble drugs (eg, diazepam, lidocaine) and decrease the volume of water-soluble drugs (eg, acetaminophen, alcohol). Plasma albumin concentrations may be decreased in the elderly (Cooper and Gardner, 1989; Veering et al, 1990), although data from a large number of healthy subjects fail to support this conclusion (Campion et al, 1988). Poor nourishment and disease are probably contributing factors in those elderly patients with decreased albumin concentrations. A decrease in the plasma protein concentration may influence the pharmacologic response or elimination kinetics for drugs that are highly protein bound.

Hepatic Clearance: Between the ages of 20 and 85, there is an approximate 25% decrease in hepatic size and a somewhat greater decrease in hepatic blood flow (Woodhouse and Wynne, 1988). These percentage changes are similar to the reduction in clearance noted for many drugs in the elderly. The relationship between aging and hepatic enzyme metabolic capacity is complex and depends on the type of metabolic reaction (oxidative versus conjugation reactions) and the patient's sex. Oxidative capacity declines with age, but the decline is greater in elderly men than in elderly women (Greenblatt et al, 1984) and there is considerable intersubject variability (Vestal et al, 1975). Environmental factors such as cigarette smoking may have a greater influence than age per se. The effect on oxidative metabolism is consistent for most drugs with low hepatic extraction ratios. The rate of hepatic conjugation appears to be unaffected by age. The data are less clear regarding drugs with high extraction ratios, because their rate of metabolism depends on hepatic blood flow in addition to hepatic metabolic enzyme activity. Liver size is a significant determinant in the elimination of drugs with high extraction ratios regardless of age.

It is important to note that the usual tests of hepatic function do not necessarily reflect drug metabolizing capacity.

Excretion: Between the ages of 20 and 90, the glomerular filtration rate and tubular secretion decline almost linearly by 35% to 50%. At age 30, the glomerular filtration rate is approximately 140 ml/min/1.73 M^2 and declines at an average rate of 8 ml/min/1.73 M^2 every decade (Anderson and Brenner, 1986). The normal decline in glomerular filtration rate that occurs during the aging process is not reflected in the serum creatinine because of the parallel loss in muscle mass, which decreases production of creatinine. This is accompanied by a similar decrease in renal blood flow. In addition, many patients over age 60 have some renal pathology, which further reduces renal function. A re-examination of the formula (Equation 4) for estimating creatinine clearance from serum creatinine led to the conclusion that the error inherent in assuming that the renal function decreases an average of 1 ml/min/yr after age 40 can be substantial (Goldberg and Finkelstein, 1987). Thus, in slightly obese, muscle-wasted geriatric patients with renal insufficiency, estimates of creatinine clearance may be falsely elevated (Lonergan, 1988). Up to one-third of older healthy patients demonstrate well-preserved glomerular function (Lindeman et al, 1985). The usual estimates of creatinine clearance in this group are falsely low. Therefore, it is important to consider the geriatric patient's renal function when determining the dose of certain drugs. The patient should be monitored carefully; determination of plasma drug concentrations may be useful.

Drugs excreted by the kidney that are used commonly in elderly patients and that may require reduction of the maintenance dose include digoxin, aminoglycosides, colistin, ethambutol, tetracyclines (except doxycycline), amantadine, and lithium. The evaluations on these drugs should be consulted for dosages in patients with decreased renal function. See also the section on Renal Impairment.

The clearance of drugs that are eliminated by active tubular secretion (eg, organic bases [procainamide]) also is decreased with age independently of the glomerular filtration rate (creatinine clearance). Thus, the elderly require smaller doses than middle-aged adults, just as the young may require larger doses.

Pharmacodynamics: Drug receptor response may be altered in elderly patients. There may be an increased or diminished pharmacodynamic response. However, in the absence of pathologic changes, the impact of aging per se on receptor-mediated processes is unclear (Lamy, 1989).

Neuromuscular blocking agents are among the drugs to which the elderly appear to be more "sensitive." Neuromuscular blockade is more intense and prolonged with advanced age. In general, these patients are more sensitive to drugs that act within the central nervous system. Thus, barbiturates, benzodiazepines, lithium, opioid analgesics, tricyclic antidepressants, and phenothiazines demonstrate therapeutic and toxic effects at lower doses. Antihistamines and cardiac glycosides can increase confusion and disorientation in the elderly. In the autonomic nervous system, beta receptor responses to both agonists and antagonists appear to be blunted.

Orthostatic hypotension is more common in elderly patients. The risk of orthostatic hypotension from antihypertensive, antidepressant, and antipsychotic drugs is increased in elderly patients with volume depletion caused by diuretic therapy. Diuretics also produce orthostatic hypotension more often, which may result from impaired compensatory mechanisms. Potassium-wasting diuretics may cause hypokalemia more frequently in the elderly, which potentiates the effects of digitalis. The incidence of hyperkalemia is higher in older patients taking potassium-sparing diuretics, ACE inhibitors, and NSAIDs, possibly because renal function is impaired in these individuals. The elderly may be more susceptible to hypoglycemia with use of sulfonylureas. With aspirin or other nonsteroidal anti-inflammatory agents, the incidence of occult blood loss may be higher and may lead to iron deficiency anemia; larger than usual doses of supplemental iron may be required because of decreased absorption.

Additional factors that affect drug response in the elderly are various disease states, the simultaneous use of a number of drugs, a marginal diet, drug-induced nutritional deficits, and, very importantly, *uneven compliance* with the medication schedule. As a general rule, both the effective dose and the toxic dose decline with advancing age.

When prescribing drugs for the elderly, special attention should be given to the following general principles:

(1) The physician should ascertain what other medications, including OTC products, the patient is taking. Elderly people often take many drugs, some of which may not be needed and should be discontinued. The patient should receive as few drugs as possible, and contraindications, potential drug interactions, and desired outcome should be evaluated whenever a new drug is added to an existing regimen.

(2) The dosage schedule should be as simple as possible, and the dosage form should be easily self-administered. Directions for taking the medication should be understood by the patient; it is estimated that more than one-half of Americans over 65 desire written instructions.

(3) Patients should be followed closely to determine compliance, drug efficacy, and adverse effects. Prescription of drugs on an as-needed basis for minor symptoms should be minimized, and automatic refills of prescriptions without adequate follow-up should be discouraged.

(4) Any physiologic or pathologic changes that may affect the dosage and response to the drug must be considered. However, these factors are often difficult to identify. Many adverse drug reactions in the elderly have a pharmacokinetic basis. A need to reduce the daily dosage should be anticipated for some drugs (Beers and Ouslander, 1989). Failure to take into account alterations in hepatic clearance, renal excretion, protein binding, and drug distribution may lead to the accumulation of toxic levels if standard doses are administered. Concurrent diseases or medications may accentuate pharmacokinetic differences.

Influence of Other Conditions

PREGNANCY. Physiologic changes during pregnancy affect the disposition of many drugs. Although the study of pharmacokinetic changes during pregnancy is necessarily limited to drugs that may be prescribed to treat an attendant condition, several generalizations can be made (Boobis and Lewis, 1982; Mattison, 1986; Rayburn and Andresen, 1986).

Absorption: The increase in progesterone during pregnancy causes a delay in gastric emptying and a decrease in intestinal motility. Gastric acidity decreases during the first few months of pregnancy and then increases. Although these physiologic alterations theoretically affect drug absorption, the clinical impact is probably negligible.

Distribution: Increases in body weight and expansion of the plasma, extracellular, and total body water volumes tend to increase the Vd of drugs during pregnancy. The expansion of blood volume may contribute to the decrease in plasma protein concentrations (eg, albumin, AAG). The decrease in plasma proteins may result in an increase in the free fraction of drugs that are protein bound (eg, nonsteroidal anti-inflammatory drugs, phenytoin, warfarin, theophylline). The increase in free fatty acids that occurs during pregnancy also may displace some drugs from albumin (eg, valproate).

Metabolism: The metabolism of some drugs is markedly increased during pregnancy. For drugs that are subject to restrictive hepatic elimination, an increase in free fraction results in an increase in clearance and a subsequent decline in the total plasma concentration. For most drugs with high extraction ratios that are eliminated by the liver, significant changes in pharmacokinetics are not observed during pregnancy. For some drugs with low or intermediate hepatic clearance (eg, clorazepate, phenytoin, oxazepam), clearance is increased, but for others (eg, caffeine, diazepam, meperidine) clearance is decreased.

Renal Elimination: During pregnancy, renal blood flow increases at least 35% while the glomerular filtration rate may more than double. The elimination rates of drugs that are predominantly cleared by the kidneys usually are increased during pregnancy; many antibiotics (eg, ampicillin, cefuroxime, ceftazidime, aminoglycosides) are included in this category.

Dosage adjustments may be necessary to ensure adequate plasma concentrations.

OBESITY. In obesity, the increased amount of adipose tissue and lean body mass may increase the apparent Vd of some drugs. Modest increases in Vd have been noted for hydrophilic drugs (eg, aminoglycosides, vancomycin, ibuprofen, prednisone, heparin, theophylline) (Abernethy and Greenblatt, 1986). The increased Vd for the aminoglycosides (30% to 50%) is similar to the estimated increase in lean body mass. This increment over the ideal body weight may be considered when determining loading doses in obese patients. Increases in the Vd of theophylline in obese individuals are the result of drug distribution into the excess body weight. Therefore, calculation of the theophylline loading dose should be based on total body weight. Lipophilic drugs (eg, benzodiazepines, thiopental, phenytoin, verapamil, lidocaine) may have substantially greater distribution volumes. Consequently, loading doses may need to be higher (eg, phenytoin). For certain drugs, it has been suggested that the loading or maintenance dose be calculated on the basis of ideal body weight (IBW), which can be calculated using the following equations:

IBW (male) = 50 kg + 2.3 kg/inch over 5 feet
IBW (female) = 45 kg + 2.3 kg/inch over 5 feet

The Vd of digoxin, cimetidine, and procainamide is unchanged in obese patients.

The plasma concentration of AAG has been reported to be increased in obese patients, which alters the protein binding of certain basic drugs (eg, lidocaine, propranolol, disopyramide). The plasma concentration of albumin is relatively unchanged. The hepatic clearance of ibuprofen and prednisone is directly related to body weight, but the rate of oxidative metabolism for most other drugs studied is unchanged. Drug conjugation (eg, acetaminophen, lorazepam, oxazepam) appears to increase as a function of body weight.

Renal clearance of drugs in obese patients may be unchanged (eg, cimetidine) or increased (eg, aminoglycosides, procainamide).

Influence of Pharmacogenetics

Variability among individuals in their response to drugs is due, in part, to genetic differences (Weinshilboum, 1984; Vesell, 1985). In normal subjects, the extent of such interindividual variability ranges from 4- to 40-fold depending on the particular drug and population. Individuals with genetic variants may not respond to or may experience adverse effects with usual therapeutic doses. Approximately 60 pharmacogenetic entities have been described. Selected disorders appear in Table 4.

Genetic Differences in Drug Biotransformation: Because most drugs are biotransformed, genetic variations in metabolic pathways or rate of biotransformation may have important clinical implications.

The disposition of tricyclic antidepressants, phenytoin, metoprolol, alprenolol, tolbutamide, and phenylbutazone has been studied in twins and in families, and a major contributor to the variability in disposition of these drugs is genetically controlled.

Oxidation of most drugs is mediated by enzymes of hepatic cytochrome P450, some of which exhibit polymorphism. The P450 gene superfamily contains at least three dozen families (designated by Arabic numerals) that are classified on the basis of amino acid similarities, 12 of which exist in all mammals (Nelson et al, 1993). For the gene and cDNA corresponding to human families, the root symbol "CYP", representing *cy*tochrome *P*450 is used. Subfamilies are designated by capital letters and individual P450 proteins are designated by Arabic numerals. Families 1, 2, and 3 are probably responsible for most xenobiotic mono-oxygenation in humans. Members of family 1 (1A1 and 1A2) are responsible for the metabolic activation of many carcinogens and toxic chemicals; certain endogenous substrates (eg, estrogens) may be hydroxylated as well. 1A1 is found constitutively in lung and placenta tissue; hepatic forms are not constitutive but are inducible.

Family 2 is the largest and most diverse of the P450 families. Some isoforms in this family are induced by phenobarbital-type compounds and ethanol (2E1); this latter isoform often converts compounds to reactive intermediates. Two closely related isoforms in family 3, A3, and A4, are induced by rifampin, barbiturates, and phenytoin and are involved in the biotransformation of steroid hormones and other large nonplanar substrates (eg, cyclosporine, macrolides), terfenadine and astemizole, nifedipine and other calcium channel blockers, triazolam and midazolam, and lovastatin. Inhibitors include ketoconazole and other azole antifungals and certain substrates (eg, nifedipine). 3A3 and 3A4 are the most abundant isoforms in the human liver; 3A4 also is present in high concentrations in the gastrointestinal villi. Consequently, substrates for 3A4 often demonstrate a significant first-pass effect. Characteristically, there is a five- to tenfold interindividual variation in clearance, but enzyme activity in the population is normally distributed. Activity generally is reduced in the elderly and in patients with liver disease and may be increased in females.

Certain pathways of drug metabolism are under monogenic control and exhibit polymorphism within the population (ie, enzyme activity is lacking or is greatly reduced in a given percentage of the population). Based on these differences, the population can be divided into poor (slow) or extensive (rapid) metabolizers.

Two well-described polymorphisms in drug oxidation occur with isoforms in family 2: the debrisoquin/sparteine and mephenytoin phenotypes (Relling, 1989). The former results from the absence or deficient production of CYP2D6 in the liver. The poor-metabolizer phenotype, which is inherited as an autosomal recessive trait, occurs in 5% to 10% of Caucasians but in 1% or less of Orientals (and is probably due to a distinct genotype in the latter population). More than 25 drugs (eg, propafenone, flecainide, tricyclic antidepressants, phenothiazines) with a wide range of indications are at least partially eliminated via oxidation by CYP2D6 (Brosen, 1990). CYP2D6 is inhibited by other drugs, most notably quinidine, propoxyphene, and haloperidol (Sanz and Bertilsson, 1990).

TABLE 4.
INHERITED DISORDERS ALTERING PATIENT RESPONSE TO DRUGS

Disorder	Drugs Affected	Enzyme and Location	Frequency
Acatalasia	Hydrogen peroxide	Catalase in erythrocytes	Primarily in Japan and Switzerland (incidence 1% of population in certain areas of Japan)
Slow acetylators	Isoniazid, sulfamethazine, phenelzine, dapsone, hydralazine, procainamide	Acetylase in liver	Nearly 50% of U.S. population
Atypical pseudocholinesterase	Succinylcholine	Pseudocholinesterase in plasma	1 in 2,500 people
Phenytoin toxicity	Phenytoin	Mixed function oxidase (MFO) that parahydroxylates phenytoin	Only small number of pedigrees
Deficient N-hydroxylation of amobarbital	Amobarbital	? MFO in liver microsomes that N-hydroxylates amobarbital	Only 1 small pedigree; screening of more than 100 unrelated normal volunteers revealed that nearly 2% were homozygously affected
Warfarin resistance	Warfarin	? Altered receptor or enzyme in liver with increased affinity for vitamin K	2 large pedigrees
Glucose-6-phosphate dehydrogenase (G6PD) deficiency	Many drugs	G6PD	Nearly 100,000,000 worldwide; high frequency where malaria is endemic
Hemoglobin Zurich	Sulfonamides	Arginine substitution for histidine at the 63rd position of the beta-chain of hemoglobin	2 small pedigrees
Hemoglobin H	Many drugs	Hemoglobin composed of 4 beta chains	———
Glaucoma due to abnormal response of intraocular pressure to corticosteroids	Corticosteroids	Unknown	Approximately 5% of U.S. population
Malignant hyperthermia	Various anesthetics, especially halothane	Unknown	Nearly 1 in 20,000 anesthetized patients
Methemoglobin reductase deficiency	Many drugs	Methemoglobin reductase	Approximately 1 in 100 people are heterozygous carriers
Porphyrias	Many drugs	Enzymatic deficiencies in the pathway of heme synthesis	———
Debrisoquine 4-hydroxylation polymorphism	Many drugs	Debrisoquine 4-hydroxylase in liver	Approximately 5% to 10% of whites
Mephenytoin hydroxylation polymorphism	Omeprazole	Mephenytoin hydroxylase in liver	Approximately 5% of whites and 20% of Japanese

Adapted from Vesell, 1979.

The mephenytoin polymorphism (also inherited as an autosomal recessive trait) involves a CYP2C isoform, which hydroxylates this antiepileptic drug (Wilkinson et al, 1989). Mephenytoin is used clinically as a racemic mixture of S- and R-enantiomers. The hydroxylation of the S-enantiomer is deficient in 3% of Caucasians and in 17% to 22% of Orientals. Other agents whose metabolism cosegregates with this trait are mephobarbital, omeprazole, and possibly warfarin and diazepam and its main metabolite, desmethyldiazepam.

Numerous hydrazine and aryl and other amines (eg, isoniazid, hydralazine, procainamide, dapsone, aminoglutethimide, sulfasalazine and other sulfonamides, clonazepam) are biotransformed by acetylation; the metabolite may be inactive (eg, N-acetylisoniazid) or active (eg, N-acetylprocainamide). The general population can be divided into slow or fast acetylators. Low acetylation capacity is related to decreased amount (low or absent) of two similar acetylating enzymes (NAT-2) in the liver (Grant et al, 1990). Individuals who are slow acetylators may experience exaggerated pharmacologic or toxic responses to conventional doses of some drugs (eg, isoniazid neuropathy, hydralazine lupus), whereas the effectiveness of such doses may be reduced in fast acetylators. The slow-acetylator phenotype, which is inherited as an autosomal recessive trait, is present in about 50% of Caucasians and blacks but is much less prevalent in Orientals (10%) and Canadian Eskimos (5%). These interethnic differences are due to different distribution of polymorphic N-acetyltransferase alleles. The slow acetylation characteristic of humans is due to multiple (at least three) alleles. The most common "slow" allele in Caucasians is not present in the Japanese populations.

A number of drugs produce *hemolytic anemia* in individuals with an inherited deficiency of glucose-6-phosphate dehydrogenase (G6PD). Enzyme-deficient cells cannot protect themselves as efficiently as normal erythrocytes against oxidant drugs or metabolites; in the presence of these agents, essential cell components are oxidized and hemolysis occurs. This inborn error of metabolism is frequently called "primaquine sensitivity," because it was originally observed in patients receiving antimalarial drugs (primaquine, pamaquine, pentaquine). Hemolytic anemia also has developed in susceptible individuals after administration of some sulfonamides, nitrofurans, sulfones, antipyretic-analgesics (acetanilid, phenacetin, and, in some extreme variants, aspirin), chloramphenicol, aminosalicylic acid, quinidine, methylene blue, and vitamin K. It also has occurred after contact with naphthalene or ingestion of fava beans. Most individuals with G6PD deficiency do not experience hematologic symptoms unless they are exposed to these agents.

The geographical distribution of G6PD deficiency closely follows the distribution of *Plasmodium falciparum* malaria, which suggests that the trait provides some selective advantage against this disease. It appears most frequently in populations of African and Mediterranean descent and occurs in about 10% to 13% of black American males. Oxidant drugs or metabolites often cause more severe symptoms in Caucasians with G6PD deficiency than in affected blacks. Also, hemolysis may be induced in Caucasians by agents that have no hemolytic effect on enzyme-deficient blacks (eg, chloramphenicol, aminosalicylic acid, fava beans).

Influence of Diet and Environmental Chemicals

Chemical determinants of the response to drugs include food, other drugs, and other xenobiotics (chemicals associated with household products, incidental environmental exposure, occupation, and social activities).

Drug interaction is a term used broadly by some authors to describe alterations of drug effects caused by other drugs, food, or an environmental chemical. For more detailed information on interactions, especially drug-drug interactions encountered in clinical practice, see index entry Drug Interactions.

Food: The effects of food on drug response are explained primarily by alterations in bioavailability (eg, absorption, presystemic clearance) and in drug metabolism. The distribution and renal excretion of drugs also may be affected. Serious vitamin and protein deficiencies can affect drug binding or biotransformation or the patient's response.

Most food-drug interactions decrease the rate or extent of drug absorption (Welling, 1984). Some are clinically relevant (eg, tetracycline and milk) but most are not. Variation in absorption can be minimized in adults by taking drugs on an empty stomach with an adequate volume (150 to 200 ml) of fluid. In a few instances, however, giving certain drugs with food may avoid gastrointestinal irritation (eg, iron preparations, metronidazole, nitrofurantoin, potassium salts, nonsteroidal anti-inflammatory agents) or even enhance absorption (eg, griseofulvin, isotretinoin). For some highly extracted drugs (eg, propranolol), food may decrease hepatic extraction, thus increasing bioavailability. When applicable, this information is included in the drug evaluations.

The diet can influence hepatic drug metabolism (Anderson, 1988). Hepatic clearances for some drugs (eg, theophylline) are greater during a high-protein diet while decreased protein intake can reduce the renal clearance of some drugs (eg, allopurinol).

Adverse food-drug interactions also may occur. For example, headache and occasional hypertensive crisis may follow the ingestion of tyramine-rich foods (eg, cheddar cheese, chicken liver, aged or tenderized meats, Chianti or sherry wine, broad beans) by patients receiving monoamine oxidase inhibitors (isocarboxazid, tranylcypromine, phenelzine).

Nondrug Chemicals: The average individual in the United States is exposed to numerous nondrug chemicals in the form of food additives and contaminants. In addition, occupational or household chemical exposures orally, dermally, or by inhalation must be taken into account. The clinical relevance of this chemical burden is unknown, but the physician should be aware that patients are exposed to nondrug chemicals. Since exposure to most nondrug chemicals does not appear in patient histories or drug profiles, the suspicion and identification of an occupational or household chemical exposure may help explain therapeutic failure or an adverse drug reaction (eg, the disulfiram-like response to alcohol-containing preparations by workers exposed to cyanamide or tetramethylthiuram disulfide).

Cigarette smoke contains polycyclic hydrocarbons that induce mixed-function hepatic oxidases, particularly in the young (Vestal and Wood, 1980). This enhancement of metabolism increases the dosage requirement for theophylline. The plasma level of imipramine also is decreased in smokers. (For further information, see index entry Nicotine, Drug Interactions.) Other hydrocarbons (eg, chlorinated hydrocarbons in pesticides such as DDT and lindane; the flame retardant polychlorinated biphenyls; polycyclic hydrocarbons in charcoal-broiled meat) also can increase the biotransformation of theophylline.

Alcohol has numerous actions that can alter the response to many drugs. Because of its widespread use, alcohol has the most clinically significant drug interaction capacity of any single nondietary nondrug chemical (see index entry Alcohol, Drug Interactions).

Influence of Biological Rhythms

The pharmacologic activity of a drug is affected by inherent biological rhythms in physiologic sensitivity (chronesthesy) and drug disposition (chronopharmacokinetics) (Reinberg and Smolensky, 1982). *Chronopharmacology* is the study of drug effects in relation to biological rhythms. Agents that have been reported to demonstrate chronopharmacokinetic variability include several antiepileptic drugs, aspirin, cisplatin, corticosteroids, cyclosporine, heparin, indomethacin, verapamil, methylprednisolone, ketoprofen, lithium, nortriptyline, propranolol, and theophylline (Matzke and St. Peter, 1990; Hla et al, 1992; Fisher et al, 1992). The apparent toxicity and efficacy of certain cytotoxic agents vary, depending on the time of administration (Hrushesky, 1985; Rivard et al, 1985; Guthrie, 1989).

The benefit of routine application of chronopharmacology to drug therapy remains to be established. However, advances in automated programmable drug delivery systems and the growing number of drugs for which significant circadian variations in disposition or response occur suggest that clinical interest in this area is likely to grow.

Selected References

Processes in Drug Disposition

Belknap SM, et al: Theophylline distribution kinetics analyzed by reference to simultaneously injected urea and inulin. *J Pharmacol Exp Ther* 243:963-969, 1987.

Chetkowski RJ, et al: Biologic effects of transdermal estradiol. *N Engl J Med* 314:1615-1620, 1986.

Gibaldi M: Prolonged-release medication. *Perspect Clin Pharmacol* 2:17-20, 25-27, 33-35, 41-43, 49-53, 1984.

Gonzalez FJ: The molecular biology of cytochrome P450s. *Pharmacol Rev* 40:243-276, 1989.

Gugler R, Allgayer H: Effects of antacids on the clinical pharmacokinetics of drugs: An update. *Clin Pharmacokinet* 18:210-219, 1990.

Langer R: New methods of drug delivery. *Science* 249:1527-1533, 1990.

van Ginneken CAM, Russel FGM: Saturable pharmacokinetics in the renal excretion of drugs. *Clin Pharmacokinet* 16:38-54, 1989.

van Hoogdalem EJ, et al: Pharmacokinetics of rectal drug administration, part I: General considerations and clinical applications of centrally acting drugs. *Clin Pharmacokinet* 21:11-26, 1991.

Winstanley PA, Orme ML'E: The effects of food on drug bioavailability. *Br J Clin Pharmacol* 28:621-628, 1989.

Wyllie E, et al: Increased seizure frequency with generic primidone. *JAMA* 258:1216-1217, 1987.

Pharmacokinetics

Atkinson AJ Jr, et al: Physiological basis of multicompartmental models of drug distribution. *Trend Pharmacol Sci* 12:96-101, (March) 1991.

Benet LZ, Galeazzi RL: Noncompartmental determination of the steady-state volume of distribution. *J Pharm Sci* 68:1971-1974, 1979.

Benet LZ, Massoud N: Pharmacokinetics, in Benet LZ, et al (eds): *Pharmacokinetic Basis for Drug Treatment*. New York, Raven Press, 1984, 1-28.

Blaschke TF: Protein binding and kinetics of drugs in liver diseases. *Clin Pharmacokinet* 2:32-44, 1977.

Bowman WC, Rand MJ: *Textbook of Pharmacology*, ed 2. London, Blackwell Scientific, 1980, 40.1-40.58.

Brosen K: Recent developments in hepatic drug oxidation: Implications for clinical pharmacokinetics. *Clin Pharmacokinet* 18:220-239, 1990.

Committee for Pharmacokinetic Nomenclature: *Manual of Symbols, Equations & Definitions in Pharmacokinetics*. Philadelphia, Committee for Pharmacokinetic Nomenclature, 1982.

Friedman H, Greenblatt DJ: Rational therapeutic drug monitoring. *JAMA* 256:2227-2233, 1986.

Gibaldi M: Basic concept: Clearance. *J Clin Pharmacol* 26:330-331, 1986.

MacKichan JJ: Pharmacokinetic consequences of drug displacement from blood and tissue proteins. *Clin Pharmacokinet* 9(suppl 1):32-41, 1984.

Riegelman S, Collier P: Application of statistical moment theory to evaluation of in vivo dissolution time and absorption time. *J Pharmacokinet Biopharm* 8:509-534, 1980.

Rowland M, Tozer TN: *Clinical Pharmacokinetics: Concepts and Applications*, ed 2. Philadelphia, Lea & Febiger, 1989.

Tozer TN, Winter ME: Phenytoin, in Evans WE, et al (eds): *Applied Pharmacokinetics: Principles of Therapeutic Drug Monitoring*, ed 2. Spokane, Wash, Applied Therapeutics, 1986, 493-539.

Therapeutic Drug Monitoring

Bryson SM, et al: Comparison of a bayesian forecasting technique with a new method for estimating phenytoin dose requirements. *Ther Drug Monit* 10:80-84, 1988.

Cridland JS: The value of therapeutic drug monitoring, letter. *Br J Clin Pharmacol* 29:278-279, 1990.

Evans WE, et al (eds): *Applied Therapeutics: Principles of Therapeutic Drug Monitoring*, ed 2. Spokane, Wash, Applied Therapeutics, 1986.

Friedman H, Greenblatt DJ: Rational therapeutic drug monitoring. *JAMA* 256:2227-2233, 1986.

Garattini S: Active drug metabolites: Overview of their relevance in clinical pharmacokinetics. *Clin Pharmacokinet* 10:216-227, 1985.

Gibson TP: Influence of renal disease on pharmacokinetics, in Evans WE, et al (eds): *Applied Pharmacokinetics: Principles of Therapeutic Drug Monitoring*, ed 2. Spokane, Wash, Applied Therapeutics, 1986, 83-115.

Godley PJ, et al: Comparison of a bayesian program with three microcomputer programs for predicting gentamicin concentrations. *Ther Drug Monit* 10:287-291, 1988.

Gugler R, Azarnoff DL: Clinical use of plasma drug concentrations. *Ration Drug Ther* 10:1-7, (Nov) 1976.

Kauffman RE: Clinical interpretation and application of drug concentration data. *Pediatr Clin North Am* 28:35-45, 1981.

Koch-Weser J: Serum level approach to individualization of drug dosage. *Eur J Clin Pharmacol* 9:1-8, 1975.

Matzke GR, St. Peter WL: Clinical pharmacokinetics 1990. *Clin Pharmacokinet* 18:1-19, 1990.

McCoy HG, Cipolle RJ: Toward optimal drug therapy: Benefits of therapeutic drug monitoring. *Postgrad Med* 74:121-134, (Oct) 1983.

Peck CC, Rodman JH: Analysis of clinical pharmacokinetic data for individualizing drug dosage regimens, in Evans WE, et al (eds): *Applied Pharmacokinetics: Principles of Therapeutic Drug Monitoring*, ed 2. Spokane, Wash, Applied Therapeutics, 1986, 55-82.

Perucca E, et al: Interpretation of drug levels in acute and chronic disease states. *Clin Pharmacokinet* 10:498-513, 1985.

Pryka RD, et al: Individualizing vancomycin dosage regimens: One-versus two-compartment bayesian models. *Ther Drug Monit* 11:450-454, 1989.

Uematsu T, et al: Prediction of individual dosage requirements for lignocaine: A validation study for bayesian forecasting in Japanese patients. *Ther Drug Monit* 11:25-31, 1989.

Wilkinson GR: Clearance approaches in pharmacology. *Pharmacol Rev* 39:1-47, 1987.

Zaske DE, et al: Gentamicin dosage requirements: Wide interpatient variations in 242 surgery patients with normal renal function. *Surgery* 87:164-169, 1980.

Renal Impairment

Anders MW: Metabolism of drugs by the kidney. *Kidney Int* 18:636-647, 1980.

Bennett WM: Guide to drug dosage in renal failure. *Clin Pharmacokinet* 15:326-354, 1988.

Brater DC: Pharmacological role of the kidney. *Drugs* 19:31-48, 1980.

Cockcroft DW, Gault MH: Prediction of creatinine clearance from serum creatinine. *Nephron* 16:31-41, 1976.

Dettli L: Drug dosage in renal disease. *Clin Pharmacokinet* 1:126-134, 1976.

Fillastre J-P, Singlas E: Pharmacokinetics of newer drugs in patients with renal impairment (part I). *Clin Pharmacokinet* 20:293-310, 1991.

Gambertoglio JG: Effects of renal disease: Altered pharmacokinetics, in Benet LZ, et al (eds): *Pharmacokinetic Basis for Drug Treatment*. New York, Raven Press, 1984, 149-171.

Gibson TP: Renal disease and drug metabolism: Overview. *Am J Kidney Dis* 8:7-17, 1986.

Reidenberg MM, Drayer DE: Drug therapy in renal failure. *Annu Rev Pharmacol Toxicol* 20:45-54, 1980.

Schwartz GJ, Gauthier B: Simple estimate of glomerular filtration rate in adolescent boys. *J Pediatr* 106:522-526, 1985.

Schwartz GJ, et al: Simple estimate of glomerular filtration rate in children derived from body length and plasma creatinine. *Pediatrics* 58:259-263, 1976.

Siersbaek-Nielsen K, et al: Rapid evaluation of creatinine clearance. *Lancet* 1:1133-1134, 1971.

Singlas E, Fillastre J-P: Pharmacokinetics of newer drugs in patients with renal impairment (part II). *Clin Pharmacokinet* 20:389-410, 1991.

Spring P: Calculation of drug dosage regimens in patients with renal disease: A new nomographic method. *Int J Clin Pharmacol Biopharm* 11:76-80, 1975.

Hepatic Impairment and Other Disease States

Bass NM, Williams RL: Guide to drug dosage in hepatic disease. *Clin Pharmacokinet* 15:396-420, 1988.

Bennett WM: Altering drug dose in patients with diseases of the kidney and liver, in Anderson RJ, Schrier RW (eds): *Clinical Use of Drugs in Patients with Kidney and Liver Disease*. Philadelphia, WB Saunders, 1981, 16-29.

Bircher J: Altered drug metabolism in liver disease: Therapeutic implications, in Thomas HC, Macsween RNM (eds): *Recent Advances in Hepatology*. London, Churchill-Livingston, 1983, 101-113.

O'Connor P, Feely J: Clinical pharmacokinetics and endocrine disorders: Therapeutic implications. *Clin Pharmacokinet* 13:345-364, 1987.

Pacifici GM, et al: Conjugation pathways in liver disease. *Br J Clin Pharmacol* 30:427-435, 1990.

Piper DW, et al: Gastrointestinal and hepatic diseases, in Speight TM (ed): *Avery's Drug Treatment: Principles and Practice of Clinical Pharmacology and Therapeutics,* ed 3. Sydney, ADIS Press, 1987, 732-811.

Shammas FV, Dickstein K: Clinical pharmacokinetics in heart failure: An updated review. *Clin Pharmacokinet* 15:94-113, 1988.

Shenfield GM: Influence of thyroid dysfunction on drug pharmacokinetics. *Clin Pharmacokinet* 6:275-297, 1981.

Wedlund PJ, Branch RA: Adjustment of medications in liver failure, in Chernow B, Lake CR (eds): *The Pharmacologic Approach to the Critically Ill Patient*. Baltimore, Williams & Wilkins, 1983, 84-114.

Wilkinson GR, Shand DG: Physiological approach to hepatic drug clearance. *Clin Pharmacol Ther* 18:377-390, 1975.

Williams RL, Benet LZ: Drug pharmacokinetics in cardiac and hepatic disease. *Annu Rev Pharmacol Toxicol* 20:389-413, 1980.

Pediatric Patients

Crom WR, et al: Age-related differences in hepatic drug clearance in children: Studies with lorazepam and antipyrine. *Clin Pharmacol Ther* 50:132-140, 1991.

Done AK: Drugs for children, in Modell W (ed): *Drugs of Choice 1972-1973*. St Louis, CV Mosby, 1982.

George SL, Gehan EA: Methods for measurement of body surface area. *J Pediatr* 94:342, 1979.

Green TP, Mirkin BL: Clinical pharmacokinetics: Pediatric considerations, in Benet LZ, et al (eds): *Pharmacokinetic Basis for Drug Treatment*. New York, Raven Press, 1984, 269-282.

Haycock GB, et al: Geometric method for measuring body surface area: Height-weight formula validated in infants, children, and adults. *J Pediatr* 93:62-66, 1978.

Kearns GL, Reed MD: Clinical pharmacokinetics in infants and children: A reappraisal. *Clin Pharmacokinet* 17 (suppl 1):29-67, 1989.

Milsap RL, Szefler SJ: Special pharmacokinetic considerations in children, in Evans WE, et al (eds): *Applied Pharmacokinetics: Principles of Therapeutic Drug Monitoring,* ed 2. Spokane, Wash, Applied Therapeutics, 1986.

Morselli PL: Clinical pharmacology of the perinatal period and early infancy. *Clin Pharmacokinet* 17 (suppl 1):13-28, 1989.

Morselli PL, et al: Clinical pharmacokinetics in newborns and infants: Age-related differences and therapeutic implications. *Clin Pharmacokinet* 5:485-527, 1980.

Nation RL: Drug kinetics in childbirth. *Clin Pharmacokinet* 5:340-364, 1980.

Roberts RJ: Pharmacologic principles in therapeutics in infants, in: *Drug Therapy in Infants: Pharmacologic Principles and Clinical Experience*. Philadelphia, WB Saunders, 1984, 3-24.

Triggs EJ, et al: Influence of age on drug metabolism. *Med J Aust* 141:823-827, 1984.

Geriatric Patients

Anderson S, Brenner BM: Effects of aging on the renal glomerulus. *Am J Med* 80:435-442, 1986.

Beers MH, Ouslander JG: Risk factors in geriatric drug prescribing: A practical guide to avoiding problems. *Drugs* 37:105-112, 1989.

Bortz WM: Redefining human aging. *J Am Geriatr Soc* 37:1092-1096, 1989.

Campion EW, et al: The effect of age on serum albumin in healthy males: Report from the normative aging study. *J Gerontol* 43:M18-M20, 1988.

Col N, et al: The role of medication noncompliance and adverse drug reactions in hospitalizations of the elderly. *Arch Intern Med* 150:841-845, 1990.

Cooper JK, Gardner C: Effect of aging on serum albumin. *J Am Geriatr Soc* 37:1039-1042, 1989.

Goldberg TH, Finkelstein MS: Difficulties in estimating glomerular filtration rate in the elderly. *Arch Intern Med* 147:1430-1433, 1987.

Goldberg PB, Roberts J: Pharmacologic basis for developing rational drug regimens for elderly patients. *Med Clin North Am* 67:315-331, 1983.

Greenblatt DJ, et al: Drug disposition in old age. *N Engl J Med* 306:1081-1088, 1982.

Greenblatt DJ, et al: Pharmacokinetic risk factors in the elderly, in Moore SR, Teal TW (eds): *Geriatric Drug Use: Clinical and Social Perspectives*. New York, Pergamon Press, 1984, 153-159.

Lamy PP: Age-related pharmacodynamic changes. *Elder Care News* 5:25-32, (Fall) 1989.

Lindeman RD, et al: Longitudinal studies on the rate of decline in renal function with age. *J Am Geriatr Soc* 33:278-285, 1985.

Lonergan ET: Aging and the kidney: Adjusting treatment to physiologic change. *Geriatrics* 43:27-33, (March) 1988.

Massoud N: Pharmacokinetic considerations in geriatric patients, in Benet LZ, et al (eds): *Pharmacokinetic Basis for Drug Treatment*. New York, Raven Press, 1984, 283-310.

Mayersohn M: "Xylose test" to assess gastrointestinal absorption in the elderly: Pharmacokinetic evaluation of literature. *J Gerontol* 37:300-305, 1982.

Veering BT, et al: The effect of age on serum concentrations of albumin and α_1-acid glycoprotein. *Br J Clin Pharmacol* 29:201-206, 1990.

Vestal RE, Dawson GW: Pharmacology and aging, in Finch CE, Schneider EL (eds): *Handbook of the Biology of Aging*, ed 2. New York, Van Nostrand, 1985, 744-819.

Vestal RE, et al: Antipyrine metabolism in man: Influence of age, alcohol, caffeine, and smoking. *Clin Pharmacol Ther* 18:425-432, 1975.

Woodhouse KW, Wynne HA: Age-related changes in liver size and hepatic blood flow: The influence on drug metabolism in the elderly. *Clin Pharmacokinet* 15:287-294, 1988.

Pregnancy and Obesity

Abernethy DR, Greenblatt DJ: Drug disposition in obese humans: An update. *Clin Pharmacokinet* 11:199-213, 1986.

Boobis AR, Lewis P: Drugs in pregnancy: Altered pharmacokinetics. *Br J Hosp Med* 28:566-573, 1982.

Dean M, et al: Serum protein binding of drugs during and after pregnancy in humans. *Clin Pharmacol Ther* 28:253-261, 1980.

Krauer B, Krauer F: Drug kinetics in pregnancy. *Clin Pharmacokinet* 2:167-181, 1977.

Mattison DR: Physiologic variations in pharmacokinetics during pregnancy, in Fabro S, Scialli AR (eds): *Drugs and Chemical Action in Pregnancy*. New York, Marcel Dekker, 1986, 37-102.

Perucca E, Crema A: Plasma protein binding of drugs in pregnancy. *Clin Pharmacokinet* 7:336-352, 1982.

Rayburn WF, Andresen BD: Principles of perinatal pharmacology, in Rayburn WF, Zuspan FP (eds): *Drug Therapy in Obstetrics and Gynecology*. Norwalk, Appleton-Century-Crofts, 1986, 3-12.

Ruprah M, et al: Decreased serum protein binding of phenytoin in late pregnancy. *Lancet* 2:316-317, 1980.

Influence of Pharmacogenetics

Bertilsson L, et al: Importance of genetic factors in the regulation of diazepam metabolism: Relationship to *S*-mephenytoin, but not debrisoquin, hydroxylation phenotype. *Clin Pharmacol Ther* 45:348-355, 1989.

Eichelbaum M: Polymorphic drug oxidation in humans. *Federation Proc* 43:2298-2302, 1984.

Grant DM, et al: Acetylation pharmacogenetics: The slow acetylator phenotype is caused by decreased or absent arylamine *N*-acetyltransferase in human liver. *J Clin Invest* 85:968-972, 1990.

Nelson DR, et al: The P450 superfamily: Update on new sequences, gene mapping, accession numbers, early trivial names of enzymes, and nomenclature. *DNA Cell Biol* 12:1-51, 1993.

Relling MV: Polymorphic drug metabolism. *Clin Pharm* 8:852-863, 1989.

Sanz EJ, Bertilsson L: *d*-propoxyphene is a potent inhibitor of debrisoquine, but not *S*-mephenytoin 4-hydroxylation in vivo. *Ther Drug Monit* 12:297-299, 1990.

Vesell ES: Pharmacogenetics: Multiple interactions between genes and environment as determinants of drug response. *Am J Med* 66:183-187, 1979.

Vesell ES: Genetic host factors: Determinants of drug response, editorial. *N Engl J Med* 313:261-262, 1985.

Weinshilboum RM: Human pharmacogenetics. *Federation Proc* 43:2295-2297, 1984.

Wilkinson GR, et al: Genetic polymorphism of S-mephenytoin hydroxylation. *Pharmacol Ther* 43:53-76, 1989.

Influence of Diet and Environmental Chemicals

Alvares AP: Interactions between environmental chemicals and drug biotransformation in man. *Clin Pharmacokinet* 3:462-477, 1978.

Alvares AP, et al: Regulation of drug metabolism in man by environmental factors. *Drug Metab Rev* 9:185-205, 1979.

Anderson KE: Influences of diet and nutrition on clinical pharmacokinetics. *Clin Pharmacokinet* 14:325-346, 1988.

Dollery CT, et al: Contribution of environmental factors to variability in human drug metabolism. *Drug Metab Rev* 9:207-220, 1979.

George CF: Food, drugs, and bioavailability. *BMJ* 289:1093-1094, 1984.

Iber FL: Drug metabolism in heavy consumers of ethyl alcohol. *Clin Pharmacol Ther* 22:735-742, 1977.

Lieber CS: Interaction of ethanol with drugs and vitamin therapy. *Ration Drug Ther* 19:1-7, (Nov) 1985.

Vestal RE, Wood AJJ: Influence of age and smoking on drug kinetics in man: Studies using model compounds. *Clin Pharmacokinet* 5:309-319, 1980.

Welling PG: Interactions affecting drug absorption. *Clin Pharmacokinet* 9:404-434, 1984.

Influence of Biological Rhythms

Fisher LE, et al: Pharmacokinetics and pharmacodynamics of methylprednisolone when administered at 8 AM versus 4 PM. *Clin Pharmacol Ther* 51:677-688, 1992.

Guthrie TH: Circadian chemotherapy of advanced squamous cell carcinoma of the head and neck. *Clin Res* 37:23A, 1989.

Hla KK, et al: Influence of time of administration on verapamil pharmacokinetics. *Clin Pharmacol Ther* 51:366-370, 1992.

Hrushesky WMJ: Circadian timing of cancer chemotherapy. *Science* 228:73-75, 1985.

Hrushesky WJM, Rushing D: Circadian chronopharmacokinetics and chronotoxicology of doxorubicin and cisplatin in human beings with cancer. *Proceedings of the First International Montreux Conference of Chronopharmacology*. Montreux, Switzerland, March 26-30, 1984, 305.

Reinberg A: Clinical chronopharmacology: Experimental basis for chronotherapy. *Arzneim Forsch* 28:1861-1867, 1978.

Reinberg A, Smolensky MH: Circadian changes of drug disposition in man. *Clin Pharmacokinet* 7:401-420, 1982.

Rivard GE, et al: Maintenance chemotherapy for childhood acute lymphoblastic leukaemia: Better in the evening. *Lancet* 2:1264-1266, 1985.

Adverse Drug Events

3

ADVERSE DRUG REACTIONS

Definition

The World Health Organization's broad definition of an adverse drug reaction (ADR) is "any response to a drug that is noxious and unintended and that occurs at doses used in man for prophylaxis, diagnosis or therapy of disease, or for the modification of physiological function." Drug abuse and accidental or suicidal poisoning are not classified as ADRs, although they are considered in the broad context of the overall risk associated with use of a drug. Adverse drug interactions can be classified as ADRs when the circumstances and clinical outcome meet the criteria specified in the WHO definition. The WHO definition does not explicitly include the concept of failure to accomplish the intended purpose, but it is a part of the discussion of ADRs by the WHO. Failure to accomplish an intended purpose is referred to as therapeutic failure. Reasons for therapeutic failure can be drug- or patient-related. Drug-related therapeutic failures can occur because the drug selected for the clinical situation is ineffective, errors occur in prescribing or dispensing medication, an interaction with concomitant drug therapy affects the drug's action, bioavailability is decreased because of factors related to the drug product (product defect, improper formulation), or the selected route of administration is ineffective. Patient-related therapeutic failures usually result from poor patient compliance or decreased bioavailability due to disease state(s) (eg, disorders that affect gastrointestinal absorption or result in decreased drug concentration at the intended site of effect). Although ADRs often occur because too much drug is present for the clinical situation, therapeutic failures frequently are associated with too little drug for the clinical situation. Since progression of the disease is a confounding factor in many instances, therapeutic failures often are difficult to verify. Nevertheless, in studies that have verified therapeutic failures, their incidence approximated that of ADRs (Bero et al, 1991). In terms of drug-related adverse events, drug-related therapeutic failures are as important as ADRs; however, much less data on their cause and management are available.

Occurrence and Relevance

Drug-related adverse events are the most common type (19%) of all adverse events in hospitalized patients (Brennan et al, 1991; Leape et al, 1991 A) and also are prominent in ambulatory patients. Prescription drugs are responsible for about 90% of all established ADRs (Tatro, 1991), and about 7% of ADRs are the result of adverse drug interactions (Edlavitch, 1988). ADRs constitute a considerable clinical problem in terms of both human suffering and increased health care costs (Ray et al, 1990; Dukes, 1992). Because studies have indicated that about 75% of drug-related adverse events are preventable (Bero et al, 1991), early identification and reporting of significant ADRs and identification of therapeutic failures, followed by preventive measures, can greatly facilitate resolution of the problem and have great relevance for both patients and physicians, including reduction of the costs of medical care (Leape et al, 1991 B; Tatro, 1991).

Information on ADRs is always incomplete when a drug is first introduced into clinical use. Premarketing exposure to an investigational drug usually is limited to 1,000 to 3,000 persons. Therefore, the probability of identifying ADRs with a frequency of less than 1:1,000 is remote. In addition, patient exclusion criteria associated with controlled trials do not allow a good estimate of the frequency of some ADRs in subgroups of patients who have complications or other illnesses and/or are receiving multiple drugs. The full range of ADRs may not be known until a drug has been used (1) in patients with a wide variety of diseases, disorders, or conditions, (2) in hundreds of thousands of patients, especially for adverse events with an incidence of less than 1 in 10,000, and (3) for a prolonged period. In addition, an ADR may not be evident until long after exposure to the drug has ceased (eg, development of vaginal cancer in daughters of women who received diethylstilbestrol during pregnancy). Therefore, the full range and frequency of ADRs can only be determined after the drug is marketed. At least two to three years and often a longer period are required to establish the actual incidence of most ADRs for a drug.

Classification

ADRs are divided into four categories based on their prevalence and severity: (1) rare/not serious, which are of little concern clinically; (2) rare/serious, which usually are identified only after the drug is marketed and large numbers of patients are exposed; (3) common/not serious; and (4) common/serious. Reactions in the latter two categories are frequently identified in clinical trials prior to Food and Drug Administration (FDA) approval, are listed on the labeling, and often are part of the benefit/risk equation in drug selection.

ADRs also can be classified as effects that produce predictable (Type A) minor and major toxicity, as well as unpredictable (Type B) idiosyncracy (Park et al, 1992) or hypersensitivity. In one study of 36,653 hospitalized patients, 731 verified ADRs occurred, of which 664 were type A and the remainder type B (Classen et al, 1991).

Another ADR classification system divides reactions on the basis of organ system involvement. In one study of 367 hospitalized patients for which an ADR was reported, the distribution of reaction types was as follows: hematologic (68), allergic (62), cardiovascular (48), gastrointestinal (48), neurologic (39), renal (22), infusion-related (20), metabolic (19), respiratory (12), special sensory (6), hepatic (6), psychiatric (5), dermatologic (3), and unclassified (9) (Hartwig et al, 1992).

Assessment of Risk

The following factors increase the risk of ADRs: Use of drugs that have a narrow therapeutic index or, for a limited number of agents, drug disposition that is characterized by saturable kinetics; use of drugs that interact adversely with one another or with food or environmental chemicals; or use of drugs in patients in whom vulnerability to ADRs is increased (ie, the elderly; neonates; immunocompromised patients; patients with debilitating diseases; patients in whom the ability to absorb, distribute, biotransform, and/or eliminate drugs is compromised; pregnant or lactating women; probably patients with a history of hypersensitivity to one or more drugs).

The elderly are especially at risk for ADRs for several reasons: The presence of multiple diseases, prescription of multiple medications, age-related changes in physiologic function, and/or atypical drug-induced disease presentations (Griffin et al, 1991; Beard, 1992; Higbee, 1992). Multiple medications and patient-specific physiologic and functional characteristics (eg, the frail elderly) are more significant risk factors than chronologic age (Gurwitz and Avorn, 1991, Chrischilles et al, 1992). An estimated 2% to 6% of hospital admissions in all patients result from ADRs, but this percentage may be as high as 10% to 30% in the elderly. The long-term use of cardiovascular, psychotropic, and nonsteroidal anti-inflammatory drugs, alone or in combination, in this population is of special concern.

Prescribing a drug for a pregnant woman or a woman who is breast feeding presents a unique problem to the physician (Mucklow, 1986). Not only must ADRs in the mother be considered, but the fetus or infant must be regarded as potentially at risk. Because of the significance of timing of drug administration for the mother and the complex mechanisms of drug transfer across the placenta, as well as drug transfer into breast milk, ADRs in pregnant and lactating women are discussed in greater detail in a separate section in this chapter.

Rarely, ADRs are not caused by the primary active ingredient of a drug. Impurities formed during manufacture, dyes, preservatives, vehicles, degradation products, and excipients, which are considered therapeutically inactive, may produce adverse effects.

Assessment of Causality

The FDA does not require a formal assessment of causality prior to submission of a suspected ADR. The FDA and/or the manufacturer will provide expertise to determine causality.

Proving that a specific drug is responsible for an adverse event in an individual may be difficult because of multiple drug exposures and underlying illness. A number of algorithms have been advanced to evaluate causality. See the Figure for one example. Most algorithms include the following criteria: (1) a *temporal* relationship between the suspected drug and the adverse reaction; (2) the presence of a positive *dechallenge*, ie, improvement after removal of the drug; (3) the presence of a positive *rechallenge,* ie, recurrence of the adverse reaction when administration of the drug is resumed;

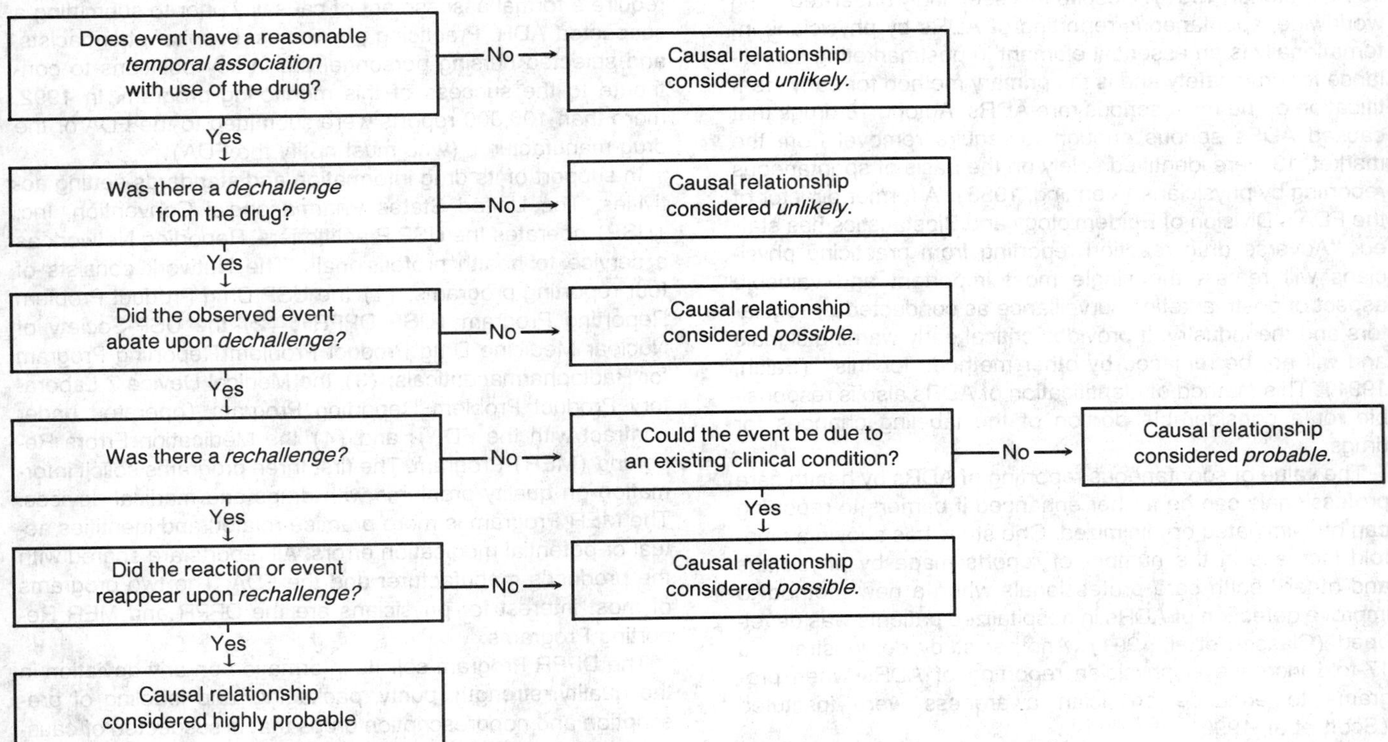

* Each drug is carried through independently; if more than one drug was dechallenged or rechallenged simultaneously, causality for all is considered to be unlikely or possible.

QUESTIONS:
1. Did the reaction follow a reasonable temporal sequence?
2. Was there a history of previous exposure (ie, sensitizing dose) or sufficient duration of exposure to the drug to suggest a hypersensitivity reaction?
3. Did the reaction vary in intensity in relation to dose or serum levels?
4. Did the patient improve after stopping the drug?
5. Did the reaction appear on repeated exposure (rechallenge)?
6. Could the reaction be reasonably explained by the known characteristics of the patient's clinical state?

Adapted from Jones, 1982.

and (4) the lack of a confounding effect (eg, concomitant drug or disease is not likely to cause the same type of disorder). If all of the above criteria are satisfied, the ADR under consideration would be highly probable.

Reporting Adverse Drug Reactions

Postmarketing surveillance methods to identify ADRs include the following: (1) Specific controlled studies (Phase IV Postmarketing Studies) recommended by the FDA and conducted by the manufacturer for selected drugs. The manufacturer's agreement to carry out such studies is a requirement for drug approval. These studies are usually performed when concerns about the safety of a drug remain despite completion of premarketing controlled clinical trials. (2) Pharmacoepidemiologic studies for selected drugs utilizing large computer databases that link medical records with drug treatment (Strom, 1990; Strom and Tugwell, 1990; Hartzema et al, 1991). These studies are especially useful for the determination of rare, delayed, serious ADRs. Such studies also provide denominator data to better estimate the true frequency of an ADR during general use rather than under premarket clinical trial conditions. (3) Spontaneous reporting of ADRs by physicians and other health professionals.

The number of spontaneous reports of ADRs by physicians is extremely limited in the United States and internationally (Waller, 1992). The figure was as low as 2% in a United

Kingdom study of 44,000 patients involving 8,000 physicians. Unfortunately, the reporting rate in the United States generally is about one-half that of the United Kingdom (Rawlins et al, 1989; Fletcher, 1991). Despite this seemingly under-reporting worldwide, spontaneous reporting of ADRs by physicians internationally is an essential element in postmarketing surveillance for drug safety and is the primary method for early identification of the most serious rare ADRs. Among 18 drugs that caused ADRs serious enough to require removal from the market, 13 were identified solely on the basis of spontaneous reporting by physicians (Venning, 1983). A former director of the FDA's Division of Epidemiology and Biostatistics has stated: "Adverse drug reaction reporting from practicing physicians will remain the single most important and valuable aspect of postmarketing surveillance as conducted by regulators and the industry. It provides critical early warning signals and will not be replaced by other methods for this" (Faich, 1991). This method of identification of ADRs also is responsible for a considerable portion of the labeling changes for drugs.

The value of spontaneous reporting of ADRs by health care professionals can be further enhanced if barriers to reporting can be eliminated or minimized. One study has shown a ninefold increase in the number of reports made by physicians and other health care professionals when a new method to improve detection of ADRs in hospitalized patients was developed (Classen et al, 1991). Another study demonstrated a 17-fold increase in physician reporting of ADRs when programs to enhance physician awareness were instituted (Scott et al, 1990).

MEDWatch, the FDA Medical Products Reporting Program for voluntary reporting by health professionals of adverse events and product problems associated with drugs, biologics, or medical devices, has been established (Kessler, 1993 A, 1993 B). MEDWatch is especially interested in receiving three types of reports: (1) serious ADRs that are not currently included in the drug's labeling; (2) all serious events (labeled and unlabeled) associated with new drugs during their first three years on the market (Kennedy et al, 1991); and (3) previously reported reactions if they are serious and occur in clusters within a hospital or clinic. A serious ADR is defined as one that results in or prolongs hospitalization; is life-threatening; contributes to significant disability; or results in death of the patient.

A reporting form is distributed by MEDWatch, Food and Drug Administration, 5600 Fishers Lane, Rockville, MD 20852-9787; Fax 1-800/FDA-0178. A mailer copy of this form with accompanying instructions appears at the end of this publication for convenience in order to promote this important activity. A copy of this form also usually is available in the *Physicians Desk Reference* and the United States Pharmacopeial Convention's text entitled *Drug Information for the Health Professional* (USP DI).

The completed form can be mailed or faxed to the FDA. The information from reported ADRs is used to update the labeling for adverse reactions and occasionally to modify a drug's indications for use or its precautions. The identity of the patient and reporter is held in confidence by the FDA and will not be disclosed in response to a request from the public. The hospital pharmacist can serve as an important resource to coordinate the information requested in the report. Attachment of other relevant data is encouraged. The FDA does not require a formal assessment of causality prior to submitting a suspected ADR. Practicing physicians, hospital pharmacists, and selected nursing personnel are in key positions to contribute to the success of this monitoring program. In 1992, more than 100,000 reports were submitted to the FDA or the drug manufacturer (who must notify the FDA).

In support of its drug information and standards-setting activities, The United States Pharmacopeial Convention, Inc. (USP) operates the USP Practitioners' Reporting Network as a service to health professionals. The Network consists of four reporting programs: (1) the USP Drug Product Problem Reporting Program (USP DPPR); (2) the USP-Society of Nuclear Medicine Drug Product Problem Reporting Program for Radiopharmaceuticals; (3) the Medical Device 7 Laboratory Product Problem Reporting Program (operated under contract with the FDA); and (4) the Medication Errors Reporting (MER) Program. The first three programs solicit information on quality problems with drugs and medical devices. The MER Program is more practice-related and identifies actual or potential medication errors. All reports are shared with the product's manufacturer and the FDA. The two programs of most interest for physicians are the DPPR and MER Reporting Programs.

The DPPR Program solicits information on any deviation in the quality, strength, purity, packaging, and labeling of prescription and nonprescription drugs that is suspected of causing an ADR. These reports have identified problems such as suspected counterfeiting, sub- or superpotency, and therapeutic ineffectiveness including lot-to-lot variations and product-to-product substitutions.

The MER Program is a nationwide system that collects reports from health care practitioners on actual and potential medication errors. The program encompasses a wide variety of problems with drug nomenclature; prescription writing (eg, use of abbreviations and look-alike drug names); and containers or packaging. Because of liability concerns of physicians and others, medication error reports may be submitted in complete anonymity by telephone (1-800/23ERROR), which operates on an automatic answering device. Reports also may be submitted in writing.

Further information on all of the programs in the USP Practitioners' Reporting Network can be obtained by calling 1-800/638-6725 24 hours a day, seven days a week.

Adverse Drug Reactions During Pregnancy

In the United States, the frequency of major defects noted at birth is 2% to 4% or about 120,000 births per year. The causes of 65% to 70% of these birth defects are unknown; 25% are ascribed to genetic factors, 3% to chromosomal aberrations, and 3% (range, 1% to 5%) to environmental factors (ie, maternal infection, radiation, drug administration). The incidence of major defects of prenatal origin that become apparent later in life is about 10% of infants affected.

Prescribing a drug for pregnant women presents a unique problem to the physician. Both the mother and the fetus must be regarded as potential targets.

The type of reaction produced in the fetus depends on the stage of development in which drug exposure occurs (Beeley, 1986 A, 1986 B; Miller, 1981). Although not strictly a part of gestation, ova may lie dormant for decades and are exposed to drugs and other environmental chemicals before conception. Four major stages of human gestation are recognized: (1) Preimplantation lasts about 12 days from conception to implantation. (2) Organogenesis occurs during days 13 to 56. Together, preimplantation and organogenesis comprise that period of embryonic development occurring in the first quarter of pregnancy (ie, the first two-thirds of the first trimester). (3) During the remaining three-quarters of pregnancy, growth and development occur, especially in the central nervous, endocrine, and musculoskeletal systems. (4) The relatively short labor-delivery stage completes the time during pregnancy when maternal drug administration may have direct and indirect effects on the fetus.

TERATOGENS. Teratology is the study of congenital malformations that are grossly visible at birth and are induced by exogenous agents (teratogens) in the first trimester, especially during organogenesis. (It is probable that harmful drug effects during the first week of pregnancy either kill the embryo or damage cells, which are then replaced by undifferentiated cells and do not have long-term sequelae [Beeley, 1986 A].) The definition of teratogenesis may be extended to include any birth defect (ie, morphologic, biochemical, behavioral) induced at any stage of gestation and detected at birth or later in life. The incidence of congenital malformations does not appear to have increased during the last 30 years despite the dramatic increase in the number of new chemical entities. Congenital abnormalities are increasing as a proportion of infant mortality, but this reflects a greater salvage rate for infants who previously died from other causes.

The presence and severity of a drug-induced congenital malformation depend on many factors: the drug's nature (ie, whether it is a potent, weak, or nonteratogen), its accessibility to the embryo or fetus, the period of gestation during which it is administered, the dose and duration of action, the synergistic or antagonistic effects of concomitantly administered drugs, and the genetic constitution and susceptibility of the fetus, which, in turn, is dependent on the age, nutritional status, and health of the mother (Iams and Rayburn, 1982).

There are only a few drugs or classes of drugs that are *proven* teratogens with a high level of risk; they include thalidomide; retinoids such as isotretinoin and etretinate; and certain antineoplastic drugs, especially DNA-damaging agents (eg, cyclophosphamide, busulfan, ifosfamide, procarbazine). Teratogenic and other adverse effects on fetal development also have been associated with the use during pregnancy of methotrexate, antiepileptic drugs (eg, valproate, phenytoin, carbamazepine), lithium, warfarin, estrogens (particularly potent synthetic agents such as diethylstilbestrol [DES]), antithyroid drugs (eg, propylthiouracil, methimazole, radioactive iodine), penicillamine, tetracyclines, and alcohol. See the evaluations on these agents and index entry Teratogenicity for further information on the use of specific drugs that are teratogens or may otherwise adversely effect fetal development.

Teratogen Testing: The identification of a teratogen in humans is exceedingly difficult (Rosa, 1992). Consequently, identification of teratogens has been limited to unique defects or patterns of defects caused by many of the drugs noted above. Because of this, it is wise to avoid using any drug during pregnancy unless definite benefits are anticipated. Therefore, the most appropriate question on whether to employ drug therapy during pregnancy may be does the treatment have important benefits rather than does the treatment have known risks (Rosa, 1992).

The doses used in experimental teratology are usually much greater than those used clinically. Furthermore, species susceptibility varies, which makes it very difficult to predict clinical effects. Despite this inability to extrapolate, the medical community is conservative about using drugs that are teratogenic in animals, even when no such effect has been documented in humans after prolonged use.

Individual case reports and epidemiologic surveys usually provide the initial suggestion of teratogenicity (Goldberg and Golbus, 1986). Although individual case reports have limitations (ie, dependence on voluntary reporting, incompleteness of data, unreliability of recall), most of the drugs that are known to be teratogenic in humans have been first identified by the astute observations of practicing physicians. Thus, case reports are the primary mechanism for alerting the medical community to potent teratogens. Epidemiologic studies are desirable for confirmation; however, an almost impractically large number of pregnant women must be monitored to distinguish between congenital malformations induced by a weak teratogen and those due to other mechanisms. An association between a congenital malformation and a drug does not necessarily imply causality. The drug may be used to treat a disorder that causes the malformation, the fetal malformation may lead to a maternal disorder requiring treatment with a certain drug, a drug may inhibit the spontaneous abortion of an already malformed fetus, or a drug may be used commonly in combination with another drug, the latter causing the malformation (Goldberg and Golbus, 1986).

FDA PREGNANCY CATEGORIES. Five categories of prescription drugs for use in pregnant women have been established by the FDA for inclusion in the precautions section of the package insert (Doering, 1992). Prescription drugs absorbed systemically or those known to have a potential for harm to the fetus are categorized according to the level of risk as follows:

FDA Pregnancy Category A: Controlled studies in women fail to demonstrate a risk to the fetus in the first trimester (and there is no evidence of a risk in later trimesters), and the possibility of fetal harm appears remote.

FDA Pregnancy Category B: Either animal reproduction studies have not demonstrated a fetal risk but there are no controlled studies in pregnant women, or animal reproduction studies have shown an adverse effect (other than decreased fertility) that was not confirmed in controlled studies on women in the first trimester (and there is no evidence of a risk in later trimesters).

FDA Pregnancy Category C: Either studies in animals have revealed adverse effects on the fetus (teratogenic, embryocidal, or other effects) and there are no controlled studies in women, or studies in women and animals are not available. Drugs in this category should be given only if safer alternatives are not available and if the potential benefit justifies the *known* risk(s) to the fetus.

FDA Pregnancy Category D: There is positive evidence of human fetal risk, but the benefits for pregnant women may be acceptable despite the risk, as in life-threatening or serious diseases for which safer drugs cannot be used or are ineffective. An appropriate statement must appear in the "warnings" section of the labeling of drugs in this category.

FDA Pregnancy Category X: Studies in animals or humans have demonstrated fetal abnormalities, there is evidence of fetal risk based on human experience, or both, and the risk of using the drug in pregnant women clearly outweighs any possible benefit. The drug is contraindicated in women who are or may become pregnant. An appropriate statement must appear in the "contraindications" section of the labeling of drugs in this category.

ADVERSE DRUG REACTIONS DURING LATER STAGES OF PREGNANCY. A substantial proportion of ADRs occur after the first trimester. For example, the excessive and prolonged maternal use of opioids, benzodiazepines, and barbiturates during pregnancy up to the time of delivery causes withdrawal symptoms (eg, hyperirritability, vomiting, shrill cry) in many exposed infants at delivery. Similarly, administration of large doses of opioids and most central nervous system depressants during labor will impair respiration in many infants at birth. Angiotensin-converting enzyme (ACE) inhibitors administered during the last half of pregnancy can cause potentially lethal fetal and neonatal renal failure (Rosa et al, 1989). Nonsteroidal anti-inflammatory drugs (NSAIDs) also can inhibit fetal renal function and can endanger fetal circulation through closure of the ductus arteriosus (Briggs et al, 1990). Thus, use of ACE inhibitors and NSAIDs should be avoided during pregnancy.

The labeling described above for teratogens also includes available information on maternal and fetal effects of drugs that have a recognized use during labor or delivery, whether or not the use is stated in the indications section of the labeling.

PHYSICIANS' RESPONSIBILITIES IN DRUG EXPOSURE DURING PREGNANCY. The physician's four responsibilities concerning drug exposures during pregnancy are (1) to avoid unnecessary drug use and choose the drug with the least hazardous risk/benefit ratio; (2) to inform patients about the implications of drug exposures during pregnancy; (3) with necessary or inadvertent drug exposures, to advise patients on the priority for pregnancy avoidance measures; and (4) when birth defects are observed, to determine unusual exposures and report these.

The physician is often faced with the need to advise patients on the risk of conception during drug therapy and on inadvertent or necessary drug exposures during pregnancy, particularly the first trimester. Concerns are magnified by widespread publicity regarding teratogenic controversies, uncertainty of risks, and legal and moral issues. From the preceding discussion, it is apparent that *unnecessary* drug exposures should be avoided. However, this should not be misconstrued to indicate that necessary treatment should be avoided or that necessary or inadvertent drug exposure is a reason for interrupting a pregnancy, except possibly for the few instances in which the maternal risk is high and well established (see previous discussion).

Mothers will be exposed to numerous environmental chemicals in every pregnancy, and little risk can be attributed to most of these. On the other hand, when reassuring pregnant patients regarding drug exposures, the inherent risks during pregnancy should always be conveyed and the physician should never suggest that an adverse outcome is not possible in the absence of drug exposure. However, the risk associated with exposure to a drug not known to be a human teratogen is probably small.

The causal association between cigarette smoking and fetal growth retardation is unequivocal, and this avoidable risk should be emphasized.

Questions regarding preconception drug exposures to the father are also raised. Birth defects resulting from preconception drug exposure have not been confirmed in the limited number of epidemiologic studies available and are unlikely to be found unless effects persist into the period of embryogenesis. This question needs further study.

It is desirable for the physician to have information on a drug's potential risk to the fetus so that the risk can be weighed against the potential benefit to the mother. Unfortunately, this information is seldom complete; however, review articles are available on drugs that might be used in pregnancy (Briggs et al, 1990; Hays, 1981; Lewis et al, 1985; Miller, 1981; Niebyl, 1988; Rayburn and Zuspan, 1982) as well as on agents that are of greatest concern (Golbus, 1980; Wood and Beeley, 1981; Shepard, 1986; Dicke, 1989).

Absolute safety from drug exposure for the fetus can be guaranteed only by practicing therapeutic nihilism for all women between the ages of 14 and 45; however, this approach would deny women the medications necessary to treat many serious disorders. Failure to treat a serious condition in the mother may be more hazardous to the fetus than the drug. An appreciation by the physician of the scope of potential effects of drugs on the embryo and fetus, together with curtailment in drug prescribing, appears to be a more sensible approach. In this publication, an effort has been made to include information on known or reasonably assumed hazards of drugs given during pregnancy. For many drugs, particularly recently marketed agents, little or no information is available on use during pregnancy. Accordingly, it often is necessary to warn that a drug should be given only if the expected benefits exceed the risks to mother and fetus. Even when data are inadequate to specify what risks, if any, are present, a warning serves as a reminder that, unless a systemically absorbed drug has been studied extensively in pregnant women, it should be given only if the need exists, and the possibility of fetal toxicity should be borne in mind.

Adverse Drug Reactions During Breast Feeding

The number of mothers who breast-feed has increased from 28% in 1975 to approximately 50% at present. This has led to increased questioning of the physician concerning the potential toxicity of drugs taken by lactating women that may appear in breast milk. Unfortunately, data on the short- and long-term effects and safety of many maternally ingested drugs on the suckling infant are incomplete.

The mechanisms that determine the concentration of a drug in breast milk are similar to those existing elsewhere within the organism. Drugs generally traverse membranes by passive diffusion, and the ultimate concentration achieved depends on the existing concentration gradient, molecular weight, degree of ionization, lipid solubility, and extent of drug-maternal plasma protein binding (Atkinson et al, 1988; Welch and Findlay, 1981). Breast milk (pH, 7.0 to 7.6; mean pH, 7.2) is more acid than plasma (pH, 7.4), and weak bases become more ionized as the pH decreases; thus, these drugs generally have higher concentrations in milk than in plasma as the relatively membrane-impermeable ionized form is retained or "trapped" within breast milk. The opposite occurs with weak acids. However, the influence of molecular weight (eg, sulfasalazine, heparin), lipid solubility, rate of metabolism, and protein binding (eg, warfarin) may be more significant than the coefficient of ionization (pKa) (Sim and McNeil, 1992).

Milk/plasma ratios signify only that the drug is present in milk. They indicate nothing about the total amount absorbed by the infant or the possibility of adverse effects, which are of concern to the individual patient. It is now clear that, with very few exceptions, all drugs present in the maternal circulation are transferred into milk; however, the maximum amount secreted into milk seldom exceeds 1% to 2% of the maternal dose. Thus, the decision to breast-feed is based primarily on the incidence and types of adverse reactions reported rather than the presence of the drug in breast milk.

Drugs that are ingested by nursing infants in milk are most often placed in one of four general categories throughout this publication. The information is located in the Precautions or Adverse Reactions and Precautions section for individual drugs or drug classes when appropriate. These categories include situations when breast-feeding is contraindicated, when periodic monitoring of the nursing infant is recommended, when no significant adverse reactions in the nursing infant have been reported, or when available data are insufficient to evaluate and recommend the safety of the drug during breast-feeding.

Antimetabolites, chloramphenicol, cocaine, bromocriptine, cyclosporine, phencyclidine, radioactive pharmaceuticals, and phenindione are contraindicated during breast-feeding. Lithium is considered to be contraindicated by most authorities, because high concentrations can occur in the plasma of nursing infants. Isotretinoin also is contraindicated during breast feeding; although the amount excreted in milk is unknown, the drug is a known teratogen, and exposure in infants should be minimized. Some authorities also express concern about the use of isoniazid because of the possible hepatotoxic action of its acetylated metabolite in the infant. Other drugs that are relatively contraindicated include sulfonamides; dapsone and nitrofurantoin, which may produce hemolytic anemia, especially in G6PD-deficient infants; and antithyroid drugs (especially methimazole) and iodides, which may inhibit thyroid function. However, propylthiouracil does not appear to be present in clinically significant concentrations in human milk (Kampmann et al, 1980).

The use of low-dose combination or progestin only-minipill oral contraceptives is generally considered safe. The amount of estrogen ingested by a suckling infant is similar whether the estrogen is exogenous from a combination oral contraceptive or endogenously produced by a lactating mother. The progestin component of combination oral contraceptives is also found in breast milk, whereas endogenous progesterone is not (Committee on Drugs, American Academy of Pediatrics, in press).

Physical signs in the infant should be monitored to identify serious adverse reactions when certain agents or drugs are used by the nursing mother, eg, drowsiness with alcohol, barbiturates, benzodiazepines, certain antihistamines, and other agents with a sedative action; diarrhea and candidiasis with ampicillin; dependence with prolonged use of large doses of opioids.

Evidence supports the contention that milk is produced continuously rather than stored. The area under the curve (AUC) of the maternal plasma drug concentration-time plot reflects the milk concentration; therefore, the concentration of drug in milk will be a relative reflection of the AUC of the maternal plasma drug concentration-time plot over time from the previous feeding. If the nursing mother waits for one half-life of the drug to elapse before nursing, the amount of drug in breast milk decreases by about 50%.

The major decision to be considered is whether medication is necessary in mothers who must or desire to nurse their infants rather than whether the medicated mother should nurse. Drugs should not be prescribed for the nursing mother to relieve trivial symptoms.

ADVERSE DRUG INTERACTIONS

Drug-drug interaction refers specifically to interactions between prescription or nonprescription drugs; the broader term, drug interactions, often is substituted. Drugs also may interact with food or environmental chemicals. Their influence on the response to drugs is discussed elsewhere; see index entry Drug Response Variation.

Many drug interactions cause undesirable effects and account for about 7% of adverse reactions (Edlavitch, 1988). They also can limit bioavailability or block desired effects. However, some drug interactions are clinically valuable (Dipalma, 1986). For example, probenecid prolongs the activity and thereby increases the effectiveness of penicillin, diuretics enhance the action of other antihypertensive drugs, and certain drugs are used as antidotes to overdosage of other agents (eg, chelating agents for metals, leucovorin for methotrexate, protamine for heparin).

Some authorities limit the scope of drug interactions that result in increased pharmacologic or toxicologic effect to those in which synergism of one drug's effect by another occurs and exclude interactions in which the final effect is related to summation (additive effect) of a similar action possessed by both drugs (McInnes and Brodie, 1988). Since both synergistic and additive drug interactions can be serious or life-threatening, the broader definition is preferred for examples used throughout this publication. Additive central nervous system depression, anticholinergic activity, nephrotoxicity, ototoxicity, hypotension, gastric irritation, and neuromuscular depression are well-documented examples. Less common but often more serious reactions result from potentiation of toxicity. Usually these reactions have a pharmacokinetic basis (eg, one drug interferes with biotransformation and/or excretion of a second drug), especially when liver or kidney function is already compromised by age or disease.

Throughout this publication, specific information on clinically relevant drug interactions is included in the introductions to the chapters and in the drug evaluations, and specific adverse drug interactions are indexed.

Mechanisms

Drug interactions are chemically based (ie, one drug is physically or chemically incompatible with another drug), pharmacokinetically based (ie, one drug affects the absorption, distribution, biotransformation, or excretion of a second drug), physiologically based (ie, one drug alters the overt activity of a second drug at a separate site of action), or pharmacodynamically based (ie, one drug alters the activity of a second drug at or near the receptor site). Most drug interactions are classified according to the mechanism of the interaction (Gibaldi 1991 A, 1991 B, 1992 A, 1992 B).

Drug interactions can cause therapeutic failure by pharmacokinetic (eg, decreasing bioavailability, inducing biotransformation enzymes, increasing clearance) or pharmacodynamic (eg, antagonizing the desired effect) mechanisms.

INACTIVATION. This includes the direct physical or chemical inactivation of drugs: the degradation of sodium nitroprusside by light, the adsorption of insulin onto glass, the binding of nitroglycerin by intravenous tubing, and the neutralization or precipitation of drugs that are mixed in the same intravenous container (eg, tobramycin and carbenicillin). Inactivation or incompatibility reduces bioavailability by decreasing the amount of available drug. Most hospital pharmacies have reference sources, such as the *Handbook on Injectable Drugs* (Trissel, 1992), on the inactivation of parenteral drugs.

ABSORPTION. A drug may affect the rate and/or extent of absorption (ie, bioavailability) of another drug through physical or chemical binding in the gastrointestinal tract, slowing or accelerating gastrointestinal motility, elevating gastric pH, or altering bacterial flora. Generally, interactions due to drug binding decrease bioavailability. For example, cholestyramine resin adsorbs a number of drugs, including digoxin and thyroid hormone, thus decreasing their bioavailability. This type of interaction can be minimized by separating the time of administration by at least four hours. Drug binding in the gastrointestinal tract also can be used for therapeutic purposes. Activated charcoal is commonly administered to counteract an acute drug overdose by binding the toxic agent in the gastrointestinal tract, thereby decreasing the amount of toxin absorbed. This type of drug interaction has been termed "gastrointestinal dialysis" (Levy, 1982).

Drugs that alter gastrointestinal motility modify the bioavailability of agents that are absorbed poorly, slowly, or by saturable carrier proteins. Fortunately, this type of interaction rarely is clinically relevant.

Drugs also can modify the bioavailability of other drugs by elevating gastric pH or altering the bacterial flora. Elevating the gastric pH by administering sodium bicarbonate decreases the absorption of some forms of tetracycline and clorazepate. Oral neomycin changes the bacterial flora and, in most patients, decreases the rate and extent of absorption of concomitantly administered digoxin. However, in a small segment of the population (less than 10%), the natural bacterial flora extensively degrade digoxin to inactive metabolites. By changing the bacterial flora, neomycin increases the bioavailability of digoxin in these individuals. Iron and zinc bind to ciprofloxacin and reduce its bioavailability.

DISTRIBUTION. The concentration of free drug in the plasma is that fraction that is most readily available for distribution to the drug's site of action. The plasma concentration of free drug, rather than the total plasma concentration, correlates best with the clinical response; however, the total drug plasma concentration correlates reasonably well with the clinical response for most drugs. Drugs that are bound to plasma proteins may be displaced by chemicals or other drugs, but clinically relevant interactions are unlikely unless the original drug is at least 98% bound. With this high degree of binding, small changes in the bound fraction can temporarily double or triple the free drug concentration and increase pharmacologic activity until re-equilibration occurs. The rate and extent of compensation depend on biotransformation and/or excretion of the drug. For example, equilibration occurs quickly if excess free drug is eliminated rapidly or distributed widely (ie, has a large volume of distribution). Most protein-binding displacement interactions are not very serious clinically, unless the displaced drug is not widely distributed, has a low systemic clearance, or the primary route of elimination (ie, hepatic metabolism, renal excretion) is impaired or inhibited.

A serious interaction may occur even when a less highly bound drug (eg, at least 85% bound) that is not widely distributed and that requires biotransformation for inactivation is displaced by a drug that also impairs hepatic or renal function. For example, phenylbutazone not only displaces warfarin but also inhibits its hepatic metabolism; therefore, severe bleeding may result from impaired elimination of the increased concentration of free warfarin.

For further information, see index entry Pharmacokinetics, Therapeutic Drug Monitoring.

BIOTRANSFORMATION. Biotransformation of drugs is usually a process of detoxification, but toxicity may occur when the metabolite is more toxic than the parent molecule (MacLeod, 1990, 1991, 1992; Gibaldi, 1992 C, 1992 D). For example, the quinone formed by oxidation of acetaminophen is hepatotoxic, especially when the amount of glutathione available is limited.

Biotransformation of drugs (most of which are fat soluble) frequently involves two phases. In the first phase, the metabolic process is oxidation; resulting metabolites often are more soluble (polar) and excreted more readily than the parent drug. Some metabolites are further transformed by processes that occur during the second phase, which consists largely of conjugation reactions (eg, glucuronidation, acetylation, sulfation) that further enhance water solubility and promote excretion. Most oxidations in the first phase are performed by a family of isoenzymes known as P450 cytochrome enzymes or hepatic microsomal mixed-function oxidases (Murray, 1992). The type and degree of biotransformation of any given drug vary among individuals, primarily because of genetic and environmental differences that affect the availability and activity of metabolizing enzymes, particularly the first-phase type (Horai and Ishizaki, 1988) (see index entry Drug Response Variation, Influence of Pharmacogenetics).

Chronic exposure to many environmental chemicals and drugs increases the synthesis or activity of drug metabolizing enzymes, ie, *enzyme induction* (Gibaldi, 1991 A, 1992 A). Because enzyme activity is in part determined genetically, the degree of enzyme induction may vary considerably. Many drugs are not given for sufficient periods in large enough doses to produce clinically significant enzyme induction. Nevertheless, those that are potent enzyme inducers (ie, barbiturates, especially phenobarbital; phenytoin; rifampin) markedly alter the response to a second drug that is metabolized by the liver, especially when they are used for prolonged periods. Carbamazepine, alcohol, glutethimide, phenylbutazone, nicotine, and some constituents of the diet also induce enzymes.

Drug metabolizing processes (ie, oxidation, reduction, hydrolysis, conjugation) also are susceptible to *enzyme inhibition* (Gibaldi, 1991 B, 1992 B). Some drugs act by inhibiting enzymes that detoxify drugs. The therapeutic use of disulfiram is based on its ability to block the oxidation of acetaldehyde. Allopurinol blocks the metabolism of purines to uric acid by xanthine oxidase and increases serum concentrations of mercaptopurine by the same mechanism.

Erythromycin, quinidine, ketoconazole, chloramphenicol, dicumarol, disulfiram, cimetidine, phenylbutazone, and propoxyphene may cause serious adverse drug interactions clinically by inhibiting one or more hepatic microsomal mixed-function oxidases, especially if metabolism of the second drug is dependent on one isoform or exhibits zero-order (dose-dependent) or nonlinear biotransformation kinetics (eg, alcohol, phenytoin, aspirin, dicumarol, theophylline). The monoamine oxidase inhibitors do not affect the hepatic mixed-function oxidases but do inhibit the monoamine oxidase enzymes that terminate the action of some sympathomimetic amines, thus enhancing the magnitude of their effects (Blackwell, 1991).

Mild or moderate liver dysfunction generally does not affect drug biotransformation; thus, a clinically significant effect occurs only in individuals with severe liver impairment (as determined by routine laboratory tests). Other determinants of hepatic function (age, genetic profile, nutritional status, disease, hepatic blood flow) may predispose to interactions when one drug is a hepatotoxin and the second drug is biotransformed in the liver. Unfortunately, there are few correlations between any of the routine laboratory liver function tests and changes in the rate of hepatic drug biotransformation. The best correlation is that between prothrombin time and drug metabolism. As prothrombin time increases (ie, a sign of decreased hepatic synthesis), drug metabolism decreases. However, monitoring of the patient, determination of plasma drug concentrations (if indicated), and individualization of dosage are also necessary to avoid such interactions.

EXCRETION. Drug-induced alterations in renal blood flow, glomerular filtration, tubular reabsorption, or tubular secretion can result in drug interaction. Tubular reabsorption can be especially sensitive to tubular fluid pH, and both reabsorption and secretion are affected by competing normal metabolites (eg, uric acid) or exogenous chemicals. Tubular secretory mechanisms are either anionic or cationic; the cationic transport system has greater specificity. Many anionic metabolites or drugs (eg, uric acid, salicylates, sulfonamides, sulfates, glycine and glucuronide conjugates, penicillin, probenecid, thiazides) are eliminated by the same transport system and thus can competitively block each other's excretion.

PHARMACODYNAMIC RECEPTOR ACTION. Certain drug responses are mediated by the activation of specific receptors. When two drugs are given concurrently, activation of one drug's receptor may enhance or decrease the response of the second drug's receptor. This type of interaction may involve the same or different receptors and is categorized as pharmacodynamic rather than pharmacokinetic.

There are many examples of pharmacodynamic drug interactions. Additive pharmacologic or toxicologic effects are generally considered to be more common than antagonistic effects. However, a less than anticipated therapeutic response resulting from drug interaction-induced antagonism is often subtle and difficult to detect; therefore, many antagonistic drug interactions are missed. The anticholinergic effects of tricyclic antidepressants, quinidine, antihistamines, and certain phenothiazines operate through the same muscarinic cholinergic receptor, while the potentiation of central nervous system depression with combined administration of an opioid and a benzodiazepine or barbiturate operates through different receptors. Naloxone's ability to antagonize opioid-induced respiratory depression is a beneficial drug interaction in which the same receptor is affected by the antagonist and agonist.

AVOIDING ADVERSE DRUG EVENTS

Almost all drugs cause reasonably predictable toxic reactions when given in excessive doses; however, some drugs must be given in doses that approach or reach the toxic range for some patients. When more than one drug must be administered and an interaction is likely, appropriate observation is needed to detect the onset of toxicity, to reverse it, and to avoid its progression to intolerable proportions. Drugs often have not been tested in seriously ill patients, the elderly, pregnant women, and infants before marketing. When prescribing newly marketed drugs, particular attention must be given to dosage and adverse effects.

The most important information that a physician can have about ADRs is knowing which reactions to anticipate with each drug prescribed. When a drug is known to cause severe organ damage, relevant baseline studies and periodic surveillance for specific toxic endpoints are recommended. Serious toxicity often can be avoided by teaching patients to be alert for its early signs. In this publication, the usual custom has been to warn of reactions but not to attempt detailed advice on monitoring them. Suggestions for periodic evaluation of symptoms, signs, and laboratory tests are ordinarily reserved for situations in which these are of definite value. More commonly, reliance is placed on the physician's judgment to determine the details of monitoring. Even when laboratory tests are recommended, it seldom has been practical to specify frequency, because it is impossible to devise a precise routine that is ideal for all patients.

When toxic reactions occur gradually or their overt manifestations appear slowly, abnormal laboratory test results may precede the appearance of symptoms and warn of toxicity. For example, drugs that cause megaloblastic anemia with prolonged use, such as some anticonvulsants and folic acid antagonists, warrant the periodic performance of blood studies. On the other hand, much routine laboratory testing done in the absence of symptoms or signs is wasteful and may lead to a false sense of security, as when efforts are made to anticipate reactions that occur precipitously. For example, warning the patient to alert the physician to any significant untoward event (eg, infection) is more important in preventing agranulocytosis than prodigious numbers of hemograms. If such an event occurs, immediate laboratory evaluation is indicated, even when a recent hemogram was normal.

Drug-induced liver disease of an allergic or hypersensitivity type presents the greatest problem in early detection. Some drugs produce liver damage (without apparent relation to dosage) in hypersensitive patients, and serious hypersensitivity reactions tend to develop precipitously. A number of cofactors increase the likelihood or severity of drug-induced liver damage, including continued use of the causative drug after the development of hepatitis and administration to elderly patients. Unfortunately, there is little evidence that such reactions can be diagnosed routinely by performing frequent liver function tests before symptoms develop. Minor abnormalities in these tests are often difficult to assess in terms of cause or importance, and striking ones seldom precede symptoms by a significant length of time. The most important precaution is to observe the patient for malaise, abdominal discomfort, anorexia, dark urine, and jaundice and to perform appropriate laboratory studies if any of these reactions occur. Cholestatic reactions are typically less dangerous than the hepatocellular type, but both must be regarded as potentially serious.

Occasionally, drug-induced nephrotoxicity occurs with dramatic suddenness. Usually, however, kidney damage develops subtly well before symptoms appear. When a nephrotoxic drug is given for prolonged periods, routine urinalyses and measurements of serum creatinine may be useful.

The following suggestions may lessen the incidence or minimize the severity of ADRs, including those that arise from interactions. (See the sections on Adverse Drug Reactions During Pregnancy and Adverse Drug Reactions During Breast Feeding for similar recommendations for these special situations.)

Individualize drug therapy by assessing the endogenous and exogenous determinants that alter drug responsiveness. An adequate history and physical examination identify hereditary diseases and health status. Identifying important exogenous factors requires determination of occupational or environmental chemical exposures, dietary intake, and the use of alcohol, tobacco, and other drugs (prescription and nonprescription).

Refer to the literature for information on potentially serious drug interactions (Dukes, 1988; Hansten, 1987; Hansten and Horn, 1992), particularly if the drug(s) intended for use has not been prescribed recently. Avoid compilations that make no attempt to establish the clinical relevance of the drug interactions listed. The clinical relevance of drug interactions requires perspective; a considerable number of reported interactions have little clinical relevance because they are based on (1) animal studies not confirmed in humans, (2) limited studies (eg, case reports) not substantiated by well-controlled studies, (3) hypothetical situations, or (4) clinically insignificant changes. Even when drug interactions are confirmed and clinically relevant, the benefit/risk ratio must be evaluated in each individual case rather than a combination avoided altogether.

Anticipate that patients requiring prolonged drug therapy (eg, those with heart disease, hypertension, diabetes, epilepsy, or psychoses) are most likely to react adversely when new therapy is initiated or terminated. Most reported ADRs occur within two weeks of initial exposure to a drug (Faich et al, 1986). ADRs occurring at termination of part or all of a therapeutic regimen are often overlooked (eg, loss of metabolic enzyme induction or enzyme inhibition, withdrawal from drug dependence). During such periods, it may be important to schedule more frequent visits, offer additional patient education, and monitor symptoms, signs, and laboratory tests.

Teach patients to identify early signs and symptoms associated with potentially serious ADRs and to contact the physician as soon as possible when these are noted. Serious toxicity often can be avoided when the patient knows what to anticipate.

Optimize drug therapy by giving the smallest number of drugs that achieves the desired effect; the risk of an ADR is proportional to the number of drugs prescribed.

Suspect drug-induced disease. It is not always possible to prevent every ADR, but early detection will minimize morbidity and mortality. A high index of suspicion is required to detect and distinguish ADRs from other clinical events. Suspicion of drug-induced disease coupled with an understanding of the major criteria for assessing drug association (eg, selective monitored dechallenge and, in selected cases, rechallenge) can sometimes resolve this question promptly (Jones, 1982).

Cited References

Atkinson HC, et al: Drugs in human milk: Clinical pharmacokinetic considerations. *Clin Pharmacokinet* 14:217-240, 1988.

Beard K: Adverse reactions as a cause of hospital admission in the aged. *Drugs Aging* 2:356-367, 1992.
Beeley L: Adverse effects of drugs in the first trimester of pregnancy. *Clin Obstet Gynaecol* 13:177-195, 1986 A.
Beeley L: Adverse effects of drugs in later pregnancy. *Clin Obstet Gynaecol* 13:197-214, 1986 B.
Bero LA, et al: Characterization of geriatric drug-related hospital readmissions. *Med Care* 29:989-1003, 1991.
Blackwell B: Monoamine oxidase inhibitor interactions with other drugs. *J Clin Psychopharmacol* 11:55-59, 1991.
Brennan TA, et al: Incidence of adverse events and negligence in hospitalized patients: Results of the Harvard Medical Practice Study I. *N Engl J Med* 324:370-376, 1991.
Briggs GG, et al: *Drugs in Pregnancy and Lactation,* ed 3. Baltimore, Williams & Wilkins, 1990.
Chrischilles EA, et al: Self-reported adverse drug reactions and related resource use: A study of community-dwelling persons 65 years of age and older. *Ann Intern Med* 117:634-640, 1992.
Classen DC, et al: Computerized surveillance of adverse drug events in hospital patients. *JAMA* 266:2847-2851, 1991.
Committee on Drugs, American Academy of Pediatrics: The transfer of drugs and other chemicals into human milk. *Pediatrics,* In press.
Dicke JM: Teratology: Principles and practice. *Med Clin North Am* 73:567-582, 1989.
Dipalma JR: Desirable drug combinations. *Am Fam Physician* 33:189-192, (June) 1986.
Doering PL: Drug use during pregnancy. *NARD J* 53-57, (Sept) 1992.
Dukes MNG (ed): *Meyler's Side Effects of Drugs,* ed 11. New York, Elsevier Science Publishers, 1988.
Dukes MNG: Economic costs of adverse drug reactions. *Pharmacoeconomics* 1:153-154, 1992.
Edlavitch SA: Adverse drug event reporting: Improving the low US reporting rates, editorial. *Arch Intern Med* 148:1499-1503, 1988.
Faich GA: Postmarketing surveillance: Lessons learned. *Drug Info J* 25:531-535, 1991.
Faich GA, et al: National adverse drug reaction surveillance: 1985. *JAMA* 257:2068-2070, 1986.
Fletcher AP: Spontaneous adverse drug reaction reporting versus event monitoring: A comparison. *J R Soc Med* 84:341-344, 1991.
Gibaldi M: Induction of drug-metabolizing enzymes. *Perspect Clin Pharm* 9:41-48, 1991 A.
Gibaldi M: Inhibition of drug metabolism and excretion. *Perspect Clin Pharm* 9:49-56, 1991 B.
Gibaldi M: Drug Interactions: Part I. *Ann Pharmacother* 26:709-713, 1992 A.
Gibaldi M: Drug Interactions: Part II. *Ann Pharmacother* 26:829-834, 1992 B.
Gibaldi M: Adverse drug effect—Reactive metabolites and idiosyncratic drug reactions: Part I. *Ann Pharmacother* 26:416-421, 1992 C.
Gibaldi M: Adverse drug effects: Part II. *Ann Pharmacother* 26:550-554, 1992 D.
Golbus MS: Teratology for obstetrician: Current status. *Obstet Gynecol* 55:269-277, 1980.
Goldberg JD, Golbus MS: Value of case reports in human teratology. *Am J Obstet Gynecol* 154:479-482, 1986.
Griffin MR, et al: Nonsteroidal anti-inflammatory drug use and increased risk for peptic ulcer disease in elderly persons. *Ann Intern Med* 114:257-263, 1991.
Gurwitz JH, Avorn J: The ambiguous relation between aging and adverse drug reactions. *Ann Intern Med* 114:956-966, 1991.
Hansten PD: *Drug Interactions: Decision Support Tables.* Spokane, Wash, Applied Therapeutics, 1987.
Hansten PD, Horn JR: *Drug Interactions & Updates.* Malvern, Penn, Lea & Febiger, 1992.
Hartwig SC, et al: Preventability and severity assessment in reporting adverse drug reactions. *Am J Hosp Pharm* 49:2229-2232, 1992.
Hartzema AG, et al (eds): *Pharmacoepidemiology: An Introduction,* ed 2. Cincinnati, Harvey Whitney Books, 1991.
Hays DP: Teratogenesis: Review of basic principles with discussion of selected agents, parts I and II. *Drug Intell Clin Pharm* 15:444-450, 542-561, 1981.
Higbee MD: Geriatric drug therapy: An overview. *Clin Trends Pharm Pract* 6:17-26, 1992.
Horai Y, Ishizaki T: Pharmacogenetics and its clinical implications: Part II. Oxidation polymorphism. *Ration Drug Ther* 22:1-8, (June) 1988.
Iams JD, Rayburn WF: Drug effects on fetus, in Rayburn WF, Zuspan FP (eds): *Drug Therapy in Obstetrics and Gynecology.* Norwalk, Conn, Appleton-Century-Crofts, 1982, 9-17.
Jones JK: Adverse drug reactions in community health setting: Approaches to recognizing, counseling, and reporting. *Fam Commun Health* 5:58-67, 1982.
Kampmann JP, et al: Propylthiouracil in human milk: Revision of dogma. *Lancet* 1:736-738, 1980.
Kennedy DL, et al: Monitoring of adverse drug events in hospitals. *JAMA* 266:28-78, 1991.
Kessler DA: Introducing MEDWatch: A new approach to reporting medication and device adverse effects and product problems. *JAMA* 269:2765-2768, 1993 A.
Kessler DA: Med *Watch*: The new FDA medical products reporting program. *Am J Hosp Pharm* 50:1151-1152, 1993 B.
Leape LL, et al: Adverse events and negligence in hospitalized patients. *Iatrogenics* 1:17-21, 1991 A.
Leape LL, et al: The nature of adverse events in hospitalized patients: Results of the Harvard Medical Practice Study II. *N Engl J Med* 324:377-384, 1991 B.
Levy G: Gastrointestinal clearance of drugs with activated charcoal, editorial. *N Engl J Med* 307:676-678, 1982.
Lewis JH, et al: Use of gastrointestinal drugs during pregnancy and lactation. *Am J Gastroenterol* 80:912-923, 1985.
MacLeod CM: Clinical implications of drug metabolism: Part I: Active drugs with active metabolites. *Resident Staff Physician* 36:53-58, (Dec) 1990.
MacLeod CM: Clinical implications of drug metabolism: Part II: Active drugs with active metabolites. *Resident Staff Physician* 37:53-58, (Jan) 1991.
MacLeod CM: Clinical implications of drug metabolism: Toxic metabolites. *Resident Staff Physician* 38:77-84, (April) 1992.
McInnes GT, Brodie MJ: Drug interactions that matter: Critical reappraisal. *Drugs* 36:83-110, 1988.
Miller RK: Drugs during pregnancy: Therapeutic dilemma. *Ration Drug Ther* 15:1-9, (July) 1981.
Mucklow JC: Fate of drugs in pregnancy. *Clin Obstet Gynaecol* 13:161-175, 1986.
Murray M: P450 enzymes: Inhibition mechanisms, genetic regulation and effects of liver disease. *Clin Pharmacokinet* 23:132-146, 1992.
Niebyl JR: *Drug Use in Pregnancy*, ed 2. Philadelphia, Lea & Febiger, 1988.
Park BK, et al: Idiosyncratic drug reactions: A mechanistic evaluation of risk factors. *Br J Clin Pharmacol* 34:377-395, 1992.
Rawlins MD, et al: National adverse drug reaction reporting: A silver jubilee. *Adverse Drug React Bull* 138:516-519, 1989.
Ray WA, et al: Adverse drug reactions and the elderly. *Health Affairs* 114-122, (Fall) 1990.
Rayburn WF, Zuspan FP: *Drug Therapy in Obstetrics and Gynecology.* Norwalk, Conn, Appleton-Century-Crofts, 1982.
Rosa F: Epidemiology of drugs in pregnancy, in Yaffe SJ, Aranda JV (eds): *Pediatric Pharmacology.* Philadelphia, WB Saunders, 1992, 97-106.
Rosa F, et al: Neonatal anuria with maternal angiotensin-converting enzyme inhibition. *Obstet Gynecol* 74:371-373, 1989.
Scott HD, et al: Physician reporting of adverse drug reactions: Result of the Rhode Island Adverse Drug Reaction Reporting Project. *JAMA* 263:1785-1788, 1990.
Shepard TH: Human teratogenicity. *Adv Pediatr* 33:225-268, 1986.
Sim MR, McNeil JJ: Monitoring chemical exposure using breast milk: A methodological review. *Am J Epidemiol* 136:1-11, 1992.
Strom B (ed): *Pharmacoepidemiology.* New York, Churchill Livingstone, 1990.

Strom BL, Tugwell P: Pharmacoepidemiology: Current status, prospects, and problems. *Ann Intern Med* 113:179-181, 1990.

Tatro DS: Adverse drug reactions: Surveillance and reporting. *Facts Comparisons Drug News Lett* 10:1-3, 1991.

Trissel LA: *Handbook on Injectable Drugs,* ed 7. Bethesda, Md, American Society of Hospital Pharmacists, 1992.

Venning GR: Identification of adverse reactions to new drugs, I-IV. *BMJ* 286:199-202; 289-292; 365-368; 458-460; 544-547, 1983.

Waller PC: Measuring the frequency of adverse drug reactions. *Br J Clin Pharmacol* 33:249-252, 1992.

Welch RM, Findlay JWA: Excretion of drugs in human breast milk. *Drug Metab Rev* 12:261-277, 1981.

Wood SM, Beeley L (eds): Prescribing in pregnancy. *Clin Obstet Gynaecol* 8:248-528, 1981.

Drugs Used in the Management of Poisoning

4

PRINCIPLES OF THERAPY

AGENTS AND PROCEDURES USED TO TERMINATE EXPOSURE TO POISONS

Topical Exposure

Ingestion

DRUG EVALUATIONS

Agents for General Management

Activated Charcoal

Agents Affecting Urinary Excretion

Agents for Specific Therapy

Metal Antagonists

Miscellaneous Specific Antidotes

Naloxone Hydrochloride (Opioid Overdose)

Naltrexone Hydrochloride (Opioid Abuse)

Cyanide Antidote

Physostigmine Salicylate (Anticholinergic Toxicity)

Pralidoxime Chloride (Organophosphate Poisoning)

Ethanol (Methanol and Ethylene Glycol Poisoning)

PRINCIPLES OF THERAPY

There are four basic elements in the treatment of poisoning: supportive care, assessment, termination of exposure, and specific therapy. Estimates of the dose, the time elapsed since exposure, and the physical status of the patient determine whether supportive care (particularly hydration), induced vomiting, gastric lavage, or specific therapy is required and the priority of the steps in management. Care must be exercised when assessing the hazard, since the experience of poison control centers and emergency rooms has shown that approximately 50% of all histories taken in this situation are incorrect regarding substance, quantity, and even actual exposure. Factors that may affect the patient's response to the poison (ie, age, presence of hereditary and other diseases, current drug therapy, allergy to drugs) also should be considered.

Supportive Care: Hypoventilation can be avoided by ensuring an adequate airway with suction, humidified oxygen, insertion of an airway, and mechanical ventilation as required. Antiepileptic drugs may be necessary if seizures are prolonged or recurrent or interfere with ventilation; intravenous diazepam [Valium] 5 to 10 mg or lorazepam [Ativan] 4 to 8 mg usually is effective. A reliable venous access with a venous catheter should be established in comatose patients. Volume depletion secondary to vomiting, diarrhea, and sweating must be corrected promptly with normal saline or Ringer's solution, particularly in young children. Hypotension severe enough to require correction, whether due to volume depletion or peripheral pooling, frequently necessitates monitoring of central venous or pulmonary wedge pressure to determine fluid needs.

Any adult in coma of unknown etiology should receive at least 50 ml (25 g) of dextrose 50% intravenously immediately, without waiting for the blood glucose determination, to prevent brain damage if the coma is due to hypoglycemia. If alcoholism or malnutrition is suspected, thiamine 100 mg should be injected simultaneously to avoid precipitating acute Wernicke's encephalopathy. Naloxone [Narcan] is given empirically (2 mg as an intravenous bolus repeated at five-minute intervals up to a total of 10 mg). Flumazenil [Mazicon], a benzodiazepine receptor antagonist, may be given empirically to reverse benzodiazepine-induced obtundation. (See index entry Flumazenil.) For children in coma of unknown etiology, dextrose 20% to 25% (0.5 g/kg) is administered over a five- to ten-minute period (dextrose 50% is too irritating to children's small veins).

Individual Assessment: An immediate evaluation of the putative intoxication must be made to determine if the exposure (1) is life-threatening and compromises vital functions, (2) poses a potential hazard, or (3) is harmless or essentially so. A poison control center, particularly a regional center, can provide information and advice. This is useful because early identification of the ingredients and their potential toxicity can facilitate early intervention and lessen the chance of complications.

Ingestion of a toxic substance is not the same as ingestion of a toxic dose. It is important to remember that hazard is associated not only with the potency of a poison, but also with the quantity ingested, the extent of exposure, and the presence of other ingredients, including solvents. See the references for information on the general management of poisoning.

Blood and urine samples to determine a baseline for monitoring elimination of the toxin and glucose, electrolyte, and acid-base status may aid in assessing therapy. Identification of the suspected toxin in the blood, urine, and/or gastric contents may be necessary to verify an exposure for which a specific intervention is required. Quantitative determinations should be requested only if the therapy may be altered by the result. This is needed for relatively few substances (eg, acetaminophen, salicylate, iron, lead, methanol, ethylene glycol, theophylline, lithium); for some of these, two plasma samples obtained one or more hours apart, depending on half-life, may be required to determine if the concentration of the toxic substance is rising or falling before deciding whether specific therapy is needed or can be discontinued. Quantitative determinations also are useful for carboxyhemoglobin and methemoglobin.

Termination of Exposure: Eliminating the poison from the gut, skin, or eyes before extensive absorption or damage can occur usually avoids the necessity for further therapeutic intervention. The elimination of some drugs may be increased by altering the pH of the urine (ion trapping). The excretion of basic drugs (eg, amphetamine, phencyclidine) is promoted by acidifying the urine and that of acidic drugs (eg, aspirin, phenobarbital) by making the urine more alkaline. Diuretics generally do not increase clearance significantly.

Dialysis and charcoal hemoperfusion may be useful for elimination of some drugs. Apparent volume of distribution, rate of intercompartmental transfer, and protein binding determine the degree to which a drug can be removed by dialysis (eg, methanol, ethylene glycol). Otherwise, these procedures usually are reserved for patients whose renal function has been affected by the intoxication.

Specific Drug Therapy: It is estimated that specific drug therapy is required in no more than 2% of poisonings. Some of these (eg, glucagon for beta-adrenergic blocking agents, acetylcysteine for acetaminophen, digoxin-immune Fab fragments [Digibind]) are discussed in other chapters; see index entries.

AGENTS AND PROCEDURES USED TO TERMINATE EXPOSURE TO POISONS

Topical Exposure

Initially, contaminated clothing should be removed and all routes of exposure should be determined. When the eyes are involved, the lids should be retracted and the eyes flushed immediately with lukewarm tap water poured from a container to avoid mechanical injury from a high-force stream. When instructions are given by telephone, adequate compliance may be achieved by specifying that flushing of the eyes be maintained for at least 15 minutes "by the clock." When the skin is affected, water and, if the poison and/or solvent is lipid soluble, soap may aid in removal. The hair should be shampooed if it is contaminated (eg, pesticide spray) and the nails should be cleaned.

Ingestion

Detoxification can be accomplished by induced emesis, gastric lavage, adsorption of the toxin on activated charcoal, administration of cathartic drugs, whole bowel irrigation, or removal by gastroscopy or surgery.

Induced emesis and lavage generally are of little benefit if not instituted within the first hour following toxic ingestion; exceptions are drugs that delay stomach emptying (salicylates, drugs with anticholinergic activity such as tricyclic antidepressants), drugs with poor solubility or slow dissolution time, or after limited mastication of plants. In these instances, the administration of activated charcoal without gastric emptying may be preferred, at least in adults (Kulig et al, 1985; Park et al, 1986; Rodgers and Matyunas, 1986; Albertson et al, 1989). In children, the choice between charcoal alone or after induced emesis or lavage has not been established. There is a perception that syrup of ipecac, particularly for children in the home, is preferable because compliance is obtained more readily (Lovejoy, 1987; Banner and Veltri, 1988).

Activated Charcoal: This adsorbent should be given as soon after ingestion of the poisonous substance as possible or after emesis has ceased if syrup of ipecac has been given, although effectiveness has been demonstrated even after several hours, particularly in cases involving drugs that delay gastric emptying or intestinal passage. If activated charcoal is being given repetitively, it may be started at any time and continued for days.

Although the efficacy of charcoal has not been determined for many drugs in vivo, it is known to reduce the gastrointestinal absorption of drugs that commonly cause poisoning, such as analgesics (salicylates, acetaminophen, propoxyphene), antianxiety agents, hypnotics, and tricyclic antidepressants. Activated charcoal is less effective in poisoning caused by rapidly absorbed agents. Activated charcoal does not affect the absorption of mineral acids, alkalis, inorganic salts, aliphatic hydrocarbons, and drugs that are insoluble in aqueous acidic solution; adsorption of ferrous sulfate is low. Cyanide is partially adsorbed but then released slowly in the intestine; however, the addition of activated charcoal to lavage fluid may be useful. Administration of a smaller dose than initially employed at two- to four-hour intervals may be effective for drugs that are absorbed slowly or recycled through the enterohepatic system or by gastric secretion (Pond, 1986).

Charcoal is mildly constipating. Therefore, when multiple doses are to be administered, a cathartic (eg, magnesium citrate, sorbitol) can be added and the combination given intermittently; this does not affect charcoal's binding capacity and does decrease the risk of intestinal obstruction. However, the charcoal-cathartic combination must be used cautiously, *if at all,* in the very young or old because significant fluid loss may occur. Usually there appears to be little desorption of poison from charcoal during its passage through the gastrointestinal tract provided that the quantity of activated charcoal is large compared to the toxin (Neuvonen, 1982). Repeated doses of charcoal also may reduce the desorption of the toxin (Neuvonen and Olkkola, 1988). Charcoal, particularly multiple doses, should be used with care if bowel sounds are absent.

Children do not accept charcoal readily. If charcoal with water is refused, commercial preparations containing activated charcoal in 70% sorbitol can be given as a single dose in children weighing more than 16 kg. (See the evaluation for available preparations.) This suspension has less gritty oral residue and its sweetness is attractive to children. The combination also has the advantage of inducing an exceptionally rapid intestinal transit time: In fasted subjects, the mean transit time of activated charcoal is about 25 hours; transit time is reduced to 1.1 hours with activated charcoal in sorbitol (Krenzelok and Hall, 1985). However, transit time is not reduced by the charcoal and sorbitol combination following intoxication by drugs usually associated with marked prolongation of transit (eg, opioids, tricyclic antidepressants) (Harchelroad et al, 1989). Sorbitol limits the quantity of charcoal that can be administered, causes liquid stools (Mayersohn et al, 1977), may evoke spontaneous emesis, and may induce serious dehydration and volume depletion, especially in children.

Induced Emesis and Lavage: Induced emesis is more convenient than lavage in alert patients with an active gag reflex and also may partially empty the upper small intestine.

Ipecac syrup is the emetic of choice (Easom and Lovejoy, 1979). The quantity of gastric contents removed by vomiting varies considerably, so activated charcoal is indicated after vomiting has ceased. Effectiveness may be increased by the concomitant ingestion of water, but the amount should be limited to 300 ml in adults and 10 ml/kg in children to avoid pyloric emptying.

Other procedures for inducing emesis are *not* recommended. Mechanically induced gagging is ineffective and hazardous. Hypertonic sodium chloride solutions should never be used to induce vomiting or as an irrigant for lavage since fatal hypernatremia may develop. Apomorphine offers no advantage over syrup of ipecac, is less convenient to prepare for use, and may depress the central nervous system.

If vomiting cannot be induced by emetics, gastric lavage with a large bore orogastric tube (adults, 36 to 42 French; children, 26 to 28 French) should be started, preferably within two hours after ingestion (see Contraindications). Lavage sometimes may be effective more than two hours after ingestion, depending on the rate of disintegration and dissolution of the formulation ingested, the formation of bezoars, and whether gastrointestinal transit time is prolonged by the poison.

To minimize the chances of aspiration and to maximize the amount of gastric emptying, the patient should be placed on his left side in the Trendelenburg position with the face near the edge of the table. In comatose patients, a cuffed endotracheal tube should be inserted before gastric intubation to reduce the risk of pulmonary aspiration. Stomach contents should be removed by suction before instilling the lavage solution. Tap water may be used as the lavage irrigant but 0.9% or 0.45% sodium chloride solution is preferred in young children, because even a 5% increase in body fluid volume of electrolyte-free water may cause dilutional hyponatremia. Lavage fluid should be at room temperature because cooled fluid may produce hypothermia. Warmed lavage fluid (not exceeding 46°C) is useful for more rapid dissolution of tablets and capsules (McDougal and Maclean, 1981). Lavage with small amounts of fluid (about 300 ml in adults and 10 ml/kg in small children) should be repeated until at least 2 liters of fluid in children and 5 liters in adults have been employed and returns are clear. The lavage tube should be repositioned frequently. Thereafter, activated charcoal should be instilled through the lavage tube and allowed to remain in the stomach. Activated charcoal also may be instilled prior to lavage and given again after lavage is complete.

Contraindications. Emetics are contraindicated in the presence of convulsions, shock, coma or imminent coma, altered sensorium, or inadequate gag reflex. They should not be used after ingestion of strongly caustic substances, such as strong alkalis (lye) or acids, since additional injury (eg, perforated esophagus with mediastinitis) may occur. Alkali ingestions should be diluted with water or milk, and the patient should be examined for esophageal ulceration.

Emesis and gastric lavage generally are not indicated after the ingestion of petroleum distillates, since most are not systemically toxic. These procedures are contraindicated after the ingestion of low-viscosity aliphatic hydrocarbons (eg, mineral seal or signal oils present in furniture polish and other oil-containing polishes) because of the risk of aspiration pneumonia. A gastric emptying procedure is indicated for those few agents that are systemically toxic (halogenated hydrocarbons) or in the presence of a toxic solute (eg, a pesticide).

Lavage with boluses of 300 ml of fluid initially, especially on a full stomach, may force material through the pylorus where it cannot be recovered. Aspiration of vomitus into the bronchial tree is a potential hazard of both gastric lavage and drug-induced vomiting; however, in conscious patients, the hazard is less with use of emetics.

Whole Bowel Irrigation: This promising detoxification technique is similar to the procedure used to prepare a patient for colonoscopy or large bowel surgery. It is recommended for patients presenting late after ingestion, following ingestion of prolonged-release or enteric-coated preparations, or for the removal of toxins not absorbed by activated charcoal (Tenenbein, 1988), and it has been employed safely for the treatment of oral overdose during pregnancy (Van Ameyde and Tenenbein, 1989). Polyethylene glycol electrolyte lavage solution (Co-Lyte, Go-LYTELY) is employed to avoid alteration of fluid or electrolyte balance. The irrigation fluid is introduced by gravity through a nasogastric tube at a rate of 2 L/hr in adults and 500 ml/hr in preschool age children. The infusion is discontinued when the effluent has the same appearance as the infusate or when 5 to 10 L has been given to adults or 2 to 3 L to children; this usually takes four to six hours. Bowel perforation, obstruction, ileus, and hemorrhage are contraindications. Active vomiting may interfere with irrigation, and pretreatment with syrup of ipecac should be avoided. The instillation of activated charcoal prior to irrigation is acceptable.

Gastroscopy or Surgery: Gastroscopy or surgical decontamination has been required in a few cases of ferrous sulfate poisoning in children in whom there was radiologic evidence of adherence of the tablets to the gastric or intestinal mucosa and in some cases of ingestion of cocaine-filled packets.

Hemodialysis, Hemoperfusion, and Plasmapheresis: For those toxins that are cleared effectively by one of these methods, the following are indications for their application:

the patient's condition is deteriorating despite maximal supportive care; the usual route of elimination is impaired (eg, renal failure); the patient has been exposed to a known lethal dose or has a lethal blood concentration of the toxin; or the patient has underlying medical problems that could increase the hazard of prolonged coma or other manifestations of the intoxication (Pond, 1984).

Dialysis or hemoperfusion is indicated only if it adds significantly to other modes of elimination (Pond, 1984; Cutler et al, 1987). For most drugs, hemodialysis is more effective than peritoneal dialysis. Dialysis is useful for drugs that have a molecular weight below 500, are water soluble, are not bound extensively to protein or tissue, and have a low volume of distribution (less than 1 L/kg). Hemoperfusion differs from hemodialysis in that the blood is passed through a column containing an adsorbent. A drug's molecular weight, water solubility, and protein binding are less severe limiting factors than with hemodialysis. Systemic anticoagulation is required. Drugs and toxins for which hemodialysis may be considered are the alcohols (methanol, ethanol, isopropanol, ethylene glycol), salicylates, and lithium. Hemoperfusion is preferred for theophylline and phenobarbital and for massive doses of the herbicide, paraquat.

Plasmapheresis should be considered an unproven and potentially hazardous procedure for detoxification (Jones and Dougherty, 1986). It is reserved for toxins that are highly protein bound and are not removed effectively by hemodialysis or hemoperfusion. Single case reports on its use for phenytoin and propranolol toxicity have appeared.

Drug Evaluations

AGENTS FOR GENERAL MANAGEMENT

ACTIVATED CHARCOAL

Charcoals from different sources vary in adsorption capacity. The most effective are those of small particle size (large total surface area) and low mineral content. Petroleum-based charcoals with a high surface area, eg, charcoal PX-21 (AX-21) [Actidose], have about three times the adsorptive capacity of standard activated charcoal while retaining a similar adsorption rate (Cooney and Kane, 1980; Cooney, 1980). See the Introduction for specific uses.

DOSAGE AND PREPARATIONS. Commercial aqueous preparations of activated charcoal may require mixing with additional water to improve fluidity for administration. When giving repeated doses of charcoal, preparations containing cathartics (particularly sorbitol) should be used only intermittently. Such combinations should not be used in children under 16 kg and they should be used with caution in the elderly.

Oral: *Adults*, 50 to 100 g, and *children*, 25 to 50 g (approximately 1 g/kg), administered with water orally or through the lavage tube after gastric lavage. Charcoal is not toxic and, therefore, there is no maximum dose limit. Doses 50% or less of those given initially can be repeated at two- to four-hour intervals for poisons that undergo enterohepatic circulation (eg, digitoxin, theophylline, *Amanita phalloides* toxin) or are resecreted into the stomach or intestine (eg, phencyclidine, phenobarbital, tricyclic antidepressants).

(All forms nonprescription)

Generic. Liquid; powder.

Available Trademarks.

Powder: ***Acta-Char*** (Med-Corp).

Powder in water: ***Acta-Char Liquid*** (Med-Corp), ***Actidose-Aqua*** (Paddock), ***Charcoaid*** (Requa), ***Insta-Char*** (Kerr), ***Liqui-Char*** (Jones Medical).

Powder in sorbitol: ***Acta-Char Liquid*** (Med-Corp).

Liquid (PX-21; AX-21) in water or sorbitol: ***Actidose with Sorbitol*** (Paddock).

SYRUP OF IPECAC

ACTIONS AND USES. Ipecac alkaloids act locally on the gastric mucosa and centrally on the chemoreceptor trigger zone to induce vomiting. Vomiting occurs within 30 minutes in about 90% of patients (average time, less than 20 minutes). Emesis may be more effective, although not more rapid, if water is taken immediately after administration of the syrup. About 10% of patients will vomit again if fluids are ingested within two hours after the initial induction of emesis. Repetitive nonproductive vomiting after this interval may be ascribed to the intoxicant rather than to ipecac.

Ipecac syrup is available without prescription in a maximum amount of 30 ml. Physicians often recommend that an ounce of the syrup be stored in the home and in the houses of grandparents and babysitters when children become 1 year old so that this emetic is readily available for immediate administration when a physician or poison control center recommends its use by telephone.

ADVERSE REACTIONS AND PRECAUTIONS. Adverse effects caused by syrup of ipecac are not significant if the recommended dose is not exceeded. In children under 3 years, drowsiness may be anticipated in about 20% and diarrhea in about 25%. Less than 4% experience coughing or choking in association with emesis.

Ipecac is classified in FDA Pregnancy Category C.

For contraindications, see the Introduction.

DOSAGE AND PREPARATIONS.

Oral: *Children over 1 year and adults,* 15 or 30 ml (the lower dose usually is adequate); *infants 9 to 11 months*, 10 ml (two teaspoonsful), but accumulating evidence shows that a dose of 15 ml probably is both safe and effective; *infants 6 to 8 months*, 5 ml (one teaspoonful). (The administration of syrup of ipecac to infants 6 to 8 months old should be conducted under medical supervision and not in the home.) In patients older than 1 year, doses may be repeated once after 30 minutes if vomiting has not occurred. If vomiting does not occur within 45 minutes after the first dose, gastric lavage may be indicated to remove the toxin.

Generic. Syrup in 15 and 30 ml containers (alcohol 1.5%, nonprescription; alcohol 2%, prescription).

Agents Affecting Urinary Excretion

AMMONIUM CHLORIDE

This acidifying salt temporarily reduces urinary pH, which increases the degree of ionization of organic bases, and impedes the renal tubular reabsorption of these bases, which enhances their urinary excretion. However, significant enhancement of urinary excretion requires that the base have a pKa close to neutral, a small volume of distribution, and be appreciably eliminated via the kidney. Only a few organic bases (eg, amphetamines) have these properties. Routine use of ammonium chloride to treat overdose of an organic base is neither safe nor advisable. Moreover, use of this agent with forced diuresis to hasten excretion of poisons is associated with considerable risk and is not generally recommended. Tolerance to ammonium chloride develops within two to three days.

ADVERSE REACTIONS AND PRECAUTIONS. Adequate doses frequently cause gastric irritation, nausea, and vomiting. Absorption also may be erratic, depending on the toxic substance ingested. Ammonium chloride is relatively contraindicated in patients with impaired hepatic or renal function, because of the risk of ammonium toxicity, and in patients with convulsions or in prolonged coma (Penn et al, 1971) to avoid complications of an acid urine if myoglobinuria is present.

DOSAGE AND PREPARATIONS.
Intravenous Infusion: This route is required only rarely in the management of intoxications. The rate of infusion in adults usually should not exceed 0.4 mEq/min. Repeated determinations of the serum bicarbonate concentration are required.

Generic. Solution 26.75% (5 mEq/ml) in 20 ml containers for dilution in 0.9% sodium chloride injection.

SODIUM BICARBONATE

ACTIONS AND USES. Sodium bicarbonate is used to treat metabolic acidosis. It also is used to alkalize the urine, which increases the degree of ionization of organic acids (eg, aspirin, phenobarbital), and interferes with renal tubular reabsorption of these acids, which enhances their excretion. However, the alkalization of the urine, particularly when combined with forced diuresis, is hazardous and should be undertaken only after careful consideration of the risk-benefit ratio.

PRECAUTIONS. Excessive bicarbonate may result in tetany and cardiac arrhythmias. Potassium depletion caused by aspirin poisoning also may be aggravated.

The maximum sodium tolerance is 250 mEq/M^2/24 hours in healthy persons (1 g of sodium bicarbonate contains 11.9 mEq of sodium). Sodium bicarbonate must be used with caution in patients with congestive heart failure or liver disease. Patients with renal insufficiency given usual doses or those with normal renal function receiving prolonged therapy may experience systemic alkalosis manifested by irritability, neuromuscular excitability, and tetany.

Parenteral sodium bicarbonate is classified in FDA Pregnancy Category C.

DOSAGE AND PREPARATIONS.
Intravenous: *Adults*, 2 to 5 mEq/kg, and *children*, 1 to 2 mEq/kg administered over a four- to eight-hour period and adjusted by monitoring. Large amounts may be required. For treatment of metabolic acidosis, the specific amount depends on the degree of acidosis. See index entry on this subject.

Generic. Solution 4.2% (0.5 mEq/ml) in 1, 5, and 10 ml containers, 5% (0.595 mEq/ml) in 500 ml containers, 7.5% (0.892 mEq/ml) and 8.4% (1 mEq/ml) in 10 and 50 ml containers.

AGENTS FOR SPECIFIC THERAPY

Metal Antagonists

Heavy metal poisoning continues to be a serious toxicologic problem. Metal ions enter the body following ingestion or inhalation, absorption through the skin, or parenteral administration of metal-containing drugs.

Heavy metal ions produce toxicity by combining with reactive groups (ligands) on physiologically important cellular components such as enzymes. Metal antagonists compete with cellular binding sites for the metal ion and incorporate the metal into a chelate or complex that can pass through the organs of excretion. The metal is usually bound into a five- or six-member heterocyclic ring structure (a chelate) or a less stable, nonheterocyclic compound (a complex). Useful heavy metal antagonists are nonionic, water soluble, form stable nontoxic chelates, do not undergo biotransformation, and are eliminated in the urine and/or feces via the bile. The stability constant of a metal antagonist-chelate indicates the affinity of the antagonist for the toxic metal or, conversely, its tendency to dissociate. If the metal antagonist-chelate has a higher stability constant than the physiologic complex or chelate in vivo, the metal will be removed from tissue binding sites. The ideal metal antagonist specifically binds the toxic metal cation, but long-term use of these agents may lead to trace element deficiencies due to binding of other metal ions by the antagonist. The type and degree of the deficiency depend on the nature of the metal antagonist.

Heavy Metal Poisoning: The primary approach to treatment of heavy metal poisoning is to terminate exposure to the toxic metal when and to whatever extent possible. A metal antagonist then can be used to enhance excretion of the previously absorbed metal. The agents administered for this purpose are edetate calcium disodium (EDTA) [Calcium Disodium Versenate] and succimer (DMSA) [Chemet] for lead; deferoxamine [Desferal] for iron and aluminum; dimercaprol [BAL in oil] for arsenic, inorganic mercury salts, or gold and, in conjunction with edetate calcium disodium, for the initial management of lead encephalopathy; and penicillamine [Cuprimine, Depen] for arsenic, copper, lead, gold, mercury, and possibly antimony. (Edetate calcium disodium should not be confused with edetate disodium [Endrate]. The latter has high affinity for calcium and is used in the treatment of severe hypercalcemia. It should not be used to treat heavy metal poisoning because it may produce severe hypocalcemia.)

It has been recognized for some time that chelation therapy can move toxic metals from storage tissue sites (eg, in bone) to more critical organs and tissues. The approach to therapy of lead encephalopathy in children is dictated by concern about too rapid mobilization during infusion of edetate calcium disodium and the resultant redistribution of lead to the brain. This concern now extends to the treatment of children with moderate and low levels of blood lead because there is relatively little information on the overall efficacy of chelation in reversing the more subtle neurologic effects of lead. Results of animal studies suggest that redistribution to critical organs such as the brain and kidney may not occur with succimer (meso-2,3-dimercapto-succinic acid), a water-soluble analogue of dimercaprol. Furthermore, this agent is administered orally and does not appear to produce any severe reactions (Fournier et al, 1988; Graziano et al, 1988). Succimer also complexes with and enhances the excretion of arsenic and mercury, but clinical experience is limited.

No specific therapy can be recommended for acute poisoning by cadmium or thallium but, of the chelating agents that have been evaluated in experimental cadmium poisoning, succimer was the most effective antagonist.

Chelation therapy is most effective when it is begun immediately after exposure to the heavy metal. Prolonged treatment will be needed if the time elapsed between ingestion of the toxic material and the initiation of therapy is sufficient to allow incorporation of the metal into metal-binding sites in tissue and bone.

Radioactive Isotope Poisoning: Because of the increasing use of radioactive isotopes in biomedical and industrial research, the possibility of accidental ingestion of a radioactive heavy metal is increasing. Poisoning with a conventional radioactive isotope, such as iron, can be treated with deferoxamine to hasten excretion. However, treatment is more difficult if a more exotic metal, such as uranium, radium, strontium, plutonium, or yttrium, is involved. Neither radium nor strontium can be removed from the body because their stability constants with various metal antagonists are about the same as those of calcium. However, their rate of excretion can be increased by infusion of calcium salts in conjunction with oral administration of ammonium chloride. The excretion of plutonium, thorium, uranium, yttrium, and some other radioactive isotopes can be increased considerably by chelation with edetate calcium disodium. Pentetic acid (trisodium zinc diethylenetriaminepentaacetate, DTPA), currently available only as an investigational drug in this country, may increase the rate of excretion of the lanthanides (cerium, lanthanum, and prometheum) and the actinides (americium, californium, curium, and plutonium) (NCRPM, 1980). It is not useful for polonium, strontium, or uranium poisoning. The daily dose is 1 g (30 micromole/kg) administered intravenously over one hour.

Miscellaneous Indications: Some metal antagonists have been tried in conditions other than heavy metal poisoning or in diseases associated with heavy metal retention (eg, penicillamine in Wilson's disease, primary biliary cirrhosis, cystinuria, rheumatoid arthritis, chronic active hepatitis; deferoxamine in hemochromatosis). Metal antagonists are ineffective in porphyria, scleroderma, angina pectoris, nephrocalcinosis, calcified mitral stenosis, otosclerosis, atherosclerosis, and sarcoidosis.

Drug Evaluations

DEFEROXAMINE MESYLATE

[Desferal]

$$\overset{+}{H_3N}(CH_2)_5\underset{\underset{OH}{|}}{N}\overset{\overset{O}{\|}}{C}(CH_2)_2\overset{\overset{O}{\|}}{C}NH(CH_2)_5\underset{\underset{OH}{|}}{N}\overset{\overset{O}{\|}}{C}(CH_2)_2\overset{\overset{O}{\|}}{C}NH(CH_2)_5\underset{\underset{OH}{|}}{N}\overset{\overset{O}{\|}}{C}CH_3 \quad CH_3SO_3^-$$

ACTIONS. Deferoxamine, a compound obtained from *Streptomyces pilosus*, is a potent and highly specific iron chelating agent. It readily complexes with ferric ion to form ferrioxamine, a stable, water-soluble chelate; it also has limited affinity for ferrous ion. In addition to combining with free ionic iron, deferoxamine can remove iron from ferritin and hemosiderin, except in bone marrow. It is much less effective against transferrin and does not remove iron from cytochromes, myoglobin, or hemoglobin. Deferoxamine 100 mg binds 8.5 mg of iron.

USES. Deferoxamine is used in severe, acute iron intoxication. Primary management should include gastric emptying and control of metabolic acidosis and shock. Patients with severe iron poisoning require serial monitoring of blood pressure, central venous pressure, and cardiac output. If primary myocardial depression is present, fluid replacement, inotropic agents, and afterload reduction should be considered (Tenenbein et al, 1988).

Deferoxamine also promotes iron excretion in secondary hemochromatosis (Weatherall et al, 1983; Mossey et al, 1988). It usually is administered intramuscularly or by slow subcutaneous infusion in patients with chronic anemia and iron overload secondary to multiple blood transfusions. A negative net accumulation of iron may be demonstrated in some patients and these patients also should receive supplemental intravenous deferoxamine during blood transfusion (the drug should be given separately from the blood). No tolerance to deferoxamine was demonstrated over a period of two years. Total dose and duration of therapy must be individualized on the basis of an initial dose-response curve. The goal is to use the minimum amount of deferoxamine that prevents net iron accumulation.

Deferoxamine is less effective in primary hemochromatosis than phlebotomy (Young et al, 1979; Halliday and Bassett, 1980). However, it is useful when venesection is contraindicated (eg, when the patient is hypoproteinemic or too anemic to tolerate blood loss).

Urinary excretion of ferrioxamine accounts for two-thirds of the iron eliminated; the remainder is excreted in bile. Ferrioxamine has a characteristic orange-red color; thus, the appearance of an orange-red urine after injection of deferoxamine is presumptive evidence of elevated serum iron levels and an indication for further therapy. However, the absence of this color *does not rule out* severe, acute iron poisoning.

DIAGNOSIS OF IRON POISONING. Most cases of excessive iron ingestion do not require deferoxamine. However, in severe poisoning, the shorter the interval between the ingestion of iron and the administration of deferoxamine, the greater the probability of recovery without sequelae. In the first phase of acute iron intoxication (30 to 120 minutes), signs and symptoms are caused principally by gastrointestinal irritation and necrosis. Although infrequent, a phase of apparent improvement may then ensue that can be misleading. Therefore, the patient must continue to be monitored closely, and deferoxamine may have to be administered to avoid or reduce the later development of acidosis, hepatic failure, oliguria, pulmonary edema, and vasomotor collapse.

Therapy with deferoxamine is determined on the basis of clinical evidence. It is inappropriate to initiate therapy solely on the basis of the serum iron concentration, but the determination provides supportive evidence. Administration of deferoxamine may confound some laboratory serum iron determinations; therefore, blood samples should be obtained prior to initiation of therapy. Samples should be obtained within four to six hours after ingestion because iron undergoes rapid redistribution into tissue. Iron in excess of total iron binding capacity is indicated by a serum iron concentration greater than 300 to 350 mcg/dL. Serum iron concentrations greater than 500 mcg/dL are generally associated with severe poisoning and immediate chelation therapy is required. A serum concentration in excess of 1,000 mcg/dL is potentially lethal.

While the serum iron concentration is being determined, an estimate of potential severity may be based on history and other findings. If diarrhea, vomiting, leukocytosis, or hyperglycemia is present and an abdominal radiograph demonstrates the presence of iron tablets, the serum iron concentration will usually exceed 300 mcg/dL and chelation therapy is indicated. If vomiting is absent or the patient remains asymptomatic for at least six hours after ingestion or if an enteric-coated preparation has not been ingested, the serum iron concentration is usually below this value (Lacouture et al, 1981).

In young children, the dose producing mild to moderate poisoning is 20 to 60 mg/kg elemental iron; serious poisoning is produced by ingestion of more than 60 mg/kg. Minimum toxic doses for adolescents and adults are not known. The ingested dose (mg/kg) equals the number of tablets ingested multiplied by the milligrams of elemental iron per tablet divided by the child's weight (kg). To calculate milligrams of elemental iron in solid preparations of iron salts, see Table 1. Compilations of the elemental iron content in liquid formulations of iron salts and in multicomponent drug products are available (Krenzelok and Hoff, 1979; Engle et al, 1987). Although uncommon, toxicity has been reported following the ingestion of children's multivitamin preparations containing iron.

TABLE 1.
ELEMENTAL IRON CONTENT OF SOLID FERROUS SALT PREPARATIONS

Component	% Elemental Iron	To Obtain Approximate mg Elemental Iron Divide mg of Iron Salt by
Ferrous sulfate (anhydrous)	36.77	2.7
Ferrous sulfate monohydrate*	32.87	3
Ferrous sulfate heptahydrate†	20.01	5
Ferrous gluconate (anhydrous)	12.52	8
Ferrous gluconate dihydrate	11.58	8.6
Ferrous fumarate	32.87	3

**Synonym: Dried ferrous sulfate*
†Synonym: Ferrous Sulfate, U.S.P.

ADVERSE REACTIONS AND PRECAUTIONS. Deferoxamine generally is well tolerated. Rapid intravenous injection can cause hypotension, tachycardia, erythema, and urticaria. Some patients experience a local histamine-like reaction or induration following subcutaneous administration for chronic iron overload (hemochromatosis); this reaction is rare when the drug is given intramuscularly. Severe, transient pain at the site of injection may occur. Adequate hydration and repeated determinations of renal function are recommended during intravenous administration (Koren et al, 1989).

Patients receiving long-term therapy to treat chronic iron storage disease have experienced mild allergic-type dermatologic reactions (wheals, pruritus), diarrhea, dysuria, abdominal discomfort, leg cramps, tachycardia, and fever. Visual and auditory neurotoxicity can be produced, particularly with larger doses (greater than 50 to 60 mg/kg) in younger patients, but usually is reversible when the dosage is reduced (Olivieri et al, 1986; Freedman et al, 1988; Bene et al, 1989; Wonke et al, 1989). Growth retardation may be induced if deferoxamine therapy is instituted before age 3 in children with transfusion-dependent thalassemia; in children over 3 years, even large doses do not appear to affect longitudinal growth (de Virgiliis et al, 1988).

There are no absolute contraindications to the use of deferoxamine in acute iron intoxication or hemochromatosis. Since the drug and the ferrioxamine complex are excreted primarily by the kidneys, deferoxamine generally is contraindicated in patients with severe renal disease, except those on dialysis. Exchange transfusion or hemodialysis may be required in patients with acute renal failure or life-threatening symptoms (especially shock) refractory to treatment or when the amount of iron is so large that maximum recommended doses of deferoxamine cannot be expected to complex with more than a fraction of the free iron available.

Chelation therapy, except that for acute iron intoxication, should be withheld, if possible, during pregnancy (FDA Pregnancy Category C).

Deferoxamine enhances the growth of *Yersinia enterocolitica*. Yersiniosis should be considered in chronically iron-overloaded patients with gastroenteric, pulmonary, or dermal problems. It is recommended that scheduled therapy with deferoxamine be withheld until treatment with trimethoprim/sulfamethoxazole or another appropriate chemotherapeutic agent has been initiated (Gallant et al, 1986; Eggleston, 1987). The incidence of septicemia is higher in dialysis patients with iron overload than in those with iron levels near the normal range. Such infections must be managed appropriately, but there is no need to defer deferoxamine therapy in these patients if yersiniosis, a relatively rare condition, is absent (Seifert et al, 1987). Opportunistic fungal infections (mucormycosis) also have been associated with prolonged deferoxamine therapy (Daly et al, 1989).

PHARMACOKINETICS. Deferoxamine has an apparent volume of distribution of about 60% of body weight. It is metabolized rapidly by tissues and plasma. The half-life following intravenous administration is about one hour.

DOSAGE AND PREPARATIONS.

Acute Iron Poisoning:

Intravenous: This route is employed *only* for *adults and children* with signs of cardiovascular shock or a serum iron level greater than 500 mcg/dL, indicating free iron in the plasma. There is no standard dose schedule. A dose of 10 to 15 mg/kg/hr may be infused until the serum iron level falls to 100 mcg/dL or less and the urine is no longer orange colored. (However, whether deferoxamine is given or not, in the absence of continuing absorption and/or an enormous overdose, serum iron will fall rapidly four to ten hours after ingestion.) Faster rates of administration or bolus injections may cause hypotension, especially if the rate of infusion exceeds 15 mg/kg/hr. In general, the total dose should not exceed 240 mg/kg/24 hr (6 g/24 hr).

Intramuscular: Deferoxamine should be prepared by adding 2 ml of sterile water for injection to each vial. A dose of 1 g is given initially, followed by 0.5 g at four-hour intervals for two doses. Subsequent doses of 0.5 g may be administered every 4 to 12 hours, as necessary. The total dose should not exceed 6 g/24 hr.

Chronic Iron Overload (Hemochromatosis):

Continuous subcutaneous or slow intravenous infusion is recommended for iron overload associated with hemochromatosis, because more iron is eliminated per unit dose of deferoxamine than with intramuscular or rapid intravenous injection. The concomitant oral administration of ascorbic acid (0.5 to 1 g twice daily) may improve the chelating action of deferoxamine in hemochromatosis. Its use should be discontinued, however, if signs and symptoms of cardiac decompensation occur. Since there is considerable dose-response variation, the dosage and duration of therapy should be adjusted by monitoring the urinary excretion of iron.

Intraperitoneal deferoxamine was superior to intravenous administration for the management of hemosiderosis in a patient undergoing continuous ambulatory peritoneal dialysis (Gomez et al, 1987). In this patient, the total weekly removal of iron following intravenous administration of 15 mg/kg once a week was 11 mg/week. In contrast, the same dose administered intraperitoneally (250 mg/L, every other bag) increased iron removal fivefold (57 mg). However, the patient developed leukopenia during therapy, a previously unreported side effect. This was abolished when the dose was halved, but iron removal decreased to 45 mg/week.

Intramuscular, Intravenous: *Adults*, 0.5 to 1 g daily is administered intramuscularly. In addition, 2 g is administered by slow infusion (not to exceed 15 mg/kg/hr) over a 12-hour period with each unit of blood transfused. Deferoxamine can be administered at the same time as blood but must not be mixed in the same container.

Subcutaneous: *Adults and children*, 20 to 40 mg/kg/day is slowly infused by pump, usually in the anterior abdominal wall over a 12-hour period during the night.

Aluminum in Dialysis Patients:

Although no specific protocol or dosage has been established, a number of nephrologists have found deferoxamine to be useful for aluminum-associated encephalopathy or osteomalacia (Hood et al, 1984; Malluche et al, 1984; Pierides and Pierce Myli, 1984; Tsuru et al, 1987). Part of the deferoxamine-aluminum complex is removed in the dialysate, but the primary route of excretion appears to be in the feces (McCarthy et al, 1987). In one study, patients managed by hemodialysis were given intravenous deferoxamine 14.25 mg/kg/hr for two hours three times a week; patients undergoing long-term ambulatory peritoneal dialysis received 85 mg/kg once a week at a rate of 14.25 mg/kg/hr (Malluche et al, 1984).

Desferal (CIBA). Powder for solution (lyophilized, sterile) 500 mg.

DIMERCAPROL
[BAL in Oil]

$$\underset{SH}{CH_2}-\underset{SH}{CH}-\underset{OH}{CH_2}$$

ACTIONS AND USES. Dimercaprol antagonizes the toxic effects of arsenic, mercury, and gold by forming chelates or complexes. Therapy is most effective when begun within one or two hours after ingestion. Retrospective clinical studies reveal that dimercaprol removes mercury when given within four hours after ingestion, but efficacy is reduced after six hours; thus, dimercaprol is used only in acute mercury poisoning.

Although this drug increases the urinary and fecal excretion of lead, edetate calcium disodium, succimer, or penicillamine is preferred. However, for severe lead poisoning in *children* (lead encephalopathy), the combination of dimercaprol and edetate calcium disodium is preferred, since some studies suggest that this regimen hastens excretion of lead and reduces the incidence of brain damage. Dimercaprol may accelerate the excretion of copper in Wilson's disease (hepatolenticular degeneration), but penicillamine is the drug of choice.

Dimercaprol is not beneficial in arsine (AsH_3), antimony, or bismuth poisoning and should *not* be used in iron, cadmium, or selenium poisoning because the complexes formed are more nephrotoxic than the metal alone.

This drug is not effective orally for systemic intoxications.

ADVERSE REACTIONS AND PRECAUTIONS. Adverse reactions are generally mild and transitory. In addition to pain at the site of injection sometimes associated with sterile abscesses, they include, in approximate order of frequency, nausea with occasional vomiting; headache; mild conjunctivitis, lacrimation, rhinorrhea, and salivation; burning sensation in the lips, mouth, and throat and feeling of constriction or pain in the throat, chest, or hands; tingling or burning paresthesias in the hands and penis; sweating; and abdominal pain (Klaassen, 1985). Many of these effects, as well as symptoms of serum sickness, are relieved by an antihistamine. Dimercaprol imparts an unpleasant odor to the breath. Drug-induced fever may persist throughout therapy in children.

Dimercaprol consistently causes moderate to marked increases in both systolic and diastolic blood pressure accompanied by tachycardia. It also may induce metabolic acidosis with elevated serum lactate levels. Continued use of large doses damages capillaries, resulting in loss of protein and fluid from the circulation. Dimercaprol may induce hemolysis in patients with glucose-6-phosphate dehydrogenase deficiency and should be utilized in such patients only in life-threatening situations.

Dimercaprol is contraindicated in patients with impaired liver function. It has been recommended for use in lead poisoning in patients with severe renal impairment because of the belief that dimercaprol and its complex with lead can be excreted in the bile and/or removed by hemodialysis (Chisolm, 1968); however, this supposition has not been verified in investigational studies and dimercaprol is potentially nephrotoxic. If acute renal failure develops during therapy, dimercaprol should be continued with extreme caution, since toxic serum concentrations may accumulate, and it is not known whether dimercaprol or the metal complex is removed by dialysis. Because the chelate rapidly dissociates in an acid medium, releasing the bound metal, *the urine should be kept alkaline.*

Dimercaprol forms a toxic complex with and should not be used in conjunction with medicinal iron.

PHARMACOKINETICS. Peak plasma concentrations of dimercaprol are obtained 30 to 60 minutes after intramuscular administration. About 50% of the drug is excreted in the bile and urine; the remainder is metabolized rapidly. A single dose is eliminated completely in 6 to 24 hours.

DOSAGE AND PREPARATIONS. *Dimercaprol in oil must never be given intravenously.* Doses in excess of 5 mg/kg should be avoided since vomiting, seizures, and coma may be induced. The injection sites should be rotated and a map of the injection sites should be part of the medical record.

Intramuscular: *Adults and children,* for mild arsenic or gold poisoning, 2.5 mg/kg four times daily for two days, two times on the third day, then once daily for ten days; for severe arsenic or gold poisoning, 3 mg/kg every four hours for two days, four times on the third day, then twice daily for ten days.

For acute mercury poisoning, 5 mg/kg initially, followed by 2.5 mg/kg one or two times daily for ten days. The suggested dosage based on body surface area is: for very severe poisoning, 750 mg/M^2/day in divided doses every four hours; for less severe poisoning, 500 mg/M^2/day in divided doses every four hours; for mild poisoning, 333 mg/M^2/day in divided doses every four to six hours. Dosage is adjusted as described above.

For dosage used in lead poisoning, see Table 2.

BAL in Oil (Becton Dickinson). Solution (sterile) 100 mg/ml in peanut oil in 3 ml containers.

EDETATE CALCIUM DISODIUM (EDTA)

[Calcium Disodium Versenate]

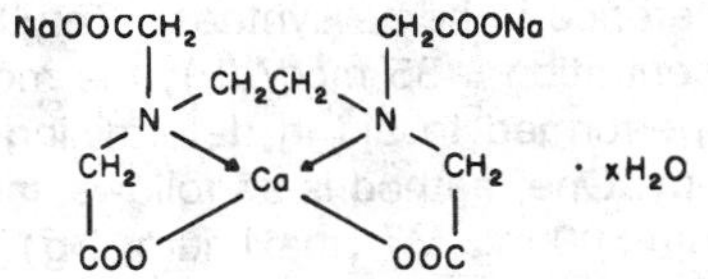

NaOOCCH$_2$ — N — CH$_2$CH$_2$ — N — CH$_2$COONa; CH$_2$ — Ca — CH$_2$; COO — OOC · xH$_2$O

ACTIONS AND USES. This drug is used primarily to treat lead poisoning (plumbism). The chelates formed are water soluble, not easily dissociated, and readily excreted by the kidney. Edetate calcium disodium does not produce negative calcium balance. It is capable of binding and increasing the excretion of zinc, but these actions are thought to be clinically insignificant if therapy is limited to five days, followed by a two- to five-day drug-free interval to permit recovery from the zinc depletion.

Edetate calcium disodium is of questionable or unproved value in poisoning caused by cadmium, chromium, manganese, nickel, vanadium, and zinc. It is ineffective in poisoning caused by mercury, gold, or arsenic.

The optimal pH range for the combination of edetate calcium disodium with lead includes all physiologic values. When treating lead poisoning in *adults,* the drug is given intravenously for three to five days to allow continued chelation and excretion of the heavy metal as it is released from tissues into extracellular fluid. Peak excretion of chelated lead occurs within 24 to 48 hours.

Too rapid mobilization of lead results in deposition in lead-avid soft tissues (brain, kidney) at a rate faster than its urinary clearance, which may exacerbate toxicity. Thus, the preferred treatment for severe lead poisoning (blood lead concentration greater than 70 mcg/dL), especially lead encephalopathy in children, is combined therapy with edetate calcium disodium and dimercaprol. This combination increases the excretion of lead and is less toxic than either agent alone. The first dose of dimercaprol should *always* precede the first dose of edetate calcium disodium by at least four hours.

Succimer may be administered orally for follow-up therapy when necessary (see the evaluation).

DIAGNOSIS OF LEAD POISONING. Guidelines established by the Centers for Disease Control for the diagnosis and treatment of lead poisoning were revised in 1991 (Centers for Disease Control, 1991). No definition of lead poisoning in terms of a specific blood lead level is given, but the "intervention level" has been lowered. Universal screening using the determination of blood lead rather than the erythrocyte protoporphyrin test is now recommended. If a large number of children in a community have blood lead levels >10 mcg/dL, community agencies should consider preventive intervention. Individual environmental evaluation and educational and nutritional intervention are suggested when blood lead levels equal or exceed 15 mcg/dL. More detailed evaluation of the patient's environment and potential sources of exposure should be undertaken and chelation therapy considered when the level is 25 mcg/dL. (See Table 2.)

With the availability of the safer, orally effective chelating agent, succimer, some clinicians question the usefulness of the lead mobilization test. However, when the blood lead concentration is between 25 and 45 mcg/dL and there is evidence of interference in heme synthesis (erythrocyte protoporphyrin concentration >35 mcg/dL), the mobilization test is sometimes performed to aid in determining the need for chelation therapy. One method is as follows: initially, edetate calcium disodium 500 mg/M^2 (maximum, 1 g) diluted in 250 ml/M^2 of dextrose 5% is infused intravenously over at least one hour. An eight-hour urine sample is collected. The concentration of lead in the urine (mcg/ml) is multiplied by the urine volume (ml) to obtain the total excretion of lead (mcg). This figure is divided by the quantity of edetate calcium disodium (mg) to obtain the "lead excretion ratio." Chelation therapy is recommended if the ratio is greater than 0.5. The result of this test is valid only when renal function is normal and lead-free glass or plastic ware is used during urine collection and analysis.

The mobilization test is omitted and appropriate chelation therapy is given immediately to symptomatic patients or to those with confirmed lead concentrations greater than 45 mcg/dL of whole blood.

In children under 6 years who have received chelation therapy, lead and protoporphyrin determinations should be performed five to seven days and two weeks after therapy is initiated. If the reduction is maintained, laboratory determinations may be scheduled at two- to four-week intervals for six months and then at three-month intervals until the child is 6 years old.

TABLE 2.
CHELATION THERAPY IN CHILDREN WITH LEAD TOXICITY

Condition	Management
Acute encephalopathy Blood lead concentration usually >100 mcg/dL	Dimercaprol 75 mg/M^2 is given by deep intramuscular injection every four hours. Four hours after the initial dose of dimercaprol, intravenous infusion of edetate calcium disodium 1.5 g/M^2/24 hours is begun.* The first course of therapy is of 5 days' duration. Therapy is discontinued for 2 days, then resumed for an additional 5 days if the blood lead concentration remains elevated. One or more additional courses may be indicated, with 5- to 7-day drug-free intervals until the patient is clinically stable. Oral succimer then can be substituted in a dose of 10 mg/kg or 350 mg/M^2 every 8 hours for 5 days, followed by the same dose every 12 hours for 14 days. The blood lead concentration should be monitored to determine the need for further therapy.
Symptomatic intoxication without encephalopathy or Asymptomatic with blood lead concentration >60 mcg/dL	Dimercaprol 50 mg/M^2 is given by deep intramuscular injection every four hours. Four hours after the initial dose of dimercaprol, intravenous infusion of edetate calcium disodium 1 g/M^2/24 hours is begun. This combined therapy is continued for 72 hours; oral succimer is then substituted and the patient monitored as above.
Asymptomatic with blood lead concentration between 45-60 mcg/dL	Oral succimer 10 mg/kg or 350 mg/M^2 is given every 8 hours for 5 days followed by the same dose every 12 hours for 14 days. (The patient should be hospitalized during the initial 72 hours of therapy to facilitate monitoring.) Further therapy should be based on the results of blood lead determinations after allowing 2 weeks for re-equilibration.
Asymptomatic with blood lead concentration between 25-45 mcg/dL	Active measures to reduce environmental sources of lead, correct iron deficiency, and maintain adequate nutrition constitute the primary approach. The value of chelation therapy at this level of toxicity is not established. In the past, an edetate calcium disodium lead mobilization test would be done to evaluate response to chelation therapy and identify the subgroup of patients in whom the quantity of lead eliminated would balance the discomfort and risks of the therapy. Since the toxicity of succimer appears to be minimal and its use avoids the discomfort and adverse effects of edetate calcium disodium and/or penicillamine, the value of the mobilization test is debatable. The dosage of succimer and monitoring is as above. See text for further discussion.
Asymptomatic with blood lead concentration <25 mcg/dL	No chelation therapy needed.

* *Less desirably, edetate calcium disodium 175 mg/M^2 may be given every four hours by slow intravenous infusion over 15 to 20 minutes or by deep intramuscular injection at a site separate from dimercaprol.*

Adapted and modified from Centers for Disease Control, 1991.

ADVERSE REACTIONS AND PRECAUTIONS. Pain at the site of intramuscular injection, hypotension, chills, fever, and histamine-like reactions (sneezing, nasal congestion, and lacrimation) may occur. Transient bone marrow depression and cheilosis may develop with prolonged administration of large doses. Occasionally, proteinuria, microscopic hematuria, and large epithelial cells in the urinary sediment are observed. The most serious reaction is acute necrosis of the proximal renal tubules.

Patients who are dehydrated from repeated vomiting should receive intravenous fluids before chelation to ensure an adequate urine flow; however, excessive fluid must be avoided in patients with encephalopathy.

Edetate calcium disodium should be used cautiously and in reduced doses in patients with pre-existing mild renal disease, and it is contraindicated in patients who are or who become anuric or severely oliguric. If anuria develops during therapy, edetate calcium disodium should be discontinued immediately. Urinalysis and blood urea nitrogen, serum creatinine, calcium, and phosphorus levels should be measured before treatment is begun and on the third and fifth days of therapy.

Since steroids enhance the renal toxicity of edetate calcium disodium in animals, they should not be used to prevent or relieve the cerebral edema that may accompany lead encephalopathy. Repeated doses of mannitol are recommended for this purpose.

Some patients may develop hypercalcemia, since lead displaces calcium from the chelate. Edetate calcium disodium interferes with the duration of action of zinc insulin preparations by forming a chelate with zinc.

PHARMACOKINETICS. Edetate calcium disodium is not metabolized and is excreted within 24 hours exclusively by glomerular filtration. Therefore, adequate urine flow should be established before initiating therapy. This agent is eliminated from the plasma by first-order kinetics (half-life, 20 to 60 minutes). Excretion is unaffected by the urinary pH. The clearance of edetate calcium disodium is significantly correlated with creatinine clearance; however, urinary lead excretion does not correlate with either edetate calcium disodium kinetics or with measures of renal function (Osterloh and Becker, 1986).

Edetate calcium disodium is poorly absorbed from the gastrointestinal tract. Furthermore, the absorption of any lead present in the intestine may be increased, because the lead chelate formed is more soluble than the lead itself. After absorption, the chelate dissociates and releases free lead ions, which can produce toxic reactions. Thus, oral administration for prophylaxis may enhance lead absorption in workers exposed to this metal (an oral preparation is no longer marketed). The most effective way to prevent chronic exposure is to maintain proper industrial hygiene.

DOSAGE AND PREPARATIONS.

Intravenous Infusion: This is the preferred route of administration in adults. Since edetate calcium disodium is eliminated by the kidneys and renal function is related to body surface area, the dosage is calculated on this basis.

Adults, 1.5 g/M^2/day in two divided doses for three to five days. For those who are mildly symptomatic or with whole blood lead levels of 50 to 70 mcg/dL, the total daily dose may be reduced to 1 g/M^2. Each dose is diluted in 250 or 500 ml of sodium chloride injection or 5% dextrose injection and administered over six to eight hours. Therapy is then interrupted for at least two days (preferably two weeks) to allow redistribution of lead from inaccessible storage sites, and a second course is then given if necessary. The maximum 24-hour dose in adults should not exceed 50 mg/kg (1.75 g/M^2), even in severe poisoning.

For *children,* intramuscular injection is preferred to avoid extravasation or excessive fluid load in encephalopathy. If the intravenous route is chosen, treatment courses and doses are the same as for adults with the following exceptions: The maximum 24-hour dose may be increased to 75 mg/kg in very severe poisoning, but the total amount of fluid administered per dose must be reduced as required and the concentration of edetate must not exceed 0.5% in the parenteral fluid. If intake volume must be decreased further, the drug should be given intramuscularly. Children may require more than two courses of therapy when mobilization of lead from labile skeletal stores approaches the critical blood level of 70 mcg/dL. Therapy should be continued intermittently until the blood lead concentration remains below 50 mcg/dL.

Intramuscular (deep): *Adults,* the dose and treatment schedule are the same as for intravenous use. The drug is administered as a 20% solution. Generally, lidocaine or procaine is added to a final concentration of 0.5% to minimize pain following injection. It is important to rotate the sites of injection, especially in children. A map of injection sites should be part of the medical record. *Children,* see Table 2.

Calcium Disodium Versenate (3M Pharmaceuticals). Solution (sterile) 200 mg/ml in 5 ml containers.

PENICILLAMINE

[Cuprimine, Depen]

$$CH_3-\underset{\underset{CH_3}{|}}{\overset{\overset{SH}{|}}{C}}-\underset{\underset{H}{|}}{\overset{\overset{NH_2}{|}}{C}}-\overset{\overset{O}{\|}}{C}OH$$

ACTIONS. Penicillamine, an inactive degradation product of penicillin, is now manufactured synthetically to avoid contamination with trace amounts of penicillin. It combines with copper, iron, mercury, lead, gold, and arsenic to form soluble complexes that are readily excreted by the kidneys. Penicillamine itself is oxidized to a disulfide derivative and is also excreted by the kidneys.

USES. This orally effective agent is superior to other metal antagonists for chelating copper and is used primarily to remove excess copper in patients with Wilson's disease (see index entry Wilson's Disease).

Penicillamine chelates lead less effectively than edetate calcium disodium or dimercaprol but has been used in asymptomatic patients with moderately elevated blood levels because it is effective orally and may enhance absorption of lead from the gastrointestinal tract. The availability of succimer will limit the use of penicillamine in the therapy of lead intoxication.

Dimercaprol is the standard therapy for arsenic poisoning, but penicillamine has also been used (Peterson and Rumack, 1977; Shannon et al, 1988); however, there is little evidence of its effectiveness. Penicillamine has been substituted for dimercaprol in acute inorganic mercury poisoning.

ADVERSE REACTIONS AND PRECAUTIONS. Although the adverse reactions associated with short-term administration are generally acceptable, penicillamine can produce serious and even fatal reactions. Side effects, precautions, and contraindications for the use of this drug are described in detail elsewhere; see the index entry Penicillamine, Uses, Urolithiasis.

DOSAGE AND PREPARATIONS.

Oral: Penicillamine should be given on an empty stomach at least one hour before meals and at bedtime; the last dose should be given at least three hours after the evening meal. Patients also should be maintained on a low-copper diet.

For lead poisoning, *adults and children,* 600 mg/M^2 daily until the concentration of lead remains below 50 mcg/dL of whole blood (usually after four weeks to several months). Side effects can be minimized by initiating therapy with 25% of the calculated dose; the amount is increased to 50% after one week and the full dose is given after another week with monitoring for possible toxicity. A low-calcium diet augments lead sequestration.

For acute arsenic poisoning, the following regimen has been used for *adults and children:* 100 mg/kg/day is given in four divided doses before meals to a maximum of 1 g/day for five days. After a drug-free interval of three to five days, therapy may be reinstituted if symptoms reappear. When the total urinary excretion of arsenic falls below 50 mcg/24 hours, further chelation therapy is unnecessary (Peterson and Rumack, 1977).

For acute mercury poisoning, *adults*, 250 mg four times a day; *children*, 100 mg/kg/day for 3 to 10 days guided by the urinary excretion of mercury (Rumack and Peterson, 1980).

Cuprimine (Merck Sharp & Dohme). Capsules 125 and 250 mg. If necessary, these capsules may be opened and the drug suspended in any liquid except milk.

Depen (Wallace). Tablets 250 mg.

SUCCIMER (DMSA)

[Chemet]

```
        COOH
         |
    H — C — SH
         |
    H — C — SH
         |
        COOH
```

ACTIONS AND USES. This meso isomer of dimercaptosuccinic acid represents a new molecular entity and is a significant addition to the available therapeutic choices of metal mobilizing agents. It is indicated for the treatment of children with blood lead concentrations above 45 mcg/dL and is probably also effective in adults. Succimer can produce lead diuresis similar to that produced by edetate calcium disodium, and the decrease in blood lead concentration is similar or slightly greater. Because succimer is administered orally and has few adverse effects, some physicians may use it inappropriately for prophylaxis of chronic lead exposure. However, prophylaxis is properly based on removal of sources of lead exposure.

Succimer complexes with and enhances the excretion of arsenic and mercury, but clinical experience is limited. It appears to have little effect on excretion of essential minerals such as zinc, magnesium, copper, and iron.

ADVERSE REACTIONS AND PRECAUTIONS. The most common adverse effects are nausea, vomiting, anorexia, and diarrhea. Pain in the back, abdominal cramps, chills, and headache also have been reported. Skin rash occurs in about 4% of patients and may require cessation of therapy. Alternative causes of rash should be considered, and if use of the drug is essential, rechallenge may be indicated. Transient, low-grade elevations of liver enzymes have been noted.

Patients should be monitored after completion of a course of therapy to evaluate rebound blood concentrations of lead caused by redistribution. The degree and duration of rebound is related to the severity of poisoning and the pretreatment lead level.

Succimer is classified in FDA Pregnancy Category C.

PHARMACOKINETICS. Succimer appears to be rapidly but incompletely absorbed from the gastrointestinal tract. A sizable portion of the dose appears in the feces and probably represents unabsorbed drug. Of the portion absorbed, most is metabolized and the products are excreted in the urine. In one study in adults, about 20% of the oral dose was recovered in the urine. Of the urinary material, 12% was unaltered succimer and the remainder was mixed disulfides of succimer with L-cysteine. Since it is generally believed that an effective chelating agent must be metabolically stable, these findings suggest that a metabolite, rather than the parent drug, is the actual binding agent (Aposhian et al, 1989). Peak excretion of succimer in urine occurs about two to four hours after administration. The elimination half-life of radio-labeled material in blood is approximately two days.

DOSAGE AND PREPARATIONS. The combined use of succimer with edetate calcium disodium with or without dimercaprol is not recommended because of lack of clinical information about this regimen. For young children who cannot swallow capsules, the contents may be removed from the capsule and mixed with food.

Oral: *Children,* a course of therapy is 19 days. A dose of 10 mg/kg or 350 mg/M^2 is given every eight hours for the first five days; this amount then is administered every 12 hours for an additional 14 days. Blood lead concentrations should be monitored following therapy to evaluate the response. An interval of 14 days between courses is recommended unless blood lead rebound indicates the need for earlier retreatment. The patient must be hydrated and renal function must be adequate for therapy to be successful.

Chemet (McNeil). Capsules 100 mg.

Miscellaneous Specific Antidotes

NALOXONE HYDROCHLORIDE

[Narcan]

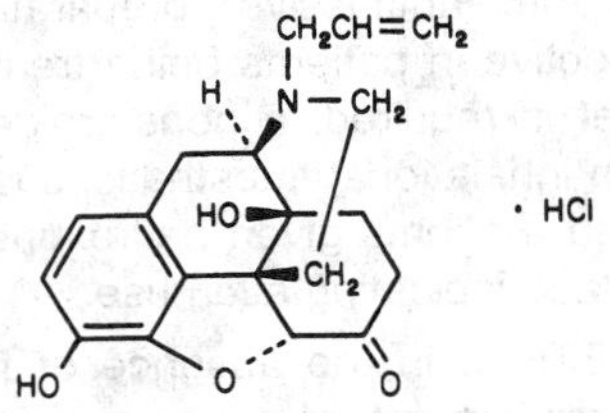

ACTIONS AND USES. Naloxone is the drug of choice to treat respiratory depression known or suspected to be caused by opioid overdose; it promptly increases the respiratory rate and reverses coma. Since naloxone does not cause respiratory depression or affect that produced by barbiturates or other respiratory depressants, lack of response suggests that the depression is not the result of opioid overdose.

Naloxone reverses the agonist effects of pentazocine and other mixed agonist-antagonists and terminates the psychotogenic and dysphoric effects sometimes caused by these drugs. It also terminates coma and convulsions associated with large doses of propoxyphene or meperidine in drug abusers (Martin, 1976) or after overdose in children (Lovejoy et al, 1974). In addition, naloxone counteracts other actions of the opioids, such as analgesia, cardiovascular and gastrointestinal effects, biliary duct spasm, pupillary response, release of antidiuretic hormone, and hyperglycemia. Even large doses of naloxone only partially reverse the actions of buprenorphine.

Naloxone may be administered postoperatively to reverse severe respiratory depression caused by opioids. However, since it also decreases the analgesic and sedative effects of these drugs, the dose must be selected carefully. Too rapid reversal may cause nausea and vomiting or tachycardia and hypertension; these reactions may be due to catecholamine release, since they sometimes occur following administration of naloxone to opioid- and pain-free subjects. Pulmonary edema and disturbances of cardiac rhythm are extremely rare. It is recommended that small, incremental doses of naloxone be given when intravenous bolus doses are employed (Partridge and Ward, 1986; Mariani, 1989).

Naloxone is effective in neonatal respiratory depression caused by large doses of morphine-like drugs administered to the mother during labor and delivery. If respiratory depression is present in the infant, naloxone may be administered into the umbilical artery or given either subcutaneously or intramuscularly. If the mother is dependent on morphine-like drugs, the infant is also dependent and may exhibit withdrawal symptoms after birth (hypertonia, sweating, continuous shrill cry, failure to feed). Because an antagonist will precipitate a withdrawal reaction in these infants, careful monitoring is essential after the desired effect is achieved.

The pupillography test using naloxone has been employed to diagnose opioid addiction, but small doses must be administered cautiously to avoid precipitating a severe withdrawal syndrome in opioid-dependent individuals.

ADVERSE REACTIONS AND PRECAUTIONS. Naloxone may precipitate a withdrawal syndrome in opioid-dependent patients. Although the syndrome is self-limited (15 to 60 minutes), hypertension and agitation may be difficult to manage; therefore, in dependent patients, naloxone should be administered in 0.1 to 0.2 mg increments until respiratory depression is reversed.

This drug has been notably free from adverse reactions. Tolerance and psychic or physical dependence do not develop. Naloxone is not subject to provisions of the Controlled Substances Act.

Naloxone is classified in FDA Pregnancy Category B.

PHARMACOKINETICS. Naloxone must be given parenterally because of extensive first-pass metabolism during absorption from the gastrointestinal tract. The onset of action is rapid; an effect usually is noted within two minutes after intravenous injection and only slightly later after intramuscular, subcutaneous, sublingual, or endotracheal administration, but the intravenous route is preferred. The apparent volume of distribution is 2.77 ± 0.16 L/kg. The duration of action may be shorter than that of most opioids. *Thus, repeated doses may be necessary to treat respiratory depression.* The half-life is 48.6 ± 7.3 minutes in normal subjects and 29.9 ± 2.6 minutes when hepatic microsomal enzymes have been induced (eg, after use of barbiturates or prolonged intake of alcohol). The pharmacokinetic parameters of naloxone in the premature neonate are: half-life 70.5 ± 35.2 minutes, clearance 39.13 ± 14.53 ml/kg/min, and apparent volume of distribution 3.52 ± 1.2 L/kg (Stile et al, 1987). Although there is evidence that the metabolic disposition differs from that of the adult, the difference in half-life is not of clinical significance.

DOSAGE AND PREPARATIONS. *Naloxone is given to antagonize opioid-induced respiratory depression only after the establishment of a clear airway and adequate assistance of respiration.* Although the intravenous route is preferred, the same dosage is effective almost as rapidly following sublingual, endotracheal, intramuscular, or subcutaneous administration.

Intravenous: For respiratory depression caused by opioid overdosage, *adults and children over 5 years or weighing more than 20 kg,* 2 mg (five ampuls) as a bolus. Larger doses (as much as 20 times the usual quantity) may be required for poisoning with propoxyphene [Darvon] or pentazocine [Talwin] or massive overdoses of other analgesics. In patients with suspected opioid tolerance, 0.1- to 0.2-mg increments are used initially to avoid an abrupt opioid withdrawal syndrome. If a single dose of 2 mg fails to reverse symptoms in suspected opioid overdosage, additional 2-mg bolus doses should be administered at two- to three-minute intervals. Because of its short half-life, additional doses of naloxone may be required at 20- to 60-minute intervals, especially with overdose of long-acting opioids such as methadone. Alternatively, after a satisfactory response to the initial dose, approximately 60% of the amount necessary for reversal may be given hourly: Ten times the hourly dose is added to 1 L of dextrose 5% in water and infused at the rate of about 100 ml/hr, adjusted to maintain a satisfactory ventilatory response without producing withdrawal symptoms (Goldfrank et al, 1986).

For postoperative respiratory depression caused by opioids, *adults,* 0.1 to 0.2 mg (1.5 mcg/kg) at two- to three-minute intervals until the desired effect is achieved. Smaller aliquots, 0.04 mg at three- to five-minute intervals, have been recommended to avoid potential postoperative cardiovascular and respiratory complications (Partridge and Ward, 1986). The drug also has been given by continuous infusion (3.66 mcg/kg/hr) to counteract respiratory depression induced by morphine anesthesia (Johnstone et al, 1974).

Intravenous, Intramuscular, Subcutaneous: To reverse opioid-induced respiratory depression in *newborn infants*, initially, 0.1 mg/kg of the 0.4 mg/ml solution; if there is no response, this dose may be repeated as necessary. The 0.02 mg/ml solution should not be used because of possible volume loading.

Generic. Solution 0.02, 0.4, and 1 mg/ml.

Narcan (DuPont). Solution 0.02 mg/ml in 2 ml containers, 0.4 mg/ml in 1 and 10 ml containers; 1 mg/ml in 1, 2, and 10 ml containers with methylparaben and propylparaben as preservatives; and 0.02 and 1 mg/ml in 2 ml containers (paraben free).

NALTREXONE HYDROCHLORIDE

[Trexan]

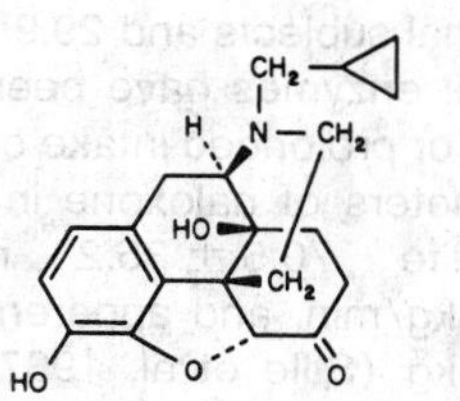

ACTIONS AND USES. Naltrexone resembles naloxone in its ability to competitively antagonize opioid drugs. An oral dose suppresses the psychological and physical effects of opioids for 48 to 72 hours. The sole indication for naltrexone is maintenance of an opioid-free state in abusers. Unlike methadone, which also is used for this purpose, it has no agonist activity. Therefore, it is not a scheduled drug and may be prescribed by physicians outside of specialized clinics and drug abuse programs. Compliance is essential to efficacy; verification of regular naltrexone use and urinalysis are essential; job counseling, psychotherapy, and physician and family support enhance compliance. Drug therapy to lessen anxiety, depression, or insomnia may be required during initial use of naltrexone.

ADVERSE REACTIONS AND PRECAUTIONS. Shortly after beginning therapy with naltrexone, minor disturbances, particularly nausea, loss of energy, mental depression, and dysphoria, may develop. These effects usually diminish in 30 to 60 days and also occur in normal volunteers. It has been speculated that this response may be ascribed to blockade of endogenous opioids (Hollister et al, 1981).

The most serious adverse reaction is dose-related hepatotoxicity. This appears to be reversible and is most common in obese patients (Ginzburg and MacDonald, 1987). Since liver dysfunction is common in many drug abusers, it is recommended that serum transaminases be measured before initiating therapy, monthly during the first six months, and periodically thereafter. A threefold or greater increase in the transaminase level is an indication for discontinuation of the medication.

Naltrexone is classified in FDA Pregnancy Category C.

Antidiarrheal and antitussive preparations containing opioids are ineffective in patients being treated with naltrexone. If pain relief is required, a nonsteroidal drug, regional anesthesia, or an inhalational anesthetic, such as nitrous oxide, must be used. Patients given naltrexone should wear a bracelet or necklace indicating such use.

PHARMACOKINETICS. In the absence of food, absorption following oral administration of naltrexone is rapid and complete; a maximum concentration is attained in the plasma within one hour. However, there is extensive first-pass metabolism in the liver, and only about 5% of a dose reaches the systemic circulation. The variability in hepatic extraction among individuals probably accounts for the discrepancies reported in pharmacokinetic data.

The principal metabolite, 6-β-naltrexol, exhibits only weak antiopioid activity and, despite its longer elimination half-life, it is presumed that this metabolite does not contribute to the clinical effect of naltrexone. The volume of distribution of naltrexone at steady state is 16.1 ± 5.2 L/kg (Verebey et al, 1976). The clearance (total) is approximately 94 L/hr and the elimination half-life is approximately four hours (Meyer et al, 1984). There is no evidence that prolonged administration results in accumulation of naltrexone or its metabolites.

DOSAGE AND PREPARATIONS. Naltrexone should not be administered unless the patient has been opioid-free for seven to ten days as confirmed by chemical urinalysis and a naloxone challenge test.

Oral: To prevent readdiction in former opioid abusers, initially, 25 mg. If no signs of an opioid withdrawal syndrome become apparent within one hour, the remainder of the daily dose may be administered. Doses of 100 to 150 mg three times per week usually are employed. However, dose schedules may be tailored to the probable compliance of the patient, eg, 50 mg per day, 100 mg every other day, 150 mg every third day, 100 mg on Monday and Wednesday and 150 mg on Friday.

Trexan (DuPont). Tablets 50 mg.

Subcutaneous (Investigational): Because of notoriously poor compliance with the oral route, studies are in progress utilizing a biodegradable bead containing naltrexone that would require subcutaneous implantation only once a month (Chiang et al, 1985).

CYANIDE ANTIDOTE

ACTIONS AND USES. Cyanide ion combines principally with ferricytochrome oxidase to produce tissue hypoxia. A cyanide antidote kit is available and contains amyl nitrite for inhalation and sodium nitrite and sodium thiosulfate for intravenous injection. Nitrite ion converts hemoglobin to methemoglobin. It is postulated that the ferric ion formed competes with ferricytochrome oxidase for available cyanide ion, but this may not be the antidotal mechanism. Cyanide ion is biotransformed to the relatively nontoxic thiocyanate ion by transfer of sulfur from donor compounds in a physiologic sulfane sulfur pool. The central position of rhodanase as enzymatic mediator of this process has been questioned. Sodium thiosulfate increases the biotransformation of cyanide to thiocyanate more than thirtyfold (Sylvester et al, 1983).

Oxygen is an important adjunct in the treatment of cyanide poisoning. It permits the saturation of hemoglobin not converted to methemoglobin and may reactivate cyanide-depressed enzymatic processes (eg, carbohydrate metabolism) (Way et al, 1984). No benefit is gained from hyperbaric oxygenation.

ADVERSE REACTIONS. Adverse reactions are seldom clinically significant with recommended doses of cyanide antagonists in the cyanide antidote kit; however, they may be clinically relevant in some situations (eg, smoke inhalation with elevated carboxyhemoglobin, in which instance-induced methemoglobinemia may worsen hypoxia). Large amounts of methemoglobin decrease the quantity of oxygen available for tissues, and nitrites also can produce cardiovascular instability, usually manifested as hypotension, especially during anesthesia.

ALTERNATIVE THERAPY. The use of the traditional cyanide antagonists is being re-evaluated in light of investigations using alternative antagonists, such as cobalt edetate and hydroxocobalamin (Graham et al, 1977; Cottrell et al, 1978; Ballantyne and Marrs, 1987). Intravenous cobalt edetate 600 mg forms a relatively nontoxic complex with cyanide; an additional 300 mg is administered if recovery is delayed. Although some physicians in England consider cobalt edetate to be the treatment of choice, it is associated with vomiting, anaphylactic reactions, chest pains, facial edema, and ventricular arrhythmias.

Hydroxocobalamin [Codroxomin] combines with cyanide ion to form cyanocobalamin (vitamin B_{12}). Hydroxocobalamin is given intravenously, but no commercial parenteral preparation is available in the United States that contains the concentration of drug required to treat cyanide toxicity without administering excessive quantities of fluid. Clinical experience using a French kit containing 4 g hydroxocobalamin and 8 g sodium thiosulfate has been reviewed (Hall and Rumack, 1987). No significant adverse reactions were reported.

Results of animal experiments in which stroma-free methemoglobin solutions are injected intravenously have been promising (Ten Eyck et al, 1984). The advantages of administering exogenous methemoglobin over endogenous conversion are that the onset of action is immediate and the patient's oxygen-carrying capacity is not compromised.

DOSAGE AND PREPARATIONS.

Inhalation, Intravenous: *Adults,* oxygen therapy should be initiated and amyl nitrite inhaled from the crushable ampuls for 30 seconds of every minute until an intravenous route is established. Amyl nitrite then is discontinued and all of the sodium nitrite (300 mg) in the 10-ml ampul is administered over a period of five minutes intravenously. The 12.5 g of sodium thiosulfate contained in the 50-ml ampul is then administered intravenously. If symptoms persist, a second dose of sodium nitrite (one-half the amount of the first dose) should be given 30 minutes later. *Children,* oxygen therapy is initiated; 0.33 ml/kg of sodium nitrite solution is administered, followed immediately by 1.65 ml/kg of sodium thiosulfate solution.

If nitrite-induced methemoglobinemia becomes severe, whole blood may be given. The methemoglobin concentration should not exceed 40% in adults or 30% in children (Hall, 1986). *Under no circumstances* should methylene blue be used to treat the methemoglobinemia. This will cause release of cyanide ion, and its use in these circumstances has resulted in fatalities (Arena, 1983).

Cyanide Antidote Package (Lilly). Each kit contains 12 crushable ampuls containing amyl nitrite inhalant 0.3 ml, two 10-ml containers of sodium nitrite 300 mg, two 50-ml containers of sodium thiosulfate 12.5 g, disposable syringes, stomach tube, tourniquet, and instructions. The expiration date on the kit must be observed.

PHYSOSTIGMINE SALICYLATE

[Antilirium]

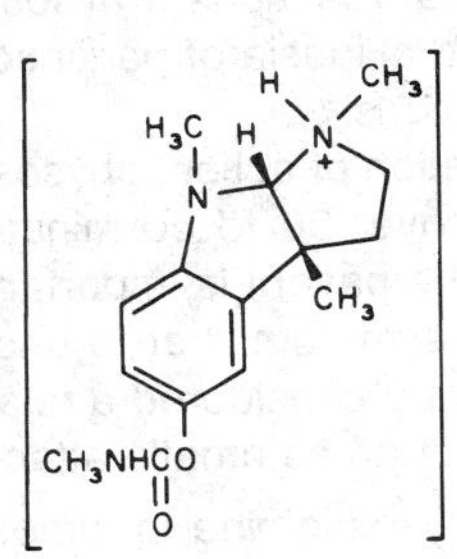

H_3C H N H CH_3 N+ CH_3 CH_3NHCO O O CO^- OH

ACTIONS AND USES. This tertiary amine alkaloid is an anticholinesterase. Its ability to penetrate the central nervous system is useful adjunctively in the treatment of severe central anticholinergic toxicity characterized by anxiety, disorientation, delirium, hyperactivity, hallucinations, illusions, impaired consciousness, and impaired memory.

This spectrum of anticholinergic toxicity is most characteristic of poisoning with atropine and scopolamine. Drugs with secondary anticholinergic activity include antihistamines, tricyclic antidepressants, certain antiemetics, some antiparkinson drugs (centrally acting anticholinergics), and phenothiazines. Physostigmine should *not* be used routinely to treat overdosage with these drugs, especially antidepressants, for it may exacerbate bradyarrhythmias and AV conduction blocks.

Physostigmine should be reserved for serious situations, because it is potentially dangerous; *its routine use for the management of anticholinergic delirium is not recommended.* Treatment of acidosis with sodium bicarbonate and correction of inadequate tidal volume usually are more appropriate. If the diagnosis of anticholinergic overdose is well documented, if supportive care has improved and stabilized vital signs, and if urine output is adequate, there may be little value in using physostigmine for arousal.

In some instances (ie, presence of hypertension, significant supraventricular arrhythmias, severe agitated delirium or hallucinations), documented anticholinergic toxicity may demand aggressive therapy. Physostigmine may improve ventilation in marginal situations, thus avoiding the necessity for endotracheal intubation and mechanical ventilation.

ADVERSE REACTIONS AND PRECAUTIONS. Hypersensitivity to physostigmine is uncommon. Slight to moderate bradycardia may occur; severe bradyarrhythmias are more likely to develop if physostigmine is given to overcome the effects of orphenadrine and tricyclic antidepressants. Convulsions have been observed, particularly with too rapid administration. Excessive salivation, bronchospasm, vomiting, urination, and defecation also may occur. The most dangerous sequela of vomiting may be aspiration, and adequate suction should always be available. In such instances, administration of atropine may be necessary.

A dystonic extrapyramidal reaction should not be mistaken for central anticholinergic toxicity. The akinesia, akathisia, and dyskinesia of the former can be confused with the signs and symptoms of hyperactivity caused by the latter; however, there is little or no impairment of consciousness associated with dystonic extrapyramidal reactions. Physostigmine worsens the rigidity, tremor, and akinesia of parkinsonism and extrapyramidal dystonic reactions.

Because of its short duration of action, physostigmine gradually becomes ineffective over 30 to 60 minutes; therefore, continued observation of the patient is important.

Any cholinergic sign or symptom that is undesirable in a given clinical situation may be considered a relative contraindication (eg, precipitation of an asthmatic attack).

PHARMACOKINETICS. Physostigmine is almost completely hydrolyzed by cholinesterase. It is relatively short acting (half-life, one to two hours). Renal impairment does not alter dosage.

DOSAGE AND PREPARATIONS.

Intravenous: *Adults,* 0.5 to 1 mg given slowly (1 mg/min). The dose may be repeated if life-threatening signs and symptoms recur. Frequent surveillance is essential to determine the appropriate dosage in any given individual. The response to a single dose seldom lasts longer than 30 to 60 minutes. Monitoring of blood pressure, heart rate, and autonomic nervous system function is required. *Children,* 0.5 mg given slowly. If toxic effects persist and no cholinergic effects are produced, the drug should be given at five-minute intervals to a maximum dose of 2 mg. The lowest total effective dose should be repeated if life-threatening signs and symptoms recur.

Antilirium (Forest). Solution 1 mg/ml in 2 ml containers.

PRALIDOXIME CHLORIDE

[Protopam Chloride]

CH_3 N^+ $CH{=}NOH$ Cl^-

ACTIONS AND USES. Pralidoxime (2-PAM) is a cholinesterase reactivator used primarily as an adjunct to atropine in the treatment of severe poisoning caused by pesticides that are organophosphate cholinesterase inhibitors.

In organophosphate poisoning, pralidoxime competes with the phosphorylated inhibited enzyme to form an oxime-phosphonate complex that liberates active cholinesterase. This occurs primarily at the neuromuscular junction in skeletal muscle and also at autonomic effector sites.

Pralidoxime is particularly useful to reverse muscular paralysis, especially that of the respiratory muscles. After the airway is secured and respiratory assistance is provided as required, atropine is given prior to pralidoxime to reduce bronchopulmonary secretions, bronchospasm, hypersalivation, lacrimation, hyperhidrosis, nausea, vomiting, abdominal cramps, and bradycardia. One of the best indices for monitoring atropine therapy is the amount of salivary secretion.

If dermal exposure has occurred, clothing should be removed as soon as possible and the hair and skin washed thoroughly with soapy water. Emergency room personnel should protect themselves from exposure.

Pralidoxime is most effective if administered immediately after poisoning. Generally, little is accomplished if the drug is given more than 36 hours after termination of exposure. However, exposure may continue for some time due to slow absorption from skin, from the lower bowel, or from fat depots in the case of highly fat-soluble organophosphates (eg, fenthion). Fatal relapses have been reported after initial improvement. Continued administration for several days may be useful in such patients. Close supervision is indicated for at least 48 to 72 hours.

Pralidoxime is not equally useful against all cholinesterase inhibitors. It has been most effective in poisoning caused by the organophosphate pesticide, parathion. Pralidoxime also has been effective in poisoning caused by the related agents, Mevinphos, Isoflurophate, Diazinon, Dursban, EPN, Guthion, methyl parathion, Phosdrin, Systox, and TEPP. (See the manufacturer's literature for additional substances.) Pralidoxime does *not* antagonize the effects of carbamate-type cholinesterase inhibitors (eg, neostigmine, pyridostigmine, ambenonium, which are used in the treatment of myasthenia gravis; the pesticides, Aldicarb, Baygon, Carbaryl, Metalkamate, Oxyamyl, and Sevin). For these drugs or insecticides, only atropine is employed.

DIAGNOSIS OF POISONING. Known exposure associated with compatible symptoms is sufficient evidence to initiate atropine therapy. If nicotinic effects persist, pralidoxime should be administered (Murphy, 1986; Minton and Murray, 1988). Therapy should not be delayed pending the results of laboratory tests; red blood cell and plasma cholinesterase and, in parathion exposure, urinary paranitrophenol measurements help to confirm the diagnosis. Depression of the plasma cholinesterase activity does not necessarily reflect nerve cholinesterase activity. The red blood cell cholinesterase activity provides a more accurate index in acute intoxication; a level less than 50% of normal has been seen only with organophosphate ester poisoning. Chronic exposure to these pesticides may depress red blood cell cholinesterase activity to less than 50% with no apparent symptoms. When pralidoxime is administered soon after the onset of poisoning, the red blood cell cholinesterase activity may be restored more rapidly than the plasma level. However, both plasma and red blood cell activities may remain depressed for a month or longer after intoxication; they also may be depressed in patients with subclinical chronic exposures. Therefore, exposure to anticholinesterase inhibitors, including organic phosphate pesticides, should be avoided for several weeks after poisoning. Pneumonitis and/or atelectasis has been observed in infants and children who ingested a pesticide containing petroleum distillate (Zwiener and Ginsburg, 1988).

ADVERSE REACTIONS AND PRECAUTIONS. Pralidoxime may cause dizziness, diplopia, impaired accommodation, headache, drowsiness, nausea, tachycardia, increased systolic and diastolic blood pressure, hyperventilation, and muscle weakness when it is given parenterally to individuals not exposed to anticholinesterase poisons.

The dose of pralidoxime should be reduced in patients with impaired renal function because blood concentrations are increased in these patients.

Pralidoxime is classified in FDA Pregnancy Category C.

DOSAGE AND PREPARATIONS. Pralidoxime should be used only in conjunction with atropine in moderate or severe organophosphate intoxications.

Intravenous: For severe poisoning (coma, cyanosis, respiratory depression) caused by organophosphate-containing substances, the following treatment program should be instituted: A patent airway is secured and, if necessary, artificial respiration with oxygen is begun. In *adults,* atropine 2 to 4 mg is given intravenously *after* adequate oxygenation is assured, and this dose is repeated at 5- to 10-minute intervals until secretions are inhibited or signs of atropine toxicity appear. For *children,* atropine 0.02 mg/kg is given initially and repeated at 5- to 10-minute intervals until salivary secretions are inhibited. Some degree of atropinization should be maintained for at least 48 hours. *Adults,* after atropine, pralidoxime 1 g, preferably diluted in 100 ml of sodium chloride injection, is infused over a 30-minute period or injected at a rate not exceeding 200 mg/min. If the response is inadequate, this dose may be repeated in one hour. Better steady-state concentrations can be maintained by the continuous infusion of 0.5 g/hr (Thompson et al, 1987). *Children* may be given 25 mg/kg (maximum, 1 g) using the same procedure. If infusion is not feasible, a 5% solution may be injected over a five-minute period.

Protopam Chloride (Wyeth-Ayerst). Powder (sterile) 1 g in 20 ml containers.

ETHANOL

ACTIONS AND USES. The toxicity of methanol (methyl or wood alcohol) and ethylene glycol (antifreeze) is caused by the metabolites of these compounds. Both are metabolized by the enzyme, alcohol dehydrogenase. Ethanol has a greater affinity for this enzyme and retards the rate of formation of toxic metabolites to a level at which they can be eliminated safely.

To avoid gastritis, an ethanol concentration no greater than 20% (40 proof) is recommended for oral use, but any blended whiskey can be substituted if necessary. In comatose patients, ethanol can be administered by orogastric tube.

For intravenous administration, a solution containing ethanol 10% in 5% dextrose in water is used (calculation errors result from failure to consider the specific gravity of ethanol [0.8 g/ml]. A 10% v/v solution of ethanol in 5% dextrose in water contains approximately 80 mg/ml ethanol.) Intravenous therapy obviates the concerns for absorption, concurrent drug administration (eg, activated charcoal), and airway management.

In adults, an oral or intravenous loading dose of 0.4 to 0.7 g/kg is given, followed by a maintenance dose of about 125 mg/kg/hr. Blood ethanol concentrations should be monitored and the maintenance dose adjusted to maintain a concentration between 100 and 150 mg/dL (Peterson, 1981). If rapid determinations of alcohol concentrations are not possible, the maintenance dose may be set arbitrarily at 125 to 150 mg/kg/hr.

The concurrent use of single-pass (not recirculating) hemodialysis readily removes both methanol and ethylene glycol (Peterson et al, 1981 A) after metabolism has been blocked by ethanol. For methanol poisoning, hemodialysis should be instituted in severely acidotic or intoxicated patients or when blood methanol concentrations exceed 50 mg/dL. Ethanol alone may be adequate therapy for methanol ingestion when it is administered early. However, the elimination half-life of methanol in the presence of ethanol is prolonged to more than 50 hours, and hemodialysis is needed to hasten removal.

Hemodialysis should be instituted for ethylene glycol poisoning when the volume ingested is greater than 100 ml or signs and symptoms of poisoning (eg, oxalate crystalluria, acidosis) are present. The ethanol maintenance dose must be increased to approximately 250 mg/kg/hr; however, because the specific amount depends on flow and extraction efficiency, the dose should be adjusted on the basis of serial blood alcohol determinations. An alternative is to add ethanol to the dialysate to give a dialysate level of 100 mg/dL (Peterson et al, 1981 B); however this method is difficult to control and very costly.

Because poisoning by these compounds also is associated with severe metabolic acidosis (formic, lactic, and glycolic), parenteral sodium bicarbonate must be administered if the serum bicarbonate concentration is below 15 mEq/L and the plasma pH is below 7.35 (see the index entry, Acid-Base Disturbances). Elimination of formic acid may be dependent on the pH, which suggests that aggressive correction of acidosis may hasten the elimination of this compound (Jacobsen et al, 1988).

ALTERNATIVE THERAPY. In methanol poisoning, acidosis and ocular damage result from accumulation of formic acid. A folate-dependent enzyme system is responsible for the oxidation of formic acid to carbon dioxide. Man and certain monkeys are relatively deficient in this system. In animals, the administration of the folate analogue, leucovorin calcium (citrovorum factor), increases the rate of metabolism of formic acid, which markedly reduces blood levels of the toxin (Noker et al, 1980). If the value of leucovorin calcium is substantiated in man, this drug would be extremely useful to treat methanol poisoning, particularly when hemodialysis is difficult (eg, in young children). Leucovorin calcium is essentially nontoxic (see the index entry, Folates). Currently, intravenous folic acid (50 mg every six hours) is recommended as adjunctive therapy.

The alcohol dehydrogenase inhibitor, fomepizole (methylpyrazole), is relatively nontoxic. Animal experiments and some clinical trials suggest that it may be a satisfactory alternative to ethanol for use in methanol and ethylene glycol poisoning, since monitoring of the serum concentration is not required and additive central nervous system depression does not occur (Blomstrand and Ingemansson, 1984; Baud et al, 1987, 1988).

References

General Management

Ellenhorn MJ, Barceloux DG: *Medical Toxicology: Diagnosis and Treatment of Human Poisoning.* New York, Elsevier, 1988.

Gleason MN, et al: *Clinical Toxicology of Commercial Products*, ed 5. Baltimore, Williams & Wilkins, 1984.

Goldfrank LR, et al: *Toxicologic Emergencies,* ed 3. New York, Appleton-Century-Crofts, 1986.

Haddad LM, Winchester JF: *Clinical Management of Poisoning and Drug Overdose*, ed 2. Philadelphia, WB Saunders, 1990.

Klaassen CD, et al (eds): *Casarett and Doull's Toxicology: The Basic Science of Poisons,* ed 3. New York, Macmillan, 1986.

Rumack BH, et al (eds): *POISINDEX®*: A Microfiche emergency poison management system. Denver, Micromedex, Inc (issued quarterly).

Charcoal, Induced Emesis, Lavage, Urinary pH, Dialysis

Albertson TE, et al: Superiority of activated charcoal alone compared with ipecac and activated charcoal in the treatment of acute toxic ingestions. *Ann Emerg Med* 18:56-59, 1989.

Banner W Jr, Veltri JC: Case for ipecac syrup. *Am J Dis Child* 142:596, 1988.

Cooney DO: *Activated Charcoal: Antidotal and Other Medical Uses.* New York, Marcel Dekker, 1980.

Cooney DO, Kane RP: "Superactive" charcoal adsorbs drugs as fast as standard antidotal charcoal. *Clin Toxicol* 16:123-125, 1980.

Cutler RE, et al: Extracorporeal removal of drugs and poisons by hemodialysis and hemoperfusion. *Ann Rev Pharmacol Toxicol* 27:169-191, 1987.

Easom JM, Lovejoy FH Jr: Efficacy and safety of gastrointestinal decontamination in treatment of oral poisoning. *Pediatr Clin North Am* 26:827-836, 1979.

Harchelroad F, et al: Gastrointestinal transit times of a charcoal/sorbitol slurry in overdose patients. *Clin Toxicol* 27:91-99, 1989.

Jones JS, Dougherty J: Current status of plasmapheresis in toxicology. *Ann Emerg Med* 15:474-482, 1986.

Krenzelok EP, et al: Gastrointestinal transit times of cathartics combined with charcoal. *Ann Emerg Med* 14:1152-1155, 1985.

Kulig K, et al: Management of acutely poisoned patients without gastric emptying. *Ann Emerg Med* 14:562-567, 1985.

Lovejoy FH Jr: Is it time to abandon ipecac? *Pediatr Alert* 12:9-10, (Jan 29) 1987.

Mayersohn M, et al: Evaluation of charcoal-sorbitol mixture as antidote for oral aspirin overdose. *Clin Toxicol* 11:561-567, 1977.

McDougal CB, Maclean MA: Modifications in the technique of gastric lavage. *Ann Emerg Med* 10:514-517, 1981.

Neuvonen PJ: Clinical pharmacokinetics of oral activated charcoal in acute intoxications. *Clin Pharmacokinet* 7:465-489, 1982.

Neuvonen PJ, Olkkola KT: Oral activated charcoal in the treatment of intoxications: Role of single and repeated doses. *Med Toxicol* 3:33-58, 1988.

Park GD, et al: Expanded role of charcoal therapy in the poisoned and overdosed patient. *Arch Intern Med* 146:969-973, 1986.

Penn AS, et al: Drugs, coma, and myoglobinuria. *Neurology* 21:453, 1971.

Pond SM: Diuresis, dialysis, and hemoperfusion. *Emerg Med Clin North Am* 2:29-45, 1984.

Pond SM: Role of repeated oral doses of activated charcoal in clinical toxicology. *Med Toxicol* 1:3-11, 1986.

Rodgers GC Jr, Matyunas NJ: Gastrointestinal decontamination for acute poisoning. *Pediatr Clin North Am* 33:261-285, 1986.

Tenenbein M: Whole bowel irrigation as a gastrointestinal decontamination procedure after acute poisoning. *Med Toxicol* 3:77-84, 1988.

Van Ameyde KJ, Tenenbein M: Whole bowel irrigation during pregnancy. *Am J Obstet Gynecol* 160:646-647, 1989.

Metal Antagonists

Aposhian HV, et al: Urinary excretion of meso-2,3-dimercaptosuccinic acid in human subjects. *Clin Pharmacol Ther* 45:520-526, 1989.

Bene C, et al: Irreversible ocular toxicity from single "challenge" dose of deferoxamine. *Clin Nephrol* 31:45-48, 1989.

Campbell JR, et al: Therapeutic use of 2,3-dimercaptopropane-1-sulfonate in two cases of inorganic mercury poisoning. *JAMA* 256:3127-3130, 1986.

Catsch A, Harmuth-Hoene AE: Pharmacology and therapeutic applications of agents used in heavy metal poisoning, in Levine WG (ed): *International Encyclopedia of Pharmacology and Therapeutics, Section 70, Chelation of Heavy Metals.* Oxford, Pergamon Press, 1979, 107-224.

Centers for Disease Control: *Preventing Lead Poisoning in Young Children.* Atlanta, Department of Health and Human Services, (Jan) 1991.

Chisolm JJ Jr: Use of chelating agents in treatment of acute and chronic lead intoxication in childhood. *J Pediatr* 73:1-38, 1968.

Daly AL, et al: Mucormycosis: Association with deferoxamine therapy. *Am J Med* 87:468-471, 1989.

de Virgiliis S, et al: Deferoxamine-induced growth retardation in patients with thalassemia major. *J Pediatr* 113:661-669, 1988.

Eggleston AM: Comment: Deferoxamine-induced sepsis, letter. *DICP* 21:835-836, 1987.

Engle JP, et al: Acute iron intoxication: Treatment controversies. *DICP* 21:153-159, 1987.

Epstein O, et al: Reduction of immune complexes and immunoglobulins induced by D-penicillamine in primary biliary cirrhosis. *N Engl J Med* 300:274-278, 1979.

Fleming CR, et al: Asymptomatic primary biliary cirrhosis: Presentation, histology, and results with D-penicillamine. *Mayo Clin Proc* 53:587-593, 1978.

Fournier L, et al: 2,3-dimercaptosuccinic acid treatment of heavy metal poisoning in humans. *Med Toxicol* 3:499-504, 1988.

Freedman MH, et al: Neurotoxicity associated with deferoxamine therapy. *Toxicology* 49:283-290, 1988.

Gallant T, et al: Yersinia sepsis in patients with iron overload treated with deferoxamine, letter. *N Engl J Med* 314:1643, 1986.

Gomez RA, et al: Deferoxamine for the treatment of hemosiderosis during CAPD. *Int J Pediatr Nephrol* 8:21-24, 1987.

Graziano JH, et al: Dose-response study of oral 2, 3-dimercaptosuccinic acid in children with elevated blood lead concentration. *J Pediatr* 113:751-757, 1988.

Halliday JW, Bassett ML: Treatment of iron storage disorders. *Drugs* 20:207-215, 1980.

Hood SA, et al: Successful treatment of dialysis osteomalacia and dementia, using desferrioxamine infusions and oral 1-alpha hydroxycholecalciferol. *Am J Nephrol* 4:369-374, 1984.

Jain S, et al: Controlled trial of D-penicillamine therapy in primary biliary cirrhosis. *Lancet* 1:831-834, 1977.

Klaassen CD: Heavy metals and heavy-metal antagonists, in Gilman AG, et al (eds): *The Pharmacological Basis of Therapeutics*, ed 7. New York, Macmillan, 1985, 1605-1627.

Koren G, et al: Acute changes in renal function associated with deferoxamine therapy. *Am J Dis Child* 143:1077-1080, 1989.

Krenzelok EP, Hoff JV: Accidental childhood iron poisoning: Problem of marketing and labeling. *Pediatrics* 63:591-596, 1979.

Lacouture PG, et al: Emergency assessment of severity in iron overdose by clinical and laboratory methods. *J Pediatr* 99:89-91, 1981.

Maiorino RM, et al: Determination and metabolism of dithiol chelating agents: VI, Isolation and identification of the mixed disulfides of *meso*-2,3-dimercaptosuccinic acid with L-cysteine in human urine. *Toxicol Appl Pharmacol* 97:338-349, 1989.

Malluche HH, et al: Use of deferoxamine in the management of aluminum accumulation in bone in patients with renal failure. *N Engl J Med* 311:140-144, 1984.

McCarthy JT, et al: Deferoxamine-enhanced fecal losses of aluminum and iron in a patient undergoing continuous ambulatory peritoneal dialysis. *Am J Med* 82:367-370, 1987.

Mossey RT, et al: Reduction in liver iron in hemodialysis patients with transfusional iron overload by deferoxamine mesylate. *Am J Kidney Dis* 12:40-44, 1988.

NCRPM (National Council on Radiation Protection and Measurements): *Management of Persons Accidentally Contaminated with Radionuclides.* Washington, NCRP Report 65, 1980.

Olivieri NF, et al: Visual and auditory neurotoxicity in patients receiving subcutaneous deferoxamine infusions. *N Engl J Med* 314:869-873, 1986.

Osterloh J, Becker CE: Pharmacokinetics of $CaNa_2EDTA$ and chelation of lead in renal failure. *Clin Pharmacol Ther* 40:686-693, 1986.

Peterson RG, Rumack BH: D-penicillamine therapy of acute arsenic poisoning. *J Pediatr* 91:661-666, 1977.

Pierides AM, Pierce Myli M: Therapy of aluminum overload (I). *Contr Nephrol* 38:65-77, 1984.

Piomelli S, et al: Management of childhood lead poisoning. *J Pediatr* 105:523-532, 1984.

Rumack BH, Peterson RG: Clinical toxicology, in Doull J, et al (eds): *Toxicology: The Basic Science of Poisons,* ed 2. New York, Macmillan, 1980, 677-698.

Seifert A, et al: Iron overload, but not treatment with desferrioxamine favours development of septicemia in patients on maintenance hemodialysis. *Q J Med* 65(NS):1015-1024, 1987.

Shannon M, et al: Efficacy and toxicity of D-penicillamine in low-level lead poisoning. *J Pediatr* 112:799-804, 1988.

Tenenbein M, et al: Myocardial failure and shock in iron poisoning. *Hum Toxicol* 7:281-284, 1988.

Tsuru N, et al: Recognition and management of aluminum intoxication in children. *Int J Pediatr Nephrol* 8:177-186, 1987.

Weatherall DJ, et al: Iron loading in thalassemia: Five years with the pump, editorial. *N Engl J Med* 308:456-458, 1983.

Wonke B, et al: Reversal of deferoxamine induced auditory neurotoxicity during treatment with Ca-DTPA. *Arch Dis Child* 64:77-82, 1989.

Young N, et al: Treatment of primary hemochromatosis with deferoxamine. *JAMA* 241:1152-1154, 1979.

Opioid Antagonists

Chiang CN, et al: Clinical evaluation of naltrexone sustained-release preparation. *Drug Alcohol Depend* 16:1-8, 1985.

Ginzburg HM, MacDonald MG: Role of naltrexone in the management of drug abuse. *Med Toxicol* 2:83-92, 1987.

Goldfrank LR, et al: Dosing nomogram for continuous infusion intravenous naloxone. *Ann Emerg Med* 15:566-570, 1986.

Hollister LE, et al: Aversive effects of naltrexone in subjects not dependent on opiates. *Drug Alcohol Depend* 8:37-41, 1981.

Johnstone RE, et al: Reversal of morphine anesthesia with naloxone. *Anesthesiology* 41:361-367, 1974.

Lovejoy FH Jr, et al: Management of propoxyphene poisoning. *J Pediatr* 85:98-100, 1974.

Mariani PJ: Seizure associated with low-dose naloxone, letter. *Am J Emerg Med* 7:127-129, 1989.

Martin WR: Naloxone. *Ann Intern Med* 85:765-768, 1976.

Meyer MC, et al: Bioequivalence, dose-proportionality, and pharmacokinetics of naltrexone after oral administration. *J Clin Psychiatry* 45(9, Sec 2):15-19, 1984.

Partridge BL, Ward CF: Pulmonary edema following low-dose naloxone administration. *Anesthesiology* 65:709-710, 1986.

Stile IL, et al: Pharmacokinetics of naloxone in the premature newborn. *Dev Pharmacol Ther* 10:454-459, 1987.

Verebey K, et al: Naltrexone: Disposition, metabolism and effects after acute and chronic dosing. *Clin Pharmacol Ther* 20:315-328, 1976.

Cyanide Antagonists

Arena JM: Cyanide, in Haddad LM, Winchester JF (eds): *Clinical Management of Poisoning and Drug Overdose.* Philadelphia, WB Saunders, 1983, 744-747.

Ballantyne B, Marrs TC (eds): *Clinical and Experimental Toxicology of Cyanides.* Bristol, United Kingdom, Wright, 1987.

Cottrell JE, et al: Prevention of nitroprusside-induced cyanide toxicity with hydroxocobalamin. *N Engl J Med* 298:809-811, 1978.

Graham DL, et al: Acute cyanide poisoning complicated by lactic acidosis and pulmonary edema. *Arch Intern Med* 137:1051-1055, 1977.

Hall AH: Cyanide poisoning: Dealing with an unexpected menace. *Emerg Med* 18:191-206, (Aug 15) 1986.

Hall AH, Rumack BH: Hydroxycobalamin/sodium thiosulfate as a cyanide antidote. *J Emerg Med* 5:115-121, 1987.

Sylvester DM, et al: Effects of thiosulfate on cyanide pharmacokinetics in dogs. *Toxicol Appl Pharmacol* 69:265-271, 1983.

Ten Eyck RP, et al: Stroma-free methemoglobin solution as antidote for cyanide poisoning: Preliminary study. *Clin Toxicol* 21:343-358, 1984.

Way JL, et al: Recent perspectives on toxicodynamic basis of cyanide antagonism. *Fund Appl Toxicol* 4:S231-S239, 1984.

Pralidoxime

Minton NA, Murray VSG: Review of organophosphate poisoning. *Med Toxicol* 3:350-375, 1988.

Murphy SD: Toxic effects of pesticides, in Klaassen CD, et al (eds): *Casarett and Doull's Toxicology: The Basic Science of Poisons,* ed 3. New York, Macmillan, 1986.

Thompson DF, et al: Therapeutic dosing of pralidoxime chloride. *DICP* 21:590-593, 1987.

Zwiener RJ, Ginsburg CM: Organophosphate and carbamate poisoning in infants and children. *Pediatrics* 81:121-126, 1988.

Methanol and Ethylene Glycol Poisoning

Baud FJ, et al: 4-Methylpyrazole may be an alternative to ethanol therapy for ethylene glycol intoxication in man. *Clin Toxicol* 24:463-483, 1987.

Baud FJ, et al: Treatment of ethylene glycol poisoning with intravenous 4-methylpyrazole. *N Engl J Med* 319:97-100, 1988.

Blomstrand R, Ingemansson SO: Studies on effect of 4-methylpyrazole on methanol poisoning using the monkey as animal model: With particular reference to ocular toxicity. *Drug Alcohol Depend* 13:343-355, 1984.

Jacobsen D, et al: Methanol and formate kinetics in late diagnosed methanol intoxication. *Med Toxicol* 3:418-423, 1988.

Noker PE, et al: Methanol toxicity: Treatment with folic acid and 5-formyl tetrahydrofolic acid. *Alcoholism Clin Exp Res* 4:378-383, 1980.

Peterson CD: Oral ethanol doses in patients with methanol poisoning. *Am J Hosp Pharm* 38:1024-1027, 1981.

Peterson CD, et al: Ethylene glycol poisoning: Pharmacokinetics during therapy with ethanol and hemodialysis. *N Engl J Med* 304:21-23, 1981 A.

Peterson CD, et al: Ethanol for ethylene glycol poisoning. *N Engl J Med* 304:977-978, 1981 B.

Swartz RD, et al: Epidemic methanol poisoning: Clinical and biochemical analysis of recent episode. *Medicine (Baltimore)* 60:373-382, 1981.

Orphan Drugs

5

ORPHAN DRUG ACT

Rare diseases have always been a problem for the medical profession because of the difficulty of diagnosis, the lack of treatment options, and, sometimes, the ethical considerations that may arise with regard to counseling about genetic advice and prognosis. Results of a survey (Department of Survey Design and Analysis, 1988 A, 1988 B) conducted for the National Commission on Orphan Diseases showed that more than 78% of the physicians queried reported seeing at least some patients with rare diseases, and it has been estimated that up to 10% of the population in the United States may be affected. The fact that there were few or no drugs commercially available for treatment of rare diseases was brought to the attention of Congress and, for the first time, the federal government, medical profession, academia, industry, private foundations, and organizations representing patients combined in a joint effort to facilitate the research, development, and marketing of such products. The following is an overview of the government's commitment to the development of orphan products and the roles that industry and the private sector have in facilitating that goal.

It is estimated that the majority of the approximately 5,000 rare diseases remain untreated since potentially useful products have not been developed. Often knowledge of the underlying pathophysiology or biochemistry of rare diseases is not sufficient to devise meaningful therapies. Furthermore, potential products for treatment of these diseases are usually of limited commercial value. The drug approval process has become more complex and costly because of regulations concerning the demonstration of a drug's safety and efficacy. In the case of orphan drugs, the situation is even more complicated because a chemical or biological may not be patentable, the number of patients requiring the drug is limited, and production costs may be enormous. In addition, evaluating effectiveness and assessing drug risk/benefit ratios in patients with rare diseases require interpretive adjustments in the drug approval process because of the small number of subjects available for statistical analysis.

In 1982, the Office of Orphan Products Development was established within the Food and Drug Administration, an agency of the Department of Health and Human Services (HHS). The Orphan Drug Act (Public Law 97–414) to encourage the development of drugs to treat rare diseases became law in January 1983 and was amended in 1984, 1985, and 1988. The Act defines an orphan drug as one used for the diagnosis, treatment, or prevention of a disease or condition affecting less than 200,000 people in the United States. If more than 200,000 people are affected, a drug has orphan status when the cost of developing and making it available would not be expected to be covered by sales in the United States. Application for an orphan designation must be made prior to filing a New Drug Application (NDA) or Product License Application (PLA). More than 400 products have been given orphan designations.

In addition to drugs and biologicals (including those used for in vivo diagnostic purposes), a study is under way to determine if recommendations should be made that special foods and medical devices be given an orphan designation.

Although the Orphan Drug Act was primarily designed to promote development of products by pharmaceutical companies, individual investigators or small laboratories also may act as sponsors. The Office of Orphan Products Development offers a grant program for orphan drug research in the area of clinical trials. The FDA reviews the proposed studies to determine whether they qualify the product for an Investigational New Drug (IND) or an Investigational Device Exemption (IDE) application. The grants are awarded for up to $100,000 per year for up to three years. A total of 120 grants have been funded, and 70 are currently active. Request for Applications (RFA) is published in the *Federal Register*. The Office of Orphan Product Development acts as an ombudsman for orphan products during the approval process. The FDA is required to give written protocol assistance, if requested, and to publish a list of designated orphan products. Sponsors are encouraged to design protocols that may permit patients to use orphan drugs for treatment while the products are under investigation.

The sponsor of a designated orphan drug that is the first to be approved for a specific rare disease or condition has seven years for exclusive marketing regardless of the patent status provided that there is assurance that sufficient quantities of the drug will be available to meet the needs of patients with the disease or condition for which the drug is approved. The sponsor may consent to the approval of other applications (eg, L-carnitine). As of January 1992, 60 orphan products have been approved for the treatment of 74 rare conditions. Tax incentives are included in the Act to encourage research and development (*Federal Register*, 1988). Companies have received $12 million in tax credits for clinical research on orphan products.

An Orphan Products Board chaired by the Assistant Secretary for Health of HHS and composed of representatives from those agencies within the Department and other governmental departments with activities relating to orphan drugs or devices has been established. The primary function of the Board is to promote the development of orphan products and to coordinate the activities of federal, public, and private agencies in achieving this goal.

In 1991, the Consortium on Rare Diseases (CORD) was formed under the auspices of the orphan Products Board. The members are representatives of organizations concerned about improving the health of people with rare diseases. This Consortium will not act as an advisory committee to the Board but will address rare disease issues that might be appropriately resolved by their various organizations.

The Orphan Drug Amendments of 1985 established the National Commission on Orphan Diseases to evaluate the research, development, and clinical activities of the National Institutes of Health; the Alcohol, Drug Abuse and Mental Health Administration; the Food and Drug Administration; other public agencies; and industry as they relate to rare diseases.

The final report of the Commission (US Department of Health and Human Services, 1989) was presented to Congress in 1989. The Commission concluded that the needs of patients with rare diseases are not being met adequately. The creation of a Central Office of Orphan and Rare Diseases was proposed. Among the responsibilities of this Office would be implementing the 54 recommendations of the Commission; responding to new needs and issues as they arise; collecting, developing, and disseminating information on rare diseases; subsuming the current responsibilities of the Orphan Products Board; and reporting to Congress on federal activities related to rare diseases.

Recommendations of the Commission concerning orphan product development included increasing incentives by (1) prolonging the period of exclusive marketing rights for the orphan indication; (2) extending tax credits to all developmental activities; (3) extending the patent on currently marketed products under certain conditions; (4) creating intellectual property protection for orphan biotechnology products not protected under the current Patent and Food, Drug and Cosmetic Acts; (5) seeking general solutions to liability issues as they apply to orphan products and the treatment of persons with rare diseases; and (6) amending the Orphan Drug Act to include devices and medical foods.

The Commission recommended that the FDA initiate an educational program for review personnel regarding problems unique to the development of products for rare diseases and that the agency should maintain flexibility with respect to regulatory requirements for protocol design and the numbers and kinds of preclinical and clinical studies needed. In addition to increased FDA funding for more review personnel, the approval process could be expedited by classifying all orphan products as 1A and eligible for a treatment IND or an open protocol. Sponsors should be encouraged to develop draft labeling and seek early inspection of manufacturing facilities. The addition of new rare disease indications to the labeling of appropriate marketed products should be encouraged.

Congress became concerned over what they perceived as abuses of the Orphan Drug Act by some companies. The proposed Orphan Drug Act Amendments of 1990 would have limited marketing exclusivity if the patient population of a previously designated rare disease or condition exceeded 200,000 and would have permitted shared exclusivity for products developed simultaneously. The proposed amendments also followed the recommendations of the National Commission in creating an Office for Orphan Conditions and Diseases in the Office of the Assistant Secretary of Health and Human Services to replace the Orphan Products Board. This bill was not signed by President Bush (Asbury, 1991). New legislation will probably be introduced during the current congressional session.

Since 1983 the Orphan Drug Act and its amendments have been implemented by existing administrative practices with no formal regulations adopted. The FDA has now published the Orphan Drug Regulations; Proposed Rule 21 CFR part 316 (*Federal Register*, 1991). The most controversial section is concerned with the criteria that would be used to determine whether one drug is the same as another with respect to orphan-drug exclusive marketing. In the past, when there was any difference in the chemical structure of a drug's active moiety (other than salts or esters), the drug was classified as a new chemical entity. This distinction was satisfactory as it applied to small molecules. However, for macromolecules, slight differences may not affect the pharmacologic activity or the active site may be only a small part of the molecule; clearly some other criteria would be needed. The following four prossible criteria are suggested by the FDA:

(1) Two drugs would be considered different if they had any defined structural difference (other than being different salts or esters of the same active moiety), such as a different amino acid sequence or glycosylation pattern, or if they had heterogeneous structures (eg, a polysaccharide with an array of molecules having different numbers of the same repeating saccharide unit and various different chain lengths) or, for other reasons, had a structure that could not be precisely defined.

(2) Two drugs would be considered different if they could be shown to have a defined structural difference, as noted above. However, they would not be considered different simply because of uncertainty about their precise structure or because the drugs are somewhat indeterminate mixtures. For example, two polypeptide or protein molecules that had the same primary, secondary, and tertiary structures, insofar as could be determined, or had uncertain or mixed chemical structures that could not be distinguished, would be considered the same drug unless the subsequent drug could be shown to be clinically superior.

(3) Two drugs would be considered the same drug if the principal, but not necessarily all, structural features of the two drugs were the same unless the subsequent drug were shown to be clinically superior. This criterion would apply as follows to different kinds of macromolecules:

(a) Two protein drugs would be considered the same if the only difference between them was due to post-transitional events; infidelity of transcription or translation; or minor differences in amino acid sequence. Other potentially important differences, such as different glycosylation patterns or different tertiary structures, would not cause the drugs to be considered different unless the subsequent drug were shown to be clinically superior.

(b) Two polysaccharide drugs would be considered the same if they had identical saccharide repeating units, even if the number of units were to vary and even if there were post-polymerization modifications, unless the subsequent drug were shown to be clinically superior.

(c) Two polynucleotide drugs consisting of two or more distinct nucleotides would be considered the same if they had an identical sequence of purine and pyrimidine bases (or their derivatives) bound to an identical sugar backbone (ribose, oxyribose, or modifications of these sugars) unless the subsequent drug were shown to be clinically superior.

(d) Closely related complex partly definable drugs with similar therapeutic intent, such as two live viral vaccines for the same indication or some other traditional biological, would be considered the same unless the subsequent drug were shown to be clinically superior or to depend on different mechanisms of action.

(4) Two similar macromolecules would be considered the same unless their structures differed in ways that could reasonably be expected to influence relevant pharmacologic activity. Other structural differences would not cause the second drug to be considered a different drug unless the subsequent drug were shown to be clinically superior.

Clinical superiority could be considered if a drug were more effective, safer, or made a major contribution to patient care. Effectiveness would be determined by direct comparative clinical trials with the approved orphan drug. Safety would be demonstrated by the second drug having fewer side effects or less severe adverse reactions. An example of a major contribution to patient care would be an effective oral preparation when the original drug could be given only parenterally. The FDA has not been charged with making decisions on the approval of drugs based on cost; therefore, the agency will rule out cost considerations in determining a contribution to patient care. This is unfortunate in the current era of medical cost containment efforts by Congress.

Other Programs Supporting Orphan Drug Development

In addition to the Orphan Drug Act, the Federal Technology Transfer Act of 1986 (Public Law 99-502) allows for commercial development of products originating in U.S. government laboratories. The federal laboratories may enter into cooperative research and development agreements with state or local governments, business and industry, private profit and nonprofit foundations, and universities.

The Small Business Innovation Research (SBIR) program (Public Law 97–219) is designed to encourage for-profit small businesses (less than 500 employees) to develop products with the help of various governmental agencies. Examples of orphan products supported by SBIR funds are vaccines, lung surfactant, and diagnostic agents.

The pharmaceutical industry, represented by the Pharmaceutical Manufacturers Association (PMA) (202/835-3550), established a Commission on Drugs for Rare Diseases in 1981. This Commission invites proposals on drugs and devices for rare diseases from scientific investigators, voluntary and government health agencies, research institutions, and other interested persons. The proposals are screened and information on promising products or other research efforts is disseminated to prospective sponsors. The Pharmaceutical Manufacturers Association Foundation (202/835-3470) provides grant support in 11 different research areas, including the study of orphan diseases and product research. The Orphan Drug Institute of the Generic Pharmaceutical Industry Association (GPIA) (212/683-1881) was founded in 1982 to foster development of treatment for rare diseases and to secure sponsorship for orphan products among its membership. Other organizations interested in orphan products are the Association of Biotechnology Companies (202/234-3330) and the Orphan Developers Coalition (708/806-7680).

Sources of Information on Rare Diseases and Orphan Drugs

The Office of Orphan Product Development of FDA (301/443-4903) can provide information and guidance on applying for sponsorship of an orphan product or grant support for research on orphan products.

Questions concerning the Public Health Service Small Business Innovation Research Program should be directed to the SBIR Program Coordinator (301/496-1968).

The National Organization for Rare Disorders (NORD) (203/746-6518) is a nonprofit organization created by a group of voluntary agencies, medical researchers in both academia and the pharmaceutical industry, and individuals concerned about rare disease and orphan drugs. NORD acts as a clearinghouse for current information on rare diseases. It provides patients and their families with accurate, comprehensible explanations of their condition and offers a networking program to link together people with the same disorder for mutual support. Assistance in forming new support groups and voluntary agencies also is available. A research program has been developed to award grants to scientists performing research on new treatments for rare disorders.

In addition, physicians can obtain information on treatment and investigators or on centers involved in clinical research on specific diseases. A Physicians Guide to NORD Services is available. The NORD Services Section available through the CompuServe Electronic Information System provides the following information: (1) Rare Disease Data Base (name of disorder, synonyms, general description, symptomatology, etiology, affected population, related disorders, standard therapies, resources, and references). (2) Newsletters (publications from several national voluntary health agencies). (3) Information on more Prevalent Health Conditions. (4) Feedback Section (sending messages and questions to NORD). (5) Orphan Drug Data Base (orphan drugs, devices, or medical foods).

The National Information Center for Orphan Drugs and Rare Diseases (NICODARD) (800/456-3505), sponsored by the Office of Orphan Product Development and currently part of the Office of Disease Prevention and Health Promotion, provides physicians and pharmacist with orphan drug sponsors' names and telephone numbers. Questions from the public concerning diseases are referred to the appropriate voluntary support group or, where none exist, to NORD. When detailed information is requested, the caller is referred to the local medical library for a MedLine or CompuServe search.

The Metabolic Information Network (MIN) (800/945-2188) is an information resource and retrieval system for physicians and researchers interested in inborn errors of metabolism. Currently, the system covers ten disorders. As a separate initiative, a cross reference database contains information on an additional several hundred inborn errors of metabolism and has resulted in the development of a directory that identifies physicians by geographic area for any given disorder (for further information, see the chapter on Therapy for Inborn Errors of Metabolism).

The Pharmaceutical Manufacturers Association (202/835-3400) provides an information kit for researchers and potential sponsors of orphan drug research. The kit may be obtained by written request from the PMA Commission on Drugs for Rare Diseases, 1100 Fifteenth Street NW, Washington, DC 20005.

For further information on orphan product grants or ongoing research on rare diseases, the following agencies may be useful: Alcohol, Drug Abuse and Mental Health Administration (301/443-4797), National Institutes of Health (301/496-4000), and Centers for Disease Control (404/639-3311). State medical associations and local medical societies often can provide physicians with information on regional availability of patient support groups and research or treatment centers. The American Medical Association has a Division of Information Services (312/645-4818) that provides general information and makes referrals.

CLASSIFICATION OF ORPHAN DRUGS

Orphan drugs are organized in the Table according to therapeutic indication. Conditions that affect multiple systems (eg, AIDS, infections, cancer) appear first; those that affect single organ systems (eg, bone, eye, skin) follow. Drugs or biologicals used for diagnostic purposes and other nontherapeutic agents are not listed because they are not generally evaluated in this publication. Products that sponsors indicated are no longer actively being investigated also are not included in the Table. When the original sponsor is no longer involved in developing the product, the current sponsor, investigator, or agency is given. Drugs that are mentioned in other chapters are identified by a footnote.

DRUGS DESIGNATED FOR ORPHAN INDICATIONS

Drug/Biological	Sponsor[1] [Tradename]
AIDS AND AIDS-RELATED DISORDERS	
Acquired Immunodeficiency Syndrome (AIDS)	
aldesleukin[2] (interleukin-2)	Cetus Corporation [Proleukin]
CD4 (recombinant)[2]	Biogen Genentech, Inc.
CD4 recombinant human immunoglobulin G	Genentech, Inc.
CD4 human truncated 369 polypeptide	SmithKline Beecham

** Approved marketing rights*
1 See listing at end of table for address
2 Appears in another chapter; see index
3 Approved New Drug Application (NDA) for orphan indication
4 Compassionate Investigational Drug Application (CIND)
5 Treatment Investigational Drug Application (TIND)
6 Marketed for other indications

Drug/Biological	Sponsor[1] [Tradename]
dextran sulfate sodium[2] (UA 001)	Ueno Fine Chemicals Industry, Ltd.
diethyldithiocarbamate[2] (DTC)	Connaught Laboratories, Inc. [Imuthiol]
interferon beta[2]	Berlex Laboratories, Inc. [Betaseron]
poly I:poly $C_{12}U$	HEM Pharmaceuticals Corporation [Ampligen]
zalcitabine[2] (2′,3′-dideoxycytidine, DDC)	Hoffmann-LaRoche Inc. National Cancer Institute
zidovudine[2,3] (AZT)	Burroughs Wellcome Co.* [Retrovir]
AIDS-Related Complex (ARC)	
zidovudine[2,3] (AZT)	Burroughs Wellcome Co.* [Retrovir]
HIV Infection with CD4 Count Less Than 200 mm[3]	
human immunodeficiency immune gobulin	Abbott Laboratories
HIV Infection with CD4 Count Less Than 400 mm[3]	
human T-lymphotropic virus type III group 160 antigens	MicroGeneSys, Inc.
Anemia, Associated with Zidovudine Therapy	
epoetin alfa[2,3]	Ortho Biotech [Procrit] Amgen, Inc. [Epogen]
Anorexia, Cachexia, or Significant Weight Loss in AIDS Patients	
megestrol acetate[6]	Bristol-Myers Squibb U.S. [Megace]
oxandrolone	Gynex Pharmaceuticals, Inc. [Oxandrin]
sermorelin acetate (injection)	Serono Laboratories [Geref]
Anorexia and Weight Loss	
dronabinol[2,6]	Unimed, Inc. [Marinol]
Cytomegalovirus (CMV) Infection, Prevention and Treatment	
anti cytomegalovirus monoclonal antibodies	Biomedical Research Institute
Cytomegalovirus (CMV) Infections, Severe Retinitis	
ganciclovir[2,3] (DHPG)	Syntex (USA), Inc.* [Cytovene]
Leukopenia Secondary to Ganciclovir Therapy for Cytomegalovirus Retinitis	
filgrastim	Amgen, Inc. [Neupogen]
Diarrhea	
bovine colostrum	Donald H. Hastings, D.V.M.
lactobin	Roxane Laboratories, Inc.

Drug/Biological	Sponsor[1] [Tradename]
***Cryptosporidium parvum* Diarrhea**	
cryptosporidium hyperimmune bovine colostrum IgG	Immucell Corporation
Herpes Simplex Encephalitis	
PR-225 (redox acyclovir)	Pharmatec, Inc.
Kaposi's Sarcoma	
interferon alfa-nl[2]	Burroughs Wellcome Co. [Wellferon]
interferon alfa-2a[2,6]	Hoffmann-LaRoche Inc. [Roferon-A]
interferon alfa-2b[2,6]	Schering Corporation [Intron A]
interferon beta	Biogen, Inc. [r-IFN-beta]
Neurosyphilis	
PR-239 (redox penicillin G)	Pharmatec, Inc.
Neutropenia	
molgramostim (granulocyte macrophage colony stimulating factor [GM/CSF])	Schering Corporation [Leucomax]
***Pneumocystis carinii* Pneumonia**	
clindamycin[6]	Upjohn Company [Cleocin]
pentamidine isethionate[2,3]	Fujisawa Pharmacal Company* [Pentam 300]
piritrexim isethionate[2]	Burroughs Wellcome Co.
trimetrexate glucuronate[2,5]	U.S. Bioscience, Inc.
566C80	Burroughs Wellcome Co.
***Pneumocystis carinii* Pneumonia in High-Risk Patients, Prevention**	
clindamycin[6]	Upjohn Company [Cleocin]
dapsone	Jacobus Pharmaceutical Company
566C80	Burroughs Wellcome Co.
pentamidine isethionate[2,3] (inhalation)	Fisons Corporation [Pneumopent] Fujisawa Pharmaceutical Co. [NebuPent]
Toxoplasmosis	
poloxamer 331	CytRx Corporation [Protox]

Drug/Biological	Sponsor[1] [Tradename]
CANCER	
Carcinomas	
Adrenal Cortex	
gossypol	Marcus M. Reidenberg, M.D.
Breast, Metastatic	
6-methylenenandrista-1,4-diene-3,17-dione	Adria Laboratories, Inc.
toremifene	Adria Laboratories, Inc.
Cervix, Invasive	
interferon alfa-2b[2,6]	Schering Corporation [Intron A]
Colorectal, Advanced	
fluorouracil with interferon alfa-2a[2]	Hoffmann-LaRoche Inc.
Colorectal, Metastatic	
anti-TAP-72 immunotoxin	Xoma Corporation [XOMAZYME-791]
disaccharide tripeptide glycerol dipalmitoyl	ImmunoTherapeutics, Inc. [Immther]
leucovorin adjunct with fluorouracil[2,3]	Burroughs Wellcome Co. Lederle Laboratories*
levoleucovorin with fluorouracil	Lederle Laboratories [Isovorin]
trimetrexate glucuronate[2,5]	U.S. Bioscience, Inc.
Esophageal	
dihematoporphyrin esters	QLT Phototherapeutics, Inc. [Photofrin]
fluorouracil with interferon alfa-2a[2]	Hoffmann-LaRoche Inc.
Head and Neck, Metastatic (buccal cavity, pharynx, and larynx)	
trimetrexate glucuronate[2,5]	U.S. Bioscience, Inc.
Hepatocellular and Hepatoblastoma	
iodine I 131 murine monoclonal antibody to human alphafetoprotein	Immunomedics, Inc.
Lung, Small Cell	
anti-N901-bR (blocked ricin murine antibody)	ImmunoGen, Inc.
Lung, Advanced Nonsmall Cell	
trimetrexate glucuronate[2,5]	U.S. Bioscience, Inc.

Drug/Biological	Sponsor[1] [Tradename]
Melanoma, Cutaneous	
interferon beta	Biogen, Inc. [r-IFN-beta]
Melanoma, Metastatic	
amifostine (chemoprotection with cisplatin)[2]	U.S. Bioscience, Inc. [Ethyol]
interferon alfa-2a with teceleukin[2]	Hoffmann-LaRoche Inc.
teceleukin[2]	Hoffmann-LaRoche Inc.
Melanoma, Stage III	
antimelanoma antibody XMMME-001-RTA	Xoma Corporation
melanoma vaccine	RIBI Immunochem Research, Inc. [Melacine]
Ovarian	
amifostine (chemoprotection with cisplatin and cyclophosphamide)	U.S. Bioscience, Inc. [Ethyol]
BMS-181339	Bristol-Myers Squibb
oncoRad OV	Cytogen Corporation
Ovarian, Advanced	
altretamine[2,3] (hexamethylmelamine)	U.S. Bioscience, Inc.* [Hexalen]
Ovarian, Germ Cell	
interferon alfa-2b[2,6]	Schering Corporation [Intron A]
Pancreatic	
monoclonal antibody 17-1A	Centocor, Inc. [Panorex]
trimetrexate glucuronate	U.S. Bioscience, Inc.
Renal Cell	
poly I:poly $C_{12}U$	HEM Pharmaceuticals Corporation [Ampligen]
Renal Cell, Metastatic	
aldesleukin[2] (interleukin-2, IL-2)	Cetus Corporation [Proleukin]
interferon alfa-2a[2,6]	Hoffmann-LaRoche Inc. [Roferon-A]
interferon alfa-2a with teceleukin[2]	Hoffmann-LaRoche Inc.
interferon alfa-2b[2,6]	Schering Corporation [Intron A]

Drug/Biological	Sponsor[1] [Tradename]
interferon beta	Biogen, Inc. [r-IFN-beta]
teceleukin[2]	Hoffmann-LaRoche Inc.
Testicular	
ifosfamide[2,3]	Bristol-Myers Squibb U.S.* [Ifex]
Thyroid, Suppression of Thyroid Stimulating Hormone	
tiratricol with levothyroxine	Medgenix Group
Urinary Bladder, in situ	
interferon alfa-2b[2,6]	Schering Corporation [Intron A]
dihematoporphyrin ethers	QLT Phototherapeutics, Inc. [Photofrin]
Sarcomas	
Leukemias	
Acute (Unspecified)	
decitabine (5-AZA-2′-deoxycytidine, DAC)	Pharmachemie B.V.
Acute, Adult (Unspecified)	
amsacrine[2]	Warner-Lambert Company [Amsidyl]
B Cell	
iodine I 131 murine monoclonal antibody IGG2A to B cell	Immunomedics, Inc. [Immurait]
Hairy Cell	
2-chlorodeoxyadenosine[2]	R.W. Johnson Pharmaceutical Research
pentostatin[2,3]	Warner-Lambert Company*
Lymphoblastic, Acute (ALL)	
Erwinia L-asparaginase[2]	Porton Products, Ltd. [Erwinase]
pegaspargase[2] (PEG-L-asparaginase)	Enzon, Inc.
teniposide[2] (VM-26)	Bristol-Myers Squibb
Lymphocytic, B-cell	
anti-B4-bR (blocked ricin murine monoclonal antibody)	ImmunoGen, Inc.
Lymphocytic B-Cell, Ex Vivo Treatment of Autologus Bone Marrow	
anti-B4-bR	ImmunoGen, Inc.
Lymphocytic, Chronic	
2-chlorodeoxyadenosine[2]	R.W. Johnson Pharmaceutical Research

Drug/Biological	Sponsor[1] [Tradename]
fludarabine phosphate[2]	Berlex Laboratories, Inc.
molgramostim[2] (granulocytic macrophage colony stimulating factor [GM/CSF])	Schering Corporation [Leucomax]
pentostatin	Warner-Lambert Company
Myelogenous, Acute (AML, Acute Nonlymphocytic ANLL)	
2-chloro-2′-deoxy adenosine[2]	St. Jude Children's Hospital
idarubicin hydrochloride[2,3]	Adria Laboratories*
mitoxantrone hydrochloride[2,3]	Lederle Laboratories* [Novantrone]
Myelogenous, Acute, Adjunctive Therapy	
monoclonal antibody PM-81	Medarex, Inc.
Myelogenous, Acute, Pediatric	
idarubicin hydrochloride	Adria Laboratories
Myelogenous, Acute, Ex Vivo Treatment of Autologous Bone Marrow	
anti-My9-bR (blocked ricin murine monoclonal antibody)	ImmunoGen, Inc.
4-hydroperoxycyclo-phosphamide	Nova Pharmaceutical Corp. [Pergamid]
monoclonal antibodies PM-81 and AML-2-23	Medarex, Inc.
Myelogenous, Chronic (CML)	
interferon alfa-2a[2,6]	Hoffmann LaRoche Inc. [Roferon-A]
interferon alfa-2b[2,6]	Schering Corporation [Intron A]
Promyelocytic, Acute	
all-trans retinoic acid[2]	Hoffman-LaRoche Inc.
Lymphomas	
B-cell	
iodine I 131 Lym-1 monoclonal antibody	Lederle Laboratories
iodine I 131 murine monoclonal antibody IGG2A to B cell	Immunomedics, Inc. [Immurait]
monoclonal antibodies (murine or human) recognizing B-cell lymphoma idiotypes	IDEC Pharmaceutical Corp.
anti-B4-bR (blocked ricin murine monoclonal antibody)	ImmunoGen, Inc.
T-Cell, Cutaneous	
interferon beta	Biogen, Inc. [r-IFN-beta]

Drug/Biological	Sponsor[1] [Tradename]
Non-Hodgkin's	
fludarabine phosphate[2]	Berlex Laboratories, Inc.
prednimustine	Kabi Pharmacia, Inc. [Sterecyt]
Mycosis fungoides	
methotrexate with laurocapram	Whitby Research, Inc.
Osteogenic	
methotrexate sodium[3,6] with leucovorin	Lederle Laboratories*
methotrexate sodium with levoleucovorin	Lederle Laboratories
Soft Tissue and Bone	
ifosfamide[2,6]	Bristol-Myers Squibb U.S.* [Ifex]
Miscellaneous Cancers	
Alphafetoprotein-Producing Germ Cell	
iodine I 131 murine monoclonal antibody to human alphafeto-protein	Immunomedics, Inc.
Brain Tumors, Primary Malignant	
adenosine (adjunct to carmustine [BiCNU])	Medco Research, Inc.
diaziquone[2]	U.S. Bioscience, Inc.
interferon alfa-2b[2,6]	Schering Corporation [Intron A]
Serratia marcescens extract (ribosomes and vesicles)	Cell Technology [ImuVert]
Glioma, Recurrent Malignant	
carmustine, biodegradable polymer implant	Nova Pharmaceutical Co. [Gliadel]
Human Chorionic Gonadotropin (hCG)-Producing Tumors (eg, germ cell and trophoblastic cell tumors)	
iodine I 131 murine monoclonal antibody to hCG	Immunomedics, Inc.
Conditions Associated with Malignancy	
Bone Resorbtion, Increased	
disodium clodronate tetrahydrate	Leiras, Oy [Bonefos]
Hypercalcemia	
etidronate disodium[2] (intravenous)	MGI Pharma, Inc. [Didronel IV]
gallium nitrate[2,3]	Fujisawa Pharmaceutical Co. [Ganite]
Neutropenia, Secondary to Hairy Cell Leukemia	
molgramostim (granulocytic macrophage colony stimulating factor [GM/CSF])	Schering Corporation [Leucomax]
Thrombocytosis in Chronic Myelogenous Leukemia	
anagrelide[2]	Roberts Pharmaceutical Corp. [Agrelin]
Conditions Induced by Antineoplastic Agents	
Chemoprotection	
amifostine (ovarian with cisplatin and cyclophosphamide) (melanoma, metastatic with cisplatin)	U.S. Bioscience, Inc. [Ethyol]
Cytoprotection	
adenosine (brain tumors with BCNU)	Medco Research, Inc.
Prevention of Cardiomyopathy	
dexrazoxane (with doxorubicin therapy)	Adria Laboratories
Rescue with Antifolate Therapy	
leucovorin calcium[2] (osteosarcoma with methotrexate)[2,3]	Lederle Laboratories*
Inhibition of Urotoxic Effects	
mesna (with ifosfamide)[2,3]	Degussa Corporation* distributed by Bristol-Myers Squibb U.S. [Mesnex]
Conditions Associated with Bone Marrow Transplant	
ABO Incompatability	
trisaccharides A and B	CHEMBIOMED, Ltd.
Cytomegalovirus Infections	
cytomegalovirus immune globulin IV with ganciclovir	Cutter Biological/Miles
ganciclovir	Syntex (USA), Inc. [Cytovene]
IgM monoclonal antibody (C-58) to cytomegalovirus	Centocor, Inc. [Centovir]

Drug/Biological	Sponsor[1] [Tradename]
Graft vs Host Disease and Transplant Rejection	
CD5-T lymphocyte immunotoxin	Xoma Corporation [XOMAZYME-CD5 Plus]
ST1-RTA immunotoxin (SR-44163)	Sanofi Pharmaceuticals, Inc.
thalidomide	Andrulis Research Corporation Pediatric Pharmaceuticals
Neutropenia	
filgrastim (G/CSF)[2,6]	Amgen, Inc. [Neupogen]
molgramostim (granulocytic macrophage colony stimulating factor [GM/CSF])	Schering Corporation [Leucomax]
sargramostim[2,3] (GM/CSF)	Hoechst-Roussel* Pharmaceuticals Inc. [Prokine]
	Immunex Corporation [Leukine]*
Oral Mucositis Associated with Cytoreductive Therapy	
sulcralfate	Naska Pharmacal Company
Conditions Associated with Radiation of the Head and Neck	
Xerostomia	
pilocarpine hydrochloride (oral)	MGI Pharma, Inc. [Salogen]

GENETIC DISEASES AND DISORDERS

Drug/Biological	Sponsor[1] [Tradename]
Enzyme Deficiencies	
Alpha$_1$ - Antitrypsin Deficiency in ZZ Phenotype Population	
recombinant secretory leucocyte protease inhibitor	Synergen, Inc.
Alpha$_1$ - Proteinase Inhibitor Deficiency (Pulmonary Emphysema)	
alpha$_1$ - proteinase inhibitor[2,3]	Cutter Biological/Miles* [Prolastin]
Alpha$_1$ - Proteinase Inhibitor Deficiency	
alpha$_1$ - proteinase[6] inhibitor	Cutter Biological/Miles [Prolastin]
Carnitine Deficiency	
levocarnitine[2,3] (L-carnitine)	McGaw, Inc.* [VitaCarn] Sigma Tau Pharmaceuticals, Inc.* [Carnitor]
Fabry's Disease	
alpha-galactosidase A[2]	David H. Calhoun, Ph.D. [CC-Glacosidase] Genzyme Corporation Robert J. Desnick, M.D., Ph.D. [FABRase]
Gaucher's Disease	
alglucerase[2,3] (glucocerebrosidase/beta-glucosidase)	Genzyme Corporation [Ceredase]
levcycloserine[2]	Meir Lev, Ph.D.
Immunodeficiency, Severe Combined (SCID)	
pegademase bovine[2,3] (PEG-ADA)	Enzon, Inc.* [Adagen]
Lactic Acidosis	
sodium dichloroacetate	Peter W. Stacpoole, M.D., Ph.D.
Urea Cycle Enzymopathy (Adjunct in Prevention and Treatment of Hyperammonemia)	
sodium benzoate/ sodium phenylacetate[2,3]	McGaw, Inc.* [Ucephan]
Disorders of Transport	
Cystinuria, Homozygous, Prevention of in Cystine Nephrolithiasis	
tiopronin[2,3]	Charles Y. C. Pak, M.D. Mission Pharmacal [Thiola]
succimer[2,6] (DMSA)	McNeil Consumer Products Co. [Chemet]
Cystinosis, Nephropathic	
cysteamine[2] (mercaptamine)	Jess G. Thoene, M.D. Warner-Lambert Company
phosphocysteamine[2]	Medea Research Laboratories, Inc.
Genetic Hematologic Disorders	
Antithrombin III (AT III) Deficiency (Prevention and Treatment of Thrombosis or Emboli)	
antithrombin III[2,3] (AT III)	Cutter Biological/Miles Hoechst-Roussel Pharmaceuticals, Inc. Hyland Division, Baxter Healthcare Corporation [Kybernin] Kabi Pharmacia, Inc.* [ATnativ] American National Red Cross

Drug/Biological	Sponsor[1] [Tradename]
Treatment of Surgical (Dental) Patients with Congenital Coagulopathies	
tranexamic acid[2,3]	Kabi Pharmacia, Inc.* [Cyklokapron]
Diamond Blackfan Anemia (Pure Red Cell Aplasia)	
interleukin 3 (human recombinant)	Immunex Corporation
Factor XIII Deficiency	
factor XIII[2]	Cutter Biological/Miles Hoechst-Roussel [Fibrogammin]
Hemophilia A and B	
factor VIIa (recombinant DNA)[2]	Novo Nordisk Biolabs, Inc.
Hemophilia A, Mild	
desmopressin acetate[2,6] (nasal spray)	Rhone-Poulenc Rorer [DDAVP Concentrate]
Hemophilia B	
coagulation factor IX (human)[2,3]	Alpha Therapeutics Corporation* [AlphaNine]
factor IX (monoclonal)	Armour Pharmaceutical Co.
Porphyria, Acute Intermittent; Porphyria Variegata; and Hereditary Coproporphyria	
hemin[2,3]	Abbott Laboratories* [Panhematin]
heme arginate	Leiras, Oy [Normosang]
histrelin	Karl E. Anderson, M.D.
Sickle Cell Anemia	
hydroxyurea[6]	Bristol-Myers Squibb [Hydrea]
Sickle Cell Disease Crisis	
BW 12C	Burroughs Wellcome Co.
cetiedil citrate	Baker Cummins Pharmaceuticals
lysine acetylsalicylate	G.D. Searle & Co. [Aspegic]
poloxamer 188	Burroughs Wellcome Co. [RheothRx]
von Willebrand's Disease	
factor VIIa (recombinant DNA origin)[2]	Novo Nordisk Biolabs, Inc.
desmopressin (nasal spray)	Rhone-Poulenc Rorer [DDAVP Concentrate]

Drug/Biological	Sponsor[1] [Tradename]
Miscellaneous Genetic Disorders	
Cystic Fibrosis	
amiloride HCl solution for inhalation	Glaxo, Inc.
dextran sulfate aerosolized	Thomas P. Kennedy, M.D. and J. Hoidal, M.D. [Aerodex]
recombinant human deoxyribonuclease	Genentech, Inc. [DNase]
recombinant secretory leucocyte protease inhibitor	Synergen, Inc.
Cystic Fibrosis, Prevention and Treatment of Pseudomonas aeruginosa	
immune globulin, pooled aerosolized	Pediatric Pharmaceuticals
mucoid exopolysaccharide pseudomonas hyperimmune globulin	Univax Biologics, Inc. [MEPIG]
Duchenne Muscular Dystrophy (DMD)	
mazindol	Platon J. Collipp, M.D. Sandoz [Sanorex]
Epidermolysis Bullosa, Oral Ulceration and Dysphagia	
sucralfate suspension	Naska Pharmacal Company
Friedreich's and Other Inherited Ataxias	
physostigmine salicylate[2,6]	Forest Pharmaceuticals, Inc. [Antilirium]
Hypercholesterolemia, Homozygous Familial	
sodium dichloroacetate	Peter W. Stacpoole, M.D., Ph.D.
Immunodeficiency, Primary	
aldesleukin	Cetus Corporation [Proleukin]
PEG interleukin-2	Cetus Corporation
Retinitis Pigmentosa	
gangliosides (as sodium salts)	Fidia Pharmaceutical Corp. [Cronassial]
Wilson's Disease	
trientine hydrochloride[2,3]	Merck Sharp & Dohme* [Syprine]
zinc acetate[2]	Lemmon Company

DISORDERS AFFECTING NEONATES

Drug/Biological	Sponsor[1] [Tradename]
Anemia of Prematurity, Treatment	
epoetin alfa[6]	Ortho Biotech [Procrit]
Apnea of Prematurity, Treatment	
caffeine[2]	Pediatric Pharmaceuticals

Drug/Biological	Sponsor[1] [Tradename]
Bronchopulmonary Dysplasia in Premature Neonates (<1500 g)	
recombinant human superoxide dismutase	Bio-Technology General Corporation
Hemolytic Disease Caused by Placental Transfer of Antibodies Against Blood Group Substances A and B	
trisaccharides A and B	CHEMBIOMED, Ltd.
Hyperbilirubinemia Unresponsive to Phototherapy	
flumecinol	Farmacon, Inc. [Zixoryn]
Nutrition, Total Parenteral in Very Low-Birth-Weight Infants	
MVI neonatal formula	Armour Pharmaceuticals
Respiratory Distress Syndrome (RDS), Treatment and Prevention	
beractant[2,3] (modified bovine lung surfactant extract)	Ross Laboratories* [Survanta]
calf lung surfactant	ONY, Inc. [Infasurf]
colfosceril palmitate/cetyl alcohol/tyloxapol[2,3]	Burroughs Wellcome Co.* [Exosurf Neonatal]
surfactant (human) (amniotic fluid)	T. Allen Merritt, M.D. [Human Surf]
surfactant (human recombinant DNA)	California Biotechnology
surfactant (synthetic) dipalmitoylphosphatidylcholine [DPPC]/ phosphatidylglycerol [PG]	Britannia Pharmaceuticals, Ltd. [ALEC]
Respiratory Syncytial Virus, Prophylaxis and Treatment	
respiratory syncytial virus immune globulin	Medimmune, Inc. [Hyperimmune RSV]
immune globulin (pooled, aerosolized)	Pediatric Pharmaceuticals
Streptococcal Infection, Group B Disseminated	
group B streptococcal hyperimmune globulin	Univax Biologics, Inc.

INFECTIONS

Bacterial

Drug/Biological	Sponsor[1] [Tradename]
Acne Rosacea	
metronidazole (topical)[2,3]	Curatek Pharmaceuticals, Inc.* [MetroGel]
Anaerobic Decubitus Ulcers (Grade III and IV)	
metronidazole (topical)[2,6]	Curatek Pharmaceuticals, Inc. [MetroGel]
Clostridium botulinum (Infant Botulism)	
botulism immune globulin (human)	California Dept. of Health Services: SIDS-Infant Botulism Prevention Program
Clostridium difficile (Antibiotic-Associated Pseudomembranous Enterocolitis)	
bacitracin[2,6]	A.L. Laboratories, Inc. [Altracin]
Endotoxic Shock Secondary to Gram-Negative Bacteremia	
nebacumab (anti-J5mAb)	Centocor, Inc.
Neurosyphilis (AIDS-Associated)	
PR-239 (redox penicillin G)	Pharmatec, Inc.
Pseudomonas aeruginosa, Prevention and Treatment in Cystic Fibrosis Patients	
mucoid exopolysaccharide pseudomonas hyperimmune globulin	Univax Biologics, Inc. [MEPIG]
Streptococcal Neonatal Infection, Group B Disseminated	
group B streptococcal hyperimmune globulin	Univax Biologics, Inc. [Neogam]

Mycobacterial

Drug/Biological	Sponsor[1] [Tradename]
Leprosy	
clofazimine[2,3]	Ciba-Geigy Corporation* [Lamprene]
thalidomide[2]	Pediatric Pharmaceuticals
Mycobacterium avium-intracellulare infection	
gentamicin liposome injection (TLC G-65)	Liposome Company
piritrexim isethionate	Burroughs Wellcome Co.
rifabutin	Adria Laboratories
Tuberculosis	
aconiazide	Lincoln Diagnostics
rifampin (injection)[2,3]	Marion Merrell Dow, Inc.* [Rifadin I.V.]

Mycosis, Systemic

Drug/Biological	Sponsor[1] [Tradename]
Cryptococcal Meningitis	
amphotericin B lipid complex	Bristol-Myers Squibb

Protozoal

Drug/Biological	Sponsor[1] [Tradename]
Cryptosporidium parvum Diarrhea (AIDS-Associated)	
cryptosporidium hyperimmune bovine colostrum IgG	Immucell Corporation
Gambian Sleeping Sickness Produced by Trypanosoma brucei	
eflornithine hydrochloride[2,3] (DFMO)	Marion Merrell Dow, Inc.* [Ornidyl]

Drug/Biological	Sponsor[1] [Tradename]
Plasmodium falciparum Malaria, Chloroquine-Resistant	
mefloquine hydrochloride[2, 3]	Mepha, Ltd. [Mephaquin]
	Hoffmann-LaRoche Inc.* [Lariam]
Plasmodium falciparum, Acute and P. vivax Malaria, Prophylaxis	
mefloquine hydrochloride[2,3]	Hoffmann-LaRoche Inc.* [Lariam]
Plasmodium falciparum and P. virax Malaria, Treatment	
halofantrine	SmithKline Beecham [Halfan]
Pneumocystis carinii Pneumonia	
clindamycin[6]	Upjohn Company [Cleocin]
pentamidine isethionate[2,3]	Fujisawa Pharmacal Company* [Pentam 300]
piritrexim isethionate[2]	Burroughs Wellcome Co.
trimetrexate glucuronate[2,5]	U.S. Bioscience, Inc.
Pneumocystis carinii Pneumonia, Prevention in High-Risk Patients	
dapsone	Jacobus Pharmaceutical Company
pentamidine isethionate[2,3] (inhalation)	Fisons Corporation [Pneumopent]
	Fujisawa Pharmacal Company [NebuPent]
Toxoplasmosis	
piritrexim isethionate	Burroughs Wellcome Co.
Viral	
Cytomegalovirus (CMV) Infection in AIDS and Transplant Patients, Prevention and Treatment	
anti cytomegalovirus monoclonal antibodies	Biomedical Research Institute
SDZ MSL-109	Sandoz Pharmaceutical Corp.
Cytomegalovirus Infections, Severe	
ganciclovir[2,3] (DHPG)	Syntex (USA), Inc.* [Cytovene]
Hepatitis B, Acute	
interferon alfa-2b[6]	Schering Corporation [Intron A]
Hepatitis B, Chronic	
thymosin alpha 1	Alpha 1 Biomedical, Inc.
Hepatitis Delta, Chronic	
interferon alfa-2b	Schering Corporation [Intron A]

Drug/Biological	Sponsor[1] [Tradename]
Herpes Simplex Encephalitis in AIDS patients	
PR-225 (redox acyclovir)	Pharmatec, Inc.
Papillomavirus, Human (HPV) (Juvenile Laryngeal Papillomatosis, Condyloma Acuminatum)	
interferon alfa-nl[2]	Burroughs Wellcome Co. [Wellferon]
interferon alfa-2b[2,6]	Schering Corporation [Intron A]
Respiratory Syncytial Virus, Prophylaxis and Treatment	
respiratory syncytial virus immune globulin	Medimmune, Inc. [Hyperimmune RSV]
immune globulin, pooled aerosolized	Pediatric Pharmaceuticals

POISONING

Drug/Biological	Sponsor[1] [Tradename]
Acetaminophen Overdose	
acetylcysteine (intravenous)[2]	Apothecon [Mucomyst 10 IV]
Alcohols (methanol, ethylene glycol, 2-methoxyethanol, 2-butoxyethanol)	
fomepizole[2] (4-methylpyrazole)	Kenneth McMartin, Ph.D.
***Amanita phalloides* (Mushroom) Hepatotoxicity**	
disodium silibinin dihemisuccinate	Pharmaquest Corporation and Dr. Madaus, GmbH and Co. [Legalon]
Cardiac Glycoside Intoxication	
digoxin immune Fab (ovine)[2,3]	Burroughs-Wellcome Co.* [Digibind]
Envenomation by Rattlesnakes (Crotalidae)	
antivenin (Crotalidae) purified (avian)	Orphidian Pharmaceuticals, Inc.
Cyanide Poisoning, Severe Acute	
hydroxocobalamin/sodium thiosulfate[2]	Alan H. Hall, M.D.
Iron Poisoning, Acute	
dextran and deferoxamine	Biomedical Frontiers, Inc. [Bio-Rescue]
Lead Poisoning in Children	
succimer[2,3] (DMSA)	McNeil Consumer Products Co.* [Chemet]
Mercury Poisoning	
succimer[6] (DMSA)	McNeil Consumer Products Co. [Chemet]
Oral Drug Overdose	
cascara sagrada (fluid extract, injectable)	Intramed Corp.

Drug/Biological	Sponsor[1] [Tradename]
ADDICTION	
Pharmacotherapeutics in the Management of Opioid Dependence	
alphacetylmethadol (LAAM)[2]	National Institute on Drug Abuse
naltrexone hydrochloride[2,3]	Du Pont Merck Pharmaceutical Company* [Trexan]
ORGAN TRANSPLANT AND TRANSPLANT AIDS	
ABO-Incompatible Solid Organ Transplantation (kidney, heart, liver, and pancreas)	
trisaccharides A and B	CHEMBIOMED Ltd.
Cyclosporine-Induced Nephrotoxicity	
ketoconazole	Pharmedic Company [Nizoral]
Cytomegalovirus Infection in Immunosuppressed Recipients, Prevention or Attenuation	
cytomegalovirus immune globulin (human)[2,3]	Massachusetts Public Health Biologic Laboratories*
Cytomegalovirus Infection, Prevention and Treatment	
anti cytomegalovirus monoclonal antibodies	Biomedical Research Institute
SDZ MSL-109	Sandoz Pharmaceutical Corp.
Hepatitis B Reinfection Prophylaxis	
tuvirumab (human monoclonal antibody against hepatitis B virus)	Sandoz Research Institute
Organ Rejection	
CD-45 monoclonal antibodies	Baxter Healthcare Corporation
BONE DISORDERS	
Metabolic Bone Disease Secondary to Parenteral Nutrition, Prevention, and Treatment	
etidronate (intravenous)	MGI Pharma, Inc. [Didronel IV]
Paget's Disease (Osteitis Deformans)	
calcitonin (human)[2,3]	Ciba-Geigy Corporation* [Cibacalcin]
Osteomyelitis, Chronic	
gentamicin impregnated PMMA beads on surgical wire	E. Merck, Darmstadt
secalciferol	TAG Pharmaceuticals, Inc. c/o Lemmon Company

Drug/Biological	Sponsor[1] [Tradename]
CARDIAC DISORDERS	
Ventricular Fibrillation, Primary, Treatment and Prevention	
bethanidine sulfate	Medco Research, Inc.
Ventricular Tachyarrhythmias, Treatment and Prevention	
D,L-sotalol hydrochloride[2]	Bristol-Myers Squibb
Automatic Implantable Cardioverter Defibrilator Therapy, Adjunct to	
N-acetylprocainamide	Medco Research, Inc [NAPA]
ENDOCRINE DISORDERS	
Constitutional Delay of Growth and Puberty	
oxandrolone[5]	Gynex Pharmaceuticals, Inc. [Oxandrin]
testosterone (sublingual)	Gynex, Pharmaceuticals, Inc. [Androtest-SL]
Growth Failure	
human growth hormone releasing factor	Hoffmann-LaRoche Inc.
sermorelin acetate (GRF(1-29)NH_2)	Serono Laboratories, Inc. [Geref]
SK&F 110679	SmithKline Beecham
somatrem[2,3]	Genentech, Inc.* [Protropin]
somatropin[2,3]	Eli Lilly & Company* [Humatrope] Genentech, Inc. Novo Nordisk Pharmaceuticals, Inc. [Norditropin] Serono Laboratories, Inc. [Saizen]
Infertility (induction of ovulation)	
luteinizing hormone releasing hormone (GnRH)	Ortho Pharmaceutical Corp.
somatropin[2]	Novo Nordisk Pharmaceuticals, Inc. [Norditropin]
urifollitropin[2,3]	Serono Laboratories, Inc.* [Metrodin]
Myxedema Coma	
liothyronine sodium injection	SmithKline Beecham
Precocious Puberty	
histrelin[2]	Ortho Pharmaceutical Corp.
leuprolide acetate[2]	TAP Pharmaceuticals Inc. [Lupron injection]

Drug/Biological	Sponsor[1] [Tradename]
deslorelin[2]	Roberts Pharmaceutical Corp. [Somagard Injection]
nafarelin acetate[2,6]	Syntex (USA), Inc.
Turner's Syndrome	
ethinyl estradiol[2]	Gynex Pharmaceuticals, Inc. [Estrafem]
oxandrolone	Gynex Pharmaceuticals, Inc. [Oxandrin]
somatrem[2,6]	Genentech, Inc. [Protropin]
somatropin[2,6]	Genentech, Inc. Eli Lilly & Company [Humatrope] Novo Nordisk Pharmaceuticals, Inc. [Norditropin]

EYE DISORDERS

Drug/Biological	Sponsor[1] [Tradename]
Acceleration of Corneal Epithelial Regeneration and Healing of Stromal Tissue	
fibronectin[2] (human plasma)	Chiron Ophthalmics New York Blood Center
Blepharospasm, Essential	
botulinum F toxin	Porton Products, Ltd.
Corneal Erosion, Recurrent	
dehydrex	Holles Labs
Corneal Melting Syndromes	
cyclosporine 2% ophthalmic	Sandoz Pharmaceutical Corp. [Sandimmune]
Corneal Ulcers	
GM 6001	Glycomed, Inc.
Corneal Ulcers, Bacterial	
ofloxacin	Allergan, Inc.
Keratoconjunctivitis Sicca	
bromhexine	Boehringer Ingelheim Pharmaceuticals, Inc.
cyclosporine ophthalmic	Sandoz Research Institute [Sandimmune]
Keratoconjunctivitis, Vernal (VKC)	
cromolyn sodium[2,3] (4% ophthalmic solution)	Fisons Corporation* [Opticrom 4%]
levocabastine hydrochloride (0.05% ophthalmic solution)	Iolab Corporation
Mydriasis, Phenylephrine-Induced in Patients with Narrow Anterior Angles at Risk of Developing Acute Glaucoma	
moxisylyte (thymoxamine hydrochloride) (0.1% ophthalmic solution)	Iolab Corporation
Penetrating Keratoplasty, Graft Rejection	
cyclosporine 2% ophthalmic	Sandoz Pharmaceutical Corp. [Sandimmune]
Retinitis Pigmentosa	
gangliosides (as sodium salts)	Fidia Pharmaceutical Corp. [Cronassial]
Squamous Metaplasia of Ocular Surface Epithelia (Conjunctiva and/or Cornea) with Mucus Deficiency and Keratinization	
tretinoin[2]	Spectra Pharmaceutical Services, Inc.
Strabismus and Blepharospasm	
botulinum A toxin[2,3]	Allergan Pharmaceutical Corp.* [Oculinum] Porton International [Dysport]

HEMATOLOGIC DISORDERS

Drug/Biological	Sponsor[1] [Tradename]
ABO Incompatible Transfusion Reactions	
trisaccharides A and B	CHEMBIOMED, Ltd.
Anemia Associated with End Stage Renal Disease	
epoetin alfa[2,3]	Amgen, Inc.* [Epogen] Ortho Biotech [Procrit]
epoetin beta[2]	Chugai Pharmaceutical Co., Ltd. [Marogen]
Antithrombin III (AT III) Deficiency (Prevention and Treatment of Thrombosis or Emboli)	
antithrombin III[2,3] (AT III)	Cutter Biological/Miles Hoechst-Roussel Pharmaceuticals, Inc. [Kybernin] Hyland Division, Baxter Healthcare Corporation Kabi Pharmacia, Inc.* [ATnativ] American National Red Cross
Aplastic Anemia	
interleukin 1 alpha	Immunex Corporation
molgramostim (granulocytic macrophage colony stimulating factor [GM/CSF])	Schering Corporation [Leucomax]

Drug/Biological	Sponsor[1] [Tradename]
Diamond Blackfan Anemia (Pure Red Cell Aplasia)	
interleukin 3 (human recombinant)	Immunex Corporation
Congenital Coagulopathies, Treatment of Surgical (Dental) Patients	
tranexamic acid[2,3]	Kabi Pharmacia, Inc.* [Cyklokapron]
Factor XIII Deficiency	
factor XIII[2]	Hoechst-Roussel Pharmaceuticals, Inc. [Fibrogammin]
	Cutter Biological/Miles
Factor IX Deficiency	
coagulation factor IX (human)[2,3]	Alpha Therapeutic Corp. [AlphaNine]
factor IX (monoclonal)	Armour Pharmaceutical Co.
Hemophilia A, Mild	
desmopressin acetate (nasal spray)	Rhone-Poulenc Rorer [DDAVP Concentrate]
Hemophilia A and B	
factor VIIa (recombinant DNA)	Novo Nordisk Biolabs, Inc.
Heparin Replacement in Hemodialysis Patients at Increased Risk of Hemorrhage	
epoprostenol (prostacyclin, PGI_2, PGX)	Burroughs Wellcome Co. [Flolan]
Myelodysplastic Syndrome	
filgrastim[2,6] (recombinant granulocyte colony stimulating factor [G/CSF])	Amgen, Inc. [Neupogen]
molgramostim (granulocytic macrophage colony stimulating factor [GM-CSF])	Schering Corporation [Leucomax]
Neutropenia, Severe Chronic	
filgrastim (G/CSF)[2,6]	Amgen, Inc. [Neupogen]
Polycythemia Vera	
anagrelide[2]	Roberts Pharmaceutical Corp. [Agrelin]
Purpura, Thrombotic Thrombocytopenic	
defibrotide	Crinos International
Sickle Cell Anemia	
hydroxyurea[6]	Bristol-Myers Squibb [Hydrea]
Sickle Cell Disease Crisis	
BW 12C	Burroughs Wellcome Co.

Drug/Biological	Sponsor[1] [Tradename]
poloxamer 188	Burroughs Wellcome Co.
cetiedil citrate	Baker Cummins Pharmaceuticals
lysine acetylsalicylate	G.D. Searle & Co.
Thrombocythemia, Essential (ET)	
anagrelide[2]	Roberts Pharmaceutical Corp. [Agrelin]
Thrombocytopenia, Heparin-Associated	
iloprost	Berlex Laboratories
Thrombocytopenia Requiring Anticoagulation, Heparin-Induced	
ancrod	Knoll Parmaceuticals [Arvin]
Thrombocytosis	
anagrelide[2]	Roberts Pharmaceutical Corp. [Agrelin]
von Willebrand's Disease	
desmopressin acetate (nasal spray)	Rhone-Poulenc Rorer [DDAVP Concentrate]

GASTROINTESTINAL DISORDERS

Drug/Biological	Sponsor[1] [Tradename]
Biliary Cirrhosis, Primary	
ursodiol[6]	Ciba-Geigy Corporation [Actigall]
	Interfalk U.S., Inc. [Ursofalk]
Esophageal Varices	
ethanolamine oleate[3]	Block Drug Company* [Ethamolin]
sodium tetradecyl sulfate	Elkins-Sinn, Inc. [Sotradecol]
terlipressin	Ferring AB [Glypressin]
Fistulas, Secreting Enterocutaneous	
somatostatin	Ferring Laboratories, Inc. [Zecnil]
Gallstones	
chenodiol[2,3]	Solvay Pharmaceuticals* [Chenix]
monoctanoin[2,3]	Ethitek Pharmaceuticals Co.* [Moctanin]
Ulcerative Colitis, Mild to Moderate	
4-aminosalicylic acid	Warren L. Beeker, M.D.
Ulcerative Colitis, Active Phase, Left Side	
Short chain fatty acid solution	Richard Breuer, M.D.

Drug/Biological	Sponsor[1] [Tradename]
DISORDERS AFFECTING THE KIDNEY AND URINARY TRACT	
Calcium Renal Stone Formation and Uric Acid Nephrolithiasis, Prevention	
potassium citrate[2,3]	Charles Y.C. Pak, M.D. Mission Pharmacal Co.* [Urocit-K]
Calculii, Apatite and Struvite	
citric acid, gluco-delta-lactone, and magnesium carbonate[2,3]	United-Guardian, Inc.* [Renacidin]
Cystine Nephrolithiasis	
succimer[6] (DMSA)	McNeil Consumer Products Co. [Chemet]
tiopronin[2,3]	Charles Y.C. Pak, M.D. Mission Pharmacal Co.* [Thiola]
Cystitis, Interstitial	
nifedipine	Johnathan Fleischmann, M.D.
pentosan polysulfate sodium[2]	Baker Cummins Pharmaceuticals [Elmiron]
End Stage Renal Disease (ESRD)	
Anemia	
epoetin alfa[2,3]	Amgen, Inc.* [Epogen] Ortho Biotech [Procrit]
epoetin beta[2]	Chugai Pharmaceutical Co., Ltd. [Marogen]
Carnitine Deficiency	
levocarnitine[2,3] (L-carnitine)	McGaw, Inc.* [VitaCarn] Sigma Tau Pharmaceuticals, Inc.* [Carnitor]
Hyperphosphatemia	
calcium acetate[2,3]	Braintree Laboratories* [Phos-Lo] Pharmedic Company
calcium carbonate	R & D Laboratories [R & D Calcium Carbonate]
Growth Retardation Secondary to Chronic Renal Failure	
somatropin	Genentech, Inc.
NEUROLOGIC DISORDERS	
Amyotrophic Lateral Sclerosis (ALS)	
insulin-like growth factor-1, recombinant human	Cephalon, Inc. [Myotrophin]

Drug/Biological	Sponsor[1] [Tradename]
L-leucine, L-isoleucine, and L-valine[2]	Andreas Plaitakis, M.D.
L-threonine	Tyson & Associates [Threostat]
Blepharospasm, Essential	
botulinum F toxin	Porton Products, Ltd.
Cerebral Palsy, Dynamic Muscle Contraction in Pediatric Patients	
botulinum A toxin	Allergan Pharmaceuticals [Oculinum]
Encephalitis, Herpes Simplex in AIDS Patients	
PR-225 (redox acyclovir)	Pharmatec, Inc.
Epilepsy (Lennox-Gastaut Syndrome)	
felbamate	Wallace Laboratories
Epilepsy, Generalized Tonic-Clonic (GTC)	
antiepilepsirine	Philip Walson, M.D.
Status Epilepticus	
fosphenytoin	Warner-Lambert Company
PR-122 (redox phenytoin)	Pharmatec, Inc.
PR-320 (cyclodextran carbamazepine)	Pharmatec, Inc. [Molecusol carbamazepine]
Duchenne Muscular Dystrophy (DMD)	
mazindol[2]	Platon J. Collipp, M.D. Sandoz [Sanorex]
Friedreich's and Other Inherited Ataxias	
physostigmine salicylate[2,6]	Forest Pharmaceuticals, Inc. [Antilirium]
Lambert-Eaton Myasthenic Syndrome	
3,4-diaminopyridine	Jacobus Pharmaceutical Company Mayo Foundation [Dynamine]
Multiple Sclerosis	
4-aminopyridine[2]	Rush-Presbyterian-St. Luke's Medical Center Elan Pharmaceutical Research
chimeric M-T 412 (human murine IgG monoclonal anti-CD4)	Centocor, Inc.
copolymer 1[2] (COP 1)	TAG Pharmaceuticals, Inc. c/o Lemmon Company
interferon beta[2]	Berlex Laboratories, Inc. [Betaseron]
myelin	Autoimmune, Inc.

Drug/Biological	Sponsor[1] [Tradename]
Myoclonus	
piracetam	UCB Secteur Pharmaceutique [Nootropil]
Myoclonus, Postanoxic	
L-5-hydroxytryptophan[2] (L-5HTP)	Bolar Pharmaceutical Co., Inc.
Narcolepsy and Cataplexy	
sodium oxybate (sodium gamma hydroxybutyrate)	Sigma F and D Division, Ltd. Biocraft Laboratories, Inc.
viloxazine hydrochloride	Stuart Pharmaceuticals, ICI [Catatrol]
Neuroleptic Malignant Syndrome	
dantrolene sodium[2,6]	Norwich Eaton Pharmaceuticals, Inc. [Dantrium]
Neurosyphilis (AIDS-Associated)	
PR-239 (redox penicillin G)	Pharmatec, Inc.
Parkinson's Disease (Adjuvant to Levodopa or Levodopa/Carbidopa Treatment)	
selegiline hydrochloride[2,3] (deprenyl)	Somerset Pharmaceuticals* [Eldepryl]
Spasticity, Intractable, Caused by Multiple Sclerosis or Spinal Cord Injury	
baclofen (intrathecal)[2,5,6]	Medtronic, Inc. [Lioresal]
baclofen[6]	Infusaid, Inc.
L-baclofen	Mericon Industries, Inc. [Neuralgon]
Strabismus and Blepharospasm	
botulinum A toxin[2,3]	Allergan Pharmaceuticals* [Oculinum]
	Porton International [Dysport]
Torticollis, Spasmodic	
botulinum A toxin	Allergan Pharmaceuticals
Trigeminal Neuralgia	
L-baclofen	Gerhard H. Fromm, M.D.
SKIN DISORDERS	
Acne Rosacea	
metronidazole (topical)[2,3]	Curatek Pharmaceuticals, Inc.* [MetroGel]
Anaerobic Decubitus Ulcers (Grade III and IV)	
metronidazole (topical)[2,6]	Curatek Pharmaceuticals, Inc. [MetroGel]
Cutaneous Wound Healing in Burn Patients	
epidermal growth factor (human)	Ethicon, Inc.

Drug/Biological	Sponsor[1] [Tradename]
molgramostim (granulocyte macrophage colony stimulating factor [GM-CSF])	Schering Corporation [Leucomax]
poloxamer 188	Burroughs Wellcome Co. [Rheothrx]
Hydrofluric Acid Burns, Emergency Treatment	
calcium gluconate gel 2.5%	LTR Pharmaceuticals, Inc. [H-F Gel]
	Paddock Laboratories, Inc.
Prevention of Graft Loss on Burn Wounds	
mafenide acetate	Sterling Drugs, Inc. [Sulfamylon]
Dermatitis Herpetiformis	
sulfpyridine	Jacobus Pharmaceutical Company
Xeroderma Pigmentosum	
T4 endonuclease V, liposome encapsulated	Applied Genetics, Inc. [T4N5]
MISCELLANEOUS CONDITIONS	
Angioedema, Treatment and Prevention	
C1-inhibitor	Immuno Clinical Research Corp. [C1 inhibitor (human) vapor treated, IMMUNO]
Arthritis, Juvenile	
interleukin 1 receptor antagonist (human recombinant)	Synergen, Inc. [Antril]
Asthma, Severe, Requiring Steroid	
troleandomycin[6]	Stanley J. Szefler, M.D. Roerig [TAO]
Burn Patients, Nitrogen Retention	
somatropin	Serono Laboratories, Inc. [Saizen]
Granulomatous Disease, Chronic (CGD)	
interferon gamma-1b[3]	Genentech, Inc.* [Actimmune]
Hemorrhagic Fever with Renal Syndrome	
ribavirin[6]	ICN Pharmaceuticals, Inc. [Virazole]
Hirsutism	
cyproterone acetate	Berlex Laboratories [Cyproreron/Androcure]
Hypertension, Primary Pulmonary (PPH)	
epoprostenol[2] (prostacyclin, PGI_2, PGX)	Burroughs Wellcome Co. [Flolan]

Drug/Biological	Sponsor[1] [Tradename]
Hypotension, Idiopathic Orthostatic	
midodrine hydrochloride[2]	Roberts Pharmaceutical Corp. [Amatine]
Mastocytosis	
cromolyn sodium[3]	Fisons Corporation* [Gastrocrom]
Microsurgical Peripheral Nerve Repair, Adjunct	
leupeptin	Lawrence C. Hurst, M.D.
Pain	
clonidine hydrochloride (epidural)	Fujisawa Pharmaceutical Co.
morphine sulfate preservative-free[2] (epidural or intrathecal administration via microinfusion devices)	Elkins-Sinn, Inc. [Infumorph]
Raynaud's Phenomenon Secondary to Systemic Sclerosis	
iloprost	Berlex Laboratories
Reflex Sympathetic Dystrophy and Causalgia, Moderate to Severe	
guanethidine monosulfate[6]	Ciba-Geigy Corporation [Ismelin I.V.]
Vulvar Dystrophies	
testosterone propionate ointment 2%	Star Pharmaceuticals, Inc.

Sponsors

Abbott Laboratories, One Abbott Park Road, Abbott Park, IL 60064 (708/937-6100): *hemin; human immunodeficiency immune globulin.*

Adria Laboratories, Division of Erbamont, Inc., P.O. Box 16529, Columbus, OH 43216-6529 (614/764-8100): *dexrazoxane; idarubicin hydrochloride; rifambutin; 6-methylenenandrista-1,4-diene-3,17-dione; toremifene.*

A.L. Laboratories, Inc., 1 Executive Drive, P.O. Box 1399, Fort Lee, NJ 07024 (201/947-7774): *bacitracin.*

Allergan Pharmaceuticals, 2525 Dupont Drive, Irvine, CA 92715 (714/752-4500): *botulinum A toxin; ofloxacin.*

Alpha 1 Biomedical, Inc., 77 14th Street NW, Suite 400, Washington, DC 20005 (202/628-9898): *thymosin alpha 1.*

Alpha Therapeutic Corp., 5555 Valley Boulevard, Los Angeles, CA 90032 (213/225-2221): *coagulation factor IX.*

American National Red Cross, National Headquarters, 17th and E Street, NW, Washington, DC 20006 (Doris Menache-Aronson, M.D., 202/639-3009): *antithrombin III.*

Amgen, Inc., Amgen Center, 1900 Oak Terrace Lane, Thousand Oaks, CA 91320-1789 (805/499-5725): *epoetin alfa; filgrastim.*

Karl E. Anderson, M.D., University of Texas Medical School at Galveston, 301 University Boulevard, Galveston, TX 77550 (409/772-4661): *historelin.*

Andrulis Pharmaceuticals Corporation, 11800 Baltimore Avenue, Beltsville, MD 20705 (301/953-1003): *thalidomide.*

Apothecon, P.O. Box 4000, Princeton, NJ 08543-4000 (609/987-6800): *acetylcysteine (intravenous).*

Applied Genetics, Inc., 205 Buffalo Avenue, Freeport, NY 11520 (516/868-9026): *T4 endonuclease V.*

Armour Pharmaceutical Co., 500 Arcola Drive, P.O. Box 1200, Collegeville, PA 19426 (Garnett E. Bergman, M.D., 215/454-3756): *factor IX (monoclonal); MVI neonatal formula.*

Autoimmune, Inc., Reservoir Office Park, 822 Boylston Street, Chestnut Hill, MA 02167 (617/738-5538): *myelin.*

Baker Cummins Pharmaceuticals, 8800 NW 36 Street, Miami, FL 30178 (305/590-2200): *cetiedil citrate; pentosan polysulfate sodium.*

Baxter Healthcare Corporation, One Baxter Parkway, Deerfield, IL 60015-4633 (Dr. John Moran 708/270-5235): *CD-45 monoclonal antibodies.*

Warren L. Beeker, M.D., University of Vermont, Burlington, VT 05405 (802/656-3480): *4-aminosalicylic acid.*

Berlex Laboratories, Inc., 300 Fairfield Road, Wayne, NJ 07470 (201/694-4100): *cyproterone acetate; iloprost.* 1501 Harbor Bay Parkway, Alameda, CA 94501 (415/769-5200): *fludarabine phosphate; interferon beta.*

Biocraft Laboratories, Inc., 18-01 River Road, Fairlawn, NJ 07410 (201/703-0400): *sodium oxybate.*

Biogen Inc., Fourteen Cambridge Center, Cambridge, MA 02142 (Dr. John Alam 617/252-9721): *CD4 recombinant; interferon beta.*

Biomedical Frontiers, Inc., 1025 10th Avenue SE, Minneapolis, MN 55414 (612/378-0228): *dextran and deferoxamine.*

Biomedical Research Institute, 345 North Smith Avenue, St. Paul, MN 55102 (612/220-6900): *anticytomegalovirus monoclonal antibodies.*

Bio-Technology General Corporation, 1250 Broadway, 20th Floor, New York, NY 10001 (212/239-4050): *human recombinant superoxide dismutase.*

Block Drug Company, 257 Cornelison Avenue, Jersey City, NJ 07320 (201/434-3000): *ethanolamine oleate.*

Boehringer Ingelheim Pharmaceuticals, Inc., 90 East Ridge, P.O. Box 368, Ridgefield, CT 06877 (203/798-9988): *bromhexine.*

Bolar Pharmaceutical Co., Inc., 33 Ralph Avenue, Copiague, NY 11726 (516/842-8383): *L-5-hydroxytryptophan (L-5HTP).*

Braintree Laboratories, 60 Columbian Street, P.O. Box 361, Braintree, MA 02184 (617/843-2202): *calcium acetate.*

Richard Breuer, M.D., 2650 Ridge Avenue, Evanston, IL 60601 (708/869-5646): *short chain fatty acid solution.*

Bristol-Myers Squibb, Pharmaceutical Research Institute, 5 Research Parkway, P.O. Box 5100, Wallingford, CT 06492 (203/284-6000): *amphotericin B lipid complex; BMS-181339; DL-sotalol hydrochloride; hydroxyurea; teniposide.*

Bristol-Myers Squibb U.S., Pharmaceutical Group, 2400 West Lloyd Expressway, Evansville, IN 47721-0001 (812/429-5000): *megestrol acetate: ifosfamide/mesna combination package.*

Britannia Pharmaceuticals, Ltd., Forum House, Brighton Road, Redhill, Surrey RH1 6YS U.K.: *surfactant (synthetic) dipalmitoylphosphatidylcholine (DPPC)/phosphatidylglycerol (PG).*

Burroughs Wellcome Co., 3030 Corwallis Road, Research Triangle Park, NC 27709 (919/248-3000): *BW 12C; colfosceril palmitate/cetyl alcohol/tyloxapol; digoxin immune Fab (ovine); epoprostenol (prostacyclin); interferon alfa-nl; leucovorin calcium; piritrexim isethionate; poloxamer 188; zidovudine (AZT); 566C80.*

David H. Calhoun, Ph.D., City College of New York Medical School, Department of Chemistry, Convent Avenue and 138th Street, New York, NY 10013 (212/650-6934): *glactosidase A.*

California Biotechnology, 2450 Bayshore Pkwy., Mountain View, CA 94043 (415/966-1550): *surfactant (human, recombinant DNA).*

California Dept. of Health Services, SIDS-Infant Botulism Prevention Program, 2151 Berkeley Way, Berkeley, CA 94704 (Stephen S. Arnon, M.D., 415/540-2646): *botulism immune globulin (human).*

Cell Technology, 1668 Valtec Lane, Boulder, CO 80301 (303/443-8155): *Serratia marcescens extract.*

Centocor, Inc., 244 Great Valley Parkway, Malvern, PA 19355 (215/269-4488): *human IgM monoclonal antibody (C-58) to cytomegalovirus; chimeric M-T412 (human murine) IgG monoclonal anti-CD4; monoclonal antibody 17-1A; nebacumab (anti-J5mA6).*

Cephalon, Inc., 145 Brandywine Parkway, West Chester, PA 19380 (215/344-0200): *insulin-like growth factor-1, recombinant human.*

Cetus Corporation, 1400 Fifty-third Street, Emeryville, CA 94608 (415/420-3300): *aldesleukin (interleukin-2); PEG interleukin-2.*

CHEMBIOMED, Ltd., P.O. Box 8050, Edmonton, Alberta, Canada, T6H4N9 (403/450-6800): *trisaccharides A and B.*

Chiron Ophthalmics, 9342 Jeronimo Road, Irvine, CA 92718-9925 (714/768-4690): *fibronectin.*

Chugai Pharmaceutical Co., Ltd., C/O Chugai Pharma, U.S.A., Inc., 520 Madison Avenue, New York, NY 10022 (212/486-7780): *epoetin beta.*

Ciba-Geigy Corporation, Pharmaceuticals Division, 556 Morris Avenue, Summit, NJ 07901 (201/277-5753): *calcitonin (human); clofazimine; guanethidine monosulfate; ursodiol.*

Platon J. Collipp, M.D., 176 Memorial Drive, Jesup, GA 31545 (912/427-9378): *mazindol.*

Connaught Laboratories, Inc., Route 611, Swiftwater, PA 18370 (717/839-4340): *diethyldithiocarbamate (DTC).*

Crinos International, Via Belvedere 1., 22079 Villa Guardia, (Como), Italy: *defibrotide.*

Curatek Pharmaceuticals, Inc., 1965 Pratt Blvd., Elk Grove Village, IL 60007 (708/806-7680): *metronidazole.*

Cutter Biological/Miles, P.O. Box 1986, Berkeley, CA 94701 (415/420-5000): *alpha$_1$-proteinase inhibitor* (see Miles Pharmaceuticals): *antithrombin III (AT-III); cytomegalovirus immune globulin; factor XIII.*

Cytogen Corporation, 600 College Road East, Princeton, NJ 08540 (609/987-8000): *oncoRad OV.*

CytRx Corporation, 150 Technology Parkway, Norcross, GA 30092 (404/368-9500); *poloxmer 331.*

Degussa Corporation, 65 Challenger Road Ridgefield Park, NJ 07660 (201/641-6100): *mesna* (marketed by Bristol-Myers Squibb US).

Robert J. Desnick, M.D., Ph.D., Mount Sinai School of Medicine, New York, NY 10029-6574 (212/241-6944): *alpha galactosidase A.*

Du Pont Merck Pharmaceutical Company, E.I. du Pont de Nemours & Company (Inc.), Wilmington, DE 19898 (302/992-4714): *naltrexone hydrochloride.*

Elan Pharmaceutical Research, 1300 Gould Avenue, Gainsville, GA 30501 (404/534-8239): *4-aminopyridine.*

Elkins-Sinn., Inc., 2 Esterbrook Lane, Cherry Hill, NJ 08003-4099 (215/971-5539): *morphine sulfate preservative-free; sodium tetradecyl sulfate.*

Enzon, Inc., 40 Cragwood Road, South Plainfield, NJ 07080-2480 (201/668-1800): *pegademase (PEG/ADA); pegaspargase (PEG-L-asparaginase).*

Ethicon, Inc., Route 22, P.O. Box 151, Somerville, NJ 08876 (908/218-0707): *epidermal growth factor.*

Ethitek Pharmaceuticals, Inc., 7855-L Gross Point Road, Skokie, IL 60077 (708/675-6611): *monoctanoin.*

Farmacon, Inc., 90 Grove Street, Suite 109, Ridgefield, CT 06877 (203/438-7331): *flumecinol.*

Ferring AB, Soldattorspvagen 5, Box 30651, 200 62 Malmo, Sweden: *terlipressin.*

Ferring Laboratories, Inc., Montebello Park, 75 Montebello Road, Suffern, NY 10901 (914/368-2244): *somatostatin.*

Fidia Pharmaceutical Corp., 1775 K Street, NW, Suite 800, Washington, DC 20006 (202/466-7066): *gangliosides (as sodium salts).*

Fisons Corporation, 755 Jefferson Road, P.O. Box 1710, Rochester, NY 14603 (716/475-9000): *cromolyn sodium; cromolyn sodium (ophthalmic); pentamidine isethionate (inhalation).*

Johnathan Fleischmann, M.D., 3395 Scranton Road, Cleveland, OH 44109 (216/459-4257); *nifedipine.*

Forest Pharmaceuticals, Inc., 2510 Metro Boulevard, Maryland Heights, MO 64043-9979 (314/569-3610): *physostigmine salicylate.*

Gerhard H. Fromm, M.D., University of Pittsburgh, Pittsburgh, PA 15261 (412/648-9200): *L-baclofen.*

Fujisawa Pharmaceutical Co., 3 Parkway North, Deerfield, IL 60015-2548 (708/317-8800): *Clonidine hydrochloride; gallium nitrate; pentamidine isethionate.*

Genentech, Inc., 460 Point San Bruno Blvd., South San Francisco, CA 94080 (415/266-1000): *CD4, recombinant; CD4 recombinant human immunogobulin G; interferon gamma-1b; recombinant human deoxyribonuclease; somatrem; somatropin.*

Genzyme Corporation, 1 Kendall Square, Cambridge, MA 02139-1562 (617/876-9405): *alglucerase; ceremide trihexosidase/alpha-galactosidase A.*

Glaxo, Inc., Five Moore Drive, Research Triangle Park, NC 27709 (919/248-2100): *amiloride hydrochloride solution for inhalation.*

Glycomed, Inc., 860 Atlantic Avenue, Alameda, CA 94501 (415/523-5555): *GM 6001.*

Gynex Pharmaceuticals, Inc., 1175 Corporate Woods Parkway, Vernon Hills, IL 60061 (708/913-1144): *ethinyl estradiol; oxandrolone; testosterone.*

Alan H. Hall, M.D. and Barry Rumack, M.D., Clinical Toxicology, 600 Grant Street, Denver, CO 80203-3527 (303/831-1400): *hydroxocobalamin/sodium thiosulfate.*

Donald H. Hastings, D.V.M., 1030 North Parkview Drive, Bismarck, ND 58501 (701/223-3036): *bovine colostrum.*

HEM Pharmaceuticals Corporation, One Penn Center, 1617 JFK Boulevard, Philadelphia, PA 19103 (215/988-0080): *poly I:poly $C_{12}U$.*

Hoechst-Roussel Pharmaceuticals Inc., Route 202-206 North, P.O. Box 2500, Somerville, NJ 08876-1258 (800/445-4774): *antithrombin III; factor XIII; sargramostim.*

Hoffmann-LaRoche Inc., 340 Kingsland Street, Nutley, NJ 07110 (201/235-2355): *fluorouracil; human growth hormone releasing factor; interferon alfa-2a; mefloquine hydrochloride; teceleukin, zalcitabine.*

Holles Labs, 30 Forest Notch, Cohasset, MA 02025 (617/383-0741): *dehydrex.*

Lawrence C. Hurst, M.D., Dept of Orthopaedics, S.U.N.Y. at Stoney Brook, H.S.C. T-18-080, Stoney Brook, NY 11794-8181 (516/444-3145): *leupeptin.*

Hyland Division, Baxter Healthcare Corporation, 444 West Glenoaks Boulevard, Glendale, CA 91202 (800/423-2090): *antithrombin III.*

ICN Pharmaceuticals, Inc., 3300 Hyland Avenue, Costa Mesa, CA 92626 (714/545-0100): *ribavirin.*

IDEC Pharmaceutical Corp., 219 North Bernardo Ave, Mountain View, CA 94043 (415/940-1200): *monoclonal antibodies recognizing B-cell lymphoma idiotypes.*

Immucell Corporation, 966 Riverside Street, Portland, ME 04103 (207/878-2770): *cryptosporidium hyperimmune bovine colostrum IgG.*

Immunex Corporation, 51 University Street, Seattle, WA 59840 (206/587-0430): *interleukin 1 alpha; interleukin 3; sargramostim (GM/CSF).*

Immuno Clinical Research Corp., 750 Lexington Avenue, New York, NY 10022 (212/759-3875): *C1-inhibitor.*

ImmunoGen, Inc., 148 Sidney Street, Cambridge, MA 02139 (617/661-9312): *anti-B4-bR (ricin blocked murine antibody); anti-My9-bR (ricin blocked murine antibody).*

Immunomedics, Inc., 150 Mt Bethel Rd., CN 4918, Warren, NJ 07060 (201/647-5400): *iodine I 131 murine monoclonal antibody to human alphafetoprotein; iodine I 131 murine monoclonal antibody to human chorionic gonadotropin; iodine I131 murine monoclonal antibody IGG2A to B cell.*

ImmunoTherapeutics, Inc., 3505 Riverview Circle, Moorhead, MN 56560-5560 (701/232-9575): *disaccharide tripeptide glycerol dipalmitoyl.*

Infusaid, Inc., 1400 Providence Highway, Norwood, MA 02062 (617/769-8330): *baclofen.*

Interfalk U.S., Inc., 25 Margaret Street, Plattsburgh, NY 12901 (518/563-7354): *ursodiol.*

Intramed Corp., 102 Tremont Way, Augusta, GA 30907 (404/863-2879): *cascara sagrada (injectable).*

Iolab Corporation, 500 Iolab Drive, Claremont, CA 91711 (714/624-2020): *levocabastine; moxisylate (thymoxamine hydrochloride).*

Jacobus Pharmaceutical Company, P.O. Box 5290, Princeton, NJ 08540 (609/921-7447): *dapsone; 3,4-diaminopyridine; sulfpyridine.*

R.W. Johnson Pharmaceutical Research, Route 202, P.O. Box 300, Raritan, NJ 08869-0602 (201/524-0400): *2-chlorodeoxyadenosine.*

Kabi Pharmacia, Inc., 800 Centennial Avenue, Piscataway, NJ 08855-1327 (201/457-8265): *prednimustine.* 160 Industrial Drive, Franklin, OH 45005 (513/743-6200): *antithromin III; predmustine; tranexamic acid.*

Thomas P. Kennedy, M.D. and J. Hoidal, M.D., 7702 Parham Road, Richmond, VA 23294 (804/346-1548): *dextran sulfate aerosolized.*

Knoll Pharmaceuticals, 30 North Jefferson Road, Whippany, NJ 07981 (201/887-8300): *ancrod.*

Lederle Laboratories Division, American Cyanamide Company, Pearl River, NY 10965 (914/735-2815): *fluorouracil; iodine I 131 Lym-1 monoclonal antibody; leucovorin calcium; levoleucovorin; methotrexate sodium; mitoxantrone hydrochloride.*

Leiras, Oy, P.O. Box 415, SF-20101 Turku, Finland: (358-21-63321) *disodium clondronate tetrahydrate; heme arginate.*

Lemmon Company, 650 Cathill Road, Sellersville, PA 18960 (215/723-5544): *zinc acetate.*

Meir Lev, Ph.D., City of New York Medical School, Convent Avenue and 138 Street, New York, NY 10013 (212/650-7788): *levcycloserine.*

Eli Lilly and Company, Lilly Corporate Center, Indianapolis, IN 46285 (317/276-5302): *somatropin.*

Lincoln Diagnostics, P.O. Box 1139, Decatur, IL 62525 (217/877-2531): *aconiazide.*

Liposome Company, One Research Way, Princeton, NJ 08540 (609/452-7060): *gentamicin liposome injection (TLC G-65).*

LTR Pharmaceuticals, Inc., 145 Sakonnet Boulevard, Narraganset, RI 02882 (401/789-1865): *calcium gluconate gel.*

Dr. Madaus, GmbH and Co., Ostmetheimer Str. 198, 5000 Koln 91, Federal Republic of Germany (0221-9898-451): *disodium silibinin dihemisuccinate.*

Marion Merrell Dow, Inc., Medical Information Department, P.O. Box 9627, Kansas City, MO 64134-0627 (800/633-1610): *eflornithine hydrochloride; rifampin injection.*

Massachusetts Public Health Biologic Laboratories, 305 South Street, Jamaica Plain, MA 02130 (617/522-3700, ext. 264): *cytomegalovirus immune globulin (human).*

Mayo Foundation, 200 S.W. First Street, Rochester, MN 55905 (Kathleen MacEvoy, M.D., 507/284-2511): *3,4-diaminopyridine.*

McGaw, Inc., P.O. Box 19791, Irvine, CA 92713-9791 (714/660-2000): *sodium benzoate/sodium phenylacetate; levocarnitine.*

Kenneth McMartin, Ph.D., Louisiana State University Medical Center, P.O. Box 33932, Shreveport, LA 71130-3932 (318/674-7871): *fomepizole (4-methylpyrazole).*

McNeil Consumer Products Co., Camp Hill Road, Fort Washington, PA 10934 (215/233-7000): *succimer (DMSA).*

Medarex, Inc., 12 Commerce Avenue, West Lebanon, NH 03784 (603/298-8456): *monoclonal antibodies PM-81 and AML-2-23.*

Medco Research, Inc., 8733 Beverly Blvd., Los Angeles, CA 90048 (213/854-1954): *adenosine; bethanidine sulfate; N-acetylprocainamide.*

Medea Research Laboratories, Inc., 200 Wilson Street, Building D-6, Port Jefferson, NY 11776 (516/331-7718): *phosphocysteamine.*

Medgenix Group, Rue du Moulin A Papier 51 Box 2, Brussels B-1160 EU: *tiratricol.*

Medimmune, Inc., 19 Firstfield Road, Gaithersburg, MD 20878 (301/590-2622): *respiratory syncytial virus immune globulin.*

Medtronic, Inc., 7000 Central Avenue, N.E., Minneapolis, MN 55432 (612/574-4925): *baclofen (intrathecal).*

Mepha AG, 4143 Dornach, Postfach 137, Aesch Basel, Switzerland (061-7014343): *mefloquine hydrochloride.*

E. Merck, Darmstadt, Frankfurterstrasse 250, 6100 Darmstadt, Germany: *gentamicin-impregnated PMMA beads on surgical wire.*

Merck Sharp & Dohme Research Laboratories, Division of Merck and Co., West Point, PA 19488 (215/661-5000): *trientine hydrochloride.*

Mericon Industries, Inc., 8819 Pioneer Road, Peoria, IL 61615 (309/693-2150): *L-baclofen.*

T. Allen Merritt, M.D., University of California, San Diego Medical Center, 225 W. Dickinson Street, 8774, San Diego, CA 92103 (619/543-3800): *surfactant human.*

MGI Pharma, Inc., 9900 Bren Road East, Suite 300 E, Minneapolis, MN 55343-9667 (612/935-7335): *etidronate disodium (intravenous); pilocarpine hydrochloride (oral).*

MicroGeneSys, Inc., 1000 Research Parkway, Meriden, CT 06450-7159 (203/686-0800; 800/541-8315): *human T-lymphotropic virus type III gp160 antigens.*

Miles Pharmaceuticals, 400 Morgan Lane, West Haven CT 06516 (800-Cutter-1): *alpha$_1$-proteinase inhibitor.*

Mission Pharmacal Co., 1325 E. Durango Street, P.O. Box 1676, San Antonio, TX 78296 (800/531-3333): *potassium citrate; tiopronin.*

Naska Pharmacal Company, Riverview Road, P.O. Box 898, Lincolnton, NC 28093 (704/735-5700): *sucralfate.*

National Cancer Institute, Division of Cancer Treatment, Bldg. 31., Room 3A49, National Institutes of Health, Bethesda, MD 20892 (301/496-6138): *zalcitabine.*

National Institute on Drug Abuse, 5600 Fishers Lane 10A-31, Rockville, MD 20852 (Frank Vocci, M.D., 301/443-6270): *alphacetylmethadol (LAAM).*

New York Blood Center, 310 East 67th Street, New York, NY 10021 (212/570-3418): *fibronectin.*

Norwich Eaton Pharmaceuticals, Inc., P.O. Box 191, Norwich, NY 13815 (607/335-2590): *dantrolene sodium.*

Nova Pharmaceutical Corporation, 6200 Freeport Centre, Baltimore, MD 21224-2788 (301/558-7000): *carmustine biodegradable polymer implant; 4-hydroperoxycyclophosphamide (4HC).*

Novo Nordisk Biolabs, Inc., 33 Turner Rd., Danbury, CT 06810-5101 (203/790-2600): *factor VIIa.*

Novo Nordisk Pharmaceuticals, Inc., 100 Overlook Center, Suite 200, Princeton, NJ 08540 (609/987-5800): *somatropin.*

ONY Inc., Baird Research Park, 1576 Sweet Home Road, Amherst, NY 14221 (716/636-9096): *calf lung surfactant.*

Ophidian Pharmaceuticals, Inc., 2800 South Fish Hatchery Road, Madison, WI 53701 (608/271-0878): *antivenin (Crotalidae) purified (avian).*

Ortho Biotech, Route 202, Box 300, Raritan, NJ 08869-0602 (908/218-6000): *epoetin alfa.*

Ortho Pharmaceutical Corp., Route 202, P.O. Box 300, Raritan, NJ 08869-0602 (908/218-6000): *histrelin; luteinizing hormone releasing hormone.*

Paddock Laboratories, Inc., 3101 Louisiana Avenue North, Minneapolis, MN 55427 (616/546-4676): *calcium gluconate gel 2.5%.*

Charles Y. C. Pak, M.D., The University of Texas, Health Science Center at Dallas, 5323 Harry Hines Blvd., Dallas, TX 75235 (214/688-3111): *potassium citrate; tiopronin.*

Pediatric Pharmaceuticals, 718 Bradford Avenue, Westfield, NJ 07090 (908/225-0989): *caffeine; immune globulin (pooled, aerosolized); thalidomide.*

Pharmachemie B.V., Swensweg 5, P.O. Box 552, 2003 RN Haarlem, Holland (023-154154): *decitabine (5-AZA-2'-deoxycytidine).*

Pharmaquest Corporation, 201 Tamal Vista Blvd., Corte Madera, CA 94925 (415/924-7122): *disodium silibinin dihemisuccinate.*

Pharmatec, Inc., P.O. Box 730, Alachua, FL 32615 (904/462-1210): *PR-122 (redox phenytoin), PR-225 (redox acyclovir), PR-239 (redox penicillin G), PR-320 (cyclodextran-carbamazepine).*

Pharmedic Company, 417 Harvester Court, Wheeling, IL 60090 (708/215-6603): *calcium acetate; ketoconazole.*

Andreas Plaitakis, M.D., Mount Sinai Medical Center, One Gustave Levy Place, New York, NY 10029 (212/241-4534): *L-leucine, L-isoleucine, and L-valine.*

Porton International, 816 Connecticut Avenue, N.W., Washington, DC 20006 (202/223-3737): *botulinum A toxin.*

Porton Products, Ltd., 30401 Agoura Road, Suite 102, Agoura Hills, CA 91301 (818/879-2200): *botulinum F toxin; Erwinia L-asparaginase.*

QLT Phototherapeutics, Inc., North Middletown Road, Pearl River, NY 10965 (K.A. Sutherland, M.D., 800/321-0339): *dihematoporphyrin esters.*

R & D Laboratories, Inc., 4204 Glencoe Avenue, Marina Del Rey, CA 90292 (213/305-8053): *calcium carbonate.*

Marcus M. Reidenberg, M.D., 1300 York Avenue, Box 70, New York, NY 10021 (212/746-6227): *gossypol.*

Rhone-Poulenc Rorer, 500 Arcola Drive, Collegeville, PA 19426-0107 (215/454-8000): *desmopressin acetate (nasal spray).*

RIBI Immunochem Research, Inc., 553 Old Corvallis Road, Hamilton, MT 59840 (406/363-6214): *melanoma vaccine.*

Roberts Pharmaceutical Corp., 6 Industrial Way West, Meridian Center III, Eatontown, NJ 07724 (908/389-1182): *anagrelide; deslorelin; midodrine hydrochloride.*

Ross Laboratories, Division of Abbott Laboratories, 625 Cleveland Avenue, Columbus, OH 43216 (614/227-3333): *beractant (surfactant TA).*

Roxane Laboratories, Inc., 1809 Wilson Road, P.O. Box 16532, Columbus, OH 43216 (614/276-4000): *lactobin.*

Rush-Presbyterian-St. Luke's Medical Center, 1753 West Congress Parkway, Chicago, IL 60612 (Dusan Stefonski, M.D., 312/942-8011): *4-aminopyridine.*

Sandoz Pharmaceutical Corp., 59 Route 10, East Hanover, NJ 07936 (201/503-7500): *calcitonin salmon nasal spray; cyclosporine (ophthalmic); SDZ MSL-109; tuvirumab (human monoclonal antibody against hepatitis B virus).*

Sanofi Pharmaceuticals, Inc., 40 East 52nd Street (13th Floor), New York, NY 10022 (Robert F. Reder, M.D. 212/754-4700): *ST1-RTA immunotoxin.*

Schering Corporation, 2000 Galloping Hill Road, Kenilworth, NJ 07033 (201/298-4000): *interferon alfa-2b; molgramostim (granulocyte macrophage colony stimulating factor).*

G.D. Searle & Co., 4901 Searle Parkway, Skokie, IL 60077 (708/982-4638): *lysine acetylsalicylate.*

Serono Laboratories, Inc., 100 Longwater Circle, Norwell, MA 02061 (800/283-8088): *somatropin; sermorelin acetate; urofollitropin.*

Sigma F and D Division Ltd., Sigma Chemical Co., 3050 Spruce Street, St. Louis, MO 63103 (314/771-5765): *sodium oxybate.*

Sigma Tau Pharmaceuticals, Inc., 200 Orchard Ridge Drive, Gaithersburg, MD 20878 (301/948-1041): *levocarnitine.*

SmithKline Beecham, 1500 Spring Garden Street, Philadelphia, PA 19101 (215/751-4000): *CD4 human truncated 369AA polypeptide; halofantrine; liothyronine sodium; SK&F 110679.*

Solvay Pharmaceuticals, 901 Sawyer Road, Marietta, GA 30062 (404/578-9000): *chenodiol.*

Somerset Pharmaceuticals, 400 Morris Avenue, Suite 7S, Denville, NJ 07834 (201/586-2310): *selegiline hydrochloride.*

Spectra Pharmaceutical Services, Inc., Hanover Business Park, 155 Webster Street, Hanover, MA 02339 (617/871-3991): *tretinoin.*

St. Jude Children's Hospital, 332 North Lauderdale, Memphis, TN 38101-0318 (901/522-0300): *2-chloro-2'-deoxyadenosine.*

Peter Stacpoole, M.D., Ph.D., University of Florida, Box J-226, Gainsville, FL 32610 (904/342-2321): *sodium dichloroacetate.*

Star Pharmaceuticals, Inc., 1990 NW 44th Street, Pompano Beach, FL 33064 (800/845-7827): *testosterone propionate ointment 2%.*

Sterling Drugs, Inc., 90 Park Avenue, New York, NY 10016 (212/907-2000): *mafenide acetate.*

Stuart Pharmaceuticals: A business unit of ICI Americas, Inc., Wilmington, DE 19897 (301/886-2231): *viloxazine hydrochloride.*

Synergen, Inc., 1885 33rd Street, Boulder CO 80301 (303/938-6200): *interleukin-1 receptor antagonist (human recombinant); recombinant secretory leucocyte protease inhibitor.*

Syntex (USA), Inc., 3401 Hillview Avenue, Palo Alto, CA 94304 (415/855-5050): *ganciclovir (DHPG); nafarelin acetate.*

Stanley J. Szefler, M.D., 1400 Jackson Street, Denver, CO (303/398-1193): *troleandomycin.*

TAG Pharmaceuticals, Inc., c/o Lemmon Company, Sellersville, PA 18960 (215/723-5544): *copolymer 1; secalciferol.*

TAP Pharmaceuticals, Inc., 2355 Waukegan Road, Deerfield, IL 60015 (800/662-2011): *leuprolide acetate.*

Jess G. Thoene, M.D., Department of Pediatrics, 2612 SPH # 1, 109 Observatory Street, University of Michigan, Ann Arbor, MI 48109 (313/763-3427): *cysteamine (mercaptamine).*

Tyson & Associates, 12832 Chadron Avenue, Hawthorne, CA 90250 (310/675-1080): *L-threonine.*

UCB Secteur Pharmaceutique, 326 Avenue, Louise, 1050, Brussels, Belgium: *piracetam.*

Ueno Fine Chemicals Industry, Ltd., C/O Arthur Checci, Inc., 1730 Rhode Island, Washington, DC 20036 (202/452-8666): *dextran sulfate sodium.*

Unimed, Inc., 35 Columbia Road, Sommerville, NJ 08876 (908/526-6894): *dronabinol.*

United-Guardian, Inc., P.O. Box 2500, Smithtown, NY 11787 (516/273-0900): *citric acid, gluco-delta-lactone, magnesium carbonate.*

Univax Biologics, Inc., 12280 Parklawn Drive, Rockville, MD 20852 (M. Lauren Macturk, 301/770-3099): *group B streptococcal hyperimmune globulin; mucoid exopolysaccharide pseudomonas hyperimmune globulin.*

Upjohn Company, 301 Henrietta Street, Kalamazoo, MI 49001 (616/329-8216): *clindamycin.*

U.S. Bioscience, Inc., One Tower Bridge, 100 Front Street, West Conshohocken, PA 19428 (William McCullock, M.D., 215/832-0570): *altretamine; amifostine; diaziquone; trimetrexate glucuronate.*

Wallace Laboratories, P.O. Box 1001 Half Acre Road, Cranbury, NJ 08512 (609/656-6000): *felbamate.*

Philip Walson, M.D., Children's Hospital, 700 Children's Drive, Columbus, OH 43205 (614/461-2000): *antiepilepsirine.*

Warner-Lambert Company, Parke-Davis Pharmaceutical Research Division, 2800 Plymouth Road, P.O. Box 1047, Ann Arbor, MI 48106 (Howard Holden, 313/996-5141): *amsacrine; cysteamine hydrochlordide; fosphenytoin; pentostatin.*

Whitby Research, Inc., P.O. Box 27426, Richmond, VA 23261-7426 (804/254-4400): *methotrexate with laurocapram.*

Xoma Corporation, 2910 Seventh Street, Berkeley, CA 94710 (415/644-1170): *antimelanoma antibody XMMME-001-RTA; anti-TAP-72 immunotoxin; CD5-T lymphocyte immunotoxin.*

Cited References

Income tax; credit for clinical testing expenses for certain drugs for rare diseases or conditions, final regulations. *Federal Register* 53:33708-38715, 1988.

Orphan drug regulations; proposed rule. *Federal Register* 56:3338-3351, 1991.

Asbury CH: The Orphan Drug Act: the first 7 years. *JAMA* 265:893-897, 1991.

Department of Survey Design and Analysis: *Final Report on the Survey of Physicians and Information About Research on Rare Diseases,* prepared for the National Commission on Orphan Diseases. Chicago, Ill, American Medical Association, (Aug) 1988 A, 1-102.

Department of Survey Design and Analysis: Supplementary report to *Final Report on the Survey of Physicians and Information About Research on Rare Diseases.* Chicago, Ill, American Medical Association, (Aug) 1988 B.

US Department of Health and Human Services: *Report of the National Commission on Orphan Diseases: Executive Summary and Recommendations.* Washington, DC, Public Health Service, (Feb) 1989, 1-10 and preface.

Other Selected References

Asbury CH: *Orphan Drugs: Medical Versus Market Value.* Lexington, Mass, Lexington Books, 1985.

Scheinberg IH, Walshe JM (eds): *Orphan Diseases and Orphan Drugs.* London, Manchester University Press, 1985.

Information Directory 5

The following directory prepared by the Consortium on Rare Diseases (1992) is intended as a starting point for individuals or groups seeking information on rare diseases/disorders. For further information regarding this directory, contact the Office of Orphan Products Development listed below.

RARE DISEASE INFORMATION DIRECTORY

Category	Information Desired	Source*
Disease/Education	General Information	AGSG, NIH, NORD, March of Dimes
	Prevalence Data	MIN, OPD, NORD
Research	Funding Sources	NIH, NORD, OPD *See Voluntary/Patient Organizations*
	Source of Subjects for Enrollment in Trials	GCRC, MIN, NORD *See Voluntary/Patient Organizations*
	Current Funded Research	ABC, IBA, DRG/NIH, GCRC, OPD, PMA
	Current Research Results	NIH, NORD
Voluntary/Patient Organizations	Networking/Patient/Family Interactions	AGSG, CHDCT, NCEMCH, NICODARD, NORD, WLF
	Travel Assistance	WLF, NORD
Treatment/Patient Care	Drug/Product Information	NICODARD, PMA, ABC, IBA *See Research*
	Physicians	GCRC, MIN *See Voluntary/Patient Organizations*

**The complete names and addresses of sources appear below.*

(ABC) Association of Biotechnology Companies
1666 Connecticut Ave., N.W.
Suite 330
Washington, D.C. 20009
(202) 234-3330

(AGSG) Alliance of Genetic Support Groups
35 Wisconsin Circle
Suite 440
Chevy Chase, MD 20815
(800) 336-GENE

(CHDCT) Coalition for Heritable Disorders of Connective Tissue
382 Main Street
Port Washington, NY 11050
(516) 883-8712

(DRG/NIH) Division of Research Grants
National Institutes of Health
Westwood Building
533 Westbard Avenue
Bethesda, MD 20892
(301) 496-7543

(GCRC) General Clinical Research Centers
Rare Disease Network
AA 3223 MCN
Vanderbilt University Medical Center
Nashville, TN 37232-2195
(615) 343-0124 or (800) 428-6626

(IBA) Industrial Biotechnology Association*
1625 K. Street, N.W.
Suite 1100
Washington, DC 20006
(202) 857-0244
*Inquiries from organizations only

March of Dimes
1275 Mamaroneck Avenue
White Plains, NY 10605
(914) 428-7100

(MIN) Metabolic Information Network
P.O. Box 670847
Dallas, TX 75367-0847
(214) 696-2188 or (800) 945-2188

National Library of Medicine
8600 Rockville Pike, Bldg. 38
Bethesda, MD 20894
(301) 496-6095 or (800) 272-4787

(NCEMCH) National Center for Education in Maternal and Child Health
38th and R Streets, N.W.
Washington, D.C. 20057
(202) 625-8400

(NICODARD) National Information Center for Orphan Drugs and Rare Diseases
P.O. Box 1133
Washington, D.C. 20013-1133
(800) 456-3505

(NIH) National Institutes of Health
9000 Rockville Pike
Bethesda, MD 20892
General Information Telephone Number:
(301) 496-4000

(NORD) National Organization of Rare Disorders
P.O. Box 8923
New Fairfield, CT 06812-1783
(203) 746-6518 or (800) 999-NORD

(OPD) Office of Orphan Products Development
Food and Drug Administration
5600 Fishers Lane (HF 35)
Rockville, MD 20857
(301) 443-4903

(PMA) Pharmaceutical Manufacturers Association
Commission on Drugs for Rare Diseases
1100 15th Street, N.W.
Washington, D.C. 20005
(202) 835-3550

(WLF) World Life Foundation
P.O. Box 571
Bedford, TX 76095
(817) 282-1405 or (800) 289-5433

Analgesics 6

The analgesics discussed in this chapter are divided into two groups: (1) the opioids (morphine-like drugs), which primarily affect the central nervous system (CNS), and (2) the nonopioids (analgesic-antipyretics), which have a predominantly peripheral site of action. Although drugs in both groups relieve pain, their other pharmacologic actions differ; therefore, the two groups are discussed separately. Mixtures containing drugs from each group are discussed in a third section.

OPIOID ANALGESICS

The opioid analgesics can be classified either as morphine-like opioid agonists or agonist-antagonists; the latter act as agonists at one type of opioid receptor and as competitive antagonists at another or as partial agonists (see Table 1). The agonists include the natural opium alkaloids (morphine, codeine, a mixture of opium alkaloids [Pantopon]), their analogues (hydrocodone in mixtures), hydromorphone [Dilaudid], oxycodone [Roxicodone], oxymorphone [Numorphan], and the following synthetic compounds: a phenylpiperidine derivative (meperidine [Demerol]), a morphinan derivative (levorphanol [Levo-Dromoran]), and diphenylheptane derivatives (methadone [Dolophine], propoxyphene [Darvon, Dolene]). The agonist-antagonists include a morphinan derivative, butorphanol [Stadol]; a phenanthrene derivative, nalbuphine [Nubain]; the benzomorphan derivatives, pentazocine [Talwin] and dezocine [Dalgan]; and an oripavine derivative, buprenorphine [Buprenex].

Pharmacodynamics

The concept that the opioid compounds interact with receptors to produce analgesia was proposed many years ago, but it was not until 1973 that specific opioid binding sites were identified as receptors and their anatomical distribution determined. The density of opioid binding sites varies markedly in different regions of the CNS. Densities are high in anatomical areas associated with physiologic functions affected by opioids, which indicates a correlation between site of binding and effect. Opioid receptors also are found outside the CNS (eg, vagus nerve, gastrointestinal tract), where they mediate opioid effects on heart rate and intestinal motility.

Neurochemical evidence indicates that the receptors are associated with the presynaptic nerve terminals of the brain, and they appear to function by decreasing the release of excitatory neurotransmitters. Endogenous polypeptides that bind to opioid receptor sites and mimic some of the actions of opioids have been found in the brain and other tissues. The first polypeptides that were isolated and sequenced were two pentapeptides, met (methionine)-enkephalin and leu (leucine)-enkephalin. A larger peptide with similar activity, beta-endorphin, is present in the pituitary and arcuate body of the hypothalamus. Beta-endorphin is composed of the amino

TABLE 1. EQUIVALENT ANALGESIC DOSES OF OPIOID DRUGS

Drug	Intramuscular/ Subcutaneous (mg)	Oral (mg)
AGONISTS		
Morphine sulfate	10	20-30*
Codeine phosphate, Codeine sulfate	†	200
Hydromorphone hydrochloride [Dilaudid]	1.5	7.5
Levorphanol tartrate [Levo-Dromoran]	2	4
Meperidine hydrochloride [Demerol]	75-100	(300)‡
Methadone hydrochloride [Dolophine]	10	20
Oxycodone hydrochloride [Roxicodone]	10-15	30
Oxymorphone hydrochloride [Numorphan]	1.0-1.5	§
AGONIST-ANTAGONISTS		
Buprenorphine hydrochloride [Buprenex]	0.3-0.4	§
Butorphanol tartrate [Stadol]	2	§
Dezocine [Dalgan]	10	§
Nalbuphine hydrochloride [Nubain]	10	§
Pentazocine hydrochloride [Talwin Nx]	§	180
Pentazocine lactate [Talwin]	50-60	§

* *60 mg in single-doses*
† *Not a recommended route of administration*
‡ *This estimated equieffective dose is not recommended. Its use to estimate the dose conversion to oral meperidine from another opioid may result in a potentially toxic dose.*
§ *No commercial preparation available*

acid sequence 61-91 of the pituitary peptide, beta-lipotropin, and, although the met-enkephalin sequence is contained in the amino acid sequence 61-65 of beta-lipotropin, the enkephalins are *not* derived from beta-endorphin. Another peptide, designated dynorphin, was identified later. Several possible functions, including neurotransmission, have been suggested for the endogenous opioid peptides and enkephalins, but their mechanism of analgesic action is not clear.

The opioids have various chemical structures, and their relative analgesic potency appears to be related to several factors, including their affinity for specific binding sites, intrinsic activity at receptors, and pharmacokinetic properties. For example, morphine has a greater affinity for opioid binding sites than does codeine.

Different types and subtypes of opioid receptors have been postulated to explain the various actions of the opioids. The μ (mu) receptor mediates morphine-like analgesia, respiratory depression, miosis, reduction of gastrointestinal motility, and euphoria; the κ (kappa) receptor probably mediates pentazocine-like analgesia. A σ (sigma) receptor may, together with a phencyclidine site, mediate psychotomimetic effects produced by pentazocine and other agonist-antagonists. The δ (delta) receptor also has been found in the CNS and is selective for enkephalins. There is evidence that this receptor plays a role in opioid-induced respiratory depression. Activation of δ receptors probably induces effects similar to those of the μ receptor; however, the link has been difficult to study in intact animals or in humans, since the only available specific agonists are peptides that do not gain access to the CNS through the blood-brain barrier. Studies in rats support the view that the μ receptor is associated with reduced tidal volume and the δ receptor with reduced respiratory rate. The μ receptor may exist as two subtypes, μ_1 and μ_2. The μ_1 receptor is present only in the CNS and is associated with supraspinal analgesia, prolactin release, hypothermia, and catalepsy. The μ_2 receptor is associated with bradycardia and reduced tidal volume. Analgesic agents acting at the spinal level presumably interact with δ and κ receptors. Although results of various studies suggest that different receptors mediate different effects, more research is needed to determine their exact nature and role (Akil and Lewis, 1987; Pasternak, 1988).

Indications and Drug Selection

Morphine is the prototype of the opioid agonists, all of which have qualitatively similar actions on the CNS. The relative usefulness of the morphine-like opioid analgesics is determined by the type and severity of pain, the onset and duration of action by different routes of administration, and the severity of adverse reactions. The availability of a number of analgesics permits considerable latitude in the selection of an agent for a specific situation.

ACUTE PAIN. Opioids are indicated for relief of moderate to severe acute pain. When administered systemically, they alter the psychological response to pain as well as the nociceptive sensation. They act on higher centers of the CNS to produce analgesia without loss of consciousness, although, at least initially, fully effective doses often cause sedation. The pure agonists, and often the agonist-antagonists as well, are useful for short-term therapy for severe, acute pain (trauma, burns, surgery). In this setting, they should be administered in sufficient doses to relieve pain and at sufficiently frequent intervals to prevent its recurrence. The patient should be evaluated frequently to determine the need for dosage adjustment.

Agents such as codeine, opioid-nonopioid combinations, and drugs that appear to have a ceiling effect for analgesia (nonopioid analgesics and agonist-antagonists) should be used for mild or moderate pain.

CHRONIC PAIN. The treatment of chronic pain of *nonmalignant* origin depends on its cause and severity. When analgesics are indicated for mild to moderate pain, adequate relief usually can be attained initially with a nonopioid (eg, acetaminophen, aspirin, another nonsteroidal anti-inflammatory agent [NSAID]). If pain is not controlled by one of these drugs, concurrent use of an opioid may be appropriate. When given in combination, opioids and nonopioids have additive analgesic effects since their mechanisms of action are different. Similarly, adverse effects may be reduced because smaller doses of each drug are required.

The prolonged administration of opioids for chronic pain of nonmalignant etiology is usually discouraged because of the potential for psychological dependence, and such use remains controversial. However, good relief is observed in some patients with chronic nonmalignant pain without the problem of dose escalation or development of psychological dependence or abuse. In these patients, the diagnosis, treatment history, management plan, and inadequacy of alternative approaches (eg, nonopioid analgesia, use of adjunctive agents, physical therapy) should be documented. The physician should consult pain specialists and other physician specialists when appropriate and, after discussion of potential problems, the informed consent of the patient should be obtained. Frequent, well-documented follow-up care is essential. Various guidelines for use of these agents have been developed (France et al, 1984; Portenoy and Foley, 1986).

The selection of an opioid should be based on the severity of the pain and the patient's response. Usually, therapy is initiated with an opioid such as codeine plus a salicylate or acetaminophen. Oral administration is preferred. The opioid preparation should not be used primarily to relieve anxiety or depression. Patients should be advised to use alcoholic beverages and drugs with additive side effects (benzodiazepines or sedative-hypnotic drugs) cautiously.

Neuropathic pain may follow injury to peripheral nerves, spinal cord, soft tissues, or visceral structures. The injury may be caused by compression, surgery, viral infection (eg, herpes), or neoplastic disease. Neuropathic pain is typically a dysesthesia (abnormal burning, shooting pain) that is less responsive to opioid analgesics than other types of pain. Nonopioid drugs, including selected antidepressants and anticonvulsants, may be useful. See index entries Headache; Neuralgias.

It may be necessary to refer some patients to a pain clinic where multidisciplinary attention is available. Additional discussions of management are included in several reviews (Foley, 1985; Foley and Inturrisi, 1987; Tollison, 1989).

CHRONIC PAIN ASSOCIATED WITH SPECIFIC CONDITIONS. ***Neoplastic Disease:*** The management of patients with chronic pain associated with neoplastic disease requires special consideration (Portenoy, 1988). The primary concern is maintenance of the patient's overall comfort, and nonmedical aspects (eg, physical, social, mental, spiritual) must be taken into account in the total care program.

The choice of analgesic depends on the status of the disease, the pain syndrome (nociceptive versus neuropathic), and the severity of the pain. It may be necessary to try several compounds, and the drug regimen should be changed as required to obtain relief. A nonopioid (acetaminophen, aspirin or another NSAID) should be tried initially if the pain is mild to moderate. These drugs may be particularly effective in pain due to metastatic bone disease. If pain is not controlled, one of the agonist opioids (eg, codeine) should be added. Agonist-antagonists (eg, pentazocine hydrochloride), with or without a nonopioid, are of limited value in neoplastic disease because of their unacceptable psychotomimetic effects. In addition, the agonist-antagonists may precipitate withdrawal symptoms in opioid-dependent patients. These drugs also exhibit a ceiling effect for analgesic activity.

The oral route is preferred and is usually adequate; oral morphine is currently the opioid of choice for long-term administration in cancer patients. The oral/parenteral effectiveness ratio of morphine and other opioids (eg, codeine, methadone, levorphanol, hydrocodone, oxycodone) are quite different (see Table 1), a fact that should be taken into account when routes of administration are changed. In general, oral medication provides analgesia equivalent to that provided by parenteral administration if the dose is adjusted appropriately.

Parenteral administration is required only if there is persistent nausea and vomiting, the patient cannot swallow or absorb medication, or if severe pain requires rapid relief. Suppositories are effective but often impractical. Intravenous injection may result in a prominent bolus effect (side effects at peak concentration and/or pain breakthrough at the trough), and administration may be required at intervals of two hours or less. Intermittent intravenous injection by catheter may be effective in some patients, but the need for careful and frequent monitoring often limits its usefulness. Continuous intravenous administration with a flow-calibrated infusion pump also can be considered. Although any opioid can be employed, morphine and hydromorphone generally are preferred because of their favorable pharmacokinetic properties. The intramuscular and subcutaneous routes reduce the bolus effect observed with intermittent intravenous administration. Intramuscular administration may be unsatisfactory in patients with diminished muscle mass or in those who may not tolerate repeated injections (eg, the terminally ill, children).

The synthetic opioid, fentanyl, is available in transdermal patches [Duragesic] that deliver 25, 50, 75, or 100 mcg/hr over 72 hours. Patches are used for long-term management of cancer-related and chronic pain. Transdermal administration of fentanyl is the noninvasive equivalent of a constant-rate infusion. Because the drug has a four-hour half-life, plasma levels increase gradually for 12 to 14 hours and then remain relatively constant for about 72 hours. Supplemental intravenous doses may be required to control pain initially. The disappearance half-time of fentanyl is prolonged to 17 to 21 hours after removal of the patch because of absorption of residual drug in the skin. As a result, respiratory depression due to high drug levels may persist even after the patch is removed; prolonged observation and treatment with antagonists may be required. See also index entry Fentanyl.

The use of epidural or intrathecal opioids in cancer patients is discussed later in this introductory section.

Small doses of antidepressants may be useful as an adjunct to opioids, particularly in patients with neuropathic pain. Their analgesic action is independent of their antidepressant activity, and they must be taken regularly for full benefit. Administration at bedtime takes advantage of their sedative side effects; however, their anticholinergic activity may exacerbate the constipating effect of the opioids. Other drugs commonly used in neuropathic pain include phenothiazines, anticonvulsants, antihistamines, antiarrhythmic drugs (eg, mexiletine), and corticosteroids (Foley, 1985). Nitrous oxide 25% to 75% in oxygen, administered by a nonrebreathing face mask, may be used to supplement opioids in the dying patient. It is very useful for short periods to manage acute procedure-related or movement-precipitated pain ("incident pain"). Palliative radiation therapy, chemotherapy, or hormonal therapy, if appropriate, should be instituted as early as practical rather than after pain becomes difficult to control. Amphetamines may be used to reduce opioid-induced sedation. Neuroleptic drugs (eg, methotrimeprazine, haloperidol [Haldol]) are sometimes given on an empiric basis, particularly when pain is associated with nausea, agitation, or anxiety.

Opioids should be administered on a fixed schedule rather than as needed when treating continuous pain. The dose, route, and schedule *must be individualized* according to the efficacy and duration of action of the analgesic and the response of the patient. Dosage requirements should be reviewed frequently. Increasing the dose usually is preferable to increasing the frequency of administration. The absolute dose is irrelevant, and some patients require very high doses. Larger or supplemental doses may be required for short periods when increased pain is associated with specific physical activities. In such cases, the additional doses should be given in anticipation of the activity.

Dosage requirements usually increase because of progression of the disease and the patient should be evaluated with this in mind. Although tolerance may develop, it seldom is a problem in patients with stable disease. Tolerance usually is manifested initially as a decrease in the duration of action. Since cross-tolerance is not complete, when the need for larger doses (whether induced by pharmacologic tolerance, progression of disease, or other reasons) becomes difficult to manage, substitution of another opioid may be helpful. Other approaches, such as continuous subcutaneous infusions or epidural or intrathecal administration, may be considered.

Concern about the development of psychological dependence should never interfere with treatment of the severe pain of neoplastic disease and must never be a reason to withhold analgesics from any patient who may benefit from them (McGivney and Crooks, 1984; Foley, 1985).

Myocardial Infarction: The aim in treating the severe pain of acute myocardial infarction is to provide adequate relief without producing untoward effects on the respiratory and cardiovascular systems. Morphine is generally considered the preferred drug for this use. When prompt relief is required, a dilute solution may be given slowly intravenously in divided doses. Hemodynamic effects may be beneficial (eg, reduction of left ventricular work index). Although morphine may cause nausea, vomiting, and some degree of respiratory depression, it relieves pain and reduces anxiety. Excessive bradycardia caused by vagotonic effects may be treated with small doses of atropine. Excessive hypotension due to venous dilation responds to leg elevation or administration of fluids.

Meperidine also is used in myocardial infarction, particularly that associated with bradycardia. In appropriate doses, its effects are similar to those of morphine. The hemodynamic effects of nalbuphine appear to resemble those of morphine, but blood pressure is not reduced. However, greater experience is needed to determine whether nalbuphine has advantages over conventional drugs. Pentazocine and butorphanol increase left ventricular workload and myocardial oxygen demands and are not recommended to relieve the pain of myocardial infarction.

Acute Pulmonary Edema: Patients with dyspnea of pulmonary edema secondary to acute left ventricular failure may benefit from administration of morphine if ventilation is adequately controlled or equipment for artificial ventilation is readily available. Morphine allays the anxiety caused by hypoxemia and produces peripheral pooling of blood, which reduces cardiac preload. Other measures (eg, oxygen, intermittent positive pressure breathing [IPPB] combined with etiologic management) also are essential. Although acute left ventricular failure is the most common cause of pulmonary edema, the specific etiology should be determined and treatment instituted accordingly. Morphine generally should not be given when pulmonary edema is caused by a chemical respiratory irritant. It should be used very cautiously if at all in patients with bronchial asthma.

Obstetric Analgesia: Use of opioids in obstetric patients requires considerable experience and judgment to provide adequate analgesia for the mother while avoiding interference with the progress of labor and preventing respiratory depression in the newborn infant. Meperidine is widely used for this purpose; however, it crosses the placenta and may depress fetal respiration (see the evaluation). If opioid-induced respiratory depression is suspected in the neonate, naloxone should be given as an adjunct to mechanical ventilatory support. Administration of an antagonist to the mother before delivery to counteract fetal depression is not recommended.

Pre- and Postanesthetic Medication and Anesthesia: Opioids are useful for preanesthetic medication because their sedative, antianxiety, and analgesic properties afford smoother induction and maintenance of anesthesia and reduce excitement during emergence. In the absence of preoperative pain, antianxiety agents (eg, diazepam [Valium], lorazepam

[Ativan]) may be preferred to avoid opioid-induced postoperative nausea and vomiting and postoperative respiratory depression (see index entry Adjuncts to Anesthesia).

Certain opioid analgesics (meperidine, morphine, fentanyl and its derivatives, and hydromorphone) are used to supplement the hypnotic and analgesic effects of nitrous oxide. Morphine or fentanyl and its derivatives may be used in very large intravenous doses as the primary agent for general anesthesia in cardiac and other surgery, particularly in poor-risk patients. See index entry Anesthetics, General.

Although aspirin and other nonopioid analgesics and orally administered opioids may relieve postoperative pain, oral administration in the immediate postoperative period often is not practical. The intramuscular preparation of the NSAID, ketorolac tromethamine [Toradol], alone or with an opioid, may be a useful substitute for an opioid alone in selected patients.

The intravenous administration of morphine 1 to 3 mg (or more if required) provides rapid pain relief. Maximal respiratory depression after this route of administration can be observed and evaluated in seven to ten minutes. Additional doses can be given every 15 to 30 minutes. Other approaches, such as a larger dose given less frequently (eg, 5 to 10 mg of morphine every three to four hours intramuscularly or subcutaneously) can be effective in many patients. Monitoring of the patient's response, followed by appropriate changes in dose, interval, and route, are essential for successful management of postoperative pain.

In selected patients, the use of a patient-controlled infusion pump may be appropriate. This technique, called patient-controlled analgesia (PCA), is a new approach to opioid administration. The infusion device can be set to deliver small intravenous doses of opioids at intervals that are determined by the patient but are limited by a preset "lockout" period following each dose and other safety features designed to preclude overdose. In a typical program, injections of morphine 1 mg or nalbuphine 3 mg are followed by a six-minute lockout period. Potential advantages include lessened patient anxiety about delays in receiving pain medication, adaptability to differing analgesic requirements, reduction of sedation and other side effects, and maintenance of continuous near-optimal analgesia. Because the required equipment is expensive, cost effectiveness must be assessed. The combination of continuous opioid infusions and PCA using intermittent bolus doses also is being evaluated (Parker et al, 1991). Patient-initiated opioid doses also may be administered subcutaneously.

In pediatric patients over 6 months, an intravenous loading dose of 0.2 mg/kg of preservative-free morphine (less if opioids have been given prior to or during surgery) can be followed by continuous infusion, by pump, of 0.02 mg/kg/hr. Additional bolus doses of 0.1 mg/kg may be administered at four-hour intervals if required (Bray, 1983).

The fentanyl transdermal patch has been investigated for use in management of postoperative pain but currently is not recommended for this purpose.

The epidural or intrathecal administration of opioids for postoperative pain relief is described elsewhere in this introductory section.

Sickle Cell Vaso-occlusive Crisis Pain: Pain relief depends on an assessment of the severity of the pain and the age of the patient. Acute pain lasts for a few days to a week and often is followed by dull, aching pain that may persist for several weeks. Chronic persistent pain also occurs. In children, the abdomen may be the primary site of the pain; the pathophysiology is obscure but may involve tonic spasm and gaseous distension. General support is indicated regardless of the nature of the pain and includes rest, warmth, increased fluid intake, and continuing reassurance. It has been observed repeatedly that most patients receive inadequate analgesia and assurance, which diminishes their ability to cope with subsequent episodes (Vichinsky et al, 1982; Cole et al, 1986; Friedman et al, 1986).

Many patients with moderate pain experience adequate relief with supportive measures and treatment with acetaminophen or an NSAID. Aspirin can be used in adults, but it is not satisfactory for children already suffering from abdominal pain. Severe pain requires administration of an opioid. Although intramuscular meperidine is used widely in the United States for sickle cell crisis pain, it is inferior to morphine for patients who experience prolonged episodes or crises at frequent intervals because it has a short duration and accumulation of its metabolite, normeperidine, may lead to CNS toxicity.

Protocols have been developed for the use of oral morphine in adolescents and adults with sickle cell crisis (Friedman et al, 1986) and for continuous intravenous infusion of morphine or meperidine in children (Cole et al, 1986) and morphine in adults (Ives and Guerra, 1987). In the first instance, 60 mg of morphine is administered orally; when pain recurs, 15 mg is administered every 20 minutes until analgesia or sedation is attained to establish a maintenance dosage, usually 30 to 60 mg. This maintenance dose is given every two to four hours as necessary. The morphine is supplemented with an antipyretic-analgesic. Prochlorperazine [Compazine] in suppository form is given to patients who become nauseated or vomit, and the antiemetic is given prophylactically to these patients at subsequent intervals. Patients who cannot tolerate morphine can be managed similarly with equivalent oral doses of hydromorphone, levorphanol, or oxycodone (see Table 1).

For intravenous infusion in children, a bolus dose of 0.15 mg/kg of morphine (or 1 mg/kg of meperidine) is given. This is followed by infusion, by pump, of 0.07 to 0.1 mg/kg/hr of morphine (or 0.5 to 0.7 mg/kg/hr of meperidine). If needed, the dosage is increased by approximately 25% every three to four hours until pain is relieved. Preservative-free morphine is recommended for continuous intravenous infusion in children. Continuous infusion of morphine also has been reported to relieve pain in adults (Ives and Guerra, 1987).

Cough: The cough reflex is depressed or abolished by opioids, but use of opioid analgesics other than codeine for this purpose should be restricted to patients with painful cough that cannot be controlled by codeine or nonopioid agents (see index entry Cough) or when cough suppression is required during certain procedures, eg, bronchoscopy.

When an active cough reflex is desired, meperidine may be a preferred analgesic because it lacks an antitussive effect.

Gastrointestinal and Urinary Tract Disorders: Acute severe pain associated with biliary colic or pancreatitis presents a problem in drug selection. Because morphine-like opioids cause an increase in the tone of the sphincter and increase intravesical pressure, theoretically they could worsen the underlying process or increase pain; the existence of this effect awaits confirmation.

The administration of anticholinergic drugs, direct smooth muscle relaxants, or calcium channel blocking agents, alone or with opioids, has had limited success. Meperidine and agonist-antagonists have less effect on smooth muscle than morphine and generally are selected for that reason.

Acute ureteral obstruction causes a rapid increase in renal pelvic pressure accompanied by intense pain. If an opioid is required, morphine is usually effective but, again, drugs with minimal action on smooth muscle tone (eg, meperidine) are often preferred. Butorphanol 4 mg intramuscularly was found to be equivalent to meperidine 80 mg intramuscularly in patients with renal colic (Henry et al, 1987).

Intrathecal and Epidural Opioid Analgesia

The epidural or intrathecal administration of an opioid can provide effective analgesia of prolonged duration. The epidural route is used most commonly. Various opioids have been employed, but a preservative-free solution of morphine is used most frequently. The primary differences among opioids are rate of onset of action, segmental spread, and duration. Onset is fastest with the most lipophilic agents, whereas spread and duration are increased as the hydrophilic property of the opioid is increased. An epidural dose of morphine 5 mg, one of the most hydrophilic opioids, potentially can provide good to excellent pain relief for 24 hours or more.

Single-dose, intermittent, and continuous epidural administration of opioids are used for chronic pain (cancer or trauma) and postoperative pain, particularly in high-risk patients following thoracic, upper abdominal, or hip surgery. The intrathecal route is employed for long-term administration to relieve the pain of cancer and postoperatively in other orthopedic procedures and in urologic surgery. These techniques are not used for intraoperative pain; only meperidine is effective by these routes for surgical pain, perhaps because of its local anesthetic property.

The advantages of these techniques include the long duration of action and the fact that, unlike spinal or epidural local anesthesia, there is no sympathetic blockade (permitting ambulation), loss of motor tone, or loss of sensitivity to temperature or pinprick.

Different types of pain may respond differently to epidural morphine. In one study, all patients with continuous somatic cancer pain or continuous visceral pain obtained complete relief; however, if both were involved, response was variable (Arnér and Arnér, 1985). Intermittent pain of visceral origin (eg, acute pancreatitis, intestinal obstruction) was mostly unaffected. Epidural morphine also failed to relieve neuropathic pain and was variably effective for intermittent somatic pain. Experience suggests that patients who have developed pronounced adverse effects, particularly sedation or confusion, after use of systemic opioids may benefit from the epidural route (Gustafsson and Wiesenfeld-Hallin, 1988).

Drug selection and comparison of the epidural and intrathecal routes are discussed in greater detail in Cousins and Mather, 1984; Hughes et al, 1984; Kotelko et al, 1984; and Stenseth et al, 1985. Limitations of the technique in patients with chronic pain, particularly the development of tolerance, are described by Max et al, 1985, and Payne, 1987.

The most serious adverse effect is respiratory depression. This adverse reaction may be somewhat more common in the elderly and occurs much less frequently with epidural than intrathecal administration. It is more pronounced with hydrophilic opioids (eg, morphine) than lipophilic drugs, such as fentanyl. Because its onset may be delayed, monitoring is required for 12 hours after administration of epidural morphine (Rawal et al, 1987). When these techniques are utilized for postoperative pain, respiratory depression may be minimized by avoiding the concomitant use of systemic opioids or sedatives and perhaps by maintaining the patient in a 30° head-up position. Intrathecal morphine in doses below 0.5 mg or epidural administration in doses below 5 mg rarely causes respiratory depression (Rawal and Sjöstrand, 1986), but these amounts may be inadequate following intrathoracic or upper abdominal surgery, for which 10 mg of morphine epidurally may be required (Cousins and Bridenbaugh, 1986).

Other side effects of intrathecal or epidural administration of opioids include pruritus, nausea and vomiting, and urinary retention. Pruritus, which can be regional or generalized, and nausea and vomiting may respond to systemic doses of naloxone too small to affect analgesia. Postoperative nausea associated with epidural morphine also can be reduced by application of transdermal scopolamine patches [Transderm-Scōp] four to six hours before the antiemetic effect is required (Loper et al, 1989).

Urinary retention generally is associated only with the initial use of opioids by these routes. It occurs in 20% to 40% of postoperative patients following doses of 4 to 6 mg of extradural morphine.

Large doses of intrathecal or epidural morphine may produce paradoxical pain in some patients.

Partial agonist or agonist-antagonist opioids should not be used epidurally or intrathecally in patients who have received pure agonist opioids systemically for a prolonged period because severe opioid withdrawal may develop. If the epidural or intrathecal route is used, the parenteral dose must be reduced simultaneously.

Adverse Reactions and Precautions

Opioids cause adverse reactions that limit their usefulness: respiratory depression, nausea, vomiting, constipation, orthostatic hypotension, urinary retention, diaphoresis, pruritus, sedation, and confusion. Constipation may be a problem, particularly with prolonged use, but may be reduced by concomitant administration of a laxative. Stimulant laxatives counteract the opioid-induced reduction in bowel motility.

Nausea and vomiting occur frequently with single-dose opioid administration, particularly in the ambulatory patient. When instituting therapy with opioids for chronic pain, small doses of an antiemetic (eg, prochlorperazine, haloperidol) may be given concomitantly for the first one or two weeks. Opioid-induced nausea and vomiting occasionally persist beyond this period, and prolonged antiemetic therapy or substitution of an alternative drug may be required. Opioids also can decrease gastric emptying, which may contribute to nausea and vomiting in some patients. This effect may be lessened by use of metoclopramide [Reglan]. During surgery, delayed gastric emptying can result in retention of secretions and create the potential for aspiration.

Other reactions include miosis, spasm of the biliary and urinary tracts, and, rarely, inappropriate secretion of antidiuretic hormone and hypersensitivity phenomena (urticaria, rash, and anaphylactic reactions with intravenous administration). Pruritus is more common with the epidural or intrathecal routes.

Respiratory depression is the most dangerous acute reaction produced by the morphine-like analgesics, although it is rarely severe with usual doses. Opioids decrease the respiratory rate, tidal volume, and minute ventilation and decrease the sensitivity to carbon dioxide. Severe hypoventilation or apnea is most likely to develop in elderly debilitated patients and in those with respiratory disorders characterized by chronic hypoxia. If severe respiratory depression occurs or appears to be imminent, intravenous naloxone [Narcan] should be given (see index entry Naloxone). Mechanical support of respiration should be provided as required to assure an adequate minute volume. The duration of action of naloxone is shorter than that of most opioids. Thus, repeated doses or infusion of this drug may be required in patients with symptomatic respiratory depression.

Opioids should be used cautiously in patients with excessive respiratory secretions (eg, chronic obstructive lung disease), because they decrease ciliary activity, reduce the cough reflex, and increase bronchomotor tone.

Opioids should be given in reduced doses or withheld from patients in shock or those with decreased blood volume, for severe hypotension may develop. Because these analgesics may cause hypoventilation, the resulting hypercapnia produces cerebrovascular dilatation and increased intracranial pressure; therefore, they must be used with extreme caution (unless mechanical ventilation is provided) in patients with head injuries, intracranial lesions or tumors, or other conditions in which increased intracranial pressure should be avoided. Because morphine and other analgesics may produce miosis, their use in patients with suspected head injuries or in those undergoing intracranial surgery may mask the dilation of one or both pupils that is an important sign of increased intracranial pressure.

Drowsiness and clouding of the sensorium and mental processes are prominent central effects of opioids. Although these effects are often desirable, impairment of the ability to concentrate limits the usefulness of these agents in some ambulatory patients. Increasing somnolence in a patient receiving opioids for chronic pain may indicate excessive dosage, either because of reduced analgesic requirement once initial control of severe pain has been achieved or because of a gradual decline in hepatic or renal clearance leading to the accumulation of the opioid or an active metabolite (Tuttle, 1985).

Since opioid analgesics are metabolized by the liver, their effects should be monitored closely in patients with hepatic insufficiency, for their duration of action may be prolonged.

Opioid analgesics are not contraindicated in patients with impaired renal function, but individualization of dosage may be required since prolonged respiratory depression and sedation have been reported after morphine was given to patients with uremia or various other disorders of renal function (Sear et al, 1985). This may be due to the accumulation of an active metabolite, morphine-6-glucuronide (Moore et al, 1987; Portenoy et al, 1991). Its elimination is dependent on renal function (Osborne et al, 1988).

Opioids decrease urine production directly by acting on the kidney and indirectly by stimulating the release of antidiuretic hormone. There may be a diminished sensory urge to urinate. An increase in the tone of the "internal" sphincter of the urinary bladder may cause acute urinary retention, particularly in patients with prostatic hypertrophy or urethral stricture.

The initial dose of analgesic should be reduced in patients with myxedema, hypothyroidism, or hypoadrenalism; subsequent doses should be determined by the patient's response.

Drug Interactions: The dose of opioids should be reduced in patients receiving other drugs that depress the CNS (eg, antipsychotic agents, barbiturates, antianxiety agents), or the dose of the latter agents should be adjusted. Severe adverse reactions have occurred following the administration of meperidine to patients receiving monoamine oxidase inhibitors; these have not been observed with morphine.

Tolerance and Dependence: Tolerance may develop after prolonged use of morphine-like drugs. Therefore, any substantial increase in the dosage requirement should be evaluated to determine if it is caused by worsening of pain due to progression of the pathologic process or by the development of tolerance. In many instances, during the long-term management of cancer pain, both processes occur simultaneously.

The opioid analgesics produce subjective effects other than analgesia (eg, euphoria, relaxation), which may contribute to abuse by some patients. The dependence occurring with use of these drugs is referred to generally as morphine-type dependence to distinguish it from that produced by alcohol, barbiturates, and other CNS depressants. Studies in former opioid addicts designed to determine dependence liability indicated that butorphanol, nalbuphine, pentazocine, propoxyphene, and codeine have less abuse potential than morphine.

Psychological dependence is extremely unlikely following the short-term use of even large doses of potent parenteral analgesics in patients with acute pain. Anxiety about dependence should never result in undermedication for acute pain and thereby cause unnecessary suffering. The great majority of patients given an opioid for analgesia are able to discontinue its use without difficulty. However, it should be kept in mind that physical dependence will develop after use of an opioid analgesic (eg, multiple daily doses for several days); therefore, the dose should be decreased gradually after the drug is no longer needed to avoid the discomfort of a withdrawal syndrome. Administration of an antagonist (eg, naloxone) may precipitate a withdrawal syndrome after only a few doses of an opioid agonist.

If a patient has been receiving very large doses, one dose reduction technique is to decrease the total daily dose by one-half to three-quarters every second or third day. When the dosage has been reduced to 10 to 15 mg of morphine (or its equivalent, see Table 1), this amount is given for two days and then the drug is discontinued.

Although it is difficult to identify patients who are prone to psychological dependence on opioids, physicians should make every effort to do so. Patients with a history of dependence or abuse of other psychotropic agents (including alcohol) and those with affective disorders may be predisposed to analgesic abuse. Opioid use should be monitored very carefully in these individuals, but they should not be deprived of necessary analgesics.

In those known to be recovering from opioid or other chemical dependency syndromes, the following approaches may help to prevent relapse when opioids are required for treatment of pain: Use scheduled adequate analgesic doses given at appropriate intervals rather than "as needed" doses to prevent periods of drug "craving." If possible, discontinue opioids prior to hospital discharge and substitute nonopioid analgesics and other methods of pain control. If opioids are required on an outpatient basis, carefully control available quantities and prescription refills. Encourage the patient's increased involvement in recovery program activities during this period. (See also index entry Drug Dependence.) The use of methadone for the management of opioid abusers is discussed later in this chapter; for the use of naltrexone [Trexan] for this purpose, see index entry Naltrexone.

Dosage and Routes of Administration

Dosage of the potent analgesics should be titrated individually. For rapid onset of effect, these agents must be given parenterally; however, oral administration can produce analgesia equivalent to that achieved after intramuscular injection if the dose is increased in accordance with the oral/parenteral potency ratio for the particular drug. Some analgesics (eg, codeine, levorphanol, methadone) have a more favorable oral/parenteral potency ratio than morphine (see Table 1), but this has little clinical significance if doses are titrated until the desired effect is achieved. Indeed, oral morphine is currently the preferred drug for long-term administration in cancer patients despite the larger doses required when the drug is given by this route. Rectal suppository preparations of morphine, hydromorphone, and oxymorphone are available commercially. This route is useful if the patient cannot be given medication orally but often is impractical for cancer-related pain. Dosage for oral and rectal use is equivalent. Transdermal administration provides another alternative.

Onset of action is most rapid with intravenous administration. Since rapid intravenous injection may produce transient, profound respiratory depression and possibly hypotension, a dilute solution should be injected over several minutes; a narcotic antagonist (eg, naloxone) and equipment for mechanical ventilation must be available. In patients confined to bed, the incidence of hypotension, dizziness, nausea, and vomiting is minimized.

In children, the initial dose of opioids for the management of acute or chronic cancer pain usually is determined by age and size as well as by the severity of the pain and the degree of opioid tolerance. The following initial doses have been recommended: children 12 years or older should receive the usual adult dose; from age 7 to 12, 50% of the adult dose; from age 2 to 6, 20% to 25% of the adult dose; for children under 2, 0.1 mg/kg of morphine (American Pain Society, 1987). As in adults, these initial doses should then be adjusted to determine the optimal amount for the relief of pain with minimal side effects.

The relief of pain in the neonate has not been studied extensively (Hatch, 1987). Because newborn infants are very sensitive to the respiratory depressant effects of opioids, brief pain from minor surgical procedures should be managed by inhalation or regional anesthesia. Opioids may be employed for pain of prolonged duration if facilities are available for continuous monitoring of respiration and heart rate. A dose of 0.1 mg/kg of morphine was well tolerated in a small number of spontaneously breathing neonates (Purcell-Jones et al, 1987). Continuous intravenous infusion of 10 mcg/kg/hr in the spontaneously breathing neonate probably is preferable to bolus dosing (Duncan, 1985). The elimination half-lives of morphine and meperidine are markedly prolonged in the neonate (see the evaluations).

Except for opioids for which appropriate pharmacokinetic data are available, it is difficult to make initial dose recommendations for the elderly. Most clinicians administer one-half to two-thirds of the amount usually given to younger patients. Two extensive studies (Belleville et al, 1971; Kaiko et al, 1982) have shown that, in the adult, age is the most important determinant of dose response to opioids. Pain relief provided by 8 mg of morphine intramuscularly in the aged was equivalent to that provided by 16 mg in middle-aged patients. As a generalization, response is more prolonged because of slower body clearance in the elderly. For this reason, to avoid the hazards of drug accumulation it is essential to evaluate the patient's response for several days when opioids are used in conditions requiring repeated dosing. The dose of methadone is particularly difficult to manage in the elderly, since the prolonged half-life of this drug, together with the added risks in this age group, necessitate close monitoring for several weeks after each change in dosage.

If an opioid is required for pain relief after surgery or trauma in a patient who has been receiving this type of drug for more than six days (because surgery had been deferred, because of cancer pain, or because of substance abuse), larger doses may be required to produce analgesia. Because of the development of tolerance, respiratory depression is usually not a problem. If possible, the prior dose and administration schedule should be ascertained to provide an appropriate initial dose.

In patients receiving methadone maintenance therapy, acute pain should be treated with supplemental doses of opioids added to the usual daily dose of methadone. Opioids should not be withheld or given in inadequate amounts.

Drug Evaluations

AGONISTS

Opium Alkaloids and Derivatives

MORPHINE SULFATE

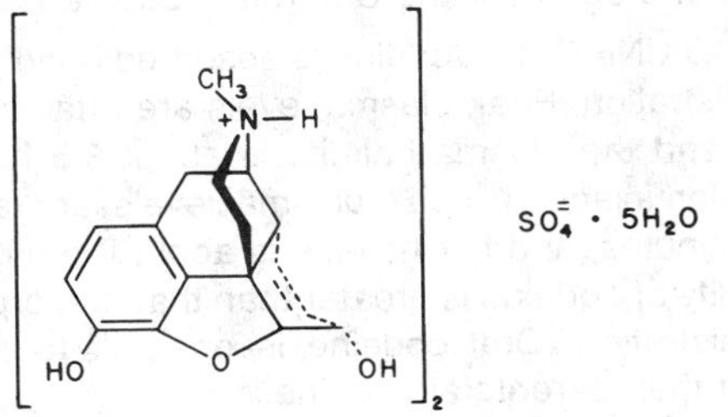

Morphine is the prototype of the strong analgesics (see the Introduction for actions, uses, adverse reactions, and precautions). It is classified as a Schedule II drug under the Controlled Substances Act.

This agent is usually given intramuscularly or subcutaneously in the management of acute pain. Its bioavailability after oral administration is low because of rapid metabolism in the intestinal wall and liver; thus, only a small percentage of an oral dose reaches the systemic circulation. However, this does not preclude use of the oral route, since analgesia equivalent to that achieved after parenteral administration can be obtained if the dose is increased in accordance with the oral/parenteral bioavailability ratio.

Maximal analgesic action usually occurs within one hour after intramuscular or subcutaneous administration; analgesia persists for approximately four hours (range, two and one-half to seven hours). The peak effect occurs later and the duration of action is longer after oral use than after intramuscular injection.

Morphine is given intravenously for analgesia in acute myocardial infarction, for control of cancer pain, by the patient-controlled analgesia technique for postoperative and other pain, and as an alternative to skeletal muscle relaxants to suppress the spontaneous respiratory effort of patients on ventilators (eg, in status asthmaticus). Oral morphine is currently the drug most commonly used for long-term administration to alleviate cancer pain.

Morphine also is given by the epidural and intrathecal routes to control acute and chronic pain in a variety of situations, including postoperative, trauma-related, and cancer pain. See the section on Intrathecal and Epidural Opioid Analgesia in the Introduction.

Morphine is classified in FDA Pregnancy Category C.

ADVERSE REACTIONS AND PRECAUTIONS. See the Introduction.

PHARMACOKINETICS. The volume of distribution is 3.2 ± 0.3 L/kg, the elimination half-life is 2.9 ± 0.5 hours, and the clearance rate is 14.7 ± 0.9 ml/min/kg (Stanski et al, 1978). Elderly patients may be more sensitive to morphine and have higher, more variable serum levels than younger patients. This may be reflected as increased duration rather than increased effect; thus, age should be considered when determining the dose and dosing interval (Kaiko et al, 1982).

There are only minor differences in the kinetic patterns of morphine in pediatric patients (1 month to 15 years) and no differences in their sensitivity to morphine (Dahlström et al, 1979). However, in infants under 1 week, the elimination half-life is prolonged to 6.8 hours (range, 4.6 to 8.9) and the clearance is less than 50% that of older infants (6.3 ml/min/kg; range, 3.6 to 7.6) (Lynn and Slattery, 1985).

The response to morphine may be enhanced in patients with uremia, various renal disorders, and renal ischemia (Sear et al, 1985). This may be due to accumulation of an active metabolite, morphine-6-glucuronide, that is eliminated by the kidney. The mean elimination half-life and clearance of the parent drug are similar in patients with renal failure and in normal subjects (Aitkenhead et al, 1983).

DOSAGE AND PREPARATIONS. Unless otherwise specified, all doses listed are appropriate for nontolerant patients.

Intramuscular, Subcutaneous: *Adults,* 10 mg (range, 5 to 20 mg) every three to four hours, depending on the cause of the pain and the response of the patient; *children* (subcutaneous), 0.1 to 0.2 mg/kg (maximal dose, 15 mg).

Intravenous: This route is indicated for severe pain when rapid control is required (eg, sickle cell crisis, acute pulmonary edema, or myocardial infarction). *Adults*, a bolus dose of 1 to 2 mg is given every 6 to 10 minutes and the patient should be monitored closely to determine the analgesic effect and appearance of toxicity. Otherwise, except in general anesthesia or for the management of postoperative pain, bolus intravenous administration is indicated infrequently.

The application and dosage recommendations for continuous infusion of morphine for postoperative pain and in the dying patient with severe cancer pain are discussed in the Introduction.

Epidural (Lumbar): *Adults,* 4 to 5 mg. Smaller doses are effective in the elderly (Ready, 1987).

Intrathecal: *Adults,* 0.2 to 1 mg.

Generic. Solution 1 mg/ml in 60 ml containers; 2 mg/ml in 1, 5, 10, 100, and 500 ml containers; 4 mg/ml in 1, 100, and 500 ml containers; 8 mg/ml in 2 ml containers; 10 mg/ml in 1 ml containers; 15 mg/ml in 1 and 20 ml containers; and 25 mg/ml in 4, 10, 20, and 40 ml containers.

Astramorph PF (Astra), ***Duramorph PF*** (Elkins-Sinn). Solution (sterile) 0.5 and 1 mg/ml in 10 ml containers (preservative-free).

Infumorph (Wyeth-Ayerst). Solution (sterile) 10 mg/ml (***Infumorph 200***) and 25 mg/ml (***Infumorph 500***) in 20 ml containers (preservative-free). For use in continuous microinfusion devices.

NOTE: Only preservative-free morphine sulfate should be employed for epidural or intrathecal administration.

Oral: In total effect, the initial doses of morphine are one-third to one-sixth as potent orally as intramuscularly. The dose must be individualized because of variation in bioavailability; 20 to 25 mg may be sufficient for some patients, but those who have been receiving opioids chronically may require doses as large as several grams per day. The prolonged-release preparation usually is administered every 12 hours or, if necessary, every eight hours.

Generic. Tablets 15 and 30 mg; tablets (soluble) 10, 15, and 30 mg; solution 10 and 20 mg/5 ml.

M S Contin (Purdue Frederick). Tablets (prolonged-release) 15, 30, 60, and 100 mg.

MSIR (Purdue Frederick). Solution 2 and 4 mg/ml in 5 ml containers and 20 mg/ml in 1 ml containers; tablets 15 and 30 mg.

OMS (Upsher-Smith). Solution 20 mg/ml in 30 and 120 ml containers.

Oramorph SR (Roxane). Tablets (prolonged-release) 30, 60, and 100 mg.

Roxanol (Roxane). Solution 4 mg/ml (***Rescudose***) and 20 mg/ml.

Rectal: The dose must be individualized but is usually the same amount as that given orally. *Adults,* 10 to 20 mg every four hours.

RMS (Upsher-Smith), ***Roxanol*** (Roxane), ***Generic***. Suppositories 5, 10, 20, and 30 mg.

CODEINE PHOSPHATE

$H_2PO_4^- \cdot \frac{1}{2}H_2O$

CODEINE SULFATE

ACTIONS AND USES. In the doses usually employed, codeine relieves mild to moderate pain; most commonly, it is administered orally in combination with nonopioid analgesics (see the section on Mixtures).

Results of controlled studies have shown that oral codeine 65 mg is approximately equivalent to aspirin 650 mg or acetaminophen 650 mg. In this dose range, codeine has been reported to be less effective than aspirin in postpartum, uterine, or dental pain; inhibition of prostaglandin synthesis and an anti-inflammatory action may play a role in aspirin's superiority.

When administered intramuscularly, codeine 120 to 130 mg is approximately equivalent to morphine sulfate 10 mg but causes more adverse reactions.

See also index entry Codeine, As Antitussive.

ADVERSE REACTIONS AND PRECAUTIONS. The adverse reactions of codeine resemble those of other morphine-like drugs. Constipation occurs frequently, but nausea, vomiting, and drowsiness are minimal after usual oral doses. Dizziness may occur in ambulatory patients. The larger doses necessary to relieve more severe pain cause most of the adverse effects observed with morphine, including respiratory depression. Naloxone alleviates these adverse effects, including the respiratory depression caused by overdosage.

Histamine released after large doses of parenteral codeine may produce hypotension, cutaneous vasodilation, pruritus and urticaria, and, more rarely, bronchoconstriction. This histamine-releasing action appears to be stronger than that of morphine in equianalgesic doses; therefore, codeine should not be administered intravenously.

Codeine is classified in FDA Pregnancy Category C.

DEPENDENCE LIABILITY. The dependence liability of codeine is somewhat less than that of morphine, and physical dependence occurs only rarely when typical analgesic doses are administered orally. Abuse of the drug as part of a pattern of multidrug abuse, particularly in the form of cough syrup, is not uncommon. Codeine (except in mixtures) is classified as a Schedule II drug under the Controlled Substances Act.

PHARMACOKINETICS. Codeine is absorbed rapidly following oral administration. Peak plasma levels are attained in about one hour, and the plasma half-life is about 3.5 hours. After intramuscular injection, peak plasma levels are attained in about 30 minutes, and the half-life is about three hours. The bioavailability of codeine is greater than that of morphine after oral administration. Oral codeine is one-half to three-fifths less potent than parenteral codeine.

Codeine is metabolized primarily by conjugation with glucuronic acid. A small amount (10%) is O-demethylated to form morphine, and recent evidence supports the longstanding hypothesis that the analgesic effect of codeine is produced primarily by this metabolite. Codeine O-demethylation cosegregates with the genetic sparteine-debrisoquin polymorphism; accordingly, morphine essentially is not formed in poor metabolizers. In one study, codeine increased experimental pain thresholds (ie, produced analgesia) in extensive metabolizers but had no effect in poor metabolizers. This finding may explain the inadequate analgesic response to codeine in some patients.

DOSAGE AND PREPARATIONS.

Oral, Subcutaneous, Intramuscular: For analgesia in nontolerant patients, *adults,* 30 to 60 mg four to six times daily as needed; *children,* 0.5 mg/kg four to six times daily.

For antitussive use, see index entry Codeine, As Antitussive.

CODEINE PHOSPHATE:

Generic. Solution (for injection) 30 and 60 mg/ml in 1 ml containers; solution (oral) 3 mg/ml in 500 ml containers; tablets (soluble, oral) 30 and 60 mg.

CODEINE SULFATE:

Generic. Tablets (soluble, oral) 15, 30, and 60 mg.

HYDROCHLORIDES OF OPIUM ALKALOIDS

[Pantopon]

This preparation is a mixture of purified opium alkaloids in solution as the hydrochloride salts (20 mg of the mixture contains the equivalent of 15 mg of morphine sulfate). The indications are the same as for morphine, and it is used most commonly for postoperative pain. Claims that the analgesic and sedative effects of morphine are enhanced while adverse effects are minimized by other constituents in the preparation have not been substantiated. It has no proven advantage over an equivalent amount of morphine.

This product is classified as a Schedule II drug under the Controlled Substances Act and in FDA Pregnancy Category C.

DOSAGE AND PREPARATIONS.

Intramuscular, Subcutaneous: The manufacturer's suggested dosage for nontolerant patients is: *Adults,* 5 to 20 mg.

Pantopon (Roche). Solution 20 mg/ml in 1 ml containers (alcohol 6%).

HYDROMORPHONE HYDROCHLORIDE

[Dilaudid]

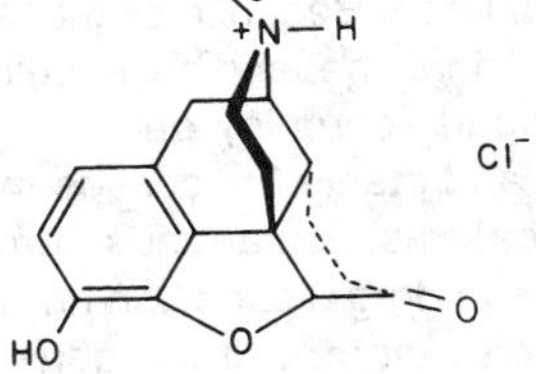

Hydromorphone, a derivative of morphine, has the same actions and uses (see the Introduction). It is about eight times more potent on a milligram basis (when given parenterally, 1.5 mg of hydromorphone is equivalent to 10 mg of morphine) and has a slightly shorter duration. The oral dose required for an equivalent analgesic effect is five times higher than the parenteral dose. The elimination half-life is about 2.5 hours after intravenous and four hours after oral administration (Ritschel et al, 1987).

Hydromorphone is more soluble than morphine; thus, higher concentrations may be injected if necessary. The greater solubility permits a smaller intramuscular or subcutaneous injection volume. This is an advantage if multiple daily doses are required in patients with diminished tissue mass due to terminal illness or when the drug is administered by continuous subcutaneous infusion.

Adverse reactions are the same as those produced by morphine in equianalgesic doses (see the Introduction).

Hydromorphone is classified as a Schedule II drug under the Controlled Substances Act and in FDA Pregnancy Category C.

DOSAGE AND PREPARATIONS. The following doses are appropriate for nontolerant patients.

Intramuscular, Intravenous (slow), Subcutaneous: *Adults,* 1 to 1.5 mg every three to four hours as required; the dose may be increased for severe pain.

Concentrated solutions of hydromorphone [Dilaudid-HP] are intended only for opioid-tolerant patients.

Generic. Solution 1 and 4 mg/ml in 1 and 2 ml containers; 2 mg/ml in 1, 2, and 20 ml containers; and 3 mg/ml in 1 ml containers.

Dilaudid (Knoll). Solution 1 and 4 mg/ml in 1 ml containers and 2 mg/ml in 1 and 20 ml containers.

Dilaudid-HP (Knoll). Solution 10 mg/ml in 1 and 5 ml containers.

Oral: *Adults,* 2 to 4 mg every four hours as required; the dose may be increased if necessary.

Generic. Tablets 2 and 4 mg.

Dilaudid (Knoll). Tablets 1, 2, 3, and 4 mg.

Rectal: *Adults,* 3 mg every six to eight hours. There is significant interpatient variability in the bioavailability of hydromorphone after rectal administration (range, 10% to 65%) (Ritschel et al, 1987).

Dilaudid (Knoll). Suppositories 3 mg.

OXYCODONE HYDROCHLORIDE

[Roxicodone]

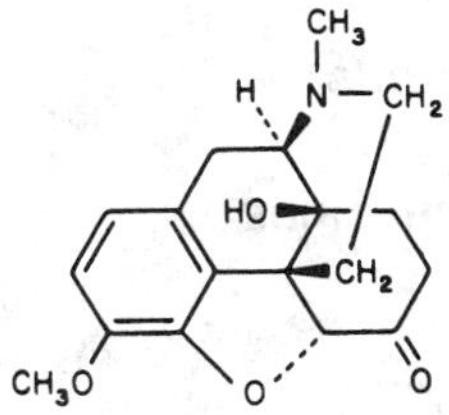

Oxycodone is similar to morphine in efficacy and duration of action, but it has a more favorable oral to parenteral potency ratio (see Table 1). The commercial preparation is for oral use only and is indicated for relief of moderate to severe pain. The drug also is available in combination with acetaminophen or aspirin.

Oxycodone is classified as a Schedule II drug under the Controlled Substances Act and in FDA Pregnancy Category C.

DOSAGE AND PREPARATIONS.

Oral: *Adults (nontolerant),* 5 to 10 mg every four to six hours.

Roxicodone (Roxane). Tablets 5 mg; solution (oral) 5 mg/5 ml and 20 mg/ml (***Intensol***).

OXYMORPHONE HYDROCHLORIDE

[Numorphan]

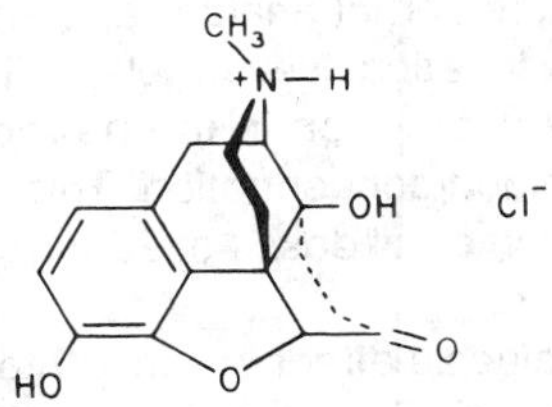

Oxymorphone is a derivative of morphine and is closely related chemically to hydromorphone. When administered parenterally, this analgesic is about ten times as potent as morphine. Its actions, uses, and duration of effect are similar to those of hydromorphone and morphine, except that oxymorphone appears to possess little antitussive activity. When administered by rectal suppository, it is about one-tenth as potent as when injected intramuscularly.

Adverse reactions are similar to those produced by morphine and other opioid analgesics in equianalgesic doses. See the Introduction for indications and adverse reactions.

Oxymorphone is classified as a Schedule II drug under the Controlled Substances Act and in FDA Pregnancy Category C.

DOSAGE AND PREPARATIONS. These doses are appropriate for nontolerant patients.

Intramuscular, Subcutaneous: *Adults,* 1 to 1.5 mg every four to six hours. For obstetric analgesia, 0.5 to 1 mg intramuscularly.

Intravenous: *Adults,* 0.5 mg initially.

Numorphan (DuPont). Solution 1 mg/ml in 1 ml containers and 1.5 mg/ml in 1 and 10 ml containers.

Rectal: *Adults,* 5 mg every four to six hours.

Numorphan (DuPont). Suppositories 5 mg.

Synthetic Compounds

MEPERIDINE HYDROCHLORIDE

[Demerol]

ACTIONS AND USES. Meperidine, a phenylpiperidine derivative, is a synthetic opioid analgesic. Many of its pharmacologic properties and indications are similar to those of morphine, but meperidine has no antitussive effect. It is one-eighth as potent as morphine when administered parenterally. Meperidine is about one-third to one-fourth as potent orally as parenterally.

This analgesic is widely used in anesthetic premedication, in balanced anesthesia, and in obstetric analgesia. Meperidine is preferred to morphine for obstetric use because its rapid onset of action and shorter duration usually permit greater flexibility in maternal analgesia, possibly with less effect on neonatal respiration. Nevertheless, it can produce significant respiratory depression in the newborn infant proportional to the fetal blood concentration. This can be minimized by giving small incremental doses of 25 mg intravenously during labor.

The maximal analgesic effect occurs 30 to 50 minutes after intramuscular injection. The duration of action (two to four hours) is shorter than that of morphine. The dose should be adjusted based on the response of the individual.

ADVERSE REACTIONS, PRECAUTIONS, AND INTERACTIONS. The most commonly observed adverse reactions include dizziness, nausea, and vomiting (especially in ambulatory patients). Its sedative effect is comparable to that of morphine. As with other opioids, extreme asthenia, hyperhidrosis, syncope, dysphoria, and nightmares have occurred. Equianalgesic doses of meperidine and morphine produce a similar degree of respiratory depression, which can be reversed by an opioid antagonist.

With prolonged administration of meperidine, large amounts of an active metabolite, normeperidine, may accumulate, particularly in patients with decreased renal function. Normeperidine, which is a potent CNS stimulant but a weak analgesic, causes excitatory phenomena, such as twitches, tremors, multifocal myoclonus, confusion, hallucinations, and grand mal seizures. A definite relationship between blood concentration of the metabolite and these reactions has not been established (Austin et al, 1981); however, the severity of the excitatory phenomena appears to be related to both the absolute concentration of normeperidine and the ratio of normeperidine (excitatory) to meperidine (predominantly depressant) (Kaiko et al, 1983). Naloxone may precipitate seizures in patients who received multiple large doses of meperidine. If there is evidence of a developing excitatory response to meperidine, the drug should be discontinued, an alternative opioid (eg, morphine) should be administered to control pain, and a benzodiazepine with anticonvulsant properties (eg, diazepam) given if indicated. Because of these problems and its short duration of action, meperidine should not be used for treatment of prolonged (chronic) pain.

Pain, induration, and sterile abscesses may occur at injection sites after repeated subcutaneous administration.

Because changes in drug disposition have been reported in patients with liver disease and the elderly, dosage must be reduced in these individuals (Mather and Meffin, 1978). The dose of meperidine also should be reduced when antipsychotic agents, sedative-hypnotics, or other drugs that depress the CNS are given concurrently. Severe toxic reactions (eg, restlessness, excitement, fever, death) have followed the use of meperidine in patients receiving monoamine oxidase inhibitors.

Contraindications to the use of meperidine are similar to those for morphine and other opioid analgesics.

Meperidine is classified as a Schedule II drug under the Controlled Substances Act.

PHARMACOKINETICS. Following intravenous administration of meperidine in healthy individuals, the volume of distribution at steady state was 269 L (range, 198 to 333 L); plasma clearance was 1.06 L/min (range, 0.71 to 1.32), and the elimination half-life was 3.6 hours (range, 3.1 to 4.1) (Mather and Meffin, 1978). Liver disease, eg, cirrhosis, acute viral hepatitis, doubles the half-life (Mather, 1986). There is evidence that the disposition of meperidine varies between day and night, with the elimination half-life being shorter and the plasma clearance greater at night. This suggests that larger doses might be required at night (Ritschel et al, 1983). Bioavailability after oral administration is about 50% due to first-pass metabolism in the liver but increases to 80% to 90% in patients with cirrhosis (Edwards et al, 1982). The elimination half-life in the neonate is 22.7 hours (range, 12 to 39 hours) (Caldwell et al, 1978).

Approximately 5% of the dose is excreted by the kidney as unchanged drug. A portion of the parent drug undergoes hydrolysis of the ester group to form meperidinic acid. In part, meperidine is N-demethylated initially to form normeperidine. Some normeperidine is hydrolyzed to normeperidinic acid. The renal clearance of normeperidine is correlated with creatinine clearance, whereas that of meperidine is not (Boréus et al, 1986). The clearance of meperidine is enhanced by an acid urine; the clearance of normeperidine is significantly less dependent on pH. The renal clearance of both compounds is independent of urinary flow. The half-life of normeperidine is 15 to 30 hours, depending on renal function. With repeated dosing, therefore, this toxic metabolite accumulates more than meperidine and its concentration may exceed that of meperidine in the plasma (Inturrisi and Umans, 1986).

DOSAGE AND PREPARATIONS. These doses are appropriate for nontolerant patients.

Intramuscular, Intravenous (slow), Oral, Subcutaneous: *Adults,* 100 mg (range, 50 to 150 mg), repeated at intervals of three to four hours if required. If repeated administration is anticipated, the intramuscular route is preferred to subcutaneous injection; the injection site should be rotated. For obstetric analgesia, 50 to 100 mg intramuscularly or subcutaneously, repeated three or four times at one- to three-hour intervals if necessary. *Children,* 1 to 1.5 mg/kg (maximal dose, 100 mg) intramuscularly, orally, or subcutaneously, repeated at intervals of three to four hours if necessary.

Generic. Solution (for injection) 10 mg/ml in 30 ml containers, 25 and 75 mg/ml in 1 and half-filled 2 ml containers, 50 mg/ml in 1 and 30 ml containers, and 100 mg/ml in 1 and 20 ml containers; syrup 50 mg/5 ml; tablets 50 and 100 mg.

Demerol (Sanofi Winthrop). Solution (for injection) 25 mg/ml in 0.5 and 2 ml containers, 50 mg/ml in 1, 2, and 30 ml containers, 75 mg/ml in 1.5 and 2 ml containers, and 100 mg/ml in 1, 2 (half-filled and filled), and 20 ml containers; syrup 50 mg/5 ml; tablets 50 and 100 mg.

LEVORPHANOL TARTRATE

[Levo-Dromoran]

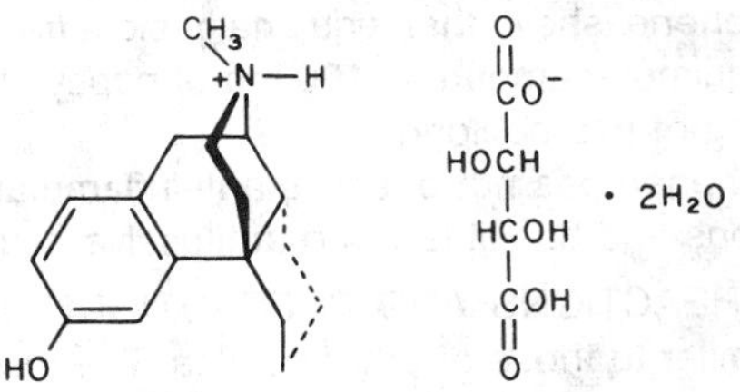

CH_3 +N—H HO · $2H_2O$ (structure: O=C(O⁻)–HOCH–HCOH–C(=O)OH)

This synthetic analgesic is a morphinan derivative related chemically and pharmacologically to morphine, and it has the same indications (see the Introduction). Levorphanol is four to eight times more potent than morphine after intramuscular injection and has a similar duration of action. It is about one-half as potent orally as intramuscularly.

The adverse reactions and precautions of levorphanol are similar to those of morphine. Although some reports suggest that levorphanol is less likely to cause nausea, vomiting, and constipation, any difference in the incidence of adverse reactions is slight. (See the Introduction.) Levorphanol is classified as a Schedule II drug under the Controlled Substances Act.

PHARMACOKINETICS. Minimal information is available. One study in a limited number of patients with advanced malignant disease or chronic intractable pain has been reported (Dixon, 1986). Following intravenous administration of levorphanol, the following approximations can be made: apparent volume of distribution is 10.5 L/kg, total body clearance is 10.6 ml/kg/min, and half-life is 11.4 hours. Because the half-life is long in relation to the duration of analgesia, repeated dosing leads to substantial accumulation and may result in excessive sedation.

DOSAGE AND PREPARATIONS.

Oral, Subcutaneous, Intravenous: *Adults (nontolerant),* 2 to 3 mg.

Generic. Tablets 2 mg.

Levo-Dromoran (Roche). Solution (for injection) 2 mg/ml in 1 and 10 ml containers; tablets 2 mg.

METHADONE HYDROCHLORIDE

[Dolophine Hydrochloride]

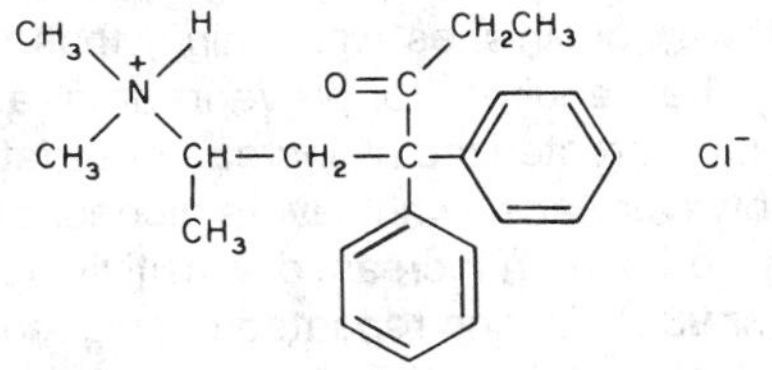

CH_3, H, +N, CH_3, CH—CH_2—C, CH_3, O=C, CH_2CH_3, Cl^-

ACTIONS AND USES. Methadone is a synthetic analgesic that differs chemically from morphine, although the actions and analgesic potency of the two drugs are similar.

Methadone is employed to relieve severe pain. Repeated doses result in accumulation of the drug. Following a single intramuscular injection of an equivalent dose, the duration of analgesia and subjective effects are the same as with morphine. With repeated doses, these responses become prolonged, which may allow less frequent administration in some patients and fewer interruptions of the patient's sleep. However, more frequent assessment of the dosage is required to avoid adverse effects that may result from accumulation, particularly sedation and respiratory depression.

Methadone can prevent or relieve acute withdrawal symptoms produced by morphine-like drugs. It is used orally in the detoxification of patients dependent on opioid drugs because the withdrawal of methadone itself produces symptoms that are less intense, although more prolonged, than those of heroin or morphine withdrawal and the syndrome develops more slowly. Methadone also is used orally in maintenance programs for individuals dependent on heroin or other morphine-like drugs.

Although methadone depresses the cough reflex, labeling for use as an antitussive is no longer permitted.

Methadone is classified as a Schedule II drug under the Controlled Substances Act.

PHARMACOKINETICS. Numerous studies have been conducted on methadone disposition following single-dose administration in normal subjects and postoperative patients and following steady-state dosing in patients with chronic pain or in methadone maintenance programs.

In single doses, urinary pH has a profound effect on both the distribution and elimination kinetics of methadone. In subjects with a mean urinary pH of 5.2, the mean half-life was

19.5 hours, the mean volume of distribution was 3.51 L/kg, and the mean clearance was 2.1 ml/min/kg. The corresponding values when the mean urinary pH was 7.8 were half-life 42.1 hours, volume of distribution 5.24 L/kg, and clearance 1.5 ml/min/kg (Nilsson et al, 1982). When urinary pH remains above 6, renal excretion is not a major route of elimination of unchanged methadone; at a pH of 5.2, however, 35% of the total clearance of methadone can be attributed to renal excretion (Inturrisi and Colburn, 1986). In anuric patients, fecal elimination of methadone and its metabolites is adequate to keep methadone blood concentrations within desirable limits following doses of 40 to 50 mg/day (Kreek et al, 1980).

Methadone is metabolized by oxidative N-demethylation in the liver, which results in two active metabolites, normethadone and nornormethadone. This is followed by cyclization to form a pyrrolidine metabolite, which can be excreted in the urine or feces or further metabolized. The effectiveness of the oxidative pathway diminishes with aging; thus, longer dose intervals may be required to prevent drug accumulation, which is usually characterized by increased sedation, in elderly patients. However, those with severe alcoholic liver disease do not appear to have an increased sensitivity to methadone (Novick et al, 1985). During repeated dosing, concurrent administration of phenytoin or rifampin induces oxidative enzymes, which accelerates metabolism of methadone and may provoke the opioid withdrawal syndrome.

More than 90% of an oral dose of methadone is absorbed. The oral to parenteral potency ratio is 1 to 2. Oral administration of subsequent identical doses produces almost equivalent analgesic activity, but the amount should be adjusted to the individual patient's response. Methadone is about 90% bound to plasma protein.

ADVERSE REACTIONS AND PRECAUTIONS. Nausea, vomiting, constipation, dizziness, dryness of the mouth, and mental depression occur most frequently in ambulatory patients. Contraindications are the same as for morphine. Because methadone accumulates with repeated administration, careful monitoring and dosage adjustments are essential during the accumulation period (about ten days), particularly in the elderly and debilitated (Foley and Inturrisi, 1987). Subcutaneous injection may be irritating.

DOSAGE AND PREPARATIONS. These doses are appropriate for nontolerant patients.

Intramuscular, Subcutaneous: *Adults,* for relief of pain, 2.5 to 10 mg, repeated every six to eight hours when necessary. Dosage should be individualized; the amount depends on the severity of pain and the response of the patient. When multiple parenteral doses are required, the intramuscular route is preferred.

Dolophine Hydrochloride (Lilly). Solution 10 mg/ml in 1 and 20 ml containers.

Oral: For relief of pain, dosage should be individualized according to the severity of pain and the response of the patient. *Adults,* (tablets) 2.5 to 10 mg every six to eight hours; (solution) 5 to 20 mg every six to eight hours. (This dose interval differs from the three- to four-hour interval cited in the manufacturers' labeling.) After pain relief is maintained for three to five days, the dose may need to be reduced or the interval increased to prevent accumulation and toxic effects; administration every 8 to 12 hours may be adequate in some patients (Hansen et al, 1982).

Dolophine Hydrochloride (Lilly). Tablets 5 and 10 mg.

Methadone Hydrochloride (Lilly). Tablets (dispersible) 40 mg (for detoxification and maintenance treatment only).

Methadone Hydrochloride (Roxane). Solution (oral) 1, 2, and 10 mg/ml (alcohol 8%); tablets 5 and 10 mg.

PROPOXYPHENE HYDROCHLORIDE

[Darvon, Dolene]

PROPOXYPHENE NAPSYLATE

[Darvon-N]

ACTIONS AND USES. Propoxyphene is related chemically to methadone and is used orally to relieve mild to moderate pain. Although this drug is an opioid, its analgesic efficacy at typical doses is limited. The potency of propoxyphene hydrochloride is one-half to two-thirds that of codeine, and 65 mg is no more (and usually less) effective than 650 mg of aspirin or acetaminophen. Results of studies comparing the two salts of propoxyphene show that equianalgesic effects are produced by equimolar amounts (100 mg of napsylate is equivalent to 65 mg of hydrochloride).

Propoxyphene does not possess anti-inflammatory or antipyretic actions and has little or no antitussive activity.

ADVERSE REACTIONS AND PRECAUTIONS. Adverse effects are similar to those of other opioids. The most common are dizziness, drowsiness, nausea, and vomiting, which are more prominent in ambulatory patients. Some reactions may be alleviated if the patient is recumbent. Less common untoward effects include constipation, abdominal pain, rash, and headache. Asthenia, euphoria, dysphoria, and minor visual disturbances have been reported rarely. Concomitant ingestion of alcohol or other central nervous system depressants produces additive effects.

Propoxyphene should not be prescribed for pregnant women since adverse effects on fetal development have not been ruled out. Withdrawal symptoms have occurred in the neonate when the drug was used by the mother near term.

DEPENDENCE LIABILITY. The dependence liability of propoxyphene is comparable to that of codeine, and abuse with development of morphine-type dependence has been reported. Propoxyphene preparations are classified as Schedule IV drugs under the Controlled Substances Act.

POISONING. Propoxyphene alone in doses of 1 g or more or lower amounts used with alcohol and other CNS depressants has caused a number of deaths from drug overdose. Most of these fatalities were associated with suicide or abuse, but some apparently resulted from accidental overdose.

Overdosage is manifested by respiratory depression; extreme somnolence, which may be followed by coma; pupillary constriction; and acute circulatory failure. In addition to these symptoms, which are characteristic of opioid poisoning, focal and generalized convulsions usually are prominent. Arrhythmias and pulmonary edema are reported occasionally and have been ascribed to the accumulation of norpropoxyphene; apnea, cardiac arrest, and death have occurred. The opioid antagonist, naloxone, overcomes severe respiratory depression and should be given following airway management and initiation of respiratory support.

PHARMACOKINETICS. Propoxyphene is completely absorbed after oral administration, but systemic availability is reduced because of the first-pass elimination by the liver of 30% to 70% of a dose. The major metabolite is the mono-N-demethylated product, norpropoxyphene, which is largely eliminated in the urine. The oral clearance is 1.3 to 3.6 L/min, and systemic clearance is 0.6 to 1.2 L/min. The apparent volume of distribution is 700 to 1,800 L. The half-life of propoxyphene is 14.6 hours (range, 8 to 24) and that of norpropoxyphene is 22.9 hours (range, 18 to 29) (Gram et al, 1979). Because of its long half-life, norpropoxyphene can accumulate if propoxyphene is given repeatedly. The neurotoxic effects described above may result from excessive doses. Studies utilizing single and multiple doses do not indicate saturation kinetics (Brøsen et al, 1985). The half-lives of propoxyphene and norpropoxyphene are prolonged in the elderly.

DOSAGE AND PREPARATIONS. This drug should be given only to nontolerant patients.

Oral: *Adults,* 65 mg (hydrochloride) every three to four hours or 100 mg (napsylate) every four hours as needed.

PROPOXYPHENE HYDROCHLORIDE:

Darvon (Lilly), ***Dolene*** (Lederle), ***Generic.*** Capsules 65 mg.

Additional Trademark.

Doxaphene (Major).

PROPOXYPHENE NAPSYLATE:

Generic. Tablets 50 and 100 mg.

Darvon-N (Lilly). Suspension 50 mg/5 ml; tablets 100 mg.

AGONIST-ANTAGONISTS

PENTAZOCINE HYDROCHLORIDE

[Talwin Nx]

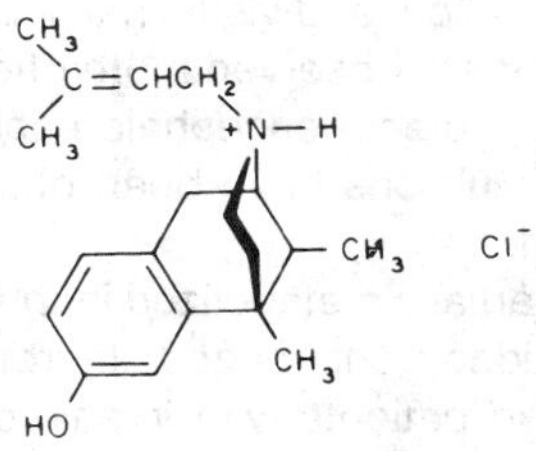

CH_3 $C=CHCH_2$ CH_3 $+N-H$ CH_3 Cl^- CH_3 HO

PENTAZOCINE LACTATE

[Talwin]

ACTIONS. Pentazocine was the first mixed agonist-antagonist analgesic to be marketed. It is an agonist at the κ opioid receptor and has a weak antagonist action at the μ receptor. Results of controlled clinical studies have shown that parenteral pentazocine is one-fourth to one-sixth as potent as morphine, and it is about one-third as potent orally as parenterally. It differs from morphine-like drugs in its subjective actions and is therefore less effective when a prominent antianxiety effect is required.

Pentazocine has a more rapid onset and a shorter duration of action than morphine; thus, its time-effect curve resembles that of meperidine. Following intramuscular injection, maximal analgesia usually occurs within 30 to 60 minutes and lasts two to three hours. After oral ingestion, the peak effect occurs in one to three hours; the duration is somewhat longer than after intramuscular injection.

USES. Pentazocine relieves moderate pain but is less effective than morphine in severe pain. Its usefulness in chronic pain is limited because of its short duration of action and the problems associated with repeated injection (see below). This drug also is administered for preoperative medication. When used for obstetric analgesia, pentazocine causes fetal respiratory depression comparable to that produced by meperidine.

ADVERSE REACTIONS AND PRECAUTIONS. Adverse reactions are generally similar to those produced by other opioid analgesics, except as indicated below. Nausea, vomiting, and dizziness occur frequently. The degree of drowsiness and sedation produced by pentazocine is approximately the same or greater than that produced by analgesic doses of morphine or meperidine, but the patient may be aroused easily to an alert and cooperative state. The detached state characteristic of morphine use is much less prominent with pentazocine. Constipation is uncommon. Pentazocine increases sphincter resistance to bile flow; therefore, it is not recommended prior to endoscopic procedures of the bile duct or in patients with biliary disease (Staritz et al, 1986).

As with other opioids, pentazocine produces respiratory depression. The severity of respiratory depression following parenteral administration of 20 mg of pentazocine is equivalent to that produced by 10 mg of morphine. However, unlike morphine, increasing the dose of pentazocine above 30 mg does not cause a proportionate increase in respiratory depression.

Dysphoria is a prominent adverse effect. Nightmares, feelings of depersonalization, and visual hallucinations may occur with usual doses but are observed more often following larger doses. Epileptiform electroencephalographic abnormalities and grand mal convulsions have been observed rarely after large intravenous doses.

Pentazocine is partially metabolized in the liver and partially excreted by the kidney unchanged; therefore, it should be used with caution in patients with impaired renal or hepatic function.

Pentazocine should not be used to relieve the pain of myocardial infarction because it tends to increase pulmonary arterial and central venous pressure and therefore cardiac workload.

Repeated injection into a single area can produce sterile abscess, ulceration, and scarring of the subcutaneous tissue and muscle. If long-term administration is required and oral pentazocine cannot be utilized, the intramuscular route should be employed and the injection site rotated. Inadvertent intra-arterial administration of pentazocine hydrochloride produces extreme pain followed by cyanosis and edema of the distal extremity. The edema is persistent and may be associated with blistering of the skin and necrosis of the tips of the digits. The immediate administration of an arterial vasodilator is recommended.

This drug is classified in FDA Pregnancy Category C.

DEPENDENCE LIABILITY. Like other opioids with agonist-antagonist properties, pentazocine has less liability for abuse than opioid agonists; nevertheless, psychological dependence has been reported, primarily after parenteral administration. In most of these individuals, prior dependence or abuse of other drugs had been established. Thus, pentazocine should be used with caution and treatment should be carefully monitored in dependence prone or emotionally unstable individuals.

Pentazocine plus the antihistamine, tripelennamine [Pyribenzamine], a combination known as "T's and blues," has been employed as a heroin substitute by drug abusers. Usually two tablets of pentazocine (50 mg each) and one of tripelennamine (50 mg) are crushed and injected intravenously. This combination appears to increase the euphoriant and suppress the dysphoric effects of pentazocine. Coadministration had no effect on the pharmacokinetic profile of either drug (Yeh et al, 1986). Because of such abuse, the oral preparation of pentazocine was reformulated to contain a parenterally effective antagonist dose of naloxone. First-pass inactivation of naloxone by the liver is extensive following oral administration and the analgesic effect of pentazocine is not diminished significantly; however, when injected intravenously naloxone reduces the euphoriant effect. The addition of naloxone has not eliminated such abuse entirely (Reed and Schnoll, 1986).

Abrupt withdrawal following prolonged parenteral administration can cause abdominal cramps, fever, lacrimation, rhinorrhea, anxiety, and restlessness in some patients. These symptoms rarely require treatment; if they are severe, administration of pentazocine can be resumed and the dose reduced gradually or an opioid agonist can be given. A benzodiazepine controls withdrawal symptoms in some patients.

Pentazocine, like other opioid antagonists, can precipitate an acute withdrawal syndrome in physically dependent patients; the severity of the reaction depends on previous experience with opioids and the dose of pentazocine.

Pentazocine is classified as a Schedule IV drug under the Controlled Substances Act. In some states, it is included in Schedule II.

POISONING. The most common toxic effects of pentazocine are dysphoria, delusions, and hallucinations. Massive overdose is characterized by unconsciousness, depressed respiration, and generalized seizures. Oxygen and mechanical support of ventilation, correction of acidosis, and other supportive measures should be employed as needed. Naloxone is effective as an antagonist, but larger than usual doses are often required. In one case report, a patient who had ingested 2.5 g of pentazocine became unconscious and had spontaneous but irregular respiration and status grand mal seizures. No further seizures occurred after the administration of naloxone 1.6 mg and diazepam 10 mg (Roytblat et al, 1986).

PHARMACOKINETICS. Pentazocine is well absorbed by all routes of administration, but there is considerable individual variation. Bioavailability after oral administration is 18.4% ± 7.8%; the reduction is due to first-pass metabolism. The elimination half-life is 203 ± 71 minutes following intravenous administration and 177 ± 34 minutes following oral administration. The volume of distribution at steady state is 396 ± 136 L. In cirrhotic patients, the elimination half-life is doubled and the rate of clearance halved. Oral bioavailability in these patients is increased from about 20% to approximately 70% (Bullingham et al, 1983). Pentazocine is metabolized extensively and is excreted in urine as conjugated and unchanged drug (Ehrnebo et al, 1977).

DOSAGE AND PREPARATIONS. (Strengths are expressed in terms of the base.) This drug should be used only in nontolerant, nonphysically dependent patients.

Oral: *Adults,* 50 mg every three or four hours as needed, increased to 100 mg if necessary (maximum, 600 mg daily). *Children under 12 years,* dosage not established.

PENTAZOCINE HYDROCHLORIDE:

Talwin Nx (Sanofi Winthrop). Tablets 50 mg with naloxone hydrochloride 0.5 mg.

Intramuscular, Intravenous, Subcutaneous: *Adults,* 30 mg every three to four hours as necessary; single doses in excess of 30 mg intravenously or 60 mg intramuscularly or subcutaneously are not advisable, and the total daily dose should not exceed 360 mg. The subcutaneous route should not be used unless essential because of possible tissue damage. (Pentazocine should not be mixed in the same syringe with soluble barbiturates because precipitation will occur.) *Children under 12 years,* dosage not established.

For obstetric analgesia, 20 or 30 mg as a single intramuscular dose. When contractions become regular, 20 mg may be given intravenously and repeated two or three times at two- to three-hour intervals as needed.

PENTAZOCINE LACTATE:

Talwin (Sanofi Winthrop). Solution 30 mg/ml in 1, 1.5, 2, and 10 ml containers.

BUPRENORPHINE HYDROCHLORIDE
[Buprenex]

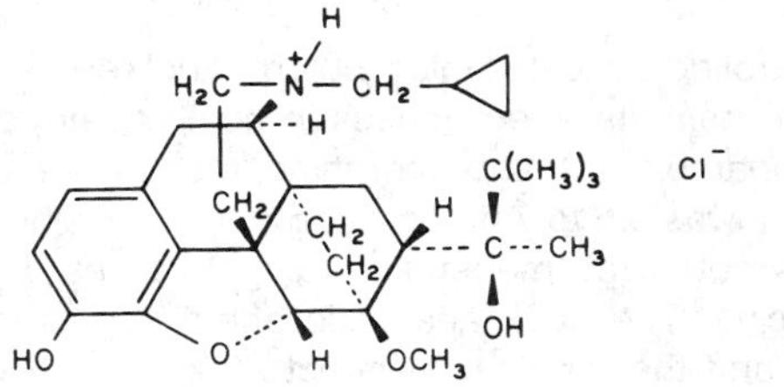

ACTIONS AND USES. Buprenorphine is a derivative of the opium alkaloid, thebaine. This potent opioid analgesic possesses both a partial agonist action at the μ and κ receptors and an antagonist property at the δ receptor, which account for some of its unique actions. The drug essentially is free from dysphoric and psychotomimetic actions. Buprenorphine is 20 to 30 times more potent than morphine; 0.3 mg buprenorphine is approximately equivalent to 10 mg morphine. It has a longer duration of action (up to six hours) than morphine, pentazocine, and meperidine. This prolonged duration is related to slow dissociation of buprenorphine from the opioid receptors rather than to slow plasma clearance. Onset of analgesia occurs within 15 minutes after intramuscular injection and sooner after intravenous administration.

In numerous clinical trials, as well as in clinical use, buprenorphine has relieved moderate to severe pain associated with surgical procedures (eg, abdominal, thoracic, orthopedic, hysterectomy), cancer, neuralgias, labor, renal colic, and myocardial infarction. When this drug was used to treat chronic pain for several months, efficacy varied with the nature of the pain, but tolerance to the analgesic effect did not develop.

Buprenorphine can be given intravenously or intramuscularly. This drug undergoes extensive first pass hepatic metabolism and thus is not useful for oral administration. This can be circumvented by giving the drug sublingually, but this dosage form is not available in the United States. It also has been given extradurally but should not be used by this route in patients who have received systemic opioids for prolonged periods because severe hypotension may occur (Christensen and Andersen, 1982).

When used with nitrous oxide and flunitrazepam in balanced anesthesia, buprenorphine produced satisfactory analgesia for minor surgery but was usually inadequate when used alone. When it was given intravenously or intramuscularly after induction of anesthesia with nitrous oxide and fentanyl, the anesthetic and respiratory depressant effects of fentanyl were reversed but the analgesic effects were prolonged. Buprenorphine apparently acted as an opioid antagonist, but its agonist effect extended the duration of analgesia. Additional studies are necessary to determine the usefulness of buprenorphine in balanced anesthesia.

The drug's cardiovascular effects are similar to those produced by morphine in equianalgesic doses. Slight reductions in heart rate and systolic blood pressure with little or no change in diastolic pressure were observed. Myocardial contractility was not affected. Buprenorphine has been used to relieve the pain of myocardial infarction in a limited number of patients and no clinically significant hemodynamic effects have been observed; however, additional studies are needed to establish the efficacy of this drug in this condition.

ADVERSE REACTIONS AND PRECAUTIONS. In general, the adverse reactions of buprenorphine resemble those of other opioid analgesics. Drowsiness occurs most frequently (50% to 85%) and is most pronounced during the first hour after administration. The incidence of nausea and vomiting is 10% to 20%. Other reactions include constipation, diaphoresis, dizziness, dryness of the mouth, miosis, bradycardia, and hypotension.

Like other opioid analgesics, buprenorphine can produce respiratory depression resembling that caused by morphine at equianalgesic doses, but the onset is delayed and the duration is longer. Maximal respiratory depression in adults is evoked by doses of 0.3 to 0.6 mg intramuscularly. Severe respiratory depression has not been reported, even with doses up to 7 mg intravenously. Large doses of naloxone (10 mg) are required to reverse the depression produced by buprenorphine, possibly because of the slow dissociation of buprenorphine from the opioid receptor; reversal does not occur immediately but rather appears to shorten buprenorphine's duration of action (Gal, 1989). Doxapram, a respiratory stimulant, has been reported to reverse the decreased respiration; however, mechanical ventilation is preferred for management. As with other opioids, buprenorphine should be used with caution in patients receiving other CNS depressants and in those with head injuries or respiratory disorders unless mechanical support of respiration is provided.

This drug is classified in FDA Pregnancy Category C.

DEPENDENCE LIABILITY. Results of studies to determine the dependence liability of buprenorphine indicate that its abuse potential is low in animals and humans and may be less than that of codeine or propoxyphene. In studies in former addicts, buprenorphine produced typical subjective morphine-like effects following single doses or long-term administration. The intensity of abstinence symptoms after prolonged administration was less than with morphine and similar to codeine, propoxyphene, nalorphine, pentazocine, and butorphanol. Symptoms develop gradually and do not reach maximum intensity for 14 to 15 days.

Buprenorphine blocks the effects of large doses of morphine for about 30 hours. On the basis of these findings, it was suggested that this analgesic could be used for maintenance therapy in the treatment of opioid addiction (Jasinski et al, 1978). Buprenorphine suppresses the self-administration of heroin or other opioids in addicts, but further studies are needed to determine whether it is useful for maintenance therapy for heroin dependence (Mello and Mendelson, 1980; Kosten and Kleber, 1988). Preliminary reports suggested that low doses of buprenorphine also decreased cocaine use in addicts who use both opioids and cocaine. However, more recent reports suggest that higher doses increase rather than decrease craving for cocaine.

Dependence on or abuse of buprenorphine was not reported in a postmarketing surveillance study (Harcus et al, 1979) in the United States, but there are documented episodes of abuse of the sublingual tablets (which are not available in the United States) in western Europe. Its abuse potential assessed after wider clinical use in the United States appears minimal. Buprenorphine should be prescribed with the same care as other opioids.

Buprenorphine is classified as a Schedule V drug under the Controlled Substances Act.

PHARMACOKINETICS. Buprenorphine is absorbed rapidly after intramuscular injection. Peak plasma concentrations occur in two to five minutes; after five minutes, concentrations are equal to those achieved with intravenous injection. After intramuscular administration, buprenorphine is excreted unchanged, mainly in the feces (68%), with smaller amounts (27%) excreted in the urine as conjugates of the unchanged drug and the dealkylated derivative.

Absorption is variable and delayed following sublingual administration; the peak blood level occurs in about three hours (range, 90 to 360 minutes) and absorption is essentially complete within five hours. Analgesia is attained in 15 to 45 minutes. There appears to be no direct relationship between plasma concentration and pharmacologic effect. Bioavailability was about 50% after sublingual administration and about 16% after oral administration. The drug is highly protein bound (about 96%).

Following intravenous administration, buprenorphine has a volume of distribution of 187.8 ± 35.3 L at steady state, a plasma clearance of 1275 ± 88.9 ml/min, and an elimination half-life of approximately five hours (Bullingham et al, 1983). Renal failure does not affect the kinetics of intravenous buprenorphine (McQuay et al, 1986).

DOSAGE AND PREPARATIONS.

Intramuscular, Intravenous (slow): *Adults,* 0.3 to 0.6 mg every six to eight hours as required. *Children under 13 years,* dosage has not been established.

Buprenex (Reckitt and Colman). Solution 0.3 mg/ml in 1 ml containers.

Sublingual, Oral: Preparations for these routes are *not* available commercially in the United States. The usual sublingual dosage for chronic pain in adults is 0.4 mg three times a day. The corresponding oral dose is 1 to 2 mg (McQuay et al, 1986).

BUTORPHANOL TARTRATE

[Stadol, Stadol NS]

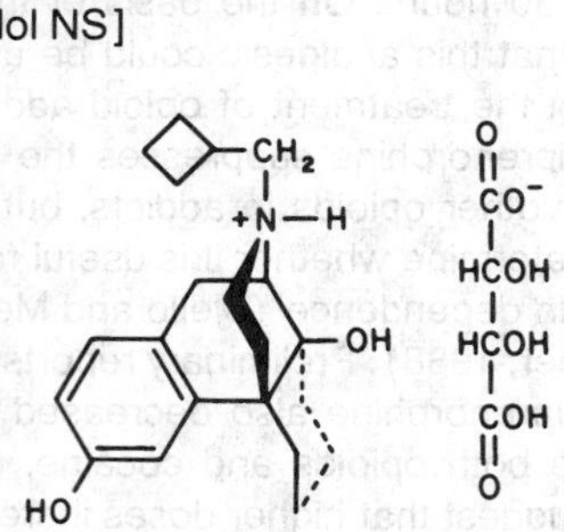

ACTIONS AND USES. Although butorphanol is related chemically to levorphanol, its actions resemble those of pentazocine. The antagonist potency of butorphanol at the μ receptor is about 10 to 30 times that of pentazocine and about one-tenth to one-fortieth that of naloxone, as determined by animal studies.

In controlled clinical studies, butorphanol relieved moderate to severe pain; its effectiveness in acute postoperative pain was comparable to that of morphine, meperidine, or pentazocine, but it was 3.5 to 7 times as potent as morphine, 30 to 40 times as potent as meperidine, and 20 times as potent as pentazocine. The peak analgesic effect occurs in about 30 minutes and the duration of effect after intramuscular injection is three to four hours. When administered as the nasal spray, onset of analgesia may be delayed and peak analgesic effect occurs within one to two hours. The duration of action is also prolonged (four to five hours).

When given in increments of 1 mg to women in active labor, butorphanol generally resembles meperidine with respect to pain relief and effects on the neonate. This dose can produce transient sinusoidal heart rate (resembling that associated with Rh-sensitization) in 75% of the fetuses (Hatjis and Meis, 1986). This also has been observed with meperidine and alphaprodine, but the incidence is much lower with these opioids. The arrhythmia is apparently benign and, in the case of meperidine, can be reversed by naloxone.

Butorphanol also appears to be comparable to meperidine when used for preanesthetic medication, except that it produces more sedation. It is not as effective as morphine as a supplement to balanced anesthesia because it exhibits a ceiling analgesic activity.

The hemodynamic effects of butorphanol, as determined in a relatively small number of patients, appear to resemble those of pentazocine more than those of morphine. Butorphanol increases pulmonary arterial pressure and pulmonary vascular resistance, left ventricular end-diastolic pressure, systemic arterial pressure, and the workload of the heart. It should not be used for the pain associated with acute myocardial infarction.

Results of animal studies have demonstrated that butorphanol has antitussive activity. It is marketed for this application in veterinary medicine, but this effect has not been studied in humans.

ADVERSE REACTIONS AND PRECAUTIONS. Adverse reactions are similar to those produced by other opioid analgesics; effects reported most frequently are sedation, nausea, and sweating. Other reactions with an incidence of more than 1% include headache, vertigo, feeling of floating, dizziness, lethargy, confusion, and lightheadedness. Psychotomimetic effects (eg, hallucinations, unusual dreams, depersonalization) reported with other antagonists (particularly pentazocine) have occurred only rarely with butorphanol. Cardiovascular (eg, palpitation) and dermatologic (eg, rash) effects also have been observed only rarely.

The respiratory depressant effects of butorphanol are similar to those of morphine in equianalgesic doses. Depression does not increase proportionally with larger doses, as with morphine, but lasts longer. Maximal respiratory depression occurs at doses above 4 mg in adults. Naloxone antagonizes respiratory depression.

Butorphanol may induce withdrawal reactions in patients who are physically dependent on opioids. It also produced a high incidence of dysphoric and psychotomimetic reactions in cancer patients who had been exposed to other opioids (Houde, 1979). Butorphanol should be used cautiously in those with respiratory depression or in conjunction with other drugs that cause respiratory depression. This drug also should be administered cautiously in reduced doses to patients with hepatic or renal impairment, for these conditions may affect its metabolism and elimination.

DEPENDENCE LIABILITY. Studies in animals and a small number of human volunteers designed to determine dependence liability indicated that butorphanol has a low potential for dependence. Symptoms resembling those of opioid withdrawal were observed when the drug was discontinued or an antagonist was administered to individuals who received large doses for several weeks; however, drug-seeking behavior was not exhibited. Subjective effects were similar to those produced by nalorphine rather than morphine. Former addicts given butorphanol tend to identify it as a barbiturate rather than as morphine and express indifference or dislike for it.

Butorphanol is not classified under the Controlled Substances Act.

PHARMACOKINETICS. Butorphanol is absorbed rapidly and completely after intramuscular injection. Bioavailability after use of the nasal spray is 60% to 70%. Peak plasma levels occur 20 to 40 minutes after intramuscular administration and 30 to 60 minutes after intranasal administration, and the elimination half-life is four to six hours. The volume of distribution is about 400 L, and the total body clearance has been reported to be 10 to 80 L/hr. This agent is metabolized primarily to the inactive hydroxybutorphanol, which is excreted mainly in the urine; some is eliminated in the bile. When butorphanol was administered to women in labor, unchanged drug and glucuronide were found in the serum of the neonate. Although the drug is excreted in human milk, the amounts are insufficient to be hazardous to a nursing infant (Pittman et al, 1980).

The nasal spray formulation of butorphanol is classified in FDA Pregnancy Category C.

DOSAGE AND PREPARATIONS. Butorphanol should be used only in nontolerant, nonphysically dependent patients.

Topical (intranasal): *Adults*, initially, 1 mg (one spray in one nostril). If pain relief is not achieved in 1 to 1.5 hours, an additional 1 mg may be applied in the other nostril. The dose may be repeated in three to four hours as needed.

For severe pain, initially, 2 mg (one spray in each nostril) in patients who will be recumbent if drowsiness or dizziness occurs. Single additional 2-mg doses may be repeated in three to four hours. For patients with impaired hepatic or renal function or who are receiving other CNS-active agents, the manufacturer recommends that the initial dose interval be increased to six to eight hours; the patient's response should determine subsequent doses. For geriatric patients, an initial dose of 1 mg should be used and a second 1-mg dose may be given if needed in 1.5 to 2 hours.

Stadol NS (Mead Johnson). Solution (spray) 10 mg/ml in 2.5 ml containers.

Intramuscular: *Adults,* 2 mg every three to four hours as necessary (range, 1 to 4 mg), depending on the severity of the pain. *Children,* dosage has not been established; 0.01 to 0.02 mg/kg has provided postoperative analgesia for approximately five hours in *children age 4 to 12* (Rodgers and Lasada, 1981). The quality and duration of analgesia as well as the degree of sedation were greater in the younger patients.

Intravenous: *Adults,* 1 mg, push; an additional dose may be given immediately if needed. The dose can be repeated every three to four hours.

Stadol (Mead Johnson). Solution 1 mg/ml in 1 ml containers and 2 mg/ml in 1, 2, and 10 ml containers.

DEZOCINE

[Dalgan]

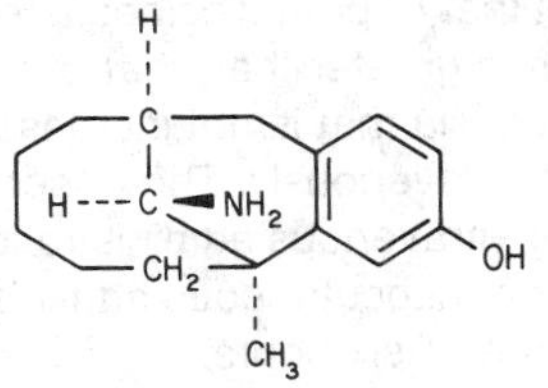

This agonist-antagonist appears to be similar to morphine in analgesic potency and duration of action after parenteral administration. In clinical trials in patients with postoperative pain, cancer pain, and other types of severe pain, dezocine was at least as effective as morphine, meperidine, and butorphanol.

ADVERSE REACTIONS AND PRECAUTIONS. Gastrointestinal distress, sedation, and dizziness occur frequently. Dezocine also may cause anxiety, headache, confusion, and delusions. Whether this drug has significant adverse cardiovascular effects is not known at present. Like the other opioid agonist-antagonist analgesics, there is a ceiling to its respiratory depressant effects, and these effects can be reversed by adequate doses of naloxone.

Dezocine is assumed to have low abuse potential and is not classified under the Controlled Substances Act; however, unlike some agonist-antagonists (eg, nalbuphine, pentazocine), dezocine produced morphine-like subjective effects in nondependent drug abusers. Further experience is required to determine its abuse liability. Because of its antagonist properties, dezocine should not be given to opioid-dependent patients.

Dezocine is classified in FDA Pregnancy Category C.

DOSAGE AND PREPARATIONS.

Intramuscular: *Adults,* initially, 10 mg; this dose is adjusted on the basis of response. For maintenance, 5 to 20 mg is given every three to six hours. *Children under 18 years,* not recommended.

Intravenous: *Adults,* 2.5 to 10 mg every two to four hours.

Dalgan (Astra). Solution (for injection) 5 and 15 mg/ml in 2 ml containers and 10 mg/ml in 2 and 10 ml containers.

NALBUPHINE HYDROCHLORIDE
[Nubain]

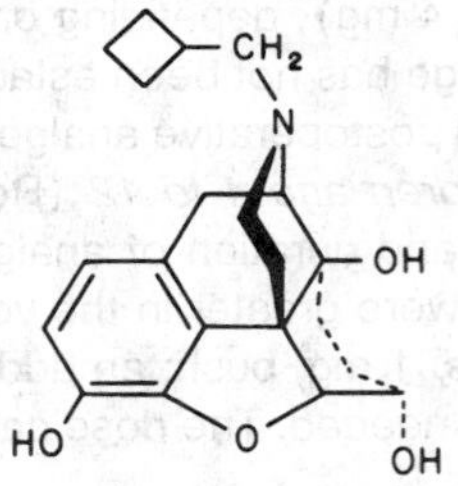

ACTIONS. Nalbuphine is related chemically to oxymorphone and the opioid antagonist, naloxone. It has both agonist and antagonist properties (Errick and Heel, 1983).

The analgesic potency of parenteral nalbuphine is approximately 0.5 to 0.9 that of morphine and about three to four times greater than that of pentazocine; its antagonistic potency is about ten times greater than that of pentazocine. There is a ceiling for analgesia that is not increased by doses greater than 0.4 mg/kg intravenously. The onset of action is two to three minutes after intravenous administration and 15 minutes after intramuscular or subcutaneous administration. The duration of effect is three to six hours.

USES. In clinical studies, nalbuphine relieved moderate to severe pain from a variety of causes (eg, postoperative, trauma, cancer, renal or biliary colic). Nalbuphine 10 to 15 mg was compared with meperidine 75 to 100 mg as an obstetric analgesic during labor and had similar effects on the mother and neonate. When used for preanesthetic medication, nalbuphine's analgesic and sedative effects were comparable to those of morphine. It is not useful as a component of balanced anesthesia because of its ceiling analgesic action.

Results of comparative studies on the hemodynamic effects of nalbuphine and morphine in patients with acute myocardial infarction indicated that nalbuphine does not increase cardiac work or pulmonary artery pressure and produces a slight but acceptable fall in heart rate and blood pressure.

ADVERSE REACTIONS AND PRECAUTIONS. In general, the adverse reactions of nalbuphine are the same as those of morphine and other opioid analgesics. The most common reaction is sedation, which occurs in about one-third of patients.

Less frequent reactions include a sweaty clammy feeling, nausea and vomiting, dizziness and vertigo, dryness of the mouth, and headache. Other CNS effects (incidence, 1% or less) include nervousness, depression, crying, confusion, hallucinations, and dysphoria. The incidence of psychotomimetic effects is very much lower than with pentazocine.

Respiratory depression may occur with usual doses of nalbuphine and is comparable to that produced by an equianalgesic dose of morphine. However, unlike the latter, depression is not increased by larger doses (greater than 30 mg) of nalbuphine. Naloxone reverses respiratory depression.

Cardiovascular reactions (hypertension, hypotension, bradycardia, tachycardia), gastrointestinal effects (dyspepsia, cramps), and dermatologic reactions (pruritus, burning, urticaria) have been reported infrequently.

Because of its antagonist property, nalbuphine may precipitate withdrawal symptoms in opioid-dependent patients. Other precautions are the same as for other opioid analgesics (see the Introduction).

DEPENDENCE LIABILITY. The abrupt withdrawal of nalbuphine following prolonged administration causes abstinence symptoms, which are milder than those of morphine but more intense than those of pentazocine. The abuse potential is low and is similar to that of pentazocine. Nalbuphine is not classified under the Controlled Substances Act.

PHARMACOKINETICS. In the manufacturer's literature, the elimination half-life is reported to be five hours after intravenous administration. Nalbuphine is metabolized to inactive conjugates by the liver. Elimination of unchanged drug and conjugates is primarily by secretion in the bile with fecal excretion. Only about 7% of unchanged drug is excreted in the urine. The potency after oral administration (not a utilized route) is about 20% of that after intramuscular use. For a summary of reported plasma concentrations as a function of time following administration, see Bullingham et al, 1983.

DOSAGE AND PREPARATIONS. This drug should be used only in nontolerant, nonphysically dependent patients.

Subcutaneous, Intramuscular, Intravenous: *Adults,* 10 mg every three to six hours as necessary, depending on the severity of the pain (maximum, 20 mg single dose and 160 mg total daily dose). *Children,* dosage has not been established.

Nubain (DuPont), ***Generic.*** Solution 10 and 20 mg/ml in 1 and 10 ml containers.

NONOPIOID ANALGESICS

The drugs discussed in this section do not bind to opioid receptors and are not classified under the Controlled Substances Act. They principally have analgesic, antipyretic, and anti-inflammatory actions.

PHARMACODYNAMICS. The exact mechanism of action of nonopioid analgesics is not known. Data from animal studies have shown that the analgesic effect of aspirin and acetaminophen on induced pain is principally peripheral (blockade of pain impulse generation); however, acetaminophen also may have a central action on transmission of nociceptive impulses (Piletta et al, 1991). The primary clinical effects of nonopioid analgesics appear to be related to inhibition of prostaglandin synthesis, since the actions of the prostaglandins have been reported to include hyperalgesia (pain), fever, edema, and erythema. They do not inhibit 5-lipoxygenase and therefore do not affect the formation of leukotrienes.

INDICATIONS. In general, nonopioid analgesics alleviate headache, myalgia, arthralgia, and other pain arising from integumental structures. Mild to moderate postoperative and postpartum pain, pain from neoplasms, and some other types of visceral pain also may respond to these drugs. They are generally not useful in severe pain and should not be substituted for opioids, but some newer NSAIDs have been effective in moderate to severe postoperative pain and can reduce the requirement for opioids. The intramuscular preparation of ketorolac tromethamine [Toradol] is useful for patients requiring parenteral medication in the immediate postoperative period. Aspirin and some other NSAIDs may be particularly useful as adjunctive agents in pain due to metastatic bone disease.

The antipyretic action of the nonopioid analgesics presumably results from inhibition of prostaglandin E_2 production within the preoptic division of the anterior hypothalamus. Reduction of elevated body temperature (more than 102° F) is indicated in young children with a history of febrile seizures, fever secondary to head trauma or CNS disease, fever-induced hallucinations in psychotic patients, and fever in patients with coronary artery and other cardiovascular disease and during early pregnancy (Gray and Blaschke, 1985). Because of the epidemiologic association of Reye's syndrome and the use of aspirin during the prodromal phase of influenza A or B and varicella (chickenpox) infections, only acetaminophen or ibuprofen is recommended as an antipyretic for fever of unknown etiology in children and adolescents. Either drug or aspirin may be employed in adults and are preferred to other nonopioid analgesics for this purpose.

Primary dysmenorrhea may be caused by increased endometrial production of prostaglandin and decreased prostacyclin. Several drugs that inhibit prostaglandin synthesis have been effective in this condition and are the preferred therapy. These include fenoprofen [Nalfon], ibuprofen, ketoprofen [Orudis], naproxen [Naprosyn], naproxen sodium [Anaprox], and piroxicam [Feldene]. Aspirin is a weak inhibitor of prostaglandin synthesis in the uterus and is almost ineffective for dysmenorrhea (Chan, 1983), as is acetaminophen. Oral contraceptives may be needed if the patient does not respond satisfactorily, and they are preferred if the patient has ulcers. For use of endocrine therapy in the management of dysmenorrhea, see index entry Dysmenorrhea, Etiology, Treatment.

DRUG SELECTION. The choice of analgesic depends on the effectiveness and adverse reactions of a particular preparation in the individual patient. The most widely used agents of this group are aspirin and acetaminophen. These drugs have equivalent analgesic and antipyretic potency, but their pharmacologic actions and adverse effects differ. If no anti-inflammatory activity is required, acetaminophen is preferred. Newer analgesic/anti-inflammatory drugs (eg, diflunisal, fenoprofen, ibuprofen, ketoprofen, naproxen, naproxen sodium, flurbiprofen, ketorolac) are equally or more effective than aspirin, acetaminophen, or codeine (see the evaluations). If oral administration cannot be employed, the intramuscular preparation of ketorolac tromethamine may be considered. Evidence supporting the analgesic efficacy of mefenamic acid [Ponstel] is limited. It has not been shown to be more effective than aspirin or similar mild analgesics and has caused a number of serious adverse reactions. The concomitant use of two NSAIDs offers no therapeutic advantage.

Etodolac [Lodine] is used in osteoarthritis and for the treatment of pain. Its analgesic effectiveness compared with other NSAIDs has not been determined. Adverse effects, primarily abdominal pain and dyspepsia, also are similar. However, animal data suggest that etodolac is less potent than some other NSAIDs in suppressing the cytoprotective effect of prostaglandins on the gastric mucosa, and gastrointestinal ulceration occurs in less than 0.3% of patients. In trials comparing etodolac with ibuprofen, indomethacin, and naproxen, fecal blood loss and gastrointestinal erosions observed by endoscopy occurred less frequently with etodolac. The drug is much more expensive than generic ibuprofen, acetaminophen, and salicylates. For the evaluation, see index entry Etodolac.

Other NSAIDs possess analgesic and antipyretic properties (see Table 2), but they are not used as general purpose mild analgesics because of their potential to cause serious adverse reactions; for discussion of these drugs, see index entry Antiarthritic Drugs.

ADVERSE REACTIONS AND PRECAUTIONS. Although some of the therapeutic actions of these drugs may be related to the inhibition of prostaglandin synthesis, many adverse reactions also are due to this pharmacologic property. Generally, serious adverse responses are associated with long-term drug use, but a few life-threatening reactions have been reported after a single exposure to the drug.

Gastrointestinal: Aspirin and all the NSAIDs cause gastroenteric side effects (Ivey, 1986; Semble and Wu, 1987; Carson et al, 1987 A, 1987 B). However, acetaminophen is not considered to be damaging to the gastric or duodenal mucosa or to cause fecal occult blood loss (Graham and Smith, 1986), and the nonacetylated salicylates, choline magnesium trisalicylate and salsalate, cause gastroenteric intolerance much less frequently. The severity of gastrointestinal side effects is related to dosage, frequency of use, and alcohol intake, but does not appear to be related to a history of ulcer disease. The incidence is greatest after use of aspirin; the other NSAIDs used as analgesics produce far less symptomatic injury. However, there is concern that the NSAIDs may aggravate damage in patients with pre-existing inflammatory bowel disease (Rampton, 1987). To minimize injury, patients receiving large doses or prolonged therapy should be asked to report black or bloody stools or faintness promptly. Such patients should be monitored for signs and symptoms of ulceration and bleeding. Although concomitant use of antacids usually prevents injury, the resulting alkalization of the urine may reduce the serum concentration of aspirin and most other NSAIDs below an effective level. Certain synthetic prostaglandins (eg, misoprostol [Cytotec]) may prevent peptic ulcers when used with aspirin or other NSAIDs (Semble and Wu, 1987) (see index entry Misoprostol for information on indications and precautions).

Renal: Renal toxicity associated with sporadic use of NSAIDs as analgesics is extremely rare. Adverse renal effects with even continuous use is uncommon. Nevertheless, since renal failure may develop, particularly in high-risk patients and the elderly, renal function should be assessed periodically with such use of these drugs (Blackshear et al, 1985; Epstein, 1986; Dunn and Patrono, 1986; Kinkaid-Smith, 1986).

In adequately hydrated patients with normal renal function and sodium intake, NSAIDs may produce sodium and water retention with edema initially, but this effect is transient. Sodium restriction, concurrent diuretic use, and conditions that diminish the circulatory volume or otherwise increase endogenous vasoconstrictor release (congestive heart failure, hepatic cirrhosis with ascites, renal disease, or nephrotic syndrome) make the kidney dependent on vasodilator prostaglandins to maintain adequate renal blood flow. If prostaglandin synthesis is inhibited by these analgesics, renal insufficiency due to hypoperfusion or acute tubular necrosis may result. Patients over 60 years; those with systemic lupus erythematosus, gout, or pre-existing renal vascular disease; and those undergoing general anesthesia also are at increased risk. If the adverse reaction is detected early and the NSAID is discontinued promptly, the nephropathy resolves gradually.

Prostaglandins stimulate the production of renin, which, in turn, enhances the release of aldosterone. Inhibition of prostaglandin production can lead to hyperkalemia, particularly in the presence of renal insufficiency or diabetes or with the coadministration of a potassium-sparing diuretic. This adverse effect can be corrected immediately by discontinuing the analgesic.

An interstitial nephritis, usually associated with nephrotic syndrome, has been reported with use of several NSAIDs. Usually patients exhibit proteinuria that may suggest nephrotoxicity, hypoalbuminemia, and edema. The severity of interstitial nephritis determines the degree of impairment in renal function, if any. The reaction may be associated with the inhibition of prostaglandin synthesis (Henrich, 1988). It is unpredictable and usually occurs only after several months of therapy. Recovery generally occurs when the drug is discontinued; however, intervention with steroids may be warranted.

The long-term use of aspirin and other NSAIDs can produce a papillary necrosis attributed to impaired blood supply to the renal medulla. Microscopic or gross hematuria suggests developing papillary necrosis (Allen et al, 1986). The previously noted association of renal papillary necrosis and long-term daily use of aspirin *as a single agent* was not confirmed in another large study, but there was suggestive evidence implicating acetaminophen (Bennett and DeBroe, 1989; Sandler et al, 1989).

Hepatic: Aspirin and the other salicylates administered regularly in doses greater than 50 mg/kg can produce mild, reversible hepatic damage. This is usually manifested as a slight but persistent increase in aminotransferase values, but biopsies reveal focal hepatocellular necrosis, hepatocytic swelling, intracellular and extracellular acidophilic bodies, and portal inflammation (Cersosimo and Matthews, 1987). A small number of patients experience more severe hepatic damage with jaundice, prolonged prothrombin time with bleeding, or intravascular coagulation. Aspirin also may precipitate hepatic encephalopathy in patients with chronic liver disease (Prescott, 1986). The role of aspirin in Reye's syndrome is described in the evaluation.

Potentially serious hepatotoxicity occurs infrequently with the remaining NSAIDs; the mechanisms are unknown. Hepatotoxicity associated with ibuprofen occurs mainly in women and appears to be a hypersensitivity reaction; symptoms include fever, rash, malaise, and usually minimal elevations of aminotransferases, bilirubin, and alkaline phosphatase values. Hepatotoxicity associated with naproxen, fenoprofen, and the antiarthritic, diclofenac [Voltaren], also primarily affects women. The hepatotoxicity generally occurs only after several months of treatment and appears as cholestatic jaundice with markedly elevated values in hepatic function tests and histologic evidence of necrosis, portal infiltrates, and cholestasis.

Studies in laboratory animals indicate that aspirin, ibuprofen, and naproxen do not induce delta-aminolevulinic acid (ALA) synthetase activity and presumably are safe for use in patients with hepatic porphyrias (McColl et al, 1987).

Acetaminophen can produce fatal hepatotoxicity after overdose in patients with normal hepatic function (see the evaluation). Usual doses only rarely are implicated as a cause of hepatotoxicity, and deterioration does not occur in patients with chronic liver disease (Prescott, 1986).

Hypersensitivity: A variety of cutaneous drug reactions have been reported. In the first review of NSAIDs by the American Academy of Dermatology (Bigby and Stern, 1985), some specificity of reaction type was associated with the chemical class to which the NSAID belongs: eg, urticaria with salicylates, photosensitivity with piroxicam, pruritus with meclofenamate [Meclomen]. For the prevalence and nature of reactions to each drug, see the individual evaluations.

Two distinct nonimmunologic syndromes characterized by bronchospasm and rhinitis or angioedema and urticaria may follow a single dose or may occur in patients who previously received these drugs without incident (Settipane, 1983; Zeitz and Jarmoszuk, 1985; Szczeklik, 1986). These syndromes are described in greater detail in the evaluation on Aspirin. Manifestation of sensitivity to one of these drugs implies sensitivity to all.

Hematologic: Acetaminophen and the nonacetylated salicylates, choline magnesium trisalicylate and salsalate, do not affect platelet aggregation, but aspirin and the NSAIDs exert a pronounced inhibitory effect. This effect is more prominent in patients with inborn disorders of platelet function (von Willebrand or Bernard-Soulier disease) and in patients receiving heparin or oral anticoagulants. For most NSAIDs, inhibition of platelet aggregation is reversible; 9 to 12 days are required for sufficient platelet synthesis to restore normal function. Inhibition by aspirin is irreversible.

Blood dyscrasias caused by acetaminophen, aspirin, or other NSAIDs employed for analgesia are rare (Miescher and Pola, 1986). Both aspirin and acetaminophen are considered safe in usual therapeutic dosage for patients with glucose-6 phosphate dehydrogenase deficiency without nonspherocytic hemolytic anemia (Beutler, 1978). Although these agents have not undergone systematic examination, the lack of case reports for NSAIDs seems to indicate that they also are safe in this regard.

Pregnancy and Lactation: Only salicylates and acetaminophen have been examined extensively for their potential adverse effects on the pregnant woman, the fetus, and on the nursing neonate whose mother is receiving one of these drugs (Heymann, 1986). It is presumed that, like aspirin, the other NSAIDs prolong gestation and labor, increase maternal blood loss during delivery, and may cause fetal intracranial hemorrhage. Fetal growth retardation may be related to inhibi-

TABLE 2.
ANALGESIC-ANTIPYRETICS AND NONSTEROIDAL ANTI-INFLAMMATORY AGENTS

Drug	Adult Analgesic Dose*
SALICYLATES	
† Aspirin	650 mg every 4 hours
Sodium salicylate	650 mg every 4 hours
Choline magnesium trisalicylate [Trilisate]	1 to 1.5 g twice daily
† Diflunisal [Dolobid]	1 g initially, 500 mg every 8 to 12 hours
‡ Salsalate [Disalcid, Mono-Gesic, Salflex]	
PARA-AMINOPHENOL DERIVATIVE	
Acetaminophen	650 mg every 4 hours
ANTHRANILIC ACID DERIVATIVES	
Mefenamic acid [Ponstel]	see evaluation
‡ Meclofenate sodium [Meclomen]	50 mg every 4 to 6 hours
PHENYLPROPIONIC ACID DERIVATIVES AND RELATED DRUGS	
‡ Carprofen [Rimadyl]	
† Fenoprofen calcium [Nalfon]	200 mg every 4 to 6 hours
† Ibuprofen [Advil, Medipren, Midol IB, Motrin, Nuprin, Rufen]	400 mg every 4 to 6 hours
† Naproxen [Naprosyn]	500 mg initially, 250 mg every 6 to 8 hours
Naproxen sodium [Anaprox]	550 mg initially, 275 mg every 6 to 8 hours
‡ Ketoprofen [Orudis]	50 mg every 6 to 8 hours
‡ Flurbiprofen [Ansaid]	
‡ Nabumetone [Relafen]	
PYRAZOLONE	
‡ Phenylbutazone [Butazolidin]	
INDOLES AND RELATED DRUGS	
‡ Etodolac [Lodine]	
‡ Indomethacin [Indocin]	
Ketorolac tromethamine [Toradol]	see evaluation
‡ Sulindac [Clinoril]	
‡ Tolmetin [Tolectin]	
OXICAM	
‡ Piroxicam [Feldene]	
ACETIC ACID DERIVATIVE	
‡ Diclofenac [Voltaren]	

** Some patients may benefit from the use of larger doses of some drugs; see text. OTC labeling may be more restrictive.*
† For additional discussion, see index entry Antiarthritic Drugs.
‡ For discussion, see index entry Antiarthritic Drugs.

tion of glucose-induced insulin release. No teratogenic effects have been substantiated.

Large doses of aspirin in the mother can induce bleeding or rash in a nursing infant. Usual therapeutic doses of other NSAIDs are presumed to be without effect. Insignificant quantities of acetaminophen are excreted in breast milk.

Summary: In summary, all nonopioid analgesics can produce serious toxicity. If only an analgesic or antipyretic action is required, acetaminophen is preferred in adolescents and children. Ibuprofen may be substituted for acetaminophen as an antipyretic and may be the drug of choice for primary dysmenorrhea in adolescent patients. The dosage of NSAIDs may require reduction in the elderly, in patients with asthma or congestive heart failure, and in those receiving diuretics or lithium. Aspirin and other NSAIDs should be avoided, if possible, in pregnant women, particularly those near term. In patients with chronic pain requiring long-term therapy, the minimum effective dose should be selected. For additional recommendations for long-term, high-dose therapy with these agents, see index entry Antiarthritic Drugs.

ACUTE OVERDOSE. Following acute or subacute overdosage, aspirin and acetaminophen produce severe and sometimes fatal intoxication despite aggressive therapy. The mechanism, signs, and management of the poisoning differ and are discussed in the evaluations. The oxicam, piroxicam, also may have a potential for serious acute toxicity. Serious intoxication with use of other nonopioid analgesics is uncommon. These analgesics are unlikely to cause significant morbidity or mortality unless they are ingested in massive overdose. A number of index cases have been reviewed (Meredith and Vale, 1986; Vale and Meredith, 1986).

Drug Evaluations

SALICYLIC ACID DERIVATIVES

ASPIRIN

USES. This prototype nonopioid analgesic is a drug of choice for the treatment of mild to moderate pain. Aspirin is more useful in the treatment of headache, neuralgia, myalgia, arthralgia, and other pain arising from integumental structures than in acute severe pain of visceral origin. However, it may relieve moderate postoperative, postpartum, or other visceral pain, such as that secondary to trauma or cancer. In the latter, aspirin may provide adequate relief and, if the pain is mild to moderate, should be tried prior to use of opioid analgesics. It is considered particularly effective for pain associated with bone metastases. Aspirin can be given with an opioid to increase the analgesic effect.

Large doses that are sufficient to provide a blood salicylate concentration of 20 to 30 mg/dL have an anti-inflammatory action, which may contribute to relief of pain when inflammation is a factor. This drug is the primary agent in the management of some rheumatic diseases (see index entry Aspirin, Uses). Aspirin is much less effective than the newer NSAIDs in dysmenorrhea.

When therapy is indicated to reduce fever, aspirin is one of the most effective drugs. However, epidemiologic evidence suggests an association between the use of aspirin to treat fever in children during the prodromal phase of varicella (chickenpox) or influenza B or A infections and the subsequent development of Reye's syndrome. Because of this risk, the use of aspirin in children and adolescents has decreased significantly. For simple analgesia, acetaminophen may be substituted; either acetaminophen or ibuprofen may be substituted if an antipyretic effect is desired.

In rheumatic fever, the amount of aspirin required to relieve pain and joint swelling exceeds usual analgesic doses. The inflammatory process is suppressed, but progression of the disease is not affected. Antibiotics and other appropriate therapy should be administered concomitantly.

Because aspirin inhibits platelet function, it has been tried in various thromboembolic diseases. For discussion, see index entry Aspirin, Uses, Myocardial Infarction.

ADVERSE REACTIONS AND PRECAUTIONS. Serious adverse reactions occur infrequently with usual analgesic doses. Gastrointestinal symptoms (gastric distress, heartburn, or nausea) are most common. Gastric distress may be diminished by taking aspirin with food or a full glass of water. Occult gastrointestinal bleeding occurs in many patients but apparently is not correlated with gastric distress. The amount of blood lost is usually insignificant clinically but, with prolonged administration, iron deficiency anemia may result. Massive gastrointestinal hemorrhage occurs rarely in relation to the frequency of aspirin use. This effect may be due to the action of aspirin on the stomach mucosa, platelet dysfunction, or both in susceptible individuals (ie, those with ulcer, bleeding problems). Aspirin may cause gastric ulcers after long-term use. There is no evidence that it produces duodenal ulcers. Aspirin should not be used in patients with a recent history of peptic ulcer or gastrointestinal bleeding. Patients should be advised that alcohol may increase gastrointestinal bleeding when ingested with aspirin.

Large doses of aspirin taken for several days can cause hypoprothrombinemia, which may be reversed by phytonadione (vitamin K_1). This effect usually is not significant except in susceptible patients (eg, those receiving anticoagulants, patients with severe liver disease). Usual analgesic doses of aspirin inhibit platelet aggregation and increase bleeding time. Because of the role of platelets in hemostasis, this effect may be an important factor in gastrointestinal and other bleeding. Aspirin is contraindicated in patients with bleeding disorders (eg, hemophilia). The drug should be discontinued one week prior to surgery to prevent or minimize postoperative bleeding. Because anti-inflammatory doses suppress both thromboxane A_2 and prostaglandin I_2, bleeding time is usually normal.

Reversible, usually mild, hepatotoxicity has been associated with the large doses given to children with rheumatic disease and adults with lupus erythematosus or rheumatoid arthritis (see index entry Aspirin, Uses, Arthritis).

An acute intolerance to aspirin occurs in about 0.3% of the population, usually adults, and is slightly (3:2) more common in women, many of whom have taken the drug without incident for many years. The reaction is nonimmunologic. Although the mechanism is not known, it is postulated to relate to prostaglandin inhibition with enhanced metabolism of arachidonic acid through the leukotriene pathway (Oates et al, 1988). Two subgroups may be distinguished in the intolerant population: one demonstrates primarily a bronchospastic response and the other are patients with chronic urticaria who demonstrate primarily exacerbation of urticaria and angioedema.

Between 10% and 50% of patients with chronic urticaria, angioedema, or both report exacerbations after ingesting aspirin or NSAIDs. Many patients who experience bronchospasm have associated chronic rhinitis, sinusitis, nasal polyps, or asthma. A typical reaction occurs between 15 minutes and three hours after ingestion; symptoms may include profuse and inappropriate rhinorrhea, macular erythema, nausea, vomiting, intestinal cramps, and diarrhea. Shortly after rhinorrhea begins, an acute asthmatic attack occurs. The reaction may be severe and there are many reports in the older medical literature of death following administration of one or two aspirin tablets. Epinephrine or theophylline may be required to counteract bronchospasm. The acute reaction normally terminates after about two hours (Zeitz and Jarmoszuk, 1985).

Intolerance to aspirin does not extend to sodium salicylate, salicylic acid esters, choline salicylate, or thiosalicylate. However, most patients who cannot tolerate aspirin also cannot tolerate other NSAIDs. Most sensitive patients can take acetaminophen, which is only 4% to 6% cross-reactive; however, only one-half of a tablet should be given initially and the patient should be observed for two to three hours. Cross-intolerance also extends to sulfinpyrazone and tartrazine (FD&C Yellow No 5), a dye often used in food, cosmetics, and pharmaceuticals.

Aspirin does not appear to have any teratogenic effects in humans. Prolonged pregnancy and labor with increased bleeding before and after delivery may be correlated with chronic ingestion of aspirin that produces high blood salicylate concentrations during the week preceding parturition. Aspirin is classified in FDA Pregnancy Category D.

POISONING. ***Acute Intoxication:*** Acute toxicity from overdosage of aspirin is a common cause of fatal drug poisoning in children, although the number of deaths has declined in recent years as a result of safety closures on bottles, public education, and increased substitution of acetaminophen for aspirin as an antipyretic or analgesic for children.

Toxic doses disturb the acid-base balance, which is manifested as metabolic acidosis in infants and young children and as compensated respiratory alkalosis in older children and adults. Salicylates uncouple oxidative phosphorylation, which is manifested as hypoglycemia and hyperpyrexia, particularly in infants and young children. Marked hyperpnea and tachypnea, tachycardia, nausea and vomiting, and reversible deafness occur; stupor and coma may develop.

The severity of intoxication can be determined by measuring the blood salicylate concentration six hours or more after acute ingestion. Serial determinations should be conducted because serum concentrations may continue to increase for as long as 24 hours. A serum salicylate concentration of 50 mg/dL indicates mild toxicity; amounts above 75 mg/dL are potentially fatal. Plasma salicylate measurements may be unreliable when enteric-coated preparations have been ingested and are misleading in chronic overdosage, particularly if associated with severe acidosis. As a general rule, the acute oral dose causing serious intoxication is 100 mg/kg in a child and 10 g in an adult.

The sequence of management in salicylate overdosage depends on the severity of intoxication. Primary resuscitation is begun if needed. Dehydration and acidosis should be corrected. Dextrose is given empirically since blood glucose determinations may not reflect the status of glucose in the CNS. Hyperthermia is managed by external cooling.

Salicylate may be retained in the stomach for up to 24 hours as the result of prostaglandin inhibition and should be removed by induced emesis or lavage as indicated. In salicylate-intoxicated alert patients with an intact glottic reflex, emesis may provide better gastric emptying in children and lavage in adults. This should be followed by gastric instillation of activated charcoal to bind salicylate and prevent further absorption. Administration of charcoal every four to six hours enhances clearance. Seizures may be controlled with intravenous doses of diazepam 1 to 2 mg/kg. Thereafter, management is directed toward reducing the body burden of salicylate. This is most readily accomplished by increasing the pH of the urine with bicarbonate. (If systemic alkalosis with an alkaline urine is present, bicarbonate is not indicated.) If the urine remains very acidic in spite of bicarbonate administration and if the flow is adequate, potassium chloride should be added to the intravenous fluids. If urine flow is markedly diminished in the presence of adequate hydration; if pulmonary edema, progressive deterioration of the patient's status (CNS abnormalities, coma, convulsions), or persistent aciduria or acid-base abnormalities are present; or if the salicylate concentration exceeds 100 to 150 mg/dL, hemodialysis or hemoperfusion is indicated. Following treatment of massive overdosage, the prophylactic administration of phytonadione (vitamin K_1) may be appropriate.

DRUG INTERACTIONS. Because aspirin is widely used, its interaction with other drugs must be considered, although few interactions are clinically important. Large doses of aspirin (over 3 g/day) taken for several days decrease prothrombin production, thus increasing the prothrombin time; even smaller doses may increase bleeding time by inhibiting platelet aggregation. Because of this, patients receiving oral anticoagulants should be instructed to avoid aspirin. (See index entry Antiplatelet Drugs.)

In noninsulin-dependent diabetics, large doses of salicylates decrease the blood glucose concentration by inhibiting prostaglandin E synthesis and may enhance the effect of the oral hypoglycemics, particularly chlorpropamide, by displacement from protein binding sites. These drugs should not be given concomitantly unless the dosage of the hypoglycemic agent is reduced as indicated by determinations of blood glucose concentrations.

Although large doses of a salicylate have a uricosuric effect, usual analgesic doses cause uric acid retention, which produces hyperuricemia in some patients. Salicylates also antagonize the activity of the uricosuric agents, probenecid and sulfinpyrazone. Patients with gout should avoid aspirin and other salicylates.

The incidence of gastric ulceration may be increased if aspirin is given with other ulcerogenic agents, such as corticosteroids or any of the NSAIDs. Concurrent use of these agents should be avoided.

Aspirin has been reported to reduce methotrexate clearance by 30% and to decrease methotrexate binding to protein by 20% to 60%. Although the clinical significance is uncertain, the patient should be monitored closely if the two drugs are used together.

Aspirin displaces valproate from protein binding sites and also interferes with its metabolism. Concomitant ingestion has been implicated in a few cases of valproate toxicity. Aspirin also can displace phenytoin from protein binding sites, but the relevance of this effect is uncertain because unbound phenytoin is cleared rapidly by the kidney.

PHARMACOKINETICS. Aspirin is absorbed primarily from the small intestine and secondarily from the stomach. Absorption is rapid following oral administration of conventional tablets or capsules, but the rate is affected by gastric emptying time and the release characteristics of the dosage form. Absorption is most rapid when aspirin is given in solution.

Aspirin is rapidly hydrolyzed, partly by esterases during absorption and partly by the liver, to salicylic acid before entering the systemic circulation. Both aspirin and salicylic acid enter the CNS. Hydrolysis by plasma esterases is rapid. Salicylic acid is cleared by renal excretion and by metabolism. It is conjugated with glycine (forming salicyluric acid) and glucuronic acid (forming salicylphenolic glucuronide and salicylacyl glucuronide). A small fraction of salicylic acid is oxidized to gentisic acid.

The enzymes forming salicyluric acid and salicylphenolic glucuronide are saturable and follow Michaelis-Menten kinetics. Therefore, the pharmacokinetics of salicylate elimination are complex, since both the ratio of metabolites and clearance are dose dependent. Approximately 70% to 90% of salicylic acid is bound to serum albumin, and the apparent volume of distribution ranges from 0.1 to 0.35 L/kg, depending on drug concentration. The half-life of salicylate increases with the dose: 3.1 to 3.2 hours with 300 to 650 mg, 5 hours with 1 g, and 9 hours with 2 g. As the dose and half-life increase, a larger portion is excreted unchanged.

Increasing the dose without increasing the dosage interval may result in accumulation with toxic effects. However, there is marked variation in the rate of elimination among individuals, possibly because of differences in salicyluric acid-forming capacity. Therefore, the dosage must be individualized when large amounts are required (Levy, 1981; Netter et al, 1985; Needs and Brooks, 1985). In adults, age and sex have little influence on the disposition of salicylates (Montgomery et al, 1986).

FORMULATIONS. The rate of absorption or bioavailability of aspirin depends on its rate of dissolution from the dosage form, the most common of which is plain (unbuffered) tablets. Several studies have shown that differences among various formulations affect the rate of dissolution and absorption and thus the levels achieved in the blood. However, the relationship of blood levels to the onset and intensity of analgesic effect is uncertain.

Antacids or buffering ingredients are combined with aspirin (buffered aspirin) to reduce gastric irritation. The relatively small amount of antacid present in most products does not increase the gastric pH significantly but does increase the dissolution rate of aspirin, resulting in more rapid absorption. Some individuals claim that they tolerate buffered preparations better than plain aspirin, but there are no controlled clinical studies to support this claim. As with plain tablets, buffered aspirin products have variable dissolution rates, and certain preparations may be less bioavailable than some unbuffered tablets. Furthermore, it has not been demonstrated conclusively that buffered aspirin has a faster onset of action, greater peak intensity, or longer analgesic effect.

Aspirin also is available in highly buffered effervescent preparations; when dissolved, the aspirin is present as sodium acetylsalicylate. Results of studies have shown that this form has a more rapid rate of absorption. In addition, highly buffered sodium acetylsalicylate solution causes less gastric irritation and gastrointestinal bleeding, although the effect on platelets is unchanged. Because effervescent preparations contain more absorbable antacid, repeated use of large doses alkalizes the urine, resulting in faster excretion and decreased salicylate blood concentration. Nevertheless, because of the rapid absorption of aspirin from effervescent preparations, they are an effective form for occasional use. These preparations should not be used by patients who must restrict sodium intake.

Enteric-coated preparations may be used to avoid gastric reactions. The incidence of gastrointestinal mucosal lesions is reduced with these preparations, but absorption of aspirin is delayed and the degree varies among different products. Although this type of preparation may be useful when administered repeatedly to treat rheumatoid arthritis, it does not relieve pain promptly. Prolonged-release preparations offer no advantage over conventional tablets.

Rectal suppositories are used in patients unable to take oral medication. However, the rectal absorption of aspirin is variable; it may be slow and incomplete or rapid and cause adverse reactions. Also, aspirin may cause rectal irritation. For these reasons, suppositories are of questionable usefulness.

DOSAGE AND PREPARATIONS.

Oral: For analgesia and antipyresis, *adults and children over 12 years,* 650 mg every four hours as necessary or 500 mg to 1 g initially, followed by 500 mg every three hours or 1 g every six hours as necessary (maximum, 4 g daily). *Children under 12 years,* 10 to 15 mg/kg. Doses may be repeated every four hours as necessary.

For acute rheumatic fever, *adults,* 6 to 8 g daily; *children,* 3 g daily (optimum salicylate level, 25 to 30 mg/dL).

NOTE: Because most manufacturers express dosage sizes of aspirin in grains rather than milligrams, the grain sizes with *approximate* milligram equivalents are given.

Generic. Tablets 5, 7 1/2, and 10 gr (325, 500, and 650 mg); tablets (buffered) 5 gr (325 mg); tablets (enteric-coated) 5, 10, and 15 gr (325, 650, and 975 mg); suppositories 1, 2, 3, 5, 10, and 20 gr (60, 130, 195, 325, and 650 mg and 1.2 g) (all forms nonprescription).

Available Trademarks.

(Examples of various formulations; all nonprescription)

Alka-Seltzer (Miles). Tablets (highly buffered, effervescent) 324 mg with sodium bicarbonate 1.9 g and citric acid 1 g (sodium 567 mg/tablet).

Ascriptin (Rhone-Poulenc Rorer). Tablets (buffered) 325 mg with magnesium and aluminum hydroxide and calcium carbonate 100 or 150 mg (***Ascriptin A/D***) and 500 mg with magnesium and aluminum hydroxide and calcium carbonate 160 mg (***Ascriptin ES***).

Bayer (Glenbrook). Tablets (prolonged-release) 650 mg.

Bufferin (Bristol-Myers). Tablets (buffered) 324 mg with aluminum glycinate and magnesium carbonate.

Cama (Sandoz). Tablets (buffered) 500 mg with magnesium oxide 150 mg and aluminum hydroxide 150 mg.

Ecotrin (SmithKline Beecham Consumer). Tablets 325 mg.

CHOLINE MAGNESIUM TRISALICYLATE
[Trilisate]

This preparation is a mixture of choline salicylate and magnesium salicylate. It may be used as a substitute for aspirin for its anti-inflammatory, analgesic, or antipyretic effects. It is generally similar to aspirin in its side effects but appears to be better tolerated by patients who experience gastric distress with aspirin. Choline magnesium trisalicylate does not affect platelet function.

DOSAGE AND PREPARATIONS.
Oral: For mild to moderate pain or as an antipyretic, *adults,* 1 to 1.5 g twice daily; some patients benefit from larger doses (eg, up to 2 to 2.5 g twice daily); *children under 37 kg,* 25 mg/kg twice daily; *over 37 kg,* a maximum of 2.25 g/day.

Trilisate (Purdue Frederick). Liquid 500 mg salicylate/5 ml; tablets 500 and 750 mg and 1 g.

SODIUM SALICYLATE

Sodium salicylate is less effective than equal doses of aspirin in relieving pain and reducing fever. However, individuals who are hypersensitive to aspirin may tolerate sodium salicylate.

In general, this salicylate produces the same adverse reactions as aspirin (see that evaluation), but there is less occult gastrointestinal bleeding. Platelet function is not affected but, as with aspirin, prothrombin time is increased. Patients on a low-sodium diet should not take this drug.

DOSAGE AND PREPARATIONS.
Oral: 650 mg every four hours as necessary (range, 325 mg to 4 g daily).

Generic. Tablets (plain, enteric-coated) 325 and 650 mg (nonprescription).

DIFLUNISAL
[Dolobid]

For chemical formula, see index entry Diflunisal, Uses, Rheumatoid Arthritis.

ACTIONS AND USES. Diflunisal has analgesic, anti-inflammatory, and antipyretic properties and also inhibits prostaglandin synthetase.

Diflunisal is useful for the acute or long-term symptomatic treatment of mild to moderate pain. In controlled clinical studies, this drug relieved postoperative pain of meniscectomy, episiotomy, and dental, orthopedic, and various other procedures. It also controlled the pain of musculoskeletal conditions, such as sprains and strains, trauma, low back disorders, and anterior knee pain. It may be employed as an initial analgesic in cancer patients.

In various comparative studies, single doses of diflunisal 500 mg were comparable in analgesic effect to aspirin 650 mg, acetaminophen 600 or 650 mg, and propoxyphene napsylate 100 mg with acetaminophen 650 mg. A single dose of diflunisal 1 g was as effective as the combination of codeine 60 mg and acetaminophen 600 mg. When administered repeatedly, diflunisal 500 mg twice daily was comparable in analgesic effect to codeine 25 mg four times daily, pentazocine 50 mg four times daily, propoxyphene 65 mg with acetaminophen 650 mg three times daily, or propoxyphene napsylate 100 mg with aspirin 650 mg four times daily. In most patients, the duration of analgesic action of diflunisal (up to 12 hours) was notably longer than that of other drugs. The onset of analgesia usually occurs within one hour and the maximum effect within two to three hours.

Diflunisal also is effective in arthritis (see index entry Diflunisal, Uses, Rheumatoid Arthritis). Although it has antipyretic activity, this drug has not been effective in febrile patients.

Diflunisal has a uricosuric effect. Analgesic doses increased renal clearance of uric acid and decreased serum uric acid (Dresse et al, 1979; van Loenhout et al, 1981). It is not known whether diflunisal interferes with the activity of other uricosuric agents or has a useful uricosuric action in the treatment of gout.

ADVERSE REACTIONS AND PRECAUTIONS. Diflunisal is generally well tolerated. The most common adverse reactions are nausea, dyspepsia, gastrointestinal pain, and diarrhea. Rash and headache are observed in 3% to 9% of patients. Other reactions with an incidence of 1% to 3% include vomiting, constipation, flatulence, dizziness, tinnitus, fatigue, somnolence, and insomnia.

In comparative studies, the incidence of gastrointestinal reactions, as well as dizziness, edema, and tinnitus, was lower than with aspirin. In addition, comparative studies in normal volunteers showed that fecal blood loss with diflunisal 1 g twice daily was about one-half that with aspirin 1.3 g twice daily (no significant differences in fecal blood loss were observed with diflunisal 500 mg twice daily and placebo). However, gastrointestinal bleeding and peptic ulceration (incidence, less than 1 in 100) have been reported, and patients with a history of upper gastrointestinal tract disease should be monitored carefully during therapy. In those with active peptic ulcer or gastrointestinal bleeding, the benefit/risk ratio should be considered and appropriate ulcer therapy instituted if diflunisal is administered.

The effect of diflunisal on platelet function and bleeding time is dose related but reversible, even when large doses (1 g twice daily) are used. However, patients at risk should be observed carefully.

Acute interstitial nephritis and acute renal failure have been reported with diflunisal therapy (Wharton et al, 1982). These reactions and nephrotic syndrome also have been observed with other NSAIDs and may be associated with inhibition of prostaglandin synthesis (Bailie, 1986). Because diflunisal is eliminated primarily by the kidney and its half-life is increased in the presence of renal insufficiency, patients with significantly impaired renal function should be monitored carefully and lower doses should be used.

Since peripheral edema has been observed, the drug should be used with caution in patients with compromised cardiac function, hypertension, or other conditions predisposing to fluid retention.

As with other NSAIDs, borderline elevations of one or more liver function tests may occur in up to 15% of patients receiving diflunisal. In controlled clinical trials, significant elevations (three times the upper limit of normal) of ALT or AST occurred in less than 1% of patients. Although severe hepatic reactions are rare, jaundice and fatal hepatitis have been reported with other NSAIDs. If signs or symptoms suggesting liver dysfunction develop or liver function tests are abnormal, the patient should be evaluated for evidence of more severe hepatic reactions; if abnormalities persist or worsen, the drug should be discontinued.

Because cross-sensitivity may occur, diflunisal should not be given to patients who experienced rhinitis, acute asthmatic attacks, urticaria, or angioedema with aspirin or other NSAIDs.

Since no adequate, well-controlled studies have been conducted in pregnant women, diflunisal should not be used during the first two trimesters unless it is clearly indicated (FDA Pregnancy Category C). It should not be administered during the third trimester because of the potential effects of prostaglandin inhibitors on the fetal cardiovascular system (premature closure of ductus arteriosus). See index entry Ductus Arteriosus, Patent.

DRUG INTERACTIONS. When diflunisal and indomethacin were given to normal volunteers, the renal clearance of indomethacin was decreased and the plasma levels were increased. Since fatal gastrointestinal hemorrhage has been associated with the concomitant use of these drugs, they should not be administered concurrently.

Clinical data on the concomitant use of diflunisal and other NSAIDs are not available; thus, their combined administration cannot be recommended. However, studies on some of these drugs have been carried out in normal volunteers with the following results: When multiple doses of aspirin and diflunisal are administered together, the effect is dose dependent. No significant effect occurs with aspirin doses below 1.2 g/day. At doses above 2.4 g/day, the plasma concentrations of diflunisal were decreased significantly. Concomitant administration of diflunisal and naproxen did not affect plasma concentrations of either drug but significantly decreased the urinary excretion of naproxen and its glucuronide metabolite. The administration of sulindac with diflunisal did not significantly affect plasma concentrations of the active sulfide metabolite of sulindac. Diflunisal increases the plasma concentration of acetaminophen.

Concomitant administration of antacids and diflunisal may reduce the bioavailability of the latter drug; the effect is slight with occasional doses of antacids, but may be clinically significant during repeated administration.

Prothrombin time was prolonged in normal volunteers when diflunisal was administered with an oral anticoagulant because of competition for protein binding sites. Thus, the dosage of oral anticoagulants may need adjustment when diflunisal is given concomitantly.

When hydrochlorothiazide and diflunisal were given to normal volunteers, the plasma levels of the thiazide were increased and its hyperuricemic effect was decreased. A similar decrease in hyperuricemic effect but not diuretic activity was observed when furosemide and diflunisal were given together.

POISONING. The most common signs and symptoms observed with overdosage are drowsiness, nausea, vomiting, diarrhea, hyperventilation, tachycardia, diaphoresis, tinnitus, disorientation, stupor, and coma. Most patients recover without permanent sequelae, but fatalities have been reported. When used alone, the lowest dose of diflunisal at which death has been reported was 15 g. In one mixed-drug overdose, ingestion of diflunisal 7.5 g was fatal. Treatment should include emptying the stomach, symptomatic and supportive measures, and careful observation of the patient. The effectiveness of forced (alkaline) diuresis has not been established. Because of extensive protein binding, hemodialysis may not be effective.

PHARMACOKINETICS. Diflunisal is well absorbed following oral administration; peak plasma levels are reached within two to three hours. When given with food, absorption of the drug is delayed slightly but not decreased.

Like salicylic acid, diflunisal exhibits dose-dependent nonlinear pharmacokinetics, ie, doubling the dose more than doubles drug plasma concentrations. The time required to reach steady state and the plasma half-life increase with larger doses. The plasma half-life of diflunisal is three to four times longer than that of salicylic acid. Its elimination half-life ranged from 8 hours with doses of 125 mg twice daily to 15 hours with doses of 500 mg twice daily. The volume of distribution is 0.1 L/kg. Clearance of a single 500-mg dose is 8 ml/min. Steady-state plasma levels were attained in three to four days with doses of 125 mg twice daily and in seven to nine days with doses of 500 mg twice daily. The half-life is increased as the creatinine clearance is reduced.

About 90% of a dose of diflunisal is converted to two soluble glucuronides, the phenol and acyl conjugates, which are excreted in the urine. Less than 10% is excreted as the sulfate conjugate following the initial dose, but with repeated administration, this increases to about 30% in one week and remains at that level thereafter. The drug is more than 99% bound to plasma proteins (Steelman et al, 1978; Verbeeck et al, 1983; Loewen et al, 1986). Approximately 2% to 7% of the concentration in plasma appears in the milk of lactating mothers.

DOSAGE AND PREPARATIONS.

Oral: The dosage should be individualized depending on the severity of pain, the presence of other disorders, and the patient's weight, age, and renal function. *Adults,* for mild to moderate pain, an initial loading dose of 1 g, followed by 500 mg every 8 to 12 hours. Doses of 500 mg initially, followed by 250 mg every 8 to 12 hours, may be appropriate for some patients. *Children,* dosage has not been established.

Dolobid (Merck). Tablets 250 and 500 mg.

PARA-AMINOPHENOL DERIVATIVE

ACETAMINOPHEN

$$\text{HO}-\bigcirc-\text{NH}\overset{\text{O}}{\overset{\|}{\text{C}}}\text{CH}_3$$

USES. Acetaminophen may be considered the drug of choice when a mild analgesic is indicated. It is as effective as aspirin when used for analgesia and antipyresis, is equipotent, and has a similar time-effect curve. It is used to treat tension-type headache, mild to moderate myalgia, arthralgia, chronic pain of cancer, postpartum pain, postoperative pain, and fever. The ceiling analgesic effect is obtained with a dose of 1 g.

Acetaminophen is the preferred alternative to aspirin for patients who cannot tolerate the latter, those with a coagulation disorder, or individuals with a history of peptic ulcer or reflux esophagitis. In children requiring only analgesia or antipyresis, acetaminophen may be preferred to aspirin because it is less toxic if an accidental overdose occurs. (Interestingly, acetaminophen overdosage in children under 6 is rarely, if ever, associated with hepatotoxicity, but such protection is lost by adolescence.) Further, no epidemiologic association has been demonstrated between acetaminophen and Reye's syndrome in children or adolescents with influenza A or B or varicella (chickenpox).

Acetaminophen is unsatisfactory for conditions that require potent anti-inflammatory activity (rheumatic disease, juvenile arthritis, dysmenorrhea, sunburn). Unlike aspirin, acetaminophen does not antagonize the effects of uricosuric agents and may be used in patients with gouty arthritis who are taking a uricosuric.

ADVERSE REACTIONS. Adverse reactions occur infrequently and hypersensitivity only rarely. Acetaminophen is a metabolite of phenacetin and acetanilid but, unlike these drugs, produces little or no methemoglobinemia and reports of hemolytic anemia have been rare. It does not cause gastrointestinal bleeding.

Although large doses have been reported to potentiate the action of oral anticoagulants, small doses have no effect on prothrombin time. There is some evidence that the prolonged use of acetaminophen as a single agent can cause the type of renal injury (renal papillary necrosis and interstitial nephritis) associated with abuse of analgesic mixtures that contained phenacetin (Bennett and DeBroe, 1989; Sandler et al, 1989). (Such mixtures are no longer available.) Care should be observed when using large doses of acetaminophen in malnourished patients or those with a history of chronic alcohol abuse because they may be more susceptible to hepatic damage similar to that observed with toxic overdosage.

POISONING. Large doses (15 g as a single dose or 5 to 8 g/day for several weeks) of acetaminophen may cause severe hepatic damage and death. The first signs of toxicity occur about 12 to 24 hours after acute overdose and include nausea, vomiting, diarrhea, diaphoresis, pallor, and abdominal pain. Hepatic injury is manifested 24 to 48 hours after overdose by increased serum transaminases, lactic dehydrogenase, prothrombin time, and serum bilirubin concentrations. Severe hepatic damage may progress to hepatic failure, encephalopathy, coma, and death.

The hepatic injury appears to be produced by a reactive metabolite of acetaminophen. This metabolic intermediate is inactivated by conjugation with glutathione. Overdosage, with subsequent hepatic injury, occurs when 70% or more of the glutathione is depleted. Regardless of the initial acetaminophen concentration, liver damage is minimal when acetylcysteine is administered orally within eight hours after ingestion of acetaminophen (Smilkstein et al, 1988). Because of the low incidence of side effects associated with acetylcysteine, therapy should be initiated immediately without waiting for plasma acetaminophen determinations if less than 24 hours have elapsed since the ingestion. The decision to continue therapy may then be guided by the reported value. The incidence of hepatotoxicity is 100% when plasma acetaminophen concentrations exceed 300 mcg/ml.

After the stomach is emptied by lavage or induced emesis, a loading dose of 140 mg/kg acetylcysteine is given as a 5% solution in iced water, grapefruit juice, or a cola drink. Additional doses of 70 mg/kg, similarly diluted, then are administered at four-hour intervals for 17 doses. Acetylcysteine has an extremely disagreeable odor and taste. To improve patient compliance, the drug may be ingested through a straw inserted through a plastic cap on an opaque cup. If frequent vomiting interferes, the drug may be instilled through an oroduodenal tube. An intravenous preparation of acetylcysteine [Mucomyst 10 IV] is available as an orphan drug. For further information on the diagnosis and management of acetaminophen poisoning, see Hall and Rumack, 1986, and Smilkstein et al, 1988.

PHARMACOKINETICS. Acetaminophen is rapidly and almost completely absorbed from the gastrointestinal tract following oral administration. Peak plasma concentrations of 5 to 20 mcg/ml occur in 30 to 60 minutes with usual analgesic doses, but there is no correlation between serum concentration and analgesic effect. Significant serum protein binding does not occur with therapeutic doses. The apparent volume of distribution is about 1 L/kg. The plasma half-life in healthy subjects ranges from 1 to 2.5 hours (Forrest et al, 1982).

Acetaminophen is metabolized in the liver, largely to glucuronide and sulfate conjugates, and is eliminated in the urine. In healthy young adults, about 85% to 95% of the usual oral dose can be recovered from the urine within 24 hours. In patients with impaired renal function, the conjugated metabolites accumulate in the blood but the unchanged drug does not. A minor fraction is metabolized to hydroxylates and deacetylated derivatives. It has been suggested that the hydroxylated metabolite is responsible for the hepatotoxicity produced by overdosage (Levy, 1981). There is evidence that some forms of liver disease decrease the conjugation of acetaminophen and increase its half-life; however, it is not known if this increases the incidence or severity of hepatotoxicity. In one study in patients with stable chronic liver disease, no adverse effects occurred with usual doses of acetaminophen (Benson, 1983). Nevertheless, patients with pre-existing liver disorders should be monitored closely.

DOSAGE AND PREPARATIONS.

Oral: *Adults and children over 12 years,* 325 to 650 mg at four-hour intervals, if needed, or 500 mg to 1 g initially, followed by 500 mg every three hours or 1 g every four to six hours as needed (maximum, 4 g daily). *Children under 12 years,* 10 to 15 mg/kg every four hours as necessary (maximum, five times daily).

Rectal: The relative potency of the suppository formulation is about one-half that of the oral tablet; however, as with other drugs, the bioavailability of acetaminophen may vary, depending on the composition of the suppository base. Since comparative data are not available, no dosage is recommended.

Generic. Capsules 500 mg; drops 100 mg/ml; elixir 80, 120, 130, 160, and 325 mg/5 ml; tablets 80 (chewable), 325, 500, and 650 mg; suppositories 120, 325, and 650 mg (all forms nonprescription).

Available Trademarks.

Anacin-3 (Whitehall), ***Liquiprin*** (Menley & James), ***Panadol*** (Glenbrook), ***Phenaphen*** (Robins), ***St. Joseph Tablets*** (Schering-Plough), ***Tempra*** (Mead Johnson), ***Tylenol*** (McNeil) (all nonprescription).

ANTHRANILIC ACID DERIVATIVE

MEFENAMIC ACID

[Ponstel]

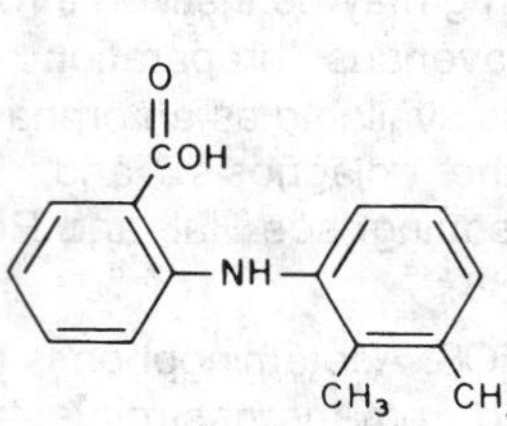

ACTIONS AND USES. Mefenamic acid is related chemically to meclofenamate, an antiarthritic drug. It has analgesic, antipyretic, and anti-inflammatory actions and is claimed to relieve mild to moderate pain, but therapy should not exceed one week. Results of comparative studies have shown that mefenamic acid is no more effective than aspirin and other nonopioid analgesics. Because it has been associated with a number of serious adverse reactions, other NSAIDs are preferred.

Results of several studies have indicated that mefenamic acid relieves the pain of primary dysmenorrhea and that associated with intrauterine devices. Comparative studies with other prostaglandin inhibitors (eg, ibuprofen, naproxen) have not been performed but, since the latter agents are better tolerated, they are preferred for this use.

ADVERSE REACTIONS AND PRECAUTIONS. Gastrointestinal symptoms are the most common adverse effects. Diarrhea occurs in a significant number of patients and usually recurs when mefenamic acid is given a second time. Occult gastrointestinal bleeding is noted less frequently than with aspirin. Dyspepsia, constipation, nausea, abdominal pain, vomiting, headache, drowsiness, vertigo, and dizziness have been observed. Elevated blood urea nitrogen levels were reported in one study. Hemolytic anemia, agranulocytosis, thrombocytopenic purpura, and megaloblastic anemia also have been reported.

If diarrhea or rash occurs, the drug should be discontinued and not used thereafter. Mefenamic acid is contraindicated in patients with gastrointestinal inflammation or ulceration and in those with impaired renal function and should be used with caution in asthmatic patients because it may exacerbate this condition.

The safety of mefenamic acid during pregnancy or in children under 14 years has not been established (FDA Pregnancy Category C).

POISONING. An overdose of mefenamic acid can produce generalized seizures. The minimum convulsive dose was 2.5 g in a 12-year-old child. There are four additional reports of convulsions with a dose of 5 g or less. The time between ingestion and seizures was between 0.5 and 12 hours (Court and Volans, 1984). The seizures may recur and can be suppressed by intravenous diazepam. However, seizures in one 18-year-old woman who ingested 22.5 g were resistant to intravenous diazepam 80 mg infused over 15 minutes; the seizures did respond to intravenous anesthesia with etomidate 20 mg (Shipton and Müller, 1985). Subconvulsive doses may produce muscle twitching and vomiting. Although it has not been established that this drug is contraindicated in epileptic patients, use of a different NSAID probably is advisable.

PHARMACOKINETICS. Mefenamic acid is metabolized to 3'-hydroxymethyl and 3'-carboxylate derivatives. These metabolites are excreted in the urine as their acyl glucuronides with unchanged drug. About 20% of the dose is eliminated as the unconjugated 3'-carboxyl derivative in the feces. The elimination half-life is three to four hours. The volume of distribution and clearance is unknown. The drug is extensively bound to plasma protein (Verbeeck et al, 1983).

DOSAGE AND PREPARATIONS.

Oral: *Adults and children over 14 years,* 500 mg initially, followed by 250 mg every six hours as needed for no longer than one week. The drug should be taken with food.

Ponstel (Parke-Davis). Capsules 250 mg.

PHENYLPROPIONIC ACID DERIVATIVES AND RELATED DRUGS

FENOPROFEN CALCIUM

[Nalfon]

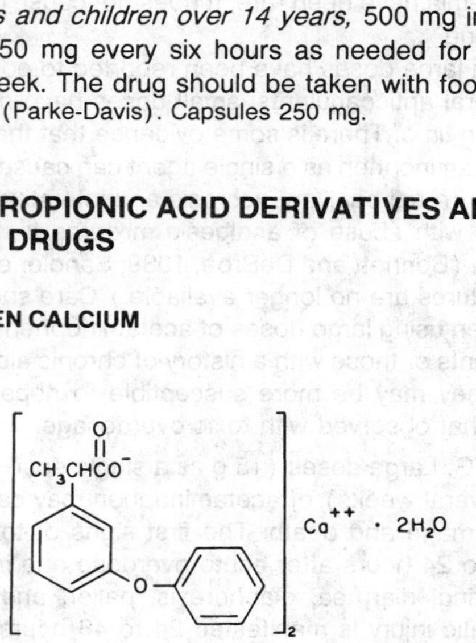

ACTIONS AND USES. Fenoprofen is chemically and pharmacologically similar to ibuprofen. Like aspirin, it has anti-inflammatory, analgesic, and antipyretic properties. Results of several controlled studies indicated that fenoprofen 200 mg was similar in effectiveness to aspirin 650 mg, codeine 60 mg, or propoxyphene napsylate 100 mg in patients with various painful conditions (eg, trauma, episiotomy, postpartum and postoperative pain). Single or repeated doses of 400 mg reduce fever associated with acute and chronic respiratory disease, but additional studies are needed to establish the optimum dose for this use.

ADVERSE REACTIONS. The most common adverse reactions are drowsiness, dizziness, sweating, and asthenia. Gastrointestinal effects (eg, dyspepsia, constipation, nausea, vomiting) also have occurred. Gastrointestinal bleeding is less than with aspirin. However, since a few cases of ulceration have been observed, fenoprofen should be used with caution in patients with a history of peptic ulcer. Patients with aspirin-sensitive asthma also may be sensitive to fenoprofen.

For information on other adverse reactions, drug interactions, and pharmacokinetics, see index entry Fenoprofen, In Arthritis.

DOSAGE AND PREPARATIONS.
Oral: *Adults*, 200 mg every four to six hours as needed. *Children,* dosage has not been established.

Generic. Capsules and tablets 200, 300, and 600 mg.
Nalfon (Dista). Capsules 200 and 300 mg; tablets 600 mg (strengths expressed in terms of the base).

IBUPROFEN
[Advil, Medipren, Midol IB, Motrin, Nuprin, PediaProfen, Rufen]

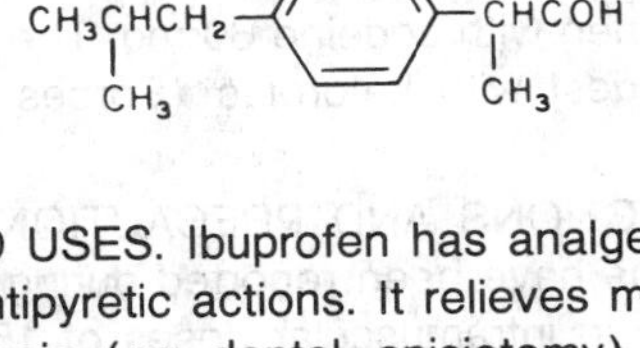

CH_3CHCH_2–(C₆H₄)–CHCOOH with CH_3 substituents

ACTIONS AND USES. Ibuprofen has analgesic, anti-inflammatory, and antipyretic actions. It relieves mild to moderate postoperative pain (eg, dental, episiotomy), dysmenorrhea, and tension-type headache. Its analgesic effectiveness is comparable to or greater than that of acetaminophen, aspirin, codeine, aspirin with codeine, or propoxyphene.

ADVERSE REACTIONS AND PRECAUTIONS. The overall incidence of adverse reactions is low, and this agent is tolerated better than aspirin. The most common reactions are nausea and vomiting; diarrhea, constipation, heartburn, and epigastric pain occur less frequently. Patients receiving ibuprofen experienced less gastrointestinal bleeding than those receiving aspirin. However, since ulcer can occur, it is advisable to use this agent with caution in those with peptic ulcer or a history of such ulcers. Patients with aspirin-sensitive asthma also may be sensitive to ibuprofen. (For other adverse reactions, see index entry Ibuprofen.)

PHARMACOKINETICS. About 80% of an oral dose is absorbed. Peak plasma concentrations are attained within 0.5 to 1.5 hours if the drug is taken on an empty stomach. When the drug is taken immediately after meals, absorption is delayed but the total amount absorbed is not decreased. The drug is highly bound (99%) to plasma protein; significant amounts do not appear in breast milk. This agent is rapidly metabolized by hydroxylation, carboxylation, and conjugation and is excreted in the urine almost exclusively as four inactive metabolites. The half-life after single or multiple doses is 1.8 to 2.6 hours. Pharmacokinetics do not appear to be appreciably altered in elderly patients or in the presence of alcoholic liver disease.

DOSAGE AND PREPARATIONS. This drug may be taken with meals or milk to reduce gastrointestinal distress.

Oral: *Adults*, 200 to 400 mg every four to six hours as necessary. Some patients may benefit from larger doses (eg, up to 800 mg every four hours). For primary dysmenorrhea, 400 mg every four to six hours. For fever, 200 mg every four to six hours. *Children 12 months to 12 years*, for relief of fever of ≤102.5° F, 5 mg/kg; for fever >102.5° F, 10 mg/kg every six to eight hours; the maximum recommended dose is 40 mg/kg.

Generic. Tablets 200 (nonprescription), 300, 400, 600, and 800 mg.
Advil (Whitehall), ***Medipren*** (McNeil), ***Midol IB*** (Sterling), ***Nuprin*** (Bristol-Myers). Tablets 200 mg (nonprescription).
Children's Advil Suspension (Wyeth-Ayerst), ***PediaProfen*** (McNeil). Suspension 100 mg/5 ml.
Motrin (Upjohn). Tablets 200 (***Motrin IB***, nonprescription), 300, 400, 600, and 800 mg.
Rufen (Boots). Tablets 400, 600, and 800 mg.

NAPROXEN
[Naprosyn]

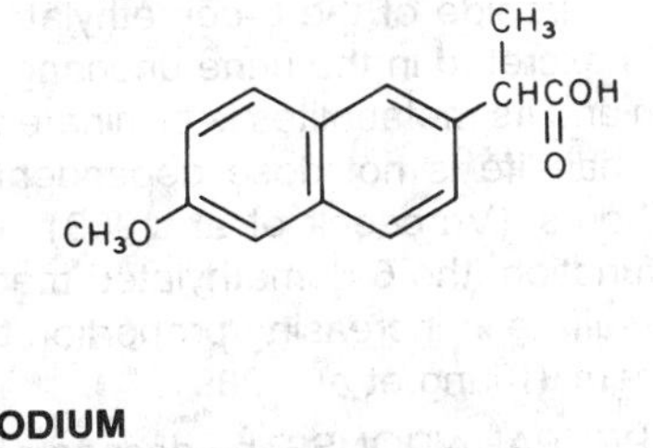

CH_3O–(naphthalene)–CHCOOH with CH_3 substituent

NAPROXEN SODIUM
[Anaprox]

ACTIONS AND USES. Like aspirin, naproxen has analgesic, anti-inflammatory, and antipyretic actions. The sodium salt is absorbed more rapidly and produces a higher peak plasma level than the acid. Otherwise, the properties and actions of the two forms are the same.

The analgesic activity of naproxen has been demonstrated in postoperative pain, including orthopedic and dental, as well as in postpartum uterine cramps, acute or chronic musculoskeletal and soft tissue inflammation, tension-type headache, and primary and secondary dysmenorrhea. Results of several comparative studies showed that the analgesic effect of naproxen is comparable to or greater than that of aspirin, aspirin with codeine, acetaminophen, or pentazocine and is of longer duration. Naproxen was as effective as indomethacin in relieving the pain of musculoskeletal disorders and trauma. The analgesic effects from a single dose become apparent in one hour and persist for seven to eight hours.

In animal studies, naproxen was a more potent antipyretic than aspirin. In children, naproxen 7.5 mg/kg was as effective as aspirin 15 mg/kg and had a much longer duration of action. Naproxen has been employed as an aid to the differential diagnosis of fever of unknown origin in cancer patients. In these patients, fevers due to infection were not responsive, but fever associated with the neoplasm responded completely within 24 hours (Chang and Gross, 1984).

ADVERSE REACTIONS AND PRECAUTIONS. The most common adverse reactions are nausea, dizziness, heartburn, headache, abdominal discomfort, pruritus, and drowsiness. Less gastrointestinal bleeding has been observed than with aspirin; however, this reaction occasionally may be severe and ulceration has been reported. Therefore, naproxen should be used with caution in patients with a history of peptic ulcer. Naproxen can induce peripheral edema and weight gain. The drug should be used with caution in patients with impaired renal function, congestive failure, or those receiving diuretics. It should not be given to patients who are sensitive to aspirin or other prostaglandin inhibitors. (For other adverse reactions, see index entry Naproxen.)

This drug is classified in FDA Pregnancy Category B.

PHARMACOKINETICS. Naproxen is completely absorbed following oral or rectal administration. The sodium salt differs only in being absorbed more rapidly. Binding to plasma protein is concentration dependent: 99.6% at 23 to 40 mcg/ml and 97.4% at 473 mcg/ml. The apparent volume of distribution is approximately 0.1 L/kg.

In normal subjects, about 60% of a dose is eliminated by the kidney, primarily as glucuronide. An additional 28% is excreted as the glucuronide of the 6-demethylated metabolite. Less than 5% is excreted in the urine unchanged. Less than 3% of naproxen and its metabolites is eliminated in the feces. The elimination half-life is not dose dependent and ranges from 12 to 15 hours (Verbeeck et al, 1983). In those with impaired renal function, the 6-demethylated metabolite is excreted as the 6-sulfate in increasing proportion to the degree of renal impairment (Kiang et al, 1989).

DOSAGE AND PREPARATIONS. The dosage of naproxen or naproxen sodium should be reduced in those with renal or hepatic insufficiency (cirrhosis) and in the elderly.

Oral: *Adults,* for mild to moderate pain and primary dysmenorrhea (naproxen sodium) 550 mg initially, followed by 275 mg every six to eight hours as needed, or (naproxen) 500 mg initially, followed by 250 mg every six to eight hours as required. The daily dose should not exceed 1.375 g (naproxen sodium) or 1.25 g (naproxen).

For mild to moderately severe acute or chronic musculoskeletal and soft tissue inflammation, (naproxen sodium) 275 mg twice daily or 275 mg in the morning and 550 mg in the evening, or (naproxen) 250 or 375 mg twice daily. During long-term administration, the dose should be adjusted in accordance with the patient's response.

NAPROXEN:
Naprosyn (Syntex). Suspension 125 mg/5 ml; tablets 250, 375, and 500 mg.

NAPROXEN SODIUM:
Anaprox (Syntex). Tablets 275 mg equivalent to 250 mg naproxen base (sodium 1 mEq/tablet) and 550 mg equivalent to 500 mg naproxen base (sodium 2 mEq/tablet) (***Anaprox DS***).

INDOLE DERIVATIVE

KETOROLAC TROMETHAMINE
[Toradol]

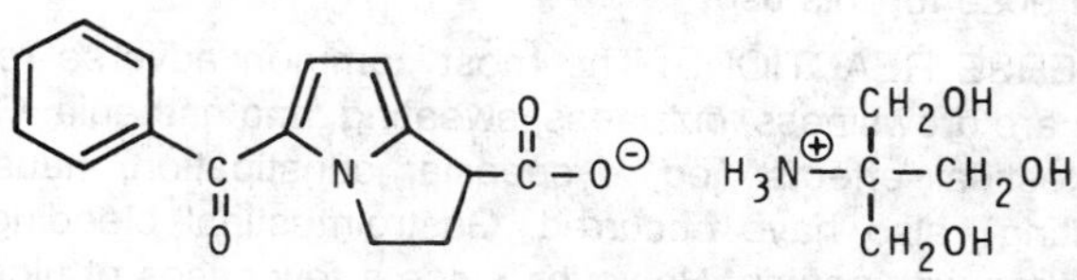

ACTIONS AND USES. Although this NSAID exhibits the anti-inflammatory and antipyretic activities of this class, it is given orally or intramuscularly in the management of moderate to severe pain, particularly in postoperative patients (Buckley and Brogden, 1990).

When given in single intramuscular doses of 30 to 90 mg, the analgesic effect of ketorolac is equivalent or superior to that of morphine 6 to 12 mg (Yee et al, 1986 A; O'Hara et al, 1987) or meperidine 50 to 100 mg (Yee et al, 1986 B; Fricke and Angelocci, 1987; Brown et al, 1988). Ketorolac may be used as the sole agent for analgesia or with opioids to permit reduction in the total dose of the opioid (Gillies et al, 1987; Kenny et al, 1989). In its recommended dosage range (15 to 60 mg), the duration of analgesia, but not the peak analgesic effect, is increased as the amount is increased.

In dental surgery studies, oral ketorolac 10 mg provided pain relief in the first hour comparable to that produced by ibuprofen 400 mg, aspirin 650 mg, acetaminophen 600 mg, and acetaminophen with codeine 60 mg. The duration of analgesia was longest with ketorolac (Forbes et al, 1990 A, 1990 B).

ADVERSE REACTIONS AND PRECAUTIONS. No serious adverse reactions have been reported during the short-term use of ketorolac in intramuscular doses of 15 to 60 mg. Its lack of psychomotor effects makes this NSAID suitable for use as an analgesic for outpatient surgery (MacDonald et al, 1989). An intramuscular dose of 30 mg administered during anesthesia produced no change in the respiratory rate, end-tidal carbon dioxide partial pressure, arterial oxygen saturation, heart rate, or systemic arterial blood pressure (Murray et al, 1989); doses of 10 and 90 mg did not change the ventilatory response to carbon dioxide in nonanesthetized subjects (Brandon Bravo et al, 1988).

In a controlled endoscopic study to determine the degree of mucosal injury produced by ketorolac, intramuscular administration produced the same degree of injury as the equivalent oral dose. Increasing intramuscular doses resulted in corresponding increases in the amount of mucosal injury; however, doses of 10 to 30 mg given four times a day for five days produced less mucosal injury than oral aspirin 650 mg using the same dose schedule. Invasive antral ulceration occurred in four of five subjects receiving ketorolac 90 mg intramuscularly four times a day for five days; because of this finding, the 90-mg dose has not been investigated further (Lanza et al, 1987).

Ketorolac inhibits platelet function reversibly, and this effect depends on the presence of the drug in plasma. Bleeding time is prolonged because of the inhibition of platelet aggregation and thromboxane production (Roe et al, 1981; Spowart et al, 1988). Ketorolac does not affect prothrombin time or partial thromboplastin time (Conrad et al, 1988). No interaction has been demonstrated between this drug and heparin (Spowart et al, 1988).

This drug should not be given to women in labor or about to begin labor, for small quantities of ketorolac administered for analgesia during labor appear in the fetal circulation. In one study employing a single 10-mg intramuscular dose, samples of blood were taken at delivery from the umbilical vein and from a maternal vein for analysis. Concentrations of ketorolac in the maternal plasma ranged from 0.233 to 0.873 mcg/ml and in cord blood from 0.017 to 0.119 mcg/ml. The ratio of the concentration of umbilical:maternal vein was 0.116 (Walker et al, 1988). Although small, the concentration of ketorolac that crosses the placenta is sufficient to inhibit neonatal platelet aggregation (Greer et al, 1988).

The appearance of ketorolac in breast milk when multiple doses are administered in the postpartum period is negligible. The amount of measurable concentrations of the drug in the milk ranged from 5.2 to 7.9 ng/ml; the ratio of ketorolac in milk to that in maternal plasma was 0.015:0.037 (Wischnik et al, 1989).

Ketorolac is classified in FDA Pregnancy Category C.

This drug should not be given to patients with a history of aspirin-sensitive asthma or similar reactions to other NSAIDs.

PHARMACOKINETICS. Absorption of ketorolac following intramuscular administration is rapid (t_{max} 45 to 60 min) and its bioavailability is complete. Following absorption, the drug dissociates irreversibly to release the ketorolac anion. In plasma, more than 99% of a dose of ketorolac is protein-bound. Ketorolac and its metabolites are excreted primarily (92%) by the kidney. The major component in the urine is the glucuronide conjugate. Since the conjugate cannot be demonstrated in the plasma, it is presumed to form in the kidney (Mroszczak et al, 1987). A small quantity of unchanged ketorolac and an essentially inactive metabolite, p-hydroxyketorolac, also are excreted.

Single doses in healthy young men (mean age, 32 years) had a terminal half-life of five hours, an apparent volume of distribution at steady state of 0.111 L/kg, and a clearance of 0.35 ml/kg/min (Jung et al, 1988). The mean plasma half-life is independent of dose. Mean C_{max} for intramuscular doses of 30, 60, and 90 mg increased proportionally and were 2.24, 4.48, and 6.88 mcg/ml, respectively. The mean total AUC also increased linearly with dose. The pharmacokinetic parameters for p-hydroxyketorolac, the only metabolite found in the plasma, also have been determined (Jung et al, 1989).

Plasma clearance and the elimination half-life apparently are not affected by hepatic impairment (Pages et al, 1987), but renal impairment prolongs the half-life and reduces the plasma clearance significantly. In one comparative study, the elimination half-life was increased from 4.45 hr to 9.62 hr and the plasma clearance was reduced from 0.44 to 0.27 ml/kg/min (Martinez et al, 1987). In subjects with a mean age of 72.3 years, the elimination half-life was increased to 7.01 hr and the clearance was decreased to 0.32 ml/kg/min; in comparison, in a young male control group with a mean age of 27.5 years, the $t_{1/2}$ was 4.5 hr and the cl_{tot} was 0.45 ml/kg/min. Renal function in the subject population was not specified (Montoya-Iraheta et al, 1986). There is no evidence that ketorolac accumulates with multiple doses (Buckley and Brogden, 1990).

DOSAGE AND PREPARATIONS. Since the clearance of this drug is reduced in those with renal disease and in the elderly, the lower end of the suggested dose range should be employed in these patients. The lower dose also has been recommended for patients weighing less than 50 kg.

Intramuscular: *Adults,* an initial loading dose of 30 to 60 mg, then 15 to 30 mg every six hours. The maximal total daily dose recommended by the manufacturer is 150 mg the first day and 120 mg/day thereafter. Therapy should not exceed five days.

Toradol (Syntex). Solution 15 mg/ml in 1 ml and 30 mg/ml in 1 and 2 ml single-dose containers.

Oral: *Adults,* 10 mg as needed every four to six hours (maximum, 40 mg/day) for a limited duration. On the day of transition from intramuscular to oral therapy, a total combined dose of 120 mg, including a maximum of 40 mg orally, should not be exceeded. Subsequent oral doses should be limited to 40 mg daily.

Toradol (Syntex). Tablets 10 mg.

MIXTURES

Mixtures of Nonopioid (Analgesic-Antipyretic) Drugs

Some products contain two or more analgesic-antipyretic drugs, eg, aspirin and acetaminophen. The analgesic effect of such a combination is theoretically no greater than the sum of effects of the individual drugs, and no advantage has been demonstrated by combining them.

Although results of some studies have suggested that caffeine may increase the analgesic effect of aspirin or acetaminophen, others have not substantiated the claim that pain relief is enhanced. An analysis of 30 clinical studies involving 10,000 patients given aspirin or acetaminophen with or without caffeine showed the relative potency of the combination with caffeine to be greater than optimal doses of the individual components (Laska et al, 1984; Beaver, 1984).

Mixtures of a Nonopioid with an Opioid

The combination of an opioid with a nonopioid (analgesic-antipyretic) appears to be rational because the mechanism of action of each drug differs and the analgesic effects of the individual drugs are additive. Since the nonopioids have a ceiling analgesic effect and the dosage of opioids should be limited to prevent adverse effects, a combination of this type may provide greater pain relief with a minimum of adverse effects in a form that is convenient for the patient. Preparations containing acetaminophen lack the anti-inflammatory action produced by those containing aspirin, although such combinations have an antipyretic action.

Codeine and propoxyphene are the most common opioid ingredients in such mixtures; however, few comparative studies have been performed to determine the relative potencies of the various combinations. Since propoxyphene is usually less effective than codeine in the same doses, combinations containing propoxyphene may be less effective than similar combinations containing codeine.

Hydrocodone, a semisynthetic analogue of codeine, also is an ingredient in some mixtures and has the same action as other opioids. It is more potent than codeine and its dependence liability is similar to that of other opioids given orally.

Combinations of meperidine with acetaminophen are available for use as oral analgesics. However, meperidine is less effective orally than parenterally, and no well-controlled studies have been performed to demonstrate the contribution of each ingredient.

Oxycodone, a codeine analogue, has pharmacologic properties similar to those of the morphine-like drugs. It is effective orally and its analgesic potency and dependence liability are similar to those of morphine. In the United States, it is available as an ingredient of mixtures with acetaminophen or aspirin. Dependence on products containing oxycodone has been reported; thus, these mixtures should be prescribed with the same caution as other opioids.

The combination of pentazocine with aspirin is indicated to relieve moderate pain. In one controlled study, this combination provided greater relief of pain in patients with cancer than aspirin alone; effectiveness was comparable to that of combinations of codeine and aspirin or oxycodone and aspirin. Similar results are obtained with the combination of pentazocine with acetaminophen.

The adverse reactions and precautions of these combinations are those of the individual ingredients. More serious untoward effects are usually caused by the opioid component.

The following analgesic mixtures are divided into groups on the basis of their opioid component. The quantitative formula of the most widely used products in each group is listed for information; this does not imply that such products have merit over similar products not listed.

MIXTURES CONTAINING CODEINE. These mixtures are classified in Schedule III of the Controlled Substances Act (unless indicated otherwise).

Acetaminophen with Codeine (Generic). Each tablet contains acetaminophen 300 mg and codeine 15, 30, or 60 mg; each 5 ml of elixir contains acetaminophen 120 mg and codeine 12 mg (Schedule V).

Aspirin with Codeine (Generic). Each tablet contains aspirin 325 mg and codeine phosphate 15, 30, or 60 mg.

Empirin with Codeine (Burroughs Wellcome). Each tablet contains aspirin 325 mg and codeine phosphate 15 mg (No. 2), 30 mg (No. 3), or 60 mg (No. 4).

Phenaphen with Codeine (Robins). Each capsule contains acetaminophen 325 mg and codeine phosphate 15 mg (No. 2), 30 mg (No. 3), or 60 mg (No. 4).

Phenaphen-650 with Codeine (Robins). Each tablet contains acetaminophen 650 mg and codeine phosphate 30 mg.

Tylenol with Codeine (McNeil). Each tablet contains acetaminophen 300 mg and codeine phosphate 7.5 mg (No. 1), 15 mg (No. 2), 30 mg (No. 3), or 60 mg (No. 4); each 5 ml of elixir contains acetaminophen 120 mg and codeine phosphate 12 mg (alcohol 7%) (Schedule V).

MIXTURES CONTAINING HYDROCODONE. These mixtures are classified in Schedule III of the Controlled Substances Act.

Generic. Tablets containing hydrocodone bitartrate 5 mg and acetaminophen 500 mg.

Lorcet (UAD). Each capsule contains hydrocodone bitartrate 5 mg and acetaminophen 500 mg (***Lorcet-HD***); each tablet contains hydrocodone bitartrate 7.5 mg and acetaminophen 650 mg (***Lorcet Plus***).

Lortab (Whitby). Each 5 ml of liquid contains hydrocodone bitartrate 2.5 mg and acetaminophen 120 mg (alcohol 7%); each tablet contains hydrocodone bitartrate 2.5 mg (***Lortab 2.5***), 5 mg (***Lortab 5***) or 7.5 mg (***Lortab 7.5***) and acetaminophen 500 mg.

Vicodin (Knoll). Each tablet contains hydrocodone bitartrate 5 mg and acetaminophen 500 mg or hydrocodone bitartrate 7.5 mg and acetaminophen 750 mg (***Vicodin ES***).

MIXTURE CONTAINING MEPERIDINE. This mixture is classified in Schedule II of the Controlled Substances Act.

Demerol APAP (Sanofi Winthrop). Each tablet contains meperidine hydrochloride 50 mg and acetaminophen 300 mg.

MIXTURES CONTAINING OXYCODONE. These mixtures are classified in Schedule II of the Controlled Substances Act.

Percocet (DuPont), ***Generic.*** Each tablet contains oxycodone hydrochloride 5 mg and acetaminophen 325 mg.

Percodan (DuPont), ***Generic.*** Each tablet contains oxycodone hydrochloride 4.5 mg, oxycodone terephthalate 0.38 mg, and aspirin 325 mg; each ***Percodan-Demi*** tablet contains oxycodone hydrochloride 2.25 mg, oxycodone terephthalate 0.19 mg, and aspirin 325 mg.

Tylox (McNeil). Each capsule contains oxycodone hydrochloride 5 mg and acetaminophen 500 mg.

MIXTURES CONTAINING PENTAZOCINE. These mixtures are classified in Schedule IV of the Controlled Substances Act.

Talacen (Sanofi Winthrop). Each tablet contains pentazocine hydrochloride equivalent to 25 mg of the base and acetaminophen 650 mg.

Talwin Compound (Sanofi Winthrop). Each tablet contains pentazocine hydrochloride equivalent to 12.5 mg of the base and aspirin 325 mg.

MIXTURES CONTAINING PROPOXYPHENE. These mixtures are classified in Schedule IV of the Controlled Substances Act.

Darvocet-N 50, 100 (Lilly), ***Generic.*** Each tablet contains propoxyphene napsylate 50 or 100 mg and acetaminophen 325 or 650 mg.

Darvon Compound-65 (Lilly), ***Generic.*** Each capsule contains aspirin 389 mg, caffeine 32.4 mg, and propoxyphene hydrochloride 65 mg.

Dolene AP-65 (Lederle), ***Wygesic*** (Wyeth-Ayerst). Each tablet contains propoxyphene hydrochloride 65 mg and acetaminophen 650 mg.

Propacet 100 (Lemmon), ***Generic.*** Each tablet contains propoxyphene napsylate 100 mg and acetaminophen 650 mg.

Mixtures Containing Analgesics With Nonanalgesics

Drugs with a sedative action (sedative-hypnotics, antianxiety agents, centrally acting skeletal muscle relaxants, antihistamines) are components of several widely used analgesic mixtures. They allegedly enhance analgesic effectiveness and relieve muscle spasm or anxiety accompanying pain.

On theoretical grounds, a sedative might be expected to alter a patient's reaction to pain, and a muscle relaxant might be useful in patients with certain musculoskeletal problems. It has not been definitely shown that the skeletal muscle relaxants have a selective muscle relaxant action or that antihistamines have activity separate from their sedative effect. (See index entry Muscle Spasm.) Results of some studies have suggested that a combination of a muscle relaxant and an analgesic provides greater benefit in patients with acute musculoskeletal problems than similar doses of analgesic alone. However, since few properly controlled studies have been designed to determine the relative efficacy of the various products, it cannot be concluded that one is superior to another.

There is some evidence that a combination containing a barbiturate is more effective in tension headache than the analgesic component alone (see index entry Headache). It should be kept in mind that the duration of action of the sedative may differ from that of the mild analgesic, that the actions of the drugs with repeated use might not coincide, and that abuse of a preparation containing a barbiturate may occur. When dependence on barbiturates comes to medical attention, there is a high probability that the source is Fiorinal, a combination of aspirin, butalbital, and caffeine.

It has been reported that meprobamate augments pain but, when given with aspirin, the latter drug antagonizes this effect.

Cited References

Aitkenhead AR, et al: Pharmacokinetics of single dose I.V. morphine in normal volunteers and patients with end stage renal failure. *Br J Anaesth* 55:905P, 1983.

Akil H, Lewis JW (eds): *Neurotransmitters & Pain Control.* New York, S. Karger, 1987.

Allen RC, et al: Renal papillary necrosis in children with chronic arthritis. *Am J Dis Child* 140:20-22, 1986.

American Pain Society: Principles of analgesic use in the treatment of acute pain and chronic cancer pain. *Clin Pharm* 6:523-532, 1987.

Arnér S, Arnér B: Differential effects of epidural morphine in the treatment of cancer-related pain. *Acta Anaesthesiol Scand* 29:32-36, 1985.

Austin KL, et al: Rate of formation of norpethidine from pethidine. *Br J Anaesth* 53:255-257, 1981.

Bailie MD: Renal papillary necrosis in children with chronic arthritis, editorial. *Am J Dis Child* 140:16-17, 1986.

Beaver WT: Caffeine revisited, editorial. *JAMA* 251:1732-1733, 1984.

Belleville JW, et al: Influence of age on pain relief from analgesics: Study of postoperative patients. *JAMA* 217:1835-1841, 1971.

Bennett WM, DeBroe ME: Analgesic nephropathy—A preventable renal disease, editorial. *N Engl J Med* 320:1269-1271, 1989.

Benson GD: Acetaminophen in chronic liver disease. *Clin Pharmacol Ther* 33:95-101, 1983.

Beutler E: *Hemolytic Anemia in Disorders of Red Cell Metabolism.* New York, Plenum, 1978.

Bigby M, Stern R: Cutaneous reactions to nonsteroidal anti-inflammatory drugs: Review. *J Am Acad Dermatol* 12:866-876, 1985.

Blackshear JL, et al: Renal complications of nonsteroidal anti-inflammatory drugs: Identification and monitoring of those at risk. *Semin Arthritis Rheum* 14:163-175, 1985.

Boréus LO, et al: Elimination of meperidine and its metabolites in old patients compared to young patients, in Foley KM, Inturrisi CE (eds): *Advances in Pain Research and Therapy.* New York, Raven Press, 1986, vol 8, 167-169.

Brandon Bravo LJC, et al: Effects on ventilation of ketorolac in comparison with morphine. *Eur J Clin Pharmacol* 35:491-494, 1988.

Bray RJ: Postoperative analgesia provided by morphine infusion in children. *Anaesthesia* 38:1075-1078, 1983.

Brøsen K, et al: Dextropropoxyphene kinetics after single and repeated oral doses in man. *Eur J Clin Pharmacol* 29:79-84, 1985.

Brown CR, et al: Efficacy of intramuscular (I.M.) ketorolac and meperidine in pain following major oral surgery, abstract. *Clin Pharmacol Ther* 43:161, 1988.

Buckley MM-T, Brogden RN: Ketorolac: Review of its pharmacodynamic and pharmacokinetic properties, and therapeutic potential. *Drugs* 39:86-109, 1990.

Bullingham RES, et al: Clinical pharmacokinetics of narcotic agonist-antagonistic drugs. *Clin Pharmacokinet* 8:332-343, 1983.

Caldwell J, et al: Maternal and neonatal disposition of pethidine in childbirth: Study using quantitative gas chromatography-mass spectrometry. *Life Sci* 22:589-596, 1978.

Carson JL, et al: Association of nonsteroidal anti-inflammatory drugs with upper gastrointestinal tract bleeding. *Arch Intern Med* 147:85-88, 1987 A.

Carson JL, et al: Relative gastrointestinal toxicity of the nonsteroidal anti-inflammatory drugs. *Arch Intern Med* 147:1054-1059, 1987 B.

Cersosimo RJ, Matthews SJ: Hepatotoxicity associated with choline magnesium trisalicylate: Case report and review of salicylate-induced hepatotoxicity. *Drug Intell Clin Pharm* 21:621-625, 1987.

Chan WY: Prostaglandins and nonsteroidal antiinflammatory drugs in dysmenorrhea. *Ann Rev Pharmacol Toxicol* 23:131-149, 1983.

Chang JC, Gross HM: Utility of naproxen in the differential diagnosis of fever of undetermined origin in patients with cancer. *Am J Med* 76:597-603, 1984.

Christensen FR, Andersen LW: Adverse reaction to extradural buprenorphine, letter. *Br J Anaesth* 54:476, 1982.

Cole TB, et al: Intravenous narcotic therapy for children with severe sickle cell pain crisis. *Am J Dis Child* 140:1255-1259, 1986.

Conrad KA, et al: Effects of ketorolac tromethamine on hemostasis in volunteers. *Clin Pharmacol Ther* 43:542-546, 1988.

Court H, Volans GN: Poisoning after overdose with non-steroidal anti-inflammatory drugs. *Adverse Drug React Acute Poisoning Rev* 3:1-21, 1984.

Cousins MJ, Bridenbaugh PO: Spinal opioids and pain relief in acute care, in Cousins MJ, Phillips GD (eds): *Acute Pain Management.* New York, Churchill Livingstone, 1986, 151-185.

Cousins MJ, Mather LE: Intrathecal and epidural administration of opioids. *Anesthesiology* 61:276-310, 1984.

Dahlström B, et al: Morphine kinetics in children. *Clin Pharmacol Ther* 26:354-365, 1979.

Dixon R: Pharmacokinetics of levorphanol, in Foley KM, Inturrisi CE (eds): *Advances in Pain Research and Therapy.* New York, Raven Press, 1986, vol 8, 217-224.

Dresse A, et al: Uricosuric properties of diflunisal in man. *Br J Clin Pharm* 7:267-272, 1979.

Duncan A: Postoperative period. *Clin Anaesth* 3:619-632, 1985.

Dunn MJ, Patrono C (eds): Renal effects of nonsteroidal anti-inflammatory drugs. *Am J Med* 81 (suppl 2B):1-132, 1986.

Edwards DJ, et al: Clinical pharmacokinetics of pethidine: 1982. *Clin Pharmacokinet* 7:421-433, 1982.

Ehrnebo M, et al: Bioavailability and first-pass metabolism of oral pentazocine in man. *Clin Pharmacol Ther* 22:888-892, 1977.

Epstein M (ed): Prostaglandins and the kidney. *Am J Med* 80 (suppl 1A):1-84, 1986.

Errick JK, Heel RC: Nalbuphine: Preliminary review of its pharmacological properties and therapeutic efficacy. *Drugs* 26:191-211, 1983.

Foley KM: Treatment of cancer pain. *N Engl J Med* 313:84-95, 1985.

Foley KM, Inturrisi CE: Analgesic drug therapy in cancer pain: Principles and practice. *Med Clin North Am* 71:207-232, 1987.

Forbes JA, et al: Evaluation of ketorolac, aspirin, and an acetaminophen-codeine combination in postoperative oral surgery pain. *Pharmacotherapy* 10(6, part 2):77S-93S, 1990 A.

Forbes JA, et al: Evaluation of ketorolac, ibuprofen, and acetaminophen-codeine combination in postoperative oral surgery pain. *Pharmacotherapy* 10(6, part 2):94S-105S, 1990 B.

Forrest JAH, et al: Clinical pharmacokinetics of paracetamol. *Clin Pharmacokinet* 7:93-107, 1982.

France RD, et al: Long-term use of narcotic analgesics in chronic pain. *Soc Sci Med* 19:1379-1382, 1984.

Fricke J, Angelocci D: Analgesic efficacy of I.M. ketorolac and meperidine for the control of postoperative dental pain, abstract. *Clin Pharmacol Ther* 41:181, 1987.

Friedman EW, et al: Oral analgesia for treatment of painful crisis in sickle cell anemia. *Ann Emerg Med* 15:787-791, 1986.

Gal TJ: Naloxone reversal of buprenorphine-induced respiratory depression. *Clin Pharmacol Ther* 45:66-71, 1989.

Gillies GWA, et al: Morphine sparing effect of ketorolac tromethamine: Study of a new, parenteral non-steroidal anti-inflammatory agent after abdominal surgery. *Anaesthesia* 42:727-731, 1987.

Graham DY, Smith JL: Aspirin and the stomach. *Ann Intern Med* 104:390-398, 1986.

Gram LF, et al: d-Propoxyphene kinetics after single oral and intravenous doses in man. *Clin Pharmacol Ther* 26:473-482,1979.

Gray JD, Blaschke TF: Fever: To treat or not to treat. *Ration Drug Ther* 19:1-6, (Dec) 1985.

Greer IA, et al: Effect of maternal ketorolac administration on platelet function in the newborn. *Eur J Obstet Gynecol Reprod Biol* 29:257-260, 1988.

Gustafsson LL, Wiesenfeld-Hallin Z: Spinal opioid analgesia: Critical update. *Drugs* 35:597-603, 1988.

Hall AH, Rumack BH: Management of acute acetaminophen overdose. *Am Fam Physician* 33:107-114, (May) 1986.

Hansen J, et al: Clinical evaluation of oral methadone in treatment of cancer pain. *Acta Anaesth Scand* suppl 74:124-127, 1982.

Harcus AW, et al: Methodology of monitored release of new preparation: Buprenorphine. *BMJ* 2:163-165, 1979.

Hatch DJ: Analgesia in the neonate. *BMJ* 294:920, 1987.

Hatjis CG, Meis PJ: Sinusoidal fetal heart rate pattern associated with butorphanol administration. *Obstet Gynecol* 67:377-380, 1986.

Henrich WL: Southwestern internal medicine conference: Analgesic nephropathy. *Am J Med Sci* 295:561-568, 1988.

Henry H II, et al: Comparison of butorphanol tartrate and meperidine in moderate to severe renal colic. *Urology* 29:339-345, 1987.

Heymann MA: Non-narcotic analgesics: Use in pregnancy and fetal and perinatal effects. *Drugs* 32(suppl 4):164-176, 1986.

Houde RW: Analgesic effectiveness of the narcotic agonists-antagonists. *Br J Clin Pharmacol* 7(suppl):297S-308S, 1979.

Hug CC Jr: Improving analgesic therapy. *Anesthesiology* 53:441-443, 1980.

Hughes SC, et al: Maternal and neonatal effects of epidural morphine for labor and delivery. *Anesth Analg* 63:319-324, 1984.

Inturrisi CE, Colburn WA: Pharmacokinetics of methadone, in Foley KM, Inturrisi CE (eds): *Advances in Pain Research and Therapy.* New York, Raven Press, 1986, vol 8, 191-199.

Inturrisi CE, Umans JG: Meperidine biotransformation and central nervous system toxicity in animals and humans, in Foley KM, Inturrisi CE (eds): *Advances in Pain Research and Therapy.* New York, Raven Press, 1986, vol 8, 143-153.

Ives TJ, Guerra MF: Constant morphine infusion for severe sickle cell crisis pain. *Drug Intell Clin Pharm* 21:625-627, 1987.

Ivey KJ: Gastrointestinal intolerance and bleeding with non-narcotic analgesics. *Drugs* 32(suppl 4):71-89, 1986.

Jasinski DR, et al: Human pharmacology and abuse potential of analgesic buprenorphine: Potential agent for treating narcotic addiction. *Arch Gen Psychiatry* 35:501-516, 1978.

Jung D, et al: Pharmacokinetics of ketorolac tromethamine in humans after intravenous, intramuscular and oral administration. *Eur J Clin Pharmacol* 35:423-425, 1988.

Jung D, et al: Pharmacokinetics of ketorolac and *p*-hydroxyketorolac following oral and intramuscular administration of ketorolac tromethamine. *Pharm Res* 6:62-65, 1989.

Kaiko RF, et al: Narcotics in the elderly. *Med Clin North Am* 66:1079-1089, 1982.

Kaiko RF, et al: Central nervous system excitatory effects of meperidine in cancer patients. *Ann Neurol* 13:180-185, 1983.

Kenny GNC, et al: Morphine sparing effect of continuous and intermittent ketorolac, abstract. *Anesthesiology* 71(3A):A766, 1989.

Kiang C-H, et al: Isolation and identification of 6-desmethylnaproxen sulfate as a new metabolite of naproxen in human plasma. *Drug Metab Dispos* 17:43-48, 1989.

Kincaid-Smith P: Effects of non-narcotic analgesics on the kidney. *Drugs* 32(suppl 4):109-128, 1986.

Kosten TR, Kleber HD: Buprenorphine detoxification from opioid dependence: Pilot study. *Life Sci* 42:635-641, 1988.

Kotelko DM, et al: Epidural morphine analgesia after cesarean delivery. *Obstet Gynecol* 63:409-413, 1984.

Kreek MJ, et al: Methadone use in patients with chronic renal disease. *Drug Alcohol Depend* 5:197-205, 1980.

Lanza FL, et al: Double-blind placebo controlled endoscopic study comparing the mucosal injury seen with an orally and parenterally administered new nonsteroidal analgesic ketorolac tromethamine at therapeutic and supratherapeutic doses, abstract. *Am J Gastroenterol* 82:939, 1987.

Laska EM, et al: Caffeine as an analgesic adjuvant. *JAMA* 251:1711-1718, 1984.

Levy G: Comparative pharmacokinetics of aspirin and acetaminophen. *Arch Intern Med* 141:279-281, 1981.

Loewen GR, et al: Isolation and identification of new major metabolite of diflunisal in man: The sulfate conjugate. *Drug Metab Dispos* 14:127-131, 1986.

Loper KA, et al: Prophylactic transdermal scopolamine patches reduce nausea in postoperative patients receiving epidural morphine. *Anesth Analg* 68:144-146, 1989.

Lynn AM, Slattery JT: Pharmacokinetics of morphine sulfate in early infancy. *Anesthesiology* 63:A349, 1985.

MacDonald FC, et al: Psychomotor effects of ketorolac in comparison with buprenorphine and diclofenac. *Br J Clin Pharmacol* 27:453-459, 1989.

Martinez JJ, et al: Single dose pharmacokinetics of ketorolac in healthy young and renal impaired subjects, abstract. *J Clin Pharmacol* 27:722, 1987.

Mather LE: Pharmacokinetic studies of meperidine, in Foley KM, Inturrisi CE (eds): *Advances in Pain Research and Therapy.* New York, Raven Press, 1986, vol 8, 155-165.

Mather LE, Meffin PJ: Clinical pharmacokinetics of pethidine. *Clin Pharmacokinet* 3:352-368, 1978.

Max MB, et al: Epidural and intrathecal opiates: Cerebrospinal fluid and plasma profiles in patients with chronic cancer pain. *Clin Pharmacol Ther* 38:631-641, 1985.

McColl KEL, et al: Studies in laboratory animals to assess the safety of anti-inflammatory agents in acute porphyria. *Ann Rheum Dis* 46:540-542, 1987.

McGivney WT, Crooks GM (eds): Care of patients with severe chronic pain in terminal illness. *JAMA* 251:1182-1188, 1984.

McQuay HJ, et al: Buprenorphine kinetics, in Foley KM, Inturrisi CE (eds): *Advances in Pain Research and Therapy.* New York, Raven Press, 1986, vol 8, 271-278.

Mello NK, Mendelson JH: Buprenorphine suppresses heroin use by heroin addicts. *Science* 207:657-659, 1980.

Meredith TJ, Vale JA: Non-narcotic analgesics: Problems of overdose. *Drugs* 32(suppl 4):177-205, 1986.

Miescher PA, Pola W: Haematological effects of non-narcotic analgesics. *Drugs* 32(suppl 4):90-108, 1986.

Montgomery PR, et al: Salicylate metabolism: Effects of age and sex in adults. *Clin Pharmacol Ther* 39:571-576, 1986.

Montoya-Iraheta C, et al: Pharmacokinetics of single dose oral and intramuscular ketorolac tromethamine in elderly vs young healthy subjects, abstract. *J Clin Pharmacol* 26:545, 1986.

Moore RA, et al: Serum concentrations of morphine and its major metabolites after oral doses in normal volunteers and IV doses in renal failure, abstract. *Pain* suppl 4:S253, 1987.

Mroszcak EJ, et al: Ketorolac tromethamine absorption, distribution, metabolism, excretion, and pharmacokinetics in animals and humans. *Drug Metab Dispos* 15:618-626, 1987.

Murray AW, et al: Comparison of the cardiorespiratory effects of ketorolac and alfentanil during propofol anaesthesia. *Br J Anaesth* 63:601-603, 1989.

Needs CJ, Brooks PM: Clinical pharmacokinetics of salicylates. *Clin Pharmacokinet* 10:164-177, 1985.

Netter P, et al: Salicylate kinetics in old age. *Clin Pharmacol Ther* 38:6-11, 1985.

Nilsson MI, et al: Effect of urinary pH on the disposition of methadone in man. *Eur J Clin Pharmacol* 22:337-342, 1982.

Novick DM, et al: Effect of severe alcoholic liver disease on the disposition of methadone in maintenance patients. *Alcohol Clin Exp Res* 9:349-354, 1985.

Oates JA, et al: Clinical implications of prostaglandin and thromboxane A_2 formation. *N Engl J Med* 319:689-698; 761-767, 1988.

O'Hara DA, et al: Ketorolac tromethamine as compared with morphine sulfate for treatment of postoperative pain. *Clin Pharmacol Ther* 41:556-561, 1987.

Osborne R, et al: Analgesic activity of morphine-6-glucuronide. *Lancet* 1:828, 1988.

Pages LJ, et al: Pharmacokinetics of ketorolac tromethamine in hepatically impaired vs. young healthy subjects, abstract. *J Clin Pharmacol* 27:724, 1987.

Parker RK, et al: Patient-controlled analgesia: Does a concurrent opioid infusion improve pain management after surgery. *JAMA* 266:1947-1952, 1991.

Pasternak GW: Multiple morphine and enkephalin receptors and the relief of pain. *JAMA* 259:1362-1367, 1988.

Payne R: Role of epidural and intrathecal narcotics and peptides in management of cancer pain. *Med Clin North Am* 71:313-327, 1987.

Piletta P, et al: Central analgesic effect of acetaminophen but not aspirin. *Clin Pharmacol Ther* 49:350-354, 1991.

Pittman KA, et al: Human perinatal distribution of butorphanol. *Am J Obstet Gynecol* 138:797-800, 1980.

Portenoy RK: Practical aspects of pain control in the patient with cancer. *CA* 38:327-352, 1988.

Portenoy RK, Foley KM: Chronic use of opioid analgesics in non-malignant pain: Report of 38 cases. *Pain* 25:171-186, 1986.

Portenoy RK, et al: Chronic morphine therapy for cancer pain. *Neurology* 41:1457-1461, 1991.

Prescott LF: Effects of non-narcotic analgesics on the liver. *Drugs* 32(suppl 4):129-147, 1986.

Purcell-Jones G, et al: Use of opioids in neonates. Retrospective study of 933 cases. *Anaesthesia* 42:1316-1320, 1987.

Rampton DS: Non-steroidal anti-inflammatory drugs and the lower gastrointestinal tract. *Scand J Gastroenterol* 22:1-4, 1987.

Rawal N, Sjöstrand UH: Clinical application of epidural and intrathecal opioids for pain management. *Int Anesthesiol Clin* 24:43-57, 1986.

Rawal N, et al: Present state of extradural and intrathecal opioid analgesia in Sweden. *Br J Anaesth* 59:791-799, 1987.

Ready LB: Age alters effective dose of epidural morphine following abdominal hysterectomy, abstract. *Pain* suppl 4:S71, 1987.

Reed DA, Schnoll SH: Abuse of pentazocine-naloxone combination. *JAMA* 256:2562-2564, 1986.

Ritschel WA, et al: Pilot study on disposition and pain relief after intramuscular administration of meperidine during day or night. *Int J Clin Pharmacol Ther Toxicol* 21:218-223, 1983.

Ritschel WA, et al: Absolute bioavailability of hydromorphone after peroral and rectal administration in humans: Saliva/plasma ratio and clinical effects. *J Clin Pharmacol* 27:647-653, 1987.

Roe RL, et al: Effects of new nonsteroidal anti-inflammatory agent on platelet function in male and female subjects, abstract. *Clin Pharmacol Ther* 29:277, 1981.

Rodgers GC Jr, Lasada M: Use of butorphanol for post operative pain in children, abstract. *Pediatr Res* 15:501, 1981.

Roytblat L, et al: Seizures after pentazocine overdose. *Isr J Med Sci* 22:385-386, 1986.

Sandler DP, et al: Analgesic use and chronic renal disease. *N Engl J Med* 320:1238-1243, 1989.

Sear J, et al: Morphine kinetics and kidney transplantation: Morphine removal is influenced by renal ischemia. *Anesth Analg* 64:1065-1070, 1985.

Semble EL, Wu WC: Anti-inflammatory drugs and gastric mucosal damage. *Semin Arthritis Rheum* 16:271-286, 1987.

Settipane GA: Aspirin and allergic diseases: Review. *Am J Med* 74(suppl 6A):102-109, 1983.

Shipton EA, Müller FO: Severe mefenamic acid poisoning: Case report. *S Afr J Med* 67:823-824, 1985.

Smilkstein MJ, et al: Efficacy of oral N-acetylcysteine in the treatment of acetaminophen overdose: Analysis of the National Multicenter Study (1976 to 1985). *N Engl J Med* 319:1557-1562, 1988.

Spowart K, et al: Haemostatic effects of ketorolac with and without concomitant heparin in normal volunteers. *Thromb Haemost* 60:382-386, 1988.

Stanski DR, et al: Kinetics of intravenous and intramuscular morphine. *Clin Pharmacol Ther* 24:52-59, 1978.

Staritz M, et al: Effect of modern analgesic drugs (Tramadol, pentazocine, and buprenorphine) on the bile duct sphincter in man. *Gut* 27:567-569, 1986.

Steelman SL, et al: Chemistry, pharmacology and clinical pharmacology of diflunisal. *Curr Med Res Opin* 5:506, 1978.

Stenseth R, et al: Epidural morphine for postoperative pain: Experience with 1085 patients. *Acta Anaesthesiol Scand* 29:148-156, 1985.

Szczeklik A: Analgesics, allergy and asthma. *Drugs* 32(suppl 4):148-163, 1986.

Tollison CD (ed): *Handbook of Chronic Pain Management.* Baltimore, Williams & Wilkins, 1989.

Tuttle CB: Drug management of pain in cancer patients. *Can Med Assoc J* 132:121-134, 1985.

Vale JA, Meredith TJ: Acute poisoning due to non-steroidal anti-inflammatory drugs: Clinical features and management. *Med Toxicol* 1:12-31, 1986.

van Loenhout JWA, et al: Persistent hypouricemic effect of long term diflunisal administration. *J Rheumatol* 8:639-642, 1981.

Verbeeck RK, et al: Clinical pharmacokinetics of non-steroidal anti-inflammatory drugs. *Clin Pharmacokinet* 8:297-331, 1983.

Vichinsky EP, et al: Multidisciplinary approach to pain management in sickle cell disease. *Am J Pediatr Hematol Oncol* 4:328-333, 1982.

Walker JJ, et al: Transfer of ketorolac tromethamine from maternal to foetal blood. *Eur J Clin Pharmacol* 34:509-511, 1988.

Wharton JG, et al: Acute renal failure associated with diflunisal. *Postgrad Med J* 58:104-105, 1982.

Wischnik A, et al: Excretion of ketorolac tromethamine into breast milk after multiple oral dosing. *Eur J Clin Pharmacol* 36:521-524, 1989.

Yee JP, et al: Comparison of intramuscular ketorolac tromethamine and morphine sulfate for analgesia of pain after major surgery. *Pharmacotherapy* 6:253-261, 1986 A.

Yee JP, et al: Comparison of analgesic efficacy of intramuscular ketorolac tromethamine and meperidine in postoperative pain, abstract. *Clin Pharmacol Ther* 39:237, 1986 B.

Yeh SY, et al: Pharmacokinetics of pentazocine and tripelennamine. *Clin Pharmacol Ther* 39:669-676, 1986.

Zeitz JK, Jarmoszuk I: Nasal polyps, bronchial asthma, and aspirin sensitivity: Samter syndrome. *Compr Ther* 11:21-26, (June) 1985.

Drugs Used for Headache and Neuralgias

7

HEADACHE

Headache, one of the most common symptoms, can be precipitated by a great variety of stimuli: emotional stress; fatigue; sensitivity to certain foods and beverages, including alcohol; medications; and acute illness. There may be no apparent underlying cause. In some individuals, headaches occur frequently but irregularly; however, they are usually acute and short lived and can be relieved by over-the-counter preparations containing aspirin, acetaminophen, or ibuprofen. This type of headache is usually not debilitating and does not require physician consultation.

In contrast, chronic recurrent headache, for which patients most often consult physicians, is associated with various medical, neurologic, or psychogenic disorders. Appropriate therapy depends on an accurate diagnosis of the type of headache.

The Headache Classification Committee of the International Headache Society (1988) has developed diagnostic criteria for classification of headache disorders, cranial neuralgias, and facial pain; the criteria include painful and nonpainful disorders of the entire head and are based on the diagnosis rather than on the underlying pain mechanisms.

A major type of headache that must be considered in differential diagnosis is that caused by underlying disease: intracranial disturbances (eg, vascular anomalies, infections, tumors, trauma); diseases involving the head and neck but not the brain (eg, cervical osteoarthritis; disorders of eye, ear, nose, sinuses, and throat; cranial neuralgias); and systemic diseases (eg, sudden and severe hypertension, hyperthyroidism). These headaches usually can be relieved by specific therapy for the underlying disorder, eg, surgical correction of tumors, antibiotics for infections, antiarthritic drugs for osteoarthritis. Drug treatment for cranial neuralgias is discussed in that section in this chapter.

Considerations in the management of recurrent migraine, cluster, or tension-type headache include the following: (1) No single therapy is effective in all patients with the same type of headache, which serves to underscore the uncertainty about the pathophysiology of these disorders and the variability among individuals. Therefore, drug therapy must be individualized, and trials of different therapies and drugs may be required to establish an effective regimen. (2) In addition to treatment, some patients should receive prophylactic therapy; these individuals should be monitored closely and adjustments made in choice of therapy or dosage when necessary. (3) Many patients with chronic headaches have received drugs that may cause drug dependence (eg, barbiturates, antianxiety agents, ergotamine, narcotics, analgesic and caffeine mixtures), and their withdrawal along with instruction regarding their proper use is necessary. This last consideration may be a primary obstacle in the long-term relief of headache.

Migraine Headache

Migraine headaches can begin during childhood, but 60% to 70% of patients are women in their late teens, twenties, and thirties. Headache pain is usually characterized as steady or throbbing and is most severe in the temporal and frontal regions. The headache usually is unilateral, frequently occurs on awakening, and typically is associated with nausea, vomiting, photophobia, phonophobia, and irritability. Diarrhea, local or generalized edema, pallor, dizziness, sweating, and many other symptoms also may occur (Solomon et al, 1988).

Migraine headaches with sharply defined aura (visual, sensory, motor, or any combination) are considered "classic"; those with no aura are considered "common." The vast majority of individuals with migraine have the common type. A patient may experience classic migraine headache at one time and the common type at other times. Combined tension-type/migraine headache is not unusual. Severe subtypes of classic migraine, including hemiplegic, ophthalmoplegic and basilar, are rare but should be considered in differential diagnosis, especially in children. Status migrainosus refers to repeated migraine attacks that persist for more than 72 hours.

Although vascular and central nervous system precipitating factors have been identified (eg, tyramine-containing foods, alcohol, glare, menses, anxiety, fatigue, stress), the precise pathophysiology of migraine remains to be determined (Lance, 1986; Raskin, 1988). A family history exists in 65% to 70% of affected patients and aids in diagnosis. Migraine patients may be genetically predisposed to headache by variant patterns of monoamine metabolism, which make them vulnerable to changes in monoamine transmitters in the central nervous system, as well as to platelet-released serotonin (Lance et al, 1989).

The effective management of recurrent migraine may require combined medical and nonmedical therapy, including the control or elimination of underlying factors that precipitate an attack. Among the nonpharmacologic techniques, some headache specialists have found that biofeedback can reduce the intensity and frequency of headaches (Sargent et al, 1986). Its beneficial effect may be mediated through generalized reduction of sympathetic tone, which produces a relaxation response (Dalessio et al, 1979). A reduction in catecholamines and decreased monoamine oxidase activity also have been observed (Mathew et al, 1980). However, in a review of the data, the American College of Physicians concluded that biofeedback may be useful adjunctively in mixed migraine and tension-type headaches, but it is no more effective than other relaxation techniques (Health and Public Policy Committee, American College of Physicians, 1985).

Migraine probably is the most frequent recurring headache in childhood. It differs from migraine in adults in that it is more common in males and possibly has somewhat better-defined triggering factors (Prensky, 1976; Barlow, 1984; Fenichel, 1985; Raskin, 1988). Nonpharmacologic measures, such as avoidance of triggering factors (glare or dim lighting, hunger, cold weather, prolonged physical exertion) and relaxation techniques, may be much more useful in children than in adults (Diamond, 1983; Barlow, 1984; Fentress et al, 1986).

Drug Selection for Acute Migraine: Pharmacotherapy consists of symptomatic treatment of the acute attack (abortive) and prophylactic (interval) therapy to reduce the frequency and severity of headaches. The goal of drug therapy for acute migraine headache is to relieve pain and reduce or prevent accompanying nausea and vomiting. Drugs should be administered during the earliest stages of an attack to obtain the greatest therapeutic effect. The early stages of classic migraine are the easiest to identify; the aura serves as a signal to begin abortive measures. Once the headache has been established, oral drugs generally are absorbed poorly due to the gastric stasis, nausea, or both often present in severe headaches. This may be circumvented by the use of rectal suppositories or inhalation preparations.

Nonspecific symptomatic relief of mild attacks may be obtained with over-the-counter analgesics (aspirin, acetaminophen, ibuprofen). If these agents are ineffective, aspirin with codeine or propoxyphene [Darvon] may be employed, but their effectiveness is limited once the attack has begun because of gastric stasis. Some mixtures containing sedatives and analgesics (eg, Axotal, Fiorinal) may be helpful but may be habituating. Metoclopramide [Reglan] 10 to 20 mg orally has been recommended to restore gastric motility, permit absorption of analgesics, and prevent nausea and vomiting (Selby, 1983; Kunkel, 1985). However, metoclopramide alone does not affect the pain component of the attack. This drug should be used cautiously in children and young adults because of the potential for severe drug-induced dystonic-dyskinetic reactions. These reactions are most common within 24 hours after starting treatment and only rarely occur after 72 hours (Bateman et al, 1985).

If symptoms of migraine headache cannot be managed with analgesics, subsequent attacks should be aborted with an ergot alkaloid. Of the available ergot alkaloids, ergotamine tartrate has the most prolonged effect and most consistently aborts migraine headache when an adequate dose is administered as soon as possible after the onset of the migraine aura or attack. It is available as a sublingual [Ergomar, Ergostat] or inhalation [Medihaler Ergotamine] preparation or in combination with caffeine [Cafergot, Wigraine] in oral or rectal preparations. Caffeine is believed to increase the absorption and effectiveness of ergotamine (Schmidt and Fanchamps, 1974), but no controlled trial has been conducted to document this impression. Pharmacokinetic considerations favor administration of ergotamine 1 mg in suppository form for the initial trial of an ergot preparation in a new patient (Bülow et al, 1986). The rectal, sublingual, or inhalation route may be most practical when nausea occurs. When used properly, the rectal and inhalation preparations of ergotamine provide rapid systemic availability of the drug. The major side effects and contraindications (eg, coronary artery disease, pregnancy, peripheral vascular disease, hepatic and/or renal disease) for the use of ergotamine should be borne in mind (see the evaluation).

Concomitant oral administration of metoclopramide may prevent the severe nausea and vomiting caused by ergotamine (or the migraine attack) and enhance ergotamine's absorption (Tfelt-Hansen et al, 1980; Bradfield, 1976). Alternatives to metoclopramide include phenothiazine antiemetics, such as prochlorperazine [Compazine] or promethazine [Phenergan], which can be administered orally, rectally, or intramuscularly.

In patients who cannot tolerate ergotamine, the mixture of the vasoconstrictor, isometheptene mucate; the mild sedative, dichloralphenazone; and the analgesic, acetaminophen [Midrin] may be an effective alternative but it is available only orally. Clinical trials indicate that Midrin is superior to acetaminophen alone (Diamond, 1976). Contraindications to the use of this preparation are hypertension, coronary artery disease, or peripheral vascular disease.

The ergotamine derivative, dihydroergotamine [D.H.E. 45], also may be a useful alternative to ergotamine when high serum concentrations are needed. This drug is administered intramuscularly or intravenously and is considered by some clinicians to be the agent of choice in physicians' offices and hospital emergency rooms for patients with severe, refractory migraine headache.

Severe headaches that fail to respond to ergot preparations may be relieved by an opioid analgesic (eg, meperidine [Demerol]). Chlorpromazine [Thorazine] 25 mg intramuscularly or 5 to 50 (mean, 22) mg by slow intravenous bolus injections is an alternative (Edmeads, 1988). In a controlled clinical trial, chlorpromazine 1 mg/kg intramuscularly was safe and effective for nausea and provided some relief from pain in a significant number of patients (McEwen et al, 1987). More recently, prochlorperazine edisylate [Compazine] in an intravenous dose of 10 mg injected slowly at a rate not to exceed 5 mg/min also was effective for acute headache in adults (Jones et al, 1989).

Although parenteral administration of a corticosteroid (eg, dexamethasone acetate 16 mg intramuscularly) has been reported to be useful in some patients with status migrainosus (Diamond and Dalessio, 1986), the lack of an experimental model prevents study of the mechanism. One investigator (Edmeads, 1988) believes that if the corticosteroid has not terminated the headache within 24 hours, additional doses are unlikely to be beneficial.

In children, acute attacks may respond to acetaminophen suppositories. Aspirin suppositories also are effective but usually are avoided in pediatric patients because of concern for the development of Reye's syndrome. Ergot alkaloids almost never are used as the initial drug to treat migraine in young patients.

A new selective serotonin agonist on the 5-HT_{1D} receptor, sumatriptan, is being investigated for treatment of the acute migrane attack. Preliminary results in Phase III trials have been promising (Peroutka, 1990).

Drug Selection for Prophylactic (Interval) Therapy: The decision to begin prophylactic therapy for migraine headaches is based on the frequency and severity of the attacks, the response to abortive therapy, and coexisting medical conditions. Usually, patients who experience two or more disabling attacks per month are candidates for prophylactic therapy. However, if the attacks respond well to abortive therapy with ergotamine and the dose does not exceed recommended safety limits, prophylactic therapy may not be required. Conversely, if treatment is inadequate or contraindicated, preventive therapy is the only alternative. Since spontaneous remissions occur, prolonged, uninterrupted prophylactic treatment without a drug-free interval is not advisable.

Ergotamine is generally not recommended for prophylaxis because its potent peripheral vasoconstrictor action may produce arterial insufficiency, and dependence may result from prolonged daily use. In dependent patients, a self-sustaining headache-medication cycle is established in which drug withdrawal precipitates a rebound headache that necessitates readministration of ergotamine. Certain patients may be predisposed to this rebound syndrome. The headache that follows ergotamine withdrawal is debilitating and lasts longer than a typical migraine headache (Saper, 1987; Saper and Jones, 1986). Nevertheless, withdrawal must be attempted to reestablish headache control, since prophylactic agents are often ineffective in ergotamine-dependent patients. Some neurologists still favor intermittent use of ergotamine to prevent predictable migraine attacks, such as those occurring on weekends, in association with menstruation, or resulting from a known stressful situation. Caution should be exercised when ergotamine is used in these circumstances.

Methysergide [Sansert] and beta-adrenergic blocking agents are the most effective agents for migraine prophylaxis. Beta blocker therapy generally is preferred because of the potential occurrence of serious fibrotic adverse reactions with prolonged methysergide therapy. Most experience has been gained with propranolol [Inderal]. Other beta blockers that have been effective in controlled clinical trials include atenolol [Tenormin], metoprolol [Lopressor], nadolol [Corgard], and timolol [Blocadren]. No significant difference in effectiveness between these beta blockers and propranolol has been demonstrated. Propranolol and nadolol probably are the agents most widely employed for migraine prophylaxis. A prolonged-release preparation of propranolol is available, and it may enhance compliance.

Prophylactic therapy with beta blockers is particularly useful in patients who cannot take ergot preparations (eg, those with hypertension, cerebrovascular disease, angina pectoris, severe peripheral vascular disease, thyrotoxicosis). However, they should not be used when beta blockade would be harmful (see the evaluation on Propranolol Hydrochloride). If the patient fails to respond to beta blockers or these drugs are contraindicated, alternative agents may be tried.

Methysergide is considered to be the most effective prophylactic drug available but, because of its potential serious adverse reactions, this drug must be used with caution and treatment should be interrupted for one month after four to six months. Methysergide may be reserved for patients in whom beta-adrenergic blocking agents, calcium channel blocking agents, and nonsteroidal anti-inflammatory drugs (NSAIDs) (eg, naproxen [Naprosyn]) have failed. Methysergide is not effective in an acute migraine attack or tension-type headache and should be restricted to short-term use in patients under age 50 who are not at risk for vascular disease.

Although the use of calcium channel blocking drugs for migraine prophylaxis is limited, these drugs reduced the frequency and, in some cases, the severity of attacks of both common and classic migraine in controlled clinical trials (Olesen, 1988; Schuler et al, 1988; Spierings, 1988). They may be useful substitutes for beta-adrenergic blocking agents. Most experience has been obtained with verapamil [Calan, Isoptin] and nifedipine [Adalet, Procardia].

Cyproheptadine [Periactin], an antihistamine with antiserotonin and calcium antagonist activity, was considered to be effective for prophylaxis in some patients, but results of controlled studies have shown that it is only slightly better than placebo in adults. Adverse effects include drowsiness and increased appetite with weight gain. A related compound, pizotyline [Sandomigran], reduced the frequency and severity of migraine attacks in clinical trials (Louis and Spierings, 1982; Selby, 1983). This drug is not available in the United States but is used in Canada, Australia, and Europe; it has the same spectrum of adverse reactions as cyproheptadine, but is considered superior to the latter for migraine prophylaxis.

In a limited number of studies, amitriptyline [Elavil], a tricyclic antidepressant, was effective prophylactically for some patients with migraine and/or tension-type headache. In one controlled study, amitriptyline was more effective than placebo in preventing migraine, and its action did not appear to be related to the antidepressant effect (Couch and Hassanein, 1979). The beneficial effect observed with amitriptyline also has been observed with its metabolite, nortriptyline [Aventyl]. Either drug may be used when a beta blocking agent is not tolerated or is ineffective.

Another antidepressant, the monoamine oxidase inhibitor, phenelzine [Nardil], has been beneficial in some patients refractory to other prophylactic therapy. However, because the response is variable and the adverse effects are potentially severe, it should be reserved for patients with severe migraine or chronic mixed migraine/tension-type headache that does not respond to prophylactic therapy with other drugs.

There is some indirect evidence that prostaglandins play a role in the development of a migraine attack. Thus, several inhibitors of prostaglandin synthetase and platelet aggregation have been studied as prophylactic drugs. The results from studies with aspirin, indomethacin [Indocin], and dipyridamole [Persantine] were not encouraging. However, a controlled double-blind trial with naproxen [Anaprox, Naprosyn] demonstrated that this drug moderately reduced the frequency and duration of migraine attacks (Ziegler and Ellis, 1985). Since then, a number of studies have supported the usefulness of naproxen (Sargent et al, 1988 A). Other NSAIDs that inhibit prostaglandin synthesis (eg, ibuprofen [Advil, Motrin, Nuprin, Rufen], fenoprofen [Nalfon], mefenamic acid [Ponstel]) also may prevent migraine, but further studies are needed to determine their ultimate role. The usefulness of NSAIDs in migraine prophylaxis and the favorable role they have in the prophylaxis of menstrual migraine have been reviewed (Diamond and Freitag, 1989). Gastritis and/or gastric bleeding can occur in some patients receiving long-term prophylactic treatment with these agents.

For children, the use of continuous medication to prevent intermittent headaches (eg, three or four per month) should be weighed carefully. Prophylactic therapy may be instituted for frequent, severe headaches in children. Cyproheptadine in a single bedtime dose of 4 to 8 mg is considered the drug of choice in young patients (Saper, 1983; Raskin, 1988); children appear to tolerate this drug better than adults. Some of these patients also respond well to phenytoin or phenobarbital, even in the absence of underlying electroencephalographic abnormalities (Barlow, 1984; Fenichel, 1985). Despite some early favorable reports, and unlike its favorable effect in adults, propranolol generally is not useful in most pediatric patients (Forsythe et al, 1984; Olness et all, 1987). Phenothiazines, particularly prochlorperazine and metoclopramide, generally should be avoided in younger patients because these individuals are more susceptible to acute dystonic reactions and neuroleptic malignant syndrome.

Cluster Headache and Chronic Paroxysmal Hemicrania

Cluster headache (also known as Horton's syndrome, histaminic cephalalgia, migrainous neuralgia, and by many other names) is related to migraine but differs sufficiently in triggering factors, presentation, and selectivity of response to therapeutic agents to be considered a separate type (Sjaastad, 1986). The typical form, classified as *episodic*, is characterized by excruciating, nonthrobbing, unilateral, and oculofrontal or oculotemporal pain that lasts 15 to 120 minutes and occurs in a series or "cluster" of closely spaced attacks (one or more per day), often at night. Clusters generally last 4 to 12 weeks, with remissions of months or years. Associated symptoms are conjunctival injection, lacrimation, nasal congestion, facial sweating, and, occasionally, ptosis and miosis, all on the side of the pain. Unlike classic migraine headaches, prodromata or aura do not precede the headache, and nausea and vomiting are absent. There is usually no family history of cluster headache (Kudrow, 1979).

In *chronic cluster headache*, the periods of remission are very brief. In one, very *rare* form (chronic paroxysmal hemicrania [CPH]), attacks occur as often as six times daily. Although cluster headaches are observed more frequently in men than in women (5:1), CPH is distinguished from chronic or episodic cluster headache by its greater occurrence in women, the great frequency of attacks, and its response to indomethacin.

The pathogenesis of cluster headache is unknown, but numerous studies indicate that certain changes in cephalic blood flow, as well as biochemical changes (eg, histamine, serotonin, and hormone levels), result from a neurogenic mechanism. Unilateral increase in blood flow is usually associated with the onset of pain, and it has been postulated that vascular changes are initiated by a vasodilator pathway involving the greater superficial petrosal nerve and trigeminal nerve arc (Drummond and Lance, 1984).

Drug Selection: Preventive therapy is the treatment of choice of most headache specialists, but treatment of the acute attack also may be required. The primary prophylactic medications are methysergide, lithium carbonate, and corticosteroids. Ergotamine tartrate also has been effective for attacks that occur at predictable times (Lance, 1982; Raskin, 1986). Indomethacin, phenelzine, divalproate, and other antimigraine drugs are effective in some patients. Calcium channel blockers also may have prophylactic activity; nimodipine was reported to be the most effective (Meyer and Hardenberg, 1983; Mullally and Livingstone, 1984; Raskin, 1988). Recently, results of an uncontrolled study demonstrated that high-dose verapamil may be beneficial (Gabai and Spierings, 1989).

Lithium is effective in the prophylactic management of episodic and chronic cluster headache (Ekbom, 1981; Manzoni et al, 1983; Mathew, 1984); blood levels must be monitored. Lithium is regarded by some authorities as a second-line drug and is preferred to corticosteroids when methysergide and calcium channel blocking agents fail. Corticosteroids are very effective in preventing cluster headache, but attacks generally return when these drugs are discontinued. Because of the self-limited nature of cluster headache and the side effects of the corticosteroids, the recommended course of therapy is limited to about three weeks. In one regimen, oral prednisone 60 mg is given daily for four days followed by a ten-day stepwise reduction of the dose to zero (Saper, 1989).

Individual cataclysmic attacks that break through preventive therapy or that occur before prophylactic therapy becomes effective may be terminated by an ergot preparation; unless contraindicated, parenteral dihydroergotamine is preferred by some clinicians for prompt relief but is not practical for regular use. As an alternative, use of ergotamine/caffeine suppositories has been recommended. Because the attacks are brief, oral and sublingual preparations of ergotamine are usually less effective. The inhalant form of ergotamine provides fast relief in selected patients, but variability in dosing and constriction of pulmonary arteries require patient education in its use. When a large number of attacks occur daily, overmedication may result.

Cluster headache also may be aborted by inhaling 100% oxygen (6 to 9 L/min for 15 minutes or less) through a nonrebreathing face mask. The mechanism of action is unknown. This form of therapy has been reported to be useful in 57% to 93% of patients (Kudrow, 1981) and is supported by results of double-blind controlled studies in which oxygen was significantly superior to compressed air.

CPH responds completely to oral indomethacin 25 to 50 mg three times daily (Mathew, 1984; Saper, 1989).

Tension-Type and Combined Headaches

Tension-type (muscle-contraction) headaches are characterized by mild to moderate nonthrobbing pain, tightness, or pressure around the head and neck unassociated with autonomic disturbances. The episodic tension-type headache is the most common one for which a physician is consulted. It may develop in response to stress of everyday life, aggravation, frustration, eye strain, or positional effects.

Many patients with tension-type headache have associated depressive symptoms. Pain is often worse in the morning than in the evening, is generalized rather than localized, is accompanied by scalp formication, and is associated with symptoms common in depression, such as sleep disturbances with early and frequent awakening.

Tension-type and migraine headaches often occur together (Anderson and Franks, 1981; Cohen and McArthur, 1981; Joffe et al, 1983; Saper, 1986), and a significant portion of patients with chronic headache have "mixed" headaches with features of both (Ziegler, 1985). Current physiologic, psychological, and clinical studies have blurred the traditional distinction between tension-type and common migraine headaches (Featherstone, 1984; Saper, 1986).

Most difficult to treat is the chronic headache syndrome that often begins in early years as migraine headache and evolves later in life into a relatively constant tension-type headache (Mathew et al, 1987). This type of headache is most common in women and frequently is accompanied by depression, anxiety, and sleep disturbances. The chronic nature of this pain increases the potential for analgesic abuse, which in turn perpetuates headache by a rebound mechanism.

Tension-type headaches also have been referred to as psychogenic headaches. Although these headaches may be precipitated by emotional factors, especially anxiety, they must be differentiated from headaches accompanying severe psychological disorders. To avoid confusion, it is proposed that the class, psychogenic, be restricted to headaches that have no known physiologic pain-producing mechanisms. In psychogenic headaches, the pain represents the primary expression of an underlying psychiatric disorder. The psychogenic class includes conversion, delusional, and hypochondriacal headaches (Packard, 1976; Weatherhead, 1980).

Tension-type headaches also must be differentiated from those caused by certain disorders of muscles or joints (inflammation of the muscles of the head and neck, cervical osteoarthritis, disorders of the temporal-mandibular joint). Treatment or correction of the underlying condition is important in the management of these headaches, although many headache experts consider treatment on the jaw in an effort to alleviate headaches to be excessive.

Drug Selection: Acute tension-type headaches with mild to moderate pain may be treated with a nonopiate analgesic such as aspirin, acetaminophen, ibuprofen (Diamond, 1983), naproxen (Sargent et al, 1988 B), other nonsteroidal anti-inflammatory analgesics, or an antidepressant. The tricyclic antidepressants are more effective than analgesics if depressive symptoms are present; there is evidence to indicate that these drugs reduce headache pain independent of the presence of depression. A nighttime dose may relieve both sleep disturbances and headache. Drugs with high dependence liability should be avoided. Certain combination products containing a barbiturate (eg, Fiorinal) or other sedative (eg, meprobamate [Micrainin]) with an analgesic are useful in this type of episodic headache (see Table). However, because these mixtures have high abuse potential, they should be avoided in patients with chronic headaches.

Therapy for chronic combined headache represents a therapeutic challenge to the headache specialist. Withdrawal of analgesics taken daily is mandatory (Saper, 1989). Some patients require hospitalization for this purpose. Chlorpromazine (or another phenothiazine) has been given during analgesic withdrawal; antianxiety agents may also be useful. A multidisciplinary approach that includes physical therapy, biofeedback, relaxation techniques, psychotherapy, and drug therapy is usually required (Martin, 1978; Nuechterlein and Holroyd, 1980; Ziegler, 1978).

The combination of propranolol (or another appropriate beta blocker) and amitriptyline has been useful for prophylaxis (Dexter et al, 1980; Mathew, 1981). Antidepressants, such as amitriptyline, are useful because of their analgesic activity and their effect on the depression commonly associated with chronic tension-type and combined headaches. Monoamine oxidase inhibitors also are reported to be effective (Saper, 1989).

An acute attack of combined tension-type/migraine headache is usually managed by treating the symptoms of the dominant headache type (eg, ergotamine for migraine, analgesics or antidepressants for tension-type headache). Combined administration of ergotamine and simple analgesics and/or antidepressants may be required.

Drug Evaluations

ERGOT ALKALOIDS

ERGOTAMINE TARTRATE

[Medihaler Ergotamine, Ergomar, Ergostat]

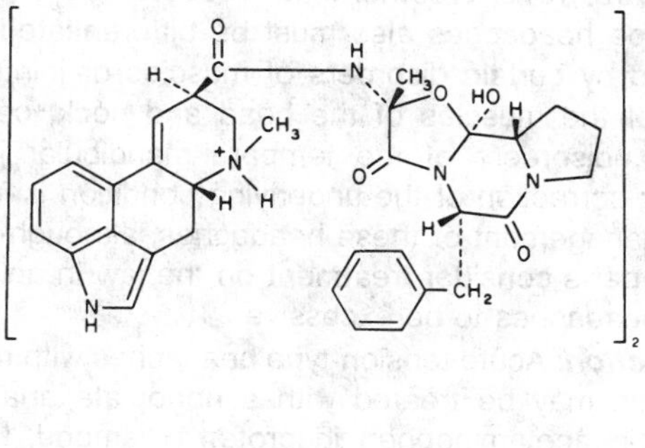

ACTIONS AND USES. Ergotamine is the drug of choice in the treatment of acute attacks of migraine. It also may be used to alleviate or prevent acute attacks of cluster headache.

The long-term prophylactic use of ergotamine is generally inadvisable because ergotamine dependence may develop with ergotism resulting from dosage escalation. However, short-term daily use may be appropriate in certain cases. For example, patients experiencing daily attacks of cluster headaches may receive the drug regularly for 10- to 14-day periods.

Ergotamine causes peripheral vasoconstriction, especially in the dilated external carotid arterial bed. It acts as a vasoconstrictor if the tonus of the vessel is low and as a vasodilator if the tonus is high. Ergotamine also may act by depressing central serotonergic neurons mediating pain transmission or circulatory regulation (Perrin, 1985). In therapeutic doses, it potentiates the action of epinephrine and norepinephrine and inhibits the reuptake of these amines after nerve stimulation (Fozard, 1975).

To be most effective, an adequate dose must be taken immediately after the onset of the aura or the headache. It may be helpful to determine a subnauseating dose during a headache-free period (Raskin, 1988). This individualized dose may be the appropriate dose by the selected route of administration for subsequent attacks. Ergotamine may not be well absorbed when given orally (available only in combination products) or sublingually, and there is considerable variation among individuals; if these routes are ineffective, rectal suppositories (available only in combination products) should be tried since higher plasma concentrations have been reported after administration by this route than after oral use. The drug also may be given by inhalation, which produces a more rapid effect than the oral route.

ADVERSE REACTIONS AND PRECAUTIONS. Ergotamine may produce nausea, vomiting, epigastric discomfort, diarrhea, polydipsia, and restlessness. More serious adverse reactions include paresthesias of the extremities, cramps and weakness of the legs, myalgia (eg, stiffness of thigh and neck muscles), angina-like precordial pain and distress, transient sinus tachycardia and bradycardia, and, in sensitive patients, localized edema, pruritus, and peripheral vasoconstriction. There have been case reports of ergotamine-induced myocardial or cerebral infarction.

Symptoms of chronic overdosage (eg, malaise, nausea, headache) have occurred when 7 to 10 mg per week was taken continuously (Hokkanen et al, 1978). These effects may be followed by severe vasoconstriction, usually affecting the lower extremities. It generally is accompanied by distal paresthesia, coldness of the toes, and exertional pain affecting the calves and heels. Patients should be warned to discontinue the drug at the first appearance of such symptoms and to notify the treating physician. Gangrene secondary to the ischemia is rare when usual doses are given to patients who do not have peripheral vascular disease, hepatic disease, or other disorders in which this drug is contraindicated. If persistent ergotamine-induced peripheral ischemia occurs, it may be relieved by the intravenous or intra-arterial infusion of sodium nitroprusside. The latter route may be preferred because it permits the use of lower doses of nitroprusside (Dierckx et al, 1986). Infusion is continued until sufficient clearance of ergotamine and its metabolites has occurred (about 24 to 48 hours).

Ergotamine is contraindicated in patients with peripheral vascular disease (eg, Raynaud's disease, thromboangiitis obliterans, thrombophlebitis, marked arteriosclerosis), severe hypertension, ischemic heart disease or anginal pain, peptic ulcer, renal or hepatic disease, malnutrition, or hypersensitivity to ergot preparations. It should not be used in the presence of infections. Since ergotamine has oxytocic properties and may be embryotoxic as the result of diminished uterine blood flow, it should not be given to pregnant women (FDA Pregnancy Category X). Ergotamine preparations should be used cautiously in children.

Physical dependence on ergotamine may occur (Saper and Jones, 1986). In most patients, it is characterized by a predictable withdrawal syndrome that consists of an irresistible, self-sustaining headache-medication cycle (Saper, 1987), nausea and vomiting, and restlessness that mimics a migraine attack. Patients receiving more than 10 mg in a week (Mathew, 1987) or any dose more than two days a week (Saper, 1987) are at particular risk. There is a trend toward limiting the dosage of inhalation or rectal ergotamine to 1 to 2 mg per attack and no more than 4 mg per week (Wilkinson, 1988). Alternative pharmacotherapy for headache is frequently ineffective until ergotamine is discontinued and the cycle is broken. Hospitalization may be required for the symptomatic treatment of the withdrawal syndrome. In some patients, naproxen 500 mg twice a day, begun one day before the planned ergotamine withdrawal, reduces the incidence or severity of headache, nausea, vomiting, and restlessness (Mathew, 1987). The biochemical basis for dependence has not been clearly determined, but may involve altered aminergic receptor sensitivity in the hypothalamic-pituitary axis and locus ceruleus as a result of the inhibition of norepinephrine and serotonin (Saper and Jones, 1986; Saper, 1987).

DRUG INTERACTIONS. The use of ergotamine to abort breakthrough migraine headaches in patients receiving propranolol for prophylaxis is usually well tolerated. A potential exists for this combination to cause excessive vasoconstriction, but this effect has not been conclusively documented.

PHARMACOKINETICS. The absorption of ergotamine following oral, sublingual, or rectal administration varies considerably. Bioavailability estimates and other pharmacokinetic studies differ widely depending on the analytical technique and, in early studies, the inability to distinguish between unchanged ergotamine in the plasma and its long-lived, pharmacologically active metabolites. Some difference in pharmacokinetic parameters exists between healthy subjects, headache-free patients, and patients experiencing headache. Representative pharmacokinetic data through 1984 have been reviewed (Perrin, 1985).

Following intravenous administration of ergotamine tartrate 0.5 mg (preparation not available in the United States) to migraine patients free of headache, the initial distribution half-life was three minutes (Ibraheem et al, 1982). The investigators calculated that the mean elimination half-life is 1.86 hours (range, 90 to 155 min), total plasma clearance is 11 ml/kg/min, and the volume of distribution is 1.85 L/kg.

In a crossover study using healthy volunteers, the bioavailability after oral and rectal administration of ergotamine tartrate 2 mg and caffeine 100 mg was compared by mass spectrographic analysis of the plasma; the mean peak concentration of ergotamine following rectal administration was approximately 20 times that following oral administration (Sanders et al, 1986). The comparative differences in the mean after rectal and oral administration, respectively, were AUC (hr x pg/ml) 1,216 and 61, the mean plasma concentration (C_{max}pg/ml) 454 and 21.4, and the time to maximum concentration (T_{max}min) 50 and 69.

Sublingual (Tfelt-Hansen et al, 1982) and buccal absorption are poor, in part due to low solubility. The serum concentrations achieved with inhalation may approximate those with rectal administration (Graham et al, 1984), but this has not been confirmed.

Total body clearance of ergotamine and its metabolites is primarily by biliary excretion into the feces. Administration of tritium-labeled ergotamine to subjects with normal hepatic, renal, and gastroenteric function showed that only 4.3% of the total dose following oral and 6.7% following intravenous administration was excreted in the urine (Aellig and Nüesch, 1977).

Since the biological half-life of ergotamine is significantly greater than the elimination half-life, it is probable that some or all of this drug's biological activity is due to persistent metabolites. Only limited studies on ergotamine have been performed, but dihydroergotamine has been studied more thoroughly; see the evaluation on the latter drug.

DOSAGE AND PREPARATIONS.

Inhalation: *Adults,* a single inhalation (0.36 mg) at the onset of an attack, repeated if necessary at intervals of no less than five minutes to a total of six inhalations in 24 hours (maximum, 15 inhalations in one week). The risk of provoking bronchospasm in asthmatic patients should be kept in mind when ergotamine is administered by this route.

Medihaler Ergotamine (3M Riker). Solution 9 mg/ml in 2.5 ml containers. Each dose (a single inhalation) contains approximately 0.36 mg of ergotamine tartrate.

Sublingual: *Adults,* 2 mg at the onset of an attack, followed by 2 mg every 30 minutes if necessary (maximum, 6 mg in 24 hours and 10 mg in one week).

Ergomar (Fisons), ***Ergostat*** (Parke-Davis). Tablets 2 mg.

Oral, Rectal: Ergotamine for oral or rectal administration is present only in mixtures with other drugs. See the following table for available trademarks and recommended dosage.

MIXTURES

Preparation	Ingredients	Comment
Cafergot (Sandoz), Wigraine (Organon), Generic	Each tablet contains ergotamine tartrate 1 mg and caffeine 100 mg	Clinical experience and comparative trials indicate that caffeine increases the effectiveness of ergotamine, probably by increasing its enteral absorption (Schmidt and Fanchamps, 1974); however, it may interfere with sleep. (FDA Pregnancy Category X)
Cafergot (Sandoz), Wigraine (Organon), Generic	Each suppository contains ergotamine tartrate 2 mg and caffeine 100 mg	
Bellergal-S (Sandoz)	Each prolonged-release tablet contains ergolamine tartrate 0.6 mg, phenobarbital 40 mg, and levorotatory belladonna alkaloids as malates 0.2 mg	Bellergal-S is claimed to be useful in migrane prophylaxis. This preparation is not useful for aborting acute attacks since the amount of ergotamine is insufficient. Most authorities believe that prolonged administration of an ergot preparation is not advisable, because peripheral vasoconstriction and ergot habituation may occur. Also, the potential abuse of the barbiturate component may compound the problems. (FDA Pregnancy Category X)
Axotal (Adria)	Each tablet contains butalbital 50 mg and aspirin 650 mg	These mixtures may be indicated to relieve tension-type headache and may be helpful as analgesics in migraine headache. Fixed-dose combinations do not permit adjustment of dose to suit the needs of individual patients. It may be preferable to prescribe the sedative separately; however, butalbital is not available as a single-entity agent. If a sedative is required for tension-type or migraine headache, an agent other than butalbital must be prescribed. Frequent use may lead to abuse.
Esgic (Forest), Fioricet (Sandoz), Generic	Each capsule (Esgic only) or tablet contains butalbital 50 mg, acetaminophen 325 mg, and caffeine 40 mg	
Fiorinal (Sandoz), Generic	Each capsule or tablet contains butalbital 50 mg, aspirin 325 mg, and caffeine 40 mg	
Micrainin (Wallace), Generic	Each tablet contains aspirin 325 mg and meprobamate 200 mg	For adverse reactions and precautions, see index entries on individual ingredients.
Phrenilin, Phrenilin Forte (Carnrick)	Each tablet or capsule contains butalbital 50 mg and acetaminophen 325 mg or 650 mg (Forte capsule)	
Midrin (Carnrick)	Each capsule contains isometheptene mucate 65 mg, dichloralphenazone 100 mg, and acetaminophen 325 mg	Midrin is effective for abortive treatment and may be useful in patients who cannot tolerate ergotamine. However, absorption is delayed with the oral route compared with inhalation or rectal administration of ergotamine. The results of a few controlled studies indicate that the combination is no more effective than isometheptene, the active ingredient, which is not available alone. Isometheptene is claimed to act as a cerebral vasoconstrictor, and results of studies show that Midrin reduces regional cerebral blood flow in migraine patients (Yamamoto and Meyer, 1980). This mixture is more effective than placebo (Diamond, 1976). Adverse reactions include insomnia or drowsiness, dizziness, feeling of weakness, paresthesias, and palpitations. This mixture should not be used in patients with hypertension, coronary artery, or peripheral vascular disease.

Usual Dosage

Oral: Adults, two tablets at onset of migraine attack, then if needed, one additional tablet every 30 minutes. Total dose should not exceed six tablets/attack or ten/week.
Children, one-half tablet initially, then if needed, one-half tablet every 30 minutes (maximum, three tablets).

Rectal: Adults, appropriate tolerated dose should be determined for each patient between headache attacks (usually one-half suppository at the beginning of an attack, but some patients require only 0.25 to 0.5 mg). If necessary, dose is repeated after one hour. Total amount should not exceed two suppositories/attack or five suppositories/week.

Oral: Adults, two prolonged-release tablets daily (one in the morning and one in the evening).

Oral: Adults, one or two tablets or capsules every four hours maximum, six tablets or capsules daily. (Phrenilin Forte, one capsule every four to six hours with maximum of three capsules daily.) No dosage has been established for *children under 12 years.*

Oral: Adults, two capsules at the onset of attack, followed by one capsule every hour until pain is relieved (maximum, five capsules in 12-hour period).

DIHYDROERGOTAMINE MESYLATE
[D.H.E. 45]

USES. Dihydroergotamine, given intramuscularly or intravenously, is considered by some to be the drug of choice for terminating a migraine or cluster headache attack in the emergency room or office setting. These routes are inconvenient if repeated self-administration is required. Intravenous dihydroergotamine has terminated status migrainosus, and repeated intravenous administration has terminated the cycles of attacks (Raskin, 1986).

ADVERSE REACTIONS AND PRECAUTIONS. The arterial vasoconstrictor effect of dihydroergotamine is much less pronounced than that of ergotamine and therefore this drug is less likely to produce vascular reactions. However, the same general precautions should be observed as with ergotamine. Electrocardiographic monitoring during the first two parenteral doses has been recommended in patients over age 60 (Raskin, 1988). Unlike ergotamine, dihydroergotamine does not appear to produce physical dependence. Diarrhea is a prominent side effect but responds well to diphenoxylate with atropine [Lomotil].

PHARMACOKINETICS. Dihydroergotamine is not administered orally because it undergoes extensive first-pass metabolism in the liver. Only about 1% of the initial dose reaches the systemic circulation (Bobik et al, 1981; Little et al, 1982). The drug is eliminated primarily by metabolism; less than 0.01% is excreted in the urine in unchanged form (Maurer and Frick, 1984). In man, 8'-hydroxy-dihydroergotamine is the principal metabolite, but at least four other major metabolites have been characterized chemically and evaluated pharmacologically (Aellig, 1984; Müller-Schweinitzer, 1984). The activity of the principal metabolite is comparable to that of dihydroergotamine, as determined by measuring its affinity for dihydroergotamine receptor sites in mammalian brain tissue (Maurer and Frick, 1984) and by the quantitatively similar activity observed on human veins in vitro (Müller-Schweinitzer, 1984) and in vivo (Aellig, 1984). The concentration of this metabolite is five- to sevenfold higher than that of dihydroergotamine in plasma and urine, and it is presumed to have a longer plasma elimination half-life.

The elimination half-life of dihydroergotamine *and* its metabolites following either oral or intravenous administration of radioactive-labeled dihydroergotamine is 21 hours (Aellig and Nüesch, 1977). Using a radioimmunoassay that distinguishes between the parent drug and its metabolites, the intravenous administration of a single dose of 1 mg of dihydroergotamine in healthy volunteers yielded an elimination half-life of the parent drug of about 30 minutes, an apparent volume of distribution at steady state of 0.33 L/kg, and a clearance rate of 1055.7 ml/min (Kanto et al, 1981). Pharmacokinetic data in healthy volunteers also have been reported following oral (Little et al, 1982) and subcutaneous (Schran and Tse, 1985) administration.

DOSAGE AND PREPARATIONS.

Intramuscular: *Adults,* 1 mg at the onset of an attack, repeated if necessary at hourly intervals to a total of 3 mg. This route is preferred.

Intravenous: For rapid effect, *adults,* 1 mg, repeated if necessary once after one hour. The total dose should not exceed 2 mg.

Subcutaneous: *Adults,* 1 to 2 mg for patients outside of medical facilities (Raskin, 1988).

D.H.E. 45 (Sandoz). Solution 1 mg/ml in 1 ml containers.

METHYSERGIDE MALEATE
[Sansert]

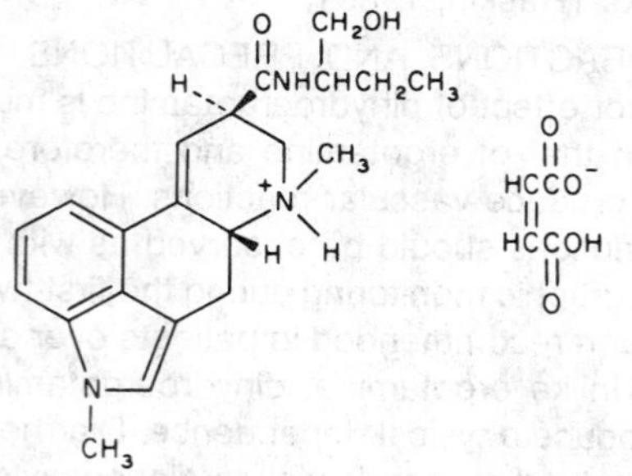

USES. This agent is a semisynthetic ergot alkaloid that is related chemically to the oxytocic agent, methylergonovine. It is not useful in aborting acute migraine headaches or in preventing or treating tension-type headache. Methysergide is an effective prophylactic agent for migraine and cluster headaches. However, since serious fibrotic reactions occur rarely with prolonged therapy, this drug is reserved for the management of severe disabling migraine headaches that do not respond to other prophylactic agents, such as propranolol. Careful supervision is required, and the daily dose should not exceed 8 mg. Some authorities suggest that a four-week drug holiday be instituted after four to six months of therapy in order to reduce the incidence of serious adverse reactions.

There is no evidence to indicate that methysergide is more effective in preventing classic than common migraine (Selby, 1983). Methysergide may be used as the initial drug in the prophylaxis of episodic cluster headache, since the duration of treatment is usually brief (2 to 10 weeks). Younger patients with episodic cluster headaches may be most responsive (Mathew, 1984).

ACTIONS. The mechanism of action of this agent in preventing migraine has not been established. Although methysergide potentiates the vasoconstrictor effects of catecholamines, it has only mild vasoconstrictor properties, which may explain its failure to abort acute migraine or a cluster attack. The drug is a potent peripheral serotonin antagonist and acts centrally as a serotonin agonist. One hypothesis suggests that migraine headache results from disruption of the serotonin/endorphin control of the pain suppressor system during an attack; disruption of nociceptive function results from decreased serotonin in the midbrain (Salmon et al, 1982). Methysergide may mimic the actions of serotonin centrally in regulating pain. Additional actions include inhibition of histamine release and stabilization of platelets against spontaneous release of serotonin.

ADVERSE REACTIONS. Adverse reactions occur with moderate frequency. Many are mild and disappear with continued use of methysergide, but the appearance of serious reactions necessitates discontinuation of therapy.

Among the serious but uncommon adverse reactions are fibrotic changes in retroperitoneal, pleuropulmonary, and cardiac tissues that may occur with long-term administration. Retroperitoneal fibrosis may obstruct the urinary tract. Early clinical manifestations are flank pain and dysuria; typical deviation and obstruction of one or both ureters may be demonstrated by intravenous pyelography. The drug may cause vascular insufficiency of the lower limbs with pain, edema, muscular atrophy, and thrombophlebitis. Involvement of the aorta, vena cava, and common iliac vessels by the fibrotic tissue also may occur.

Usual signs of pleuropulmonary fibrosis are dyspnea, chest pain, and pleural friction rubs or effusion. Murmurs and dyspnea are signs of fibrosis of the aortic valve, mitral valve, and root of the aorta.

Partial and even complete regression of retroperitoneal, pleuropulmonary, or cardiac fibrosis may occur after the drug is discontinued, but surgery may be necessary. Incompetent valves may require replacement.

Although methysergide has only weak vasoconstrictor properties, vascular insufficiency may occur. Angina-like pain has been precipitated or increased. Symptoms of peripheral vascular insufficiency include cold, numb, painful extremities with or without paresthesias and diminished or absent pulse. If these symptoms occur, the drug should be discontinued to prevent severe tissue ischemia.

Central nervous system reactions include insomnia, nervousness, euphoria, dizziness, ataxia, rapid speech, difficulty in thinking, feeling of depersonalization, nightmares, and hallucinations. Drowsiness, lethargy, and mental depression also have been reported.

Gastrointestinal reactions (eg, nausea, vomiting, diarrhea, abdominal pain) are common during early therapy. Administration of methysergide to patients with peptic ulcer has caused pronounced elevations in gastric hydrochloric acid levels. Other adverse reactions include dermatitis, alopecia, peripheral and localized edema, weight gain, arthralgia, and myalgia. Neutropenia and eosinophilia have occurred rarely.

PRECAUTIONS. Patients should be seen frequently during therapy with methysergide, and they should be instructed to report symptoms such as chest pain, leg cramps, edema of ankles or hands, change in skin color, or paresthesias in the extremities. These symptoms can be evaluated by repeated examination of the blood supply to the extremities to avoid dangerous sequelae. However, retroperitoneal fibrosis can develop without symptoms or positive results from laboratory studies. Some authorities advocate periodic abdominal and pelvic imaging to detect ureteral compression.

Contraindications are the same as for ergotamine (see that evaluation). In addition, methysergide should not be used in patients with pulmonary disease, valvular heart disease, rheumatoid arthritis or other collagen diseases, and conditions that may progress to fibrosis.

The manufacturer recommends that methysergide not be used continuously for more than six months without imposing a reasonable drug-free period (three to four weeks). However, the dosage should be reduced gradually during the two to three weeks preceding discontinuation of the drug to avoid rebound headache.

PHARMACOKINETICS. The ability to measure nanogram quantities of methysergide independently from its metabolites became possible only in the early 1980s. In previous studies, results were flawed because it could not be determined that methysergide undergoes N(1)-demethylation to form methylergonovine (methylergometrine). This metabolite has significantly greater activity and a much longer elimination half-life. It has been proposed that methysergide is a prodrug and that its metabolite is responsible for the desired therapeutic activity (Müller-Schweinitzer and Tapparelli, 1986; Bredberg et al, 1986).

Pharmacokinetic data for methysergide and its metabolite, methylergometrine, were determined in five healthy volunteers (Bredberg et al, 1986). Methysergide undergoes extensive first-pass metabolism ($F = 13\%$). The maximum concentration (C_{max}) of methysergide after oral administration of 2.67 mg was approximately 1.4 ng/ml and was reached after about one hour. The C_{max} for methylergometrine was about three times higher, 4.2 ng/ml, and this concentration was obtained in about three hours. The elimination half-life of methysergide was about one hour, which was significantly shorter than the elimination half-life of methylergometrine (about 3.5 hours). Following intravenous administration of 1 mg of methysergide maleate, plasma clearance of the parent drug was 1.09 L/min and the apparent volume of distribution was 0.93 L/kg.

DOSAGE AND PREPARATIONS.
Oral: *Adults,* for prophylaxis of migraine or cluster headache, initially, 2 mg with meals on the first day, increased by 2 mg on days two and three until 4 to 8 mg daily is administered.

Sansert (Sandoz). Tablets 2 mg.

BETA-ADRENERGIC BLOCKING DRUGS

Clinical trials have demonstrated the efficacy of propranolol in the prevention of migraine headache. Other studies have shown that atenolol, timolol, metoprolol, and nadolol also are effective for prophylaxis (Steiner et al, 1988). However, oxprenolol, pindolol, practolol, and alprenolol were ineffective, which suggests that beta blockade does not account for the activity of these drugs in migraine prophylaxis. Nonselective and $beta_1$-selective adrenergic blocking drugs are equally effective for migraine prophylaxis. All of the active drugs lack intrinsic sympathomimetic activity and antagonize $beta_1$ receptors. They are generally well tolerated. The initial doses of metoprolol, timolol, and atenolol used investigationally are similar to those given for the treatment of hypertension.

PROPRANOLOL HYDROCHLORIDE

[Inderal]

For chemical formula, see index entry Beta-Adrenergic Blocking Agents.

ACTIONS AND USES. Many neurologists consider propranolol the preferred drug for the prophylaxis of migraine in adults in whom it is not contraindicated. Although only a very small number of patients become headache-free, over 60% experience a reduction in the frequency and severity of attacks. The mechanism by which propranolol prevents migraine attacks is not known. Its efficacy in the treatment of an acute attack has not been established, and this drug does not prevent cluster headache.

ADVERSE REACTIONS AND PRECAUTIONS. Propranolol is generally well tolerated. Fatigue and lack of energy are common, especially with larger doses. Nausea, lightheadedness, insomnia, and diarrhea have been reported occasionally. Cold extremities are common. Mild mental dulling also occurs rarely. Heart rate and blood pressure are reduced. The heart rate should be monitored; in general, when full beta-blocking doses are used, the pulse rate should not fall below 50.

Propranolol should not be used in patients with asthma, chronic obstructive lung disease, congestive heart failure, or atrioventricular conduction disturbances.

For other adverse reactions and precautions, see index entry Beta-Adrenergic Blocking Agents.

DOSAGE AND PREPARATIONS.
Oral: Since doses vary widely (80 to 240 mg daily), the dosage must be individualized. *Adults*, initially, usually 20 to 40 mg two or three times per day, increased gradually by 20 to 40 mg every third or fourth week until a therapeutic effect is observed or adverse reactions occur. Once the maintenance dose has been achieved, the prolonged-release formulation may be considered for convenience and compliance. If the drug must be discontinued, the dose should be reduced gradually over two weeks, for abrupt withdrawal may precipitate headache, arrhythmia, or angina pectoris in patients with preexisting coronary disease. *Children*, dosage must be individualized but approximates 0.6 to 1.5 mg/kg/day (Lai et al, 1982). See references related to its use in pediatric migraine in the Introduction.

Inderal (Wyeth-Ayerst), ***Generic.*** Tablets 10, 20, 40, 60, 80, and 90 (***Generic*** only) mg.
Inderal LA (Wyeth-Ayerst), ***Generic.*** Capsules (prolonged-release) 60, 80, 120, and 160 mg.

CALCIUM CHANNEL BLOCKING DRUGS

Calcium antagonists are used in the treatment of cardiovascular disorders such as hypertension, dysrhythmias, Raynaud's disease, and vasospastic angina. Diltiazem [Cardizem], flunarizine (not available in the United States), nimodipine [Nimotop], nifedipine [Adalat, Procardia], and verapamil [Calan, Isoptin] have been reported to be useful for the prophylaxis of migraine, cluster, and mixed headaches. The basis for their prophylactic activity in these headaches is unknown (Spierings, 1988). Controlled trials on use of calcium antagonists in headache compared with placebo or with other prophylactic agents have been reviewed (Olesen, 1988; Spierings, 1988). Only a few studies have compared the efficacy or adverse reactions of the various calcium channel blocking agents in headache prophylaxis (Jónsdóttir et al, 1987; Greenberg, 1987). Tolerance may develop during their use but this depends on the specific agent.

Flunarizine has been studied most extensively in controlled trials. This drug appeared to be equally effective for common and classic migraine and was similar to propranolol in efficacy and in the relative severity of side effects (Lücking et al, 1988; Ludin, 1989). It is useful in pediatric patients, in whom propranolol has limited efficacy (Sorge et al, 1988). However, the potential for inducing extrapyramidal side effects limits flunarizine's value (Chouza et al, 1986).

Verapamil, in daily doses ranging from 240 to 480 mg, is effective and has been used most extensively in the United States (Raskin, 1988; Solomon, 1989). To lessen adverse effects, the total dose should be divided for administration three times a day. As with other drugs of this class, several weeks may be required to attain maximal effectiveness. When substituting the prolonged-release preparation, the manufacturer states that the total daily dose may remain the same. However, careful titration is advised; a higher dose of the prolonged-release preparation may be required. The most common adverse reaction during migraine prophylaxis is constipation. For information on other reactions and contraindications, see index entry Calcium Channel Blocking Agents.

A more recently introduced agent, nimodipine, has been of considerable interest in migraine and cluster headache prophylaxis. Its very high partition coefficient permits rapid entry across the blood-brain barrier; thus, it can be used in doses smaller than those that affect the peripheral circulation. Troublesome side effects have not yet been reported, presumably because of the low doses required. Nimodipine also has a shorter latent period than verapamil. This drug is too expensive for routine prophylactic use in migraine but may be used advantageously in patients with intractable cluster headache who require short-term therapy (Raskin, 1988).

The frequency of side effects has limited the use of nifedipine in migraine. This drug has considerable promise, however, in the prophylactic therapy of cluster headache. Initial daily doses of 40 mg, increased to 120 mg daily if necessary or decreased if a satisfactory response is obtained, have been employed (Mullally and Livingstone, 1984; Raskin, 1988).

Some established migraine prophylactic drugs also act by antagonizing calcium channel influx. Cyproheptadine, for example, has significant nonspecific calcium channel blocking activity at doses used for migraine prophylaxis (Peroutka and Allen, 1984). Experimentally, amitriptyline inhibits basilar artery contraction induced by serotonin and norepinephrine.

The initial results of clinical trials with calcium antagonists indicate that these drugs may become useful alternatives to established prophylactic agents.

NIMODIPINE
[Nimotop]

For chemical formula, see index entry Calcium Channel Blocking Agents.

ACTIONS AND USES. This calcium channel blocking drug possesses potent cerebrovascular dilating properties. Pharmacodynamic and early clinical studies of this agent have been reviewed (Scriabine and van den Kerckhoff, 1988; Langley and Sorkin, 1989). Investigation of nimodipine's use in the prevention of ischemic damage following intracranial hemorrhage was prompted by its ability to cross the blood-brain barrier. This easily produces intracerebral arterial vasodilation in a dose range that generally does not affect the systemic blood pressure; however, this mechanism may not be related to this drug's effectiveness in preventing neurologic deficits.

Similarly, the mechanism of action of nimodipine as a prophylactic agent for common or classic migraine and cluster headache, like that of other calcium channel blocking drugs that have been useful for these purposes, is unknown. Although its prophylactic administration in migraine headache remains investigational, a number of studies have shown that nimodipine was modestly effective for this purpose in oral doses of 40 mg three times a day and had a greater effect in doses of 60 mg three times a day (Bussone et al, 1987; Stewart et al, 1988). About four weeks of daily therapy are required before the drug is maximally effective for migraine prophylaxis.

ADVERSE REACTIONS AND PRECAUTIONS. At a dose of 60 mg three times a day, nimodipine is well tolerated; hypotension usually is the only side effect severe enough to require discontinuation of therapy. In patients with impaired hepatic function, the dosage should be reduced to 30 mg every four hours. The blood pressure and heart rate should be evaluated at intervals until tolerance to the drug is established.

PHARMACOKINETICS. Nimodipine undergoes extensive hepatic metabolism. Less than 0.1% of unchanged drug is excreted by the kidney (Lettieri et al, 1988). The principal metabolites have been identified and quantified (Meyer et al, 1983). Investigation of these on isolated tissue preparations shows that they have no calcium channel blocking activity (Towart et al, 1982).

Following oral administration, nimodipine undergoes rapid and nearly complete absorption, with maximum concentrations appearing in the circulation within 30 to 60 minutes. Oral bioavailability is low (only 13% in one study) (Rämsch et al, 1987) and there is significant individual variability. This is attributed to extensive first-pass metabolism. More than 95% of a dose is bound to plasma proteins. Binding is independent of the concentration over the therapeutic dose range. When administered intravenously, nimodipine has an apparent volume of distribution at steady state of 121 L and a clearance rate of 124 L/hr (Rämsch et al, 1987). The elimination half-life following oral administration is approximately five hours, but there is considerable variation among individuals.

As anticipated, bioavailability after oral administration is increased significantly in patients with cirrhosis; there is up to a fourfold increase in the AUC related to an approximately 50%

decrease in clearance (Gengo et al, 1987). However, the diminished clearance and markedly prolonged elimination half-life in patients with renal insufficiency (Kirch et al, 1984) requires verification in age-matched controls and measurement of potential variables (eg, protein binding).

DOSAGE AND PREPARATIONS.

Oral: *Adults,* to reduce neurologic deficits following subarachnoid hemorrhage (administration initiated within 96 hours of hemorrhage), 60 mg every four hours for 21 consecutive days. For migraine prophylaxis, 30 to 60 mg three times a day.

Nimotop (Miles). Capsules 30 mg.

ANTIDEPRESSANTS

AMITRIPTYLINE HYDROCHLORIDE

[Elavil, Endep]

For chemical formula, see index entry Amitriptyline, In Mood Disorders.

ACTIONS AND USES. This tricyclic compound is useful in the prophylaxis of migraine. Results of one controlled study indicated that amitriptyline was most effective in nondepressed patients with severe migraine and depressed patients with less severe migraine (Couch and Hassanein, 1979). In some studies, amitriptyline was as effective as methysergide but, in others, the drug was no better than placebo (Diamond and Medina, 1980). Patient selection appears to be important for optimum results.

Amitriptyline inhibits the reuptake of norepinephrine and serotonin at nerve endings, but its mechanism of action in migraine is not known. Its effect is relatively independent of antidepressant action.

This drug also is quite effective in patients with chronic tension-type headache as well as in patients with mixed migraine and episodic tension-type headache.

ADVERSE REACTIONS AND PRECAUTIONS. The usual adverse effects are dryness of the mouth, drowsiness, blurred vision, constipation, urinary retention, weight gain, and tachycardia. Amitriptyline should be used with caution in patients with angle-closure glaucoma, urinary retention or obstruction, and cardiac disease.

For other uses and a more complete discussion of adverse reactions and precautions, see index entry Amitriptyline, In Mood Disorders.

DOSAGE AND PREPARATIONS.

Oral: For migraine prophylaxis, *adults*, initially, 25 mg daily at bedtime, increased by 25 mg every one to two weeks to a daily dose of 100 to 200 mg, if necessary (Diamond and Medina, 1980). Tolerance may be improved by giving three or four doses daily rather than one dose at bedtime.

For tension-type headaches, initially, 50 to 75 mg at bedtime, increased every two to three weeks to 200 to 250 mg daily (Diamond, 1983). The drug can be discontinued after the patient has been headache-free for one or two months. If headaches recur, the course may be repeated.

Elavil (Merck Sharp & Dohme), ***Endep*** (Roche), ***Generic***. Tablets 10, 25, 50, 75, 100, and 150 mg.

LITHIUM CARBONATE

[Eskalith, Lithane, Lithobid, Lithonate, Lithotabs]

ACTIONS AND USES. The mechanism of action of lithium carbonate in preventing cluster headache is unknown. The use of this agent for cluster headache was based on its effectiveness in another cyclical neurologic disorder, manic depressive psychosis. Few agents prevent chronic cluster headache, and lithium is now regarded by some authorities as a second-line drug and is preferred to corticosteroids when methysergide and calcium channel blocking agents fail. Patients have reported dramatic relief in the first week of treatment, but approximately 60% of initial responders experienced breakthrough attacks, which were claimed to be less severe and of short duration. Lithium may be effective in episodic cluster headache, and some neurologists use it when verapamil or methysergide are not effective or are contraindicated. The apparent effectiveness of lithium decreases with long-term administration but can be re-established by providing a two-week drug holiday before readministering the drug (Saper, 1983).

Patients receiving lithium must be closely monitored for side effects and toxicity; repeated measurement of lithium blood levels is necessary (see index entry Lithium, In Mania). This drug is classified in FDA Pregnancy Category D.

DOSAGE AND PREPARATIONS.

Oral: *Adults,* 300 mg two to four times daily (Mathew, 1984). Prolonged-release tablets are usually given twice daily at approximately 12-hour intervals.

Generic. Capsules 150, 300, and 600 mg; tablets 300 mg.
Eskalith (Smith Kline & French). Capsules, tablets 300 mg; tablets (prolonged-release) 450 mg (***Eskalith CR***).
Lithane (Miles), ***Lithotabs*** (Reid-Rowell). Tablets 300 mg.
Lithobid (CIBA). Tablets (prolonged-release) 300 mg.
Lithonate (Reid-Rowell). Capsules 300 mg.

CRANIAL NEURALGIAS

A variety of drugs with antiepileptic, antispastic, or antidepressant activity are used to manage cranial neuralgias. These compounds are usually more useful than agents with general analgesic properties, but the mechanisms by which they alleviate pain are not well understood. Some of these agents may exert their analgesic activity by inhibiting polysynaptic pain transmission.

Evaluating the efficacy of agents used to manage the pain of cranial neuralgias is difficult because of the spontaneous remissions that occur, inadequate follow-up of drug therapy, and the subjective nature of the pain.

Trigeminal and Glossopharyngeal Neuralgias

Trigeminal neuralgia, an episodic facial pain syndrome, occurs most often in elderly patients. Unilateral paroxysms of severe shooting pain within one or more divisions of the trigeminal nerve are followed by a period of relief and then by another paroxysm of severe pain. This pain is characteristically triggered by tactile stimuli on the face and by using the jaws or mouth (eg, chewing, talking, brushing teeth). A proposed model for the pathogenesis of this neuralgia and for the mechanisms of alleviating pain has been proposed (Fromm, 1989).

Carbamazepine [Epitol, Tegretol] is the drug of choice. If attacks are not controlled completely by carbamazepine or the patient cannot tolerate this agent, the addition of baclofen [Lioresal] has been effective (Fromm et al, 1980, 1984 A). Phenytoin [Dilantin] also may be administered when results are suboptimal with carbamazepine. Both drugs may be given alone, with carbamazepine, or with each other, but phenytoin is less effective than baclofen.

A recent limited but controlled study indicated that pimozide [Orap] was more effective than carbamazepine (Lechin et al, 1989). However, the potential for severe extrapyramidal adverse effects with pimozide is considerable, and it is not a drug of choice.

Clonazepam [Klonopin], a benzodiazepine anticonvulsant, has been useful in a limited number of patients, but controlled studies comparing this drug with carbamazepine and baclofen have never been performed.

Remissions are not unusual in trigeminal neuralgia and a drug holiday should be tried by gradually reducing the dose of carbamazepine and other drugs over one to two weeks following a pain-free period of several months. If pain recurs, drug treatment can be reinstituted.

Between 25% and 50% of patients receiving drug therapy for trigeminal neuralgia experience a relapse (Dalessio, 1982). When drug therapy fails to control pain or produces unacceptable side effects, surgery should be recommended. Although a permanent sensory deficit and anesthesia dolorosa may result, surgical treatment is usually effective. For a review of surgical interventions, see Sweet, 1986.

Glossopharyngeal neuralgia is much less common than trigeminal neuralgia and is characterized by similar paroxysms of lancinating pain in the pharynx, tonsils, and ear. Pain is often triggered by swallowing. It may be accompanied by syncope that is thought to be due to increased vagal activity and usually is responsive to atropine. Carbamazepine is the drug of choice, but the other agents employed in trigeminal neuralgia may be substituted or used concomitantly. If pain persists, cocainization of the pharynx may provide temporary relief. When glossopharyngeal neuralgia is refractory to drug therapy, microvascular decompression of the glossopharyngeal nerve or surgical section of the ninth and tenth cranial nerve roots is recommended (Bruyn, 1983).

Drug Evaluations

BACLOFEN

[Lioresal]

For chemical formula, see index entry Baclofen, In Muscle Spasticity.

ACTIONS. Baclofen is an analogue of gamma aminobutyric acid (GABA) and interacts with a bicuculline-insensitive presynaptic GABA receptor. This drug antagonizes excitatory neurotransmission, possibly by blocking the release of the putative excitatory transmitters, glutamic and aspartic acids, from primary afferent fibers and substance P from cutaneous nociceptive afferent nerve endings. In experimental animals, baclofen has depressed excitatory transmission and enhanced segmental inhibition in the spinal trigeminal nucleus (Fromm et al, 1980; Fromm, 1989).

USES. This drug sometimes is effective alone for long-term control in newly diagnosed patients with trigeminal neuralgia who cannot tolerate carbamazepine. However, because it appears to have a synergistic action with carbamazepine and phenytoin, baclofen is more commonly used with these drugs in previously uncontrolled patients (Baker et al, 1985). Baclofen alone appears to be less effective than carbamazepine but more effective than phenytoin (Fromm et al, 1984 A). The L-stereoisomer of baclofen (not commercially available) is five times more active than the commercial racemic preparation, since the D-isomer partially antagonizes the L-isomer (Fromm and Terrence, 1987; Fromm, 1989).

ADVERSE REACTIONS. Baclofen appears to be well tolerated in responsive patients treated for trigeminal neuralgia (Fromm et al, 1984 B). Drowsiness, nausea, and vomiting are the most common adverse effects and occur more frequently when baclofen is administered with carbamazepine. Hallucinations, seizures, or both may develop after abrupt dosage reduction or discontinuation of treatment after more than two months.

See index entry Baclofen, In Muscle Spasticity, for a more detailed discussion of adverse reactions and pharmacokinetics.

DOSAGE AND PREPARATIONS.

Oral: *Adults,* initially, 10 mg three times daily; the amount is increased by 10 mg/day every other day to 60 to 80 mg/day in three or four divided doses by the end of the second week. The average maintenance dose is 50 to 60 mg/day for patients receiving baclofen alone and 30 to 40 mg/day when baclofen is given with carbamazepine or phenytoin (Fromm et al, 1984 A; Ringel and Roy, 1987). A lower initial dose (5 mg three times daily) that is increased more gradually should be given to elderly patients and those taking other central nervous system depressants.

Lioresal (Geigy), ***Generic.*** Tablets 10 and 20 mg.

CARBAMAZEPINE

[Epitol, Tegretol]

For chemical formula, see index entry Carbamazepine, In Epilepsy.

ACTIONS AND USES. Carbamazepine, a primary antiepileptic drug, is related chemically to the tricyclic compounds. Its antineuralgic action may result from reduced excitatory synaptic transmission in the spinal trigeminal nucleus produced by an increase in the latency of trigeminal neuronal response and a decrease in the number of neuronal discharges (Fromm, 1989); blockade of sodium channels in rapidly firing neurons is the most likely cellular action. Similar actions have been reported for phenytoin and baclofen. Carbamazepine-10,11-epoxide, a major metabolite of carbamazepine, also has considerable antineuralgic activity (Tomson and Bertilsson, 1984).

Carbamazepine is the drug of choice for trigeminal and glossopharyngeal neuralgia. Satisfactory relief of pain is obtained in 70% to 90% of patients within 24 to 72 hours and effectiveness may persist for many years; however, in one study, 19% of patients developed resistance (Taylor et al, 1981). When a relapse occurs during therapy, the dose may be increased; if this is ineffective or not tolerated, the concomitant administration of baclofen and/or phenytoin may be helpful. Patients who do not respond to drug therapy may require surgery.

Carbamazepine also is effective in the lightning pains of tabes dorsalis, although clinical experience is more limited than in trigeminal neuralgia. It has been used to relieve pain in multiple sclerosis, acute idiopathic polyneuritis (Guillain-Barré syndrome), peripheral diabetic neuropathy, phantom limb pain, post-traumatic paresthesia, and superior laryngeal neuralgia. It should be kept in mind that carbamazepine is not a general analgesic but is specific for certain types of pain; thus, it should not be used to treat trivial facial pain or minor pain at other sites.

ADVERSE REACTIONS AND PRECAUTIONS. The adverse reactions that occur most commonly during early treatment are drowsiness, dizziness, lightheadedness, ataxia, nausea, and vomiting; they usually subside spontaneously within a week or after a reduction in dose. Their incidence may be minimized by utilizing a small dose initially and increasing the amount gradually.

Dermatologic reactions occur occasionally and include pruritic and erythematous rashes, urticaria, Stevens-Johnson syndrome, exfoliative dermatitis, erythema multiforme, erythema nodosum, and aggravation of systemic lupus erythematosus. These effects may be severe enough to necessitate discontinuation of therapy.

Hematopoietic reactions (leukopenia, agranulocytosis, eosinophilia, leukocytosis, purpura, aplastic anemia, and thrombocytopenia) develop rarely but may be serious. Aplastic anemia and thrombocytopenia may be fatal. Therefore, patients should be advised to notify their physician if signs of hematologic toxicity appear (eg, fever, sore throat, aphthous stomatitis, easy bruising, petechial or purpuric hemorrhage).

Cardiovascular, genitourinary, metabolic, hepatic, and other reactions have been reported rarely. Although the antidiuretic action of carbamazepine rarely causes water intoxication and hyponatremia, caution should be used when treating elderly patients with cardiovascular disease. If symptoms of water intoxication occur, the plasma sodium level and osmolality should be measured. If hyponatremia develops, carbamazepine should be discontinued or the dosage reduced.

It is advisable to perform blood and platelet counts, liver function tests, urinalysis, and blood urea nitrogen determinations prior to treatment and to repeat these tests at regular intervals during treatment.

Since carbamazepine is related chemically to the tricyclic antidepressants, it should not be administered to patients sensitive to these compounds. The possibility of activating latent psychosis or, in elderly patients, of precipitating confusion or agitation also exists.

This drug is classified in FDA Pregnancy Category C.

For other adverse reactions, see index entry Carbamazepine, In Epilepsy.

PHARMACOKINETICS. The pharmacokinetics of carbamazepine have been reviewed (Bertilsson and Tomson, 1986). Because carbamazepine induces its own metabolism, the established steady-state concentration may be subtherapeutic and attacks of pain may recur. A positive correlation between drug plasma concentrations and pain relief has been demonstrated; concentrations between 5.7 and 10.1 mcg/ml were most effective. Side effects were not observed with plasma concentrations below 7.9 mcg/ml (Tomson et al, 1980). For further information, see index entry Carbamazepine, In Epilepsy.

DRUG INTERACTIONS. Carbamazepine enhances the metabolism of phenytoin through enzyme induction, and plasma concentrations of phenytoin may be reduced when these drugs are given concomitantly. Conversely, carbamazepine serum concentrations may be reduced by phenytoin.

There is evidence that erythromycin, isoniazid, and propoxyphene inhibit carbamazepine metabolism and thus may cause toxic effects (dizziness, drowsiness, nausea). Patients receiving carbamazepine should be monitored for signs of toxicity when these drugs are administered. The dosage of carbamazepine may have to be reduced.

If carbamazepine is given with warfarin, the half-life of the latter is reduced and the dose must be increased to maintain the anticoagulant effect. See also index entry Carbamazepine, In Epilepsy.

DOSAGE AND PREPARATIONS.

Oral: *Adults*, 200 mg to a maximum of 1.2 g daily; small doses should be used initially and the amount increased gradually (eg, 100 mg of the tablet form twice on the first day, increased by 100 mg every 12 hours, or 50 mg of oral suspension four times daily until freedom from pain is achieved or toxicity occurs). A pain-free state usually can be maintained with 400 to 800 mg daily.

Carbamazepine should be administered in the minimal effective dose with meals. Since many individuals experience spontaneous prolonged remissions every few months, an attempt should be made to discontinue therapy. If pain recurs when the drug is withdrawn, reinstitution of therapy is effective.

Generic. Tablets (chewable) 100 mg; tablets 200 mg.
Epitol (Lemmon). Tablets 200 mg.
Tegretol (Geigy). Tablets (chewable) 100 mg; tablets 200 mg; suspension 100 mg/5 ml.

PHENYTOIN
[Dilantin]

PHENYTOIN SODIUM
[Dilantin]

For chemical formula, see index entry Phenytoin, In Epilepsy.

Phenytoin is sometimes used in trigeminal and glossopharyngeal neuralgia, although it is less effective than carbamazepine and baclofen. It may be tried in patients who do not respond to carbamazepine or baclofen or it may be given with these drugs.

Phenytoin has been reported to be effective in several other pain syndromes (eg, peripheral neuralgia, phantom limb pain, Fabry's disease, thalamic pain, dysesthesia, postherpetic neuralgia), but adequate controlled studies to establish its usefulness are lacking (Walson et al, 1975). In one double-blind crossover study, phenytoin did not significantly improve symptoms of diabetic symmetric polyneuropathy (Saudek et al, 1977).

The most common adverse reactions include nausea, dizziness, ataxia, dyspepsia, and nystagmus. See index entry Phenytoin, In Epilepsy, for a more detailed discussion of adverse reactions.

DOSAGE AND PREPARATIONS.

Oral: For trigeminal neuralgia, *adults,* 300 to 400 mg daily. Since relief of pain does not correlate with drug blood concentrations, dosage may be increased until pain is relieved or toxic effects occur (Loeser, 1977).

PHENYTOIN:

Generic. Suspension 30 and 125 mg/5 ml (alcohol ≤0.6%).

Dilantin (Parke-Davis). Suspension 30 and 125 mg/5 ml (alcohol ≤0.6%); tablets (chewable) 50 mg.

PHENYTOIN SODIUM:

Generic. Capsules (prompt, extended) 100 mg; suspension 125 mg/5 ml.

Dilantin (Parke-Davis). Capsules (extended) 30 and 100 mg.

Additional Trademark:

Diphenylan (Lannett).

NEUROPATHIC PAIN

Postherpetic Neuralgia

Postherpetic neuralgia is a complication of acute herpes zoster that occurs almost exclusively in individuals over 60 years. It is commonly associated with ophthalmic or spinal segment involvement due to zoster infections (Loeser, 1986). Chronic pain characterized as severe and sharp or sometimes as a burning sensation is often associated with hyperesthesia. Unlike the episodic pain of trigeminal neuralgia, the constant pain of postherpetic neuralgia usually is not alleviated by carbamazepine or phenytoin, although their trial may be justified. Intralesional and subcutaneous injection of long-acting corticosteroids in conjunction with tricyclic antidepressants has been useful (Stein and Warfield, 1982).

Results of clinical trials have shown that amitriptyline [Elavil, Endep] or its metabolite, nortriptyline [Aventyl], is effective in the management of 60% of patients with postherpetic neuralgia (Watson et al, 1988 A). The analgesic action of amitriptyline appears to be independent of its antidepressant action because analgesia occurs rapidly at doses below those employed to treat depression. The drug has been given initially in a single dose of 12.5 to 25 mg at bedtime, with the amount increased by 12.5 mg every two to five days to a mean daily dose of 70 mg (range, 25 to 138 mg) (Watson et al, 1982, 1988 A). It has been suggested that a "therapeutic window" effect occurs in some patients treated with amitriptyline, which implies that a dosage range may exist below and above which pain relief is not achieved and within which analgesia occurs. Since this effect may occur at a lower dosage range than for depression, amitriptyline should be administered in small amounts with reassessment and gradual incremental increases until analgesia is achieved (Watson, 1984).

Capsaicin [Axsain, Zostrix], derived from the hot pepper, has shown promise in refractory cases of postherpetic neuralgia. It is too early to determine if it will provide long-term benefit.

Drug Evaluation

CAPSAICIN

[Axsain, Zostrix]

ACTIONS AND USES. Capsaicin reduces the pain of postherpetic neuralgia and diabetic neuropathy (see the following section) by interfering with substance P-mediated pain transmission. The mechanism for this action is being investigated. Capsaicin may decrease the sensitivity by depleting and inhibiting the reuptake of substance P in the peripheral neuron (Buck and Burks, 1986).

The topical application of capsaicin 0.025% for four to six weeks has been shown to provide either complete or significant relief of chronic postherpetic pain (Watson et al, 1988 B; Bernstein et al, 1989). In refractory cases, the 0.075% concentration may be tried. This higher concentration is used more commonly for diabetic and postsurgical neuropathies.

ADVERSE REACTIONS AND PRECAUTIONS. A mild to moderate burning sensation is experienced following application and, in some patients, can be pronounced enough to require discontinuation of treatment. It can be mitigated in some individuals by the application of 5% lidocaine ointment prior to the use of capsaicin, by covering smaller areas of skin surface, and by use of analgesics (Watson et al, 1988 A).

Care must be exercised to prevent capsaicin from entering the eyes, open lesions, or mucous membranes.

DOSAGE AND PREPARATIONS.

Topical: *Adults and children 2 years or older,* the preparation is applied to the affected area three or four times daily.

Axsain (GalenPharma). Cream 0.075% in 60 g containers (nonprescription).

Zostrix (GenDerm). Cream 0.025% in 45 g containers (nonprescription).

Diabetic Neuropathy

Peripheral nerve disorders are complications of diabetes mellitus. Disabling spontaneous pains, dysesthesias, and paresthesias are common in sensory polyneuropathy. The pain of diabetic neuropathy often does not respond to drug therapy.

The management of painful diabetic neuropathy should begin with the control of blood glucose concentrations and the administration of nonopiate analgesics, although their effect on pain of this nature is limited. Shooting or stabbing pains can be multifocal and may respond to carbamazepine or phenytoin (Brown and Asbury, 1984). The deep, constant, aching pain may be relieved by tricyclic antidepressants. Results of a small controlled clinical trial with imipramine [Janimine, Tofranil] demonstrated this drug's effectiveness in reducing pain, paresthesia, dysesthesia, and numbness (Kvinesdal et al, 1984). Patients received 50 mg/day the first week and 100 mg/day for the remaining four weeks. Amitriptyline 25 to 150 mg taken orally at bedtime also may be beneficial (Brown and Asbury, 1984; Max et al, 1987). The use of phenothiazines, such as fluphenazine [Permitil, Prolixin], in combination with tricyclic antidepressants is based on anecdotal reports, and their effectiveness remains to be determined by controlled clinical trial (Mendel et al, 1986). However, the prolonged use of phenothiazines is associated with potential risks of extrapyramidal and cardiovascular side effects, particularly tardive dyskinesia, which may develop after drug withdrawal. The use of aldolase reductase inhibitors for the arrest, prevention, or reversal of diabetic neuropathy remains investigational (Asbury, 1988).

Initial results of a multicenter controlled trial with topical capsaicin cream 0.075% [Axsain] suggest that this preparation produced more relief of the pain associated with diabetic neuropathy than placebo (Tandan et al, 1990). Approximately 75% of patients claimed pain relief from capsaicin compared with 45% of patients treated with cream containing the vehicle only; however, a significant difference was noted only after four weeks of treatment. More studies on efficacy will be needed to determine the role of this local analgesic agent in diabetic neuropathy. About one-half of patients receiving capsaicin experienced a burning sensation at the application site, especially when more than a thin film is applied or the preparation is rubbed too hard into warm skin (eg, after a hot bath). Capsaicin was otherwise well tolerated.

Cited References

Aellig WH: Investigation of the venoconstrictor effect of 8' hydroxydihydroergotamine, the main metabolite of dihydroergotamine, in man. *Eur J Clin Pharmacol* 26:239-242, 1984.

Aellig WH, Nüesch E: Comparative pharmacokinetic investigations with tritium-labeled ergot alkaloids after oral and intravenous administration in man. *Int J Clin Pharmacol* 15:106-112, 1977.

Anderson CD, Franks RD: Migraine and tension headache: Is there a physiologic difference? *Headache* 21:63-71, 1981.

Asbury AK: Understanding diabetic neuropathy, editorial. *N Engl J Med* 319-577-578, 1988.

Baker KA, et al: Treatment of trigeminal neuralgia: Use of baclofen in combination with carbamazepine. *Clin Pharm.* 4:93-96, 1985.

Barlow CF: Treatment of juvenile migraine, in: *Headaches and Migraine in Childhood.* Oxford, Blackwell Scientific, 1984, 155-171.

Bateman DN, et al: Extrapyramidal reactions with metoclopramide. *Br Med J* 291:930-932, 1985.

Bernstein JE, et al: Topical capsaicin treatment of chronic postherpetic neuralgia. *J Am Acad Dermatol* 21:265-270, 1989.

Bertilsson L, Tomson T: Clinical pharmacokinetics and pharmacological effects of carbamazepine and carbamazepine-10, 11-epoxide: Update. *Clin Pharmacokinet* 11:177-198, 1986.

Bobik A, et al: Low oral bioavailability of dihydroergotamine and first-pass extraction in patients with orthostatic hypotension. *Clin Pharmacol Ther* 30:673-679, 1981.

Bradfield JM: New look at use of ergotamine. *Drugs* 12:449-453, 1976.

Bredberg U, et al: Pharmacokinetics of methysergide and its metabolite methylergometrine in man. *Eur J Clin Pharmacol* 30:75-77, 1986.

Brown MJ, Asbury, AK: Diabetic neuropathy. *Ann Neurol* 15:2-12, 1984.

Bruyn GW: Glossopharyngeal neuralgia. *Cephalalgia* 3:143-157, 1983.

Buck SH, Burks TF: Neuropharmacology of capsaicin: Review of some recent observations. *Pharmacol Rev* 38:179-226, 1986.

Bülow PM, et al: Comparison of pharmacodynamic effects and plasma levels of oral and rectal ergotamine. *Cephalalgia* 6:107-111, 1986.

Bussone G, et al: Nimodipine versus flunarizine in common migraine: Controlled pilot study. *Headache* 27:76-79, 1987.

Chouza C, et al: Parkinsonism, tardive dyskinesia, akathisia, and depression induced by flunarizine. *Lancet* 1:1303-1304, 1986.

Cohen MJ, McArthur DL: Classification of migraine and tension headache from survey of 10,000 headache diaries. *Headache* 21:25-29, 1981.

Couch JR, Hassanein RS: Amitriptyline in migraine prophylaxis. *Arch Neurol* 36:695-699, 1979.

Dalessio DJ: Trigeminal neuralgia: Practical approach to treatment. *Drugs* 24:248-255, 1982.

Dalessio DJ, et al: Conditioned adaptation-relaxation reflex in migraine therapy. *JAMA* 242:2102-2104, 1979.

Dexter JD, et al: Concomitant use of amitriptyline and propranolol in intractable headache, abstract. *Headache* 20:157, 1980.

Diamond S: Treatment of migraine with isometheptene, acetaminophen, and dichloralphenazone combination: Double-blind, crossover trial. *Headache* 15:282-287, 1976.

Diamond S: Rational approach to diagnosing and treating headache. Part III: Therapy. *Fam Med Rep* 1:39-44, (Sept 26) 1983.

Diamond S, Dalessio DJ: Migraine headache, in Diamond S, Dalessio DJ (eds): *The Practicing Physician's Approach to Headache,* ed 4. Baltimore, Williams & Wilkins, 1986, 44-65.

Diamond S, Freitag FG: Do non-steroidal anti-inflammatory agents have a role in the treatment of migraine headache? *Drugs* 37:755-760, 1989.

Diamond S, Medina JL: Current thoughts on migraine. *Headache* 20:208-212, 1980.

Dierckx RA, et al: Intraarterial sodium nitroprusside infusion in the treatment of severe ergotism. *Clin Neuropharmacol* 9:542-548, 1986.

Drummond PD, Lance JW: Thermographic changes in cluster headache. *Neurology* 34:1292-1298, 1984.

Edmeads JG: Migraine. *Can Med Assoc J* 138:107-113, 1988.

Ekbom K: Lithium for cluster headache: Review of literature and preliminary results of long-term treatment. *Headache* 21:132-139, 1981.

Featherstone HJ: Migraine and muscle contraction headaches: A continuum. *Headache* 25:194-198, 1984.

Fenichel GM: Migraine in children. *Neurol Clin* 3:77-94, 1985.

Fentress DW, et al: Biofeedback and relaxation-response training in the treatment of pediatric migraine. *Dev Med Child Neurol* 28:139-146, 1986.

Forsythe WI, et al: Propranolol (Inderal) in the treatment of childhood migraine. *Dev Med Child Neurol* 26:737-741, 1984.

Fozard JR: Animal pharmacology of drugs used in treatment of migraine. *J Pharm Pharmacol* 27:297-321, 1975.

Fromm GH: Pharmacology of trigeminal neuralgia. *Clin Neuropharmacol* 12:185-194, 1989.

Fromm GH, Terrence CF: Comparison of L-baclofen and racemic baclofen in trigeminal neuralgia. *Neurology* 37:1725-1728, 1987.

Fromm GH, et al: Baclofen in trigeminal neuralgia: Effect on spinal trigeminal nucleus: Pilot study. *Arch Neurol* 37:768-771, 1980.

Fromm GH, et al: Baclofen in treatment of trigeminal neuralgia: Double blind study and long-term follow-up. *Ann Neurol* 15:240-244, 1984 A.

Fromm GH, et al: Trigeminal neuralgia: Current concepts regarding etiology and pathogenesis. *Arch Neurol* 41:1204-1207, 1984 B.

Gabai IJ, Spierings ELH: Prophylactic treatment of cluster headache with verapamil. *Headache* 29:167-168, 1989.

Gengo FM, et al: Nimodipine disposition and haemodynamic effects in patients with cirrhosis and age-matched controls. *Br J Clin Pharm* 23:47-53, 1987.

Graham AN, et al: Systemic availability of ergotamine tartrate given by three different routes of administration to healthy volunteers, in Rose FC (ed): *Progress in Migraine Research.* London, Pitman, 1984, vol 2, 283-292.

Greenberg DA: Calcium channels and calcium channel antagonists. *Ann Neurol* 21:317-330, 1987.

Headache Classification Committee of the International Headache Society: Classification and diagnostic criteria for headache disorders, cranial neuralgias and facial pain. *Cephalalgia* 8 (suppl 7): 1-96, 1988.

Health and Public Policy Committee, American College of Physicians: Position paper: Biofeedback for headaches. *Ann Intern Med* 102:128-131, 1985.

Hokkanen E, et al: Toxic effects of ergotamine used for migraine. *Headache* 18:95-98, 1978.

Ibraheem JJ, et al: Kinetics of ergotamine after intravenous and intramuscular administration to migraine sufferers. *Eur J Clin Pharmacol* 23:235-240, 1982.

Joffe R, et al: Self-observation study of headache symptoms in children. *Headache* 23:20-25, 1983.

Jones J, et al: Randomized double-blind trial of intravenous prochlorperazine for the treatment of acute headache. *JAMA* 261:1174-1176, 1989.

Jónsdóttir M, et al: Efficacy, side effects and tolerance compared during headache treatment with three different calcium blockers. *Headache* 27:364-369, 1987.

Kanto J, et al: Pharmacokinetics of dihydroergotamine in healthy volunteers and in neurological patients after a single intravenous injection. *Int J Clin Pharmacol Ther Toxicol* 19:127-130, 1981.

Kirch W, et al: Clinical pharmacokinetics of nimodipine in normal and impaired renal function. *Int J Clin Pharmacol Res* 4:381-384, 1984.

Kudrow L: Cluster headache: Diagnosis and management. *Headache* 19:142-150, 1979.

Kudrow L: Response of cluster headache attacks to oxygen inhalation. *Headache* 21:1-4, 1981.

Kunkel RS: Pharmacologic management of migraine--1985. *Cleve Clin Q* 52:95-101, (Spring) 1985.

Kvinesdal B, et al: Imipramine treatment of painful diabetic neuropathy. *JAMA* 251:1727-1730, 1984.

Lai C-W, et al: Hemiplegic migraine in childhood: Diagnostic and therapeutic aspects. *J Pediatr* 100:696-699, 1982.

Lance JW: Pathogenesis of migraine, in: *Mechanism and Management of Headache*, ed 4. Boston, Butterworth Scientific, 1982, 152-177.

Lance JW: Pharmacotherapy of migraine. *Med J Aust* 144:85-88, 1986.

Lance JW, et al: 5-hydroxytryptamine and its putative aetiological involvement in migraine. *Cephalalgia* 9 (suppl 9): 7-13, 1989.

Langley MS, Sorkin EM: Nimodipine: Review of its pharmacodynamic and pharmacokinetic properties, and therapeutic potential in cerebrovascular disease. *Drugs* 37:669-699, 1989.

Lechin F, et al: Pimozide therapy for trigeminal neuralgia. *Arch Neurol* 46:960-963, 1989.

Lettieri J, et al: Pharmacokinetics and metabolism of radiolabeled nimodipine. *Ann NY Acad Sci* 522:719, 1988.

Little PJ, et al: Bioavailability of dihydroergotamine in man. *Br J Clin Pharm* 13:785-790, 1982.

Loeser JD: Management of tic douloureux. *Pain* 3:155-162, 1977.

Loeser JD: Herpes zoster and postherpetic neuralgia. *Pain* 25:149-164, 1986.

Louis P, Spierings ELH: Comparison of flunarizine (Sibelium) and pizotifen (Sandomigran) in migraine treatment: Double-blind study. *Cephalalgia* 2:197-203, 1982.

Lücking CH, et al: Flunarizine vs propranolol in the prophylaxis of migraine: Two double-blind comparative studies in more than 400 patients. *Cephalalgia* 8 (suppl 8): 21-26, 1988.

Ludin H-P: Flunarizine and propranolol in the treatment of migraine. *Headache* 29:219-223, 1989.

Manzoni GC, et al: Lithium carbonate in cluster headache: Assessment of its short- and long-term therapeutic efficacy. *Cephalalgia* 3:109-114, 1983.

Martin MJ: Psychogenic factors in headache. *Med Clin North Am* 62:559-570, 1978.

Mathew NT: Prophylaxis of migraine and mixed headache: Randomized controlled study. *Headache* 21:105-109, 1981.

Mathew NT: Prophylactic pharmacotherapy of cluster headache, in: *Cluster Headache.* New York, Spectrum Publications, 1984, 97-109.

Mathew NT: Amelioration of ergotamine withdrawal symptoms with naproxen. *Headache* 27:130-133, 1987.

Mathew RJ, et al: Catecholamines and migraine: Evidence based on biofeedback induced changes. *Headache* 20:247-252, 1980.

Maurer G, Frick W: Elucidation of the structure and receptor binding studies of the major primary metabolite of dihydroergotamine in man. *Eur J Clin Pharmacol* 26:463-470, 1984.

Max MB, et al: Amitriptyline relieves diabetic neuropathy pain in patients with normal or depressed mood. *Neurology* 37:589-596, 1987.

McEwen JI, et al: Treatment of migraine with intramuscular chlorpromazine. *Ann Emerg Med* 16:758-762, 1987.

Mendel CM, et al: Trial of amitriptyline and fluphenazine in treatment of painful diabetic neuropathy. *JAMA* 255:637-639, 1986.

Meyer JS, Hardenberg J: Clinical effectiveness of calcium entry blockers in prophylactic treatment of migraine and cluster headache. *Headache* 23:266-277, 1983.

Meyer H, et al: Nimodipine: Synthesis and metabolic pathway. *Arzneim-Forsch/Drug Res* 33:106-112, 1983.

Mullally WJ, Livingstone IR: Treatment of chronic cluster headache with nifedipine. *Headache* 24:164-165, 1984.

Müller-Schweinitzer E: Pharmacological actions of the main metabolites of dihydroergotamine. *Eur J Clin Pharmacol* 26:699-705, 1984.

Müller-Schweinitzer E, Tapparelli C: Methylergometrine, an active metabolite of methysergide. *Cephalalgia* 6:35-41, 1986.

Nuechterlein KH, Holroyd JC: Biofeedback in treatment of tension headache: Current status. *Arch Gen Psychiatry* 37:866-873, 1980.

Olesen J: Calcium entry blockers in the prophylaxis of migraine. *Ann NY Acad Sci* 522:720-722, 1988.

Olness K, et al: Comparison of self-hypnosis and propranolol in treatment of juvenile classic migraine. *Pediatrics* 79:593-597, 1987.

Orton DA, Richardson RJ: Ergotamine absorption and toxicity. *Postgrad Med J* 58:6-11, 1982.

Packard RC: What is psychogenic headache? *Headache* 16:20-23, 1976.

Peroutka SJ: The pharmacology of current anti-migraine drugs. *Headache* 5-11, (Jan) 1990.

Peroutka SJ, Allen GS: Calcium antagonist properties of cyproheptadine: Implications for antimigraine action. *Neurology* 34:304-309, 1984.

Perrin VL: Clinical pharmacokinetics of ergotamine in migraine and cluster headache. *Clin Pharmacokinet* 10:334-352, 1985.

Prensky AL: Migraine and migrainous variants in pediatric patients. *Pediatr Clin North Am* 23:461-471, 1976.

Rämsch K-D, et al: Pharmacokinetics of intravenous and orally administered nimodipine, abstract. *Clin Pharmacol Ther* 41:216, 1987.

Raskin NH: Repetitive intravenous dihydroergotamine as therapy for intractable migraine. *Neurology* 36:995-997, 1986.

Raskin NH: *Headache,* ed 2. New York, Churchill Livingstone, 1988.

Ringel RA, Roy EP III: Glossopharyngeal neuralgia: Successful treatment with baclofen. *Ann Neurol* 21:514-515, 1987.

Salmon S, et al: Putative S-HT central feedback in migraine and cluster headache attacks. *Adv Neurol* 33:265-274, 1982.

Sanders SW, et al: Pharmacokinetics of ergotamine in healthy volunteers following oral and rectal dosing. *Eur J Clin Pharmacol* 30:331-334, 1986.

Saper JR (ed): *Headache Disorders: Current Concepts and Treatment Strategies.* Boston, John Wright, 1983.

Saper JR: Changing perspectives on chronic headache. *Clin J Pain* 2:19-28, 1986.

Saper JR: Ergotamine dependency: Review. *Headache* 27:435-438, 1987.

Saper JR: Chronic headache syndromes. *Neurologic Clinics* 7:387-411, 1989.

Saper JR, Jones JM: Ergotamine tartrate dependency: Features and possible mechanisms. *Clin Neuropharmacol* 9:244-256, 1986.

Sargent J, et al: Results of controlled, experimental, outcome study of nondrug treatments for the control of migraine headaches. *J Behav Med* 9:291-323, 1986.

Sargent JD, et al: Aborting a migraine attack: Naproxen sodium vs ergotamine plus caffeine. *Headache* 28:263-266, 1988 A.

Sargent JD, et al: Naproxen sodium for muscle contraction headache treatment. *Headache* 28:180-182, 1988 B.

Saudek CD, et al: Phenytoin in treatment of diabetic symmetrical polyneuropathy. *Clin Pharmacol Ther* 22:196-199, 1977.

Schmidt R, Fanchamps A: Effect of caffeine on intestinal absorption of ergotamine in man. *Eur J Clin Pharmacol* 7:213-216, 1974.

Schran HF, Tse FLS: Pharmacokinetics of dihydroergotamine following subcutaneous administration in humans. *Int J Clin Pharmacol Ther Toxicol* 23:1-4, 1985.

Schuler ME, et al: Role of calcium channel blocking agents in the prevention of migraine. *Drug Intell Clin Pharm* 22:187-191, 1988.

Scriabine A, van den Kerckhoff W: Pharmacology of nimodipine: Review. *Ann NY Acad Sci* 522:698-706, 1988.

Selby G: Treatment, in: *Migraine and Its Variants.* Boston, ADIS Health Science Press, 1983, 107-149.

Sjaastad O: On the classification of cluster headache, editorial. *Cephalalgia* 6:65-68, 1986.

Solomon GD: Verapamil in migraine prophylaxis: Five-year review. *Headache* 29:425-427, 1989.

Solomon S, et al: Common migraine: Criteria for diagnosis. *Headache* 28:124-129, 1988.

Sorge F, et al: Flunarizine in prophylaxis of childhood migraine: Double-blind, placebo-controlled, crossover study. *Cephalalgia* 8:1-6, 1988.

Spierings ELH: Clinical and experimental evidence for a role of calcium entry blockers in the treatment of migraine. *Ann NY Acad Sci* 522:676-689, 1988.

Stein JM, Warfield CA: Herpes zoster and postherpetic neuralgia. *Hosp Pract* 17:96A-96O, (Sept) 1982.

Steiner TJ, et al: Metoprolol in the prophylaxis of migraine: Parallel-groups comparison with placebo and dose-ranging follow-up. *Headache* 28:15-23, 1988.

Stewart DJ, et al: Effect of prophylactic administration of nimodipine in patients with migraine. *Headache* 28:260-262, 1988.

Sweet WH: Treatment of trigeminal neuralgia (tic douloureux). *N Engl J Med* 315:174-177, 1986.

Tandan R, et al: Topical capsaicin in painful diabetic polyneuropathy. *Neurology* 40:4 (suppl 1), 1990.

Taylor JC, et al: Long-term treatment of trigeminal neuralgia with carbamazepine. *Postgrad Med J* 57:16-18, 1981.

Tfelt-Hansen P, et al: Double blind study of metoclopramide in treatment of migraine attacks. *J Neurol Neurosurg Psychiatry* 43:369-371, 1980.

Tfelt-Hansen P, et al: Bioavailability of sublingual ergotamine. *Br J Clin Pharmacol* 13:239-240, 1982.

Tomson T, Bertilsson L: Potent therapeutic effect of carbamazepine-10,11-epoxide in trigeminal neuralgia. *Arch Neurol* 41:598-601, 1984.

Tomson T, et al: Carbamazepine therapy in trigeminal neuralgia: Clinical effects in relation to plasma concentration. *Arch Neurol* 37:699-703, 1980.

Towart R, et al: Effects of nimodipine, its optical isomers and metabolities, on isolated vascular smooth muscle. *Arzneim Forsch/Drug Res* 32:338-346, 1982.

Walson P, et al: New uses for phenytoin. *JAMA* 233:1385-1389, 1975.

Watson CPN: Therapeutic window for amitriptyline analgesia. *Can Med Assoc J* 130:105-106, 1984.

Watson CP, et al: Amitriptyline versus placebo in postherpetic neuralgia. *Neurology* 32:671-673, 1982.

Watson CPN, et al: Post-herpetic neuralgia: 208 cases. *Pain* 35:289-297, 1988 A.

Watson CPN, et al: Post-herpetic neuralgia and topical capsaicin. *Pain* 33:333-340, 1988 B.

Weatherhead AD: Psychogenic headache. *Headache* 20:47-54, 1980.

Wilkinson M: Treatment of migraine. *Headache* 28:659-661, 1988.

Yamamoto M, Meyer JS: Hemicranial disorders of vasomotor adrenoreceptors in migraine and cluster headache. *Headache* 20:321-335, 1980.

Ziegler DK: Tension headache. *Med Clin North Am* 62:495-505, 1978.

Ziegler DK: Headache symptom: How many entities? *Arch Neurol* 42:273-274, 1985.

Ziegler DK, Ellis DJ: Naproxen in prophylaxis of migraine. *Arch Neurol* 42:582-584, 1985.

New Evaluation

SUMATRIPTAN SUCCINATE

[Imitrex]

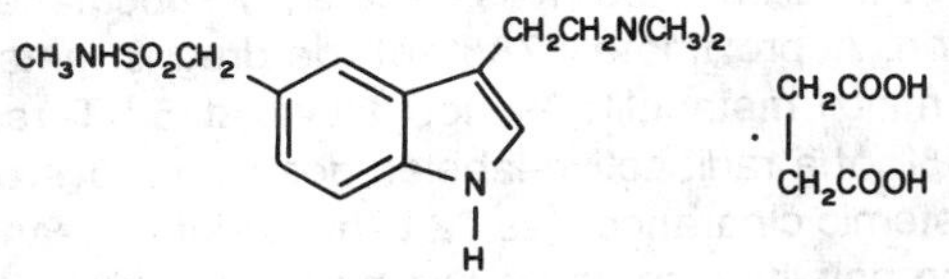

$CH_3NHSO_2CH_2$ — $CH_2CH_2N(CH_3)_2$ · CH_2COOH / CH_2COOH (N–H)

ACTIONS AND USES. Sumatriptan is a serotonin (5-HT_1) receptor agonist. At least four types of serotonin receptors and subtypes of several have been described; when activated, these produce either vasoconstriction or vasodilation, depending on the particular vascular bed affected or the preexisting state of vascular tone. Sumatriptan displays a high degree of selectivity for the 5-HT_{1D} receptor binding site, which is located predominantly on cranial blood vessels. The antimigraine action of sumatriptan is thought to derive from vasoconstriction of cranial blood vessels, which is consistent with the vascular concept of migraine pathophysiology that relates the throbbing headache phase of the migraine syndrome to vasodilation of cranial vessels, particularly the basilar artery and arteries of the dura mater.

Sumatriptan is useful for the acute treatment of migraine headache with or without aura. It should not be used for subtypes of migraine that are associated with persistent neurologic phenomena (hemiplegic), ophthalmoplegic, basilar migraine, or complicated migraine. It also may be useful for cluster headaches.

To be most effective, the drug should be administered as soon as possible after headache begins; however, in contrast to ergotamine tartrate, sumatriptan is reported to be effective well after the headache has started. Sumatriptan should be given after onset of headache rather than during the aura. There is some evidence that it may prolong the migraine aura.

At present, the drug is available only for subcutaneous administration. Oral and intranasal spray formulations are being tested clinically.

Results of controlled clinical trials indicate that subcutaneous administration of sumatriptan 6 mg is effective for moderately severe or severe migraine headache. One hour after administration, 70% to 77% of 60 patients who received 6-mg doses had complete or almost complete resolution of headache compared with 22% to 31% of patients treated with placebo. After two hours, the response increased to 81% to 87% in those who received sumatriptan. Little additional benefit is derived from 8-mg doses or from repeating the 6-mg dose at one hour, although the second dose is well tolerated (Ensink, 1991). Onset of pain relief is rapid and may begin within 10 minutes. The drug is equally effective in patients with and without aura.

A randomized, double-blind, placebo-controlled study of 639 patients with migraine was reported from an international study group. One hour after administration of sumatriptan, the severity of headache was decreased in 72% of patients given 6 mg and 79% of patients given 8 mg; improvement occurred in 25% of those given placebo. At two hours, pain was relieved in 86% to 92% of patients given 6 or 8 mg of sumatriptan compared with 37% of those receiving placebo. Adverse effects were minor and transient. Patients treated early (up to four hours) in the course of the headache and those treated later responded equally well. Headache-associated nausea, vomiting, photophobia, and phonophobia also were relieved. However, 34% to 38% of sumatriptan-treated patients who reported relief of headache reported recurrence within 24 hours. This headache was usually relieved by another 6-mg dose of sumatriptan without further recurrence. The administration of a second dose at one hour in those with residual initial headache had no influence on the recurrence rate (The Subcutaneous Sumatriptan International Study Group, 1991).

In 1,104 adults given either sumatriptan 6 mg subcutaneously or placebo, 70% of those receiving the drug experienced reduction in headache pain from moderate or severe to mild or no pain at one hour compared with 22% of those receiving placebo. Complete relief of headache occurred in 49% of sumatriptan recipients and in 9% of placebo-treated patients. Sumatriptan also was more effective in relieving associated nausea and photophobia than placebo. A second injection of sumatriptan at one hour in those without complete relief conferred no additional benefit. Adverse effects (tingling, dizziness, sensations of warmth, and local reactions at the injection site) were mild and well tolerated (Cady et al, 1991).

In a dose-ranging study in 242 adults with migraine, headache pain was reduced from moderate or severe to mild or no pain at one hour in 73% of those given sumatriptan 6 mg.

There was a clear dose-response relationship between 1 and 6 mg and an insignificantly greater response (80%) at 8 mg. Adverse effects were dose-related through the 8-mg dose, leading the investigators to suggest that the 6-mg dose is optimal (Mathew et al, 1992).

A randomized, double-blind, placebo-controlled crossover study in 49 patients was conducted to assess the effectiveness of sumatriptan in cluster headache. Patients received in random order a subcutaneous injection of sumatriptan 6 mg for one cluster headache episode and placebo for another. In 39 evaluable patients, headache severity decreased to mild or was completely eliminated in 74% of episodes treated with sumatriptan compared with 26% of episodes treated with placebo. Relief of headache was complete within 10 minutes in 36% of episodes treated with sumatriptan compared with 3% after placebo; by 15 minutes, the percentages were 46% and 10%, respectively. Use of ancillary medication was less and relief of associated symptoms was greater after administration of sumatriptan. Adverse events were mild or tolerable in all patients (The Sumatriptan Cluster Headache Study Group, 1991).

ADVERSE REACTIONS AND PRECAUTIONS. The most common adverse effects are local reactions at the site of injection, including pain and erythema and local or generalized paresthesias, including sensations of warmth, cold, numbness, tightness, or burning. Flushing; fatigue; dizziness; drowsiness; and sensations of chest pain, pressure, or tightness also may occur but are usually transient. Because of coronary ischemic events that occurred during earlier experience with this drug and the potential of sumatriptan to produce coronary vasospasm, the drug is contraindicated in patients with ischemic heart disease (angina pectoris, history of myocardial infarction, asymptomatic ischemic episodes documented by electrocardiography), or Prinzmetal's angina. It also is contraindicated in those with uncontrolled hypertension because it may increase the blood pressure. Sumatriptan should be used with caution in patients with asthma. It should never be given intravenously.

Because of its potential for inducing coronary vasospasm the manufacturer suggests that the first dose be administered in the physician's office to any patient in whom unrecognized coronary disease is thought to be comparatively likely. Those considered to be at risk include postmenopausal women, males over age 40, and any patient with a risk factor for coronary atherosclerotic disease (CAD) (eg, hypertension, hypercholesterolemia, obesity, diabetes, smoking, family history of CAD). There is no evidence that susceptible individuals will experience this adverse effect at first injection. The prudent course, however, may be to give each new patient a test dose under observation. This would also provide an opportunity to instruct the patient in the use of the autoinjector device for self-administration.

In rabbits, sumatriptan was teratogenic and embryolethal at doses producing plasma levels several times higher than those produced in humans. Even higher doses (and resultant plasma levels) were not teratogenic in rats. There is no evidence of teratogenicity in humans at this time, but the available data are limited. The question of teratogenicity will be addressed in a postmarketing study. At the present time, women who are pregnant or likely to become pregnant should consider the risk versus benefit before using sumatriptan (FDA Pregnancy Category C).

Because of the potential for additive vasoconstrictive effects, sumatriptan should not be administered within 24 hours of ergotamine or ergot-containing preparations.

PHARMACOKINETICS. Pharmacokinetic information is limited and preliminary. In healthy volunteers, single subcutaneous 6-mg doses in the deltoid area produced peak plasma levels of 74 ng/ml 12 minutes after administration. Injection into skin over the thigh or with use of the autoinjector produced lower peak plasma levels but did not influence the total amount of drug absorbed. Sumatriptan is 14% to 21% bound to plasma proteins and has a volume of distribution of approximately 170 L. Bioavailability is 97% after subcutaneous administration. Approximately 78% of the drug is metabolized, and the major metabolite is not active at 5-HT receptors. About 75% of a radioactive-labeled dose is recovered in the urine. Systemic clearance was 72 L/hr, and the mean plasma elimination half-life was about two hours. The drug does not accumulate if no more than two doses are taken per day. Because metabolism is the predominant process of disposition, it may be appropriate to reduce the dose in patients with liver disease. The pharmacokinetics are reported to be similar in the elderly and in younger patients with migraine.

An oral preparation is expected to be available soon. Oral bioavailability is only 14%, probably due to a combination of presystemic metabolism and erratic absorption. Plasma levels after oral doses have multiple peaks, which may be caused by drug effects influencing gastrointestinal absorption. Approximately 87% is metabolized and 38% of an oral radiolabeled dose appears in the feces, 9% as unchanged drug; in contrast, less than 1% appears as unchanged drug in the feces after parenteral injection. Gastric stasis, which may occur during a migraine attack, reduces the extent of oral absorption up to 20%.

DOSAGE AND PREPARATIONS.

Subcutaneous: *Adults*, the maximum single dose is 6 mg; lower doses may be used if side effects occur. In patients receiving less than 6 mg, only the single-dose vial should be used. An autoinjection device is available to facilitate self-administration by patients who have responded to a 6-mg dose. A second 6-mg dose may be administered one or more hours later, but no more than two doses should be given in a 24-hour period. Controlled clinical trials have not demonstrated conclusively that a second dose is beneficial in patients who did not respond to the first injection.

Imitrex (Cerenex). Solution 6 mg/0.5 ml in 1 and 2 ml (single-dose) containers. A kit (self-dose system) also is available containing two 6-mg unit-dose syringes, an autoinjector, and instructions for use.

Cited References

Cady RK, et al: Treatment of acute migraine with subcutaneous sumatriptan. *JAMA* 265:2831-2835, 1991.

Ensink F-BM: Subcutaneous sumatriptan in the acute treatment of migraine. *J Neurol* 238:S66-S69, 1991.

Mathew NT, et al: Dose ranging efficacy and safety of subcutaneous sumatriptan in the acute treatment of migraine. *Arch Neurol* 49:1271-1276, 1992.

The Subcutaneous Sumatriptan International Study Group: Treatment of migraine attacks with sumatriptan. *N Engl J Med* 325:316-321, 1991.

The Sumatriptan Cluster Headache Study Group: Treatment of acute cluster headache with sumatriptan. *N Engl J Med* 325:322-326, 1991.

Local Anesthetics 8

Local anesthetics produce loss of sensation and prevent muscle activity in circumscribed areas of the body by reversibly blocking nerve conduction (regional anesthesia). Local anesthetics (other than benzocaine) are amines. They are classified as esters or amides depending on whether they are derivatives of para-aminobenzoic acid (eg, procaine) or aniline (eg, lidocaine). This chemical classification is clinically significant in that it indicates the principal site of biotransformation and the potential for allergic sensitization. Certain antihistaminic, anticholinergic, and adrenergic agents having a similar configuration also exhibit local anesthetic activity. The intrathecal (subarachnoid) or epidural administration of opioids in conjunction with local anesthetics to relieve pain is discussed in the evaluation on bupivacaine; see also index entry Opioids.

Local anesthetic bases are relatively insoluble in water but are soluble in lipid vehicles (eg, ointments). Salts of local anesthetic bases are water soluble and stable. In tissue water, the ratio of the nonionized base to the cationic (ionized) form depends on the pKa of the compound (range, 7.7 to 9.05) (Kamaya et al, 1983; Tucker and Mather, 1988) and tissue fluid pH (see Table 1). The nonionized base penetrates the nerve sheath and membrane more readily than the cation. After re-equilibration at the internal pH of the axon, the cation is quantitatively the principal form that blocks nerve conduction.

The cationic form attaches to the internal axoplasmic membrane, possibly a phospholipid receptor, to decrease ion flux, particularly sodium. The rate of increase and the amplitude of the nerve action potential are depressed to the degree that depolarization is not sufficient to initiate a propagated action potential. At least 1 cm of nerve should be exposed to the local anesthetic to ensure conduction blockade, because the impulse in myelinated fibers is capable of skipping over two or three nodes of Ranvier.

The nonionized base also blocks nerve conduction, but this action is less prominent. The site appears to be the lipophilic areas of the nerve membrane, and the mechanism is believed to be similar to that of the general anesthetics, which are thought to act through a physicochemical mechanism rather than through specific receptors. After the anesthetic occupies a critical volume fraction of the nerve membrane, the membrane expands; this interferes with the conformational changes of the protein necessary for ion flux and depolarization. There also is substantial evidence to suggest that anesthetics block transmission of a wave of depolarization by membrane stabilization. Both concepts—expansion and stabilization—are of equal merit and are equally controversial. Topical anesthetics that possess a very low pKa (eg, benzocaine: pKa 3.5) or certain non-nitrogenous local anesthetic alcohols (eg, benzyl alcohol) may produce nerve block almost exclusively through the physicochemical mechanism.

The onset of anesthesia (essentially the rate and degree of penetration into individual nerves) depends on the lipid solubility, molecular weight, and quantity of available nonionized form of the local anesthetic (see Table 1). Thus, those with a high lipid solubility and/or a low pKa have a more rapid onset of action. The anesthetic's vasoactive action, the blood flow and pH at the site of injection, and the total volume and concentration of the anesthetic solution also are important determinants of onset of action.

TABLE 1.
PHYSICOCHEMICAL PROPERTIES OF LOCAL ANESTHETIC AGENTS

Local Anesthetic	Partition Coefficient*	Protein Binding %	pKa	% Free Base pH 6.8	7.0	7.2	7.4	7.6
ESTERS								
Chloroprocaine	0.14	NA†	8.97	0.7	1.1	1.7	2.6	4.1
Procaine	0.02	5.8‡	9.05	0.6	0.9	1.4	2.2	3.4
Tetracaine	4.1	75.6§	8.46	2.1	3.4	5.2	8.0	12
AMIDES								
Bupivacaine	27.5	95.6§	8.16	4.2	6.5	9.9	15	22
Etidocaine	141	94§	7.7	11	17	24	33	44
Lidocaine	2.9	64.3§	7.91	7.2	11	16	24	33
Mepivacaine	0.8	77.5§	7.76	9.9	15	22	30	41
Prilocaine**	0.9	55 approx.	7.9	7.4	11	17	24	33

** n-heptane/buffer, pH 7.4* *† NA = Not available* *‡ Nerve homogenate binding* *§ Plasma protein binding*
*** See individual evaluation for adverse effects.*

It is believed that nerves generally are blocked in sequence according to their size. Thus, small nonmyelinated autonomic C fibers, thinly myelinated sensory delta A fibers (carrying pain, pressure, fine touch, and temperature sensations), and myelinated autonomic preganglionic B fibers are blocked before larger myelinated A fibers that transmit motor functions. The clinical appearance of sensory or motor loss may vary from this order in larger nerves because of the geographical location of fibers (either near the surface or core of the nerve). The concentration of drug required to block large nerve trunks is greater than that needed for smaller peripheral nerves. The duration of the block depends on all of the factors listed for onset of anesthesia, as well as on the extent of protein binding and whether or not a vasoconstrictor is added to the solution.

Pharmacokinetics: After the local anesthetic is absorbed from its site of administration into the systemic circulation, it is redistributed to other tissues and cleared from the body by metabolism and excretion. The anesthetic is redistributed to the various body tissues in proportion to its tissue-blood partition coefficient and the mass and perfusion of the tissue. In vivo, the partition coefficient is affected by the extent to which the agent is bound to tissue and erythrocyte proteins, by its nonspecific binding to albumin and specific binding to alpha$_1$-acid glycoproteins in the plasma, and by the pH gradient. These factors determine the amount of free drug available for crossing membranes and the extent of ion trapping.

Ester-type local anesthetics are partly or completely hydrolyzed by plasma cholinesterase and, to a much lesser extent, by hepatic cholinesterase; the inert metabolites are excreted in the urine. After regional block with usual doses, hydrolysis is so rapid that only small concentrations of the ester anesthetics may be detected in the plasma. An exception is cocaine, 10% to 12% of which is excreted unchanged. The elimination half-life ($t_{1/2\beta}$) for chloroprocaine is less than four minutes (Zsigmond and Kothary, 1979) and that of procaine is 7.7 minutes (Seifen et al, 1979). The $t_{1/2\beta}$ is not available for tetracaine. The half-life of cocaine is dose dependent and may be determined by using the equation, $t_{1/2\beta} = 13.5 + 24.5 \times \text{dose (mg/kg)}$ (Barnett et al, 1981).

The amide anesthetics are metabolized in the liver by microsomal enzymes; the small quantity of unchanged amide that is excreted in the urine is not relevant in patients with impaired renal function. In contrast to the esters, appreciable concentrations of the amide anesthetics may appear in the plasma and may accumulate after multiple administrations.

Pharmacokinetic data in adults for the commonly employed amide anesthetics are given in Table 2 (Tucker and Mather, 1988). The metabolism of both the esters and amides may be reduced in patients with severe hepatic disease, and the metabolism of the esters is decreased in patients in whom esterase activity is suppressed or genetically atypical. Conditions that decrease the volume of distribution (eg, congestive heart failure) may increase the plasma concentration of the local anesthetic and thus increase the likelihood of side effects. Factors that diminish protein binding can significantly elevate the plasma concentrations of the pharmacologically active form of those agents that are usually bound in excess of 90% (see Table 1). The specific binding capacity of the alpha$_1$-acid glycoproteins is limited. Thus, the greater the vascular concentration of a local anesthetic, such as bupivacaine [Marcaine, Sensorcaine], the greater will be the unbound fraction. For bupivacaine (Rothstein et al, 1986) and probably other anesthetics, there is a significant relationship between the blood:plasma concentration ratio and the hematocrit. Following prolonged epidural infusion of bupivacaine

TABLE 2.
AMIDE LOCAL ANESTHETICS: MEAN PHARMACOKINETIC DATA IN ADULTS

	$t_{1/2\beta}$ minutes	Vdss liters	Cltot liters/minute	% Excreted Unchanged
Bupivacaine	162	73	0.58	5
Etidocaine	162	134	1.11	1
Lidocaine	96	91	0.95	10
Mepivacaine	114	84	0.78	16
Prilocaine	96	191	2.37	NA*

* *NA = Not available*

0.25% to young healthy adults (age 20 to 35 years), the elimination half-life was increased to 257 min and the volume of distribution to 107 L, and the clearance was decreased to 0.29 L/min (Perkins, 1989).

For most local anesthetics, the perineural concentration is several hundredfold greater than the plasma concentration associated with side effects; therefore, the drug should be injected precisely at the appropriate site to avoid systemic toxicity. In general, the most rapid rate of absorption, and hence the amount in the plasma, is achieved by use of large volumes or high concentrations. Plasma concentrations are relatively unaffected by the speed of injection except with intravenous administration. Thus, the least volume of the most dilute solution that is effective should be administered. Injection into highly vascular sites (eg, head and neck region, intercostal and caudal blocks) and topical application to respiratory mucous membranes must be conducted with care.

Except for those intended for use in spinal anesthesia, solutions of local anesthetics are usually isotonic to avoid edema, local irritation, and inflammation at the site of injection.

REGIONAL ANESTHETIC TECHNIQUES

Regional (conduction) anesthetic techniques are classified according to the site of application: (1) infiltration (local), including extravascular and intravascular (intravenous regional anesthesia, Bier block); (2) peripheral nerve block (nerve or field block); (3) central neural block, ie, epidural (peridural, extradural, caudal), spinal (subarachnoid, intrathecal); and (4) topical (surface). The agents most commonly employed for these applications are listed in Tables 3 and 4.

To prevent accidental intravascular injection, needle placement *always* must be verified by gentle aspiration in several planes with a syringe before injection and periodically during injection. An intravenous infusion *always* should be started prior to injecting a substantial dose of a local anesthetic. Apparatus for administering oxygen and artificial ventilation, diazepam [Valium], vasopressors, intravenous fluids, succinylcholine [Anectine, Quelicin, Sucostrin], thiopental [Pentothal], and any additional drugs and equipment that may be useful for resuscitation should be available.

TABLE 3.
LOCAL ANESTHETICS PRINCIPALLY EMPLOYED FOR INJECTION

	Infiltration	Nerve Block	Intravenous Regional	Epidural	Spinal
AMIDES					
Bupivacaine [Marcaine, Sensorcaine]	0.25%	0.25-0.5%	NR	0.25-0.75%	0.5-0.75%
Etidocaine [Duranest]	0.5%	0.5-1%	—	0.5-1.5%	—
Lidocaine [Xylocaine]	0.5%	0.5-1.5%	0.5%†	1.5-2%	1.5-5%
Mepivacaine [Carbocaine]	0.5-1%	1-1.5%	—	1.5-2%	—
Prilocaine [Citanest]‡	4%‡	—	—	—	—
AMINOBENZOATE ESTERS					
Chloroprocaine [Nesacaine]	1%	2-3%	NR	2-3%	NR*
Procaine [Novocain]	0.25-0.5%	1-2%	—	NR	10%*
Tetracaine [Pontocaine]	NR	NR	—	NR	1%

* = *Infrequent application* — = *Not in current use or ineffective* NR = *Not recommended* † = *Without epinephrine*
‡ *No longer used.*

Infiltration Anesthesia: This is the conventional technique of injecting the anesthetic in the immediate area of surgery.

Peripheral Nerve Block Anesthesia: In *field block anesthesia*, the solution is injected close to the nerves around the area to be anesthetized. In *nerve block anesthesia*, a localized perineural injection is made at an access point along the course of a nerve proximal to the operative site. More concentrated solutions of drug often are required with nerve blocks because the nerves being blocked have a sheath and relatively large diameters.

The drugs most commonly used for infiltration and peripheral nerve block anesthesia include chloroprocaine [Nesacaine], lidocaine [Xylocaine], mepivacaine [Carbocaine], and procaine [Novocain]. Bupivacaine [Marcaine, Sensorcaine] and etidocaine [Duranest] are indicated if a more prolonged block is desired. Because methemoglobinemia has been associated with the use of prilocaine [Citanest], clinical use of this local anesthetic has virtually ceased.

Intravascular Anesthesia: This term is synonymous with *intravenous regional anesthesia* or *Bier block*. Usually the entire distal portion of an extremity is anesthetized. Initially, a double pneumatic tourniquet is applied to the upper arm or leg but is not inflated. For surgery on the hand, the tourniquet almost always is applied to the upper arm; for the foot, it is applied below the knee. Bier blocks on the leg are done infrequently because of the possibility of producing a neuropathy of the common peroneal nerve. A needle is inserted into a distal peripheral vein and secured in place. The extremity then is exsanguinated by gravity or with an elastic wrap (eg, Esmarch). The proximal cuff is inflated first to a pressure that occludes arterial flow. If this tourniquet fails, the other cuff can be inflated promptly to prevent dangerously high concentrations of anesthetic. Double tourniquets now are considered the standard of practice. The tourniquet must be in place before the intravenous administration of anesthetic is started. A dilute solution of local anesthetic without preservatives or epinephrine is then injected and diffuses via the veins and capillaries to produce an evenly distributed anesthesia of all nerves in the occluded limb. This technique is not applicable to the entire leg because of the large quantity of anesthetic that would be required.

Epidural Anesthesia: Epidural anesthesia is accomplished by injecting a local anesthetic into the epidural space (Bromage, 1978; Cousins and Bridenbaugh, 1988). In lumbar epidural anesthesia, the injection is usually made in an interspace between the second and fifth lumbar vertebrae to avoid injury to the spinal cord, which ends at the first lumbar vertebra in 95% of individuals. In caudal anesthesia, the solution is introduced into the caudal canal (a continuation of the epidural space) through the sacral hiatus.

In general, the number of spinal segments blocked is determined by the site of injection (lumbar or caudal), the position of the patient, the quantity of drug injected (more segments with larger dose), possibly the age of the patient (more segments in children and the elderly), and pregnancy (more segments). Increasing the concentration of the anesthetic shortens the onset time and increases the degree of motor block. Cephalad spread of anesthetic occurs more readily than sacral spread following lumbar epidural injection; a significant delay in onset or even the absence of anesthesia at the first and second sacral segments is observed occasionally (Concepcion and Covino, 1984). Onset of block of these dermatomes can be shortened and the degree intensified by alkalization of the local anesthetic (Benzon et al, 1993). Physiologic changes are slower in onset with epidural anesthesia than with spinal anesthesia.

A test dose should be administered at least five minutes before the main dose in an attempt to detect inadvertent intravenous or spinal (subarachnoid) injection. The addition of 1:200,000 epinephrine to the test dose aids in the recognition of an intravascular injection. The relatively large dose needed and the great vascularity of the epidural space also increase the possibility of systemic reactions. Repeated fractional injections or continuous infusion of a dilute solution through an in situ catheter (continuous epidural anesthesia) may be used to prolong epidural anesthesia.

The drugs most commonly employed for epidural anesthesia are chloroprocaine, lidocaine, or mepivacaine for surgical procedures of one to two hours and bupivacaine or etidocaine for procedures lasting longer than two hours. Selection is based on the degree of motor block desired, if any, and the required duration of sensory block (see the evaluations). The anesthetics differ in the degree of motor nerve block produced. This is least marked with bupivacaine, which, in a concentration of 0.125% to 0.25%, produces adequate analgesia for obstetric or postoperative pain relief with minimal motor block. On the other hand, etidocaine blocks motor nerves more readily than sensory nerves.

To minimize the danger of injecting a solution contaminated by chemicals or bacteria, only single-dose containers should be used. Epinephrine reduces the peak blood concentration of most local anesthetics.

Spinal Anesthesia: With this technique, the local anesthetic agent is injected into the subarachnoid space, usually in an interspace between the second and fifth lumbar vertebrae. The level of anesthesia is determined by the site of injection, density and volume of the solution, and position of the patient during and immediately after administration of the anesthetic. Extreme obesity or abdominal tumors decrease spinal fluid volume, resulting in a significant reduction in the dosage requirement. Dosage reduction may be necessary during pregnancy due to altered sensitivity of nerve roots. Factors that do not affect the spread of spinal anesthetic solutions are the dose (if the volume and density are constant), the age or body weight (if the length and volume of the subarachnoid space are the same), sudden increases in cerebrospinal fluid pressure (eg, occurring during coughing, straining, Valsalva's maneuver), or the presence of a vasoconstrictor in the anesthetic solution (Greene, 1985; Lambert, 1989; Burm, 1989). The rate of injection has an unpredictable but minor effect on spread.

In addition to isobaric solutions for use in spinal anesthesia, hyperbaric (with dextrose) solutions that possess a density greater than 1.0010 or hypobaric (in distilled water) solutions with a density less than 1.0003 are available to assure that the local anesthetic solution is heavier or lighter, respectively, than that of cerebrospinal fluid. The hypobaric (light) solutions gravitate upward and the hyperbaric (heavy) solutions gravitate downward. The extent of this effect depends on the volume of solution and the length of time the patient remains in the position in which the injection was made.

Consciousness is preserved at all times unless profound arterial hypotension develops secondary to the sympathetic block that is always produced. The degree of sympathetic block is determined by the level of anesthesia but extends further cephalad than either sensory or motor block (Greene, 1986).

Hypotension is the most important side effect commonly associated with spinal anesthesia; individual tolerance varies. Hypotension is intensified by changes in position that promote diminished venous return and by pre-existing hypertension or hypovolemia. Pregnancy, old age, and use of drugs that depress sympathetic activity (antihypertensive agents, phenothiazines, haloperidol [Haldol]) also increase the likelihood of hypotension. The patient is at greatest risk during the first 30 minutes after spinal anesthesia is induced. Oxygen should be administered. The cardiac output can be increased by administration of ephedrine and a judicious increase in fluid administration.

The duration of anesthesia depends on the rate at which the anesthetic leaves the subarachnoid space by diffusion across the dura into the epidural space and by vascular absorption. Enzymatic hydrolysis of the drugs in cerebrospinal fluid does not occur. The duration of action, particularly that of tetracaine, may be increased 50% to 100% by adding epinephrine to the solution. The repeated injection of a local anesthetic often is associated with diminished effectiveness and duration of action (tachyphylaxis). If the concentration of the anesthetic in solution is increased, the duration is increased, but not proportionally.

Tetracaine, bupivacaine, and lidocaine are most widely used for spinal anesthesia; procaine also can be administered. The anesthetic profiles of tetracaine and bupivacaine are similar. However, tetracaine causes a greater degree and duration of motor block. In contrast, there is hypotension and a lower incidence of tourniquet pain with bupivacaine (Stewart et al, 1988). To minimize the danger of injecting a contaminated solution, only single-dose containers should be employed, and only local anesthetics specifically prepared for spinal anesthesia (ie, without preservatives or antioxidants, such as methylparaben, sodium bisulfite, or sodium metabisulfite) should be used.

The dose administered for spinal anesthesia generally is too small, even if injected intravascularly, to produce systemic toxicity or to exert any direct depressant effects on the fetus when given during labor and delivery.

Topical (Surface) Anesthesia: This may be defined as the production of anesthesia by direct application of the local anesthetic to the skin or mucous membranes lining the body cavities. The agent may be applied as a solution, jelly, ointment, cream, or paste. Mucous membranes and the intact skin differ in penetrability. The skin is impermeable to local anesthetic salts, but their corresponding unionized bases can penetrate to a limited degree. As a result, only certain agents (see Table 4) are utilized for the skin. Topical anesthetics are not effective on the ear canal or drum.

Mucous membranes of the nose, mouth, pharynx, larynx, trachea, bronchi, vagina, and urethra are readily anesthetized by both cationic and nonionized forms. However, since absorption from certain of these areas may be quite rapid, the smallest dose required for adequate analgesia should be administered to minimize the possibility of systemic reactions. The addition of a vasoconstrictor generally does not lessen the incidence of these reactions.

The use of local anesthetics on conjunctival and corneal tissues represents a form of topical application. Because proparacaine [Ak-Taine, Alcaine, Ophthaine, Ophthetic] is used topically only on the eye, it is discussed in the chapter on Mydriatics, Cycloplegics, Local Anesthetics, and Intraocular Miotics; see index entry Proparacaine. The ophthalmologic use of cocaine and tetracaine also is discussed in that chapter; however, in view of their more widespread local anesthetic use, evaluations appear in this chapter as well.

ADJUNCTS TO REGIONAL ANESTHETICS

Vasoconstrictors may be added to local anesthetic solutions used for infiltration, peripheral nerve block, epidural, and spinal anesthesia to decrease the rate of absorption. In general, this prolongs the anesthetic effect and reduces the risk of systemic reactions, while increasing the frequency of complete conduction blocks at low anesthetic concentration. The addition of a vasoconstrictor is more appropriate than increasing the concentration to prolong the duration. Epinephrine is the vasoconstrictor most commonly used for infiltration, nerve block, epidural, and spinal anesthesia.

Local anesthetic solutions containing epinephrine should not be used for nerve blocks in areas supplied by end-arteries (eg, digits, ears, nose, penis) because they may cause ischemia, which could progress to necrosis. The total dosage of epinephrine should not exceed 0.2 mg, and concentrations exceeding 1:200,000 are not recommended except in dentistry. Solutions containing epinephrine for infiltration and nerve blocks should be used with caution in patients in labor because of the danger of producing vasoconstriction in uterine blood vessels, which may decrease placental circulation, diminish the intensity of uterine contractions, and prolong labor. It also is undesirable to use solutions containing epinephrine in patients with thyrotoxicosis. The risk of using vasoconstrictor-containing solutions in patients with severe cardiovascular disease must be assessed individually. The systemic effects of epinephrine may be potentiated in patients receiving tricyclic antidepressants or monoamine oxidase inhibitors. Epinephrine should not be injected into areas with diminished blood flow resulting from severe peripheral vascular disease.

Cocaine is the only local anesthetic that exhibits an inherent vasoconstrictor action, although there is some evidence that low concentrations of mepivacaine and lidocaine may also possess this effect (Blair, 1975). Moderate to high concentrations of all local anesthetics, except cocaine, have a vasodilator effect.

TABLE 4.
LOCAL ANESTHETICS EMPLOYED FOR TOPICAL (SURFACE) APPLICATION

	Eye	Ear	Nose	Throat	Urethra	Rectum	Skin
AMIDES							
Dibucaine [Nupercainal]	−	+	−	−	−	+	+*
Lidocaine [Xylocaine]	−	−	−	−	−	−	+*
Lidocaine Hydrochloride [Xylocaine]	−	+	+	+	+	−	−
ESTERS							
*Benzoic Acid Esters**							
Cocaine Hydrochloride	NR*	+	+	+	−	−	−*
Proparacaine Hydrochloride [Ak-Taine, Alcaine,* Ophthaine, Ophthetic]	+	−	−	−	−	−	−*
*Aminobenzoate Esters**							
Benzocaine [Americaine]	−	+	+	+	+	+	+*
Butamben Picrate [Butesin Picrate]	−	−	−	−	−	−	+*
Tetracaine Hydrochloride [Pontocaine]	+	+	+	+	−	+	+
MISCELLANEOUS							
Dyclonine Hydrochloride [Dyclone]	−	−	−	+	+	+	+*
Pramoxine Hydrochloride [Tronolane, Tronothane]	−	−	−	−	−	+	+

+ = In current use *− = Not in current use or ineffective* *NR = Not recommended* ** See text.*

ADVERSE REACTIONS AND PRECAUTIONS

Hypersensitivity Reactions: Unpredictable adverse reactions (ie, hypersensitivity, including anaphylaxis) are extremely rare. Use of a test dose to determine hypersensitivity may not be reliable. If a patient is known to be hypersensitive to a particular local anesthetic, a drug from a different chemical group should be substituted.

Systemic Reactions: The most common cause of toxic reactions to local anesthetics is unintentional intravascular injection. Predictable central nervous system reactions occur when plasma concentrations reach a critical level and are qualitatively similar for all local anesthetics. In general, the dose required to produce central nervous system toxicity is proportional to the inherent anesthetic potency of each agent (Covino, 1986). However, when absorption is slow, the peak plasma concentration (and presumably the possibility of prolonged systemic reactions) may not be observed for 20 to 30 minutes after the drug is injected. Because of accumulation, systemic reactions are more likely to occur after repeated doses. The reactions primarily involve the central nervous system and, at higher plasma concentrations, the cardiovascular system.

Signs and symptoms of central nervous system toxicity are restlessness, lightheadedness and dizziness, confusion, circumoral paresthesias, tinnitus, difficulty in focusing, and tremors involving the face and distal extremities. Tonic clonic convulsions may follow. Subconvulsive doses of lidocaine [Xylocaine] and procaine [Novocain] are often associated with sedation or sleep; this has not been reported with other local anesthetics (Covino and Vassallo, 1976). If the plasma concentration is high, seizure activity ceases and ventilatory depression progressing to respiratory arrest and coma may develop as a result of generalized central nervous system depression.

The initial and most important treatment is to ensure and maintain a patent airway and to support ventilation with oxygen and assisted or controlled respiration if required.

Some authorities suggest that adequate doses of benzodiazepines or succinylcholine be given to permit controlled ventilation. Usual preoperative doses of benzodiazepines have little or no value in averting central nervous system reactions.

Cardiovascular toxicity is characterized by bradycardia, hypotension, and heart block that may ultimately progress to cardiac arrest. Cardiovascular symptoms (hypertension and tachycardia) usually begin after signs of central nervous system toxicity are established and may reflect hypoxia more than a direct action of the anesthetic. Further increases in blood concentration lead to cardiovascular depression caused by a negative inotropic action and by direct peripheral vasodilation. Rapid unintentional intravenous injection can produce an abrupt hypotensive episode.

In animal studies, administration of bupivacaine and etidocaine has been associated with nodal or ventricular arrhythmias before or at the onset of convulsions and in the absence of such predisposing factors as hypoxemia, acidemia, and hyperkalemia. It appears that the enhanced sensitivity of the myocardium may be due to greater myocardial uptake with these agents (Covino, 1986). It is recommended that injection of large doses of all local anesthetics be made in fractional increments at two-minute intervals with monitoring for symptoms of overdosage (Marx, 1984).

Acute circulatory failure is treated with fluids and vasopressors (eg, ephedrine) administered intravenously. If respiratory arrest occurs or asystole is suspected, artificial ventilation and external cardiac massage must be instituted immediately.

Systemic effects (anxiety, restlessness, tremors, palpitations, tachycardia, anginal pain, dizziness, headache, and hypertension) may be produced by the vasoconstrictor that is added to local anesthetics for parenteral use. These reactions occur most frequently in office dentistry and are usually mild and transient.

Local Reactions: The most common local adverse reaction caused by local anesthetics is contact dermatitis characterized by erythema and pruritus that may progress to vesiculation and oozing. This occurs most commonly in individuals (eg, physicians, dentists) who are frequently exposed to ester-type local anesthetics or in patients following prolonged self-medication (eg, hemorrhoidal preparations). Allergic reactions are more common with ester-type agents, which are derivatives of p-aminobenzoic acid (a potent sensitizer). If rash, urticaria, edema, or other manifestations of allergy develop during use of a topical anesthetic, the drug should be discontinued. To minimize the possibility of a serious allergic reaction, topical preparations should not be applied for prolonged periods except under continual supervision. These reactions have become rare since the amides were introduced.

Repeated corneal application of topical anesthetics should be avoided since keratitis, which occasionally may lead to permanent reduction in visual acuity, can occur.

Effects on Newborn Infants: Local anesthetics diffuse readily through the placenta and reports have appeared of diminished muscle strength and tone and decreased rooting behavior in the newborn infant, although Apgar scores are normal. If used in excessive quantities, particularly in paracervical block, the increased absorption of these agents may cause fetal bradycardia and central nervous system depression after birth.

Drug Evaluations

Selected uses of currently available local anesthetics appear in Tables 3 and 4. When allergic, pharmacokinetic, or individual factors necessitate use of a different agent, selection of an alternative drug will depend on the factor or factors involved. Some topical preparations may contain a small quantity of antimicrobial agent as a preservative, but no claim is made for antimicrobial action.

Suggested maximum single doses appear in the evaluations for those local anesthetics recommended for injection; however, there is considerable evidence that these amounts may be excessive in some clinical situations (Covino, 1978) and inadequate or arbitrary in others (Scott, 1989). Therefore, suggested doses should be considered only as guidelines.

BENZOCAINE

[Americaine]

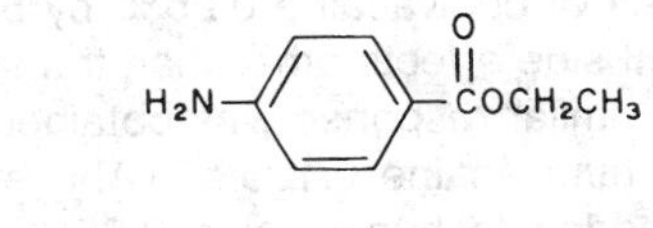

Benzocaine is used for surface anesthesia of the skin and mucous membranes. It is one of the most widely used agents for relief of sunburn, pruritus, and minor burns. Ointments containing less than 10% benzocaine or acidic preparations are ineffective on intact or mildly sunburned skin.

Since benzocaine is poorly soluble in water and poorly absorbed, the incidence of systemic toxic reactions is low. The possibility of sensitization should always be considered. Preparations containing benzocaine may cause methemoglobinemia in susceptible infants. For additional information on adverse reactions and precautions, see the Introduction.

DOSAGE AND PREPARATIONS.

Topical: The appropriate preparation is applied as required.

Generic. Cream 5% (nonprescription); bulk (crystals, powder).

Americaine Anesthetic Spray (CIBA Consumer). Aerosol containing benzocaine 20% in a water-dispersible base in 20, 60, and 120 ml containers (nonprescription).

Americaine First Aid Ointment (Fisons). Gel containing benzocaine 20% and benzethonium chloride 0.1% in a water-soluble polyethylene glycol base in 23 g containers.

Additional Trademark:

Benzocol (Hauck).

BUPIVACAINE HYDROCHLORIDE

[Marcaine, Sensorcaine]

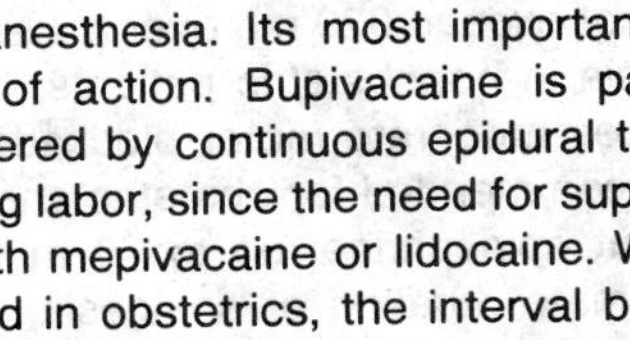

ACTIONS AND USES. This amide, which is related chemically to mepivacaine, is used for infiltration, nerve block, spinal, and epidural anesthesia. Its most important property is its long duration of action. Bupivacaine is particularly useful when administered by continuous epidural techniques to relieve pain during labor, since the need for supplemental doses is less than with mepivacaine or lidocaine. When the 0.25% solution is used in obstetrics, the interval between doses is usually two to three hours. Although bupivacaine may accumulate in the mother during continuous epidural anesthesia, few systemic toxic reactions have been reported, since delivery usually occurs before toxic plasma levels are attained. It is contraindicated for paracervical block and is not recommended for intravenous regional block.

Bupivacaine is sometimes combined with an opioid for epidural or intrathecal administration during labor. An opioid alone provides insufficient analgesia for most patients, but its combination with bupivacaine appears to induce analgesia of more rapid onset and duration and to reduce the dose of anesthetic required; with the decrease in dosage, anesthetic-associated hypotension and muscle weakness are lessened. Studies suggest that sulfentanil 20 to 30 mcg increases the duration of analgesia of bupivacaine 0.25% by 50% without producing significant side effects other than transient pruritus (Phillips, 1987). A similar response was obtained with alfentanil 500 mcg and bupivacaine 0.125% (Ahn et al, 1989). Fentanyl 50 mcg added to bupivacaine 0.25% as a single epidural administration provided no demonstrable benefit (Cohen et al, 1987), but the addition of fentanyl in a continuous epidural infusion produced consistent and sustained analgesia during labor (Jones et al, 1989). Perioperative administration of fentanyl 6.25 mcg with intrathecal hyperbaric bupivacaine 0.75% for caesarean section provided postoperative pain relief for three to four hours (Hunt et al, 1989). This anesthetic is classified in FDA Pregnancy Category C.

Data on use of bupivacaine in children under 12 years are limited.

The potency of bupivacaine is similar to that of etidocaine (ie, four times greater than that of mepivacaine and lidocaine). In general, the onset of action is slower and the interval to maximal anesthesia is longer with bupivacaine than with lidocaine. The duration of action is two to three times longer than with mepivacaine and lidocaine. Some peripheral nerve blocks may last more than 24 hours.

ADVERSE REACTIONS AND PRECAUTIONS. The systemic reactions produced by bupivacaine are qualitatively similar to those produced by other local anesthetics. However, ventricular arrhythmias have been observed following intravenous administration (Clarkson and Hondeghem, 1985). For additional information on adverse reactions and precautions, see the Introduction.

DOSAGE AND PREPARATIONS.

Injection: As a general guide, the maximal single dose in healthy *adults* should not exceed 175 mg without epinephrine and 225 mg with epinephrine 1:200,000. This dose should not be repeated at intervals of less than three hours. A maximal total dosage of 400 mg (8 mg/kg) in 24 hours generally should not be exceeded.

If the 0.25% solution without epinephrine is used for continuous epidural anesthesia in obstetric patients, the total dose probably should not exceed 320 mg over a 12-hour period. In epidural anesthesia in nonobstetric patients, the 0.5% concentration produces moderate motor blockade. Solutions of 0.75% are not recommended for obstetric anesthesia.

Infiltration: Without epinephrine, up to 70 ml of the 0.25% solution (approximate duration of analgesia, 200 minutes); with epinephrine, up to 90 ml of the 0.25% solution (approximate duration of analgesia, 400 minutes).

Intravenous regional: Bupivacaine is not recommended for intravenous regional anesthesia.

Nerve block: Without epinephrine, up to 70 ml of the 0.25% solution or 35 ml of the 0.5% solution; with epinephrine, up to 90 ml of the 0.25% solution or 45 ml of the 0.5% solution. The 0.5% solution is required to produce a consistent complete motor block of the larger nerves. Onset of anesthesia is slow (approximately 10 to 20 minutes). The duration of analgesia with either concentration is about 400 minutes and is little affected by epinephrine. A concentration of 0.75% is employed for retrobulbar block, but this concentration is not recommended for other nerve blocks.

Caudal: With or without epinephrine, for obstetric analgesia and perineal surgery, up to 30 ml of the 0.25% solution; for surgery of the lower extremities, up to 30 ml of the 0.5% solution. A single dose of either the 0.25% or 0.5% solution does not reliably produce motor block and, when used for a continuous technique, supplemental doses of the 0.25% or 0.5% solution are necessary. Only single-dose containers should be used.

Lumbar epidural: For obstetric analgesia, 0.25% solution is adequate; for surgery of the lower extremities, up to 20 ml of the 0.5% solution with or without epinephrine. When used for a continuous technique, supplemental 5- to 10-ml doses of the 0.25% or 0.5% solution usually produce excellent sensory analgesia. Motor block, such as that required for abdominal surgery, usually can be obtained by use of up to 20 ml of the 0.75% solution. Repeated use of the 0.75% solution for continuous epidural anesthesia is inadvisable because of the possibility of accumulation. Only single-dose containers should be used.

Spinal anesthesia: Bupivacaine is used almost as often as tetracaine for spinal anesthesia. Plain solutions are approximately equivalent to isobaric solutions. Heavy solutions with dextrose also are available [Marcaine Spinal, Sensorcaine MPF]. Onset of action is relatively rapid (about three to eight minutes). The duration of anesthesia is 90 to 110 minutes. Motor blockade usually is profound. The recommended dosage is 8 to 10 mg for the lower extremities and perineal surgery and 15 to 20 mg for upper abdominal surgery.

Generic. Solution 0.25%, 0.5%, and 0.75%.

Marcaine (Sanofi Winthrop), ***Sensorcaine*** (Astra). Solution 0.25% and 0.5% with and without epinephrine 1:200,000 in 3 (0.5% with epinephrine only [***Marcaine***], 5 (0.5% without epinephrine only [***Sensorcaine***]), 10, 30, and 50 ml containers; 0.75% with and without epinephrine 1:200,000 in 10 and 30 ml containers; and 0.75% with 8.25% dextrose in 2 ml containers for spinal anesthesia [***Marcaine Spinal, Sensorcaine MPF***]. Solutions that do not contain epinephrine may be autoclaved. Solutions in multiple-dose (50 ml) containers also contain methylparaben.

BUTAMBEN PICRATE

[Butesin Picrate]

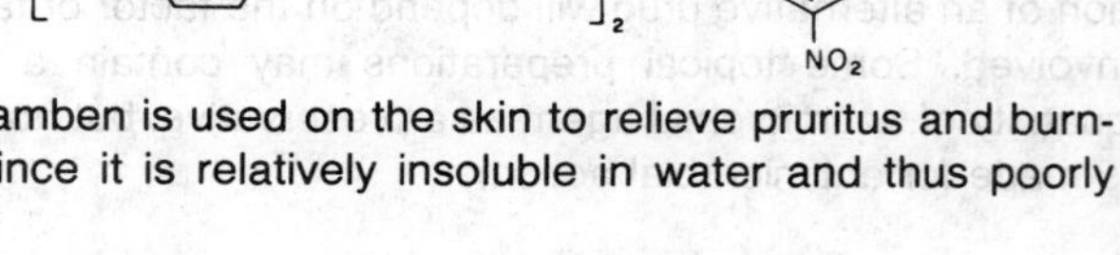

Butamben is used on the skin to relieve pruritus and burning. Since it is relatively insoluble in water and thus poorly absorbed, this drug may remain in contact with the skin for a prolonged period with a low incidence of systemic reactions.

Butamben picrate may cause a rash in sensitive individuals. For additional information on adverse reactions and precautions, see the Introduction.

DOSAGE AND PREPARATIONS.

Topical: The ointment is applied to affected areas as required.

Butesin Picrate (Abbott). Ointment 1% in 30 g containers (nonprescription).

CHLOROPROCAINE HYDROCHLORIDE

[Nesacaine]

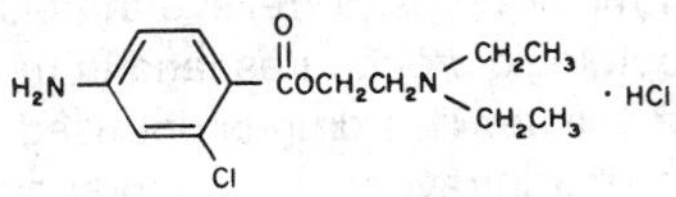

ACTIONS AND USES. Chloroprocaine, a chlorinated analogue of procaine, is used for infiltration, peripheral nerve block, caudal, and epidural anesthesia. The drug is not effective topically and has not been studied sufficiently to be used for spinal anesthesia. Its anesthetic potency is slightly greater than that of procaine; its onset of action is more rapid and the duration is slightly shorter. Nerve blocks last an average of one hour. The addition of epinephrine 1:200,000 prolongs the duration to as much as one and one-half hours.

ADVERSE REACTIONS AND PRECAUTIONS. The systemic toxicity of chloroprocaine is less than that of all other local anesthetics because of its rapid hydrolysis by plasma cholinesterase (even in the presence of decreased maternal and fetal cholinesterase activity at term), which shortens the plasma half-life. This anesthetic is classified in FDA Pregnancy Category C.

Neural irritation after accidental subarachnoid administration of a large volume of chloroprocaine solution has been reported (Gissen et al, 1984; Wang et al, 1984). This was ascribed to the presence of sodium bisulfite utilized as a preservative and the low pH of the preparation. Chlorprocaine distributed after October 1, 1987, contains ethylene diaminetetracetic acid instead of sodium bisulfite.

For additional information on adverse reactions and precautions, see the Introduction.

DOSAGE AND PREPARATIONS.

Injection: As a general guide, the maximal single dose is 800 mg (20 mg/kg) without epinephrine and 1 g with epinephrine 1:200,000. Repeated doses of up to 300 mg without epinephrine and 600 mg with epinephrine 1:200,000 may be given at 50-minute intervals.

Infiltration: Without epinephrine, up to 80 ml of the 1% solution; with epinephrine 1:200,000, 100 ml of the 1% solution. Three ml of 1% chloroprocaine is injected at each of four sites for paracervical block; 3 to 4 ml of the 1% solution without epinephrine may be used for digital blocks.

Peripheral nerve block: The dose of the 1% or 2% solution, with or without epinephrine 1:200,000, depends on the type of block and intensity and duration of effect needed: 10 ml of a 2% solution on each side for pudendal nerve block, 30 to 40 ml of a 2% solution for brachial plexus block, 2 to 3 ml of a 2% solution for mandibular block, and 0.5 to 1 ml of a 2% solution for infraorbital block.

Caudal: Initially, 15 to 25 ml (depending on the size of the patient) of the 2% or 3% *Nesacaine-MPF* solution. Repeated doses may be given at 30- to 40-minute intervals as required; epinephrine 1:200,000 may be used to prolong the action.

Lumbar and sacral epidural: The usual total initial dose, with or without epinephrine 1:200,000, is 15 to 25 ml of the 2% or 3% *Nesacaine-MPF* solution. Supplemental doses of 10 to 20 ml may be given at 30- to 40-minute intervals.

Chloroprocaine Hydrochloride (Abbott). Solution 2% and 3% in 30 ml containers.

Nesacaine (Astra). Solution 1% and 2% in 30 ml containers (2% not for caudal or epidural anesthesia); solution 2% and 3% in 30 ml containers for caudal or epidural anesthesia (***Nesacaine MPF***) (contains no preservative).

COCAINE HYDROCHLORIDE

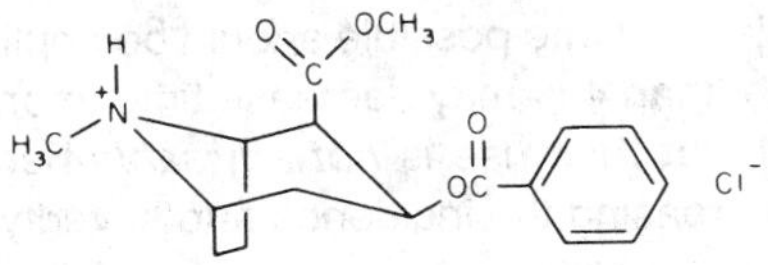

ACTIONS AND USES. Cocaine is a naturally occurring alkaloid that produces excellent topical anesthesia and intense vasoconstriction when applied to mucous surfaces. It is used for anesthesia in the ear, nose, and throat and in bronchoscopy. The addition of epinephrine is not only unnecessary (it does not delay absorption), but it may increase the likelihood of arrhythmias. The moistening of dry cocaine powder with epinephrine solution to form so-called "cocaine mud" for use on the nasal mucosa is particularly dangerous and is not recommended. Cocaine should not be used parenterally.

Onset of action is rapid (one minute) with an anesthetic duration of approximately one hour, depending on the dose and concentration applied.

ADVERSE REACTIONS AND PRECAUTIONS. Toxic symptoms may occur when cocaine is absorbed rapidly after topical application, in spite of its vasoconstrictor action, and dosage is difficult to monitor carefully. The toxic signs differ slightly from those observed with other local anesthetics in that pronounced central and peripheral sympathetic activities occur concurrently. The central nervous system effects include euphoria and cortical stimulation manifested by excitement, restlessness, and tremors followed by grand mal seizures. Tachycardia and elevated blood pressure also are observed initially.

Repeated use results in psychological dependence and physical tolerance; therefore, cocaine is classified as a Schedule II drug under the Controlled Substances Act. It is classified in FDA Pregnancy Category C.

Cocaine exerts an indirect adrenergic effect by interfering with the tissue reuptake of catecholamines. This effect also will potentiate the action of exogenous epinephrine and norepinephrine. Ventricular fibrillation caused by absorption of excessive amounts of cocaine may occur, particularly if a general anesthetic that sensitizes the myocardium to catecholamines also is being administered. For this reason, cocaine should be used with extreme caution, if at all, in patients with hypertension, severe cardiovascular disease, or thyrotoxicosis or in patients taking drugs that also potentiate catecholamines (eg, guanethidine, monoamine oxidase inhibitors). For additional information on adverse reactions and precautions, see the Introduction.

Solutions of cocaine are unstable and deteriorate on standing; boiling and autoclaving cause decomposition.

DOSAGE AND PREPARATIONS.

Topical: For the ear, nose, and throat and for bronchoscopy, concentrations of 4% are used. A 0.25% to 0.5% solution is satisfactory for corneal anesthesia, but cocaine has largely been replaced by other agents because of its tendency to produce transient irregularity of the corneal epithelium (see also index entry Cocaine, As Ocular Anesthetic). As a general guide, the maximal dose is 150 mg. The lowest concentration and smallest volume possible should be applied. Concentrations greater than 4% may decrease time to onset of anesthesia slightly, but their use is *not advisable* because of the potential for increasing the incidence and severity of systemic toxic reactions.

Generic. Tablets (soluble) 135 mg; solution (topical) 40 and 100 mg/ml; bulk (crystals, powder).

DIBUCAINE

[Nupercainal]

Dibucaine is applied to the skin and rectal mucocutaneous junction for long-acting surface anesthesia.

For adverse reactions and precautions, see the Introduction.

DOSAGE AND PREPARATIONS.

Topical:

Skin: The 0.5% cream or 1% ointment is applied as required.

Rectum: The ointment is used morning and night, preferably following bowel movements.

Generic. Ointment 1% (nonprescription).

Nupercainal (CIBA Consumer). Cream 0.5% in 45 g containers; ointment 1% in 30 and 60 g containers (both forms nonprescription).

DYCLONINE HYDROCHLORIDE

[Dyclone]

Dyclonine is used topically to anesthetize mucous membranes prior to endoscopy, to suppress the gag reflex, to relieve the pain of minor burns, to relieve the discomfort of gynecologic or proctologic procedures, and in the management of pruritus ani or vulvae. This drug is not used in cystoscopic procedures following intravenous pyelography with contrast media containing iodine because of formation of a precipitate that interferes with visualization.

The potency of dyclonine is comparable to that of cocaine. Generally, up to 10 minutes are required for onset of action and the duration is up to one hour.

The toxicity of dyclonine is presumed to be low. For additional information on adverse reactions and precautions, see the Introduction. Dyclonine is classified in FDA Pregnancy Category C.

DOSAGE AND PREPARATIONS. Either the 0.5% or the 1% solution may be used for most of the indications described below. When continuous or repetitive application is anticipated, as in some oral or anogenital uses, the 0.5% solution may be preferred to reduce transmucosal absorption and the attendant possibility of cumulative systemic toxicity.

Topical: As a general guide, the maximal single dose is 200 mg.

Skin: 0.5% or 1% solution is applied as required.

Mouth, esophagus, oral endoscopy: For relief of oral pain, 5 to 10 ml of the 0.5% or 1% solution is swabbed, gargled, or sprayed and then expectorated. For esophagoscopy after pharyngeal anesthesia, 10 to 15 ml of the 0.5% solution is swallowed. For relief of esophageal pain, 5 to 15 ml of the 0.5% solution is swallowed.

Bronchoscopy: The tongue is pulled forward and the larynx and trachea are sprayed with 2 ml of the 1% solution every five minutes until the laryngeal reflex is abolished. This usually requires two or three applications of spray. Five minutes should be allowed before instrumentation.

Urologic endoscopy: 6 to 30 ml of the 0.5% to 1% solution (usually 10 to 15 ml) is instilled into the urethra and retained for five to ten minutes before instrumentation.

Gynecology: 0.5% or 1% solution is used as a wet compress or spray.

Proctology: A cotton pledget saturated with the 0.5% or 1% solution is applied for relief of pain and discomfort.

Dyclone (Astra). Solution 0.5% and 1% with chlorobutanol in 30 ml containers.

ETIDOCAINE HYDROCHLORIDE
[Duranest]

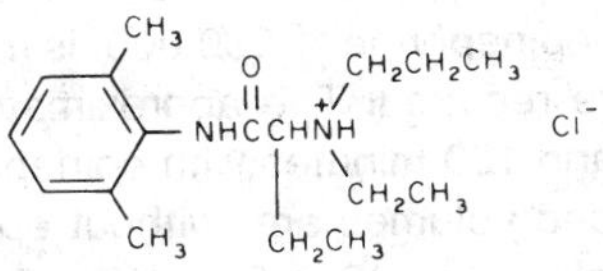

ACTIONS AND USES. Etidocaine is currently employed for infiltration, peripheral nerve block, and epidural (but not spinal) anesthesia. A 0.5% concentration, with or without epinephrine, is generally adequate for infiltration anesthesia. Solutions of 0.5%, with or without epinephrine, are used for peripheral nerve blocks. The addition of epinephrine does not prolong the duration of analgesia but maintains lower plasma concentrations of the anesthetic. A 1% or 1.5% concentration is suggested for epidural anesthesia; onset of sensory block is rapid (about five minutes) with complete block in 12 minutes.

This agent differs from other local anesthetics in that it produces a profound motor nerve block after epidural administration; this may be preferred for abdominal surgery but is undesirable for normal obstetric delivery. Regression of anesthesia following epidural administration is similar to that seen with spinal anesthesia, ie, the patient may experience pain at the operative site while motor block is still present.

The onset of action of this amide is more rapid than that of bupivacaine and, at equipotent levels of anesthesia, the duration is comparable to that of bupivacaine and usually at least twice as long as that of lidocaine.

Although etidocaine and bupivacaine elicit seizures at the same plasma concentration, the decreased rate of absorption, more rapid plasma decay, and increased volume of distribution are probably responsible for the fact that, experimentally, etidocaine is less toxic than bupivacaine after injection of the same dose.

Like other amides, etidocaine is metabolized primarily by the liver, and metabolic products are excreted in the urine; little unchanged drug is excreted.

ADVERSE REACTIONS AND PRECAUTIONS. See the Introduction. This anesthetic is classified in FDA Pregnancy Category B.

DOSAGE AND PREPARATIONS.

Injection: A 0.5% solution is recommended for infiltration and peripheral nerve block; however, this concentration is no longer available commercially. The 1% solution may be more appropriate for major peripheral nerve blocks and is recommended for epidural blocks in various gynecologic and obstetric procedures. A total dose of the 0.5%, 1%, or 1.5% solution for infiltration and nerve blocks should not exceed 5.5 mg/kg (400 mg) for solutions with epinephrine and 4 mg/kg (300 mg) for solutions without epinephrine.

The 1.5% solution may be required in epidural anesthesia for intra-abdominal procedures and cesarean sections. The usual dose is 100 to 300 mg for intra-abdominal or pelvic surgery, 150 to 300 mg for lower limb surgery and cesarean section, and 50 to 150 mg for vaginal obstetric procedures.

Duranest (Astra). Solution (sterile) 1% with and without epinephrine 1:200,000 in 30 ml (single-dose) containers and 1.5% with epinephrine 1:200,000 in 20 ml containers. Single-dose (30 ml) containers without epinephrine may be autoclaved.

LIDOCAINE

[Xylocaine]

LIDOCAINE HYDROCHLORIDE
[Xylocaine]

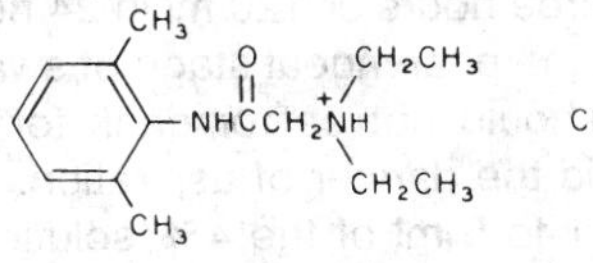

ACTIONS AND USES. This amide is one of the most widely used local anesthetics for infiltration, intravenous regional, nerve block, epidural, and spinal anesthesia; it also is commonly used for topical anesthesia.

Compared to procaine, the action of lidocaine is more rapid in onset, more intense, and of longer duration. This anesthetic has excellent powers of diffusion and penetration. It has a local vasodilator action but is usually administered with epinephrine. When used alone, anesthesia after perineural injection lasts 60 to 75 minutes; with epinephrine, anesthesia lasts up to two hours.

ADVERSE REACTIONS AND PRECAUTIONS. When administered by extravascular injection, lidocaine is approximately one and one-half times as toxic as procaine. When given intravenously, lidocaine is twice as toxic as procaine. Rapid absorption of large amounts generally causes convulsions, but central nervous system depression rather than apparent stimulation may occur in some patients. Even therapeutic doses may cause drowsiness, lassitude, and amnesia. Other systemic reactions are similar to those produced by local anesthetics in general.

Lidocaine is not irritating and produces relatively little sensitization when used topically.

This anesthetic is classified in FDA Pregnancy Category B. For additional information on adverse reactions and precautions, see the Introduction.

DOSAGE AND PREPARATIONS. As a general guide, in healthy *adults* with normal hepatic function and hepatic blood flow, the maximal single dose recommended by the manufacturer for topical use is 300 mg and for injection (excluding spinal anesthesia) is 300 mg (4.5 mg/kg) without epinephrine or 500 mg (7 mg/kg) with epinephrine. This dose should not be repeated at intervals of less than two hours. The vascularity of tissue at the site of injection also should be considered when estimating total dose. In healthy *children,* the dose (preferably of the 0.5% or 1% solution) should be reduced according to the type of block and the age of the child (see index entry Drug Response Variation).

Topical: The 2% solution is generally recommended for topical anesthesia, particularly in infants. The 4% solution is used principally for laryngotracheal anesthesia. The maximal recommended dose is 10 ml of the 2% or 5 ml of the 4% concentration.

Skin: The maximal dose is 35 g of the 2.5% or 5% ointment daily.

Nose and nasopharynx: 1 to 5 ml of a 1% to 4% solution is sprayed or used on cotton applicators, depending on the procedure. *Mouth, pharynx, and upper digestive tract:* The 2% viscous solution is used. The preparation can be moved around the mouth and pharynx by the cheeks and tongue and then swallowed. The adult dose should not exceed 15 ml (300 mg) every three hours or 120 ml in 24 hours. This anesthetic may obtund the pharyngeal stage of swallowing. Therefore, the patient should not eat or drink for one hour after application to avoid the danger of aspiration.

Respiratory tract: 1 to 5 ml of the 4% solution is sprayed or used by applicator or pack to produce anesthesia of the pharynx, larynx, and trachea for laryngoscopy, endotracheal intubation, and bronchoscopy. In addition, 2 to 3 ml of the 4% solution may be injected through the cricothyroid membrane (transtracheal), but a total dose of 5 ml generally should not be exceeded. Endotracheal tubes may be lubricated with 2% lidocaine hydrochloride jelly or 5% lidocaine ointment.

Urology: A 2% aqueous solution or 2% jelly may be used. *Men*, prior to catheterization, 5 to 10 ml of the 2% jelly is instilled slowly into the urethra and retained by penile clamp for five to ten minutes. For sounding or cystoscopy, 10 to 15 ml is given initially; an additional 15 ml is instilled after the clamp is removed. The maximal dose is 30 ml in 12 hours. In *women,* the dose is 3 to 5 ml. Several minutes should be allowed to elapse prior to performing urologic procedures.

LIDOCAINE:

Xylocaine (Astra). Ointment 2.5% (nonprescription) and 5% in 35 g containers.

LIDOCAINE HYDROCHLORIDE:

Generic. Ointment 5%; solution 4%.

Xylocaine (Astra). Jelly 2% with methylparaben and propylparaben in 30 g containers; solution (viscous) 2% in 100 and 450 ml containers; solution (sterile) 4% with methylparaben in 50 ml containers.

Additional Trademark:

Anestacon (Webcon).

Injection:

Infiltration: Onset of anesthesia is almost immediate. Without epinephrine, for extensive procedures, 25 to 60 ml of a 0.5% solution (duration of analgesia, approximately 75 minutes) or 10 to 30 ml of a 1% solution (duration of analgesia, approximately 90 minutes); for minor surgery and relief of pain, 2 to 50 ml of a 0.5% solution. With epinephrine 1:200,000, the duration of analgesia is approximately 150 minutes for the 0.5% solution and 240 minutes for the 1% solution. For dentistry, a 2% solution with epinephrine 1:100,000 is employed; the approximate duration of analgesia or anesthesia is 150 minutes. The maximum single dose is 7 mg/kg.

Intravenous regional: 40 to 50 ml of a 0.5% solution without epinephrine is used for the arm and approximately 60 ml for the leg.

Nerve block: For minor nerve blocks (eg, ulnar, intercostal), a 0.5% solution is adequate. For major nerve blocks (eg, pudendal, brachial plexus), a 0.5% or 1% solution is used. The addition of epinephrine 1:200,000 is recommended if large volumes are required. The approximate duration is 60 minutes without and 120 minutes with epinephrine. The maximum recommended volumes are, without epinephrine, up to 30 ml of a 1% solution or 25 to 35 ml of a 2% solution; with epinephrine 1:200,000, up to 50 ml of a 1% or 25 ml of a 2% solution. The usual doses are 25 to 35 ml of a 1.5% solution for brachial plexus, 1 to 5 ml of a 2% solution for mandibular, 3 ml of a 1% solution for intercostal, 3 to 5 ml of a 1% solution for paravertebral, and 10 ml of a 1% solution on each side for pudendal nerve block; for cervical nerve (stellate ganglion) block, the dose is 5 to 10 ml of a 1% solution; for lumbar sympathetic block, 5 to 10 ml of a 1% solution.

Caudal: Without epinephrine, for obstetric analgesia, up to 30 ml of the 1% solution; for surgical anesthesia, up to 20 ml of the 1.5% solution. With epinephrine 1:200,000, for surgical anesthesia, up to 30 ml of the 1.5% solution or 25 ml of the 2% solution. Analgesia during labor may be obtained with 20 to 30 ml of a 0.5% solution. Only single-dose containers should be used.

Lumbar epidural: Without epinephrine, for obstetric or postoperative analgesia, 8 to 15 ml of the 1% solution; for surgical anesthesia, 15 to 20 ml of the 1.5% or 10 to 15 ml of the 2% solution. The dose depends on the level of analgesia required but cannot be predicted accurately. With epinephrine 1:200,000, up to 20 ml of the 1%, 1.5%, or 2% solution. Analgesia during labor may be obtained with 8 to 10 ml of a 0.5% solution. Only single-dose containers should be used.

Spinal: The 1.5% and 5% solutions with 7.5% dextrose (hyperbaric) are used for spinal anesthesia. For vaginal delivery, 0.8 or 1 ml (40 or 50 mg) of the 5% solution or 2 ml (30 mg) of the 1.5% solution will provide perineal anesthesia for about one hour; analgesia lasts an additional 40 minutes. For cesarean section, 1.5 ml (75 mg) of the 5% solution may be used.

LIDOCAINE HYDROCHLORIDE:

Generic. Solution 1%, 1.5%, and 2%; 1.5% with epinephrine.

Xylocaine (Astra). Solution 0.5% with or without epinephrine 1:200,000 and methylparaben in 50 ml containers; 1% with methylparaben in 2, 5, 20, 30, and 50 ml containers, with epinephrine 1:100,000 and methylparaben in 20 and 50 ml containers, and with epinephrine 1:200,000 in 30 ml containers; 1.5% in 20 ml containers and with epinephrine 1:200,000 in 10 and 30 ml containers and with dextrose 7.5% in 2 ml containers; 2% with methylparaben in 2, 5, 10, 20, and 50 ml containers and 1.8 ml dental cartridges and with epinephrine 1:50,000 in 1.8 ml dental cartridges, with epinephrine 1:100,000 and methylparaben in 20 and 50 ml containers and 1.8 ml dental cartridges and with epinephrine 1:200,000 in 20 ml containers; 4% in 5 ml containers; 5% with dextrose 7.5% in 2 ml containers. Aqueous solutions without epinephrine can be autoclaved repeatedly if necessary; preparations containing dextrose should not be autoclaved more than once or twice.

Additional Trademarks:

Dilocaine (Hauck), ***Lidoject-1*** (Mayrand), ***Nervocaine*** (Keene).

MEPIVACAINE HYDROCHLORIDE
[Carbocaine, Polocaine]

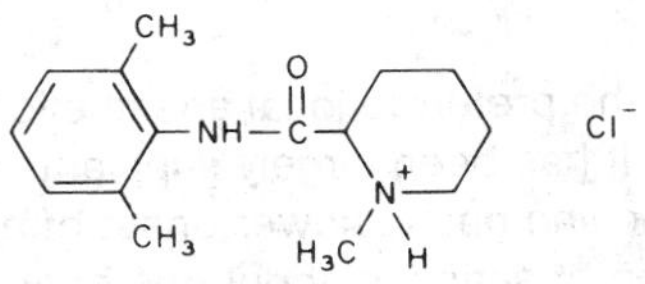

ACTIONS AND USES. This amide is chemically related to bupivacaine but pharmacologically is related to lidocaine. It is indicated for infiltration, nerve block, and epidural anesthesia. Mepivacaine is effective topically only in large doses and therefore should not be used by this route.

The potency of mepivacaine is similar to that of lidocaine. Anesthesia develops in three to five minutes and lasts two to two and one-half hours. Conventional doses may be used without epinephrine for most purposes. Unless contraindicated, epinephrine should be added to reduce plasma concentrations of mepivacaine when larger doses must be given.

ADVERSE REACTIONS. The systemic reactions produced by mepivacaine are similar to those caused by other local anesthetics.

Because the potentially high maternal blood concentration and rapid placental transfer can produce a high blood level in the fetus, utilization of mepivacaine in pudendal or paracervical nerve blocks for obstetric analgesia is not recommended (FDA Pregnancy Category C).

For additional information on adverse reactions and precautions, see the Introduction.

DOSAGE AND PREPARATIONS.
Injection: *Adults,* as a general guide, the doses of mepivacaine are similar to those of lidocaine. The maximal single dose is 7 mg/kg or 400 mg, whichever is less. This dose should not be repeated at intervals of less than 90 minutes, and no more than 1 g should be administered during any 24-hour period. The dose should be reduced in elderly or debilitated patients. The *pediatric* dose should be carefully measured as a percentage of the total adult dose based on weight and should not exceed 5 to 6 mg/kg (2.5 to 3 mg/lb). In children under 3 years or weighing less than 30 lb, concentrations less than 2% (eg, 0.5% to 1.5%) should be employed.
Infiltration: Up to 80 ml of a 0.5% or 40 ml of the 1% solution.
Nerve block: 5 to 40 ml of the 1% or 5 to 20 ml of the 1.5% solution.
Epidural: 15 to 25 ml of the 1% solution, 10 to 20 ml of the 1.5% solution, or 10 to 20 ml of the 2% solution. Only single-dose containers should be used.

Carbocaine (Sanofi Winthrop). Solution 1% with methylparaben in 30 and 50 ml containers and 1.5% in 30 ml containers.
Polocaine (Astra). Solution 1% and 2% in 30 and 50 ml containers and 1.5% in 30 ml containers.

PRAMOXINE HYDROCHLORIDE
[Tronolane, Tronothane]

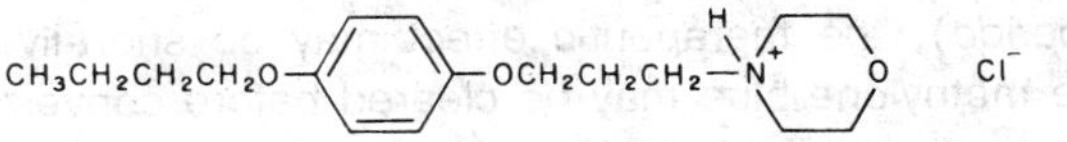

Pramoxine is derived from morpholine and, since it is chemically different from ester- or amide-type compounds, may be useful in patients who are sensitive to these classes of drugs. The potency of pramoxine is comparable to that of benzocaine. Onset of action is within three to five minutes.

Pramoxine is applied topically to the skin or mucous membranes to relieve pain caused by minor burns and wounds and to relieve pruritus secondary to dermatoses or hemorrhoids. This anesthetic should not be applied to the nasal mucosa, for it may irritate the tissue, and it should not be used for bronchoscopy or gastroscopy.

For adverse reactions and precautions, see the Introduction.

DOSAGE AND PREPARATIONS.
Topical:
Skin, mucous membranes: The 1% cream is applied as required, usually every three or four hours. For severe discomfort, preparations may be applied every two or three hours for one or two days; applications should be decreased thereafter to every four hours.

Tronolane (Ross). Cream 1% in 30 and 60 g containers; suppositories 1% (both forms nonprescription).
Tronothane (Abbott). Cream (water-miscible) 1% in 30 g containers (nonprescription).
Additional Trademark:
Prax (Ferndale).

PRILOCAINE HYDROCHLORIDE
[Citanest]

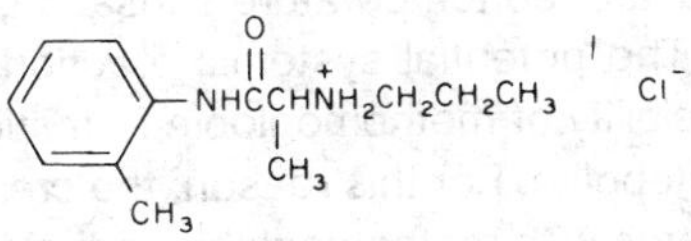

ACTIONS AND USES. Prilocaine is similar pharmacologically to lidocaine. Its clinical use has virtually ceased. The evaluation is retained primarily because of prilocaine's characteristic adverse effects and its presence in the eutectic mixture with lidocaine for topical application (see following evaluation).

The effectiveness of prilocaine and lidocaine in equivalent doses is comparable, but the action of prilocaine is slightly slower in onset and is of slightly longer duration. Epinephrine prolongs its effect.

ADVERSE REACTIONS AND PRECAUTIONS. Two metabolites of prilocaine, ortho-toluidine and nitroso-toluidine, form methemoglobin. Doses in excess of 600 mg may produce a grayish or slate-blue cyanosis of the lips, mucous membranes, and nail beds, but respiratory and circulatory distress apparently do not occur. In one study, there were no signs of inadequate oxygen transport in healthy individuals who received prilocaine 1.2 g. Although methemoglobinemia is readily reversed by the intravenous administration of methylene blue (1 to 2 mg/kg of a 1% solution injected over a five-minute period), the therapeutic effect may be short-lived because methylene blue may be cleared before conversion of all the methemoglobin to hemoglobin. Prilocaine should not be administered to patients with idiopathic or congenital methemoglobinemia, anemia, or cardiac or ventilatory failure with hypoxia; it should be used with caution for continuous epidural anesthesia since the methemoglobinemic effect of individual doses is additive.

This anesthetic is classified in FDA Pregnancy Category B. For additional information on adverse reactions and precautions, see the Introduction.

PRILOCAINE HYDROCHLORIDE AND LIDOCAINE HYDROCHLORIDE
[EMLA]

ACTIONS AND USES. A local anesthetic cream, a eutectic mixture of lidocaine and prilocaine in a 1:1 (2.5% each) oil/water emulsion, is useful for anesthesia of the intact skin (eg, in preparation for venipuncture, superficial surgical procedures, laser therapy). The mixture may be particularly useful for prevention of venipuncture pain in children.

Systemic absorption is limited, although variable, and is dependent on the dose and site and duration of application. Absorption is greater, for example, from the skin of the face than from the skin of the thigh.

ADVERSE REACTIONS AND PRECAUTIONS. This preparation should not be used on open wounds, mucous membranes, genital skin or mucosa, or in or near the eye. Local reactions occur in 50% to 60% of patients and include redness, blanching, altered temperature sensation, edema, pruritus, and rash. The potential systemic reaction of main concern is the possibility of methemoglobin formation induced by a prilocaine metabolite. For this reason, the cream should not be used in patients with methemoglobin reductase deficiency, in infants under 6 months, or in those 6 to 12 months old who are receiving other methemoglobin-inducing agents (eg, sulfonamides).

DOSAGE AND PREPARATIONS.

Topical: The cream is applied on the skin in a thick layer at the site of the procedure and covered with an occlusive dressing. Anesthesia efficacy and depth depend on the duration of application. The duration of anesthesia after a one- to two-hour application is about two hours; shorter application periods may be appropriate in certain circumstances.

EMLA (Astra). Cream containing prilocaine hydrochloride 2.5% and lidocaine hydrochloride 2.5% in 5 and 30 g tubes (5 g tubes also supplied with occlusive dressings).

PROCAINE HYDROCHLORIDE
[Novocain]

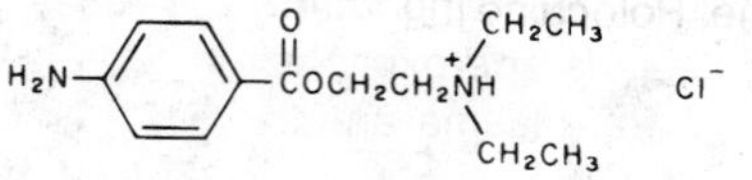

Procaine was the preferred local anesthetic for injection for many years, but it has been largely supplanted by other local anesthetics. Procaine has a slower onset of action than lidocaine; its duration of action is about one hour. It is ineffective topically.

Procaine is metabolized rapidly, which accounts for its safety. Much of it is hydrolyzed by plasma cholinesterase; the remainder is metabolized in the liver. The adverse reactions produced by procaine are similar to those of other synthetic local anesthetics. This anesthetic is classified in FDA Pregnancy Category C.

For additional information on adverse reactions and precautions, see the Introduction.

DOSAGE AND PREPARATIONS.

Injection: As a general guide, the maximal single dose for *adults* (excluding spinal anesthesia) is 500 or 600 mg with epinephrine 1:200,000.

Infiltration: With or without epinephrine 1:200,000, up to 100 ml of a 0.25% or 0.5% solution.

Nerve block: With or without epinephrine 1:200,000, up to 50 ml of the 1% or 25 ml of the 2% solution.

Caudal, lumbar epidural: Procaine is not indicated for caudal or epidural anesthesia.

Spinal: The 10% solution diluted with 10% dextrose prepared for spinal anesthesia (hyperbaric) is used. For saddle block (perineum), 0.5 ml of the 10% solution diluted with 0.5 ml of 10% dextrose injection; for lower extremities, 1 ml of the 10% solution diluted with 1 ml of 10% dextrose injection; for level to costal margin, 2 ml of the 10% solution diluted with 1 ml of 10% dextrose injection. Onset is rapid and the duration of analgesia is 30 to 45 minutes.

Generic. Solution 1% and 2%.

Novocain (Sanofi Winthrop). Solution 1% (isotonic) in 2, 6, and 30 ml containers; solution (isotonic) 2% in 30 ml containers; solution 10% in 2 ml containers (for spinal anesthesia; autoclaving more than once is not recommended).

TETRACAINE HYDROCHLORIDE
[Pontocaine]

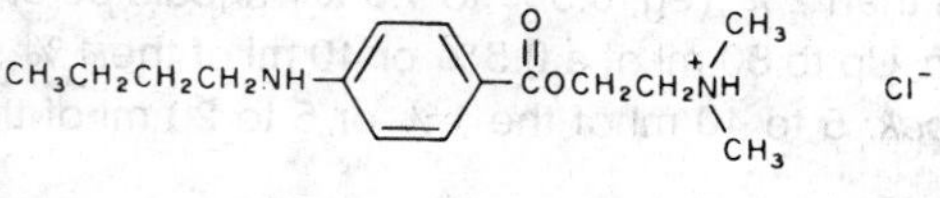

Tetracaine is most widely used for spinal anesthesia but is being replaced to some extent by bupivacaine. It is not recommended for infiltration or epidural block because of its slow onset of action and great systemic toxicity. Tetracaine is approximately ten times more potent and toxic than procaine. The onset of action is slow (approximately five minutes) after injection, but the duration of anesthesia is more than twice as long as that of procaine (two to three hours). Onset of action also develops slowly following topical application, and the duration of anesthesia is approximately 45 minutes. Tetracaine is metabolized in the plasma and liver at a slower rate than procaine.

This anesthetic is classified in FDA Pregnancy Category C. For information on adverse reactions and precautions, see the Introduction.

DOSAGE AND PREPARATIONS.

Topical:

Skin, anus: The 0.5% ointment or 1% cream is used. No more than 30 g for *adults* or 7.5 g for *children* should be applied in a 24-hour period.

Nose, pharynx: Up to 2 ml of a 1% solution.

Esophageal and laryngeal reflexes: 2 ml of a 1% solution effectively abolishes reflexes in preparation for esophagoscopy, bronchoscopy, and bronchography. These doses should not be exceeded because of the risk of systemic toxicity caused by rapid absorption of the drug.

Pontocaine (Sanofi Winthrop). Cream 1% in 30 g containers (nonprescription); ointment 0.5% in 30 g containers (nonprescription); solution 2% in 30 and 118 ml containers (rhinolaryngology).

Injection:

Spinal: The 1% solution diluted with an equal volume of 10% dextrose prepared for spinal anesthesia (hyperbaric) is used. For obstetric saddle block, 2 to 4 mg; for lower extremities and perineal operations, 3 to 6 mg; for most cesarean sections and lower abdominal surgery, 9 to 12 mg; for upper abdominal surgery, 12 to 20 mg. Epinephrine 1:1,000 (0.1 to 0.2 mg) may be added to prolong the duration of anesthesia by 30% to 50% in the average adult.

Pontocaine (Sanofi Winthrop). Solution 0.2% with dextrose 6% in 2 ml containers, 0.3% with dextrose 6% in 5 ml containers (saddle block, perineal), and 1% in 2 ml containers (subarachnoid).

Cited References

Ahn NN, et al: Epidural alfentanil and bupivacaine for analgesia during labor. *Anesthesiology* 71(3A):A845, 1989.

Barnett G, et al: Cocaine pharmacokinetics in humans. *J Ethnopharmacol* 3:353-366, 1981.

Benzon HT, et al: Onset, intensity of blockade and somatosensory evoke potential changes of the lumbrosacral dermatomes after epidural anesthesia with alkalinized lidocaine. *Anesth Analg* 76:328-332, 1993.

Blair MA: Cardiovascular pharmacology of local anaesthetics. *Br J Anaesth* 47:247-252, 1975.

Bromage PR: *Epidural Analgesia*. Philadelphia, WB Saunders, 1978.

Burm AGL: Clinical pharmacokinetics of epidural and spinal anaesthesia. *Clin Pharmacokinet* 16:283-311, 1989.

Clarkson CW, Hondeghem LM: Mechanism for bupivacaine depression of cardiac conduction: Fast block of sodium channels during the action potential with slow recovery from block during diastole. *Anesthesiology* 62:396-405, 1985.

Cohen SE, et al: Epidural fentanyl/bupivacaine mixtures for obstetric analgesia. *Anesthesiology* 67;403-407, 1987.

Concepcion M, Covino BG: Rational use of local anesthetics. *Drugs* 27:256-270, 1984.

Cousins MJ, Bridenbaugh PO (eds): *Neural Blockade in Clinical Anesthesia and Management of Pain*, ed 2. Philadelphia, JB Lippincott, 1988.

Covino BG: Systemic toxicity of local anesthetic agents. *Anesth Analg* 57:387-388, 1978.

Covino BG: Toxicity of local anesthetics. *Adv Anesth* 3:37-65, 1986.

Covino BG, Vassallo HG: *Local Anesthetics: Mechanisms of Action and Clinical Use.* New York, Grune & Stratton, 1976.

Gissen AJ, et al: Chloroprocaine controversy II. Is chloroprocaine neurotoxic? *Reg Anesth* 9:135-145, 1984.

Greene NM: Distribution of local anesthetic solutions within the subarachnoid space. *Anesth Analg* 64:715-730, 1985.

Greene NM: New look at sympathetic denervation during spinal anesthesia. *Anesthesiology* 65:137-138, 1986.

Hunt CO, et al: Perioperative analgesia with subarachnoid fentanyl-bupivacaine for cesarean delivery. *Anesthesiology* 71:535-540, 1989.

Jones G, et al: Comparison of bupivacaine and bupivacaine with fentanyl in continuous epidural analgesia during labor. *Br J Anaesth* 63:254-259, 1989.

Kamaya H, et al: Dissociation constants of local anesthetics and their temperature dependence. *Anesth Analg* 62:1025-1030, 1983.

Lambert DH: Factors influencing spinal anesthesia. *Int Anesthesiol Clin* 27:13-20, (Spring) 1989.

Marx GF: Cardiotoxicity of local anesthetics: The plot thickens. *Anesthesiology* 60:3-5, 1984.

Perkins FM: Pharmacokinetics of bupivacaine following prolonged administration. *Anesthesiology* 71(3A):A714, 1989.

Phillips GH: Epidural sufentanil/bupivacaine combinations for analgesia during labor: Effect of varying sufentanil doses. *Anesthesiology* 67:835-838, 1987.

Rothstein P, et al: Bupivacaine for intercostal nerve blocks in children: Blood concentrations and pharmacokinetics. *Anesth Analg* 65:625-632, 1986.

Scott DB: "Maximum recommended doses" of local anaesthetic drugs, editorial. *Br J Anaesth* 63:373-374, 1989.

Seifen AB, et al: Pharmacokinetics of intravenous procaine infusion in humans. *Anesth Analg* 58:382-386, 1979.

Stewart A, et al: Decreased incidence of tourniquet pain during spinal anesthesia with bupivacaine: A possible explanation. *Anesth Analg* 67:833-837, 1988.

Tucker GT, Mather LE: Properties, absorption, and disposition of local anesthetic agents, in Cousins MJ, Bridenbaugh PO (eds): *Neural Blockade in Clinical Anesthesia and Management of Pain,* ed 2. Philadelphia, JB Lippincott, 1988, 47-110.

Wang BC, et al: Chronic neurological deficits and Nesacaine-CE: Effect of the anesthetic, 2-chloroprocaine, or the antioxidant, sodium bisulfite? *Anesth Analg* 63:445-447, 1984.

Zsigmond EK, Kothary SP: *2-Chloroprocaine: Clinical Pharmacology, Pharmacokinetics and its Safety in Regional Anesthesia* (exhibit). International Anesthesia Research Society, Hollywood, Fla, March 11-15, 1979.

Other Selected References

Local anesthetic human prescription drugs class labeling guideline for professional labeling. *Federal Register Notice* 47 FR: 41636, September 21, 1982.

Katz RL (ed): Regional anesthesia. *Semin Anesth* 2:1-80, 1983.

Ralston DH, Shnider SM: Fetal and neonatal effects of regional anesthesia in obstetrics. *Anesthesiology* 48:34-64, 1978.

Yaster M, Maxwell LG: Pediatric regional anesthesia. *Anesthesiology* 70:324-338, 1989.

General Anesthetics

9

General anesthetics induce various degrees of analgesia; depression of consciousness, circulation, and respiration; relaxation of skeletal muscle; reduction of reflex activity; and amnesia. There are two types of general anesthetics, inhalation and intravenous. With either type, the arterial concentration of drug required to induce anesthesia varies with the condition of the patient, the desired depth of anesthesia, and the concomitant use of other drugs.

Anesthesia almost always is induced by administration of an intravenous anesthetic and maintained with an inhalation or intravenous agent or a combination. A muscle relaxant also may be required during induction for intubation of the trachea or during the intraoperative period. Thus, for most procedures, a number of drugs are administered. The concomitant use of certain inhalation and intravenous anesthetics, often in conjunction with opioid analgesics, neuroleptic drugs, or muscle relaxants, is referred to as combination anesthesia. Special types of combination anesthesia (ie, balanced anesthesia, neuroleptanesthesia) are discussed later in this chapter.

INHALATION ANESTHETICS. These are gases or volatile liquids that vary in the rate at which they induce anesthesia; potency; the degree of circulatory, respiratory, or neuromuscular depression they produce; and analgesic effects (see the Table). Inhalation anesthetics have advantages over intravenous agents in that the depth of anesthesia can be changed rapidly by altering the inhaled concentration. Because of their rapid elimination, any postoperative respiratory depression is of relatively short duration.

The rate at which the partial pressure of an inhalation anesthetic in the arterial blood approaches that in the inspired gas depends largely on the drug's solubility in blood (the blood gas partition coefficient at 37° C). When solubility is low, equilibrium is approached rapidly and induction, changes in anesthetic depth, and recovery times are rapid. The observed recovery time for halothane and methoxyflurane is more rapid than the partition coefficient would suggest. This may reflect an additional factor, the significant clearance by metabolism of these agents (Carpenter et al, 1986 A). The newest agent, desflurane, promises to give the best control among the volatile liquid agents because of its low solubility in blood (Tinker, 1992).

The clinical potency of an inhalation anesthetic is often defined in terms of MAC: the minimum alveolar concentration necessary to prevent movement in 50% of individuals subjected to a painful stimulus, usually skin incision. For clinical purposes, MAC is an additive function; thus, 0.5 MAC nitrous oxide plus 0.5 MAC halothane will suppress movement in 50% of patients subjected to a painful stimulus. The volatile anesthetics (volatility is expressed as vapor pressure [VP] in mm Hg at 20° C) usually are given with 40% to 70% nitrous oxide, which reduces the required dose of a volatile anesthetic. Anesthetic requirements (MAC) are not affected by the sex of the patient; the duration of the procedure; clinically

PHYSICAL CONSTANTS OF INHALATION ANESTHETIC AGENTS

	Anesthetic	Blood/Gas Partition Coefficient (37° C)	Minimum Alveolar Concentration (MAC) vols %	Vapor Pressure (mm Hg; 20° C)	Metabolism %*
VOLATILE LIQUIDS					
Hydrocarbon	Halothane [Fluothane]	2.54**	0.8	243	20
Ethers	Desflurane [Suprane]	0.424	7.3	669	0.02
	Enflurane [Ēthrane]	2.11**	1.7	172	2.4
	Isoflurane [Forane]	1.46**	1.2	240	0.17
	Methoxyflurane [Penthrane]	15.44**	0.2	23	50
GAS					
Inorganic	Nitrous Oxide	0.5	100†	gas	0

**Expressed as percent of absorbed anesthetic recovered as metabolites.*
***Eger and Eger, 1985*
†Hornbein et al, 1982

acceptable variations in the arterial pH, PaO_2, or $PaCO_2$; the basal metabolic rate; or the usual doses of atropine or scopolamine given preoperatively. MAC decreases with increasing age and also is reduced by hypothermia, pregnancy, hypotension (mean blood pressure, less than 40 to 50 mm Hg), and the concurrent administration of other central nervous system depressants (opioids, including those given intrathecally; sedative-hypnotics; or neuroleptic agents).

The only commercially available anesthetic *gas* is nitrous oxide. The *volatile liquids*, halothane [Fluothane], methoxyflurane [Penthrane], enflurane [Ēthrane], desflurane [Suprane], and isoflurane [Forane], are halogenated compounds. Methoxyflurane is employed only rarely as a general anesthetic, but it may be used as an on-demand, intermittent analgesic, particularly in obstetric patients.

INTRAVENOUS ANESTHETICS. The ultrashort-acting barbiturates, thiopental [Pentothal], methohexital [Brevital], and thiamylal [Surital], are used for induction. Loss of consciousness is rapid and induction is pleasant, but there is no muscle relaxation and reflexes frequently are not reduced adequately. Repeated administration results in accumulation and prolongs the recovery time. Since these agents have little if any analgesic activity, they are seldom used alone except in brief minor procedures.

Ketamine [Ketalar], a short-acting nonbarbiturate anesthetic, may be given intravenously or intramuscularly. It induces a dissociative state in which the patient may appear to be awake but is unconscious and does not respond to pain. Ketamine has been used in various diagnostic procedures; in brief, minor surgical procedures that do not require substantial skeletal muscle relaxation; and for changing dressings in burn patients. It also may be used as an induction agent, especially when cardiovascular or sympathetic depression is undesirable. When combined with nitrous oxide, diazepam [Valium] or lorazepam [Ativan], and a muscle relaxant, ketamine may be employed for major surgical procedures. Ketamine is not widely used, however, because it increases cerebral blood flow and postoperative hallucinations occur occasionally. The psychic disturbances during emergence can be reduced substantially by the administration of diazepam or midazolam [Versed] prior to ketamine induction (Ramasubramanian et al, 1988).

Diazepam and midazolam are benzodiazepines given intravenously for induction. Large doses produce amnesia that is useful, particularly in opioid/nitrous oxide anesthesia. These drugs are used alone to produce basal (conscious) sedation for diagnostic procedures (eg, endoscopy). Because it has a rapid onset, causes less pain during intravenous administration, and produces a lower incidence of thrombophlebitis, midazolam is replacing diazepam for this indication. Care must be exercised, however, for it has a greater propensity to produce respiratory depression and hypotension, particularly in older patients.

Etomidate [Amidate] may be given intravenously to induce anesthesia or as a supplement to nitrous oxide or an analgesic in combination anesthesia. It can be used as a substitute for thiopental in patients with asthma, severe cardiovascular disease, or peripheral circulatory failure. Because etomidate is metabolized by hydrolysis, presumably it could be used in patients with acute intermittent porphyria. This agent may find specific applications in neurosurgery because cerebral vascular flow and intracranial pressure are decreased.

Propofol [Diprivan] is the most recently introduced intravenous anesthetic. Advantages of propofol include rapid awakening and orientation, noncumulative action, and lack of suppression of steroidogenesis, which permit its use for long-term sedation in the intensive care unit. This drug's primary disadvantage is its pronounced hypotensive effect after induction dosage without a compensatory increase in heart rate; thus, its use is limited in patients with severe coronary artery disease, in hypovolemic patients, and in those classified as ASA III or IV patients. Although propofol has been employed satisfactorily for obstetric anesthesia and in children, dosages in these patients have not been established.

Opioids, particularly fentanyl [Sublimaze], sufentanil [Sufenta], or alfentanil [Alfenta], may be given with oxygen and muscle relaxants for induction and maintenance of anesthesia in selected high-risk patients (see the section on Combination Anesthesia).

Adverse Reactions and Precautions

INHALATION ANESTHETICS. Delirium may develop during induction and recovery, but drugs given for preanesthetic medication, particularly scopolamine, may be responsible. Gastroesophageal reflux or vomiting with aspiration may occur during induction, and nausea and vomiting may develop postoperatively.

Enflurane and halothane produce dose-related myocardial depression when present in useful anesthetic concentrations. Myocardial depression is less when isoflurane and nitrous oxide are used. Enflurane, isoflurane, desflurane, and nitrous oxide may increase the heart rate; halothane does not have this effect. Arrhythmias may develop during administration of any inhalation anesthetic. Supraventricular arrhythmias are common and usually benign except when cardiac output and arterial pressure are reduced. Loss of the P wave (junctional rhythm, nodal rhythm, isorhythmic AV dissociation) is very common during inhalation anesthesia. If myocardial function is borderline from any cause, decreased arterial pressure and cardiac output are likely. Therefore, the blood pressure should be determined immediately if the P wave disappears; conversely, a rapid fall in blood pressure requires immediate assessment of the electrocardiogram. Ventricular arrhythmias occur only rarely unless hypoxia or hypercapnia is present but are more likely to occur with use of the halogenated hydrocarbon, halothane, than with the ethers, enflurane, isoflurane, or methoxyflurane. Halothane sensitizes the heart to the actions of catecholamines. Therefore, use of epinephrine, norepinephrine [Levophed], or isoproterenol [Isuprel] during halothane anesthesia may increase the risk of ventricular arrhythmias. Drugs that indirectly stimulate sympathetic activity (eg, ephedrine) and the theophyllines (eg, aminophylline) also have been associated with arrhythmias during halothane anesthesia. Administration of halothane also may increase the risk of ventricular arrhythmias in patients with high levels of endogenous catecholamines (eg, pheochromocytoma, severe anxiety). Isoflurane, desflurane, and, to a lesser extent, enflurane reduce systemic vascular resistance; halothane has no effect. Isoflurane decreases coronary vascular resistance and may produce a steal of myocardial blood flow in patients with severe coronary artery disease. Whether this causes appreciable myocardial ischemia remains controversial.

Respiratory depression occurs at all levels of general anesthesia with inhalation anesthetics. At a given level, the most profound depression is produced by enflurane. Controlled ventilation is recommended if normocapnia must be assured. The ventilatory response to hypoxia is depressed by subanesthetic concentrations and is lost at anesthetic concentrations of all inhalation agents. The ventilatory response to hypercapnia is depressed at anesthetizing concentrations and is lost at 1.5 to 3 times MAC.

The cause of transient, slight abnormalities in the results of liver function tests is uncertain, but such changes are relatively common after any general anesthetic technique; serious liver damage is rare. All volatile anesthetics have been shown to decrease hepatic blood flow; this may have some relationship to the abnormal liver function postoperatively. Although halothane apparently is associated with hepatitis, no cause-and-effect relationship has been established and the diagnosis remains one of exclusion under normal circumstances (Stock and Strunin, 1985). Experimentally, the oxidative metabolism of the inhalational anesthetics (halothane >> enflurane >> isoflurane) leads to the formation of immunoreactive protein complexes. These proteins, acting as antigens, may induce an immune response against the liver. There is a suggestion that sensitization to halothane may result in cross-sensitization to enflurane (Christ et al, 1988; Hubbard et al, 1988).

Reversible oliguria results from reduced renal blood flow and glomerular filtration during general anesthesia. This may be minimized if the patient is hydrated adequately and deep levels of anesthesia are avoided. However, methoxyflurane can produce direct, dose-related tubular injury with high-output renal failure and is contraindicated in patients with impaired renal function and in those receiving other potentially nephrotoxic agents (eg, aminoglycosides, tetracyclines). Because this complication is dose related and caused by the free fluoride ion produced by metabolism of the drug, methoxyflurane must be administered in diminishing concentrations during prolonged procedures. In comparison to methoxyflurane, enflurane produces substantially less free fluoride ion, isoflurane and desflurane produce minimal amounts, and halothane produces essentially none. Metabolism of enflurane may be increased appreciably in patients taking isoniazid.

Body temperature tends to fall during anesthesia because of exposure, vasodilation, and suppression of thermoregulation. However, the postoperative shivering or tremor commonly seen after anesthesia with the potent inhalation agents does not resemble thermoregulatory shivering (Sessler et al, 1988). Various mechanisms have been suggested (Sessler et al, 1988; Hammel, 1988). Risks with postanesthetic shivering-like activity include hypoxia, wound dehiscence, and dental damage.

Malignant hyperthermia is a rare, often fatal complication that may be triggered by the potent inhalation anesthetics in genetically susceptible individuals (see index entry Adjuncts to Anesthesia for a more detailed discussion).

Nitrous oxide, enflurane, halothane, isoflurane, desflurane, and methoxyflurane elevate intracranial pressure by increasing cerebral blood flow, but this appears to be significant only in patients with intracranial lesions. Halothane increases cerebral blood flow more than enflurane or isoflurane. Cerebral autoregulation is lost during halothane anesthesia but not during isoflurane anesthesia. Hypocapnia induced by hyperventilation usually eliminates the increase in intracranial pressure, most reliably during isoflurane anesthesia. Patients with intracranial lesions should not receive halothane until measures to produce hyperventilation have been instituted. In contrast, isoflurane can be administered at the same time that hyperventilation is instituted. Enflurane should be used with care in these patients, because it may produce seizures in the presence of hypocapnia; convulsions are less likely if concentrations are maintained below 1.5% to 2%. Thiopental constricts cerebral vessels and also may be used to attenuate the increase in intracranial pressure during the use of volatile anesthetics.

Although enflurane, halothane, isoflurane, and nitrous oxide were teratogenic in some animal studies, they are not known to affect the human fetus. However, it is inadvisable to administer these agents during the first trimester unless such use is unavoidable. General anesthesia per se is not teratogenic. Neonatal depression can be anticipated if high concentrations of potent inhalation agents are administered during a prolonged delivery. However, general anesthesia is not used routinely for vaginal deliveries because of the advantages of regional anesthesia in this situation. During cesarean section, fetal exposure to anesthesia is generally very short. Nitrous oxide does not relax uterine muscle or increase uterine bleeding. Anesthetizing concentrations of enflurane, halothane, and isoflurane relax the uterus and may increase postpartum bleeding. Equipotent doses of volatile anesthetics have the same effect. Volatile anesthetic concentrations ranging from 0.5 to 1.5 MAC produced no significant change in myometrial contractility or response to oxytocics (Paull and Ziccone, 1980). The use of high concentrations of volatile anesthetics for uterine surgery during the first trimester of pregnancy (eg, dilation and curettage) also is associated with increased blood loss.

The dose of nondepolarizing neuromuscular blocking agents (tubocurarine, metocurine [Metubine], pancuronium [Pavulon], atracurium [Tracrium], vecuronium [Norcuron], and gallamine [Flaxedil]) should be reduced when these agents are used with the volatile anesthetics because the latter potentiate the muscle relaxant effects. Halothane is the least and enflurane, isoflurane, and desflurane are the most potent in this regard.

INTRAVENOUS ANESTHETICS. Yawning, coughing, and laryngeal spasm may occur during induction of anesthesia with barbiturates. Hypotension may develop, particularly in hypovolemic patients or in those with diminished cardiac contractility. Undesirably light anesthesia due to rapid redistribution from the central nervous system can occur, particularly in young patients. Pronounced respiratory depression and apnea usually develop immediately after rapid injection of anesthetic dosages. Shivering or excitement and delirium in the presence of pain may be observed during recovery.

The barbiturates may exacerbate acute intermittent porphyria and are *contraindicated* in patients with this disease. Care should be taken to avoid extravasation or intra-arterial injection of these drugs, particularly thiopental, for tissue necrosis and gangrene caused by their extreme alkalinity may occur.

See the evaluations for adverse reactions and precautions to be observed with the nonbarbiturate anesthetics.

Drug Evaluations

INHALATION ANESTHETICS

Gas

NITROUS OXIDE

ACTIONS AND USES. Nitrous oxide (blood/gas solubility, 0.5; MAC, 104% at one atmosphere) (Hornbein et al, 1982) is nonexplosive, but combustible items will burn in nitrous oxide. It must always be administered with at least 25% to 30% oxygen during induction and maintenance. Induction with 70% nitrous oxide is facilitated by premedication with an opioid analgesic or barbiturate.

For surgical anesthesia, nitrous oxide must be supplemented with other agents (eg, thiopental, benzodiazepines, opioid analgesics, more potent inhalation agents). It reduces the requirement for other inhalation anesthetics, and thus is included as one of the inhalation agents in most patients undergoing general anesthesia. A neuromuscular blocking agent often is given concomitantly if muscle relaxation is necessary.

Nitrous oxide has good analgesic properties and thus is useful in the second stage of labor. It also is employed as a sedative in regional anesthesia with local anesthetics.

ADVERSE REACTIONS AND PRECAUTIONS. Serious adverse effects on the cardiovascular or ventilatory systems, liver, kidneys, or metabolic function rarely occur when the inhalation mixture contains an adequate concentration of oxygen and ventilation is maintained. Severe hypotension may occur when hypovolemia, shock, or significant heart disease exists. Nitrous oxide may be detrimental to patients with pulmonary vascular occlusive disease.

Because nitrous oxide is 35 times more soluble in blood than nitrogen, more nitrous oxide diffuses into a closed air-containing cavity than nitrogen diffuses out. If the cavity has rigid walls, the pressure within it rises; if the cavity does not have rigid walls, the volume increases. Therefore, nitrous oxide should be used with extreme caution in the presence of conditions such as air embolism, pneumothorax, pulmonary air cysts, or acute intestinal obstruction and during or after recent pneumoencephalography. Nitrous oxide should not be employed in patients in whom poorly soluble gases (sulfur hexafluoride, nitrogen [in air], or a mixture of these) is injected into the vitreal cavity of the eye during retinal reattachment surgery (Stinson and Donlon, 1982). Because nitrous oxide also can diffuse into the cuff of the endotracheal tube, periodic deflation is recommended. To avoid the diffusion hypoxia that may develop after discontinuing prolonged anesthesia with nitrous oxide, oxygen should be employed briefly during emergence and during recovery.

Recovery from anesthesia is rapid unless large doses of supplemental agents have been used. Postoperative nausea and vomiting may occur in a substantial number of patients. The observation that nausea and vomiting occur more frequently if nitrous oxide is used to supplement a more potent anesthetic is controversial (Kottila et al, 1987; Muir et al, 1987; Melnick and Johnson, 1987).

Nitrous oxide inactivates the vitamin B_{12} cofactor of methionine synthase; thus, serum tetrahydrofolate and methionine concentrations are reduced during and after anesthesia. The reduction of tetrahydrofolate can cause leukopenia and megaloblastic anemia. Frequent repeated exposure to nitrous oxide can cause neurologic injury, and this mechanism may be responsible for the fetotoxic action of nitrous oxide in operating room personnel (Nunn, 1984). In an extensive survey of dental personnel exposed to nitrous oxide as the sole inhalational anesthetic and in whom exposure is greater than would be experienced in a hospital operating room, an increase in spontaneous abortion was noted in both the wives of the dentists and in female chairside assistants; there was no increase, however, in the number of birth defects (Cohen et al, 1980). Nitrous oxide should not be used to produce analgesia or light narcosis for longer than 48 hours (eg, in patients receiving artificial ventilation). However, the use of nitrous oxide anesthesia in prolonged surgical procedures, up to 13 hours, is not associated with leukopenia (Tyson et al, 1987).

DOSAGE AND PREPARATIONS.

Inhalation: There is considerable variability in response to nitrous oxide. Generally, sedation is produced by nitrous oxide 25%, analgesia requires 25% to 50%, and laryngeal incompetence may develop with use of the 50% concentration. For maintenance, 30% to 70% nitrous oxide may be used, depending on the patient's condition and the type and amount of supplemental agents used. Because of its low potency, nitrous oxide cannot be used as the sole agent for induction without large doses of a narcotic for premedication.

Generic. Available in metal cylinders color-coded with blue paint.

Volatile Liquids

DESFLURANE

[Suprane]

```
     F   H       F
     |   |       |
 F — C — C — O — C — H
     |   |       |
     F   F       F
```

ACTIONS AND USES. This new inhalation anesthetic, the first to become available in almost 20 years (Tinker, 1992), is a nonflammable liquid administered via a special heated vaporizer (Saidman, 1991). Structurally, it differs from isoflurane only in having a fluorine atom substituted for the chlorine atom in the isoflurane molecule. Desflurane is a chemically stable, colorless, volatile liquid below 22.8° C.

The MAC of desflurane in young (25 years) adults is 7.3% (Rampil et al, 1991 A) and decreases with increasing age or in combination with opioids or benzodiazepines. The VP is 660 mm Hg at 20° C with a blood/gas solubility of 0.424 at 37° C (Fletcher et al, 1991).

Desflurane has respiratory irritant properties that can produce secretions, coughing, breath holding, apnea, and laryngospasm during the inhalational induction in both children and adults (Taylor et al, 1990; Rampil et al, 1991 A; Van Hamelrijck et al, 1991; Wrigley et al, 1991). This probably will limit its use as an induction agent (Lerman, 1991). Administration of intravenous induction agents plus desflurane for maintenance results in a smoother anesthetic course.

A rapid wash in and wash out profile produces fast changes in the anesthetic depth or level and an impression, on the part of the anesthesiologist, of good "control" of the agent and patient status. Rapid induction and emergence were observed with concentrations of 3% to 7% (Wrigley et al, 1991) in a nitrous oxide/oxygen mixture. Loss of eyelash reflex occurred in 1.6 to 2 minutes. The wash in was faster for desflurane (0.91) than for isoflurane (0.74) and halothane (0.58). The wash out at five minutes also was more rapid for desflurane (0.12) than for isoflurane (0.22) and halothane (0.25). Recovery/emergence times following cessation of desflurane (1 MAC or less/oxygen anesthesia until patients opened their eyes and responded verbally) was five to seven minutes (Ghouri et al, 1991; Wrigley et al, 1991). "Street-ready" or "home-ready" time was about the same as with propofol anesthesia (average, 3.3 hours). Recovery/emergence time was reported to be more prolonged when intravenous agents (ie, sodium pentothal, fentanyl and propofol) were used with desflurane (Fletcher et al, 1991).

ADVERSE REACTIONS, PRECAUTIONS, AND DRUG INTERACTIONS. As with other volatile anesthetics, the effects of desflurane potentiate the action of neuromuscular blocking drugs, and the dose of the latter should be reduced when they are used with desflurane (Caldwell et al, 1991).

Desflurane increases the heart rate and decreases arterial pressure and systemic vascular resistance. Cardiac output tends to remain stable. In general, the hemodynamic effects during induction and maintenance anesthesia are the same as those of isoflurane (Cahalan et al, 1991). Desflurane, like other volatile anesthetics, can increase cerebral blood flow and intracranial pressure.

Headaches have been reported following desflurane anesthesia (Rampil et al, 1991 B). Compared with propofol, the duration of psychomotor impairment following surgery was less. There was, however, a higher incidence of nausea and vomiting with desflurane than with propofol anesthesia (Ghouri et al, 1991; Wrigley et al, 1991).

Malignant hyperthermia was observed in a genetically susceptible pig model (Wedel et al, 1991). Although no cases in humans have been reported at this time, it is recommended that desflurane not be used for patients who have a history of malignant hyperthermia or expected susceptibility to the syndrome. No cases of nephrotoxicity have been reported. Desflurane may be less likely to induce tissue toxicity, since its biotransformation to fluoride metabolites is minimal (0.02%) (Sutton et al, 1991). Results of liver function studies after desflurane anesthesia reveal no evidence of hepatotoxicity (Jones et al, 1990; Ray and Drummond, 1991).

The safety of desflurane during pregnancy and delivery has not been established (FDA Pregnancy Category B). When this anesthetic is used during therapeutic abortion, blood loss may be increased due to smooth muscle relaxation.

DOSAGE AND PREPARATIONS.

Inhalation: For induction, the concentration of anesthetic must be individualized based on the patient's responses. In *adults*, a frequent initial concentration is 3% desflurane, with incremental increases of 0.5% to 1% every two to three breaths to concentrations of 4% to 11% with and without concomitant nitrous oxide. For maintenance, surgical levels of anesthesia can be provided by concentrations of 2.5% to 8.5% desflurane with or without nitrous oxide. In *children*, surgical levels of anesthesia may be maintained with concentrations of 5.2% to 10% with or without nitrous oxide.

Suprane (Anaquest). Liquid in 240 ml containers.

ENFLURANE

[Ēthrane]

```
 F  F F
 |  | |
HCOCCH
 |  | |
 F  F Cl
```

ACTIONS, USES, AND INTERACTIONS. Enflurane (VP, 172 mm Hg; blood/gas solubility, 2.11; MAC, 1.7%) is a nonflammable, halogenated ether anesthetic that provides rapid induction with little or no excitement. The rapidity of induction, however, may be limited due to breath holding or coughing caused by the pungency of this agent. Although salivary and bronchial secretions are increased slightly, use of atropine-like drugs for premedication is not essential. Enflurane, like halothane and isoflurane, dilates constricted bronchial muscles and is useful in the management of asthmatic patients or patients with chronic obstructive pulmonary disease in whom there is a bronchospastic component. To avoid the cardiovascular depression and central nervous system stimulation produced by high concentrations, this agent usually is given in a low concentration (1% to 2%) with nitrous oxide. Enflurane provides better muscle relaxation than halothane. Neuromuscular blocking agents may be used to enhance the muscle relaxation, but the usual dosage of nondepolarizing drugs must be reduced significantly (see index entry Neuromuscular Blocking Drugs).

With low concentrations, the cardiovascular system remains relatively stable, although blood pressure is often reduced and the pulse rate is increased; cardiac rhythm is only slightly affected. Results of some studies in humans suggest that this anesthetic does not sensitize the heart to catecholamines; however, other studies show that enflurane does sensitize the heart but considerably less than does halothane. Enflurane has been used during resection of pheochromocytoma, and it appears to be useful when increased catecholamine concentrations are anticipated.

Enflurane 1% with nitrous oxide, oxygen, and controlled ventilation significantly decreases intraocular pressure and is useful for eye surgery.

Relaxation of the uterus is dose related, but concentrations below 3% do not prevent the uterine response to oxytocic agents. Analgesic concentrations (0.25% to 1.25%) do not interrupt spontaneous uterine activity or produce excessive bleeding.

Enflurane is suitable for both induction and maintenance of anesthesia in children, although most anesthesiologists find that its pungency makes this anesthetic less acceptable than halothane.

Recovery from anesthesia is usually very rapid and uneventful; postoperative tremor is relatively common, but restlessness, delirium, nausea, and vomiting are infrequent. The speed of recovery may necessitate the earlier administration of larger doses of analgesics to relieve postoperative pain.

ADVERSE REACTIONS AND PRECAUTIONS. Enflurane causes profound respiratory depression. The ventilatory rate remains essentially constant or slightly elevated, but the tidal volume is decreased with resulting depression of minute volume. In adults, spontaneous ventilation may be sufficient at light levels of anesthesia but, as the depth increases, controlled ventilation is required to avoid hypercapnia.

Transient, slight abnormalities in the results of liver function tests similar to those observed after use of other volatile anesthetics have been noted. There have been several reports of hepatic damage related to enflurane anesthesia, but analysis of these cases does not support a causal relationship.

The clinical implications of the biotransformation of enflurane to free fluoride ion require further study. Plasma concentrations of fluoride ion are considerably below the nephrotoxic threshold in normal individuals, but may approach toxic levels in patients receiving isoniazid. The renal excretion of fluoride ion is promoted by an alkaline urine.

Central nervous system stimulation, manifested by increased electrical activity and seizure-like electroencephalographic patterns, occurs as anesthesia deepens; these changes usually appear when inspired concentrations exceed 3%. Paroxysms of tonic-clonic or twitching movements of the facial muscles and extremities develop in a few patients, usually in association with deep anesthesia *and* hypocapnia. These can be terminated without sequelae by lightening anesthesia and reducing minute ventilation or by substituting another anesthetic agent. Children are more sensitive to this effect and may exhibit grand mal seizures at concentrations in excess of 4%. These seizures are not harmful if oxygenation is sustained. Seizure activity is not exacerbated in patients with pre-existing convulsive disorders if normocapnia is maintained.

This anesthetic agent is classified in FDA Pregnancy Category B.

DOSAGE AND PREPARATIONS.

Inhalation: For induction, 2% to 4.5% vaporized by a flow of oxygen or a nitrous oxide-oxygen mixture. Generally, a 0.5% to 3% concentration is administered for maintenance.

Ēthrane (Anaquest). Liquid in 125 and 250 ml containers.

HALOTHANE
[Fluothane]

$$CF_3CH(Br)Cl$$

ACTIONS, USES, AND INTERACTIONS. Halothane (VP, 243 mm Hg; blood/gas solubility, 2.54; MAC, 0.8%) is a nonflammable, halogenated, hydrocarbon anesthetic that provides relatively rapid induction with little or no excitement. Analgesia may not be adequate. Nitrous oxide is generally given concomitantly. Because halothane may not produce sufficient muscle relaxation, supplemental neuromuscular blocking agents may be required.

Halothane is far less irritating to the respiratory tract than enflurane or isoflurane. It depresses pharyngeal and laryngeal reflexes, dilates the bronchioles, and reduces salivation and bronchial secretions. It depresses the depth of respiration, produces tachypnea, and increases the alveolar-arterial oxygen difference; controlled ventilation may be needed to avoid respiratory acidosis.

Halothane diminishes sympathetic activity, augments vagal tone, depresses the contractility of the heart, and induces venodilation. Cardiac output, arterial pressure, and pulse rate are reduced, usually in proportion to the depth of anesthesia. Severe hypotension and circulatory failure may occur with overdosage. Supraventricular arrhythmias or nodal rhythm may be observed during induction or deep anesthesia. Small doses of epinephrine (1 to 1.5 mcg/kg) may be administered subcutaneously or submucosally with halothane when adequate ventilation is assured. Exceeding this dose is potentially hazardous, however, since this anesthetic sensitizes the heart to catecholamines. The administration of lidocaine during epinephrine use decreases the risk of arrhythmias.

Transient, slight abnormalities in the results of liver function tests have been observed after a single administration. The changes are similar to those noted following administration of other anesthetics, all of which decrease hepatic blood flow, but the abnormalities are noted more frequently than with enflurane or isoflurane. Although many cases of liver damage, ranging from mild hepatitis to massive hepatic necrosis, have been reported after such use, the incidence of unexplained cases of massive hepatic necrosis is about 1 in 35,000 anesthetic administrations. There is evidence suggesting that liver damage is more likely to develop if there is intraoperative or postoperative hypoxia. Halothane should not be given to patients who developed jaundice or acute liver damage after previous exposure to this drug unless other obvious causes for the hepatic damage have been demonstrated. It also may be unwise to give halothane to patients who developed a similar response after exposure to methoxyflurane and possibly to other halogenated anesthetics, although there is no evidence to substantiate this precaution.

Dose-dependent, reversible effects on the kidney (eg, decreased renal blood flow, glomerular filtration rate, and urine volume) have been observed during anesthesia, particularly in dehydrated patients or those with intraoperative hypotension. No significant metabolic disturbances have been noted. Renal oxygen consumption is reduced.

Controlled studies have indicated that low concentrations of halothane may increase uterine hemorrhage when this agent is used during therapeutic abortions in early pregnancy. Concentrations of halothane above 0.5% relax the uterus, thus inhibiting natural or induced uterine contractions and delaying delivery. Concentrations above 1% interfere with the action of the oxytocic drugs, oxytocin and ergonovine, and considerable uterine hemorrhage may occur.

Recovery from anesthesia is usually rapid and uneventful, although usually less rapid than with enflurane and isoflurane. Postoperative tremor is common. Restlessness, delirium, nausea, and vomiting are infrequent.

DOSAGE AND PREPARATIONS.

Inhalation: For induction, a 1% to 4% concentration vaporized by a flow of oxygen or a nitrous oxide-oxygen mixture. For maintenance, a 0.5% to 2% concentration.

Generic. Liquid in 250 ml containers.

Fluothane (Wyeth-Ayerst). Liquid in 125 and 250 ml containers.

ISOFLURANE
[Forane]

$$HCF_2—O—CHClCF_3$$

ACTIONS AND USES. Isoflurane (VP, 240 mm Hg; blood/gas solubility, 1.46; MAC, 1.2%) is a nonflammable, halogenated ether anesthetic. Although it is a structural isomer of enflurane, there are many pharmacologic differences between the two agents.

This anesthetic has a pungent odor, which limits the rate of increase in the inspired concentration that is acceptable to the patient; coughing and breath holding may occur. Induction is smoother and excitement is decreased when premedication is given and when nitrous oxide and oxygen are administered concomitantly. However, induction is more often accomplished with intravenous agents. Relaxation of the jaw, although not as profound as with halothane, is satisfactory for endotracheal intubation. The effects of nondepolarizing neuromuscular blocking drugs are markedly potentiated in the presence of isoflurane; therefore, their dose must be reduced by one-third to two-thirds (see index entry Neuromuscular Blocking Drugs).

With concentrations of 1 to 2 MAC, limited myocardial depression is observed in normocapnic patients. Reduction of blood pressure is dose related and secondary to peripheral vasodilation rather than decreased cardiac output. There is little tendency to develop arrhythmias and the myocardium is not sensitized to catecholamines. The pulse rate may increase, and occasional patients experience tachycardia that is not suppressed by increasing the concentration of isoflurane. After ruling out hypoxia or malignant hyperthermia and providing adequate fluid replacement, the pulse rate usually can be decreased with small doses of an opioid (eg, fentanyl 0.1 mg, morphine 8 to 10 mg), using care to compensate for the greater ventilatory depression.

Depression of minute volume can be counteracted by adjusting the dose. Controlled ventilation may be required to assure normocapnia and is required for hypocapnia.

Isoflurane is metabolized minimally; the major metabolites are trifluoroacetic acid and fluoride ion in a ratio of about 2:1. In one study, serum fluoride ion concentrations were dose related (maximum, 5.5 micromoles [mcM]/L). In another study, serum fluoride ion concentrations at the end of anesthesia averaged 3.6 mcM/L (maximum, 12 mcM/L). In comparative studies, methoxyflurane produced serum fluoride ion concentrations as high as 200 mcM/L (average, 60 mcM/L) and enflurane produced concentrations as high as 80 mcM/L (average, 20 mcM/L). Laboratory evidence of subtle defects in renal concentrating ability occurs at serum fluoride ion concentrations above 50 mcM/L, and overt damage is observed at concentrations greater than approximately 100 mcM/L. There is no evidence of renal dysfunction following use of isoflurane. Likewise, no alterations in hepatic function due to isoflurane itself have been observed.

Unlike enflurane, no central nervous system stimulation is evident with deep anesthesia. Isoflurane increases cerebral blood flow at concentrations exceeding 1.1 MAC and may increase intracranial pressure. However, hyperventilation may be used to decrease cerebral blood flow and pressure since hypocapnia does not induce seizure activity during isoflurane anesthesia. At 1 MAC, cerebral blood flow is significantly greater with halothane. Autoregulation of cerebral blood flow is maintained with isoflurane but not with halothane. Cerebral protrusion is less with isoflurane or enflurane than with halothane. Increases in blood pressure minimally increase brain protrusion during isoflurane or enflurane anesthesia, whereas increases in blood pressure may more than double brain protrusion during halothane anesthesia. The cerebral metabolic rate is decreased by 30% to 50%; this decrease is directly proportional to the concentration of isoflurane. Therefore, isoflurane may be preferable for neurosurgery when an inhalation anesthetic is required.

The safety of isoflurane during pregnancy and delivery has not been established (FDA Pregnancy Category C). Analgesic concentrations of 0.3% to 0.7% do not depress the frequency or force of uterine contractions or increase maternal blood loss.

Mental alertness is depressed for two to three hours after anesthesia; however, postoperative nausea, vomiting, and excitation are uncommon.

DOSAGE AND PREPARATIONS.

Inhalation: For induction, a 1.5% to 3% concentration vaporized in oxygen or in a nitrous oxide-oxygen mixture. Concentrations between 0.5% and 3% are satisfactory for maintenance. Rarely is more than 3% required when isoflurane is given with oxygen alone.

Forane (Anaquest). Liquid containing no additives or chemical stabilizers in 100 ml containers.

METHOXYFLURANE

[Penthrane]

$$\begin{array}{cc} \text{Cl} & \text{F} \\ | & | \\ \text{HC} - & \text{COCH}_3 \\ | & | \\ \text{Cl} & \text{F} \end{array}$$

ACTIONS AND USES. Currently, methoxyflurane is rarely used for surgical, obstetric, or dental anesthesia. If so employed, it should be administered with nitrous oxide to achieve a relatively light level of anesthesia, and a neuromuscular blocking agent usually is given concurrently to obtain the desired degree of muscular relaxation. The upper MAC-hour limit described (see Precautions) should be observed. Since methoxyflurane augments the neuromuscular blocking effects of nondepolarizing muscle relaxants, the dose of the latter should be markedly reduced (see index entry Neuromuscular Blocking Agents).

ADVERSE REACTIONS, PRECAUTIONS, AND INTERACTIONS. Methoxyflurane depresses the cardiovascular system to approximately the same degree as halothane. Cardiac contractility is reduced and cardiac output and arterial pressure are decreased in proportion to the concentration of inhaled vapor. The heart rate is relatively unchanged, although atropine-responsive sinus bradycardia may occur and nodal escape rhythm may develop during deep anesthesia. The drug may sensitize the heart to catecholamines and may stimulate the sympathetic nervous system if adequate ventilation and depth of anesthesia are not maintained.

Methoxyflurane should not be administered to patients who developed acute unexplained liver damage after previous exposure to this drug. It also may be unwise to give methoxyflurane to patients who responded similarly to halothane.

This anesthetic should not be used in patients with renal damage, since impaired renal function has been associated with its use. The symptoms are usually those of vasopressin-resistant, high-output renal failure and include output of a large volume of dilute urine; dehydration; weight loss; increased serum osmolality; significantly increased blood sodium, urea nitrogen, and creatinine levels; elevated serum and urine concentrations of inorganic fluoride; and increased excretion of oxalic acid. Some patients develop oliguric renal failure, a few develop chronic renal failure, and, rarely, a patient dies. High-output renal failure is dose related and is caused by the free fluoride ion produced by metabolism of the drug; fluoride ion interferes with sodium transport necessary for concentrating urine and also may render the appropriate renal tubules unresponsive to antidiuretic hormone.

The severity of nephrotoxicity depends primarily on the dose (ie, concentration and time or MAC-hours) of methoxyflurane and secondarily on the degree of metabolism, the presence of enzyme induction (eg, from barbiturates), and variations in sensitivity to fluoride ion. Subclinical nephropathy occurs after about 2.5 MAC-hours of methoxyflurane, which results in about 50 to 60 mcM/L serum fluoride. As much as 75% of methoxyflurane taken up during the course of anesthesia is metabolized by the liver (Carpenter et al, 1986 B).

Normal arterial pressure does *not* indicate that a light level of anesthesia is being maintained. Methoxyflurane should not be given to patients receiving other potentially nephrotoxic drugs (eg, aminoglycosides, tetracyclines), because concurrent use of these agents has been associated with irreversible renal failure.

Nausea and vomiting may occur postoperatively. Recovery from anesthesia is prolonged, but there is a good analgesic effect in the immediate postoperative period.

This anesthetic is classified in FDA Pregnancy Category C.

DOSAGE AND PREPARATIONS.

Inhalation: For analgesia, 0.3% to 0.8% in air. A draw-over device is acceptable when the drug is inhaled only to produce analgesia. It may be wise to limit the amount of drug used for self-administration during labor to 15 ml.

An intravenous agent should be used for induction of anesthesia. For maintenance, at least 50% nitrous oxide is employed and supplemental neuromuscular blocking agents are used, if required, so that the lowest effective total dose of methoxyflurane is given. See the manufacturer's literature for tables indicating stepwise dose reductions with exposure duration. Since subclinical nephrotoxicity has been detected after the administration of one MAC (0.16%) for 2.5 hours, *the total dose of methoxyflurane should not exceed this MAC-hour limit.* This restricts this drug's usefulness to relatively few indications.

When methoxyflurane is administered to produce anesthesia, a vaporizer calibrated for methoxyflurane must be used, and it must be placed outside the anesthesia delivery circle.

Penthrane (Abbott). Liquid in 15 and 125 ml containers. Also available for self-administered analgesia by inhaler (***Analgizer***).

INTRAVENOUS ANESTHETICS

Barbiturates

THIOPENTAL SODIUM
[Pentothal]

H O N S^- CH_3CH_2 N Na^+ $CH_3CH_2CH_2CH$ O CH_3

ACTIONS AND USES. This ultrashort-acting barbiturate is useful to induce general anesthesia, since loss of consciousness occurs within 30 to 60 seconds after intravenous administration. Thiopental usually is not employed for maintenance (even with nitrous oxide) for procedures lasting longer than 15 to 20 minutes, because the cumulative dose results in delayed awakening. It has poor analgesic properties. The use of nitrous oxide 67% decreases requirements for thiopental by two-thirds. Depending on the type of surgery, opioid analgesics and neuromuscular blocking agents also may be required. Usual doses have no significant effects at the myoneural junction. Uterine muscle tone is not affected.

Although this anesthetic may be administered rectally for basal sedation or anesthesia, absorption of a thiopental suspension from the rectum is unpredictable.

ADVERSE REACTIONS AND PRECAUTIONS. In some instances, the arterial pressure is only slightly affected by thiopental. Frequently, a reduction in cardiac output and arterial pressure caused by myocardial depression and peripheral vasodilation occurs immediately after rapid intravenous injection of enough thiopental to produce deep anesthesia. In hypovolemic patients and those with myocardial disease or untreated hypertension, the drug must be administered more slowly, in dilute solution, and incrementally, if at all.

Thiopental is a potent respiratory depressant, and apnea frequently occurs immediately after intravenous injection, particularly in the presence of hypovolemia, cranial trauma, or preanesthetic medication with opioid drugs. Tidal volume is depressed to a greater extent than the respiratory rate. Respiratory depression may be prolonged in patients with myasthenia gravis.

Rapid redistribution of thiopental out of the brain can result in light anesthesia characterized in part by reflex hyperactivity of the airway to mechanical stimulation (eg, intubation, instrumentation, secretions, blood). Therefore, an adequate depth of anesthesia should be assured in asthmatic patients sensitive to bronchospasm; in those with upper airway obstruction; when coughing, hiccupping, or straining is undesirable; and to avoid laryngospasm, which might otherwise occur at any time from direct or indirect stimulation (eg, rectal dilation). Introduction of an artificial airway or painful stimulus also may cause hypertension and tachycardia in lightly anesthetized patients. This may increase myocardial oxygen demand profoundly, which is undesirable in patients with coronary artery disease.

Transient, slight alterations in the results of liver function tests similar to those observed following administration of other anesthetics may occur after use of thiopental. Pre-existing liver disease is not a contraindication to the usual induction dose.

Thiopental decreases urine output by reducing perfusion pressure, constricting renal arteries, and releasing antidiuretic hormone, but it does not cause renal damage.

Thiopental is contraindicated in patients with acute intermittent porphyria or other hepatic porphyrias.

Anaphylaxis has been reported following injection of thiopental, but this response is *very* rare. It is associated most often with prior exposure to the agent. Thiopental-reactive IgE antibodies can be demonstrated following anaphylaxis. Thiopental frequently causes histamine release resulting in truncal flushing.

Care should be taken to avoid extravasation or intra-arterial injection, for neuritis and skin slough may occur with the former (especially with concentrations exceeding 25 mg/ml) and arteritis, followed by vasospasm, edema, thrombosis, and gangrene, with the latter. Damage is reduced when dilute solutions are administered; concentrations should not exceed 2.5%. Intra-arterial injection usually produces immediate intense pain prior to loss of consciousness. The injection must be discontinued immediately and a vasodilator (eg, nitroprusside) or a local anesthetic without epinephrine (eg, lidocaine) must be injected locally (preferably through the needle used for the thiopental). If the needle has been removed from the artery, the vasodilator should be injected into the subclavian artery, since the affected artery will be in spasm. Local injection of heparin may reduce thrombosis, and sympathetic block or general anesthesia with halothane may relieve pain and vascular spasm and assist in opening collateral circulation. Infiltration of the area with a local anesthetic not containing epinephrine (eg, 1% lidocaine) may ameliorate the consequences of extravasation.

Consciousness returns rapidly unless large doses have been given. Postoperative nausea and vomiting are uncommon, but shivering occurs often and excitement and delirium may develop during recovery in the presence of pain.

This drug is classified in FDA Pregnancy Category C.

PHARMACOKINETICS. The duration of unconsciousness after a single dose of thiopental is determined by the rate of redistribution from the central nervous system into muscle. Factors that diminish blood flow into muscle (eg, hypovolemia) delay awakening. Thiopental is almost completely metabolized (more than 99%) in the liver. The half-life is 11.5 hours, the apparent volume of distribution at steady state is 1.4 L/kg, and the clearance is 150 ml/min. These values are increased during pregnancy; at term, the half-life is 26.1 hours, the apparent volume of distribution is 4.1 L/kg, and the clearance rate is 286 ml/min (Morgan et al, 1981). The elimination half-life in pediatric patients is one-half that in adults; the clearance values are 6.6 ml/kg/min in children and 3.1 ml/kg/min in adults (Sorbo et al, 1984). Morbid obesity markedly increases the volume of distribution to 7.9 L/kg and the half-life to 27.85 hours (Jung et al, 1982).

DOSAGE AND PREPARATIONS.

Intravenous: The dose required to induce and maintain anesthesia varies with premedication, concurrent nitrous oxide administration, physical status, pre-existing disease, and adequacy of the respiratory and circulatory systems. Sex and weight have little effect on thiopental requirements. Adherence to a strict "usual" dose regimen is discouraged. Tolerance has been reported following repeated use (eg, in burn patients).

For induction, *adults,* after a 2-ml test dose of a freshly prepared 2.5% solution, a single injection of 3 to 5 mg/kg is given. A few clinicians prefer to inject 50 to 100 mg intermittently every 30 to 40 seconds until the desired effect is obtained. For maintenance, 50 to 100 mg of a 2.5% solution is injected as required. *Children 5 to 15 years,* a 2.5% solution is injected at 30-second intervals. The total dose for induction is 4 to 5 mg/kg in relatively healthy, unpremedicated patients. For maintenance, the usual total dose for *children weighing 30 to 50 kg* is 25 to 50 mg injected intermittently.

Pentothal (Abbott), ***Generic.*** Powder (for solution) 0.25, 0.4, 0.5, 1, 2.5, and 5 g.

Rectal: For basal anesthesia in *children,* 30 mg/kg in a 40% suspension.

Pentothal (Abbott). Suspension 400 mg/g in 2 g containers.

METHOHEXITAL SODIUM

[Brevital Sodium]

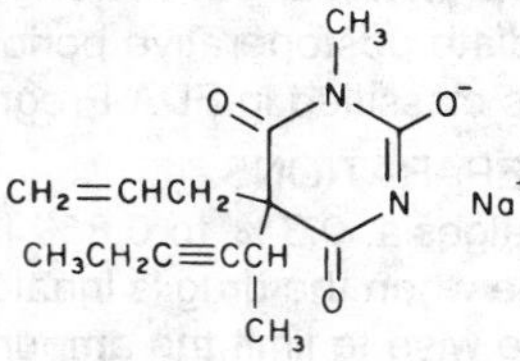

Methohexital has a shorter duration of action than thiopental because hepatic clearance is more rapid. It may be used for induction or for procedures in which momentary loss of consciousness is desirable (eg, electroshock therapy).

ADVERSE REACTIONS. Adverse effects are similar to those noted with thiopental. Unlike thiopental or thiamylal, methohexital does not induce the release of histamine from mast cells. Hiccups may occur after rapid intravenous injection. Involuntary muscle movements, tremor, and rigidity have been observed more frequently with methohexital than with thiopental. This is more pronounced following use of promethazine for preanesthetic medication but is reduced when fentanyl or meperidine is used for this purpose.

Methohexital can induce psychomotor seizures in susceptible patients. It is recommended that thiopental be utilized in place of methohexital in such patients except when activation of the epileptogenic focus is desirable for diagnostic purposes or during temporal lobectomy with EEG recording from the exposed tissue.

PHARMACOKINETICS. The short duration of action of methohexital results largely from its rapid redistribution out of the central nervous system. The distribution, half-life, volume of distribution, and protein binding for methohexital and thiopental are similar; however, this barbiturate is cleared more rapidly (9.9 ± 2.9 ml/kg/min) than thiopental (3.4 ± 0.5 ml/kg/min). The elimination half-life of methohexital is 4 ± 2.5 hours, and its apparent volume of distribution is 2.1 ± 0.7 L/kg (Hudson et al, 1982).

DOSAGE AND PREPARATIONS.

Intravenous: *Adults,* for induction, after a 2-ml test dose, 5 to 12 ml of a 1% solution is injected at the rate of 1 ml every five seconds. For maintenance, 2 to 4 ml of a 1% solution injected as required.

Brevital Sodium (Lilly). Powder (for solution) 0.5, 2.5, and 5 g.

Rectal: *Children,* for basal anesthesia, 25 mg/kg in a 1% solution in lukewarm tap water. More concentrated solutions (conventionally, 2% and 10%) are associated with higher failure rates (Khalil et al, 1988).

Dosage form not commercially available. Compounding required for prescription.

THIAMYLAL SODIUM
[Surital]

$$CH_2{=}CHCH_2,\ CH_3CH_2CH_2CH(CH_3)\text{-substituted thiobarbiturate, } S^-\ Na^+$$

The uses and adverse effects of this rapid-acting barbiturate are similar to those of thiopental sodium.

DOSAGE AND PREPARATIONS.

Intravenous: *Adults,* for induction, after a 2-ml test dose of a freshly prepared 2.5% solution, a single injection of 3 to 5 mg/kg is given. A few clinicians prefer to inject 2 to 4 ml every 30 to 40 seconds until the desired effect is obtained. For maintenance, 2 to 4 ml of a 2.5% solution is injected as required.

Surital (Parke-Davis). Powder (for solution) 1, 5, and 10 g.

Benzodiazepines

DIAZEPAM
[Valium]

For chemical formula, see index entry Diazepam, In Anxiety.

ACTIONS AND USES. Diazepam is administered intravenously to produce basal sedation during regional anesthesia, for cardioversion, and in endoscopic and dental procedures. It also is used occasionally as an induction agent. Otherwise, it is considered less satisfactory than the ultrashort-acting barbiturates for induction because of its slightly slower onset of action (at least one minute) and especially because the recovery period is substantially more prolonged. Sleep and altered consciousness usually are preceded by nystagmus and slurred speech but not excitement. Diazepam also is used for preanesthetic medication (see index entry Diazepam), as a component of neuroleptanalgesia, and to control convulsions caused by local anesthetics.

Since diazepam has no analgesic action, concurrent use of local or topical anesthetics improves anesthetic management in some patients (eg, prior to endoscopy). Diazepam will not enhance the analgesic action of opioid drugs or potentiate the effects of neuromuscular blocking agents. However, it does significantly enhance the sedative action of opioids.

ADVERSE REACTIONS, PRECAUTIONS, AND INTERACTIONS. The intravenous administration of diazepam may cause mild tachycardia and slight respiratory depression, but acute circulatory failure has occurred in a healthy adult and respiratory arrest was observed in a healthy elderly patient after intravenous injections of 20 mg and 10 mg, respectively. Such effects may be anticipated if the drug is administered too rapidly. Respiratory arrest also has been noted after use of the drug during anesthesia, particularly if an opioid analgesic was included in the premedication. It is advisable to decrease the dose of opioid drugs used for premedication by at least one-third and to administer them in small increments. In high-dose opioid anesthesia, even small amounts (2.5 to 5 mg) of intravenous diazepam can decrease blood pressure and cardiac output profoundly. Smaller doses of diazepam (usually 2 to 5 mg) should be used for elderly or debilitated patients or when other sedative drugs are administered.

The half-life of diazepam is 20 or more hours; thus, outpatients must be accompanied home because of the slow recovery of psychomotor skills. Cimetidine decreases diazepam clearance, resulting in more pronounced and prolonged sedation.

Superficial, painless venous thrombosis develops at the site of injection in 15% of patients; the incidence increases with age. A high incidence of phlebitis has been reported following the intravenous use of diazepam. Injection into small veins (such as on the back of the hand) frequently causes pain and is not recommended. Care should be taken to avoid intra-arterial injection, which can cause extensive tissue necrosis.

Although Apgar scores are little affected when diazepam is used for vaginal delivery, hypotonicity, hypoactivity, and hypothermia may occur in infants after doses of 20 to 50 mg are given to the mother. Therefore, diazepam is *not* recommended for obstetric patients.

The administration of heparin during cardiopulmonary bypass to patients who have received diazepam for preanesthetic medication, induction, or in conjunction with opioid anesthesia may result in transient but significant hypotension.

PHARMACOKINETICS. Diazepam is metabolized to active derivatives. The half-life of diazepam depends on age, ranging from 20 hours at age 20 years to 90 hours at age 80 years, a relationship that parallels the age-related increase in the initial volume of distribution. However, the plasma clearance remains nearly constant (20 to 32 ml/min) regardless of age. The apparent volume of distribution at steady state is 1.1 L/kg.

DOSAGE AND PREPARATIONS.

Intravenous: Diazepam should not be mixed with solutions of other drugs. To prevent prolonged exposure of the vein to a high concentration of the solvent and to reduce venous thrombosis, diazepam is injected through the intravenous tubing with the intravenous fluid flowing rapidly.

For induction of anesthesia, 0.1 to 1.5 mg/kg is required. Although some healthy patients may fall asleep with doses of 0.4 mg/kg, or even 0.2 mg/kg if an opioid analgesic is used for preanesthetic medication, 0.8 to 1.5 mg/kg is required if anesthesia is to be assured. This combination is dangerous in poor-risk patients because of the possibility of cardiovascular depression. Diazepam should be injected slowly (no more than 5 mg [1 ml]/min in adults and no more than 0.25 mg/kg/3 min in children).

For basal sedation, increments of 2.5 mg are given until the patient falls into a light sleep or nystagmus, ptosis, or slurred speech develops. Ptosis covering half of the pupil is a reproducible endpoint. Generally, 5 to 30 mg is required.

Valium (Roche), ***Generic.*** Solution 5 mg/ml in 2 and 10 ml containers.

MIDAZOLAM HYDROCHLORIDE
[Versed]

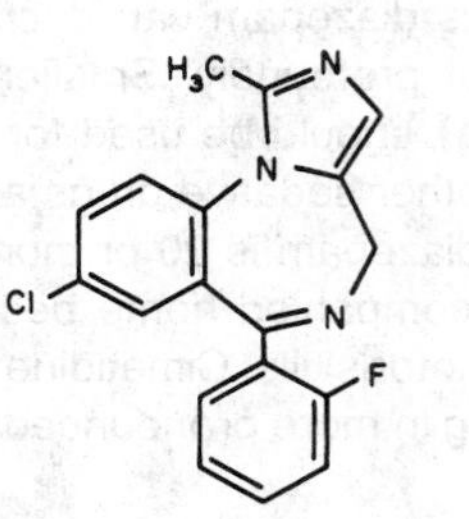

ACTIONS AND USES. This induction agent differs from other benzodiazepines in that it is water soluble. Induction (approximately 80 seconds) is more rapid than with diazepam or flunitrazepam but slower than with thiopental (30 to 60 seconds).

Midazolam amnesia may be related to the duration of the sedative action. It has no analgesic action and will not enhance the analgesic effect of opioids.

The degree of respiratory depression produced by midazolam is similar to that observed with diazepam but may be more severe in the older patient. *Midazolam should not be given intravenously to elderly patients unless facilities for tracheal intubation and ventilation are present.* A brief period of apnea may occur about two minutes after intravenous administration. The incidence and duration of apnea are less than with an equivalent dose of thiopental and its onset is later. Oxygen should be employed during spontaneous ventilation. The minute volume is decreased following intravenous administration in about 25% of patients. As with diazepam, slightly increased airway resistance is noted occasionally.

The cardiovascular system remains stable during induction. There is a slight, dose-dependent reduction in blood pressure, but the heart rate, cardiac output, and rhythm usually are not affected in normal subjects. Significant hypotensive episodes are more common in the older patient or after administration of meperidine. The drug appears to be satisfactory for induction in patients with ischemic heart disease.

Midazolam has no effects on gastrointestinal smooth muscle. It does not affect the response to muscle relaxants. Intraocular pressure is reduced, but the increase in intraocular pressure produced by succinylcholine or intubation is not prevented. The cerebral blood flow in healthy volunteers was reduced by one-third, suggesting that midazolam might be appropriate for induction in neurosurgical patients with intracranial hypertension.

Fetal transfer of midazolam is significantly less than that of diazepam, and it may be possible to employ this agent in obstetric patients without producing fetal hypotonia or hypothermia. Midazolam is classified in FDA Pregnancy Category D.

No renal, hepatic, or other complications have been reported. Intravenous administration rarely causes pain or thrombophlebitis.

PHARMACOKINETICS. Midazolam is metabolized in the liver to two hydroxylated derivatives that are excreted by the kidney. Neither metabolite possesses a soporific action. The duration of hypnotic action is approximately 4.5 minutes. Midazolam is extensively protein bound (more than 95%). With an intravenous dose of 0.075 mg/kg, the half-life is 68 minutes, the apparent volume of distribution is 0.23 L/kg, and the clearance is 13 ml/kg/min (Kanto et al, 1984). The half-life is prolonged in patients with cirrhosis (Chauvin et al, 1987; Trouvin et al, 1988).

DOSAGE AND PREPARATIONS.

Intravenous: *Adults*, as sole agent for conscious sedation, according to response: approximately 10 to 10.5 mg in adults to age 45, decreasing to about 7 to 7.5 mg at ages 55 to 64, 5 to 5.5 mg at ages 65 to 74, 3.6 mg at ages 75 to 84, and 2.3 mg at age 85 and older (Bell et al, 1987).

For induction, 0.2 mg/kg over two to three minutes if an opioid analgesic is used for preanesthetic medication. There is considerable variation in the dose required for induction; some adults are resistant to 30 mg. Since these patients readily accept a mask after the administration of midazolam, induction may be completed with the planned maintenance agent.

No dosage has been established for *children* or for *obstetric procedures*.

Versed (Roche). Solution (buffered, aqueous) 1 and 5 mg/ml in 1, 2, 5, and 10 ml containers.

Miscellaneous Agents

ETOMIDATE
[Amidate]

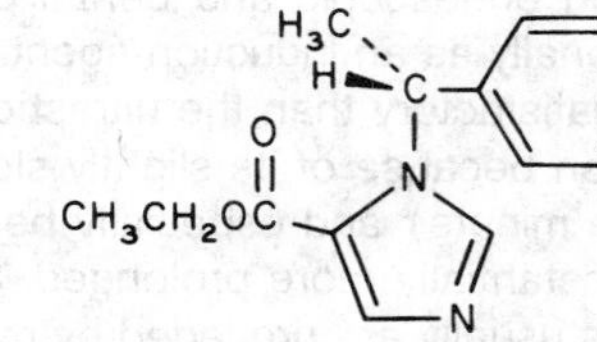

ACTIONS AND USES. Etomidate is a nonbarbiturate anesthetic (Giese et al, 1985) used primarily to induce surgical anesthesia. It does not produce analgesia, but can be employed in a totally intravenous technique in which continuous infusion is combined with intermittent or continuous administration of fentanyl.

The advantages of etomidate are its minimal effects on the cardiovascular system and respiration during induction. It does not cause the release of histamine. An induction dose reduces cardiac output, stroke volume, and arterial pressure and produces a small compensatory increase in heart rate. All of these alterations are within acceptable limits. Arrhythmias are uncommon. No significant changes in pulmonary or vascular resistance are noted, although peripheral blood flow may be increased. The effects are similar in normal patients and in those with severe cardiovascular disease. The cardiovascular stability of etomidate during administration is not affected by nitrous oxide or opioids. Etomidate decreases cerebral blood flow (by 35% to 50%), cerebral metabolic rate, and intracranial pressure and may be useful in neurosurgery.

ADVERSE REACTIONS AND PRECAUTIONS. Pain at the injection site is common during administration but can be reduced by slow injection into a large vein, premedication with an analgesic (eg, fentanyl), or instillation of 25 to 100 mg of lidocaine in the intravenous line about 30 seconds prior to administration of etomidate. In marked contrast to the barbiturates, etomidate produces no adverse effects following inadvertent intra-arterial injection.

Spontaneous muscle movements occur during induction in about 60% of patients not given premedication. These movements are myoclonic, not epileptic, and their severity is not clearly dose related. They subside rapidly, and premedication with an opioid or benzodiazepine may lessen their severity.

Since etomidate lacks analgesic action, intubation of the trachea following its use for induction may be accompanied by pronounced tachycardia and hypertension. These effects usually can be prevented by analgesic premedication in patients at risk.

Transient apnea (15 to 20 seconds) may occur during induction, particularly in elderly patients, and this may be prolonged if an analgesic (eg, fentanyl) or benzodiazepine is used for preanesthetic medication. Coughing and hiccupping also have been observed, but their incidence is not dose related. Laryngospasm is uncommon.

Postoperative nausea and vomiting are more common with etomidate than with thiopental and occur more frequently (in up to 50% of patients) following multiple doses. Hypersensitivity reactions apparently are infrequent. Rash has been reported occasionally, but anaphylactic responses (eg, hypotension, bronchospasm) have not been observed.

Etomidate reversibly suppresses adrenocortical function. Prolonged infusion may produce hypotension, oliguria, and electrolyte disturbances that respond to glucocorticoids. For this reason, etomidate is not recommended for long surgical procedures or for prolonged sedation in intensive care patients.

This drug is classified in FDA Pregnancy Category C.

PHARMACOKINETICS. After administration of the usual induction dose (0.3 mg/kg), unconsciousness occurs within one minute and responsiveness returns within two to three minutes. Recovery time is dependent on dose, redistribution, and metabolism. Etomidate is hydrolyzed rapidly in the plasma and liver to an inactive metabolite. The plasma elimination half-life after a single intravenous dose is 2.9 ± 1.1 hours. Systemic clearance is 1.074 L/kg/hr. The volume of distribution (Vdss) is 2.5 L/kg. Clearance was 0.699 ± 0.177 L/kg/hr when induction was followed by nitrous oxide anesthetic maintenance, probably due to the effect of the gaseous agent on liver blood flow (Van Hamme et al, 1978). The drug is 78% bound to serum albumin. Age-dependent changes in etomidate pharmacokinetics (ie, a lower initial volume of distribution rather than an increase in CNS sensitivity) has been proposed as the reason for a decrease in the dosage requirement in the elderly (Arden et al, 1986).

DOSAGE AND PREPARATIONS.

Intravenous: *Adults and children over 10 years*, the usual dose is 0.3 mg/kg (range, 0.2 to 0.6 mg/kg) injected over a period of 30 to 60 seconds. This dose should be reduced in the older patient. This drug is not recommended during pregnancy or lactation or for children under 10 years.

Amidate (Abbott). Solution 2 mg/ml in 10 and 20 ml containers.

KETAMINE HYDROCHLORIDE

[Ketalar]

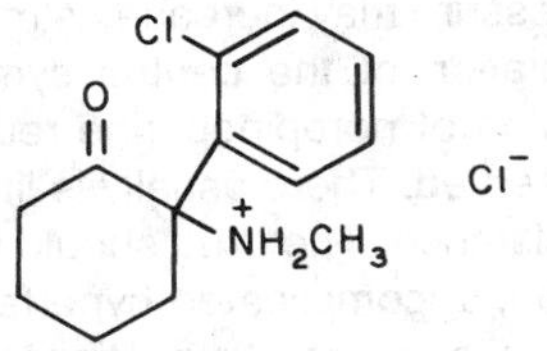

ACTIONS AND USES. Ketamine is a nonbarbiturate anesthetic that can be administered intravenously or intramuscularly. It induces a state of sedation and amnesia during which the patient may appear to be awake but is dissociated from the environment, immobile, and unresponsive to pain. Induction of anesthesia is rapid, even after intramuscular injection. Like thiopental, ketamine's anesthetic action is terminated by redistribution out of the central nervous system in approximately 10 minutes. Recovery from the postanesthetic psychic effects is more prolonged and may depend on elimination.

Because this anesthetic is rapidly effective when administered intramuscularly, it is particularly useful for repeated anesthesia in burn patients, for diagnostic studies, for sedating uncontrollable patients (eg, the mentally retarded), and for minor surgical procedures in young children. A small dose (0.5 to 1 mg/kg intramuscularly) can be used to calm agitated children and facilitate insertion of an intravenous cannula; a dose of 2 mg/kg can be used for induction in young children (age 1 to 3) who refuse a face mask (Hannallah and Patel, 1988). The analgesic properties of ketamine may contribute to its usefulness for these purposes.

Ketamine also may be of value to induce anesthesia, particularly when a barbiturate cannot be used or cardiovascular depression must be avoided (eg, shock, severe dehydration, severe anemia, cardiac tamponade, constrictive pericarditis, nonischemic cardiomyopathies). It is particularly useful in the presence of bronchospasm and as an induction agent in asthmatic patients. When given in combination with diazepam and a muscle relaxant, it is an alternative to inhalation agents for one-lung anesthesia in patients with pre-existing pulmonary disease and abnormal preoperative blood gas values. It is not satisfactory as the sole agent for abdominal or other major surgical procedures because skeletal muscle relaxation is inadequate and adverse effects occur.

An anticholinergic drug should be given for premedication to reduce the hypersalivation produced by ketamine. The concomitant use of diazepam, hydroxyzine, or a barbiturate increases recovery time. Another general anesthetic and a neuromuscular blocking agent can be used with ketamine if required. Ketamine potentiates the neuromuscular blocking effects of tubocurarine but not of pancuronium or succinylcholine. The analgesic effect of ketamine may continue postoperatively when ketamine is administered intraoperatively.

ADVERSE REACTIONS AND PRECAUTIONS. Muscular rigidity, athetoid motions of the mouth and tongue, swallowing, random movements of the extremities, vocalization, laryngospasm, fasciculations, tremors, and generalized extensor spasm have occurred occasionally. Frank convulsions are extremely rare.

Ketamine usually increases heart rate and cardiac output, and the arterial pressure may increase as much as 25%, principally from stimulation of the central sympathetic nervous system and inhibition of norepinephrine reuptake. Arrhythmias are seldom observed. There usually is little change in systemic vascular resistance. The drug should be used with care in patients with mild, uncomplicated hypertension and is contraindicated when a significant elevation of blood pressure would constitute a serious hazard (in patients with aneurysms, angina, heart failure, cerebral trauma, or thyrotoxicosis) and in those who are hypersensitive to the drug. Ketamine may produce an unacceptable increase in myocardial oxygen consumption in patients with ischemic heart disease. Premedication with a benzodiazepine will attenuate ketamine-induced hypertension and tachycardia. Intravenous labetalol, 1 mg/kg, also can be employed to manage an unacceptable increase in blood pressure and heart rate (White, 1988 A). (See also Dosage and Preparations.) The indirect cardiovascular stimulant properties of ketamine are blocked when halothane or enflurane is given concomitantly and the direct myocardial depressant action of ketamine then becomes evident. Hypotension also may be observed in severely ill patients (eg, septic shock) or in patients with chronic congestive heart failure. There is some evidence that the drug interacts with thyroid medication to produce severe hypertension and tachycardia.

Transient respiratory depression may occur immediately after intravenous administration of anesthetic doses, and respiratory arrest has occurred in neonates. Laryngeal reflexes are obtunded but retained during anesthesia. Aspiration of stomach contents has been reported, and an endotracheal tube should be used when any doubt exists concerning gastric content. Upper airway infection may increase the incidence of laryngospasm after use of ketamine, but there are no controlled studies to substantiate this finding. Tracheobronchial secretions are increased. Pre-existing bronchospasm usually is abolished by the smooth muscle relaxant action of ketamine.

Ketamine increases cerebrospinal fluid pressure and intracranial blood flow and should be used with extreme caution in patients with evidence of increased intracranial pressure or a space-occupying lesion. It has been suggested that ketamine does not always produce satisfactory analgesia in patients with cerebral cortical disease; the mechanism is unknown.

Ketamine may increase intraocular pressure slightly; thus, its use for some intraocular surgical procedures is inappropriate. It may be wise to avoid this anesthetic in patients with pre-existing elevation of intraocular pressure.

Ketamine may cause vomiting, lacrimation, shivering, and transient cutaneous reactions.

Recovery from anesthesia sometimes takes up to several hours. Psychic disturbances during emergence (unpleasant dreams, irrational behavior, excitement, disorientation, illusions, delirium, hallucinations) may occur more frequently in adults (particularly women) than in children. The reported incidence varies between 3% and 50%. Several techniques can reduce the incidence of such reactions: (1) oral premedication with lorazepam 4 mg or diazepam 10 mg; (2) intravenous administration of diazepam 0.15 to 0.3 mg/kg at the end of anesthesia or midazolam 125 mcg/kg three minutes prior to induction; (3) use of no more than 2 mg/kg as the induction dose and maintenance of anesthesia with doses of 0.5 to 1 mg/kg; (4) use of a low-dose microdrip intravenous infusion; (5) use of glycopyrrolate instead of atropine or scopolamine for premedication; and (6) maintenance of anesthesia with other agents. Although there is no evidence that psychic disturbances have any residual effect, it may be advisable to avoid ketamine in patients with preoperative psychiatric problems.

Studies on ketamine's effects on the fetus when used during delivery indicate that doses greater than 2 mg/kg are likely to cause fetal depression. Although smaller doses (0.25 to 0.5 mg/kg) appear to be safe for analgesia, caution is advised.

PHARMACOKINETICS. Ketamine is metabolized in the liver. The half-life is 2.5 to 4 hours, the apparent volume of distribution is 3.3 L/kg, and the clearance rate is 1.3 L/min.

DOSAGE AND PREPARATIONS. Tachyphylaxis has been observed when ketamine is given for repeated operative, diagnostic, or therapeutic procedures.

Intravenous: For induction, single-dose method, 2 mg/kg (range, 1 to 4.5 mg/kg) administered over 60 seconds. Unconsciousness persists for 10 to 15 minutes and analgesia persists for an additional 30 minutes. For maintenance, one-half of the full induction dose, repeated as necessary.

Using the low-dose, microdrip technique, a 0.1% concentration is administered at a rate of 20 ml/min as needed for induction. The rate is adjusted according to the patient's blood pressure, pulse rate, and response to surgical stimulation. When this technique is employed for maintenance with nitrous oxide and a muscle relaxant, the total dose of ketamine required is only one-third to one-half of the amount employed for bolus administration.

An anesthetic technique that minimizes the adverse cardiovascular response to ketamine may be accomplished by premedication with diazepam 10 mg orally 30 to 120 minutes prior to induction and atropine sulfate 0.4 mg intravenously at induction. Induction is initiated by infusing ketamine 0.1% in a dose of 1.5 mg/kg in three minutes; at the beginning of each minute, 5 mg of diazepam is given for a total of 15 mg. During the second minute, 0.6 mg/kg of tubocurarine or atracurium (pancuronium is not satisfactory because of the tachycardia produced by the drugs in combination) is given intravenously as a bolus. After intubation, ventilation is maintained with nitrous oxide and oxygen. Maintenance doses of ketamine during the first hour are 0.2 mg/kg/hr by infusion with intermittent boluses of diazepam 5 mg every 30 minutes. For the second and subsequent hours, the dose of ketamine is reduced to 0.1 mg/kg/hr and of diazepam to 2.5 mg every 30 minutes. Additional amounts of tubocurarine are given as needed (Aldrete and McDonald, 1980; Wilson et al, 1980).

Intravenous: For induction, 1 to 2 mg/kg over 60 seconds. For maintenance, infusion of 0.1 to 0.5 mg/min or one-half of the induction dose as required.

Intramuscular: For induction, 5 to 10 mg/kg. For maintenance, one-half of the full induction dose, repeated as necessary. For analgesia (eg, burn patients), 2 mg/kg.

Ketalar (Parke-Davis). Solution (equivalent to base) 10 mg/ml in 20 and 50 ml containers, 50 mg/ml in 10 ml containers, and 100 mg/ml in 5 ml containers.

PROPOFOL

[Diprivan]

OH
$(CH_3)_2HC$ — benzene ring — $CH(CH_3)_2$

ACTIONS AND USES. Propofol, an intravenously administered anesthetic agent, is employed for induction, as a maintenance agent in balanced techniques with opioids (eg, alfentanil) or inhalation anesthetics (eg, nitrous oxide), as a sedative or light general anesthetic to supplement regional anesthetics, or as a sole agent for selected procedures not requiring analgesia, such as endoscopy (Sebel and Lowdon, 1989). Pharmacodynamic studies of propofol in humans have been reviewed (Kanto, 1988; Langley and Heel, 1988; White, 1988 B).

Induction time with propofol does not differ from that for thiopental, methohexital, or etomidate. Excitatory effects and spontaneous movement during induction are infrequent but somewhat more common than with thiopental (Stark et al, 1985). Emergence depends on redistribution from the central nervous system. Awakening and reorientation following an induction dose of propofol are more rapid than with thiopental and are similar to etomidate; postoperative nausea and vomiting are uncommon.

There is considerable interest in the use of propofol for long-term sedation in the intensive care unit (Grounds et al, 1987; Newman et al, 1987; Beller et al, 1988; Aitkenhead et al, 1989). Cumulative effects, tachyphylaxis, or delayed awakening are not observed after administration of propofol as they are after prolonged infusion of thiopental, diazepam, or midazolam. Unlike etomidate, propofol does not inhibit adrenal steroidogenesis (Fragen et al, 1988).

There is insufficient information on the use of this anesthetic for obstetric anesthesia, including cesarean section, or for nursing mothers. However, in two investigations comparing propofol with thiopental for induction of anesthesia in cesarean section, there were no significant differences in effects on Apgar score, neonatal blood gas analysis, or uterine bleeding or relaxation (Moore et al, 1989; Valtonen et al, 1989 A). In a third study, propofol was employed as an induction agent (bolus dose of 2.5 mg/kg followed by maintenance infusion of 5 mg/kg/hr) in patients undergoing cesarean section; the quantity of propofol subsequently found in the milk/colostrum was considered to be negligible compared with that from direct placental exposure. No adverse effects on the neonate, as determined by Apgar or Neurologic and Adaptive Capacity (NACS) scores, were observed (Dailland et al, 1989). This agent is classified in FDA Pregnancy Category B.

ADVERSE REACTIONS AND PRECAUTIONS. Aberrant uncomfortable sensations such as tingling, numbness, feeling of warmth or cold, and mild to moderate pain may be produced at the injection site. These responses are more common if the venous catheter is placed in a small vein (eg, in the dorsum of the hand rather than the antecubital fossa). The pain can be reduced or abolished in most patients by adding 1 ml of lidocaine 1% to the propofol emulsion immediately prior to administration (Helbo-Hansen et al, 1988). When this combination was used in children 3 years or older, pain during administration was reduced significantly (Valtonen et al, 1989 B). The incidence of thrombosis or phlebitis is less than 1% (Mattila and Koski, 1985).

There appears to be only a single report on the inadvertent arterial administration of propofol, although the risk of this is increased with administration into the antecubital fossa. In this report (Chong and Davis, 1987), propofol 4 ml without lidocaine was injected into the left brachial artery. Blanching at the injection site and severe pain radiating down the forearm into the palm occurred. Injection was stopped and anesthesia was induced using the other forearm. Postoperatively, 30 minutes after the first injection the forearm and palm were hyperemic and these areas felt slightly stiff to the patient. No residual effects were observed on follow-up.

Propofol decreases arterial pressure more than other intravenous induction agents. Changes in heart rate are variable but usually there is no compensatory increase. Systemic hypotension results from a reduction in systemic vascular resistance; the cardiac index is not affected consistently. The results of a number of clinical studies suggest that propofol should be used with caution in patients with compromised myocardial function, in the elderly, and in hypovolemic patients (Gallently and Short, 1988; Larsen et al, 1988; Perry et al, 1988; Sebel and Lowdon, 1989). Propofol was reported to be unsatisfactory for induction in patients with severe coronary artery disease who were undergoing coronary artery surgery; even a dose of 1.5 mg/kg resulted in pronounced hypotension, which occasionally required intervention with vasopressors (Russell et al, 1989). However, these investigators reported that induction with fentanyl and diazepam, followed by large doses of propofol (10 mg/kg/hr) plus fentanyl during sternotomy and sternal spread provided excellent hemodynamic stability. Following the intense surgical stimulation, a maintenance dose of 3 mg/kg/hr was satisfactory for the remainder of the cardiopulmonary bypass procedure.

Propofol is a respiratory depressant and will produce apnea of greater than 30 seconds duration in a substantial number of patients following an induction dose, but it does not differ from thiopental in this regard. Propofol is considered "possibly safe" in patients susceptible to malignant hyperthermia based on limited experience (Marks et al, 1988) and "probably safe" in patients with hepatic porphyrias (McLoughlin, 1989). There are no known interactions with agents used in general anesthesia. Appropriate reductions in dosage will be required when propofol is used with other central nervous system depressants, including opioids.

PHARMACOKINETICS. In male volunteers, only 0.3% of an administered dose of ^{14}C-labeled propofol was eliminated in unchanged form. The remainder was excreted, primarily in the urine, as more polar inactive metabolites. The major metabolite is propofol glucuronide (about 50%). Lesser quantities of the sulfate and glucuronide conjugates of the para-hydroxylated derivative of propofol also are excreted. A high percentage of a single dose is eliminated by the kidney within eight hours; the remainder clears more slowly, probably because of slow release from poorly perfused tissues (Simons et al, 1988).

Following intravenous administration, the concentration of propofol in blood at different times can be described best with a three-compartment open model. Since there is no evidence of accumulation during long-term infusion of propofol, the value for the beta half-life can be employed to describe the elimination of the drug. Sex (Kay et al, 1986) or obesity (White, 1988 B) does not appear to affect the elimination half-life of propofol, and, in a single study, no clinically significant difference in clearance was noted in patients with impaired and normal renal function (Morcos and Payne, 1985). The pharmacokinetics of propofol and its protein binding following a single induction dose in patients with uncomplicated cirrhosis of the liver are not markedly affected (Servin et al, 1988). There have been no reports on the use of propofol in patients with acute hepatic disease.

Both dosage and awakening times are influenced by age. In age-comparative studies, the mean age of children was 5.5 years (range, 4 to 7 years); young adults, 27.5 years (range, 18 to 35 years); and elderly patients, 71.4 years (range, 65 to 80 years). The corresponding pharmacokinetic parameters, mean and standard deviation (SD), were: *children:* $t_{1/2\beta}$ (min) 56.1 (6.3), $t_{1/2\gamma}$ (min) 735 (82.7), Vd $_{ss}$(L/kg) 10.9 (1.2), Cl (ml/kg/min) 30.6 (2.9); *young adults:* $t_{1/2\beta}$ 52.4 (9.2); $t_{1/2\gamma}$ 674 (122), Vd_{ss} 11.9 (3.5), Cl 27.7 (2.3); *elderly:* $t_{1/2\beta}$ 69.3 (8.7), $t_{1/2\gamma}$ 834 (170), Vd_{ss} 12.4 (3.3), Cl 23.3 (1.1) (Kirkpatrick et al, 1988; Saint-Maurice et al, 1989).

In one study comparing the influence of age on dose requirements in unpremedicated young adults (25 to 40 years) and older adults (65 to 80 years), the younger patients required a mean induction dose of 2.2 mg/kg and a maintenance dose (with vecuronium and fentanyl) of 10 mg/kg/hr, and they had a mean awakening time of 7.8 minutes. In contrast, the older patients required only 1.7 mg/kg for induction and a maintenance dose of 8.6 mg/kg/hr, and they had a mean awakening time of 14.3 minutes (Scheepstra et al, 1989).

A dosage schedule for children has not been established. In the few reported studies on children, it was concluded that they required proportionally larger induction doses than adults and that even 2.5 mg/kg was insufficient in some patients (Purcell-Jones et al, 1987; Valtonen et al, 1988). However, light anesthesia in children (0 to 3 years) that was satisfactory for computerized tomography could be produced by propofol 1.8 mg/kg combined with diazepam 0.2 mg/kg (Valtonen, 1989).

Pharmacokinetic studies of propofol in man have been reviewed (Kanto and Gepts, 1989).

DOSAGE AND PREPARATIONS.

Intravenous: *Adults,* for induction, increments of approximately 40 mg every 10 seconds until adequate anesthesia is achieved. The usual total dose for *adults 55 years or younger* is 2 to 2.5 mg/kg. For *elderly, debilitated, hypovolemic, and/or ASA III or IV patients,* 1 to 1.5 mg/kg; ie, approximately 20 mg every 10 seconds until anesthesia is achieved, is adequate (Langley and Heel, 1988). See the section on Adverse Reactions and Precautions for information on use in patients with severe coronary artery disease. For maintenance, 25 to 50 mg as required is given by intermittent bolus or 0.1 to 0.2 mg/kg/min is infused. This dose is reduced approximately 50% for *elderly, debilitated, hypovolemic, and/or ASA III and IV patients.*

Diprivan (Stuart). Solution 10 mg/ml in 20 and 50 ml containers.

COMBINATION ANESTHESIA

Balanced Anesthesia

Components: Because of its low potency, nitrous oxide must be supplemented with other agents to produce conditions suitable for surgery. The use of more potent inhalation or intravenous agents to achieve this goal has been discussed. The intravenous use of an ultrashort-acting barbiturate, an opioid analgesic, a neuromuscular blocking agent, and nitrous oxide to produce general anesthesia is termed "balanced anesthesia." Morphine, fentanyl [Sublimaze], sufentanil [Sufenta], and, more recently, alfentanil [Alfenta] are the most widely employed analgesics and, in combination with a barbiturate, supplement the hypnotic and analgesic effects of nitrous oxide. Meperidine was the first opioid analgesic used in this manner but is not satisfactory because of its tendency to produce myocardial depression, vasodilation, and tachycardia when given in large doses. Various agonist-antagonist opioids have been examined but generally these have been of limited value because they possess an analgesic ceiling.

An opioid analgesic often is included in the preanesthetic medication and anesthesia is induced with a barbiturate and nitrous oxide. The opioid then is given intravenously in increments over five to ten minutes until adequate analgesia has been produced. Additional small amounts may be required during surgery if the patient reacts to painful stimuli (eg, increasing pulse rate and arterial pressure, pupillary dilation, sweating, muscle movement). If used judiciously in this manner and if avoided during the last one to two hours of *prolonged* surgery, adequate intraoperative analgesia usually can be achieved without the need for postoperative ventilatory support.

Morphine became popular in balanced anesthesia for cardiac surgery and for poor-risk patients in general because it usually did not affect myocardial function or cardiovascular dynamics. Large intravenous doses (0.5 to 3 mg/kg) were administered with nitrous oxide or halothane. However, later studies indicated that the administration of nitrous oxide in concentrations greater than 60% or halothane 0.21% to 0.23% after use of morphine 1 mg/kg produced cardiovascular depression (eg, decreased arterial pressure and cardiac index). Anesthetic concentrations of sufentanil and fentanyl maintain hemodynamic stability. The doses of these drugs should be titrated on the basis of the desired effect, and the total dose should be based on the need to extubate the patient at the end of the procedure. For cardiovascular surgery, the dose of sufentanil ranges from 8 to 40 mcg/kg and of fentanyl from 50 to 120 mcg/kg. For procedures such as neurosurgery, in which postoperative awakening and extubation are desirable, sufentanil can be used in a dose equal to 1 mcg/kg/hr or less and fentanyl in a dose between 10 and 20 mcg/kg/hr. Neither should be administered during the last 30 to 45 minutes prior to the desired awakening time. Postoperative ventilation must be monitored closely.

When large doses of opioids are used with 100% oxygen, controlled ventilation must be given postoperatively. The easy transition from intraoperative to postoperative analgesia and ventilatory support is one of the major advantages of this technique in these poor-risk patients. Amnesia may not be achieved with large doses of opioids alone. Anterograde amnesia can be provided by the concurrent administration of a benzodiazepine; however, the combination with the opioid may cause hemodynamic alteration secondary to the decrease in circulating endogenous catecholamines. This can be minimized by maintaining appropriate preload as a primary maneuver. Additional hemodynamic support is required only rarely but may be needed in very ill patients. A small number of patients may become hypertensive, which can be managed by increasing the opioid dosage or using vasodilators or volatile anesthetics.

The opioid antagonist, naloxone [Narcan], may be administered to overcome the residual effects of the opioid analgesic at the end of surgery. However, this reduces or eliminates postoperative analgesia and sometimes increases sympathetic stimulation, which results in arrhythmias and increased myocardial work. It also can be hazardous if the effect of the antagonist ends before that of the analgesic. If an opioid antagonist is used in this manner, the patient must be observed carefully and additional doses of the antagonist given as necessary. (See index entry Naloxone.)

In practice, the technique of balanced anesthesia remains somewhat empirical: The choice of opioid analgesic, the dose used, and the frequency of administration differ and always must be individualized. The adequacy of spontaneous ventilation always must be evaluated carefully and objectively during the postoperative period.

Advantages and Disadvantages: Clinical experience and data from some controlled trials indicate that properly administered balanced anesthesia minimizes intraoperative cardiovascular depression and may increase peripheral resistance; there is an early return of consciousness, and the incidence of postoperative nausea, vomiting, excitement, and pain is low.

Balanced anesthesia is not recommended when an FIO_2 of 0.25 to 0.4 cannot be tolerated or in patients with anemia that limits the oxygen-carrying capacity of the blood. Care must be taken not to "cover up" inadequate analgesia with muscle relaxants. Patient awareness during surgery has been reported.

Neuroleptanalgesia and Neuroleptanesthesia

Neuroleptanalgesia historically refers to administration of both an opioid analgesic and droperidol [Inapsine], a neuroleptic (antipsychotic) drug, to produce an altered state of consciousness and awareness. Alternative combinations used in clinical studies include diazepam [Valium], ketamine [Ketalar], or droperidol with meperidine [Demerol], morphine, fentanyl [Sublimaze], or sufentanil [Sufenta].

Consciousness is not lost during neuroleptanalgesia and the technique may be useful for diagnostic and therapeutic procedures performed under local anesthesia (eg, cardiac catheterization, repeated burn dressings).

When nitrous oxide is used to supplement these combinations, the term neuroleptanesthesia is employed. A muscle relaxant also may be included. This technique often provides satisfactory general anesthesia and may be particularly valuable when the patient's cooperation is required during the procedure, for consciousness returns soon after the flow of nitrous oxide is terminated.

The opioid analgesic, fentanyl, has been used most commonly with the butyrophenone, droperidol, in neuroleptanesthesia. Droperidol and fentanyl are available as single-entity products or in a fixed-dose combination [Innovar].

Drug Evaluations

ALFENTANIL
[Alfenta]

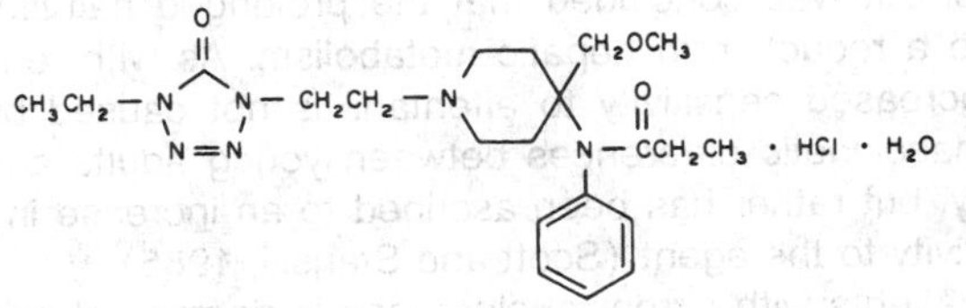

ACTIONS AND USES. Alfentanil is the newest fentanyl analogue introduced into anesthetic practice. Anesthesia with this agent is characterized by a very rapid onset and short duration of action. As with fentanyl and sufentanil, recovery time from a single dose is determined by redistribution rather than by elimination.

Alfentanil may be used for induction, as an anesthetic adjunct, or as the sole anesthetic agent. Since it has a short duration, this anesthetic can be administered by a variable rate of infusion determined by patient response in a manner analogous to that for an inhalation anesthetic agent. Alfentanil is used most frequently as a supplement to nitrous oxide in a balanced anesthesia technique.

ADVERSE REACTIONS AND PRECAUTIONS. As with the other potent opioids, particularly of the fentanyl class, the rapid intravenous administration of alfentanil induces skeletal muscle rigidity ("frozen chest syndrome"), which can interfere with thoracic compliance. The effect develops more rapidly than with fentanyl; it is dose related and will occur consistently with induction doses unless certain precautions are taken. The incidence can be reduced if large doses of alfentanil are administered slowly (over at least a three-minute interval) and if approximately 25% of a paralyzing dose of a neuromuscular blocking agent is given before induction, with the remainder given after loss of consciousness.

Alfentanil differs from fentanyl and sufentanil in its tendency to produce hypotension. This effect can be ameliorated by a slow infusion rate and adequate fluid loading. The combination of diazepam and a large dose of alfentanil may cause bradycardia and profound hypotension. Alfentanil alone also may produce bradycardia, which is responsive to atropine. The likelihood of this adverse effect may be minimized by use of a vagolytic muscle relaxant (eg, pancuronium).

The dose requirements of alfentanil are reduced in the elderly or in patients with impaired liver function (see Pharmacokinetics and Dosage).

Alfentanil is classified in FDA Pregnancy Category C.

PHARMACOKINETICS. The activity of low doses of alfentanil is terminated by redistribution. The repeated administration of large doses may make recovery more dependent on elimination. The drug is more than 99% metabolized by the liver.

A number of pharmacokinetic studies of alfentanil have been reviewed (Davis and Cook, 1986). In adults, a common elimination half-life is 83 minutes, the apparent volume of distribution is 0.46 L/kg, and the clearance is 6.5 ml/kg/min (Helmers et al, 1984). The same investigators reported that in the elderly (mean age, 77), the half-life increased to 137 minutes, the volume of distribution did not differ significantly (0.54 L/kg), and the clearance decreased to 4.4 ml/min/kg. Since the volume of distribution and protein binding were not different, it was concluded that the prolonged half-life was due to a reduction in hepatic metabolism. As with fentanyl, the increased sensitivity to alfentanil is not caused by the pharmacokinetic differences between young adults and the elderly, but rather has been ascribed to an increase in CNS sensitivity to the agent (Scott and Stanski, 1985).

In patients with cirrhosis, clearance is decreased approximately 50% and half-life is increased more than twofold (Ferrier et al, 1985). Although the volume of distribution is markedly altered, the elimination of alfentanil is not affected in patients with chronic renal failure (Van Peer et al, 1986; Chauvin et al, 1987). Obesity may double the elimination half-life of alfentanil. To achieve a desired steady-state concentration, the loading dose, but not the maintenance dose, will require adjustment according to the patient's weight (Maitre et al, 1987).

The volume of distribution is much smaller in children 4 to 8 years. Therefore, even though the clearance and extent of protein binding are not significantly different, the half-life is only about 50% that in adults. Therefore, awakening time is expected to be shorter in children (Meistelman et al, 1987). The pharmacokinetics of the drug in neonates and children less than 4 years has not been examined.

DOSAGE AND PREPARATIONS. There is a wide disparity in response to alfentanil and thus individualization of dosage is required. In obese patients (greater than 20% ideal body weight), the dose should be calculated on the basis of lean body weight. Minimal doses should be given to elderly patients until the response can be determined. Dosage has not been established for children under 12 years. In prolonged procedures, it is recommended that alfentanil be discontinued approximately 15 minutes prior to completion of surgery. The following dosages are recommended by the manufacturer.

Intravenous: *Adults,* for short (30-minute) procedures in patients breathing spontaneously or with assisted ventilation and with nitrous oxide/oxygen, a slow (two-minute) bolus injection of 8 to 20 mcg/kg is administered prior to induction with a barbiturate; a maintenance dose of 3 to 5 mcg/kg is then given. For long procedures, the loading dose may be increased to 50 to 75 mcg/kg. A variable-rate, continuous infusion (approximately 0.5 to 3 mcg/kg/min) is recommended for maintenance. In the absence of signs of lightening anesthesia (increased heart rate, increased blood pressure, movement, tearing), infusion rates always should be decreased. If additional opioid is required during the final 15 minutes of surgery, bolus doses of 7 mcg/kg are preferred to continuing or increasing the infusion rate.

Alfenta (Janssen). Solution 500 mcg/ml in 2, 5, 10, and 20 ml containers (preservative free).

DROPERIDOL
[Inapsine]

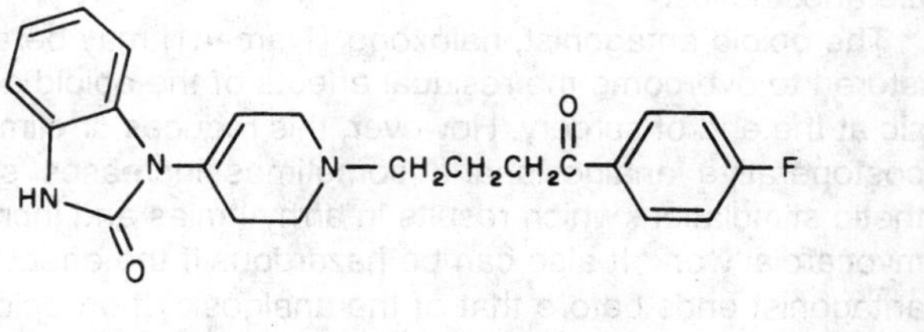

ACTIONS AND USES. Droperidol, a butyrophenone, produces an altered state of awareness, sedation, and, in many patients, dysphoria. It causes little or no amnesia and is not an analgesic. Intravenous administration causes a slight, transient fall in arterial pressure secondary to peripheral vasodilation that may be due to block of alpha-adrenergic receptors, direct vasodilation, or both. Droperidol may potentiate the respiratory depressant action of fentanyl. A dose of 10 mg reduces total body oxygen consumption by approximately 25%.

Droperidol has an antiemetic action and when it was not used previously during the procedure, intravenous administration of a dose not exceeding 1.25 mg in an adult at the termination of general anesthesia reduced the incidence of postoperative vomiting. However, because this drug may produce untoward effects and the incidence of severe, protracted postoperative vomiting is less than 3%, its prophylactic use to produce an antiemetic effect should be reserved for procedures in which vomiting could interfere with the results of surgery (eg, intraocular surgery, laparoscopy)

ADVERSE REACTIONS AND PRECAUTIONS. Droperidol occasionally produces extrapyramidal reactions (protrusion and uncontrolled movements of the tongue, dysphagia, lateral movements of the head, torticollis, twitching of limbs, restlessness, agitation, and parkinsonian crises) within 24 to 48 hours. Signs and symptoms can be relieved rapidly by diphenhydramine or benztropine (see index entries Diphenhydramine; Benztropine). Patients occasionally have reported dysphoric reactions when droperidol was given for preanesthetic medication.

Droperidol is classified in FDA Pregnancy Category C.

DRUG INTERACTIONS. Anecdotal evidence suggests that droperidol may antagonize the effects of levodopa resulting in reappearance of parkinsonian symptoms. Because of the drug's prolonged action (usually 12 to 24 hours), other central nervous system depressants should be given cautiously and in reduced doses during the early postoperative period.

PHARMACOKINETICS. Droperidol has an elimination half-life of approximately 2.2 hours (Cressman et al, 1973). Other pharmacokinetic parameters have not been reported.

DOSAGE AND PREPARATIONS. See the evaluation on Droperidol and Fentanyl Citrate.

Inapsine (Janssen), ***Generic.*** Solution 2.5 mg/ml in 1, 2, 5, and 10 ml containers.

DROPERIDOL AND FENTANYL CITRATE
[Innovar]

ACTIONS AND USES. This fixed-dose combination contains the opioid analgesic, fentanyl (0.05 mg/ml), and the neuroleptic butyrophenone, droperidol (2.5 mg/ml). These drugs usually provide satisfactory amnesia and analgesia, and the mixture has been used to produce neuroleptanalgesia and neuroleptanesthesia. As with all combinations, its use is appropriate only when both drugs would be administered at the same time and in the dosage ratio present in the mixture; otherwise, the two drugs should be administered separately as necessary.

Droperidol and fentanyl are safe for use in patients who have previously experienced malignant hyperpyrexia under general anesthesia.

ADVERSE REACTIONS AND PRECAUTIONS. Cardiac output is reduced and systemic vascular resistance is increased initially (due to the fentanyl component) but returns to normal as surgery continues. The arterial pressure and pulse rate tend to remain stable, but the heart rate may decrease. Ventricular arrhythmias are uncommon unless the sympathetic nervous system is stimulated by accumulation of carbon dioxide due to inadequate ventilation. Profound depression of the ventilatory rate and minute volume and apnea (caused by fentanyl) are to be expected. Apnea may result from central nervous system depression or peripheral muscle rigidity and can be treated by controlled ventilation. Muscle rigidity ("frozen chest syndrome") can be overcome by neuromuscular blocking agents.

Transient, slight abnormalities in the results of liver function tests similar to those observed after other anesthetic techniques have developed. Hyperglycemia occurs, but there is no evidence of metabolic acidosis. Pupils are constricted, intraocular tension is unchanged, and, if hypercapnia is avoided, cerebrospinal fluid pressure is reduced in patients with and without space-occupying lesions. In contrast, the volatile agents may increase pressure, even with normocapnia.

Consciousness and spontaneous ventilation return rapidly when nitrous oxide and controlled ventilation are stopped if large doses have not been administered repeatedly. Postoperative nausea and vomiting are extremely rare; shivering due to hypothermia also is rare, and restlessness or delirium is uncommon. Extrapyramidal reactions may develop if a large dose of droperidol has been used (see the evaluation on Droperidol).

Evidence that the combination reduces laryngeal competence suggests that this mixture should be used only with great caution and in small quantities to facilitate "awake intubation" indicated for a full stomach.

Droperidol has caused significant dysphoria when given alone. When Innovar was used for preanesthetic medication in an intramuscular dose of 1 to 2 ml, patients sometimes developed dysphoria and occasionally disorientation during the preoperative period, probably caused by the much shorter duration of action of fentanyl.

See also the evaluations on Fentanyl Citrate and Droperidol.

This combination is classified in FDA Pregnancy Category C.

DOSAGE AND PREPARATIONS.

Intravenous: Neuroleptanesthesia can be induced with 1 ml/9 to 12 kg (smaller doses may be adequate) administered slowly (1 ml every one to two minutes), followed by nitrous oxide and oxygen when drowsiness develops. Thiopental 100 mg also may be used to hasten induction. Anesthesia can be maintained with nitrous oxide or with fentanyl alone (usual dose, 0.05 to 0.1 mg every 30 to 60 minutes) when clinical signs indicate that anesthesia may be too light (voluntary movements, rapid or irregular ventilation, increasing pulse rate and arterial pressure, lacrimation). The mixture should not be used for maintenance unless the patient specifically requires the pharmacologic effects of both drugs.

Neuromuscular blocking agents and controlled ventilation should be utilized as indicated. If the former are not required, assisted ventilation may be adequate if the total dose of fentanyl does not exceed approximately 3 mcg/kg. A narcotic antagonist can be given to reverse severe respiratory depression but, unless carefully titrated to a satisfactory level of depression, it will antagonize the analgesic effect as well. The patient must be observed carefully after use of the narcotic antagonist in case the effect of the antagonist ends before that of fentanyl.

Because droperidol is long acting and has a relatively slow onset (10 to 15 minutes) and fentanyl has a relatively rapid onset (one to two minutes) but a short duration of action, an alternative technique that avoids the use of Innovar has been described: Induction is started with a single dose of droperidol

0.15 mg/kg; six to eight minutes later, fentanyl 0.002 to 0.003 mg/kg is given incrementally over six to eight minutes. Nitrous oxide is started when drowsiness develops and anesthesia is maintained as described above.

Innovar (Janssen), ***Generic***. Each milliliter of solution contains fentanyl citrate 0.05 mg and droperidol 2.5 mg in 2 and 5 ml containers.

FENTANYL CITRATE

[Sublimaze]

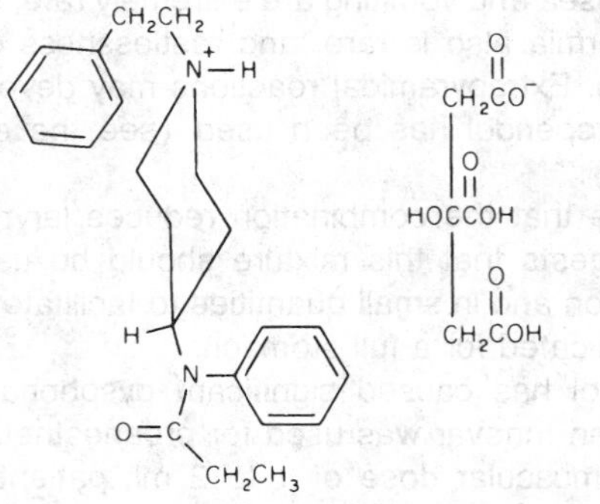

ACTIONS. On a milligram basis, fentanyl is 50 to 100 times more potent than morphine; however, the analgesia produced by morphine lasts two to three times longer. Moderate single doses are short acting due to redistribution from the central nervous system. Multiple doses or large amounts accumulate and prolong recovery time.

USES. For balanced anesthesia with nitrous oxide or another inhalation agent and a muscle relaxant, repeated doses of 0.05 to 0.1 mg of fentanyl can be used instead of morphine in poor-risk patients. Fentanyl does not cause the moderate to marked vasodilation produced by morphine and meperidine and, unlike morphine, does not cause release of histamine. Fentanyl can be used for induction of surgical anesthesia and as the sole anesthetic agent with oxygen and a muscle relaxant for any kind of surgery in selected (usually critically ill) patients.

Fentanyl is used with the butyrophenone, droperidol, in neuroleptanalgesia and with both droperidol and nitrous oxide in neuroleptanesthesia (see the evaluation on Droperidol and Fentanyl).

ADVERSE REACTIONS AND PRECAUTIONS. If an intravenous dose of fentanyl is administered rapidly, a generalized increase in muscle tone, including chest wall rigidity, may develop; such rigidity also can occur with use of meperidine or morphine. The incidence of rigidity increases with age and is believed to be caused by a central action of fentanyl. Thoracic compliance, the so-called "frozen chest syndrome," decreases markedly, which impairs the ability to assist or control ventilation. The incidence and severity of rigidity can be decreased by preanesthetic medication with a small dose of a nondepolarizing muscle relaxant (eg, pancuronium, 1 to 1.5 mg in the adult). Rigidity also is exacerbated by nitrous oxide but can be relieved or prevented by intravenous or volatile anesthetic agents. Controlled ventilation must be established but may be difficult while rigidity is present. A delayed effect of fentanyl that occurs rarely two to six hours after surgery has been reported; it is characterized by muscle rigidity, decreased chest wall compliance, and impaired ventilation leading to acidosis, hypotension, and respiratory arrest (Klausner et al, 1988). This condition responds to mechanical ventilation and the intravenous administration of naloxone 0.4 mg. It is postulated to be caused by re-entry of fentanyl into the circulation from sequestering sites in the gastrointestinal tract, muscle, and fat.

Slowing of the heart rate, which is easily reversed by atropine, may occur when fentanyl is given. The incidence and severity of bradycardia are lessened by the concomitant use of a vagolytic muscle relaxant (eg, pancuronium, even in a defasciculating dose [about 1 mg in adults]).

Fentanyl is classified in FDA Pregnancy Category C.

PHARMACOKINETICS. Fentanyl 6.4 mcg/kg given intravenously has an elimination half-life of 3.6 hours, an apparent volume of distribution of 4 L/kg, and a clearance of 0.96 L/min. It is 81% protein bound (McClain and Hug, 1980). The pharmacokinetic data from several sources have been reviewed (Mather, 1983). The decrease in fentanyl dose requirement with age has been thought to be related to an increased sensitivity of the central nervous system rather than to altered pharmacokinetics (Scott and Stanski, 1985); however, an alternative explanation is the appearance of a higher initial fentanyl concentration in the circulation secondary to the diminished volume of distribution (Singleton et al, 1988).

DOSAGE AND PREPARATIONS.

Intramuscular: *Adults,* for premedication, 0.05 to 0.1 mg (1 to 2 ml) 30 to 60 minutes prior to surgery. This dose should be decreased in the elderly or poor-risk patient.

Intravenous: *Adults,* for induction, 0.05 to 0.1 mg (1 to 2 ml) initially, repeated at two- to three-minute intervals until satisfactory induction is achieved. If attenuation of sympathetic activity is desired (eg, coronary artery disease), a total dose of 50 to 120 mcg/kg is required. The dose should be reduced to 0.025 to 0.05 mg (0.5 to 1 ml) in elderly or poor-risk patients. For maintenance, 0.025 mg to one-half the loading dose may be administered if lightening of anesthesia is manifested by movement. Change in vital signs may or may not occur. *Children 2 to 12 years,* for induction and maintenance, 2 to 3 mcg/kg. See also the evaluation on Droperidol and Fentanyl Citrate.

Sublimaze (Janssen), ***Generic.*** Solution 0.05 mg/ml in 2, 5, 10, and 20 ml containers.

SUFENTANIL CITRATE

[Sufenta]

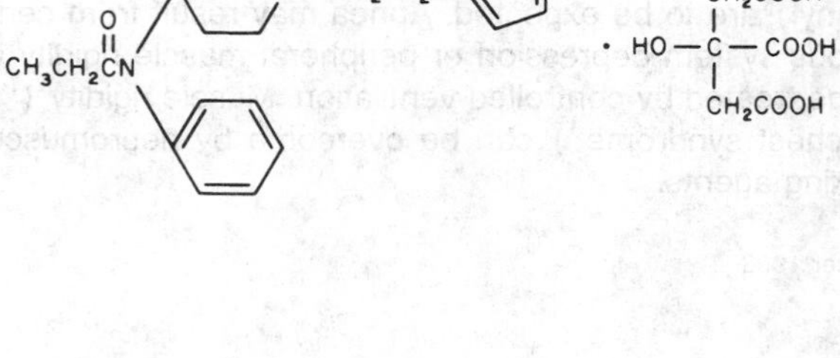

ACTIONS. This opioid is a derivative of fentanyl and is pharmacologically similar. On a weight basis, sufentanil is about 10 times more potent than fentanyl and 625 times more potent than morphine. When given in equipotent doses to induce anesthesia, the onset of action of sufentanil is equal to or more rapid than that of fentanyl. After induction of general anesthesia, recovery is significantly more rapid than with an equivalent anesthetic dose of fentanyl. The duration of action, like that of fentanyl, is determined by redistribution from the central nervous system. Because sufentanil is cleared more rapidly from tissue storage sites, there presumably is less tendency for accumulation.

USES. Sufentanil is used for balanced anesthesia in general surgery as an adjunct to nitrous oxide and oxygen. It also may be used for induction of surgical anesthesia and as the sole anesthetic agent with a muscle relaxant and oxygen for cardiovascular, neurosurgical, and other procedures.

ADVERSE REACTIONS AND PRECAUTIONS. Like fentanyl, the rapid intravenous administration of sufentanil may produce a general increase in skeletal muscle tone, including chest wall rigidity, the "frozen chest syndrome." The incidence of this response can be reduced by the prior or concomitant administration of a nondepolarizing muscle relaxant. A delayed postoperative respiratory depression associated with increased muscle tone and decreased chest wall compliance is observed rarely. It responds to mechanical ventilation and administration of naloxone.

Bradycardia occurs in about 3% of patients and responds to atropine. The combined use of sufentanil and succinylcholine also can produce significant bradycardia. Both hypotension and hypertension have been reported. Significant hypotension and bradycardia have been observed during induction in patients who received a benzodiazepine for premedication. Whether this is a specific drug interaction has not been determined.

Postoperative recovery may be delayed in the elderly, even after small doses, and the use of naloxone may be considered. Doses in the elderly should be limited to 10 to 20 mcg/min and administered only as required to meet the anesthetic need.

Sufentanil is classified in FDA Pregnancy Category C.

PHARMACOKINETICS. In adults, sufentanil 5 mcg/kg given intravenously is metabolized rapidly (elimination half-life, 2.7 hours). The apparent volume of distribution is 2.8 L/kg and the clearance is 12.7 L/kg/min (Bovill et al, 1984). The pharmacokinetics of sufentanil in patients over age 70 do not differ from those in young adults (Spielvogel et al, 1987).

In the neonate (0 to 1 month), the elimination half-life is about 12 hours, the volume of distribution is 4.2 L/kg, and the clearance is 6.7 ml/kg/min. By age 1 year, the pharmacokinetic parameters are not significantly different from those in the adult (Greeley et al, 1987). Sufentanil is bound primarily to α1-acid glycoprotein. This is reflected in its degree of plasma protein binding, which increases with age in parallel with the increase in α1-acid glycoprotein. Sufentanil is 81% bound in the newborn, 88.5% at age 1 to 12 months, 91.9% at age 3 to 10 years, and 92.2% at age 25 to 50 years (Meistelman et al, 1987).

DOSAGE AND PREPARATIONS.

Intravenous: For general surgery requiring intubation and mechanical ventilation, *adults*, 1 to 2 mcg/kg with nitrous oxide/oxygen; for maintenance, 10 to 25 mcg (0.2 to 0.5 ml) as needed or by continuous infusion.

For major surgical procedures requiring some attenuation of sympathetic response to surgical stimuli, *adults*, 2 to 8 mcg/kg with nitrous oxide/oxygen; for maintenance, 25 to 50 mcg (0.5 to 1 ml) as needed or by continuous infusion of 0.3 to 1 mcg/kg/min.

For induction in patients undergoing cardiovascular procedures, *adults*, 8 to 30 mcg/kg or more with oxygen and a nondepolarizing muscle relaxant; for maintenance, 25 to 50 mcg (0.5 to 1 ml) as needed or continuous infusion at the higher dose range. Postoperative mechanical ventilation will be required with these doses. *Children 2 to 12 years undergoing cardiovascular surgery*, 10 mcg/kg or more with oxygen only; *newborn to 2 years*, no dosage has been established. However, sufentanil appears to be safe for cardiovascular procedures in this population (Davis et al, 1987).

For induction for neurosurgical procedures, *adults*, 1 to 2 mcg/kg with a benzodiazepine or small doses of thiopental and oxygen and a nondepolarizing muscle relaxant; for maintenance, incremental doses not exceeding 1 mcg/kg/hr or a continuous infusion not exceeding that rate.

Sufenta (Janssen). Solution 50 mcg/ml in 1, 2, and 5 ml containers (preservative free).

Cited References

Aitkenhead AR, et al: Comparison of propofol and midazolam for sedation in critically ill patients. *Lancet* 2:704-709, 1989.

Aldrete JA, McDonald JS: Low-dose ketamine-diazepam prevents adverse reactions, in Aldrete JA, Stanley TH (eds): *Trends in Intravenous Anesthesia*. Chicago, Year Book Medical Publishers, 1980, 331-341.

Arden JR, et al: Increased sensitivity to etomidate in the elderly: Initial distribution versus altered brain response. *Anesthesiology* 65:19-27, 1986.

Bell GD, et al: Intravenous midazolam for upper gastrointestinal endoscopy: Study of 800 consecutive cases relating dose to age and sex of patient. *Br J Clin Pharmacol* 23:241-243, 1987.

Beller JP, et al: Prolonged sedation with propofol in ICU patients: Recovery and blood concentration changes during periodic interruptions in infusion. *Br J Anaesth* 61:583-588, 1988.

Bovill JG, et al: Pharmacokinetics of sufentanil in surgical patients. *Anesthesiology* 61:502-506, 1984.

Cahalan MK, et al: Hemodynamic effects of desflurane/nitrous oxide anesthesia in volunteers. *Anesth Analg* 73:157-164, 1991.

Caldwell JE, et al: The neuromuscular effects of desflurane, alone and combined with pancuronium or succinylcholine in humans. *Anesthesiology* 74:412-418, 1991.

Carpenter RL, et al: Pharmacokinetics of inhaled anesthetics in humans: Measurements during and after the simultaneous administration of enflurane, halothane, isoflurane, methoxyflurane, and nitrous oxide. *Anesth Analg* 65:575-582, 1986 A.

Carpenter RL, et al: Extent of metabolism of inhaled anesthetics in humans. *Anesthesiology* 65:201-205, 1986 B.

Chauvin M, et al: Pharmacokinetics of midazolam in anesthetized cirrhotic patients, abstract. *Anesthesiology* 67(suppl 3A):A290, 1987.

Chong M, Davis TP: Accidental intra-arterial injection of propofol, letter. *Anaesthesia* 42:781, 1987.

Christ DD, et al: Potential metabolic basis for enflurane hepatitis and the apparent cross-sensitization between enflurane and halothane. *Drug Metab Disp* 16:135-140, 1988.

Cohen EN, et al: Occupational disease in dentistry and chronic exposure to trace anesthetic gases. *J Am Dent Assoc* 101:21-31, 1980.

Cressman WA, et al: Absorption, metabolism and excretion of droperidol by human subjects following intramuscular and intravenous administration. *Anesthesiology* 38:363-369, 1973.

Dailland P, et al: Intravenous propofol during cesarean section: Placental transfer, concentrations in breast milk, and neonatal effects: Preliminary study. *Anesthesiology* 71:827-834, 1989.

Davis PJ, Cook DR: Clinical pharmacokinetics of the newer intravenous anaesthetic agents. *Clin Pharmacokinet* 11:18-35, 1986.

Davis PJ, et al: Pharmacodynamics and pharmacokinetics of high-dose sufentanil in infants and children undergoing cardiac surgery. *Anesth Analg* 66:203-208, 1987.

Eger RR, Eger EI II: Effect of temperature and age on solubility of enflurane, halothane, isoflurane, and methoxyflurane in human blood. *Anesth Analg* 64:640-642, 1985.

Ferrier C, et al: Alfentanil pharmacokinetics in patients with cirrhosis. *Anesthesiology* 62:480-484, 1985.

Fletcher JE, et al: Psychomotor performance after desflurane anesthesia: A comparison with isoflurane. *Anesth Analg* 73:260-265, 1991.

Fragen RJ, et al: Adrenocortical effects of Diprivan (propofol), etomidate, and thiopental. *Semin Anesth* 7 (suppl 1):108-111, 1988.

Gallently DC, Short TG: Total intravenous anaesthesia using propofol infusion: 50 consecutive cases. *Anaesth Intens Care* 16:150-157, 1988.

Ghouri AF, et al: Recovery profile after desflurane-nitrous oxide versus isoflurane-nitrous oxide in outpatients. *Anesthesiology* 74:419-424, 1991.

Giese JL, et al: Etomidate versus thiopental for induction of anesthesia. *Anesth Analg* 64:871-876, 1985.

Greeley WJ, et al: Sufentanil pharmacokinetics in pediatric cardiovascular patients. *Anesth Analg* 66:1067-1072, 1987.

Grounds RM, et al: Acute ventilatory changes during IV induction of anaesthesia with thiopentone or propofol in man: Studies using inductance plethysmography. *Br J Anaesth* 59:1098-1102, 1987.

Hammel HT: Anesthetics and body temperature regulation, editorial. *Anesthesiology* 68:833-835, 1988.

Hannallah RS, Patel RI: Low dose intramuscular ketamine for anesthesia induction in young children undergoing brief outpatient procedures, abstract. *Anesth Analg* 67:S85, 1988.

Helbo-Hansen S, et al: Reduction of pain on injection of propofol: Effect of addition of lignocaine. *Acta Anaesthesiol Scand* 32:502-504, 1988.

Helmers H, et al: Alfentanil kinetics in the elderly. *Clin Pharmacol Ther* 36:239-243, 1984.

Hornbein TF, et al: Minimum alveolar concentration of nitrous oxide in man. *Anesth Analg* 61:553-556, 1982.

Hubbard AK, et al: Halothane hepatitis patients generate an antibody response toward a covalently bound metabolite of halothane. *Anesthesiology* 68:791-796, 1988.

Hudson PJ, et al: Comparative pharmacokinetics of methohexital and thiopental. *Anesthesiology* 57:A240, 1982.

Jones RM, et al: Biotransformation and hepato-renal function in volunteers after exposure to desflurane (I-653). *Br J Anaesth* 64:482-487, 1990.

Jung D, et al: Thiopental disposition in lean and obese patients undergoing surgery. *Anesthesiology* 56:269-274, 1982.

Kanto JH: Propofol, the newest induction agent of anesthesia. *Int J Clin Pharmacol Ther Toxicol* 26:41-57, 1988.

Kanto J, Gepts E: Pharmacokinetic implications for the clinical use of propofol. *Clin Pharmacokinet* 17:308-326, 1989.

Kanto J, et al: Pharmacokinetics and sedative effect of midazolam in connection with Caesarean section performed under epidural anesthesia. *Acta Anaesthiol Scand* 28:116-118, 1984.

Kay NH, et al: Disposition of propofol in patients undergoing surgery: Comparison in men and women. *Br J Anaesth* 58:1075-1079, 1986.

Khalil SN, et al: Sigmoidorectal methohexital as inducing agent for general anesthesia in children, abstract. *Anesth Analg* 67:S113, 1988.

Kirpatrick T, et al: Pharmacokinetics of propofol (Diprivan) in elderly patients. *Br J Anaesth* 60:146-150, 1988.

Klausner JM, et al: Delayed muscular rigidity and respiratory depression following fentanyl anesthesia. *Arch Surg* 123:66-67, 1988.

Kottila K, et al: Omission of nitrous oxide does not decrease the incidence or severity of emetic symptoms after isoflurane anesthesia, abstract. *Anesth Analg* 66:S98, 1987.

Langley MS, Heel RC: Propofol: Review of its pharmacodynamic and pharmacokinetic properties and use as an intravenous anaesthetic. *Drugs* 35:334-372, 1988.

Larsen R, et al: Effects of propofol on cardiovascular dynamics and coronary blood flow in geriatric patients: Comparison with etomidate. *Anaesthesia* 43 (suppl):25-31, 1988.

Lerman J: Desflurane: The dawn of a new era? *Can J Anaesth* 38:954-957, 1991.

Maitre PO, et al: Population pharmacokinetics of alfentanil: Average dose-plasma concentration relationship and interindividual variability in patients. *Anesthesiology* 66:3-12, 1987.

Marks LF, et al: Propofol during cardiopulmonary bypass in a patient susceptible to malignant hyperpyrexia. *Anaesth Intens Care* 16:482-485, 1988.

Mather LE: Clinical pharmacokinetics of fentanyl and its newer derivatives. *Clin Pharmacokinet* 8:422-446, 1983.

Mattila MAK, Koski EMJ: Venous sequelae after intravenous propofol ('Diprivan'): Comparison with methohexitone in short anaesthesia. *Postgrad Med J* 61 (suppl 3):162-164, 1985.

McClain DA, Hug CC Jr: Intravenous fentanyl kinetics. *Clin Pharmacol Ther* 28:106-114, 1980.

McLoughlin C: Use of propofol in a patient with porphyria, letter. *Br J Anaesth* 62:114, 1989.

Meistelman C, et al: Comparison of alfentanil pharmacokinetics in children and adults. *Anesthesiology* 66:13-16, 1987.

Melnick BM, Johnson LS: Effects of eliminating nitrous oxide in outpatient anesthesia. *Anesthesiology* 67:982-984, 1987.

Moore J, et al: Comparison between propofol and thiopentone as induction agents in obstetric anaesthesia. *Anaesthesia* 44:753-757, 1989.

Morcos WE, Payne JP: Induction of anaesthesia with propofol ('Diprivan') compared in normal and renal failure patients. *Postgrad Med J* 61 (suppl 3):62-63, 1985.

Morgan DJ, et al: Pharmacokinetics and plasma binding of thiopental. I. Studies in surgical patients. II. Studies at cesarean section. *Anesthesiology* 54:468-473, 474-480, 1981.

Muir JJ, et al: Role of nitrous oxide and other factors in postoperative nausea and vomiting: Randomized and blinded prospective study. *Anesthesiology* 66:513-518, 1987.

Newman LH, et al: Propofol infusion for sedation in intensive care. *Anaesthesia* 42:929-937, 1987.

Nunn JF: Interaction of nitrous oxide and vitamin B_{12}. *Trends Pharmacol Sci* 5:225-227, 1984.

Paull J, Ziccone S: Halothane, enflurane, methoxyflurane, and isolated human uterine muscle. *Anaesth Intens Care* 8:397-401, 1980.

Perry SM, et al: Comparison of propofol and thiopental for the induction of anesthesia. *South Med J* 81:611-615, 1988.

Purcell-Jones G, et al: Comparison of the induction characteristics of thiopentone and propofol in children. *Br J Anaesth* 59:1431-1436, 1987.

Ramasubramanian R, et al: Attenuation of psychological effects of ketamine anesthesia by midazolam: Dose-response study, abstract. *Anesth Analg* 67:S182, 1988.

Rampil IJ, et al: Clinical characteristics of desflurane in surgical patients: Minimum alveolar concentration. *Anesthesiology* 74:429-433, 1991 A.

Rampil IJ, et al: The electroencephalographic effects of desflurane in humans. *Anesthesiology* 74:434-439, 1991 B.

Ray DC, Drummond GB: Halothane hepatitis. *Br J Anaesth* 67:84-99, 1991.

Russell GN, et al: Propofol-fentanyl anaesthesia for coronary artery surgery and cardiopulmonary bypass. *Anaesthesia* 44:205-208, 1989.

Saidman LJ: The role of desflurane in the practice of anesthesia, editorial. *Anesthesiology* 74:399-401, 1991.

Saint-Maurice C, et al: Pharmacokinetics of propofol in young children after a single dose. *Br J Anaesth* 63:667-670, 1989.

Scheepstra GL, et al: Propofol for induction and maintenance of anaesthesia: Comparison between younger and older patients. *Br J Anaesth* 62:54-60, 1989.

Scott JC, Stanski DR: Decreased fentanyl/alfentanil dose requirements with increasing age: Pharmacokinetic basis, abstract. *Anesthesiology* 63 (suppl 3A):A374, 1985.

Sebel PS, Lowdon JD: Propofol: New intravenous anesthetic. *Anesthesiology* 71:260-277, 1989.

Servin F, et al: Pharmacokinetics and protein binding of propofol in patients with cirrhosis. *Anesthesiology* 69:887-891, 1988.

Sessler DI, et al: Spontaneous post-anesthetic tremor does not resemble thermoregulatory shivering. *Anesthesiology* 68:843-850, 1988.

Simons PJ, et al: Disposition in male volunteers of a subanaesthetic intravenous dose of an oil in water emulsion of ^{14}C-propofol. *Xenobiotica* 18:429-440, 1988.

Singleton MA, et al: Pharmacokinetics of fentanyl in the elderly. *Br J Anaesth* 60:619-622, 1988.

Sorbo S, et al: Pharmacokinetics of thiopental in pediatric surgical patients. *Anesthesiology* 61:666-670, 1984.

Spielvogel C, et al: Pharmacokinetics of sufentanil in the elderly, abstract. *Anesthesiology* 67 (suppl 3A):A389, 1987.

Stark RD, et al: Review of the safety and tolerance of propofol ('Diprivan'). *Postgrad Med J* 61 (suppl 3):152-156, 1985.

Stinson TW III, Donlon JV Jr: Interaction of intraocular air and sulfur hexafluoride with nitrous oxide: Computer simulation. *Anesthesiology* 56:385-388, 1982.

Stock JGL, Strunin L: Unexplained hepatitis following halothane. *Anesthesiology* 63:424-439, 1985.

Sutton TS, et al: Fluoride metabolites after prolonged exposure of volunteers and patients to desflurane. *Anesth Analg* 73:180-185, 1991.

Taylor R, et al: Induction and recovery characteristics of desflurane in infants and children, abstract. *Anesthesiology* 73:A1246, 1990.

Tinker JH: Desflurane: First new volatile anesthetic in almost 20 years. *Anesth Analg* 75:S1-S2, 1992.

Trouvin J-H, et al: Pharmacokinetics of midazolam in anaesthetized cirrhotic patients. *Br J Anaesth* 60:762-767, 1988.

Tyson G, et al: Prolonged anesthesia with nitrous oxide: Is it hazardous? abstract. *Anesth Analg* 66:S182, 1987.

Valtonen M: Anaesthesia for computerized tomography of the brain in children: Comparison of propofol and thiopentone. *Acta Anaesthesiol Scand* 33:170-173, 1989.

Valtonen M, et al: Comparison between propofol and thiopentone for induction of anaesthesia in children. *Anaesthesia* 43:696-699, 1988.

Valtonen M, et al: Comparison of propofol and thiopentone for induction of anaesthesia for elective Caesarean section. *Anaesthesia* 44:758-762, 1989 A.

Valtonen M, et al: Propofol as an induction agent in children: Pain on injection and pharmacokinetics. *Acta Anaesthesiol Scand* 33:152-155, 1989 B.

Van Hamelrijck J, et al: Use of desflurane for outpatient anesthesia: A comparison with propofol and nitrous oxide. *Anesthesiology* 75:197-203, 1991.

Van Hamme MJ, et al: Pharmacokinetics of etomidate, new intravenous anesthetic. *Anesthesiology* 49:274-277, 1978.

Van Peer A, et al: Alfentanil kinetics in renal insufficiency. *Eur J Clin Pharmacol* 30:245-247, 1986.

Wedel DJ, et al: Desflurane is a trigger of malignant hyperthermia in susceptible swine. *Anesthesiology* 74:508-512, 1991.

White PF: Ketamine update: Its clinical uses in anesthesia. *Semin Anesth* 7:113-126, 1988 A.

White PF: Propofol: Pharmacokinetics and pharmacodynamics. *Semin Anesth* 7 (suppl 1):4-20, 1988 B.

Wilson RD, et al: Cardiovascular effects of ketamine infusion, in Aldrete JA, Stanley TH (eds): *Trends in Intravenous Therapy*. Chicago, Year Book Medical Publishers, 1980, 343-354.

Wrigley SR, et al: Induction and recovery characteristics of desflurane in day case patients: A comparison with propofol. *Anaesthesiology* 46:615-622, 1991.

Other Selected References

Miller RD (ed): *Anesthesia,* ed 2. New York, Churchill Livingstone, 1986.

Smith NT, Corbascio AN (eds): *Drug Interactions in Anesthesia,* ed 2. Philadelphia, Lea & Febiger, 1986.

Stanley TH: Opiate anaesthesia. *Anaesth Intens Care* 15:38-59, 1987.

Stoelting RK: *Pharmacology and Physiology in Anesthetic Practice.* Philadelphia, JB Lippincott, 1987.

Swerdlow BN, Holley FO: Intravenous anesthetic agents: Pharmacokinetic-pharmacodynamic relationships. *Clin Pharmacokinet* 12:79-110, 1987.

Adjuncts to Anesthesia 10

A number of drugs commonly used as adjuncts to anesthesia have additional therapeutic indications and may be discussed in more detail in other chapters. Agents given to reduce the incidence of postoperative nausea and vomiting are discussed elsewhere; see index entry Antiemetics. For discussion of drugs used in the prevention and management of aspiration pneumonitis, see index entry Pneumonitis, Aspiration.

AGENTS USED FOR PREMEDICATION

Generally, a patient's usual medication need not be altered when surgery is indicated, but potential complications or drug interactions must be evaluated. Medications that must be continued (eg, antianginal, antiepileptic, antihypertensive drugs) may necessitate modification of the anesthetic technique. The dose of insulin may require adjustment to avoid intraoperative hypoglycemia or hyperglycemia and ketosis. Glucocorticoids should be continued and may need to be supplemented in patients who have received high-dose therapy in the preceding six months or in those with chronic asthma. Opioid analgesics frequently are required in patients with moderate to severe preoperative pain and in opioid-dependent individuals. Defects in hydration, electrolyte balance, hemoglobin levels, and nutritional status should be corrected before surgery if possible.

Historically, drugs were administered before the induction of anesthesia with diethyl ether to sedate the patient, reduce apprehension, facilitate induction, diminish the dose of anesthetic, inhibit salivary and airway secretions, and prevent bradycardia. Morphine was used to achieve the first four effects, and atropine or scopolamine was given to achieve the remaining two. During the last several decades, other analgesics, hypnotics, benzodiazepines, and neuroleptics have been used instead of morphine, but definitive comparative studies have not been conducted.

Analgesics: There are few important differences among the individual analgesics. Euphoria is not a characteristic of the preanesthetic use of opioids. These agents should be reserved for relief of preoperative pain. Most opioids increase the incidence of pre- and postoperative nausea and vomiting. Other adverse effects include dizziness, tachycardia, sweating, and, less commonly, hypotension, restlessness or excitement, and respiratory depression with a marked reduction in the respiratory response to increases in PCO_2.

If scopolamine is given with morphine or meperidine [Demerol], the incidence of sedation and delayed awakening may be increased, while that of apprehension and pre- and postoperative nausea and vomiting may be reduced.

Intramuscular fentanyl [Sublimaze] has an inappropriate onset and too short a duration of action for routine preanesthetic use. When administered intravenously just prior to induction of general or regional anesthesia, it produces good to profound sedation.

See also Table 1 for dosages and index entries Analgesics; Opioids.

Barbiturates: In an attempt to avoid the adverse effects of opioid analgesics, secobarbital [Seconal] and pentobarbital [Nembutal] have been administered. However, preanesthetic doses of these drugs may depress respiration and do not provide analgesia; disorientation or delirium may develop in the presence of pain. Circulation is only slightly affected and nausea or vomiting is rare. Barbiturates must not be used in patients with a hepatic porphyria.

Barbiturates now are being replaced by benzodiazepines, which produce more anterograde amnesia and less respiratory depression. See also Table 1 for dosages and index entry Barbiturates, Uses.

Benzodiazepines: The benzodiazepines may be preferred to the opioid analgesics and the short-acting barbiturates for premedication. These drugs provide sedation and anterograde amnesia and reduce anxiety to varying degrees.

TABLE 1.
AGENTS USED FOR PREMEDICATION

Drug	Route	Dosage
ANALGESICS		
Fentanyl Citrate [Sublimaze]	Intramuscular Intravenous	*Adults,* 0.05 to 0.1 mg.
Morphine Sulfate	Subcutaneous Intramuscular Intravenous	*Adults,* 10 mg (range, 5 to 12 mg); *children 1 year and over,* 0.1 mg/kg (maximum, 10 mg).
Meperidine Hydrochloride [Demerol Hydrochloride]	Subcutaneous Intramuscular Intravenous	*Adults,* 100 mg (range, 50 to 150 mg); *children 1 year and over,* 1 mg/kg (maximum, 100 mg).
Pentazocine Lactate [Talwin Lactate]	Subcutaneous Intramuscular	*Adults,* 20 to 40 mg.
BARBITURATES		
Pentobarbital Sodium [Nembutal Sodium]	Intramuscular Intravenous	*Adults,* 100 to 150 mg (range, 75 to 200 mg); *children 6 months and over,* 2 to 4 mg/kg (maximum, 100 mg).
Secobarbital Sodium [Seconal Sodium]	Intramuscular Intravenous	*Adults,* 100 to 150 mg (range, 75 to 200 mg); *children 6 months and over,* 2 to 4 mg/kg (maximum, 100 mg).
BENZODIAZEPINES		
Chlordiazepoxide Hydrochloride [Librium]	Oral Intravenous	*Adults,* 50 to 100 mg.
Diazepam [Valium, Valrelease]	Oral Intravenous	*Adults,* 10 mg; *children 2 years and over,* 0.25 mg/kg. *Adults,* 10 to 20 mg; *children,* 0.4 to 0.5 mg/kg.
Lorazepam [Ativan]	Oral Intramuscular Intravenous	*Adults,* 4 mg. *Adults,* * 0.05 mg/kg (maximum, 4 mg) two hours prior to surgery. *Adults,* * 0.044 mg/kg (maximum, 2 mg).
Midazolam Hydrochloride [Versed]	Intravenous Intramuscular	*Adults,* 5 mg. *Adults,* 0.07 to 0.08 mg/kg.
Temazepam [Restoril]	Oral	*Adults,* 20 to 30 mg.
Triazolam [Halcion]	Oral	*Adults,* 0.125 to 0.25 mg (maximum, 0.5 mg).
NEUROLEPTIC DRUGS		
Droperidol [Inapsine]	Intramuscular Intravenous	*Adults,* 2.5 to 5 mg.
Droperidol and Fentanyl Citrate [Innovar]	Intramuscular Intravenous	*Adults,* 0.5 to 2 ml (fentanyl 0.05 mg/ml and droperidol 2.5 mg/ml).
ANTICHOLINERGIC DRUGS		
Atropine Sulfate	Oral Intramuscular Intravenous	*Adults,* 2 mg. *Adults,* 0.4 to 0.6 mg; *newborn infants,* 0.1 mg; *4 to 12 months,* 0.2 mg; *children 1 to 3 years,* 0.3 mg; *3 to 14 years,* 0.4 mg.
Glycopyrrolate [Robinul Injectable]	Intramuscular Intravenous	*Adults,* 0.0044 mg/kg; *children up to 12 years,* 4.4 to 8.8 mcg/kg 60 minutes prior to induction.
Scopolamine Hydrobromide	Oral Intramuscular Intravenous	*Adults,* 1 mg. *Adults,* 0.4 to 0.6 mg; *infants 4 to 7 months,* 0.1 mg; *7 months to 3 years,* 0.15 mg; *children 3 to 8 years;* 0.2 mg; *8 to 12 years,* 0.3 mg.

Subcutaneous or intramuscular doses are administered 45 to 60 minutes and oral doses one to four hours before anesthesia. The amounts should be reduced in elderly or debilitated patients.

Intravenous administration should be slow and cautious, ie, titrated to effect. Intravenous doses are generally smaller than those recommended for other parenteral routes.

**Not recommended for patients under 18 years.*

Excitement, dizziness, tachycardia, hypotension, and pre- or postoperative nausea and vomiting are uncommon, although the combined use of lorazepam and scopolamine may produce pronounced restlessness. Benzodiazepines slightly reduce lower esophageal sphincter pressure, which increases the possibility of reflux. Following premedication with intravenous diazepam 0.14 mg/kg, the minute ventilation, respiratory frequency, and mean inspiratory flow rate were reduced by 17%, 12%, and 19%, respectively (Clergue et al, 1981). The other benzodiazepines are presumed to cause equivalent respiratory depression.

Since benzodiazepines are absorbed reliably from the gastrointestinal tract, the oral route often is used. The onset of action is rapid after parenteral administration, but absorption following intramuscular injection of diazepam may be erratic because of this drug's low water solubility. Absorption is more rapid following injection into the upper thigh or deltoid rather than the buttock. Pain may persist at the injection site. In general, the water-soluble benzodiazepine, midazolam, is now used instead of diazepam when intramuscular or intravenous administration is preferred for premedication.

In children, benzodiazepines produce effective sedation, few nightmares, and, possibly, better acceptance of the anesthetic face mask; the incidence of postoperative vomiting also is lower than with opioids.

See also Table 1 for dosages and index entry Benzodiazepines, Uses.

Neuroleptic Drugs: When used as the sole preanesthetic medication in adults, intramuscular droperidol [Inapsine] 5 mg causes drowsiness significantly more often than secobarbital 100 mg but less often than 10 mg of either morphine or diazepam. In addition, the incidence of extrapyramidal reactions (dystonia, akathisia, and oculogyric crises), dysphoria, tachycardia, and hypotension is higher than with a placebo.

Droperidol alone does not always lessen postoperative nausea and vomiting more than a placebo, and the severity of preoperative nausea and vomiting may be similar to that experienced with morphine 10 mg. It has a significant pre- and postoperative antiemetic action when given with meperidine. In general, droperidol alone is unsatisfactory for preanesthetic medication in adults unless an analgesic is given concomitantly to prevent dysphoria. When droperidol 2.5 mg/ml is given with fentanyl citrate 0.05 mg/ml (available in this ratio as the fixed-dose combination Innovar) for premedication, the quality of sedation may be better than that produced by 10 mg of morphine. The incidence of preoperative nausea and vomiting with the combination is low and that of postoperative nausea and vomiting is significantly less than with 10 mg of morphine. See Table 1 for dosages and index entry Neuroleptanesthesia.

Controlled studies comparing the phenothiazine derivatives, chlorpromazine [Thorazine] and promethazine [Phenergan], with meperidine plus atropine showed that, at doses inducing comparable sedation, apprehension was relieved to a greater degree by the phenothiazines; however, the incidence of preoperative tachycardia and/or hypotension and restlessness appeared to be greater with their use. Some phenothiazines also produce postoperative dyskinesia. The usefulness of most phenothiazines for premedication is severely curtailed by these adverse effects and by their potential hazard of causing intraoperative hypotension. See also index entry Neuroleptic Drugs.

Anticholinergic Drugs: Atropine, scopolamine, or glycopyrrolate [Robinul Injectable] is given to reduce excessive salivary and other airway secretions caused by some inhalation anesthetics and ketamine [Ketalar]. They also are used to protect against bradycardia, sinus arrest, and hypotension induced by succinylcholine [Anectine, Quelicin, Sucostrin] during tracheal intubation or certain surgical manipulations (eg, stimulation of the peritoneum, pressure on the eye, traction of ocular muscles).

Atropine is preferred to scopolamine for preventing reflex bradycardia because it has a more sustained accelerating effect on the heart rate. However, usual preanesthetic doses (0.4 or 0.6 mg intramuscularly) do not block the cardiac vagal nerves (this requires 1.5 to 2 mg), and the vagolytic action of an intramuscular or intravenous dose is usually brief (30 minutes). Small doses (up to 0.4 mg) of scopolamine may slow rather than accelerate the heart rate; therefore, this drug is preferred to atropine when tachycardia must be avoided (eg, in patients with mitral stenosis).

Scopolamine is a more potent antisialagogue than atropine. It has a significant sedative effect and may reduce the incidence of postoperative nausea and vomiting. However, scopolamine also may produce dizziness, delay awakening, and prolong postoperative confusion, especially in the elderly. Scopolamine alone does not produce anterograde amnesia as effectively as lorazepam, but it does cause significant additive amnesia when used with a benzodiazepine or opioid analgesic.

The quaternary ammonium anticholinergic, glycopyrrolate, is a more potent antisialagogue than atropine and often is used for preanesthetic medication because it lacks central anticholinergic activity. The duration of parasympathetic blockade is two to three hours, and secretions are reduced for up to seven hours.

Anticholinergic drugs inhibit heat loss, presumably by suppressing perspiration, and should be given cautiously to patients with fever, particularly children, to avoid hyperpyrexia. All anticholinergic drugs reduce the tone of the lower esophageal sphincter, which may increase gastric reflux.

If anticholinergic premedication is required in patients predisposed to increased intraocular pressure, the hazard of inducing acute glaucoma can be minimized by instilling one drop of 1% pilocarpine in each eye. Anticholinergic drugs can be given safely to patients with open-angle glaucoma (80% of glaucoma patients have the open-angle type), particularly if they are being treated with miotics, and to patients who have undergone peripheral iridectomy.

Atropine and scopolamine, but not glycopyrrolate, readily cross the blood-brain barrier and can cause confusion, particularly in children and the elderly. The intraoperative use of atropine or scopolamine may prolong postanesthetic somnolence or cause emergence delirium postoperatively, especially in elderly individuals or patients in pain.

Physostigmine salicylate [Antilirium] administered intravenously is the specific antidote for central anticholinergic intoxication; doses of 1 mg reduce delirium and 2 mg may be required to lessen somnolence (see the discussion on Respiratory Stimulants in this chapter and index entry Physostigmine, In Anticholinergic Toxicity).

See Table 1 for dosages.

NEUROMUSCULAR BLOCKING DRUGS

Nondepolarizing (competitive) or depolarizing neuromuscular blocking agents are used to provide skeletal muscle relaxation during surgical procedures, particularly abdominal surgery. These drugs also are employed to facilitate endotracheal intubation, relieve laryngospasm, provide adequate muscle relaxation during diagnostic procedures performed under general anesthesia, prevent dislocations and fractures during electroconvulsive shock therapy, produce apnea to facilitate controlled ventilation during thoracic surgery and neurosurgery, control muscle spasms in tetanus, and facilitate controlled ventilation by eliminating inadequate spontaneous efforts in patients with ventilatory failure. Because neuromuscular blocking drugs have no anesthetic or analgesic properties, they should not be used to compensate for inadequate anesthesia.

Ventilation must be controlled whenever neuromuscular blocking agents are used. An objective evaluation of residual muscular paralysis (ie, the ability of the patient to breathe adequately, maintain an open airway, take a deep breath and cough, lift the head for five seconds, exhibit hand grip strength) must be conducted on completion of surgery. In infants, the ability to keep the eyes open or hold up the legs indicates restoration of neuromuscular function. For patients who are not sufficiently awake to permit satisfactory evaluation of ventilatory recovery, a peripheral nerve stimulator can be used to determine residual paralysis more precisely. Nerve stimulators also are commonly used to assess the magnitude of neuromuscular blockade during surgery.

Nondepolarizing (Competitive) Blocking Drugs

The nondepolarizing blocking drugs (tubocurarine, metocurine [Metubine], gallamine [Flaxedil], pancuronium [Pavulon], atracurium [Tracrium], vecuronium [Norcuron], doxacurium [Nuromax], mivacurium [Mivacron], and pipecuronium [Arduan]) compete with acetylcholine for cholinergic receptor sites on the postjunctional membrane but lack the transmitter action of acetylcholine. They also may have significant presynaptic depressant activities.

The nondepolarizing muscle relaxants display multicompartment pharmacokinetics. Schedules for loading doses, infusions, and use in various pathologic states and obstetrics have been designed, but these cannot substitute for monitoring of neuromuscular function. The pharmacokinetic properties of the nondepolarizing muscle relaxants are compared in Table 2.

Antagonists: The competitive block can be antagonized by anticholinesterases, such as neostigmine [Prostigmin] (adults, 2.5 to 5 mg; children, 0.08 mg/kg), pyridostigmine [Mestinon, Regonol] (adults, 10 to 20 mg; children, 0.4 mg/kg), or edrophonium [Enlon, Tensilon] (adults, 30 to 50 mg; children, 1 mg/kg).

Pyridostigmine has a slower onset (13 minutes) than edrophonium (three minutes) or neostigmine (six to eight minutes), but a longer duration of action than either. The pharmacokinetic properties of anticholinesterase agents employed to reverse neuromuscular blockade appear in Table 3.

Anticholinesterase drugs have undesirable vagal and muscarinic properties; thus, atropine (adults and children, 0.015 to 0.02 mg/kg) or glycopyrrolate (adults and children, 0.2 mg for each 1 mg of neostigmine or 5 mg of pyridostigmine) must be administered prior to or with these cholinesterase inhibitors. Atropine 0.01 mg/kg must be given with edrophonium to prevent bradycardia; a larger dose (0.015 mg/kg) is recommended during nitrous oxide/opioid anesthesia in pediatric patients. The anticholinesterase drugs must be used cautiously in patients with cardiac rhythm or conduction disturbances. Bronchial asthma does not present a problem.

The effectiveness of anticholinesterases in reversing skeletal muscle paralysis depends on the dose of the nondepolarizing blocking agent used and, more important, on the extent of neuromuscular block (percentage of spontaneous recovery from block) at the time of reversal. Neostigmine is more effective than pyridostigmine or edrophonium if little spontaneous recovery has occurred. If no response is elicited, additional quantities of the anticholinesterase should not be given until more spontaneous recovery can be demonstrated.

Depolarizing Blocking Drug

The depolarizing drug, succinylcholine [Anectine, Quelicin, Sucostrin], is believed to depolarize the postsynaptic membrane in a manner similar to the normal neurotransmitter, acetylcholine. Initially, muscle fasciculations occur and are usually visible. Continued occupation of the receptors by succinylcholine (which dissociates less readily from the receptor than acetylcholine) results in persistent blockade (phase I) and paralysis. Phase I block is not antagonized by anticholinesterase drugs; indeed, since anticholinesterase agents inhibit plasma cholinesterase (the enzyme responsible for the primary metabolism of succinylcholine), as well as acetylcholinesterase, these drugs may prolong the block.

A desensitization block (dual, antidepolarizing, or phase II block), which superficially is similar to that produced by the nondepolarizing drugs, may occur after a single large dose, repeated administration, or prolonged infusion of succinylcholine. The safest treatment of phase II block is maintenance of controlled ventilation until the block reverses spontaneously. However, antagonism of phase II block with an anticholinesterase drug may be a reasonable alternative when succinylcholine is not present in the circulation. Thus, succinylcholine can produce two types of block with different characteristics, durations, and responses to antagonists.

TABLE 2.
PHARMACOKINETICS OF NONDEPOLARIZING NEUROMUSCULAR BLOCKING AGENTS

Agent	t½β min	Vdss L/kg	Cl ml/kg/min	Reference
NORMOTHERMIC ADULTS				
Atracurium	21	0.16	5.3	Ward and Neill, 1983
Doxacurium	87	0.15	2.2	Dresner et al, 1990
Gallamine	150	0.29	1.6	Ramzan et al, 1980
Metocurine	269	0.45	1.1	Matteo et al, 1985
Mivacurium	3	0.20	54.5	deBros et al, 1987 A
Pancuronium	107	0.28	1.8	Duvaldestin et al, 1982
Pipecuronium	127	0.31	2.5	Caldwell et al, 1987 A
Tubocurarine	173	0.43	1.7	Matteo et al, 1985
Vecuronium	57.7	0.18	4.5	Arden et al, 1988
ELDERLY PATIENTS (> 65 years)				
Atracurium	19	0.17	6.4	deBros et al, 1987 A
Doxacurium	96	0.22	2.5	Dresner et al, 1990
Metocurine	530	0.28	0.4	Matteo et al, 1985
Pancuronium	201	0.32	1.2	Duvaldestin et al, 1982
Tubocurarine	268	0.28	0.8	Matteo et al, 1985
NEONATES (0-1 month)				
Tubocurarine	311	0.51	1.1	Matteo et al, 1984
INFANTS (1-12 months)				
Atracurium	14	0.18	9.1	Brandom et al, 1986 A
Metocurine	162	0.77	3.3	Weinstein et al, 1987
Tubocurarine	306	0.47	1.0	Matteo et al, 1984
Vecuronium	65	0.36	5.6	Fisher et al, 1982
PATIENTS WITH RENAL FAILURE				
Atracurium	18	0.17	6.3	de Bros et al, 1985
Metocurine	10.7 hrs	—	0.4	Brotherton and Matteo, 1980
Pancuronium	257	0.30	0.9	Somogyi et al, 1977 A
Pipecuronium	275	0.45	1.5	Caldwell et al, 1987 A
Tubocurarine	330	—	—	Miller et al, 1977
Vecuronium	83	0.24	3.1	Lynam et al, 1988
PATIENTS WITH HEPATIC FAILURE OR CIRRHOSIS				
Atracurium	24.9	0.16	4.7	Cook et al, 1984
Pancuronium	208	0.42	1.5	Duvaldestin et al, 1978
Vecuronium	51.4	0.22	4.2	Arden et al, 1988
PATIENTS WITH HEPATIC AND RENAL FAILURE				
Atracurium	22	0.21	6.5	Ward and Neill, 1983
PATIENTS WITH BILIARY OBSTRUCTION				
Gallamine	220	0.26	0.9	Westra et al, 1981
Pancuronium	224	0.43	1.5	Westra et al, 1981
Vecuronium	270	0.31	0.97	Somogyi et al, 1977 B

TABLE 3.
PHARMACOKINETICS OF ANTICHOLINESTERASE AGENTS EMPLOYED FOR REVERSAL OF NEUROMUSCULAR BLOCKADE

Agent	t½β min	Vdss L/kg	Cl ml/kg/min	Reference
NORMOTHERMIC ADULTS				
Edrophonium	110	1.1	9.6	Morris et al, 1981 A
Neostigmine	104	1.0	9.4	Cronnelly and Morris, 1982
Pyridostigmine	112	1.1	8.6	Cronnelly et al, 1980
PATIENTS WITH RENAL FAILURE				
Edrophonium	206	0.7	2.7	Morris et al, 1981 B
Neostigmine	183	0.78	3.4	Cronnelly and Morris, 1982
Pyridostigmine	379	1.0	2.1	Cronnelly et al, 1980

Drug Selection

The choice between the two classes of neuromuscular blocking drugs is determined by the expected duration of the operative procedure, the possibility of interactions between the blocking agent and the general anesthetic or other drugs, and the presence of pathologic conditions that may influence the drug's pharmacokinetics or the patient's response. Generally, a single dose of succinylcholine is used to produce brief relaxation or to facilitate endotracheal intubation. For longer surgical procedures and to facilitate controlled ventilation, repeated intravenous doses or infusions of nondepolarizing agents are used.

Adverse Reactions and Precautions

Prolonged paralysis may occur with succinylcholine if the plasma cholinesterase level is low or atypical. The dose should be reduced when plasma cholinesterase levels are low (eg, in those with severe parenchymatous liver disease or malnutrition; after administration of anticholinesterase miotic drugs or exposure to organophosphate insecticides).

Succinylcholine is a triggering agent for malignant hyperthermia in susceptible patients and is contraindicated when there is a history or suspicion of this syndrome and in children with Duchenne muscular dystrophy. Succinylcholine should be avoided in patients recovering from burns, in paraplegic and quadriplegic patients, in those with tetanus, and in others in whom muscle denervation may have occurred (eg, massive crush injury), because it may induce significant hyperkalemia leading to cardiac arrest.

Gallamine, pancuronium, metocurine, pipecuronium, doxacurium, and tubocurarine depend on renal function for clearance (see Table 2), but succinylcholine, mivacurium, atracurium, and, to some extent, vecuronium do not. The latter three are the nondepolarizing muscle relaxants of choice in patients with renal failure.

The main hazard with use of all neuromuscular blocking agents is inadequate postoperative ventilation. Their actions are prolonged by overdose, by interactions between the blocking agent and other drugs (including potent inhalation anesthetics, calcium channel blocking drugs, lithium, magnesium, procainamide, quinidine, and certain antibiotics, especially the aminoglycosides and polymyxins), or by certain pathologic conditions (eg, myasthenia gravis, Eaton-Lambert syndrome, amyotrophic lateral sclerosis). Respiratory acidosis, hypomagnesemia, hypocalcemia, and hypokalemia enhance the action of nondepolarizing drugs and make the block resistant to reversal. Dosage requirements may be reduced by 50% in hypothermic procedures. Use of a peripheral nerve stimulator should prevent an absolute or relative overdose.

Tachycardia and a slight increase in arterial pressure due to a vagolytic action follow administration of gallamine and, to a lesser extent, pancuronium. In contrast, tubocurarine induces histamine release and ganglionic blockade, thus reducing arterial pressure and producing bradycardia. The muscarinic effects of succinylcholine can cause bradycardia, sinus arrest, and severe arrhythmias, particularly after repeated doses in children; atropine may be used to counteract these effects.

Any nondepolarizing muscle relaxant is safe for use in patients with penetrating wounds of the eye, but succinylcholine generally is not recommended because intraocular pressure may increase. The mechanism of this increase has not been clearly defined (see the evaluation).

Histamine release induced by tubocurarine, metocurine, atracurium, and mivacurium may cause or exacerbate bronchospasm. This mechanism or the pressor action of succinylcholine may be responsible for increased intracranial pressure.

The use of muscle relaxants in patients with neuromuscular disorders has been reviewed (Azar, 1984; Hunter, 1987). Since the response of any particular patient is unpredictable, continuous monitoring of neuromuscular function during the use of muscle relaxants in these patients is strongly recommended. Patients with myasthenia gravis that is not in remission are extremely sensitive to nondepolarizing blocking agents. It is recommended that anticholinesterase therapy for the myasthenia patient be continued until induction and that the shorter acting nondepolarizing muscle relaxants (atracurium, mivacurium, or vecuronium) be utilized. Although the response to succinylcholine is abnormal (somewhat greater doses occasionally may be required and a phase II block develops early), a single dose usually provides safe and satisfactory conditions for intubation.

In patients with myasthenic syndrome associated with small cell carcinoma of the lung and other malignancies, there is increased sensitivity to both depolarizing and nondepolarizing muscle relaxants. Prolonged respiratory impairment may occur in patients receiving a single dose of succinylcholine as the sole relaxant for brief procedures (eg, bronchoscopy).

Succinylcholine should be avoided in patients with myotonia congenita, since it may cause spasm of the respiratory muscles.

Drug Evaluations

NONDEPOLARIZING (COMPETITIVE) BLOCKING DRUGS

ATRACURIUM BESYLATE

[Tracrium]

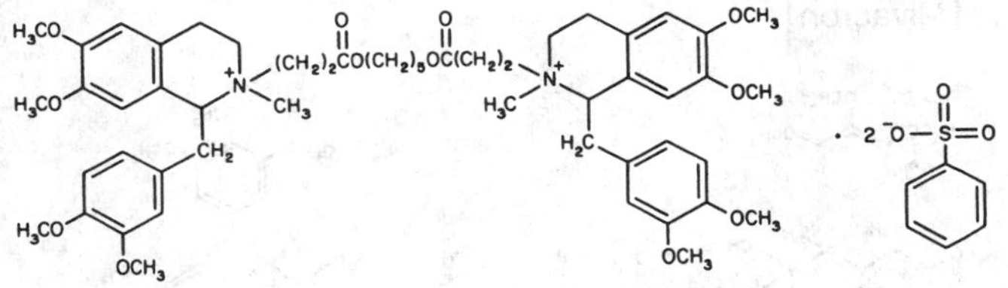

ACTIONS AND USES. This symmetrical bis-quaternary isoquinoline compound is approximately 2.5 times more potent than tubocurarine, but its duration of action is shorter. Atracurium is of particular value in patients with renal and/or hepatic impairment because neither condition alters the duration of block. Cardiovascular effects are minimal when recommended doses are given. The duration of action is similar in young adults and the elderly (Lowry et al, 1985), and obesity does not affect recovery time. Paralysis is antagonized readily by neostigmine, edrophonium, or pyridostigmine.

ADVERSE REACTIONS AND PRECAUTIONS. Urticaria, rash, local erythema, wheezing, and hypotension occur occasionally. Histamine release can be minimized by slow administration or by giving divided doses over at least one minute. Atracurium is classified in FDA Pregnancy Category C.

PHARMACOKINETICS. Atracurium is presumed to be inactivated by two degradative pathways, hydrolysis of an ester group and Hofmann elimination, both of which lead to breaks in the chain between the two quaternary nitrogen atoms. The relative contributions of these pathways have not been determined. Metabolites have no muscle relaxant action. The recovery rate after a single bolus dose is determined by spontaneous degradation, ester hydrolysis, and to a lesser extent redistribution. See Table 2 for the pharmacokinetic profile of atracurium.

DOSAGE AND PREPARATIONS. Dosage requirements vary, and a peripheral nerve stimulator aids in determining the appropriate amount. Enflurane, isoflurane, and, to a lesser extent, halothane decrease the dosage requirement.

Intravenous: *Adults and children 2 years or older,* initially, 0.4 to 0.5 mg/kg administered slowly; subsequent doses, 0.08 to 0.1 mg/kg titrated on the basis of patient response following spontaneous partial recovery from the initial bolus or a continuous infusion of 5 to 9 mcg/kg/min. If atracurium is given after succinylcholine-assisted intubation, 0.3 to 0.4 mg/kg is recommended initially. This reduced dose also is recommended for patients with cardiovascular disease, a history of asthma, or anaphylactoid reactions. *Infants 1 month to 2 years,* initially, 0.3 to 0.4 mg/kg. Infants appear to be more sensitive to atracurium than older children and may require lower doses. However, recovery in infants occurs at the same rate as in older children and adults (Goudsouzian, 1988).

Tracrium (Burroughs Wellcome). Solution 10 mg/ml in 5 ml containers and in 10 ml containers with benzyl alcohol.

DOXACURIUM CHLORIDE

[Nuromax]

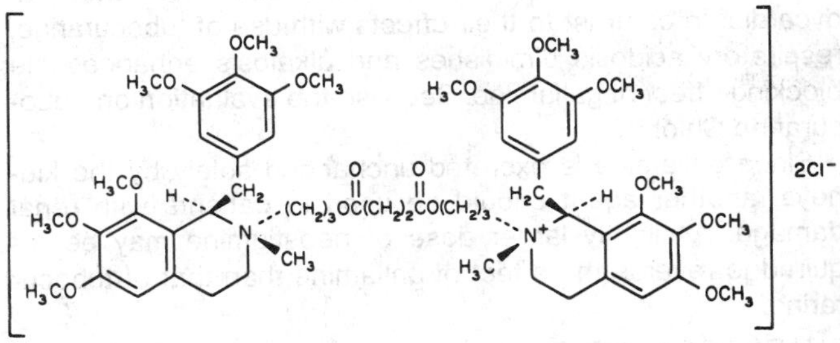

ACTIONS AND USES. This long-acting nondepolarizing muscle relaxant is a bis-benzylisoquinoline derivative. At two times the ED_{95} dosage (0.05 mg/kg), the drug appears to have minimal hemodynamic effects in patients with coronary or valvular heart disease or in other ASA physical status class III and IV patients (Konstadt et al, 1987; Stoops et al, 1987; Basta et al, 1988).

The onset to 100% twitch inhibition following an intubating dose of doxacurium (0.05 to 0.08 mg/kg) is four to five minutes; the duration of neuromuscular block is approximately 90 to 110 minutes after administration of 0.05 mg/kg. Onset and recovery from equipotent doses are somewhat more rapid in children 2 to 12 years old than in adults (Sarner et al, 1988).

This drug is classified in FDA Pregnancy Category C.

PHARMACOKINETICS. The pharmacokinetics of doxacurium are similar in healthy young adults and elderly patients. After a dose of 0.025 mg/kg, the clearance was identical in the two groups (Dresner et al, 1990). The major route of elimination of doxacurium is renal excretion of the unchanged compound (Dresner et al, 1990).

DOSAGE AND PREPARATIONS.

Intravenous: The ED_{95}, two times ED_{95}, and three times ED_{95} dose of doxacurium is 0.025, 0.05, and 0.08 mg/kg, respectively. Residual neuromuscular blockade can be antagonized readily by usual doses of neostigmine or edrophonium (Basta et al, 1988).

Nuromax (Burroughs Wellcome). Solution 1 mg/ml with benzyl alcohol 9% in 5 ml containers.

GALLAMINE TRIETHIODIDE
[Flaxedil]

ACTIONS AND USES. This synthetic agent has a longer duration of action than tubocurarine at equipotent doses; very large doses may have a prolonged effect. The actions of gallamine are similar to those of tubocurarine, but this agent blocks the cardiac vagus and may cause sinus tachycardia and, occasionally, hypertension and increases cardiac output; therefore, it should be used cautiously in patients at risk from increased heart rate but may be preferred for those with bradycardia. In contrast to their effects with use of tubocurarine, respiratory acidosis diminishes and alkalosis enhances the blocking effect of gallamine. See also the evaluation on Tubocurarine Chloride.

Since gallamine is excreted unchanged solely by the kidneys, another agent should be used in patients with renal damage. A slightly larger dose of neostigmine may be required to reverse the effect of gallamine than that of tubocurarine.

PHARMACOKINETICS. See Table 2.

DOSAGE AND PREPARATIONS. The required dose varies greatly, and a peripheral nerve stimulator aids in determining the appropriate amount. The doses listed are for use with nitrous oxide as the only inhalation agent; they must be reduced if gallamine is used with more potent inhalation agents. The size of subsequent doses depends on the anticipated duration of the procedure.

Intravenous: *Adults and children,* initially, 1 mg/kg; subsequent doses, 0.3 to 0.5 mg/kg. *Infants up to 1 month,* initially, 1 mg/kg; subsequent doses, 0.5 mg/kg.

Flaxedil (Davis & Geck). Solution 20 mg/ml in 10 ml containers.

METOCURINE IODIDE (Dimethyl Tubocurarine Iodide)
[Metubine]

This semisynthetic derivative of tubocurarine is approximately twice as potent as the parent drug and, at equipotent dosage, has a similar or slightly longer duration of action (about 60 minutes). Obese patients experience slower recovery. Since metocurine causes less histamine release and less ganglionic blockade, its effect on the circulatory system is not as prominent as that of tubocurarine. It is a suitable muscle relaxant for patients who cannot tolerate hypotension or tachycardia. Differences in pharmacokinetic profile are shown in Table 2.

For uses and adverse reactions, see the evaluation on Tubocurarine Chloride. Metocurine is classified in FDA Pregnancy Category C.

DOSAGE AND PREPARATIONS. The required dose varies greatly, and a peripheral nerve stimulator may aid in determining the appropriate amount. The doses listed are for use with nitrous oxide as the only inhalation agent; they must be reduced if metocurine is used with more potent inhalation agents. The size of subsequent doses depends on the anticipated duration of the procedure.

Intravenous: *Adults,* initially, 0.1 to 0.3 mg/kg; subsequent doses, 0.02 to 0.05 mg/kg.

Metubine (Lilly). Solution (sterile) 2 mg/ml in 20 ml containers.

MIVACURIUM CHLORIDE
[Mivacron]

ACTIONS AND USES. This short-acting, nondepolarizing muscle relaxant is a bis-benzylisoquinoline derivative. Mivacurium has a relatively short onset, does not accumulate, and the duration of action is not increased with an increase in dose (Savarese et al, 1988).

This drug is classified in FDA Pregnancy Category C.

PHARMACOKINETICS. Mivacurium is hydrolyzed by plasma cholinesterase and perhaps by other esterases. It has a half-life of two to five minutes (de Bros et al, 1987 B; Cook et al, 1987). The pharmacokinetics of mivacurium are complicated by the fact that this drug consists of three stereoisomers; two are the active components and the third is much less active with a long half-life.

DOSAGE AND PREPARATIONS.

Intravenous: *Adults,* doses of 0.15 to 0.25 mg/kg are effective in facilitating tracheal intubation. Cardiovascular side effects do not occur with doses of 0.15 mg/kg or less or when the drug is infused. Transient hypotension and tachycardia caused by histamine release may occur in some patients with higher doses of 0.2 to 0.25 mg/kg. As with atracurium, these effects may be reduced or abolished by injecting the drug slowly over 30 to 60 seconds (Saverese et al, 1985).

The ED_{95} is 0.07 mg/kg. Intubation conditions comparable to those achieved with succinylcholine may occur in about 90 to 120 seconds with a dose of 0.25 mg/kg or with a priming dose of 0.03 mg/kg followed by 0.22 mg/kg 90 to 120 seconds later (Savarese et al, 1986). Following single bolus doses of two to three times ED_{95} in adults, 5% twitch recovery occurs in approximately 15 minutes and 95% twitch recovery in approximately 30 minutes (Choi et al, 1987; Lee et al, 1987; Savarese et al, 1988). *Children* require a higher mg/kg dose than adults (Brandom et al, 1988; Miler et al, 1988; Woelfel et al, 1988).

Because it does not accumulate and has a short duration of action, mivacurium may be given by continuous infusion. A dose of 7 to 8 mcg/kg/min is required to maintain approximately 95% twitch suppression during nitrous oxide/opioid anesthesia (Ali et al, 1986; Brandom et al, 1986 B; Powers et al, 1987). Lower doses are required during nitrous oxide/isoflurane anesthesia (Weber et al, 1988).

Spontaneous recovery from 5% to 95% occurs approximately 15 minutes after cessation of infusion. Neostigmine may be given to reverse the effects of mivacurium but this may not be necessary with appropriate discontinuation of the infusion.

Mivacron (Burroughs Wellcome). Solution (sterile) 0.5 mg/ml in 5% dextrose (premixed) in 50 and 100 ml containers; solution 2 mg/ml in 5 and 10 ml containers and with benzyl alcohol 9% in 20 and 50 ml containers.

PANCURONIUM BROMIDE

[Pavulon]

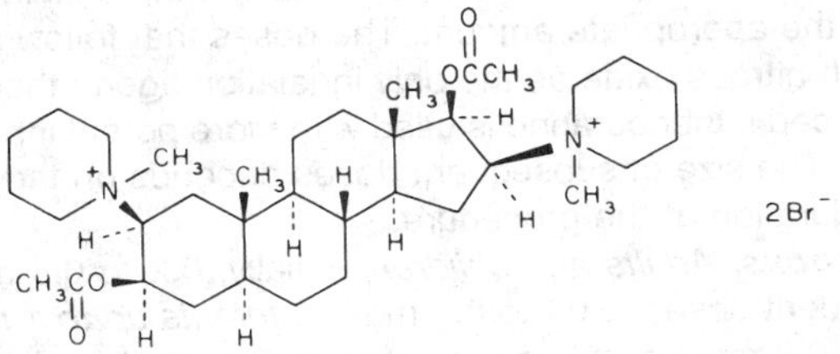

ACTIONS AND USES. The effects and indications for pancuronium appear to be similar to those for tubocurarine; however, there are some important differences in actions. Pancuronium is approximately five times more potent than tubocurarine. The onset of action of the two drugs is comparable. Endotracheal intubation is accomplished with ease in approximately three minutes. At equipotent dosage, pancuronium has a shorter duration of action than tubocurarine.

Unlike tubocurarine, pancuronium does not cause hypotension, presumably because it lacks ganglionic blocking action and rarely, if ever, causes release of histamine. It may increase heart rate, cardiac output, and arterial pressure, primarily because of its vagolytic action and secondarily because it blocks the neuronal reuptake of norepinephrine. Atrioventricular conduction is accelerated, but cardiac contractility and total peripheral resistance are unaffected. Ventricular extrasystoles occur occasionally. In the elderly, neuromuscular block may be prolonged with delayed recovery of normal tone (Duvaldestin et al, 1982). The use of pancuronium and halothane in patients receiving tricyclic antidepressants may result in ventricular arrhythmia. This reaction does not occur if enflurane is used in place of halothane. For other adverse reactions, see the evaluation on Tubocurarine Chloride.

Only insignificant quantities of pancuronium enter the fetal blood stream, which suggests that the drug may be used safely in obstetrical anesthesia.

Pancuronium is classified in FDA Pregnancy Category C.

PHARMACOKINETICS. See Table 2.

DOSAGE AND PREPARATIONS. The required dose varies greatly, and a peripheral nerve stimulator aids in determining the appropriate amount. The doses listed are for use with nitrous oxide as the only inhalation agent; they must be reduced if pancuronium is used with more potent inhalation agents. The size of subsequent doses depends upon the anticipated duration of the procedure.

Intravenous: *Adults and children*, initially, 0.04 to 0.1 mg/kg; for intubation, 0.1 mg/kg; subsequently, 0.01 to 0.02 mg/kg, repeated as required (generally every 20 to 40 minutes).

Pavulon (Organon). Solution 1 mg/ml in 10 ml containers and 2 mg/ml in 2 and 5 ml containers.

PIPECURONIUM BROMIDE

[Arduan]

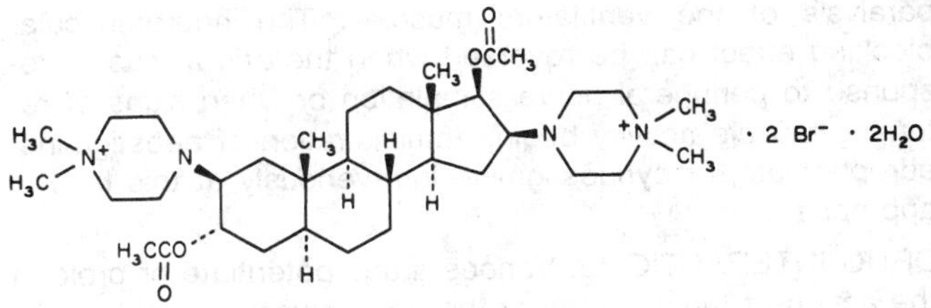

ACTIONS AND USES. This nondepolarizing muscle relaxant is similar, chemically and clinically, to pancuronium. The onset, duration, recovery time, and reversibility of the two agents are equivalent (Caldwell et al, 1987 B). However, pipecuronium lacks the cardiovascular side effects of pancuronium, even at doses three or four times the ED_{95} (Tassonyi et al, 1986; Wierda et al, 1987). Residual neuromuscular block can be antagonized readily by the usual dose of neostigmine.

This drug is classified in FDA Pregnancy Category C.

PHARMACOKINETICS. The principal route of elimination is by renal excretion. In patients with normal renal function, the half-life is approximately two hours. In patients with renal failure, the elimination half-life is prolonged, but the clinical duration of action does not differ significantly. In the virtual absence of renal function, clearance remains at 60% of normal (Caldwell et al, 1987 A). See also Table 2.

DOSAGE AND PREPARATIONS.

Intravenous: A dose of 0.07 mg/kg of pipecuronium is equivalent to 0.1 mg/kg of pancuronium. The effective dose is similar in young adults and in the elderly (65 to 80 years) (Azad et al, 1987).

Arduan (Organon). Powder (for injection, lyophilized) 10 mg.

TUBOCURARINE CHLORIDE

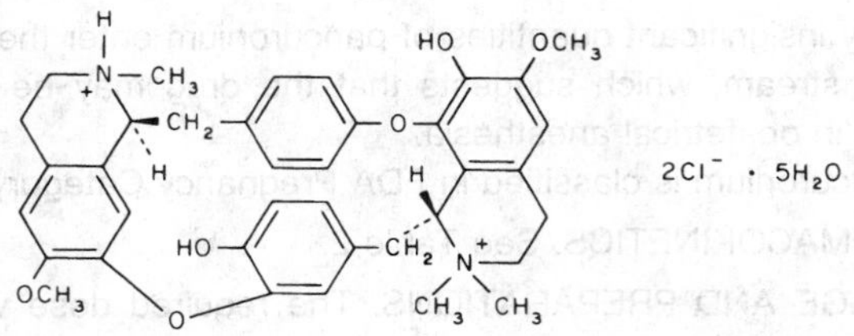

ACTIONS AND USES. Tubocurarine (curare) is used to produce muscle relaxation during surgical procedures of moderate or long duration, to reduce the severity of muscle spasms in severe tetanus, to facilitate controlled ventilation, and, occasionally, in the diagnosis of myasthenia gravis (see index entry Myasthenia Gravis, Diagnosis). Tubocurarine does not readily cross the placenta in significant quantities and does not affect the tone of the uterus; therefore, it may be used in obstetric anesthesia. However, repeated use of large doses may result in fetal paralysis (FDA Pregnancy Category C).

Tubocurarine causes flaccid paralysis of all skeletal muscles. The muscles of the eyes are affected first, followed by those of the face, limbs, and trunk; then the intercostal muscles and, finally, the diaphragm become paralyzed. Paralysis of abdominal muscles cannot be achieved without substantial paralysis of the ventilatory muscles. The neuromuscular blocking effect can be reversed when there is a muscle response to peripheral nerve stimulation or when signs of returning muscle activity begin; administration of neostigmine, edrophonium, or pyridostigmine intravenously at this time is appropriate.

DRUG INTERACTIONS. Various drugs potentiate or prolong the action of tubocurarine at the neuromuscular junction. Of the volatile anesthetics, enflurane and isoflurane cause the greatest potentiation, methoxyflurane somewhat less, and halothane the least. When tubocurarine is given with enflurane or isoflurane, the dose of the blocking agent should be reduced to one-third to one-half that used with nitrous oxide and one-half to two-thirds that used with halothane.

Many antibiotics (eg, streptomycin, neomycin, polymyxin B, colistin, kanamycin, bacitracin, gentamicin, amikacin, lincomycin, clindamycin) enhance the neuromuscular block produced by tubocurarine and other nondepolarizing agents. If extremely large doses of these drugs have been used recently, especially in patients with renal failure, controlled ventilation may be required postoperatively. Quinidine, magnesium sulfate, and trimethaphan (but not sodium nitroprusside) also have been reported to potentiate the neuromuscular blocking action of tubocurarine.

ADVERSE REACTIONS AND PRECAUTIONS. Tubocurarine may cause hypotension when large doses are given intravenously. This effect tends to be transient and is directly related to the depth of anesthesia and the volemic status; it is due to peripheral vasodilatation, which, in turn, is believed to be caused by release of histamine and ganglionic blockade. The hypotensive effect can be minimized by administering incremental doses.

Tubocurarine has been reported to cause bronchospasm as a result of the release of histamine. Although this effect is considered to be clinically unimportant in normal patients, pancuronium may be preferred in those with asthma.

Respiratory acidosis and hypokalemia enhance and respiratory alkalosis diminishes the blocking effect of tubocurarine. Patients with myasthenia gravis are sensitive to the blocking effects of nondepolarizing agents; therefore, the dose of these drugs should be reduced considerably in these patients.

Tubocurarine does not readily penetrate the blood-brain barrier; therefore, it is devoid of central nervous system effects when administered in therapeutic doses. However, adequate ventilation must be assured, for hypoventilation may result in hypercarbia, cerebral vasodilation, and increased intracranial pressure. Intracranial pressure also may be increased as the result of histamine release, which causes cerebral vasodilation.

PHARMACOKINETICS. A single intravenous dose of tubocurarine produces maximum paralysis in three to five minutes, and the clinical effect may persist for more than 60 minutes. About 40% of the dose is excreted unchanged by the kidneys over 24 hours. When repeated doses are used, the amount of each succeeding fraction generally should be reduced. See Table 2 for this drug's pharmacokinetic profile.

DOSAGE AND PREPARATIONS. The required dose varies greatly, and a peripheral nerve stimulator is of value in determining the appropriate amount. The doses that follow are for use with nitrous oxide as the only inhalation agent; they must be reduced if tubocurarine is used with more potent inhalation agents. The size of subsequent doses depends on the anticipated duration of the procedure.

Intravenous: *Adults and children,* initially, 0.2 to 0.5 mg/kg; subsequent doses, 0.04 to 0.1 mg/kg. *Infants up to 1 month,* initially, 0.3 mg/kg; subsequent doses, 0.1 mg/kg.

Generic. Solution 3 mg/ml in 5, 10, and 20 ml containers.

VECURONIUM BROMIDE
[Norcuron]

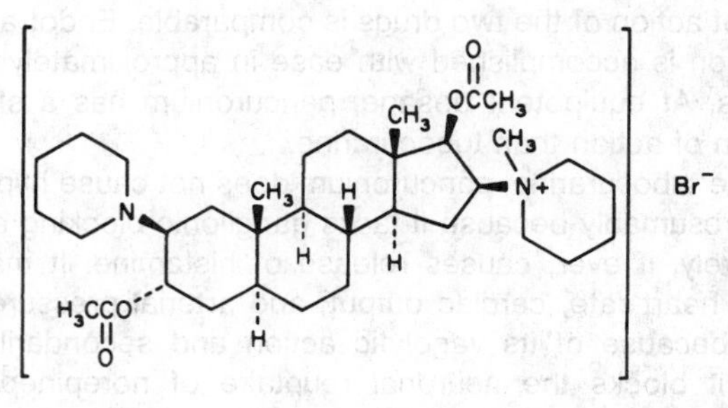

ACTIONS AND USES. This monoquaternary analogue of pancuronium has equivalent potency and a similar rate of onset, but the duration of vecuronium's effect is about one-third to one-half that of pancuronium. Recovery time is not linear with dose if the usual clinical dose range is exceeded. Following a single dose of 0.1 mg/kg, recovery to 90% of the initial twitch is achieved in 40 to 50 minutes. The duration of action is similar in young adults and the elderly (Lowry et al, 1985), but recovery time in infants is approximately twice as long (73 minutes) as in young children (35 minutes) (Fisher et al, 1982). Recovery is significantly prolonged in obese patients. Vecuronium does not produce significant ganglionic or vagal block or interfere with the uptake of norepinephrine, and it is essentially free of histamine-releasing action. Therefore, it does not affect the heart rate or blood pressure. Intracranial and intraocular pressures are unaffected.

Vecuronium is used during endotracheal intubation and surgery. Unlike pancuronium, it does not increase the esophageal sphincter pressure. The block produced by vecuronium is readily reversed by neostigmine, pyridostigmine, or edrophonium.

This drug is classified in FDA Pregnancy Category C.

PHARMACOKINETICS. About 10% to 25% of a dose is eliminated by the kidney; the major portion is excreted in the bile (Bencini et al, 1986 A, 1986 B). In patients with chronic renal failure, clearance is reduced by 40% and neuromuscular block is prolonged by 40% (Lynam et al, 1988). In patients with impaired hepatic function, both the intensity and duration of neuromuscular block are increased (Durant et al, 1979; Lebrault et al, 1985; Arden et al, 1988). For further information on pharmacokinetics, see Table 2.

DOSAGE AND PREPARATIONS. The required dose varies greatly, and a peripheral nerve stimulator may be of value in determining the appropriate amount. The doses that follow are for use with nitrous oxide and/or halothane as inhalation agents; they may be reduced 20% to 30% if vecuronium is used with enflurane or isoflurane. Vecuronium does not accumulate under usual circumstances of use.

Intravenous: *Adults,* for intubation, 0.08 to 0.1 mg/kg; subsequent intraoperative doses, 0.01 to 0.015 mg/kg, repeated as required or a maintenance infusion of approximately 1 mcg/kg/min. If vecuronium is given after succinylcholine-assisted intubation, 0.04 to 0.06 mg/kg is recommended as the initial dose.

Children 1 to 10 years may require a slightly larger initial dose and more frequent supplemental doses than adults; *infants under 1 year* are more sensitive to vecuronium than adults, and recovery time may be more prolonged.

Norcuron (Organon). Powder (for solution) 1 mg/ml in 10 ml containers with diluent.

DEPOLARIZING BLOCKING DRUG

SUCCINYLCHOLINE CHLORIDE

[Anectine, Quelicin, Sucostrin]

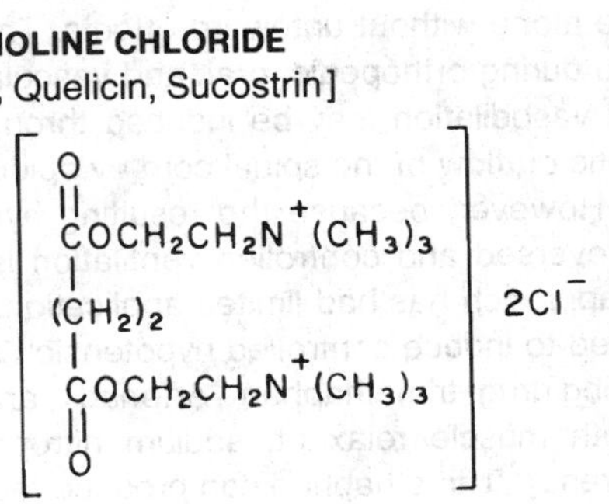

$$\left[\begin{array}{l} \overset{\displaystyle O}{\overset{\|}{C}}OCH_2CH_2\overset{+}{N}(CH_3)_3 \\ | \\ (CH_2)_2 \\ | \\ \underset{\displaystyle O}{\underset{\|}{C}}OCH_2CH_2\overset{+}{N}(CH_3)_3 \end{array}\right] 2Cl^-$$

ACTIONS AND USES. Succinylcholine has a rapid onset (one minute) and short duration of action (five to ten minutes) after doses of 1 mg/kg. It undergoes rapid hydrolysis by plasma cholinesterase. A single dose usually causes transient, visible muscle fasciculations, followed by profound flaccid paralysis of all skeletal muscles.

Succinylcholine is used primarily during brief procedures, such as endotracheal intubation, to relieve laryngospasm, in endoscopy, in orthopedic manipulation, and in electroconvulsive therapy.

Since succinylcholine is almost completely hydrolyzed by plasma cholinesterase, prolonged postoperative apnea can occur in patients with abnormal plasma cholinesterase activity caused by a genetically determined variant of plasma cholinesterase or diminished hepatic synthesis of normal cholinesterase. The plasma cholinesterase level also can be reduced significantly after exposure to organophosphorus pesticides or topical use of long-acting anticholinesterase agents (eg, echothiophate) for open-angle glaucoma or accommodative esotropia. Complications can be avoided by using a small test dose and observing the response to a peripheral nerve stimulator.

Prolonged postoperative apnea caused by phase II block also can develop in normal patients receiving repeated or increasing doses. The dose-response curve is quite steep for succinylcholine (1 to 3 mg/kg for phase I block; 3 to 5 mg/kg for phase II block), and a peripheral nerve stimulator aids in monitoring the block when succinylcholine is used to provide continuous muscle relaxation. Prolonged postoperative apnea can be avoided if the infusions are interrupted frequently to evaluate the rate of return of neuromuscular function. Airway management and monitoring for respiratory adequacy should be continued for at least one hour thereafter.

The response to succinylcholine may be prolonged in the presence of hypokalemia. Patients with myasthenia gravis may be resistant to depolarizing agents and have a predisposition to phase II block.

Succinylcholine does not cross the placenta in appreciable quantities and is safe for administration in obstetric anesthesia, including use in parturients with eclampsia who are receiving magnesium, unless the patient has atypical or depressed plasma cholinesterase activity (FDA Pregnancy Category C).

ADVERSE REACTIONS AND PRECAUTIONS. Succinylcholine has been reported to cause nodal and ventricular arrhythmias, decreased or increased heart rate, and increased arterial pressure. Nodal arrhythmias, bradycardia, and sinus arrest have occurred after intravenous injection (particularly in children) or after fractional doses were given intravenously at three- to ten-minute intervals to patients also receiving halothane. These effects usually can be avoided by administering atropine prior to the repeated doses. Induction with thiopental and, to some extent, midazolam affords significant protection against rhythm disturbances produced by the second dose of succinylcholine in adults. Etomidate offers no protection (Abdul-Rasool et al, 1987). Intravenous administration can produce bradyarrhythmia. The complex cardiovascular effects of this blocking agent have been attributed in part to autonomic ganglionic stimulation.

Severe ventricular arrhythmias and cardiac arrest have followed administration of succinylcholine to patients with severe burns, major crush injuries, upper motor neuron lesions due to stroke or tumor, spinal cord injuries, multiple sclerosis of recent onset, tetanus, or diffuse lower motor neuron disease. These adverse effects have been attributed to a pronounced increase in plasma potassium levels following depolarization of the supersensitive denervated muscle. This sensitivity develops one to two weeks after the onset of motor paralysis and persists for several months, sometimes up to a year or more. Sensitivity may begin somewhat sooner in those with lower motor neuron disease and lasts until recovery of neuromuscular function or atrophy of the muscle occurs. The vulnerable period following burns is 5 to 120 days after injury. Succinylcholine should be avoided in these patients.

Succinylcholine increases intraocular pressure markedly within one minute. This effect lasts five to ten minutes and occurs during the stage of generalized muscle fasciculations. It can be attenuated by the prior administration of a nondepolarizing relaxant. Succinylcholine should not be used alone after the eye has been opened surgically or is already open at the beginning of anesthesia (eg, penetrating wounds, iris prolapse). Since the effect on intraocular pressure is brief, succinylcholine is not contraindicated in patients with open-angle glaucoma or those predisposed to angle closure. In these patients, one or two drops of pilocarpine may be instilled prior to surgery.

Patients with myotonia congenita (Thomsen's disease) or myotonia dystrophica (Steinert's disease) respond to succinylcholine with contracture that ranges from clenched fists to a whole body response with legs drawn up, back arched, spasm of masseter muscles, laryngospasm, and contraction of the diaphragm. Contracture also is an immediate or early sign of succinylcholine-induced malignant hyperthermia, a rare complication of general anesthesia that may have a genetic basis. Its management is discussed later in this chapter.

Postoperative pain and stiffness in the neck, shoulder, subcostal, and back muscles are common after use of succinylcholine, particularly in patients aged 20 to 50; these effects apparently do not occur in children under 3 years. The incidence varies from 10% in patients maintained on bed rest for one day to 70% in ambulatory patients. Symptoms generally appear 12 to 24 hours after administration and last for several hours to a few days. The incidence of pain and stiffness may be reduced by giving tubocurarine 3 mg or gallamine 20 mg three minutes prior to succinylcholine; however, the dose of succinylcholine should be increased by approximately 50% to produce an equal degree of relaxation.

When the angle of the cardioesophageal sphincter is normal, the increase in pressure required to open the sphincter is 28 cm/water. Succinylcholine-induced abdominal muscle fasciculations increase intragastric pressure: 1 mg/kg increases pressure to 40 cm/water and larger doses may increase pressure to 85 cm/water, which may result in regurgitation, particularly in young adults. Pretreatment with nondepolarizing relaxants may prevent this complication.

About 40% of prepubertal children exhibit myoglobinuria. This effect is not related to the apparent severity of the fasciculations. Myoglobinuria occurs only rarely in adults.

DOSAGE AND PREPARATIONS. The dose required varies greatly, and a peripheral nerve stimulator aids in regulating the rate of infusion and in the diagnosis of phase II block.

Intravenous: *Adults,* initially, 0.3 to 1.5 mg/kg; subsequent doses, 0.01 to 0.05 mg/kg. For continuous infusion, a 0.1% (1 mg/ml) or 0.2% (2 mg/ml) solution is administered at an average rate of 2.5 to 7.5 mg/min. The dose necessary to maintain paralysis is reduced in pregnant women.

Infants, 2 mg/kg. *Children,* 1 mg/kg. Continuous infusion is not recommended for neonates and infants since tachyphylaxis occurs with a cumulative dose of 4 mg/kg and phase II block at about 6 mg/kg.

Intramuscular: *Adults, infants, and older children*, when a suitable vein is not accessible, a dose of up to 3 to 4 mg/kg (not to exceed a total dose of 150 mg) may be administered.

Generic. Solution 20 mg/ml in 10 ml containers.

Anectine (Burroughs Wellcome). Powder (sterile) 500 mg and 1 g; solution 20 mg/ml in 10 ml containers.

Quelicin (Abbott). Solution 20 mg/ml in 5 and 10 ml containers and 50 and 100 mg/ml in 10 ml containers.

Sucostrin (Apothecon). Solution (aqueous) 20 and 100 mg/ml in 10 ml containers.

MISCELLANEOUS ADJUNCTIVE DRUGS

Vasodilators Used for Controlled Hypotension

Hypotensive drugs may be given during certain surgical procedures (eg, plastic, vessel, or neurosurgery) to reduce bleeding that would interfere with the technique. They may be used during intracerebral aneurysm ligation to decrease transmural pressure and reduce the risk of rupture during manipulation prior to clipping. Controlled hypotension also may be appropriate to reduce large volume blood losses during hip replacement, insertion of the Harrington rod, prostatectomy, or radical neck or pelvic surgery and in threatened hemorrhage. In addition, hypotensive drugs can improve myocardial performance by decreasing cardiac preload and afterload.

In some instances, an adequate hypotensive effect can be accomplished by deepening general anesthesia. For example, a mean blood pressure of 60 to 70 torr can be maintained by isoflurane alone without untoward effects. This technique may be used during orthopedic, oral, and vascular surgery.

Peripheral vasodilation may be induced through blockade of sympathetic outflow of the spinal cord by epidural or spinal anesthesia. However, because the resulting hypotension is not readily reversed and controlled ventilation is usually required, this approach has had limited application.

Agents used to induce controlled hypotension are the ganglionic blocking drug, trimethaphan [Arfonad], and the direct-acting smooth muscle relaxant, sodium nitroprusside [Nipride, Nitropress]. Trimethaphan can produce tachycardia by blockade of vagal ganglia; it also depresses cardiac sympathetic tone, which reduces organ perfusion as the cardiac output is diminished at mean arterial pressures of 50 mm Hg. However, there is evidence that trimethaphan may produce direct cerebral toxic effects at doses required to induce a mean arterial pressure of 50 mm Hg. Thus, trimethaphan is used less often than sodium nitroprusside, which lacks direct autonomic and cardiac effects and has a shorter duration of action. Sodium nitroprusside may not decrease perfusion at 50 mm Hg. However, some patients are resistant to its effects, and fatal cyanide poisoning may occur if the drug is not administered as indicated. Since sodium nitroprusside tends to increase cardiac output reflexly, it has been speculated that it may not produce as dry a surgical field as trimethaphan.

Hypotension should be induced gradually over five to ten minutes. The blood pressure (measured directly via an indwelling catheter attached to a pressure transducer), arterial blood gas levels, electrocardiogram, and urinary output must be monitored continuously. Scrupulous attention to respiration is essential. Hyperventilation must be avoided, since normocarbia is required for autoregulation of cerebral perfusion. Although positive fluid balance opposes induced hypotension, hypovolemia can produce irreversible shock. If inadequate circulatory volume is suspected, infusion of the hypotensive agent should be discontinued at intervals until the pressure rises in order to assess the reversibility of hypotension. Overdosage usually results in an undesirable fall in blood pressure before the effect on recovery time becomes significant. Diuretics, antihypertensive agents, and beta blockers enhance the action of the hypotensive agents. Consideration should be given to the risk/benefit ratio of this technique in patients with hypertension, anemia, coronary artery disease, renal insufficiency, Addison's disease, or deficient cerebral circulation. This technique is not recommended during pregnancy.

Induced hypotension should be performed only by anesthesiologists familiar with the interrelationships between blood volume, blood pressure, muscle relaxants, anesthetics, and end-expiratory pressure with the perfusion of the brain, heart, kidney, and liver.

Other Indications: In addition to inducing controlled hypotension, vasodilators are used to control pre- or intraoperative hypertension during surgery, to treat myocardial ischemia or ventricular failure, and to improve forward flow in patients with valvular insufficiency. These effects are achieved by reducing preload (venous dilation) or afterload (arteriolar dilation).

The selection of an appropriate agent permits a whole range of vasodilating activity from predominant dilation of the venous vascular bed to predominant arteriolar dilation according to the following sequence: morphine, nitroglycerin, spinal anesthesia, fentanyl, general anesthesia with enflurane or isoflurane, sodium nitroprusside, phentolamine. Nitroglycerin is a venodilator and sodium nitroprusside is an arteriolar dilator, but these agents dilate both venous and arterial beds to some extent. The dominant vascular response may be matched to the clinical situation.

Drug Evaluations

NITROGLYCERIN

[Nitro-Bid IV, Nitrostat IV, Tridil]

For chemical formula, see index entry Nitroglycerin, In Heart Failure.

ACTIONS AND USES. Nitroglycerin relaxes vascular, bronchial, gastrointestinal, ureteral, and uterine smooth muscle. Following rapid intravenous administration, transient arteriolar dilation occurs in association with increased stroke volume, cardiac output, and coronary flow. This is followed within one minute by reflex arteriolar constriction. Venous capacitance increases, left ventricular filling pressure declines markedly, and ventricular volume and cardiac work are reduced. With continuous infusion, preload is affected more than afterload, usually with little change in cardiac output. Discontinuation of the infusion is followed by restoration of baseline vascular parameters within nine minutes (Hill et al, 1981).

ADVERSE REACTIONS. Side effects of intravenous nitroglycerin include bradycardia (of vagal origin), hypoxemia (due to increased pulmonary ventilation-perfusion abnormalities), and, perhaps, methemoglobinemia. (This has not been reported during intraoperative use of nitroglycerin.) Hypotension and bradycardia are managed by discontinuing the infusion, assuring an adequate airway and oxygenation, and administering a vasoconstrictor if required.

Nitroglycerin is classified in FDA Pregnancy Category C.

DOSAGE AND PREPARATIONS.

Intravenous Infusion: (An infusion pump is preferred.) 0.1 to 1 mg/kg/min.

Generic. Solution 5 mg/ml in 5, 10, and 20 ml containers; solution 25, 50, and 100 mg in 5% dextrose in 250 ml containers.

Nitro-Bid IV (Marion Merrell Dow). Solution 5 mg/ml in 1, 5, and 10 ml containers (alcohol 70%).

Nitrostat IV (Parke-Davis). Solution 0.8, 5, and 10 mg/ml in 10 ml containers with or without delivery set (alcohol 5%, 30%, and 50%, respectively).

Tridil (DuPont). Solution 0.5 mg/ml in 10 ml containers (alcohol 10%) and 5 mg/ml in 5, 10, and 20 ml containers (alcohol 30%).

SODIUM NITROPRUSSIDE

[Nitropress]

$$Na_2\left[Fe(CN)_5NO\right] \cdot 2H_2O$$

ACTIONS AND USES. Sodium nitroprusside acts directly to dilate resistance and, in larger doses, capacitance vessels. Peripheral resistance, central venous pressure, and pulmonary artery pressure are reduced. The drug has no direct action on the myocardium or on the central and autonomic nervous systems. The fall in blood pressure is dose dependent and, therefore, is related to the rate of infusion. There may be a reflex increase in heart rate and a variable increase in cardiac output, sometimes as great as 30%, depending on the type and depth of anesthesia. When the infusion is slowed or stopped, the blood pressure usually increases immediately and returns to pretreatment levels in one to ten minutes.

The dose response is extremely variable and the infusion rate requires individual titration; some patients are relatively resistant to the drug's action. Tachyphylaxis is rare. Increasing tolerance and metabolic acidosis are early indications of toxicity.

See also the discussion on Controlled Hypotension.

PHARMACOKINETICS AND ADVERSE REACTIONS. Nitroprusside is metabolized to cyanide. The major elimination pathway of cyanide is conversion to thiocyanate, which is excreted by the kidney. If the rate of conversion is adequate, no toxic effects are observed with short-term treatment. If the production of cyanide is excessive, a reaction with cellular cytochrome oxidase interferes with cellular respiration, which decreases A-VO_2 difference and causes lactic acidosis. The infusion of nitroprusside should be stopped and a 25% solution of sodium thiosulfate in dextrose 5% in water should be injected over a 10- to 15-minute period to a total dose of 150 mg/kg. Sodium nitrite 3% then should be injected at a rate of 2.5 to 5 ml/min to a total dose of 5 mg/kg. (Sodium thiosulfate is a cofactor for the conversion of cyanide to thiocyanate, and sodium nitrite forms methemoglobin, which produces an inactive cyanide derivative.)

The administration of a 0.1% solution of hydroxocobalamin in 5% dextrose in water at a rate of 25 mg/hour during nitroprusside administration reduces the accumulation of cyanide ion (Cottrell et al, 1979) and significantly decreases the tendency toward lactic acidosis. Experimental data suggest that sodium thiosulfate 75 mg/kg also prevents cyanide accumulation (Krapez et al, 1981). If prolonged exposure to maximum doses of sodium nitroprusside is anticipated, the prophylactic use of an antagonist should be considered.

The precautions for the use of nitroprusside are those common to the induction of hypotensive anesthesia (see the discussion on Controlled Hypotension).

Sodium nitroprusside is classified in FDA Pregnancy Category C.

DOSAGE AND PREPARATIONS.

Intravenous Infusion: (An infusion pump is preferred.) *Adults and children,* 0.5 to a maximum of 10 mcg/kg/min.

Nitropress (Abbott), ***Generic.*** Powder equivalent to sodium nitroprusside dihydrate 50 mg in 5 ml containers for dilution in dextrose injection 5% in water to 1,000 ml (50 mcg/ml), 500 ml (100 mcg/ml), or 250 ml (200 mcg/ml).

TRIMETHAPHAN CAMSYLATE

[Arfonad]

ACTIONS AND USES. Trimethaphan reduces peripheral resistance, primarily by ganglionic blockade; it also has direct peripheral dilating activity. It is a weak histamine liberator. The usual rate of administration produces maximal hypotension in two to ten minutes. After discontinuation of the infusion, blood pressure increases in three to five minutes with return to a systolic pressure greater than 100 mm Hg within ten minutes. Occasionally, return to prehypotensive levels may be delayed for as long as 30 minutes, particularly when large doses are used for prolonged periods.

Some patients are resistant to the hypotensive effect of ganglionic blocking agents, and repeated administration of large doses is not recommended. In many patients, an appropriate hypotensive response occurs initially but tachyphylaxis then develops. The mechanism of this response has not been determined.

About one-third of the dose is excreted unchanged by the kidneys. The fate of the remainder is unknown.

See also the discussion on Controlled Hypotension.

ADVERSE REACTIONS AND PRECAUTIONS. In elderly patients, the usual response to trimethaphan-induced hypotension is bradycardia. In contrast, some degree of tachycardia usually occurs in children and young adults. The resulting increase in cardiac output reduces the hypotensive effect, which may necessitate the administration of increased amounts of the drug or augmentation with halothane. If the patient's condition permits, treatment with small incremental intravenous doses of a beta-blocking agent (eg, propranolol 0.01 to 0.05 mg/kg) also may prevent the increase in heart rate.

The precautions for the use of trimethaphan are those common to the induction of hypotensive anesthesia (see the discussion on Vasodilators Used for Controlled Hypotension). Ganglionic blocking agents may conceal the signs of hypoglycemia in diabetic patients and interfere with sympathetically mediated gluconeogenesis.

Trimethaphan is classified in FDA Pregnancy Category D.

DOSAGE AND PREPARATIONS.

Intravenous Infusion: *Adults,* a 0.1% solution (1 mg/ml) in dextrose injection 5% is infused at a rate of 3 to 4 mg/min initially; the amount is titrated to maintain the desired level of hypotension.

Arfonad (Roche). Solution 50 mg/ml in 10 ml containers for dilution in dextrose 5% to 500 ml.

Agents Used in Pheochromocytoma

The alpha-adrenergic blocking agents, phenoxybenzamine [Dibenzyline] and phentolamine [Regitine]; the beta-adrenergic blocking agents, esmolol [Brevibloc], propranolol [Inderal], and metoprolol [Lopressor]; and sodium nitroprusside are used in the surgical management of patients with pheochromocytoma. Phenoxybenzamine and propranolol also are used preoperatively, the former to control hypertension and sometimes to estimate the intravascular volume for volume replacement and the latter to control sinus tachycardia and frequent premature ventricular contractions. Since the beta-adrenergic blocking agents may increase peripheral vascular resistance significantly as a result of unopposed alpha-adrenergic activity, they should not be used alone. Since labetalol [Normodyne, Trandate] has both alpha- and beta-blocking activity, it may be useful in this regard.

Paroxysms of severe hypertension may be controlled during anesthesia by infusion of sodium nitroprusside, by intravenous injection of 1 to 5 mg of phentolamine, or by infusion of a 0.01% (0.1 mg/ml) solution of phentolamine. Severe ventricular arrhythmias may be controlled by the slow intravenous injection of propranolol in increments of 0.5 to 1 mg to a total of 3 to 5 mg in adults or by continuous intravenous infusion of esmolol 0.05 to 0.3 mg/kg/min after a bolus dose of 0.1 to 0.2 mg/kg.

If severe hypotension develops after removal of the tumor, the infusion of norepinephrine may be indicated (see also index entry Norepinephrine, Uses, Shock).

Agents Used in Malignant Hyperthermia

This potentially fatal syndrome may develop in genetically susceptible individuals receiving general anesthesia (Steward, 1979) and can develop in patients who have undergone previous surgery uneventfully. It is more common in males, and the incidence declines after puberty. The syndrome may be induced by any volatile anesthetic, but the onset is usually more abrupt when succinylcholine is used, either alone or in conjunction with volatile agents.

Signs: The earliest and most consistent sign of malignant hyperthermia in susceptible patients usually is unexplained tachycardia or tachyarrhythmia. Other early signs may include tachypnea, labile blood pressure (usually a moderate increase), and flushing followed by cyanotic mottling. Blood pH falls quickly due to production of carbon dioxide and later to formation of lactic acid. Serum potassium levels become elevated. Muscle rigidity may develop and usually is noted first in the jaw muscles but does not occur in all patients.

Hyperthermia is a late sign. Heat produced in the skeletal muscle elevates core temperature rapidly, which ultimately may rise to more than 110° F (42° C). Disseminated intravascular coagulation and oozing of blood at the surgical site may develop. Acute pulmonary edema secondary to left ventricular failure often appears in the terminal stage. Creatine phosphokinase may increase during the crisis but reaches maximal levels (20,000 to 100,000 IU) 12 to 24 hours later.

Treatment: An operating room protocol should be established to guide therapy (Ryan, 1979; Gronert, 1983). Appropriate steps are: (1) discontinue anesthesia immediately; (2) administer 100% oxygen with hyperventilation; (3) administer dantrolene [Dantrium] by continuous, rapid intravenous push, beginning with a minimum of 2 mg/kg and continuing until symptoms subside or a total dose of 10 mg/kg has been reached; (4) correct acidosis with sodium bicarbonate 1 to 2 mEq/kg immediately, thereafter guided by measurements of arterial pH and PCO_2; (5) control hyperkalemia by administering 10 units of regular insulin in 50 ml of dextrose injection 50%; (6) initiate cooling until the temperature is 38° to 39° C (surface cooling with ice in children; intravenous iced saline in adults, 1 L every ten minutes to a maximum of 3 L); and (7) maintain urinary output above 2 ml/kg/hour to protect against renal damage from myoglobinuria. The electrocardiogram, temperature, and urinary output should be monitored. In addition, an arterial line for measuring blood gases, electrolytes, and blood pressure should be inserted. If the physiologic and metabolic abnormalities reappear, the drug regimen should be repeated. It has been recommended that dantrolene 1 to 2 mg/kg be administered every 6 hours for 12 hours after termination of the acute episode. Frequent monitoring should be continued for 24 to 48 hours after the acute episode.

Anesthesia for the Susceptible Patient: No anesthetic technique is completely safe for patients susceptible to malignant hyperthermia, since even stress may trigger an attack. The incidence can be reduced by selecting techniques that are rarely associated with an unfavorable reaction, administering prophylactic doses of dantrolene preoperatively (see evaluation), monitoring the patient closely, and instituting remedial measures immediately if necessary (Relton, 1979). The practice of administering oral dantrolene for two to four days prior to anesthesia is no longer recommended (Harrison, 1988).

Balanced anesthesia is the preferred technique (see index entry Neuroleptanalgesia). A barbiturate or benzodiazepine may be used for premedication with or without an opioid. Nondepolarizing muscle relaxants may be used as needed, but succinylcholine and potent inhalation anesthetics should not be given.

Drug Evaluation

DANTROLENE SODIUM
[Dantrium]

For chemical formula, see index entry Dantrolene, In Muscle Spasticity.

USES. See above discussion on malignant hyperthermia.

ADVERSE REACTIONS AND PRECAUTIONS. The use of dantrolene in hyperthermic emergencies or for the preoperative preparation of patients susceptible to malignant hyperthermia is not associated with the hepatotoxicity that can occur during prolonged administration. However, large doses may produce nausea, diarrhea, blurred vision, muscle weakness, and incoordination.

Intravenous dantrolene is classified in FDA Pregnancy Category C.

DOSAGE AND PREPARATIONS.

Intravenous: For malignant hyperthermia, the dose for *adults* and *children* is the same: Intravenous push, beginning with a minimum dose of 2 mg/kg and continuing until symptoms subside or a cumulative dose of 10 mg/kg has been reached. If the physiologic and metabolic abnormalities reappear, administration of dantrolene and the other drugs (oxygen, sodium bicarbonate) should be repeated.

For prophylaxis, 2.5 mg/kg during induction of anesthesia.

Dantrium Intravenous (Procter & Gamble). Powder (sterile, lyophilized) 20 mg for reconstitution to 60 ml.

Oral: For prophylaxis, 4 to 8 mg/kg/day in four divided doses for one to two days prior to surgery, with the last dose given three to five hours prior to surgery. The larger dose may cause considerable weakness.

Dantrium (Proctor & Gamble). Capsules 25, 50, and 100 mg.

Agent Used in Pre-eclampsia and Eclampsia

MAGNESIUM SULFATE

ACTIONS AND USES. Magnesium sulfate is used to prevent or control convulsions in patients with pre-eclampsia or eclampsia. It acts at the myoneural junction to prevent the presynaptic release of acetylcholine and to decrease the amplitude of the motor endplate potential. Uterine contractions are inhibited and uterine blood flow is enhanced. Although magnesium sulfate causes some peripheral vasodilation, its antihypertensive action is slight and unpredictable; therefore, an antihypertensive drug (usually hydralazine) must be used concomitantly to reduce blood pressure (Pritchard, 1980).

Magnesium should be reserved for patients who experienced a significant increase in blood pressure with imminent or existing eclampsia (Lubbe, 1984). Less severe hypertensive change usually responds to combination therapy with alpha- and beta-adrenergic blocking agents.

ADVERSE REACTIONS AND PRECAUTIONS. Magnesium sulfate is classified in FDA Pregnancy Category A. Magnesium ion rapidly crosses the placenta but rarely causes hypermagnesemia in the neonate. Toxicity in the mother is indicated by loss of deep tendon reflexes, which occurs with magnesium plasma concentrations of 7 to 10 mEq/L. Plasma concentrations exceeding 10 mEq/L affect the respiratory muscles. This action can be antagonized by calcium gluconate or calcium chloride (10 ml of 10% solution infused over a three-minute period). High plasma levels of magnesium also produce heart block.

Magnesium sulfate potentiates the neuromuscular blocking effects of the nondepolarizing muscle relaxants. It should be given cautiously to patients with impaired renal function.

DOSAGE AND PREPARATIONS.

Intravenous (by constant infusion pump): *Adults*, a loading dose of 2 to 4 g (4 to 8 ml of a 50% solution) is infused over a five-minute period; for constant infusion, 1 to 2 g/hr (8 ml of 50% solution in 230 ml of dextrose injection 5% = 1 g magnesium sulfate/60 ml). Intravenous bolus injections are not recommended for maintenance. Magnesium is eliminated by renal excretion; if the urine output is below 30 ml/hr, the rate of administration must be reduced (Barford and Sokol, 1981).

Intramuscular administration no longer is recommended in patients with pre-eclampsia or eclampsia because absorption is unpredictable due to vasospasm and abnormal extracellular fluid distribution.

Generic. Solution 50% in 2, 5, 10, 20, 30, and 50 ml containers.

Respiratory Stimulants (Analeptics)

Analeptics are general central nervous system stimulants; they stimulate respiration, enhance the response to sensory stimulation, and hasten the return of normal reflexes. However, studies have demonstrated that analeptics are of limited usefulness in the supportive treatment of ventilatory insufficiency or arrest caused by anesthetics or other drugs with hypnotic activity. None of these drugs have the high specificity of action of the narcotic antagonists or anticholinesterase agents and should not be substituted for these agents when respiratory depression is caused by opioids or neuromuscular blocking drugs. They are ineffective in ventilatory depression caused by cardiac arrest, airway obstruction, bronchospasm, or overdosage of other central nervous system depressants.

Analeptics act directly on nervous tissue. When ventilation is improved, their site of action is in the brain stem, particularly the medulla; certain analeptics (eg, doxapram [Dopram]) act on the carotid chemoreceptors as well. Reflex activity is improved when the spinal cord is stimulated in addition to the brain stem. Arousal occurs when higher centers are stimulated. Any improvement in cardiovascular reflexes results from improved central nervous system function rather than direct myocardial stimulation.

Convulsions may occur with increasing doses of any analeptic. Large doses given frequently may depress respiration. The margin between the analeptic and convulsant dose is narrow with the older analeptics (picrotoxin, nikethamide, pentylenetetrazol). Doxapram is safer and has supplanted the older agents when analeptic therapy is elected to stimulate ventilation; its usefulness in hastening arousal is less established.

The xanthines, caffeine and theophylline, are not recommended for general analeptic use, but they are given to treat apnea in premature infants.

Analeptics, particularly caffeine sodium benzoate and the amphetamines, have been promoted to overcome the "hangover" effects of drug-induced coma. However, their administration for this purpose is neither logical nor advisable.

Physostigmine [Antilirium] reduces the arousal time in postoperative patients who received anticholinergic drugs, antihistamines, benzodiazepines, and droperidol and alleviates the disorientation and agitation occasionally caused by these agents, but its routine use is not recommended. Physostigmine also has been administered to arouse patients for brief periods during neuroleptanesthesia when their cooperation is required (eg, in certain neurosurgical procedures). Central depression produced by inhalation anesthetics, opioids, ketamine, or barbiturates is not affected by physostigmine. See index entry Physostigmine, In Anticholinergic Toxicity, for adverse reactions, precautions, and dosage.

Drug Evaluations

DOXAPRAM HYDROCHLORIDE

[Dopram]

H

CH_2CH_2—N+ O Cl^-

O N

CH_2CH_3

ACTIONS AND USES. Animal studies have demonstrated that this analeptic causes arousal, stimulates ventilation, and increases arterial pressure. Studies in patients with normal central nervous and respiratory systems confirmed that doxapram increased the ventilatory response to carbon dioxide and the minute ventilation by increasing tidal volume and, to a lesser extent, the ventilatory rate. However, the drug also increased oxygen uptake, reduced carbon dioxide tension, and elevated pH, oxygen tension, and oxygen saturation. The adverse effects did not necessitate reducing the rate of administration.

Controlled double-blind studies reveal that doxapram hastens arousal when administered during the immediate postoperative period. It is not widely used, however, perhaps because the clinical usefulness and possible hazards remain unclear.

The availability of other simple tests (eg, measurement of inspiratory and expiratory airway pressures, evaluation of the ventilatory rate and pattern, ability of the patient to lift his head, response to peripheral nerve stimulation) renders the diagnostic use of doxapram in postanesthetic apnea or hypoventilation of minimal clinical value.

ADVERSE REACTIONS AND PRECAUTIONS. Generalized warmth, sweating, dyspnea, restlessness, hyperreflexia, laryngospasm, coughing, breathholding, retching, tachycardia, hypertension, nausea, lightheadedness, headache, and tremor may occur, particularly if large doses are given. Agitation and hallucinations are rare.

Doxapram is contraindicated in patients with convulsive disorders, hypertension, cerebral edema, hyperthyroidism, or pheochromocytoma and in those taking monoamine oxidase inhibitors or adrenergic agents. It is not recommended in patients with known or suspected pulmonary embolism, pneumothorax, or airway obstruction. Because controlled ventilation and standard supportive therapy are effective in ventilatory failure, doxapram *should not be used* in patients with drug-induced coma.

This drug is classified in FDA Pregnancy Category B.

PHARMACOKINETICS. Doxapram is extensively metabolized; less than 5% of an intravenous dose is excreted unchanged in the urine. The mean half-life is 3.4 hours. The apparent volume of distribution is 1.5 L/kg, and the clearance is 370 ml/min (Robson and Prescott, 1978).

DOSAGE AND PREPARATIONS. The manufacturer's suggested dosages are:

Intravenous: *Adults,* for ventilatory depression following anesthesia, 0.5 to 1 mg/kg is injected as a single dose and repeated at five-minute intervals until a maximum of 2 mg/kg has been given. Alternatively, 1.5 to 2 mg/kg is infused. The calculated total dose is added to dextrose 5% or 10% or sodium chloride injection and administered at an initial rate of approximately 5 mg/min until a satisfactory response is observed; for maintenance, an infusion rate of 1 to 3 mg/min is suggested. The maximal dosage by infusion is 4 mg/kg or 300 mg for adults of average weight.

To hasten arousal during the recovery period, 1 to 1.5 mg/kg is injected. The total amount is given as a single dose or in divided doses at five-minute intervals.

Doxapram is not labeled for use in *children* or during pregnancy.

Dopram (Robins), ***Generic***. Solution 20 mg/ml in 20 ml containers.

METHYLXANTHINES

ACTIONS AND USES. The methylxanthines, caffeine and theophylline, are effective in the treatment of primary apnea of prematurity (Higbee and Bosso, 1979; Aranda et al, 1981). This disorder has been defined as an absence of respiratory effort lasting more than 20 seconds; cyanosis and/or bradycardia also may be present.

The methylxanthines decrease the frequency of apneic episodes, probably through a central action. Regularization of breathing is associated with increased alveolar ventilation and increased sensitivity of the medullary respiratory center to carbon dioxide. Lung compliance, PaO_2, pH, respiratory rate, and blood pressure usually are not affected by methylxanthine therapy, although $PaCO_2$ often is decreased when apneic episodes are reduced (Davi et al, 1978).

Premature infants undergoing general anesthesia during their first 12 months are at risk for postoperative apnea and/or bradycardia. It is recommended that the respiratory and heart rates be monitored during the postanesthetic period. The incidence of postoperative ventilatory dysfunction can be reduced by the slow intravenous administration of 5 to 10 mg/kg of caffeine following induction (Welborn et al, 1988).

ADVERSE REACTIONS AND PRECAUTIONS. The frequency and severity of adverse reactions to methylxanthines are minimal if care is taken to maintain the serum concentration of the stimulant, particularly theophylline, within the recommended range (Howell et al, 1981). Both caffeine and theophylline increase central nervous system activity. Two times the recommended serum concentration of theophylline (more than 20 mcg/ml) has been associated with tachypnea, tachycardia, jitteriness, and vomiting, while four times the recommended serum concentration (more than 40 to 60 mcg/ml) has produced seizures. Too rapid intravenous administration of either agent can induce hypotension. Caffeine has a much greater therapeutic index than theophylline and there are fewer reports of toxicity with its use in apnea of prematurity. Both caffeine and theophylline may increase serum glucose.

PHARMACOKINETICS. The plasma clearance of methylxanthines, especially caffeine, is markedly prolonged in premature infants and may change significantly during therapy as the infant matures. There also is wide variability in plasma clearance among infants, and dosage is best determined by monitoring the drug plasma concentration. This is especially important in premature infants.

Unlike adults, premature infants metabolize theophylline in part to caffeine (Tserng et al, 1983; Aranda et al, 1984). The fraction of the dose excreted as caffeine and other metabolites is a function of gestational age and birth weight and decreases with postnatal maturation. It has been recommended that the total plasma concentration of methylxanthines (caffeine plus theophylline) be determined in order to adjust the dose of theophylline.

In a summary of pharmacokinetic studies in premature infants (Roberts, 1984), theophylline was reported to have an approximate half-life of 28 hours (range, 12 to 58 hours) and a volume of distribution of 0.7 L/kg; clearance was about 17 ml/kg/hr in premature infants 6 to 11 days old and increased to about 31 ml/kg/hr by the ninth week. There have been fewer studies on the pharmacokinetics of caffeine in the premature infant. The values reported in most available studies (Gorodischer and Karplus, 1982) are: half-life, 60 to 100 hours; volume of distribution, 0.8 to 0.9 L/kg; and clearance, 8 to 9 ml/kg/hr (Roberts, 1984).

DOSAGE AND PREPARATIONS. Theophylline is administered orally by nasogastric tube, preferably as a nonalcoholic syrup, and also may be given intravenously. Caffeine usually is administered orally as a solution of caffeine citrate; however, an intravenous solution of caffeine citrate can be prepared by the hospital pharmacy.

THEOPHYLLINE:

Doses are given as theophylline base.

Oral (nasogastric tube): A loading dose of 5 mg/kg is followed by a maintenance dose of 2 mg/kg every 12 hours. Plasma concentrations of total methylxanthines should be monitored, with the first determination made within 24 hours after starting the maintenance dose. Generally, 5 to 12 mcg/ml are effective theophylline plasma concentrations. The smallest effective dose should be used; many premature infants respond satisfactorily to plasma concentrations of 3 to 5 mcg/ml. Toxicity often occurs at methylxanthine concentrations greater than 20 mcg/ml. Smaller doses may be given more frequently to maintain a more constant, effective concentration without high, possibly toxic, peak concentrations. It may be necessary to increase the daily dose occasionally to maintain therapeutic blood concentrations, because the clearance of theophylline increases with age during the first month of life.

Intravenous: The loading dose is 2.5 to 5 mg/kg of theophylline (commercial preparations of aminophylline may contain 79% or 85% theophylline equivalent); this is followed by the constant intravenous infusion of 2 mg/kg every 12 hours, *with frequent monitoring of serum concentrations,* until a serum theophylline concentration of 2 to 12 mcg/ml is attained. Infants who do not benefit from serum concentrations of 12.7 mcg/ml will not benefit from higher concentrations. These infants will require additional management with doxapram or continuous positive airway pressure (Muttitt et al, 1988).

See index entry Theophylline, Uses, Bronchial Disorders, for a list of available theophylline products.

CAFFEINE:

Preparations containing sodium benzoate should not be employed in the neonate.

Oral (nasogastric tube): The loading dose is 10 mg/kg (caffeine citrate contains 50% caffeine), followed by 2.5 mg/kg once daily. Serum levels should be monitored if possible; generally, 5 to 12 mcg/ml of caffeine is effective. Toxic signs may develop at plasma concentrations above 20 mcg/ml and are common with concentrations above 50 mcg/ml.

Intravenous: A loading dose of 10 mg/kg (as caffeine base) is followed by 2.5 mg/kg/day beginning 24 hours after the loading dose.

Generic. Powder.

Benzodiazepine Antagonist

FLUMAZENIL
[Mazicon]

ACTIONS. Flumazenil is a benzodiazepine receptor antagonist that attenuates or reverses the cognitive, psychomotor, hypnogenic, and electroencephalographic effects of benzodiazepines. This agent also competitively blocks benzodiazepine receptor inverse agonists (eg, beta carbolines), which produce effects opposite those of the benzodiazepines. Results of some studies on animals and human volunteers suggest that flumazenil may have weak partial agonist or inverse agonist actions, but it is unlikely that these effects are important clinically.

USES. Results of several controlled trials have confirmed the ability of flumazenil to partially or completely reverse most central effects of the benzodiazepines (for review, see Votey et al, 1991; Brogden and Goa, 1991). These studies included patients in whom general anesthesia was induced and/or maintained with benzodiazepines (eg, cardiac surgery, arterial surgery); patients sedated with benzodiazepines who had undergone various surgical procedures (eg, lower abdominal, urologic, orthopedic, dental) under local, regional, or spinal anesthesia; and patients in whom sedation was produced with benzodiazepines for diagnostic and therapeutic procedures (eg, cardioversion, cardiac catheterization, endoscopy, dental procedures).

In patients who received midazolam for induction of general anesthesia, postoperative administration of flumazenil shortened recovery time. Flumazenil also improves postoperative performance following total intravenous anesthesia. In either case, residual sedation may require repeated administration. Amnesia for the operative procedure is not eliminated by the postoperative administration of flumazenil, but further amnesia is usually prevented unless there is significant residual sedation. The effects of midazolam on resting ventilation and ventilatory drive in anesthetized patients, especially in the presence of an opioid, are controversial (Mora et al, 1987; Tolksdorf et al, 1990), and flumazenil has not been established as an effective treatment in these patients.

Flumazenil is more effective than doxapram or physostigmine in enhancing recovery following general anesthesia supplemented with benzodiazepines (Bill et al, 1989; Schneider et al, 1988; Breimer et al, 1988). In some studies, patients recovered earlier if they had been sedated or anesthetized with propofol rather than treated with flumazenil following midazolam-based anesthesia (Kestin et al, 1990; Norton and Dundas, 1990).

Results of double-blind controlled studies indicate that intravenous administration of flumazenil increases the level of consciousness in patients who received an overdose of benzodiazepines alone or benzodiazepines with alcohol or other drugs (Aarseth et al, 1988; Hojer et al, 1990; Ritz et al, 1990). Accordingly, the use of flumazenil may facilitate the differential diagnosis of comatose patients, and the need for supportive interventions (eg, gastric lavage, intubation, artificial ventilation) may be reduced; however, flumazenil is intended as an adjunct to, not a substitute for, adequate clinical evaluation and appropriate supportive care in these patients. Symptoms of poisoning with barbiturates, alcohol, tricyclic antidepressants, or phenothiazines are not affected, and toxicity due to tricyclic antidepressants may be exacerbated.

There is some evidence that flumazenil may be useful in portal systemic encephalopathy (PSE), a complex neuropsychiatric syndrome most commonly associated with acute or chronic hepatocellular failure. PSE frequently accompanies liver failure caused by viral hepatitis, drug overdose, or alcohol abuse. Although the disorder does not alter the central nervous system architecture, it impairs mentation and neuromuscular function. Because increased GABAergic activity is observed, benzodiazepine antagonists have been used to reduce functional central nervous system impairment (Basile and Gammal, 1988; Rothstein et al, 1989). In two small controlled studies that excluded patients who had recently received benzodiazepines, use of flumazenil (0.2 to 15 mg) resulted in distinct but transient improvement in 60% to 70% of patients (Grimm et al, 1988; Bansky et al, 1989). However, in a preliminary report of another controlled study, flumazenil was no more effective than standard treatment (Van der Rijt et al, 1989). Further study is required to clarify the role of flumazenil in the treatment of PSE.

ADVERSE REACTIONS AND PRECAUTIONS. Generally, flumazenil is well tolerated. Adverse effects may be related to flumazenil or to reversal of the effects of benzodiazepines. The incidence of adverse effects is higher when flumazenil is given after general anesthesia than for conscious sedation. Following general anesthesia, the most common adverse effects were nausea, vomiting, agitation, and shivering. Agitation, anxiety, and emotional lability also may occur in patients treated with flumazenil for benzodiazepine intoxication. Dizziness, cutaneous vasodilation, pain at the injection site, fatigue, visual abnormalities, hypoesthesia, and headache also have been reported. Because flumazenil has not been established as an effective treatment for hypoventilation, patients should be monitored for recurrence of sedation and respiratory depression for an appropriate period based on the dose and duration of action of the benzodiazepine.

Deaths have occurred after administration of flumazenil, primarily in patients with serious underlying disease or those who were intoxicated with nonbenzodiazepine drugs, particularly tricyclic antidepressants. Seizures have occurred most frequently in patients physically dependent on benzodiazepines and in those with severe tricyclic antidepressant overdose, in whom the use of flumazenil is contraindicated. Withdrawal symptoms may develop in patients who are physically dependent on benzodiazepines; the use of lower doses of flumazenil may reduce emergent confusion and agitation. This drug is contraindicated in patients who have been given a benzodiazepine to control a potentially life-threatening condition (eg, seizures).

Flumazenil is classified in FDA Pregnancy Category C.

PHARMACOKINETICS. After oral administration, flumazenil is well absorbed, but bioavailability is low due to high hepatic clearance. After intravenous administration, the peak concentration of flumazenil is proportional to the dose; the apparent initial volume of distribution is 0.5 L/kg. The volume of distribution at steady state (V_{ss}) ranges from 0.8 to 1.6 L/kg, and protein binding is approximately 50%. Clearance occurs primarily by hepatic metabolism and is dependent on hepatic blood flow. The de-ethylated free acid and its glucuronide metabolite are the major end products. Because flumazenil has a short half-life (0.7 to 1.3 hours), recurrence of sedation due to residual benzodiazepine may occur and repeated administration or continuous intravenous infusion of flumazenil may be required. Clearance is reduced 40% to 60% in patients with mild to moderate hepatic disease and up to 75% in those with severe hepatic dysfunction.

DOSAGE AND PREPARATIONS. Flumazenil is recommended for intravenous use only and is compatible with 5% dextrose in water, lactated Ringer's solution, and normal saline.

Reversal of Conscious Sedation or in General Anesthesia:

Intravenous: Initially, 0.2 mg (2 ml) administered over 15 seconds; if the desired level of consciousness is not reached within 45 seconds, 0.2 mg can be injected at 60-second intervals to a maximum dose of 1 mg (10 ml). Most patients respond to doses of 0.6 to 1 mg. In the event of recurrence of sedation, no more than 1 mg (given at a rate of 0.2 mg/min) is administered at 20-minute intervals; no more than 3 mg should be given in any one hour.

Suspected Benzodiazepine Overdose:

Intravenous: Initially, 0.2 mg (2 ml) administered over 30 seconds. If the desired level of consciousness is not obtained after another 30 seconds, an additional 0.3 mg can be administered over 30 seconds, followed by 0.5 mg over 30 seconds at one-minute intervals up to a cumulative dose of 3 mg. Rarely, patients with a partial response to 3 mg will require additional titration up to a total dose of 5 mg. If the patient does not respond within five minutes after receiving a cumulative dose of 5 mg, benzodiazepines are probably not the major cause of sedation. In the event of recurrence of sedation, no more than 1 mg administered at a rate of 0.5 mg/min may be given at 20-minute intervals to a maximum of 3 mg in one hour.

Mazicon (Roche). Solution 0.1 mg/ml in 5 and 10 ml containers.

Cited References

Aarseth HP, et al: Benzodiazepine-receptor antagonist, a clinical double blind study. *Clin Toxicol* 26:283-292, 1988.

Abdul-Rasool IH, et al: Effect of second dose of succinylcholine on cardiac rate and rhythm following induction of anesthesia with etomidate or midazolam. *Anesthesiology* 67:795-797, 1987.

Ali HH, et al: Clinical pharmacology of BW B1090U continuous infusion, abstract. *Anesthesiology* 65(3A):A282, 1986.

Aranda JV, et al: Pharmacologic considerations in therapy of neonatal apnea. *Pediatr Clin North Am* 28:113-133, 1981.

Aranda JV, et al: Ontogeny of human caffeine and theophylline metabolism. *Dev Pharmacol Ther* 7(suppl 1):18-25, 1984.

Arden JR, et al: Vecuronium in alcoholic liver disease: Pharmacokinetic and pharmacodynamic analysis. *Anesthesiology* 68:771-776, 1988.

Azad S, et al: Dose-response evaluation of pipecuronium bromide in the elderly population under balanced anesthesia, abstract. *Anesthesiology* 67(suppl 3A):A370, 1987.

Azar I: Response of patients with neuromuscular disorders to muscle relaxants: Review. *Anesthesiology* 61:173-187, 1984.

Bansky G, et al: Effects of the benzodiazepine receptor antagonist flumazenil in hepatic encephalopathy in humans. *Gastroenterology* 97:744-750, 1989.

Barford DAG, Sokol RJ: Modern approach to severe preeclampsia. *Drug Ther* 6:31-35, (Feb) 1981.

Basile AS, Gammal SH: Evidence for the involvement of the benzodiazepine receptor complex in hepatic encephalopathy: Implications for treatment with benzodiazepine receptor antagonists. *Clin Neuropharmacol* 11:401-422, 1988.

Basta SJ, et al: Clinical pharmacology of doxacurium chloride: New long-acting nondepolarizing muscle relaxant. *Anesthesiology* 69:478-486, 1988.

Bencini AF, et al: Disposition and urinary excretion of vecuronium bromide in anesthetized patients with normal renal function or renal failure. *Anesth Analg* 65:245-251, 1986 A.

Bencini AF, et al: Hepatobiliary disposition of vecuronium bromide in man. *Br J Anaesth* 58:988-995, 1986 B.

Bill KM, et al: Antagonism of midazolam-induced sedation with flumazenil or doxapram. *Br J Anaesth* 63:627P, 1989.

Brandom BW, et al: Pharmacokinetics of atracurium in anaesthetized infants and children. *Br J Anaesth* 58:1210-1213, 1986 A.

Brandom BW, et al: Comparison of the effects of BW B1090U and succinylcholine administered by bolus and infusion in anesthetized patients, abstract. *Anesthesiology* 65(3A):A288, 1986 B.

Brandom BW, et al: Mivacurium chloride (BW B1090U) infusion requirements in children during halothane or narcotic anesthesia, abstract. *Anesth Analg* 67:S20, 1988.

Breimer LTM, et al: The efficacy of flumazenil versus physostigmine after midazolam-alfentanil anaesthesia in man. *Eur J Anaesthesiol Suppl* (2)109-116, 1988.

Brogden RN, Goa KL: Flumazenil: A reappraisal of its pharmacological properties and therapeutic efficacy as a benzodiazepine antagonist. *Drugs* 42:1061-1089, 1991.

Brotherton WP, Matteo RS: Pharmacokinetics of metocurine in man with renal failure, abstract. *Anesthesiology* 53(suppl):268, (Sept) 1980.

Caldwell JE, et al: Influence of renal failure on the pharmacokinetics and duration of action of pipecuronium bromide, abstract. *Anesthesiology* 67(suppl 3A):A612, 1987 A.

Caldwell JE, et al: Pipecuronium and pancuronium: Comparison of their pharmacokinetics and durations of action, abstract. *Anesthesiology* 67(suppl 3A):A611, 1987 B.

Choi WW, et al: Neuromuscular effects of BW B1090U during narcotic nitrous oxide anesthesia, abstract. *Anesthesiology* 67 (3A):A355, 1987.

Clergue F, et al: Depression of respiratory drive by diazepam as premedication. *Br J Anaesth* 53:1059-1063, 1981.

Cook DR, et al: Pharmacokinetics of atracurium in normal and liver failure patients, abstract. *Anesthesiology* 61(suppl 3A):A433, 1984.

Cook DR, et al: In vitro metabolism of BW B1090U, abstract. *Anesthesiology* 67(3A):A610, 1987.

Cottrell JE, et al: Prevention of nitroprusside-induced cyanide toxicity with hydroxocobalamin. *N Engl J Med* 298:809-811, 1979.

Cronnelly R, Morris RB: Antagonism of neuromuscular blockade. *Br J Anaesth* 54:183-194, 1982.

Cronnelly R, et al: Pyridostigmine kinetics with and without renal function. *Clin Pharmacol Ther* 28:78-81, 1980.

Davi MJ, et al: Physiologic changes induced by theophylline in treatment of apnea in preterm infants. *J Pediatr* 92:91-95, 1978.

de Bros FM, et al: Pharmacokinetics and pharmacodynamics of atracurium under isoflurane anesthesia in normal and anephric patients, abstract. *Anesth Analg* 64:207, 1985.

de Bros F, et al: Pharmacokinetics and pharmacodynamics of atracurium in the elderly, abstract. *Anesthesiology* 67(suppl 3A):A604, 1987 A.

de Bros F, et al: Pharmacokinetics and pharmacodynamics of BW B1090U in healthy surgical patients receiving $N_20/0_2$ isoflurane anesthesia, abstract. *Anesthesiology* 67(suppl 3A):A609, 1987 B.

Dresner DL, et al: Pharmacokinetics and pharmacodynamics of doxacurium in young and elderly patients during isoflurane anesthesia. *Anesth Analg* 71:498-502, 1990.

Durant NN, et al: Hepatic elimination of Org-NC45 and pancuronium, abstract. *Anesthesiology* 51(suppl):267, (Sept) 1979.

Duvaldestin P, et al: Pancuronium pharmacokinetics in patients with liver cirrhosis. *Br J Anaesth* 50:1131-1136, 1978.

Duvaldestin P, et al: Pharmacokinetics, pharmacodynamics, and dose-response relationships of pancuronium in control and elderly subjects. *Anesthesiology* 56:36-40, 1982.

Fisher DM, et al: Pharmacokinetics and pharmacodynamics of d-tubocurarine in infants, children, and adults. *Anesthesiology* 57:203-208, 1982.

Gorodischer R, Karplus M: Pharmacokinetic aspects of caffeine in premature infants with apnea. *Eur J Clin Pharmacol* 22:47-52, 1982.

Goudsouzian NG: Atracurium infusion in infants. *Anesthesiology* 68:267-269, 1988.

Grimm G, et al: Improvement of hepatic encephalopathy treated with flumazenil. *Lancet* 2:1392-1394, 1988.

Gronert GA: Malignant hyperthermia. *Semin Anesth* 2:197-204, 1983.

Harrison GG: Dantrolene: Dynamics and kinetics. *Br J Anaesth* 60:279-286, 1988.

Higbee MD, Bosso JA: Apnea of prematurity. *Drug Intell Clin Pharm* 13:24-29, 1979.

Hill NS, et al: Intravenous nitroglycerin: Review of pharmacology, indications, therapeutic effects and complications. *Chest* 79:69-76, 1981.

Hojer J, et al: Diagnostic utility of flumazenil in coma with suspected poisoning: A double blind, randomized controlled study. *BMJ* 301:1308-1311, 1990.

Howell J, et al: Adverse effects of caffeine and theophylline in newborn infant. *Semin Perinatol* 5:359-369, 1981.

Hunter JM: Adverse effects of neuromuscular blocking drugs. *Br J Anaesth* 59:46-60, 1987.

Kestin IG, et al: Psychomotor recovery after three methods of sedation during spinal anaesthesia. *Br J Anaesth* 64:675-681, 1990.

Konstadt S, et al: Study of the hemodynamic effects of BW A938U: New long acting nondepolarizing muscle relaxant, abstract. *Anesthesiology* 67(suppl 3A):A369, 1987.

Krapez JR, et al: Effects of cyanide antidotes used with sodium nitro prusside infusions: Sodium thiosulphate and hydroxocobalamin given prophylactically to dogs. *Br J Anaesth* 53:793-804, 1981.

Lebrault C, et al: Pharmacokinetics and pharmacodynamics of vecuronium (ORG NC 45) in patients with cirrhosis. *Anesthesiology* 62:601-605, 1985.

Lee C, et al: Dose-duration relationship of BW1090U by bolus injections, abstract. *Anesthesiology* 67(3A):A353, 1987.

Lowry KG, et al: Vecuronium and atracurium in the elderly: Clinical comparison with pancuronium. *Acta Anaesthesiol Scand* 29:405-408, 1985.

Lubbe WF: Hypertension in pregnancy: Pathophysiology and management. *Drugs* 28:170-188, 1984.

Lynam DP, et al: Pharmacodynamics and pharmacokinetics of vecuronium in patients anesthetized with isoflurane with normal renal function or with renal failure. *Anesthesiology* 69:227-231, 1988.

Matteo RS, et al: Distribution, elimination, and action of d-tubocurarine in neonates, infants, children, and adults. *Anesth Analg* 63:799-804, 1984.

Matteo RS, et al: Pharmacokinetics and pharmacodynamics of d-tubocurarine and metocurine in the elderly. *Anesth Analg* 64:23-29, 1985.

Miler V, et al: Dose response of mivacurium in pediatric patients, abstract. *Anesth Analg* 67:S149, 1988.

Miller RD, et al: Pharmacokinetics of d-tubocurarine in man with and without renal failure. *J Pharmacol Exp Ther* 202:1-7, 1977.

Mora CT, et al: Sedative and ventilatory effects of midazolam and flumazenil. *Anesthesiology* 67:A534, 1987.

Morris RB, et al: Pharmacokinetics of edrophonium and neostigmine when antagonizing d-tubocurarine neuromuscular blockade in man. *Anesthesiology* 54:399-402, 1981 A.

Morris RB, et al: Pharmacokinetics of edrophonium in anephric and renal transplant patients. *Br J Anaesth* 53:1311-1314, 1981 B.

Muttitt SC, et al: Dose response of theophylline in the treatment of apnea of prematurity. *J Pediatr* 112:115-121, 1988.

Norton AC, Dundas CR: Induction agents for day-case anaesthesia: A double-blind comparison of propofol and midazolam antagonised by flumazenil. *Anaesthesia* 45:198-203, 1990.

Powers D, et al: BW B1090U infusion requirements in adults during isoflurane anesthesia, abstract. *Anesthesiology* 67 (suppl 3A): A359, 1987.

Pritchard JA: Management of preeclampsia and eclampsia. *Kidney Int* 18:259-266, 1980.

Ramzan MJ, et al: Pharmacokinetic studies in man with gallamine triethiodide. II. Single 4 and 6 mg/kg IV doses. *Eur J Clin Pharmacol* 17:145-152, 1980.

Relton JES: Anesthesia for elective surgery in patients susceptible to malignant hyperthermia. *Int Anesthesiol Clin* 17:141-151, (Winter) 1979.

Ritz R, et al: Use of flumazenil in intoxicated patients with coma: A double-blind placebo-controlled study in ICU. *Intensive Care Med* 16:242-247, 1990.

Roberts RJ: *Drug Therapy in Infants: Pharmacologic Principles and Clinical Experience*. Philadelphia, WB Saunders, 1984, 119-137.

Robson RH, Prescott LF: Pharmacokinetic study of doxapram in patients and volunteers. *Br J Clin Pharmacol* 7:81-87, 1978.

Rothstein JD, et al: Cerebrospinal fluid content of diazepam binding inhibitor in chronic hepatic encephalopathy. *Ann Neurol* 26:57-62, 1989.

Ryan JF: Treatment of acute hyperthermia crises. *Int Anesthesiol Clin* 17:153-168, (Winter) 1979.

Sarner JB, et al: Clinical pharmacology of doxacurium chloride (BW A938U) in children. *Anesth Analg* 67:303-306, 1988.

Savarese JJ, et al: Neuromuscular and cardiovascular effects of BW B1090U in anesthetized children, abstract. *Anesth Analg* 64:278, 1985.

Savarese JJ, et al: Ninety and 120-second tracheal intubation with BW B1090U: Clinical conditions with and without priming after fentanyl-thiopental induction, abstract. *Anesthesiology* 65 (3A):A283, 1986.

Savarese JJ, et al: Clinical neuromuscular pharmacology of mivacurium chloride (BW B1090U): Short-acting nondepolarizing ester neuromuscular blocking drug. *Anesthesiology* 68:723-732, 1988.

Schneider I, et al: Flumazenil for midazolam reversal: Dose-effect relationships compared with doxapram in a placebo-controlled study. *Eur J Anaesthesiol Suppl* (2) 117-121, 1988.

Somogyi AA, et al: Effect of renal failure on disposition and neuromuscular blocking action of pancuronium bromide. *Eur J Clin Pharmacol* 12:23-29, 1977 A.

Somogyi AA, et al: Disposition kinetics of pancuronium bromide in patients with total biliary obstruction. *Br J Anaesth* 49:1103-1108, 1977 B.

Steward DJ: Malignant hyperthermia: Acute crisis. *Int Anesthesiol Clin* 17:1-9, (Winter) 1979.

Stoops CM, et al: Hemodynamic effects of BW A938U in coronary artery bypass graft and valve replacement patients receiving oxygen sufentanil anesthesia, abstract. *Anesthesiology* 67 (suppl 3A):A368, 1987.

Tassonyi E, et al: Hemodynamic effects of pipecuronium bromide during fentanyl-midazolam anesthesia induction for coronary artery bypass grafting, abstract. *Anesthesiology* 65 (suppl 3A):A284, 1986.

Tolksdorf W, et al: The influence of flumazenil on respiration after midazolam and/or fentanyl. *Anesth Analg* 70:S409, 1990.

Tserng K-Y, et al: Developmental aspects of theophylline metabolism in premature infants. *Clin Pharm Ther* 33:522-528, 1983.

Van der Rijt CD, et al: Flumazenil therapy for hepatic encephalopathy: A double blind crossover study. *Hepatology* 10:590, 1989.

Votey SR, et al: Flumazenil: A new benzodiazepine antagonist. *Ann Emerg Med* 20:181-188, 1991.

Ward S, Neill EAM: Pharmacokinetics of atracurium in acute hepatic failure (with acute renal failure). *Br J Anaesth* 55:1169-1172, 1983.

Weber S, et al: Mivacurium chloride (BW B1090U)-induced neuromuscular blockade during nitrous oxide-isoflurane and nitrous oxide-narcotic anesthesia in adult surgical patients. *Anesth Analg* 67:495-499, 1988.

Weinstein JA, et al: Pharmacokinetics and pharmacodynamics of metocurine in infants, children and adults, abstract. *Anesthesiology* 67 (suppl 3A):A615, 1987.

Welborn LG, et al: Control of postoperative apnoea in the ex-premature infant: Experience with a high caffeine dose, abstract. *Can J Anaesth* 35:S140-S141, 1988.

Westra P, et al: Hepatic and renal disposition of pancuronium and gallamine in patients with extrahepatic cholestasis. *Br J Anaesth* 53:331-338, 1981.

Wierda JMKH, et al: Pharmacokinetics and cardiovascular effects of pipecuronium bromide (Arduan) in C.A.G.B. patients, abstract. *Anesthesiology* 67 (suppl 3A):A613, 1987.

Woelfel SK, et al: Potency of mivacurium chloride (BW B1090U) during halothane-nitrous oxide anesthesia in children. *Anesth Analg* 67:S261, 1988.

Drugs Used for Anxiety and Sleep Disorders

11

ANXIETY

Description and Classification

Anxiety is apprehension, tension, or uneasiness related to anticipated danger (American Psychiatric Association, 1987). It may be a response to stress associated with environmental stimuli or it may be devoid of any apparent cause. Anxiety that is related to stressful circumstances is normal and reflects biologically determined tendencies as well as cognitive and learned factors. Only when anxiety is disproportionate to a presenting or anticipated situation or when it occurs without an identifiable stimulus does it become pathologic. The decision on when to initiate treatment usually is made on the basis of a careful history combined with consultation between the physician, the patient, and, in some instances, the family.

The diagnosis of a primary anxiety disorder is made by assessing symptom criteria. Attempts should be made to identify medical disorders (eg, hyperthyroidism, pheochromocytoma), substance abuse (eg, intoxication, withdrawal), or psychiatric disorders (eg, mood [affective] disorders, somatoform disorders) that may be causative or contributory (Schuckit, 1983). A primary anxiety disorder also must be differentiated from situational anxiety, which can be precipitated by psychosocial stressors (eg, unpleasant social interactions, bereavement, business losses, marital conflict).

The anxiety disorders described in the revised third edition of the *Diagnostic and Statistical Manual of Mental Disorders (DSM-III-R)* (American Psychiatric Association, 1987) are characterized by anxiety, phobia, and other related symptoms. These disorders have a lifetime prevalence of 10% to 20% in the general population. The anxiety states are classified as panic disorder with and without agoraphobia, generalized anxiety disorder, obsessive-compulsive disorder, posttraumatic stress disorder, and anxiety disorders not otherwise specified in the above classifications. Phobic disorders include simple phobia, social phobia, and agoraphobia, which usually occurs as a complication of panic disorder.

ANXIETY STATES. *Panic disorder* is characterized by spontaneous, recurrent attacks of anxiety (panic) accompanied by feelings of terror, autonomic manifestations, and morbid anticipation of death. For diagnostic purposes, at least four panic attacks must have occurred within a four-week period, or one or more attacks must have been followed by a fear of having another attack that persists for at least one month. Also, at least four of the following symptoms must have occurred during at least one of the attacks: dyspnea or smothering sensation; choking; palpitations or tachycardia; chest pain or discomfort; sweating; dizziness, unsteady feeling, or faintness; nausea or abdominal distress; depersonalization or derealization; numbness or tingling sensations (paresthesias); hot flashes or chills; trembling or shaking; fear of dying, going crazy, or doing something uncontrolled. Usually, several of these symptoms appear suddenly and increase to peak intensity within ten minutes of the first symptom becoming apparent. Major depression and alcohol or drug abuse are present in many patients with panic disorder (Otto et al, 1992; Pollack et al, 1992). Personality disorders also are present in some patients.

Generalized anxiety disorder may be diagnosed when anxiety persists for six months or longer during which an individual is bothered on most days by unrealistic or excessive worry about two or more life circumstances, such as possible misfortune to a child or concern about finances, that is unwarranted. In children or adolescents, the anxiety may be about academic, athletic, or social performance. However, patients sometimes develop symptoms of generalized anxiety that require treatment but do not meet these criteria (eg, symptoms lasting less than six months) (Dubovsky, 1990).

At least 6 of the following 18 symptoms are required for the diagnosis of generalized anxiety disorder: Symptoms of *motor tension* include trembling, twitching, or feeling shaky; muscle tension, aches, or soreness; restlessness; or easy fatigability. Symptoms of *autonomic hyperactivity* include dyspnea or smothering sensation; palpitations or tachycardia; sweating or cold clammy hands; dry mouth; dizziness or lightheadedness; nausea, diarrhea, or other abdominal distress; hot flashes or chills; frequent urination; and trouble swallowing or lump in the throat. Finally, *vigilance and scanning* symptoms include feeling keyed up or on edge; exaggerated startle response, difficulty concentrating, or mind going blank; trouble falling or staying asleep; and irritability.

Results of recent surveys suggest that *obsessive-compulsive disorder* (OCD) develops in 1% to 2% of the general population (Regier et al, 1988; Swedo et al, 1989). Onset usually occurs during late adolescence or early adulthood. The disorder is characterized by anxiety arising from either (1) recurrent and persistent obsessive ideas, images, or impulses that are experienced as intrusive, unwanted, and senseless and which the individual attempts to ignore, suppress, or counter; (2) repetitive, purposeful, and intentional ritualistic behaviors (eg, hand washing) or thoughts (mental rituals) that decrease discomfort or anxiety associated with obsessions. Most often there is a logical link between the obsession and the ritualistic behavior, but some rituals are performed simply because they relieve stress and not because of any clear connection to the problem they address. Depression is common in these patients and other conditions sometimes coexist (eg, Tourette's syndrome, panic and phobic disorders).

Post-traumatic stress disorder follows a unique and psychologically traumatic experience (eg, serious threat to life or physical integrity; destruction of home or community). Responsiveness to the environment may begin to decline soon after the event; however, a latency period of months or even years may follow the traumatic experience. There is a persistent avoidance of stimuli (eg, thoughts, feelings, activities, situations) associated with the trauma or a decrease (numbing) of general responsiveness (eg, restricted range of emotions, feeling of detachment or estrangement). The patient with post-traumatic disorder also has persistent symptoms of increased arousal (eg, insomnia, irritability, exaggerated startle response).

Anxiety disorder not otherwise specified represents a residual category for disorders involving prominent anxiety or phobic symptoms that are not classified as a specific anxiety disorder or as an adjustment disorder with anxious mood.

PHOBIC DISORDERS. The lifetime prevalence of phobic disorders is about 6% in the United States. These disorders are characterized by irrational fear of objects, activities, or situations and by the compelling desire to avoid them. The affected individual clearly recognizes that the fear is disproportionate to any real threat. Three phobic disorders are identified in the current classification (American Psychiatric Association, 1987).

Agoraphobia is characterized by a marked fear of being in places or situations from which escape might be difficult or embarrassing or in which help might not be available in the event of sudden incapacitation. Normal activities become increasingly curtailed, and avoidant behavior interferes with, and sometimes dominates, the individual's life. Common agoraphobic situations include being outside the home alone, being in a crowd or standing in a line, being on a bridge or in a tunnel, traveling on public transportation, or attending events in an auditorium. Clinically, agoraphobia usually occurs as a complication of panic disorder.

Social phobia consists of a persistent and irrational fear of social situations in which the individual feels he may be scrutinized by others and may behave in a humiliating or embarrassing manner. The individual recognizes that the fear is excessive and unreasonable. Some patients have a general fear of social situations; the generalized form often is chronic and can be incapacitating. Often, social phobia is limited to one activity, such as public speaking, eating in front of others, urinating in a public lavatory, or writing in the presence of others. Performance anxiety (ie, fear related to public speaking or performance) is considered a specific subtype of social phobia.

Simple phobia is a persistent and irrational fear of an object or situation (eg, fear of spiders, snakes, heights) that does not involve spontaneous panic attacks or potentially embarrassing social situations. Simple phobia represents a residual category for the phobic disorders that cannot be classified either as agoraphobia or social phobia. Simple phobias seldom are incapacitating despite the fact that the feared objects or situations are avoided or endured with intense anxiety. Simple phobia responds to behavioral therapy (exposure) but is generally unresponsive to pharmacotherapy.

Management

Therapy is based principally on the type and degree of anxiety (Lader, 1987 A; Frazier, 1988). The goal is to control anxiety in order to reduce social impairment and to prevent complications (eg, alcohol and other substance abuse, depression, suicide, sexual dysfunction, physical illness) (Pasnau, 1988).

PANIC AND PHOBIC DISORDERS. Anticipatory fear of having more attacks, followed by avoidance of situations of vulnerability, occurs in most patients with panic disorder. The disorder often is chronic. Factors that contribute to the severity and persistence of panic disorder include phobic subtype, coexisting anxiety or mood disorders, and personality disorders (Noyes et al, 1991; Pollack et al, 1992).

Behavioral therapy involving the alteration of catastrophic cognitions and graded exposure to the feared situation to reduce symptoms of panic is effective. Exposure-based behavioral therapy is especially helpful for those with phobic avoidance. Drug therapy also is useful. Either modality may be successful alone, and results of some studies suggest that a combination of medication and behavioral therapy results in more rapid and complete response (Lydiard and Ballenger, 1987). Their effectiveness, either alone or together, should be evaluated on the basis of patient acceptance and tolerance, reduction or resolution of panic attacks, diminution of phobic avoidance and anxiety, amelioration of other conditions (eg, depression), and prevention of relapse (National Institutes of Health, 1991).

Panic disorder with or without agoraphobia is commonly treated with antidepressants (ie, imipramine [Janimine, Tofranil] or other tricyclic agents, monoamine oxidase [MAO] inhibitors), or high-potency benzodiazepines (eg, alprazolam [Xanax], clonazepam [Klonopin]). Results of comparative studies suggest that the short-term efficacy of these drugs is similar; long-term efficacy is less clear. It has been recommended that responsive patients be maintained on medication for at least 6 to 12 months before reducing the dose or discontinuing the drug (Salzman, 1989). Many patients who discontinue drug therapy may experience a return of panic or phobic symptoms. If the anxiety state recurs, indefinite drug therapy may be indicated.

Of the tricyclic compounds that have been used to treat panic disorder, imipramine has been studied most thoroughly. Clomipramine [Anafranil] has been used primarily in Europe, where its efficacy has been demonstrated in controlled trials. The usefulness of imipramine or clomipramine is often limited by the anticholinergic side effects of these drugs, orthostatic hypotension, weight gain, or by an initial "activation syndrome" (restlessness, agitation, exacerbation of anxiety). In those who cannot tolerate the anticholinergic effects, desipramine [Norpramin, Pertofrane] (Kalus et al, 1991) or fluoxetine [Prozac] (Schneier et al, 1990) may be beneficial; nortriptyline [Aventyl, Pamelor] may be useful in patients who experience orthostatic hypotension (Roy-Byrne, 1992). Overall, up to one-third of patients may discontinue therapy because of side effects (Noyes et al, 1989). Thus, dose escalation with antidepressants should be individualized and flexible. Another disadvantage of tricyclic therapy in some individuals is delayed onset of action. Advantages of tricyclic compounds include once-daily dosing, a low risk of dependence, lack of dietary restrictions, and effectiveness for the treatment of concurrent depression. For further information, see the evaluation on Imipramine Hydrochloride in this chapter.

Of the MAO inhibitors, phenelzine [Nardil] has been evaluated most frequently in panic disorder. It is widely believed to be effective in blocking panic attacks, although the ability of this or other MAO inhibitors to decrease the actual frequency of panic attacks has not been documented by placebo-controlled studies. In one open study, phenelzine (mean dose, 53.5 mg/day) significantly reduced the frequency of panic attacks in patients with agoraphobia during a 12-week period (Lydiard and Ballenger, 1987). In another open study, complete blockage of attacks was reported in 16 patients with panic disorder (Buigues and Vallejo, 1987). Phenelzine may be effective in individuals resistant to other therapy, and some authorities consider it the preferred therapy for patients with severe, crippling panic disorder (Salzman, 1989). The average effective daily dose of phenelzine is between 45 and 60 mg (range, 45 to 90 mg). Amounts exceeding 90 mg can be administered if side effects do not become a problem. Because of phenelzine's potential for serious interactions with some foods and drugs, the patient or the person supervising drug administration should receive written instructions regarding appropriate dietary and drug restrictions.

Alprazolam and other benzodiazepines (eg, clonazepam) have assumed an increasingly important role in the treatment of panic disorder. Results of short-term studies (6 to 12 weeks) indicate that alprazolam is effective in reducing both panic attacks and phobic avoidance and also substantially reduces anticipatory anxiety (Ballenger et al, 1988; Tesar, 1990). In most controlled trials, doses of 1 to 10 mg were employed (mean dose, 5 to 6 mg); however, patients often respond satisfactorily to lower doses and many clinicians prefer not to exceed a daily dosage of approximately 6 mg, especially if the initial response has been inadequate (see the evaluation). The efficacy of alprazolam is comparable to that of antidepressants, but it acts more rapidly and is better tolerated. Thus, it may be the drug of choice for patients with significant disability who require immediate relief (Roy-Byrne, 1992).

Some clinicians have prescribed alprazolam with either a tricyclic antidepressant or MAO inhibitor to achieve rapid control of panic symptoms and to minimize any initial increase in anxiety that may be attributable to the antidepressant (*Med Lett Drugs Ther*, 1991). Alprazolam then may be discontinued gradually as the antidepressant becomes effective. Combination therapy also may be utilized in refractory patients or in those who respond partially. However, in one controlled trial, there was no benefit of the drug combination after the first two weeks compared with imipramine alone, and the condition of patients receiving the combination deteriorated after alprazolam was discontinued (Woods et al, 1992). It must be noted that, by most standards, the doses of imipramine and alprazolam employed in this study were low and the rate of alprazolam's withdrawal (0.5 mg every three days) was rapid.

Adverse reactions usually are infrequent and mild with short-term alprazolam therapy. The major concern is development of physical dependence and subsequent withdrawal symptoms on discontinuation; about one-third of patients with panic disorder experience difficulty when alprazolam is discontinued over a four-week period (Pecknold et al, 1988). In patients who completed a four-month combined drug and behavioral treatment program and continued to receive alprazolam (mean dose, 3.1 mg/day), only 30% had discontinued the drug at long-term follow-up (mean, 2.5 years). The majority (60%) continued use of alprazolam but at a lower dosage (Nagy et al, 1989). The potential for physical dependence and difficulties encountered with discontinuation of alprazolam may make a tricyclic antidepressant or MAO inhibitor a better choice in those patients who can tolerate the adverse effects and dietary restrictions, respectively (*Med Lett Drugs Ther*, 1991).

Alprazolam's short duration of action can lead to interdose anxiety symptoms, which may be prevented by administering the same total daily amount in multiple doses. However, the requirement for frequent dosing with alprazolam has led to consideration of alternative benzodiazepines with more favorable pharmacokinetic properties. Several open trials have demonstrated the efficacy of clonazepam in the treatment of panic attacks. In one regimen, clonazepam 0.5 mg or less is given once daily initially and the amount is increased gradually until 1 to 2 mg daily in two divided doses is reached. A placebo-controlled, six-week trial comparing clonazepam (mean dose, 2.5 mg/day) with alprazolam (mean dose, 5.4 mg/day) revealed no significant differences in effects. Approximately 50% of patients treated with either drug were free of panic attacks during the last two weeks of the trial (Tesar et al, 1991). Since clonazepam has a slower onset and longer duration of action, it may be useful in patients who experience rebound or interdose recurrence of symptoms with alprazolam therapy (Tesar, 1990; Herman et al, 1987). After the patient begins to respond to either alprazolam or clonazepam, the lowest effective dose should be determined.

Evidence is accumulating that lorazepam [Ativan] also is useful in the treatment of panic disorder (for review see Tesar, 1990). Results of several open studies suggest that lorazepam compares favorably with phenelzine and alprazolam and, in two controlled trials, the efficacy of lorazepam was comparable to that of alprazolam (Charney and Woods, 1989; Schweizer et al, 1990 A).

Phenelzine is the drug of choice for social phobia, especially the generalized type; in controlled trials it was superior to atenolol [Tenormin] and alprazolam (Gelernter et al, 1991; Liebowitz et al, 1992). Results of open trials and pilot studies suggest that clonazepam, buspirone [BuSpar], and fluoxetine also may be beneficial in some patients with social phobia (Davidson et al, 1991; Munjack et al, 1991). Cognitive and behavioral therapy also have been reported to be effective (Heimberg and Barlow, 1991). A beta blocker or benzodiazepine (eg, clonazepam, alprazolam) administered as needed may be useful for performance anxiety or situational social phobia (Liebowitz et al, 1991).

Behavioral therapy alone is the treatment of choice for simple phobia. Exposure to the feared object or situation often eliminates the tendency to avoid, which then extinguishes anticipatory anxiety.

GENERALIZED ANXIETY DISORDER. Before treatment of generalized anxiety disorder is begun, it is necessary to exclude other psychiatric or physical disorders that may be obscured by prominent anxiety symptoms. A comprehensive treatment plan should then be formed that includes pharmacotherapy and/or supportive psychotherapy (eg, advice, counseling, relaxation training, stress management, cognitive behavioral therapy).

Antianxiety agents can play an important role in controlling anxious feelings that could prevent the patient from participating more fully in psychotherapeutic treatment. In most individuals, the benzodiazepines are the drugs of choice. Patients for whom benzodiazepine therapy is particularly suitable may have precipitating stress and acute symptoms characterized by pronounced somatic and psychic distress but not clinically significant depression (Dubovsky, 1990).

Results of studies focusing on the long-term efficacy of benzodiazepines (Rickels et al, 1983 A) indicate that patients with persistent chronic anxiety of this type may require continuous therapy for six months or more. During long-term treatment, it may be possible to reduce the dosage or discontinue the drug during periods of reduced stress. Intermittent, variable-dose therapy reduces the risk of physical dependence on benzodiazepines (Marks, 1990). However, in patients with unrelenting stress or those unable to resolve conflict, discontinuation of therapy may result in a return of symptoms or impaired functioning or may be otherwise inadvisable (eg, arrhythmias exacerbated by anxiety), and long-term uninterrupted therapy with these drugs may be appropriate (Greenblatt et al, 1983 A; Uhlenhuth et al, 1988; Dubovsky, 1990).

Buspirone is a nonbenzodiazepine antianxiety agent (Rakel, 1987; Schnabel, 1987; Jann, 1988). In generalized anxiety disorder, the antianxiety action of this azaspirone is comparable to that of diazepam [Valium, Valrelease] and other benzodiazepines, but the onset of action is more gradual (Goldberg and Finnerty, 1982; Rickels et al, 1982; Cohn and Wilcox, 1986; Cohn and Rickels, 1989; Strand et al, 1990). In some studies, diazepam was more effective in reducing somatic symptoms and buspirone appeared to be more effective in reducing cognitive symptoms and interpersonal problems (Gershon and Eison, 1983; Pecknold et al, 1989). Buspirone lacks the sedative-hypnotic, muscle relaxant, and antiepileptic properties of the benzodiazepines; does not potentiate the central nervous system (CNS) depressant effects of alcohol or other drugs; and produces less psychomotor impairment, lethargy, and depression (Schuckit, 1987). Also, studies in animals and humans have failed to demonstrate abuse potential, dependency syndromes, or significant withdrawal reactions (Lader, 1987 B). Buspirone appears to be most beneficial in patients without acute precipitants of anxiety who do not require the immediate relief offered by the benzodiazepines (Rickels, 1990). Other patients who are potentially suitable for buspirone therapy include the elderly, those with a history of substance abuse, and those with conditions or employment in which sedation or psychomotor impairment would be dangerous (eg, airline pilots, those with sleep apnea). Further studies are necessary to define the role of this drug in the treatment of other anxiety disorders.

Some patients with chronic generalized anxiety may benefit from long-term administration. For reassessment of therapy, buspirone can be withheld periodically without the problems associated with chronic benzodiazepine therapy (ie, distinguishing between withdrawal reactions and recurrence of symptoms) (Rickels, 1990).

Antidepressants may be beneficial in the treatment of some patients with generalized anxiety disorder. In several studies in patients with mixed anxiety and depression, doxepin [Adapin, Sinequan] was reported to be more effective than placebo (for review see Liebowitz et al, 1988). Doxepin also may be effective in primarily anxious outpatients (Kahn et al, 1981). Limited data also support the use of amitriptyline [Elavil, Endep], imipramine, or desipramine (Liebowitz et al, 1988). Further controlled, comparative trials in patients with generalized anxiety disorder, but without significant symptoms of depression or panic disorder, are needed to clarify the potential role of these agents.

OBSESSIVE-COMPULSIVE DISORDER (OCD). Some antidepressants are effective in many patients with OCD. Depression is not a prerequisite for an effective response, and no clear relationship exists between the antidepressant and antiobsessional actions of these drugs. All of the antiobsessional drugs characteristically inhibit the neuronal reuptake of serotonin, and this observation lends partial support to the hypothesis that alteration of serotonin neurotransmission is involved in OCD (Benkelfat et al, 1989; Goodman et al, 1989; March et al, 1989; Rapoport, 1989). Although a few patients respond completely to medication, a 35% to 60% decrease in obsessions and compulsions after 10 to 12 weeks of treatment is more common. If patients do not respond to one agent, a trial with a different serotonin-uptake blocker is warranted.

Several controlled trials have established the antiobsessional efficacy of clomipramine (see the evaluation) and the investigational drug, fluvoxamine (Pato, 1990; The Clomipramine Collaborative Study Group, 1991; Goodman et al, 1992). In controlled trials, fluvoxamine 50 mg initially was given either nightly or in divided doses. The dosage may be increased by 25 to 50 mg every three to four days as tolerated and on the basis of clinical response to a maximum of 300 mg daily in three divided doses (Perse et al, 1987; Price et al, 1987; Goodman et al, 1989).

The efficacy of fluoxetine has been demonstrated in several uncontrolled trials and in a small crossover, comparative trial with clomipramine; in the latter study, the therapeutic efficacy of fluoxetine (mean dose, 75 mg daily) did not significantly differ from that of clomipramine (mean dose, 209 mg daily) statistically, although in approximately 50% of patients the degree of response to clomipramine was at least 20% greater (Pigott et al, 1990). However, detection of differences between treatment groups was difficult due to the small number of patients studied. Thus, the efficacy of fluoxetine in the treatment of OCD is unresolved. In open trials, the most common daily dosage of fluoxetine also was 75 or 80 mg (Turner et al, 1985; Jenike et al, 1989 A; Levine et al, 1989; Frenkel et al, 1990).

In a large multicenter double-blind study, eight weeks of treatment with sertraline [Zoloft] was reported to be significantly more effective than placebo in reducing symptoms of OCD (Chouinard et al, 1990).

Unlike the uptake blockers that globally influence serotonergic neurotransmission, buspirone primarily affects the $5HT1_A$ receptor and, in a small open trial, was ineffective in OCD (Jenike and Baer, 1988). In a controlled comparison of buspirone and clomipramine, both drugs produced a similar reduction in OCD symptoms (Pato et al, 1991); however, the study lasted only six weeks, and changes in the severity of symptoms in the clomipramine recipients were not of the same magnitude that normally occur in longer (eg, ten-week) trials. Although use of buspirone alone may be ineffective, anecdotal reports and small open trials suggest that buspirone as well as other agents (eg, lithium, trazodone [Desyrel], pimozide [Orap]) may be beneficial as adjunctive agents in refractory patients (Markovitz et al, 1990; Jenike et al, 1990). However, in controlled trials, adjunctive use of lithium or buspirone did not substantially reduce symptoms of OCD in patients treated with fluvoxamine and clomipramine, respectively (McDougle et al, 1991; Pigott et al, 1992), although a few patients with a partial response to clomipramine may have benefitted from the addition of buspirone. Therefore, a trial of adjunctive use of buspirone may be considered in refractory patients (Pigott et al, 1992). MAO inhibitors may be useful in patients suffering concomitant panic attacks (Jenike et al, 1987).

There are no adequate guidelines on the optimal length of therapy, and currently it is not possible to predict which patients will maintain improvement without medication (Jenike, 1990). Relapse is unfortunately common when drug therapy is discontinued. Therapy probably should continue for at least one year, and withdrawal of medication should be gradual (ie, over three to six months).

The techniques of exposure therapy plus response prevention are the mainstay of behavioral treatment. Comprehensive treatment, involving both medication and behavioral therapy either in sequence or concurrently, is recommended for most patients (Greist, 1990). Behavioral therapy is unlikely to be effective unless concurrent psychiatric disorders (eg, depression) are well controlled initially. It was formerly believed that behavioral therapy also is not effective in patients with severe obsessions who do not also perform compulsive rituals, but it is now apparent that many patients confuse mental rituals with obsessions. Once the distinction is understood, many "pure obsessionals" are found to perform anxiolytic mental rituals and thus are good candidates for behavioral therapy.

SLEEP DISORDERS

Description and Classification

The essential function of sleep is still unknown, although it is generally recognized to have a restorative quality that diminishes fatigue and dysphoria. The onset and duration of sleep correlate with circadian body temperature rhythms but also depend on other factors such as the length of prior wakefulness. There is no recommended daily optimum amount of sleep for any age group, but it is possible to determine the optimum quantity required by an individual. A shortened or lengthened total sleep time is not considered pathologic in the absence of other symptoms, and some individuals are unaware of daytime sequelae. Shortened and fragmented sleep periods are common in the elderly.

In *DSM-III-R,* disorders of sleep and arousal are divided into two major subgroups, dyssomnias and parasomnias. The International Classification of Sleep Disorders includes a third subgroup, medical/psychiatric sleep disorders (American Sleep Disorders Association, 1990). The most common sleep disorders encountered clinically are the dyssomnias (eg, insomnia, hypersomnia, sleep-wake schedule disorders) in which the amount, quality, or timing of sleep is disturbed. Insomnia, which may be the primary symptom of a variety of sleep, medical, and psychiatric disorders, is encountered most frequently. In the parasomnias, the predominant complaint is an abnormal event that occurs during sleep and is associated with abrupt but usually incomplete arousal.

DYSSOMNIAS. Insomnia: Insomnia encompasses a broad spectrum of disorders with diverse underlying causes. It may be associated with a psychiatric disorder; the use of drugs or alcohol; medical (eg, arthritis, Parkinson's disease), toxic, or environmental conditions; and occasionally respiratory impairment, periodic limb movements in sleep (nocturnal myoclonus), or "restless legs syndrome."

Inability to fall asleep, remain asleep, and experience restorative sleep at night are frequent complaints associated with insomnia. During the course of a year, 35% of adults report episodes of insomnia, and about half of them consider it to be serious (Mellinger et al, 1985). Common subjective daytime complaints that correlate with nighttime sleeplessness include drowsiness, fatigue, lack of energy, dysphoria, and lack of alertness.

The temporal classification of insomnia as transient, short-term, or long-term (National Institutes of Health, 1983) is useful for diagnosis and determination of appropriate therapeutic measures. In transient insomnia, acute situational stress (eg, hospitalization, jet travel) may adversely affect sleep. This condition usually lasts only a few days.

Short-term insomnia usually is also associated with situational stress but can last up to three weeks. Sleep difficulty may be caused by such factors as the loss of a loved one; job pressures; concerns regarding examinations; nightshift work and travel across time zones (jet lag), which upset internal circadian rhythms; use of certain drugs (eg, amphetamines, caffeine); or withdrawal of some drugs (eg, alcohol, nicotine).

Long-term insomnia persists for more than three weeks and, in one-third to two-thirds of patients, it is due to an underlying psychiatric disorder, especially major depressive disorder. Chronic drug abuse (eg, alcohol) or dependence causes long-term insomnia in a second major group of patients. Other causes include medical conditions, such as arthritis, neurogenic pain, and various types of headache. The daytime pain experienced by the latter patients may be magnified greatly at night when sleep is attempted, environmental stimuli are decreased, and more attention is focused internally. In patients with malignancies, pain can be severe, and fear and anxiety about the ultimate consequences of the illness often are overwhelming. Patients with angina pectoris or arrhythmias often are afraid to sleep because of fear that an attack may occur during the night when they feel most vulnerable and helpless. Other causes of long-term insomnia include sleep apnea; periodic movements in sleep, sometimes associated with restless legs syndrome; 24-hour rhythm disturbances (eg, advanced and delayed sleep phase); or undefined psychological or physiologic stress (National Institutes of Health, 1983).

Hypersomnias: About 85% of cases of hypersomnia seen in sleep disorder centers are related to a known organic factor (eg, sleep apnea, narcolepsy, periodic movements in sleep). Regardless of etiology, the primary symptoms of hypersomnias are inappropriate and undesirable sleepiness during waking hours, decreased cognitive and motor performance, excessive tendency to sleep, unavoidable napping, increase in total 24-hour sleep, and difficulty in achieving full arousal on awakening. Because patients often use the terms interchangeably, chronic persistent sleepiness must be distinguished from chronic fatigue. Most people who are seen in sleep disorder clinics for hypersomnia have sleep apnea and, less frequently, narcolepsy. Hypersomnias, like the insomnias, also may be associated with other medical or psychiatric disorders (eg, atypical or major depression, substance abuse associated with tolerance to or withdrawal from CNS stimulants, use of CNS depressants, including manifestations after both long- or short-term use).

Sleep Apnea. Sleep apnea is characterized by episodic reductions or complete cessation in ventilation during sleep. Hypopneic and apneic episodes are defined as a more than 50% reduction in air flow or the complete cessation of air flow, respectively, for at least 10 seconds, typically in association with a fall in oxyhemoglobin saturation and arousal from sleep (Schwartz and Smith, 1989). Central apnea is characterized by the complete cessation of respiratory efforts, while obstructive apnea is characterized by the presence of continued paradoxical thoracoabdominal respiratory efforts against an occluded pharyngeal airway. Apneas that include both central and obstructive components are termed mixed apneas (Chokroverty and Sharp, 1981). The obstructive and mixed types are the most common; the central type is relatively rare prior to old age. Episodes may occur hundreds of times each night. Severe bradycardia, hypoxemia, hypercapnia, and life-threatening arrhythmias may develop during the apneic episodes. Apnea is terminated by reflex arousal from sleep.

The apneic patient usually has no memory of these difficulties and consequently complains only of daytime fatigue and sleepiness. Questioning the patient's bed partner and observing the sleeping infant or child may be necessary for a presumptive diagnosis when all the classical features of the disorder are not present. Diagnosis is confirmed by polysomnographic recordings.

The obstructive disorders are more common in middle-aged obese men who snore; however, infants and children can be affected quite severely (Brouillette et al, 1982), and increased awareness is necessary to provide earlier treatment and reduce morbidity in this age group. A special subset of individuals susceptible to sleep apnea include those with the obesity-hypoventilation (pickwickian) syndrome. These patients are predominantly male and demonstrate extreme obesity, hypoventilation (which results in hypoxemia and hypercapnia), polycythemia, and cor pulmonale.

Narcolepsy. The classical diagnostic tetrad of the primary symptoms of narcolepsy (Parkes, 1977; Ferriss, 1982) is (1) excessive daytime sleepiness with a history of falling asleep episodically, rapidly, and often inappropriately while performing a daily task; (2) episodic cataplectic attacks of muscular weakness precipitated by emotional stimulation (ie, humor, anger, fear, surprise); momentary (partial) attacks are most common and may cause patients to drop objects, sit down, or stop walking; (3) hypnagogic hallucinations, which may be visual, auditory, or tactile, occurring during the transition from wakefulness to sleep; and (4) sleep paralysis characterized by consciousness and inability to move or cry out during the transition from wakefulness to sleep. Sleep paralysis and hypnagogic hallucinations occur in about 60% of narcoleptic patients.

All narcoleptics have sleep attacks and 50% to 70% experience cataplexy, which is pathognomonic of the disorder. Less than 25% of patients have all four symptoms (Browman et al, 1983). Most authorities agree that increasing drowsiness precedes episodes of sleep (Aldrich, 1990). Common secondary signs and symptoms include automatic behavior with complete retrograde amnesia, disturbed nocturnal sleep characterized by frequent awakenings, and disturbances of vision. In the absence of cataplexy, the Multiple Sleep Latency Test is the most useful diagnostic technique (Aldrich, 1990). A polysomnograph showing a transition from wakefulness directly into REM (rapid eye movement) rather than NREM (nonrapid eye movement) sleep helps to confirm the diagnosis. Multiple occurrences of REM at the onset or within 10 minutes of sleep is characteristic.

Narcolepsy usually develops between ages 15 and 25; it rarely appears after age 40. Susceptibility appears to be genetic, based on 98% to 100% association with HLA-DR2 and HLA-DQwl antigens. The disorder generally persists for life, although some adaptation occurs. Effects on the patient's life are substantial; 60% to 80% have fallen asleep while driving or at work or both.

Sleep-Wake Schedule Disorder: This disorder represents a mismatch between the normal sleep-wake schedule for a patient's environment and his or her circadian sleep pattern that results in a complaint of either insomnia or hypersomnia (eg, jet lag, shift working when the chronological night does not consistently coincide with the biologic sleep period). Approximately 25% of the work force have variable-shift schedules.

PARASOMNIAS. Nightmares: Individuals with this disorder experience repeated awakenings from REM sleep with detailed recall of extended and extremely frightening dreams that usually involve threats to survival, security, or self-esteem. On awakening, the person rapidly becomes oriented and alert, although the dream experience may cause significant distress.

Sleep Terrors: Diagnostic criteria include recurrent episodes associated with abrupt apparent awakening from non-REM sleep lasting from one to ten minutes; they usually occur during the first third of a major sleep period and begin with a panicky scream, although no details may be recalled. Anxiety and signs of autonomic effects, such as tachycardia, rapid breathing, and sweating, are intense. Initially, the individual is relatively unresponsive to being comforted by others. Almost invariably several minutes of confusion, disorientation, and perseveration, ie, repetitive motor movements (eg, picking at a pillow), are observed.

Sleepwalking Disorder: Affected individuals arise during sleep (usually during the first third of a major sleep episode) and walk about. While sleepwalking, a person has a blank, staring face and is relatively unresponsive to attempts to communicate. A sleepwalker usually can be awakened only with great difficulty and on awakening may experience a short period of confusion or disorientation with little or no recall of the episode.

A number of other manifestations occur that are not classified in the three categories above. Functional enuresis during sleep is a parasomnia. Similarly, although rare, nocturnal seizure disorders may mimic the symptoms of other parasomnias.

Management

A sleep complaint, whether it is nighttime sleeplessness, daytime sleepiness, decreased daytime performance, or excessive daytime sleep, requires careful diagnostic evaluation prior to therapy.

DYSSOMNIAS. Insomnia: An accurate diagnosis of insomnia requires that the underlying cause be determined. A medical history, including a detailed sleep, drug, and psychiatric history; physical examination; and appropriate laboratory procedures may be needed for differential diagnosis. Taking a sleep history, including input from the patient's bed partner, also is helpful. In some cases, polysomnography may be required. A survey suggests that some physicians place inadequate emphasis on history-taking in the evaluation of insomnia (Everitt et al, 1990).

The treatment of an insomnia depends on the underlying cause and the duration of the complaint. Assessment of the duration of insomnia and of the impact of sleep disruption on daytime functioning provides the most reliable indication of severity (Czeisler and Richardson, 1991).

Transient insomnia most often will disappear once the underlying stressful situation has been resolved; drug treatment may or may not be needed. When a drug is prescribed, a small dose may be adequate. Treatment may be needed for one to three nights.

Short-term insomnia often can be treated by eliminating the underlying stressful situation if possible or improving the coping skills of the individual. Counseling, training in relaxation techniques, and education in sleep hygiene (eg, regular sleep routines and waking time; avoiding long periods of wakefulness in bed; not reading or working in bed; avoiding naps, alcohol, caffeine-containing beverages, and strenuous exercise three to four hours before bedtime) are beneficial. If a hypnotic is needed despite good sleep hygiene, the smallest effective dose should be prescribed for no more than three weeks and intermittent use is advisable during this period. If administration for one or two nights results in good sleep, the dose for the next night can be skipped. Use of the drug then can be resumed for one- or two-day periods.

The causes of long-term insomnia require special medical, physiologic, and psychiatric evaluations. Conditioned anxiety about falling asleep may perpetuate the disorder to varying degrees in all patients with chronic insomnia. If a major psychiatric disorder is present, it should be treated appropriately. In drug abusers, the offending agent(s) must be identified and detoxification and rehabilitation started. When pain causes loss of sleep, analgesics should be administered.

Periodic movements in sleep, a disorder characterized by rhythmic myoclonic jerks that occur during sleep, may be relieved by clonazepam or an equivalent benzodiazepine. Although benzodiazepines may not significantly decrease the frequency of the movements, they increase the arousal threshold so that the patient's sleep is less disturbed. Dopaminergic compounds, such as levodopa/carbidopa [Sinemet] or bromocriptine [Parlodel], may directly decrease the frequency of myoclonic jerks.

In many patients with long-term insomnia, counseling, stress management, psychotherapy, and behavior modification may obviate or complement the use of drugs. Regular exercise; decreased caffeine intake; slow withdrawal of excessive, inappropriate, or ineffective medications; and a trial of various stress reduction techniques should be employed initially. A concomitant short trial (less than one month) of sleep-promoting medication also may be indicated (National Institutes of Health, 1983). However, it must be kept in mind that a hypnotic is only an adjunct to achieving the main therapeutic goal of breaking the vicious cycle of insomnia, fear of sleeplessness, subsequent emotional and physiologic arousal, and insomnia. Symptoms of sleep apnea (ie, daytime sleepiness, heavy snoring) are contraindications to use of sleep-promoting medications.

Perceived benefits of hypnotic drugs include an increase in total sleep time, reduced sleep fragmentation, and reduced night-to-night variability. Although hypnotics often alleviate insomnia, they do not induce normal sleep as defined by objective sleep parameters. Sleep laboratory studies have demonstrated that hypnotic doses of most of these agents reduce the amount of REM sleep. The benzodiazepines, the usual drugs of choice, may produce less disruption; however, they reduce stage 3 and 4 sleep. The clinical significance of this alteration is unknown, and emphasis is now on the patient's subjective evaluation of sleep, objective measurements of wakefulness as obtained in the sleep laboratory, and the impact of the drug on daytime performance (eg, memory, excessive sedation).

When hypnotics are indicated for patients with sleep disorders, appropriate guidelines should be followed: (1) Special caution is required for patients with respiratory difficulties; suicidal tendencies; or a history of alcoholism, drug dependence, or substance abuse. (2) The potential for impairment of daytime performance, including anterograde amnesia or memory impairment, should be discussed with the patient. It should be stressed that the patient may be unaware of his impairment. (3) Because of individual response variation, conservative therapy is especially necessary to avoid drug interactions in the elderly, in patients with associated illnesses, in those who drink alcohol, or in those taking other medication, especially antihistamines. (4) The minimum effective amount should be administered, and dose escalation should be avoided. (5) Hypnotics generally should not be prescribed beyond a period of about one month. If longer use is deemed necessary, drug therapy should be restricted to every second or third night to avoid drug accumulation or tolerance. (Recently, the manufacturer of triazolam [Halcion] and the FDA agreed on revision in the drug's labeling specifying that prescriptions should be written for short-term use [7 to 10 days], that the drug should not be prescribed in quantities exceeding a one-month supply, and that use for more than two to three weeks requires complete re-evaluation of the patient. Similar changes in the product labeling have been requested from the manufacturers of other hypnotics.) (6) Periodic monitoring is necessary to reassess drug effectiveness, minimize nightly reliance on medication, and determine toxic or other factors that would alter the risk of continuing hypnotic use. (7) Drug therapy should be discontinued when goals have been met. Gradual dosage reduction is essential after long-term administration to minimize rebound insomnia and possible withdrawal signs.

Hypersomnias: *Sleep Apnea.* Specific therapy may not be required for sleep apnea unless there is evidence of clinically significant gas exchange abnormalities, cardiopulmonary compromise, or daytime hypersomnolence (Schwartz and Smith, 1989). Avoidance of sedatives, including alcohol, is critically important. When indicated, weight loss and training to sleep in the lateral position may be the only management strategy required in patients with mild to moderate sleep apnea. In children, particular attention should be given to the possibility of anatomic obstruction of the upper airways, such as tonsillar or adenoid hypertrophy and deviated nasal septum, which can be corrected surgically.

Although not typically effective, drug therapy is an alternative in patients with less severe sleep apnea (Schott et al, 1989). Apnea during REM sleep is longer lasting and is associated with greater oxygen desaturation than NREM apnea; therefore, the use of a tricyclic antidepressant that decreases the amount of REM sleep results in fewer episodes of apnea during REM sleep per night. Although both imipramine and protriptyline have been effective, the latter is preferred because it tends to produce less sedation. Protriptyline also sometimes converts the apneas during NREM sleep to hypopneas with a corresponding decrease in duration; this improves nocturnal oxygenation. The effective dose range is 5 to 30 mg daily.

Endogenous progesterone stimulates respiration during the menstrual luteal phase and pregnancy. Medroxyprogesterone acetate (MPA) administered to normal men has the same effect. MPA stimulates respiration and improves blood gases in awake patients but does not benefit those with mechanical airway obstruction during sleep (Block, 1985). This drug appears to be most effective in the obesity-hypoventilation (pickwickian) syndrome in the presence of chronic hypercapnia (Wiggins and Schmidt-Nowara, 1987).

Uvulopalatopharyngoplasty has improved obstructive apnea in approximately 50% of patients, but its long-term effectiveness has not been established. Continuous positive airway pressure (CPAP) administered by nasal mask is the treatment of choice for severe sleep apnea and is effective in less severe forms as well. With proper patient selection, virtually all patients will benefit from this form of therapy, but 20% to 30% cannot tolerate the device. Tracheostomy remains a last resort for the refractory apneic patient and in those with life-threatening arrhythmias or severe cor pulmonale.

Respiratory stimulants, theophylline, and acetazolamide have not been sufficiently or consistently effective in the therapy of sleep apnea, and their use is not recommended until further data become available.

Narcolepsy. For most narcoleptic patients, treatment usually includes use of stimulant medication and a schedule of deliberate napping for the hypersomnia and use of nonsedating tricyclic antidepressants for the cataplexy, hypnagogic hallucinations, and sleep paralysis. Such treatment must meet the specific needs of the individual; a small proportion of patients with mild narcolepsy prefer to take no medications.

Methylphenidate, dextroamphetamine, and pemoline are the CNS stimulants most commonly prescribed to control the excessive daytime sleepiness characteristic of the disorder. The tricyclic antidepressants, protriptyline [Vivactil] and imipramine, also may diminish daytime sleepiness, but the consistency of this effect is controversial.

Methylphenidate and dextroamphetamine have a duration of action of two to five hours; pemoline's therapeutic effects persist for eight to ten hours. For the patient whose narcolepsy is almost controlled by adhering to a regular nocturnal sleep schedule plus a convenient schedule of napping, an average daily dose of 20 mg of methylphenidate (10 mg twice daily) may be sufficient (Regestein et al, 1983). If cataplexy is severe, protriptyline or imipramine can be added in small doses initially and the amount increased gradually over two to four weeks while the maintenance dose that maximizes therapeutic effect and minimizes adverse effects is determined. The therapeutic actions of these drugs in narcolepsy are immediate, unlike their antidepressant activities. Protriptyline or imipramine is effective in most patients, but fluoxetine or the investigational drug, viloxazine, also may be useful in the treatment of cataplexy and have fewer anticholinergic side effects (Guilleminault et al, 1986; Langdon et al, 1986).

In severe narcolepsy, it is difficult to control daytime sleepiness with doses of CNS stimulants that do not interfere with nighttime sleep. The dose and schedule of administration should be adjusted to provide the minimal useful amount during periods demanding concentrated effort and sustained activity. Naps are often used as an adjunct to medications. Three or more 15- to 20-minute naps daily improve alertness and do not interfere with nocturnal sleep.

Tolerance often develops to the CNS stimulants and may be minimized by instituting drug holidays one day a week. Another approach is gradual withdrawal, followed by resumption of therapy at a lower dose. The patient should be cautioned not to drive or engage in other potentially hazardous activities during withdrawal.

See also index entries Dextroamphetamine; Methylphenidate, In Narcolepsy.

PARASOMNIAS. Drug therapy is seldom indicated for parasomnias (eg, childhood enuresis, childhood night terrors, sleepwalking at any age). Behavioral modification, reassurance, and injury prevention techniques, respectively, are the modalities of choice. Rarely, an antidepressant may be appropriate for unresponsive childhood enuresis (see index entry Enuresis) or a benzodiazepine may be effective for severe, persistent night terrors (published clinical data are available only for diazepam).

SLEEP DISORDERS IN THE ELDERLY. As an individual ages, the sleep pattern typically becomes more fragmented with increased arousals and reduced total deep sleep time. The development of discrete sleep disorders appears to be a consequence of concomitant medical and psychosocial problems. Diagnosis and management are guided by the general principles previously discussed. In particular, a careful review of all drug use, including over-the-counter preparations, is warranted to determine possible effects on sleep and cardiopulmonary status. Insomnia usually is a consequence of underlying psychosocial, psychiatric, and medical disorders. Therapy for insomnia should be determined by the cause and severity of symptoms, with the establishment of good sleep hygiene practices and other nonpharmacologic alternatives taking precedence over pharmacologic treatment (Gillin and Byerley, 1990). If drug therapy is indicated, the lowest dose should be prescribed initially.

ANTIANXIETY AND HYPNOTIC DRUGS

Antianxiety and hypnotic drugs are listed in Table 1. Principles of use and drug selection follow.

Benzodiazepines

ACTIONS. Knowledge about the site and mechanism of action mediating the antianxiety, sedative, hypnotic, muscle relaxant, and antiepileptic effects of the benzodiazepines has progressed remarkably (Brogden and Goa, 1988; Teicher, 1988; Saano, 1988; Snyder, 1989). Cardiovascular and respiratory effects generally are minor except in severe intoxication or with parenteral use (eg, preanesthetic doses).

Gamma aminobutyric acid (GABA) is the principal inhibitory neurotransmitter in the CNS. There appear to be at least two types of GABA receptors in the brain: $GABA_A$ and $GABA_B$. The inhibitory effects of GABA are mediated in part by the $GABA_A$ receptor, which is a hetero-oligomer that is believed to be pentameric in structure (Costa, 1991). Activation of the receptor by GABA increases inward chloride conductance resulting in membrane hyperpolarization and neuronal inhibition. A number of subunits have been cloned and sequenced, and it is generally believed that there are multiple

TABLE 1. ANTIANXIETY AND HYPNOTIC DRUGS

DRUG: CONTROLLED SUBSTANCE SCHEDULE	PRINCIPAL USES			
	Generalized Anxiety Disorder	Panic/Phobic Disorders	Obsessive-Compulsive Disorder	Insomnia
BENZODIAZEPINES				
Compounds with Active Metabolites				
Chlordiazepoxide [Libritabs, Librium]: IV	+			
Clorazepate [Gen-XENE, Tranxene]: IV	+			
Diazepam [Valium, Valrelease]: IV	+	+		+
Flurazepam [Dalmane]: IV				+
Halazepam [Paxipam]: IV	+			
Prazepam [Centrax]: IV	+			
Quazepam [Doral]: IV				+
Compounds with Weakly Active, Short-lived, or Inactive Metabolites				
Alprazolam [Xanax]: IV	+	+		
Clonazepam [Klonopin]: IV	+	+		+
Estazolam [ProSom]: IV				+
Lorazepam [Ativan]: IV	+	+		+
Oxazepam [Serax]: IV	+			+
Temazepam [Restoril]: IV				+
Triazolam [Halcion]: IV				+
BENZODIAZEPINE RECEPTOR AGONIST				
Zolpidem [Ambien]: IV				+
BARBITURATES				
Phenobarbital: IV	+			+
Amobarbital [Amytal]: II				+
Pentobarbital [Nembutal]: II				+
Secobarbital [Seconal]: II				+
NONBENZODIAZEPINE-NONBARBITURATES				
Antianxiety Agents				
Buspirone [BuSpar]: NONE	+			
Imipramine [Janimine, Tofranil]: NONE		+		
Meprobamate [Equanil, Meprospan, Miltown]: IV	+			
Phenelzine [Nardil]: NONE		+		
Antiobsessional Agent				
Clomipramine [Anafranil]: NONE			+	
Hypnotic Agents				
Chloral Hydrate: IV				+
Ethchlorvynol [Placidyl]: IV				+
Glutethimide: II				+
Hypnotic Agents (antihistamines [nonprescription])				
Diphenhydramine [Nervine, Nytol, Sleep-Eze 3, Sominex 2]: NONE				+
Doxylamine [Unisom]: NONE				+
Pyrilamine [Dormarex]: NONE				+

$GABA_A$ receptor subtypes. This macromolecular complex also contains binding sites for the benzodiazepines, barbiturates, and numerous other substances (eg, steroid anesthetics). The major modulatory site of the $GABA_A$ receptor complex is located on its alpha subunit. The benzodiazepine (or omega) receptor is located on this subunit. Benzodiazepine agonists that bind to this site augment the inhibitory action of GABA through an allosteric mechanism.

Relatively high densities of benzodiazepine central receptors are found in the cortex and limbic system (ie, hippocampus, amygdala). Studies on binding support the existence of at least two central benzodiazepine receptor subtypes: a type I receptor enriched in the cerebellum and some other brain regions and a type II receptor enriched in the hippocampus, cortex, and spinal cord. The antianxiety action of the benzodiazepines is believed to be mediated principally through interactions with receptors in the limbic system. In addition, benzodiazepines, acting through receptors in the hypothalamic-pituitary-adrenocortical axis, inhibit the secretion of ACTH, cortisol, thyroid-stimulating hormone, and prolactin that occurs during the major endocrine response to stress (Cole, 1988).

Three other classes of substances interact with benzodiazepine receptors. Imidazopyridines (eg, zolpidem [Ambien]) show selectivity for binding to the type I receptor. Inverse agonists (eg, some beta-carbolines) have opposite effects on the benzodiazepine receptor resulting in reduced affinity of the GABA receptor and having anxiogenic and proconvulsant effects. Specific antagonists (eg, flumazenil) bind to benzodiazepine receptors and block all types of modulatory agonists.

INDICATIONS. The benzodiazepines are often the drugs of choice when an antianxiety, sedative, or hypnotic action is needed. Other indications for selected benzodiazepines include alcohol withdrawal, seizure disorders, spasticity, localized skeletal muscle spasm, preanesthetic medication, induction of sedation or amnesia prior to certain procedures (eg, endoscopy, cardioversion), and reduction of periodic movements in sleep. The benzodiazepines have distinct advantages over older drugs (eg, barbiturates, meprobamate) when their respective adverse reactions, abuse or dependence liability, drug interactions, and lethality in overdose are compared. The pharmacokinetic parameters of these drugs affect their onset, intensity, and duration of action and thus influence drug selection (Greenblatt and Shader, 1987).

Anxiety Disorders: For most patients, the benzodiazepines are the drugs of choice for uncomplicated generalized anxiety disorder. The decision to prescribe a benzodiazepine should be made only after the physician and patient have discussed the drug's clinical and side effects. In addition, the patient's age and concomitant diseases and the drug's potential for abuse and dependency, as well as the strategies to be utilized for tapering the dose and withdrawing the drug, must be considered (Bowden, 1990). The selection of a short- or long-acting benzodiazepine will depend on the individual patient and the clinical situation, as well as on the side effect profile of drugs in these two groups. When treating situational anxiety or intermittent anxiety secondary to other medical or psychiatric disorders for a brief period of time or in the elderly, a short-acting benzodiazepine may be the drug of choice.

Of the benzodiazepines used in agoraphobia and panic disorder, alprazolam has been studied most extensively; however, other benzodiazepines have been effective (eg, clonazepam, diazepam, lorazepam) and can be considered in the drug selection process for these disorders. Sedation is a problem with the high doses of diazepam required in the treatment of panic disorder. When used in chronically symptomatic patients, the risks of long-term administration of benzodiazepines must be weighed against the benefits. These drugs do not possess antiobsessional properties.

Insomnia: Flurazepam [Dalmane], triazolam [Halcion], temazepam [Restoril], quazepam [Doral], and estazolam [ProSom] are used most commonly to treat insomnia. Clonazepam, diazepam, oxazepam [Serax], and lorazepam also are effective hypnotic agents. Flurazepam, quazepam, and temazepam are most effective in preventing repeated awakenings because of the longer duration of their hypnotic effect. When impairment of daytime skills (eg, alertness, manual dexterity) is especially undesirable, triazolam and temazepam are preferred. However, rebound insomnia upon abrupt discontinuation of therapy has been reported with these two benzodiazepines, especially triazolam (Bixler et al, 1985; Gillin et al, 1989), the first or second night of withdrawal, possibly after only brief and intermittent use (Kales et al, 1991). However, rebound insomnia is dose related (Roth and Roehrs, 1991), and gradual reduction of the dose largely eliminates this problem (Greenblatt et al, 1987). Based on pharmacokinetic characteristics, estazolam is most similar to temazepam.

As with all drugs, there is a need for clear directions and warnings to the patient about the use of benzodiazepines; frequent reappraisal of efficacy and vigilant monitoring for side effects or risk factors that would make continued use of the drug hazardous (eg, renal or hepatic disease, alcoholism, depression) also are essential.

PHARMACOKINETICS. The pharmacokinetic properties of the benzodiazepines often provide the rationale for proper selection of these compounds. Absorption, volume of distribution, and metabolic route are prime determinants of onset of action, duration of effect, and the need for special caution in certain patients (eg, the elderly, those with hepatic disease, the debilitated).

As previously discussed, onset of action has significant implications for the pharmacologic management of insomnia (disorders of initiating sleep) and, to a lesser extent, the short-term treatment of anxiety. Benzodiazepines with a rapid onset are particularly useful when temporary relief of symptoms is adequate. After oral administration, a drug's onset of action is determined mainly by the rapidity of absorption from the gastrointestinal tract (see Table 2). All benzodiazepines are essentially completely absorbed, except clorazepate [Gen-XENE, Tranxene], which is converted in the stomach to nordiazepam. Alprazolam, clorazepate, diazepam, flurazepam, temazepam, triazolam, and estazolam are absorbed most rapidly, while halazepam, oxazepam, and prazepam

[Centrax] are absorbed slowly. Prazepam and flurazepam appear in the systemic circulation largely as metabolites.

Chlordiazepoxide [Librium], diazepam, and lorazepam also are available for parenteral use, and midazolam [Versed], a water-soluble benzodiazepine used for induction of anesthesia, is available only in a parenteral formulation in the United States. Since chlordiazepoxide is absorbed erratically after intramuscular injection, intravenous use is preferred when parenteral therapy is required. Lorazepam is absorbed rapidly and reliably after intramuscular administration. The site of injection also may affect the absorption rate. For example, the probability of rapid and complete absorption of intramuscular diazepam is enhanced by injection into the deltoid muscle area (Greenblatt et al, 1983 B).

Duration of action after a single dose is related largely to the lipophilic properties of the benzodiazepines. Drugs that are highly lipophilic have a more rapid onset and a shorter duration of action than compounds that have low lipid solubility. Highly lipophilic drugs, such as diazepam, enter brain tissue rapidly but also redistribute rapidly to other regions of the body (Greenblatt et al, 1989 A). Effective concentrations of less lipophilic drugs may persist longer in the brain because of reduced peripheral distribution. The effect of a drug's volume of distribution becomes less apparent when multiple doses are given over a one- or two-week period.

With multiple doses, the direct relationship between the degree of lipophilic properties and duration of action is confounded somewhat by the biotransformation of certain benzodiazepines to active metabolites. Clorazepate, chlordiazepoxide, diazepam, halazepam [Paxipam], flurazepam, prazepam, and quazepam are transformed to active metabolites, primarily by oxidation to N-dealkylated products with half-lives longer than those of the parent drugs. Alprazolam, estazolam, and triazolam undergo hydroxylation to weakly active or inactive metabolites. Lorazepam, oxazepam, and temazepam are conjugated to inactive metabolites. For those benzodiazepines that are biotransformed principally by oxidation, hepatic clearance is typically reduced in the elderly or newborn, in individuals with liver disease, and by other drugs that inhibit hepatic microsomal oxidation. In many studies, the decrease in clearance noted in the elderly is more evident in males (Greenblatt et al, 1991 A).

The elimination half-life of a benzodiazepine also may be prolonged in elderly patients because the proportion of fat to total body weight increases with age, which increases the volume of distribution of lipid-soluble drugs, including benzodiazepines. The effect on volume of distribution also explains in part the more rapid elimination half-life of some benzodiazepines in men, who have a lower proportion of fat to total body weight than women. The elderly also may be more sensitive to the pharmacodynamic effects of benzodiazepines (Greenblatt et al, 1991 B).

Since monitoring benzodiazepine concentrations in blood is not clearly established as a guide to therapy, dosage adjustments and multiple daily doses may be necessary initially until the desired response and acceptable level of untoward effects are established. After the optimum total daily dosage is determined, single daily doses may be sufficient for some patients, whereas other patients will require multiple daily doses even when benzodiazepines with long half-lives are prescribed.

For specific pharmacokinetic data, see Table 2.

ADVERSE REACTIONS. Daytime sedation and hangover are the most common initial untoward effects of the benzodiazepines, but they appear to occur less frequently than with the barbiturates. Other common adverse effects with oral use are dizziness, incoordination, and ataxia, which are dose related.

Blurred vision, diplopia, hypotension, confusion, anterograde amnesia and memory impairment, slurred speech, tremor, fatigue, urinary incontinence, and constipation occur occasionally. Recently, concern has been raised about the potential for triazolam [Halcion] to cause certain adverse reactions involving the CNS (eg, hyperexcitability, cognitive and behavioral effects, amnesia). For information on this controversy, see the evaluation. Numerous anecdotal reports of disinhibition (increased anger and hostility, violent and aggressive behavior, rage reactions) occurring in association with use of a number of benzodiazepines also have been cited (Rothschild, 1992). Other behavioral changes that have been observed rarely include bizarre behavior, agitation, depersonalization, and hallucinations. In depressed patients, worsening of depression, including suicidal ideation, has occurred in association with use of these agents.

Rash, chills, fever, and, rarely, blood dyscrasias have developed after use of benzodiazepines. Dysarthria, muscle weakness, dryness of the mouth, and gastrointestinal discomfort (nausea and vomiting) also have been reported, but a causal relationship has not been definitely established. The gastrointestinal disturbances may be reduced by administering the drug with or immediately after meals.

Respiratory depression, apnea, and cardiac arrest have occurred rarely, usually following intravenous administration. These reactions are most common in elderly or severely ill patients, in those receiving other CNS depressants, or in those with limited ventilatory reserve. Intravenous injection of diazepam may cause local pain and thrombophlebitis; the solvent may contribute to these effects. There also is tentative evidence that benzodiazepines may further suppress respiration in patients with undiagnosed sleep apnea or chronic lung disease.

PRECAUTIONS. Sedation may be lessened by prescribing relatively small doses initially and increasing the amount gradually; however, if tolerance develops, the dosage and continued use of the benzodiazepine should be reassessed. Activities that require mental alertness, judgment, and physical coordination (eg, driving a car, operating dangerous machinery) should be undertaken with caution during initial therapy when sedation may be pronounced. If benzodiazepines are to be used with other psychotropic agents or antiepileptic drugs, the possibility of potentiation of their effects should be considered carefully (see Drug Interactions). The concomitant use of alcohol or other drugs with a sedative effect is usually hazardous.

Ataxia, dizziness, and headache often are observed during the early period of dosage adjustment. Elderly and debilitated patients develop drowsiness and ataxia more often than younger individuals. Case-control studies have linked the use

TABLE 2.
ANTIANXIETY AND HYPNOTIC DRUGS: PHARMACOKINETIC DATA*

Drug	Oral Absorption: t max hours (Relative Rate)	Most Significant Biologically Active Compounds in Blood	Mean (Range) Elimination Half-life† (hours)	Apparent Volume of Distribution (L/kg)	Clearance (ml/kg/min)
BENZODIAZEPINES					
Compounds With Active Metabolites					
Chlordiazepoxide	0.5-4	Chlordiazepoxide Desmethylchlor-diazepoxide	10 (5-30) (24-96)	0.3 ± 0.03	0.54 ± 0.49
Clorazepate	1-2	Desmethyldiazepam	73 (30-100)	0.78 ± 0.12	0.14 ± 0.05
Diazepam	1.5-2	Diazepam Desmethyldiazepam	43 (20-70) 73 (30-100)	1.1 ± 0.3	0.38 ± 0.06
Flurazepam	0.5-2	Desalkylflurazepam	74 (36-120)		
Halazepam	1-3	Halazepam Desmethyldiazepam	14 (30-100)		
Prazepam	6	Desmethyldiazepam	(30-100)		
Quazepam	2	Quazepam Oxoquazepam Desalkylflurazepam	39 39 74 (36-120)		
Compounds With Weakly Active, Short-lived, or Inactive Metabolites					
Alprazolam	1-2	Alprazolam	11 (6-16)	0.72 ± 0.12	0.74 ± 0.14
Clonazepam	1-4	Clonazepam	23 (18-50)	3.2 ± 1.1	0.92 ± 0.25
Estazolam	2	Estazolam	14 (10-24)		
Lorazepam	2	Lorazepam	14 (10-20)	1.3 ± 0.2	1.1 ± 0.4
Oxazepam	1-4	Oxazepam	7 (5-15)	0.6 ± 0.2	1.05 ± 0.36
Temazepam	1-1.5	Temazepam	13 (8-38)	1.06 ± 0.31	0.87 ± 0.18
Triazolam	1-2	Triazolam	2.9 (1.5-.5)	1.1 ± 0.4	5.6 ± 2
BENZODIAZEPINE RECEPTOR AGONIST					
Zolpidem	1-2	Zolpidem	2.5	0.54	4.3
BARBITURATES					
Phenobarbital	6-18	Phenobarbital	79 (53-118)	0.54 ± 0.03	0.06 ± 0.01
Amobarbital	2	Amobarbital	25 (14-42)		
Pentobarbital	2	Pentobarbital	(15-50)		
Secobarbital	2	Secobarbital	30 (15-40)		
NONBENZODIAZEPINE-NONBARBITURATES					
Antianxiety Agents					
Buspirone	0.7-1.5	Buspirone 1-(2-pyrimidinyl)-piperazine	2.5 (2-11)	5.3 ± 2.6	28
Imipramine	1-2	Imipramine Desipramine	7.6 (4-17.6)	21	16
Meprobamate	2-3	Meprobamate	(10-24)		

(table continued on next page)

TABLE 2 (continued)

Drug	Oral Absorption: t max hours (Relative Rate)	Most Significant Biologically Active Compounds in Blood	Mean (Range) Elimination Half-life (hours)	Apparent Volume of Distribution (L/kg)	Clearance (ml/kg/min)
Antiobsessional Agent					
Clomipramine	2-6	Clomipramine Desmethylclomipramine	31-37	12	12.5
Hypnotic Agents					
Chloral Hydrate		Trichloroethanol	(4-9.5)		
Ethchlorvynol		Ethchlorvynol	(10-25)		
Glutethimide		Glutethimide	(5-22)		
Hypnotic Agents (antihistamines [nonprescription])					
Diphenhydramine	2-3	Diphenhydramine	8.4	4.5	6.2
Doxylamine		Doxylamine	9.3 (4-12)		
Pyrilamine		Pyrilamine			

* *Adapted from Mandelli et al, 1978; Greenblatt et al, 1978, 1983 B, 1987, 1988; Benet and Williams, 1990; and information supplied by manufacturers.*

† *Values for mean and range reflect those usually obtained in healthy (male) adults. For compounds eliminated by hepatic oxidation, values for elimination half-life in the elderly may be considerably larger. For example, the mean half-life of desalkylflurazepam in elderly males is approximately 160 hours.*

of benzodiazepines with long elimination half-lives (chlordiazepoxide, clorazepate, diazepam, flurazepam, halazepam, quazepam, prazepam) to an increased incidence of confusion, falls, and hip fractures in the elderly (Ray et al, 1989). In addition, symptoms of organic brain disease in the elderly may be aggravated if they receive the larger doses appropriate for younger patients.

Many benzodiazepines accumulate until steady-state concentrations are reached (several days to two weeks). Drugs and active metabolites with long elimination half-lives are most likely to accumulate excessively. Cumulative clinical effects do not always occur, possibly because of tolerance or the widely variable response among individuals. The dosage should be limited to the smallest effective amount to preclude the development of ataxia or oversedation, which may be a particular problem in elderly or debilitated patients. Some patients, particularly the elderly, may be subjectively unaware of sedation or impairment of performance.

Caution is required when prescribing benzodiazepines for patients with severely impaired hepatic function. This is especially important when administering agents with long-acting active metabolites and those eliminated by microsomal oxidation. In these patients, it may be advisable to use a benzodiazepine that is conjugated and not converted to an active metabolite (eg, lorazepam, oxazepam). Caution also is advised in patients with impaired renal or pulmonary function. Benzodiazepines may exacerbate ventilatory failure in patients with severe, chronic obstructive pulmonary disease (COPD) and generally should not be used in patients with sleep apnea. These agents are also contraindicated in patients with acute angle-closure glaucoma.

PREGNANCY AND BREAST FEEDING. An association between the use of benzodiazepines during the first trimester of pregnancy and the development of cleft lip with or without cleft palate has been reported. Some data suggest that such exposure to diazepam does not materially increase the risk of cleft lip with or without cleft palate or of cleft palate alone (Rosenberg et al, 1983). Dysmorphogenic changes in rib formation were observed in two animal species given 50 to 100 times the human dose. Overall, data are not adequate to assess the safety of the benzodiazepines during pregnancy (Jick, 1988; Shader and Greenblatt, 1989). Therefore, unless a pressing need exists, it is advisable to avoid using these agents during pregnancy, especially the first trimester. If patients become pregnant during therapy or intend to become pregnant, the desirability of discontinuing the drug should be emphasized. Alprazolam, halazepam, and lorazepam (parenteral) are classified in FDA Pregnancy Category D. Temazepam, estazolam, quazepam, and triazolam are classified in FDA Pregnancy Category X.

Diazepam and desmethyldiazepam cross the placenta during labor, and fetal concentrations exceed those in the mother. Available evidence suggests that intramuscular or intravenous administration of more than 30 mg of diazepam during the final 15 hours of labor can produce low Apgar scores, apnea, hypothermia, and poor sucking in newborn infants (the floppy-infant syndrome). Hypothermia and delayed feeding, particularly in preterm infants, also were associated with large doses of intravenous lorazepam given before delivery.

Full-term neonates whose mothers received oral lorazepam had no complications other than delayed feeding associated with relatively large doses in 7 of 29 infants (Whitelaw et al, 1981).

Withdrawal symptoms and signs can be expected in infants born to mothers who have a history of benzodiazepine use during the last trimester.

Detectable amounts of diazepam appear in breast milk. If it is essential to prescribe any benzodiazepine for a nursing mother, the infant should be monitored closely.

POISONING. When alcohol or other CNS depressants are not used concomitantly, the benzodiazepines are the safest of the antianxiety and hypnotic agents and have a wide margin of safety with overdosage; in combination with alcohol or other CNS depressants, these agents become substantially more toxic. When overdose occurs, adjunctive use of flumazenil [Mazicon] and usual supportive measures, including gastric lavage, often are adequate. However, in more severe cases (eg, acute circulatory failure and coma), treatment is similar to that for barbiturate overdose, except that hemodialysis is of limited value; flumazenil is useful as an adjunct. (For further information on the use of flumazenil in the treatment of benzodiazepine overdose, see index entry on this drug.) The benzodiazepine blood concentration may remain well above the range associated with sleep or even anesthesia during recovery from overdose even though the patient is awake and vital signs are stable.

TOLERANCE. Tolerance to the sedation and ataxia produced by benzodiazepines develops with continued administration of the same dosage. If tolerance to the antianxiety effect develops, it occurs much more slowly and has minor consequences (Rickels et al, 1983 A; Greenblatt et al, 1983 A). A rapidly developing tolerance (tachyphylaxis) to the hypnotic, respiratory, and cardiovascular actions occurs with overdosage. Metabolic tolerance (liver enzyme induction) does not appear to be of clinical significance.

ABUSE AND DEPENDENCE LIABILITY. The potential for abuse of benzodiazepines is much less than with drugs such as barbiturates, opioid analgesics, and cocaine. The benzodiazepines are classified under Schedule IV of the Controlled Substances Act. Physical dependence occurs with administration of larger than usual doses and often develops with regular daily use of therapeutic doses (American Psychiatric Association, 1990). Such dependency may lead to more prolonged use than is therapeutically necessary but generally is not associated with dosage escalation or drug-seeking behavior. Withdrawal symptoms may be uncomfortable but are rarely severe unless the drug is discontinued abruptly.

Abuse occurs most often in those who have a history of abuse of alcohol or other psychoactive drugs. Consequently, the risks and benefits of benzodiazepine use must be carefully considered in these individuals. Abuse in other patients can be minimized by careful patient selection, administration of low daily doses given intermittently and graded to the level of stress, and timely discontinuation of use when clinically warranted.

Following discontinuation of long-term benzodiazepine therapy, three distinct but overlapping clinical syndromes may occur and can be differentiated on the basis of the time course and intensity of the signs and symptoms produced. All three syndromes may occur in the same individual. Symptom *recurrence or recrudescence* develops slowly over a period of days to weeks (or months); signs and symptoms are typically those that the patient observed prior to therapy and are of no greater intensity. Sleep disturbance and an increase in anxiety are frequently initial signs. *Rebound* signs and symptoms develop within hours or days. The time course of rebound is related in part to the pharmacokinetic parameters, dose, and duration of use of the benzodiazepine. The signs and symptoms are qualitatively similar to those of the anxiety disorder under treatment but are more severe. The rebound syndrome is of relatively short duration, usually a week or two but no longer than a month even with a long-acting benzodiazepine. (Rebound insomnia following abrupt discontinuation of nightly therapy for insomnia typically lasts only one or two days and can be minimized by tapering the dosage.) The *benzodiazepine withdrawal syndrome* usually persists for about seven days but may last two to three weeks and includes symptoms that were not present when the drug was originally prescribed. Although some of the signs and symptoms are typical of generalized anxiety disorder, autonomic-like signs and symptoms (eg, tachycardia, tremulousness, abdominal distress, mild systolic hypertension, sweating) are more prevalent and/or intense; "flu-like" signs and symptoms (eg, muscle ache, malaise), disturbances in equilibrium, sensory disturbances (eg, excessive sensitivity to light, sound paresthesias, metallic taste), depersonalization, or perceptual distortion also may occur. Seizures and delirium are infrequent. Both the rebound and benzodiazepine withdrawal syndromes are self-limited.

The intensity of symptoms after discontinuation of benzodiazepines is related to the (1) duration of treatment, (2) daily dose, (3) half-life of the benzodiazepine and active metabolites, and (4) rate of tapering of the dose. Patient characteristics also are influential. Dependent personality traits, severe initial psychopathology, and a high level of neurosis may increase the severity of withdrawal reactions (Rickels et al, 1990; Schweizer et al, 1990 B). Review of the evidence for benzodiazepine withdrawal symptoms is complicated by the use of different criteria by investigators for the definition of withdrawal and the overlap of anxiety and withdrawal symptoms. The applicability of most studies to the general patient population also is unclear because of the extensive reliance on drug-dependent subjects. Nevertheless, some aspects of the benzodiazepine withdrawal syndrome seem clearly established.

Benzodiazepines should not be discontinued abruptly. Rebound anxiety occurs in almost 50% of anxious patients who have received therapeutic doses of alprazolam for 3 to 34 weeks (Noyes et al, 1988). Results of some studies have indicated that, with abrupt discontinuation, symptoms of withdrawal can occur after only four to six weeks of treatment (Fontaine et al, 1984; Murphy et al, 1984; Power et al, 1985). In prospective studies, a withdrawal syndrome occurred in approximately 40% of patients when a long-acting benzodiazepine administered for six months was discontinued (Rickels et al, 1988); about 50% of patients had symptoms of withdrawal when treated for at least eight months (Rickels et al, 1983 A; Sellers, 1988). A withdrawal syndrome occurred in virtually all patients when the drug was discontinued abruptly after even therapeutic doses were taken for more than one year (Rickels et al, 1990). With abrupt discontinuation, withdrawal symptoms occur earlier and are more severe with benzodiazepines with a short half-life or when daily dosage is high.

Outpatient management of discontinuation of benzodiazepines should be considered for any patient taking these agents regularly for more than a few weeks. There is no single best technique (Marks, 1988), but gradual and flexible tapering of the dose is often adequate to decrease the intensity of the withdrawal syndrome (Murphy and Tyrer, 1991). In long-term users, a discontinuation syndrome can be expected, even when low to moderate therapeutic doses of benzodiazepines are reduced gradually at a rate of 25% or less per week (Schweizer et al, 1990 B). In some patients receiving a short-acting benzodiazepine, substitution of a long-acting agent with a variety of dosage forms may facilitate gradual dosage reduction. Although the issue is complex, approximate empirical dose equivalents to diazepam 5 mg are oxazepam 30 mg, chlordiazepoxide 25 mg, flurazepam 15 mg, clorazepate 7.5 mg, lorazepam or estazolam 1 mg, alprazolam 0.5 mg, and triazolam 0.125 mg. However, gradual tapering tends to lessen the importance of half-life with respect to the severity of withdrawal reactions; thus, this type of substitution may not be necessary. The majority of withdrawal symptoms occur during the final phase of dosage reduction. More than 50% of patients, especially those taking larger daily doses, require a more gradual reduction of the dose (ie, beyond four weeks). An extended tapering schedule (eg, six to eight weeks), adjusted on the basis of signs and symptoms, and the occasional use of antidepressants or hypnotics may facilitate discontinuation in some patients (Schweizer et al, 1990 B).

Results of a pilot study suggest that administration of carbamazepine [Tegretol] prior to withdrawal of the benzodiazepine may decrease the intensity of symptoms and enhance outcome (Schweizer et al, 1991). Further controlled studies are needed to determine the role of carbamazepine in the treatment of benzodiazepine withdrawal.

Patients who are already in acute, severe withdrawal will probably require hospitalization. This is especially true if the individual has a history of seizures. Oral diazepam should be given at a rate of 20 mg hourly until symptoms are suppressed. On an outpatient basis, the dosage can be decreased gradually and terminated in six to eight weeks (eg, 20% to 30% reduction weekly); however, a 5% to 10% daily reduction in dose can be safely undertaken in hospitalized patients.

Optimum overall management of the benzodiazepine withdrawal syndrome requires that the physician discuss the management plan with the patient. This therapeutic alliance will do much to minimize apprehension, set realistic expectations, and assure patient cooperation. Counseling and relaxation training can make the withdrawal syndrome much more tolerable.

DRUG INTERACTIONS. Additive CNS depression may occur with concomitant use of a benzodiazepine and other CNS depressants (eg, other antianxiety and hypnotic drugs, alcohol, tricyclic antidepressants, opioid analgesics, anticonvulsants, antipsychotics [neuroleptics], antihistamines including nonprescription sleep aids and cold remedies). The combination of a benzodiazepine and another CNS depressant is not necessarily contraindicated, although the dose of the benzodiazepine may require reduction. Close follow-up of the patient may be necessary initially, and precautionary advice about activities that require alertness should be stressed.

The sedative effects of benzodiazepines may be antagonized by stimulant drugs, including caffeine and theophylline.

Concurrent use of erythromycin may inhibit the elimination of benzodiazepines that are subject to hepatic oxidative metabolism. Cimetidine [Tagamet] inhibits the hepatic microsomal enzymes responsible for the N-dealkylation and hydroxylation of benzodiazepines metabolized by oxidation, but this interaction appears to be of minimal clinical importance (Greenblatt et al, 1984 A). Omeprazole [Prilosec] also appears to inhibit the oxidative metabolism of benzodiazepines.

Isoniazid inhibits the elimination of diazepam and triazolam, probably through inhibition of hepatic microsomal enzymes. (A reduced clearance would be expected for other benzodiazepines affected similarly by cimetidine [see above].) However, if the patient also is receiving rifampin, the enzyme-inducing action of this latter drug usually overwhelms the effect of isoniazid; as a result, clearance is increased and the elimination half-life of diazepam is shortened (Ochs et al, 1981). Dosage adjustment of diazepam may be necessary.

Low-dose estrogen-containing oral contraceptives prolong the elimination half-life of diazepam, presumably through inhibition of hepatic microsomal enzymes (Abernethy et al, 1982). Because a direct relationship between diazepam's plasma concentration and clinical effect has not been clearly delineated, the clinical significance of these interactions has not been established.

Hypothermia has developed when diazepam was administered with lithium. Administration of benzodiazepines with clozapine [Clozaril] may cause respiratory depression.

ISSUES IN PRESCRIBING BENZODIAZEPINES. In recent years, the medical use of benzodiazepines has received much attention because of concern that these drugs, when used as antianxiety agents and hypnotics, are overprescribed both in terms of the absolute number of people receiving them and in the length of time that patients take them. Questions also have arisen about prescription practices in certain segments of the population, such as women and the elderly.

The charge that the benzodiazepines are overprescribed in this country has not been borne out by analyses of prescription practices (Mellinger and Balter, 1983), which have characterized the prescription of psychotherapeutic agents as moderate if not conservative, especially when the number of medical and psychiatric conditions for which they are effective is considered. Short-term and infrequent use of antianxiety agents and hypnotics are more common than long-term daily use. A total of 1.6% of all adults between 18 and 79 years used these drugs daily for one year or longer. Further analysis of this figure indicated that the long-term use was appropriate and associated with bona fide health problems being treated within the health care system (Mellinger et al, 1984).

Nonmedical use of benzodiazepines in the general population is rare; their abuse primarily is limited to those who also abuse other psychoactive drugs. Patients for whom benzodiazepines are appropriately prescribed for psychopathology do not exhibit drug-seeking or drug-taking behavior; the tendency is to reduce usage with time. Thus, the available evidence regarding nonmedical use of benzodiazepines fails to match a traditional drug abuse model (Woods et al, 1988). Nevertheless, there are patients who become dependent on benzodiazepines, for whom further prescribing is ill-advised and who may require assistance in discontinuing these drugs. Therefore, physicians must remain alert for signs and symptoms of abuse and be ready to take appropriate action.

More women use antianxiety agents than men, but a study of indications for such use also has deemed such therapy appropriate. Gender differences may reflect a male's reluctance to admit to being sick and to seek medical care. Also, men are more likely to use alcohol to relieve anxiety. Men and women are equally likely to use benzodiazepines for long periods, and the tendency for long-term use increases with age in association with the treatment of significant medical problems.

SUMMARY. The benzodiazepines are effective antianxiety and hypnotic agents that should be reserved for patients with significant subjective distress whose ability to function normally has been compromised. The physician's role in controlling benzodiazepine overuse and abuse is to scrutinize his or her own prescribing practices. It is often recommended that these agents be used in the smallest dose and for the shortest time necessary and that patients be re-evaluated frequently with regard to their continued need for the medication. However, conventional wisdom about "lowest dose required" and "short-term" use may conflict with the need for prolonged treatment of patients with panic disorder and other conditions that may be marked by significant, long-term impairment. Data indicate that patients with panic disorder who are maintained on low doses frequently have residual symptoms; this suggests that these patients may be undertreated. Therefore, in patients with chronic disorders, the rational use of benzodiazepines requires careful determination of dosages that maintain effectiveness and minimize adverse reactions. Finally, physicians must attempt to ascertain prior and current drug use patterns and be wary of drug scams. Benzodiazepines should be used only for short-term, specific indications in patients with a history of sedative-hypnotic, alcohol, or other drug abuse, and they should be used with caution in pregnant women.

Barbiturates

ACTIONS. The barbiturates reversibly depress the activity of excitable tissue; the CNS is especially sensitive. With nonanesthetic doses, facilitation is diminished and inhibition, primarily at GABAergic synapses, is enhanced. Barbiturates bind at or near the chloride channel of the $GABA_A$/benzodiazepine chloride ionophore complex and promote GABA-induced chloride currents. Whereas the benzodiazepines increase the frequency of channel openings, the barbiturates appear to increase the duration of channel opening (Twyman et al, 1989). At concentrations similar to those that potentiate GABA, glutamate-induced depolarizations are reduced. At higher concentrations, impairment of Ca^+ and Na^+ ion fluxes can be demonstrated. These nonspecific depressant effects contribute to the low degree of selectivity and the low therapeutic index of the barbiturates. The known actions of barbiturates on membrane lipids, protein synthesis, neurotransmitters other than GABA, and ion regulation have been reviewed (Ho and Harris, 1981).

INDICATIONS. Derivatives of barbituric acid possess hypnotic and antiepileptic activity. Except for a few specialized uses, the barbiturates have been replaced by the benzodiazepines. The longer-acting barbiturate, phenobarbital, is administered principally for seizure disorders. It also is used as a sedative and may be useful during withdrawal after prolonged use of barbiturates and certain nonbenzodiazepine-nonbarbiturate hypnotic drugs (chloral hydrate, ethchlorvynol [Placidyl], glutethimide, meprobamate [Equanil, Meprospan, Miltown], paraldehyde). (See also the discussion on Dependence in this section.)

Phenobarbital is prescribed in some cases of congenital hyperbilirubinemia because it enhances the metabolism of bilirubin by enzyme induction.

Amobarbital [Amytal], pentobarbital [Nembutol], and secobarbital [Seconal] are shorter acting barbiturates and are occasionally used as hypnotics. Daytime sedation (hangover) is common. All three drugs also are administered orally or parenterally as preanesthetic medication (see index entry Barbiturates, Uses) and intravenously as an adjunct for regional anesthesia.

The ultrashort-acting barbiturates, thiopental, methohexital, and thiamylal, are used intravenously to induce anesthesia. Barbiturate-induced anesthesia decreases brain oxygen utilization by approximately 50% and increases glycogen and high energy phosphate. Because of these actions, barbiturates have a limited role for brain resuscitation in metabolic, toxic, or infectious encephalopathy (Rogers and Kirsch, 1989).

PHARMACOKINETICS. All barbiturates are weak acids that are well absorbed orally and intramuscularly, especially their salts. Distribution, in turn, is related to lipid solubility and plasma and protein binding. Phenobarbital, which has the longest onset and duration of action clinically, also has the lowest degree of lipid solubility and protein binding.

All barbiturates are metabolized principally to inactive derivatives by the microsomal enzyme system of the liver. The inactive metabolites are conjugated with glucuronic acid and excreted in the urine, but 25% to 50% of a dose of phenobarbital also is eliminated unchanged in the urine. See also Table 2 and Breimer, 1977.

ADVERSE REACTIONS AND PRECAUTIONS. Drowsiness and lethargy are common in sensitive individuals (eg, the elderly, those with severe liver disease) or in patients taking large doses; residual sedation ("hangover") is common after hypnotic doses. Ambulatory patients should be specifically warned to avoid activities that require mental alertness, judgment, and physical coordination (eg, driving a vehicle, operating dangerous machinery) and to avoid concomitant ingestion of alcohol.

Reactions noted infrequently include skin eruptions (eg, urticaria, angioedema, generalized morbilliform rash, Stevens-Johnson syndrome, discrete violaceous macules) and gastrointestinal disturbances (eg, nausea and vomiting). Paradoxical restlessness or excitement and exacerbation of the symptoms of certain organic brain disorders may develop, especially in elderly patients and children.

Because barbiturates may aggravate acute intermittent porphyria by inducing the enzymes responsible for porphyrin synthesis, their use is contraindicated in patients with this disease (Smith and DeMatteis, 1980).

Since the liver is the major site of barbiturate degradation, caution should be observed when these drugs are given to patients with hepatic disease. Drug-induced hepatitis has been reported with use of phenobarbital (Lane and Peterson, 1984). Pulmonary insufficiency is a relative contraindication.

Great caution should be taken to avoid intra-arterial injection or extravasation of the highly alkaline sodium salts of barbiturates. Injection into an artery provokes intense, prolonged, spastic vasoconstriction and ischemia and has caused gangrene of the extremities. Acute excruciating pain, edema, erythema, inflammation, and obliteration of the distal pulse are rapidly evident in the affected limb. For treatment of this complication, see index entry Thiopental.

Physicians should assess a patient's susceptibility to drug abuse before prescribing a barbiturate.

PREGNANCY AND BREAST FEEDING. Reproductive studies in animals reveal no evidence of impaired fertility or harm to the fetus; no adequate controlled studies in pregnant women are available. Results of retrospective, case-controlled studies in pregnant women have suggested that there is an association between maternal consumption of phenobarbital and a higher than expected incidence of fetal abnormalities, but this has not been established. Barbiturates are classified in FDA Pregnancy Category D.

Barbiturates readily cross the placenta and can depress the neonate's respiration and central nervous system. Withdrawal symptoms and signs are likely to occur in infants born to mothers who are physically dependent on barbiturates during the last trimester.

Cautions concerning the special use of phenobarbital in epileptic patients who become pregnant are discussed elsewhere; see index entry Antiepileptic Drugs.

Small amounts of most barbiturates appear in breast milk; caution should be used when a barbiturate is administered to a nursing mother.

POISONING. Overdosage of the barbiturates can cause hypotension, tachycardia, profound shock, ventilatory depression, areflexia, coma, and death due to cardioventilatory failure secondary to depression of the vital medullary centers.

If the patient is still completely alert and less than four hours have elapsed since ingestion, vomiting may be induced by syrup of ipecac. Gastric lavage and activated charcoal are used in comatose patients only after an open airway has been secured, if necessary by endotracheal intubation. An adequate airway should be maintained, arterial blood gases should be monitored, and sufficient oxygen should be given to prevent hypoxemia. Controlled ventilation must be instituted if ventilatory failure develops.

Alkalization of the urine significantly increases the renal excretion of phenobarbital. In severe poisoning, hemodialysis or charcoal hemoperfusion may be lifesaving, especially if vigorous diuresis cannot be maintained.

Complications can be avoided by changing the patient's position hourly to prevent pressure sores and hypostatic pneumonia, maintaining adequate hydration and nutrition with parenteral administration of fluids, and providing all standard supportive therapy.

TOLERANCE. Two types of tolerance may be observed with the barbiturates. Metabolic tolerance may occur when a barbiturate or other drug accelerates the hepatic inactivation of the barbiturate by enzyme induction; this is most common with barbiturates that have relatively short half-lives. Pharmacodynamic tolerance results when the depressant effect on the CNS decreases after repeated administration. This cellular tolerance is noted most frequently with the long-acting barbiturate, phenobarbital, and with large doses of the shorter acting barbiturates. Cross tolerance develops among the barbiturates and between these drugs and alcohol. Although tolerance develops to the hypnotic effects of barbiturates, it is important to remember that the lethal dose does not increase significantly.

DEPENDENCE. Acute intoxication occurs most commonly with use of the short-acting barbiturates, and symptoms are similar to those of alcohol intoxication (eg, disorientation, ataxia, euphoria). Prolonged, uninterrupted use of escalating doses of barbiturates, particularly the short-acting drugs, may result in physical and psychological dependence. Withdrawal reactions have been reported in neonates after maternal ingestion of these drugs.

If a barbiturate appears to have lost its effectiveness after long-term administration, it should be withdrawn slowly. The patient should be warned that unpleasant symptoms (eg, increased frequency and intensity of dreaming, nightmares) may occur. Abrupt withdrawal after administration of pentobarbital 400 mg for three months or secobarbital 600 mg for one month may be followed within 24 hours by a severe withdrawal syndrome that usually lasts approximately one week. Multiple seizures or status epilepticus may occur between 12 hours and six days after withdrawal. A psychosis resembling delirium tremens and, sometimes, progressive hyperpyrexia, coma, and death may occur.

Gradual withdrawal of the offending agent (nonsubstitutive treatment) over ten days to three weeks, depending on the severity of dependence, is necessary to minimize the signs and symptoms of withdrawal. Because of its long duration of action, phenobarbital is sometimes used for substitutive treatment. In this procedure, phenobarbital dosage equivalents are substituted for the offending drug (eg, chloral hydrate, ethchlorvynol, glutethimide, paraldehyde, meprobamate) until signs and symptoms have stabilized. The dose of phenobarbital then is reduced by 10% every 24 hours. Alternatively, the degree of drug dependence is assessed, and plasma levels of the offending drug are permitted to fall. A loading dose of phenobarbital sufficient to produce signs of barbiturate intoxication is then administered. The long half-life of phenobarbital allows gradual adaptation of the central nervous system. (For details and inclusion criteria, see Robinson et al, 1981, and Sellers, 1988.) Pentobarbital also has been used for this procedure.

Amobarbital, pentobarbital, and secobarbital are classified as Schedule II agents, and phenobarbital is classified as a Schedule IV agent. (See index entry Controlled Substances Act for additional information.)

DRUG INTERACTIONS. The dosage of barbiturates must be reduced when these drugs are given with other CNS depressants (eg, alcohol, other hypnotic and antianxiety agents, tricyclic antidepressants, opioid analgesics, antipsychotics, antihistamines).

Phenobarbital increases the synthesis and activity of hepatic microsomal enzymes involved in the metabolism of warfarin and dicumarol; the shorter acting barbiturates are less likely to produce this effect. The benzodiazepines are preferred in patients who are also receiving anticoagulants.

Barbiturates may enhance the metabolism of tricyclic antidepressants, phenytoin, griseofulvin, and adrenal corticosteroids. For example, the administration of phenobarbital to asthmatic patients dependent on corticosteroids has been reported to exacerbate asthma; this effect was reversed when phenobarbital was discontinued. It may be necessary to adjust the dosage schedule of these drugs to maintain control of the disorder. For other drug interactions, see index entry Phenobarbital.

SUMMARY. The use of the barbiturates as antianxiety agents and sedative-hypnotics has many disadvantages; therefore, the benzodiazepines are preferred in most patients. The benzodiazepines exhibit less abuse and dependence liability and have a greater therapeutic index.

Nonbenzodiazepine-Nonbarbiturates

ANXIETY. Drugs in this group are used to treat a variety of anxiety disorders. Buspirone represents a novel anxiolytic chemical used to treat generalized anxiety disorder. Tricyclic antidepressants, especially imipramine, and the MAO inhibitors, especially phenelzine, are used to treat panic and phobic disorders. Clomipramine, fluvoxamine (investigational), and possibly fluoxetine and sertraline possess antiobsessional activity and are used to treat obsessive-compulsive disorder. The comparative usefulness of these nonbenzodiazepines is discussed in the management section of this chapter under the specific anxiety disorder. Evaluations of buspirone, clomipramine, and imipramine appear in this chapter; for evaluations of monoamine oxidase inhibitors and fluoxetine, see those index entries.

Additional antianxiety drugs in this group include meprobamate and propranolol [Inderal] and other beta-adrenergic blocking agents. Meprobamate is less effective than the benzodiazepines in the treatment of anxiety. Long-term use of larger than usual doses produces physical dependence and this further limits its use. Propranolol and other beta blockers are not as effective as benzodiazepines in the treatment of anxiety (Rickels et al, 1983 A; Lader, 1988). When somatic symptoms of anxiety (eg, tremor, palpitations, tachycardia) are more prominent than psychological symptoms, beta blockers may be useful alone or adjunctively in carefully selected patients with anxiety disorders, particularly those with social phobias or performance anxiety. Controlled studies have suggested that, when psychological symptoms are predominant, beta blockers usually produce little improvement.

The remainder of the drugs in this group include various "sedating" antihistamines and miscellaneous hypnotics and sedatives. The benzodiazepines have largely replaced these compounds. Pharmacokinetic data on these agents are fragmentary (see Table 2). Adverse reactions, precautions, and poisoning are discussed in the evaluations. For information on dependence, see the evaluations and the discussion of Dependence in the section on Barbiturates.

INSOMNIA. Chloral hydrate is an effective sedative and hypnotic. Because of its rapid onset of action and short half-life, it is especially useful when there is difficulty in falling asleep. Some tolerance to the hypnotic action generally develops within five weeks. Although the benefit/risk ratio is not as desirable as that of the benzodiazepines, this drug may be the preferred alternative among the nonbenzodiazepine hypnotics in selected patients.

Ethchlorvynol and glutethimide have very limited or variable antianxiety action and are marketed only for the treatment of insomnia. Ethchlorvynol has low potency and, like chloral hydrate, has a rapid onset and brief duration of action. In some studies, its hypnotic effect was reported to be less predictable than that of chloral hydrate. Its overall safety is comparable to that of the barbiturates.

The effect of the piperidinedione derivative, glutethimide, on electroencephalographic sleep patterns is similar to that of the barbiturates. Management of overdosage with this drug can be very difficult, especially the cardiovascular manifestations. Glutethimide rarely, if ever, should be considered for treatment of insomnia.

Since serotonin is believed to play a role in inducing and maintaining normal sleep, tryptophan has been administered orally to increase brain levels of serotonin. Although a dose of 1 g significantly decreased sleep latency and total time awake without altering sleep patterns, the hypnotic action is observed only during the early part of the sleep cycle, is unpredictable, and is not characterized by a satisfactory dose-response relationship (Hartmann, 1977). Because of recent reports associating administration of tryptophan with eosinophilia, myalgia, and other symptoms, it should not be employed until further evidence establishes its safety. In order to avoid central serotonergic toxicity, tryptophan should be used with great caution in patients also receiving an MAO inhibitor or drugs that are potent inhibitors of the neuronal uptake of 5-HT (ie, clomipramine, fluoxetine, sertraline).

An OTC Sedative, Sleep-Aid and Tranquilizer Panel appointed by the FDA concluded that short-term use of certain antihistamines as sleep aids may be acceptable, but the Panel urged that better controlled studies be conducted to establish their usefulness and safety. Subsequent studies (Rickels et al, 1983 B, 1984) demonstrated that diphenhydramine and doxylamine produced significantly more improvement than placebo in several sleep parameters, including sleep latency, the target symptom for OTC sleep aids. However, these effects were less pronounced than with the benzodiazepines.

Drug Evaluations

BENZODIAZEPINE AGONISTS

ALPRAZOLAM
[Xanax]

H_3C N N N Cl N

USES. Alprazolam, a triazolobenzodiazepine compound with antianxiety and sedative-hypnotic actions, is efficacious in the treatment of panic disorder with or without agoraphobia and in generalized anxiety disorder. Results from open (Lydiard et al, 1988; Reich and Yates, 1988) and controlled (Gelernter et al, 1991) trials suggest that alprazolam may be beneficial in some patients with social phobia, although phenelzine is more effective. Anxiety associated with depression also responds to alprazolam (see index entry Alprazolam, In Depression).

ADVERSE REACTIONS AND PRECAUTIONS. Drowsiness is the most common side effect reported. Other reactions associated with antianxiety dosages are similar to those observed with other benzodiazepines. Although these occasionally may be severe, most are mild and seldom require discontinuation of therapy. Caution should be observed when other drugs possessing central nervous system depressant or sedative actions are given with alprazolam.

At the higher dosages that are sometimes necessary to produce a therapeutic response in panic disorder, sedation, fatigue, incoordination, and dysarthria are more prominent. Sedation and ataxia are common during the first one to three weeks of treatment, but, after five to six weeks, their incidence is similar to that reported by patients receiving placebo. Memory impairment, cognitive dysfunction, and confusion also may be more likely to occur with higher doses. Some patients may have changes in libido, appetite, and body weight. Hallucinations, depersonalization, taste alteration, diplopia, and hepatic enzyme elevation have been reported rarely.

Some patients may experience considerable difficulty in reducing the dose or discontinuing alprazolam therapy. The incidence and severity of withdrawal phenomena appear to be related to the dose and duration of treatment and are more prominent after a rapid decrease in dosage or abrupt discontinuation of alprazolam; use of large doses increases the likelihood of physical dependence. Withdrawal reactions can range from mild dysphoria and insomnia to a major syndrome that may include abdominal and muscle cramps, vomiting, sweating, tremors, and seizures. The risk of withdrawal seizures may be increased at doses above 4 mg daily. For patients receiving large doses of alprazolam for longer periods, an eight-week tapering period with dosage reduction of no greater than 0.5 mg every three days has been suggested. Dosage reduction by 0.25 to 0.125 mg every three days may be more appropriate, especially when the daily dose falls below 2 mg (Noyes et al, 1991). Some patients may require even slower tapering over several weeks or a period of months in order to minimize rebound anxiety (Ciraulo et al, 1990; *Med Lett Drugs Ther*, 1991).

See the Introduction for additional information on adverse reactions, precautions, interactions, use during pregnancy, poisoning, and dependence. This drug is classified in FDA Pregnancy Category D.

PHARMACOKINETICS. Alprazolam is rapidly and well absorbed orally. The time to peak blood level is one to two hours. Protein binding is about 80%, generally less than for other benzodiazepines. Although this benzodiazepine is biotransformed, the range of half-life in many patients overlaps the ranges for lorazepam, oxazepam, and temazepam. In healthy adults, the mean half-life is 11 hours (range, 6 to 16 hours); in geriatric patients, the half-life is prolonged to approximately 16 hours (range, 9 to 27 hours). The half-life of alprazolam also may be increased in obese patients and in those with alcoholic liver disease. Likewise, oral contraceptives, cimetidine, and dextropropoxyphene (Abernethy et al, 1985) may increase the half-life of the drug, while alprazolam may increase the steady-state concentrations of desipramine and imipramine. Mean values for apparent volume of distribution are approximately 0.72 L/kg and for clearance are 0.74 ml/kg/min.

Plasma levels appear to be linearly related to dose, with 1-mg increments in daily dosage causing approximately a 10 ng/ml increase. Preliminary data support the observation that there is a positive correlation between plasma levels and therapeutic response in panic disorder (Ciraulo et al, 1990). The major metabolites, alphahydroxyalprazolam and 4-hydroxyalprazolam, are conjugated and excreted rapidly in the urine. With chronic therapy, steady-state levels of alprazolam are attained in two to five days.

DOSAGE AND PREPARATIONS.

Oral: For anxiety, *adults,* initially, 0.25 to 0.5 mg three times a day; if necessary, the dosage may be increased at intervals of three to four days to a maximum of 4 mg given in divided doses; in *elderly or debilitated patients or those with severe liver disease,* the initial dosage is 0.25 mg two or three times daily.

For panic disorder, *adults,* 0.5 mg three times daily initially. Depending on the response, the dose may be increased in increments of no more than 1 mg per day at intervals of three or four days. Slower titration to the higher dose levels may be advisable. In controlled clinical trials, many patients tolerated doses greater than 4 mg daily. Some patients required doses of 6 mg daily, and a few required as much as 10 mg daily. To lessen the possibility of interdose symptoms, the daily amount should be divided into three or four doses. Although the manufacturer recommends a maximum of 10 mg/day, many clinicians are reluctant to exceed 6 mg/day, particularly if continued improvement is not demonstrated during the upward titration of dosage. However, patients who have a positive but incomplete response to 6 mg/day may benefit from a higher daily dosage. As the daily dosage increases, the risk of physical dependence becomes greater, and it may be difficult to reduce the dose for maintenance therapy. Thus, in general the upward titration should cease when an acceptable therapeutic response is achieved (ie, substantial reduction or elimination of panic attacks), intolerance occurs, or a maximum of about 6 mg is achieved. See the Introduction for a discussion on duration of therapy and discontinuation of treatment.

Children under 18 years, safety and effectiveness have not been established.

Xanax (Upjohn). Tablets 0.25, 0.5, 1, and 2 mg.

CHLORDIAZEPOXIDE

[Libritabs]

CHLORDIAZEPOXIDE HYDROCHLORIDE

[Librium]

USES. Chlordiazepoxide is effective in the management of generalized anxiety disorder and also is used to ameliorate the symptoms of alcohol withdrawal and preoperative apprehension and anxiety. It is more useful in relieving anxiety than most nonbenzodiazepines; however, chlordiazepoxide has not been extensively compared with buspirone in generalized anxiety disorder. Its anticonvulsant and muscle relaxant actions are less pronounced than those of diazepam.

ADVERSE REACTIONS AND PRECAUTIONS. Drowsiness, confusion, and ataxia have been reported, particularly in the elderly. Syncope, increased or decreased libido, agranulocytosis, jaundice, and extrapyramidal symptoms have been observed rarely. Large doses have caused hypotension.

Long-term use of larger than usual doses may produce psychological and physical dependence. Withdrawal symptoms were reported in twin neonates during the third week of life when the mother had taken 20 to 30 mg daily throughout pregnancy.

Chlordiazepoxide has a wide margin of safety unless taken with alcohol or other central nervous system depressants. Although coma has been reported after ingestion of 300 mg, it has not developed after ingestion of 1 g, and patients have recovered after taking as much as 2.5 g in a single dose.

See the Introduction for additional information on adverse reactions, precautions, interactions, use during pregnancy, poisoning, and dependence.

PHARMACOKINETICS. Chlordiazepoxide is well absorbed orally. Absorption after intramuscular administration may be slow and erratic. The drug is metabolized to active (eg, desmethyldiazepam, desmethylchlordiazepoxide, oxazepam, demoxepam) as well as inactive metabolites before final inactivation as glucuronide conjugates. Clearance (0.54 ± 0.49 ml/min/kg) is decreased in patients with hepatic dysfunction and in the elderly and tends to be higher in females. The half-life of chlordiazepoxide is approximately 10 hours (range, 5 to 30 hours), but the major metabolite, desmethyldiazepam, is long lasting; therefore, cumulative effects can occur with repeated daily administration.

DOSAGE AND PREPARATIONS.

Oral: *Adults,* for anxiety, 15 to 100 mg divided into three or four doses or once daily at bedtime; *elderly or debilitated patients* and *children over 6 years,* 5 mg two to four times daily. *Children under 6 years,* information is inadequate to establish a dose.

CHLORDIAZEPOXIDE:
Libritabs (Roche). Tablets 5, 10, and 25 mg.

CHLORDIAZEPOXIDE HYDROCHLORIDE:
Librium (Roche), ***Generic.*** Capsules 5, 10, and 25 mg.

Intravenous: For severe withdrawal symptoms in acute alcoholism, *adults,* 50 to 100 mg given cautiously over at least one minute, repeated, if necessary, in two to four hours. The dose may be reduced to 25 to 50 mg three or four times daily if necessary. The total daily dose should not exceed 300 mg. Oral administration should be substituted as soon as possible. The dose should be reduced by one-half in *elderly or debilitated patients.*

CHLORDIAZEPOXIDE HYDROCHLORIDE:
Librium (Roche). Powder 100 mg in 5 ml containers.

CLORAZEPATE DIPOTASSIUM

[Gen-XENE, Tranxene]

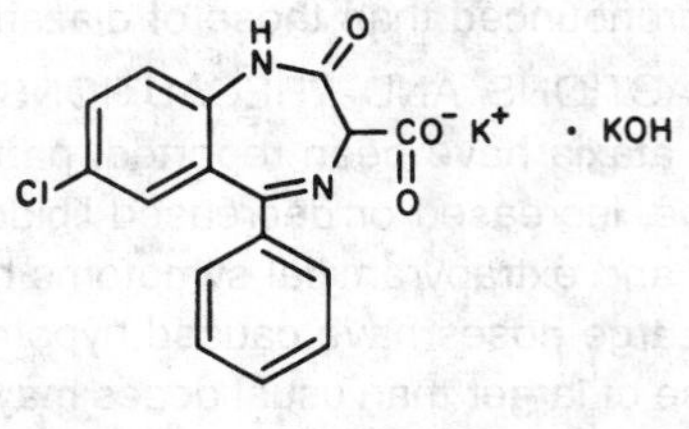

USES. Clorazepate is used in the treatment of generalized anxiety disorders, alcohol withdrawal, and as adjunctive treatment for partial seizures. Its antianxiety efficacy is equal to that of diazepam and depends on conversion of the parent compound to the active metabolite, desmethyldiazepam.

ADVERSE REACTIONS AND PRECAUTIONS. The most common adverse effects are similar to those of the other benzodiazepines. Blurred vision, confusion, and depression occur occasionally.

Long-term therapy with larger than usual doses may produce psychological and physical dependence. See the Introduction for additional information on adverse reactions, precautions, interactions, use during pregnancy, poisoning, and dependence.

PHARMACOKINETICS. Clorazepate undergoes decarboxylation to desmethyldiazepam in liquid, and the rate of conversion is accelerated at low pH; however, in bioavailability studies in normal subjects, the concomitant administration of antacids did not significantly interfere with the bioavailability of clorazepate. The drug is almost totally converted to desmethyldiazepam in the stomach and is absorbed rapidly by the gastrointestinal tract, primarily in this form. Accumulation occurs with repeated administration until steady-state plasma concentrations of desmethyldiazepam are reached (one to two weeks).

DOSAGE AND PREPARATIONS.

Oral: *Adults,* for anxiety, 15 to 60 mg in two to four divided doses or a single dose at bedtime; *elderly or debilitated patients,* initially, 7.5 to 15 mg daily.

Generic. Capsules and tablets 3.75, 7.5, and 15 mg.

Gen-XENE (Alra). Tablets 3.75, 7.5, and 15 mg.

Tranxene (Abbott). Tablets 3.75, 7.5, and 15 mg; tablets (single-dose) 11.25 and 22.5 mg (***Tranxene-SD***).

DIAZEPAM

[Valium, Valrelease]

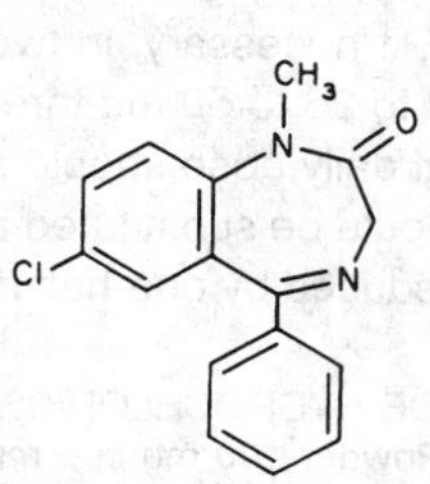

USES. Diazepam is effective in the management of generalized anxiety disorder. It also may be useful in the treatment of panic disorder and insomnia, but other benzodiazepines are preferred. Its use preoperatively or prior to endoscopy or cardioversion relieves anxiety and diminishes the patient's recall of the procedure. Additional uses include the treatment of skeletal muscle spasms due to inflammation or trauma, spasticity (eg, multiple sclerosis, cerebral palsy, paraplegia, stiff-man syndrome), seizure disorders (eg, status epilepticus, febrile seizures), and alleviation of abstinence symptoms during alcohol withdrawal. See the Introduction and index entry Diazepam for additional information.

ADVERSE REACTIONS AND PRECAUTIONS. The most common adverse reactions are similar to those of other benzodiazepines (see the Introduction). Untoward effects noted occasionally are blurred vision, diplopia, hypotension, amnesia, slurred speech, tremor, urinary incontinence, and constipation. Rarely, diazepam causes paradoxical rage and excitement. Depression may be observed but may represent a previously masked condition. Although suicidal impulses have been reported in several patients taking 40 to 60 mg daily, it is uncertain whether this is a drug-induced side effect. Apnea and cardiac arrest have occurred rarely, usually after intravenous administration, in elderly or severely ill patients, in those receiving other central nervous system depressant drugs, or in those with limited ventilatory reserve. Intravenous injection may cause local pain and thrombophlebitis.

Like other benzodiazepines, in certain patients diazepam is subject to abuse and may produce physical dependence after prolonged administration. It is classified as a Schedule IV agent under the Controlled Substances Act.

PREGNANCY AND LACTATION. Cleft lip, with or without cleft palate, has been reported when diazepam was used during the first trimester of pregnancy. More recent data suggest that exposure to diazepam during the first trimester does not materially affect the risk of cleft lip with or without cleft palate or of cleft palate alone. Diazepam and desmethyldiazepam cross the placenta during labor, and fetal concentrations may exceed those in the mother. Available evidence suggests that intramuscular or intravenous administration of more than 30 mg during the final 15 hours of labor can produce low Apgar scores, apnea, hypothermia, and poor sucking in the newborn infant (floppy-infant syndrome).

Although detectable amounts of diazepam appear in breast milk, effects on the nursing infant are insignificant if doses do not exceed 10 mg daily.

PHARMACOKINETICS. Diazepam is absorbed rapidly and predictably after oral administration. Injection into the deltoid muscle area increases the likelihood of rapid and complete absorption after intramuscular administration (Divoll et al, 1983). Cumulative effects can occur with repeated administration until steady-state plasma concentrations are achieved (one to two weeks). The half-life ranges from 20 to 70 hours; however, the major active metabolite of diazepam, desmethyldiazepam, has a half-life ranging from 30 to 100 hours. Another active metabolite, temazepam, has a relatively short half-life and is clinically unimportant after usual therapeutic doses of diazepam are administered. The clearance of diazepam and its major active metabolites is usually decreased in neonates, the elderly, and those with severe hepatic disorders; age-related decreases in clearance may be more significant in males than in females (Greenblatt et al, 1991 A).

DOSAGE AND PREPARATIONS.

Oral: *Adults,* for anxiety, 4 to 40 mg daily in two to four divided doses or a single dose of 2.5 to 10 mg at bedtime; *elderly or debilitated patients and those taking other central nervous system depressants concomitantly,* initially, 2 to 2.5 mg once or twice daily, increased gradually as needed or tolerated. A prolonged-release preparation [Valrelease] is recommended for adults only when it has been determined that the optimal dose of diazepam is at least 5 mg three times daily. The usual daily dose is one or two capsules, depending on the severity of symptoms. *Children,* 0.12 to 0.8 mg/kg daily in three or four divided doses.

Generic. Tablets 2, 5, and 10 mg; solution (oral) 1 and 5 mg/ml.
Valium (Roche). Tablets 2, 5, and 10 mg.
Valrelease (Roche). Capsules (prolonged-release) 15 mg.

Intravenous, Intramuscular (deep): When used intravenously, the solution should be injected slowly; at least one minute should elapse for each 5 mg (1 ml) given. Small veins, such as those on the dorsum of the hand or wrist, should not be used. Extreme care should be taken to avoid intra-arterial administration or extravasation in order to reduce the possibility of venous thrombosis, phlebitis, and local irritation. Diazepam should not be mixed with other solutions or drugs or added to intravenous fluids. If it is not feasible to administer diazepam directly, it may be injected slowly through the infusion tubing as close as possible to the vein insertion.

For severe anxiety, *adults,* initially, 5 to 10 mg, repeated in three to four hours if necessary. *Elderly or debilitated patients,* initially, 2 to 5 mg, with the dosage increased gradually as needed and tolerated.

Generic, Valium (Roche). Solution 5 mg/ml in 2 and 10 ml containers.

ESTAZOLAM
[ProSom]

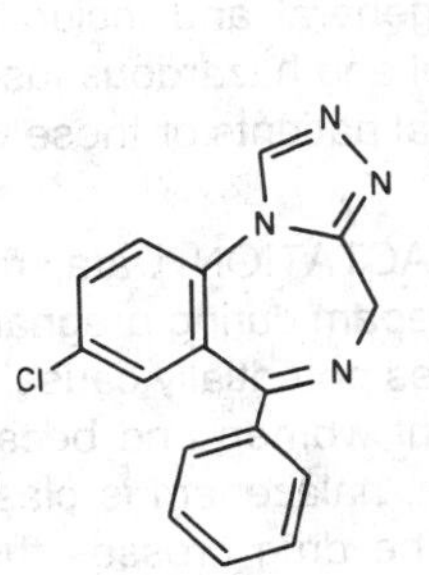

USES. Estazolam is useful in the treatment of insomnia characterized by difficulty in falling asleep, frequent nocturnal awakenings, or early-morning awakenings. Doses of 1 or 2 mg reduce sleep latency, increase sleep duration, and reduce the number of nocturnal awakenings. Efficacy also has been demonstrated in situational insomnia (eg, presurgical hospitalized patients), in the elderly, and in insomnia associated with anxiety or depression (Pierce and Shu, 1990; Post et al 1991). In short-term outpatient studies, 2 mg was somewhat more effective than 1 mg and was equivalent to flurazepam 30 mg by most measures of hypnotic efficacy (Pierce and Shu, 1990). The 2-mg dosage appears to retain its effectiveness for at least six weeks (Pierce and Shu, 1990), but data are lacking on the long-term effectiveness of estazolam and possible drug dependence or withdrawal phenomena.

ADVERSE REACTIONS AND PRECAUTIONS. The adverse effects reported for estazolam appear to be similar to those reported with other benzodiazepines. The most frequent reactions are somnolence, hypokinesia, dizziness, and abnormal coordination. Precautions for the use of estazolam are those for the benzodiazepines in general. See the Introduction for additional information on adverse reactions, precautions, interactions, use during pregnancy, poisoning, and dependence. Estazolam is contraindicated in pregnant women (FDA Pregnancy Category X).

PHARMACOKINETICS. Based on pharmacokinetic characteristics, estazolam is most similar to temazepam. Pharmacokinetic studies in healthy male subjects indicate that estazolam is rapidly absorbed; peak plasma concentrations that are proportional to the dose are reached in less than two hours (Gustavson and Carrigan, 1990). The drug appears to be eliminated according to linear kinetics, primarily by hepatic oxidative metabolism, to yield the 4-hydroxylated metabolite. The mean half-life is 14 hours (range, 10 to 24 hours). Based on limited data, the mean half-life in elderly patients appears to be 18 hours (range, 13 to 34 hours).

DOSAGE AND PREPARATIONS.

Oral: For sleep induction, *adults*, 1 mg at bedtime; 2 mg may be required in some patients. *Elderly patients*, 0.5 mg to 1 mg, with the lower dose recommended for small or debilitated individuals. *Children under 18 years*, information is inadequate to establish a dose.

ProSom (Abbott). Tablets 1 and 2 mg.

FLURAZEPAM HYDROCHLORIDE
[Dalmane]

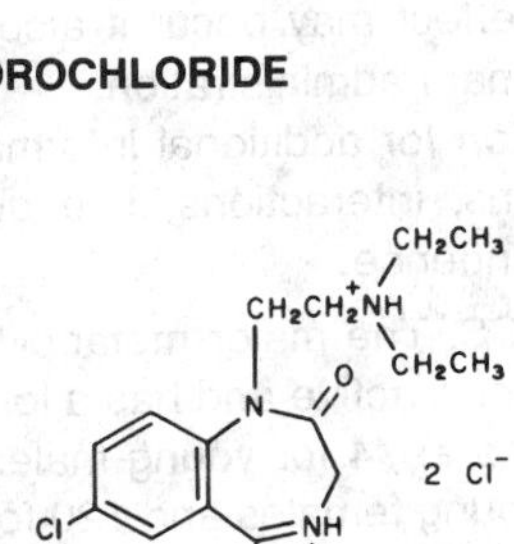

USES. Flurazepam is chemically and pharmacologically similar to the other benzodiazepines. This drug is marketed exclusively for use in insomnia. Results of well-controlled clinical and sleep laboratory studies have shown that flurazepam significantly reduces sleep-induction time, number of awakenings, and time spent awake and increases the duration of sleep. Hypnotic effects begin approximately 20 minutes after oral administration and last seven to eight hours. In a small controlled sleep laboratory study, flurazepam was reported to maintain its effectiveness for up to four weeks. As with other benzodiazepines, the percentage of REM sleep is slightly reduced during therapy because total sleep time is increased significantly without a proportional increase in the amount of REM sleep. Like other benzodiazepines, flurazepam reduces sleep in Stages 3 and 4. After discontinuing therapy, the sleep stage pattern returns to normal. The clinical significance of the alteration in sleep pattern has not been established.

Flurazepam produces, at least initially, residual daytime sedation in most patients due to the production of a long-acting metabolite. In four comparative trials, three of which involved elderly patients, flurazepam produced more residual daytime sedation than triazolam, temazepam, or quazepam (Conrad, 1990; Dement, 1991). Therefore, the drug is most appropriate for the intermittent treatment of long-term insomnia and for short-term therapy when a benzodiazepine with a long elimination half-life and a resulting daytime antianxiety effect is desirable (Mitler et al, 1984).

Sleep disturbances after withdrawal of flurazepam occur infrequently and are mild compared with shorter acting benzodiazepines.

ADVERSE REACTIONS AND PRECAUTIONS. The most common adverse reactions are a consequence of excessive central nervous system depression (eg, drowsiness, dizziness, fatigue, lightheadedness, ataxia) (Greenblatt et al, 1984 B). These effects may contribute to accidental falls, especially in elderly or debilitated patients. Paradoxical reactions (eg, excitement, hyperactivity) also have been observed. In clinical studies, neurologic reactions (eg, headache, paresthesias, visual disturbances, tinnitus) and orolingual complaints were reported in more than 1% of patients (Roth and Roehrs, 1991).

Flurazepam is contraindicated in pregnant women. Also, patients should be cautioned that an additive central nervous system depressant effect may occur if alcohol is consumed the day after flurazepam administration.

See the Introduction for additional information on adverse reactions, precautions, interactions, use during pregnancy, poisoning, and dependence.

PHARMACOKINETICS. The major metabolite of flurazepam, N-desalkylflurazepam, is active and has a long half-life. Mean half-lives (in hours) are: 74 for young males and 160 for elderly males; 90 for young females and 120 for elderly females (Greenblatt et al, 1981). Accumulation of this metabolite may be responsible for some degree of drowsiness or impairment of daytime skills, especially with doses of 30 mg. However, these effects do not consistently parallel the actual increase in plasma concentration of N-desalkylflurazepam, possibly because of adaptation. Slow elimination of this metabolite on termination of therapy probably accounts for minimal rebound insomnia.

DOSAGE AND PREPARATIONS.

Oral: For sleep induction, *adults,* 30 mg at bedtime (15 mg may be adequate in some patients); *elderly or debilitated patients,* 15 mg. *Children under 15 years,* information is inadequate to establish a dose.

Dalmane (Roche), ***Generic.*** Capsules 15 and 30 mg.

HALAZEPAM

[Paxipam]

USES. Halazepam is indicated for generalized anxiety disorder or for the short-term relief of anxiety symptoms associated with other disorders. Observation in humans has shown that tolerance does not develop to the antianxiety action after four months.

See the Introduction for additional information on anxiety and its management.

ADVERSE REACTIONS, PRECAUTIONS, AND DRUG INTERACTIONS. The most common side effect is drowsiness. Other central nervous system effects include dizziness, headache, apathy, ataxia, psychomotor retardation, disorientation, confusion, euphoria, dysarthria, depression, and syncope. Gastrointestinal disturbances, fatigue, and paradoxical agitation or rage reaction also have occurred.

Like other benzodiazepines, halazepam has a low order of acute toxicity. Overdosage is characterized by confusion, impaired coordination, respiratory depression, hypotension, and coma.

No adverse drug interactions peculiar to halazepam have been reported. Additive sedation with alcohol and other central nervous system depressant drugs occurs (see the Introduction).

Precautions for the use of halazepam include those for the benzodiazepines in general and include instructions to patients to avoid alcohol and hazardous tasks. This drug should not be given to suicidal patients or those with a history of drug abuse.

PREGNANCY AND LACTATION. Data are insufficient to evaluate the use of halazepam during pregnancy or lactation. Because benzodiazepines potentially cause fetal harm when administered to pregnant women and because of its chemical similarity to diazepam, halazepam is classified in FDA Pregnancy Category D. The drug crosses the placenta and appears in breast milk.

Until more data become available, it is assumed that the use of halazepam just prior to delivery is likely to produce CNS depression in the neonate (neonatal flaccidity or floppy-infant syndrome). Mothers dependent on halazepam during the third trimester are likely to deliver dependent infants who require additional management.

PHARMACOKINETICS. Oral bioavailability is good, and the rate of absorption is rapid (time to peak effect, one to three hours). Protein binding is at least 90%. The elimination half-life of the parent compound is 14 hours but that of desmethyldiazepam ranges from 30 to 100 hours. Accumulation can occur with repeated doses, especially in the elderly or in those with significant hepatic (but not renal) impairment.

DOSAGE AND PREPARATIONS.
Oral: For anxiety, *adults,* 20 to 40 mg three or four times a day; *elderly or sensitive patients,* 20 mg once or twice a day. *Children under 18 years*, information is inadequate to establish a dose.

Paxipam (Schering). Tablets 20 and 40 mg.

LORAZEPAM
[Ativan]

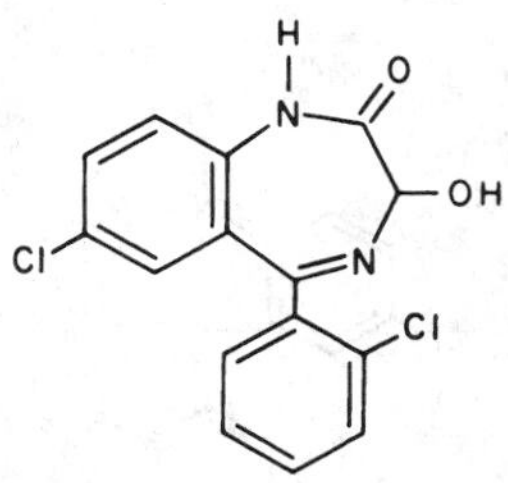

USES. Lorazepam is an effective antianxiety and hypnotic agent (Ameer and Greenblatt, 1981) and is useful in the treatment of the acute alcohol abstinence syndrome (Solomon et al, 1983). It also may be beneficial in panic disorder and neuroleptic-induced catatonia (Fricchione et al, 1983). Because of its sedative and anterograde amnesic actions when given parenterally, lorazepam is used as a preanesthetic medication and also prior to certain procedures (eg, endoscopy, cardioversion). It also is effective when given parenterally in the treatment of status epilepticus and as an adjunct in the relief of nausea and vomiting due to cancer chemotherapy (see index entry Lorazepam).

ADVERSE REACTIONS AND PRECAUTIONS. The most common untoward effects of lorazepam are sedation, dizziness, weakness, and ataxia. These reactions abate in over 50% of patients during continued administration; the remainder usually respond to reduction of the dose. Other reactions are similar to those of benzodiazepines in general (see the Introduction). Only minimal effects on respiration and cardiovascular reflexes have been noted, even when large doses were given.

Based on lorazepam's pharmacokinetics and pharmacodynamics, dependence liability is expected to be similar to that of other rapidly eliminated benzodiazepines. Abrupt discontinuation may be associated with severe rebound or withdrawal symptoms.

Until sufficient clinical experience accumulates, the drug should be avoided in pregnant and nursing women and in children younger than 12 years. The parenteral form of lorazepam is classified in FDA Pregnancy Category D.

See the Introduction for additional information on adverse reactions, precautions, interactions, use during pregnancy, poisoning, and dependence.

PHARMACOKINETICS. Like oxazepam, lorazepam is not metabolized to an active derivative. It is eliminated principally as the inactive glucuronide, and cumulative effects are not likely after daily administration. This drug has a relatively short half-life of 14 hours (range, 10 to 25 hours). Lorazepam also resembles oxazepam in that the half-life, volume of distribution, and systemic clearance are reported to be unaltered by age (up to the seventh decade), alcoholic cirrhosis, or acute viral hepatitis. The drug should be used cautiously in elderly patients and in those with impaired renal function.

Although it is absorbed almost completely, absorption after oral administration is somewhat slow (the peak effect and peak plasma concentrations occur in about two hours). The parenteral formulation is reliably absorbed intramuscularly; however, pain at the injection site has been reported occasionally.

DOSAGE AND PREPARATIONS.
Oral: *Adults,* for anxiety, initially, 1 to 2 mg two or three times daily; the usual range is 2 to 6 mg daily in divided doses. The dose can be increased gradually if needed to a maximum of 10 mg daily in two or three divided doses. For insomnia associated with anxiety or transient situational stress, a single dose of 2 to 4 mg is given at bedtime. These doses should be reduced by one-half initially in *elderly or debilitated patients.*

Generic. Tablets 0.5, 1, and 2 mg; solution (oral) 2 mg/ml.
Ativan (Wyeth-Ayerst). Tablets 0.5, 1, and 2 mg.

Intravenous: *Adults,* for anxiety, 2 mg or 0.044 mg/kg, whichever is smaller. This dose will sedate most adults and generally should not be exceeded in patients over age 50.

Ativan Injection (Wyeth-Ayerst). Solution 2 and 4 mg/ml in 1 and 10 ml containers.

OXAZEPAM
[Serax]

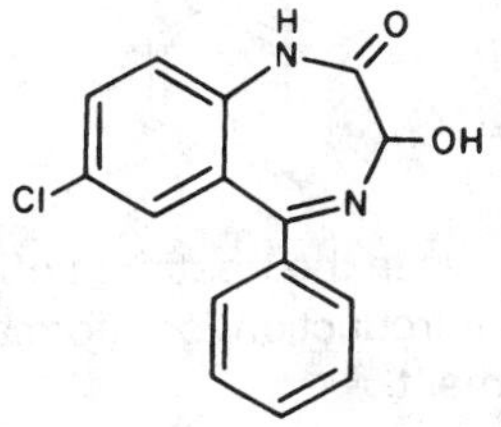

This drug is similar to the other benzodiazepines in its effectiveness in generalized anxiety disorder, alcohol withdrawal, and insomnia.

ADVERSE REACTIONS AND PRECAUTIONS. The incidence of adverse reactions is low. Drowsiness is most common and may occur after a daily dose of 60 mg. Reactions noted occasionally include rash, nausea, dizziness, syncope, hypotension, tachycardia, edema, nightmares, lethargy, slurred speech, and such paradoxical reactions as excitement and confusion. The incidence of ataxia is less than with related drugs. Hepatic dysfunction has occurred rarely. The long-term use of larger than usual doses may result in psychological and physical dependence.

See the Introduction for additional information on adverse reactions, precautions, interactions, use during pregnancy, poisoning, and dependence.

PHARMACOKINETICS. Oxazepam has a short elimination half-life (5 to 15 hours) and, like lorazepam and temazepam, is metabolized to inactive glucuronide metabolites; thus, accumulation is less likely. The inactive glucuronide is eliminated by the kidney. The rate of glucuronidation appears to be relatively unaffected by aging. The pharmacokinetic parameters of oxazepam are not altered significantly by liver disease (alcoholic cirrhosis, acute viral hepatitis). Nevertheless, until more data are available on the disposition of oxazepam in the elderly and those with hepatic and renal disorders, this drug should be used cautiously in these patients.

DOSAGE AND PREPARATIONS.

Oral: For anxiety, *adults,* 30 to 120 mg daily divided into three or four doses. *Elderly patients,* initially, 30 mg daily divided into three doses; if necessary, the dose may be increased cautiously to 45 to 60 mg daily divided into three or four doses. *Children 6 to 12 years,* information is inadequate to establish a dosage; this agent should not be used in *children under 6 years.*

Serax (Wyeth-Ayerst), ***Generic.*** Capsules 10, 15, and 30 mg; tablets 15 mg.

PRAZEPAM

[Centrax]

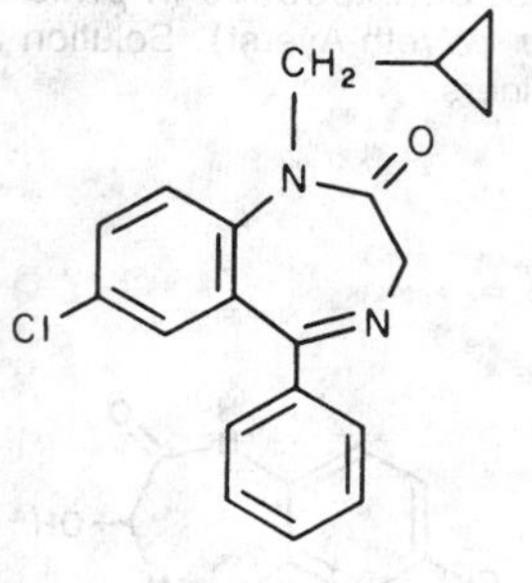

Prazepam is effective in the treatment of generalized anxiety disorder. See the Introduction for information on this disorder and its management.

ADVERSE REACTIONS AND PRECAUTIONS. The untoward effects of prazepam are similar to those of other benzodiazepines. Reactions observed most frequently are fatigue, dizziness, weakness, drowsiness, lightheadedness, and ataxia.

Prazepam is excreted in breast milk and should be avoided in nursing mothers. It is not recommended for use during pregnancy or in children.

Based on prazepam's chemical structure, metabolism, and available data, tolerance, intoxication, dependence, and interactions are expected to resemble those of other benzodiazepines. (See the Introduction.)

PHARMACOKINETICS. Like diazepam, halazepam, and clorazepate, prazepam is converted primarily to desmethyldiazepam, which appears to be the principal active metabolite. This conversion occurs relatively slowly in the liver, and peak levels of desmethyldiazepam are observed approximately six hours after oral administration. A mean half-life of 73 hours (range, 30 to 100 hours) has been reported, which represents desmethyldiazepam.

DOSAGE AND PREPARATIONS.

Oral: For anxiety, *adults,* initially, 20 mg as a single dose; if necessary, the dose may be increased to 40 to 60 mg daily given in divided amounts or as a single dose, usually at bedtime. *Elderly or debilitated patients,* 10 to 15 mg.

Generic. Capsules and tablets 5 and 10 mg.

Centrax (Parke-Davis). Capsules 5, 10, and 20 mg; tablets 10 mg.

QUAZEPAM

[Doral]

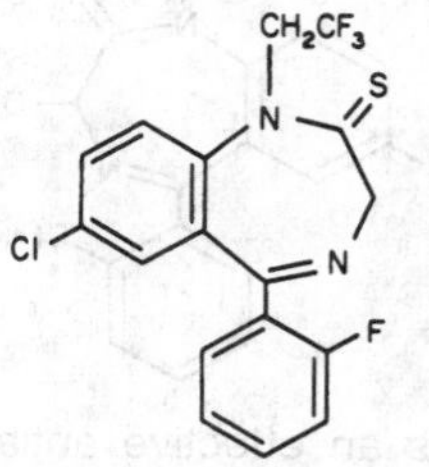

ACTIONS AND USES. Quazepam and one of its active metabolites (2-oxoquazepam) bind preferentially to the type I benzodiazepine receptor. The clinical significance of this is unknown.

Quazepam is useful in the treatment of insomnia characterized by difficulty in falling asleep, frequent nocturnal awakenings, or early morning awakenings. In short-term studies, it has decreased sleep latency and increased total sleep time. Several studies have demonstrated that this drug maintains its effectiveness for 14 consecutive days (Kales, 1990). One long-term study (28 days) demonstrated that the effectiveness of the 15-mg dose continued, but flurazepam 30 mg was more effective (Kales et al, 1982). In double-blind comparative trials, after two weeks of nightly use, quazepam 15 mg was more effective than temazepam 15 mg or triazolam 0.125 mg in inducing and/or maintaining sleep (Kales et al, 1986 A, 1986 B), and it produced less daytime somnolence than flurazepam (Dement, 1991).

ADVERSE REACTIONS AND PRECAUTIONS. The most frequent side effect associated with quazepam is daytime drowsiness. The incidence of headache, fatigue, dizziness, dry mouth, and dyspepsia was greater than 1%. Paradoxical reactions (eg, excitement, nervousness, agitation, hallucinations) have been observed infrequently.

Quazepam is contraindicated in patients with known hypersensitivity to it or other benzodiazepines or in those with established or suspected sleep apnea. This drug also should not be used during pregnancy because the potential risks outweigh the possible benefits (FDA Pregnancy Category X). Patients should be cautioned about the potential for an additive central nervous system depressant effect if alcohol is consumed within several days of quazepam administration.

See the Introduction for additional information on adverse reactions, precautions, interactions, use during pregnancy, poisoning, and dependence.

PHARMACOKINETICS. Quazepam is rapidly absorbed after oral administration with peak plasma concentrations achieved in about two hours. The active parent compound is metabolized in the liver to 2-oxoquazepam and N-desalkyl-2-oxoquazepam (desalkylflurazepam), both of which have central nervous system activity. Quazepam is approximately 95% bound to plasma protein. The mean elimination half-life is 39 hours. Its two active metabolites have half-lives of 39 and 74 hours. The half-life of desalkylflurazepam is prolonged in the elderly (see evaluation on Flurazepam).

DOSAGE AND PREPARATIONS.
Oral: *Adults,* initially, 15 mg until the response is determined. In some patients, the dose may be reduced to 7.5 mg. In *elderly and debilitated patients*, an attempt should be made to reduce the nightly dose after the first one or two nights of therapy. *Children under 18 years*, information is inadequate to establish a dose.

Doral (Wallace). Tablets 7.5 and 15 mg.

TEMAZEPAM
[Restoril]

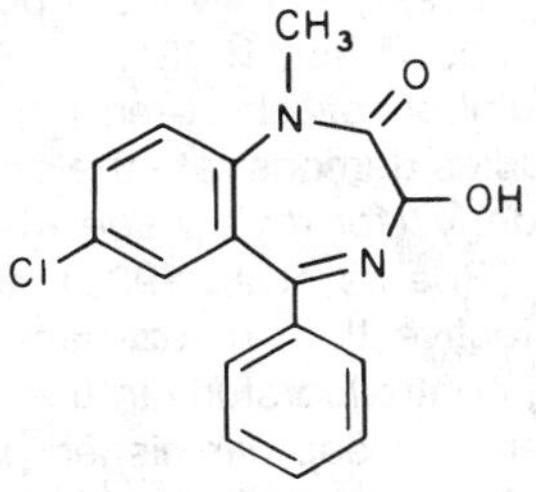

USES. Temazepam, a hydroxylated minor metabolite of diazepam, is indicated for the treatment of transient insomnia or prolonged sleep latency and insomnia associated with frequent nocturnal or early morning awakenings. The drug decreases sleep latency and the total number of awakenings, increases total sleep time, and improves the subjective quality of sleep.

The former hard-capsule formulation of temazepam was shown in double-blind, placebo-controlled, clinical trials to relieve complaints of difficulty in falling asleep, frequent awakenings, and early morning wakenings (Fillingim, 1979, 1982; Heffron and Roth, 1979), but sleep latency (time to onset of sleep) was not affected in some sleep laboratory studies (Bixler et al, 1978; Mitler et al, 1979). The slow absorption rate that characterized the earlier formulation may account for these observations. Data obtained from studies using the new formulation suggest that absorption of temazepam is now relatively rapid (see section on Pharmacokinetics). In a laboratory model of transient insomnia, temazepam (7.5, 15, and 30 mg) reduced sleep latency in a dose-related fashion. Total sleep time was increased by the 15- and 30-mg dose; the number of awakenings was decreased only by the 30-mg dose (Roehrs et al, 1990).

Suggested adult doses of 30 mg (elderly, 15 mg) may impair daytime performance. Hypnotic doses of 15 mg do not affect daytime functioning, except in some elderly patients; in these patients, doses of 15 to 20 mg may cause a reduction in blood pressure, which may be greater in the standing position (Ford et al, 1990).

See the Introduction for additional information on insomnia and its management.

ADVERSE REACTIONS AND PRECAUTIONS. Side effects are usually mild and diminish with continued administration. Those reported most frequently are morning drowsiness, dizziness, lethargy, confusion, and gastrointestinal disturbances (anorexia, diarrhea). Reactions with an incidence of less than 1% include vertigo, dryness of the mouth, paresthesias, tachycardia, panic reaction, nystagmus, paradoxical excitement, and hallucinations.

Like other benzodiazepines, temazepam has a low order of acute toxicity. Overdosage is characterized principally by confusion, impaired coordination, respiratory depression, coma, and hypotension.

Precautions for the use of temazepam include those for benzodiazepines in general and include instructions to patients to avoid alcohol and hazardous tasks. This drug should not be given to patients with a history of drug abuse or suicidal tendencies.

Tolerance or withdrawal reactions have been mild to moderate after nightly administration for one month. However, patients should be advised that sleep may be somewhat disturbed for a night or two following termination of therapy. Rebound insomnia after abrupt discontinuation of 14 nights of therapy with the 30-mg dose has been reported.

No adverse drug interactions peculiar to temazepam have been reported. Additive sedation with alcohol and other central nervous system depressant drugs would be anticipated, but not that reported with cimetidine (see the Introduction).

Dysmorphogenic changes in rib formation were observed in two animal species given 50 to 100 times the human dose. Use of temazepam during pregnancy should be avoided (FDA Pregnancy Category X).

PHARMACOKINETICS. Oral bioavailability is 100%, and the absorption rate of the newer formulation of temazepam is relatively rapid (mean time to peak concentration in young adults, 1 to 1.5 hours) (Greenblatt et al, 1989 B; Locniskar and Greenblatt, 1990). The volume of distribution and clearance are approximately 1.06 L/kg and 0.87 ml/kg/min, respectively.

Temazepam is principally conjugated and excreted in the urine as the glucuronide. A much smaller fraction is converted to oxazepam by N-demethylation and also is subsequently conjugated with glucuronic acid and excreted in the urine. The mean elimination half-life is 13 hours (range, 8 to 20 hours). As with lorazepam and oxazepam, the hepatic clearance of temazepam is not substantially altered in patients with hepatic dysfunction or in the elderly. With usual hypnotic use, accumulation is generally not a problem.

DOSAGE AND PREPARATIONS.
Oral: For sleep induction, *adults,* 30 mg at bedtime; in some patients, 15 mg may be sufficient. *Elderly or sensitive patients,* 15 mg. *Children under 18 years*, information is inadequate to establish a dose.

Restoril (Sandoz), ***Generic***. Capsules 15 and 30 mg.

TRIAZOLAM
[Halcion]

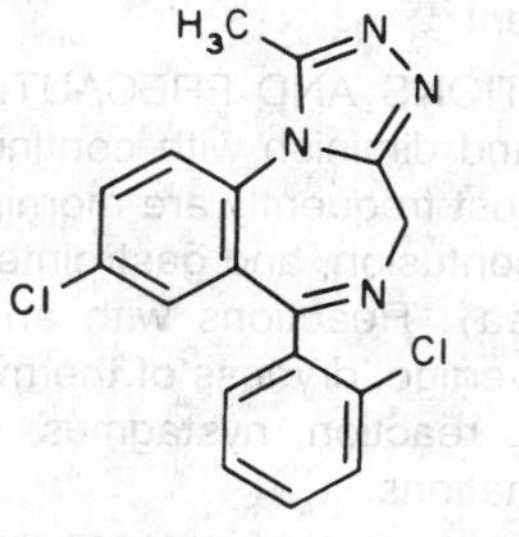

In 1983, the Food and Drug Administration approved triazolam for marketing for the treatment of insomnia in dosage strengths of 0.5 mg (for healthy adults) and 0.25 mg or 0.125 mg (for elderly and debilitated patients). The drug had been withdrawn from the market in Holland four years earlier after reports of central nervous system adverse reactions of varying severity associated with use of a 1-mg dosage (this ban was reversed in 1985). In the intervening years, the 0.5 mg dosage strength was banned by several other countries because of concerns about dose-related adverse reactions. In 1988, this dosage strength also was withdrawn from the market in the United States, and the recommended starting dose was reduced (0.25 mg for most adults and 0.125 mg for the elderly and debilitated). After review of the data, the FDA recently reaffirmed its approval for marketing of the 0.25-mg and 0.125-mg dosage strengths but with stronger warnings and more stringent criteria for its use. Current labeling states that complete re-evaluation of the patient is required if use is continued for more than two to three weeks.

ACTIONS AND USES. Triazolam is indicated for the short-term treatment of insomnia (generally 7 to 10 days). The sleep induced by this agent is characterized by (1) shortened sleep-onset time, (2) delay in onset and slight decrease in total percentage of REM sleep, (3) reduction of Stage 4 sleep but increased total sleep time, (4) decreased number of nocturnal awakenings, (5) a quality of sleep described as good in controlled studies, and (6) absence of REM rebound.

The effectiveness of triazolam 0.5 mg is well established for the treatment of insomnia characterized by difficulty in falling asleep, frequent nocturnal awakenings, or early morning awakenings when daytime sedation and an antianxiety action are not needed. In controlled studies, a single dose of 0.5 mg at bedtime was equivalent to 30 mg of flurazepam; however, many individuals experienced daytime impairment with this amount. Currently, it is recommended that this dose be reserved for patients who do not respond to a lower amount.

Results of some studies indicate that effectiveness may diminish within the first two weeks of uninterrupted use. Early morning awakening and daytime anxiety have been reported in some studies (Kales et al, 1983; Adam and Oswald, 1989), but these findings have not been consistent (Mamelak et al, 1984; Puech et al, 1991). The design and interpretation of studies that purported to indicate that triazolam causes early morning insomnia and produces anxiogenic effects have been criticized and their clinical relevance has been questioned by the manufacturer (Jonas, 1992; Jonas et al, 1992). Rebound insomnia after abrupt discontinuation of triazolam has been reported with use of the 0.5-mg dose but can be attenuated by tapering the dose (Greenblatt et al, 1987).

There are several short-term polysomnographic studies comparing triazolam 0.25 mg with placebo in patients with insomnia, patients with chronic obstructive pulmonary disease (Timms et al, 1988), and normal adult volunteers (for review see Klett, 1992). Results of most studies, especially in insomniac patients, indicate that this dose increases total sleep time; effects on sleep latency and number of awakenings are variable. Some negative results have been obtained in normal adult volunteers using sleep deprivation or phase-shift models (Seidel et al, 1986; Balkin et al, 1989; Schweitzer et al, 1991); however, another study involving a larger number of subjects produced positive results (Bonnet et al, 1988).

In studies lasting less than seven days that relied on the patient's subjective estimates, 0.25 mg was judged to be effective in improving sleep in insomniacs (Chatwin and Johns, 1977; Bowen, 1978; Moon et al, 1985; Klett, 1992). Results of questionnaire studies that exceeded seven days are more variable, but those that involved insomniac patients, including one that lasted 84 days, generally were positive on at least two outcome measures (Klett, 1992).

Results of a number of short-term, placebo-controlled sleep laboratory studies demonstrate the efficacy of triazolam 0.125 mg in the elderly (for review see Klett, 1992). In one comparative study (Roehrs et al, 1985), this dose of triazolam was more effective than nitrazepam 5 mg. In a nine-week, double-blind, controlled study in the elderly, triazolam-induced improvement in sleep diminished progressively after one week and the drug eventually had little effect (Bayer et al, 1986); however, results of another long-term study in the elderly (Bonnet and Arand, 1991) indicated continued effectiveness. Thus, although there are fewer studies on the 0.125-mg dose in elderly patients, this amount appears to be useful for short-term administration in this population. This dose consistently increases objective measurements and subjective estimates of total sleep time. Effects on sleep latency and number of awakenings are less consistent. Further study is required to determine whether clinically significant tolerance develops during its long-term (ie, three weeks or more) use in elderly patients.

See the Introduction for additional information on insomnia and its management.

ADVERSE REACTIONS AND PRECAUTIONS. The most common side effects are drowsiness, incoordination/ataxia, dizziness, light headedness, and amnesia (see below). These reactions appear to be dose-related. There have been several anecdotal reports of more severe central nervous system adverse reactions (eg, hallucinations, paranoid ideation, delirium, moderate to marked confusion, agitation). Many adverse effects occurred in the elderly or in patients with a history of psychiatric disorders. Worsening of insomnia or the emergence of new abnormalities of thinking or behavior may be the consequence of an unrecognized psychiatric or physical disorder. Evidence from spontaneous postmarketing reports to the FDA suggests that these reactions also may be dose related; however, the data are inconclusive.

No unusual or excessive adverse reactions had been reported during controlled trials involving more than 2,700 patients in the United States (Greenblatt et al, 1984 B). The manufacturer's analysis of results of controlled clinical trials and epidemiologic studies of triazolam use indicate that efficacy and adverse effects are similar to those of other short-acting hypnotic drugs (Jonas et al, 1992). Based on data collected throughout the FDA's spontaneous reporting system, adverse reactions involving the central nervous system (eg, hyperexcitability, cognitive and behavioral effects, withdrawal reactions, amnesia) were reported much more frequently with triazolam than with temazepam or flurazepam (Bixler et al, 1987; Wysowski and Barash, 1991). However, it is important to note that these reports cannot be used to calculate incidence or to estimate drug risk, and comparisons of drug safety cannot be made from these data.

As with some other benzodiazepines, anterograde amnesia of varying severity has been reported following therapeutic doses of triazolam. Data from several sources suggest that this adverse effect may occur at a higher rate with triazolam than with other benzodiazepine hypnotics (Bixler et al, 1987; Scharf et al, 1988; Greenblatt et al, 1989 B; Bixler et al, 1991). However, with repeated administration of (the longer acting) flurazepam (but not triazolam), the amnesic effect may increase (Roehrs et al, 1983). In one study, next-day anterograde amnesia occurred more frequently in patients who received flurazepam than in those who received triazolam (Juhl et al, 1984).

Amnesia may occur in healthy subjects taking therapeutic doses. Patients should be advised about the possibility of temporary memory loss and warned against taking triazolam when the time would be too short (ie, seven to eight hours) to permit clearance of the drug prior to their need to be active and functional. Increased daytime anxiety has been reported to be associated with the use of triazolam in some patients; this may occur after as few as 10 days of continuous use. If this effect is observed during triazolam therapy, discontinuation of the drug may be advisable. However, there is no consistent evidence that use of triazolam as a hypnotic causes daytime anxiety (Bliwise et al, 1988; Jonas et al, 1992).

Intrahepatic cholestasis has been observed in patients using triazolam, but a causal relationship has not been demonstrated conclusively.

Additive sedation with alcohol and other central nervous system depressant drugs would be anticipated.

Overdosage is characterized principally by somnolence, confusion, impaired coordination, respiratory depression, hypotension, and ultimately coma.

Precautions for the use of triazolam include those for benzodiazepines in general: avoidance of alcohol and hazardous tasks, as well as avoidance in depressed and potentially suicidal patients and those with a history of drug abuse or other psychiatric disorders.

Data are inadequate to evaluate the use of this drug during pregnancy, but triazolam is classified in FDA Pregnancy Category X. Administration of triazolam to nursing mothers is not recommended.

PHARMACOKINETICS. Triazolam is rapidly and well absorbed orally. Time to peak concentration is within two hours after oral administration. Plasma concentrations achieved are proportional to the dose. Protein binding is about 90%. Volume of distribution is approximately 1.1 L/kg. Clearance is 5.6 ± 2 ml/min/kg and may be decreased in the elderly (especially males), in obese individuals, and in those with cirrhosis (Garzone and Kroboth, 1989). The elimination half-life ranges from 1.5 to 5.5 hours (mean, 2.9 hours). Following hydroxylation and subsequent glucuronide conjugation, metabolites of triazolam are eliminated in the urine. Hydroxylated metabolites of triazolam have little if any hypnotic activity, and their elimination half-lives are less than four hours.

DOSAGE AND PREPARATIONS.

Oral: For insomnia, *adults*, initially, 0.25 mg or less; a dose of 0.125 mg may be sufficient for some patients (eg, low body weight). A dose of 0.5 mg should not be exceeded and should be reserved for those patients who are unresponsive to a lower dose. *Elderly, debilitated, or sensitive patients*, initially, 0.125 mg until individual response is determined; up to 0.25 mg may be given for the occasional patient who does not respond to the lower dose. *Children under 18 years*, information is inadequate to establish a dose.

Halcion (Upjohn). Tablets 0.125 and 0.25 mg.

ZOLPIDEM TARTRATE

[Ambien]

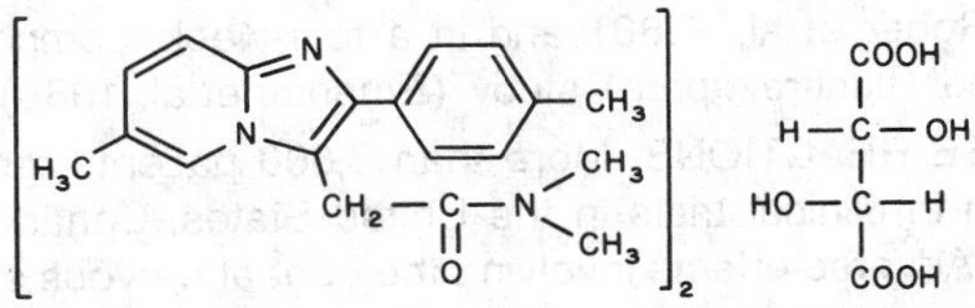

ACTIONS. Zolpidem is an imidazopyridine derivative that binds preferentially to benzodiazepine (omega) type I receptors. The clinical significance of this is unclear. Compared with benzodiazepines, zolpidem has only weak anxiolytic, skeletal muscle relaxant, and anticonvulsant actions at sedative doses. The drug has a rapid onset and relatively short duration of action. Psychomotor effects, including memory impairment, may occur but generally are minor and transient. Results of most studies indicate that in recommended doses (ie, 5 to 10 mg) deep sleep (stages 3 and 4) are preserved and zolpidem has only minor and inconsistent effects on REM sleep. Doses that exceed 10 mg slightly delay onset of REM sleep and decrease total time spent in this sleep stage. Zolpidem does not produce respiratory depression in hospitalized patients with transient insomnia or chronic obstructive pulmonary disease.

USES. Zolpidem is indicated for the short-term treatment of insomnia. Data provided by the manufacturer indicate that in a double-blind, placebo-controlled, five-week trial of adult outpatients with chronic insomnia, zolpidem 10 mg was superior to placebo in reducing sleep latency for the first four weeks and in increasing sleep efficiency for weeks two and four on objective (polysomnographic) measures. In another study on adult outpatients with chronic insomnia, zolpidem 10 mg was superior to placebo on subjective measures of sleep latency for four weeks and on subjective measures of total sleep time, number of awakenings, and sleep quality for the first week of treatment; these findings confirm European observations in the same patient population (Wheatley, 1988). In the treatment of short-term insomnia in adults, zolpidem 10 mg significantly reduced sleep latency and the number of awakenings and increased total sleep time compared with placebo (Ochs et al, 1992 A). Similar results were reported in European studies (Oswald and Adam, 1988). In normal adults experiencing transient insomnia, both the 10-mg dose and a lower dose (7.5 mg) were effective in placebo-controlled, one-night trials.

A few studies to determine the efficacy of lower doses in elderly patients have been conducted. Results of one randomized study using questionnaires in hospitalized geriatric patients indicated that the effects of zolpidem 5 mg were similar to those of placebo; however, the placebo response was very high in this study. Results of another study that used polysomnographic criteria indicated that 5 mg was efficacious in elderly noninsomniac volunteers (Scharf et al, 1991 A). Preliminary reports of other studies in healthy elderly volunteers (Scharf et al, 1991 B) and elderly patients with chronic insomnia (Ochs et al, 1992 B) also indicate that 5 mg is efficacious and compares favorably with triazolam 0.125 mg and temazepam 15 mg. The results confirm the hypnotic efficacy reported in a single-dose, placebo-controlled European study (Roger et al, 1988) and in a four-week, comparator-controlled (flunitrazepam) study (Emeriau et al, 1988).

ADVERSE REACTIONS. More than 3,600 patients received zolpidem in clinical trials in the United States, Canada, and Europe. Adverse effects involving the central nervous system and gastrointestinal tract appear to be dose related. In short-term controlled trials, the most common adverse events associated with doses up to 10 mg were drowsiness (2%), dizziness (1%), and diarrhea (1%). In long-term (28 to 35 days), placebo-controlled, clinical trials, the most common adverse events associated with administration of zolpidem 5 to 10 mg in excess of those reported in placebo recipients were dizziness (4%); allergy, drowsiness, and "drugged" feeling (3%); influenza-like symptoms, palpitations, dry mouth, lethargy, and sinusitis (2%). Reactions that exceeded those reported in placebo recipients by 1% included chest pain, lightheadedness, amnesia, depression, diarrhea, constipation, and rash. In addition to the reactions listed above, the following adverse events involving the central nervous system were reported in at least 1% of individuals who received zolpidem: ataxia, confusion, euphoria, vertigo, diplopia, and abnormal vision. Given the relatively small number of patients involved in the long-term studies, only the incidence rates for dizziness and "drugged feeling" were significantly different in zolpidem recipients than in placebo recipients.

Adverse events most commonly associated with discontinuation of zolpidem in clinical trials in the United States were drowsiness (0.5%), dizziness (0.4%), headache (0.5%), nausea (0.6%), and vomiting (0.5%).

Based on measures of daytime sleepiness and psychomotor performance in normal subjects, administration of recommended doses of zolpidem appears unlikely to cause significant residual next-day effects (Merlotti et al, 1989; Scharf et al, 1991 A). In one controlled trial, use of zolpidem for up to 35 consecutive nights was not associated with loss of hypnotic effect (Vogel et al, 1989). Further study is required to determine whether the therapeutic use of zolpidem is associated with development of tolerance or whether its discontinuation causes the onset of sleep disturbance.

PRECAUTIONS. Zolpidem should not be used during hazardous activities that require mental alertness, judgment, and/or physical coordination. It should be used with caution in elderly and/or debilitated patients; in those with concomitant illness (eg, respiratory, renal, hepatic impairment); and in those with depression and other psychiatric disorders. Other general precautions that apply to use of benzodiazepine hypnotics also apply to use of zolpidem (see the Introduction).

This drug is classified in FDA Pregnancy Category B.

PHARMACOKINETICS. Zolpidem is rapidly and well absorbed; first-pass metabolism results in an oral bioavailability of approximately 70% (Langtry and Benfield, 1990). The drug is oxidized and hydroxylated by the liver to inactive metabolites that are eliminated primarily by renal excretion. After oral administration, peak plasma concentrations are achieved in less than two hours. Food decreases the rate and extent of oral absorption. The mean elimination half-life is approximately 2.5 hours; elimination kinetics are linear within a dose range of 5 to 20 mg. Peak plasma concentrations are larger and elimination half-life is prolonged in elderly patients and in those with chronic hepatic insufficiency; dosage should be modified accordingly. No dosage adjustment is necessary in patients with impaired renal function.

DRUG INTERACTIONS. Concomitant use of zolpidem may additively increase the effects of other drugs that cause sedation (eg, tricyclic antidepressants, antihistamines, antipsychotic agents) or depress central nervous system function (ie, alcohol, other hypnotic agents). Pharmacokinetic interactions have not been identified.

DOSAGE AND PREPARATIONS.

Oral: *Adults,* for sleep induction, 10 mg at bedtime. In *elderly or debilitated patients and patients with hepatic insufficiency,* 5 mg initially; the total dose should not exceed 10 mg.

Ambien (Searle). Tablets 5 and 10 mg.

BARBITURATES

PHENOBARBITAL

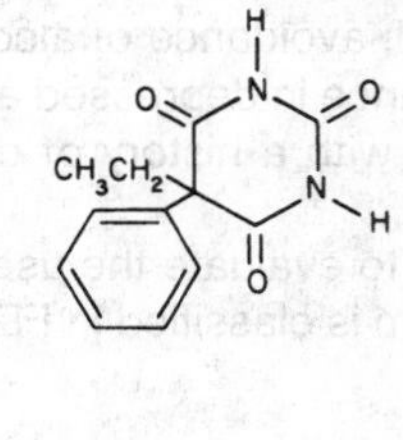

CH_3CH_2 H N O O N H O

PHENOBARBITAL SODIUM

ACTIONS AND USES. Phenobarbital differs from shorter acting analogues in that it is used in seizure disorders and has been employed as a daytime sedative or for mild anxiety. However, the benzodiazepines are now preferred for the latter indications. Phenobarbital is generally given orally but may be administered parenterally if necessary. This drug also is employed to treat barbiturate and certain nonbenzodiazepine drug withdrawal syndromes (see the Introduction).

Since phenobarbital decreases serum bilirubin levels, it has been used in newborn infants to prevent physiologic jaundice and to treat hyperbilirubinemia, but a hemorrhagic diathesis has been observed occasionally. Phenobarbital also reduces elevated serum bilirubin levels in older children and adults with Gilbert's disease (familial nonhemolytic nonobstructive jaundice). This action may be mediated, at least in part, by the enhanced formation of bilirubin glucuronide. Phenobarbital also is given to control signs and symptoms of withdrawal in infants of mothers addicted to opioids and short-acting barbiturates.

PRECAUTIONS. Long-term use of larger than usual doses may result in physical and psychological dependence. Pharmacodynamic tolerance may develop in the central nervous system, but the mechanism is unknown; this is observed primarily when large doses are taken. Death can occur after ingestion of several grams. The fatal blood level in nontolerant individuals is usually 8 to 12 mg/dL. See the Introduction and index entry Phenobarbital, Uses, Epilepsy, for further information on adverse reactions, precautions, interactions, and pharmacokinetics.

The safety of this agent during pregnancy has not been established, but barbiturates are classified in FDA Pregnancy Category D.

DOSAGE AND PREPARATIONS.

PHENOBARBITAL:

Oral: For anxiety, *adults,* 30 to 120 mg daily in two or three divided doses; *children,* 6 mg/kg daily in three divided doses. For sleep induction, *adults,* 100 to 320 mg.

Generic. Elixir 20 mg/5 ml; tablets 15, 30, 60, and 100 mg.

Available Trademark.

Solfoton (Poythress).

PHENOBARBITAL SODIUM:

Intramuscular, Intravenous: These routes should be used only when oral administration is impossible or impractical. For sleep induction, *adults,* 100 to 320 mg; for sedation, same as oral dosage. Patients should be observed carefully during intravenous injection; the rate must not exceed 100 mg (2 ml of 5% solution)/min. Relaxation, drowsiness, yawning, and slowing of speech and motor activity usually indicate that only a small additional amount is necessary; 15 minutes or longer may be required before a peak concentration is attained in the brain.

Generic. Powder (for injection) 120 mg; solution 30, 60, 65, and 130 mg/ml in 1 ml containers.

Available Trademark.

Luminal Sodium (Sanofi Winthrop).

AMOBARBITAL

[Amytal]

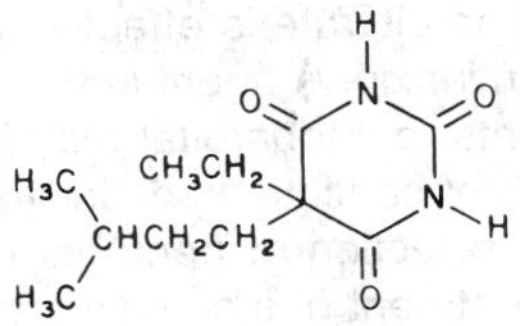

AMOBARBITAL SODIUM

[Amytal Sodium]

Amobarbital is effective as a sedative and hypnotic (but not antianxiety) agent and is usually given orally. Its action is comparable to that of secobarbital or pentobarbital but, like these agents, its effectiveness may be diminished by the second week of continued administration. Clinical situations that warrant selection of amobarbital over a benzodiazepine for the treatment of insomnia are extremely rare.

Amobarbital sodium is sometimes used parenterally to produce relaxation to facilitate a psychiatric interview, especially for the diagnosis of catatonia ("Amytal interview").

The fatal blood level is usually 40 to 80 mcg/ml. See the Introduction for information on adverse reactions, precautions, poisoning, dependence, and interactions.

DOSAGE AND PREPARATIONS. The parenteral routes should be used only when oral administration is impossible or impractical.

AMOBARBITAL:

Oral: Same as oral dosage for sodium salt.

Amytal (Lilly). Tablets 30 mg.

AMOBARBITAL SODIUM:

Intramuscular: For sleep induction, *adults,* 65 to 500 mg. No more than 5 ml should be injected at any one site.

Intravenous (10% aqueous solution): For sleep induction, *adults and children over 6 years,* 65 to 500 mg; the injection rate should not exceed 1 ml/min. The final dosage is determined largely by the patient's response as the dose is adjusted.

Generic. Powder.

Amytal Sodium (Lilly). Powder (sterile) 250 and 500 mg.

Oral: For sedation, *adults and children over 12 years,* 50 to 300 mg daily in divided doses; *children under 12 years,* 6 mg/kg/day divided into three doses. For sleep induction, *adults and children over 12 years,* 65 to 200 mg at bedtime.

Amytal Sodium (Lilly). Capsules 200 mg.

PENTOBARBITAL

[Nembutal]

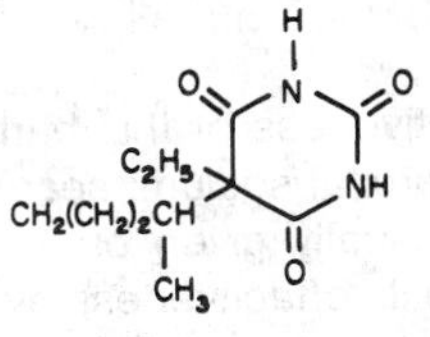

PENTOBARBITAL SODIUM
[Nembutal Sodium]

This short-acting barbiturate is effective as a sedative and hypnotic (but not antianxiety) agent and is usually given orally. Like similar agents, pentobarbital may lose effectiveness by the second week of continued administration. Clinical situations that warrant selection of pentobarbital over a benzodiazepine for the treatment of insomnia are extremely rare.

Pentobarbital is frequently abused by drug-dependent individuals. Death can occur after ingestion of more than 3 g; the fatal blood level usually is 1 to 2.5 mg/dL.

Pentobarbital is classified in FDA Pregnancy Category D.

See the Introduction for information on adverse reactions, precautions, poisoning, dependence, and interactions.

DOSAGE AND PREPARATIONS. The parenteral routes should be used only when oral administration is impossible or impractical.

PENTOBARBITAL:

Oral: Same as oral dosage for sodium salt.

Nembutal (Abbott). Elixir 18.2 mg/5 ml (strength expressed in terms of sodium salt) (alcohol 18%).

PENTOBARBITAL SODIUM:

Intramuscular: For sleep induction, *adults,* 150 to 200 mg. No more than 250 mg (5 ml) should be injected at any one site because of possible tissue irritation. Injection should be made only into a large muscle mass, preferably the upper outer quadrant of the gluteus maximus. *Children*, 2 to 6 mg/kg (maximum, 100 mg).

Intravenous: For sleep induction, *adults*, 100 mg initially; when the effect is determined (after at least one minute), additional small incremental doses to a total of 500 mg may be given slowly until the desired effect is obtained. *Children*, 50 mg initially.

Nembutal Sodium (Abbott), ***Generic***. Solution 50 mg/ml in 2, 20, and 50 ml containers.

Oral: For sedation, *adults,* 30 mg three or four times daily or 100 mg in the morning; *children,* 6 mg/kg daily in three divided doses. For sleep induction, *adults,* 100 mg.

Generic. Capsules and tablets 100 mg.

Nembutal Sodium (Abbott). Capsules 50 and 100 mg.

Rectal: For sedation or sleep induction, *adults,* 120 or 200 mg; for sedation, *children,* 6 mg/kg daily in three divided doses.

Nembutal Sodium (Abbott). Suppositories 30, 60, 120, and 200 mg.

SECOBARBITAL SODIUM
[Seconal Sodium]

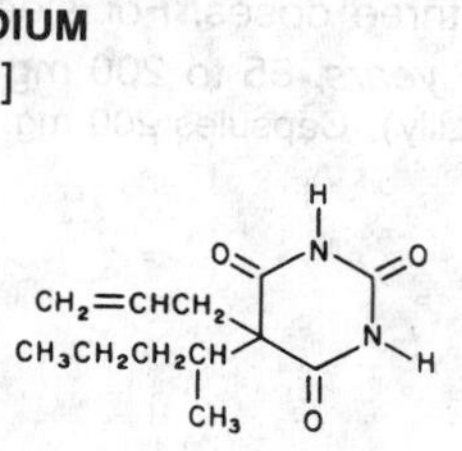

The hypnotic effectiveness of this barbiturate is comparable to that of pentobarbital sodium; secobarbital has no antianxiety action. It is usually given orally. Like similar drugs, secobarbital may lose its effectiveness by the second week of continued administration. Clinical situations that warrant selection of secobarbital over a benzodiazepine for the treatment of insomnia are extremely rare.

Secobarbital is subject to abuse by drug-dependent individuals. The fatal blood level is usually 1.5 to 4 mg/dL.

Secobarbital is classified in FDA Pregnancy Category D.

See the Introduction for information on adverse reactions, precautions, poisoning, dependence, and interactions.

DOSAGE AND PREPARATIONS. The parenteral routes should be used only when oral administration is impossible or impractical. An aqueous solution is preferred to preparations containing polyethylene glycol, because the latter may be irritating to the kidney, especially in patients with renal insufficiency.

Intramuscular: For sleep induction, *adults,* 100 to 200 mg; *children,* 3 to 5 mg/kg (maximum, 100 mg).

Intravenous: For sleep induction, *adults,* 50 to 250 mg; the injection rate should not exceed 50 mg/15 seconds. Administration should be discontinued as soon as the desired effect is attained.

Generic. Solution 50 mg/ml in 2 ml containers.

Oral: For sleep induction, *adults,* 100 mg at bedtime. For sedation, *children,* 6 mg/kg daily in three divided doses.

Seconal Sodium (Lilly), ***Generic.*** Capsules 100 mg.

NONBENZODIAZEPINE-NONBARBITURATES

BUSPIRONE HYDROCHLORIDE
[BuSpar]

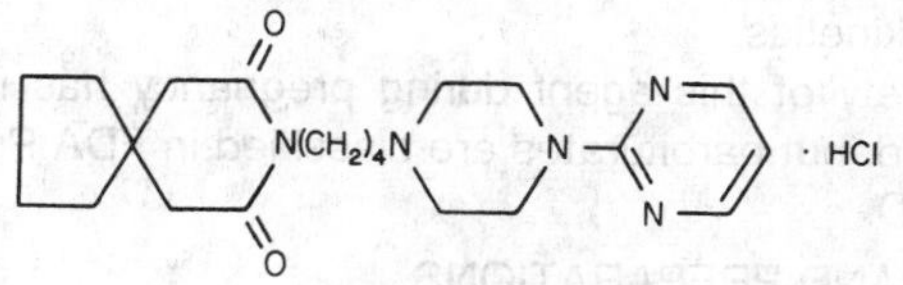

ACTIONS AND USES. Buspirone is the first novel antianxiety drug to be developed for clinical use in the United States since the benzodiazepines were introduced 30 years ago (Jann, 1988). This drug does not act directly on the GABA receptor. It appears to be a 5-HT_{1A} partial agonist (Taylor, 1988). It also has moderate to weak affinity for DA_2, 5-HT_2, and $alpha_2$ adrenergic receptors, respectively.

In most comparative double-blind studies, the efficacy of buspirone in relieving anxiety was comparable to that of diazepam and other benzodiazepines. However, patients who had previously taken benzodiazepines often indicate that buspirone is less effective, and many experts in the treatment of anxiety disorders feel that the therapeutic response to buspirone is less reliable than that produced by the benzodiazepines. In some studies, buspirone appeared to be more effective than benzodiazepines in reducing cognitive symptoms and interpersonal problems. In open pilot studies, buspirone was effective in some patients with social phobia (Liebowitz et al, 1991; Munjack et al, 1991). Antidepressant activity also has been demonstrated in some studies. This drug has not been shown to be useful in panic disorder.

Most attempts to use buspirone as the sole agent in the treatment of patients with obsessive-compulsive disorder (OCD) have failed. In open trials, it was reported to augment the effect of fluoxetine (Markovitz et al, 1990; Jenike et al, 1991). However, in a double-blind controlled trial of the adjunctive use of buspirone in OCD patients stabilized on clomipramine, buspirone did not substantially reduce OCD (or depressive) symptoms more than clomipramine alone (Pigott et al, 1992).

Unlike diazepam, buspirone has no hypnotic, anticonvulsant, or muscle relaxant properties, and it does not potentiate the central nervous system depressant effects of alcohol and other commonly used depressant medications; therefore, it may be particularly appropriate in anxious elderly patients, who tolerate the drug well (Robinson et al, 1988) and in those with suspected or proven sleep apnea.

The dependence liability of buspirone appears to be negligible (Lader, 1987 B; Rickels et al, 1988); therefore, it also may be especially beneficial in anxious patients with a history of substance abuse or in the long-term treatment of chronic anxiety. In one study of patients with generalized anxiety who abused alcohol, buspirone was superior to placebo in reducing anxiety and decreased the number of days that patients desired alcohol (Tollefson et al, 1992).

In contrast to the benzodiazepines, one to two weeks of administration are required for onset of antianxiety action; single doses usually are not effective. Since response to buspirone may be impeded in those who previously received benzodiazepines (Schweizer et al, 1986), patients should be informed that buspirone is less sedating and has a more gradual onset of action than benzodiazepines (Rickels, 1990). Reassurance can be provided about the lack of dependency.

ADVERSE REACTIONS AND PRECAUTIONS. Nervousness, restlessness, sleep disturbance, headache, weakness, lightheadedness, dizziness, depression or excitement, paresthesia, sweating/clamminess, dry mouth, nausea, and diarrhea have been reported with use of buspirone (Schnabel, 1987). When diazepam and buspirone were compared, the incidence of drowsiness, depression, confusion, decreased libido, fatigue, and weakness was significantly higher among diazepam-treated patients. Conversely, tachycardia/palpitations, nervousness, nausea, diarrhea, and paresthesia occurred significantly more frequently in those receiving buspirone (Newton et al, 1982; Schnabel, 1987). Buspirone produced less psychological impairment than diazepam and did not affect driving skills. Larger doses (eg, 40 mg) caused dysphoric effects (Cole et al, 1982). Concern that buspirone's interaction with the brain's dopamine receptors might produce tardive dyskinesia has not been borne out by clinical observation.

Buspirone is classified in FDA Pregnancy Category B.

DRUG INTERACTIONS. The administration of buspirone to a patient taking a monoamine oxidase inhibitor may cause an elevation of blood pressure. Buspirone also may increase the plasma concentration of haloperidol.

PHARMACOKINETICS. When administered orally, buspirone is rapidly and completely absorbed. Because of extensive first-pass metabolism, the mean bioavailability is 4% (Gammans et al, 1986). Plasma concentrations vary about tenfold among individuals after oral administration. Food increases bioavailability. Buspirone is 95% bound to plasma protein (Bullen et al, 1985). The apparent volume of distribution is 5.3 L/kg ± 2.6; clearance is approximately 28 ml/kg/min, and the mean elimination half-life is 2.5 hours (range, 2 to 11 hours). The drug is eliminated primarily by oxidative metabolism with only 0.1% or less appearing in the urine as unchanged drug (Gammans et al, 1986). In humans, metabolism of buspirone occurs by three major pathways; hydroxylation to yield 6-OH-buspirone and N-dealkylation and hydroxylation to yield 1-(2-pyrimidinyl)-piperazine (1-PP) and 5-OH-1-PP; 1-PP is the major active metabolite. In animal models, 1-PP has about 25% of the activity of buspirone. Age has no significant impact on the pharmacokinetics of this agent (Gammans et al, 1989). Liver disease may decrease clearance.

DOSAGE AND PREPARATIONS.

Oral: Initially, 5 mg is given three times daily; the amount is increased by increments of 5 mg every two to four days until the desired response is achieved. The usual effective dose is 15 to 30 mg daily, although some individuals may require up to 60 mg daily in divided doses (Rakel, 1987). Onset of improvement in some symptoms of anxiety occurs in about one week and the full effect usually is evident by four weeks. Results of one study in patients with impaired renal function indicated that doses may not have to be reduced in individuals with mild to moderate renal impairment (Caccia et al, 1988). Dosage schedules for patients with renal impairment have not yet been developed.

BuSpar (Mead Johnson). Tablets 5 and 10 mg.

CHLORAL HYDRATE

```
     Cl  OH
     |   |
Cl—C—C—OH
     |   |
     Cl  H
```

USES. Chloral hydrate is a relatively safe, rapidly effective, reliable sedative and hypnotic agent for short-term use. It is especially useful in insomnia characterized by difficulty in falling asleep. The lethal to therapeutic dose ratio is much lower than with the barbiturates. Some tolerance to the hypnotic action generally develops within five weeks. The antianxiety action of chloral hydrate is too limited and variable to be useful.

The unpleasant taste and odor of chloral hydrate can be minimized by the use of chilled vehicles, the capsule form, or rectal administration.

ADVERSE REACTIONS AND PRECAUTIONS. Gastric irritation occurs in some patients. Paradoxical excitement is observed rarely. The continued use of large doses causes peripheral vasodilation, hypotension, ventilatory depression, arrhythmias, and myocardial depression.

Overdosage may result in coma, and pinpoint pupils are observed occasionally. The narcotic antagonist, naloxone, does not overcome these symptoms.

Long-term use of larger than usual doses may result in psychological and physical dependence. Chloral hydrate is contraindicated in patients with marked hepatic or renal impairment, severe cardiac disease, and gastritis.

This drug is classified in FDA Pregnancy Category C.

See the Introduction and Tables 1 and 2 for more information on hypnotic drugs.

DRUG INTERACTIONS. Chloral hydrate may transiently potentiate the action of oral anticoagulants, because its major metabolite displaces the anticoagulants from their protein binding sites. A benzodiazepine may be preferred in patients who are also receiving oral anticoagulants. Clinically relevant enzyme induction does not occur. Intravenous furosemide has been reported to cause transient episodes of flushing, tachycardia, diaphoresis, and anxiety when given less than 24 hours after chloral hydrate (Dean et al, 1991).

PHARMACOKINETICS. Trichloroethanol is the active metabolite of chloral hydrate; it is formed rapidly by a large first-pass hepatic effect and has a mean half-life of 8 (range, 4 to 9.5) hours. Chloral hydrate is excreted in the urine, in part as trichloroethanol glucuronide, which may give false-positive results on tests for glucose.

DOSAGE AND PREPARATIONS.

Oral, Rectal: For sedation, *adults,* 250 mg three times daily after meals; *children,* 25 mg/kg daily divided into three or four doses. For sleep induction, *adults,* 500 mg to 1 g 15 to 30 minutes before bedtime; *children,* 50 mg/kg. The daily dose for adults should not exceed 2 g, and no more than 1 g should be given as a single dose in children.

Generic. Capsules 500 mg; syrup 250 and 500 mg/5 ml; suppositories 500 mg.

Available Trademarks.

Aquachloral (Webcon), ***Noctec*** (Apothecon).

CLOMIPRAMINE HYDROCHLORIDE

[Anafranil]

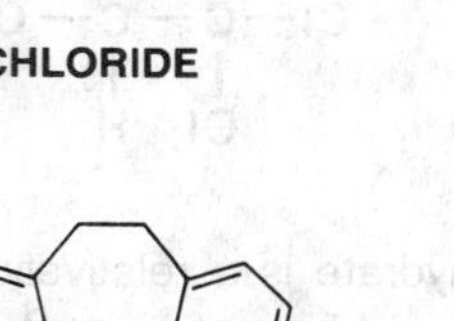

N Cl

$CH_2CH_2CH_2N(CH_3)_2$

ACTIONS. Clomipramine, a tricyclic antidepressant related to imipramine, has more potent 5-HT uptake blocking properties than imipramine. It has been widely used as an antidepressant in Europe for many years. Approximately a decade ago, open and controlled studies demonstrated that clomipramine has an antiobsessional action as well. This action correlates with the plasma level of clomipramine rather than that of the major metabolite, desmethylclomipramine, which is more potent in blocking the uptake of norepinephrine (Mavissakalian et al, 1990). Available evidence suggests that the antiobsessional action is relatively independent of clomipramine's antidepressant action but is probably related to its ability to block reuptake of 5-HT (Benkelfat et al, 1989).

USES. Results of controlled studies show that clomipramine is effective in the treatment of depressive disorders, panic disorder with and without agoraphobia, phobic disorders, and obsessive-compulsive disorder (OCD) (Swedish National Board of Health and Welfare, 1988; McTavish and Benfield, 1990; Peters et al, 1990).

About 40% to 75% of patients (both children and adults) with OCD respond favorably but seldom completely (Flament et al, 1985; Mavissakalian et al, 1985; DeVeaugh-Geiss et al, 1989; Jenike et al, 1989 B; Leonard et al, 1989; Greist et al, 1990). In a multicenter clinical trial of clomipramine in children and adolescents with OCD (DeVeaugh-Geiss et al, 1992), results (37% reduction in symptoms, lack of placebo response) were consistent with those reported in two similarly designed trials in adults with OCD. Behavioral therapy is helpful to maximize the effect (Jenike, 1983). In most controlled studies that employed a ten-week treatment period, improvement continued throughout therapy. Behavioral and drug therapy for six months to a year is recommended in responsive patients, but relapse is common following discontinuation of therapy.

ADVERSE REACTIONS AND PRECAUTIONS. The adverse reactions, drug interactions, and precautions of clomipramine are similar to those observed with other tricyclic antidepressants (see index entry Tricyclic Drugs). Thus, sedation, orthostatic hypotension, and cardiac conduction abnormalities are usually of most concern. The incidence of seizures (0.7% based on 3,000 patients) tends to be higher than with other tricyclic antidepressants. Anticholinergic effects (dry mouth, constipation, urinary retention, and blurred vision), weight gain, reversible elevation of serum aminotransferase, nausea, and vomiting are more common but usually of less significance than cardiac abnormalities and seizures.

This drug is classified in FDA Pregnancy Category C.

PHARMACOKINETICS. Clomipramine is well absorbed orally but probably undergoes significant first-pass metabolism. Metabolism may be dose related (capacity limited), which should be kept in mind when using large doses (eg, more than 150 mg/day). Time to peak plasma concentration is two to six hours. Protein binding is about 95%, and the apparent volume of distribution is 12 L/kg. The major hepatic metabolite, desmethylclomipramine, has biologic activity. Both active compounds are hydroxylated; the rate is determined by the debrisoquin phenotype. The elimination half-lives of clomipramine and desmethylclomipramine are 31 to 37 hours and 96 hours, respectively.

DOSAGE AND PREPARATIONS.

Oral: For obsessive-compulsive disorder, *adults,* initially 25 mg once daily in the evening; the amount is increased as tolerated in 25-mg increments to 75 mg, 100 mg, 150 mg, and 200 mg daily in the first through the fourth week. The maximum dosage recommended is 250 mg. *Children and adolescents,* initially 25 mg, gradually increased during the first two weeks, as tolerated, to a maximum of 3 mg/kg or 100 mg, whichever is smaller. Thereafter, the dosage may be increased gradually, if necessary, to a daily maximum of 3 mg/kg or 200 mg, whichever is smaller.

Titration of dosage to maximize the favorable effect with minimal drug exposure is recommended during long-term therapy. A daily dose of 300 mg or more should be avoided because of an increased risk of seizures. During initial titration, the drug should be given in divided doses with meals to reduce gastrointestinal side effects. After titration, the total daily dose may be given once daily at bedtime to minimize daytime sedation.

Anafranil (Basel). Capsules 25, 50, and 75 mg

ETHCHLORVYNOL
[Placidyl]

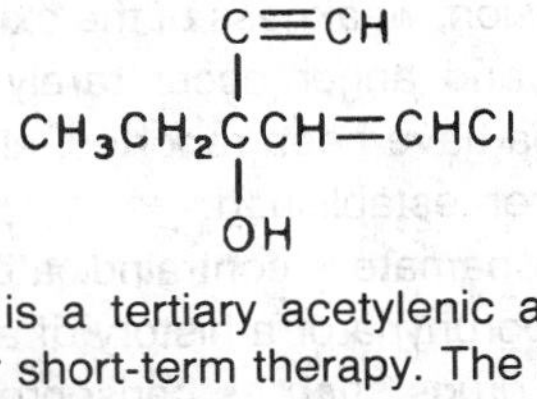

$$\begin{array}{c} C\equiv CH \\ | \\ CH_3CH_2CCH{=}CHCl \\ | \\ OH \end{array}$$

USES. This drug is a tertiary acetylenic alcohol used as a hypnotic agent for short-term therapy. The hypnotic action of ethchlorvynol may be less predictable than that of the benzodiazepines, barbiturates, or chloral hydrate. The elimination half-life is 10 to 25 hours. Clinical situations that warrant selection of ethchlorvynol over a benzodiazepine are extremely rare.

ADVERSE REACTIONS AND PRECAUTIONS. Hypotension, nausea or vomiting, aftertaste, blurred vision, dizziness, facial numbness, urticaria, and toxic amblyopia have been reported occasionally. One case of fatal immune thrombocytopenia has been described.

Long-term use of larger than usual doses may result in psychological and physical dependence. A daily dose of 1.5 g may be sufficient to induce the latter. Withdrawal symptoms, including convulsions, may occur when ethchlorvynol is discontinued abruptly.

This drug is classified in FDA Pregnancy Category C.

POISONING. Overdose with ethchlorvynol can produce prolonged unconsciousness. Pancytopenia and hemolysis also have been reported. Because large amounts of ethchlorvynol are taken up by adipose tissue, the blood concentration does not accurately indicate the magnitude of overdose.

Intravenous overdosage of ethchlorvynol causes primarily noncardiac pulmonary edema in contrast to the central nervous system depression produced by large oral doses (Schottstaedt et al, 1981). Experimentally, the drug has been shown to exert a direct toxic action on the alveolar-capillary membrane.

Charcoal and/or amberlite hemoperfusion may be most effective for removing this drug.

See the Introduction and Tables 1 and 2 for further information on hypnotic drugs.

DOSAGE AND PREPARATIONS.

Oral: For sleep induction, *adults,* 500 mg to 1 g at bedtime. The 1-g dose is usually reserved for unusually severe insomnia. This drug should not be used in *children*.

Placidyl (Abbott). Capsules 200, 500, and 750 mg.

GLUTETHIMIDE

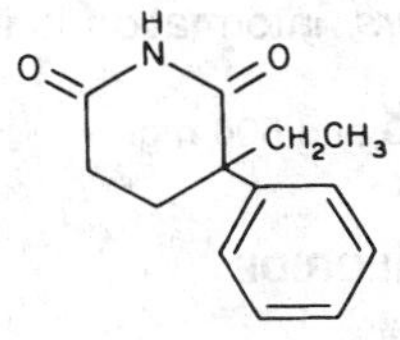

USES. Glutethimide is a hypnotic drug but, like similar agents, loses its effectiveness by the second week of continued administration. This agent has no therapeutic advantage over the benzodiazepines, barbiturates, or chloral hydrate, and clinical situations that warrant selection of glutethimide over a benzodiazepine are extremely rare. The elimination half-life ranges from 5 to 22 hours.

ADVERSE REACTIONS, PRECAUTIONS, AND DRUG INTERACTIONS. Generalized rash may occur but usually disappears within two or three days after withdrawal of the drug. Nausea, residual sedation, paradoxical excitement, blurred vision, acute hypersensitivity reactions, acute intermittent porphyria, thrombocytopenic purpura, aplastic anemia, urticaria, exfoliative dermatitis, and leukopenia have been reported rarely.

If coumarin anticoagulants are used with glutethimide, their metabolism is increased and their dosage may require adjustment, because glutethimide induces hepatic microsomal enzymes. Concurrent ingestion of glutethimide and alcohol may increase blood levels of the latter by approximately 10%, resulting in greater central nervous system depression than when either agent is used alone.

Long-term use of larger than usual doses may result in psychological and physical dependence. A daily dose of more than 2.5 g may be sufficient to cause the latter. Withdrawal symptoms, including convulsions, may occur when glutethimide is discontinued abruptly. The drug is contraindicated in patients with porphyria.

Glutethimide is classified in FDA Pregnancy Category C.

POISONING. Overdosage (20 to 30 times the usual dose) has caused areflexia, fever, and prolonged coma. Toxic doses produce less respiratory depression than the barbiturates, but circulatory depression is more profound. The long duration and fluctuating depth of the coma are partly due to the production of a potent active metabolite. Although death has been reported after ingestion of 12 g, patients have recovered after doses as large as 15 g. The fatal blood level is usually 1.5 to 3 mg/dL.

This agent is very insoluble in water, and catharsis removes residual amounts from the intestines. Most authorities feel that peritoneal dialysis or hemodialysis is ineffective in treating overdosage but, because of the drug's low water solubility, lipid dialysis may be more effective. Intensive supportive therapy alone frequently is satisfactory.

See the Introduction and Tables 1 and 2 for further information on hypnotic drugs.

DOSAGE AND PREPARATIONS.

Oral: For sleep induction, *adults,* 250 to 500 mg at bedtime; *children under 12 years,* information is inadequate to establish a dose.

Generic. Tablets 250 and 500 mg.

IMIPRAMINE HYDROCHLORIDE

[Janimine, Tofranil]

For chemical formula, see index entry Imipramine, Uses, Depression.

USES. Imipramine is the most thoroughly studied tricyclic antidepressant for the treatment of agoraphobia and panic disorder. Several small, placebo-controlled studies and open trials have confirmed the panic-blocking effects of this drug (Lydiard and Ballenger, 1987); however, many of these studies also employed behavioral therapy, thus obscuring the relative contribution of imipramine. A recent placebo-controlled, dose-response study confirmed that imipramine alone has significant antipanic and antiphobic effects (Mavissakalian and Perel, 1989). The best response was obtained at a dosage of 150 to 200 mg/day (mean, 185 mg/day). Most other studies also emphasize titrating the dosage to establish plasma concentrations within the range used for the treatment of depression (Zitrin et al, 1983; Garakani et al, 1984). However, some patients may respond to doses below 100 mg/day (Garakani et al, 1984). Imipramine also has been given with high-potency benzodiazepines for panic disorder (see the discussion in the Introduction).

For other uses of this drug, see index entry Imipramine.

ADVERSE REACTIONS AND PRECAUTIONS. The ability of patients to tolerate effective doses of imipramine may be limited by the anticholinergic side effects. An initial increase in anxiety and delayed onset of action also may limit patient acceptance. In a fixed-dose study employing 225 mg of imipramine, only 50% of patients completed an eight-week trial (Uhlenhuth et al, 1989).

For a detailed discussion on the adverse effects and pharmacokinetics of imipramine, see the discussion on Tricyclic Drugs and the evaluation on Imipramine Hydrochloride in the chapter on Drugs Used in Mood Disorders.

DOSAGE AND PREPARATIONS.

Oral: Dosage titration should be individualized and flexible. *Adults,* initially 25 mg at bedtime, with the amount increased every two to three nights up to 150 mg (Zitrin et al, 1983; Garakani et al, 1984). Other experience suggests that an initial dosage of 10 mg daily enhances patient tolerance (Lydiard and Ballenger, 1987). If panic attacks do not cease, the dosage may be increased to 225 mg daily and then to a maximum of 300 mg daily as tolerated. Once improvement is sustained, the daily dose may be decreased by 25 mg at monthly intervals to ascertain the lowest effective maintenance dose and lessen side effects. Eventually discontinuation of the medication may be attempted. However, relapse commonly occurs. The optimum duration and dosage for maintenance therapy are not known.

For preparations, see index entry Imipramine, Uses, Depression.

MEPROBAMATE

[Equanil, Meprospan, Miltown]

$$H_2N\overset{\overset{O}{\|}}{C}OCH_2\overset{CH_3}{\underset{CH_2CH_2CH_3}{C}}CH_2O\overset{\overset{O}{\|}}{C}NH_2$$

Meprobamate is useful in the treatment of anxiety, but it is less effective than the benzodiazepines.

ADVERSE REACTIONS AND PRECAUTIONS. The most common untoward effect is drowsiness, which develops with doses larger than 1.2 g daily. Thrombocytopenia, leukopenia, dermatitis, urticaria, anaphylactic reactions, hypotension and syncope, blurred vision, weakness of the extremities, and paradoxical euphoria and anger occur rarely. Agranulocytosis and aplastic anemia have been reported, although no causal relationship has been established.

The use of meprobamate is contraindicated in patients with acute intermittent porphyria or a history of allergic or idiosyncratic reactions to drugs such as carisoprodol, because the latter drug is metabolized in part to meprobamate.

Long-term use of larger than usual doses may result in psychological and physical dependence. Withdrawal symptoms may occur when meprobamate is discontinued abruptly after the prolonged daily administration of 1.6 to 2.4 g. Generalized seizures develop in about 10% of patients during withdrawal. Death has occurred during withdrawal. Death from poisoning has been reported after ingestion of 12 g, but patients have survived after ingestion of 40 g.

Meprobamate appears in breast milk in concentrations two to four times that in maternal plasma. Therefore, the risks to the infant should be considered when this drug is used in a nursing mother.

See the Introduction and Tables 1 and 2 for additional information on antianxiety drugs.

PHARMACOKINETICS. Efficacy coincides with the peak plasma concentration, which is attained two to three hours after ingestion. Induction of hepatic microsomal enzymes occurs but does not appear to be a problem with usual doses. Consistent bioavailability of the prolonged-release preparation has been demonstrated; however, because meprobamate has a mean half-life of 10 to 24 hours, prolonged-release preparations do not offer any significant advantage over ordinary dosage forms for most patients.

DOSAGE AND PREPARATIONS.

Oral: *Adults,* 1.2 to 1.6 g (maximum, 2.4 g) daily divided into three or four doses. *Children 6 to 12 years,* 100 to 200 mg two or three times daily; *children under 6 years,* not recommended.

Equanil (Wyeth-Ayerst), ***Generic.*** Tablets 200 and 400 mg.

Meprospan (Wallace). Capsules (prolonged-release) 200 and 400 mg.

Miltown (Wallace). Tablets 200, 400, and 600 mg.

MIXTURES

Mixtures containing one or more barbiturates, most commonly amobarbital, butabarbital, pentobarbital, phenobarbital, or secobarbital (eg, Tuinal), or other hypnotic and antianxiety agents have been used extensively for many years, but any alleged advantage of such combination products is hypothetical. The effects of these mixtures may only be additive, often without any compensating advantage to the patient. Furthermore, fixed-ratio combinations do not permit careful adjustment of the dosage of each drug, which may be important when administering two or more drugs with different durations of action. For these reasons, use of this type of mixture is not recommended.

For the same reasons, fixed-ratio combinations of two or more antianxiety agents or antianxiety agents with anorexiants, antihypertensive agents, estrogens, mild analgesics, antianginal agents, or antispasmodics are not recommended. Such mixtures are marketed for the treatment of anxiety, pain, menopausal symptoms, angina pectoris, obesity, hypertension, and musculoskeletal and gastrointestinal disorders.

Cited References

Alprazolam for panic disorder. *Med Lett Drugs Ther* 33:30-31, 1991.

Benzodiazepine Dependence, Toxicity, and Abuse: A Task Force Report of the American Psychiatric Association. Washington, DC, American Psychiatric Association, 1990.

Diagnostic and Statistical Manual of Mental Disorders, ed 3 (revised). Washington, DC, American Psychiatric Association, 1987.

Drugs and Insomnia Consensus Development Conference Summary. Bethesda, Md, National Institutes of Health, 1983, vol 4, number 10.

The International Classification of Sleep Disorders: Diagnostic and Coding Manual. Rochester, Minn, American Sleep Disorders Association, 1990.

Panic: Consensus Statement: NIH Consensus Development Conference, September 25-27, 1991. Bethesda, Md, National Institutes of Health, 1991, vol 9, number 2.

Abernethy DR, et al: Impairment of diazepam metabolism by low-dose estrogen-containing oral-contraceptive steroids. *N Engl J Med* 306:791-792, 1982.

Abernethy DR, et al: Interaction of propoxyphene with diazepam, alprazolam and lorazepam. *Br J Clin Pharmacol* 19:51-57, 1985.

Adam K, Oswald I: Can a rapidly-eliminated hypnotic cause daytime anxiety? *Pharmacopsychiatry* 22:115-119, 1989.

Aldrich MS: Narcolepsy. *N Engl J Med* 323:389-394, 1990.

Ameer B, Greenblatt DJ: Lorazepam: Review of its clinical pharmacological properties and therapeutic uses. *Drugs* 21:161-200, 1981.

Balkin TJ, et al: Administration of triazolam prior to recovery sleep: Effects on sleep architecture, subsequent alertness and performance. *Psychopharmacology* 99:526-531, 1989.

Ballenger JC, et al: Alprazolam in panic disorder and agoraphobia: Results from a multicenter trial: I. Efficacy in short-term treatment. *Arch Gen Psychiatry* 45:413-422, 1988.

Bayer AJ, et al: A double-blind controlled study of chlormethiazole and triazolam as hypnotic in the elderly. *Acta Psychiatr Scand* 73(suppl 329):104-111, 1986.

Benet LZ, Williams RL: Design and optimization of dosage regimens: Pharmacokinetic data, in Gilman AG, et al (eds): *Goodman and Gilman's The Pharmacological Basis of Therapeutics*, ed 8. New York, Pergamon Press, 1990, 1650-1735.

Benkelfat C, et al: Clomipramine in obsessive-compulsive disorder: Further evidence for a serotonergic mechanism of action. *Arch Gen Psychiatry* 46:23-28, 1989.

Bixler ED, et al: Effectiveness of temazepam with short-, intermediate-, and long-term use: Sleep laboratory evaluation. *J Clin Pharmacol* 18:110-118, 1978.

Bixler EO, et al: Rebound insomnia and elimination half-life: Assessment of individual subject response. *J Clin Pharmacol* 25:115-124, 1985.

Bixler EO, et al: Adverse reactions to benzodiazepine hypnotics: Spontaneous reporting system. *Pharmacology* 35:286-300, 1987.

Bixler EO, et al: Next-day memory impairment with triazolam use. *Lancet* 337:827-831, 1991.

Bliwise DL, et al: Profile of mood state changes during and after 5 weeks of nightly triazolam administration. *J Clin Psychiatry* 49:349-355, 1988.

Block AJ: *Sleep Apnea and Related Disorders.* Chicago, Year Book Medical Publishers, 1985, 6-53.

Bonnet MH, Arand DL: The use of triazolam in patients with periodic leg movements, fragmented sleep and daytime sleepiness. *Aging* 3:313-324, 1991.

Bonnet MH, et al: The use of triazolam in phase-advanced sleep. *Neuropsychopharmacology* 1:225-234, 1988.

Bowden CL: Clinical management of anxiety. *Hosp Pract* 25(suppl 2):19-30, 1990.

Bowen AJ: Comparison of triazolam, flurazepam and placebo in outpatient insomniacs. *J Int Med Res* 6:337-342, 1978.

Breimer DD: Clinical pharmacokinetics of hypnotics. *Clin Pharmacokinet* 2:93-109, 1977.

Brogden RN, Goa KL: Flumazenil: Preliminary review of its benzodiazepine antagonist properties, intrinsic activity and therapeutic use. *Drugs* 35:448-467, 1988.

Brouillette RT, et al: Obstructive sleep apnea in infants and children. *J Pediatr* 100:31-40, 1982.

Browman CP, et al: Hypersomnia: Diagnosis and management. *Compr Ther* 9:67-74, (June) 1983.

Buigues J, Vallejo J: Therapeutic response to phenelzine in patients with panic disorder and agoraphobia with panic attacks. *J Clin Psychiatry* 48:55-59, 1987.

Bullen WW, et al: Binding of buspirone to human plasma proteins. *Fed Proc* 44:1123, 1985.

Caccia S, et al: Clinical pharmacokinetics of oral buspirone in patients with impaired renal function. *Clin Pharmacokinet* 14:171-177, 1988.

Charney DS, Woods SW: Benzodiazepine treatment of panic disorder: A comparison of alprazolam and lorazepam. *J Clin Psychiatry* 50:418-423, 1989.

Chatwin JC, Johns WL: Triazolam: An effective hypnotic in general practice. *Curr Ther Res* 21:207-214, 1977.

Chokroverty S, Sharp JT: Primary sleep apnea syndrome. *J Neurol Neurosurg Psychiatry* 44:970-982, 1981.

Chouinard G, et al: Results of a double-blind placebo controlled trial of a new serotonin uptake inhibitor, sertraline, in the treatment of obsessive-compulsive disorder. *Psychopharmacol Bull* 26:279-284, 1990.

Ciraulo DA, et al: The relationship of alprazolam dose to steady-state plasma concentrations. *J Clin Psychopharmacol* 10:27-32, 1990.

The Clomipramine Collaborative Study Group: Clomipramine in the treatment of patients with obsessive-compulsive disorder. *Arch Gen Psychiatry* 48:730-738, 1991.

Cohn JB, Rickels K: A pooled, double-blind comparison of the effects of buspirone, diazepam and placebo in women with chronic anxiety. *Curr Med Res Opin* 11:304-320, 1989.

Cohn JB, Wilcox CS: Low-sedation potential of buspirone compared with alprazolam and lorazepam in the treatment of anxious patients: A double-blind study. *J Clin Psychiatry* 47:409-412, 1986.

Cole J: Drug treatment of anxiety and depression. *Med Clin North Am* 72:815-830, 1988.

Cole JO, et al: Assessment of abuse liability of buspirone in recreational sedative users. *J Clin Psychiatry* 43(12, sec 2):69-74, 1982.

Conrad KA: Sedative hypnotic drug use in the elderly. *Drug Ther* 20:22-28, 1990.

Costa E: The allosteric modulation of GABA receptors. *Neuropsychopharmacology* 4:225-235, 1991.

Czeisler CA, Richardson GS: Detection and assessment of insomnia. *Clin Ther* 13:663-679, 1991.

Davidson JRT, et al: Long-term treatment of social phobia with clonazepam. *J Clin Psychiatry* 52 (suppl) :16-20, (Nov) 1991.

Dean RP, et al: Interaction of chloral hydrate and intravenous furosemide in a child. *Clin Pharm* 10:385-387, 1991.

Dement WC: Objective measurements of daytime sleepiness and performance comparing quazepam with flurazepam in two adult populations using the multiple sleep latency test. *J Clin Psychiatry* 52 (suppl) :31-37, (Sept) 1991.

DeVeaugh-Geiss J, et al: Treatment of obsessive compulsive disorder with clomipramine. *Psychiatr Ann* 19:97-101, 1989.

DeVeaugh-Geiss J, et al: Clomipramine hydrochloride in childhood and adolescent obsessive-compulsive disorder: A multicenter trial. *J Am Acad Child Adolesc Psychiatry* 31:45-49, 1992.

Divoll M, et al: Absolute bioavailability of oral and intramuscular diazepam: Effects of age and sex. *Anesth Analg* 62:1-8, 1983.

Dubovsky SL: Generalized anxiety disorder: New concepts and psychopharmacologic therapies. *J Clin Psychiatry* 51 (suppl) :3-10, 1990.

Emeriau JP, et al: Zolpidem and flunitrazepam: A multicenter trial in elderly hospitalized patients, in Sauvanet JP, et al (eds): *Imidazopyridines in Sleep Disorders: A Novel Experimental and Therapeutic Approach*. New York, Raven Press, 1988, vol 6 (LERS Monograph Series), 317-326.

Everitt DE, et al: Clinical decision-making in the evaluation and treatment of insomnia. *Am J Med* 89:357-362, 1990.

Ferriss GS: Narcolepsy. *Cont Educ* 16:41-48, (May) 1982.

Fillingim JM: Double-blind evaluation of the efficacy and safety of temazepam in outpatients with insomnia. *Br J Clin Pharmacol* 8:73S-77S, 1979.

Fillingim JM: Double-blind evaluation of temazepam, flurazepam, and placebo in geriatric insomniacs. *Clin Ther* 4:369-380, 1982.

Flament MF, et al: Clomipramine treatment of childhood obsessive-compulsive disorder. *Arch Gen Psychiatry* 42:977-983, 1985.

Fontaine R, et al: Rebound anxiety in anxious patients after abrupt withdrawal of benzodiazepine treatment. *Am J Psychiatry* 141:848-852, 1984.

Ford GA, et al: Effect of temazepam on blood pressure regulation in healthy elderly subjects. *Br J Clin Pharmacol* 29:61-67, 1990.

Frazier SH (ed): Anxiety and depression. *Med Clin North Am* 72:745-977, (July) 1988.

Frenkel A, et al: Efficacy of long-term fluoxetine treatment of obsessive-compulsive disorder. *Mt Sinai J Med* 57:348-352, 1990.

Fricchione GL, et al: Intravenous lorazepam in neuroleptic-induced catatonia. *J Clin Psychopharmacol* 3:338-342, 1983.

Gammans RE, et al: Metabolism and disposition of buspirone. *Am J Med* 80 (suppl 3B) :41-51, 1986.

Gammans RE, et al: Pharmacokinetics of buspirone in elderly subjects. *J Clin Pharmacol* 29:72-78, 1989.

Garakani H, et al: Treatment of panic disorder with imipramine alone. *Am J Psychiatry* 141:446-448, 1984.

Garzone PD, Kroboth PD: Pharmacokinetics of the newer benzodiazepines. *Clin Pharmacokinet* 16:337-364, 1989.

Gelernter CS, et al: Cognitive-behavioral and pharmacological treatments of social phobia. *Arch Gen Psychiatry* 48:938-945, 1991.

Gershon S, Eison AS: Anxiolytic profiles. *J Clin Psychiatry* 44 (11, sec 2) :45-56, 1983.

Gillin JC, Byerley WF: The diagnosis and management of insomnia. *N Engl J Med* 322:239-248, 1990.

Gillin JC, et al: Rebound insomnia: Critical review. *J Clin Psychopharmacol* 9:161-172, 1989.

Goldberg HL, Finnerty R: Comparison of buspirone in two separate studies. *J Clin Psychiatry* 43 (12, sec 2) :87-91, 1982.

Goodman WK, et al: Efficacy of fluvoxamine in obsessive-compulsive disorder: Double-blind comparison with placebo. *Arch Gen Psychiatry* 46:36-44, 1989.

Goodman WK, et al: Pharmacotherapy of obsessive compulsive disorder. *J Clin Psychiatry* 53 (suppl) :29-37, (April) 1992.

Greenblatt DJ, Shader RI: Pharmacokinetics of antianxiety agents, in Meltzer HY (ed): *Psychopharmacology: The Third Generation of Progress.* New York, Raven Press, 1987, 1377-1386.

Greenblatt DJ, et al: Clinical pharmacokinetics of chlordiazepoxide. *Clin Pharmacokinet* 3:381-394, 1978.

Greenblatt DJ, et al: Kinetics and clinical effects of flurazepam in young and elderly noninsomniacs. *Clin Pharmacol Ther* 30:475-486, 1981.

Greenblatt DJ, et al: Current status of benzodiazepines, parts 1 and 2. *N Engl J Med* 309:354-358, 410-415, 1983 A.

Greenblatt DJ, et al: Clinical pharmacokinetics of the newer benzodiazepines. *Clin Pharmacokinet* 8:233-252, 1983 B.

Greenblatt DJ, et al: Clinical importance of interaction of diazepam and cimetidine. *N Engl J Med* 310:1639-1643, 1984 A.

Greenblatt DJ, et al: Adverse reactions to triazolam, flurazepam, and placebo in controlled clinical trials. *J Clin Psychiatry* 45:192-195, 1984 B.

Greenblatt DJ, et al: Effect of gradual withdrawal on the rebound sleep disorder after discontinuation of triazolam. *N Engl J Med* 317:722-728, 1987.

Greenblatt DJ, et al: Desmethyldiazepam pharmacokinetics: Studies following intravenous and oral desmethyldiazepam, oral clorazepate, and intravenous diazepam *J Clin Pharmacol* 28:853-859, 1988.

Greenblatt DJ, et al: Kinetic and dynamic study of intravenous lorazepam: Comparison with intravenous diazepam. *J Pharmacol Exp Ther* 250:134-140, 1989 A.

Greenblatt DJ, et al: Pharmacokinetic determinants of dynamic differences among three benzodiazepine hypnotics: Flurazepam, temazepam, and triazolam. *Arch Gen Psychiatry* 46:326-332, 1989 B.

Greenblatt DJ, et al: Clinical pharmacokinetics of anxiolytics and hypnotics in the elderly: Therapeutic considerations (part I). *Clin Pharmacokinet* 21:165-177, 1991 A.

Greenblatt DJ, et al: Clinical pharmacokinetics of anxiolytics and hypnotics in the elderly: Therapeutic considerations (part II). *Clin Pharmacokinet* 21:262-273, 1991 B.

Greist JH: Treatment of obsessive compulsive disorder: Psychotherapies, drugs, and other somatic treatment. *J Clin Psychiatry* 51 (8, suppl) :44-50, 1990.

Greist JH, et al: Clomipramine and obsessive compulsive disorder: A placebo-controlled double-blind study of 32 patients. *J Clin Psychiatry* 51:292-297, 1990.

Guilleminault C, et al: Viloxazine hydrochloride in narcolepsy: A preliminary report. *Sleep* 9:275-279, 1986.

Gustavson LE, Carrigan PJ: The clinical pharmacokinetics of single doses of estazolam. *Am J Med* 88 (suppl 3A) :2S-5S, 1990.

Hartmann E: *L*-tryptophan: Rational hypnotic with clinical potential. *Am J Psychiatry* 134:366-370, 1977.

Heffron WA, Roth P: Double-blind evaluation of the safety and hypnotic efficacy of temazepam in insomniac outpatients. *Br J Clin Pharmacol* 8:69S-72S, 1979.

Heimberg RG, Barlow DH: New developments in cognitive-behavioral therapy for social phobia. *J Clin Psychiatry* 52 (suppl) :21-30, 1991.

Herman JB, et al: The alprazolam to clonazepam switch for the treatment of panic disorder. *J Clin Psychopharmacol* 7:175-178, 1987.

Ho IK, Harris RA: Mechanism of action of barbiturates. *Ann Rev Pharmacol* 21:83-111, 1981.

Jann MW: Buspirone: Update on a unique anxiolytic agent. *Pharmacotherapy* 8:100-116, 1988.

Jenike MA: Obsessive compulsive disorder. *Compr Psychiatry* 24:99-115, (March/April) 1983.

Jenike MA: Approaches to the patient with treatment-refractory obsessive compulsive disorder. *J Clin Psychiatry* 51 (2, suppl) :15-21, 1990.

Jenike MA, Baer L: Open trial of buspirone in obsessive-compulsive disorder. *Am J Psychiatry* 145:1285-1286, 1988.

Jenike MA, et al: Disabling obsessive thoughts responsive to antidepressants. *J Clin Psychopharmacol* 7:33-35, 1987.

Jenike MA, et al: Open trial of fluoxetine in obsessive-compulsive disorder. *Am J Psychiatry* 146:909-911, 1989 A.

Jenike MA, et al: Obsessive-compulsive disorder: A double-blind, placebo-controlled trial of clomipramine in 27 patients. *Am J Psychiatry* 146:1328-1330, 1989 B.

Jenike MA, et al: Sertraline in obsessive-compulsive disorder: A double-blind comparison with placebo. *Am J Psychiatry* 147:923-928, 1990.

Jenike MA, et al: Buspirone augmentation of fluoxetine in obsessive-compulsive disorder. *J Clin Psychiatry* 52:13-14, 1991.

Jick H: Early pregnancy and benzodiazepines, editorial. *J Clin Psychopharmacol* 8:159-160, 1988.

Jonas JM: Idiosyncratic side effects of short half-life benzodiazepine hypnotics: Fact or fancy? *Human Psychopharmacol* 7:205-216, 1992.

Jonas JM, et al: Comparative clinical profiles of triazolam versus other shorter-acting hypnotics. *J Clin Psychiatry* 53(12, suppl):19-31, 1992.

Juhl RP, et al: Incidence of next-day anterograde amnesia caused by flurazepam hydrochloride and triazolam. *Clin Pharm* 3:622-625, 1984.

Kahn RJ, et al: Effects of psychotropic agents on high anxiety subjects. *Psychopharmacol Bull* 17:97-100, 1981.

Kales A: Quazepam: Hypnotic efficacy and side effects. *Pharmacotherapy* 10:1-12, 1990.

Kales A, et al: Quazepam and flurazepam: Long-term use and extended withdrawal. *Clin Pharmacol Ther* 32:781-788, 1982.

Kales A, et al: Rebound insomnia and rebound anxiety: A review. *Pharmacology* 26:121-137, 1983.

Kales A, et al: Quazepam and temazepam: Effects of short- and intermediate-term use and withdrawal. *Clin Pharmacol Ther* 39:345-352, 1986 A.

Kales A, et al: Comparison of short and long half-life benzodiazepine hypnotics: Triazolam and quazepam. *Clin Pharmacol Ther* 40:378-386, 1986 B.

Kales A, et al: Rebound insomnia after only brief and intermittent use of rapidly eliminated benzodiazepines. *Clin Pharmacol Ther* 49:468-476, 1991.

Kalus O, et al: Desipramine treatment in panic disorder. *J Affect Disord* 21:239-244, 1991.

Klett CJ: Review of triazolam data. *J Clin Psychiatry* 53(12, suppl): 61-67, 1992.

Lader MH: Rational use of anxiolytic drugs. *Ration Drug Ther* 21:1-5, (Sept) 1987 A.

Lader M: Assessing the potential for buspirone dependence or abuse and effects of its withdrawal. *Am J Med* 82(suppl 5A):20-26, 1987 B.

Lader M: Beta-adrenoceptor antagonists in neuropsychiatry: Update. *J Clin Psychiatry* 49:213-223, 1988.

Lane T, Peterson EA: Hepatitis as manifestation of phenobarbital hypersensitivity, letter. *South Med J* 77:94, 1984.

Langdon N, et al: Fluoxetine in the treatment of cataplexy. *Sleep* 9:371-373, 1986.

Langtry HD, Benfield P: Zolpidem: A review of its pharmacodynamic and pharmacokinetic properties and therapeutic potential. *Drugs* 40:291-313, 1990.

Leonard HL, et al: Treatment of obsessive-compulsive disorder with clomipramine and desipramine in children and adolescents: A double-blind crossover comparison. *Arch Gen Psychiatry* 46:1088-1092, 1989.

Levine R, et al: Long-term fluoxetine treatment of a large number of obsessive-compulsive patients. *J Clin Psychopharmacol* 9:281-283, 1989.

Liebowitz MR, et al: Tricyclic therapy of the DSM-III anxiety disorders: A review with implications for further research. *J Psychiatr Res* 22(suppl 1):7-31, 1988.

Liebowitz MR, et al: Treatment of social phobia with drugs other than benzodiazepines. *J Clin Psychiatry* 52(suppl):10-15, 1991.

Liebowitz MR, et al: Phenelzine vs atenolol in social phobia: A placebo-controlled comparison. *Arch Gen Psychiatry* 49:290-300, 1992.

Locniskar A, Greenblatt DJ: Oxidative versus conjugative biotransformation of temazepam. *Biopharm Drug Dispos* 11:499-506, 1990.

Lydiard RB, Ballenger JC: Antidepressants in panic disorder and agoraphobia. *J Affective Disord* 13:153-168, 1987.

Lydiard RB, et al: Alprazolam in the treatment of social phobia. *J Clin Psychiatry* 49:17-19, 1988.

Mamelak M, et al: A comparative 25-night sleep laboratory study on the effects of quazepam and triazolam on chronic insomniacs. *J Clin Pharmacol* 24:65-75, 1984.

Mandelli M, et al: Clinical pharmacokinetics of diazepam. *Clin Pharmacokinet* 3:72-91, 1978.

March JS, et al: Obsessive-compulsive disorder. *Am Fam Physician* 39:175-182, (May) 1989.

Markovitz PJ, et al: Buspirone augmentation of fluoxetine in obsessive-compulsive disorder. *Am J Psychiatry* 147:798-800, 1990.

Marks J: Techniques of benzodiazepine withdrawal in clinical practice: A consensus workshop report. *Med Toxicol* 3:324-333, 1988.

Marks J: Introduction, in benzodiazepines: A 1990 update. *Hosp Pract* 25(suppl 2):5-7, 1990.

Mavissakalian MR, Perel JM: Imipramine dose-response relationship in panic disorder with agoraphobia: Preliminary findings. *Arch Gen Psychiatry* 46:127-131, 1989.

Mavissakalian M, et al: Tricyclic antidepressants in obsessive-compulsive disorder: Antiobsessional or antidepressant agents? II. *Am J Psychiatry* 142:572-576, 1985.

Mavissakalian MR, et al: Clomipramine in obsessive-compulsive disorder: Clinical response and plasma levels. *J Clin Psychopharmacol* 10:261-268, 1990.

McDougle CJ, et al: A controlled trial of lithium augmentation in fluvoxamine-refractory obsessive-compulsive disorder: Lack of efficacy. *J Clin Psychopharmacol* 11:175-184, 1991.

McTavish D, Benfield P: Clomipramine: An overview of its pharmacological properties and a review of its therapeutic use in obsessive compulsive disorder and panic disorder. *Drugs* 39:136-153, 1990.

Mellinger GD, Balter MB: Psychotherapeutic drugs: Current assessment of prevalence and patterns of use, in Morgan JP, Kagan DV (eds): *Society and Medication: Conflicting Signals for Prescribers and Patients.* Lexington, Mass, Lexington Books, 1983, 137-154.

Mellinger GD, et al: Prevalence and correlates of long-term regular use of anxiolytics. *JAMA* 251:375-379, 1984.

Mellinger GD, et al: Insomnia and its treatment: Prevalence and correlates. *Arch Gen Psychiatry* 42:225-232, 1985.

Merlotti L, et al: The dose effects of zolpidem on the sleep of healthy normals. *J Clin Psychopharmacol* 1:9-14, 1989.

Mitler MM, et al: Hypnotic efficacy of temazepam: A long-term sleep laboratory evaluation. *Br J Clin Pharmacol* 8:63S-68S, 1979.

Mitler MM, et al: Comparative hypnotic effects of flurazepam, triazolam, and placebo: Long-term simultaneous nighttime and daytime study. *J Clin Psychopharmacol* 4:2-16, 1984.

Moon CA, et al: Early morning insomnia and daytime anxiety: A multicentre general practice study comparing loprazolam and triazolam. *Br J Clin Pract* 39:352-358, 1985.

Munjack DJ, et al: A pilot study of buspirone in the treatment of social phobia. *J Anxiety Disord* 5:87-98, 1991.

Murphy SM, Tyrer P: A double-blind comparison of the effects of gradual withdrawal of lorazepam, diazepam and bromazepam in benzodiazepine dependence. *Br J Psychiatry* 158:511-516, 1991.

Murphy SM, et al: Withdrawal symptoms after six weeks' treatment with diazepam. *Lancet* 2:1389, 1984.

Nagy LM, et al: Clinical and medication outcome after short-term alprazolam and behavioral group treatment in panic disorder: 2.5-Year naturalistic follow-up study. *Arch Gen Psychiatry* 46:993-999, 1989.

Newton RE, et al: Side effect profile of buspirone in comparison to active controls and placebo. *J Clin Psychiatry* 43(12, sec 2):100-102, 1982.

Noyes R Jr, et al: Benzodiazepine withdrawal: Review of the evidence. *J Clin Psychiatry* 49:382-389, 1988.

Noyes R Jr, et al: Problems with tricyclic antidepressant use in patients with panic disorder or agoraphobia: Results of a naturalistic follow-up study. *J Clin Psychiatry* 50:163-169, 1989.

Noyes R Jr, et al: Controlled discontinuation of benzodiazepine treatment for patients with panic disorder. *Am J Psychiatry* 148:517-523, 1991.

Ochs HR, et al: Diazepam kinetics in relation to age and sex. *Pharmacology* 23:24-30, 1981.

Ochs RF, et al: An evaluation of the effects of zolpidem in patients with short-term insomnia. *Sleep Res* 21:191, 1992 A.

Ochs R, et al: The effect of zolpidem in elderly patients with chronic insomnia, abstract. *Sleep Res* 21:190, 1992 B.

Oswald I, Adam K: A new look at short-acting hypnotics, in Sauvanet JP, et al (eds): *Imidazopyridines in Sleep Disorders: A Novel Experimental and Therapeutic Approach*. New York, Raven Press, 1988, vol 6 (LERS Monograph Series), 253-259.

Otto MW, et al: Alcohol dependence in panic disorder patients. *J Psychiatr Res* 26:29-38, 1992.

Parkes JD: The sleepy patient. *Lancet* 1:990-993, 1977.

Pasnau RO (chairman): Consequences of anxiety, symposium. *J Clin Psychiatry* 49 (suppl):1-29, 1988.

Pato MT: Treatment of obsessive-compulsive disorder with serotonergic agents. *Drug Ther Suppl* 122-128, (Aug) 1990.

Pato MT, et al: Controlled comparison of buspirone and clomipramine in obsessive-compulsive disorder. *Am J Psychiatry* 148:127-129, 1991.

Pecknold JC, et al: Alprazolam in panic disorder and agoraphobia: Results from a multicenter trial: III. Discontinuation effects. *Arch Gen Psychiatry* 45:429-436, 1988.

Pecknold J, et al: Evaluation of buspirone as an antianxiety agent: Buspirone and diazepam versus placebo. *Can J Psychiatry* 34:766-771, 1989.

Perse TL, et al: Fluvoxamine treatment of obsessive-compulsive disorder. *Am J Psychiatry* 144:1543-1548, 1987.

Peters MD II, et al: Clomipramine: An antiobsessional tricyclic antidepressant. *Clin Pharm* 9:165-178, 1990.

Pierce MW, Shu VS: Efficacy of estazolam: The United States clinical experience. *Am J Med* 88 (suppl 3A):6S-11S, 1990.

Pigott TA, et al: Controlled comparisons of clomipramine and fluoxetine in the treatment of obsessive-compulsive disorder. *Arch Gen Psychiatry* 47:926-932, 1990.

Pigott TA, et al: A double-blind study of adjuvant buspirone hydrochloride in clomipramine-treated patients with obsessive-compulsive disorder. *J Clin Psychopharmacol* 12:11-17, (Feb) 1992.

Pollack MH, et al: Personality disorders in patients with panic disorder: Association with childhood anxiety disorders, early trauma, comorbidity, and chronicity. *Compr Psychiatry* 33:78-83, (March/April) 1992.

Post GL, et al: Estazolam treatment of insomnia in generalized anxiety disorder: A placebo-controlled study. *J Clin Psychopharmacol* 11:249-253, 1991.

Power KG, et al: Controlled study of withdrawal symptoms and rebound anxiety after six week course of diazepam for generalised anxiety. *BMJ* 290:1246-1248, 1985.

Price LH, et al: Treatment of severe obsessive-compulsive disorder with fluvoxamine. *Am J Psychiatry* 144:1059-1061, 1987.

Puech AJ, et al: Comparison of efficacy and safety of triazolam with three other hypnotics in three different populations of insomniacs. *Sleep Res* 20A:378, 1991.

Rakel R: Assessing the efficacy of antianxiety agents. *Am J Med* 82 (suppl 5A):1-6, 1987.

Rapoport JL: The biology of obsessions and compulsions. *Sci Am* 83-89, (March) 1989.

Ray WA, et al: Benzodiazepines of long and short elimination half-life and the risk of hip fracture. *JAMA* 262:3303-3307, 1989.

Regestein QR, et al: Narcolepsy: Initial clinical approach. *J Clin Psychiatry* 44:166-172, 1983.

Regier DA, et al: One-month prevalence of mental disorders in the United States: Based on five epidemiologic catchment area sites. *Arch Gen Psychiatry* 45:977-986, 1988.

Reich J, Yates W: A pilot study of treatment of social phobia with alprazolam. *Am J Psychiatry* 145:590-594, 1988.

Rickels K: Buspirone in clinical practice. *J Clin Psychiatry* 5 (suppl):51-54, 1990.

Rickels K, et al: Buspirone and diazepam in anxiety: Controlled study. *J Clin Psychiatry* 43 (12, sec 2):81-86, 1982.

Rickels K, et al: Long-term diazepam therapy and clinical outcome. *JAMA* 250:767-771, 1983 A.

Rickels K, et al: Diphenhydramine in insomniac family practice patients: Double blind study. *J Clin Pharmacol* 23:235-242, 1983 B.

Rickels K, et al: Doxylamine succinate in insomniac family practice patients: Double-blind study. *Curr Ther Res* 35:532-540, 1984.

Rickels K, et al: Long-term treatment of anxiety and risk of withdrawal: Prospective comparison of clorazepate and buspirone. *Arch Gen Psychiatry* 45:444-450, 1988.

Rickels K, et al: Long-term therapeutic use of benzodiazepines: I. Effects of abrupt discontinuation. *Arch Gen Psychiatry* 47:899-907, 1990.

Robinson GM, et al: Barbiturate and hypnosedative withdrawal by multiple oral phenobarbital loading dose technique. *Clin Pharmacol Ther* 30:71-76, 1981.

Robinson D, et al: Safety and usefulness of buspirone as an anxiolytic drug in elderly versus young patients. *Clin Ther* 10:740-746, 1988.

Roehrs T, et al: Effects of hypnotics on memory. *J Clin Psychopharmacol* 3:310-313, 1983.

Roehrs T, et al: Efficacy of a reduced triazolam dose in elderly insomniacs. *Neurobiol Aging* 6:293-296, 1985.

Roehrs T, et al: Dose effects of temazepam in transient insomnia. *Drug Res* 40:859-862, 1990.

Roger M, et al: Hypnotic effect of zolpidem in geriatric patients: A dose-finding study, in Sauvanet JP, et al (eds): *Imidazopyridines in Sleep Disorders: A Novel Experimental and Therapeutic Approach*. New York, Raven Press, 1988, vol 6 (LERS Monograph Series), 279-287.

Rogers MC, Kirsch JR: Current concepts in brain resuscitation. *JAMA* 261:3143-3147, 1989.

Rosenberg L, et al: Lack of relation of oral clefts to diazepam use during pregnancy. *N Engl J Med* 309:1282-1285, 1983.

Roth T, Roehrs TA: A review of the safety profiles of benzodiazepine hypnotics. *J Clin Psychiatry* 52 (suppl):38-41, 1991.

Rothschild AJ: Disinhibition, amnestic reactions, and other adverse reactions secondary to triazolam: A review of the literature. *J Clin Psychiatry* 53 (12, suppl):69-79, 1992.

Roy-Byrne PP: Integrated treatment of panic disorder. *Am J Med* 92 (suppl 1A):1A-49S-1A-54S, 1992.

Saano V: Central-type and peripheral-type benzodiazepine receptors. *Ann Clin Res* 20:348-355, 1988.

Salzman C: Treatment with antianxiety agents, in: *Treatment of Psychiatric Disorders: A Task Force Report of the American Psychiatric Association.* Washington, DC, American Psychiatric Association, 1989, vol 3, 2036-2051.

Scharf MB, et al: Comparative amnestic effects of benzodiazepine hypnotic agents. *J Clin Psychiatry* 49:134-137, 1988.

Scharf MB, et al: Dose response effects of zolpidem in normal geriatric subjects. *J Clin Psychiatry* 52:77-83, 1991 A.

Scharf M, et al: Dose-response of zolpidem in elderly patients with chronic insomnia, abstract. *Sleep Res* 20:84, 1991 B.

Schnabel T Jr: Evaluation of safety and side effects of antianxiety agents. *Am J Med* 82 (suppl 5A):7-13, 1987.

Schneier FR, et al: Fluoxetine in panic disorder. *J Clin Psychopharmacol* 10:119-121, 1990.

Schott WJ, et al: Drug treatment for sleep apnea. *Ann Pharmacother* 23:308-315, 1989.

Schottstaedt MW, et al: Placidyl abuse: Dimorphic picture. *Crit Care Med* 9:677-679, 1981.

Schuckit MA: Anxiety related to medical disease. *J Clin Psychiatry* 44 (11, sec 2):31-36, 1983.

Schuckit MA: Alcohol and drug interactions with antianxiety medications. *Am J Med* 82 (suppl 5A):27-33, 1987.

Schwartz AR, Smith PL: Sleep apnea in the elderly. *Clin Geriatr Med* 5:315-329, 1989.

Schweitzer PK, et al: Effects of estazolam and triazolam on transient insomnia associated with phase-shifted sleep. *Hum Psychopharmacol* 6:99-107, 1991.

Schweizer E, et al: Resistance to the anti-anxiety effect of buspirone in patients with a history of benzodiazepine use, correspondence. *N Engl J Med* 314:719-720, 1986.

Schweizer E, et al: Lorazepam versus alprazolam in the treatment of panic disorder. *Pharmacopsychiatry* 23:90-93, 1990 A.

Schweizer E, et al: Long-term therapeutic use of benzodiazepines: II. Effects of gradual taper. *Arch Gen Psychiatry* 47:908-915, 1990 B.

Schweizer E, et al: Carbamazepine treatment in patients discontinuing long-term benzodiazepine therapy: Effects on withdrawal severity and outcome. *Arch Gen Psychiatry* 48:448-452, 1991.

Seidel WF, et al: Dose-related effects of triazolam and flurazepam on a circadian rhythm insomnia. *Clin Pharmacol Ther* 40:314-320, 1986.

Sellers EM: Alcohol, barbiturate and benzodiazepine withdrawal syndromes: Clinical management. *Can Med Assoc J* 139:113-118, 1988.

Shader RI, Greenblatt DJ: Benzodiazepines and pregnancy: More to say and more to learn, editorial. *J Clin Psychopharmacol* 9:237, 1989.

Smith AG, DeMatteis F: Drugs and hepatic porphyrias. *Clin Haematol* 9:399-424, 1980.

Snyder SH: Drug and neurotransmitter receptors: New perspectives with clinical relevance. *JAMA* 261:3126-3129, 1989.

Solomon J, et al: Double-blind comparison of lorazepam and chlordiazepoxide in treatment of acute alcohol abstinence syndrome. *Clin Ther* 6:52-58, 1983.

Strand M, et al: A double-blind, controlled trial in primary care patients with generalized anxiety: A comparison between buspirone and oxazepam. *J Clin Psychiatry* 51 (suppl):40-45, 1990.

Swedish National Board of Health and Welfare: Pharmacological treatment of anxiety, workshop. Uppsala, Sweden (Nov 1987), 1988, 7-178.

Swedo SE, et al: Obsessive-compulsive disorder in children and adolescents: Clinical phenomenology of 70 consecutive cases. *Arch Gen Psychiatry* 46:335-341, 1989.

Taylor DC: Buspirone: New approach to the treatment of anxiety. *FASEB J* 2:2445-2452, 1988.

Teicher MH: Biology of anxiety. *Med Clin North Am* 72:791-814, 1988.

Tesar GE: High-potency benzodiazepines for short-term management of panic disorder: The U. S. experience. *J Clin Psychiatry* 51 (suppl):4-10, 1990.

Tesar GE, et al: Double-blind, placebo-controlled comparison of clonazepam and alprazolam for panic disorder. *J Clin Psychiatry* 52:69-76, 1991.

Timms RM, et al: Effect of triazolam on sleep and arterial oxygen saturation in patients with chronic obstructive pulmonary disease. *Arch Intern Med* 148:2159-2163, 1988.

Tollefson GD, et al: Treatment of comorbid generalized anxiety in a recently detoxified alcoholic population with a selective serotonergic drug (buspirone). *J Clin Psychopharmacol* 12:19-26, 1992.

Turner SM, et al: Fluoxetine treatment of obsessive-compulsive disorder. *J Clin Psychopharmacol* 5:207-212, 1985.

Twyman RE, et al: Differential regulation of γ-aminobutyric acid receptor channels by diazepam and phenobarbital. *Ann Neurol* 25:213-220, 1989.

Uhlenhuth EH, et al: Risks and benefits of long-term benzodiazepine use. *J Clin Psychopharmacol* 8:161-167, 1988.

Uhlenhuth EH, et al: Response of panic disorder to fixed doses of alprazolam or imipramine. *J Affective Disord* 17:261-270, 1989.

Vogel G, et al: Effects of chronically administered zolpidem on the sleep of healthy insomniacs. *Sleep Res* 18:80, 1989.

Wheatley D: Zolpidem and placebo: A study in general practice in patients suffering from insomnia, in Sauvanet JP, et al (eds): *Imidazopyridines in Sleep Disorders: A Novel Experimental and Therapeutic Approach*. New York, Raven Press, 1988, vol 6 (LERS Monograph Series), 305-316.

Whitelaw AGL, et al: Effect of maternal lorazepam on neonate. *BMJ* 282:1106-1108, 1981.

Wiggins RV, Schmidt-Nowara WW: Treatment of the obstructive sleep apnea syndrome. *West J Med* 147:561-568, 1987.

Woods JH, et al: Use and abuse of benzodiazepines: Issues relevant to prescribing. *JAMA* 260:3476-3480, 1988.

Woods SW, et al: Controlled trial of alprazolam supplementation during imipramine treatment of panic disorder. *J Clin Psychopharmacol* 12:32-38, 1992.

Wysowski DK, Barash D: Adverse behavioral reactions attributed to triazolam in the Food and Drug Administration's spontaneous reporting system. *Arch Intern Med* 151:2003-2008, 1991.

Zitrin CM, et al: Treatment of phobias: I. Comparison of imipramine hydrochloride and placebo. *Arch Gen Psychiatry* 40:125-138, 1983.

Antipsychotic Drugs

12

Psychoses are characterized by one or more of the following: diminished and distorted capacity to process information and draw logical conclusions, impaired judgment, hallucinations, incoherence or marked loosening of associations, delusions, catatonic or disorganized behavior, excitement, and aggression or violence. Most psychotic syndromes are idiopathic; however, when the underlying disorder is an acute organic mental syndrome (eg, delirium), fluctuating levels of consciousness, disorientation, and loss of recent memory also are observed.

Antipsychotic drugs ameliorate the symptoms of psychosis regardless of the underlying cause. They are useful in mania, acute exacerbations of schizophrenia, schizoaffective disorder, delusional disorder, psychotic disorder Not Otherwise Specified (NOS), brief reactive psychosis that develops in critical care units following surgery or myocardial infarction, psychotic symptoms induced by amphetamine and other stimulants, rage reactions, major depression with psychotic features, and sensory deprivation syndromes, as well as in acute psychotic episodes associated with either delirium or complex partial seizures. In chronic schizophrenia, maintenance therapy with antipsychotic drugs reduces the rate of exacerbations. For other uses of antipsychotic drugs, see the section on Other Indications.

CLASSIFICATION. Antipsychotic drugs also are referred to as *neuroleptics*. Originally, this term was introduced to describe the syndrome of central effects caused by chlorpromazine [Thorazine], which includes suppression of spontaneous motor movements and modification of complex behavior (eg, reduced initiative and interest in the environment, blunted emotional display). Currently, there is a tendency to use this term to refer to the neurologic aspects of these central effects, especially the extrapyramidal reactions that may be associated with use of antipsychotic drugs (Baldessarini, 1990). Neurologic reactions and increased serum prolactin concentrations are predictable effects of the so-called *typical* antipsychotic agents. The risk of extrapyramidal effects is low with *atypical* agents such as clozapine [Clozaril], and this provides a clear distinction between antipsychotic and neuroleptic effects.

Currently available antipsychotic drugs include the phenothiazines, thioxanthenes, butyrophenones, dihydroindolones, dibenzoxazepines, dibenzodiazepines, and diphenylbutylpiperidines (see Table 1). Phenothiazines are classified on the basis of their chemistry (aliphatic, piperidine, or piperazine compounds), pharmacologic actions, and potency. The thioxanthene derivatives, chlorprothixene [Taractan] and thiothixene [Navane], are related chemically to the aliphatic and piperazine phenothiazines, respectively. Haloperidol [Haldol], a butyrophenone; molindone [Moban], a dihydroindolone; loxapine [Loxitane], a dibenzoxazepine; and clozapine, a dibenzodiazepine, are the only representatives of their respective chemical classes available in the United States that are commonly used to treat psychiatric patients. Droperidol [Inapsine], a short-acting butyrophenone used in neuroleptanalgesia and neuroleptanesthesia, has potent sedative and antipsychotic actions and may be useful in drug-induced (eg, amphetamine) psychosis. The diphenylbutylpiperidine, pimozide [Orap], also has an antipsychotic action, but it is principally used in the treatment of Tourette's syndrome (see index entry Pimozide).

Awareness of these categories can be useful in choosing specific drugs for therapy. Results of comparative studies indicate that the typical antipsychotic drugs are approximately equally efficacious, but a patient who does not respond to one drug may respond to or have better tolerance for an agent from a different chemical class. Current evidence suggests that the atypical agent, clozapine, may have relatively greater usefulness in treatment-resistant patients (Kane et al, 1988; Baldessarini and Frankenburg, 1991; Pickar et al, 1992).

The antipsychotic drugs can be divided into high- and low-potency categories based on the dose needed for efficacy. Regardless of chemical class, high-potency compounds tend to produce less sedation and hypotension but more acute extrapyramidal effects. Clinically, it is useful to divide antipsychotic drugs into oral versus depot forms and into agents with atypical versus typical pharmacologic profiles.

The decanoate and enanthate esters of fluphenazine [Prolixin] and the decanoate ester of haloperidol are marketed as long-acting depot preparations for intramuscular or subcutaneous administration (see Table 2). The decanoate esters are used most commonly.

MECHANISM OF ACTION. The etiology of schizophrenia and most other forms of psychosis is unknown. The specific mechanism by which antipsychotic drugs exert their therapeutic effects is not completely understood; however, research has shown that antipsychotic drugs block dopaminergic receptors of the forebrain mesolimbic-mesocortical and nigrostriatal areas, as well as the mammotropic cells of the anterior pituitary. These systems are associated with higher mental and emotional functions, posture and movement, and neuroendocrine functions, respectively. The affinity of antipsychotic drugs for dopaminergic receptors parallels the milligram-dose potency.

Historically, the dopaminergic receptor systems have been classified as follows: (1) D_1 receptors that are associated with stimulation of dopamine-sensitive adenyl cyclase and are blocked by most phenothiazine and thioxanthene antipsychotic agents and clozapine (roughly in proportion to their clinical efficacy) but only weakly by butyrophenone or diphenylbutylpiperidine compounds, and (2) D_2 receptors that may inhibit dopamine-sensitive adenylate cyclase in some tissues and are blocked by nearly all types of antipsychotic agents, including butyrophenones, but only weakly by clozapine. The clinical potency of the antipsychotic drugs correlates well with their affinity for D_2 receptors, which exist in two isoforms; however, the correlation becomes less significant when corrected for plasma:brain drug concentration ratios.

More recently, molecular cloning procedures have revealed the existence of three other types of dopamine receptors, which are termed D_3, D_4, and D_5 (Sokoloff et al, 1990; Sunahara et al, 1991; Van Tol et al, 1991). The D_5 receptor bears a strong homology to D_1, but it has a tenfold higher affinity for the endogenous agonist, dopamine, and is localized primarily to neurons in limbic regions. The D_3 and D_4 receptors are highly homologous to the D_2 receptor. The D_3 receptor is mainly expressed in limbic brain areas or discrete areas of the ventral striatum (eg, olfactory tubercle, nucleus accumbens) that receive afferents from prefrontal, amygdalar, or allocortical areas. Whereas typical antipsychotic agents have a ten- to twentyfold greater affinity for D_2 receptors, the atypical antipsychotic, clozapine, has only a two- to threefold binding preference for D_2 compared with D_3 receptors. The D_4 receptor, which exists in multiple variants (Van Tol et al, 1992) and is found in the frontal cortex, amygdala, and midbrain, has a tenfold higher affinity for clozapine compared with the D_2 receptor. Determination of the relative importance of the D_1, D_3, D_4, and D_5 receptors for mediating the therapeutic effects of antipsychotic drugs will require the development of more specific antagonists.

The antagonism of dopamine in the mesolimbic-mesocortical pathways probably contributes to the therapeutic actions of the antipsychotic drugs. Antagonism of dopamine's action in the striatum (caudate and putamen) probably contributes to many of the characteristic neurologic side effects (eg, parkinsonism, dystonia, akathisia, tardive dyskinesias) of antipsychotic agents. Antagonism of dopamine's neurohormonal action at D_2 receptors in the anterior pituitary to prevent release of prolactin accounts for the hyperprolactinemia associated with antipsychotic and other antidopaminergic agents. The site of the antiemetic action of the antipsychotic drugs is probably the chemoreceptor trigger zone of the medulla.

Antipsychotic drugs affect other transmitter systems, which may contribute to their antipsychotic and antimanic actions as well as produce adverse reactions. They have variable antagonistic actions on muscarinic, alpha-adrenergic, histaminergic, and serotonergic receptors in the brain and peripheral tissues. The antimuscarinic activities of the antipsychotic drugs, especially the low-potency agents, cause blurred vision, dry mouth, and urinary retention and may contribute to excessive sedation or confusion. The alpha-adrenergic blocking actions may cause sedation, orthostatic hypotension, and lightheadedness, especially with low-potency drugs. The antihistaminergic activities of antipsychotic drugs probably contribute to drowsiness and sedation as well. Phenothiazines may weakly inhibit the neuronal uptake of norepinephrine.

TABLE 1.
ANTIPSYCHOTIC DRUGS

Drug	Chemical Classification	Therapeutically Equivalent Oral Dose (mg)	Side Effects: Sedation	Side Effects: Autonomic[1]	Side Effects: Extrapyramidal Reactions[2]
Fluphenazine[3] Permitil (Schering) Prolixin (Apothecon)	Phenothiazine: Piperazine Compound	2	+	+	+++
Haloperidol[3] Haldol (McNeil)	Butyrophenone	2	+	+	+++
Pimozide[4] Orap (Gate)	Diphenylbutylpiperidine	2	+	+	+++
Thiothixene[3] Navane (Roerig)	Thioxanthene	5	+	+	+++
Trifluoperazine[3] Stelazine (SmithKline Beecham)	Phenothiazine: Piperazine Compound	5	++	+	+++
Perphenazine[3] Trilafon (Schering)	Phenothiazine: Piperazine Compound	10	++	+	++/+++
Molindone Moban (Gate)	Dihydroindolone	10	++	+	++
Loxapine[3] Loxitane (Lederle)	Dibenzoxazepine	15	++	+/++	++/+++
Prochlorperazine[3, 4] Compazine (SmithKline Beecham)	Phenothiazine: Piperazine Compound	15	++	+	+++
Triflupromazine Vesprin (Apothecon)	Phenothiazine: Aliphatic Compound	25[5]	+++	++/+++	++
Chlorprothixene Taractan (Roche)	Thioxanthene	50	+++	+++	+/++
Mesoridazine Serentil (Boehringer)	Phenothiazine: Piperidine Compound	50	+++	++	+
Clozapine Clozaril (Sandoz)	Dibenzodiazepine	75	+++	+++	+/−
Chlorpromazine[3] Thorazine (SmithKline Beecham)	Phenothiazine: Aliphatic Compound	100	+++	+++	++
Thioridazine[3] Mellaril (Sandoz)	Phenothiazine: Piperidine Compound	100	+++	+++	+

[1] *Alpha-antiadrenergic and anticholinergic effects*

[2] *Excluding tardive dyskinesia, which appears to be produced to the same degree and frequency by all agents except clozapine with equieffective antipsychotic doses. Clozapine has produced agranulocytosis; therefore, recommendations for its use are limited (see text).*

[3] *Available generically.*

[4] *Pimozide is used principally in the treatment of Tourette's syndrome; prochlorperazine is used rarely, if ever, as an antipsychotic agent.*

[5] *Available only as parenteral product.*

Investigational antipsychotic agents include risperidone [Risperdal] and olanzepine, which inhibit D_2 and 5-HT_2 receptors, and remoxipride, a substituted benzamide that is a weak but selective D_2 receptor antagonist and also antagonizes sigma receptors. Antagonists of 5-HT_3 receptors (eg, ondansetron [Zofran]) also are being investigated for antipsychotic activity.

Results of controlled comparative studies indicate that risperidone (which has received FDA Advisory Committee approval) is equal or superior to haloperidol in patients with chronic schizophrenia (Borison et al, 1992; Claus et al, 1992; Chouinard et al, 1993), most of whom were not treatment-resistant. In a dose range of 4 to 8 mg, risperidone appears to produce less frequent and severe extrapyramidal effects and

TABLE 2.
LONG-ACTING ANTIPSYCHOTIC DRUGS

Drug	Chemical Classification	Route of Administration	Duration of Action
Fluphenazine Decanoate Prolixin Decanoate (Apothecon)	Phenothiazine: Piperazine	Intramuscular Subcutaneous	2-4 weeks
Fluphenazine Enanthate Prolixin Enanthate (Apothecon)	Phenothiazine: Piperazine	Intramuscular Subcutaneous	2 weeks
Haloperidol Decanoate Haldol Decanoate (McNeil)	Butyrophenone	Intramuscular	3-4 weeks

is better tolerated than haloperidol. It is superior to placebo in reducing symptoms of tardive dyskinesia, but further study is required to determine whether this drug will produce less tardive dyskinesia than typical antipsychotic drugs. Like the latter, risperidone increases serum prolactin concentrations.

Schizophrenia (Schizophrenic Disorders)

ETIOLOGY AND DIAGNOSIS. Psychotic symptoms are common and nonspecific, and they may be present in such conditions as delirium, anticholinergic poisoning, hypoglycemia, Wernicke's and Korsakoff's syndromes, mania, melancholia, dementia, and drug intoxication (eg, phencyclidine, cocaine), as well as in schizophrenia. Thus, alternative diagnoses must be considered in the differential diagnosis of schizophrenia if appropriate treatment is to be selected (Manschreck, 1983).

Schizophrenia represents a group of heterogeneous, chronic, idiopathic, psychotic disorders. Symptoms are diverse and include disturbances in perception, attention, affect, and motor behavior and distinctive changes in reasoning. The pattern and outcome of illness are variable. Genetic factors contribute to the etiology. Behavioral and cognitive deficits may occur during early childhood in patients who subsequently develop schizophrenia (DeLisi, 1992; Ambelas, 1992). Overt psychotic symptoms typically become evident during adolescence or early adulthood. This age of onset, combined with evidence derived from epidemiologic, brain imaging, and microscopic pathologic studies (Bracha et al, 1992; Waldman, 1992; Bloom, 1993; Waddington, 1993), suggests that neurodevelopmental anomalies are important etiologic factors.

Ventricular enlargement and corresponding atrophic or cytoarchitectural abnormalities of temporal lobe structures and other related limbic regions have been reported in several studies of schizophrenic patients (Reynolds, 1989; Mesulam, 1990; Andreasen et al, 1990; Suddath et al, 1990; Young et al, 1991), and both asymmetrical and bilateral changes have been noted (Crow, 1990; Conrad et al, 1991). Hypoperfusion or hypometabolism of the frontal cortex and temporal lobe has been a frequent finding in regional studies (Buchsbaum, 1990; Andreasen et al, 1992). Although these findings are not universal and may not be specific, their presence in combination with subtle neurologic deficits indicates that deviation in the brain's structure may be associated with emotional and cognitive disabilities in some patients with schizophrenia (Roberts, 1991). Psychosocial stressors are not considered causal, but they can influence the timing of onset and relapse (Mesulam, 1990).

According to the revised edition of the *Diagnostic and Statistical Manual of Mental Disorders (DSM-III-R)* (American Psychiatric Association, 1987), for a diagnosis of schizophrenia to be made, psychotic symptoms must persist for at least one week (unless the symptoms have responded to therapy). The presence of two of the following symptoms is required for diagnosis: (1) delusions, (2) prominent hallucinations lasting longer than a few moments throughout the day for several days or several times a week for several weeks, (3) incoherence or marked loosening of associations, (4) catatonic behavior, and (5) flat or grossly inappropriate affect. Alternatively, the diagnosis can be made if the delusions are bizarre (ie, involving a phenomenon that the person's culture would regard as totally implausible, such as thought broadcasting or being controlled by another person) or the hallucinations are prominent and auditory (ie, a voice with content having no apparent relation to depression or elation, a voice commenting on the person's behavior or thoughts, two or more voices conversing with each other). In addition to psychotic symptoms, the diagnosis requires marked disturbance of function in areas such as work, social relations, and self-care. Symptoms and signs of disturbance must be present for at least six months.

Prodromal or residual phases may be present when the individual is not in an active phase of the disorder. To identify these phases, at least two of the following symptoms must be present: Marked social isolation or withdrawal; marked impairment in vocational functioning; peculiar behavior (eg, talking to oneself in public, collecting garbage); marked impairment in personal hygiene; blunted or inappropriate affect; manifestations of thought disorder (eg, overelaborate or vague speech, poverty of speech content, metaphorical speech); odd beliefs or magical thinking (eg, severe superstitiousness, belief in telepathy or clairvoyance); unusual perceptual experiences (eg, recurrent illusions); and marked lack of initiative, interests, or energy. Additionally, the diagnosis requires exclusion of an organic mental syndrome (especially delirium, dementia), mental retardation (IQ <85), and other organic factors. If a mood disorder coexists, its duration must be brief in relation to the duration of the active and residual phases of schizophrenia. If there is a history of autism, the added diagnosis of schizophrenia is made only if delusions or hallucinations are prominent.

In an attempt to bring some coherence to their broad range, symptoms of schizophrenia have been divided into two major categories: positive and negative (deficit). Positive symptoms are those that can be regarded as an abnormality, distortion, or exaggeration of normal function (eg, delusions, hallucinations, incoherent speech, agitation). Antipsychotic drugs are often most effective in controlling such symptoms. Negative symptoms are those that indicate a loss or diminution of function, such as poverty of speech content, blunted affect, emotional or social withdrawal, and lack of initiative. Some investigators believe that negative or deficit symptoms represent a distinct pathophysiologic process; however, there is little consensus about what specifically are regarded as negative symptoms or how best to measure their severity (Fenton and McGlashan, 1992). During prolonged observation, both positive and negative features will be apparent in most patients. Furthermore, interpretation of negative symptoms may be obscured because (1) the severity of positive symptoms can influence negative symptoms, and (2) certain negative symptoms may be secondary to positive features, such as depression, anxiety, use of antipsychotic drugs, or environmental deprivation. Thus, although negative symptoms are reportedly more chronic and persistent, less responsive to antipsychotic drugs, and possibly associated with structural abnormalities, they are not necessarily irreversible (Healy, 1989; Kay, 1990).

Although a schizophrenic disorder may undergo partial remission, persistent dysfunction and exacerbations are common and signify the presence of chronic schizophrenia. Patients with chronic schizophrenic disorder may experience stabilization of impairments of affect, volition, insight, and judgment over a prolonged period (years). Suicide rates among schizophrenic individuals are comparable to those for persons with major affective disorders; depression is an important factor in both disorders (Caldwell and Gottesman, 1990).

The principal goals with use of antipsychotic drugs in a chronic schizophrenic disorder are to minimize symptoms and prevent exacerbations; however, not all patients respond to the same degree or at all times. Whether antipsychotic drugs play a therapeutic or prophylactic role, results of controlled studies demonstrate that they reduce the exacerbation rate in chronic schizophrenia by about two and one-half times (Davis and Andriukaitis, 1986).

MANAGEMENT. Active Phase Schizophrenia: The pharmacologic treatment of active phase schizophrenia is indicated when symptoms significantly disrupt the patient's ability to perform important daily routines at work and at home. In more severe and critical cases, loss of behavioral control may threaten the well-being of the individual (including suicide) or of others. Generally, an antipsychotic drug should be tried in every patient who experiences an exacerbation of schizophrenia; however, drug therapy should be undertaken with caution if severe adverse effects were experienced during past episodes.

When agitation and combativeness are present in severe active phase schizophrenia, they often are managed by parenteral (usually intramuscular) administration of an antipsychotic drug. Parenteral therapy may hasten the onset of the sedative if not antipsychotic effect but, more important, bioavailability is assured. Some psychiatrists employ benzodiazepines initially to reduce the dose of antipsychotic drug required, thus lessening the risk of toxicity, especially extrapyramidal and hypothalamic symptoms (Rifkin and Siris, 1987). In one comparative study, intramuscular administration of lorazepam [Ativan] 2 mg was as effective as haloperidol 5 mg in controlling disruptive and aggressive psychotic behavior and caused less severe adverse effects (Salzman et al, 1991). In another study, acutely psychotic patients treated with alprazolam [Xanax] required significantly smaller doses of haloperidol and experienced fewer dystonic reactions during the first 72 hours after hospitalization (Barbee et al, 1992).

When intramuscular administration is indicated, haloperidol, fluphenazine hydrochloride [Prolixin], or an equivalent drug is injected at intervals of four to eight hours until the patient is calm. Total daily doses of 5 to 20 mg of haloperidol usually are sufficient. However, not all patients respond satisfactorily.

The value and safety of more rapid escalation of dosage in those with active psychosis are not proved (Donaldson et al, 1986; Baldessarini et al, 1988). Many controlled studies have concluded that improvement in severe psychosis is not expedited by use of unusually large or rapidly increased doses of potent antipsychotic drugs, and the incidence of acute dystonic reactions increases when larger doses of antipsychotics are given more frequently (especially in young men); rarely, deaths have been associated with such aggressive, rapid dosing.

Some authorities recommend the prophylactic use of a centrally acting anticholinergic drug (eg, oral benztropine [Cogentin] 2 mg once or twice daily) beginning with the first dose of antipsychotic drug and continuing during the initial weeks of treatment to minimize the risk of acute dystonic reactions as well as of other extrapyramidal effects commonly associated with large doses of potent antipsychotic agents. Since these side effects are a major cause of noncompliance leading to relapse, the use of anticholinergic drugs could minimize this problem. Other physicians oppose this practice as being unnecessarily complicated and reserve prophylactic use of anticholinergic drugs for patients who cannot be monitored closely or for those in whom large doses of potent antipsychotic drugs are required, especially young males. Use of an anticholinergic drug then is initiated when clinically significant acute extrapyramidal reactions develop during antipsychotic drug therapy.

If psychotic symptoms are not severe and cooperation or safety is not a problem, the oral route is preferred. Liquid preparations are more reliably administered and are absorbed somewhat more readily but may be inconvenient. Since the nominal half-life of most antipsychotic drugs is at least 20 hours and may be more than several days for some drugs (eg, haloperidol), prolonged-release oral preparations are not needed and may decrease drug absorption. Oral doses of a low-, mid-, or high-potency antipsychotic drug are given daily after assessment of the individual situation. Although too gradual an increase in dosage and administration of inadequate amounts sometimes cause early treatment failure, excessive dosing and too rapid increase of dose during the first days and weeks of treatment are more common errors. For acute episodes, daily dosages generally should not exceed the equivalent of 15 to 20 mg of haloperidol during the initial phase of treatment (Kane and Marder, 1993). The lowest dose that achieves a therapeutic effect with minimal extrapyramidal signs should be used.

In newly diagnosed patients, some degree of response to an antipsychotic drug may be evident within one to two days of adequate treatment, although, for some individuals, substantial improvement is not observed until the drug has been given for several weeks. In the great majority of patients, after the initial response, improvement of many symptoms (eg, agitation, combativeness, hallucinations, paranoia) continues over the next six to eight weeks (and in many cases even longer). Identifying predictors of outcome in first episodes of schizophrenia has received considerable attention (for review, see Lieberman, 1993). Variables that have been associated with unfavorable outcome include poor premorbid adjustment, significant cognitive or memory impairment, young age or gradual mode of onset, positive family history, long duration of psychosis before treatment, absence of affective features, and male gender.

The therapeutic alliance between physician and patient is important to optimize compliance and appropriate dosage adjustment. In some psychotic patients, side effects of antipsychotic drugs may masquerade as worsening of the disorder or contribute to symptoms. For example, akathisia can resemble or exacerbate agitation, and anxiety or akinesia can be mistaken for depression or "negative" symptoms. In such instances, improvement may occur if the dose is decreased.

If the desired therapeutic effect is not attained after an adequate trial (generally considered to be about six weeks with daily oral doses equivalent to a maximum of 800 mg of chlorpromazine or 20 mg of a high-potency agent), a drug from a different chemical class can be substituted. If the new drug is as potent as the previous drug, substitution of a near-equivalent dose of the new drug usually can be made quickly. However, equivalent doses of high-potency and low-potency agents cannot be substituted rapidly because of the different pattern of side effects. Alternative strategies (eg, decreasing the dose, allowing more time for response, administering clozapine) are equally important measures to consider (see discussion on Treatment Resistance).

Maintenance Therapy: The goal in management is to limit the duration of acute psychotic episodes and prevent relapses. The relapse or exacerbation rate after successful medical treatment of an acute episode of schizophrenia is about 5% of patients per month for at least 6 to 12 months, but the course in individual patients is quite variable. For many, even though treatment for relapses may be adequate, recovery from each episode may be incomplete. Maintenance therapy decreases the exacerbation rate two- to threefold, but also increases the risk of extrapyramidal side effects and tardive dyskinesia. However, in view of the success of prophylactic antipsychotic therapy, the use of these drugs generally is justified for at least one year after remission (Kane and Lieberman, 1987), and many patients continue drug therapy for two to three years or longer. The antipsychotic drugs may be required indefinitely or at least intermittently if two or more exacerbations occur. As in active phase schizophrenia, the maintenance dose should be the lowest amount that maintains the therapeutic response, causes the least troublesome side effects, allows optimal function, and prevents relapse.

In recent years, a number of studies have focused on strategies to improve the benefit-to-risk ratio of long-term pharmacotherapy in schizophrenia. In many studies that compared usual with unusually large doses, no correlation was found between dose and efficacy in preventing relapse (Aubree and Lader, 1980; Baldessarini et al, 1988). Other investigators reported that dosage reduction can improve objective and subjective measures of well-being but that the risk of exacerbation of psychoses rises as doses decrease, particularly with daily doses equivalent to less than 100 mg of chlorpromazine (Kane et al, 1986; Marder et al, 1987; Baldessarini et al, 1988). However, most exacerbations were readily controlled by increasing the dosage temporarily, and the patients rarely required rehospitalization. Thus, relapse and rehospitalization rates may be reduced in some individuals by an early intervention strategy involving (1) education of patients and family members about prodromal symptoms, (2) close monitoring, (3) continuous use of moderate doses of an antipsychotic drug, and (4) prompt increase of dose in combination with supportive interventions if predictable stress or prodromal signs of exacerbation appear (Herz et al, 1991). Gradual reduction of dose to a minimum effective amount should be attempted whenever careful monitoring of the patient is possible or when past history indicates that the consequences of relapse do not lead to behavior that would be dangerous to the patient or others (Kane and Lieberman, 1987; Baldessarini et al, 1988).

Intermittent prophylaxis has been suggested as a viable strategy for maintenance treatment. This approach involves gradually reducing the dose and extending the time that the patient is not receiving medication, careful monitoring for prodromal signs of exacerbation, and reinstituting medication when early signs of relapse are detected. Although results of open studies indicate that some patients tolerate this approach (Herz et al, 1982; Carpenter et al, 1987), continuous maintenance therapy has been superior for prevention of psychotic symptoms in most individuals (Baldessarini, 1985; Jolley et al, 1990; Herz et al, 1991); thus, intermittent prophylaxis is not recommended.

Both the parenteral depot and oral routes are useful for maintenance therapy. With oral administration, the drug is given daily; depot subcutaneous or intramuscular preparations are administered at intervals, usually of two to four weeks.

When the oral route is selected, the daily dose can be given in divided amounts initially to minimize adverse reactions until a satisfactory maintenance dose has been established. Thereafter, one, or occasionally two, doses are administered daily unless adverse reactions increase. A single dose at bedtime is preferred to take advantage of the sedation produced, to minimize drowsiness during the day, to decrease the incidence of orthostatic hypotension, and to facilitate compliance.

Depot formulations, which utilize high-potency drugs that are eliminated very gradually, produce more consistent drug concentrations and often are preferred for patients suspected of being poorly compliant or when response to oral medication is otherwise unsatisfactory. Other patients also can benefit from their use. Clinicians in the United States underutilize the depot route compared with physicians in Europe and Asia, apparently because of concern about extrapyramidal reactions. However, the risks of major side effects or intolerance do not appear to be greater than with standard oral preparations when the lowest effective dosage is used (Glazer and Kane, 1992).

Traditional insight-oriented psychotherapy offers little demonstrated benefit for schizophrenia, although education and support by health professionals can help both patient and family understand the nature and treatment of the disorder and facilitate rehabilitation and cooperation. Social support systems (family, social services, occupational therapy) and well-designed, individualized, behaviorally oriented rehabilitative efforts of limited intensity in a sheltered environment may help develop coping skills. Initial as well as repeated periods of treatment in an institutional setting may be necessary.

For guidelines on the prevention of relapse in chronic schizophrenic patients, see Hogarty, 1993.

DRUG SELECTION. Numerous controlled studies have determined that patterns of response to any standard antipsychotic drug are similar among patients with various types of schizophrenia (eg, disorganized, paranoid, catatonic, undifferentiated). Thus, despite differences in potency, all commonly used antipsychotic drugs are about equally effective in equivalent doses; however, an individual patient may be more responsive to, or tolerant of, one drug than another (Rifkin and Siris, 1987). Clozapine in particular has been effective in some severely disturbed, treatment-resistant patients. The incidence of most acute extrapyramidal effects is low with this drug; however, large doses can cause seizures as well as agranulocytosis, which has been fatal. Thus, clozapine is recommended for patients who have not responded to or who have experienced severe extrapyramidal reactions or tardive dyskinesia with other antipsychotic drugs (Marder and Van Putten, 1988; Weintraub and Evans, 1989).

Drug selection is determined mainly by past response and potential adverse effects. The incidence and severity of untoward effects produced by each drug should be taken into account, because the potential adverse reactions that the patient accepts are essential considerations in compliance. The history of a favorable response to a particular antipsychotic agent by the patient or family members suggests its use initially. Conversely, a previously unfavorable response to adequate doses tends to militate against use of that drug. The patient's age and physical condition and the cost of the drug are other significant factors. Since sensitivity or tolerance varies among patients and in a given patient over time, individualization of dosage and treatment procedures is required.

Antipsychotic drugs are arranged in decreasing order of potency in Table 1. Sedative and autonomic effects are less prominent with high-potency drugs, but these agents are more likely to produce acute extrapyramidal reactions (dystonia, akathisia, parkinsonism). With minor exceptions, the reverse is noted as potency decreases. Allergic, systemic (cholestatic jaundice and bone marrow depression), cutaneous, and ophthalmic reactions are more prominent with low-potency drugs. With the exception of clozapine, there is no evidence that a given antipsychotic drug is more or less likely than another to produce tardive dyskinesia (Baldessarini and Frankenburg, 1991). A rational approach is for the physician to become proficient in the use of at least one low-potency, one high-potency, and one atypical antipsychotic drug.

Antipsychotic drugs also are about equally efficacious when administered parenterally. Fluphenazine hydrochloride, trifluoperazine [Stelazine], thiothixene, loxapine, and haloperidol are often given parenterally, although this route is relatively costly. These high-potency antipsychotic drugs are preferred for injection because less discomfort and tissue damage are observed and the incidence of hypotensive reactions is considerably reduced compared with chlorpromazine and other low-potency drugs given by this route. However, the risk of extrapyramidal signs and symptoms is increased.

The phenothiazines, thioxanthenes, loxapine, molindone, and pimozide are extensively metabolized, and haloperidol is biotransformed via oxidation to inactive compounds and via reduction to a much less active metabolite. Monitoring the plasma concentration is not useful routinely; its benefits are limited to assessing compliance and bioavailability in clinical studies and evaluating patients who are not responding to treatment. The most established standard is for haloperidol, therapeutic blood concentrations of which typically are 5 to 15 ng/ml (Baldessarini et al, 1988). Therapeutic plasma levels that offer the best risk-benefit ratio also have been tentatively identified for perphenazine [Trilafon] (0.8 to 2.4 ng/ml), fluphenazine (0.2 to 2 ng/ml), and chlorpromazine (30 to 100 ng/ml) (Van Putten et al, 1991). Standardization of optimal therapeutic plasma levels is difficult because of wide individual variance and the presence of active metabolites for most agents.

TREATMENT RESISTANCE. Despite adequate trials (ie, dosage, duration, compliance) with no less than two standard antipsychotic drugs, at least moderate positive and negative symptoms, as well as impaired social function, persist in perhaps 25% of schizophrenic patients (Meltzer, 1992).

Treatment-resistant patients who are compliant and have access to an adequate system of care generally should receive clozapine alone for up to six months. It has been suggested that pimozide may be an alternative in those who are particularly disabled by treatment-resistant negative symptoms (Opler and Feinberg, 1991); preliminary evidence derived from open trials suggests that the "activating" antidepressants (ie, tranylcypromine, fluoxetine) also may be of value in the treatment of negative symptoms (Bucci, 1987; Goff et al, 1990).

Combinations of antipsychotic drugs are no more effective than adequate doses of a single agent. The addition of lithium to an antipsychotic drug regimen in patients refractory to the antipsychotic alone may enhance the therapeutic response, especially if there is evidence that an affective illness or agitation also is present. In several double-blind studies, carbamazepine [Tegretol] was moderately beneficial as an adjunct in the treatment of schizophrenic patients with aggressive or violent behavior or agitation that did not respond satisfactorily to an antipsychotic drug (Klein et al, 1984; Dose et al, 1987; Okuma et al, 1989). However, concomitant therapy with carbamazepine can decrease the plasma concentration of antipsychotic drugs. Carbamazepine also may be useful in schizophrenic patients with EEG abnormalities of the temporal lobe (Neppe, 1983). Alprazolam and other benzodiazepines may enhance the effect of antipsychotic drugs (see Wolkowitz and Pickar, 1991). Adjunctive therapy with other types of medication occasionally may be helpful in patients whose response to antipsychotic drugs is only partial.

For reviews of drugs other than antipsychotics in the treatment of schizophrenia and therapeutic options for treatment-resistant patients, see Christison et al, 1991; Meltzer, 1992.

Other Indications

MANIA. Lithium is a relatively selective agent for mania. However, because it has a longer latent period than the antipsychotic drugs, one of the latter often is administered alone or with lithium in initial treatment, especially for severe manifestations or temporarily when alternative treatments fail to control treatment-resistant or rapidly cycling bipolar disorder. Once behavior has been controlled and lithium has become effective, the dosage of the antipsychotic drug may be reduced and, in some patients, the drug eventually may be discontinued (see index entry Lithium).

SCHIZOAFFECTIVE DISORDER. Diagnosis of this poorly validated disorder requires that a major depressive or manic syndrome be present in addition to psychotic symptoms. Schizoaffective disorder responds to antipsychotic drugs; however, lithium, an antidepressant, or antiepileptic drug (eg, carbamazepine, valproate) may have to be added to the regimen for more complete control. Lithium may be preferred for long-term prophylaxis in some patients.

DELUSIONAL DISORDER. This disorder is characterized by an organized, persistent, nonbizarre delusion in an otherwise relatively intact personality without features of schizophrenia or significant affective symptoms (American Psychiatric Association, 1987). Some patients respond adequately to antipsychotic drugs but may require prolonged treatment. However, paranoia of this type often is resistant to antipsychotic drugs, especially in elderly patients, and the efficacy of alternative treatments is not established.

Paranoid features may be found in many psychiatric, neurologic, metabolic, and endocrine disorders, as well as in substance-induced psychoses (eg, alcohol, amphetamine, cocaine, phencyclidine). The antipsychotic drug regimens described for schizophrenia are used for other forms of psychosis with predominant or extensive paranoid features.

ORGANIC MENTAL SYNDROMES. Antipsychotic drugs can be useful in acute psychotic episodes associated with organic mental syndromes, including substance-induced syndromes (toxic psychoses or delirium) and acute idiopathic psychoses. However, the low-potency drugs may compound some forms of toxicity (eg, toxic delirium caused by drugs with considerable anticholinergic activity may be exacerbated and prolonged by low-potency antipsychotic agents, which also have anticholinergic properties). The cautious administration of small doses of a higher potency antipsychotic drug may be justified and may reduce confusion, agitation, and hyperactivity in patients with delirium or dementia with psychotic features; they may help control behavioral problems that impair management and in those who do not respond to appropriate nursing care (see index entries Delirium; Dementia). However, concern is mounting that the antipsychotic drugs are overprescribed, especially in patients in custodial and intermediate long-term care facilities. The consequences of antipsychotic-induced oversedation, orthostatic hypotension, and anticholinergic side effects that lead to mental deterioration, falls and fractures, and bowel and bladder dysfunction in frail, elderly patients are well documented (Riesenberg, 1988).

PERVASIVE DEVELOPMENTAL DISORDER (AUTISM). Antipsychotic drug therapy can be useful in the treatment of some autistic individuals as one component of a comprehensive program that includes behavior modification and education in a highly structured environment (Campbell, 1989). The low-potency agents probably are not as well tolerated as high-potency agents. In some studies, haloperidol has been effective in children with prominent symptoms of withdrawal, hyperactivity, and aggressive and stereotyped behavior (Campbell et al, 1984). When combined with behavioral therapy, this drug also improved the acquisition of language. Other clinical experience suggests that only the overt behavioral manifestations improve (Biederman and Jellinek, 1984).

MENTAL RETARDATION. High-potency antipsychotic agents sometimes are used in agitated patients with severe mental retardation. These drugs may alleviate irritability, disturbed sleep, agitation, hostility, and combativeness and may improve social behavior and concentration. However, they do not improve speech, communication, or the mental deficiency. No high-potency agent is more effective than another. Low-potency drugs are not preferred due to excessive sedation and other side effects. Because of the danger of tardive dyskinesia, use of antipsychotic drugs in children and adolescents with behavior disorders other than schizophrenia or autism should be approached cautiously and reviewed critically on a regular basis.

HUNTINGTON'S DISEASE. Although antipsychotic drugs do not reverse or halt the progression of dementia or other neurologic deficits in Huntington's disease, they ameliorate and control chorea and agitation, especially in earlier stages. Dopamine-depleting drugs, such as tetrabenazine and reserpine, also are being investigated (see index entry Huntington's Disease).

TOURETTE'S SYNDROME. Antipsychotic agents can be effective in Tourette's syndrome, a heterogenous neurobehavioral disorder associated with motor and vocal tics of variable form and severity. Precise dosage adjustment is difficult in these patients. Most clinical experience has been obtained with haloperidol, although evidence of its specificity is limited. The development of a school avoidance syndrome in young patients or a social phobia in older patients is an unusual adverse reaction produced by haloperidol (Mikkelsen et al, 1981). The effectiveness of pimozide also has been demonstrated, and it is an alternative for those who do not respond to or cannot tolerate haloperidol. Clonidine [Catapres] is another alternative; it is effective in about two-thirds of such patients (Cohen et al, 1980). (See index entry Tourette's Syndrome.)

BALLISM (BALLISMUS). This disorder is characterized by continual, usually unilateral (hemiballism), purposeless, "flinging" movements of the extremities (particularly the arms). Antipsychotic drugs are the agents of choice for treatment. For further information, see index entry Ballism, Description, Etiology, Treatment.

MISCELLANEOUS USES. Chlorpromazine is indicated (and other antipsychotic drugs have been used) in the treatment of *intractable hiccups*.

Although all antipsychotic drugs potentiate the effects of hypnotic, analgesic, and anesthetic agents, the antipsychotic drug, droperidol (a butyrophenone related to haloperidol), is used mainly as an *adjunct to anesthesia*. (See index entry Droperidol.)

With the exception of mesoridazine [Serentil], molindone, thioridazine [Mellaril], and clozapine, most antipsychotic drugs have a pronounced *antiemetic* action (see index entry Vomiting).

Results of some placebo-controlled studies indicate that low doses of high-potency antipsychotics may be effective for a broad spectrum of symptoms (eg, anger and hostility, impulsiveness, paranoid ideation, ideas of reference) in patients with *borderline personality disorder* (Soloff et al, 1986; Goldberg et al, 1986; Cowdry and Gardner, 1988; Soloff et al, 1993). They may be used in this condition and other severe personality disorders, such as *schizotypal personality*, when a benefit-risk ratio is clearly established in individual patients. Antipsychotic drugs are of no value in *uncomplicated acute or chronic alcoholism,* but they may be useful when hallucinations or psychoses complicate such disorders. However, because antipsychotic drugs may lower the seizure threshold, they should be used with caution during acute alcohol withdrawal reactions.

All antipsychotic drugs produce varying degrees of sedation. They have been inappropriately termed major tranquilizers and prescribed for patients with *anxiety.* Benzodiazepines are more effective and better tolerated by most anxious patients than even small doses of an antipsychotic drug. An antidepressant usually is preferred when anxiety is associated with depression, panic disorder, or obsessive-compulsive disorder; however, concurrent use of an antidepressant and an antipsychotic drug is indicated in major depression with psychotic features.

Adverse Reactions

Antipsychotic drugs are characterized by a high therapeutic index with respect to mortality, but side effects occur routinely at therapeutic doses. Overdose is seldom fatal in adults, and most adverse reactions are not life-threatening. However, the characteristic neurologic side effects of these drugs are particularly troublesome, often limit the tolerated dose, and may interfere with therapeutic effects and compliance. Close and critical clinical observation is essential to monitor the patient's progress and detect adverse reactions promptly. Although selected laboratory tests based on individual patient characteristics are advisable to establish baseline values, frequent laboratory tests are unnecessary and have little predictive value.

CENTRAL EFFECTS. Sedation is common after use of all antipsychotic drugs and is especially pronounced after large doses of the low-potency phenothiazines (chlorpromazine, triflupromazine, mesoridazine, thioridazine, chlorprothixene, and clozapine). (See Table 1.) It can be minimized by reducing the dose or substituting a less sedating agent. However, sedation decreases during long-term treatment and many patients become tolerant to this effect. Daytime somnolence usually can be minimized by giving a single dose at bedtime.

Toxic delirium generally occurs with agents that have a pronounced anticholinergic effect (see Table 1) and may be difficult to differentiate from deterioration in schizophrenia. Reactions are characterized by exacerbation of psychotic symptomatology, confusion, marked sedation or insomnia associated with bizarre dreams, dysarthria, extrapyramidal signs, and general impairment of psychomotor activity. Dosage reduction usually ameliorates the condition, although nonspecific withdrawal symptoms may follow discontinuation of treatment, especially with low-potency agents. Substituting an antipsychotic drug with less anticholinergic activity also may be helpful, particularly if an anticholinergic drug is being prescribed simultaneously.

EXTRAPYRAMIDAL REACTIONS. Two of these common reactions, acute dystonia and akathisia, occur early during treatment (within hours to days). The risk of developing dystonia diminishes after one to two weeks. A third reaction, parkinsonism, tends to evolve gradually over days to weeks. All three reactions are especially characteristic of the high-potency antipsychotic drugs (see Table 1). In one recent study, 62% of a group of patients experiencing their first episode of schizophrenia developed acute extrapyramidal symptoms during eight weeks of treatment with fluphenazine 20 to 40 mg/day (Chakos et al, 1992). The low-potency aliphatic and piperidine phenothiazines (chlorpromazine, mesoridazine, and thioridazine) are less likely to cause these reactions. The dibenzodiazepine, clozapine, is least likely to produce dystonia and parkinsonism but occasionally can cause akathisia.

A fourth reaction, tardive (late) dyskinesia, is a global term that encompasses orobuccal-lingual dyskinetic syndromes and widespread choreoathetosis. Other late-occurring movement disorders include tardive dystonia, tardive akathisia, tardive tic, and tardive myoclonus syndromes (Kang and Fahn, 1988; Teoh, 1988). Tardive dyskinesias usually are not observed for months to years after initiation of therapy, and all commonly used antipsychotic drugs have been associated with these reactions. To date, no cases of tardive dyskinesia have been reported when clozapine is used as the sole antipsychotic agent. (See discussion on Tardive Dyskinesia below.)

Although anticholinergic drugs reduce the severity of some acute extrapyramidal effects (especially dystonia and parkinsonism), there is both support and concern about their routine prophylactic use with antipsychotic drugs. Those who oppose routine concomitant administration emphasize the risks, which include additive anticholinergic toxicity, complexity of management, and cost. Those who favor prophylactic use note that some extrapyramidal side effects are subtle, easy to miss, and tend to continue indefinitely. Furthermore, avoidance of side effects can improve compliance, and some outpatients may not have ready access to a physician. Some authorities suggest that routine prophylactic use of an anticholinergic compound is most appropriate for young males receiving a high-potency antipsychotic drug (Arana et al, 1988). The physician must weigh these issues with each individual patient.

Initial treatment with an antipsychotic alone (adding an anticholinergic later if necessary) or with both classes of drugs is acceptable, particularly for hospitalized or otherwise closely supervised, cooperative patients. When the latter regimen is selected, it is important to remember that acute dystonia, akathisia, and parkinsonism can occur early in treatment. Therefore, if these side effects do not occur within one month, the dose of the anticholinergic should be reduced gradually and the drug discontinued if possible. In many patients, bradykinesia or parkinsonism and akathisia continue after many months or even years of treatment. If slow withdrawal of the anticholinergic leads to worsening of extrapyramidal symptoms, the anticholinergic drug may be added again. Anticholinergic drugs are often difficult to withdraw. It is important to realize that their half-life is much shorter than that of antipsychotics; thus, when both are to be discontinued, the anticholinergic should be withdrawn more gradually and continued for at least one week after withdrawal of the antipsychotic drug.

Acute Dystonia: Acute dystonic reactions are noted most frequently following administration of a high-potency antipsychotic drug, and patients should be warned of this possibility. Young males are at increased risk; this may, in part, reflect use of larger doses in males (Chakos et al, 1992). Acute reactions often are bizarre and abrupt in onset; they may be confused with tetanus, hysteria, epilepsy, meningitis, encephalitis, or stroke, and patients have been treated for these disorders erroneously.

Acute dystonia generally occurs within several hours to days of initial therapy or increases in dosage. It is characterized primarily by abnormal, sustained, posturing movements of the neck, jaw, trunk, and eyes (ie, spastic torticollis, opisthotonus, grimacing, blepharospasm, perioral spasms, dysphagia, impaired respiration) often with protrusion of the tongue, masseter spasms, and oculogyric crisis. Hyperhidrosis, pallor, fever, marked anxiety or tremor, laryngeal and pharyngeal spasm with dysphagia or dyspnea, asphyxia, and cyanosis also have been reported, and fatalities have occurred rarely, presumably due to asphyxia.

Dystonia should be treated by temporarily discontinuing antipsychotic therapy and administering a centrally acting anticholinergic agent (eg, benztropine 1 to 2 mg intramuscularly or intravenously, trihexyphenidyl [Artane] 5 mg initially orally) or an antihistamine (eg, diphenhydramine [Benadryl] 25 to 50 mg intramuscularly or intravenously) to alleviate symptoms during the adaptive phase. Parenteral administration is preferable to oral therapy for more rapid termination of abnormal movements, especially when life-threatening pharyngeal or laryngeal spasm develops.

Akathisia: This disorder is characterized by a feeling of intense restlessness, and the resultant uncomfortable pacing and agitation may mimic an anxiety disorder. It can appear immediately but most commonly occurs within a few weeks to a few months after initiation of therapy, and it typically persists. Akathisia is a frequent cause of noncompliance and also may contribute to behavioral deterioration. Because this condition is frequently mistaken for psychotic agitation, the dose of the antipsychotic agent may be increased unnecessarily, and thus exacerbate the akathisia. Attempts should be made to reduce the dose or substitute a low-potency antipsychotic drug. Anticholinergic agents may be administered, although their efficacy in relieving akathisia is inconsistent and limited at best. Propranolol [Inderal] can be given in low doses (eg, 10 mg three times daily) and the amount gradually increased to a maximum of 90 to 120 mg daily. Alternatively, or if subjective distress continues, a benzodiazepine (eg, lorazepam 1 to 3 mg in divided doses, clonazepam [Klonopin] 0.5 to 1 mg daily, diazepam [Valium] 15 mg daily) may be used. If these agents do not provide relief, there are limited data to suggest that clonidine and amantadine [Symmetrel] may be beneficial. The pharmacologic treatment of neuroleptic-induced akathisia has been reviewed (Fleischhacker et al, 1990).

Parkinsonism: Symptoms similar to those of Parkinson's disease (rigidity, bradykinesia, shuffling gait, postural abnormalities, mask-like facies, and hypersalivation, but variable tremor) may develop gradually over a few days to a few weeks after initiating therapy. Clinically, this syndrome is indistinguishable from postencephalitic or idiopathic Parkinson's disease, although tremor tends to be a minor feature in the antipsychotic drug-induced form.

It is important not to confuse the bradykinesia, mask-like facies, and apathy of parkinsonism with the diminished affect of major depression or the apathy of schizophrenia. Oral administration of a central anticholinergic drug or amantadine often controls this condition; the dose of antipsychotic drug may be reduced if psychotic symptoms do not worsen.

Tardive Dyskinesia: This late-occurring condition (months to years) is characterized classically by choreiform movements of the face, jaw, tongue, trunk, and extremities. Each choreiform movement is a single muscle jerk (tic); however, novel patterns of movement emerge because the patient attempts to mask the tics by incorporating them into semipurposeful movements. A to-and-fro pattern of trunk movement and sustained posturing movements can complicate the differentiation of this condition from other dystonic syndromes. The disorder ranges in severity from mild isolated dyskinesias, usually of the choreiform type, to widespread disabling dystonias and akathisia that interfere with walking, eating, and skilled motor control. Tardive dyskinesias disappear during sleep and worsen with heightened arousal or anxiety; they also tend to respond poorly or to worsen on exposure to anticholinergic agents.

Differential diagnosis of tardive dyskinesia can be complex. For example, minor movements may be difficult to distinguish from habit spasms, mannerisms, or the spontaneous chewing movements seen in many normal elderly patients (senile chorea). Supersensitivity of postsynaptic dopamine receptors may be a pathophysiologic factor in tardive dyskinesia (Stahl et al, 1982; Friedman et al, 1983; Tarsy and Baldessarini, 1984), but the cause of this condition remains unclear.

One disturbing recent observation involves the adverse effects of some antipsychotics on complex I of the mitochondrial electron transport chain (Burkhardt et al, 1993). Haloperidol is structurally similar to the neurotoxin, 1-methyl-4-phenyl-1,2,3,6-tetra-hydropyridine (MPTP), which destroys dopaminergic neurons and can cause parkinsonism. Like MPTP, haloperidol, chlorpromazine, and thiothixene inhibit complex I in vitro in mitochondria. It remains to be determined whether inhibition of complex I causes or contributes to the extrapyramidal side effects of these drugs.

The incidence of tardive dyskinesia is greatest during the first five years of treatment with antipsychotic drugs, although the disorder can develop many years after the first exposure (Glazer et al, 1993). In young adults, the average incidence is approximately 5% per year of antipsychotic drug therapy with a five-year risk of 20% (American Psychiatric Association, 1992; Glazer et al, 1993). Most cases are mild, but some are seriously disabling. Results of long-term studies indicate that the course of tardive dyskinesia can be intermittent, with remission and exacerbation observed in patients who continue to receive antipsychotic therapy (Glazer et al, 1991). As many as two out of three patients receiving maintenance therapy for 25 years may develop tardive dyskinesia (Glazer et al, 1993).

The elderly and possibly those with a major affective disorder are at increased risk. The early occurrence of drug-induced parkinsonism may indicate increased vulnerability for the development of tardive dyskinesia. In the elderly, tardive dyskinesias are more frequent, severe, and less readily reversible (Tarsy and Baldessarini, 1984; Saltz et al, 1991). Similar reactions also have been reported in children, who develop chorea and sometimes behavioral changes that are especially evident when an antipsychotic is discontinued temporarily. At all ages, symptoms characteristically are unmasked or aggravated by the abrupt discontinuation of antipsychotic drugs. If the symptoms gradually disappear over days to weeks after medication is withdrawn, they usually are termed "withdrawal-emergent dyskinesias." Many patients with persistent tardive dyskinesia, especially younger persons, improve significantly within months, while some patients require one year or more (Glazer et al, 1984); rates of remission probably increase if the dose is reduced.

Drugs available to treat tardive dyskinesia are not satisfactory (see also index entry Extrapyramidal Movement Disorders). Therefore, prevention of the disorder is critical and the following guidelines have been recommended: (1) Educate the patient and family regarding benefits and risks. Obtain informed consent for long-term treatment and document this in the medical records. (2) In acute psychoses, antipsychotic drugs should be reserved for time-limited treatment, including first attacks of schizophrenia, paranoia, mania, some cases of toxic or organic psychoses, childhood psychoses, and as adjuncts in psychotic depression. (3) The use of these drugs for longer than three months is indicated only in chronic psychotic disorders, primarily schizophrenia; for the follow-up phase of recovery from an acute psychotic episode when risk of relapse remains high; and when no safer alternative (eg, lithium in bipolar disorder) is available. (4) Antipsychotic therapy should be evaluated at least every three to six months to determine ongoing need and benefit and to examine the patient for early signs of dyskinesia. The use of a rating instrument such as the Abnormal Involuntary Movement Scale (AIMS) during these examinations is recommended. The lowest dose that reduces the exacerbation rate should be established, and changes in dosage should be made as the situation warrants. When using depot antipsychotics, the lowest dose and longest interval between injections compatible with control of symptoms should be determined (Kane et al, 1986).

Because there is no proven alternative therapy for idiopathic psychoses, the American Psychiatric Association Task Force concluded that the clinician, in consultation with the patient and family, must balance the risks of continuing treatment in a patient who develops tardive dyskinesia against the benefits of antipsychotic therapy. The Task Force stressed that tardive dyskinesia usually is neither relentless nor progressive and that continuing treatment, at least in the short term, is usually justifiable if the patient has an active psychosis, particularly if relatively low doses of an antipsychotic are adequate. Undertreatment of chronic psychoses carries high risks, including death. If the antipsychotic drug is continued, an attempt should be made to reduce the dosage. If dyskinesia worsens but continued antipsychotic drug therapy is required, substitution of clozapine may be considered. Adjunctive treatment specifically for the dyskinesia may be considered, although the efficacy of various agents remains largely unproven. Benzodiazepines, calcium channel blockers, clonidine, vitamin E, or propranolol may provide partial benefit in some patients (American Psychiatric Association, 1992; Egan et al, 1992; Adler et al, 1993).

NEUROLEPTIC MALIGNANT SYNDROME (NMS). This syndrome is a relatively rare reaction associated with antipsychotic agents. A similar syndrome has been reported in a few patients after discontinuation of long-term therapy with central dopaminergic stimulants (eg, levodopa). NMS is characterized by *hyperthermia* (oral temperature of at least 38°C); *diffuse muscular rigidity*, often with severe extrapyramidal effects (eg, dyskinetic or choreiform movements, coarse fluctuating tremor, dysphagia, retrocollis, oculogyric crisis, sialorrhea, opisthotonus, trismus, flexor-extensor posturing, festinating gait), muteness, or catatonic signs; *autonomic dysfunction* (eg, tachycardia, hypertension, hypotension, tachypnea, prominent diaphoresis, incontinence); and *fluctuating levels of consciousness*, including stupor. Because many patients receiving antipsychotics often have some degree of rigidity or other extrapyramidal side effects, the most helpful clues to diagnose NMS may be impairment of consciousness and hyperthermia; in patients with NMS, these occur acutely and in temporal relation to one another. Altered laboratory values may include increased creatine kinase, leukocytosis, mildly elevated hepatic transaminase, and increased myoglobin and myoglobinuria; the tests are sensitive but results are nonspecific. Rapid escalation of dosage, especially of parenterally administered high-potency drugs; physical exhaustion; dehydration; and pneumonia or emboli may be predisposing or complicating factors. NMS is twice as common in males as in females, and 80% of cases occur in patients under 40 years. The prevalence is uncertain, but as many as 1% to 2% of patients treated with antipsychotic drugs may be at risk. The reported mortality rate has been as high as 20% (Caroff, 1980); in more recent studies, the mortality rate was reported to be 5% to 12% (Rosenberg and Green, 1989; Shalev et al, 1989).

Specific treatment for NMS consists of immediate discontinuation of antipsychotic drugs and any other medication that may have dopamine receptor-blocking activity (Rosenberg and Green, 1989; Olmsted, 1988) and specific antagonist therapy: Dantrolene [Dantrium] is given intravenously in doses of 0.8 to 2.5 mg/kg every six hours (maximum, 10 mg/kg daily) until symptoms subside and the patient can swallow; it then is given orally in doses of 100 to 200 mg daily. Oral bromocriptine [Parlodel] is then added (up to 80 mg [mean, 20 to 30 mg] daily in four divided doses). Amantadine may be helpful if the other agents are not adequate, but daily doses above 300 mg can cause central intoxication. The duration of therapy is usually five to ten days unless a depot preparation of a potent antipsychotic drug was used, particularly in an elderly patient. In addition, expert management is essential (ie, control of hyperthermia with antipyretics and cooling blankets, administration of intravenous fluids, maintenance of respiratory ventilation if required, monitoring for renal failure due to rhabdomyolysis, vigilance for development of infection and embolism). Because of the danger of recurrence if antipsychotics are reintroduced, some authorities recommend an interval of at least two weeks before therapy is resumed with relatively low doses of a less potent drug than the precipitating agent (Rosebush et al, 1989; Ayd, 1990).

AUTONOMIC EFFECTS. Most antipsychotic agents have both alpha-antiadrenergic and some anticholinergic actions, especially the low-potency drugs (see Table 1). Antihistaminergic and antiserotonergic actions contribute to the autonomic effects of some of these agents. Although these effects are common after oral administration, they are most pronounced after parenteral administration of low-potency antipsychotic drugs. Autonomic reactions rarely necessitate drug withdrawal, but reduced doses may be advisable if effects are severe.

Hypotension is an especially troublesome autonomic reaction; patients with cardiovascular disease or autonomic nervous system disorders associated with diabetes or Parkinson's disease may be most susceptible. Acute hypotensive crises, with the risk of falls and injuries, may occur in elderly or debilitated patients or after large parenteral doses in younger patients. Rarely, the cautious administration of intravenous fluids is required to correct hypovolemia. Norepinephrine [Levophed] or phenylephrine [Neo-Synephrine] is required only rarely. Agents with beta$_2$-adrenergic agonist activity (eg, epinephrine, isoproterenol) are contraindicated, for they may worsen hypotension.

Patients often find anticholinergic side effects particularly bothersome (Breslin, 1992). These include dryness of the mouth, tachycardia, blurred vision, urinary retention, and constipation. Death has resulted from adynamic ileus or fulminating infection of the bladder. Antipsychotic agents impair central thermoregulatory mechanisms, which may be a problem when temperatures are high and is a risk factor for development of NMS. Anticholinergic drugs should be used cautiously with antipsychotic drugs to avoid additive anticholinergic toxicity.

ALLERGIC AND IDIOSYNCRATIC EFFECTS. Cholestatic jaundice is noted infrequently, but most often with use of aliphatic phenothiazines and usually during the first few weeks of treatment. This may be a hypersensitivity reaction and is usually mild and self-limited; however, if hyperbilirubinemia or jaundice is detected, the drug should be withdrawn immediately and an agent from a different chemical group administered.

Cutaneous allergic reactions, manifested as urticarial, maculopapular, or petechial lesions, occur infrequently. Serious reactions (eg, exfoliative dermatitis) have been reported occasionally. If these effects are noted, the drug should be discontinued and therapy resumed later with a drug from a different chemical class.

Photosensitivity usually is manifested as an acute hypersensitivity reaction to sun with severe sunburn or rash. A chronic skin reaction manifested by dark purplish brown pigmentation also may develop. These idiosyncratic reactions are generally mild and seldom require dosage adjustment. They have been associated most often with the aliphatic phenothiazines, especially chlorpromazine, when these agents were given for prolonged periods in large doses (800 mg or more daily). The risk of photosensitivity may be minimized by administering the lowest effective dose, avoiding exposure to ultraviolet light, and using sunscreen preparations.

NEUROENDOCRINE EFFECTS. All antipsychotic drugs except clozapine produce hyperprolactinemia by blocking the inhibitory action of dopamine on prolactin secretion. Although some human metastatic breast carcinomas are prolactin-dependent, results of several epidemiologic studies have indicated that there is no association between the long-term administration of antipsychotic or other antidopaminergic drugs and the development of mammary tumors in humans.

Weight gain is common. Delayed ovulation and menstruation, amenorrhea, and galactorrhea in women and gynecomastia and edema in men have been reported occasionally. These effects are generally transient. They are considered manifestations of hyperprolactinemia and other neuroendocrine imbalances caused by altered hypothalamic and pituitary function.

Sexual dysfunction in both men and women has been reported with the use of antipsychotic drugs (Pollack et al, 1992). In women, these drugs can cause loss of libido and inability to achieve orgasm. In men, erectile and ejaculatory dysfunction, as well as loss of libido, have been reported. Thioridazine has been associated with painful, delayed, or retrograde ejaculation. Most types of sexual dysfunction disappear when the drugs are discontinued. Priapism, although rare, may persist and eventually may require surgical intervention.

Chlorpromazine, and possibly other antipsychotic drugs, may interfere with the control of blood glucose levels and the efficacy of oral hypoglycemic agents in patients with diabetes mellitus.

CARDIAC EFFECTS. Chlorpromazine has a direct negative inotropic action and quinidine-like effects on the heart. Thioridazine may produce sinus tachycardia, and both thioridazine and pimozide may produce electrocardiographic alterations resembling hypokalemia (ie, prolonged QT interval, appearance of U waves). Similar disturbances in ventricular repolarization have been reported in patients receiving large doses of low-potency antipsychotic drugs.

RESPIRATORY EFFECTS. Respiratory dysfunction has been reported rarely and may be due to the sedative or extrapyramidal actions of these drugs. The sedative effects may exacerbate acute problems in patients with a history of chronic obstructive lung disease. Extrapyramidal actions may result in acute pharyngeal and laryngeal paralysis leading to dysphagia and asphyxiation. Respiratory dyskinesias and distress also may be associated with tardive dyskinesia (Young and Patel, 1984).

OPHTHALMIC EFFECTS. Dose-related pigmentary keratopathy, conjunctival melanosis, and possibly glaucoma have been observed when large doses of chlorpromazine were employed for long periods. Opacities of the cornea and lens due to deposition of fine particulate matter were detectable on slit-lamp examination. Generally, vision is not impaired and changes regress slowly after withdrawal of therapy. However, chlorpromazine has been implicated in one case of optic atrophy.

Large doses of thioridazine have caused pigmentary retinopathy, and the patchy loss of visual acuity (scotoma) sometimes is irreversible. For this reason, the maximal recommended dose of thioridazine is 800 mg daily.

HEMATOLOGIC EFFECTS. Although these reactions appear to be most frequent with low-potency antipsychotic drugs, they may be associated with any of these agents. Mild depression of leukopoiesis is detectable in some patients, particularly with large doses of low-potency phenothiazines (eg, chlorpromazine, thioridazine), but rarely persists or progresses. Agranulocytosis is a potentially catastrophic idiosyncratic reaction that usually appears within the first three months of phenothiazine therapy. Although the incidence is extremely low (about 1 in 10,000 with most antipsychotic drugs other than clozapine), mortality is high. Therefore, appearance of fever, sore throat, or cellulitis is an indication for discontinuing the phenothiazine and performing white blood cell and differential counts immediately. After recovery, low doses of a high-potency antipsychotic drug can be substituted cautiously.

The risk of developing agranulocytosis is highest with clozapine (perhaps in up to 1% to 2% of infrequently monitored patients). The risk may be higher in certain ethnic groups (eg, Finns, Jews of Eastern European origin). Most commonly, this reaction develops between the sixth and eighteenth week of treatment. When agranulocytosis is detected promptly and clozapine is discontinued, the condition is usually reversible; therefore, careful monitoring to detect any signs of infection promptly and periodic (at least weekly for the first four to five months) blood counts may be advisable. Currently, the availability of clozapine is linked to mandatory weekly monitoring of the white blood cell count (see the evaluation).

Precautions

Patient Reassurance: After discharge from the hospital, both patient and family should be advised that antipsychotic medication must be continued for awhile, even though the patient feels better; reassurance about needless fears of addiction is important. The effects of drowsiness on such tasks as driving or operating machinery should be stressed, and dosage schedules that minimize interference with the patient's ability to perform daily tasks should be employed. The patient should be further warned about the possible additive effects of other central nervous system depressants (eg, antianxiety agents, hypnotics, centrally acting anticholinergics, tricyclic antidepressants) and specifically about the additive depressant effects of alcoholic beverages.

Informed Consent: The principles of informed consent govern antipsychotic drug treatment as they do other therapies and procedures in medicine, and the establishment of an active therapeutic alliance between physician and patient should underlie the process. Despite the presence of psychotic symptoms, most patients are considered legally competent to participate in informed consent procedures. However, most patients are never evaluated for competency, and there is no standard for determination of competency to receive informed consent for treatment with antipsychotic drugs. The physician also may wish to inform relatives or other responsible members of the patient's household of the risks and benefits of treatment.

In the acute phases of illness, it is generally considered sufficient to give reasonable indication of the purposes, anticipated benefits, and both short- and long-term (eg, tardive dyskinesia) risks of antipsychotic drug therapy. The medical record should document that this information has been discussed. When treatment lasts more than six months, repeated, explicit discussion of the risks (eg, tardive dyskinesia) and benefits (eg, prevention of relapse) is indicated and the patient should be evaluated at least every 6 to 12 months for clinical response and signs of adverse effects. The patient also should be advised of the risks (eg, exacerbation of symptoms) and benefits associated with discontinuation of therapy. Alternative strategies for using antipsychotic drugs may be reviewed. The record should reflect the fact that these matters have been discussed and that the patient has consented to the treatment strategy used.

Some clinicians believe that written and signed informed consent may provide better documentation that the patient has been advised of risks, benefits, and alternative treatment strategies, particularly when evidence of dyskinesia has been observed. Others recommend that written forms not be used in the belief that the therapeutic alliance may be threatened and the physician misled into thinking that the issue has been addressed adequately (Glazer and Kane, 1992).

A continued effort to gain the patient's cooperation is desirable; however, overriding the patient's right to refuse treatment by court order or guardianship is indicated when necessary to protect the patient, family, and society. Guidelines for defining emergencies that permit forcible medication of the psychotic patient vary among states and federal jurisdictions. The physician faced with this dilemma must be familiar with local medical practice and legal standards.

Use in Children: Antipsychotic drugs are used in children when normal functioning is significantly impaired (eg, behavioral, psychological, educational) (Oyewumi, 1983). Most clinicians prefer low doses of high-potency antipsychotic drugs. The lowest effective dose should be employed for an adequate period. Tardive dyskinesia can occur in children, and they may be at increased risk of developing parkinsonism.

Use in Older Patients: The incidence of adverse effects, especially hypotension, sedation, anticholinergic effects, and neurologic reactions, is higher in patients over 60 years; therefore, antipsychotic drugs should be prescribed cautiously. To minimize these reactions, the dose should be reduced to the lowest effective level, the patient should be observed closely, and the maintenance regimen should be reviewed periodically.

Since sleep disturbances are more common in elderly patients, the administration of antipsychotic agents once daily at bedtime may be appropriate. However, when higher dosage levels are indicated, smaller amounts at more frequent intervals may be necessary because the drug may not be eliminated quickly enough to avoid excessive tissue concentrations. Some clinicians prefer medium-potency drugs, such as perphenazine, in geriatric patients to balance extrapyramidal and autonomic risks.

Psychiatric syndromes in the elderly frequently are caused by many drugs or organic (brain or systemic) diseases. In these instances, withdrawal of the precipitating drug or treatment of the medical condition should supersede antipsychotic medication and may obviate the need for these agents.

Coexisting Medical Problems: A history of liver disease is not an absolute contraindication to use of antipsychotic agents, but smaller doses may be required because metabolic clearance is decreased. The more potent antipsychotic drugs (piperazine phenothiazines, thiothixene, or haloperidol) are preferred in these patients.

Antipsychotic agents may be given to epileptic patients receiving adequate antiepileptic drug therapy. The increased incidence of seizures that has been observed occasionally may be averted by increasing the dose of the antiepileptic drug. Patients with a family history of seizures or febrile convulsions are more likely to develop seizures than those without such history. Clozapine is associated with an increased risk of seizures, especially when doses exceed 600 mg daily. Thioridazine, mesoridazine, fluphenazine, and molindone may be relatively less epileptogenic. Specific guidelines for antipsychotic drug selection and management of epileptic patients have been reviewed (Itil and Soldatos, 1980).

Pregnancy: Data on the teratogenicity of antipsychotic drugs are fragmentary. Antipsychotic drugs have been identified in maternal and fetal plasma, amniotic fluid, and the urine of newborn infants. Prolonged extrapyramidal effects may appear in the infant. Behavioral developmental abnormalities have been observed in laboratory animals but not in humans. Thus, the use of antipsychotic drugs should be avoided during the first trimester if possible, and therapy should be discontinued one or two weeks before delivery to avoid extrapyramidal signs in the neonate due to impaired drug clearance. The uncertain but small risk of teratogenicity may be outweighed by the need for treatment (Edlund and Craig, 1984). When treatment is necessary during pregnancy, divided doses of the high-potency antipsychotic drugs are preferred (Cohen et al, 1989).

Lactation: Antipsychotic drugs are secreted in low concentrations into breast milk (Oyewumi, 1983). If a mother who needs continuous therapy nurses her infant, close supervision of the infant is recommended; however, bottle feeding is preferred.

Drug Interactions: Obviously, antipsychotic drugs will inhibit the actions of dopamine agonists and levodopa. The action of other central nervous system depressants (eg, alcohol, benzodiazepines, barbiturates, other sedative-hypnotics, opioid analgesics) may be enhanced. Concomitant use of lithium may increase the risk of neurotoxicity. The doses of preanesthetic drugs having a sedative action and general anesthetics may need to be reduced with concomitant use. Antipsychotic drugs should be discontinued temporarily in patients receiving spinal or epidural anesthesia to allow time for the remaining drug to be metabolized.

Several pharmacokinetic drug interactions with antipsychotic drugs have been identified (Goff and Baldessarini, 1993). Concurrent use of imipramine-like tricyclic antidepressants or other agents with anticholinergic activity may cause additive central nervous system dysfunction as well as peripheral anticholinergic effects. Tricyclic antidepressants and several antipsychotic drugs also inhibit the hepatic metabolism of each other. The hypotensive effects of a drug may be increased by diuretics, methyldopa, captopril, and presumably other antihypertensive medications. Propranolol increases the plasma concentrations of chlorpromazine and thioridazine. Antiepileptic drugs that induce hepatic metabolism (ie, phenytoin, carbamazepine, phenobarbital) accelerate the elimination of many antipsychotic agents; cigarette smoking has a similar effect, while fluoxetine has the opposite effect (Goff et al, 1991).

For other specific interactions, see the individual evaluations.

Tolerance, Dependence, and Withdrawal Symptoms: Some tolerance to the sedative, anticholinergic, hypotensive, and other effects of antipsychotic drugs develops within weeks to months. Little tolerance to the antipsychotic action occurs in spite of the adaptive dopamine supersensitivity that develops and that is postulated to contribute to withdrawal-emergent tardive dyskinesia.

Although drug dependence does not occur with antipsychotic drugs, some physiologic adaptation is evident, because abrupt withdrawal after prolonged therapy results in the following cluster of symptoms in about one-third of patients: nausea, vomiting, diaphoresis, headache, restlessness, and insomnia (Lacoursiere et al, 1976; Luchins et al, 1980). The mechanism may be related to altered sensitivity of cholinergic neurons following prolonged anticholinergic blockade, because the low-potency antipsychotic drugs with stronger anticholinergic effects are more likely to produce the phenomenon. Similar withdrawal symptoms also are produced by the concomitant withdrawal of anticholinergic drugs given to alleviate extrapyramidal reactions.

Withdrawal signs and symptoms commonly occur in two to three days and may persist for about two weeks. A gradual (over one to two weeks) reduction in dosage is recommended when terminating antipsychotic drug therapy. An anticholinergic drug given concomitantly also should be withdrawn gradually and later than the antipsychotic drug. Drug "holidays" should be utilized cautiously for patients sensitive to withdrawal symptoms or at high risk of relapse based on past history.

Drug Evaluations

The efficacy of most antipsychotic agents in current clinical use in the United States is similar, and doses may be equated with approximately 100 mg of chlorpromazine (see Table 1). Differences among compounds are related to the presence of other pharmacologic properties, to the prevalence of particular adverse reactions, and possibly to variation in individual response.

The pharmacologic properties and the prevalence of particular adverse reactions depend principally on the chemical class; therefore, the following evaluations are arranged by chemical class. Information on dosage is given for each member of a class, but information pertaining to the class is included in the first evaluation (ie, prototype drug) in each category.

PHENOTHIAZINE DERIVATIVES

Aliphatic Compounds

CHLORPROMAZINE HYDROCHLORIDE

[Thorazine]

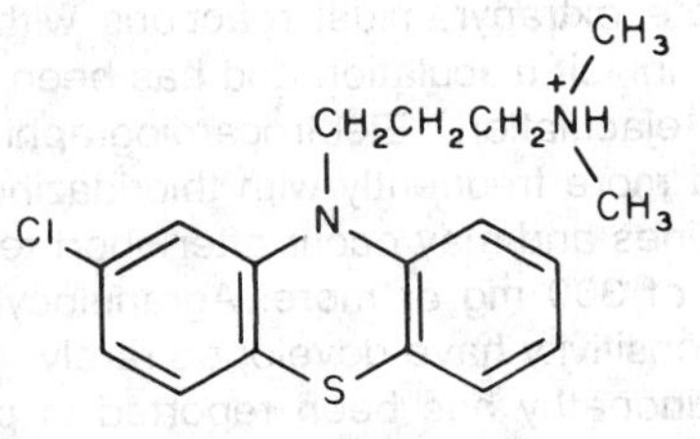

$CH_2CH_2CH_2\overset{+}{N}H(CH_3)_2$ Cl^-

ACTIONS AND USES. Chlorpromazine was the first antipsychotic agent marketed and is the prototype of the aliphatic phenothiazines. This agent is used primarily to treat schizophrenia, other psychoses, or mania; it is employed less commonly in schizoaffective disorder or major depression with psychotic features, delusional disorder, intractable hiccups, severe behavioral problems in children marked by combativeness and disturbed behavior associated with mental retardation, and nausea and vomiting.

Chlorpromazine also is sometimes used to treat ballism, Tourette's syndrome, and the chorea of Huntington's disease (see the Introduction).

This phenothiazine has a relatively low potency. It is one of the most sedative antipsychotic drugs, but tolerance to this effect usually develops. Chlorpromazine probably is best tolerated by patients under 40 years. In older patients, the incidence of dizziness, hypotension, ocular changes, and extrapyramidal side effects increases, although the latter are more commonly associated with the more potent antipsychotic agents.

ADVERSE REACTIONS. Chlorpromazine is less likely to cause acute dystonia and parkinsonism than piperazine phenothiazines.

Because chlorpromazine has pronounced antiadrenergic and anticholinergic properties, orthostatic hypotension, dryness of the mouth, blurred vision, urinary retention, and constipation are common. These reactions tend to diminish after the first week of continual therapy. Chlorpromazine appears to have the greatest propensity among the phenothiazines to produce agranulocytosis and cholestatic jaundice, but both are rare. Allergic skin reactions are uncommon, but mild photosensitivity occurs relatively often and the patient should be so informed. A lupus-like illness with a lupus-like coagulation inhibitor has been reported (Alberti-Flor, 1983; Tollefson et al, 1984). Patients should be examined periodically for conjunctival melanosis, pigmentary opacities in the cornea and lens, and pigmentary retinopathy. Menstrual irregularities, galactorrhea, gynecomastia, and impotence have been reported occasionally.

DRUG INTERACTIONS. Antacids and aluminum-containing antidiarrheal drugs may impair gastrointestinal absorption of chlorpromazine. Chlorpromazine may increase the plasma concentration of valproate. Concomitant administration of chlorpromazine and propranolol, especially in large doses, results in elevated plasma levels of both drugs. In doses larger than 100 mg daily, chlorpromazine can reverse the antihypertensive effects of guanethidine.

For further information on indications, adverse reactions, precautions, and drug interactions, see the Introduction.

PHARMACOKINETICS. Although intestinal absorption is complete, the oral bioavailability is 32% ± 19% because of variable metabolism in the intestinal wall and liver (marked first-pass effect). Time to peak plasma concentration is two to four hours. After intramuscular administration, peak plasma concentrations are four to ten times higher than after oral administration; onset of action occurs within 20 to 30 minutes, and the peak levels are noted in two to three hours. Volume of distribution (21 ± 9 L/kg) is high, and plasma binding (95% to 98%) is extensive. Clearance after intramuscular administration averages 8.6 ± 2.9 ml/min/kg. Less than 1% of the drug is excreted unchanged by the kidney. The mean elimination plasma half-life of the parent drug is 30 ± 7 hours; however, some metabolites are eliminated slowly (months) in the urine. Hepatic enzyme induction with increased clearance usually is a minor effect that varies considerably among individuals.

At least 100 metabolites of chlorpromazine appear in humans; most are minor. Several, including 7-hydroxychlorpromazine, 11-hydroxychlorpromazine, norchlorpromazine, and possibly chlorpromazine N-oxide, are neuropharmacologically active.

DOSAGE AND PREPARATIONS.

Intramuscular: For psychoses in hospitalized *adults,* 25 to 100 mg initially, repeated in one to four hours as necessary until control is achieved. Most patients respond to 300 to 600 mg daily. *Elderly or debilitated patients,* doses 50% to 25% of the lower range for adults are usually adequate and tolerated. *Children,* 0.5 mg/kg every six to eight hours, gradually increased until symptoms are controlled; the total daily dose should not exceed 40 mg in children under 5 years or 75 mg in older children. This drug generally should not be used in infants under 6 months. Oral administration should be substituted when symptoms are controlled.

Thorazine (SmithKline Beecham), ***Generic***. Solution (aqueous) 25 mg/ml in 1, 2, and 10 ml containers.

Oral: *Adults and adolescents,* the usual initial dose is 10 to 25 mg two to four times daily, increased by 20 to 50 mg daily every three to four days as needed and tolerated. *Elderly or debilitated patients,* one-third to one-half the usual adult dose, increased more gradually (20- to 25-mg increments). The response of older patients seldom improves with doses exceeding 300 mg daily, and higher doses are not likely to be well tolerated. *Children,* 0.5 mg/kg every four to six hours. For all patients, when symptoms have been controlled, the dosage should be reduced gradually to the minimum effective level for maintenance.

For severe psychoses, *adults,* initially, 200 to 600 mg daily, increased if necessary until symptoms are controlled or adverse reactions intervene. The rate of increase in dosage depends on the patient's age and weight and the severity of symptoms. A dose of 300 to 600 mg/day usually is adequate after several days of treatment (Donaldson et al, 1986). Although the maximum recommended daily dose is 2 g, amounts exceeding 800 mg rarely increase the response and produce a higher incidence of adverse reactions. The average dose in patients under 40 years is 300 to 600 mg daily.

Generic. Concentrate 30 and 100 mg/ml; tablets 10, 25, 50, 100, and 200 mg; syrup 10 mg/5 ml.

Thorazine (SmithKline Beecham). Capsules (prolonged-release) 30, 75, 150, 200, and 300 mg; concentrate 30 and 100 mg/ml; syrup 10 mg/5 ml; tablets 10, 25, 50, 100, and 200 mg.

Rectal: *Children,* 1 mg/kg every six to eight hours.

Thorazine (SmithKline Beecham). Suppositories 25 and 100 mg (equivalent to base).

TRIFLUPROMAZINE HYDROCHLORIDE

[Vesprin]

$CH_2CH_2CH_2\overset{+}{N}H(CH_3)_2$ F_3C N S Cl^-

Triflupromazine has the same actions and indications as chlorpromazine and is equally effective (see Table 1). Only a parenteral preparation is available. For information on indications, adverse reactions, drug interactions, and precautions, see the Introduction and the evaluation on Chlorpromazine Hydrochloride.

DOSAGE AND PREPARATIONS.

Intramuscular: For psychoses in hospitalized patients, *adults,* initially, 60 to 150 mg daily; *elderly or debilitated patients,* 10 to 75 mg daily; *children over 2 1/2 years,* 0.2 to 0.25 mg/kg (maximum, 10 mg daily).

Vesprin (Apothecon). Solution 10 mg/ml in 10 ml containers and 20 mg/ml in 1 ml containers.

Piperidine Compounds

THIORIDAZINE HYDROCHLORIDE

[Mellaril]

H_3C $\overset{+}{N}$ H CH_2CH_2 N SCH_3 S Cl^-

ACTIONS AND USES. This low-potency phenothiazine is widely used. Its efficacy is similar to that of chlorpromazine in equal doses (see Table 1). The effectiveness of thioridazine may be due both to the parent compound and to the formation of the active metabolite, mesoridazine, which is commercially available and commonly used.

Thioridazine is administered primarily to treat schizophrenia and other psychoses, and thioridazine and mesoridazine have been employed in schizoaffective disorders or major depression with psychotic features. See the Introduction for other indications.

ADVERSE REACTIONS. Risks of sedation and orthostatic hypotension are similar to those of chlorpromazine. The pronounced anticholinergic activity of thioridazine (and its relatively weak antidopaminergic action) may explain the low incidence of acute extrapyramidal reactions with this drug. Thioridazine may inhibit ejaculation and has been associated with retrograde ejaculation. Electrocardiographic changes have been noted more frequently with thioridazine than with other phenothiazines and may occur after short-term therapy with daily doses of 300 mg or more. Agranulocytosis, jaundice, and photosensitivity have developed rarely.

Pigmentary retinopathy has been reported in patients receiving more than 800 mg/day of thioridazine; diminished visual acuity may be irreversible. Smaller daily doses have impaired vision without detectable retinal changes. Because of these ocular reactions, 800 mg/day is the maximum dose; the manufacturer recommends that doses exceeding 300 mg/day be used only in patients with severe psychoses. Thus, if large doses are required for long periods or if 800 mg/day is inadequate, another antipsychotic agent should be substituted.

Rarely, the combination of thioridazine and lithium has produced severe neurotoxicity manifested by seizures, delirium, encephalopathy, and EEG abnormalities. The risk of cardiac conduction problems is increased when thioridazine is given with a tricyclic antidepressant.

For further information on indications, adverse reactions, drug interactions, and precautions, see the Introduction.

PHARMACOKINETICS. Pharmacokinetic data are limited (Chakraborty et al, 1989), but thioridazine produces peak plasma concentrations within two hours after oral administration. The drug is sulfoxidized principally to mesoridazine (elimination $t_{1/2}$ 9 to 12 hours) and small amounts of sulforidazine ($t_{1/2}$ 10 hours), which are pharmacologically active, and thioridazine-5-sulfoxide, which is inactive. The $t_{1/2}$ of thioridazine is approximately seven to nine hours. Both thioridazine and mesoridazine are widely distributed, and the ratio of bound to free drug is 3:1 and 2:1, respectively. Both drugs have equal receptor-binding affinity, but the concentration of free mesoridazine is relatively higher.

DOSAGE AND PREPARATIONS.

Oral: *Adults,* initially, 150 to 300 mg daily in divided doses; this may be increased gradually to a maximum of 800 mg daily in hospitalized patients. For maintenance therapy, the dose should be reduced gradually to the minimum effective level. *Elderly or debilitated patients,* one-third to one-half the usual adult dosage. *Children 2 years or older,* 1 mg/kg daily in divided doses; *under 2 years,* information is inadequate to establish a dosage.

Generic. Concentrate 30 and 100 mg/ml; tablets 10, 15, 25, 50, 100, 150, and 200 mg.

Mellaril (Sandoz). Concentrate 30 mg/ml (alcohol 3%) and 100 mg/ml (alcohol 4.2%); suspension 25 and 100 mg/5 ml (equivalent to hydrochloride) (***Mellaril-S***); tablets 10, 15, 25, 50, 100, 150, and 200 mg.

MESORIDAZINE BESYLATE
[Serentil]

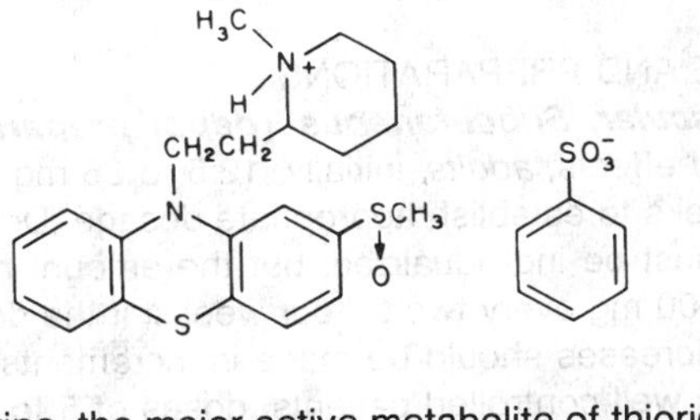

Mesoridazine, the major active metabolite of thioridazine, is an effective low-potency antipsychotic agent (see Table 1).

For information on indications, adverse reactions, drug interactions, precautions, and pharmacokinetics, see the Introduction and the evaluation on Thioridazine Hydrochloride.

DOSAGE AND PREPARATIONS.

Intramuscular: For psychoses, *adults and children over 12 years,* 25 to 200 mg daily in divided doses. Since intramuscular injection is irritating, oral administration should be substituted when symptoms are controlled.

Serentil (Boehringer). Solution 25 mg/ml in 1 ml containers.

Oral: *Adults and children over 12 years,* initially, 150 mg daily in divided doses, increased gradually in 50-mg increments until symptoms are controlled, then reduced gradually to the minimum effective amount for maintenance (range, 100 to 400 mg daily). *Elderly or debilitated patients,* one-third to one-half the usual adult dosage. *Children under 12 years,* information is inadequate to establish a dosage.

Serentil (Boehringer). Concentrate 25 mg/ml (alcohol 0.61%); tablets 10, 25, 50, and 100 mg.

Piperazine Compounds

TRIFLUOPERAZINE HYDROCHLORIDE
[Stelazine]

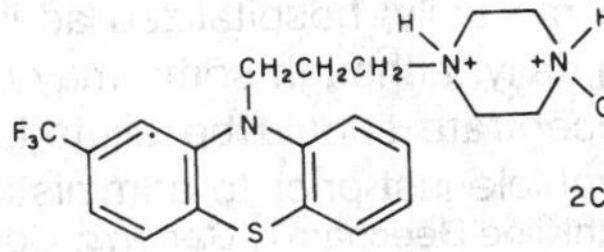

ACTIONS AND USES. Trifluoperazine, a piperazine phenothiazine, is a high-potency antipsychotic drug (see Table 1). It is used primarily to treat schizophrenia and other psychoses. It also is administered in schizoaffective disorder or major depression with psychotic features, delusional disorder, and mental retardation with disturbed behavior (see the Introduction). Trifluoperazine has been used to treat ballism and Tourette's syndrome.

ADVERSE REACTIONS AND PRECAUTIONS. The piperazines have less sedative effect than other phenothiazines. The incidence of autonomic effects (eg, orthostatic hypotension) also is lower, but acute extrapyramidal reactions occur more frequently, particularly when large doses are used.

Piperazine compounds are less likely to produce blood dyscrasias or jaundice, although transient leukopenia has been reported occasionally. Ocular changes have developed rarely with trifluoperazine but have not yet been noted with other piperazine compounds.

Since no marked electrocardiographic changes have been observed, piperazine compounds may be preferred for patients with cardiovascular disease. However, a few patients with angina pectoris have reported increased pain during therapy with trifluoperazine. Therefore, patients with angina should be observed carefully and the drug withdrawn if an unfavorable response occurs.

For further information on indications, adverse reactions, drug interactions, and precautions, see the Introduction.

PHARMACOKINETICS. Pharmacokinetic data on trifluoperazine are limited, but bioavailability, onset of action, time to peak effect, first-pass effect, metabolism, and elimination half-lives appear to resemble those of chlorpromazine. Plasma concentrations of 1 to 2 ng/ml are typical with clinical doses (Janicak et al, 1989).

DOSAGE AND PREPARATIONS.

Intramuscular: For psychoses, *adults*, 1 to 2 mg by deep intramuscular injection every four to six hours, as needed. *Elderly and debilitated patients,* one-third to one-half of the usual adult dose given at longer intervals. *Children 6 years and older,* 1 mg once or twice daily; *under 6 years,* information is inadequate to establish a dosage. When symptoms are controlled, oral administration should be substituted.

Stelazine (SmithKline Beecham), ***Generic.*** Solution 2 mg/ml in 10 ml containers.

Oral: Initially, *adults (outpatients),* 2 to 4 mg daily in divided doses; *(hospitalized),* 5 to 25 mg daily in divided doses, increased gradually to the optimum amount. *Elderly or debilitated patients,* one-third to one-half the usual adult dose. *Children 6 years or older,* 1 to 2 mg daily, gradually increased to the optimum amount (rarely more than 15 mg daily).

When symptoms are controlled, the dosage should be reduced gradually for all patients to the minimum effective amount for maintenance. Adult outpatients often can be maintained on 5 to 15 mg daily; hospitalized adults generally require 15 to 20 mg daily, although some may require up to 40 mg/day. The concentrate should be diluted in fruit juice or another suitable vehicle just prior to administration.

Stelazine (SmithKline Beecham), ***Generic.*** Concentrate 10 mg/ml; tablets 1, 2, 5, and 10 mg.

FLUPHENAZINE DECANOATE
[Prolixin Decanoate]

FLUPHENAZINE ENANTHATE
[Prolixin Enanthate]

FLUPHENAZINE HYDROCHLORIDE
[Permitil, Prolixin]

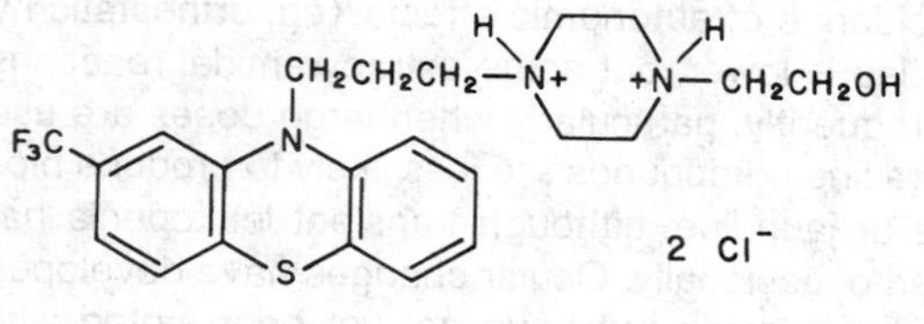

ACTIONS AND USES. Fluphenazine has the highest milligram potency of the phenothiazines (see Table 1).

The duration of action of the depot forms, fluphenazine decanoate and fluphenazine enanthate, usually is two to three weeks. An interval of four weeks or longer between injections may be adequate for maintenance therapy in selected patients, particularly with the decanoate ester. Depot forms are useful in outpatients with a history of poor compliance, inadequate absorption of oral medication, poor response to oral therapy, or frequent relapses (Glazer, 1984).

Close supervision and individualization of dosage are required during the conversion from a short-acting oral form to the depot preparation. Initial doses of a depot form and the intervals between doses then should be determined carefully, based on the patient's personal and family drug history. Since steady-state plasma concentrations are not achieved until approximately three dosage intervals after depot injections of fluphenazine are initiated, supplementation with oral fluphenazine may be necessary initially (Marder et al, 1989). There is no precise formula for conversion from oral to depot preparations, but results of multicenter studies suggest that for each 10 mg of fluphenazine hydrochloride required daily, fluphenazine decanoate 12.5 mg be given intramuscularly every three weeks, with the dose then adjusted to produce the desired effect.

In physically healthy patients with refractory chronic schizophrenia, optimal doses of parenteral preparations have been used successfully for years without producing severe extrapyramidal reactions. For patients in whom extrapyramidal reactions have occurred previously, see regimen under Dosage and Preparations.

ADVERSE REACTIONS AND PRECAUTIONS. With the exception of tardive dyskinesia, extrapyramidal reactions usually appear during the first few weeks of therapy but they may occur even after the patient's condition is stabilized. Occasionally, usual doses of anticholinergic drugs do not adequately control extrapyramidal symptoms, and increased amounts may precipitate toxic psychosis. In such cases, smaller doses or less frequent administration of fluphenazine generally controls symptoms.

Depending on dosage and individual sensitivity, sedation, anticholinergic side effects, and hypotensive episodes have been observed. Usually these reactions are mild and subside spontaneously. Rarely, jaundice occurs with oral use of fluphenazine; the depot forms have not yet been reported to cause this reaction. Only the risk of extrapyramidal reactions appears to be increased by use of the depot form (Glazer, 1984).

For further information on indications, adverse reactions, precautions, and drug interactions, see the Introduction.

PHARMACOKINETICS. Time to maximum blood concentration after intramuscular injection of the decanoate ester is 4 to 24 hours, and the plasma half-life ranges from 6.8 to 9.6 days. Time to maximum blood concentration after intramuscular injection of fluphenazine enanthate is two to four days, and the plasma half-life is 3.7 days compared with two to four hours and about 12 hours, respectively, for fluphenazine hydrochloride.

DOSAGE AND PREPARATIONS.

Intramuscular, Subcutaneous (depot preparations): For sustained effects, *adults,* initially, 12.5 to 25 mg every two to three weeks to establish appropriate dosage. Dosage and intervals must be individualized, but the amount rarely should exceed 100 mg every two to four weeks; if the dose exceeds 50 mg, increases should be made in increments of 12.5 mg. For many well-controlled patients, doses of 5 to 6.25 mg every two weeks are sufficient (Burnett et al, 1993).

Debilitated patients or those with a history of extrapyramidal reactions (particularly following use of high-potency drugs or a chemical class that produces a lower incidence of these symptoms), it is advisable to give a test dose (usually, 2.5 mg) and increase the amount every 10 to 14 days during the first month until a therapeutic response has been attained. Oral supplements also may be required with this regimen. After the patient has been stabilized on the optimum dose, the amount should be adjusted to provide the minimum effective maintenance dose as infrequently as possible. This period usually varies between three and six weeks. Continued supervision and a flexible dosage regimen, including the use of oral supplements during mild exacerbations, usually are necessary for optimum response. *Children,* information is inadequate to establish a dosage.

FLUPHENAZINE DECANOATE:
Prolixin Decanoate (Apothecon), ***Generic.*** Solution 25 mg/ml (in sesame oil) in 1 and 5 ml containers.

FLUPHENAZINE ENANTHATE:
Prolixin Enanthate (Apothecon). Solution 25 mg/ml (in sesame oil) in 5 ml containers.

Intramuscular (regular preparation): For psychoses, *adults,* initially, 1.25 to 2.5 mg every six to eight hours until symptoms are controlled; dosages >10 mg/day should be used cautiously. When symptoms are controlled, oral administration should be substituted. *Elderly or debilitated patients,* one-third to one-half the usual adult dose. *Children,* information is inadequate to establish a dosage.

FLUPHENAZINE HYDROCHLORIDE:
Prolixin (Apothecon), ***Generic.*** Solution 2.5 mg/ml in 10 ml containers.

Oral: *Adults,* initially, 2.5 to 10 mg daily. A therapeutic effect often is achieved with less than 20 mg daily. The manufacturers' literature indicates that daily doses up to 40 mg may be necessary in some patients. When symptoms are controlled, the maintenance dosage generally can be reduced gradually to 1 to 5 mg daily (maintenance doses exceeding 5 mg are rarely necessary). *Elderly or debilitated patients,* initially, 1 to 2.5 mg daily, adjusted on the basis of response. *Children,* information is inadequate to establish a dosage, although 0.75 to 10 mg/day has been used in *children 5 to 12 years.* The concentrate should be diluted with water, fruit juice, or another suitable vehicle before administration.

FLUPHENAZINE HYDROCHLORIDE:
Generic. Tablets 1, 2.5, 5, and 10 mg.
Permitil (Schering). Concentrate 5 mg/ml (alcohol 1%); tablets 2.5, 5, and 10 mg.
Prolixin (Apothecon). Concentrate 5 mg/ml (alcohol 14%); elixir 2.5 mg/5 ml (alcohol 14%); tablets 1, 2.5, 5, and 10 mg.

PERPHENAZINE
[Trilafon]

$CH_2CH_2CH_2-N \quad N-CH_2CH_2OH$, Cl, N, S

See the Introduction and the evaluation on Trifluoperazine Hydrochloride.

DOSAGE AND PREPARATIONS.
Intramuscular: *Adults,* for psychoses, initially, 5 to 10 mg; 5 mg may be given every six hours thereafter, but the total amount should not exceed 15 mg/day in outpatients or 30 mg/day in hospitalized patients. *Elderly or debilitated patients,* one-third to one-half the usual adult dose. *Children under 12 years,* information is inadequate to establish a dosage; *over 12 years,* lowest limit of adult dose. When symptoms are controlled, oral administration should be substituted.

Trilafon (Schering). Solution 5 mg/ml in 1 ml containers.

Oral: *Adults,* 8 to 32 mg daily in divided doses. Daily doses >64 mg should be used very cautiously. When symptoms are controlled, the dosage should be reduced gradually to the minimum effective level. *Elderly or debilitated patients,* one-third to one-half the usual adult dose. Pediatric dosage has not been established, but the following amounts have been given in divided doses: *Children 1 to 6 years,* 4 to 6 mg daily; *6 to 12 years,* 6 mg daily; *over 12 years,* 6 to 12 mg daily. The concentrate should be diluted in fruit juice or another suitable liquid vehicle (tea, coffee, cola, and apple juice are not recommended) prior to administration.

Generic. Tablets 2, 4, 8, and 16 mg.
Trilafon (Schering). Concentrate 16 mg/5 ml (alcohol <0.1%); tablets 2, 4, 8, and 16 mg.

THIOXANTHENE DERIVATIVES

CHLORPROTHIXENE
[Taractan]

$CHCH_2CH_2N(CH_3)_2$, Cl, S

The pharmacologic actions of chlorprothixene, a low-potency xanthene compound, are very similar to those of chlorpromazine.

For information on indications and adverse reactions, see the Introduction and the evaluation on Chlorpromazine Hydrochloride.

DOSAGE AND PREPARATIONS.
Intramuscular: For psychoses, *adults and children over 12 years,* 75 to 200 mg daily in divided doses. *Elderly or debilitated patients,* 30 to 100 mg daily in divided doses. When symptoms are controlled, oral administration should be substituted. *Children under 12 years,* information is inadequate to establish a dosage.

Taractan (Roche). Solution 12.5 mg/ml in 2 ml containers (as hydrochloride).

Oral: *Adults,* 75 to 200 mg daily in divided doses, increased gradually until symptoms are controlled or adverse reactions intervene. The optimum dose rarely exceeds 600 mg daily. *Elderly or debilitated patients and children over 6 years,* 30 to 100 mg daily in divided doses. When symptoms are controlled, the dosage should be reduced gradually to the minimum effective level. *Children under 6 years,* information is inadequate to establish a dosage.

Taractan (Roche). Concentrate 100 mg of base/5 ml (as lactate and hydrochloride); tablets 10, 25, 50, and 100 mg.

THIOTHIXENE
[Navane]

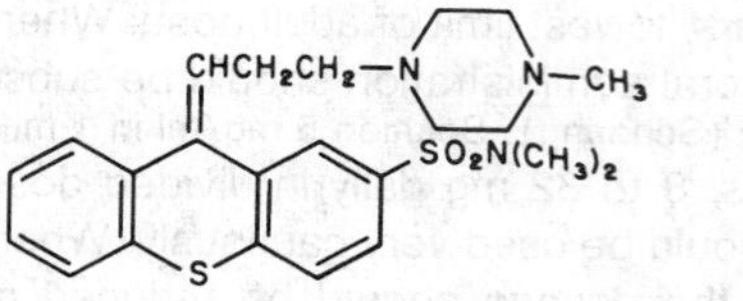

THIOTHIXENE HYDROCHLORIDE
[Navane]

The chemical structure and pharmacologic actions of thiothixene, a high-potency compound, are very similar to those of the piperazine phenothiazines. For information on indications, adverse reactions, and precautions, see the Introduction and the evaluation on Trifluoperazine Hydrochloride.

PHARMACOKINETICS. Thiothixene undergoes oxidative metabolism by the liver. Hepatic clearance is increased by carbamazepine and cigarette smoking; clearance is decreased by cimetidine and also is lower in females and in patients over 50 years (Ereshefsky et al, 1991).

DOSAGE AND PREPARATIONS.

Intramuscular: For psychoses, *adults and children 12 years or older,* initially, 4 mg two to four times daily, increased gradually until symptoms are controlled (maximum, 30 mg daily). *Elderly or debilitated patients*, one-third to one-half the usual adult dose. When symptoms are controlled, oral administration should be substituted. *Children under 12 years,* use not recommended because the drug's safety in pediatric patients has not been established.

THIOTHIXENE HYDROCHLORIDE:
Navane (Roerig). Solution 5 mg/ml (equivalent to base) after reconstitution.

Oral: *Adults,* 6 to 10 mg daily in divided doses, increased gradually if necessary. The usual optimal dose is 20 to 30 mg daily, and amounts in excess of 60 mg daily rarely enhance the response. *Elderly or debilitated patients,* initially, one-third to one-half the usual adult dosage. When symptoms are controlled, the dose should be reduced gradually to the minimum effective level. *Children under 12 years,* use not recommended because the drug's safety in pediatric patients has not been established.

THIOTHIXENE:
Navane (Roerig), ***Generic.*** Capsules 1, 2, 5, 10, and 20 mg.
THIOTHIXENE HYDROCHLORIDE:
Navane (Roerig), ***Generic.*** Concentrate 5 mg/ml (alcohol 7%) (equivalent to base).

BUTYROPHENONE DERIVATIVE

HALOPERIDOL
[Haldol]

HALOPERIDOL LACTATE
[Haldol]

HALOPERIDOL DECANOATE
[Haldol Decanoate]

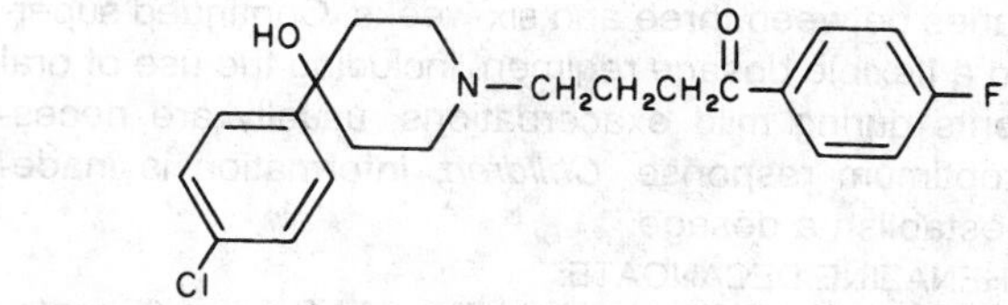

ACTIONS AND USES. Haloperidol is pharmacologically, but not chemically, related to the high-potency piperazine phenothiazines. This drug is used primarily to treat schizophrenia and other psychoses; it also is used in schizoaffective disorder, delusional disorder, ballism, and Tourette's syndrome (a drug of choice) and occasionally as adjunctive therapy in mental retardation and the chorea of Huntington's disease (see the Introduction). It is a potent antiemetic and is effective in the treatment of intractable hiccups.

Haloperidol decanoate is a long-acting injectable depot preparation for the prophylactic treatment of chronic schizophrenia (Hemstrom et al, 1988).

ADVERSE REACTIONS. Like the piperazine phenothiazines, haloperidol is relatively nonsedating and is likely to produce extrapyramidal reactions (see Table 1), especially if there is a history of such reactions to other antipsychotic agents. Akathisia and acute dystonias occasionally are severe. Persistent extrapyramidal symptoms usually are dose related but have also occurred following use of relatively small amounts.

Haloperidol causes fewer autonomic effects than the phenothiazines, although transient orthostatic hypotension has been reported occasionally. Torsades de pointes has been reported after intravenous administration of very large doses of haloperidol (Wilt et al, 1993).

Dermatologic reactions are rare, and the risk of adverse hepatic effects is minimal. Mild, transient hematologic changes have occurred.

Epidemiologic studies have not confirmed a teratogenic effect of haloperidol. Haloperidol decanoate is classified in FDA Pregnancy Category C.

For further information on indications, adverse reactions, drug interactions, and precautions, see the Introduction.

PHARMACOKINETICS. Haloperidol is well absorbed orally; however, a first-pass effect results in 60% (range, 44% to 74%) oral bioavailability. Time to peak effect after intramuscular and oral administration is one and three hours, respectively. Volume of distribution (Vd) is 20 L/kg, and plasma protein binding is 92%. Clearance (11.8 ± 2.9 ml/min/kg) is greater in children and smokers and is reduced in the elderly. The metabolism of haloperidol involves cleavage by oxidative N-dealkylation to piperidine metabolites and 4-fluorobenzoylpropionic acid; less than 1% of unchanged haloperidol is excreted in the urine. The nominal early plasma half-life after oral administration of single doses varies from 14 to 24 hours (Froemming et al, 1989). After multiple doses, the apparent half-life may be much longer and is characterized by multiexponential kinetics. Haloperidol (ketone) also undergoes reversible metabolism to reduced haloperidol (alcohol); the reduced metabolite is much less active than the parent compound. Although the clearance of reduced haloperidol is similar, its Vd and early half-life (67 ± 51 hours) are considerably longer. The accumulation and slow reconversion of reduced haloperidol to parent compound increases the apparent plasma elimination half-life of haloperidol (three to ten days) with repeated dosing.

Because of the lack of active metabolites, several studies have investigated the relationship between plasma levels and clinical response. Data from fixed-dose studies suggest that therapeutic responses to haloperidol are associated with plasma concentrations between 3 and 22 ng/ml. A commonly quoted range for the optimal plasma concentration of haloperidol is 5 to 15 ng/ml. In a study of newly hospitalized schizophrenic men, optimal response occurred with concentrations of 5 to 12 ng/ml (Van Putten et al, 1992). These figures may not be applicable to chronic, treatment-refractory, or acutely agitated patients. In smokers, higher doses of haloperidol may be required to establish effective plasma concentrations (Perry et al, 1993).

Dopamine (D_2) receptors in the brain appear to be approximately 90% saturated at plasma concentrations of 15 to 20 ng/ml (Cannon et al, 1988; Wolkin et al, 1989). In reviews (Perry et al, 1988; Baldessarini et al, 1988) and in one study of the dose-response relationship (Coryell et al, 1990), plasma levels >15 to 20 ng/ml were associated with no improvement in and possibly with decreased efficacy. Concomitant administration of phenytoin, carbamazepine, or phenobarbital decreases the steady-state plasma concentrations of haloperidol; fluoxetine has the opposite effect (Goff et al, 1991).

The activity of haloperidol decanoate, a depot preparation, depends on the enzymatic hydrolysis of the ester to free haloperidol. Monthly injection has reduced the exacerbation rate in patients with chronic schizophrenia.

DOSAGE AND PREPARATIONS.

Intramuscular (regular preparation): For psychoses with marked agitation, *adults,* initially, 2 to 10 mg. Depending on response, subsequent doses may be administered as often as every hour (although four- to eight-hour intervals are satisfactory in most patients) until symptoms are controlled. A dose of 5 to 15 mg daily usually is sufficient, and doses >25 mg daily are seldom required. Oral administration should then be substituted and the dosage individualized. *Elderly or debilitated patients and children under 12 years,* information is inadequate to establish a dosage.

HALOPERIDOL LACTATE:
Haldol (McNeil), ***Generic.*** Solution 5 mg/ml in 1 and 10 ml containers.

Intramuscular (depot formulation): Maintenance depot injections are administered monthly. The manufacturer suggests the following: For chronic psychoses, patients should be stabilized on a safe and effective oral dose of haloperidol before conversion to haloperidol decanoate. Close clinical supervision is required during initial dose adjustment to minimize overdosage or reappearance of psychotic symptoms before the next injection.

For patients maintained on oral doses >10 mg/day and in those who are at risk of relapse, up to 20 times the daily oral dose should be used initially. The maximum volume per injection site should not exceed 3 ml. During initial conversion, the first injection should not exceed 100 mg; the balance of the first month's dosage can be administered in a second injection three to seven days later. Supplementation with oral haloperidol can be used during dosage adjustment or exacerbation of psychoses. For patients who are elderly, debilitated, or stabilized on oral doses <10 mg/day, the initial dose should be 10 to 15 times the daily oral dose.

The usual monthly maintenance dose for all patients is 10 to 15 times the daily oral dose, depending on clinical response. If 20 times the daily oral dose is used initially, the monthly dose should be reduced by approximately 25% each month for two months based on clinical response until an appropriate maintenance dose is reached. Results of one multicenter trial indicate that monthly maintenance doses of 200 mg prevent relapse more consistently than doses of 25, 50, or 100 mg (Davis et al, 1993). The total monthly dose should not exceed 450 mg.

HALOPERIDOL DECANOATE:
Haldol Decanoate (McNeil). Solution (in sesame oil) 70.5 mg (equivalent to 50 mg of base)/ml (***Haldol Decanoate 50***) and 141.04 mg (equivalent to 100 mg of base)/ml (***Haldol Decanoate 100***) in 1 and 5 ml containers.

Oral: For psychoses, *adults and children over 12 years,* initially, 0.5 to 2 mg for moderate symptoms and 3 to 5 mg for severe symptoms; this amount is given every 8 to 12 hours until psychotic symptoms are controlled. Doses of 10 mg daily are usually sufficient and doses >20 mg daily are seldom required. When control has been achieved, the dose should be reduced gradually to the minimum effective maintenance level (usually, 2 to 8 mg daily). *Elderly or debilitated patients,* initially, 0.5 to 2 mg, gradually increased in increments of 0.5 mg.

For chronic schizophrenia, *adults and children over 12 years,* initially, 5 to 15 mg in divided doses, gradually increased until control is achieved (usually no more than 20 mg) and then gradually reduced to maintenance levels (usually, 5 to 15 mg daily). *Elderly or debilitated patients,* initially, 0.5 to 1.5 mg, increased gradually in small increments; the usual maintenance dose is 2 to 8 mg daily. *Children 3 to 12 years,* initially, 0.5 mg daily, increased by 0.5 mg at five- to seven-day intervals until the desired therapeutic effect is obtained. The total daily dose may be given in two or three divided amounts. Maintenance doses usually range from 0.05 to 0.15 mg/kg/day for psychotic disorders. *Children under 3 years,* information is inadequate to establish dosage.

HALOPERIDOL:
Haldol (McNeil), ***Generic.*** Tablets 0.5, 1, 2, 5, 10, and 20 mg.
HALOPERIDOL LACTATE:
Haldol (McNeil), ***Generic.*** Concentrate 2 mg/ml.

DIBENZOXAZEPINE DERIVATIVE

LOXAPINE HYDROCHLORIDE

[Loxitane C, Loxitane IM]

LOXAPINE SUCCINATE
[Loxitane]

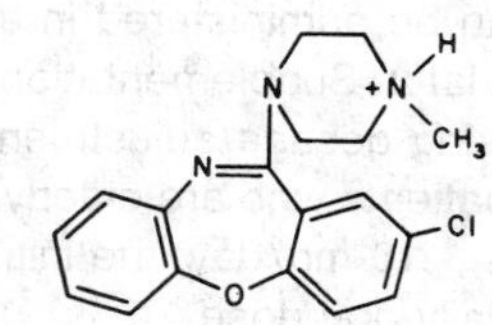

ACTIONS AND USES. This dibenzoxazepine derivative represents a class of antipsychotic agents that is chemically distinct from the phenothiazines, butyrophenones, thioxanthenes, and dihydroindolone compounds. However, the major pharmacologic actions of loxapine do not differ appreciably from those of the other antipsychotic drugs. Loxapine has antiemetic, sedative, anticholinergic, and alpha-antiadrenergic actions.

This compound is effective in the treatment of schizophrenia and other psychoses. A closely related derivative, the antidepressant, amoxapine [Asendin], is actually norloxapine.

ADVERSE REACTIONS AND PRECAUTIONS. The incidence of extrapyramidal reactions, other than tardive dyskinesia, is only slightly lower than that of piperazine phenothiazines (see Table 1). Pigmentary retinopathy and skin pigmentation have not been reported. Loxapine, like other antipsychotic drugs, decreases the seizure threshold and should be used with caution in patients with a history of convulsive disorders. Hepatitis has been associated rarely with use of loxapine.

For further information on indications, adverse reactions, drug interactions, and precautions, see the Introduction.

PHARMACOKINETICS. Loxapine is well absorbed orally, but its bioavailability is approximately 33% due to rapid and extensive hepatic metabolism. Major active metabolites include 7- and 8-hydroxyloxapine (antipsychotic) and 8-hydroxyamoxapine (antidepressant). Several other hydroxylated and N-oxidized metabolites also are formed; these are conjugated and excreted in the urine along with the active metabolites. Mean elimination half-lives of loxapine, 8-hydroxyloxapine, and 8-hydroxyamoxapine are 4, 9, and 30 hours, respectively.

DOSAGE AND PREPARATIONS.

Oral: *Adults and adolescents 16 years or older,* initially, 10 mg twice daily; a maximum of 50 mg daily may be given to severely psychotic patients. Dosage should be increased rapidly over the next week to ten days until control is achieved. For maintenance, dosage should be reduced gradually to the minimum effective level. The usual therapeutic range is 60 to 100 mg daily; however, many patients have been maintained satisfactorily on dosages of 20 to 60 mg daily. *Elderly and debilitated patients,* initially, one-third to one-half the usual adult dose. *Children under 16 years,* information is inadequate to establish a dosage. The concentrate should be diluted in fruit juice prior to administration.

LOXAPINE HYDROCHLORIDE:
Loxitane C (Lederle). Concentrate 25 mg/ml (equivalent to base).

LOXAPINE SUCCINATE:
Loxitane (Lederle), ***Generic.*** Capsules 5, 10, 25, and 50 mg (equivalent to base).

Intramuscular: 12.5 to 50 mg every four to six hours or at longer intervals, depending on the response. Once symptoms are controlled, oral therapy should be substituted. This preparation should *not* be injected intravenously.

LOXAPINE HYDROCHLORIDE:
Loxitane IM (Lederle). Solution 50 mg/ml (equivalent to base) in 1 and 10 ml containers.

DIBENZODIAZEPINE DERIVATIVE

CLOZAPINE
[Clozaril]

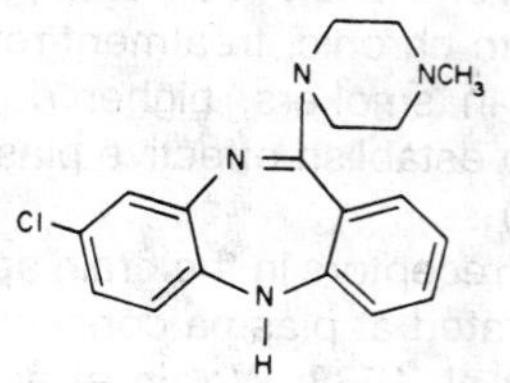

ACTIONS. This low-potency agent is related chemically, but not pharmacologically, to loxapine. Its pharmacologic profile is atypical compared with those of other currently available antipsychotic drugs. Most notably, the risk of producing most extrapyramidal effects is minimal with clozapine. No cases of tardive dyskinesia have been reported among patients receiving the drug to date, some of whom have been treated for up to ten years, although mild akathisia or muscle stiffness occurs occasionally (Baldessarini and Frankenburg, 1991) and neuroleptic malignant syndrome has been reported. Serum prolactin concentrations also are not elevated in humans.

Clozapine is further distinguished from other antipsychotic drugs by low affinity for D_1, D_2, and D_3 receptors but higher affinity for the D_4 receptor (Van Tol et al, 1991). Neurochemical and electrophysiologic studies in animals suggest that the drug may have some specificity for altering the function of dopamine neurons that project to the forebrain mesolimbic-mesocortical system in contrast to dopamine neurons in the extrapyramidal system. Clozapine also antagonizes muscarinic cholinergic, $alpha_1$ adrenergic, 5-hydroxytryptaminergic (especially 5-HT_2), and possibly histamine receptors. These actions may contribute to the clinical and behavioral effects of the drug.

USES. Clozapine is effective in controlling both positive (irritability, hallucinations, delusions) and negative (social disinterest and incompetence, personal neatness) symptoms of schizophrenia and other psychoses (Kane et al, 1988; Weintraub and Evans, 1989; Kay and Lindenmayer, 1991). A beneficial effect is often observed within two weeks, with additional gradual improvement over many weeks. Compared with other antipsychotic drugs, clozapine appears to be particularly useful in the treatment of severely disturbed, treatment-refractory patients (Kane et al, 1988; Pickar et al, 1992). Depending on trial duration and response criteria, between 30% and 60% of previously unresponsive patients appear to benefit significantly from use of clozapine (Kane, 1992). This drug also may be effective in otherwise unresponsive psychotic mood or schizoaffective disorders (McElroy et al, 1991). In addition, because of the very low risk of most extrapyramidal effects with this agent, a trial of clozapine is clearly indicated for patients in whom extrapyramidal signs and symptoms (including tardive dyskinesia) are severe and intolerable with other agents. It also has been used to treat psychosis and agitation in patients with Parkinson's disease. Case reports suggest clozapine may be useful in the treatment of bipolar patients with mixed, dysphoric mania (Suppes et al, 1992).

Because there is greater risk of agranulocytosis with clozapine than with any other antipsychotic drug, its use should be limited to treatment-resistant patients who are unresponsive to or cannot tolerate the other drugs (Marder and Van Putten, 1988). Currently, clozapine is administered only through "treatment systems" that are established by individual physicians, community health centers, or hospitals in conjunction with a designated pharmacy and are registered with the manufacturer, Sandoz Pharmaceuticals. This distribution system is designed to ensure weekly monitoring of white blood cell (WBC) counts.

ADVERSE REACTIONS AND PRECAUTIONS. The most significant reaction associated with clozapine therapy is agranulocytosis. Although this also occurs with other antipsychotic drugs, it is more prominent with clozapine and resulted in several deaths before careful monitoring procedures were defined. In preapproval studies in the United States, the cumulative incidence of agranulocytosis was 1.3%, and this adverse reaction developed most frequently 4 to 18 weeks after treatment began. Over 40,000 patients have received clozapine therapy in the United States. Through October 1992, seven deaths from complications attributable to agranulocytosis had been reported in this country. According to the manufacturer, approximately 0.5% of patients exposed to clozapine in the United States developed agranulocytosis and 1% discontinued therapy due to development of serious leukopenia or neutropenia. In one postmarketing study, results of a survival analysis on 11,555 patients who received clozapine indicate that the cumulative incidence of agranulocytosis is 0.8% at 12 months and 0.91% at 18 months; the risk increased with age and was higher among women (Alvir et al, 1993). Sixty-one (83%) of these patients developed the complication within three months and 96% within six months. Several cases of eosinophilia also have been reported.

The manufacturer recommends that the treatment period not exceed six weeks unless some improvement in psychotic symptoms has been observed. Concurrent administration of other drugs that suppress bone marrow function is contraindicated. Therapy generally should not be initiated if the WBC count is $<3,500/mm^3$, the patient has a history of myeloproliferative disorder, or clozapine-induced leukopenia previously required discontinuation of therapy. For suggested strategies if there is a progressive fall in the total WBC count to between $3,000/mm^3$ and $2,000/mm^3$, see the manufacturer's literature. The availability of clozapine is currently linked to mandatory weekly hematologic testing. Hematologic status should be monitored periodically but, based on recent experience in other countries (eg, United Kingdom), not necessarily weekly, particularly after the first several months of therapy. The relaxation of the weekly monitoring requirement in the United States awaits results of further prospective studies and possible revision in the product labeling.

Clozapine can produce benign hyperthermia, most commonly within the first three weeks of treatment. This appears to have no deleterious physiologic consequences and is quite distinct from neuroleptic malignant syndrome (NMS). (However, NMS associated with clozapine has been reported [see discussion of this adverse reaction in the Introduction]. Whether clozapine alone can cause NMS has not been established [Weller and Kornhuber, 1993].) Because temperature elevation can be an initial sign of agranulocytosis, the hyperthermia should be evaluated. The WBC count should be determined as an aid in differential diagnosis.

Dose-dependent tachycardia has occurred; in some patients, the rate can increase by 20 to 25 beats per minute. Like other low-potency agents, clozapine also produces orthostatic hypotension and should be used cautiously in patients with cardiovascular disorders. Orthostatic hypotension is more likely to occur soon after initiation of therapy when the dosage is escalated rapidly and may even occur after the first dose; rarely (approximately 1/3,000 patients), collapse can be accompanied by respiratory and/or cardiac arrest.

Clozapine may cause seizures in 3% to 5% of patients. Because this side effect is dose-related, greater than usual caution should be exercised in selecting the initial dose and the rate of dose escalation in any patient with a history of seizures. Some clinicians prescribe an antiepileptic drug (eg, valproate) in these patients or when clozapine is given in doses >500 mg daily (Baldessarini and Frankenburg, 1991).

Sedation, dizziness, hypersalivation, and weight gain occur frequently. Weight gain may be substantial (Cohen et al, 1990; Leadbetter et al, 1992). Hypersalivation is dose-dependent and often is relieved by dosage reduction. Nausea and vomiting, constipation, headache, tremor, restlessness, dry mouth, and sweating also may occur. Urinary disorders, hyponatremia, hypertension, confusion, agitation, priapism, and abdominal discomfort are uncommon.

Symptoms of overdosage include drowsiness, lethargy, coma, areflexia, confusion, disorientation, delirium, tachycardia, hypotension, respiratory depression, arrhythmias, heart block, mydriasis, blurred vision, restlessness, hyperreflexia, convulsions, and hyperthermia. The pronounced central anticholinergic effects of clozapine increase the likelihood of the occurrence of confusion and delirium; these effects have been counteracted by the cautious administration of physostigmine, but immediately decreasing the dose of clozapine is an appropriate initial step (Baldessarini and Frankenburg, 1991). In one case, death occurred in a physically emaciated man who ingested 3 g. Tonic-clonic seizures occurred in two frail women who received 1.2 and 1.5 g.

Clozapine is classified in FDA Pregnancy Category B.

PHARMACOKINETICS. Following oral administration, clozapine is rapidly and completely absorbed; bioavailability averages 50% to 60%. Peak plasma concentrations are linearly related to dose and are attained an average of two hours after administration. Plasma concentrations are higher in women and the elderly and are lower in smokers (Haring et al, 1990). More than 95% of the drug is bound to plasma proteins; apparent Vd is 5 L/kg. Clozapine is almost completely metabolized prior to excretion in the urine and, to a minor extent, in the feces. The main metabolites are N-desmethyl and N-oxide derivatives and they have little pharmacologic activity. The mean half-life is approximately 12 hours (range, 6 to 33 hours).

Preliminary evidence suggests that there is greater likelihood of response in treatment-refractory schizophrenic patients when plasma concentrations exceed 350 ng/ml (Perry et al, 1991).

DRUG INTERACTIONS. Excessive sedation and respiratory depression may occur when benzodiazepines or other psychotropic drugs are administered concomitantly. Phenytoin or carbamazepine may decrease plasma concentrations of clozapine and lead to clinical deterioration, while cimetidine and fluoxetine may increase plasma concentrations and cause toxicity (Szymanski et al, 1991; Miller, 1991).

DOSAGE AND PREPARATIONS.

Oral: *Adults,* because clozapine initially may be sedating, the recommended initial dose is 12.5 mg once or twice daily. The amount is increased in increments of 25 to 50 mg daily, if well tolerated, to 300 to 450 mg daily within two weeks. Efficacy is less likely with doses lower than 100 mg/day. The optimal therapeutic dose is usually 300 to 600 mg/day. If necessary, the dose can be increased to a maximum of 900 mg/day, providing no limiting adverse reactions occur, but the risk of seizures increases significantly when the dosage exceeds 600 mg daily. When symptoms are controlled, the dose should be gradually reduced to the minimum effective maintenance level (usually approximately 300 mg daily). Although no significant withdrawal reactions have occurred on termination of treatment, gradual withdrawal is always preferred if possible. Monitoring of WBC counts should continue during the withdrawal period and for at least one month following termination of treatment. In patients who have discontinued therapy for two days or more, the manufacturer recommends that treatment be reinitiated with 12.5 mg once or twice daily. If that amount is well tolerated, it may be possible to titrate the dose to the therapeutic amount more rapidly than for initial treatment.

Only general dosage guidelines are available for converting a patient from standard antipsychotic drug therapy to clozapine. Patients receiving depot formulations (eg, haloperidol decanoate) should first be converted to oral forms. To lessen the likelihood of adverse drug reactions but avoid early relapse, oral doses of standard antipsychotic drugs should be tapered and clozapine therapy initiated before the discontinuation of the former is complete.

Clinical experience with clozapine in *children, the elderly, or debilitated patients* is not sufficient to provide dosage guidelines.

Clozaril (Sandoz). Tablets 25 and 100 mg.

DIHYDROINDOLONE DERIVATIVE

MOLINDONE HYDROCHLORIDE

[Moban]

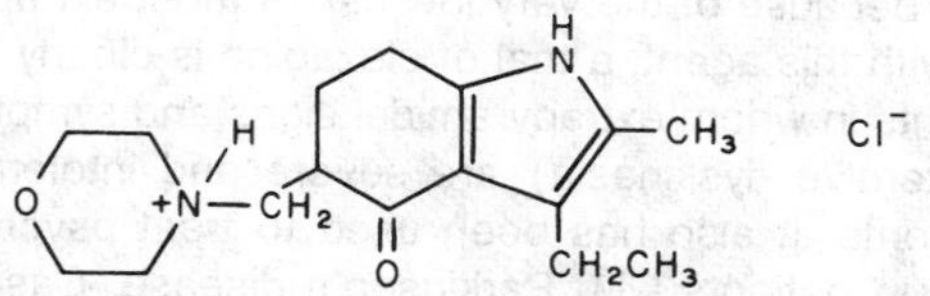

ACTIONS AND USES. Molindone is chemically unrelated to the phenothiazines, butyrophenones, thioxanthenes, dibenzoxazepines, or dibenzodiazepines. It is effective in schizophrenia and other psychoses and may be useful in the treatment of the aggressive type of undersocialized conduct disorder (Owen and Cole, 1989). Molindone has much lower affinity for D_2 receptors than most antipsychotic agents and has a relatively low affinity for D_1 receptors. It has only low to moderate affinity for cholinergic and alpha-adrenergic receptors. Some electrophysiologic data from animals indicate that molindone has certain characteristics that resemble those of clozapine.

ADVERSE REACTIONS AND PRECAUTIONS. The anticholinergic and antiadrenergic effects of molindone generally are less severe than those of the other antipsychotic drugs. The sedative effects are intermediate between those of the aliphatic and piperazine phenothiazines (see Table 1). Extrapyramidal effects generally are less prominent, but molindone has been associated with tardive dyskinesia. Lens opacities and pigmentary retinopathy have not been reported.

For further information on adverse reactions and precautions, see the Introduction.

PHARMACOKINETICS. The pharmacokinetics of molindone are distinct from those of other antipsychotic agents. Peak plasma levels are reached in approximately 0.6 and 1.1 hours following intramuscular and oral administration, respectively. Molindone is rapidly converted to numerous metabolites by the liver. The half-life is approximately two hours. However, the clinical duration of action is at least 24 hours, which suggests the presence of an active metabolite.

DOSAGE AND PREPARATIONS.

Oral: *Adults,* initially, 50 to 75 mg daily in divided doses, gradually increased if necessary until symptoms are controlled; doses as high as 225 mg daily have been used. When symptoms are controlled, the dose should be reduced gradually to the minimum effective level for maintenance. *Elderly or debilitated patients,* initially, one-third to one-half the usual adult dosage. *Children under 12 years,* information is inadequate to establish a dosage.

Moban (Gate). Concentrate 20 mg/ml as the hydrochloride; tablets 5, 10, 25, 50, and 100 mg.

Cited References

Diagnostic and Statistical Manual of Mental Disorders, ed 3, revised. Washington, DC, American Psychiatric Association, 1987, 113-118.

Tardive Dyskinesia: A Task Force Report of the American Psychiatric Association. Washington, DC, American Psychiatric Association, 1992.

Adler LA, et al: Vitamin E treatment of tardive dyskinesia. *Am J Psychiatry* 150:1405-1407, 1993.

Alberti-Flor JJ: Chlorpromazine-induced lupus-like illness. *Am Fam Physician* 27:151-152, (April) 1983.

Alvir JMJ, et al: Clozapine-induced agranulocytosis: Incidence and risk factors in the United States. *N Engl J Med* 329:162-167, 1993.

Ambelas A: Preschizophrenics: Adding to the evidence, sharpening the focus. *Br J Psychiatry* 160:401-404, 1992.

Andreasen NC, et al: Magnetic resonance imaging of the brain in schizophrenia: The pathophysiologic significance of structural abnormalities. *Arch Gen Psychiatry* 47:35-44, 1990.

Andreasen NC, et al: Hypofrontality in neuroleptic-naive patients and in patients with chronic schizophrenia: Assessment with xenon 133 single-photon emission computed tomography and the Tower of London. *Arch Gen Psychiatry* 49:943-958, 1992.

Arana GW, et al: Efficacy of anticholinergic prophylaxis for neuroleptic-induced acute dystonia. *Am J Psychiatry* 145:993-996, 1988.

Aubree JC, Lader MH: High and very high dosage antipsychotics: Critical review. *J Clin Psychiatry* 41:341-350, 1980.

Ayd FJ Jr: Neuroleptic rechallenge for patients with a history of neuroleptic malignant syndrome (NMS). *Int Drug Ther Newslett* 25:1-4, (Jan) 1990.

Baldessarini RJ: *Chemotherapy in Psychiatry: Principles and Practice,* ed 2. Cambridge, Mass, Harvard University Press, 1985.

Baldessarini RJ: Drugs and the treatment of psychiatric disorders, in Gilman AG, et al (eds): *Goodman and Gilman's The Pharmacological Basis of Therapeutics*, ed 8. New York, Pergamon Press, 1990, 383-435.

Baldessarini RJ, Frankenburg FR: Clozapine: A novel antipsychotic agent. *N Engl J Med* 324:746-754, 1991.

Baldessarini RJ, et al: Significance of neuroleptic dose and plasma level in the pharmacological treatment of psychoses. *Arch Gen Psychiatry* 45:79-91, 1988.

Barbee JG, et al: Alprazolam as a neuroleptic adjunct in the emergency treatment of schizophrenia. *Am J Psychiatry* 149:506-510, 1992.

Biederman J, Jellinek MS: Psychopharmacology in children. *N Engl J Med* 310:968-971, 1984.

Bloom FE: Advancing a neurodevelopmental origin for schizophrenia. *Arch Gen Psychiatry* 50:224-227, 1993.

Borison RL, et al: Risperidone: Clinical safety and efficacy in schizophrenia. *Psychopharmacol Bull* 28:213-218, 1992.

Bracha HS, et al: Second-trimester markers of fetal size in schizophrenia: A study of monozygotic twins. *Am J Psychiatry* 149:1355-1361, 1992.

Breslin NA: Treatment of schizophrenia: Current practice and future promise. *Hosp Community Psychiatry* 43:877-885, 1992.

Bucci L: The negative symptoms of schizophrenia and the monoamine oxidase inhibitors. *Psychopharmacology* 91:104-108, 1987.

Buchsbaum MS: The frontal lobes, basal ganglia, and temporal lobes as sites for schizophrenia. *Schizophr Bull* 16:379-389, 1990.

Burkhardt C, et al: Neuroleptic medications inhibit complex I of the electron transport chain. *Ann Neurol* 33:512-517, 1993.

Burnett PL, et al: Low-dose depot medication in schizophrenia. *Schizophr Bull* 19:155-164, 1993.

Caldwell CB, Gottesman II: Schizophrenics kill themselves too: A review of risk factors for suicide. *Schizophr Bull* 16:571-589, 1990.

Campbell M: Pharmacotherapy, in: *Treatment of Psychiatric Disorders: A Task Force Report of the American Psychiatric Association.* Washington, DC, American Psychiatric Association, 1989, vol 1, 226-248.

Campbell M, et al: Psychopharmacological treatment of children with syndrome of autism. *Pediatr Ann* 13:309-316, 1984.

Cannon D, et al: Serum haloperidol and neuroleptic receptor levels in chronic psychosis. *Ann Clin Lab Sci* 18:378-383, 1988.

Caroff S: The neuroleptic malignant syndrome. *J Clin Psychiatry* 41:79-83, 1980.

Carpenter WT Jr, et al: A comparative trial of pharmacologic strategies in schizophrenia. *Am J Psychiatry* 144:1466-1470, 1987.

Chakos MH, et al: Incidence and correlates of acute extrapyramidal symptoms in first episode of schizophrenia. *Psychopharmacol Bull* 28:81-86, 1992.

Chakraborty BS, et al: Single dose kinetics of thioridazine and its two psychoactive metabolites in healthy humans: A dose proportionality study. *J Pharmaceut Sci* 78:796-801, 1989.

Chouinard G, et al: A Canadian multicenter placebo-controlled study of fixed doses of risperidone and haloperidol in the treatment of chronic schizophrenic patients. *J Clin Psychopharmacol* 13:25-40, (Feb) 1993.

Christison GW, et al: When symptoms persist: Choosing among alternative somatic treatments for schizophrenia. *Schizophr Bull* 17:243-245, 1991.

Claus A, et al: Risperidone versus haloperidol in the treatment of chronic schizophrenic inpatients: A multicentre double-blind comparative study. *Acta Psychiatr Scand* 85:295-305, 1992.

Cohen DJ, et al: Clonidine ameliorates Gilles de la Tourette syndrome. *Arch Gen Psychiatry* 37:1350-1357, 1980.

Cohen LS, et al: Treatment guidelines for psychotropic drug use in pregnancy. *Psychosomatics* 30:25-33, 1989.

Cohen S, et al: Weight gain associated with clozapine. *Am J Psychiatry* 147:503-504, 1990.

Conrad AJ, et al: Hippocampal pyramidal cell disarray in schizophrenia as a bilateral phenomenon. *Arch Gen Psychiatry* 48:413-417, 1991.

Coryell W, et al: Haloperidol plasma levels and acute clinical change in schizophrenia. *J Clin Psychopharmacol* 10:397-402, 1990.

Cowdry RW, Gardner DL: Pharmacotherapy of borderline personality disorder: Alprazolam, carbamazepine, trifluoperazine and tranylcypromine. *Arch Gen Psychiatry* 45:111-119, 1988.

Crow TJ: Temporal lobe asymmetries as the key to the etiology of schizophrenia. *Schizophr Bull* 16:433-443, 1990.

Davis JM, Andriukaitis S: Natural course of schizophrenia and effective maintenance drug treatment. *J Clin Psychopharmacol* 6:2S-10S, 1986.

Davis JM, et al: Dose response of prophylactic antipsychotics. *J Clin Psychiatry* 54 (suppl 3):24-30, 1993.

DeLisi LE: The significance of age of onset for schizophrenia. *Schizophr Bull* 18:209-215, 1992.

Donaldson S, et al: Alternative treatments for schizophrenic psychoses, in Berger P, Brodie HKH (eds): *American Handbook of Psychiatry.* New York, Academic Press, 1986, vol 8, 513-535.

Dose M, et al: Carbamazepine as an adjunct of antipsychotic therapy. *Psychiatry Res* 22:303-310, 1987.

Edlund MJ, Craig TJ: Antipsychotic drug use and birth defects: Epidemiologic reassessment. *Compr Psychiatry* 25:32-37, (Jan/Feb) 1984.

Egan MF, et al: Treatment of tardive dyskinesia with vitamin E. *Am J Psychiatry* 149:773-777, 1992.

Ereshefsky L, et al: Thiothixene pharmacokinetic interactions: A study of hepatic enzyme inducers, clearance inhibitors, and demographic variables. *J Clin Psychopharmacol* 11:296-301, 1991.

Fenton WS, McGlashan TH: Testing systems for assessment of negative symptoms in schizophrenia. *Arch Gen Psychiatry* 49:179-184, 1992.

Fleischhacker WW, et al: The pharmacologic treatment of neuroleptic-induced akathisia. *J Clin Psychopharmacol* 10:12-21, (Feb) 1990.

Friedman E, et al: Chronic fluphenazine and clozapine elicit opposite changes in brain muscarinic receptor binding: Implications for understanding tardive dyskinesia. *J Pharmacol Exp Ther* 226:7-12, 1983.

Froemming JS, et al: Pharmacokinetics of haloperidol. *Clin Pharmacokinet* 17:396-423, 1989.

Glazer WM: Depot fluphenazine: Risk/benefit ratio. *J Clin Psychiatry* 45 (5, sec 2):28-35, 1984.

Glazer WM, Kane JM: Depot neuroleptic therapy: An underutilized treatment option. *J Clin Psychiatry* 53:426-433, 1992.

Glazer WM, et al: Tardive dyskinesia. *Arch Gen Psychiatry* 41:623-627, 1984.

Glazer WM, et al: The prediction of chronic persistent versus intermittent tardive dyskinesia: A retrospective follow-up study. *Br J Psychiatry* 158:822-828, 1991.

Glazer WM, et al: Predicting the long-term risk of tardive dyskinesia in outpatients maintained on neuroleptic medications. *J Clin Psychiatry* 54:133-139, 1993.

Goff DC, Baldessarini RJ: Drug interactions with antipsychotic agents. *J Clin Psychopharmacol* 13:57-67, 1993.

Goff DC, et al: Trial of fluoxetine added to neuroleptics for treatment-resistant schizophrenic patients. *Am J Psychiatry* 147:492-494, 1990.

Goff DC, et al: Elevation of plasma concentrations of haloperidol after the addition of fluoxetine. *Am J Psychiatry* 148:790-792, 1991.

Goldberg SC, et al: Borderline and schizotypal personality disorders treated with low-dose thiothixene vs placebo. *Arch Gen Psychiatry* 43:680-686, 1986.

Haring C, et al: Influence of patient-related variables on clozapine plasma levels. *Am J Psychiatry* 147:1471-1475, 1990.

Healy D: Neuroleptics and psychic indifference: A review. *J R Soc Med* 82:615-619, 1989.

Hemstrom CA, et al: Haloperidol decanoate: Depot antipsychotic. *DICP* 22:290-295, 1988.

Herz MI, et al: Intermittent medication for stable schizophrenic: An alternative to maintenance medication. *Am J Psychiatry* 139:918-922, 1982.

Herz MI, et al: Intermittent vs maintenance medication in schizophrenia: Two-year results. *Arch Gen Psychiatry* 48:333-339, 1991.

Hogarty GE: Prevention of relapse in chronic schizophrenic patients. *J Clin Psychiatry* 54(suppl):18-23, (March) 1993.

Itil TM, Soldatos C: Epileptogenic side effects of psychotropic drugs: Practical recommendations. *JAMA* 244:1460-1463, 1980.

Janicak PG, et al: Trifluoperazine plasma levels and clinical response. *J Clin Psychopharmacol* 9:340-346, 1989.

Jolley AG, et al: Trial of brief intermittent neuroleptic prophylaxis for selected schizophrenic outpatients: Clinical and social outcome at two years. *BMJ* 301:837-842, 1990.

Kane JM: Clinical efficacy of clozapine in treatment-refractory schizophrenia: An overview. *Br J Psychiatry* 160(suppl 17):41-45, 1992.

Kane JM, Lieberman JA: Maintenance pharmacotherapy in schizophrenia, in Meltzer HY (ed): *Psychopharmacology: The Third Generation of Progress*. New York, Raven Press, 1987, 1103-1109.

Kane JM, Marder SR: Psychopharmacologic treatment of schizophrenia. *Schizophr Bull* 19:287-302, 1993.

Kane JM, et al: Depot neuroleptics: Comparative review of standard, intermediate, and low-dose regimens. *J Clin Psychiatry* 47(suppl):30-33, (May) 1986.

Kane J, et al: Clozapine for the treatment-resistant schizophrenic: Double-blind comparison with chlorpromazine. *Arch Gen Psychiatry* 45:789-796, 1988.

Kang UJ, Fahn S: Management of tardive dyskinesia. *Ration Drug Ther* 22:1-7, (Aug) 1988.

Kay SR: Significance of the positive-negative distinction in schizophrenia. *Schizophr Bull* 16:635-652, 1990.

Kay SR, Lindenmayer J-P: Stability of psychopathology dimensions in chronic schizophrenia: Response to clozapine treatment. *Compr Psychiatry* 32:28-35, (Jan/Feb) 1991.

Klein E, et al: Carbamazepine and haloperidol versus placebo and haloperidol in excited psychotics: A controlled study. *Arch Gen Psychiatry* 41:165-170, 1984.

Lacoursiere RB, et al: Medical effects of abrupt neuroleptic withdrawal. *Compr Psychiatry* 17:285-293, (March-April) 1976.

Leadbetter R, et al: Clozapine-induced weight gain: Prevalence and clinical relevance. *Am J Psychiatry* 149:68-72, 1992.

Lieberman JA: Prediction of outcome in first-episode schizophrenia. *J Clin Psychiatry* 54(suppl 3):13-17, 1993.

Luchins DJ, et al: Role of cholinergic supersensitivity in medical symptoms associated with withdrawal of antipsychotic drugs. *Am J Psychiatry* 137:1395-1398, 1980.

Manschreck TC: Drug treatment of schizophrenia: Principles and limitations. *Drug Ther* 13:185-204, (Sept) 1983.

Marder SR, Van Putten T: Who should receive clozapine? *Arch Gen Psychiatry* 45:865-867, 1988.

Marder SR, et al: Low- and conventional-dose maintenance therapy with fluphenazine decanoate: Two-year outcome. *Arch Gen Psychiatry* 44:518-521, 1987.

Marder SR, et al: The pharmacokinetics of long-acting injectable neuroleptic drugs: Clinical implication. *Psychopharmacology* 98:433-439, 1989.

McElroy SL, et al: Clozapine in the treatment of psychotic mood disorders, schizoaffective disorder, and schizophrenia. *J Clin Psychiatry* 52:411-414, 1991.

Meltzer HY: Treatment of the neuroleptic-nonresponsive schizophrenic patient. *Schizophr Bull* 18:515-542, 1992.

Mesulam M-M: Schizophrenia and the brain. *N Engl J Med* 322:842-845, 1990.

Mikkelsen EJ, et al: School avoidance and social phobia triggered by haloperidol in patients with Tourette's syndrome. *Am J Psychiatry* 138:1572-1576, 1981.

Miller DD: Effect of phenytoin on plasma clozapine concentrations in two patients. *J Clin Psychiatry* 52:23-25, 1991.

Neppe VM: Carbamazepine as adjunctive treatment in nonepileptic chronic patients with EEG temporal lobe abnormalities. *J Clin Psychiatry* 44:326-331, 1983.

Okuma T, et al: A double-blind study of adjunctive carbamazepine versus placebo on excited states of schizophrenic and schizoaffective disorders. *Acta Psychiatr Scand* 80:250-259, 1989.

Olmsted TR: Neuroleptic malignant syndrome: Guidelines for treatment and reinstitution of neuroleptics. *South Med J* 81:888-891, 1988.

Opler LA, Feinberg SS: The role of pimozide in clinical psychiatry: A review. *J Clin Psychiatry* 52:221-233, 1991.

Owen RR Jr, Cole JO: Molindone hydrochloride: A review of laboratory and clinical findings. *J Clin Psychopharmacol* 9:268-276, 1989.

Oyewumi LK: Neuroleptics under high risk conditions. *Can J Psychiatry* 28:398-403, 1983.

Perry P, et al: The relationship of haloperidol concentrations to therapeutic response. *J Clin Psychopharmacol* 8:38-43, 1988.

Perry PJ, et al: Clozapine and norclozapine plasma concentrations and clinical response of treatment-refractory schizophrenic patients. *Am J Psychiatry* 148:231-235, 1991.

Perry PJ, et al: Haloperidol dosing requirements: The contribution of smoking and nonlinear pharmacokinetics. *J Clin Psychopharmacol* 13:46-51, 1993.

Pickar D, et al: Clinical and biologic response to clozapine in patients with schizophrenia: Crossover comparison with fluphenazine. *Arch Gen Psychiatry* 49:345-353, 1992.

Pollack MH, et al: Genitourinary and sexual adverse effects of psychotropic medication. *Int J Psychiatry Med* 22:305-327, 1992.

Reynolds GP: Beyond the dopamine hypothesis: The neurochemical pathology of schizophrenia. *Br J Psychiatry* 155:305-316, 1989.

Riesenberg D: Drugs in the institutionalized elderly: Time to get it right? *JAMA* 260:3054, 1988.

Rifkin A, Siris S: Drug treatment of acute schizophrenia, in Meltzer HY (ed): *Psychopharmacology: The Third Generation of Progress*. New York, Raven Press, 1987, 1095-1101.

Roberts GW: Schizophrenia: A neuropathological perspective. *Br J Psychiatry* 158:8-17, 1991.

Rosebush P, et al: Twenty neuroleptic rechallenges after neuroleptic malignant syndrome in 15 patients. *J Clin Psychiatry* 50:295-298, 1989.

Rosenberg MR, Green M: Neuroleptic malignant syndrome: Review of response to therapy. *Arch Intern Med* 149:1927-1931, 1989.

Saltz BL, et al: Prospective study of tardive dyskinesia incidence in the elderly. *JAMA* 266:2402-2406, 1991.

Salzman C, et al: Parenteral lorazepam versus parenteral haloperidol for the control of psychotic disruptive behavior. *J Clin Psychiatry* 52:177-180, 1991.

Shalev A, et al: Mortality from neuroleptic malignant syndrome. *J Clin Psychiatry* 50:18-25, 1989.

Sokoloff P, et al: Molecular cloning and characterization of a novel dopamine receptor (D_3) as a target for neuroleptics. *Nature* 347:146-151, 1990.

Soloff PH, et al: Progress in pharmacotherapy of borderline disorders. *Arch Gen Psychiatry* 43:691-697, 1986.

Soloff PH, et al: Efficacy of phenelzine and haloperidol in borderline personality disorder. *Arch Gen Psychiatry* 50:377-385, 1993.

Stahl SM, et al: Neuropharmacology of tardive dyskinesia, spontaneous dyskinesia, and other dystonias. *J Clin Psychopharmacol* 2:321-328, 1982.

Suddath RL, et al: Anatomical abnormalities in the brains of monozygotic twins discordant for schizophrenia. *N Engl J Med* 322:789-794, 1990.

Sunahara RK, et al: Cloning of the gene for a human dopamine D_5 receptor with higher affinity for dopamine than D_1. *Nature* 350:614-619, 1991.

Suppes T, et al: Clozapine in the treatment of dysphoric mania. *Biol Psychiatry* 32:270-280, 1992.

Szymanski S, et al: A case report of cimetidine-induced clozapine toxicity. *J Clin Psychiatry* 52:21-22, 1991.

Tarsy D, Baldessarini RJ: Tardive dyskinesia. *Am Rev Med* 35:605-623, 1984.

Teoh R: Tardive dyskinesia. *Adverse Drug React Bull* 132:496-499, 1988.

Tollefson G, et al: Circulating lupus-like coagulation inhibitor induced by chlorpromazine. *J Clin Psychopharmacol* 4:49-51, 1984.

Van Putten T, et al: Neuroleptic plasma levels. *Schizophr Bull* 17:197-216, 1991.

Van Putten T, et al: Haloperidol plasma levels and clinical response: A therapeutic window relationship. *Am J Psychiatry* 149:500-505, 1992.

Van Tol HHM, et al: Cloning of the gene for a human dopamine D_4 receptor with high affinity for the antipsychotic clozapine. *Nature* 350:610-614, 1991.

Van Tol HHM, et al: Multiple dopamine D4 receptor variants in the human population, letter. *Nature* 358:149-152, (July) 1992.

Waddington JL: Schizophrenia: Developmental neuroscience and pathobiology. *Lancet* 341:531-536, 1993.

Waldman AJ: Neuroanatomic/neuropathologic correlates in schizophrenia. *South Med J* 85:907-916, 1992.

Weintraub M, Evans P: Clozapine: Neuroleptic agent for selected schizophrenics and patients with tardive dyskinesia. *Hosp Formul* 24:16-27, 1989.

Weller M, Kornhuber J: Does clozapine cause neuroleptic malignant syndrome, letter. *J Clin Psychiatry* 54:70-71, 1993.

Wilt JL, et al: Torsade de pointes associated with the use of intravenous haloperidol. *Ann Intern Med* 119:391-394, 1993.

Wolkin A, et al: Dopamine receptor occupancy and plasma haloperidol levels. *Arch Gen Psychiatry* 46:482-483, 1989.

Wolkowitz OM, Pickar D: Benzodiazepines in the treatment of schizophrenia: A review and reappraisal. *Am J Psychiatry* 148:714-726, 1991.

Young LK, Patel MM: Respiratory complications of antipsychotic drugs in medically ill patients. *Res Staff Physician* 30:73-80, (Nov) 1984.

Young AH, et al: A magnetic resonance imaging study of schizophrenia: Brain structure and clinical symptoms. *Br J Psychiatry* 158:158-164, 1991.

New Evaluation

RISPERIDONE

[Risperdal]

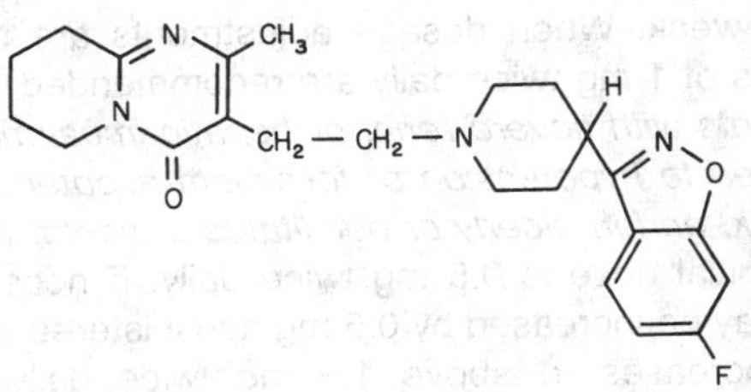

ACTIONS. Risperidone is the first available member of a new chemical class of antipsychotic agents, the benzisoxazole derivatives. The antipsychotic activity of this drug is believed to be related to its ability to competitively block dopamine (D_2) and serotonin (5-HT_2) receptors. Risperidone and its major metabolite, 9-hydroxyrisperidone, bind with high affinity to these and other receptors, including the α_1 and α_2 adrenergic and H_1 histaminergic receptors (Schotte et al, 1993). Risperidone has a much lower affinity for other 5-HT receptors and only weakly antagonizes the dopamine D_1 receptor and the haloperidol-sensitive sigma receptor. Cholinergic, muscarinic, and beta-adrenergic receptors are unaffected by risperidone.

USES. Risperidone was approved by the FDA for the "manifestations of psychotic disorders." Its antipsychotic efficacy was established in short-term (six- to eight-week) controlled trials in schizophrenic inpatients. In controlled comparative studies with a duration of 6 to 12 weeks, risperidone was superior to placebo in patients with chronic schizophrenia (Borison et al, 1992; Claus et al, 1992; Müller-Spahn and The International Risperidone Research Group, 1992; Chouinard et al, 1993; Meibach and the Risperidone Study Group, 1993). Its efficacy was equal or superior to that of haloperidol 10 or 20 mg in several studies. Comparative studies that incorporate a range of haloperidol doses are required before risperidone's relative efficacy and propensity to cause extrapyramidal side effects can be established. Further studies also are required to determine whether the risk of developing tardive dyskinesia is lower with long-term use of risperidone than with typical antipsychotic drugs. Risperidone is superior to placebo in reducing the symptoms of tardive dyskinesia.

Risperidone has not been tested extensively in patients who are resistant to treatment, and only limited data comparing it with clozapine are available. In one small double-blind study on patients with acute exacerbations of schizophrenia, risperidone 4 to 8 mg was comparable to clozapine 400 mg during the first month of treatment (Heinrich et al, 1994).

ADVERSE REACTIONS AND PRECAUTIONS. Administration of risperidone increases prolactin concentrations. Because this drug antagonizes alpha-adrenergic receptors, it may cause orthostatic hypotension (dizziness, tachycardia, and, in some patients, syncope), especially during the initial dose titration period. An increase in the QT interval was reported in some risperidone recipients during clinical trials. Risperidone has not been evaluated or used to any appreciable extent in patients with a recent history of myocardial infarction or unstable heart disease. Risperidone should be used with caution in individuals with cardiovascular or cerebrovascular disease and other conditions that could affect metabolism or hemodynamics.

Seizures were reported in 0.3% of patients who received risperidone during clinical trials. Single cases of priapism and thrombotic thrombocytopenic purpura also were reported.

In Phase II and III studies, approximately 9% of risperidone recipients discontinued treatment because of an adverse event; these included extrapyramidal symptoms (2.1%), dizziness (0.7%), hyperkinesia (0.6%), somnolence (0.5%), and nausea (0.3%). Dose-related adverse events probably include extrapyramidal symptoms, somnolence, increased duration of sleep, accommodation disturbances, orthostatic dizziness, palpitations, weight gain, erectile dysfunction, ejaculatory dysfunction, orgastic dysfunction, asthenia/lassitude/increased fatigability, and increased pigmentation.

In two six- to eight-week placebo-controlled trials, other adverse events (not noted above) that were reported spontaneously or detected by checklist in at least 5% of risperidone recipients and at a rate at least twice that of placebo recipients included anxiety, increased dreaming, reduced salivation, dyspepsia, diarrhea, constipation, rhinitis, rash, tachycardia, micturition disturbances, weight gain, menorrhagia, and diminished libido.

PREGNANCY AND LACTATION. There are no adequate, well-controlled studies on the use of risperidone in pregnant women. However, one case of agenesis of the corpus callosum in an infant exposed to risperidone in utero was reported; the causal relationship to risperidone therapy is unknown. This drug should be used during pregnancy only if the benefit justifies the potential risk to the fetus (FDA Pregnancy Category C). Patients taking risperidone should not breast feed.

DRUG INTERACTIONS. Metabolism of risperidone is inhibited by drugs that inhibit cytochrome P450IID_6 (CYP2D6), also known as debrisoquin hydroxylase. However, the pharmacokinetics and adverse reactions of the active moiety (defined as the sum of the plasma concentrations of risperidone and 9-hydroxyrisperidone) appear to be similar in both extensive and poor metabolizers. Based on in vitro data, risperidone is only a weak inhibitor of CYP2D6 and is not expected to have a significant effect in inhibiting the clearance of drugs that are metabolized by this enzyme. Pharmacokinetic studies in humans to confirm this expectation have not been conducted. Carbamazepine may increase and clozapine may decrease the clearance of risperidone.

Pharmacodynamically, risperidone would be expected to enhance the effects of drugs that depress the central nervous system or that decrease blood pressure and to antagonize the effects of levodopa and dopamine agonists. Because risperidone and/or 9-hydroxyrisperidone appears to lengthen the QT interval in some patients, concomitant use with other drugs that prolong the QT interval may increase the risk of development of torsades de pointes.

PHARMACOKINETICS. Risperidone is rapidly absorbed after oral administration; absolute oral bioavailability is 70%. Peak plasma concentrations are achieved within one hour. Food does not affect the rate or extent of absorption.

Risperidone is metabolized in the liver to a major equipotent active metabolite, 9-hydroxyrisperidone, and clinical effects are determined by the total plasma concentration of both compounds. Hydroxylation of risperidone is mediated by CYP2D6. The hepatic content and activity of this isoform are subject to genetic polymorphism. Accordingly, the apparent half-life of risperidone is three hours in extensive metabolizers and 20 hours in poor metabolizers; corresponding values for 9-hydroxyrisperidone are 21 and 30 hours, respectively. However, the pharmacokinetics of the active moiety are similar in patients with different phenotypes (mean elimination half-life of the active moiety is approximately 20 hours in both groups). Therefore, the clinical relevance of risperidone's metabolic polymorphism is probably minimal. In analyses comparing the rate of adverse reactions in extensive and poor metabolizers in open and controlled studies, no important differences were seen.

Plasma protein binding of risperidone is 90% and is correlated with the plasma concentration of alpha$_1$ acid glycoprotein. 9-Hydroxyrisperidone is 77% protein bound, but binding sites for the parent compound and metabolite appear to be distinct.

Clearance of the active moiety is decreased by 60% in patients with moderate to severe renal disease; renal clearance also is decreased in the elderly. The free fraction of risperidone may increase in patients with hepatic disease.

DOSAGE AND PREPARATIONS. In clinical trials, doses of 4 to 6 mg generally produced the best overall response. Daily doses >6 mg have not been shown to be more efficacious and are associated with a higher incidence of extrapyramidal effects and other adverse reactions.

Oral: *Adults*, initially, 1 mg twice daily; the dosage may be increased to 2 mg twice daily on the second day and 3 mg twice daily on the third day as tolerated. Further dosage increases, if required, should be limited to intervals of not less than one week. When dosage adjustments are necessary, increments of 1 mg twice daily are recommended.

In *patients with severe renal or hepatic impairment, those predisposed to hypotension or for whom hypotension would pose a risk, and in elderly or debilitated patients,* the recommended initial dose is 0.5 mg twice daily. If necessary, the dosage may be increased by 0.5 mg administered twice daily; dosage increases to above 1.5 mg twice daily generally should be limited to intervals of not less than one week.

Risperdal (Janssen). Tablets 1, 2, 3, and 4 mg.

Cited References

Borison RL, et al: Risperidone: Clinical safety and efficacy in schizophrenia. *Psychopharmacol Bull* 28:213-218, 1992.

Chouinard G, et al: A Canadian multicenter placebo-controlled study of fixed doses of risperidone and haloperidol in the treatment of chronic schizophrenic patients. *J Clin Psychopharmacol* 13:25-40, (Feb) 1993.

Claus A, et al: Risperidone versus haloperidol in the treatment of chronic schizophrenic inpatients: A multicentre double-blind comparative study. *Acta Psychiatr Scand* 85:295-305, 1992.

Heinrich K, et al: Risperidone versus clozapine in the treatment of schizophrenic patients with acute symptoms: A double blind, randomized trial. *Prog Neuropsychopharmacol Biol Psychiatry* 18:129-137, 1994.

Meibach RC, Risperidone Study Group: A fixed-dose, parallel group study of risperidone vs. haloperidol vs. placebo, abstract. *Schizophr Res* 9:245, 1993.

Müller-Spahn F, The International Risperidone Research Group: Risperidone in the treatment of chronic schizophrenic patients: An international double-blind parallel-group study versus haloperidol. *Clin Neuropharm* 15(suppl 1, part A):90A-91A, 1992.

Schotte A, et al: Occupancy of central neurotransmitter receptors by risperidone, clozapine, and haloperidol measured ex vivo by quantitative autoradiography. *Brain Res* 631:191-202, 1993.

Drugs Used in Mood Disorders 13

MOOD DISORDERS

- **Description and Classification**
- **Etiology**
- **Treatment Modalities**
- **Drug Selection**

CLASS EVALUATIONS

- **Tricyclic Antidepressants**
- **Serotonin (5-HT) Uptake Inhibitors**
- **Monoamine Oxidase (MAO) Inhibitors**
- **Antimanic Drugs**

DRUG EVALUATIONS

- **Tricyclic Compounds**
- **Serotonin (5-HT) Uptake Inhibitors**
- **Other Cyclic Agents**
- **Monoamine Oxidase (MAO) Inhibitors**
- **Antimanic Drug**
- **Mixtures**

Depression usually is diagnosed and treated initially by a primary care physician. Treatment by a psychiatrist generally is required if initial drug therapy fails; if the patient is unable to function at work or at home, neglects self-care, or is severely anxious or agitated; or if the patient is suicidal, has bipolar disorder, or has accompanying psychotic symptoms.

Many patients treated by primary care physicians have depressive symptoms, including mood disturbance, that do not meet *DSM-III-R* criteria for diagnosis of major depression or dysthymia (Barrett et al, 1988) (see following section on Description and Classification). These milder forms of depression are often characterized by coexisting anxiety or may be "masked" depressions, in which vague discomfort or nonspecific somatic complaints dominate. Although symptoms may be relieved by antidepressants, the placebo response is high and data on which to base optimal treatment of these patients are very limited. However, these individuals are at increased risk of developing major depression within one year (Broadhead et al, 1990).

Symptoms of depression can be caused by or occur in response to diverse diseases, including endocrinopathies (eg, hypothyroidism, Cushing's or Addison's disease, hyperparathyroidism), immunologic (eg, multiple sclerosis) and collagen/vascular (eg, systemic lupus erythematosus, vasculopathies) disorders, neurodegenerative diseases and stroke, vitamin B_{12} or folate deficiency, postviral syndromes, acquired immunodeficiency syndrome, and carcinoma, especially of the pancreas.

Depression also may be associated with various drug therapies. Although certain drugs (eg, reserpine, methyldopa, clonidine, corticosteroids, oral contraceptives, and possibly beta-adrenergic blocking agents) are more likely to affect mood, many others have been implicated (*Med Lett Drugs Ther*, 1989). The physician also should attempt to identify possible substance abuse or other coexisting psychiatric conditions, since successful treatment of the depression is less likely if such disorders are not recognized.

Diagnosis of major depression in the elderly may be confounded by the presence of chronic illnesses and use of medications. Because depression often is associated with deficits in attention and concentration, it may exacerbate or mimic dementia. (For differential diagnosis of dementia and depression see Kokmen, 1988; also see index entry Dementia.)

MOOD DISORDERS

Clinically significant disturbances in affect define the major characteristic of the mood disorders. Such disturbances are manifested as depressive and/or manic episodes in the major mood disorders (major depression and bipolar disorder) or as less severe but chronic aberrations in affect in other mood disorders, such as cyclothymic disorder and dysthymic disorder.

DESCRIPTION AND CLASSIFICATION. The criteria for the diagnosis and classification of mood disorders have been established by the American Psychiatric Association in the revised third edition of the *Diagnostic and Statistical Manual of Mental Disorders (DSM-III-R)* (American Psychiatric Association, 1987). It is important to distinguish among mood disorders because their prognosis, management, and, especially, responsiveness to drug therapy differ.

Major Depression: For a diagnosis of major depression, at least five of the following symptoms must be present nearly every day for at least a two-week period and one of the symptoms must be depressed mood or loss of interest or pleasure: (1) depressed mood (may be irritable mood in children or adolescents), (2) markedly decreased interest or pleasure in nearly all activities, (3) significant weight loss (when not dieting) or weight gain, (4) insomnia or hypersomnia, (5) psychomotor agitation or retardation, (6) fatigue or loss of energy, (7) feelings of worthlessness or excessive or inappropriate guilt, (8) diminished ability to think or concentrate or indecisiveness, (9) recurrent thoughts of death. The depression may be a single episode or recurrent. When recurrent, the episodes may have a seasonal pattern.

Major depressive episodes may be *chronic*, if the current episode has lasted two years without a remission of at least two months, and *melancholic*. Their severity is variable, and psychotic symptoms also may be present in some patients.

Diagnosis of melancholic depression requires the presence of at least five of the following symptoms: (1) loss of interest or pleasure in almost all activities; (2) no reactivity, even temporarily, when something good happens; (3) depression worse in the morning; (4) early morning awakening, at least two hours before normal wakeup time; (5) psychomotor retardation or agitation; (6) significant anorexia or weight loss; (7) no significant personality disturbance before the first major depressive episode; (8) previous depressive episode(s) followed by recovery; (9) previous good response to somatic antidepressant therapy.

Another subtype of major depression is not defined in the *DSM-III-R* but is frequently discussed in the clinical research literature as *atypical depression.* In contrast to those with the melancholic type, the person with atypical depression has a depressed mood that temporarily remits in response to pleasurable stimuli but worsens significantly following disappointment or rejection; often experiences hyperphagia, fatigue, and hypersomnia; feels worse at night; may complain of a leaden feeling in the limbs; and often has significant anxiety. An individual may have the melancholic type of depression during one episode and atypical depression during another (Gold et al, 1988).

Dysthymia: The essential feature of this disorder is the presence of a chronic depressed mood (or possibly an irritable mood in children or adolescents), usually lasting at least two years (one year in children and adolescents). In addition, at least two of the following symptoms are present: poor appetite or overeating; insomnia or hypersomnia; low energy or fatigue; low self-esteem; poor concentration or difficulty in making decisions; and feelings of hopelessness (Finlayson, 1989). A major depressive episode may be superimposed on dysthymia, resulting in so-called double depression.

Bipolar Disorder: The essential feature of bipolar disorder is the occurrence of one or more manic episodes interspersed with one or more major depressive episodes.

A manic episode is a distinct period of abnormally and persistently expansive or irritable mood, during which at least three of the following seven symptoms are present: (1) inflated self-esteem or grandiosity, (2) decreased need for sleep, (3) unusual talkativeness, (4) flight of ideas or racing thoughts, (5) distractibility, (6) increase in goal-directed activity, (7) excessive involvement in pleasurable activities that have a high potential for painful consequences (eg, buying sprees, sexual indiscretions, foolish investments). In addition, the mood disturbance is severe enough to impair work and social functioning. When this last criterion is not met, the episode is designated as hypomanic.

Patients with bipolar disorder may be either in the manic or the depressive phase when they see a physician.

Compared with unipolar depression, the depressive phase of bipolar disorder is more likely to be characterized by reversed vegetative signs (eg, hypersomnia, hyperphagia and weight gain, decreased energy). Occasionally, both manic and depressive symptoms will be intermixed or rapidly cycling. Also, in a small percentage of patients, only manic episodes are experienced. Thus, only history and/or monitoring of the patient over time allows definitive diagnosis of bipolar disorder.

Cyclothymia: When patients experience chronic cycles of hypomania interspersed with periods of depressed mood, the disorder is called cyclothymia. Although the intensity of each episode is not as great as in a full manic or major depressive disorder, the chronicity of the mood changes (two years or more) makes this disorder distressing to patients and families.

Secondary Mood Disorders: Primary disorders must be differentiated from *reactive* or *secondary depression* that occurs during the course of some other primary psychiatric or medical disorder.

Adjustment reaction with depressed mood is one of the more common secondary mood disorders. This disorder is a reaction to an identifiable psychosocial stressor (or multiple stressors) and occurs within three months of onset of the stressors. Either impairment in occupational (including school) functioning or in usual social activities or relationships with others, or symptoms that are in excess of a normal and expected reaction to stressors, or both, may be present.

Alcoholism is a common cause of *substance-induced depression*; street drug abuse or adverse reactions to prescription drugs also cause this type of depression.

Uncomplicated bereavement after a significant loss (eg, spouse, employment, friend, position) is not classified as a depressive disorder but is considered a normal, self-limited grief reaction. It is much more common than all of the primary and secondary depressive disorders; however, clinical depression can follow bereavement.

ETIOLOGY. Although neurochemical research has produced many promising leads, definitive characterization of the underlying causes of the major mood disorders remains elusive. Most clinicians support a risk factor model that reflects the varying contributions of biological (including genetic), psychological, and environmental factors.

The biogenic amine hypothesis of affective disorders asserts that abnormal function in central noradrenergic or serotonergic neurotransmission forms the biological basis of major mood disorders. This hypothesis is based on the observation that drugs that deplete (eg, reserpine) or elevate (eg, monoamine oxidase inhibitors) the neuronal concentrations of norepinephrine and 5-hydroxytryptamine (5-HT) cause depression and mood elevation, respectively. Additional support is derived from the fact that most antidepressant drugs act on neurons that utilize these neurotransmitters. For example, antidepressant drugs cause down-regulation of central beta-adrenergic receptors and decreased expression in the brain of the rate-limiting biosynthetic enzyme (eg, tyrosine hydroxylase) for norepinephrine. Serotonergic mechanisms also are implicated based on the observation that antidepressant-induced remission is reversed by rapid depletion of plasma tryptophan (Delgado et al, 1990).

Depression also is often accompanied by changes in circadian rhythms or basal concentrations of cortisol, ACTH, and growth hormone and, in some patients, suppression of central ACTH release in response to administration of glucocorticoids (eg, dexamethasone) may be diminished. Involvement of the hypothalamic-pituitary-thyroid axis is suggested by recognition of the fact that hypothyroidism is a risk factor for major mood disorders and that, in some patients, the plasma thyroid-stimulating hormone response to thyrotropin-releasing hormone is subnormal. Some data also suggest that combining liothyronine (T_3) with a tricyclic antidepressant accelerates the onset of the therapeutic effect of the latter and may improve the condition of patients (especially females) who had not responded adequately to tricyclic antidepressants (see Drug Selection).

Cholinergic mechanisms also may play a causative role in the development of mood disorders (Janowsky and Risch, 1987). The endogenous opioid, dopamine, gamma-aminobutyric acid, and other peptide systems have been implicated as well (Jimerson, 1987; Berger and Nemeroff, 1987). Recent studies on the neurochemical effects of lithium suggest that its primary site of action may be at the level of neurohumoral signal transduction, where it has the potential to affect a broad range of neuronal activities.

In summary, many individuals with major mood disorders appear to be genetically vulnerable. Current evidence suggests that dysregulation among neuromodulatory systems in combination with behavioral and environmental factors may be causative.

TREATMENT MODALITIES. Drug therapy and psychotherapy are effective in the treatment of the major mood disorders and are the major treatment modalities in use today. A combination of both modalities often is required to achieve a maximal response (Weissman et al, 1987; Gold et al, 1988). Counseling that embodies nonjudgmental listening, empathy, and reassurance is essential in all patients and may improve compliance with drug therapy. Electroconvulsive therapy (ECT) is particularly effective in major depression, but it generally is reserved for patients who are potentially suicidal, also have severe psychotic symptoms, or are unresponsive to drug therapy; ECT is safe for use in geriatric and pregnant patients.

Drug therapy for the major mood disorders utilizes tricyclic antidepressants, monoamine oxidase (MAO) inhibitors, selective serotonin (5-HT) uptake inhibitors (ie, fluoxetine [Prozac], sertraline [Zoloft]), other cyclic agents (ie, bupropion [Wellbutrin], trazodone [Desyrel]), or lithium. Except for lithium, antidepressants are most useful in both the acute treatment and prophylaxis of major unipolar depressive disorders; they also are probably effective in dysthymia. Lithium alone or with an antidepressant is effective in the treatment of depressive episodes of bipolar disorders. Mania can be treated with lithium alone or in combination with an antipsychotic if severe psychotic symptoms are also present. High-potency benzodiazepines (eg, lorazepam [Ativan], clonazepam [Klonopin]) also may be useful in agitated manic patients. Carbamazepine [Tegretol] and valproic acid [Depakene] have been used as alternatives or adjuncts for patients who cannot tolerate or do not respond adequately to lithium and in patients with rapid cycling or mixed bipolar states.

Anxiety often accompanies depression, and antidepressants usually resolve anxiety and insomnia along with the depressive symptoms. Adjunctive antianxiety drugs need not be prescribed routinely and should not be substituted inappropriately for antidepressants or given for longer than two to three weeks without re-evaluation of the disorder.

Although psychomotor stimulants (eg, dextroamphetamine [Dexedrine], methylphenidate [Ritalin]) generally are ineffective, they have been reported to be helpful in carefully selected patients with mood disorders (eg, hospitalized, physically ill individuals who cannot tolerate or do not respond to standard regimens) (Satel and Nelson, 1989). These findings have not been confirmed in controlled studies. Self-escalation of the dose is rare unless the patient has a history of substance abuse. Compared with the tricyclic agents and MAO inhibitors, the psychomotor stimulants produce few adverse cardiovascular effects (most common, tachycardia), especially in the elderly. The diagnostic use of dextroamphetamine to determine the probable efficacy of tricyclic antidepressant therapy has not been demonstrated to be beneficial in any controlled study. For additional information on these drugs, see index entry Stimulants, Central Nervous System.

Psychotherapy interventions for the major mood disorders that have been systematically studied include cognitive-behavior therapy and interpersonal psychotherapy. The National Institute of Mental Health initiated and coordinated a multi-institutional trial comparing the effectiveness of imipramine [Janimine, Tofranil] with brief (16 to 20 sessions) interpersonal psychotherapy and cognitive-behavior therapy (Elkin et al, 1989). At the end of the study period, between 50% and 60% of patients who completed active treatment were virtually symptom-free compared with 29% in the control population (ie, placebo plus clinical management but neither form of brief psychotherapy). No significant differences between the two brief psychotherapies and drug use or between the two forms of psychotherapy were observed in those with mild to moderate depression. However, improvement was more rapid with imipramine plus clinical management and was significantly more pronounced than with either of the two forms of brief psychotherapies in the more severe forms of depression (ie, Hamilton Rating Scale Depression scores of greater than 20).

DRUG SELECTION. In most patients with depression, initial drug selection is determined by the type of mood disorder, personal or family history of response to a particular antidepressant, the pharmacologic profile of the drug (especially the degree of sedative action; see Table 1), the patient's susceptibility to side effects, and compatibility of the antidepressant with other medications taken concurrently.

TABLE 1.
MAJOR SELECTION CRITERIA FOR USE OF ANTIDEPRESSANTS IN MOOD DISORDERS

Drug	Initial Amine(s) Affected[1]	Sedative/ Stimulant Activity[2]	Anticholinergic Activity	Orthostatic Hypotension
TRICYCLIC ANTIDEPRESSANTS				
Amitriptyline	NE +			
Elavil (Stuart)	5HT +	↓↓↓	+++	+++
Endep (Roche)				
Amoxapine	NE ++			
Asendin (Lederle)	5HT o/+	↓	+	++
Clomipramine	5HT +++	↓↓	+++	++
Anafranil (CIBA)	NE +			
Desipramine	NE +++			
Norpramin (Marion Merrell Dow)	5HT o/+	↓	+	+
Pertofrane (Rhone-Poulenc Rorer)				
Doxepin	NE +			
Sinequan (Roerig)	5HT o/+	↓↓↓	+++	+++
Imipramine	NE +			
Janimine (Abbott)	5HT +	↓↓	++	++
Tofranil (Geigy)				
Maprotiline	NE ++			
Ludiomil (CIBA)	5HT o	↓↓	++	++
Nortriptyline	NE ++			
Aventyl (Lilly)	5HT o/+	↓	+	+/−
Pamelor (Sandoz)				
Protriptyline	NE ++			
Vivactil (Merck Sharp & Dohme)	5HT o/+	↓	++	+
Trimipramine	NE +			
Surmontil (Wyeth-Ayerst)	5HT o/+	↓↓↓	+++	
SELECTIVE SEROTONIN (5-HT) UPTAKE INHIBITORS				
Fluoxetine	5HT +++			
Prozac (Dista)	NE o	↑↓[3]	o	o
Sertraline	5HT +++			
Zoloft (Roerig)	NE o	↑↓	o	o
OTHER CYCLIC AGENTS				
Bupropion	DA o/+			
Wellbutrin (Burroughs Wellcome)	5HT o	↑	o	o
	NE o			
Trazodone	5HT[4] +			
Desyrel (Mead Johnson)	NE o	↓↓↓	+/−	+
MONOAMINE OXIDASE INHIBITORS				
Isocarboxazid	5HT ++			
Marplan (Roche)	NE ++	o/↑	o	++
	DA ++			

Cardiac Toxicity	Seizure Risk	Weight Gain	Comments
+ + +	+ +	+ +	
+ +	+ +	+ /o	Metabolite blocks dopamine receptors; infrequently, extrapyramidal reactions develop. Incidence of seizures in patients who have taken excessive amounts is relatively high.
+ + +	+ + +	+	Threshold for increased risk of seizures is approximately 250 mg daily.
+ +	+	+	Active metabolite of imipramine
+ +	+ +	+	
+ + +	+ +	+	
+ +	+ + +	+	Incidence of skin rash is 3%. Incidence of seizures is highest among the tricyclic compounds, which are pharmacologically quite similar to maprotiline, a tetracyclic compound.
+ +	+ +	+	
+ + +	+ +	+	
+ + +	+ +	+	
+ /−	+	o/ −	
+ /−	+	o/ −	
+ /−	+ + + +	o/ −	Preferable dose is ≤300 mg daily; maximum is 450 mg daily. Incidence of seizures approximately 0.4% in patients receiving up to 450 mg; the estimated incidence of seizures increases almost tenfold when the dosage is between 450 and 600 mg daily. Extrapyramidal reactions and worsening of psychoses have been noted rarely.
+	+	+ /o	Prolonged priapism may occur (incidence, 1:6,000) within one to two weeks after initiating therapy; medical intervention may be required.
o	o	+	Food and drug interactions require education of the patient and vigilant monitoring by the physician to minimize toxicity.

(table continued on next page)

TABLE 1 (continued)

Drug	Initial Amine(s) Affected[1]	Sedative/ Stimulant Activity[2]	Anticholinergic Activity	Orthostatic Hypotension
Phenelzine Nardil (Parke-Davis)	5HT + + NE + + DA + +	↓ ↑[3]	o	+ + +
Tranylcypromine Parnate (Nova/SmithKline Beecham)	5HT + + NE + + DA + +	↑[3]	o	+ + +

1 5-HT = serotonin; NE = norepinephrine; DA = dopamine. The number of symbols represents a relative estimate of the intensity of the effect.

2 Sedative activity is indicated by ↓ and stimulant activity by ↑. The number of symbols represents a relative estimate of the intensity of the effect within columns, but does not reflect the absolute incidence of side effects across columns.

3 Causes somnolence in some patients.

4 Although trazodone inhibits 5-HT uptake, it also possesses other biochemical properties and thus cannot be considered a selective 5-HT uptake inhibitor.

Type of Mood Disorder: Initial therapy of major depressive disorder is likely to involve a tricyclic agent, a 5-HT uptake inhibitor, trazodone, or bupropion. Tricyclic agents may be the drugs of choice for most hospitalized or severely ill patients with melancholic depression whose symptoms have persisted for at least six weeks (Potter et al, 1991). The efficacy and onset of action of the antidepressant agents are essentially equivalent in uncomplicated, nondelusional depression, but the efficacy of the newer (5-HT uptake inhibitors, trazodone, bupropion) agents has not been established in severe depression. Patients with associated panic disorder are often treated with imipramine, desipramine [Norpramine, Pertofrane], or MAO inhibitors; those with associated obsessive-compulsive disorder should be treated with clomipramine [Anafranil] or fluoxetine. MAO inhibitors are efficacious in the treatment of depression with social phobia, but other antidepressants also are effective when these disorders coexist.

Because of their side effects, MAO inhibitors have long been considered second-line drugs in the treatment of mood disorders. However, recognition of their usefulness has increased with refinement of the definition and classification of the mood disorders and with greater understanding of the need to titrate doses carefully. Nevertheless, the risk of hypertensive crises due to drug-food or drug-drug interaction is significant with MAO inhibitors, and the need to avoid certain foods and drugs must receive due consideration when they are prescribed. In addition, their prolonged duration of action makes it difficult to substitute most other antidepressants readily if treatment fails. As with other antidepressants, the therapeutic response to MAO inhibitors is delayed.

Although the results of a few controlled trials suggest that alprazolam [Xanax] has antidepressant effects, many authorities believe it is most beneficial in patients with mild to moderate depression when pronounced anxiety coexists. Further studies are required to establish the role of this potent anxiolytic in major depression. In addition, the long-term usefulness of alprazolam in most patients is limited by the potential for dependence.

Clinicians have tended to employ the more sedating antidepressants for patients with agitation, anxiety, and insomnia and less sedating agents when lethargy and psychomotor retardation are prominent. Similarly, the desire to promote weight gain or loss may dictate drug choice; most tricyclic compounds promote weight gain (desipramine is least likely). Fluoxetine, sertraline, and bupropion may promote moderate weight loss initially, but this effect may not be sustained. For some patients, the anticholinergic effects of tricyclic agents may be particularly troublesome, thus requiring the use of an agent with less pronounced anticholinergic activity (eg, desipramine, nortriptyline [Aventyl, Pamelor]) or an agent that lacks these effects (eg, a 5-HT uptake inhibitor, trazodone, bupropion). These agents also are less likely to produce orthostatic hypotension, cardiotoxic effects, and drug interactions. Thus, they may be preferred in selected patients with certain coexisting conditions or diseases, in patients taking other drugs concomitantly, and in patients who have compliance problems with tricyclic agents.

The pharmacologic actions that are useful in the process of drug selection for mood disorders appear in Table 1. Since these values change with increasing dosage and frequency of administration, they are only relative. However, they offer an approximate comparison of the currently known major benefits and risks associated with each antidepressant. Supportive references for these comparative values are available (Baldessarini, 1989; Potter et al, 1991; Richelson, 1991).

Approximately 30% to 40% of patients with *major depression* do not respond to a trial of the selected antidepressant, even though an appropriate dose is given for an adequate period of time. After evaluation of compliance with drug therapy and reassessment of the diagnosis, the initial drug can be withdrawn gradually and another drug with a different spectrum of activity can be tried. For example, preliminary uncontrolled evidence indicates that some patients who were unresponsive to tricyclic agents may respond to fluoxetine (Beasley et al, 1990). There is increasing clinical and empiric support for substituting an MAO inhibitor (Devlin and Walsh,

Cardiac Toxicity	Seizure Risk	Weight Gain	Comments
o	o	+ −	Food and drug interactions require education of the patient and vigilant monitoring by the physician to minimize toxicity; hepatotoxicity may occur.
o	o	+/o	Food and drug interactions require education of the patient and vigilant monitoring by the physician to minimize toxicity.

1990) in patients who do not respond to an adequate therapeutic trial with a tricyclic or other antidepressant.

Alternatively, some clinicians believe that augmentation is the most viable initial option before another type of antidepressant is substituted. This strategy eliminates the delay necessary when discontinuing the initial agent. Lithium or liothyronine [Cytomel] may be considered for addition to the antidepressant regimen when therapeutic blood levels have been achieved but clinical response is inadequate. Although some patients respond to daily doses of lithium 600 to 900 mg, other resistant patients require 0.8 to 1.2 mEq/L (Nierenberg and White, 1990). Use of liothyronine (25 to 50 mcg) in the morning has been beneficial in 20% to 40% of patients. Women may be more likely to respond to this agent (Nierenberg and White, 1990). If these measures fail, electroconvulsive therapy (ECT) is an alternative.

If the patient refuses ECT, a combination of a tricyclic compound and an MAO inhibitor is sometimes effective, although caution should be exercised and the clinician should be experienced with their combined use (White and Simpson, 1984). Small doses of the tricyclic agent should be given initially, after which the MAO inhibitor is added. The reverse is not advisable. However, results of the few controlled studies on use of these combinations have failed to demonstrate an advantage in refractory depression (Niereneberg and White, 1990). Carbamazepine also has been used in resistant patients (Post et al, 1986). Although the evidence for efficacy of psychomotor stimulants (eg, dextroamphetamine) is weak, they may be of value in some patients (Schwartz et al, 1990; Fawcett et al, 1991).

The response to drug therapy is highly variable in patients with *atypical depression.* Certain subtypes, such as atypical depression with panic attacks and hysteroid dysphoria, seem to be more responsive to MAO inhibitors (Brotman et al, 1987; Liebowitz et al, 1988; Quitkin et al, 1989) and fluoxetine than to other antidepressants. Antidepressants also may be useful in some patients with *dysthymia* (Kocsis et al, 1988; Howland, 1991), although few controlled studies have been done. In general, patients with dysthymic or atypical depressive disorders may be less responsive to antidepressants than those with major depression.

In the *manic phase of bipolar disorder* (manic-depressive illness), 60% to 80% of patients respond to lithium. Treatment of *acute mania* is often initiated with an antipsychotic agent, alone or in combination with lithium, particularly if mania is severe (eg, agitation, psychotic symptoms). (Patients with bipolar disorder may be at increased risk for the development of tardive dyskinesia.) High-potency benzodiazepines (eg, lorazepam, clonazepam) also have been used in acute mania to control agitation or sleeplessness, and their administration may decrease the required dose of the antipsychotic. Carbamazepine or valproic acid has been used as an alternative or adjunct to lithium in patients with acute mania who cannot tolerate or do not respond to an adequate course of lithium. Preliminary results suggest that calcium channel blockers (eg, verapamil [Calan, Isoptin]) may be useful in manic patients who do not respond adequately to these regimens. ECT is an alternative in those with severe mania.

The signs and symptoms of the *depressed phase of bipolar disorder* are essentially the same as those of major depression, although these patients have anergic symptoms more frequently. The combination of lithium and an antidepressant is frequently used for long-term maintenance therapy in those with bipolar disorder; however, this regimen has not been fully evaluated. Results of some studies have indicated that there is no decided advantage of the combination over lithium alone (Johnstone et al, 1990), and the tricyclic may induce cycling in some patients. In one trial, tranylcypromine [Parnate] was more effective than imipramine in patients with anergic bipolar depression (Himmelhoch et al, 1991).

Carbamazepine or valproic acid may be used alone or in combination with lithium for maintenance therapy in patients who respond inadequately to lithium. There is some evidence that carbamazepine may be beneficial in patients who exhibit *rapid cycling, dysphoric mania,* or *mixed states*, all of which correlate with poor response to lithium and pose significant treatment problems (Post et al, 1990; Prien and Potter, 1990). In one series of patients with rapid cycling, bupropion relieved depression and decreased cycling. Whether this drug is more effective than other antidepressants in preventing recurrences of manic episodes when treatment with an antidepressant is required remains to be established (Prien and Potter, 1990; Haykal and Akiskal, 1990).

A limited number of studies indicate that lithium may be useful in treating *cyclothymia.*

Simultaneous treatment with antipsychotic drugs and/or antidepressants and/or lithium is necessary for patients with *major depression with psychotic features* and *schizoaffective disorder*. MAO inhibitors generally are not first-choice antidepressants, because of side effects and other risks associated with their use.

Uncomplicated bereavement requires drug therapy infrequently; counseling is usually adequate. A few patients may benefit from the temporary use of antianxiety agents to reduce anxiety and/or promote sleep without interfering with the normal grief reaction. Antidepressants should relieve relatively persistent depressive symptoms. Complicated bereavement with the full syndrome of major depression, including suicidal ideation, may require both counseling and antidepressant therapy.

The dosage and available preparations for each antidepressant appear in the evaluations. Table 2 summarizes the usual initial and maximum recommended daily dose used for outpatients.

Class discussions on the tricyclic antidepressants, serotonin uptake inhibitors, monoamine oxidase inhibitors, and antimanic drugs follow. Information on other cyclic antidepressants appears in the evaluations.

TRICYCLIC ANTIDEPRESSANTS

Uses: The tricyclic antidepressants (amitriptyline, amoxapine, clomipramine, desipramine, doxepin, imipramine, nortriptyline, protriptyline, and trimipramine) and the tetracyclic compound, maprotiline, elevate mood, increase physical activity and activities of daily living, improve appetite and sleep patterns, and reduce morbid preoccupation in 60% to 70% of patients with major depression. The antidepressant response to these agents often is gradual (one to six weeks or more) and is not accelerated appreciably by parenteral administration. Therefore, ECT may be the treatment of choice in melancholic suicidal patients.

In addition to their usefulness in treating acute depressive episodes, tricyclic antidepressants are effective for maintenance therapy to prevent recurrence of major depressive episodes, which typically have a duration of six months or longer. Selected tricyclic compounds also have been somewhat beneficial in atypical and dysthymic depression, as well as in postherpetic neuralgia, attention deficit hyperactivity disorder, cataplexy associated with narcolepsy, headache (tension, migraine), enuresis, anorexia nervosa, and bulimia. Protriptyline may be beneficial in conditions associated with nocturnal oxygen desaturation (sleep apnea, chronic obstructive pulmonary disease). Imipramine, desipramine, and clomipramine are useful in the treatment of panic or phobic disorders and clomipramine in the treatment of obsessive-compulsive disorder (see index entries on these disorders).

Low-dose sedative tricyclic antidepressants also have been used in primary care settings for adjustment reaction with mixed depression and anxiety. Results are often excellent but may be unrelated to the plasma levels achieved; the nonspecific sedative action of the drugs may play a significant role. Few well-controlled studies on this application have been undertaken in primary care settings (Klerman, 1989).

The tricyclic antidepressants are effective and may have an adjunctive role in the treatment of chronic pain of both malignant and nonmalignant origin; they often are preferred drugs in neuropathic (deafferentation) pain (eg, diabetic neuropathy). See index entry Neuropathy, Diabetic.

Other indications for tricyclic antidepressants remain controversial or incompletely established. These include hysteroid dysphoria, peptic ulcer, acute delusional disorder, and to decrease craving and depression during abstinence from cocaine.

Mechanism of Action: The mechanism of action of the tricyclic antidepressants has not been established despite the large body of data that has accumulated (Garrattini and Samanin, 1988). Initially, the tricyclic antidepressants usually nonselectively block the reuptake of norepinephrine and serotonin into their respective nerve terminals within the central nervous system. They also block serotonergic (5-HT_{1A}, 5-HT_2), noradrenergic ($alpha_1$), histaminergic (H_1 more than H_2), and muscarinic receptors to varying degrees. These combined effects on reuptake and receptor occupation acutely reduce the synthesis and turnover of norepinephrine and serotonin and reduce the discharge rates of the neurons of these two transmitters.

Correlation of specific neurochemical actions of the tricyclic compounds with their therapeutic effects must take into consideration the several weeks that elapse before such effects are apparent. After prolonged administration, blockade of the neuronal reuptake of norepinephrine and serotonin continues, and turnover and discharge rates gradually return to normal. A decrease in beta- and $alpha_2$-adrenergic receptor sensitivity, tyrosine hydroxylase concentration, and in the number of 5-HT receptors occurs in animals following long-term administration of most of the antidepressants and ECT. Probably no change or a slight increase occurs in $alpha_1$-adrenergic receptor sensitivity and in the number of muscarinic receptors. The selective receptor changes that are produced support the hypothesis that depression is caused by dysregulation of neurotransmitter systems. However, direct evidence in humans is lacking.

Pharmacokinetics: All tricyclic compounds are well absorbed orally, extensively metabolized, highly protein-bound in plasma and tissue, and eliminated slowly. Mean half-lives and/or ranges (in hours) are: desipramine 21 (12 to 30), nortriptyline 31 (13 to 79), imipramine 18 (4 to 34), amitriptyline 21 (10 to 36), doxepin 17 (8 to 24), protriptyline 78 (55 to 127), maprotiline 43, and amoxapine 8. The half-life of 8-hydroxyamoxapine formed from amoxapine is approximately 30 hours. Because half-lives are prolonged in individuals over 55 years, the initial dose for older patients may require modification.

There has been much speculation regarding the value of monitoring plasma levels of the tricyclic antidepressants. If a therapeutic plasma range can be established, dosing could take into account individual variation in metabolism. Reliable data exist only for imipramine, nortriptyline, and, to a lesser extent, desipramine (Task Force on the Use of Laboratory Tests in Psychiatry, 1985; Orsulak, 1989). For imipramine, a relationship exists between plasma concentrations and clinical response. The suggested plasma range of the drug and its metabolite, desipramine, is 200 to 300 ng/ml; for desipramine alone, a threshold of 115 to 125 ng/ml appears to be necessary to produce a favorable clinical response. For nortriptyline, a curvilinear relationship is reported with a "therapeutic window" of 50 to about 150 ng/ml; however, these data were obtained primarily from severely depressed inpatients. Little data are available for outpatients or those less severely depressed. Thus, the Task Force recommended that plasma monitoring be limited to those who do not respond to usual dosage regimens or to high-risk patients who need the lowest possible dose. For other patients, dosage should be adjusted on the basis of side effects and therapeutic response.

Administration and Dosage: The *initial treatment* period is considered to be the four to eight weeks needed for most patients to respond. Many signs and symptoms often may not completely resolve for months (ie, during maintenance therapy). Outpatient treatment usually is instituted with the smaller dose of the range listed in Table 2, and the amount is increased gradually. The initial two to three weeks of drug therapy are critical. Common causes of inadequate treatment in outpatients are oversedation and intolerance to anticholinergic side effects during the first few days because of an excessive initial dose, which may result in noncompliance.

In hospitalized patients, closer monitoring is possible; the initial daily dose generally can be larger and the time needed to attain a maximum daily dose shorter.

For most individuals with recurrent depression, effective preventive treatment requires long-term therapy. To prevent relapse, pharmacologic treatment of an episode of depression must continue for four to five months after the symptoms have responded to antidepressant medication (Prien and Kupfer, 1986).

Daily doses of imipramine 50 (in the elderly) to 150 mg or comparable doses of another tricyclic compound are reported to have prophylactic value (National Institutes of Health Consensus Development Conference, 1984). Results of a randomized three-year maintenance trial in patients with recurrent depression who had responded to combined short-term and continuation treatment with imipramine (mean daily dose 215 mg) and interpersonal psychotherapy demonstrated that recurrent depression was prevented in 80% of patients (Frank et al, 1990). Thus, patients with multiple recurrences within a relatively recent period (eg, three to five years) should be considered candidates for long-term treatment with adequate dosage (at least 200 mg of imipramine); regular sessions of interpersonal psychotherapy also may provide substantial prophylactic benefit (Klerman, 1990; Frank et al, 1991). Tranylcypromine has been reported to be of value in imipramine-resistant, recurrent depression (Thase, 1992). Long-term prophylactic benefits also have been reported with phenelzine (Robinson et al, 1991) and fluoxetine (Montgomery et al, 1988).

If a patient remains free of recurrence for a period equal to several previous cycle lengths, therapy may be discontinued provided that a family member or friend is available to alert the physician to signs of relapse. Early treatment intervention shortens the duration of recurrent episodes (Kupfer et al, 1988). In general, the stronger the indications for instituting maintenance therapy, the longer its duration should be (National Institutes of Health Consensus Development Conference, 1984).

Since the rates of metabolism and, hence, plasma concentrations of these drugs vary widely, individualization of dose on the basis of clinical effect is more important than strict adherence to recommendations for initial, maintenance, and maximum doses. Some patients may require more than the usual maximum dose.

Drug therapy should be discontinued gradually over a few weeks whenever possible. This avoids a withdrawal syndrome and allows minimum dosage alteration if symptoms of relapse occur.

Adverse Reactions: Differences in activity at norepinephrine and serotonin reuptake sites and/or adrenergic, serotonergic, histaminergic, muscarinic, and dopaminergic receptors account for the differences in adverse reactions among the tricyclic agents. The most common adverse reactions that limit treatment are anticholinergic effects, orthostatic hypotension, sedation, sexual dysfunction, and weight gain. In some patients, hypomania or mania may be triggered. The anticholinergic activity of the tricyclic antidepressants is variable; tertiary amines, such as amitriptyline and doxepin, have greater activity than secondary amines. Anticholinergic side effects are dose related. The severity of reactions ranges from minor (eg, sedation, dry mouth, dizziness) to moderate (blurred vision, constipation, tachycardia, urinary hesitancy), to intolerable/unacceptable (paralytic ileus, delirium). Some tolerance to these side effects generally develops with continued use. Gradual increases in dosage may facilitate patient acceptance. The frequency of reactions also must be considered (see Nierenberg and Cole, 1991).

Allergic skin reactions, photosensitivity, agranulocytosis, cholestatic jaundice, leukopenia, leukocytosis, Loeffler's syndrome, eosinophilia, and thrombocytopenia are relatively uncommon. Delayed, inhibited, or retrograde ejaculation can occur.

Central nervous system effects include sedation (see Table 1), fine tremor, speech blockage, cognitive dysfunction, and anxiety or insomnia. Increased appetite with weight gain occurs in some patients. These drugs may produce seizures, particularly in patients with a history of such disorders, including those with a history of severe alcoholism or head trauma. Among these agents, maprotiline lowers the seizure threshold to the greatest degree and desipramine the least.

Parkinsonism occurs rarely, especially on abrupt withdrawal of the drug; antidepressants with minimal anticholinergic activity are implicated most commonly. Tricyclic drugs are reported to produce tardive dyskinesia very rarely and only after prolonged use of large doses, but there are no controlled studies to substantiate this finding; amoxapine, a derivative of the antipsychotic, loxapine, has been cited most often. Hyponatremia resulting from the syndrome of inappropriate secretion of antidiuretic hormone (SIADH) has been observed rarely.

Serious cardiac reactions are uncommon unless overdosage occurs or these drugs are used in patients with pre-existing cardiac dysfunction. Sinus tachycardia (minor) and quinidine-like effects (eg, delayed conduction, impaired contractility) may occur. Peripheral vascular effects include orthostatic hypotension caused by central vasomotor system effects or pe-

TABLE 2.
COMPARATIVE DAILY DOSES OF ANTIDEPRESSANT DRUGS FOR OUTPATIENTS (ADULTS)[1]

	Usual Initial Dose Range[2,3] (mg)	Maximum Recommended Dose (mg)
TRICYCLIC ANTIDEPRESSANTS		
amitriptyline	50-150	300[4]
amoxapine	50-200	400[4]
clomipramine	50-150	250
desipramine	50-150	300
doxepin	50-150	300
imipramine	50-150	300
maprotiline	50-100	225
nortriptyline	25-100	150
protriptyline	15-40	60
trimipramine	75-150	250[5]
SEROTONIN (5-HT) UPTAKE INHIBITORS		
fluoxetine	20	80
sertraline	50-100	200
OTHER CYCLIC AGENTS		
bupropion	200	450
trazodone	150-200	200[4]
MONOAMINE OXIDASE INHIBITORS		
isocarboxazid	20-30	30
phenelzine	45-75	75[6]
tranylcypromine	20-30	30[6]

[1] *Adapted from Baldessarini, 1989.*

[2] *Treatment usually is initiated with the smaller dose of the range listed and gradually increased to the larger dose or more, if required, over approximately a two- to three-week period (see the following footnote). Initial treatment is regarded as the four- to eight-week period needed for most patients to respond. The optimal daily dose will vary for each individual within the range established by the initial dosage target and the maximum recommended dose. Larger doses often are required in severely depressed inpatients or in treatment-resistant patients. Inpatients often receive higher initial doses with a more rapid escalation of the daily dosage (see the evaluations). Continuation treatment at the optimal daily dose (or somewhat less) determined during initial treatment usually is then instituted.*

[3] *One initial schedule that lessens the intensity of sedative, hypotensive, and anticholinergic effects in outpatients and makes dosage adjustment easier follows: Imipramine or an equivalent dose of another tricyclic antidepressant 25 mg twice daily for three days, 50 mg twice daily for three days, and 75 mg twice daily for the next ten days. (Some patients may require even lower doses initially (eg, 25 mg/day) with subsequent dosage increments made after the patient adapts to side effects.) A minimum of five days between dosage adjustments may be more appropriate and particularly desirable in the elderly, the debilitated, or patients with cardiac disease to avoid undue sedation and hypotension that may result in injury. If insomnia is prominent, it may be preferable to give the initial daily amount as a single dose at bedtime to obtain the full benefit of sedation and minimize functional impairment and drowsiness during the day. With a large single dose at bedtime, however, hypotension may occur when the patient awakens during the night because of nocturia and goes to the toilet unassisted, thereby placing the patient at risk for falls and injury. After two to three weeks of therapy, a single daily dose is commonly given at bedtime. If limited benefit is observed by the third week, the daily dose is increased, usually weekly, until satisfactory improvement, intolerable adverse reactions, or the recommended maximum dose is reached (see the evaluations for dosing information on serotonin uptake inhibitors, bupropion, trazodone, and monoamine oxidase inhibitors and further information on the tricyclic antidepressants).*

[4] *Maximum daily dose of 600 mg may be necessary for the treatment of inpatients with severe depression.*

[5] *Maximum daily dose of 300 mg may be necessary for the treatment of inpatients with severe depression.*

[6] *Maximum daily dose of phenelzine 90 mg and tranylcypromine 60 mg may be necessary for the treatment of inpatients with severe depression; higher doses have been used rarely for treatment-resistant depression.*

ripheral alpha-adrenergic receptor blockade. Thus, a baseline ECG, periodic monitoring, and especially determination of the width of the QRS complex are recommended for elderly patients and those with prior or existing cardiac disease, particularly those receiving quinidine, procainamide, or disopyramide. In addition, pretreatment measurement with regular monitoring of supine and standing blood pressure should be undertaken to minimize unrecognized orthostatic hypotension.

For information on the etiology and management of specific adverse drug reactions to antidepressants, see Tollefson, 1991.

Precautions: The tricyclic antidepressants should not be used in acutely agitated schizophrenic patients, and they should be used cautiously in those with bipolar disorder, since they may trigger mania. The possibility of a suicide attempt is inherent in depression and may persist until significant remission occurs. Physicians should carefully monitor patients receiving antidepressants for any evidence of suicidal ideation and behavior.

These compounds should be used with caution in elderly patients and in those with a history of seizure disorders (especially maprotiline). Sedation and orthostatic hypotension may increase an elderly patient's risk of falling and sustaining fractures (Ray et al, 1991). Close supervision is advised if treatment is considered in patients with angle-closure glaucoma, urinary retention or obstruction, or those at risk of developing adynamic ileus.

The risks should be weighed carefully in patients with cardiac disease. It is also important to monitor the blood pressure, for hypotensive side effects are common and serious, especially in elderly patients with hypertension or orthostatic hypotension. Relative contraindications to the use of the tricyclic antidepressants include bundle branch block, the postmyocardial infarction period, and arrhythmias being treated with Class I antiarrhythmic drugs.

Routine precautions should be followed when these drugs are used during pregnancy and breast feeding (see index entries Pregnancy; Breast Feeding).

Poisoning: The most serious complications of tricyclic antidepressant overdosage are arrhythmias, hypotension, seizures, and coma. A single oral dose of 1 g of amitriptyline, imipramine, or doxepin produces severe toxic reactions in adults, and doses exceeding 2 g can be fatal. Death is usually due to cardiotoxicity. Based on case reports from the 1960s and early 1970s, many clinicians became concerned about the possibility of delayed complications. This possibility, in conjunction with uncertainty about predictors of outcome, caused most patients to be hospitalized for continuous cardiac monitoring, regardless of their early symptoms. Somewhat more flexible management algorithms have now been proposed (Callaham and Krassel, 1985; Frommer et al, 1987; Tokarski and Young, 1988; Banahan and Schelkun, 1990) that may help determine whether the patient actually needs admission.

Cardiac complications (eg, conduction defects, decreased inotropy) are usually caused by blockade of the fast inward sodium current (quinidine-like effect) in Purkinje and other cardiac fibers. Although a variety of conduction defects and supraventricular arrhythmias (including bradycardia) may occur, a typical pattern of cardiac changes includes rightward terminal vector and P-R and Q-T prolongation, followed by progressive QRS increase, ventricular ectopy, and ventricular tachycardia with subsequent decrement to a slow, very wide (preterminal) idioventricular rhythm. Loss of effective inotropy and systemic hypotension complicate management. Sinus tachycardia due to anticholinergic effects may contribute to cardiotoxicity but is not in itself life-threatening.

Neurologic effects of overdosage may include dilated pupils, nystagmus, hyperactive tendon reflexes, tremors, myoclonus, choreoathetosis, agitation, ataxia, delirium, seizures, respiratory depression, and coma. Anticholinergic toxicity may contribute to bladder and bowel paralysis and hyperthermia.

Treatment consists of general supportive measures. Crystalloid infusion can be used to treat hypotension; alpha agonists (eg, norepinephrine [Levophed]) also may be required. Hyperpyrexia is managed by physical cooling procedures and the stomach should be emptied. The patient also should receive multiple doses of activated charcoal (hourly) and a cathartic, even as late as six to eight hours following ingestion of an overdose. Continued instillation of activated charcoal by nasogastric tube (with appropriate endotracheal intubation) is indicated for comatose patients, because the parent drug and its active metabolites may undergo enterohepatic recirculation.

Alkalization of the serum to pH 7.45 to 7.55 is recommended to reduce cardiotoxicity if the QRS is greater than 100 msec; right axis deviation is another early warning signal. Sodium bicarbonate is preferred if the QRS is approaching 140 to 160 msec or there is evidence of hemodynamic instability, imminent hypotension, or seizures. Hyperventilation, which avoids the risk of excessive sodium bicarbonate, may be most useful if the patient is already intubated and stable and the QRS is only slightly prolonged (Groleau et al, 1990; Smilkstein, 1990).

If alkalization does not correct ventricular arrhythmias, lidocaine can be administered, but toxic levels may lead to myocardial depression. Type 1A agents (eg, quinidine, procainamide, disopyramide) are contraindicated. Cardioversion also may be useful. The use of phenytoin is controversial but probably represents the next best choice; bretylium has not been studied. Severe bradycardia and prolonged intraventricular conduction delays or torsades de pointes ventricular tachycardia may benefit from treatment with beta agonists (eg, isoproterenol), but overdrive pacing may be required; magnesium sulfate also may be beneficial in the latter condition.

Physostigmine [Antilirium] (1 to 3 mg intravenously in divided doses) has been administered to help control central nervous system reactions and some arrhythmias, but this agent is no longer recommended for routine use because it can cause serious cholinergic effects, including excessive salivation requiring suction, bradycardia, bronchoconstriction, and convulsions and can worsen cardiotoxicity.

Drug Interactions: Since drugs used to treat cardiovascular disease, hypertension, and depression have numerous effects on biogenic amines, there are many interactions between drugs in these classes. Adrenergic neuronal blocking agents (eg, guanethidine, guanadrel) should not be given to patients receiving the tricyclic compounds because these antidepressants interfere with the action of the antihypertensive agents. The effect of clonidine [Catapres] and other alpha$_2$ agonists also may be antagonized by some tricyclic antidepressants.

The pressor effect of direct-acting adrenergic drugs (eg, epinephrine, certain sympathomimetic amines) may be potentiated by tricyclic antidepressants. Methylphenidate [Ritalin] may inhibit the metabolism of tricyclic drugs and increase their blood concentrations.

The prominent anticholinergic effects of the tricyclic drugs are additive with those produced by other drugs having a similar action (eg, centrally acting anticholinergic drugs, antihistamines, antipsychotic agents). A toxic confusional and delirious state may result, particularly in the elderly.

Gastric emptying may be delayed in some individuals, thus limiting the bioavailability of some concurrently administered drugs (eg, levodopa). It is advisable to administer other agents one to two hours before or after the tricyclic drugs.

Extreme caution should be exercised if a tricyclic compound is given with or soon after an MAO inhibitor, for their concomitant use rarely may produce tremors, excitability, hyperpyrexia, muscle rigidity, generalized clonic convulsions, delirium, and death. Based on theoretical considerations, if possible an interval of at least seven days is suggested after a tricyclic compound is discontinued before the MAO inhibitor is given, and a two-week interval after an MAO inhibitor is discontinued before a tricyclic compound is given. Some specialists have concluded that concurrent administration of tricyclic agents and MAO inhibitors may not be dangerous if the dosage of each drug is titrated carefully and if the MAO inhibitor is begun after the tricyclic antidepressant is started, but not vice versa. Combined therapy should be undertaken only by clinicians experienced with the procedure.

Tricyclic drugs that cause significant sedation (ie, doxepin, amitriptyline, trimipramine, nortriptyline, imipramine, maprotiline) interact additively with alcohol and other central nervous system depressants. Adynamic ileus and excessive hepatic lipid concentrations also have been reported after use of such combinations. Moderate to heavy alcohol consumption should be avoided, especially if the patient drives or works in a hazardous occupation. The anorexiant, fenfluramine [Pondimin], has sedative properties and markedly potentiates this effect of some tricyclic antidepressants; therefore, the combination should be avoided.

Tricyclic compounds that are structurally similar to antipsychotic drugs also are metabolized by cytochrome P450IID6; therefore, antipsychotic drugs may impair the hepatic metabolism of tricyclic antidepressants and vice versa. Quinidine inhibits the metabolism of tricyclic agents in individuals who extensively metabolize debrisoquin. Other drugs that reduce the hepatic clearance of tricyclic antidepressants include fluoxetine, cimetidine [Tagamet], propoxyphene [Darvon, Dolene], and labetalol [Normodyne, Trandate].

The long-term administration of drugs that induce hepatic microsomal enzymes (eg, barbiturates, carbamazepine, phenytoin) hastens the elimination of the tricyclic agents.

The plasma concentration of the tricyclic drugs may be reduced by heavy smoking.

SEROTONIN (5-HT) UPTAKE INHIBITORS

Evidence that dysfunction in central serotonergic and noradrenergic neurotransmission may underlie the biologic basis of mood disorders led to efforts to develop agents that selectively affect the function of these systems. This resulted in the development of a class of agents that inhibit the neuronal uptake of serotonin (5-HT) with little or no effect on the neuronal uptake of norepinephrine. These agents include fluoxetine [Prozac], sertraline [Zoloft], and several investigational agents, including fluvoxamine and paroxetine. Both fluvoxamine and paroxetine are marketed outside the United States.

Trazodone [Desyrel] inhibits the neuronal uptake of 5-HT but also binds to 5-HT and alpha adrenergic receptors. Clomipramine [Anafranil] inhibits the neuronal uptake of 5-HT but also significantly inhibits norepinephrine uptake and has other properties commonly associated with tricyclic agents.

Actions and Uses. The antidepressant action of selective serotonin 5-HT inhibitors is presumed to be related to inhibition of the neuronal uptake of serotonin. Their efficacy has been established primarily in moderately and severely depressed outpatients; fluvoxamine also has been studied in more severely depressed inpatients (Feighner et al, 1989). Like the tricyclic drugs, the antidepressant effect is delayed. The selective serotonin uptake inhibitors may be particularly useful in patients with concurrent illness such as hypertension, coronary artery disease, prostatic enlargement, or narrow-angle glaucoma; in those who cannot tolerate the adverse effects of tricyclic agents; and in the elderly (Winbow, 1991). Serotonin uptake inhibitors have been useful in obsessive-compulsive disorder, panic disorder, and, possibly in bulimia nervosa and obesity, and they also are being investigated for use in the treatment of alcohol abuse (see index entries on these disorders).

Adverse Effects. Unlike the tricyclics, selective 5-HT uptake inhibitors do not possess significant sedative, anticholinergic, or hypotensive effects; do not have significant effects on cardiac conduction; and do not cause weight gain. Overdose also appears to be less hazardous. Side effects associated with these agents include nausea; anorexia; sweating; dry mouth; tremor; headache; and sexual dysfunction, including anorgasmia (women) and ejaculatory delay. Restlessness, anxiety, agitation, and insomnia also may occur, although some patients may experience somnolence. Rarely, extrapyramidal reactions (eg, akathisia, dystonia) have developed.

For information on pharmacokinetics, drug interactions, more specific adverse reactions and precautions, and dosage and administration, see the evaluations on Fluoxetine and Sertraline.

MONOAMINE OXIDASE (MAO) INHIBITORS

The MAO inhibitors, isocarboxazid, phenelzine, and tranylcypromine, have similar efficacy in major depression and are useful when psychomotor agitation or anxiety are present or when tricyclic and other antidepressants have failed (Kayser et al, 1988). They also may be effective in patients with atypical depression (Liebowitz et al, 1984; Robinson, 1986; Quitkin et al, 1989) dysthymia, and panic or phobic disorders (Sheehan, 1984). Phenelzine is the MAO inhibitor that has been studied most thoroughly for the latter disorders. Because they do not lower the seizure threshold, MAO inhibitors may be preferred in patients with seizure disorders (Richardson and Richelson, 1984). Preliminary evidence suggests that the MAO inhibitors may be effective in the treatment of bulimia, post-traumatic stress disorder, and borderline personality disorder (Kurtz and Robinson, 1988).

Since the efficacy of MAO inhibitors is generally equivalent to that of the tricyclic antidepressants, the choice is most often based on the drugs' safety profile. Patients who cannot adhere to dietary restrictions; those who overuse alcohol; those with severe cardiovascular, hepatic, or renal disease; and those with pheochromocytoma should not receive MAO inhibitors. Asthmatic patients and others who require pressor agents also should not be given these agents.

Mechanism of Action: The mechanism of action of the MAO inhibitors has not been established definitively. However, as with the tricyclic antidepressants, much is known about the acute and chronic pharmacologic actions of these drugs (Murphy et al, 1987).

Tranylcypromine, phenelzine, and isocarboxazid irreversibly inhibit both monoamine oxidase A and B. Selegiline [Deprenyl] causes a dose-dependent inhibition of monoamine oxidase B; antidepressant activity has been demonstrated at dosages that inhibit monoamine oxidase nonselectively. Reversible type A inhibitors are being investigated. Monoamine oxidase A preferentially deaminates norepinephrine and serotonin, while monoamine oxidase B selectively degrades benzylamine and phenethylamine. When administered initially, MAO inhibitors transiently elevate the cytoplasmic and vesicular concentrations of norepinephrine, dopamine, and serotonin. This activates a feedback loop that reduces the synthesis of these monoamines. If administration continues, there is a reduction in the number and sensitivity of beta-adrenergic receptors, as well as in the number of alpha$_2$-adrenergic and serotonergic receptor sites. The relationship between the specific long-term pharmacologic actions of MAO inhibitors and the delayed therapeutic response is unclear.

Administration and Dosage: The MAO inhibitors are well absorbed orally and widely distributed. The effects of currently available MAO inhibitors are irreversible, and the inhibited enzyme requires several weeks for regeneration.

These drugs should be reserved for patients who can be observed closely. It may be prudent to monitor blood pressure to detect significant orthostatic hypotension (Robinson et al, 1982). The dose that relieves symptoms without causing undesirable effects is given daily, usually in divided amounts. Because of tranylcypromine's mild stimulant effect, this drug is not given in the evening. Paradoxically, phenelzine and tranylcypromine may cause daytime sedation in some patients.

The duration of therapy is based on response. Maintenance doses may be necessary for patients with chronic or recurrent depressive episodes. If the recurrences are part of a manic-depressive illness, concurrent administration of lithium should be considered. As with tricyclic antidepressants, abrupt discontinuation of MAO inhibitors may precipitate mild autonomic rebound. The recommended drug and dietary restrictions should be adhered to for two to three weeks after discontinuation of the drug.

Adverse Reactions: The most common side effects of the MAO inhibitors are orthostatic hypotension, sexual disturbances, hypomania (usually in patients with bipolar disorder), and insomnia. Orthostatic hypotension is seldom severe enough to require discontinuation of therapy. Sexual dysfunction includes relative impotence and delayed ejaculation in males and loss of libido or difficulty in achieving orgasm in women. Edema of the extremities is infrequent but may not respond to thiazide or loop diuretics; if it does not, the dose of the MAO inhibitor should be reduced or, if possible, therapy discontinued. Periodic movements during sleep (nocturnal myoclonus) occur infrequently. Leukopenia, skin eruptions, photosensitivity, hepatotoxicity, hallucinations, and polyneuropathy have been reported rarely.

These drugs may differ in the severity of the various side effects. Therefore, if discontinuation of a particular drug is required because of an adverse reaction, a different MAO inhibitor may be tried. However, a ten-day period should elapse before tranylcypromine is administered following use of another MAO inhibitor (Perry et al, 1988).

These drugs may have a clinically detectable psychostimulant effect, usually manifested only with larger doses. Insomnia associated with euphoria, tremors, and hypomanic agitated behavior may reflect overdosage or sensitivity to these drugs. If headache, tachycardia, palpitation, nausea, vomiting, and hypertension occur together, the symptoms may indicate a hypertensive crisis caused by a food- or a drug-drug interaction (see the section on Drug Interactions).

Precautions: It is important to educate patients in detail about the untoward effects produced by MAO inhibitors, especially the potential for severe interactions with certain foods and drugs. Physicians also should be alert for signs of severe hypotension. Like other antidepressants, MAO inhibitors may exacerbate acute schizophrenic conditions and thus generally should be avoided in patients with these disorders. However, some schizophrenic patients in remission who are receiving maintenance antipsychotic drug therapy have a superimposed endogenous depression and may benefit from treatment with antidepressants. Patients should be instructed to inform other physicians treating them and pharmacists that they are taking MAO inhibitors. They also should carry a card stating that they are taking these drugs; information on potential food and drug interactions may be included.

Food and Drug Interactions: Hypertensive crises have been associated with the concomitant use of MAO inhibitors and foods or beverages containing a large amount of tyramine, a naturally occurring pressor amine. These hypertensive crises are characterized by headache, tachycardia, palpitation, nausea, and vomiting. Occasionally, pulmonary edema or subarachnoid or intracranial hemorrhage manifested by stiffness of the neck, decreasing consciousness, and syncope results from severe hypertension. Therefore, patients should be instructed to avoid foods and beverages with a high tyramine content (eg, cheese, most wines, vermouth, most dried meats and fish, canned figs, broad beans [fava beans], concentrated yeast products). It has been suggested that other foods containing tyramine may be consumed in moderation and need not be prohibited (Brown and Bryant, 1988); however, differences in food processing can influence tyramine content. Alcohol intake also should be limited to one or two drinks daily. A recently updated list of foods and beverages to avoid should be given to any patient receiving MAO inhibitors.

The effects of other direct and indirect-acting sympathomimetic amines (eg, amphetamines; methylphenidate [Ritalin]; ephedrine; cocaine; including sympathomimetic amines in cold or asthma remedies) are markedly potentiated, and these drugs also should be avoided. Phentolamine, parenteral and oral chlorpromazine, and nifedipine (10 mg) have been used to counteract the hypertensive crises.

Levodopa should be withdrawn two to four weeks prior to institution of MAO inhibitor therapy. Methyldopa [Aldomet], tryptophan, and 5-hydroxytryptophan also are relatively contraindicated.

Excitation, hyperpyrexia, seizures, and delirium also are features of the "serotonin" syndrome that may be associated with the combination of MAO inhibitors with tryptophan or 5-HT uptake inhibitors such as fluoxetine, sertraline, or clomipramine. At least five weeks should elapse before an MAO inhibitor is used after fluoxetine has been discontinued due to the long half-life of fluoxetine and norfluoxetine. This syndrome also may occur when dextromethorphan (a common ingredient of over-the-counter cough preparations) or meperidine [Demerol] and related analgesics are given to patients receiving MAO inhibitors. If emergency surgery is necessary, meperidine should be avoided and the dose of any opioid chosen should be reduced by at least one-fourth to one-half. The central nervous system depressant action of anesthetics and alcohol is also markedly potentiated.

Furazolidone [Furoxone], an antimicrobial drug, and procarbazine [Matulane], an antineoplastic agent, act as MAO inhibitors when given for more than five days; therefore, caution should be observed if these drugs are administered with other MAO inhibitors.

Enhanced hypoglycemic responses have been reported in patients receiving MAO inhibitors in combination with insulin or sulfonylurea hypoglycemic agents. Insulin-dependent patients should be monitored for hypoglycemia at the start of MAO inhibitor therapy; the dosage of insulin may require adjustment.

Tranylcypromine should be administered with caution to patients receiving disulfiram [Antabuse], because severe toxicity, including convulsions and death, has been noted in animals.

For interactions between MAO inhibitor and tricyclic antidepressants, see the section on Tricyclic Antidepressants. MAO inhibitors should not be used with buspirone.

Poisoning: Currently, little data are available on the mean lethal dose of the MAO inhibitors. Death has been reported with doses of 170 to 650 mg of tranylcypromine and 375 mg to 1.5 g of phenelzine. Toxic effects may not appear for 12 hours or more after ingestion and are largely adrenergic in nature: agitation, increased ventilatory and cardiac rates, dilated pupils, hyperreflexia, tremors, ataxia, sweating, hyperthermia, heart block, hypotension, delirium, convulsions, and coma. Aggressive supportive therapy to maintain vital functions, physical cooling procedures, forced diuresis, and acidification of the urine are indicated. Because MAO inhibitors decrease gut motility, gastric lavage should be performed up to several hours after ingestion.

ANTIMANIC DRUGS

Lithium is effective in 60% to 80% of all acute hypomanic and manic episodes. Onset of its therapeutic effect is slow (five days to three weeks), but larger doses may shorten the time to clinical response. Alternatively, antipsychotic agents alone or with lithium usually are employed in the initial treatment of highly agitated, hyperactive manic patients. High-potency benzodiazepines (eg, lorazepam) also may be used to control agitation and sleeplessness (Lenox et al, 1992). When the acute episode is controlled, the antipsychotic agent or benzodiazepine may be withdrawn gradually and lithium continued as the sole therapeutic agent. Careful dosage adjustment of both drugs is essential for optimum effectiveness and to lessen any additive central nervous system toxicity.

Lithium decreases the intensity and frequency of successive episodes of cyclic mania and depression and, thus, is clearly indicated in the prophylaxis of bipolar disorder. However, it is not effective in all patients and should be given prophylactically only when it does reduce the frequency and/or intensity of the episodes. Patients with a history of dysphoric mania or rapid cycling appear to be less responsive to prophylactic lithium therapy.

Administration of an antidepressant with lithium may be required in breakthrough depression. Likewise, if mania is observed during use of antidepressants in patients with recurring depressive episodes, combination therapy with lithium may be helpful. However, the evidence indicates that long-term use of lithium plus an antidepressant is no more effective than lithium alone (Johnson, 1987; Johnstone et al, 1990).

Several controlled studies have compared the effects of carbamazepine and its keto congener, oxcarbazepine, with those of antipsychotic agents and placebo in patients with acute mania; carbamazepine has been directly compared with lithium in only two small controlled trials (for review see Post, 1990; Chou, 1991). In most studies, carbamazepine was used in combination with other agents in patients who had had an inadequate response to lithium. Approximately 70% of patients improved with the regimen containing carbamazepine, which is similar to the improvement rate reported in uncontrolled trials. Onset of action and efficacy of carbamazepine and antipsychotic drugs in acute mania appear to be roughly equivalent. Carbamazepine may be more effective than lithium in a limited subgroup of manic patients (eg, those with severe or dysphoric mania, rapid cycling, mixed affective states) (Post et al, 1987), but specific predictors of response have not been determined (Cook and Winokur, 1990). Further study is required to establish the efficacy of carbamazepine when it is used alone in the treatment of acute mania and to clarify whether its use should be confined to patients who are resistant to or cannot tolerate lithium (Prien and Potter, 1990). Doses of 600 mg to 1.2 g/day have been given to acutely ill patients; rapid cyclers may require 1.2 to 2 g/day. (See also index entry Carbamazepine, Uses.)

Controlled trials of prophylaxis with carbamazepine in patients with bipolar disorder have been limited. In uncontrolled studies involving approximately 500 patients, the response rate was 64% (Post, 1990). In seven partially controlled trials (blinded or randomized), the response rate was 72%, but in double-blind studies the response rate was 45% to 67% (Small, 1990). In one comparative trial, which included both unipolar and bipolar patients, those receiving lithium experienced longer remissions than those receiving carbamazepine (Watkins et al, 1987). It is generally believed that carbamazepine is more effective in mania than in depression but evidence from controlled studies is lacking.

Valproic acid also is being studied as an alternative to lithium for the treatment of mania. In open studies on its value for acute therapy and prophylaxis, valproic acid's antimanic properties were moderate to marked (response rate 57%). The drug was used primarily with other therapy and often in patients described as lithium-resistant; however, formal diagnostic criteria frequently were not specified (McElroy et al, 1989). Few patients have received valproic acid alone; the majority have been treated with concurrent lithium and/or intermittent antidepressant or antipsychotic therapy. In three small studies that used patients as their own controls, 71% (10/14) responded to valproic acid. In a parallel design study involving 36 lithium-resistant subjects, 53% responded to valproic acid; most or all of the observed clinical response appeared one to four days after serum valproate concentrations of at least 50 mcg/ml were reached (Pope et al, 1991). A level of 75 mcg/ml may be necessary for patients with schizoaffective disorder.

In a comparative trial that included many patients with mixed bipolar disorder, the response to valproic acid (64%) was less than that to lithium (90%). In a larger prospective open trial involving 55 patients with rapid-cycling bipolar disorder, both acute and prophylactic therapy were beneficial in over 90% of patients; the response was less pronounced in those with depression (Calabrese and Delucchi, 1990). Almost two-thirds of the patients in this study received combination therapy with lithium, antidepressants, or carbamazepine. These results differ somewhat from those reported in a randomized, double-blind, parallel-group trial in which both lithium and valproic acid relieved manic symptoms, although lithium was slightly more efficacious (Freeman et al, 1992). However, unlike lithium, a favorable response to valproic acid was associated with high pretreatment depression scores, which suggests that valproic acid may be more effective in manic patients with mixed affective states.

For patients who are resistant to lithium, the addition or substitution of valproic acid may be considered. The initial dosage of valproic acid in these disorders is 250 mg two or three times daily. The dose should be increased in increments of 250 mg every two to three days as side effects permit until plasma trough levels determined 12 hours after the nighttime dose are within the proposed therapeutic range (usually 50 to 120 mcg/ml) (Chou, 1991). Because it produces less gastrointestinal upset, the enteric-coated form, divalproex sodium [Depakote], may be preferred. For additional information on adverse reactions, precautions, interactions, use during pregnancy, and pharmacokinetics, see index entry Valproic Acid.

Preliminary evidence suggests that verapamil [Calan, Isoptin] may be beneficial in acute mania. In one small comparative trial, verapamil (mean dose, 295 mg daily) was reported to be as effective as chlorpromazine alone (mean dose, 375 mg daily) or chlorpromazine (mean dose, 344 mg daily) combined with lithium (mean level, 0.75 mEq/L), although these doses of the latter agents are comparatively low (Hoschl and Kozeny, 1989). Favorable results in those with acute mania also were reported in three small placebo-controlled trials and one crossover trial with lithium (for review see Chou, 1991).

In a recent randomized, double-blind trial comparing verapamil (320 mg daily) with lithium (serum levels 0.75 to 1.5 mEq/L) in acutely manic patients, patients in both treatment groups improved significantly (Garza-Treviño et al, 1992). More patients in the verapamil group required the addition of haloperidol [Haldol] or lorazepam [Ativan] for optimal control of agitation. Thus, although verapamil appears to be effective in some patients with mania, further study is required to determine whether this or other calcium channel blockers are effective alternatives in patients who do not respond adequately to lithium.

Drug Evaluations

TRICYCLIC COMPOUNDS

IMIPRAMINE HYDROCHLORIDE
[Janimine, Tofranil]

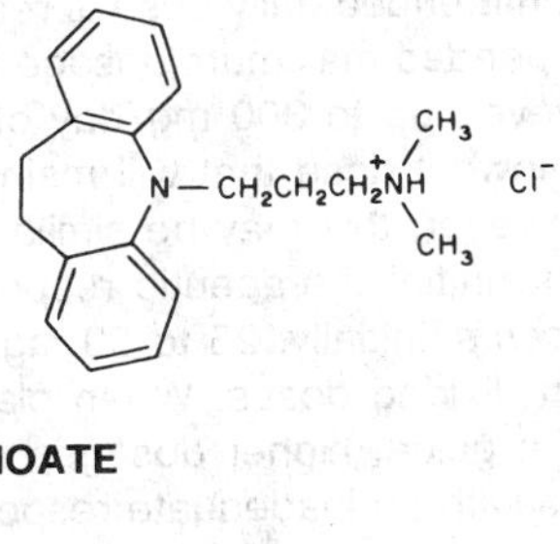

IMIPRAMINE PAMOATE
[Tofranil-PM]

USES. Imipramine is the prototype of the tricyclic antidepressants and is effective in the treatment of depressive episodes of major depression and bipolar, atypical, and dysthymic disorders. For other uses of this drug, see index entry Imipramine.

The pamoate form offers no advantage over the hydrochloride salt; both salts are inherently long acting.

ADVERSE REACTIONS AND PRECAUTIONS. The untoward effects of imipramine are characteristic of all tricyclic antidepressants. Sedation, orthostatic hypotension, and anticholinergic effects are most common. Tremor, nervousness, and excessive perspiration are troublesome in some patients; quinidine-like properties may be detrimental in patients with pre-existing conduction deficits. Allergic reactions, blood dyscrasias, endocrine effects, and jaundice are uncommon. Cardiac and central nervous system toxicity may be prominent with overdosage.

Abrupt cessation of treatment after long-term therapy may produce withdrawal symptoms (eg, headache, malaise, increased salivation, diarrhea, anorexia, fatigue). An akathisia-like syndrome also has been reported when administration of large doses (300 mg or more daily) was stopped suddenly. Although most fatal cases of poisoning have occurred after ingestion of more than 1.5 g, individual sensitivity varies; death has been reported after as little as 500 mg and recovery has occurred after ingestion of 5.4 g.

See the Introduction for a more complete discussion on adverse reactions, precautions, pharmacokinetics, and the use of imipramine with other drugs.

DOSAGE AND PREPARATIONS. Dosage should be individualized on the basis of clinical response. See Table 2.

Intramuscular: *Adults,* initially, up to 100 mg daily in divided doses. The oral route should be substituted as soon as possible.

IMIPRAMINE HYDROCHLORIDE:

Tofranil (Geigy). Solution 12.5 mg/ml in 2 ml containers.

Oral: *Adults (hospitalized),* initially, 50 to 100 mg daily in divided doses, increased gradually to 200 mg daily; 250 to 300 mg daily may be given if there is no response after two weeks. *Adults (outpatients),* initially, 50 mg increased to 150 mg daily in divided doses; a schedule to minimize sedation and anticholinergic effects is described in the footnote to Table 2. A single daily dose or the major portion of the daily dose may be given at bedtime if insomnia is prominent or undue sedation occurs during the day. If little benefit is noted by the third week, the dose may be increased (eg, by 50 mg daily every week) until clinical improvement, intolerable side effects, or the maximum recommended daily dose is reached. The manufacturers' recommended maximum dosage for outpatients is 200 mg/day; however, up to 300 mg/day often is used. For maintenance, the lowest dose that will maintain remission is recommended; however, this may be similar to the dose required to attain the initial therapeutic response. *Elderly patients and adolescents,* initially, 25 to 50 mg daily, increased to 100 mg daily in divided doses. When plasma concentrations are used as a guide, higher dosages may be administered to individuals with an inadequate response.

IMIPRAMINE HYDROCHLORIDE:

Janimine (Abbott), ***Tofranil*** (Geigy), ***Generic***. Tablets 10, 25, and 50 mg.

IMIPRAMINE PAMOATE:

Tofranil-PM (Geigy). Capsules equivalent to 75, 100, 125, and 150 mg of imipramine hydrochloride.

AMITRIPTYLINE HYDROCHLORIDE

[Elavil, Endep]

$$=CHCH_2CH_2\overset{+}{N}H(CH_3)_2\quad Cl^-$$

USES. Amitriptyline is as effective as imipramine in the treatment of depressive episodes of major depression, bipolar disorder, dysthymic disorder, and atypical depression. As with any tricyclic agent, concomitant administration of amitriptyline with an antipsychotic drug can be beneficial in schizoaffective disorder and depression with psychotic features.

Amitriptyline may control abnormal eating behavior in bulimic patients (Mitchell and Groat, 1984), but its long-term effectiveness has not been established. Amitriptyline (mean dose, 65 mg) also may be beneficial in the treatment of postherpetic neuralgia (Max et al, 1988). For other uses of this drug, see index entry Amitriptyline.

ADVERSE REACTIONS AND PRECAUTIONS. Effective doses have a moderate to marked sedative action. Because anticholinergic activity may be pronounced, confusional episodes can occur with amitriptyline, especially in elderly patients. Increased appetite for carbohydrates with resultant weight gain often occurs with prolonged treatment. Leukopenia has been reported.

Although most fatal cases of poisoning have resulted from ingestion of more than 1.3 g, death has been reported after ingestion of 500 mg and recovery after ingestion of almost 4 g.

Amitriptyline is classified in FDA Pregnancy Category C.

See the Introduction for a more complete discussion on indications, adverse reactions, precautions, and the use of tricyclic antidepressants with other drugs.

DOSAGE AND PREPARATIONS.

Intramuscular: *Adults,* initially, 20 to 30 mg four times a day. The oral route should be substituted as soon as possible.

Elavil (Stuart), ***Generic***. Solution 10 mg/ml in 10 ml containers.

Oral: *Adults (hospitalized),* initially, 50 to 100 mg daily in divided doses, increased gradually to 200 mg daily if necessary; some patients may require as much as 300 mg daily. *Adults (outpatients),* initially, 50 mg increased to 150 mg daily in divided doses; a schedule to minimize sedation and anticholinergic effects is described in the footnote to Table 2. A single daily dose or the major portion of the daily dose may be given at bedtime if insomnia is prominent or undue sedation occurs during the day. If little benefit is noted by the third week, the dose may be increased (eg, by 50 mg daily every week) until clinical improvement, intolerable side effects, or the maximum recommended daily dose is reached. The manufacturers' recommended maximum dosage for outpatients is 150 mg/day; however, up to 300 mg/day may be required in some individuals. For maintenance, the lowest dose that will maintain remission is recommended. *Elderly patients and adolescents,* initially, 25 to 50 mg daily, increased to 100 mg daily in divided doses; some may require and tolerate higher dosages.

Elavil (Stuart), ***Endep*** (Roche), ***Generic***. Tablets 10, 25, 50, 75, 100, and 150 mg.

AMOXAPINE

[Asendin]

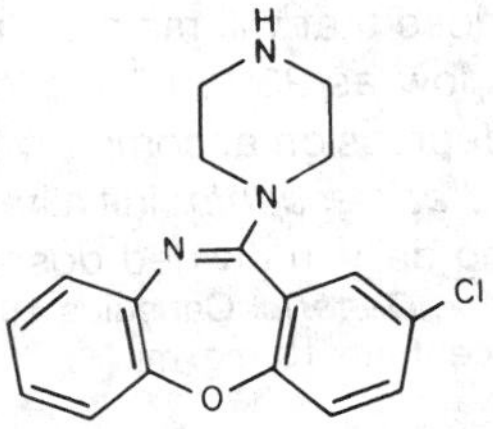

The chemical structure of amoxapine is similar to that of the antipsychotic drug, loxapine. Amoxapine and its metabolites, 7-hydroxyamoxapine and 8-hydroxyamoxapine, have dopamine receptor (D_2) antagonist action (Lydiard and Gelenberg, 1981).

USES. Results of controlled studies show that the antidepressant action of amoxapine is comparable to that of imipramine and amitriptyline. As with other tricyclic drugs, amoxapine generally is more effective in major depression than in dysthymic or atypical depression. It has relatively weak sedative and anticholinergic activities compared to imipramine or amitriptyline. Amoxapine has been claimed to have a more rapid onset of action, but this finding has not been observed consistently.

ADVERSE REACTIONS AND PRECAUTIONS. Although sedation and anticholinergic effects are less common than with other tricyclics, caution is advised when prescribing this drug for patients who perform hazardous tasks that require alertness or for those with a history of urinary retention or angle-closure glaucoma.

Extrapyramidal effects have been observed infrequently and are caused by amoxapine and its hydroxylated metabolites, which are dopamine antagonists. Hyperprolactinemia, galactorrhea, and amenorrhea have been reported and also probably are linked to dopamine receptor blockade. Dyskinesias have developed, but it is not clear whether they are tardive or withdrawal dyskinesias. Neuroleptic malignant syndrome also has been observed (Hunt-Fugate et al, 1984, Madakasira, 1989).

Tachycardia and arrhythmias have occurred less frequently than anticipated on the basis of experience with amitriptyline and imipramine; nevertheless, caution is advised when amoxapine is used in individuals with cardiac abnormalities, and use of the drug is not recommended during the immediate period following myocardial infarction.

A high incidence of seizures has been reported, most often after overdose or use of large therapeutic doses. Amoxapine should be employed with caution in epileptic patients. Skin rashes occur infrequently. Agranulocytosis has developed (Christenson, 1983).

DRUG INTERACTIONS. Drug interactions with amoxapine are similar to those observed with traditional tricyclic drugs.

PREGNANCY AND LACTATION. Embryotoxic and fetotoxic effects, as well as decreased postnatal survival (intrauterine death, stillbirth, decreased weight gain), occurred in animals given three to ten times the human dose, but no teratogenic effects were observed. Amoxapine should be used during pregnancy only if the benefit justifies the risk to the fetus (FDA Pregnancy Category C).

Amoxapine and 8-hydroxyamoxapine are detectable in human breast milk and this drug is not recommended for nursing women.

See the Introduction for a more complete discussion of indications, adverse reactions, interactions, pharmacokinetics, and management of overdose.

DOSAGE AND PREPARATIONS.

Oral: *Adults,* initially, 50 mg, increased to 200 mg daily in divided doses; a schedule is described in the footnote to Table 2. A single daily dose or the major portion of the daily dose may be given at bedtime if insomnia is prominent or undue sedation occurs during the day. If little benefit is noted by the third week, the dose may be increased (eg, by 50 mg daily every week) until clinical improvement, intolerable side effects, or the maximum recommended daily dose is reached (ie, *outpatients*, 400 mg; *inpatients*, 600 mg). For maintenance, the lowest dose that will maintain remission is recommended. *Elderly patients and adolescents,* initially, 25 to 50 mg daily, increased to 100 mg daily in divided doses; some may require and tolerate higher doses.

Asendin (Lederle), ***Generic.*** Tablets 25, 50, 100, and 150 mg.

DESIPRAMINE HYDROCHLORIDE

[Norpramin, Pertofrane]

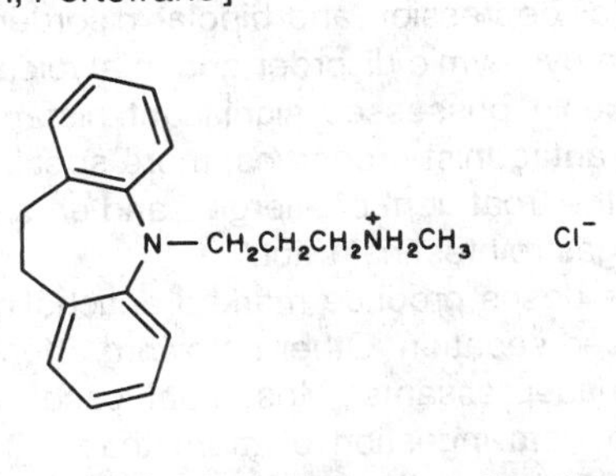

N—$CH_2CH_2CH_2\overset{+}{N}H_2CH_3$ Cl^-

Desipramine, a metabolite of imipramine, has actions and uses similar to those of the parent compound and is as effective as imipramine in the treatment of mood disorders.

Untoward effects are similar to those produced by imipramine, but anticholinergic and sedative actions are less pronounced. Thus, desipramine may be especially useful in patients who are particularly sensitive to these effects (eg, the elderly).

See the Introduction for more complete information on indications, adverse reactions, precautions, pharmacokinetics, and the use of tricyclic antidepressants with other drugs.

DOSAGE AND PREPARATIONS.

Oral: *Adults (hospitalized),* initially, 75 mg daily in divided doses, increased gradually to 200 mg daily. If necessary, after two weeks the dosage may be increased gradually to a maximum of 300 mg daily. *Adults (outpatients),* initially, 50 to 75 mg increased to 150 mg daily in divided doses; a schedule is described in the footnote to Table 2. A single daily dose or the major portion of the daily dose may be given at bedtime if insomnia is prominent or undue sedation occurs during the day. If little benefit is noted by the third week, the dose may be increased (eg, by 50 mg daily every week) until clinical improvement, intolerable side effects, or the maximum recommended daily dose is reached (ie, 300 mg). For maintenance, the lowest dose that will maintain remission is recommended. *Elderly patients and adolescents,* initially, 25 to 50 mg daily, increased to 100 mg daily in divided doses. When plasma concentrations are used as a guide, higher dosages may be administered to individuals with an inadequate response.

Norpramin (Marion Merrell Dow), ***Generic.*** Tablets 10, 25, 50, 75, 100, and 150 mg.

Pertofrane (Rhone-Poulenc Rorer). Capsules 25 and 50 mg.

DOXEPIN HYDROCHLORIDE

[Sinequan]

$=CHCH_2CH_2\overset{+}{N}H(CH_3)_2 \quad Cl^-$

The usefulness of this tricyclic antidepressant is comparable to that of imipramine in the treatment of depressive episodes of major depression and bipolar disorder. It also may be effective in dysthymic disorder and in atypical depression. Although doxepin possesses significant histamine receptor (H_1 and H_2) antagonist properties, more specific agents are preferred for the treatment of allergies and erosive conditions of the upper gastrointestinal tract.

Therapeutic doses produce marked anticholinergic effects and pronounced sedation. Other untoward effects are typical of tricyclic antidepressants. Most fatal cases of poisoning have resulted from ingestion of more than 1.5 g; however, recovery has occurred after ingestion of 5 g.

See the Introduction for additional information on indications, adverse reactions, precautions, pharmacokinetics, and the use of tricyclic antidepressants with other drugs.

DOSAGE AND PREPARATIONS.

Oral: *Adults (hospitalized),* initially, 75 mg daily in divided doses for patients with mild to moderate illness. Larger doses may be required in more severely ill patients, but the dose must be titrated carefully to avoid undue sedation. The usual optimum dosage is 75 to 150 mg daily. The dosage may be increased gradually after two weeks to a maximum of 300 mg daily. *Adults (outpatients),* initially, 50 to 75 mg daily in divided doses; the usual optimum dosage is 75 to 150 mg daily. A schedule to minimize sedation and anticholinergic effects is described in the footnote to Table 2. A single daily dose or the major portion of the daily dose may be given at bedtime if insomnia is prominent or undue sedation occurs during the day. If little benefit is noted by the third week, the dose may be increased (eg, by 50 mg daily every week) until clinical improvement, intolerable side effects, or the maximum recommended daily dose is reached (ie, 300 mg). For maintenance, the lowest dose that will maintain remission is recommended. Doses as low as 25 to 50 mg/day have controlled mild symptoms or depression accompanying organic disease. *Elderly patients and adolescents,* initially, 25 to 50 mg daily, increased to 100 mg daily in divided doses.

Sinequan (Roerig), ***Generic.*** Capsules 10, 25, 50, 75, 100, and 150 mg; oral concentrate 10 mg/ml.

MAPROTILINE HYDROCHLORIDE

[Ludiomil]

$CH_2CH_2CH_2\overset{+}{N}H_2CH_3 \quad Cl^-$

ACTIONS AND USES. Maprotiline is a tetracyclic antidepressant; however, its pharmacologic and clinical profiles, as well as efficacy, resemble those of imipramine (see that evaluation).

ADVERSE REACTIONS AND PRECAUTIONS. Drowsiness and anticholinergic effects are the most common reactions reported. They are less severe than with amitriptyline. Skin rashes occur in approximately 3% of patients after two weeks of therapy. Hypotension and tachycardia are less severe than with imipramine or amitriptyline, but the incidence is similar for all three drugs. Therefore, maprotiline also should be used cautiously in patients with a history of myocardial infarction or cardiac disorders.

Seizures are observed more often than with tricyclic compounds and have occurred over a broad dose range, after even modest increases in the daily dosage, and during stabilized dosing regimens (Mendelis, 1983). They also have been reported on initiation of therapy and during prolonged treatment. Their incidence in patients who ingested overdoses is 25%. Therefore, maprotiline should not be used in patients with known or suspected seizure disorders. The risk may be minimized by starting therapy at a low dose for two weeks before gradually increasing the amount to recommended levels.

See the Introduction for a more complete discussion of indications, adverse reactions, drug interactions, pharmacokinetics, and management of overdose.

PREGNANCY AND LACTATION. No teratogenic, embryotoxic, or fetotoxic effects have been observed in animals. Because no adequate, well-controlled studies have been performed in pregnant women, maprotiline should be administered during pregnancy only if the benefit justifies the risk to the fetus (FDA Pregnancy Category B).

Concentrations of maprotiline in breast milk are similar to those in the blood; therefore, its use should be discouraged in nursing women.

DOSAGE AND PREPARATIONS.

Oral: *Adults (hospitalized)*, initially, 100 to 150 mg daily in divided doses, gradually increased as required and tolerated. Most hospitalized patients with moderate to severe depression respond to 150 mg daily, although as much as 225 mg may be required. Doses above 225 mg are not recommended because of the risk of seizures.

Adults (outpatients), initially, 50 to 75 mg daily in single or divided doses for two weeks. If little benefit is noted by the third week, the dose may be increased gradually (eg, by 25 mg daily every week) until clinical improvement, intolerable side effects, or the maximum recommended daily dose is reached (ie, 225 mg). For maintenance, the lowest dose that will maintain remission is recommended. *Elderly patients,* initially, 25 to 50 mg daily; 50 to 75 mg daily is usually satisfactory for maintenance, but some patients require higher doses.

Ludiomil (CIBA), ***Generic.*** Tablets 25, 50, and 75 mg.

NORTRIPTYLINE HYDROCHLORIDE

[Aventyl Hydrochloride, Pamelor]

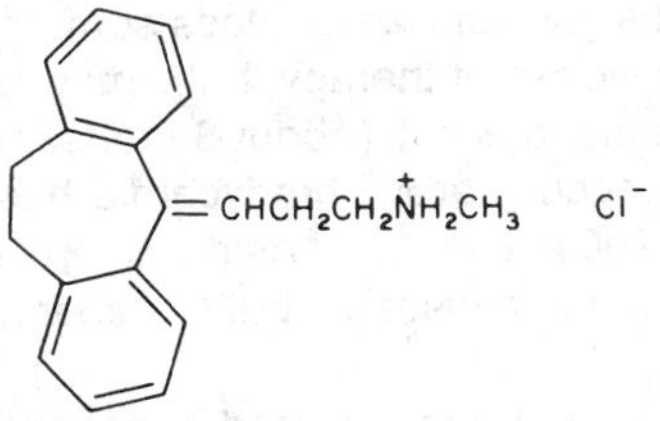

$=CHCH_2CH_2\overset{+}{N}H_2CH_3 \quad Cl^-$

Nortriptyline, the N-demethylated metabolite of amitriptyline, is as effective as imipramine in the treatment of depressive episodes of major depression and bipolar disorder. It also may be useful in dysthymic disorder and atypical depression.

Plasma concentrations below 50 ng/ml are thought to be ineffective and those exceeding 150 to 175 ng/ml often are associated with a suboptimal response in patients with major depression; therefore, excessive dosage may diminish responsiveness. In addition, active metabolites of nortriptyline may accumulate in elderly patients, and toxic side effects may develop despite plasma nortriptyline concentrations below 150 ng/ml. However, in one study, the pharmacokinetic parameters of nortriptyline in frail elderly patients were similar to those in younger individuals.

Nortriptyline may be less likely than other tricyclic agents to produce orthostatic hypotension, particularly in the elderly. It also may be relatively safer than other tricyclic antidepressants in cardiac patients, including those who have received a transplant.

See the Introduction for additional information on indications, adverse reactions, precautions, and the use of tricyclic antidepressants with other drugs.

DOSAGE AND PREPARATIONS.

Oral: *Adults (hospitalized),* initially, 25 mg daily in two or three divided doses, increased to a maximum of 150 mg daily after two weeks, if necessary. After adjustment as needed, the total dose can be given once daily at bedtime.

Adults (outpatients), initially, 25 mg daily, increased as required to 25 mg three or four times daily. Some patients may require lower doses initially (eg, 10 mg). A schedule to minimize sedation and anticholinergic effects is described in the footnote to Table 2. Doses above 150 mg are not recommended unless plasma concentrations indicate that a higher dose is needed. For maintenance, the lowest dose that maintains remission should be given. *Adolescents and elderly patients,* 30 to 50 mg daily in divided doses.

Aventyl Hydrochloride (Lilly). Capsules 10 and 25 mg; liquid 10 mg/5 ml (alcohol 4%).

Pamelor (Sandoz). Capsules 10, 25, 50, and 75 mg; oral solution 10 mg/5 ml (alcohol 4%).

PROTRIPTYLINE HYDROCHLORIDE

[Vivactil]

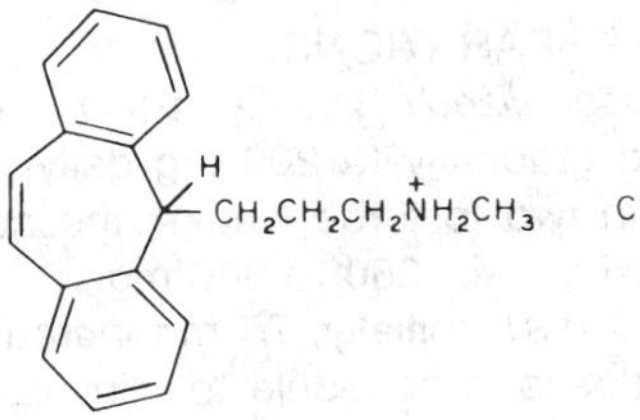

$H \quad CH_2CH_2CH_2\overset{+}{N}H_2CH_3 \quad Cl^-$

This tricyclic antidepressant is effective in the treatment of major depression and the depressed phase of bipolar disorder and also may be useful in the treatment of dysthymic disorder and atypical depression.

Unlike most of the other tricyclic antidepressants, protriptyline causes little, if any, sedation. Because of this, it may be particularly useful in depression associated with psychomotor retardation, apathy, and extreme fatigue. It also may reduce nocturnal oxygen desaturation in patients with sleep apnea (see index entry Sleep Apnea, Treatment) or chronic obstructive pulmonary disease (Sériès and Cormier, 1990).

See the Introduction for additional information on indications, adverse reactions, precautions, pharmacokinetics, and the use of tricyclic antidepressants with other drugs.

DOSAGE AND PREPARATIONS.

Oral: *Adults (hospitalized),* 15 mg daily in one or two doses, increased to a maximum of 60 mg daily after two weeks, if necessary. After adjustment as needed, the total dose can be given once daily, usually in the morning. *Adults (outpatients),* initially, 15 to 40 mg daily in three or four doses. Doses should begin at a low level and be increased gradually. A schedule to minimize anticholinergic effects is described in the footnote to Table 2. Doses above 60 mg daily are not recommended. For maintenance, the lowest amount that maintains remission should be given. *Adolescents and elderly patients,* initially, 10 to 15 mg daily in one or two divided doses, increased gradually if necessary. In elderly patients, the cardiovascular system must be monitored closely if the daily dose exceeds 20 mg.

Vivactil (Merck Sharp & Dohme). Tablets 5 and 10 mg.

TRIMIPRAMINE MALEATE
[Surmontil]

Trimipramine is an effective antidepressant that resembles the other dibenzazepines (ie, desipramine, imipramine); however, the sedation produced is equivalent to that observed with amitriptyline and doxepin. Therapeutic doses have intermediate anticholinergic activity.

The indications, adverse reactions, and precautions of trimipramine are similar to those of the other tricyclic compounds (see the Introduction). The potential risk to the fetus is unknown (FDA Pregnancy Category C).

DOSAGE AND PREPARATIONS.
Oral: *Adults (hospitalized),* initially, 100 mg daily in divided doses, increased gradually to 200 mg daily; if improvement does not occur in two to three weeks, the dose may be increased to a maximum of 250 to 300 mg.

Adults (outpatients), initially, 75 mg increased to 150 mg daily in divided doses; a schedule to minimize sedation and anticholinergic effects is described in the footnote to Table 2. A single daily dose or the major portion of the daily dose may be given at bedtime if insomnia is prominent or undue sedation occurs during the day. If little benefit is noted by the third week, the dose may be increased (eg, by 50 mg daily every week) until clinical improvement, intolerable side effects, or the maximum recommended daily dose is reached (ie, 250 mg). For maintenance, dosage should be adjusted to the lowest level required to prevent relapse; however, this may be similar to the dose needed to attain the initial therapeutic response. *Elderly patients and adolescents,* initially, 25 to 50 mg daily, increased to 100 mg daily in divided doses.

Surmontil (Wyeth-Ayerst), ***Generic.*** Capsules 25, 50, and 100 mg.

SEROTONIN (5-HT) UPTAKE INHIBITORS

FLUOXETINE HYDROCHLORIDE
[Prozac]

ACTIONS. Fluoxetine, a phenylpropylamine, inhibits the neuronal uptake of serotonin, which is presumed to be related to its antidepressant action. This compound has little effect on the neuronal uptake of norepinephrine or on dopamine dynamics following short- or long-term administration. In addition, fluoxetine does not bind to cholinergic, histaminergic, or alpha-adrenergic receptors, which are thought to be associated with the undesirable side effects of tricyclic antidepressant drugs.

USES. The efficacy of fluoxetine in the treatment of nondelusional, moderately depressed patients is comparable to that of the tricyclic agents; its efficacy in severely depressed hospitalized patients has not been established. In limited studies, fluoxetine was useful in treating patients with atypical depression, panic disorder, and the depressed component of bipolar disorder. Fluoxetine may be indicated as initial therapy in patient's with concurrent obsessive-compulsive disorder. Its efficacy in obesity and bulimia is being explored.

The selection of fluoxetine appears to be most appropriate for patients who are at special risk from sedative, hypotensive, and anticholinergic side effects caused by other antidepressants. In addition, it appears to be relatively safe for use in the elderly, although its very long elimination half-life may pose special problems for these individuals.

ADVERSE REACTIONS AND PRECAUTIONS. The most frequent side effects of fluoxetine are nausea, nervousness/agitation, and insomnia (incidence 20% to 40%); these effects are generally mild and seldom require discontinuation of treatment. Less frequently reported reactions include headache, tremor, anxiety, drowsiness, dry mouth, sweating, and diarrhea. Small but significant weight loss sometimes occurs during the first few weeks of therapy, but it may not be sustained.

In some patients, a slight (about 3 beats/min) decrease in heart rate may occur; rarely, bradycardia has been reported (Ellison et al, 1990). The drug has not been tested specifically in those with cardiac disease, but it probably is safe in such patients.

Hyponatremia has been reported in patients taking fluoxetine, especially older patients and those taking diuretics or who were otherwise volume-depleted.

Sexual dysfunction, including anorgasmia, may occur. Extrapyramidal reactions (eg, acute dystonia) have been noted rarely; akathisia also may develop (Lipinski et al, 1989).

Based on a series a case reports, attention has focused on the possibility that use of fluoxetine may be associated with the development of intense suicidal preoccupation in patients who were previously free of such thoughts. These patients were characterized by nonresponse to earlier treatment with fluoxetine or other drugs, escalation of fluoxetine dosage despite severe side effects (eg, marked agitation, anxiety), and concurrent treatment with other psychoactive drugs (Teicher et al, 1990). However, reanalysis of clinical trial data supports the contention that serious suicidal thoughts occurred less often in patients receiving fluoxetine than in those receiving other antidepressants or placebo (Beasley et al, 1991). In another retrospective analysis (Fava and Rosenbaum, 1991), no significant difference in the incidence of treatment-emergent suicidal ideation was observed among patients treated with fluoxetine alone compared with those treated with other antidepressants. It has been suggested that the emergence of akathisia during treatment may be an important risk factor for the development of suicidal ideation in response to fluoxetine. Three patients who had previously attempted suicide while receiving fluoxetine also developed suicidal ideation in association with akathisia after reexposure to this agent (Rothschild and Locke, 1991). The akathisia and suicidal ideation abated upon discontinuation of fluoxetine or after the addition of propranolol. Further study is required to support this theory. After reviewing the available data, the FDA has concluded that fluoxetine is not associated with unreasonable or unexpected risk.

Fluoxetine is classified in FDA Pregnancy Category B.

DRUG INTERACTIONS. Concomitant administration of fluoxetine and MAO inhibitors, including selegiline, is not recommended. Fourteen days should elapse between discontinuation of an MAO inhibitor and initiation of treatment with fluoxetine; at least five weeks should elapse between discontinuation of fluoxetine and initiation of therapy with an MAO inhibitor in order to avoid the "serotonergic" syndrome. This syndrome also can occur in patients receiving fluoxetine and tryptophan. Both fluoxetine and norfluoxetine inhibit cytochrome P450IID6 and therefore increase the plasma concentrations of desipramine and nortriptyline and other tricyclic agents that depend on this isozyme for elimination. Carbamazepine and some antipsychotic agents (eg, haloperidol and possibly the phenothiazines) are similarly affected.

POISONING. Drug overdose has been fatal in two patients who also were receiving other drugs. In other patients, ingestion of up to 3 g has produced generally mild symptoms, such as agitation and vomiting, but seizures have occurred. Treatment is symptomatic and supportive.

PHARMACOKINETICS. Fluoxetine is well absorbed after oral administration, whether or not food is present, and peak plasma concentrations are attained six to eight hours after a dose. Steady-state plasma concentrations are reached after two to four weeks. Fluoxetine is widely distributed throughout the body, and about 94% of a dose is bound to plasma protein. The drug is metabolized in the liver to norfluoxetine, which also selectively inhibits serotonin reuptake, and other unidentified metabolites. Fluoxetine is excreted in the urine primarily as inactive metabolites. Renal impairment does not appear to alter the pharmacokinetics, although alcohol-induced cirrhosis does prolong the half-life.

The elimination half-life is long: one to four days for fluoxetine and seven to ten days for norfluoxetine. Because of the long half-life, the drug can be administered once daily, efficacy is unaffected by an occasional missed dose, and abrupt termination of therapy results in gradual cessation of effects. This drug's pharmacokinetic profile is similar in elderly and younger patients.

DOSAGE AND PREPARATIONS.

Oral: *Adults*, initially, 20 mg given once daily in the morning. The liquid formulation may be used to provide a lower (eg, 5 to 10 mg) dose in patients who cannot tolerate 20 mg. A study comparing the effects of 20, 40, or 60 mg daily found no significant differences in efficacy, but fewer side effects were observed with the 20-mg dose (Fabre and Putman, 1987). If no therapeutic effect is obtained after several weeks, the dose can be increased in 20-mg increments to a maximum of 80 mg daily in younger patients; a lower maximum dose may suffice in the elderly. Doses higher than 20 mg should be given in divided amounts in the morning and at noon. Because of the drug's long half-life, several weeks are required to establish a new steady state, and this must be considered when adjusting the dose.

Prozac (Dista). Capsules 20 mg; solution (oral) 20 mg/5 ml.

SERTRALINE HYDROCHLORIDE

[Zoloft]

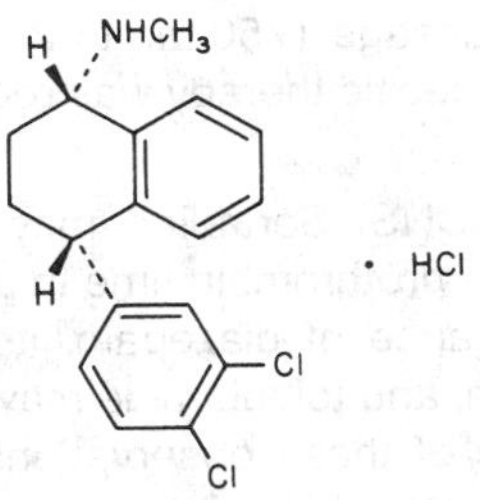

ACTIONS. Sertraline, a naphthylamine, selectively inhibits the neuronal uptake of serotonin, and this action is presumed to underlie its antidepressant action. Only very weak effects are exerted on the neuronal uptake of norepinephrine and dopamine, and sertraline does not bind significantly to adrenergic, dopaminergic, serotonergic, cholinergic, histaminergic, or GABAergic receptors. Sertraline has a weak uricosuric effect.

USES. In controlled trials, sertraline was more effective than placebo (Amin et al, 1989) and was comparable (dose range, 150 to 200 mg) to amitriptyline (dose range, 50 to 150 mg) in the treatment of moderately depressed adult outpatients (Reimherr et al, 1990; Cohn et al, 1990). Its efficacy in severely depressed hospitalized patients has not been adequately studied. Sertraline appears to be most appropriate for patients who are at special risk from the sedative, hypotensive, and anticholinergic side effects produced by other antidepressants. In addition, it appears to be relatively safe for use in the elderly.

In a double-blind trial, sertraline (50 to 200 mg daily) was more effective than placebo on most outcome measures in patients with OCD who were not depressed (Chouinard et al, 1990). Further study is required to determine its role in the treatment of this disorder.

ADVERSE REACTIONS AND PRECAUTIONS. In clinical trials, the most frequent side effects of sertraline were gastrointestinal disturbances (nausea, dyspepsia, diarrhea/loose stools), autonomic nervous system dysfunction (dry mouth, increased sweating), and central nervous system effects (dizziness, tremor, insomnia, somnolence). Sexual dysfunction in males, primarily ejaculatory delay, also may occur. Other side effects that led to discontinuation of sertraline in clinical trials were agitation, headache, anorexia, and fatigue. Like fluoxetine, sertraline may cause modest weight loss during initial therapy.

The use of sertraline in patients with recent myocardial infarction, unstable heart disease, significant hepatic or renal dysfunction, and seizure disorders has not been adequately studied; thus, this agent should be used with caution in such patients.

During premarketing testing, hypomania or mania occurred in approximately 0.4% of patients treated with sertraline.

Sertraline should not be used in combination with an MAO inhibitor or within 14 days after discontinuing treatment with an MAO inhibitor. Similarly, at least 14 days should elapse before initiating therapy with an MAO inhibitor after sertraline has been discontinued.

Sertraline is classified in FDA Pregnancy Category B.

POISONING. Overdosage (750 mg to 2.1 g) has occurred in three patients; no specific therapy was required and all recovered completely.

DRUG INTERACTIONS. Sertraline may cause a slight increase (8%) in the prothrombin time in patients treated with warfarin. The clearance of diazepam, its active metabolite, desmethyldiazepam, and tolbutamide may be decreased. The clinical significance of these observations has not been established. Because of its high degree of protein binding, sertraline may interact with other drugs that also are highly protein bound.

PHARMACOKINETICS. Sertraline appears to be well absorbed. Peak plasma concentrations are dose-related and occur four to eight hours after administration. Based on limited data, food appears to increase both the rate and extent of bioavailability; plasma protein binding is 98%.

Sertraline undergoes first-pass metabolism, primarily via N-demethylation. This metabolite has a long half-life (62 to 104 hours) but is substantially less active than the parent compound. Both sertraline and N-desmethylsertraline undergo further metabolism, eventually forming glucuronide conjugates. Clearance is reduced by approximately 40% in elderly patients.

DOSAGE AND PREPARATIONS.

Oral: *Adults*, initially, 50 mg once daily. In patients with an inadequate response, the dose may be increased up to a maximum of 200 mg. At least one week should elapse between adjustments in dosage.

Zoloft (Roerig). Tablets 50 and 100 mg.

OTHER CYCLIC AGENTS

BUPROPION HYDROCHLORIDE

[Wellbutrin]

$NHC(CH_3)_3$

$COCHCH_3$

Cl

ACTIONS AND USES. Bupropion, a phenylaminoketone structurally related to amphetamine and diethylpropion, has unique actions compared with other antidepressants (Benfield et al, 1986; Weintraub and Evans, 1989). This compound weakly inhibits dopamine reuptake; metabolites of the drug also are active. Bupropion is reported to reduce the total body turnover of norepinephrine and may down-regulate beta-adrenergic receptors after prolonged administration, an effect seen with many tricyclic antidepressants. This drug has no anticholinergic activity, and it does not inhibit either form (A or B) of monoamine oxidase.

The antidepressant action of bupropion has been established in both inpatients and outpatients with major depression and the depressive component of bipolar disorder. Its efficacy is comparable to that of tricyclic antidepressants; the serotonin uptake inhibitor, fluoxetine (Feighner et al, 1991); and MAO inhibitors. Because it has mild stimulant rather than sedative activity, this drug is most beneficial in major depression associated with psychomotor retardation. The lower than expected incidence of cycling in patients with rapid cycling bipolar disorder suggests that bupropion is less likely than the tricyclics to precipitate mania (Gardner, 1983; Haykal and Akiskal, 1990) and therefore may be useful in patients with rapid cycling.

ADVERSE REACTIONS. Bupropion was approved by the FDA in 1985. Just prior to marketing, a high incidence of seizures was observed in patients being treated for bulimia. Marketing was delayed and further studies were initiated to evaluate this adverse reaction. Investigations have since determined that the approximate incidence of generalized seizures is 0.4% (4/1,000) at doses up to 450 mg daily. The incidence increases almost tenfold at doses between 450 and 600 mg daily; therefore, the maximum recommended dose is 450 mg. (See Precautions.)

A substantial proportion of patients experience increased restlessness, agitation, anxiety, and insomnia; these side effects were sufficiently severe in clinical trials to require discontinuation of treatment in about 2% of patients. Other common side effects are dry mouth, headache/migraine, nausea and vomiting, constipation, and tremor. Side effects reported in at least 1/100 patients include stomatitis, nonspecific rashes, nocturia, ataxia/incoordination, myoclonus, dyskinesia, and hallucinations. Neuropsychiatric symptoms (dysphoria, depersonalization, psychosis, paranoia, and bizarre thought disorder) occurred less frequently (1/100 to 1/1,000 patients). Weight loss of about 2.5 kg occurred in approximately 25% of patients; weight gain was less frequent than that observed with tricyclic antidepressants. Bupropion produces no significant orthostatic hypotension or cardiac abnormalities, even in patients with cardiac disease (Wenger and Stern, 1983; Roose et al, 1987), although exacerbation of hypertension has been observed infrequently in these patients (Roose et al, 1991).

DRUG INTERACTIONS. A higher incidence of adverse reactions may occur with concurrent administration of levodopa and possibly other dopaminergic agents. Since bupropion is extensively metabolized, drugs that affect hepatic metabolism could cause adverse interactions. In animal studies, bupropion was a weak inducer of drug metabolizing enzymes.

PRECAUTIONS. Retrospective analysis of clinical experience gained during the development of bupropion suggests that the risk of seizures may be minimized if (1) the total daily dose does not exceed 450 mg, (2) the daily dose is administered three times daily with a maximum single dose of 150 mg to avoid high peak concentrations of bupropion and/or its metabolites, and (3) the rate of incrementation of dose is very gradual. Extreme caution should be used when bupropion is (1) administered to patients with a history of seizures, cranial trauma, or other predisposition(s) toward seizure, or (2) prescribed or used with other agents (eg, antipsychotics, alcohol, other antidepressants) or treatment regimens (eg, abrupt discontinuation of a benzodiazepine, alcohol withdrawal) that lower seizure threshold. Since a higher incidence of seizures occurred in patients with bulimia and anorexia nervosa, bupropion is not recommended for use in such patients until further clinical data are available.

At least 14 days should elapse between discontinuation of an MAO inhibitor and initiation of treatment with bupropion.

Bupropion should be used during pregnancy only if it is clearly needed (FDA Pregnancy Category B).

PHARMACOKINETICS. Bupropion is rapidly absorbed after oral administration; peak concentrations are attained in the plasma within two hours. It is widely distributed to body tissues and is highly (80% to 85%) protein bound. The elimination half-life is biphasic, with a beta phase of approximately 14 (range, 8 to 24) hours. Bupropion undergoes extensive first-pass metabolism in the liver. Six metabolites have been identified, two of which have antidepressant activity. Their potency is less than half that of the parent compound; however, the steady-state plasma concentrations of these metabolites (ie, the morpholinol and *threo*-amino alcohol derivatives) are 10 to 100 times that of the parent drug. High plasma concentrations of these metabolites may be associated with ineffectiveness and toxicity (Rudorfer and Potter, 1989). Most of the dose of bupropion is excreted in the urine as inactive metabolites. The effects of liver or kidney disorders on bupropion kinetics are not currently known, but it is possible that such diseases might prolong the half-life of the drug and its metabolites.

DOSAGE AND PREPARATIONS.

Oral: *Adults,* the initial dosage is 100 mg twice daily. Based on clinical response, this amount may be increased to 300 mg/day, *given in three divided doses,* no sooner than three days after beginning therapy. As with other antidepressants, the full antidepressant effect may not be evident until four or more weeks of treatment. An increase in dosage to a maximum of 450 mg/day, *given in divided doses of no more than 150 mg* each, may be considered for patients in whom no clinical improvement is noted after several weeks of treatment at 300 mg/day. Dosage above 300 mg/day may be accomplished using the 75- or 100-mg tablets. *The 100-mg tablet must be administered four times daily with at least four hours between successive doses in order not to exceed the limit of 150 mg in a single dose.* Bupropion should be discontinued in patients who do not demonstrate an adequate response after an appropriate period of treatment at 450 mg/day. The lowest dose that maintains remission is recommended.

Wellbutrin (Burroughs Wellcome). Tablets 75 and 100 mg.

TRAZODONE HYDROCHLORIDE

[Desyrel]

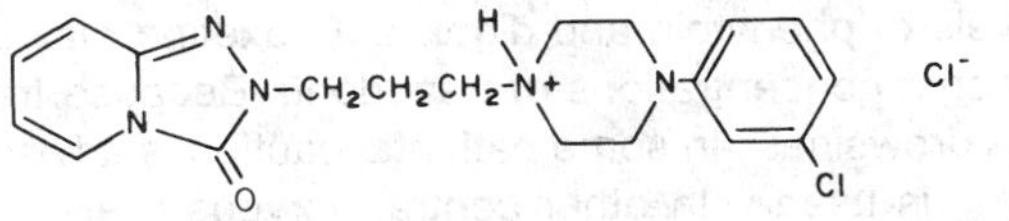

ACTIONS. Trazodone is a phenylpiperazine propyl derivative of triazolopyridine and is chemically unrelated to tricyclic or tetracyclic antidepressants. It has no monoamine oxidase inhibiting or amphetamine-like properties and little, if any, anticholinergic activity. Its alpha-adrenergic blocking activity may account for the adverse reactions of dryness of the mouth and hypotension. In therapeutic doses, trazodone inhibits the neuronal uptake of serotonin in man. Trazodone and its metabolite, *m*-chlorophenylpiperazine, are serotonin agonists as well. Experimentally, prolonged administration decreases the number of serotonin receptors; the uptake of norepinephrine and dopamine is essentially unaffected. After long-term administration, the number of presynaptic alpha$_2$-adrenergic receptors may be decreased.

USES. Controlled studies have demonstrated that trazodone is as effective as amitriptyline and imipramine in patients with major depressive disorders and other subsets of depressive disorders (Feighner and Boyer, 1988; Cazzullo and Silvestrini, 1989). Because of its sedative effect, trazodone is generally more useful in depressive disorders associated with insomnia and anxiety. This drug does not aggravate psychotic symptoms in patients with schizophrenia or schizoaffective disorders.

ADVERSE REACTIONS AND PRECAUTIONS. Trazodone is well tolerated. Drowsiness is the most common side effect (incidence, 15% to 20%). Nausea and vomiting occur less frequently and are mild. Dizziness and lightheadedness also may be noted. Dryness of the mouth, constipation, and urinary retention are infrequent. Like the tricyclic drugs, trazodone can cause orthostatic hypotension. However, this effect generally lasts only four to six hours and can be lessened by administering each dose with food. Agitation is noted in less than 1% of patients. The risk of seizures is no greater than with any of the tricyclics. Extrapyramidal reactions and hepatotoxicity are rare.

Priapism has been associated with trazodone therapy (incidence 1:6,000) and, if surgery is required, may lead to permanent impotence. Male patients should be alerted to the warning signs. Sometimes progressively prolonged erections occur before the episode of priapism. Injection of a dilute solution of epinephrine 1:100,000 directly into the corpus cavernosa has been effective and minimizes permanent sequelae (Molina et al, 1989).

The neurotoxicity and respiratory depression commonly encountered after an overdose of tricyclic antidepressants are less severe with trazodone. Overdosage is relatively safe compared with the tricyclics; however, cardiac toxicity is an increasing concern as more experience has accumulated (Blackwell and Simon, 1988).

DRUG INTERACTIONS. Trazodone antagonizes the hypotensive effects of clonidine and methyldopa and increases plasma levels of phenytoin and digoxin. Fluoxetine may increase the plasma concentrations of trazodone. Because trazodone causes drowsiness in some patients, caution is advised when this drug is used with other central nervous system depressants, including alcohol.

PREGNANCY AND LACTATION. Trazodone is classified in FDA Pregnancy Category C because it is associated with increased fetal resorption in rats and congenital anomalies in rabbits. Small amounts of trazodone and its metabolites have been found in the milk of lactating rats, suggesting that the drug may be secreted in human milk; therefore, caution is advised when prescribing this drug during pregnancy and for nursing mothers.

PHARMACOKINETICS. When given orally, trazodone is absorbed rapidly, bioavailability is essentially complete, and the mean time to peak absorption is about 1.5 (range, 0.5 to 2) hours in fasting and 2.5 hours in nonfasting patients. However, the manufacturer recommends that the drug be taken after a light meal or snack to improve total absorption and diminish the incidence of dizziness and lightheadedness. The volume of distribution is approximately 1 L/kg; protein binding is 96% (at 1 ng/ml).

Trazodone is extensively metabolized by hepatic microsomal enzymes, but enzyme induction has not been observed. Major metabolites include *m*-chlorophenylpiperazine (active) and oxotriazolopyridin propionic acid. Two-thirds of the drug and its metabolites are excreted in the urine and one-third appears in the feces. The mean plasma elimination half-life of parent drug is six hours. Based on the limited data available at this time, it is not clear whether there is a direct relationship between trazodone plasma levels and its therapeutic effects.

DOSAGE AND PREPARATIONS.

Oral: *Adults (hospitalized),* initially, 150 mg daily in divided doses, increased by 50 mg daily every three to four days. Those who are severely depressed may require 400 to 600 mg daily.

Adults (outpatients), initially, the manufacturers recommend 150 mg daily in divided doses; however, this amount may not be tolerated by some patients and lower doses may be required. A single daily dose or a major portion of the daily dose may be given at bedtime if insomnia is prominent or undue sedation occurs during the day. If little benefit is noted by the third week, the dose may be increased (eg, by 50 mg daily every three to four days) until clinical improvement, intolerable side effects, or the maximum recommended daily dose is reached (ie, 400 mg). For maintenance, the lowest dose that will maintain remission is recommended. *Elderly patients and adolescents,* initially, 25 to 50 mg daily, increased to 100 to 150 mg daily in divided doses, depending on the response and tolerance.

Desyrel (Mead Johnson), ***Generic.*** Tablets 50, 100, 150, and (***Desyrel*** only) 300 mg.

MONOAMINE OXIDASE (MAO) INHIBITORS

PHENELZINE SULFATE

[Nardil]

$$C_6H_5\text{-}CH_2CH_2\overset{+}{N}H_2NH_2 \quad HSO_4^-$$

USES. Phenelzine is effective in the treatment of major depression, dysthymic disorder, and atypical depression. Some patients refractory to the tricyclic drugs respond to phenelzine, especially those with atypical depression or severe anxiety.

Phenelzine has improved eating behavior in some patients with bulimia; however, its definitive role in this disorder awaits the results of controlled clinical trials. Phenelzine also is effective in panic and phobic disorders.

For other uses of this drug, see index entry Phenelzine.

PRECAUTIONS. Because all MAO inhibitors have the potential to produce serious adverse reactions, patients should be supervised closely. Dietary restrictions and precautions regarding concomitant medication should be adhered to, and vasoactive drugs should be avoided or administered in reduced dosage.

Although several fatal cases of poisoning have occurred after ingestion of 375 mg to 1.5 g, recovery was reported after ingestion of doses within this range.

See the Introduction for a discussion on adverse reactions, precautions, and the use of MAO inhibitors with other drugs.

PHARMACOKINETICS. There is evidence that acetylation is not a major metabolic pathway for phenelzine, and no relationship has been demonstrated between acetylator phenotype and therapeutic or adverse effects.

DOSAGE AND PREPARATIONS. The dose must be individualized to achieve adequate therapeutic results with minimal adverse effects.

Oral: *Adults (outpatients),* initially, 45 to 75 mg daily in two or three divided doses; alternatively, 1 mg/kg daily. The dose can be increased to 90 mg if there is no response after 21 days. Most patients require at least 60 mg to inhibit monoamine oxidase by about 80%, but the dose should be decreased if untoward effects develop. It often is useful to maintain patients on a therapeutic dose for at least six months after improvement is noted. If long-term maintenance therapy is indicated for recurrent illness, the total daily dose should be reduced to the lowest effective amount, usually 45 to 60 mg daily. Information is inadequate to establish a dosage for *children under 16 years.*

Nardil (Parke-Davis). Tablets 15 mg.

ISOCARBOXAZID
[Marplan]

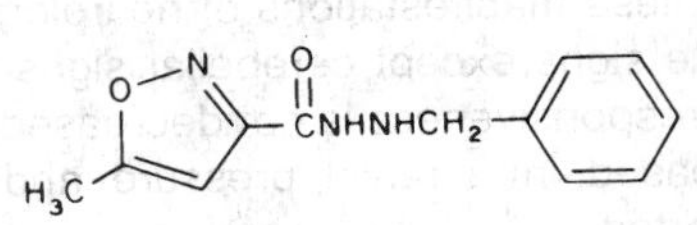

Isocarboxazid is effective in the treatment of major depression, dysthymic disorder, and atypical depression. It also is useful in the treatment of panic disorder and the phobic disorders.

Because all MAO inhibitors can produce serious adverse reactions, patients should be supervised closely. Recovery has been reported after ingestion of 300 to 500 mg of isocarboxazid.

See the Introduction for additional information on indications, adverse reactions, precautions, and the use of MAO inhibitors with other drugs.

DOSAGE AND PREPARATIONS.
Oral: *Adults (outpatients),* initially, 20 to 30 mg daily in divided doses. The dosage should be reduced as soon as clinical improvement is observed; 10 to 20 mg daily or less is the usual amount given for maintenance. However, the actual maintenance dose has not been established in controlled trials, and a larger dose may be necessary. Information is inadequate to establish dosage for *children under 16 years.*

Marplan (Roche). Tablets 10 mg.

TRANYLCYPROMINE SULFATE
[Parnate]

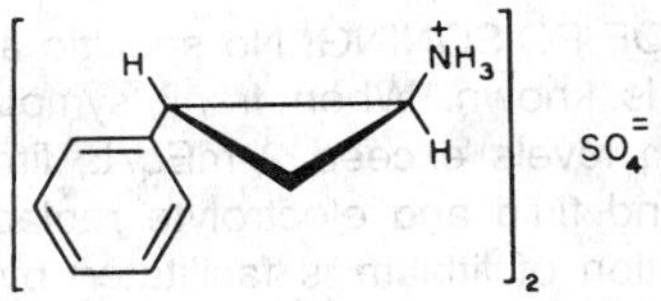

Tranylcypromine differs structurally from the hydrazines, phenelzine and isocarboxazid, in that it is formed from cyclization of the side chain of amphetamine. This MAO inhibitor is effective in the treatment of major depression, dysthymic disorder, and atypical depression. It also is useful in panic and phobic disorders.

Adverse reactions are generally comparable to those of other MAO inhibitors; tranylcypromine is least likely to cause weight gain. Because of its amphetamine-like structure, this drug may cause psychomotor stimulation, (usually at doses larger than those used for depression), although fatigue and somnolence also have been reported (Joffe, 1990). The incidence of intracranial hemorrhage (sometimes fatal) associated with paradoxical hypertension and severe occipital headache appears to be greater than with phenelzine or isocarboxazid. Dependence has been reported occasionally; therefore, tranylcypromine should be used with care in patients prone to drug abuse.

A small number of deaths have resulted from ingestion of more than 350 mg; however, recovery also has occurred after ingestion of this amount.

See the Introduction for additional information on indications, adverse reactions, precautions, and the use of MAO inhibitors with other drugs.

DOSAGE AND PREPARATIONS.
Oral: *Adults (outpatients),* initially, 20 to 30 mg daily in two equally divided doses in the morning and afternoon for two weeks. Subsequent doses should be adjusted according to the patient's response; the lowest effective dose should be given in divided amounts. Doses exceeding 30 mg daily are rarely necessary, although 60 to 90 mg has been used in hospitalized patients with severe depression. Information is inadequate to establish a dosage for *children under 16 years.*

Parnate (Nova/SmithKline Beecham). Tablets 10 mg.

ANTIMANIC DRUG

LITHIUM CARBONATE
[Eskalith, Eskalith CR, Lithane, Lithobid, Lithonate, Lithotabs]

LITHIUM CITRATE
[Cibalith-S]

ACTIONS AND USES. Although its antimanic mechanism of action has not been fully determined, lithium is known to affect a variety of neurohumoral signal transduction mechanisms. It may influence neurotransmitter systems by interfering with guanine nucleotide binding (G) protein function (Risby et al, 1991). Lithium counteracts mood changes and is considered the most specific antimanic drug for the prophylaxis and treatment of bipolar disorder. Acute hypomanic and manic episodes respond to this drug, but combined therapy with an antipsychotic agent or high potency benzodiazepines may be preferred to control behavior initially. Lithium also has been used to augment the action of tricyclic antidepressants (in depression) and antipsychotics (in schizophrenia and schizoaffective disorder) in patients who responded inadequately to these agents. Lithium may be effective for maintenance therapy in those with major depression, but other antidepressants are preferred. For other uses, see index entry Lithium.

Lithium has little effect on otherwise healthy patients except for mild sedation, and it has no antiadrenergic or anticholinergic actions.

ADVERSE REACTIONS. Patients receiving lithium require close clinical observation, careful dosage adjustment, and frequent monitoring of blood levels to avoid toxic effects. To prevent toxicity, the dosage should be maintained within a critical and narrow range, for adverse reactions may occur at doses that are close to therapeutic levels. Patients can tolerate larger doses of lithium during acute manic episodes. However, as the attack subsides, the dose should be reduced rapidly to prevent accumulation. *Serum lithium levels should not exceed 2 mEq/L (preferably 0.75 to 1.5 for most pa-*

tients) during initial treatment and should be kept within a range of 0.4 to 1 mEq/L during maintenance.

The following clinical manifestations are useful guidelines for evaluating most patients, and serum lithium levels alone should not be substituted for clinical observation:

Transient mild to moderate side effects occur in most patients at serum levels of 1.5 to 2 mEq/L but may be observed at lower levels, depending on the patient's tolerance. The most common reactions include nausea, diarrhea, malaise, and fine hand tremor. Other common untoward effects are thirst, polyuria, polydipsia, weight gain, and fatigue, which may persist throughout treatment but are reversible when the drug is discontinued. Hand tremor occasionally can be modified by the elimination of caffeine or treated with propranolol if it is necessary to maintain the dosage for antimanic effectiveness.

Drowsiness, vomiting, muscle weakness, ataxia, dryness of the mouth, abdominal pain, lethargy, dizziness, slurred speech, and nystagmus are early symptoms of intoxication. These reactions may occur at concentrations above 1.5 mEq/L and are common at concentrations of 2 mEq/L.

Moderate to severe adverse reactions may occur at serum concentrations above 2 mEq/L. At levels of 2 to 2.5 mEq/L, symptoms include anorexia, persistent nausea and vomiting, blurred vision, fasciculations, clonic movements of whole limbs, hyperactive deep tendon reflexes, choreoathetoid movements, epileptiform convulsions, toxic psychosis, syncope, electroencephalographic changes, acute circulatory failure, stupor, and coma. At serum levels above 2.5 mEq/L, symptoms may progress rapidly to generalized convulsions, oliguria, and death.

When the serum lithium level exceeds 1.5 mEq/L or adverse reactions become bothersome regardless of the serum level, the drug generally should be discontinued for 24 hours and therapy then resumed at a lower dose. The patient and those living in the household should be cautioned to notify the physician immediately if untoward symptoms or unexplained illnesses occur.

Prolonged administration of lithium has resulted in impaired renal function. However, the risk of impairment may be reduced when patients take single rather than multiple daily doses (Mellerup er al, 1987). Of greatest clinical significance is a reduction in urine concentrating ability that may present as nephrogenic diabetes insipidus. The impairment usually is reversed when lithium is withdrawn; it cannot be corrected by vasopressin. Salt restriction or diuretic therapy should not be instituted, since these measures only enhance lithium toxicity (Waller and George, 1984).

Diffuse thyroid enlargement with no change in thyroid function or, occasionally, hypothyroidism also may occur after long-term treatment. Hyperthyroidism also has been reported. The administration of thyroid hormones controls the glandular enlargement, and thyroid function generally returns to normal when lithium is withdrawn. Thyroid function tests should be performed periodically in all patients receiving long-term therapy.

Mild cognitive and memory impairment and, rarely, persistent neurologic deficits may be associated with the use of lithium. Manifestations include an akinetic hypertonic state with cogwheel rigidity, tremor, dysarthria, mask-like facies, and mutism. These manifestations of neurologic damage are similar to acute signs except cerebellar signs are more conspicuous and responsiveness is not decreased. Pseudotumor cerebri (increased intracranial pressure and papilledema) has been reported.

A wide range of cutaneous adverse effects has been associated with lithium therapy (Deandrea et al, 1982). Maculopapular, follicular, and acneiform eruptions occur. The first two may clear despite continued lithium therapy, but the acneiform reaction may necessitate decreasing the dose or discontinuing therapy. Lithium also may induce or exacerbate psoriasis and, more rarely, may be associated with exfoliative dermatitis.

Mild leukocytosis (white blood count, 10,000 to 18,000) occurs frequently throughout therapy, but it is reversible when lithium is discontinued. Reversible electrocardiographic alterations (flattening and inversion of T waves, occasional bradycardia, disturbance in sinus node function, or sinoatrial block and widening of the QRS complex) that do not respond to potassium therapy also have been noted (Mitchell and MacKenzie, 1982). Transient hyperglycemia, headache, peripheral edema, weight gain, hair loss, metallic taste, and hypertension have been reported infrequently.

An acute brain syndrome occurs infrequently and is characterized by a toxic confusional state, convulsions, and changes in the electroencephalogram, but signs of lithium toxicity and toxic serum levels are not present. This reaction is observed most commonly within three weeks after initiating therapy and responds rapidly to discontinuation of the drug or reduction of the dose. Patients with schizophrenia and organic brain disease may be hypersensitive to this action of lithium.

TREATMENT OF POISONING. No specific antidote for lithium poisoning is known. When frank symptoms of toxicity occur or serum levels exceed 2 mEq/L, lithium should be discontinued and fluid and electrolyte replacement therapy initiated. Excretion of lithium is facilitated by alkalization of urine and administration of osmotic diuretics (urea, mannitol), acetazolamide, and theophylline. Electrocardiograms and measurements of serum hematocrit should be performed periodically. Antiepileptic drugs may be necessary if seizures occur.

The most important object of management of overdose is removal of lithium from the body as rapidly as possible. Hemodialysis is most effective for this purpose (Amdisen, 1988). If the overdose occurred very recently, gastric lavage can be performed but is not adequate alone. Hemodialysis should be used routinely when lithium levels exceed 2.5 mEq/L or when renal function is impaired.

PRECAUTIONS. If the clinical situation indicates, a complete physical examination and selected laboratory studies are useful before initiating therapy; this should include tests for cardiovascular, hepatic, thyroid, and renal function; total and differential white blood counts; hemoglobin levels; and complete urinalysis.

Recommendations for the frequency of monitoring serum lithium concentrations have varied. All blood samples should be drawn 8 to 12 hours after the last dose to produce comparable results. During the acute manic phase, lithium levels probably should be determined twice weekly until the target concentration is established and once weekly after any dosage changes. During long-term therapy, lithium levels should be determined every three months and whenever the risk of toxicity is increased (eg, illness producing fever, vomiting, diarrhea; prolonged unconsciousness; excessive weight loss; low salt intake; dehydration; treatment with diuretics or NSAIDs).

Long-term use of lithium should be restricted to responsive patients, but the risk of renal dysfunction attributable to chronic therapy is lower than formerly believed. According to the results of one longitudinal study, renal tubular function remained stable in patients treated continuously for up to 20 years. Dysfunction is related more to age, intoxication episodes, pre-existing renal disease, and treatment schedule than to duration of prophylactic therapy (Hetmar et al, 1991). Once-daily dosing may cause less polyuria (Bowen et al, 1991). The possibility of renal dysfunction can be minimized by (1) judicious monitoring of lithium serum levels to avoid acute intoxication and establish the lowest effective maintenance dose, (2) adequate fluid intake (at least 2 L daily) distributed evenly throughout the day, and (3) establishment of baseline renal function, followed by periodic testing as indicated by the clinical situation.

Since lithium is excreted mainly by the kidneys, its elimination depends on normal renal function and adequate salt and fluid intake. Lithium usually is relatively contraindicated in patients with renal or cardiac disease (eg, sick sinus syndrome), when interference with excretion is likely (eg, in those with decreased renal blood flow), or when electrolyte imbalance is present. In the presence of sodium deficiency, lithium ion is selectively reabsorbed in the renal tubules and may accumulate to toxic levels because of dehydration and sodium and potassium depletion. Therefore, lithium should be used cautiously in patients receiving diuretics or in those on a "crash" or low-salt diet. If lithium must be used with diuretics, the serum lithium and electrolyte levels should be monitored closely and the dosage of lithium reduced as indicated. Loop diuretics may be preferable to other diuretics. If excessive and prolonged diarrhea, profuse perspiration, or vomiting occurs, lithium should be discontinued and supplemental salt and fluid administered. The drug should not be given to debilitated or dehydrated individuals or to those with severe infections.

Special precautions are necessary when lithium is used in the elderly, since the rate of renal excretion tends to decline with age. Use of small doses with very gradual increases and frequent determination of serum lithium levels generally are necessary.

Although lithium is not contraindicated in diabetic patients, it has increased serum insulin levels. Blood sugar and electrolyte levels should be monitored periodically.

PREGNANCY AND LACTATION. An increase in the rate of congenital abnormalities, especially heart defects, has been reported in infants exposed to lithium during early pregnancy. Therefore, its use is relatively contraindicated during the first trimester. Carbamazepine is an alternative, since data on 94 infants exposed in utero indicate an absence of major malformations. However, minor craniofacial defects, fingernail hypoplasia, and developmental delay have been linked to prenatal exposure to carbamazepine (Perry et al, 1988; Jones et al, 1989). There is more experience with chlorpromazine during pregnancy, and its use can be considered; additional alternatives include clonazepam and ECT (Sitland-Marken, 1989).

If lithium is considered for use after the third month of pregnancy to avoid postpartum psychosis, the risk to the fetus or infant should be weighed against the expected benefits (FDA Pregnancy Category D). Lithium crosses the placenta and is present in equivalent concentrations in the mother and fetus. Since the half-life of lithium is prolonged in newborn infants, it may be advisable to discontinue this agent two to three days before the expected delivery date in order to lower concentrations of the drug in the newborn and to prevent lithium accumulation in the mother caused by derangement of fluid and water balance during delivery (Schou, 1990). Water deprivation, infusion of hypertonic sodium chloride, or injection of pituitary hormones should be avoided during delivery. Additionally, the concentration of lithium in breast milk is one-third to one-half that in maternal plasma; therefore, mothers taking lithium probably should not breast-feed their infants.

DRUG INTERACTIONS. The combined use of lithium and iodine should be avoided, for synergistic antithyroid effects have been reported; patients receiving lithium should be warned to avoid medications that contain iodides (eg, cough medicines, multivitamin preparations).

Nonsteroidal anti-inflammatory drugs increase plasma lithium concentrations (possible exception, sulindac [Clinoril]) and therefore may cause toxicity when they are used with lithium. Thiazide diuretics and indapamide also increase serum lithium concentrations, usually after several days of use, especially if there is dehydration, hyponatremia, or pre-existing renal disease; loop diuretics appear less likely to interact with lithium. Concomitant use of lithium with carbamazepine may depress thyroid function. Lithium reverses the normal depressant effect of carbamazepine on the white blood cell count. Case reports suggest that ACE inhibitors may increase lithium plasma concentrations.

PHARMACOKINETICS. Lithium is completely absorbed six to eight hours after oral administration. Since the onset of action is slow (five to ten days), parenteral administration is of no advantage. The plasma half-life is 17 to 36 hours, and this drug is eliminated almost entirely by the kidneys. Lithium clearance averages approximately 20% of creatinine clearance, but significant variability exists among patients.

Lithium ion is not protein bound, is distributed in total body water, and is concentrated in various tissues to different degrees. After a steady state has been achieved, the lithium level in cerebrospinal fluid is about 40% of that in serum, and renal clearance for an individual remains relatively constant.

In general, a good correlation exists between the serum concentration of lithium ion and therapeutic efficacy and toxicity. However, some patients who show no therapeutic benefit have adequate serum concentrations of lithium but low erythrocyte concentrations. Since lithium works intracellularly, the erythrocyte concentration of the drug may be more relevant than levels in serum. Therefore, in unresponsive patients, doses that produce higher than usual serum concentrations can be used if erythrocyte concentrations are lower.

DOSAGE AND PREPARATIONS. Dosage should be individualized on the basis of serum levels and response, and the drug should be discontinued if a satisfactory response is not obtained in three to six weeks.

Oral: *Adults,* for acute mania, initially, 0.6 to 1.8 g daily in three divided doses, increased or decreased daily or every other day by 0.3 g (maximum, 2.4 g daily) to produce a serum level of 0.75 to 1.5 mEq/L. During acute manic episodes, some patients show increased tolerance to ordinarily toxic blood levels. When the acute attack subsides, the dose should be reduced rapidly to obtain a serum level of 0.4 to 1 mEq/L. In one study, maintenance concentrations of 0.8 to 1 mEq/L were more effective in reducing the number of relapses than concentrations of 0.4 to 0.6 mEq/L (Gelenberg et al, 1989). For many patients, concentrations of 0.6 to 0.8 mEq/L may provide prophylactic protection with a minimum of side effects. Lithium should be used cautiously in *debilitated or elderly patients,* who may require or tolerate lower doses (eg, serum concentrations of 0.4 mEq/L). *Children under 12,* information is inadequate to establish safety and efficacy in this age group.

LITHIUM CARBONATE:

Generic. Capsules 150, 300, and 600 mg; tablets 300 mg.

Eskalith (Nova/SmithKline Beecham). Capsules, tablets 300 mg; tablets (prolonged-release) 450 mg (***Eskalith CR***).

Lithane (Miles), ***Lithotabs*** (Solvay). Tablets 300 mg.

Lithobid (CIBA). Tablets (prolonged-release) 300 mg.

Lithonate (Solvay). Capsules 300 mg.

LITHIUM CITRATE:

Cibalith-S (CIBA), ***Generic***. Syrup 300 mg (8 mEq)/5 ml (equivalent to lithium carbonate).

MIXTURES

MIXTURES CONTAINING AN ANTIDEPRESSANT AND ANTIPSYCHOTIC DRUG

Combination products containing amitriptyline and perphenazine are available purportedly for use in patients with schizoaffective disorders. Some of these patients require only an antipsychotic drug, although amitriptyline occasionally is useful adjunctively to control symptoms of depression. However, the amounts supplied in fixed-ratio combinations usually are not suitable for most patients. Tardive dyskinesia has been reported with the antipsychotics, and their use should be restricted to patients with clear-cut indications for these drugs.

DOSAGE AND PREPARATIONS. See the manufacturers' labeling for dosage.

Etrafon (Schering), ***Triavil*** (Merck Sharp & Dohme), ***Generic.*** Tablets containing perphenazine 2 mg and amitriptyline hydrochloride 10 mg (***Etrafon 2-10, Triavil 2-10***) or 25 mg (***Etrafon 2-25, Triavil 2-25***); tablets containing perphenazine 4 mg and amitriptyline hydrochloride 10 mg (***Etrafon-A, Triavil 4-10***), 25 mg (***Etrafon-Forte, Triavil 4-25***), or 50 mg (***Triavil 4-50***).

MIXTURE CONTAINING AN ANTIDEPRESSANT AND ANTIANXIETY DRUG

The combination product, Limbitrol, contains amitriptyline and chlordiazepoxide and is promoted for patients with moderate to severe depression associated with moderate to severe anxiety. Since most anxiety accompanying depression is ultimately relieved during the course of treatment with an antidepressant alone, antianxiety drugs are not required routinely. Thus, combined use for initial therapy is not recommended. Further, antidepressant drugs require individual titration of dose to obtain optimum response, and this is less easily accomplished with a fixed-dose combination. Safe use of Limbitrol during pregnancy and lactation has not been established.

See the section on Tricyclic Antidepressants in this chapter and index entry Chlordiazepoxide, Uses, for additional information on adverse reactions and precautions.

DOSAGE AND PREPARATIONS. See the manufacturer's labeling for dosage.

Limbitrol (Roche), ***Generic.*** Tablets containing amitriptyline hydrochloride 12.5 or 25 mg and chlordiazepoxide 5 or 10 mg (***Limbitrol, Limbitrol DS).***

Cited References

Drugs that cause psychiatric symptoms. *Med Lett Drugs Ther* 31:113-118, (Dec) 1989.

Amdisen A: Clinical features and management of lithium poisoning. *Med Toxicol* 3:18-32, 1988.

American Psychiatric Association: *Diagnostic and Statistical Manual of Mental Disorders,* ed 3 (revised) *(DSM-III-R)*. Washington, DC, American Psychiatric Association, 1987.

Amin M, et al: A double-blind, placebo controlled dose finding study with sertraline. *Psychopharmacol Bull* 25:164-167, 1989.

Baldessarini RJ: Current status of antidepressants: Clinical pharmacology and therapy. *J Clin Psychiatry* 50:117-126, 1989.

Banahan BF Jr, Schelkun PH: Tricyclic antidepressant overdose: Conservative management in a community hospital with cost-saving implications. *J Emerg Med* 8:451-454, 1990.

Barrett JE, et al: The prevalence of psychiatric disorders in a primary care practice. *Arch Gen Psychiatry* 45:1100-1106, 1988.

Beasley CM Jr, et al: Fluoxetine in tricyclic refractory major depressive disorder. *J Affective Disord* 20:193-200, 1990

Beasley CM Jr, et al: High-dose fluoxetine: Efficacy and activating-sedating effects in agitated and retarded depression. *J Clin Psychopharmacol* 11:166-174, 1991.

Benfield P, et al: Fluoxetine: Review of its pharmacodynamic and pharmacokinetic properties, and therapeutic efficacy in depressive illness. *Drugs* 32:481-508, 1986.

Berger PA, Nemeroff CB: Opioid peptides in affective disorders, in Meltzer HY (ed): *Psychopharmacology: The Third Generation of Progress.* New York, Raven Press, 1987, 637-646.

Blackwell B, Simon JS: Antidepressant drugs, in Dukes MNG (ed): *Myeler's Side Effects of Drugs,* ed 11. New York, Elsevier, 1988, 27-70.

Bowen RC, et al: Less frequent lithium administration and lower urine volume. *Am J Psychiatry* 148:189-192, 1991.

Broadhead WE, et al: Depression, disability days, and days lost from work in a prospective epidemiologic survey. *JAMA* 264:2524-2528, 1990.

Brotman AW, et al: Pharmacologic treatment of acute depressive subtypes, in Meltzer HY (ed): *Psychopharmacology: The Third Generation of Progress.* New York, Raven Press, 1987, 1031-1040.

Brown CS, Bryant SG: Monoamine oxidase inhibitors: Safety and efficacy issues. *Drug Intell Clin Pharm* 22:232-235, 1988.

Calabrese JR, Delucchi GA: Spectrum of efficacy of valproate in 55 patients with rapid-cycling bipolar disorder. *Am J Psychiatry* 147:431-434, 1990.

Callaham M, Kassel D: Epidemiology of fatal tricyclic antidepressant ingestion: Implications for management. *Ann Emerg Med* 14:1-9, 1985.

Cazzullo C, Silvestrini B (eds): Trazodone: Antidepressant with adrenolytic activity, symposium. *Clin Pharmacol* 12 (suppl 1): S1-S59, 1989.

Chou JC-Y: Recent advances in treatment of acute mania. *J Clin Psychopharmacol* 11:3-21, 1991.

Chouinard G, et al: Results of a double-blind, placebo-controlled trial of a new serotonin uptake inhibitor, sertraline, in the treatment of obsessive compulsive disorder. *Psychopharmacol Bull* 26:279-284, 1990.

Christenson BC: Agranulocytosis associated with amoxapine. *Am J Psychiatry* 140:921-922, 1983.

Cohn CK, et al: Double-blind, multicenter comparison of sertraline and amitriptyline in elderly depressed patients. *J Clin Psychiatry* 51 (12, suppl B): 28-33, 1990.

Cook BL, Winokur G: Perspectives on bipolar illness. *Compr Ther* 16:18-23, (Dec) 1990.

Deandrea D, et al: Dermatological reactions to lithium: Critical review of literature. *J Clin Psychopharmacol* 2:199-204, 1982.

Delgado PL, et al: Serotonin function and the mechanism of antidepressant action. *Arch Gen Psychiatry* 47:411-418, 1990.

Devlin MJ, Walsh BT: Use of monoamine oxidase inhibitors in refractory depression, in Tasman A, et al (eds): *American Psychiatric Press Review of Psychiatry*. Washington, DC, American Psychiatric Press, 1990, vol 9, 74-90.

Elkin I, et al: National Institute of Mental Health Treatment of Depression Collaborative Research Program: General effectiveness of treatments. *Arch Gen Psychiatry* 46:971-982, 1989.

Ellison JM, et al; Fluoxetine-induced bradycardia and syncope in two patients. *J Clin Psychiatry* 51:385-386, 1990.

Fabre LF, Putman HP III: A fixed-dose clinical trial of fluoxetine in outpatients with major depression. *J Clin Psychiatry* 48:406-408, 1987.

Fava M, Rosenbaum JF: Suicidality and fluoxetine: Is there a relationship? *J Clin Psychiatry* 52:108-111, 1991.

Fawcett J, et al: CNS stimulant potentiation of monoamine oxidase inhibitors in treatment-refractory depression. *J Clin Psychopharmacol* 11:127-132, 1991.

Feighner JP, Boyer WF: Overview of USA controlled trials of trazodone in clinical depression. *Psychopharmacology* 95:S50-S53, 1988.

Feighner JP, et al: A placebo-controlled inpatient comparison of fluvoxamine maleate and imipramine in major depression. *Int Clin Psychopharmacol* 4:239-244, 1989.

Feighner JP, et al: Double-blind comparison of bupropion and fluoxetine in depressed outpatients. *J Clin Psychiatry* 52:329-335, 1991.

Finlayson R: Recognition and management of dysthymic disorder. *Am Fam Physician* 40:229-238, (Oct) 1989.

Frank E, et al: Three-year outcomes for maintenance therapies in recurrent depression. *Arch Gen Psychiatry* 47:1093-1099, 1990.

Frank E, et al: Efficacy of interpersonal psychotherapy as a maintenance treatment of recurrent depression: Contributing factors. *Arch Gen Psychiatry* 48:1053-1059, 1991.

Freeman TW, et al: A double-blind comparison of valproate and lithium in the treatment of acute mania. *Am J Psychiatry* 149:108-111, 1992.

Frommer DA, et al: Tricyclic antidepressant overdose: A review. *JAMA* 257:521-526, 1987.

Garattini S, Samanin R: Biochemical hypotheses on antidepressant drugs: Guide for clinicians or toy for pharmacologists? *Psychol Med* 18:287-304, 1988.

Gardner EA: Long-term preventive care in depression: Use of bupropion in patients intolerant of other antidepressants. *J Clin Psychiatry* 44 (sec 2): 157-162, 1983.

Garza-Treviño ES, et al: Verapamil versus lithium in acute mania. *Am J Psychiatry* 149:121-122, 1992.

Gelenberg AJ, et al: Comparison of standard and low serum levels of lithium for maintenance treatment of bipolar disorder. *N Engl J Med* 321:1489-1493, 1989.

Gold PW, et al: Clinical and biochemical manifestations of depression: Relation to the neurobiology of stress. *N Engl J Med* 319:348-353; 413-420, 1988.

Groleau G, et al: The electrocardiographic manifestations of cyclic antidepressant therapy and overdose: A review. *J Emerg Med* 8:597-605, 1990.

Haykal RF, Akiskal HS: Bupropion as a promising approach to rapid cycling bipolar II patients. *J Clin Psychiatry* 51:450-455, 1990.

Hetmar O, et al: Lithium: Long-term effects on the kidney: A prospective follow-up study ten years after kidney biopsy. *Br J Psychiatry* 158:53-58, 1991.

Himmelhoch JM, et al: Tranylcypromine versus imipramine in anergic bipolar depression. *Am J Psychiatry* 148:910-916, 1991.

Hoschl C, Kozeny J: Verapamil in affective disorders: A controlled double-blind study. *Biol Psychiatry* 25:128-140, 1989.

Howland RH: Pharmacotherapy of dysthymia: A review. *J Clin Psychopharmacol* 11:83-92, 1991.

Hunt-Fugate AK, et al: Adverse reactions due to dopamine blockade by amoxapine: Case report and review of literature. *Pharmacotherapy* 4:35-39, 1984.

Janowsky DS, Risch SC: Role of acetylcholine mechanisms in the affective disorders, in Meltzer HY (ed): *Psychopharmacology: The Third Generation of Progress*. New York, Raven Press, 1987, 527-533.

Jenike MA, et al: Sertraline in obsessive compulsive disorder: A double-blind comparison with placebo. *Am J Psychiatry* 147:923-928, 1990.

Jimerson DC: Role of dopamine mechanisms in the affective disorders, in Meltzer HY (ed): *Psychopharmacology: The Third Generation of Progress*. New York, Raven Press, 1987, 505-511.

Joffe RT: Afternoon fatigue and somnolence associated with tranylcypromine treatment. *J Clin Psychiatry* 51:92-93, 1990.

Johnson GF: Lithium in depression: Review of the antidepressant and prophylactic effects of lithium. *Aust NZ J Psychiatry* 21:356-365, 1987.

Johnstone EC, et al: Combination tricyclic antidepressant and lithium maintenance medication in unipolar and bipolar depressed patients. *J Affective Disord* 20:225-233, 1990.

Jones KL, et al: Pattern of malformations in children of women treated with carbamazepine during pregnancy. *N Engl J Med* 320:1661-1666, 1989.

Kayser A, et al: Influence of panic attacks on response to phenelzine and amitriptyline in depressed outpatients. *J Clin Psychopharmacol* 8:246-253, 1988.

Klerman GL: Depressive disorders: Further evidence for increased medical morbidity and impairment of social functioning. *Arch Gen Psychiatry* 46:856-858, 1989.

Klerman GL: Treatment of recurrent unipolar major depressive disorder: Commentary on the Pittsburgh study. *Arch Gen Psychiatry* 47:1158-1162, 1990.

Kocsis JH, et al: Imipramine treatment for chronic depression. *Arch Gen Psychiatry* 45:253-257, 1988.

Kokmen E: Etiology, diagnosis, and management of dementia. *Compr Ther* 15:59-69, (Sept) 1988.

Kupfer DJ, et al: Possible role of antidepressants in precipitating mania and hypomania in recurrent depression. *Am J Psychiatry* 145:804-808, 1988.

Kurtz NM, Robinson DS: Monoamine oxidase inhibitors, in Georgatas A, Cancro R (eds): *Depression and Mania*. New York, Elsevier, 1988, 358-371.

Lenox RH, et al: Adjunctive treatment of manic agitation with lorazepam versus haloperidol: A double-blind study. *J Clin Psychiatry* 53:47-52, 1992.

Liebowitz MR, et al: Phenelzine versus imipramine in atypical depression: Preliminary report. *Arch Gen Psychiatry* 41:669-677, 1984.

Liebowitz MR, et al: Antidepressant specificity in atypical depression. *Arch Gen Psychiatry* 45:129-137, 1988.

Lipinski JF Jr, et al: Fluoxetine-induced akathisia: Clinical and theoretical implications. *J Clin Psychiatry* 50:339-342, 1989.

Lydiard RB, Gelenberg AJ: Amoxapine: Antidepressant with some neuroleptic properties? Review of its chemistry, animal pharmacology and toxicology, human pharmacology, and clinical efficacy. *Pharmacotherapy* 1:163-178, 1981.

Madakasira S: Amoxapine-induced neuroleptic malignant syndrome. *DICP* 23:50-55, 1989.

Max MB, et al: Amitriptyline, but not lorazepam, relieves postherpetic neuralgia. *Neurology* 38:1427-1432, 1988.

McElroy SL, et al: Valproate in psychiatric disorders: Literature review and clinical guidelines. *J Clin Psychiatry* 50 (suppl) :23-29, 1989.

Mellerup ET, et al: Renal and other controversial adverse effects of lithium, in Meltzer HY (ed): *Psychopharmacology: The Third Generation of Progress*. New York, Raven Press, 1987, 1443-1448.

Mendelis PS: Maprotiline and convulsions. *ADR Highlights* 83:1-10, (Oct 11) 1983.

Mitchell JE, Groat R: Placebo-controlled, double-blind trial of amitriptyline in bulimia. *J Clin Psychopharmacol* 4:186-193, 1984.

Mitchell JE, MacKenzie TB: Cardiac effects of lithium therapy in man: Review. *J Clin Psychiatry* 43:47-51, 1982.

Molina L, et al: Diluted epinephrine solution for the treatment of priapism. *J Urol* 141:1127-1128, 1989.

Montgomery SA, et al: The prophylactic efficacy of fluoxetine in unipolar depression. *Br J Psychiatry* 153 (suppl 3) :69-76, 1988.

Murphy DL, et al: Monoamine oxidase inhibitors as antidepressants: Implications for the mechanism of action of antidepressants and the psychobiology of the affective disorders and some related disorders, in Meltzer HY (ed): *Psychopharmacology: The Third Generation of Progress*. New York, Raven Press, 1987, 545-552.

National Institutes of Health Consensus Development Conference: *Mood Disorders: Pharmacologic Prevention of Recurrences*. Bethesda, Mass, National Institutes of Health, vol 5, 1984.

Nierenberg AA, Cole JO: Antidepressant adverse drug reactions. *J Clin Psychiatry* 52 (suppl) :40-47, (June) 1991.

Nierenberg AA, White K: What next? A review of pharmacologic strategies for treatment resistant depression. *Psychopharmacol Bull* 26:429-460, 1990.

Orsulak PJ: Therapeutic monitoring of antidepressant drugs: Guidelines updated. *Ther Drug Monit* 11:497-507, 1989.

Perry PJ, et al: *Psychotropic Drug Handbook,* ed 5. Cincinnati, Harvey Whitney Books, 1988.

Pope HG Jr, et al: Valproate in the treatment of acute mania: A placebo-controlled study. *Arch Gen Psychiatry* 48:62-68, 1991.

Post RM: Non-lithium treatment for bipolar disorder. *J Clin Psychiatry* 51 (8, suppl) :9-16, 1990.

Post RM, et al: Antidepressant effects of carbamazepine. *Am J Psychiatry* 143:29-34, 1986.

Post RM, et al: Correlates of antimanic response to carbamazepine. *Psychiatry Res* 21:71-83, 1987.

Post RM, et al: Treatment of rapid cycling bipolar illness. *Psychopharmacol Bull* 26:37-47, 1990.

Potter WZ, et al: The pharmacologic treatment of depression. *N Engl J Med* 325:633-642, 1991.

Prien RF, Kupfer DJ: Continuation drug therapy for major depressive episodes: How long should it be maintained? *Am J Psychiatry* 143:18-23, 1986.

Prien RF, Potter WZ: NIMH workshop report on treatment of bipolar disorder. *Psychopharmacol Bull* 26:409-427, 1990.

Quitkin FM, et al: Phenelzine and imipramine in mood reactive depressives: Further delineation of the syndrome of atypical depression. *Arch Gen Psychiatry* 46:787-793, 1989.

Ray WA, et al: Cyclic antidepressants and the risk of hip fracture. *Arch Intern Med* 151:754-756, 1991.

Reimherr FW, et al: Antidepressant efficacy of sertraline: A double-blind, placebo- and amitriptyline-controlled, multicenter comparison study in outpatients with major depression. *J Clin Psychiatry* 5 (12, suppl B) :18-27, 1990.

Richardson JW III, Richelson E: Antidepressants: Clinical update for medical practitioners. *Mayo Clin Proc* 59:330-337, 1984.

Richelson E: Biological basis of depression and therapeutic relevance. *J Clin Psychiatry* 52 (6, suppl) :4-10, 1991.

Risby ED, et al: The mechanisms of action of lithium, II: Effects on adenylate cyclase activity and β-adrenergic receptor binding in normal subjects. *Arch Gen Psychiatry* 48:513-524, 1991.

Robinson DS: New perspectives on long-standing issues: Monoamine oxidase inhibitors. *Psychopharmacol Bull* 22:12-15, 1986.

Robinson DS, et al: Cardiovascular effects of phenelzine and amitriptyline in depressed outpatients. *J Clin Psychiatry* 43:8-15, 1982.

Robinson DS, et al: Continuation and maintenance treatment of major depression with the monoamine oxidase inhibitor phenelzine: A double-blind placebo-controlled discontinuation study. *Psychopharmacol Bull* 27:31-39, 1991.

Roose SP, et al: Cardiovascular effects of imipramine and bupropion in depressed patients with congestive heart failure. *J Clin Psychopharmacol* 7:247-251, 1987.

Roose SP, et al: Cardiovascular effects of bupropion in depressed patients with heart disease. *Am J Psychiatry* 148:512-516, 1991.

Rothschild AJ, Locke CA: Reexposure to fluoxetine after serious suicide attempts by three patients: The role of akathisia. *J Clin Psychiatry* 52:491-493, 1991.

Rudorfer MV, Potter WZ: Antidepressants: Comparative review of the clinical pharmacology and therapeutic use of the 'newer' versus the 'older' drugs. *Drugs* 37:713-738, 1989.

Satel SL, Nelson JC: Stimulants in the treatment of depression: A critical overview. *J Clin Psychiatry* 50:241-249, 1989.

Schou M: Lithium treatment during pregnancy, delivery, and lactation: An update. *J Clin Psychiatry* 51:410-413, 1990.

Schwartz J, et al: Antidepressants in the medically ill: Prediction of benefits. *Int J Psychiatry* 19:363-369, 1990.

Sériès F, Cormier Y: Effects of protriptyline on diurnal and nocturnal oxygenation in patients with chronic obstructive pulmonary disease. *Ann Intern Med* 113:507-511, 1990.

Sheehan DV: Delineation of anxiety and phobic disorders responsive to monoamine oxidase inhibitors: Implications for classification. *J Clin Psychiatry* 45 (7, sec 2) :29-36, 1984.

Sitland-Marken PA: Pharmacologic management of acute mania during pregnancy. *J Clin Psychopharmacol* 9:78-87, 1989.

Small JG: Anticonvulsants in affective disorders. *Psychopharmacol Bull* 26:25-36, 1990.

Smilkstein MJ: Reviewing cyclic antidepressant cardiotoxicity: Wheat and chaff, editorial. *J Emerg Med* 8:645-648, 1990.

Task Force on the Use of Laboratory Tests in Psychiatry: Tricyclic antidepressant-blood level measurements and clinical outcome. APA task force report. *Am J Psychiatry* 142:155-162, 1985.

Teicher MH, et al: Emergence of intense suicidal preoccupation during fluoxetine treatment. *Am J Psychiatry* 147:207-210, 1990.

Thase ME, et al: Treatment of imipramine-resistant recurrent depression, III: Efficacy of monoamine oxidase inhibitors. *J Clin Psychiatry* 53:5-11, 1992.

Tokarski GF, Young MJ: Criteria for admitting patients with tricyclic antidepressant overdose. *J Emerg Med* 6:121-124, 1988.

Tollefson GD: Antidepressant treatment and side effect considerations. *J Clin Psychiatry* 52 (5, suppl) :4-13, 1991.

Waller DG, George CF: Lithium and the kidney. *Adv Drug React Acc Pois Rev* 3:65-89, 1984.

Watkins SE, et al: The effect of carbamazepine and lithium on remission from affective illness. *Br J Psychiatry* 150:180-182, 1987.

Weintraub M, Evans P: Bupropion: Chemically and pharmacologically unique antidepressant. *Hosp Formul* 24:254-259, 1989.

Weissman MM, et al: Psychotherapy and its relevance to the pharmacotherapy of major depression: A decade later (1976-1985), in Meltzer HY (ed): *Psychopharmacology: The Third Generation of Progress*. New York, Raven Press, 1987, 1059-1069.

Wenger TL, Stern WC: Cardiovascular profile of bupropion. *J Clin Psychiatry* 44:176-182, 1983.

White K, Simpson G: The combined use of MAOIs and tricyclics. *J Clin Psychiatry* 45:67-69, (July) 1984.

Winbow A: New hope for depression? *Practitioner* 235:532-534, 1991.

New Evaluation

PARAXETINE HYDROCHLORIDE
[Paxil]

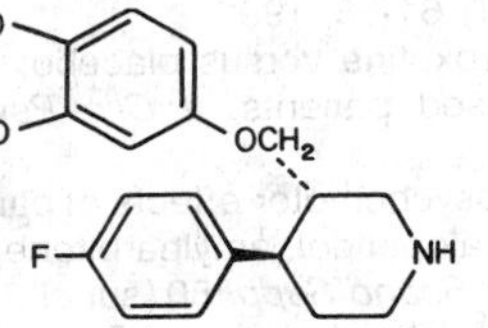

ACTIONS. Paroxetine, a phenylpiperidine derivative, selectively inhibits the neuronal uptake of serotonin, and this action is presumed to underlie its antidepressant effects. Paroxetine does not bind significantly to adrenergic, dopaminergic, serotonergic, cholinergic, or histaminergic receptors and exerts only very weak effects on the neuronal uptake of norepinephrine and dopamine. Compared with fluoxetine and sertraline, paroxetine inhibits the neuronal uptake of 5-HT more selectively in vitro (Tulloch and Johnson, 1992); the clinical significance of this is unknown.

USES. Results of several short-term, double-blind, placebo-controlled trials, some of which compared paroxetine with imipramine, demonstrated the clinical efficacy of paroxetine (Peselow et al, 1989; Dunbar et al, 1991; Claghorn et al, 1992; *J Clin Psychiatry*, 1992). Most of these trials involved outpatients, predominantly those who were moderately depressed. With the exception of two trials (Miller et al, 1989; Smith and Glaudin, 1992), the efficacy of paroxetine was superior to that of placebo; the former trial lasted only four weeks and in the latter trial, subgroup analysis indicated that paroxetine was effective in patients whose depression had persisted for more than one year. In most of these trials, paroxetine's efficacy was equal or superior to that of imipramine. Paroxetine also has been compared with amitriptyline (Laursen et al, 1985; Battegay et al, 1985; Bascara, 1989), doxepin (Dunner et al, 1992), and clomipramine (Guillibert et al, 1989) in the treatment of moderately depressed adult and elderly outpatients. In virtually all of these studies, paroxetine was better tolerated and its overall efficacy was equal or superior to that of the tricyclic agent. Paroxetine has not been adequately studied in more severely depressed hospitalized patients but, in one comparative trial, inpatients treated with clomipramine improved more than those treated with paroxetine (Danish University Antidepressant Group, 1990).

There is some evidence that maintenance therapy with paroxetine for at least one year is well tolerated and reduces the rate of recurrence of major depressive episodes (Jakovljevic and Mewett, 1991).

ADVERSE REACTIONS AND PRECAUTIONS. In placebo-controlled clinical trials, the most frequently reported adverse reactions were gastrointestinal disturbances (nausea, constipation, decreased appetite, diarrhea), urogenital effects (ejaculatory dysfunction, other genital disorders in males), autonomic nervous system dysfunction (sweating, dry mouth), central nervous system effects (somnolence, dizziness, insomnia, tremor, nervousness, anxiety), and asthenia. Other adverse events that led to discontinuation of paroxetine in clinical trials were agitation and vomiting. Like fluoxetine and sertraline, paroxetine may cause modest weight loss during initial therapy, but patients in controlled trials experienced only minimal weight loss (an average of 1 lb).

At therapeutic doses, paroxetine does not significantly impair psychomotor skills (Cooper et al, 1989) and does not appear to significantly affect the cardiovascular system (Boyer and Blumhardt, 1992). However, use of this drug in patients with recent myocardial infarction or unstable heart disease has not been adequately studied; thus, it should be used cautiously in such patients.

During clinical trials, mania occurred in approximately 1% of patients treated with paroxetine. However, in patients with bipolar disorder, the incidence of mania associated with use of paroxetine (2%) was lower than in those treated with other antidepressants (11%). Patients randomized to receive paroxetine also were at no greater risk for suicidal ideation or suicidal behavior than patients randomized to other antidepressants.

Generally, adverse events in elderly patients appear to be similar to those reported in patients under age 65. However, several cases of hyponatremia have been reported, most of which occurred in elderly patients who also were taking diuretics or who were otherwise volume-depleted.

Paroxetine is classified in FDA Pregnancy Category B.

POISONING. Overdose (up to 850 mg) occurred in 10 patients during preclinical testing; all recovered fully after routine supportive care.

DRUG INTERACTIONS. Preliminary data suggest that administration of paroxetine with warfarin may result in an increased bleeding tendency, although prothrombin time is unchanged. Drugs that induce cytochrome P450 isozymes (eg, phenytoin, phenobarbital) may decrease the plasma concentration of paroxetine. Drugs that inhibit these isozymes (eg, cimetidine) may increase the plasma concentration of paroxetine. Dosage adjustments should be guided by clinical response. Administration of paroxetine with other drugs that (1) are metabolized by $P450IID_6$, including most tricyclic antidepressants, phenothiazines, and Class 1C antiarrhythmics (eg, propafenone, flecainide), or (2) inhibit $P450IID_6$ (eg, quinidine, propoxyphene, haloperidol) is likely to result in pharmacokinetic interactions, and combined therapy should be undertaken with caution.

Paroxetine should not be used with a monoamine oxidase (MAO) inhibitor or within 14 days after discontinuing treatment with an MAO inhibitor. Similarly, at least 14 days should elapse before initiating therapy with an MAO inhibitor after paroxetine has been discontinued.

PHARMACOKINETICS. Paroxetine is well absorbed after oral administration; absorption appears to be unaffected by the presence of food. Plasma protein binding is approximately 95%. Elimination occurs primarily by hepatic oxidation, followed by methylation and conjugation with glucuronic acid and sulfate. Compared with paroxetine, all metabolites lack significant pharmacologic activity. Initial oxidative metabolism is performed by at least two enzymes (Bloomer et al, 1992), one of which is cytochrome $P450IID_6$, an isozyme under monogenic control that exhibits polymorphism within the population. Steady-state concentrations may vary 25-fold between patients with the extensive and poor metabolizer phenotype (Sindrup et al, 1992 A). Saturation of $P450IID_6$ probably explains the dose-dependent (ie, nonlinear) pharmacokinetics of paroxetine in extensive metabolizers (Sindrup et al, 1992 B). In these patients, bioavailability increases with increasing dose and duration of treatment. The elimination half-life is approximately 24 hours, but there is wide individual variability. In one study, the half-life was 41 hours in poor metabolizers but only 16 hours in extensive metabolizers (Sindrup et al, 1992 B). Steady-state plasma concentrations are established within 4 to 14 days.

Increased plasma concentrations of paroxetine occur in the elderly (eightfold) and in patients with renal or hepatic impairment (two to fourfold).

DOSAGE AND PREPARATIONS.

Oral: *Adults*, initially, 20 mg once daily, usually in the morning. Administration of the daily dose in the evening may be beneficial in those who experience daytime somnolence. If the response is inadequate, the dose may be increased in 10-mg increments at intervals of at least one week to a maximum of 50 mg/day. In elderly or debilitated patients and those with severe renal or hepatic impairment, the recommended initial dose is 10 mg/day (maximum, 40 mg/day).

Paxil (SmithKline Beecham). Tablets 20 and 30 mg.

Cited References

A clinical profile of paroxetine: A novel selective serotonin reuptake inhibitor (SSRI). *J Clin Psychiatry* 53:3-68, 1992.

Bascara L: A double-blind study to compare the effectiveness and tolerability of paroxetine and amitriptyline in depressed patients. *Acta Psychiatr Scand Suppl* 80 (suppl 350):141-142, 1989.

Battegay R, et al: Double-blind comparative study of paroxetine and amitriptyline in depressed patients of a university psychiatric outpatient clinic. *Neuropsychobiology* 13:31-37, 1985.

Bloomer JC, et al: The role of cytochrome P4502D6 in the metabolism of paroxetine by human liver microsomes. *Br J Clin Pharmacol* 33:521-523, 1992.

Boyer WF, Blumhardt CL: The safety profile of paroxetine. *J Clin Psychiatry* 53 (2, suppl):61-66, 1992.

Claghorn JL, et al: Paroxetine versus placebo: A double-blind comparison in depressed patients. *J Clin Psychiatry* 53:434-438, 1992.

Cooper SM, et al: The psychomotor effects of paroxetine alone and in combination with haloperidol, amylbarbitone, oxazepam, or alcohol. *Acta Psychiatr Scand Suppl* 80 (suppl 350):53-55, 1989.

Danish University Antidepressant Group: Paroxetine: A selective serotonin reuptake inhibitor showing better tolerance, but weaker antidepressant effect than clomipramine in a controlled multicenter study. *J Affect Disord* 18:289-299, 1990.

Dunbar GC, et al: A comparison of paroxetine, imipramine and placebo in depressed out-patients. *Br J Psychiatry* 159:394-398, 1991.

Dunner DL, et al: Two combined, multicenter double-blind studies of paroxetine and doxepin in geriatric patients with major depression. *J Clin Psychiatry* 53 (2, suppl):57-60, 1992.

Guillibert E, et al: A double-blind, multi-centre study of paroxetine versus clomipramine in depressed elderly patients. *Acta Psychiatr Scand Suppl* 80 (suppl 350):132-134, 1989.

Jakovljevic M, Mewett S: Comparison between paroxetine, imipramine, and placebo in preventing recurrent major depressive episodes. *Eur Neuropsychopharmacol* 1:440, 1991.

Laursen AL, et al: Paroxetine in the treatment of depression: A randomized comparison with amitriptyline. *Acta Psychiatr Scand* 71:249-255, 1985.

Miller SM, et al: A double-blind comparison of paroxetine and placebo in the treatment of depressed patients in a psychiatric outpatient clinic. *Acta Psychiatr Scand Suppl* 80 (suppl 350):143-144, 1989.

Peselow ED, et al: The short- and long-term efficacy of paroxetine HCl: A. Data from a 6-week double-blind parallel design trial vs. imipramine and placebo. *Psychopharmacol Bull* 25:267-271, 1989.

Sindrup SH, et al: Pharmacokinetics of the selective serotonin reuptake inhibitor paroxetine: Nonlinearity and relation to the sparteine oxidation polymorphism. *Clin Pharmacol Ther* 51:288-295, 1992 A.

Sindrup SH, et al: The relationship between paroxetine and the sparteine oxidation polymorphism. *Clin Pharmacol Ther* 51:278-287, 1992 B.

Smith WT, Glaudin V: A placebo-controlled trial of paroxetine in the treatment of major depression. *J Clin Psychiatry* 53 (2, suppl):36-39, 1992.

Tulloch IF, Johnson AM: The pharmacologic profile of paroxetine, a new selective serotonin reuptake inhibitor. *J Clin Psychiatry* 53 (2, suppl):7-12, 1992.

Drugs Used in Other Mental Disorders

14

The abuse of psychoactive drugs exacts an enormous human and monetary toll. Excessive alcohol intake and cigarette smoking cause hundreds of thousands of premature deaths, contribute billions of dollars to the total national health expenditure, and account for billions more in lost productivity. Excessive drinking and cigarette smoking are recognized substance abuse disorders and, for many abusers of these drugs, constitute an addiction. Treatment primarily involves professional counseling, which may include psychological and behavioral modification therapy and/or participation in self-help programs (eg, Alcoholics Anonymous). Pharmacologic intervention is available to relieve withdrawal symptoms and, for alcoholism, to prevent relapse.

ALCOHOL (ETHANOL, ETHYL ALCOHOL)

Properties of Alcohol

Because alcohol is nonionized, lipid soluble, and completely miscible in water, every human cell is subject to interaction with it. In the liver, alcohol is oxidized to acetaldehyde, an even more toxic compound; consequently, the ratio of reduced nicotinamide adenine dinucleotide (NADH) to the oxidized form (NAD+) is increased, thereby altering the metabolism of compounds that depend on the NADH:NAD+ system. Alcohol has caloric but no nutritive value. Although it is not a carcinogen, alcohol may enhance the carcinogenic activity of other compounds.

PHARMACOLOGIC ACTIVITY. Acute Effects. Alcohol exerts both central and peripheral effects. There probably are many molecular and cellular sites of action because relatively high (eg, millimolar) concentrations of ethanol are required for biological actions. In the central nervous system, alcohol causes dose-dependent depression. The depression and disinhibition induced contribute to the feelings of relaxation, confidence, and euphoria that often accompany use of alcohol.

The mechanism by which alcohol affects neuronal activity and synaptic transmission is uncertain. The effects of alcohol on the central nervous system had been attributed to nonspecific membrane actions (eg, membrane fluidization, disordering of the lipid matrix). However, receptor-gated ion channels may be selective targets for alcohol (Gonzales and Hoffman, 1991). Pharmacologically relevant concentrations of alcohol enhance gamma-aminobutyric acid (GABA)-stimulated chloride ion flux and inhibit N-methyl-D-aspartate (NMDA)-activated ion currents in some neurons. Similar concentrations enhance the function of 5-hydroxytryptamine (5-HT_3) receptor-gated channels (Lovinger et al, 1990). Acute effects on voltage-gated calcium channels require somewhat higher concentrations. Effects on a variety of other neurotransmitters, neuropeptides, and secondary messenger systems also have been reported (Deitrich et al, 1989).

As blood alcohol concentrations rise, reasoning, memory, and coordination deteriorate. Loss of inhibitions and impaired judgment may lead to disregard for social norms or even dangerous or violent behavior. Susceptibility to the effects of alcohol varies widely and is based partly on genetic and constitutional factors, nutritional status, and degree of tolerance. Thus, it is difficult to associate particular blood alcohol concentrations with specific degrees of impairment. However, alcohol blood concentrations of 50 to 100 mg/dL produce deficits in attention and coordination. Concentrations of 100 to 200 mg/dL generally are associated with slurred speech and ataxia, and concentrations of 200 to 300 mg/dL may produce stupor, anesthesia, and coma. Levels exceeding 400 to 500 mg/dL generally produce dangerous or lethal depression of respiration, although chronic alcoholics rarely may tolerate blood concentrations of 500 to 600 mg/dL.

Although moderate amounts of alcohol produce vasodilation of cutaneous vessels, larger amounts may cause tachycardia and increase blood pressure. A diuretic effect is mediated by inhibition of the release of antidiuretic hormone and decreased tubular reabsorption of water.

Gastric and salivary secretions usually are stimulated. Alcohol alters intestinal motility; causes inflammation of the mucosa; and contributes to development of lesions of the esophagus, stomach, duodenum, and pancreas. Mucosal damage can impair the digestion of food and the absorption of nutrients into the blood stream.

PHARMACOKINETICS. In the fasting state, up to 20% of ingested alcohol may be absorbed from the stomach. Intestinal absorption is very rapid; thus, the gastric emptying time is a major factor in determining absorption rates. Approximately 90% to 98% of ingested alcohol is oxidized in a dose-dependent fashion (primarily by hepatic cytosolic alcohol dehydrogenase and microsomal enzymes) to acetaldehyde, which is converted to acetyl CoA for oxidation via the citric acid cycle. The microsomal oxidation is mediated by an inducible isoform (cytochrome P4502EI) that also may contribute to the accelerated metabolism of other drugs that occurs as a consequence of chronic alcohol consumption (Lieber, 1988). Significant first-pass metabolism of ethanol by gastric alcohol dehydrogenase also has been reported after ingestion of smaller amounts (Frezza et al, 1990). Enzyme activity is lower in females and alcoholics; thus, the bioavailability of alcohol also may be increased in these individuals. Coupled with the lower volume of distribution in women, the lower enzyme activity causes higher blood alcohol concentrations to be achieved in women than in men. This sex-related difference in gastric alcohol dehydrogenase may diminish as individuals age (Seitz et al, 1990).

In nontolerant individuals, the liver can metabolize the alcohol contained in approximately 1 to 1.5 ounces of 80 to 100 proof whiskey, a 4-ounce glass of wine, or 12 ounces of beer per hour (ie, about 10 ml of 100% alcohol/hour), although this is at least partially a function of body size. Ingestion in excess of an individual's ability to metabolize alcohol leads to accumulation. The rate of metabolism often is increased in alcoholics who have been drinking recently and in smokers, perhaps because of enzyme induction. The increase in metabolism and the development of pharmacodynamic tolerance may be masked by hepatitis, advanced cirrhosis of the liver, or nutritional deficiencies. Hyperthyroid patients may metabolize alcohol twice as rapidly as normal individuals. In the elderly, blood alcohol concentrations may be 10% to 15% higher than those in younger patients who have ingested identical amounts of alcohol.

INGESTION OF ALCOHOL DURING PREGNANCY. Alcohol readily crosses the placenta, and its use during pregnancy can produce the fetal alcohol syndrome (Clarren and Smith, 1978; Iosub et al, 1981). This syndrome represents the extreme end of a continuum of disabilities caused by maternal alcohol use during pregnancy. Prenatal and postnatal growth retardation, microcephaly, neurologic abnormalities, facial dysmorphology, and other congenital anomalies are characteristic of affected infants. The risk of fetal alcohol syndrome is increased if alcohol is consumed during the first trimester, but development of the most severe manifestations may require sustained heavy drinking throughout pregnancy (Rosett and Weiner, 1985).

The incidence of various other malformations of the cutaneous, cardiac, urogenital, and musculoskeletal systems (fetal alcohol effects) is increased by exposure to alcohol, as are more subtle cognitive/behavioral deficits. Maladaptive behaviors, learning disabilities, and hyperactivity may persist (Ernhart et al, 1987; Streissguth et al, 1991).

Even moderate alcohol consumption during pregnancy increases the risk of spontaneous abortion and low birth weight. Since a safe level of alcohol intake during pregnancy has not been established, physicians should advise pregnant women not to consume alcohol.

DRUG INTERACTIONS. Numerous interactions occur between alcohol and other drugs (Linnoila et al, 1979; Lieber, 1980). The most important of these is enhanced central nervous system depression induced by the concomitant use of alcohol and other compounds with a similar action. These agents include general anesthetics, opioid analgesics, hypnotic and antianxiety drugs, antihistamines, antipsychotic agents, antidepressants, central skeletal muscle relaxants, centrally acting anticholinergic agents, antiepileptic drugs, and certain antihypertensive agents (reserpine, methyldopa, clonidine).

The mechanism may be pharmacodynamic or pharmacokinetic. The latter type of interaction occurs because alcohol competes with many endogenous and exogenous chemicals that utilize a common biotransformation pathway, ie, oxidation by hepatic microsomal enzymes. Some adaptive tolerance occurs gradually to both alcohol and other central nervous system depressants (eg, general anesthetics, hypnotics, antianxiety agents) and diminishes the sedative effect. Nevertheless, patients should be cautioned to avoid alcohol intake in conjunction with any other central nervous system depressant or while performing tasks requiring alertness (eg, operation of a motor vehicle or other machinery).

Additive orthostatic hypotension is less common but significant. This interaction results from concomitant use of alcohol and drugs with vasodilator activity (eg, alpha adrenergic blockers, methyldopa, hydralazine, calcium channel blockers, organic nitrates). The bioavailability of alcohol may be increased by aspirin, cimetidine, and verapamil (Caballeria et al, 1989; Roine et al, 1990; Bauer et al, 1992).

Concomitant ingestion of alcohol and aspirin or ingestion of alcohol by those receiving high-dose aspirin therapy should be avoided because the combination promotes gastrointestinal bleeding. Severe hypoglycemia may occur when alcohol is taken with insulin or oral hypoglycemic agents. Alcohol interferes with the metabolism of the oral hypoglycemic drugs and rarely may produce hypoglycemia even when consumed alone. Alcohol also interferes with the metabolism of oral anticoagulants, antiepileptic drugs, and nifedipine, and higher than expected plasma concentrations of these agents may result when they are given to individuals also imbibing alcohol. Conversely, chronic intake of alcohol can induce microsomal enzymes and accelerate the clearance of warfarin, phenytoin, tolbutamide, propranolol, and rifampin (Lieber, 1988). The effect of enzyme induction can be offset by the liver damage induced by alcohol or nutritional deficiency, which may affect the capacity of the liver to detoxify drugs. Accordingly, the dosage of these agents and presumably other drugs subject to hepatic oxidation may require adjustment on initiation and termination of therapy in chronic alcoholics. Careful monitoring of the patient is essential.

The enhanced susceptibility of chronic alcoholics to hepatitis induced by acetaminophen, isoniazid, and carbon tetrachloride also is explained by enzyme induction because the biotransformation to toxic metabolites is enhanced. The hypertensive reaction that occurs when monoamine oxidase inhibitors are taken with alcoholic beverages appears to result from dihydroxyphenylalanine and/or tyramine rather than from alcohol itself.

Chronic Excessive Alcohol Ingestion

ETIOLOGY. Alcohol-related problems are heterogenous, and individuals who experience them are diverse. The most recent estimate of the lifetime prevalence rate for alcohol dependence or abuse in the U.S. population is 13.5% (Regier et al, 1990). A growing body of evidence suggests that biological, psychological, and social factors interact to cause a drinking problem. In some individuals, alcohol-related problems develop from attempts to alleviate symptoms of anxiety, depression, or insomnia. Two other major risk factors are a family history of alcoholism (although a wide range of familial risk rates have been reported) and male sex. Various etiologic subtypes have been proposed that consider pattern of drinking, type of dependence, genetic vulnerability, personality profile, and the role of psychopathologic dysfunction (Jellinek, 1960; Morey and Skinner, 1986; Cloninger, 1987; von Knorring et al, 1987; Babor and Dolinsky, 1988). Although the relative contribution of genetic and environmental factors is controversial, genetic components may most strongly influence development of alcohol dependence in men (Pickens et al, 1991), particularly those with early-onset alcoholism (McGue et al, 1992; Babor et al, 1992). Females are at lower risk for alcoholism, although the difference between the sexes is narrowing (Kendler et al, 1992).

DIAGNOSIS. It is difficult to define alcoholism adequately. The National Council on Alcoholism and Drug Dependence and the American Society of Addiction Medicine define alcoholism as a "primary chronic disease with genetic, psychosocial, and environmental factors influencing its development and manifestations. The disease is often progressive and fatal. It is characterized by continuous or periodic impaired control over drinking, preoccupation with the drug alcohol, use of alcohol despite adverse consequences, and distortions in thinking, most notably denial." Each of these symptoms may be continuous or periodic (Morse and Flavin, 1992). Previous definitions have emphasized medical and psychosocial consequences and have differentiated alcohol abuse (eg, problem drinking) from alcoholism (Rinaldi et al, 1988).

In the *Diagnostic and Statistical Manual of Mental Disorders,* Revised (*DSM-III-R*), the diagnosis of alcohol dependence emphasizes the pattern of alcohol consumption, the primacy of alcohol use in relationship to other behavioral options, and impaired control over drinking behavior. At least three of the following characteristic symptoms are necessary to make a diagnosis of alcohol dependence (American Psychiatric Association, 1987): (1) Alcohol is often consumed in larger amounts or over a longer period than the person intended. (2) The individual either has a persistent desire or has made one or more unsuccessful efforts to reduce or control alcohol intake. (3) A great deal of time is spent in activities necessary to procure alcohol, consume it, or recover from its effects. (4) Frequent intoxication or withdrawal symptoms occur when the individual is expected to fulfill major role obligations at work, school, or home. (5) Important social, occupational, or recreational activities are given up or reduced because of alcoholism. (6) With heavy and prolonged alcohol use, a variety of social, psychological, and physical problems occur and are exacerbated by continued use of alcohol. (7) A markedly diminished effect (tolerance) with the same amount of alcohol occurs. (8) Characteristic withdrawal symptoms of alcohol are present. (9) Alcohol is often consumed to relieve or avoid withdrawal symptoms. In addition, the diagnosis of this dependence syndrome requires that some symptoms have persisted for at least one month or have occurred repeatedly over a longer period of time, as in binge drinking.

Because treatment of individuals with alcohol problems cannot realistically be the sole responsibility of specialized treatment programs, primary care physicians are urged to play an increased role in the identification, intervention, and/or referral of patients with alcohol problems (see discussion on Rehabilitation) (Institute of Medicine, 1990).

MANIFESTATIONS. Although certain psychiatric disturbances can be risk factors for the development of alcoholism, chronic alcohol intoxication also is accompanied by increased psychopathology (eg, anxiety, panic, depression, belligerence) and a high lifetime prevalence of associated psychiatric disorders (Meyer, 1989; Regier et al, 1990; Kushner et al, 1990).

Alcohol, unlike other drugs, contains 7.1 calories per gram; ingestion of a pint of 86 proof whiskey daily (not unusual for an alcoholic) provides approximately one-half the daily caloric requirement for the average adult. Chronic consumption of alcohol may inhibit the absorption of amino acids, vitamins, and other nutritive substances in the gastrointestinal tract. Inadequate dietary intake or malabsorption is responsible for the malnutrition that may be present in chronic alcoholics. Folic acid and protein deficiencies, pancreatic insufficiency, abnormal biliary secretions, and gastrointestinal mucosal abnormalities are induced directly by alcohol and cause malabsorption of fat, amino acids, glucose, sodium, water, thiamine, folic acid, zinc, and vitamin B_{12}. Hematologic abnormalities, which may include megaloblastic anemia, thrombocytopenia, and neutropenia, are primarily due to folate deficiency. A nutritious diet with little or no alcohol intake reverses many of these abnormalities (Green and Tall, 1979).

Prolonged malnutrition, especially thiamine deficiency, produces Wernicke's encephalopathy and cerebral atrophy, possibly as direct effects of alcohol and its metabolic products on the central nervous system. The classic triad of encephalopathy, ophthalmoplegia, and ataxia may not be apparent in some individuals. A subset of patients may have inherited or acquired abnormalities that reduce the affinity of transketolase for thiamine. Accordingly, effective treatment may require parenteral administration of thiamine (100 mg) for at least five days. Deficiencies of other vitamins, minerals, and electrolytes, especially the transketolase cofactor, magnesium, should be corrected simultaneously (Charness et al, 1989). Patients may develop Korsakoff's syndrome, a disabling memory disorder characterized by selective amnesia that is manifested by recent memory loss and impairment of new learning. Confabulation and polyneuropathy are often associated with this syndrome. Alcohol-induced neurotoxicity also causes other neuropathologic events that may contribute to chronic cognitive dysfunction. Enlargement of the cerebral ventricles and sulci is apparent on CT or MRI in most alcoholics.

The harmful effects in the liver observed with chronic ingestion of alcohol appear to result principally from alcohol metabolism; these include accumulation of fat (steatosis), alcoholic hepatitis, and cirrhosis (Lieber, 1988). However, only 15% to 20% of alcoholics develop severe liver damage (Zetterman, 1990). Elevated gamma glutamyl transpeptidase and AST levels may indicate hepatic injury, but enzyme levels do not correlate with the degree of functional impairment or histologic changes in the liver. Only liver biopsy accurately ascertains the type and extent of damage. Malnutrition can intensify the damage, but fatty liver and more serious hepatic lesions can occur despite adequate nutrition (Lieber, 1978). Direct toxic effects of acetaldehyde, enhanced lipid peroxidation, perivenular hypoxia, and a variety of subcellular or biochemical alterations have been proposed. Even therapeutic doses of acetaminophen (ie, 4 g daily) may cause synergistic hepatotoxicity (Wootton and Lee, 1990). Autoimmune mechanisms may play a role in some patients (Laskin et al, 1990). Corticosteroids may improve short-term mortality in patients with acute alcoholic hepatitis and hepatic encephalopathy who do not have active gastrointestinal bleeding (Carithers et al, 1989; Imperiale and McCullough, 1990; Ramond et al, 1992). In patients with moderate to severe alcoholic hepatitis and moderate malnutrition, treatment with oxandrolone [Oxandrin] also appears to improve short-term mortality.

Although regular excessive consumption of alcohol is a risk factor for the development of hypertension and stroke (Regan, 1990), chronic use of moderate amounts (eg, one to three drinks daily) may favorably affect the balance of HDL- and LDL-cholesterol fractions, possibly decreasing the incidence of coronary heart disease (Steinberg et al, 1991). However, long-term excessive use increases the risk of coronary artery disease and may cause direct cardiac injury leading to cardiomyopathy and atrial or ventricular arrhythmias (Urbano-Marquez et al, 1989; Regan, 1990). Skeletal myopathy also may occur.

Hyperlipidemia, hyperuricemia, hypomagnesemia, pancreatitis, increased risk of cancer (tongue, mouth, oropharynx, hypopharynx, esophagus, larynx, and liver), sexual and reproductive dysfunction, depression and suicide, traffic and industrial accidents, and sociopathology (eg, family violence, child abuse, rape, assault) are additional complications of alcoholism and alcohol abuse (Lieber, 1976; West, 1984).

TOLERANCE AND PHYSICAL DEPENDENCE. Chronic use of alcohol results in the development of tolerance and physical dependence. Initially, tolerance appears to be related to both increased metabolism (drug-disposition) and adaptive changes in neuronal constituents (pharmacodynamic) that serve to counteract the short-term effects of alcohol. Metabolic tolerance may decrease temporarily in the presence of hepatitis or permanently with severe cirrhosis.

Cellular adaptation in the central nervous system eventually establishes a state of physical dependence. Such dependence becomes apparent when reduction of intake or abstention from alcohol causes subjective distress and objective signs of withdrawal. Withdrawal syndromes of varying severity can be distinguished. The earliest and most common symptoms include autonomic and somatic hyperactivity (eg, anxiety, tachycardia, diaphoresis, hypertension, arrhythmias, increased muscle tone and tremors, nausea and vomiting), insomnia, and a mild confusional state with irritability or agitation. More pronounced symptoms of neuronal excitation include perceptual disorders (eg, erethism, visual or auditory illusions, hallucinations) and hyperreflexia; a small percentage of patients have one or more tonic-clonic seizures. The most serious manifestation of alcohol withdrawal is delirium tremens, a severe confusional state characterized by profound agitation, delusions, severe autonomic hyperactivity, hyperpyrexia, tremors, and seizures.

TREATMENT. Alcoholism is a chronic disease. Continuity of care with a goal of relapse prevention is central to its management. Treatment can be divided into three phases: acute intoxication, the withdrawal syndrome, and long-term rehabilitation.

Acute Intoxication: Therapy for severe acute intoxication is solely supportive, and drugs usually are not required. The essential elements of management include mechanical ventilatory support; maintenance of normal body temperature; correction of dehydration, acid-base abnormalities, electrolyte imbalance, and/or hypoglycemia; and lavage (rarely indicated).

Withdrawal Syndrome: The goals of treating alcohol withdrawal are to relieve symptoms, to prevent progressive, severe withdrawal reactions, and to prepare the alcoholic for long-term rehabilitation (Reed and Liskow, 1987; Romach and Sellers, 1991).

In 95% of alcoholic patients, withdrawal is expressed as a mild to moderate abstinence syndrome. Onset and peak of withdrawal symptoms usually occur 6 to 8 and 24 to 36 hours, respectively, after cessation of drinking. For the remaining 5% of alcoholics, symptoms are more severe and may even be life-threatening; these usually peak in 96 to 120 hours and then gradually subside over the next 72 hours. Delirium tremens occurs in less than 5% of hospitalized patients. The mortality rate is less than 2% in those with severe withdrawal who receive treatment but is 15% to 20% in untreated patients.

Detoxification may not require the use of psychoactive drugs, but no validated criteria have been developed to identify individuals who require only supportive care as opposed to those who require hospitalization. Although supportive care decreases the general symptoms associated with withdrawal, it does not prevent hallucinations, seizures, or arrhythmias; hence, drugs are required in patients with late or severe withdrawal reactions or in those in whom treatment may be complicated (eg, presence of malnutrition, fever, trauma, abnormalities in fluid and electrolyte balance) (Romach and Sellers, 1991). These patients should be hospitalized for management.

When drug therapy is needed, the benzodiazepines are preferred because they are as efficacious and less toxic than barbiturates, chloral hydrate, paraldehyde, hydroxyzine and other antihistamines, and antipsychotic drugs (Lewis and Femino, 1982). Ethanol has a short duration of action and a narrow range of safety; therefore, since cross-tolerance exists between ethanol and the benzodiazepines, the long-acting derivatives, diazepam [Valium] and chlordiazepoxide [Librium], are preferred as substitutes in the management of moderate to severe withdrawal from alcohol. Other long-acting benzodiazepines (eg, flurazepam [Dalmane], clorazepate [Tranxene]) are effective, but they have been used less extensively. Because of pharmacokinetic considerations, benzodiazepines that possess relatively shorter half-lives and are converted to inactive glucuronide metabolites (eg, oxazepam [Serax], lorazepam [Ativan], temazepam [Restoril]) may be preferred in older patients or in those with severe liver disease (Sellers and Kalant, 1976). The elimination of these benzodiazepines usually is not prolonged, even in the presence of severe liver damage. Approximate dosage equivalents to diazepam 20 mg are chlordiazepoxide 100 mg, clorazepate 15 mg, flurazepam and temazepam 60 mg, lorazepam 4 mg, and oxazepam 120 mg.

The management of patients with moderate to severe withdrawal reactions is improved when a benzodiazepine loading dose is administered. Chlordiazepoxide 100 mg every two hours or diazepam 20 mg every one to two hours is given orally until the patient is mildly sedated or until clinical observation indicates that withdrawal signs and symptoms are controlled, preferably verified by employing an objective, quantitative assessment scale to monitor therapeutic efficacy (Sellers, 1988). The usual dose required is diazepam 60 mg or chlordiazepoxide 300 mg. When withdrawal symptoms are severe, diazepam 20 mg can be given slowly intravenously, followed by infusion of 20 mg/hr until the patient is mildly sedated. The mean time to sedation is about three hours.

A single dose of thiamine 100 mg also is given intramuscularly or intravenously, but 100 mg of thiamine daily for at least five days may be necessary to prevent Wernicke's encephalopathy in some patients. The longer treatment period or parenteral administration may be necessary if thiamine absorption is impaired due to alcohol-induced mucosal injury or in patients who have transketolase variants. Multivitamin preparations may be given daily; however, their value has not been proved. If prothrombin time is prolonged more than three seconds, phytonadione (vitamin K_1) 5 to 10 mg should be administered intramuscularly.

Fluid and electrolyte balance also must be maintained. Fluid volume depletion usually is not a problem with alcoholics unless there has been protracted vomiting or diarrhea. With delirium tremens, large volumes of fluid can be lost through the skin.

Potassium and magnesium supplements may be needed. Patients with a serum potassium concentration below 3 mEq/L should be given 10% potassium chloride (20 mEq/15 ml) diluted with fruit juice or other fluid and taken orally two or three times daily. Replacement of more than 100 mEq of potassium daily is not advised. In patients with normal renal function and magnesium levels below 1.4 mEq/L, 2 ml of 50% magnesium sulfate (1 g) may be given intramuscularly every six to eight hours on the first day of treatment. This dosage usually corrects total body deficits and controls seizures caused by low magnesium levels. Low serum phosphorus concentrations (less than 2 mg/dL) should be treated with oral phosphate supplements or a diet rich in milk.

Since autonomic hyperactivity is a prominent feature of the alcohol withdrawal syndrome, drugs that decrease sympathetic tone (eg, beta blockers, clonidine [Catapres]) also have been investigated. Beta blockers reduce some symptoms (eg, tremor, tachycardia) but do not prevent seizures or delirium. Results of preliminary studies suggest that they may allow reduction in benzodiazepine dosage and help to ameliorate symptoms of mild to moderate withdrawal when administered with benzodiazepines (Kraus et al, 1985; Horwitz et al, 1989).

Clonidine reduces alcohol withdrawal symptoms compared with placebo and, in two studies of patients with mild to moderate alcohol withdrawal, was reported to be equivalent or superior to chlordiazepoxide (Baumgartner and Rowen, 1987, 1991). Further comparative studies are necessary to determine whether clonidine is an alternative to benzodiazepines for the initial management of mild to moderate alcohol withdrawal. There is no evidence that this drug prevents the more serious complications of severe withdrawal, and it should not be used as sole treatment in patients with a history of seizures (Robinson et al, 1989).

Usually, hallucinations associated with alcoholism are a type of self-limiting psychosis that lasts from a few hours to a few days. In the milder forms, sedation is sufficient to overcome them; in more severe cases, an antipsychotic drug may be indicated. Haloperidol [Haldol] 0.5 to 2 mg (or equivalent) can be administered intramuscularly every two hours until hallucinations are controlled. Usually, it is not necessary to give more than five doses in a 24-hour period.

During withdrawal, the alcoholic may experience tonic-clonic (grand mal) seizures. Prolonged alcohol abuse may increase the risk of new-onset seizures independent of withdrawal (Ng et al, 1988). Most often, withdrawal seizures are self-limited, and the patient needs only supportive care and continued benzodiazepine therapy. If seizures are repeated or continuous, intravenous diazepam or lorazepam can be administered until they are controlled. Only if the patient has epilepsy, focal seizures, or a history of alcohol withdrawal seizures should an agent other than a benzodiazepine be used. In epileptic patients, phenytoin [Dilantin] can be given prophylactically during withdrawal in a dose of 300 mg orally followed by 100 mg every eight hours. For focal or other acute seizures not controlled by diazepam, rapid intravenous loading doses of phenytoin generally are recommended. In nonepileptic patients, intravenous phenytoin was not significantly more effective than placebo in the prevention of subsequent seizures when it was administered within six hours of the onset of seizures induced by alcohol withdrawal (Alldredge et al, 1989).

The risk of inducing seizure activity (ie, kindling) may increase with recurrent alcohol detoxification (Brown et al, 1988; Lechtenberg and Worner, 1990). Accordingly, antiepileptic drugs that inhibit kindling phenomena may be useful, not only in suppressing acute withdrawal symptoms, but also in reducing long-term sequelae. Several controlled trials in Europe concluded that carbamazepine [Tegretol] is superior to placebo and equivalent to various central nervous system depressants in the management of alcohol withdrawal. Results of a controlled comparative trial indicated that carbamazepine was as effective as oxazepam in relieving the symptoms of moderate to severe alcohol withdrawal (Malcolm et al, 1989), and this and another study (Agricola et al, 1982) found that carbamazepine was more effective in reducing associated psychiatric symptoms. Further comparative studies of carbamazepine are warranted, particularly in individuals with coexisting psychiatric disorders.

Delirium tremens is a medical emergency. Management includes monitoring of vital signs, correction of fluid and electrolyte imbalances, and medication to control the agitation and delirium. Intravenous diazepam in a dose of 10 mg initially, followed by 5 mg every five minutes, may be necessary to achieve rapid sedation. If the patient does not become calm within 30 minutes, the dose of diazepam can be increased progressively. When sedation is achieved, the patient can be maintained on oral diazepam or chlordiazepoxide in the amount necessary to maintain mild sedation. Neuroleptic agents may be required to control perceptual disturbances, thought disorders, or severe agitation. Haloperidol usually is the drug of choice because it causes less sedation and hypotension.

Lidocaine [Xylocaine] or intravenous procainamide [Procan, Pronestyl] may be needed to treat arrhythmias; propranolol [Inderal] also is useful and may be especially effective for uncontrolled, severe tremor.

Rehabilitation: In the long-term management of alcoholic patients, pharmacotherapy is much less important than counseling of the patient and family and a program of rehabilitation (Whitfield, 1988). It is important to make an early diagnosis and focus on the process by which the patient achieves control over drinking. Rehabilitation encompasses all activities designed to change the pattern of excessive alcohol consumption and prevent relapse. It includes the development of an individualized treatment strategy (evaluation and assessment) aimed at eliminating or reducing alcohol consumption, as well as primary and extended care (Institute of Medicine, 1990). In most studies, no significant differences between inpatient and outpatient programs have been identified. However, in one randomized trial of treatment options in alcohol abusers, inpatient treatment was more effective in reducing drinking and other drug use (Walsh et al, 1991). The earlier the diagnosis is made and intervention begins, the better the prognosis for recovery; people do not have to "hit bottom" before they can accept help.

The physician who is already known and trusted by the patient has an advantage in eliciting and understanding the history, helping the patient recognize the problem, encouraging some patients to begin specialized treatment, and providing ongoing support. A range of options from single questions (eg, Do you drink now and then? When was your last drink?) to brief (eg, CAGE [Ewing, 1984]) or multi-item (eg, Michigan Alcoholism Screening Test [MAST]) questionnaires (Selzer, 1971) can help identify patients with alcohol problems (most of the latter tests are designed to identify individuals with severe problems). The CAGE questionnaire consists of the following four questions and can be easily incorporated into the patient interview: Have you ever: (1) thought about Cutting down? (2) felt Annoyed when others criticize your drinking? (3) felt bad or Guilty about drinking? (4) used alcohol in the morning to steady your nerves or get rid of a hangover (Eye opener)? Two affirmative responses are suggested as constituting a positive indication of alcohol abuse or dependence. Although patients cannot be divided into "either/or" groups because alcohol-related problems actually lie along a continuum of severity, the CAGE test is remarkably accurate in identifying outpatients with alcohol abuse or dependence as defined by *DSM-III-R* criteria.

In the majority of patients, the drinking problem is not severe. Many individuals either do not require intensive, specialized treatment or would not accept referral for such treatment but can benefit from the physician's encouragement to reduce or eliminate alcohol consumption (Wallace et al, 1988). The brief intervention can be accomplished in several ways (see Babor et al, 1986; Institute of Medicine, 1990).

The most severely affected patients may have the greatest difficulty confronting their problem. Many have tried to quit repeatedly, without success. Because these individuals are often highly sensitive to rebuff, it is important that physicians accept them with the same concern they would give patients suffering from any chronic disease, accept relapses, and encourage continuation of treatment. Relapse prevention includes support of activities designed to maintain therapeutic gains achieved through intervention and avoid a return to previous drinking patterns. Continued patient and family contact with the primary care physician can be an important stabilizing force while the alcoholic is receiving specialized care.

Cognitive/behavioral models for relapse prevention have been described but not extensively tested (Marlatt and Gordon, 1985; Annis, 1986; Littman, 1986). Other relapse prevention strategies have been publicized, and training programs are available for practitioners (Gorski, 1986). Relapse prevention strategies are an integral part of Alcoholics Anonymous, the major nonmedical referral resource available to patients. Al-Anon and Alateen are self-help groups for spouses and adolescents. Finally, disulfiram [Antabuse] may be used for one to two months as an adjunct to behavior modification or psychotherapy.

Alcohol-Sensitizing Drugs: The interaction between alcohol and disulfiram can be used therapeutically to control alcohol intake. The threatened or actual occurrence of a severe, unpleasant physiologic response to alcohol after disulfiram has been ingested may condition behavior to the avoidance of alcohol consumption; however, the efficacy of this approach to improve behavioral or medical problems is questionable (Peachey and Naranjo, 1984). Some investigators (Fuller et al, 1986) have concluded that disulfiram may help reduce drinking frequency after relapse in a minority of alcoholics, but it does not enhance counseling or delay the resumption of drinking.

Disulfiram or calcium carbimide (not available in the United States) produce an aversive effect by inhibiting the conversion of acetaldehyde, a metabolite of alcohol, to acetic acid by aldehyde dehydrogenase. Elevation of blood acetaldehyde concentrations is believed to cause the aversive effect. The enzymatic inhibition produced by disulfiram is irreversible and, thus, persists longer than that produced by calcium carbimide. Compared with disulfiram, calcium carbimide's side effects appear to be less frequent and less severe. Use of alcohol-sensitizing drugs should be restricted to recovering alcoholics who clearly seek abstinence, wish to take one of these drugs, and have no illnesses that preclude their use (Peachey and Naranjo, 1984) (see evaluation on Disulfiram).

Metronidazole [Flagyl, Protostat], procarbazine [Matulane], monoamine oxidase inhibitors, chloramphenicol, certain cephalosporins, quinacrine [Atabrine], furazolidone [Furoxone], and chlorpropamide [Diabinese] have been reported to produce mild disulfiram-like actions when alcohol is ingested. Controlled studies have not substantiated this finding for metronidazole. Further, acetaldehyde blood levels are not always significantly elevated following use of alcohol and chlorpropamide. Flushing as a result of a chlorpropamide-alcohol interaction may be a genetic marker for noninsulin-dependent diabetes even before the onset of glucose intolerance (Hansten, 1981). The disulfiram-like reactions produced by these drugs are considered to be of minor significance, since they are much less severe than disulfiram-alcohol and calcium carbimide-alcohol reactions.

Drug Evaluation

DISULFIRAM

[Antabuse]

ACTIONS AND USES. Disulfiram, a thiuram derivative, interferes with the conversion of acetaldehyde to acetic acid by aldehyde dehydrogenase (Eneanya et al, 1981). When taken with alcohol, this drug increases the blood acetaldehyde concentration and produces several uncomfortable symptoms. The unpleasantness of this interaction is the basis for disulfiram's adjunctive use to decrease alcohol consumption.

Although some controlled clinical trials support the short-term effectiveness of disulfiram when employed with behavioral and psychological counseling, the drug's efficacy in the long-term treatment of chronic alcoholism has not been established (Sellers et al, 1981; Fuller et al, 1986), and compliance with long-term therapy is a major problem. Supervised, voluntary short-term use of the drug in outpatients probably reduces alcohol consumption and improves behavior (American College of Physicians, 1989). There is no evidence that use of disulfiram without accompanying education, counseling, therapy, or rehabilitation is beneficial (American College of Physicians, 1989).

The alcohol-disulfiram reaction usually is manifested by flushing, dyspnea, nausea, thirst, abdominal or chest pain, palpitation, and vertigo; hyperventilation, tachycardia, vomiting, hyperhidrosis, hypotension, syncope, and confusion also may occur. Blood pressure can fall to shock level. The reaction lasts 30 minutes to several hours, and drowsiness and sleep follow. The intensity of the reaction varies among individuals but generally is proportional to the amount of alcohol ingested, the dose of disulfiram, and the time elapsed since its administration.

The true incidence of mild reactions is a subject of controversy (Gragg, 1982). Severe reactions, which include respiratory depression, acute circulatory failure, arrhythmias, myocardial infarction, acute congestive heart failure, syncope, and convulsions, may be fatal. During severe reactions, individuals should be treated as for shock (see index entry Shock). Inhalation of 95% oxygen with 5% carbon dioxide, as well as other symptomatic treatment, may be useful. The serum potassium level should be monitored and maintained, particularly in patients receiving digitalis, since hypokalemia has been reported. Aldehyde dehydrogenase activity generally returns to normal in about one week (but may take two weeks or more) after termination of disulfiram therapy. Patients should be advised not to ingest alcohol during this period and warned about the accidental consumption of alcohol in unexpected forms (see Precautions).

ADVERSE REACTIONS. In the absence of alcohol, disulfiram may cause transient mild drowsiness, fatigue, impotence, headache, acneiform eruptions, allergic dermatitis, or a metallic or garlic-like aftertaste, especially during the first two weeks of therapy. These effects usually disappear spontaneously with continued therapy, but sometimes dosage reduction is required.

Psychotic reactions or mood disorders (eg, severe depression, mania) have been noted rarely. Polyneuropathy, peripheral neuritis, and, rarely, optic neuropathy also have occurred. These reactions may be caused by carbon disulfide, a metabolite of disulfiram.

Disulfiram has been reported to be hepatotoxic in a few patients (Mason, 1989). A latent period of 2 to 25 weeks may elapse before symptoms of liver disease occur. Hepatotoxicity may be masked by the natural tendency to attribute any hepatic impairment to alcohol.

PRECAUTIONS. Disulfiram should be used cautiously in patients with diabetes mellitus, hypothyroidism, epilepsy, cerebral damage, chronic or acute nephritis, severe hepatic cirrhosis or insufficiency, and during pregnancy. It is contraindicated in patients with symptomatic ischemic heart disease, coronary thrombosis, psychosis, neuropathy, or hypersensitivity and in those recently treated with paraldehyde or who have a measurable blood alcohol concentration due to recent ingestion of alcohol or an alcohol-containing product (eg, foods, elixirs, cough syrups). Lotions with a high alcohol content that are liberally applied topically also should be used cautiously. Before treatment commences, the patient and the patient's family or social support network should be fully informed of the purpose, procedure, and consequences of disulfiram administration. It may be advisable for those undergoing treatment with this agent to carry identification cards describing the most common symptoms of the disulfiram-alcohol reaction and designating the attending physician. (Identification cards may be obtained from the manufacturer.)

DRUG INTERACTIONS. Disulfiram inhibits the metabolism of several drugs other than alcohol, and the consequences should be borne in mind. In particular, toxic levels of phenytoin, warfarin, isoniazid, rifampin, theophylline, and benzodiazepines with active long-acting metabolites (eg, clorazepate, diazepam, flurazepam, chlordiazepoxide, halazepam, prazepam) may accumulate when disulfiram is given concomitantly. It may be necessary to adjust the dosage of such drugs during or on discontinuation of disulfiram therapy.

PHARMACOKINETICS. With oral administration, 70% to 90% of a dose is absorbed rapidly, and the time to peak serum concentration is one to two hours. Disulfiram first is reduced rapidly to diethyldithiocarbamate, which is methylated, glucuronidated, or sulfated and undergoes oxidation to diethylamine and carbon disulfide. Half-life data are unavailable for most metabolites; however, the inhibition of aldehyde dehydrogenase by disulfiram develops slowly over 12 hours and is irreversible. The duration of action is the six days or more required for resynthesis of the enzyme.

DOSAGE AND PREPARATIONS. When initiating disulfiram therapy, the patient must not have significant withdrawal signs and symptoms and should not have a measurable blood alcohol content; abstention from alcohol generally is required for at least 12 hours before disulfiram treatment is begun.

Oral: *Adults,* initially, 250 mg daily (maximum, 500 mg daily) as a loading dose for one week. For maintenance, 250 mg daily (range, 125 to a maximum of 500 mg) is given for months to years, depending on the individual. However, because of potential hepatotoxicity, the presence of the carbon disulfide metabolite, and unproved efficacy, administration for more than two months should be undertaken with caution. Liver enzymes should be monitored periodically during long-term therapy.

Antabuse (Wyeth-Ayerst), ***Generic.*** Tablets 250 and 500 mg.

CIGARETTE SMOKING

Although the prevalence of smoking is declining (Pierce et al, 1989), perhaps due to educational efforts and increasing restrictions on tobacco use in public and in the workplace, it is estimated that almost 50 million Americans still smoke cigarettes (*MMWR*, 1992). Three of every five smokers have tried to quit, and nine of ten smokers say they want to quit (Richmond, 1983). Only one in ten smokers have five or fewer cigarettes daily. Most heavy smokers are physically dependent on nicotine and psychologically dependent on the behavior of smoking (US Department of Health and Human Services, 1988).

Properties of Nicotine

Nicotine activates acetylcholine (nicotinic) receptors. The brain, sympathetic ganglia, peripheral chemoreceptors, and adrenal medulla are affected by the plasma concentrations of nicotine typically produced by cigarette smoking. The central effects of nicotine are critical for maintaining the behavior of cigarette smoking (US Department of Health and Human Services, 1988). The pharmacologic response is dose dependent and is modified by the development of tolerance. Initial exposure to nicotine typically causes nausea and dizziness. The sympathetic nervous system is activated through a combination of central and peripheral effects, including the release of adrenal catecholamines. The result is an increase in heart rate, cardiac output, and skeletal muscle blood flow; cutaneous vessels are constricted and the venous circulation is decreased. Salivary and bronchial secretions are stimulated initially but later are inhibited. Nicotine causes tremor and respiratory stimulation, and toxic doses (eg, ingestion of nicotine-containing pesticides or tobacco products) may cause seizures and respiratory arrest.

Tolerance to nausea and cardiovascular effects develops rapidly, and a lower degree of cardiovascular stimulation is apparent in chronic smokers. The heart rate and blood pressure may increase when the first few cigarettes of the day are smoked. The average heart rate is five to seven beats/min higher in smokers, but blood pressure in smokers is comparable to or lower than that in nonsmokers (Green et al, 1986). Modulation of neuroendocrine function (eg, release of vasopressin, beta-endorphin, and cortisol) also may contribute to the effects of nicotine (Seyler et al, 1986). Nicotine appears to suppress appetite and increase energy expenditure both at rest and during exercise (Perkins et al, 1989).

PHARMACOKINETICS. Nicotine is absorbed readily from the respiratory tract, buccal mucosa, and skin. After oral administration, it is absorbed largely from the intestine. Pulmonary absorption after inhalation of cigarette smoke is rapid.

Nicotine is metabolized primarily in the liver; pulmonary metabolism occurs to a limited extent. The major metabolites excreted in urine are cotinine and *trans*-3-hydroxycotinine; they cause little or no cardiovascular or subjective effects. Alkalization of the urine decreases the renal excretion of these metabolites; acidification increases the proportion of nicotine that is excreted unchanged. Because the half-life of cotinine (15 to 20 hours) is considerably longer than that of nicotine (about two hours), it has been used as an index of exposure to nicotine.

CIGARETTE SMOKING DURING PREGNANCY. Smoking during pregnancy decreases birth weight and increases the risk of abortion, premature birth, and stillbirth. Fetal breathing time is decreased. At present, there is no definitive evidence that cigarette smoking during pregnancy produces congenital malformations, although results of some studies suggest that the risk is increased (US Department of Health and Human Services, 1989). Nicotine is excreted in breast milk.

DRUG INTERACTIONS. Cigarette smoking can alter the pharmacokinetics and activity of many drugs. The mechanism of such interactions usually is induction of liver microsomal enzyme activity by the polycyclic hydrocarbons in cigarette smoke. This enzyme induction differs qualitatively and quantitatively from that produced by phenobarbital.

Compared with nonsmokers, smokers tend to have lower blood concentrations after administration of theophylline; pentazocine; propranolol; propoxyphene; imipramine and other tricyclic antidepressants; haloperidol and phenothiazines; and desmethyldiazepam, the active metabolite of several benzodiazepines. The hemodynamic effects of nicotine, including nicotine derived from replacement therapies, may result in impairment of the subcutaneous absorption of insulin and of the antihypertensive and antianginal effects of beta blockers and nifedipine. Blood coagulates more easily in smokers; consequently, smoking increases the potential for serious adverse effects in women taking oral contraceptives (see index entry Contraceptives, Oral) and may inhibit the anticoagulant effect of heparin. Sedative or analgesic effects of drugs also may be diminished.

Chronic Cigarette Smoking

Nicotine dependence is considered a psychoactive substance use disorder in *DSM-III-R* (American Psychiatric Association, 1987). Most commonly, nicotine dependence is associated with cigarette smoking. The use of chewing tobacco or snuff, cigar or pipe smoking, and long-term use of nicotine gum also are associated with dependence. Because nicotine does not cause intoxication akin to that produced by alcohol, there is little impairment of occupational or social function. Nevertheless, because of persistent withdrawal symptoms, some people with nicotine dependence have difficulty remaining in either occupational or social situations in which smoking is prohibited.

Chronic cigarette smoking is a major cause of coronary artery disease and arteriosclerotic peripheral vascular disease. It is a causative factor in cancer of the lung, mouth, larynx, and esophagus and is a contributory factor in cancer of the bladder, pancreas, and kidney. The premature mortality rate in smokers is greater than 25% (Mattson et al, 1987). Approximately 90% of cases of chronic bronchitis and emphysema are caused by cigarette smoking (US Department of Health, Education and Welfare, 1979).

TOLERANCE AND PHYSICAL DEPENDENCE. The dizziness, nausea, and vomiting that often are reported by first-time users do not occur in experienced smokers. This is in part due to the tobacco user learning to regulate the intake of nicotine and avoid such effects. In addition, a considerable degree of tolerance develops to some of the effects of nicotine. Such tolerance probably is pharmacodynamic in nature.

The severity of nicotine dependence is demonstrated by the low success rate (<10%) of any given attempt to stop smoking; however, after repeated attempts, 40% to 45% of smokers eventually stop (US Department of Health and Human Services, 1990).

Physical dependence on nicotine is manifested by the rapid onset of a withdrawal syndrome after abrupt cessation or marked reduction in the use of nicotine-containing substances. Nicotine withdrawal is considered an organic mental disorder (American Psychiatric Association, 1987). Diagnosis is usually self-evident based on a history of tobacco use and the disappearance of symptoms when smoking is resumed. The diagnostic criteria for nicotine withdrawal include the daily use of nicotine for at least several weeks and the occurrence within 24 hours (sometimes as soon as six hours) following discontinuation of smoking of at least four of the following signs: craving for nicotine; irritability, frustration, or anger; anxiety; difficulty concentrating; restlessness; decreased heart rate; increased appetite. Impairment in cognitive performance may occur within four hours of smoking cessation and persist for several days. Other symptoms may include impatience, insomnia, and physical complaints. Most of the withdrawal symptoms peak within four days and resolve within four weeks, but increased appetite and craving for nicotine may persist for months (Hughes, 1992). In one study, 21% of former smokers reported craving cigarettes at least intermittently five to nine years after cessation (Jarvik, 1979). Major weight gain (eg, >25 lb) occurs in approximately 10% of individuals who quit smoking for at least one year (Williamson et al, 1991). The role withdrawal symptoms play in smoking relapse has not been established (Hughes et al, 1991 A).

Nicotine intake, whether measured by plasma cotinine level or by number of cigarettes smoked, is a determinant of the severity of nicotine withdrawal symptoms, difficulty in discontinuing smoking, and the total daily dose level of nicotine required in replacement therapy (Killen et al, 1988; US Department of Health and Human Services, 1988). Sex, age at smoking initiation, length of smoking history, cigarette nicotine concentration, and number of attempts to quit smoking do not appear to be related to severity of withdrawal symptoms. In addition to quantity of cigarettes smoked per day, the score on the Fagerström Tolerance Questionnaire may be helpful to predict severity of withdrawal effects (Fagerström and Schneider, 1989; Sachs, 1991).

Both tolerance to the adverse effects of cigarette smoking and physical dependence on nicotine contribute to maintenance of the smoking behavior. Physical dependence also appears to be a significant obstacle to achievement of short-term abstinence after cessation of smoking (US Department of Health and Human Services, 1990).

TREATMENT. Long-term cessation of smoking requires mastery of both the short-term and residual effects of the psychological and physical dependence that contribute to preservation of the addiction. A variety of techniques, including counseling programs, educational campaigns, proprietary or public service clinics, hypnosis, sensory deprivation, behavior modification, and aversion therapy, have achieved modest success in producing long-term abstinence. These techniques have been reviewed elsewhere (US Department of Health and Human Services, 1988; Sachs, 1991).

Most cigarette smokers try to quit on their own. However, the vast majority of these individuals fail; those who succeed tend to be less dependent and are aided by circumstances, such as smoking-related disease or workplace restrictions, or are encouraged by a friend's or spouse's success in quitting (US Department of Health and Human Services, 1990). Physician advice, including the personalization of risks, is a key element in motivation (Fiore et al, 1990). Physicians should take a brief smoking history (eg, how long and how much the patient has smoked, when and how the patient has tried to quit), explicitly advise the smoker to stop, and determine if the patient would like to quit smoking. A firm quit date should be agreed on for those who are sufficiently motivated, and follow-up consultation to promote continued abstention should be provided. A manual (Glynn and Manley, 1989) that explains an effective protocol and provides educational support materials for patients is available from the National Cancer Institute at no charge (1-800/422-6237).

Pharmacologic intervention (eg, nicotine gum [nicotine polacrilex] [Nicorette], transdermal nicotine [Habitrol, Nicoderm, Nicotrol, Prostep]) in conjunction with behavioral intervention and training for relapse prevention can substantially contribute to success (for reviews see Covey and Glassman, 1990; Hughes, 1991; Fiore et al, 1992). The adjunctive use of antidepressants and sedative-hypnotics has not been shown to be an effective aid in achieving success. One-year cessation rates average 30%, but the rates vary considerably in the reported trials. Typically, those achieved with combined treatment strategies that include nicotine replacement are approximately double those achieved with placebo. Nicotine replacement therapy may be particularly effective in smokers who score high on a dependence scale. The transdermal nicotine system is easier to use and may enhance patient compliance. Use of the gum requires specialized instructions and is more difficult, but it can be employed as needed in acute, high-stress situations to enhance coping responses that may prevent relapse.

Nicotine Gum: Use of nicotine gum without behavioral skills training has had only limited benefit in patients seen in general practice (Lam et al, 1987; Hughes et al, 1989), and relapse rates are higher than in specialized smoking clinics (Goldstein et al, 1989).

Use of nicotine polacrilex substitutes a much less hazardous vehicle and route of administration (eg, chewing gum with buccal absorption) for more dangerous ones (eg, inhalation of cigarette smoke including chemical and particulate matter). Venous blood concentrations of nicotine generally are lower with the gum than with smoking but are sufficient to reduce withdrawal symptoms. Craving is not consistently reduced; however, by reducing withdrawal symptoms, use of the gum may enable the patient to focus on behavioral aspects of the dependence. As coping mechanisms develop and the urge to smoke diminishes, patients gradually reduce the number of pieces of gum chewed each day. Gradual withdrawal from nicotine gum should be initiated within two to three months.

Transdermal Nicotine: With the transdermal nicotine patch, the average plasma nicotine concentration is lower than that produced by smoking; however, patches that deliver a 21- or 22-mg dose produce concentrations similar to trough concentrations of serum nicotine in moderate to heavy smokers (Mulligan et al, 1990; Benowitz et al, 1991).

The short-term success rates of smoking cessation with use of the nicotine patch vary depending on the population, how abstinence and "success" are defined, adjuvant interventions, length of follow-up, and dose/duration of therapy (Fiore et al, 1992). Unlike nicotine gum, effective use of transdermal nicotine appears to require only brief advice (Abelin et al, 1989; Hurt et al, 1990; Sachs, 1991; Tønnesen et al, 1991). In four placebo-controlled trials that lasted 4 to 12 weeks and lacked (or used only brief) behavioral intervention, 39% to 77% of the transdermal nicotine recipients remained abstinent compared with 10% to 39% of those in the placebo group (Abelin et al, 1989; Hurt et al, 1990; Daughton et al, 1991; Tønnesen et al, 1991). In studies that employed more extensive behavioral intervention, higher cessation rates were achieved at six weeks (47% to 77%) compared with placebo (15% to 27%) (Transdermal Nicotine Study Group, 1991; Buchkremer et al, 1991; Mulligan et al, 1990).

As with other smoking cessation therapy, there is a decline in long-term efficacy. Overall success rates at six months (22% to 42%) are lower than those noted shortly after patch treatment is discontinued but still are significantly better than those achieved by placebo users (2% to 28%) (Abelin et al, 1989; Tønnesen et al, 1991; Transdermal Nicotine Study Group, 1991; Hurt et al, 1990; Daughton et al, 1991).

Use of transdermal nicotine has been associated with reduction in craving in most studies. In heavy smokers, amelioration of withdrawal symptoms has been reported (Rose et al, 1990). In a recent study, combined use of nicotine gum and nicotine patches decreased withdrawal symptoms more than use of the patch alone (Fagerström et al, in press).

Transdermal Clonidine: Clonidine [Catapres] also has been evaluated in several clinical trials of smoking cessation. Short-term cessation was reported in six of nine controlled trials (including two with six-month follow-up) using oral or transdermal patch preparations (Covey and Glassman, 1990). However, in the most recent study, use of the transdermal patch for six weeks (accompanied by only minimal behavioral intervention) did not increase the smoking cessation rate (Prochazka et al, 1992). Clonidine appears to relieve irritability, anxiety, restlessness, and, in some subjects, craving when abstinence is attempted (Ornis et al, 1988; Prochazka et al, 1992). However, it may worsen the difficulty in concentration often associated with smoking cessation. A meta-analysis of double-blind, placebo-controlled trials showed that the early cessation rate was significantly greater with clonidine than with placebo (Covey and Glassman, 1991).

In contrast to nicotine replacement therapy, use of clonidine is preferably initiated before cessation of smoking. Low oral doses (eg, 0.1 mg daily) are prescribed initially, and the amount is increased to 0.2 to 0.4 mg daily before the planned date of quitting. Transdermal clonidine patches have been used in a similar manner. Gradual increase in dosage may enable the patient to adapt to side effects (eg, sedation); however, adverse effects still may be the limiting factor in the use of clonidine for this indication. A typical pattern of use involves four weeks of clonidine therapy followed by gradual tapering of dose over the next eight weeks. Like nicotine gum, it is most effective with concomitant behavioral support.

Drug Evaluations

NICOTINE POLACRILEX (Nicotine Resin Complex)

[Nicorette]

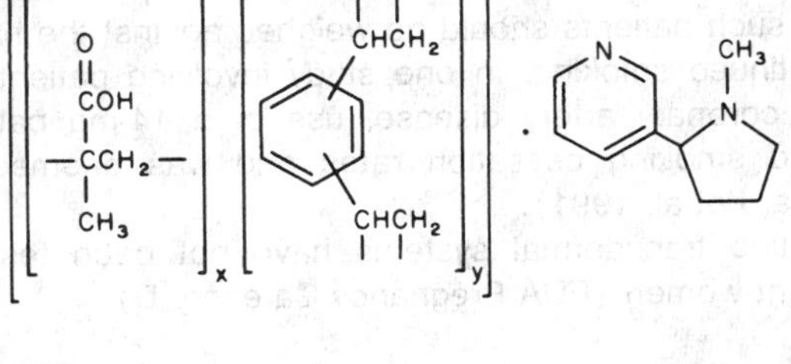

Nicotine polacrilex (gum) is of therapeutic value as an adjunct to behavioral or psychological therapy for smokers who are physically dependent on nicotine and wish to quit smoking. Use of the gum reduces many withdrawal symptoms but does not alleviate all of them, especially craving. Weight gain may be reduced. The degree of reduction of withdrawal signs and symptoms is directly related to the dose actually delivered; improper use or inadequate dosage may yield no beneficial effect.

ADVERSE REACTIONS AND PRECAUTIONS. Adverse effects associated with use of nicotine polacrilex gum generally are mild and transient. Gastrointestinal and central nervous system disturbances and effects related to chewing and absorption (ie, traumatic injury to oral mucosa or teeth, jaw muscle ache, eructation secondary to air swallowing) are most prevalent. In clinical trials in the United States, nonspecific gastrointestinal distress was reported in 10% and nausea or vomiting in 10% to 18% of patients. Soreness in the mouth (including ulcers) and throat has been reported in about 37% of patients. Jaw muscle ache and hiccups were noted in 18% and 15% of patients, respectively. Lightheadedness, insomnia, irritability, and headache occur in less than 2% of individuals. Anorexia and excessive salivation also are noted in a small percentage of patients. Other reactions are characteristic of those associated with smoking.

Abuse potential is minimal. However, it should be kept in mind that use of the gum can maintain the patient's physical dependence on nicotine, and a few patients may have difficulty discontinuing the gum. After one year, 7% to 9% of patients are still using nicotine gum; after two years, approximately 3% persist in its use (Hughes, 1988). In two studies, 17% to 25% of abstinent smokers were long-term users of nicotine gum (Hajek et al, 1988; Hughes et al, 1991 B). In terms of health consequences, prolonged use of the gum still represents a vast improvement over smoking. Withdrawal from gum use generally can be accomplished over a period of several months by decreasing the daily dose by one piece of gum every four to seven days (or as tolerated by the patient without development of an intolerable desire to resume smoking). Alternatively, the amount of time each piece of gum is chewed can be decreased (eg, from 30 to 15 minutes) or sugarless gum can be substituted with increasing frequency.

The use of nicotine gum is contraindicated in nonsmokers, during the immediate postmyocardial infarction period, in those with life-threatening arrhythmias, in patients with severe or worsening angina pectoris, in those with active temporomandibular joint disease, and during pregnancy (FDA Pregnancy Category C).

Caution should be exercised when the gum is used by patients with coronary artery disease, hypertension, vasospastic diseases, hyperthyroidism, pheochromocytoma, insulin-dependent diabetes, and peptic ulcer, but the risk of continued smoking also should be considered when deciding whether to prescribe the gum. It should be used cautiously in patients with oral or pharyngeal inflammation, a history of esophagitis, or dental problems that may be exacerbated by chewing gum. During lactation, consideration should be given to discontinuing either the nursing or the gum after evaluation of the risk to the infant and the benefit derived by the mother.

POISONING. The minimal oral lethal dose of nicotine is approximately 40 to 60 mg (MacArthur and Williams, 1983). However, the likelihood of overdose by accidental swallowing of the gum is small.

Two factors prevent serious adverse sequelae following oral overdose: First, the nicotine in the gum is bound to an ion exchange resin and is released only during chewing. Second, nicotine absorbed from the gastrointestinal tract is largely inactivated by gastric acid and the microsomal enzyme system on first pass through the liver. Notwithstanding this, the patient should be instructed to contact a physician or the local poison control center immediately in case of accidental overdose or if a child chews or swallows one or more pieces of the gum.

PHARMACOKINETICS. The nicotine in the gum is bound to an ion exchange resin, and the gum must be chewed to release nicotine. After release, absorption of nicotine through the buccal mucosa depends on the oral pH. The gum contains a bicarbonate/carbonate buffer that raises the oral pH to about 8.0; therefore, absorption is significantly increased. Chewing sugar-containing gum or consuming acidic beverages (eg, coffee, carbonated soft drinks) immediately prior to or during use of nicotine polacrilex may block the buffering action of polacrilex and reduce nicotine absorption. Attainment of effective blood concentrations of nicotine depends on proper use of the gum. In one study, chewing one piece of gum containing 2 mg of nicotine for one hour produced a mean steady-state plasma nicotine level of 11.8 ng/ml. This compared with a mean plasma nicotine trough concentration of 15.7 ng/ml during usual smoking.

DOSAGE AND PREPARATIONS. The patient must be motivated to give up smoking and should be instructed to stop smoking immediately prior to initiation of therapy.

Buccal: The gum should be chewed slowly. Patients should stop chewing when they experience a peppery taste or slight tingling, at which point the gum is stored between the cheek and gum. Chewing is resumed when the taste or tingling almost ceases (usually after about one minute). The cycle is repeated until most of the nicotine is released (after about 30 minutes). The gum should be placed in a different part of the mouth after each cycle. Although usually used as needed, the gum may be prescribed by number of pieces per day according to a fixed time interval (eg, one piece per hour) and tailored to the number of cigarettes normally smoked. Preliminary results suggest that use of the gum at fixed intervals may increase efficacy (Sachs, 1991). Patients should be instructed not to exceed 30 2-mg pieces or 20 4-mg pieces per day. Use for more than six months is not recommended, except when relapse to smoking appears likely if the prescription for gum is withheld.

Nicorette (Marion Merrell Dow). Chewing gum containing 2 or 4 mg (***Nicorette DS***) nicotine (as resin complex) per square (sugar-free).

NICOTINE TRANSDERMAL SYSTEMS

[Habitrol, Nicoderm, Nicotrol, Prostep]

Nicotine transdermal systems are effective as an adjunct to brief physician advice or behavioral/psychological therapy for smokers who are physically dependent on nicotine and wish to stop smoking. Use of a transdermal system has been reported to reduce some withdrawal symptoms including craving. Although studies have not been conducted, transdermal nicotine also may be of value as an adjunct to alleviate acute nicotine withdrawal symptoms in hospitalized patients when such symptoms may exacerbate the patient's illness (Fiore et al, 1992). Use of the patches does not appear to significantly affect the weight gain frequently observed following smoking cessation (Palmer et al, 1992). Three brands of the patches marketed for use in the United States [Habitrol, Nicoderm, Prostep] are designed for 24-hour delivery of nicotine; steady-state plasma concentrations are achieved after about three days of use. The fourth brand [Nicotrol] is designed for 16-hour application and is removed prior to bedtime. Nicotine-induced sleep disturbances may occur more frequently with the 24-hour patches; however, early morning craving for cigarettes may be lessened with use of these patches compared with the 16-hour patches.

ADVERSE EFFECTS AND PRECAUTIONS. Adverse effects associated with use of nicotine transdermal systems generally are mild. However, assessment of these effects is complicated by overlap in symptoms that may be attributable to either nicotine replacement (ie, excess) or nicotine withdrawal. In clinical trials, the most common side effect was minor local skin irritation reported in 37% to 54% of patients. Local erythema and edema also may be noted after system removal; contact sensitization occurs in 2% to 3% of patients. In clinical trials, therapy was discontinued because of skin reactions more frequently with use of Prostep (7%) and Habitrol (6%) than with Nicoderm (2%) and Nicotrol (1%). In clinical trials, 1% to 23% of patients reported mild to moderate insomnia and 1% to 9% reported abnormal dreaming (Fiore et al, 1992). Other side effects noted more frequently in patch than in placebo users were dizziness, arthralgia, sweating, abdominal pain, somnolence, sweating, diarrhea, dyspepsia, myalgia, and nervousness.

The use of transdermal nicotine is contraindicated in nonsmokers, during the immediate postmyocardial infarction period, in those with severe arrhythmias, and in patients with severe or worsening angina pectoris. Although nicotine may aggravate certain other pre-existing conditions (eg, coronary artery disease, peripheral vascular disease, hyperthyroidism, pheochromocytoma, insulin-dependent diabetes, peptic ulcer disease, hypertension), the use of nicotine replacement therapy in such patients should be weighed against the hazards of continued smoking. In one study involving patients with stable coronary artery disease, use of a 14-mg patch increased smoking cessation rates and was deemed safe (Rennard et al, 1991).

Nicotine transdermal systems have not been tested in pregnant women (FDA Pregnancy Category D).

TABLE 1.
STEADY-STATE PHARMACOKINETIC DATA FOR NICOTINE TRANSDERMAL SYSTEMS

Product Name	Duration (hrs)	Delivered Dose (mg)	C_{max} (ng/ml)	C_{avg} (ng/ml)	C_{min} (ng/ml)	T_{max} (hrs)
Habitrol	24	21	17	13	9	6
	24	14	12	9	6	5
Nicoderm	24	21	23	17	11	4
	24	14	17	12	7	4
	24	7	8	6	4	4
Prostep	24	22	16	11	5	9
Nicotrol	16	15	13	9.4	2.5	8
	16	10	6.9	4.9	1.4	9

C_{max} = mean observed peak plasma concentration
C_{avg} = average plasma concentration
C_{min} = minimum observed plasma concentration
T_{max} = time of maximum plasma concentration

PHARMACOKINETICS. See Table 1 for a summary of pharmacokinetic data reported by the manufacturers. Plasma nicotine concentrations are proportional to dose. Depending on the product, peak plasma concentrations are achieved within four to nine hours and decline slowly during the remaining time that the patch is in place; steady-state concentrations are achieved within two days. Following patch removal, plasma nicotine concentrations decline gradually (apparent half-life, three to four hours) due to release of residual nicotine from the skin. No significant skin metabolism occurs.

DOSAGE AND PREPARATIONS. Patients should be advised to stop smoking immediately prior to application of the nicotine patch and to read the instruction sheet that accompanies the product.

Topical: A summary of the manufacturers recommended dosing schedule appears in Table 2.

A recent review that considered outcome rates in long- and short-term clinical trials concluded that there was little basis for empirical use of nicotine patch therapy beyond six to eight weeks. Because different dosage regimens and durations of patch use have not been extensively tested, individualization of therapy may be beneficial (see Fiore et al, 1992).

Habitrol (Basel), ***Nicoderm*** (Marion Merrell Dow). Nicotine transdermal system providing systemic delivery of 21, 14, or 7 mg/24 hours.

Prostep (Lederle). Nicotine transdermal system providing systemic delivery of 22 or 11 mg/24 hours.

Nicotrol (Parke-Davis). Nicotine transdermal system providing systemic delivery of 15, 10, or 5 mg/16 hours.

DEMENTIA

In dementia, cognitive impairment is multifaceted and typically involves memory, language, and reasoning. In many dementing disorders, behavioral disturbances also are present. Dementia is classified as a subset of organic mental syndromes (American Psychiatric Association, 1987).

TABLE 2.
RECOMMENDED DOSING SCHEDULE FOR NICOTINE TRANSDERMAL SYSTEMS

Trade Name	Patch Duration	Dosing Schedule (mg/day)		Reduced Dosing Schedule[1] (mg/day)	
Habitrol	24 hrs	21 mg:	4-8 wks	14 mg:	4-8 wks
		14 mg:	2-4 wks	7 mg:	2-4 wks
		7 mg:	2-4 wks		
Nicoderm	24 hrs	21 mg:	6 wks	14 mg:	6 wks
		14 mg:	2 wks	7 mg:	2-4 wks
		7 mg:	2 wks		
Prostep	24 hrs	22 mg:	4-8 wks	11 mg:	4-8 wks
		11 mg:	2-4 wks		
Nicotrol	16 hrs	15 mg:	4-12 wks	10 mg[2]	
		10 mg:	2-4 wks		
		5 mg:	2-4 wks		

[1] *Patients with cardiovascular disease, weighing less than 100 pounds, or smoking fewer than 10 cigarettes daily.*
[2] *If patient has signs or symptoms suggesting nicotine excess, the 10 mg/day system may be tried.*

About one-half to two-thirds of all cases of dementia are due to Alzheimer's disease. Multi-infarct dementia is the next most common type, followed by dementia associated with Parkinson's disease. Pick's disease, a frontal lobe degenerative syndrome with dementia, is rare. The estimated prevalence of dementia has varied; however, it does increase dramatically with advancing age. According to some estimates, 3.5% of all persons over age 65 may be demented; among those over age 85, the prevalence is 20% to 30% (Kokmen et al, 1989; Skoog et al, 1993). Other studies suggest that the prevalence of the condition may be much higher, possibly affecting up to 50% of those 85 years or older (Evans et al, 1989). Potentially reversible causes of dementia occur in approximately 20% of patients and include depression, infection, neoplasm, subdural hematoma, substance abuse or drug toxicity, trauma, nutritional or thyroid deficiency, and normal pressure hydrocephalus. Thus, accurate diagnosis of the cause of dementia is critical.

Dementia is associated in part with deterioration of both cortical and subcortical neurons, but the precise etiology has not been determined (Chui, 1989). In Alzheimer's disease, there is marked loss of larger neurons in the neocortex, hippocampus, basal nucleus of Meynert, and locus coeruleus. As a result, there is a substantial decrease in brain concentrations of several neurotransmitters, including norepinephrine, 5-hydroxytryptamine, glutamate, somatostatin, substance P, and, especially, acetylcholine (ACh). At autopsy, the brains of patients with Alzheimer's disease reveal three other major neuropathologic lesions: (1) neurofibrillary tangles that contain paired helical filaments consisting principally of hyperphosphorylated *tau* protein; this protein normally functions to stabilize the neuronal "skeleton" and enhance the intraneuronal movement of substrates and nutrients to nerve endings; (2) neuritic plaques consisting of dystrophic nerve endings, a core of β-amyloid peptide, plus microglia, astrocytes, and other less abundant components; β-amyloid is the proteolytic product of a larger precursor (amyloid precursor protein [APP]), a membrane-spanning glycoprotein expressed in most mammalian cells; and (3) β-amyloid deposits in the walls of small pia blood vessels ("angiopathy").

Neuritic plaques and neurofibrillary tangles occur mainly in the association areas of the neocortex, hippocampus, and certain deeper gray areas, and the brain is shrunken. Bilateral parietotemporal hypoperfusion and hypometabolism are typical findings with positron emission tomography (PET). The amount of synaptic loss in the neocortex correlates with the degree of cognitive deficit.

Circumstantial evidence suggests that the deposition of β-amyloid may trigger the pathogenic process in Alzheimer's disease. The gene for APP is located on chromosome 21. Many individuals with Down's syndrome (trisomy 21) develop diffuse plaques during adolescence, and these adults have changes characteristic of Alzheimer's disease in their brains by age 40. Mutations in the APP gene and in adjacent linkage sites on chromosome 21 have been identified in a small number of patients with familial, early-onset Alzheimer's disease. Recently, a genetic linkage site for early-onset Alzheimer's disease has been located on chromosome 14 in a large number of families. The specific gene mutation has not been identified, but two genes whose products (c-fos and heat shock protein) act as promoters for APP are found near the linkage site.

Whether β-amyloid or related protein fragments are directly neurotoxic is still unresolved. The β-amyloid fragment consists of parts of the transmembrane domain and a short portion of the extracellular domain of APP. Two pathways, secretory and endosomal/lysosomal, for APP metabolism have been described; only the latter results in the formation of fragments that contain the entire β-amyloid sequence. β-amyloid is produced in soluble form in vitro and in vivo during normal cellular metabolism (Haass et al, 1992; Seubert et al, 1992; Shoji et al, 1992); the cellular and biochemical nature of this process is unknown. The relationship of this soluble peptide (40 amino acids long) to the predominant component of β-amyloid (usually 42 to 43 amino acids) in plaques is not established. Results of some in vitro studies suggest that soluble β-amyloid exerts trophic effects on immature neurons; however, the resultant neuritic growth is dystrophic (Pike et al, 1992). Aggregated β-amyloid is toxic to mature neuronal cell cultures (Pike et al, 1991); morphologic changes mimic those found in "programmed" cell death.

DIAGNOSIS. The diagnosis of dementia is based on a combined exclusionary and inclusionary approach. Multi-infarct dementia associated with cerebrovascular atherosclerosis and ischemia is more abrupt in onset than Alzheimer's disease and progresses incrementally rather than gradually as new infarcts destroy cortical or subcortical tissue. The Hachinski Ischemic Scale is a helpful distinguishing test. Dementia must be differentiated from delirium, which is characterized by the acute onset (hours to days) of altered consciousness that fluctuates irregularly and unpredictably (Lipowski, 1989), and from depression (Wells, 1979; Kokmen, 1989). In contrast to patients with dementia, depressed individuals may have a past history of mood disorder, project a hopeless appearance, and have a negative outlook. The differential diagnosis of dementia has been reviewed (Small et el, 1981; Dahl, 1983; NIH Consensus Development Conference, 1987; Chui, 1989).

Alzheimer's disease is accurately diagnosed in 85% to 90% of patients based on criteria established in the *DSM-III-R* (see Table 3) and by the Work Group of the National Institute of Neurological and Communicative Disorders and Stroke and the Alzheimer's Disease and Related Disorders Association (NINCDS/ADRDA) (McKhann et al, 1984). All patients suspected of having Alzheimer's disease should receive a comprehensive physical examination, including hearing and vision tests, to rule out other pathology and should undergo a battery of tests, including CT or MRI; complete blood count; serum chemistries; vitamin B_{12}, folic acid, and thyroid profiles; and a test for syphilis. A collateral source of information may be needed for adequate history taking. The neurologic examination is used primarily to exclude focal neurologic deficits.

Definitive diagnosis of Alzheimer's disease requires histopathologic confirmation. In the absence of systemic disorders or other brain diseases that could account for progressive deficits, the clinical diagnosis of probable Alzheimer's disease can be made in patients with a normal level of consciousness between the ages of 40 and 90 (most often after age 65) based on (1) documentation by examination of mental status (Mini-Mental State, Blessed Dementia Scale, or similar test) with confirmation by neuropsychological testing; (2) deficits in two or more areas of cognition; (3) insidious onset with progressive worsening of memory and other cognitive functions; plateaus are permitted and deterioration may occur in a specific cognitive function (eg, aphasia, apraxia, agnosia); and (4) impaired activities of daily living and altered patterns of behavior. Associated symptoms may include depression, delusions, illusions and hallucinations, insomnia, sexual disorders, weight loss, and catastrophic outbursts. Other neurologic abnormalities may occur in patients with advanced disease, but gait disturbances and focal neurologic deficits are unusual.

TABLE 3. THE DSM-III-R DIAGNOSTIC CRITERIA[1] FOR DEMENTIA[2]

A. Demonstrable evidence of impairment in short- and long-term memory
B. At least one of the following:
  1. impairment in abstract thinking
  2. impaired judgment
  3. other disturbances of higher cortical function (eg, aphasia, apraxia, agnosia, constructional difficulty)
  4. personality change
C. Impairment or disturbance that significantly interferes with work, social activities, or interpersonal relationships
D. Impairment or disturbance that does not occur exclusively during delirium
E. Either of the following:
  1. Evidence from history, physical examination, or laboratory tests of a specific, etiologically related organic factor
  2. In the absence of such evidence, an etiologic organic factor can be presumed if the disturbance cannot be accounted for by a nonorganic mental disorder (eg, major depression)

[1]*Adapted from* Diagnostic and Statistical Manual of Mental Disorders, *ed 3 (revised). American Psychiatric Association, 1987.*

[2]*For the diagnosis of Alzheimer's disease, there must be insidious onset with a generally progressive deteriorating course and other specific causes of dementia must be excluded.*

MANAGEMENT. The treatment of dementia presents a significant challenge to the medical community. Optimal care for the patient requires that the physician and others providing such care understand a broad spectrum of medical, scientific, and psychosocial issues.

The long-term management of dementia differs in several respects from that of other chronic illnesses. The following focuses on devising a framework for optimal long-term care of patients with Alzheimer's disease, although much of this information also applies to patients with multi-infarct dementia. Several principles of these disorders and their impact on family and societal relationships must be recognized:

1. No interventions are known that will alter the course of the disease.

2. The disease is of long duration and total disability occurs late in its course. For most of the duration, the patient is ambulatory and able to aid in daily living activities to some extent. Furthermore, the patient is apparently able to experience some interpersonal emotions.

3. Many families choose to provide care at home for as long as possible prior to placement of the patient in an institution.

4. In most other disorders, the patient's response to the illness is the focus for psychological intervention, but this is much less true in dementia.

5. The social milieu of demented patients should remain as fixed as possible. These patients are very sensitive to changes in residence and in caregivers. A demented patient is much more likely to retain functional effectiveness in a familiar environment.

Given these principles, management of the demented patient in a noninstitutional setting, most likely the home, will be the first approach to long-term care. Before the decision for home management can be endorsed, however, the health, emotional state, and coping skills of the primary caregiver should be assessed. Support in the form of day care, respite care, adult companions, home health aids, "meals on wheels," and visiting nurses often makes it possible for the patient to remain in the home. When home management becomes impractical, even with the above assistance, institutionalization is the sole option. Agitation, combativeness, aggression, and incontinence are common complaints of caregivers that lead to residential care of the patient. For the demented patient in a nursing home, requirements similar to those of home management must be met (eg, competent staff, optimization of physical environment, availability of physicians). The level of expertise must be higher than at home, since the magnitude of the nursing problems will be greater.

The uncertain etiology of Alzheimer's disease has precluded the development of specific therapy to prevent the disease or impede progression. Thus, treatment regimens focus on amelioration of symptoms.

Nondrug Therapy: Nondrug therapy is most important and includes environmental management, family counseling and support, and psychotherapy. These behavioral and psychological approaches seek both to maintain the patient's optimal awareness of the time, place, and composition of his/her environment and to enhance the family's understanding of the patient's needs and their own limitations as caregivers.

Awareness of the environment is best maintained by the constant and continuous presentation of cues to aid and orient the patient. Management of that environment should include: (1) Prominent color-coded displays of calendars, clocks, and checklists to facilitate orientation; (2) nightlights to minimize nocturnal sensory deprivation; (3) photographs and other objects to help create a familiar and, therefore, stable environment; (4) appraisal of the need for corrective glasses and hearing aids; (5) routine hygienic measures to minimize the effects of minor illnesses and prevent bedsores; (6) adequate nutrition and fluid intake to minimize constipation and prevent nutritional deficiencies and dehydration that may aggravate the disorder; and (7) accident prevention techniques to minimize falls and burns. Referral of the patient's family to the Alzheimer's Association, a national voluntary health association, is often beneficial. The Association has its headquarters in Chicago (312/335-8700) and has more than 200 chapters nationwide.

Drug Therapy: Pharmacologic treatment of dementia is limited, primarily because of poor understanding of its etiology and pathogenesis. Although considerable progress has been made in understanding certain aspects of the neurodegenerative process in Alzheimer's disease, at present there is no cure or satisfactory restorative treatment. Until more specific information is available, drug therapy is investigational and is aimed at (1) facilitating function in remaining neural elements that may be involved in memory and other cognitive processes, (2) inhibiting or reversing neuronal degeneration, and (3) increasing cerebral metabolism in a nonspecific way.

Ergoloid mesylates are among the most widely used agents in the treatment of Alzheimer's disease and other dementia syndromes. In more than 20 double-blind, placebo-controlled trials, the mixture of ergoloid mesylates [Hydergine] has been claimed to produce modest improvement in confusional states, depressed mood, dizziness, unsociability, and self-care (Hollister and Yesavage, 1984). These agents were initially thought to act as cerebral vasodilators, but they are now considered to have effects on multiple neurotransmitter systems and possibly to act as metabolic enhancers (Krassner et al, 1984). There also is some evidence that ergoloid mesylates may slow the rate of cognitive decline (Gaitz et al, 1977; van Loveren-Huyben et al, 1984). However, most clinicians remain skeptical of the clinical importance of these observed beneficial effects (Thompson et al, 1990). The daily dose used in most clinical trials in the United States for treatment of dementia has been 3 mg; 7.5 mg daily has also been used (van Loveren-Huyben et al, 1984). In a recent study, which utilized a new dosage form with increased bioavailability [Hydergine-LC], 3 mg daily for six months was ineffective. Additional studies are in progress to evaluate the efficacy of higher dosages.

Cholinomimetic agents (eg, anticholinesterase inhibitors, cholinergic agonists, enhancers of acetylcholine release) are being investigated intensively, based on the observation that the concentrations of choline acetyltransferase and acetylcholinesterase are markedly reduced in the brains of patients with Alzheimer's disease and the number of cholinergic (muscarinic) receptors is normal or only slightly decreased. These enzymatic markers for cholinergic neurons roughly parallel the severity of neuronal loss, density of neuritic plaques, and cognitive decline (especially in memory).

There has been considerable controversy concerning the efficacy of the cholinesterase inhibitor, tacrine (tetrahydroaminoacridine, THA) [Cognex], either alone or in combination with lecithin. Striking beneficial effects were reported in one study (Summers et al, 1986), but this study has been criticized by the FDA (Food and Drug Administration, 1991; for reply see Summers et al, 1991). Subsequently, no significant benefit was demonstrated in three controlled clinical trials of tacrine in combination with lecithin (Gauthier et al, 1990; Chatellier et al, 1990; Molloy et al, 1991). These studies used lower doses (up to 125 mg/daily) than the first trial (up to 200 mg/daily) to reduce the occurrence of hepatotoxicity observed with larger doses. However, in another trial in which up to 150 mg of tacrine plus 10.8 g of lecithin was administered, 45% of the recipients improved by 3 or more points on the Mini-Mental State Examination compared with 11% who received placebo. However, no significant effect of treatment was observed when the caregiver assessed the activities of daily living (Eagger et al, 1991).

There appears to be a subpopulation of tacrine-responsive patients. This would explain the generally negative results reported using fixed doses but may account for the occasional dramatic improvement noted in individual patients. One clinical trial (Davis et al, 1992) studied only patients who had demonstrated significant improvement on the cognitive subscale of the Alzheimer's Disease Assessment Scale (ADAS COG) during a dose-finding (40 or 80 mg) phase before rerandomization to a six-week double-blind phase with placebo. Treatment of patients with their "best dose" resulted in a statistically significant reduction in the decline in cognitive function; continued decline in the placebo group was the basis of the assessment of tacrine's advantage. No improvement in global assessments was reported by the study physician. In another randomized controlled trial (12 weeks) sponsored by the manufacturer (Warner-Lambert) as part of its New Drug Application, patients treated with a daily dose of 80 mg (for the final six weeks) achieved a 4-point or greater cognitive improvement on the ADAS COG; global assessment by the physician also favored tacrine (Farlow et al, 1992). The degree of improvement roughly corresponded to the average decline that normally occurs every six months. In these studies, 18% to 25% of patients had to discontinue use of tacrine because of side effects, most commonly elevation in ALT. Other adverse effects included dyspepsia, nausea, vomiting, diarrhea, abdominal pain, and headache.

Additional safety and efficacy data collected by the manufacturer in a 30-week double-blind, dose-titration study in 663 patients indicate that tacrine significantly improved patient performance on the ADAS COG and the Clinician Interview-Based Impression of Change (CIBIC) compared with placebo (*F-D-C Reports*, 1993). This study was important because it examined the effect of tacrine in doses as high as 160 mg/day. Twenty percent of patients who completed the trial showed at least a 4-point improvement on the ADAS COG. The percentage of evaluable patients who improved increased in a dose-dependent manner; 42% of patients in the 160 mg/day group were rated as improved.

In most patients, tacrine's clinical benefit is modest. A combination of intolerance and lack of response may limit significant cognitive improvement to ≤15% of patients with mild to moderate Alzheimer's disease (*F-D-C Reports*, 1993). It is estimated that 60% to 75% of patients with Alzheimer's disease will be able to tolerate tacrine in clinical practice. Potential hepatotoxicity and other serious adverse events probably can be minimized with regular monitoring.

Tacrine has been available as a Treatment IND since December 1991. It was recommended for approval by the FDA's Peripheral and Central Nervous System Advisory Committee in March 1993.

The efficacy of a tacrine analogue, velnacrine [Mentane], has been evaluated in three clinical trials sponsored by the manufacturer. In one study on 35 patients, velnacrine demonstrated significant acute effects on the core symptoms of Alzheimer's disease. In a large, dose-finding study that used a crossover design, 43% of patients improved by 4 points on the ADAS COG and the drug was well tolerated; the doses were 150 mg or 225 mg. Effects were replicated in a subsequent double-blind study of this enriched sample. However, in a long-term fixed-dose study that compared daily doses of 15 mg with 150 mg, no significant difference in the effects of the two doses on various psychometric variables was detected.

Similarly, some patients with Alzheimer's disease may respond temporarily to physostigmine [Antilirium]. In early trials of this agent, intravenous administration improved recall, but results using oral preparations were equivocal (Mayeux, 1990). An oral prolonged-release formulation of physostigmine is being studied in a large, multicenter trial.

More recent studies have reinforced the belief that the response of patients with Alzheimer's disease to acetylcholinesterase inhibitors is quite variable and that a subgroup may benefit (Stern et al, 1988; Jenike et al, 1990; Harrell et al, 1990). Efficacy is improved in some patients in dose-finding studies, but overall the data are not impressive, especially in studies using fixed-dose schedules (Jenike et al, 1990). Oral dosage forms of muscarinic agonists and oral enhancers of acetylcholine release are being studied in preclinical trials.

Other investigational approaches to improving the function of surviving neuronal cells include the use of metabolic enhancers (eg, acetyl-l-carnitine) or nootropic agents (eg, oxiracetam, pramiracetam). Results of a small placebo-controlled study that used an enrichment-type trial design suggest that pramiracetam does not confer significant symptomatic benefit in Alzheimer's disease patients (Claus et al, 1991); findings from another trial of oxiracetam in patients with probable Alzheimer's disease indicate that this nootropic agent also is ineffective in reducing cognitive impairment (Green et al, 1992).

Two randomized placebo-controlled trials of acetyl levocarnitine in patients with Alzheimer's disease have been reported (Spagnoli et al, 1991; Sano et al, 1992). Patients who received the drug or placebo continued to worsen but, in both studies, a modest reduction in the rate of deterioration on some outcome measures was reported in those receiving the drug. No cognitive enhancement over baseline was noted.

Ultimately, strategies to slow or reverse neuronal degeneration are required. Investigational approaches include the use of growth factors (eg, nerve growth factor), neuroprotective agents (eg, nimodipine, sabeluzole, glutamate antagonists, adenosine analogues, selegiline), and cell membrane stabilizers (eg, phosphatidylserine). A 5-hydroxytryptamine receptor antagonist (ie, ondansetron) and angiotensin-converting enzyme (ACE) inhibitors also are being investigated.

Although specific drug therapy for the disease process is lacking, disruptive and debilitating symptoms (eg, psychotic behavior, depression, anxiety, insomnia) are amenable to treatment with drugs (see index entries Antipsychotic Drugs; Antidepressants; Antianxiety Drugs; and Hypnotics). However, serious consideration of the pharmacodynamic and pharmacokinetic alterations characteristic of the elderly is critical before drug therapy is initiated. Generally, drugs should be administered in doses lower than those given to younger patients. A drug's spectrum and potential for producing adverse effects, as well as its potential for interaction with other drugs the patient is taking, must be considered. Finally, the individual supervising administration of the drug must fully understand the appropriate dosing schedule, the expectation for improvement, the potential for adverse drug reactions, and the possibility of multiple prescribers.

ATTENTION-DEFICIT HYPERACTIVITY DISORDER

This condition is first recognized principally in elementary school-age children and is characterized by developmentally inappropriate inattentiveness, impulsiveness, and usually hyperactivity. Its nosology has undergone extensive changes over the past century (Zametkin and Rapoport, 1987; Shaywitz and Shaywitz, 1988).

The *DSM-III-R* (American Psychiatric Association, 1987) places equal emphasis on the presence of motor overactivity and inattentiveness, and this clinical condition is now termed *attention-deficit hyperactivity disorder* (ADHD). A smaller number of patients without signs of hyperactivity are classified as having *undifferentiated attention-deficit disorder*—a condition that may be quite difficult to distinguish from learning disabilities or other neuropsychiatric disorders.

ADHD occurs in approximately 2% to 6% of prepubertal children in the United States (Costello, 1989); males predominate in clinical samples (6:1) and in epidemiologic studies (3:1) of symptomatic children. In one regional survey, the percentage of students treated with medication for hyperactivity/inattentiveness was reported to have doubled every four to seven years from 1971 to 1987 and in 1987 was nearly 6% in students in public schools (Safer and Krager, 1988). Therefore, concern exists that these stimulants are being prescribed inappropriately, especially for children who may have a learning disability, which, unlike ADHD, does not respond to medication. Concern also exists that older postpubertal adolescents are responsible for the increase in stimulant use. However, evidence from a number of studies supports the concept that in approximately one-third to one-half of all children with ADHD, the disorder persists with varying degrees of severity into adolescence and adulthood and includes manifestations of antisocial behavior, underachievement, lack of emotional control, and substance abuse (Cantwell, 1985; Wender et al, 1985; Thorley, 1988; Mannuzza et al, 1991).

DIAGNOSIS. The diagnosis of ADHD is based on the major criteria of inattention, impulsivity, and hyperactivity. At least eight of the following signs of inattention must be present (American Psychiatric Association, 1987): the patient often fidgets with hands or feet or squirms in seat (in adolescents, may be limited to subjective feelings of restlessness); has difficulty remaining seated when required to do so; is easily distracted by extraneous stimuli; has difficulty awaiting turn in group situations; often blurts out answers to questions before they have been completed; has difficulty following through on instructions from others (not due to oppositional behavior or failure of comprehension), eg, fails to finish chores; has difficulty sustaining attention in tasks or play activities; often shifts from one uncompleted activity to another; has difficulty playing quietly; often talks excessively; often interrupts or intrudes on others, eg, butts into other children's games; often does not seem to listen to what is being said; and often loses things necessary for tasks or activities at school or at home (eg, toys, pencils, books, assignments). Onset of the disorder must occur before age 7, and the disorder must have persisted for at least six months.

ADHD must be differentiated from age-appropriate overactivity, learning disability, severe and profound mental retardation, conduct disorder, schizophrenia, affective disorder with mania, pervasive developmental disorder, absence seizures, and hyperthyroidism (American Psychiatric Association, 1987). Emerging evidence suggests that ADHD often is observed in children with conduct, depressive, anxiety, and other disorders (Biederman et al, 1991). The use of questionnaires that can identify classic symptoms of the disease can increase confidence in the diagnosis. A learning disability is usually detectable as a more selective lag in development for a particular element of academic performance. Mental retardation is characterized by a more uniform and broad deficiency in academic performance than that usually seen with ADHD. Some patients with mental retardation present with the characteristic symptoms of ADHD. In such cases, the additional diagnosis of ADHD is warranted. Many patients with conduct disorder have signs of impulsivity, inattention, and hyperactivity, and the additional diagnosis of ADHD also frequently is warranted in these patients. Schizophrenia and mood disorders with mania may be characterized by features of ADHD; however, these diagnoses pre-empt that of the latter. Finally, a child who experiences frequent absence seizures may exhibit inattentiveness; further clinical evaluation may be necessary to establish the correct diagnosis.

MANAGEMENT. ADHD has a profound impact on the child's emotional life, and counseling may be required. Adjunctive therapy, such as remedial education, behavior modification, and counseling the child's parents and teachers, also is indicated (Committee on Children with Disabilities, 1987). Parents and teachers must establish an environment of predictable structure with experiences of manageable intensity for the child; such an environment will diminish anxiety and facilitate normal maturation.

Drug Therapy: The goal of pharmacotherapy is to reduce abnormal behavior to permit a greater degree of normal functioning. Many studies employing both subjective and objective criteria to judge outcome indicate that central nervous system stimulants decrease symptoms. These agents improve short-term learning; prolong attention span; improve goal-directed activity, concentration, and classroom behavior; and reduce impulsiveness, hyperactivity, and aggressive behavior. Questionnaires used by teachers and parents to evaluate the effects of medication on behavior can be helpful, and the physician should monitor the effects of the drug and adjust dosage.

Stimulant drugs relieve symptoms but are not curative (Biederman and Jellinek, 1984), and only limited data are available to demonstrate that they improve learning. In long-term studies, improvement has not been a consistent finding. Onset of adolescence alone is not a sufficient reason to discontinue pharmacotherapy in responsive patients because children with ADHD may continue to have difficulty in school, exhibit behavioral disorders, and have poor self-esteem into adolescence or even adulthood (Milman, 1979; Weiss, 1981; Amado and Lustman, 1982; Cantwell, 1985; Thorley, 1988; Mannuzza et al, 1991).

Dextroamphetamine [Dexedrine], methylphenidate [Ritalin], and pemoline [Cylert] are useful. Methylphenidate is most commonly prescribed, although dextroamphetamine is equally effective. Use of prolonged-release preparations of these drugs may improve acceptability in children with ADHD by eliminating the need for administration of medication during school hours (Bowen et al, 1991). Pemoline is less frequently considered the drug of choice because improvement may occur more slowly with recommended initial doses than with methylphenidate or dextroamphetamine and rarely the drug is hepatotoxic. However, its longer duration of action allows once-daily dosing in some children.

Because amphetamine sulfate, the racemic form of amphetamine, has less central nervous system activity and a more pronounced effect on the cardiovascular system than the dextrorotatory isomer, dextroamphetamine, the latter is preferred. Another form, methamphetamine [Desoxyn], is essentially equivalent to dextroamphetamine in its central nervous system and cardiovascular effects but has been extensively abused in nonmedical settings and is prescribed less frequently.

Although dextroamphetamine and methylphenidate facilitate dopamine and norepinephrine release by different mechanisms (Lawson-Wendling et al, 1981), their mechanism of action in ADHD remains speculative. Their ability to increase attention span is nonspecific and has been reported in normal children as well (Weingartner et al, 1980; Rapoport et al, 1978). The latter observation has led these investigators to conclude that clinical response to amphetamines and methylphenidate has no diagnostic significance.

The prolonged use of dextroamphetamine, methylphenidate, and pemoline may limit linear growth and weight, presumably because of appetite suppression, decreased food intake, and altered secretion of growth hormone. Therefore, weight gain and linear growth must be monitored closely. However, results of many studies suggest that these drugs have no effect on ultimate height and weight (Klein and Mannuzza, 1988). One two-year study on prepubertal children showed that methylphenidate depressed linear growth slightly in the first year of therapy, but this was offset by a greater than expected growth rate in the second year (Satterfield et al, 1979). Early adolescent growth appears to be unaffected by methylphenidate (Vincent et al, 1990). Total dosage and summer drug holidays were reported to influence weight, but not height, deficits. The goal is to use doses that reduce ADHD without suppressing weight. The decision to provide drug holidays on weekends or during the summer should be made on the basis of individual functional requirements. Pemoline also was reported to depress longitudinal growth for up to 18 months; however, children treated with this drug caught up with their normal peers in subsequent months (Friedmann et al, 1981).

Central nervous system stimulants can precipitate tics in susceptible children (Lowe et al, 1982). Those with a history of tics or a diagnosis of Tourette's syndrome should not receive these stimulants unless extreme behavioral difficulties due to ADHD are present and the tics and syndrome are mild in degree. Those with a family history of similar disorders should be given a stimulant only under careful supervision (Morgan, 1988).

As many as 25% of patients do not respond to or cannot tolerate stimulant medication. In those who are unresponsive, antidepressants may be appropriate alternatives. Results of controlled trials generally show that tricyclic antidepressants are superior to placebo but are not always as effective as methylphenidate. Disadvantages include potential cardiotoxicity and delayed onset of action. Potential advantages include added benefit in depressed or anxious patients and the convenience of once-daily dosing prior to bedtime. Imipramine [Janimine, Tofranil] was used most often in early clinical trials. More recent controlled trials have employed desipramine [Norpramin, Pertofrane] (Garfinkel et at, 1983; Donnelly et al, 1986; Biederman et al, 1989). Comparison of clinical trials from different time periods is complicated by changing diagnostic criteria and differences in dosage. Mean daily dosages in the trials with desipramine ranged from 3.4 to 4.6 mg/kg.

The report of sudden death in three 8- to 9-year-old children receiving desipramine underscores the need to individualize treatment, monitor plasma drug concentrations, and employ electrocardiograms, especially when larger dosages are utilized (*Med Lett Drugs Ther*, 1990). Treatment with desipramine (or a comparable tricyclic agent) should be preceded by a baseline ECG and initiated at a dosage of approximately 1 mg/kg. The daily dosage may be increased by 20% to 30% every four to five days to the lowest effective amount (maximum, 5 mg/kg) (Biederman, 1991). Daily doses above 3.5 mg/kg or plasma concentrations above 150 ng/ml may increase the risk of electrocardiographic changes. Determination of the steady-state plasma concentrations (desipramine plasma concentrations >300 ng/ml) and periodic ECGs (PR interval <200 ms, QRS duration <120 ms) may help maximize benefits and avoid toxicity (Biederman, 1991).

Another antidepressant, bupropion [Wellbutrin], may be useful and is well tolerated. Controlled trials in children and one open trial in adults demonstrated its efficacy (Simeon et al, 1986; Casat et al, 1987; Wender and Reimherr, 1990), but further comparative trials are necessary to define the role of this agent in the treatment of ADHD. Available data indicate that monoamine oxidase inhibitors, such as tranylcypromine [Parnate], also may be useful in children with ADHD (Zametkin et al, 1985). However, the risk of hypertensive reactions due to interaction with a wide variety of foods and medications (including over-the-counter products) is a deterrent to use of these agents.

Results of controlled and open trials indicate that clonidine 3 to 10 mcg/kg daily may be an effective alternative medication in ADHD (Hunt et al, 1985; Hunt, 1987). Some investigators have recommended this drug's use in patients who have ADHD and tics or Tourette's syndrome (Stevenson and Wolraich, 1989; Steingard et al, 1993). Further comparative trials are necessary to clarify the role of clonidine in these disorders.

Antipsychotic drugs (eg, haloperidol) also have been employed. Because of their potential to produce significant extrapyramidal movement disorders and tardive dyskinesia, use of antipsychotic drugs for the treatment of ADHD is rarely if ever indicated.

Diet Therapy: Diet therapy has been advocated for children with ADHD. The Feingold diet is essentially free of artificial flavors and colors that are purported to be etiologic agents. Although synthetic food dyes adversely affect learning (Swanson and Kinsbourne, 1980) and behavior (Weiss et al, 1980) in some children with ADHD, the results achieved with this diet are not encouraging (Conners, 1980). A National Institutes of Health Consensus Conference (1982) agreed that additive-free diets are not effective for most children but did not object to their use on a trial basis because they may be beneficial adjuncts to drugs and other therapies. Considerable effort is required by parents if this type of dietary intervention is chosen (Kaplan et al, 1989).

Drug Evaluations

DEXTROAMPHETAMINE SULFATE
[Dexedrine]

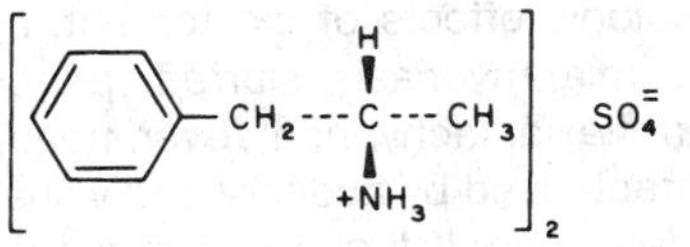

$$\left[C_6H_5-CH_2-\overset{H}{\underset{+NH_3}{C}}-CH_3 \right]_2 SO_4^{=}$$

USES. Dextroamphetamine is useful when combined with remedial measures in the management of children and adolescents with attention-deficit hyperactivity disorder (ADHD) (see the Introduction) and as an alternative to methylphenidate in patients with narcolepsy (see index entry Narcolepsy). Dextroamphetamine generally is preferred to amphetamine because it has less effect on the cardiovascular system. All amphetamines are classified as Schedule II drugs under the Controlled Substances Act.

The use of amphetamines to allay fatigue is unjustifiable except under the most extraordinary circumstances. These agents are dangerous for motor vehicle drivers and those engaged in comparable activities, and they have no legitimate role in athletics. Indeed, their use may contribute to increased athletic injuries.

For other uses, see index entry Dextroamphetamine.

ADVERSE REACTIONS AND PRECAUTIONS. Untoward effects of the amphetamines, particularly their sympathomimetic effects, are related to their pharmacologic actions. These agents may cause nervousness, restlessness, tremors, insomnia, cardiovascular disturbances (eg, tachycardia, arrhythmias, hypertension), dizziness, mydriasis, dryness of the mouth, and gastrointestinal disturbances (eg, nausea, constipation, diarrhea). Anorexia and temporary growth retardation have been observed in children. Dosage should not be increased unnecessarily because larger amounts may produce marked restlessness, irritability, and aggressiveness.

More serious central nervous system reactions occur rarely and include psychic changes and dystonic movements of the head, neck, and extremities. Serious depressive reactions and psychoses have followed prolonged use, especially of large doses.

Generally, the amphetamines should not be prescribed for patients with cardiovascular disease or hyperthyroidism because their sympathomimetic effect may aggravate these conditions. They also should not be given to those known to be susceptible to drug abuse. These drugs should be used with caution in patients who are sensitive to adrenergic agents.

Reproduction studies employing large multiples of the human dose in mammals have suggested that the amphetamines have both an embryotoxic and a teratogenic potential. Fetal malformations also have been reported clinically but have not been established conclusively (see index entry Pregnancy). One retrospective study of offspring of women who took dextroamphetamine during pregnancy showed no effect on neonatal birth weight when the drug was taken before the third trimester and only a small effect when it was taken during the third trimester. Neither length nor head circumference was affected (Naeye, 1983) (FDA Pregnancy Category C).

POISONING. In general, acute overdosage accentuates the usual pharmacologic effects of excitement, agitation, hypertension, tachycardia, mydriasis, slurred speech, ataxia, tremor, chills, hyperreflexia, tachypnea, fever, headache, and toxic psychoses characterized by auditory and visual hallucinations and paranoid delusions. If these symptoms develop, lavage, sedatives, custodial care, and psychotherapy should be employed when indicated. Chlorpromazine may block the central nervous system effects but aggravates similar signs and symptoms produced by anticholinergic drugs if these have been taken concurrently. Excretion can be hastened by acidification of the urine.

In severe cases, overdosage may cause hyperpyrexia, chest pain, acute circulatory failure, convulsions, and coma. Fatalities have occurred in adults after doses of only 100 to 500 mg.

ABUSE. Susceptible patients may develop marked psychological dependence on amphetamines. Individuals who abuse these Schedule II drugs frequently inject as much as several grams daily (parenteral amphetamine preparations are not available commercially). In general, the toxic features of chronic abuse include a distinctive amphetamine psychosis that resembles schizophrenia and is characterized by paranoia, stereotyped behavior, picking at the skin, preoccupation with one's own thoughts, and auditory and visual hallucinations.

Abrupt termination of large doses of amphetamines may unmask symptoms of chronic fatigue, mental depression, paranoid psychosis, tremor, and gastrointestinal disturbances. Fatigue may be followed by drowsiness and prolonged sleep. Such reactions often are considered to be a type of abstinence syndrome.

DRUG INTERACTIONS. Amphetamines interfere with the hypotensive effect of methyldopa; therefore, amphetamines should not be used with this drug.

Amphetamines are contraindicated in patients receiving monoamine oxidase inhibitors, because their use may precipitate a hypertensive crisis. Although the amphetamines are resistant to monoamine oxidase, their actions are potentiated by the monoamine oxidase inhibitors, presumably as a result of the release of biogenic amines. Amphetamines may precipitate arrhythmias through their catecholamine-releasing effect in patients receiving general anesthetics that sensitize the heart to epinephrine.

Amphetamines can increase blood levels of the tricyclic antidepressants by interfering with their metabolism. Neuroleptic drugs antagonize most of the central nervous system actions of the amphetamines.

PHARMACOKINETICS. The amphetamines are well absorbed orally, are not highly bound to protein, and are excreted largely by the kidney. Their half-lives range from 7 to 14 hours (10 ± 1.7 hours) if the urine is acid; this may be extended to 30 hours if the urine is alkaline.

DOSAGE AND PREPARATIONS.

Oral: For attention-deficit hyperactivity disorder, dextroamphetamine is usually administered three times daily with or after meals during the waking hours. Individualization of dosage is very important; optimal amounts for morning, noon, and late afternoon administration need not be the same. A few children will require only one or the first two doses per day. *Children 3 to 5 years,* 2.5 mg daily initially, increased by 2.5 mg at weekly intervals until satisfactory improvement is reported, intolerable side effects occur, or the child becomes withdrawn, tearful, suspicious, or dulled in interactions with others; *6 years and older,* 5 mg once or twice daily or 2.5 mg three times a day initially, increased by 5 mg at weekly intervals until an optimum response is obtained. The usual effective dosage range is 5 to 20 mg daily, but up to 1 mg/kg may be needed in some children. Once the dosage schedule is stabilized, use of the prolonged-release preparation may be considered, but it is not always as effective as the standard preparation (Pelham et al, 1987).

For narcolepsy, *adults and children over 6 years,* 5 to 60 mg daily in divided doses, depending on the patient's requirements. Tolerance is a major problem when large doses are administered daily for prolonged periods. An occasional drug holiday or withholding therapy during nonworking periods restores sensitivity to dextroamphetamine and allows the dosage to be decreased when therapy is reinstituted.

Generic. Tablets 5 and 10 mg.

Dexedrine (SmithKline Beecham). Capsules (prolonged-release) 5, 10, and 15 mg; tablets 5 mg.

Similar Drug.

METHAMPHETAMINE HYDROCHLORIDE:
Generic. Tablets 5 and 10 mg.
Desoxyn (Abbott). Tablets 5 mg; tablets (prolonged-release) 5, 10, and 15 mg.

METHYLPHENIDATE HYDROCHLORIDE
[Ritalin]

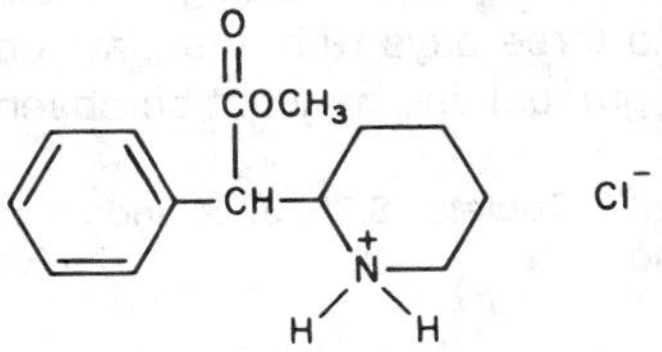

ACTIONS AND USES. This central nervous system stimulant is useful as an adjunct to remedial measures (psychological, educational, or social) in the management of children with attention-deficit hyperactivity disorder (ADHD). Methylphenidate was statistically superior to dextroamphetamine and pemoline in some measurements of improvement in a few but not most studies. Behavioral improvement appeared to be sustained for at least two years as judged by subjective criteria.

Methylphenidate also may be useful in narcolepsy (see index entry Narcolepsy) and idiopathic edema.

ADVERSE REACTIONS AND PRECAUTIONS. The most common adverse reactions are nervousness and insomnia. Anorexia, weight loss, and growth retardation may occur during prolonged therapy, but ultimate height is not affected. Occasional reactions include dizziness, dyskinesia, rash, nausea, abdominal pain, hypertension, hypotension, palpitation, changes in the pulse rate, tachycardia, arrhythmias, and headache. Toxic psychosis has been reported rarely.

Psychological dependence has occurred after long-term use of large doses but has not been reported during treatment of ADHD in children. Misuse of methylphenidate does not appear to be a problem in patients under adequate medical supervision when recommended dose levels are maintained, but the drug should be given cautiously to patients with a history of substance abuse. Methylphenidate has been substituted for amphetamines by individuals who abuse drugs and is classified as a Schedule II drug under the Controlled Substances Act.

Methylphenidate is contraindicated in patients with marked anxiety, tension, agitation, or glaucoma, and it should be used cautiously in hypertensive patients. The manufacturers caution against the use of methylphenidate in children with seizures and recommend that the drug be discontinued if seizures occur. However, in a four-week trial, methylphenidate 0.6 mg/kg/day produced no significant changes in the electroencephalogram or seizure activity in patients with epilepsy (Feldman et al, 1989).

DRUG INTERACTIONS. Methylphenidate may increase the plasma concentration of antiepileptic drugs (phenytoin, phenobarbital, and primidone), coumarin anticoagulants, phenylbutazone, and tricyclic antidepressants if these drugs are administered concurrently. The drug should be used cautiously with pressor agents, and the dosage of these agents should be adjusted when they are given with methylphenidate.

PHARMACOKINETICS. Methylphenidate is rapidly and well absorbed after oral administration. Peak plasma concentrations are attained in one to two hours. In one study, oral administration of the drug with breakfast accelerated rather than impeded absorption compared with administration 30 minutes before breakfast, and no significant differences were noted in behavioral, cognitive, or electrophysiologic effects (Swanson et al, 1983; Chan et al, 1983). The plasma half-life is reported to be one to two hours.

The duration of action usually is no more than four to six hours, but there is considerable individual variation. Methylphenidate is principally (80%) hydrolyzed to ritalinic acid, which is excreted in the urine.

DOSAGE AND PREPARATIONS.
Oral: For attention-deficit hyperactivity disorder, individualization of the dose is very important; optimal amounts for morning, afternoon, and evening administration need not be the same. Some children may require only two doses per day, and a few may require an extra dose at 4 PM. If equally satisfactory results are achieved, use of the prolonged-release preparation improves compliance. *Children 6 years and older,* initially, 5 mg twice daily (with or after breakfast and lunch); this dose may be gradually increased by 5 or 10 mg at weekly intervals. The usual effective dosage range is 0.5 to 1 mg/kg daily (10 to 20 mg daily for the average child). The maximum daily dose is 2 mg/kg. If adequate improvement at tolerated doses is not observed after one month, the drug should be discontinued.

Since the effects of a single dose usually do not persist for more than four hours, the following alternative schedule utilizes administration three times daily during the waking hours. This often improves behavior and interpersonal relationships at home as well as in school. *Children 6 years and older,* initially, 5 mg three times a day, usually after meals, increased by 5 mg/dose every three or four days until satisfactory improvement is reported, intolerable side effects occur, or the child becomes withdrawn, tearful, suspicious, or dulled in interactions with others. The maximum recommended dose is 60 mg/day.

For narcolepsy, *adults,* 10 mg two or three times daily (range, 10 to 60 mg daily). Tolerance is a major problem when large doses are administered daily for prolonged periods. An occasional drug holiday or withholding therapy during nonworking periods restores sensitivity to the drug and allows the dosage to be decreased when therapy is reinstituted.

Ritalin (CIBA), ***Generic.*** Tablets 5, 10, and 20 mg; tablets (prolonged-release) 20 mg ***(Ritalin-SR)***.

PEMOLINE
[Cylert]

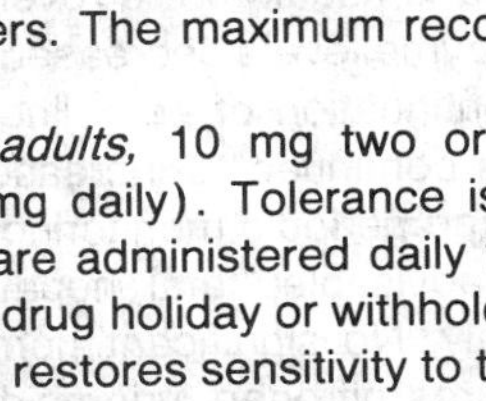

ACTIONS AND USES. This central nervous system stimulant is an oxazolidine. It is indicated as an adjunct to remedial measures in the management of children with ADHD. In controlled clinical studies, it improved the condition of children with this disorder as judged by physicians, parents, and teachers and by the results of psychological test scores.

In comparative studies, pemoline, dextroamphetamine, and methylphenidate appear to be equally effective. The beneficial effects occurred more rapidly with the other stimulants than with pemoline; however, pemoline was administered once daily while the other drugs were given twice daily. As with methylphenidate and dextroamphetamine, subjective improvement appeared to be sustained over a period of two years.

The effectiveness of pemoline in combating depression and fatigue and enhancing performance has not been demonstrated.

ADVERSE REACTIONS AND PRECAUTIONS. The most common adverse effects of pemoline are insomnia and anorexia. The insomnia may be transient or severe enough to necessitate adjustment of dosage. Anorexia may result in weight loss, particularly during the early weeks of therapy, but weight gain occurs after three to six months of continued administration and the weight curve approximates normal. A decrease in expected linear growth has been reported after long-term use, but the effect appears to be only temporary (see the Introduction to this section). Onset of puberty was not delayed in the limited number of patients studied to determine this effect.

Other reported adverse reactions include dizziness, drowsiness, headache, depression, hallucinations, rash, nausea, and gastrointestinal distress. No clinically significant sympathomimetic effects (increased pulse rate or blood pressure) were observed with pemoline.

Elevated AST, ALT, and LDH levels occurred in a few patients, and jaundice and hepatitis have been reported. The hepatic dysfunction appears to be a delayed hypersensitivity reaction. These reactions generally developed after several months of therapy and usually were reversible on withdrawal of the drug. The enzyme levels decreased within three to nine months after discontinuation of pemoline. In a few patients, liver enzyme levels continued to increase after cessation of therapy. Baseline and periodic monitoring of hepatic function during therapy is advisable; fatal hepatic dysfunction has been reported rarely. No significant hematologic effects or changes in blood urea nitrogen, uric acid, or bilirubin values were observed in long-term studies.

Although no potential for abuse was found in studies in primates, psychotic symptoms have been reported in adults and children who misused the drug. However, its abuse potential is low. Because pemoline has properties similar to those of other central nervous system stimulants, it is classified as a Schedule IV drug.

Pemoline is classified in FDA Pregnancy Category B.

PHARMACOKINETICS. Pemoline is well absorbed orally and has a half-life of approximately 12 hours. It is excreted principally by the kidney.

DOSAGE AND PREPARATIONS.

Oral: For attention-deficit hyperactivity disorder, *children 6 years and over,* initially, 37.5 mg daily as a single dose in the morning, increased by 18.75 mg at one-week intervals until the desired response is observed. The usual effective range is 56.25 to 75 mg daily (maximum, 112.5 mg daily). For *older children and adolescents,* weight-corrected doses of 1 to 3 mg/kg daily may be required. Although effects have been observed in one to three days with adequate dosage, improvement usually is gradual and may not be observed for three to four weeks.

Cylert (Abbott). Tablets 18.75, 37.5, and 75 mg; tablets (chewable) 37.5 mg.

Cited References

Cigarette smoking among adults—United States, 1990. *MMWR* 41:354-355, 1992.

Sudden death in children treated with a tricyclic antidepressant. *Med Lett Drugs Ther* 32:53, 1990.

Warner-Lambert's *Cognex* tolerated by up to three-quarters of Alzheimer's patients, firm estimates; advisory committee unanimously supports approval. *F-D-C Reports* 7-9, (March) 1993.

Abelin T, et al: Controlled trial of transdermal nicotine patch in tobacco withdrawal. *Lancet* 1:7-10, 1989.

Agricola R, et al: Treatment of acute alcohol withdrawal with carbamazepine: A double-blind comparison with tiapride. *J Int Med Res* 10:160-165, 1982.

Alldredge BK, et al: Placebo-controlled trial of intravenous diphenylhydantoin for short-term treatment of alcohol withdrawal seizures. *Am J Med* 87:645-648, 1989.

Amado H, Lustman PJ: Attention deficit disorders persisting in adulthood: Review. *Compr Psychiatry* 23:300-314, (July-Aug) 1982.

American College of Physicians: Disulfiram treatment of alcoholism. *Ann Intern Med* 111:943-945, 1989.

American Psychiatric Association: *Diagnostic and Statistical Manual of Mental Disorders,* ed 3 (revised) *(DSM-III-R)*. Washington, DC, American Psychiatric Press, 1987.

Annis HM: A relapse prevention model for treatment of alcoholics, in Miller WR, Heather N (eds): *Treating Addictive Behaviors.* New York, Plenum Press, 1986, 407-433.

Babor TF, Dolinsky ZS: Alcoholic typologies: Historical evolution and empirical evaluation of some common classification schemes, in Rose RM, Barrett J (eds): *Alcoholism: Origins and Outcome*. New York, Raven Press, 1988, 245-266.

Babor TF, et al: Alcohol-related problems in the primary health care setting: A review of early intervention strategies. *Br J Addict* 81:23-46, 1986.

Babor TF, et al: Types of alcoholics, I: Evidence for an empirically derived typology based on indicators of vulnerability and severity. *Arch Gen Psychiatry* 49:599-608, 1992.

Bauer LA, et al: Verapamil inhibits ethanol elimination and prolongs the perception of intoxication. *Clin Pharmacol Ther* 52:6-10, 1992.

Baumgartner GR, Rowen RC: Clonidine vs chlordiazepoxide in the management of acute alcohol withdrawal syndrome. *Arch Intern Med* 147:1223-1226, 1987.

Baumgartner GR, Rowen RC: Transdermal clonidine versus chlordiazepoxide in alcohol withdrawal: A randomized, controlled clinical trial. *South Med J* 84:312-321, 1991.

Benowitz NL, et al: Stable isotope method for studying transdermal drug absorption: The nicotine patch. *Clin Pharmacol Ther* 50:286-293, 1991.

Biederman J: Sudden death in children treated with a tricyclic antidepressant. *J Am Acad Child Adolesc Psychiatry* 30:495-498, 1991.

Biederman J, Jellinek MS: Psychopharmacology in children. *N Engl J Med* 310:968-972, 1984.

Biederman J, et al: A double-blind placebo controlled study of desipramine in the treatment of ADD: I. Efficacy. *J Am Acad Child Adolesc Psychiatry* 28:777-784, 1989.

Biederman J, et al: Comorbidity of attention deficit hyperactivity disorder with conduct, depressive, anxiety, and other disorders. *Am J Psychiatry* 148:564-577, 1991.

Bowen J, et al: Stimulant medication and attention deficit-hyperactivity disorder: The child's perspective. *Am J Dis Child* 145:291-295, 1991.

Brown ME, et al: Alcoholic detoxification and withdrawal seizures: Clinical support for a kindling hypothesis. *Biol Psychiatry* 24:507-514, 1988.

Buchkremer G, et al: Smoking cessation treatment combining transdermal nicotine substitution with behavioral therapy. *Pharmacopsychiatry* 24:96-102, 1991.

Caballeria J, et al: Effects of cimetidine on gastric alcohol dehydrogenase activity and blood ethanol levels. *Gastroenterology* 96:388-392, 1989.

Cantwell DP: Pharmacotherapy of ADD in adolescents: What do we know, where should we go, how should we do it? *Psychopharmacol Bull* 21:251-257, 1985.

Carithers RL Jr, et al: Methylprednisolone therapy in patients with severe alcoholic hepatitis: A randomized multicenter trial. *Ann Intern Med* 110:685-690, 1989.

Casat CD, et al: A double-blind trial of bupropion in children with attention deficit disorder. *Psychopharmacol Bull* 23:120-122, 1987.

Chan Y-PM, et al: Methylphenidate hydrochloride given with or before breakfast: II. Effects on plasma concentration of methylphenidate and ritalinic acid. *Pediatrics* 72:56-59, 1983.

Charness ME, et al: Ethanol and the nervous system. *N Engl J Med* 321:442-454, 1989.

Chatellier G, et al: Tacrine (tetrahydroaminoacridine; THA) and lecithin in senile dementia of the Alzheimer type: A multicentre trial. *BMJ* 300:495-499, 1990.

Chui HC: Dementia: A review emphasizing clinicopathologic correlation and brain-behavior relationships. *Arch Neurol* 46:806-814, 1989.

Clarren SK, Smith DW: Fetal alcohol syndrome. *N Engl J Med* 298:1063-1067, 1978.

Claus JJ, et al: Nootropic drugs in Alzheimer's disease: Symptomatic treatment with pramiracetam. *Neurology* 41:570-574, 1991.

Cloninger CR: Neurogenetic adaptive mechanism in alcoholism. *Science* 236:1341-1345, 1987.

Committee on Children with Disabilities, American Academy of Pediatrics: Medication for children with an attention deficit disorder. *Pediatrics* 80:758-760, 1987.

Conners CK: *Food Additives and Hyperactive Children.* New York, Plenum Press, 1980.

Costello EJ (ed): Developments in child psychiatric epidemiology. *Am Acad Child Adolesc Psychiatry* 28:836-841, 1989.

Covey LS, Glassman AH: New approaches to smoking cessation. *Drug Ther* 20:55-58, 61, 1990.

Covey LS, Glassman AH: A meta analysis of double-blind, placebo-controlled trials of clonidine for smoking cessation. *Br J Addict* 86:991-998, 1991.

Dahl DS: Diagnosis of Alzheimer's disease. *Postgrad Med* 73:217-221, (April) 1983.

Daughton DM, et al: Effect of transdermal nicotine delivery as an adjunct to low-intervention smoking cessation therapy: A randomized, placebo-controlled, double-blind study. *Arch Intern Med* 151:749-752, 1991.

Davis KL, et al: A double-blind, placebo-controlled multicenter study of tacrine for Alzheimer's disease. *N Engl J Med* 327:1253-1259, 1992.

Deitrich RA, et al: Mechanism of action of ethanol: Initial central nervous system actions. *Pharmacol Rev* 41:489-537, 1989.

Donnelly M, et al: Treatment of childhood hyperactivity with desipramine: Plasma drug concentration, cardiovascular effects, plasma and urinary catecholamine levels, and clinical response. *Clin Pharmacol Ther* 39:72-81, 1986.

Eagger SA, et al: Tacrine in Alzheimer's disease. *Lancet* 337:989-992, 1991.

Eneanya DI, et al: Actions and metabolic fate of disulfiram. *Annu Rev Pharmacol Toxicol* 21:575-596, 1981.

Ernhart CB, et al: Alcohol teratogenicity in the human: A detailed assessment of specificity, critical period, and threshold. *Am J Obstet Gynecol* 156:33-39, 1987.

Evans DA, et al: Prevalence of Alzheimer's disease in a community population of older persons: Higher than previously reported. *JAMA* 262:2551-2556, 1989.

Ewing JA: Detecting alcoholism: The CAGE questionnaire. *JAMA* 252:1905-1907, 1984.

Fagerström KO, Schneider NG: Measuring nicotine dependence: A review of the Fagerstrom tolerance questionnaire. *J Behav Med* 12:159-182, 1989.

Fagerström KO, et al: Effectiveness of nicotine patch and nicotine gum as individual vs. combined treatments for tobacco withdrawal symptoms. *Psychopharmacology* In press.

Farlow M, et al: A controlled trial of tacrine in Alzheimer's disease. *JAMA* 268:2523-2529, 1992.

Feldman H, et al: Methylphenidate in children with seizures and attention-deficit disorder. *Am J Dis Child* 143:1081-1086, 1989.

Fiore MC, et al: Methods used to quit smoking in the United States: Do cessation programs help? *JAMA* 263:2760-2765, 1990.

Fiore MC, et al: Tobacco dependence and the nicotine patch: Clinical guidelines for effective use. *JAMA* 268:2687-2694, 1992.

Food and Drug Administration: An interim report from the FDA. *N Engl J Med* 324:349-352, 1991.

Frezza M, et al: High blood alcohol levels in women: The role of decreased gastric alcohol dehydrogenase activity and first-pass metabolism. *N Engl J Med* 322:95-99, 1990.

Friedmann N, et al: Effect on growth in pemoline-treated children with attention deficit disorder. *Am J Dis Child* 135:329-332, 1981.

Fuller RK, et al: Disulfiram treatment of alcoholism: Veterans Administration cooperative study. *JAMA* 256:1449-1455, 1986.

Gaitz CM, et al: Pharmacotherapy for organic brain syndrome in late life: Evaluation of an ergot derivative vs placebo. *Arch Gen Psychiatry* 34:839-845, 1977.

Garfinkel BD, et al: Tricyclic antidepressants and methylphenidate treatment of attention deficit disorder in children. *J Am Acad Child Adolesc Psychiatry* 22:343-348, 1983.

Gauthier S, et al: Tetrahydroaminoacridine-lecithin combination treatment in patients with intermediate-stage Alzheimer's disease: Results of a Canadian double-blind, crossover, multicenter study. *N Engl J Med* 322:1272-1276, 1990.

Glynn TJ, Manley MW: *How to Help Your Patients Stop Smoking: A National Cancer Institute Manual for Physicians.* Bethesda, Md, US Dept. of Health and Human Services, 1989. National Institutes of Health publication 89-3064.

Goldstein MG, et al: Effects of behavioral skills training and schedule of nicotine gum administration on smoking cessation. *Am J Psychiatry* 146:56-60, 1989.

Gonzales R, Hoffman P: Receptor gated ion channels may be selective CNS target for ethanol. *Trends Pharmacol Sci* 12:1-3, 1991.

Gorski TT: Relapse prevention planning: A new recovery tool. *Alcohol Health Res World* 10(No. 63):6-11, 1986.

Gragg DM: Drugs to decrease alcohol consumption, letter. *N Engl J Med* 306:747, 1982.

Green PHR, Tall AR: Drugs, alcohol and malabsorption. *Am J Med* 67:1066-1076, 1979.

Green MS, et al: Blood pressure in smokers and nonsmokers: Epidemiologic findings. *Am Heart J* 111:932-940, 1986.

Green RC, et al: Treatment trial of oxiracetam in Alzheimer's disease. *Arch Neurol* 49:1135-1136, 1992.

Haass C, et al: Amyloid β-peptide is produced by cultured cells during normal metabolism, letter. *Nature* 359:322-325, 1992.

Hajek P, et al: Long-term use of nicotine chewing gum: Occurrence, determinants, and effect on weight gain. *JAMA* 260:1593-1596, 1988.

Hansten PD: Chlorpropamide and alcohol. *Drug Interact Newslett* 1:39-40, (Oct) 1981.

Harrell LE, et al: The effect of long-term physostigmine administration in Alzheimer's disease. *Neurology* 40:1350-1354, 1990.
Hollister LE, Yesavage J: Ergoloid mesylates for senile dementias: Unanswered questions. *Ann Intern Med* 100:894-898, 1984.
Horwitz RI, et al: The efficacy of atenolol in the outpatient management of the alcohol withdrawal syndrome. *Arch Intern Med* 149:1089-1093, 1989.
Hughes JR: Dependence potential and abuse liability of nicotine replacement therapies. *Prog Clin Biol Res* 261:261-277, 1988.
Hughes JR: Combining psychological and pharmacological treatment for smoking. *J Subst Abuse* 3:337-350, 1991.
Hughes JR: Tobacco withdrawal in self-quitters. *J Consult Clin Psychol* 60:689-697, 1992.
Hughes JR, et al: Nicotine vs placebo gum in general medical practice. *JAMA* 261:1300-1305, 1989.
Hughes JR, et al: Symptoms of tobacco withdrawal: A replication and extension. *Arch Gen Psychiatry* 48:52-59, 1991 A.
Hughes JR, et al: Long-term use of nicotine versus placebo gum. *Arch Intern Med* 151:1993-1998, 1991 B.
Hunt RD: Treatment effects of oral and transdermal clonidine in relation to methylphenidate: An open pilot study in ADD-H. *Psychopharmacol Bull* 23:111-114, 1987.
Hunt RD, et al: Clonidine benefits children with attention deficit disorder and hyperactivity: Report of a double-blind placebo-crossover therapeutic trial. *J Am Acad Child Psychiatry* 24:617-629, 1985.
Hurt RD, et al: Nicotine-replacement therapy with use of a transdermal nicotine patch: A randomized double-blind placebo-controlled trial. *Mayo Clin Proc* 65:1529-1537, 1990.
Imperiale TF, McCullough AJ: Do corticosteroids reduce mortality from alcoholic hepatitis? A meta-analysis of the randomized trials. *Ann Intern Med* 113:299-307, 1990.
Institute of Medicine: *Broadening the Base of Treatment for Alcohol Problems*. Washington, DC, National Academy Press, 1990.
Iosub S, et al: Fetal alcohol syndrome revisited. *Pediatrics* 68:475-479, 1981.
Jarvik ME: Biological influences on cigarette smoking, in: *The Behavioral Aspects of Smoking.* NIDA Monograph, vol 26, 1979.
Jellinek EM: Alcoholism: A genus and some of its species. *Can Med Assoc J* 83:1341-1345, 1960.
Jenike MA, et al: Oral physostigmine treatment for patients with presenile and senile dementia of the Alzheimer's type: A double-blind placebo-controlled trial. *J Clin Psychiatry* 51:3-7, 1990.
Kaplan BJ, et al: Dietary replacement in preschool-aged hyperactive boys. *Pediatrics* 83:7-17, 1989.
Kendler KS, et al: A population-based twin study of alcoholism in women. *JAMA* 268:1877-1882, 1992.
Killen JD, et al: Are heavy smokers different from light smokers? Comparison after 48 hours without cigarettes. *JAMA* 260:1581-1585, 1988.
Klein RG, Mannuzza S: Hyperactive boys almost grown up: III. Methylphenidate effects on ultimate height. *Arch Gen Psychiatry* 45:1131-1134, 1988.
Kokmen E: Etiology, diagnosis, and management of dementia. *Compr Ther* 15:59-69, (Sept) 1989.
Kokmen E, et al: Prevalence of medically diagnosed dementia in a defined US population. *Neurology* 39:773-776, 1989.
Krassner MB, et al: Mechanism of action of Hydergine (ergoloid mesylates) in relation to organic brain disorders. *Adv Ther* 1:172-188, 1984.
Kraus MI, et al: Randomized clinical trial of atenolol in patients with alcohol withdrawal. *N Engl J Med* 313:905-909, 1985.
Kushner MG, et al: The relation between alcohol problems and the anxiety disorders. *Am J Psychiatry* 147:685-695, 1990.
Lam W, et al: Meta-analysis of randomised controlled trials of nicotine chewing-gum. *Lancet* 2:27-30, 1987.
Laskin CA, et al: Autoantibodies in alcoholic liver disease. *Am J Med* 89:129-133, 1990.
Lawson-Wendling KL, et al: Differential effects of (*d*)-amphetamine, methylphenidate, and amfonelic acid on catecholamine synthesis in selected regions of rat brain. *J Pharm Pharmacol* 33:803-804, 1981.
Lechtenberg R, Worner TM: Seizure risk with recurrent alcohol detoxification. *Arch Neurol* 47:535-538, 1990.
Lewis DC, Femino J: Management of alcohol withdrawal. *Ration Drug Ther* 16:1-5, (Feb) 1982.
Lieber CS: Metabolism of alcohol. *Sci Am* 234:25-33, (March) 1976.
Lieber CS: Pathogenesis and early diagnosis of alcoholic liver injury. *N Engl J Med* 298:888-893, 1978.
Lieber CS: Interaction of ethanol with drug toxicity. *Am J Gastroenterol* 74:313-320, 1980.
Lieber CS: Biochemical and molecular basis of alcohol-induced injury to liver and other tissues. *N Engl J Med* 319:1639-1650, 1988.
Linnoila M, et al: Drug interactions with alcohol. *Drugs* 18:299-311, 1979.
Lipowski ZJ: Delirium in the elderly patient. *N Engl J Med* 320:578-582, 1989.
Littman GK: Alcoholism survival: The prevention of relapse, in Miller WR, Heather N (eds): *Treating Addictive Behaviors*. New York, Plenum Press, 1986, 294-303.
Lovinger DM, et al: Ethanol inhibition of neuronal glutamate receptor function. *Ann Med* 22:247-252, 1990.
Lowe TL, et al: Stimulant medications precipitate Tourette's syndrome. *JAMA* 247:1168-1169, 1982.
MacArthur DR, Williams GW: Nicotine gum in smoking cessation. *Pharmaceut J* 230:45-46, (Jan 15) 1983.
Malcolm R, et al: Double-blind controlled trial comparing carbamazepine to oxazepam treatment of alcohol withdrawal. *Am J Psychiatry* 146:617-621, 1989.
Mannuzza S, et al: Hyperactive boys almost grown up: V. Replication of psychiatric status. *Arch Gen Psychiatry* 48:77-83, 1991.
Marlatt GA, Gordon JR (eds): *Relapse Prevention: Maintenance Strategies in the Treatment of Addictive Behaviors*. New York, Guildford Press, 1985.
Mason NA: Disulfiram-induced hepatitis: Case report and review of the literature. *DICP* 23:872-875, 1989.
Mattson ME, et al: What are the odds that smoking will kill you? *Am J Public Health* 77:425-431, 1987.
Mayeux R: Therapeutic strategies in Alzheimer's disease. *Neurology* 40:175-180, 1990.
McGue M, et al: Sex and age effects on the inheritance of alcohol problems: A twin study. *J Abnorm Psychol* 101:3-17, (Feb) 1992.
McKhann G, et al: Clinical diagnosis of Alzheimer's disease: Report of the NINCDS-ADRDA Work Group under the auspices of Department of Health and Human Services Task Force on Alzheimer's disease. *Neurology* 34:939-944, 1984.
Meyer RE: Prospects for a rational pharmacotherapy of alcoholism. *J Clin Psychiatry* 50:403-412, 1989.
Milman D: Minimal brain dysfunction in childhood: Outcome in late adolescence and early adult years. *J Clin Psychiatry* 40:371-380, 1979.
Molloy DW, et al: Effect of tetrahydroaminoacridine on cognition, function and behaviour in Alzheimer's disease. *Can Med Assoc J* 144:29-34, 1991.
Morey LC, Skinner HA: Empirically derived classifications of alcohol-related problems, in Galanter M (ed): *Recent Developments in Alcoholism,* ed 5. New York, Plenum Publishing, 1986, 145-168.
Morgan AM: Use of stimulant medications in children. *Am Fam Physician* 38:197-202, (Oct) 1988.
Morse RM, Flavin DK: The definition of alcoholism. *JAMA* 268:1012-1014, 1992.
Mulligan SC, et al: Clinical and pharmacokinetic properties of a transdermal nicotine patch. *Clin Pharmacol Ther* 47:331-337, 1990.
Naeye RL: Maternal use of dextroamphetamine and growth of fetus. *Pharmacology* 26:117-120, 1983.
Ng SKC, et al: Alcohol consumption and withdrawal in new-onset seizures. *N Engl J Med* 319:666-673, 1988.
NIH (National Institutes of Health) Consensus Conference: Defined diets and childhood hyperactivity. *JAMA* 248:290-292, 1982.
NIH (National Institutes of Health) Consensus Development Conference: Differential diagnosis of dementing diseases. *NIH Consensus Development Conference Statement,* vol 6, July 6-8, 1987 (US Government Printing Office 1987-181-296:61128).

Ornis SA, et al: Effects of transdermal clonidine treatment on withdrawal symptoms associated with smoking cessation. *Arch Intern Med* 148:2027-2031, 1988.

Palmer KJ, et al: Transdermal nicotine: A review of its pharmacodynamic and pharmacokinetic properties, and therapeutic efficacy as an aid to smoking cessation. *Drugs* 44:498-529, 1992.

Peachey JE, Naranjo CA: Role of drugs in treatment of alcoholism. *Drugs* 27:171-182, 1984.

Pelham WE Jr, et al: Sustained release and standard methylphenidate effects on cognitive and social behavior in children with attention deficit disorder. *Pediatrics* 80:491-501, 1987.

Perkins KA, et al: The effect of nicotine on energy expenditure during light physical activity. *N Engl J Med* 320:898-903, 1989.

Pickens RW, et al: Heterogeneity in the inheritance of alcoholism: A study of male and female twins. *Arch Gen Psychiatry* 48:19-28, 1991.

Pierce JP, et al: Trends in cigarette smoking in the United States: Educational differences are increasing. *JAMA* 261:56-60, 1989.

Pike C, et al: Aggregation-related toxicity of synthetic beta-amyloid protein in hippocampal cultures. *Eur J Pharmacol* 207:367-368, 1991.

Pike C, et al: Beta-amyloid induces neuritic dystrophy in vitro: Similarities with Alzheimer pathology. *Neural Rep* 3:769-772, 1992.

Prochazka AV, et al: Transdermal clonidine reduced some withdrawal symptoms but did not increase smoking cessation. *Arch Intern Med* 152:2065-2069, 1992.

Ramond M-J, et al: A randomized trial of prednisolone in patients with severe alcoholic hepatitis. *N Engl J Med* 326:507-512, 1992.

Rapoport J, et al: Dextroamphetamine: Cognitive and behavioral effects in normal prepubertal boys. *Science* 199:560-563, 1978.

Reed JS, Liskow BI: Current treatment of alcohol withdrawal. *Ration Drug Ther* 21:1-6, (Feb) 1987.

Regan TJ: Alcohol and the cardiovascular system. *JAMA* 264:377-381, 1990.

Regier DA, et al: Comorbidity of mental disorders with alcohol and other drug abuse: Results from the Epidemiologic Catchment Area (ECA) Study. *JAMA* 264:2511-2518, 1990.

Rennard S, et al: Transdermal nicotine enhances smoking cessation in coronary artery disease patients. *Chest* 100:5S, 1991.

Richmond JB: Ending the cigarette pandemic. *NY State J Med* 83:1259, 1983.

Rinaldi RC, et al: Clarification and standardization of substance abuse terminology. *JAMA* 259:555-557, 1988.

Robinson BJ, et al: Is clonidine useful in the treatment of alcohol withdrawal? *Alcoholism Clin Exp Res* 13:95-98, 1989.

Roine R, et al: Aspirin increases blood alcohol concentrations in humans after ingestion of ethanol. *JAMA* 264:2406-2408, 1990.

Romach MK, Sellers EM: Management of the alcohol withdrawal syndrome. *Annu Rev Med* 42:323-340, 1991.

Rose JE, et al: Transdermal nicotine facilitates smoking cessation. *Clin Pharmacol Ther* 47:323-330, 1990.

Rosett HL, Weiner L: Alcohol and pregnancy: A clinical perspective. *Ann Rev Med* 36:73-80, 1985.

Sachs DP: Advances in smoking cessation treatment. *Curr Pulmonology* 12:139-198, 1991.

Safer DJ, Krager JM: Survey of medication treatment for hyperactive/inattentive students. *JAMA* 260:2256-2258, 1988.

Sano M, et al: Double-blind parallel design pilot study of acetyl levocarnitine in patients with Alzheimer's disease. *Arch Neurol* 49:1137-1141, 1992.

Satterfield JH, et al: Growth of hyperactive children treated with methylphenidate. *Arch Gen Psychiatry* 36:212-217, 1979.

Seitz HK, et al: High blood alcohol levels in women, editorial. *N Engl J Med* 323:58-59, 1990.

Sellers EM: Alcohol, barbiturate and benzodiazepine withdrawal syndromes: Clinical management. *Can Med Assoc J* 139:113-118, 1988.

Sellers EM, Kalant H: Alcohol intoxication and withdrawal. *N Engl J Med* 294:757-762, 1976.

Sellers EM, et al: Drugs to decrease alcohol consumption. *N Engl J Med* 305:1255-1262, 1981.

Selzer ML: The Michigan Alcoholism Screening Test: The quest for a new diagnostic instrument. *Am J Psychiatry* 127:1653-1658, 1971.

Seubert P, et al: Isolation and quantification of soluble Alzheimer's β-peptide from biological fluids, letter. *Nature* 359:325-327, 1992.

Seyler LE, et al: Pituitary hormone response to cigarette smoking. *Pharmacol Biochem Behav* 24:159-162, 1986.

Shaywitz SE, Shaywitz BA: Increased medication use in attention-deficit hyperactivity disorder: Regressive or appropriate? editorial. *JAMA* 260:2270-2272, 1988.

Shoji M, et al: Production of the Alzheimer amyloid β protein by normal proteolytic processing. *Science* 258:126-129, 1992.

Simeon JG, et al: Bupropion effects in attention deficit and conduct disorders. *Can J Psychiatry* 31:581-585, 1986.

Skoog I, et al: A population-based study of dementia in 85-year-olds. *N Engl J Med* 328:153-158, 1993.

Small GW, et al: Diagnosis and treatment of dementia in the aged. *West J Med* 135:469-481, 1981.

Spagnoli A, et al: Long-term acetyl-L-carnitine treatment in Alzheimer's disease. *Neurology* 41:1726-1732, 1991.

Steinberg D (moderator), et al: Alcohol and atherosclerosis. *Ann Intern Med* 114:967-976, 1991.

Steingard R, et al: Comparison of clonidine response in the treatment of attention-deficit hyperactivity disorder with and without comorbid tic disorders. *J Am Acad Child Adolesc Psychiatry* 32:350-353, (March) 1993.

Stern Y, et al: Long-term administration of oral physostigmine in Alzheimer's disease. *Neurology* 38:1837-1841, 1988.

Stevenson RD, Wolraich ML: Stimulant medication therapy in the treatment of children with attention deficit hyperactivity disorder. *Clin Pharmacol* 36:1183-1197, 1989.

Streissguth AP, et al: Fetal alcohol syndrome in adolescents and adults. *JAMA* 265:1961-1967, 1991.

Summers WK, et al: Oral tetrahydroaminoacridine in long-term treatment of senile dementia, Alzheimer type. *N Engl J Med* 315:1241-1245, 1986.

Summers WK, et al: A response from Summers et al. *N Engl J Med* 324:352, 1991.

Swanson JM, Kinsbourne M: Artificial colors and hyperactive behavior, in Knights R, Bakker D (eds): *Treatment of Hyperactive and Learning Disabled Children: Current Research.* Baltimore, University Park Press, 1980, 131-150.

Swanson JM, et al: Methylphenidate hydrochloride given with or before breakfast: I. Behavioral, cognitive, and electrophysiologic effects. *Pediatrics* 72:49-55, 1983.

Thompson TL II, et al: Lack of efficacy of Hydergine in patients with Alzheimer's disease. *N Engl J Med* 323:445-448, 1990.

Thorley G: Adolescent outcome for hyperactive children. *Arch Dis Child* 63:1181-1183, 1988.

Tønnesen P, et al: A double-blind trial of a 16-hour transdermal nicotine patch in smoking cessation. *N Engl J Med* 325:311-325, 1991.

Transdermal Nicotine Study Group: Transdermal nicotine for smoking cessation: Six-month results from two multicenter controlled trials. *JAMA* 266:3133-3138, 1991.

Urbano-Marquez A, et al: The effects of alcoholism on skeletal and cardiac muscle. *N Engl J Med* 320:409-415, 1989.

US Department of Health and Human Services: *The Health Consequences of Smoking: Nicotine Addiction: A Report of the Surgeon General, 1988.* US Department of Health and Human Services, Public Health Service, Centers for Disease Control, Center for Health Promotion and Education, Office on Smoking and Health. DHHS Publication No. (CDC) 88-8406, 1988.

US Department of Health and Human Services: *Reducing the Health Consequences of Smoking: 25 Years of Progress. A Report of the Surgeon General, 1988.* US Department of Health and Human Services, Public Health Service, Centers for Disease Control, Center for Chronic Disease Prevention and Health Promotion, Office on Smoking and Health. DHHS Publication No. (CDC) 89-8411, prepublication version. January 11, 1989.

US Department of Health and Human Services: *The Health Benefits of Smoking Cessation: A Report of the Surgeon General.* Rockville, Md, Office on Smoking and Health. Publication No. (CDC) 90-8416, 1990.

US Department of Health, Education and Welfare: *Surgeon General's Report on Smoking and Health*. Washington, DC, HEW, 1979.

van Loveren-Huyben CMS, et al: Double-blind clinical and psychologic study of ergoloid mesylates (Hydergine) in subjects with senile mental deterioration. *J Am Geriatr Soc* 32:584-588, 1984.

Vincent J, et al: Effects of methylphenidate on early adolescent growth. *Am J Psychiatry* 147:501-502, 1990.

von Knorring L, et al: Personality traits in subtypes of alcoholics. *J Stud Alcohol* 48:523-527, 1987.

Wallace P, et al: Randomised controlled trial of general practitioner intervention in patients with excessive alcohol consumption. *BMJ* 297:663-668, 1988.

Walsh DC, et al: A randomized trial of treatment options for alcohol-abusing workers. *N Engl J Med* 325:775-782, 1991.

Weingartner H, et al: Cognitive processes in normal and hyperactive children and their response to amphetamine treatment. *J Abnorm Psychol* 89:25-37, 1980.

Weiss G: Controversial issues of pharmacotherapy of hyperactive child. *Can J Psychiatry* 26:385-392, 1981.

Weiss B, et al: Behavioral responses to artificial food colors. *Science* 107:1487-1488, 1980.

Wells CE: Pseudodementia. *Am J Psychiatry* 136:895-900, 1979.

Wender PH, Reimherr FW: Bupropion treatment of attention-deficit hyperactivity disorder in adults. *Am J Psychiatry* 147:1018-1020, 1990.

Wender PH, et al: Pharmacological treatment of attention deficit disorder, residual type (ADD, RT, "minimal brain dysfunction," "hyperactivity") in adults. *Psychopharmacol Bull* 21:222-231, 1985.

West LJ (moderator): UCLA Conference, Alcoholism. *Ann Intern Med* 100:405-416, 1984.

Whitfield CL: Advances in alcoholism and chemical dependence, editorial. *Am J Med* 85:465, 1988.

Williamson DF, et al: Smoking cessation and severity of weight gain in a national cohort. *N Engl J Med* 324:739-745, 1991.

Wootton FT, Lee WM: Acetaminophen hepatotoxicity in the alcoholic. *South Med J* 83:1047-1049, 1990.

Zametkin AJ, Rapoport JL: Neurobiology of attention deficit disorder with hyperactivity: Where have we come in 50 years? *J Am Acad Child Adolesc Psychiatry* 26:676-686, 1987.

Zametkin A, et al: Treatment of hyperactive children with monoamine oxidase inhibitors: I. Clinical efficacy. *Arch Gen Psychiatry* 42:962-966, 1985.

Zetterman RK: Autoimmunity and alcoholic liver disease, editorial. *Am J Med* 89:127-128, 1990.

New Evaluation 14

TACRINE HYDROCHLORIDE

[Cognex]

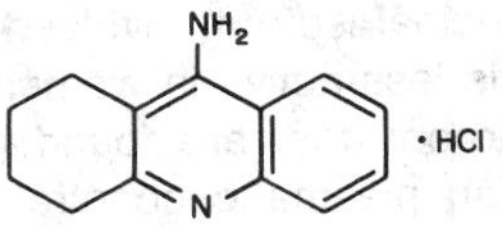

NH_2 ·HCl

ACTIONS. Tacrine hydrochloride (1,2,3,4-tetrahydro-9-acridinamine monohydrochloride monohydrate) is a centrally active, noncompetitive, reversible cholinesterase inhibitor. The use of cholinesterase inhibitors and other cholinomimetic agents in the treatment of Alzheimer's disease (AD) is based on observations that choline acetyltransferase and acetylcholinesterase activity are markedly reduced in the brains of these patients. The decrease in enzymatic markers for cholinergic neurons roughly parallels the severity of neuronal loss, density of neuritic plaques, and cognitive decline (especially memory) in patients with dementia of the Alzheimer's type.

Tacrine presumably acts by inhibiting the hydrolysis of acetylcholine released from remaining cholinergic neurons in the cerebral cortex, although many other neuropharmacologic effects have been described (eg, partial agonist activity at muscarinic receptors, inhibition of monoamine reuptake, inhibition of monoamine oxidase, sodium and potassium channel blockade) (Freeman and Dawson, 1991; Adem, 1992). This drug's ability to enhance cholinergic function may lessen as more cholinergic neurons are lost and the disease progresses. There is no evidence that tacrine alters the course of the underlying disease in patients with AD.

USES. The development of tacrine for treatment of AD has not been without controversy ever since striking beneficial effects were reported in one study on a small number of patients who received large doses (up to 200 mg/day) in combination with lecithin (Summers et al, 1986; Food and Drug Administration, 1991; Summers et al, 1991). Subsequently, no significant benefit was demonstrated in three small controlled trials that used smaller doses of tacrine (up to 125 mg/day) in combination with lecithin (Gauthier et al, 1990; Chatellier et al, 1990; Molloy et al, 1991). In another trial in which up to 150 mg of tacrine plus 10.8 g of lecithin was administered daily, 45% of recipients improved by three or more points on the Mini-Mental State Examination, compared with 11% who received placebo; however, no significant effect was observed when caregivers assessed the activities of daily living (Eagger et al, 1991).

Some investigators have speculated that there is a subpopulation of tacrine-responsive patients. This may explain the generally negative results reported using fixed doses and could account for the occasional dramatic improvement observed in some patients with AD. One clinical trial (Davis et al, 1992) studied only patients who had demonstrated significant improvement on the Alzheimer's Disease Assessment Scale (ADAS) during a six-week dose finding (40 or 80 mg) phase before rerandomization to a six-week double-blind placebo-controlled phase. Treatment of patients with their "best dose" resulted in a statistically significant reduction in the decline in cognitive function as assessed by the ADAS cognitive subscale (ADAS COG), whereas patients in the placebo group continued to decline. No improvement in global function was reported by the study physicians. In another randomized controlled trial (12 weeks) sponsored by the manufacturer as part of its New Drug Application, 51% of 37 patients who received a daily dose of 80 mg (for the final six weeks) achieved a four-point or greater improvement on the ADAS COG compared with 18% of those on placebo; in global assessment by the physician, tacrine also was favored (Farlow et al, 1992). The degree of improvement roughly corresponded to the average decline that normally occurs over six months in patients with mild to moderate AD. In these studies, 18% to 25% of patients had to discontinue use of tacrine because of side effects, most commonly elevation in ALT.

Additional safety and efficacy data collected by the manufacturer in a 30-week double-blind, dose-titration study in 663 patients indicate that tacrine significantly improved patient performance on the ADAS COG and the Clinician Interview Based Impression of Change (CIBI) compared with placebo (Knapp et al, 1994). This study was important because it examined the effect of tacrine in doses as high as 160 mg/day. Twenty percent of patients who completed the trial had at least a four-point improvement on the ADAS COG. The percentage of evaluable patients who improved increased in a dose-dependent manner; 42% of those in the 160 mg/day group were rated as improved on the CIBI.

It is estimated that 60% to 75% of patients with AD will be able to tolerate tacrine in clinical practice, although many may not be able to tolerate the maximum dosage of 160 mg/day. Potential hepatotoxicity and other serious adverse events probably can be minimized with regular monitoring. However, in most patients, tacrine's benefit is modest. A combination of intolerance and lack of response may limit noticeable cognitive improvement to ≤15% of patients with mild to moderate AD (*F-D-C Reports*, 1993). The relationship between tacrine-induced cognitive improvement as detected by standardized rating instruments and clinically useful functional improvement is not clearly established. Nevertheless, in the 30-week trial (Knapp et al, 1994), significant effects of treatment were noted subjectively by both the treating clinician and the caregiver in patients who received tacrine 160 mg/day.

ADVERSE REACTIONS AND PRECAUTIONS. Because tacrine is an inhibitor of cholinesterase and has both central and peripheral actions, it may (1) have vagotonic effects on the heart, (2) increase gastric acid secretion, (3) cause nausea, vomiting, and diarrhea or loose stools, (4) cause bladder outflow obstruction, and (4) exacerbate asthmatic conditions.

In clinical trials sponsored by the manufacturer, tacrine was discontinued in 17% of patients because of adverse events, most commonly increases in serum ALT concentrations that exceeded three times the upper limit of normal (ULN). The other most frequent causes of discontinuation of therapy were nausea and/or vomiting, agitation, rash, anorexia, and confusion. Diarrhea, dyspepsia, myalgia, and ataxia also were reported frequently. Other adverse events observed in controlled trials included weight decrease, chills, fever, malaise, peripheral edema, hypotension or hypertension, arthralgia, hypertonia, convulsions, vertigo, syncope, hyperkinesia, paresthesia, nervousness, dyspnea, increased sweating, conjunctivitis, tremor, and facial flushing.

Because of the possibility of hepatotoxicity, serum concentrations of ALT should be monitored weekly for at least the first 18 weeks following initiation of tacrine treatment, after which monitoring may be decreased to every three months. Weekly monitoring should be resumed for a minimum of six weeks whenever the dose is increased. Continued weekly monitoring (beyond 18 weeks) may be indicated in patients with modest increases (greater than two times the ULN).

Nearly 50% of patients experience an increase in ALT; in approximately 25%, the increases exceed three times the ULN and in 7% the increases exceed 10 times the ULN. The initial increase in ALT usually occurs 4 to 12 weeks after initiation of therapy (median, six weeks), and concentrations usually return to normal four to six weeks after discontinuation of the drug. Tacrine is contraindicated in patients who developed treatment-associated jaundice confirmed by elevated total bilirubin concentrations >3 mg/dL during previous therapy with this drug.

Abrupt discontinuation of tacrine or a large reduction in total daily dose (80 mg/day or more) may be associated with a rapid decline in cognitive function and increased behavioral disturbances. A full monitoring sequence should be repeated if administration is resumed after being discontinued for more than four weeks.

DRUG INTERACTIONS. Additive or synergistic effects may occur when tacrine is combined with succinylcholine, cholinergic agonists, or other cholinesterase inhibitors, and, conversely, this drug may interfere with the action of anticholinergic medications. Tacrine also may inhibit the metabolism of other drugs that are metabolized by cytochrome P450IA2 (CYP1A2). For example, steady-state theophylline concentrations may be doubled in patients who receive theophylline and tacrine concurrently. In addition, steady-state tacrine concentrations may be doubled in patients who receive cimetidine and tacrine concurrently.

PHARMACOKINETICS. Tacrine is rapidly absorbed after oral administration; peak plasma concentrations are achieved within two hours. Absolute bioavailability of tacrine is low (17%), and plasma concentrations are highly variable. Food reduces bioavailability by 30% to 40%; this effect on absorption can be avoided by administering the drug at least one hour before meals.

Tacrine's mean volume of distribution far exceeds total body water (349 L or approximately 5 L/kg); plasma protein binding is 55%. Data obtained from studies using radiolabeling indicate that approximately 20% of tacrine and/or its metabolite(s) may be retained at an extravascular site.

Tacrine is extensively metabolized by the cytochrome P450 system and multiple metabolites are formed, only some of which have been identified (1-, 2-, and 4-hydroxytacrine); CYP1A2 is the principal isoform involved in tacrine metabolism. This isoform is less active in women and is induced by polycyclic hydrocarbons that are found in cigarette smoke. Consequently, mean plasma concentrations of tacrine are higher in women and lower in smokers. Because CYP1A2 is saturated with relatively low doses, systemic availability of tacrine increases disproportionately with increasing oral doses. However, elimination of tacrine from the plasma is independent of dose or plasma concentration ($t_{1/2}$ = two to four hours).

The systemic clearance of tacrine is relatively normal in elderly patients and in those with renal disease. Although studies have not been done, hepatic impairment probably reduces the clearance of tacrine and its metabolites.

DOSAGE AND ADMINISTRATION. Tacrine should be taken between meals unless administration with meals is required to improve tolerability.

Oral: Initially, 10 mg four times daily for a minimum of six weeks. If there is no significant increase in ALT and the patient is tolerating treatment, the daily dose should be increased to 80 mg in four divided doses. If this amount is tolerated, daily dosage should be increased at six-week intervals to 120 mg and then to 160 mg in four divided doses.

If ALT increases but remains within three times the ULN, normal upward dosage titration may be continued. If increases in ALT are between three and five times the ULN, the daily dose should be reduced by 40 mg. The normal schedule for dosage titration may be resumed when ALT concentrations return to normal limits. If ALT concentrations exceed five times the ULN, tacrine should be discontinued; administration may be resumed when the ALT concentrations return to normal limits. The risks associated with rechallenge in patients who experienced elevations greater than 10 times the ULN are not well characterized. In patients who are rechallenged, the initial dose should not exceed 40 mg/day and ALT concentrations should be monitored weekly for six weeks. If ALT values remain within normal limits, the recommended dose-titration schedule can be resumed.

Cognex (Parke-Davis). Capsules 10, 20, 30, and 40 mg.

Cited References

Warner-Lambert's *Cognex* tolerated by up to three-quarters of Alzheimer's patients, firm estimates; advisory committee unanimously supports approval. *F-D-C Reports* 7-9, (March) 1993.

Adem A: Putative mechanisms of action of tacrine in Alzheimer's disease. *Acta Neurol Scand* (suppl 139):69-74, 1992.

Chatellier G, et al: Tacrine (tetrahydroaminoacridine; THA) and lecithin in senile dementia of the Alzheimer type: A multicentre trial. *BMJ* 300:495-499, 1990.

Davis KL, et al: A double-blind, placebo-controlled multicenter study of tacrine for Alzheimer's disease. *N Engl J Med* 327:1253-1259, 1992.

Eagger SA, et al: Tacrine in Alzheimer's disease. *Lancet* 337:989-992, 1991.

Farlow M, et al: A controlled trial of tacrine in Alzheimer's disease. *JAMA* 268:2523-2529, 1992.

Food and Drug Administration: An interim report from the FDA. *N Engl J Med* 324:349-352, 1991.

Freeman SE, Dawson RM: Tacrine—A pharmacological review. *Prog Neurobiol* 36:257-277, 1991.

Gauthier S, et al: Tetrahydroaminoacridine-lecithin combination treatment in patients with intermediate-stage Alzheimer's disease: Results of a Canadian double-blind, crossover, multicenter study. *N Engl J Med* 322:1272-1276, 1990.

Knapp MJ, et al: A 30-week randomized controlled trial of high-dose tacrine in patients with Alzheimer's disease. *JAMA* 271:985-991, 1994.

Molloy DW, et al: Effect of tetrahydroaminoacridine on cognition, function and behaviour in Alzheimer's disease. *Can Med Assoc J* 144:29-34, 1991.

Summers WK, et al: Oral tetrahydroaminoacridine in long-term treatment of senile dementia, Alzheimer type. *N Engl J Med* 315:1241-1245, 1986.

Summers WK, et al: A response from Summers et al. *N Engl J Med* 324:352, 1991.

Antiepileptic Drugs 15

SEIZURES

Seizures are the clinical expression of abnormal, hypersynchronous brain activity. The manifestations of a seizure reflect the function of the brain area involved and may include impairment of cognition or consciousness, involuntary movements, behavioral automatisms, and sensory, psychic, or autonomic features. In infants and children, seizures may be caused by perinatal insults, congenital or developmental defects, cerebrovascular disease, metabolic disorders, head injuries, infection, or fever. In adolescents and adults, important causes include head trauma, neoplasms, vascular lesions, infection, and drug or alcohol abuse (including withdrawal from central nervous system depressants). In adults and elderly patients, degenerative processes and cerebrovascular disease are important causes of seizures. In most patients, seizures occur in the absence of any diagnosable condition. When an acute or pre-existing condition causing the seizure can be determined, treatment is directed at the underlying cause, and antiepileptic drugs are used as needed to control the seizures.

Seizures are classified on the basis of distinctive behavioral features as well as on ictal and interictal electroencephalographic (EEG) findings (Commission on Classification and Terminology of the International League Against Epilepsy, 1981) and are divided broadly into two groups: partial and generalized (see Table 1). Partial seizures arise in part of one cerebral hemisphere and are often accompanied by focal EEG abnormalities. They are subdivided according to whether consciousness is maintained (simple) or impaired (complex). The manifestations of partial seizures are determined by the particular brain area involved. Either type of partial seizure may become secondarily generalized.

Generalized seizures are characterized by impaired consciousness with clinical or EEG evidence indicating involvement of both hemispheres initially; they are classified as nonconvulsive or convulsive subtypes.

Neonatal seizures differ greatly from those in older patients and often represent the initial symptom of a serious neurologic disorder. A range of behaviors (including apnea and autonomic phenomena) may be seizures, but not all are reflected in the EEG findings (electroclinical dissociation). Thus, neonatal seizures may be difficult to diagnose and classify (Mizrahi, 1987; Volpe, 1989).

EPILEPSIES AND EPILEPTIC SYNDROMES

Spontaneous recurrent seizures are the presenting symptom of the neurologic disorder, epilepsy. Because the International Classification of Epileptic Seizures (ICES) is limited to a description of individual seizure types, epileptic syndromes, which permit the appropriate classification of patients, are classified separately (Commission on Classification and Terminology of the International League Against Epilepsy, 1989). An epileptic syndrome is characterized by a clustering of

TABLE 1.
EPILEPTIC SEIZURES: CLASSIFICATION AND CHARACTERISTICS*

Seizure Classification	Clinical Characteristics
I. PARTIAL SEIZURES (FOCAL SEIZURES)	
A. Simple partial seizures 1. with motor signs 2. with somatosensory or special sensory symptoms 3. with autonomic symptoms 4. with psychic symptoms	Most common in older children and adults. Consciousness is not impaired. Paroxysmal attacks limited to functional disturbances of sensory, motor, and/or autonomic nerves and to anatomic regions of the brain, depending on the particular cortical area of involvement. Seizures with motor and special sensory symptoms (odor, taste) are most common. Partial motor seizures may spread in a sequential fashion to adjacent cortical areas causing an epileptic "march" (Jacksonian seizure). Following partial seizure activity, localized weakness (Todd's paresis) may occur for a variable period of time.
B. Complex partial seizures 1. simple partial onset followed by impairment of consciousness 2. with impairment of consciousness at the onset	Most common in older children and adults. Daily to monthly episodes of impaired consciousness (eg, amnesia, unresponsiveness), usually characterized by brief (1 to 2 minutes) episodes. Clinical manifestations varied; most commonly consist of automatisms (eg, staring, chewing movements or smacking of lips, gestures, purposeless motor movements, bizarre behavior, mumbled speech or unintelligible sounds). Confusion may persist for several minutes after attack subsides. EEG is helpful for diagnosis, because unusual variants of this disorder may be difficult to distinguish from purely functional psychiatric disorders.
C. Partial seizures evolving to secondarily generalized seizures 1. simple partial seizures (A) evolving to generalized seizures 2. complex partial seizures (B) evolving to generalized seizures 3. simple partial seizures evolving to complex partial seizures evolving to generalized seizures	Partial seizures may evolve into generalized tonic-clonic seizures. Prior to treatment, partial seizures may spread to generalized tonic-clonic seizures so rapidly that the partial nature of the seizure is not recognized.
II. GENERALIZED SEIZURES (CONVULSIVE OR NONCONVULSIVE)	
A. 1. Typical absence seizures (petit mal seizures)	Onset usually between age 4 and 8 years; rarely occurs before age 3 or after age 15. An absence attack is an abrupt, brief episode of loss of consciousness, amnesia, or unawareness characterized by staring and a 3 Hertz spike-and-wave pattern in the EEG, which may be associated with mild clonic movements (eye blinking, twitching movements), automatisms, or changes in postural tone or tonic components. No postictal or confused state follows attack. Duration of attack is 3 to 30 seconds, and attacks may occur as frequently as 50 to 100 times a day.
2. Atypical absence seizures	EEG pattern is more heterogenous. May have changes in tone that are more pronounced than typical absence seizures. Onset and/or cessation may be less abrupt.
B. Myoclonic seizures	Single or multiple sudden, brief, "shock-like" contractions may be generalized or confined to the face and trunk or individual muscles or groups of muscles. They are frequently associated with the sleep-wake cycle. Many types of myoclonic jerks and action myoclonus are not classified as epileptic seizures.
C. Clonic seizures	Clonic seizures are characterized by repetitive clonic jerks that lack a tonic component. Clonic jerks may be symmetrical, asymmetrical, rhythmic, or arrhythmic; these seizures are relatively rare, occurring primarily in early childhood.
D. Tonic seizures	Tonic contraction of certain muscle groups is accompanied by altered consciousness, but there is no progression to clonic phase. Duration of seizures is brief (10 seconds). Ocular phenomena are common and include fixation of the eyes, eyelid retraction, superior ocular deviation, nystagmus, and mydriasis.

(table continued on next page)

TABLE 1 (continued)

Seizure Classification	Clinical Characteristics
E. Tonic-clonic seizures (grand mal)	These are the most commonly encountered generalized seizures and can occur at any age. While some patients experience a vague warning, the majority lose consciousness without premonitory signs. Seizures begin with a sudden tonic contraction of muscles (if respiratory muscles are affected, there is stridor); the patient falls to the ground and remains rigid (10 to 30 seconds). The tonic phase gives way to the clonic phase (30 to 50 seconds) and muscle relaxation interrupts tonic contraction. Muscle tone returns primarily during extensor spasms that become less frequent as the seizure subsides. Following this, the patient remains unconscious for variable periods. Seizures usually last 2 to 3 minutes. Urinary and fecal incontinence may occur after the clonic phase.
F. Atonic seizures	Sudden reduction of muscle tone may selectively affect muscle groups, leading to head drop with slackening of the jaw, the dropping of a limb, or loss of all muscle tone leading to slumping or falling to the ground. When attacks are brief, they are called "drop attacks." Other conditions, such as narcolepsy, cataplexy syndrome, and brainstem ischemia, also cause "drop attacks."
III. UNCLASSIFIED EPILEPTIC SEIZURES	Inadequate data for classification. This category includes some neonatal seizures (eg, rhythmic eye movements, chewing and swimming movements).

**Adapted from Commission on Classification and Terminology of the International League Against Epilepsy, 1981.*

signs and symptoms that regularly occur together; the seizure type(s), etiology, precipitating factors, hereditary components, associated clinical features (eg, mental impairment), and natural history (eg, age of onset, chronicity, severity) are considered in this classification. Delineating epileptic syndromes permits a greater precision of diagnosis and prognosis than simply classifying seizure types, because the same type of seizure can occur in various syndromes (Aicardi, 1988). Some syndromes are well defined and unequivocal while others are heterogenous. For many patients, data are inadequate to assign a specific syndrome based on the current classification system (Manford et al, 1992).

The epilepsies are classified on the basis of seizure type (localization-related or generalized) and seizure etiology (idiopathic or symptomatic) (see Table 2). Idiopathic epilepsies have no definable cause; they often are familial, and onset is age-related. Benign familial neonatal convulsions and juvenile myoclonic epilepsy are two of the idiopathic epilepsies with putative gene assignments (Delgado-Escueta et al, 1989; Leppert et al, 1989), although genetic heterogeneity may exist (Lewis et al, 1993; Grünewald and Panayiotopoulos, 1993). In general, idiopathic epilepsies are more likely than symptomatic epilepsies to be associated with normal development, responsiveness to antiepileptic drugs, and remission. Symptomatic epilepsies and syndromes are caused by diagnosable central nervous system (CNS) disorders, although, in some patients with presumed symptomatic epilepsy, the underlying cause remains obscure (cryptogenic). In these epilepsies, the interictal EEG is more likely to be abnormal, the prognosis is less favorable, and the response to antiepileptic drugs is variable.

The age-adjusted prevalence of epilepsy among whites in this country is 6.8/1,000 population (Hauser et al, 1991). The prevalence is probably higher in urban minority populations (Locke et al, 1989). Symptomatic partial epilepsies and idiopathic generalized epilepsy are the most common syndromes observed in adults. In the pediatric population, the spectrum of syndromes is large and is age dependent. Prevalence increases with age during childhood and adolescence, is stable in adult years, and increases again in elderly individuals (Hauser et al, 1991).

PATHOPHYSIOLOGY. Regardless of the diversity of epileptic syndromes, seizures are caused by the abnormal, synchronous activation of a localized (partial epilepsy) or more diffuse (generalized epilepsy) population of neurons. In experimental models of partial epilepsy, freezing the neocortex or applying certain chemicals topically (eg, penicillin, bicuculline, cobalt, alumina cream) leads to spontaneous epileptiform discharge. Cells within the seizure focus display paroxysmal depolarizing shifts (PDS) of the membrane potential with superimposed trains or bursts of action potentials (Dichter, 1989). A number of factors, including intrinsic neuronal mechanisms and specific alterations in synaptic events (enhanced excitation, disinhibition), may contribute to the PDS. The PDS usually is followed by a prolonged after-hyperpolarization (AHP) that limits the duration and propagation of the after-discharge. Failure of mechanisms that generate the AHP appears to be a critical factor in the transition from interictal spiking to seizure in some models. Propagation of burst discharges to other brain regions involves other mechanisms.

Dysfunction of inhibitory influences is considered important for the development and spread of epileptiform activity. Gamma-aminobutyric acid (GABA) is believed to be the major inhibitory neurotransmitter in the mammalian CNS and, indeed, antagonists of the GABA receptor are potent convulsants in experimental models of epilepsy. Recently, the role of excitatory amino acids in the CNS, in particular glutamate, has been studied most intensely. Ionotropic glutamate receptors mediate rapid excitatory synaptic transmission at many sites in the CNS. These glutamate receptors include N-

TABLE 2.
EPILEPSIES AND EPILEPTIC SYNDROMES: CLASSIFICATION*

I. LOCALIZATION-RELATED (FOCAL, LOCAL, PARTIAL) EPILEPSIES AND SYNDROMES
- A. Idiopathic (with age-related onset)
  1. Benign childhood epilepsy with centrotemporal spike (Rolandic)
  2. Childhood epilepsy with occipital paroxysms
  3. Primary reading epilepsy
- B. Symptomatic
  1. Chronic progressive epilepsia partialis continua of childhood (Kojewnikow's syndrome)
  2. Syndromes characterized by seizures with specific modes of precipitation (eg, reflex, startle epilepsy)
  3. Temporal lobe epilepsies
  4. Frontal lobe epilepsies
  5. Parietal lobe epilepsies
  6. Occipital lobe epilepsies
- C. Cryptogenic

II. GENERALIZED EPILEPSIES AND SYNDROMES
- A. Idiopathic (with age-related onset—listed in order of age)
  1. Benign neonatal familial convulsions
  2. Benign neonatal convulsions
  3. Childhood absence epilepsy (pyknolepsy)
  4. Juvenile myoclonic epilepsy (impulsive petit mal of Janz)
  5. Epilepsy with grand mal (GTCS) seizures on awakening
  6. Epilepsies with seizures precipitated by specific modes of activation
- B. Cryptogenic or symptomatic (in order of age)
  1. West syndrome (infantile spasms, Blitz-Nick-Salaam Krämpfe)
  2. Lennox-Gastaut syndrome
  3. Epilepsy with myoclonic-astatic seizures
  4. Epilepsy with myoclonic absences
- C. Symptomatic
  1. Nonspecific etiology
     a. Early myoclonic encephalopathy
     b. Early infantile epileptic encephalopathy with suppression burst
  2. Specific syndromes
     Epileptic seizures may complicate many disease states. Diseases in which seizures are a presenting or predominant feature are included in this category.

III. EPILEPSIES AND SYNDROMES UNDETERMINED WHETHER FOCAL OR GENERALIZED
- A. With both generalized and focal seizures
  1. Neonatal seizures
  2. Severe myoclonic epilepsy of infancy
  3. Epilepsy with continuous spike waves during slow-wave sleep
  4. Acquired epileptic aphasia (Landau-Kleffner syndrome)
- B. Without unequivocal generalized or focal features
  All cases with generalized tonic-clonic seizures in which clinical and EEG findings do not permit classification as clearly generalized or localization-related, such as in many cases of sleep-grand mal

IV. SPECIAL SYNDROMES
- A. Situation-related seizures
  1. Febrile convulsions
  2. Isolated seizures or isolated status epilepticus
  3. Seizures occurring only when there is an acute metabolic or toxic event associated with factors such as alcohol, drugs, eclampsia, nonketotic hyperglycemia

**Adapted from Commission on Classification and Terminology of the International League Against Epilepsy, 1989.*

methyl-d-aspartate (NMDA) and non-NMDA types (eg, kainate, AMPA). Both NMDA and non-NMDA receptors exist as subtypes. Activation of a second class of glutamate receptors (metabotropic), which is G protein-linked, also may increase neuronal excitability, at least in the hippocampus (Miller, 1991). NMDA receptors gate a high conductance ion channel (Ca^{2+}, Na^{+}, K^{+}) that is blocked in a voltage-dependent manner by Mg^{2+}; glycine increases the affinity of NMDA receptors for glutamate and is required for activation. Activation of kainate, AMPA, as well as NMDA receptors also produces depolarization that is sufficient to open voltage-dependent Ca^{2+} channels, which allows glutamate-triggered calcium influx to occur indirectly. Entry of Ca^{2+} is believed to be critical for synaptic plasticity (eg, learning and development, kindling, long-term potentiation [LTP]). Activation of the NMDA receptor system occurs when synaptic inhibition is depressed, especially during high-frequency stimulation. The NMDA receptor-mediated excitatory postsynaptic potential (EPSP) has a long duration, which promotes high-frequency neuronal firing. Similar responses in target neurons may encourage the spread of epileptiform activity.

Intense activation of NMDA receptors (prolonged seizure activity, ischemia, trauma) provokes excessive Ca^{2+} entry, which may trigger biochemical mechanisms causing neuronal death; kainate also causes neurodegeneration. In the hippocampus, the pathology produced by excitatory amino acid toxicity resembles the degeneration associated with periods of prolonged seizure activity. Hippocampal cell degeneration also occurs following intense stimulation of the perforant pathway or kindling involving hippocampal structures. The neuronal loss and synaptic reorganization that occur in these models are similar to those cellular events associated with human temporal lobe epilepsy (hippocampal sclerosis).

A focal area of abnormal electrical activity, manifested as the interictal EEG spike, is present in many patients with partial epilepsy; however, the etiology and self-perpetuating discharge observed in humans with idiopathic epilepsy are less well understood. Multiple cerebral sites may be capable of generating interictal epileptiform discharges. Results of studies utilizing positron emission tomography with ^{18}F-deoxyglucose reveal an interictal zone of hypometabolism that becomes hypermetabolic during seizures. Thus, neurons in the interictal state in an epileptogenic zone in humans may have decreased firing rates, or this may reflect "surround inhibition" similar to that apparent in models of partial epilepsy (Engel, 1989).

Much less is known about the pathogenesis of generalized epilepsies, in which abnormalities of cortex and/or subcortical structures are diffuse. Generalized seizures can be provoked by stimulation of subcortical structures. Other evidence supports the view that these seizures are initiated in the cortex. Data from animal models suggest that subcortical initiating (deep prepyriform cortex) and "gating" sites (mammillary bodies, anterior thalamic nuclei, substantia nigra) are important in the secondary generalization of partial seizures (Dichter and Ayala, 1987; Gale, 1989).

In animal models of absence seizures, thalamocortical circuits are involved in the genesis of the spike-and-wave discharge. This oscillatory pattern is generated during a state of diffuse cortical hyperexcitability and is synchronized by thalamic nuclei (Gloor and Fariello, 1988). Thalamic bursts seem to depend on deinactivation of the low-threshold (T) calcium current and may involve activation of $GABA_B$ receptors (Steriade and Llinas, 1988).

In experimental models, the intermittent application of brief trains of subconvulsive electrical stimuli to a single area of the brain results in the development of seizures that become longer and more intense; eventually, widespread independent epileptiform discharges arise from sites remote but connected synaptically to the original site of stimulation. This process, known as kindling, can be achieved from most forebrain gray matter structures; the amygdala is most sensitive. The neuronal reorganization underlying kindling may explain the latency, repetitive discharge, and progression of some forms of epilepsy (Morrell, 1991). Antiepileptic drugs are variably effective in suppressing the kindling process or controlling kindled seizures. Activation of NMDA receptors appears to be critical for inducing the kindled state. NMDA antagonists reduce seizures in many animal models of epilepsy, including kindled seizures; however, their clinical efficacy and safety have not been established (Rogawski, 1992).

DRUG THERAPY

Mechanism of Action

The efficacy of antiepileptic drugs in treating different types of seizures varies (see Table 3). Carbamazepine [Tegretol] and phenytoin [Dilantin] are most effective in partial and generalized tonic-clonic seizures. Felbamate [Felbatol], gabapentin [Neurontin], and lamotrigine [Lamictal] (investigational) have reduced the frequency of partial and generalized seizures. Felbamate also is effective in seizures associated with Lennox-Gastaut syndrome (eg, atonic). Ethosuximide [Zarontin] is useful in generalized absence seizures. Valproate (valproic acid [Depakene]; divalproex sodium [Depakote], a compound containing sodium valproate and valproic acid); and some benzodiazepines have a broad range of action that includes myoclonic seizures. Barbiturates also have a broad range of action but are relatively ineffective against absence, myoclonic, and atonic seizures. These clinical results suggest that there are at least three basic principles of antiepileptic drug action.

Based on results of in vitro studies, therapeutic concentrations of phenytoin and carbamazepine produce a voltage- and frequency-dependent blockade of sodium channels and slow their recovery from inactivation. These effects prevent development of sustained, high-frequency bursts of action potentials. Valproate and felbamate also have been reported to inhibit the occurrence of sustained bursts of potentials, but their effects on sodium channels have not been determined directly (White et al, 1992; Macdonald and Kelly, 1993). Lamotrigine inhibits voltage-dependent sodium channels and may preferentially decrease depolarization-induced release of excitatory amino acids such as glutamate. Phenobarbital and

TABLE 3.
DRUG SELECTION FOR SEIZURE TYPES

Seizure Type	Drug(s) of Choice	Alternative(s)/Adjunct	Infrequently Used
PARTIAL, INCLUDING SECONDARILY GENERALIZED TONIC-CLONIC	Carbamazepine Phenytoin Valproate	Clorazepate Felbamate[3] Gabapentin Lamotrigine Phenobarbital Primidone	Acetazolamide Ethotoin Mephenytoin Methsuximide Phenacemide
GENERALIZED			
Absence	Ethosuximide Valproate[1,2]	Clonazepam	Acetazolamide Clorazepate Methsuximide Phensuximide Paramethadione Trimethadione
Tonic-Clonic	Carbamazepine Phenytoin Valproate	Phenobarbital Primidone	Acetazolamide Bromides, inorganic Ethotoin Mephenytoin Mephobarbital
Myoclonic, Atonic	Valproate	Clonazepam Felbamate[3]	Bromides, inorganic Carbamazepine Clorazepate Ethosuximide Methsuximide Phenobarbital Phenytoin

[1] Drug of choice if generalized tonic-clonic seizures also present; ethosuximide plus phenytoin may be effective if valproate is contraindicated, although phenytoin may exacerbate absence seizures.

[2] Valproate is preferred in atypical absence seizures.

[3] Because of the increased risks of aplastic anemia and acute liver failure, use of felbamate should be restricted to patients who do not respond adequately to alternative therapy and whose epilepsy is so severe that the potential benefits of felbamate outweigh these risks.

benzodiazepines (eg, diazepam [Valium]) reduce action potential bursts at the high concentrations typical of those achieved in the treatment of status epilepticus. Thus, blockade of sustained, high-frequency repetitive firing of action potentials may contribute to preventing generalized tonic-clonic and partial seizures (Macdonald and Kelly, 1993). Unlike other antiepileptic drugs, ethosuximide and the trimethadione metabolite, dimethadione, inhibit the low threshold (T) calcium current in thalamic neurons (Coulter et al, 1989). It has been suggested that the T calcium current is important in the thalamic bursting that underlies cortical synchronization and the typical spike-and-wave pattern of absence seizures (Gloor and Fariello, 1988). Valproate and clonazepam [Klonopin] also inhibit absence seizures; valproate may affect the T current but to a lesser extent than ethosuximide (Kelly et al, 1990).

Antagonism of GABA receptors provokes seizures, and, at least in partial seizures, failure of inhibition at postsynaptic receptors has been thought to be an important contributing factor for ictal transition (Gloor and Fariello, 1988). Benzodiazepines (eg, clonazepam) and barbiturates enhance postsynaptic GABA-receptor current; barbiturates also may activate chloride conductance directly (see index entries Benzodiazepines; Barbiturates). Valproate also may enhance GABA-ergic function. This enhancement may contribute to its broad antiepileptic efficacy and especially to reduction of myoclonic seizures.

Accordingly, some investigational agents have been designed to enhance GABA-mediated inhibition. Vigabatrin [Sabril] (gamma vinyl GABA) inhibits GABA transaminase, thus increasing the neuronal concentration of GABA. Investigation of vigabatrin, which had been slowed in the United States because of concern about its potential neurotoxicity, has resumed (Browne et al, 1991). Vacuolation limited to myelinated tracts and edema of white matter has been observed in animals who received this agent. However, postmortem and operative specimens from humans given the drug have revealed no evidence of vacuolation (Butler, 1989). In controlled trials in Europe, vigabatrin reduced seizures by 25% to 50% in most adults with therapy-resistant epilepsy (Reynolds, 1990). Patients with partial seizures, including those with secondary generalization, responded best.

Felbamate and gabapentin appear to have novel actions. In animal models, felbamate increases the seizure threshold and prevents spread of seizure activity; its unique anticonvulsant profile is accompanied by a high margin of safety. Gabapentin does not have a major effect on standard ligand- or voltage-gated channels in neurons; however, it increases

TABLE 4.
DRUG SELECTION IN EPILEPTIC SYNDROMES[1]

Syndrome	Antiepileptic Drug (in order of choice)
LOCALIZATION-RELATED	
Idiopathic	
· Benign rolandic[2]	Carbamazepine, phenytoin, or valproate or no treatment if seizures are few
Symptomatic	
· Temporal, frontal, parietal, occipital lobe epilepsies	Valproate, clonazepam, phenobarbital, methsuximide
· Reflex epilepsy	Carbamazepine, phenytoin, felbamate[4]
GENERALIZED	
Idiopathic	
· Childhood absence	Ethosuximide or valproate
· Juvenile myoclonic	Valproate, primidone
· Epilepsy with generalized tonic-clonic seizures	Valproate, carbamazepine, phenytoin
Cryptogenic or Symptomatic	
· West syndrome (infantile spasms)	ACTH/corticosteroids, valproate, clonazepam, nitrazepam[3]
· Lennox-Gastaut	Valproate, clonazepam, felbamate[4]
· Epilepsy with myoclonic-astatic seizures	Valproate and/or clonazepam
· Epilepsy with myoclonic absences	Valproate plus ethosuximide
UNDETERMINED WHETHER PARTIAL OR GENERALIZED	
With generalized and partial seizures	
· Neonatal seizures	Phenobarbital, phenytoin

[1] Adapted from Ogunyemi and Dreifuss, 1988; Dodson, 1989; and Engel, 1989.
[2] Syndromes labeled as benign frequently remit spontaneously or do not require antiepileptic drug therapy. The symptomatic epileptic syndromes not identified in this table typically respond very poorly to antiepileptic drug therapy. Antiepileptic drugs also are generally ineffective in the treatment of severe myoclonic epilepsy of infancy and epilepsy with continuous spike waves during slow-wave sleep. Seizures are easily controlled and almost always remit in patients with acquired epileptic aphasia.
[3] Available on a compassionate-use basis.
[4] Because of the increased risks of aplastic anemia and acute liver failure, use of felbamate should be restricted to patients who do not respond adequately to alternative therapy and whose epilepsy is so severe that the potential benefits of felbamate outweigh these risks.

GABA turnover and binds with high affinity to a novel synaptic membrane site that also recognizes the potent convulsant, 3-isobutyl-GABA.

Many other effects of antiepileptic drugs on neurotransmitter dynamics and on synaptic transmission have been demonstrated. Effects on Na^+-K^+-ATPase, voltage dependent K^+ and Ca^{2+} channels, calmodulin target enzymes, cyclic nucleotide metabolism, and energy metabolism also have been identified for antiepileptic drugs. Some of these effects occur at concentrations exceeding normal therapeutic ranges.

Drug Selection

EPILEPTIC SEIZURES AND SYNDROMES. Initial drug therapy is based principally on seizure type (see Tables 1 and 3). If an epileptic syndrome can be diagnosed and prognosis determined, selection among agents with comparable efficacy is guided by differences in untoward effects (see Table 4). However, certain neonatal or infantile seizures and syndromes, as well as status epilepticus, require different specific therapy. Monotherapy is preferred in newly diagnosed patients; in others, response to previous therapy influences drug selection.

Partial and Secondarily Generalized Seizures: Partial (focal) seizures are the most common epileptic disorder. Almost 55% of seizures in adults are complex partial seizures, and approximately 80% of these originate in the temporal lobe (Cascino et al, 1990). For the initial treatment of partial seizures, monotherapy with phenytoin or carbamazepine is currently recommended (Mattson, 1989). The antiepileptic activity of these agents is similar, but differences in toxicity influence selection.

More than 50% of patients with partial seizures experience secondarily generalized tonic-clonic seizures. Comparative data in clinical trials indicate that the efficacy of carbamazepine, phenytoin, phenobarbital, primidone [Mysoline], and valproate are similar in these seizures (Mattson et al, 1991).

Many neurologists choose carbamazepine, especially in women and children over 5 years, because it does not cause the coarsening of facial features, hirsutism, and gingival hyperplasia induced in some patients by phenytoin. Carbamazepine often is effective alone, but the pharmacokinetics of this agent are complicated by a concentration-dependent autoinduction of its metabolism on initiation of treatment. Concern about carbamazepine's potentially serious hematologic toxicity has decreased in recent years.

Many other neurologists prefer phenytoin for initial treatment of adults and older children because of the long experience with its use and its effectiveness when used alone. Mephenytoin [Mesantoin] and ethotoin [Peganone] are rarely used alternatives to phenytoin. Mephenytoin is effective but may be toxic to the bone marrow. The use of ethotoin has been limited because of its reputation for poor efficacy. However, in some studies ethotoin was effective and did not produce the side effects of hirsutism and gingival hyperplasia associated with phenytoin (Carter et al, 1984). In a retrospective study, adjunctive use of ethotoin reduced seizure frequency by at least 50% in one-half of patients with intractable partial seizures (Biton et al, 1990). Prospective controlled trials are needed to confirm the usefulness of this drug.

Phenobarbital is more often reserved for initial use in children under 5 years. However, there is growing evidence that barbiturates exert adverse effects on cognitive ability in both children and adults. Therefore, these drugs may be less desirable than carbamazepine or phenytoin except in the neonatal period (during which orally administered phenytoin may be poorly absorbed). The actions of mephobarbital [Mebaral] resemble those of phenobarbital, but it is less potent and appears to have no advantages over the latter. The short-acting barbiturates are not useful prophylactically, because their hypnotic action tends to parallel their antiepileptic effect.

Primidone is associated with poorer patient acceptance than phenytoin, phenobarbital, or carbamazepine because of a greater incidence of side effects during initial therapy, even with low doses. However, in patients who can tolerate the drug, seizure control is similar to that with carbamazepine or phenytoin. Patient acceptance may be improved by initiating treatment with phenobarbital until a plasma concentration of 20 mg/L is reached and then substituting primidone.

The role of valproate in partial seizures is becoming more clearly defined. In a prospective, controlled multicenter trial of carbamazepine and valproate in partial seizures, the efficacy of carbamazepine was somewhat better as determined by several measures. Patients treated with valproate had twice as many complex partial seizures as those treated with carbamazepine, although overall the number of seizures was low (Mattson et al, 1991). More patients treated with valproate complained of weight gain and tremor, while 11% of those treated with carbamazepine had idiosyncratic (hypersensitivity) reactions. For these reasons, valproate has been considered a secondary drug in the treatment of complex partial seizures. However, other prospective and retrospective data indicate that valproate is comparable to carbamazepine and phenytoin in patients with partial seizures and secondarily generalized tonic-clonic seizures (Callaghan et al, 1985; Chadwick, 1987; Dean and Penry, 1988; Mattson et al, 1991). Although there is concern about possible hepatotoxicity, this effect is rare (see the evaluation).

Phenacemide [Phenurone] occasionally is effective in complex partial seizures (temporal lobe epilepsy), but it often produces severe adverse reactions and therefore is not recommended unless the benefit justifies the considerable risk. Clorazepate [Tranxene] is used adjunctively in the management of partial seizures.

The newer drugs, felbamate, gabapentin, and lamotrigine, have been studied extensively as adjunctive therapy in patients with refractory partial seizures with or without secondary generalization. All three drugs may be useful when partial seizures are not adequately controlled by monotherapy or by combinations of other antiepileptic drugs. Felbamate also can be used as primary monotherapy in patients with partial seizures; it generally is well tolerated, and discontinuation of other antiepileptic drugs may be feasible in some patients. However, the future use of this drug is uncertain pending investigation of its potential to cause aplastic anemia and acute liver failure (see the evaluation). Studies directly comparing felbamate or gabapentin with carbamazepine, phenytoin, valproate, or phenobarbital in the treatment of newly diagnosed patients with partial seizures have not been conducted. The manufacturer of lamotrigine has sponsored clinical trials comparing lamotrigine and phenytoin as monotherapy in patients with newly diagnosed epilepsy and lamotrigine and carbamazepine as monotherapy in patients with newly diagnosed or recurrent partial or generalized tonic-clonic seizures. Results of these studies have not yet been published.

Tonic-Clonic Seizures: Tonic-clonic seizures associated with idiopathic generalized epilepsy occur alone or in association with absence and/or myoclonic seizures. Results of earlier studies suggested that carbamazepine, phenobarbital, phenytoin, primidone, and valproate had similar efficacy. The same principles govern selection of the appropriate agent as discussed above; thus, carbamazepine, phenytoin, and valproate have been considered primary choices by most neurologists, with phenobarbital and primidone available as alternative agents. Combination therapy is occasionally more effective than monotherapy, but monotherapy with valproate has been successful in many patients with idiopathic generalized epilepsy not controlled by other antiepileptic drugs, singly or in combination (Bourgeois et al, 1987). Based on this observation, valproate is now the drug of choice in those with primary generalized tonic-clonic seizures associated with absence or myoclonic seizures.

Benzodiazepines (eg, clonazepam, clorazepate) are variably effective, but sedation and tolerance limit their use. Inorganic bromides (eg, sodium or potassium bromide) have antiepileptic activity in generalized tonic-clonic seizures. However, they are not commonly employed because of their significant side effects, which include sedation associated with prolonged administration. In addition, because the FDA has classified the bromides as investigational, their use requires a Treatment IND. Acetazolamide [Diamox] is used only occasionally as a temporary adjunct in generalized tonic-clonic or partial seizures because of the development of tolerance. It has been administered to treat clustering of seizures in women with catamenial epilepsy. The succinimides and oxazolidinediones are ineffective in generalized tonic-clonic seizures and rarely may precipitate them.

Absence Seizures: Drugs that are effective in absence seizures include ethosuximide, valproate, clonazepam, and trimethadione [Tridione]. Ethosuximide is the drug of choice when absence seizures are not associated with generalized tonic-clonic seizures. Some clinicians prefer valproate initially for absence seizures, but, because of the possibility of severe idiosyncratic hepatotoxicity associated with this drug, others reserve it for use when therapeutic failure or intolerance to ethosuximide occurs. If seizure control is not complete with either drug alone, they can be given together. Clonazepam represents an alternative; it is very effective, but tolerance develops, seizures may recur, and the drug is sedating (Aird et al, 1984). The other succinimides, methsuximide [Celontin] and phensuximide [Milontin], also may be effective but are less commonly used. Of the oxazolidinediones, trimethadione is more effective than paramethadione [Paradione]; however, because of toxicity, both should be reserved for patients who do not respond to safer drugs. Acetazolamide can be used as an adjunct to other drugs in selected patients.

Approximately 25% of patients with absence seizures also develop generalized tonic-clonic seizures. Most neurologists prefer to treat such patients with valproate monotherapy, which usually is effective in both types of primary generalized seizures. Some clinicians employ carbamazepine or phenytoin in addition to ethosuximide for the generalized tonic-clonic seizures, but phenytoin and carbamazepine may increase the frequency of absence attacks. Phenobarbital and primidone are not usually employed because side effects are more common with these drugs and they also may increase the frequency of absence attacks.

Atypical absence seizures have been treated with the benzodiazepines, (eg, clonazepam, clorazepate) with variable success. These agents should be considered in patients who do not respond to ethosuximide or valproate. When atypical absence seizures are accompanied more frequently by other generalized seizures, valproate is generally preferred (Holmes et al, 1987).

Myoclonic Seizures: These are associated with many epileptic syndromes; response to antiepileptic drugs is more often based on the syndrome than the seizure type (Mattson, 1989). Valproate is the drug of choice in idiopathic epilepsies, such as juvenile myoclonic epilepsy; it may fully control seizures in 90% of these patients. This drug is less effective in epilepsy with myoclonic-astatic seizures. Myoclonic seizures associated with other symptomatic epilepsies or degenerative conditions are generally refractory to drug therapy. Clonazepam is an alternative drug for myoclonic seizures. In susceptible patients with the juvenile form, it may control myoclonic jerks but does not suppress generalized tonic-clonic seizures (Obeid and Panayiotopoulos, 1989). Ethosuximide is less effective, but methsuximide has been useful in some patients who do not respond to other drugs. Valproate and clonazepam may be combined in the treatment of severe progressive myoclonus epilepsy (Iivanainen and Himberg, 1982). Although phenytoin, phenobarbital, primidone, and carbamazepine have been employed as second-line therapy for myoclonic seizures, response to these agents is poor. In fact, these drugs may exacerbate myoclonic seizures in some individuals.

West Syndrome: This syndrome usually occurs within the first year of life, with a peak onset at age 4 to 8 months. It consists of the characteristic triad of infantile spasms, developmental delay, and associated EEG pattern (hypsarrhythmia). Both symptomatic and cryptogenic forms are recognized; the latter is characterized by normal neurologic and cognitive development before the onset of spasms and by the absence of identifiable causes.

The most effective treatment is generally believed to be corticotropin (ACTH) or corticosteroids (eg, prednisone) (Hrachovy et al, 1983). However, because few well-controlled studies have been done, there is considerable controversy regarding the preferred dosage schedule and long-term effectiveness. Two therapeutic approaches to the intramuscular use of ACTH have been advocated. Either larger doses (40 to 160 units daily) for 3 to 12 months or relatively low doses (5 to 40 units daily) for brief periods (two to six weeks) have been given (Lombroso, 1983; Snead et al, 1983). In a typical low-dose, short-term regimen, 20 units of ACTH or 2 mg/kg of prednisone is administered daily for two weeks and the dose then is reduced if seizure control is achieved. If patients do not respond to one agent, they may benefit from the other. In more aggressive high-dose regimens, ACTH 150 units/M^2 is given daily for one week, followed by 75 units daily for one week and 75 units every other day for the third week, with the amount reduced gradually over the next ten weeks. Alternatively, prednisone 3 mg/kg daily in four divided doses is given for two weeks followed by withdrawal over ten weeks (Snead, 1990).

In one study, long-term monitoring of patients treated with ACTH or prednisone indicated that response to therapy is an all-or-none phenomenon (Glaze et al, 1988). The major factor affecting long-term outcome is whether the disorder is cryptogenic or symptomatic. Cryptogenic variants have a considerably better prognosis; approximately 25% of patients experience spontaneous remission within one year of onset (Snead, 1990; Hrachovy et al, 1991). Results of the largest prospective study on cryptogenic patients suggest that ACTH is more beneficial than prednisone, and outcome is more favorable if treatment is initiated within one month (Lombroso, 1983; Hrachovy et al, 1991). The side effects of ACTH or corticosteroids that may require discontinuation of therapy include hypertension, electrolyte imbalance, cardiac hypertrophy or congestive heart failure, and immunosuppression.

Benzodiazepines and valproate also have been effective in West syndrome. Of the benzodiazepines, clonazepam is used most frequently. In one short-term study, nitrazepam [Mogadon] was comparable to ACTH in reducing seizure frequency (Dreifuss et al, 1986). In an open prospective study using large doses (eg, 40 to 100 mg/kg daily) of valproate, patients with cryptogenic infantile spasms became seizure-free within five weeks. Considerable reduction in seizure frequency also was noted in patients with the symptomatic form; however, as in other studies, moderate to very severe retar-

TABLE 5.
PARENTERAL THERAPY FOR CONVULSIVE STATUS EPILEPTICUS

Drug	Intravenous Dosage	Usual Rate	Usual Maximum Dose*	Comment
ACUTE MANAGEMENT				
Lorazepam	*Adults*, 0.1 mg/kg	2 mg/min	8 mg	Initial doses may be repeated in 5 to 10 minutes if seizures persist. *Usual* maximum dosage is based on a decision to follow acute management of seizures with loading doses of phenytoin (when indicated) or, if necessary, phenobarbital. Some neurologists may recommend more liberal use of the benzodiazepine throughout the initial 24-hour period if seizures persist, resulting in higher maximum dosages. If intravenous access is difficult or delayed, rectal or intraosseous administration can be used.
or	*Children*, 0.05 to 0.1 mg/kg	Over 2 min	0.2 mg/kg	
Diazepam	*Adults*, 0.2 mg/kg	5 mg/min	20 mg	
	Children, 0.15 to 0.3 mg/kg	Over 2 min	5 to 10 mg	
PREVENTIVE MANAGEMENT				
Phenytoin	*Adults*, 15 to 20 mg/kg *Elderly patients*, 15 mg/kg	Not to exceed 50 mg/min	30 mg/kg	Preferred initial dosage in adults is 20 mg/kg by infusion. If cardiovascular depression results, the infusion rate should be slowed. This is usually the only dose required. If the loading dose does not terminate seizures during administration (approximately 30 minutes) or if seizures recur, additional phenytoin in increments of 5 mg/kg can be administered to a maximal dose of 30 mg/kg.
	Children, 15 to 20 mg/kg	1 mg/kg/min	25 mg/kg	
Phenobarbital	*Adults*, 15 to 20 mg/kg; alternatively, 10 mg/kg followed by another 10 mg/kg if necessary	Not to exceed 100 mg/min	20 mg/kg	Although most neurologists recommend that phenytoin follow the initial use of a benzodiazepine, phenobarbital is occasionally used, especially in infants and children. The risk of respiratory depression is increased with concomitant benzodiazepine and phenobarbital therapy. *Additional* doses of phenobarbital (5 to 10 mg/kg at 20-minute intervals) may be considered for refractory seizures before other measures are employed.
	Children, 15 to 20 mg/kg; alternatively, 10 mg/kg followed by another 10 mg/kg if necessary	1 to 2 mg/kg/min	20 mg/kg	
REFRACTORY MANAGEMENT				
Pentobarbital	Initially, 5 to 15 mg/kg	For maintenance, 0.5 to 3 mg/kg/hr		See text

* *The usual maximum dose reflects the amount anticipated in an orderly progression from acute management to preventive management in patients who are responsive. The upper limit for dosage may be much higher in a 24-hour period, depending on the therapeutic strategy* (Med Lett Drugs Ther, *1989*).

dation was observed in most patients on long-term follow-up (Siemes et al, 1988).

Lennox-Gastaut Syndrome: This is a severe form of childhood epilepsy characterized by frequent seizures (usually tonic, atonic, and atypical absences), mental retardation, and diffuse, slow spike and wave pattern in the EEG (Livingston, 1988). Thirty to fifty percent of patients with West syndrome eventually develop Lennox-Gastaut syndrome. Seizure control in these patients often is exceedingly difficult. As in other epilepsies with mixed seizure types, valproate is the drug of choice. Felbamate may be useful adjunctively, especially to reduce atonic and generalized tonic-clonic seizures (The Felbamate Study Group in Lennox-Gastaut Syndrome, 1993). Additional antiepileptic drugs (eg, clonazepam) may be required.

A ketogenic diet has been recommended as adjunctive therapy for older children when drug refractoriness is a problem (Livingston et al, 1979) or for children with severe static-encephalopathy and intractable seizures (Kinsman et al, 1992). However, the value of such diets remains to be assessed by controlled clinical trials.

Atonic Seizures: Valproate and clonazepam also are given for atonic seizures. Ethosuximide and trimethadione are drugs of second choice or adjuncts, especially when the preferred agents are ineffective. However, most patients respond poorly. Felbamate reduces atonic seizures in children with Lennox-Gastaut syndrome, but its efficacy in other patients with atonic seizures has not been studied.

STATUS EPILEPTICUS. Status epilepticus can be defined as a state in which seizures last more than 30 minutes as either (1) one continuous seizure or (2) two or more sequential seizures without full recovery of consciousness between attacks. Status epilepticus can occur with any seizure type. Tonic-clonic (convulsive) status epilepticus is the most common form and is an emergency requiring prompt, vigorous treatment. In epileptic patients, most episodes occur in those with symptomatic epilepsy. Although noncompliance or abrupt withdrawal of medication can cause status epilepticus, low plasma concentrations or withdrawal of antiepileptic drugs explains only some cases (Barry and Hauser, 1994). In patients who have not experienced a prior seizure, metabolic disorders (eg, hypoglycemia, hypocalcemia, hyponatremia), stroke, infections, encephalopathy, trauma, neoplasia, drug intoxication (eg, cocaine, tricyclic antidepressants), or withdrawal of alcohol or hypnotic drugs may be causative (Lowenstein and Alldredge, 1992). In all patients, acute or prior disease of the brain is an important factor in development of status epilepticus (Barry and Hauser, 1993). Nonconvulsive status epilepticus, while less common, is important in the differential diagnosis of acute confusional states and other unusual neurologic syndromes.

Initial diagnostic and therapeutic measures should be conducted simultaneously. If possible, the underlying cause should be determined and treated. General principles of acute treatment include restoration of homeostasis, prompt management of seizures, and prevention of seizure recurrence. Basic life support, including establishment of an adequate airway and intravenous lines and cardiovascular monitoring and ventilatory support if needed, are required initially for management. To avoid injuring the patient when endotracheal intubation is required, convulsive activity first must be stopped by administration of diazepam or lorazepam or, if necessary, a short-acting barbiturate or neuromuscular blocker (Working Group on Status Epilepticus, 1993). Systolic blood pressure should be maintained at normal or high-normal levels. A blood sample should be obtained for a complete blood count, serum chemistry, determination of antiepileptic drug concentrations, and toxicologic screening. If hypoglycemia is documented or if it is not possible to measure blood glucose, an intravenous bolus of dextrose 50% (50 ml or 1 g/kg) is commonly administered to adolescents and adults. Dextrose 25% (2 ml/kg) is given to infants and children. Administration of thiamine (100 mg for adults) or pyridoxine (infants) also may be advisable.

Only three prospective, randomized studies of the management of status epilepticus, each employing a different protocol, have been reported (Leppik et al, 1983; Treiman et al, 1985; Shaner et al, 1988); thus, recommendations for the treatment of this condition vary. (For recent reviews, see Treiman, 1993; Working Group on Status Epilepticus, 1993.) In recent years, attention has been given to control of seizures as soon as possible after onset in an effort to minimize neuronal damage. The use of lorazepam, diazepam, phenytoin, and phenobarbital in the initial management of generalized convulsive status epilepticus is being studied in a prospective, randomized, double-blind trial (Treiman, 1990); results should provide definitive data for the selection of the optimal regimen.

Administration of antiepileptic drugs should be considered whenever a seizure has lasted 10 minutes or longer and in anyone who is convulsing on arrival at the place of treatment. Attention to the possibility of drug-induced hypoventilation is necessary regardless of which agent is used.

Specific management of convulsive status epilepticus (see Table 5) is usually begun with intravenous administration of lorazepam or diazepam. Other benzodiazepines, notably midazolam [Versed], also have been used (Galvin and Jelinek, 1987; Rivera et al, 1993). The efficacy of diazepam and lorazepam in controlling seizures is similar, but the latter may be preferred because it has a longer duration of action (Leppik et al, 1983; Treiman, 1990) and thus seizures do not recur as rapidly. Larger doses may be needed in patients who have been treated with benzodiazepines for long periods (Reincke et al, 1988). In children, rectal or intraosseous administration of diazepam or lorazepam may be employed if intravenous access is difficult or delayed.

When indicated, the benzodiazepine is followed by a loading dose of phenytoin to provide sustained protection and to allow a smooth transition to maintenance therapy. (If lorazepam was used initially, it may not be necessary to administer subsequent loading doses of phenytoin at the maximum rate.) Phenytoin is preferred to phenobarbital because it causes less depression of sensorium and respiration. In some patients (eg, those withdrawing from ethanol, those experiencing seizures caused by drug toxicity), phenytoin may not be desirable. In patients with cardiac conduction disturbances (eg, sinus arrest and second- or third-degree AV block, those with severe heart failure), phenytoin is contraindicated. If significant hypotension develops, the infusion should be slowed or stopped.

If the patient is not actively convulsing or if seizures are separated by prolonged periods of stupor, intravenous phenytoin has been recommended as the initial drug (Leppik, 1986). If seizures subsequently occur during the administration of phenytoin, lorazepam 4 to 8 mg or diazepam 5 to 20 mg may be given. The intravenous preparation of phenytoin currently available is cardiotoxic (pH 12; propylene glycol solvent) and the rate of administration in adults should not exceed 50 mg/min. A phenytoin prodrug (fosphenytoin) that is water soluble is undergoing Phase III clinical trials (Smith et al, 1989; Leppik et al, 1990). Another phenytoin derivative, redox phenytoin, and a carbamazepine derivative, cyclodextran carbamazepine, also are being investigated for use in status epilepticus; all three agents have been accorded orphan drug status.

If seizures persist or recur, intravenous phenobarbital should be added to the regimen to produce a therapeutic plasma concentration as rapidly as possible (Leppik, 1986). At this point, intubation and respiratory assistance are required. Although phenytoin is generally administered before phenobarbital in adults, some clinicians prefer phenobarbital in very young children.

Phenobarbital also may be used initially during barbiturate or primidone withdrawal and following benzodiazepine treatment when phenytoin is relatively or absolutely contraindicated.

Paraldehyde may be tried if seizures do not respond to diazepam or lorazepam, phenytoin, and phenobarbital (see the evaluation). Although paraldehyde has several disadvantages, it can be given rectally.

If status epilepticus persists, pentobarbital coma or general anesthesia with neuromuscular paralysis can be instituted under the supervision of an anesthesiologist or intensivist; EEG monitoring is essential during either of these procedures, and vasopressors usually are required (Yaffe and Lowenstein, 1993). For pentobarbital, a loading dose (5 to 15 mg/kg) followed by infusion of 0.5 to 2 mg/kg/hr to maintain burst suppression in the EEG has been recommended (Lowenstein et al, 1988; Treiman, 1990; Working Group on Status Epilepticus, 1993). The objective is to minimize the brain damage that may result from prolonged seizures. After electrical seizure activity subsides, the rate of pentobarbital infusion is slowed periodically to determine if a remission has been induced. Other clinicians favor induction of coma with phenobarbital because continuous infusion is not needed, although the duration of the coma may be longer.

The results of a small retrospective study suggest that midazolam may be an effective and safe alternative to induction of coma with large doses of barbiturates to terminate refractory status epilepticus (Kumar and Bleck, 1992). After seizure activity is controlled, diagnostic studies can be completed and antiepileptic drug therapy instituted to prevent recurrence.

Treatment of partial and complex partial status epilepticus is generally the same as for the tonic-clonic type except that induction of coma usually is not required. For absence status epilepticus, intravenous diazepam or lorazepam is usually preferred initially. If possible, oral ethosuximide or valproate then should be administered to establish an effective plasma concentration as rapidly as possible. If stupor prevents oral administration, the nasogastric or rectal route may be utilized. Valproate is the drug of choice to prevent recurrence of absence status epilepticus (Berkovic et al, 1989).

POST-TRAUMATIC/POSTSURGICAL EPILEPSY. The use of antiepileptic drugs in the prophylaxis of post-traumatic epilepsy is controversial. Epilepsy complicates head trauma in approximately 7% of civilian patients. Intracranial hematoma seems especially critical for the development of post-traumatic epilepsy. Patients who may benefit most from therapy are those who have (1) penetrating head injuries, (2) closed brain injuries with neurologic symptoms of brain contusion or abnormal EEG, and (3) closed brain injuries without contusion when coma lasts more than three hours and epilepsy is present in family members. Early administration of loading doses of intravenous phenytoin to patients with head injury may be warranted to prevent seizures and their complications during the first week, but prolonged therapy does not seem justified (Temkin et al, 1990). Similarly, prophylaxis with phenytoin or carbamazepine reduces the number of seizures in the first week following craniotomy but does not reduce the incidence of subsequent epilepsy (Foy et al, 1992). Whether other antiepileptic agents (eg, phenobarbital, benzodiazepines, valproate) or drugs of different classes can provide prophylactic protection is not known.

NEONATAL SEIZURES. Neonatal seizures are associated with a high risk of mortality or permanent neurologic morbidity. These seizures have been grouped into four types based on clinical description (Volpe, 1989). However, dissociation between clinically observed seizures and discharges observed on the EEG is common, especially with "subtle" neonatal seizures, the most frequent type. This electroclinical dissociation may lead to either overestimation (movements or behaviors that are not truly epileptic) or underestimation (EEG evidence without observed clinical activity) of epileptic seizures. A revised classification of seizure and nonseizure behavior based on synchronized video-EEG correlation has been proposed (Mizrahi and Kellaway, 1987).

Although there are difficulties in establishing the etiology, seizures in neonates are usually symptomatic. Major causes include perinatal asphyxia, hemorrhage, infection, hypoglycemia, hypocalcemia, and developmental and metabolic defects. The time of seizure onset is closely related to the etiology. The prognosis frequently depends on the etiology, clinical variables (eg, age, seizure type, severity, recurrence), and findings on the interictal EEG.

Despite uncertainty regarding the efficacy of antiepileptic drugs and their effect on CNS development, the current practice is to treat neonatal seizures. Phenobarbital (initially, 20 mg/kg followed by 3 to 4 mg/kg/day) and phenytoin (initially, 15 to 20 mg/kg followed by 3 to 4 mg/kg/day) are the most widely used drugs (Legido et al, 1988). Diazepam, lorazepam, and primidone may be effective adjunctively; diazepam or lorazepam also may be used initially. The decision on when to discontinue medication is controversial. Antiepileptic drug therapy is discontinued in many infants prior to or within two months after discharge from neonatal intensive care units (Novotny, 1990). However, many neurologists continue therapy for three to six months and discontinue it completely after this period only if the child remains seizure-free and appears to be developmentally and neurologically normal (Legido et al, 1988).

OTHER SEIZURES. Febrile Seizures: A febrile seizure most often occurs in children between 6 months and 5 years of age; the average age is 18 to 22 months (Hirtz, 1989). These seizures are associated with rectal temperature of at least 101° F in the absence of intracranial infection or any other cause of convulsions. A Consensus Development Conference of the National Institutes of Health (Freeman, 1980) concluded that two significant sequelae are associated with a febrile seizure: a 30% to 40% risk of recurrent febrile seizures and a very small risk of epilepsy.

The Consensus Conference also developed guidelines for the prophylactic use of antiepileptic drugs in children with febrile seizures and identified the limited circumstances under which prophylaxis (usually with phenobarbital) may be appropriate. These include (1) in a child in whom recurrences are frequent, particularly at a young age; (2) in dangerous situations (eg, when a febrile seizure lasts longer than 15 minutes, is partial, or is followed by persistent neurologic abnormalities); or (3) when the child is isolated from timely access to emergency medical care (National Institutes of Health, 1981). However, of these factors, only young age at onset has been consistently associated with an increased risk of recurrence (Berg et al, 1990). History of febrile seizures in a first-degree relative, short duration of fever before seizure onset, and seizure onset at a lower temperature appear to increase the risk of recurrence to a lesser extent (Berg et al, 1992). Data on the relationship between the occurrence of a complex febrile seizure or family history of epilepsy and risk of recurrence are inconsistent (Berg et al, 1992). The association between complex febrile seizures and subsequent epilepsy may reflect predisposition to both conditions.

Although results of some controlled studies in which compliance was verified by determination of plasma concentration indicate that both phenobarbital and valproate reduced the recurrence of febrile seizures (Mikati and Browne, 1988), there is no evidence that prophylaxis of febrile seizures decreases the subsequent development of epilepsy. Thus, consensus has developed that chronic prophylaxis usually is not indicated in patients with simple febrile seizures. The trend to eliminate prophylactic therapy was reinforced by the results of a study involving children at higher risk for febrile seizure recurrence (Farwell et al, 1990). Based on an intent-to-treat analysis, assignment to the phenobarbital regimen did not decrease recurrences, but almost one-third of those in the phenobarbital group were not taking the drug at the time of seizure recurrence and compliance was not documented by plasma drug concentration. In children receiving long-term phenobarbital therapy, there was a mild decrease in measured intelligence that exceeded the duration of drug administration by several months.

A rational alternative to prophylaxis is the rectal (or oral if the child is old enough) administration of diazepam during febrile episodes (Knudsen, 1985; Camfield et al, 1989). Results of a recent randomized, double-blind, placebo-controlled trial on children who experienced at least one febrile seizure confirmed that oral diazepam reduces the risk of recurrent febrile seizures when administered in this fashion (Rosman et al, 1993). Although approximately one-third of these patients developed significant side effects (eg, ataxia, drowsiness), this approach appears to be safe and in most cases is preferred to chronic prophylaxis for treatment of high-risk children. See the evaluation on Diazepam.

Drug Withdrawal Syndrome: Convulsive seizures are sometimes associated with the drug withdrawal syndrome in persons physically dependent on the barbiturates, alcohol, benzodiazepines, and other nonbarbiturate-nonbenzodiazepine antianxiety and hypnotic drugs. Phenobarbital or benzodiazepines are used most often to alleviate moderate to severe signs and symptoms, depending on the etiology of the syndrome. Since these drugs have an anticonvulsant action, additional antiepileptic drugs usually are not required; however, carbamazepine and valproate have been used adjunctively. Carbamazepine's ability to attenuate mood swings in bipolar disorders may be of value in selected patients (see index entry Carbamazepine, Uses, Mania).

Phenothiazines are usually avoided because most of these agents lower the seizure threshold; however, when psychotic signs and symptoms occur during withdrawal, haloperidol [Haldol] is efficacious and does not increase the frequency of seizures or cause extensive vasodilation with hypotension.

General Principles of Drug Therapy

The objective of drug therapy is to control seizures as completely as possible without causing intolerable adverse reactions. Antiepileptic therapy must be individualized. The appropriate dosage of a drug or combination of drugs depends on the size, age, and condition of the patient; the response to treatment; and the interactions between concomitantly administered medications.

Antiepileptic drugs are initiated in most patients only after two or more seizures have occurred. However, estimates of the risk of recurrence within the first year after the initial diagnosis vary widely (21% to 67%); selection bias, definitions used for case ascertainment, referral patterns, timing of assessment, and diagnostic uncertainty contribute to the disparity. In studies that enter patients at the time of their first seizure, the recurrence rate after two years was reported to be approximately 42% (Berg and Shinnar, 1991). Results of one recent randomized study suggest that treatment after the first unprovoked seizure is useful in gaining an eventual remission (First Seizure Trial Group, 1993).

The decision on whether to initiate therapy may be modified based on neurologic findings (eg, focal brain lesion, epileptiform EEG) after a single seizure, the seizure type, or, when recurrent, the interval between seizures. Properly individualized monotherapy controls approximately 80% of the more common forms of epilepsy and avoids drug interactions. Treatment is initiated with a dose calculated to establish a therapeutic plasma concentration. If seizures recur, the dosage may be increased until they are controlled or toxicity makes further increases inadvisable. The dose for children is usually 50% to 100% larger on a weight basis than that for adults because of higher clearance values.

Enough time must be allowed for the drug to reach steady state before evaluating its effectiveness (see Table 6). The occurrence of frequent seizures may mandate a more immediate attainment of steady-state antiepileptic plasma concentrations; this may be achieved by giving a loading dose at the onset of therapy or larger doses at any stage before the steady state is reached. Loading doses may be given intravenously, intramuscularly, or orally depending on the drug. However, even though valproate has a relatively short half-life, full therapeutic response may lag several days to weeks behind establishment of steady state.

Initially, antiepileptic drugs may cause CNS depression or gastrointestinal disturbances, but the effects may be transient and are not indications to discontinue treatment. If untoward effects continue, the amount should be reduced to the tolerated level. Medication should not be withdrawn abruptly unless serious adverse reactions develop; prompt substitution of another drug is mandatory if these occur (Reynolds and Shorvon, 1981). The patient should be hospitalized for observation and for immediate treatment if status epilepticus develops. Lorazepam may be useful for prophylaxis. Patients must be warned of the dangers of discontinuing any medication, informed of possible adverse reactions, and advised of the need to report any untoward effects to the physician.

If the initial drug does not control seizures and compliance is verified, a trial with at least one other agent should be attempted before considering a multidrug regimen. The second drug should be introduced before the first is discontinued. Effectiveness of the second drug should be judged over a period of sufficient length to detect a significant change in seizure frequency.

In some patients, polytherapy may be superior to monotherapy; treatment must be individualized to determine the optimal dosage of the second drug and possible drug interactions should be considered.

Most treatment failures are caused by noncompliance (Leppik and Schmidt, 1988). Therefore, it is important for the patient to understand and accept his disorder. It is also important for the physician to appreciate the patient's social, psychological, and economic needs, which may require a multidisciplinary approach (Leppik and Schmidt, 1988). Office visits should be scheduled regularly to evaluate the efficacy and adverse reactions of the medication, to measure drug plasma concentrations when indicated, and to adjust the dose if necessary. Other steps to improve compliance include simplification of the dosage schedule, maintenance of a medication calendar, use of individualized medicine containers, and patient education.

Uncontrolled epilepsy may lead to intractable epilepsy. Data from kindling experiments in animals support the view that seizures are self-perpetuating and repetitive brain stimulation leads to neuronal changes that cause spontaneous electrical discharge. If seizures remain poorly controlled after two years despite an adequate trial of drug therapy, the patient should be referred to a specialized epilepsy center. (The names and addresses of these centers in the United States can be obtained from the Epilepsy Foundation of America, 4351 Garden City Drive, Suite 406, Landover, MD 20785 [patient information, 1-800/332-1000; physician information, 1-800/332-4050]).

Patients with certain epileptic conditions may be candidates for early surgical intervention (National Institutes of Health, 1990; see Engel, 1993). In particular, surgical resection may be indicated in those with mesial temporal lobe epilepsy or partial seizures caused by a well-defined cerebral lesion. Infants and small children with diffuse hemispheric syndromes or Lennox-Gastaut syndrome may benefit from hemispheric resection and corpus callosotomy, respectively, shortly after the diagnosis is confirmed.

WITHDRAWAL OF MEDICATION. Although the following discussion evaluates the average probability of seizure recurrence after discontinuation of antiepileptic drug therapy, individual factors (eg, the patient's seizure type and age, the requirement for vehicle operator's license, the social or employment consequences of seizure recurrence) weigh heavily in the decision to attempt withdrawal of antiepileptic drug therapy.

A number of factors influence the risk of relapse when antiepileptic drug therapy is discontinued (Chadwick, 1988). In conditions such as juvenile myoclonic epilepsy, virtually all patients will relapse if drug treatment is discontinued. However, unless a progressive underlying disease is involved, spontaneous remissions may occur, especially with idiopathic epilepsies that usually begin during childhood (eg, benign epilepsy with centrotemporal spikes, absence epilepsy in children). Because of the heterogenous nature of epilepsy, determination of precise individual prognoses is not possible. Nevertheless, in patients who have remained seizure-free for extended periods, the eventual discontinuation of an antiepileptic drug regimen may be considered.

Results of retrospective studies (Emerson et al, 1981; Thurston et al, 1982) suggest that 70% or more of children who originally experienced only a few seizures, who have remained seizure-free for four years with antiepileptic medication, and who have a normal or mildly abnormal EEG will remain seizure-free after withdrawal of antiepileptic medication. In two prospective studies, a seizure-free interval of two to four years was associated with a good prognosis, and persistence of EEG abnormalities was predictive of recurrence (Shinnar et al, 1985; Matricardi et al, 1989).

In another prospective study, children who had remained seizure-free for two years with normalization of the EEG demonstrated a relapse rate of 25% after withdrawal of medication (Arts et al, 1988). Patients with partial seizures had a higher relapse rate. Within this group, neurologic deficit, a positive family history, and number of drugs necessary for control were predictive of recurrence. Thus, successful withdrawal of therapy may be achieved in up to 75% of selected pediatric or adolescent patients. Factors favoring discontinuation of antiepileptic drugs include single type of primary generalized seizure, onset of epilepsy after age 2 years, lack of neurologic deficit or EEG abnormality, and a seizure-free period of at least two years (Dean and Penry, 1989).

Many neurologists have been reluctant to apply these data to older patients (Pedley, 1988). In general, relapse rates have tended to be higher in adults (22% to 66%) than in children (21% to 34%). Most studies in adults have been retrospective; in prospective studies, relapse rates of 35% to 66% have been reported (Overweg et al, 1987; Callaghan et al, 1988; Medical Research Council Antiepileptic Drug Withdrawal Study Group, 1991). In one of these studies, the relapse rate among adults and children was similar (35% and 31%, respectively) (Callaghan et al, 1988). Prior to withdrawal of medication, these patients were controlled by monotherapy with carbamazepine, phenytoin, or valproate and had been seizure-free for two years.

As in children, persistent EEG abnormalities and neurologic dysfunction militate against discontinuation of therapy. Patients with a higher frequency of seizures may require longer periods before withdrawal is attempted (Overweg et al, 1987). Seizure type may be helpful for predicting relapse. A history of myoclonic seizures, partial seizures with secondary generalization, or of a combination of seizure types may increase the risk of relapse compared with primary generalized seizures, although data obtained from a randomized, prospective study indicate that a history of primary generalized tonic-clonic seizures also increases the risk of recurrence (Chadwick, 1988; Medical Research Council Antiepileptic Drug Withdrawal Study Group, 1993). Results of a recent meta-analysis support the concept that patients with symptomatic partial seizures are more likely to relapse than those with idiopathic seizures (Berg and Shinnar, 1994).

Results of most studies suggest that continued remission after withdrawal of antiepileptic drugs is less likely in patients with adolescent- or adult-onset epilepsy than in children (Berg and Shinnar, 1994). Fewer seizures with prompt control by monotherapy and a seizure-free condition for two to five years (with normal EEG) increase the probability of success.

In patients receiving polytherapy, the dose of one drug at a time should be reduced very gradually while the plasma concentration of the second drug is maintained in the therapeutic range, since sudden withdrawal may precipitate seizures and is one of the most common causes of status epilepticus. Adjunctive (eg, acetazolamide) or sedative (eg, barbiturate, benzodiazepine) drugs may be withdrawn first. In some patients, the goal of drug "withdrawal" is to convert to monotherapy. Various protocols, particularly those leading to valproate monotherapy, have been devised (Wilder and Rangel, 1988; Mattson and Cramer, 1988). Withdrawal of carbamazepine, phenytoin, or phenobarbital may be associated with significant elevation in the plasma concentrations of concomitant antiepileptic drugs because of the reversal of hepatic enzyme induction.

The optimal length of time for withdrawal of medication has not been established; a minimum of a few months (eg, 25% reduction in dosage every two to three weeks) and a maximum of 12 months (eg, 25% reduction in dosage every three months) have been advocated (Chadwick and Reynolds, 1985). Until these issues are resolved, the physician is urged to seek consultant opinion before discontinuing drug therapy.

MONITORING THERAPEUTIC DRUG CONCENTRATIONS. Monitoring concentrations of antiepileptic drugs in plasma is a valuable aid in patient management. Therapeutic or "target" ranges have been determined for most antiepileptic drugs. However, although plasma monitoring can help decision-making in therapy, it is not a substitute for clinical judgment; the ultimate determinants of dosage are frequency of seizures and dose-related adverse effects. There is considerable variability in the plasma concentrations necessary to control certain seizure types and at which adverse effects occur in individual patients (Schmidt et al, 1986).

Drug monitoring improves the overall management of epileptic patients by (1) identifying the baseline concentration of antiepileptic drugs associated with optimal therapeutic response; (2) guiding dosage adjustments required because of poor seizure control or dose-related toxicity; (3) confirming compliance; and (4) guiding dosage adjustments caused by changing physiologic status, disease states, or drug interactions. It also may be of value in infants or mentally retarded patients in whom assessment of toxicity is more difficult (Chadwick, 1988).

The relative value of plasma monitoring for individual antiepileptic drugs is quite variable; however, monitoring generally is considered essential for phenytoin because of the wide interindividual variation in the rate of metabolism of this drug, the existence of nonlinear elimination kinetics, and the relatively low therapeutic ratio. Similarly, monitoring is very useful for carbamazepine because of autoinduction and this drug's narrow therapeutic range. For valproate, a poor correlation exists between plasma concentrations and therapeutic response. Wide variability in the relative distribution of valproate between the brain and blood may be an underlying factor (Shen et al, 1992). Both valproate and carbamazepine have short half-lives, which make standardization of sampling time relative to dose administration necessary. For the barbiturates and benzodiazepines, development of tolerance diminishes the value of monitoring. For ethosuximide, most evidence suggests that monitoring is useful, but correlation between plasma concentrations and adverse effects is weaker. Clinically useful plasma concentration ranges appear to be between 30 and 100 mcg/ml for felbamate and 2 to 6 mcg/ml for lamotrigine and gabapentin; however, further study is needed.

Some investigators have considered the more specific issue of monitoring free (unbound) plasma concentrations for those drugs that are highly protein bound and demonstrate significant variability (eg, phenytoin, carbamazepine, valproate). These antiepileptic drugs are extensively metabolized and have low hepatic extraction ratios. Under these conditions, when the free fraction increases (eg, displacement from protein, hypoalbuminemia) the total concentration decreases; since free concentration is independent of the degree of plasma protein binding and remains unchanged, total drug concentrations may be unreliable therapeutic guides. On the other hand, elevation of the free fraction *and* inhibition of metabolism (decreased clearance) may lead to a new steady-state characterized by increased free but unchanged total concentrations. Neither clinical nor pharmacologic considerations warrant the *routine* monitoring of free phenytoin or valproate concentrations. However, it may be a valuable adjunct in special situations when changes in free fraction may occur (eg, renal or hepatic disease, pregnancy, hypoalbuminemia, aging, drug interactions). Monitoring free carbamazepine concentrations is virtually never warranted (Porter, 1989; Lenn and Robertson, 1992).

Because of the importance of drug plasma concentrations in determining adequate therapy, considerable pharmacokinetic data are available for all commonly used antiepileptic drugs (see Table 6 and Hvidberg and Dam, 1976; Levy et al, 1989). Three observations are of special interest: (1) Within the first few weeks of administration, carbamazepine can induce hepatic enzymes that are responsible for its own biotransformation. The degree of autoinduction is variable, but an increase in dosage frequently is required. Autoinduction

TABLE 6.
PHARMACOKINETIC DATA ON SELECTED ANTIEPILEPTIC DRUGS

Drug	Usually Effective Plasma Concentration (Range, mcg/ml)	Time to Steady State (Days)	Plasma Half-Life (Hours): Adults Range	Adults Mean	Children Range	Children Mean
Carbamazepine [Tegretol]	4-12	4-5[a]	5-26	15[b]	3-25	11
Clonazepam [Klonopin]	0.02-0.08	6	18-50		22-33	
Ethosuximide [Zarontin]	40-100	7-10	40-60	54	15-68	33
Felbamate [Felbatol]	30-100[c]	4	14-23	20		
Gabapentin [Neurontin]	2-6[c]	1-2	5-7	6		
Lamotrigine [Lamictal]	2-6[c]	5-8		25.4 (monotherapy) 12.6 (polytherapy[d])		7 (polytherapy[d])
Phenobarbital	15-40	>21	53-140	96	37-133	70[e]
Phenytoin [Dilantin]	10-20	variable (6-8)[f]	8-59	25[g]	Somewhat less than adults. Higher doses required to maintain similar plasma concentrations	
Primidone [Mysoline]	10-14	3	4-22 (monotherapy)	15	(monotherapy)	10
	5-12		3-11 (polytherapy[d])	9	(polytherapy[d])	8
Valproate [Depakene, Depakote]	40-120	1-4	12-16 (monotherapy)		8-12 (monotherapy)	
			5-10 (polytherapy[d])	8	5-9 (polytherapy[d])	8[h]

[a] *In patients in whom clearance of carbamazepine increases as a result of autoinduction, steady-state may not be achieved until three to four weeks after initiation of therapy.*

[b] *Initially the average half-life is 30 to 35 hours; values listed are obtained after three to four weeks as a result of autoinduction.*

[c] *Tentative ranges; further data required to establish clinical significance.*

[d] *Polytherapy with enzyme-inducing drugs.*

[e] *Values are shorter in infants and longer in neonates.*

[f] *May be two to three weeks if plasma concentrations are in the high range.*

[g] *Dose-dependent (eg, 20 hours at 4 mg/kg/day, 40 hours at 6.5 mg/kg/day). Half-life increases with dose, exhibits large interindividual variation, and is better described by Michaelis-Menten kinetics. At doses given for status epilepticus, the apparent half-life ranges from 20 to 70 hours but may be much higher in some patients.*

[h] *Although the range of half-lives is similar for adults and children receiving polytherapy, larger doses are required in children to establish similar plasma concentrations due to larger volume of distribution.*

[i] *Dose-dependent; percent bound decreases with increases in total plasma concentration.*

Volume of Distribution (L/kg)	Plasma Protein Binding (Percent)	Clearance (ml/kg/min)	Elimination Site (Percent)	Biologically Active Compounds in Blood
0.8-1.4	75	0.58 ± 0.12	hepatic 98%	carbamazepine 10,11 epoxide of carbamazepine (shorter half-life than parent)
1.5-4.4	85	0.92 ± 0.25	hepatic 98%	clonazepam
0.67	nil	0.26 ± 0.05	hepatic 80%-90%	ethosuximide
0.75	22-25	0.5	hepatic 50%-60% renal 40%-50%	felbamate
0.7	0	1.3	renal 80% fecal 20%	gabapentin
0.9-1.4	55	0.58	hepatic 92% renal 8%	lamotrigine
0.5-1	40-60	0.09 ± 0.04	hepatic 50%-80% renal unchanged 20%-50%	phenobarbital
0.5-1	90	V_{max} = 6.5 mg/kg/day (adults) 11.7 mg/kg/day (children)	hepatic 95%	phenytoin
0.8	20	0.78 ± 0.62	hepatic 30%-90% renal 15%-65%	primidone phenobarbital phenylethyl malonamide ($t\frac{1}{2}$ about 15 hours)
0.15	80-94[i]	0.12 ± 0.04	hepatic 97%	valproate 2-en-valproate

and heteroinduction also contribute to drug interactions. (2) The biotransformation of phenytoin is characterized by dose-dependent kinetics; thus, as the metabolism of phenytoin approaches saturation, even small dosage increases may cause unexpected toxicity as a result of disproportionately large increases in the plasma concentration and the apparent half-life of the drug. The enzymatic biotransformation of phenytoin also is inhibited by a number of drugs, resulting in unexpected toxicity. (3) The plasma protein binding of valproate is saturable within the usual therapeutic range; thus, plasma concentrations may not increase proportionately with the dose because clearance increases.

ADVERSE REACTIONS AND PRECAUTIONS. Because of the chronicity of epilepsy and the longstanding availability of the commonly used agents, the adverse reactions produced by the older antiepileptic drugs have been extensively reported. Some common characteristics of reactions to antiepileptic drugs are considered below. During clinical trials, much of the data on the safety of gabapentin, lamotrigine, and felbamate were derived from patients who were also receiving other antiepileptic agents. Adverse reactions that are directly attributable to gabapentin and lamotrigine have not been clearly determined; however, sufficient numbers of patients received felbamate as monotherapy to provide some indication of its safety profile as a single agent. For details on individual drugs, see the evaluations.

When loading doses are not necessary, initiation of the maintenance dose is most commonly limited by gastrointestinal or CNS reactions. Carbamazepine, ethosuximide, primidone, and valproate may cause dose-related nausea or abdominal discomfort; thus, a gradual increase in dosage is required. Phenytoin and phenobarbital often can be introduced at maintenance dosage levels; however, several days are still required to achieve steady-state (Scheuer and Pedley, 1990).

Central Nervous System: Sedation has been reported with all antiepileptic drugs, most noticeably during initial therapy, but tolerance usually develops. Usual doses of carbamazepine, phenytoin, ethosuximide, and valproate are less sedating than barbiturates and benzodiazepines. The sedative effects of lamotrigine and gabapentin probably are only minor. Although somnolence has been reported with adjunctive use of felbamate, some patients receiving monotherapy with this drug complain of insomnia.

Dizziness, blurred vision, and diplopia have been reported with use of many antiepileptic drugs, especially carbamazepine. These effects, as well as ataxia, also appear to be dose-related effects of lamotrigine and occur more frequently in patients who receive both lamotrigine and carbamazepine.

Symptoms of cerebellar and brainstem dysfunction (standing or gait imbalance, vertigo, dysarthria, nystagmus) are dose-related side effects of phenytoin, carbamazepine, valproate, and phenobarbital. Extrapyramidal dysfunction (eg, tremors, bradykinesia, dyskinesia) has been associated with most antiepileptic drugs but occurs infrequently, usually only at high plasma concentrations. Adjunctive therapy with felbamate, lamotrigine, and gabapentin may increase the occurrence of many of these central nervous system reactions.

Paradoxical excitement may occur with the benzodiazepines (diazepam and clonazepam) and phenobarbital, especially in young children and the elderly. Phenacemide may cause profound personality changes, including psychoses and suicidal depression.

Antiepileptic drugs, especially in combination, may impair attention, concentration, memory, and mental or motor speed (Reynolds and Trimble, 1985). In children and adults, behavioral problems occur most frequently with phenobarbital and least often with valproate and carbamazepine (Dodrill, 1991). Although disinhibition also occurs in children treated with clonazepam or diazepam, only a few studies have examined the behavioral effects of benzodiazepines in epileptic patients.

Available data suggest that felbamate, lamotrigine, and gabapentin do not cause significant cognitive impairment. However, there are limited data comparing these antiepileptic drugs with the older commonly used agents. The following discussion is based on published studies on the effects of barbiturates, valproate, carbamazepine, and phenytoin on cognitive functioning.

Results of studies that compared (1) treated with nontreated patients, (2) patients before and after initiation of drug therapy, (3) patients after conversion to monotherapy or after withdrawal of all antiepileptic drugs indicate that these agents may impair cognitive ability. Results of most studies in children indicate that impairment usually is less evident with valproate and carbamazepine (Vining et al, 1987; Pellock et al, 1988; Trimble, 1990), although elevated plasma concentrations of these drugs impair performance of some tasks (O'Dougherty et al, 1987; Aman et al, 1987, 1990). In one study in epileptic children, long-term treatment with phenobarbital, but not valproate, significantly impaired learning ability as measured by IQ scores (Calandre et al, 1990); use of phenobarbital for prophylaxis of febrile seizures also is associated with a decrease in measured intelligence (Farwell et al, 1990). However, other data indicate that the cognitive side effects of these drugs may have been overstated (Mitchell et al, 1993).

In adults, results of several nonrandomized studies suggest that patients treated with carbamazepine experience less cognitive and motor impairment than those receiving phenytoin, phenobarbital, or primidone (Andrewes et al, 1986; Smith et al, 1987; Gallassi et al, 1988). However, when plasma concentrations are controlled and patients with high levels are excluded from analysis, significant differences between carbamazepine and phenytoin are not apparent (Meador et al, 1990; Dodrill and Troupin, 1991). In other studies, monotherapy with carbamazepine, phenytoin, or valproate had little effect on overall cognitive function in patients tolerating treatment (Gillham et al, 1990), but motor performance improved in patients also treated with other antiepileptic drugs when these agents were discontinued (Duncan et al, 1990). Thus, the effects of antiepileptic drugs on cognition and motor performance may be subtle and whether important differences exist among the commonly used agents is controversial.

The American Academy of Pediatrics (Committee on Drugs, 1985) recommends that careful attention be given to parental, teacher, and clinical observations of cognitive function, mood, and behavior. If significant changes occur, consideration should be given to reducing the dose or substituting another antiepileptic drug. The results of repeated neuropsychological screening tests may be useful in detecting subtle behavioral and intellectual effects.

A frequently cited paradoxical effect of antiepileptic drugs is the tendency of agents effective in relieving one type of seizure to aggravate or precipitate seizures of another type. However, the apparent aggravation of one seizure type frequently is a manifestation of the natural course of disease and reflects the ineffectiveness of the particular drug for that type of seizure. Rarely, the aggravation may be due to multiple drug therapy. Carbamazepine has been reported to exacerbate atypical absence seizures in children with mixed partial and generalized epilepsy (Snead and Hosey, 1985). Some authorities believe that plasma phenytoin concentrations in excess of approximately 25 mcg/ml may exacerbate seizures and that seizure control may be obtained by reducing the dose. In general, precipitation of seizures by antiepileptic drugs probably is rare. There is no question, however, that abrupt withdrawal of most antiepileptic drugs can precipitate seizures. When a drug is to be discontinued, the dose should be reduced gradually. If rapid withdrawal and substitution of another drug is mandatory because of a serious adverse reaction or is otherwise therapeutically warranted, it should be accomplished only under carefully controlled conditions in the hospital.

Dermatologic: Antiepileptic drugs cause rash as a hypersensitivity reaction. Such sensitivity reactions cannot be predicted, but they usually become apparent after 10 to 14 days of therapy (within 28 days for lamotrigine). Most skin reactions are morbilliform and mild. If it is necessary to continue the causative medication to maintain seizure control, a short course of prednisone with or without adjunctive use of antihistamines may lessen the reaction in some patients (Murphy et al, 1991). A skin reaction may rarely precede the development of a more serious exfoliative dermatitis (eg, Stevens-Johnson syndrome) or systemic lupus erythematosus, dermatomyositis, serum sickness, or polyarteritis nodosa. Immediate or accelerated urticarial reactions with angioedema and bullous or severe morbilliform eruptions require discontinuation of the drug. Anaphylaxis is extremely rare.

Hematologic: The adverse effects of antiepileptic drugs on the hematopoietic system include reactions secondary to altered folate metabolism, coagulation defects, immune-mediated phenomena, and bone marrow suppression.

Macrocytic, and, rarely, megaloblastic anemias have been observed with several antiepileptic drugs, particularly the hydantoins, some barbiturates, and primidone. Therapy usually can be continued if the anemia responds to folic acid. Even in the absence of anemia, there is some evidence that reduction of folic acid concentrations precipitated by these antiepileptic drugs may cause reversible symptoms of mental deterioration. Lamotrigine is a weak inhibitor of dihydrofolate reductase in vitro, but it does not appear to affect serum concentrations of folate or hematologic parameters in humans. Poor memory, inattentiveness, lethargy, and slow learning may result from other effects of antiepileptic drugs or may indicate brain damage. However, if such symptoms occur in the presence of low folate blood concentrations, treatment with folic acid may be warranted.

Clotting defects have occurred in neonates born to mothers receiving phenobarbital, primidone, or phenytoin and are secondary to depletion of vitamin K-dependent clotting factors. Valproate may interfere with the secondary phase of platelet aggregation. Thrombocytopenia has been associated with antiepileptic drugs. Phenytoin and carbamazepine may provoke generalized lymphadenopathy with multisystem involvement.

Baseline studies should be performed in patients receiving these drugs. Although periodic blood studies detect leukopenias, they usually do not predict the more serious reactions that occur precipitously (eg, agranulocytosis, thrombocytopenia, aplastic anemia). Since early recognition of the dyscrasia and discontinuance of the offending drug are essential, the patient should be advised to report promptly such symptoms as sore throat, fever, easy bruising, petechiae, epistaxis, or other signs of infection or bleeding tendency. Clinical and laboratory evaluations are necessary if such symptoms occur.

Among older antiepileptic drugs, severe blood dyscrasias occur most commonly with phenacemide and mephenytoin; they are rare with other antiepileptic drugs, including paramethadione, trimethadione, phenytoin, and carbamazepine. Recent data suggest that the use of felbamate may be associated with a marked increase in the incidence of aplastic anemia (see the evaluation). Although the risk is diminished after the first year of treatment, the physician should be alert to their possible occurrence. Mortality from aplastic anemia is particularly high, and recovery is slow in surviving patients.

Hepatic: Baseline liver function studies should be performed before antiepileptic drug treatment is initiated, and patients should be instructed to report promptly any symptoms of hepatotoxicity, such as anorexia, abdominal discomfort or other gastrointestinal symptoms, jaundice, or dark urine. Severe, sometimes fatal, hepatotoxicity has occurred with valproate and, more rarely, with other antiepileptic drugs, including the hydantoins, carbamazepine, phenacemide, trimethadione, and phenobarbital. Patients at high risk of toxicity induced by valproate must be identified, and therapy with this drug should be avoided in these individuals (see the evaluation). Since drug-induced hepatitis is probably idiosyncratic, the value of performing periodic laboratory studies in asymptomatic patients is doubtful. Serious hepatotoxicity has not been associated with use of gabapentin or lamotrigine. Barbiturates, phenytoin, and carbamazepine exacerbate acute intermittent porphyria. Recently, eight cases of acute liver failure, including four deaths, have been reported in association with use of felbamate; one of the four survivors received a liver transplant. See the evaluation for recommendations concerning the appropriate use of felbamate and for monitoring liver function tests in patients receiving felbamate.

Renal: Nephropathies have developed occasionally during antiepileptic therapy, especially with trimethadione and paramethadione. These reactions usually develop insidiously. The appearance of any significant renal abnormality is an indication for discontinuing the drug.

Musculoskeletal: The long-term use of phenobarbital and phenytoin has been associated with a decrease in bone mineral content and an increased frequency of rickets (Iivanainen and Savolainen, 1983). These effects have been explained, at least in part, by induction of vitamin D metabolism with subsequent lowering of active metabolite concentrations. They are most prominent in institutionalized patients (especially children) in whom inactivity, diet, and lack of sun exposure may be contributing factors. They also have been noted in outpatients, although results of one study did not demonstrate any effect of phenobarbital or phenytoin therapy (for up to ten years) on bone mineral density in epileptic outpatients 5 to 20 years old (Timperlake et al, 1988).

The results of some retrospective studies have linked the use of antiepileptic drugs, in particular the barbiturates, to the development of a variety of connective tissue disorders. In a prospective controlled study, approximately 6% of male patients treated with phenobarbital or primidone for at least six months developed a connective tissue disorder (eg, Dupuytren's contracture, frozen shoulder, Peyronie's disease, arthralgias) (Mattson et al, 1989). Use of an alternative antiepileptic drug may be advisable in these patients.

Endocrine: Antiepileptic drugs may act on endocrine systems at various levels. Generally, these effects are subclinical

TABLE 7.
PLASMA CONCENTRATIONS, TOXIC SYMPTOMS, AND RELATED DRUG INTERACTIONS OF COMMONLY USED ANTIEPILEPTIC DRUGS

Drug	Average Daily Maintenance Dose: Adults	Average Daily Maintenance Dose: Children (mg/kg)	Usually Effective Plasma Concentration Range (mcg/ml)	Signs and Symptoms Usually Associated with Elevated Plasma Concentrations or Toxicity of Cited Drugs
Carbamazepine [Tegretol]	600 mg-1.2 g	15-30	4-12	Diplopia, nystagmus, blurred vision, ataxia, vertigo, lethargy, confusion, stupor
Clonazepam [Klonopin]	0.05-0.2 mg/kg	0.1-0.2	0.02-0.08	Sedation, confusion, slurred speech, somnolence, respiratory depression, coma, hypotension
Ethosuximide [Zarontin]	750 mg-2 g	20-40	40-100	Nausea, vomiting, gastric distress, drowsiness, ataxia
Phenobarbital	120-250 mg	3-5	15-40	Drowsiness, slurred speech, nystagmus, confusion, somnolence, ataxia, respiratory depression, coma, hypotension
Primidone [Mysoline]	750 mg-1.5 g	10-25	5-12	Similar to phenobarbital; crystalluria
Phenytoin [Dilantin]	300-400 mg	4-7	10-20	Vertigo, ataxia, slurred speech, nystagmus, diplopia, somnolence, stupor, coma (arrhythmias with rapid intravenous administration)
Valproate [Depakene, Depakote]	10-20 mg/kg (monotherapy)	15-60 (monotherapy)	40-120	Sedation, gastric disturbance, diarrhea, tremor, ataxia, somnolence, coma, thrombocytopenia, platelet dysfunction
	30-60 mg/kg (combination therapy)	30-100 (combination therapy)		
Felbamate [Felbatol]	2.4 g	30	30-100	Anorexia, nausea, vomiting, insomnia, headache
Gabapentin [Neurontin]	900 mg-1.8 g	—	2-6	Somnolence, dizziness, ataxia, fatigue, nystagmus

Other Antiepileptic Drugs Whose Plasma Concentration is Altered by Cited Antiepileptic Drug		Antiepileptic Drugs that Alter Plasma Concentration of Cited Drug		Nonantiepileptic Drugs that Alter Plasma Concentration of Cited Drug	
Increase	**Decrease**	**Increase**	**Decrease**	**Increase**	**Decrease**
	Clonazepam Ethosuximide Felbamate Phenobarbital[1] Phenytoin[1] Primidone Valproate	Acetazolamide	Phenobarbital[1] Phenytoin[1]	Cimetidine Clarithromycin Danazol Diltiazem Erythromycin Fluoxetine Isoniazid Propoxyphene Troleandomycin Verapamil	
No consistent change in other antiepileptic plasma concentrations noted			Carbamazepine Phenobarbital Primidone	Cimetidine Disulfiram Oral contraceptives	
Phenytoin[2]			Carbamazepine Phenobarbital Phenytoin Primidone		
	Carbamazepine[1] Clonazepam Phenytoin[1]	Valproate	Carbamazepine Phenytoin[1]	Chloramphenicol Propoxyphene	
Same as phenobarbital		Same as phenobarbital		Isoniazid	
	Carbamazepine[1] Felbamate Phenobarbital[1] Primidone[1] Valproate[1]	Felbamate	Carbamazepine[1] Phenobarbital[1] Valproate[1]	Allopurinol Amiodarone Chloramphenicol Chlorpheniramine Cimetidine Dicumarol Disulfiram Fluconazole Isoniazid Phenylbutazone Sulfonamides Trazodone Trimethoprim	Antineoplastics Diazoxide Loxapine Rifampin
Carbamazepine[4] Phenobarbital	Ethosuximide[1] Phenytoin[3]	Felbamate	Carbamazepine Phenobarbital Phenytoin Primidone	Erythromycin Fluoxetine Salicylates	
Phenytoin Valproate	Carbamazepine[4]	Valproate	Carbamazepine Phenytoin		
				Aluminum-containing antacids Cimetidine	

(table continued on next page)

TABLE 7. (continued)

Drug	Average Daily Maintenance Dose: Adults	Average Daily Maintenance Dose: Children (mg/kg)	Usually Effective Plasma Concentration Range (mcg/ml)	Signs and Symptoms Usually Associated with Elevated Plasma Concentrations or Toxicity of Cited Drugs
Lamotrigine [Lamictal]	200-400 mg	1.3-10[5]	2-6	Dizziness, diplopia, ataxia, blurred vision

[1]*Variable effects (increase, decrease, no change) reported. See text for explanation.*
[2]*Possibly; clinical importance not established.*
[3]*Variable effects on free and total plasma concentrations. See text for explanation.*
[4]*Increases the concentration of carbamazepine epoxide or the carbamazepine epoxide/carbamazepine ratio.*
[5]*Dose in children depends on age and concomitant therapy.*

(eg, diminished thyroid function, decreased anterior pituitary responsiveness), although they can cause drug interactions (eg, with oral contraceptives). Hyponatremia can occur with carbamazepine therapy because of inappropriate release of antidiuretic hormone, but symptoms may not develop for as long as one year after treatment is initiated.

DRUG INTERACTIONS. The potential for antiepileptic drug interactions is considerable, since many of these agents possess a relatively narrow therapeutic range, and they are usually administered for long periods. In addition, many of the commonly used antiepileptic drugs are weak acids, they significantly bind to plasma proteins, and they either induce or inhibit hepatic enzymes involved in biotransformation.

Most drug interactions are pharmacokinetic, but some are pharmacodynamic. Thus, drugs that produce CNS depression (eg, antihistamines, centrally acting alpha agonists or muscle relaxants, opioid analgesics, sedative-hypnotics) can exacerbate the sedative or neurotoxic effects of antiepileptic drugs, and concomitant use should be avoided. Drugs that decrease seizure threshold (eg, phenothiazines and other antipsychotic agents, tricyclic antidepressants, reserpine) also should be avoided, if possible. The pharmacokinetically based drug interactions commonly increase (promote toxicity) or decrease (result in therapeutic failure) drug plasma concentrations. Monitoring for signs and symptoms of toxicity and to determine plasma drug concentrations provides the clinical basis on which to evaluate drug interactions.

Table 7 summarizes the average daily maintenance doses and therapeutic plasma concentrations of selected antiepileptic drugs, signs and symptoms of acute toxicity, and drug interactions that affect drug plasma concentrations. For interactions of antiepileptic drugs with other drugs, see the evaluations and index entry Drug Interactions.

USE IN PREGNANCY AND LACTATION. Childbearing Age: Guidelines for the care of women of childbearing age with epilepsy are available (Commission on Genetics, Pregnancy, and the Child, International League Against Epilepsy, 1993).

Prepregnancy counseling should include the information that the effectiveness of oral contraceptives may be impaired in women receiving phenytoin, phenobarbital, primidone, carbamazepine, and possibly ethosuximide. A combination oral contraceptive preparation containing at least 50 mcg of estrogen may be required for effective contraception in patients who are receiving drugs that induce hepatic cytochrome P450 (O'Brien and Gilmour-White, 1993) or a different method of contraception may be employed.

Pregnancy: Recommendations for antiepileptic drug use during pregnancy are complicated by several interrelated factors, including the influence of pregnancy on epilepsy and antiepileptic drug disposition, the impact of epilepsy on pregnancy outcome, and the question of teratogenesis produced by antiepileptic drugs. Several studies have found that the risk of complications is increased in pregnant women with epilepsy, but the effect of pregnancy on seizure frequency is unpredictable. In most patients, the seizure frequency is unchanged; however, some women experience either a decrease or an increase. Plasma concentrations of antiepileptic drugs tend to decrease during pregnancy (Levy and Yerby, 1985; Lander and Eadie, 1991). Although this in itself does not justify an increase in dosage, it is a common reason for an increase in seizure frequency that does require an increase in dosage. The concentrations should be monitored throughout pregnancy and the dosage adjusted according to clinical circumstances.

The type of antiepileptic drug, dosage, and treatment regimen should be considered carefully in women of childbearing age. Withdrawal of drug therapy can be considered for patients without evidence of cerebral lesions who have remained seizure-free for two to three years before they plan to become pregnant. Otherwise, patients should be treated with the lowest effective dose and, if possible, with a single agent. A single daily dose is not advisable because peak plasma concentrations are higher, and this may increase the risk of adverse effects.

At present, there is no evidence to indicate that the risk to the fetus differs significantly following monotherapy with phenytoin, phenobarbital, carbamazepine, or primidone; thus, it has been argued that in a well-controlled patient, there is no reason to change the medication.

Infants born to mothers with epilepsy may be at increased risk for prematurity, low birth weight, low Apgar scores, hypoxia, hemorrhage, and congenital malformations. Congenital anomalies occur with increased frequency among the offspring of epileptic women, whether the mothers were treated or untreated. In general, the risk of seizures outweighs the risk of teratogenesis produced by antiepileptic drugs. Women

Other Antiepileptic Drugs Whose Plasma Concentration is Altered by Cited Antiepileptic Drug		Antiepileptic Drugs that Alter Plasma Concentration of Cited Drug		Nonantiepileptic Drugs that Alter Plasma Concentration of Cited Drug	
Increase	**Decrease**	**Increase**	**Decrease**	**Increase**	**Decrease**
Carbamazepine	Valproate	Valproate	Carbamazepine Phenobarbital Phenytoin Primidone		

of childbearing age who are receiving these drugs as monotherapy may be informed that the chance of having a normal child is greater than 90% but that the risk of a congenital malformation may be about two to three times higher (ie, 6%) than in the general population. It is uncertain whether malformations result from epilepsy in general, genetic predisposition to both epilepsy and these birth defects, antiepileptic drugs, or drug-induced deficiency states (eg, folate). All these factors may be contributory, but antiepileptic drugs probably play a major role. The risk is increased with use of more than one antiepileptic drug during pregnancy.

Both valproate and carbamazepine have been reported to increase the risk of spina bifida (Rosa, 1991). The risk of neural tube defects associated with valproate justifies special consideration. Several case-control studies indicate that the incidence of spina bifida or neural tube defect may be 1% to 2% in offspring of women taking this drug; however, treatment with valproate may be necessary to control seizures in pregnant women with some epileptic syndromes.

Felbamate, gabapentin, and lamotrigine have not been linked with human teratogenesis, and results of animal studies suggest that they have little effect on the developing fetus. Nevertheless, experience with these agents is very limited. All of the older commonly used antiepileptic drugs have been implicated in human teratogenesis. The most common major malformations are congenital heart disease and cleft lip and/or palate. In children born to epileptic women taking antiepileptic drugs, the combined incidence of both defects is approximately 18/1,000 (Committee on Maternal and Fetal Medicine, American College of Obstetricians and Gynecologists, 1984).

Although most congenital malformations generally are mild and have been observed most frequently with use of phenytoin and/or phenobarbital, this probably reflects the wider use of these agents. Plasma folate levels are inversely correlated with plasma concentrations of phenytoin and phenobarbital; this may be related to fetal outcome (Hiilesmaa et al, 1983; Dansky et al, 1987). Reduced folate concentrations may contribute to congenital malformations, especially neural tube defects. There is evidence that supplemental doses of folic acid during the periconceptional period may reduce the incidence of neural tube defects (Milunsky et al, 1989; MRC Vitamin Study Research Group, 1991; Czeizel and Dudas, 1992) both in normal women and those who are receiving antiepileptic drugs (Biale and Lewenthal, 1984).

Current guidelines recommend daily consumption of folic acid 0.4 mg by all women capable of becoming pregnant and of 4 mg by women who have previously had an infant or fetus with a neural tube defect and are planning another pregnancy (*MMWR*, 1992). However, a firm recommendation for the appropriate supplemental dose in women receiving antiepileptic drugs is not established. Case reports and uncontrolled studies suggest that folic acid may antagonize the effects of phenytoin, but results of controlled studies have not demonstrated adverse effects on seizure control. On the other hand, phenytoin can induce folate deficiency. Women who are receiving antiepileptic drugs that increase the incidence of neural tube defects (ie, valproate, carbamazepine) or other antiepileptic drugs that may influence folate metabolism (ie, phenytoin, phenobarbital, primidone) might benefit from doses larger than 0.4 mg; however, this has not been studied directly.

The pattern of some abnormalities initially thought to be caused by phenytoin now is termed the "fetal antiepileptic drug syndrome," and reports linking it to phenobarbital, carbamazepine, and valproate also have been published. Prenatal and postnatal growth deficiencies, microencephaly, developmental delay, short nose, hypoplastic fingernails and distal phalanges, and congenital heart defects have been observed after exposure to alcohol as well. The phenotypic overlay may be explained by different teratogens exerting cytotoxic effects during the same stage of development (Dow and Riopelle, 1989). Low activity of epoxide hydrolase in the fetus may be a risk factor for phenytoin-induced abnormalities (Buehler et al, 1990).

Trimethadione is rarely used but is a very potent teratogen; birth defects or spontaneous abortions have occurred in 80% of pregnancies in women exposed to this agent. Therefore, trimethadione should not be prescribed for females of childbearing age unless absolutely necessary, and women receiving the drug should be counseled regarding the risks.

Close obstetrical supervision to assess fetal well-being, including prenatal diagnosis by ultrasound and maternal serum alpha-fetoprotein (AFP) screening for detection of neural tube defects and other fetal malformations, is essential during pregnancy (Burton, 1989). Women with elevated serum concentrations of AFP should have ultrasonographic evaluation and diagnostic amniocentesis to assess the AFP and acetylcholinesterase concentrations in the amniotic fluid (Cunningham and Gilstrap, 1991; American Academy of Pediatrics, Committee on Genetics, 1991).

Antiepileptic drugs that induce hepatic enzymes can reduce vitamin K-dependent clotting factors. To decrease the risk of bleeding in the perinatal period, pregnant women who take enzyme-inducing antiepileptic drugs should receive phytonadione (vitamin K_1) 20 mg daily for at least one week prior to delivery, and 2 mg should be administered to the infant immediately after birth (O'Brien and Gilmour-White, 1993). Bleeding and coagulation studies should be performed periodically during the first 24 to 48 hours, and additional vitamin K should be administered if required.

Although the plasma concentration of antiepileptic drugs tends to decrease during pregnancy, the opposite generally occurs during the postpartum period. Therefore, monitoring should continue to prevent development of dose-related toxicity.

Lactation: Nursing is not contraindicated in mothers receiving most antiepileptic medications. However, if symptoms such as sedation develop in an infant whose mother is receiving phenobarbital, primidone, or the benzodiazepines, breast feeding may need to be discontinued; occasionally, this may provoke withdrawal symptoms in the infant.

Drug Evaluations

ACETAZOLAMIDE

[Diamox]

For chemical formula, see index entry Acetazolamide, Uses, Glaucoma.

This carbonic anhydrase inhibitor has been used in absence, generalized tonic-clonic, and partial seizures. It is most often administered as an adjunct to other drugs, but its usefulness is limited by the rapid development of tolerance in some patients. Acetazolamide is often helpful when intermittent administration is required (eg, in women whose seizure frequency increases with menstruation).

For adverse reactions and other uses, see index entry Acetazolamide.

DOSAGE AND PREPARATIONS.

Oral: *Adults and children,* 8 to 30 mg/kg daily in divided doses (range, 250 mg to 1 g daily).

Diamox (Lederle), ***Generic.*** Tablets 125 and 250 mg.

CARBAMAZEPINE

[Tegretol]

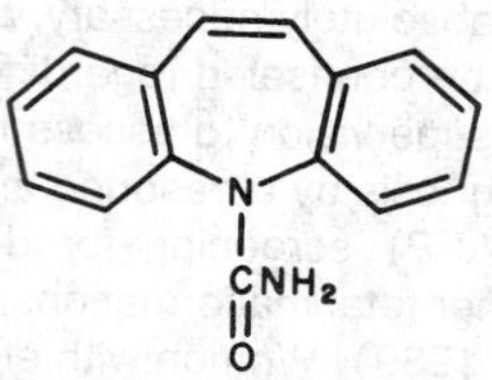

ACTIONS AND USES. This heterocyclic (iminostilbene) compound has potent antiepileptic properties and is effective alone or with other antiepileptic drugs in partial seizures, especially complex partial seizures, generalized tonic-clonic seizures, and combinations of these seizure types. Carbamazepine generally is ineffective for absence, myoclonic, and atonic seizures. In children with symptomatic generalized epilepsy and continuous spike-and-wave discharge, these seizure types may develop or tonic-clonic seizures may increase in frequency with use of carbamazepine (Snead and Hosey, 1985).

Comparative clinical trial data indicate that patients with partial seizures may tolerate carbamazepine better than phenobarbital and primidone, but individual responses vary (Mattson et al, 1985). Many clinicians consider carbamazepine a drug of choice for initial therapy in idiopathic and symptomatic localization-related epilepsies, especially in children and women. This drug is increasingly preferred to phenobarbital in pediatric patients because it has less effect on cognition and behavior. It is reported to have psychotropic activity that may increase alertness and elevate mood in depressed epileptic patients, but not in otherwise normal patients. Mental improvements may be due to substitution of carbamazepine for sedative drugs, control of seizures, or a direct psychotropic effect.

ADVERSE REACTIONS AND PRECAUTIONS. Reactions that occur most commonly during early treatment are drowsiness, dizziness, lightheadedness, diplopia, ataxia, nausea, and vomiting. These side effects usually subside spontaneously within one week or after a reduction in dose. They may be minimized by initiating therapy with a small dose and increasing it gradually. Less common neurologic reactions include confusion, headache, fatigue, blurred vision, oculomotor disturbances, dysphasia, abnormal involuntary movements, peripheral neuritis and paresthesias, depression with agitation, talkativeness, nystagmus, and tinnitus.

Gastrointestinal reactions include gastric distress and abdominal pain, diarrhea, constipation, and anorexia. Dryness of the mouth, glossitis, and stomatitis also occur.

Dermatologic reactions (pruritic and erythematous rashes, urticaria, Stevens-Johnson syndrome, photosensitivity, altered skin pigmentation, exfoliative dermatitis, alopecia, hyperhidrosis, erythema multiforme, erythema nodosum, and aggravation of systemic lupus erythematosus) occur in 6% of patients and usually necessitate discontinuation of carbamazepine. Skin rash accompanied by fever, generalized lymphadenopathy, hepatomegaly, splenomegaly, and pulmonary symptoms also have been reported.

Transient leukopenia occurs in approximately 10% of patients treated with carbamazepine. Discontinuance of the drug is not required unless the leukopenia is accompanied by evidence of infection. Other hematopoietic reactions (eosinophilia, leukocytosis, purpura, and thrombocytopenia) are rare, and aplastic anemia and agranulocytosis are very rare (Pellock, 1987; Tohen et al, 1991). All of these reactions may be serious. Since their onset is gradual and reversible on dosage reduction, patients should be advised to notify their physician if fever, sore throat, aphthous stomatitis, easy bruising, petechial or purpuric hemorrhage, or other signs of hematologic toxicity appear.

Cardiovascular, genitourinary, metabolic, hepatic, and other reactions have been reported rarely. These include aggravation of hypertension or ischemic heart disease, arrhythmias, hypotension, syncope, edema, congestive heart failure, recurrence of thrombophlebitis, urinary frequency, acute urinary retention, albuminuria, glycosuria, decreased total and free thyroxine, elevated blood urea nitrogen levels, microscopic deposits in the urine, impotence, cholestatic and hepatocellular jaundice, fever and chills, myalgia and arthralgia, leg cramps, and conjunctivitis.

Carbamazepine increases the release of antidiuretic hormone and this effect may be troublesome, particularly in cardiac or elderly patients. Mild, symptomless hyponatremia is an established side effect. Serious water intoxication with sodium concentrations below 120 mEq/L and characterized by confusion, lethargy, neurologic dysfunction, and seizures is uncommon. The risk increases with age (all cases have been reported in individuals over 25 years) and with elevated carbamazepine plasma concentrations. Other conditions or drugs predisposing to water intoxication should be avoided (Hansten and Horn, 1987).

Baseline blood and platelet counts, urinalysis, and hepatic and renal function studies should be performed before initiating treatment. However, excessively frequent and specialized monitoring is unwarranted and costly (Hart and Easton, 1982; Pellock and Willmore, 1991). Careful clinical evaluation is probably more effective in preventing serious complications (Camfield et al, 1986; Evans et al, 1989; Pellock and Willmore, 1991). Some physicians prefer to perform blood counts once or twice during the first few months of therapy and when plasma drug concentrations are measured. Patients should be instructed to contact their physician immediately if petechiae, pallor, weakness, fever, or infection occurs.

PREGNANCY. Assessing the teratogenic potential of carbamazepine is difficult because of its use with other agents and because the epileptic disorder also contributes to this effect. The risk of major malformations is not measurably different from that associated with phenytoin and phenobarbital. Craniofacial defects, nail hypoplasia, and developmental delay have been noted in children exposed to this agent in utero (Jones et al, 1989). The results of one retrospective study (Rosa, 1991) suggest that the risk of spina bifida may be increased, but this has not been confirmed. The potential for birth defects is increased when carbamazepine is used with other antiepileptic drugs, and the risks and benefits should be weighed. This drug is classified in FDA Pregnancy Category C. Concentrations of carbamazepine and its epoxide metabolite in breast milk are 25% to 60% of those in the serum.

DRUG INTERACTIONS. Clinically important drug interactions with carbamazepine have been reviewed (Ketter et al, 1991 A, 1991 B).

Since carbamazepine is chemically related to the tricyclic compounds, it should not be administered to patients who are sensitive to these drugs or who are receiving monoamine oxidase inhibitors. The possibility of activating latent psychosis or inducing confusion or agitation in elderly patients exists.

Approximately 75% of carbamazepine is bound to plasma albumin, but it is not displaced by acidic drugs as is phenytoin, and it does not displace the latter. Terfenadine may increase the free fraction of carbamazepine (Hirschfeld and Jarosinski, 1993). As a result of enzyme induction, carbamazepine increases the hepatic metabolism of clonazepam, diazepam, ethosuximide, valproate, felbamate, and lamotrigine. In patients treated with phenobarbital, phenytoin, or primidone concomitantly, a small increase or, more commonly, a decrease in the plasma concentration of one or both agents may occur. Valproate also has a variable effect on carbamazepine steady-state concentration, depending on whether displacement from protein binding sites or inhibition of carbamazepine metabolism exerts the greatest influence. Valproate, felbamate, and lamotrigine increase the concentration of carbamazepine epoxide, which may have therapeutic or toxic significance.

Acetazolamide, cimetidine, danazol, diltiazem, erythromycin, fluoxetine, isoniazid, propoxyphene, troleandomycin, and verapamil increase the plasma concentration of carbamazepine. The effect of cimetidine is transient. In pediatric patients, large doses of niacinamide may increase carbamazepine plasma concentrations. Carbamazepine increases the hepatic clearance and may decrease the effectiveness of oral anticoagulants, certain anti-infective agents (doxycycline, mebendazole, praziquantel), cyclosporine, haloperidol, theophylline, oral contraceptives, methadone, pancuronium, and tricyclic antidepressants (Leinonen et al, 1991; Brøsen and Kragh-Sørensen, 1993). This drug also may reduce the plasma concentration and therapeutic response to corticosteroids or thyroid hormones. Other drug interactions (eg, with quinidine) related to hepatic enzyme induction that have been reported for other antiepileptic drugs conceivably could occur with carbamazepine. The combination of carbamazepine and lithium may increase the risk of neurotoxicity.

PHARMACOKINETICS. The pharmacokinetics of carbamazepine have been reviewed (Bertilsson and Tomson, 1986). Oral absorption is variable; peak plasma concentrations after use of solid dosage forms occur in 4 to 12 hours. Bioavailability is estimated at 85% but may be less when the drug is taken with meals. Carbamazepine undergoes significant enterohepatic cycling. With monotherapy, the usual therapeutic plasma concentration is 4 to 12 mcg/ml, but concentrations as high as 17 mcg/ml rarely may be required to control seizures without producing unacceptable adverse reactions or toxicity. With concomitant use of other antiepileptic drugs, concentrations as low as 4 mcg/ml may be associated with toxicity.

Carbamazepine is metabolized in the liver to its 10,11-epoxide, which has a half-life of about six hours. The 10,11-epoxide also has therapeutic and toxic effects. In some patients, carbamazepine induces its own metabolism to a significant degree; as a result, the usual initial half-life (18 to 55 hours) is reduced considerably after three or four weeks of administration. Because of autoinduction of metabolism, plasma concentrations should be monitored at least twice during the first month of treatment. Also, because concomitant use with phenytoin or phenobarbital may further induce this metabolic pathway, significantly larger doses of carbamazepine often are required when it is used in combination with these drugs. Pregnancy may alter plasma steady-state concentrations, although clearance does not seem to be greatly affected (Battino et al, 1985). Children metabolize carbamazepine more rapidly than adults.

For other pharmacokinetic data, see Table 6.

DOSAGE AND PREPARATIONS. Because carbamazepine tablets can be degraded by moisture, patients should be advised to store them away from heat and areas of high moisture (eg, the bathroom) and to keep the containers closed tightly. The suspension formulation of carbamazepine is absorbed more rapidly than the tablet formulation to yield a higher peak plasma concentration; therefore, when the suspension formulation is substituted for the tablet formulation, the same total daily dosage should be divided into smaller amounts given at more frequent intervals.

Oral: *Children 6 to 12 years,* initially, 5 to 10 mg/kg in two divided doses. The amount is increased by 5 mg/kg/day at appropriate intervals (usually one to two weeks) and given in three or four divided doses until the desired response is obtained (usual maximum dose, 1 g). The usual maintenance dose is 20 to 40 mg/kg (400 to 800 mg) daily; the frequency of administration must be individualized. *Children 4 to 6 years,* 5 mg/kg in two or three divided doses, increased by 5 mg/kg/day at weekly intervals to a dose of 15 to 20 mg/kg/day in two or three divided doses. Subsequent increases in dosage are made as needed and tolerated and may be guided by plasma drug concentrations. *Children under 4 years,* an initial dose of 20 to 60 mg is recommended (Porter, 1987).

Adults and adolescents, initially, 400 mg divided into two doses on the first day, increased by 200 mg daily at appropriate intervals (usually one to two weeks) and administered in three or four divided doses. When the drug is used as monotherapy, some epileptologists consider a twice-daily regimen acceptable in the absence of dose-related side effects (Porter, 1987). The usual daily maintenance dose is 600 mg to 1.2 g in monotherapy but may be as high as 1.6 g with combination therapy. The usual maximum dose is 1 g daily in *children 12 to 15 years* and 1.2 g in patients *over 15 years.* Up to 2 g daily has been given to *adults* when necessary, and even larger doses may be required in heavy individuals.

Generic. Tablets 200 mg; tablets (chewable) 100 mg.

Tegretol (Basel). Tablets 200 mg; tablets (chewable) 100 mg; suspension 100 mg/5 ml.

Additional Trademarks:

Atretol (Athena Neurosciences), ***Epitol*** (Lemmon).

CLONAZEPAM

[Klonopin]

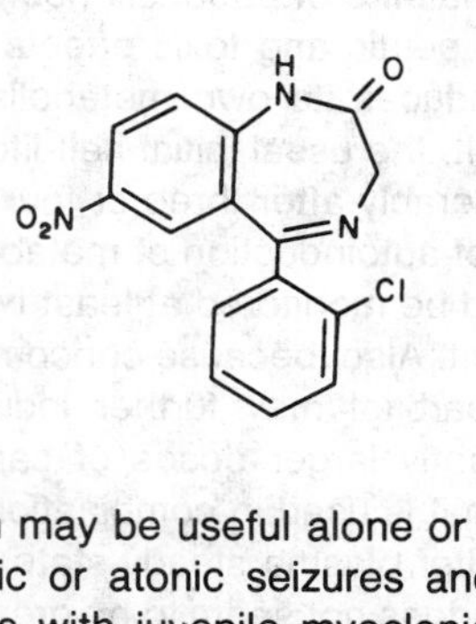

H
O
O_2N
N
Cl

USES. Clonazepam may be useful alone or with other drugs to control myoclonic or atonic seizures and photosensitive epilepsy. In patients with juvenile myoclonic epilepsy, myoclonic jerks may be controlled but generalized tonic-clonic seizures are not (Obeid and Panayiotopoulos, 1989). Although this drug also is effective in absence seizures, tolerance develops and breakthrough seizures often occur after one or two months. Increasing the dose may re-establish partial control in some patients. For this reason, ethosuximide or valproate is preferred. In addition, the incidence of drowsiness and ataxia is higher with prolonged use of clonazepam than with ethosuximide. Limited data suggest that clonazepam may be useful in the treatment of some neonatal seizures that are unresponsive to phenobarbital (André et al, 1991). It is seldom effective in generalized tonic-clonic or partial seizures.

Clonazepam may be helpful in status epilepticus, but parenteral forms are not available in the United States.

ADVERSE REACTIONS AND PRECAUTIONS. The most common adverse reactions of clonazepam affect the central nervous system. Approximately one-half of patients experience drowsiness; about one-third, ataxia; and up to one-quarter, behavioral and personality changes, including irritability and aggression, and, in children, hyperactivity. These effects appear to be dose related, occur early in the course of therapy, and may partially subside with long-term administration. The sedation may limit clonazepam's usefulness and may be minimized by initiating therapy with a small dose and increasing the amount gradually. Other neurologic effects include nystagmus, slurred speech, tremor, vertigo, confusion, fatigue, and hypotonia. Weight gain also may occur.

Minor, but sometimes troublesome, reactions involving the cardiovascular, gastrointestinal, and genitourinary systems have been observed. Skin rashes, anemia, leukopenia, thrombocytopenia, and eosinophilia also have occurred. Clonazepam causes respiratory depression and hypersecretion in the upper respiratory passages; therefore, it should be used with caution in individuals with respiratory tract disease. In young children, sialorrhea and difficulty in swallowing can be troublesome. This drug is contraindicated in those with a history of sensitivity to the benzodiazepines, significant liver disease, or acute angle-closure glaucoma.

Both psychological and physical dependence have been reported. If tolerance develops after long-term therapy, attempts to discontinue clonazepam abruptly may be complicated by withdrawal symptoms and seizures even in patients who do not experience continued therapeutic benefit (Specht et al, 1989). The withdrawal symptoms are similar to those observed with the barbiturates. Rapid withdrawal also may precipitate status epilepticus. This drug is classified as a Schedule IV substance under the Controlled Substances Act.

The effects of clonazepam on the fetus and nursing infant are not known; therefore, this drug should be used during pregnancy only if the expected benefits outweigh the potential hazards (see the Introduction). Nursing infants should be monitored for excessive sedation.

DRUG INTERACTIONS. Interactions between clonazepam and other antiepileptic drugs usually are not significant. Clonazepam does not consistently alter the plasma concentrations of carbamazepine, phenobarbital, phenytoin, or primidone, but these drugs may decrease the plasma concentration of clonazepam. Additive central nervous system depression may occur when clonazepam is given with another drug that has this action, especially barbiturates. The combination of clonazepam and primidone may provoke or exacerbate behavioral disorders. The combination of clonazepam and valproate rarely has been associated with increased neurotoxicity or nonconvulsive spike-wave stupor (absence status). Cimetidine, oral contraceptives, and disulfiram may increase the plasma concentration of clonazepam.

PHARMACOKINETICS. Clonazepam is well absorbed; peak plasma concentrations occur one to four hours after oral administration. This drug is virtually completely biotransformed to inactive metabolites via nitroreduction and acetylation. The half-life ranges reported are similar for adults (19 to 50 hours) and children (22 to 33 hours), but the mean ratio of plasma level to oral dose generally is considerably lower in children (Sato, 1989). A relationship between seizure control and plasma concentration has not been clearly established, although the usual range at which seizures are controlled is 0.02 to 0.08 mcg/ml. Clonazepam reduces the frequency of absence seizures at plasma concentrations of 0.013 to 0.072 mcg/ml. Steady-state concentrations during long-term therapy rarely exceed 0.1 mcg/ml. For other pharmacokinetic data, see Table 6.

DOSAGE AND PREPARATIONS.

Oral: *Adults,* initially, 1.5 mg daily in three divided doses, increased by 0.5 to 1 mg every third day until seizures are adequately controlled or adverse effects intervene (maximum, 20 mg daily). The usual daily maintenance dose is 0.05 to 0.2 mg/kg. *Infants and children up to 10 years or 30 kg,* 0.01 to 0.03 (maximum, 0.05) mg/kg daily in two or three divided doses, increased by 0.25 to 0.5 mg every third day until a maintenance dose of 0.1 to 0.2 mg/kg/day has been reached.

Klonopin (Roche). Tablets 0.5, 1, and 2 mg.

CLORAZEPATE DIPOTASSIUM

[Gen-Xene, Tranxene]

For chemical formula, see index entry Clorazepate, In Anxiety.

USES. Clorazepate has been studied primarily in open trials involving patients with refractory epilepsy. This benzodiazepine may be effective as adjunctive therapy in selected patients with partial or generalized seizures (Wilensky and Friel, 1989). In those with partial seizures treated with phenytoin, clorazepate was equivalent to phenobarbital as an adjunct and was preferred by more patients. This drug may be useful in patients in whom seizures occur frequently or in those with complex partial seizures (Griffith and Murray, 1985); however, tolerance to the anticonvulsant effects develops frequently.

ADVERSE REACTIONS AND PRECAUTIONS. The adverse effects of clorazepate are similar to those of other benzodiazepines (see index entry Benzodiazepines). Behavioral changes or irritability may be provoked, especially when this agent is administered with primidone (Feldman, 1976).

PHARMACOKINETICS. Clorazepate is a prodrug that is decarboxylated in the stomach or plasma to desmethyldiazepam. Hepatic clearance is accelerated in patients treated concomitantly with hepatic enzyme-inducing drugs. Cimetidine is reported to decrease hepatic clearance. The half-life is prolonged during the last trimester of pregnancy. For more information on the disposition of clorazepate, see index entry Clorazepate, In Anxiety.

DOSAGE AND PREPARATIONS.

Oral: *Adults,* initially, up to 7.5 mg three times a day (0.4 mg/kg). The dose may be increased weekly by 7.5 mg to a maximum of 90 mg based on clinical response. The usual amount is 0.5 to 1 mg/kg/day, but up to 3 mg/kg/day has been used in refractory epilepsy. The pediatric dosage is not firmly established, but is adjusted for body weight; the usual daily dose is higher than for adults. *Children 9 to 12 years,* initially, up to 7.5 mg two times a day, increased weekly by no more than 7.5 mg to a maximum of 60 mg, has been recommended.

Generic. Capsules and tablets 3.75, 7.5, and 15 mg.

Gen-Xene (Alra). Tablets 3.75, 7.5, and 15 mg.

Tranxene (Abbott). Tablets 3.75, 7.5, 11.25 (***Tranxene-SD Half Strength***), 15 (***Tranxene T-Tab***), and 22.5 mg (***Tranxene-SD***).

DIAZEPAM

[Valium]

For chemical formula, see index entry Diazepam, In Anxiety.

ACTIONS AND USES. Intravenous diazepam is used for initial control of seizures in patients with convulsive status epilepticus because of its rapid onset of action. Therapeutic plasma concentrations are achieved in two to six minutes (Woodbury et al, 1982). Its duration of action is short due to rapid redistribution from the brain; therefore, a loading dose of intravenous phenytoin sodium or phenobarbital should be given concomitantly or immediately after control of seizures is achieved in order to maintain antiepileptic activity. Intravenous diazepam also may be useful with or as an alternative to magnesium sulfate to control the seizures of eclampsia (see index entry Eclampsia, Pre-eclampsia).

The rectal administration of the parenteral solution of diazepam is useful as an alternative to intravenous therapy in children with status epilepticus and in patients who tend to have clusters of seizures (Albano et al, 1989; Kriel et al, 1991; Remy et al, 1992). This route can be employed in the home or by emergency medical services personnel when intravenous access is difficult or delayed. Rectal administration also is effective for the short-term prophylaxis of febrile seizures in children (Camfield et al, 1989; Knudsen, 1991); oral administration is an alternative in children in whom this route can be used (Rosman et al, 1993). Respiratory depression occasionally may complicate rectal use. A viscous solution of diazepam for rectal administration [Diastat] (Athena Neurosciences) has been granted orphan drug status and is undergoing clinical trials for the treatment of febrile and other acute seizures.

ADVERSE REACTIONS AND PRECAUTIONS. When diazepam is given parenterally for status epilepticus, the patient must be observed for signs of respiratory and central nervous system depression and hypotension, especially when it is administered with other antiepileptic agents. Young and elderly patients are most vulnerable. However, the overall safety of the drug appears to compare favorably with that of other agents used for this emergency.

For further information on adverse reactions, precautions, drug interactions, and other uses, see index entry Diazepam. This drug is classified as a Schedule IV substance under the Controlled Substances Act.

PHARMACOKINETICS. Onset of action is almost immediate after intravenous administration. The volume of distribution is reported to be 0.95 to 2 L/kg. The half-lives of diazepam and its active derivative, desmethyldiazepam, are 27 to 37 and 50 to 100 hours, respectively; however, rapid redistribution out of the brain occurs within 30 minutes after injection, which reduces effectiveness.

Effective plasma concentrations of diazepam and desmethyldiazepam have not been determined definitively, but minimal concentrations of about 0.5 mcg/ml are required to terminate status epilepticus. The plasma concentration of diazepam exceeds 0.5 mcg/ml immediately after intravenous injection of 10 mg in adults.

For complete pharmacokinetic data, see index entry Diazepam, In Anxiety.

DOSAGE AND PREPARATIONS.

Intravenous (slow): For status epilepticus, see Table 5.

Rectal: The parenteral solution can be injected into the rectal lumen using a 1-ml disposable insulin syringe. Introduction of the enema 4 to 5 cm within the rectum is easily achieved with this length syringe; alternatively, a syringe with a soft plastic or rubber catheter can be used, but this may create a dead space in the administration apparatus. For short-term prophylaxis of febrile seizures, a dose of 5 mg in *children less than 3 years* and 7.5 mg in those *3 years or older* is administered every 12 hours during febrile illness. For *children* with status epilepticus, the initial recommended dose is 0.5 mg/kg, followed by 0.25 mg/kg in ten minutes if seizures continue. For patients with cluster, serial, or prolonged seizures, 0.3 to 0.5 mg/kg may be administered to terminate the seizure(s) and prevent development of status epilepticus.

Generic. Solution 5 mg/ml in 1, 2, 5, and 10 ml containers.

Valium (Roche). Solution 5 mg/ml in 2 and 10 ml containers.

Oral: For short-term prophylaxis of febrile seizures in *children*, 0.33 mg/kg every eight hours during febrile illness.

Valium (Roche), ***Generic.*** Tablets 2, 5, and 10 mg.

ETHOSUXIMIDE

[Zarontin]

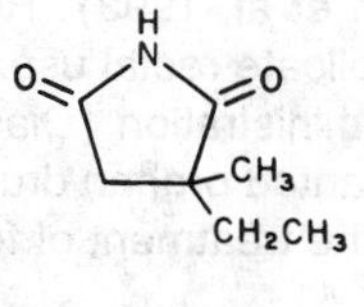

ACTIONS AND USES. Ethosuximide is the drug of choice for absence seizures unaccompanied by other types of seizures; its use avoids the potential hepatotoxicity of valproate. This drug abolishes seizures in 60% of such patients, and practical control is achieved in 80% to 90% of newly diagnosed patients. Ethosuximide is preferred to other succinimides because it is more effective and less likely to produce drowsiness and gastrointestinal upset. In patients with absence seizures resistant to ethosuximide or valproate monotherapy, concomitant use frequently is successful.

Ethosuximide also may be effective in myoclonic seizures and akinetic epilepsy but is ineffective in complex partial or generalized tonic-clonic seizures. Patients with a combination of absence and tonic-clonic seizures must receive combination therapy (eg, carbamazepine, phenytoin) if ethosuximide is used. Valproate monotherapy is preferred in these patients, however.

ADVERSE REACTIONS AND PRECAUTIONS. The most common adverse reactions are gastrointestinal disturbances (eg, nausea, vomiting, anorexia). Drowsiness, ataxia, headache, dizziness, euphoria, hiccup, rash, urticaria, and behavioral changes have been observed occasionally. Psychotic reactions with hallucinations may occur at high plasma concentrations, but they seldom develop in young children with typical absence seizures who have no previous history of psychiatric disturbances. Systemic lupus erythematosus, Stevens-Johnson syndrome, aplastic anemia, thrombocytopenia, leukopenia, pancytopenia, and eosinophilia have been reported rarely. (See also the Introduction.)

Psychometric studies on the effect of ethosuximide in children of normal intelligence who had absence seizures and minimal or no evidence of nervous system abnormalities have shown that reduction in the number of seizures by the drug had a positive effect on test results in approximately 50% (Browne and Feldman, 1983).

DRUG INTERACTIONS. Ethosuximide does not consistently alter the plasma concentration of other antiepileptic drugs. Carbamazepine, phenytoin, phenobarbital, and primidone may decrease the plasma concentration of ethosuximide. Isoniazid may inhibit metabolism, thus increasing plasma concentrations of ethosuximide.

PHARMACOKINETICS. Ethosuximide is well absorbed orally, and the peak plasma concentration occurs in one to four hours. It is minimally bound to plasma protein and eliminated primarily via hepatic metabolism with 10% to 20% of the administered dose excreted unchanged in the urine. The half-life is variable but averages 52 to 56 hours in adults and 32 to 41 hours in children. Breast milk concentrations are slightly less than corresponding plasma concentrations, but problems related to breast-feeding in humans have not been documented. Control of absence seizures usually is achieved with plasma concentrations of 40 to 100 mcg/ml, but concentrations up to 160 mcg/ml may be required and are tolerated in some patients. For other pharmacokinetic data, see Table 6.

DOSAGE AND PREPARATIONS.

Oral: *Adults and children over 6 years,* initially, 500 mg daily, increased, if necessary, by 250 mg every four to seven days until seizures are controlled or untoward effects develop. The daily maintenance dose is usually 15 to 40 mg/kg. Doses exceeding 1.5 g daily are seldom more effective than smaller amounts. *Children 3 to 6 years,* initially, 250 mg daily with incremental increases in dosage as for older patients. The daily maintenance dose is usually 15 to 40 mg/kg (usual maximum, 1 g daily).

Zarontin (Parke-Davis). Capsules 250 mg; syrup 250 mg/5 ml.

FELBAMATE
[Felbatol]

CH_2OCNH_2 (O)
CH
CH_2OCNH_2 (O)

In early August 1994, the FDA and the manufacturer, Wallace Laboratories, recommended suspending the use of felbamate following two deaths among ten reported cases of aplastic anemia. As of August 18, 1994, there were 21 reported cases (three fatalities) of aplastic anemia associated with the administration of felbamate, representing a crude incidence rate of approximately 1/5,000 (based on estimates of prescriptions written). The true risk may be closer to $\geq$1/2,000 among patients remaining on the drug for more than a few weeks.

The time to onset of the aplastic anemia after initiation of felbamate therapy ranged from 5 to 30 weeks (mean, 128 days) among those for whom that information is available. The effects of the dose, duration of exposure, age, gender, and concomitant antiepileptic drugs on the risk of developing aplastic anemia cannot be assessed at this time.

Recently, ten cases of acute liver failure, including four deaths, have been reported in association with use of felbamate; one of the four survivors received a liver transplant. Patients were of both sexes and ranged in age from 5 to 78 years. Most of those affected also were taking other drugs, including other antiepileptic and nonprescription drugs. In several instances, there were nonspecific premonitory signs but, in others, the patients were already in frank liver failure at the time their illness was detected. The time between initiation of treatment with felbamate and diagnosis of liver failure ranged from 14 to 257 days.

After reviewing the data, the FDA recommended that felbamate remain available as second-line therapy for patients who do not respond adequately to alternative therapy and whose epilepsy is so severe that a substantial risk of aplastic anemia is deemed acceptable in light of the benefits conferred by use of felbamate. The information on potentially fatal liver injury gives further reason to limit the use of felbamate to those with the most severe, refractory seizures.

ACTIONS AND USES. The mechanism of action by which felbamate reduces seizure activity is not established; however, this drug has been reported to interact with the glycine modulatory site on N-methyl-D-aspartate (NMDA) receptors (McCabe et al, 1993) and to inhibit NMDA responses in vitro (Rho et al, 1993). Blockade of NMDA responses may contribute to the neuroprotective effects of felbamate (Wallis et al, 1992; Wasterlain et al, 1993).

Felbamate is used as monotherapy or adjunctive therapy in the treatment of partial seizures with or without secondary generalization in adults and as adjunctive therapy in the treatment of partial and generalized seizures associated with Lennox-Gastaut syndrome in children. Studies directly comparing felbamate with other antiepileptic drugs have not been conducted. In one trial on patients undergoing surgical evaluation for intractable partial seizures, the dosage of standard antiepileptic drugs was reduced prior to treatment with felbamate 3.6 g or placebo (Bourgeois et al, 1993). Forty-six percent of felbamate recipients (13 of 28) experienced a fourth seizure within 28 days (primary end point) compared with 88% of placebo recipients. Of the remaining 15 felbamate recipients who completed four weeks of treatment, all experienced at least a 50% reduction in seizure frequency and four were seizure-free. In a double-blind, placebo-controlled crossover trial on patients with refractory partial seizures, adjunctive administration of felbamate (average dose, 2.3 g) with phenytoin and carbamazepine reduced seizure frequency 19% compared with a 4% increase in seizure frequency in placebo recipients (Leppik et al, 1991). Overall, seizures were reduced by 63% in patients receiving polytherapy.

The efficacy of felbamate monotherapy (3.6 g) in patients with refractory partial seizures (with or without secondary generalization) was assessed in two trials that employed low-dose valproate (15 mg/kg/day) as the control (Sachdeo et al, 1992; Faught et al, 1993). During the treatment phase, other standard antiepileptic drugs were discontinued over a one-month period. Study end points were completion of 112 study days or fulfillment of "escape criteria," which included (1) doubling of the monthly or highest two-day seizure frequency and (2) appearance or significant prolongation of generalized tonic-clonic seizures. In these studies, 60% to 82% of the felbamate recipients completed the treatment phase compared with only 9% to 22% of the valproate recipients.

Results of a placebo-controlled trial on patients with Lennox-Gastaut syndrome indicate that adjunctive administration of felbamate significantly reduces the frequency of seizures, including atonic and generalized tonic-clonic seizures (The Felbamate Study Group in Lennox-Gastaut Syndrome, 1993). In addition, in global evaluations completed by parents or guardians that considered alertness, verbal responsiveness, and general well-being, felbamate recipients were rated more favorably than placebo recipients. Children with intractable partial seizures also may respond to adjunctive therapy with felbamate (Carmant et al, 1993).

ADVERSE REACTIONS AND PRECAUTIONS. See comments at beginning of this evaluation. Because of the uncertain risk of acute liver failure, once treatment with felbamate is initiated, ALT, AST, and bilirubin should be monitored weekly. Whether prompt discontinuation of felbamate at the first sign of liver injury can reduce the risk of subsequent fulminant liver failure has not been established; nevertheless, treatment should be discontinued immediately if laboratory findings indicate liver injury. Use of felbamate should be avoided in any patients with pre-existing liver impairment.

In general, felbamate was well tolerated in clinical trials; 6% of children and 12% of adults discontinued therapy because of adverse effects. In adults, the most common adverse reactions during felbamate monotherapy were anorexia, nausea, vomiting, insomnia, and headache. The incidence of these reactions, as well as somnolence and dizziness, was considerably greater when felbamate was administered as adjunctive therapy; this probably reflects drug interactions between felbamate and other antiepileptic drugs. The spectrum of adverse reactions appears to be similar in children.

Weight loss may occur in both adults and children, and some children who receive felbamate do not achieve predicted weight in the short-term (Parks et al, 1993). Whether weight loss is caused by associated nausea or is attributable to a central anorexiant effect is not known. Further study on the mechanism of weight loss and its clinical importance, particularly in children, is warranted.

Felbamate does not affect cardiovascular parameters. No serious adverse reactions have been reported after overdose.

PREGNANCY. Although placental transfer of felbamate occurs in rats, the incidence of malformations was not increased compared with controls in teratogenicity experiments in animals. There are no studies on use of felbamate in pregnant women, and the effect of this drug on labor and delivery in humans is unknown (FDA Pregnancy Category C). Felbamate has been detected in human milk; however, the effect on the nursing infant also is unknown.

DRUG INTERACTIONS. Felbamate causes a dose-related increase in steady-state plasma concentrations of phenytoin and valproate. It decreases the steady-state concentration of carbamazepine but increases the steady-state plasma concentration of carbamazepine epoxide. A 20% to 33% reduction in the dose of phenytoin, valproate, and carbamazepine is recommended when treatment with felbamate is initiated. Both phenytoin and carbamazepine increase the clearance of felbamate; steady-state trough concentrations of felbamate may decline 40% to 45% (Wagner et al, 1990).

PHARMACOKINETICS. Felbamate is well absorbed after oral administration, and peak plasma concentrations are achieved within two to six hours. Neither food nor antacids affect absorption. Protein binding (22% to 25%) is independent over a wide range of plasma concentrations (10 to 310 mcg/ml). Average trough plasma concentrations were 83 mcg/ml after multiple daily doses of 3.6 g in adults. Corresponding values were lower in children; peak concentrations of 49 mcg/ml occurred after daily doses of 45 mg/kg. Peak and trough plasma concentrations are proportional to dose.

Forty to fifty percent of the absorbed dose is excreted unchanged in the urine; the remainder is converted to parahydroxyfelbamate, 2-hydroxyfelbamate, felbamate monocarbamate, and other unidentified metabolites. Metabolites do not contribute significantly to the antiepileptic action of this drug. The terminal half-life is 20 to 23 hours in adults. See also Table 6.

DOSAGE AND PREPARATIONS. When felbamate is added to a regimen that includes carbamazepine, phenytoin, or valproate, the dosage of these drugs should be reduced 20% to 33% to minimize the occurrence of adverse reactions caused by drug interactions.

Oral: *Adults, monotherapy*, initially, 1.2 g in divided doses three or four times daily. The dosage may be increased in 600-mg increments every two weeks to 2.4 g/day based on clinical response and thereafter to 3.6 g/day if necessary.

Adults, adjunctive therapy, initially, 1.2 g in divided doses three or four times daily with reduction of the dosage of other antiepileptic drugs by 20% to 33%; further reductions in the dosage of other antiepileptic drugs may be required in some patients. The dosage of felbamate may be increased in increments of 1.2 g at weekly intervals to a maximum of 3.6 g daily.

Adults, conversion to monotherapy, initially, 1.2 g/day in divided doses three or four times daily with reduction of the dosage of other antiepileptic drugs by 33%. After one week, the dosage of felbamate may be increased to 2.4 g daily and the dosage of other antiepileptic drugs reduced by 33%. At week 3, the felbamate dosage may be increased to 3.6 g/day and other antiepileptic drugs discontinued or dosage further reduced in stepwise fashion as clinically indicated.

Children 2 to 14 years with Lennox-Gastaut syndrome, as adjunctive therapy, initially, 15 mg/kg/day in divided doses three or four times daily; the dosage of other antiepileptic drugs is reduced by 20%. The amount of felbamate may be increased in increments of 15 mg/kg/day at weekly intervals to 45 mg/kg/day. Further reduction in the dosage of other antiepileptic drugs may be necessary to minimize adverse reactions caused by drug interactions.

Felbatol (Wallace). Tablets 400 and 600 mg; suspension 600 mg/5 ml.

GABAPENTIN

[Neurontin]

CH_2NH_2 / CH_2COOH (cyclohexane ring)

ACTIONS AND USES. Gabapentin is an analogue of gamma-aminobutyric acid (GABA). The mechanism of its antiepileptic action is unknown. Gabapentin increases GABA turnover but does not bind to GABA or other established neurotransmitter receptors, GABA neuronal uptake sites, or ligand-gated ion channels. High-affinity binding sites have been described on synaptic membranes, but their function is unknown (Taylor et al, 1993); they may correspond to a peptide component of the membrane transport system for L-amino acids. In animal models of epilepsy, gabapentin potentiates the action of phenytoin, carbamazepine, and valproate.

Gabapentin is used as adjunctive therapy in patients with partial seizures with or without secondary generalization. A dose-related antiepileptic effect was observed during a double-blind, crossover study that compared daily gabapentin doses of 300, 600, and 900 mg given for two months each plus one or more other antiepileptic drugs in 25 patients with severe partial or generalized epilepsy (Crawford et al, 1987); the frequency of partial seizures was reduced by 45% in those who received gabapentin 900 mg daily.

Subsequently, data from four large controlled trials on patients with partial seizures refractory to other antiepileptic drugs indicated that seizure frequency decreased when this drug was given in doses ranging from 600 mg to 1.8 g/day

(UK Gabapentin Study Group, 1990; Bruni et al, 1991; Browne, 1993; The US Gabapentin Study Group No. 5, 1993). In approximately 18% to 26% of patients treated with 900 mg to 1.8 g, the number of partial seizures decreased by at least 50%. The magnitude of this effect is comparable to that reported with other antiepileptic drugs given adjunctively in patients with refractory partial seizures. In one study, daily doses of 600 mg and 1.2 g were comparable, but, in general, the antiepileptic effects of larger doses appear to be more pronounced. Compared with placebo, gabapentin was more effective in patients with refractory complex partial seizures and secondarily generalized partial seizures. Results of open studies suggest that the efficacy of gabapentin is maintained over periods of 12 to 24 months (Browne, 1993; Ojemann et al, 1992).

Its low apparent toxicity and lack of interactions with other antiepileptic drugs (see below) make gabapentin an attractive candidate for adjunctive use in patients with refractory partial seizures. Gabapentin has not been directly compared with other antiepileptic drugs as monotherapy in newly diagnosed patients with partial seizures. It is ineffective in the treatment of absence seizures.

ADVERSE REACTIONS AND PRECAUTIONS. In premarketing clinical trials, dosages up to 2.4 g/day were generally well tolerated; approximately 7% of individuals discontinued treatment because of an adverse event. Adjunctive therapy with gabapentin may increase the frequency of adverse events that often occur with other antiepileptic drugs, particularly symptoms affecting the central nervous system (eg, somnolence, dizziness, ataxia, fatigue, diplopia, blurred vision, amnesia, nystagmus, tremor); in many patients, these symptoms resolve after a few weeks. The other most commonly reported adverse events were weight increase, dysarthria, dry mouth, dyspepsia, constipation, and depression. Use of gabapentin does not appear to be associated with significant hematologic, hepatic, pancreatic, renal, or hypersensitivity reactions.

This drug is classified in FDA Pregnancy Category C.

DRUG INTERACTIONS. No clinically significant drug interactions have been observed with phenytoin, valproate, carbamazepine, or phenobarbital. Aluminum-containing antacids decrease absorption by 20% and cimetidine decreases renal clearance by 12%, but these interactions are probably not clinically significant.

PHARMACOKINETICS. Gabapentin is rapidly absorbed after oral administration; absorption is generally unaffected by food, and maximum plasma concentrations are achieved within three hours. Oral bioavailability appears to be dose-dependent and ranges from approximately 73% (single 100-mg dose) to 35% (single 1.6-g dose); this is consistent with saturable carrier-mediated absorption (Stewart et al, 1993). However, after administration of therapeutic doses (ie, 900 mg to 1.8 g daily in three divided doses), plasma concentrations are approximately proportional to dose. Bioavailability over this dose range is approximately 60%. Gabapentin does not bind significantly to plasma proteins and is not appreciably metabolized in humans. At steady state, concentrations of gabapentin in the cerebrospinal fluid are approximately 20% of those in the plasma. Systemic and renal clearance are linearly correlated with creatinine clearance and thus are decreased in the elderly and in patients with impaired renal function. The elimination half-life is five to seven hours.

DOSAGE AND PREPARATIONS. Because gabapentin is eliminated primarily by renal excretion, the dose should be adjusted for patients with compromised renal function.

Patients over 12 years of age, 900 mg to 1.8 g/day administered as adjunctive therapy in three divided doses. Titration to an effective dose normally can be achieved within three days by initiating therapy with 300 mg and then increasing the dose in 300-mg increments on the next two days to establish a dosage of 900 mg/day administered in three divided doses. If necessary, the dosage may be increased to 1.8 g/day. Dosages of 2.4 to 3.6 g/day also have been well tolerated.

Patients with compromised renal function or undergoing hemodialysis, the following adjustment in dosage is recommended:

Renal Function Creatinine Clearance (ml/min)	Total Daily Dose (mg/day)	Dose Regimen (mg)
>60	1200	400 three times daily
30-60	600	300 twice daily
15-30	300	300 once daily
<15	150	300 once every other day
Hemodialysis	—	200-300[1]

[1] *Loading dose of 300 to 400 mg in patients who have never received gabapentin, then gabapentin 200 to 300 mg following each four hours of hemodialysis.*

Neurontin (Parke-Davis). Capsules 100, 300, and 400 mg.

LAMOTRIGINE (Investigational drug)
[Lamictal]

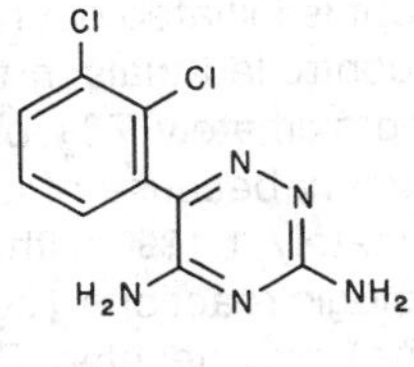

ACTIONS AND USES. Lamotrigine is a phenyltriazine compound that was originally synthesized as a folic acid antagonist. In animal models, its anticonvulsant profile is similar to that of phenytoin. The antiepileptic effect of lamotrigine may be due to inhibition of voltage-dependent sodium currents and reduction of sustained repetitive neuronal activity. Inhibition of glutamate release also has been reported.

Lamotrigine is indicated in the treatment of patients with partial seizures and secondarily generalized tonic-clonic seizures that are not satisfactorily controlled with other antiepileptic drugs. In several small (<50 patients) 8- to 12-week, placebo-controlled crossover studies conducted in the United Kingdom and one larger 14-week trial conducted in the United States, lamotrigine 150 to 400 mg decreased seizure frequency by 17% to 59% in adults with refractory partial seizures.

Approximately 25% of patients experienced at least a 50% reduction in seizure frequency (Risner, 1990; Brodie, 1992; Schapel et al, 1993; Messenheimer et al, 1994).

A large six-month parallel-design study evaluated the efficacy of lamotrigine 300 and 500 mg as adjunctive therapy in 216 patients with refractory partial seizures; the frequency of seizures decreased by a median of 36% in the group that received the larger dose and by a median of 8% in patients who received placebo (Matsuo et al, 1993).

In open-label extension studies, 50 adults with partial seizures were successfully converted to lamotrigine monotherapy (300 to 700 mg/day); 15 of these patients remained seizure-free during treatment periods lasting up to four years (Pellock et al, 1993). Lamotrigine monotherapy has been compared with carbamazepine in an open study and with phenytoin in a parallel group, double-blind trial in adults with newly diagnosed epilepsy or recurrent seizures; however, results have not yet been published.

Experience in children is limited; results from open studies indicate that lamotrigine may be beneficial in the treatment of absence and generalized tonic-clonic seizures and Lennox-Gastaut syndrome (Schlumberger et al, 1994). Data from controlled trials are required to assess the benefit of lamotrigine in childhood epilepsy and its potential usefulness as monotherapy.

ADVERSE REACTIONS AND PRECAUTIONS. Lamotrigine is a weak inhibitor of dihydrofolate reductase in vitro; however, it does not affect serum folate concentrations or hematologic parameters in humans.

The most common adverse reactions (reported in at least 10% of patients also receiving other antiepileptic drugs) were nausea, headache, diplopia, blurred vision, dizziness, ataxia, somnolence, and rash. Dizziness, diplopia, ataxia, and blurred vision appear to be dose related and may occur more frequently in patients receiving lamotrigine and carbamazepine. Skin rashes may develop in some patients within four to six weeks after treatment is initiated but resolve on discontinuation of the drug. In controlled trials in the United Kingdom and United States, approximately 7% of lamotrigine recipients discontinued treatment because of adverse events; rash accounted for approximately 1.1% of the drug withdrawals. Rarely, severe dermatologic reactions (eg, angioedema, Stevens-Johnson syndrome) may develop. Patients who acutely develop any combination of rash, fever, influenza-like symptoms, drowsiness, or worsening of seizure control should be closely monitored.

No clinically significant changes in ophthalmologic, neurologic, or electrocardiographic parameters have been associated with use of lamotrigine.

DRUG INTERACTIONS. Lamotrigine does not cause clinically significant induction or inhibition of hepatic cytochrome P450. Inhibition of carbamazepine metabolism with accumulation of carbamazepine 10,11-epoxide has been reported in a few patients, but data on this possible interaction are conflicting.

Antiepileptic drugs that induce cytochrome P450 (eg, carbamazepine, phenytoin, phenobarbital, primidone) enhance the metabolism of lamotrigine and decrease its half-life by approximately 50% (mean, 12.6 hours). Although valproate inhibits the hepatic metabolism of lamotrigine and approximately doubles its half-life (mean, 58.8 hours), the half-life of lamotrigine may be relatively unaffected in patients also taking valproate plus an enzyme-inducing drug. Acetaminophen increases lamotrigine clearance by 15%, but this probably is not clinically significant. Lamotrigine does not affect the efficacy of oral contraceptives.

PHARMACOKINETICS. After oral administration to normal volunteers, lamotrigine is well absorbed with a bioavailability of 98%. Pharmacokinetics appear to be linear in a daily dosage range of 100 to 700 mg. A therapeutic range in plasma concentration has not been established for lamotrigine. Peak plasma concentrations are achieved one to four hours after administration. Food slightly delays the rate but not the extent of absorption. The apparent volume of distribution is 0.9 to 1.4 L/kg; plasma protein binding is approximately 55% and is independent of plasma concentration up to 10 mcg/ml.

Lamotrigine is extensively metabolized; less than 10% of a dose is excreted unchanged. Elimination is primarily by hepatic metabolism to glucuronide conjugates. In healthy volunteers, the elimination half-life of lamotrigine after single doses is approximately 33 hours; clearance increased and the half-life decreased by 25% following administration of multiple doses, suggesting that autoinduction occurs. There was no evidence from clinical trials that lamotrigine induces its own metabolism.

Results from open studies indicate that pediatric patients, especially those 2 to <6 years, in general eliminate lamotrigine more rapidly than adults. The half-life of lamotrigine is 7 to 7.7 hours in children receiving other enzyme-inducing drugs, 45 to 66 hours in children receiving valproate, and approximately 19 hours in children receiving enzyme-inducing drugs plus valproate.

DOSAGE AND PREPARATIONS.

Oral: *Adults,* initially, 50 mg twice daily for the first two weeks followed by maintenance doses of 200 to 400 mg daily in two divided doses. In patients also taking valproate, the initial dose of lamotrigine is 50 mg every other day for the first two weeks, 50 mg daily for the next two weeks, followed by maintenance doses of 100 to 200 mg daily in two divided doses.

Children, precise dosage has not been established. Dosage has ranged from 1.3 to 10 mg/kg/day depending on concomitant therapy (ie, enzyme-inducing drugs, valproate).

Lamictal (Burroughs Wellcome). Tablets 100, 150, and 200 mg.

LORAZEPAM

[Ativan]

For chemical formula, see index entry Lorazepam, In Anxiety.

USES. Lorazepam is an effective agent for the initial treatment of status epilepticus and is regarded as a drug of choice for initial control of continuous generalized tonic-clonic or partial seizures. Lorazepam and diazepam are equally effective for the initial control of seizures in status epilepticus, but the duration of action of lorazepam is considerably longer (Leppik et al, 1983; Treiman, 1990).

ADVERSE REACTIONS AND PRECAUTIONS. When lorazepam is administered intravenously for status epilepticus, the patient must be observed for signs of cardiorespiratory depression, especially when this drug is given with other antiepileptic agents. Results of a controlled study and a retrospective analysis suggest that lorazepam and diazepam are similar in their tendency to cause respiratory depression (Leppik et al, 1983; Giang and McBride, 1988). The respiratory depression may be severe enough to require ventilatory support, particularly in children under 2 years who also received phenobarbital and in the elderly (Giang and McBride, 1988).

For further information on adverse reactions, precautions, drug interactions, and other uses, see index entry Lorazepam, In Anxiety.

PHARMACOKINETICS. Seizure control after intravenous administration is usually achieved within three to five minutes; however, as long as ten minutes may be required in children, particularly if a lower dose (eg, 0.05 mg/kg) is used. Plasma concentrations above 30 ng/ml are required (range, 30 to 100 ng/ml). In adults, intravenous administration of 5 mg will maintain plasma concentrations above 30 ng/ml for approximately 18 hours.

For complete pharmacokinetic data, see index entry Lorazepam, In Anxiety.

DOSAGE AND PREPARATIONS.

Intravenous: For status epilepticus, see Table 5.

Ativan Injection (Wyeth-Ayerst). Solution 2 mg/ml in 0.5, 1, and 10 ml containers and 4 mg/ml in 1 and 10 ml containers.

MEPHOBARBITAL

[Mebaral]

CH_3, O, N, O, CH_3CH_2, N, H, O

Mephobarbital is metabolized to phenobarbital and thus has similar properties and uses, but larger doses must be given. There is no evidence that it has any advantage over phenobarbital. (See the Introduction and the evaluation on Phenobarbital.)

This drug is classified in FDA Pregnancy Category D.

DOSAGE AND PREPARATIONS. The plasma concentrations given for phenobarbital (see that evaluation) may be used as a guide to adjust the dosage of mephobarbital.

Oral: *Adults,* 400 to 600 mg daily in divided doses. *Children under 5 years,* 16 to 32 mg three or four times daily; *over 5 years,* 32 to 64 mg three or four times daily.

Mebaral (Sanofi Winthrop). Tablets 32, 50, and 100 mg.

PARALDEHYDE

[Paral]

H_3C, CH_3, O, O, O, CH_3

This drug is used rectally in status epilepticus when other agents are not effective. (Parenteral dosage forms have been discontinued.) Rectal administration is employed most commonly in children; however, the dose is difficult to control by this route and absorption is very slow.

Fatalities have occurred with use of paraldehyde. Bronchopulmonary disease is a relative contraindication, since a significant amount is excreted by the lungs. The sedative effect may be intensified and prolonged in patients with liver disease.

Paraldehyde is classified in FDA Pregnancy Category C.

DOSAGE AND PREPARATIONS. Outdated drug may be toxic. Plastic devices must be avoided; only glass syringes and containers and rubber tubing are advised.

Rectal: *Children,* 0.3 ml/kg dissolved in one or two parts of olive oil or cottonseed oil and administered every four to six hours.

Paral (Forest), ***Generic.*** Liquid 1 g/ml in 30 ml containers.

PHENOBARBITAL

[Solfoton]

H, O, N, O, CH_3CH_2, N, H, O

PHENOBARBITAL SODIUM

[Luminal Sodium]

USES. Phenobarbital, a long-acting barbiturate, is effective in generalized tonic-clonic and simple partial seizures. Higher plasma concentrations may be required to control the latter. Complex partial seizures do not respond as well, and absence seizures are not relieved and may be exacerbated. Phenobarbital frequently is used in the treatment of neonatal seizures and may be the initial drug employed in young children. However, because of increasing concern about adverse neuropsychological reactions to sedative/hypnotic antiepileptic drugs, many neurologists prefer less sedating drugs, such as carbamazepine, phenytoin, or valproate (Porter and Theodore, 1983). The prophylactic use of phenobarbital in infants with febrile seizures has been challenged (Farwell et al, 1990).

Phenobarbital also is useful in seizures caused by barbiturate withdrawal in dependent individuals. The sodium salt is administered parenterally as part of the treatment regimen for status epilepticus (see Table 5).

ADVERSE REACTIONS AND PRECAUTIONS. With the exception of significant behavioral and more subtle cognitive effects (Vining et al, 1987), phenobarbital may cause the least systemic toxicity of all antiepileptic drugs. Neurotoxicity is its major adverse effect. Drowsiness is the most common adverse reaction and, although tolerance usually develops, a significant percentage of patients continue to be bothered by sedation. Memory, perceptual motor performance, and tasks requiring sustained performance may be affected. In pediatric patients at risk for recurrent febrile seizures, prophylaxis with phenobarbital resulted in minor cognitive impairment as revealed by lower scores on intelligence testing. This impairment outlasted the period of drug administration by several months (Farwell et al, 1990). However, in some studies, cognitive impairments in school-age children were not detected (Mitchell and Chavez, 1987; Trimble, 1987). There is more general agreement that phenobarbital markedly influences behavior. Irritability may be provoked, and existing behavioral problems, particularly hyperkinesia, may be exacerbated (Herranz et al, 1988; Trimble and Cull, 1988).

A substantial number of adults develop depression. An occasional patient may become excitable; children and the elderly are most susceptible. Ataxia sometimes occurs; if it persists, a reduction in dosage is required.

Barbiturates are contraindicated in patients with acute intermittent porphyria. Abrupt termination of therapy may exacerbate seizures, but drug dependence is unlikely with usual antiepileptic doses. (See the Introduction.)

Skin eruptions are uncommon but rarely progress to exfoliative dermatitis. Megaloblastic anemia also is uncommon.

When phenobarbital is given during pregnancy, the possibility of congenital malformations or a coagulation defect and hemorrhage in the newborn must be considered (FDA Pregnancy Category D). Nursing infants whose mothers are receiving phenobarbital should be monitored for excessive sedation, since phenobarbital concentrations in milk may be significant (Nau et al, 1982).

DRUG INTERACTIONS. Although phenobarbital induces hepatic enzymes, it also may competitively inhibit drug biotransformation. Thus, mutual enzyme induction or inhibition in patients treated with phenobarbital and phenytoin may result in an increase, decrease, or no change in the plasma concentration of one or both drugs. Plasma concentrations tend to be somewhat higher during monotherapy, however. Similarly, with concomitant administration of carbamazepine, plasma concentrations of both drugs are only moderately affected but tend to be reduced. Valproate inhibits phenobarbital metabolism, thus increasing plasma concentrations.

Because phenobarbital induces hepatic enzymes, it also may enhance the hepatic clearance and diminish the clinical effectiveness of oral anticoagulants, oral contraceptives, anti-infectives (chloramphenicol, doxycycline, griseofulvin), lipophilic beta blockers (eg, propranolol, metoprolol), corticosteroids, cyclosporine, tricyclic antidepressants (eg, desipramine, nortriptyline), haloperidol, phenothiazines, quinidine, and theophylline. The effectiveness of digitoxin, doxorubicin, guanfacine, and verapamil may be similarly modified.

Chloramphenicol and propoxyphene increase phenobarbital plasma concentrations. Combination of phenobarbital with other drugs that depress the central nervous system may increase sedative or neurotoxic side effects.

See also Table 7.

PHARMACOKINETICS. Phenobarbital is almost completely absorbed orally, but one to six hours may be necessary to achieve peak plasma concentrations. The drug also is well absorbed after intramuscular injection. Protein binding is about 45%; in adults, the Vd is 0.5 to 1 L/kg. In neonates, protein binding is lower and the Vd is higher. Phenobarbital is eliminated by hepatic metabolism and renal filtration. Because the pKa (7.3) of phenobarbital is close to body pH, the rate of renal excretion is increased significantly in alkaline urine. Interestingly, there are little data to support autoinduction of phenobarbital metabolism in humans. The average plasma half-life is three days in children and four days in adults; consequently, three or more weeks may be required to attain steady-state plasma concentrations. The half-life is somewhat longer in neonates. Doubling the dose for the first four days of therapy provides effective plasma concentrations more promptly, but sedation is prominent.

Plasma concentrations of 15 to 40 mcg/ml are usually optimal for the control of epilepsy; concentrations greater than 40 mcg/ml are often accompanied by symptoms of toxicity, but higher concentrations, which may be necessary for control of partial seizures, are tolerated by some patients. For other pharmacokinetic data, see Table 6.

DOSAGE AND PREPARATIONS.

PHENOBARBITAL:

Oral: *Adults,* 120 to 250 mg; alternatively, 2 to 3 mg/kg daily. *Children,* 30 to 100 mg daily; alternatively, 3 to 5 mg/kg daily. These amounts are taken at bedtime. Administration more than once a day is unnecessary.

Recurrent febrile seizures have been treated with an oral loading dose of 6 to 8 mg/kg, followed by a maintenance dose of 3 to 4 mg/kg to maintain plasma concentrations of 15 to 30 mcg/ml (Painter, 1989).

Generic. Elixir 15 and 20 mg/5 ml; tablets 8, 15, 30, 60, and 100 mg.

Solfoton (ECR). Capsules and tablets 16 mg.

PHENOBARBITAL SODIUM:

Intramuscular, Intravenous (slow): For status epilepticus, see Table 5.

Neonates, for treatment of neonatal seizures, a loading dose of 15 to 20 mg/kg intravenously, followed by a maintenance dose of 3 to 4 mg/kg to maintain a plasma concentration of 20 to 40 mcg/ml.

Generic. Powder in 120 mg containers; solution 30, 60, 65, and 130 mg/ml in 1 ml containers.

Luminal Sodium (Sanofi Winthrop). Solution 130 mg/ml in 1 ml containers.

PHENYTOIN
[Dilantin]

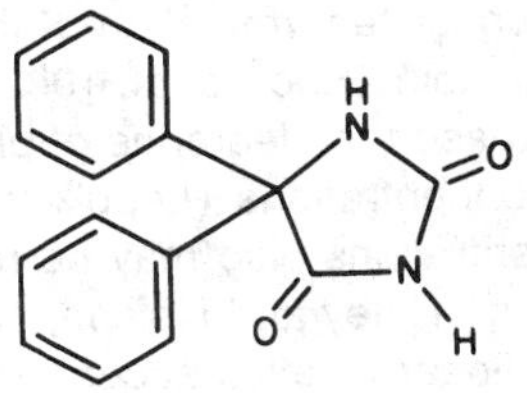

PHENYTOIN SODIUM
[Dilantin Sodium]

USES. Phenytoin is useful in generalized tonic-clonic, complex partial, and simple partial seizures and frequently is chosen for initial therapy, particularly in adults. Because of phenytoin's potential adverse reactions (hirsutism, gingival hyperplasia, coarsening of facial features), other antiepileptic drugs are often prescribed for infants and young children. Phenytoin is commonly given with phenobarbital, primidone, carbamazepine, or valproate when monotherapy fails. It is ineffective in absence, myoclonic, and atonic seizures and is not recommended for the treatment of infantile spasms, Lennox-Gastaut syndrome, and epileptic syndromes in older children and adolescents when absence seizures or myoclonus is present (Wilder and Rangel, 1989).

Intravenous phenytoin sodium is effective for status epilepticus (see Table 5) and can be used as the initial drug to manage recurrent seizures if they are widely spaced.

This drug also may prevent seizures initially in high-risk patients with head trauma (see the Introduction).

Phenytoin has been advocated for many other disorders, but conclusive evidence of effectiveness is inadequate for most proposed indications. For other uses, see index entry Phenytoin.

ADVERSE REACTIONS AND PRECAUTIONS. In usual amounts, phenytoin produces little or no sedation. Anorexia, dyspepsia, and nausea occur occasionally. As plasma concentrations increase progressively above 20 mcg/ml, nystagmus, ataxia, and lethargy may occur. Many patients tolerate plasma concentrations between 20 and 30 mcg/ml if the increase into this range has been gradual.

Ataxia is a common effect of all hydantoins and requires dosage reduction. Although the evidence is conflicting, these drugs probably cause permanent cerebellar damage if toxic concentrations are maintained for prolonged periods. In very young patients, drug-induced ataxia may be confused with the natural unsteadiness of the toddler.

Ocular signs and symptoms, such as nystagmus and diplopia, may necessitate reduction of dosage. Peripheral neuropathy may develop after years of use. Skin eruptions occur in 8% of patients but are only rarely serious and are unrelated to the initial dosage or the plasma concentration (Leppik et al, 1985). Extravasation during intravenous administration may cause tissue necrosis.

Gingival hyperplasia is common and sometimes severe. Scrupulous oral hygiene may prevent secondary inflammation and possibly reduce the severity of this complication. Repeated gingivectomies may be required if use of the drug is continued. (In children, gingival hyperplasia seldom occurs with mephenytoin and has not been reported with ethotoin.) Hypertrichosis and hirsutism are less common but do occur.

Rare but serious idiosyncratic reactions include hepatitis, bone marrow depression, systemic lupus erythematosus, Stevens-Johnson syndrome, and lymphadenopathy resembling malignant lymphomas. Usually lymphadenopathy begins to disappear one to two weeks after therapy is discontinued. A few cases of true lymphoma and Hodgkin's disease have been reported.

Folic acid depletion may occur and sometimes causes megaloblastic anemia. Interference with vitamin D metabolism may cause hypocalcemia and osteomalacia, but this usually occurs in institutionalized patients who do not receive adequate sunshine.

When phenytoin is given during pregnancy, the possibility of congenital malformations and coagulation defect with hemorrhage in the newborn infant must be considered. This drug is classified in FDA Pregnancy Category C. Low concentrations of phenytoin appear in breast milk. See also the section on Adverse Reactions in the Introduction.

DRUG INTERACTIONS. Phenytoin may reduce the plasma concentration of carbamazepine, valproate, ethosuximide, felbamate, lamotrigine, and primidone by enzyme induction. When combined use of phenytoin and carbamazepine is necessary, plasma concentrations of both drugs should be monitored to ensure that adequate concentrations of each agent are maintained. Phenytoin and phenobarbital exert variable, reciprocal effects. The interaction of valproate with phenytoin is complex. Valproate displaces phenytoin from protein binding sites but inhibits metabolism. Plasma concentrations may be increased or decreased (see Table 7 and the evaluation on Valproate). Other drugs that may displace phenytoin include phenylbutazone, salicylates, and tolbutamide. The total plasma concentration of phenytoin may decrease, but the total free concentration may be relatively unchanged as a result of the increase in free fraction. Phenytoin may displace warfarin from protein binding sites causing acute toxicity (Panegyres and Rischbieth, 1991).

Drugs that significantly increase the plasma concentration of phenytoin include chloramphenicol, cimetidine, dicumarol, disulfiram, fluconazole, isoniazid, sulfonamides, and trimethoprim. Amiodarone, allopurinol, chlorpheniramine, and trazodone may possibly increase the plasma phenytoin concentration. Folic acid, prolonged ingestion of alcohol, and rifampin may decrease the phenytoin plasma concentration. In patients with tuberculosis, the effects of rifampin and isoniazid may cancel one another when these drugs are used with phenytoin. Certain antineoplastic agents (bleomycin, cisplatin, vinblastine, carboplatin) also may reduce plasma concentrations of phenytoin.

Phenytoin is a relatively potent enzyme inducer and may decrease the effectiveness of oral anticoagulants, certain antibiotics (doxycycline, rifampin, chloramphenicol), praziquantel, oral contraceptives, antiarrhythmic agents (disopyramide, mexiletine, quinidine), verapamil, digitoxin, analgesics (meperidine, methadone), cyclosporine, corticosteroids, and theophylline. Pharmacodynamically, phenytoin has been reported to impair blood pressure control by dopamine and to decrease the response to nondepolarizing skeletal muscle relaxants.

See also Table 7.

PHARMACOKINETICS. Oral absorption is variable but averages 85% to 90%. Time to peak plasma concentration is variable and increases with the dose but normally occurs within 1.5 to 3 hours for prompt-release capsules and somewhat later (4 to 12 hours) for the extended-release preparations. Plasma protein binding is 90%.

Phenytoin is eliminated almost entirely by hepatic metabolism. Oxidative metabolism proceeds via an epoxide intermediate, which probably represents the rate-limiting step. The epoxide may have toxic or teratogenic significance.

Plasma concentrations are not related linearly to the daily dose due to saturable metabolism, and small increases in dose may greatly increase the plasma concentration throughout the therapeutic range. Plasma concentrations of 10 to 20 mcg/ml are usually optimal. Concentrations required to control partial seizures may be higher (eg, 25 mcg/ml). Since phenytoin demonstrates nonlinear elimination kinetics, clearance and apparent half-life are dose-dependent. In addition to Vd, the more useful kinetic parameters are V_{max} and K_m. However, there is significant intersubject variability with these Michaelis-Menten parameters.

Methods used to guide phenytoin dose adjustments include graphic, which employs a linear transformation of the Michaelis-Menten equation; nomograms; estimates using population clearance values; and bayesian procedures. Although the latter are most accurate, appropriate computer programs and facilities must be available (Welty et al, 1986; Privitera et al, 1989). One simple method is to increase the daily dosage by 100 mg when the initial steady-state plasma concentration is <7 mcg/ml and by 50 mg/day when this concentration is between 7 and 12 mcg/ml; dosage increases should be restricted to 30 mg/day when initial plasma concentrations are ≥12 mcg/ml. This may represent a reasonable balance between avoiding toxicity and achieving a substantial increase in the plasma concentration of phenytoin in patients who do not respond adequately (Privitera, 1993). As with any approach, sound clinical judgment is required to account for variables that may alter the response of individual patients.

Another simple method using a semilogarithmic plot of steady-state drug concentrations versus corresponding maintenance doses also has been described (Wagner, 1985). However, adjustments in the equation for different patient populations may be required (Bryson et al, 1988).

There is little clinical evidence that the plasma concentration of free phenytoin is a better indicator of toxicity than total concentrations in healthy subjects (Levine and Chang, 1990); however, since the plasma concentration of free phenytoin can be increased by hyperbilirubinemia (eg, in neonates, in those with liver disease), hypoalbuminemia (eg, in the elderly, in those with liver disease), uremia, and concomitant administration of valproate, monitoring free concentrations may be more useful in these patients (Peterson et al, 1991). Salivary monitoring using appropriate precautions is a reproducible and consistent reflection of the plasma concentration of free phenytoin (Knott et al, 1982). Febrile illnesses may markedly increase the clearance of phenytoin leading to lowered plasma concentrations (Leppik et al, 1986). Phenytoin plasma concentrations also may be reduced by concurrent enteral feeding (Haley and Nelson, 1989).

Phenytoin's nonlinear kinetics accentuate the variations in the rates of dissolution and absorption among the various dosage forms and products. Thus, the phenytoin plasma concentrations attained may differ significantly from one product to another. It may not be cost effective to change products, because plasma concentrations should be determined and adjustments in dosage made to maintain optimum plasma concentrations after the substitution (Nuwer et al, 1990).

For other pharmacokinetic data, see Table 6.

DOSAGE AND PREPARATIONS.

Oral: The dosage must be individualized according to the patient's response and the drug plasma concentrations. Initially, phenytoin may be administered in divided doses (usually twice daily). In adults, once-daily administration usually is sufficient to maintain plasma concentrations in the therapeutic range once steady state has been achieved; it also improves compliance. However, once-daily dosage may not be practical in patients who are bothered by adverse reactions at peak plasma concentrations, in patients in whom good seizure control is not achieved, and in children because they metabolize phenytoin more rapidly. Prompt-release products (capsule, tablet, or suspension) are not suitable for once-daily dosing.

Adults, initially, 300 mg daily in two divided doses; the maintenance dose is usually 300 to 400 mg or 3 to 5 mg/kg daily (maximum, usually 600 mg). Incremental increases can be made using chewable 50-mg tablets or 30-mg capsules. The tablets can be halved to provide further refinement of the dosage increment. Formulation differences between tablet and capsules may cause problems due to nonlinear kinetics. The tablets (free acid phenytoin) contain 8% more phenytoin than the phenytoin sodium capsules. Many physicians avoid these difficulties by using only 100- and 30-mg capsules (Porter, 1989). *Children,* initially, 5 mg/kg daily in two divided doses with the maintenance dose individualized. A suggested initial maintenance dose is 5 to 7 mg/kg daily.

PHENYTOIN:

Generic. Suspension 125 mg/5 ml (alcohol ≤0.6%).

Dilantin (Parke-Davis). Suspension 30 (pediatric) and 125 mg/5 ml (alcohol ≤0.6%) ***[Dilantin-30, Dilantin-125]***; tablets (chewable) 50 mg.

PHENYTOIN SODIUM:

Generic. Capsules (prompt, extended-release) 100 mg.

Dilantin (Parke-Davis). Capsules (extended-release) 30 and 100 mg.

Intravenous: For status epilepticus, see Table 5.

PHENYTOIN SODIUM:

Dilantin (Parke-Davis), ***Generic.*** Solution 50 mg/ml in 2 and 5 ml containers.

Intramuscular: Intramuscular injection is not recommended because it is painful, crystals are precipitated at the site of injection, and absorption is very erratic.

PRIMIDONE
[Mysoline]

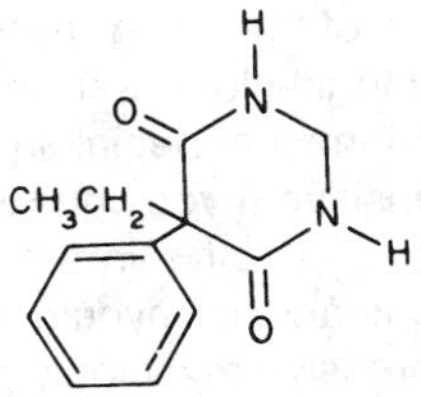

USES. This deoxybarbiturate is closely related chemically to the barbiturates. It is converted to two active metabolites, phenobarbital and phenylethylmalonamide (PEMA). Primidone is used principally in generalized tonic-clonic and complex and simple partial seizures; some clinicians believe that the drug has specific usefulness for complex partial seizures. It is as effective as carbamazepine or phenytoin in controlling partial or generalized tonic-clonic seizures, although a greater incidence of adverse reactions, especially during initial therapy, limits patient acceptance (Mattson et al, 1985). Primidone is commonly given with phenytoin but monotherapy is preferred. The conversion of primidone to phenobarbital is significantly increased when this drug is used with other enzyme-inducing antiepileptic medication. It is not effective in absence seizures.

ADVERSE REACTIONS AND PRECAUTIONS. Sedation is common but often diminishes with continued administration. As with phenobarbital, if the dose is increased gradually, incapacitating drowsiness may be avoided. Neurotoxic side effects are dose-related and initially parallel the plasma concentrations of primidone. Skin eruptions, such as maculopapular or morbilliform rash, are noted occasionally. Megaloblastic anemia, which responds to folic acid, has been reported.

In general, drug interactions are similar to those described for phenobarbital (see the evaluation). When the drug is given during pregnancy, the same precautions should be observed as with use of barbiturates (see the Introduction). Primidone, like the barbiturates, is contraindicated in patients with acute intermittent porphyria.

PHARMACOKINETICS. Primidone is rapidly and completely absorbed after oral administration; peak plasma concentrations are attained in an average of four hours, but there is wide interpatient variation. Although primidone is metabolized to phenobarbital and PEMA, a considerable percentage of the administered dose is excreted unchanged. There is a poor correlation between the dose of primidone and steady-state concentrations of primidone or phenobarbital. Because the half-life of primidone (9 to 22 hours) is considerably shorter than that of phenobarbital, plasma concentrations of phenobarbital are generally higher than those of primidone. The phenobarbital/primidone ratio, which averages 1.3 to 2 during monotherapy, may approach 4 during polytherapy. Concentrations of PEMA are intermediate. Since both phenobarbital and, to a much lesser degree, PEMA contribute to the therapeutic and toxic response, some clinicians believe that it is important to adjust the dose of primidone on the basis of both primidone and phenobarbital concentrations (Smith, 1989). However, because of the considerable interdosage fluctuation in steady-state primidone concentrations, other clinicians find it more convenient to adjust the dosage according to the plasma concentrations of phenobarbital and the patient's response. Significant ataxia and lethargy usually occur when primidone concentrations acutely exceed 12 mcg/ml (usual effective range, 5 to 12 mcg/ml). A primidone plasma concentration of 12 mcg/ml may be optimal when phenobarbital concentrations are 15 mcg/ml (Smith, 1989); however, concentrations of primidone in excess of 20 mcg/ml may be well tolerated if phenobarbital concentrations are low. Primidone concentrations are sensitive to enzyme induction produced by other antiepileptic drugs and derived phenobarbital. Under these conditions, both phenobarbital and PEMA concentrations may rise relative to those of primidone.

For other pharmacokinetic data, see Table 6.

DOSAGE AND PREPARATIONS.

Oral: *Adults and older children,* initially, 125 mg at bedtime for three days, with the dose increased by 125 mg every three days until a maintenance dose of 250 mg three times a day is established on the tenth day. The amount may be adjusted to a maximum of 2 g/day administered in three or four divided doses, based on clinical response. Alternatively, 10 to 25 mg/kg daily is given in two or three divided doses. *Children under 8 years,* initially, one-half of the adult dosage. For maintenance, 125 mg to 250 mg is given three times a day; alternatively, 10 to 25 mg/kg daily is given in two or three divided doses.

Generic. Tablets 250 mg.
Mysoline (Wyeth-Ayerst). Suspension 250 mg/5 ml; tablets 50 and 250 mg.

TRIMETHADIONE
[Tridione]

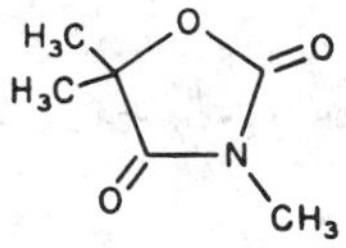

This drug is effective in absence seizures but should be reserved for refractory cases because of toxicity.

ADVERSE REACTIONS AND PRECAUTIONS. Serious reactions, some of which were fatal, include rash that may progress to exfoliative dermatitis or erythema multiforme, nephropathy, hepatitis, and bone marrow depression with aplastic anemia, neutropenia, or agranulocytosis. Pseudolymphomas, systemic lupus erythematosus, and a myasthenia gravis-like syndrome also have been reported. Drowsiness, alopecia, and hiccups may occur during early treatment. Reversible visual disturbances, particularly hemeralopia (defective vision in bright light), have been reported.

A high incidence of congenital abnormalities has been associated with the use of trimethadione during pregnancy. Accordingly, this drug should be avoided in females of childbearing age. (See the Introduction.)

PHARMACOKINETICS. Trimethadione is rapidly and well absorbed orally; time to peak plasma concentration is 0.5 to 2 hours. Protein binding is insignificant, and the volume of distribution is 60% of body weight. Trimethadione is demethylated by hepatic microsomal enzymes to the active metabolite, dimethadione, which has a half-life of 6 to 13 days. Plasma concentrations of trimethadione average 0.6 mcg/ml per mg/kg of daily dose. The plasma concentration of dimethadione averages 12 mcg/ml per mg/kg of daily dose and is used to guide dosage adjustment. Adequate seizure control is usually obtained with dimethadione concentrations above 700 mcg/ml.

DOSAGE AND PREPARATIONS.

Oral: *Adults,* initially, 900 mg daily in three or four divided doses, increased by 300 mg daily at weekly intervals to a maximum of 2.4 g daily. *Children,* initially, 40 mg/kg (300 to 900 mg) daily in three or four divided doses.

Tridione (Abbott). Capsules 300 mg; solution 40 mg/ml; tablets (chewable) 150 mg.

Valproate

VALPROIC ACID
[Depakene]

$$CH_3CH_2CH_2CH(CH_2CH_2CH_3)C(=O)OH$$

DIVALPROEX SODIUM
[Depakote]

$$(CH_3CH_2CH_2)_2CH{-}C(=O)OH \cdot Na^{+}\,{}^{-}O{-}C(=O){-}CH(CH_2CH_2CH_3)_2$$

USES. Valproate (valproic acid; divalproex sodium, a compound containing sodium valproate and valproic acid) controls absence, myoclonic, and tonic-clonic seizures in generalized, idiopathic, and symptomatic epilepsy. Valproate is as effective as ethosuximide in patients with absence seizures alone and is variably effective in atypical absence seizures. Although some clinicians prefer valproate for absence seizures, the American Academy of Pediatrics (Committee on Drugs, 1982) recommended that it be reserved for use when therapeutic failure or intolerance to ethosuximide occurs, because valproate has been associated with rare but potentially fatal hepatotoxicity. Many neurologists consider valproate the drug of choice for patients with both absence and other generalized seizure types, including tonic-clonic convulsions. Its efficacy is about the same as in patients with the latter type alone.

Valproate is an alternative drug in the treatment of complex partial seizures but may be considered for initial therapy in patients with partial and secondarily generalized seizures.

Valproate is the drug of choice in myoclonic epilepsy, with or without generalized tonic-clonic seizures, including juvenile myoclonic epilepsy of Janz that begins in adolescence or early adulthood. Photosensitive myoclonus is usually easily controlled. Valproate also is effective in the treatment of benign myoclonic epilepsy, postanoxic myoclonus, and, with clonazepam, in severe progressive myoclonic epilepsy that is characterized by tonic-clonic seizures as well (Bourgeois, 1989). It also may be preferred in certain stimulus-sensitive (reflex, startle) epilepsies.

Although valproate may be effective for infantile spasms, it is relatively contraindicated in children whose spasms are due to hyperglycinemia or other underlying metabolic (mitochondrial) abnormalities. In general, atonic and akinetic seizures in patients with Lennox-Gastaut syndrome are difficult to control, but valproate is the drug of choice for treatment of mixed seizure types. Since this drug has been useful in some patients who are refractory to all other antiepileptic drugs, it may warrant a trial in nearly all nonresponsive patients regardless of seizure type.

ADVERSE REACTIONS AND PRECAUTIONS. Adverse reactions generally appear early in the course of therapy and are mild and transient. Hematologic and gastrointestinal reactions, sedation, minimal elevation in liver function tests, and hyperammonemia usually are not major concerns when considering the benefit of valproate therapy. However, fatal hepatotoxicity has developed and is most common in children under 2 years who have congenital anomalies and metabolic and neurologic disorders and who are receiving polytherapy.

The incidence of gastrointestinal disturbances (nausea, vomiting, anorexia, heartburn) ranges from 6% to 45% (Turnbull, 1983). Symptoms are transient and require drug withdrawal in only 0.9% of adults and 2.9% of children (Schmidt, 1984). Discomfort can be avoided in the majority of patients by administering the delayed-release preparation [Depakote] (Wilder et al, 1983). Diarrhea, abdominal cramps, and constipation are reported occasionally. Increased appetite with weight gain is common and may be controlled by diet; however, in some cases excessive weight gain may require drug withdrawal (Turnbull, 1983).

Rarely, severe or fatal pancreatitis has been reported, and the physician should be prepared to treat this complication if severe abdominal pain and vomiting occur (Wyllie et al, 1984; Lott et al, 1990; Asconapé et al, 1993).

Hand tremor, resembling benign essential tremor, is the most common neurologic adverse reaction and occasionally is severe enough to interfere with writing. Tremor occurs more frequently with doses greater than 750 mg/day and may improve with dosage reduction (Turnbull, 1983).

Sedation and drowsiness develop infrequently in patients receiving valproate alone. Conversely, central nervous system stimulation and excitement have been observed, and aggressiveness and hyperactivity are sometimes noted in children. Other central nervous system effects reported rarely include ataxia, headache, and stupor. For discussion of cognitive effects, see the section on Adverse Reactions and Precautions, Central Nervous System, in the Introduction.

Alopecia, thinning, or changes in hair texture occur in some patients, but these effects usually are temporary and do not necessitate withdrawal of the drug. One case of persistent hair curliness has been described (Gupta, 1988). Rash occurs rarely.

Valproate inhibits the secondary phase of platelet aggregation, but this is unlikely to be of clinical significance unless patients are receiving other drugs that affect coagulation. The benefit of determining bleeding time before initiating therapy is unproven. Dose-related, reversible thrombocytopenia has been observed; this reaction is related to secondary destruction of mature platelets rather than to bone marrow suppression. Platelet counts should be monitored in patients receiving large doses of valproate, especially when the platelet count may be further reduced (eg, during viral infections). Rarely, hematomas, epistaxis, and increased bleeding after surgery have been reported; thus, platelet function should be monitored before surgery. Caution is recommended when administering drugs that affect coagulation to patients receiving valproate, and dosage adjustments should be made when necessary.

Transient elevations of liver transaminases (eg, AST and ALT) are common. The elevations usually are not related to serious liver dysfunction, and levels often return to normal with or without dosage adjustment. However, severe hepatotoxicity has occurred rarely during valproate therapy. Prodromal illness characterized by vomiting, lethargy, anorexia, and muscle weakness often may be present. Hepatotoxicity usually develops after an average of two months (range, three days to six months) of therapy.

In the United States, 37 fatalities associated with valproate hepatotoxicity were reported between 1978 and 1984. Most occurred in children receiving polytherapy and in patients with mental retardation, congenital abnormalities, organic brain disease, or other neurologic disorders. Children with partial seizures that cause recurrent status epilepticus and that are associated with progressive neurologic signs are at high risk. Other disorders associated with valproate hepatotoxicity include G_{M2} gangliosidosis, spinocerebellar degeneration, Friedreich's ataxia, Lafora's disease, Alper's disease, and the myoclonic epilepsy and ragged-red fibers syndrome (Dreifuss et al, 1987). Specific biochemical abnormalities associated with valproate hepatotoxicity include urea cycle defects, organic aciduria, multiple carboxylase deficiency, and mitochondrial or respiratory-chain dysfunction.

Based on retrospective analysis, the following risks for fatal hepatotoxicity were identified: Overall, 1:10,000. Polytherapy: children <2 years, 1:500; >2 years, 1:12,000. Monotherapy: overall, 1:37,000; children 0 to 2 years, 1:7,000; >2 years, 1:45,000 (Dreifuss et al, 1987). Since 1984, hepatic fatalities associated with the use of valproate have decreased. During 1985 and 1986, five fatalities (none in individuals over 10 years) among 198,000 treated patients were reported (incidence, 1:49,000). This can be attributed to a change in the prescribing patterns for valproate, including increased use of monotherapy and decreased use in high-risk patients (Dreifuss et al, 1989). Analysis of hepatic fatalities associated with valproate therapy in West Germany through 1986 failed to identify specific "high-risk" groups (Scheffner et al, 1988). In this study, only 12% of individuals were under 3 years and 25% of the patients were receiving monotherapy.

Guidelines recommended by the American Academy of Pediatrics and others (Committee on Drugs, 1982; Dreifuss et al, 1987) include: (1) Avoid administering valproate as polytherapy in children under 3 years unless monotherapy has failed. (2) Use other effective therapy initially whenever possible (eg, in absence and febrile seizures), although valproate is effective in many of these and other types of seizures. (3) Avoid administering valproate to patients with pre-existing hepatic disease or a family history of childhood hepatic disease or to critically ill children and children receiving other medication that affects mitochondrial function or coagulation. (4) Since laboratory monitoring alone may be inadequate to diagnose valproate-induced hepatotoxicity, instruct patients and their parents to report symptoms, such as loss of appetite, lethargy, nausea, vomiting, abdominal pain, jaundice, edema, easy bruising, and loss of seizure control. (5) Maintain dosage at the lowest amount that produces optimal seizure control.

Tests of liver synthetic function (eg, one-stage prothrombin time and fibrinogen levels) may be more helpful than routine monitoring of liver function (eg, AST levels) in detecting hepatic dysfunction (Dreifuss et al, 1989). Some current guidelines include the recommendation that liver function be assessed prior to therapy, approximately once monthly during the first six months of use, and periodically thereafter (Committee on Drugs, 1982; Dreifuss et al, 1987). Other authorities recommend that vigilant clinical assessment supplant reliance on routine laboratory monitoring for most patients (Willmore et al, 1991). As an alternative strategy, young children within the risk groups noted above and those who require polytherapy should have routine chemistry screening and hepatic synthetic function tests, as well as metabolic evaluation including determination of arterial blood gases and, to assess mitochondrial function, ammonia, lactate and pyruvate, carnitine, and urinary organic acids. Careful attention to the early clinical signs of valproate-induced hepatic dysfunction (eg, vomiting, lethargy, increased number of seizures, influenza-like symptoms), particularly during the first six months of therapy, would indicate the need for appropriate detailed metabolic assessment in these and other patients.

Valproate therapy commonly produces reversible hyperammonemia, but the clinical significance of this reaction in the absence of liver dysfunction is unknown. Valproate occasionally causes acute confusional states that may progress to stupor or coma. The encephalopathy is most common in pediatric patients and, like hyperammonemia, may be manifested in the absence of other indices of hepatic failure; however, there is little correlation between serum ammonia concentrations and valproate-induced encephalopathy, and most patients with hyperammonemia are asymptomatic. In mitochondrial pathways, sequential utilization of acetyl-CoA and carnitine inhibits beta oxidation of long-chain fatty acids and may interfere with intermediary metabolism or rarely may induce secondary carnitine deficiency. Patients treated with valproate usually have a mild dicarboxylic aciduria. The accumulation may inhibit urea cycle enzymes; a direct inhibitory effect of valproate or its metabolites on urea cycle enzymes also may contribute to the hyperammonemia. Administration of carnitine has been recommended to ameliorate metabolic defects and to avoid carnitine depletion (Coulter, 1991).

Isolated cases of systemic lupus erythematosus associated with valproate therapy have been reported, but a definite cause-and-effect relationship has not been established (Bleck and Smith, 1990).

Since valproate is partly eliminated as a ketone-containing metabolite, the urine ketone test may produce false-positive results.

TERATOGENICITY. Valproate has teratogenic effects in mice, rats, and rabbits, usually manifested as increased fetal resorption, retarded fetal growth, and major developmental abnormalities, including skeletal defects. The incidence was about the same as with phenytoin at similar dose levels. Neural tube abnormalities occurred in about 1% to 2% of infants whose mothers received valproate alone or with other antiepileptic drugs during pregnancy (Turnbull, 1983; Jeavons, 1984). In one study, there was a significant relationship between development of spina bifida and use of larger doses of valproate (ie, >1 g/day), suggesting a dose-dependent effect (Omtzigt et al, 1992). Although a precise estimate of risks cannot be determined, physicians should carefully weigh the risks and benefits when prescribing valproate to women of childbearing age (FDA Pregnancy Category D). Low concentrations (1% to 10% of maternal plasma concentration) of valproate appear in breast milk. (See the Introduction.)

DRUG INTERACTIONS. When valproate is given with phenobarbital, the plasma phenobarbital concentration is increased by 25% to 68% (Rimmer and Richens, 1985); this can cause marked sedation or intoxication. Therefore, a 30% to 75% reduction in phenobarbital dosage is required when valproate is added to the regimen, and two to three weeks must elapse before a new steady-state level is achieved.

Valproate inhibits the hepatic metabolism of lamotrigine and approximately doubles its half-life; however, the half-life may be relatively unaffected in patients who also are taking an enzyme-inducing drug. Felbamate causes a dose-related increase in the steady-state plasma concentration of valproate; a 20% to 33% reduction in the dose of valproate is recommended when treatment with felbamate is initiated.

The interaction between valproate and phenytoin is complex (Hansten and Horn, 1989). Valproate displaces phenytoin from plasma albumin, which temporarily increases the ratio of free/bound drug; toxicity may result if phenytoin concentrations were high prior to administration of valproate. The total plasma concentration may decrease by about 30% during the first several weeks of therapy but usually does not result in recurrence of seizures because the free phenytoin concentration does not change. However, valproate also may inhibit the biotransformation of phenytoin, which, over the next 4 to 16 weeks, produces a gradual return of total phenytoin plasma concentrations to previous values. Free phenytoin measurements may be useful to explain the onset of central nervous system toxicity when the total plasma phenytoin concentration is in the therapeutic range. Careful patient monitoring rather than aggressive therapeutic drug monitoring is recommended. (See also Table 7.)

Valproate displaces diazepam from protein binding sites and may augment its sedative action.

Other interactions between valproate and phenobarbital, primidone, phenytoin, and carbamazepine result from the enzyme-inducing effects of the latter drugs, which reduce the half-life of valproate. The half-life is not consistently affected by ethosuximide or the benzodiazepines. Valproate does not induce liver enzymes but may increase the relative concentration of carbamazepine epoxide. In some patients, aspirin or other salicylates may displace valproate from protein binding sites and cause a sufficient increase in free valproate concentrations to result in toxicity. Fluoxetine may inhibit the metabolism of valproate (Sovner and Davis, 1991).

PHARMACOKINETICS. Valproate is absorbed rapidly and completely following oral administration; peak plasma concentrations usually occur within two hours after ingestion of liquid preparations and three to four hours after ingestion of the delayed-release tablet preparation, divalproex sodium, which contains sodium valproate and valproic acid. Food delays absorption but does not affect bioavailability.

The plasma protein binding of valproate is saturable within the usual therapeutic range (approximately 90% at 75 mcg/ml). Usual effective plasma concentrations range from 40 to 120 mcg/ml, but concentrations exceeding 150 mcg/ml may be required and tolerated in some patients. With a daily dose of more than 500 mg, plasma concentrations may not increase proportionately because clearance increases with an increase in the free fraction. Daily fluctuations (up to two times higher) in free fraction and clearance also occur as a result of displacement by free fatty acids or circadian influences; thus, when plasma concentrations are being monitored, samples should be taken at a uniform time. Many neurologists recommend measuring trough concentrations.

Valproate is eliminated almost exclusively by hepatic metabolism. The metabolic fate is complex. A variety of conjugation and oxidative processes are involved, including entry into pathways (eg, beta oxidation) normally reserved for endogenous fatty acids. As the dose is increased, mitochondrial beta oxidation becomes saturated and increased glucuronidation occurs.

Metabolites may contribute to both antiepileptic and hepatotoxic effects. The antiepileptic activity of valproate (including the time course) is poorly correlated with steady-state valproate plasma concentrations. One unsaturated metabolite, 2-n-propyl-4-pentenoic acid (4-ene-VPA), has been proposed as a key hepatotoxic metabolite (see Adverse Reactions). The formation of this metabolite is increased with larger doses of valproate (Anderson et al, 1992) and with concomitant use of phenytoin, phenobarbital, carbamazepine, and other drugs that induce cytochrome P450 (Levy et al, 1990).

The half-life of valproate in adults is 12 to 16 hours. In epileptic patients receiving polytherapy, the half-life is approximately nine hours, although five hours also has been reported. Although hepatic clearance is reduced, the half-life in geriatric patients is approximately 15 hours. This has been attributed to the larger free fraction observed in this age group, especially in those with hypoalbuminemia. The half-lives in school-age children and young adolescents are well within the range of values in adults (Levy and Shen, 1989). Elimination half-lives are longer in neonates and generally shorter during middle and late infancy.

For other pharmacokinetic data, see Table 6.

DOSAGE AND PREPARATIONS.

Oral: *Adults*, initially, 5 to 15 mg/kg daily; usual maintenance dose, 10 to 20 mg/kg/day. When used with other antiepileptic drugs, the initial dose is 10 to 30 mg/kg/day and the usual maintenance dose is 30 to 60 mg/kg/day. *Children 1 to 12 years*, initially, 10 to 30 mg/kg/day; maintenance dose, 20 to 30 mg/kg/day. When used with other antiepileptic drugs that induce hepatic metabolism, the initial dose is 15 to 45 mg/kg/day. With polytherapy, some pediatric patients require doses larger than the manufacturer's recommended maximum maintenance dose (60 mg/kg/day) in order to maintain plasma concentrations >50 mcg/ml (Suzuki et al, 1991). In all populations, dosage increases in increments of 5 to 10 mg/kg weekly are recommended according to clinical response. If the total daily dose is more than 250 mg, it should be divided into two daily doses to minimize gastrointestinal irritation. Depakote Sprinkle may be preferable for use in children and elderly patients. It tastes better than the syrup form and can be sprinkled over food.

VALPROIC ACID:

Depakene (Abbott), ***Generic.*** Capsules 250 mg; syrup 250 mg/5 ml (as sodium valproate).

DIVALPROEX SODIUM:

Depakote (Abbott). Tablets (delayed-release) 125, 250, and 500 mg.

Depakote Sprinkle (Abbott). Capsules 125 mg.

Cited References

Drugs for epilepsy. *Med Lett Drugs Ther* 31:1-4, 1989.

NIH Consensus Development Conference on Surgery for Epilepsy. Bethesda, Md, National Institutes of Health, (March) 1990, vol 8.

Recommendations for the use of folic acid to reduce the number of cases of spinal bifida and other neural tube defects. *MMWR* 41:1-7, 1992.

Aicardi J: Epileptic syndromes in childhood. *Epilepsia* 29(suppl 3):S1-S5, 1988.

Aird RB, et al: *The Epilepsies: A Critical Review.* New York, Raven Press, 1984.

Albano A, et al: Rectal diazepam in pediatric status epilepticus. *Am J Emerg Med* 70:168-172, 1989.

Aman MG, et al: Effect of sodium valproate on psychomotor performance in children as a function of drug concentration, fluctuations in concentration and diagnosis. *Epilepsia* 28:115-124, 1987.

Aman MG, et al: Effects of carbamazepine on psychomotor performance in children as a function of dose, concentration, seizure type, and time of medication. *Epilepsia* 31:51-60, 1990.

American Academy of Pediatrics, Committee on Genetics: Maternal serum α-fetoprotein screening. *Pediatrics* 88:1282-1283, 1991.

Anderson GD, et al: Effect of valproate dose on formation of hepatotoxic metabolites. *Epilepsia* 33:736-742, 1992.

André M, et al: Clonazepam in neonatal seizures: Dose regimens and therapeutic efficacy. *Eur J Clin Pharmacol* 40:193-195, 1991.

Andrewes DG, et al: Comparative study of the cognitive effects of phenytoin and carbamazepine in new referrals with epilepsy. *Epilepsia* 27:128-134, 1986.

Arts WFM, et al: Follow-up of 146 children with epilepsy after withdrawal of antiepileptic therapy. *Epilepsia* 29:244-250, 1988.

Asconapé JJ, et al: Valproate-associated pancreatitis. *Epilepsia* 34:177-183, 1993.

Barry E, Hauser WA: Status epilepticus: The interaction of epilepsy and acute brain disease. *Neurology* 43:1473-1478, 1993.

Barry E, Hauser WA: Status epilepticus and antiepileptic medication levels. *Neurology* 44:47-50, 1994.

Battino D, et al: Plasma concentrations of carbamazepine and carbamazepine-10,11-epoxide during pregnancy and after delivery. *Clin Pharmacokinet* 10:279-284, 1985.

Berg AT, Shinnar S: The risk of seizure recurrence following a first unprovoked seizure: A quantitative review. *Neurology* 41:965-972, 1991.

Berg AT, Shinnar S: Relapse following discontinuation of antiepileptic drugs: A meta-analysis. *Neurology* 44:601-608, 1994.

Berg AT, et al: Predictor of recurrent febrile seizures: A metaanalytic review. *J Pediatr* 116:329-337, 1990.

Berg AT, et al: A prospective study of recurrent febrile seizures. *N Engl J Med* 327:1122-1127, 1992.

Berkovic SF, et al: Valproate prevents the recurrence of absence status. *Neurology* 39:1294-1297, 1989.

Bertilsson L, Tomson T: Clinical pharmacokinetics and pharmacological effects of carbamazepine and carbamazepine-10, 11,-epoxide: Update. *Clin Pharmacokinet* 11:177-198, 1986.

Biale Y, Lewenthal M: Effect of folic acid supplementation on congenital malformations due to anticonvulsant drugs. *Eur J Obstet Gynaecol Reprod Biol* 18:211-216, 1984.

Biton V, et al: Adjunctive therapy for intractable epilepsy with ethotoin. *Epilepsia* 31:433-437, 1990.

Bleck TP, Smith MC: Possible induction of systemic lupus erythematosus by valproate. *Epilepsia* 31:343-345, 1990.

Bourgeois BFD: Valproate: Clinical use, in Levy RH, et al (eds): *Antiepileptic Drugs,* ed 3. New York, Raven Press, 1989, 633-642.

Bourgeois B, et al: Monotherapy with valproate in primary, generalized epilepsies. *Epilepsia* 28(suppl 2):S8-S11, 1987.

Bourgeois B, et al: Felbamate: A double-blind controlled trial in patients undergoing presurgical evaluation of partial seizures. *Neurology* 43:693-696, 1993.

Brodie MJ: Lamotrigine. *Lancet* 339:1397-1400, 1992.

Brøsen K, Kragh-Sørensen P: Case report: Concomitant intake of nortriptyline and carbamazepine. *Ther Drug Monit* 15:258-260, 1993.

Browne TR, Feldman RG (eds): *Epilepsy: Diagnosis and Management.* Boston, Little Brown, 1983.

Browne TR for the International, UK, and US Gabapentin Study Groups, in Chadwick D (ed): *New Trends in Epilepsy Management: The Role of Gabapentin.* London, Royal Society of Medicine Services, 1993, 47-57.

Browne TR, et al: Multicenter long-term safety and efficacy study of vigabatrin for refractory complex partial seizures: An update. *Neurology* 41:363-364, 1991.

Bruni J, et al: Efficacy and safety of gabapentin (neurontin): A multicenter, placebo-controlled, double-blind study. *Neurology* 41(suppl 1):330-331, 1991.

Bryson SM, et al: Comparison of a bayesian forecasting technique with a new method for estimating phenytoin dose requirements. *Ther Drug Monit* 10:80-84, 1988.

Buehler BA, et al: Prenatal prediction of risk of the fetal hydantoin syndrome. *N Engl J Med* 322:1567-1572, 1990.

Burton BK: Maternal serum α-fetoprotein screening. *Pediatr Ann* 18:687-697, 1989.

Butler WH: Neuropathology of vigabatrin. *Epilepsia* 30(suppl 3):S15-S17, 1989.

Calandre EP, et al: Cognitive effects of long-term treatment with phenobarbital and valproic acid in school children. *Acta Neurol Scand* 81:504-506, 1990.

Callaghan N, et al: A prospective study between carbamazepine, phenytoin and sodium valproate as monotherapy in previously untreated and recently diagnosed patients with epilepsy. *J Neurol Neurosurg Psychiatry* 48:639-644, 1985.

Callaghan N, et al: Withdrawal of anticonvulsant drugs in patients free of seizures for two years: Prospective study. *N Engl J Med* 318:942-946, 1988.

Camfield C, et al: Asymptomatic children with epilepsy: Little benefit from screening for anticonvulsant-induced liver, blood, or renal damage. *Neurology* 36:838-841, 1986.

Camfield CS, et al: Home use of rectal diazepam to prevent status epilepticus in children with convulsive disorders. *J Child Neurol* 4:125-126, 1989.

Carmant L, et al: Felbamate is effective against intractable partial seizures in children, abstract. *Epilepsia* 34 (suppl 6):99, 1993.

Carter AC, et al: Ethotoin in seizures of childhood and adolescence. *Neurology* 34:791-795, 1984.

Cascino GD, et al: Stereotactic resection of intra-axial cerebral lesions in partial epilepsy. *Mayo Clin Proc* 65:1053-1060, 1990.

Chadwick DW: Valproate monotherapy in the management of generalized and partial seizures. *Epilepsia* 28 (suppl 2):S12-S17, 1987.

Chadwick D: Drug withdrawal and epilepsy: When and how? *Drugs* 35:579-583, 1988.

Chadwick D, Reynolds EH: When do epileptic patients need treatment? Starting and stopping medication. *BMJ* 290:1885-1888, 1985.

Commission on Classification and Terminology of the International League Against Epilepsy: Proposal for revised clinical and electroencephalographic classification of epileptic seizures. *Epilepsia* 22:489-501, 1981.

Commission on Classification and Terminology of the International League Against Epilepsy: Proposal for revised classification of epilepsies and epileptic syndromes. *Epilepsia* 30:389-399, 1989.

Commission on Genetics, Pregnancy, and the Child, International League Against Epilepsy: Guidelines for the care of women of childbearing age with epilepsy. *Epilepsia* 34:588-589, 1993.

Committee on Drugs, American Academy of Pediatrics: Valproic acid: Benefits and risks. *Pediatrics* 70:316-319, 1982.

Committee on Drugs, American Academy of Pediatrics: Behavioral and cognitive effects of anticonvulsants. *Pediatrics* 76:644-647, 1985.

Committee on Maternal and Fetal Medicine, American College of Obstetricians and Gynecologists: Anticonvulsants and pregnancy. *ACOG Committee Statement*. Washington, DC, ACOG, 1984.

Coulter DL: Carnitine, valproate, and toxicity. *J Child Neurol* 6:7-14, 1991.

Coulter DA, et al: Specific petit mal anticonvulsants reduce calcium currents in thalamic neurons. *Neurosci Lett* 98:74-78, 1989.

Crawford P, et al: Gabapentin as an antiepileptic drug in man. *J Neurol Neurosurg Psychiatry* 50:682-686, 1987.

Cunningham FG, Gilstrap LC: Maternal serum alpha-fetoprotein screening, editorial. *N Engl J Med* 325:55-57, 1991.

Czeizel A, Dudas I: Prevention of the first occurrence of neural tube defects by periconceptional vitamin supplementation. *N Engl J Med* 327:1832-1835, 1992.

Dansky LV, et al: Anticonvulsants, folate levels, and pregnancy outcome: A prospective study. *Ann Neurol* 21:176-182, 1987.

Dean JC, Penry JK: Valproate monotherapy in 30 patients with partial seizures. *Epilepsia* 29:140-144, 1988.

Dean JC, Penry JK: Discontinuation of antiepileptic drugs, in Levy RH, et al (eds): *Antiepileptic Drugs,* ed 3. New York, Raven Press, 1989, 133-142.

Delgado-Escueta AV, et al: Mapping the gene for juvenile myoclonic epilepsy. *Epilepsia* 30 (suppl 4):S8-S18, 1989.

Dichter MA: Cellular mechanisms of epilepsy and potential new treatment strategies. *Epilepsia* 30 (suppl 1):S3-S12, 1989.

Dichter MA, Ayala GF: Cellular mechanisms of epilepsy: A status report. *Science* 237:157-164, 1987.

Dodrill CB: Behavioral effects of antiepileptic drugs. *Adv Neurol* 55:213-224, 1991.

Dodrill CB, Troupin AS: Neuropsychological effects of carbamazepine and phenytoin: A reanalysis. *Neurology* 41:141-143, 1991.

Dodson WE: Medical treatment and pharmacology of antiepileptic drugs. *Pediatr Clin North Am* 36:421-434, 1989.

Dow KE, Riopelle RJ: Teratogenic effects of carbamazepine, letter. *N Engl J Med* 321:1481, 1989.

Dreifuss FE, et al: Infantile spasms: Comparative trial of nitrazepam and corticotropin. *Arch Neurol* 43:1107-1110, 1986.

Dreifuss FE, et al: Valproic acid hepatic fatalities: A retrospective review. *Neurology* 37:379-385, 1987.

Dreifuss FE, et al: Valproic acid hepatic fatalities, II: US experience since 1984. *Neurology* 39:201-207, 1989.

Duncan JS, et al: Effects of removal of phenytoin, carbamazepine, and valproate on cognitive function. *Epilepsia* 31:584-591, 1990.

Emerson R, et al: Stopping medication in children with epilepsy: Predictors of outcome. *N Engl J Med* 304:1125-1129, 1981.

Engel J Jr: Epileptic syndrome, in: *Seizures and Epilepsy.* Philadelphia, FA Davis, 1989, 179-220.

Engel J Jr: Update on surgical treatment of the epilepsies: Summary of The Second International Palm Desert Conference on the Surgical Treatment of the Epilepsies (1992). *Neurology* 43:1612-1617, 1993.

Evans OB, et al: Hematologic monitoring in children with epilepsy treated with carbamazepine. *J Child Neurol* 4:286-290, 1989.

Farwell JR, et al: Phenobarbital for febrile seizures: Effects on intelligence and on seizure recurrence. *N Engl J Med* 322:364-369, 1990.

Faught E, et al: Felbamate monotherapy for partial-onset seizures: An active-control trial. *Neurology* 43:688-692, 1993.

The Felbamate Study Group in Lennox-Gastaut Syndrome: Efficacy of felbamate in childhood epileptic encephalopathy (Lennox-Gastaut syndrome). *N Engl J Med* 328:29-33, 1993.

Feldman RG: Clorazepate in temporal lobe epilepsy, letter. *JAMA* 236:2603, 1976.

First Seizure Trial Group: Randomized clinical trial of the efficacy of antiepileptic drugs in reducing the risk of relapse after a first unprovoked tonic-clonic seizure. *Neurology* 43:478-483, 1993.

Foy PM, et al: Do prophylactic anticonvulsant drugs alter the pattern of seizures after craniotomy? *J Neurol Neurosurg Psychiatry* 55:753-757, 1992.

Freeman JM: Febrile seizures: Consensus of significance, evaluation, and treatment. *Pediatrics* 66:1009-1012, 1980.

Gale K: GABA in epilepsy: Pharmacologic basis. *Epilepsia* 30 (suppl 3):S1-S11, 1989.

Gallassi R, et al: Carbamazepine and phenytoin: Comparison of cognitive effects in epileptic patients during monotherapy and withdrawal. *Arch Neurol* 45:892-894, 1988.

Galvin GM, Jelinek GA: Midazolam: An effective agent for seizure epilepsy control. *Arch Emerg Med* 4:169-172, 1987.

Giang DW, McBride MC: Lorazepam versus diazepam for the treatment of status epilepticus. *Pediatr Neurol* 4:358-361, 1988.

Gillham RA, et al: Cognitive function in adult epileptic patients established on anticonvulsant monotherapy. *Epilepsy Res* 7:219-225, 1990.

Glaze DG, et al: Prospective study of outcome of infants with infantile spasms treated during controlled studies of ACTH and prednisone. *J Pediatr* 112:389-396, 1988.

Gloor P, Fariello RG: Generalized epilepsy: Some of its cellular mechanisms differ from those of focal epilepsy. *Trends Neurosci* 11:63-68, 1988.

Griffith JL, Murray GB: Clorazepate in the treatment of complex partial seizures with psychic symptomatology. *J Nerv Ment Dis* 173:185-186, 1985.

Grünewald RA, Panayiotopoulos CP: Juvenile myoclonic epilepsy. *Arch Neurol* 50:594-598, 1993.

Gupta AK: 'Perming' effects associated with chronic valproate therapy. *Br J Clin Pract* 42:75-77, 1988.

Haley CJ, Nelson J: Phenytoin-enteral feeding interaction. *Ann Pharmacother* 23:796-798, 1989.

Hansten PD, Horn JR: Carbamazepine-induced water intoxication: Drugs that may increase the risk. *Drug Interact Newslett* 7:53-56, 1987.

Hansten PD, Horn JR: *Drug Interactions: Clinical Significance of Drug-Drug Interactions,* ed 6. Philadelphia, Lea & Febiger, 1989, 149.

Hart RG, Easton JD: Carbamazepine and hematological monitoring. *Ann Neurol* 11:309-312, 1982.

Hauser WA, et al: Prevalence of epilepsy in Rochester, Minnesota: 1940-1980. *Epilepsia* 32:429-445, 1991.

Herranz JL, et al: Clinical side effects of phenobarbital, primidone, phenytoin, carbamazepine, and valproate during monotherapy in children. *Epilepsia* 29:794-804, 1988.

Hiilesmaa VK, et al: Serum folate concentrations during pregnancy in women with epilepsy: Relation to antiepileptic drug concentrations, number of seizures, and fetal outcome. *BMJ* 287:577-579, 1983.

Hirschfeld S, Jarosinski P: Drug interaction of terfenadine and carbamazepine, letter. *Ann Intern Med* 118:907-908, 1993.

Hirtz DG: Generalized tonic-clonic and febrile seizures. *Pediatr Clin North Am* 36:365-382, 1989.

Holmes GL, et al: Absence seizures in children: Clinical and electroencephalographic features. *Ann Neurol* 21:268-273, 1987.

Hrachovy RA, et al: Double-blind study of ACTH vs prednisone therapy in infantile spasms. *J Pediatr* 103:641-645, 1983.

Hrachovy RA, et al: A retrospective study of spontaneous remission and long-term outcome in patients with infantile spasms. *Epilepsia* 32:212-214, 1991.

Hvidberg EF, Dam M: Clinical pharmacokinetics of anticonvulsants. *Clin Pharmacokinet* 1:161-188, 1976.

Iivanainen M, Himberg J-J: Valproate and clonazepam in treatment of severe progressive myoclonus epilepsy. *Arch Neurol* 39:236-238, 1982.

Iivanainen M, Savolainen H: Side effects of phenobarbital and phenytoin during long-term treatment of epilepsy. *Acta Neurol Scand* 68 (suppl 97):49-67, 1983.

Jeavons PM: Non-dose-related side effects of valproate. *Epilepsia* 25 (suppl 1):S50-S55, 1984.

Jones KL, et al: Pattern of malformations in the children of women treated with carbamazepine during pregnancy. *N Engl J Med* 320:1661-1666, 1989.

Kelly KM, et al: Valproic acid selectivity reduces the low-threshold (T) calcium current in rat nodose neurons. *Neurosci Lett* 116:233-238, 1990.

Ketter TA, et al: Principles of clinically important drug interactions with carbamazepine, part I. *J Clin Psychopharmacol* 11:198-203, 1991 A.

Ketter TA, et al: Principles of clinically important drug interactions with carbamazepine, part II. *J Clin Psychopharmacol* 11:306-313, 1991 B.

Kinsman SL, et al: Efficacy of the ketogenic diet for intractable seizure disorders: Review of 58 cases. *Epilepsia* 33:1132-1136, 1992.

Knott C, et al: Phenytoin-valproate interaction: Importance of saliva monitoring in epilepsy. *BMJ* 284:13-16, 1982.

Knudsen FU: Effective short-term diazepam prophylaxis in febrile convulsions. *J Pediatr* 106:487-490, 1985.

Knudsen FU: Intermittent diazepam prophylaxis in febrile convulsions. *Acta Neurol Scand Suppl* 83 (No. 135):1-24, 1991.

Kriel RL, et al: Home use of rectal diazepam for cluster and prolonged seizures: Efficacy, adverse reactions, quality of life, and cost analysis. *Pediatr Neurol* 7:13-17, 1991.

Kumar A, Bleck TP: Intravenous midazolam for the treatment of refractory status epilepticus. *Crit Care Med* 20:483-488, 1992.

Lander CM, Eadie MJ: Plasma antiepileptic drug concentrations during pregnancy. *Epilepsia* 32:257-266, 1991.

Legido A, et al: Recent advances in the diagnosis, treatment and prognosis of neonatal seizures. *Pediatr Neurol* 4:79-86, 1988.

Leinonen E, et al: Effects of carbamazepine on serum antidepressant concentrations in psychiatric patients. *J Clin Psychopharmacol* 11:313-318, 1991.

Lenn NJ, Robertson M: Clinical utility of unbound antiepileptic drug blood levels in the management of epilepsy. *Neurology* 42:988-990, 1992.

Leppert M, et al: The gene for benign familial neonatal convulsions maps to human chromosome 20. *Nature* 337:647-648, 1989.

Leppik IE: Status epilepticus. *Neurol Clin North Am* 4:633-643, 1986.

Leppik IE, Schmidt D: Consensus statement on compliance in epilepsy. *Epilepsy Res* (suppl 1):179-182, 1988.

Leppik IE, et al: Double-blind study of lorazepam and diazepam in status epilepticus. *JAMA* 249:1452-1454, 1983.

Leppik IE, et al: Seasonal incidence of phenytoin allergy unrelated to plasma levels. *Arch Neurol* 42:120-122, 1985.

Leppik IE, et al: Altered phenytoin clearance during febrile illness. *Neurology* 36:1367-1370, 1986.

Leppik IE, et al: Pharmacokinetics and safety of a phenytoin prodrug given IV or IM in patients. *Neurology* 40:456-460, 1990.

Leppik IE, et al: Felbamate for partial seizures: Results of a controlled clinical trial. *Neurology* 41:1785-1789, 1991.

Levine M, Chang T: Therapeutic drug monitoring of phenytoin: Rationale and current status. *Clin Pharmacokinet* 19:341-358, 1990.

Levy RH, Shen DD: Absorption, distribution, and excretion, in Levy RH, et al (eds): *Antiepileptic Drugs,* ed 3. New York, Raven Press, 1989, 583-600.

Levy RH, Yerby MS: Effects of pregnancy on antiepileptic drug utilization. *Epilepsia* 26 (suppl 1):S52-S57, 1985.

Levy RH, et al (eds): *Antiepileptic Drugs,* ed 3. New York, Raven Press, 1989.

Levy RH, et al: Effects of polytherapy with phenytoin, carbamazepine, and stiripentol on formation of 4-ene-valproate, a hepatotoxic metabolite of valproic acid. *Clin Pharmacol Ther* 48:225-235, 1990.

Lewis TB, et al: Genetic heterogeneity in benign familial neonatal convulsions: Identification of a new locus on chromosome 8q. *Am J Hum Genet* 53:670-675, 1993.

Livingston JH: Lennox-Gastaut syndrome. *Dev Med Child Neurol* 30:536-540, 1988.

Livingston S, et al: Medical treatment of epilepsy: Introduction. *Pediatr Ann* 8:210-274, 1979.

Locke GE, et al: Prevalence of epilepsy and seizure disorders in an urban minority population: A feasibility study. *Epilepsia* 30:747-755, 1989.

Lombroso CT: A prospective study of infantile spasms: Clinical and therapeutic correlations. *Epilepsia* 24:135-158, 1983.

Lott JA, et al: Valproic-acid associated pancreatitis: Report of three cases and a brief review. *Clin Chem* 36:395-397, 1990.

Lowenstein D, Alldredge B: Status epilepticus at an urban public hospital. *Neurology* 42:483-488, 1992.

Lowenstein DH, et al: Barbiturate anesthesia in the treatment of status epilepticus: Clinical experience with 14 patients. *Neurology* 38:395-400, 1988.

Macdonald RL, Kelly KM: Antiepileptic drug mechanisms of action. *Epilepsia* 34 (suppl 5):S1-S8, 1993.

Manford M, et al: The National General Practice Study of Epilepsy: The syndromic classification of the International League Against Epilepsy applied to epilepsy in a general population. *Arch Neurol* 49:801-808, 1992.

Matricardi M, et al: Outcome after discontinuation of antiepileptic drug therapy in children with epilepsy. *Epilepsia* 30:582-589, 1989.

Matsuo F, et al: Placebo-controlled study of the efficacy and safety of lamotrigine in patients with partial seizures. *Neurology* 43:2284-2291, 1993.

Mattson RH: Selection of antiepileptic drug therapy, in Levy RH, et al (eds): *Antiepileptic Drugs,* ed 3. New York, Raven Press, 1989, 103-116.

Mattson RH, Cramer JA: Crossover from polytherapy to monotherapy in primary generalized epilepsy. *Am J Med* 84 (suppl 1A):23-28, 1988.

Mattson RH, et al: Comparison of carbamazepine, phenobarbital, phenytoin, and primidone in partial and secondarily generalized tonic-clonic seizures. *N Engl J Med* 313:145-151, 1985.

Mattson RH, et al: Barbiturate-related connective tissue disorders. *Arch Intern Med* 149:911-914, 1989.

Mattson RH, et al: Comparison between carbamazepine and valproate for complex partial and secondarily generalized tonic clonic seizures, abstract. *Epilepsia* 32 (suppl 3):18, 1991.

McCabe RT, et al: Evidence for anticonvulsant and neuroprotectant action of felbamate mediated by strychnine-insensitive glycine receptors. *J Pharmacol Exp Ther* 264:1248-1252, 1993.

Meador KJ, et al: Comparative cognitive effects of anticonvulsants. *Neurology* 40:391-394, 1990.

Medical Research Council Antiepileptic Drug Withdrawal Study Group: Randomised study of antiepileptic drug withdrawal in patients in remission. *Lancet* 337:1175-1180, 1991.

Medical Research Council Antiepileptic Drug Withdrawal Study Group: Prognostic index for recurrence of seizures after remission of epilepsy. *BMJ* 306:1374-1378, 1993.

Messenheimer J, et al: Lamotrigine for partial seizures: A multicenter, placebo-controlled, double blind cross-over trial. *Epilepsia* 35:113-121, 1994.

Mikati MA, Browne TR: Comparative efficacy of antiepileptic drugs. *Clin Neuropharmacol* 11:130-140, 1988.

Miller RJ: Metabotropic excitatory amino acid receptors reveal their true colors. *Trends Pharmacol Sci* 12:365-367, 1991.

Milunsky A, et al: Multivitamin/folic acid supplementation in early pregnancy reduces the prevalence of neural tube defects. *JAMA* 262:2847-2852, 1989.

Mitchell WG, Chavez JM: Carbamazepine versus phenobarbital for partial onset seizures in children. *Epilepsia* 28:56-60, 1987.

Mitchell WG, et al: Effects of antiepileptic drugs on reaction time, attention, and impulsivity in children. *Pediatrics* 91:101-105, 1993.

Mizrahi EM: Neonatal seizures: Problems in diagnosis and classification. *Epilepsia* 28 (suppl 1):S46-S55, 1987.

Mizrahi EM, Kellaway P: Characterization and classification of neonatal seizures. *Neurology* 37:1837-1844, 1987.

Morrell F: The role of secondary epileptogenesis in human epilepsy, editorial. *Arch Neurol* 48:1221-1224, 1991.

MRC Vitamin Study Research Group: Prevention of neural tube defects: Results of the Medical Research Council Vitamin Study. *Lancet* 338:131-137, 1991.

Murphy JM, et al: Suppression of carbamazepine-induced rash with prednisone. *Neurology* 41:144-145, 1991.

National Institutes of Health: Consensus development conference on febrile seizures. *Epilepsia* 22:377-381, 1981.

Nau H, et al: Anticonvulsants during pregnancy and lactation: Transplacental, maternal, and neonatal pharmacokinetics. *Clin Pharmacokinet* 7:508-543, 1982.

Novotny EJ Jr: Seizures and other abnormal behavior in the newborn. *Resident Staff Physician* 36:71-74, (Nov) 1990.

Nuwer MR, et al: Generic substitutions for antiepileptic drugs. *Neurology* 40:1647-1651, 1990.

Obeid T, Panayiotopoulos CP: Clonazepam in juvenile myoclonic epilepsy. *Epilepsia* 30:603-606, 1989.

O'Brien MD, Gilmour-White S: Epilepsy and pregnancy. *BMJ* 307:492-495, 1993.

O'Dougherty M, et al: Carbamazepine plasma concentration: Relationship to cognitive impairment. *Arch Neurol* 44:863-867, 1987.

Ogunyemi AO, Dreifuss FE: Syndromes of epilepsy in childhood and adolescence. *J Child Neurol* 3:214-224, 1988.

Ojemann LM, et al: Long term treatment with gabapentin for partial seizures. *Epilepsy Res* 13:159-165, 1992.

Omtzigt JGC, et al: The risk of spina bifida aperta after first-trimester exposure to valproate in a prenatal cohort. *Neurology* 42 (suppl 5):119-125, 1992.

Overweg J, et al: Clinical and EEG prediction of seizure recurrence following antiepileptic drug withdrawal. *Epilepsy Res* 1:272-283, 1987.

Painter MJ: Phenobarbital: Clinical use, in Levy RH, et al (eds): *Antiepileptic Drugs,* ed 3. New York, Raven Press, 1989, 329-340.

Panegyres PK, Rischbieth RH: Fatal phenytoin warfarin interaction. *Postgrad Med J* 67:98, 1991.

Parks BR, et al: Weight loss in pediatric patients treated with felbamate, abstract. *Epilepsia* 34 (suppl 6):44, 1993.

Pedley TA: Discontinuing antiepileptic drugs, editorial. *N Engl J Med* 318:982-984, 1988.

Pellock JM: Carbamazepine side effects in children and adults. *Epilepsia* 28 (suppl 3):S64-S70, 1987.

Pellock JM, Willmore LJ: A rational guide to routine blood monitoring in patients receiving antiepileptic drugs, editorial. *Neurology* 41:961-964, 1991.

Pellock JM, et al: Significant differences of cognitive and behavioral effects of antiepileptic drugs in children. *Ann Neurol* 24:325-326, 1988.

Pellock JM, et al: Lamotrigine efficacy and safety update: U.S. experience, abstract. *Epilepsia* 34 (suppl 6):42, 1993.

Peterson GM, et al: Clinical response in epilepsy in relation to total and free serum levels of phenytoin. *Ther Drug Monit* 13:415-419, 1991.

Porter RJ: How to initiate and maintain carbamazepine therapy in children and adults. *Epilepsia* 28 (suppl 3):S59-S63, 1987.

Porter RJ: *Epilepsy: 100 Elementary Principles: Major Problems in Neurology.* Philadelphia, WB Saunders, 1989, vol 20.

Porter RJ, Theodore WH: Nonsedative regimens in treatment of epilepsy. *Arch Intern Med* 143:945-947, 1983.

Privitera MD: Clinical rules for phenytoin dosing. *Ann Pharmacother* 27:1169-1173, 1993.

Privitera MD, et al: Clinical utility of a bayesian dosing program for phenytoin. *Ther Drug Monit* 11:285-294, 1989.

Reincke HM, et al: High-dose lorazepam therapy for status epilepticus in a pediatric patient. *Drug Intell Clin Pharm* 22:889-890, 1988.

Remy C, et al: Intrarectal diazepam in epileptic adults. *Epilepsia* 33:353-358, 1992.

Reynolds EH: Vigabatrin: Rational treatment for chronic epilepsy. *BMJ* 300:277-278, 1990.

Reynolds EH, Shorvon SD: Single drug or combination therapy for epilepsy? *Drugs* 21:374-382, 1981.

Reynolds EH, Trimble MR: Adverse neuropsychiatric effects of anticonvulsants. *Drugs* 29:570-581, 1985.

Rho JM, et al: Felbamate inhibits NMDA responses and potentiates GABA responses in cultured rat hippocampal neurons, abstract. *Epilepsia* 34 (suppl 6):119, 1993.

Rimmer EM, Richens A: Update on sodium valproate. *Pharmacotherapy* 5:171-184, 1985.

Risner ME for Lamictal Study Group: Multicenter, double-blind, placebo-controlled, add-on crossover study of lamotrigine in epileptic outpatients with partial seizures. *Epilepsia* 31:619-620, 1990.

Rivera R, et al: Midazolam in the treatment of status epilepticus in children. *Crit Care Med* 21:991-994, 1993.

Rogawski MA: The NMDA receptor, NMDA antagonists and epilepsy therapy: A status report. *Drugs* 44:279-292, 1992.

Rosa FW: Spina bifida in infants of women treated with carbamazepine during pregnancy. *N Engl J Med* 324:674-677, 1991.

Rosman NP, et al: A controlled trial of diazepam administered during febrile illnesses to prevent recurrence of febrile seizures. *N Engl J Med* 329:79-84, 1993.

Sachdeo R, et al: Felbamate monotherapy: Controlled trial in patients with partial onset seizures. *Ann Neurol* 32:386-392, 1992.

Sato S: Clonazepam, in Levy RH, et al (eds): *Antiepileptic Drugs,* ed 3. New York, Raven Press, 1989, 765-784.

Schapel GJ, et al: Double-blind, placebo controlled, crossover study of lamotrigine in treatment resistant partial seizures. *J Neurol Neurosurg Psychiatry* 56:448-453, 1993.

Scheffner D, et al: Fatal liver failure in 16 children with valproate therapy. *Epilepsia* 29:530-542, 1988.

Scheuer ML, Pedley TA: The evaluation and treatment of seizures. *N Engl J Med* 323:1468-1474, 1990.

Schlumberger E, et al: Lamotrigine in treatment of 120 children with epilepsy. *Epilepsia* 35:359-367, 1994.

Schmidt D: Adverse effects of valproate. *Epilepsia* 25 (suppl 1):S44-S49, 1984.

Schmidt D, et al: The influence of seizure type on the efficacy of plasma concentrations of phenytoin, phenobarbital, and carbamazepine. *Arch Neurol* 43:263-265, 1986.

Shaner DM, et al: Treatment of status epilepticus: A prospective comparison of diazepam and phenytoin versus phenobarbital and optional phenytoin. *Neurology* 38:202-207, 1988.

Shen DD, et al: Low and variable presence of valproic acid in human brain. *Neurology* 42:582-585, 1992.

Shinnar S, et al: Discontinuing antiepileptic medication in children with epilepsy after two years without seizures: Prospective study. *N Engl J Med* 313:976-980, 1985.

Siemes H, et al: Therapy of infantile spasms with valproate: Results of a prospective study. *Epilepsia* 29:553-560, 1988.

Smith DB: Primidone: Clinical use, in Levy RH, et al (eds): *Antiepileptic Drugs,* ed 3. New York, Raven Press, 1989, 423-438.

Smith DB, et al: Results of a nationwide Veterans Administration Cooperative Study comparing the efficacy and toxicity of carbamazepine, phenobarbital, phenytoin, and primidone. *Epilepsia* 28(suppl 3):S50-S58, 1987.

Smith RD, et al: Pharmacology of ACC-9653 (phenytoin prodrug). *Epilepsia* 30(suppl 2):S15-S21, 1989.

Snead OC III: Treatment of infantile spasms. *Pediatr Neurol* 6:147-150, 1990.

Snead OC III, Hosey LC: Exacerbation of seizures in children by carbamazepine. *N Engl J Med* 313:916-921, 1985.

Snead OC, et al: ACTH and prednisone in childhood seizure disorders. *Neurology* 33:966-970, 1983.

Sovner R, Davis JM: A potential drug interaction between fluoxetine and valproic acid, letter. *J Clin Psychopharmacol* 11:389, (Dec) 1991.

Specht U, et al: Discontinuation of clonazepam after long-term treatment. *Epilepsia* 30:458-463, 1989.

Steriade M, Llinas RR: The functional states of the thalamus and the associated neuronal interplay. *Physiol Rev* 68:649-742, 1988.

Stewart BH, et al: A saturable transport mechanism in the intestinal absorption of gabapentin is the underlying cause of the lack of proportionality between increasing dose and drug levels in plasma. *Pharm Res* 10:276-281, 1993.

Suzuki Y, et al: Valproic acid dosages necessary to maintain therapeutic concentrations in children. *Ther Drug Monit* 13:314-317, 1991.

Taylor CP, et al: Potent and stereospecific anticonvulsant activity of 3-isobutyl GABA relates to in vitro binding at a novel site labeled by tritiated gabapentin. *Epilepsy Res* 14:11-15, 1993.

Temkin NR, et al: A randomized, double-blind study of phenytoin for the prevention of post-traumatic seizures. *N Engl J Med* 323:497-502, 1990.

Thurston JH, et al: Prognosis in childhood epilepsy: Additional follow-up of 148 children 15 to 23 years after withdrawal of anticonvulsant therapy. *N Engl J Med* 306:831-836, 1982.

Timperlake RW, et al: Effects of anticonvulsant drug therapy on bone mineral density in a pediatric population. *J Pediatr Orthopaed* 8:467-470, 1988.

Tohen M, et al: Thrombocytopenia associated with carbamazepine: A case series. *J Clin Psychiatry* 52:496-498, 1991.

Treiman DM: The role of benzodiazepines in the management of status epilepticus. *Neurology* 40(suppl 2):32-42, 1990.

Treiman DM: Generalized convulsive status epilepticus in the adult. *Epilepsia* 34(suppl 1):S2-S11, 1993.

Treiman DM, et al: Lorazepam vs phenytoin in the treatment of generalized convulsive status epilepticus: Report of an ongoing study, abstract. *Neurology* 35(suppl 1):284, 1985.

Trimble MR: Anticonvulsant drugs and cognitive function: A review of the literature. *Epilepsia* 28(suppl 3):S37-S45, 1987.

Trimble MR: Antiepileptic drugs, cognitive function, and behavior in children: Evidence from recent studies. *Epilepsia* 31(suppl 4):S30-S34, 1990.

Trimble MR, Cull C: Children of school age: The influence of antiepileptic drugs on behavior and intellect. *Epilepsia* 29(suppl 3):S15-S19, 1988.

Turnbull DM: Adverse effects of valproate. *Adv Drug React Acc Pois Rev* 2:191-216, 1983.

UK Gabapentin Study Group: Gabapentin in partial epilepsy. *Lancet* 335:1114-1117, 1990.

The US Gabapentin Study Group No. 5: Gabapentin as add-on therapy in refractory partial epilepsy: A double-blind, placebo-controlled, parallel-group study. *Neurology* 43:2292-2298, 1993.

Vining EPG, et al: Psychologic and behavioral effects of antiepileptic drugs in children: A double-blind comparison between phenobarbital and valproic acid. *Pediatrics* 80:165-174, 1987.

Volpe JJ: Neonatal seizures: Current concepts and revised classification. *Pediatrics* 84:422-428, 1989.

Wagner JG: New and simple method to predict dosage of drugs obeying simple Michaelis-Menten elimination kinetics and to distinguish such kinetics from simple first order and from parallel Michaelis-Menten and first order kinetics. *Ther Drug Monit* 7:377-386, 1985.

Wagner ML, et al: Felbamate serum concentrations: Effect of valproate, carbamazepine, phenytoin and phenobarbital, abstract. *Epilepsia* 31(suppl 6):642, 1990.

Wallis RA, et al: Protective effects of felbamate against hypoxia in the rat hippocampal slice. *Stroke* 23:547-551, 1992.

Wasterlain CG, et al: Felbamate has potent neuroprotective effects in a rat model of incomplete hypoxia-ischemia, abstract. *Epilepsia* 34(suppl 6):84, 1993.

Welty TC, et al: A comparison of phenytoin dosing methods in private practice seizure patients. *Epilepsia* 27:76-80, 1986.

White HS, et al: A neuropharmacological evaluation of felbamate as a novel anticonvulsant. *Epilepsia* 33:564-572, 1992.

Wilder BJ, Rangel RJ: Review of valproate monotherapy in the treatment of generalized tonic-clonic seizures. *Am J Med* 84(suppl 1A):7-14, 1988.

Wilder BJ, Rangel RJ: Clinical use, in Levy RH, et al (eds): *Antiepileptic Drugs,* ed 3. New York, Raven Press, 1989, 233-240.

Wilder BJ, et al: Gastrointestinal tolerance of divalproex sodium. *Neurology* 33:808-811, 1983.

Wilensky AJ, Friel PN: Clorazepate, in Levy RH, et al (eds): *Antiepileptic Drugs,* ed 3. New York, Raven Press, 1989, 805-820.

Willmore LJ, et al: Valproate toxicity: Risk-screening strategies, editorial. *J Child Neurol* 6:3-6, 1991.

Woodbury DM, et al (eds): *Antiepileptic Drugs,* ed 2. New York, Raven Press, 1982.

Working Group on Status Epilepticus: Treatment of convulsive status epilepticus: Recommendations of the Epilepsy Foundation of America's Working Group on Status Epilepticus. *JAMA* 270:854-859, 1993.

Wyllie E, et al: Pancreatitis associated with valproic acid therapy. *Am J Dis Child* 138:912-914, 1984.

Yaffe K, Lowenstein DH: Prognostic factors of pentobarbital therapy for refractory generalized status epilepticus. *Neurology* 43:895-900, 1993.

Drugs Used in Extrapyramidal Movement Disorders

16

Anatomically, the term extrapyramidal includes the central nervous system except for the corticospinal (pyramidal) tract. In current use, this term refers to "motor systems," which implies a functional unit consisting of multisynaptic neurons located in the cerebral cortex, basal ganglia and related nuclei (thalamus, subthalamus, substantia nigra), red nucleus, and parts of the reticular formation and cerebellum. Functionally, such a "system" is thoroughly intertwined with the pyramidal tract.

Many clinicians use the term "extrapyramidal disorders" as a synonym for basal ganglia disorders. Such disorders are characterized by abnormal movements and increased muscle tone (rigidity) in contrast to pyramidal (upper motor neuron) disorders, which are characterized by loss of voluntary movements, weakness, spasticity, increased stretch reflexes, and presence of the Babinski sign. Extrapyramidal movement disorders include conditions with either hyperkinetic (eg, chorea, athetosis, dystonia, ballism, myoclonus, tremors, tics) or hypokinetic (eg, akinesia, bradykinesia) symptoms.

The functional organization of the basal ganglia, of which the striatum (caudate nucleus and putamen) is the major afferent component, has undergone considerable reassessment. The caudate nucleus processes input from virtually the entire cerebral cortex. The putamen receives input primarily from the motor and premotor cortex, as well as from somatic sensory and supplementary motor areas (Leigh, 1989). Extending the boundaries of the striatum ventrally to include the nucleus accumbens and olfactory tubercle has been proposed (Alheid and Heimer, 1988). Allocortical areas project to the ventral striatum and provide a link among motor, cognitive, and affective functions of the basal ganglia. The compartmental organization of the striatum is arranged as a mosaic ("patches" and "matrix"), which differs in its neurochemical and neuroanatomical properties. The compartmental organization of corticostriatal inputs is related to both laminar and cortical areas of origin (Gerfen, 1989). The output nuclei (ie, globus pallidus interna, substantia nigra pars reticularis) transmit signals to the thalamus and, by this route, project back on the cortex resulting in the creation of multiple open and closed loops, each focused on a particular region of the frontal cortex. Topographic segregation of corticostriatal terminals is at least partially maintained in output pathways. Thus, in contrast to the classical view, the striatum appears to consist of discrete populations of projection neurons, each with relatively restricted inputs and outputs (Albin et al, 1989; Hoover and Strick, 1993). It seems likely that the diversity of symptoms and signs of movement disorders may be related to involvement of topographically and functionally discrete populations of striatal, pallidal, subthalamic, and nigral neurons (Leigh, 1989).

PARKINSON'S DISEASE

Idiopathic Parkinson's disease has generally been considered to be a nonhereditary, progressive, neurologic disorder of the extrapyramidal system, although reports of small familial clusters and two kindreds with autosomal dominant disease have appeared in the literature (Golbe et al, 1990; Waters and Miller, 1994). Based on reanalysis of twin studies, emerging evidence of mitochondrial enzyme dysfunction in patients with Parkinson's disease, and preliminary findings with use of positron emission tomography to detect preclinical manifestations in unaffected twins, some investigators believe that genetic factors may play a more important role than previously recognized (Brooks, 1991; Johnson, 1991; Burn et al, 1992; Sawle et al, 1992; Lazzarini et al, 1994).

Neuropathologically, loss of pigmented neurons in the substantia nigra and the presence of intraneuronal inclusion bodies (Lewy bodies) are apparent. The etiology of Parkinson's disease is still unknown. Extrapyramidal manifestations result largely from a deficiency of dopamine in the putamen and, to a lesser degree, in the caudate nucleus that is caused by degeneration of the dopaminergic nigrostriatal pathway. Degeneration also may occur in the dopaminergic mesocortical, mesolimbic, and hypothalamic pathways, noradrenergic locus coeruleus, the dorsal motor nucleus of the vagus, and cholinergic nucleus basalis, all of which probably contribute to clinical dysfunction.

The discovery that the parkinsonian symptoms observed in some drug addicts were caused by 1-methyl-4-phenyl-1, 2, 3, 6-tetrahydropyridine (MPTP), a neurotoxic byproduct of the synthesis of some meperidine analogues, has stimulated research on the underlying mechanism of Parkinson's disease. MPTP is metabolized to MPP+ by monoamine oxidase type B in a two-stage process; MPP+ accumulates in and destroys dopaminergic neurons in the substantia nigra. The cytotoxicity is probably related to impairment of mitochondrial respiration via inhibition of complex I (Sayre, 1989). In patients with Parkinson's disease, defects in mitochondrial oxidative phosphorylation have been detected in the substantia nigra and, in some studies, in platelets and skeletal muscle (Parker et al, 1989; Schapira et al, 1990; Shoffner et al, 1991).

Delineation of the mode of action of MPTP has led to speculation about the possible role of environmental substances in the etiology of Parkinson's disease, but results of epidemiologic studies are equivocal. Some possible positive associations with Parkinson's disease include rural residence, use of private well water, agricultural occupation, and exposure to pesticides or herbicides; an inverse association has been noted between Parkinson's disease and cigarette smoking (Butterfield et al, 1993).

Attention also has focused on the role of "oxidative stress" as an important neuropathologic factor (for reviews, see Olanow, 1990; Furtado and Mazurek, 1991). This theory suggests that an interplay of dopamine oxidation, formation of hydrogen peroxide, deficient protective mechanisms (eg, glutathione, glutathione peroxidase), and elevated iron (with decreased ferritin buffering) and increased neuromelanin concentrations in the brains of parkinsonian patients may increase the generation of free radicals leading to lipid peroxidation of membranes and accelerated neuronal cell death.

In addition to the classic motor abnormalities (resting tremor, cogwheel rigidity, bradykinesia, loss of normal postural reflexes, and impaired gait), patients with Parkinson's disease often perform poorly on many neuropsychological tests. Because some of these tests do not distinguish between motor and mental impairments, the extent of cognitive dysfunction may be difficult to determine. Nevertheless, multiple mild cognitive defects have been identified in areas of memory, language, problem-solving, perceptual motor, and visuospatial skills (Gibb, 1989). These neuropsychological deficits may result from disruption of basal ganglia and frontal lobe interactions, but they are distinct from global dementia. Results of some studies indicate that the incidence of moderate to severe dementia in these patients is 10% to 25% or approximately twice that in the general population (Gibb, 1989; Ebmeier et al, 1991). Cognitive slowing (bradyphrenia), motor impairment, and depression are closely related in patients with Parkinson's disease (Starkstein et al, 1990). Depression occurs in approximately 40% of these individuals and may require specific treatment with antidepressant agents (Dooneief et al, 1992; Cummings, 1992). Impaired speech, gastrointestinal dysfunction (sialorrhea, dysphagia, impaired gastric emptying, constipation), and seborrheic dermatitis also are present in some patients with Parkinson's disease (Edwards et al, 1992).

It is important to recognize that the neurologic signs produced by Parkinson's disease may be difficult to differentiate from those produced by a variety of less common neurodegenerative disorders (eg, progressive supranuclear palsy and the multiple system atrophies, striatonigral degeneration, Shy-Drager syndrome). Certain drugs (eg, neuroleptic agents, metoclopramide, reserpine), toxins (eg, MPTP, manganese, carbon disulfide), metabolic disorders (eg, Wilson's disease), and encephalitis (eg, postencephalitic parkinsonism) also may produce symptoms resembling those of Parkinson's disease (Jankovic, 1989). In addition, case reports suggest that verapamil and fluoxetine may unmask or intensify symptoms in some patients with Parkinson's disease (García-Albea et al, 1993; Steur, 1993).

Management must be individualized. The goal of therapy for Parkinson's disease is to relieve functional disability with the lowest dosage of antiparkinsonian medication possible. The patient's ability to carry out daily activities, such as arising from a bed or chair, walking, dressing, eating, and working, should serve as the primary determinant for dosage adjustments. Impairment of these functional capabilities generally is manifested as bradykinesia, gait disturbance, and postural instability. Other parkinsonian signs, such as tremor and rigidity, may be less disabling. Therapy is symptomatic, not curative, and it is directed toward replenishing striatal dopamine or stimulating striatal dopamine receptors.

Although pharmacotherapy is the basis for the management of Parkinson's disease, nondrug measures also are important. Exercise, physical therapy, and psychotherapy may be beneficial. Family support and involvement are important for optimal care.

Drug Selection

The choice of drugs (see Table 1) is based principally on the severity of the disease and may change as a result of the

TABLE 1. DRUGS USED IN THE MANAGEMENT OF PARKINSON'S DISEASE

Drugs	Comment
EARLY STAGES OF DISEASE	
Selegiline [Eldepryl]	Use in newly diagnosed patients *may* slow progression of the clinical disease and delay the requirement for levodopa therapy. This strategy is used for protective rather than symptomatic purposes, although a slight symptomatic effect may be observed.
Anticholinergic Agents Benztropine [Cogentin] Biperiden [Akineton] Diphenhydramine [Benadryl] Procyclidine [Kemadrin] Trihexyphenidyl [Artane]	If symptoms are mild, symptomatic drug therapy may not be necessary. If treatment is elected, an anticholinergic may be useful in younger patients and in those in whom tremor is the major complaint. Because of age-related central nervous system adverse reactions, these drugs are used with caution in the elderly.
Amantadine [Symmetrel]	When bradykinesia is the major symptom and patients have only mild disability, some neurologists consider use of amantadine to be beneficial; signs and symptoms may improve temporarily in many patients.
ONSET OF DISABILITY*	
Levodopa and Carbidopa [Atamet, Sinemet, Sinemet CR, generic] Levodopa [Dopar, Larodopa] Dopamine Receptor Agonists Bromocriptine [Parlodel] Pergolide [Permax] Selegiline [Eldepryl] Amantadine [Symmetrel] Anticholinergic Agents	Levodopa therapy is the most effective treatment and is usually begun when disability threatens employment or a reasonable lifestyle. The combination of levodopa/carbidopa is preferred. Dosage should be individualized so that the minimal amount that will allow performance of daily activities can be determined. Amantadine, anticholinergic drugs, dopamine agonists, and/or selegiline may be given concomitantly; the latter *may* slow progression of the disease. After one to five years of levodopa therapy, problems such as early morning akinesia, "wearing off" of drug effect, and peak-dose dyskinesias often occur. Substitution of the prolonged-release preparation [Sinemet CR], manipulation of the levodopa dosage regimen, and/or adjunctive use of dopamine agonists often is helpful. Use of selegiline may prolong the duration of levodopa's effects and increase "on" time. Early combination therapy with levodopa and dopamine agonists may decrease the prevalence of later motor complications. Some neurologists advocate an initial trial of a dopamine agonist followed by introduction of levodopa. See text for further discussion.
ADVANCED DISEASE	
Levodopa and Carbidopa [Atamet, Sinemet, Sinemet CR, generic] Levodopa [Dopar, Larodopa] Dopamine Receptor Agonists Bromocriptine [Parlodel] Pergolide [Permax] Amantadine [Symmetrel] Selegiline [Eldepryl]	More complex motor fluctuations may develop in association with chronic levodopa therapy; these include "on-off" fluctuations, start hesitation, "freezing," and diphasic dyskinesias. Rapid and unpredictable motor fluctuations are less responsive to dosage changes. Adjunctive use of a direct-acting dopamine agonist may enhance efficacy and decrease dyskinesia and motor fluctuations. Amantadine and selegiline also may be used adjunctively but usually are less beneficial in patients with advanced disease.

** The degree of disability requiring the use of levodopa will vary according to the occupational, social, and subjective needs of the patient.*

disease's progression or the patient's ability to tolerate adverse reactions (Calne, 1993; Stacy and Jankovic, 1993; *Med Lett Drugs Ther,* 1993).

Early Stages: In the early stages of Parkinson's disease, asymmetrical tremor and bradykinesia may predominate, and medication for symptomatic relief usually is not required if the patient functions relatively well.

Anticholinergic drugs are useful in some individuals, especially younger patients who will require long-term therapy and those who are particularly troubled by tremor. Tremor, rigidity, and drooling may be diminished by anticholinergic drugs, but bradykinesia and loss of postural reflexes are less responsive. The benefit of these drugs can be temporary or long lasting but may be additive at any stage of disease. Unfortunately, their use often is associated with significant central nervous system side effects (ie, memory loss, confusion, paranoia, hallucinations) and autonomic effects (constipation, urinary retention), particularly in older patients, in whom they should be used with great caution.

When tremor is not predominant, some neurologists prescribe amantadine [Symmetrel] for patients with mild disability; this drug may relieve signs and symptoms for limited periods. Because amantadine is excreted primarily unchanged by the kidney, the renal function of older patients should be monitored to prevent toxicity. The combination of amantadine and an anticholinergic drug may have additive therapeutic and adverse effects.

A variety of oxidative mechanisms involving the activity of monoamine oxidase and the formation of free radicals have been implicated in the degeneration of neurons in the substantia nigra. The possible pathogenic role of such mechanisms and evidence that the neurotoxin, MPTP, requires enzymatic activation by monamine oxidase B (MAO-B) led to clinical trials on therapy designed to slow the progression of clinical disability in Parkinson's disease (Parkinson Study Group, 1989). In patients with early, untreated disease, selegiline 10 mg/day was found to delay the onset of disability requiring levodopa therapy by approximately nine months, whereas tocopherol (vitamin E) 2,000 IU/day had no effect (The Parkinson Study Group, 1993). (The lack of results with vitamin E are in contrast to those reported in an uncontrolled pilot study [Fahn, 1989].)

Selegiline's mechanism of action in delaying progression of disability is unclear. This drug modestly improved clinical ratings of patients with Parkinson's disease during the first three months of therapy, and in some individuals motor performance worsened slightly after it was withdrawn at the end of the study. Results of other small controlled studies also have attributed minor symptomatic improvement to selegiline (Tetrud and Langston, 1989; Teravainen, 1990; Myllylä et al, 1992). Although the observed benefit of selegiline in delaying disability is at least partly due to symptomatic improvement, the degree of improvement is unlikely to be significant enough to be perceived as beneficial by most patients. Furthermore, this "delay" in the requirement for levodopa must be balanced with the expense of the drug. In addition, use of selegiline may provoke anxiety in some patients, which can exacerbate tremor.

It is not known whether selegiline affects the neuropathology of Parkinson's disease. Whether this agent or other antioxidants may be beneficial in patients with presymptomatic disease has not been studied. In contrast to an earlier recommendation that untreated patients with early Parkinson's disease receive selegiline (Parkinson Study Group, 1989), final results of the DATATOP indicate that the scientific basis for its use as a neuroprotectant is tenuous.

Onset of Disability: Levodopa is the most effective drug to relieve symptoms of Parkinson's disease, especially bradykinesia and rigidity. Tremor may be refractory to levodopa. Patients who are beginning to experience symptoms that interfere with daily activities usually are given levodopa combined with carbidopa, a peripheral decarboxylase inhibitor. Either the standard [Atamet, Sinemet, generic] or prolonged-release formulation [Sinemet CR] is prescribed. These preparations contain carbidopa and levodopa in a ratio of 1:4 or 1:10 and are preferred to levodopa alone because more levodopa is available to penetrate the central nervous system and the peripheral adverse reactions of the latter, especially nausea and vomiting, are minimized. (See the evaluation.) Another combination, which contains the decarboxylase inhibitor, benserazide, and levodopa in a ratio of 1:4, is used widely in Europe [Madopar] and Canada [Prolopa].

The lowest effective dosage of levodopa that permits adequate performance of daily activities and provides patient comfort should be administered (Kurlan, 1987; Ahlskog and Wilkinson, 1990). Unless side effects intervene, many neurologists advocate that the dosage of carbidopa/levodopa be increased to the level that is most beneficial. Therapeutic effects should be ascertained on the basis of repeated examinations by the physician rather than on subjective reports by the patient. Those who are depressed may deny any benefit even though improvement is apparent on examination. Dosage requirements vary from patient to patient, but optimal control typically is achieved with a daily levodopa (in combination with carbidopa) dosage of 300 to 600 mg administered in three or four divided doses. Clinical response generally is quite satisfactory in Parkinson's disease of recent onset, and a poor response to therapy should raise the possibility that the patient has another neurologic disorder with parkinsonian features. Newly diagnosed patients who have not responded to 1.2 g daily over a period of two to three months probably do not have Parkinson's disease (Ahlskog and Wilkinson, 1990).

Fluctuations in motor function and dyskinesias in response to levodopa emerge gradually and affect more than one-half of patients within five years after initiation of therapy. The dyskinesias often occur at peak plasma concentrations of levodopa and take the form of chorea but dystonia also is common. Some patients experience painful dystonia that occurs when the antiparkinsonian effects of levodopa are not apparent, most commonly in the morning when the patient has been without medication overnight; hence, the term "early-morning dystonia" is sometimes used. Symptoms that recur in the afternoon or significant early-morning akinesia may necessitate the use of an additional dose. In later stages, a clear pattern of end-of-dose deterioration ("wearing off" effect) may develop. The fluctuations can be lessened by shortening the dosage intervals; sometimes individual doses also may have to be reduced with possible loss of efficacy. Alternatively, Sinemet CR may be substituted. The more uniform delivery of levodopa with use of this formulation may reduce clinical fluctuations, particularly in patients with simple "wearing off." Based on the hypothesis that some of these later-stage motor complications occur secondary to postsynaptic changes induced by *intermittent* stimulation of dopamine receptors, studies are underway to determine whether administration of Sinemet CR initially may decrease the incidence of fluctuations and dyskinesias during long-term therapy.

The addition of dopamine receptor agonists (bromocriptine [Parlodel], pergolide [Permax]) also may alleviate these hypokinetic manifestations, especially if manipulation of the levodopa dosage regimen is inadequate. Some neurologists advocate an initial trial of a dopamine agonist followed by introduction of levodopa or early combination therapy (see the section on Dopamine Receptor Agonists).

Although the relatively specific type B monoamine oxidase inhibitor, selegiline, generally produces no perceptible benefits when used without levodopa in patients who are experiencing significant symptoms, it may prolong the action of dopamine. Clinical evaluation of its effectiveness as an adjunct to levodopa/carbidopa has indicated that selegiline ameliorates the "wearing-off" of levodopa's effects in 50% to 70% of patients, and a 10% to 30% reduction in levodopa dosage is usually possible (Golbe, 1988). Amantadine and/or anticholinergic drugs may be given as well in an attempt to enhance control, although at this stage they may provide only minimal benefit and can provoke significant side effects.

Advanced Disease: Once patients begin experiencing "wearing off" effects, the required dosage interval for levodopa generally continues to shorten, and eventually more complex response variations may develop. Patients may alternate between periods of good mobility ("on" time), often accompanied by dyskinesias, and periods of immobility with painful dystonia in some patients ("off" time). The dyskinesias may occur primarily at the time of greatest improvement in mobility ("peak dose") or, less commonly, they may be diphasic, emerging immediately before levodopa's therapeutic effect occurs and reappearing prior to loss of therapeutic benefit. Rarely, one-half of the body may be "on" and dyskinetic, while parkinsonian symptoms persist in the other half. The addition of dopamine agonists can decrease the incidence of fluctuations, dyskinesias, and dystonia, although effectiveness decreases with time. These adjunctive medications also may have adverse mental effects or may exacerbate dyskinesias, especially if the dose of levodopa is not decreased.

In some patients, "freezing" (sudden onset of short-stepped gait or inability to walk) may occur. This generally is regarded as a component of Parkinson's disease. It is unrelated to treatment and, in some patients, may develop earlier in the course of the disease. Episodes may be associated with activities other than walking. Patients also may experience "start hesitation" (eg, after standing), which is characterized by prolonged hesitation before taking a first step followed by the sudden onset of a short-stepped gait. Similar disturbances in gait are commonly observed when changing direction or turning. Different types of motor fluctuations can appear in the same patient. These symptoms differ from the "off" periods that occur during motor fluctuations and that respond to dopaminergic drugs. However, those patients who have freezing in the "off" periods will respond to changes in drug regimens that are designed to lessen the motor fluctuations. Other patients experience freezing in the "on" or "off" periods. "On" period freezing generally is not relieved, and may be aggravated, by levodopa (Obeso et al, 1989).

The final type of motor problem associated with levodopa therapy in advanced Parkinson's disease is diminution of efficacy; this is secondary to progression of the underlying disease. Although complete lack of responsiveness rarely occurs even after 20 years of treatment, the quality of motor response deteriorates and symptoms appear that do not respond to levodopa therapy (eg, postural instability, speech dysfunction, freezing). Dyskinesias occurring in response to dopaminergic drugs may further impair function, and side effects (eg, hallucinations, confusion) may prevent administration of full therapeutic doses. Formerly, some authorities recommended hospitalization with temporary supervised withdrawal of levodopa in an effort to eliminate or reduce adverse drug effects (eg, hallucinations) and to reverse down-regulation of dopamine receptors, thus restoring the effectiveness of levodopa (Direnfeld et al, 1980; Weiner et al, 1980). However, many patients become extremely akinetic and are essentially paralyzed when levodopa is withdrawn completely. These patients are at risk for aspiration pneumonia and pulmonary emboli. Since benefits gained by this maneuver last no more than a few months, its primary use is limited to the relief of specific (usually psychiatric) toxicity (Kurlan et al, 1994).

Prevention and Management of Fluctuations in Motor Performance

Although levodopa in combination with a dopa decarboxylase inhibitor is the most effective symptomatic treatment for patients with Parkinson's disease, long-term therapy often is associated with oscillations in motor performance, emergence of involuntary movements, and psychotoxicity. Most treatment regimens developed to alleviate these problems (ie, changes in dose or dosage interval; adjunctive use of dopamine agonists, selegiline) were designed to manage complications after they become manifest. Measures to forestall levodopa-associated complications now are being studied.

Some neurologists believe that progression of Parkinson's disease and development of adverse reactions correlate with the duration and/or cumulative dosage of levodopa (Lesser et al, 1979; Fahn and Bressman, 1984; Melamed, 1986; de Jong et al, 1987), and they recommend that this drug not be used until patients develop significant functional disability. Those opposing this view believe that late management problems with levodopa result from progression of the disease (Markham and Diamond, 1986; Muenter, 1984) and thus therapy should begin earlier. Results of several longitudinal studies indicate that levodopa prolongs life expectancy and reduces disability in patients with Parkinson's disease. In addition, the results of several retrospective studies (Roos et al, 1990; Caraceni et al, 1991; Cedarbaum et al, 1991) are consistent with the hypothesis that motor fluctuations are due to progression of the disease rather than to effects attributable to levodopa. In practice, most clinicians initiate levodopa therapy on the basis of degree of disability and the social and occupational needs of the patient. If symptoms preclude a normal work or social life, it is generally agreed that levodopa therapy is indicated.

Some data indicate that so-called low-dose levodopa therapy is associated with a lower incidence of motor fluctuations (Rajput et al, 1984; Poewe et al, 1988). Clinical observations, but not controlled studies, suggest that early combination therapy (ie, a dopamine agonist and levodopa) induces a motor response similar to that of levodopa monotherapy (while utilizing lower doses of levodopa) and dyskinesias and motor fluctuations are lessened (Rinne, 1987; Kurlan, 1988). For example, therapy is initiated with levodopa/carbidopa and the dosage adjusted as needed to supply 300 to 600 mg of levodopa daily. If further dopaminergic therapy is required, bromocriptine or pergolide is gradually added to the regimen in stepwise fashion. Most patients require 20 mg/day or less of bromocriptine. Alternatively, some neurologists initiate therapy with bromocriptine or pergolide and add levodopa later as needed. Although the use of bromocriptine as initial dopaminergic therapy may be associated with a lower incidence of fluctuations in response, the control of Parkinson's disease is generally less than that obtainable with levodopa and the potential value of this approach in most patients is limited (Hely et al, 1989; Montastruc et al, 1989; Parkinson's Disease Research Group in the United Kingdom, 1993).

Since use of a dopamine agonist with levodopa offers no immediate symptomatic benefit compared with levodopa alone in patients with Parkinson's disease of recent onset, further prospective evaluation is required to determine whether long-term benefits (ie, slower rate of disease progression) are sufficient to warrant the expense and potential adverse effects of this combination therapy for early treatment (Zimmerman and Sage, 1991). The major indications for dopamine agonists currently are as adjuncts to levodopa early in therapy and for patients experiencing problems with long-term levodopa therapy.

Because motor fluctuations and dyskinesias develop primarily in patients with advanced Parkinson's disease and long-term exposure to levodopa, they may be related to *both* natural disease progression and the pharmacokinetics and pharmacodynamics of levodopa (Nutt, 1990). It is hypothesized that progressive degeneration of dopaminergic terminals diminishes central dopamine synthesis capability and storage capacity (ie, "buffering ability") and renders the striatum dependent on minute-to-minute variations in levodopa delivery. Erratic gastric emptying of levodopa and competition between the drug and dietary amino acids for cerebral transport are two factors that might interfere with steady delivery of levodopa to the brain. Redistribution of protein in the diet ($\leq$7 g prior to the evening meal) may benefit some patients with motor fluctuations, presumably by limiting competition between levodopa and dietary amino acids for transport across the blood-brain barrier (Pincus and Barry, 1987). Therefore, patients should understand the relationship between dietary protein and levodopa. Administration of levodopa on an empty stomach and avoidance of high-protein meals, especially before social events and physical activities, can enhance the response (Ahlskog and Wilkinson, 1990).

The relevance of peripheral levodopa pharmacokinetics to motor fluctuations following oral ingestion is emphasized by the finding that prompt correction of wearing-off fluctuations can be achieved by continuous intravenous infusion of levodopa (Chase et al, 1989; Mouradian et al, 1990). "Off" episodes are rarely observed with continuous infusion if the dosage is well above the motor threshold, but dyskinesias usually occur (Marion et al, 1986). Thus, drugs or strategies capable of providing a relatively constant level of central dopamine receptor stimulation may minimize wearing-off phenomena and mitigate on-off fluctuations.

Considerable experience has been obtained with Sinemet CR (Duvoisin, 1989). In patients without motor fluctuations, Sinemet CR may produce the same therapeutic benefit as the standard preparation, but less frequent dosing is required. The prolonged-release formulation may be most beneficial in (1) patients with simple wearing-off problems who had been on a complex Sinemet regimen, or (2) a subgroup of patients who experience a short duration of response to Sinemet and have less severe motor fluctuations (Factor et al, 1989). In those with mild to moderate disease, conversion from a standard preparation to Sinemet CR increases the amount but decreases the number of daily doses. In some patients, early morning dystonia resolves, "off" time is decreased, and sleep is improved (Pahwa et al, 1993).

Fewer patients with moderate to severe motor fluctuations experience quantitatively significant reductions in "off-time" compared with those taking standard Sinemet, but the safety profile of the two forms is similar (Hutton et al, 1989). In one study, the percentage of "on" time remained stable for at least three years with Sinemet CR, although this was associated (as with standard preparations) with an increase in dyskinesias (Hutton and Morris, 1991). The onset of action of Sinemet CR tends to be slow, especially in the morning. In one study, the bioavailability of Sinemet CR was lowest when it was administered after fasting overnight (Wilding et al, 1991); therefore, some patients receiving Sinemet CR may require a dose of a standard preparation in the morning (ie, first daily dose) in order to achieve a satisfactory (ie, faster) onset of action. The bioavailability of Sinemet CR is approximately 30% less than that of levodopa.

In patients with established fluctuations in response to levodopa, drugs that would rapidly reverse "off" periods would be very useful. One investigational approach to management includes the use of continuous intraduodenal administration of levodopa (Kurlan, 1990). Results of an open pilot study on four patients experiencing severe motor fluctuations suggest that oral administration of an infusion solution containing levodopa, carbidopa, and ascorbic acid at timed intervals reduces bradykinesia, decreases dyskinesias, and increases functional "on" time compared with use of the tablet formulations (Kurth et al, 1993). Subcutaneous or sublingual administration of apomorphine also has been employed (Lees, 1989). In some patients, injection of single doses of apomorphine (not available in the United States) produces motor responses comparable to those produced by levodopa (Kempster et al, 1990). Intermittent subcutaneous injection or continuous infusion and sublingual or intranasal delivery have been effective in reducing incapacitating "off" periods (Stibe et al, 1988;

Poewe et al, 1988; Kempster et al, 1991; van Laar et al, 1992; Durif et al, 1993; Deffond et al, 1993).

Drug Evaluations

ANTICHOLINERGIC AGENTS

ACTIONS AND USES. The efficacy of these drugs in Parkinson's disease is limited and appears to be related to their central muscarinic cholinergic blocking action. Inhibition of dopamine reuptake into presynaptic nerve terminals also may be involved. Anticholinergic medications appear most helpful early in the course of Parkinson's disease, particularly in younger patients who have minimal disability but are bothered by prominent resting tremor. Anticholinergic drugs also may be useful in patients with drooling.

The belladonna alkaloids, atropine and scopolamine, were the first of these agents to be used in Parkinson's disease. They now have been replaced by synthetic drugs that are equally effective but produce fewer peripheral side effects. The synthetic drugs include the piperidyl compounds (trihexyphenidyl [Artane]), their analogues (biperiden [Akineton], procyclidine [Kemadrin]), and the tropanol derivative, benztropine [Cogentin]. The antihistamine, diphenhydramine [Benadryl], also has some antiparkinsonian activity attributable to its anticholinergic properties. The durations of action of these anticholinergic drugs differ, and patients may tolerate one drug better than another. Otherwise, none has any advantages over the others.

Trihexyphenidyl, biperiden, or benztropine is usually preferred. Diphenhydramine is used primarily as an adjunct; however, it may be used alone for initial therapy in mild Parkinson's disease and for adjunctive therapy in elderly patients who cannot tolerate the more potent anticholinergic drugs.

After long-term administration of anticholinergic agents, patients frequently become refractory to their effects. Increasing the dose or substituting a drug from another class sometimes restores responsiveness.

ADVERSE REACTIONS AND PRECAUTIONS. Most untoward effects are related to the peripheral or central cholinergic blocking activity of these drugs. Adverse reactions occur least often with diphenhydramine because of its milder anticholinergic activity. However, some undesirable effects can be expected when therapeutic doses of any of these agents are administered, particularly in the elderly. Thus, these agents are used primarily in younger patients.

Adverse reactions are common and include dryness of the mouth, mydriasis, cycloplegia, tachycardia, constipation, urinary retention, and psychiatric disturbances. Dry mouth may contribute to chewing, swallowing, or speech difficulties. Patients with prostatic hypertrophy should be observed carefully for signs of urinary retention, and those with hypomotile gastrointestinal disorders should be monitored for signs of constipation or intestinal obstruction. A decrease in the rate of gastric emptying may contribute to erratic absorption of other drugs. Fatal adynamic ileus has occurred in patients receiving combinations of drugs with anticholinergic properties. It should be remembered that amantadine also has significant anticholinergic effects. Patients with a tendency to develop tachycardia should receive the smallest effective dose. Anticholinergic agents inhibit sweating, thus reducing the ability of the body to dissipate heat. Large doses can markedly elevate body temperature.

Because of their mydriatic effect, anticholinergic drugs can precipitate an attack of acute glaucoma in patients predisposed to angle closure. This has occurred occasionally after parenteral administration but only rarely after oral use. As a rule, anticholinergic drugs can be given safely to patients with open-angle glaucoma who are receiving miotics. Reduced accommodation may contribute to dizziness.

Confusion, excitement, impaired memory, and mental slowing may occur in susceptible patients (eg, the elderly, patients with dementia, those taking tricyclic antidepressants with anticholinergic activity). More serious mental disturbances (agitation, disorientation, delirium, paranoid reaction, and hallucinations) are usually drug-induced and do not represent an intensification of the existing symptoms of Parkinson's disease. Anticholinergic drugs occasionally cause dyskinesias but more often exacerbate levodopa-induced dyskinesias.

Great care must be taken when administering anticholinergic agents to elderly patients, especially those with any degree of dementia (Kurlan and Como, 1988). Many neurologists avoid their use in these patients because of possible mental changes and other adverse effects. Anticholinergic drug-induced impairment of memory is very common in this group, and the mental changes can be mistaken for dementia. Susceptible patients should be observed carefully. In one comparative study, benztropine (but not amantadine) impaired memory and perception (Gelenberg et al, 1989).

Diphenhydramine also has adverse effects unrelated to its anticholinergic action. Drowsiness and dizziness are common with therapeutic doses. Anorexia, nausea, and vomiting may occur. Other reactions reported occasionally include euphoria, hypotension, headache, weakness, tingling, and heaviness of the hands.

DOSAGE AND PREPARATIONS. Therapy with anticholinergic drugs should be initiated with a small amount that is increased gradually until satisfactory benefits are attained or unacceptable untoward effects occur. Younger patients and those with postencephalitic parkinsonism tolerate these drugs better than older patients with idiopathic Parkinson's disease. If the anticholinergic drug must be discontinued, a stepwise reduction of dose should be employed (unless acute toxicity occurs) to avoid exacerbating parkinsonian symptoms. This exacerbation may be marked and out of proportion to the apparent benefit achieved when anticholinergic therapy was initiated.

See Table 2 for dosage and preparations.

TABLE 2.
CENTRALLY ACTIVE ANTICHOLINERGIC DRUGS

Drug and Chemical Structure	Usual Dosage	Preparations
PIPERIDYL COMPOUNDS		
Biperiden Hydrochloride	*Oral:* For Parkinson's disease and postencephalitic parkinsonism, *adults,* initially, 2 mg three times daily. The dose may be gradually increased up to 16 mg daily if required and tolerated. For drug-induced extrapyramidal reactions, *adults,* 2 mg one to three times daily.	*Akineton* (Knoll). Tablets 2 mg.
Procyclidine Hydrochloride	*Oral:* For Parkinson's disease and postencephalitic parkinsonism, *adults,* initially, 2.5 mg three times daily after meals. The dose may be increased gradually to 20 to 30 mg daily if required and tolerated. For drug-induced extrapyramidal reactions, except tardive dyskinesia, *adults,* initially, 2.5 mg three times daily. The dose then may be increased by 2.5 mg daily until symptoms are controlled. Generally, symptomatic relief is obtained with 10 to 20 mg daily.	*Kemadrin* (Burroughs Wellcome). Tablets 5 mg.
Trihexyphenidyl Hydrochloride	*Oral:* (Tablets or elixir is preferred, as the efficacy of prolonged-release capsules has not been established.) For Parkinson's disease and postencephalitic parkinsonism, *adults,* initially, 2 mg two or three times daily. The dose is gradually increased until the desired therapeutic effect is obtained or until severe adverse reactions preclude a further increase. Doses larger than 10 to 20 mg daily are rarely required or tolerated and are not recommended for Parkinson's disease. Larger doses have been used for patients with dystonia. For drug-induced extrapyramidal reactions, except tardive dyskinesia, *adults,* initially, 1 mg. If symptoms are not controlled within a few hours, subsequent doses are increased until symptoms subside. The usual total daily dose is 5 to 15 mg.	*Generic.* Tablets 2 and 5 mg. *Artane* (Lederle). Capsules (prolonged-release) 5 mg; elixir 2 mg/5 ml; tablets 2 and 5 mg.
TROPANOL DERIVATIVE		
Benztropine Mesylate	*Oral:* For Parkinson's disease and postencephalitic parkinsonism, *adults,* initially, 0.5 to 1 mg at bedtime. Patients with postencephalitic parkinsonism often tolerate an initial dosage of 2 mg/day, administered in single or divided doses. The dosage may be gradually increased to 4 to 6 mg daily if required and tolerated. *Oral, Intramuscular, Intravenous:* For drug-induced extrapyramidal reactions, except tardive dyskinesia, *adults,* 1 to 4 mg once or twice daily. In acute dystonic reactions, initially, 1 to 2 mg intramuscularly or intravenously; to prevent recurrence, 1 to 2 mg orally twice daily.	*Generic.* Tablets 0.5, 1, and 2 mg. *Cogentin* (Merck). Tablets 0.5, 1, and 2 mg; solution (for injection) 1 mg/ml in 2 ml containers.

(table continued on next page)

TABLE 2 (continued)

Drug and Chemical Structure	Usual Dosage	Preparations
ANTIHISTAMINE		
Diphenhydramine Hydrochloride	*Oral:* For Parkinson's disease and postencephalitic parkinsonism, *adults,* initially, 25 mg three times daily. The dosage may be gradually increased to 50 mg four times daily if required. For extrapyramidal reactions, *children,* 5 mg/kg daily in divided doses at six-hour intervals.	*Generic.* Capsules, tablets 25 and 50 mg; elixir, syrup 12.5 mg/5 ml (without alcohol). *Benadryl* (Parke-Davis). Capsules 25 and 50 mg; elixir 12.5 mg/5 ml (alcohol 5.6%); tablets 25 mg.
$(C_6H_5)_2CH\text{–}OCH_2CH_2\overset{+}{N}H(CH_3)_2\ Cl^-$	*Intramuscular (deep), Intravenous:* For drug-induced extrapyramidal reactions, except tardive dyskinesia, *adults,* 10 to 50 mg. The maximal single dose is 100 mg and the total daily dose should not exceed 400 mg. *Children* (intramuscular), 5 mg/kg daily. The maximal daily dose should not exceed 300 mg in 24 hours.	*Generic.* Solution (for injection) 10 and 50 mg/ml. *Benadryl* (Parke-Davis). Solution (for injection) 10 mg/ml in 10 and 30 ml containers and 50 mg/ml in 1 and 10 ml containers.

DRUGS AFFECTING BRAIN DOPAMINE

AMANTADINE HYDROCHLORIDE
[Symmetrel]

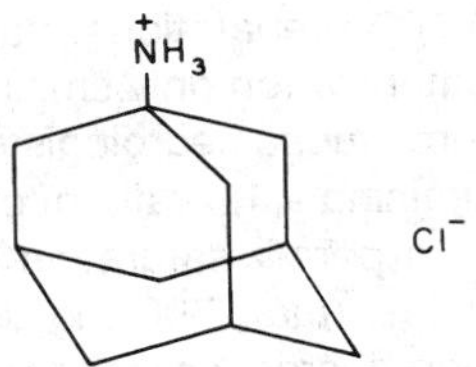

ACTIONS AND USES. This antiviral agent reduces signs and symptoms and improves functional capacity in some patients with Parkinson's disease. Its precise mechanism of action is not established. Amantadine is believed to act by augmenting the release of dopamine from neurons, by delaying the reuptake of dopamine into the presynaptic terminal, and by exerting anticholinergic effects. It also may be a weak dopamine receptor agonist.

Amantadine may be effective when used alone for initial therapy in patients with mild disability, but it also is useful when given with anticholinergic drugs or as adjunctive therapy with levodopa in some individuals who cannot tolerate maximally effective doses of levodopa or in whom the response to levodopa fluctuates. Amantadine is much less effective than levodopa, although a small proportion of patients may have a striking initial response. Initial clinical improvement may not be sustained, and performance may deteriorate after three to six months.

ADVERSE REACTIONS AND PRECAUTIONS. Amantadine is usually well tolerated. Some adverse effects are similar to those produced by anticholinergic agents: changes in mood, dizziness, nervousness, inability to concentrate, ataxia, slurred speech, insomnia, lethargy, blurred vision, urinary retention, dryness of the mouth, gastrointestinal hypomotility, and rash.

Some patients develop difficulty in thinking, confusion, lightheadedness, hallucinations, and anxiety. These symptoms are usually mild, occur shortly after therapy is initiated, are reversible following withdrawal of the drug, and often cease even when administration is continued. Activities requiring mental alertness (eg, driving) should be avoided until it is reasonable to assume that this cluster of symptoms will not recur.

Livedo reticularis (mottling of the skin) is relatively common in patients (particularly women) receiving amantadine for one month or longer. This reaction may subside during continued administration but can persist throughout therapy. It disappears gradually within days or weeks after amantadine is discontinued. There is no association between livedo reticularis and any underlying systemic disorder.

Edema of the feet, ankles, and legs (usually associated with livedo reticularis) has been noted in some patients. Orthostatic hypotension may accompany amantadine therapy.

Large doses of amantadine are embryotoxic and teratogenic in certain laboratory animals; therefore, the drug should not be used during pregnancy unless the benefits to the mother outweigh the risks to the fetus (FDA Pregnancy Category C). Amantadine is excreted in milk and should not be given to nursing mothers. As with anticholinergic drugs, withdrawal should be gradual because patients may experience a pronounced worsening of parkinsonian symptoms if amantadine is discontinued abruptly.

DRUG INTERACTIONS. Both the peripheral and central adverse effects of anticholinergic drugs are increased by amantadine. Combined therapy has induced acute psychotic reactions identical to those caused by atropine poisoning. If signs of central toxicity occur during combined therapy, the dose of the anticholinergic drug should be reduced. Visual hallucinations are not uncommon in patients receiving amantadine with levodopa. Amantadine may exacerbate levodopa-induced dyskinesias.

PHARMACOKINETICS. The clinical pharmacokinetics of amantadine have been reviewed (Aoki and Sitar, 1988). Absorption is relatively complete, but bioavailability appears to be lower and the time to peak plasma concentrations longer in elderly patients. A volume of distribution of 6 L/kg and plasma protein binding of 67% have been reported.

Elimination is based primarily on renal function; 85% to 90% of the dose is excreted unchanged in the urine. Enzymatic acetylation may represent a minor elimination pathway. The half-life in young adults (14 hours) is doubled in healthy elderly patients (29 hours). The renal clearance of amantadine exceeds creatinine clearance, which indicates that the drug is actively secreted by the renal tubules. There is an inverse correlation between creatinine clearance and the plasma half-life; thus, the dosage must be adjusted in those with renal impairment, preferably by extension of the dosage interval (Bennett, 1988). Hemodialysis is relatively ineffective in removing amantadine.

DOSAGE AND PREPARATIONS.

Oral: For Parkinson's disease or postencephalitic parkinsonism, initially, 25 to 50 mg daily of the syrup, with the amount increased gradually to 200 mg/day. The syrup preparation allows smaller initial dosage and helps lessen the risk of early side effects. The capsule preparation is useful for daily dosages of 100 to 200 mg. Amounts exceeding 200 mg daily generally provide little additional relief and may be associated with increasing toxicity.

Generic. Capsules 100 mg.

Symmetrel (DuPont). Capsules 100 mg; syrup 50 mg/5 ml.

CARBIDOPA

[Lodosyn]

LEVODOPA

[Dopar, Larodopa]

LEVODOPA AND CARBIDOPA

[Atamet, Sinemet, Sinemet CR]

ACTIONS AND USES. Although dopamine does not enter the brain in sufficient quantities to be of value in the treatment of Parkinson's disease, levodopa, its immediate precursor, penetrates the blood-brain barrier and is then converted to dopamine by the enzyme, L-aromatic amino acid decarboxylase. The amount of this enzyme in peripheral tissues is far in excess of that in the brain; therefore, in the absence of peripheral decarboxylase inhibition, large doses of levodopa are required to achieve therapeutic levels of dopamine in the central nervous system.

Except in rare circumstances (eg, allergy, intolerance to carbidopa), levodopa is administered in combination with the dopa decarboxylase inhibitor, carbidopa, which does not cross the blood-brain barrier and therefore does not prevent the central conversion of levodopa to dopamine. By preventing the extracerebral metabolism of levodopa, carbidopa increases the amount of levodopa available in the brain for decarboxylation to dopamine, thereby enhancing the therapeutic response and reducing side effects caused by peripheral actions of dopamine and other catecholamines. The combination of carbidopa and levodopa increases the plasma concentrations of levodopa, reduces dosage requirements for levodopa by approximately 75%, and decreases the incidence of nausea and vomiting significantly. Therefore, the dosage can be increased more rapidly and the response is somewhat smoother.

This combination is the most effective drug therapy for symptoms of Parkinson's disease. The standard [generic, Atamet, Sinemet] or prolonged-release formulation [Sinemet CR] is used when symptoms interfere with normal daily activities. Carbidopa and levodopa are supplied in ratios of 1:4 (25-100, 50-200) and 1:10 (10-100, 25-250).

Most adults require 75 to 150 mg daily of carbidopa for maximum inhibition of peripheral dopa decarboxylase, and the 1:10 ratio of 10-100 preparations may deliver less than the minimum requirement when only small doses of levodopa are desired. Therefore, most neurologists prescribe one of the preparations containing a 1:4 ratio of carbidopa/levodopa (25-100 or 50-200) to permit saturation of peripheral dopa decarboxylase when less than 700 mg daily of levodopa is needed. This regimen increases responsiveness and decreases adverse reactions.

In patients who do not have motor fluctuations, the prolonged-release formulation, Sinemet CR, produces the same therapeutic benefit as standard preparations but requires less frequent dosing. Patients with severe motor fluctuations may not experience a significant decrease in "off" time, but the reduction in dosing frequency may be beneficial. Use of the prolonged-release formulation does not decrease any of the adverse effects attributable to levodopa.

Carbidopa alone [Lodosyn] is available to physicians on request from the distributor, DuPont Pharma, and may be useful when given with the combination for patients experiencing adverse gastrointestinal symptoms at initiation of therapy.

When administered in gradually increasing doses for an adequate period of time, levodopa relieves symptoms and significantly improves functional capacity in about 75% of patients with Parkinson's disease. In 50% of patients, the quality of life is improved markedly for many years. Levodopa is so specific and effective in Parkinson's disease that an initial lack of response is cause to question the accuracy of diagnosis;

some unresponsive patients have atypical parkinsonian syndromes involving brain sites in addition to the dopaminergic nigrostriatal pathway.

Levodopa does not halt progression of the underlying disease, but symptoms improve substantially and life expectancy is prolonged. This may be attributed partially to better medical care, more frequent monitoring that identifies complications early, and better control of complications, such as infections. All major parkinsonian symptoms may be ameliorated, particularly bradykinesia and rigidity. Tremor may respond well, but patients often are aware of even the slightest dysfunction in this regard; balance and gait are less likely to be improved. Mood may be elevated, and seborrhea and drooling may diminish. Although intellectual function may improve initially, this effect often is transient. Mental deterioration and dementia may develop in about one-third of patients with moderate to advanced disease. There are probably multiple causes for the development of dementia in different subsets of patients with Parkinson's disease (Gibb, 1989).

Although levodopa is far more effective than the central anticholinergic drugs and amantadine, many neurologists reserve it for patients with some degree of functional impairment (see the Introduction). When initiating therapy in patients already receiving anticholinergic drugs or amantadine, dosage adjustment may be necessary to minimize adverse effects. If treatment is initiated with levodopa/carbidopa, anticholinergic drugs, amantadine, dopamine agonists, or selegiline may be added later to achieve optimal effects.

Levodopa generally is very effective in the treatment of parkinsonian syndromes caused by neural damage resulting from MPTP intoxication. It also may be beneficial in postencephalitic parkinsonism and usually provides some benefit in the early stages of progressive supranuclear palsy and the multiple system atrophies. Levodopa may be beneficial in the treatment of some children with dystonia (see discussion on Dystonias in the section on Other Dyskinetic Disorders in this chapter).

ADVERSE REACTIONS AND PRECAUTIONS. ***Gastrointestinal:*** Nausea, vomiting, and anorexia occur in most patients if the initial daily dose is large or increased too rapidly. To avoid nausea and vomiting, levodopa should be administered in combination with carbidopa and smaller doses taken more frequently with slow titration of the dose. Some clinicians prefer to give levodopa with meals initially to lessen gastrointestinal upset. However, in those receiving long-term therapy, the relationship between high-protein meals and motor fluctuations usually requires separation of dosing and meals (Nutt et al, 1984). Approximately 2% to 5% of patients treated with levodopa/carbidopa experience persistent nausea and vomiting. Antiemetics should be avoided because they may counteract the therapeutic effect of levodopa. The investigational dopamine antagonist, domperidone, blocks dopamine receptors in the medullary chemoreceptor trigger zone outside the blood-brain barrier and may diminish nausea and vomiting (see index entry Domperidone).

Other gastrointestinal disturbances occasionally reported but questionably related to levodopa therapy include abdominal pain, diarrhea, constipation, activation of peptic ulcer, and gastrointestinal bleeding.

Neurologic: Abnormal involuntary movements sometimes occur just before or soon after the optimal therapeutic response is obtained and may be the major dose-limiting factor in levodopa therapy. Combined therapy with carbidopa does not significantly decrease the dyskinesias and psychiatric disturbances induced by levodopa alone. Mild, intermittent dyskinesias (usually choreiform movements) involving the mouth, tongue, face, and neck are common in the first years of therapy if larger doses of levodopa are used. Dyskinesias of the limbs also are common. Many patients are willing to tolerate them in order to obtain the beneficial effects of levodopa. The incidence of peak-dose dyskinesias is as high as 80% in patients receiving prolonged levodopa therapy (Shaw et al, 1980).

Choreiform, choreoathetoid, dystonic, myoclonic, or a combination of these movements may occur. They may disappear when the dose is reduced, although parkinsonian symptoms then may increase. In some patients, abnormal involuntary movements recur at progressively lower doses.

Episodes of motor fluctuations often are seen in patients after more than one year of levodopa therapy (see the Introduction). Akathisia (eg, sensation of inner restlessness) may be a parkinsonian symptom and may persist if the dose is inadequate or, conversely, it may be an early indication of excessive dosage. Undertreated parkinsonian patients also may experience unsteadiness and may refer to this as dizziness; this symptom also can be confused with orthostatic hypotension.

Headache occasionally has been associated with levodopa therapy.

A condition similar to neuroleptic malignant syndrome has been reported in patients after rapid reduction in dosage or discontinuation of levodopa.

Respiratory: Respiratory abnormalities may develop during levodopa therapy. Symptoms include cough, hoarseness, postnasal drip, tachypnea, bradypnea, gasping, panting, sniffing, and feelings of pressure in the chest. These phenomena may represent dyskinesias of the diaphragm and intercostal muscles. Respiratory symptoms in patients with Parkinson's disease also may be due to thoracodiaphragmatic dystonia or rigidity during "off" phases or to concurrent cardiopulmonary disease.

Psychiatric: Psychiatric disturbances are common, particularly in elderly patients receiving other psychoactive drugs (eg, anticholinergic agents, amantadine, selegiline, dopamine agonists, antidepressants) concomitantly. Some neurologists prefer to reduce the dosage or discontinue these drugs before levodopa therapy is initiated. Euphoria, anxiety, irritability, hyperactivity, hallucinations, and vivid dreams are common. Agitation, hypomanic and paranoid reactions, delirium, psychosis, and severe depression, including aggressive or suicidal behavior, have developed occasionally, most often in patients with pre-existing dementia or a history of mental illness. In some cases, levodopa may unmask a previously unrecognized dementia. To the extent that mental changes are due to levodopa, they may respond to a reduction in dose with possible loss of efficacy. Occasionally, discontinuation of levodopa is required. Case reports and results of several open studies indicate that clozapine (25 to 150 mg) may be effective in the treatment of levodopa- and dopamine agonist-induced psychosis in patients with Parkinson's disease (Friedman, 1991; Wolk and Douglas, 1992; Factor et al, 1994); phenothiazines, thioxanthenes, and butyrophenones should be avoided.

Cardiovascular: If the initial daily dose of levodopa is large or is increased too rapidly, the standing systolic and diastolic blood pressures may fall. This effect usually is well tolerated, but significant orthostatic hypotension with syncope may occur, especially in patients taking diuretics and/or tricyclic antidepressants concomitantly. This reaction tends to diminish in time and often can be alleviated by wearing elastic stockings, temporarily reducing the dose of levodopa, increasing the intake of salt, or administering a salt-retaining steroid. When the latter measures are employed, the patient should be monitored for symptoms of hypervolemia, hypokalemia, and congestive heart failure.

Palpitations may occur but often disappear with continued therapy. Minor disturbances of cardiac rate and rhythm (tachycardia and premature ventricular contractions) and severe arrhythmias have developed occasionally. It is not clear whether levodopa was a causal factor or whether the arrhythmia was related to underlying heart disease. Antiarrhythmic therapy usually is not required, and it is seldom necessary to discontinue levodopa therapy. No significant difference in the severity of ventricular arrhythmias or in the incidence of orthostatic hypotension was noted in patients receiving levodopa/carbidopa compared with levodopa alone (Leibowitz and Lieberman, 1975).

Hypertension, myocardial infarction, and venous thrombosis have been reported occasionally, but there is no evidence that these complications are more common in patients receiving levodopa than in a comparable age group not receiving the drug. If myocardial infarction occurs during therapy, modification of the treatment program may be required.

Miscellaneous: Transient flushing of the skin is common during levodopa therapy. The product labeling cautions against use of this drug in patients with a history of melanoma or a suspicious, undiagnosed skin lesion and in those with angle-closure glaucoma. However, current evidence suggests that levodopa/carbidopa can be used safely in patients with Parkinson's disease and a history of melanoma (Weiner et al, 1993).

No adverse reactions have been attributed to carbidopa alone.

LABORATORY FINDINGS. Results of laboratory studies have not revealed evidence of serious hematologic, renal, hepatic, or thyroid dysfunction due to levodopa. Large doses may cause hypokalemia associated with increased plasma levels of aldosterone; this effect is substantially reduced by adding carbidopa to the regimen. The white blood cell count has decreased temporarily in a few patients. Positive Coombs' tests occur occasionally, and there have been a few reports of reduced hemoglobin and hematocrit levels unrelated to a hemolytic process.

Mild, transient elevations of blood urea nitrogen occur and usually can be controlled by increasing fluid intake. Elevation of AST activity has been noted in a few patients, but this usually returned to normal despite continued drug administration. Increased blood lactic acid dehydrogenase activity and bilirubin and alkaline phosphatase concentrations are rare. Elevations of uric acid have been noted using the colorimetric method of measurement but have not been reported in tests using the uricase method.

Levodopa increases plasma growth hormone levels and may produce mild carbohydrate intolerance, but signs of acromegaly or diabetes mellitus have not occurred during long-term therapy. Dark-colored sweat and changes in urine color (red-tinged when voiding, black when exposed to air) have been reported but are not indications for discontinuing the drug.

TERATOGENICITY. Levodopa has caused visceral and skeletal malformations in rabbits and has depressed fetal and postnatal growth and viability in rodents. This drug is not recommended during pregnancy or in nursing mothers unless motor function would otherwise be significantly compromised; however, there is no evidence of teratogenic effects in humans.

DRUG INTERACTIONS. The effectiveness of levodopa may be reduced by antipsychotic drugs (eg, phenothiazines), rauwolfia alkaloids, phenytoin, papaverine, and metoclopramide. In a few patients, parkinsonian symptoms were apparently exacerbated when benzodiazepines were given concomitantly; however, a causal relationship has not been established (Hansten and Horn, 1990). Dopamine agonists, amantadine, or selegiline may accentuate levodopa-induced adverse motor and mental effects.

Since a hypertensive crisis may occur if levodopa is given with a nonspecific monoamine oxidase inhibitor, these drugs should be discontinued two weeks prior to initiation of levodopa therapy.

Methyldopa may decrease the antiparkinson effect of levodopa. Additive hypotensive effects also have been noted in patients receiving levodopa and other antihypertensive drugs.

If general anesthesia is required, levodopa may be continued as long as the patient is permitted to take fluids and medication by mouth. If therapy is interrupted temporarily, the usual daily dosage may be administered as soon as the patient is able to take oral medication. When therapy is interrupted for longer periods, the dosage should be adjusted gradually.

The therapeutic response to levodopa alone may be reduced or abolished by pyridoxine (vitamin B_6) in doses as low as 5 mg daily, but not when levodopa is combined with sufficient amounts of carbidopa (approximately 75 mg/day). This has been attributed to the pyridoxine-induced accelerated decarboxylation of levodopa in peripheral tissues. Patients receiving levodopa alone should avoid multiple vitamin preparations containing more than the recommended daily allowance of pyridoxine (see index entry Pyridoxine).

PHARMACOKINETICS. Levodopa is well absorbed by the amino acid transport system in the small bowel. Approximately 95% of an oral dose is decarboxylated in the liver and peripheral tissue. The concomitant administration of a decarboxylase inhibitor markedly increases the amount of levodopa available to enter the systemic circulation and brain. The plasma concentration of levodopa peaks approximately 30 minutes and two hours after administration of Sinemet and Sinemet CR, respectively. The bioavailability of levodopa in Sinemet CR is 25% to 30% lower than that in Sinemet; peak plasma concentrations achieved with Sinemet CR are lower, but trough plasma concentrations are higher. Because of the lower bioavailability of levodopa in Sinemet CR, the daily dosage of levodopa necessary to produce a clinical response comparable to that with Sinemet will be higher with the prolonged-release formulation.

Levodopa has a relatively short plasma half-life (one to two hours) in the presence of carbidopa. The apparent half-life of levodopa administered as Sinemet CR is prolonged because of continuous absorption.

DOSAGE AND PREPARATIONS. Levodopa is almost never administered without the benefit provided by peripheral decarboxylase inhibition. Dosage must be titrated carefully to obtain the desired therapeutic response with minimal adverse effects. The patient should be observed closely during dosage adjustment and, if adverse reactions occur, the dose should be reduced or, rarely, temporarily discontinued. When initiating therapy with levodopa/carbidopa, patients in good general health who have only moderate neurologic impairment are treated as outpatients if they are seen at regular intervals and good compliance is anticipated. Rarely, hospitalization may be required for patients with marked disability, those with coexisting systemic disorders that should be monitored daily, or those for whom drug administration cannot be properly supervised on an outpatient basis. All patients should be seen at regular intervals and the dosage modified as necessary for optimal results.

STANDARD PREPARATIONS:

Oral: Therapy is usually initiated with one-half tablet of a 25-100 preparation given two to four times daily; subsequent increments depend on the therapeutic response and side effects. The dosage may be increased by one-half to one tablet/day every two to three days to minimize adverse effects. Patients who experience nausea should receive dosage increments more slowly and only after the nausea is attenuated at a given dose (Ahlskog, 1989). Relatively complete inhibition of peripheral decarboxylase requires at least 75 mg of carbidopa daily. Thus, patients generally benefit from the 25-100 (1:4 ratio) rather than the 10-100 (1:10 ratio) preparation; the former ensures an adequate daily intake of the decarboxylase inhibitor. If a larger daily dose of levodopa is needed, the 25-250 tablets may be given, with the amount increased by one-half to one tablet daily or every other day if necessary. The usual dosage range for levodopa when combined with carbidopa is 300 mg to 1 g. Patients with mild disease usually require 200 to 400 mg daily. Those with more advanced disease may require more. If no improvement occurs at a daily levodopa dosage of 2 g, it is unlikely that further increments will be helpful (Ahlskog, 1989). Combination with a dopamine agonist or selegiline permits smaller doses of levodopa to be employed.

PROLONGED-RELEASE PREPARATION (SINEMET CR):

Oral: In patients with mild to moderate disease not currently receiving the standard preparation, therapy is usually initiated with one tablet of Sinemet CR 50-200 twice daily at intervals of not less than six hours; subsequent dosage adjustments are based on the therapeutic response. An interval of at least three days between dosage adjustments is recommended. In clinical trials, most patients responded adequately to two to eight tablets daily, administered at intervals ranging from four to eight hours during the waking day. Shorter dosage intervals may be required for patients with moderate to severe disease. Cutting the scored 50-200 tablet in half enhances short-term activity but decreases long-term release (Sinemet CR 25-100 tablets are not scored and should not be halved.) Chewing or crushing either prolonged-release tablet abolishes long-term activity.

For patients currently receiving the standard preparation, initially, Sinemet CR should be substituted at an amount that provides approximately 10% more levodopa per day; the amount may need to be increased subsequently to provide approximately 30% more levodopa than with the standard preparation, depending on clinical response. The interval between doses generally should be four to eight hours during the waking day; some patients may require a shorter dosage interval. A dose of the standard preparation can be added to this regimen if further adjustment is indicated in those patients already receiving carbidopa 200 mg or in those who need additional levodopa in the morning or for brief periods during the day; however, combined use of Sinemet CR and a standard preparation can be associated with unpredictable and prolonged dyskinesias.

For further information on suggested guidelines for initial conversion from the standard preparation to Sinemet CR, see the product labeling.

CARBIDOPA:

Lodosyn (DuPont Pharma). Tablets 25 mg. Available by prescription directly from the manufacturer.

LEVODOPA:

For information on the use of levodopa alone, see the manufacturer's package literature.

Dopar (Roberts). Capsules 100, 250, and 500 mg.

Larodopa (Roche). Tablets 100, 250, and 500 mg.

LEVODOPA AND CARBIDOPA:

Atamet (Athena Neurosciences). Tablets containing carbidopa 25 mg and levodopa 100 or 250 mg.

Sinemet (DuPont Pharma), ***Generic.*** Tablets containing carbidopa 10 mg and levodopa 100 mg or carbidopa 25 mg and levodopa 100 or 250 mg.

Sinemet CR (DuPont Pharma). Tablets (prolonged-release) containing carbidopa 25 mg and levodopa 100 mg (unscored) or carbidopa 50 mg and levodopa 200 mg (scored).

SELEGILINE HYDROCHLORIDE (Deprenyl)

[Eldepryl]

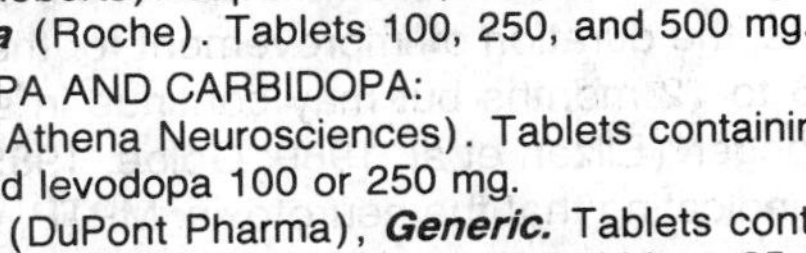

$$C_6H_5-CH_2-CH(CH_3)-N(CH_3)-CH_2-C\equiv CH$$

ACTIONS. Early clinical trials revealed that monoamine oxidase inhibitors potentiated the antiparkinsonian actions of levodopa, presumably by inhibiting the degradation of dopamine, but the concomitant use of these agents produced hypertension. Monoamine oxidase occurs as two isozymes, types A and B, which are differentiated by relative substrate and inhibitor selectivity. Norepinephrine and serotonin are preferentially metabolized by type A, whereas phenylethylamine is a preferred substrate for type B. Dopamine is a substrate for both forms. Noncompetitive ("suicide") inhibition of type A may produce hypertensive crises in response to dietary intake of tyramine. Type B predominates in the human brain; however, the exact cellular localization of types A and B and their contribution to neuronal dopamine metabolism is still unclear. Monoamine oxidase type A has been localized in dopaminergic neurons of nonhuman primates (Westlund et al, 1985), while type B has been localized in glial cells and midbrain serotonergic neurons (Levitt et al, 1982).

Several studies in animals show that selegiline, a relatively specific type B monoamine oxidase inhibitor, has no effect on dopamine catabolism in the striatum, but it potentiates the response to levodopa (Paterson et al, 1991). Prolonged administration of selegiline also has been observed to cause an up-regulation in the neuronal uptake of dopamine (Wiener et al, 1989).

USES. Selegiline may provide minor symptomatic benefit when used alone in early, untreated Parkinson's disease (Myllylä et al, 1992; The Parkinson Study Group, 1993). In patients with advanced disease, the addition of selegiline to levodopa therapy lessens end-of-dose "wearing-off" effects. Sudden "on-off" or "freezing" motor fluctuations are generally unaffected (Lees et al, 1977; Yahr et al, 1983; Rinne, 1983; Golbe et al, 1988) and only a modest increase in "on" time is noted. With combined use, potentiation of dyskinesias is common. This and other dopaminergic effects may be minimized by reducing the levodopa dosage 10% to 30%. Thus, selegiline is indicated as an adjunct in the management of parkinsonian patients who exhibit deterioration in their response to levodopa/carbidopa therapy. Overall, the benefit observed has been only slight to moderate. In those experiencing wearing-off effects, the duration of improvement for the majority of patients is 6 to 12 months but may continue in some for 24 months or longer (Elizan et al, 1989; Golbe, 1989).

Evidence indicating that the neurotoxin, MPTP, requires enzymatic activation by monoamine oxidase B (MAO-B) has increased interest in the possible neuroprotective effects of selegiline. This and other specific MAO-B inhibitors prevent MPTP-induced parkinsonism in animals (Langston et al, 1984; Heikkila et al, 1984). In a retrospective study, patients with parkinsonism who took selegiline and levodopa lived longer than those who took only levodopa (Birkmayer et al, 1985). Administration of selegiline 10 mg daily delays the onset of disability requiring levodopa therapy by approximately nine months in patients with early, otherwise untreated Parkinson's disease (The Parkinson Study Group, 1993). Because selegiline has a slight effect in relieving symptoms, further study, perhaps on presymptomatic individuals, is required before it can be determined whether treatment with this drug spares nigral neurons in patients with Parkinson's disease (see the discussion on Drug Selection in the Introduction).

Selegiline is metabolized extensively to N-desmethylselegiline, L-methamphetamine, and L-amphetamine (Reynolds et al, 1978). The L isomers are three to ten times less potent than the D form. Methamphetamine and amphetamine interfere with neuronal uptake of dopamine and potentiate the release of dopamine and other neurotransmitters. Results of animal studies indicate that metabolites may contribute to the effects of selegiline within the striatum (Engberg et al, 1991). In one controlled study on a small group of patients, the conversion of selegiline to amphetamine was confirmed; amphetamine also counteracted the dose-related fluctuations in response to optimal levodopa therapy without causing serious side effects (Schachter et al, 1980). Results of another small trial failed to confirm any contributory role of amphetamine metabolites (Elsworth et al, 1982). Thus, while inhibition of MAO-B is of primary importance, selegiline or its metabolites also may act through other mechanisms to improve responsiveness to levodopa.

ADVERSE REACTIONS. When selegiline is added to levodopa/carbidopa, an increase in dopaminergic side effects (dyskinesias, nausea, hallucinations) commonly occurs. These often may be controlled by reducing the levodopa/carbidopa dosage. Confusion, dizziness, and insomnia also occur. Other adverse reactions reported more than once as a cause for discontinuation of the drug when used adjunctively with levodopa include orthostatic hypotension, arrhythmias, hypertension, angina pectoris, and syncope.

When selegiline was administered by itself to patients with early, untreated Parkinson's disease, symptoms related to excessive dopaminergic activity were not observed. Transient elevations in alanine aminotransferase (ALT) and aspartate aminotransferase (AST) occurred infrequently. In the DATATOP study, arrhythmias developed in a few patients (The Parkinson Study Group, 1993).

Selegiline is classified in FDA Pregnancy Category C.

DRUG INTERACTIONS. Stupor, muscular rigidity, severe agitation, and elevated temperature have been reported in one patient receiving selegiline and meperidine, as well as other medications. These symptoms are compatible with the well-recognized interaction of meperidine with nonselective monoamine oxidase inhibitors. Thus, combination of selegiline with meperidine and other opioids should be avoided, if possible. A possible interaction with fluoxetine also has been reported (Suchowersky and deVries, 1990; Montastruc et al, 1993). The combined use of other monoamine oxidase inhibitors and 5-HT uptake inhibitors has caused serious reactions; thus, it is prudent to avoid use of the latter in patients receiving selegiline.

DOSAGE AND PREPARATIONS.

Oral: As an adjunct in the treatment of parkinsonian patients who exhibit deterioration in their response to therapy with levodopa/carbidopa, a total of 10 mg per day is administered in divided doses of 5 mg at breakfast and lunch. Insomnia occurs less frequently with this dosage schedule. After two to three days, an attempt may be made to reduce the dose of levodopa/carbidopa, especially if signs of dopaminergic activity (eg, dyskinesias) worsen. Doses of selegiline greater than 10 mg/day should be avoided to preserve the selective nature of MAO-B inhibition. Hypertension in response to dietary tyramine has not been observed with this dosage of selegiline. Daily dosage lower than 10 mg has not been adequately studied.

Eldepryl (Somerset). Tablets 5 mg.

DOPAMINE RECEPTOR AGONISTS

The motor fluctuations that develop one to five years after initiation of levodopa therapy may be caused in part by a decreasing capacity of nigrostriatal neurons to synthesize, store, and release dopamine. This assumption has reinforced the search for specific agonists that act directly on striatal dopamine receptor sites. Natural and semisynthetic ergolines derived from ergot alkaloids are the primary sources of such agonists.

In the central nervous system, dopaminergic neurotransmission is mediated through receptors belonging to the G protein-coupled family. On the basis of their homology, several different types have been cloned, the most abundant of which are termed D_1 and D_2. The D_1 receptor stimulates adenylate cyclase and exists in at least two forms, D_{1A} (formerly termed D_1) and D_{1B}; these forms are pharmacologically similar but differ in their distribution in the brain. The D_2 receptor, which inhibits adenylate cyclase or possibly is linked to other transduction mechanisms, exists in two isoforms that appear to be pharmacologically identical but differ in relative distribution.

In general, the distribution of D_1 and D_2 receptors overlaps and coincides with brain regions known to have dopaminergic input. In the substantia nigra, D_2 receptors are present on cell bodies or dendrites of neurons, whereas a large proportion of D_1 receptors appears to be located on terminals of fibers originating in the striatum. In the striatum, both receptors are located primarily on cell bodies.

Recently, molecular cloning procedures have identified three other types of dopamine receptors, D_3, D_4, and D_5. The D_3 and D_4 receptors are homologous to the D_2 receptor. The D_3 receptor is mainly expressed in limbic brain areas or discrete areas of the ventral striatum (eg, olfactory tubercle, nucleus accumbens) that receive afferents from prefrontal, amygdalar, or allocortical areas (Sokoloff et al, 1990). The D_4 receptor is found in the frontal cortex, amygdala, midbrain, and, to a lesser extent, in the striatum (Van Tol et al, 1991). The D_5 receptor (Sunahara et al, 1991) bears a strong homology to D_1 but has a tenfold higher affinity for dopamine and is localized in the striatum and limbic regions.

Most investigators believe that stimulation of D_2 receptors is primarily responsible for the beneficial effects of dopamine receptor agonists in Parkinson's disease. Selective D_1 receptor agonists are not very effective in patients with idiopathic or MPTP-induced parkinsonism. However, experiments in animals indicate that stimulation of D_1 receptors may potentiate the action of D_2 receptor agonists (Waddington and O'Boyle, 1989). It is unclear whether this is relevant to dopaminergic function in Parkinson's disease. However, results of one uncontrolled study suggest that D_1 receptor stimulation enhances antiparkinsonian responses but also increases choreiform side effects of dopaminergic therapy (Ahlskog et al, 1992), and several investigators have noted that patients who exhibit deteriorating responses to the D_2 agonist, bromocriptine, improve after substitution of pergolide (Lieberman et al, 1983; Goetz et al, 1984; Factor et al, 1987).

Bromocriptine and pergolide are the only clinically useful direct-acting dopamine receptor agonists currently available in the United States for the treatment of Parkinson's disease (Vance et al, 1984; Ahlskog and Muenter, 1988 A; Olanow et al, 1994). Both drugs have D_2 and D_3 receptor activity; pergolide weakly activates D_1 receptors as well. Like dopamine, pergolide appears to be a relatively more potent D_3 receptor agonist; the clinical significance of this is unknown. It has a longer duration of action than bromocriptine.

Other D_2 receptor agonists (eg, cabergoline, pramipexol) are being evaluated for efficacy in the treatment of Parkinson's disease (Ahlskog et al, 1992; Hutton et al, 1993; Lera et al, 1993).

BROMOCRIPTINE MESYLATE

[Parlodel]

For chemical formula, see index entry Bromocriptine, In Female Hyperprolactinemia.

USES. Bromocriptine is more effective than the anticholinergic drugs and amantadine but less effective than levodopa in the symptomatic treatment of Parkinson's disease. Its primary indications are (1) as an adjunct to levodopa/carbidopa in patients experiencing fluctuations in therapeutic response, end-of-dose akinesia, and painful dystonia; the decrease in fluctuations may be related to bromocriptine's longer duration of action or bromocriptine and levodopa may affect different dopamine receptors and/or sites; (2) as an adjunct to levodopa/carbidopa early in the course of illness because current evidence suggests that early combination therapy may decrease the prevalence of levodopa-induced dyskinesias and motor fluctuations; and (3) as an alternative to levodopa if that drug is contraindicated or is not tolerated.

When bromocriptine is added, the dose of levodopa/carbidopa can be reduced as the amount of bromocriptine is increased. This may reduce the incidence of dyskinesias and dystonias induced by levodopa because bromocriptine appears to have less tendency to produce these involuntary movements (Olsson et al, 1989; Bergamasco et al, 1990).

There is less experience with bromocriptine as the initial drug for long-term management of Parkinson's disease. In controlled trials of bromocriptine monotherapy, there has been considerable variation in the percentage of patients responding (30% to 80%), the daily dosage given (11 to 50 mg), and the degree and duration of improvement (Hely et al, 1989; Montastruc et al, 1989; UK Bromocriptine Research Group, 1989). Although some patients with functional disability respond adequately to bromocriptine, the number experiencing marked improvement is low, cost to the patient is increased, and it may take several weeks to months to reach the dose that produces an acceptable degree of improvement because the dosage must be escalated slowly to decrease adverse effects.

ADVERSE REACTIONS AND PRECAUTIONS. There is considerable individual variation in response to bromocriptine. Thus, careful titration of dosage to determine the maximum benefit/risk ratio is required.

Transient dizziness and nausea often occur with initiation of bromocriptine therapy. Administering the drug with food or antacids, reducing individual doses, and increasing the daily dosage more gradually may alleviate nausea if it is severe. Domperidone, a peripheral dopamine antagonist, also has controlled marked nausea and vomiting (see index entry Domperidone).

Orthostatic hypotension occurs frequently and can be severe, even with doses of 2.5 mg, especially when initiating therapy. Colicky abdominal pain, constipation, blurred vision with or without diplopia, nasal stuffiness, and Raynaud's phenomena are observed occasionally. Hepatotoxicity is rare and resolves with discontinuation of the drug.

Mental disturbances also can occur at low doses, especially when bromocriptine is added to levodopa. Such disturbances may be limited to confusion and vivid dreams or, less frequently, paranoid delusions and visual hallucinations.

Other adverse reactions generally occur with total daily doses of 50 to 100 mg (but can develop even at lower dosages) and include erythromelalgia, which is characterized by red, tender, warm, edematous lower extremities. Dyskinesias are rare in patients receiving only bromocriptine, particularly at low doses, although use of bromocriptine lowers the threshold for dyskinesias produced by levodopa. These effects are reversible upon decreasing the dose or discontinuing the drug. Pulmonary infiltrates and thickening of the pleura (pleuropulmonary disease) are observed in 2% to 3% of patients with Parkinson's disease being treated with bromocriptine, especially those with a history of smoking (McElvaney et al, 1988).

Asymptomatic elevations of serum transaminase and alkaline phosphatase levels have been reported. No other liver function or routine laboratory tests appear to be affected.

DRUG INTERACTIONS. Concomitant administration of erythromycin may decrease the hepatic clearance of bromocriptine.

PHARMACOKINETICS. Following oral administration, absorption is rapid and peak effect and peak concentration are achieved within one to two hours. The drug is 90% to 96% bound to serum albumin.

Bromocriptine is almost completely metabolized in the liver to at least two inactive metabolites that are excreted in the feces. Less than 5% of the administered dose is excreted in the urine. The half-life of bromocriptine is approximately three hours (Schran et al, 1980).

DOSAGE AND PREPARATIONS.

Oral: It is important to initiate treatment with a low dosage and increase the amount slowly until a maximum therapeutic response is achieved. Initially, 1.25 mg once daily is suggested to lessen nausea and hypotensive effects. The dose can be increased weekly by 1.25 to 2.5 mg until beneficial effects or intolerable adverse reactions are noted. The drug usually is administered three or four times daily, but more frequent intervals may be necessary in patients with motor fluctuations. Most patients respond to 10 to 20 mg daily, but in advanced disease a daily dosage of up to 100 mg may be used.

Parlodel (Sandoz), ***Generic***. Capsules 5 mg; tablets 2.5 mg.

PERGOLIDE MESYLATE

[Permax]

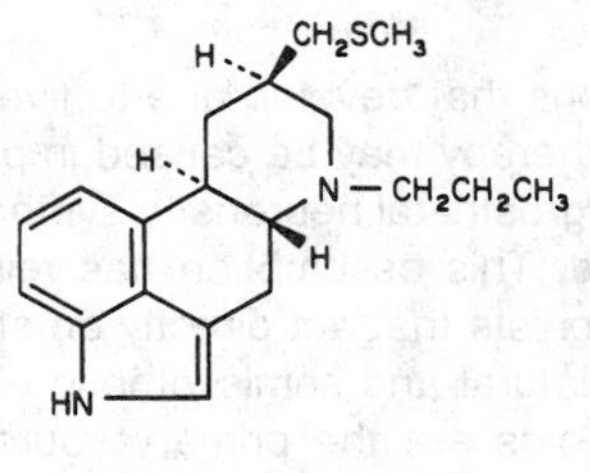

ACTIONS AND USES. This drug is a synthetic ergoline with direct dopaminergic activity. Unlike bromocriptine, pergolide has both D_1 and D_2 receptor activity. It is more potent than bromocriptine and has a longer half-life. However, its overall efficacy in combination with levodopa/carbidopa in advanced Parkinson's disease is similar to that of bromocriptine (LeWitt et al, 1983). Most experience with pergolide has been in parkinsonian patients experiencing moderate to severe dyskinesia and/or on-off phenomena. Results of short-term studies have shown that, when given with levodopa, this drug is useful in managing the motor fluctuations that typically develop during long-term levodopa therapy (LeWitt et al, 1983; Ahlskog and Muenter, 1988 B; Olanow et al, 1994). In some studies, efficacy declined after six months, but subgroups of patients experienced continued benefit for up to three years (Lieberman et al, 1984; Jankovic, 1985; Ahlskog and Muenter, 1988 B). Results of one retrospective analysis involving a small number of patients indicate that the beneficial effects of adjunctive therapy with pergolide can be maintained for more than seven years (Zimmerman and Sage, 1991).

Restoration of the effect of levodopa/carbidopa/dopamine agonist therapy has been reported following substitution of pergolide for bromocriptine (Goetz et al, 1984). Thus, failure of one dopaminergic agonist may not rule out response to an alternative agonist.

ADVERSE REACTIONS AND PRECAUTIONS. Adverse reactions are similar to those of bromocriptine. At optimal dosage, the most common reactions are dyskinesias, hallucinations, nausea and other gastrointestinal disturbances, and lightheadedness. The use of pergolide in patients receiving levodopa may cause or exacerbate dyskinesias, hallucinations, and confusional states. Abrupt cessation of therapy has provoked an acute worsening of symptoms (McHale and Sage, 1988). Hypotension has occurred and can be reduced during initiation of therapy by increasing the dosage gradually (see Dosage and Preparations). Patients receiving pergolide have experienced significantly more episodes of atrial premature contractions and sinus tachycardia than those on placebo.

Therefore, caution should be exercised when administering pergolide to patients with a history of arrhythmias.

Pergolide is classified in FDA Pregnancy Category B.

PHARMACOKINETICS. Little pharmacokinetic information on pergolide is available. A significant portion of a dose appears to be absorbed, although the absolute bioavailability and volume of distribution are not established. Pergolide is approximately 90% bound to plasma proteins. The drug is extensively metabolized. At least ten metabolites have been detected, including sulfoxide and sulfone derivatives, which retain dopamine agonist activity.

DOSAGE AND PREPARATIONS.

Oral: Initially, 0.05 mg daily for the first two days, increased by 0.1 to 0.15 mg daily at three-day intervals for 12 days and then increased by 0.25 mg daily every three days until the antiparkinson effect is optimum or a maximum of 5 mg daily is reached. In clinical studies, the mean therapeutic daily dosage of pergolide was 3 mg, but some patients may achieve maximal therapeutic benefit with a lower dosage. Pergolide can be administered in two or three divided doses daily. The drug also can be given on an alternate-day schedule, usually in patients with milder disease (Kurlan et al, 1985). The dosage of concurrent levodopa/carbidopa therapy may be reduced gradually during titration of the pergolide dosage.

Permax (Athena Neurosciences). Tablets 0.05, 0.25, and 1 mg.

OTHER DYSKINETIC DISORDERS

MYOCLONUS. This disorder is characterized by brief, shock-like muscular contractions of sudden onset. Jerks can occur singly or repetitively and with focal, segmental, or generalized distribution. The regularity and degree of synchronization of repetitive contractions vary. Sensory stimuli or voluntary motor activity can activate or influence the pattern. Pathologically, myoclonus is associated with epilepsy or is symptomatic of a variety of metabolic, degenerative, or focal central nervous system disorders (Fahn et al, 1986). Essential myoclonus refers to a disorder in which myoclonus is the sole neurologic abnormality; its etiology is hereditary or unknown.

Physiologically, myoclonus may be tentatively classified as cortical, reticular (subcortical), or spinal. Observations in humans and animals suggest that dysfunction in 5-hydroxytryptaminergic or GABAergic neurotransmission may be important (Jenner et al, 1986). *Cortical myoclonus* can be secondary to many types of focal cortical lesions. In some cases, the lesions may not be in the cortex but the myoclonus emanates from that location (ie, cortex is disinhibited). Cortical myoclonus currently is considered a subset of epilepsy and responds best to polytherapy with drugs such as clonazepam [Klonopin], valproate [Depakene], and primidone [Mysoline] (Obeso et al, 1989).

Reticular (reflex) myoclonus is characterized by generalized jerks induced by external stimuli or voluntary movement. It is most frequently caused by anoxia or acute encephalopathies and responds best to clonazepam, valproate, or L-5-hydroxytryptophan (L-5HTP).

Posthypoxic myoclonus is a symptomatic myoclonic syndrome that occurs after hypoxic coma. The characteristic feature is the induction of myoclonic jerks associated with voluntary motor activity. It may respond to L-5HTP used with the peripherally acting aromatic amino acid decarboxylase inhibitor, carbidopa, to minimize adverse reactions (Van Woert and Hwang, 1978; Thal et al, 1980). A relative deficiency of serotonin (the decarboxylation product of L-5HTP) has been suggested as the cause of the myoclonus. The optimal dosage of L-5HTP must be determined by gradual titration to avoid severe gastrointestinal side effects (nausea, diarrhea, anorexia, vomiting). The initial recommended dosage is 25 mg four times daily. This may be increased in 100 mg-increments every three to five days as tolerated. A reduction in myoclonus may be observed at a daily dosage of 600 mg to 1 g; the optimal response usually occurs at a daily dosage of 1 to 2 g. L-5HTP is available from Bolar Pharmaceutical under a Treatment IND. (Because of this agent's structural similarity to tryptophan, which has been reported to cause the eosinophilia myalgia syndrome, determinations of eosinophil aldolase and platelet counts must be performed weekly in patients receiving L-5HTP.) Among the antiepileptic drugs, clonazepam or valproate may be effective (Fahn, 1986).

Some patients with essential myoclonus may benefit from clonazepam (Bressman and Fahn, 1986). Drugs used in the treatment of myoclonic seizures are discussed elsewhere; see index entry Antiepileptic Drugs.

TICS. Tics are involuntary brief movements (motor tics) or sounds (vocal tics) that occur intermittently and unpredictably out of a background of normal motor activity. Motor and vocal tics are further classified as *simple* or *complex* (The Tourette Syndrome Classification Study Group, 1993). Simple motor tics are often repetitive and stereotyped. Although tics are involuntary, they usually can be temporarily suppressed voluntarily. Tics occasionally are induced by drugs and are commonly accentuated by emotional stress. Most tic disorders appear to have a hereditary etiology.

Tourette syndrome is a heterogenous neurobehavioral disorder associated with motor and vocal tics of variable form and severity. Results of functional and imaging studies suggest that morphologic abnormalities and dysfunction of the basal ganglia are involved in the pathogenesis of this syndrome (Riddle et al, 1992; Peterson et al, 1993; Singer et al, 1993). Chronic multiple motor or vocal tic disorder and transient tic disorder probably represent milder expressions (Kurlan, 1989). Tourette syndrome is thought to have an autosomal dominant pattern of inheritance with incomplete penetrance and variable expression (van de Wetering and Heutink, 1993).

Obsessive-compulsive symptoms, attention-deficit hyperactivity disorder (ADHD), behavioral difficulties, anxiety, depression, and learning disabilities are commonly associated with tic disorders (Singer and Walkup, 1991). For many patients, these associated problems are the most severe or predominant feature that requires appropriate treatment. The obsessive-compulsive disorder is often alleviated by clomipramine [Anafranil] or, possibly, by fluoxetine [Prozac] (Riddle et al, 1990; Como and Kurlan, 1991). See index entry Obsessive-Compulsive Disorder, Treatment. The treatment of the associated ADHD may be more problematic because stimulants can provoke or intensify tics.

In some studies, clonidine [Catapres] reduced tics and behavioral symptoms associated with Tourette syndrome (Hunt et al, 1985; Leckman et al, 1991); it may be most helpful in patients with milder tics in whom behavioral disturbances predominate. In general, clonidine therapy is initiated with low doses (eg, 0.05 mg/day) and the dose is increased over several weeks to 0.15 to 0.3 mg daily (Cohen et al, 1992). Daily doses larger than 0.3 mg (up to 0.5 mg) sometimes are indicated. At higher doses, hypotension and dizziness may occur, especially if these amounts are given early in treatment. Desipramine [Norpramin] also is recommended by some clinicians (Singer and Walkup, 1991). Results of one open pilot study suggest that selegiline (mean dose, 8.1 mg/day) may be useful in children with ADHD and Tourette syndrome (Jankovic, 1993). (See also index entry Attention-Deficit Hyperactivity Disorder.)

Vocal and motor tics in patients with Tourette syndrome may be suppressed with the antipsychotic drugs, haloperidol [Haldol] or pimozide [Orap] (see the evaluations). Other antipsychotic drugs (eg, fluphenazine [Prolixin], perphenazine [Trilafon], trifluoperazine [Vesprin]) may be equally effective in controlling disabiling tics.

Dystonic tics may be treated with local injections of botulinum toxin type A (Jankovic, 1994).

Not all tic disorders require treatment. Patients with mild disability should not receive dopamine antagonists, which may provoke tardive dyskinesia or other extrapyramidal motor disorders. Periodic attempts should be made to reduce the dose of drugs used for suppression of tics.

DYSTONIAS. Dystonia is a syndrome of sustained muscle contraction(s) that frequently causes twisting and repetitive movements or abnormal postures (Fahn, 1988). Classification is based on age at onset, etiology, and distribution of the abnormal movements. Age is prognostically important since dystonia that begins during childhood is likely to become more severe and eventually involve a number of body parts.

Approximately 25% of patients have symptomatic dystonia due to various degenerative neurologic disorders and environmental causes (Marsden and Quinn, 1990). The remainder of cases are classified as idiopathic and may be either familial or sporadic. Dystonia is inherited in an autosomal dominant form with reduced penetrance (Bressman et al, 1989). In both Ashkenazi Jewish (Kramer et al, 1990) and some non-Jewish families (Ozelius et al, 1989), the causative genes are located on chromosome 9; it is not known whether the same genetic defect exists in both groups. In other non-Jewish familial cases, the gene is probably not located on chromosome 9; thus, there appears to be genetic heterogeneity.

Typically the disorder is manifested in one body region as a focal dystonia. In idiopathic dystonia, initially the abnormal movements and postures may be provoked only during a specific motor act. The dystonia may be aggravated by attempts to move (action dystonia) (Marsden and Quinn, 1990); tremor also may be superimposed. Later, the initial action dystonia may occur at rest and in many patients eventually spreads to involve other body regions (see index entry Dystonias).

The most common form of focal dystonia for which a patient seeks treatment affects the muscles of the neck (spasmodic torticollis). Focal dystonia affecting the hand (writer's cramp) may be more common, but does not cause the same degree of disability. Slightly less common are focal dystonias affecting the muscles of the upper face (blepharospasm) and face and/or jaw (oromandibular dystonia [cranial dystonia includes both types of disorder]) (Marsden and Quinn, 1990). Focal dystonias that affect the larynx (spasmodic dysphonia), pharynx (dystonic dysphagia), and other muscles are least common. The pathophysiologic basis for these disorders is unclear; dysfunction in neurotransmitter pathways of the basal ganglia may be involved.

Additional classifications that are based on distribution include segmental (two or more adjacent parts), multifocal (two or more noncontiguous parts), hemi (one body half), and generalized (one or both legs plus some other body region) (Marsden and Quinn, 1990).

Drug Therapy: Patients with segmental, generalized, and, occasionally, focal dystonia may benefit from anticholinergic drugs; large doses often are required (Fahn, 1983). Approximately 50% of children and 20% to 40% of adults with dystonia experience moderate to marked improvement (Lang, 1989). Most studies of high-dose anticholinergic therapy have employed trihexyphenidyl [Artane]. Both peripheral and central adverse effects may limit dosage, however (see the evaluation on Anticholinergic Agents in the section on Parkinson's Disease). Children and adolescents tolerate larger doses than adults; in these patients, therapy may be initiated with trihexyphenidyl 5 mg daily in two divided doses. The dose is increased by 2.5 to 5 mg every one to two weeks until improvement occurs or intolerance develops (mean responsive dose, 40 mg). Once a dosage of 30 to 40 mg daily is attained, this may be given for one month to allow evaluation of therapeutic response (Burke et al, 1986). Occasionally, more than 100 mg daily is required (Marsden and Quinn, 1990). Other drugs that have been beneficial in some patients include baclofen [Lioresal] (Greene and Fahn, 1992), carbamazepine [Tegretol], and diazepam [Valium] or clonazepam [Klonopin] (Greene et al, 1988). No drug has been effective consistently.

Injection of botulinum toxin type A [Botox] may provide relatively long-term relief (several weeks to months) in focal dystonias and other conditions marked by repetitive or tonic muscle contractions. Because the effect is temporary, the injection must be repeated periodically to maintain the therapeutic response. Chemodenervation by botulinum toxin is the treatment of choice for most patients with hemifacial spasm, blepharospasm, strabismus, and laryngeal dystonia. Patients with spasmodic torticollis and segmental dystonias may be given anticholinergic drugs. In those who respond inadequately, periodic injections of botulinum toxin may enhance the therapeutic response. However, many clinicians now prefer to use botulinum toxin as initial therapy in patients with spasmodic torticollis. Individuals with other focal dystonias and some other neurologic conditions (eg, spasticity, tremor) may respond as well (see the evaluation).

Approximately 5% to 10% of patients with idiopathic juvenile-onset dystonia have a distinct form that may respond to levodopa (dopa-responsive dystonia) (Nygaard et al, 1991). All children and adolescents with dystonia, particularly that which begins in the legs, should be given a trial of levodopa; most of these patients can be managed with Sinemet 25-100 two or three times daily (Marsden and Quinn, 1990), although some may require as little as 50 mg of levodopa (Nygaard et al, 1991).

Acute dystonia is a common adverse reaction to the initial administration of antipsychotic drugs and other antidopaminergic agents, such as the antiemetics, metoclopramide [Reglan] and prochlorperazine [Compazine]. These dystonias generally respond rapidly to parenteral administration of an antihistamine (eg, diphenhydramine [Benadryl]) or a centrally acting anticholinergic agent (eg, benztropine [Cogentin]; see index entry Antipsychotic Drugs, Adverse Reactions.

BALLISM. Ballism is characterized by continual, usually unilateral (hemiballismus), purposeless, flinging movements of the upper extremities. It is most often produced by acute vascular infarction of the subthalamic nucleus, but other subcortical structures and disorders other than stroke may be involved in the pathogenesis (Dewey and Jankovic, 1989). Some authorities believe that this disorder represents a severe form of chorea. Although the movement disorder often improves spontaneously or with therapy with antipsychotic drugs, reserpine, or tetrabenazine [Nitoman] (not available in the United States), in some patients the underlying disease may produce serious consequences (Dewey and Jankovic, 1989).

TREMOR. Tremor is most simply defined as a rhythmical oscillation of a body part caused by involuntary contraction of antagonistic muscles. It may occur at rest or with movement (action tremor). Resting tremor is primarily associated with Parkinson's disease. Tremor associated with movement may occur during maintained posture (postural tremor), with movement from point to point (kinetic tremor), or only with a specific type of movement (task-specific tremor) (Hallett, 1991). The term "intention" has been used to describe movement tremors, especially those associated with cerebellar disease such as multiple sclerosis. Classifications based on the physiologic characteristics of the tremor, the response to drug therapy, or family history have been proposed (Findley and Cleeves, 1989; Hubble et al, 1989), but they are largely unvalidated (Lou and Jankovic, 1991; Koller et al, 1992).

Essential tremor is most common. It presents as a monosymptomatic postural and movement tremor; most commonly affects the hands, head, and voice and, more rarely, the legs and trunk; and may be associated with dystonia. The frequency is usually 5 to 9 Hz but the range may be wider (Koller and Huber, 1989). The etiology is unknown, but the incidence increases with age, and 40% to 50% of cases are familial. Late-onset or senile tremor that occurs in patients over 65 years is probably the same disorder. More recent electrophysiologic data do not support the earlier suggestion that essential tremor is simply an exaggerated physiologic tremor (Hubble et al, 1989).

Although alcohol cannot be recommended for control of essential tremor due to its abuse potential, under certain circumstances it may be the most effective agent for some patients (Koller and Biary, 1984 A). Alcohol usually acts within a few minutes, but efficacy decreases with continued use (Larsen and Calne, 1983).

Short-term studies have demonstrated that beta-adrenergic blocking drugs and primidone are effective for the symptomatic treatment of essential tremor. Although propranolol [Inderal] (see evaluation) has been used most extensively, nadolol [Corgard], metoprolol [Lopressor] (100 to 200 mg daily), timolol [Blocadren], and sotalol [Betapace] also are effective (Hubble et al, 1989). Most investigators believe that peripheral $beta_2$ receptor blockade mediates the antitremor effect. Cardioselective beta blockers (eg, metoprolol) may not be effective until the dose is large enough to provide some degree of $beta_2$ receptor blockade. More recently, longer term studies have demonstrated that the effectiveness of propranolol and primidone can persist for at least one year. However, 20% to 30% of patients experience no benefit. In some of these patients, the combination of propranolol and primidone is beneficial (Hubble et al, 1989). Acute adverse reactions with primidone and side effects with prolonged use of propranolol hamper therapy, however (Koller and Vetere-Overfield, 1989; Sasso et al, 1990).

Results of two open-label studies suggested that treatment with carbonic anhydrase inhibitors (eg, acetazolamide [Diamox], methazolamide [Neptazane]) may reduce symptoms in some patients with essential tremor (Muenter et al, 1991; Busenbark et al, 1992). A subsequent double-blind study on methazolamide failed to confirm its efficacy, however (Busenbark et al, 1993).

In an open study, 67% of patients with disabling tremor involving the head or hand benefitted from injections of botulinum toxin type A; many of these patients had dystonic tremors (Jankovic and Schwartz, 1991).

CHOREA. The term "chorea" refers to continuous, random flow of involuntary movements from one muscle group to another that interrupts normal movement. The face, trunk, or extremities may be involved.

Chorea may be caused by many disorders affecting the basal ganglia (Kurlan and Shoulson, 1988). It occurs as a component of Huntington's disease and after lacunar infarction in the basal ganglia, rarely with hyperthyroidism or systemic lupus erythematosus, after rheumatic fever (Sydenham's chorea) or encephalitis, and during pregnancy (chorea gravidarum). Drug therapy also is an important cause of chorea. Choreiform, and occasionally dystonic, movements are a component of antipsychotic drug-induced tardive dyskinesia. Therapy with levodopa also is a common cause of choreiform movements. Chorea may occur with use of contraceptive drugs, amphetamine, methylphenidate [Ritalin], and phenytoin [Dilantin] as well.

Athetosis consists of slow, writhing, involuntary movements of the limb muscles that often accompany chorea (choreoathetosis) as a sequel of birth injury (eg, cerebral palsy).

Huntington's Disease: Huntington's disease is a progressive, autosomal-dominant, genetic disorder characterized by choreiform movements, dementia, and behavioral abnormalities (Shoulson, 1986 A). Widespread degenerative changes in striatal projection neurons produce a relative excess of dopamine in nigrostriatal neurotransmission and striatal reductions in GABA, acetylcholine, substance P, and enkephalins. Corticostriatal glutamate projections and afferent glutaminergic inputs to the hippocampus also may be affected (Carter et al, 1989). The overall lesion in terminal stages also reflects extensive cortical atrophy. A loss of *N*-methyl-D-aspartate receptors has been detected in patients with both presymptomatic and established Huntington's disease, which supports the hypothesis that excitotoxins mediate cell death in this disease (Albin et al, 1990). A preferential loss of striatal neurons projecting to the external segment of the globus pallidus or substantia nigra also was reported in one presymptomatic patient carrying the Huntington's disease allele (Albin et al, 1992).

Symptoms usually develop in the third to fifth decade of life. Juvenile-onset (first or second decade) Huntington's disease (akinetic-rigid form) is characterized by bradykinesia and hypertonicity resembling parkinsonism more than chorea. Seizures and ataxia are present in some juvenile patients. Localization of the gene for Huntington's disease to the dorsal short arm of chromosome 4 now allows reliable genetic testing. The affected gene contains a sequence of tandemly repeated trinucleotides (CAG) at one end. This repeat sequence varies in length in normal subjects but is much longer in virtually all patients with Huntington's disease (Huntington's Disease Collaborative Research Group, 1993). The mechanism by which the expanded repeat sequence causes cellular dysfunction in Huntington's disease is not known.

Drug therapy is only a small part of the overall management of adults with Huntington's disease (Folstein and Folstein, 1981; Shoulson, 1986 B). Pharmacotherapy is limited to symptomatic treatment of the movement disorder, depression, and psychosis but provides only transient relief and does not alter the functional decline.

The goal of therapy in patients with Huntington's disease is to reduce brain dopaminergic transmission by administration of agents that inhibit the presynaptic synthesis and storage of dopamine or that antagonize dopamine receptors postsynaptically. Antichoreic therapy is usually reserved for patients with disabling features, but attempts to mask choreic movements completely are not recommended. The minimum dosage usually is administered.

Levodopa may be of short-term palliative value in juvenile-onset Huntington's disease. However, this drug markedly increases choreiform activity in the adult-onset form and may aggravate behavioral abnormalities. Antipsychotic agents antagonize dopamine and usually lessen the chorea temporarily in adult-onset Huntington's disease. The use of larger doses may restore control, but prolonged administration may increase the incidence of tardive dyskinesia and may impair speech and swallowing function (Shoulson, 1979). Clozapine [Clozaril] may be of value in some patients with Huntington's disease who have severe psychotic and depressive symptoms that have not responded to treatment with standard antipsychotic drugs (Sajatovic et al, 1991).

The administration of various agents to increase GABA or mimic its action (eg, muscimol, gamma-vinyl GABA, baclofen, isoniazid) has been of little clinical value (Foster et al, 1983; Scigliano et al, 1984; Perry et al, 1982).

TARDIVE DYSKINESIA. Classic tardive dyskinesia is characterized by involuntary, repetitive, stereotypic movements of the cheek, mouth, and tongue. Lip smacking, chewing, tongue thrusting or protruding, lateral jaw movements, and sucking maneuvers result and are frequently termed the buccolingual masticatory or oral masticatory syndrome. As with most other movement disorders, the dyskinesia disappears during sleep and is aggravated by stress. Tardive dyskinesia may take other forms, including choreiform movements of the hands and feet, athetoid movements of the extremities, dystonic posturing of the neck and trunk, tics, and myoclonus.

Tardive dystonia is a condition secondary to chronic use of drugs with dopamine receptor blocking activity. The condition is treated by removal of the offending agent whenever possible and institution of therapy for dystonia as outlined above (Burke and Kang, 1988). Dopamine receptor antagonists usually are more effective in patients with tardive dystonia than in those with idiopathic dystonia.

A Task Force of the American Psychiatric Association has reviewed the late neurologic effects of antipsychotic drugs (American Psychiatric Association, 1992). A summary of their findings on the risk factors, pathogenesis, differential diagnosis, and prognosis appears elsewhere; see index entry, Antipsychotic Drugs, Adverse Reactions. That section also includes guidelines to reduce the incidence of this type of tardive dyskinesia. The risk of developing tardive dyskinesia is similar for all antipsychotic drugs with the exception of clozapine [Clozaril]. (See index entry Clozapine.)

No treatment programs to date uniformly relieve all signs of dyskinesia, and most produce only slight to moderate improvement in fewer than one-half of patients treated (Tarsy, 1989). Therefore, emphasis must be placed on prevention, early detection, and management of potentially reversible cases.

When disabling tardive dyskinesia persists for years after antipsychotic drug withdrawal, treatment with a dopamine depletor may be attempted, although the success of such therapy is limited. Improvement has been reported with reserpine (1 to 5 mg daily), and this drug may be helpful as initial therapy (Kang and Fahn, 1988). Tetrabenazine [Nitoman], which is not commercially available in the United States, is probably the most effective drug for this form of treatment (Jankovic and Orman, 1988).

Bromocriptine and levodopa also have been given to modify dopaminergic function. Low doses of bromocriptine are postulated to act on dopamine presynaptic autoreceptors to inhibit dopamine synthesis and release. Approximately 20 mg daily improved symptoms in 20% of patients (Jeste and Wyatt, 1982). Similar results were obtained using lower doses (eg, 0.75 to 7.5 mg daily) (Lenox et al, 1985). Large doses (eg, 30 to 60 mg) generally are not useful, but moderate improvement in dystonic symptoms may occur (Lieberman et al, 1989 A). Administration of levodopa is based on the hypothesis that a temporary increase in dopamine levels would reduce receptor supersensitivity. Results of studies have shown that although improvement may be achieved in some patients, this approach is more likely to aggravate the condition (Jeste and Wyatt, 1982; Burke, 1984; Shoulson, 1983).

In patients with persistent and disabling dyskinesia, cautious use of antipsychotic drugs may be required. Undertreatment of chronic psychoses carries high risks, including death. If the antipsychotic drug is continued, an attempt should be made to reduce the dosage. If dyskinesia worsens but continued antipsychotic drug therapy is required, substitution of clozapine may be considered (Lieberman et al, 1989 B).

Adjunctive treatment specifically for the dyskinesia may be considered, although, in general, drugs available to treat tardive dyskinesia are not satisfactory. Benzodiazepines, calcium channel blockers, clonidine, vitamin E, or propranolol may provide partial benefit in some patients (American Psychiatric Association, 1992; Egan et al, 1992; Adler et al, 1993). Anecdotal reports and open studies also indicate that choline, lecithin, lithium, baclofen, methyldopa [Aldomet], valproate, and amantadine may partially relieve symptoms in some patients, but controlled studies are necessary (Simpson et al, 1982; Jeste and Wyatt, 1982; Meltzer and Luchins, 1984; Kushnir and Ratner, 1989).

Drug Evaluations

BOTULINUM TOXIN TYPE A
[Botox]

ACTIONS. Botulinum toxin type A, one of seven immunologically distinct neurotoxins produced by *Clostridium botulinum*, blocks neuromuscular function by preventing the release of acetylcholine from nerve endings. Botulinum toxin type A acts as a zinc-dependent protease that selectively cleaves SNAP-25, a synaptic protein believed to play a key role in exocytosis. This probably accounts for the blockade in neurotransmitter release (Blasi et al, 1993). The resulting chemical denervation of muscle produces local paralysis and allows individual muscles to be weakened selectively.

USES. Hemifacial spasm, which is characterized by sudden, unilateral, synchronous contractions of muscles innervated by the facial nerve, is effectively relieved in more than 90% of patients by injection of botulinum toxin type A into facial muscles. Because facial weakness may be especially noticeable in the lower face, some clinicians limit injections to the eyelid muscles depending on the patient's complaints. As with other palliative uses of the toxin, injection must be repeated periodically to maintain the therapeutic response. Surgical decompression to relieve mechanical irritation of the facial nerve is a therapeutic alternative.

This toxin also appears to provide relatively long-term relief in a number of focal dystonias. Assessments by both the American Academy of Neurology (AAN) and the National Institutes of Health (NIH) concluded that botulinum toxin injection is safe and effective for cervical dystonia (ie, spasmodic torticollis), laryngeal dystonia (ie, adductor spasmodic dysphonia), and jaw-closing oromandibular dystonia (*Neurology*, 1990; *Arch Neurol*, 1991). Both the AAN and NIH consider injection of this toxin promising therapy for the management of other oromandibular dystonias and abductor spasmodic dysphonia, and the NIH concluded that botulinum toxin also is promising therapy for stuttering and vocal and other tremors. Results obtained in a small number of patients suggest that injections of botulinum toxin may be useful for the treatment of other focal or segmental dystonias (eg, pharyngeal, urinary and rectal sphincter, limb, palatal) and spasticity, as well as for palliation of certain deformities associated with cerebral palsy (Das and Park, 1990; Snow et al, 1990; *Arch Neurol*, 1991; Koman et al, 1993).

Spasmodic Torticollis (Cervical Dystonia): This condition is characterized by dystonia affecting the nuchal muscles, which may cause the head to deviate, most often rotated and/or tilted to the side. Studies on the natural progression of idiopathic torticollis indicate that approximately 10% to 12% of patients experience spontaneous remission (Jahanshahi et al, 1990; Chan et al, 1991); however, remissions may be short-lived. In controlled trials, subjective improvement was reported by 75% to 80% of patients with spasmodic torticollis (Tsui et al, 1986; Gelb et al, 1989; Lorentz et al, 1991) after treatment with botulinum toxin type A. Objective improvement after this form of therapy has been more difficult to establish. This may be due, in part, to the difficulty encountered in reliably rating the severity of torticollis. In most controlled trials, objective improvement has been reported in 60% to 65% of patients (Greene et al, 1990; Lorentz et al, 1991; Moore and Blumhardt, 1991). Pain usually is reduced or eliminated. Results in open trials indicate that 40% to 90% of patients experience significant relief (*Neurology*, 1990; Jankovic et al, 1990; Berardelli et al, 1993).

Some disagreement exists about the manner in which the muscle to be injected should be determined (electromyography [EMG] or clinical observation), the injection technique (number and distribution of injections per muscle), and the optimal dose. The sites of injection can be determined by the nature of head deviation. When the contracting muscles cannot be identified by inspection and palpation, EMG is used to select the most appropriate muscles for injection. Results of one randomized study confirm that use of EMG may enhance identification and treatment of deep cervical muscles. In particular, patients with retrocollis, head tilt, and shoulder elevation may experience greater benefit when injection of botulinum toxin injection is guided by EMG (Comella et al, 1992 A).

The average dose appears to be 50 to 100 units per neck or shoulder muscle, depending on the specific muscle and type of torticollis (Greene et al, 1990; Jankovic et al, 1990; Lorentz et al, 1991). The maximum total dose employed in most investigational studies was 150 to 300 units per treatment, but there is no consensus in this regard. The optimal dose varies considerably among patients. In order to achieve an optimal response, the dose and site of injection may need to be adjusted at each visit on the basis of the patient's response to previous injections.

Adverse effects generally are transient and include dysphagia, neck weakness, pain at the site of injection or in nearby muscles, paresthesias, fatigue, malaise, headache, and enhanced head tremor (*Neurology*, 1990; Greene et al, 1990). Results of one prospective study indicate that up to one-third of patients treated with botulinum toxin for spasmodic torticollis develop dysphagic symptoms within 10 days after injection (Comella et al, 1992 B). In one study, the use of EMG for guidance decreased the incidence of postinjection neck weakness and dysphagia (Dubinsky et al, 1991). A few patients have difficulty swallowing for four to six weeks following the injection.

Some patients who received repeated injections did not respond with the typical muscle wasting, perhaps due to antibody formation. In patients who have become resistant to the type A toxin as indicated by the development of antibodies, injection of botulinum toxin type F has been effective (Ludlow et al, 1992).

Single-fiber EMG and fiber density determinations reveal that muscles far from the injection site (eg, extensor digitorum communis) are affected by the usual treatment for torticollis (Tsui et al, 1988; Lange et al, 1987; *Neurology*, 1990; Girlanda et al, 1992). However, objective weakness has not been documented, and laboratory findings indicate that this minor systemic effect of botulinum toxin type A is entirely subclinical. Results of one long-term follow-up study indicate that chronic treatment with botulinum toxin type A in patients with cervical dystonia is not associated with decreasing effectiveness and that efficacy may improve slightly when injections are repeated (Jankovic and Schwartz, 1993).

Spasmodic Dysphonia: The adductor-type focal laryngeal dystonia is characterized by slow, effortful, harsh, strained speech with uncontrollable voice and pitch breaks. In open studies, almost all patients with adductor spasmodic dysphonia have benefited from injections of botulinum toxin type A (Blitzer et al, 1988; Ludlow, 1990; *Neurology*, 1990; Whurr et al, 1993). Speech pattern is usually improved by at least 75% and often normalizes. Laryngeal EMG is used for proper localization of the thyroarytenoid muscle where injections should be placed. An indirect perioral approach also has been used (Ford et al, 1990). Two injection techniques are effective. In one, a total dose of 15 to 30 units is injected at multiple sites along the muscle on one side. Unilateral vocal fold paralysis must occur before a therapeutic effect is observed. In the other technique, 1.25 to 5 units is injected into the thyroarytenoid muscles on both sides. A therapeutic effect is noted without complete vocal fold paralysis. Bilateral injections have the advantage of keeping the dose low. There is some concern that chronic exposure to toxin may ultimately result in irreversible atrophy and fibrosis; however, no long-term problems have been identified.

Transient adverse reactions include dysphagia; hoarseness; breathy dysphonia; and, occasionally, aspiration of fluids. Reflex laryngeal stridor has occurred rarely during EMG.

Botulinum toxin also has been used to treat patients with abductor spasmodic dysphonia (Brin et al, 1990). EMG-guided injections are administered with the needle placed posterior to the thyroid lamina, which directly impales the posterior cricoarytenoid muscle overlying the cricoid cartilage. Potential serious risks include dysphagia and laryngeal stridor that necessitate temporary tracheostomy. Special training is required and therapy is available at only a limited number of medical centers.

Case reports indicate that in patients with Gerhardt's syndrome, stridor can be abolished by injection of botulinum toxin type A into overactive thyroarytenoid muscles (Marion et al, 1992).

Oromandibular Dystonia: This disorder is characterized by dystonic movements involving the jaw, tongue, and lower facial muscles. Injection of botulinum toxin type A 10 to 50 units into the masseter and temporalis muscles improves jaw-closing dystonia by approximately 70% (*Neurology*, 1990; Jankovic et al, 1990). Ten percent of patients do not respond. Jaw opening and lateral deviation dystonia are more complicated and resistant to therapy, but up to 50% of patients may respond to injection, usually into a combination of the submental muscle complex and the pterygoid muscles. Mild dysphagia may occur. Lingual dystonia also may respond to botulinum toxin type A injection, but there is a risk of significant dysphagia and aspiration.

Limb Dystonias: Results of open studies indicate that patients with occupational cramps (eg, writer's and musician's cramp) may benefit from injection of botulinum toxin type A (Cohen et al, 1989). In a prospective, placebo-controlled, blinded dose response study, most patients with limb dystonia (due to various causes) in association with transient focal weakness experienced subjective improvement after at least one injection of botulinum toxin type A; however, there was no significant objective evidence of improvement following treatment (Yoshimura et al, 1992). In a double-blind, placebo-controlled study on patients with writer's cramp, improvement in pen control was reported in 60% of patients but improvement in writing occurred in only 20%. Botulinum toxin was most beneficial in patients with pronounced deviation of the wrist joint (Tsui et al, 1993).

Strabismus, Blepharospasm: See index entry Botulinum A Toxin, In Ocular Disorders.

PRECAUTIONS. Therapy with botulinum toxins is not recommended for patients who are receiving aminoglycosides because these agents may interfere with neuromuscular transmission. Although patients with disorders that affect the function of the neuromuscular junction have been treated with botulinum toxin, caution is recommended in treating those with conditions such as myasthenia gravis, Eaton-Lambert syndrome, and motor neuron disease, particularly when large doses are required (eg, treatment of cervical dystonia). Systemic exposure is generally believed to be limited; however, the potential for exacerbation of neuromuscular disease should be weighed against the severity of the hyperkinetic (dystonic) symptoms.

PREPARATIONS.

Botox (Allergan). Powder 100 units.

HALOPERIDOL
[Haldol]

HALOPERIDOL LACTATE
[Haldol]

For chemical formula, see index entry Haloperidol, Uses, Psychosis.

ACTIONS AND USES. This butyrophenone neuroleptic has been used extensively for the treatment of Tourette syndrome. Haloperidol binds more specifically to the dopamine D_2 receptor, but it is unclear if this actually confers any therapeutic benefit compared with phenothiazine derivatives in this disorder. Approximately 75% to 80% of patients treated with haloperidol experience a tolerable suppression of symptoms (Kurlan, 1989). In one controlled study, haloperidol was slightly more effective than pimozide in reducing the severity of symptoms; the frequency of adverse effects was similar (Shapiro et al, 1989). However, results of other studies suggest that akinetic or sedative effects may be greater with haloperidol (Ross and Moldofsky, 1978; Regeur et al, 1986).

ADVERSE REACTIONS. Akathisia is a common but frequently overlooked side effect of haloperidol therapy that may cause a variety of symptoms, including increased tics in some children. It may be difficult to recognize akathisia in young children who are unable to adequately verbalize the symptoms.

For further information, see index entry Haloperidol, Uses, Psychosis.

DOSAGE AND PREPARATIONS.

Oral: *Adults,* initially 0.25 to 2.5 mg at bedtime, increased, if necessary, until improvement is noted or intolerable adverse effects occur (Kurlan, 1989). Most patients respond to 5 mg or less, although a larger dose may be required (Ross and Moldofsky, 1978; Shapiro et al, 1989). Smaller initial doses and more gradual adjustment are recommended for *elderly or debilitated patients. Children 3 to 12 years,* initially 0.25 to 0.5 mg, increased by 0.25 to 0.5 mg at five- to seven-day intervals until the desired therapeutic effect is obtained, intolerable adverse effects occur, or a maximal daily dose of 0.075 mg/kg is given. The total dose may be administered at bedtime or in two or three divided doses. *Children under 3 years,* information is inadequate to establish dosage.

HALOPERIDOL:
Haldol (McNeil), ***Generic.*** Tablets 0.5, 1, 2, 5, 10, and 20 mg.
HALOPERIDOL LACTATE:
Haldol (McNeil), ***Generic.*** Concentrate 2 mg/ml.

PIMOZIDE
[Orap]

ACTIONS AND USES. This diphenylbutylpiperidine derivative has neuroleptic activity and is employed as an alternative to haloperidol (Shapiro et al, 1989) for the suppression of vocal and motor tics in patients with Tourette syndrome. In short-term studies, its efficacy was similar (Ross and Moldofsky, 1978) or slightly less than that of haloperidol (Shapiro et al, 1989) and significantly greater than that of placebo (Shapiro and Shapiro, 1984). Although the precise mechanism of action is unknown, blockade of postsynaptic dopamine receptors has been postulated.

ADVERSE REACTIONS. The incidence of adverse reactions is similar to that of other neuroleptics, although sedation is usually less apparent than with haloperidol therapy. Anticholinergic reactions, such as dry mouth, constipation, and blurred vision, also may occur. Extrapyramidal reactions, including akathisia and tardive dyskinesia, are a risk with long-term use.

Significant cardiac effects have been associated with higher dosages. Ventricular arrhythmias are rare but may be serious. An electrocardiogram should be performed before initiation of therapy and again in one month. Prolongation of the QT interval may necessitate withdrawal of the drug. Pimozide is contraindicated in patients with congenital long QT syndrome, in patients with a history of significant arrhythmias, or in patients taking other drugs that prolong the QT interval.

Pimozide is classified in FDA Pregnancy Category C.

PHARMACOKINETICS. Approximately 50% of an oral dose is bioavailable. Peak absorption time is variable and ranges from 4 to 12 hours. Pimozide is widely distributed, but no data are available on the apparent volume of distribution or protein binding. The drug is extensively metabolized, primarily by N-dealkylation in the liver; there is a significant first-pass effect. The antipsychotic activity of the two major metabolites has not been established. The elimination half-life in patients with psychoses averaged 55 hours, but individual variation is considerable. Some unchanged drug and metabolites are found in the urine and, to a lesser extent, in feces; enterohepatic cycling has been observed.

DOSAGE AND PREPARATIONS. The dose should be individualized so that the suppression of motor and vocal tics is balanced against adverse reactions. Data on the use of pimozide in children under 12 years are limited.

Oral: *Adults,* initially, 1 to 2 mg daily in divided doses, increased gradually every other day; most patients are maintained by dosages of <0.2 mg/kg or 10 mg daily, whichever is less; larger doses are not recommended by the manufacturer. As with other drugs used to suppress tics, periodic attempts should be made to reduce the dosage to determine whether tics persist at the original frequency and severity. *Children under 12 years,* initially, 0.05 mg/kg, preferably taken once at bedtime. The dose may be increased every third day to a maximum of 0.2 mg/kg or 10 mg daily.

Orap (Gate). Tablets 2 mg.

PRIMIDONE
[Mysoline]

For chemical formula, see index entry Primidone, Uses, Epilepsy.

ACTIONS AND USES. In short-term comparative studies, primidone has been similar to or more effective than propranolol in decreasing essential tremor (Gorman et al, 1986; Koller and Royse, 1986). In the only long-term comparative study, primidone and propranolol were comparable in improving symptoms and in the percentage of patients responding (Koller and Vetere-Overfield, 1989). Thirteen percent of patients demonstrated some loss of effectiveness over one year of therapy. It is unclear if this represents development of tolerance or disease progression. Thus, primidone may be a useful alternative to propranolol in elderly patients who cannot tolerate prolonged therapy with beta blockers. However, the incidence of initial adverse reactions is higher with primidone, which may limit patient acceptance.

The therapeutic response to primidone is probably due to the parent compound and not to metabolically derived phenobarbital. Primidone decreases tremor when no detectable level of phenobarbital is apparent, although the contribution of phenobarbital during long-term therapy cannot be ruled out. The effectiveness and role of the latter in essential tremor is controversial. In comparative studies, it has been variably judged as comparable to propranolol, less effective than primidone, better than placebo, or ineffective (Hubble et al, 1989). Phenobarbital may be considered in patients who do not respond to propranolol or primidone or who cannot tolerate primidone.

ADVERSE REACTIONS. The incidence of initial toxicity (dizziness, headache, ataxia, nausea, and vomiting) is high with primidone. These adverse effects may resolve after the first few days and should not be a reason to discontinue the drug; however, patients who experience significant neurologic side effects initially often cannot tolerate continued use of primidone.

DOSAGE AND PREPARATIONS.

Oral: Therapy should be initiated with small doses (eg, 50 to 62.5 mg) and the amount gradually increased to a therapeutic level over a period of two to three weeks. The dose ranges utilized have been quite wide. In one study employing doses of 50 mg to 1 g/day, 250 mg/day was as effective as larger doses (Koller and Royse, 1986). In studies on long-term efficacy, larger doses (350 to 750 mg/day) have been used (Sasso et al, 1990). Thus, the following dosage schedule has been recommended (Hubble et al, 1989): Initially, 50 mg at night, increased to 125 mg at night and, if necessary, to 250 mg at night. If tremor is not controlled, further increases may be attempted in the absence of limiting adverse effects; alternatively, propranolol 80 mg may be added in the morning, with the amount increased in stepwise fashion to 320 mg if necessary.

Generic. Tablets 250 mg

Mysoline (Wyeth-Ayerst). Suspension 250 mg/5 ml; tablets 50 and 250 mg.

PROPRANOLOL HYDROCHLORIDE

[Inderal]

For chemical formula, see index entry Beta-Adrenergic Blocking Agents: Chemical Structures (Figure).

ACTIONS AND USES. Most neurologists consider propranolol the drug of choice for the management of essential tremor when it is not contraindicated. Therapy is usually initiated when tremor disrupts or limits occupational and social activities. Hand tremor responds best; head tremor also has responded (Koller, 1984). Voice tremor may be more resistant (Larsen and Calne, 1983). The response to propranolol is variable and often incomplete. It is generally estimated that up to 70% of patients will experience beneficial effects characterized by an average reduction in tremor amplitude of 50% to 60% (Hubble et al, 1989). No definite predictive factors have been identified to aid in selecting those who will receive satisfactory symptomatic relief. However, younger patients with tremor of short duration (Dupont et al, 1973), older patients, and those with slow tremor frequencies (Teravainen et al, 1976) appear to respond best. In general, those more severely affected are refractory to therapy.

Patients who do not respond to propranolol are unlikely to benefit from another beta blocker. In asthmatic patients who cannot tolerate propranolol, metoprolol has been an effective alternative (Koller and Biary, 1984 B).

The mechanism of action of propranolol in this disorder is unknown, although most available evidence supports the concept that the primary effect is mediated by peripheral $beta_2$ receptors (Teravainen et al, 1986; Jefferson et al, 1987).

For adverse reactions, precautions, and pharmacokinetics, see index entry Beta-Adrenergic Blocking Agents.

DOSAGE AND PREPARATIONS.

Oral: Initially, 40 mg twice daily with the dosage subsequently titrated according to clinical response. Although propranolol blood concentrations do not appear to correlate with effectiveness, clinical improvement is related to dosage and is generally achieved when 120 to 240 mg is given daily in three divided doses, although some patients require 320 mg to achieve optimal response (Koller, 1986). A few patients respond to as little as 60 mg daily (Sorensen et al, 1981). The prolonged-release preparation provides equivalent or better therapeutic response (Koller, 1985; Cleeves and Findley, 1988).

Generic. Tablets 10, 20, 40, 60, 80, and 90 mg; capsules (prolonged-release) 60, 80, 120, and 160 mg; solution (oral) 20 and 40 mg/5 ml and 80 mg/ml.

Inderal (Wyeth-Ayerst). Tablets 10, 20, 40, 60, and 80 mg; capsules (prolonged-release) 60, 80, 120, and 160 mg ***[Inderal LA]***.

Cited References

Assessment: The clinical usefulness of botulinum toxin-A in treating neurologic disorders: Report of the Therapeutics and Technology Assessment Subcommittee of the American Academy of Neurology. *Neurology* 40:1332-1336, 1990.

Clinical use of botulinum toxin: National Institutes of Health Consensus Development Conference Statement, November 12-14, 1990. *Arch Neurol* 48:1294-1298, 1991.

Drugs for Parkinson's disease. *Med Lett Drugs Ther* 35:31-34, 1993.

Tardive Dyskinesia: A Task Force Report of the American Psychiatric Association. Washington, DC, American Psychiatric Association, 1992.

Adler LA, et al: Vitamin E treatment of tardive dyskinesia. *Am J Psychiatry* 150:1405-1407, 1993.

Ahlskog JE: Medical treatment of Parkinson's disease. *Compr Ther* 15:53-59, (March) 1989.
Ahlskog JE, Muenter MD: Treatment of Parkinson's disease with pergolide: Double-blind study. *Mayo Clin Proc* 63:969-978, 1988 A.
Ahlskog JE, Muenter MD: Pergolide: Long-term use in Parkinson's disease. *Mayo Clin Proc* 63:979-987, 1988 B.
Ahlskog JE, Wilkinson JM: New concepts in the treatment of Parkinson's disease. *Pract Ther* 41:574-584, 1990.
Ahlskog JE, et al: Dopamine agonist treatment of fluctuating parkinsonism: D-2 (controlled-release MK-458) vs combined D-1 and D-2 (pergolide). *Arch Neurol* 49:560-568, 1992.
Albin RL, et al: The functional anatomy of basal ganglia disorders. *Trends Neurosci* 12:366-375, 1989.
Albin RL, et al: Abnormalities of striatal projection neurons and *N*-methyl-D-aspartate receptors in presymptomatic Huntington's disease. *N Engl J Med* 322:1293-1298, 1990.
Albin RL, et al: Preferential loss of striato-external pallidal projection neurons in presymptomatic Huntington's disease. *Ann Neurol* 31:425-430, 1992.
Alheid FG, Heimer L: New perspectives in basal forebrain organization of special relevance for neuropsychiatric disorders: The striatopallidal, amygdaloid, and corticopetal components of the substantia innominata. *Neuroscience* 27:1-40, 1988.
Aoki FY, Sitar DS: Clinical pharmacokinetics of amantadine hydrochloride. *Clin Pharmacokinet* 14:35-51, 1988.
Bennett WM: Guide to drug dosage in renal failure. *Clin Pharmacokinet* 15:326-354, 1988.
Berardelli A, et al: Botulinum toxin treatment in patients with focal dystonia and hemifacial spasm: A multicenter study of the Italian movement disorder group. *Ital J Neurol Sci* 14:361-367, 1993.
Bergamasco B, et al: Long-term bromocriptine treatment of *de novo* patients with Parkinson's disease: A seven-year follow-up. *Acta Neurol Scand* 81:383-387, 1990.
Birkmayer W, et al: Increased life expectancy resulting from addition of L-deprenyl to Madopar treatment in Parkinson's disease: Long-term study. *J Neural Transm* 64:113-127, 1985.
Blasi J, et al: Botulinum neurotoxin A selectively cleaves the synaptic protein SNAP-25, letter. *Nature* 365:160-163, 1993.
Blitzer A, et al: Clinical and laboratory characteristics of focal laryngeal dystonia: Study of 110 cases. *Laryngoscope* 98:636-640, 1988.
Bressman S, Fahn S: Essential myoclonus. *Adv Neurol* 43:287-294, 1986.
Bressman SB, et al: Idiopathic dystonia among Ashkenazi Jews: Evidence for autosomal dominant inheritance. *Ann Neurol* 26:612-620, 1989.
Brin MF, et al: Botulinum toxin: Now for abductor laryngeal dystonia. *Neurology* 40 (suppl 1):381, 1990.
Brooks DJ: Detection of preclinical Parkinson's disease with PET. *Neurology* 41 (suppl 2):24-27, 1991.
Burke RE: Tardive dyskinesia: Current clinical issues. *Neurology* 34:1348-1358, 1984.
Burke RE, Kang UJ: Tardive dystonia: Clinical aspects and treatment. *Adv Neurol* 49:199-210, 1988.
Burke RE, et al: Torsion dystonia: Double-blind, prospective trial of high dosage trihexyphenidyl. *Neurology* 36:160-164, 1986.
Burn DJ, et al: Parkinson's disease in twins studied with ^{18}F-dopa and positron emission tomography. *Neurology* 42:1894-1900, 1992.
Busenbark K, et al: The effect of acetazolamide on essential tremor: An open-label trial. *Neurology* 42:1394-1395, 1992.
Busenbark K, et al: Double-blind controlled study of methazolamide in the treatment of essential tremor. *Neurology* 43:1045-1047, 1993.
Butterfield PG, et al: Environmental antecedents of young-onset Parkinson's disease. *Neurology* 43:1150-1158, 1993.
Calne DB: Treatment of Parkinson's disease. *N Engl J Med* 329:1021-1027, 1993.
Caraceni T, et al: The occurrence of motor fluctuations in parkinsonian patients treated long term with levodopa: Role of early treatment and disease progression. *Neurology* 41:380-384, 1991.
Carter CJ, et al: The biochemistry of Huntington's chorea, in Quinn NP, Jenner PG (eds): *Disorders of Movement: Clinical, Pharmacological and Physiological Aspects.* London, Academic Press, 1989, 469-494.
Cedarbaum JM, et al: 'Early' initiation of levodopa treatment does not promote the development of motor response fluctuations, dyskinesias, or dementia in Parkinson's disease. *Neurology* 41:622-629, 1991.
Chan J, et al: Idiopathic cervical dystonia: Clinical characteristics. *Mov Disord* 6:119-126, 1991.
Chase TN, et al: Rationale for continuous dopaminomimetic therapy of Parkinson's disease. *Neurology* 39 (suppl 2):7-10, 1989.
Cleeves L, Findley LJ: Propranolol and propranolol-LA in essential tremor: A double blind comparative study. *J Neurol Neurosurg Psychiatry* 51:379-384, 1988.
Cohen LG, et al: Treatment of focal dystonias of the hand with botulinum toxin injections. *J Neurol Neurosurg Psychiatry* 52:355-363, 1989.
Cohen DJ, et al: Pharmacotherapy of Tourette's syndrome and associated disorders. *Psychiatric Clin North Am* 15:109-129, 1992.
Comella CL, et al: Botulinum toxin injection for spasmodic torticollis: Increased magnitude of benefit with electromyographic assistance. *Neurology* 42:878-882, 1992 A.
Comella CL, et al: Dysphagia after botulinum toxin injections for spasmodic torticollis: Clinical and radiologic findings. *Neurology* 42:1307-1310, 1992 B.
Como PG, Kurlan R: An open-label trial of fluoxetine for obsessive-compulsive disorder in Tourette's syndrome. *Neurology* 41:872-874, 1991.
Cummings JL: Depression and Parkinson's disease: A review. *Am J Psychiatry* 149:443-454, 1992.
Das TK, Park DM: Effect of treatment with botulinum toxin on spasticity. *Postgrad Med J* 65:208-210, 1990.
Deffond D, et al: Apomorphine in treatment of Parkinson's disease: Comparison between subcutaneous and sublingual routes. *J Neurol Neurosurg Psychiatry* 56:101-103, 1993.
de Jong GJ, et al: Factors that influence the occurrence of response variations in Parkinson's disease. *Ann Neurol* 22:4-7, 1987.
Dewey RB Jr, Jankovic J: Hemiballism-hemichorea: Clinical and pharmacologic findings in 21 patients. *Arch Neurol* 46:862-867, 1989.
Direnfeld LK, et al: Is L-dopa drug holiday useful? *Neurology* 30:785-788, 1980.
Dooneief G, et al: An estimate of the incidence of depression in idiopathic Parkinson's disease. *Arch Neurol* 49:305-307, 1992.
Dubinsky RM, et al: Electromyographic guidance of botulinum toxin treatment in cervical dystonia. *Clin Neuropharmacol* 14:262-267, 1991.
Dupont E, et al: Treatment of benign essential tremor with propranolol. *Acta Neurol Scand* 49:75-84, 1973.
Durif F, et al: Relation between clinical efficacy and pharmacokinetic parameters after sublingual apomorphine in Parkinson's disease. *Clin Neuropharmacol* 16 (2):157-166, 1993.
Duvoisin RC (ed): New strategies in dopaminergic therapy of Parkinson's disease: The use of a controlled-release formulation. *Neurology* 39 (suppl 2):1-106, 1989.
Ebmeier SA, et al: Dementia in idiopathic Parkinson's disease: Prevalence and relationship with symptoms and signs of parkinsonism. *Psychol Med* 21:69-76, 1991.
Edwards LL, et al: Gastrointestinal dysfunction in Parkinson's disease: Frequency and pathophysiology. *Neurology* 42:726-732, 1992.
Egan MF, et al: Treatment of tardive dyskinesia with vitamin E. *Am J Psychiatry* 149:773-777, 1992.
Elizan TS, et al: Selegiline as an adjunct to conventional levodopa therapy in Parkinson's disease: Experience with this type B monoamine oxidase inhibitor in 200 patients. *Arch Neurol* 46:1280-1283, 1989.
Elsworth JD, et al: The contribution of amphetamine metabolites of (-)-deprenyl to its antiparkinsonian properties. *J Neural Transm* 54:105-110, 1982.
Engberg G, et al: Deprenyl (selegiline), a selective MAO-B inhibitor with active metabolites; effects on locomotor activity, dopaminergic neurotransmission and firing rate of nigral dopamine neurons. *J Pharmacol Exp Ther* 259:841-847, 1991.

Factor SA, et al: Parkinson's disease: An open-label study of pergolide in 63 patients failing bromocriptine therapy, abstract. *Neurology* 37 (suppl 1):37, 1987.
Factor SA, et al: Efficacy of Sinemet CR4 in subgroups of patients with Parkinson's disease. *J Neurol Neurosurg Psychiatry* 52:83-88, 1989.
Factor SA, et al: Clozapine: A 2-year open trial in Parkinson's disease patients with psychosis. *Neurology* 44:544-546, 1994.
Fahn S: High dosage anticholinergic therapy in dystonia. *Neurology* 33:1255-1261, 1983.
Fahn S: Posthypoxic action myoclonus: Literature review update. *Adv Neurol* 43:157-169, 1986.
Fahn S: Concept and classification of dystonia. *Adv Neurol* 50:1-8, 1988.
Fahn S: The endogenous toxin hypothesis of the etiology of Parkinson's disease and a pilot trial of high-dosage antioxidants in an attempt to slow the progression of the illness. *Ann NY Acad Sci* 570:186-196, 1989.
Fahn S, Bressman SB: Should levodopa therapy for parkinsonism be started early or late? Evidence against early treatment. *Can J Neurol Sci* 11:200-206, 1984.
Fahn S, et al: Definition and classification of myoclonus. *Adv Neurol* 43:1-5, 1986.
Findley LJ, Cleeves L: Classification of tremor, in Quinn NP, Jenner PG (eds): *Disorders of Movement: Clinical, Pharmacological and Physiological Aspects.* London, Academic Press, 1989, 505-519.
Folstein S, Folstein M: Diagnosis and treatment of Huntington's disease. *Compr Ther* 7:60-66, (April) 1981.
Ford CN, et al: Indirect laryngoscopic approach for injection of botulinum toxin in spasmodic dysphonia. *Otolaryngol Head Neck Surg* 103:752-758, 1990.
Foster NL, et al: THIP treatment of Huntington's disease. *Neurology* 33:637-639, 1983.
Friedman JH: The management of the levodopa psychoses. *Clin Neuropharmacol* 14:283-295, 1991.
Furtado JCS, Mazurek MF: MPTP-induced neurotoxicity and the quest for a preventative therapy for Parkinson's disease. *Can J Neurol Sci* 18:77-82, 1991.
García-Albea E, et al: Parkinsonism unmasked by verapamil. *Clin Neuropharmacol* 16:263-265, 1993.
Gelb DJ, et al: Controlled trial of botulinum toxin injections in the treatment of spasmodic torticollis. *Neurology* 39:80-84, 1989.
Gelenberg AJ, et al: Anticholinergic effects on memory: Benztropine versus amantadine. *J Clin Psychopharmacol* 9:180-185, 1989.
Gerfen CR: The neostriatal mosaic: Striatal patch-matrix organization is related to cortical lamination. *Science* 246:385-388, 1989.
Gibb WRG: Dementia and Parkinson's disease. *Br J Psychiatry* 154:596-614, 1989.
Girlanda P, et al: Botulinum toxin therapy: Distant effects on neuromuscular transmission and autonomic nervous system. *J Neurol Neurosurg Psychiatry* 55:844-845, 1992.
Goetz CG, et al: Chronic agonist therapy for Parkinson's disease: 5-year study of bromocriptine and pergolide. *Neurology* 34 (suppl 12):218, 1984.
Golbe LI: Deprenyl as symptomatic therapy in Parkinson's disease. *Clin Neuropharmacol* 11:387-400, 1988.
Golbe LI: Long-term efficacy and safety of deprenyl (selegiline) in advanced Parkinson's disease. *Neurology* 39:1109-1111, 1989.
Golbe LI, et al: Deprenyl in the treatment of symptom fluctuations in advanced Parkinson's disease. *Clin Neuropharmacol* 11:45-55, 1988.
Golbe LI, et al: A large kindred with autosomal dominant Parkinson's disease. *Ann Neurol* 27:276-282, 1990.
Gorman WP, et al: A comparison of primidone, propranolol, and placebo in essential tremor, using quantitative analysis. *J Neurol Neurosurg Psychiatry* 49:64-68, 1986.
Greene PE, Fahn S: Baclofen in the treatment of idiopathic dystonia in children. *Mov Disord* 7:48-52, 1992.
Greene PE, et al: Analysis of open-label trials in torsion dystonia using high dosages of anticholinergics and other drugs. *Mov Disord* 3:46-60, 1988.
Greene P, et al: Double-blind, placebo-controlled trial of botulinum toxin injections for the treatment of spasmodic torticollis. *Neurology* 40:1213-1218, 1990.
Hallett M: Classification and treatment of tremor. *JAMA* 266:1115-1117, 1991.
Hansten PD, Horn JR: *Drug Interactions & Updates.* Malvern, Penn, Lea & Febiger, 1990.
Heikkila RE, et al: Protection against dopaminergic neurotoxicity of 1-methyl-4-phenyl-1, 2, 3, 6-tetrahydropyridine by monoamine oxidase inhibitors. *Nature* 311:467-469, 1984.
Hely MA, et al: The Sydney multicentre study of Parkinson's disease: A report on the first 3 years. *J Neurol Neurosurg Psychiatry* 52:324-328, 1989.
Hoover JE, Strick PL: Multiple output channels in the basal ganglia. *Science* 259:819-821, 1993.
Hubble JP, et al: Essential tremor. *Clin Neuropharmacol* 12:453-482, 1989.
Hunt RD, et al: Clonidine benefits children with attention deficit disorder and hyperactivity. *J Am Acad Adolesc Psychiatry* 24:617-629, 1985.
Huntington's Disease Collaborative Research Group: A novel gene containing a trinucleotide repeat that is expanded and unstable on Huntington's disease chromosomes. *Cell* 72:971-983, 1993.
Hutton JT, Morris JL: Long-term evaluation of Sinemet CR in parkinsonian patients with motor fluctuations. *J Can Neurol Sci* 18:467-471, 1991.
Hutton JT, et al: Multicenter controlled study of Sinemet CR vs Sinemet (12/100) in advanced Parkinson's disease. *Neurology* 39 (suppl 2):67-72, 1989.
Hutton JT, et al: Controlled study of the antiparkinsonian activity and tolerability of cabergoline. *Neurology* 43:613-616, 1993.
Jahanshahi M, et al: Natural history of adult-onset idiopathic torticollis. *Arch Neurol* 47:548-552, 1990.
Jankovic J: Long-term study of pergolide in Parkinson's disease. *Neurology* 35:296-299, 1985.
Jankovic J: Parkinsonism plus syndromes. *Mov Disord* 4:S95-S119, 1989.
Jankovic J: Deprenyl in attention deficit associated with Tourette's syndrome. *Arch Neurol* 50:286-288, 1993.
Jankovic J: Botulinum toxin in the treatment of dystonic tics. *Mov Disord* 9:347-349, 1994.
Jankovic J, Orman J: Tetrabenazine therapy of dystonia, chorea, tics, and other dyskinesias. *Neurology* 38:391-394, 1988.
Jankovic J, Schwartz K: Botulinum toxin treatment of tremors. *Neurology* 41:1185-1188, 1991.
Jankovic J, Schwartz KS: Longitudinal experience with botulinum toxin injections for treatment of blepharospasm and cervical dystonia. *Neurology* 43:834-836, 1993.
Jankovic J, et al: Dystonia, spasmodic dysphonia, other focal dystonias and hemifacial spasm. *J Neurol Neurosurg Psychiatry* 53:633-639, 1990.
Jefferson D, et al: The comparative effects of ICI 118551 and propranolol on essential tremor. *Br J Clin Pharmacol* 24:729-734, 1987.
Jenner P, et al: Mechanism of action of clonazepam in myoclonus in relation to effects on GABA and 5-HT. *Adv Neurol* 43:629-643, 1986.
Jeste DV, Wyatt RJ: Therapeutic strategies against tardive dyskinesia: Two decades of experience. *Arch Gen Psychiatry* 39:803-816, 1982.
Johnson WG: Genetic susceptibility to Parkinson's disease. *Neurology* 41 (suppl 2):82-87, 1991.
Kang UJ, Fahn S: Management of tardive dyskinesia. *Ration Drug Ther* 22:1-7, (Aug) 1988.
Kempster PA, et al: Comparison of motor response to apomorphine and levodopa in Parkinson's disease. *J Neurol Neurosurg Psychiatry* 53:1004-1007, 1990.
Kempster PA, et al: Intermittent subcutaneous apomorphine injection treatment of parkinsonian motor oscillations. *Aust N Z J Med* 21:314-318, 1991.
Koller WC: Propranolol therapy for essential tremor of the head. *Neurology* 34:1077-1079, 1984.

Koller WC: Long-acting propranolol in essential tremor. *Neurology* 35:108-110, 1985.

Koller WC: Dose-response relationship of propanolol in the treatment of essential tremor. *Arch Neurol* 43:42-43, 1986.

Koller WC, Biary N: Effect of alcohol on tremors: Comparison with propranolol. *Neurology* 34:221-222, 1984 A.

Koller WC, Biary N: Metoprolol compared with propranolol in treatment of essential tremor. *Arch Neurol* 41:171-172, 1984 B.

Koller WC, Huber SJ: Tremor disorders of aging: Diagnosis and management. *Geriatrics* 44:33-41, 1989.

Koller WC, Royse VL: Efficacy of primidone in essential tremor. *Neurology* 36:121-124, 1986.

Koller WC, Vetere-Overfield BV: Acute and chronic effects of propranolol and primidone in essential tremor. *Neurology* 39:1587-1588, 1989.

Koller WC, et al: Classification of essential tremor. *Clin Neuropharmacol* 15(2):81-87, 1992.

Koman LA, et al: Management of cerebral palsy with botulinum-A toxin: Preliminary investigation. *J Pediatr Orthop* 13:489-495, 1993.

Kramer PL, et al: Dystonia gene in Ashkenazi Jewish population is located on chromosome 9q32-34. *Ann Neurol* 27:114-120, 1990.

Kurlan R: Practical therapy of Parkinson's disease. *Semin Neurol* 7:160-166, 1987.

Kurlan R: International symposium on early dopamine agonist therapy of Parkinson's disease. *Arch Neurol* 45:204-208, 1988.

Kurlan R: Tourette's syndrome. *Neurology* 39:1625-1630, 1989.

Kurlan R: Duodenal administration of levodopa, in Koller WC, et al (eds): *Therapy of Parkinson's Disease.* New York, Marcell Dekker, 1990, 223-237.

Kurlan R, Como P: Drug-induced alzheimerism. *Arch Neurol* 45:356-357, 1988.

Kurlan R, Shoulson I: Differential diagnosis of facial chorea. *Adv Neurol* 49:225-237, 1988.

Kurlan R, et al: Long-term experience with pergolide therapy of advanced parkinsonism. *Neurology* 35:738-742, 1985.

Kurlan R, et al: Levodopa drug holiday versus drug dosage reduction in Parkinson's disease. *Clin Neuropharmacol* 17:117-127, 1994.

Kurth MC, et al: Oral levodopa/carbidopa solution versus tablets in Parkinson's patients with severe fluctuations: A pilot study. *Neurology* 43:1036-1039, 1993.

Kushnir SL, Ratner JT: Calcium channel blockers for tardive dyskinesia in geriatric psychiatric patients. *Am J Psychiatry* 146:1218-1219, 1989.

Lang AE: Drug treatment of dystonia. *Adv Neurol* 50:313-321, 1989.

Lange DJ, et al: Distant effects of local injection of botulinum toxin. *Muscle Nerve* 10:552-555, 1987.

Langston JW, et al: Pargyline prevents MPTP-induced parkinsonism in primates. *Science* 225:1480-1482, 1984.

Larsen TA, Calne DB: Essential tremor. *Clin Neuropharmacol* 6:185-206, 1983.

Lazzarini AM, et al: A clinical genetic study of Parkinson's disease: Evidence for dominant transmission. *Neurology* 44:499-506, 1994.

Leckman JF, et al: Clonidine treatment of Gilles de la Tourette's syndrome. *Arch Gen Psychiatry* 48:324-328, 1991.

Lees AJ: The on-off phenomenon. *J Neurol Neurosurg Psychiatry* (suppl) 29-37, 1989.

Lees AJ, et al: Deprenyl in Parkinson's disease. *Lancet* 2:791-795, 1977.

Leibowitz M, Lieberman A: Comparison of dopa decarboxylase inhibitor (carbidopa) combined with levodopa and levodopa alone on cardiovascular system of patients with Parkinson's disease. *Neurology* 25:917-921, 1975.

Leigh PN: Functional organization of the basal ganglia, in Quinn NP, Jenner PG (eds): *Disorders of Movement: Clinical, Pharmacological and Physiological Aspects.* London, Academic Press, 1989, 11-32.

Lenox RH, et al: Tardive dyskinesia: Clinical and neuroendocrine response to low dose bromocriptine. *J Clin Psychopharmacol* 5:286-292, 1985.

Lera G, et al: Cabergoline in Parkinson's disease: Long-term follow-up. *Neurology* 43:2587-2590, 1993.

Lesser RP, et al: Analysis of the clinical problems in parkinsonism and the complications of long-term levodopa therapy. *Neurology* 29:1253-1260, 1979.

Levitt P, et al: Immunocytochemical demonstration of monoamine oxidase B in brain astrocytes and serotonergic neurons. *Proc Natl Acad Sci USA* 79:6385-6389, 1982.

LeWitt PA, et al: Comparison of pergolide and bromocriptine therapy in parkinsonism. *Neurology* 33:1009-1014, 1983.

Lieberman AN, et al: Comparative efficacy of pergolide and bromocriptine in patients with advanced Parkinson's disease. *Adv Neurol* 37:95-108, 1983.

Lieberman AN, et al: Long-term treatment with pergolide: Decreased efficacy with time. *Neurology* 34:223-226, 1984.

Lieberman JA, et al: Treatment of tardive dyskinesia with bromocriptine: Test of the receptor modification strategy. *Arch Gen Psychiatry* 46:908-913, 1989 A.

Lieberman J, et al: Clozapine pharmacology and tardive dyskinesia. *Psychopharmacology* 99(suppl):54-59, 1989 B.

Lorentz IT, et al: Treatment of idiopathic spasmodic torticollis with botulinum toxin A: A double-blind study on twenty-three patients. *Mov Disord* 6:145-150, 1991.

Lou J-S, Jankovic J: Essential tremor: Clinical correlates in 350 patients. *Neurology* 41:234-238, 1991.

Ludlow CL: Treatment of speech and voice disorders with botulinum toxin. *JAMA* 264:2671-2675, 1990.

Ludlow CL, et al: Therapeutic use of type F botulinum toxin. *N Engl J Med* 326:349-350, 1992.

Marion MH, et al: Repeated levodopa infusions in fluctuating Parkinson's disease: Clinical and pharmacokinetic data. *Clin Neuropharmacol* 9:165-181, 1986.

Marion M-H, et al: Stridor and focal laryngeal dystonia. *Lancet* 339:457-458, 1992.

Markham CH, Diamond SG: Modification of Parkinson's disease by long-term levodopa treatment. *Arch Neurol* 43:405-407, 1986.

Marsden CD, Quinn NP: The dystonias. *BMJ* 300:139-144, 1990.

McElvaney NG, et al: Pleuropulmonary disease during bromocriptine treatment of Parkinson's disease. *Arch Intern Med* 148:2231-2236, 1988.

McHale DM, Sage JI: Hallucinations and confusion after pergolide withdrawal. *Clin Neuropharmacol* 11:545-548, 1988.

Melamed E: Initiation of levodopa therapy in parkinsonian patients should be delayed until the advanced stages of the disease. *Arch Neurol* 43:402-405, 1986.

Meltzer HY, Luchins DJ: Effect of clozapine in severe tardive dyskinesia: Case report. *J Clin Psychopharmacol* 4:286-287, 1984.

Montastruc JL, et al: A randomised controlled study of bromocriptine versus levodopa in previously untreated Parkinsonian patients: A 3 year follow-up. *J Neurol Neurosurg Psychiatry* 52:773-775, 1989.

Montastruc JL, et al: Pseudophaeochromocytoma in parkinsonian patient treated with fluoxetine plus selegiline. *Lancet* 341:555, 1993.

Moore AP, Blumhardt LD: A double blind trial of botulinum toxin 'A' in torticollis, with one year follow up. *J Neurol Neurosurg Psychiatry* 54:813-816, 1991.

Mouradian MM, et al: Modification of central dopaminergic mechanisms by continuous levodopa therapy for advanced Parkinson's disease. *Ann Neurol* 27:18-23, 1990.

Muenter MD: Should levodopa be started early or late? *Can J Neurol Surg* 11:195-199, 1984.

Muenter MD, et al: Treatment of essential tremor with methazolamide. *Mayo Clin Proc* 66:991-997, 1991.

Myllylä VV, et al: Selegiline as initial treatment in de novo parkinsonian patients. *Neurology* 42:339-343, 1992.

Nutt JG: Levodopa-induced dyskinesia: Review, observations, and speculations. *Neurology* 40:340-345, 1990.

Nutt JG, et al: "On-off" phenomenon in Parkinson's disease: Relation to levodopa absorption and transport. *N Engl J Med* 310:483-488, 1984.

Nygaard TG, at al: Dopa-responsive dystonia: Long-term treatment response and prognosis. *Neurology* 41:174-181, 1991.

Obeso JA, et al: The physiology of myoclonus in man, in Quinn NP, Jenner PG (eds): *Disorders of Movement: Clinical, Pharmacological and Physiological Aspects.* London, Academic Press, 1989, 437-444.

Olanow CW: Oxidation reactions in Parkinson's disease. *Neurology* 40(suppl 3):32-39, 1990.

Olanow CW, et al: A multicenter double-blind placebo-controlled trial of pergolide as an adjunct to Sinemet in Parkinson's disease. *Mov Disord* 9:40-47, 1994.

Olsson JE, et al: Early treatment with a combination of bromocriptine and levodopa compared with levodopa monotherapy in the treatment of Parkinson's disease. *Curr Ther Res* 46:1002-1014, 1989.

Ozelius L, et al: Human gene for torsion dystonia located on chromosome 9q32-34. *Neuron* 3:1427-1434, 1989.

Pahwa R, et al: Clinical experience with controlled-release carbidopa/levodopa in Parkinson's disease. *Neurology* 43:677-681, 1993.

Parker WD, et al: Abnormalities of the electron transport chain in idiopathic Parkinson's disease. *Ann Neurol* 26:719-723, 1989.

Parkinson Study Group: Effect of deprenyl on the progression of disability in early Parkinson's disease. *N Engl J Med* 321:1364-1371, 1989.

The Parkinson Study Group: Effects of tocopherol and deprenyl on the progression of disability in early Parkinson's disease. *N Engl J Med* 328:176-183, 1993.

Parkinson's Disease Research Group in the United Kingdom: Comparisons of therapeutic effects of levodopa, levodopa and selegiline, and bromocriptine in patients with early, mild Parkinson's disease: Three year interim report. *BMJ* 307:469-472, 1993.

Paterson IA, et al: Inhibition of monoamine oxidase-B by (-)-deprenyl potentiates neuronal responses to dopamine agonists but does not inhibit dopamine catabolism in the rat striatum. *J Pharmacol Exp Ther* 258:1019-1026, 1991.

Perry TL, et al: Double-blind clinical trial of isoniazid in Huntington's disease. *Neurology* 32:354-358, 1982.

Peterson B, et al: Reduced basal ganglia volumes in Tourette's syndrome using three-dimensional reconstruction techniques from magnetic resonance images. *Neurology* 43:941-949, 1993.

Pincus JH, Barry K: Influence of dietary protein on motor fluctuations in Parkinson's disease. *Arch Neurol* 44:270-272, 1987.

Poewe W, et al: Subcutaneous apomorphine in Parkinson's disease, letter. *Lancet* 1:943, 1988.

Rajput AH, et al: Chronic low dose therapy in Parkinson's disease: An argument for delaying levodopa therapy. *Neurology* 34:991-996, 1984.

Regeur L, et al: Clinical features and long-term treatment with pimozide in 65 patients with Gilles de la Tourette's syndrome. *J Neurol Neurosurg Psychiatry* 49:791-795, 1986.

Reynolds GP, et al: Deprenyl is metabolized to methamphetamine and amphetamine in man. *Br J Clin Pharmacol* 6:542-544, 1978.

Riddle MA, et al: Fluoxetine treatment of children and adolescents with Tourette's and obsessive compulsive disorders: Preliminary clinical experience. *J Am Acad Child Adolesc Psychiatry* 29:45-48, 1990.

Riddle MA, et al: SPECT imaging of cerebral blood flow in Tourette syndrome, in Chase TN, et al (eds): *Advances in Neurology.* New York, Raven Press, 1992, vol 58, 213-226.

Rinne UK (ed): New approach to the treatment of Parkinson's disease. *Acta Neurol Scand* 68(suppl 95):1-144, 1983.

Rinne UK: Early combination of bromocriptine and levodopa in the treatment of Parkinson's disease: A five-year follow-up study. *Neurology* 37:826-828, 1987.

Roos RAC, et al: Response fluctuations in Parkinson's disease. *Neurology* 40:1344-1346, 1990.

Ross MS, Moldofsky H: Comparison of pimozide and haloperidol in treatment of Gilles de la Tourette's syndrome. *Am J Psychiatry* 135:585-587, 1978.

Sajatovic M, et al: Clozapine treatment of psychiatric symptoms resistant to neuroleptic treatment in patients with Huntington's chorea. *Neurology* 41:156, 1991.

Sasso E, et al: Primidone in the long-term treatment of essential tremor: A prospective study with computerized quantitative analysis. *Clin Neuropharmacol* 13:67-76, 1990.

Sawle GV, et al: The identification of presymptomatic parkinsonism: Clinical and [^{18}F]dopa positron emission tomography studies in an Irish kindred. *Ann Neurol* 32:609-617, 1992.

Sayre LM: Biochemical mechanism of action of the dopaminergic neurotoxin 1-methyl-4-phenyl-1,2,3,6-tetrahydropyridine (MPTP). *Toxicol Lett* 48:121-149, 1989.

Schachter M, et al: Deprenyl in management of response fluctuations in patients with Parkinson's disease on levodopa. *J Neurol Neurosurg Psychiatry* 43:1016-1021, 1980.

Schapira AH, et al: Anatomic and disease specificity of NADH CoQ1 reductase (complex I) deficiency in Parkinson's disease. *J Neurochem* 55:2142-2145, 1990.

Schran HF, et al: The pharmacokinetics of bromocriptine in man, in Goldstein M, et al (eds): *Ergot Compounds and Brain Function: Neuroendocrine and Neuropsychiatric Aspects.* New York, Raven Press, 1980, 125-139.

Scigliano G, et al: Gamma-vinyl GABA treatment of Huntington's disease. *Neurology* 34:94-96, 1984.

Shapiro AK, Shapiro E: Controlled study of pimozide vs placebo in Tourette's syndrome. *J Am Acad Child Psychiatry* 23:161-173, 1984.

Shapiro E, et al: Controlled study of haloperidol, pimozide, and placebo for the treatment of Gilles de la Tourette's syndrome. *Arch Gen Psychiatry* 46:722-730, 1989.

Shaw KM, et al: Impact of treatment with levodopa on Parkinson's disease. *Q J Med* 49:283-293, 1980.

Shoffner JM, et al: Mitochondrial oxidative phosphorylation defects in Parkinson's disease. *Ann Neurol* 30:332-339, 1991.

Shoulson I: Huntington's disease: Overview of experimental therapeutics, in Chase TN, et al: *Huntington's Disease.* New York, Raven Press, 1979.

Shoulson I: Levodopa therapy of coexistent drug-induced parkinsonism and tardive dyskinesias, in Fahn S, et al (eds): *Experimental Therapeutics of Movement Disorders.* New York, Raven Press, 1983, 51-60.

Shoulson I: On chorea. *Clin Neuropharmacol* 9(suppl 2):585-599, 1986 A.

Shoulson I: Huntington's disease, in Asbury AK, et al (eds): *Diseases of the Nervous System.* Philadelphia, WB Saunders, 1986 B, 1258-1267.

Simpson GM, et al: Management of tardive dyskinesia: Current update. *Drugs* 23:381-393, 1982.

Singer HS, Walkup JT: Tourette syndrome and other tic disorders: Diagnosis, pathophysiology, and treatment. *Medicine* 70:15-32, 1991.

Singer HS, et al: Volumetric MRI changes in basal ganglia of children with Tourette's syndrome. *Neurology* 43:950-956, 1993.

Snow BJ, et al: Treatment of spasticity with botulinum toxin: A double-blind study. *Ann Neurol* 28:512-515, 1990.

Sokoloff P, et al: Molecular cloning and characterization of a novel dopamine receptor (D3) as a target for neuroleptics. *Nature* 347:146-151, 1990.

Sorensen PS, et al: Essential tremor treated with propranolol: Lack of correlation between clinical effect and plasma propranolol levels. *Ann Neurol* 9:53-57, 1981.

Stacy M, Jankovic J: Current approaches in the treatment of Parkinson's disease. *Annu Rev Med* 44:431-440, 1993.

Starkstein SE, et al: Cognitive impairments and depression in Parkinson's disease: A follow up study. *J Neurol Neurosurg Psychiatry* 53:597-602, 1990.

Steur ENHJ: Increase of Parkinson disability after fluoxetine medication. *Neurology* 43:211-213, 1993.

Stibe CMH, et al: Subcutaneous apomorphine in parkinsonian on-off oscillations. *Lancet* 1:403-406, 1988.

Suchowersky O, deVries JD: Interaction of fluoxetine and selegiline. *Can J Psychiatry* 35:571-572, 1990.

Sunahara RK, et al: Cloning of the gene for a human dopamine D_5 receptor with higher affinity for dopamine than D_1, letter. *Nature* 350:614-619, 1991.

Tarsy D: Neuroleptic-induced movement disorders, in Quinn NP, Jenner PG (eds): *Disorders of Movement: Clinical, Pharmacological and Physiological Aspects.* London, Academic Press, 1989, 361-394.
Teravainen H: Selegiline in Parkinson's disease. *Acta Neurol Scand* 81:333-336, 1990.
Teravainen H, et al: Effect of propranolol on essential tremor. *Neurology* 26:27-30, 1976.
Teravainen H, et al: Selective adrenergic beta-2-receptor blocking drug, ICI-118.551 is effective in essential tremor. *Acta Neurol Scand* 74:34-37, 1986.
Tetrud JW, Langston JW: Effect of deprenyl (selegiline) on the natural history of Parkinson's disease. *Science* 245:519-521, 1989.
Thal LJ, et al: Treatment of myoclonus with L-5-hydroxytryptophan and carbidopa: Clinical, electrophysiological, and biochemical observations. *Ann Neurol* 7:570-576, 1980.
The Tourette Syndrome Classification Study Group: Definitions and classification of tic disorders. *Arch Neurol* 50:1013-1016, 1993.
Tsui JKC, et al: Double-blind study of botulinum toxin in spasmodic torticollis. *Lancet* 2:245-247, 1986.
Tsui JKC, et al: Production of circulating antibodies to botulinum-A toxin in patients receiving repeated injections for dystonia. *Ann Neurol* 23:181, 1988.
Tsui JKC, et al: Botulinum toxin in the treatment of writer's cramp: A double-blind study. *Neurology* 43:183-185, 1993.
UK Bromocriptine Research Group: Bromocriptine in Parkinson's disease: A double-blind study comparing "low-slow" and "high-fast" introductory dosage regimens in de novo patients. *J Neurol Neurosurg Psychiatry* 52:77-82, 1989.
van de Wetering BJM, Heutink P: The genetics of the Gilles de la Tourette syndrome: A review. *J Lab Clin Med* 121:638-645, 1993.
van Laar T, et al: Intranasal apomorphine in parkinsonian on-off fluctuations. *Arch Neurol* 49:482-484, 1992.
Van Tol HHM, et al: Cloning of the gene for a human dopamine D_4 receptor with high affinity for the antipsychotic clozapine, letter. *Nature* 350:610-614, 1991.
Van Woert MH, Hwang EC: Biochemistry and pharmacology of myoclonus, in Klawans HL (ed): *Clinical Neuropharmacology.* New York, Raven Press, 1978, vol 3, 167-184.
Vance ML, et al: Bromocriptine. *Ann Intern Med* 100:78-91, 1984.
Waddington JL, O'Boyle KM: Drugs acting on brain dopamine receptors: A conceptual re-evaluation five years after the first selective D-1 antagonist. *Pharmacol Ther* 43:1-52, 1989.
Waters CH, Miller CA: Autosomal dominant Lewy body parkinsonism in a four-generation family. *Ann Neurol* 35:59-64, 1994.
Weiner WJ, et al: Drug holiday and management of Parkinson disease. *Neurology* 30:1257-1261, 1980.
Weiner WJ, et al: Levodopa, melanoma, and Parkinson's disease. *Neurology* 43:674-677, 1993.
Westlund KN, et al: Distinct monoamine oxidase A and B populations in primate brain. *Science* 230:181-183, 1985.
Whurr R, et al: The use of botulinum toxin in the treatment of adductor spasmodic dysphonia. *J Neurol Neurosurg Psychiatry* 56:526-530, 1993.
Wiener L, et al: Chronic L-deprenyl induced up-regulation of the dopamine uptake carrier. *Eur J Pharmacol* 193:191-194, 1989.
Wilding IR, et al: Characterisation of the in vivo behaviour of a controlled-release formulation of levodopa (Sinemet CR). *Clin Neuropharmacol* 14:305-321, 1991.
Wolk SI, Douglas CJ: Clozapine treatment of psychosis in Parkinson's disease: A report of five consecutive cases. *J Clin Psychiatry* 53:373-376, (Oct) 1992.
Yahr MD, et al: Treatment of Parkinson's disease in early and late phases: Use of pharmacological agents with special reference to deprenyl (selegiline). *Acta Neurol Scand* (suppl 95):95-102, 1983.
Yoshimura DM, et al: Botulinum toxin therapy for limb dystonias. *Neurology* 42:627-630, 1992.
Zimmerman T, Sage JI: Comparison of combination pergolide and levodopa to levodopa alone after 63 months of treatment. *Clin Neuropharmacol* 14:165-169, 1991.

Drugs Used in Immunologic Neuromuscular Disorders

17

MYASTHENIA GRAVIS

Etiology

Myasthenia gravis is an autoimmune disorder characterized by fluctuating weakness and rapid fatigability of skeletal muscle due to impaired neuromuscular transmission. The muscle weakness is of variable severity and sometimes is exacerbated by infection, stress, and loss of sleep. When involvement is limited, those muscles innervated by the cranial nerves (ie, extraocular, facial, pharyngeal, laryngeal) often are among the first affected. With moderate to severe involvement, axial and limb muscles may be affected. The Osserman classification, which is based on a combination of age, rate of progression, distribution of symptoms, and severity, is a useful guide to prognosis and management (Osserman and Genkins, 1971). Another classification, which is based on the pattern of immunologic abnormalities, provides evidence for disease heterogeneity (Compston et al, 1980). About 15% of patients with myasthenia gravis also have other autoimmune disorders.

Myasthenia gravis is caused by a reduction in the number of functional acetylcholine receptors at the neuromuscular junction as a result of antibody-mediated autoimmunity. The acetylcholine (nicotinic) receptor monomer found in skeletal muscle consists of five subunits: two alpha, one beta, one delta, and one gamma (fetal or denervated muscle) or epsilon (adult muscle). The native receptor exists as a dimer. The main immunogenic region of the receptor is believed to be in the alpha subunit that is apart from the acetylcholine binding site.

Antibodies to acetylcholine receptors reduce synaptic transmission by (1) accelerating the breakdown of receptors, (2) blocking acetylcholine binding, and (3) initiating complement-mediated lysis of the postsynaptic membrane (Drachman et al, 1988). A combination of these actions reduces the number of functional acetylcholine receptors in the involved muscles by as much as 70% to 90%. In addition, the neuromuscular junctional folds become simplified or are destroyed. Hence, the number of interactions between the acetylcholine released by nerve impulses and the receptors is decreased; this causes progressive failure of contraction from repeated nerve stimulation and thus reduces muscle strength.

Circulating antibodies to the receptor have been demonstrated in 85% to 90% of patients with generalized myasthenia with or without thymoma (Drachman et al, 1987). Abnormal antibody titers occur in about 50% of patients with purely ocular manifestations. In general, clinical severity does not correlate with antibody titer levels; however, there may be a relationship between titer and the clinical state in an individual. Since myasthenic antibodies are polyclonal (Hohlfeld, 1989), the lack of correlation may reflect the differing capacities of antibody idiotypes to cause receptor loss. Further, there are patients in whom circulating antibodies are not detected by standard radioimmunoassay (RIA), but even in these "seronegative" patients, the number of acetylcholine receptors is decreased.

A thymic abnormality is found in approximately 75% of patients with myasthenia under the age of 45; of these, 85% have thymic hyperplasia, which is characterized by germinal centers in the medulla. The other 15% have a thymoma.

In addition to generalized and purely ocular myasthenia (symptoms confined to extraocular muscles), myasthenia can be induced by penicillamine [Cuprimine, Depen] in patients with rheumatoid arthritis or Wilson's disease who are being treated with this drug. Neonatal myasthenia occurs in one of six infants born to women with myasthenia. In these infants, there usually is a good correlation between antibody titers in the mother and child. In contrast, acetylcholine receptor antibodies are not found in congenital myasthenia, which occurs in infants of healthy mothers and is associated with a diverse group of nonautoimmune disorders caused by phenotypic expression of different defects in acetylcholine biosynthesis, metabolism, and receptor function (Misulis and Fenichel, 1989).

The Lambert-Eaton syndrome is another myasthenic disorder of autoimmune pathogenesis (O'Neill et al, 1988). It is characterized by muscle weakness, hyporeflexia, and autonomic dysfunction. Two-thirds of cases are associated with a malignancy, usually a small cell carcinoma of the lung. The defect in neurotransmission is due to impaired calcium-dependent release of acetylcholine from nerve terminals. Autoantibodies appear to recognize a specific subtype of voltage-gated calcium channel in neurons that is involved in neurotransmitter secretion (Sher et al, 1989).

Diagnosis

The diagnosis of myasthenia gravis usually can be made on the basis of the patient's history and signs observed during physical examination and can be substantiated by several tests, in particular the assay of antiacetylcholine receptor antibody in plasma. Computerized tomography (CT) or magnetic resonance imaging (MRI) of the anterior mediastinum is part of the evaluation of all newly diagnosed patients to determine if a thymoma is present.

Typically, repetitive, mixed nerve stimulation of proximal muscles (eg, biceps, deltoid) produces a decremental response in amplitude of the muscle compound action potential. Single-fiber electromyography (EMG) may improve diagnostic sensitivity (Sanders, 1987). In doubtful cases, myasthenia can be differentiated from other neuromuscular diseases by the parenteral administration of the short-acting anticholinesterase, edrophonium [Enlon, Reversol, Tensilon], or the longer acting agent, neostigmine methylsulfate [Prostigmin]. When these drugs are used for diagnosis, cranial muscle signs (eg, ptosis, ocular movements, speech) can be evaluated more reliably than limb strength or diplopia, which may be influenced by subjective attributes. An appropriate focal deficit, such as ptosis, diplopia, or weakness of a specific muscle group, should be selected as an endpoint for evaluation and the effect of drug administration followed closely and quantitatively, if possible. Muscle strength improves in patients with myasthenia gravis and in some patients with congenital myasthenia, whereas individuals with other disorders experience either no increase or even a slight weakness and also may develop fasciculations, especially in the eyelids. Some physicians routinely administer saline initially as a placebo to improve interpretation of the test results, but this generally is not necessary for evaluation of cranial muscles. The edrophonium and neostigmine tests are almost specific for autoimmune myasthenia gravis. Botulinum intoxication is another disorder that reliably improves when these drugs are administered.

Management

The primary goal in the management of myasthenia gravis is to reduce or eliminate symptoms; this usually involves strategies to reduce the titer of acetylcholine receptor-targeted antibody. Management varies according to the severity of the disease, the age of the patient, and the type of myasthenia. Controversy exists as to the most effective sequence and combination of the main therapeutic modalities, which include anticholinesterase drugs, corticosteroids, other immunosuppressants, thymectomy, and plasmapheresis. Data from well-controlled, comparative, clinical trials to guide management are lacking. Close supervision by the physician is required to assess the patient's symptoms and psychological status.

When myasthenic patients must be treated for other disorders or infection, it should be noted that certain drugs may exacerbate their condition, although this need not preclude use of these agents when necessary. Antibiotics that depress neuromuscular transmission (eg, aminoglycosides; polymyxins; possibly norfloxacin [Noroxin], ciprofloxacin [Cipro], and erythromycin), antiarrhythmic agents (eg, procainamide [Procan, Pronestyl], quinidine, propranolol [Inderal]), chlorpromazine [Thorazine], lithium, phenytoin [Dilantin], thyroid hormones, and methoxyflurane [Penthrane] aggravate or unmask myasthenia gravis (Adams et al, 1984; Argov and Mastaglia, 1979; Rauser et al, 1990; Mumford and Ginsberg, 1990; May and Calvert, 1990). Since myasthenic patients may have depressed respiration, central nervous system depressants should be used with caution because of their inhibitory effects on the respiratory drive.

Most neurologists advocate thymectomy for the majority of patients with generalized myasthenia without thymoma. The decision may be influenced by the age of the patient, the duration and severity of the disease, and the response to medication. However, since there have been no prospective controlled trials, the precise therapeutic benefit of thymectomy is unresolved. This procedure appears to benefit 75% to 85% of patients with generalized myasthenia, especially young adults, with remissions observed in 20% to 50% of these patients; another 30% require drug therapy (ie, anticholinesterase and/or prednisone or other immunosuppressive drugs) to remain asymptomatic following thymectomy. Some neurologists advocate surgery within the first year of diagnosis or reserve it for those with disease of relatively short duration (eg, two to five years) in order to achieve the greatest benefit (Havard and Fonseca, 1990). Others reserve thymectomy for patients with disabling myasthenia or for those unresponsive to anticholinesterase and, occasionally, immunosuppressive therapy (Oosterhuis, 1984; Lanska, 1990). The time to maximum response (clinical improvement and reduction of antibody titer) may be a few weeks or as long as five years. Some patients with chronic disabling myasthenia gravis may benefit from a second thymectomy, especially if the first operation was performed by cervical incision or if it is uncertain whether the thymic tissue was completely removed during the initial procedure (Miller et al, 1991 A).

The decision to perform thymectomy in elderly patients, those with ocular disease, and children must be individualized. Thymectomy in patients aged 50 to 70 years is controversial unless a thymoma is present, because, in general, the response is less favorable than in younger individuals. Other treatment options (eg, prednisone, other immunosuppressive agents) may be more suitable in these patients. Although concern has been expressed about removing the thymus in children, thymectomy has been performed on many juvenile patients (some as young as 2 years) with excellent results and no apparent immunologic complications (Olanow et al, 1987; Adams et al, 1990). The lower age limit for thymectomy remains controversial; age recommendations range from 1 year to puberty (median, 7.5 years) (Lanska, 1990).

Thymectomy occasionally is advocated for patients with disabling ocular myasthenia (Lanska, 1990).

With rare exceptions (eg, limited life expectancy, evidence of metastasis), thymectomy is recommended for all patients with thymoma to eliminate the possibility of local invasion as well as possibly improve myasthenic symptoms. For further information on patient selection, see Rowland, 1980; Snead et al, 1980; Craven et al, 1981; Grob, 1981; Mulder et al, 1983; and Olanow et al, 1987.

Anticholinesterase drugs may be given initially to enhance the function of remaining normal acetylcholine receptors. Their use alone is limited to the treatment of mild myasthenia (before and after thymectomy).

Corticosteroids may be effective in patients of all ages with moderate to severe myasthenia, especially elderly men, those with purely ocular symptoms, and patients over age 40 at disease onset (Cosi et al, 1991 A). A long-term trial of corticosteroids to reduce antibodies and anticholinesterase drugs as necessary to improve residual weakness may lead to marked improvement in 60% to 80% of patients, but side effects (eg, cushingoid appearance, weight gain, compression fracture, aseptic necrosis of the hip) complicate therapy (Snead et al, 1980; Pascuzzi et al, 1984).

Other immunosuppressants are commonly used adjunctively with corticosteroids or in those who cannot tolerate corticosteroids. Azathioprine [Imuran] is most often chosen and may be combined with prednisone in many individuals with severe disease (Oosterhuis, 1984). Use of azathioprine often permits the dose of prednisone to be lowered and, in some patients, discontinued (Scherpbier and Oosterhuis, 1987; Miano et al, 1991). The doses of azathioprine used to treat severe myasthenia are similar to those used to maintain allografts (2 to 2.5 mg/kg). The incidence of severe adverse reactions also is similar, and, since significant improvement usually takes months to appear, the risks associated with long-term administration should be considered carefully before initiating therapy. Some neurologists reserve corticosteroids and other immunosuppressive drugs for patients who are disabled after thymectomy or for those who have a crisis before thymectomy and then become disabled.

Plasmapheresis is useful in refractory patients with severe myasthenia gravis. It should be employed only in conjunction with other treatment modalities, especially corticosteroids and other immunosuppressive drugs (Seybold, 1987). When used for its anticoagulant effect, citrate may reduce the ionized calcium concentration and thus aggravate myasthenic weakness during or immediately after plasmapheresis (Wirguin et al, 1990). Although improvement is transient, plasmapheresis in combination with prednisone has been recommended for emergencies, such as respiratory crisis, to avoid tracheostomy (Oosterhuis, 1984). It also may be used to prepare patients for thymectomy.

Results of open trials suggest that treatment with intravenous immune globulin (IGIV) (0.4 to 1 g/kg/day for five days) may significantly improve symptoms for up to three months in patients with either acute or chronic disease (Arsura et al, 1986; Cosi et al, 1991 B).

3,4-Aminopyridine may be useful as an adjunct to immunosuppression in the treatment of Lambert-Eaton syndrome (McEvoy et al, 1989) and also may be beneficial in the treatment of congenital myasthenia (Palace et al, 1991). Aminopyridines enhance the release of acetylcholine by prolonging the activation of voltage-gated calcium channels at the nerve terminal. An average maintenance dose of 80 mg/day increases muscle strength by 10% to 20%, most notably in the lower extremities. Neurologic disability scores are decreased, and some autonomic deficits (eg, dry mouth, erectile function) also may be improved. Administration of pyridostigmine [Mestinon, Regonol] produces additional benefit in some patients.

Drug Therapy

ANTICHOLINESTERASE AGENTS. The cholinesterase inhibitors, pyridostigmine bromide, neostigmine bromide, and, less often, ambenonium chloride [Mytelase], are used alone for mild symptoms of myasthenia gravis and as adjuncts in patients not adequately controlled by other measures (eg, thymectomy, corticosteroids, other immunosuppressive agents). These drugs act by reversibly inhibiting acetylcholinesterase, the enzyme that hydrolyzes acetylcholine, thereby increasing the duration of action of acetylcholine released at the motor endplate. Thus, the number of interactions between the transmitter and receptors is increased and muscular strength and response to repetitive nerve stimulation improve.

Although the anticholinesterases may improve the condition of some patients, muscle strength remains below normal in others. In any given patient, strength may improve in some muscle groups, while no improvement or even deterioration may occur in others. The optimal dose and timing of administration must be determined empirically for each individual, taking into account fluctuations in strength and variations in the patient's needs. A beneficial effect is dose dependent, but the improvement with larger doses must be weighed against the danger of overdosage. The potency of individual anticholinesterase agents varies, but the maximal achievable muscle strength in any one patient is approximately equivalent with these drugs.

There are no adequately controlled studies that unequivocally document differences in the efficacy of the available anticholinesterase agents. However, many physicians regard pyridostigmine as the drug of choice for maintenance when the symptoms are mild to moderate because it is reputed to cause fewer adverse effects than neostigmine or ambenonium and has a longer half-life.

The dose often must be increased in the presence of infection and, occasionally, premenstrually and during stress. Mild exacerbations of myasthenia are treated by increasing the dose of oral medication very gradually and carefully; dosage adjustment should continue as long as symptomatic improvement results.

Pharmacokinetics: These quaternary ammonium derivatives are poorly and variably absorbed orally, especially with regard to extent compared with rate of absorption. The ratio of effectiveness of a parenteral to an oral dose is about 30:1. The volume of distribution and plasma half-life of pyridostigmine are approximately 1.4 L/kg and 1.5 hours, respectively. The compounds are extensively metabolized by plasma esterases and hepatic enzymes to inactive metabolites; unchanged drug and metabolites are excreted in the urine. Severely impaired renal function prolongs the effect of pyridostigmine and neostigmine (Aquilonius and Hartvig, 1986). Therapeutic drug monitoring is not useful; dosage alterations are based on clinical response.

Adverse Reactions: The most common adverse reactions to anticholinesterase agents are caused by excessive cholinergic stimulation and include both muscarinic and nicotinic effects. The former consist of abdominal cramps, nausea, vomiting, diarrhea, hypersalivation, increased bronchial secretions, lacrimation, miosis, and diaphoresis. Nicotinic effects include muscle cramps, fasciculations, and weakness. Only the muscarinic effects can be counteracted by atropine. However, atropine or other anticholinergic agents should not be administered routinely to control the anticholinesterase side effects because these reactions are warning signs and masking them may inadvertently lead to toxicity. Use of atropine also may result in drying and inspissation of bronchial secretions. Many neurologists use anticholinergic agents to minimize abdominal cramps *after* the anticholinesterase dosage has been stabilized.

Precautions: Myasthenic weakness may worsen suddenly, often without recognizable cause. Such exacerbations are characterized by decreased responsiveness to drug therapy that cannot be overcome by administration of larger doses and may progress to a *myasthenic crisis,* which is characterized by severe muscular weakness with dysphagia and ventilatory insufficiency that requires mechanical support.

Myasthenic crises and respiratory failure may occur postoperatively (eg, thymectomy, cesarean section) and also can be precipitated by upper respiratory tract infections, hyperthyroidism, stress, and certain drugs (see Introduction). Monitoring of the patient's ability to clear secretions, maximum sustainable expired pressure, and vital capacity may be useful in detecting impending respiratory failure (Bennett and Bleck, 1988). Institution of high-dose corticosteroid therapy or reduction in the dose of these and other immunosuppressive agents also can cause a crisis (Linton and Philcox, 1990).

In patients with myasthenic crisis, anticholinesterase therapy should be temporarily discontinued because of side effects and uncertainty about the existence of cholinergic crisis, but optimal doses of immunosuppressive agents should be given. Plasmapheresis should be considered once the diagnosis is established. After 24 to 48 hours of respiratory support, anticholinesterase therapy can be cautiously reintroduced (eg, no more than 60 mg of pyridostigmine every eight hours) until gastrointestinal function is restored. With appropriate intensive care, most patients can be weaned from mechanical ventilatory support within 10 days (Perlo, 1983).

Rarely, overdosage of anticholinesterase agents may occur when patients in a refractory phase of myasthenia gravis receive increasing amounts of the drug in an attempt to control symptoms. In these patients, the maximal obtainable strength is below normal and the administration of excessive doses may convert a myasthenic crisis into a *cholinergic crisis*. Fasciculations and cholinergic side effects, which are common symptoms of overdosage in normal individuals (eg, organophosphate poisoning), may be mild or absent in myasthenic patients; instead, generalized weakness may be the principal sign. Ventilation must be supported and the patient observed until a diagnosis is possible. A dose of 1 to 2 mg of atropine should be given intravenously to counteract the muscarinic effects.

The anticholinesterase compounds are contraindicated in the presence of mechanical obstruction of the intestinal or urinary tract. They should be used with extreme caution in patients with bronchial asthma. Pyridostigmine bromide and neostigmine bromide should not be used in patients with a history of sensitivity to the bromide ion. Neostigmine is classified in FDA Pregnancy Category C.

ADRENAL CORTICOSTEROIDS. Adrenal corticosteroids are beneficial in patients with moderate to severe myasthenic muscle weakness. There is general agreement that their indications include (1) inadequate control with anticholinesterase drugs (ie, most patients with more than mild involvement, those with rapidly progressing disease); (2) older adults (usually >40 years) with moderate to severe involvement, whether or not they have undergone thymectomy; (3) possibly for an interim period following thymectomy because of the delayed response often associated with this procedure; (4) patients who refuse or do not respond to thymectomy; (5) maintenance therapy after surgical removal of an invasive thymoma; and (6) possibly to prepare patients for thymectomy, although the increased risk of infection and delay in postoperative healing often make this use of steroids inadvisable. The use of corticosteroids for ocular myasthenia gravis that cannot be managed with anticholinesterase drugs or lid-crutches, occlusion, or prism has been recommended (Oosterhuis, 1984), but this use is controversial.

Steroids probably act by suppressing the immune system. Therapy is not curative, as evidenced by recurrence of symptoms within three months after these drugs are discontinued.

Therefore, their administration may be required indefinitely or reinstituted periodically when needed.

Use of a high-dose, alternate-day maintenance regimen has minimized adverse effects while improving muscular strength. This regimen may prevent lethal weakness and permanent damage to the neuromuscular system as long as it is continued. A short-acting corticosteroid (eg, prednisone) is preferred for the alternate-day regimen because there is less interference with the normal ACTH-cortisol circadian rhythm and no accumulation of drug, thus reducing the likelihood of deleterious effects on the tissues. It has been suggested that patients on an alternate-day regimen receive a high-protein, low-carbohydrate diet supplemented with potassium and possibly antacids.

When large doses of corticosteroids are used initially, weakness is exacerbated in about 80% of patients. Therefore, some neurologists initiate treatment with relatively small doses (eg, 25 mg of prednisone daily), which are then increased gradually, even though this may slow the rate of improvement. Maximum response is usually noted in about five months. Optimal doses of anticholinesterase medication can be continued with this regimen, especially during initiation of steroid therapy. The need for anticholinesterase drugs usually decreases as the patient improves. Alternatively, some neurologists prefer to use larger doses of prednisone initially (eg, 60 to 80 mg or 1 mg/kg daily) to achieve a more rapid response. A further exacerbation of weakness may occur in patients who are also taking anticholinesterase drugs. Hence, patients should be hospitalized before high-dose regimens are employed.

OTHER IMMUNOSUPPRESSIVE AGENTS. A number of other immunosuppressive drugs (eg, azathioprine, chlorambucil [Leukeran], cyclophosphamide [Cytoxan, Neosar], cyclosporine [Sandimmune], methotrexate [Folex]) have been employed in the treatment of myasthenia gravis. Only azathioprine is commonly used. The therapeutic effect is characteristically delayed with immunosuppressive agents. With azathioprine, clinical benefit may not be observed for three to eight months.

The effectiveness of azathioprine is difficult to evaluate, since thymectomy and corticosteroids are commonly used in conjunction with this agent. Although there are no prospective controlled studies comparing azathioprine with placebo, several studies have demonstrated its effectiveness based on withdrawal and reintroduction, thereby using patients as their own controls (Mertens et al, 1981; Witte et al, 1984; Hohlfeld et al, 1985).

Cyclophosphamide has been reported to produce early improvement in more than 75% of patients (Niakan et al, 1986), but azathioprine is preferred to this and other alkylating or cytotoxic agents because adverse effects occur less frequently (Matell, 1987).

In a preliminary trial, patients with progressively worsening generalized myasthenia gravis of recent onset who were treated with cyclosporine 5 mg/kg/day experienced an increase in muscle strength (Tindall et al, 1987). In those with generalized severe myasthenia gravis not well controlled by other therapy, eight of ten patients benefited from cyclosporine therapy (peak serum levels <200 ng/ml) over a 12-month period (Goulon et al, 1988). In an initial trial comparing cyclosporine and azathioprine, no difference in clinical response was noted (Schalke et al, 1988). In other small open trials, cyclosporine produced moderate to marked improvement in 12 of 14 patients, most of whom were also receiving prednisone (Nyberg-Hansen and Gjerstad, 1988; Antonini et al, 1990). The preliminary results of cyclosporine therapy in myasthenia gravis are encouraging, but its role in the management of these patients remains to be established. It may be useful in individuals who cannot tolerate prednisone or in those who are taking prednisone and require additional immunosuppressive therapy but cannot tolerate azathioprine because of an idiosyncratic reaction.

Drug Evaluations

ANTICHOLINESTERASE AGENTS

AMBENONIUM CHLORIDE

[Mytelase]

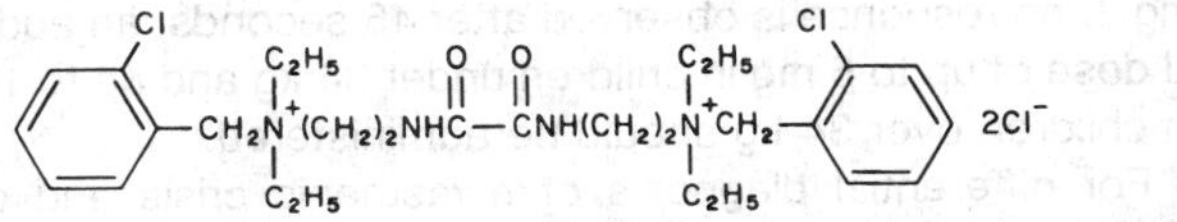

$$\text{Cl-C}_6\text{H}_4\text{-CH}_2\overset{+}{\text{N}}(\text{C}_2\text{H}_5)_2(\text{CH}_2)_2\text{NHC(=O)-C(=O)NH(CH}_2)_2\overset{+}{\text{N}}(\text{C}_2\text{H}_5)_2\text{CH}_2\text{-C}_6\text{H}_4\text{-Cl} \quad 2\text{Cl}^-$$

Although ambenonium is widely employed in other countries to treat myasthenia, it is not used frequently in this country. However, it may be preferred to pyridostigmine or neostigmine in patients who cannot tolerate these drugs because of sensitivity to the bromide ion. The oral route is employed. Ambenonium was originally believed to produce fewer cholinergic side effects than neostigmine, but it may have a longer duration of action and a greater tendency to accumulate.

For adverse reactions and precautions, see the Introduction to this section.

DOSAGE AND PREPARATIONS.

Oral: The dose and frequency of administration vary greatly and must be individualized according to the response of the patient (see the evaluation on Pyridostigmine Bromide). *Adults,* initially, 5 mg three or four times daily, increased as required; the dosage should be adjusted at intervals of one to two days to avoid accumulation. *Children,* initially, 0.3 mg/kg daily in divided doses, increased, if necessary, to 1.5 mg/kg daily in divided doses.

Mytelase (Sanofi Winthrop). Tablets 10 mg.

EDROPHONIUM CHLORIDE

[Enlon, Reversol, Tensilon]

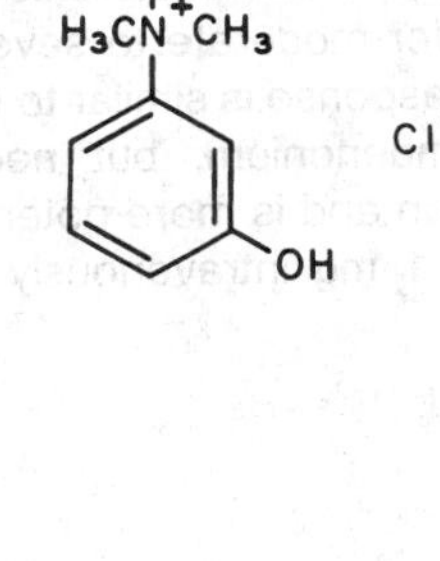

$$\text{H}_3\text{C}\overset{+}{\text{N}}(\text{C}_2\text{H}_5)\text{CH}_3\text{-C}_6\text{H}_4\text{-OH} \quad \text{Cl}^-$$

USES. Edrophonium is used in the diagnosis of myasthenia gravis. It has a more rapid onset and shorter duration of action than pyridostigmine. Administration of atropine is usually unnecessary, but this agent should be readily available, especially for older patients. After intravenous administration of edrophonium, muscle strength increases in myasthenic patients within one to three minutes and lasts for five to ten minutes.

Although not considered a reliable test, a smaller dose of edrophonium can be used to differentiate a myasthenic crisis from a rare cholinergic crisis: A carefully administered intravenous dose produces a brief remission of symptoms if these are caused by an exacerbation of the illness but further weakens patients suffering from an overdose of medication.

For untoward effects, see the Introduction to this section.

DOSAGE AND PREPARATIONS.

Intravenous: For diagnosis, *adults,* 2 mg injected within 15 to 30 seconds; if no response occurs within 45 seconds, an additional 8 mg should be given. The test may be repeated after one to two hours (see manufacturer's labeling for details). Atropine should be readily available, although it is not administered routinely. *Children under 34 kg,* 1 mg; *over 34 kg,* 2 mg. If no response is observed after 45 seconds, an additional dose of up to 5 mg in children under 34 kg and up to 10 mg in children over 34 kg should be administered.

For differential diagnosis of myasthenic crisis and cholinergic crisis, *adults,* 1 to 2 mg. This test should be undertaken only if facilities for endotracheal intubation and controlled ventilation are immediately available.

Intramuscular: For diagnosis, *infants,* 0.5 mg as a single dose. *Children under 34 kg,* 2 mg; *over 34 kg,* 5 mg. There is a delay of two to ten minutes before a response is noted with this route of administration.

Enlon (Anaquest), ***Reversol*** (Organon), ***Tensilon*** (ICN). Solution (sterile) 10 mg/ml in 15 ml containers (***Enlon***), 10 ml containers (***Reversol***), and 1 and 10 ml containers (***Tensilon***).

NEOSTIGMINE BROMIDE
[Prostigmin]

NEOSTIGMINE METHYLSULFATE
[Prostigmin]

$\overset{+}{N}(CH_3)_3$ … $OCN(CH_3)_2$

USES. Neostigmine bromide is used orally alone to treat mild myasthenia gravis and with corticosteroids and other immunosuppressive agents for moderate to severe muscle weakness. The therapeutic response is similar to that obtained with pyridostigmine and ambenonium, but neostigmine has a shorter duration of action and is more potent than pyridostigmine; 15 mg orally or 1 mg intravenously is approximately equivalent to pyridostigmine 60 mg. The methylsulfate salt is given parenterally to patients who are unable to swallow; the intravenous route is preferred. It also is an alternative to edrophonium for diagnosis.

ADVERSE REACTIONS AND PRECAUTIONS. Adverse effects after therapeutic doses occur more frequently with neostigmine than with pyridostigmine or ambenonium. For adverse reactions and precautions, see the Introduction to this section.

DOSAGE AND PREPARATIONS.

NEOSTIGMINE BROMIDE:

Oral: The dose and frequency of administration must be individualized according to the response of the patient (see evaluation on Pyridostigmine Bromide). *Adults,* initially, 15 mg every three to four hours; the dose and frequency of administration are then adjusted in accordance with the patient's requirements. *Children,* 2 mg/kg daily in divided doses as required.

Prostigmin (ICN), ***Generic.*** Tablets 15 mg.

NEOSTIGMINE METHYLSULFATE:

Intramuscular, Subcutaneous: For treatment of exacerbations of myasthenia gravis when oral therapy is impractical, *adults,* 0.5 mg. Subsequent dosage should be adjusted according to the patient's response. *Infants and children,* 0.01 to 0.04 mg/kg every two to three hours.

Atropine (0.01 mg/kg intramuscularly or subcutaneously) should not be used routinely but should be available to control adverse effects.

Intravenous: The intravenous route may be employed for the treatment of exacerbations of myasthenia gravis or when the patient cannot take anticholinesterase agents orally (eg, difficulty in swallowing, following thymectomy). The rate of infusion by intravenous pump should parallel the rate at which oral medication is given. For example, if the patient normally takes 60 mg of pyridostigmine four times a day, neostigmine 4 mg should be infused over the 24-hour period (neostigmine 1 mg intravenously is equivalent to pyridostigmine 60 mg orally).

Generic. Solution 0.5 and 1 mg/ml in 10 ml containers.

Prostigmin (ICN). Solution 0.25 mg/ml in 1 ml containers, 0.5 mg/ml in 1 and 10 ml containers, and 1 mg/ml in 10 ml containers.

PYRIDOSTIGMINE BROMIDE
[Mestinon, Regonol]

CH_3 N^+ Br^- $OCN(CH_3)_2$

USES. Pyridostigmine, given orally, is the most widely used anticholinesterase agent for the treatment of myasthenia gravis. It is given alone for mild muscle weakness and is combined with corticosteroids for moderate to severe impairment. The drug also may be administered parenterally with great caution to treat neonatal myasthenia, exacerbations of myasthenia, and as an alternative to edrophonium for diagnosis.

The therapeutic response is similar to that observed with neostigmine, but pyridostigmine has a slightly longer duration of action.

ADVERSE REACTIONS AND PRECAUTIONS. Adverse effects after therapeutic doses occur less frequently with pyridostigmine than with neostigmine. For further discussion of adverse reactions and precautions, see the Introduction to this section.

DOSAGE AND PREPARATIONS. Dosage requirements vary widely among patients because of differences in absorption, metabolism, and excretion of the drug; thus, the dose and timing of administration must be determined empirically. Careful record keeping by the patient is helpful in adjusting the schedule.

Oral: *Adults,* initially, 30 to 60 mg every three to four hours; the intervals are altered as necessary on the basis of response. As a general rule, 120 mg every two hours during waking hours may be considered the maximum dosage. In severe myasthenia, as much as 600 mg to 1.5 g daily has been recommended by the manufacturer. Doses above 800 mg/day increase the risk of severe side effects or cholinergic crisis. *Children,* 7 mg/kg daily in divided doses and timed as required. The syrup is useful for infants, young children, and patients who cannot swallow tablets or when the dose is in fractions of tablet size; it may be given by nasogastric tube if necessary.

The prolonged-release preparation is not recommended for use during the day but is useful at night if the patient has difficulties during the night or is weak in the morning. The usual dose is 90 to 360 mg once or twice daily. Because of the delayed onset of action, regular tablets or syrup may be needed in addition. Use of prolonged-release preparations may increase the risk of cholinergic crises.

Mestinon (ICN). Syrup 60 mg/5 ml (alcohol 5%); tablets 60 mg; tablets (prolonged-release) 180 mg.

Intramuscular, Intravenous: For exacerbations of myasthenia gravis or when oral administration is impractical, *adults,* approximately one-thirtieth of the oral dose. For *newborn infants* of myasthenic mothers, 0.05 to 0.15 mg/kg.

Mestinon (ICN). Solution 5 mg/ml in 2 ml containers.

Regonol (Organon). Solution 5 mg/ml in 2 and 5 ml containers.

IMMUNOSUPPRESSIVE AGENTS

AZATHIOPRINE

[Imuran]

For chemical formula, see index entry Azathioprine, Uses, Immune Disorders.

ACTIONS AND USES. Azathioprine can provide some degree of benefit to more than 90% of patients with myasthenia gravis and has restored muscle control to a near normal state in some patients (Drachman, 1987). The mechanism by which this drug modulates the immune response in myasthenia gravis is not completely understood. Azathioprine suppresses T-cell activity more than B-cell activity. See index entry Azathioprine, Uses, Immune Disorders, for details on the immunosuppressive actions of azathioprine.

In most patients, azathioprine exerts its therapeutic effect in severe myasthenia gravis only after three to four months of treatment, but improvement may continue for up to two years after the initially observed benefit (Matell, 1987). The best results with azathioprine have been noted in late-onset, rapidly progressive myasthenia gravis in older patients or in those in all age groups with thymoma (Matell, 1987). Corticosteroids are commonly given concomitantly.

ADVERSE REACTIONS. Since significant improvement requires months of therapy, the risks of long-term administration should be considered carefully before initiating therapy. Gastrointestinal disturbances and reversible, dose-related bone marrow depression are the most common adverse reactions observed (Hohlfeld et al, 1988). Gastrointestinal discomfort with nausea and vomiting occur during initial therapy and are reported to decrease with time. If it occurs, bone marrow depression usually is observed during the initial phases of therapy but can appear at any time.

Severe hepatotoxicity has developed in approximately 1% of patients, and the drug should be discontinued in those experiencing this reaction. The patient should be instructed to report any acute symptoms of malaise, epigastralgia, or fever immediately. The frequency of infections also may increase in treated patients.

Although the number of neoplasms in myasthenia gravis patients treated with azathioprine has been reported to be low (Matell, 1987), long-term experience with the development of cancer secondary to treatment with this agent is less extensive than with its use in allotransplantation.

For a more complete discussion of side effects, see index entry Azathioprine, Uses, Immune Disorders.

PHARMACOKINETICS. Azathioprine is well absorbed. Peak plasma concentrations are obtained two hours after an oral dose. This agent is metabolized to mercaptopurine, which is eliminated by metabolic degradation. See index entry Azathioprine, Uses, Immune Disorders, for details on the metabolism of azathioprine.

DOSAGE AND PREPARATIONS. Azathioprine should be used under the direction of a physician familiar with the risks associated with immunosuppressive therapy. The patient should be monitored carefully during treatment.

Oral: The usual dose is 2 to 2.5 mg/kg/day. A test dose of 50 mg/day may be given for the first week to screen for idiosyncratic reactions. The white blood cell count can be monitored to guide adjustments in dosage. A fall below 3,500/mm^3 has been recommended as an indication to reduce dosage by 50% (Matell, 1987), while a count of 2,800 to 3,200/mm^3 may be considered the end point of dosage adjustment (Drachman, 1985). In patients also taking prednisone, a lymphocyte count below 1,000/mm^3 may be a useful alternative measurement of sufficient immunosuppression (Drachman, 1985; Matell, 1987).

Imuran (Burroughs Wellcome). Tablets 50 mg.

PREDNISONE

Oral administration of a short-acting corticosteroid, such as prednisone, is beneficial in approximately 80% of patients with moderate to severe myasthenia gravis, but treatment may have to be continued indefinitely and the patient must be observed closely for adverse effects. Anticholinesterase agents or azathioprine may be given concomitantly. Concomitant use of the latter drug often permits the dose of prednisone to be reduced. Prednisone also has been reported to produce dramatic improvement in both myasthenic symptoms and tumor burden in one patient with disseminated thymoma (Taylor et al, 1989).

ADVERSE REACTIONS AND PRECAUTIONS. The adverse reactions usually associated with prolonged use of steroids occur frequently and must be treated appropriately. The most common adverse reactions, cushingoid appearance and weight gain, are related to dose and duration of therapy and can be minimized by alternate-day therapy and a reduction in dosage. For a more detailed discussion, see the Introduction to this section and index entry Prednisone, In Immune Disorders. This drug is classified in FDA Pregnancy Category C.

DOSAGE AND PREPARATIONS. The following oral dosages should serve only as a guide. The patient's status should be evaluated carefully before each dosage change. If there is an exacerbation of myasthenic weakness following an increase in the dose of prednisone, the amount should be reduced or maintained without further increases until the patient's condition stabilizes.

Oral: Initially, 25 mg daily for two days, increased by 5 mg every two days until an optimal response occurs (usually, 50 to 60 mg daily). An alternate-day program is gradually substituted by adding 10 mg to the first day's dose (60 mg) and subtracting 10 mg from the second day's dose (40 mg) each week until improvement reaches a plateau (ie, the patient experiences weakness on the "off" day) or until 100 mg is given every other day. The dosage then should be reduced very gradually over many months to establish a minimal maintenance dose to be given on alternate days (often as much as 30 to 60 mg).

Alternatively, in hospitalized patients, a relatively large dose of prednisone (eg, 60 to 80 mg daily) may be administered until improvement is observed on each of three consecutive days ("sustained improvement") (Johns, 1987). Thereafter, an equivalent alternate-day schedule is initiated with a 10-mg reduction every one to two months if improvement is sustained. The dosage of anticholinesterase inhibitors can be reduced as rapidly as tolerated.

Patients with severe myasthenia gravis who do not respond to 100 mg every other day usually do not respond to dosage increases. In these individuals, it may be preferable to add another immunosuppressive drug, such as azathioprine (see that evaluation). The dosage of anticholinesterase drugs should be adjusted as necessary during steroid therapy.

For preparations, see index entry Prednisone, In Immune Disorders.

INFLAMMATORY MYOPATHIES

ETIOLOGY. The causes of the three major acquired inflammatory myopathies, polymyositis (PM), dermatomyositis (DM), and inclusion body myositis (Plotz et al, 1989; Dalakas, 1991), are unknown; however, these rare disorders appear to result from an autoimmune response that may be triggered by an environmental agent in a genetically susceptible host. PM and inclusion body myositis appear to result from cell-mediated cytotoxicity, while muscle damage in DM appears to result from complement-mediated microvasculopathy (Kissel et al, 1991). There has been considerable interest in retroviruses, enteroviruses, or other novel picornaviruses as causative agents, but results of studies are conflicting and the role of these agents is unclear (Leff et al, 1992).

PM typically occurs after the second decade of life, whereas inclusion body myositis usually occurs after age 50 and is more common in white males. DM occurs in both children and adults and is more common in females. The inflammatory muscle lesions in these myopathies vary in severity, pattern of involvement, pathologic characteristics, and response to therapy (see Lotz et al, 1989; Dalakas, 1991). PM, DM, and rarely inclusion body myositis may be associated with other connective tissue diseases.

PM frequently occurs with other systemic autoimmune diseases and may develop in response to infection with bacteria, HIV or HTLV-1 (and possibly other viruses), or infestation with parasites, or it may be drug-induced (eg, penicillamine, zidovudine [Retrovir]). DM also may be associated with HIV or *Toxoplasma* infection and the use of penicillamine. Treatment of the underlying disorder or discontinuation of the offending drugs usually corrects myopathies produced by infections or drugs. Both DM and PM are probably associated with an increased risk of malignancy, although the association is stronger and better established with DM (Sigurgeirsson et al, 1992).

DIAGNOSIS. Muscle weakness and the presence of inflammatory infiltrates within the skeletal muscles are the principal clinical and histologic findings of these myopathies. PM is diagnosed by exclusion of other possible causes of inflammatory myopathy (see Bohan and Peter, 1975); a probable diagnosis is made if three of the following criteria are met: symmetrical proximal weakness, elevation of muscle enzymes in serum, myopathic electromyographic findings, and evidence from biopsy (ie, muscle fiber necrosis, regeneration, interstitial mononuclear infiltration with or without muscle fiber atrophy) (Bohan and Peter, 1975).

In addition to the above, DM is marked by characteristic cutaneous manifestations that accompany, or more often precede, muscle weakness (Caro, 1988). These include erythematous papules and small plaques over the knuckles (Gottron's papules) and a bilaterally symmetrical, dusky red to lilac ("heliotrope") periorbital skin eruption with edema of the upper eyelids and periorbital tissue, which is virtually pathognomonic. In blacks, edema is the main feature. An erythematous, finely scaling macular eruption also may appear on the face, most commonly in a "butterfly" pattern, or on the scalp, neck, upper torso, and extremities. Accentuation on sun-exposed areas may be noted. Other cutaneous manifestations of DM may include poikiloderma and capillary changes in the nailbed. Subcutaneous calcifications also may be associated with DM, particularly in juveniles.

The diagnosis of inclusion body myositis is made on the basis of the characteristic findings on muscle biopsy (see Calabrese et al, 1987; Dalakas, 1991). Involvement of distal muscles, especially foot extensors and finger flexors, may be an early diagnostic clue.

Creatine kinase levels usually are elevated on presentation in patients with inflammatory myopathies but rarely may be normal. Elevation is observed at some time during the course of the disease in most patients. Although alterations may not be clearly associated with corresponding changes in weakness or disability, most clinicians monitor creatine kinase concentrations because this often is a good barometer of disease activity in individual patients. Improvement in muscle strength generally lags behind normalization of creatine kinase concentrations by several weeks. A rise in the creatine kinase level may herald an impending exacerbation, and persistent elevation often is predictive of persistent disease activity. Creatine kinase levels usually are not elevated in corticosteroid-induced myopathy; thus, normal creatine kinase levels in patients who weaken during prolonged corticosteroid therapy may be helpful in diagnosis.

Systemic complications also occur in patients with these disorders, and symptoms may be more obvious if the myositis is brought under control. In some patients, systemic involvement may be the presenting feature. Generalized symptoms include fatigue, malaise, fever, and weight loss. Esophageal (dysphagia), gastric, and intestinal disorders often are present, and joint involvement and thyroid dysfunction may occur. Cardiopulmonary manifestations (eg, interstitial lung disease, conduction abnormalities, heart failure) contribute substantially to morbidity and mortality (Plotz et al, 1989).

Various autoantibodies are found in approximately 30% of patients with PM and DM but are not diagnostic; they occur less frequently in those with inclusion body myositis. The autoantibodies include antinuclear and antimuscle antibodies, antibodies associated with coexisting or related connective tissue disorders, and, in patients with PM or DM, myositis-specific antibodies. A number of myositis-specific autoantibodies are targeted to aminoacyl-tRNA synthetases (eg, anti-Jo-1, anti-PL-7) and appear to be present in a genetically restricted group of patients who are prone to develop interstitial lung disease. Other autoantibodies (eg, anti-Mi-2, anti-SRP) may be characteristic of different genetically restricted patient subsets (Plotz et al, 1989).

DRUG THERAPY. Because the idiopathic inflammatory myopathies are rare and clinically heterogenous, optimal therapy and factors that influence response to treatment have not been established.

Inclusion body myositis generally is believed to be refractory to standard therapy. However, case reports (Lane et al, 1985; Cohen et al, 1989) and results of a case series (Sayers et al, 1992) indicate that therapy with prednisone and another immunosuppressive agent, in particular methotrexate, may stabilize function and slow the rate of disease progression in some patients.

Adrenal Corticosteroids: The primary indication for treatment is muscle weakness severe enough to cause disability. Although controlled trials have not been conducted, prednisone often is chosen as the initial agent used to treat PM or DM and produces at least partial improvement in approximately 75% to 90% of patients. Results of a retrospective analysis indicate that patients treated within three months after diagnosis are most responsive (Joffe et al, 1993). Patients who are less likely to respond adequately include those with a delay of more than 18 months between onset of muscle weakness and diagnosis, those with systemic complications (eg, acute pulmonary infiltration, cardiac involvement, fever, dysphagia), and possibly those with certain myositis-specific autoantibodies (eg, antisynthetase, anti-SRP [Joffe et al, 1993]).

The course of myositis is variable, and therapy generally is required for one to two years or longer. Only general guidelines are available; the optimal initial dose or duration of therapy and the usefulness of alternate-day therapy remain to be determined. Currently, the recommended initial dosage of prednisone in adults is at least 60 mg/day or 1 mg/kg/day (Oddis and Medsger, 1988; Plotz et al, 1989). Lower doses (eg, 40 mg) may be effective in those with less severe disease, but some patients may require doses as large as 1.5 mg/kg (Oddis and Medsger, 1989). In children, the recommended initial dosage is 1 to 2 mg/kg/day (Pachman, 1986).

Various schedules for dosage reduction have been employed when clinical improvement (reduction in muscle pain, objective increase in muscle strength, normalization of serum enzyme levels, clearing of skin lesions) occurs. Based on a retrospective study, the initial dosage of prednisone should be given for two to four weeks after the creatine kinase concentration returns to normal (Oddis and Medsger, 1988). Depending on the dosage at which clinical improvement occurs, a 20% to 25% reduction at monthly intervals may be possible until a maintenance dose of 5 to 10 mg/day or 10 to 20 mg on alternate days is achieved (Mastaglia and Ojeda, 1985; Caro, 1988; Oddis and Medsger, 1989; Targoff, 1990). Alternatively, a large dose of prednisone (eg, 80 to 100 mg) is given once daily for three to four weeks, after which the amount is tapered over a ten-week period so that a total of 80 to 100 mg is given on alternate days (Dalakas, 1991). This can be accomplished by gradually reducing the alternate "off-day" dose by 10 mg/week (or more rapidly if necessary). Patients who do not respond to this regimen can be considered to be unresponsive to prednisone. In those with objective evidence of efficacy, the dosage may continue to be reduced gradually by 5 to 10 mg at three- to four-week intervals until the lowest effective maintenance dose is reached.

In most recommended regimens, the rate of tapering decreases as the amount is lowered (Targoff, 1990). In some patients, a slower rate of reduction may be necessary to prevent disease flareup. Unless attempts to taper the dosage have been unsuccessful, further reduction below the 5- to 10-mg maintenance dose is justified. However, prolonged maintenance is often required. In patients with increasing weakness, corticosteroid-induced myofibril atrophy can mimic active myositis; dosage reduction may be prudent in these individuals.

Intravenous administration of large doses of methylprednisolone ("pulse therapy") has been employed in acutely ill patients and in those with juvenile DM (Yanagisawa et al, 1983; Laxer et al, 1987).

Other Immunosuppressive Agents: Other immunosuppressive agents have been used (1) in severe acute disease, (2) when no improvement is observed with prednisone within approximately three months, (3) when the corticosteroid dosage cannot be reduced without exacerbation of disease, or (4) when severe adverse reactions are associated with corticosteroid therapy. Methotrexate or azathioprine has been used most frequently for DM or PM. In patients with resistant disease, one of these agents usually is given with prednisone. No prospective comparative studies have been performed, and firm guidelines for maintenance therapy are lacking (Tuffanelli and Lavoie, 1988; Caro, 1989; Plotz et al, 1989; Targoff, 1990). However, results of a recent retrospective study suggest that methotrexate is more beneficial than azathioprine or continued corticosteroid therapy in refractory patients (Joffe et al, 1993).

Methotrexate can be administered intravenously or orally. Intravenous therapy may be initiated with doses of 10 mg weekly with a gradual increase to 0.4 to 0.8 mg/kg/week (maximum, 30 to 50 mg/week). Intramuscular administration should be avoided because it may increase creatine kinase concentrations and interfere with monitoring of disease activity. Oral therapy may be initiated with doses of 7.5 to 10 mg weekly, increased gradually by 2.5-mg increments, if necessary, to a maximum of 20 (Targoff, 1990) to 30 mg/week (Oddis and Medsger, 1989). Once the patient has responded, the weekly dosage of oral or intravenous methotrexate can be reduced by 25% or the interval can be extended to two weeks and later to four weeks. Because of pulmonary toxicity induced by methotrexate, caution should be exercised when administering the drug to patients with interstitial lung disease or anti-Jo-1 (or related) autoantibodies. For other precautions, see index entries Methotrexate, Uses, Arthritis, Cancer.

Azathioprine is most often given in doses of 1.5 to 2 mg/kg/day (maximum, 2.5 mg/kg/day). After the patient responds (usually in three to six months), the amount can be reduced by approximately 25 mg monthly to a maintenance dose of 50 mg daily (Oddis and Medsger, 1989).

In refractory patients, other cytotoxic or immunosuppressive agents that have been utilized include cyclosporine, cyclophosphamide, and chlorambucil. Investigational approaches include total body irradiation and administration of intravenous immune globulin (Lang et al, 1991; Cherin et al, 1991; Jann et al, 1992). Plasmapheresis is ineffective (Miller et al, 1992 A).

MULTIPLE SCLEROSIS

ETIOLOGY. Multiple sclerosis (MS) is an inflammatory disease of the central nervous system characterized by primary destruction of myelin and manifested by motor, sensory, and visual dysfunction. In the United States, an estimated 250,000 to 350,000 individuals have been diagnosed with MS (Anderson et al, 1992). The risk of developing the disease is increased in young adults, females, and persons of northern European descent who spent their childhood in temperate latitudes and who have a first-degree relative with MS.

Circumstantial evidence supports the hypothesis that MS is an autoimmune disorder triggered in a genetically susceptible host by an environmental exposure. The importance of environmental factors is supported by migration pattern studies that confirm latitude-dependent and age-associated geographic risk regions and by the occurrence of sporadic disease-cluster outbreaks.

The central nervous system (CNS) autoantigen is unknown. Monozygotic twins are more likely to be concordant for MS (26% to 50%) than dizygotic twins (2.3% to 9%) (McFarland et al, 1984; Ebers et al, 1986; Kinnunen et al, 1988); however, susceptibility to MS appears to be polygenic. HLA, T-cell receptor, and immunoglobulin heavy-chain genes all have been linked with susceptibility. Evidence is accumulating that subclinical forms of the disease occur, and abnormalities typical of MS have been detected by MRI in the clinically unaffected twin of a monozygotic pair when the other twin has obvious signs of the disease and in asymptomatic siblings of MS patients with familial disease (Uitdehaag et al, 1989; Tienari et al, 1992).

Cellular immune responses are implicated in the pathogenesis of MS (Martin et al, 1992). Initially, permeability of the blood-brain barrier increases, accompanied by edema, perivascular orientation of inflammatory cells (principally macrophages), and infiltration of activated T-cells. The characteristic plaques of MS form as a result of primary demyelination and death of myelin-producing oligodendrocytes, followed by formation of extensive astrocyte-mediated scar tissue and incomplete remyelination by oligodendrocytes at the margins of the plaque (Rodriguez, 1989). Plaques are found throughout the CNS but primarily are localized to periventricular white matter and the brain stem, spinal cord, and optic nerves. Macrophages are the primary lymphoid population at the site of active demyelination, and, based on ultrastructural studies, they appear to remove myelin directly (Prineas et al, 1984). The antigenic signal that triggers T-cell mediated activation of macrophages has not been determined. When the inflammatory component resolves, chronic lesions show depletion of oligodendrocytes and loss of axons.

Secretion of cytokines and a local immune activation result in the synthesis of oligoclonal immunoglobulin by plasma cells within the CNS; however, the precise relationship between these elevated immunoglobulin levels and the disease state has not been established conclusively.

In addition to alteration in lymphocyte subsets within the CNS during active stages of MS (Chofflon et al, 1989; Salonen et al, 1989; Hartung et al, 1990; Matsui et al, 1990), immune abnormalities in the peripheral blood (an increase in activated T-cells, including those targeted to myelin; a decrease in suppressor inducer cells; and a decrease in the number or function of suppressor cells) have been reported. However, it is not known whether these changes are causative or secondary to the disease process.

Except for patients with benign forms, a pattern of disease activity generally emerges. Following the initial attack, recovery with recurrent exacerbations occurs in most individuals. In some patients, symptoms remit partially or totally after an exacerbation, and the periods of stability are relatively long (relapsing-remitting disease). In others, a progressive phase evolves after a number of relapses, and disability increases slowly (relapsing-progressive disease). Less commonly, symptoms progress without remission to chronic paraparesis or hemiparesis (chronic progressive disease). In about 5% of patients, the disease progresses rapidly from the onset with very severe early disability, and potentially fatal complications occur within a few weeks to months.

DIAGNOSIS. Initial attacks or early relapses of MS are likely to involve the ocular (reversible vision loss, optic neuritis) and/or motor or sensory (weakness, tingling of an extremity) systems. Approximately 50% to 75% of patients with isolated optic neuritis have other brain lesions detectable by MRI (Jacobs et al, 1991; Städt et al, 1990). Symptoms also may be related to dysfunction of movement, coordination, and sensory perception.

Diagnosis of MS is based on clinical history, neurologic examination, and chemical analysis of cerebrospinal fluid (CSF). For research purposes, including clinical trials (Poser et al, 1983), *clinically definite MS* is indicated if two episodes of neurologic dysfunction have occurred that represent at least two CNS lesions; evidence for one of these lesions may be based on the results of paraclinical studies. *Laboratory-supported definite MS* is indicated if two attacks have occurred, one CNS lesion is apparent, and CSF testing reveals immunoglobulin abnormalities. Alternatively, one attack and the presence of two CNS lesions plus abnormal immunoglobulins also satisfy this diagnostic criteria.

In clinical settings, the Schumacher criteria (Schumacher et al, 1965) are most widely used in the United States for the diagnosis of MS. In patients 10 to 50 years with signs and symptoms that cannot be accounted for by other conditions, a diagnosis of clinically definite MS is indicated when the neurologic examination reveals objective abnormalities that predominantly involve white matter. There must be evidence on examination or in the history of two or more separate lesions of the CNS. The pattern of CNS involvement must include at least two episodes separated by at least one month and lasting at least 24 hours or, if the disease is progressive, deterioration must have persisted for at least six months. Even though the specificities of most of the IgG antibodies in the CSF are unknown, the presence of electrophoretically restricted IgG (oligoclonal bands) and quantitative IgG abnormalities can be used to confirm the diagnosis of MS (Rudick et al, 1989).

Paraclinical studies permit the clinician to probe or visualize brain and spinal cord abnormalities that may be clinically silent (Gilmore et al, 1989). More than 95% of patients with clinically definite MS have periventricular and focal abnormalities in the white matter. Although MRI is the most sensitive method to detect lesions in MS, the lesions are not diagnostically specific and also can be seen in patients with migraine, vascular disease, sarcoidosis, multiple emboli, and CNS infections (eg, chronic meningitis, Lyme disease, neurosyphilis, HTLV-1). This emphasizes the need to exclude other differential diagnoses before making a diagnosis of MS (McDonald, 1988; Noakes et al, 1990). Evoked potential methods may be more widely available and enable assessment of areas not currently imaged effectively by MRI (Gilmore et al, 1989).

Several investigators have reported the frequent occurrence of "new," "enlarging," or asymptomatic lesions (as detected by gadolinium-enhancing MRI), which suggests that disease activity may be more pronounced, even in mildly affected patients, than was previously suspected (Isaac et al, 1988; Willoughby et al, 1989; Harris et al, 1991; Thompson et al, 1992). Pathologic correlations with MRI findings remain largely undocumented, but stereotactic biopsy of an active MS lesion in one patient revealed that histologic demyelination was closely correlated with MRI results (Estes et al, 1990). Since serial gadolinium-enhancing MRI can apparently detect clinically silent disease in both early relapsing-remitting and progressive MS, it has a potentially important role in monitoring the effects of therapy. Accordingly, guidelines have been offered for using MRI to monitor treatment trials in these patients (Miller et al, 1991 B; Goodkin et al, 1992).

DRUG THERAPY. Currently, no therapeutic or prophylactic measure has been shown to reverse the course of MS, although treatment with interferon beta reduces the exacerbation rate and thus alters the natural history of the disease in patients with the relapsing-remitting form.

Symptomatic Treatment: Relief of symptoms is directed toward reducing spasticity, bladder dysfunction, fatigue, and pain (Carter and Rodriguez, 1990; Rudick et al, 1992). Baclofen [Lioresal] and other antispastic drugs (eg, diazepam [Valium, Valrelease], dantrolene [Dantrium]) are employed to relieve spasticity and may reduce painful flexor spasms. Patients who cannot tolerate or do not respond adequately to oral baclofen may benefit from intrathecal administration (Latash et al, 1990). In individuals with spastic contraction of adductor muscles that interferes with sitting, positioning, hygiene, or urethral catheterization, botulinum A toxin injection [Botox] may reduce spasticity significantly (Snow et al, 1990) (see index entry Spasticity).

Hyperreflexic bladder usually is treated with an anticholinergic agent (eg, propantheline [Pro-Banthīne], oxybutynin [Ditropan], hyoscyamine [Levsin]), but these drugs can aggravate changes in mental status.

Chronic pain is a common feature of well-established MS and usually is associated with myelopathy (Moulin et al, 1988). Therapy must be individualized for each specific pain syndrome. Chronic back pain may respond to nonsteroidal anti-inflammatory agents and physical therapy. Myofascial trigger points can be treated locally (Moulin et al, 1988). Paroxysmal pain of CNS origin may respond to carbamazepine [Tegretol] 200 mg or phenytoin 100 mg two to four times daily. Paresthetic pain can be managed with tricyclic antidepressants (eg, amitriptyline [Elavil, Endep] 25 to 150 mg daily).

Psychiatric and cognitive abnormalities (Rao et al, 1991) are common in MS and add considerably to distress and disability. Antidepressants can relieve affective symptoms (Schiffer and Wineman, 1990).

Fatigue occurs in a majority of patients with MS and may be independent of neurologic disability. Amantadine [Symmetrel] 100 mg twice daily (given in the morning and early afternoon to avoid insomnia) may benefit many patients with significant fatigue (Cohen and Fisher, 1989). Pemoline [Cylert] (up to 75 mg daily) also may be employed to relieve fatigue, but approximately 25% of patients do not tolerate the drug well (Weinshenker et al, 1992).

Long-term controlled trials have confirmed the preliminary results of small open, single-dose studies indicating that treatment with 4-aminopyridine (mean daily dose, 31 mg) can produce significant improvement in approximately one-third of patients (van Diemen et al, 1992); approximately 75% improved on some measures in another short-term trial (Stefoski et al, 1991). Temperature-sensitive patients and those with a longer duration of disease may be more likely to benefit.

Results of a number of controlled studies demonstrated that no significant benefit is achieved with the use of hyperbaric oxygen therapy (Aita, 1988; Barnes et al, 1987; Wiles et al, 1986).

Marked variations in the severity of MS in any one patient and increased scarring and disabilities as the illness progresses make effectiveness of therapy difficult to evaluate. Evaluation thus far has been limited largely to subjective rating of clinical signs and symptoms. The Kurtzke Disability Status Scale and the Expanded Disability Status Scale are the most widely used measures of disability in MS (Kurtzke, 1970; Kurtzke, 1983). The assessment of trials utilizing these scales as functional measures can be hampered by their low test/retest reliability and the potential bias of unblinded observers. Thus, a more sensitive and reliable measure of outcome is needed.

Disease Suppression: Based on the assumption that MS is an autoimmune disease, a number of clinical trials have been conducted to evaluate therapy designed to suppress or alter the immune response. Therapeutic goals depend on manifestations of the disease and include improving the rate or extent of recovery from acute attacks, preventing or decreasing the number of relapses, and halting the progressive phase (Weiner and Hafler, 1988).

Corticosteroids. In acute relapsing MS, a 14-day course of intramuscular corticotropin (ACTH) (80 units for seven days, 40 units for four days, and 20 units for three days) was more effective than placebo in increasing the rate but not the extent of short-term recovery (Rose et al, 1970). However, although the results of this large multicenter study have been widely cited as evidence for the effectiveness of ACTH in treating acute relapses, 69% of patients receiving placebo also improved. Furthermore, the reliability of the blinded assessment may have been affected by the frequent occurrence of side effects in the group receiving active treatment.

In more recent studies, high-dose intravenous methylprednisolone (500 mg daily for five days or 1 g daily for three to seven days) has been reported to be superior to placebo (Milligan et al, 1987) and equivalent or superior to ACTH in enhancing short-term recovery from acute attacks of MS (Barnes et al, 1985; Thompson et al, 1989). Similar conclusions were reached in a retrospective study using a 5-g cumulative dose that was followed by oral administration of prednisone (Lyons et al, 1988). (Prednisone has not been directly compared with ACTH.) Thus, some investigators conclude that high-dose, intravenous ("pulse") methylprednisolone is the current treatment of choice for acute exacerbations of MS (Troiano et al, 1987; Compston, 1988; Myers and Ellison, 1990).

The appropriateness of treating acute relapsing MS with corticosteroids is not universally accepted (Goodin, 1991); however, it is agreed that high-dose intravenous methylprednisolone has caused a rapid reduction in abnormalities of the blood-brain barrier that are characteristic of an acute stage of lesion development in MS (Burnham et al, 1991; Miller et al, 1992 B). Although short intensive courses of adrenal corticosteroids hasten recovery from acute attacks, they have no effect on progressive MS and confer no lasting benefit.

Administration of intravenous methylprednisolone followed by oral prednisone hastens recovery of the visual loss caused by optic neuritis and results in slightly improved vision at six months. In contrast, oral prednisone alone is ineffective and may actually increase the risk of new episodes of optic neuritis (Beck et al, 1992).

Interferons. Three forms of interferon (alpha, beta, and gamma) have been investigated for use in MS. The rationale for the administration of interferons is their antiviral and immunomodulatory properties. The latter effects vary with the interferon type, dose, and route of administration. In clinical trials with the alpha form, beneficial effects have been modest. In a randomized, double-blind, placebo-controlled trial involving patients with chronic progressive MS, treatment with lymphoblastoid interferon (primarily alpha, some beta) for six months did not retard disease progression after two years (Kastrukoff et al, 1990).

In one study, interferon beta reduced exacerbation rates when administered intrathecally to patients with relapsing-remitting disease (Jacobs et al, 1985). In another study in patients with relapsing-remitting or progressive forms of the disease, intrathecal administration of interferon beta was without benefit and appeared to increase the frequency of relapses (Milanese et al, 1990). In a recent large multicenter, randomized, double-blind, placebo-controlled trial on patients with relapsing-remitting disease, the exacerbation rates and severity of attacks decreased in those who received subcutaneous interferon beta-1b 1.6 or 8 million IU every other day for two years (The IFNB Multiple Sclerosis Study Group, 1993). Disease activity, as detected by serial MRIs, also was significantly reduced in the group receiving high-dose interferon beta (Paty et al, 1993). On the basis of these results, interferon beta-1b was approved for marketing for the treatment of patients with relapsing-remitting MS. Its effect on chronic progressive MS is not known. One large controlled study employing intramuscular interferon beta is currently under way.

Administration of interferon gamma increases the number of exacerbations in MS patients (Panitch et al, 1987).

Immunosuppressive Agents. Some clinicians believe that immunosuppressive agents, such as azathioprine and cyclophosphamide, may retard chronic deterioration in chronic progressive MS. However, their effectiveness is disputed by others (Tourtellote and Pick, 1989). In relapsing-remitting MS, monthly pulse doses of intravenous cyclophosphamide (750 mg/M^2) plus ACTH appear to reduce the exacerbation rate (Killian et al, 1988). Lower doses without concomitant ACTH therapy were not beneficial (Likosky et al, 1987). There is evidence that progressive MS may be stabilized for at least 12 months by short-term, intensive immunosuppression with cyclophosphamide plus ACTH, after which disease progression resumes (Hauser et al, 1983; Goodkin et al, 1987). Maintenance therapy with pulse cyclophosphamide (700/M^2 every other month for two years) after induction therapy with cyclophosphamide/ACTH can prolong the duration to treatment failure, especially in younger patients (Weiner et al, 1993 A).

Another regimen employs methylprednisolone (1 g intravenously daily for five days) followed by a single intravenous dose of cyclophosphamide (800 mg to 1.4 g/M^2) adjusted to produce leukopenia, plus methylprednisolone 1 g administered monthly for one year, every six weeks in the following year, and every two months in the third year. Results of a pilot study suggest that this regimen is more efficacious than similar treatment schedules using methylprednisolone alone, is less toxic than other regimens, and may be given as outpatient therapy (Hohol et al, 1992). However, since long-term administration of cyclophosphamide is required to maintain effectiveness, less toxic agents for use during remission must be found. (For this drug's actions and adverse reactions, see index entry Cyclophosphamide, Uses, Cancer.)

Azathioprine has had some beneficial effect in patients with a component of relapsing disease (Patzold et al, 1982; Ellison et al, 1989; Goodkin et al, 1991), but there have been little data to support use of this agent in other controlled trials (Milanese et al, 1988; Minderhoud et al, 1988; British and Dutch Multiple Sclerosis Azathioprine Trial Group, 1988). Meta-analysis of randomized, blinded, controlled trials in which azathioprine was used as a single agent indicates that this drug's effect on disability scores is small and any improvement in the patient's condition is not apparent until the second or third year of treatment and is unlikely to be clinically relevant (Yudkin et al, 1991). Use of azathioprine does appear to be associated with a modest decrease in the frequency of relapse over a three-year period, but this probably does not outweigh the risks of drug-induced reactions for most patients.

Theoretically, the specificity of cyclosporine for T-cells suggests that the action of this agent would be more specific than that of cyclophosphamide or azathioprine. In a study that lacked placebo control, cyclosporine 5 mg/kg/day and azathioprine 2.5 mg/kg/day appeared to provide some degree of stabilization in patients with relapsing-remitting and relapsing-progressive disease (Kappos et al, 1988). In another two-year controlled trial, cyclosporine 5 mg/kg/day was not beneficial in patients with relapsing (remitting or progressive) disease. Larger doses (eg, 7.2 mg/kg/day) reduced disease progression but were not well tolerated (Rudge et al, 1989). In a recently completed multicenter controlled trial, cyclosporine delayed progression of disease for a short period in patients with moderately severe and progressive MS. Nephrotoxicity and hypertension were common adverse effects even though dosage was adjusted individually to provide a blood concentration of 310 to 430 ng/ml (The Multiple Sclerosis Study Group, 1990).

Cop 1, a synthetic analogue of myelin basic protein, was developed as a nontoxic agent that would be an antigen-specific form of therapy. It was effective in an animal model of MS and in experimental allergic encephalomyelitis (EAE); in a preliminary clinical trial, Cop 1 decreased the number of relapses in patients with early relapsing-remitting disease (Bornstein et al, 1987). On the basis of this trial, Cop 1 has been granted Treatment IND status for patients with relapsing-remitting MS. Although Cop 1 had a positive effect on disability scores in patients with minor neurologic impairment, it had little effect on those with more severe impairment (Bornstein at al, 1987; Weiner, 1987). In a large study in patients with chronic progressive disease, no effect on overall survival curves was noted (Bornstein et al, 1991). A larger multicenter study in which patients with relapsing-remitting disease receive Cop 1 20 mg daily by injection is in progress.

Other immunosuppressive approaches under investigation include plasma exchange and total lymphoid irradiation. In a Canadian study of plasmapheresis in conjunction with cyclophosphamide and prednisone in progressive MS, no significant benefit was observed (Noseworthy, 1990). In two other studies, two to five months of plasma exchange performed at least once weekly appeared to enhance recovery from acute exacerbations in patients with relapsing-remitting disease when used with cyclophosphamide and ACTH or prednisone, although the data were not wholly persuasive (Khatri et al, 1985; Weiner et al, 1989). Because the effect is transient, the authors of one study consider the technique warranted only in patients with relapsing-remitting disease who experience a severe attack and in whom a more rapid recovery may significantly lessen morbidity (Weiner et al, 1989). Plasmapheresis regimens that do not include concomitant immunosuppression do not appear to be beneficial (Weiner and Hafler, 1988). In a double-blind study, the potent immunosuppressive effects of total lymphoid irradiation were reported to be useful in patients with chronic progressive MS, although 50% of patients experienced disease progression within 36 months and there were several delayed deaths in the treated group (Cook et al, 1986).

Research continues on more specific immunosuppressive measures. One such approach is induction of tolerance by oral administration of antigen. In a one-year, double-blind pilot study involving 30 patients with relapsing-remitting disease, 6 of 15 patients who received bovine myelin 300 mg daily experienced a major relapse compared with 12 of 15 patients who received a placebo (Weiner et al, 1993 B).

Monoclonal antibodies targeted to helper/inducer and cytotoxic T-cells, activated T-cells (expressing interleukin-2 receptors), class II major histocompatibility complex (MHC) and immune response (Ia) gene products, and T-cell adhesion molecules have been used successfully to treat EAE. It is hoped that similar approaches in humans will enhance understanding of the pathogenesis of MS and provide eventual therapeutic applications.

Drug Evaluation

INTERFERON BETA-1b
[Betaseron]

ACTIONS AND USES. Interferon beta-1b (IFN_β-1b) is a nonglycosylated protein containing 165 amino acids produced in *E. coli* by recombinant DNA techniques; a serine has been substituted for the cysteine residue found at position 17 in the human form. IFN_β-1b possesses antiviral, antiproliferative, and immunomodulating effects. The mechanism of action in reducing exacerbations in patients with relapsing-remitting MS is unknown but may involve decreases in T-cell proliferation, inhibition of interferon gamma synthesis, inhibition of cytokine release, or increases in suppressor T-cell activity (Arnason, 1993).

IFN_β-1b is indicated for use in ambulatory patients with relapsing-remitting MS to reduce the frequency of clinical exacerbations. Its effectiveness was evaluated in a double-blind, randomized, placebo-controlled, multicenter two-year study (The INFB Multiple Sclerosis Study Group, 1993). Subcutaneous self-administration of 0.25 mg (8 million IU) every other day decreased the number of exacerbations 31% compared with placebo. After two years, more IFN_β-1b recipients (25%) were free of exacerbations than placebo recipients (16%) and the exacerbations that occurred in the other IFN_β-1b recipients were less severe and resulted in fewer MS-related hospitalizations. Patients who received a lower dose (0.05 mg) of IFN_β-1b also benefited on most outcome measures compared with placebo recipients, but the degree of improvement was not as pronounced as that in the high-dose group. Total lesion area as determined by annual MRI increased 16.5% in placebo recipients but did not change significantly in patients who received the higher dose (Paty et al, 1993).

ADVERSE REACTIONS AND PRECAUTIONS. In general, IFN_β-1b is well tolerated. Complete and differential white blood cell counts, platelet counts, blood chemistries including hemoglobin, and liver function tests are recommended prior to initiating therapy and periodically thereafter.

The most common adverse reactions associated with use of IFN_β-1b are injection site reactions (85%) and flu-like symptoms (76%) (eg, fever, chills, myalgia, malaise, sweating, asthenia). Other reactions include increase in ALT (19% of patients), decrease in absolute neutrophil count (<1500/mm^3) (18%), menstrual disorders (17%), decrease in white blood cell count (<3000/mm^3) (16%), dyspnea (8%), palpitation (8%), and increase in AST (4%). Therapy should be discontinued if the absolute neutrophil count falls below 750/mm^3 or if AST/ALT levels exceed 10 times the upper limit of normal. Therapy may be resumed with one-half the dose when these parameters are reestablished.

One suicide and four attempted suicides were observed in IFN_β-1b recipients during a three-year period. Patients should be informed that depression and suicidal ideation may occur and advised to report their development to the prescribing physician.

IFN_β-1b causes a dose-related increase in spontaneous abortions in rhesus monkeys when administered at 2.8 to 40 times the recommended human dose. Spontaneous abortions were reported by four patients who received IFN_β-1b during clinical trials. IFN_β-1b is classified in FDA Pregnancy Category C.

DRUG INTERACTIONS. No clinically significant interactions between IFN_β-1b and other drugs have been reported.

PHARMACOKINETICS. Serum concentrations of IFN_β-1b are very low or undetectable following subcutaneous administration of 0.25 mg. Data obtained after subcutaneous administration of higher doses indicate that bioavailability is at least 50%. The elimination half-life reported after intravenous administration of 2 mg is highly variable (range, 8 minutes to 4.3 hours).

DOSAGE AND ADMINISTRATION. Patients should be instructed in the use of aseptic technique. Appropriate instructions for reconstitution of IFN_β-1b and self-injection should be given, including careful review of the Patient Information sheet.

Subcutaneous: *Adults,* 0.25 mg (8 million IU) injected every other day.

Betaseron (Berlex). Powder (lyophilized) containing 0.3 mg (9.6 million IU) with human albumin 15 mg and dextrose 15 mg in a single-use vial for reconstitution with sodium chloride 0.54%.

Cited References

Adams SL, et al: Drugs that may exacerbate myasthenia gravis. *Ann Emerg Med* 13:532-538, 1984.

Adams C, et al: Thymectomy in juvenile myasthenia gravis. *J Child Neurol* 5:215-218, 1990.

Aita JF: Hyperbaric oxygen and multiple sclerosis: Review. *Nebr Med J* 73:266-268, 1988.

Anderson DW, et al: Revised estimate of the prevalence of multiple sclerosis in the United States. *Ann Neurol* 31:333-336, 1992.

Antonini G, et al: Results of an open trial of cyclosporine in a group of steroidodependent myasthenic subjects. *Clin Neurol Neurosurg* 92:317-321, 1990.

Aquilonius S-M, Hartvig P: Clinical pharmacokinetics of cholinesterase inhibitors. *Clin Pharmacokinet* 11:236-249, 1986.

Argov Z, Mastaglia FL: Disorders of neuromuscular transmission caused by drugs. *N Engl J Med* 301:409-413, 1979.

Arnason BGW: Interferon beta in multiple sclerosis, editorial. *Neurology* 43:641-643, 1993.

Arsura EL, et al: High-dose intravenous immunoglobulin in the management of myasthenia gravis. *Arch Intern Med* 146:1365-1368, 1986.

Barnes MP, et al: Intravenous methylprednisolone for multiple sclerosis in relapse. *J Neurol Neurosurg Psychiatry* 48:157-159, 1985.

Barnes MP, et al: Hyperbaric oxygen and multiple sclerosis: Final results of a placebo-controlled, double-blind trial. *J Neurol Neurosurg Psychiatry* 50:1402-1406, 1987.

Beck RW, et al: A randomized, controlled trial of corticosteroids in the treatment of acute optic neuritis. *N Engl J Med* 326:581-588, 1992.

Bennett DA, Bleck TP: Recognizing impending respiratory failure from neuromuscular causes. *J Crit Illness* 3:46-60, 1988.

Bohan A, Peter JB: Polymyositis and dermatomyositis (first of two parts). *N Engl J Med* 292:344-347, 1975.
Bornstein MB, et al: A pilot trial of Cop 1 in exacerbating-remitting multiple sclerosis. *N Engl J Med* 317:408-414, 1987.
Bornstein MB, et al: A placebo-controlled, double-blind, randomized, two center, pilot trial of Cop 1 in chronic progressive multiple sclerosis. *Neurology* 41:533-539, 1991.
British and Dutch Multiple Sclerosis Azathioprine Trial Group: Double-masked trial of azathioprine in multiple sclerosis. *Lancet* 2:179-183, 1988.
Burnham JA, et al: The effect of high-dose steroids on MRI gadolinium enhancement in acute demyelinating lesions. *Neurology* 41:1349-1354, 1991.
Calabrese LH, et al: Inclusion body myositis presenting as treatment-resistant polymyositis. *Arthritis Rheum* 30:397-403, 1987.
Caro I: A dermatologist's view of polymyositis/dermatomyositis. *Clin Dermatol* 6:9-14, 1988.
Caro I: Dermatomyositis as a systemic disease. *Med Clin North Am* 73:1181-1192, 1989.
Carter JL, Rodriguez M: Newer drug therapies for multiple sclerosis. *Drug Ther* 31-43, (March) 1990.
Cherin P, et al: Efficacy of intravenous gammaglobulin therapy in chronic refractory polymyositis and dermatomyositis: An open study with 20 adult patients. *Am J Med* 91:162-168, (Aug) 1991.
Chofflon M, et al: Decrease of suppressor inducer (CD4+2H4+) T cells in multiple sclerosis cerebrospinal fluid. *Ann Neurol* 25:494-499, 1989.
Cohen RA, Fisher M: Amantadine treatment of fatigue associated with multiple sclerosis. *Arch Neurol* 46:676-680, 1989.
Cohen MR, et al: Clinical heterogeneity and treatment response in inclusion body myositis. *Arthritis Rheum* 32:734-740, 1989.
Compston A: Methylprednisolone and multiple sclerosis. *Arch Neurol* 45:669-670, 1988.
Compston DAS, et al: Clinical, pathological, HLA antigen and immunological evidence for disease heterogeneity in myasthenia gravis. *Brain* 103:579-601, 1980.
Cook SD, et al: Effect of total lymphoid irradiation in chronic progressive multiple sclerosis. *Lancet* 1:1405-1409, 1986.
Cosi V, et al: Effectiveness of steroid treatment in myasthenia gravis: A retrospective study. *Acta Neurol Scand* 84:33-39, 1991 A.
Cosi V, et al: Treatment of myasthenia gravis with high-dose intravenous immunoglobulin. *Acta Neurol Scand* 84:81-84, 1991 B.
Craven C, et al: Effect of corticosteroids on thymus in myasthenia gravis. *Muscle Nerve* 4:425-428, 1981.
Dalakas MC: Polymyositis, dermatomyositis, and inclusion-body myositis. *N Engl J Med* 325:1487-1498, 1991.
Drachman DB: Neuromuscular junction and muscle disease: Myasthenia gravis, in Johnson RT (ed): *Current Therapy in Neurologic Disease.* Philadelphia, BC Decker, 1985, 366-371.
Drachman DB: Present and future treatment of myasthenia gravis, editorial. *N Engl J Med* 316:743-745, 1987.
Drachman DB, et al: Humoral pathogenesis of myasthenia gravis. *Ann NY Acad Sci* 505:90-104, 1987.
Drachman DB, et al: Strategies for the treatment of myasthenia gravis. *Ann NY Acad Sci* 540:176-186, 1988.
Ebers GC, et al: A population-based study of multiple sclerosis in twins. *N Engl J Med* 315:1638-1642, 1986.
Ellison GW, et al: A placebo-controlled, randomized, double-masked, variable dosage, clinical trial of azathioprine with and without methylprednisolone in multiple sclerosis. *Neurology* 39:1018-1026, 1989.
Estes ML, et al: Stereotactic biopsy of an active multiple sclerosis lesion: Immunocytochemical analysis and neuropathologic correlation with magnetic resonance imaging. *Arch Neurol* 47:1299-1303, 1990.
Gilmore RL, et al: Comparative impact of paraclinical studies in establishing the diagnosis of multiple sclerosis. *Electroencephalogr Clin Neurophysiol* 73:433-442, 1989.
Goodin DS: The use of immunosuppressive agents in the treatment of multiple sclerosis: A critical review. *Neurology* 41:980-985, 1991.
Goodkin DE, et al: Cyclophosphamide in chronic progressive multiple sclerosis: Maintenance vs nonmaintenance therapy. *Arch Neurol* 44:823-827, 1987.
Goodkin DE, et al: The efficacy of azathioprine in relapsing-remitting multiple sclerosis. *Neurology* 41:20-25, 1991.
Goodkin DE, et al: Magnetic resonance imaging lesion enlargement in multiple sclerosis: Disease-related activity, chance occurrence, or measurement artifact? *Arch Neurol* 49:261-263, 1992.
Goulon M, et al: Results of a one-year open trial of cyclosporine in ten patients with severe myasthenia gravis. *Transplant Proc* 20(suppl 4):211-217, 1988.
Grob D (ed): Myasthenia gravis: Pathophysiology and management. *Ann NY Acad Sci* 377:1-902, 1981.
Harris JO, et al: Serial gadolinium-enhanced magnetic resonance imaging scans in patients with early, relapsing-remitting multiple sclerosis: Implications for clinical trials and natural history. *Ann Neurol* 29:548-555, 1991.
Hartung H-P, et al: T cell activation in Guillain-Barré syndrome and in MS: Elevated serum levels of soluble IL-2 receptors. *Neurology* 40:215-218, 1990.
Hauser SL, et al: Intensive immunosuppression in progressive multiple sclerosis: A randomized, three-arm study of high-dose intravenous cyclophosphamide, plasma exchange, and ACTH. *N Engl J Med* 308:173-180, 1983.
Havard CWH, Fonseca V: New treatment approaches to myasthenia gravis. *Drugs* 39:66-73, 1990.
Hohlfeld R: Neurological autoimmune disease and the trimolecular complex of T-lymphocytes. *Ann Neurol* 25:531-538, 1989.
Hohlfeld R, et al: Myasthenia gravis: Reactivation of clinical disease and of autoimmune factors after discontinuation of long-term azathioprine. *Ann Neurol* 17:238-242, 1985.
Hohlfeld R, et al: Azathioprine toxicity during long-term immunosuppression of generalized myasthenia gravis. *Neurology* 38:258-261, 1988.
Hohol MJ, et al: Pilot study of three-year intermittent pulse cyclophosphamide/methylprednisolone therapy in multiple sclerosis. *Ann Neurol* 32:256-257, 1992.
The IFNB Multiple Sclerosis Study Group: Interferon beta-1b is effective in relapsing-remitting multiple sclerosis: I. Clinical results of a multicenter, randomized, double-blind, placebo-controlled trial. *Neurology* 43:655-661, 1993.
Isaac C, et al: Multiple sclerosis: A serial study using MRI in relapsing patients. *Neurology* 38:1511-1515, 1988.
Jacobs L, et al: Intrathecal interferon in the treatment of multiple sclerosis: Patient follow-up. *Arch Neurol* 42:841-847, 1985.
Jacobs L, et al: Clinical and magnetic resonance imaging in optic neuritis. *Neurology* 41:15-19, 1991.
Jann S, et al: High-dose intravenous human immunoglobulin in polymyositis resistant to treatment. *J Neurol Neurosurg Psychiatry* 55:60-66, 1992.
Joffe MM, et al: Drug therapy of the idiopathic inflammatory myopathies: Predictors of response to prednisone, azathioprine, and methotrexate and a comparison of their efficacy. *Am J Med* 94:379-387, 1993.
Johns TR: Long-term corticosteroid treatment of myasthenia gravis. *Ann NY Acad Sci* 505:568-583, 1987.
Kappos L, et al: Cyclosporine versus azathioprine in the long-term treatment of multiple sclerosis: Results of the German multicenter study. *Ann Neurol* 23:56-63, 1988.
Kastrukoff LF, et al: Systemic lymphoblastoid interferon therapy in chronic progressive multiple sclerosis: I. Clinical and MRI evaluation. *Neurology* 40:479-486, 1990.
Khatri BO, et al: Chronic progressive multiple sclerosis: Double-blind controlled study of plasmapheresis in patients taking immunosuppressive drugs. *Neurology* 35:312-319, 1985.
Killian JM, et al: Controlled pilot trial of monthly intravenous cyclophosphamide in multiple sclerosis. *Arch Neurol* 45:27-30, 1988.
Kinnunen E, et al: Genetic susceptibility to multiple sclerosis: A co-twin study of a nationwide series. *Arch Neurol* 45:1108-1111, 1988.

Kissel JT, et al: The relationship of complement-mediated microvasculopathy to the histologic features and clinical duration of disease in dermatomyositis. *Arch Neurol* 48:26-30, 1991.

Kurtzke JF: Neurologic impairment in multiple sclerosis and the disability status scale. *Acta Neurol Scand* 46:493-512, 1970.

Kurtzke JF: Rating neurologic impairment in multiple sclerosis: An expanded disability status scale (EDSS). *Neurology* 33:1444-1452, 1983.

Lane RM, et al: Inclusion body myositis: A case with associated collagen vascular disease responding to treatment. *J Neurol Neurosurg Psychiatry* 48:270-273, 1985.

Lang BA, et al: Treatment of dermatomyositis with intravenous gammaglobulin. *Am J Med* 91:169-172, (Aug) 1991.

Lanska DJ: Indications for thymectomy in myasthenia gravis. *Neurology* 40:1828-1829, 1990.

Latash ML, et al: Effects of intrathecal baclofen on voluntary motor control in spastic paresis. *J Neurosurg* 72:388-392, 1990.

Laxer RM, et al: Intravenous pulse methylprednisolone treatment of juvenile dermatomyositis. *Arthritis Rheum* 30:328-334, 1987.

Leff RL, et al: Viruses in idiopathic inflammatory myopathies: Absence of candidate viral genomes in muscle. *Lancet* 339:1192-1195, 1992.

Likosky WH, et al: Intensive cyclophosphamide immunosuppression in multiple sclerosis: A randomized blinded multicenter clinical trial. *Neurology* 37 (suppl 1):108, 1987.

Linton DM, Philcox D: Myasthenia gravis. *Dis Mon* 35:597-637, 1990.

Lotz BP, et al: Inclusion body myositis: Observations in 40 patients. *Brain* 112:727-747, 1989.

Lyons PR, et al: Methylprednisolone therapy in multiple sclerosis: A profile of adverse effects. *J Neurol Neurosurg Psychiatry* 51:285-287, 1988.

Martin R, et al: Immunological aspects of demyelinating diseases. *Annu Rev Immunol* 10:153-187, 1992.

Mastaglia FL, Ojeda VJ: Inflammatory myopathies, part 2. *Ann Neurol* 17:317-323, 1985.

Matell G: Immunosuppressive drugs: Azathioprine in the treatment of myasthenia gravis. *Ann NY Acad Sci* 505:588-594, 1987.

Matsui M, et al: Cellular immunoregulatory mechanisms in the central nervous system: Characterization of noninflammatory and inflammatory cerebrospinal fluid lymphocytes. *Ann Neurol* 27:647-651, 1990.

May EF, Calvert PC: Aggravation of myasthenia gravis by erythromycin. *Ann Neurol* 28:577-579, 1990.

McDonald WI: The role of NMR imaging in the assessment of multiple sclerosis. *Clin Neurol Neurosurg* 90:3-9, 1988.

McEvoy KM, et al: 3,4-Diaminopyridine in the treatment of Lambert-Eaton myasthenic syndrome. *N Engl J Med* 321:1567-1571, 1989.

McFarland HF, et al: Family and twin studies in multiple sclerosis. *Ann NY Acad Sci* 436:118-124, 1984.

Mertens HG, et al: Effect of immunosuppressive drugs (azathioprine). *Ann NY Acad Sci* 377:691-698, 1981.

Miano MA, et al: Factors influencing outcome of prednisone dose reduction in myasthenia gravis. *Neurology* 41:919-921, 1991.

Milanese C, et al: Double blind controlled randomized study on azathioprine efficacy in multiple sclerosis. *Ital J Neurol Sci* 9:53-57, 1988.

Milanese C, et al: Double blind study of intrathecal beta-interferon in multiple sclerosis: Clinical and laboratory results. *J Neurol Neurosurg Psychiatry* 55:554-557, 1990.

Miller RG, et al: Repeat thymectomy in chronic refractory myasthenia gravis. *Neurology* 41:923-924, 1991 A.

Miller DH, et al: Magnetic resonance imaging in monitoring the treatment of multiple sclerosis: Concerted action guidelines. *J Neurol Neurosurg Psychiatry* 54:683-688, 1991 B.

Miller FW, et al: Controlled trial of plasma exchange and leukapheresis in polymyositis and dermatomyositis. *N Engl J Med* 326:1380-1384, 1992 A.

Miller DH, et al: High dose steroids in acute relapses of multiple sclerosis: MRI evidence for a possible mechanism of the therapeutic effect. *J Neurol Neurosurg Psychiatry* 55:450-453, 1992 B.

Milligan NM, et al: A double-blind controlled trial of high dose methylprednisolone in patients with multiple sclerosis: I, Clinical effects. *J Neurol Neurosurg Psychiatry* 50:511-516, 1987.

Minderhoud JM, et al: A long-term double-blind controlled study on the effect of azathioprine in the treatment of multiple sclerosis. *Clin Neurol Neurosurg* 90:25-28, 1988.

Misulis KE, Fenichel GM: Genetic forms of myasthenia gravis. *Pediatr Neurol* 5:205-210, 1989.

Moulin DE, et al: Pain syndromes in multiple sclerosis. *Neurology* 38:1830-1834, 1988.

Mulder DG, et al: Thymectomy for myasthenia gravis. *Am J Surg* 146:61-66, 1983.

The Multiple Sclerosis Study Group: Efficacy and toxicity of cyclosporine in chronic progressive multiple sclerosis: A randomized, double-blinded, placebo-controlled clinical trial. *Ann Neurol* 27:591-605, 1990.

Mumford CJ, Ginsberg L: Ciprofloxacin and myasthenia gravis. *BMJ* 301:818, 1990.

Myers LW, Ellison GW: The peculiar difficulties of therapeutic trials for multiple sclerosis. *Neurol Clin* 8:119-141, 1990.

Niakan E, et al: Immunosuppressive drug therapy in myasthenia. *Arch Neurol* 43:155-156, 1986.

Noakes JB, et al: Magnetic resonance imaging in clinically-definite multiple sclerosis. *Med J Aust* 152:136-140, 1990.

Noseworthy JH: The Canadian cooperative study of cyclophosphamide and plasma exchange in progressive multiple sclerosis. *Neurology* 40 (suppl 1): 284, 1990.

Nyberg-Hansen R, Gjerstad L: Myasthenia gravis treated with ciclosporin. *Acta Neurol Scand* 77:307-313, 1988.

Oddis CV, Medsger TA Jr: Relationship between serum creatine kinase level and corticosteroid therapy in polymyositis-dermatomyositis. *J Rheumatol* 15:807-811, 1988.

Oddis CV, Medsger TA: Current management of polymyositis and dermatomyositis. *Drugs* 37:382-390, 1989.

Olanow CW, et al: Thymectomy as primary therapy in myasthenia gravis. *Ann NY Acad Sci* 505:595-606, 1987.

O'Neill JH, et al: The Lambert-Eaton myasthenic syndrome: A review of 50 cases. *Brain* 111:577-596, 1988.

Oosterhuis HJGH: Treating the myasthenic patient, in: *Myasthenia Gravis: Clinical Neurology and Neurosurgery Monographs*. Edinburgh, Churchill Livingstone, 1984, vol 5, 175-261.

Osserman KE, Genkins G: Studies in myasthenia gravis: Review of a twenty-year experience in over 1,200 patients. *Mt Sinai J Med* 38:497-537, 1971.

Pachman LM: Juvenile dermatomyositis. *Pediatr Clin North Am* 33:1097-1117, 1986.

Palace J, et al: 3,4-Diaminopyridine in the treatment of congenital (hereditary) myasthenia. *J Neurol Neurosurg Psychiatry* 54:1069-1072, 1991.

Panitch HS, et al: Treatment of multiple sclerosis with gamma interferon: Exacerbations associated with activation of the immune system. *Neurology* 37:1097-1102, 1987.

Pascuzzi RM, et al: Long-term corticosteroid treatment of myasthenia gravis: Report of 116 patients. *Ann Neurol* 15:291-298, 1984.

Paty DW, et al: Interferon beta-1b is effective in relapsing-remitting multiple sclerosis: II. MRI analysis results of a multicenter, randomized, double-blind, placebo-controlled trial. *Neurology* 43:662-667, 1993.

Patzold U, et al: Azathioprine in treatment of multiple sclerosis: Final results of a 4½-year controlled study of its effectiveness covering 115 patients. *J Neurol Sci* 54:377-394, 1982.

Perlo VP: Treatment of the critically ill patient with myasthenia, in Ropper AH, et al (eds): *Neurology and Neurological Intensive Care*. Baltimore, University Park Press, 1983, 157-161.

Plotz PH, et al: Current concepts in the idiopathic inflammatory myopathies: Polymyositis, dermatomyositis, and related disorders. *Ann Intern Med* 111:143-157, 1989.

Poser CM, et al: New diagnostic criteria for multiple sclerosis: Guidelines for research protocols. *Ann Neurol* 13:227-231, 1983.

Prineas JW, et al: Continual breakdown and regeneration of myelin in progressive multiple sclerosis plaques. *Ann NY Acad Sci* 436:11-32, 1984.

Rao SM, et al: Cognitive dysfunction in multiple sclerosis: I. Frequency, patterns, and prediction. *Neurology* 41:685-691, 1991.

Rauser EH, et al: Exacerbation of myasthenia gravis by norfloxacin, letter. *DICP* 24:207-208, 1990.

Rodriguez M: Multiple sclerosis: Basic concepts and hypothesis. *Mayo Clin Proc* 64:570-576, 1989.

Rose AS, et al: Cooperative study in the evaluation of therapy in multiple sclerosis: ACTH vs. placebo—Final report. *Neurology* 20 (part II):1-59, 1970.

Rowland LP: Controversies about treatment of myasthenia gravis. *J Neurol Neurosurg Psychiatry* 43:644-659, 1980.

Rudge P, et al: Randomised double blind controlled trial of cyclosporin in multiple sclerosis. *J Neurol Neurosurg Psychiatry* 52:559-565, 1989.

Rudick RA, et al: Relative diagnostic value of cerebrospinal fluid kappa chains in MS: Comparison with other immunoglobulin tests. *Neurology* 39:964-968, 1989.

Rudick RA, et al: Pharmacotherapy of multiple sclerosis: Current status. *Cleve Clin J Med* 59:267-277, 1992.

Salonen R, et al: Lymphocyte subsets in the cerebrospinal fluid in active multiple sclerosis. *Ann Neurol* 25:500-502, 1989.

Sanders DB: The electrodiagnosis of myasthenia gravis. *Ann NY Acad Sci* 505:539-556, 1987.

Sayers ME, et al: Inclusion body myositis: Analysis of 32 cases. *J Rheumatol* 19:1385-1389, 1992.

Schalke B, et al: Cyclosporin A treatment of myasthenia gravis: Initial results of a double-blind trial of cyclosporin A versus azathioprine. *Ann NY Acad Sci* 505:872-875, 1988.

Scherpbier HJ, Oosterhuis HJGH: Factors influencing the relapse risk at steroid dose reduction in myasthenia gravis. *Clin Neurol Neurosurg* 89:145-150, 1987.

Schiffer RB, Wineman NM: Antidepressant pharmacotherapy of depression associated with multiple sclerosis. *Am J Psychiatry* 147:1493-1497, 1990.

Schumacher GA, et al: Problems of experimental trials of therapy in multiple sclerosis: Report by the panel on evaluation of experimental trials of therapy in multiple sclerosis. *Ann NY Acad Sci* 122:552-568, 1965.

Seybold ME: Plasmapheresis in myasthenia gravis. *Ann NY Acad Sci* 505:584-587, 1987.

Sher E, et al: Specificity of calcium channel autoantibodies in Lambert-Eaton myasthenic syndrome. *Lancet* 2:640-643, 1989.

Sigurgeirsson B, et al: Risk of cancer in patients with dermatomyositis or polymyositis: A population-based study. *N Engl J Med* 326:363-367, 1992.

Snead OC III, et al: Juvenile myasthenia gravis. *Neurology* 30:732-739, 1980.

Snow BJ, et al: Treatment of spasticity with botulinum toxin: A double-blind study. *Ann Neurol* 28:512-515, 1990.

Städt D, et al: Occurrence of MRI abnormalities in patients with isolated optic neuritis. *Eur Neurol* 30:305-309, 1990.

Stefoski D, et al: 4-Aminopyridine in multiple sclerosis: Prolonged administration. *Neurology* 41:1344-1348, 1991.

Targoff IN: Diagnosis and treatment of polymyositis and dermatomyositis. *Compr Ther* 16:16-24, 1990.

Taylor R, et al: Disseminated thymoma and myasthenia gravis: Dramatic response to prednisone, letter. *Ann Neurol* 24:208, 1989.

Thompson AJ, et al: Relative efficacy of intravenous methylprednisolone and ACTH in the treatment of acute relapse in MS. *Neurology* 39:969-971, 1989.

Thompson AJ, et al: Serial gadolinium-enhanced MRI in relapsing/remitting multiple sclerosis of varying disease duration. *Neurology* 42:60-63, 1992.

Tienari PJ, et al: Familial multiple sclerosis: MRI findings in clinically affected and unaffected siblings. *J Neurol Neurosurg Psychiatry* 55:883-886, 1992.

Tindall RS, et al: Preliminary results of a double blind, randomized, placebo-controlled trial of cyclosporine in myasthenia gravis. *N Engl J Med* 316:719-724, 1987.

Tourtellote WW, Pick PW: Current concepts about multiple sclerosis, editorial. *Mayo Clin Proc* 64:592-596, 1989.

Troiano R, et al: Steroid therapy in multiple sclerosis: Point of view. *Arch Neurol* 44:803-807, 1987.

Tuffanelli DL, Lavoie PE: Prognosis and therapy of polymyositis/dermatomyositis. *Clin Dermatol* 6:93-104,1988.

Uitdehaag BMJ, et al: Magnetic resonance imaging studies in multiple sclerosis twins. *J Neurol Neurosurg Psychiatry* 52:1417-1419, 1989.

van Diemen HAM, et al: The effect of 4-aminopyridine on clinical signs in multiple sclerosis: A randomized, placebo-controlled, double-blind, cross-over study. *Ann Neurol* 32:123-130, 1992.

Weiner HL: Cop 1 therapy for multiple sclerosis, editorial. *N Engl J Med* 317:442-444, 1987.

Weiner HL, Hafler DA: Immunotherapy of multiple sclerosis. *Ann Neurol* 23:211-222, 1988.

Weiner HL, et al: Double-blind study of true vs. sham plasma exchange in patients treated with immunosuppression for acute attacks of multiple sclerosis. *Neurology* 39:1143-1149, 1989.

Weiner HL, et al: Intermittent cyclophosphamide pulse therapy in progressive multiple sclerosis: Final report of the Northeast Cooperative Multiple Sclerosis Treatment Group. *Neurology* 43:910-918, 1993 A.

Weiner HL, et al: Double-blind pilot trial of oral tolerization with myelin antigens in multiple sclerosis. *Science* 259:1321-1324, 1993 B.

Weinshenker BG, et al: A double-blind, randomized, crossover trial of pemoline in fatigue associated with multiple sclerosis. *Neurology* 42:1468-1471, 1992.

Wiles CM, et al: Hyperbaric oxygen in multiple sclerosis: Double blind trial. *BMJ* 292:367-371, 1986.

Willoughby EW, et al: Serial magnetic resonance scanning in multiple sclerosis: A second prospective study in relapsing patients. *Ann Neurol* 25:43-49, 1989.

Wirguin I, et al: Citrate-induced impairment of neuromuscular transmission in human and experimental autoimmune myasthenia gravis. *Ann Neurol* 27:328-330, 1990.

Witte AS, et al: Azathioprine in treatment of myasthenia gravis. *Ann Neurol* 15:602-605, 1984.

Yanagisawa T, et al: Methylprednisolone pulse therapy in dermatomyositis. *Dermatologica* 167:47-51, 1983.

Yudkin PL, et al: Overview of azathioprine treatment in multiple sclerosis. *Lancet* 338:1051-1055, 1991.

Drugs Used for Spasticity and Muscle Spasm

18

SPASTICITY

Spasticity is a frequent component of the upper motor neuron syndrome and has been defined as a motor disorder characterized by a velocity-dependent increase in tonic stretch reflexes (muscle tone) with exaggerated tendon jerks resulting from hyperexcitability of the stretch reflex. Depending on the site and extent of central nervous system (CNS) damage, *positive* signs that can occur with spasticity include the Babinski response, flexor and extensor spasms, increased or exaggerated deep tendon reflexes, and clonus (Young, 1989). *Negative* symptoms, such as weakness, fatigue, lack of dexterity, and paralysis, may be caused by damage to upper or lower motor neurons. The combination of positive and negative signs and symptoms creates the various clinical syndromes collectively known as spastic paresis (Young, 1989).

Closed head injuries, cerebral palsy, and stroke are common causes of spasticity. Other causes include multiple sclerosis (two-thirds of patients experience moderate to severe spasticity), spinal cord trauma, and other neurologic disorders. The therapy of true reflex spasticity is at times complicated by dystonias (eg, rigidity following subcortical brain injury or athetosis that is associated with cerebral palsy). Both spasticity and dystonia lead to rigidity and increased tone as measured on the Ashworth scale. Problems that are related to dystonia do not respond as well to antispastic medications.

Antispastic drugs are used in conjunction with physical therapy, including an exercise program that emphasizes daily stretching, and education to ensure confidence and full use of residual capabilities. Reduction of pain is important because afferent input from lesions that would normally be painful tends to exacerbate spasticity and may provoke flexor spasms. Control of decubitus ulcers and infections (eg, bladder) also is very important.

Clinical and functional assessment of the musculoskeletal system are used to monitor drug therapy. However, reduction in spasticity does not necessarily correlate with overall functional improvement, since paralysis and other motor deficits are often associated with this condition. Drugs relieve positive symptoms only. In some patients, function improves when spasticity diminishes. Those with spastic and dystonic hemiplegias from cerebral lesions are less responsive (Rice, 1987). Drug therapy that diminishes spasticity may unmask underlying weakness and consequently hinder ambulation or jeopardize functional ability in some individuals, including those who rely on increased tone as an aid in standing or ambulation.

Drug Selection: The three primary antispastic drugs for oral administration are diazepam [Valium] and baclofen [Lioresal], which act centrally, and dantrolene [Dantrium], which acts peripherally (Davidoff, 1978; Young and Delwaide, 1981). Results of double-blind controlled studies confirm that these drugs are superior to placebo in reducing positive spastic symptoms and pain. The choice among them depends on the condition being treated, its initial or presenting status, associated illness, and the drugs' other pharmacologic actions. Continuous intrathecal infusion of baclofen is effective in patients who do not respond adequately to oral medication. Other drugs, in particular opioids (eg, morphine, hydromorphone [Dilaudid]), also can be administered intrathecally to decrease symptoms in patients with spinal cord spasticity (Erickson et al, 1989).

Response rates to oral antispastic drugs are higher in patients with traumatic spinal cord lesions (65% to 75%) or multiple sclerosis (30% to 65%) than in those with purely cerebral lesions. Baclofen appears to be most effective in relieving spasticity due to increased cutaneous or flexor reflexes in patients with multiple sclerosis and spinal cord injury.

Dantrolene appears to be most effective in spasticity of cerebral origin, but the incidence of dose-related hepatotoxicity limits its long-term use (see the evaluation). Dantrolene occasionally is beneficial in spasticity caused by stroke; diazepam and baclofen are of limited usefulness in this disorder. These drugs are not effective in rigidity associated with parkinsonism or Huntington's disease.

The antispastic action of diazepam does not appear to differ from that of other benzodiazepines, but there are few controlled clinical studies using related benzodiazepines for comparison. Baclofen may be preferred to diazepam in patients who are already experiencing considerable sedation, poor coordination, and/or ataxia associated with marginal cerebellar function, although this drug also may have considerable effects on the CNS, and tolerance may develop with prolonged administration. Dantrolene weakens muscle and therefore tends to be less satisfactory than diazepam and baclofen in patients with borderline strength.

Clonidine [Catapres] has been effective in the treatment of spinal cord spasticity when used alone (mean dose, 0.37 mg) or as an adjunct (median dose, 0.2 mg) to baclofen (Maynard, 1986; Donovan et al, 1988; Stewart et al, 1991). In a double-blind, placebo-controlled crossover study on nine patients with spinal cord injury, clonidine (mean dose, 0.2 mg) improved locomotion in one paretic patient and reduced spasticity in paraplegic patients (Stewart et al, 1991). Transdermal administration of clonidine (0.1 to 0.3 mg) also has decreased spasticity in those with spinal cord injury and may be better tolerated than oral administration (Weingarden and Belen, 1992; Yablon and Sipski, 1993). The hypotensive reactions observed in normal individuals may not occur in patients with complete spinal cord injuries. Clonidine's effectiveness is currently being evaluated in a multicenter clinical trial involving patients with spasticity associated with multiple sclerosis.

Phenothiazines with alpha-adrenergic blocking activity (eg, aliphatic and piperidine compounds) also have been used to treat spasticity. Although chlorpromazine [Thorazine] has been effective in some patients, the response is unpredictable and sedation and lethargy have limited its use. In addition, the increase in extrapyramidal adverse reactions, including tardive dyskinesia, with chlorpromazine therapy introduces significant risk in a patient who already has neurologic deficits. In animal studies, phenytoin [Dilantin] enhanced the antispastic action of chlorpromazine; the mechanism is not understood. Results of one controlled clinical study confirmed that concomitant administration of chlorpromazine and phenytoin was more effective than either agent alone (Cohan et al, 1980), but comparative studies are needed to establish the role of this combination in spastic disorders.

L-threonine, a precursor of glycine, is an orphan drug product for treatment of familial spastic paresis. Limited data indicate that it also may provide modest antispastic effects in patients with multiple sclerosis or spinal cord injury (Growdon et al, 1991; Hauser et al, 1992; Lee and Patterson, 1993). Published case reports suggest that treatment with intrathecal baclofen also may be effective in patients with familial spastic paresis (Meythaler et al, 1992).

Intramuscular injections of botulinum toxin type A [Botox] are very effective in the treatment of certain focal dystonias (eg, spastic dysphonia) and are being investigated for use in other types of spasticity (eg, cerebral palsy, multiple sclerosis). See index entry Botulinum A Toxin.

Local injection of dilute solutions of absolute alcohol or phenol into affected muscle "motor points" (intramuscular neurolysis) and intrathecal injection (chemical neurolysis) also have been tried to relieve spasticity. Intramuscular neurolysis may be of value if only one extremity or joint is affected. The effect of intrathecal injection often does not persist for more than several months; however, in some instances, the destruction may be irreversible. In fact, autopsy examination of both the spinal cord and the spinal nerve roots in patients treated with either intrathecal alcohol or phenol infusions shows evidence of widespread and unpredictable damage; this makes justification for the procedure questionable except in those with intractable, continuous pain.

Depolarizing or nondepolarizing neuromuscular blocking drugs and the central skeletal muscle relaxant drugs that are given for localized muscle spasm are of no value in spastic disorders.

Surgery: In addition to nerve blocks or neurectomies, ablative treatments for spastic paresis include selective posterior rhizotomies and myelotomies (Putty and Shapiro, 1991; Park and Owen, 1992). Posterior rhizotomy is appropriate for patients with spastic diplegia, especially children with cerebral palsy, and for those with severe lower extremity spasticity. Relief of spasticity is evident immediately after successful surgery, and the reduction in lower extremity spasticity is probably permanent (Albright, 1992). Range of motion and function also are improved in some patients (Berman et al, 1989; Peacock and Staudt, 1991). This procedure is not beneficial in individuals who depend on their spasticity to sit, stand, or walk; for these patients, intrathecal baclofen may be more appropriate.

Drug Evaluations

CENTRALLY ACTING DRUGS

BACLOFEN
[Lioresal]

$H_2NCH_2CHCH_2COH$ (C=O on terminal carbon; 4-chlorophenyl substituent on CH)

ACTIONS. Baclofen is a chemical analogue of the inhibitory neurotransmitter, gamma aminobutyric acid (GABA). It has no direct effect on the neuromuscular junction but diminishes monosynaptic and polysynaptic transmission in the spinal cord. The mechanism of baclofen's antispastic action is not fully understood. Stimulation of presynaptic $GABA_B$ receptors may decrease the release of excitatory transmitters from primary afferent terminals within the spinal cord (Dolphin and Scott, 1986) or from cutaneous nociceptive afferent nerve endings involved in flexor reflexes (Bowery et al, 1980). Postsynaptic effects also may be contributory (Azouvi et al, 1993). During intrathecal infusion, concentrations of the drug are high in superficial layers of the spinal cord dorsal horn, while cerebral side effects are minimized.

Analgesic effects have been observed in animals after both systemic and intrathecal administration; however, it is not known whether these effects contribute to the relief of painful flexor spasms observed clinically with baclofen.

USES. Baclofen relieves some of the primary components of spinal spasticity: involuntary flexor and extensor spasms and resistance to passive movements. Spasticity induced by spinal lesions is much more responsive to oral baclofen than that of cerebral origin.

Results of a controlled study comparing oral baclofen, dantrolene, and diazepam in patients with multiple sclerosis showed baclofen to be the most effective (response rate, up to 65% compared with placebo response rate of 10% to 30%) (Hedley et al, 1975). Other controlled studies comparing placebo and baclofen confirm the latter's efficacy in multiple sclerosis and spinal cord injury (Duncan et al, 1976; Levine et al, 1977; Feldman et al, 1978). The degree of response is limited but clinically relevant in terms of improved comfort, progression to a more independent state of self-care, less disruption of sleep, and ability to participate in a more aggressive rehabilitation program.

Unlike dantrolene, baclofen has no peripheral muscle relaxant activity; consequently, this drug theoretically may be a more appropriate choice for patients with borderline strength. However, some individuals may experience loss of strength while receiving baclofen (see Adverse Reactions).

In clinical studies, continuous intrathecal infusion of baclofen reduced flexor spasms and hypertonia in patients with severe spasticity associated with spinal cord injury or multiple sclerosis (Ochs et al, 1989; Penn et al, 1989; Lazorthes et al, 1990; Coffey et al, 1993). Activities of daily living, sleep patterns, and bladder and sphincter function also may improve (Nanninga et al, 1989; Tallala et al, 1990; Steers et al, 1992). Experience in patients with cerebral lesions is limited, but intrathecal infusion has been effective in those with intractable axial dystonia and in pediatric patients with cerebral palsy (Narayan et al, 1991; Albright et al, 1993).

Continuous intrathecal administration of baclofen may be an alternative to destructive neurosurgical procedures when (1) patients do not respond adequately to oral medication, (2) side effects of oral medications are intolerable, or (3) the probable gain in function justifies the implementation and long-term maintenance of this specialized drug delivery system. Experience indicates that continuous intrathecal infusion can be maintained satisfactorily for most patients (Penn, 1992; Coffey et al, 1993), although technological problems, especially with the catheter component, may interrupt drug delivery. Pump or catheter malfunction usually can be managed by replacing the defective part under local anesthesia.

Stiff-man syndrome is associated with autoantibodies specific for glutamic acid decarboxylase, an enzyme important for the synthesis of GABA (Solimena et al, 1988; Darnell et al, 1990). Baclofen is reported to be effective in this syndrome, but diazepam is the drug of choice (Miller and Korsvik, 1981; Lorish et al, 1989). Oral baclofen has been reported to provide partial relief in patients with intractable hiccups (Ramirez and Graham, 1992). Baclofen is not effective in the rigidity of parkinsonism or Huntington's disease.

ADVERSE REACTIONS. ***Oral:*** Baclofen is relatively well tolerated, and severe adverse reactions are uncommon. Drowsiness, lassitude, and dizziness occur most frequently, especially if the initial dosage is too high. Ataxia may develop even at therapeutic dose levels. These effects often are transient and may disappear with continued treatment. Their incidence is reported to be less than with diazepam at equieffective doses and can be reduced appreciably by using a small initial dose and increasing it gradually. Patients over 40 years and those with cerebral lesions appear to be most susceptible.

Severe muscle weakness does not appear to be a direct effect of the drug and probably represents paresis that is unmasked when muscle tone is reduced. This phenomenon has required dosage reduction or discontinuation of therapy.

Side effects with a reported incidence of 1% to 10% are nausea, mild gastrointestinal upset, constipation or diarrhea, insomnia, headache, fatigue, confusion, symptomatic hypotension, and urinary dysfunction (eg, dysuria, urgency, retention). Reduced bowel responsiveness is more common in patients with paraplegia. Allergic skin reactions and adverse effects on renal, hepatic, cardiac, and bone marrow function are extremely rare. Neuropsychiatric signs and symptoms (eg, euphoria, depression, paresthesias, muscle pain, impaired coordination, tremor, nystagmus, accommodation disorders, hallucinations, seizures, enuresis) occur rarely and often are difficult to differentiate from those of the underlying disease.

Intrathecal: Intrathecal administration in the lumbar region is generally well tolerated. The dosage can be titrated to reduce spasticity but maintain sufficient motor power and tone for transfers and ambulation. Continuous infusion of drugs into the lumbar subarachnoid space creates a lumbar-to-cisternal concentration gradient in the cerebrospinal fluid (CSF). During dosage titration, drowsiness, weakness or fatigue, dizziness, lightheadedness, and nausea and/or vomiting may occur. During maintenance therapy, adverse reactions may include drowsiness, dizziness, nausea, hypotension, headache, weakness or fatigue, blurred vision, slurred speech, numbness or paresthesias, and constipation. Confusion, memory impairment, or dysmetria have been rare (Penn, 1992). Seizures have occurred in patients with traumatic brain injury (Kofler et al, 1994). Reversible respiratory depression and coma have occurred rarely, especially in patients who received bolus injections and continued self-medication with oral baclofen or in those with upper limb spasticity when the site of infusion was too rostral. Some individuals who previously were able to walk may have difficulty standing if extensor tone is reduced too much.

PRECAUTIONS. There are no absolute contraindications to baclofen therapy other than hypersensitivity. This drug should be used with caution when spasticity actually sustains upright posture and balance in locomotion or sustains function. Dosage reduction should be considered in patients with impaired renal function and in those receiving other CNS depressants concurrently. When the intrathecal pump system is used, complications can result either from the pump or the catheters.

There have been reports that baclofen adversely affected seizure control in a few epileptic patients, but in one study employing therapeutic doses, there was no effect on seizures controlled by antiepileptic drugs (Terrence et al, 1983).

Rarely, asymptomatic elevations of the AST, alkaline phosphatase, and blood glucose levels have occurred; therefore, appropriate laboratory tests should be performed periodically in patients with liver disease or diabetes.

Baclofen has not been a drug of abuse but tolerance has developed, especially when the intrathecal route was used. In one large clinical trial, the daily dose required to maintain a therapeutic effect increased from 187 mcg/day (mean) to 405 mcg/day over six months to two years and then tended to stabilize (Coffey et al, 1993).

Because abrupt withdrawal causes a rebound increase in the number of flexor spasms, gradual reduction of the dose over a one- to two-week period is recommended. In addition, auditory and visual hallucinations, paranoid ideation, agitated behavior, and seizures (especially in patients with cerebral lesions) have been reported after abrupt termination of intrathecal therapy that had exceeded two months. Abrupt discontinuation of oral therapy also can precipitate hallucinations and seizures. Therefore, the drug should be used cautiously in patients with schizophrenia, other psychotic disorders, or confusional states. Intrathecal baclofen also should be used with caution in patients with autonomic dysreflexia because abrupt changes in the intensity of nociceptive stimuli can trigger a dysreflexic episode.

Baclofen crosses the placenta. Its safety during pregnancy has not been established (FDA Pregnancy Category C). Baclofen is excreted in breast milk after oral administration; there are no data on nursing mothers who have received the drug intrathecally.

TOXICITY. Symptoms of CNS depression are most prominent during acute intrathecal overdose. Central effects, notably mild drowsiness and respiratory depression, may respond to intravenous physostigmine (1 to 2 mg) (Müller-Schwefe and Penn, 1989); additional doses of 1 mg may be administered at 30- to 60-minute intervals in responsive patients. Drainage of CSF (30 to 40 ml) by lumbar puncture combined with symptomatic treatment has been used for the management of intrathecal overdose, but experience with this approach is limited (Delhaas and Brouwers, 1991).

Severe intoxication is characterized by seizures, coma, more severe respiratory depression, and muscular hypotonia with absent limb reflexes. Bradycardia and hypotension also have been observed. Emergency management of acute oral baclofen intoxication includes respiratory support followed by gastric lavage and diuresis (Haubenstock et al, 1983). No specific antidote is available; intravenous physostigmine is inadequate for management of severe intoxication. During the recovery phase, seizures and myoclonic tics have been reported in some patients. Seizures have been managed with diazepam or clonazepam (Haubenstock et al, 1983), although these drugs may prolong unconsciousness.

Patients with underlying cardiovascular disease should be observed for the occurrence of late-onset tachycardia and/or hypertension.

PHARMACOKINETICS. ***Oral:*** Baclofen is rapidly and well absorbed; however, absorption may be reduced as dosage is increased. The peak serum concentration is attained in two to three hours (Brogden et al, 1974). Protein binding is about 30%. The plasma:brain distribution ratio is about 10:1 following systemic administration, and the drug is cleared slowly from the brain. About 70% to 85% of a dose is eliminated unchanged in the urine within one day, and complete elimination takes three days. The mean half-life is three to four hours, but there is considerable individual variation.

Intrathecal bolus: Onset of action generally is within 30 to 60 minutes following injection. Peak spasmolytic effects occur approximately four hours after administration, and effects may last four to eight hours; however, as with the oral route, there is considerable individual variation. The half-life of baclofen after intrathecal bolus administration is approximately 90 minutes.

Continuous infusion: The antispastic action is usually apparent within six to eight hours after initiation of the infusion. A lumbar-cisternal concentration gradient is established during continuous infusion in which cisternal concentrations are approximately 20% of those of the lumbar region. Maximum activity associated with a particular intrathecal infusion rate usually is observed within 24 to 48 hours. Clearance of baclofen from the CSF approximates CSF turnover, which suggests that the drug is eliminated through bulk flow.

DOSAGE AND PREPARATIONS.

Oral: The initial daily dose should be low and increased gradually. Administration several times daily appears to control spasticity more evenly with fewer side effects.

Adults, some authorities prefer to initiate therapy with 5 or 10 mg daily for the first three days to minimize drowsiness, dizziness, and ataxia. However, the manufacturers recommend 5 mg three times daily for three days, increased by 5 mg three times daily every three days until the optimum effect has been achieved or a maximum of 80 mg daily has been reached; the usual optimal dose ranges from 40 to 80 mg daily, but some patients may require up to 120 mg daily to achieve beneficial effects. When therapy is to be terminated, the dosage should be reduced gradually over one or two weeks. A more gradual reduction in dosage (eg, over three to four weeks) may be required to minimize exacerbation of symptoms. The safety of baclofen in *children* has not been established, but 1 to 1.5 mg/kg daily has been reported to be effective. Treatment should begin with 5 mg/day, and the amount should be increased gradually (Melnick and Shellenberger, 1982).

Lioresal (Geigy), ***Generic.*** Tablets 10 and 20 mg.

Intrathecal: *Screening phase:* Prior to pump implantation and initiation of continuous infusion, patients must demonstrate a positive response to an intrathecal bolus injection of baclofen via a catheter placed in the lumbar intrathecal space or by lumbar puncture. Patients must be monitored closely in a hospital setting to detect alterations in vital signs and/or neurologic status. Baclofen injection for intrathecal administration must be diluted with sterile, preservative-free 0.9% sodium chloride injection to a concentration of 50 mcg/ml; no other diluent should be used. Initially, a bolus of 50 mcg/ml is administered into the intrathecal space by barbotage over a period of not less than one minute, and the patient is observed for four to eight hours. In those who do not respond adequately, a second bolus injection containing 75 mcg/1.5 ml can be administered 24 hours later and, if necessary, a final bolus of 100 mcg/2 ml may be administered 24 hours later. Patients who do not respond to 100 mcg are not candidates for an implanted pump for continuous infusion.

Post-implant dose titration: After the response is verified, baclofen is administered by implantable pumps approved by the FDA specifically for the intrathecal administration of this drug. (See manufacturer's literature and the manual provided by the manufacturer of the implantable intrathecal infusion pump for (1) specific instructions and precautions for programming the pump or refilling the reservoir, (2) specifications for drug delivery, and (3) warnings, precautions, adverse reactions, and instructions for administration and dosage.)

To determine the initial daily dose, the bolus dose that produced a positive effect is doubled and administered over 24 hours, unless the efficacy of that dose had been maintained for >12 hours, in which case the initial daily dose is the same as the bolus dose. The dose is not increased in the first 24 hours (ie, until steady-state is achieved). After the first 24 hours, the dose may be increased in increments of 10% to 30% once every 24 hours until the desired effect is achieved.

Maintenance therapy: During periodic refills of the pump, the daily dose may be increased by 10% to 40% to maintain adequate control of symptoms or reduced 10% to 20% to alleviate side effects. Most patients require gradual increases in dosage over time to maintain optimal response. Maintenance dosage for continuous infusion has ranged from 12 mcg to 1.5 mg/day; most patients are maintained adequately on 300 to 800 mcg/day. Some patients may become refractory during long-term treatment. Sensitivity to baclofen can be re-established by institution of a "drug holiday" during which the dosage is gradually reduced over a two-week period and an alternative method of spasticity management (eg, intrathecal morphine) is used. After a variable period ranging from several days to a few weeks, sensitivity to baclofen returns and intrathecal administration may be resumed at the initial continuous infusion dose.

For patients with programmable pumps who have achieved relatively satisfactory control on continuous infusion, further benefit may be attained using more complex schedules of delivery. For example, those who experience an increase in spasms at night may benefit from an increase (eg, 20%) in the hourly infusion rate. Changes in flow rate should be programmed to start two hours before the time of desired effect.

Lioresal (Medtronic). Solution 500 mcg/ml (10 mg/20 ml) and 2 mg/ml (10 mg/5 ml) in single-use containers.

DIAZEPAM

[Valium]

For chemical formula, see index entry Diazepam, In Anxiety.

ACTIONS. Diazepam has an antispastic action in addition to its antianxiety, hypnotic, and antiepileptic properties. The muscle relaxant action of this drug is thought to result from its ability to enhance GABA-mediated presynaptic inhibition in the CNS and to depress neurons in the descending lateral reticular system that facilitate the gamma motor neurons; however, neither the spinal nor supraspinal site of action has been established conclusively. Unfortunately, diazepam also depresses neurons in the ascending reticular activating system that mediate wakefulness. The resulting sedation and lethargy generally detract from its antispastic effect and may be the most common reason for discontinuation of administration. Diazepam does not alter the synthesis, release, reuptake, or enzymatic degradation of GABA.

USES. Diazepam may be useful in a variety of chronic upper motor neuron disorders in which spasticity is a component. It is superior to placebo in spasticity associated with spinal cord lesions, multiple sclerosis, and cerebral disorders, although improvement is less pronounced in the latter. Other benzodiazepines may have similar activity but few controlled, comparative clinical studies have been published.

The CNS side effects of diazepam may make this drug less useful in patients with pre-existing sedation and marginal cerebellar function. Unlike dantrolene, diazepam has no peripheral muscle relaxant activity; consequently, this drug may be appropriate for patients with borderline strength.

Diazepam is beneficial adjunctively in acute, localized traumatic disorders associated with painful muscle spasm (see the section on Spasm), and it relieves some symptoms of athetosis as a result of its antianxiety and sedative actions.

This drug is moderately effective in alleviating the rigidity, spasms, and pain of the stiff-man syndrome, a rare autoimmune disorder characterized by intermittent spasms and stiffness of the axial muscles in which a pattern of continuous motor unit activity is observed by electromyography; patients with severe disease may not respond adequately.

Diazepam may be useful in the motor restlessness of akathisia, although its antianxiety action is probably of greater significance than its antispastic action in this condition.

When given intravenously, diazepam is a useful adjunct in muscle spasms caused by tetanus toxin (Alfery and Rauscher, 1979) or strychnine, although its anticonvulsant rather than its antispastic action may play some role.

ADVERSE REACTIONS AND PRECAUTIONS. Drowsiness is the primary side effect of diazepam, but some adaptation occurs with long-term therapy. Alcohol enhances central sedation. Oversedation in elderly patients may be a problem, even at the lower limits of the dosage range. Impairment of coordination (hand coordination and speed, walking speed, station stability) has been observed. Prolonged uninterrupted use of diazepam may lead to physical and psychological dependence.

For a more complete discussion of the mechanism of action, pharmacokinetics, adverse reactions, precautions, and dosage of the benzodiazepines, see index entry Diazepam, In Anxiety.

DOSAGE AND PREPARATIONS.

Oral: *Adults,* for spasticity or severe localized muscle spasms, 2 to 10 mg three or four times daily; *children and infants over 6 months,* 0.12 to 0.8 mg/kg daily divided into three or four doses. A prolonged-release preparation [Valrelease] should be used only when it has been determined that the optimal daily dose of diazepam is at least 5 mg three times a day.

For the stiff-man syndrome, the usual daily dose is 20 to 100 mg, but individual dosage titration is required to minimize excessive sedation (Lorish et al, 1989).

Generic. Tablets 2, 5, and 10 mg; solution (oral) 1 and 5 mg/ml (concentrate).

Valium (Roche). Tablets 2, 5, and 10 mg; capsules (prolonged-release) 15 mg (***Valrelease***).

Intravenous: The solution should be injected slowly, allowing at least one minute for each 5 mg (1 ml). Intravenous infusion has been used, but since diazepam is significantly absorbed by plastic containers and intravenous administration sets, large-volume glass containers and careful dose titration are necessary. Diazepam should not be mixed with other drugs for intravenous use (Mason et al, 1981).

For spasticity or severe localized muscle spasm, *adults,* 2 to 10 mg, repeated in three to four hours, if necessary. *Children,* initially, 0.04 to 0.2 mg/kg (maximum, 0.6 mg/kg in an eight-hour period).

Intravenous diazepam should not be used in spastic patients with impaired respiratory function.

Valium (Roche), ***Generic.*** Solution 5 mg/ml in 1 (***Generic*** only), 2, and 10 ml containers.

PERIPHERALLY ACTING DRUG

DANTROLENE SODIUM

[Dantrium]

O_2N–(C₆H₄)–(furan)–CH=N–N(hydantoin) Na^+ · $4H_2O$

ACTIONS. This unique skeletal muscle relaxant reduces muscle contractility. It acts at a site beyond the neuromuscular junction and interferes with the intracellular release of calcium ions from the sarcoplasmic reticulum (Ward et al, 1986). The maximal decrease in contractile activity is 75% to 80%.

Therapeutic doses have no effect on cardiac and smooth muscles and minimal effects on neurons. Dantrolene does not have GABAergic actions.

USES. Dantrolene is superior to placebo in spasticity induced by spinal cord and cerebral injuries or lesions associated with multiple sclerosis, cerebral palsy, and possibly stroke. It can be used in spastic patients, especially those with cerebral spasticity, who are in a stable neurologic state and in whom spasticity causes pain, discomfort, or distress. This drug may be most useful in patients with limited function to decrease adductor tone for hygienic reasons. Dantrolene must be given cautiously to ambulatory patients, because relief of spasticity may be associated with weakness that may worsen the patient's overall functional capacity. The benefit of reducing muscle stiffness versus the possible disadvantage of reducing muscle strength must be weighed individually; however, dantrolene generally is less useful in patients with borderline strength, many of whom cannot tolerate the sense of fatigue or weakness.

Intravenous administration is useful in the treatment of neuroleptic malignant syndrome (see index entry Dantrolene, In Neuroleptic Malignant Syndrome). It also is indicated intraoperatively when a presumptive diagnosis of malignant hyperthermia has been made and is used prophylactically in patients with a history of this disorder (see index entry Hyperthermia, Malignant). Dantrolene also has been given to treat heat stroke; the rigidity occurring as a result of toxicity from cocaine, carbon monoxide, and other substances; and to relieve exercise-induced pain in Duchenne's muscular dystrophy. In general, however, dantrolene should never be used in any muscular or neuromuscular disorder in which weakness is a prominent symptom.

Dantrolene is not indicated in fibrositis, rheumatoid spondylitis, bursitis, arthritis, or acute muscle spasm of local origin. It should not be given to patients with amyotrophic lateral sclerosis because these individuals have a very low tolerance for the muscle weakness induced by this drug.

ADVERSE REACTIONS AND PRECAUTIONS. Muscle weakness, drowsiness, dizziness, general malaise, and diarrhea are the most common reactions. Severe persistent diarrhea may require treatment with antidiarrheal agents, reduction in dose, or temporary cessation of therapy. Anorexia, nausea, vomiting, and an acne-like rash are also significant side effects. Less frequently, headache, nervousness, insomnia, depression, and visual disturbances have occurred. Pleuropericardial reactions, including eosinophilic pleural effusion, develop rarely.

The most serious adverse reaction is idiosyncratic or hypersensitivity-mediated hepatocellular injury, which occurs rarely and has been fatal. The risk appears to be greatest in patients over 35 years and in women, especially those receiving estrogen therapy. Hepatotoxicity has been observed more frequently in patients with multiple sclerosis, which may reflect the fact that this disease is more common in women (Chan, 1990). Hepatotoxicity rarely has been reported in children under 10 years; no fatalities have occurred in those under age 20 (Chan, 1990).

Hepatotoxicity occurs most frequently 3 to 12 months after initiation of therapy. Therefore, routine baseline hepatic function studies should be performed prior to treatment, and AST or ALT and alkaline phosphatase levels should be determined at appropriate intervals during therapy. Most cases of hepatotoxicity are reversible if the drug is withdrawn. Dantrolene is contraindicated in patients with active hepatic disease.

The lowest effective dose (preferably no more than 400 mg daily) should be prescribed. Therapy should not be continued for more than 45 days unless symptoms are adequately relieved, there is no evidence of hepatic impairment, and the patient's ability to function is significantly improved by the drug.

Dantrolene should be given cautiously to patients with impaired respiratory function; frequent monitoring is essential.

The safety of dantrolene during pregnancy has not been established, although in one study no adverse effects were observed in neonates born to mothers who received the drug prophylactically (Shime et al, 1988). Dantrolene (intravenous) is classified in FDA Pregnancy Category C.

No clinically significant drug interactions have been confirmed; however, in one diabetic patient, intravenous dantrolene may have interacted with verapamil (but not nifedipine) to produce cardiovascular depression (Rubin and Zablocki, 1987).

PHARMACOKINETICS. ***Oral:*** More than 70% of a 100-mg dose of dantrolene is absorbed. Peak serum concentrations are reached after one to four hours. Dantrolene is metabolized to 5-hydroxydantrolene (major), which is less potent than the parent compound, and acetylamino dantrolene (minor), which is only weakly active. The blood concentrations of dantrolene and 5-hydroxydantrolene after dosages of 400 mg/day for several weeks are not significantly different from those obtained after a single dose of 100 mg. This finding does not appear to be related to enzyme induction but rather to capacity-limited absorption or protein binding (Meyler et al, 1981).

In healthy volunteers, the plasma half-life of dantrolene is six to nine hours and that of 5-hydroxydantrolene is 15.5 hours. After two weeks of therapy, a linear dose-concentration relationship is observed in the therapeutic dose range (daily doses of 50, 100, and 200 mg), but not with doses of 400 mg daily. There is no correlation between blood concentration and clinical improvement; doses exceeding 100 mg daily often do not increase the drug's effect.

Approximately 15% to 25% of an oral dose of dantrolene is excreted in the urine; 5-hydroxydantrolene (79%) and reduced acetylated dantrolene (17%) are the major excretion products.

DOSAGE AND PREPARATIONS.

Oral: Dosage must be individualized. *Adults,* initially, 25 mg once or twice daily, increased to 25 mg three or four times daily, and then, by increments, to 50 to 100 mg four times daily. Each dosage level should be maintained for four to seven days to determine response. The dose should not be increased beyond the amount that produces maximal benefit with an acceptable level of adverse effects. (The manufacturer's literature indicates that most patients respond to 400 mg/day or less; 100 to 200 mg daily often is adequate.) *Children,* a similar schedule should be utilized, starting with 0.5 mg/kg once or twice daily (maximum, 100 mg four times daily or 3 mg/kg four times daily).

Dantrium (Procter & Gamble). Capsules 25, 50, and 100 mg.

Intravenous: See index entry Hyperthermia, Malignant.

SPASM

Spasm is an involuntary contraction of a muscle or group of muscles, usually accompanied by pain and limited function. Reflex muscle spasm (splinting) often occurs as a protective response to local injury but may be exaggerated and require therapy. Drug therapy depends on the etiology of the spasm (eg, antiepileptic drugs for epileptic myoclonic seizures, calcium for hypocalcemic muscle spasm, analgesics and/or central skeletal muscle relaxants for spasm associated with acute pain syndromes). Acetazolamide [Diamox] and phenytoin [Dilantin] have been useful in treating myotonia congenita.

Most muscle strains and minor injuries are self-limited and respond rapidly to rest and physical therapy. Initial immobilization of the affected part with casts, pressure bandages, neck collars, arm slings, or crutches; cold compresses; and whirlpool baths often obviate the need for drugs other than mild analgesics. Occasionally, an anti-inflammatory drug may be prescribed when there is considerable tissue damage and edema, although there is no evidence that these drugs reduce the healing time.

Cramps are a form of muscle spasm that are abrupt in onset and last for minutes at a time. Common precipitating factors include hyponatremia and dehydration (eg, after vigorous exercise, excessive sweating, vomiting, diarrhea), hypotension, and hypokalemia associated with use of diuretics or corticosteroids; in some patients, cramps may be provoked by drug therapy (eg, beta$_2$ agonists, cimetidine, clofibrate, lithium, opioids) (Eaton, 1989). Cramps usually involve the calf or foot and are treated by rubbing and stretching the affected muscle. Night cramps are common in elderly patients, pregnant women, diabetics, and patients with peripheral vascular disease. For frequent nocturnal leg cramps, quinine [Quinamm] is most commonly used despite the paucity of controlled studies documenting its effectiveness (see the evaluation). There is less experience with other agents for this condition. However, the results of one double-blind study suggest that orphenadrine citrate [Norflex] may be a useful alternative to quinine (Latta and Turner, 1989). In a small open trial, seven of eight patients improved when verapamil [Calan, Isoptin, Verelan] was substituted for quinine (Baltodano et al, 1988).

More severe acute or chronic local spasms may be produced by strains and sprains, trauma, and cervical or lumbar radiculopathy resulting from degenerative osteoarthritis, herniated disc, spondylolysis, chemonucleolysis, or laminectomy. These spasms are characterized by local pain, tenderness on palpation, muscle firmness, and limitation of motion and daily activities. However, these physical findings may be difficult to reproduce, especially in those with low back pain (McCombe et al, 1989). In an extensive randomized study (Wiesel et al, 1980), bedrest decreased absence from work by 50%, whereas analgesic and anti-inflammatory agents had no effect on work attendance, although they did provide adjunctive pain relief. Results of two subsequent randomized trials did not demonstrate any advantage of bedrest (Gilbert et al, 1985; Deyo et al, 1986). The use of chymopapain [Chymodiactin] for herniated disc is discussed in the section on Chemonucleolysis for Sciatica Caused by Herniated Lumbar Disc.

DRUG THERAPY. Central skeletal muscle relaxants are used in the treatment of spasm. These drugs include carisoprodol [Soma]; chlorphenesin [Maolate]; chlorzoxazone [Paraflex, Parafon Forte DSC]; methocarbamol [Robaxin]; orphenadrine; and cyclobenzaprine [Flexeril], which is chemically related to the tricyclic antidepressants. Diazepam also is used in muscle spasms associated with injury (see the evaluation in the section on Spasticity).

Actions: Experimentally, central skeletal muscle relaxants depress spinal polysynaptic reflexes preferentially over monosynaptic reflexes as well as facilitative and neuronal activity affecting muscle stretch reflexes, primarily in the lateral reticular area of the brainstem. In addition, the activity of these drugs within the substantia nigra may enhance the depressant effect (Turski et al, 1990). Most of these drugs produce sedation, which may reflect depression of neuronal activity in the medial reticular ascending system that is essential for wakefulness. In humans, the oral doses of all these drugs are well below the amount required experimentally to elicit effects directly on muscle; thus, some investigators conclude that their muscle relaxant activity is related only to their sedative effect. However, relief of muscle spasm is not always associated with sedation, which may contribute to overall improvement in some patients but is considered a side effect in others.

Uses: All spasmolytic drugs are superior to placebo in alleviating the symptoms and signs of localized muscle spasm. However, none of these agents is more effective than analgesic/anti-inflammatory drugs in relieving the pain of acute or chronic localized muscle spasm.

Methocarbamol and orphenadrine can be administered intravenously to relieve severe, acute muscle spasm of local origin caused by inflammation or trauma. Intravenous methocarbamol also reduces spasticity in selected patients being prepared for physical therapy.

Oral administration of skeletal muscle relaxant drugs is ineffective in spasticity induced by cerebrospinal trauma, cerebral palsy, or demyelinating disorders, such as multiple sclerosis. In general, skeletal muscle relaxants are not useful in rheumatoid arthritis, but they have been given with anti-inflammatory agents.

Drug Selection: Comparative, controlled, crossover studies to identify drugs of choice to treat spasm are difficult to conduct because of the subjective, variable, and self-limited nature of these disorders. Extensive reviews of the literature support this view and further emphasize the numerous errors in design and interpretation of clinical studies (Elenbaas, 1980; Deyo, 1983). No one central skeletal muscle relaxant appears to be more effective than another in acute disorders. Available data support the use of cyclobenzaprine, carisoprodol, and diazepam in skeletal muscle spasms (Basmajian, 1978; Deyo, 1983).

Some central skeletal muscle relaxants are available in combination with analgesics, and the following two mixtures are classified as effective by the Drug Efficacy and Safety Implementation Program of the Food and Drug Administration: carisoprodol with aspirin [Soma Compound] and methocarbamol with aspirin [Robaxisal]. The combination of orphenadrine with aspirin and caffeine [Norgesic, Norgesic Forte] is classified as possibly effective.

Adverse Reactions: The adverse reactions and precautions listed below can occur with use of all skeletal muscle relaxants; in addition, cyclobenzaprine has significant anticholinergic activity. For specific adverse reactions and precautions, see the evaluations.

Drowsiness, lightheadedness, and dizziness may be observed. Occasionally, nausea, vomiting, heartburn, abdominal distress, constipation, diarrhea, or ataxia may develop. Blurred vision, flushing, asthenia, lethargy, and lassitude are more common after intravenous administration than after oral use and are usually transient. With the exception of methocarbamol, respiratory depression, tachycardia, and hypotension occur occasionally after large oral doses.

The centrally acting agents should be discontinued if rash, pruritus, or other evidence of hypersensitivity occurs. Serious allergic manifestations (eg, anaphylactic reactions, leukopenia) have been observed rarely.

Acute poisoning is rarely fatal. Vomiting may be induced or gastric lavage and/or saline catharsis may be employed. Supportive therapy is adequate in most instances of excessive dosage. Dialysis is probably of no value in overdosage of diazepam or cyclobenzaprine.

Precautions: Patients receiving these drugs should not undertake activities that require mental alertness, judgment, and physical coordination (eg, driving a vehicle, operating dangerous machinery) until it is known that drowsiness or other incapacitating effects will not develop. Caution is necessary if skeletal muscle relaxants and other CNS depressants (eg, alcohol, hypnotics, antianxiety drugs, antipsychotic drugs, antidepressants) are used concomitantly, since their effects may be additive. Symptoms of organic brain disease in elderly patients may be aggravated.

Physical dependence may develop after long-term administration of large doses of some of these agents, especially in patients with a tendency to abuse drugs. Abrupt discontinuance after prolonged use of large amounts may produce severe withdrawal symptoms, including seizures.

Routine precautions should be followed if these drugs are given during pregnancy (see index entry Pregnancy). Unless specifically stated in the evaluations, there is no information on the presence of these compounds in the milk of lactating women.

Drug Evaluations

CARISOPRODOL

[Soma]

$$H_2N\overset{O}{\overset{\|}{C}}OCH_2\overset{CH_3}{\overset{|}{\underset{\underset{CH_2CH_2CH_3}{|}}{C}}}CH_2O\overset{O}{\overset{\|}{C}}NH\overset{CH_3}{\overset{|}{C}}HCH_3$$

ACTIONS AND USES. Carisoprodol is chemically related to meprobamate. It is useful as an adjunct to rest, physical therapy, and other appropriate measures to treat the pain of local muscle spasm. This drug is not effective in spastic or dyskinetic movement disorders.

ADVERSE REACTIONS AND PRECAUTIONS. The most common untoward effect is drowsiness. Idiosyncratic reactions (eg, extreme asthenia, transient quadriplegia, dizziness, ataxia, diplopia, agitation, confusion, disorientation) have occurred rarely after initial administration. Carisoprodol is contraindicated in patients with acute intermittent porphyria. See the Introduction to this section for additional information on adverse reactions and precautions.

PHARMACOKINETICS. The onset of action is rapid and the duration is four to six hours. The elimination half-life is eight hours. (The manufacturer's unpublished data indicate the drug has a half-life of 1 to 1.5 hours.) The compound is metabolized in the liver to its principal metabolite, meprobamate; the products formed are eliminated in the urine. Carisoprodol is present in the milk of lactating women.

DOSAGE AND PREPARATIONS.
Oral: *Adults,* 350 mg four times daily; *children under 12 years,* information is inadequate to establish a dosage.
Soma (Wallace), ***Generic***. Tablets 350 mg.

CHLORPHENESIN CARBAMATE
[Maolate]

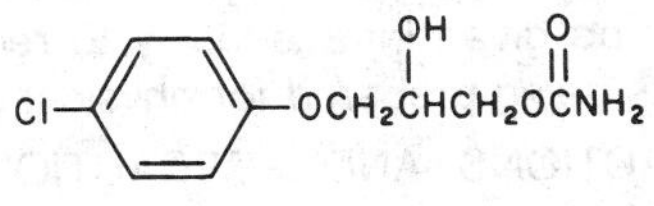

$Cl-C_6H_4-OCH_2CH(OH)CH_2OC(O)NH_2$

USES. This analogue of mephenesin is useful as an adjunct to rest, physiotherapy, and other appropriate measures for the relief of discomfort associated with acute painful musculoskeletal conditions. It is not effective in spastic or dyskinetic movement disorders.

ADVERSE REACTIONS AND PRECAUTIONS. Adverse reactions noted occasionally include paradoxical stimulation, nervousness, insomnia, headache, and asthenia. Drowsiness, dizziness, confusion, nausea, and epigastric distress have been reported infrequently. Reduction in dose usually controls many of these adverse reactions. Anaphylactoid reactions, drug fever, and other symptoms of hypersensitivity have been observed occasionally; if they develop, the medication should be discontinued. Rash, pruritus, and blood dyscrasias (leukopenia, thrombocytopenia, agranulocytosis, pancytopenia) occur rarely. Two cases of gastrointestinal bleeding have been reported, but these have not been established as being drug related. The tablet contains tartrazine, which may produce allergic reactions in asthmatics, aspirin-sensitive individuals, and other susceptible patients.

Chlorphenesin should be used with caution in patients with pre-existing liver disease or impaired hepatic function. Use of this drug during pregnancy, lactation, or in women who may become pregnant is not recommended unless the potential benefits outweigh the possible hazards. See the Introduction to this section for additional information on adverse reactions and precautions.

PHARMACOKINETICS. The half-life of chlorphenesin is 3.5 ± 0.2 (2.3 to 5.1) hours. The compound is conjugated, principally with glucuronic acid, and eliminated in the urine.

DOSAGE AND PREPARATIONS.
Oral: *Adults,* initially, 800 mg three times daily until the desired effect is obtained; for maintenance, 400 mg four times daily or less frequently, as required. The safety of chlorphenesin when used for periods exceeding eight weeks has not been established. *Children,* information is inadequate to establish a dosage, and the drug is not recommended in this age group.
Maolate (Upjohn). Tablets 400 mg.

CHLORZOXAZONE
[Paraflex, Parafon Forte DSC]

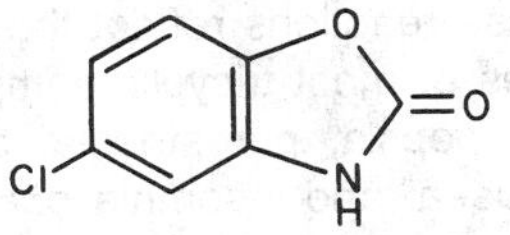

(Structure: 5-chloro-benzoxazol-2(3H)-one; Cl, O, =O, N–H)

USES. Chlorzoxazone, a benzoxazolinone, is chemically distinct from all other muscle relaxants. It is useful as an adjunct to rest, physical therapy, and other appropriate measures to treat the pain of local muscle spasm. Chlorzoxazone is not effective in spastic or dyskinetic movement disorders.

ADVERSE REACTIONS AND PRECAUTIONS. Drowsiness, dizziness, lightheadedness, malaise, or paradoxical stimulation may occur occasionally. Other adverse reactions include headache, gastrointestinal irritation, and, rarely, gastrointestinal bleeding and hypersensitivity reactions.

Hepatic dysfunction and jaundice have been reported, but a causal relationship cannot be established. Nevertheless, chlorzoxazone should be used cautiously in patients with a history of liver disease. Patients should be monitored closely for signs of liver damage, and the drug should be discontinued if hepatic dysfunction develops.

See the Introduction to this section for additional information on adverse reactions and precautions.

PHARMACOKINETICS. Chlorzoxazone is absorbed rapidly after oral administration, and peak blood concentrations may be attained in one to two hours. It is extensively metabolized in the liver, conjugated with glucuronic acid, and excreted by the kidney. The elimination half-life is 1.1 hours.

DOSAGE AND PREPARATIONS.
Oral: *Adults,* 250 to 750 mg three or four times daily; *children,* 125 to 500 mg three or four times daily.
Generic. Tablets 250 and 500 mg.
Paraflex (McNeil). Tablets 250 mg.
Parafon Forte DSC (McNeil). Tablets 500 mg.

Additional Trademark.
Remular (International Ethical).

CYCLOBENZAPRINE HYDROCHLORIDE
[Flexeril]

CH_3
$CHCH_2CH_2\overset{+}{N}H$
CH_3
Cl^-

ACTIONS AND USES. Cyclobenzaprine is structurally and pharmacologically related to the tricyclic antidepressants. It is useful as an adjunct to rest, physical therapy, and other appropriate measures in the short-term treatment of painful local muscle spasm. Results of the few comparative controlled studies that have been published suggest that a total daily dose of 30 mg is necessary to distinguish this drug's effects on muscle spasm from those of a placebo. Oral doses of 60 mg daily do not affect spasticity of spinal or cerebral origin.

ADVERSE REACTIONS AND PRECAUTIONS. The most common side effects are drowsiness, dryness of the mouth, and dizziness. These reactions reflect the sedative and anticholinergic activities of most tricyclic compounds. Tachycardia, weakness, dyspepsia, paresthesia, blurred vision, unpleasant taste, nausea, and insomnia occur less frequently. Sweating, myalgia, dyspnea, abdominal pain, constipation, coated tongue, tremors, dysarthria, euphoria, nervousness, disorientation, confusion, headache, urinary retention, decreased bladder tonus, ataxia, and allergic reactions are rare.

Short-term studies to assess uses other than for muscle spasm usually employed somewhat larger doses than those recommended for spasm, and some of the more serious CNS reactions noted with the tricyclic antidepressants occurred.

Because of its anticholinergic properties, caution is advised when administering cyclobenzaprine to patients with angle-closure glaucoma or a history of urinary retention or prostatic hypertrophy. Its sedative effects may be additive with those of other CNS depressants.

Cyclobenzaprine is contraindicated during the acute recovery phase of myocardial infarction and in patients with hyperthyroidism, arrhythmias, heart block, conduction disturbances, or congestive heart failure.

For general adverse reactions, precautions, and management of overdosage for tricyclic antidepressants, see index entry Tricyclic Drugs.

The safe use of cyclobenzaprine during pregnancy has not been established (FDA Pregnancy Category B). Its safety in nursing mothers and children younger than 15 years also has not been determined.

DRUG INTERACTIONS. Cyclobenzaprine may interact with monoamine oxidase inhibitors when given concomitantly or within 14 days after their discontinuation. It may enhance the effects of alcohol, other CNS depressants, and drugs with anticholinergic actions. The antihypertensive action of guanethidine and related drugs may be antagonized.

PHARMACOKINETICS. Doses of 5 to 30 mg are absorbed rapidly, but absorption may be saturated with these amounts. A considerable first-pass effect occurs in the intestine and/or liver of some individuals.

Cyclobenzaprine is highly bound to plasma proteins (93%) and is extensively metabolized to derivatives that are excreted by the kidney, principally as glucuronide conjugates. These effects probably account, in part, for the large variation in plasma concentrations observed among patients.

An elimination half-life of one to three days and a duration of action of 12 to 24 hours have been reported; however, postmarketing surveillance studies suggest that administration three times daily is appropriate for most patients.

DOSAGE AND PREPARATIONS.

Oral: *Adults,* 10 mg three times daily (maximum, 60 mg daily). The manufacturers recommend that treatment be limited to two or three weeks.

Flexeril (Merck), ***Generic.*** Tablets 10 mg.

METHOCARBAMOL
[Robaxin]

$H_2NCOCH_2CHCH_2O$ (O, OH)
CH_3O

USES. This analogue of mephenesin is useful as an adjunct to rest and physical therapy to alleviate the pain of local muscle spasm. The drug can be given parenterally in severe cases or when oral administration is not feasible. Methocarbamol is not effective orally in spastic or dyskinetic movement disorders, but it may be given intravenously to reduce spasm in selected patients being prepared for physical therapy.

ADVERSE REACTIONS AND PRECAUTIONS. Dizziness, drowsiness, headache, anorexia, vertigo, and mild nausea occur occasionally after oral administration, and skin eruptions have been reported rarely. Flushing, metallic taste, nausea, nystagmus, diplopia, mild ataxia, hypotension, and bradycardia have been observed after parenteral administration of methocarbamol. These untoward effects may be lessened by giving the injection at a rate not exceeding 3 ml/min. Because the polyethylene glycol 300 vehicle may be nephrotoxic, parenteral administration is contraindicated in patients with impaired renal function.

The safety of methocarbamol during pregnancy or lactation is not established.

PHARMACOKINETICS. Data are limited, but time to peak blood concentration is two hours after administration of the tablet form. Methocarbamol is largely metabolized. The elimination half-life is 0.9 to 2.2 hours.

DOSAGE AND PREPARATIONS.

Oral: *Adults,* initially, 1.5 to 2 g four times daily for 48 to 72 hours; for maintenance, 1 g four times daily. *Children under 12 years,* safety and efficacy are not established.

Robaxin (Robins), ***Generic.*** Tablets 500 and 750 mg.

Intramuscular: *Adults,* 500 mg alternately in each gluteal region every eight hours.

Intravenous: *Adults,* 1 to 3 g daily at a rate not exceeding 3 ml/min; some physicians substitute oral administration after 1 or 2 g has been administered. The drug should not be given by this route for more than three days.

Generic. Solution 100 mg/ml in 10 ml containers.
Robaxin (Robins). Solution (aqueous) 100 mg/ml with polyethylene glycol 300 50% in 10 ml containers.

ORPHENADRINE CITRATE
[Norflex]

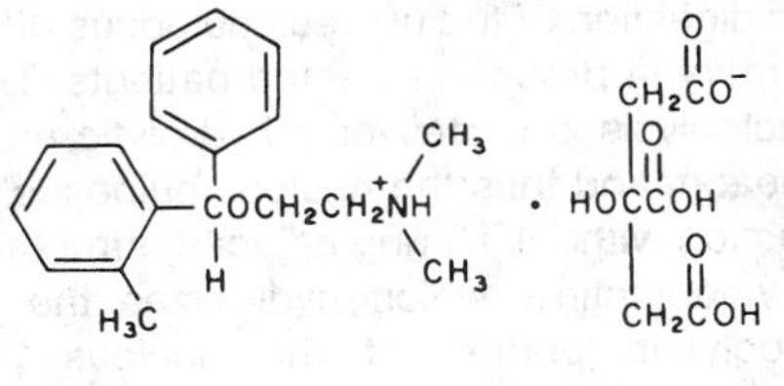

This analogue of the antihistamine, diphenhydramine, is useful as an adjunct to rest, physiotherapy, and other appropriate measures to relieve the pain of local muscle spasm. In one double-blind study involving 59 patients with nocturnal leg cramps, a single bedtime oral dose of orphenadrine citrate reduced the frequency of painful episodes by more than 50%; adverse effects were minor, and relief was sustained in those continuing therapy for up to 28 months (Latta and Turner, 1989). The drug can be given parenterally in severe cases or when oral administration is not feasible. Orphenadrine is not effective in spastic or dyskinetic movement disorders.

ADVERSE REACTIONS AND PRECAUTIONS. The most common side effects of orphenadrine reflect its anticholinergic activity and include blurred vision, dryness of the mouth and skin, and mild excitation. This agent is contraindicated in patients with angle-closure glaucoma or myasthenia gravis, and it should be used with caution in those with tachycardia, cardiac decompensation, or urinary retention. Dosage reduction may be required in the elderly to avoid intolerable side effects. Some patients experience transient dizziness, lightheadedness, or syncope, which may impair their ability to perform potentially hazardous activities. Hypersensitivity reactions are uncommon. Hypoglycemic reactions have developed rarely when propoxyphene or a phenothiazine was given concomitantly.

For a more complete discussion of the adverse reactions and precautions of centrally acting anticholinergic drugs, see index entry Anticholinergic Agents.

PHARMACOKINETICS. Data in humans are limited; orphenadrine is almost completely metabolized to at least eight metabolites that have not been fully characterized. The elimination half-life of the parent compound is about 14 hours.

DOSAGE AND PREPARATIONS.

Oral: *Adults,* 100 mg twice daily.

Generic. Tablets 100 mg.
Norflex (3M Pharmaceuticals). Tablets (prolonged-release) 100 mg.

Intramuscular, Intravenous: *Adults,* 60 mg twice daily.

Generic. Solution 30 mg/ml in 2 and 10 ml containers.
Norflex (3M Pharmaceuticals). Solution (aqueous) 30 mg/ml in 2 ml containers.

Additional Trademarks.
Banflex (Forest), ***Mio-Rel*** (International Ethical).

QUININE SULFATE
[Quinamm]

For chemical formula, see index entry Quinine, Uses, Malaria.

ACTIONS AND USES. Quinine is used to prevent nocturnal leg cramps. It has a long history of use for this indication, based primarily on uncontrolled data collected more than 50 years ago (Moss and Herrmann, 1940). The effects on skeletal muscle attributed to quinine include (1) increased refractory period, (2) decreased excitability of the motor endplate to acetylcholine (curare-like effect), and (3) redistribution of calcium in muscle fiber. However, the degree to which these effects occur with therapeutic doses has not been determined.

Although this drug is widely believed to be effective, the results of controlled trials are conflicting and the Food and Drug Administration has stated that quinine generally should not be regarded as safe and effective for nocturnal leg cramps (*Federal Register,* 1985). Two small controlled clinical trials on nine patients each demonstrated that quinine was significantly more effective than placebo in reducing the number and severity of associated muscle cramps (Kaji et al, 1976; Jones and Castleden, 1983). The earlier trial included only patients who were maintained on hemodialysis for chronic renal failure. Considerable benefit from quinine was reported in another small controlled trial (Fung and Holbrook, 1989). In larger controlled studies, quinine was reported to be ineffective in general (Lim, 1986; Warburton et al, 1987). However, one of these studies was flawed by randomization of the same patient on successive nights to a new treatment arm with no washout period; in the other study, a significant relationship between quinine blood level and reduced frequency of cramps in responsive patients was observed. More recently, in a placebo-controlled crossover trial with quinine and vitamin E, quinine (200 mg at the evening meal and 300 mg at bedtime), but not vitamin E (800 U at bedtime), was judged to be superior to placebo in the treatment of nocturnal leg cramps. Nearly one-half of the quinine recipients experienced at least a 50% reduction in the frequency but not the severity of cramps (Connolly et al, 1992).

ADVERSE REACTIONS. The dose used for nocturnal leg cramps (about one-fourth that given for malaria) usually does not produce symptoms of cinchonism (eg, tinnitus, headache, altered auditory acuity, blurred vision, nausea, diarrhea). Two deaths due to suspected quinine-induced thrombocytopenia have occurred in patients taking the drug to treat nocturnal leg cramps (Freiman, 1990). In Australia, quinine-related thrombocytopenia was reported in 75 patients (most of whom had been treated for nocturnal leg cramps) through 1989; three fatalities occurred and many cases were considered life-threatening (Boyd, 1991).

For other adverse reactions, see index entry Quinine, Uses,

PRECAUTIONS. Quinine should not be given to patients who are hypersensitive to this agent or to individuals with glucose-6-phosphate dehydrogenase deficiency. Thrombocytopenic purpura may follow its administration in highly sensitive individuals. Quinine should be avoided in patients with optic neuritis and tinnitus or a history of blackwater fever. It should be discontinued if the patient experiences ringing in the ears, deafness, skin rash, visual disturbances, or nausea and vomiting.

Because this drug readily crosses the placenta and has been associated with fetal malformations (eg, auditory nerve hypoplasia, limb anomalies, visceral defects), it should not be taken during pregnancy (FDA Pregnancy Category X). The manufacturer advises caution when it is given to nursing mothers.

DRUG INTERACTIONS. Alkalization of the urine with acetazolamide or sodium bicarbonate may lead to toxic serum concentrations of quinine by decreasing its urinary excretion. Antacids containing aluminum may decrease quinine's effectiveness by delaying or decreasing absorption.

Quinine decreases the therapeutic effectiveness of anticholinesterase drugs, such as pyridostigmine, and should be given with caution to myasthenic patients.

Increased plasma concentrations of digoxin and digitoxin have been demonstrated after concomitant administration of quinine. Therefore, plasma digoxin and digitoxin concentrations should be determined periodically for individuals taking either of these glycosides and quinine.

Quinine has the potential to depress hepatic enzyme systems and thus vitamin K factors. The action of warfarin and other oral anticoagulants may be enhanced by the resulting hypoprothrombinemia.

PHARMACOKINETICS. This drug is well absorbed, and peak plasma concentrations are attained one to three hours after ingestion of a single oral dose. The elimination half-life ranges from 5 to 16 hours but may be longer in elderly patients (Warburton et al, 1987). Approximately 70% of a dose is bound to plasma protein, and degradation primarily occurs in the liver. Quinine and its metabolites are eliminated mainly by renal excretion; only 5% of the dose is excreted unaltered in the urine.

DOSAGE AND PREPARATIONS.

Oral: *Adults*, 200 to 300 mg once daily at bedtime (Webster, 1985) or twice daily (after the evening meal and at bedtime) if necessary. Treatment should be interrupted after several days to determine whether continued therapy is required.

Generic. Capsules 200, 260, 300, and 325 mg; tablets 260, 300, and 325 mg.

Quinamm (Marion Merrell Dow). Tablets 260 mg.

CHEMONUCLEOLYSIS FOR SCIATICA CAUSED BY HERNIATED LUMBAR DISC

Lumbar nerve root compression caused by a ruptured intervertebral disc is characterized primarily by leg (including buttock) pain and back pain, with the former being the dominant complaint. The pain is usually felt in one leg and follows a typical sciatic nerve distribution. The most common forms of treatment for lumbar disc herniation with radicular signs and symptoms include conservative therapy (bedrest, physiotherapy), open surgery, percutaneous discectomy, and enzymatic digestion of the disc material (ie, chemonucleolysis).

Disc prolapse causes persistent symptoms in less than 10% of patients with back pain and sciatica (Fraser, 1985). In the long term (eg, ten years), the improvement obtained with conservative therapy is similar to that with open surgery (Weber, 1983). Comparative, retrospective analysis indicates that the outcome ten years after chemonucleolysis or open discectomy is similar (Weinstein et al, 1986).

Enzymatic digestion of the nucleus pulposus offers an alternative to surgery in properly selected patients. The objective of chemonucleolysis is to deliver a hydrolytic enzyme to the intradiscal space, and thus the nucleus pulposus, by transcutaneous injection without injuring adjacent structures. Chymopapain [Chymodiactin], which hydrolyzes the noncollagenous proteoglycan portion of the nucleus pulposus, is effective for chemonucleolysis.

Intradiscal injection of collagenase [Nucleolysin] (investigational) hydrolyzes the Type I and II collagen matrix of the nucleus pulposus and may be effective in the treatment of ruptured lumbar discs (Brown and Tompkins, 1986), but there is less experience with this agent than with chymopapain. Collagenase may offer an alternative to surgery in patients previously treated with chymopapain who may be sensitized to this enzyme. However, it is not used in the United States at this time for chemonucleolysis. The rate of anaphylaxis with collagenase has not been determined.

Drug Evaluation

CHYMOPAPAIN

[Chymodiactin]

ACTIONS. Chymopapain, a proteolytic enzyme, hydrolyzes the noncollagenous proteoglycan portion of the nucleus pulposus of the intervertebral disc. Disruption of the proteoglycan complex significantly decreases the water-binding capacity, which reduces the volume of the nucleus pulposus and intradiscal pressure. It is hypothesized that pain relief and improvements in neurologic deficits result from reduction of the mass of herniated material pressing on the nerve roots. Results of several imaging studies indicate that the size of the herniated nucleus pulposus may or may not decrease in patients who obtain pain relief from the procedure. Shrinkage also can occur during the natural history of the disease in those who are treated conservatively (Delauche-Cavallier et al, 1992). Another proposed mode of action of chymopapain is a reduction in tension on the affected nerve root resulting from a narrowing of the disc space (Spencer and Miller, 1983). Significant proteolytic activity outside the disc appears to be limited by the inhibitory activity of plasma α_2-macroglobulin and kininogen (Buttle et al, 1986).

USES. Intradiscal chymopapain has been used in patients with sciatica caused by documented compression of a lumbar nerve root by protrusion of an intervertebral disc. Sciatic pain rather than back pain is dominant in patients who benefit from intradiscal chymopapain. In addition, they should have the following signs: radicular pain and paresthesias localized to specific dermatomal distribution and affecting one leg or rarely both legs; positive straight leg raising of less than 50 degrees with pain below the knee that is increased by dorsiflexion of the foot (positive nerve root tension sign); two of the following neurologic signs: sensory alteration, depressed reflex activity, muscle weakness; and diagnosis of herniated disc confirmed by a myelogram, CT, and/or MRI scan.

Intradiscal injection of chymopapain is indicated only in patients with documented herniated lumbar intervertebral discs who have not responded to an adequate period of conservative therapy. Radiculopathy of nondiscogenic origin, such as impingement of the nerve root by hypertrophic bony spurs, spondylolisthesis or spinal stenosis, intraspinal tumor, spinal arteriovenous malformation, and arachnoiditis are contraindications to chemonucleolysis (Ramirez and Javid, 1984). Patients with lateral recess syndrome, facet arthropathy, instability syndrome, or sequestered disc also are not suitable candidates. The latter may be difficult to identify by CT or MRI scan in some patients.

When these strict criteria for patient inclusion are followed, the results of randomized, double-blind studies indicate that chymopapain is more effective than placebo in the treatment of sciatica caused by lumbar intervertebral disc herniation (Javid et al, 1983; Fraser, 1984; Dabezies et al, 1988). Six months after injection, improvement was moderate to marked in 71% to 80% of chymopapain recipients; in comparison, approximately 46% of placebo recipients improved. The percentage of patients who experienced moderate to marked relief was similar in prospective open trials (71% to 83%) (Onofrio, 1975; Maroon et al, 1976; McCulloch, 1981; McDermott et al, 1985). Results of a ten-year follow-up of patients in one double-blind study (Fraser, 1984) indicate that the therapeutic effect of chymopapain in the treatment of classic lumbar intervertebral disc herniation is sustained (Gogan and Fraser, 1992). Eighty percent of the chymopapain recipients regarded the injection as successful compared with 34% of placebo recipients. Laminectomy was required in 20% of the chymopapain recipients within two years after injection and in 47% of placebo recipients.

The significant placebo response emphasizes the importance of suitable outcome criteria. In most studies of sciatica, criteria for determining the effectiveness of any form of treatment are the subjective satisfaction of the patient, pain relief, improvement of neurologic symptoms, and resumption of work. In general, less favorable results are reported when patients with compensable injury are involved or objective signs primarily are measured (Howe and Frymoyer, 1985; Javid, 1988). The variation in reported success with chemonucleolysis in open trials (44% to 98%) is probably due to differences in patient selection and outcome criteria (van Alphen et al, 1989). Thus, randomization in comparative studies is critical.

In prospective, randomized trials comparing results achieved with open surgery and chymopapain, patients fared better with surgery (85% to 89% success rate) than with chymopapain (48% to 63% success rate) (Crawshaw et al, 1984; van Alphen et al, 1989). Another small trial was discontinued when more than one-half of the chymopapain-treated patients (8 of 15) required surgery (Ejeskär et al, 1983). However, four of these patients had sequestered disc fragment, a condition that does not respond to chymopapain injection. In most prospective, nonrandomized studies, patients with simple disc protrusion who received chymopapain did as well as or better than those who had surgery (Watts et al, 1975; Leavitt et al, 1980; Alexander et al, 1989; Javid, 1992). Results reported in earlier retrospective comparisons of chymopapain injection with open surgery were more favorable for chymopapain (71% to 77% versus 48% to 63%) (Nordby and Lucas, 1973; Dabezies and Brunet, 1978).

Results were comparable in another retrospective comparison of chemonucleolysis and open discectomy (Weinstein et al, 1986). In a retrospective analysis comparing chymopapain injection with microsurgical discectomy, surgery was more successful (80% to 90% versus 58% to 60%) (Maroon and Abla, 1985; Zeiger, 1987). In one randomized multicenter clinical trial on patients with sciatica, the success rate at six months was higher after chemonucleolysis (61%) than after automated percutaneous lumbar discectomy (44%) (Revel et al, 1993).

The most commonly reported causes of failure of chemonucleolysis as demonstrated at subsequent surgery are extruded/sequestered disc and lateral stenosis (Deburge et al, 1985; McCulloch and MacNab, 1983). To be effective, chymopapain must reach and digest the herniated portion of the nucleus pulposus. This can be more readily achieved after assessment by CT discography. In a retrospective analysis, successful chemonucleolysis was reported in 95% of patients when intradiscally injected contrast medium extended into a defect previously seen on myelography or plain CT scanning (Edwards et al, 1987).

Despite the apparent benefit derived from chymopapain in carefully selected patients, use of the technique has declined sharply. Even though the mortality and morbidity rates associated with chemonucleolysis compare favorably with those for surgery (Bouillet, 1990), some physicians are apparently concerned about efficacy and the potential for anaphylaxis or severe, unpredictable neurologic complications (eg, paraplegia, acute transverse myelitis, hemorrhage) (Thomas, 1989; Brown and Currier, 1990). Although no serious complications were associated with use of chymopapain from 1989 to 1991 (Nordby et al, 1993), controversy about the proper interventional treatment for lumbar disc disease continues. When conservative methods of treatment have failed, those who fulfill criteria for patient selection may be offered a choice between chemonucleolysis and surgical intervention.

Although a patient who has a radicular syndrome caused by lumbar disc herniation can benefit from chemonucleolysis, pain may persist or recur and surgery may be required in approximately 15% to 20% of the patients. The final results obtained with chymopapain injection can occasionally take three months or longer to become apparent, but surgery may be indicated if sciatica fails to improve or worsens within four to six weeks after injection. Paravertebral muscle spasm and back pain occur in some patients and occasionally may result in a prolonged convalescent period. Therefore, it has been argued that short-term results are inferior and the clinical course may be more complicated when chemonucleolysis rather than surgery is chosen as the primary treatment (van Alphen et al, 1989; Muralikuttan et al, 1992). Proponents argue that since chemonucleolysis is less invasive than surgery, is similar in efficacy and long-term outcome, and overall is safer, it should be used as a therapeutic intervention before disc excision is considered when conservative measures have failed (Fraser, 1984; Alexander et al, 1989). Use of chemonucleolysis does not appear to jeopardize the results of later surgery (Gogan and Fraser, 1992).

ADVERSE REACTIONS. Serious but rare adverse reactions caused by chymopapain are anaphylaxis and neurologic complications due to subarachnoid injection. Mild to severe anaphylaxis has been reported in approximately 0.3% to 1% of patients not known to have been previously sensitized (Watts, 1977; Boots Pharmaceuticals, 1991). Data indicate that the overall incidence is higher in females, particularly black females, than in males. In more recent reports, the incidence has been reduced to 0.29%; this may reflect improvements in preoperative screening and possibly the use of local rather than general anesthesia.

The risk of hypersensitivity reactions can be minimized by screening for chymopapain-specific IgE antibodies by immunoassay (ChymoFAST [Immugenex, Palo Alto, California]) prior to injection. However, approximately 0.2% of patients with negative test results (IgE concentration <0.06 IU/ml) experience adverse reactions (Tsay et al, 1984). If the test is considered to be positive when any trace of IgE antibody to chymopapain is detected, the incidence of allergic reactions decreases to 0.05%, but this excludes 13% of patients from injection. Skin sensitivity testing also has been used to detect patients who might be hypersensitive (McCulloch et el, 1985).

Almost all anaphylactic reactions occur immediately but may be observed up to two hours after injection. Since the intervertebral disc is avascular, release of chymopapain into the blood stream is delayed. Thus, the patient should be observed closely for 30 minutes after injection and for an additional 90 minutes in the recovery room. The signs and symptoms of anaphylaxis include almost immediate tachycardia and hypotension. Bronchospasm, a less common component of the anaphylactic reaction to chymopapain, may lead to laryngeal edema, tachycardia, arrhythmia, cardiac arrest, coma, and death.

Careful placement of the needle is essential because neurologic complications may result from injection or leakage of contrast media and enzyme into the subarachnoid space. The enzyme hydrolyzes the basement membranes of the small vessels in the pia-arachnoid, and the resulting subarachnoid hemorrhage may cause headache, anxiety, hypertension, nuchal rigidity, unconsciousness, convulsions, paraplegia, and, occasionally, death.

Serious neurologic complications, such as paraplegia/paraparesis and CNS hemorrhage, have been observed within hours or days following chymopapain injection (incidence <1 in 2,000 patients). Onset of paraplegia/paraparesis also has been reported two to three weeks after chymopapain injection (incidence <1 in 20,000 patients).

Temporary back pain, stiffness, and soreness are observed in 50% of patients. Muscle spasm occurs in 20% to 30% of patients immediately following injection. Back pain from muscle spasm may be incapacitating and occasionally may prolong convalescence, but it does not appear to affect the outcome of chymopapain treatment.

Rash, urticaria, or pruritus may occur as late as two weeks after chymopapain injection (incidence <1%). Rash may occur alone or as part of the anaphylactic reaction and is associated with pruritus, which may be managed with diphenhydramine (Ramirez and Javid, 1984). Urticaria with pruritus may develop suddenly seven to ten days after injection and is twice as common as anaphylaxis.

PRECAUTIONS. Safe and effective use of chymopapain requires specialized training in chemonucleolysis. Since nerve root compression may result from conditions other than herniated disc, extensive training and experience in the diagnosis and management of all spinal disorders are required for proper patient selection. Additionally, physicians and support personnel should be aware of and trained to manage the potential complications from the use of chymopapain, including anaphylaxis.

Chymopapain is extremely toxic when injected intrathecally, as are some radio-opaque contrast media used for discography. In many of the reported cases of serious neurologic complications, discography was performed as part of the procedure. Great care must be taken to assure that the dura is not penetrated and that chymopapain or contrast medium does not enter the subarachnoid space. If there is any question regarding needle tip location within the nucleus of the disc or if contrast medium extravasates into the subarachnoid space, the procedure should be halted and chymopapain should not be injected (Boots Pharmaceuticals, 1992).

A history of allergy to papaya or its extracts precludes the use of chymopapain. This enzyme is immunogenic; thus, repeat injections are contraindicated. The determination of chymopapain-specific IgE plasma levels and skin sensitivity testing using inactivated chymopapain may help identify high-risk patients (Tsay et al, 1984; McCulloch et al, 1985; Bernstein et al, 1985).

Because of the possibility of an anaphylactic reaction to chymopapain, some surgeons advocate the preoperative administration of corticosteroids and antihistamines (Brown, 1983); other authorities feel that routine premedication has not been proven to be beneficial (McCulloch and MacNab, 1983). Whether or not patients are pretreated with antihistamines and steroids, if anaphylaxis occurs, the physician must be prepared to make an immediate diagnosis and administer epinephrine and large amounts of fluids.

Opinions have differed among surgeons regarding the choice of anesthesia (general versus local) for chemonucleolysis (Brown, 1983; *FDC Rep,* 1985; McCulloch, 1984), but it is now generally accepted that local anesthesia is the method of choice because the patient is able to report pain due to a misplaced injection needle, because it allows early detection of anaphylactic reactions, and because it does not interfere with subsequent treatment (Brown and Currier, 1990). Halothane should not be used for general anesthesia because of the potential for arrhythmias if epinephrine is required to treat an anaphylactic reaction.

Previous surgery at the same level may increase the possibility of neurologic complications from chemonucleolysis. Therefore, this enzyme should not be injected at the level of previous surgery. Because patients receiving injections at two or more disc spaces appear to be at increased risk of developing serious neurologic adverse effects, most authorities believe that only a single disc should be injected.

Because its safety during any phase of pregnancy also remains to be determined, chemonucleolysis with chymopapain is contraindicated during pregnancy or suspected pregnancy (FDA Pregnancy Category C).

PHARMACOKINETICS. Fragments of chymopapain immunoreactive to protein and keratan sulfate (Block et al, 1989), a degradation product of nuclear glycoprotein, have been detected in plasma shortly after intradiscal injection. The inhibitory activity of α_2-macroglobulin is believed to prevent significant chymopapain activity outside the disc.

DOSAGE AND PREPARATIONS. Some protocols for chemonucleolysis recommend the administration of a test dose of chymopapain to assess the potential for anaphylaxis, but the predictive value has been questioned (Bernstein, 1984).

Intradiscal Injection: *Adults*, 2,000 to 4,000 picoKatal units per disc; 3,000 picoKatal units is usually used. The value of doses <2,000 picoKatal units has not been established. The maximal dose in a patient with multiple disc herniation is 8,000 picoKatal units.

Chymodiactin (Boots). Powder (lyophilized) 4,000 picoKatal units/vial (2 ml).

Cited References

Spasticity and Muscle Spasm

Internal analgesic, antipyretic, and antirheumatic drug products for over-the-counter human use; tentative final monograph for drug products for treatment and/or prevention of nocturnal leg cramps. *Federal Register* 50:46588-46954, 1985.

Albright AL: Neurosurgical treatment of spasticity: Selective posterior rhizotomy and intrathecal baclofen. *Stereotact Funct Neurosurg* 58:3-13, 1992.

Albright AL, et al: Continuous intrathecal baclofen infusion for spasticity of cerebral origin. *JAMA* 270:2475-2477, 1993.

Alfery DD, Rauscher LA: Tetanus: Review. *Crit Care Med* 7:176-181, 1979.

Azouvi P, et al: Effect of intrathecal baclofen on the monosynaptic reflex in humans: Evidence for a postsynaptic action. *J Neurol Neurosurg Psychiatry* 56:515-519, 1993.

Baltodano N, et al: Verapamil vs quinine in recumbent nocturnal leg cramps in the elderly. *Arch Intern Med* 148:1969-1970, 1988.

Basmajian JV: Cyclobenzaprine hydrochloride effect on skeletal muscle spasm in lumbar region and neck: Two double-blind controlled clinical and laboratory studies. *Arch Phys Med Rehabil* 59:58-63, 1978.

Berman B, et al: The effect of rhizotomy on movement in patients with cerebral palsy. *Am J Occup Ther* 44:511-516, 1989.

Bowery NG, et al: Baclofen decreases neurotransmitter release in mammalian CNS by action at novel GABA receptor. *Nature* 283:92-93, 1980.

Boyd IW: Nocturnal cramps, quinine, and thrombocytopenia. *Arch Intern Med* 151:1021, 1991.

Brogden RN, et al: Baclofen: Preliminary report of its pharmacological properties and therapeutic efficacy in spasticity. *Drugs* 8:1-14, 1974.

Chan CH: Dantrolene sodium and hepatic injury. *Neurology* 40:1427-1432, 1990.

Coffey RJ, et al: Intrathecal baclofen for intractable spasticity of spinal origin: Results of a long-term multicenter study. *J Neurosurg* 78:226-232, 1993.

Cohan SL, et al: Phenytoin and chlorpromazine in treatment of spasticity. *Arch Neurol* 37:360-364, 1980.

Connolly PS, et al: Treatment of nocturnal leg cramps: A crossover trial of quinine vs vitamin E. *Arch Intern Med* 152:1877-1880, 1992.

Darnell RB, et al: Stiff-man syndrome-80: A variant associated with abnormal visual processing and a new antineuronal antibody. *Ann Neurol* 28:219-220, 1990.

Davidoff RA: Pharmacology of spasticity. *Neurology* 28:46-51, 1978.

Delhaas EM, Brouwers JRBJ: Intrathecal baclofen overdose: Report of 7 events in 5 patients and review of the literature. *Int J Clin Pharmacol Ther Toxicol* 29:274-280, 1991.

Deyo RA: Conservative therapy for low back pain: Distinguishing useful from useless therapy. *JAMA* 250:1057-1062, 1983.

Deyo RA, et al: How many days of bed rest for acute low back pain? A randomized clinical trial. *N Engl J Med* 315:1064-1070, 1986.

Dolphin AC, Scott RY: Inhibition of calcium currents in cultured rat dorsal root ganglion neurons by baclofen. *Br J Pharmacol* 88:213-220, 1986.

Donovan WH, et al: Clonidine effect on spasticity: A clinical trial. *Arch Phys Med Rehabil* 69:193-194, (March) 1988.

Duncan GW, et al: Evaluation of baclofen treatment for certain symptoms in patients with spinal cord lesions. *Neurology* 26:441-446, 1976.

Eaton JM: Is this really a muscle cramp? *Postgrad Med* 86:227-232, (Sept) 1989.

Elenbaas JK: Centrally acting oral skeletal muscle relaxants. *Am J Hosp Pharm* 37:1313-1323, 1980.

Erickson DL, et al: Control of intractable spasticity with intrathecal morphine sulfate. *Neurosurgery* 24:236-238, 1989.

Feldman RG, et al: Baclofen for spasticity in multiple sclerosis: Double-blind crossover and three-year study. *Neurology* 28:1094-1098, 1978.

Freiman J: Fatal quinine-induced thrombocytopenia. *Ann Intern Med* 112:308-309, 1990.

Fung MC, Holbrook JH: Placebo-controlled trial of quinine therapy for nocturnal leg cramps. *West J Med* 151:42-44, 1989.

Gilbert JR, et al: Clinical trial of common treatments for low back pain in family practice. *Br Med J* 291:791-794, 1985.

Growdon JH, et al: L-threonine in the treatment of spasticity. *Clin Neuropharmacol* 14:403-412, 1991.

Haubenstock A, et al: Baclofen (Lioresal) intoxication: Report of 4 cases and review of literature. *Clin Toxicol* 20:59-68, 1983.

Hauser SI, et al: An antispastic effect of threonine in multiple sclerosis. *Arch Neurol* 49:923-926, 1992.

Hedley DW, et al: Evaluation of baclofen (Lioresal) for spasticity in multiple sclerosis. *Postgrad Med J* 51:615-618, 1975.

Jones K, Castleden CM: A double-blind comparison of quinine sulphate and placebo in muscle cramps. *Age Ageing* 12:155-158, 1983.

Kaji DM, et al: Prevention of muscle cramps in haemodialysis patients by quinine sulphate. *Lancet* 2:66-67, 1976.

Kofler M, et al: Epileptic seizures associated with intrathecal baclofen application. *Neurology* 44:25-27, 1994.

Latta D, Turner E: Alternative to quinine in nocturnal leg cramps. *Curr Ther Res* 45:833-837, 1989.

Lazorthes Y, et al: Chronic intrathecal baclofen administration for control of severe spasticity. *J Neurosurg* 72:393-402, 1990.

Lee A, Patterson V: A double-blind study of L-threonine in patients with spinal spasticity. *Acta Neurol Scand* 88:334-338, 1993.

Levine IM, et al: Lioresal, new muscle relaxant in treatment of spasticity: Double-blind quantitative evaluation. *Dis Nerv Syst* 38:1011-1015, 1977.

Lim SH: Randomised double-blind trial of quinine sulphate for nocturnal leg cramp. *Br J Clin Pract* 40:462, 1986.

Lorish TR, et al: Stiff-man syndrome updated. *Mayo Clin Proc* 64:629-636, 1989.

Mason NA, et al: Factors affecting diazepam infusion: Solubility, administration-set composition, and flow rate. *Am J Hosp Pharm* 38:1449-1454, 1981.

Maynard FM: Early clinical experience with clonidine in spinal spasticity. *Paraplegia* 24:175-182, 1986.

McCombe PF, et al: Reproducibility of physical signs in low-back pain. *Spine* 14:908-918, 1989.

Melnick ME, Shellenberger MK: Management of pediatric spasticity. *Compr Ther* 8:20-26, (Oct) 1982.

Meyler WJ, et al: Effect of dantrolene sodium in relation to blood levels in spastic patients after prolonged administration. *J Neurol Neurosurg Psychiatry* 44:334-339, 1981.

Meythaler JM, et al: Intrathecal baclofen in hereditary spastic paraparesis. *Arch Phys Med Rehabil* 73:794-797, 1992.

Miller F, Korsvik H: Baclofen in treatment of stiff-man syndrome. *Ann Neurol* 9:511-512, 1981.

Moss HK, Herrmann LG: Use of quinine for relief of "night cramps" in the extremities. *JAMA* 115:1358-1359, 1940.

Müller-Schwefe G, Penn RD: Physostigmine in the treatment of intrathecal baclofen overdose. *J Neurosurg* 71:273-275, 1989.

Nanninga JB, et al: Effect of intrathecal baclofen on bladder and sphincter function. *J Urol* 142:101-105, 1989.

Narayan RK, et al: Intrathecal baclofen for intractable axial dystonia. *Neurology* 41:1141-1142, 1991.

Ochs G, et al: Intrathecal baclofen for long-term treatment of spasticity: A multi-centre study. *J Neurol Neurosurg Psychiatry* 52:933-939, 1989.

Park TS, Owen JH: Surgical management of spastic diplegia in cerebral palsy. *N Engl J Med* 326:745-749, 1992.

Peacock WJ, Staudt LA: Functional outcomes following selective posterior rhizotomy in children with cerebral palsy. *J Neurosurg* 74:370-375, 1991.

Penn RD: Intrathecal baclofen for spasticity of spinal origin: Seven years of experience. *J Neurosurg* 77:236-240, 1992.

Penn RD, et al: Intrathecal baclofen for severe spinal spasticity. *N Engl J Med* 320:1517-1521, 1989.

Putty TK, Shapiro SA: Efficacy of dorsal longitudinal myelotomy in treating spinal spasticity: A review of 20 cases. *J Neurosurg* 75:397-401, 1991.

Ramirez FC, Graham DY: Treatment of intractable hiccup with baclofen: Results of a double-blind randomized, controlled, cross-over study. *Am J Gastroenterol* 87:1789-1791, 1992.

Rice GPA: Pharmacotherapy of spasticity: Some theoretical and practical considerations. *Can J Neurol Sci* 14:510-512, 1987.

Rubin AS, Zablocki AD: Hyperkalemia, verapamil, and dantrolene. *Anesthesiology* 66:246-249, 1987.

Shime J, et al: Dantrolene in pregnancy: Lack of adverse effects on the fetus and newborn infant. *Am J Obstet Gynecol* 159:831-834, 1988.

Solimena M, et al: Autoantibodies to glutamic acid decarboxylase in a patient with stiff-man syndrome, epilepsy, and type I diabetes mellitus. *N Engl J Med* 318:1012-1020, 1988.

Steers WD, et al: Effects of acute bolus and chronic continuous intrathecal baclofen on genitourinary dysfunction due to spinal cord pathology. *J Urol* 148:1849-1855, 1992.

Stewart JE, et al: Modulation of locomotor patterns and spasticity with clonidine in spinal cord injured patients. *Can J Neurol Sci* 18:321-332, (Aug) 1991.

Tallala A, et al: The effect of intrathecal baclofen on the lower urinary tract in paraplegia. *Paraplegia* 28:420, 1990.

Terrence CF, et al: Baclofen: Effect on seizure frequency. *Arch Neurol* 40:28-29, 1983.

Turski L, et al: Substantia nigra: A site of action of muscle relaxant drugs. *Ann Neurol* 28:341-348, 1990.

Warburton A, et al: A quinine a day keeps the leg cramps away? *Br J Clin Pharm* 23:459-465, 1987.

Ward A, et al: Dantrolene: Review of its pharmacodynamic and pharmacokinetic properties and therapeutic use in malignant hyperthermia, neuroleptic malignant syndrome, and update of its use in muscle spasticity. *Drugs* 32:130-168, 1986.

Webster LT: Drugs used in chemotherapy of protozoal infections: Malaria, in Gilman AG, et al (eds): *The Pharmacological Basis of Therapeutics*, ed 8. New York, Macmillan, 1985, 944.

Weingarden SI, Belen JG: Clonidine transdermal system for treatment of spasticity in spinal cord injury. *Arch Phys Med Rehabil* 73:876-877, 1992.

Wiesel SW, et al: Acute low-back pain: Objective analysis of conservative therapy. *Spine* 5:324-330, 1980.

Yablon SA, Sipski ML: Effect of transdermal clonidine on spinal spasticity: A case series. *Am J Phys Med Rehabil* 72:154-157, (June) 1993.

Young RR: Treatment for spastic paresis. *N Engl J Med* 320:1553-1555, 1989.

Young RR, Delwaide PJ: Spasticity, parts I and II. *N Engl J Med* 304:28-33, 96-99, 1981.

Herniated Lumbar Disc

Chemonucleolysis Update: Patient Selection. Lincolnshire, Ill, Boots Pharmaceuticals, (June) 1991.

Full Prescribing Information. Lincolnshire, Ill, Boots Pharmaceuticals, 1992.

General anesthesia should remain option for chemonucleolysis. *FDC Rep* April 15, 1985.

Alexander AH, et al: Chymopapain chemonucleolysis *versus* surgical discectomy in a military population. *Clin Orthop* 244:158-165, 1989.

Bernstein IL: Anaphylaxis from chymopapain, letter reply. *JAMA* 251:1953-1954, 1984.

Bernstein DI, et al: Prospective evaluation of chymopapain sensitivity in patients undergoing chemonucleolysis. *J Allergy Clin Immunol* 76:458-465, 1985.

Block JA, et al: Effect of chemonucleolysis on serum keratan sulfate levels in humans. *Arthritis Rheum* 32:100-104, 1989.

Bouillet R: Treatment of sciatica: A comparative survey of complications of surgical treatment and nucleolysis with chymopapain. *Clin Orthop* 251:144-152, (Feb) 1990.

Brown MD: *Intradiscal Therapy: Chymopapain or Collagenase*. Chicago, Year Book Medical Publishers, 1983.

Brown MD, Currier BL: Chemonucleolysis, in Weinstein JN, Wiesel SW (eds): *The Lumbar Spine.* Philadelphia, WB Saunders, 1990, 441-448.

Brown MD, Tompkins JS: Chemonucleolysis (discolysis) with collagenase. *Spine* 11:123-130, 1986.

Buttle DJ, et al: The biochemistry of action of chymopapain in relief of sciatica. *Spine* 11:688-694, 1986.

Crawshaw C, et al: A comparison of surgery and chemonucleolysis in the treatment of sciatica: A prospective randomized trial. *Spine* 9:195-198, 1984.

Dabezies EJ, Brunet M: Chemonucleolysis vs. laminectomy. *Orthopedics* 1:26-29, 1978.

Dabezies EJ, et al: Safety and efficacy of chymopapain (Discase) in the treatment of sciatica due to a herniated nucleus pulposus: Results of a randomized, double-blind study. *Spine* 13:561-565, 1988.

Deburge A, et al: Surgical findings and results of surgery after failure of chemonucleolysis. *Spine* 10:812-815, 1985.

Delauche-Cavallier M-C, et al: Lumbar disc herniation: Computed tomography scan changes after conservative treatment of nerve root compression. *Spine* 17:927-933, 1992.

Edwards WC, et al: CT discography: Prognostic value in the selection of patients for chemonucleolysis. *Spine* 12:791-795, 1987.

Ejeskär A, et al: Surgery *versus* chemonucleolysis for herniated lumbar discs: A prospective study with random assignment. *Clin Orthop* 174:236-242, 1983.

Fraser RD: Chymopapain for the treatment of intervertebral disc herniation: The final report of a double-blind study. *Spine* 9:815-818, 1984.

Fraser RD: Treatment of intervertebral disc prolapse by intradiscal injection of chymopapain. *Med J Aust* 142:431-434, 1985.

Gogan WJ, Fraser RD: Chymopapain: A 10-year, double-blind study. *Spine* 17:388-394, 1992.

Howe J, Frymoyer JW: The effects of questionnaire design on the determination of end results in lumbar spinal surgery. *Spine* 10:804-805, 1985.

Javid MJ: Signs and symptoms after chemonucleolysis: Detailed evaluation of 214 worker's compensation and noncompensation patients. *Spine* 13:1428-1437, 1988.

Javid MJ: A 1- to 4-year follow-up review of treatment of sciatica using chemonucleolysis or laminectomy. *J Neurosurg* 76:184-190, 1992.

Javid MJ, et al: Safety and efficacy of chymopapain (Chymodiactin) in herniated nucleus pulposus with sciatica: Results of a randomized double-blind study. *JAMA* 249:2489-2494, 1983.

Leavitt F, et al: A comparison of patients treated by chymopapain and laminectomy for low back pain using a multidimensional pain scale. *Clin Orthop* 146:136-143, 1980.

Maroon JC, Abla A: Microdiscectomy versus chemonucleolysis. *Neurosurgery* 16:644-649, 1985.

Maroon JC, et al: Chymopapain in the treatment of ruptured lumbar discs: Preliminary experience in 48 patients. *J Neurol Neurosurg Psychiatry* 39:508-513, 1976.

McCulloch JA: Chemonucleolysis for relief of sciatica due to a herniated intervertebral disc. *Can Med Assoc J* 124:879-882, 1981.

McCulloch JA: Chemonucleolysis: State of the art, in Genant HK (ed): *Spine Update 1984: Perspectives in Radiology, Orthopaedic Surgery, and Neurosurgery*. San Francisco, University of California, 1984, 127-130.

McCulloch JA, MacNab I: *Sciatica and Chymopapain.* Baltimore, Williams & Wilkins, 1983.

McCulloch J, et al: Skin tests for chymopapain allergy. *Ann Allergy* 55:609-611, 1985.

McDermott DJ, et al: Chymodiactin in patients with herniated lumbar intervertebral disc(s): An open-label, multicenter study. *Spine* 10:242-249, 1985.

Muralikuttan KP, et al: A prospective randomized trial of chemonucleolysis and conventional disc surgery in single level lumbar disc herniation. *Spine* 17:381-387, 1992.

Nordby EJ, Lucas GL: A comparative analysis of lumbar disc disease treated by laminectomy or chemonucleolysis. *Clin Orthop* 90:119-129, 1973.

Nordby EJ, et al: Safety of chemonucleolysis: Adverse effects reported in the United States, 1982-1991. *Clin Orthop* 293:122-134, 1993.

Onofrio BM: Injection of chymopapain into intervertebral discs. *J Neurosurg* 42:384-388, 1975.

Ramirez LF, Javid MJ: Chymopapain: A new alternative for herniated discs. *Drug Ther (Hosp)* 9:169-181, (March) 1984.

Revel M, et al: Automated percutaneous lumbar discectomy versus chemonucleolysis in the treatment of sciatica: A randomized multicenter trial. *Spine* 18:1-7, 1993.

Spencer DL, Miller JAA: The mechanism of sciatic pain relief by chemonucleolysis. *Orthopedics* 6:1600-1603, 1983.

Thomas P: Interest in chymopapain low despite reported successes. *Med World News* 13, (June 26) 1989.

Tsay Y-G, et al: A preoperative chymopapain sensitivity test for chemonucleolysis candidates. *Spine* 9:764-768, 1984.

van Alphen HAM, et al: Chemonucleolysis versus discectomy: A randomized multicenter trial. *J Neurosurg* 70:869-875, 1989.

Watts C: Complications of chemonucleolysis for lumbar disc disease. *Neurosurgery* 1:2-5, 1977.

Watts C, et al: Comparison of intervertebral disc disease treatment by chymopapain injection and open surgery. *J Neurosurg* 42:397-400, 1975.

Weber H: Lumbar disc herniation: A controlled, prospective study with ten years of observation. *Spine* 8:131-140, 1983.

Weinstein J, et al: Lumbar disc herniation: A comparison of the results of chemonucleolysis and open discectomy after ten years. *J Bone Joint Surg* 68-A:43-54, 1986.

Zeiger HE Jr: Comparison of chemonucleolysis and microsurgical discectomy for the treatment of herniated lumbar disc. *Spine* 12:796-799, 1987.

Drugs Used for Motion Disorders and Vomiting

19

Dizziness, vertigo, nausea, and vomiting are only symptomatic indications of altered function; they are not diseases. Rational therapy depends on diagnosis of the underlying disorder and may or may not include drugs (Barbezat, 1981). Therapy should be initiated when symptoms are severe even if the cause has not been identified.

Nausea and vomiting are idiopathic or are associated with motion sickness, pregnancy, the postoperative period, toxins (metabolic toxins [eg, uremia], microbial toxins), radiation therapy, and drugs used for cancer chemotherapy. Nausea and vomiting induced by other drugs (eg, opioids, digitalis, estrogens, aminophylline, levodopa, iron preparations) are obviated by reducing the dose, altering the route or time of administration, giving the drug with food, or substituting another agent if possible. Although reducing the dosage of an opioid alleviates drug-induced nausea and vomiting, analgesic activity may be decreased; therefore, use of an antiemetic may be preferred. Because tolerance to the emetic effects of opioids often occurs, the dose of the antiemetic agent can be gradually reduced to the minimum amount required to control symptoms.

Nausea and vomiting related to pathology of the abdominal organs, increased intraluminal pressure in the intestine, food allergies, hypo- or hyperglycemia, increased intracranial pressure, or of psychogenic origin are reduced by correcting the underlying disorder (when possible).

PHARMACOLOGIC CLASSIFICATION. The pharmacodynamic classification (see Table 1) of drugs used to prevent and treat motion disorders and vomiting is of more value in defining anticipated side effects than efficacy. Useful drugs include (1) the anticholinergic agent, scopolamine, which appears to act by depressing conduction in vestibular cerebellar pathways or preventing recruitment of impulses at the vomiting center; (2) H_1 antihistamines (buclizine, cyclizine, dimenhydrinate, diphenhydramine, hydroxyzine, meclizine, promethazine), which also have anticholinergic activity that may account for their antiemetic effects; (3) dopamine receptor antagonists, which include metoclopramide, domperidone (investigational), the aliphatic and piperazine phenothiazines (eg, chlorpromazine, perphenazine, thiethylperazine), and the butyrophenones, droperidol and haloperidol; and (4) the serotonin antagonists (5-HT_3 receptor antagonists), ondansetron and granisetron.

Drugs in the third and fourth categories act primarily on the chemoreceptor trigger zone (CTZ) and/or by inhibiting peripheral autonomic afferent impulses to the vomiting center via the vagus nerve. In addition to their antidopaminergic activity at the CTZ, metoclopramide and domperidone also appear to act by stimulating upper gastrointestinal motility (but not secretion), which enhances gastric emptying. Both drugs increase lower esophageal sphincter pressure. Antiserotoninergic drugs block 5-HT_3 receptors involved in the emetic response. When given in large doses, metoclopramide also blocks these receptors, which may be its primary mechanism of action as an antiemetic agent.

Unlike the aliphatic and piperazine phenothiazines, the piperidine phenothiazines (eg, thioridazine [Mellaril]) are *not* effective antiemetics. Although promethazine is an aliphatic

TABLE 1. ANTIVERTIGO AND ANTIEMETIC DRUGS

Drug Classification	AVAILABLE PREPARATIONS: Parenteral	Suppository	Oral
ANTICHOLINERGIC			
Scopolamine Hydrobromide	x		
Scopolamine [Transderm-Scōp]	x (dermal)		
ANTIHISTAMINIC			
Buclizine Hydrochloride [Bucladin-S]			x
Cyclizine Hydrochloride [Marezine]			x
Dimenhydrinate [Dramamine]	x		x
Diphenhydramine Hydrochloride [Benadryl]	x		x
Hydroxyzine Hydrochloride [Atarax, Vistaril]	x		x
Hydroxyzine Pamoate [Vistaril]			x
Meclizine Hydrochloride [Antivert, Bonine, Dramamine II]			x
Promethazine Hydrochloride [Phenergan]	x	x	x
ANTIDOPAMINERGIC			
Aliphatic Phenothiazines			
Chlorpromazine [Thorazine]		x	
Chlorpromazine Hydrochloride [Thorazine]	x		x
Promazine Hydrochloride‡ [Sparine]	x		x
Triflupromazine Hydrochloride [Vesprin]	x		
Piperazine Phenothiazines			
Fluphenazine Hydrochloride [Permitil, Prolixin]	x		x
Perphenazine [Trilafon]	x		x
Prochlorperazine [Compazine]		x	
Prochlorperazine Edisylate [Compazine]	x		x
Prochlorperazine Maleate [Compazine]			x
Thiethylperazine Malate [Torecan]	x		
Thiethylperazine Maleate [Torecan]		x	x
Butyrophenones			
Droperidol [Inapsine]	x		
Haloperidol [Haldol]			x
Haloperidol Lactate [Haldol]	x		x
Miscellaneous Antidopaminergic Agents			
Domperidone‡ [Motilium]			x
Metoclopramide Hydrochloride [Maxolon, Octamide PFS, Reglan]	x		x
ANTISEROTONINERGIC			
5-Hydroxytryptamine$_3$ (5-HT$_3$) Receptor Antagonists			
Ondansetron Hydrochloride [Zofran]	x		
Granisetron Hydrochloride [Kytril]	x		
MISCELLANEOUS			
Benzquinamide Hydrochloride [Emete-Con]	x		
Diphenidol Hydrochloride [Vontrol]			x

PRINCIPAL USES

Vertigo	Motion Sickness	Pregnancy*	Postoperative Emesis	Cancer Chemotherapy	Toxins† Radiation Therapy
	++		+		
+	++				
±	+				
+	+	+	++		
++	++	+			
+	+	+		+	
±	+		+		
±	+				
++	+	+			+
+	++	+	+	+	+
				+	±
				+	±
			+		±
			+	±	±
			+	±	+
			+	±	+
			+		+
			++	+	++
+			++	+	
			++	+	+
			++	+	+
			+	+	++
			+	++	+‡
			+++	+++	++
				+++	
			+	+	
+			+	+	+

(table continued on next page)

TABLE 1 (continued)

Drug Classification	AVAILABLE PREPARATIONS Parenteral	Suppository	Oral
MISCELLANEOUS (continued)			
Trimethobenzamide Hydrochloride [Tigan]	x	x	x
Benzodiazepines			
Diazepam [Valium, Valrelease]	x		x
Lorazepam [Ativan]	x		x
Cannabinoid			
Dronabinol (delta-9-tetrahydrocannabinol) [Marinol]			x
Corticosteroids			
Dexamethasone‡ [Decadron] Dexamethasone Sodium Phosphate‡ [Decadron Phosphate]	x		x
Methylprednisolone Sodium Succinate [Solu-Medrol]	x		

* *Antiemetics generally are not recommended during pregnancy (see text).*
† *Toxins include metabolic toxins (eg, uremia, hypercalcemia) and other exogenous toxins (eg, microbial, chemicals).*
‡ *Investigational drug or indication*
+, + +, + + + = *relative effectiveness based on available data*
± *equivocal/inconsistent effects*

phenothiazine, it has only weak dopamine antagonist activity, possesses considerable antihistaminic and anticholinergic activity, and, like H_1 antihistamines, its effectiveness in vertigo and motion sickness may be due to its anticholinergic action.

The miscellaneous agents used to prevent or treat vomiting include the corticosteroids, dexamethasone and methylprednisolone, which help control cancer chemotherapy-induced nausea and vomiting by a mechanism that is unclear; the benzodiazepines, diazepam and lorazepam, and the cannabinoid, dronabinol, which inhibit cortical transmission; and diphenidol, trimethobenzamide, and benzquinamide. Diphenidol is thought to act on the aural vestibular apparatus, and the latter two drugs act primarily on the CTZ.

DIZZINESS AND VERTIGO

Complaints of dizziness account for 2.6% of visits to primary care physicians (Bowen, 1993), and almost 30% of patients older than 60 years complain of current or prior episodes of significant dizziness. Extensive diagnostic testing is usually unnecessary, since most causes are benign and the symptom resolves without treatment in about two weeks in approximately one-third of patients. Serious disorders such as cardiovascular disease or tumors rarely cause dizziness, and chronic dizziness is seldom the presenting symptom of these or other serious organic diseases (Kroenke, 1993).

Generally acceptable criteria are not available for diagnosis of many conditions that cause dizziness. Psychiatric disturbances play a significant role as the primary cause or as a major complication that aggravates other causes (Bowen, 1993; Kroenke et al, 1993; Sullivan et al, 1993) in approximately 25% of patients who complain of being dizzy. Estimates of hyperventilation as a cause of dizziness range from 1% to 23% (Bowen, 1993), and no cause can be determined in up to 10% of patients (Kroenke, 1993).

Vertigo (usually of vestibular origin) accounts for approximately 50% of cases of dizziness. In most patients, the disorder is benign and can be managed easily. Careful history and physical examination will usually identify those individuals with more serious disease who require more extensive diagnostic testing. Vertigo related to tumors of the central nervous system, infection, migraine, vascular insufficiency, or diabetes is reduced by correction of the underlying disorder if possible.

The major types of vertigo include true (objective) vertigo and near-syncope (subjective vertigo); the terms "objective" and "subjective" are obsolete. *True vertigo* is associated with a hallucination of movement (commonly, but not exclusively, rotational). Patients may feel that everything is moving while they remain stationary or the reverse; the distinction has no clinical significance. True vertigo can be produced by any lesion or process affecting the brain, the eighth cranial nerve, or the labyrinthine system. Benign positional paroxysmal vertigo caused by a sudden change in body or head position is most common; because of varying definitions of disease and variations in patient populations, its reported prevalence varies from 6.5% to 52%. Other causes of true vertigo (episodic or prolonged) include cerebral ischemia, vestibular or labyrinthine neuronitis, and Meniere's disease. True vertigo also may be associated with migraine headache or hearing loss. Nausea and vomiting are not always present, although they are more likely to be associated with true vertigo rather than near-syncope (see below). The diagnosis (Turner, 1975; Baloh, 1989; Kerr, 1990; Samuels, 1990) and management (String-

PRINCIPAL USES

Vertigo	Motion Sickness	Pregnancy*	Postoperative Emesis	Cancer Chemotherapy	Toxins† Radiation Therapy
			+		+
+	±				
				+	
				+	
				+	+
				+	+

er and Meyerhoff, 1990; Kumar and Petchenik, 1990) of true vertigo, including selection of appropriate drug therapy if indicated, depend on the etiology, rapidity of onset, and character (episodic or prolonged) of the disorder.

Near-syncope is characterized by a feeling of lightheadedness, faintness, or altered consciousness, sometimes associated with a vague sensation of motion described as being within the head. A sensation of unsteadiness (episodic or prolonged) characterizes near-syncope much more than dizziness, although patients may use the latter term to describe their discomfort (Kerr, 1990). Near-syncope may be associated with disorders that result in inadequate blood supply to the cochlea and/or vestibular apparatus (eg, severe anemia, heart block, hypersensitive carotid sinus syndrome, sick sinus syndrome, transient ischemic attack, stroke, trauma). The latter three disorders also may cause true vertigo, depending on the location of the impairment. In addition, near-syncope may be associated with psychiatric disturbances, especially when hyperventilation or panic disorder is present. Some drugs with anticholinergic activity used to treat vertigo may exacerbate near-syncope.

Drug-induced vertigo occurs most frequently after use of agents that damage the eighth nerve (eg, aminoglycoside antibiotics, ethacrynic acid [Edecrin], furosemide [Lasix]) or produce orthostatic hypotension (eg, some antihypertensive agents, phenothiazines).

DRUG SELECTION. Management of the underlying disorder usually is more important than use of antivertigo drugs to treat the patient's discomfort. In many individuals, compensatory mechanisms take effect over time and vertigo resolves without treatment. Drug therapy may interfere with these mechanisms.

Pharmacotherapy has little value in patients with benign positional paroxysmal vertigo; exercise therapy is curative in more than 90% of these individuals (Troost and Patton, 1992).

The value of scopolamine in vertigo is markedly limited by it's side effects, especially those associated with chronic use. The antihistaminic drugs (dimenhydrinate, meclizine, and promethazine) occasionally are beneficial in patients with mild to moderate vertigo (Baloh, 1989; Stringer and Meyerhoff, 1990; Kumar and Petchenik, 1990). If vertigo is severe enough to produce intolerable anxiety or major depression, patients may benefit from the use of antianxiety agents or antidepressants (see index entries Antianxiety Drugs; Mood Disorders, respectively). Diazepam may reduce the anxiety that can accompany vertigo, but care must be taken to avoid drug dependence with chronic use. Its effectiveness is not dependent on its sedative action.

Acute incapacitating vertigo is often treated with intravenous diazepam or fentanyl citrate combined with droperidol [Innovar]; these agents appear to act centrally to block vestibular responses. If severe vomiting is associated with vertigo, antidopaminergic agents or diphenidol may be required. Use of preparations containing droperidol or diphenidol generally is limited to hospitalized patients or closely supervised outpatients because of the potential severity of their adverse effects.

In drug-induced vertigo, withdrawing the offending drug or reducing the dose is preferred to administering labyrinthine suppressants; however, drug withdrawal is not possible in some patients.

Meniere's Disease: In this disorder, an attempt is made to suppress the vestibular symptoms and to treat the underlying pathologic feature of endolymphatic hydrops. The therapeutic efficacy of drugs used to manage vertigo associated with this disorder is difficult to evaluate because spontaneous remission occurs in 60% of patients (Brookes, 1983; Stringer and Meyerhoff, 1990).

Oral diazepam controls symptoms of Meniere's disease in 60% to 70% of patients. In refractory cases, meclizine 25 to 100 mg orally, dimenhydrinate 50 mg orally or intramuscularly, scopolamine hydrobromide 0.6 mg subcutaneously, droperidol 5 mg intravenously, or diazepam 5 to 20 mg *slowly* intravenously may be required. Prochlorperazine 5 to 10 mg orally and cinnarizine 15 to 30 mg orally every eight hours also have been reported to alleviate vertigo resulting from Meniere's disease (Brookes, 1983) (the latter drug is not available in the United States). Dehydration and electrolyte imbalance caused by vomiting should be corrected. Symptoms are relieved in many patients by administration of diuretics and by restriction of salt intake. Patients with vertigo also are usually advised to restrict intake of caffeine, nicotine, and alcohol.

The use of papaverine, histamine, betahistine, and nylidrin and other vasodilators to improve blood flow to the labyrinth and brainstem has temporarily relieved vertigo, tinnitus, and deafness, but their role in symptomatic treatment and in arresting progression of Meniere's disease has not been defined adequately.

VOMITING

Vomiting is a complex reflex that is coordinated by the vomiting center (VC) in the medulla. Stimuli are relayed to this center from peripheral areas (eg, gastric mucosa, peritoneum). Major sensory stimuli also arise within the central nervous system itself (ie, cerebral cortex, otic vestibular apparatus) and may be transmitted through the CTZ sensory nucleus in the medulla to the VC. The VC frequently is stimulated directly. The efferent arc is completed by excitatory impulses transmitted to the salivary glands and the muscles of the diaphragm, anterior abdominal wall, gastric antrum, and duodenum. Inhibitory impulses to the muscles of the gastric fundus, gastroesophageal sphincter, and esophagus arrive simultaneously (Andrews et al, 1988).

Nausea and vomiting may be symptoms of serious organic disturbances of almost any of the viscera of the chest or abdomen or may be produced by infections, neoplasms, drug therapy, radiation, painful or noxious stimuli, metabolic and emotional disturbances (eg, stage fright), exposure to unfamiliar environmental forces, audiovisual-proprioceptive sensory mismatch phenomena (eg, air or ship travel, amusement park rides, prolonged car or train travel, exposure to strong centrifugal forces), or vertigo. Whenever possible, the underlying cause should be corrected. The use of antiemetics is justified only when no alternative therapy exists and the benefits outweigh the risks of adverse reactions or of masking more serious underlying conditions.

In general, drug therapy is more effective for prophylaxis than for treatment of vomiting, especially that caused by motion sickness, radiation, or chemotherapy. Oral dosage forms and adhesive units for transdermal application are most useful for prophylaxis; suppository and parenteral forms are preferred for treatment.

NAUSEA. Unlike vomiting, the mechanism of nausea is poorly understood. Because subemetic doses of emetic agents can cause nausea and nausea usually precedes vomiting, it is possible that nausea represents low-level activation of the vomiting pathway. It is difficult to direct therapy for nausea to any system because of the dearth of understanding of its mechanism. Therapy for vomiting has some effect in relieving nausea, but the effectiveness of treatment for nausea can only be assessed subjectively.

VOMITING ASSOCIATED WITH GASTROENTERITIS. Because nausea and vomiting associated with acute gastroenteritis is self-limited, antiemetics may be required only when intravenous hydration and nutrition, electrolyte replenishment, rest, and fasting do not improve the patient's condition.

VOMITING ASSOCIATED WITH MOTION SICKNESS. Motion sickness includes sea, air, car, and space sickness. Nausea is the most common symptom; other subjective components of the motion sickness syndrome are vomiting, pallor, and cold sweating, which occur on exposure to certain types of real or apparent motion. Tolerance develops in two or three days if the intensity of the stimulus does not increase. The prophylactic use of drugs (usually one to two hours before travel) is more effective than treatment (Ruckenstein and Harrison, 1991).

The most effective single drug for the prophylaxis and treatment of motion sickness is scopolamine. An adhesive unit containing scopolamine [Transderm-Scōp] for placement behind the ear delivers a sufficient dose at a constant rate transdermally to prevent motion sickness in most patients. Although it has been claimed that transdermal delivery decreases the incidence, type, and severity of most side effects (primarily drowsiness, dryness of the mouth, and blurred vision) observed with parenteral scopolamine (Price et al, 1979; Clissold and Heel, 1985), this does not appear to be true (Parrott, 1989). The primary advantages of the transdermal route are ease of administration and prolonged duration of action (72 hours). Disadvantages include delayed onset of action (six to eight hours), increasing visual problems on continuing or repeated use, and the variability of scopolamine's effects on different kinds of motion and in different individuals (Parrott, 1989).

The subcutaneous form of scopolamine may be useful for severe motion sickness of brief duration when only a few small doses are required. Repeated doses may have a cumulative effect or may produce toxicity.

The first-generation antihistamines, buclizine, cyclizine, dimenhydrinate, meclizine, diphenhydramine, promethazine, and hydroxyzine, prevent mild to moderate motion sickness. Thay are less effective than parenteral scopolamine but are available in oral preparations and produce fewer adverse effects; their anticholinergic activity varies. Results of controlled studies comparing transdermal scopolamine with dimenhydrinate found both drugs to be about equally effective, but neither was as effective as subcutaneous scopolamine. The duration of action of antihistamines ranges from four to six hours; the action of meclizine is claimed to persist for 24 hours. The second-generation (nonsedating) antihistamines (eg, terfenadine [Seldane], astemizole [Hismanal]) do not enter the central nervous system and have no value in motion sickness or other conditions associated with nausea and vomiting

Promethazine is the most effective antihistamine for the prophylaxis of moderate to severe motion sickness and also is usually beneficial in the treatment of vomiting associated with this disorder. The considerable sedative action of promethazine and the other first-generation antihistamines may limit their use. However, promethazine has been used by astronauts in the space program.

Dextroamphetamine sulfate and ephedrine sulfate, which appear to potentiate the prophylactic effects of scopolamine, also may be useful in combination with one of the first-generation antihistamines for intense forms of motion or for patients who respond inadequately to transdermal scopolamine or other single-drug therapy (Wood and Graybiel, 1972; Wood, 1979; Wood et al, 1987). However, this use of dextroamphetamine may be legally prohibited. Promethazine is especially useful when combined with ephedrine.

Antidopaminergic phenothiazines may be required for intractable vomiting; they are ineffective in the prophylaxis of motion sickness.

VOMITING DURING PREGNANCY. Drugs should not be used to treat vomiting during pregnancy unless absolutely necessary. Although morning sickness may occur in 50% to 80% of pregnant patients during the sixth to fourteenth weeks of gestation, a very small percentage experience nausea and vomiting of sufficient severity to necessitate antiemetic drug therapy. Nondrug therapy (eg, alteration of diet and time of eating, rest) should always be tried before antiemetics are prescribed. Emetrol (a mixture of fructose, dextrose, and orthophosphoric acid) and cola syrup frequently are employed for morning sickness. However, the use of cola syrup, which contains caffeine, should be avoided during pregnancy. If an antiemetic is necessary, cyclizine or meclizine may be used initially. If persistent vomiting compromises maternal nutrition, promethazine or an antidopaminergic drug (see Table 1) may be considered.

Despite lack of data from controlled studies, claims have been made that pyridoxine (vitamin B_6) is effective in relieving the nausea and vomiting of pregnancy, and it has been used for this purpose for many years. In one double-blind study, significant relief of severe nausea occurred with use of pyridoxine compared with placebo in pregnant women (Sahakian et al, 1991).

POSTOPERATIVE VOMITING. Postoperative vomiting has many causes and thus may be particularly difficult to prevent. The *routine* postoperative use of antiemetics is unwarranted. Their administration to prevent postoperative vomiting is indicated in only a few clinical situations: when vomiting would endanger the results of surgery (eg, intraocular, ear, or oral surgery [when the jaws have been wired together]), in debilitated patients at risk of dehydration or electrolyte imbalance, or when labyrinthine activity is increased, which occurs during almost all ear surgery.

Prochlorperazine, perphenazine, promethazine, benzquinamide, haloperidol, and droperidol are useful for the treatment of postoperative vomiting. In a study comparing intramuscular antiemetics, haloperidol 2 mg, droperidol 5 mg, and prochlorperazine 10 mg all had a significant antiemetic effect but differed in onset and duration of action. Both haloperidol and prochlorperazine became effective within 30 minutes and had a duration of four hours; droperidol reached peak effectiveness in three to four hours and the antiemetic effect lasted 24 hours (Loeser et al, 1979).

Although droperidol is very effective for postoperative vomiting, it probably should be reserved for preoperative prophylaxis because of the disturbing mental effects that sometimes occur during the recovery period when doses greater than 5 mg are used. Droperidol, promethazine, prochlorperazine, or benzquinamide usually is administered to patients undergoing ear surgery. Some physicians use promethazine or hydroxyzine for preoperative medication in patients with a history of nausea and vomiting after general anesthesia.

Ondansetron is effective, safe, and well tolerated in the prophylaxis and treatment of vomiting associated with surgery (Leeser and Lip, 1991; Dershwitz et al, 1992; *FDC Reports*, 1992; Woodward and Gora, 1993) and radiation therapy (Priestman et al, 1990); thus, it is now preferred by many practitioners because the adverse reactions of the other agents used for this purpose are poorly tolerated by many patients.

VOMITING ASSOCIATED WITH CANCER CHEMOTHERAPY. Nausea and vomiting are major adverse reactions in patients receiving cancer chemotherapy; when severe, they can cause dehydration, anorexia, malnutrition, or esophageal tears and may lead to discontinuation of chemotherapy.

The mechanism(s) by which antineoplastic agents induce nausea and vomiting is not well understood. The existence of an emetic reflex arc has been hypothesized to explain chemotherapy-induced emesis and the action of antiemetic agents (Gralla, 1991; Hesketh and Gandara, 1991). Neuroreceptors in the emetic reflex arc have been identified in the VC, which is located in the lateral reticular formation of the medulla and coordinates the act of vomiting. In chemotherapy-induced emesis, predominant sources of sensory input to the VC include the CTZ, cerebral cortex, and afferent vagal impulses from the gastrointestinal tract. The CTZ also is located in the medulla in the area postrema and is an important relay station in the reflex arc. The CTZ is sensitive to chemical stimuli from both blood and cerebrospinal fluid. Chemotherapeutic agents that produce vomiting or their metabolites stimulate CTZ receptors; these in turn generate impulses to the VC that initiate vomiting. Emetic chemical irritants also stimulate enterochromaffin cells in the intestinal mucosa; these cells are the primary storage sites for serotonin.

Serotonin (5-hydroxytryptamine [5-HT]) receptors in the central and peripheral nervous systems are believed to be involved in the emetic response. Neurons in the VC and CTZ, as well as in the enterochromaffin cells, release large amounts of serotonin during the first two to three hours after chemotherapy; the released serotonin acts as a neurotransmitter to initiate vomiting. For these reasons, serotonin blockade has received increasing attention as a mechanism to prevent or treat nausea and vomiting in patients receiving emetogenic drugs.

Acute vomiting refers to episodes that occur within the first 24 hours after chemotherapy. Episodes that begin 24 to 120 hours following chemotherapy (peak incidence, 48 to 72 hours) are referred to as delayed vomiting (Tortorice and O'Connell, 1990). Delayed vomiting is usually less severe but

TABLE 2.
EMETIC POTENTIAL OF ANTINEOPLASTIC DRUGS

High (>90%)	Moderately High (60%-90%)	Moderate (30%-60%)	Moderately Low (10%-30%)	Low (<10%)
Cisplatin	Semustine	Fluorouracil	Bleomycin	Busulfan
Dacarbazine	Carmustine	Doxorubicin	Hydroxyurea	Chlorambucil
Mechlorethamine	Lomustine	Daunorubicin	Melphalan	Thioguanine
Streptozotocin	Cyclophosphamide	Asparaginase	Etoposide	Vincristine
Cytarabine[1]	Dactinomycin	Mitomycin	Cytarabine[3]	Estrogens
	Plicamycin	Azacitidine	Mercaptopurine	Progestins
	Procarbazine	Hexamethylmelamine	Methotrexate[3]	Corticosteroids
	Methotrexate[2]	Carboplatin	Thiotepa	Androgens
			Vinblastine	
			Ifosfamide	
			Mitoxantrone	

From Tortorice and O'Connell, 1990. Reprinted with permission.
[1]*High-dose therapy (>500 mg/M²)*
[2]*High-dose therapy (>200 mg/M²)*
[3]*Standard or low-dose therapy*

also is less responsive to drug therapy. Complete control of an episode of acute vomiting does not preclude the subsequent occurrence of delayed vomiting.

Vomiting often develops within 1.5 to 3.5 hours after administration of emetogenic antineoplastic drugs in previously untreated patients; however, episodes may occur later (Borison and McCarthy, 1983) with cyclophosphamide (9 to 18 hours) (Fetting et al, 1982) and carboplatin (6 to 10 hours) (Harvey et al, 1991). This delay suggests that drug metabolites or cellular material released as a result of tissue toxicity may be partly responsible.

A number of patient characteristics determine the likelihood of nausea and vomiting and the pattern of antiemetic-related adverse effects following administration of antineoplastic agents (Gralla et al, 1987; Morrow, 1989; Grunberg and Hesketh, 1993): (1) A history of heavy alcohol intake enhances the response to antiemetic drugs. (2) Prior exposure to antineoplastic agents, particularly if associated with poor response to antiemetic drugs, increases the likelihood of nausea and vomiting. (3) Susceptibility to motion sickness increases the incidence of nausea and vomiting. (4) The incidence of anticipatory nausea and vomiting may be increased in younger patients. (5) Dystonic reactions are more likely to occur in younger patients (<30 years old) receiving dopamine antagonists. (6) Males are more responsive to antiemetic drug therapy than females.

Antiemetics are indicated to prevent medical complications (esophageal tearing [Mallory-Weiss syndrome], anorexia, malnutrition, dehydration), to alleviate patient discomfort, and to improve compliance with therapy and overall quality of life. They are more useful prophylactically than in the treatment of vomiting. The response to prophylactic therapy, for the most part, depends on (1) the effectiveness of the antiemetic agents and (2) the emetogenic potential of the antineoplastic agents (see Table 2); when less emetogenic agents are used in combination, they may have the emetogenic potential of monotherapy with a highly emetogenic agent.

Effective management of vomiting also should consider the patient's physiologic condition (eg, maintenance of hydration); provide emotional support; and, possibly, utilize behavioral relaxation techniques, especially for anticipatory nausea and vomiting (Triozzi and Laszlo, 1987; Gralla et al, 1987; Morrow, 1989; Cotanch, 1991; Morrow et al, 1991).

DRUG SELECTION FOR CHEMOTHERAPY-INDUCED EMESIS. The primary agents used for the management of nausea and vomiting associated with cancer chemotherapy are the 5-HT_3 receptor antagonists (ondansetron, granisetron), metoclopramide, dexamethasone, phenothiazines (prochlorperazine), droperidol, lorazepam, and dronabinol. The complex nature of the sensory and stimulatory input underlying chemotherapy-induced nausea and vomiting and the large number of different steps in the reflex nausea and vomiting pathway susceptible to emetogenic stimuli may explain why single-agent antiemetic therapy usually provides incomplete relief. Antiemetics with different mechanisms of action, such as dopamine antagonists (eg, metoclopramide, phenothiazines, butyrophenones) or 5-HT_3 receptor antagonists in combination with corticosteroids (eg, methylprednisolone, dexamethasone) and/or antihistamines (eg, promethazine, diphenhydramine), generally are more effective than single agents in preventing and treating chemotherapy-induced nausea and vomiting (Merrifield and Chaffee, 1989; Tortorice and O'Connell, 1990; Gralla, 1991; Smith et al, 1991; Roila et al, 1991; Latreille et al, 1993).

Highly Emetogenic Antineoplastic Drug Regimens: In controlled trials conducted prior to the availability of the 5-HT_3 receptor antagonists, the most active single drug in preventing acute nausea and vomiting in patients receiving cisplatin was high-dose intravenous metoclopramide (1 to 3 mg/kg), which prevents vomiting completely in approximately 40% of patients (Gralla et al, 1981, 1984). However, single-drug therapy is often inadequate, and combination therapy is necessary for more complete protection in the majority of patients receiving cisplatin alone, cisplatin in combination with other drugs (Gralla, 1983; Strum et al, 1982; Eyre and Ward, 1984; Kris et al, 1985; Sridhar and Donnelly, 1988; Graves, 1991; Gralla, 1991), and moderate to highly emetogenic regimens not containing cisplatin (Fortner et al, 1985; Strum et al, 1984, 1985). Prior to the introduction of the 5-HT_3 receptor antagonists, the most useful combinations included high-dose metoclopramide, dexamethasone, and either diphenhydramine or lorazepam.

The concurrent administration of metoclopramide and intravenous dexamethasone afforded complete protection in more than 60% of patients receiving high-dose cisplatin. Although nausea and vomiting were substantially reduced in some of the remaining patients, a significant number (more than 30%) continued to experience an unacceptable degree of vomiting. In controlled trials, most patients preferred this combination to metoclopramide alone (Cersosimo and Karp, 1986; Allan et al, 1984; Kris et al, 1985; Strum et al, 1985). Diphenhydramine often is added to this antiemetic regimen to prevent metoclopramide-induced extrapyramidal reactions (Sridhar and Donnelly, 1988). Some authorities believe diphenhydramine enhances the antiemetic effect of high-dose metoclopramide/dexamethasone in addition to reducing the incidence of extrapyramidal reactions. Diazepam, lorazepam, or benztropine also rapidly reverse extrapyramidal reactions; however, there is little clinical experience with diazepam. Lorazepam is regarded by a number of oncologists (and by more than 90% of treated patients) as a useful adjunct to the metoclopramide/dexamethasone regimen (Kris et al, 1987; Merrifield and Chaffee, 1989). It produces antegrade amnesia that lasts four to six hours, and this ability to diminish or prevent the recall of chemotherapy apparently is the basis for patient acceptance. Lorazepam also can eliminate the need for diphenhydramine (Tortorice and O'Connell, 1990); intravenous doses greater than 1.5 mg/M^2 can prevent akathisia in patients taking dopamine antagonists (Laszlo et al, 1985; Kris et al, 1987). For specific doses and the schedule of administration employed with an intravenous regimen containing metoclopramide, dexamethasone, and either diphenhydramine or lorazepam, see the evaluation of Metoclopramide.

The 5-HT_3 receptor antagonists appear to be effective and safe in the control of acute cisplatin-induced nausea and vomiting and have now replaced metoclopramide as drugs of choice in both single-drug and combination therapy in patients receiving highly emetogenic regimens. In contrast to use of metoclopramide, adverse reactions have been mild and transient and extrapyramidal reactions have not occurred with these drugs (Hesketh et al, 1989; Kris et al, 1989 A; Plosker and Goa, 1991). The addition of dexamethasone significantly increases the efficacy of these agents (Cunningham et al, 1989; Smith et al, 1990, 1991; Roila et al, 1991); other drugs such as lorazepam and/or diphenhydramine are not needed. For specific doses and schedules suggested for combination therapy with ondansetron and dexamethasone, see the evaluation on Dexamethasone.

The results of animal and clinical studies suggest that the investigational 5-HT_3 receptor antagonists, tropisetron, bemesetron, and dolasetron, have actions, indications, and adverse reactions generally similar to those of ondansetron and granisetron (Merrifield and Chaffee, 1989; Plosker and Goa, 1991; Hunter-Johnson, 1991; Wade-Evans, 1991; Hesketh and Gandara, 1991; Madej et al, 1993).

Two investigational substituted benzamides, alizapride and clebopride, have been evaluated in clinical trials. Like metoclopramide, these agents produce extrapyramidal reactions; it is unclear if they offer any advantages over presently available therapy. A third substituted benzamide, batanopride, also appears to block serotonin receptors. This investigational agent does not bind to dopamine receptors and does not produce dystonic reactions; however, the occurrence of dose-related hypotension has limited interest in the drug's development (Gralla, 1992).

The usual recommended dose of prochlorperazine (10 mg given orally or intramuscularly every four to six hours) is considered by most authorities to provide the greatest antiemetic effect of the phenothiazines. For a discussion on use of high-dose intravenous prochlorperazine (40 mg), see the evaluation.

Intravenous butyrophenones (haloperidol and droperidol) are less effective than metoclopramide for acute cisplatin-induced nausea and vomiting (Saller and Hellenbrecht, 1986) but can provide complete protection in some patients (30% with haloperidol) (Neidhart et al, 1981; Wilson et al, 1981; Grunberg et al, 1984). There is less experience with intravenous butyrophenone/dexamethasone combinations than with metoclopramide/dexamethasone regimens. In one study, the combination of metoclopramide, dexamethasone, droperidol, and diphenhydramine was highly efficacious in preventing nausea and vomiting in high-dose cisplatin chemotherapy, and toxicity was negligible (Sridhar and Donnelly, 1988).

Dronabinol has limited activity against cisplatin-induced vomiting and is less effective than high-dose metoclopramide (Gralla et al, 1984).

Domperidone has been investigated to alleviate nausea and vomiting induced by a variety of chemotherapeutic combinations, including those containing cisplatin (Brogden et al, 1982; Triozzi and Laszlo, 1987); however, interest in its use for this purpose is waning (see the evaluation).

Moderately to Mildly Emetogenic Antineoplastic Drug Regimens: Useful prophylactic agents for acute nausea and vomiting induced by mildly or moderately emetogenic agents include phenothiazines, ondansetron, granisetron, butyrophenones, metoclopramide, dronabinol, and dexamethasone.

Phenothiazines (prochlorperazine, thiethylperazine) are most commonly used, but few patients prefer them to other effective agents (Markman et al, 1984). Intravenous dexamethasone followed by oral administration is more effective than low-dose prochlorperazine; more than two-thirds of patients were completely protected from nausea and vomiting (Markman et al, 1984).

The role of 5-HT_3 receptor antagonists in relieving nausea and vomiting induced by moderately emetogenic agents is unclear. In some trials, ondansetron had no greater efficacy than dexamethasone (Jones et al, 1991; *Lancet*, 1991). In two studies (one of which was open-label) in patients receiving a regimen containing cyclophosphamide, oral ondansetron had significantly more antiemetic activity than placebo

(Beck et al, 1993; Fraschini et al, 1991). Ondansetron also was effective in patients receiving carboplatin or doxorubicin combination regimens who had been refractory to antiemetic combinations containing metoclopramide (Mitchell et al, 1992). The efficacy of ondansetron or granisetron in moderately emetogenic chemotherapeutic regimens has been supported by the results of other studies (Marty et al, 1990 A; Warr et al, 1991; Jantunen et al, 1993), and use of ondansetron plus a phenothiazine may be beneficial in these patients (Herrstedt et al, 1993).

In clinical trials, the antiemetic activity of the antihistamines, cyclizine and cinnarizine (investigational agent), was inadequate (Morran et al, 1979; Moertel et al, 1963). Although meclizine and dimenhydrinate have not been thoroughly studied, most oncologists consider them ineffective.

Delayed Nausea and Vomiting: Delayed emesis can occur with a number of antineoplastic drugs and is common 48 to 72 hours after administration of cisplatin in doses >90 mg/M². Therapy should be designed to protect patients at times when the delayed effect occurs. Antiemetics are used orally for prophylaxis. Combinations of metoclopramide/dexamethasone and prochlorperazine/dexamethasone have provided a high degree of protection in a regimen continued for four to six days (Strum et al, 1985; Kris et al, 1989 B; Gralla, 1991). For one recommended regimen employing metoclopramide/dexamethasone to prevent delayed nausea and vomiting in patients receiving high-dose cisplatin, see the evaluation on Metoclopramide.

Although ondansetron is safer than metoclopramide, initial studies indicated that it may not be more effective than the latter for delayed nausea and vomiting. Some investigators postulated that the mechanism responsible for delayed nausea and vomiting may differ from that for acute nausea and vomiting and that serotonin receptors may not play a predominant role. However, in more recent studies in patients treated with regimens containing cyclophosphamide, ondansetron alone was very effective in preventing delayed emesis (Beck et al, 1993); moreover, the combined use of dexamethasone and ondansetron probably will increase the efficacy of the latter for delayed effects experienced with a number of emetogenic cancer chemotherapeutic regimens (*Lancet*, 1991; Plosker, 1992; Navari et al, 1993). The addition of prophylactic doses of prochlorperazine to ondansetron/dexamethasone may provide further control (Navari et al, 1993). The value of combinations containing ondansetron for cisplatin-induced delayed nausea and vomiting is being investigated.

Anticipatory Nausea and Vomiting: With repeated cycles of chemotherapy, patients may experience nausea and vomiting before the administration of chemotherapeutic drugs. This is a conditioned response in individuals who responded poorly to antiemetic drugs during previous exposure to chemotherapy. The onset of emesis may be triggered by the hospital environment or any treatment-related association (eg, sight, smell, touch, sound).

Prevention of anticipatory emesis is more successful than treatment. Aggressive prophylactic therapy with antiemetic agents, which prevents the initial episode of nausea and vomiting, and lorazepam can inhibit the development of anticipatory emesis (Gralla et al, 1987; Morrow, 1989). Nonpharmacologic behavioral therapy, such as hypnosis and deep muscle relaxation, have been investigated; the latter technique can be useful (Morrow, 1989; Cotanch, 1991; Morrow et al, 1991).

ADVERSE REACTIONS AND PRECAUTIONS

Caution is required with use of all antiemetics because they may mask the symptoms of organic disease (eg, gastrointestinal or central nervous system disorders) or the toxic effects of other drugs. Because the actions of other central nervous system depressants may be potentiated, individuals receiving antiemetic drugs should be cautioned about activities that require alertness, such as operating vehicles or machinery. Antiemetic agents that cause significant sedation may increase the risk of pulmonary aspiration.

Concomitant use of agents that exacerbate nausea and vomiting (eg, beta-adrenergic agonists, opioids) generally should be avoided in patients receiving antiemetics. However, opioids should be continued in patients who require these agents for relief of pain.

Although it may be wise to avoid concurrent administration of metoclopramide with other dopamine antagonists (eg, phenothiazines, butyrophenones) to prevent additive dystonic reactions (*Med Lett Drugs Ther*, 1988), such combinations are probably safe if diphenhydramine, benztropine, or lorazepam is included in the regimen (Sridhar and Donnelly, 1988).

ANTICHOLINERGIC AND ANTIHISTAMINIC DRUGS. Drowsiness is the most common untoward effect observed with these agents; anticholinergic side effects also may be anticipated, even with the antihistamines. Promethazine [Phenergan] is relatively free of the extrapyramidal reactions observed with the phenothiazines and other antidopaminergic drugs.

Buclizine, cyclizine, hydroxyzine, and meclizine are teratogenic in animals when given in very large doses. After review of the existing epidemiologic data on pregnant women, the Food and Drug Administration concluded that these data do not support a restriction on the use of meclizine or cyclizine or a pregnancy warning (*Federal Register,* 1979). (See also index entry Pregnancy, Adverse Drug Reactions During.)

ANTIDOPAMINERGIC DRUGS. The incidence of reactions is quite low when phenothiazines are used as antiemetics, since the duration of administration is short and the dosage relatively small. Phenothiazines in the piperazine group (fluphenazine, perphenazine, prochlorperazine, and thiethylperazine) are less likely to cause drowsiness, orthostatic hypotension, dryness of the mouth, and nasal congestion than those in the aliphatic group (chlorpromazine, promazine, and triflupromazine). Cholestatic jaundice, urticaria, dermatitis, thrombocytopenia, galactorrhea, edema of the extremities, purpura, and gastroenteritis have occurred after use of all phenothiazines. Photosensitivity is less common. Rarely observed adverse reactions include granulocytopenia, leukopenia, agranulocytosis, and pancytopenia.

Phenothiazines lower the seizure threshold; they should be used cautiously in patients with brain metastases who are receiving chemotherapy.

Extrapyramidal reactions, including akathisia, dystonia, parkinsonian syndrome, and dysarthria, have been associated with use of all phenothiazines, the butyrophenones, and metoclopramide, and they may occur after a single dose. Their incidence is higher with phenothiazines in the piperazine group than with those in the aliphatic group. In patients treated with the butyrophenones, the incidence of extrapyramidal reactions may be relatively high with larger doses (Morrow, 1989). The most common extrapyramidal adverse effects produced by short-term therapy with antidopaminergic drugs are dystonic reactions, which are usually rapidly reversed by parenteral administration of diphenhydramine, benztropine (Morrow, 1989; Gralla et al, 1987), or lorazepam.

The extrapyramidal symptoms and signs that may occur, particularly after parenteral administration of large doses, may be confused with the central nervous system signs of an undiagnosed primary disease responsible for the vomiting (eg, Reye's syndrome, other encephalopathy, brain metastases). Thus, use of these drugs and other hepatotoxic agents should be avoided in children and adolescents with signs and symptoms suggesting Reye's syndrome.

Phenothiazines are contraindicated in patients with a history of hypersensitivity to any phenothiazine. Although they are usually contraindicated in patients with bone marrow depression, which is a common consequence of chemotherapy, their intermittent administration to prevent vomiting due to cancer chemotherapy should not be precluded on this basis. Phenothiazines should be used with caution in individuals with a history of dyskinetic reactions and, since these drugs are detoxified primarily in the liver, in those with moderate to severe hepatic dysfunction. Patients with severe pulmonary disorders should not receive these agents.

The action of phenothiazines and butyrophenones may be potentiated if other central nervous system depressants are used concomitantly. Sedation may be desirable in some patients (eg, those with malignancies) but undesirable in others. Phenothiazines are contraindicated when marked central nervous system depression or hypotension is present. They also may augment the fall in blood pressure when given to patients receiving spinal or epidural anesthesia or adrenergic blocking agents. Caution should be used in pregnant women with pre-eclampsia, since some of these patients have labile blood pressure and may experience a significant fall in pressure. See also index entry Antipsychotic Drugs and the evaluation on Haloperidol.

ANTISEROTONINERGIC DRUGS. Adverse reactions produced by the 5-HT_3 receptor antagonists are generally mild and well tolerated. In most clinical trials, these agents caused headache; the incidence of other adverse reactions was similar to that reported with placebo. Extrapyramidal adverse reactions have been reported rarely but are not clearly documented (Chaffee and Tankanow, 1991; Plosker and Goa, 1991). See the evaluations on Ondansetron and Granisetron for additional information.

MISCELLANEOUS DRUGS. See the evaluations.

Drug Evaluations

SCOPOLAMINE
[Transderm-Scōp]

SCOPOLAMINE HYDROBROMIDE

$Br^- \cdot 3H_2O$

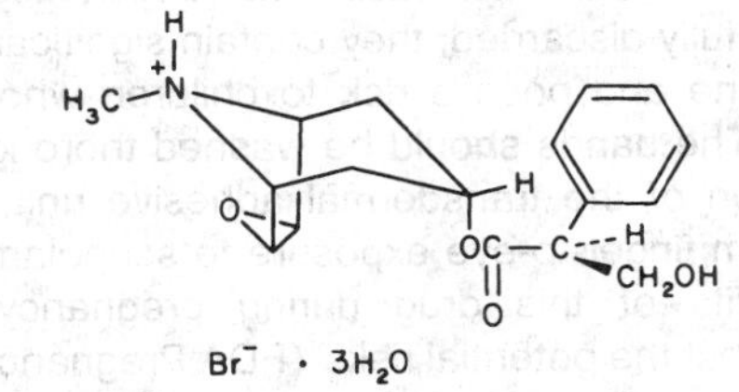

ACTIONS AND USES. Scopolamine is the most effective single agent for motion sickness, especially when it is given subcutaneously and the disorder is severe and of brief duration. This drug acts primarily by reducing the excitability of the labyrinthine receptors and by depressing conduction in the vestibular cerebellar pathway.

When the transdermal adhesive unit is applied postauricularly, scopolamine is released at a uniform rate for 72 hours, which protects most individuals susceptible to motion sickness. However, there is some evidence to suggest that the therapeutic effect of this system of delivery decreases before 72 hours in some individuals. The chief advantages of transdermal administration are ease of administration and prolonged duration of action. Disadvantages include the slow onset of action (six to eight hours), increasing visual problems with continuing or repeated use, and variability of effects for different kinds of motion and different individuals (Parrott, 1989; Clissold and Heel, 1985).

The effect of scopolamine is enhanced when ephedrine sulfate, dextroamphetamine sulfate, or promethazine is given concomitantly; however, these combinations are indicated only for intense conditions of motion (eg, storms at sea, aerobatics, severe rotary experimental circumstances) or for patients who respond inadequately to transdermal scopolamine or other single-drug therapy (Wood and Graybiel, 1972). Furthermore, the use of dextroamphetamine with scopolamine may be legally prohibited.

Scopolamine hydrobromide also has been used to prevent postoperative nausea and vomiting (see index entry Scopolamine, As Anesthetic Premedication), and transdermal scopolamine is superior to placebo in reducing the number of vertigo attacks.

ADVERSE REACTIONS AND PRECAUTIONS. Anticholinergic side effects (blurred vision, mydriasis, dryness of the mouth, changes in pulse rate, drowsiness, amnesia, and fatigue) often occur with use of scopolamine, especially in large doses. Less frequent but more severe effects (urinary retention, constipation, disorientation) may develop, especially in children and elderly patients. Scopolamine should not be used in patients with glaucoma and should be used cautiously in those with prostatic enlargement.

Although it has been claimed that transdermal administration is associated with fewer and milder adverse reactions than other routes of administration, this does not appear to be true (Parrott, 1989). A toxic psychosis consisting of excitement, restlessness, hallucinations, or delirium occurs infrequently. The transdermal form of scopolamine should be avoided in children because the dose delivered by this system may produce serious intoxication. Moreover, used patches must be carefully discarded; they contain significant amounts of scopolamine and pose a risk to children who handle or chew them. The hands should be washed thoroughly following application of the transdermal adhesive unit to prevent mydriasis from finger-to-eye exposure to scopolamine.

The benefits of this drug during pregnancy must be weighed against the potential risks (FDA Pregnancy Category C).

DOSAGE AND PREPARATIONS.

SCOPOLAMINE:

Topical: *Adults,* one transdermal adhesive unit is applied to clean dry skin in the postauricular area six to eight hours before antiemetic protection is required. The unit delivers 1.5 mg over a period of 72 hours. This system is not suitable for use in *children* and may not be suitable for use in *elderly patients.*

Transderm-Scōp (CIBA). Adhesive unit 2.5 cm^2 containing 1.5 mg scopolamine.

SCOPOLAMINE HYDROBROMIDE:

Subcutaneous: *Adults,* for prevention and treatment of motion sickness, initially, 0.6 mg, then 0.3 mg every six hours if required; *children,* 0.006 mg/kg.

Generic. Solution 0.3, 0.4, and 1 mg/ml in 1 ml containers.

ANTIHISTAMINIC DRUGS

BUCLIZINE HYDROCHLORIDE

[Bucladin-S]

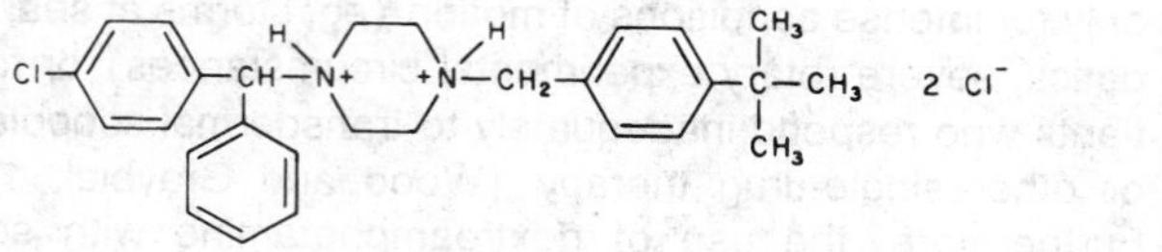

USES. Buclizine, a piperazine antihistamine, is useful in preventing motion sickness; controlled studies are insufficient to evaluate its effectiveness in vertigo. The duration of action is four to six hours.

ADVERSE REACTIONS AND PRECAUTIONS. Drowsiness, dryness of the mouth, headache, and agitation may occur. Buclizine is contraindicated during early pregnancy; see the Introduction for a discussion of the drug's teratogenic effects in animals. This product contains tartrazine, which may cause allergic-type reactions (including bronchial asthma) in susceptible individuals.

DOSAGE AND PREPARATIONS.

Oral: For motion sickness, *adults,* 50 mg at least one-half hour before departure and four to six hours later, if necessary. For vertigo, the usual dosage that has been given is 50 mg twice daily. *Children,* dosage has not been established.

Bucladin-S Softab (Stuart). Tablets (chewable) 50 mg.

CYCLIZINE HYDROCHLORIDE

[Marezine]

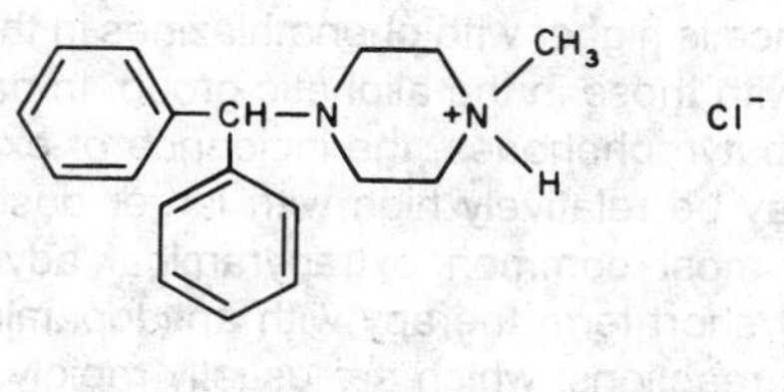

USES. Cyclizine prevents and relieves motion sickness, vertigo, and symptoms of aural vestibular disorders. The duration of action is about four hours. Cyclizine generally does not relieve vomiting associated with cancer chemotherapeutic agents (Morran et al, 1979).

ADVERSE REACTIONS AND PRECAUTIONS. Recommended doses may cause drowsiness and dryness of the mouth. In a large-scale study that included pregnant women who received cyclizine during the first trimester, no teratogenic effects were demonstrated with the doses employed (Milkovich and van den Berg, 1976). After review of the existing epidemiologic data on pregnant women, the Food and Drug Administration concluded that these data do not support a restriction on the use of cyclizine or a pregnancy warning (*Federal Register,* 1979). This drug is classified in FDA Pregnancy Category B.

DOSAGE AND PREPARATIONS.

Oral: For motion sickness, *adults,* 50 mg one-half hour before departure, then every four to six hours as necessary (maximum, 200 mg daily); *children 6 to 10 years,* 3 mg/kg divided into three doses during a 24-hour period.

Marezine (Himmel). Tablets 50 mg (nonprescription).

DIMENHYDRINATE

[Dramamine]

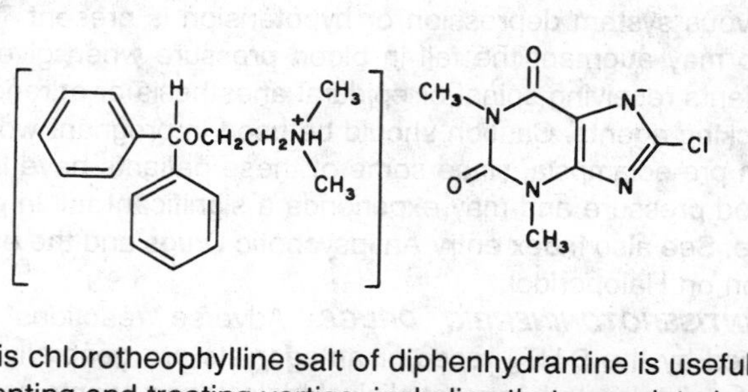

This chlorotheophylline salt of diphenhydramine is useful in preventing and treating vertigo, including that associated with Meniere's disease, and motion sickness; it also is effective in nausea and vomiting during pregnancy. The duration of action is four to six hours. As with other antihistamines, dimenhydrinate generally is ineffective in relieving nausea and vomiting induced by cancer chemotherapeutic agents.

Marked drowsiness may occur. Dimenhydrinate is classified in FDA Pregnancy Category B.

DOSAGE AND PREPARATIONS.
Intramuscular: *Adults,* 50 mg every three to four hours as needed; *children,* 1 to 1.5 mg/kg every six hours (maximum, 300 mg/day).
Intravenous: *Adults,* 50 mg diluted in 10 ml of sodium chloride injection administered over a period of two minutes; *children,* no dosage has been established.

Generic. Solution 50 mg/ml in 1 and 10 ml containers.

Oral: *Adults,* 50 to 100 mg every four to six hours (maximum, 400 mg/day); *children 2 to 6 years,* 12.5 to 25 mg every six to eight hours (maximum, 75 mg/day); *6 to 12 years,* 25 to 50 mg every six to eight hours (maximum, 150 mg/day).

Generic. Liquid 12.5 mg/5 ml; tablets 50 mg (both forms nonprescription).

Dramamine (Upjohn). Liquid 12.5 mg/5 ml (alcohol 5%); tablets (plain, chewable) 50 mg (all forms nonprescription).

DIPHENHYDRAMINE HYDROCHLORIDE
[Benadryl]

For chemical formula, see index entry Diphenhydramine, As Antihistamine.

USES. This antihistamine has actions similar to those of cyclizine. It is effective in the prevention and treatment of vertigo, motion sickness, and nausea and vomiting during pregnancy. When given intravenously, it is a drug of choice for the treatment of dystonic reactions induced by the dopaminergic blocking agents used as antiemetics because of its high degree of effectiveness. Primarily for this reason, it has become a component of antiemetic regimens containing metoclopramide. Diphenhydramine is not effective in relieving akathisia. The duration of action is four to six hours.

ADVERSE REACTIONS AND PRECAUTIONS. In recommended doses, the incidence of drowsiness is high. Individuals whose activities require alertness, such as those operating vehicles or machinery, should not use diphenhydramine.

This drug is classified in FDA Pregnancy Category B.

DOSAGE AND PREPARATIONS.
Intramuscular (deep), Intravenous: *Adults,* 10 mg initially; if sedation is not severe, the subsequent dose may be increased to 20 to 50 mg every two or three hours (maximum, 400 mg/day). For dystonic reactions (oculogyric crises, torticollis) produced by phenothiazines, butyrophenones, and metoclopramide, 50 mg is administered intravenously over two to three minutes. When used with metoclopramide and dexamethasone in antineoplastic regimens containing cisplatin, this dose is given 30 to 40 minutes prior to chemotherapy and can be repeated in four hours.
Intramuscular (deep): *Children,* 1 to 1.5 mg/kg every six hours (maximum, 300 mg/day).

Generic. Solution 10 mg/ml in 30 ml containers and 50 mg/ml in 1 and 10 ml containers.

Benadryl (Parke-Davis). Solution (sterile) 10 mg/ml in 10 and 30 ml containers and 50 mg/ml in 1 and 10 ml containers.

Oral: For motion sickness, *adults,* 50 mg one-half hour before departure and 50 mg before each meal; *children,* 1 to 1.5 mg/kg every six hours (maximum, 300 mg/day).

Generic. Capsules and tablets 25 and 50 mg; elixir and syrup 12.5 mg/5 ml.

Benadryl (Parke-Davis). Capsules 25 and 50 mg; elixir 12.5 mg/5 ml (alcohol 14%).

(Some oral preparations may be nonprescription depending on manufacturer's labeling.)

HYDROXYZINE HYDROCHLORIDE
[Atarax, Vistaril]

HYDROXYZINE PAMOATE
[Vistaril]

For chemical formula, see index entry Hydroxyzine, As Antihistamine.

Hydroxyzine has reduced nausea and vomiting when given intramuscularly after induction of anesthesia (McKenzie et al, 1981). It also is useful for the treatment of motion sickness and, possibly, vertigo. The duration of action is four to six hours. The incidence of drowsiness is low.

Hydroxyzine potentiates the central nervous system depressant actions of opioids and barbiturates; therefore, when hydroxyzine is used concurrently, the dose of these drugs should be individualized (usually reduced by 50% or more). It was demonstrated in one study that hydroxyzine enhances opioid analgesia (Beaver and Feise, 1976), which allows reduction of the opioid dosage, but this finding is not universally accepted.

Very large doses of hydroxyzine are teratogenic in animals.

DOSAGE AND PREPARATIONS.
Intramuscular: To reduce postoperative vomiting, *adults,* 25 to 100 mg; *children,* 1 mg/kg, repeated every six hours if necessary.

HYDROXYZINE HYDROCHLORIDE:
Generic. Solution 25 and 50 mg/ml in 1, 2, and 10 ml containers.
Vistaril (Roerig). Solution 25 mg/ml in 10 ml containers and 50 mg/ml in 1 and 2 ml unit-dose and 10 ml containers.

Oral: *Adults,* 25 to 100 mg three or four times daily; *children under 6 years,* 12.5 mg every six hours; *over 6 years,* 12.5 to 25 mg every six hours.

HYDROXYZINE HYDROCHLORIDE:
Atarax (Roerig), ***Generic.*** Syrup 10 mg/5 ml (alcohol 0.5%); tablets 10, 25, 50, and 100 mg.

HYDROXYZINE PAMOATE:
Generic. Capsules 25, 50, and 100 mg.
Vistaril (Pfizer). Capsules 25, 50, and 100 mg; suspension 25 mg/5 ml (strengths expressed in terms of the hydrochloride salt).

MECLIZINE HYDROCHLORIDE
[Antivert, Bonine, Dramamine II]

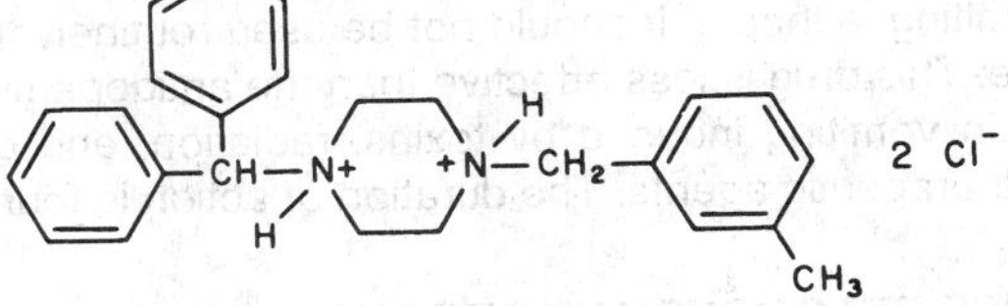

Cl
CH—N+ H
H +N—CH₂
2 Cl⁻
CH₃

USES. Meclizine is effective in preventing and treating motion sickness. It has a slower onset and longer duration of action

(24 hours) than most other antihistamines used for motion sickness. Meclizine also is one of the most useful antiemetics to prevent and treat nausea and vomiting associated with vertigo of vestibular origin (eg, labyrinthitis, Meniere's disease) and occasionally prevents vomiting associated with radiation sickness. It helps alleviate nausea and vomiting associated with pregnancy when conservative measures are ineffective (see the Introduction).

ADVERSE REACTIONS AND PRECAUTIONS. Drowsiness, blurred vision, dryness of the mouth, and fatigue have occurred following administration of this drug. After review of the existing epidemiologic data on pregnant women, the Food and Drug Administration concluded that these data do not support a restriction on use of meclizine or a pregnancy warning (*Federal Register,* 1979) (FDA Pregnancy Category B).

DOSAGE AND PREPARATIONS.

Oral: *Adults,* for motion sickness, 25 to 50 mg once daily; the initial dose should be taken one hour prior to departure. For vertigo and radiation sickness, 25 to 100 mg daily in divided doses, depending on clinical response. *Children,* dosage has not been established.

Antivert (Roerig), ***Generic.*** Tablets 12.5, 25, and 50 mg; tablets (chewable) 25 mg. (Generic preparations may be nonprescription depending on manufacturers' labeling.)

Bonine (Roerig). Tablets (plain, chewable) 25 mg (nonprescription).

Dramamine II (Upjohn). Tablets 25 mg (nonprescription).

PROMETHAZINE HYDROCHLORIDE
[Phenergan]

ACTIONS AND USES. Unlike other phenothiazines, promethazine has pronounced antihistaminic activity in addition to strong central cholinergic blocking activity. It is effective in the prevention and treatment of vertigo and motion sickness but has limited, if any, effect on vomiting caused by stimulation of the chemoreceptor trigger zone. The central cholinergic blocking action may account for promethazine's effectiveness in motion sickness. Results of controlled studies in individuals subjected to severe motion indicate that a synergistic effect occurs when promethazine 25 mg is combined with ephedrine 12.5 mg (Wood, 1979).

Promethazine is useful in preventing postoperative nausea and vomiting, although it should not be used routinely for this purpose. This drug is less effective than the antidopaminergic agents in vomiting induced by toxins, radiation, and cancer chemotherapeutic agents. The duration of action is four to six hours.

ADVERSE REACTIONS AND PRECAUTIONS. The most frequent and prominent side effect of promethazine is sedation. Anticholinergic and antiadrenergic adverse reactions occur infrequently after oral administration.

In the usual antiemetic dose, promethazine is relatively free of the extrapyramidal reactions associated with some phenothiazine and other antidopaminergic derivatives. For other adverse reactions and precautions, see the Introduction.

DOSAGE AND PREPARATIONS.

Intramuscular, Rectal: For treatment of nausea and vomiting, *adults,* initially, 25 mg, then 12.5 to 25 mg as needed every four to six hours. A dose of 12.5 mg (which is usually effective) should be tried initially in selected high-risk postoperative patients, because hypotension is observed more frequently when the 25-mg dose is given parenterally postoperatively. *Children 2 to 12 years,* the dose should be adjusted on the basis of the age and weight of the patient and severity of the condition, and no more than one-half the suggested adult dose should be administered; if given as an adjunct to premedication, the suggested dose is 1.1 mg/kg. This drug is not recommended for use in *children under 2 years.*

Generic. Solution 25 and 50 mg/ml in 1 and 10 ml containers; suppositories 50 mg.

Phenergan (Wyeth-Ayerst). Solution 25 and 50 mg/ml in 1 ml containers; suppositories 12.5, 25, and 50 mg.

Oral, Rectal: For motion sickness, *adults,* 25 mg twice daily. Administration one-half to one hour before anticipated travel is most beneficial. *Children,* 12.5 to 25 mg twice daily. Tablets, syrup, or rectal suppositories may be used.

Generic. Syrup 6.25 and 25 mg/5 ml; tablets 12.5, 25, and 50 mg; suppositories 50 mg.

Phenergan (Wyeth-Ayerst). Syrup 6.25 and (***Fortis***) 25 mg/5 ml (alcohol 7% and 1.5%); tablets 12.5, 25, and 50 mg; suppositories 12.5, 25, and 50 mg.

ANTIDOPAMINERGIC DRUGS

CHLORPROMAZINE
[Thorazine]

CHLORPROMAZINE HYDROCHLORIDE
[Thorazine]

For chemical formula, see index entry Chlorpromazine, As Antipsychotic Drug.

ACTIONS AND USES. Chlorpromazine is the prototype of the aliphatic phenothiazines. This drug's antiemetic activity is based on its antagonism of dopamine receptors in the chemoreceptor trigger zone, which reduces neural impulses to the vomiting center.

This phenothiazine is less potent as an antiemetic than prochlorperazine, thiethylperazine, and perphenazine; however, the incidence of dystonic reactions is less with chlorpromazine than with the latter drugs, especially with intramuscular administration. As with other phenothiazines, chlorpromazine is useful to alleviate nausea and vomiting associated with mildly emetogenic chemotherapy regimens but does not effectively control these symptoms after administration of potent emetogenic agents, such as cisplatin, doxorubicin, mechlorethamine, dacarbazine, or dactinomycin. Because a greater degree of sedation and a higher incidence of orthostatic hypotension is encountered with chlorpromazine than with prochlorperazine, most specialists prefer the latter or thiethylperazine to prevent chemotherapy-induced nausea and vomiting.

Chlorpromazine does not prevent vertigo or motion sickness, although it may be useful to treat severe vomiting produced by these disorders.

ADVERSE REACTIONS AND PRECAUTIONS. Unacceptable drowsiness may occur, although tolerance usually develops after continued use. Chlorpromazine prolongs postanesthesia sleeping time.

The untoward effects that may occur after long-term use or administration of large doses include extrapyramidal reactions, orthostatic hypotension, cholestatic jaundice, and leukopenia. Because of the severity of these adverse reactions, chlorpromazine should be considered only when vomiting cannot be controlled by less toxic antiemetics. For other adverse reactions and precautions, see the Introduction and index entry Chlorpromazine, As Antipsychotic Drug.

DOSAGE AND PREPARATIONS. This drug generally should not be used in *infants under 6 months* except when it is potentially lifesaving. The manufacturers' suggested dosages are:

CHLORPROMAZINE:

Rectal: *Adults,* 50 to 100 mg every six to eight hours; *children,* 1 mg/kg every six to eight hours.

Thorazine (SmithKline Beecham). Suppositories 25 and 100 mg.

CHLORPROMAZINE HYDROCHLORIDE:

Intramuscular: *Adults,* initially, 25 mg. If hypotension does not occur, 25 to 50 mg is given every three or four hours until vomiting stops; the drug is then given orally. *Children,* 0.5 mg/kg every six to eight hours; maximum daily doses: *up to 5 years* (22.5 kg), 40 mg; *5 to 12 years* (22.5 to 45 kg), 75 mg.

Thorazine (SmithKline Beecham), ***Generic.*** Solution (aqueous) 25 mg/ml in 1, 2, and 10 ml containers.

Oral: *Adults,* 10 to 25 mg every four to six hours; *children,* 0.5 mg/kg every four to six hours. Since all phenothiazines have prolonged half-lives (12 to 20 hours), the prolonged-release preparation has no significant advantage over the ordinary oral dosage forms for most patients.

Generic. Concentrate 30 and 100 mg/ml; syrup 10 mg/5 ml; tablets 10, 25, 50, 100, and 200 mg.

Thorazine (SmithKline Beecham). Capsules (prolonged-release) 30, 75, and 150 mg; concentrate 30 and 100 mg/ml; syrup 10 mg/5 ml; tablets 10, 25, 50, 100, and 200 mg.

DOMPERIDONE (Investigational drug)

[Motilium]

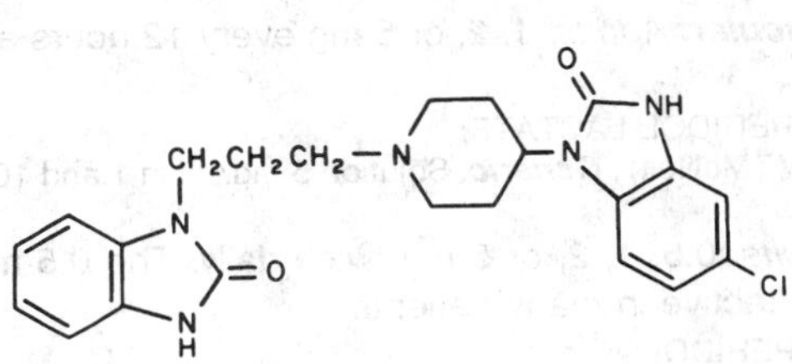

ACTIONS AND USES. Interest in this investigational antidopaminergic drug as an antiemetic agent may wane with the continued development of the serotonin antagonists and other useful agents. The antiemetic actions of domperidone are similar to those of metoclopramide, although the incidence of extrapyramidal side effects is lower, perhaps because this drug is poorly distributed to the central nervous system and does not block dopaminergic receptors in the basal ganglia. Oral administration increases lower esophageal sphincter pressure, the duration of antral and duodenal contractions, and the gastric emptying of liquids and semisolids (Brogden et al, 1982).

In open and placebo-controlled studies in adults and children (Dhondt et al, 1978; Reyntjens, 1979; Hoffbrand, 1979), domperidone appeared to be particularly effective in chronic postprandial dyspepsia, postprandial nausea and vomiting, and that associated with gastroenteritis. Domperidone also has been useful for nausea and vomiting associated with dysmenorrhea, migraine, head injury, hemodialysis, and radiation therapy. It has little value for nausea and vomiting induced by opioids. In postoperative vomiting, this drug was effective when given after the first vomiting episode but not when given before induction or at the end of anesthesia. Domperidone has been investigated to alleviate nausea and vomiting induced by cancer chemotherapy (Brogden et al, 1982; Triozzi and Laszlo, 1987), but few studies have been conducted in recent years.

Domperidone, like metoclopramide, may increase serum prolactin concentrations. A few cases of galactorrhea have been reported after prolonged use (Cann et al, 1983).

PHARMACOKINETICS. Domperidone is well absorbed when given orally; peak plasma concentrations are attained in 10 to 30 minutes. Domperidone undergoes extensive hepatic biotransformation and is excreted in the bile (60%). The half-life is approximately seven hours.

DOSAGE AND PREPARATIONS.

Oral: *Adults,* 20 to 40 mg three or four times daily; *children,* 0.6 mg/kg three or four times daily (Brogden et al, 1982).

For chronic postprandial dyspepsia, the usual *adult* dose is 10 mg three times a day 15 to 30 minutes before meals and at bedtime. *Children,* 0.3 mg/kg three times a day 15 to 30 minutes before meals and, if necessary, at bedtime. The daily dose for adults and children may be doubled if there is no significant improvement after two weeks of therapy.

Motilium (Janssen).

DROPERIDOL

[Inapsine]

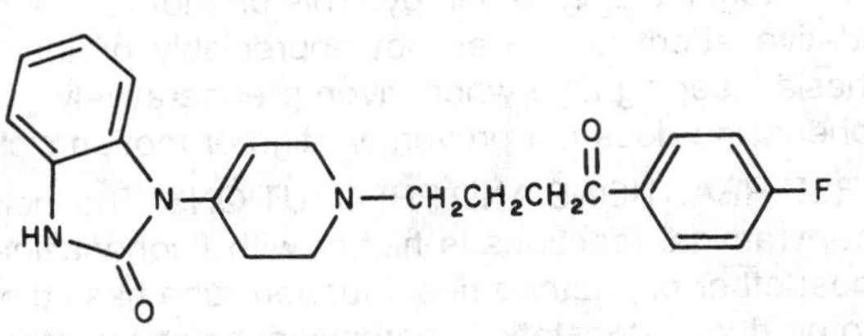

Because extrapyramidal reactions, hypotension, and sedation occur less frequently and are less severe with low doses of droperidol than with phenothiazines and because of its longer duration of action, this drug may be preferred for prophylaxis of nausea and vomiting associated with surgery. This butyrophenone has been used occasionally to alleviate nausea and vomiting in Meniere's syndrome. An intravenous loading dose of droperidol followed by either continuous infusion or repeated intravenous administration has been effective in some patients with cisplatin-induced nausea and vomiting. However, with the large doses used for control of cancer chemotherapy-induced vomiting, the incidence of dystonic reactions may be relatively high (Morrow, 1989).

Droperidol is classified in FDA Pregnancy Category C.

For a more detailed discussion on droperidol, see index entry Droperidol, In Combination Anesthesia.

DOSAGE AND PREPARATIONS.

Intramuscular: For premedication, *adults,* 2.5 to 10 mg (1 to 4 ml). The dosage must be individualized according to the physical status of the patient and is reduced in the elderly or when other depressant drugs are used concomitantly. *Children 2 to 12 years,* 1 to 1.5 mg (0.4 to 0.6 ml)/9 to 11 kg.

Intravenous: For Meniere's syndrome, *adults,* 5 mg. To prevent postoperative nausea and vomiting, *adults,* 1.25 mg to 2.5 mg five minutes prior to termination of anesthesia, repeated intramuscularly during the first 24 hours after surgery if the patient complains of nausea, retches, or vomits; *children 1 to 15 years,* 0.05 mg/kg.

As an antiemetic in cancer chemotherapy, *adults,* 2.5 to 5 mg 30 to 60 minutes prior to treatment; the same or one-half the dose is given intramuscularly after therapy on request but no more than once every hour; *children,* 1.25 mg (0.5 ml)/20 kg repeated intramuscularly as necessary, but no more than once every hour. For nausea and vomiting induced by cisplatin or other potent emetogenic agents, *adults,* a loading dose of 15 mg, followed by 7.5 mg every two hours for seven doses (Citron et al, 1984).

Inapsine (Janssen), ***Generic.*** Solution 2.5 mg/ml in 1 (***Inapsine*** only), 2, 5, and 10 ml containers.

FLUPHENAZINE HYDROCHLORIDE

[Permitil, Prolixin]

For chemical formula, see index entry Fluphenazine, As Antipsychotic Drug.

USES. Fluphenazine, a piperazine phenothiazine, is effective in the management of postoperative nausea and vomiting and that caused by toxins and radiation. There is little evidence to support its use in cancer chemotherapy, but fluphenazine probably can be used for nausea and vomiting induced by mildly emetogenic chemotherapy. This phenothiazine has little sedative effect and does not appreciably prolong postanesthesia sleeping time when given preoperatively.

Fluphenazine does not prevent vertigo or motion sickness.

ADVERSE REACTIONS AND PRECAUTIONS. The incidence of extrapyramidal reactions is higher with fluphenazine than with most other phenothiazines. Fluphenazine has little tendency to produce orthostatic hypotension; however, other anticholinergic effects (blurred vision, dryness of the mouth, and urinary retention) have been reported. See also the Introduction and index entry Fluphenazine, As Antipsychotic Drug.

DOSAGE AND PREPARATIONS.

Intramuscular, Oral: *Adults,* 1.25 mg repeated at six- to eight-hour intervals if needed. *Children < 12 years,* 0.25 to 3.5 mg daily in four to six divided doses administered orally; alternatively, one-third to one-half of the oral dose may be administered intramuscularly in divided doses.

Permitil (Schering). Concentrate (oral) 5 mg/ml (alcohol 1%); tablets 2.5, 5, and 10 mg.

Prolixin (Apothecon), ***Generic.*** Concentrate (oral) 5 mg/ml (alcohol 14%); elixir 2.5 mg/5 ml (alcohol 14%); tablets 1, 2.5, 5, and 10 mg; solution (for injection, aqueous, sterile) 2.5 mg/ml in 10 ml containers.

HALOPERIDOL

[Haldol]

HALOPERIDOL LACTATE

[Haldol]

For chemical formula, see index entry Haloperidol, Uses, Psychosis.

ACTIONS AND USES. The antiemetic action of this antidopaminergic butyrophenone is achieved mainly through inhibition of stimuli at the chemoreceptor trigger zone. The duration of action of haloperidol is longer than that of droperidol. It has been administered to alleviate nausea and vomiting associated with opioids and surgery, radiation therapy, cancer chemotherapy, and gastrointestinal disorders. It does not prevent vertigo or motion sickness and is not recommended for use as an antiemetic during pregnancy until more clinical data are available.

ADVERSE REACTIONS AND PRECAUTIONS. The adverse reactions produced by haloperidol closely resemble those of the piperazine phenothiazines (see the Introduction and index entry Haloperidol, Uses), but they occur only rarely with small doses and the short-term therapy employed to relieve nausea and vomiting.

As with other antiemetics, haloperidol must be given with great caution to patients with gastrointestinal disorders to avoid masking the development of life-threatening conditions that may be amenable to surgery. Because large doses of haloperidol have a marked potential to produce acute dystonia and other extrapyramidal reactions, this drug should be avoided in children and adolescents. Elderly or debilitated patients also may be more sensitive to the effects of haloperidol.

DOSAGE AND PREPARATIONS.

Intramuscular: *Adults,* 1, 2, or 5 mg every 12 hours as needed.

HALOPERIDOL LACTATE:

Haldol (McNeil), ***Generic.*** Solution 5 mg/ml in 1 and 10 ml containers.

Oral: *Adults,* 0.5, 1, 2, or 5 mg twice daily. The 0.5-mg dose may be effective in many patients.

HALOPERIDOL:

Haldol (McNeil), ***Generic.*** Tablets 0.5, 1, 2, 5, 10, and 20 mg.

HALOPERIDOL LACTATE:

Haldol (McNeil), ***Generic.*** Concentrate 2 mg/ml in 15, 120, and 240 ml (***Haldol*** only) containers.

METOCLOPRAMIDE HYDROCHLORIDE
[Octamide PFS, Maxolon, Reglan]

For chemical formula, see index entry Metoclopramide, In Gastrointestinal Disorders.

ACTIONS AND USES. Like the phenothiazines, metoclopramide has an antidopaminergic effect at the chemoreceptor trigger zone, but it also increases gastrointestinal motility. Its antiemetic effects may be more related to its antagonism of 5-HT_3 receptors than to blockade of dopamine receptors (Andrews et al, 1988).

Until the introduction of the 5-HT_3 antagonists, ondansetron and granisetron, intravenous metoclopramide was regarded by many authorities as the initial drug of choice in preventing nausea and vomiting induced by cisplatin (especially at doses >100 mg/M^2) and other highly emetogenic antineoplastic agents, such as dacarbazine, dactinomycin, mechlorethamine, and doxorubicin (Kris et al, 1985; Strum et al, 1984, 1985). Results of recent trials comparing metoclopramide with ondansetron or granisetron for control of cisplatin-induced acute emesis indicate that the latter two drugs are safer and more effective (De Mulder et al, 1990; Marty et al, 1990 B; Hainsworth et al, 1991; Warr et al, 1992; Chevallier, 1990).

The theoretical pharmacokinetic advantage of continuous infusion of metoclopramide over intermittent infusion has not been documented in clinical trials; no greater efficacy or decreased toxicity was observed (Merrifield and Chaffee, 1989). Oral administration may be as efficacious as intravenous administration in preventing acute vomiting in patients receiving cisplatin; however, the incidence of extrapyramidal reactions and diarrhea may be significantly higher with this route (Merrifield and Chaffee, 1989).

Optimal control of acute nausea and vomiting is obtained with a combination of intravenous metoclopramide, dexamethasone, and diphenhydramine or lorazepam (Strum et al, 1985; Gralla et al, 1987; Morrow, 1989; Merrifield and Chaffee, 1989). Oral metoclopramide/dexamethasone is used for delayed nausea and vomiting in patients receiving high-dose cisplatin (see Dosage and Preparations for specific regimens employed). It is unclear if the combined use of ondansetron or granisetron with dexamethasone is superior to metoclopramide/dexamethasone combinations for delayed nausea and vomiting.

As with other antiemetics, the efficacy of metoclopramide is reduced in the presence of anticipatory nausea and vomiting.

Metoclopramide also may alleviate nausea and vomiting induced by toxins and radiation. Gastric stasis induced by morphine is reversed by metoclopramide, and this antiemetic is effective in relieving opioid-induced postoperative vomiting. There is evidence that metoclopramide may be useful preoperatively to empty the stomach prior to emergency surgery. Additionally, it tightens the lower esophageal sphincter to prevent aspiration when emergency general anesthesia must be given. Like other antidopaminergic agents, this drug does *not* prevent motion sickness.

ADVERSE REACTIONS AND PRECAUTIONS. The principal adverse effects of metoclopramide are sedation and diarrhea, which develop in most patients given the larger doses needed to alleviate vomiting induced by antineoplastic agents.

Extrapyramidal reactions are more prominent when metoclopramide is used for many months or years, but they also can occur with short-term use for nausea and vomiting (Kataria et al, 1978). Symptoms usually resolve in a few weeks following drug withdrawal but may persist for several months. Dystonic reactions (oculogyric crises, trismus, torticollis, opisthotonos) and akathisia are more likely to occur within the first 72 hours of treatment. They are more common in children, young adults, and patients with renal impairment. In one study, the incidence of extrapyramidal effects in cancer patients receiving metoclopramide to control nausea and vomiting induced by anticancer drugs was 2% in those over age 30 but 27% in younger patients (Gralla, 1991). Usually, extrapyramidal reactions are readily reversed by diphenhydramine, benztropine, or lorazepam.

Metoclopramide may increase the sedative actions of central nervous system depressants and may increase the severity and frequency of extrapyramidal reactions produced by medications given concurrently, particularly phenothiazines. It is contraindicated in the presence of gastrointestinal obstruction, hemorrhage, or perforation; convulsive disorders; and pheochromocytoma.

Occasional reactions include agitation, irritability, urticarial or maculopapular rash, dryness of the mouth, glossal or periorbital edema, and neck pain and rigidity. Methemoglobinemia has been reported in neonates who received excessive doses.

This drug is classified in FDA Pregnancy Category B.

PHARMACOKINETICS. The elimination half-life is 4.5 to 8.8 hours in patients receiving intravenous metoclopramide and is not dose dependent. This drug is eliminated by hepatic conjugation (80%) with sulfate and glucuronic acid; 20% is excreted unchanged in the urine. Total clearance is reduced in patients with renal disease (McGovern et al, 1986). In one study, blood concentrations of metoclopramide that exceeded 850 ng/ml before the third intravenous dose correlated with antiemetic efficacy (Meyer et al, 1984), but this finding was not substantiated in a second study (Strum et al, 1985).

DOSAGE AND PREPARATIONS. Dosage should be reduced by approximately 60% in patients with severe renal impairment.

Intravenous: *Adults*, to alleviate nausea and vomiting induced by moderately emetogenic cancer chemotherapeutic agents, 0.5 to 0.75 mg/kg diluted in 50 ml of a large-volume parenteral solution and infused slowly over a 15-minute period 30 minutes prior to chemotherapy and at intervals of two, five, and eight hours after the first dose. When used with dexamethasone, 0.5 mg/kg given intravenously at the same intervals is effective.

For highly emetogenic regimens containing cisplatin, 2 to 3 mg/kg is administered 30 minutes before and 90 minutes after the antineoplastic drug; if 2 mg/kg is used, an additional dose is given in 3.5 hours (Gralla et al, 1987). Dexamethasone 20 mg and diphenhydramine 50 mg also are given intravenously 35 to 40 minutes prior to chemotherapy; the dose of diphenhydramine can be repeated in four hours. For highly emetogenic noncisplatin-containing regimens, 1 mg/kg of metoclopramide is given intravenously 30 minutes before chemotherapy and two hours later; subsequent doses are given orally. Dexamethasone and diphenhydramine are administered in the same dosage as for cisplatin-containing regimens (see above).

Single-dose regimen (with dexamethasone and lorazepam) prior to chemotherapy, 4 mg/kg infused over 20 minutes (Gralla, 1991). In one study, metoclopramide 4 to 6 mg/kg was infused intravenously as a single dose in a combination regimen with dexamethasone and lorazepam just prior to chemotherapy. This higher dose of metoclopramide was as effective and safe as the lower amount usually infused intermittently, was less expensive, and required less intensive nursing care (Clark et al, 1989).

Children, the incidence of extrapyramidal reactions is unacceptably high with doses of 1 to 2 mg/kg (even with concomitant use of diphenhydramine). Further studies are needed to determine a safe and effective dosage.

Solutions may be diluted more than one hour prior to use, but partially used material should not be stored for later administration.

Generic. Solution 5 mg/ml in 2, 10, 20, 30, 50, and 100 ml containers and 10 mg/ml in 2 ml containers.

Octamide PFS (Adria), ***Reglan*** (Robins). Solution 5 mg/ml (monohydrochloride) in 2, 10, and 30 ml containers.

Oral: *Adults,* for delayed-onset nausea and vomiting caused by cisplatin, 0.5 mg/kg is given four times a day for four days beginning 24 hours after chemotherapy. Another suggested regimen: At 24 and 48 hours (days 1 and 2) after cisplatin administration, patients receive oral metoclopramide 0.5 mg/kg four times daily and dexamethasone 8 mg two times daily. On days 3 and 4, oral dexamethasone 4 mg is administered twice daily. Additional metoclopramide is given if nausea and vomiting occur (Gralla, 1991).

Concomitant use with oral dexamethasone is most effective with a four- to six-day regimen (Strum et al, 1985; Kris et al, 1989 B) (see that evaluation).

Generic. Solution (oral) 10 mg/ml in 30 ml containers; syrup 1, 5, and 15 mg/ml (monohydrochloride); tablets and capsules (monohydrochloride) 5 and 10 mg.

Maxolon (SmithKline Beecham). Tablets 10 mg.

Reglan (Robins). Syrup 1 mg/ml; tablets 5 and 10 mg.

PERPHENAZINE
[Trilafon]

For chemical formula, see index entry Perphenazine, As Antipsychotic Drug.

This piperazine phenothiazine is effective in the management of postoperative nausea and vomiting and for that caused by opioids, toxins, and radiation. It is not widely used as an antiemetic in cancer chemotherapy regimens, but its effectiveness appears to be similar to that of other antidopaminergic agents. Perphenazine does *not* prevent vertigo or motion sickness.

Untoward effects include extrapyramidal reactions, blurred or double vision, nasal congestion, dryness of the mouth, salivation, headache, and, occasionally, drowsiness. For other adverse reactions and precautions, see the Introduction and index entry Perphenazine, As Antipsychotic Drug.

DOSAGE AND PREPARATIONS. No dosage has been established for *children under 12 years.*

Intramuscular: *Adults,* 5 or, rarely, 10 mg.

Intravenous: *Adults,* the solution is diluted to 0.5 mg/ml and is administered at a rate of 1 mg over one to two minutes (maximum dose, 5 mg).

Trilafon (Schering). Solution 5 mg/ml in 1 ml containers.

Oral: *Adults,* 2 to 4 mg every four to six hours.

Generic. Tablets and capsules 2, 4, 8, and 16 mg.

Trilafon (Schering). Concentrate 16 mg/5 ml (alcohol <0.1%); tablets 2, 4, 8, and 16 mg.

PROCHLORPERAZINE
[Compazine]

PROCHLORPERAZINE EDISYLATE
[Compazine]

PROCHLORPERAZINE MALEATE
[Compazine]

USES. Prochlorperazine is effective in the management of postoperative nausea and vomiting in adults and that caused by toxins and radiation. It is the most widely studied phenothiazine for management of mild chemotherapy-induced nausea and vomiting and is especially useful when minimal sedation is desired. When used alone in the usual recommended doses, prochlorperazine is less useful for vomiting caused by moderately to severely emetogenic antineoplastic agents. A dose of 10 mg every four to six hours, orally or intramuscularly, generally has been considered to provide the greatest antiemetic efficacy. Results of a number of studies suggest that, with intravenous doses of 40 mg or more, the antiemetic efficacy of this drug is comparable to that of metoclopramide (Carr et al, 1987; Merrifield and Chaffee, 1989). Although such doses have a greater potential for producing orthostatic hypotension than the usual doses used orally or intramuscularly, some authorities believe that large doses of this drug are safe (Akhtar et al, 1991). Hypotension can be avoided at these and lower doses by administering the drug as a slow intravenous infusion over 15 to 20 minutes.

In a small, well-controlled study in patients receiving high-dose cisplatin (100 mg/M^2), the combination of intravenous prochlorperazine and dexamethasone was reported to be as effective as metoclopramide and dexamethasone (Akhtar et al, 1991). Prochlorperazine also has been used with metoclopramide/dexamethasone or ondansetron/dexamethasone combinations for prophylaxis of delayed nausea and vomiting in patients receiving moderately emetogenic antineoplastic regimens (Navari et al, 1993).

Prochlorperazine does *not* prevent vertigo or motion sickness.

ADVERSE REACTIONS AND PRECAUTIONS. This piperazine phenothiazine frequently causes extrapyramidal reactions. Although these effects are most likely to occur with large doses, signs may appear abruptly in patients taking only moderate doses. Consideration should be given to the increased potential for extrapyramidal side effects when prochlorperazine is used in repeated cycles of radiation therapy.

With oral or intramuscular doses, drowsiness, dizziness, cutaneous reactions, and amenorrhea occur occasionally, and orthostatic hypotension, neutropenia, and cholestasis have been reported rarely. Large intravenous doses (40 mg) were generally well tolerated; sedation was the most common adverse effect (Carr et al, 1987; Merrifield and Chaffee, 1989).

Particular caution is necessary in patients who are sensitive to other phenothiazines, in those with hepatic disease, and in children. The drug should be avoided in children undergoing surgery and in children and adolescents whose symptoms and signs suggest Reye's syndrome (see the Introduction). Prochlorperazine also should not be used in children under 2 years or weighing less than 9 kg unless it is potentially lifesaving. See also index entry Prochlorperazine, As Antipsychotic Drug.

DOSAGE AND PREPARATIONS.

PROCHLORPERAZINE:

Rectal: *Adults,* 25 mg twice daily; *children 9 to 14 kg,* 2.5 mg every 12 to 24 hours; *14 to 18 kg,* 2.5 mg every 8 to 12 hours; *18 to 39 kg,* 2.5 mg every eight hours or 5 mg every 12 hours.

Compazine (SmithKline Beecham). Suppositories 2.5, 5, and 25 mg.

PROCHLORPERAZINE EDISYLATE:

Intramuscular (deep): *Adults,* 5 to 10 mg every three or four hours (maximum, 40 mg daily); *children over 10 kg,* 0.13 mg/kg; intramuscular administration usually is not repeated in children.

Intravenous: *Adults,* 2.5 to 10 mg administered at a rate not to exceed 5 mg/min (maximum total daily dose, 40 mg).

Generic. Solution 5 mg/ml in 1, 2, and 10 ml containers.

Compazine (SmithKline Beecham). Solution (aqueous) 5 mg/ml in 2 and 10 ml containers.

Oral: *Adults,* 5 to 10 mg three or four times daily; *children 9 to 14 kg,* 2.5 mg every 12 to 24 hours; *14 to 18 kg,* 2.5 mg every 8 to 12 hours; *18 to 39 kg,* 2.5 mg every eight hours or 5 mg every 12 hours.

Compazine (SmithKline Beecham). Syrup 5 mg/5 ml.

PROCHLORPERAZINE MALEATE:

Oral: Same as oral dosage for edisylate salt. Since all phenothiazines have prolonged half-lives (12 to 20 hours), the prolonged-release preparation has no significant advantage over ordinary oral dosage forms for most patients.

Generic. Tablets 5, 10, and 25 mg.

Compazine (SmithKline Beecham). Capsules (prolonged-release) 10 and 15 mg; tablets 5, 10, and 25 mg.

PROMAZINE HYDROCHLORIDE

[Sparine]

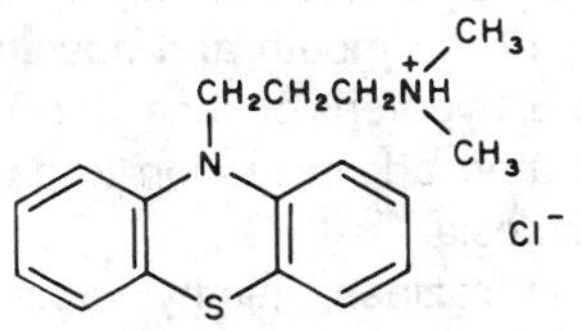

USES. Promazine, an aliphatic phenothiazine, is effective in preventing postoperative nausea and vomiting. It has not been studied extensively to prevent vomiting caused by cancer chemotherapeutic agents, radiation sickness, or toxins. However, as with most phenothiazine antiemetics, promazine is unlikely to prevent nausea and vomiting associated with moderately or severely emetogenic chemotherapy.

ADVERSE REACTIONS AND PRECAUTIONS. The incidence of adverse reactions (eg, drowsiness, orthostatic hypotension) is similar to that of the other aliphatic phenothiazines, especially after parenteral administration. The hypotensive action may be detrimental in patients with cardiac or cerebrovascular insufficiency, and the anticholinergic actions may be detrimental in patients with ileus, angle-closure glaucoma, or urinary retention.

Extrapyramidal reactions are infrequent. Although relatively rare, agranulocytosis is reported to occur more frequently than with chlorpromazine or prochlorperazine. For other adverse reactions and precautions, see the Introduction.

DOSAGE AND PREPARATIONS.

Oral: *Adults,* 25 to 50 mg every four to six hours.

Sparine (Wyeth-Ayerst). Tablets 25, 50, and 100 mg.

Intramuscular: *Adults,* 50 mg.

Generic. Solution 25 and 50 mg/ml in 10 ml containers.

Sparine (Wyeth-Ayerst). Solution 50 mg/ml in 2 and 10 ml containers.

THIETHYLPERAZINE MALATE

[Torecan]

THIETHYLPERAZINE MALEATE

[Torecan]

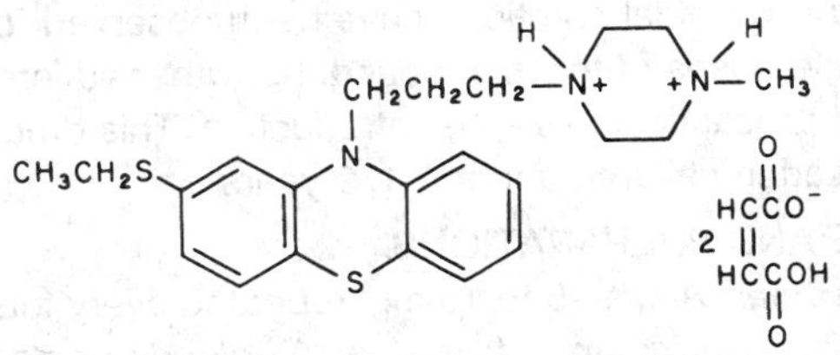

USES. Thiethylperazine is particularly useful to treat nausea and vomiting associated with anesthesia; it also relieves nausea and vomiting caused by mildly emetogenic cancer chemotherapeutic agents, radiation therapy, and toxins. This piperazine phenothiazine does *not* prevent vertigo or motion sickness.

ADVERSE REACTIONS AND PRECAUTIONS. Untoward effects are infrequent, mild, and transitory with usual doses. Adverse reactions noted occasionally include drowsiness, dizziness, dryness of the mouth and nose, tachycardia, and anorexia. Moderate hypotension has occurred occasionally within 30 minutes after administration to patients recovering from general anesthesia.

Like other phenothiazines, thiethylperazine may produce extrapyramidal reactions. Symptoms may appear even after a single dose but abate if therapy is discontinued. For severe dystonic reactions, such as oculogyric crisis and torticollis, diphenhydramine 50 mg given intravenously usually abolishes symptoms within minutes. For other adverse reactions and precautions, see the Introduction.

DOSAGE AND PREPARATIONS. No dosage has been established for *children*.

Intramuscular: *Adults,* 10 mg one to three times daily.

THIETHYLPERAZINE MALATE:

Torecan (Roxane). Solution (aqueous) 5 mg/ml in 2 ml containers.

Oral, Rectal: *Adults,* 10 mg one to three times daily.

THIETHYLPERAZINE MALEATE:

Torecan (Roxane). Tablets 10 mg; suppositories 10 mg.

TRIFLUPROMAZINE HYDROCHLORIDE

[Vesprin]

For chemical formula, see index entry Triflupromazine, As Antipsychotic Drug.

USES. This aliphatic phenothiazine is effective in preventing postoperative nausea and vomiting. Its effectiveness in preventing nausea and vomiting induced by cancer chemotherapeutic agents, radiation, or toxins has not been well studied. Like other phenothiazine antiemetics, triflupromazine may be useful to alleviate vomiting due to mildly emetogenic agents. It is less effective when more potent antineoplastic drugs are used. Triflupromazine does *not* prevent vertigo or motion sickness.

ADVERSE REACTIONS AND PRECAUTIONS. Triflupromazine produces less sedation than some other phenothiazines (eg, promazine), but it prolongs the postanesthesia sleep time. Extrapyramidal reactions have been observed following even single doses of this compound. For other adverse reactions and precautions, see the Introduction. This drug should not be used in children under 2 1/2 years.

DOSAGE AND PREPARATIONS.

Intramuscular: *Adults,* 5 to 15 mg, repeated every four hours if necessary (maximum, 60 mg daily); *elderly or debilitated patients,* 2.5 mg every four hours if necessary (maximum, 15 mg daily); *children over 2½ years,* 0.07 mg/kg three times a day (maximum, 10 mg daily).

Intravenous: *Adults,* 1 mg to a maximum total daily dose of 3 mg.

Vesprin (Apothecon). Solution 10 mg/ml in 10 ml containers and 20 mg/ml in 1 ml containers.

ANTISEROTONINERGIC DRUGS

GRANISETRON HYDROCHLORIDE

[Kytril]

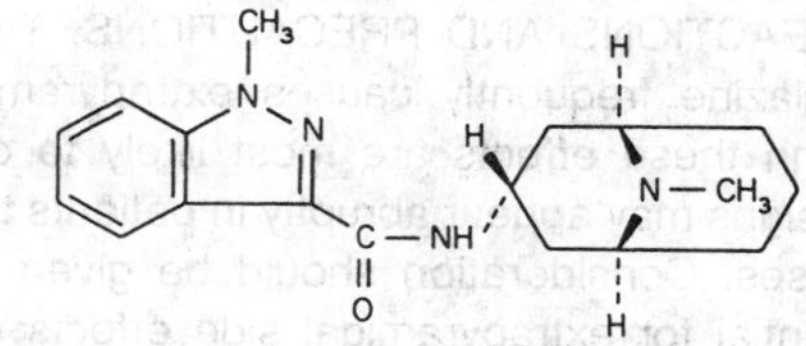

ACTIONS AND USES. The actions, indications, and efficacy of this 5-HT_3 serotonin receptor antagonist are similar to those of ondansetron (Plosker and Goa, 1991). Like the latter drug, monotherapy with granisetron is superior to metoclopramide/dexamethasone combinations for prevention and control of acute nausea and vomiting associated with cisplatin and other highly emetogenic cancer chemotherapeutic regimens (Plosker and Goa, 1991; Robinson, 1993). Experience with granisetron/dexamethasone combinations is limited but this combination appears to be more efficacious than granisetron alone (Latreille et al, 1993). Preliminary data indicate that this drug also is effective in moderately emetogenic chemotherapeutic regimens (Jantunen et al, 1993; Marty et al, 1990 A; Warr et al, 1991) and is effective and safe in children. The advantages and cost effectiveness of granisetron for delayed emesis have not been clearly established.

ADVERSE REACTIONS. Granisetron is well tolerated; constipation, diarrhea, headache, and transient hypotension have occurred in some patients. Extrapyramidal adverse reactions have not been reported (Plosker and Goa, 1991; Hunter-Johnson, 1991; Robinson, 1993).

This drug is classified in FDA Pregnancy Category B.

PHARMACOKINETICS. Granisetron is extensively metabolized in the liver. Its elimination half-life (approximately 9 hours) is longer than that of ondansetron.

Granisetron does not inhibit or stimulate the cytochrome P450 enzyme system.

DOSAGE AND PREPARATIONS.

Intravenous: *Adults,* for acute nausea and vomiting, 10 mcg/kg infused over five minutes, beginning within 30 minutes before initiation of chemotherapy. *Children 2 to 16 years,* 10 mcg/kg.

Kytril (SmithKline Beecham). Solution (sterile) 1 mg/ml in 1 ml single-use containers.

ONDANSETRON HYDROCHLORIDE

[Zofran]

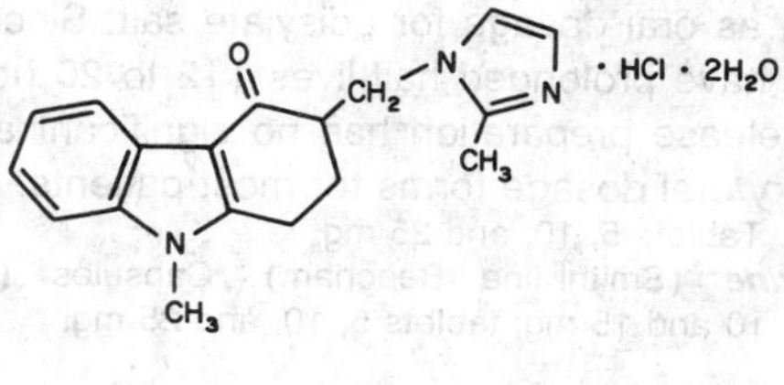

ACTIONS. This carbazole derivative binds competitively to 5-HT_3 receptors in the chemoreceptor trigger zone of the central nervous system and gastrointestinal tract. Blockade of these receptors by ondansetron prevents the action of serotonin and inhibits emesis. This agent does not bind dopamine receptors.

USES. Ondansetron has replaced metoclopramide as the agent of choice for nausea and vomiting induced by cisplatin and other highly emetogenic antineoplastic drugs. The primary advantage of ondansetron over metoclopramide is its lack of significant adverse reactions, particularly extrapyramidal effects and sedation. Ondansetron is especially useful for patients younger than 30 years, who are more susceptible to extrapyramidal reactions (Gralla, 1991).

In numerous controlled and uncontrolled studies, this agent was superior to placebo and equal or superior to metoclopramide in the prevention of acute vomiting episodes induced by an initial course of chemotherapy employing a single dose of cisplatin plus other antineoplastic drugs (Marty et al, 1990 B; De Mulder et al, 1990; Hainsworth et al, 1991; Bonneterre et al, 1990; Kaasa et al, 1990; Figg et al, 1993). Although ondansetron is clearly beneficial prior to the initial course of chemotherapy, it is unclear whether this drug is equally effective when used to prevent or treat nausea and vomiting produced by repeated doses of an antineoplastic drug in a course of chemotherapy (Chaffee and Tankanow, 1991; Milne and Heel, 1991). Ondansetron is presently being studied in clinical trials to assess its efficacy for delayed nausea and vomiting induced by cisplatin.

As with metoclopramide, the addition of dexamethasone to the antiemetic regimen enhances protection against acute as well as delayed nausea and vomiting (Cunningham et al, 1989; Smith et al, 1990; Roila et al, 1991; *Lancet*, 1991; Navari et al, 1993). The advantages and cost effectiveness of ondansetron/dexamethasone combinations for moderately emetogenic chemotherapy regimens have not been established (Plosker and Milne, 1992), although some data support its efficacy (Jantunen et al, 1993). At present, some authorities recommend that this combination be reserved for patients in whom better control of vomiting will decrease the incidence of anticipatory emesis during subsequent courses of chemotherapy and for those who are refractory to other antiemetic regimens.

Ondansetron alone is effective in controlling postoperative nausea and vomiting and vomiting caused by radiation therapy (Leeser and Lip, 1991; Priestman et al, 1990; Dershwitz et al, 1992; *FDC Reports*, 1992; Woodward and Gora, 1993).

Ondansetron is considerably more expensive than metoclopramide, but its greater acceptance by patients, its contribution to improved chemotherapy outcomes and quality of life, and the potential for outpatient management contribute to cost effectiveness of this agent and combinations containing it compared with metoclopramide combinations (Plosker and Milne, 1992; Beck et al, 1993). The finding that a single 8- or 32-mg dose of intravenous ondansetron administered just prior to chemotherapy is as effective as three intravenous doses will decrease nursing and other costs and permit outpatient management for many patients (Beck et al, 1992). The use of three oral doses for less emetogenic regimens has similar advantages.

ADVERSE REACTIONS AND PRECAUTIONS. Ondansetron is well tolerated and few adverse reactions have been reported. In most clinical trials, the incidence of headache, dizziness, lightheadedness, sedation, diarrhea, and constipation was similar to that reported with placebo. In multidrug clinical trials, headache and constipation have occurred more frequently than with placebo. Extrapyramidal adverse reactions, which have been reported rarely, are not clearly documented (Chaffee and Tankanow, 1991).

Careful analysis of reports of thrombosis, thrombocytopenia, angina, and renal dysfunction in cancer patients receiving cisplatin and ondansetron does not indicate that there is any relationship between these reactions and use of the latter drug (Castle et al, 1992; Palmer et al, 1992).

Chemotherapy with cisplatin produces transient reversible elevations in bilirubin and serum transaminases that appear to be clinically insignificant; previously these changes were attributed to ondansetron (Hesketh et al, 1990; Beck et al, 1993).

Ondansetron is classified in FDA Pregnancy Category B.

PHARMACOKINETICS. This drug is rapidly absorbed after oral administration and undergoes extensive first-pass metabolism. Peak plasma concentrations occur 1 to 1.5 hours after an oral dose. Bioavailability is about 60% and plasma protein binding is 70% to 75%.

Ondansetron is extensively metabolized in the liver, and less than 10% of the parent compound is recovered in the urine. The major route of metabolism is hydroxylation, followed by glucuronidation or sulfate conjugation. Almost one-half of the metabolites are recovered in the urine and one-half in the feces (Chaffee and Tankanow, 1991). The drug may not be metabolized in patients with severe hepatic dysfunction and high serum levels may result.

The plasma half-life is about 3.5 hours in adults and is slightly shorter in children (Saynor and Dixon, 1989; Blackwell and Harding, 1989); it may increase to about eight hours in elderly patients (Chaffee and Tankanow, 1991). No correlation exists between plasma concentrations and antiemetic efficacy.

DRUG INTERACTIONS. Limited data are available on possible interactions with other agents; no significant drug interactions have been reported.

DOSAGE AND PREPARATIONS.

Intravenous: *Adults and children over 4 years,* for acute nausea and vomiting, a total of 0.15 mg/kg is given in three doses. The first dose is infused over a 15-minute period 30 minutes before chemotherapy. The next two doses are given four and eight hours after the first dose. Alternatively, a single dose of 8 or 32 mg administered 30 minutes before chemotherapy is as effective as the three-dose regimen (Beck et al, 1992). For suggested doses in combination with dexamethasone, see the evaluation on the latter drug. The optimal dose and schedule when ondansetron is given alone or in combination with dexamethasone and other agents have not been determined.

Zofran (Cerenex). Solution 2 mg/ml in 20 ml containers. The drug should be diluted in 50 ml of 5% dextrose injection or 0.9% sodium chloride injection before administration.

Oral: *Adults and children over 12 years*, for acute nausea and vomiting with less emetogenic antineoplastic regimens, 8 mg 30 minutes before chemotherapy and repeated four and eight hours after the first dose (total daily dose 24 mg) (Beck et al, 1992). *Children 4 to 12 years,* 4 mg three times daily as above.

Zofran (Cerenex). Tablets 4 and 8 mg.

MISCELLANEOUS DRUGS

BENZQUINAMIDE HYDROCHLORIDE

[Emete-Con]

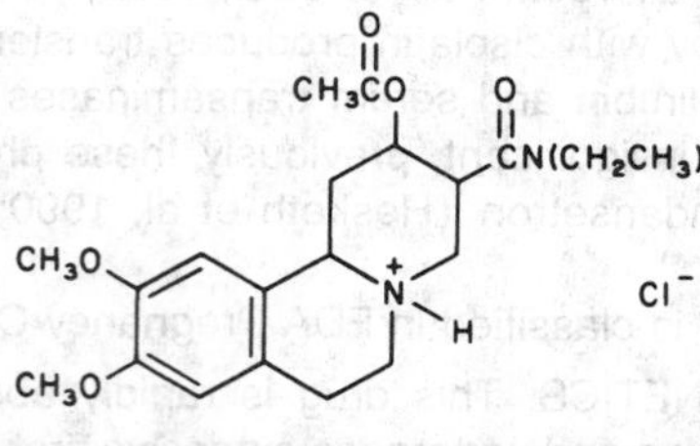

ACTIONS AND USES. Like the antidopaminergic drugs, this short-acting benzquinoline derivative apparently inhibits stimuli at the chemoreceptor trigger zone. Benzquinamide is used primarily to prevent and treat postoperative nausea and vomiting. It may be useful in some patients to prevent nausea and vomiting produced by cancer chemotherapy; however, benzquinamide has rarely been effective against cisplatin- or mechlorethamine-induced emesis, and it eliminated vomiting in only 20% of patients receiving doxorubicin (Neidhart et al, 1981). Data are not sufficient to justify the use of benzquinamide during pregnancy or in children.

ADVERSE REACTIONS AND PRECAUTIONS. Results of a few controlled studies suggest that benzquinamide produces fewer serious adverse reactions than the phenothiazines; however, there is less overall experience with this agent. Drowsiness is noted most frequently. Shivering, chills, and other anticholinergic reactions (eg, dry mouth, blurred vision) also have been reported. Other reactions include hypertension, hypotension, atrial fibrillation, and premature atrial and ventricular contractions.

A sudden increase in blood pressure has occurred with rapid intravenous administration. Arrhythmias may develop in anesthetized patients regardless of the route of administration, even at doses below those required for antiemetic effect. Use of benzquinamide in patients with moderate to severe hypertension or severe cardiovascular disease is questionable, particularly if the drug is given intravenously during anesthesia.

DOSAGE AND PREPARATIONS.

Intramuscular (preferred route): *Adults,* 0.5 to 1 mg/kg at least 15 minutes prior to administration of antineoplastic drugs or emergence from anesthesia. (The plasma half-life is approximately 40 minutes.) This dose may be repeated in one hour and then every three to four hours as required.

Intravenous: The powder must be reconstituted with 2.2 ml of sterile water for injection or bacteriostatic water for injection with benzyl alcohol or methylparaben and propylparaben. To achieve therapeutic concentrations in less than 15 minutes, a single dose of 0.2 to 0.4 mg/kg is given to *adults*; the drug may be diluted in 5% dextrose in water, sodium chloride injection, or lactated Ringer's injection and administered over one to three minutes or given as an intravenous infusion. Subsequent doses should be given intramuscularly.

Emete-Con (Roerig). Powder equivalent to benzquinamide 50 mg.

DIPHENIDOL HYDROCHLORIDE

[Vontrol]

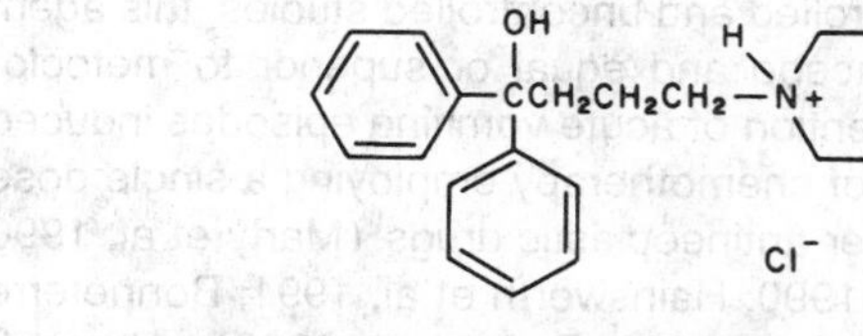

ACTIONS AND USES. Diphenidol acts on the aural vestibular apparatus and is useful in nausea and vomiting associated with general anesthesia, toxins, radiation therapy, and cancer chemotherapeutic agents. In adults, this drug also is effective in vertigo following surgery of the middle and inner ear and in Meniere's disease. Its use in the treatment of vertigo in children has not been investigated.

ADVERSE REACTIONS AND PRECAUTIONS. Because of its central anticholinergic actions, diphenidol rarely may induce visual or auditory hallucinations, disorientation, or confusion. Therefore, it should be used only when close supervision is possible. These effects usually occur within a few days after initiation of therapy (incidence, about 1 in 350 patients) and subside spontaneously within three days after the drug is discontinued.

Diphenidol occasionally has produced drowsiness, dryness of the mouth, tachycardia, and dizziness. Untoward effects reported rarely include rash, heartburn, headache, nausea, indigestion, blurred vision, malaise, and mild, transient hypotension.

Since over 90% of diphenidol is eliminated by the kidney, the drug is contraindicated in patients with severe renal impairment.

DOSAGE AND PREPARATIONS.

Oral: *Adults,* 25 to 50 mg four times daily; *children weighing 23 to 45 kg,* 25 mg. This drug should not be used in *children weighing <23 kg.*

Vontrol (SmithKline Beecham). Tablets 25 mg.

TRIMETHOBENZAMIDE HYDROCHLORIDE

[Tigan]

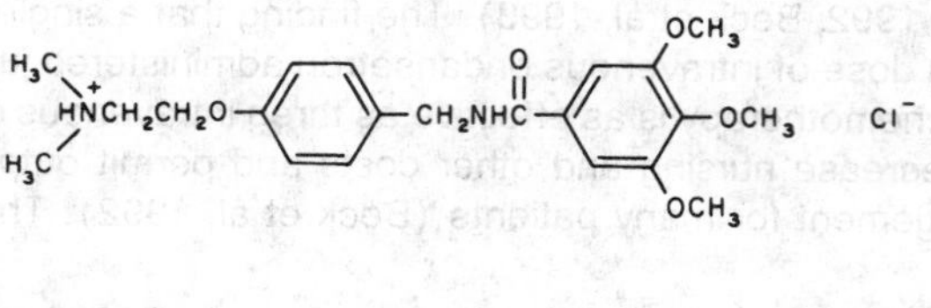

ACTIONS AND USES. This drug inhibits stimuli at the chemoreceptor trigger zone in animals and has been promoted for use in alleviating nausea and reducing the frequency of vomiting during the immediate postoperative period, in radiation sickness, and in gastroenteritis. It is not as effective as the phenothiazines postoperatively. Trimethobenzamide has little or no value in the prevention or treatment of vertigo, motion sickness, or nausea and vomiting due to cancer chemotherapy.

In general, the effectiveness of the oral form appears to be somewhat unpredictable.

ADVERSE REACTIONS AND PRECAUTIONS. With usual doses, the incidence of adverse effects is low; with larger doses, drowsiness, vertigo, diarrhea, and cutaneous hypersensitivity reactions may occur. Extrapyramidal reactions or convulsions also have been noted; the latter occur more often in children and the elderly.

Pain at the site of injection and local irritation after rectal administration have been noted. Although the association between Reye's syndrome and trimethobenzamide has not been proved, this drug should be avoided in children with signs and symptoms suggesting this disorder.

DOSAGE AND PREPARATIONS.

Intramuscular: *Adults,* 200 mg three or four times daily. To prevent postoperative vomiting, a single dose of 200 mg may be given before or during surgery; this dose may be repeated three hours after termination of anesthesia if needed. This route should not be used in *children.*

> ***Tigan*** (SmithKline Beecham), ***Generic.*** Solution 100 mg/ml in 2 and 20 ml containers.

Oral: *Adults,* 250 mg three or four times daily; *children,* 4 to 5 mg/kg every six to eight hours.

> ***Tigan*** (SmithKline Beecham), ***Generic***. Capsules 100 and 250 mg.

Rectal: *Adults,* 200 mg three or four times daily; *children,* 4 to 5 mg/kg every six to eight hours. This route should not be used in *premature or newborn infants.*

> ***Tigan*** (SmithKline Beecham), ***Generic***. Suppositories 100 (pediatric) and 200 mg with benzocaine 2% (***Tigan*** only).

Cannabinoid

DRONABINOL (delta-9-tetrahydrocannabinol, THC)
[Marinol]

USES. This agent is the principal psychoactive component of marijuana. Although its antiemetic efficacy when given orally during cancer chemotherapy has been confirmed in a number of controlled studies (Cocchetto et al, 1981), superiority over other antiemetics has not been proved (Carey et al, 1983).

Dronabinol may be indicated for patients who do not respond to metoclopramide, serotonin antagonists, butyrophenones, or phenothiazines or who develop tolerance to their antiemetic effect. It may be used initially in those who are less likely to be troubled by the drug's central nervous system adverse reactions. Younger patients who are previous drug users may enjoy the psychological "high" produced by the cannabinoids. The side effects of loss of control and altered sensation are not tolerated well by older individuals. Dronabinol is useful in selected patients receiving methotrexate. It has reduced nausea and vomiting caused by high doses of cisplatin; in one study, the number of vomiting episodes was reduced to less than two in approximately one-third of patients (Gralla et al, 1984). This drug is less effective during chemotherapy with cyclophosphamide, doxorubicin, and mechlorethamine (Gralla et al, 1984).

There is little experience with the use of dronabinol for nausea and vomiting associated with anesthesia and surgery, radiation therapy, and toxins.

ADVERSE REACTIONS AND PRECAUTIONS. Psychoactive effects occur with the antiemetic use of dronabinol; the durations of these effects and of the antiemetic action are similar (about two to three hours). These effects (eg, mood changes, distortions in visual and time sense, somnolence) are dose related and may be unacceptable to some patients, especially the elderly. Occasional dysphoria or hallucinations limit the usefulness of this drug in individuals with psychiatric disorders. Since dronabinol may enhance seizure activity, it should be administered with caution to epileptic patients.

Dronabinol may produce transient tachycardia and large doses may cause orthostatic hypotension; these effects should be considered before the drug is used in patients with angina, mitral stenosis, and similar cardiovascular disorders.

In some clinical trials, the adverse effects of the cannabinoids were significantly decreased by combined use with a phenothiazine (Tortorice and O'Connell, 1990; Lane et al, 1990).

The safety of dronabinol during pregnancy has not been determined (FDA Pregnancy Category B).

PHARMACOKINETICS. Dronabinol is slowly and erratically absorbed from the intestine. The peak plasma concentration is attained in approximately two to three hours. The systemic bioavailability is 10% to 20%. Dronabinol is 97% to 99% protein bound.

Following oral administration, dronabinol is converted to a number of metabolites, including 11-hydroxy-dronabinol (Lemberger et al, 1973), which possesses equivalent activity. This, in turn, is converted into even more polar and acidic compounds. The metabolites and their conjugates are eliminated in the feces and urine. The terminal elimination half-life of 11-hydroxy-dronabinol is approximately 15 to 18 hours (Anderson and McGuire, 1981).

There are no formulations of dronabinol for intravenous or inhalational use.

DOSAGE AND PREPARATIONS.
Oral: Initially, 5 mg/M^2 one to three hours prior to chemotherapy and every two to four hours after chemotherapy to a total of four to six doses in 24 hours. The amount may be increased by 2.5 mg/M^2 increments to a maximum of 15 mg/M^2/dose.

Marinol (Roxane). Capsules (liquid, in sesame seed oil) 2.5, 5, and 10 mg.

Benzodiazepines

DIAZEPAM

[Valium, Valrelease]

For chemical formula, see index entry Diazepam, In Anxiety.

Diazepam acts as a vestibular depressant. It may be useful in vertigo (particularly when associated with anxiety), Meniere's disease, and nausea and vomiting of psychogenic origin. Although it may be beneficial in combination with metoclopramide and dexamethasone or other antiemetic agents to prevent nausea and vomiting caused by cisplatin and other highly emetogenic antineoplastic agents, it has been used infrequently for this indication; experience with lorazepam is much more extensive.

For adverse reactions, precautions, and pharmacokinetics, see index entry Diazepam, In Anxiety.

DOSAGE AND PREPARATIONS.
Oral: *Adults,* for Meniere's disease, 5 mg every three hours.

Generic. Solution (oral) 1 and 5 mg/ml; tablets 2, 5, and 10 mg.
Valium (Roche). Tablets 2, 5, and 10 mg.
Valrelease (Roche). Capsules (prolonged-release) 15 mg.

Intravenous: *Adults,* for Meniere's disease, 5 mg initially (maximum dose, 20 mg).

Valium (Roche), ***Generic.*** Solution 5 mg/ml in 1 (***Generic*** only), 2, and 10 ml containers.

LORAZEPAM

[Ativan]

For chemical formula, see index entry Lorazepam, In Anxiety.

This drug is one of the primary agents used in combination with metoclopramide/dexamethasone or other antiemetic agents to prevent nausea and vomiting caused by cisplatin and other highly emetogenic antineoplastic agents. Lorazepam alone has weak antiemetic activity. Its primary effect may be induction of antegrade amnesia for four to six hours in approximately 50% of patients receiving 2 mg and in almost 100% of those receiving 4 mg. In intravenous doses exceeding 1.5 mg/M^2, lorazepam can prevent or diminish akathisia in patients taking dopamine antagonists (Laszlo et al, 1985; Kris et al, 1987). Antiemetic therapy also is enhanced by the antianxiety and sedative effects of lorazepam. This drug has a high degree of subjective acceptance even in patients whose vomiting is not relieved. Further clinical studies are needed to determine the optimal dose and use of this agent.

Mild to marked sedation is the most common side effect.

The injectable form of lorazepam is classified in FDA Pregnancy Category D.

DOSAGE AND PREPARATIONS.
Intravenous, Intramuscular, Oral: *Adults,* a single dose of 0.025 to 0.05 mg/kg injected slowly intravenously or given intramuscularly 30 to 35 minutes before chemotherapy (*Oncol Times*, 1985; Gralla et al, 1987). The maximum dose is 4 mg. The initial intravenous or intramuscular dose may be supplemented with oral lorazepam 1 to 2 mg hourly as needed to maintain mild to moderate sedation.

Generic. Tablets 0.5, 1, and 2 mg.
Ativan (Wyeth-Ayerst). Solution (for injection) 2 and 4 mg/ml in 1 and 10 ml containers; tablets 0.5, 1, and 2 mg.

Corticosteroids

DEXAMETHASONE

DEXAMETHASONE SODIUM PHOSPHATE

For chemical formula, see index entry Adrenal Corticosteroids, Chemistry.

USES. Studies have shown that dexamethasone is superior to prochlorperazine (10 mg/dose) in reducing nausea and vomiting caused by moderately emetogenic cancer chemotherapeutic regimens (eg, cyclophosphamide, methotrexate, fluorouracil) (Cassileth et al, 1983; Markman et al, 1984). In one study, it relieved or significantly reduced nausea and vomiting induced by cisplatin (50 to 75 mg/M^2) in approximately 65% of patients undergoing repeated courses of chemotherapy (Aapro and Alberts, 1981). This effect has not been demonstrated universally, but subjective patient preference for this agent has been noted (Strum et al, 1985). It also may prevent radiation-induced vomiting.

Dexamethasone has significant additive effects when used with intravenous ondansetron, granisetron, or metoclopramide to alleviate vomiting caused by cisplatin and other highly emetogenic antineoplastic agents (see the Introduction) (Cunningham et al, 1989; Smith et al, 1990; Roila et al, 1991). It decreases the incidence of diarrhea caused by large doses of metoclopramide.

The intermittent, short-term use of glucocorticoids generally is not associated with toxicity. Rapid intravenous administration can cause intense perineal discomfort.

DOSAGE AND PREPARATIONS. The optimal dose and schedule for the use of dexamethasone in the treatment of nausea and vomiting caused by cancer chemotherapeutic agents have not been determined.

Intravenous: *Adults,* for mild vomiting caused by chemotherapy (eg, methotrexate, fluorouracil, vinblastine, vincristine, etoposide), 10 mg administered over three to five minutes 30 minutes before chemotherapy, followed by oral administration (if needed) of 8 mg 6, 12, and 18 hours after therapy.

A dose of 10 to 20 mg (Markman et al, 1984) 30 minutes before chemotherapy plus metoclopramide 0.5 mg/kg (see the evaluation on Metoclopramide) is given for moderately severe vomiting caused by chemotherapy (eg, cyclophosphamide 500 mg to 1.1 g/M^2, doxorubicin $>$50 mg/M^2, carmustine 100 to 200 mg/M^2, lomustine <60 mg/M^2). Dexamethasone 8 mg is then given orally every six hours for three doses (Strum et al, 1985).

For severe vomiting caused by cancer chemotherapy (eg, cisplatin, mechlorethamine, cyclophosphamide >1.2 g/M^2, dactinomycin, dacarbazine >300 mg/M^2, carmustine >300 mg/M^2, lomustine >60 mg/M^2), dexamethasone 20 mg is administered over ten minutes or longer 35 to 40 minutes before chemotherapy plus either (1) concomitant intravenous administration of metoclopramide 1 to 3 mg/kg and diphenhydramine 50 mg (Strum et al, 1985; Kris et al, 1985, 1987) or lorazepam 1.5 mg/M^2 (Kris et al, 1987); (2) concomitant intravenous administration of ondansetron 0.15 mg/kg infused 30 minutes before chemotherapy and four and eight hours after the first antiemetic dose; alternative schedules include administration of a single intravenous 8- or 32-mg dose of ondansetron once daily 30 minutes before chemotherapy and oral doses of ondansetron 8 mg 30 minutes before chemotherapy and four and eight hours after the first antiemetic dose (Beck et al, 1992, 1993); or (3) concomitant intravenous administration of granisetron 10 mcg/kg infused over five minutes within 30 minutes before chemotherapy. The optimal doses and schedule have not been determined. See also the evaluations on Metoclopramide, Ondansetron, and Granisetron.

Oral: *Adults,* for delayed nausea and vomiting caused by cisplatin, beginning 24 hours after chemotherapy, 4 mg is given every eight hours for three days, then 2 mg every eight hours for three days; oral metoclopramide 0.5 mg/kg is given concomitantly every six hours for six days. Alternatively, dexamethasone 8 mg is given every 8 hours on day 1 and every 12 hours on day 2, then 4 mg every 12 hours for three days. Oral prochlorperazine is given concomitantly in the following dosage: 20 to 30 mg every eight hours on day 1, 30 mg twice on day 2, and 15 mg twice daily for three days (Strum et al, 1985).

For preparations, see index entry Dexamethasone, In Immune Disorders.

METHYLPREDNISOLONE SODIUM SUCCINATE

[Solu-Medrol]

For chemical formula, see index entry Adrenal Corticosteroids, Chemistry.

Methylprednisolone has been used as an antiemetic in cancer chemotherapy. The mechanism of action is unknown, although it has been postulated that inhibition of prostaglandin formation may be responsible for the antiemetic effect of corticosteroids.

Sequential intravenous administration of large doses of methylprednisolone in combination with droperidol and chlorpromazine has been reported to relieve vomiting induced by cisplatin 120 mg/M^2 (Mason et al, 1982). No data are available on the compatibility of intravenous solutions of these drugs with their concurrent use.

The intermittent, short-term use (<14 days) of glucocorticoids generally is not associated with toxicity. Rapid intravenous administration can cause intense perineal discomfort.

DOSAGE AND PREPARATIONS.

Intravenous: The definitive dosage has not been determined. Doses of 125 to 500 mg (administered over ten minutes or longer) have been given before chemotherapy and once or twice at six-hour intervals after chemotherapy.

Generic. Powder 40, 125, and 500 mg and 1 g.

Solu-Medrol (Upjohn). Powder 40, 125, and 500 mg and 1 and 2 g.

Mixture

No controlled studies exist to support the contention that fixed-ratio combinations are as effective as single-entity preparations.

Emetrol (Bock). Solution (oral) containing balanced amounts of fructose, dextrose, and orthophosphoric acid with controlled hydrogen ion concentration (nonprescription). The manufacturer's recommended dose is one to two tablespoonsful, repeated every 15 minutes as needed.

Cited References

Antiemetic drug products for over-the-counter human use; tentative final order. *Federal Register* 44:41064-41073, (July 13) 1979.

Glaxo's *Zofran* recommended for approval in prevention and treatment of post-op nausea and vomiting; Zofran use not advised for all procedures. *FDC Reports* 12-13, (Sept 7) 1992.

Nabilone and other antiemetics for cancer patients. *Med Lett Drugs Ther* 29:2-4, 1988.

Ondansetron *vs* dexamethasone for chemotherapy-induced emesis. *Lancet* 338:478-479, 1991.

Proceedings of investigational review--June 10, 1983: Lorazepam as adjunct in cancer chemotherapy. *Oncol Times* 7(suppl):1-27, (Feb) 1985.

Aapro MS, Alberts DS: High-dose dexamethasone for prevention of *cis*-platin-induced vomiting. *Cancer Chemother Pharmacol* 7:11-14, 1981.

Akhtar SS, et al: A double-blind randomized cross-over comparison of high-dose prochlorperazine with high-dose metoclopramide for cisplatin-induced emesis. *Oncology* 48:226-229, 1991.

Allan SG, et al: Dexamethasone and high dose metoclopramide: Efficacy in controlling cisplatin-induced nausea and vomiting. *BMJ* 289:878-879, 1984.

Anderson PO, McGuire GG: Delta-9-tetrahydrocannabinol as antiemetic. *Am J Hosp Pharm* 38:639-646, 1981.

Andrews PLR, et al: Neuropharmacology of emesis induced by anticancer therapy. *TIPS* 9:334-341, 1988.

Baloh RW: Managing dizziness: Symptomatic treatment of vertigo. *Drug Ther* 15-40, (April) 1989.

Barbezat GO: The vomiting patient: Rational approach. *Drugs* 22:246-253, 1981.

Beaver WT, Feise G: Comparison of analgesic effects of morphine, hydroxyzine, and their combination in patients with postoperative pain. *Adv Pain Res Ther* 1:553-557, 1976.

Beck TM, et al: Stratified, randomized, double-blind comparison of intravenous ondansetron administered as a multiple-dose regimen versus two single-dose regimens in the prevention of cisplatin-induced nausea and vomiting. *J Clin Oncol* 10:1969-1975, 1992.

Beck TM, et al: Efficacy of oral ondansetron in the prevention of emesis in outpatients receiving cyclophosphamide-based chemotherapy. *Ann Intern Med* 118:407-413, 1993.

Blackwell CP, Harding SM: The clinical pharmacology of ondansetron. *Eur J Cancer Clin Oncol* 25(suppl 1):21-24, 1989.

Bonneterre J, et al: A randomized double-blind comparison of ondansetron and metoclopramide in the prophylaxis of emesis induced by cyclophosphamide, fluorouracil, and doxorubicin or epirubicin chemotherapy. *J Clin Oncol* 8:1063-1069, 1990.

Borison HL, McCarthy LE: Neuropharmacology of chemotherapy-induced emesis. *Drugs* 25(suppl 1):8-17, 1983.

Bowen J: Dizziness and psychiatric disease, editorial. *J Gen Intern Med* 8:581-582, (Oct) 1993.

Brogden RN, et al: Domperidone: Review of pharmacological activity, pharmacokinetics and therapeutic efficacy in symptomatic treatment of chronic dyspepsia and as antiemetic. *Drugs* 24:360-400, 1982.

Brookes GB: Meniere's disease: Practical approach to management. *Drugs* 25:77-89, 1983.

Cann PA, et al: Galactorrhoea as side effect of domperidone. *BMJ* 286:1395-1396, 1983.

Carey MP, et al: Delta-9-tetrahydrocannabinol in cancer chemotherapy: Research problems and issues. *Ann Intern Med* 99:106-114, 1983.

Carr BI, et al: High doses of prochlorperazine for cisplatin induced emesis. *Cancer* 60:2165-2169, 1987.

Cassileth PA, et al: Antiemetic efficacy of dexamethasone therapy in patients receiving cancer chemotherapy. *Arch Intern Med* 143:1347-1349, 1983.

Castle WM, et al: Ondansetron is not associated with vascular adverse events, thrombocytopenia or renal failure. *Ann Oncol* 3:773-774, 1992.

Cersosimo RJ, Karp DD: Adrenal corticosteroids as antiemetics during cancer chemotherapy. *Pharmacol Ther* 6:118-127, 1986.

Chaffee BJ, Tankanow RM: Ondansetron: The first of a new class of antiemetic agents. *Clin Pharm* 10:430-446, 1991.

Chevallier B: Efficacy and safety of granisetron compared with high-dose metoclopramide plus dexamethasone in patients receiving high-dose cisplatin in a single-blind study: The Granisetron Study Group. *Eur J Cancer* 26(suppl 1):s33-s36, 1990.

Citron ML, et al: Droperidol: Optimal dose and time of initiation, abstract. *Proc Am Assoc Cancer Res/Am Soc Clin Oncol* 25:106, 1984.

Clark RA, et al: Exploring very high doses of metoclopramide (4-6 mg/kg): Preservation of efficacy and safety with only a single dose in a combination antiemetic regimen. *Proc Am Soc Clin Oncol* 8:330, 1989.

Clissold SP, Heel RC: Transdermal hyoscine (scopolamine): Preliminary review of its pharmacodynamic properties and therapeutic efficacy. *Drugs* 29:189-207, 1985.

Cocchetto DM, et al: Critical review of safety and antiemetic efficacy of delta-9-tetrahydrocannabinol. *Drug Intell Clin Pharm* 15:867-875, 1981.

Cotanch PH: Use of nonpharmacological techniques to prevent chemotherapy-related nausea and vomiting. *Recent Results Cancer Res* 121:101-107, 1991.

Cunningham D, et al: Ondansetron with and without dexamethasone to treat chemotherapy-induced emesis. *Lancet* 1:1323, 1989.

De Mulder PHM, et al: Ondansetron compared with high-dose metoclopramide in prophylaxis of acute and delayed cisplatin-induced nausea and vomiting: A multicenter, randomized, double-blind, crossover study. *Ann Intern Med* 113:834-840, 1990.

Dershwitz M, et al: Ondansetron is effective in decreasing postoperative nausea and vomiting. *Clin Pharmacol Ther* 52:96-101, 1992.

Dhondt F, et al: Domperidone (R33 812) suppositories: Effective antiemetic agent in diverse pediatric conditions: Multicenter trial. *Curr Ther Res* 24:912-923, 1978.

Eyre HJ, Ward JH: Control of cancer chemotherapy-induced nausea and vomiting. *Cancer* 54:2642-2648, 1984.

Fetting JH, et al: Course of nausea and vomiting after high-dose cyclophosphamide. *Cancer Treat Rep* 66:1487-1493, 1982.

Figg WD, et al: Ondansetron: A novel antiemetic agent. *South Med J* 86:497-502, (May) 1993.

Fortner CL, et al: Combination antiemetic therapy in control of chemotherapy-induced emesis. *Drug Intell Clin Pharm* 19:21-24, 1985.

Fraschini G, et al: Evaluation of three oral dosages of ondansetron in the prevention of nausea and emesis associated with cyclophosphamide-doxorubicin chemotherapy. *J Clin Oncol* 9:1268-1274, 1991.

Gralla RJ: Metoclopramide: Review of antiemetic trials. *Drugs* 25(suppl 1):63-73, 1983.

Gralla RJ: Controlling emesis in patients receiving cancer chemotherapy. *Recent Results Cancer Res* 121:68-85, 1991.

Gralla RJ: Antiemetic drugs for chemotherapeutic support: Current treatment and rationale for development of newer agents. *Cancer Suppl* 70:1003-1006, 1992.

Gralla RJ, et al: Antiemetic efficacy of high-dose metoclopramide: Randomized trials with placebo and prochlorperazine in patients with chemotherapy-induced nausea and vomiting. *N Engl J Med* 305:905-909, 1981.

Gralla RJ, et al: Antiemetic therapy: Review of recent studies and report of random assignment trial comparing metoclopramide with delta-9-tetrahydrocannabinol. *Cancer Treat Rep* 68:163-172, 1984.

Gralla RJ, et al: Management of chemotherapy-induced nausea and vomiting. *Med Clin North Am* 71:289-301, 1987.

Graves T: Chemotherapy-induced nausea and vomiting: Treatment options. *Hosp Formul* 26:474-488, 1991.

Grunberg SM, Hesketh PJ: Control of chemotherapy-induced emesis. *N Engl J Med* 329:1790–1796, 1993.

Grunberg SM, et al: Comparison of antiemetic effect of high-dose intravenous metoclopramide and high-dose intravenous haloperidol in randomized double-blind crossover study. *J Clin Oncol* 2:782-787, 1984.

Hainsworth J, et al: A single-blind comparison of intravenous ondansetron, a selective serotonin antagonist, with intravenous metoclopramide in the prevention of nausea and vomiting associated with high-dose cisplatin chemotherapy. *J Clin Oncol* 9:721-728, 1991.

Harvey VJ, et al: Reduction of carboplatin induced emesis by ondansetron. *Br J Cancer* 63:942-944, 1991.

Herrstedt J, et al: Ondansetron plus metopimazine compared with ondansetron alone in patients receiving moderately emetogenic chemotherapy. *N Engl J Med* 328:1076-1080, 1993.

Hesketh PJ, Gandara DR: Serotonin antagonists: A new class of antiemetic agents. *J Natl Cancer Inst* 83:613-620, 1991.

Hesketh PJ, et al: GR 38032F (GR-C507/75): A novel compound effective in the prevention of acute cisplatin-induced emesis. *J Clin Oncol* 7:700-705, 1989.

Hesketh PJ, et al: A possible role for cisplatin (DDP) in the transient hepatic enzyme elevations noted after ondansetron administration, abstract. *Proc Am Soc Clin Oncol* 9:323, 1990.

Hoffbrand BI (ed): Domperidone in treatment of upper gastrointestinal symptoms, symposium. *Postgrad Med J* 55(suppl):1-54, 1979.

Hunter-Johnson P: Granisetron—The antiemetic battle has begun. *INPHARMA* 12-13, (Nov 23) 1991.

Jantunen IT, et al: 5-HT_3 receptor antagonists in the prophylaxis of acute vomiting induced by moderately emetogenic chemotherapy–A randomised study. *Eur J Cancer* 29A:1669-1672, 1993.

Jones AL, et al: Comparison of dexamethasone and ondansetron in the prophylaxis of emesis induced by moderately emetogenic chemotherapy. *Lancet* 338:483-487, 1991.

Kaasa S, et al: A comparison of ondansetron with metoclopramide in the prophylaxis of chemotherapy-induced nausea and vomiting: A randomized, double-blind study. *Eur J Cancer* 26:311-314, 1990.

Kataria M, et al: Extrapyramidal side-effects of metoclopramide. *Lancet* 2:1254-1255, 1978.

Kerr AG: Aspects of vertigo. *J R Soc Med* 83:348-351, 1990.

Kris MG, et al: Improved control of cisplatin-induced emesis with high-dose metoclopramide and with combinations of metoclopramide, dexamethasone, and diphenhydramine: Results of consecutive trials in 255 patients. *Cancer* 55:527-534, 1985.

Kris MG, et al: Antiemetic control and prevention of side-effects of anticancer therapy with lorazepam or diphenhydramine when used in combination with metoclopramide plus dexamethasone: Double-blind, randomized trial. *Cancer* 60:2816-2822, 1987.

Kris MG, et al: Phase II trials of the serotonin antagonist GR 38032F for control of vomiting caused by cisplatin. *J Natl Cancer Inst* 81:42-46, 1989 A.

Kris MG, et al: Controlling delayed vomiting: Double-blind, randomized trial comparing placebo, dexamethasone alone, and metoclopramide plus dexamethasone in patients receiving cisplatin. *J Clin Oncol* 7:108-114, 1989 B.

Kroenke K: Practical office workup and management recommendations. *Consultant* 80-90, (Jan) 1993.

Kroenke K, et al: Psychiatric disorders and functional impairment in patients with persistent dizziness. *J Gen Intern Med* 8:530-535, 1993.

Kumar A, Petchenik L: The diagnosis and management of vertigo. *Compr Ther* 16:56-66, (Dec) 1990.

Lane M, et al: Dronabinol and prochlorperazine alone and in combination as antiemetic agents for cancer chemotherapy. *Am J Clin Oncol* 13:480-484, 1990.

Laszlo J, et al: Lorazepam in cancer patients treated with cisplatin: A drug with antiemetic, amnestic, and anxiolytic effects. *J Clin Oncol* 3:864-869, 1985.

Latreille J, et al: Dexamethasone (DEX) improves the efficacy of granisetron (GRAN) in the first 24 hours following high-dose cisplatin (HDCP) chemotherapy, in: *Program/Proceedings at American Society of Clinical Oncology in Orlando, FL May 16-18, 1993*, Abstract 330, 1993.

Leeser J, Lip H: Prevention of postoperative nausea and vomiting using ondansetron, a new, selective, 5-HT_3 receptor antagonist. *Anesth Analg* 72:751-755, 1991.

Lemberger L, et al: Comparative pharmacology of Δ^9-tetrahydrocannabinol and its metabolite, 11-OH-Δ^9-tetrahydrocannabinol. *J Clin Invest* 52:2411-2417, 1973.

Loeser EA, et al: Comparison of droperidol, haloperidol and prochlorperazine as postoperative antiemetics. *Can Anaesth Soc J* 26:125-127, 1979.

Madej G, et al: A comparative study of the use of navoban (ICS 205-930), a 5-HT_3 antagonist, versus a standard antiemetic regimen of dexamethasone and metoclopramide in the treatment of cisplatin-containing chemotherapy. *Drug Invest* 6:162-169, 1993.

Markman M, et al: Antiemetic efficacy of dexamethasone: Randomized, double-blind, crossover study with prochlorperazine in patients receiving cancer chemotherapy. *N Engl J Med* 311:549-552, 1984.

Marty M, et al: A comparative study of the use of granisetron, a selective 5-HT_3 antagonist, versus a standard anti-emetic regimen of chlorpromazine plus dexamethasone in the treatment of cytostatic-induced emesis. *Eur J Cancer* 26(suppl 1):S28-S32, 1990 A.

Marty M, et al: Comparison of the 5-hydroxytryptamine$_3$ (serotonin) antagonist ondansetron (GR 38032F) with high-dose metoclopramide in the control of cisplatin-induced emesis. *N Engl J Med* 322:816-821, 1990 B.

Mason BA, et al: Effective control of cisplatin-induced nausea using high-dose steroids and droperidol. *Cancer Treat Rep* 66:243-245, 1982.

McGovern EM, et al: Pharmacokinetics of high-dose metoclopramide in cancer patients. *Clin Pharmacokinet* 11:415-424, 1986.

McKenzie R, et al: Antiemetic effectiveness of intramuscular hydroxyzine compared with intramuscular droperidol. *Anesth Analg* 60:783-788, 1981.

Merrifield KR, Chaffee BJ: Recent advances in the management of nausea and vomiting caused by antineoplastic agents. *Clin Pharm* 8:187-199, 1989.

Meyer BR, et al: Optimizing metoclopramide control of cisplatin-induced emesis. *Ann Intern Med* 100:393-395, 1984.

Milkovich I, van den Berg BJ: Evaluation of teratogenicity of certain antinauseant drugs. *Am J Obstet Gynecol* 125:244-248, 1976.

Milne RJ, Heel RC: Ondansetron: Therapeutic use as an antiemetic. *Drugs* 41:574-595, 1991.

Mitchell PLR, et al: Ondansetron reduces chemotherapy induced nausea and vomiting refractory to standard antiemetics. *N Z Med J* 105:73-75, (March) 1992.

Moertel CG, et al: Controlled clinical evaluation of antiemetic drugs. *JAMA* 186:116-118, 1963.

Morran C, et al: Incidence of nausea and vomiting with cytotoxic chemotherapy: Prospective randomised trial of antiemetics. *BMJ* 1:1323-1324, 1979.

Morrow GR: Chemotherapy-related nausea and vomiting: Etiology and management. *Cancer J Physicians* 39:89-104, 1989.

Morrow GR, et al: Predicting development of anticipatory nausea in cancer patients: Prospective examination of eight clinical characteristics. *J Pain Symptom Management* 6:215-223, 1991.

Navari RM, et al: Comparison of intermittent ondansetron versus continuous infusion metoclopramide used with standard combination antiemetics in control of acute nausea induced by cisplatin chemotherapy. *Cancer* 72:583-586, 1993.

Neidhart JA, et al: Specific antiemetics for specific cancer chemotherapeutic agents: Haloperidol versus benzquinamide. *Cancer* 47:1439-1443, 1981.

Palmer JBD, et al: Ondansetron and chest pain. *Lancet* 340:1410, 1992.

Parrott AC: Transdermal scopolamine: Review of its effects upon motion sickness, psychological performance, and physiological functioning. *Aviat Space Environ Med* 60:1-9, 1989.

Plosker G: 5HT_3 antagonists and corticosteroids—Powerful partners in antiemesis. *INPHARMA* 5-6, (Nov 21) 1992.

Plosker GL, Goa KL: Granisetron: A review of its pharmacological properties and therapeutic use as an antiemetic. *Drugs* 42:805-824, 1991.

Plosker GL, Milne RJ: Ondansetron: A pharmacoeconomic and quality-of-life evaluation of its antiemetic activity in patients receiving cancer chemotherapy. *PharmacoEconomics* 2:285-304, 1992.

Price N, et al: Transdermal delivery of scopolamine for prevention of motion-induced nausea in rough seas. *Clin Ther* 2:258-262, 1979.

Priestman TJ, et al: Results of a randomized, double-blind comparative study of ondansetron and metoclopramide in the prevention of nausea and vomiting following high-dose upper abdominal irradiation. *Clin Oncol* 2:71-75, 1990.

Reyntjens A: Domperidone as antiemetic: Summary of research reports. *Postgrad Med J* 55:50-54, 1979.

Robinson B: Control of emesis associated with cancer chemotherapy. *N Z Med J* 106:52-54, 1993.

Roila F, et al: Prevention of cisplatin-induced emesis: A double-blind multicenter randomized crossover study comparing ondansetron and ondansetron plus dexamethasone. *J Clin Oncol* 9:675-678, 1991.

Ruckenstein MJ, Harrison RV: Motion sickness: Helping patients tolerate the ups and downs. *Postgrad Med* 89:139-142, 144, 1991.

Sahakian V, et al: Vitamin B_6 is effective therapy for nausea and vomiting of pregnancy: A randomized, double-blind placebo-controlled study. *Obstet Gynecol* 78:33-36, 1991.

Saller R, Hellenbrecht D: High doses of metoclopramide or droperidol in prevention of cisplatin-induced emesis. *Eur J Cancer Clin Oncol* 22:1199-1203, 1986.

Samuels MA: Vertigo: *Harvard Med School Health Lett* 6-8, (Mar) 1990.

Saynor DA, Dixon CM: The metabolism of ondansetron. *Eur J Cancer Clin Oncol* 25(suppl 1):75-77, 1989.

Smith DB, et al: Ondansetron (GR38032F) plus dexamethasone: Effective anti-emetic prophylaxis for patients receiving cytotoxic chemotherapy. *Br J Cancer* 61:323-324, 1990.

Smith DB, et al: Comparison of ondansetron and ondansetron plus dexamethasone as antiemetic prophylaxis during cisplatin-containing chemotherapy. *Lancet* 338:487-490, 1991.

Sridhar KS, Donnelly E: Combination antiemetics for cisplatin chemotherapy. *Cancer* 61:1508-1517, 1988.

Stringer SP, Meyerhoff WL: Diagnosis, causes, and management of vertigo. *Compr Ther* 16:34-41, (Mar) 1990.

Strum SB, et al: Intravenous metoclopramide: Effective antiemetic in cancer chemotherapy. *JAMA* 247:2683-2686, 1982.

Strum SB, et al: Intravenous metoclopramide: Prevention of chemotherapy-induced nausea and vomiting; preliminary evaluation. *Cancer* 53:1432-1439, 1984.

Strum SB, et al: Control of acute onset and delayed-onset chemotherapy-induced nausea and emesis with metoclopramide-based regimens. *Int Med* 6:104-117, 1985.

Sullivan M, et al: Psychiatric and otologic diagnoses in patients complaining of dizziness. *Arch Intern Med* 153:1479-1484, 1993.

Tortorice PV, O'Connell MB: Management of chemotherapy-induced nausea and vomiting. *Pharmacotherapy* 10:129-145, 1990.

Triozzi PL, Laszlo J: Optimum management of nausea and vomiting in cancer chemotherapy. *Drugs* 34:136-149, 1987.

Troost BT, Patton JM; Exercise therapy for positional vertigo. *Neurology* 42:1441-1444, 1992.

Turner JS Jr: Practical approach to patient with vertigo: Outline of diagnosis and management for nonspecialist. *South Med J* 68:241-245, 1975.

Wade-Evans V (ed): Conference focus on tropisetron. *INPHARMA* 12-13, (Nov 9) 1991.

Warr D, et al: Superiority of granisetron to dexamethasone plus prochlorperazine in the prevention of chemotherapy-induced emesis. *J Natl Cancer Inst* 83:1169-1173, 1991.

Warr D, et al: A randomised, double-blind comparison of granisetron with high-dose metoclopramide, dexamethasone and diphenhydramine for cisplatin-induced emesis: An NCI Canada Clinical Trials Group Phase III Trial. *Eur J Cancer* 29A:33-36, 1992.

Wilson J, et al: Continuous infusion droperidol: Antiemetic therapy for cis-platinum (DDP) toxicity, abstract. *Proc Am Assoc Cancer Res/Am Soc Clin Oncol* 22:241, 1981.

Wood CD: Antimotion sickness and antiemetic drugs. *Drugs* 17:471-479, 1979.

Wood CD, Graybiel A: Theory of antimotion sickness drug mechanisms. *Aerospace Med* 43:249-252, 1972.

Wood CD, et al: Mechanisms of antimotion sickness drugs. *Aviat Space Environ Med* 58 (suppl 9):A262-A265, 1987.

Woodward M, Gora ML: Ondansetron for postoperative nausea and vomiting. *Ann Pharmacother* 27:188, 1993.

Drugs Used to Treat Upper Respiratory Tract Disorders

20

COUGH

Cough is a protective respiratory reflex by which foreign matter can be expelled from the tracheobronchial tree. As such, cough is usually helpful and occurs when needed in healthy people. However, in many disorders, coughing increases in frequency and severity and becomes troublesome rather than helpful, particularly when it is painful or disturbs sleep.

The cough reflex is initiated by stimulation of mechanical receptors or chemoreceptors and is mediated by efferent pathways along the vagus, glossopharyngeal, and superior laryngeal nerves to a cough center located near the respiratory and vomiting centers in the hindbrain. An effective cough reflex requires an intact peripheral nerve pathway to the abdomen, thoracic muscles, diaphragm, and glottis, and the muscles of these organs must be functional. Cough is severely impaired if any component in the reflex arc is inhibited, depressed, or malfunctioning.

Cough can be caused by disorders within the upper as well as the lower respiratory tracts. Irritation of the trigeminal and glossopharyngeal nerves in the nose, sinuses, or pharynx; the vagal nerve supplying the ears, pleura, or stomach; or the phrenic nerve adjacent to the pericardium or in the diaphragm also can produce coughing. Thus, cough can result from disorders in the head and abdomen as well as in the chest. Accordingly, an accurate diagnosis is required to determine the most appropriate measures to correct the causes as well as to select the most appropriate agents for cough therapy.

The self-limited character of most coughs associated with acute respiratory infection accounts for the popular conception that many cough preparations are effective, and this explains their corresponding widespread use. Accordingly, patients who seek treatment for a cough usually expect some form of medication. Symptomatic treatment is employed primarily for the self-limited acute nonproductive cough that accompanies mild upper respiratory infection or a common cold.

Chronic cough can be defined as that persisting for at least three weeks. A specific cause can be identified in more than 95% of patients, and specific therapy is successful in most of these individuals (Irwin et al, 1990, 1993). Postnasal drip (probably related to chronic sinusitis), asthma, or both may account for approximately 70% of chronic coughs (Irwin and Curley, 1988; Irwin et al, 1990); cough may be the only symptom in some patients with asthma (eg, cough-variant asthma). A significant percentage of other cases of chronic cough may be due to silent gastrointestinal reflux, with or without aspiration (Irwin and Curley, 1989; Fitzgerald et al, 1989). Chronic bronchitis and smoking are other causes. In adults, bronchiectasis, tracheitis, sarcoidosis, congestive heart failure, chronic pulmonary infections, pulmonary tumors, psychogenic factors, and therapy with beta-adrenergic blocking agents or angiotensin-converting enzyme (ACE) inhibitors also produce cough. Up to 25% of patients treated with

ACE inhibitors develop a chronic cough (Simon et al, 1992), and the incidence may increase with continued therapy (Keogh, 1993). Consequently, discontinuation of therapy may be required in up to 10% of patients (Goldszer et al, 1988; Sebastian et al, 1991).

For a comprehensive discussion of the management of psychogenic cough in children, see Lavigne et al, 1991.

Drug Therapy

Cough suppressants should be considered when their action will not compromise resolution of the underlying disease or when complications (eg, rib fracture, cough syncope) produce discomfort or pose a danger to the patient (Irwin and Curley, 1991). Patients with productive cough generally should not be given cough suppressants, particularly if they are elderly, not fully alert, or neurologically impaired. However, in general, cough suppressants do not impair voluntary coughing to clear secretions.

Over-the-counter remedies, such as cough drops, lozenges, troches, rock candy, and preparations of traditional remedies (eg, horehound), are generally considered to be relatively ineffective but are usually harmless. They may offer symptomatic relief for episodes of self-limited cough or cough induced reflexly by pharyngeal or laryngeal irritation.

The numerous prescription and nonprescription products available for the treatment of cough may contain a single ingredient or a combination of agents designed to suppress cough (antitussives), increase mucus excretion (expectorants), or liquefy secretions (hydrating or mucolytic agents). Antihistamines, vasoconstrictors, analgesics, local antitussives or anesthetics, flavoring agents, and placebos often are added. For a listing of selected combination products containing antitussives, see the section on Mixtures.

Antitussives are usually classified as centrally or peripherally acting, depending on whether they act on the medullary cough center or on the peripheral receptors in the tracheobronchial tree. The centrally acting group includes opioids (eg, codeine, hydrocodone, hydromorphone [Dilaudid]) and the nonopioid agents, dextromethorphan (most commonly present as an ingredient in mixtures) and caramiphen and carbetapentane, which are available only in combination products. Some antihistamines (eg, diphenhydramine [Benadryl], promethazine [Phenergan]) also have central antitussive effects. The peripherally acting group includes agents with local anesthetic or analgesic activity, anti-inflammatory agents, bronchodilators, and expectorants. Demulcents have a soothing effect on the pharynx that can provide symptomatic relief.

Reports on the effectiveness of various antitussive agents frequently conflict because of the difficulties in assessing their effects. Most currently available evaluations of single-entity antitussive drugs are based on subjective rather than objective methods, and the placebo effect is an important factor. Results of studies on patients with chronic cough are not necessarily applicable to those with acute cough, which often improves spontaneously within a few days.

CENTRALLY ACTING ANTITUSSIVES. Opioids: These agents decrease the sensitivity of the cough center to incoming stimuli. Results of experimental and clinical studies and many years of experience have shown that codeine is very efficacious for cough caused by a variety of disease states or irritants. The related agent, hydrocodone, also is effective and is three times more potent as an antitussive than codeine on a milligram basis, but it has greater dependence liability. Hydrocodone (available only as an ingredient in mixtures) and codeine have been used to suppress acute cough in patients with irritative, nonproductive cough associated with many disorders, including subacute congestive heart failure. However, the opioids can cause gastrointestinal upset, constipation, and drying of the mucosa, and they may release histamine that can result in bronchospasm and urticaria. In addition, because of the danger of depression of the respiratory center, the opioids must be used with great care in patients with pulmonary insufficiency. This is especially true of the cough that accompanies acute asthma; therapy should be directed at the asthma rather than the cough. The dependence potential of the opioids also must be considered.

The more potent opioid analgesics (eg, morphine, hydromorphone, oxycodone, methadone, meperidine [Demerol]) probably have antitussive activity, but they may produce more adverse reactions and have a greater dependence liability with continued use than codeine and hydrocodone. Thus, these opioid analgesics are seldom used as general antitussives but are reserved for conditions in which cough is associated with pain, anxiety, and restlessness and for severe, nonproductive, or stressful cough.

Nonopioids: Dextromethorphan, a synthetic agent structurally related to codeine, is as effective as codeine except for severe acute cough. Usual doses generally have no analgesic, sedative, or respiratory depressant effects. This drug has had more extensive clinical study than other nonopioid antitussives and is the safest antitussive available for use by adults and adolescents. Adverse effects are usually mild and may be similar to those produced by opioids (eg, nausea, drowsiness, dizziness) except that dextromethorphan does not have neuropsychiatric effects. The efficacy of this drug in younger children has not been established.

Some antihistamines, particularly diphenhydramine, may have antitussive as well as local anesthetic properties. The mechanism of diphenhydramine's antitussive action is unclear. Promethazine, a phenothiazine antihistamine, is an ingredient of some combination products for cough, but whether it has a specific antitussive effect has not been established.

PERIPHERALLY ACTING ANTITUSSIVES. Expectorants: In experimental studies, large doses of expectorants stimulate the flow of respiratory tract fluid and facilitate the movement of loosened material toward the pharynx by ciliary motion and coughing. These agents should be most useful when secretions thicken or become dry. Increasing the quantity of secretion facilitates removal of irritants and has a demulcent effect on the irritated mucosa, thus diminishing the tendency to cough. However, satisfactory techniques to prove that these drugs increase the secretion of respiratory tract fluid when administered in recommended doses are not available. Their use is based primarily on tradition and the widespread subjective impression among both patients and physicians that they are effective.

Commonly used expectorants probably produce some of their effects through a local or reflex irritant action or an emetic effect that activates the vagus to stimulate the secretion of respiratory tract fluid. Of the many agents promoted for their expectorant action, guaifenesin is currently the most widely used and is a common ingredient of many cough mixtures. Its efficacy in doses recommended by manufacturers is questionable, although some clinicians believe that there is a response to larger doses.

Other ingredients often present in cough mixtures (eg, ammonium salts, electrolytes, iodides, ipecac syrup, guaiacol sulfonate potassium) may stimulate the secretion of respiratory tract fluid when subemetic doses are given, but little evidence on their effectiveness is available.

Although few controlled studies have evaluated the efficacy of iodides as expectorants for minor upper respiratory disorders, many clinicians believe that iodide salts may be beneficial in adults with acute upper respiratory infection when used judiciously. However, prolonged administration of the iodides can suppress thyroid function in susceptible patients. Although these agents appear to be safe as expectorants if administered for less than six weeks, it is recommended that they not be used in pregnant women (to avoid risk to the fetus) and children (Galina et al, 1962; Committee on Drugs, American Academy of Pediatrics, 1976; Schatz et al, 1988).

In the multicenter National Mucolytic Study, the investigators concluded that iodinated glycerol is a safe and effective expectorant in patients with stable chronic obstructive bronchitis (Petty, 1990) and that its effectiveness is maintained in those with less severe disease. Although many clinicians agreed with the conclusions of this study, the FDA questioned its design. A possible increase in the incidence of tumors was observed in animal studies after administration of iodinated glycerol (*FDC Reports*, 1992 A); it is unclear whether this agent causes tumors in humans. Because of lack of adequate data on safety and efficacy, the FDA has ordered its withdrawal from the market and supplies are being depleted (*FDC Reports,* 1993; *Dickinson's FDA,* 1993).

Mucolytics: The solubilizing action of a mucolytic agent may make tenacious or inspissated secretions easier to eliminate. Acetylcysteine [Mucomyst, Mucosil] aerosol can loosen secretions, thus leading to a more effective cough. A 5% to 10% solution also can be instilled into the tracheobronchial tree to treat atelectasis; its mucolytic action coupled with its cough-inducing effect may dislodge mucous plugs. In addition, the free radical scavenging action of this drug may be beneficial in smokers with chronic obstructive pulmonary disease. A major disadvantage of acetylcysteine is its sulfurous odor; a European product, which lacks this disadvantage, is given orally. Hypertonic saline in aerosol form is usually less effective than acetylcysteine. Some physicians prefer to use hypertonic sodium bicarbonate as an aerosol or by direct instillation to loosen viscous secretions. (This agent also may be useful as a diluent for acetylcysteine.) These aerosol agents are irritating and frequently trigger reflex bronchospasm; the bronchospasm can be decreased by the concomitant use of bronchodilators.

Hydrating Agents: The demulcent action of hydrating agents diminishes the frequency, severity, and duration of cough and also alleviates the discomfort of laryngotracheobronchitis. Hydrating agents are thought to thin bronchial secretions and may be more beneficial than expectorants. Some clinicians suggest that the most effective hydrating agent is the glass of water taken with the cough preparation. Water given by inhalation, orally, or parenterally may be useful. However, in laboratory studies, increasing the daily intake of water in patients with chronic bronchitis had no effect on the quality or quantity of sputum (Shim et al, 1987).

The use of vaporizers is soothing for patients with upper airway, nasal, or sinus congestion and inflammation and may reduce the viscosity of secretions. However, the increase in relative humidity associated with use of these devices may be hazardous because it can promote mold growth and mite proliferation. The growth of molds can be controlled by cleaning the vaporizer with a 10% chlorine solution. Hot water steam may cause burns, especially in young children. Since little of the vaporizer mist reaches the lower airways, this treatment has limited value in bronchial disorders.

Water or saline inhaled as a hot or cold steam mist may aggravate bronchospasm in patients with asthma or chronic bronchitis. Normal and hypotonic saline solutions are occasionally preferred for cool mist when the bronchial tree is affected. Particles should be 1 to 5 microns to have a significant effect. Patients often report a beneficial effect from inhalation of water-saturated air; tap water can be used to produce steam or for direct nebulization for inhalation to relieve disorders of the upper respiratory tract. Hypertonic saline delivered by an ultrasonic nebulizer is very useful to induce sputum production for diagnostic purposes (eg, diagnosis of pneumocystis pneumonia in patients with AIDS).

Local Antitussives: Menthol is believed to have a local soothing or counterirritant effect when used in lozenge, ointment, or drop form; however, excessive amounts can inhibit ciliary activity. Camphor also is applied in ointment form; its usefulness in solution is limited by the great danger of inducing seizures, especially in children. Ointments should not be inhaled since they are irritating to the lungs.

Local Anesthetics: Topical local anesthetics may relieve irritation of pharyngeal tissue receptors, particularly in cough accompanying sore throat or postnasal drip. These agents also may enhance productive cough by blocking pain that discourages coughing, as in postoperative patients. Local anesthesia of respiratory tract mucous membranes can be achieved with nebulization of lidocaine [Xylocaine]; however, this may be impractical because the tongue and hypopharynx also are anesthetized, which increases the danger of aspiration. The local anesthetic activity of benzonatate [Tessalon] and some other cough suppressants is claimed to be the basis for their effect when taken in oral forms. In several studies, benzonatate was shown to be effective for some chronic coughs.

Bronchodilators: Since cough may be caused or aggravated by bronchospasm, use of bronchodilators (beta-adrenergic receptor agonists, ipratropium [Atrovent], or theophylline) often diminishes cough, particularly in asthmatic patients whose earliest symptom is cough alone. The cough-variant form of asthma, in which cough is the only symptom, may be difficult to diagnose because the classical feature of asthma (ie, reversible airway obstruction) is not present (Johnson and Osborn, 1991; O'Connell et al, 1991). In young children, bronchodilators often relieve the cough associated with asthma or with bronchospasm caused by viral respiratory infections.

Miscellaneous Drugs: In case studies involving small numbers of patients, cromolyn sodium [Nasalcrom] relieved the chronic cough produced by ACE inhibitors in many patients (Aldis, 1991; Barnes, 1992; Sebastian et al, 1991). Agents that inhibit prostaglandin synthesis (eg, the nonsteroidal anti-inflammatory drugs, indomethacin [Indocin], ibuprofen, and sulindac [Clinoril]) and calcium channel blockers such as nifedipine [Aladat, Procardia] also have reduced cough symptoms in patients receiving ACE inhibitors (Dales et al, 1992; Fogari et al, 1992; Irwin et al, 1993). Nedocromil sodium [Tilade] is effective in cough induced by nonallergenic stimuli (eg, sulfur dioxide).

The intranasal or inhalant aerosol preparation of the anticholinergic drug, ipratropium bromide, may relieve cough in patients with chronic bronchitis or chronic persistent cough following an upper respiratory infection (Irwin et al, 1993; Holmes et al, 1992). Antihistamines and intranasal steroids may be beneficial when coughing is a component of a generalized allergy affecting the respiratory tract.

Adverse Reactions and Precautions

Untoward effects produced by antitussives or expectorants occur infrequently, are generally mild, and usually subside promptly when the drugs are withdrawn. However, caution is indicated when opioid antitussives are used in sedated, debilitated, hypoxic, or hypercapnic patients or in those receiving other central nervous system depressants.

In patients with obstructive lung diseases, such as asthma, emphysema, chronic bronchitis, or cystic fibrosis, productive cough expels respiratory tract fluid. In addition to limiting the flow of sputum, cough suppressants may cause sedation and exacerbate retention of carbon dioxide. Therefore, individuals with obstructive lung diseases should not, in general, receive cough suppressants. The correct treatment for cough in these patients is the appropriate management of the underlying condition. Nevertheless, in some patients with hyperactive airway disease, carefully monitored cough suppression may be beneficial; moreover, the effectiveness of voluntary coughing is not lessened by use of antitussives.

It should be borne in mind that the drugs administered postoperatively to relieve pain have cough suppressant properties and may cause retention of secretions leading to bronchial obstruction, atelectasis, and pneumonia. However, opioids given appropriately for pain will not cause significant respiratory depression since the respiratory center rapidly adapts to analgesic doses of morphine and similar drugs.

Serious reactions, such as respiratory depression and excessive drowsiness, occur only rarely when usual doses of opioid preparations are given to children under 5 years, but poisoning and some deaths have followed ingestion of larger doses. Parents may be unaware that the cough preparation contains an opioid. Therefore, such cough preparations should rarely be prescribed for infants and should be used with great care in children. Tolerance to the antitussive effects of opioids may occur with prolonged use.

The safety of most of these agents in pregnant or nursing women has not been established. Iodide products should be avoided during pregnancy because they can be goitrogenic in the fetus.

Drug Evaluations

Opioids

CODEINE PHOSPHATE

CODEINE SULFATE

Codeine, the reference compound with which other antitussives are compared, acts centrally to depress cough. This opioid is effective orally for acute cough associated with a variety of diseases and irritants. Codeine is more effective than dextromethorphan for severe cough.

ADVERSE REACTIONS AND PRECAUTIONS. Antitussive doses generally are well tolerated, but nausea, vomiting, constipation, dizziness, palpitations, drowsiness, pruritus, urticaria, and, rarely, sweating and agitation have been reported.

Dependence is uncommon after antitussive use of codeine because of the short duration of therapy and the small doses required. However, codeine is sometimes abused since it is readily available in many cough mixtures. This opioid is classified as a Schedule II drug under the Controlled Substances Act; cough mixtures containing codeine are classified as Schedule III or V substances.

As with other opioid analgesics, respiratory depression occurs with overdosage; the alcohol content of some preparations may be contributory. This is a particular problem in children, especially those under 5 years. Codeine is not recommended for children under 2 years. Respiratory depression can be reversed by the opioid antagonist, naloxone (see index entry Naloxone, In Opioid Overdose).

This drug is classified in FDA Pregnancy Category C.

DOSAGE AND PREPARATIONS.

Oral: *Adults,* 10 to 20 mg every four to six hours (maximum, 120 mg/day) as necessary. Codeine is rarely indicated as a cough suppressant in children. The following doses have been used: For *children 6 to 12 years*, 5 to 10 mg or 0.5 to 1.5 mg/kg every four to six hours (maximum, 60 mg/day); *2 to 6 years*, 0.5 to 1 mg/kg daily in equally divided doses every four to six hours (maximum, 30 mg/day).

CODEINE PHOSPHATE:

Generic. Tablets 30 and 60 mg; solution (oral) 15 mg/5 ml. The phosphate salt is much more soluble in water than the sulfate salt; however, this may not have clinical relevance.

CODEINE SULFATE:

Generic. Tablets 15, 30, and 60 mg.

See the section on Mixtures for a listing of combination products containing codeine.

HYDROCODONE BITARTRATE

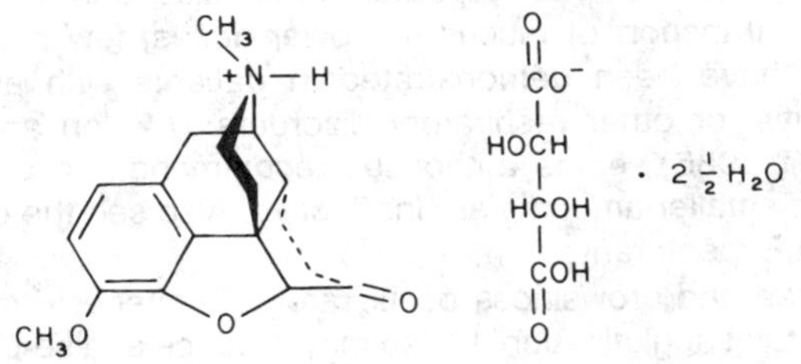

The usefulness of hydrocodone as an antitussive is similar to that of codeine; it is two to three times more potent on a milligram basis. Accordingly, the dependence liability of hydrocodone is also greater than that of codeine. This antitussive is classified as a Schedule III drug under the Controlled Substances Act.

Hydrocodone is rarely indicated as a cough suppressant in children.

This antitussive is available only in combination products.

The most common adverse reactions are nausea, dizziness, and constipation. Dryness of the pharynx and occasional tightness of the chest have been reported. Other adverse reactions and precautions are the same as those reported for codeine. This drug is classified in FDA Pregnancy Category C.

See the section on Mixtures for a listing of combination products containing hydrocodone.

Nonopioids

BENZONATATE

[Tessalon]

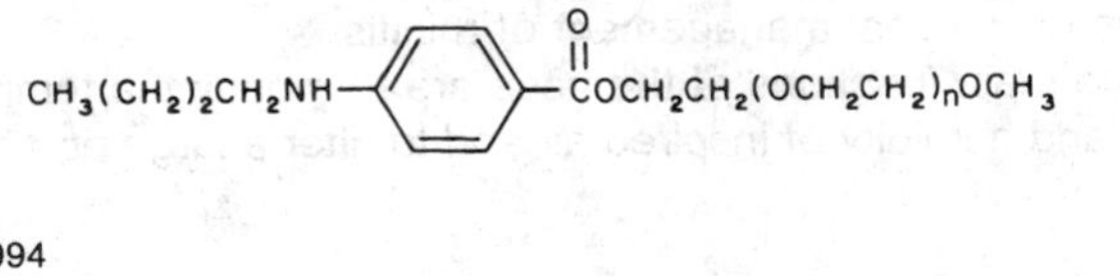

$CH_3(CH_2)_2CH_2NH-C_6H_4-COCH_2CH_2(OCH_2CH_2)_nOCH_3$

ACTIONS AND USES. Benzonatate is related structurally to tetracaine. It is believed to exert its antitussive action by anesthetizing stretch or cough receptors in the respiratory tract, as well as by a central mechanism.

Benzonatate is safe and effective in relieving acute cough associated with a variety of diseases and irritants. Onset of action is 15 to 30 minutes after oral administration, and the duration of effect is three to eight hours.

ADVERSE REACTIONS. Adverse reactions are mild; the following have been reported: constipation, nasal congestion, slight vertigo, headache, nausea, drowsiness, and hypersensitivity reactions including rash. The local anesthetic effect of benzonatate produces numbness of the mouth, tongue, and pharynx if the capsules are chewed; the numbness produced may cause difficulty in swallowing, and aspiration may result. This drug should not be used in children under 10 years. Benzonatate has a very unpleasant taste.

This drug is classified in FDA Pregnancy Category C.

DOSAGE AND PREPARATIONS.

Oral: *Adults and children over 10 years*, initially, 100 mg three times daily. If necessary, this drug may be given every four hours (maximum, 600 mg/day). *Children under 10 years*, not recommended.

Tessalon (Forest). Capsules (liquid-filled) 100 mg.

DEXTROMETHORPHAN HYDROBROMIDE

[Benylin, Delsym, Pertussin ES, Robitussin Maximum Strength Cough Suppressant, Vicks Formula 44 Cough Medicine]

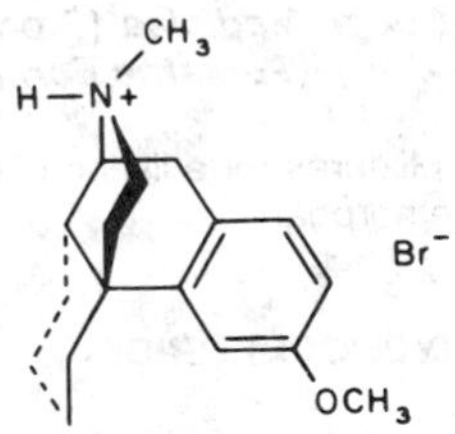

This synthetic nonopioid cough suppressant, the dextroisomer of the codeine analogue of levorphanol, appears to be as effective as codeine except for severe cough and, like codeine, acts centrally to elevate the cough threshold. It does not have addictive, analgesic, or sedative actions and does not produce respiratory depression with usual doses. Dextromethorphan is the safest antitussive available for use by adults and adolescents. It is often administered to children, but its efficacy in younger children has not been established. Dextromethorphan is present in many over-the-counter cough preparations. Prolonged-release preparations deliver the drug from liquid ion-exchange complexes over 9 to 12 hours.

ADVERSE REACTIONS AND INTERACTIONS. Adverse reactions are mild and infrequent. Nausea and dizziness can occur. Central nervous system and respiratory depression may develop after very large doses or in patients with impaired respiratory function (eg, asthma, emphysema) (Schneider et al, 1991).

Quinidine inhibits liver cytochrome P450 enzymes that metabolize dextromethorphan; concomitant administration of these drugs increases the serum concentration of the latter (Zhang et al, 1992). Pronounced central nervous system stimulation and severe respiratory depression have been reported with concomitant administration of dextromethorphan and monoamine oxidase inhibitors (*FDC Reports,* 1992 B).

Abuse of dextromethorphan by adolescents has occurred. Presumably, respiratory depression could be reversed by naloxone (Schneider et al, 1991).

DOSAGE AND PREPARATIONS.

Oral: (Regular preparation) *Adults,* 10 to 20 mg every four hours or 30 mg every six to eight hours (maximum, 120 mg/day). *Children,* 1 mg/kg daily in three or four divided doses. Alternatively, *children 6 to 12 years*, 5 to 10 mg every four hours or 15 mg every six to eight hours (maximum, 60 mg/24 hours); *2 to 6 years*, 2.5 to 5 mg every four hours or 7.5 mg every six to eight hours (maximum, 30 mg/day).

(Prolonged-release preparation) *Adults*, 60 mg twice daily. *Children 6 to 12 years*, 30 mg twice daily; *2 to 6 years*, 15 mg twice daily.

This drug is not recommended for use in *children under 2 years.*

All forms nonprescription.

Benylin (Warner Wellcome). Syrup 7.5 mg/5 ml (***Benylin Pediatric***) and 15 mg/5 ml (***Benylin Adult Formula***).

Delsym (Fisons). Suspension (prolonged-release) dextromethorphan polistirex equivalent to 30 mg/5 ml of hydrobromide (alcohol-free).

Pertussin ES (Blairex), ***Generic.*** Solution (oral) 15 mg/5 ml.

Robitussin Maximum Strength Cough Suppressant (Robins). Liquid 15 mg/5 ml.

Vicks Formula 44 Cough Medicine (Procter & Gamble). Syrup 5 mg/5 ml (alcohol-free) (***Pediatric Formula***) and 15 mg/5 ml (alcohol 10%).

See the section on Mixtures for a listing of combination products containing dextromethorphan.

DIPHENHYDRAMINE HYDROCHLORIDE

[Benadryl]

For chemical formula, see index entry Diphenhydramine, As Antihistamine.

Diphenhydramine is an amino alkyl ether antihistamine with limited central antitussive action. Like other first-generation antihistamines, it has a moderate sedative effect and some anticholinergic activity. Diphenhydramine has antitussive effects only in doses that produce significant sedation. Disturbing central nervous system reactions (ie, bizarre behavior, visual and auditory hallucinations) have been reported when a dermatologic preparation of diphenhydramine was used in patients with varicella; symptoms disappeared within 24 hours of withdrawal of the diphenhydramine-containing preparation (Chan and Wallander, 1991). These adverse effects may not occur with oral preparations.

DOSAGE AND PREPARATIONS.

Oral: *Adults,* 25 mg every four hours (maximum, 150 mg/24 hours). *Children 6 to 11 years,* 12.5 mg every four hours or 5 mg/kg/day in four divided doses (maximum, 75 mg/day); *2 to 6 years,* 6.25 mg every four hours (maximum, 25 mg/day). However, this drug is not recommended for *children under 6 years* except under the direct supervision of a physician.

Generic. Syrup 12.5 mg/5 ml (nonprescription).

Benadryl (Warner-Wellcome). Capsules 25 (nonprescription) and 50 mg; elixir 6.25 mg/5 ml (dye-free) and 12.5 mg/5 ml (nonprescription).

Expectorant

GUAIFENESIN (Glyceryl Guaiacolate)

[Breonesin, Glycotuss, Glytuss, Hytuss, Naldecon Senior EX, Robitussin]

$OCH_2CH(OH)CH_2OH$, OCH_3 (benzene ring structure)

Guaifenesin is the most widely used expectorant. Doses up to ten times the usual amount probably act as an emetic, increase the volume of respiratory tract fluids, and may facilitate the transport of mucus. At lower doses, few beneficial effects have been demonstrated in patients with asthma, bronchitis, or other respiratory disorders (Medon and Holshouser, 1985); some authorities recommend use of larger doses if smaller amounts are ineffective. Also see the discussion on Expectorants.

Nausea and drowsiness occur rarely. Guaifenesin may affect platelet agglutination. It also may produce a false-positive response for urinary 5-hydroxyindoleacetic acid (5-HIAA) and vanillylmandelic acid (VMA).

This drug is classified in FDA Pregnancy Category C.

DOSAGE AND PREPARATIONS.

Oral: Manufacturers' suggested dosage: *Adults,* 200 to 400 mg every four hours (maximum, 2.4 g/day). *Children 6 to 12 years,* 100 to 200 mg every four hours (maximum, 1.2 g/day); *2 to 6 years,* 50 to 100 mg every four hours (maximum, 600 mg/day). This drug should be given to *children under 2 years* only under the direct supervision of a physician.

All forms nonprescription.

Generic. Syrup 100 mg/5 ml.

Breonesin (Sanofi Winthrop). Capsules 200 mg.

Glycotuss (Pal-Pack). Tablets 100 mg.

Glytuss (Mayrand). Tablets 200 mg.

Hytuss (Hyrex). Tablets 100 mg; capsules 200 mg (***Hytuss 2X***).

Naldecon Senior EX (Apothecon). Syrup 200 mg/5 ml.

Robitussin (Robins). Syrup 100 mg/5 ml (alcohol 3.5%).

See the section on Mixtures for a listing of combination products containing Guaifenesin.

RHINITIS

NASAL PHYSIOLOGY. Considerations of the pertinent anatomy and physiology of the respiratory tract can serve as a basis for rational management of rhinitis.

The main functions of the nose are to modify the temperature and humidity of inspired air and to filter a large portion of inhaled foreign material. The vasculature of the nose plays an important role in regulating the patency of the nasal airway. Neural control of the vascular smooth muscle allows for delicate adjustment of capillary and arterial blood flow, which are responsible for changes in the cross-sectional diameter of the nasal airway; parasympathetic neural control is important in regulation of glandular secretion and the sneezing reflex.

The nose accounts for about one-half of total respiratory tract resistance to air flow. Resistance varies with the individual and is affected by the degree of nasal vascular congestion, anatomic variations, posture, exercise, air temperature, irritants, medications, time of day, emotional stress, and disease states. Normally, the greatest resistance to air flow occurs at the nasal valves in the anterior nares, which have the smallest cross-sectional diameter. When mucosal congestion over the turbinates becomes severe, air flow resistance increases markedly (Proctor and Anderson, 1982).

Normal variations in nasal congestion alter nasal air flow resistance, and they can be confused with alterations associated with disease. Cold air increases resistance, as does change in posture when moving from a standing or sitting position to a recumbent one. In contrast, exercise initially decreases resistance. There is a normal, reciprocal fluctuation in the patency of each side of the nose (the nasal cycle). Turning on the side while sleeping causes a reflex from the lower side, which increases the patency of the opposite side. Conditions such as the common cold, allergy, infection of the nose and sinuses, hypothyroidism, and possibly pregnancy increase nasal congestion. Certain drugs (eg, reserpine, estrogens, alpha-adrenergic blocking agents) and alcohol, as well as the rebound after prolonged administration of intranasal vasoconstrictors (rhinitis medicamentosa), also may increase nasal congestion. In contrast, spicy food and other irritants cause rhinorrhea (gustatory rhinitis).

Normal functioning of the nose is not always sufficient to protect the respiratory tract from illness, a fact attested to by the prevalence of the common cold. Colds are not only major nuisances but associated complications, including ear, throat, and sinus infections, may predispose to more severe illnesses. Upper respiratory tract infections may be associated with bronchial hyperreactivity that exacerbates bronchial asthma or chronic bronchitis. Lower airway obstruction results from bronchospasm and mucosal edema, as well as from increased and abnormal secretions. During normal breathing, the airway widens during inspiration and closes slightly during expiration. Conditions such as asthma and viral infections increase bronchial muscle reactivity and/or airway inflammation and narrow the airways, especially during expiration; this may cause wheezing, chest tightness, shortness of breath, or cough. The diameter of the larger airways can be modified by drugs that regulate autonomic function.

ACUTE AND LATE-PHASE IMMUNE RESPONSE. Both antigenic and nonantigenic stimuli can trigger the acute- and late-phase reactions in the nose that are characteristic of rhinitis (Naclerio et al, 1985; Lichtenstein, 1988; Sedgwick et al, 1991). The acute (immediate) phase occurs within 30 minutes of exposure to antigenic stimuli. The late phase begins 3 to 11 hours after exposure (average, four to six hours); a well-defined late-phase response (as determined by criteria to identify the late-phase reaction in bronchial asthma) occurs less frequently in patients with acute allergic rhinitis than in those with bronchial asthma (Mygind, 1993). These responses are triggered by the initial antigenic challenge in the absence of any further exposure.

The acute reaction occurs when antigen binds to specific IgE attached to high-affinity IgE receptors present on the surface of mast cells in the airway. This activates the cells and causes the release of histamine and other inflammatory mediators such as leukotrienes, kinins, and prostaglandins. The tight junctions between epithelial cells are breached by the inflammatory mediators, which allow antigen to penetrate deep into the mucosa and react with other mast cells. Histamine and other preformed mediators increase vascular permeability to produce edema; histamine also apparently produces sneezing. Leukotrienes and other inflammatory mediators increase the production of mucus that contributes to congestion. Reflex responses are initiated by the interaction of histamine and other mediators with afferent nerves.

Nonantigenic, nonallergenic stimuli, such as exercise, irritants, and cold dry air, also can activate mast cells, presumably by drying out the mucosa and increasing the osmolality of the nasal mucosal stroma.

Activation and degranulation of mast cells stimulate release of histamine and also are responsible for the synthesis and/or release of chemotactic factors that subsequently trigger the influx of leukocytes (eg, basophils, eosinophils, neutrophils, lymphocytes) to signal the start of the late-phase response. Infiltration of leukocytes and fluid into the nasal mucosa, along with vascular engorgement, produces congestion and obstruction.

During the late-phase response, histamine-releasing factors are produced by lymphocytes, monocytes, macrophages, platelets, and endothelial and other cells; these cells also release inflammatory mediators and chemotactic factors that participate in the inflammatory cascade of reactions leading to the allergic response. The basophil, not the mast cell, appears to be responsible for late-phase histamine release because the prostanoid, PGD_2, which is specific for mast cells, is not found in secretions obtained after the late-phase reaction.

Histamine-releasing factors may bind to specific IgE on the basophil surface to stimulate the release of histamine and other inflammatory mediators; however, these mediators may exert effects through nonIgE mechanisms as well. The renewed late-phase release appears to result in the resumption of mucus output, increased permeability, congestion, and sneezing. Eosinophil-derived products, particularly major basic protein, are a primary cause of epithelial damage associated with inflammation. Late-phase reactions occur in more than 20% of allergic patients and are predominant in chronic rhinitis. Late-phase responses also commonly occur in bronchial asthma.

Hyperreactivity: After an antigen-induced late-phase response, hyperreactivity to antigenic and nonantigenic stimuli occurs in the nose and lungs of patients with seasonal allergic rhinitis or asthma. An example is the symptoms that persist late in the season when pollen counts are falling rapidly. This hyperreactivity can increase the response to a particular antigen by a hundredfold or more and is responsible for the augmented response after repeated exposure to an allergen or nonspecific stimuli such as cold dry air, exercise, smoke, automobile exhaust, perfumes, or strong chemicals. In susceptible patients with nasal or bronchial hyperreactivity, such nonspecific nonallergenic stimuli can produce acute rhinitis and asthma.

FORMS OF RHINITIS. Signs and symptoms of noninfectious upper respiratory disorders caused by inflammatory conditions (eg, allergic and nonallergic rhinitis) often resemble those caused by infection (eg, the common cold). For proper therapy, it is necessary to distinguish between an upper respiratory infection and allergic rhinitis. The latter diagnosis is much more probable in patients with clear mucous secretions, sneezing characterized by rapid multiple bursts, and normal temperature. Considerably less malaise is associated with allergic disorders, and appetite suppression is uncommon.

Allergy frequently causes noninfectious *acute* rhinitis. It is estimated that seasonal allergic rhinitis (hay fever, pollinosis) affects more than 30 million Americans. Symptoms are caused by the release of histamine and other chemical mediators from mast cells and basophils. Sneezing, nasal stuffiness, rhinorrhea, nasal and ocular pruritus, increased lacrimation, and postnasal drip may be associated with allergic and nonallergic rhinitis, as well as with chronic nasal or sinus infection. Complications of allergic rhinitis include sinus infection (common) and otitis media in children (less frequent).

Chronic or nonseasonal rhinitis, often referred to as perennial rhinitis, usually is defined as inflammation of the nasal mucosa that results in daily episodes of rhinorrhea, nasal congestion, and sneezing that persist for several weeks at any time of the year (Simons, 1984). In a large percentage of cases, chronic rhinitis commonly is a mixed form; that is, it consists of perennial rhinitis plus a nonallergic component. Several types of chronic rhinitis can coexist in the same patient.

Common types of nonallergic chronic rhinitis include vasomotor rhinitis (VMR), a nonallergic noninfective rhinitis in which eosinophils are generally absent on nasal smear, and nonallergic noninfective rhinitis with eosinophilia (NARES) in which large numbers of eosinophils are present on nasal smear (Lieberman, 1988; Druce and Kaliner, 1988; Mikaelian, 1989). The etiology of VMR is not completely understood. It is exacerbated by emotion, airway irritants such as tobacco smoke, changes in weather or ambient temperature, or an alteration in general health. NARES resembles allergic rhinitis but there is no evidence of an IgE-mediated reaction. Some authorities believe that NARES is a form of allergic rhinitis with an obscure antigenic stimulus, whereas others regard NARES as an eosinophilic form of VMR (Jones and Lancer, 1987).

Symptoms of chronic rhinitis can be produced by drugs (eg, adrenergic blocking agents, cholinesterase inhibitors, estrogen preparations including contraceptives), pregnancy, hypothyroidism, presence of a foreign body, ciliary disorders, nasal polyps, tumors, Wegener's granulomatosis, and cerebrospinal rhinorrhea. Persistent rhinitis that does not respond to standard therapy may be due to use of inhaled cocaine (Snyder and Snyder, 1985).

For a detailed discussion of etiologic, diagnostic, and therapeutic aspects of chronic rhinitis, see Meltzer et al, 1983; deShazo and Smith, 1992. Information on allergic and nonallergic rhinitis is summarized in Table 1.

NONDRUG THERAPY. Nondrug therapy for infectious and noninfectious rhinitis is similar. Exposure to cigarette smoke, pollutants, known allergens, and other irritants should be avoided. In patients with pharyngitis, isotonic saline gargles and warm mist therapy may be helpful. (However, the latter may be hazardous to allergic patients because an increase in the relative humidity can promote mold growth and mite proliferation.)

Results of a number of limited studies indicated that local instillation of hyperheated humidified air (42° to 43° C) directly into the nasal passages significantly relieved symptoms of allergic rhinitis (Yerushalmi et al, 1982; Ophir et al, 1988; Johnston et al, 1993). In one of these studies, 102 patients with allergic rhinitis were exposed to heated, humidified air twice for 30 minutes with a 90-minute interval between treatment periods. The inhalations were repeated one week later. Symptoms of allergic rhinitis were relieved and nasal patency increased in a high proportion of patients. No adverse effects were observed and relief was maintained for one week or longer (Ophir et al, 1988). However, in subsequent randomized controlled trials, inhalation of humidified heated air provided no benefit in patients with allergic rhinitis or the common cold (Macknin et al, 1990; Oppenheimer et al, 1993; Forstall et al, 1994; Hendley et al, 1994; Monto, 1994).

When nasal congestion is severe, nasal irrigation with a saline solution prepared by dissolving one level teaspoonful each of table salt and baking soda in one pint (one quart in children) of warm (37° C) tap water may relieve the congestion and obstruction. This procedure helps liquefy secretions, cleanse allergens, and decrease mucous crust formation (Wood, 1984). It is a safe alternative in all age groups but may be especially useful in young infants, in whom nasal decongestants generally are not recommended. In addition, irrigation before use of other intranasal medications may enhance their efficacy.

Patients must be instructed on the appropriate technique for nasal irrigation. The head should be down with chin on chest. Using a small rubber bulb ear syringe, each nostril is irrigated with about one cup of solution (in small infants, a few drops is usually adequate) until thick mucus is no longer flushed out. This procedure is performed once or twice daily (Wood, 1984; Crawford and Cohen, 1985). If ear pain or excessive discomfort occurs during irrigation, the procedure should be stopped.

Some physicians recommend application of a small amount of skin moisturizer or water-based ointment (eg, K-Y jelly) under the nose to prevent and/or treat the irritation and dryness resulting from nasal discharge in patients with rhinitis. These agents should not be inhaled because they are irritating.

Patients should drink plenty of liquids. Regular exercise may reduce nasal obstruction.

TABLE 1.
TYPES OF ALLERGIC AND NONALLERGIC RHINITIS AND RESPONSE TO THERAPY[1]

	Allergic		Nonallergic (Chronic)	
Variable	**Acute (Seasonal)**	**Chronic (Nonseasonal)**	**NARES**[2]	**VMR**[3]
Onset	Childhood to young adulthood	Childhood	Nonspecific	Adult
Cause	Pollens, outdoor molds	Animal dander, house dust mites, indoor molds and spores	Unknown	Unknown
Family history of allergy	Common	Common	Coincidental	Coincidental
Occurrence of symptoms	Seasonal	Throughout the year	Sporadic; throughout the year	Worse in changing seasons
Laboratory tests				
Eosinophilia	Present	Present	Present	Absent
Serum IgE	Elevated or normal	Elevated or normal	Normal	Normal
Skin tests	Positive	Positive	Negative	Negative
Symptoms				
Sneezing	Frequent	Frequent	Sporadic	Sporadic
Rhinorrhea, watery	Profuse	Profuse	Moderate	Moderate
Nasal or eyelid pruritus	Marked	Marked	Minimal to moderate	Minimal
Nasal polyps	Occasional	Occasional	Frequent	Rare
Congestion	Moderate	Moderate	Marked	Moderate
Lacrimation	Common	Common	Variable	Rare
Therapeutic response to:				
Isotonic saline (inhalation or intranasal)	Fair	Fair	Fair	Fair to good
Antihistamines (oral)	Fair to good	Fair to good	Poor	Poor
Decongestants (oral, intranasal)	Fair	Fair	Fair	Poor to fair
Cromolyn (intranasal)	Fair to good	Fair to good	Poor	Poor
Corticosteroids (intranasal)	Good	Good	Good	Poor to fair
Anticholinergic agents (intranasal) (effects limited to reduction of watery discharge)	Fair to good	Fair to good	Fair to good	Fair to good
Immunotherapy	Good	Good	None	None

[1] *Adapted from Dushay and Johnson, 1989; Mikaelian, 1989.*
[2] *Nonallergic rhinitis with eosinophilia.*
[3] *Nonallergic rhinitis without eosinophilia (vasomotor rhinitis).*

Immunotherapy has been effective in selected patients with chronic or seasonal allergic rhinitis but should only be used when an IgE mechanism is demonstrated by in vivo or in vitro testing. Some practitioners believe that immunotherapy should be reserved for those with severe symptoms that last several months during the year and for whom allergen avoidance measures are not possible and who are refractory to or cannot tolerate drug therapy (Naclerio, 1991).

DRUG THERAPY. Most drug therapy provides symptomatic relief only and does not affect underlying inflammatory factors. No drug is likely to abolish symptoms completely. In general, drugs are more effective for allergic than nonallergic forms of rhinitis, and acute forms of allergic rhinitis usually respond more favorably than chronic allergic forms.

Severely affected patients with allergic rhinitis may require concurrent administration of an antihistamine and a nasal decongestant given separately or in a proprietary mixture. For maximal control and the smallest number of side effects, separate administration is preferred so that the dose of each agent can be titrated (see also the section on Mixtures). It is claimed that, when used in combination, the sedative effect of the first-generation antihistamines is balanced by the stimulant effect of nasal decongestants, but this action is unpredictable. The use of second-generation (ie, nonsedating) antihistamines in such mixtures obviates concern about sedative effects.

Nasal sprays containing cromolyn sodium and/or a corticosteroid may provide good control of symptoms. Corticosteroid nasal sprays are increasingly being considered first-line therapy for most types of nasal disorders (see Table 1). Patients with the eosinophilic forms of chronic rhinitis (NARES) are more responsive to intranasal corticosteroids than patients with the noneosinophilic forms (VMR) (Mullarkey, 1988).

Agents with adrenergic activity or those that block parasympathetic responses may be helpful for symptomatic treatment of VMR. Combinations of systemic adrenergic agents and antihistamines may control symptoms in some patients. The intranasal administration of ipratropium bromide, an anticholinergic preparation that is investigational for intranasal use, has shown promise in controlling watery hypersecretion in such patients.

Antihistamine/decongestant combinations are widely used in the prophylaxis of otitis media with effusion, but their value is unproved. Results of double-blind studies demonstrate that such combinations are ineffective in childhood serous otitis media (Cantekin et al, 1983; Bhambhani et al, 1983). However, they may be of some benefit in children with associated symptoms such as allergy, nasal congestion, or upper respiratory infection (*Pediatr Alert*, 1983).

Drug therapy for rhinitis has been reviewed (Lieberman, 1988; Dushay and Johnson, 1989; Simons and Simons, 1989; Naclerio, 1991; Mabry, 1992; Bernstein, 1993).

Drug Selection

Treatment of rhinitis is directed at preventing the release of inflammatory mediators or blocking their effects after they are released and inhibiting the influx of leukocytes. The rational selection of drugs requires that noninfectious forms be distinguished from infectious forms, for agents that are most useful for noninfectious allergic rhinitis (antihistamines, cromolyn sodium nasal spray, intranasal corticosteroids) have little value in patients with infectious rhinitis if appropriate antibiotic therapy is not administered concomitantly. Nasal decongestants are often beneficial in both conditions (see Table 1).

Antibiotics have no value for viral upper respiratory infections but are often used inappropriately for this purpose. They should be reserved for patients with bacterial infections; prolonged therapy (three to six weeks) may be required for sinus infections.

A variety of mixtures are available over-the-counter for rhinitis and other minor respiratory illnesses (see the section on Mixtures). Because the components are often similar to those of prescription medicines, they have the same advantages and disadvantages.

ANTIHISTAMINES. Antihistamines are the most widely used agents for allergic rhinitis and are often chosen for initial therapy. They help relieve rhinorrhea, sneezing, nasal or eyelid pruritus, and conjunctivitis; antihistamines can prevent nasal congestion but do not relieve existing congestion. They are administered alone when the disorder is mild or moderately severe and are usually effective in seasonal allergic rhinitis when sneezing and rhinorrhea predominate and edema and congestion are minimal. Antihistamines are more effective if taken before symptoms occur and should be taken regularly by sensitive patients just prior to and during the allergen-exposure period or season even when symptoms are absent. When nasal congestion and turbinate swelling are prominent, as in VMR and NARES, antihistamines are less useful than decongestants.

Some antihistamines also block the release and actions of various inflammatory mediators (Togias et al, 1989). When these actions result in significant antiallergic and anti-inflammatory effects, the drug can no longer be classified solely as an H_1-receptor blocker (See the discussion on Antiallergy Drugs in this section).

Drowsiness, the most common adverse effect of the first-generation antihistamines, is lessened in many patients after a few days to weeks of therapy. A single oral daily dose of an antihistamine with a relatively long half-life, when taken at bedtime, may relieve symptoms in adults and children the following day. The availability of the second-generation (nonsedating) antihistamines, terfenadine [Seldane], astemizole [Hismanal], loratadine [Claritin], and the expected approval of similar drugs (eg, cetirizine [Reactine]) will extend the usefulness of these drugs in rhinitis. However, serious arrhythmias have occurred rarely in patients treated with terfenadine or astemizole when these agents were used with drugs that inhibit their metabolism (eg, erythromycin, ketoconazole) or in doses exceeding the manufacturers' recommendations (see index entries on these drugs).

Levocabastine [Livostin], an extremely potent histamine$_1$ receptor antagonist, is the first antihistamine developed for topical application in the treatment of rhinitis. The efficacy of the intranasal preparation, which is still investigational, has been reported to be similar to that of oral antihistamines, and it is well tolerated (Dechant and Goa, 1991).

Some antihistamines have anticholinergic activity that has a drying effect on mucosal secretions. The long-held concept that agents with anticholinergic or antihistaminic properties should be avoided in asthmatic patients is not valid (Meltzer,

1990). Other adverse effects, such as gastrointestinal upset and hyperactivity, occur rarely in children.

For a more detailed discussion of these drugs, see index entry Antihistamines.

NASAL DECONGESTANTS. When antihistamines are ineffective, a nasal decongestant often is added to the regimen or is used alone. Nasal decongestants shrink swollen turbinates and are the most effective agents for temporary relief of nasal congestion.

Alpha-adrenergic agonists exert their sympathomimetic effects directly on receptors or indirectly by facilitating the release of norepinephrine from sympathetic nerve endings. They constrict dilated blood vessels in the nasal mucosa, reducing blood flow to engorged, edematous tissue.

These drugs provide temporary, symptomatic relief of acute rhinitis associated with the common cold and other respiratory infections, as well as seasonal or nonseasonal allergic rhinitis, NARES, and sinusitis, but they are less useful in VMR. In addition, decongestants are applied intranasally to facilitate visualization of nasal and nasopharyngeal membranes during diagnostic procedures and, in severe obstruction, to reduce mucosal swelling prior to application of intranasal corticosteroids or nasal surgery. The headache and blocked-up ears that occur during air travel in patients with colds can be decreased by the oral or intranasal administration of a decongestant at appropriate times before takeoff and landing.

Administration: Decongestants can be administered intranasally or orally. Intranasal decongestants are available as drops, sprays, pumps, and vapors. These forms have the advantages of greater efficacy and more rapid onset of action. However, their use for more than three to five days can result in rebound nasal congestion, which leads to rhinitis medicamentosa (see Adverse Reactions and Precautions). Prolonged use also can cause atrophy of nasal mucosa. Rhinitis medicamentosa rarely occurs after long-term use of oral decongestants: therefore, oral forms are preferred for prolonged treatment. Oral decongestants also may reach areas that are inaccessible with intranasal application. However, they may produce undesirable systemic effects (eg, insomnia, palpitations, increased blood pressure) and may provide only marginal symptomatic relief in many patients.

When treating barotitis by producing vasoconstriction in the mucosa near the orifices of the eustachian tubes, drops should be instilled as follows: The patient lies supine, but not hyperextended, with the head turned 15° toward the affected ear. Nose drops are instilled into the affected side and allowed to run along the floor of the nose and "puddle" at the eustachian orifice, which is positioned at the low point. The patient should remain in this position for about five minutes. If necessary, the procedure is repeated for the other side.

In children, maintaining the head in an upright position minimizes accumulation, since the spray and secretions drip anteriorly from the nostril and are not swallowed. For children under 6 years, drops or metered-dose spray bottles that deliver the drug more precisely are preferred to use of a spray because of the difficulty of controlling dosage with the latter. It is even possible to deliver enough medication to cause overdose in these patients with use of the spray. Intranasal preparations for children should always be administered by an adult. Because of the risks of systemic absorption, many physicians suggest that nasal decongestants not be used in infants and small children.

Adverse Reactions: *Oral Preparations:* The most common adverse effects of oral nasal decongestants are insomnia and irritability. Isolated reports suggest that antihistamine/decongestant combinations containing phenylpropanolamine or pseudoephedrine can cause hallucinations in children. However, most of these patients received larger doses than those usually recommended or had predisposing factors, such as febrile conditions.

Since the nasal vessels are not more sensitive to adrenergic drugs than other blood vessels, oral doses large enough to reduce nasal congestion constrict other vascular beds. In normal individuals, usual decongestant doses do not increase blood pressure; however, susceptible patients can develop marked tachycardia and arrhythmias. Negligible systemic effects on blood pressure may occur in patients with hypertension. Decongestant therapy may affect the efficacy of antihypertensive agents, however.

If antibiotics are being used for a sinus or middle ear infection, concomitant administration of a nasal decongestant may be detrimental because the resultant vasoconstriction significantly decreases access of the antibiotic to sites of action (*Health Gazette*, 1992).

Intranasal Preparations: Intranasal decongestants sometimes cause temporary local discomfort, including stinging, burning, or dryness of the mucosa. Inhaled vapors of volatile bases (eg, propylhexedrine) may dry the mucosa rapidly and interfere with ciliary action, but the latter effect usually is clinically insignificant. Moreover, the ability of inhaled vapors to reach all areas of the nose is an advantage.

Use of intranasal decongestants can produce rebound congestion, and prolonged administration can lead to rhinitis medicamentosa, a disorder characterized by chronic swelling and a red, boggy, edematous appearance of the nasal mucosa. The swelling (edema) probably results from an irritant effect on the nasal mucosa; as the decongestant effect of each application wears off, congestion recurs with increasing severity and after shorter periods of time, thereby encouraging repeated use. Swelling of the mucosa that is often worse than the original congestion then occurs. Dryness, severe soreness, and a burning sensation also can develop.

Discontinuation of the intranasal decongestant relieves soreness and burning within 48 to 72 hours, but nasal congestion and other symptoms of chronic rhinitis worsen. Some patients have great difficulty in discontinuing intranasal decongestants. Those with severe rebound congestion occasionally respond to an oral decongestant, but a short-term course of an intranasal corticosteroid is more effective. For rebound congestion resistant to this therapy, some authorities recommend treating each nostril separately; adrenergic nasal sprays are continued in one nostril and the other is treated with a cromolyn or corticosteroid nasal spray.

Intranasal decongestants also may produce systemic reactions, especially in infants and young children in whom decreased body temperature, central nervous system depression, and even coma can develop. Significant absorption from the nasal mucosa or gastrointestinal tract occurs if excess solution is swallowed. Appropriate use of metered-dose nasal sprays is the best way to avoid systemic absorption; however, misuse or overuse is common and is difficult to prevent in some patients. For these reasons, some authorities recommend that topical preparations of nasal decongestants be avoided in patients with allergic rhinitis (Bernstein, 1993; Horak, 1993).

Precautions: Overdosage of most adrenergic drugs causes transient hypertension, nervousness, insomnia, nausea, dizziness, palpitations, arrhythmias, and, occasionally, central nervous system stimulation with seizures.

Overdoses of two imidazolines, tetrahydrozoline [Tyzine] and naphazoline [Privine], have caused severe reactions characterized by hypertension or hypotension, bradycardia, sweating, drowsiness, deep sleep, and coma. Children are more at risk for these uncommon effects than adults. The possibility that such reactions may occur with other adrenergic decongestants should be kept in mind. The intranasal and oral decongestants, especially the imidazolines, should be used sparingly, if at all, and with particular caution in infants, young children, and patients with cardiovascular disease.

Adrenergic agents also should be given with caution to patients with thyroid disease and diabetes mellitus and to those receiving tricyclic antidepressants (in whom additive pressor effects can occur). Intranasal and oral decongestants should not be used in individuals whose sensitivity to even small doses is manifested by insomnia, dizziness, weakness, tremor, and arrhythmias; in patients who are receiving or have received monoamine oxidase inhibitors during the previous two weeks; or in men who have difficulty in urinating because of enlargement of the prostate.

Solutions, inhalers, and applicators used for intranasal administration quickly become contaminated after use and can serve as reservoirs for bacteria and fungi. Use of an aqueous nasal spray pump can eliminate this problem because of the design of the pump and the addition of preservatives to this form. Patients should be cautioned not to place the dropper or inhaler in the nostril or to allow more than one person to use the same dropper, inhaler, applicator, or bottle. The bottle or spray pack should be discarded when the medication is no longer needed. Discoloration or precipitation of normally clear solutions indicates decomposition. Nasal solutions of many adrenergic agents, especially naphazoline and probably the other imidazolines, should not be used in atomizers having aluminum parts because they interact with this metal.

ANTIALLERGY DRUGS. The antiallergic drugs discussed in this section prevent the release of a number of inflammatory mediators and inhibit the action of released mediators on their target cells. As a result, late-phase reactions are blocked or diminished to varying degrees and the development of hyperreactivity (priming) may be prevented.

The nasal spray preparation of cromolyn sodium [Nasalcrom] is probably as effective as an antihistamine in preventing the symptoms of allergic rhinitis, and it can be considered an alternative to these agents. Patients with seasonal allergic rhinitis may be more responsive than those with the chronic form. However, cromolyn is less effective than the intranasal corticosteroids for both seasonal and chronic allergic rhinitis. This drug is most useful if administered before exposure to antigens; it is usually of limited value in relieving established symptoms, although it may prevent progression of mild symptoms. The greatest effect is observed in patients with positive skin tests to allergens, elevated IgE levels, or nasal eosinophilia. Sneezing, nasal pruritus, and rhinorrhea are relieved more than nasal congestion; watery itchy eyes also are relieved in some patients, but the mechanism is unclear. In a double-blind study on patients with a history of moderate to severe seasonal rhinitis, intranasal cromolyn sodium was slightly more effective than the second-generation oral antihistamine, terfenadine, in reducing symptoms. Significant additive benefits occurred with the concomitant use of these two drugs (Lindsay-Miller and Chambers, 1987).

The therapeutic advantage of cromolyn sodium over other medications used for allergic rhinitis is its lack of adverse effects. A disadvantage is the need for administration three or four times daily. Cromolyn sodium also appears to be safe for use in pregnant women (FDA Pregnancy Category B).

Nasal cromolyn sodium is ineffective for nasal polyps, NARES, VMR, and other nonallergic conditions.

Nedocromil sodium and the investigational drugs, ketotifen and azelastine, are being studied for their use in allergic rhinitis. The properties of nedocromil are similar to those of cromolyn, and an intranasal preparation (investigational route) is promising for the prophylaxis and treatment of allergic rhinitis (Druce et al, 1990; Schuller et al, 1990, Donnelly and Casale, 1993). Nedocromil may inhibit not only allergen-induced sneezing and rhinorrhea but also nasal congestion. When administered intranasally with a metered-dose inhaler, the primary untoward effect appears to be a bitter taste.

Daily prophylactic administration of ketotifen, an oral antiallergic agent with antihistaminic properties, has significantly reduced symptoms of allergic rhinitis (sneezing, rhinorrhea, ocular irritation, and lacrimation) and may be useful in allergic asthma. However, adverse effects limit its value (eg, drowsiness, stimulation of appetite with weight gain). Like antihistamines, ketotifen is less effective for nasal congestion (Grant et al, 1990). In a double-blind controlled study on patients with seasonal rhinitis, astemizole, a second-generation antihistamine, was considerably more effective than ketotifen in inhibiting all these symptoms (Leclercq-Foucart et al, 1986).

Azelastine can be administered orally or intranasally. It has a relatively long half-life and, in controlled studies, has been as effective as terfenadine and cromolyn for acute and chronic allergic rhinitis (McTavish and Sorkin, 1989; Rafferty et al, 1989). Oral doses of 4 mg administered twice daily have been well tolerated; minor sedation, headache and a bitter taste or altered taste perception are the most common adverse effects.

ANTICHOLINERGIC AGENTS. Rhinorrhea, a common symptom in patients with allergic or nonallergic rhinitis, is primarily a result of glandular hypersecretion that is mediated by reflexes mainly involving cholinergic innervation of the nasal mucosa. Anticholinergic agents, which often are administered preoperatively to decrease respiratory tract secretions, can be useful in rhinitis. Some patients with severe rhinorrhea and congestion experience more relief from propantheline [Pro-Banthīne] or belladonna alkaloids than from nasal decongestants. Atropine nasal spray can relieve rhinorrhea, but adverse effects, such as dry mouth and tachycardia, decrease acceptance of this agent.

Intranasal administration of ipratropium bromide (investigational route) significantly reduces rhinorrhea in patients with all forms of rhinitis (Baroody et al, 1992), and effectiveness has been maintained in most patients for one year or longer (Borum, 1987; Dolovich et al, 1987; Kirkegaard et al, 1987). This drug also is effective for nasal hypersecretion due to the common cold and other disorders (Borum, 1987; Dockhorn et al, 1992). Other symptoms of rhinitis, such as sneezing or nasal congestion, are not relieved. Ipratropium is well tolerated when applied intranasally. For a more detailed discussion, see the evaluation.

CORTICOSTEROIDS. Intranasal corticosteroid preparations exert a marked anti-inflammatory effect on the nasal mucosa by inhibiting the release of inflammatory mediators from mast cells and basophils and blocking the recuitment and activation of leukocytes in the nose. Intranasal administration decreases the number of surface basophils, eosinophils, and mast cells; reduces vasodilatation, congestion, and edema in the inflamed mucosa; stabilizes epithelial and endothelial membranes; reduces receptor sensitivity to irritants; and decreases the effect of cholinergic stimulation on intranasal glands. If the pretreatment period is one week or longer, intranasal corticosteroids inhibit both immediate and delayed reactions to allergen challenge (Clissold and Heel, 1984; Pipkorn et al, 1987). The specific mechanisms responsible for these actions are unclear.

Intranasal corticosteroids with potent topical activity are safe and are the most effective agents available for the prophylaxis and treatment of seasonal and nonseasonal allergic rhinitis or for weaning patients with rhinitis medicamentosa from intranasal decongestants (Brogden et al, 1984; Clissold and Heel, 1984). Because of their anti-inflammatory action, corticosteroids are beneficial alone or as adjuncts to nasal decongestants or antihistamines when these drugs are ineffective or inadequate. Nasal symptoms are decreased in up to 90% of patients with allergic rhinitis after treatment with an intranasal corticosteroid alone; some patients may require an oral or parenteral form for optimal management of severe allergic rhinitis (eg, during the pollen season in ragweed areas). Intranasal corticosteroids may prevent seasonal increases in bronchial responsiveness in patients with asthma and acute allergic rhinitis (Corren et al, 1992). NARES also may respond to corticosteroids; their effectiveness for VMR is usually limited.

The efficacy of nasal spray preparations of beclomethasone dipropionate [Beconase, Vancenase]; flunisolide [Nasalide]; triamcinolone acetonide [Nasacort]; budesonide [Rhinocort]; and the investigational drugs, fluticasone propionate [Flovent] and fluocortin butyl, is similar. The effectiveness of once-daily administration of triamcinolone, budesonide, and fluticasone improves compliance. Dexamethasone [Decadron Turbinaire] may have greater potency than the other intranasal corticosteroids; however, significant absorption occurs and it can suppress adrenocortical function with usual doses. Dexamethasone is used only rarely now that safer drugs are available. Little or no evidence of systemic adverse effects or adrenocortical suppression has been reported with usual doses in patients treated with intranasal preparations of beclomethasone, flunisolide, or triamcinolone but such effects occur with larger daily doses. Systemic adverse effects and adrenocortical suppression are much less likely with either recommended or larger daily doses of budesonide, fluticasone, or fluocortin butyl (Day et al, 1990; Ross et al, 1991; Orgel et al, 1991; Bryson and Faulds, 1992).

Rhinorrhea, nasal pruritus, erythema, nasal congestion, postnasal drainage, and sneezing are relieved by corticosteroids. Occasionally, ocular symptoms are partially relieved. Patients with seasonal allergic rhinitis should be informed that, although significant relief of symptoms may be observed in one to three days, full effects may not occur for one week or longer. If no response is observed after three weeks, the corticosteroid should be withdrawn and the patient re-evaluated. In chronic rhinitis, significant relief of symptoms may require at least one week and maximal improvement may not be observed for two to three weeks. Daily administration is required.

Intranasal corticosteroids occasionally shrink nasal polyps and reduce nasal obstruction significantly; small polyps may even disappear. However, when the corticosteroid is discontinued, the polyps can regrow. When used prior to polypectomy, reduction in size of the polyps facilitates surgery. After polypectomy, continued use of an intranasal preparation may prevent recurrence or slow regrowth.

Patients with severe rhinosinusitis and polyps or persistent middle ear effusion may not respond to these drugs. In some patients with nasal polyps, rhinitis medicamentosa, or other nasal disorders, severe nasal obstruction or congestion inhibits the access of intranasal corticosteroid sprays and thus renders them ineffective. A few days of treatment with an intranasal decongestant or a short course of oral corticosteroids can reduce the obstruction and permit treatment with an intranasal steroid; the following doses have been used: prednisone 10 mg two or three times a day in adults and one-half this dose or less in children (usual maximum dose for adults and children, 0.5 to 1 mg/kg/day or 30 mg/day, whichever is less; some individuals require higher doses) for five to seven days. However, a single daily dose of oral prednisone (1 to 2 mg/kg) is effective, lessens the risk of adrenocortical suppression, and is safer than more frequent daily doses.

In patients with severe turbinate dysfunction, intraturbinate injection of triamcinolone acetonide within each nostril may relieve severe nasal congestion within one to two hours; the effect lasts four to six weeks (Mabry, 1983; Ward and Berry, 1984). Adverse effects with this route include transient nasal bleeding, flushing of the cheeks, and a vasovagal reaction. Permanent atrophy of the turbinate has been reported rarely. Many authorities are opposed to intraturbinate injection of corticosteroids because intra-arterial embolization of drug particles occurs rarely and may cause unilateral transient or permanent blindness.

Depot injections or prolonged oral therapy may be effective in unresponsive patients but can cause temporary but significant adrenocortical suppression (Phelan, 1984; Busse, 1983).

The combined use of an inhalant and intranasal corticosteroid in patients with a nasal disorder and asthma appears to be safe when recommended doses are not exceeded (Norman, 1983).

Intranasal beclomethasone and flunisolide are safer than nasal decongestants in pregnant women, but cromolyn is preferred.

Adverse Reactions and Precautions: Adverse reactions occur fairly frequently, are usually minor, and are probably due to the vehicle, since the incidence is the same as with a placebo. After initial application of an intranasal corticosteroid, stinging and burning may occur but usually dissipate with continued use. Sneezing, headache, dry nose, and nasal bleeding have been reported. Beclomethasone, triamcinolone, or budesonide aerosol that is delivered from a Freon-containing cannister has a drying, irritant effect on nasal mucous membranes. This can be avoided by using a nasal wetting agent (eg, isotonic saline solution) or a non-Freon-containing preparation (eg, beclomethasone aqueous suspension, flunisolide). However, transient stinging and burning occur more frequently with these preparations, especially with flunisolide.

The safety of long-term therapy with intranasal corticosteroids has not been established, but their use for periods beyond one year has not caused significant adverse effects. Nasal candidiasis has been reported rarely. Mucosal atrophy has not been observed in patients using intranasal beclomethasone or flunisolide for up to five years and, in some studies with beclomethasone, for up to 12 years. Patients should receive instructions on the proper application of these drugs to avoid direct deposition on the septum; they also should be told to report bleeding or other adverse effects to the physician. Septal perforation occurs rarely; it is more likely with dexamethasone or in patients who also inhale cocaine. Adrenocortical function is not affected when usual doses are employed, and even large doses of intranasal budesonide, flucortin butyl, or fluticasone are unlikely to cause adrenocortical suppression.

The intranasal corticosteroids should be used with caution in patients with active tuberculosis, untreated bacterial infections, and systemic fungal or viral infections; they can be employed adjunctively to treat bacterial sinusitis. They should be used with caution, if at all, in patients with ocular herpes simplex. See also index entry Adrenal Corticosteroids, Adverse Reactions.

Drug Evaluations

Adrenergic Drugs

EPINEPHRINE HYDROCHLORIDE
[Adrenalin Chloride]

For chemical formula, see index entry Epinephrine, In Asthma.

Epinephrine stimulates both alpha and beta receptors. It is used rarely as a nasal decongestant but can be beneficial when administered intranasally to control epistaxis or to facilitate nasal surgery. This drug should be applied by a physician.

For a more detailed discussion, see Drug Selection in the Introduction to this section.

ADVERSE REACTIONS AND PRECAUTIONS. Like other intranasal decongestants, epinephrine can cause rebound nasal congestion. Systemic adverse reactions include anxiety, tremor, vomiting, pallor, restlessness, weakness, dizziness, throbbing headache, and palpitations. Central nervous system stimulation occurs occasionally. Adverse effects disappear quickly when the drug is discontinued. Epinephrine should be used with cocaine hydrochloride only with extreme caution.

DOSAGE AND PREPARATIONS.

Intranasal: A 0.1% aqueous solution, instilled as drops or spray, is applied by the physician as needed (maximum in healthy adults, 1 ml in one hour). Drops should be instilled with the head in the lateral, head-low position. Some solutions may sting slightly due to the presence of sodium bisulfite added as an antioxidant. *Children under 6 years,* not recommended.

Adrenalin Chloride (Parke-Davis). Solution (aqueous) 0.1% in 30 ml containers (nonprescription).

NAPHAZOLINE HYDROCHLORIDE
[Privine]

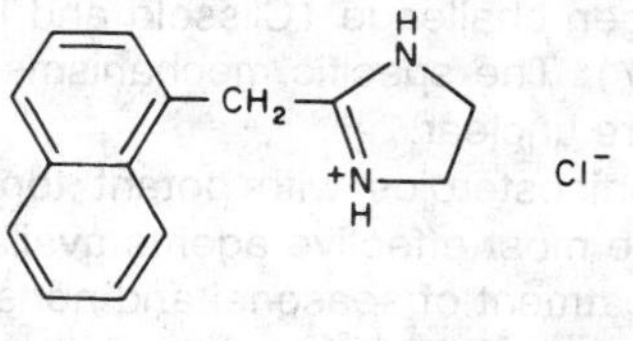

Naphazoline is an imidazoline derivative used intranasally to relieve local swelling and congestion of nasal mucous membranes. This direct-acting alpha-adrenergic agonist constricts dilated nasal arterioles and has little or no effect on beta-adrenergic receptors. The onset of action occurs in less than ten minutes, and the duration is two to six hours. Naphazoline has variable effectiveness in VMR.

For a more detailed discussion of nasal decongestants, see the section on Rhinitis, Drug Selection, in the Introduction.

ADVERSE REACTIONS AND PRECAUTIONS. Adverse reactions include severe rebound congestion with irritation and swelling of the nasal mucosa from prolonged use. Swelling is generally alleviated a few days after the medication is discontinued. Naphazoline also may cause paralysis of the nasal cilia and, occasionally, stinging and sneezing.

Systemic adverse reactions with large intranasal doses include arrhythmias and transient hypertension, bradycardia, sweating, and drowsiness; hypotension may follow hypertension and bradycardia. Systemic absorption after overdosage has caused deep sleep and, in children, coma. Because of these effects, naphazoline 0.05% is not recommended for use in children younger than 12 years and should be used with particular caution (if at all) in patients with cardiovascular disease.

The solution should not be used in atomizers containing any aluminum parts.

DOSAGE AND PREPARATIONS.

Intranasal: *Adults and children over 12 years,* two drops or two spray inhalations in each nostril no more often than every three hours (drops) or four to six hours (spray) for a maximum of three to five days. The drops should be instilled with the head in the lateral, head-low position. *Children under 12 years,* not recommended.

Privine (CIBA). Solution 0.05% in 20 and 473 ml containers; spray 0.05% in 15 ml containers (nonprescription).

OXYMETAZOLINE HYDROCHLORIDE

[Afrin, Dristan 12-Hour, Neo-Synephrine 12-Hour, Nōstrilla, NTZ, Vicks Sinex Long-Acting]

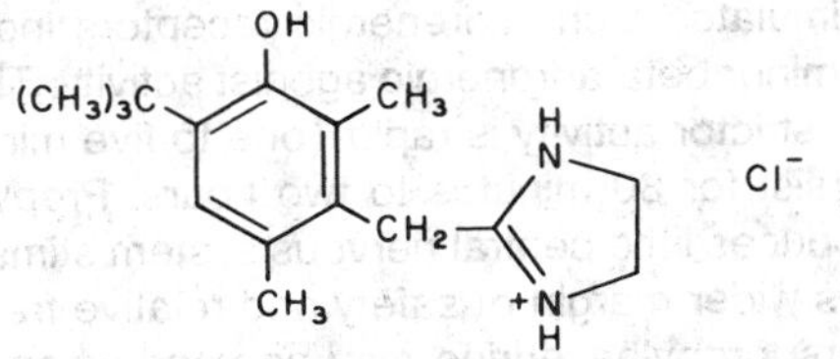

Oxymetazoline can relieve nasal congestion associated with the common cold, seasonal or nonseasonal allergic rhinitis, NARES, or sinusitis; it has variable effectiveness in VMR. The onset of action occurs in less than ten minutes, and significant effects persist for five to six hours with a gradual loss of activity over the next six hours; this duration of action is somewhat longer than that of the other topical imidazoline derivatives.

For a more detailed discussion of nasal decongestants, see Drug Selection in the Introduction to this section.

ADVERSE REACTIONS AND PRECAUTIONS. Untoward effects are milder than with shorter acting nasal decongestants and include stinging, burning, and dryness of the nasal mucosa; sneezing; headache; lightheadedness; insomnia; and palpitations. Effects on the central nervous system or blood pressure have not been reported, but overdosage is presumed to produce side effects similar to those of other imidazolines. Rebound congestion may result from prolonged or excessive use. This drug should be used with great caution in children.

DOSAGE AND PREPARATIONS.

Intranasal: *Adults and children 6 years and older,* two or three drops or two or three squeezes of spray (0.05% concentration) in each nostril every 10 to 12 hours (morning and bedtime) for no more than three to five days. *Children under 6 years,* 0.05% concentration is not recommended; the manufacturer's suggested dosage for 0.025% concentration is: *children 2 to 5 years,* two or three drops or sprays in each nostril every 10 to 12 hours.

All forms nonprescription.

Afrin (Schering-Plough). Solution (drops) 0.025% (pediatric) and 0.05% in 20 ml containers; spray 0.05% in 15 (metered pump) and 30 ml (regular) containers and 15 ml (menthol) containers.

Dristan 12-Hour Nasal Spray (Whitehall). Spray 0.05% in 15 (metered pump) and 30 ml (regular) containers and 15 ml (menthol) containers.

Neo-Synephrine Maximum Strength 12-Hour (Sterling Health). Spray 0.05% in 15 ml (metered pump or regular) containers.

Nōstrilla (CIBA). Spray 0.05% in 15 ml (metered pump) containers.

NTZ Long Acting Nasal Decongestant (Sterling Health). Solution (drops) and spray 0.05% in 15 ml containers.

Vicks Sinex Long-Acting (Procter & Gamble), ***Generic.*** Spray 0.05% in 15 and 30 ml metered pump and regular containers.

PHENYLEPHRINE HYDROCHLORIDE

[Alconefrin, Neo-Synephrine Hydrochloride, Nostril, Vicks Sinex]

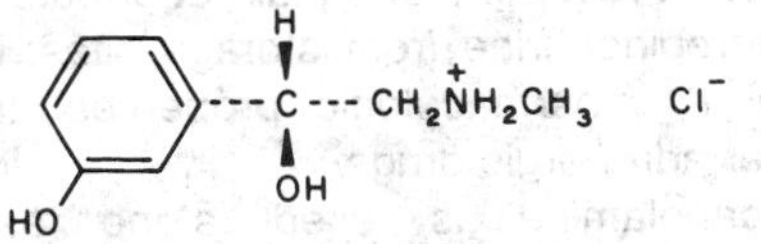

Phenylephrine is one of the most widely used intranasal decongestants. It has purely alpha-adrenergic effects (direct-acting) in contrast to epinephrine, which stimulates both alpha and beta receptors. Onset of action is rapid, and the duration ranges from 30 minutes to four hours. Oral dosage forms available in combination with antihistamines in cold remedy preparations (see Table 2) are less effective for nasal congestion than intranasal forms when the suggested dose is used.

For a more detailed discussion of nasal decongestants, see Drug Selection in the Introduction to this section.

ADVERSE REACTIONS AND PRECAUTIONS. Adverse reactions include all of the untoward effects associated with ephedrine or epinephrine, except that phenylephrine causes little or no central nervous system stimulation. A concentration of 0.25% is usually effective; stronger concentrations cause prolonged rebound swelling of the nasal mucosa within a few days and probably should not be instilled except under the direct supervision of a physician.

DOSAGE AND PREPARATIONS.

Intranasal: *Adults,* two or three drops or sprays of a 0.25% to 1% solution instilled in each nostril with the head in the lateral, head-low position. Administration may be repeated in four hours if needed. Phenylephrine is not recommended for use in *children under 2 years* and should not be used in *children under 12 years* without medical supervision. *Children 6 to under 12 years,* two or three drops or sprays of a 0.25% solution in each nostril every four hours; *2 to under 6 years,* two or three drops or sprays of a 0.125% solution in each nostril every four hours. Application should not exceed three to five days.

All forms nonprescription.

Generic. Solution 0.25% in 30 and 500 ml and gallon containers and 1% in 500 ml and gallon containers.

Alconefrin (PolyMedica). Solution (drops) 0.16% (pediatric), 0.25%, and 0.5% in 30 ml containers; spray 0.25% in 30 ml containers.

Neo-Synephrine Hydrochloride (Sterling Health). Solution (drops) 0.125% (pediatric), 0.25% (mild), 0.5% (regular), and 1% (extra strength) in 15 ml containers; spray 0.25%

(mild), 0.5% (regular), and 1% (extra strength) in 15 ml containers.

Nostril (CIBA). Spray 0.25% (mild) and 0.5% (regular) in 15 ml metered pump containers.

Vicks Sinex (Procter & Gamble). Spray 0.5% in 15 and 30 ml metered pump and regular containers.

PHENYLPROPANOLAMINE HYDROCHLORIDE

[Dexatrim, Propagest]

$$C_6H_5-\underset{OH}{CH}-\underset{CH_3}{CH}\overset{+}{N}H_3 \quad Cl^-$$

ACTIONS AND USES. This amphetamine analogue has both a direct effect on receptors and indirect effects in stimulating release of norepinephrine from storage sites, but the latter predominate. Its pharmacologic properties are similar to those of other adrenergic drugs.

Phenylpropanolamine is used alone as an orally administered nasal decongestant and also is a common ingredient in many oral cold and cough preparations. It can cause central nervous system stimulation. For a more detailed discussion of nasal decongestants, see Drug Selection in the Introduction to this section.

For use of phenylpropanolamine in weight reduction preparations, see index entry Phenylpropanolamine, In Obesity.

ADVERSE REACTIONS AND PRECAUTIONS. This agent can cause transient elevation in blood pressure. Doses moderately larger than normal may increase blood pressure significantly in an occasional individual. The possibility has been raised that, when used as a nasal decongestant or weight-reducing agent (in much larger doses), phenylpropanolamine can cause strokes and other significant sequelae of elevated blood pressure in susceptible patients. However, nearly all the evidence is anecdotal, and the results of the majority of well-controlled studies support the safety of this drug (Funderburk et al, 1993). In a double-blind study in stable hypertensive patients, therapeutic doses of a standard form of phenylpropanolamine (25 mg every four hours during waking hours) had no pressor effect (Kroenke et al, 1989). Similar results have been reported in other studies in patients with hypertension controlled by drugs (O'Connell and Gross, 1991; Petrulis et al, 1991; Sands et al, 1992). Use of caffeine with phenylpropanolamine may produce additive hypertensive effects; the mechanism of this interaction is unclear (Lake et al, 1990; Brown et al, 1991).

Concern about the safety of this agent in recommended doses is probably unwarranted (Blackburn et al, 1989; Puder and Morgan, 1987; Veltri et al, 1992). Nevertheless, it is desirable to monitor blood pressure in hypertensive patients. Some physicians feel that the questions raised concerning its safety make use of other agents preferable.

DOSAGE AND PREPARATIONS.

Oral: *Adults,* for nasal decongestion, 25 mg every four hours, 50 mg every eight hours, or 75 mg (prolonged-release form) every 12 hours (maximum, 150 mg/day). *Children 6 to 12 years,* 12.5 mg every four hours or 25 mg every eight hours (maximum, 75 mg/day); *children 2 to 6 years,* 6.25 mg every four hours or 12.5 mg every eight hours (maximum, 37.5 mg/day). Phenylpropanolamine should be used only under the direct supervision of a physician in *children under 2 years.* Use should not exceed three to five days.

Generic. Capsules (prolonged-release) 75 mg; tablets 25 and 50 mg (nonprescription).

Dexatrim Maximum Strength (Thompson Medical). Tablets (prolonged-release) 75 mg.

Propagest (Carnrick). Tablets 25 mg (nonprescription).

PROPYLHEXEDRINE

[Benzedrex, Dristan Decongestant]

$$C_6H_{11}-CH_2\underset{CH_3}{CH}NHCH_3$$

Propylhexedrine is used as a vapor for its nasal decongestant effect. This drug is believed to act similarly to amphetamine; it stimulates alpha-adrenergic receptors indirectly and has some minor beta-adrenergic agonist activity. The onset of its vasoconstrictor activity is rapid (one to five minutes), and effects persist for 30 minutes to two hours. Propylhexedrine usually produces little central nervous system stimulation. Because of its wider margin of safety and relative freedom from toxic effects, propylhexedrine may be used when an ephedrine-like pressor or stimulant action is undesirable. This nasal decongestant is considered safe for self-medication by adults, but children should not have unsupervised access to an inhaler. The vapor may dry the nasal mucosa and interfere with ciliary action.

For a more detailed discussion of nasal decongestants, see Drug Selection in the Introduction to this section.

DOSAGE AND PREPARATIONS.

Intranasal (Inhalation): *Adults and children 6 years and over,* two inhalations (0.4 to 0.5 mg) in each nostril as needed but not more often than every two hours for no more than three to five days. This drug is not recommended for *children under 6 years* except under physician supervision. The inhaler usually retains its effectiveness for two to three months after opening. If the inhaler is cold, it should be warmed in the hand before use.

Benzedrex (Menley and James), ***Dristan Decongestant*** (Whitehall). Inhaler 250 mg (nonprescription).

PSEUDOEPHEDRINE HYDROCHLORIDE

[Actifed Allergy Daytime, Dorcol Children's Decongestant, Novafed, Sudafed]

$$C_6H_5-\overset{OH}{\underset{H}{C}}-\overset{H}{\underset{\overset{+}{N}H_2CH_3}{C}}-CH_3 \quad Cl^-$$

PSEUDOEPHEDRINE SULFATE

[Afrin, Drixoral Non-Drowsy Formula]

This stereoisomer of ephedrine is used orally to relieve nasal congestion. It usually is used in combination with an antihistamine in patients with VMR, but the effectiveness of decongestants for this condition is variable.

For a more detailed discussion of nasal decongestants, see Drug Selection in the Introduction to this section.

ADVERSE REACTIONS. Adverse reactions are similar to those of other nasal decongestants, but central nervous system stimulation and transient elevations in blood pressure occur less frequently and are less severe. There have been rare reports that antihistamine/pseudoephedrine combinations produced hallucinations in adults and children, but dosages exceeding those usually recommended were administered or patients had predisposing factors, such as febrile conditions. Hallucinations also have been reported rarely with other sympathomimetic agents.

Pseudoephedrine is classified in FDA Pregnancy B.

DOSAGE AND PREPARATIONS.

Oral: *Adults and children 12 years and older,* 60 mg every four to six hours or, prolonged-release form, 120 mg every 12 hours (maximum, 240 mg/day). *Children 6 to 11 years,* 30 mg every four to six hours (maximum, 120 mg/day); *2 to 5 years*, 15 mg every four to six hours (maximum, 60 mg/day). Pseudoephedrine should not be used in *children under 2 years* without medical supervision.

PSEUDOEPHEDRINE HYDROCHLORIDE:

Generic. Liquid 30 mg/5 ml; tablets 30 and 60 mg; tablets (prolonged-release) 120 mg (all forms nonprescription).

Actifed Allergy Daytime (Warner Wellcome). Caplets 30 mg.

Dorcol Children's Decongestant (Sandoz). Liquid 15 mg/5 ml (nonprescription).

Novafed (Marion Merrell Dow). Capsules (prolonged-release) 120 mg.

Sudafed (Warner Wellcome). Liquid 30 mg/5 ml; tablets 30 and 60 mg; caplets (prolonged-release) 120 mg (***Sudafed 12 Hour***) (all forms nonprescription).

PSEUDOEPHEDRINE SULFATE:

Afrin, Drixoral Non-Drowsy Formula (Schering-Plough). Tablets (prolonged-release) 120 mg (nonprescription).

TETRAHYDROZOLINE HYDROCHLORIDE

[Tyzine]

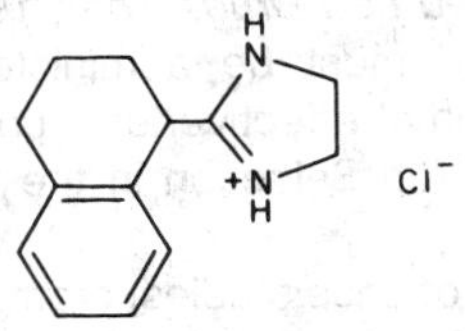

This imidazoline derivative is effective intranasally for temporary relief of nasal congestion. It acts within a few minutes, and the duration of effect is four to eight hours. Tetrahydrozoline has variable effectiveness in VMR.

For a more detailed discussion of nasal decongestants, see Drug Selection in the Introduction to this section.

ADVERSE REACTIONS. The most frequent adverse reactions are burning, stinging, and dryness of the mucosa; sneezing; headache; weakness; tremors; lightheadedness; and palpitations. Prolonged or excessive use may cause rebound congestion. Adverse effects observed especially with overdosage include hypertension, bradycardia, drowsiness with sweating, rebound hypotension, and arrhythmias. Overdosage may produce severe drowsiness in young children. Because of these effects, tetrahydrozoline should be avoided in infants under 2 years and in patients with cardiovascular disease.

Tetrahydrozoline is classified in FDA Pregnancy Category C.

DOSAGE AND PREPARATIONS.

Intranasal: *Adults and children 6 years or older,* two to four drops of the 0.1% solution instilled in each nostril no more often than every three hours for no more than three to five days. Tetrahydrozoline should be used cautiously, if at all, in *children 2 to 6 years* and should not be used in *children under 2 years.* The manufacturer's suggested dosage is: *Children 2 to 6 years,* two to three drops of the 0.05% solution instilled in each nostril, with the head in the lateral, head-low position, at intervals of four to six hours.

Tyzine (Kenwood). Solution 0.05% (pediatric) in 15 ml containers and 0.1% in 15 (spray) and 30 ml containers.

XYLOMETAZOLINE HYDROCHLORIDE

[Otrivin]

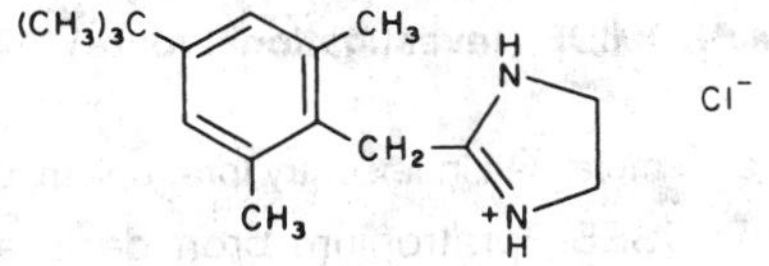

This imidazoline derivative is effective intranasally for temporary relief of nasal congestion. The onset of action is five to ten minutes, and the duration of effect is five to six hours. Xylometazoline has variable effectiveness in VMR.

For a more detailed discussion of nasal decongestants, see Drug Selection in the Introduction to this section.

ADVERSE REACTIONS. Untoward reactions generally are mild and infrequent and include local stinging or burning, sneezing, dryness of the nose, headache, and palpitations. Rebound congestion of the nasal mucosa has been reported with prolonged or excessive administration.

The solution should not be used in atomizers that have aluminum parts.

DOSAGE AND PREPARATIONS.

Intranasal: *Adults,* two or three drops of the 0.1% solution or two or three inhalations of the 0.1% nasal spray in each nostril every eight to ten hours. *Children 6 to under 12 years,* two or three drops of the 0.05% solution in each nostril every eight to ten hours; *under 6 years,* not recommended. The manufacturer's suggested dosage is: *children 2 to under 6 years*, two or three drops or sprays of a 0.05% solution in each nostril every eight to ten hours. Application should not exceed three to five days.

All forms nonprescription.

Generic. Spray 0.1%.

Otrivin (CIBA). Solution (drops) 0.05% (pediatric) and 0.1% in 20 ml containers; spray 0.1% in 15 ml containers.

Intranasal Antihistamine

LEVOCABASTINE HYDROCHLORIDE (Investigational route)
[Livostin]

For chemical formula, see index entry Levocabastine, as Antihistamine,

Levocabastine, a highly specific H_1 receptor antagonist, is more potent than other antihistamines and is the first antihistamine developed for use alone in a nasal spray preparation, which is still investigational. In clinical trials, intranasal levocabastine administered four times daily significantly relieved symptoms in patients with allergic rhinitis (Palma-Carlos et al, 1991; Schata et al, 1991). An eyedrop preparation, which is now approved, also was effective for allergic rhinoconjunctivitis (Dechant and Goa, 1991). Ocular or intranasal application in low doses did not appear to be sensitizing.

Levocabastine appears to be well tolerated (Dechant and Goa, 1991; Rombaut et al, 1991). An investigational oral preparation has caused sedation in many patients, but the intranasal preparation is nonsedating.

Livostin (Janssen).

Anticholinergic Agent

IPRATROPIUM BROMIDE (Investigational route)
[Atrovent]

For chemical formula, see index entry Ipratropium, Uses, Asthma.

ACTIONS AND USES. Ipratropium bromide is a quaternary ammonium congener of atropine that is minimally absorbed after intranasal application and does not cross the blood-brain barrier. Systemic adverse reactions characteristic of atropine and other tertiary amines have not been reported.

This anticholinergic agent significantly reduces rhinorrhea in patients with allergic and nonallergic rhinitis in doses that are well tolerated (Baroody et al, 1992). Nasal hypersecretion due to the common cold and other causes also is responsive (Borum, 1987; Dockhorn et al, 1992). The drug is particularly useful for rhinorrhea in rhinitis that persists after resolution of the common cold or in allergic and nonallergic chronic rhinitis (Holmes et al, 1992; Druce et al, 1992; Meltzer et al, 1992). Other symptoms of rhinitis, such as sneezing or nasal congestion, are not relieved. In normal volunteers, basal nasal secretion was unaffected by this drug.

For a discussion of the use of ipratropium as a bronchodilator, see index entry Ipratropium, Uses, Asthma.

ADVERSE REACTIONS. In short-term studies (three weeks or less), the only significant adverse effect produced by ipratropium was nasal dryness, which can be alleviated by a nasal saline spray. Long-term use may produce nasal congestion and bloody nasal secretions, but administration for a period of one year has not been associated with significant adverse effects in most patients (Dolovich et al, 1987).

DOSAGE AND PREPARATIONS.

Intranasal (investigational route): The wide end of a baby bottle nipple may be fitted over the mouthpiece of the metered-dose inhaler and the tip of the nipple truncated so that its open end can be inserted into the nostrils (Lieberman, 1988). A dose of 80 mcg (two puffs in each nostril) four times a day has been effective for a period of one year (Borum, 1987; Dolovich et al, 1987; Kirkegaard et al, 1987).

Atrovent (Boehringer Ingelheim).

Prophylactic Agent

CROMOLYN SODIUM
[Nasalcrom]

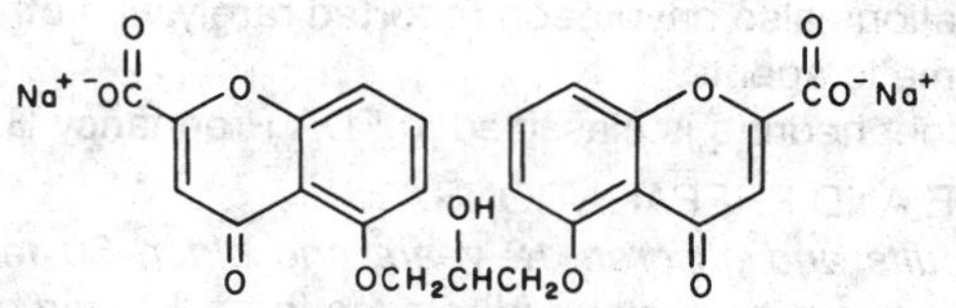

$Na^+ \ ^-OOC$ … OCH_2CHCH_2O (OH) … $COO^- \ Na^+$

ACTIONS AND USES. The mechanism of action of cromolyn sodium includes inhibition of the release of histamine and other allergic mediators from mast cells by blocking calcium transport across the mast cell membrane; its specific mode of action has not been determined. Use of the nasal spray prevents symptoms of seasonal allergic rhinitis (rhinorrhea and postnasal drip), but up to three weeks may be required before relief is obtained. Alleviation of sneezing, nasal congestion, and eye irritation is variable; throat irritation is not relieved significantly. Cromolyn sodium is usually less beneficial after symptoms have developed but, in some patients with mild symptoms, progression to more severe nasal congestion may be prevented. The presence of high preseasonal concentrations of IgE ragweed antibody may predict the drug's effectiveness (Welsh et al, 1977).

Cromolyn's effectiveness in seasonal allergic rhinitis is similar to that of the antihistamines and is less than that of the intranasal corticosteroids. Some patients with chronic allergic rhinitis may not respond well. Cromolyn is ineffective in nonallergic rhinitis and conditions such as nasal polyps in which obstruction of nasal passages prevents access of the drug to its site of action (*Med Lett Drugs Ther*, 1983).

Because cromolyn must be administered three or four times a day for maximal effectiveness, compliance can be a problem. See also Drug Selection in the Introduction to this section.

In a small number of case studies, cromolyn sodium administered by inhalation into the lungs relieved chronic cough due to ACE inhibitor therapy in most patients (Aldis, 1991; Sebastian et al, 1991; Barnes, 1992).

An oral preparation of cromolyn has been used experimentally to alleviate symptoms of food allergy (Pelikan et al, 1989), but its value is controversial.

ADVERSE REACTIONS AND PRECAUTIONS. The lack of serious adverse reactions is an advantage of cromolyn over other agents. Side effects generally are mild and rarely require discontinuation of treatment. Local effects (nasal stinging, burning, irritation, or sneezing) occur in 2.5% to 10% of patients. Headache and an unpleasant taste have been reported in about 2% of patients and postnasal drip, rash, and epistaxis in less than 1%. Allergic reactions are very rare.

Cromolyn is probably safe in pregnant and lactating women and may be preferred to intranasal corticosteroids and nasal decongestants in these patients. However, its safety has not been established unequivocally (FDA Pregnancy Category B).

PHARMACOKINETICS. Following intranasal application, about 7% of the dose is absorbed into the blood stream; when given orally, less than 2% is absorbed through the gastrointestinal tract. Cromolyn is not metabolized. Approximately 50% of the amount absorbed is recovered in the urine and the remaining one-half in the bile. Most of the unabsorbed portion is excreted in the feces. The plasma half-life is 0.75 to 1.5 hours.

DOSAGE AND PREPARATIONS.

Intranasal: *Adults and children 6 years and over,* one spray (5.2 mg) in each nostril three or four times a day at regular intervals. The patient should inhale through the nose during administration of the spray. Nasal passages should be cleared (using a nasal decongestant if needed) prior to use of cromolyn.

For seasonal allergic rhinitis, prophylactic therapy should be initiated before exposure to antigen or the expected occurrence of symptoms, and use should be continued throughout the period of exposure.

Nasalcrom (Fisons). Solution 40 mg/ml (5.2 mg/actuation) with a 13- and 26-ml metered spray device (***Nasalmatic Inhaler***).

Intranasal Corticosteroids

DEXAMETHASONE SODIUM PHOSPHATE

[Decadron Turbinaire]

Dexamethasone was the first intranasal corticosteroid available in this country and is as effective as the newer agents, beclomethasone, triamcinolone, budesonide, and flunisolide, for the treatment of rhinitis and certain other nasal disorders. However, intranasal dexamethasone is absorbed and can cause systemic adverse effects, including mild adrenocortical suppression, if used for more than 30 days. Therefore, intranasal use of this drug is limited to a maximum of 30 days. Excessive intranasal application rarely causes nasal mucosal atrophy, ulceration, or septal perforation.

The use of dexamethasone nasal spray has been greatly diminished by the availability of intranasal preparations of beclomethasone, flunisolide, budesonide, and triamcinolone, which do not suppress adrenocortical function in recommended doses (Busse, 1983). See also Drug Selection in the Introduction to this section.

DOSAGE AND PREPARATIONS.

Intranasal: *Adults,* two sprays (200 mcg) in each nostril two or three times daily (maximum, 12 sprays [1.2 mg]). *Children 6 to 12 years,* one or two sprays (100 to 200 mcg) in each nostril twice daily (maximum, eight sprays [800 mcg]). When the maximal response is obtained (usually in one to two weeks), the dose is reduced to the lowest level that maintains symptomatic control. Continued use beyond 30 days is inappropriate.

Decadron Turbinaire (Merck). Aerosol providing 84 mcg/actuation (equivalent to base).

BECLOMETHASONE DIPROPIONATE

[Beconase, Beconase AQ, Vancenase, Vancenase AQ]

For chemical formula, see index entry Beclomethasone, In Asthma.

ACTIONS AND USES. This halogenated corticosteroid has a marked local anti-inflammatory effect when applied intranasally. The nasal spray is effective and safe for seasonal and nonseasonal allergic rhinitis; for nonallergic disorders, such as nasal polyps and rhinitis medicamentosa; and for the rhinitis of pregnancy (Brogden et al, 1984). NARES also responds. Beclomethasone is more effective than antihistamines, decongestants, or cromolyn for prophylaxis and treatment of these disorders. Rhinorrhea, nasal pruritus, postnasal drainage, nasal congestion, and sneezing respond to therapy. Effectiveness is reduced when nasal congestion is severe, and a short course of an intranasal decongestant or an oral corticosteroid may be required prior to use of beclomethasone. Ocular symptoms usually are not relieved by topical nasal therapy. This drug is less useful for VMR.

Significant relief of symptoms occurs within three days in patients with seasonal allergic rhinitis, but full effects are not attained for a week or longer. In patients with nonseasonal rhinitis, relief may require one week and full effects are not observed for two to three weeks. Daily administration is required for maximal effectiveness.

No difference in efficacy has been noted between the aqueous form that contains no Freon and the conventional pressurized spray (Welsh et al, 1987).

See also Drug Selection in the Introduction to this section.

ADVERSE REACTIONS AND PRECAUTIONS. The incidence of minor adverse reactions is high in patients using the pressurized spray; these effects probably are due to the vehicle, since the incidence is the same as with a placebo. In one study, more than 50% of the patients reported nasal burning, stinging, irritation, or pressure and/or sneezing immediately after administration of the pressurized nasal spray. These symptoms usually subside with continued use. Except for nasal stinging that lasts only a few seconds after administration (and is much less pronounced than with flunisolide), symptoms were absent in most patients who used the aqueous spray form, which does not contain Freon (Orgel et al, 1986); however, some patients complain that the aqueous spray form causes postnasal drip and has an offensive flowery odor. Other adverse effects include headache, dry nose, and nasal bleeding. Nasal candidiasis has not been reported, and mucosal atrophy does not appear to develop with prolonged use.

Adrenocortical suppression does not occur with usual doses but is possible with extremely large doses.

Some authorities recommend that intranasal corticosteroids be used with caution in patients with active tuberculosis, untreated bacterial infections, and systemic fungal or viral infections. They should be administered with caution, if at all, in patients with ocular herpes simplex. If used cautiously, they can be employed adjunctively in bacterial sinusitis. Nasal polyps decrease in size during continuous use of beclomethasone but may enlarge after cessation of therapy or in the presence of a respiratory infection.

If no significant response occurs, intranasal corticosteroids should be discontinued after three to four weeks when used for chronic rhinitis or after four to six weeks when used to reduce nasal polyps (unless administered after surgery to prevent regrowth).

This drug is classified in FDA Pregnancy Category C.

PHARMACOKINETICS. Although a portion of the administered dose is absorbed from the nasal mucosa, beclomethasone dipropionate is rapidly metabolized to beclomethasone monopropionate and then to inactive metabolites; this explains in part the low incidence of systemic side effects. Little unchanged drug is recovered in the urine or feces.

DOSAGE AND PREPARATIONS.

Intranasal: (Beconase, Vancenase) *Adults and children 12 years and older,* one inhalation (42 mcg) in each nostril two to four times daily (total dose, 168 to 336 mcg/day); *children 6 to 12 years,* one inhalation in each nostril two to three times daily (total dose, 252 mcg/day). (Beconase AQ, Vancenase AQ): *Adults and children 6 years and older,* one or two inhalations (42 to 84 mcg) in each nostril twice daily (total dose, 168 to 336 mcg/day). When the maximal response is obtained (usually in one to two weeks), the dose is reduced to the lowest level that maintains symptomatic control. The intranasal spray must be directed appropriately into the nostrils to avoid local deposition of drug on the mucosa of the septum. Beclomethasone is not recommended for use in *children under 6 years.*

Beconase, Beconase AQ (Allen & Hanburys). Spray providing 42 mcg/actuation.

Vancenase, Vancenase AQ (Schering). Spray providing 42 mcg/actuation; inhaler 7 g (***Pockethaler***).

BUDESONIDE
[Rhinocort]

This intranasal corticosteroid is similar to beclomethasone dipropionate in efficacy, indications, actions, adverse reactions, and precautions (Clissold and Heel, 1984; Day et al, 1990; Ross et al, 1991). See that evaluation. Large doses of budesonide produce fewer systemic effects than comparable doses of other currently available intranasal corticosteroids. Adrenocortical suppression is unlikely, even with doses larger than those usually recommended.

PHARMACOKINETICS. Budesonide is well absorbed. It undergoes significant first-pass metabolism in the liver and is converted rapidly to compounds with little systemic activity, which explains in part the low incidence of systemic side effects. The plasma half-life is approximately two hours. Little unchanged drug is recovered in the urine.

DOSAGE AND PREPARATIONS.

Intranasal: *Adults,* the usual daily dose for rhinitis is 256 mcg (two sprays in each nostril twice daily or four sprays in each nostril once daily in the morning) (Clissold and Heel, 1984; Ross et al, 1991).

Rhinocort (Astra). Spray 32 mcg/actuation.

FLUNISOLIDE
[Nasalide]

For chemical formula, see index entry Flunisolide, In Asthma.

The efficacy, indications, actions, adverse reactions, and precautions of flunisolide are similar to those of beclomethasone dipropionate. This preparation does not contain Freon and is delivered in a propylene glycol vehicle, which does not cause dryness.

See also Drug Selection in the Introduction to this section and the evaluation on Beclomethasone Dipropionate.

ADVERSE REACTIONS. The most common adverse reactions of flunisolide nasal spray are stinging and burning (incidence, more than 40%), which last only a few seconds after application. (This is a particular complaint in children.)

This drug is classified in FDA Pregnancy Category C.

PHARMACOKINETICS. Flunisolide is well absorbed; approximately 50% of a dose reaches the systemic circulation. The drug is converted rapidly to less active metabolites and conjugates. This explains in part the low incidence of systemic side effects. The plasma half-life is one to two hours. About one-half of the absorbed drug is recovered in the urine and one-half in the feces. The onset of action is usually two to five days.

DOSAGE AND PREPARATIONS.

Intranasal: *Adults,* initially, two sprays (50 mcg) in each nostril two times daily (total dose, 200 mcg/day). The daily dose should not exceed eight sprays in each nostril (400 mcg/day). *Children 6 to 14 years,* initially, one spray (25 mcg) in each nostril three times daily or two sprays in each nostril two times daily. The dose should not exceed four sprays in each nostril (200 mcg/day). This drug is not recommended in *children under 6 years.* When the maximal response is obtained (usually in one to two weeks), the dose is reduced to the lowest level that maintains symptomatic control.

Nasalide (Syntex). Spray 0.025% providing approximately 25 mcg/actuation.

TRIAMCINOLONE ACETONIDE
[Nasacort]

For chemical formula, see index entry Triamcinolone, In Asthma.

The aerosol form of triamcinolone acetonide appears to be similar to beclomethasone dipropionate in efficacy, indications, adverse reactions, and precautions. See that evaluation.

In controlled clinical studies, signs and symptoms of seasonal and perennial allergic rhinitis were relieved significantly (Spector et al, 1990; Tinkelman et al, 1990; Storms et al, 1991). Once-daily administration enhances compliance.

This corticosteroid is well tolerated; there is no evidence of adrenocortical suppression.

Triamcinolone is classified in FDA Pregnancy Category C.

PHARMACOKINETICS. In pharmacokinetic studies of radiolabeled preparations of triamcinolone acetonide (oral and intravenous preparations), most of the drug was eliminated in the feces. Following administration of the aerosol, triamcinolone disappeared rapidly from the lungs, with virtually none remaining in the lungs or trachea 24 hours after administration. Three major metabolites, less active than the parent compound, have been identified (unpublished data, Rhone-Poulenc Rorer Pharmaceuticals).

DOSAGE AND PREPARATIONS.

Intranasal: *Adults and children 12 years and older*, initially, two sprays (approximately 55 mcg/spray) in each nostril once daily. The response should be evaluated in four to seven days. If needed, the dosage may be increased to a total of 440 mcg per day applied once or divided and applied up to four times daily. After the desired effect is obtained, some patients may be maintained on as little as one spray in each nostril once daily.

Nasacort (Rhone-Poulenc Rorer). Spray providing 55 mcg/actuation.

FLUOCORTIN BUTYL (Investigational drug)

This agent appears to be similar to beclomethasone dipropionate in efficacy, indications, actions, adverse reactions, and precautions (Hartley et al, 1985; Orgel et al, 1991). See that evaluation.

Following systemic absorption, fluocortin is metabolized rapidly by nonspecific tissue esterases to an inactive C-21 corticosteroid. Therefore, it is highly active topically and almost inactive systemically.

The potential advantage of fluocortin butyl is that larger doses are safer than with use of beclomethasone or flunisolide; daily doses 20 to 80 times larger than normal have no effect on adrenocortical function. Its disadvantages compared with budesonide, fluticasone, or triamcinolone are the need for administration three times daily in most patients and a higher incidence of local adverse reactions (Orgel et al, 1991). This compound has poor stability and can be prepared only as a dry powder for inhalation.

Fluocortin Butyl (Berlex).

FLUTICASONE PROPIONATE (Investigational route)
[Flovent]

This potent intranasal corticosteroid has low bioavailability as a result of poor absorption; fluticasone is metabolized rapidly after it reaches the systemic circulation. Its actions, indications, and efficacy are similar to those of beclomethasone dipropionate (Mabry, 1992; Bryson and Faulds, 1992; Bousquet et al, 1993). The advantages of fluticasone are its lack of systemic effects, the absence of adrenocortical suppression in doses eight times above the recommended daily dose, and improved compliance with once-daily administration.

Flovent (Glaxo).

COMMON COLD

The common cold is an acute infection of the upper respiratory tract mucosa caused by many different types of viruses, particularly rhinoviruses and coronaviruses. Bacterial diseases that cause primarily nasal symptoms are nasal diphtheria and infection by *Haemophilus* species or meningococci. Nasal discharge is often purulent from the onset in these rare infections. In infants under 18 months, nasopharyngitis may be caused by group A streptococci and presents as a purulent nasal discharge (Levin et al, 1988).

It is believed that colds are transmitted both by exposure to aerosols generated by sneezing or coughing and by direct contact (hand to hand to nose) (Dick et al, 1987; Hendley and Gwaltney, 1988). A variety of factors affect an individual's susceptibility to cold viruses (Mills, 1983; Evans et al, 1988). In one well-controlled study, psychological stress increased the susceptibility of healthy subjects to experimentally induced colds (Cohen et al, 1991).

A viral upper respiratory infection usually can be distinguished from other forms of rhinitis. The major complaints include rhinorrhea, sneezing, nasal stuffiness, and dry cough with or without mild sore throat. The chest is usually clear on auscultation. Systemic symptoms are common and include malaise, headache, and myalgia. Fever is unusual in adults, although mild to moderately high temperatures are common in children. The nasal discharge is clear initially but may become purulent.

The common cold is usually benign and self-limiting. Failure of symptoms to abate within one or two weeks or worsening symptoms suggests secondary bacterial infection of the paranasal sinuses, ears, tracheobronchial tree, or lungs. In such cases, administration of antibiotics may be warranted after appropriate evaluation. Routine administration of antimicrobial agents to patients with uncomplicated colds has been shown to be useless. However, it is reasonable to give an antibiotic to patients with chronic obstructive pulmonary disease or nasal polyps who develop a cold in order to prevent an exacerbation of bronchitis or sinusitis.

Identification of the virus is unnecessary since specific therapy does not exist. Only symptoms can be relieved. That such relief is sought very frequently is attested to by the large number of patient visits for treatment of the common cold and the widespread use of prescription and nonprescription cold remedies.

It is very difficult to establish clearly the value of any medication for the common cold because controlled, blind, randomized trials are difficult to perform. This problem occurs for a number of reasons, including the lack of objective outcome measures and suitable controls, strong placebo effect, self-limited nature of colds, inadequate randomization, and poor follow-up of patients (West et al, 1975; Lampert et al, 1974; Lowenstein and Parrino, 1987; Sperber and Hayden, 1988).

No practical methods of prevention or cure are currently available.

INVESTIGATIONAL STUDIES. Vitamin C, the subject of many clinical studies, is ineffective.

Among the experimental approaches to prevention and treatment of the common cold are the following: A number of cold vaccines administered intranasally have been effective in preventing clinical infection by specific cold viruses. However, a vaccine that would be effective against all etiologic agents appears unlikely because more than 100 viruses cause colds, and single viruses, such as rhinovirus, have more than 100 serotypes; moreover, these are constantly mutating and changing antigenic specificity (Macnaughton, 1982).

Rhinoviruses and other cold viruses initiate infection and gain entry into host cells in adenoidal or residual adenoidal tissue by attaching to host cell receptors. The development of monoclonal antibodies or synthetic agents that block binding to the receptor offers the potential to prevent and possibly treat a cold during the early stages of the infection (Sperber and Hayden, 1988; Hayden et al, 1988). Their use against the common cold virus has shown some efficacy in clinical trials; however, the immunity achieved is not long lasting.

The surface of adenoidal host cells contains a protein, intercellular adhesion molecule-1 (ICAM-1), that, when expressed, serves as a ligand for circulating leukocytes when infectious agents are present. Rhinoviruses also bind to ICAM-1 to gain intracellular access and subsequently multiply. Agents under investigation that may block viral binding to the host cell surface include capsid binders and ICAM-1 receptor antagonists. Capsid binders alter the configuration of the cell surface to prevent viral attachment. The development of ICAM-1 receptor antagonists appears to be a more practical approach; antibodies could be designed that prevent viral binding or agents could be developed that serve as synthetic ICAM-1 receptor decoys (Cecchin, 1993).

Win 51 711, an antiviral agent, binds the viral protein coat and stabilizes the virus, preventing it from shedding its coat and invading the host cell (Smith et al, 1986). Intranasal enviroxime, another antiviral drug, was particularly effective in preventing rhinovirus infection, but the incidence of adverse effects was high (Levandowski et al, 1982; Hayden and Gwaltney, 1982; Phillpotts et al, 1983). Analogues of these compounds and other antiviral agents are being investigated and continue to show promise in clinical trials (Al-Nakib et al, 1989).

Facial tissues impregnated with virucides such as citric/malic acid and sodium lauryl sulfate have been investigated as a means of preventing the transmission of colds (Dick et al, 1986; Longini and Monto, 1988). Studies have established their value in interrupting transmission for short periods in small groups, but their long-term value in large populations has not been determined (Farr et al, 1988).

In two studies, zinc gluconate lozenges were reported to reduce symptoms but did not prevent colds (Eby et al, 1984; *Pharm J*, 1987). In other studies, zinc acetate lozenges had no effect on cold symptoms (Douglas et al, 1987; Potter and Hart, 1993). Long-term use of zinc in doses that ameliorate symptoms could produce significant adverse effects (Sperber and Hayden, 1988).

Interferon, which prevents viral invasion of respiratory mucosa, has been used experimentally to prevent rhinovirus infection (Hayden and Gwaltney, 1983; Samo et al, 1983). A nasal wash or aerosol preparation of interferon has been used. In two independent studies among family members, an intranasal aerosol spray of interferon alfa-2 was administered once daily for seven days when cold symptoms first appeared in another family member. A 40% decrease in respiratory illnesses and a 79% decrease in colds due to rhinovirus were observed (Hayden et al, 1986; Douglas et al, 1986). The short-term prophylactic administration of interferon alfa-2 was effective in a third study (Douglas, 1986) but was ineffective in another study (Monto et al, 1989). Long-term use of interferon alfa-2 is not practical, primarily because this agent produces unpleasant adverse effects, such as nasal congestion and inflammation that are as bad as the cold itself, and it is expensive. Other types of interferon (beta and gamma) have been ineffective (Higgins et al, 1988; Sperber et al, 1989). The safety of interferon in children is unclear. Most physicians believe that the magnitude of the effect of interferon is not enough to justify the time, expense, and adverse reactions observed with its use (Mills, 1986). However, renewed interest in interferon has developed because of a placebo-controlled study showing that combination therapy with intranasal interferon alfa-2 and ipratropium plus oral naproxen reduced cold symptoms significantly (Gwaltney, 1992; Cecchin, 1993).

In a number of studies, inhalation of humidified warm air (43° C) into the nasal passages once or twice daily for 20 minutes significantly relieved cold symptoms and decreased nasal airway resistance for several days (Ophir and Elad, 1987; Tyrrell et al, 1989). However, in subsequent randomized controlled trials, inhalation of humidified heated air provided no benefit in patients with allergic rhinitis or the common cold (Macknin et al, 1990; Oppenheimer et al, 1993; Forstall et al, 1994; Hendley et al, 1994; Monto, 1994).

SYMPTOMATIC TREATMENT. Cold remedies are designed to relieve nasal congestion, to decrease the nasal discharge, and, less often, to relieve fever and pain (Sperber and Hayden, 1988). Since no one drug accomplishes all of these functions, various mixtures are employed, but they have the disadvantages of all mixtures: When a therapeutic amount of one agent is given, other drugs in the mixture may be administered at higher or lower than optimal therapeutic levels. In addition, some mixtures contain more than one ingredient from a pharmacologic group, often in subtherapeutic quantities of each. On the other hand, if the patient suffers from multiple symptoms, particularly during the early stages of a cold, use of a mixture provides a more convenient and sometimes less expensive means of providing relief than use of several single-entity products. In practice, both doctors and patients find mixtures convenient and without serious disadvantages (see the section on Mixtures).

No controlled studies exist that demonstrate the efficacy of nasal decongestants in treating cold symptoms. However, it is generally accepted that they relieve nasal stuffiness in the common cold and also may help to maintain patency of the eustachian tubes and sinus ostia, thereby inhibiting the development of secondary infection. Intranasal sprays provide the greatest symptomatic relief; intranasal adrenergic agonists increase nasal patency, lower nasal resistance, and provide subjective relief of nasal symptoms in patients with the common cold (Lampert et al, 1974; Lea, 1984; Lowenstein and Parrino, 1987); they do not relieve other symptoms such as rhinorrhea, cough, or earache. Intranasal sprays produce fewer side effects than systemic preparations but have the disadvantage of causing rebound congestion. Therefore, intranasal decongestants should be used for no more than three to five days. Adverse effects after systemic administration of decongestants are due to the alpha-adrenergic properties of these drugs. (See Drug Selection in the section on Rhinitis.)

Antihistamines are frequently used in cold preparations, although neither histamine nor allergy has a significant role in the common cold. Any value of antihistamines is most likely due to their anticholinergic and sedative effects. These are properties of the first-generation antihistamines; the second-generation (nonsedating) antihistamines, such as terfenadine and astemizole (which lack these actions), have little or no usefulness in the common cold.

Sneezing and rhinorrhea may respond to first-generation antihistamines, but other symptoms such as sore throat, sinus congestion, and cough usually are not relieved and nasal blockage and sinus congestion may worsen (West et al, 1975; *Med Lett Drugs Ther*, 1975; Lowenstein and Parrino, 1987; Sperber and Hayden, 1988). In a double-blind study in patients with experimentally induced rhinovirus colds, oral chlorpheniramine and intranasal diphenhydramine were ineffective in reducing nasal mucus production or other nasal symptoms. These results and those reported in other studies (Hutton et al, 1991) further demonstrate the limited role of histamine in the pathogenesis of the common cold and the general lack of value of antihistamines for infectious rhinitis (Gaffey et al, 1987).

In a review of data from clinical trials carried out between 1950 and 1991, the lack of benefit of antihistamines for children with colds was reaffirmed, but, based on results from three studies, these drugs were reported to have value for cold symptoms in adolescents and adults (Smith and Feldman, 1993). Critical analysis of the three positive studies (Luks and Anderson, 1993) indicates that they had design flaws, presented statistical data that was without clinical significance, and/or that determination of effectiveness was based on inadequate data. See index entry Antihistamines, Uses.

It has been claimed that the anticholinergic properties of some antihistamines dry and thicken lower respiratory tract secretions and eventually cause inspissation, particularly in infants and small children; however, this is probably not true. Nevertheless, it is sometimes desirable to discontinue the use of drying medications.

Acetaminophen may be preferable to aspirin for the treatment of colds because aspirin may interfere with antiviral defense mechanisms by decreasing mucociliary clearance, may enhance the spread of infection by increasing virus shedding (Stanley et al, 1975; Gerrity et al, 1983), and may be associated with Reye's syndrome in children.

Caffeine is present in some cold preparations; although it may not sufficiently counteract antihistamine-induced drowsiness, caffeine generally is not harmful. If a decongestant is present in the formulation, the additional cardiac stimulation provided by caffeine may be undesirable.

Some physicians recommend application of a small amount of skin moisturizer or water-based ointment under the nose to prevent and treat the irritation and dryness resulting from nasal discharge in patients with the common cold. Ointments should not be inhaled.

Pungent hot soups are sometimes recommended, since they enhance mucocilliary clearance from the nose and sinuses. Folk remedies employing horseradish (eg, as a gargle, in water with honey) also are popular.

See the following section on Mixtures for information on combination products used to treat cough or rhinitis and Table 2 at the end of this chapter for a listing of commonly used oral cold remedy products.

MIXTURES

Single-entity products may be preferable to mixtures for most patients with cough or rhinitis. Certain combination products are useful and convenient in patients with multiple symptoms who do not respond adequately to a single drug. If a mixture is to be used, it should meet the following criteria: (1) It contains no more than three active ingredients from different pharmacologic groups and only one active ingredient from each pharmacologic group. (2) Each active ingredient is present in an effective and safe concentration and contributes to the usefulness of the product. (3) The product is used only when multiple symptoms are present concurrently. (4) The product is therapeutically appropriate for the type and severity of symptoms being treated. (5) The possible adverse reactions of the components are taken into consideration.

Many mixtures popular with the lay public and physicians for treatment of upper respiratory tract disorders do not meet these criteria. Moreover, physicians should be aware that a product may be reformulated without a change in the brand name.

Overdoses that produced serious adverse effects have occurred when a combination of dextromethorphan, an antihistamine, and a decongestant was ingested by children under 2 years (Gadomski and Horton, 1992). Consequently, the use of such combinations probably should be avoided in infants.

The mixtures listed in the following sections and in Table 2 are representative; no attempt has been made to include all available mixtures used for rhinitis or the common cold.

Mixtures Containing Antitussives

Many of the preparations listed in this section appear to have been formulated for the symptomatic treatment of minor respiratory disorders rather than for specific relief of cough. Thus, in addition to an antitussive, these mixtures usually contain one or more ingredients classified as expectorants, one or more sympathomimetic agents as bronchodilators or nasal decongestants, and antihistamines. The effectiveness of such mixtures compared with single-entity preparations is not known. The physician should be aware of the ingredients in the formulation; for example, the brand name often does not indicate that the mixture contains codeine or other opioid antitussives. The antitussive efficacy of carbetapentane and caramiphen, which are available only in combination products, is unproven. Caramiphen has local anesthetic and anticholinergic effects, and mixtures containing this drug must be used cautiously in patients sensitive to anticholinergic complications, such as glaucoma and prostatic hypertrophy; however, reports of these complications are rare.

The following commonly used preparations are listed for information only; inclusion in the list does not indicate approval or recommendation for use.

Antitussive Mixtures Containing Codeine (All Schedule V Preparations Except As Noted)

Actifed W/Codeine (Burroughs Wellcome). Each 5 ml of syrup contains codeine phosphate 10 mg, pseudoephedrine hydrochloride 30 mg, and triprolidine hydrochloride 1.25 mg (alcohol 4.3%).

Ambenyl (Forest). Each 5 ml of syrup contains codeine phosphate 10 mg and bromodiphenhydramine hydrochloride 12.5 mg (alcohol 5%).

Calcidrine (Abbott). Each 5 ml of syrup contains codeine 8.4 mg and calcium iodide 152 mg (alcohol 6%).

Cheracol (Roberts). Each 5 ml of syrup contains codeine phosphate 10 mg and guaifenesin 100 mg (alcohol 4.75%).

Dimetane-DC (Robins). Each 5 ml of syrup contains codeine phosphate 10 mg, brompheniramine maleate 2 mg, and phenylpropanolamine hydrochloride 12.5 mg (alcohol 0.95%).

Isoclor Expectorant (Fisons). Each 5 ml of syrup contains codeine phosphate 10 mg, guaifenesin 100 mg, and pseudoephedrine hydrochloride 30 mg (alcohol 5%).

Naldecon-CX (Apothecon). Each 5 ml of suspension contains codeine phosphate 10 mg, phenylpropanolamine hydrochloride 12.5 mg, and guaifenesin 200 mg.

Novahistine-DH (SmithKline Beecham). Each 5 ml of liquid contains codeine phosphate 10 mg, chlorpheniramine maleate 2 mg, and pseudoephedrine hydrochloride 30 mg (alcohol 5%).

Novahistine Expectorant (SmithKline Beecham). Each 5 ml of liquid contains codeine phosphate 10 mg, guaifenesin 100 mg, and pseudoephedrine hydrochloride 30 mg (alcohol 7.5%).

Nucofed (Roberts). Each capsule or 5 ml of syrup contains codeine phosphate 20 mg and pseudoephedrine hydrochloride 60 mg (Schedule III).

Nucofed Expectorant (Roberts). Each 5 ml of syrup contains codeine phosphate 20 mg, guaifenesin 200 mg, and pseudoephedrine hydrochloride 60 mg (alcohol 12.5%). (Schedule III).

Nucofed Pediatric Expectorant (Roberts). Each 5 ml of syrup contains codeine phosphate 10 mg, guaifenesin 100 mg, and pseudoephedrine hydrochloride 30 mg (alcohol 6%).

Pediacof (Sanofi Winthrop). Each 5 ml of syrup contains codeine phosphate 5 mg, chlorpheniramine maleate 0.75 mg, phenylephrine hydrochloride 2.5 mg, and potassium iodide 75 mg (alcohol 5%, sodium benzoate 0.2% as preservative).

Phenergan W/Codeine (Wyeth-Ayerst). Each 5 ml of syrup contains codeine phosphate 10 mg and promethazine hydrochloride 6.25 mg (alcohol 7%).

Phenergan-VC W/Codeine (Wyeth-Ayerst). Each 5 ml of expectorant contains same formulation as ***Phenergan W/Codeine*** plus phenylephrine hydrochloride 5 mg.

Robitussin A-C (Robins). Each 5 ml of syrup contains codeine phosphate 10 mg and guaifenesin 100 mg (alcohol 3.5%).

Robitussin-DAC (Robins). Each 5 ml of syrup contains codeine phosphate 10 mg, guaifenesin 100 mg, and pseudoephedrine hydrochloride 30 mg (alcohol 1.9%).

Triaminic Expectorant with Codeine (Sandoz). Each 5 ml of syrup contains codeine phosphate 10 mg, guaifenesin 100 mg, and phenylpropanolamine hydrochloride 12.5 mg (alcohol 5%).

Tussar-2, Tussar SF (Rhone-Poulenc Rorer). Each 5 ml of syrup contains codeine phosphate 10 mg, pseudoephedrine hydrochloride 30 mg, guaifenesin 100 mg (alcohol 2.5%) (***Tussar-SF*** sugar-free).

Tussi-Organidin (Wallace). Each 5 ml of liquid contains codeine phosphate 10 mg and iodinated glycerol 30 mg.

Antitussive Mixtures Containing Hydrocodone (All Schedule III Preparations)

Hycodan (DuPont). Each tablet or 5 ml of syrup contains hydrocodone bitartrate 5 mg and homatropine methylbromide 1.5 mg.

Hycomine (DuPont). Each 5 ml of syrup or 10 ml of pediatric syrup contains hydrocodone bitartrate 5 mg and phenylpropanolamine hydrochloride 25 mg.

Hycomine Compound (DuPont). Each tablet contains hydrocodone bitartrate 5 mg, phenylephrine hydrochloride 10 mg, chlorpheniramine maleate 2 mg, acetaminophen 250 mg, and caffeine 30 mg.

Hycotuss Expectorant (DuPont). Each 5 ml of syrup contains hydrocodone bitartrate 5 mg and guaifenesin 100 mg (alcohol 10%).

P-V-Tussin (Solvay). Each 5 ml of syrup contains hydrocodone bitartrate 2.5 mg, pseudoephedrine hydrochloride 30 mg, and chlorpheniramine maleate 2 mg (alcohol 5%).

Ru-Tuss w/Hydrocodone (Boots). Each 5 ml of liquid contains hydrocodone bitartrate 1.7 mg, phenylpropanolamine hydrochloride 3.3 mg, phenylephrine hydrochloride 5 mg, pyrilamine maleate 3.3 mg, and pheniramine maleate 3.3 mg (alcohol 5%).

Tussionex (Fisons). Each 5 ml of suspension (prolonged-release) contains hydrocodone polistirex equivalent to 10 mg of hydrocodone bitartrate and chlorpheniramine polistirex equivalent to 8 mg of chlorpheniramine maleate.

Antitussive Mixtures Containing Dextromethorphan

Anatuss DM (Mayrand). Each 5 ml of syrup contains dextromethorphan hydrobromide 10 mg, pseudoephedrine hydrochloride 30 mg, and guaifenesin 100 mg (nonprescription); each tablet contains dextromethorphan hydrobromide 20 mg, pseudoephedrine hydrochloride 60 mg, and guaifenesin 400 mg.

Benylin Expectorant (Warner Wellcome). Each 5 ml of liquid contains dextromethorphan hydrobromide 5 mg and guaifenesin 100 mg (alcohol-free) (nonprescription).

Benylin Multisymptom (Warner Wellcome). Each 5 ml of liquid contains dextromethorphan hydrobromide 5 mg, pseudoephedrine 15 mg, and guaifenesin 100 mg (sugar- and alcohol-free).

Cerose-DM (Wyeth-Ayerst). Each 5 ml of liquid contains dextromethorphan hydrobromide 15 mg, phenylephrine hydrochloride 10 mg, and chlorpheniramine maleate 4 mg (alcohol 2.4%) (nonprescription).

Cheracol D (Roberts). Each 5 ml of liquid contains dextromethorphan hydrobromide 10 mg and guaifenesin 100 mg (alcohol 4.75%) (nonprescription).

Cheracol Plus (Roberts). Each 15 ml of syrup contains dextromethorphan hydrobromide 20 mg, phenylpropanolamine hydrochloride 25 mg, and chlorpheniramine maleate 4 mg (alcohol 8%) (nonprescription).

Conar (SmithKline Beecham). Each 5 ml of syrup (sugar-free) contains dextromethorphan hydrobromide 15 mg and phenylephrine hydrochloride 10 mg (nonprescription).

Dimacol (Robins). Each tablet contains dextromethorphan hydrobromide 10 mg, pseudoephedrine hydrochloride 30 mg, and guaifenesin 100 mg (nonprescription).

Dorcol Children's Cough Syrup (Sandoz). Each 5 ml of syrup contains dextromethorphan hydrobromide 5 mg, guaifenesin 50 mg, and pseudoephedrine hydrochloride 15 mg (nonprescription).

Naldecon-DX (Apothecon). Each 5 ml of liquid (sugar-free) contains dextromethorphan hydrobromide 10 mg, phenylpropanolamine hydrochloride 12.5 mg, and guaifenesin 200 mg (alcohol 0.06%); each 5 ml of pediatric syrup contains dextromethorphan hydrobromide 5 mg, phenylpropanolamine hydrochloride 6.25 mg, and guaifenesin 100 mg (alcohol 5%); each milliliter of pediatric drops (sugar-free) contains dextromethorphan hydrobromide 5 mg, phenylpropanolamine hydrochloride 6.25 mg, and guaifenesin 50 mg (alcohol 0.6%) (all forms nonprescription).

Naldecon Senior DX (Apothecon). Each 5 ml of liquid contains dextromethorphan hydrobromide 10 mg and guaifenesin 200 mg (sugar- and alcohol-free) (nonprescription).

Novahistine DMX (SmithKline Beecham). Each 5 ml of liquid contains dextromethorphan hydrobromide 10 mg, pseudoephedrine hydrochloride 30 mg, and guaifenesin 100 mg (alcohol 10%) (nonprescription).

Phenergan w/Dextromethorphan (Wyeth-Ayerst). Each 5 ml of syrup contains dextromethorphan hydrobromide 15 mg and promethazine hydrochloride 6.25 mg (alcohol 7%).

Robitussin-CF (Robins). Each 5 ml of syrup contains dextromethorphan hydrobromide 10 mg, guaifenesin 100 mg, and phenylpropanolamine hydrochloride 12.5 mg (alcohol 4.75%) (nonprescription).

Robitussin-DM (Robins). Each 5 ml of syrup contains dextromethorphan hydrobromide 10 mg and guaifenesin 100 mg (nonprescription).

Rondec-DM (Ross). Each 5 ml of syrup contains dextromethorphan hydrobromide 15 mg, carbinoxamine maleate 4 mg, and pseudoephedrine hydrochloride 60 mg; each milliliter of oral drops contains dextromethorphan hydrobromide 4 mg, carbinoxamine maleate 2 mg, and pseudoephedrine hydrochloride 25 mg.

Ru-Tuss Expectorant (Boots). Each 5 ml of liquid contains dextromethorphan hydrobromide 10 mg, guaifenesin 100 mg, and pseudoephedrine hydrochloride 30 mg (alcohol 10%) (nonprescription).

Sudafed Cough Syrup (Warner Wellcome). Each 5 ml of syrup contains dextromethorphan hydrobromide 5 mg, pseudoephedrine hydrochloride 15 mg, and guaifenesin 100 mg (alcohol 2.4%) (nonprescription).

Sudafed Severe Cold Formula (Warner Wellcome). Each caplet or tablet contains dextromethorphan hydrobromide 15 mg, pseudoephedrine hydrochloride 30 mg, and acetaminophen 500 mg (nonprescription).

Triaminic-DM (Sandoz). Each 5 ml of syrup contains dextromethorphan hydrobromide 5 mg and phenylpropanolamine hydrochloride 6.25 mg (nonprescription).

Triaminic Nite Light (Sandoz). Each 5 ml of syrup contains dextromethorphan hydrobromide 7.5 mg, chlorpheniramine maleate 1 mg, and pseudoephedrine hydrochloride 15 mg (alcohol-free) (nonprescription).

Triaminic Sore Throat Formula (Sandoz). Each 5 ml of syrup contains dextromethorphan hydrobromide 7.5 mg, acetaminophen 160 mg, and pseudoephedrine hydrochloride 15 mg (alcohol-free) (nonprescription).

Triaminicol Multi-Symptom Cold (Sandoz). Each tablet contains dextromethorphan hydrobromide 10 mg, chlorpheniramine maleate 2 mg, and phenylpropanolamine hydrochloride 12.5 mg (nonprescription).

Triaminicol Multi-Symptom Relief (Sandoz). Each 5 ml of liquid contains dextromethorphan hydrobromide 5 mg, phenylpropanolamine hydrochloride 6.25 mg, and chlorpheniramine maleate 1 mg (nonprescription).

Tussar DM (Rhone-Poulenc Rorer). Each 5 ml of syrup contains dextromethorphan hydrobromide 15 mg, chlorpheniramine maleate 2 mg, and pseudoephedrine hydrochloride 30 mg (nonprescription).

Tussi-Organidin DM (Wallace). Each 5 ml of liquid contains dextromethorphan hydrobromide 10 mg and iodinated glycerol 30 mg (sugar- and alcohol-free).

Vicks NyQuil Nighttime Cold/Flu Medicine (Procter & Gamble). Each 5 ml of liquid contains dextromethorphan hydrobromide 5 mg, pseudoephedrine hydrochloride 10 mg, doxylamine succinate 1.25 mg, and acetaminophen 167 mg (alcohol 25%) (nonprescription).

Additional Antitussive Mixtures

Rynatuss (Wallace). Each tablet contains carbetapentane tannate 60 mg, chlorpheniramine tannate 5 mg, ephedrine tannate 10 mg, and phenylephrine tannate 10 mg; each 5 ml of pediatric suspension contains carbetapentane tannate 30 mg, chlorpheniramine tannate 4 mg, ephedrine tannate 5 mg, and phenylephrine tannate 5 mg.

Tuss-Ornade (SmithKline Beecham). Each capsule (prolonged-release) contains caramiphen edisylate 40 mg and phenylpropanolamine hydrochloride 75 mg; each 5 ml of liquid contains caramiphen edisylate 6.7 mg and phenylpropanolamine hydrochloride 12.5 mg (alcohol 5%).

Mixtures Containing Guaifenesin or Other Expectorants

(See previous lists for other combination products containing guaifenesin.)

Congess Jr, Congess Sr (Fleming). Each capsule (prolonged-release) contains guaifenesin 125 mg and pseudoephedrine hydrochloride 60 mg (***Congess Jr***) or guaifenesin 250 mg and pseudoephedrine hydrochloride 120 mg (***Congress Sr***).

Entex (Procter & Gamble). Each capsule contains guaifenesin 200 mg, phenylpropanolamine hydrochloride 45 mg, and phenylephrine hydrochloride 5 mg; each 5 ml of liquid contains guaifenesin 100 mg, phenylpropanolamine hydrochloride 20 mg, and phenylephrine hydrochloride 5 mg (alcohol 5%).

Entex LA (Procter & Gamble). Each tablet (prolonged-release) contains guaifenesin 400 mg and phenylpropanolamine hydrochloride 75 mg.

Histalet X (Solvay). Each tablet contains guaifenesin 400 mg and pseudoephedrine hydrochloride 120 mg.

Naldecon-EX (Apothecon). Each 5 ml of pediatric syrup contains guaifenesin 100 mg and phenylpropanolamine hydrochloride 6.25 mg (alcohol 5%); each milliliter of pediatric drops contains guaifenesin 50 mg and phenylpropanolamine hydrochloride 6.25 mg (alcohol 0.6%) (both forms sugar-free, nonprescription).

Robitussin-PE (Robins). Each 5 ml of syrup contains guaifenesin 100 mg and pseudoephedrine hydrochloride 30 mg (alcohol 1.4%) (nonprescription).

Ru-Tuss DE (Boots). Each prolonged-release tablet contains guaifenesin 600 mg and pseudoephedrine hydrochloride 120 mg.

Triaminic Expectorant (Sandoz). Each 5 ml of liquid contains guaifenesin 50 mg and phenylpropanolamine hydrochloride 6.25 mg (alcohol-free) (nonprescription).

Mixtures Containing Nasal Decongestants

Mixtures combining a nasal decongestant with one or more other drugs are available for intranasal or oral use. Frequently, the added drug is an antihistamine, analgesic, or a second nasal decongestant. Other compounds occasionally present include atropine or other anticholinergic agents, various wetting compounds, and quaternary ammonium salts.

If relief of several respiratory symptoms is sought (eg, in hay fever), the combination of an antihistamine and adrenergic agent may be beneficial. When headache accompanies the nasal congestion, products containing an analgesic and a decongestant may be useful.

If nasal decongestion is the only desired effect, there is no good evidence that any of the available mixtures is more effective than a single-entity drug. Moreover, there is evidence that some of the other agents in the mixture may either be detrimental or do not assist in relieving nasal decongestion and often increase the cost. For example, intranasal antihistamines provide limited added relief of nasal congestion when combined with decongestants. Intranasal mixtures are used and abused widely. Careful comparative evaluation of these mixtures with single-entity decongestants has not been made. Because a mixture containing a nasal decongestant cannot be expected to be more effective than the same quantity of the decongestant drug alone, the use of a mixture for relief of nasal congestion instead of a single-entity drug should be discouraged. Rebound congestion also may occur with use of an intranasal preparation for more than three to five days.

The preparation chosen and the total duration of use must be determined by the physician on the basis of experience and the response of the patient. Since individual tolerance and the tendency to develop chronic mucosal congestion with prolonged use vary among patients, administration of these agents should be regulated on an individual basis.

The following intranasal mixtures are listed for information only. For oral mixtures, see Table 2.

Dristan Nasal (Whitehall). Spray containing phenylephrine hydrochloride 0.5% and pheniramine maleate 0.2% in 15 (regular, menthol, metered pump) and 30 (regular) ml containers (nonprescription).

4-Way Nasal (Bristol-Myers). Spray containing phenylephrine hydrochloride 0.5%, naphazoline hydrochloride 0.05%, and pyrilamine maleate 0.2% in 15 (regular, menthol, metered pump) and 30 (regular, menthol) ml containers (nonprescription).

TABLE 2.
COMPOSITION OF ORAL MIXTURES COMMONLY USED FOR RHINITIS OR THE COMMON COLD

Preparation	Decongestant†	Antihistamine†	Analgesic†
*Actifed (Warner Wellcome): tablets, syrup	pseudoephedrine HCl 60 mg (tablets), 30 mg (syrup)	triprolidine HCl 2.5 mg (tablets), 1.25 mg (syrup)	
*Actifed Allergy Nighttime (Warner Wellcome): caplets (blue)	pseudoephedrine HCl 30 mg	diphenhydramine HCl 25 mg	
*Actifed Plus (Warner Wellcome): tablets	pseudoephedrine HCl 30 mg	triprolidine HCl 1.25 mg	acetaminophen 500 mg
*Actifed Sinus (Warner Wellcome):			
tablets (daytime-white)	pseudoephedrine HCl 30 mg		acetaminophen 500 mg
tablets (nighttime-blue)	pseudoephedrine HCl 30 mg	diphenhydramine HCl 25 mg	acetaminophen 500 mg
*Benadryl Decongestant (Warner Wellcome): elixir, tablets	pseudoephedrine HCl 30 mg (elixir), 60 mg (tablets),	diphenhydramine HCl 12.5 mg (elixir), 25 mg (tablets)	
Brexin LA (Savage): capsules (prolonged-release)	pseudoephedrine HCl 120 mg	chlorpheniramine maleate 8 mg	
*Chlor-Trimeton Decongestant (Schering-Plough): tablets, tablets (prolonged-release)	pseudoephedrine sulfate 60 mg (tablets), 120 mg (prolonged-release) tablets)	chlorpheniramine maleate 4 mg (tablets), 8 mg (prolonged-release tablets)	
Comhist (Roberts): tablets	phenylephrine HCl 10 mg	phenyltoloxamine citrate 25 mg; chlorpheniramine maleate 2 mg	
Comhist LA (Roberts): capsules (prolonged-release)	phenylephrine HCl 20 mg	phenyltoloxamine citrate 50 mg; chlorpheniramine maleate 4 mg	

**Nonprescription*
†Per 5 ml of liquid (except drops)

(table continued on next page)

TABLE 2 (continued)

Preparation	Decongestant†	Antihistamine†	Analgesic†
***Comtrex Allergy-Sinus (Bristol-Myers): capsules, tablets**	**pseudoephedrine HCl 30 mg**	**chlorpheniramine maleate 2 mg**	**acetaminophen 500 mg**
*Contac 12 Hours (SmithKline Beecham): capsules (prolonged-release)	phenylpropanolamine HCl 75 mg	chlorpheniramine maleate 8 mg	
*Coricidin (Schering-Plough): tablets		chlorpheniramine maleate 2 mg	acetaminophen 325 mg
*Coricidin D (Schering-Plough): tablets	phenylpropanolamine HCl 12.5 mg	chlorpheniramine maleate 2 mg	acetaminophen 325 mg
*Coricidin Demilets (Schering-Plough): tablets	phenylpropanolamine HCl 6.25 mg	chlorpheniramine maleate 1 mg	acetaminophen 80 mg
*Coricidin Maximum Strength Sinus Headache (Schering-Plough): tablets	phenylpropanolamine HCl 12.5 mg	chlorpheniramine maleate 2 mg	acetaminophen 500 mg
Deconamine (Kenwood): tablets, syrup, capsules (prolonged-release) [Deconamine SR]	pseudoephedrine HCl 60 mg (tablets), 30 mg (syrup), 120 mg (capsules)	chlorpheniramine maleate 4 mg (tablets), 2 mg (syrup), 8 mg (capsules)	
*Dehist (Forest): capsules (prolonged-release)	phenylpropanolamine HCl 75 mg	chlorpheniramine maleate 8 mg	
*Demazin (Schering-Plough): tablets (prolonged-release), syrup	phenylpropanolamine HCl 25 mg (tablets), 12.5 mg (syrup)	chlorpheniramine maleate 4 mg (tablets), 2 mg (syrup)	
*Dimetane Decongestant (Robins): capsules, elixir	phenylephrine HCl 10 mg (capsules), 5 mg (elixir)	brompheniramine maleate 4 mg (capsules), 2 mg (elixir)	
*Dimetapp (Robins): elixir, tablets, tablets (prolonged-release)	phenylpropanolamine HCl 12.5 mg (elixir), 25 mg (tablets), 75 mg (prolonged-release tablets)	brompheniramine maleate 2 mg (elixir), 4 mg (tablets), 12 mg (prolonged-release tablets)	
*Disophrol (Schering-Plough): tablets, tablets (prolonged-release)	pseudoephedrine sulfate 60 mg (tablets), 120 mg (prolonged-release tablets)	dexbrompheniramine maleate 2 mg (tablets), 6 mg (prolonged-release tablets)	
*Dristan Cold No Drowsiness Formula (Whitehall): tablets	phenylephrine HCl 5 mg	chlorpheniramine maleate 2 mg	acetaminophen 325 mg

*Nonprescription
†Per 5 ml of liquid (except drops)

(table continued on next page)

TABLE 2 (continued)

Preparation	Decongestant†	Antihistamine†	Analgesic†
*Drixoral Cold and Allergy (Schering-Plough): syrup, tablets (prolonged-release)	pseudoephedrine sulfate 30 mg (syrup), 120 mg (tablets)	brompheniramine maleate 2 mg (syrup); dexbrompheniramine maleate 6 mg (tablets)	
*Drixoral Cold and Flu (Schering-Plough): tablets (prolonged-release)	pseudoephedrine sulfate 60 mg	dexbrompheniramine maleate 3 mg	acetaminophen 500 mg
Entex (Procter & Gamble): capsules, liquid, tablets (prolonged-release) [Entex LA]	phenylephrine HCl 5 mg (capsules, liquid); phenylpropanolamine HCl 45 mg (capsules), 20 mg (liquid), 75 mg (prolonged-release tablets)	guaifenesin 200 mg (capsules), 100 mg (liquid), 400 mg (prolonged-release tablets)	
Histalet (Solvay): syrup	pseudoephedrine HCl 45 mg	chlorpheniramine maleate 3 mg	
Histalet Forte (Solvay): tablets	phenylpropanolamine HCl 50 mg; phenylephrine HCl 10 mg	chlorpheniramine maleate 4 mg; pyrilamine maleate 25 mg	
*Isoclor (CIBA): tablets, liquid, capsules (prolonged-release)	pseudoephedrine HCl 60 mg (tablets), 30 mg (liquid); phenylpropanolamine HCl 120 mg (capsules)	chlorpheniramine maleate 4 mg (tablets), 2 mg (liquid), 8 mg (capsules)	
Naldecon (Apothecon): syrup, tablets (prolonged-release)	phenylpropanolamine HCl 20 mg (syrup), 40 mg (tablets); phenylephrine HCl 5 mg (syrup), 10 mg (tablets)	phenyltoloxamine citrate 7.5 mg (syrup), 15 mg (tablets); chlorpheniramine maleate 2.5 mg (syrup), 5 mg (tablets)	
Naldecon Pediatric (Apothecon): syrup, oral drops	phenylpropanolamine HCl 5 mg (syrup), 5 mg/ml (drops); phenylephrine HCl 1.25 mg (syrup), 1.25 mg/ml (drops)	phenyltoloxamine citrate 2 mg (syrup), 2 mg/ml (drops); chlorpheniramine maleate 0.5 mg (syrup), 0.5 mg/ml (drops)	
Nolamine (Carnrick): tablets (prolonged-release)	phenylpropanolamine HCl 50 mg	chlorpheniramine maleate 4 mg; phenindamine tartrate 24 mg	
Novafed A (Marion Merrell Dow): capsules (prolonged-release)	pseudoephedrine HCl 120 mg	chlorpheniramine maleate 8 mg	
Ornade (SmithKline Beecham): capsules (prolonged-release)	phenylpropanolamine HCl 75 mg	chlorpheniramine maleate 12 mg	

**Nonprescription*
†Per 5 ml of liquid (except drops)

(table continued on next page)

TABLE 2 (continued)

Preparation	Decongestant†	Antihistamine†	Analgesic†
Phenergan VC (Wyeth-Ayerst): syrup	phenylephrine HCl 5 mg	promethazine HCl 6.25 mg	
*Pyrroxate (Roberts): capsules	phenylpropanolamine HCl 25 mg	chlorpheniramine maleate 4 mg	acetaminophen 650 mg
Rondec (Ross): oral drops, syrup, tablets, tablets (prolonged-release) [Rondec-TR]	pseudoephedrine HCl 25 mg/ml (oral drops), 60 mg (syrup, tablets), 120 mg (prolonged-release tablets)	carbinoxamine maleate 2 mg/ml (oral drops), 4 mg (syrup, tablets), 8 mg (prolonged-release tablets)	
*Ru-Tuss (Boots): liquid	phenylephrine HCl 5 mg	chlorpheniramine maleate 2 mg	
Ru-Tuss II (Boots): capsules (prolonged-release)	phenylpropanolamine HCl 75 mg	chlorpheniramine maleate 12 mg	
Rynatan (Wallace): tablets, pediatric suspension [Rynatan-S]	phenylephrine tannate 25 mg (tablets), 5 mg (suspension)	chlorpheniramine tannate 8 mg (tablets), 2 mg (suspension); pyrilamine tannate 25 mg (tablets), 12.5 mg (suspension)	
Seldane-D (Marion Merrell Dow): tablets (prolonged-release)	pseudoephedrine HCl 120 mg	terfenadine 60 mg	
Semprex-D (Warner Wellcome): capsules	pseudoephedrine HCl 60 mg	acrivastine 8 mg	
*Singlet (SmithKline Beecham): tablets	pseudoephedrine HCl 60 mg	chlorpheniramine maleate 4 mg	acetaminophen 650 mg
*Sinulin (Carnrick): tablets	phenylpropanolamine HCl 25 mg	chlorpheniramine maleate 4 mg	acetaminophen 650 mg
*Sinutab Sinus Allergy (Warner Wellcome): caplets, tablets	pseudoephedrine HCl 30 mg	chlorpheniramine maleate 2 mg	acetaminophen 500 mg
*Sinutab Sinus Medication Without Drowsiness (Warner Wellcome): tablets (regular strength); caplets, tablets (maximum strength)	pseudoephedrine HCl 30 mg		acetaminophen 325 mg (regular strength); 500 mg (maximum strength)

Nonprescription
†Per 5 ml of liquid (except drops)
(table continued on next page)

TABLE 2 (continued)

Preparation	Decongestant†	Antihistamine†	Analgesic†
*Sudafed Plus (Warner Wellcome): tablets, liquid	pseudoephedrine HCl 60 mg (tablets), 30 mg (liquid)	chlorpheniramine maleate 4 mg (tablets), 2 mg (liquid)	
*Sudafed Sinus (Warner Wellcome): tablets, caplets	pseudoephedrine HCl 30 mg		acetaminophen 500 mg
*Tavist-D (Sandoz): tablets (prolonged-release)	phenylpropanolamine HCl 75 mg	clemastine fumarate 1.34 mg	
*Triaminic (Sandoz): cold tablets, tablets (chewable), syrup	phenylpropanolamine HCl 12.5 mg (cold tablets), 6.25 mg (chewable tablets), 6.25 mg (syrup)	chlorpheniramine maleate 2 mg (cold tablets), 0.5 mg (chewable tablets), 1 mg (syrup)	
*Triaminic-12 (Sandoz): tablets (prolonged-release)	phenylpropanolamine HCl 75 mg	chlorpheniramine maleate 12 mg	
*Triaminic Allergy (Sandoz): tablets	phenylpropanolamine HCl 25 mg	chlorpheniramine maleate 4 mg	
Trinalin (Key): tablets (prolonged-release)	pseudoephedrine sulfate 120 mg	azatadine maleate 1 mg	
*Tylenol Cold (Children's) (McNeil): tablets (chewable), liquid	pseudoephedrine HCl 7.5 mg (tablets), 15 mg (liquid)	chlorpheniramine maleate 0.5 mg (tablets), 1 mg (liquid)	acetaminophen 80 mg (tablets), 160 mg (liquid)
*Ursinus (Sandoz): tablets	pseudoephedrine HCl 30 mg		aspirin 325 mg

**Nonprescription*
†Per 5 ml of liquid (except drops)

Cited References

Carter-Wallace's Organidin should remain on market while FDA reviews efficacy data, advisory cmte. says; 'Dear doctor' letter on carcinogenicity recommended. *FDC Reports* 5-6, (March) 1992 A.

OTC dextromethorphan label warning will be proposed by FDA, CDer's Meyer says; Over-the-counter drug ADR reports would be required under Rep. Wyden proposal. *FDC Reports* 12-13, (May) 1992 B.

Carter Wallace assures clients of continued Organidin supply. *FDC Reports* 2-3, (May 3) 1993.

Cromolyn sodium nasal spray for hay fever. *Med Lett Drugs Ther* 25:89-90, 1983.

Decongestant-antihistamine judged ineffective in secretory otitis. *Pediatr Alert* 8:13-14, (Feb 17) 1983.

Don't use zinc long term. *Pharm J* 239:210, 1987.

Iodinated glycerol withdrawn because of cancer concerns. *Dickinson's FDA* (May) 1993.

Oral cold remedies. *Med Lett Drugs Ther* 17:89-92, 1975.

Problems with nasal decongestants. *Health Gazette* 15, (Feb) 1992.

Aldis WL: Cromolyn for cough due to angiotensin-converting enzyme inhibitor therapy: Preliminary observations. *Chest* 100:1741-1742, 1991.

Al-Nakib W, et al: Suppression of colds in human volunteers challenged with rhinovirus by a new synthetic drug (R61837). *Antimicrob Agents Chemother* 33:522-525, 1989.

Barnes DJ: Sodium cromoglycate for ACE inhibitor cough. *Med J Aust* 156:671, 1992.

Baroody FM, et al: Ipratropium bromide (Atrovent nasal spray) reduces the nasal response to methacholine. *J Allergy Clin Immunol* 89:1065-1075, 1992.

Bernstein JA: Allergic rhinitis: Helping patients lead an unrestricted life. *PostGrad Med* 93:124-132, (May) 1993.

Bhambhani K, et al: Acute otitis media in children: Are decongestants or antihistamines necessary? *Ann Emerg Med* 12:13-16, 1983.

Blackburn GL, et al: Determinants of the pressor effect of phenylpropanolamine in healthy subjects. *JAMA* 261:3267-3272, 1989.

Borum P: Nasal disorders and anticholinergic therapy. *Postgrad Med J* 63(suppl 1): 61-68, 1987.

Bousquet J, et al: Prevention of pollen rhinitis symptoms: Comparison of fluticasone propionate aqueous nasal spray and disodium cromoglycate aqueous nasal spray: A multicenter, double-blind, double-dummy parallel group study. *Allergy* 48:327-333, 1993.

Brogden RN, et al: Beclomethasone dipropionate: Reappraisal of its pharmacodynamic properties and therapeutic efficacy after decade of use in asthma and rhinitis. *Drugs* 28:99-126, 1984.

Brown NJ, et al: A pharmacodynamic interaction between caffeine and phenylpropanolamine. *Clin Pharmacol Ther* 50:363-371, 1991.

Bryson HM, Faulds D: Intranasal fluticasone propionate: A review of its pharmacodynamic and pharmacokinetic properties, and therapeutic potential in allergic rhinitis. *Drugs* 43:760-775, 1992.

Busse WW: Chronic rhinitis: Systematic approach to diagnosis and management. *Postgrad Med* 73:325-335, (Feb) 1983.

Cantekin EI, et al: Lack of efficacy of decongestant-antihistamine combination for otitis media with effusion ("secretory" otitis media) in children. *N Engl J Med* 308:297-301, 1983.

Cecchin A: The emergence of new clinical clues may bring us closer to a cure for the common cold. *Med World News* 30-42, (March) 1993.

Chan CYJ, Wallander KA: Diphenhydramine toxicity in three children with varicella-zoster infection. *DICP* 25:130-132, (Feb) 1991.

Clissold SP, Heel RC: Budesonide: Preliminary review of its pharmacodynamic properties and therapeutic efficacy in asthma and rhinitis. *Drugs* 28:485-518, 1984.

Cohen S, et al: Psychological stress and susceptibility to the common cold. *N Engl J Med* 325:606-612, 1991.

Committee on Drugs, American Academy of Pediatrics: Adverse reactions to iodide therapy of asthma and other pulmonary diseases. *Pediatrics* 57:272-274, 1976.

Corren J, et al: Nasal beclomethasone prevents the seasonal increase in bronchial responsiveness in patients with allergic rhinitis and asthma. *J Allergy Clin Immunol* 90:250-256, 1992.

Crawford LV, Cohen RM: Therapy for allergic rhinitis: *Compr Ther* 11:60-69, (June) 1985.

Dales R, et al: Chronic cough responsive to ibuprofen. *Pharmacotherapy* 12:331-333, 1992.

Day JH, et al: Efficacy and safety of intranasal budesonide in the treatment of perennial rhinitis in adults and children. *Ann Allergy* 64:445-450, 1990.

Dechant KL, Goa KL: Levocabastine: A review of its pharmacological properties and therapeutic potential as a topical antihistamine in allergic rhinitis and conjunctivitis. *Drugs* 41:202-224, 1991.

deShazo RD, Smith DL (eds): Primer on allergic and immunologic diseases—Third edition. *JAMA* 268:2785-3026, 1992.

Dick EC, et al: Interruption of transmission of rhinovirus colds among human volunteers using virucidal paper handkerchiefs. *J Infect Dis* 153:352-356, 1986.

Dick EC, et al: Aerosol transmission of rhinovirus colds. *J Infect Dis* 156:442-448, 1987.

Dockhorn R, et al: A double-blind, placebo-controlled study of the safety and efficacy of ipratropium bromide nasal spray versus placebo in patients with the common cold. *J Allergy Clin Immunol* 90:1076-1082, 1992.

Dolovich J, et al: Control of hypersecretion of vasomotor rhinitis by topical ipratropium bromide. *J Allergy Clin Immunol* 80:274-278, 1987.

Donnelly A, Casale TB: Nedocromil sodium is rapidly effective in the therapy of seasonal allergic rhinitis. *J Allergy Clin Immunol* 91:997-1004, 1993.

Douglas RG Jr: Common cold: Relief at last. *N Engl J Med* 314:114-115, 1986.

Douglas RM, et al: Prophylactic efficacy of intranasal alpha-$_2$-interferon against rhinovirus infections in the family setting. *N Engl J Med* 314:65-70, 1986.

Douglas RM, et al: Failure of effervescent zinc acetate lozenges to alter the course of upper respiratory tract infections in Australian adults. *Antimicrob Agents Chemother* 31:1263-1265, 1987.

Druce HM, Kaliner MA: Allergic rhinitis. *JAMA* 259:260-263, 1988.

Druce HM, et al: Multicenter placebo-controlled study of nedocromil sodium 1% nasal solution in ragweed seasonal allergic rhinitis. *Ann Allergy* 65:212-216, (Sept) 1990.

Druce HM, et al: Double-blind study of intranasal ipratropium bromide in nonallergic perennial rhinitis. *Ann Allergy* 69:53-60, (July) 1992.

Dushay ME, Johnson CE: Management of allergic rhinitis: Focus on intranasal agents. *Pharmacotherapy* 9:338-350, 1989.

Eby GA, et al: Reduction in duration of common colds by zinc gluconate lozenges in double-blind study. *Antimicrob Agents Chemother* 25:20-24, 1984.

Evans PD, et al: Minor infection, minor life events and the four day desirability dip. *J Psychosom Res* 32:533-539, 1988.

Farr BM, et al: Two randomized controlled trials of virucidal nasal tissues in the prevention of natural upper respiratory infections. *Am J Epidemiol* 128:1162-1172, 1988.

Fitzgerald JM, et al: Chronic cough and gastroesophageal reflux. *Can Med Assoc J* 140:520-524, 1989.

Fogari R, et al: Indomethacin or nifedipine for cough induced by captopril therapy. *J Cardiovasc Pharmacol* 19:670-673, 1992.

Forstall GJ, et al: Effect of inhaling heated vapor on symptoms of the common cold. *JAMA* 271:1109-1111, 1994.

Funderburk FR, et al: Untangling a safety controversy: Pressor effects of phenylpropanolamine. *J Clin Res Drug Dev* 7:3-15, 1993.

Gadomski A, Horton L: The need for rational therapeutics in the use of cough and cold medicine in infants, commentary. *Pediatrics* 89:774-776, 1992.

Gaffey MJ, et al: Intranasally and orally administered antihistamine treatment of experimental rhinovirus colds. *Am Rev Respir Dis* 136:556-560, 1987.

Galina MD, et al: Iodides during pregnancy: Apparent cause of neonatal death. *N Engl J Med* 267:1124, 1962.

Gerrity TR, et al: Effect of aspirin on lung mucociliary clearance. *N Engl J Med* 308:139-141, 1983.

Goldszer RC, et al: Prevalence of cough during angiotensin-converting enzyme inhibitor therapy. *Am J Med* 85:887, 1988.

Grant SM, et al: Ketotifen: A review of its pharmacodynamic and pharmacokinetic properties, and therapeutic use in asthma and allergic disorders. *Drugs* 40:412-448, 1990.

Gwaltney JM: Combined antiviral and antimediator treatment of rhinovirus colds. *J Infect Dis* 166:776-782, 1992.

Hartley TF, et al: Efficacy and tolerance of fluocortin butyl administered twice daily in adult patients with perennial rhinitis. *J Allergy Clin Immunol* 75:501-507, 1985.

Hayden FG, Gwaltney JM: Prophylactic activity of enviroxime against experimentally induced rhinovirus type 39 infection. *Antimicrob Agents Chemother* 21:892-897, 1982.

Hayden FG, Gwaltney JM: Intranasal interferon alpha 2 for prevention of rhinovirus infection. *J Infect Dis* 148:543-540, 1983.

Hayden FG, et al: Prevention of natural colds by contact prophylaxis with intranasal alpha$_2$-interferon. *N Engl J Med* 314:71-75, 1986.

Hayden FG, et al: Modification of experimental rhinovirus colds by receptor blockade. *Antiviral Res* 9:233-247, 1988.

Hendley JO, Gwaltney JM Jr: Mechanisms of transmission of rhinovirus infections. *Epidemiol Rev* 10:242-258, 1988.

Hendley JO, et al: Effect of inhalation of hot humidified air on experimental rhinovirus infection. *JAMA* 271:1112-1113, 1994.

Higgins PG, et al: Recombinant human interferon-gamma as prophylaxis against rhinovirus colds in volunteers. *J Interferon Res* 8:591-596, 1988.

Holmes PW, et al: Chronic persistent cough: Use of ipratropium bromide in undiagnosed cases following upper respiratory tract infection. *Respir Med* 36:425-429, 1992.

Horak F: Seasonal allergic rhinitis: Newer treatment approaches. *Drugs* 45:518-527, 1993.

Hutton N, et al: Effectiveness of an antihistamine-decongestant combination for young children with the common cold: A randomized, controlled clinical trial. *J Pediatr* 118:125-130, 1991.

Irwin RS, Curley FJ: The diagnosis of chronic cough. *Hosp Pract* 82-89, (Nov) 1988.

Irwin RS, Curley FJ: Anatomic diagnostic workup of chronic cough not all that it is hacked up to be. *Chest* 95:711-713, 1989.

Irwin RS, Curley FJ: The treatment of cough: A comprehensive review. *Chest* 99:1477-1484, 1991.

Irwin RS, et al: Chronic cough: The spectrum and frequency of causes, key components of the diagnostic evaluation, and outcome of specific therapy. *Am Rev Respir Dis* 141:640-647, 1990.

Irwin RS, et al: Appropriate use of antitussives and protussives: A practical review. *Drugs* 46:80-91, 1993.

Johnson D, Osborn LM: Cough variant asthma: A review of the clinical literature. *J Asthma* 28:85-90, 1991.

Johnston SL, et al: Respiratory pathophysiologic responses: The effect of local hyperthermia on allergen-induced nasal congestion and mediator release. *J Allergy Clin Immunol* 92:850-856, 1993.

Jones AS, Lancer JM: Vasomotor rhinitis. *BMJ* 294:1505-1506, 1987.

Keogh A: Sodium cromoglycate prophylaxis for angiotensin-converting enzyme inhibitor cough, letter. *Lancet* 341:560, 1993.

Kirkegaard J, et al: Ordinary and high-dose ipratropium in perennial nonallergic rhinitis. *J Allergy Clin Immunol* 79:585-590, 1987.

Kroenke K, et al: The safety of phenylpropanolamine in patients with stable hypertension. *Ann Intern Med* 111:1043-1044, 1989.

Lake CR, et al: Phenylpropanolamine increases plasma caffeine levels. *Clin Pharmacol Ther* 47:675-685, 1990.

Lampert RP, et al: Critical look at oral decongestants. *Pediatrics* 55:550-552, 1974.

Lavigne JV, et al: Behavioral management of psychogenic cough: Alternative to the 'bedsheet' and other aversive techniques. *Pediatrics* 87:532-537, 1991.

Lea P: Double-blind controlled evaluation of nasal decongestant effect of Day Nurse in the common cold. *J Int Med Res* 12:124-127, 1984.

Leclercq-Foucart J, et al: Double-blind trial comparing astemizole and ketotifen in suppression of hay fever symptoms. *Curr Ther Res* 39:875-883, 1986.

Levandowski RA, et al: Topical enviroxime against rhinovirus infection. *Antimicrob Agents Chemother* 22:1004-1007, 1982.

Levin RM, et al: Group A streptococcal infection in children younger than three years of age. *Pediatr Infect Dis J* 7:581-587, 1988.

Lichtenstein LM: The nasal late-phase response: An in vivo model. *Hosp Pract* 119-142, (Jan) 1988.

Lieberman P: Rhinitis, allergic and nonallergic. *Hosp Pract* 117-145, (June) 1988.

Lindsay-Miller ACM, Chambers A: Group comparative trial of cromolyn sodium and terfenadine in treatment of seasonal allergic rhinitis. *Ann Allergy* 58:28-32, 1987.

Longini IM, Monto AS: Efficacy of virucidal nasal tissues in interrupting familial transmission of respiratory agents. *Am J Epidemiol* 128:639-644, 1988.

Lowenstein SR, Parrino TA: Management of common cold. *Adv Intern Med* 32:207-234, 1987.

Luks D, Anderson M: Over-the-counter cold remedies, letter. *JAMA* 270:1812, 1993.

Mabry RL: Corticosteroids in management of allergic rhinitis. *South Med J* 76:487-489, 1983.

Mabry RL: Topical pharmacotherapy for allergic rhinitis: New agents. *South Med J* 85:149-154, (Feb) 1992.

Macknin ML, et al: Effect of inhaling heated vapor on symptoms of the common cold. *JAMA* 264:989-991, 1990.

Macnaughton MR: Structure and replication of rhinoviruses. *Curr Top Microbiol Immunol* 97:1-26, 1982.

McTavish D, Sorkin EM: Azelastine: A review of its pharmacodynamic and pharmacokinetic properties, and therapeutic potential. *Drugs* 38:778-800, 1989.

Medon PJ, Holshouser MH: Self-medication: Antitussives. *Pharmacy Times* 80-90, (Jan) 1985.

Meltzer EO: To use or not to use antihistamines in patients with asthma, editorial. *Ann Allergy* 64:183-185, 1990.

Meltzer EO, et al: Chronic rhinitis in infants and children: Etiologic, diagnostic, and therapeutic considerations. *Pediatr Clin North Am* 30:847-871, 1983.

Meltzer EO, et al: Ipratropium bromide aqueous nasal spray for patients with perennial allergic rhinitis: A study of its effect on their symptoms, quality of life, and nasal cytology. *J Allergy Clin Immunol* 90:242-249, 1992.

Mikaelian AJ: Vasomotor rhinitis. *Ear Nose Throat J* 68:207-218, 1989.

Mills J: Viral URIs: How to fight back. *Mod Med* 88-97, (Nov) 1983.

Mills J: Common cold: Old and new facts to help your patient cope. *Mod Med* 52, (Dec) 1986.

Monto AS: The common cold: Cold water on hot news, editorial. *JAMA* 271:1122-1124, 1994.

Monto AS, et al: Ineffectiveness of postexposure prophylaxis of rhinovirus infection with low-dose intranasal alpha 2b interferon in families. *Antimicrob Agents Chemother* 33:387-390, 1989.

Mullarkey MF: Eosinophilic nonallergic rhinitis. *J Allergy Clin Immunol* 82:941-949, 1988.

Mygind N: Glucocorticosteroids and rhinitis. *Allergy* 48:476-490, 1993.

Naclerio RM: Allergic rhinitis. *N Engl J Med* 325:860-869, 1991.

Naclerio RM, et al: Inflammatory mediators in late antigen-induced rhinitis. *N Engl J Med* 313:65-70, 1985.

Norman PS: Review of nasal therapy: Update. *Allergy Clin Immunol* 72:421-432, 1983.

O'Connell MB, Gross CR: The effect of multiple doses of phenylpropanolamine on the blood pressure of patients whose hypertension was controlled with β blockers. *Pharmacotherapy* 11:376-381, 1991.

O'Connell EJ, et al: Cough-type asthma: A review. *Ann Allergy* 66:278-285, (April) 1991.

Ophir D, Elad Y: Effects of steam inhalation on nasal patency and nasal symptoms in patients with the common cold. *Am J Otolaryngol* 3:149-153, 1987.

Ophir D, et al: Effects of inhaled humidified warm air on nasal patency and nasal symptoms in allergic rhinitis. *Ann Allergy* 60:239-242, 1988.

Oppenheimer J, et al: Double-blind trial of a heated nasal aerosol in the treatment of perennial allergic rhinitis. *J Allergy Clin Immunol* 92:56-60, 1993.

Orgel HA, et al: Clinical, rhinomanometric and cytologic evaluation of seasonal allergic rhinitis treated with beclomethasone dipropionate as aqueous nasal spray or pressurized aerosol. *J Allergy Clin Immunol* 77:858-864, 1986.

Orgel HA, et al: Intranasal fluocortin butyl in patients with perennial rhinitis: A 12-month efficacy and safety study including nasal biopsy. *J Allergy Clin Immunol* 88:257-264, 1991.

Palma-Carlos AG, et al: Double-blind comparison of levocabastine nasal spray with sodium cromoglycate nasal spray in the treatment of seasonal allergic rhinitis. *Ann Allergy* 67:394-398, 1991.

Pelikan Z, et al: Effects of oral cromolyn on the nasal response due to foods. *Arch Otolaryngol Head Neck Surg* 115:1238-1243, 1989.

Petrulis AS, et al: Effect of phenylpropanolamine and brompheniramine on blood pressure. *J Gen Intern Med* 6:503-506, 1991.

Petty TL: The National Mucolytic Study: Results of a randomized, double-blind, placebo-controlled study of iodinated glycerol in chronic obstructive bronchitis. *Chest* 97:75-83, 1990.

Phelan MJ: Prevention and treatment of hay fever. *Pharmaceut J* 232:711-712, (June) 1984.

Phillpotts RJ, et al: Therapeutic activity of enviroxime against rhinovirus infection. *Antimicrob Agents Chemother* 23:671-675, 1983.

Pipkorn U, et al: Topical nasal glucocorticoid pretreatment inhibits symptoms and mediator release during the early, late and rechallenge response to nasal challenge with antigen. *N Engl J Med* 316:1506-1510, 1987.

Potter YJ, Hart LL: DIAS Rounds: Drug Information Analysis Service: Zinc lozenges for treatment of common colds. *Ann Pharmacother* 27:589-592, 1993.

Proctor DF, Anderson I (eds): *The Nose, Upper Airway Physiology and the Atmospheric Environment.* Amsterdam, Elsevier Biomedical Press, 1982.

Puder KS, Morgan JP: Persuading by citation: Analysis of references of 53 published reports of phenylpropanolamine's clinical toxicity. *Clin Pharmacol Ther* 42:1-9, 1987.

Rafferty P, et al: The inhibitory actions of azelastine hydrochloride on the early and late bronchoconstrictor responses to inhaled allergen in atopic asthma. *J Allergy Clin Immunol* 84:649-657, 1989.

Rombaut N, et al: Effects of topical administration of levocabastine on psychomotor and cognitive function. *Ann Allergy* 67:75-79, 1991.

Ross JRM, et al: Budesonide once-daily in seasonal allergic rhinitis. *Curr Med Res Opin* 12:507-515, 1991.

Samo TC, et al: Efficacy and tolerance of intranasally applied recombinant leukocyte A interferon in normal volunteers. *J Infect Dis* 148:535-542, 1983.

Sands CD, et al: Effect of phenylpropanolamine hydrochloride on blood pressure in Korean patients with hypertension controlled by hydrochlorothiazide. *Clin Pharm* 11:168-173, 1992.

Schata M, et al: Levocabastine nasal spray better than sodium cromoglycate and placebo in the topical treatment of seasonal allergic rhinitis. *J Allergy Clin Immunol* 87:873-878, 1991.

Schatz M, et al: Course and management of asthma and allergic diseases during pregnancy, in Middleton E Jr, et al (eds): *Allergy Principles and Practice,* ed 3. St Louis, CV Mosby, 1988, 1093-1155.

Schneider SM, et al: Dextromethorphan poisoning reversed by naloxone. *Am J Emerg Med* 9:237-238, 1991.

Schuller DE, et al: A multicenter trial of nedocromil sodium, 1% nasal solution, compared with cromolyn sodium and placebo in ragweed seasonal allergic rhinitis. *J Allergy Clin Immunol* 86:554-561, 1990.

Sebastian JL, et al: Angiotensin-converting enzyme inhibitors and cough: Prevalence in an outpatient medical clinic population. *Chest* 99:36-39, 1991.

Sedgwick JB, et al: Immediate and late airway response of allergic rhinitis patients to segmental antigen challenge: Characterization of eosinophil and mast cell mediators. *Am Rev Respir Dis* 144:1274-1281, 1991.

Shim C, et al: Lack of effect of hydration on sputum production in chronic bronchitis. *Chest* 92:679-682, 1987.

Simon SR, et al: Cough and ACE inhibitors. *Arch Intern Med* 152:1698-1700, 1992.

Simons FER: Chronic rhinitis. *Pediatr Clin North Am* 31:801-819, 1984.

Simons FER, Simons KJ: Optimum pharmacological management of chronic rhinitis. *Drugs* 38:313-331, 1989.

Smith MBH, Feldman W: Over-the-counter cold medications: A critical review of clinical trials between 1950 and 1991. *JAMA* 269:2258-2263, 1993.

Smith TJ, et al: Site of attachment in human rhinovirus 14 for antiviral agents that inhibit uncoating. *Science* 233:1286-1293, 1986.

Snyder RD, Snyder LB: Intranasal cocaine abuse in allergists office. *Ann Allergy* 54:489-492, 1985.

Spector S, et al: Multicenter, double-blind, placebo-controlled trial of triamcinolone acetonide nasal aerosol in the treatment of perennial allergic rhinitis. *Ann Allergy* 64:300-305, 1990.

Sperber SJ, Hayden FG: Chemotherapy of rhinovirus colds. *Antimicrob Agents Chemother* 32:409-419, 1988.

Sperber SJ, et al: Ineffectiveness of recombinant human interferon-β_{serine} nasal drops for prophylaxis of natural colds. *J Infect Dis* 160:700-705, 1989.

Stanley ED, et al: Increased shedding with aspirin treatment of rhinovirus infection. *JAMA* 231:1248-1251, 1975.

Storms W, et al: Once-daily triamcinolone acetonide nasal spray is effective for the treatment of perennial allergic rhinitis. *Ann Allergy* 66:329-334, (April) 1991.

Tinkelman D, et al: Multicenter evaluation of triamcinolone acetonide nasal aerosol in the treatment of adult patients with seasonal allergic rhinitis. *Ann Allergy* 64:234-240, 1990.

Togias AG, et al: *In vivo* and *in vitro* effects of antihistamines on mast cell mediator release: A potentially important property in the treatment of allergic disease. *Ann Allergy* 63:465-469, 1989.

Tyrrell D, et al: Local hyperthermia benefits natural and experimental common colds. *BMJ* 298:1280-1283, 1989.

Veltri JC, et al: Acute exposure to phenylpropanolamine: An analysis of 5447 cases reported to poison control centers from 1984-1987. *PostMarketing Surveillance* 6:95-106, (Nov) 1992.

Ward NO, Berry DW: Intranasal steroid treatment. *Ariz Med* 41:88-90, 1984.

Welsh PW, et al: Preseasonal IgE ragweed antibody level as predictor of response to therapy of ragweed hayfever with intranasal cromolyn sodium solution. *J Allergy Clin Immunol* 60:104-109, 1977.

Welsh PW, et al: Efficacy of beclomethasone nasal solution, flunisolide, and cromolyn in relieving symptoms of ragweed allergy. *Mayo Clin Proc* 62:125-134, 1987.

West S, et al: Review of antihistamines and the common cold. *Pediatrics* 56:100-107, 1975.

Wood RP: Allergic rhinitis, in Cherniack RM (ed): *Current Therapy of Respiratory Disease, 1984-1985.* Philadelphia/St Louis, Decker/Mosby, 1984, 1-2.

Yerushalmi A, et al: Treatment of perennial allergic rhinitis by local hyperthermia. *Proc Natl Acad Sci USA* 79:4766-4769, 1982.

Zhang Y, et al: Dextromethorphan: Enhancing its systemic availability by way of low-dose quinidine-mediated inhibition of cytochrome P4502D6. *Clin Pharmacol Ther* 51:647-655, 1992.

Other Selected Reference

Establishment of monograph for OTC cold, cough, allergy, bronchodilator, and antiasthmatic products. *Federal Register* 41:38312-38424, (Sept 9) 1976.

Drugs Used in Bronchial Disorders

21

Asthma should be considered to be predominantly an inflammatory disease with associated bronchospasm. The degree of hyperresponsiveness and narrowing of the bronchi produced by stimuli is greater in asthmatic patients than in normal individuals. Persistent inflammation is a primary cause of the increased bronchial hyperresponsiveness. Mucosal edema, mucus plugging, and hypersecretion may be present; pulmonary parenchyma is normal. Airway narrowing may reverse spontaneously or with therapy. Type I (IgE-mediated) immune responses often play an important role in the development of asthma in children and many adults; however, when onset of disease occurs in adulthood, allergic factors may be more difficult to identify or may be absent. Exposure to cold dry air, exercise, upper respiratory infections, and other aggravating factors such as occupational exposure to provocative substances may trigger asthmatic exacerbations.

Emphysema and chronic obstructive bronchitis frequently coexist in what is commonly termed chronic obstructive pulmonary or lung disease (COPD or COLD). In emphysema, the primary pathology is parenchymal; airway collapse results from loss of elasticity and tissue destruction. Clinically, it is difficult to assess the relative contributions of emphysema and chronic bronchitis to airway obstruction. Smoking and other environmental irritants contribute to the etiology of COPD. Response to therapy is partial at best. In some individuals, asthma, emphysema, and chronic bronchitis coexist.

Major advances in the understanding of the pathophysiology of cystic fibrosis now make it possible to develop effective therapy. Investigational studies are underway and are designed to restore genetically deficient enzymes responsible for the disease (gene therapy) as well as to halt disease progression before irreversible lung damage has occurred (administration of alpha$_1$-proteinase inhibitor, recombinant deoxyribonuclease).

Respiratory disorders in premature infants include apnea of prematurity (AP), respiratory distress syndrome (RDS), and bronchopulmonary dysplasia (BPD). BPD appears to occur during therapy in infants with RDS. A relationship exists between the degree of prematurity and the severity of AP and RDS. RDS and BPD also occur in adults.

ASTHMA

The most common symptoms of asthma are cough, breathlessness, and chest tightness; wheezing also is prominent. Reduced pulmonary function typical of obstructive rather than restrictive airway disease is observed. Asymptomatic periods often alternate with paroxysms.

Medical management is directed toward reversing or preventing bronchospasm, inflammation, and edema, as well as eliminating mucus plugs and correcting hypoxemia. Critical for optimal management of asthma are counseling to promote patient understanding, cooperation, and compliance; early intervention at the first sign of an impending exacerbation; and avoiding pulmonary irritants, certain drugs, and allergens. In an acute exacerbation, the severity of symptoms and response to drug therapy vary considerably among patients and even in the same patient. The duration of therapy is guided as much by the patient's response to drug therapy as by the severity of symptoms. During a period of partial remission, the extent of treatment is determined by the symptoms that interfere with daily functions and the results of appropriate pulmonary function tests.

Pathophysiology

Normally the bronchial muscles are chiefly controlled by the autonomic nervous system, and parasympathetic fibers predominate in number and effect. Stimulation of parasympathetic nerves (cholinergic nerve stimulation) causes calcium-dependent constriction of the bronchi. Sympathetic nerves are absent or sparse; animal experiments have shown that, if present, these nerves may promote the local release of norepinephrine with subsequent relaxation. Stimulation of beta$_2$-adrenergic receptors by circulating epinephrine activates adenylate cyclase, an enzyme in the plasma membrane of many cells; this enzyme catalyzes the production of cyclic adenosine monophosphate (cAMP), an intracellular mediator that relaxes bronchial smooth muscle and inhibits certain inflammatory processes.

Stimuli that trigger a bronchospastic response in a susceptible individual include allergens, emotional stress, viral respiratory infections, exercise, exposure to cold air, environmental pollutants, occupational exposure, chemicals, and drugs. Inflammatory mediators and chemotactic factors released by the mast cells and eosinophils contribute to bronchospasm; they play a central role in the pathogenesis of asthma and the resulting airway hyperresponsiveness (bronchial hyperreactivity) is a characteristic of asthma. Mediators include histamine, histamine-releasing factor, interleukins, neutrophil and eosinophil chemotactic factors, platelet activating factor, prostaglandins, and leukotrienes. Other mediators and their exact roles have not yet been identified, but new information suggests that lymphocytes also may be involved in asthma.

Studies on early- and late-phase asthmatic reactions have used allergens as an asthmatic stimulus. The maximal *early-phase asthmatic response* to a stimulus occurs within 10 to 20 minutes after exposure; spontaneous recovery is observed after 60 to 90 minutes. This response is caused directly or indirectly by mast cell mediators. Activation of airway epithelial and mast cells by asthmatic stimuli releases mediators; these may directly cause the airway smooth muscle to contract, increase capillary permeability, and stimulate the release of chemotactic factors that attract inflammatory cells (eg, eosinophils, lymphocytes, neutrophils) to the lung. This early-phase response is largely bronchospastic in nature; inflammatory reactions are less important.

Based on an in vitro laboratory model, the *late-phase asthmatic response* is postulated to be primarily inflammatory and begins three to four hours after exposure to an allergen. It is maximal at four to eight hours and may persist for 12 hours. This response begins with the influx of inflammatory cells (eg, eosinophils, lymphocytes, neutrophils) into the lung. As in the nasal late-phase reaction, basophils may cause release of a second wave of mediator cells that play a similar role in the asthmatic late-phase reaction. Within one to two weeks, infiltration of macrophages, fibroblasts, and other mononuclear cells into the lung is observed; by this time the lung epithelium is significantly damaged.

The bronchial smooth muscle of patients with moderate to severe asthma is hypertrophied, which may enhance the bronchoconstrictor response to a given stimulus. The airway epithelial surface is denuded, and cilia are damaged and reduced in number. Goblet cells increase in number, and the submucosal cells are hyperplastic. Mucus plugs also are present. Inflammatory cells are observed within the bronchial mucosa and in the airway secretions (Beasley et al, 1989 A; Barnes, 1989; Bernstein and Lazarus, 1989). The inflammatory cell most characteristic of asthma is the eosinophil, and the number of eosinophils in the bronchoalveolar lavage fluid and peripheral blood is closely related to the degree of bronchial hyperresponsiveness (Barnes, 1989). The major basic protein that plays a primary role in producing lung tissue damage is derived from eosinophils (Beasley et al, 1989 B). Asthma has been defined by some as chronic desquamative eosinophilic bronchitis.

Since many of the above pathologic and biochemical changes also are observed in asymptomatic patients with mild, stable asthma, it is clear that asthma is an inflammatory disease (Barnes, 1989; Beasley et al, 1989 B). Bronchial hyperresponsiveness (and its enhancement by nonallergenic stimuli) is directly associated with the late-phase response and is a consistent marker of airway inflammation. Available evidence indicates that the degree of increase in responsiveness to nonallergenic stimuli correlates with the extent of airway inflammation and the severity of asthma (Barnes, 1989; Cockroft, 1990 A).

Although bronchospasm may appear to be totally suppressed by bronchodilators, the disease process can progress silently because of inflammatory changes that do not respond to bronchodilators alone and must be controlled by agents with anti-inflammatory effects (Barnes, 1989; Beasley et al, 1989 A, 1989 B; Cockroft, 1990 A; Hargreave et al, 1990).

For further discussion of the etiology and pathophysiology of asthma, see Kaliner et al, 1987; Jenne and Murphy, 1987; Beasley et al, 1989 A, 1989 B; Cockroft, 1990 A; Nelson, 1991; Sears et al, 1991).

Nondrug Management

Patients with asthma must understand the nature of the illness and the effect of each medication and treatment modality. Personal instruction by the physician and simple written directions are helpful. Patients and family members must play an active role in the management of this disease. Noncompliance, lack of understanding of the severity of the disorder, failure to recognize and take appropriate medication to manage early signs of an exacerbation, and delay in seeking help when self-management is inadequate are the primary factors responsible for an asthmatic patient's repeated visits to the emergency care unit (ECU) (Donnelly et al, 1989; Parker et al, 1989; Reed and Hunt, 1990). When these issues are adequately understood and the patient and family members have a clear plan of action to manage an exacerbation, the number of visits to an ECU and the number of hospitalizations decrease significantly (Mayo et al, 1990; Reed and Hunt, 1990).

Psychological support (but not hypnosis) and breathing exercises may be beneficial adjuncts to specific therapy; the value of biofeedback is controversial. Hydration has been considered an important part of management, since adequate intake of fluids may minimize inspissation of bronchial secretions; however, little data are available to support this contention. Overhydration can be harmful, particularly in infants, young children, and the elderly, and should be avoided.

Portable peak flow meters for home use are recommended for patients with moderate or severe disease so that daily physiologic records can be maintained and early signs of deterioration can be detected (Cross and Nelson, 1991). A persistent reduction from the usual reading in peak expiratory flow rate (PEFR) that exceeds 20% to 25% or a sudden worsening of PEFR are signs of serious impending difficulty. A more important indicator of sudden deterioration that requires immediate attention is a change in bronchial lability greater than 20% to 40% between morning and evening readings. However, total dependence must not be placed on measurement of PEFR. In some patients, the PEFR reading may be relatively normal despite other signs (eg, the need for more frequent administration of bronchodilators) of an impending exacerbation (Ferguson, 1988).

In moderately severe, recurrent asthmatic attacks, it is important that infectious and psychological elements be identified in order to develop a complete program of management. Management of any underlying allergic disorder also can be beneficial.

A small percentage of patients develop severe asthmatic reactions to aspirin or other nonsteroidal anti-inflammatory drugs; some physicians instruct asthma patients to avoid these drugs. An aspirin-sensitive individual also should avoid medications and foods containing tartrazine dye. Monosodium glutamate or metabisulfites also may trigger asthma in some patients.

Nonselective beta blockers, such as propranolol, administered systemically or even topically (eye drops) may increase the degree of bronchospasm in an asthmatic patient and should be avoided; if deemed essential, a $beta_1$ cardioselective agent may be used with extreme caution. Respiratory depressants should be avoided during an acute asthmatic attack.

Drug Therapy

GLOBAL TREATMENT. The goals of drug therapy for asthma are prevention of bronchospasm and long-term control of bronchial hyperresponsiveness and inflammation. Because it is usually not possible for either the patient or the physician to predict when bronchospasm may occur, patients with all but the most episodic and/or entirely seasonal attacks must realize that continuous therapy may be necessary. Observation over several months is required before it can be determined that intermittent or seasonal therapy may be sufficient.

Maintenance therapy with currently available bronchodilators is only symptomatic and does not significantly decrease bronchial hyperresponsiveness or affect the primary inflammatory reactions responsible for persistence of asthma. For maintenance, agents that inhibit bronchial hyperresponsiveness and block inflammation as well as the late-phase asthmatic reaction should supplement and/or replace bronchodilators (Barnes, 1989; Cockroft, 1990 B; Cockroft and Hargreave, 1990).

The bronchodilators include beta agonists, which stimulate $beta_2$-adrenergic receptors, increase intracellular cAMP, and may partially inhibit the release of inflammatory mediators; theophylline and other xanthine drugs, which produce bronchodilation through mechanisms that have not yet been determined; and anticholinergic drugs, which may relieve bronchospasm by blocking parasympathetic cholinergic impulses at the receptor level. Antihistamines occasionally prevent or abort mild allergic asthmatic episodes, particularly in children, but they can only be partially effective because histamine is only one of many mediators.

Agents with anti-inflammatory actions include the biscromone, cromolyn sodium [Intal], which prevents the release of mediator substances and blocks respiratory neuronal reflexes, and corticosteroids, which primarily decrease inflammation and edema.

Mild Asthma: In mild asthma, brief episodes of wheezing with or without dyspnea or cough occur; cough may be the predominant symptom in some patients. Episodes may be sporadic or occur daily and are easily controlled by inhalant $beta_2$ selective agonists (albuterol [Ventolin, Proventil]; pirbuterol [Maxair]; terbutaline [Brethaire, Bricanyl]; bitolterol [Tornalate]; metaproterenol [Alupent, Metaprel]). These drugs should be taken prior to exposure to factors that provoke asthma, at the first manifestation of symptoms, or when PEFR lability increases. (Proper use of a metered-dose inhaler is discussed in the section on Drug Selection, Beta Agonists.) Xanthine drugs have a slower onset of action after oral use; thus, they are less helpful for initial management of acute attacks.

If some signs and symptoms persist after treatment of the acute exacerbation, the combined use of an inhaled $beta_2$-adrenergic agonist and an oral theophylline preparation may be indicated. In the cromolyn-responsive patient, cromolyn sodium metered-dose inhaler is as effective as oral theophylline and may be preferable for prophylaxis in compliant patients because of its greater safety (Marks, 1987; Eigen et al, 1987; *Pediatr Alert,* 1987 A). Some physicians now advocate the use of an inhalant corticosteroid for prophylaxis of mild asthma (Juniper et al, 1990; Lorentzson et al, 1990; Haahtela et al, 1991; Reed, 1991; Waalkens et al, 1991) (see the following discussion on moderate asthma). Neither inhalant corticosteroids nor cromolyn should be used for an acute exacerbation.

Moderate Asthma: Patients with moderate asthma experience wheezing and dyspnea, with or without cough and expectoration, that interfere with daily activities and/or sleep. When this pattern is apparent, daily therapy should be instituted.

Several classes of drugs are now being prescribed for moderate asthma. Although a prolonged-release preparation of theophylline has been the primary medication used in the United States for maintenance therapy in these patients, many authorities and the expert panel of the National Education Program of the National Heart, Lung, and Blood Institute (NHLBI) have recommended replacing theophylline with an inhalant corticosteroid (*J Allergy Clin Immunol,* 1991).

Alternatively, for moderate asthma requiring daily therapy, a six-week trial of cromolyn sodium may be prescribed for children and adults. This drug may be as effective as $beta_2$ agonists and theophylline and is safer than these agents or oral steroids for prophylaxis. If cromolyn does not control symptoms, some authorities recommend substituting or adding an inhalant steroid, but data on additive actions are limited.

The greater emphasis on cromolyn and inhalant steroids, agents that significantly reduce bronchial hyperresponsiveness and inhibit late-phase reactions, has occurred in the hope that the inflammatory components of the disease will decrease and progression to severe disease can be halted. Frequent exacerbations suggest that a short course of oral corticosteroids is necessary, but inhalant steroid preparations should be substituted as soon as possible.

Long-acting inhaled $beta_2$ selective agonists also may be useful, especially in compliant patients; inhalations up to a total of 8 to 12/day may be prescribed when control is not achieved with the usual dosage, or theophylline may be added to the regimen. However, the safety of regular daily administration of inhalant $beta_2$ agonists is unresolved. (See the discussion on Drug Selection, Beta-Adrenergic Agonists.)

Nocturnal Asthma: Adequate control of nocturnal symptoms allows patients to sleep, and control during the day may help reduce symptoms at night. Two or more inhalations of a short-acting $beta_2$ agonist at bedtime may be tried (Jenne, 1984). However, their duration of action is short and affords only temporary relief in most patients. Prolonged-release albuterol may control nocturnal symptoms in many patients. The investigational long-acting $beta_2$-adrenergic agonists, salmeterol [Serevent] and formoterol [Foradil], both given twice daily, also have been effective (Fitzpatrick et al, 1990; Brogden and Faulds, 1991; Faulds et al, 1991). Alternatively, a 24-hour prolonged-release preparation of theophylline administered once daily between 6 and 8 PM may be more effective than the 8- or 12-hour preparations in protecting against a significant reduction in the PEFR that occurs between 2 and 4 AM (Fairshter et al, 1985; Arkinstall et al, 1987).

Severe Asthma: Patients with severe asthma often are incapacitated by dyspnea and usually are unable to carry out routine daily activities. These patients usually require oral steroids, often combined with inhalant corticosteroids and other medications, for maintenance to prevent acute episodes.

Acute Asthma: Signs of a potentially *life-threatening acute exacerbation* include a PaO_2 of less than 60 (at sea level) or a $PaCO_2$ of more than 45 (at sea level) with increasing respiratory acidosis; poor air exchange and breath sounds; marked retraction of the accessory muscles of respiration; cyanosis; confusion and mental obtundation; pulsus paradoxus greater than 18 mm Hg; signs of exhaustion; and a forced expiratory volume (FEV_1) <1 L. For further discussion, see Jenne and Murphy, 1987, and Bernstein, 1985 C.

A *severe acute exacerbation* of asthma is usually accompanied by hypoxemia, and oxygen should be administered routinely. A flow rate of 2 to 4 L/minute by nasal cannula usually increases the arterial saturation of oxygen to 90% or greater. To reduce the thick mucus plugs in the airways and sputum viscosity, fluids are often administered intravenously, but it is unclear if this makes a difference. Oral intake may be limited by nausea and vomiting.

Drug therapy for a *moderate to severe acute exacerbation* usually includes a beta agonist; drug delivery by metered-dose inhaler in conventional doses often is inadequate for severe acute attacks, but repeated large doses (two to six times greater than maintenance doses) delivered with a metered-dose inhaler using a spacer may be more effective and avoid the need to use nebulized doses (Lam and Newhouse, 1990). However, delivery with a nebulizer usually is required, with the dose repeated every 20 minutes for at least the first hour. If this therapy is not feasible or is inadequate, two doses of terbutaline or epinephrine may be injected subcutaneously 15 to 30 minutes apart; a third dose of epinephrine occasionally is used. Patients may respond to the injectable formulation even when oral or inhalant beta agonists were ineffective prior to the acute episode (Rossing et al, 1983; Appel et al, 1989). Ipratropium bromide [Atrovent], an anticholinergic drug administered by inhalation (an investigational route), may provide significant additional bronchodilation (Rebuck et al, 1987) if maximally tolerated doses of a $beta_2$ agonist are inadequate.

The value of xanthines for acute asthma has been questioned (Lam and Newhouse, 1990; Newhouse, 1990), but many practitioners continue to advocate the administration of intravenous aminophylline or theophylline with an inhalant beta agonist for severe acute exacerbations, particularly if the beta agonist produces a suboptimal response (Spector, 1991). Although intravenous aminophylline had no effect on objective parameters of pulmonary function when it was used adjunctively for acute exacerbations in one study, the need for hospitalization was reduced threefold in the patients who had received this drug (Wrenn et al, 1991). If these results are confirmed, intravenous xanthines once again may be generally accepted as part of the regimen for acute asthma (McFadden, 1991). When intravenous xanthines are used, therapy is usually continued for 24 to 48 hours after initial improvement has occurred.

It has generally been recommended that if three courses of a nebulized or two courses of a subcutaneous $beta_2$ agonist over one to two hours fail to achieve physiologic improvement, if patients do not respond to bronchodilator therapy within one hour with at least a 10% increase in peak flow (*J Allergy Clin Immunol*, 1991), if the FEV_1 is <1L or the PEFR <100 L, or if the patient has difficulty speaking a complete sentence, intravenous steroids should be administered without waiting for a response to the bronchodilators. Administration of intravenous steroids routinely to high-risk patients is advocated by many physicians, and some authorities recommend that all patients sick enough to seek emergency care should receive intravenous steroids without delay. They must be given early because of their slow onset of action (two to six hours) and time to maximal effects (24 to 96 hours). A fatal outcome is much more likely from inadequate or inappropriate drug treatment than from the adverse effects of the drugs themselves. Fatalities have resulted from delay in instituting parenteral corticosteroid treatment or failure to employ adequate doses (Hetzel, 1984; Clarke and Newman, 1984; Paterson et al, 1983). Mechanical respiratory support may be indicated on clinical grounds (eg, fatigue) or when consecutive arterial blood gas determinations reveal progressive hypercapnia. Clinical signs of improvement (decreased dyspnea or wheezing) are notoriously unreliable. Response to therapy must be assessed by measurement of PEFR, FEV_1, and blood gas and serial estimates of lung compliance.

For children under 16 years with impending respiratory failure, frequent or continuous inhalation by nebulization of a selective $beta_2$ agonist is used; even intravenous administration of a selective $beta_2$ agonist or isoproterenol occasionally may be required in refractory cases. Only clinicians experienced with intravenous administration of isoproterenol should employ this route.

Once a severe acute exacerbation has resolved, an inhalant $beta_2$ agonist may be prescribed, and, if needed, an oral xanthine may be given. However, many physicians feel that inhalant steroids and/or cromolyn are essential as first-line therapy. Most patients can be taught to perform home peak flow measurements in order to recognize the onset of an acute attack and institute self-care, including temporary use of oral steroids; children under 5 years are an obvious exception.

When significant inflammation, mucus plugging, and hypersecretion have developed (particularly when an attack has developed over several days), bronchodilators are less effective (or may be ineffective) alone, and oral or intravenous steroids are required. After an acute exacerbation has resolved in patients requiring intravenous steroids, use of a short-acting oral corticosteroid, such as prednisone, may decrease the rate of relapse (Chapman et al, 1991). The oral steroid may be withdrawn immediately or gradually, depending on the response of the patient, or a single morning dose then may be given on alternate days. An inhaled steroid is preferred for prophylaxis in stable, well-controlled, compliant patients but is not useful to treat acute symptoms.

Status Asthmaticus: Most practitioners do not make a distinction between status asthmaticus and acute severe asthma. Status asthmaticus is life-threatening and hospitalization is required. Treatment is difficult, and the regimen is similar to that described for acute severe asthma. It usually includes a subcutaneous or nebulized $beta_2$ agonist and intravenous aminophylline, and intravenous steroids must be given as soon as possible. All patients should receive oxygen for hypoxemia and intravenous fluids for dehydration. Antibiotics may be useful, especially if a Gram stain demonstrates the presence of a bacterial infection.

Exercise-Induced Asthma: Many patients develop asthma five minutes or more after starting exercise, but characteristically asthmatic episodes occur after cessation of strenuous exercise. Rapid loss of heat and/or water from the respiratory passages may trigger bronchoconstriction. In patients with mild asthma, an inhalant $beta_2$-adrenergic agent usually is effective if used 5 to 15 minutes before exercise and offers protection for about 45 minutes (but up to four hours in some patients) (Sly, 1984). Cromolyn sodium is effective for two hours after administration and may afford significant protection for up to four hours in some patients. An extra dose of cromolyn should be inhaled 15 minutes before exercise. In refractory cases, a combination of a $beta_2$ agonist and cromolyn may provide protection for four hours or longer in most patients (Woolley et al, 1990). Those whose wheezing prevents continuation of exercise should take medications regularly to improve their overall respiratory function.

Asthma During Pregnancy: During pregnancy, severe bronchoconstriction is a greater danger to the fetus than the drugs used to combat it. Because of its safety, cromolyn sodium is advocated as first-line therapy in pregnant women. Theophylline, corticosteroids, and beta-adrenergic agonists also are relatively safe during pregnancy. Many practitioners are reluctant to use selective $beta_2$ agonists in these patients because data demonstrating their safety are limited; of the beta agonists, physicians have most experience with terbutaline, which has not been associated with teratogenicity. Other practitioners feel that inhalant $beta_2$ agonists are preferable to systemic drugs because little of the inhalant reaches the circulation. Systemic $beta_2$ agonists may inhibit labor and are contraindicated at term.

For a more extensive discussion of treatment of asthma during pregnancy, see *J Allergy Clin Immunol*, 1991; Paterson et al, 1990; Schatz and Zeiger, 1990.

Complications and Coexisting Conditions: Cough, nasal discharge, and other signs of *sinusitis* or *rhinitis* are often present in asthmatic patients, and appropriate symptomatic treatment may prevent acute asthmatic exacerbations (see index entries Cough; Rhinitis). Acute or chronic *bacterial infection* may coexist and require appropriate antibiotic therapy based on the results of Gram stain and cultures.

Gastroesophageal reflux may accompany asthma and should be treated because it can cause or aggravate asthma

(Nelson, 1987); this may explain the occurrence and/or persistence of nocturnal symptoms in some asthmatics. Patients with a history of repeated exacerbations, lack of response to bronchodilators, or frequent need for oral steroids may have reflux or an unrecognized sinus infection. It is claimed that reflux symptoms are independent of the use of bronchodilators in the majority of asthmatic patients (Larrain et al, 1991; Sontag, 1991).

In patients with *heart disease*, the potential cardiovascular complications induced by any bronchodilator must be weighed against the greater risk of bronchoconstriction and hypoxemia.

Potassium depletion is the most common electrolyte disturbance in acute asthma. Therapy with large doses of beta agonists, theophylline, and/or steroids may lower serum levels of potassium. A potassium supplement (40 to 60 mEq/day or more) may be required, particularly in patients who are vomiting or taking steroids. However, delay in instituting intravenous steroid and/or beta agonist therapy because of infusion of potassium is likely to be more hazardous than hypokalemia.

DRUG SELECTION. Primary factors in drug selection in asthmatic patients are the severity and status of the disease (ie, acute exacerbation, persistence of signs and symptoms between exacerbations, frequency and severity of previous exacerbations, prior response to therapy, cardiovascular-renal status, age, current medications, drug allergies, associated disease). The availability of agents with different mechanisms of action and adverse reactions, as well as the availability of metered-dose inhalers, nebulizers, and prolonged-release preparations, also are important in drug selection.

A report on the management of asthma prepared by an expert panel of the National Education Program of the National Heart, Lung, and Blood Institute reflects the growing awareness that airway inflammation is a key element in all cases of asthma. The panel recommends that aggressive and early therapy with inhaled corticosteroids, cromolyn sodium, and other anti-inflammatory agents should be considered for maintenance in patients with moderate (nonsteroid-dependent) as well as severe asthma (*J Allergy Clin Immunol*, 1991).

Beta-Adrenergic Agonists: *Actions and Uses.* Beta agonists quickly reverse bronchoconstriction. These drugs also increase the rate of mucociliary clearance, which may be decreased in patients with obstructive lung disease (Clarke and Newman, 1984). Expectoration often is improved as a result of enhanced bronchodilation.

Endogenous catecholamines, such as epinephrine, are readily metabolized by enzymes that are widely distributed throughout the body. Newer $beta_2$ agonists have been designed to better withstand enzyme degradation and, thus, are longer acting and useful orally. Adrenergic drugs can stimulate both $beta_1$ and $beta_2$ receptors to varying degrees; activation of $beta_2$ receptors relaxes bronchial smooth muscle, and activation of $beta_1$ receptors stimulates the heart. Newer compounds have been modified to emphasize $beta_2$ activity and minimize $beta_1$ activity.

The prototype of the adrenergic bronchodilators, epinephrine, stimulates $beta_2$ receptors but also has significant $beta_1$ and alpha-adrenergic (vasoconstrictor) activity. Since epinephrine acts within minutes after subcutaneous injection and side effects are short-lived, it is useful for the immediate management of acute bronchospasm in younger patients. Often, tachycardia and hypertension associated with acute asthma resolve after respiratory status improves.

Ephedrine is now considered obsolete and should not be used, since selective $beta_2$ agonists are more potent and longer acting. It may be unwise, however, to withdraw the drug from patients who have been treated successfully with it for many years. Like epinephrine, this nonselective beta agonist activates $beta_1$ as well as $beta_2$-adrenergic receptors; in addition, it acts indirectly by causing release of norepinephrine. This drug can cause central nervous system stimulation and cardiovascular side effects. Isoproterenol [Isuprel, Medihaler-Iso] is a potent bronchodilator but is short acting, has significant $beta_1$ receptor activity, and can be dangerous in patients with cardiovascular disorders. Epinephrine or isoproterenol should not be used routinely by inhalation, particularly in patients with cardiac disease; longer-acting inhalant beta agonists are preferable.

Adrenergic agents with greater specificity for $beta_2$ than $beta_1$ receptors include isoetharine [Bronkometer, Bronkosol], metaproterenol [Alupent, Metaprel], terbutaline [Brethaire, Brethine, Bricanyl], albuterol [Proventil, Ventolin], bitolterol [Tornalate], and pirbuterol [Maxair]. Of these, isoetharine is the least selective for $beta_2$ receptors. Other longer-acting and more selective drugs are preferred. These drugs are effective when administered by metered-dose inhaler. (See Table for their duration of action.)

The investigational drugs, procaterol and fenoterol, also are selective $beta_2$ agonists, and their efficacy is comparable to that of albuterol; their duration of action is claimed to be slightly longer. Fenoterol has been associated with a number of deaths in New Zealand and probably will not be marketed in this country (*Lancet*, 1990). (See the section below on Adverse Reactions and Precautions for discussion on the controversy surrounding the use of this and other $beta_2$ agonists administered orally or by inhalation for asthma maintenance therapy.) A significant potential advance in therapy is offered by two additional investigational selective $beta_2$ agonists, formoterol and salmeterol. Metered-dose inhalant preparations of these agents provide bronchodilation for 12 hours or more after a single dose (Ullman and Svedmyr, 1988; Becker et al, 1989; Maesen et al, 1990).

In acute airway obstruction, rapid relief of bronchospasm may be obtained by the subcutaneous injection of epinephrine or terbutaline. Each inhalation may improve the effectiveness of subsequent inhalations (Summers and Smith, 1984; Sly, 1984). Three inhalant doses of nebulized metaproterenol or albuterol at intervals of 20 minutes (in contrast to the standard therapy of two to three doses one hour apart) may identify those patients who will not respond to bronchodilators (Nelson et al, 1990). For many patients, a metered-dose inhalant preparation of a $beta_2$ agonist may be the initial therapy chosen. Failure to respond to therapy by metered-dose

ADRENERGIC AGONISTS FOR INHALATION

Drug	Potency	$Beta_2$ Selectivity	Peak Effect (min)	Duration of Effect* (hrs)	Dosage Forms†
Epinephrine	++++	0	>2	1-1.5	MDI, Solution
Isoproterenol	++++	0	5-15	1-2	MDI, Solution
Isoetharine	+++	++	15-60	2-3	MDI, Solution
Metaproterenol	++++	+++	30-60	3-4	MDI, Solution
Terbutaline	++++	++++	60	4	MDI
Albuterol	++++	++++	30-60	4-6	MDI, Solution
Bitolterol	++++	++++	30-60	5	MDI
Pirbuterol	++++	++++	60	5	MDI

**May have longer duration of action in certain patients*
†MDI = Metered dose inhaler
Solution = Solution for nebulization

inhalation usually results from increasingly severe asthma with mucus plugging of the airways. Inhaled $beta_2$-adrenergic agonists alone are inadequate in patients with severe asthma, steroid dependence, severe coughing, mucus hypersecretion, and/or inflammation. Nebulization, which delivers larger doses and does not require the patient's cooperation for administration, is usually preferred for moderate to severe exacerbations. A subcutaneous beta agonist should be tried in patients with acute asthma who fail to respond to an inhalant form (Appel et al, 1989).

Albuterol, metaproterenol, and terbutaline have been administered orally for maintenance therapy but should be reserved for patients who cannot use the inhalant form correctly. A long-acting oral preparation, prolonged-release albuterol, may control nocturnal asthma. Oral administration requires the use of much larger doses, produces more adverse reactions, and has a slower onset of action than inhalation. When given systemically, selective $beta_2$ agonists appear to lose some $beta_2$ specificity, and they produce significant tachycardia and other adverse effects as a result of stimulation of beta receptors in cardiovascular as well as nonvascular tissues.

Metered-Dose Inhalers. Many beta-adrenergic drugs are available in pressurized metered-dose inhalers (MDI), which deliver medication directly to the lung and allow use of much smaller doses, thus reducing the incidence and severity of adverse reactions. Patients must receive instructions on the correct use of this device. Fifty percent or more of patients may use the device improperly and obtain inadequate therapy.

For best results with any MDI, actuation should begin early in inspiration. Inspiration should be slow and complete, and the breath should be held for four to ten seconds before slow exhalation. Administration is repeated once or twice at one- to five-minute intervals. This regimen may be repeated at four- to six-hour intervals. Children should be allowed to use handheld MDIs only under the supervision of a knowledgeable adult. For most patients, especially the very young and elderly, tube and reservoir spacers may be helpful (Newman and Clarke, 1983; Clarke and Newman, 1984; De Blaquiere et al, 1989; Levison, 1990). Breath-activated, nonpressurized devices (eg, Rotohaler) may be a useful alternative delivery system for elderly patients and children over age 3. Pressurized devices containing chlorocarbons or fluorohydrocarbons will become obsolete in 1994 or 1995; at that time, all medications will be delivered by nonpressurized devices.

Overuse can occur during exacerbations of asthma, and patients should be instructed to seek immediate medical attention when symptoms worsen or when more frequent use of the inhaler is needed.

Nebulizer Devices. Nebulizers have no inherent advantages over properly used MDIs in maintenance therapy. However, many practitioners prefer to administer a beta-adrenergic agonist through a nebulizer for patients with an acute exacerbation of moderate to severe asthma because the delivered dose is more consistent and often larger and the patient's coordination and cooperation are less critical. The chief disadvantages of a nebulizer are its expense, lessened portability (Newman, 1984), and the possibility of greater toxicity due to higher dosage.

A nebulizer can deliver almost any drug solution, including combinations of a beta-adrenergic drug, cromolyn, and/or other agents. Potentially, more drug is available for absorption by the lungs with nebulizers than with MDIs. The amount deposited in the lungs is up to 15% of the delivered dose; the remainder is deposited within the nebulizer walls and apparatus.

Correct use of a nebulizer depends more on the specific unit employed and its operation than on the patient's technique (Newman and Clarke, 1983). A nebulizer solution should be administered slowly and intermittently over 15 to 30 minutes. In patients with hypoxemia, compressed air or oxygen may be used to drive the unit. A final volume of 3 to 4 ml and a flow rate of 6 L/minute ensure a high aerosol outflow, small particle size, and short treatment period. Handheld bulb nebulizers (eg, DeVilbiss model #45) can be used instead of gas-driven units, but the amount of drug delivered to the lungs is variable. Ultrasonic nebulizer devices can cause bronchoconstriction and generally should be avoided.

To avoid bacterial contamination, the nebulizer unit should be cleaned frequently.

Intermittent positive pressure breathing (IPPB) has no apparent benefit over other delivery systems and introduces the potential for pneumothorax.

Adverse Reactions and Precautions. All adrenergic drugs may cause anxiety, tremor, and restlessness. Older patients and those with long-standing chronic lung disease can be given epinephrine at reduced doses, but it is difficult to avoid tachycardia and other disturbances of cardiac rhythm and rate; unless it is lifesaving, this drug should be avoided in patients with hypertension. These effects also may occur after parenteral administration or inhalation of isoproterenol or newer beta agonists.

Central nervous system stimulation manifested by nervousness, irritability, and insomnia is common after oral administration of ephedrine, especially in adults. Less frequently, similar reactions follow the subcutaneous injection of epinephrine and the inhalation of isoproterenol.

Adrenergic drugs, particularly ephedrine, may cause urinary retention severe enough to necessitate catheterization in patients with bladder neck obstruction.

Skeletal muscle tremor resulting from $beta_2$ receptor stimulation is more common with oral agents. A reduction in the dosage usually eliminates this reaction, and tolerance develops with continued use.

Inhalation of a selective $beta_2$ agonist usually has only slight effects on heart rate in normal patients. When palpitations do occur, they are generally observed within five minutes after an inhalant dose. Large doses delivered through a nebulizer or overuse of a metered-dose inhaler not uncommonly produce tachycardia and tremor; rarely, hypokalemia, hypoxemia, and arrhythmias develop. Administration of oxygen during nebulization of a beta-adrenergic agonist protects against the possibility of hypoxemia (Ziment, 1984; Williams, 1984).

Beta agonist inhalers cannot control increasingly severe asthma. Excessive inhalation causes toxicity without additional benefit. Tolerance, refractoriness, and even paradoxical bronchospastic reactions also may develop with regular or too frequent administration. Responsiveness can be restored by a five- to seven-day course of oral corticosteroids, which frequently improves respiratory status (Jenne, 1984; Sly, 1984).

Several fixed-dose oral combinations (eg, Bronkolixir, Marax, Tedral) contain sedating agent(s), as well as adrenergic drugs and other components. Since effective individual drugs are currently available, use of combinations is not advisable (see the section on Mixtures).

Hyperthyroidism aggravates asthma and tends to accentuate all adrenergic side effects, particularly those of epinephrine, and may cause an exaggerated pressor effect.

Beta agonist preparations for use in MDIs do not contain sulfites, which can precipitate bronchospasm, but some solutions for nebulization or injection may.

It has been claimed that maintenance therapy employing regular daily administration of fenoterol and other $beta_2$-adrenergic agonists increases bronchial hyperresponsiveness and may be dangerous even when used with steroids (van Schayck et al, 1990; Sears et al, 1990; Pearce et al, 1991; Burrows and Lebowitz, 1992; Spitzer et al, 1992). Many clinicians believe that beta-adrenergic agonists may produce better overall control and are safer when used as required rather than on a daily schedule (Sears et al, 1990; *Lancet*, 1990), but this assertion has not been confirmed.

It is not clear if inhalant beta-adrenergic drugs contributed to an increase in asthma deaths reported in the United States and other countries in recent years. The principal causes of these deaths were probably erroneous assessment of the severity of asthma, undertreatment (especially with corticosteroids), and delay in seeking additional therapy (Hetzel, 1984; Clarke and Newman, 1984; Sheffer and Buist, 1987; Birkhead et al, 1989; Walker et al, 1990; *WHO Drug Info*, 1989).

Interactions. Severe hypertension and, rarely, death may occur if beta agonists are administered with a monoamine oxidase (MAO) inhibitor (ie, isocarboxazid [Marplan], phenelzine [Nardil], tranylcypromine [Parnate]), because these agents block the metabolism of catecholamines. Ephedrine may antagonize the antihypertensive effect of guanethidine [Ismelin].

Adrenergic bronchodilators may be less effective in patients receiving nonselective beta blockers, such as propranolol [Inderal], which have a $beta_2$-receptor blocking action. It may be necessary to increase the dose of the $beta_2$ agonist or substitute theophylline, cromolyn, or an inhalant steroid. Cardioselective beta blockers are safer when used with $beta_2$ agonists.

Xanthine Drugs: *Actions.* Theophylline's mechanism of action is not precisely defined but may involve an increase in the level of cAMP in selective cell compartments, modulation of intracellular calcium transport, and inhibition of adenosine receptors (Weinberger, 1984; Torphy, 1988). Theophylline increases the contractility of diaphragmatic muscle and enhances its resistance to fatigue (Aubier et al, 1981). In patients with obstructive lung diseases associated with cor pulmonale, theophylline increases cardiac output and enhances right ventricular ejection fraction through its positive inotropic effects and reduction in pulmonary vascular resistance. Theophylline also may inhibit the release of inflammatory mediators. The respiratory center is stimulated primarily because the hypoxic drive is increased.

Uses. Theophylline is used to treat status asthmaticus, to prevent attacks, or to minimize signs and symptoms during periods of remission; its use for acute asthma is controversial. Extensive clinical experience has demonstrated that theophylline is effective and safe when care is taken to ensure that the optimal dose, dosing schedule, formulation, and route of administration are employed. Serum levels should be monitored in every patient.

In the United States, oral theophylline is widely used for maintenance therapy. The development of prolonged-release (sustained-release, SR) preparations and the availability of improved techniques to determine serum concentrations contribute to its popularity. Although some investigators believe that theophylline is even more effective than a $beta_2$ agonist or cromolyn sodium for maintenance therapy (Weinberger, 1984), others stress that theophylline is not as safe or as effective as inhalant $beta_2$ agonists or cromolyn and that it should be a secondary drug (Bukowskyj et al, 1984; Marks, 1987). Some authorities believe that the popularity of theophylline in this country will decline because of (1) increasing emphasis on agents that block inflammation and bronchial hyperresponsiveness, (2) the anticipated availability of long-acting inhalant $beta_2$ agonists (eg, salmeterol, formoterol), and (3) increasing evidence that raises doubt about the value of xanthines in acute asthma (Lam and Newhouse, 1990; Niewoehner, 1990; Newhouse, 1990; Jenne, 1990).

In practice, theophylline and beta agonists are commonly used together, but such use is now being questioned. Some authorities believe that optimal dosing with a $beta_2$ agonist increases the degree of bronchodilation and eliminates the need for added theophylline and/or that, for maintenance, anti-inflammatory drugs (eg, inhalant cromolyn, an inhalant steroid) are preferable (Lam and Newhouse, 1990; Newhouse, 1990). Others believe that theophylline has a useful role in selected patients, such as those with mild exacerbations, or in the severely asthmatic patient whose condition is not adequately controlled despite optimal use of steroids (Jenne, 1990). Patients maintained on bronchodilators may experience breakthrough episodes of acute asthma. If this occurs, a five- to seven-day course of oral corticosteroid therapy usually is effective.

Intravenous aminophylline or theophylline is used for the treatment of acute exacerbations of moderate to severe asthma. Since a number of studies have shown that little additional bronchodilation is produced beyond that obtained acutely with maximum $beta_2$-agonist therapy or a combination of an inhalant beta agonist and an oral or intravenous steroid, some practitioners recommend that intravenous aminophylline be given only when beta agonist drugs and steroids are inadequate (Rees, 1984 A; Self et al, 1990). However, other clinicians believe that intravenous administration probably should be employed in most patients with severe or prolonged airway obstruction because it provides sustained bronchodilation (Jenne, 1984, 1990) and may decrease the need for hospitalization (Wrenn et al, 1991). It also has been suggested that xanthine drugs enhance the contractility of the diaphragm and increase its resistance to fatigue, but recent evidence suggests that diaphragmatic fatigue may not be an important factor in obstructive lung disease (Similowski et al, 1991).

The ethylenediamine component of aminophylline occasionally may be associated with allergic reactions. A parenteral theophylline preparation diluted in 5% dextrose that contains no ethylenediamine is now available for intravenous administration.

Another xanthine, dyphylline, is much less potent than theophylline and is rarely used. An investigational xanthine, enprofylline, produces significant bronchodilation in asthma patients and appears to be safer than theophylline but still can produce headache and nausea (Boe et al, 1987). There is no xanthine preparation for inhalation.

Rectal suppositories of aminophylline are absorbed erratically and produce local irritation with prolonged use. A rectal solution is absorbed rapidly and reliably, although it too may cause local irritation. Although rectal preparations occasionally are useful, their misuse results in serious toxicity, especially when vomiting or dehydration develops, and this route should not be used.

Prolonged-Release Preparations. When standard (rapidly absorbed) tablets are administered every four to six hours, the serum concentration of theophylline can vary in the same patient from dose to dose and varies considerably in those who metabolize the drug rapidly (especially smokers and children). To correct this problem and increase compliance, prolonged-release 8-hour, 12-hour, and 24-hour formulations were developed. Unfortunately, the absorption curves of prolonged-release forms can vary in the same individual (Szefler, 1987). Also, some 24-hour preparations administered within one hour of food or other ingested substances may be released prematurely (dumped) or, conversely, absorption may be delayed (Hendeles et al, 1985; Spector, 1985 A).

The package insert for any theophylline preparation should be consulted before use for more detailed information on avoiding toxicity and obtaining optimal serum levels. See also the evaluation on Theophylline.

Standard (Rapidly Absorbed) Preparations. The availability of prolonged-release preparations has diminished the need for short-acting oral preparations (Weinberger, 1984). However, some nonsmoking adults and those who metabolize the drug slowly can be maintained on standard oral forms (Weinstein and Brokaw, 1984).

Adverse Reactions and Precautions. Although serum concentrations of 8 to 15 mcg/ml are usually efficacious and safe, and are most desirable, these levels may not be tolerated by an occasional patient. Minor adverse reactions include nausea, vomiting, and epigastric pain; these generally are preceded by headache and signs of central nervous system stimulation (dizziness, nervousness, and insomnia). Theophylline may decrease lower esophageal sphincter pressure and produce gastroesophageal reflux. Some minor reactions can be avoided if low doses are used initially and the amount increased gradually (Hendeles and Weinberger, 1983).

Serum concentrations above 15 mcg/ml provide little added benefit, increase the frequency and severity of the above reactions, and can produce tachycardia and hematemesis. At serum concentrations above 30 mcg/ml, life-threatening clonic and tonic convulsions or arrhythmias may develop. The seizures are often refractory to anticonvulsant therapy and may prove fatal.

Since the therapeutic blood level is close to the toxic one, careful evaluation of the patient is indicated and factors that alter the rate of elimination of this drug must be considered when adjusting dosage.

For a more detailed discussion of adverse reactions, precautions, factors affecting clearance, and interactions, see the evaluation on Theophylline.

Anti-inflammatory Corticosteroids: *Actions and Uses.* The specific mechanisms by which steroids exert their beneficial actions in asthma are largely unknown. Steroids inhibit the response to inflammation and decrease bronchial hyperreactivity. These drugs appear to prevent the synthesis or action of inflammatory mediators; release of mediators from mast cells may be decreased (Norn and Clementsen, 1988). Corticosteroids inhibit late-phase asthmatic reactions but have little effect on immediate hypersensitivity reactions. Neutrophil, eosinophil, and monocyte chemotaxis is inhibited. Steroids reduce the formation of mucus and lessen or block formation of edema. They also stabilize lysosomal membranes, reduce mast and basophil histamine stores, and restore the responsiveness of leukocytes and bronchial smooth muscle to beta agonists (Daniele, 1984; Spector, 1985 B; McFadden, 1988; Nelson and Lockey, 1988).

Systemic corticosteroids are the most effective antiasthmatic drugs available and should be considered in all patients with severe acute exacerbations of asthma. Because of adverse reactions, however, their long-term use should be restricted to patients who do not respond adequately to beta-adrenergic drugs, theophylline, cromolyn sodium, inhalant corticosteroids, or combinations of these drugs.

A brief course of an oral corticosteroid (eg, prednisone given as a single morning dose or in divided doses for five to eight days or until symptoms are controlled) during an acute exacerbation of asthma may prevent status asthmaticus and avoid hospitalization (Chapman et al, 1991). The total daily dose of oral prednisone usually employed for adults is 30 to 60 mg and, for children, 1 to 2 mg/kg/day; larger doses may be given if necessary. Some patients can be taught to recognize their need for additional medication and to self-administer oral steroids; they should be instructed to contact their physicians at the onset of increased dyspnea, wheezing, and/or respiratory distress.

The short-term intravenous administration of a corticosteroid may be necessary in acute severe asthma. It is generally recommended that 200 to 300 mg of hydrocortisone sodium succinate, 40 to 80 mg of methylprednisolone, or the equivalent should be administered intravenously over 20 to 30 minutes every four to six hours until improvement has occurred as determined by the results of FEV_1, pulmonary function tests, and clinical observation. Larger doses have not been more effective in most patients (Hiller and Wilson, 1983). When the patient has improved (often after 24 to 72 hours of therapy), an oral steroid (eg, prednisone 40 to 60 mg daily [or the equivalent] in divided doses) is substituted. When the overall clinical condition improves and symptoms are completely controlled, a single daily dose of prednisone or methylprednisolone is given between 7 and 8 AM if possible; the dose then should be tapered and a maintenance regimen substituted. The systemic steroid should be withdrawn as soon as possible. In some patients, the oral steroid can be withdrawn within one week.

A temporary period of stress (eg, surgery, infection) necessitates administration of larger oral or parenteral doses in patients already receiving oral steroids daily or on alternate days or in patients taking inhalant steroids (Spector, 1985 B). A larger dose also is indicated in those who have received prolonged steroid therapy within the past year.

Asthma not controlled by large doses of oral prednisone and bronchodilators may respond to the combination of oral methylprednisolone and the macrolide antibiotic, troleandomycin. Although combined administration of these agents decreases steroid metabolism and may allow considerable reduction in the dose of the steroid in both children and adults (Weinstein and Brokaw, 1984; Eitches et al, 1985; Wald et al, 1986), use of this combination is controversial.

In investigational studies, the use of low-dose methotrexate, dapsone, hydroxychloroquine, cyclosporine, or gold salts had a steroid-sparing action in asthmatic patients and permitted a significant reduction in the dose of the steroid (Mullarkey et al, 1988; Bernstein et al, 1988; Alvarez and Szefler, 1992). Of these drugs, the use of methotrexate for acute severe asthma has been evaluated most thoroughly (Mullarkey et al, 1991; Mullarkey, 1991; Dyer et al, 1991; Geddes, 1991). One negative conclusion has been criticized because the placebo effect was high, which suggested that the patients selected for the study were not steroid-dependent (Erzurum et al, 1991; Mullarkey et al, 1991). In most studies, low-dose methotrexate was well tolerated. It is unclear if the long-term toxicity associated with methotrexate, gold, or other immunosuppressive/cytotoxic drugs is less than that observed with full-dose steroid therapy or if these agents should be used at all.

Long-acting steroids (eg, dexamethasone) should not be prescribed to treat asthma, because severe withdrawal symptoms (eg, fever, myalgia, joint pain) are likely to follow their administration. Moreover, they can suppress the HPA axis even when given on alternate days. Corticotropin (ACTH) does not aid in HPA axis recovery.

Metered-dose Inhalers. A major advance in the therapy of asthma has been the development of inhalant corticosteroid preparations. Because an MDI delivers the drug directly to the lung, small doses can be employed, thus reducing the incidence and severity of adverse reactions. Increasingly, the use of inhalant steroids is being advocated as first-line therapy in patients with mild to moderate asthma (Barnes, 1989; Cockroft and Hargreave, 1990; Juniper et al, 1990; Lorentzson et al, 1990; *J Allergy Clin Immunol*, 1991).

Inhalant corticosteroids are inactivated rapidly when they are absorbed systemically from the oropharynx and gut. The efficacy of currently available corticosteroid aerosol preparations (beclomethasone dipropionate [Beclovent, Vanceril], flunisolide [AeroBid], and triamcinolone acetonide [Azmacort]) appears to be similar. All are well absorbed, rapidly metabolized to inactive compounds, and highly active within the lung, and the incidence of systemic effects is low. Recommended doses usually are safe in both adults and children.

In general, severe asthma should be controlled completely by oral steroids before a steroid inhaler is employed, and bronchodilators or other antiasthmatic agents should not be discontinued. Most patients who require less than 10 mg of prednisone or its equivalent daily can be converted to inhalant corticosteroids alone. Those who require 20 mg or more of oral prednisone a day are not easily converted to inhalant steroids, but their concomitant use may reduce the oral dose required (Tse and Bernstein, 1984).

For the patient with severe asthma who requires larger doses of inhaled steroids, a high-dose preparation would be advantageous. One such preparation, flunisolide, is available and others may soon be marketed; the latter include beclomethasone dipropionate (250 mcg/inhalation) and the investigational agent, budesonide (200 mcg/inhalation). In England and Canada, use of these preparations has allowed some patients to reduce the frequency of administration to twice daily and to reduce or discontinue oral medication (Barnes, 1989; Cockroft, 1990 B). Less frequent administration may increase patient compliance. Some patients may respond to lower-dose inhalant steroid preparations given twice daily.

Adverse Reactions and Precautions. Large oral or parenteral doses of short-acting corticosteroids can be used for up to two weeks with little risk of significant HPA axis suppression or toxicity. Serious adverse reactions also are less likely during continuous, more prolonged therapy with daily doses at or below 10 mg of prednisone (or the equivalent), but few patients respond to doses less than 10 mg/day.

Significant effects on the HPA axis and most adverse reactions may be avoided if steroid-dependent patients are converted from daily therapy with a single morning dose of a short-acting corticosteroid (prednisone, methylprednisolone) to alternate-day therapy after symptoms have been controlled (Spector, 1985 B). (Since the changeover is more difficult when divided daily doses have been used, patients usually are first converted to a single morning dose.) In alternate-day therapy, three times the total daily dose is administered as a single dose every other morning at 8 AM. It may take considerable time to wean patients from daily to alternate-day therapy. Those receiving more than 20 mg of prednisone or the equivalent per day are not easily converted to alternate-day therapy but the conversion should nevertheless be attempted. Rhinitis and atopic dermatitis may be exacerbated after withdrawal of oral steroids.

For a detailed discussion of the adverse reactions of systemic corticosteroids, see index entry Adrenal Corticosteroids, Adverse Reactions.

The only significant adverse effects of inhaled corticosteroids are oropharyngeal candidiasis (thrush), dysphonia, and coughing or wheezing. The incidence of oropharyngeal candidiasis apparently is somewhat dose-dependent. The mouth should be rinsed with water after inhalation. Slow inspiration and holding the breath for another four to ten seconds may improve delivery of the drug to the lungs and decrease adverse reactions. The use of a spacer (tube or reservoir chamber) decreases systemic absorption, increases the efficiency of drug delivery in patients using the MDI improperly (as many as 50% of patients), and may allow doses to be increased several-fold without producing oral candidiasis. The cough or wheezing produced by inhaled steroids also can be minimized with use of a spacer or inhalation of a beta agonist five minutes prior to the steroid; however, the latter must be considered in light of advice against regular use of beta agonists. As another alternative, a short course of an oral steroid may be useful.

A number of reports have indicated that in some patients treated for long periods with daily inhalant steroid therapy, bone formation may be impaired, osteoporosis may occur, and growth rate in children may be reduced (Toogood and Hodsman, 1991; Storr, 1991; Wales et al, 1991). Further studies are underway to determine the extent of these effects. Daily doses of calcium administered to maximize bone formation in children and adults usually are not beneficial.

Patients who use inhalant steroid preparations must be instructed to take steroids orally when acute attacks occur. Some patients may benefit from a few days of concomitant oral steroid therapy (burst or pulse) to improve the delivery of the inhaled drug into the bronchi.

Drug Interactions. Careful dosage adjustment is advised when barbiturates, other anticonvulsants, and rifampin are administered to asthmatic patients receiving systemic corticosteroids, since the enzyme-inducing properties of these drugs may increase the metabolism of the steroids. For other drug interactions, see index entry Adrenal Corticosteroids, Drug Interactions.

The macrolide antibiotics (eg, troleandomycin, erythromycin, clarithromycin) have a steroid-sparing action and also prolong the half-life of theophylline. When a macrolide antibiotic is used in patients receiving theophylline and methylprednisolone, particularly for chronic illness, the doses of the latter two drugs must be reduced to prevent overdosage.

Antiallergy Drugs: Drugs in this category were previously misnamed mast cell stabilizers. Evidence that inhibition of release of mast cell inflammatory mediators may not be their primary action and the fact that other agents (eg, beta agonists) have greater effects on the mast cell have led to abandonment of this term. These agents block various inflammatory cascade reactions in the late-phase asthmatic response and may diminish or inhibit bronchial hyperresponsiveness.

Cromolyn Sodium. Unlike other drugs discussed in this chapter, cromolyn sodium [Intal] is used only to prevent asthma attacks. It reduces bronchial hyperresponsiveness but has no adrenergic, antihistaminic, or corticosteroid-like actions and little bronchodilator activity. Daily administration in divided doses is required for optimal efficacy. Onset of action is delayed (generally two to six weeks), and other agents must be used in the interim. When cromolyn is used prior to challenge (eg, exercise, cold air, exposure to sulfur dioxide or animals), its effects are usually observed within 10 to 15 minutes.

In several controlled clinical trials, cromolyn sodium was as effective as theophylline in children with chronic asthma (Bernstein, 1985 A; Shapiro and König, 1985). The availability of an MDI formulation has improved compliance and has led to the recommendation that it be considered a first-line agent and the drug of choice for prophylaxis in children with mild asthma (Marks, 1987; Eigen et al, 1987; *Pediatr Alert,*

1987 A). It also has considerable value in some children with moderate asthma.

Although this drug has been used primarily in children, there is considerable evidence of its effectiveness as a first-line antiasthmatic agent in adults (Bernstein, 1985 B; Eigen et al, 1987; Blumenthal et al, 1988; Barnes, 1989; Cockroft and Hargreave, 1990; Petty et al, 1989). Cromolyn prevents allergic asthma and some cases of nonallergic asthma and should be considered for patients with frequent wheezing, seasonal or occupational asthma, animal- or exercise-induced asthma, and asthma not controlled by beta-adrenergic drugs or theophylline or in those who cannot tolerate the latter drugs (Summers and Smith, 1984). In some patients who respond to cromolyn sodium, it may be possible to reduce the dose of corticosteroids, beta agonists, and/or theophylline or eliminate their use (Daniele, 1984). Some authorities advocate a six-week trial with cromolyn sodium for initial therapy in all patients with chronic asthma (Kaliner et al, 1987). Cromolyn causes minimal adverse reactions.

Cromolyn is currently available in a 1% solution for nebulization and in MDIs. (It also has been available as an encapsulated powder administered with a special device provided by the manufacturer [Spinhaler]. Because of difficulty in obtaining raw materials for the powder, cromolyn capsules are not available at present but it is anticipated that they will be in the near future.) Rapid inhalation is efficient for delivery of the dry powder, but there is considerable deposition of drug on the walls of the oropharynx, and only about 5% of the dose may reach the lungs (Newman and Clarke, 1983). Although hand-lung coordination is not required with a dry powder inhaler, some patients find it inconvenient to load a capsule into the device before use, and improper technique can affect compliance.

Nedocromil. Like cromolyn, nedocromil [Tilade], a disodium salt of pyranoquinoline dicarboxylic acid, is not a bronchodilator; it prevents the release of inflammatory mediators from tissue mast cells, inhibits recruitment of other inflammatory cells (such as eosinophils and neutrophils) into the airway epithelium, inhibits both immediate and late bronchoconstriction, and decreases bronchial hyperresponsiveness (Holgate, 1986; Kay, 1987). In addition, this agent stabilizes other types of mediator-releasing cells and may modulate the release of tachykinins from airway sensory nerve endings (Thomson, 1991; Verleden et al, 1991); these actions may explain in part its greater spectrum of activity than cromolyn sodium. It has the same indications as inhalant cromolyn and does not appear to be more efficacious than cromolyn in most patients (*F-D-C Rep*, 1990).

A number of clinical trials have demonstrated that administration of nedocromil sodium as an aerosol twice a day is effective for prophylaxis of allergic and nonallergic asthma, exercise-induced asthma, and bronchospasm provoked by a variety of stimuli (Holgate, 1986; North American Tilade Study Group, 1990; Busse et al, 1989; Thomson, 1989; Cherniak et al, 1990). Nedocromil has been used alone and as an adjunct to therapy with beta$_2$-adrenergic agonists, steroids, or theophylline. In some patients, addition of nedocromil has produced benefits beyond those obtained by maximum doses of bronchodilators. The bronchodilator dose can sometimes be reduced or the other drugs discontinued. Nedocromil is not a substitute for inhaled or oral steroids, although it may be possible to decrease the dosage of steroid in some patients. Nedocromil is well tolerated; the most common adverse effects are unpleasant taste, nausea, and headache.

Ketotifen. Several oral biscromones with similar properties are being investigated. One of these, ketotifen, a tricyclic compound of the benzocycloheptathiopene class, is available in many countries (Grant et al, 1990). In addition to its cromolyn-like actions, it has antihistaminic activity and has been investigated as a long-acting (12 to 24 hours) oral alternative to cromolyn for maintenance in those with chronic asthma. The results of clinical studies have been variable and conflicting, and its ultimate efficacy for the prophylaxis of asthma remains to be established (Shapiro and Koñig, 1985). A few studies suggest that it may have value for prophylaxis of atopic asthma.

Sedation and weight gain may occur after prolonged administration. Other common adverse effects include dizziness, nausea, headache, dry mouth, bronchospasm, and aggravation of asthma.

Azelastine. This investigational agent appears to have a variety of antiallergic and antiasthmatic actions. In in vitro and animal studies, azelastine inhibited release of histamine and other mediators of inflammation. Possible mechanisms of action include inhibition of synthesis and antagonism of inflammatory chemical mediators of airway hyperresponsiveness (Kemp at al, 1987). In a number of clinical studies, once- or twice-daily oral administration of azelastine produced significant bronchodilation in patients with moderate to severe asthma in doses that were well tolerated (Spector et al, 1987; Kemp et al, 1987; Tinkelman et al, 1990). This drug may have value for both prophylaxis and treatment.

Anticholinergic Drugs: Some elements of asthma may be due to vagal-mediated stimulation of bronchial muscle, which increases cholinergic tone in the airways and causes bronchospasm and mucus hypersecretion. Atropine and its congeners reduce bronchospasm. Their use in asthma has received renewed attention with the availability of atropine and ipratropium in inhalant form. Some of the side effects (central nervous system stimulation, mydriasis, cycloplegia, dry mouth) that occur with subcutaneous administration of atropine are less severe after inhalation (Hemstreet, 1980); nevertheless, adverse reactions may occur after inhalation even at the lowest effective dose.

An anticholinergic agent may be used when inhaled beta-adrenergic agonists or theophylline is ineffective or when cough is prominent. Anticholinergic drugs generally are much less useful than beta$_2$ agonists in asthma. When these two classes of drugs are used together, significant additive bronchodilation beyond that obtained with either drug alone apparently occurs only in patients with severe acute asthma (Rebuck et al, 1987; Simons, 1987). Anticholinergic drugs given by inhalation also may be useful when asthma is produced by beta-adrenergic blockade or specific stimuli (eg, cold air, exercise).

Some physicians prefer atropine methonitrate as an alternative to atropine sulfate because it has a longer duration of action. A congener of atropine, ipratropium bromide [Atrovent], has been widely used overseas and in Canada and is available in this country in an MDI. It is not yet available as a solution for nebulization. When inhaled, it is as effective as atropine but produces fewer adverse effects because it is a quaternary ammonium compound and, therefore, is not well absorbed systemically. Ipratropium and other quaternary ammonium drugs, glycopyrrolate and oxyphenonium, are being investigated for use in a nebulized solution for inhalation.

H_1 Receptor Antagonists: Most early clinical trials carried out to determine the effects of oral H_1 antihistamines in asthma showed that these agents had little benefit. In a subsequent study, intravenously administered chlorpheniramine, a first-generation H_1 receptor blocker, produced bronchodilation in asthmatic patients (Popa, 1977). However, the possible value of this and other H_1 blockers in asthma is limited by the involvement of other mediators in addition to histamine in asthma pathophysiology as well as by the sedation and other adverse effects produced by the large doses needed to achieve significant bronchodilation.

The development of the second-generation (nonsedating) H_1 antihistamines has renewed interest in the possible value of these drugs in asthma. In clinical trials, second-generation antihistamines showing possible value in asthma therapy include terfenadine [Seldane] (Rafferty and Holgate, 1987; Cookson, 1987), astemizole [Hismanal] (Holgate et al, 1985), and the investigational agents, cetirizine [Reactine] (Brik et al, 1987) and loratadine [Claritin]. These agents appear to produce only modest bronchodilation in patients with mild to moderate asthma, and their role in asthma therapy remains to be determined (Meltzer, 1990).

For many years, antihistamines were contraindicated in asthmatic patients because of concern that they could dry bronchial secretions and produce bronchoconstriction and other adverse effects. It is now clear that this fear is unjustified and that antihistamines are safe for these patients (Meltzer, 1990).

Calcium Channel Blocking Drugs: Calcium antagonists (eg, verapamil [Calan, Isoptin], diltiazem [Cardizem], nifedipine [Adalat, Procardia]) selectively inhibit calcium ion influx across the cell membrane, thus suppressing calcium-dependent smooth muscle excitation. The secretion of histamine and other mediators may be initiated by movement of calcium into mast cells. Investigationally, calcium antagonists have prevented exercise-induced asthma. However, those presently available have little bronchodilating activity and do not appear likely to replace bronchodilators or anti-inflammatory agents.

Mucokinetic Agents: Mucokinetic drugs, such as acetylcysteine [Mucomyst], guaifenesin, or potassium iodide, have limited value in patients with asthma (Ziment, 1984). Acetylcysteine induces expectoration through an irritant effect on bronchial mucosa, which causes bronchorrhea and stimulates coughing, and liquifies sputum. It may be useful in patients with severe mucoid impaction of the bronchi or persistent mucus lodgment, but concomitant administration with a beta-adrenergic inhalant is necessary to protect against bronchospasm. Acetylcysteine has an unpleasant sulfurous odor and taste upon nebulization that can produce gagging, nausea, and vomiting.

In recommended doses, guaifenesin is of doubtful benefit in asthma. Although a saturated solution of potassium iodide may be a useful expectorant, iodides can cause hypothyroidism and skin lesions (usually acneiform), and they are not recommended for children or pregnant women. For use of iodinated glycerol in chronic obstructive bronchitis, see the following section.

Isotonic saline is an effective expectorant. Inhalation of hypertonic saline also is effective, but its use may be undesirable in patients who must restrict their intake of sodium and it may cause acute bronchospasm.

Patients who produce sputum chronically should be well hydrated. The value of water in inhalant therapy is considered to be due to its demulcent properties rather than its mucokinetic effects. Water can cause bronchospasm when inhaled. Some physicians do not believe that mucus becomes less viscid even with aggressive hydration.

CHRONIC BRONCHITIS AND EMPHYSEMA

BRONCHITIS. Two distinct forms of chronic bronchitis are recognizable clinically. The first is defined as the presence of cough and sputum for three or more months per year for at least two consecutive years. This form of the disease is characterized by mucus hypersecretion with hypertrophy and hyperplasia of bronchial mucus glands, but the air flow is not necessarily limited. Some investigators have coined the term, simple chronic bronchitis, to distinguish this benign entity from chronic obstructive bronchitis. It is unclear at the present time whether chronic simple bronchitis progresses to obstructive disease or is a separate entity.

In chronic obstructive bronchitis, there is significant obstruction in the small airways. Major ventilation/perfusion inequalities characterize the disease, and dyspnea, cyanosis, and cor pulmonale may ultimately result.

Management of Chronic Obstructive Bronchitis: Hypersecretion may be reduced by humidifying inspired air. Although removal of secretions markedly reduces the risk of upper respiratory infection, improved hydration to promote expectoration and postural drainage is thought to be beneficial only in patients with abundant secretions. Viral and bacterial infections increase airway hyperreactivity and sputum production and may progress to pneumonia; antibiotics should be prescribed to treat bacterial exacerbations. Stress and bronchial irritants, particularly cigarette smoke, must be avoided; even passive smoking can aggravate or precipitate bronchospasm in these patients.

In 361 patients with stable chronic obstructive bronchitis who participated in the National Mucolytic Study, iodinated glycerol improved expectoration, provided significant adjunctive relief of cough, and reduced chest discomfort as well as the duration of acute exacerbations (Petty, 1990 A). This double-blind, multicenter study demonstrated that oral administration of iodinated glycerol 60 mg four times a day for eight weeks was effective and safe as adjunctive therapy. However, there is concern about the possible increase in the incidence of tumors reported in animal studies after administration of iodinated glycerol (*F-D-C Rep*, 1992), although the data are not sufficiently strong to ban use of this drug at this time.

Chronic bronchitis responds to drug therapy, but the effect is not as great as in patients with asthma. Nevertheless, therapy with a $beta_2$ agonist, theophylline, and/or ipratropium should be tried even if results of pulmonary function tests indicate that airway obstruction is only slightly reversible. Inhalant forms of anticholinergic agents are considered among the drugs of choice in patients with chronic bronchitis (Gross and Skorodin, 1984; Gross, 1987; Chapman, 1991), particularly in patients not well controlled by beta-adrenergic drugs; because of their greater efficacy, many authorities now consider them to be the drugs of choice in such patients. They often are used with beta agonists (Gross and Skorodin, 1984; Gross, 1987); however, combined use may not produce any more bronchodilation than that achieved with larger doses of either agent alone (Easton et al, 1986).

Some physicians recommend steroid therapy for two to four weeks to identify those patients with a significant inflammatory component. A history of wheezing attacks, allergy, or increased eosinophils may be predictive of the usefulness of steroids. Responsiveness to adrenergic agents also may be predictive of their benefit (Estepan and Libby, 1982).

A severe acute exacerbation of chronic obstructive bronchitis with a rising PCO_2 and respiratory acidosis requires intravenous hydration, an inhalant or oral $beta_2$-adrenergic drug, controlled oxygen therapy, chest physical therapy with postural drainage, and usually antibiotics; the benefits of intravenous aminophylline have been questioned (Rice et al, 1987), but it is usually administered. Mechanical ventilatory support should be instituted if the blood gases continue to deteriorate and other clinical findings (eg, fatigue) worsen (Burton, 1984). Many practitioners believe that short-term steroid therapy may help reduce bronchial edema and inflammation (Ingram and Davies, 1992). Management of right heart failure may require oxygen, salt restriction, and diuretics. Continuous oxygen therapy is the only treatment that prolongs survival in patients with severe pulmonary hypertension and cor pulmonale.

EMPHYSEMA. Emphysema is characterized by irreversible destruction and coalescence of alveolar septa with enlargement of the distal air spaces and loss of lung elasticity. The terminal airways tend to collapse during expiration, increasing the work of breathing. Cor pulmonale and respiratory failure are observed less frequently in emphysema than in chronic obstructive bronchitis.

The enzyme, neutrophil elastase (NE), is a protease that cleaves the connective tissue supporting the lung parenchyma. Within the lung and plasma, a number of antiproteases exist that are able to prevent the action of NE and other proteases (Cohen, 1986; Wewers et al, 1987 A). The most important antiprotease is $alpha_1$-antitrypsin (AAT). This antiprotease is synthesized in the liver by parenchymal cells and by mononuclear phagocytes and passes various body membranes to reach the lung. AAT is present in the lung interstitium and fluid lining the epithelium of the lower respiratory tract of normal persons. In those with the homozygous form of AAT deficiency (approximately 1% to 2% of patients with emphysema), the levels of this protein in plasma and the lung are less than 15% of normal and the risk for the development of emphysema is markedly increased. Since not all individuals with this form of AAT deficiency develop emphysema, other protective mechanisms may be active in the lower respiratory tract (American Thoracic Society, 1989; Crystal et al, 1989).

AAT is responsible for more than 90% of the antineutrophil elastase activity in the lung. Weekly intravenous infusions of 60 mg/kg of $alpha_1$-proteinase inhibitor (human plasma $alpha_1$-antitrypsin) raise the plasma level to more than twice that needed to protect the lung against injury by proteases. In one study in 21 patients with the homozygous form of this deficiency, weekly infusion for up to six months increased the level of this protein in the lung epithelial fluid fourfold and doubled the capacity of the lung to inhibit NE; these effects were sustained and no serious adverse reactions were reported. This finding and others support the hypothesis that decreased antineutrophil elastase protection in the lower respiratory tract due to deficiency of AAT predisposes a patient to emphysema (Wewers et al, 1987 A, 1987 B). In addition to a simple deficiency of AAT, the activity of the protein that is present may be reduced due to a change in its chemical structure (Ogushi et al, 1987).

Long-term studies are necessary to demonstrate whether continued therapy with $alpha_1$-proteinase inhibitor slows the progression of emphysema or prevents its development in AAT-deficient individuals. Emphysema normally progresses slowly in people with this enzyme deficiency, but symptoms usually develop 15 to 20 years earlier in smokers than in nonsmokers. Appropriate therapy requires cessation of smoking and may include AAT replacement.

The commercially available product, $alpha_1$-proteinase inhibitor [Prolastin], is derived from human plasma. Monthly intravenous administration of 250 mg/kg, a dose four times larger than the weekly dose, has been effective in selected individuals (Hubbard et al, 1988; Crystal, 1991). The usefulness of an aerosol preparation that is inhaled once or twice daily is being investigated (Hubbard et al, 1989 A, 1989 B).

Since some patients with the homozygous form of AAT deficiency do not develop lung disease, many experts feel that only those with evidence of emphysema should be given the enzyme; the unknown risk of long-term therapy, the possible limited availability of the enzyme, and the high cost of this agent (approximately $50,000/year) support this position. This therapy has not been shown to be useful for patients with emphysema caused by smoking who have normal levels of AAT or for patients with the heterozygous form of ATT deficiency and normal or moderately reduced AAT levels (Cohen, 1986; American Thoracic Society, 1989; Snider, 1989). See also the evaluation on $Alpha_1$-Proteinase Inhibitor.

Emphysema in Smokers. Although the pathogenesis of pulmonary emphysema in cigarette smokers is unclear, the primary mechanism probably involves accelerated proteolysis of lung tissue. Oxidants present in cigarette smoke and alveolar macrophages can inactivate or significantly impair the activity of AAT (Hubbard et al, 1987; Ogushi, et al, 1991). The role of NE and decreased AAT activity in the pathogenesis of emphysema associated with smoking is controversial (Wewers and Gadek, 1987), but improved assay procedures have demonstrated that plasma and lung NE activity may be increased in cigarette smokers (Weitz et al, 1987; Ogushi et al, 1991). Thus, it appears that an acquired AAT deficiency or impairment in the activity of lung AAT may be a major mechanism in the pathogenesis of emphysema primarily due to smoking (Wewers and Gadek, 1987; MacNee et al, 1989; McGowan and Hunninghake, 1989; Ogushi, et al, 1991).

Compensatory mechanisms that maintain the balance of protease and antiprotease levels in many smokers and in some patients with AAT deficiency are being investigated (Glaser et al, 1987). Lung damage also is accelerated in cigarette smokers because the smoke strongly attracts macrophages and neutrophils into the lung. A search is continuing for other enzyme deficiencies and factors that could be involved in the pathogenesis of emphysema associated with smoking.

Management: Therapy for emphysema is aimed at relieving bronchospasm, reducing secretions, and managing infection, hypoxemia, and heart failure if these occur. Most patients with emphysema have an element of coexisting chronic bronchitis, and inhalant $beta_2$ agonists and/or anticholinergic drugs (eg, ipratropium) may be beneficial.

Oxygen may be required for acute episodes and/or persistent hypoxia (see the evaluation). Continuous oxygen therapy (more than 19 hours a day) has prolonged survival in patients with severe airway destruction. The effectiveness of long-term oxygen therapy has been demonstrated for emphysema patients with coexisting chronic bronchitis; oxygen has not been beneficial in patients with pure emphysema (AAT deficiency). In patients with cor pulmonale and pulmonary hypertension, continuous low-flow oxygen relieves hypoxemia, reduces pulmonary vascular resistance, and improves mental status and exercise tolerance. Home oxygen therapy should be considered for patients with a resting PaO_2 of less than 55 mm Hg with room air or a PaO_2 that falls below this level upon mild exertion. Continuous oxygen is advisable if the PaO_2 is less than 50 mm Hg.

Theophylline enhances the contractility and decreases the fatigability of diaphragmatic muscle, provides chronotropic and inotropic stimulation of cardiac muscle, and lowers pulmonary and peripheral vascular resistance. In theory, these actions should be beneficial, especially in patients with cor pulmonale; however, theophylline may not relieve symptoms subjectively even when pulmonary function improves (Jenne, 1987). A plasma concentration of 10 to 15 mcg/ml is adequate and safe in most patients (Jenne, 1984).

Exercise reconditioning improves exercise tolerance and permits performance of work with less oxygen consumption. Pursed lip breathing (inhaling through the nose with slow expiration through pursed lips) improves gas exchange and may relieve dyspnea, particularly during exercise.

Lung transplantation has become an established form of therapy for treatment of end-stage lung disease due to emphysema (AAT deficiency). One-year survival rates approaching 70% have been reported (Kaiser and Cooper, 1992). Gene therapy also is being investigated as a technique to allow replacement of the AAT gene in emphysema patients with AAT deficiency. For further discussion, see Rosenfeld et al, 1991.

Investigational Agent for Chronic Bronchitis and Emphysema. Almitrine bismesylate is commonly used in Europe for the treatment of acute and chronic hypoxemia associated with COPD (Smith et al, 1987; Watanabe et al, 1989). Unlike the traditional centrally acting respiratory stimulants, this piperazine derivative acts as an agonist of peripheral chemoreceptors located on the carotid bodies. Some physicians question the value of almitrine, and further studies are necessary.

Mucolytic agents that have been used in Europe in patients with chronic bronchitis include ambroxol and sobrerol (Castiglioni and Gramolini, 1986; Guyatt et al, 1987); the role of these and other investigational mucolytics remains to be determined.

CYSTIC FIBROSIS

In this inherited disorder, which affects about 40,000 Americans, a thick mucus is produced that damages the lungs and causes respiratory failure and death, usually before age 30. Until recently, the cause of cystic fibrosis (CF) was unclear and therapy did little more than help patients remove mucus from their lungs by coughing. In the last decade, the genetic deficit responsible for CF has been discovered and its pathophysiology defined (Davis, 1991): Congenital absence of a membrane protein, the cystic fibrosis transmembrane conductance regulator (CFTR), which serves as a chloride channel in lung cell membranes, leads to decreased chloride secretion and increased reabsorption of sodium; the thick mucus produced in the dehydrated epithelium predisposes the patient to impaired mucociliary clearance. Alterations in the lung cell membranes enhance the attachment of *Pseudomonas aeruginosa*. The resultant infection induces a host inflammatory response that, together with the bacterial products elaborated by this organism, results in destruction of the lung extracellular matrix similar to that which occurs in emphysema. The protease, neutrophil elastase (NE), is released by neutrophils recruited to the lung during the immune response and is believed to be responsible for most of the damage to lung structure. This protease also damages neutrophils and cleaves complement, resulting in an impaired ability to destroy lung pathogens.

$Alpha_1$-antitrypsin (AAT) that is present in the serum and lungs of healthy individuals serves as the primary protection against NE activity by irreversibly complexing to NE and blocking its proteolytic action. In CF patients, the levels of AAT in the lungs are insufficient and are overwhelmed by the large amounts of NE released by neutrophils (Meyer et al, 1991). Large amounts of DNA derived from damaged neutrophils and other anti-inflammatory cells in the lungs contribute significantly to the high viscosity of the thick mucus (Aitken et al, 1992).

Therapy: Aggressive use of antipseudomonal antibiotics and physical therapy have been primarily responsible for the increase in the median age of death from under 10 years to 28 years in the last three decades. This may be due to the ability of these antibiotics to partially inhibit the influx of neutrophils to the lungs, which slows the rate of progression of proteolytic lung destruction by NE (Meyer et al, 1991).

Several promising approaches in the treatment of CF are being pursued. Preliminary data suggest that daily administration of alpha$_1$-proteinase inhibitor (AAT) in aerosol form inactivates NE, improves lung function, and may slow the progressive lung damage (McElvaney et al, 1991; Meyer et al, 1991). Another potentially useful treatment is administration in aerosol form of recombinant deoxyribonuclease (DNase); this enzyme digests the DNA in the thick mucus and appears to enhance mucociliary clearance and improve lung function (Hubbard et al, 1992; Aitken et al, 1992). Aerosol AAT and DNase appear to be safe and are well tolerated.

Agents that act on ion channels and either block sodium reabsorption (eg, amiloride) or increase chloride secretion (eg, adenosine triphosphate, uridine triphosphate) (Knowles et al, 1991; Davis, 1991) are in the early stages of investigation. Genetic replacement therapy also is being explored. In animal experiments, copies of the normal gene for CFTR are inserted into genetically altered, noninfectious cold viruses (adenoviruses). The altered virus carrying the gene copies is administered as an aerosol to the lungs. The inserted gene can be detected for up to six weeks in lung epithelia (Rosenfeld et al, 1992). In this manner, it may be possible to produce significant amounts of the CFTR and thus repair the damage produced by the mutation of its gene.

As with end-stage lung disease produced by emphysema, lung transplantation is being used for treatment of cystic fibrosis; similar one-year survival rates have been reported (approximately 70%) (Kaiser and Cooper, 1992).

LUNG DISORDERS IN PREMATURE INFANTS

Respiratory disorders in premature infants that are of primary concern are the respiratory distress syndrome (RDS), bronchopulmonary dysplasia (BPD), and apnea of prematurity,

RESPIRATORY DISTRESS SYNDROME. A clear association exists between the incidence of infant RDS, a major cause of neonatal mortality, and the degree of prematurity. This disorder principally affects preterm infants of less than 37 weeks' gestation. Those delivered before 30 weeks' gestation are at greatest risk and have more severe problems. Approximately 20% of premature infants develop RDS (50,000 cases in the United States annually). In the absence of surfactant, the lungs collapse and serum proteins leak into the airway. The resulting atelectasis and fibrin formation cause hyaline membranes to form.

Pathophysiology: Surfactant, a surface-active substance present in the lungs of full-term infants, is synthesized, stored, and transported within type II pneumonocytes. It is secreted in massive amounts at the time of birth with the onset of breathing and spreads quickly and forms a monolayer at the alveolar air-liquid interface. Surfactant usually is present in inadequate amounts in premature infants, and, as a result, the surface tension at the alveolar epithelial air-liquid interface remains high throughout the respiratory cycle and predisposes the infant to alveolar collapse during expiration. Functional residual volume is substantially decreased and, as a result, lung inflation is difficult.

Soon after birth, respiratory distress becomes evident and rapid breathing, sternal retractions, expiratory grunting, and flaring of the nasal alae occur. These attempts at compensation fail, and lung collapse becomes progressive. Atelectasis leads to an uneven, low ventilation-perfusion ratio, and hypoxemia develops; fatigue in the neonate eventually results in hypoventilation and hypercapnia. Oxygen deficiency combined with an elevated CO_2 level produces respiratory and metabolic acidosis. During the acute phase, progressive hypoxia and acidosis cause pulmonary vasoconstriction and reduce blood flow. During recovery, a patent ductus arteriosus and pulmonary vasodilation may result in pulmonary edema. Indomethacin trihydrate given intravenously is frequently used to constrict the ductus arteriosus. As a result of alveolar epithelial damage, increased capillary permeability causes leakage of plasma into the alveolar air spaces. Finally, with the formation of hyaline membranes, fibrinogen is converted into fibrin. The ability of the lung to exchange gases is lost and, without treatment, the exhausted and hypoxic infant will die.

During recovery from RDS, ventilation may be impaired by bronchiolar-alveolar inflammation that occurs 48 hours to seven days after birth; proteases and reactive oxygen intermediates are released and antiproteases and antioxidants in the epithelial lining fluid are reduced. Twenty to fifty percent of infants develop BPD and require prolonged oxygen therapy. The overwhelming majority of infants survive the acute episode with careful management. However, complications may occur that alter the course of the disease. Pneumothorax, pneumomediastinum, and pulmonary interstitial emphysema are most common.

Therapy: Until exogenous surfactant preparations became available, treatment was largely supportive and included correction of acidosis, circulatory support, supplementation of oxygen, assisted ventilation with positive end-expiratory pressure (PEEP), and continuous positive pressure breathing.

Dexamethasone given to the mother at least 24 hours before delivery may prevent RDS in infants of greater than 30 weeks' gestation (Avery et al, 1986 A; Van Marter et al, 1990).

It is now clear that surfactant obtained from a number of sources (eg, human amniotic fluid at cesarean delivery, synthetic preparation, animal lungs) improves the survival of premature infants with surfactant deficiency and may reduce many complications (Merritt et al, 1986; Avery et al, 1986 B; Raju et al, 1987; Avery and Merritt, 1991; Long et al, 1991 A).

None of the surfactant preparations now available or being developed has been demonstrated to be superior (Avery and Merritt, 1991; Prevost, 1991). Two marketed preparations continue to be studied in clinical trials. The first, beractant (surfactant TA) [Survanta], is obtained from minced bovine lung supplemented with dipalmitoylphosphatidylcholine (DPPC), palmitic acid, and tripalmitin; the second, Exosurf Neonatal, is a synthetic preparation that contains colfosceril palmitate (DPPC) and two emulsifying agents, cetyl alcohol and tyloxapol, to facilitate spreading and dispersal (Dechant and Faulds, 1991; Prevost, 1991).

Both preparations are administered via an endotracheal tube directly into the infant's lungs either prophylactically immediately after intubation (before RDS develops) or after development of RDS ("rescue"). In extensive clinical trials, administration both prophylactically and for rescue decreased the severity of RDS, improved oxygenation and ventilation, lowered the incidence of pneumothorax, and decreased the death rate at 28 days by 30% to 90%. The incidence of BPD was not decreased in most trials, although the number of deaths caused by BPD may be reduced (Merritt et al, 1991). Antenatal administration of corticosteroids to the mother has synergistic beneficial effects in infants receiving surfactant (Farrell et al, 1989; Polak et al, 1989).

Surfactant is more effective in reducing the incidence or severity of most complications of RDS in larger premature infants (>26 weeks' gestation and weighing >1,250 g) than in smaller, more premature infants (<26 weeks' gestation) (Long et al, 1991 B). In most premature infants, the results achieved with rescue therapy generally are equivalent to those produced by prophylactic therapy (Dunn et al, 1991; Merritt et al, 1991). In premature infants <26 weeks' gestation, prophylactic therapy may be more beneficial than rescue therapy (Kendig et al, 1991). For both prophylaxis and rescue, multiple doses may not be needed in larger premature infants or in those with mild RDS but are clearly superior to single doses in infants with severe RDS (Hoekstra et al, 1991; Speer et al, 1992). Not all premature infants respond to surfactant, which suggests that factors other than surfactant deficiency contribute to pulmonary dysfunction in some cases of RDS.

The incidence of infections, apnea of prematurity, and pulmonary hemorrhage may be increased in premature infants receiving surfactant; however, these adverse effects may not be clinically significant and are easily managed (Long et al, 1991 B). Chronic lung disease and multiple organ deficits unrelated to RDS may be consequences in very premature infants whose lives are saved by surfactant (Merritt et al, 1991). The variable results obtained in clinical trials appear to be largely due to significant differences in dosing schedules and in the patient population (ie, different degrees of prematurity or RDS). A clear assessment of these variables, as well as of surfactant's long-term effects on neurodevelopmental performance in early childhood, is lacking. In one study, prophylactic treatment was reported to improve the neurologic outcome at 1 year of age of infants who had had extremely low birth weight (Ferrara et al, 1991).

The Committee on the Fetus and Newborn of the American Academy of Pediatrics has published specific guidelines for use of exogenous surfactant preparations (American Academy of Pediatrics, 1991).

Concern that natural surfactants obtained from animal products might be contaminated with proteins or microbes and result in immunogenicity and other problems stimulated studies of artificial surfactants that do not contain protein (Avery et al, 1986 B). Single or multiple doses of the bovine lung preparation, beractant, have not been shown to cause circulating antibodies to surfactant (Whitsett et al, 1991). Whether it is more desirable to employ an artificial surfactant is unclear, because both biologically derived and artificial surfactants may have unknown benefits as well as unknown risks.

In one controlled study, administration of inositol to premature infants with RDS who were receiving parenteral nutrition during the first week of life increased survival and decreased the incidence of retinopathy of prematurity and BPD (Hallman et al, 1992). The concomitant administration of surfactant did not produce additional benefits, which suggests that inositol may act by stimulating the synthesis of surfactant or surfactant-like compounds.

Results of randomized trials of surfactant replacement for surfactant deficiency secondary to pulmonary injury or disease (eg, adult RDS) have not yet been published, although physiologic benefits have been reported in uncontrolled studies (Nosaka et al, 1990; Avery et al, 1986 B; Morton, 1990; Petty, 1990 B).

For further information, see the evaluation on surfactant preparations at the end of this chapter.

BRONCHOPULMONARY DYSPLASIA. BPD is a multifactorial disease resulting from prematurity, lung injury, nutritional deficiencies, fluid overload, oxygen toxicity, and positive pressure ventilation. This disorder is characterized by severe damage to lung tissues; an acute phase is seen after at least 20 hours of oxygen therapy and a proliferative phase occurs after at least 50 hours of oxygen therapy.

Because of the close relationship between RDS and the development of BPD, prevention of RDS should be the primary concern. After BPD has developed, most therapy is supportive. Recovery occurs slowly through reconstruction and growth of lung tissue.

A number of agents have shown promise in alleviating BPD in infants. In most studies, dexamethasone was useful and complications were minimal (Avery et al, 1985; Mammel et al, 1987; Harkavy et al, 1989; Cummings et al, 1989). The results of one large controlled multicenter study confirm the short-term benefits of this drug (Collaborative Dexamethasone Trial Group, 1991). However, its long-term value for BPD is controversial (Frank, 1991; Harkavy, 1991; Avery, 1991). In two case studies, six infants with BPD treated with dexamethasone developed gastroduodenal perforation (Ng et al, 1991; O'Neil et al, 1992), but the incidence of this potentially life-threatening adverse effect was not significantly different from that of placebo in a multicenter trial (Collaborative Dexamethasone Trial Group, 1991). The long-term danger of the catabolic effects of dexamethasone is unknown (Brownlee et al, 1992).

Theophylline or diuretics improve pulmonary function; they have additive effects when used together (Albersheim et al, 1989; Kao et al, 1987). Bronchospasm associated with BPD can be relieved by bronchodilators, such as albuterol or ipratropium bromide (Wilkie and Bryan, 1987; Rotschild et al, 1989); combined use of these two drugs may have additive benefits (Brundage et al, 1990).

A deficiency of vitamin A (retinol) occurs in premature infants. In some studies, replacement therapy to restore plasma levels of retinol to normal decreased morbidity of BPD in premature infants (Lawson and Stiles, 1987; Shenai et al, 1987, 1990; Sharma et al, 1990). Further study is required to determine the efficacy of this treatment and the safety of higher doses of retinol.

APNEA OF PREMATURITY. For a discussion of the therapy of apnea of prematurity with methylxanthines, see index entry Methylxanthines.

Drug Evaluations

BETA-ADRENERGIC AGONISTS

ALBUTEROL
[Proventil, Ventolin]

$HOCH_2$
HO— —$CHCH_2NHC(CH_3)_3$
OH

ALBUTEROL SULFATE
[Proventil, Ventolin]

This potent, selective, $beta_2$-adrenergic agonist is closely related to terbutaline and is the most commonly used agent of this class of drugs for asthma; it is generally the $beta_2$ agonist drug with which new agents are compared. The catecholamine nucleus of albuterol has been modified to decrease the rate of its degradation by sulfatase and catechol-O-methyltransferase. This drug appears to stimulate the respiratory center.

Albuterol is commonly used by inhalation for acute asthma; a metered-dose inhaler form often has been prescribed for patients requiring regular daily maintenance therapy. In this form, albuterol and other $beta_2$ agonists are drugs of choice to prevent exercise-induced asthma (Sly, 1984). The improvement in asthmatic patients is dose dependent (Spector and Gomez, 1977). In recommended doses, the durations of action of the inhalant and regular oral forms are usually similar (about four hours), but significant relief of symptoms may persist for up to eight hours after an oral dose of the regular preparation or the inhalant powder and up to 12 hours after use of the oral prolonged-release preparation. A parenteral formulation for intravenous, intramuscular, and subcutaneous administration is available in Europe.

ADVERSE REACTIONS AND PRECAUTIONS. The most common side effect of oral or inhaled albuterol is fine finger tremor, which may interfere with precise hand work. Large doses of oral or intravenous albuterol can cause mild tachycardia and a slight fall in diastolic blood pressure, but equieffective doses may cause fewer cardiovascular side effects than with most other adrenergic bronchodilators. Thus, this drug usually is safe in patients with myocardial ischemia. With intravenous use (investigational), albuterol produces minimal arrhythmia and is less likely to cause hypoxemia than isoproterenol and other nonselective beta agonists. This and other beta agonists may increase bronchial responsiveness when used in long-term maintenance therapy. Albuterol inhibits premature labor when given intravenously or orally.

This drug is classified in FDA Pregnancy Category C.

For more information on indications, adverse reactions, and precautions, see the section on Asthma, Drug Selection, in the Introduction.

PHARMACOKINETICS. Most of an oral dose is conjugated in the intestinal mucosa and liver and excreted in the urine as unchanged drug and sulfate conjugates.

DOSAGE AND PREPARATIONS.

ALBUTEROL:

Inhalation: (metered-dose inhaler) *Adults and children over 4 years,* two or three deep inhalations of aerosol one to five minutes apart. This may be repeated every four to six hours. The total daily dosage should not exceed 12 inhalations.

Proventil (Schering), ***Ventolin*** (Allen & Hanburys). Metered aerosol 90 mcg/actuation.

ALBUTEROL SULFATE:

Inhalation (nebulization): *Adults and children over 12 years,* 2.5 mg inhaled three or four times daily.

Proventil (Schering). Solution (for nebulization) 0.083% (0.83 mg/ml) in 3 ml containers and 0.5% (5 mg/ml) in 20 ml containers.

Ventolin (Allen & Hanburys). Solution (for nebulization) 0.5% (5 mg/ml) of albuterol (as 6 mg of albuterol sulfate) in 20 ml containers.

Inhalation (dry powder): *Children over 4 years and adults,* 200 or 400 mcg every four to six hours (maximum, 2.4 mg daily).

Ventolin (Allen & Hanburys). Capsules (for inhalation) 200 mcg of microfine albuterol (as sulfate) (***Rotacaps*** administered with ***Rotohaler***).

Oral: (Tablets) *Adults and children over 12 years,* 2 to 4 mg three or four times daily; *children 6 to 12 years,* initially, 2 mg three or four times a day. (Prolonged-release tablets) *Adults and adolescents over 12 years,* 4 or 8 mg every 12 hours. (Syrup) *Adults and adolescents over 14 years,* 2 to 4 mg three or four times daily; *children 6 to 14 years,* 2 mg three or four times daily; *2 to 6 years,* 0.1 mg/kg (maximum, 2 mg) three times daily.

Generic. Tablets 2 and 4 mg; syrup 2 mg of albuterol base/5 ml.

Proventil (Schering), ***Ventolin*** (Allen & Hanburys). Syrup 2 mg of albuterol (equivalent to 2.4 mg of albuterol sulfate)/5 ml; tablets 2 and 4 mg of albuterol (equivalent to 2.4 and 4.8 mg, respectively, of albuterol sulfate); tablets (prolonged-release) 4 mg ***(Proventil Repetabs).***

BITOLTEROL MESYLATE
[Tornalate]

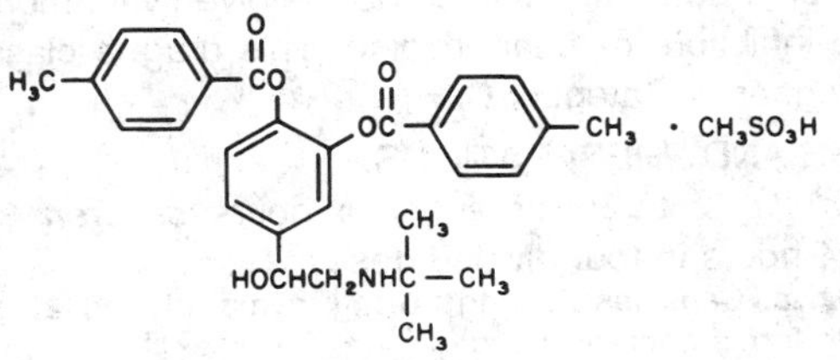

The efficacy of this inhalant $beta_2$-adrenergic agonist in asthmatic patients is similar to that of albuterol, but bitolterol is more potent (Walker et al, 1985; Orgel et al, 1985). It may be as effective as albuterol in preventing exercise-induced asthma.

When inhaled, this prodrug is activated primarily by lung esterases to the active catecholamine, colterol. Its slightly longer duration of action compared with albuterol (about five hours compared with four hours for albuterol) may be due to its greater potency and/or to the relatively slow activation process. In about 25% of patients, the duration of action of bitolterol is eight hours, which may make this drug useful in nocturnal asthma. It has been suggested that the duration of action decreases with prolonged use, but this has not been demonstrated in clinical studies.

In usual doses, bitolterol appears to produce few cardiovascular side effects. Some patients have complained about its taste. Development of tolerance is rare.

This drug is classified in FDA Pregnancy Category C.

For indications, adverse reactions, and precautions, see the section on Asthma, Drug Selection, in the Introduction.

DOSAGE AND PREPARATIONS.

Inhalation: *Adults and children over 12 years,* two or three deep inhalations one to five minutes apart. This may be repeated every four to six hours. The total daily dosage should not exceed 12 inhalations.

Tornalate (Sanofi Winthrop). Metered aerosol 370 mcg/actuation.

EPINEPHRINE
[Bronkaid Mist Solution, Primatene Mist Solution, Sus-Phrine]

EPINEPHRINE BITARTRATE
[AsthmaHaler, Bronkaid Mist Suspension, Medihaler-Epi, Primatene Mist Suspension]

EPINEPHRINE HYDROCHLORIDE
[Adrenalin Chloride]

EPINEPHRINE HYDROCHLORIDE RACEMIC
[AsthmaNefrin, microNefrin, Vaponefrin]

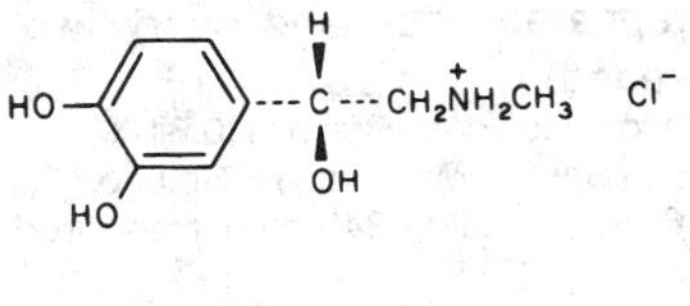

ACTIONS AND USES. The principal therapeutic effect of epinephrine in asthma is bronchodilation; vasoconstriction and relief of bronchial edema also contribute to the improvement in vital capacity.

Epinephrine is commonly administered by subcutaneous injection to relieve acute asthma. It has a short duration of action by any route and its nonspecific adrenergic actions may cause a wide variety of adverse reactions, particularly in patients with cardiac decompensation.

Effects occur immediately after subcutaneous injection, but administration may have to be repeated within 20 minutes. The duration may be extended to six to eight hours by using a suspension of crystalline epinephrine in glycerin [Sus-Phrine]. Since only about 80% of the epinephrine in this preparation is actually in suspension, the remaining 20% acts immediately. Sus-Phrine is useful after an initial dose of epinephrine hydrochloride has been administered subcutaneously and found to be effective.

A metered-dose inhaler or solution for nebulization can be employed for prophylaxis and treatment of bronchospasm, but selective $beta_2$ agonists are much longer acting. Thus, this drug should not be given routinely to prevent exacerbations during periods of remission.

ADVERSE REACTIONS AND PRECAUTIONS. Adverse reactions are relatively rare. Rapid absorption in the respiratory tract and systemic absorption of epinephrine may cause symptoms of excessive stimulation of alpha- and beta-adrenergic receptors (anxiety, tremors, palpitation, tachycardia, and headache). Such reactions are most common after intravenous administration. Rebound bronchospasm may occur, particularly after inhalation. Ventricular arrhythmias also may develop. Epinephrine generally is contraindicated in patients with hypertension, hyperthyroidism, ischemic heart disease, or cerebrovascular insufficiency. Geriatric patients and those with long-standing chronic lung disease may be given one-third to one-half the ususal dosage only with considerable caution; however, despite the risk, this drug may have to be administered, since hypoxemia from uncontrolled bronchospasm can be life-threatening.

The short duration of action of epinephrine requires repeated use, which can lead to overdosage. Refractoriness and tolerance may occur after too frequent administration, and too frequent inhalation irritates the pharyngeal and bronchial mucosa. Epinephrine should not be given with monoamine oxidase inhibitors.

Well-controlled studies have not been performed, but this drug appears to be safe in pregnant women (FDA Pregnancy Category C).

See also the section on Asthma, Drug Selection, in the Introduction.

DOSAGE AND PREPARATIONS.

Subcutaneous: *Adults,* 0.2 to 0.3 mg (0.2 to 0.3 ml of 1:1,000 solution); *children,* 0.01 mg/kg. In severe acute attacks of asthma, doses may be repeated for adults and children every 20 minutes for a maximum of three doses. Alternatively, 0.1 to 0.3 ml of an aqueous suspension of free base 1:200 [Sus-Phrine] for *adults* (maximum initial dose, 0.1 ml) or 0.005 ml/kg for *children* (maximum dose for children less than 30 kg, 0.15 ml) may be used after the initial subcutaneous dose of epinephrine hydrochloride when prolonged action is desired. Caution must be exercised, for this preparation is more concentrated than the standard preparation; administration generally should not be repeated within four hours.

EPINEPHRINE:

Generic. Solution 1:1,000 (1 mg/ml) in 1 and 30 ml containers.

Sus-Phrine (Forest). Suspension 1:200 (5 mg/ml) in 0.3 and 5 ml containers. (According to the manufacturer, this drug may be unavailable temporarily at any given time because the supply is limited.)

EPINEPHRINE HYDROCHLORIDE:

Adrenalin Chloride (Parke-Davis), ***Generic.*** Solution (sterile) 1:1,000 (1 mg/ml) in 1 and 30 ml containers.

Inhalation: 0.1% to 1% solution from a nebulizer or two inhalations from a metered-dose inhaler. However, epinephrine is not a preferred drug for this route of administration.

EPINEPHRINE:

Bronkaid Mist Solution (Winthrop Consumer). Aerosol providing 0.25 mg/inhalation (alcohol 33%) (nonprescription).

Primatene Mist Solution (Whitehall), ***Generic.*** Aerosol providing 0.2 mg/inhalation (alcohol 34%) (nonprescription).

EPINEPHRINE BITARTRATE:

AsthmaHaler (Menley & James), ***Bronkaid Mist Suspension*** (Winthrop Consumer), ***Medihaler-Epi*** (3M Pharmaceuticals), ***Primatene Mist Suspension*** (Whitehall). Aerosol providing 0.3 mg (equivalent to 0.16 mg base)/inhalation (nonprescription).

EPINEPHRINE HYDROCHLORIDE:

Generic. Solution (for inhalation) 2.25%.

Adrenalin Chloride (Parke-Davis). Solution (for nebulization) 1:100 (10 mg/ml) (nonprescription).

EPINEPHRINE HYDROCHLORIDE RACEMIC:

AsthmaNefrin (Norcliff Thayer), ***microNefrin*** (Bird), ***Vaponefrin*** (Fisons). Solution (for nebulization) 2.25% (nonprescription).

EPHEDRINE SULFATE

For chemical formula, see index entry Ephedrine, In Rhinitis.

The actions of this nonselective adrenergic agonist are similar to those of epinephrine, but its use is obsolete in most patients with asthma. Nevertheless, ephedrine should not be discontinued in patients who have been using it for a long period. Ephedrine is given orally and is not useful for severe attacks of asthma because of its weak bronchodilator action. This drug is less effective and its duration of action is shorter than that of the selective $beta_2$ agonists in patients who require continuous medication. Tachyphylaxis develops quickly.

ADVERSE REACTIONS AND INTERACTIONS. Adverse reactions are similar to those caused by epinephrine (see also the section on Drug Selection in the Introduction and the evaluation on Epinephrine). Central nervous system stimulation, manifested by nervousness, excitability, and insomnia, is common. Use of a sedative to reduce these effects is not recommended. An increase in peripheral vascular resistance may result in hypertension. The alpha-adrenergic effects of ephedrine may cause urinary retention in men with prostatic hypertrophy. Ephedrine should not be given with monoamine oxidase inhibitors or guanethidine. This drug is classified in FDA Pregnancy Category C.

DOSAGE AND PREPARATIONS.

Oral: *Adults,* 25 to 50 mg every six hours; *children,* 3 mg/kg every 24 hours in four divided doses.

Generic. Capsules 25 and 50 mg; syrup 11 and 20 mg/5 ml (both forms nonprescription).

ISOETHARINE HYDROCHLORIDE

[Bronkosol]

ISOETHARINE MESYLATE

[Bronkometer]

Isoetharine resembles isoproterenol structurally but has less $beta_1$-adrenergic activity and produces fewer adverse effects. It is widely used in metered-dose inhaler form but is less effective than the newer selective $beta_2$-adrenergic drugs. The onset of action is rapid and the duration of action is relatively short (two to three hours). Isoetharine is available only as a solution for nebulization in the United States.

This drug is classified in FDA Pregnancy Category C.

For indications, adverse reactions, and precautions, see the section on Asthma, Drug Selection, in the Introduction.

DOSAGE AND PREPARATIONS.

ISOETHARINE HYDROCHLORIDE:

Inhalation: When the 1% solution is used with a handheld nebulizer, two to four inhalations. When oxygen is used for nebulization, the usual dose is 5 mg inhaled over a period of 15 to 30 minutes. Some nebulized preparations contain sodium metabisulfate as an antioxidant. Bronkosol also contains benzalkonium chloride as a preservative. Reactions to these additives have been documented.

Generic. Solution (for nebulization) 0.08%, 0.1%, 0.125%, 0.167%, 0.17%, 0.2%, 0.25%, and 1%.

Bronkosol (Sanofi Winthrop). Solution (for nebulization) 1%.

Additional Trademark:

Arm-a-Med Isoetharine (Rhone Poulenc Rorer).

ISOETHARINE MESYLATE:

Inhalation: By handheld nebulizer, one or two inhalations. If the therapeutic response is inadequate after one minute, this dose may be repeated once and every two to four hours thereafter as needed.

Generic. Solution (for nebulization) 0.61%.

Bronkometer (Sanofi Winthrop). Solution (for nebulization, handheld) 0.61% providing 340 mcg/measured dose.

ISOPROTERENOL HYDROCHLORIDE
[Isuprel, Isuprel Mistometer, Norisodrine]

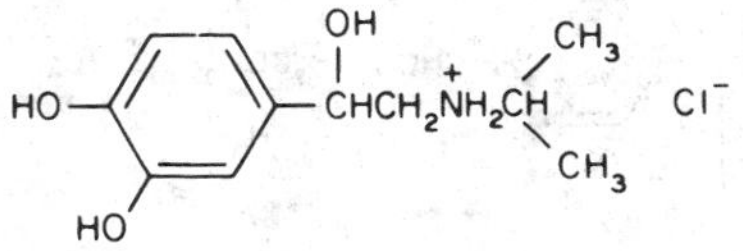

ISOPROTERENOL SULFATE
[Medihaler-Iso]

ACTIONS AND USES. Isoproterenol prevents and relieves bronchoconstriction. Because it has significant $beta_1$ activity, the rate and force of heart contractions are increased. Isoproterenol also relaxes vascular smooth muscle ($beta_2$ effect).

The duration of action (one to two hours) after inhalation is similar to that of epinephrine. For acute asthma, isoproterenol must be administered every one to two hours by inhalation. Absorption is erratic when it is given sublingually.

Intravenous isoproterenol has been used in children under 16 years in an attempt to avoid mechanical ventilation during status asthmaticus. Some physicians believe that intravenous terbutaline (investigational route) is safer and is preferable for use in pediatric patients. Isoproterenol generally should be avoided in the elderly or patients with cardiovascular disorders.

ADVERSE REACTIONS AND PRECAUTIONS. Palpitation, tachycardia and other arrhythmias, hypotension, tremor, headache, and nervousness are especially frequent with excessive use. Angina has been reported. Excessive inhalation of isoproterenol also can cause refractory bronchial obstruction that rarely is followed by sudden death, presumably from arrhythmia associated with hypoxemia. In sensitive patients, inhalation may cause a severe, prolonged attack of asthma.

Tolerance and refractoriness may develop with too frequent administration.

Isoproterenol should not be given with monoamine oxidase inhibitors or guanethidine.

This drug is classified in FDA Pregnancy Category C.

See also the section on Asthma, Drug Selection, in the Introduction.

DOSAGE AND PREPARATIONS.

Inhalation: For acute asthma, *adults,* one or two deep inhalations every one to two hours from a handheld bulb, pressure-driven nebulizer, or metered-dose inhaler; *children,* 5 to 15 deep inhalations from a handheld nebulizer containing the 1:200 solution, repeated in 10 to 30 minutes if necessary, or three to seven deep inhalations of the 1:100 dilution. Some physicians prefer to limit the dose to five inhalations of the 1:200 solution and to avoid use of the 1:100 solution. Children should be allowed to use a metered-dose inhaler only if they are instructed in proper use.

When a pressure-driven nebulizer is used, *adults,* up to 0.5 ml of the 1:200 solution or 0.3 ml of the 1:100 solution is delivered over 30 minutes with a flow of 5 to 10 L/min; however, a dilution of 1:2,000 may be preferable. Lower doses are recommended for children.

ISOPROTERENOL HYDROCHLORIDE:
Generic. Aerosol 1:400 (2.5 mg/ml); solution (for nebulization) 1:400 (2.5 mg/ml) and 1:200 (5 mg/ml).
Isuprel (Sanofi Winthrop). Solution (for nebulization) 1:100 (10 mg/ml) and 1:200 (5 mg/ml); aerosol providing 131 mcg/dose ***(Isuprel Mistometer).***
Norisodrine (Abbott). Aerosol 0.25% providing 0.12 mg/dose.
ISOPROTERENOL SULFATE:
Medihaler-Iso (3M Pharmaceutical). Aerosol 0.2% (1:500) providing 80 mcg/measured dose.

Intravenous: This route is used only in intensive care units by experienced personnel and only with great caution; it should not be used in patients over 16 years. *Children under 16 years with respiratory failure caused by asthma,* the initial infusion rate is 0.1 mcg/kg/min, increased by 0.1 mcg/kg/min at 15-minute intervals until a clinical response, a heart rate greater than 180, or an infusion rate of 0.8 mcg/kg/min is achieved.

ISOPROTERENOL HYDROCHLORIDE:
Generic. Solution 1:5,000 (0.2 mg/ml) in 5 ml containers.
Isuprel Hydrochloride (Sanofi Winthrop). Solution (sterile) 1:5,000 (0.2 mg/ml) in 1 and 5 ml containers.

Sublingual: This route is not recommended because absorption is unpredictable. The manufacturer's suggested dosage is: *Adults,* 10 to 15 mg three or four times daily (maximum, 60 mg daily); *children,* 5 to 10 mg three or four times daily (maximum, 30 mg daily).

ISOPROTERENOL HYDROCHLORIDE:
Isuprel Hydrochloride (Sanofi Winthrop). Tablets 10 and 15 mg.

METAPROTERENOL SULFATE
[Alupent, Metaprel]

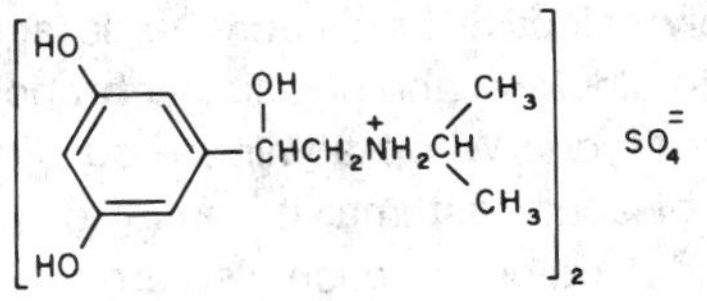

ACTIONS AND USES. This $beta_2$ agonist is widely used in nebulizers to treat acute asthma and also is available in metered-dose inhalers. Studies in animals suggest that this drug is less selective for $beta_2$ receptors than albuterol. When inhaled, metaproterenol often is as effective as albuterol; onset of action is usually within one to two minutes, and the duration is up to four hours.

Metaproterenol also can be used orally; therapy should be initiated with small doses and the amount increased gradually. Although side effects are more common when metoproterenol is given orally, this route is generally safe, and the duration of action is three to four hours.

ADVERSE REACTIONS. As with other $beta_2$ agonists, the most common adverse reactions are tremor, nervousness, and palpitations.

This drug is classified in FDA Pregnancy Category C.

For further information on indications, adverse reactions, and precautions, see the section on Asthma, Drug Selection, in the Introduction.

DOSAGE AND PREPARATIONS.

Inhalation: *Adults and children over 12 years,* two or three deep inhalations every one to five minutes. This may be repeated at four-hour intervals, but the total daily dose should not exceed 12 inhalations.

Generic. Solution (for nebulization) 0.4% and 0.6% unit dose and 5%.

Alupent (Boehringer Ingelheim). Inhaler aerosol (metered-dose) 150 mg (0.65 mg/measured dose); solution (for nebulization) 0.4% and 0.6% unit dose and 5%.

Metaprel (Sandoz). Inhaler aerosol (metered-dose) 150 mg (0.65 mg/measured dose); solution (for nebulization) 5%.

Additional Trademark:

Arm-a-Med Metaproterenol (Astra).

Oral: (Tablets and syrup) *Adults,* initially, 10 mg three or four times a day, increased gradually over two to four weeks to 20 mg three or four times daily, if needed. Limited data are available on use of the tablet form in *children.* (Syrup) *Children 6 to 9 years (under 27 kg),* 10 mg three or four times daily; *over 9 years (over 27 kg),* adult dose.

Generic, Alupent (Boehringer Ingelheim), ***Metaprel*** (Sandoz). Syrup 10 mg/5 ml; tablets 10 and 20 mg.

PIRBUTEROL ACETATE

[Maxair]

$(CH_3)_3CNCH_2CH(OH)$–[pyridine ring with N, CH_2OH, OH]

This relatively selective beta$_2$-adrenergic agonist is structurally related to albuterol and has similar bronchodilating and cardiovascular effects. When administered by inhalation for the treatment of acute asthma, its onset of action, time to peak effect, and duration of action also are similar to those of albuterol; it is less potent on a weight basis.

Minor adverse effects associated with inhalant therapy include tremors, nervousness, and headache; tachycardia, dry mouth, and palpitations have also been noted (Richards and Brogden, 1985).

Pirbuterol is classified in FDA Pregnancy Category C.

For further information on indications, adverse reactions, and precautions, see the section on Asthma, Drug Selection, in the Introduction.

DOSAGE AND PREPARATIONS.

Inhalation: *Adults and children over 12 years,* two to three inhalations (0.4 mg) repeated every four to six hours. One inhalation may be sufficient for some patients. A total daily dose of 12 inhalations should not be exceeded.

Maxair (3M Pharmaceutical). Aerosol providing 0.2 mg/inhalation.

TERBUTALINE SULFATE

[Brethaire, Brethine, Bricanyl]

$[(HO)_2C_6H_3$–$CH(OH)CH_2\overset{+}{N}H_2C(CH_3)_3]_2\ SO_4^{=}$

ACTIONS AND USES. The efficacy of this selective beta$_2$ agonist in acute asthma is similar to that of albuterol. It may be administered by metered-dose inhaler, subcutaneously, or orally. When inhaled in usual doses, terbutaline appears to have little or no effect on beta$_1$ receptors.

Inhaled terbutaline has a duration of action similar to that of albuterol (about four hours). In some studies, the oral form was reported to have a slightly longer duration of action than oral albuterol. This preparation is as effective as oral metaproterenol, but side effects are more common with the oral forms of both drugs than with the inhaled form.

Intravenous terbutaline (investigational route) has been used in children under 16 years in an attempt to avoid mechanical ventilation during status asthmaticus; some physicians believe that it is safer than intravenous isoproterenol and is preferable for use in pediatric patients.

ADVERSE REACTIONS AND PRECAUTIONS. Oral terbutaline is generally safe and well tolerated, but tremor occurs frequently, especially in the elderly. Dizziness, nervousness, fatigue, tinnitus, and palpitations are rare. When this agent is inhaled, the incidence of these adverse reactions is low. The incidence and severity of adverse reactions of subcutaneous terbutaline resemble those observed with subcutaneous epinephrine.

This is drug is classified in FDA Pregnancy Category B.

For more information on indications, adverse reactions, and precautions, see the section on Asthma, Drug Selection, in the Introduction.

DOSAGE AND PREPARATIONS. Terbutaline is not indicated for children under 12 years.

Inhalation: *Adults and children 12 years and older,* two or three deep inhalations one to five minutes apart. This may be repeated at four- to six-hour intervals. The total daily dosage should not exceed 12 inhalations.

Brethaire (Geigy). Aerosol 200 mcg/measured dose.

Oral: *Adults,* initially, 2.5 mg three times daily at approximately six-hour intervals, increased gradually over two to four weeks to 5 mg three times daily, if needed. *Children 12 years and older,* 1.25 to 2.5 mg three times daily at six- to eight-hour intervals; the dose may be increased, if needed and tolerated, to a maximum of 7.5 mg daily.

Brethine (Geigy), ***Bricanyl*** (Marion Merrell Dow). Tablets 2.5 and 5 mg (equivalent to 2.05 and 4.1 mg of free base, respectively).

Subcutaneous: *Adults,* for acute exacerbations, 0.25 mg, repeated in 15 to 30 minutes if necessary; no more than 0.5 mg should be administered in any four-hour period. *Children 12 years and older,* 0.01 mg/kg (maximum total dose, 0.25 mg). The dose may be repeated once in 30 minutes if necessary but usually is effective for four hours.

Brethine (Geigy), ***Bricanyl*** (Marion Merrell Dow). Solution (sterile) 1 mg (equivalent to 0.82 mg of free base)/ml in 2 ml containers.

XANTHINE DRUGS

THEOPHYLLINE

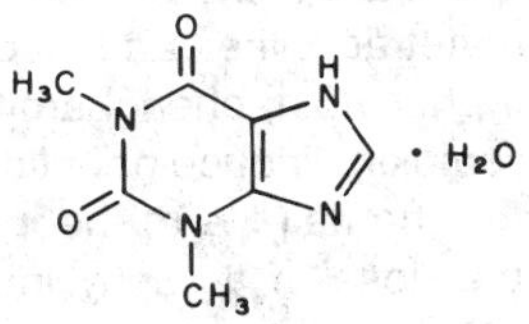

ACTIONS AND USES. In addition to its bronchodilator effect, theophylline has positive cardiac inotropic, vasodilating, and diuretic actions. This bronchodilator also stimulates diaphragmatic contraction and increases its resistance to fatigue; however, the role of diaphragmatic fatigue as a factor in obstructive lung disease has been questioned (Similowski et al, 1991). The increasing emphasis on agents that block inflammation and bronchial hyperresponsiveness, the anticipated availability of long-acting inhalant beta$_2$ agonists, and the increasing uncertainty about the value of xanthines in acute asthma suggest that the popularity of theophylline may decline in this country (Lam and Newhouse, 1990; Niewoehner, 1990; Newhouse, 1990; Jenne, 1990). However, at present theophylline remains the most widely prescribed bronchodilator in the United States for maintenance therapy in patients with moderate or severe asthma (Jenne, 1984; Weinberger, 1984; Bukowskyj et al, 1984).

Indications for use of theophylline have generally included treatment of moderate to severe exacerbations of asthma, prevention of attacks, or alleviation of signs and symptoms during periods of remission. For a discussion on its use in acute asthma, see the section on Xanthine Drugs in the Introduction.

Theophylline may be beneficial in patients with chronic bronchitis who have bronchospasm and, because of its stimulatory effects on the heart and diaphragmatic muscle, in some patients with emphysema (Jenne, 1987). Theophylline stimulates the central nervous system at the medullary level and is given to treat apnea of prematurity (see index entry Apnea of Prematurity).

The wide individual variation in theophylline plasma half-life (2 to 12 hours in adults) and the variety of factors that alter clearance (eg, drugs, age, disease, diet, fever, viral infection, smoking) necessitate frequent monitoring of serum concentrations and careful adjustment of dosage (Dwyer, 1984).

Because absorption kinetics of preparations vary, it is advisable for the physician to become familiar with only a few theophylline preparations.

ADVERSE REACTIONS AND PRECAUTIONS. Compliance may be a problem with use of theophylline, and patients should be warned that doubling a dose after missing a dose can lead to serious toxicity. Serum concentrations of 8 to 15 mcg/ml are usually efficacious and safe but may not be tolerated by an occasional patient. Side effects are primarily dose related and usually develop when serum concentrations exceed 15 mcg/ml. Serum concentrations above this level provide little added benefit and increase the frequency and severity of the above reactions.

Minor adverse effects include headache, dizziness, nervousness, insomnia, nausea, vomiting, and epigastric pain. If vomiting occurs, the serum concentration of theophylline should be measured. Patients with pre-existing multifocal atrial tachycardia have been reported to experience an increase in the frequency of arrhythmias with serum concentrations in the normal range (Marchlinski and Miller, 1985). When adverse reactions occur, the drug should be withdrawn temporarily. During initial therapy, some authorities recommend gradual increases in dose every one to three weeks to reduce minor adverse effects and improve patient compliance (Hendeles and Weinberger, 1983).

The above adverse reactions intensify and increase in number with high serum concentrations and are more frequent in the elderly. At a serum concentration above 30 mcg/ml, toxic reactions manifested by severe headache, hypokalemia, arrhythmias, persistent vomiting, agitation, hyperreflexia, fasciculations, and sometimes convulsions can occur regardless of the route of administration. Seizures, the first sign of toxicity in some patients, have rarely been reported with serum concentrations as low as 25 mcg/ml but are more common when concentrations are above 35 mcg/ml in patients receiving the drug chronically. Seizures often are refractory to therapy, and death or severe residual effects occur in a high percentage of patients. Arrhythmias usually respond to lidocaine. In children, hematemesis, central nervous system stimulation, diaphoresis, and fever may be observed with higher serum concentrations.

Theophylline may relax the gastroesophageal sphincter, leading to reflux into the esophagus and possible aggravation of asthma. Theophylline compounds increase gastric acidity and should be used cautiously, if at all, in patients with gastrointestinal ulcers or significant reflux. Bladder relaxation may cause urinary retention when outflow from the urinary tract is already compromised.

Some reports have suggested that prolonged administration of theophylline in children occasionally produces behavioral and intellectual changes that interfere with learning and adversely affect personality (Furukawa et al, 1984; Selcow et al, 1983; Rachelefsky et al, 1986). In contrast, in one study theophylline was reported to enhance fine motor coordination and did not produce significant detrimental effects on behavior or intellectual function (Joad et al, 1985). The clinical significance of effects of theophylline on learning and/or behavior in children is unclear and further studies are necessary (Weinberger et al, 1987; *Pediatr Alert*, 1987 B).

Theophylline crosses the placenta, and usual serum concentrations in the mother are well tolerated by the fetus. There is no evidence that theophylline is unsafe for pregnant women, infants of nursing mothers, or the fetus. However, neonates may sometimes show signs of theophylline toxicity such as agitation, jitteriness, tachycardia, gagging, and vomiting. This drug is classified in FDA Pregnancy Category C. Theophylline is found in breast milk; a nursing infant could receive as much as 10% of the maternal dose.

TREATMENT OF ACUTE OVERDOSE. An acute single overdose of theophylline is better tolerated than sustained high levels occurring in chronic overdosage. Aggressive treatment is necessary to prevent seizures. Initial treatment with ipecac removes theophylline from the stomach, and further absorption is prevented by administering activated charcoal. Repeated use of activated charcoal enhances elimination of the drug. Concomitant administration of a cathartic, such as sodium sulfate or sorbitol, increases the elimination of charcoal and unabsorbed theophylline.

These procedures should be instituted when the serum concentration exceeds 40 mcg/ml (Weinberger, 1984) or at lower levels when seizures or arrhythmias occur. When theophylline serum concentrations exceed 50 mcg/ml, much of the administered dose of charcoal may be lost by vomiting (Sessler et al, 1985). Extracorporeal hemoperfusion with charcoal clears theophylline more rapidly and may be used for an acute single overdose if the serum concentration of theophylline exceeds 100 mcg/ml. For chronic overdosage, hemoperfusion is recommended when serum levels exceed 60 mcg/ml and should be considered when serum levels exceed 40 mcg/ml if side effects are severe (Olson et al, 1985). However, hemoperfusion requires special equipment and services, is costly, takes time to set up, and may be hazardous to the patient.

Since intravenous phenobarbital may raise the seizure threshold in patients with dangerously high serum theophylline concentrations, prophylactic use of this drug is advisable, particularly in the agitated patient (Hendeles and Weinberger, 1983; Jenne, 1984). Arrhythmias usually respond to lidocaine.

PHARMACOKINETICS AND DRUG INTERACTIONS. Theophylline is metabolized by the liver and excreted by the kidneys. A slight alteration in the percentage of theophylline metabolized can produce large differences in clearance. Since the volume of distribution is usually constant in adults and children, changes in elimination half-life are generally inversely parallel to changes in clearance.

The mean half-life of theophylline is about 8.7 hours in nonsmoking adults, 5.5 hours in smoking adults, and 3.7 hours in children. However, the half-life varies widely among individuals and is prolonged in premature infants, elderly patients, and patients with congestive heart failure, pulmonary edema, alcoholism, liver dysfunction, obesity, viral upper respiratory infections, pneumonia, and sustained fever (Jenne, 1984).

Large doses of allopurinol and usual doses of cimetidine, oral contraceptives, fluoroquinolones (eg, ciprofloxacin, norfloxacin), and some macrolide antibiotics (eg, erythromycin, troleandomycin, clarithromycin) may reduce the clearance and prolong the plasma half-life of theophylline, possibly leading to toxicity. Influenza virus vaccine, furosemide, and beta-blocking agents also may prolong the half-life of theophylline. For concurrent use with theophylline, ranitidine is preferable to cimetidine.

The dose of theophylline may need to be decreased or the drug withdrawn in the presence of one or more of the above factors. A 50% reduction in dose of theophylline is indicated for patients receiving troleandomycin, cimetidine, or fluoroquinolones and for those with persistent high fever. The maintenance dose of theophylline should be decreased by 33% in patients also receiving erythromycin for over three days.

Antibiotics that do not affect theophylline clearance include penicillin, ampicillin, tetracycline, and cephalexin [Keflex]. Concomitant use of phenytoin, phenobarbital, rifampin, or tobacco or marijuana smoking induce hepatic drug metabolizing enzymes and shorten the half-life of theophylline by increasing its clearance; the dose of theophylline may need to be increased in these patients.

Other methylxanthines consumed in the diet, such as caffeine and theobromine, compete with theophylline at sites of metabolism. These substances appear to decrease theophylline clearance but also may provide additional bronchodilator effects. It has been estimated that two to three cups of coffee are equivalent to 200 mg of theophylline. Patients who reduce their dietary intake of methylxanthines may need increased doses of theophylline.

Most preparations of theophylline are almost completely absorbed after oral administration. Once-a-day preparations may be less completely absorbed. Some prolonged-release preparations may provide a nearly constant rate of absorption. Aminophylline suppositories are erratically and unreliably absorbed; rectal solutions are well absorbed but may be irritating.

A fatty meal may cause the premature release (dumping) of theophylline from some prolonged-release preparations (primarily Theo-24) taken within one hour of eating (Hendeles et al, 1985). Dumping apparently does not occur with Theo-Dur, a 12-hour preparation. When Uniphyl, a 24-hour preparation, is administered with a meal, absorption may be enhanced significantly (Karim et al, 1985); when it is taken on an empty stomach, absorption may not be complete. Food has been shown to decrease the bioavailability of Theo-Dur Sprinkle. Serum concentrations may fluctuate in an individual after prolonged treatment with any long-acting preparation.

Administration every 12 hours is preferable to once-daily dosing for maintenance therapy in children and in adult smokers. In rapid metabolizers, 12-hour preparations may have to be given every 8 hours and 24-hour preparations every 12 hours. Nonsmoking adults generally can be managed with either a standard (rapidly absorbed) or prolonged-release form.

MONITORING OF SERUM CONCENTRATIONS. Monitoring the serum concentrations of theophylline is important for the following reasons: (1) The safe range of serum concentrations is narrow, and individual requirements vary widely. (2) It is unclear to what extent drug interactions alter theophylline's rate of clearance. (3) The dosage can be adjusted to avoid toxicity if a serum concentration has been determined for at least the initial dose adjustment period.

Significant changes in serum concentration can result from small changes in dosage.

Steady-state levels are reached in five half-lives (two to three days), and almost 90% of steady state is reached in three half-lives. In patients receiving long-term therapy, adjustment of serum concentration should be based on response to therapy and disease status. The serum theophylline concentration should be measured when the patient's clinical condition changes or there are signs of possible toxicity (eg, vomiting).

In order to provide an adequate margin of safety and prevent toxic serum levels in both children and adults, it is generally recommended that a peak serum concentration of 8 to 15 mcg/ml be maintained (Jenne, 1984). In some individuals, lower serum levels (5 to 8 mcg/ml) are adequate. Levels above 15 mcg/ml are required occasionally in a specific patient who can tolerate the higher concentration.

DOSAGE AND PREPARATIONS. Before use, the package insert for any theophylline preparation should be consulted for more detailed information. Because absorption kinetics of preparations vary, it is advisable for the physician to become familiar with only a few theophylline preparations. Theophylline may be administered orally (as theophylline, oxtriphylline, or aminophylline), rectally (as aminophylline), or intravenously (as theophylline or aminophylline). Oral preparations containing salts of theophylline, such as aminophylline and oxtriphylline, have no advantage over oral theophylline.

A number of maintenance dosing schedules are employed. Some of the most widely quoted schedules are discussed in this section.

The standard rapidly absorbed oral preparations must be given every four to six hours to sustain effective serum concentrations in patients in whom the theophylline half-life is short (children and adult smokers); however, considerable interdose fluctuation occurs. Prolonged-release preparations increase compliance and can provide less variable serum concentrations when given every 8, 12, or 24 hours. However, since the rates of absorption and metabolism vary widely among patients and in the same patient at different times (Dederich et al, 1981), use of prolonged-release preparations does not obviate the need for clinical and laboratory monitoring. These preparations are particularly useful in patients with nocturnal symptoms. A 24-hour preparation administered in the early evening may be more useful than a 12-hour preparation to maintain the PEFR during the night (Fairshter et al, 1985; Arkinstall et al, 1987). Preparations with at least a 12-hour dosing interval are preferred by some investigators (Weinberger, 1984; Jenne, 1984). Some experts prefer 24-hour preparations.

It is generally necessary to administer prolonged-release preparations more frequently in smokers and children. *Various once-daily preparations are formulated differently; to avoid toxicity, they must be administered according to the specific instructions in the package insert.* Theo-24 is administered once daily in the morning one hour before or two hours after eating. The dose of Uniphyl should be initiated with a twice-daily schedule and the total 24-hour dose then given once daily in the evening with food.

Serum levels should be determined in all patients receiving theophylline. The following guideline is suggested: The first serum determination can be made at least 48 hours after the initial dose and subsequent dose adjustments. Ideally, the peak serum concentration should be determined 8 to 12 hours after administration of a 24-hour preparation (see package insert), four to six hours after the morning dose of a 12-hour preparation, or two hours after a standard rapidly absorbed preparation has been given. Some authorities measure only the trough concentration just before the next dose; however, this is inappropriate in children or adults who are rapid metabolizers, since the peak concentration may be more than twice that of the trough. Before serum concentrations are determined during long-term therapy, the patient should have taken the drug as prescribed with no missed or added doses for at least 48 hours.

Rapid methods now available for determination of serum theophylline levels can help determine whether a loading dose is required for immediate induction of optimal theophylline therapy. Methods for measurement in the office are available to guide dosage in ambulatory patients.

THEOPHYLLINE:

Dosages are expressed as milligrams of *anhydrous theophylline equivalents* per kilogram of ideal body weight for the elixir, syrup, liquid, oral suspension, tablet, chewable tablet, capsule, prolonged-release capsule, and tablet preparations (see below). The dose should be reduced and closely monitored in patients with liver disease or congestive heart failure; many physicians believe that the drug should be avoided altogether in these patients.

Oral: *(Standard Rapidly Absorbed Oral Formulations: Capsules, Tablets, and Liquids) Adults,* a maintenance dose of 3 mg/kg every six hours to control symptoms. In adult smokers, single doses in excess of 3 mg/kg every six hours should not be given until the theophylline serum concentration is determined. In nonsmoking adults (in whom theophylline half-lives are longer), the total daily dose is 10 to 12 mg/kg/day initially (up to a maximum of 600 mg/day, whichever is less), and a dose can be given every eight hours. This initial dosage for adults should usually result in peak theophylline serum concentrations of 8 to 15 mcg/ml. Further adjustments are made on the basis of measured serum concentrations and clinical response. The same dosages and limitations are applicable for *children*; the initial maintenance dose is 3 mg/kg every six hours.

(*Oral Formulations Including Prolonged-Release Forms*) For long-term prophylaxis, if there is no urgency and laboratory facilities for measurement of serum theophylline concentration are available, the following schedule for multistep titration of dosage has been recommended (Hendeles et al, 1992) to minimize the incidence and severity of side effects and toxic reactions.

Multistep Titration of Dosage: For *adults and children over 1 year,* the initial dose with either a standard or prolonged-release form (12- or 24-hour preparation) is 300 mg or 12 to 14 mg/kg daily (*whichever is less*) given in two or three divided doses at 8- or 12-hour intervals. This is inadequate for most patients but is unlikely to produce serious adverse effects. This dose should be increased to 400 mg after three days *if tolerated* in adults and children weighing more than 45 kg; children weighing less than 45 kg should receive 16 mg/kg/

day to a maximum of 400 mg/day. After an additional three days, *if tolerated*, the final dosage adjustment before measurement of serum concentration is as follows: the dose is increased to 600 mg/day in adults and children over 45 kg; children weighing less than 45 kg should receive 20 mg/kg/day to a maximum of 600 mg/day. For infants less than 1 year of age, the initial daily dosage can be calculated by the following regression equation: Dose (in milligrams per kilogram per day) = (0.2) (Age in weeks) + 5.0; subsequent dosage increases in this age group should be based on a peak serum concentration measurement at least three days after the start of therapy.

The final dosage adjustment (expressed as percentage change in total daily dose) is dependent on the peak theophylline serum concentration (in mcg/ml) and assessment of clinical improvement. Dosage reduction or measurement of serum concentration is indicated whenever adverse effects are present, physiologic abnormalities that can reduce theophylline clearance occur, or a drug that interacts with theophylline is added or discontinued (see the section on Pharmacokinetics and Drug Interactions). If it is not possible to measure the serum concentration, the dose should not exceed 16 mg/kg/day in children over 1 year (up to a maximum of 400 mg/day) and not more than 400 mg/day in adults.

Alternative to Multistep Titration of Dosage: Although the multistep titration of dosage described above is often quoted in the medical literature, some authorities believe that this approach is difficult to use chiefly because of intraindividual variabilities in theophylline absorption kinetics. An alternative simpler approach for adults is to begin therapy with 300 to 400 mg/24 hours (adaptation phase) for several days and then to increase to conservative full doses of 500 to 600 mg/day (depending on stature) in nonsmokers, patients with cor pulmonale, and the elderly and to 800 to 900 mg/day in smokers. Following institution of a conservative full-dose schedule, the serum concentration is measured at least 48 hours after no missed doses and a final dose adjustment is made to achieve serum levels between 8 to 15 mcg/ml (Jenne, 1984). In general, some smokers may require a slightly larger daily dose.

Serum Concentration (mcg/ml)	Dosage Adjustment
7.5 or less	Increase the dose 25%. Remeasure the serum theophylline concentration for guidance in further dosage adjustment.
7.5 to 10	If tolerated, increase the dose by 25%.
10 to 15	If tolerated, maintain the dose. Remeasure serum theophylline concentration at 6- to 12-month intervals.
15 to 20	Consider a 10% decrease in dose to provide a greater margin of safety.
20 to 25	Decrease the dose 10% to 25%. Remeasure the serum concentration after 3 days.
25 to 30	Skip the next dose and decrease subsequent doses at least 25%. Remeasure the serum concentration after 3 days.
30 or above	Skip the next 2 doses and decrease subsequent doses by 50%. Remeasure the serum theophylline concentration for guidance in further dosage adjustment. (See the section on Treatment of Acute Overdose.)

STANDARD PREPARATIONS:

Generic. Elixir and solution 26.7 mg/5 ml; tablets 100, 200, and 300 mg.

Aerolate (Fleming). Liquid 50 mg/5 ml.

Bronkodyl (Sanofi Winthrop). Capsules 100 and 200 mg.

Elixophyllin (Forest). Capsules 100 and 200 mg; elixir 26.5 mg/5 ml (alcohol 20%).

Quibron-T (Apothecon). Tablets 300 mg.

Slo-Phyllin (Rhone-Poulenc Rorer). Syrup 26.5 mg/5 ml; tablets 100 and 200 mg.

Theoclear 80 (Central), ***Theostat 80*** (Laser). Syrup 80 mg/15 ml.

Theolair (3M Pharmaceutical). Liquid 26.5 mg/5 ml; tablets 125 and 250 mg.

PROLONGED-RELEASE PREPARATIONS:

Generic. Tablets 100, 200, 300, and 450 mg (12 to 24 hours).

Aerolate (Fleming). Capsules 65 (***III***), 130 (***JR***), and 260 (***SR***) mg (8 to 12 hours).

Constant-T (Geigy). Tablets 200 and 300 mg (8 to 12 hours).

Duraphyl (Forest). Tablets 100, 200, and 300 mg (12 hours).

Elixophyllin SR (Forest). Capsules 125 and 250 mg (8 to 12 hours).

Quibron-T/SR (Apothecon). Tablets 300 mg (8 to 12 hours).

Respbid (Boehringer Ingelheim). Tablets 250 and 500 mg (8 to 12 hours).

Slo-bid (Rhone-Poulenc Rorer). Capsules 50, 75, 100, 125, 200, and 300 mg (8 to 12 hours).

Slo-Phyllin (Rhone-Poulenc Rorer). Capsules 60, 125, and 250 mg (8 to 12 hours).

Theo-24 (Whitby). Capsules 100, 200, and 300 mg (24 hours).

Theobid (Whitby). Capsules 130 (***Jr.***) and 260 mg (12 hours).

Theochron (Inwood). Tablets 100, 200, and 300 mg (12 to 24 hours).

Theoclear LA (Central). Capsules 130 and 260 mg (12 hours).

Theo-Dur (Key). Tablets 100, 200, 300, and 450 mg (8 to 24 hours).

Theo-Dur Sprinkle (Key). Capsules 50, 75, 125, and 200 mg (12 hours).

Theolair-SR (3M Pharmaceutical). Tablets 200, 250, 300, and 500 mg (8 to 12 hours).

Theo-Sav (Savage). Tablets 100, 200, and 300 mg (8 to 24 hours).

Theovent (Schering). Capsules 125 and 250 mg (12 hours).

Theox (Carnrick). Tablets 100, 200, and 300 mg (12 to 24 hours).

T-Phyl (Purdue Frederick). Tablets 200 mg (8 to 12 hours).

Uniphyl (Purdue Frederick). Tablets 400 mg (24 hours).

NOTE FOR ONCE-A-DAY FORMS: If doses of Theo-24 exceed 900 mg/day or 13 mg/kg/day (whichever is less), this product should be administered at least one hour before a meal. Uniphyl should be taken with meals and at the same time each day. Fasting patients may not absorb the total daily dose of 24-hour preparations completely. Once-a-day forms are usually administered at 8 AM or in the evening. Increasing evidence suggests that preparations other than Theo-24 given in the evening provide higher early morning serum levels of theophylline for patients with nocturnal bronchospasm (Rivington et al, 1985; Fairshter et al, 1985; Arkinstall et al, 1987).

Intravenous: See Aminophylline.

Theophylline and 5% Dextrose (Abbott). 0.4 mg/ml in 1,000 ml containers, 0.8 mg/ml in 500 and 1,000 ml containers, 1.6 mg/ml in 250 and 500 ml containers, 2 mg/ml in 100 ml containers, 3.2 mg/ml in 250 ml containers, and 4 mg/ml in 50 and 100 ml containers.

AMINOPHYLLINE:

Aminophylline formulations vary from 79% to 86% in their equivalence to anhydrous theophylline. Therefore, it is necessary to follow the manufacturers' recommended dose for the individual product or to calculate the appropriate dose on the basis of anhydrous theophylline equivalents: 100 mg of the 86% formulation = 86 mg anhydrous theophylline; 100 mg of the 79% formulation = 79 mg anhydrous theophylline. The following doses are given for milligrams of anhydrous theophylline per kilogram of body weight. Solutions of aminophylline or theophylline must be diluted properly and injected or infused very slowly; rapid intravenous infusion has caused fatal cardiovascular reactions (Jenne, 1984).

Intravenous: *Adults and children,* for an acute attack, a loading dose of 6 mg/kg aminophylline (5 mg/kg theophylline) is administered using a slow intravenous drip (rate no more than 25 mg/min). The loading dose should be reduced by 50% if the patient has received theophylline within the previous 24 hours. However, if the patient already is being maintained on theophylline and one of the new rapid methods of determining serum concentrations is available, it is advisable to determine the serum concentration first and adjust the dose as needed, keeping in mind that an additional dose of 1 mg/kg usually will raise the theophylline level about 2 mcg/ml.

After the loading dose, the following amounts of aminophylline (mg/kg/hr) are infused for maintenance: *children less than 9 years,* 1; *children over 9 years and healthy adults who smoke*, 0.8; *healthy adults who do not smoke,* 0.5; *patients with cardiac decompensation or liver dysfunction,* 0.2. The maintenance dose should be reduced if nausea, vomiting, headache, tachycardia, or other toxic effects appear or the serum theophylline concentration exceeds 20 mcg/ml. Following the loading dose, measurement of serum concentrations will indicate the need for any adjustment in dose. Levels measured at 18 to 24 hours may warn of impending toxic levels before they occur (Jenne, 1984).

Generic. Solution (intravenous) 25 mg/ml in 10, 20, 100, and 200 ml containers.

Rectal: The rectal solution is absorbed reliably and rapidly and is safe for occasional use, but routine administration cannot be recommended. *Suppositories are not recommended because of their erratic absorption.*

(*Retention Unit*) *Adults,* 5 ml (equivalent to 255 mg theophylline) one to three times daily. The total daily dose should not exceed the average therapeutic dose limits (see oral dosage for theophylline) or a serum theophylline concentration of 15 mcg/ml. *Children,* 5 mg/kg (as theophylline) administered no more often than every six hours. The total daily dose should be based on age and determined as for adults.

Generic. Suppositories 250 and 500 mg.

Oral: Dosage is based on theophylline equivalents. Because of occasional hypersensitivity to aminophylline, prolonged-release theophylline preparations are preferred for oral use.

Generic. Liquid 105 mg/5 ml; tablets (plain, enteric-coated) 100 and 200 mg.

Phyllocontin (Purdue-Frederick). Tablets (prolonged-release) 225 mg (12 hours).

OXTRIPHYLLINE (Theophylline 64% with Choline 36%):

Oral: Dosage is based on theophylline equivalents.

Generic. Elixir 100 mg/5 ml; syrup (pediatric) 50 mg/5 ml; tablets 100 and 200 mg.

Choledyl (Parke-Davis). Elixir 100 mg/5 ml (alcohol 20%); syrup (pediatric) 50 mg/5 ml; tablets 100 and 200 mg; tablets (prolonged-release) 400 and 600 mg (***Choledyl SA***).

DYPHYLLINE

[Dilor, Lufyllin, Neothylline]

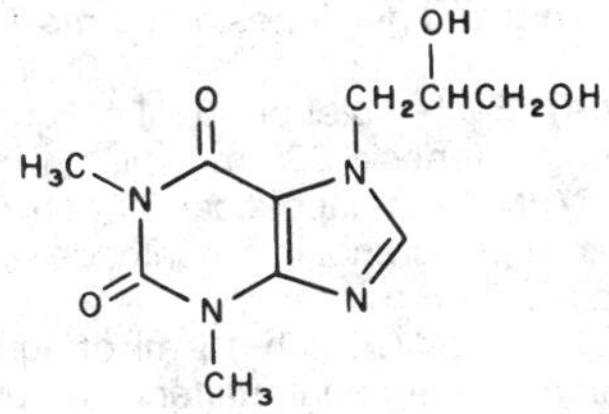

Dyphylline is much less potent than theophylline and is rarely used. Doses about five times larger than those of theophylline are required to produce equivalent serum concentrations (Lawyer et al, 1980). Theophylline serum assays cannot be used to monitor dyphylline levels (Bussey, 1981). Since the range of therapeutic plasma concentrations for dyphylline is not yet as clearly defined as that for theophylline, the latter is preferred for chronic and acute asthma, particularly when intravenous administration is required.

This drug may be administered orally, intramuscularly, or intravenously (investigational). It is rapidly eliminated unchanged in the urine; the half-life is about two hours (one-half that of theophylline). This may be extended by administering oral probenecid 1 g one-half hour before dyphylline is used (May and Jarboe, 1981).

Adverse reactions are similar to those produced by theophylline, although nervousness, dizziness, and palpitations may be less prominent.

DOSAGE AND PREPARATIONS. The following doses are recommended by the manufacturers.

Intramuscular: *Adults*, 250 to 500 mg every six hours; the dosage should be individualized on the basis of the condition and response of the patient. *Children,* dosage has not been established.

Dilor (Savage), ***Lufyllin*** (Wallace), ***Generic***. Solution (for intramuscular use only) 250 mg/ml in 2 (***Dilor, Lufyllin***) and 10 ml containers.

Oral: *Adults,* 15 mg/kg every six hours; the dosage should be individualized on the basis of the condition and response of the patient. *Children,* dosage has not been established.

Dilor (Savage). Elixir 53.3 mg/5 ml (alcohol 18%); tablets 200 and 400 mg.

Lufyllin (Wallace). Elixir 33.3 mg/5 ml (alcohol 20%); tablets 200 and 400 mg.

Neothylline (Lemmon). Tablets 200 and 400 mg.

MIXTURES

Mixtures used in asthma and bronchitis often contain an expectorant or decongestant and one or two bronchodilators.

There is no evidence that expectorants or mucolytics are effective in acute asthma. Iodides are not recommended as expectorants for children or women of childbearing age by the Committee on Drugs of the American Academy of Pediatrics. For these reasons, the use of the following combination products is not advised.

Generic. Each capsule or 15 ml of liquid contains theophylline (anhydrous) 150 mg and guaifenesin 90 mg.
Asbron G (Sandoz). Each tablet or 15 ml of elixir contains theophylline sodium glycinate 300 mg (equivalent to 137 mg theophylline) and guaifenesin 100 mg (alcohol 15%, elixir).
Brondecon (Parke-Davis). Each tablet or 10 ml of elixir contains oxtriphylline 200 mg and guaifenesin 100 mg (alcohol 20%, elixir).
Dilor-G (Savage). Each tablet or 10 ml of liquid contains dyphylline 200 mg and guaifenesin 200 mg.
Duo-Medihaler (3M Pharmaceutical). Each measured dose of aerosol contains isoproterenol hydrochloride 0.16 mg and phenylephrine bitartrate 0.24 mg.
Elixophyllin-GG (Forest). Each 15 ml of liquid contains anhydrous theophylline 100 mg and guaifenesin 100 mg.
Elixophyllin-KI (Forest), ***Generic.*** Each 15 ml of elixir contains theophylline (anhydrous) 80 mg and potassium iodide 130 mg (alcohol 10%).
Lufyllin-GG (Wallace). Each tablet or 30 ml of elixir contains dyphylline 200 mg and guaifenesin 200 mg (alcohol 17%, elixir).
Neothylline GG (Lemmon). Each tablet contains dyphylline 200 mg and guaifenesin 200 mg.
Quibron (Apothecon), ***Generic.*** Each capsule contains theophylline (anhydrous) 150 or 300 mg and guaifenesin 90 or 180 mg; each 15 ml of liquid contains theophylline (anhydrous) 150 mg and guaifenesin 90 mg.
Slo-Phyllin GG (Rhone-Poulenc Rorer), ***Generic.*** Each capsule or 15 ml of syrup contains theophylline (anhydrous) 150 mg and guaifenesin 90 mg.
Synophylate GG (Central). Each 15 ml of syrup contains theophylline sodium glycinate 300 mg and guaifenesin 100 mg (alcohol 10%).
Theo-Organidin (Wallace). Each 15 ml of elixir contains theophylline (anhydrous) 120 mg and iodinated glycerol 30 mg (alcohol 15%).

Other types of mixtures used in asthma and bronchitis contain a barbiturate or antianxiety agent, one or more bronchodilators, and, in some preparations, an expectorant. Use of such fixed-dose combinations is inadvisable because the efficacy of barbiturates and antianxiety agents in bronchial disorders is not documented, and barbiturates may increase the metabolism of corticosteroids if the latter are given concomitantly.

Adrenergic drugs available in mixtures are those with the least beta$_2$ specificity. The undesirable central nervous system stimulant action of ephedrine may be synergistic with that of theophylline. Adjustment of the dose of theophylline is especially difficult or impossible with fixed-dose combination products.

Some physicians elect not to substitute single-entity products in patients with chronic asthma who have responded satisfactorily for an extended period to one of the following combination products; however, the overall disadvantages of these types of mixtures should be considered before initiating therapy in asthmatic patients.

Bronkaid (Winthrop Consumer). Each tablet contains ephedrine sulfate 24 mg, guaifenesin 100 mg, and theophylline 100 mg (nonprescription).
Bronkolixir (Sanofi Winthrop), ***Generic.*** Each 5 ml of elixir contains theophylline 15 mg, ephedrine sulfate 12 mg, phenobarbital 4 mg, and guaifenesin 50 mg (alcohol 19%) (nonprescription).
Bronkotabs (Sanofi Winthrop). Each tablet contains theophylline 100 mg, ephedrine sulfate 24 mg, phenobarbital 8 mg, and guaifenesin 100 mg (nonprescription).
Marax (Roerig), ***Generic.*** Each tablet contains theophylline 130 mg, ephedrine sulfate 25 mg, and hydroxyzine hydrochloride 10 mg.
Marax-DF (Roerig). Each 5 ml of syrup contains theophylline 32.5 mg, ephedrine sulfate 6.25 mg, and hydroxyzine hydrochloride 2.5 mg (alcohol 5%).
Mudrane GG (Poythress). Each 5 ml of elixir contains theophylline 20 mg, ephedrine hydrochloride 4 mg, phenobarbital 2.5 mg, and guaifenesin 26 mg (alcohol 20%); each tablet contains aminophylline 130 mg, ephedrine hydrochloride 16 mg, phenobarbital 8 mg, and guaifenesin 100 mg.
Primatene Tablets (Whitehall). Each tablet contains theophylline anhydrous 130 mg and ephedrine hydrochloride 24 mg (nonprescription).
Quibron Plus (Bristol). Each capsule or 15 ml of elixir contains theophylline 150 mg, ephedrine hydrochloride 25 mg, butabarbital 20 mg, and guaifenesin 100 mg (alcohol 15%, elixir).
Tedral (Parke-Davis). Each tablet contains theophylline 118 mg, ephedrine hydrochloride 24 mg, and phenobarbital 8 mg; each tablet (prolonged-release) contains theophylline 180 mg, ephedrine hydrochloride 48 mg, and phenobarbital 25 mg ***(Tedral SA)***

ANTI-INFLAMMATORY CORTICOSTEROIDS

BECLOMETHASONE DIPROPIONATE

[Beclovent, Vanceril]

ACTIONS AND USES. Beclomethasone dipropionate is an esterified chlorinated analogue of betamethasone. This potent, lipid-soluble corticosteroid acts locally on the respiratory mucosa. Very low doses are delivered by a metered-dose inhaler (42 mcg/inhalation), and the absorbed drug is inactivated rapidly, which markedly reduces the incidence of hypothalamic-pituitary-adrenal (HPA) axis suppression or serious adverse reactions.

This potent inhalant corticosteroid is the standard with which other drugs of this class are compared (Brogden et al, 1984). Its use allows the elimination of oral steroids or a reduction in their dosage in some patients with severe steroid-dependent asthma. Symptoms of daytime or nocturnal asthma may be prevented. Most authorities now advocate use of this or other inhalant steroids as first-line therapy for maintenance in patients with mild to moderate asthma (Barnes, 1989; Cockroft and Hargreave, 1990; Juniper et al, 1990;

Lorentzson et al, 1990; Haahtela et al, 1991; Reed, 1991; Waalkens et al, 1991; *J Allergy Clin Immunol*, 1991). See the Introduction for further discussion.

Severe asthma should be brought under optimal control with an oral corticosteroid before an inhalant corticosteroid preparation is utilized. Patients who require less than 10 mg/day of oral prednisone or the equivalent often can be converted to an inhalant corticosteroid; conversion is usually much more difficult in patients who require 20 mg/day or more of the oral preparation, but the oral dose may be reduced.

Caution must be exercised in the transfer from an oral corticosteroid to an inhaled corticosteroid. Patients are at great risk from adrenal crises during the transfer; the degree of HPA axis suppression caused by the oral corticosteroid may not be appreciated. Early morning cortisol levels may be monitored after slow withdrawal of the systemic steroid, but a normal level does not always indicate adequate adrenal responsiveness.

If patients undergo stressful situations (surgery, trauma, respiratory infection, or an exacerbation of severe asthma), a short course of an oral or intravenous steroid in full therapeutic doses is indicated.

Beclomethasone inhalers are being developed that are inspiration- or actuator-activated. In England and Canada, use of a high-dose beclomethasone inhaler that provides five times more drug (250 mcg/inhalation) has allowed some patients to reduce the frequency of administration to twice daily and to reduce or discontinue oral medication (Barnes, 1989; Cockroft, 1990 B). Some patients also can use the regular beclomethasone inhaler (42 mcg per puff) twice daily.

ADVERSE REACTIONS AND PRECAUTIONS. Inhalant corticosteroids are generally safe. Patients using beclomethasone aerosol occasionally complain of throat irritation. Dysphonia, sore throat, or dryness of the mouth may limit patient compliance. Use of an adrenergic aerosol about five minutes before inhalation of the steroid has been recommended to enhance bronchial distribution and prevent cough and throat irritation; however, this practice probably should be reconsidered because the dangers of regular daily administration of $beta_2$ agonists are not known. (See the section on Drug Selection, Beta-Adrenergic Agonists.) The reported incidence of candidal infection of the oropharynx or larynx varies considerably but may be as high as 15%. To prevent candidiasis, patients should be instructed to use a spacer device and gargle with water after inhalation. Antifungal therapy and reduction of the dose may be required; discontinuation of beclomethasone therapy is rarely necessary.

Because interference with bone formation and childhood growth have been reported (Toogood and Hodsman, 1991; Storr, 1991; Wales et al, 1991), questions have arisen about the long-term safety of this and other inhalant steroids. More data are needed to determine the incidence and severity of these effects.

Although inhalant doses of beclomethasone dipropionate below 1.6 mg/day or the equivalent do not usually produce systemic adverse reactions or affect HPA axis function, these can occur at doses as low as 1 mg/day. In most patients, doses between 1.6 and 2 mg/day also may be safe, but some systemic absorption is likely (Clark, 1985).

The substitution of inhaled drug for oral corticosteroids can cause withdrawal symptoms, such as muscle and joint pain, lassitude, tiredness, headache, mental depression, nausea, vomiting, and anorexia (Brogden et al, 1984). Exacerbation of conditions previously controlled by systemic steroid therapy (eg, allergic rhinitis, eczema, nasal polyposis) has been observed. Most of these disorders respond to appropriate topical therapy.

For further discussion of indications, adverse reactions, and precautions, see the section on Asthma, Drug Selection, in the Introduction.

DOSAGE AND PREPARATIONS.

Oral Inhalation: *Adults,* two to four inhalations three or four times daily or four inhalations twice daily. The usual maximum recommended dose is 840 mcg/day, but doses up to 1.6 mg/day have been used without systemic reactions or effects on HPA axis function; higher doses (up to 2 mg/day) may be safe, but some systemic absorption is more likely (Clark, 1985). *Children 6 to 12 years,* the usual dosage is one or two inhalations three or four times daily; the maximum recommended dose is 420 mcg/day. There are insufficient data to recommend a dosage for *children under 6 years*.

The use of a spacer attachment between the mouth and the metered-dose inhaler usually increases the efficiency of drug delivery in patients with improper technique and may decrease the occurrence or severity of oral candidiasis and throat irritation.

Beclovent (Allen & Hanburys), ***Vanceril*** (Schering). Aerosol providing 42 mcg/actuation.

BUDESONIDE (Investigational drug)

[Pulmicort]

This investigational nonhalogenated corticosteroid has a higher ratio of topical to systemic activity and greater potency than beclomethasone dipropionate, triamcinolone acetonide, or flunisolide (Clissold and Heel, 1984). Inhalation of doses of 200 to 800 mcg/day is approximately as effective as doses of 400 to 800 mcg/day of beclomethasone in adults and children with moderate to severe chronic asthma. In England and Canada, use of this high-dose inhalant steroid has allowed some patients to reduce the frequency of administration to twice daily and to reduce or discontinue oral medication (Barnes, 1989; Cockroft, 1990 B). Indications, adverse reactions, and precautions resemble those of beclomethasone dipropionate.

Pulmicort (Astra).

FLUNISOLIDE
[AeroBid]

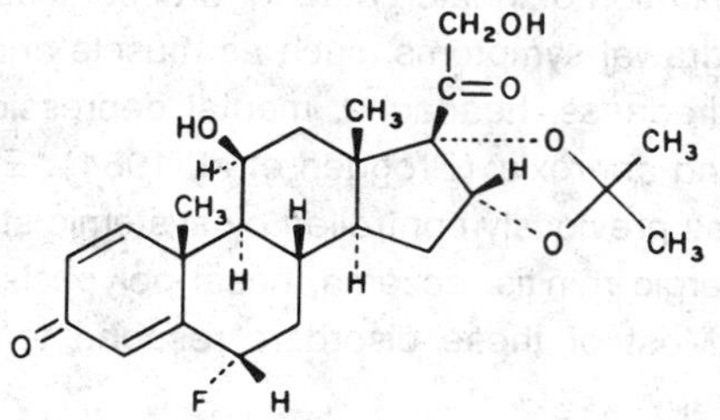

The indications for this inhalant halogenated corticosteroid are similar to those for inhaled beclomethasone. Twice-daily administration appears to be effective in most patients and the incidence of oral candidiasis and dysphonia may be less than with inhaled beclomethasone (Orgel et al, 1983).

For additional information on indications, adverse reactions, and precautions, see the evaluation on Beclomethasone Dipropionate and the section on Asthma, Drug Selection, in the Introduction. This drug is classified in FDA Pregnancy Category C.

DOSAGE AND PREPARATIONS.

Oral Inhalation: *Adults and children 6 years and older*, two to four inhalations two or three times daily. The maximum daily dose should not exceed 2 mg. There are insufficient data to recommend a dosage for *children under 6 years*.

AeroBid (Forest). Aerosol providing approximately 250 mcg/actuation.

TRIAMCINOLONE ACETONIDE
[Azmacort]

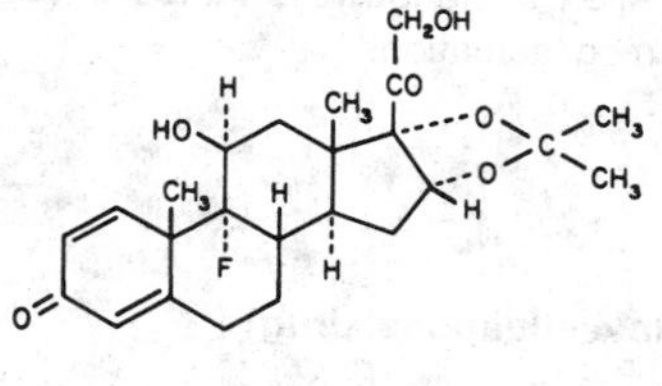

The indications for this inhalant halogenated corticosteroid are similar to those for inhaled beclomethasone. The spacer attachment provided with the unit may deliver a greater percentage of drug to the lungs and less to the oropharyngeal cavity, which may enhance the response in poorly coordinated patients who fail to show benefit when using a corticosteroid MDI without a spacer device. Fewer coughing paroxysms may occur with this preparation than with beclomethasone dipropionate (Bernstein et al, 1982).

For additional information on indications, adverse reactions, and precautions, see the evaluation on Beclomethasone Dipropionate and the section on Asthma, Drug Selection, in the Introduction. Triamcinolone is classified in FDA Pregnancy Category C.

DOSAGE AND PREPARATIONS.

Oral Inhalation: *Adults*, two to four inhalations three or four times daily. The daily dose should not exceed 1.6 mg. *Children 6 to 12 years*, one or two inhalations three or four times daily. The daily dose should not exceed 1.2 mg. There are insufficient data to recommend a dosage for *children under 6 years*.

Azmacort (Rhone-Poulenc Rorer). Aerosol providing approximately 100 mcg/actuation.

ANTIALLERGY DRUG

CROMOLYN SODIUM
[Intal]

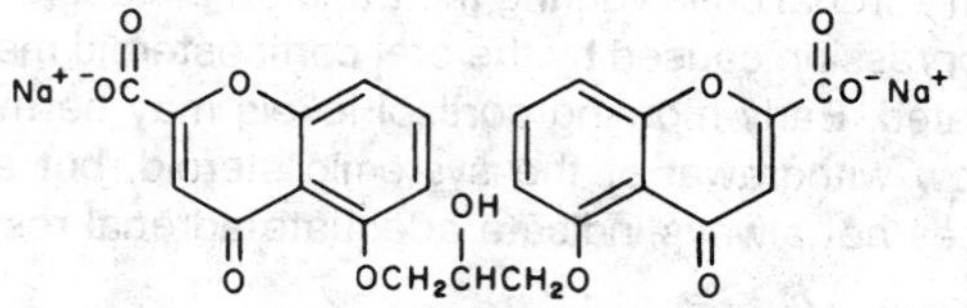

ACTIONS. Cromolyn inhibits both immediate and late asthmatic responses after exposure to a variety of allergens and appears to affect both large and small airways by a mechanism that is not clearly understood. Cromolyn has mast cell stabilizing properties. Major mechanisms may involve inhibition of mediator release from mast cells and attenuation or blockade of respiratory neuronal reflexes (Murphy, 1987). These actions may in part be due to inhibition of calcium transport. Cromolyn may also inhibit recruitment of inflammatory cells, such as eosinophils and neutrophils, to the lung epithelium (Kay, 1987; Holgate, 1986) and thus may have anti-inflammatory effects. Cromolyn reduces bronchial hyperresponsiveness; it also may diminish the effects of reflex mediated asthma and diurnal swings of bronchial lability. It has no adrenergic, antihistaminic, or corticosteroid-like actions and little bronchodilator activity.

USES. Unlike other drugs discussed in this chapter, cromolyn sodium is used only to prevent asthma attacks. It is as effective as theophylline for prophylaxis of mild to moderate asthma and, because of its greater safety, is preferred to theophylline (Marks, 1987; Eigen et al, 1987; *Pediatr Alert*, 1987 A). Numerous well-controlled clinical trials, including large multicenter studies, have demonstrated that a large proportion of children with chronic asthma experience either partial or complete protection after oral inhalation of cromolyn (Shapiro and König, 1985). Although some experts believe it is more useful for children, considerable evidence has accumulated demonstrating cromolyn's effectiveness as a first-line antiasthmatic agent in adults (Bernstein, 1985 A, 1985 B; Eigen et al, 1987; Blumenthal et al, 1988; Petty et al, 1989). Some authorities recommend that a trial of cromolyn sodium be considered in every patient with chronic mild to moderate asthma. It has been suggested that its early use for maintenance could decrease the number of exacerbations and prevent progression to severe disease (Barnes, 1989; Cockroft, 1990 B; Cockroft and Hargreave, 1990).

Cromolyn prevents allergic asthma, some cases of nonallergic asthma, and asthma induced by exercise, cold air, or sulfur dioxide. Prophylaxis for exercise- or irritant-induced bronchospasm may be enhanced by continuous therapy. Optimal effects are achieved by giving cromolyn 30 minutes before exposure to a known allergen, 15 minutes before exercise, and about one week before high allergen exposure.

In patients with severe asthma, who respond poorly to individual drugs, benefits may be enhanced by combining cromolyn with a bronchodilator (theophylline or a $beta_2$ agonist) and/or corticosteroid. If combined therapy is prescribed, the physician must individualize the dose of each drug to obtain maximal benefit with minimal adverse reactions. Patients who respond to lower doses of systemic steroid while taking cromolyn must be observed carefully when the latter drug is discontinued. If asthma worsens in these patients, the dose of systemic steroid may be increased temporarily and cromolyn therapy reinstituted for maintenance.

Cromolyn has limited value when asthma is associated with emphysema and/or chronic bronchitis. It is ineffective in acute asthma. If an acute attack occurs, conventional therapy should be instituted immediately but cromolyn should be continued.

The three forms of cromolyn available for inhalant administration have similar efficacy. The metered-dose inhaler delivers 0.8 mg of cromolyn/inhalation, which is much less than the amount delivered with the Spinhaler. Many therapeutic failures are due to incorrect inhalation technique utilizing the Spinhaler. With improved drug delivery resulting from use of other inhalant devices, cromolyn is being employed more frequently. Wheezing and bronchospasm associated with use of the Spinhaler do not occur with the metered-dose inhaler or nebulizer and compliance is enhanced. The latter devices are particularly beneficial in young children and patients who cannot tolerate the powder because of cough. The combination of cromolyn and a beta-adrenergic drug in the same nebulizing solution is commonly used.

See also the section on Drug Selection in the Introduction.

ADVERSE REACTIONS AND PRECAUTIONS. Based on the extensive clinical experience that has accumulated in many countries, cromolyn appears to have an unusual record of safety. Serious adverse effects are rare. Urticaria, maculopapular rashes, myositis, and gastroenteritis seldom occur and disappear when the drug is withdrawn. Reversible eosinophilic pneumonia has been associated with administration of cromolyn in a few patients.

Occasionally, transient coughing, bronchospasm, throat irritation, dizziness, nausea, vomiting, hoarseness, and wheezing occur after oral inhalation. However, some of these symptoms also developed in patients inhaling a placebo and may be caused by the powder rather than by cromolyn. An inhaled beta agonist used five minutes prior to inhalation of cromolyn may be helpful for patients who develop coughing or wheezing following use of this drug. Throat irritation and hoarseness can be minimized by rinsing the mouth with water after inhalation.

No alterations in the results of hematologic, urinary, hepatic and renal function tests, chest roentgenograms, or electrocardiograms have been reported in patients receiving the drug continuously for as long as five years.

The safety of cromolyn during pregnancy has not been established unequivocally, but no damaging effects on the fetus have been reported; therefore, cromolyn is advocated as first-line therapy during pregnancy. No teratogenic effects have been observed in animals, even after daily intravenous administration of enormous doses of cromolyn throughout pregnancy; however, increased fetal resorption and decreased fetal weight were observed with doses that produced toxic effects in the mother (FDA Pregnancy Category B).

Tolerance usually does not develop with long-term use.

PHARMACOKINETICS. Oral absorption of cromolyn sodium is minimal and the drug is not active by this route. After inhalation, 8% to 10% is absorbed into the blood stream (primarily by the lung but also by the gastrointestinal tract). The fraction of cromolyn absorbed following inhalation of 20 mg does not appear to exert any generalized systemic effects. Most of the absorbed portion is excreted unchanged in the bile and urine within a few days; none appears to undergo metabolic degradation. The unabsorbed portion (approximately 80%) is recovered from the feces.

Following inhalation, the maximal plasma level is attained within several minutes, and the plasma half-life is 1 to 1.5 hours. The duration of action is four to six hours.

DOSAGE AND PREPARATIONS. For prophylactic therapy in chronic asthma, daily administration in divided doses is required for optimal efficacy. Because of its slow onset of action, cromolyn may not be effective for two to six weeks after initiation of therapy and other drugs may be needed in the interim. In some patients, the total trial period can be extended from 8 to 12 weeks, and the dose can be doubled during the last six weeks (Bernstein, 1985 B). The physician must ensure that the patient is able to use the Spinhaler or metered-dose inhaler effectively, because inefficient use will reduce the amount of drug reaching the site of action. For instructions on correct use, see the manufacturer's package insert.

Inhalation: *Adults and children over 5 years,* initially, 20 mg (one Spinhaler capsule or nebulizer dose) or 1.6 mg (two inhalations from a metered-dose inhaler) should be inhaled four times per day at regular intervals. The number of doses should then be reduced to the minimum that will control symptoms. Any inhaled particulate matter may produce acute obstruction of pulmonary airflow in patients with hyperirritable airway; use of an inhaled adrenergic agonist five to ten minutes prior to cromolyn may lessen this problem.

Only power-driven nebulizer devices with a suitable face mask or mouthpiece should be used to deliver the nebulizer solution; hand-operated units are not an acceptable alternative because they deliver too small a volume. The nebulizer solution is compatible with metaproterenol sulfate, 0.25% isoetharine hydrochloride, terbutaline sulfate, or 20% acetylcysteine solution for at least one hour after their admixture. (The capsule used for the Spinhaler is currently unavailable, but, according to the manufacturer, it will soon be supplied again.)

Intal (Fisons). Capsules 20 mg (***Spinhaler*** supplied separately); solution (for nebulizer) 10 mg/ml in 2 ml containers; metered-dose inhaler 0.8 mg per actuation.

ANTICHOLINERGIC DRUGS

ATROPINE SULFATE

For chemical formula, see index entry Atropine, As Mydriatic-Cycloplegic.

ACTIONS AND USES. This parasympathetic antagonist has particularly potent antimuscarinic effects. Inhaled atropine and other anticholinergic drugs inhibit the increase in cholinergic tone that occurs during reflex bronchoconstriction.

Nebulized atropine enhances the bronchodilation produced by beta-agonist drugs and may be a useful adjunct in some patients with acute asthma or status asthmaticus who do not respond satisfactorily to theophylline and/or inhaled beta-agonist drugs (Gross and Skorodin, 1984). The response to inhaled atropine is highly individualized. The peak effect occurs in 30 to 60 minutes; the duration of action is about three hours in young adults and may be considerably longer in children and the elderly.

At present, the primary use of inhaled atropine appears to be in patients with chronic bronchitis and emphysema or asthma with a bronchitic component in which irritant-induced elevations in cholinergic tone contribute to reflex bronchoconstriction. It is more likely to be effective when cough is associated with the asthma or chronic bronchitis. Atropine sulfate 1 to 2 mg by inhalation may be as effective as 100 to 200 mcg of albuterol.

ADVERSE REACTIONS. Atropine sulfate is more effective and may produce fewer adverse reactions when administered by inhalation. However, this tertiary amine crosses the blood-brain barrier; it enters the systemic circulation more readily and produces more adverse effects than ipratropium and other quaternary ammonium agents. Dry mouth is common. Difficulty in urination and skin flushing have been reported occasionally. Other anticholinergic effects (eg, tachycardia, gastrointestinal complaints, blurred vision) are rare. Although it is often claimed that atropine increases the viscosity of bronchial secretions and impairs ciliary clearance, there is little evidence that such effects occur.

With massive overdoses, acute glaucoma, psychosis, hyperthermia, and fatalities may occur after inhalation of atropine.

Atropine is classified in FDA Pregnancy Category C.

Atropine methonitrate, a quarternary amine, is available generically and has a longer duration of action than the sulfate. Its uses, actions, adverse reactions, and precautions are the same as atropine sulfate.

For additional information, see the section on Drug Selection in the Introduction.

DOSAGE AND PREPARATIONS.

Oral Inhalation: *Adults*, 0.025 mg/kg given by nebulizer three or four times daily. This dose is provided by diluting 0.1 to 0.2 ml of a 1% solution of atropine sulfate injection with isotonic saline to 3 to 5 ml. A dose of 0.05 mg/kg results in a maximal effect but causes more adverse reactions. A total of 2.5 mg is the maximum single dose for most adults. For *children*, 0.05 mg/kg diluted in saline and given by nebulizer three or four times daily.

IPRATROPIUM BROMIDE

[Atrovent]

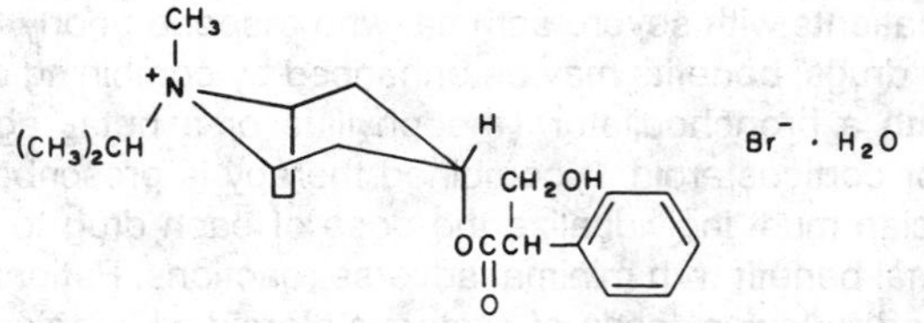

ACTIONS AND USES. This quaternary ammonium drug is as effective as atropine and is safer. An inhaled form has been used as a bronchodilator in Europe for a number of years and may be useful when theophylline and/or an inhaled $beta_2$ agonist is not adequate or not tolerated and in asthmatic patients with coexisting chronic bronchitis or cough as the predominant symptom. It is most useful in very young children and older patients; it is least useful in asthmatic patients in their teens or young adults.

In England, nebulized ipratropium has been used in acute asthma and status asthmaticus when the response to inhaled beta-adrenergic drugs was inadequate (Rees, 1984 B). However, it is not clear whether anticholinergic drugs provide a significant increase in the FEV_1 beyond that obtained with maximal beta agonist therapy (see the discussion on Anticholinergic Drugs in the Section on Asthma). A solution for nebulization is not yet available in the United States. When this form is employed, isotonic saline should be used to dilute the solution because bronchospasm has occurred when water was used as the diluent.

Ipratropium is more effective than beta agonists for the treatment of chronic bronchitis and emphysema and may be considered the drug of choice (Gross, 1987). In chronic bronchitis and emphysema, ipratropium 36 mcg delivered by metered-dose inhaler is reported to be as effective as albuterol 180 mcg or inhaled atropine 1 mg.

Inhaled ipratropium has no significant effects on mucus viscosity, production, or clearance. The drug is absorbed poorly and blood levels are very low; thus, inhalation is safe and generally free of adverse effects (Gross and Skorodin, 1984). Paradoxical bronchoconstriction occurs occasionally due to the hypotonicity of the inhalant solution but has not been observed with use of metered-dose inhalers.

Ipratropium is classified in FDA Pregnancy Category B.

Peak onset of action occurs about one to two hours after inhalation, and the duration of action is approximately three to five hours. Ipratropium does not cross the blood-brain barrier. Tolerance has not developed in patients treated for up to five years. Ipratropium is probably safe for use in patients with glaucoma or bladder neck obstruction. Patients should use a closed-mouth inhalation technique and close their eyes to avoid accidental contact of the spray with the eyes.

For additional information, see the section on Drug Selection in the Section on Asthma.

DOSAGE AND PREPARATIONS.

Inhalation: *Adults,* two inhalations (36 mcg) three or four times a day but no more often than every four hours or 12 inhalations in 24 hours. *Children under 12,* dosage has not been established.

Atrovent (Boehringer Ingelheim). Metered-dose inhaler 18 mcg per metered spray.

PROTEINASE ENZYME INHIBITOR

ALPHA$_1$-PROTEINASE INHIBITOR (HUMAN) (alpha$_1$-antitrypsin)

[Prolastin]

ACTIONS AND USES. This purified protein derived from human plasma is useful for replacement therapy for individuals with the homozygous form of alpha$_1$-antitrypsin (AAT) deficiency who have clinical evidence of panacinar emphysema. Alpha$_1$-proteinase inhibitor inhibits the activity of neutrophil elastase (NE); this prevents the severe damage to lung tissue produced by that enzyme and thus blocks the progression of emphysema. In clinical trials in patients with a pretreatment trough plasma serum concentration of 30 mg/dL, the intravenous infusion of 60 mg/kg of alpha$_1$-proteinase inhibitor over 30 minutes once a week for up to six months raised the serum concentration to 163 mg/dL, which is more than twice that required to protect the lung against NE and other proteases (Wewers et al, 1987 B). Intravenous infusion of 250 mg/kg once monthly also has been effective (Hubbard et al, 1988; Crystal, 1991). Replacement therapy is unwarranted in patients with either smoker's emphysema or the heterozygous forms of the enzyme deficiency who have normal plasma concentrations of AAT.

Investigationally, administration of alpha$_1$-antitrypsin inhibitor shows promise as a therapeutic agent to reduce lung damage produced by NE in patients with cystic fibrosis (Meyer et al, 1991; McElvaney et al, 1991).

See also the section on Chronic Bronchitis and Emphysema.

ADVERSE REACTIONS. Weekly injections for six months were well tolerated and produced few adverse reactions. A self-limited fever that did affect therapy occurred in a few patients. No long-term studies have been carried out, and the risks associated with prolonged therapy are unknown.

This drug is classified in FDA Pregnancy Category C.

DOSAGE AND PREPARATIONS.

Intravenous: *Adults,* 60 mg/kg once weekly at a rate of 0.08 ml/kg/min or greater.

Prolastin (Cutter). Powder 500 mg and 1 g with a 20- or 40-ml container of sterile water for reconstitution. Refrigerate at 35 to 46° F.

OXYGEN THERAPY

OXYGEN

Oxygen is transported in the blood primarily bound to hemoglobin. Available tissue stores are small and quickly exhausted when an increased demand for oxygen cannot be met by respiration. Tissue oxygen requirements increase during exercise and hypermetabolic states. The primary indication for oxygen therapy is to treat hypoxemia and to prevent hypoxia. As such, it should be regarded as a "drug" used to treat oxygen deficiency.

In emergencies, oxygen should be given without awaiting results of laboratory tests (arterial oxygen determination) when hypoxemia is apparent (eg, in shock, severe asthma, myocardial infarction). However, the use of oxygen is only supportive, and the cause of the hypoxemia must be determined and treated when possible.

USES. ***Chronic Obstructive Pulmonary Disease (COPD):*** Long-term home oxygen therapy is the only treatment that consistently improves survival in patients with severe emphysema and/or chronic obstructive bronchitis. Exercise tolerance improves, pulmonary hypertension and erythrocytosis decrease, and neuropsychologic function improves (Petty et al, 1979). Oxygen given for 15 hours/day has been shown to prolong survival (Medical Research Council Working Party, 1981); continuous administration for 19 hours/day prolongs survival more than treatment for 12 hours (Nocturnal Oxygen Therapy Trial Group, 1980; American Thoracic Society, 1987).

The primary aim of oxygen therapy in patients with COPD is to correct hypoxemia and thereby improve the quality of life, allow the patient to be ambulatory, and prolong survival. In COPD patients with pulmonary hypertension and cor pulmonale, oxygen is particularly useful at night to prevent hypoxemia and increased pulmonary hypertension. The value of oxygen in preventing cor pulmonale has not been established.

Long-term continuous oxygen therapy is indicated when the PaO_2 is below 55 mm Hg with the patient in the resting, nonrecumbent position, and oxygen given for more than 12 hours/day may be useful when the PaO_2 falls below 55 mm Hg during exercise or sleep. Oxygen therapy also should be considered when the PaO_2 exceeds 55 mm Hg and there is evidence of hypoxic organ dysfunction, such as cor pulmonale, pulmonary hypertension, secondary polycythemia, or impaired mental function. The need for continued oxygen should be assessed every six months for the first year and at yearly intervals thereafter.

Hypoxemic patients with COPD should receive concentrations of oxygen sufficient to raise the arterial oxygen tension to 60 mm Hg or more than 90% oxygen saturation. A PaO_2 above this range may cause excessive carbon dioxide retention and respiratory acidosis and result in ventilatory depression or failure in patients with hypercapnia. Hypercapnia and respiratory acidosis in patients with COPD are not contraindications to the initiation of prolonged oxygen therapy, but patients should be monitored carefully. The increase in carbon dioxide retention sometimes associated with chronic, controlled, low-flow oxygen is generally mild and well tolerated. Patients with COPD should discontinue cigarette smoking prior to the initiation of oxygen therapy.

Oxygen is generally safe for use in nebulizers except when hypercapnia is present (Gunawardena et al, 1984). An oxygen concentrator delivering 95% oxygen at a flow rate of 0.5 to 3 L/minute is adequate for most patients with COPD.

The sources of oxygen suitable for patient use include liquid systems, steel and aluminum cylinders containing compressed gas, and concentrators. Among these, the least expensive is the concentrator, which separates atmospheric oxygen from nitrogen. Unfortunately, this is prohibitive for ambulatory patients outside the home.

Hypoxemia: Large doses of beta$_2$-adrenergic agonists administered by an air-driven nebulizer have the theoretical risk of increasing hypoxemia. The utilization of oxygen-driven nebulizers removes this hazard.

In most hypoxemic and normoxemic patients whose PaO_2 values worsen during exercise, exercise endurance and capacity improve following oxygen therapy.

Many patients with hypoxemic lung diseases develop disordered breathing during sleep, which is characterized by apnea or hypopnea and oxygen desaturation. Nocturnal oxygen therapy prevents desaturation and relieves the elevated pulmonary arterial pressure; however, the disordered breathing is not improved. In COPD patients who develop nocturnal desaturation without severe daytime hypoxemia, nighttime administration decreases morning headache, daytime sleepiness, and nocturnal arrhythmias. The availability of oxygen for home use for patients with severe asthma may result in overuse of oxygen during a severe attack and inappropriate delay in institution of lifesaving therapy; home use should be reserved for patients with life-threatening asthma.

Acute Myocardial Infarction: Oxygen should be given to patients with uncomplicated myocardial infarction to reverse the mild hypoxemia often present. Measurement of arterial oxygen by noninvasive oximeters is preferable to determine the appropriate concentration.

Acute Anemia: In contrast to chronic anemia in which adaptive mechanisms occur, acute anemia is usually poorly tolerated. The administration of oxygen using a high FIO_2 (fraction of oxygen in inspired air) is useful temporarily until adequate blood replacement is available.

Dyspnea: Dyspnea is often present in patients without hypoxemia and is related to increased work of breathing. Any relief obtained after oxygen administration is associated with a decrease in ventilatory work rather than an increase in PaO_2.

Miscellaneous Uses: Oxygen is valuable for the treatment of carbon monoxide poisoning. Because arterial oxygen tension is often reduced in patients with hypotension and congestive heart failure, oxygen therapy is often recommended. The hypoxemia associated with adult respiratory distress syndrome is due to intrapulmonary shunting. Treatment requires a high FiO_2 and, often, mechanical ventilation. Oxygen also has been used to relieve migraine and cluster headache.

Unestablished Uses: The usefulness of oxygen therapy for angina pectoris has not been determined in controlled studies. In patients with sickle cell disease, administration of 100% oxygen has been reported to decrease the number of sickle cells. However, in controlled studies, attempts to treat sickle cell crises with oxygen have not been successful.

ADVERSE REACTIONS AND PRECAUTIONS. For acute therapy, use of the lowest concentration of oxygen for the shortest time minimizes serious lung damage (*Chest,* 1984). The dose and duration of therapy that produce toxicity vary. Breathing 100% oxygen for less than 24 hours at atmospheric pressure has little adverse effect on the lungs, and exposure to 50% oxygen for two to seven days has no clinically significant effects. No specific index to allow early detection of oxygen toxicity exists, and no therapeutically useful way to use antioxidant substances to protect against lung damage produced by oxygen radicals is currently available. The benefits of therapy must be weighed against the serious and sometimes lethal effects of excessive oxygen.

Oxygen drawn from cylinders and piping systems is anhydrous and tends to dry the mucous membranes, which thickens secretions, reduces ciliary function, and causes discomfort. Dehydrating effects are accentuated when the gas is used by tube or catheter, which bypasses the humidifying functions of the mucosal surfaces. Careful use of a heated nebulizing apparatus reduces dryness, but the heated devices may produce condensation in the delivery tubing, particularly in infants. Ultrasonic nebulizers should not be used in infants because of the risk of pulmonary edema or in COPD patients either with or without oxygen because bronchospasm occurs frequently.

Chronically high FIO_2 may decrease minute ventilation, produce absorption atelectasis, increase retention of carbon dioxide, or reverse compensatory hypoxic pulmonary vasoconstriction. Atelectasis may develop when the "nitrogen scaffold" is reduced by washout. The administration of high oxygen concentrations without mechanical support of respiration may induce apnea in patients with chronic hypercapnia, traumatic injury of the respiratory center, or barbiturate intoxication. Thus, high concentrations of supplemental oxygen may worsen hypoventilation in hypoxic patients with hypercapnia and may increase intrapulmonary shunting.

The intensity of fire in oxygen-enriched atmospheres is directly proportional to the concentration of oxygen supplied and is particularly great with oxygen tents. Smoking should be forbidden in areas in which oxygen is being used.

Cytotoxicity: Exposure to high concentrations of oxygen by lung cells can produce severe and fatal cytotoxic effects. It is generally believed that oxygen generates intracellular radicals as normal byproducts of metabolism, including the superoxide anion (O^-_2), activated hydroxyl radical (OH-), hydrogen peroxide (H_2O_2), and singlet oxygen (O_2). The most toxic is probably the hydroxyl radical (not superoxide). These radicals apparently interact with DNA, proteins, carbohydrates, and lipids and disrupt transcription, cellular membrane integrity, enzyme activity, and other cell functions that alter structure and metabolism and cause cell death.

Within 24 hours after exposure to excessive oxygen, patients experience substernal discomfort, cough, and decreased vital capacity, which predict the development of pulmonary cytotoxicity. After one to four days of 100% oxygen, progressive dyspnea and hypoxemia occur in association with productive cough and a widened alveolar-arterial oxygen tension gradient (Ryerson and Block, 1984).

With continued exposure to excessive oxygen concentrations, extensive irreversible pathologic changes in lung structure occur. The early exudative phase is characterized by edema, hemorrhage, influx of inflammatory cells, destruction of type I alveolar pneumonocytes, and necrosis of the capillary endothelium. If the patient survives this early exudative phase and more than 72 hours of exposure to oxygen, the proliferative phase begins. In this phase, early exudates are resorbed, the alveolar septa thicken, and type II alveolar pneumonocytes hypertrophy and proliferate; lung scarring is sometimes permanent but may regress. Progressive loss of lung function occurs. The clinical pattern resembles pulmonary fibrosis and emphysema. It is often difficult to differentiate the effects of oxygen from those of the underlying disease. In the newborn exposed to excessive oxygen, manifestation of these pathologic changes is termed bronchopulmonary dysplasia.

Retrolental fibroplasia occurs in premature infants treated with oxygen concentrations above ambient air levels. The exact level or duration of elevated arterial oxygen that results in injury is unknown, but arterial oxygen partial pressure should be kept below 50 to 70 mm Hg. In this disorder, the immature retinal blood vessels are damaged. Scarring, retinal detachment, and permanent blindness can result. Hyperbaric oxygen causes similar effects in adults. The risk of hypoxia must be balanced against the risk of retrolental fibroplasia.

SURFACTANT PREPARATIONS

BERACTANT (Surfactant TA)
[Survanta]

COLFOSCERIL PALMITATE, CETYL ALCOHOL, AND TYLOXAPOL
[Exosurf Neonatal]

ACTIONS. Endogenous surfactant reduces surface tension in the lungs, decreases the work of breathing, increases lung compliance, decreases the need for oxygen and assisted ventilation, and stabilizes the alveoli, which prevents atelectasis at end expiration (Reynolds and Wallander, 1989).

Natural surfactants are obtained from a variety of human and animal sources and are composed of a mixture of lipoproteins containing phospholipids and pulmonary surfactant proteins A (PSP-A), B (PSP-B), and C (PSP-C); lipid-extracted surfactant contains only PSP-B and PSP-C and may be supplemented with phospholipids and neutral lipids such as palmitic acid. The phospholipids, primarily dipalmitoylphosphatidylcholine (DPPC, lecithin, colfosceril palmitate), exert the greatest effect in lowering surface tension. PSP-B and PSP-C facilitate the absorption and spreading of the surfactant mixture; PSP-A promotes surfactant recycling but is destroyed by heat treatment during extraction.

Beractant [Survanta] is obtained from lipid extraction of minced bovine lung and is modified by the addition of DPPC, palmitic acid, and tripalmitin. Pulmonary surfactant proteins B and C also are present in the bovine extract. Another surfactant preparation, which is available as Exosurf Neonatal, contains colfosceril palmitate (DPPC) in a sodium chloride solution that contains two emulsifying agents: cetyl alcohol, which acts as a spreading agent, and tyloxapol, a nonionic detergent that acts as a dispersing agent. This synthetic preparation has been used extensively in the United States and Canada.

USES. Surfactant obtained from a variety of sources has been used in clinical trials to prevent and treat RDS in several thousand premature infants. In both prophylactic and treatment ("rescue") trials, the severity of RDS has been significantly diminished and the percentage of deaths at 28 days has been decreased by 30% to 90% (Reynolds and Wallander, 1989; Halliday, 1989; Ross Laboratories, Treatment IND; Exosurf Neonatal package insert).

For further discussion of the use of surfactant preparations, see the section on Lung Disorders in Premature Infants in the Introduction.

ADVERSE REACTIONS. After short-term administration, adverse reactions have been minimal and easily controlled. In some studies, the incidence of apnea (probably due to the early removal of assisted ventilation) is increased. Data on the effect of surfactant on intraventricular hemorrhage are conflicting (Long et al, 1991 B). Surfactant therapy unmasks the presence of patent ductus arteriosus but does not appear to increase its prevalence. Atopy (sensitization) has not been reported in humans. Up to 20 ml of surfactant solution administered through an endotracheal tube has not produced pulmonary edema. No significant long-term adverse effects have been identified in a number of follow-up studies (Reynolds and Wallander, 1989).

For further discussion of adverse reactions and precautions, see the section on Lung Disorders in Premature Infants in the Introduction.

PHARMACOKINETICS. ***Metabolism and Pool Size.*** The metabolic fate of released surfactant is unclear; it may be recycled by reuptake into type II pneumonocytes. The pool size of endogenous surfactant in full-term infants is 100 to 250 mg/kg; in contrast, infants with severe RDS may have a pool size of only 10 micromole/kg.

Clearance. Surfactant clearance is slow and may be prolonged with increasing severity of RDS. The biological half-life has been estimated to be 20 to 36 hours (Hallman et al, 1986).

DOSAGE AND PREPARATIONS. The most effective dose and schedule of administration have not been determined. Both beractant and the combination of colfosceril palmitate, cetyl alcohol, and tyloxapol are administered to high-risk or ventilator-dependent infants through an endotracheal tube. For more specific information and instructions on administration, see the manufacturers' package insert.

BERACTANT:

For prophylaxis in high-risk infants weighing 600 to 1,250 g, a single dose of 100 mg/kg phospholipids (4 ml/kg) is given within 15 minutes of birth. For established RDS in infants requiring assisted ventilation and weighing 600 to 1,750 g ("rescue"), up to four doses of 100 mg/kg phospholipids (4 ml/kg) are given at intervals of six hours or more.

Survanta (Ross Laboratories). Suspension (sterile) 25 mg phospholipids/ml in 0.9% sodium chloride solution. Reconstitution before use is not required. Available from the manufacturer or hospital pharmacies.

COLFOSCERIL PALMITATE, CETYL ALCOHOL, AND TYLOXAPOL: For prophylaxis in high-risk infants weighing less than 1,350 g, an initial dose of 80 mg/kg (5 ml/kg) is given shortly after birth; administration is repeated 12 and 24 hours later in infants who remain on mechanical ventilation. For established RDS in infants requiring assisted ventilation ("rescue"), 80 mg/kg is given twice at an interval of 12 hours.

Exosurf Neonatal (Burroughs Wellcome). Powder (lyophilized) 108 mg colfosceril palmitate. Available from the manufacturer or hospital pharmacies.

Cited References

ACCP-NHLBI National Conference on Oxygen Therapy. *Chest* 86:234-247, 1984.

β_2 agonists in asthma: Relief, prevention, morbidity, editorial. *Lancet* 336:1411-1412, 1990.

Carter-Wallace's Organidin should remain on market while FDA reviews efficacy data, advisory cmte. says; 'Dear Doctor' letter on carcinogenicity recommended. *F-D-C Rep* 5-6, (March) 1992.

Fenoterol and fatal asthma. *WHO Drug Info* 3:57-58, 1989.

Fisons' *Tilade* recommended for approval as nonbronchodilating antiasthmatic. *F-D-C Rep* 10-11, (June) 1990.

Guidelines for the Diagnosis and Management of Asthma: National Heart, Lung, and Blood Institute National Asthma Education Program Expert Panel Report. *J Allergy Clin Immunol* 88:425-534, (Sept) 1991.

Role of cromolyn in long-term management of asthma. *Pediatr Alert* 12:97-98, 1987 A.

Does theophylline cause behavior problems and poor school performance? *Pediatr Alert* 12:17-18, 1987 B.

Aitken ML, et al: Recombinant human DNase inhalation in normal subjects and patients with cystic fibrosis. *JAMA* 267:1947-1951, 1992.

Albersheim SG, et al: Randomized, double-blind, controlled trial of long-term diuretic therapy for bronchopulmonary dysplasia. *J Pediatr* 115:615-620, 1989.

Alvarez J, Szefler SJ: Alternative therapy in severe asthma. *J Asthma* 29:3-11, 1992.

American Academy of Pediatrics, Committee on Fetus and Newborn: Surfactant replacement therapy for respiratory distress syndrome. *Pediatrics* 87:946-947, 1991.

American Thoracic Society: Standards for diagnosis and care of patients with chronic obstructive pulmonary disease (COPD) and asthma. *Am Rev Respir Dis* 136:225-244, 1987.

American Thoracic Society: Guidelines for the approach to the patient with severe hereditary alpha-1-antitrypsin deficiency. *Am Rev Respir Dis* 140:1494-1497, 1989.

Appel D, et al: Epinephrine improves expiratory flow rates in patients with asthma who do not respond to inhaled metaproterenol sulfate. *J Allergy Clin Immunol* 84:90-98, 1989.

Arkinstall WW, et al: Once-daily sustained-release theophylline reduces diurnal variation in spirometry and symptomatology in adult asthmatics. *Am Rev Respir Dis* 135:316-321, 1987.

Aubier M, et al: Aminophylline improves diaphragmatic contractility. *N Engl J Med* 305:249-252, 1981.

Avery GB: The use of dexamethasone in premature infants at risk for bronchopulmonary dysplasia or who already have developed chronic lung disease: A cautionary note, letter. *Pediatrics* 88:414-415, 1991.

Avery ME, Merritt TA: Surfactant-replacement therapy. *N Engl J Med* 324:910-912, 1991.

Avery GB, et al: Controlled trial of dexamethasone in respirator-dependent infants with bronchopulmonary dysplasia. *Pediatrics* 75:106-111, 1985.

Avery ME, et al: Update on prenatal steroid for prevention of respiratory distress: Report of conference, September 26-28, 1985. *Am J Obstet Gynecol* 155:2-5, 1986 A.

Avery ME, et al: Surfactant replacement, editorial. *N Engl J Med* 315:825-826, 1986 B.

Barnes PJ: A new approach to the treatment of asthma. *N Engl J Med* 321:1517-1527, 1989.

Beasley R, et al: Cellular events in the bronchi in mild asthma and after bronchial provocation. *Am Rev Respir Dis* 139:806-817, 1989 A.

Beasley R, et al: Inflammatory processes in bronchial asthma. *Drugs* 37(suppl 1):117-122, 1989 B.

Becker AB, et al: Formoterol, a new long-acting selective B_2-adrenergic receptor agonist: Double-blind comparison with salbutamol and placebo in children with asthma. *J Allergy Clin Immunol* 84:891-895, 1989.

Bernstein IL: Cromolyn sodium. *Chest* 87(suppl):68S-73S, 1985 A.

Bernstein IL: Cromolyn sodium in the treatment of asthma: Coming of age in the United States. *J Allergy Clin Immunol* 76:381-388, 1985 B

Bernstein IL: Treatment decisions of asthma based on a paradigm of clinical severity. *J Allergy Clin Immunol* 76:357-365, 1985 C.

Bernstein MS, Lazarus SC: Diagnosis and management of asthma. *Compr Ther* 15:53-60, 1989.

Bernstein IL, et al: Efficacy and safety of triamcinolone acetonide aerosol in chronic asthma. *Chest* 81:20-26, 1982.

Bernstein DI, et al: Open study of auranofin in treatment of steroid-dependent asthma. *J Allergy Clin Immunol* 81:6-16, 1988.

Birkhead G, et al: Investigation of a cluster of deaths of adolescents for asthma: Evidence implicating inadequate treatment and poor patient adherence with medications. *J Allergy Clin Immunol* 84:484-491, 1989.

Blumenthal MN, et al: Multicenter evaluation of the clinical benefits of cromolyn sodium aerosol by metered-dose inhaler in the treatment of asthma. *J Allergy Clin Immunol* 81:681-687, 1988.

Boe J, et al: Efficacy of enprofylline, new bronchodilating xanthine, in acute asthma. *Ann Allergy* 59:155-158, 1987.

Brik A, et al: Effect of cetirizine, new histamine H_1 antagonist, on airway dynamics and responsiveness to inhaled histamine in mild asthma. *J Allergy Clin Immunol* 80:51-60, 1987.

Brogden RN, Faulds D: Salmeterol xinafoate: A review of its pharmacological properties and therapeutic potential in reversible obstructive airways disease. *Drugs* 42:895-912, 1991.

Brogden RN, et al: Beclomethasone dipropionate: Reappraisal of its pharmacodynamic properties and therapeutic efficacy after decade of use in asthma and rhinitis. *Drugs* 28:99-126, 1984.

Brownlee KG, et al: Catabolic effect of dexamethasone in the preterm baby. *Arch Dis Child* 67:1-4, 1992.

Brundage KL, et al: Bronchodilator response to ipratropium bromide in infants with bronchopulmonary dysplasia. *Am Rev Respir Dis* 142:1137-1142, 1990.

Bukowskyj M, et al: Theophylline reassessed. *Ann Intern Med* 101:63-73, 1984.

Burrows B, Lebowitz MD: The β-agonist dilemma. *N Engl J Med* 326:560-561, 1992.

Burton GG: Differential diagnosis of various obstructive pulmonary diseases and implications for therapy, in Burton GG, Hodgkin JE (eds): *Respiratory Care: A Guide to Clinical Practice*. Chicago, Year Book Medical Publishers, 1984, 787-805.

Busse WW, et al: International symposium on nedocromil sodium. *Drugs* 37(suppl 1):1-137, 1989.

Bussey HI: Theophylline toxicity after dyphylline therapy. *Am Rev Respir Dis* 124:504, 1981.

Castiglioni CL, Gramolini C: Effect of long-term treatment with sobrerol on exacerbations of chronic bronchitis. *Respiration* 50:202-217, 1986.

Chapman KR: Anticholinergic bronchodilators for adult obstructive airways disease. *Am J Med* 91(suppl 4A):4A-13S-4A-16S, 1991.

Chapman KR, et al: Effect of a short course of prednisone in the prevention of early relapse after the emergency room treatment of acute asthma. *N Engl J Med* 324:788-794, 1991.

Cherniak RM, et al: A double-blind multicentre group comparative study of the efficacy and safety of nedocromil sodium in the management of asthma. *Chest* 97:1299-1306, 1990.

Clark TJH: Inhaled corticosteroid therapy: Substitute for theophylline as well as prednisolone? *J Allergy Clin Immunol* 76:330-334, 1985.

Clarke SW, Newman SP: Therapeutic aerosols 2: Drugs available by inhaled route, editorial. *Thorax* 39:1-7, 1984.

Clissold SP, Heel RC: Budesonide: Preliminary review of its pharmacodynamic properties and therapeutic efficacy in asthma and rhinitis. *Drugs* 28:485-518, 1984.

Cockcroft DW: Airway hyperresponsiveness in asthma. *Hosp Pract* 111-129, (Jan) 1990 A.

Cockcroft DW: A stepwise approach to the outpatient management of asthma. *Mod Med* 58:50-60, 1990 B.

Cockcroft DW, Hargreave FE: Outpatient management of bronchial asthma. *Med Clin North Am* 74:797-809, 1990.

Cohen AB: Unraveling the mysteries of alpha$_1$-antitrypsin deficiency. *N Engl J Med* 314:778-779, 1986.

Collaborative Dexamethasone Trial Group: Dexamethasone therapy in neonatal chronic lung disease: An international placebo-controlled trial. *Pediatrics* 88:421-427, 1991.

Cookson WOCM: Bronchodilator action of anti-histamine terfenadine, letter. *Br J Clin Pharmacol* 24:120-121, 1987.

Cross D, Nelson HS: The role of the peak flow meter in the diagnosis and management of asthma. *J Allergy Clin Immunol* 87:120-128, 1991.

Crystal RG: α_1-Antitrypsin deficiency: Pathogenesis and treatment. *Hosp Pract* 81-94, (Feb) 1991.

Crystal RG, et al: The α_1-antitrypsin gene and its mutations: Clinical consequences and strategies for therapy. *Chest* 95:196-208, 1989.

Cummings JJ, et al: A controlled trial of dexamethasone in preterm infants at high risk for bronchopulmonary dysplasia. *N Engl J Med* 320:1505-1510, 1989.

Daniele RP: Chronic asthma, in Cherniack RM (ed): *Current Therapy of Respiratory Disease, 1984-1985*. Philadelphia/St Louis, Decker/Mosby, 1984, 107-111.

Davis PB: Cystic fibrosis from bench to bedside, editorial. *N Engl J Med* 325:575-577, 1991.

De Blaquiere P, et al: Use and misuse of metered-dose inhalers by patients with chronic lung disease. *Am Rev Respir Dis* 140:910-916, 1989.

Dechant KL, Faulds D: Colfosceril palmitate: A review of the therapeutic efficacy and clinical tolerability of a synthetic surfactant preparation (Exosurf Neonatal) in neonatal respiratory distress syndrome. *Drugs* 42:877-894, 1991.

Dederich RA, et al: Intrasubject variation in sustained-release theophylline absorption. *J Allergy Clin Immunol* 67:465-471, 1981.

Donnelly JE, et al: Inadequate parental understanding of asthma medications. *Ann Allergy* 62:337-341, 1989.

Dunn MS, et al: Bovine surfactant replacement therapy in neonates of less than 30 weeks' gestation: A randomized controlled trial of prophylaxis versus treatment. *Pediatrics* 87:377-386, 1991.

Dwyer JM: Pharmacological approach to management of asthma. *Ration Drug Ther* 18:1-8, 1984.

Dyer PD, et al: Methotrexate in the treatment of steroid-dependent asthma. *J Allergy Clin Immunol* 88:208-212, 1991.

Easton PA, et al: Comparison of the bronchodilating effects of a beta-2 adrenergic agent (albuterol) and an anticholinergic agent (ipratropium bromide), given by aerosol alone or in sequence. *N Engl J Med* 315:735-739, 1986.

Eigen H, et al: Evaluation of addition of cromolyn sodium to bronchodilator maintenance therapy in long-term management of asthma. *J Allergy Clin Immunol* 80:612-621, 1987.

Eitches RW, et al: Methylprednisolone and troleandomycin in treatment of steroid-dependent asthmatic children. *Am J Dis Child* 139:264-268, 1985.

Erzurum SC, et al: Lack of benefit of methotrexate in severe, steroid-dependent asthma: A double-blind, placebo-controlled study. *Ann Intern Med* 114:353-360, 1991.

Estepan H, Libby DM: Glucocorticoid therapy of pulmonary disease. *Drug Ther* 12:109-118, (Oct) 1982.

Fairshter RD, et al: Comparison of clinical effects and pharmacokinetics of once-daily Uniphyl and twice-daily Theo-Dur in asthmatic patients. *Am J Med* 79 (suppl 6A):48-53, 1985.

Farrell EE, et al: Impact of antenatal dexamethasone administration on respiratory distress syndrome in surfactant-treated infants. *Am J Obstet Gynecol* 161:628-633, 1989.

Faulds D, et al: Formoterol: A review of its pharmacological properties and therapeutic potential in reversible obstructive airways disease. *Drugs* 42:115-137, 1991.

Ferguson AC: Persisting airway obstruction in asymptomatic children with asthma with normal peak expiratory flow rates. *J Allergy Clin Immunol* 82:19-22, 1988.

Ferrara TB, et al: Effects of surfactant therapy on outcome of infants with birth weights 600-750 grams. *Pediatrics* 119:455-457, 1991.

Fitzpatrick MF, et al: Salmeterol in nocturnal asthma: A double-blind, placebo controlled trial of a long acting inhaled β_2 agonist. *BMJ* 301:1365-1368, 1990.

Frank L: The use of dexamethasone in premature infants at risk for bronchopulmonary dysplasia or who already have developed chronic lung disease: A cautionary note, letter. *Pediatrics* 88:413, 1991.

Furukawa CT, et al: Learning and behaviour problems associated with theophylline therapy. *Lancet* 1:621, 1984.

Geddes DM: Methotrexate in asthma. *Clin Exp Allergy* 21:541-543, 1991.

Glaser CB, et al: Studies on turnover of methionine oxidized alpha-1-protease inhibitor in rats. *Am Rev Respir Dis* 136:857-861, 1987.

Grant SM, et al: Ketotifen: A review of its pharmacodynamic and pharmacokinetic properties, and therapeutic use in asthma and allergic disorders. *Drugs* 40:412-448, 1990.

Gross NJ: Anticholinergic agents in chronic bronchitis and emphysema. *Postgrad Med J* 63 (suppl 1):29-34, 1987.

Gross NJ, Skorodin MS: Anticholinergic, antimuscarinic bronchodilators. *Am Rev Respir Dis* 129:856-870, 1984.

Gunawardena K, et al: Oxygen as driving gas for nebulizers: Safe or dangerous? *BMJ* 288:272-274, 1984.

Guyatt GH, et al: Controlled trial of ambroxol in chronic bronchitis. *Chest* 92:618-620, 1987.

Haahtela T, et al: Comparison of a β_2-agonist, terbutaline, with an inhaled corticosteroid budesonide, in newly detected asthma. *N Engl J Med* 325:388-392, 1991.

Halliday HL: Clinical experience with exogenous natural surfactant. *Dev Pharmacol Ther* 13:173-181, 1989.

Hallman M, et al: Effect of surfactant substitution on lung effluent phospholipids in respiratory distress syndrome: Evaluation of surfactant phospholipid turnover, pool size, and the relationship to severity of respiratory failure. *Pediatr Res* 20:1228-1235, 1986.

Hallman M, et al: Inositol supplementation in premature infants with respiratory distress syndrome. *N Engl J Med* 326:1233-1239, 1992.

Hargreave FE, et al (eds): The assessment and treatment of asthma: A conference report. *J Allergy Clin Immunol* 85:1098-1111, 1990.

Harkavy KL: The use of dexamethasone in premature infants at risk for bronchopulmonary dysplasia or who already have developed chronic lung disease: A cautionary note, letter. *Pediatrics* 88:414-415, 1991.

Harkavy KL, et al: Dexamethasone therapy for chronic lung disease in ventilator- and oxygen-dependent infants: A controlled trial. *J Pediatr* 115:979-983, 1989.

Hemstreet MPB: Atropine nebulization: Simple and safe. *Ann Allergy* 44:138-141, 1980.

Hendeles L, Weinberger M: Theophylline: "State of the art" review. *Pharmacotherapy* 3:2-44, 1983.

Hendeles L, et al: Food-induced "dose-dumping" from once-a-day theophylline product as cause of theophylline toxicity. *Chest* 87:758-765, 1985.

Hendeles L, et al: Safety and efficacy of theophylline in children with asthma. *J Pediatr* 120:177-183, 1992.

Hetzel M: More logical approach to asthma. *Postgrad Med J* 60:201-207, 1984.

Hiller FC, Wilson FJ Jr: Evaluation and management of acute asthma. *Med Clin North Am* 67:669-683, 1983.

Hoekstra RE, et al: Improved neonatal survival following multiple doses of bovine surfactant in very premature neonates at risk for respiratory distress syndrome. *Pediatrics* 88:10-18, 1991.

Holgate ST: Clinical evaluation of nedocromil sodium in asthma. *Eur J Respir Dis* 69 (suppl 147): 149-159, 1986.

Holgate ST, et al: Astemizole and other H_1-antihistaminic drug treatment of asthma. *J Allergy Clin Immunol* 76:375-380, 1985.

Hubbard RC, et al: Oxidants spontaneously released by alveolar macrophages of cigarette smokers can inactivate active site of alpha-1-antitrypsin, rendering it ineffective as inhibitor of neutrophil elastase. *J Clin Invest* 80:1289-1295, 1987.

Hubbard RC, et al: Biochemical efficacy and safety of monthly augmentation therapy for alpha-1-antitrypsin deficiency. *JAMA* 260:1259-1264, 1988.

Hubbard RC, et al: Recombinant DNA-produced α1-antitrypsin administered by aerosol augments lower respiratory tract antineutrophil elastase defenses in individuals with α1-antitrypsin deficiency. *J Clin Invest* 84:1349-1354, 1989 A.

Hubbard RC, et al: Anti-neutrophil-elastase defenses of the lower respiratory tract in alpha-1-antitrypsin deficiency directly augmented with an aerosol of alpha-1-antitrypsin. *Ann Intern Med* 111:206-212, 1989 B.

Hubbard RC, et al: A preliminary study of aerosolized recombinant human deoxyribonuclease I in the treatment of cystic fibrosis. *N Engl J Med* 326:812-815, 1992.

Ingram RH Jr, Davies S: Chronic obstructive diseases of the lung. *Sci Am* 1-23, (March) 1992.

Jenne JW: Theophylline use in asthma: Some current issues. *Clin Chest Med* 5:645-658, 1984.

Jenne JW: Physiology and pharmacodynamics of the xanthines, in Jenne JW, Murphy S (eds): *Drug Therapy for Asthma: Research and Clinical Practice.* New York, Marcel Dekker, 1987, 297-334.

Jenne JW: Theophylline is no more obsolete than "two puffs *qid*" of current $beta_2$ agonists, editorial. *Chest* 98:3-4, 1990.

Jenne JW, Murphy S (eds): *Drug Therapy for Asthma: Research and Clinical Practice.* New York, Marcel Dekker, 1987.

Joad J, et al: Physiological and psychological variables during maintenance therapy with inhaled albuterol and theophylline used separately and in combination, abstract. *J Allergy Clin Immunol* 75:113, 1985.

Juniper EF, et al: Effect of long-term treatment with an inhaled corticosteroid (budesonide) on airway hyperresponsiveness and clinical asthma in nonsteroid-dependent asthmatics. *Am Rev Respir Dis* 142:832-836, 1990.

Kaiser LR, Cooper JD: The current status of lung transplantation. *Adv Surg* 25:259-307, 1992.

Kaliner M, et al: Rhinitis and asthma. *JAMA* 258:2851-2873, 1987.

Kao LC, et al: Oral theophylline and diuretics improve pulmonary mechanics in infants with bronchopulmonary dysplasia. *J Pediatr* 111:439-444, 1987.

Karim A, et al: Food-induced changes in theophylline absorption from controlled-release formulations: Part I. Substantial increased and decreased absorption with Uniphyl tablets and Theo-Dur Sprinkle. *Clin Pharmacol Ther* 38:77-83, 1985.

Kay AB: Mode of action of anti-allergic drugs. *Clin Allergy* 17:153-164, 1987.

Kemp JP, et al: Dose-response study of bronchodilator action of azelastine in asthma. *J Allergy Clin Immunol* 79:893-899, 1987.

Kendig JW, et al: A comparison of surfactant as immediate prophylaxis and as rescue therapy in newborns of less than 30 weeks' gestation. *N Engl J Med* 324:865-871, 1991.

Knowles MR, et al: Activation by extracellular nucleotides of chlorine secretion in the airway epithelia of patients with cystic fibrosis. *N Engl J Med* 325:533-538, 1991.

Lam A, Newhouse MT: Management of asthma and chronic airflow limitation: Are methylxanthines obsolete? *Chest* 98:44-52, 1990.

Larrain A, et al: Medical and surgical treatment of nonallergic asthma associated with gastroesophageal reflux. *Chest* 99:1330-1335, 1991.

Lawson EE, Stiles AD: Vitamin A therapy for prevention of chronic lung disease in infants. *J Pediatr* 111:247-248, 1987.

Lawyer CH, et al: Utilization of intravenous dihydroxypropyl theophylline (dyphylline) in aminophylline-sensitive patient, and pharmacokinetic comparison with theophylline. *J Allergy Clin Immunol* 65:353-357, 1980.

Levison H: Spacers in childhood asthma: Is there one for all occasions? editorial. *Ann Allergy* 64:323-324, 1990.

Long W, et al: Effects of two rescue doses of a synthetic surfactant on mortality rate and survival without bronchopulmonary dysplasia in 700- to 1350-gram infants with respiratory distress syndrome. *J Pediatr* 118:595-605, 1991 A.

Long W, et al: A controlled trial of synthetic surfactant in infants weighing 1250 g or more with respiratory distress syndrome. *N Engl J Med* 325:1696-1703, 1991 B.

Lorentzson S, et al: Use of inhaled corticosteroids in patients with mild asthma. *Thorax* 45:733-735, 1990.

MacNee W, et al: The effect of cigarette smoking on neutrophil kinetics in human lungs. *N Engl J Med* 321:924-928, 1989.

Maesen FPV, et al: Bronchodilator effect of inhaled formoterol vs salbutamol over 12 hours. *Chest* 97:590-594, 1990.

Mammel MC, et al: Short-term dexamethasone therapy for bronchopulmonary dysplasia: Acute effects and one-year follow-up. *Dev Pharmacol Ther* 10:1-11, 1987.

Marchlinski FE, Miller JM: Atrial arrhythmias exacerbated by theophylline: Response to verapamil and evidence for triggered activity in man. *Chest* 88:931-934, 1985.

Marks MB: Theophylline: Primary or tertiary drug? Brief review. *Ann Allergy* 59:85-87, 1987.

May DC, Jarboe CH: Inhibition of clearance of dyphylline by probenecid, letter. *N Engl J Med* 304:791, 1981.

Mayo PH, et al: Results of a program to reduce admissions for adult asthma. *Ann Intern Med* 112:864-871, 1990.

McElvaney NG, et al: Aerosol α1-antitrypsin treatment for cystic fibrosis. *Lancet* 337:392-394, 1991.

McFadden ER Jr: Corticosteroids and cromolyn sodium as modulators of airway inflammation. *Chest* 94:181-184, 1988.

McFadden ER Jr: Methylxanthines in the treatment of asthma: The rise, the fall, and the possible rise again. *Ann Intern Med* 115:323-324, 1991.

McGowan SE, Hunninghake GW: Neutrophils and emphysema. *N Engl J Med* 321:968-970, 1989.

Medical Research Council Working Party: Long-term domiciliary oxygen therapy in chronic hypoxic cor pulmonale complicating chronic bronchitis and emphysema. *Lancet* 1:681-686, 1981.

Meltzer EO: To use or not to use antihistamines in patients with asthma, editorial. *Ann Allergy* 64 (part II): 183-186, 1990.

Merritt TA, et al: Prophylactic treatment of very premature infants with human surfactant. *N Engl J Med* 315:785-790, 1986.

Merritt TA, et al: Randomized, placebo-controlled trial of human surfactant given at birth versus rescue administration in very low birth weight infants with lung immaturity. *J Pediatr* 118:581-594, 1991.

Meyer KC, et al: Human neutrophil elastase and elastase/$alpha_1$-antiprotease complex in cystic fibrosis: Comparison with interstitial lung disease and evaluation of the effect of intravenously administered antibiotic therapy. *Am Rev Respir Dis* 144:580-585, 1991.

Morton NS: Exogenous surfactant treatment for the adult respiratory distress syndrome? A historical perspective, editorial. *Thorax* 45:825-830, 1990.

Mullarkey MF: Methotrexate and asthma. *J Allergy Clin Immunol* 88:272-274, 1991.

Mullarkey M, et al: Methotrexate in treatment of corticosteroid-dependent asthma. *N Engl J Med* 318:603-607, 1988.

Mullarkey MF, et al: Methotrexate for asthma, letter. *Ann Intern Med* 115:66-67, 1991.

Murphy S: Cromolyn sodium, in Jenne JW, Murphy S (eds): *Drug Therapy for Asthma: Research and Clinical Practice.* New York, Marcel Dekker, 1987, 669-717.

Nelson HS: Gastroesophageal reflux and bronchial asthma. *Airway Dis* 3:2-10, (Fall) 1987.

Nelson HS: The natural history of asthma. *Ann Allergy* 66:196-203, 1991.

Nelson RP, Lockey RF: Treatment of asthma with glucocorticosteroids. *South Med J* 81:761-769, 1988.

Nelson MS, et al: Frequency of inhaled metaproterenol in the treatment of acute asthma exacerbation. *Ann Emerg Med* 19:21-25, 1990.

Newhouse MT: Is theophylline obsolete? editorial. *Chest* 98:1-2, 1990.

Newman SP: Therapeutic inhalation agents and devices: Effectiveness in asthma and bronchitis. *Postgrad Med* 76:194-207, (Oct) 1984.

Newman SP, Clarke SW: Therapeutic aerosols 1: Physical and practical considerations, editorial. *Thorax* 38:881-886, 1983.

Ng PC, et al: Gastroduodenal perforation in preterm babies treated with dexamethasone for bronchopulmonary dysplasia. *Arch Dis Child* 66:1164-1166, 1991.

Niewoehner DE: Theophylline therapy: A continuing dilemma. *Chest* 98:5, 1990.

Nocturnal Oxygen Therapy Trial Group: Continuous or nocturnal oxygen therapy in hypoxemic chronic obstructive lung disease: Clinical trial. *Ann Intern Med* 93:391-398, 1980.

Norn S, Clementsen P: Bronchial asthma: Pathophysiological mechanisms and corticosteroids. *Allergy* 43:401-405, 1988.

North American Tilade Study Group: A double-blind multicenter group comparative study of the efficacy and safety of nedocromil sodium in the management of asthma. *Chest* 97:1299-1306, 1990.

Nosaka S, et al: Surfactant for adults with respiratory failure. *Lancet* 336:947-948, 1990.

Ogushi F, et al: Z-type alpha-1-antitrypsin is less competent than M1-type alpha-1-antitrypsin as inhibitor of neutrophil elastase. *J Clin Invest* 80:1366-1374, 1987.

Ogushi F, et al: Risk factors for emphysema: Cigarette smoking is associated with a reduction in the association rate constant of lung α1-antitrypsin for neutrophil elastase. *J Clin Invest* 87:1060-1065, 1991.

Olson KR, et al: Theophylline overdose: Acute single ingestion versus chronic repeated overmedication. *Am J Emerg Med* 3:386-394, 1985.

O'Neil EA, et al: Dexamethasone treatment during ventilator dependency: Possible life threatening gastrointestinal complications. *Arch Dis Child* 67:10-11, 1992.

Orgel HA, et al: Flunisolide aerosol in treatment of steroid-dependent asthma in children. *Ann Allergy* 51:21-25, 1983.

Orgel HA, et al: Bitolterol and albuterol metered-dose aerosols: Comparison of two long-acting beta$_2$-adrenergic bronchodilators for treatment of asthma. *J Allergy Clin Immunol* 75:55-62, 1985.

Parker SR, et al: NHLBI workshop summary: Asthma education: A national strategy. *Am Rev Respir Dis* 140:848-853, 1989.

Paterson JW, et al: Comment on β_2-agonists and their use in asthma. *TIPS* 67-69, 1983.

Patterson R, et al: Asthma and pregnancy: Responsibility of physicians and patients. *Ann Allergy* 65:469-472, 1990.

Pearce N, et al: Beta agonists and asthma mortality: Dé jà vu. *Clin Exp Allergy* 21:401-410, 1991.

Petty TL: The National Mucolytic Study: Results of a randomized, double-blind, placebo-controlled study of iodinated glycerol in chronic obstructive bronchitis. *Chest* 97:75-83, 1990 A.

Petty TL: Acute respiratory distress syndrome (ARDS). *Dis Mon* 1-52, (Jan) 1990 B.

Petty TL, et al: Outpatient oxygen therapy in chronic obstructive pulmonary disease: Review of 13 years experience and evaluation of modes of therapy. *Arch Intern Med* 139:28-32, 1979.

Petty TL, et al: Cromolyn sodium is effective in adult chronic asthmatics. *Am Rev Respir Dis* 139:694-701, 1989.

Polak MJ, et al: Perspectives on respiratory distress syndrome of the newborn. *Compr Ther* 15:28-34, (Dec) 1989.

Popa VT: Bronchodilating activity of H$_1$-blocker, chlorpheniramine. *J Allergy Clin Immunol* 59:54-63, 1977.

Prevost RR: Comparing surfactant products. *Clin Pharm* 10:909, 911, 1991.

Rachelefsky GS, et al: Behavior abnormalities and poor school performance due to oral theophylline use. *Pediatrics* 78:1133-1138, 1986.

Rafferty R, Holgate ST: Terfenadine (Seldane) is a potent and selective histamine H$_1$ receptor antagonist in asthmatic airways. *Am Rev Respir Dis* 135:181-184, 1987.

Raju TNK, et al: Double-blind controlled trial of single-dose treatment with bovine surfactant in severe hyaline membrane disease. *Lancet* 1:651-656, 1987.

Rebuck AS, et al: Nebulized anticholinergic and sympathomimetic treatment of asthma and chronic obstructive airways disease in the emergency room. *Am J Med* 82:59-64, 1987.

Reed CE: Aerosol steroids as primary treatment of mild asthma, editorial. *N Engl J Med* 325:425-426, 1991.

Reed CE, Hunt LW: The emergency visit and management of asthma, editorial. *Ann Intern Med* 112:801-802, 1990.

Rees J: Drug treatment in acute asthma. *BMJ* 288:1747-1750, 1984 A.

Rees J: Treatment of chronic asthma. *BMJ* 288:1819-1821, 1984 B.

Reynolds MS, Wallander K: Use of surfactant in the prevention and treatment of neonatal respiratory distress syndrome. *Clin Pharm* 8:559-576, 1989.

Rice KL, et al: Aminophylline for acute exacerbations of chronic obstructive pulmonary disease: Controlled trial. *Ann Intern Med* 107:305-309, 1987.

Richards DM, Brogden RN: Pirbuterol: Preliminary review of pharmacological properties and therapeutic efficacy in reversible bronchospastic disease. *Drugs* 30:6-21, 1985.

Rivington RN, et al: Comparison of morning versus evening dosing with new once-daily oral theophylline formulation. *Am J Med* 79(suppl 6A):67-71, 1985.

Rosenfeld MA, et al: Adenovirus-mediated transfer of a recombinant alpha 1-antitrypsin gene to the lung epithelium in vivo. *Science* 252:431-434, (April) 1991.

Rosenfeld MA, et al: In vivo transfer of the human cystic fibrosis transmembrane conductance regulator gene to the airway epithelium. *Cell* 68:143-155, 1992.

Rossing TH, et al: Effect of outpatient treatment of asthma with beta agonists on response to sympathomimetics in emergency room. *Am J Med* 75:781-784, 1983.

Rotschild A, et al: Increased compliance in response to salbutamol in premature infants with developing bronchopulmonary dysplasia. *J Pediatr* 115:984-991, 1989.

Ryerson GG, Block AJ: Oxygen as drug: Chemical properties, benefits, and hazards of administration, in Burton GG, Hodgkin JE (eds): *Respiratory Care: A Guide to Clinical Practice.* Philadelphia, JB Lippincott, 1984, 395-415.

Schatz M, Zeiger RS: Treatment of asthma and allergic rhinitis during pregnancy, editorial. *Ann Allergy* 65:427-428, 1990.

Sears MR, et al: Regular inhaled beta-agonist treatment in bronchial asthma. *Lancet* 336:1391-1396, 1990.

Sears MR, et al: Relation between airway responsiveness and serum IgE in children with asthma and in apparently normal children. *N Engl J Med* 325:1067-1071, 1991.

Selcow J, et al: Comparison of cromolyn and bronchodilators in patients with mild to moderately severe asthma in office practice. *Ann Allergy* 50:13-18, 1983.

Self TH, et al: Inhaled albuterol and oral prednisone therapy in hospitalized adult asthmatics: Does aminophylline add any benefit? *Chest* 98:1317-1321, 1990.

Sessler CN, et al: Treatment of theophylline toxicity with oral activated charcoal. *Chest* 87:325-329, 1985.

Shapiro GG, König P: Cromolyn sodium: Review. *Pharmacotherapy* 5:156-170, 1985.

Sharma A, et al: Retinol inhibition of in vitro human neutrophil superoxide anion release. *Pediatr Res* 27:547-579 (June) 1990.

Sheffer AL, Buist AS (eds): Proceedings of the Asthma Mortality Task Force. *J Allergy Clin Immunol* 80:1-514, 1987.

Shenai JP, et al: Clinical trial of vitamin A supplementation in infants susceptible to bronchopulmonary dysplasia. *J Pediatr* 111:269-277, 1987.

Similowski T, et al: Contractile properties of the human diaphragm during chronic hyperinflation. *N Engl J Med* 325:917-923, 1991.

Simons FER: Anticholinergic drugs and airways: "Time future contained in time past." *J Allergy Clin Immunol* 80:239-241, 1987.

Sly RM: Beta-adrenergic drugs in management of asthma in athletes. *J Allergy Clin Immunol* 73:680-685, 1984.

Smith PD, et al: Almitrine bismesylate. *Drug Intell Clin Pharm* 21:417-421, 1987.

Snider GL: Pulmonary disease in alpha-1-antitrypsin deficiency, editorial. *Ann Intern Med* 111:957-959, 1989.

Sontag SJ: Gut feelings about asthma: The burp and the wheeze. *Chest* 99:1321-1324, 1991.

Spector SL: Advantages and disadvantages of 24-hour theophylline. *J Allergy Clin Immunol* 76:302-311, 1985 A.

Spector SL: Use of corticosteroids in treatment of asthma. *Chest* 87 (suppl):73S-79S, 1985 B.

Spector S: Asthma and chronic obstructive lung disease: A pharmacologic approach. *Dis Mon* 10-58, (Jan) 1991.

Spector SL, Gomez MG: Dose-response effects of albuterol aerosol compared with isoproterenol and placebo aerosols. *J Allergy Clin Immunol* 59:280-286, 1977.

Spector SL, et al: Pharmacodynamic evaluation of azelastine in subjects with asthma. *J Allergy Clin Immunol* 80:75-80, 1987.

Speer CP, et al: Randomized European multicenter trial of surfactant replacement therapy for severe neonatal respiratory distress syndrome: Single versus multiple doses of Curosurf. *Pediatrics* 89:13-20, 1992.

Spitzer WO, et al: The use of β-agonists and the risk of death and near death from asthma. *N Engl J Med* 326:501-506, 1992.

Storr JNP: Growth of asthmatic children, letter. *BMJ* 303:719, 1991.

Summers R, Smith L: Asthma management: New perspectives, improved options. *Postgrad Med* 76:209-221, (July) 1984.

Szefler SJ: Theophylline: Pharmacokinetics and clinical applications, in Jenne JW, Murphy S (eds): *Drug Therapy for Asthma: Research and Clinical Practice.* New York, Marcel Dekker, 1987, 353-387.

Thomson NC: Nedocromil sodium: An overview. *Resp Med* 83:269-276, 1989.

Thomson NC: Anti-inflammatory therapies. *Br Med Bull* 48:205-220, 1991.

Tinkelman DG, et al: Evaluation of the safety and efficacy of multiple doses of azelastine to adult patients with bronchial asthma over time. *Am Rev Respir Dis* 141:569-574, 1990.

Toogood JH, Hodsman AB: Effects of inhaled and oral corticosteroids on bone, editorial. *Ann Allergy* 67:87-90, 1991.

Torphy TJ: Action of mediators on airway smooth muscle: Functional antagonism as a mechanism for bronchodilator drugs. *Agents Actions Suppl* 23:37-53, 1988.

Tse CST, Bernstein IL: Corticosteroid aerosols in treatment of asthma. *Pharmacotherapy* 4:334-342, 1984.

Ullman A, Svedmyr N: Salmeterol, a new long acting inhaled B_2 adrenoceptor agonist: Comparison with salbutamol in adult asthmatic patients. *Thorax* 43:674-678, 1988.

Van Marter LJ, et al: Maternal glucocorticoid therapy and reduced risk of bronchopulmonary dysplasia. *Pediatrics* 86:331-336, 1990.

Verleden GM, et al: Nedocromil sodium modulates nonadrenergic, noncholinergic bronchoconstrictor nerves in guinea pig airways *in vitro. Am Rev Respir Dis* 143:114-118, 1991.

van Schayck CP, et al: Increased bronchial hyperresponsiveness after inhaling salbutamol during 1 year is not caused by subsensitization to salbutamol. *J Allergy Clin Immunol* 86:793-800, 1990.

Waalkens HF, et al: Budesonide and terbutaline or terbutaline alone in children with mild asthma: Effects on bronchial hyperresponsiveness and diurnal variation in peak flow. *Thorax* 46:499-503, 1991.

Wald JA, et al: An improved protocol for the use of troleandomycin (TAO) in the treatment of steroid-requiring asthma. *J Allergy Clin Immunol* 78: 36-42, 1986.

Wales JKH, et al: Growth retardation in children on steroids for asthma. *Lancet* 338:1535, 1991.

Walker SB, et al: Bitolterol mesylate: Beta-adrenergic agent. *Pharmacotherapy* 5:127-137, 1985.

Walker CL, et al: Potentially fatal asthma. *Ann Allergy* 64:487-493, 1990.

Watanabe S, et al: Long-term effect of almitrine bismesylate in patients with hypoxemic chronic obstructive pulmonary disease. *Am Rev Respir Dis* 140:1269-1273, 1989.

Weinberger M: Pharmacology and therapeutic use of theophylline. *J Allergy Clin Immunol* 73:525-540, 1984.

Weinberger M, et al: Effects of theophylline on learning and behavior: Reasons for concern or concern without reason? *J Pediatr* 111:471-474, 1987.

Weinstein AM, Brokaw A: Pharmacotherapy of asthma. *Ear Nose Throat J* 63:112-120, 1984.

Weitz JI, et al: Increased neutrophil elastase activity in cigarette smokers. *Ann Intern Med* 107:680-682, 1987.

Wewers MD, Gadek JE: The protease theory of emphysema, editorial. *Ann Intern Med* 107:761-763, 1987.

Wewers MD, et al: Comparison of alpha-1-antitrypsin levels and antineutrophil elastase capacity of blood and lung in patient with alpha-1-antitrypsin phenotype null-null before and during alpha-1-antitrypsin augmentation therapy. *Am Rev Respir Dis* 135:539-543, 1987 A.

Wewers MD, et al: Replacement therapy for $alpha_1$-antitrypsin deficiency associated with emphysema. *N Engl J Med* 316:1055-1062, 1987 B.

Whitsett JA, et al: Failure to detect surfactant protein-specific antibodies in sera of premature infants treated with Survanta, a modified bovine surfactant. *Pediatrics* 87:505-510, 1991.

Wilkie RA, Bryan HM: Effect of bronchodilators on airway resistance in ventilator-dependent neonates with chronic lung disease. *J Pediatr* 111:278-282, 1987.

Williams HO: Drug treatment of asthma. *Practitioner* 228:503-508, 1984.

Woolley M, et al: Duration of protective effect of terbutaline sulfate and cromolyn sodium alone and in combination on exercise-induced asthma. *Chest* 97:39-45, 1990.

Wrenn K, et al: Aminophylline therapy for acute bronchospastic disease in the emergency room. *Ann Intern Med* 115:241-247, 1991.

Ziment I: Drugs used in respiratory therapy, in Burton GG, Hodgkin JE (eds): *Respiratory Care: A Guide to Clinical Practice.* Philadelphia, JB Lippincott, 1984, 456-492.

THIS EVALUATION WAS PREPARED AFTER COMPLETION OF THIS CHAPTER

New Evaluation 21

NEDOCROMIL SODIUM
[Tilade]

ACTIONS AND USES. This pyranoquinolone derivative has the same uses as cromolyn sodium. Like that drug, it is extremely safe and causes few adverse reactions. Nedocromil differs from cromolyn sodium in that it affects the function and inhibits the release of additional inflammatory mediators (cytokines, tachykinins); this explains nedocromil's greater potency and its classification as an anti-inflammatory agent (Rainey, 1992). Unlike bronchodilators (beta agonists, theophylline), this drug inhibits bronchial hyperresponsiveness as well as both early- and late-phase bronchoconstrictive reactions. Like cromolyn sodium, it is not a bronchodilator and is not useful in the treatment of acute asthma.

Monotherapy with nedocromil appears to be effective for maintenance therapy in adults with mild to moderate asthma. It is as effective as cromolyn in preventing asthma induced by exercise, irritants, or other stimuli. When used adjunctively with beta agonists, theophylline, or corticosteroids, nedocromil enhances their efficacy and reduces dosage requirements (Busse et al, 1989; Cherniack et al, 1990; Callaghan et al, 1992). It may replace beta agonists or theophylline in many individuals and may allow complete withdrawal of corticosteroids in some patients (ie, those receiving <600 mcg/day) (Bone, 1992).

See also the section on Drug Selection in the Introduction to this chapter.

PHARMACOKINETICS AND ADVERSE REACTIONS. Like cromolyn, this drug is not suitable for oral administration because only insignificant amounts are absorbed from the gastrointestinal tract. Nedocromil also is poorly absorbed in the lungs after inhalation and little drug reaches the systemic circulation; this probably accounts for the extremely low incidence of adverse reactions. The most common adverse effect reported (occurring in about 13% of patients) is an unpleasant taste that is generally transient (Kemp, 1992).

DOSAGE AND PREPARATIONS. For prophylactic therapy in chronic asthma, daily administration in divided doses is required for optimal therapy. Significant clinical effects can occur three days after initiation of therapy; peak effects may not be observed for two weeks and other drugs may be needed in the interim (Kemp, 1992; Cherniack et al, 1990). Inefficient or improper use of the metered-dose inhaler may reduce the amount of drug reaching the site of action; for instructions on correct use, see the manufacturer's literature.

Inhalation: *Adults and adolescents over 12 years*, initially, 3.5 mg (two inhalations) four times daily at regular intervals. The number of doses should then be reduced to the minimum that will control symptoms. Twice-daily administration may be effective in some patients (Callaghan et al, 1992). Data are insufficient to recommend use of nedocromil in *children under 12 years*.

Tilade (Fisons). Metered-dose inhaler providing 1.75 mg per actuation in 16.2 g containers.

Cited References

Bone M: Nedocromil sodium may substitute for steroids in asthma, letter. *BMJ* 305:1367-1368, 1992.

Busse WW, et al: International symposium on nedocromil sodium. *Drugs* 37(suppl 1):1-137, 1989.

Callaghan B, et al: Effects of the addition of nedocromil sodium to maintenance bronchodilator therapy in the management of chronic asthma. *Chest* 101:787-792, 1992.

Cherniack RM, et al: North American Tilade Study Group: A double-blind multicentre group comparative study of the efficacy and safety of nedocromil sodium in the management of asthma. *Chest* 97:1299-1306, 1990.

Kemp JP: Nedocromil sodium, a new bronchial anti-inflammatory agent. *Today's Ther Trends* 10(2):39-48, 1992.

Rainey DK: Evidence for the anti-inflammatory activity of nedocromil sodium, editorial. *Clin Exp Allergy* 22:976-979, 1992.

Beta-Adrenergic Blocking Drugs 22

The response to sympathetic nerve stimulation or circulating catecholamines is mediated by adrenergic receptors (eg, beta receptors) located at postsynaptic, extrasynaptic, and presynaptic sites. Drugs that selectively activate or block these beta receptors have wide therapeutic applications.

Characteristics of Beta-Adrenergic Receptors

Postsynaptic and Extrasynaptic Beta Receptors: Beta-adrenergic receptors are found in the heart, blood vessels, bronchi, kidney, liver, pancreas, adipose tissue, gastrointestinal and uterine smooth muscle, and other tissues. Activation of these receptors increases heart rate and myocardial contractility; facilitates atrioventricular (AV) conduction; stimulates insulin secretion, renin release, glycogenolysis, gluconeogenesis, and lipolysis; and relaxes bronchial, vascular, uterine, and gastrointestinal smooth muscles.

Three subtypes of beta receptor are recognized: beta$_1$, beta$_2$, and beta$_3$. All three subtypes have been cloned and described, but beta$_3$ receptors have not been characterized in humans. In some species, beta$_3$ receptors mediate lipolysis (Zaagsma and Nahorski, 1990). Beta$_1$ and beta$_2$ receptors differ in their relative sensitivity to norepinephrine and epinephrine, in their principal locations, and in the functions that they mediate. Both subtypes produce their physiologic effects by activating the enzyme, adenylyl cyclase, and increasing intracellular concentrations of cyclic adenosine monophosphate (cAMP) (Stiles et al, 1983); however, in the human heart, beta$_2$ receptors are more efficiently coupled to adenylyl cyclase than beta$_1$ receptors (Brodde, 1991). Beta$_1$ receptors are located at postsynaptic sites and have equal affinity for the neurotransmitter, norepinephrine, and for the adrenal medullary hormone, epinephrine, the principal circulating catecholamine. In contrast, beta$_2$ receptors have a greater affinity for epinephrine than norepinephrine.

Beta$_1$ and beta$_2$ receptors coexist in many organs, including the heart. Mixed populations have been identified in human atrial and ventricular tissue and the AV node (Heitz et al, 1983; Saito et al, 1988; Stiles et al, 1983). The numbers of beta receptors are similar in the atria and ventricles, but the relative proportion of beta$_1$ to beta$_2$ receptors varies in the two tissues. Ventricular beta$_2$ receptors constitute approximately 20% of total beta receptors as compared with 30% of those in the atria.

Both inotropic and chronotropic responses are mediated by beta$_1$ and beta$_2$ receptors (Brodde, 1991). In atrial tissue, both beta$_1$ and beta$_2$ receptor stimulation can cause maximal positive inotropic effects; however, in ventricular tissue, the inotropic effect of beta$_2$ receptors can be submaximal compared with that of beta$_1$ receptors. Exercise-induced tachycardia is predominantly mediated by beta$_1$ receptor stimulation, and isoprenaline-induced tachycardia is mediated by

$beta_1$ and $beta_2$ receptor stimulation to about the same degree.

Cardiac $beta_2$ receptors are thought to be activated during acute stress when circulating epinephrine concentrations are elevated. In this setting, their effects are additive to those of $beta_1$ receptors in increasing heart rate (Brown et al, 1986; Friedman et al, 1987) and myocardial contractility (Bristow et al, 1986).

Presynaptic Beta Receptors: Beta receptors also are found at presynaptic sites on sympathetic nerve endings in the heart, blood vessels, kidney, and other sympathetically innervated tissues (Langer, 1981). Unlike presynaptic alpha receptors, which, when activated, *inhibit* the subsequent release of norepinephrine, presynaptic beta receptors *enhance* norepinephrine release. This effect is independent of the alpha or beta nature of the postsynaptic receptor that mediates the response of the effector organ. Thus, activation of presynaptic beta receptors located on vasoconstrictor nerve endings potentiates the vasoconstrictor (alpha) response.

Presynaptic beta receptors are usually classified as $beta_2$ subtype, but the evidence for this is not conclusive. These receptors are activated by circulating epinephrine, which also may be incorporated into the nerve terminals and released as cotransmitter with norepinephrine (Majewski et al, 1980). Both alpha and beta mechanisms, mediated by presynaptic receptors, may play a role in the physiologic regulation of noradrenergic transmission. Low concentrations of epinephrine may enhance norepinephrine release by activating presynaptic beta receptors, while high concentrations may inhibit release of the neurotransmitter by activating presynaptic alpha receptors (Stjärne and Brundin, 1975).

Effects of Beta Blockade

Blockade of Postsynaptic and Extrasynaptic Beta Receptors: Beta-blocking drugs (see Figure for structural formulas) bind reversibly with beta receptors to block the response to sympathetic nerve impulses and circulating catecholamines. Their effects are most pronounced when sympathetic tone is increased. Blockade of myocardial $beta_1$ receptors reduces heart rate, myocardial contractility, and cardiac output. The AV nodal conduction time is prolonged, AV nodal refractoriness is increased, and sinus node automaticity is depressed. $Beta_1$ blockade also suppresses adrenergically induced renin secretion and catecholamine-induced release of free fatty acids from adipose tissue.

BETA-ADRENERGIC BLOCKING AGENTS

Acebutolol

Atenolol

Betaxolol Hydrochloride

Bisoprolol Fumarate

Carteolol

Esmolol Hydrochloride

Labetalol

BETA-ADRENERGIC BLOCKING AGENTS (continued)

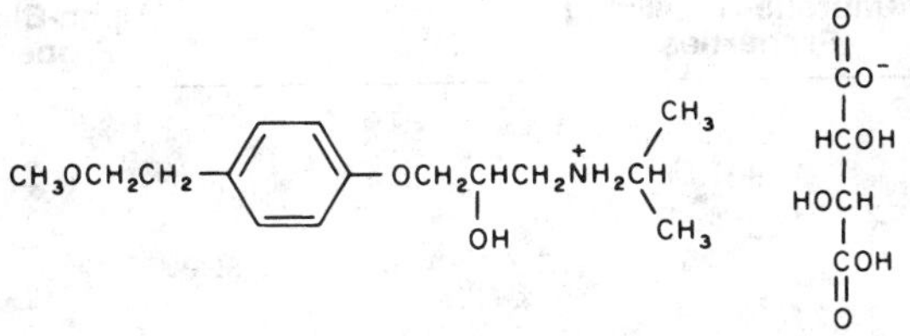

Metoprolol Tartrate

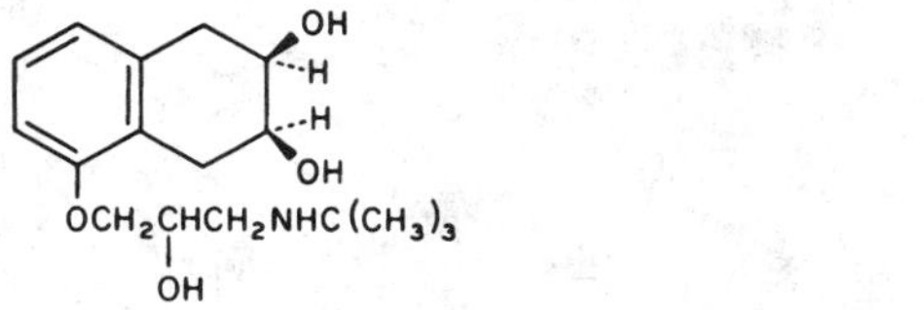

Nadolol

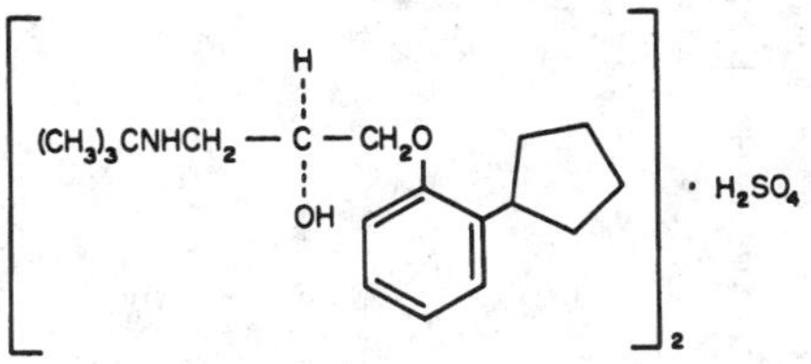

Penbutolol Sulfate

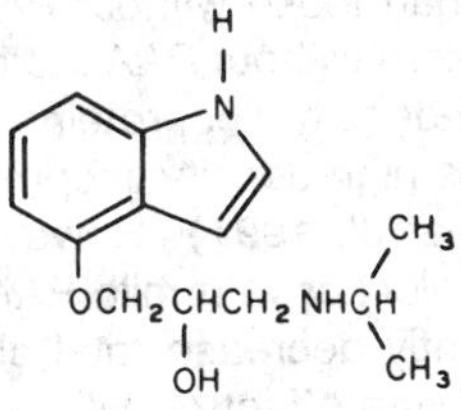

Pindolol

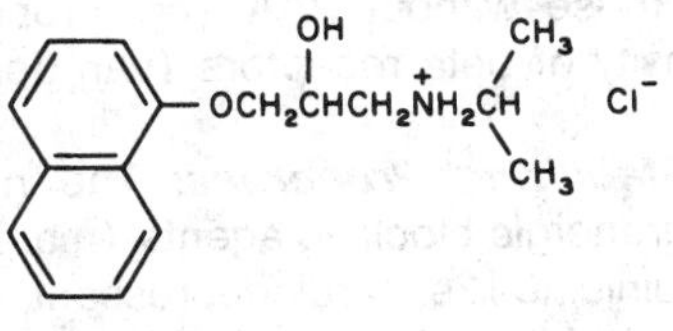

Propranolol Hydrochloride

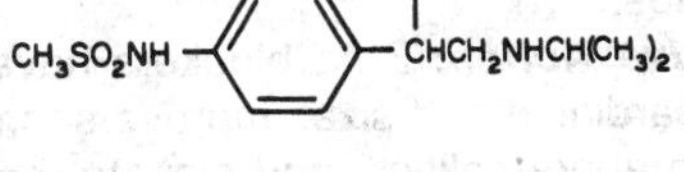

Sotalol

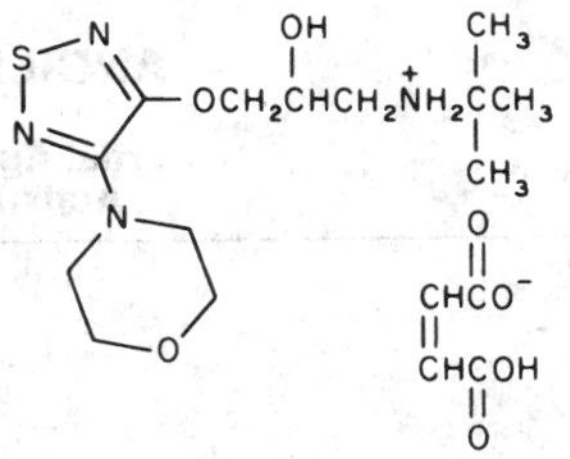

Timolol Maleate

$Beta_2$ blockade in the myocardium may attenuate the positive chronotropic and inotropic effects of circulating catecholamines. Blockade of noncardiac $beta_2$ receptors increases airway resistance; inhibits catecholamine-induced glycogenolysis, gluconeogenesis, and hypokalemia; and blocks the vasodilating effect of catecholamines on vascular smooth muscle. These noncardiac actions are responsible for some of the adverse effects of beta-blocking drugs (ie, bronchospasm, delayed recovery from hypoglycemia, interaction with sympathomimetic amines, aggravation of vasospastic peripheral vascular disease).

Blockade of Presynaptic Beta Receptors: The facilitatory effect of epinephrine on neurotransmitter release during nerve stimulation is prevented by beta blockade, particularly after long-term administration of a beta blocker. A decrease in transmitter release has been demonstrated in both vasoconstrictor (Stjärne and Brundin, 1976) and cardioaccelerator (Yamaguchi et al, 1977) nerves and thus does not depend on the alpha or beta nature of the receptors mediating the end organ response.

Ancillary Properties of Beta-Adrenergic Blocking Agents

Cardioselectivity: Beta blockers are classified as either cardioselective or nonselective on the basis of their relative affinity for $beta_1$ and $beta_2$ receptors (see Table 1). The nonselective agents (eg, propranolol, nadolol, penbutolol, pindolol, labetalol, timolol) block both $beta_1$ and $beta_2$ receptors at all sites, while the cardioselective drugs (eg, acebutolol, atenolol, esmolol, metoprolol) block $beta_1$ receptors but have less effect on $beta_2$ receptors when used in small doses. (The term cardioselectivity came into use because of the misconception that $beta_1$ receptors have only cardiac stimulant activity.) Since $beta_2$ blockade underlies some adverse effects of beta blockers, a cardioselective agent may be safer than a nonselective drug in patients with asthma and in those prone to hypoglycemia. However, all beta blockers should be used cautiously in these individuals because cardioselectivity is not absolute and may be lost at therapeutic doses.

The potential advantages of selective versus nonselective beta blockers are unclear in situations in which circulating epinephrine concentrations are elevated (eg, in acute myocardial infarction). Although cardioselective agents are less likely to enhance the pressor effect of epinephrine (Houben et al, 1982), nonselective beta blockers are more effective in

TABLE 1.
ANCILLARY PROPERTIES OF BETA BLOCKERS

Drug	Partial Agonist Activity	Membrane-Stabilizing Properties	Alpha-Blocking Properties
CARDIOSELECTIVE			
Acebutolol	+	+	–
Atenolol	–	–	–
Betaxolol	–	–	–
Bevantolol*	–	?	–
Bisoprolol	–	–	–
Esmolol	–	–	–
Metoprolol	–	–	–
NONCARDIOSELECTIVE			
Alprenolol*	+	+	–
Carteolol	+	–	–
Dilevalol*	+	–	–
Flestolol*	–	?	–
Labetalol	–	+	+
Nadolol	–	–	–
Penbutolol	+	–	–
Pindolol	+	+	–
Propranolol	–	+	–
Sotalol	–	–	–
Timolol	–	–	–

* *Investigational drug*

preventing epinephrine-induced hypokalemia (Brown et al, 1983; Reid et al, 1986; Simpson et al, 1987) and tachycardia (Brown et al, 1986; Leenen et al, 1988).

Partial Agonist Activity: Partial agonist activity (PAA) (also termed intrinsic sympathomimetic activity [ISA]) is a characteristic of some beta-adrenergic blocking agents that possess both stimulant and antagonistic properties (Table 1) (Jaillon, 1990). A beta-adrenergic blocking agent with PAA stimulates the receptor to which it is bound, leading to activation of adenylyl cyclase and formation of cAMP, while at the same time competitively opposing the stimulant effects of catecholamines. In contrast to the stimulant effect of a pure beta-adrenergic agonist (eg, isoproterenol), the response of a beta-adrenergic blocking agent with PAA is submaximal with maximal receptor occupancy. Binding sites for beta agonists may be in a high- or low-affinity state, and agonists temporarily may either adjust or maintain the beta receptors in the high-affinity form. However, it is not yet known whether partial agonists activate a small percentage of beta receptors into the high-affinity state or if they induce a partial conformational change in all receptors (Benovic et al, 1988).

PAA in a beta-adrenergic blocking agent modifies its pharmacologic effects, especially on cardiac hemodynamics, peripheral circulation, metabolic activity, and receptor density. Cardiac dynamics (heart rate and cardiac output) and peripheral circulation are decreased to a lesser degree by beta blockers with PAA than those without PAA. Long-term treatment with beta blockers without PAA increases plasma triglyceride and very-low-density lipoprotein (VLDL) cholesterol levels and decreases high-density lipoprotein (HDL) cholesterol levels (Ferrari et al, 1991). However, long-term treatment with one beta blocker with mild PAA (acebutolol) was reported to significantly decrease total cholesterol and LDL cholesterol and had little effect on HDL cholesterol (Schnaper, 1990). Pindolol, a beta blocker with more prominent PAA, tends to increase HDL levels. Finally, nonselective beta-adrenergic blocking agents with PAA have been shown to decrease and those without PAA (eg, propranolol) to increase the density of beta receptors (van den Meiracker et al, 1989).

Membrane-Stabilizing Properties: The nonspecific actions of beta-adrenergic blocking agents (manifested as antiarrhythmic or quinidine-like, cardiodepressant, local anesthetic, or membrane-stabilizing) mainly involve a physicochemical interaction between the drug and the cell membrane (Imai, 1991). This interaction is partially dependent on the lipophilicity of the beta blocker and usually is not important at usual therapeutic doses.

Cytoprotective Action: Beta blockers have been shown to reduce myocardial infarct size, improve segmental ventricular wall motion abnormalities, and elevate the threshold for ventricular fibrillation in the ischemic myocardium. These drugs also have a significant, although less striking, effect on subendocardial perfusion. Although the mechanism of action of these protective effects is not clear, beta blockers may lessen certain phenomena associated with irreversible damage during ischemia and/or reperfusion, including accumulation of intracellular and intramitochondrial calcium, deterioration of mitochondrial oxidative phosphorylation, depletion of energy-rich phosphate compounds, reduction of intracellular pH, and accumulation of intracellular free fatty acids and their metabolites.

Alpha-Blocking Properties: In addition to its nonselective effect on beta receptors, labetalol blocks alpha-adrenergic receptors and thus reduces heart rate, myocardial contractility, and total peripheral resistance. This drug is useful in some patients with hypertension, but its advantages or disadvantages in other disorders have not been established. The adverse effects of labetalol reflect both alpha blockade (eg, orthostatic hypotension) and beta blockade. It may be less likely than a conventional beta blocker to precipitate heart failure, AV conduction disturbances, or bronchospasm and to aggravate vasospastic peripheral vascular disease.

Factors Affecting Beta Receptor Density

The density of beta receptors can be altered by interventions that increase or decrease receptor activation. Reduced response to repeated administration of beta agonists is associated with a decrease in receptor density ("down-regulation") in some tissues. In patients with heart failure, plasma norepinephrine levels are increased and ventricular myocardial $beta_1$ receptors down-regulate in direct relation to the severity of ventricular dysfunction (Bristow et al, 1990). Heart failure, particularly that caused by idiopathic dilated cardiomyopathy and aortic valve disease, reduces the density of $beta_1$ receptors but that of $beta_2$ receptors remains constant. This selective loss of $beta_1$ receptors changes the proportion of $beta_1$ and $beta_2$ receptors from approximately 80%:20% in the normal heart to 60%:40% in the failing ventricular myocardium. The 60% to 70% loss in $beta_1$ receptor density leads to a marked decrease in the ability of $beta_1$ agonists (eg, denopamine) to stimulate muscle contraction. Even though the total number of $beta_2$ receptors does not differ in the failing and normal heart, the stimulation of adenylate cyclase in the failing heart by selective $beta_2$ agonists (eg, zinterol) is decreased by approximately 30%. Similarly, selective $beta_2$ stimulation of muscle contraction also is decreased by 30% in right ventricular trabeculae of failing hearts. The densities of both $beta_1$ and $beta_2$ receptors are decreased in mitral valve disease, end-stage ischemic cardiomyopathy, hypertrophic obstructive cardiomyopathy, and tetralogy of Fallot (Brodde et al, 1989). In mitral valve disease and hypertrophic obstructive cardiomyopathy, the ratio of $beta_1$ to $beta_2$ receptors in ventricular muscles was 75%:25% to 80%:20%, which is similar to that found in the left ventricles in normal hearts (Brodde, 1991).

The chronotropic response to both beta agonists and beta blockers is reduced in elderly patients. This has been attributed to a decrease in the apparent affinity rather than to a reduction in the density of beta receptors (Vestal et al, 1979).

Beta blockade also may increase beta receptor density ("up-regulation") during prolonged treatment with both cardioselective and nonselective beta blockers (Aarons et al, 1980; Hedberg et al, 1985). Beta blockers with PAA tend to decrease the density of beta receptors (van den Meiracker et al, 1989). After the drug is discontinued, receptor density returns to the pretreatment level over several days (Aarons et al, 1980).

Mechanisms of Therapeutic Actions in Cardiovascular Disorders

Antianginal Action: The beneficial effect of beta-blocking drugs in angina pectoris derives from their ability to decrease heart rate and myocardial contractility, particularly during exercise. By attenuating the cardiac response to sympathetic stimulation, beta blockade reduces myocardial oxygen demand and thereby delays the onset of ischemic pain. The oxygen-sparing action usually overrides other effects that tend to increase myocardial oxygen consumption (ie, prolonged systolic ejection period, increased ventricular volume). The reduction in blood pressure with beta blockade further decreases myocardial oxygen demand. Beta blockers also may increase coronary blood flow and oxygen supply by reducing heart rate, which prolongs the diastolic interval during which coronary flow occurs. Depending on the level of tonic alpha- and beta-adrenergic receptor activity, beta blockers theoretically could cause coronary vasoconstriction; however, quantitative coronary angiography performed on patients with stable angina revealed no significant constriction of normal or stenotic coronary arteries during beta blocker therapy (Prida et al, 1987). In another study employing angiography, beta blockade prevented the narrowing of stenotic coronary arteries induced by exercise (Gaglione et al, 1987).

Propranolol and metoprolol also may reduce platelet aggregation, and propranolol may cause a shift to the right in the oxyhemoglobin dissociation curve. The clinical importance of these actions is unclear.

Antiarrhythmic Action: The antiarrhythmic effect of beta blockers has been attributed to two actions: blockade of cardiac beta-adrenergic receptors and membrane-stabilizing activity. However, the former action is probably the most important, because the direct membrane effect occurs only at concentrations in excess of those usually employed clinically. The cardiac effects of beta blockade include a reduction in heart rate and myocardial contractility, lengthening of AV conduction time and refractoriness, and suppression of automaticity. Beta blockers may prevent the decrease in ventricular fibrillation threshold induced by catecholamines. They do not reduce the number or complexity of premature ventricular contractions.

Sotalol has additional electrophysiologic properties. In addition to its beta-blocking effects (Class 2), sotalol prolongs the effective refractory period of Purkinje fibers and atrial and ventricular muscle. Thus, it is also classified as a Class 3 antiarrhythmic drug.

Antihypertensive Action: The mechanism(s) by which beta blockers lower blood pressure remains unclear (Hansson, 1991). Blockade of $beta_1$-adrenergic receptors appears to be an important mechanism, since both nonselective and cardioselective blocking agents reduce blood pressure while $beta_2$-selective blockers do not (Dalof et al, 1983). In addition, beta blockers with PAA lower blood pressure via a slightly different mechanism than those without this activity. Generally, beta-adrenergic blocking agents cause an acute fall in cardiac output with a concomitant increase in total peripheral resistance; thus, blood pressure does not fall abruptly. During long-term therapy, cardiac output remains at a reduced level, but total peripheral resistance decreases and blood pressure falls. This dissociation of beta blockade and antihypertensive effects also can be observed on cessation of beta-adrenergic blocking agent therapy, when blood pressure gradually returns to initial levels but the heart rate increases much more rapidly. In contrast, beta blockers with marked PAA reduce total peripheral resistance without lowering cardiac output. This causes an acute fall in blood pressure that is maintained during long-term therapy.

Cardioprotective Action: Antiarrhythmic (particularly antifibrillatory), anti-ischemic, antihypertensive, and/or antiplatelet actions may explain the beneficial effects of long-term beta blockade after acute myocardial infarction. Alternatively, beta blockers may postpone plaque rupture by reducing coronary wall strain (Fitzgerald, 1987). In pronounced hyperadrenergic states, such as acute head injury, subarachnoid hemorrhage, or acute myocardial infarction, beta blockers may prevent catecholamine-induced myocardial necrosis. In one study, patients with traumatic head injury had marked elevations of plasma catecholamines that were directly correlated with increased concentrations of creatine kinase-MB isozyme, sometimes to levels indicative of myocardial infarction (Cruickshank et al, 1987). This rise in catecholamine and creatine kinase-MB isozyme levels was prevented by $beta_1$ blockade. At autopsy, no patients in the beta blocker treatment group had signs of myocardial necrosis, whereas necrotic lesions were observed in the limited number of placebo recipients who were examined.

The cardioprotective effect of beta blockers in myocardial infarction patients also may involve $beta_1$ receptors, for there is no difference between cardioselective and nonselective beta blockers in reducing mortality rates in these patients (Yusuf et al, 1985). However, beta blockers with PAA are less protective. Thus, the success of beta blockers in reducing mortality in cardiovascular disease may be due to a composite of different actions at different sites.

Pharmacokinetics

The pharmacokinetic properties of the available beta blockers are summarized in Table 2. Differences among these

TABLE 2. PHARMACOKINETICS OF AVAILABLE BETA BLOCKERS

Drug	Bioavailability (%)	Half-life (hours)	Lipid Solubility (Log Partition Coefficient Octanol/Water)*	Volume of Distribution (L/kg)	Protein Binding (%)	Urinary Excretion of Unchanged Drug (%)	Active Metabolites
Acebutolol	40	3-4 (active metabolite: 8-13)	low	1.6	26	30-40	Yes
Atenolol	40	6-7 (increased in uremia)	very low	0.7	5	85†	No
Betaxolol	89	14-22	very low	6.1	~50	15	No
Bisoprolol	>90	9-12 (increased in cirrhosis)	moderate	2.9	26-33	50†	No
Carteolol	85	6 (increased in uremia)	low	4.0	23-30	50-70†	Yes
Esmolol	—	0.15	low	3.4	55	2	Yes
Labetalol	25	6-8	moderate/high	9.4	50	5	No
Metoprolol	50	3-7 (increased in poor hydroxylators)	moderate	5.6	12	5	No
Nadolol	30	20-24 (increased in uremia)	very low	2.1	30	76†	No
Penbutolol	~100	26	high	?	50-70	<10	?
Pindolol	95	3-4	low	2.0	40	35-40	No
Propranolol	36	2-3 (increased in cirrhosis)	high	3.9	93	0.5	Yes
Sotalol	100	5-13	very low	1.3	<1	75	No
Timolol	50	4	moderate	1.8	<10	15	No

** very low: 0-1; low: 1-2; moderate: 2-3; high: >3.*

† Dosage adjustment required in patients with renal failure.

drugs relate mainly to their lipid solubility. Compared with lipophilic drugs (eg, propranolol, metoprolol), hydrophilic beta blockers (eg, atenolol, nadolol) are not as readily absorbed from the gastrointestinal tract, are not extensively metabolized, have relatively long plasma half-lives, and do not cross the blood-brain barrier as readily (Cruickshank, 1980). The more water-soluble beta blockers also are thought to cause fewer central nervous system side effects than the lipid-soluble agents (Cruickshank, 1980; Kostis and Rosen, 1987), but this has not been established conclusively (Frishman, 1982; Gengo et al, 1987). Hydrophilic beta blockers should be used in reduced dosage when renal function is impaired.

Plasma concentrations of beta blockers are not closely correlated with the clinical response and are not useful as a guide to therapy.

Major Uses and Drug Selection

Beta-adrenergic blocking agents are used in a wide variety of cardiovascular disorders, including angina pectoris, hypertension, arrhythmias, myocardial infarction, and hypertrophic cardiomyopathy. Noncardiovascular uses include hyperthyroidism, migraine, essential tremor, glaucoma, alcohol withdrawal, and anxiety. See index entries on these indications for further discussion.

All beta blockers have similar therapeutic and adverse effects; however, ancillary or pharmacokinetic properties, experience, and available formulations may influence drug selection for some indications (see Table 3) or when certain coexisting disorders are present (see Table 4).

TABLE 3.
CHOICE OF A BETA BLOCKER IN CARDIOVASCULAR DISORDERS

Indication	Drug Selection
Hypertension	All oral agents are effective in chronic hypertension. Labetalol may have additional applications in hypertensive emergencies.
Angina pectoris	All appear to be effective in stable angina.
Arrhythmias	There has been much more experience with propranolol than with the other beta-blocking drugs. It is not known whether ancillary properties of PAA* or alpha blockade are beneficial or detrimental. Propranolol, metoprolol, atenolol, and esmolol are the only pure beta blockers available in intravenous formulations. Esmolol may be used when a short-acting agent is desirable, but it is more likely to cause hypotension than propranolol.
Myocardial infarction	
Long-term therapy	Both selective and nonselective beta blockers have been effective. Agents with PAA may be less beneficial, and the cardioprotective effect of labetalol is not established.
Acute intervention	Choice is limited to beta blockers available in intravenous formulation. There has been more experience with metoprolol, but the relative merits of selective versus nonselective agents are unsettled. The benefits of esmolol and labetalol are not established.
Hypertrophic cardiomyopathy	More experience with propranolol.

**Partial agonist activity*

TABLE 4.
COEXISTING DISORDERS AFFECTING CHOICE OF A BETA BLOCKER

Coexisting Disorder	Drug Selection
Asthma, chronic obstructive pulmonary disease	Beta blockers should be avoided whenever possible. If a beta blocker must be used, a cardioselective agent or labetalol is preferred.
Diabetes mellitus	Beta blockers probably can be used safely in most patients. A cardioselective agent may be preferred in insulin-dependent diabetic patients.
Raynaud's phenomenon, peripheral occlusive vascular disease	Beta blockers should be avoided if possible. If a beta blocker is strongly indicated, labetalol may be the best choice.
Bradycardia	Agent with partial agonist activity (or a nonbeta blocker) preferred.
Depression	Hydrophilic agent may be preferred.

Adverse Reactions, Precautions, and Interactions

Cardiovascular Reactions: Beta-blocking drugs may cause pronounced bradycardia and hypotension, most commonly with the intravenous route. These drugs should be discontinued if bradycardia is pronounced and symptomatic; however, asymptomatic bradycardia (45 to 55 beats/minute) is common and should not be cause for drug withdrawal. Beta blockers with PAA may cause less resting bradycardia than those lacking this characteristic, but all beta blockers should be used cautiously in patients with slow sinus rates, and they should be avoided in those with sick sinus syndrome.

Beta blockers may precipitate heart failure in patients with inadequate cardiac reserve and should be given with extreme caution to those with frank or incipient heart failure who depend on sympathetic stimulation to remain compensated. If a beta-blocking drug must be used in such patients, therapy should be initiated with small doses, and digitalis and/or a diuretic should be given concomitantly.

Beta-blocking agents may cause fatal cardiac slowing in patients with AV block and are contraindicated in the presence of significant AV conduction disturbances (ie, greater than first-degree AV block). Beta blockers potentiate the effects of other drugs with negative inotropic, chronotropic, and dromotropic actions.

If it becomes necessary to discontinue treatment, dosage should be reduced gradually over a one- to two-week period and physical activity should be restricted during this time. Severe rebound reactions are rare in hospitalized patients with reduced activity, including those with acute myocardial infarction (Croft et al, 1986). It is neither necessary nor desirable to discontinue beta blockers before surgery. Continued intraoperative and postoperative drug administration may reduce the risk of supraventricular arrhythmias after bypass surgery.

Beta blockers often cause cold extremities and occasionally precipitate or worsen Raynaud's phenomenon. The digital vasospasm is caused by blockade of humorally activated (extrasynaptic) beta receptors that mediate dilation of arteriovenous shunts in the fingertips (Cohen and Coffman, 1981). Vasospastic reactions have been reported most commonly in patients with hypertension. Although the presence of Raynaud's phenomenon is not an absolute contraindication, beta blockers probably should be avoided whenever possible, especially in patients with coexisting hypertension (Coffman and Rasmussen, 1985). If a beta blocker is strongly indicated, one also possessing alpha-blocking properties (ie, labetalol) or PAA may be more desirable.

Beta blockers are often withheld from patients with chronic occlusive peripheral vascular disease because of reports that they may adversely affect calf blood flow and aggravate or unmask intermittent claudication. This complication is usually attributed to the reduction in cardiac output rather than $beta_2$ blockade because vascular resistance in skeletal muscle during exercise is largely controlled by local metabolites. In one prospective controlled trial in patients with chronic stable intermittent claudication, calf blood flow and treadmill walking capacity were adversely affected by beta blockers despite their ancillary properties of cardioselectivity, PAA, or alpha blockade (Roberts et al, 1987). In other studies in patients with mild to moderate occlusive vascular disease, no association between beta-blocker therapy and intermittent claudication was observed (Hiatt et al, 1985; Lepäntalo et al, 1985). Nevertheless, such patients should be carefully monitored during initiation of therapy, and beta blockers should be avoided in patients with severe occlusive vascular disease, particularly those with pain at rest.

The effects of beta blockers and ergot alkaloids on the peripheral circulation are additive.

Beta blockers with PAA may increase ventricular ectopic activity and large doses may increase blood pressure. Hypertensive reactions have occurred rarely because of an interaction between nonselective beta blockers and intravenous epinephrine. A hypertensive episode in one patient was attributed to an interaction between the methyldopa metabolite, alpha-methyl-norepinephrine, and intravenous propranolol. These interactions are caused by $beta_2$ blockade, which prevents beta-adrenergic vasodilation and thus permits unopposed alpha stimulation. An enhanced pressor response would therefore occur only with agents that have mixed alpha and beta agonist actions (eg, epinephrine). Although there have been isolated reports that beta blockade also potentiates the pressor response to the alpha agonist, phenylephrine, such an interaction would not be expected on a pharmacologic basis and was not supported by results of a controlled study (Myers, 1984).

Beta blockade may mask the cardiovascular signs of hyperthyroidism and cardiac tamponade.

Respiratory Reactions: Blockade of $beta_2$ receptors increases airway resistance and may provoke asthmatic attacks in patients with a history of asthma or chronic bronchitis. Beta blockers also may worsen respiratory function in those with nonasthmatic chronic obstructive lung disease. Although a cardioselective beta blocker may be safer than a nonselective agent in these patients, all beta blockers should be used cautiously because cardioselectivity may be lost at therapeutically effective dosage. A $beta_2$ agonist (eg, terbutaline) given with a cardioselective blocker reduces the risk of bronchospasm. If bronchospasm develops, a $beta_2$ agonist and theophylline should be administered.

Vasomotor rhinitis has occasionally been associated with use of propranolol or ophthalmic timolol. Apnea has occurred following intentional massive overdose.

Potentiation of Allergic Reactions: Beta blockade may increase the severity (and possibly the frequency) of anaphylactic reactions to drugs, biologicals, allergy injections, insect stings, and foods, and the reaction may prove resistant to treatment with epinephrine (Toogood, 1987). The American College of Allergy and Immunology has warned about the potential danger of systemic reactions to allergen extracts in patients taking beta blockers and suggested that prospective studies be initiated to clarify the magnitude of the risk (Executive Committee, American Academy of Allergy and Immunology, 1989). One prospective study on patients receiving radiographic contrast media detected no increased risk of anaphylactoid reactions in those being treated with beta blockers (Greenberger et al, 1987).

Metabolic Effects: $Beta_2$ blockade impairs the sympathetically mediated rebound response to hypoglycemia and may mask some hypoglycemic symptoms (primarily tachycardia). Although beta blockers probably are safe for use in most diabetic patients, they may potentiate and prolong insulin-induced hypoglycemia and may produce hypoglycemia in individuals recovering from anesthesia, in those on dialysis, and in children during periods of restricted food intake. Beta blockers also occasionally induce hypoglycemia during prolonged exercise. In hypertensive patients, blood pressure may increase during hypoglycemic episodes.

Beta blockers may reduce high-density lipoprotein (HDL) cholesterol and increase serum triglyceride levels, possibly by reducing lipoprotein lipase activity. Beta blockers with PAA appear to have less effect on the lipoprotein profile than those lacking this property (Northcote et al, 1986). Chronic beta blocker therapy does not prevent the elevation in HDL cholesterol induced by exercise training (Arvan and Rueda, 1988).

The effects of thiazide diuretics on blood glucose, lipid, and urate levels may be enhanced by beta blockers (Ballantyne and Ballantyne, 1983).

Neurologic, Psychiatric, and Neuromuscular Reactions: Fatigue and lethargy are the most common central side effects of beta blockers. Vivid dreams or nightmares (with or without insomnia), depression, somnolence, and memory loss also may occur. Visual hallucinations, delirium, and psychotic reactions develop rarely. These central nervous system side effects are believed to be more common with lipophilic beta blockers but also have occurred with the hydrophilic agents. PAA may contribute to sleep disturbances (Kostis and Rosen, 1987). Arthropathy, paresthesias, and reversible hearing loss have been reported rarely in patients treated with beta blockers. Seizures and coma have occurred following intentional massive overdose.

Muscle fatigue and weakness and reduced exercise capacity are common in patients treated with beta blockers. It is not clear whether these symptoms are due to cardiac, vascular, or metabolic effects, impaired neuromuscular transmission, a direct effect on the muscle fiber, or central mechanisms. Beta blockers do not interfere with the beneficial effects of exercise training in patients with coronary artery disease (see index entry Antianginal Agents).

Sexual Dysfunction: Beta-blocking drugs may cause impotence and loss of libido. The mechanism is unclear.

Dermatologic Reactions: Various dermatologic reactions have been reported, including erythematous rashes, psoriasis, pruritus, alopecia, and cheilostomatitis. The severe oculomucocutaneous syndrome caused by practolol has not been clearly associated with other beta-blocking drugs.

Sclerosing and Fibrosing Syndromes: Sclerosing peritonitis was one of the severe adverse effects of practolol that led to its withdrawal. Despite occasional reports, there is no convincing evidence that other beta blockers cause this disorder.

Retroperitoneal fibrosis has been reported in patients receiving various beta blockers, but the available evidence suggests that these drugs may have been used to treat hypertension associated with the retroperitoneal fibrosis and were not causative (Castle, 1985; Pryor et al, 1983). An association also has been reported between therapy with beta blockers and Peyronie's disease, a less severe fibrosing syndrome. It is now believed that this disorder is associated with chronic occlusive peripheral vascular disease and is not caused by beta-blocker therapy (Castle, 1985).

Hematologic Reactions: Agranulocytosis and thrombocytopenic and nonthrombocytopenic purpura have developed rarely.

Miscellaneous Reactions: Gastrointestinal disturbances, fever, sore throat, and dry eyes have been reported occasionally. Hepatic toxicity has occurred very rarely, and a cause-and-effect relationship with beta blocker therapy has not been established.

For adverse effects of labetalol unrelated to beta blockade, see index entry Labetalol, In Hypertension.

Pregnancy and Lactation: Beta blockers cross the placenta and have rarely caused bradycardia, hypotension, and hypoglycemia in the newborn. They also are excreted in breast milk. Atenolol, betaxolol, bisoprolol, carteolol, esmolol, labetalol, metoprolol, nadolol, penbutolol, propranolol, and timolol are classified in FDA Pregnancy Category C and acebutolol and pindolol in FDA Pregnancy Category B.

Interactions: See Table 5 for a summary of major interactions of beta blockers.

Treatment of Toxicity: Atropine 0.5 to 1 mg intravenously controls excessive bradycardia when pronounced vagal tone is a major contributing factor. If emetics or gastric lavage is to be employed, it is advisable to administer atropine first to counteract the associated increase in parasympathetic activity that, in the presence of beta blockade, may lead to cardiovascular collapse (Soni et al, 1983). Isoproterenol should be given in large doses by slow intravenous infusion to treat myocardial depression. Glucagon, which has positive inotropic, chronotropic, and dromotropic effects that are not counteracted by beta blockade, is more effective than isoproterenol for treating beta blocker overdose but is not always readily available. Glucagon is given intravenously (usually in conjunction with high-dose isoproterenol) in a dose of 3 mg or 0.05 mg/kg over 30 seconds followed by continuous infusion of 5 mg/hr or 0.07 mg/kg/hr (Weinstein, 1984). Volume replacement and a vasopressor, such as epinephrine or norepinephrine, have been used to treat severe hypotension. Heart failure is treated with digitalis and diuretics and bronchospasm with a $beta_2$ agonist (eg, terbutaline) and/or theophylline. Diazepam has been used to control seizures.

PREPARATIONS

ACEBUTOLOL HYDROCHLORIDE:

Sectral (Wyeth-Ayerst). Capsules 200 and 400 mg.

ATENOLOL:

Tenormin (ZENECA). Tablets 25, 50, and 100 mg; solution (injection) 0.5 mg/ml in 10 ml containers.

TABLE 5.
DRUG INTERACTIONS WITH BETA BLOCKERS

Interacting Agent	Interaction
Epinephrine	Nonselective beta blockers increase the pressor response and reduce the bronchodilator response to epinephrine but are more effective than selective beta blockers in preventing epinephrine-induced hypokalemia and tachycardia. Patients receiving a beta blocker who experience anaphylactic reactions to drugs or allergy injections may be resistant to treatment with epinephrine.
Calcium channel blocking agents and other drugs with negative inotropic, chronotropic, and dromotropic effects	Additive depressant effect on myocardium and SA and AV nodes
Insulin	Potentiation and prolongation of hypoglycemia, masking of warning symptoms, and hypertensive reactions
Thiazide diuretics	Enhanced effect on blood glucose, serum triglyceride, and urate levels
Indomethacin and possibly other nonsteroidal anti-inflammatory agents	May reduce antihypertensive effect of propranolol, pindolol, and possibly other beta blockers
Ergot alkaloids	Severe peripheral ischemia
Clonidine	Enhanced hypertensive effect following clonidine withdrawal
Methyldopa	Paradoxical hypertensive response to intravenous propranolol
Cimetidine	Reduced clearance of propranolol, labetalol, and possibly other beta blockers
Nicotine	Propranolol is more effective in preventing cardiovascular complications of hypertension in nonsmokers than in smokers
Enzyme-inducing drugs	May reduce plasma concentrations of lipophilic beta blockers (eg, smoking induces hepatic metabolism and lowers serum concentrations of propranolol)

BETAXOLOL HYDROCHLORIDE:
Kerlone (Searle). Tablets 10 and 20 mg.

BISOPROLOL FUMARATE:
Zebeta (Lederle). Tablets 5 and 10 mg.

CARTEOLOL HYDROCHLORIDE:
Cartrol (Abbott). Tablets 2.5 and 5 mg.

ESMOLOL HYDROCHLORIDE:
Brevibloc (DuPont). Solution (injection) 10 and 250 mg/ml in 10 ml containers.

LABETALOL HYDROCHLORIDE:
Normodyne (Schering), ***Trandate*** (Allen & Hanburys). Tablets 100, 200, and 300 mg; solution (injection) 5 mg/ml in 4, 8, 20, and 40 ml containers.

METOPROLOL TARTRATE:
Lopressor (Geigy). Tablets 50 and 100 mg; solution (injection) 1 mg/ml in 5 ml containers.

NADOLOL:
Corgard (Bristol). Tablets 20, 40, 80, 120, and 160 mg.

PENBUTOLOL SULFATE:
Levatol (Reed & Carnrick). Tablets 20 mg.

PINDOLOL:
Visken (Sandoz). Tablets 5 and 10 mg.

PROPRANOLOL HYDROCHLORIDE:
Generic. Tablets 10, 20, 40, 60, 80, and 90 mg; solution (oral) 4, 8, and 80 mg/ml; solution (injection) 1 mg/ml.
Inderal (Wyeth-Ayerst). Tablets 10, 20, 40, 60, and 80 mg; solution (injection) 1 mg/ml in 1 ml containers.
Inderal LA (Wyeth-Ayerst), ***Generic.*** Capsules (prolonged-release) 60, 80, 120, and 160 mg.

SOTALOL HYDROCHLORIDE:
Betapace (Berlex). Tablets 80, 160, and 240 mg.

TIMOLOL MALEATE:
Blocadren (Merck), ***Generic***. Tablets 5, 10, and 20 mg.

Cited References

Aarons RD, et al: Elevation of β-Adrenergic receptor density in human lymphocytes after propranolol administration. *J Clin Invest* 65:949-957, 1980.

Arvan S, Rueda BJ: Nonselective beta-receptor effect on high density lipoprotein cholesterol after chronic exercise. *J Am Coll Cardiol* 12:662-668, 1988.

Ballatyne D, Ballantyne FC: Thiazides, beta blockers and lipoproteins. *Postgrad Med J* 59:483-488, 1983.

Benovic JL, et al: β-Adrenergic receptor kinase: Activity of partial agonists for stimulation of adenylate cyclase correlates with ability to promote receptor phosphorylation. *J Biol Chem* 263:3893-3897, 1988.

Bristow MR, et al: β_1- and β_2-adrenergic-receptor subpopulations in nonfailing and failing human ventricular myocardium: Coupling of both receptor subtypes to muscle contraction and selective β_1-receptor down-regulation in heart failure. *Circ Res* 59:297-309, 1986.

Bristow MR, et al: β-Adrenergic pathways in nonfailing and failing human ventricular myocardium. *Circulation* 82(suppl I):I-12-I-25, 1990.

Brodde O-E: β_1-, and β_2-adrenoceptors in the human heart: Properties, function, and alterations in chronic heart failure. *Pharmacol Rev* 43:203-242, 1991.

Brodde O-E, et al: Drug and disease-induced changes of human cardiac (β_1)-1 and (β_1)-2 receptors. *Eur Heart J* 10(suppl B):38-44, 1989.

Brown MJ, et al: Hypokalemia from beta$_2$-receptor stimulation by circulating epinephrine. *N Engl J Med* 309:1414-1419, 1983.

Brown JE, et al: In support of cardiac chronotropic beta$_2$ adrenoceptors. *Am J Cardiol* 57:11F-16F, 1986.

Castle WM: Drugs and fibrotic reactions: Part 1 and 2. *Adv Drug React Bull* 113:420-423; 114:424-427, 1985.

Coffman JD, Rasmussen HM: Effects of β-adrenoreceptor-blocking drugs in patients with Raynaud's phenomenon. *Circulation* 72:466-470, 1985.

Cohen RA, Coffman JD: β-Adrenergic vasodilator mechanism in finger. *Circ Res* 49:1196-1201, 1981.

Croft CH, et al: Abrupt withdrawal of β-blockade therapy in patients with myocardial infarction: Effects on infarct size, left ventricular function, and hospital course. *Circulation* 73:1281-1290, 1986.

Cruickshank JM: Clinical importance of cardioselectivity and lipophilicity in beta blockers. *Am Heart J* 100:160-178, 1980.

Cruickshank JM, et al: Reduction of stress/catecholamine-induced cardiac necrosis by beta-1 selective blockade. *Lancet* 2:585-589, 1987.

Dalof A, et al: Antihypertensive mechanism of beta-adrenergic antagonism. *J Hypertension* 1(suppl 2):112-115, 1983.

Executive Committee, American Academy of Allergy and Immunology: Beta-adrenergic blockers, immunotherapy and skin testing. *J Allergy Clin Immunol* 84:129-130, 1989.

Ferrari P, et al: Antihypertensive agents, serum lipoproteins and glucose metabolism. *Am J Cardiol* 67:26B-35B, 1991.

Fitzgerald JD: By what means might beta blockers prolong life after acute myocardial infarction? *Eur Heart J* 8:945-951, 1987.

Friedman DB, et al: Beta adrenergic blockade with propranolol and atenolol in the exercising dog: Evidence for beta$_2$ adrenoceptors in the sinoatrial node. *Cardiovasc Res* 21:124-129, 1987.

Frishman WH: Beta-adrenoceptor blocking drugs, editorial. *Int J Cardiol* 2:165-178, 1982.

Gaglione A, et al: Is there coronary vasoconstriction after intracoronary beta-adrenergic blockade in patients with coronary artery disease. *J Am Coll Cardiol* 10:299-310, 1987.

Gengo FM, et al: Lipid-soluble and water-soluble β-blockers: Comparison of the central nervous system depressant effect. *Arch Intern Med* 147:39-43, 1987.

Greenberger PA, et al: Effects of beta-adrenergic and calcium antagonists on the development of anaphylactoid reactions from radiographic contrast media during cardiac angiography. *J Allergy Clin Immunol* 80:698-702, 1987.

Hansson L: Review of state-of-the-art beta-blocker therapy. *Am J Cardiol* 67:43B-46B, 1991.

Hedberg A, et al: Coexistence of beta-1 and beta-2 adrenergic receptors in human heart: Effects of treatment with receptor antagonists or calcium entry blockers. *J Pharmacol Exp Ther* 234:561-568, 1985.

Heitz A, et al: β-Adrenoceptors of human myocardium: Determination of β_1 and β_2 subtypes by radioligand binding. *Br J Pharmacol* 80:711-717, 1983.

Hiatt WR, et al: Effect of β-adrenergic blockers on peripheral circulation in patients with peripheral vascular disease. *Circulation* 72:1226-1231, 1985.

Houben H, et al: Effect of low-dose epinephrine infusion on hemodynamics after selective and nonselective β-blockade in hypertension. *Clin Pharmacol Ther* 31:685-690, 1982.

Imai S: Pharmacologic characterization of beta blockers with special reference to the significance of nonspecific membrane effects. *Am J Cardiol* 67:8B-12B, 1991.

Jaillon P: Relevance of intrinsic sympathomimetic activity for beta blockers. *Am J Cardiol* 66:21C-23C, 1990.

Kostis JB, Rosen RC: Central nervous system effects of β-adrenergic-blocking drugs: Role of ancillary properties. *Circulation* 75:204-212, 1987.

Langer SZ: Presynaptic regulation of release of catecholamines. *Pharmacol Rev* 32:337-362, 1981.

Leenen FHH, et al: Epinephrine and left ventricular function in humans: Effects of beta-1 vs nonselective beta-blockade. *Clin Pharmacol Ther* 43:519-528, 1988.

Lepäntalo M, et al: Does β-blockade provoke intermittent claudication? *Acta Med Scand* 218:35-39, 1985.

Majewski H, et al: Adrenaline activation of prejunctional β-adrenoceptors in guinea-pig atria. *Br J Pharmacol* 71:435-444, 1980.

Myers MG: Beta adrenoceptor antagonism and pressor response to phenylephrine. *Clin Pharmacol Ther* 36:57-63, 1984.

Northcote RJ, et al: Beta blockers and lipoproteins: Review of current knowledge. *Scott Med J* 31:220-228, 1986.

Prida XE, et al: Comparison of selective (beta-1) and nonselective (beta-1 and beta-2) beta-adrenergic blockade on systemic and coronary hemodynamic findings in angina pectoris. *Am J Cardiol* 60:244-248, 1987.

Pryor JP, et al: Do beta-adrenoceptor blocking drugs cause retroperitoneal fibrosis? *BMJ* 287:639-641, 1983.

Reid JL, et al: Epinephrine-induced hypokalemia: Role of beta adrenoceptors. *Am J Cardiol* 57:23F-27F, 1986.

Roberts DH, et al: Placebo-controlled comparison of captopril, atenolol, labetalol, and pindolol in hypertension complicated by intermittent claudication. *Lancet* 2:650-653, 1987.

Saito K, et al: Characterization of β_1 and β_2 adrenoceptor subtypes in the rat atrioventricular node by quantitative autoradiography. *Circ Res* 62:173-177, 1988.

Schnaper HW: Acebutolol effects on lipid profile. *Am J Cardiol* 66:49C-54C, 1990.

Simpson E, et al: Pre-treatment with β blockers and frequency of hypokalaemia in patients with acute chest pain. *Br Heart J* 58:499-504, 1987.

Soni N, et al: Cardiovascular collapse and propranolol overdose. *Med J Aust* 2:629-630, 1983.

Stiles GL, et al: Human cardiac beta-adrenergic receptors: Subtype heterogeneity delineated by direct radioligand binding. *Life Sci* 33:467-473, 1983.

Stjärne L, Brundin J: Dual adrenoceptor-mediated control of noradrenaline secretion from human vasoconstrictor nerves: Facilitation by β-receptors and inhibition by α-receptors. *Acta Physiol Scand* 94:139-141, 1975.

Stjärne L, Brundin J: β_2-Adrenoceptors facilitating noradrenaline secretion from human vasoconstrictor nerves. *Acta Physiol Scand* 97:88-93, 1976.

Toogood JH: Beta-blocker therapy and the risk of anaphylaxis. *Can Med Assoc J* 136:929-933, 1987.

van den Meiracker AH, et al: Hemodynamic and β-adrenergic receptor adaptations during long-term β-adrenoceptor blockade. *Circulation* 80:903-914, 1989.

Vestal RE, et al: Reduced β-adrenoceptor sensitivity in the elderly. *Clin Pharmacol Ther* 24:181-186, 1979.

Weinstein RS: Recognition and management of poisoning with beta-adrenergic blocking agents. *Ann Emerg Med* 13:1123-1131, 1984.

Yamaguchi N, et al: Regulation of norepinephrine release from cardiac sympathetic fibers in dog by presynaptic α- and β-receptors. *Circ Res* 41:108-117, 1977.

Yusuf S, et al: Beta blockade during and after myocardial infarction: Overview of randomized trials. *Prog Cardiovasc Dis* 27:335-371, 1985.

Zaagsma J, Nahorski SR: Is the adipocyte β-adrenoceptor a prototype for the recently cloned atypical -'β_3-adrenoceptor'? *TIPS* 11:1-7, 1990.

Calcium Channel Blocking Drugs 23

Calcium ions play a major role in the function of many tissues, including the myocardium and vascular smooth muscle. Excitation in atrial and ventricular muscle cells and the His-Purkinje system depends on two currents using separate transport systems: the "fast" and "slow" channels. The fast inward current is associated with a rapid influx of sodium ions and is responsible for the upstroke of the cardiac action potential. A subsequent slow inward current, which is carried by calcium, contributes to the plateau phase of the action potential and links myocardial excitation to contraction. In contrast, the pacemaker cells in the sinoatrial (SA) node and cells in the proximal region of the atrioventricular (AV) node are initially depolarized by the calcium current. However, the precise ionic mechanisms mediating the pacemaker potential in these tissues are not well understood, and the role of the calcium current is complex. Activation of the contractile process in vascular smooth muscles also depends on two major systems, one of which involves voltage-dependent calcium influx through channels that resemble those in the myocardium (Robinson, 1985).

ACTIONS

Calcium channel blocking agents are a chemically heterogeneous group of compounds that share the specific basic property of inhibition of the calcium-dependent processes (Opie et al, 1987; Triggle, 1990). By inhibiting calcium influx through the slow channel into cardiac cells and smooth muscle cells of the coronary and systemic arterial beds, calcium channel blocking agents may reduce heart rate and myocardial contractility, slow AV conduction, and reduce peripheral vascular resistance. They prevent increases in coronary artery tone but have considerably less effect than nitroglycerin on basal tone. Most are less active in veins than in arteries and do not increase venous capacitance. Calcium channel blocking agents also suppress calcium-dependent excitation of nonvascular smooth muscle in the gastrointestinal tract, bronchi, uterus, bladder, and ureter.

Calcium channel blocking agents also decrease the vasoconstriction induced by activation of postsynaptic $alpha_2$ receptors in resistance vessels (Van Zwieten et al, 1986). In addition, these drugs (especially the active metabolite of verapamil) may act as antagonists at the beta receptor and, when given for prolonged periods, may increase receptor affinity for agonists (Feldman et al, 1985) or increase the density of beta receptors (Hedberg et al, 1985).

The electrophysiologic and hemodynamic effects and clinical uses of the individual calcium channel blocking drugs vary according to their selectivity of action at different sites, their ancillary properties, and the degree to which afterload reduction and reflex increases in beta-adrenergic tone counteract their direct negative inotropic, chronotropic, and dromotropic effects. The calcium channel blocking drugs can be divided into two groups, based on the specificity of their actions.

The highly specific drugs are represented by three distinct chemical classes (Table 1). The diphenylalkylamine, verapamil [Calan, Isoptin, Verelan], and the benzothiazepine, diltiazem [Cardizem, Dilacor XR], have both cardiac and vascular actions. They depress sinus node automaticity, prolong AV nodal conduction time, increase the refractory period of the AV node, depress myocardial contractility, reduce peripheral vascular resistance, and prevent coronary artery spasm. These drugs have antiarrhythmic, antianginal, and antihypertensive properties. The dihydropyridines (isradipine [DynaCirc], nifedipine [Adalat, Procardia], nicardipine [Cardene], nimodipine [Nimotop], felodipine [Plendil], and amlodipine [Norvasc]) act primarily on vascular smooth muscle. They lack antiarrhythmic properties and usually do not have a net depressant effect on myocardial contractility because their direct negative inotropic, chronotropic, and dromotropic effects are offset by a reflex increase in sympathetic tone induced by vasodilation. In addition, dihydropyridines are such potent vasodilators that reduction in blood pressure occurs before antiarrhythmic or myocardial depressant effects are apparent and thus these effects are rarely seen clinically except in patients with congestive heart failure. Dihydropyridines reduce peripheral vascular resistance and prevent coronary artery spasm. They have antihypertensive and antianginal properties. Some dihydropyridines may demonstrate tissue selectivity (eg, nimodipine and nicardipine for the cerebral vasculature).

TABLE 1.
CALCIUM CHANNEL BLOCKING AGENTS

Chemical Class and Drug	Uses
SPECIFIC CALCIUM ANTAGONISTS	
Diphenylalkylamine	
Verapamil Calan (Searle) Isoptin (Knoll) Verelan (Lederle, Wyeth-Ayerst)	angina pectoris (oral), hypertension (oral), paroxysmal supraventricular tachycardia (intravenous), atrial flutter and fibrillation (oral, intravenous)
Benzothiazepine	
Diltiazem Cardizem (Marion Merrell Dow) Dilacor XR (Rhone-Poulenc Rorer)	angina pectoris (oral), hypertension (oral, intravenous), supraventricular tachycardia (intravenous), atrial flutter and fibrillation (intravenous)
Dihydropyridines	
Amlodipine Norvasc (Pfizer)	angina pectoris (oral), hypertension (oral)
Felodipine Plendil (Merck)	hypertension (oral)
Isradipine DynaCirc (Sandoz)	hypertension (oral)
Nicardipine Cardene (Syntex) Cardene I.V. (Wyeth-Ayerst)	angina pectoris (oral), hypertension (oral, intravenous), subarachnoid hemorrhage (intravenous)
Nifedipine Adalat (Miles) Procardia (Pratt)	angina pectoris (oral), hypertension (oral)
Nimodipine Nimotop (Miles)	subarachnoid hemorrhage (oral)
Nisoldipine* Syscor (Miles)	angina pectoris (oral), hypertension (oral)
Nitrendipine* Baypress (Miles)	hypertension (oral)
LESS SPECIFIC CALCIUM ANTAGONIST	
Bepridil Vascor (McNeil)	angina pectoris (oral)

** investigational drug*

The less specific calcium channel blocking agent, bepridil [Vascor], blocks the sodium channel as well as the myocardial calcium channel and also increases the refractoriness of atrial, His-Purkinje, and ventricular tissues. This drug has been used mainly for the treatment of angina.

USES AND DRUG SELECTION

Arrhythmias: Verapamil and diltiazem are widely used in antiarrhythmic therapy (Singh and Nademanee, 1987). Their ability to prolong AV conduction time and the refractory period of the AV node makes them useful in the treatment of supraventricular tachycardia, including atrial fibrillation, AV nodal reentrant tachycardia, AV reentrant tachycardia with concealed pathway, multifocal atrial tachycardia, and preexcitation syndrome (Wolff-Parkinson-White syndrome) that originates at or above the AV node. In patients with atrial fibrillation, verapamil and diltiazem reduce the heart rate at the onset of the syndrome and during exercise (Pritchett, 1992). These agents usually do not restore sinus rhythm and hence are not appropriate for cardioversion.

Although intravenous adenosine [Adenocard] is the preferred drug, intravenous verapamil or diltiazem can be used for acute termination of AV nodal reentrant tachycardia in adults who do not have sinus node disease or left ventricular dysfunction (Huycke et al, 1989; Morady et al, 1989). After the acute episode has been terminated, long-term oral therapy with verapamil or diltiazem can prevent recurrences if attacks have been frequent or severe.

Multifocal atrial tachycardia, which is usually attributed to enhanced automaticity or triggered activity and is encountered most frequently in patients with chronic pulmonary disease, diabetes, or advanced age, is difficult to treat. Treatment of the underlying disorder is primary. Modification of bronchodilator therapy (eg, reduction in theophylline dosage) may reduce the intensity of the tachycardia in patients with pulmonary disease. Patients also may respond to verapamil, which reduces atrial and ventricular rates and occasionally converts the arrhythmia to sinus rhythm (Levine et al, 1985; Salerno et al, 1987).

A reciprocating tachycardia is the most common arrhythmia in patients with the Wolff-Parkinson-White syndrome, and measures that prolong conduction in the AV node are used to manage an acute attack. Intravenous verapamil or diltiazem is often the preferred drug for terminating the arrhythmia (Buckley et al, 1990; McGovern et al, 1986). However, calcium channel blocking drugs should be avoided when atrial fibrillation or flutter complicates this syndrome because they may increase the ventricular response, leading to ventricular fibrillation. Under these circumstances, radiofrequency catheter ablation of the accessory pathways appears to be the therapy of choice (Ruskin et al, 1991).

See also index entry Arrhythmias.

Angina Pectoris: Angina pectoris occurs when oxygen supply is insufficient to meet the demands of the heart. This is caused by reduction in coronary blood flow and/or lack of increased blood flow at times of increased myocardial oxygen demand (eg, during exercise, in response to stress).

Angina pectoris is categorized as stable or unstable (Brown and Kloner, 1990; Betriu et al, 1992). In patients with stable angina, calcium channel blockers reduce the frequency of attacks, decrease nitrate requirements, and improve exercise performance. Their beneficial effect appears to be due primarily to reduced myocardial oxygen demand (De Servi et al, 1986; Joyal et al, 1986). They may be indicated when nitrates are ineffective or poorly tolerated or when beta-adrenergic blocking agents are contraindicated or produce intolerable side effects. Calcium channel blockers also may be used as first-line therapy. Since these agents do not adversely affect airway resistance, they are preferred to beta blockers in patients with bronchospastic disorders. Calcium channel blockers also may be better tolerated in those with peripheral vascular disease, severe hypertriglyceridemia, or insulin-dependent diabetes. These drugs should not be used for angina that develops after myocardial infarction (Held et al, 1989), except in the subset of patients with normal left ventricular function (Danish Study Group on Verapamil in Myocardial Infarction, 1990).

Calcium antagonists alleviate symptoms of unstable angina by relieving coronary artery spasm, thus increasing myocardial oxygen supply as well as reducing myocardial oxygen consumption. However, calcium channel blocking drugs did not reduce death or incidence of myocardial infarction in patients with unstable angina (Held et el, 1989). The Agency for Health Care Policy and Research and the National Heart, Lung, and Blood Institute recommend that calcium channel blocking drugs only be used as second- or third-line therapy following initiation of nitrates and beta-adrenergic blocking drugs (Braunwald et al, 1994).

Verapamil and diltiazem usually cause mild bradycardia, which is beneficial in patients with angina. Verapamil has the most pronounced effect on AV nodal conduction and is the calcium channel blocker of choice in patients with coexisting supraventricular tachycardia. Diltiazem also may be useful in these patients. Reflex tachycardia occasionally exacerbates anginal symptoms in patients taking nifedipine or nicardipine.

Bepridil depresses the sodium channel current and prolongs cardiac repolarization, which may significantly increase QT intervals and cause torsades de pointes (Flaim and Cummings, 1986). This drug is not appropriate for anginal patients with hypotension and severe left ventricular dysfunction.

See also index entry Angina.

Hypertension: Untreated hypertension can eventually damage the heart, kidneys, brain, and eyes with subsequent morbidity and mortality. The Joint National Committee on Detection, Evaluation, and Treatment of High Blood Pressure (1993) recommended the use of pharmacologic and nonpharmacologic measures to treat chronic hypertension. The aim is to lower both systolic and diastolic blood pressures to target levels using relatively low doses of one, two, or three drugs in rational additive or synergistic combinations to minimize adverse reactions and interference with the patient's lifestyle. An increasing number of drugs and drug groups, including calcium channel blocking drugs, lower blood pressure as monotherapy in patients with mild to moderate hypertension.

In double-blind, placebo-controlled trials, calcium channel blocking drugs were at least as effective in reducing systolic and diastolic blood pressure as beta-adrenergic blocking drugs, diuretics, angiotensin converting enzyme (ACE) inhibitors, labetalol [Normodyne, Trandate], and prazosin [Minipress] (Man in't Veld, 1989; Reid, 1989; Neaton et al, 1993; Materson et al, 1993). A response rate of up to 80% has been reported with some calcium channel blocking drugs (Kirkendall, 1988). These drugs are effective for initial therapy in both blacks and whites and are well tolerated by elderly and physically active patients. They are useful in those who cannot tolerate the pulmonary side effects of beta blockers and in hypertensive patients with coexisting angina. However, these agents, especially verapamil and diltiazem, should be avoided in patients with left ventricular dysfunction, especially those with overt heart failure or after myocardial infarction. Calcium channel blocking drugs also can be used in the treatment of patients with hypertensive emergencies and postoperative hypertension (Onoyama et al, 1988; Sorkin et al, 1985). In individuals with hypertension, concomitant use of a beta blocking agent or an ACE inhibitor enhances blood pressure control. Concurrent diuretic therapy also may be effective (Kaplan, 1989).

See also index entry Hypertension and Table 2 in the chapter on Antihypertensive Drugs.

Pulmonary Hypertension: Pulmonary hypertension is characterized by an increase in the pulmonary arterial pressure and pulmonary vascular resistance. Endothelial cell dysfunction and injury may be responsible for the disease process (Loscalzo, 1992). Inability of the endothelial cells to function may lead to decreased elaboration of prostacyclin, decreased production of endothelium-derived relaxing factor (nitric oxide), and increased release of endothelin, processes that promote pulmonary vasoconstriction and platelet adhesion. The increased afterload on the right ventricle impairs right heart function.

The goals in the treatment of primary pulmonary hypertension are to relieve symptoms and prevent progression of the disease (Brown, 1991; Palevsky and Fishman, 1991; Rubin, 1992). Nifedipine and diltiazem are probably the most effective oral vasodilators for long-term therapy (Rich et al, 1987; Rubin, 1992). Pronounced reduction in pulmonary artery pressure and pulmonary vascular resistance were observed in a small number of patients who received much larger than conventional oral doses of nifedipine (up to 240 mg daily) or diltiazem (up to 720 mg daily). These effects were sustained after one year and were associated with regression of right ventricular hypertrophy (Rich and Brundage, 1987). A majority of patients who responded to high-dose therapy with calcium channel blockers were alive after five years; in contrast, only 50% of patients who did not respond survived for five years (Rich et al, 1992). However, because of the occurrence of hypotension and other side effects, less than 30% of patients were able to tolerate the high-dose regimen (Rich et al, 1992). Addition of digoxin and diuretics to the regimen did not improve the overall outcome.

In a small number of patients with primary pulmonary hypertension, the combination of a calcium channel blocking agent in large doses plus adenosine further decreased pulmonary artery pressure and vascular resistance (Inbar et al, 1993).

See also index entry Pulmonary Hypertension.

High-Altitude Pulmonary Edema: Hypoxic pulmonary hypertension appears to play a role in the pathogenesis of high-altitude pulmonary edema. Transfer of the patient to sea level cures acute cases and ameliorates chronic ones. Nifedipine has been useful for the emergency treatment of this life-threatening condition; its effect has been attributed to a reduction in pulmonary artery pressure (Oelz et al, 1989; Bärtsch et al, 1991).

Peripheral Vascular Disorders: Raynaud's phenomenon is characterized by well-demarcated ischemia of the digits with pallor or cyanosis ending abruptly at one level on the digits (Coffman, 1993). One or all digits may be involved, but the thumb is usually not affected. The pallor phase is due to digital artery vasospasm. There is still some blood flow in the cyanotic phase, although it is slow. Idiopathic or primary Raynaud's phenomenon is most common in females aged 11 to 45 years. Exposure to cold is the most frequent precipitant; in addition, emotional stress has been reported to produce attacks in 9% to 60% of patients.

Nifedipine has decreased the frequency, duration, and intensity of vasospastic attacks in approximately two-thirds of patients with primary or secondary Raynaud's phenomenon (Smith and McKendry, 1982; Rodeheffer et al, 1983; Creager et al, 1984). Those with primary Raynaud's phenomenon may experience the most improvement; digital ulcers have been reported to heal in patients with scleroderma. Doses of 10 to 30 mg three times a day of the regular preparation or 30 to 90 mg once daily of the prolonged-release preparation have been used. Felodipine is as effective as nifedipine. Diltiazem 60 to 360 mg daily divided into two or three doses also was useful in patients with primary or secondary Raynaud's phenomenon in four double-blind, placebo-controlled studies (Coffman, 1993). Isradipine 2.5 to 5 mg two times daily may be effective. Verapamil, nicardipine, and nisoldipine either have been ineffective or responses have been inconsistent.

See also index entry Raynaud's Syndrome.

Stroke: Stroke is the third leading cause of death in the United States and is especially prevalent in individuals over 60 years. Vascular lesions of the brain resulting from hemorrhage, embolism, thrombosis, or rupturing aneurysm are generally involved (Marmot and Poulter, 1992; Pulsinelli, 1992). The three main types of stroke are ischemic stroke, intracerebral hemorrhage, and subarachnoid hemorrhage. Ischemic stroke occurs more frequently in Caucasians than in Asians and blacks; the opposite is true for hemorrhagic stroke. The major risk factor for stroke, whether hemorrhagic or not, is high blood pressure. Other risk factors include elevated levels of serum cholesterol and fibrinogen, diabetes, reduced ventilatory function, smoking, obesity, and use of oral contraceptives and alcohol.

Ischemic stroke results primarily from occlusion of a cerebral blood vessel that causes reduced delivery of oxygen and glucose to the affected vascular territory (Pulsinelli, 1992). The extent of damage from cerebrovascular occlusion depends on the degree and duration of impaired blood flow. Ischemia that causes persistent loss of membrane potentials and lasts at least five minutes but less than one hour results in death of some or all vulnerable neurons, such as the pyramidal neurons in the CA1 and CA4 zones of the hippocampus. When ischemia lasts more than one hour, infarction begins in the central zone receiving the least cerebral blood flow and progressively enlarges in circumference to result in death of glia and other supportive cells in addition to neurons.

Early treatment of acute ischemic stroke may reverse or limit the degree of brain dysfunction by increasing cerebral blood flow and blocking the damaging and irreversible disruption of cellular homeostasis that results from failure of energy-dependent membrane pumps. Nimodipine and nicardipine have been tested for their efficacy in the treatment of ischemic stroke (Sila, 1993). As yet there is no clear evidence that nimodipine is effective. Results of large clinical trials in patients with acute cerebral infarction were negative when nimodipine therapy was begun up to 48 hours after the onset of symptoms (Trust Study Group, 1990; The American Nimodipine Study Group, 1992). However, subgroup analysis suggested that treatment with moderate doses (up to 120 mg/day) might be effective when initiated within 12 hours, and a study in the Netherlands indicated that effects were positive when treatment was begun within 24 hours (Gelmers et al, 1989).

In a feasibility and safety study using nicardipine, treatment was more successful in a small number of patients in whom therapy was started ≤6 hours after stroke onset than in those in whom therapy was initiated 6 to 12 hours after onset; however, there was no correlation between the dose of nicardipine and outcome (Rosenbaum et al, 1991). Thus, it is advantageous to treat patients with ischemic stroke as early as possible.

Subarachnoid hemorrhage due to aneurysms affects more than 25,000 North Americans annually: it causes approximately 8% of all strokes (van Gijn, 1992). Among patients who reach major medical centers alive, the three-month mortality rate exceeds 25%; another 30% have major neurologic deficits. One of the primary causes of death or disability after aneurysmal subarachnoid hemorrhage is cerebral vasospasm, which usually develops and peaks during the first week after subarachnoid hemorrhage but can persist for up to three weeks. Cerebral vasospasm can be detected radiologically in up to 70% of patients with subarachnoid hemorrhage; it most commonly causes narrowing of the distal internal carotid and proximal anterior or middle cerebral arteries. The narrowing is usually localized to the arteries adjacent to the ruptured aneurysm, but remote vessels can be involved; the consequence is hypoperfusion. Blood flow changes may be localized to the rear of the arterial narrowing or may involve several vascular beds. If cerebral blood flow is sufficiently impaired, cerebral infarction can result and cause death or disability.

Because of their ability to dilate cerebral blood vessels and prevent cerebral ischemic complications, nimodipine and nicardipine have been used in the management of patients with subarachnoid hemorrhage. In double-blind, placebo-controlled trials, nimodipine significantly reduced the number of cerebral infarcts and deaths and the incidence of permanent neurologic deficits in these patients (Tettenborn and Dycka, 1990; Wadworth and McTavish, 1992). The incidence of death from delayed ischemic deficit also was lower in patients receiving nimodipine. Similarly, following continuous administration of intravenous nicardipine for 7 to 11 days, vasospasm was significantly reduced in those treated with this drug compared with those receiving placebo (Haley et al, 1991). A reduction of delayed ischemic deficits after treatment with nicardipine also was claimed.

Atherosclerosis: Atherosclerosis develops through numerous complex and interrelated processes involving the accumulation of cholesterol, calcium, and matrix materials (collagen, elastin, and proteoglycans) in the major arteries. Many of the intracellular and extracellular processes involved in atherosclerotic plaque formation require calcium, and it has been suggested that large deposits of cholesterol may trigger physiologic changes in membranes that favor uptake of calcium into the vascular smooth muscle (Henry, 1990). Hence, attempts have been made to modify the atherosclerotic process through modulation of the availability of calcium ions.

Results of recent controlled trials employing angiography indicate that some calcium channel blocking drugs may retard the progression of atherosclerosis in humans. In the Frankfurt trial (Kober et al, 1989), 26 patients with coronary artery disease were treated with verapamil for an average of 13 months and 17 patients in a control group received conventional antianginal therapy with beta-adrenergic blocking drugs and nitrates. Repeat angiography revealed that coronary stenoses regressed in a significantly greater proportion of patients receiving verapamil (21%) compared with those receiving conventional therapy (8%). High-grade stenoses (41%) regressed significantly more frequently than low-grade stenoses (12%) in those receiving verapamil. There also was slower progression in individual stenoses and development of overall disease and less frequent occurrence of new stenoses in the verapamil-treated patients.

In the International Nifedipine Trial on Atherosclerosis Coronary Therapy (INTACT) study (Lichtlen et al, 1990), the effect of nifedipine on the progression of mild coronary artery disease was compared with that of placebo for up to three years in 348 patients. Angiographic follow-up of patients in the two groups indicated that nifedipine therapy did not retard progression or enhance regression of pre-existing lesions. However, formation of new lesions was reduced by 28% in the group treated with nifedipine compared with the placebo group (0.59 versus 0.82 lesions per patient). Twelve deaths occurred among the nifedipine-treated patients with a history of myocardial infarction compared with two deaths in the control group (which had a similar percentage of postinfarction patients).

Administration of nicardipine for 24 months also had no effect on the progression or retardation of advanced stenoses (20% to 75%) in patients with coronary atherosclerosis as confirmed by arteriography (Waters et al, 1990). However, the drug may retard small lesions with stenosis of ≤20%.

The Multicenter Isradipine Diuretic Atherosclerosis Study (MIDAS Research Group, 1989), a three-year, double-blind, randomized trial comparing the effectiveness of isradipine and hydrochlorothiazide in retarding the progression of atherosclerotic lesions in the carotid arteries of more than 800 hypertensive patients, has been completed and the data are being evaluated.

Since the therapeutic effects of calcium channel blocking drugs in controlled clinical trials were achieved without a reduction in hypercholesterolemia, it may be assumed that mechanisms of action of these drugs differ from those of hypolipidemic agents in current use for the treatment of atherosclerosis. Limited data from the clinical trials indicate that calcium channel blocking drugs may prevent the appearance of new lesions or at least retard their growth in patients at high risk for progression of coronary artery disease; however, they do not appear to prevent worsening of symptoms of angina and perhaps may increase the risk of infarction and mortality (Lichtlen et al, 1990; Waters et al, 1990). Long-term clinical trials are needed to confirm their effect in coronary atherosclerosis (Yusuf and Garg, 1991).

Hypertrophic Cardiomyopathy: This disease is characterized by myocardial cellular enlargement in the intraventricular septum, left ventricular free wall, and/or right ventricle. The hypertrophy enhances systolic function, leading to left ventricular outflow obstruction and a decrease in the rate and duration of diastolic filling.

Verapamil is frequently beneficial in patients with hypertrophic cardiomyopathy who are refractory to or cannot tolerate beta blockers (Fananapazir et al, 1992). Oral verapamil improved exercise tolerance and reduced symptoms in a majority of patients; these improvements were maintained for a prolonged period in more than 50%. However, the electrophysiologic and hemodynamic actions of verapamil may cause severe adverse effects in individuals with the obstructive form of hypertrophic cardiomyopathy or elevated diastolic filling pressure. Fatalities have been reported, usually in patients with symptoms of pulmonary congestion or in those with pulmonary capillary wedge pressure >22 mm Hg. The concurrent administration of quinidine appeared to contribute to some hypotensive episodes (Rosing et al, 1985). Experience with other calcium channel blocking drugs is limited. Nifedipine has improved left ventricular diastolic filling; however, its vasodilating effects may cause severe adverse reactions.

Studies on the treatment of hypertrophic cardiomyopathy have not yet demonstrated that mortality is reduced with use of calcium channel blocking agents.

See also index entry Cardiomyopathy, Hypertrophic.

Heart Failure: Heart failure is precipitated by the inability of the myocardium to contract sufficiently during systole, and thus supply an inadequate volume of blood for the metabolic needs of the tissues of the body, or to distend sufficiently during diastole, which results in congestion (Kloner, 1991). Heart failure is associated with increased atrial pressure, reduced exercise tolerance, ventricular arrhythmias, and shortened life expectancy. The abnormality in cardiac function may be due to aberrations in the myocardial cells themselves or to some other structural irregularity (eg, valvular stenosis impairing ventricular ejection).

In patients with congestive heart failure, calcium channel blocking agents (nifedipine, diltiazem, nicardipine, nitrendipine, felodipine, and isradipine) appear to act predominantly on the peripheral and coronary vasculature. Acute administration of these drugs increases coronary blood flow and decreases the aortocoronary sinus oxygen difference, thus improving myocardial energetics. They also increase the cardiac index and decrease systemic vascular resistance and pulmonary capillary wedge pressure during exercise (Weiner, 1988). However, these hemodynamic benefits are not always sustained during long-term treatment, and even in patients who continue to respond, prolonged therapy is not accompanied by a lessening of symptoms or an increase in exercise tolerance (Packer, 1989). In addition, many patients with severe heart failure experience hemodynamic and symptomatic deterioration when treated with calcium channel blockers; some develop severe hypotension and cardiogenic shock. In a randomized, double-blind, cross-over study on patients with New York Association Class II/III congestive heart failure, clinical deterioration necessitated hospitalization in 24% of patients during nifedipine treatment and in 26% during combined therapy with isosorbide dinitrate [Isordil, Sorbitrate], but no patient who received isosorbide dinitrate alone required hospitalization (Elkayam et al, 1990; Jezek et al, 1990). Similarly, compared with the ACE inhibitor, enalapril [Vasotec], felodipine did not enhance treadmill exercise time and peak exercise oxygen consumption in patients with heart failure (Dusselman et al, 1990).

Although evidence is incomplete, there are indications that a cardiac tissue renin-angiotensin system may counteract the actions of the calcium channel blocking agents and other vasodilators, especially in those with heart failure, myocardial infarction, and ischemia (Lindpaintner and Ganten, 1991). This inference is supported by the fact that although most vasodilators improve symptoms of congestive heart failure, ACE inhibitors are more effective and, in the V-HeFT II and SOLVD trials, reduced mortality (Cohn et al, 1991; The SOLVD Investigators, 1991).

Since calcium channel blocking drugs are potent vasodilators, particularly on the arterial circulation, the combination of an ACE inhibitor and a calcium antagonist would appear to further augment vasodilation, improve myocardial perfusion and ejection fraction, and reduce left ventricular hypertrophy. Hence, the V-HeFT III trial is being conducted to test the efficacy of the combination of felodipine, enalapril, and a diuretic on patients with heart failure. The end points to be evaluated are exercise tolerance, quality of life, left ventricular function, plasma norepinephrine and atrial natriuretic factor levels, and reduction in occurrence of arrhythmias and mortality.

See also index entry Heart Failure.

Myocardial Infarction: Myocardial infarction occurs when one or more coronary arteries in the myocardium are blocked, resulting in an insufficient supply of oxygen to the tissues. Many large prospective double-blind placebo-controlled clinical trials of calcium channel blocking agents in acute myocardial infarction have been performed, notably with nifedipine, diltiazem, and verapamil (Gheorghiade and Goldstein, 1991; Yusuf et al, 1991). Nifedipine has no role as a secondary agent in the treatment of myocardial infarction with or without thrombolytic therapy. Not only did this drug fail to improve the clinical state of the postinfarction patients, but it also tended to increase the risk of reinfarction and mortality (Goldbourt et al, 1993).

Diltiazem and verapamil produce effects in subsets of patients: Diltiazem reduced reinfarction in patients without pulmonary congestion or in those with left ventricular ejection fraction >0.4; its efficacy was especially apparent in patients with first non-Q wave and first anterior Q-wave myocardial infarction (Boden et al, 1991). Verapamil, on the other hand, caused reduction in mortality, major cardiac events, and reinfarction only in patients without heart failure. It is unclear why calcium channel blocking agents do not consistently improve the prognosis of patients with myocardial infarction.

See also index entry Myocardial Infarction.

Renal Transplantation: Human cadaver kidneys sustain irreversible injury if kept at room temperature for 30 to 60 minutes after removal from the donor (Epstein, 1992). Flushing and immersion of the kidneys in ice-cold cardioplegic solution with an ion concentration similar to the intracellular space (high potassium, low sodium and calcium) maintains function for up to 72 hours. However, reversible acute tubular necrosis develops after transplantation in a significant number of these cadaver kidneys. Addition of a calcium channel blocking drug to the perfusate solution at the time of kidney removal maintains graft function and delays renal insufficiency. In prospective randomized trials, diltiazem was added to Eurocollins solution perfusate at the time of donor nephrectomy (Neumayer and Wagner, 1987; Wagner et al, 1987). The graft recipient also received a bolus injection of diltiazem preoperatively, followed by maintenance therapy with this drug. The group receiving diltiazem developed acute tubular necrosis less frequently and fewer hemodialysis procedures were required than in the control group. Treatment of only the recipient with diltiazem after transplantation was less effective in protecting against postgraft failure (Neumayer and Wagner, 1987). The beneficial effect of diltiazem on human cadaver kidneys may be due to the drug's cytoprotective action (Schrier et al, 1987). Calcium channel blocking drugs also dilate the preglomerular afferent arterioles, possess inherent immunosuppressive properties, and ameliorate the nephrotoxic effects of cyclosporine [Sandimmune], all of which are useful in those receiving a kidney transplant (Epstein, 1992).

In transplant recipients with initially low parenchymal diastolic blood flow velocity, administration of verapamil promptly increased flow velocity, which continued to improve throughout the course of therapy (Dawidson et al, 1989); those who did not receive verapamil had a further decrease in flow velocity. The number of both first and second rejections was lower and kidney function improved one year after transplantation in patients who had received verapamil (Palmer et al, 1991). In addition, the actuarial graft survival rate at one year was 93% in verapamil-treated patients compared with 68% in the placebo group (Dawidson et al, 1991). Similar effects also were observed with nifedipine (Palmer et al, 1991).

Cyclosporine is a cyclic endecapeptide that inhibits immune responses by inhibiting T-cell lymphokine production. This drug has improved the success rates for all forms of transplantation, but its use is frequently complicated by the occurrence of hypertension, neurologic and dermatologic reactions, endothelial proliferation, and nephrotoxicity. The nephrotoxicity may be caused by the elevated renal vascular resistance, as demonstrated by a 70% reduction in the renal parenchymal diastolic flow velocity in recipients of cadaveric

TABLE 2.
PHARMACOKINETICS OF CALCIUM CHANNEL BLOCKING AGENTS

Drug	Bioavailability (%)	Half-life (hours)	Protein Binding (%)	Volume of Distribution (L/kg)	Urinary Excretion of Unchanged Drug (%)	Active Metabolites
Amlodipine	64	34	97	21	—	No
Bepridil	59	33	99	8	<1	Yes
Diltiazem	40	3-5	70-80	3.3-5.1	2-4	Yes
Felodipine	13-16	10-18	99	0.6-1.5	0	No
Isradipine	15-24	8	95	3	0	No
Nicardipine	35	9	95	0.6	<1	No
Nifedipine	40-70	2-5	92-99	0.6-1.5	<1	No
Nimodipine	13	5	95	0.9-2.3	0.1	No
Verapamil	20-35	4.5-12	90	4.5-7	3-4	Yes

grafts undergoing cyclosporine therapy (Fry et al, 1988). Administration of calcium channel blocking agents (verapamil, isradipine) before initiation of cyclosporine therapy prevented the latter's vasoconstrictive effect (Dawidson et al, 1989, 1991). In addition, glomerular filtration rates were greater in verapamil recipients than in control subjects.

Blood levels of cyclosporine were significantly higher in transplant recipients treated with verapamil or diltiazem than in control subjects (Brockmoller et al, 1990; Dawidson et al, 1989, 1991). This may be related to the ability of verapamil and diltiazem to interfere with the cytochrome P450 enzyme system in the liver and thereby decrease the degradation of cyclosporine. Despite the higher blood levels of cyclosporine, kidney function was markedly improved and there was a lower incidence of rejection and a higher rate of graft survival (Dawidson et al, 1989, 1991). Interestingly, the beneficial effects on kidney function and graft survival did not persist when the dosage of cyclosporine was decreased to correct for the higher blood levels (Oppenheimer et al, 1992). Other calcium channel blocking agents, including dihydropyridines, have no effect on cyclosporine levels in these patients.

Cardioplegia: To limit myocardial damage caused by ischemia and reperfusion in coronary surgical procedures, the myocardium is perfused with an ice-cold cardioplegic solution that has an ion concentration similar to that of the intracellular space (ie, high potassium, low sodium and calcium) (Havel et al, 1991). Addition of diltiazem to the cardioplegic solution appeared to preserve high-energy phosphate levels at the time of cross-clamp removal and after 30 minutes of reperfusion in 40 patients undergoing aortocoronary artery bypass surgery (Christakis et al, 1986). The cardiac index improved early in the postoperative period. In a double-blind placebo-controlled study on patients undergoing percutaneous transluminal coronary angioplasty of the left anterior coronary artery (Piessens et al, 1989), intracoronary diltiazem administered distal to the stenosis greatly reduced the severity and delayed the onset of ischemic pain and ST-segment elevation. However, the number of patients in these studies was small and further assessment of the usefulness of the calcium channel blocking agents is needed.

Amaurosis Fugax: Hypoperfusion of the retinal circulation may lead to a brief loss of vision in one eye, a syndrome known as amaurosis fugax (Amaurosis Fugax Study Group, 1990). The brief loss of sight has been attributed to embolism from the heart or great vessels or to carotid occlusive disease. If attacks are prolonged, the loss of vision can be permanent. The principal treatment has been anticoagulant or antiplatelet therapy and carotid endarterectomy.

Although vasospasm of the ophthalmic blood vessels has not been considered one of the causes of this condition, retinal arterioles are constricted during the period of loss of vision (Burger et al, 1991). In a small group of patients with amaurosis but with no signs of emboli or carotid hypoperfusion, administration of aspirin or warfarin did not relieve symptoms (Winterkorn et al, 1993). However, oral doses of either verapamil or nifedipine abolished attacks. In several patients, the attacks returned when the calcium channel blocking agent was discontinued. Thus, in individuals with amaurosis fugax not caused by thromboembolic disease or carotid artery hypoperfusion, vasospasm of the ophthalmic artery should be suspected. A calcium channel blocking drug may be beneficial in these patients.

PHARMACOKINETICS

See Table 2.

ADVERSE REACTIONS, PRECAUTIONS, AND INTERACTIONS

See the evaluations on the individual drugs.

Drug Evaluations

AMLODIPINE MALEATE
[Norvasc]

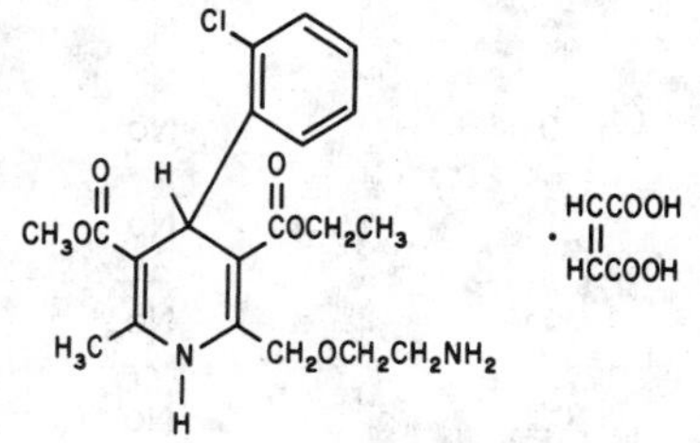

$$\text{Amlodipine: 2-chlorophenyl dihydropyridine with } CH_3OC(=O)\text{, } COCH_2CH_3\text{, } H_3C\text{, } CH_2OCH_2CH_2NH_2 \cdot \text{HCCOOH=HCCOOH}$$

ACTIONS. Like some other calcium channel blockers of the dihydropyridine class, amlodipine is more selective for vascular smooth muscle than for myocardial tissue (Murdoch and Heel, 1991). In the vascular tissue, amlodipine is an arterial vasodilator; its main site of action is in the peripheral vasculature, as indicated by a significant increase in forearm blood flow following intra-arterial infusion (Taylor et al, 1989). This drug also dilates the coronary vascular bed and increases renal blood flow and the glomerular filtration rate. Even though amlodipine inhibits the calcium channel in isolated cardiac tissue, it has no significant effect on sinus node function or cardiac conduction in humans. High concentrations of amlodipine slightly depress contractile activity in isolated cardiac tissue in humans. However, short-term intravenous administration in doses up to 20 mg does not produce evidence of negative inotropism in patients with coronary artery disease.

USES. Amlodipine is effective in the management of mild to moderate hypertension when given alone or with hydrochlorothiazide or ACE inhibitors (Julius, 1988; Murdoch and Heel, 1991). In double-blind trials comparing amlodipine (2.5 to 10 mg once daily for 4 to 12 weeks) with placebo in patients with mild to moderate hypertension, the calcium channel blocking agent reduced systolic and diastolic blood pressure; the effect was dose-dependent. The efficacy of doses of 2.5 to 10 mg was comparable to that of atenolol 50 to 100 mg, hydrochlorothiazide 25 to 100 mg, and captopril 50 to 100 mg and was superior to that of verapamil 160 to 320 mg. In patients with mild to severe hypertension that was partially responsive to hydrochlorothiazide 50 mg or captopril 25 mg, addition of amlodipine 2.5 to 10 mg further improved blood pressure control.

In placebo-controlled studies on patients with stable angina pectoris, amlodipine 10 mg once daily lengthened the period between episodes of anginal pain, increased exercise duration, and reduced nitroglycerin use (Cocco and Alfiero, 1991; Murdoch and Heel, 1991). Significant reductions in ST-segment deviation during exercise were noted. In comparative studies, the antianginal efficacy of amlodipine 10 mg was comparable to that of nadolol 100 mg and diltiazem 180 to 360 mg (Taylor, 1989). In patients with unstable angina, results of one multicenter, randomized, double-blind, placebo-controlled trial showed that amlodipine lengthened the period between anginal attacks, reduced nitroglycerin consumption, and decreased anginal symptoms (Murdoch and Heel, 1991).

ADVERSE REACTIONS AND PRECAUTIONS. The most common side effects of amlodipine are ankle edema, headache, dizziness, fatigue, nausea, and flushing; their occurrence is dose-related, and they develop more frequently in elderly than in younger patients. Muscle cramps, frequency of micturition/nocturia, cough, impotence, asthma, epistaxis, nervousness, and conjunctivitis occur less commonly.

Amlodipine is classified in FDA Pregnancy Category C.

PHARMACOKINETICS. See Table 2.

DOSAGE AND PREPARATIONS.

Oral: *Adults*, for hypertension and angina pectoris, initially, 5 mg once daily. After two weeks, the dosage may be increased to 10 mg once daily. For *patients with hepatic dysfunction*, initially, 2.5 mg once daily.

Norvasc (Pfizer). Tablets 2.5, 5, and 10 mg.

BEPRIDIL HYDROCHLORIDE
[Vascor]

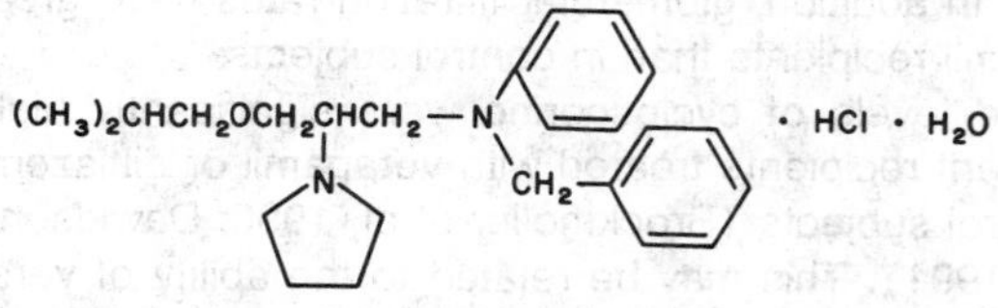

$$(CH_3)_2CHCH_2OCH_2CHCH_2-N(C_6H_5)CH_2C_6H_5 \text{ (pyrrolidinyl at CH)} \cdot HCl \cdot H_2O$$

ACTIONS. The actions of bepridil are less specific than those of verapamil, diltiazem, and the dihydropyridines (Flaim and Cummings, 1986). In addition to blocking the calcium channels of the blood vessels and the heart, bepridil inhibits the sodium current and significantly lengthens cardiac repolarization (Singh et al, 1985; Berger et al, 1989). Because this drug depresses cardiac muscle contraction much more than the calcium current, it has been suggested that bepridil has an intracellular site of action (Flaim and Cummings, 1986). This is supported by the finding that bepridil and some other calcium channel blocking agents (eg, verapamil, nitrendipine) accumulate inside vascular, intestinal, and cardiac muscle cells (Pang and Sperelakis, 1984). The additional uptake of bepridil may explain its relatively long elimination half-life of 33 hours (see Table 2).

Bepridil is more selective for the coronary than the peripheral vasculature (Flaim and Cummings, 1986).

USES. Bepridil is indicated for the treatment of stable angina pectoris in patients who do not respond adequately to other antianginal agents. Results of numerous short- and long-term studies showed that bepridil increases exercise duration, time to onset of angina, time to onset of ST-segment depression, and total workload (Flaim and Cummings, 1986). The frequency of anginal attacks and the consumption of nitroglycerin are decreased. Bepridil does not cause significant changes in the supine resting left ventricular end-diastolic volume index, end-systolic volume index, stroke volume index, cardiac index, or ejection fraction. Nitrates or beta-adrenergic blocking agents can be given concomitantly.

ADVERSE REACTIONS AND PRECAUTIONS. The most common side effects of bepridil are nausea, dyspepsia, diarrhea, dizziness, asthenia, and nervousness. Although adverse effects are frequent, most are well tolerated; however, in long-term open studies, bepridil was discontinued in about 15% of patients because of gastrointestinal disturbances, ventricular arrhythmias, dizziness, or syncope.

Bepridil differs from other calcium channel blocking agents in that it also depresses the sodium current and prolongs cardiac repolarization; significant increases in the QT-intervals occurred in 13 patients with chronic stable angina who were treated with bepridil (Hill and Pepine, 1984). Changes in T-waves also were noted; these included a characteristic notching pattern in three patients and varying degrees of flattening in the remaining ten patients. The prolonged QT interval may precipitate ventricular arrhythmias. Torsades de pointes was reported in 13 of 35,000 patients treated with bepridil. This proarrhythmic action limits the usefulness of bepridil, and the drug is contraindicated in patients with QT intervals >0.44s, conduction abnormalities, or hypokalemia. Bepridil also is inappropriate for use in patients with hypotension and severe left ventricular dysfunction.

Bepridil is classified in FDA Pregnancy Category C.

PHARMACOKINETICS. See Table 2.

DOSAGE AND PREPARATIONS.

Oral: *Adults,* for chronic stable angina pectoris, initially, 200 mg once daily. After ten days, the dosage may be increased. The long interval for dosage adjustment is needed because steady-state blood levels are not achieved until after eight days of therapy. The usual maintenance dose is 300 mg once daily, and the maximum dose is 400 mg once daily.

Vascor (McNeil). Tablets 200, 300, and 400 mg.

DILTIAZEM HYDROCHLORIDE

[Cardizem, Dilacor XR]

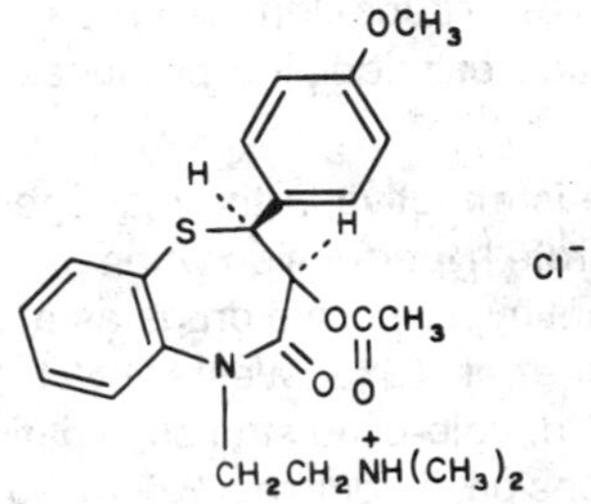

ACTIONS. Diltiazem is a benzothiazepine derivative that causes dose-dependent inhibition of the calcium currents in cardiac and smooth muscle (Buckley et al, 1990). Depression of cardiac action potentials usually results in lengthening of the intranodal conduction time, prolongation of the effective and functional refractory periods of the AV node, and an increase in Wenckebach cycle lengths. In vitro, diltiazem decreases cardiac contractility, but in vivo it is a potent vasodilator and has only mildly negative inotropic effects. The resulting reduction in blood pressure by vasodilation is not accompanied by reflex tachycardia because of the suppression of SA node stimulation by diltiazem.

The response of vascular smooth muscle to diltiazem varies with location. In humans, increased blood flow has been demonstrated in the fingers and forearm and in the splanchnic circulation only when preconstricted with digoxin. Diltiazem neither reduces renal blood flow nor alters the glomerular filtration rate despite its ability to reduce mean arterial pressure and systemic vascular resistance significantly. Renal function may improve in patients with dysfunction caused by hypertension.

USES. Diltiazem is effective in the treatment of mild to moderate hypertension (Buckley et al, 1990). In double-blind, controlled, multicenter clinical trials, the degree of reduction of diastolic and systolic blood pressure produced by diltiazem was similar to that produced by other antihypertensive drugs (eg, hydrochlorothiazide, propranolol, atenolol, captopril, enalapril, nifedipine). Diltiazem also decreased the heart rate by 8% to 10%. In studies conducted over 12 to 20 months, reductions in systolic and diastolic blood pressure of 10% to 18% and 14% to 32%, respectively, were sustained and there was no evidence of tolerance (Stallard et al, 1988).

Black hypertensive patients responded equally well to diltiazem, propranolol, and hydrochlorothiazide (Buckley et al, 1990). Generally, diltiazem was more effective in lowering the systolic blood pressure in the elderly (≥60 years) than in younger patients. In older patients, its antihypertensive effect was equivalent to that of enalapril, captopril, and hydrochlorothiazide and was more pronounced than that of propranolol and atenolol.

In hypertensive emergencies, marked reduction in systolic and diastolic blood pressure was achieved within the first hour following intravenous administration. Further gradual reductions occurred up to six hours after bolus administration of diltiazem in patients with malignant hypertension (Onoyama et al, 1987). Its infusion stabilized the blood pressure of severely hypertensive patients to a normal range within three hours (Onoyama et al, 1988).

The ability of diltiazem to lower blood pressure was compared with that of nifedipine and sodium nitroprusside in 62 patients with postoperative hypertension after coronary bypass procedures (Mullen et al, 1988). The three agents reduced blood pressure equally, but diltiazem also controlled the tachycardia and abnormal myocardial compliance associated with postoperative hypertension. Intravenous diltiazem also reduced ischemic events in patients with coronary artery disease during the pre- and postoperative periods of noncardiac surgery (Buckley et al, 1990).

In stable angina pectoris, diltiazem 240 to 360 mg/day produced consistent and significant improvement in exercise time and time of onset of 1 mm ST-segment depression, and it significantly decreased the frequency of angina attacks and use of nitroglycerin (Klinke et al, 1989). In long-term monotherapy, it was effective in patients with stable exertional angina, and tolerance did not develop (Buckley et al, 1990).

Diltiazem significantly decreased the number of transient ischemic episodes in patients with variant and unstable angina. The survival rate in patients with variant angina who did not experience myocardial infarction was approximately 80% after treatment for 1, 3, 5, and 10 years (Yasue et al, 1988).

Intravenous diltiazem converted paroxysmal supraventricular tachycardia to sinus rhythm and slowed the ventricular response when rapid conversion did not occur (Buckley et al, 1990). Ninety percent of patients with induced re-entrant supraventricular tachycardia converted to sinus rhythm within a median of two minutes (Huycke et al, 1989). Oral diltiazem slowed the ventricular rate in patients with atrial fibrillation or flutter (Steinberg et al, 1987).

ADVERSE REACTIONS, PRECAUTIONS, AND DRUG INTERACTIONS. The incidence of side effects appears to be low with diltiazem. Congestive heart failure, AV conduction disturbances, and sinus arrest have occurred rarely. Severe sinus bradycardia, hypotension, and congestive heart failure may occur during combined treatment with a beta blocker. Excessive hypotension also has occurred in patients receiving diltiazem and prolonged-release nitroglycerin. Diltiazem should be avoided in patients with sick sinus syndrome, AV conduction disturbances, and atrial fibrillation and flutter complicating the Wolff-Parkinson-White syndrome, and it should be given cautiously with other drugs that depress the myocardium or the SA or AV node (eg, beta blockers). Worsening of myocardial ischemia has been reported rarely following sudden withdrawal, but no evidence of a withdrawal reaction was found in a retrospective analysis of a crossover study.

Diltiazem occasionally causes dizziness, weakness, headache, flushing, pedal edema, and gastrointestinal disturbances (pyrosis, anorexia, nausea, diarrhea, abdominal discomfort, constipation).

Dermatologic adverse effects include acne, rash, pruritus, and, rarely, severe reactions such as Stevens-Johnson syndrome, cutaneous vasculitis, erythema multiforme, and exfoliative dermatitis. Glucose intolerance, shoulder and elbow pain, extrapyramidal disorders (akathisia), and gingival hyperplasia also have been reported.

Diltiazem may increase serum digoxin concentrations by up to 20% with concurrent administration. Cimetidine may reduce diltiazem clearance, whereas carbamazepine and other hepatic enzyme inhibitors may enhance diltiazem clearance. Diltiazem may inhibit the metabolism of carbamazepine, theophylline, and cyclosporine. When diltiazem and cyclosporine are given together, the serum cyclosporine concentration is increased significantly (Epstein, 1992). However, no cyclosporine-induced nephrotoxicity has been observed in renal transplantation patients, possibly because of the protective action of diltiazem.

Diltiazem is classified in FDA Pregnancy Category C. It is excreted in breast milk.

For treatment of overdosage or exaggerated response, see the evaluation on Verapamil.

PHARMACOKINETICS. See Table 2.

DOSAGE AND PREPARATIONS.

Oral: *Adults,* for hypertension (prolonged-release preparation), initially, 60 to 120 mg twice daily; (extended-release preparation) 180 to 240 mg once daily. The usual optimal maintenance dose is 240 to 360 mg daily.

For angina pectoris, *adults,* (regular preparation), initially, 30 mg four times daily before meals and at bedtime (maximum, 360 mg daily); (extended-release preparation) initially, 120 to 180 mg once daily (maximum, 480 mg daily).

Generic. Tablets 30, 60, 90, and 120 mg.

Cardizem (Marion Merrell Dow). Tablets 30, 60, 90, and 120 mg; capsules (prolonged-release) 60, 90, and 120 mg (***Cardizem SR***); capsules (extended-release) 120, 180, 240, and 300 mg (***Cardizem CD***).

Dilacor XR (Rhone-Poulenc Rorer). Capsules (prolonged-release) 120, 180, and 240 mg.

Intravenous: *Adults,* for atrial fibrillation and flutter and paroxysmal supraventricular tachycardia, initially, 20 mg or 0.25 mg/kg is given as a bolus over a period of two minutes. If the response is inadequate after 15 minutes, a second dose of 25 mg or 0.35 mg/kg may be administered as a bolus over a period of two minutes. For continual reduction of heart rate, the drug is infused continuously for up to 24 hours at rates of 5, 10, or 15 mg/hr.

Cardizem Injectable (Marion Merrell Dow). Solution 5 mg/ml in 5 and 10 ml containers.

FELODIPINE

[Plendil]

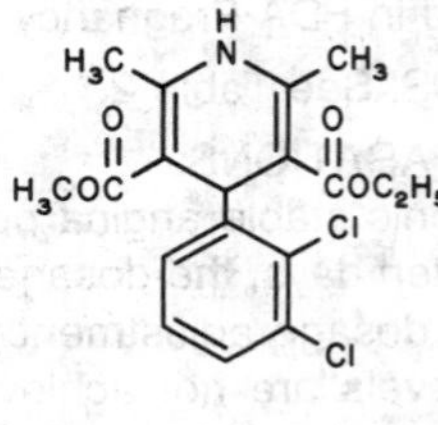

ACTIONS. This calcium channel blocker of the dihydropyridine class is more selective for vascular smooth muscle than for myocardial tissue (Saltiel et al, 1988). Felodipine is 50-fold and 430-fold more potent than nifedipine and verapamil, respectively, in relaxing isolated porcine coronary segments. The primary vascular site of action of felodipine is on the peripheral arterioles (Lund-Johansen and Omvik, 1990). Acute administration of felodipine produces reflex tachycardia.

USES. Felodipine is effective in the management of patients with mild to moderate hypertension when used as monotherapy or with other antihypertensive drugs as a second- or third-line agent (Saltiel et al, 1988; Wester et al, 1991). In short-term, randomized, double-blind studies in patients with mild to moderate hypertension, felodipine 2.5 to 20 mg twice daily was more effective than placebo in lowering blood pressure; the systolic and diastolic blood pressure was decreased up to 25 mm Hg and 20 mm Hg, respectively. Ambulatory monitoring indicated that the mean diastolic pressure in patients treated with felodipine was consistently lower than in placebo-treated patients throughout a 24-hour period. In comparative monotherapy, the efficacy of felodipine (5 to 10 mg twice daily) in mildly to moderately hypertensive patients was equivalent to that of hydrochlorothiazide 25 mg or atenolol 100 mg.

The addition of felodipine (5 to 15 mg twice daily) as a second- or third-line drug in patients who were refractory to beta-adrenergic blocker and/or diuretic therapy reduced the systolic and diastolic blood pressure significantly. When used with a beta-adrenergic blocking agent and/or diuretic, the antihypertensive effect of felodipine (5 to 20 mg twice daily) was comparable to that of minoxidil (10 to 45 mg once daily), prazosin (0.5 to 4 mg twice daily), and propranolol (80 to 160 mg twice daily) and was slightly more prominent than that of hydralazine (25 to 100 mg twice daily).

Felodipine also may be beneficial in patients with hypertension secondary to renal disease and in those with pulmonary hypertension.

ADVERSE REACTIONS, PRECAUTIONS, AND DRUG INTERACTIONS. The most common side effects following therapy with felodipine include ankle edema, headache, and flushing (Saltiel et al, 1988). Ankle edema is usually not associated with a gain in body weight and hence could be due to infiltration of fluid from blood into the local tissues. Other side effects include dizziness, fatigue, insomnia, palpitations, dyspnea, and muscle pain. The overall incidence of adverse reactions is high, although effects are usually mild.

Felodipine is classified in FDA Pregnancy Category C.

Felodipine has produced a transient increase in plasma digoxin levels, but the effect was not sustained with continued administration. Cimetidine significantly increased, while phenytoin, carbamazepine, and phenobarbital reduced, felodipine plasma concentrations. The bioavailability of felodipine was increased by 184% when it was taken with grapefruit juice (Bailey et al, 1991).

PHARMACOKINETICS. See Table 2.

DOSAGE AND PREPARATIONS.

Oral: *Adults,* for hypertension, initially, 5 mg once daily. After two weeks, the dosage may be increased to 10 mg once daily. The maximum dose is 20 mg once daily or, for *elderly patients and those with hepatic dysfunction,* ≤10 mg once daily.

Plendil (Merck). Tablets (prolonged-release) 5 and 10 mg.

ISRADIPINE

[DynaCirc]

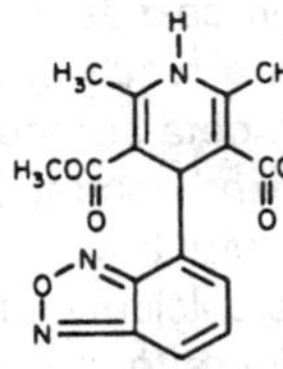

ACTIONS. This calcium channel blocker of the dihydropyridine class is more selective for vascular smooth muscle than for myocardial tissue (Fitton and Benfield, 1990; Vidt, 1990). Isradipine preferentially dilates coronary, cerebral, and skeletal muscle vasculature, particularly the arterial circulation, and has a long duration of action. It has a minimal depressant effect on sinoatrial node automaticity and negligible negative chronotropic, dromotropic, and inotropic actions.

USES. Isradipine is effective in the treatment of mild to moderate hypertension, alone and in combination therapy, regardless of the age or race of the patient (Kirkendall, 1988; Dahlof, 1989; Shepherd et al, 1989). In double-blind, controlled, multicenter clinical trials in patients with mild to moderate hypertension who received isradipine 2.5 to 10 mg administered twice daily for four to ten weeks, the degree of reduction in diastolic and systolic blood pressures was similar to that observed in those treated with hydrochlorothiazide, propranolol, prazosin, diltiazem, and nifedipine. Its antihypertensive efficacy has been maintained for up to two years with no evidence of tachyphylaxis. Isradipine also is effective when given with a diuretic, beta blocker, or ACE inhibitor.

In a study involving a small group of pregnant women with hypertension, isradipine lowered blood pressure and had no adverse effect on the fetal circulation (Ingemarsson et al, 1990).

Results of preliminary studies showed that, in patients with stable angina, isradipine reduces the frequency of angina attacks and the need to use nitroglycerin (Taylor et al, 1987). This calcium channel blocker tends to increase the exercise time to onset of angina and the duration of maximum exercise.

Isradipine has antiatherogenic properties in animal models of atherosclerosis (Weinstein and Heider, 1989). Its effect in humans is unknown. The Multicenter Isradipine Diuretic Atherosclerosis Study (MIDAS Research Group, 1989), a three-year, double-blind, randomized trial in more than 800 men and women with hypertension aged 40 years or older, compared the efficacy of isradipine with that of hydrochlorothiazide in retarding the progression of extracranial carotid atherosclerosis. This study has now been completed and the data are being evaluated.

In patients with sick sinus syndrome, isradipine did not cause negative SA or AV nodal effects (van Wijk et al, 1989). In fact, AV conduction appeared to be enhanced.

ADVERSE REACTIONS AND PRECAUTIONS. Adverse reactions of isradipine were generally dose-related and the result of vasodilation (Dahlof, 1989). Side effects can be minimized by using low doses initially and gradually increasing the amount.

Common adverse reactions are headache, edema, flushing, palpitation, and dizziness. Headache usually occurs early during therapy and is reduced substantially with continued treatment. Because there is no associated weight gain, it is thought that edema is caused by a microvascular mechanism and is not the result of fluid retention caused by heart failure or sodium retention. Isradipine does not cause rebound hypertension, orthostatic hypotension, or impotence.

Isradipine is classified in FDA Pregnancy Category C.

PHARMACOKINETICS. See Table 2.

DOSAGE AND PREPARATIONS.

Oral: *Adults,* for hypertension, the initial dose is 2.5 mg twice daily for two to four weeks; the dose is then increased in 5-mg increments every two to four weeks until the optimal response is achieved. The maximum dose is 20 mg per day. However, no additional benefit, except for longer duration of action, has been observed at dosages >10 mg per day.

DynaCirc (Sandoz). Capsules 2.5 and 5 mg.

NICARDIPINE HYDROCHLORIDE
[Cardene]

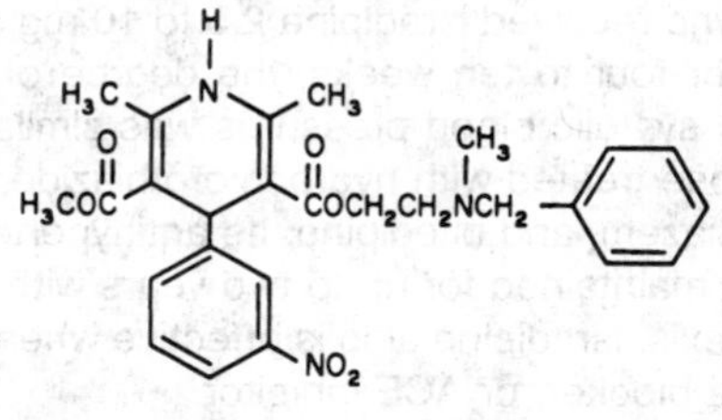

ACTIONS. This calcium channel blocker of the dihydropyridine class is more selective for vascular smooth muscle than for myocardial tissue (Sorkin and Clissold, 1987). Nicardipine is a potent vasodilator of the systemic, coronary, cerebral, and renal vasculature. Systemic and cardiac hemodynamic effects are manifested clinically by decreased systemic vascular resistance and increased cardiac output. Increased heart rate secondary to reflex adrenergic stimulation caused by the decreased systemic vascular resistance may be observed. The increase in cardiac output presumably is due to decreased afterload.

USES. Nicardipine is effective in the treatment of mild to moderate hypertension alone or in combination therapy (Sorkin and Clissold, 1987; Lessem et al, 1990). In double-blind, controlled, multicenter clinical trials, doses of 10 to 40 mg administered three times daily for 1 to 17 weeks reduced diastolic and systolic blood pressures in a dose-dependent fashion with minimal increase in heart rate.

Intravenous administration lowers elevated blood pressure in noncardiac surgical patients with postoperative hypertension (Halpern et al, 1990). In double-blind trials, a therapeutic response was observed in 93% of patients treated with nicardipine and in 30% of those treated with placebo. The heart rate was only minimally elevated.

Nicardipine also is useful in the treatment of severe hypertension that requires rapid lowering of blood pressure (Clifton and Wallin, 1990). Intravenous administration reduced both systolic and diastolic pressure, and control was maintained throughout infusion periods of up to 24 hours. Most patients did not require adjustment of the dose once initial blood pressure control (or therapeutic end point) was achieved. In 56 patients, the mean dose at the end of maintenance was 7.85 mg/hr (range, 3 to 15 mg/hr).

Nicardipine is given orally for the management of chronic stable angina; its efficacy has been reported to be similar to that of nifedipine (Armstrong et al, 1986) and beta blockers (Bjerle et al, 1986) and less than that of verapamil (Rodrigues et al, 1988).

Nicardipine has been used in the treatment of patients with ischemic stroke (Rosenbaum et al, 1991) and subarachnoid hemorrhage (Haley et al, 1991) with varying degrees of success (see the Introduction).

ADVERSE REACTIONS AND PRECAUTIONS. Most of the side effects are transient and appear to be related to the vasodilating property of the drug (Sorkin and Clissold, 1987). These include headache, lightheadedness, flushing, and hypotension. Other cardiovascular side effects are increased anginal symptoms, exercise-induced hypotension, palpitations, dyspnea, and myocardial infarction. Reactions involving the central nervous, gastrointestinal, musculoskeletal, or dermatologic systems occur infrequently and are minor.

Nicardipine is classified in FDA Pregnancy Category C.

PHARMACOKINETICS. See Table 2.

DOSAGE AND PREPARATIONS.

Oral: *Adults,* for hypertension or angina pectoris (regular preparation), initially, 20 mg three times daily. For maintenance, 20 to 40 mg three times daily. In *patients with hepatic insufficiency*, the initial dose is 20 mg two times daily. For hypertension (prolonged-release preparation), *adults*, initially 30 mg two times daily. For maintenance, 30 to 60 mg two times daily.

Cardene (Syntex). Capsules 20 and 30 mg; capsules (prolonged-release) 30, 45, and 60 mg (***Cardene SR***).

Intravenous: *Adults*, for perioperative hypertension, dosage must be individualized depending on severity of the disorder; initially, 5 mg/hour is infused continuously.

Cardene I.V. (Wyeth-Ayerst). Solution (injection) 2.5 mg/ml in 10 ml containers.

NIFEDIPINE
[Adalat, Procardia]

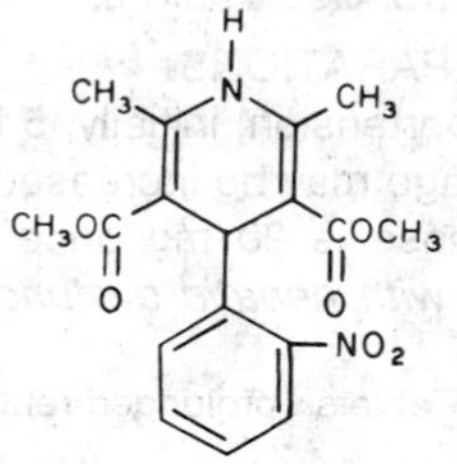

ACTIONS. Nifedipine, a dihydropyridine, inhibits the voltage-dependent calcium channel in the vascular smooth muscle. Its strong vasodilatory action causes a reduction in the systemic arterial resistance. As a result of a secondary baroreceptor-mediated increase in beta-adrenergic tone, there is a reflex increase in heart rate and contractility, leading to a significant increase in cardiac output.

Nifedipine also inhibits the calcium current in normal isolated cardiac tissues; its major effect is on the SA and AV nodes. However, compared with verapamil and diltiazem, in vivo nifedipine either has no effect on or enhances sinus or paced AV nodal conduction. The lack of a direct suppressant effect on AV nodal conduction may be due to the low doses of nifedipine used and reflex tachycardia. Thus, in patients with depressed AV nodal function, nifedipine may be preferable to diltiazem or verapamil in the treatment of symptomatic ischemic heart disease.

USES. Oral doses of nifedipine 30 to 100 mg/day reduce blood pressure in patients with mild to moderate hypertension (Sorkin et al, 1985). This drug can be used as an alternative to beta-adrenergic blocking drugs, diuretics, and ACE inhibitors. Nifedipine has been combined with methyldopa, captopril, and clonidine for the management of hypertension, especially in patients who do not respond to monotherapy with these agents. When nifedipine was given with beta-adrenergic blocking drugs (propranolol, atenolol, acebutolol, pindolol, or timolol), the reduction in blood pressure was sustained. Nifedipine also has been used as a third- or fourth-line drug to further reduce blood pressure to >95 to 105 mm Hg. Tolerance has not developed during long-term therapy.

In single-dose studies in patients with mild to severe hypertension, nifedipine 10 to 20 mg (oral) was safe and reduced blood pressure rapidly (Sorkin et al, 1985). The maximal hypotensive effect is generally observed 30 to 60 minutes after oral administration.

Nifedipine also is used for the treatment of acute episodes of severe hypertension, particularly in hypertensive crises. It is effective in the treatment of acute severe hypertension during pregnancy or the puerperium, arterial hypertension in patients undergoing coronary artery bypass surgery, in postsurgical patients, and in patients with chronic renal failure.

In double-blind, placebo-controlled studies, nifedipine 30 to 60 mg/day for up to six weeks was effective in the management of stable angina (Sorkin et al, 1985). The incidence of anginal attacks and the consumption of nitroglycerin were reduced by 50% to 60%. Exercise tolerance also improved markedly, as indicated by significant increases in the time to onset of angina, maximal exercise duration, and work performance.

Retrospective analysis indicated that nifedipine 10 to 160 mg/day was effective for up to six years in 87% of 439 patients with unstable angina (Sorkin et al, 1985). In a multicenter trial, nifedipine 40 to 160 mg/day was added to the treatment regimen of 127 patients with severe recurrent angina at rest who were refractory to conventional antianginal therapy. Complete remission of anginal attacks was reported in 63% of these patients, and, in 87% of the remaining patients, the frequency of attacks was reduced by at least 50% during a mean follow-up period of nine months; these favorable responses were observed more often in patients with unstable angina than in those with stable angina (Stone et al, 1983).

ADVERSE REACTIONS AND PRECAUTIONS. Nifedipine has been studied more extensively than the other dihydropyridines, but the side effects of all of these drugs appear to be similar.

Nifedipine may cause headache, palpitations, tachycardia, dizziness, weakness, nausea, flushing, transient hypotension, muscle cramps, and hypersensitivity reactions (rash, pruritus, urticaria). Ankle edema occurs in about 10% to 30% of patients. It usually is not caused by heart failure and may not respond to diuretics; local vasodilation has been suggested as a possible cause. Periorbital edema has been reported rarely.

Nifedipine may worsen myocardial ischemia in some patients. This complication may be caused by reflex increases in heart rate and myocardial contractility, reduced perfusion pressure, coronary steal phenomenon, or altered transmural redistribution of myocardial blood flow (Ferlinz, 1986). Concurrent administration of a beta blocker or administration of nifedipine with food may reduce the frequency of this complication when the cause is reflex activation of $beta_1$ receptors. If hypotension is the cause of the myocardial ischemia, beta blockers, nitrates, and other hypotensive drugs may increase the risk. When myocardial ischemia is worsened by nifedipine, the dose should be reduced or other antianginal drugs substituted. Nifedipine shunts blood away from exercising muscle, which may exacerbate leg fatigue during exercise (Choong et al, 1985).

Rarely, nifedipine has precipitated congestive heart failure or cerebral or retinal ischemia. Patients with advanced heart failure or aortic stenosis or those receiving beta blockers or other myocardial depressant drugs are particularly at risk for hemodynamic deterioration. There have been several reports of circulatory collapse in patients treated with nifedipine up to 12 hours prior to coronary artery bypass surgery. Withdrawal reactions (coronary artery spasm, hypertensive crisis) have been reported rarely following sudden discontinuation of nifedipine.

Nocturia has occurred in patients treated with nifedipine, and a few cases of acute urinary retention have been reported. Immune complex glomerulonephritis has occurred rarely. Menorrhagia, gingival hyperplasia, gynecomastia, dermatologic reactions (photosensitivity, erythromelalgia, erythema multiforme, exfoliative dermatitis), eye pain, neuropathies, myoclonic dystonia, and hallucinations have occurred. A possible association between use of nifedipine and an increased risk of cataract formation was observed in a retrospective study (van Heyningen and Harding, 1986).

Nifedipine is classified in FDA Pregnancy Category C.

DRUG INTERACTIONS. Nifedipine may increase serum digoxin levels, but to a lesser extent than verapamil. This drug may alter the disposition of quinidine, possibly by its hemodynamic effects, and the serum quinidine concentration may increase when nifedipine is withdrawn. An increase in plasma phenytoin levels and signs of phenytoin toxicity have been observed when nifedipine was given concurrently. Cimetidine and, to a lesser extent, ranitidine inhibit the metabolism of nifedipine. The bioavailability of nifedipine was increased by 34% when it was taken with grapefruit juice (Bailey et al, 1991).

TREATMENT OF OVERDOSAGE OR EXAGGERATED RESPONSE. There are no well-documented recommendations for treatment of overdosage, and the value of calcium salts is unknown. Excessive hypotension should be treated by elevation of the extremities with careful attention to maintaining adequate circulating fluid volume and urine output. A vasopressor, such as norepinephrine, may be indicated.

PHARMACOKINETICS. See Table 2.

DOSAGE AND PREPARATIONS.

Oral: *Adults,* for chronic hypertension (regular preparation), initially, 10 mg three times daily, followed by 20 mg three times daily. Dosage is titrated upward until the blood pressure is controlled. The usual maximum dose is 180 mg daily. Prolonged-release preparation, initially, 30 or 60 mg once daily (maximum daily dose, 120 mg).

For angina (regular preparation), initially, 10 mg three times daily (range, 10 to 20 mg three times daily). For some patients with unstable angina, 20 to 30 mg three or four times daily may be required. Doses should not exceed 180 mg daily. Prolonged-release preparation, initially, 30 or 60 mg once daily.

Generic. Capsules and tablets 10 and 20 mg.

Adalat (Miles), ***Procardia*** (Pratt). Capsules 10 and 20 mg; tablets (prolonged-release) 30, 60, and 90 mg (***Adalat CC, Procardia XL***).

NIMODIPINE

[Nimotop]

ACTIONS. This dihydropyridine derivative inhibits the voltage- and receptor-operated channels of vascular smooth muscle. It preferentially relaxes the cerebral vasculature, especially when 5-hydroxytryptamine is used as an agonist to constrict isolated blood vessels (Langley and Sorkin, 1989). Nimodipine has a more pronounced effect than other calcium channel blocking agents on cerebral blood vessels (eg, isolated intracerebral penetrating arterioles in the absence of agonist-induced constriction in the rat) (Takayasu et al, 1988). In healthy subjects and in patients with ischemic stroke, nimodipine increases cerebral blood flow without affecting the systolic and diastolic pressure and heart rate (Langley and Sorkin, 1989).

USES. Several uncontrolled and controlled studies on the use of nimodipine in patients with subarachnoid hemorrhage have been performed; the results were variable. In a randomized trial in 116 patients, 60 of whom received oral nimodipine (0.7 mg/kg loading dose followed by 0.35 mg/kg every four hours for 21 days) and 56 of whom received placebo, cerebral vasospasm caused severe ischemic neurologic deficits or death in eight patients who received placebo and in one patient given nimodipine (Allen et al, 1983); arteriographic evidence of vasospasm was similar in 16 patients who received placebo and in 13 who received nimodipine. In a second study, 214 patients received oral nimodipine 30, 60, or 90 mg every four hours, and efficacy was assessed in 170 of these patients. No patients received placebo. No major dose-dependent effect was noted; vasospasm was diagnosed in 7 of 55 patients taking 30 mg of nimodipine, in 3 of 56 patients taking 60 mg, and in 3 of 59 patients taking 90 mg. Only four patients, all of whom received one of the two larger doses, had severe vasospasm.

In a small controlled trial (Mee et al, 1988), 25 patients who were treated with nimodipine were compared with 25 who received a placebo. Six patients given a placebo died (three from ischemia) while only one patient given nimodipine died (as the result of resumption of bleeding). In a randomized multicenter Canadian study testing the efficacy of nimodipine in preventing cerebral ischemia after subarachnoid hemorrhage (Petruk et al, 1988), nimodipine was given to 72 patients and 82 received placebo. Although favorable responses were much more common in the patients given nimodipine (29% versus 9.8%), mortality was also higher in the nimodipine-treated group (47.2% vs 39%). The high mortality rate reflects the seriously ill population, but deaths were consistently more common among patients given nimodipine. The reason for this is not obvious. Permanent neurologic sequelae attributed to vasospasm were diagnosed in 5 patients given nimodipine (6.9%) and in 22 of those receiving placebo (26.8%).

In the British aneurysm nimodipine trial, 554 patients received nimodipine or placebo within 96 hours of the occurrence of subarachnoid hemorrhage (Pickard et al, 1989). The incidence of cerebral infarction and poor outcome was significantly lower in those receiving nimodipine than in the control group.

Results of a clinical trial of nimodipine in 1,064 patients with acute cerebral infarction (ischemic stroke) were unfavorable when therapy was begun up to 48 hours after the onset of symptoms (Trust Study Group, 1990; The American Nimodipine Study Group, 1992); however, subgroup analysis suggested that moderate doses (up to 120 mg/day) might be effective when administered within 12 hours after symptom onset. Results in a study in the Netherlands were positive when treatment was started within 24 hours (Gelmers et al, 1989).

ADVERSE REACTIONS AND PRECAUTIONS. Nimodipine has been well tolerated by patients with subarachnoid hemorrhage. Hypotension is the most prevalent adverse effect.

Following intravenous administration, elevated serum concentrations of gamma-glutamyl transferase and transaminase enzymes were reported in a number of studies. These returned to normal at the end of the treatment period and did not require early withdrawal of nimodipine. The mechanism underlying the rise in serum level of liver enzymes is not clear.

Nimodipine is classified in FDA Pregnancy Category C.

PHARMACOKINETICS. See Table 2.

DOSAGE AND PREPARATIONS.

Oral: For subarachnoid hemorrhage, oral administration should be started as soon as possible; 60 mg is given every four hours for 21 consecutive days. Alternatively, the contents of the capsule can be aspirated into a syringe and emptied into a nasogastric tube, followed by washing with 30 ml of normal saline (0.9%). For patients with hepatic cirrhosis, the dosage is reduced by 50% and the blood pressure and heart rate are monitored closely.

Nimotop (Miles). Capsules 30 mg.

VERAPAMIL HYDROCHLORIDE
[Calan, Isoptin, Verelan]

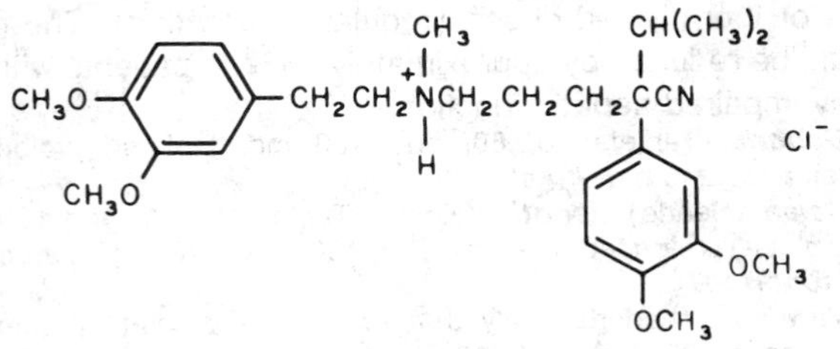

ACTIONS. Verapamil is a diphenylalkylamine that antagonizes calcium influx through the calcium channels of vascular smooth muscle and cardiac cell membranes. By reducing intracellular calcium concentrations, this agent causes coronary and peripheral vasodilation and depresses cardiac contractility and electrical activity in the AV and SA nodes.

USES. In placebo-controlled studies in patients with mild to moderate hypertension, regular or prolonged-release preparations of verapamil administered in daily oral doses of 120 to 480 mg consistently lowered supine, standing, and sitting blood pressure by up to 20% (McTavish and Sorkin, 1989). Twenty-four hour blood pressure control is similar after two or three daily doses of the regular preparation or a single dose of the prolonged-release formulation.

Verapamil's effect on blood pressure is equivalent to that of other first-line antihypertensive agents, including other calcium channel blocking agents (eg, nicardipine, diltiazem, nifedipine, nitrendipine), beta-adrenergic blocking drugs, and diuretics. In one comparative study, oral verapamil 240 to 480 mg/day was as efficacious as propranolol 80 to 480 mg/day, atenolol 50 to 100 mg/day, metoprolol 100 to 200 mg/day, or pindolol 15 mg/day (McTavish and Sorkin, 1989). During exercise, both verapamil and propranolol lower blood pressure without altering the pressor response to exercise, but only propranolol decreases exercise tolerance in hypertensive patients.

Verapamil is particularly useful in elderly patients and in those with low plasma renin activity. A four-week study showed that 320 mg/day of the regular preparation of verapamil reduced supine blood pressure by 26/18 mm Hg, compared with bendroflumethiazide 5 mg/day, which reduced blood pressure by 14/8 mm Hg (McTavish and Sorkin, 1989).

In patients who do not respond to monotherapy, verapamil is effective as a second agent. In patients with moderate to severe hypertension, captopril 100 mg/day combined with verapamil 320 mg/day significantly reduced systolic and diastolic blood pressure. Similarly, combined verapamil and prazosin regimens reduced blood pressure by up to 30/13 mm Hg compared with either drug alone, while treatment with a verapamil/chlorthalidone combination reduced diastolic blood pressure to below 95 mm Hg in patients refractory to verapamil monotherapy. Although the antihypertensive effect of verapamil and a beta-adrenergic blocking agent is beneficial in hypertensive patients, this combination should be avoided in those with impaired cardiac function because of the risk of severe cardiac depression or asystole.

Verapamil also is effective as a third agent in antihypertensive regimens. In patients with severe hypertension refractory to treatment with a diuretic and an ACE inhibitor, blood pressure fell by 37/22 mm Hg after at least seven months of therapy with these agents and verapamil.

Verapamil has been used with varying success in other hypertensive disorders. Patients with pulmonary hypertension had reduced pulmonary arterial pressure and vascular resistance after orally or intravenously administered verapamil, but adverse effects on right ventricular function have been reported. Verapamil has been effective in hypertension secondary to renal disease, in hypertension during pregnancy, and, when given intravenously, in hypertensive crises.

In angina pectoris, verapamil 120 mg three times daily is as effective as propranolol and nifedipine (Krikler, 1987). Verapamil decreased the frequency of anginal attacks and the consumption of nitroglycerin by 15% and significantly improved exercise ability. When verapamil and a beta-adrenergic blocking agent were used in combination in carefully selected, closely monitored patients with refractory, effort-induced angina, symptoms were relieved and exercise tolerance was improved.

Verapamil can be used to terminate paroxysmal supraventricular tachycardia with narrow QRS complexes due to reentry involving anterograde conduction over the AV node (Singh and Nademanee, 1987). Prompt and predictable reversion was observed in 80% to 100% of patients receiving 10 to 15 mg intravenously. The success rate for conversion of paroxysmal supraventricular tachycardia to sinus rhythm may be improved to nearly 100% by carotid sinus massage or the addition of edrophonium 5 to 10 mg given soon after verapamil. This drug is equally effective in terminating both slow-fast and fast-slow paroxysmal supraventricular tachycardia in patients of all ages.

ADVERSE REACTIONS AND PRECAUTIONS. Constipation is the most common side effect of oral verapamil. Headache, dizziness, weakness, flushing, rash, urticaria, and gastric disturbances also may occur. Orthostatic hypotension, AV block (which may lead to AV dissociation and AV junctional rhythms), pedal edema, pulmonary edema, and congestive heart failure have occurred occasionally. Rebound angina has been reported rarely following sudden withdrawal.

A transient, usually asymptomatic, fall in blood pressure is a frequent side effect of intravenous verapamil. Severe hypotension, bradycardia, and asystole have developed in patients with sick sinus syndrome or in those treated concurrently with an intravenous beta blocker. Fatigue, severe hypotension, bradycardia, cardiac failure, and heart block also have developed during combined therapy with oral verapamil and a beta blocker; these drugs should not be used together if left ventricular function is compromised or if AV conduction is impaired.

Verapamil generally should be avoided in patients with sick sinus syndrome, second- or third-degree AV block, cardiogenic shock, or severe congestive heart failure (except when cardiac failure is secondary to supraventricular tachyarrhythmia). Although verapamil is very effective in selected patients with hypertrophic cardiomyopathy, severe adverse reactions (including sinus arrest, AV block, and pulmonary edema) have occurred in others, and fatalities have been reported. Verapamil should be avoided in atrial fibrillation or flutter complicating the Wolff-Parkinson-White syndrome because it may increase the ventricular rate. Adverse hemodynamic events have occurred when verapamil was used to treat ventricular tachycardia misdiagnosed as being of supraventricular origin (Stewart et al, 1986).

Perceptual disorders (feelings of coldness and numbness), vivid dreams, myoclonic dystonia, hyperprolactinemia, galactorrhea, gynecomastia, alopecia, Stevens-Johnson syndrome, gingival hyperplasia, elevated transaminase and alkaline phosphatase levels, and hepatitis have occurred rarely.

Verapamil is classified in FDA Pregnancy Category C. It is excreted in breast milk.

DRUG INTERACTIONS. Verapamil increases serum digoxin concentrations. It reduces quinidine clearance, and hypotension has been reported to result from an interaction between oral quinidine and intravenous verapamil in patients with idiopathic hypertrophic cardiomyopathy. Rifampin (and probably other enzyme-inducing drugs) reduces the bioavailability of verapamil, and cimetidine may theoretically reduce its clearance. Verapamil inhibits the metabolism of carbamazepine and potentiates its neurotoxic effect. It also may inhibit theophylline metabolism. Calcium preparations have been effective in treating verapamil toxicity, and it is possible that the therapeutic response to verapamil (and perhaps to other calcium channel blockers) could be reduced in patients taking calcium supplements. Since calcium supplements are widely prescribed today to prevent postmenopausal osteoporosis, this is an important area for future research.

Verapamil increased the serum cyclosporine concentration in renal transplantation patients without inducing cyclosporine-related nephrotoxicity (Dawidson et al, 1989, 1991).

TREATMENT OF OVERDOSAGE OR EXAGGERATED RESPONSE. Severe hypotensive reactions should be treated with intravenous infusion of norepinephrine and complete AV block with isoproterenol, atropine, and/or pacing. Isoproterenol also is used to treat severe myocardial depression. Intravenous calcium salts (usually gluconate or chloride) also may be used to treat toxicity. Calcium may antagonize the hypotensive effect of verapamil without affecting the antiarrhythmic action (Haft and Habbab, 1986).

In patients with hypertrophic cardiomyopathy, an alpha-adrenergic agonist, such as phenylephrine, should be used to maintain blood pressure; norepinephrine and isoproterenol should be avoided. If further support is needed, dopamine or dobutamine may be used. If verapamil causes a marked increase in the ventricular rate, DC cardioversion is the treatment of choice.

PHARMACOKINETICS. See Table 2.

DOSAGE AND PREPARATIONS.

Oral: *Adults,* for chronic hypertension, 120 mg daily in three divided doses (regular preparation) or 180 mg once daily in the morning (prolonged-release preparation) (maximum daily dose, 480 mg); amounts of the latter preparation above 240 mg daily should be administered in divided doses every 12 hours. For angina and arrhythmias, 240 to 480 mg daily in three or four divided doses (regular preparation). The dose should be reduced by approximately 70% in patients with severely impaired hepatic function.

Generic. Tablets 40, 80, and 120 mg; tablets (prolonged-release) 240 mg.

Calan (Searle), ***Isoptin*** (Knoll). Tablets 40, 80, and 120 mg; tablets (prolonged-release) 120, 180, and 240 mg (***Calan SR, Isoptin SR***).

Verelan (Lederle, Wyeth-Ayerst). Capsules (prolonged-release) 120, 180, and 240 mg.

Intravenous: For paroxysmal supraventricular tachycardia, *adults,* 10 to 15 mg; *children,* 3 to 5 mg.

Isoptin (Knoll), ***Generic.*** Solution (injection) 2.5 mg/ml in 2, 4, and (generic only) 5 ml containers.

Cited References

Allen GS, et al: Cerebral arterial spasm: A controlled trial of nimodipine in patients with subarachnoid hemorrhage. *N Engl J Med* 308:619-624, 1983.

Amaurosis Fugax Study Group: Current management of amaurosis fugax. *Stroke* 21:201-208, 1990.

The American Nimodipine Study Group: Clinical trial of nimodipine in acute ischemic stroke. *Stroke* 23:3-8, 1992.

Armstrong C, et al: Comparison of the efficacy of nicardipine and nifedipine in patients with chronic stable angina. *Br J Clin Pharm* 22:325S-330S, 1986.

Bailey DG, et al: Interaction of citrus juices with felodipine and nifedipine. *Lancet* 337:268-269, 1991.

Bärtsch P, et al: Prevention of high-altitude pulmonary edema by nifedipine. *N Engl J Med* 325:1284-1289, 1991.

Berger F, et al: Effects of the calcium entry blocker bepridil on repolarizing and pacemaker currents in sheep cardiac Purkinje fibres. *Naunyn-Schmiedeberg's Arch Pharmacol* 339:638-646, 1989.

Betriu A, et al: Unstable angina: Outcome according to clinical presentation. *J Am Coll Cardiol* 19:1659-1663, 1992.

Bjerle P, et al: Nicardipine and propranolol in angina pectoris: Comparative study with special reference to ergometer working capacity tests. *Br J Clin Pharm* 22:339S-343S, 1986.

Boden WE, et al: Electrocardiographic subset analysis of diltiazem administration on long-term outcome after acute myocardial infarction. *Am J Cardiol* 67:335-342, 1991.

Braunwald E, et al: *Unstable Angina: Diagnosis and Management.* Clinical Practice Guideline Number 10. AHCPR Publication No. 94-0602. Rockville, Md, Agency for Health Care Policy and Research and the National Heart, Lung, and Blood Institute, 1994.

Brockmoller J, et al: Pharmacokinetic interaction between cyclosporine and diltiazem. *Eur J Clin Pharmacol* 38:237-242, 1990.

Brown G: Pharmacologic treatment of primary and secondary pulmonary hypertension. *Pharmacotherapy* 11:137-156, 1991.

Brown E, Kloner RA: Angina pectoris. *Cardiovasc Rev Rep* 11:21-51, 1990.

Buckley MM-T, et al: Diltiazem: A reappraisal of its pharmacological properties and therapeutic use. *Drugs* 39:757-806, 1990.

Burger SK, et al: Transient monocular blindness caused by vasospasm. *N Engl J Med* 325:870-873, 1991.

Choong CYP, et al: Effects of nifedipine on systemic and regional oxygen transport and metabolism at rest and during exercise. *Circulation* 71:787-796, 1985.

Christakis GT, et al: Diltiazem cardioplegia: A balance of risk and benefit. *J Thorac Cardiovasc Surg* 91:647-661, 1986.

Clifton CG, Wallin JD: Intravenous nicardipine: An effective new agent for the treatment of severe hypertension. *Angiology* 41:1005-1008, 1990.

Cocco G, Alfiero R: A double-blind dose-response study of amlodipine in patients with stable angina pectoris. *Eur Heart J* 12:169-174, 1991.

Coffman JD: Raynaud's phenomenon. *Curr Opin Cardiol* 8:821-828, 1993.

Cohn JN, et al: A comparison of enalapril with hydralazine-isosorbide dinitrate in the treatment of chronic congestive heart failure. *N Engl J Med* 325:303-310, 1991.

Creager MA, et al: Nifedipine-induced fingertip vasodilation in patients with Raynaud's phenomenon. *Am Heart J* 108:370-373, 1984.

Dahlof B: Hemodynamic response, safety, and efficacy of isradipine in the treatment of essential hypertension. *Am J Med* 86 (suppl 4A):19-26, 1989.

Danish Study Group on Verapamil in Myocardial Infarction: Effect of verapamil on mortality and major events after acute myocardial infarction (The Danish Verapamil Infarction Trial II-DAVIT II). *Am J Cardiol* 66:779-785, 1990.

Dawidson I, et al: Prevention of acute cyclosporine-induced renal blood flow inhibition and improved immunosuppression with verapamil. *Transplantation* 48:575-580, 1989.

Dawidson I, et al: Verapamil improves the outcome after cadaver renal transplantation. *J Am Soc Nephrol* 2:983-990, 1991.

De Servi S, et al: Effects of diltiazem on regional coronary hemodynamics during atrial pacing in patients with stable exertional angina: Implications for mechanism of action. *Circulation* 73:1248-1253, 1986.

Dusselman PHJM, et al: Different results in cardiopulmonary exercise tests after long-term treatment with felodipine and enalapril in patients with congestive heart failure due to ischemic heart disease. *Eur Heart J* 11:200-206, 1990.

Elkayam U, et al: A prospective, randomized, double-blind, crossover study to compare the efficacy and safety of chronic nifedipine therapy with that of isosorbide dinitrate and their combination in the treatment of chronic congestive heart failure. *Circulation* 82:1954-1961, 1990.

Epstein M: Calcium antagonists and renal protection: Current status and future perspectives. *Arch Intern Med* 152:1573-1584, 1992.

Fananapazir L, et al: Prognostic determinants in hypertrophic cardiomyopathy: Prospective evaluation of a therapeutic strategy based on clinical, Holter, hemodynamic, and electrophysiological findings. *Circulation* 86:730-740, 1992.

Feldman RD, et al: Interaction of verapamil and norverapamil with β-adrenergic receptors. *Circulation* 72:547-554, 1985.

Ferlinz J: Nifedipine in myocardial ischemia, systemic hypertension, and other cardiovascular disorders. *Ann Intern Med* 105:714-729, 1986.

Fitton A, Benfield P: Isradipine: A review of its pharmacodynamic and pharmacokinetic properties, and therapeutic use in cardiovascular disease. *Drugs* 40:31-74, 1990.

Flaim SF, Cummings DM: Bepridil hydrochloride: A review of its pharmacologic properties. *Curr Ther Res* 39:568-597, 1986.

Fry WR, et al: Cyclosporine A induces decreased blood flow in cadaveric kidney transplants. *Trans Proc* 20:222, 1988.

Gelmers HJ, et al: A controlled trial of nimodipine in acute ischemic stroke. *N Engl J Med* 310:203-207, 1989.

Gheorghiade M, Goldstein S: Calcium-channel blockers in postmyocardial infarction patients with special notation to the Danish Verapamil Infarction Trial II. *Prog Cardiovasc Dis* 34:37-43, (July/Aug) 1991.

Goldbourt U, et al: Early administration of nifedipine in suspected acute myocardial infarction: The Second Prevention Reinfarction Israel Nifedipine Trial 2 Study. *Arch Intern Med* 153:345-353, 1993.

Haft JI, Habbab MA: Treatment of atrial arrhythmias: Effectiveness of verapamil when preceded by calcium infusion. *Arch Intern Med* 146:1085-1089, 1986.

Haley EC, et al: Nicardipine ameliorates angiographic vasospasm following subarachnoid hemorrhage. *Neurology* 41 (suppl 1):346, 1991.

Halpern NA, et al: Postoperative hypertension: A prospective, placebo-controlled, randomized, double-blind trial, with intravenous nicardipine hydrochloride. *Angiology* 41:992-1004, 1990.

Havel M, et al: Basic principles of cardioplegic management in donor heart preservation. *Clin Ther* 13:289-303, 1991.

Hedberg A, et al: Coexistence of beta-1 and beta-2 adrenergic receptors in the human heart: Effects of treatment with receptor antagonists or calcium entry blockers. *J Pharmacol Exp Ther* 234:561-568, 1985.

Held PH, et al: Calcium channel blockers in acute myocardial infarction and unstable angina: An overview. *BMJ* 299:1187-1192, 1989.

Henry PD: Atherogenesis, calcium and calcium antagonists. *Am J Cardiol* 66:3I-6I, 1990.

Hill JA, Pepine CJ: Effects of bepridil on the resting electrocardiogram. *Int J Cardiol* 6:319, 1984.

Huycke EC, et al: Intravenous diltiazem for termination of reentrant supraventricular tachycardia: A placebo-controlled, randomized, double-blind, multicenter study. *J Am Coll Cardiol* 13:538-544, 1989.

Inbar S, et al: Effects of adenosine in combination with calcium channel blockers in patients with primary pulmonary hypertension. *Am Coll Cardiol* 21:413-418, 1993.

Ingemarsson I, et al: Maternal and fetal cardiovascular changes after intravenous injections of isradipine to pregnant women. *Drugs* 40 (suppl 2):58-59, 1990.

Jezek V, et al: Long-term effect of isosorbide dinitrate and nifedipine, singly and in association, in patients with chronic heart failure. *Eur Heart J* 11:1059-1064, 1990.

Joint National Committee on Detection, Evaluation, and Treatment of High Blood Pressure: The fifth report of the Joint National Committee on Detection, Evaluation, and Treatment of High Blood Pressure (JNC V). *Arch Intern Med* 153:154-183, 1993.

Joyal M, et al: Effects of diltiazem during tachycardia-induced angina pectoris. *Am J Cardiol* 57:10-14, 1986.

Julius S: Amlodipine in hypertension: An overview of the clinical dossier. *J Cardiovasc Pharmacol* 12 (suppl 7):S27-S33, 1988.

Kaplan NM: Calcium entry blockers in the treatment of hypertension: Current status and future prospects. *JAMA* 262:817-823, 1989.

Kirkendall WN: Comparative assessment of first-line agents for treatment of hypertension. *Am J Med* 84 (suppl 3B):32-41, 1988.

Klinke WP, et al: Usefulness of sustained-release diltiazem for stable angina pectoris. *Am J Cardiol* 64:1249-1252, 1989.

Kloner RA: Heart failure. *Cardiovasc Rev Rep* 12:19-59, 1991.

Kober G, et al: Can the progression of coronary sclerosis be influenced by calcium antagonists? *J Cardiovasc Pharmacol* 13 (suppl 4):S2-S6, 1989.

Krikler DM: Calcium antagonists for chronic stable angina pectoris. *Am J Cardiol* 59:95B-100B, 1987.

Langley MS, Sorkin EM: Nimodipine: A review of its pharmacodynamic and pharmacokinetic properties, and therapeutic potential in cerebrovascular disease. *Drugs* 37:669-699, 1989.

Lessem J, et al: Nicardipine in essential hypertension: The evaluation of different dosages of a second generation Ca-channel blocker. *Clin Trial J* 27:313-326, 1990.

Levine JH, et al: Treatment of multifocal atrial tachycardia with verapamil. *N Engl J Med* 312:21-25, 1985.

Lichtlen PR, et al: Retardation of angiographic progression of coronary artery disease by nifedipine. *Lancet* 335:1109-1113, 1990.

Lindpaintner K, Ganten D: The cardiac renin-angiotensin system: An appraisal of present experimental and clinical evidence. *Circ Res* 68:905-921, 1991.

Loscalzo J: Endothelial dysfunction in pulmonary hypertension, editorial. *N Engl J Med* 327:117-119, 1992.

Lund-Johansen P, Omvik P: Chronic hemodynamic effects of tiapamil and felodipine in essential hypertension at rest and during exercises. *J Cardiovasc Pharmacol* 15 (suppl 4):S42-S47, 1990.

Man in't Veld AJ: Calcium antagonists in hypertension. *Am J Med* 86 (suppl 4A):6-14, 1989.

Marmot MG, Poulter NR: Primary prevention of stroke. *Lancet* 339:334-347, 1992.

Materson BJ, et al: Single-drug therapy for hypertension in men. *N Engl J Med* 328:914-921, 1993.

McGovern B, et al: Precipitation of cardiac arrest by verapamil in patients with Wolff-Parkinson-White syndrome. *Ann Intern Med* 104:791-794, 1986.

McTavish D, Sorkin EM: Verapamil: An updated review of its pharmacodynamic and pharmacokinetic properties, and therapeutic use in hypertension. *Drugs* 38:19-76, 1989.

Mee E, et al: Controlled study of nimodipine in aneurysm patients treated early after subarachnoid hemorrhage. *Neurosurgery* 22:484-491, 1988.

MIDAS Research Group: Multicenter Isradipine Diuretic Atherosclerosis Study (MIDAS): Design features. *Am J Med* 86(suppl 4A):37-39, 1989.

Morady F, et al: Epinephrine-induced reversal of verapamil's electrophysiologic and therapeutic effects in patients with paroxysmal supraventricular tachycardia. *Circulation* 79:783-790, 1989.

Mullen JC, et al: Postoperative hypertension: A comparison of diltiazem, nifedipine, and nitroprusside. *J Thorac Cardiovasc Surg* 96:122-132, 1988.

Murdoch D, Heel RC: Amlodipine: A review of its pharmacodynamic and pharmacokinetic properties, and therapeutic use in cardiovascular disease. *Drugs* 41:478-505, 1991.

Neaton JD, et al: Treatment of mild hypertension study. *JAMA* 270:713-724, 1993.

Neumayer HH, Wagner K: Prevention of delayed graft function in cadaver kidney transplants by diltiazem: Outcome of two prospective, randomized clinical trials. *J Cardiovasc Pharmacol* 10(suppl):S170-S177, 1987.

Oelz O, et al: Nifedipine for high altitude pulmonary oedema. *Lancet* 2:1241-1244, 1989.

Onoyama K, et al: Effect of drip infusion or a bolus injection of intravenous diltiazem on hypertensive crisis. *Curr Ther Res* 42:1223-1231, 1987.

Onoyama K, et al: Effect of a drip infusion of intravenous diltiazem on severe systemic hypertension. *Curr Ther Res* 43:361-368, 1988.

Opie LH, et al: International Society and Federation of Cardiology: Working group on classification of calcium antagonists for cardiovascular disease. *Am J Cardiol* 60:630-632, 1987.

Oppenheimer F, et al: Influence of the calcium blocker diltiazem on the prevention of acute renal failure after renal transplantation. *Transplant Proc* 24:50-51, 1992.

Packer M: Second generation calcium channel blockers in the treatment of chronic heart failure: Are they any better than their predecessors? *J Am Coll Cardiol* 14:1339-1342, 1989.

Palevsky HI, Fishman AP: The management of primary pulmonary hypertension. *JAMA* 265:1014-1020, 1991.

Palmer BF, et al: Improved outcome of cadaveric renal transplantation due to calcium channel blockers. *Transplantation* 52:640-645, 1991.

Pang DC, Sperelakis N: Uptake of calcium antagonistic drugs into muscles as related to their lipid solubilities. *Biochem Pharmacol* 33:821-826, 1984.

Petruk KC, et al: Nimodipine treatment in poor-grade aneurysm patients: Results of a multicenter double-blind placebo controlled trial. *J Neurosurg* 68:505-517, 1988.

Pickard JD, et al: Effect of oral nimodipine on cerebral infarction and outcome after subarachnoid haemorrhage: British aneurysm nimodipine trial. *BMJ* 298:636-642, 1989.

Piessens J, et al: Effect of intravenous diltiazem on myocardial ischemia during percutaneous transluminal coronary angioplasty. *Am J Cardiol* 64:1103-1107, 1989.

Pritchett ELC: Management of atrial fibrillation. *N Engl J Med* 326:1264-1271, 1992.

Pulsinelli W: Pathophysiology of acute ischaemic stroke. *Lancet* 339:533-536, 1992.

Reid JL: First-line and combination treatment for hypertension. *Am J Med* 86(suppl 4A):2-5, 1989.

Rich S, Brundage BH: High-dose calcium channel-blocking therapy for primary pulmonary hypertension: Evidence for long-term reduction in pulmonary arterial pressure and regression of right ventricular hypertrophy. *Circulation* 76:135-141, 1987.

Rich S, et al: Primary pulmonary hypertension: National prospective study. *Ann Intern Med* 107:216-223, 1987.

Rich S, et al: The effect of high doses of calcium-channel blockers on survival in primary pulmonary hypertension. *N Engl J Med* 327:76-81, 1992.

Robinson BF: Functional differences in blood vessels determined from studies with calcium-channel blockers: Functional changes in forearm resistance vessels in men with primary hypertension. *Am J Cardiol* 55:24B-29B, 1985.

Rodeheffer RJ, et al: Controlled double-blind trial of nifedipine in the treatment of Raynaud's phenomenon. *N Engl J Med* 308:880-883, 1983.

Rodrigues EA, et al: Comparison of nicardipine and verapamil in the management of chronic stable angina. *Int J Cardiol* 18:357-369, 1988.

Rosenbaum D, et al: Early treatment of ischemic stroke with a calcium antagonist. *Stroke* 22:437-441, 1991.

Rosing DR, et al: Use of calcium channel blocking drugs in hypertrophic cardiomyopathy. *Am J Cardiol* 55:185B-195B, 1985.

Rubin LJ: Primary pulmonary hypertension: Practical therapeutic recommendations. *Drugs* 43:37-43, 1992.

Ruskin AC, et al: Catheter ablation for supraventricular tachycardia, editorial. *N Engl J Med* 324:1660-1662, 1991.

Salerno DM, et al: Intravenous verapamil for treatment of multifocal atrial tachycardia with and without calcium pretreatment. *Ann Intern Med* 107:623-628, 1987.

Saltiel E, et al: Felodipine: A review of its pharmacodynamic and pharmacokinetic properties, and therapeutic use in hypertension. *Drugs* 36:387-428, 1988.

Schrier RW, et al: Cellular calcium in ischemic acute renal failure: Role of calcium entry blockers. *Kidney Int* 32:313-321, 1987.

Shepherd AMM, et al: Efficacy and safety of isradipine in hypertension. *J Cardiovasc Pharmacol* 13:580-585, 1989.

Sila CA: Prophylaxis and treatment of stroke: The state of the art in 1993. *Drugs* 45:329-337, 1993.

Singh BN, Nademanee K: Use of calcium antagonists for cardiac arrhythmias. *Am J Cardiol* 59:153B-162B, 1987.

Singh BN, et al: Comparative electrophysiologic profiles of calcium antagonists with particular reference to bepridil. *Am J Cardiol* 55:14C-19C, 1985.

Smith CD, McKendry RVR: Controlled trial of nifedipine in the treatment of Raynaud's phenomenon. *Lancet* 2:1299-1301, 1982.

The SOLVD Investigators: Effect of enalapril on survival in patients with reduced left ventricular ejection fractions and congestive heart failure. *N Engl J Med* 325:293-302, 1991.

Sorkin EM, Clissold, SP: Nicardipine: A review of its pharmacodynamic and pharmacokinetic properties, and therapeutic efficacy, in the treatment of angina pectoris, hypertension and related cardiovascular disorders. *Drugs* 33:296-345, 1987.

Sorkin EM, et al: Nifedipine: A review of its pharmacodynamic and pharmacokinetic properties, and therapeutic efficacy, in ischaemic heart disease, hypertension and related cardiovascular disorders. *Drugs* 30:182-274, 1985.

Stallard MP, et al: Systolic blood pressure response in three subgroups of hypertensives treated with sustained-release diltiazem. *J Cardiovasc Pharmacol* 12(suppl 6):S117-S119, 1988.

Steinberg JS, et al: Efficacy of oral diltiazem to control ventricular response in chronic atrial fibrillation at rest and during exercise. *J Am Coll Cardiol* 9:405-411, 1987.

Stewart RB, et al: Wide complex tachycardia: Misdiagnosis and outcome after emergent therapy. *Ann Intern Med* 104:766-771, 1986.

Stone PH, et al: Efficacy of nifedipine therapy in patients with refractory angina pectoris: Significance of presence of coronary vasospasm. *Am Heart J* 106:644-652, 1983.

Takayasu IM, et al: Effects of calcium antagonists on intracerebral penetrating arterioles in the rat. *J Neurosurg* 69:104-109, 1988.

Taylor SH: The efficacy of amlodipine in myocardial ischemia. *Am Heart J* 118:1123-1126, 1989.

Taylor SH, et al: Efficacy of a new calcium antagonist PN 200-110 (isradipine) in angina pectoris. *Am J Cardiol* 59:123B-129B, 1987.

Taylor SH, et al: A hemodynamic comparison of verapamil, diltiazem, and amlodipine in coronary artery disease. *Am Heart J* 118:1105-1106, 1989.

Tettenborn D, Dycka, J: Prevention and treatment of delayed ischemic dysfunction in patients with aneurysmal subarachnoid hemorrhage. *Stroke* 21 (suppl IV):IV-85-IV-89, 1990.

Triggle DJ: Calcium antagonists: History and perspective. *Stroke* 21 (suppl IV):IV-49-IV-58, 1990.

Trust Study Group: Randomised, double-blind, placebo-controlled trial of nimodipine in acute stroke. *Lancet* 336:1205-1209, 1990.

van Gijn J: Subarachnoid haemorrhage. *Lancet* 339:653-655, 1992.

van Heyningen R, Harding JJ: Do aspirin-like analgesics protect against cataract? *Lancet* 1:1111-1113, 1986.

van Wijk LM, et al: Cardiac electrophysiologic properties of intravenous isradipine in patients with sick sinus syndrome. *Am J Med* 86 (suppl 4A):88-90, 1989.

Van Zwieten PA, et al: Inhibitory effect of calcium antagonist drugs on vasoconstriction induced by vascular alpha$_2$-adrenoreceptor stimulation. *Am J Cardiol* 57:11D-15D, 1986.

Vidt DG: Isradipine in the treatment of hypertension: A clinical profile. *Cleve Clin J Med* 57:677-684, 1990.

Wadworth AN, McTavish D: Nimodipine: A review of its pharmacological properties, and therapeutic efficacy in cerebral disorders. *Drugs Aging* 2:262-286, 1992.

Wagner K, et al: Prevention of post-transplant acute tubular necrosis by the calcium antagonist diltiazem: A prospective randomized study. *Am J Nephrol* 7:287-291, 1987.

Waters D, et al: A controlled clinical trial to assess the effect of a calcium channel blocker on the progression of coronary atherosclerosis. *Circulation* 82:1940-1953, 1990.

Weiner DA: Calcium channel blockers. *Med Clin North Am* 72:83-115, 1988.

Weinstein DB, Heider JG: Antiatherogenic properties of calcium antagonists: State of the art. *Am J Med* 86 (suppl 4A):27-32, 1989.

Wester A, et al: Felodipine extended release in mild to moderate hypertension. *Curr Med Res Opin* 12:275-281, 1991.

Winterkorn JMS, et al: Brief report: Treatment of vasospastic amaurosis fugax with calcium-channel blockers. *N Engl J Med* 329:396-398, 1993.

Yasue H, et al: Long term prognosis for patients with variant angina and influential factors. *Circulation* 78:1-9, 1988.

Yusuf S, Garg R: Randomized trials to assess the long-term effects of therapies on angiographic end points. *Chest* 99:1243-1247, 1991.

Yusuf S, et al: Update of effects of calcium antagonists in myocardial infarction or angina in light of the second Danish Verapamil Infarction Trial (DAVIT-II) and other recent studies. *Am J Cardiol* 67:1295-1297, 1991.

Angiotensin-Converting Enzyme Inhibitors 24

Angiotensin-converting enzyme inhibitors (ACE inhibitors) have assumed an important role in the treatment of hypertension and congestive heart failure. Seven orally active ACE inhibitors, benazepril [Lotensin], captopril [Capoten], enalapril [Vasotec], fosinopril [Monopril], lisinopril [Prinivil, Zestril], quinapril [Accupril], and ramipril [Altace], and an intravenous preparation, enalaprilat [Vasotec I.V.], are now available.

RENIN-ANGIOTENSIN SYSTEM

FUNCTIONS. Renin, a proteolytic enzyme produced and stored mainly in the kidney, is released in response to various stimuli, the most important of which is a reduction in renal perfusion pressure associated with hemorrhage, dehydration, chronic sodium depletion, or renal artery stenosis. The secretion of renin also is regulated by sodium delivery to the macula densa, sympathetic nervous system activity, and certain humoral factors.

Renin acts on angiotensinogen, a glycoprotein substrate produced by the liver, to form the inactive compound, angiotensin I. This prohormone is then hydrolyzed to the active angiotensin II by the angiotensin-converting enzyme (ACE) (kininase II) present in the lungs and other tissues. The converting enzyme also catalyzes degradation of the vasodilator, bradykinin, to inactive peptides.

Circulating angiotensin II acts on receptor sites in the vasomotor centers of the brain, vascular smooth muscle, and adrenal cortex to constrict arterioles and stimulate secretion of aldosterone, thereby increasing total peripheral resistance and enhancing reabsorption of sodium and water and excretion of potassium. The resultant rise in blood pressure, extracellular fluid volume, and angiotensin II concentration activates a negative feedback loop that reduces renin secretion and restores homeostasis. The circulating renin-angiotensin system responds rapidly to postural changes and also is of major importance in short-term maintenance of blood pressure and intravascular volume during sodium deprivation or volume depletion.

In addition to the circulating renin-angiotensin system, renin and angiotensin I and II are produced locally in many tissues, including blood vessels, brain, kidney, heart, and adrenal glands. Local generation is not reflected in the plasma concentration of angiotensin II or plasma renin activity. Tissue angiotensin-generating systems may be involved in local control of cardiac, renal, and vascular function (Campbell, 1987; Dzau, 1988). Local angiotensin II production in the heart may increase coronary vasoconstriction and myocardial contractility, contribute to the development of cardiac hypertrophy, precipitate ventricular arrhythmias, and play a role in postischemic reperfusion injury. In the kidney, a local renin-angiotensin system appears to regulate intrarenal hemodynamics and sodium homeostasis. Vascular angiotensin production is thought to increase vascular tone, an effect that may involve potentiation of adrenergic transmission. In the central nervous system, a tissue renin-angiotensin system may play a role in blood pressure control and in the autoregulation of cerebral blood flow and may induce drinking (Campbell, 1987; Dzau, 1988; Paulson et al, 1988; Unger et al, 1988). The central actions of angiotensin II may involve an effect on sympathetic and parasympathetic outflow. At present, the role of plasma and tissue ACE activity in the pathogenesis of hypertension and congestive heart failure and on the response of these conditions to ACE inhibitors remains unclear.

ROLE IN PATHOLOGIC CONDITIONS. The circulating renin-angiotensin system is one of the neurohumoral mechanisms activated in response to reduced cardiac output and renal blood flow in patients with congestive heart failure. As pump function deteriorates, the vasoconstrictor activity of angiotensin II and the sodium-retaining properties of aldosterone initially help maintain perfusion pressure, intravascular volume, and cardiac filling. In addition, locally produced angiotensin II supports glomerular filtration by an intrarenal action that appears to involve an increase in efferent arteriolar (postglomerular) resistance (Levenson and Dzau, 1987; Packer et al, 1986). Although they are initially beneficial, the hemodynamic changes induced by the renin-angiotensin system and other neurohumoral systems eventually increase the burden on the failing heart (see index entry Heart Failure).

The renin-angiotensin system is involved in some secondary forms of hypertension, but its role in the pathogenesis or prognosis of essential hypertension is not established (Alderman et al, 1991; Dzau, 1991). "Renin profiling" is of questionable value in selecting antihypertensive therapy and does not replace other methods for diagnosing renovascular hypertension (see index entry Hypertension).

CONVERTING ENZYME INHIBITORS

Actions

ACE inhibitors block the conversion of angiotensin I to the active angiotensin II by inhibiting the converting enzyme. Captopril and lisinopril, a derivative of enalaprilat, are direct ACE inhibitors, whereas benazepril, enalapril, fosinopril, quinapril, and ramipril are prodrugs that are de-esterified in the liver and probably other tissues (eg, kidney, gastrointestinal tract) to the active diacid form (benazeprilat, enalaprilat, fosinoprilat, quinaprilat, and ramiprilat, respectively).

HUMORAL EFFECTS. Administration of ACE inhibitors leads to an initial decrease in circulating angiotensin II and aldosterone levels, which is accompanied by a compensatory increase in angiotensin I concentration and plasma renin activity. Because aldosterone secretion is reduced, less sodium-potassium exchange occurs in the distal renal tubule and the serum potassium concentration may increase slightly (Cleland et al, 1985; Gavras et al, 1978; Johnston et al, 1979). ACE inhibitors reduce diuretic-induced hyperaldosteronism and hypokalemia, but they have additive effects on plasma renin activity.

During prolonged administration of an ACE inhibitor, plasma angiotensin I concentration and plasma renin activity remain elevated; the plasma concentration of angiotensin II may remain suppressed or return to baseline levels. Aldosterone secretion is influenced by other factors in addition to the renin-angiotensin system, and the aldosterone concentration returns to or exceeds the pretreatment level during long-term therapy (Jungmann et al, 1985; Lijnen et al, 1982). It has been suggested that local concentrations of ACE and angiotensin II at vascular and/or intrarenal sites may be as important as plasma concentrations in mediating the therapeutic response to ACE inhibitors.

In addition to their effects on the renin-angiotensin system, ACE inhibitors increase the renal production of kinins and prostaglandins and also may inhibit the action of angiotensin II on sympathetic nervous system activity. The clinical significance of these actions remains to be determined (Erdös, 1990).

HEMODYNAMIC EFFECTS. ACE inhibitors reduce total peripheral resistance and lower systemic blood pressure. Venodilation may occur in patients with congestive heart failure. The antihypertensive effect of ACE inhibitors, which is due to the reduction in total peripheral resistance, is not accompanied by reflex increases in heart rate, cardiac output, and myocardial contractility. The effect on blood pressure is greatly enhanced by sodium restriction or diuretic therapy. The beneficial effect of converting enzyme inhibitors in congestive heart failure is associated with a reduction in both preload and afterload.

ACE inhibitors have a relatively selective action on the renal vasculature, and the kidney plays an important role in their therapeutic and adverse effects (Ando et al, 1986; Leslie et al, 1980; Levenson and Dzau, 1987). These drugs reduce both preglomerular (afferent) and postglomerular (efferent) arteriolar resistance and reduce the glomerular capillary hydraulic pressure. ACE inhibitors may improve renal hemodynamics and the clinical course of patients with diabetic nephropathy and other renal diseases characterized by glomerular hypertension, but this has not been confirmed.

Major Uses

CHRONIC HYPERTENSION. ACE inhibitors are one of the classes of antihypertensive drugs that are recommended by the Joint National Committee on Detection, Evaluation, and Treatment of High Blood Pressure (1988) as initial agents for the management of patients with mild to severe hypertension. They are useful in both elderly (65 to 75 years) and younger patients (18 to 35 years) but are less effective in blacks than in nonblacks. ACE inhibitors generally are safe and effective in patients with renal impairment, but the dosage must be reduced when renal clearance is diminished.

Control of mild to severe hypertension usually is enhanced when ACE inhibitors are combined with diuretics. In addition, blood pressure is reduced in both blacks and nonblacks with this combination therapy.

Among the advantages of ACE inhibitors in the treatment of hypertension is their freedom from serious adverse metabolic, respiratory, or central nervous system side effects. Their use also may lead to regression of left ventricular hypertrophy. See index entry Hypertension.

CHRONIC HEART FAILURE. This syndrome is characterized by left ventricular dysfunction, reduced exercise tolerance, impaired quality of life, and markedly shortened life expectancy (Cohn, 1988). In the first multicenter Veterans Administration Cooperative Vasodilator-Heart Failure Trial (V-HeFT I), addition of the vasodilators, hydralazine and isosorbide dinitrate, to the standard treatment of digoxin and diuretics reduced mortality in patients with mild to moderate heart failure by 38% after one year, 25% after two years, and 28% over the entire follow-up period (2.3 years). In the second Vasodilator-Heart Failure Trial (V-HeFT II), the addition of the ACE inhibitor, enalapril, to the regimen of digoxin and diuretics reduced mortality to a greater extent than the combination of hydralazine and isosorbide dinitrate, especially in the first year of therapy (Cohn et al, 1991). Similar results were reported with this regimen in the Studies of Left Ventricular Dysfunction (SOLVD) (The SOLVD Investigators, 1991). However, the decrease in mortality in V-HeFT II was attributable to a lower incidence of sudden death, with no reduction in mortality or hospitalization due to pump failure, whereas in SOLVD the reduction in deaths was attributable to a decrease in the incidence of progressive heart failure.

ACE inhibitors also are effective in the long-term treatment of patients with severe heart failure. In the first Cooperative North Scandinavian Enalapril Survival Study (CONSENSUS I), enalapril not only improved signs and symptoms in patients with severe heart failure (New York Heart Association [NYHA] Class IV), but also decreased the mortality rate (CONSENSUS Trial Study Group, 1987).

In general, ACE inhibitors, including the newer compounds (benazepril, fosinopril, quinapril, and ramipril), improve overall hemodynamics, exercise tolerance, ejection fraction, and functional class; relieve symptoms; correct hyponatremia and hypokalemia; and halt progression of left ventricular hypertrophy in patients with heart failure. (See index entry Heart Failure.)

MYOCARDIAL INFARCTION. ACE inhibitors have been shown to play a role in the secondary treatment of myocardial infarction. Combined early intravenous captopril and thrombolytic therapy in patients with acute myocardial infarction decreased left ventricular end-diastolic volume, prevented further ventricular dilatation, and increased exercise capacity (Nabel et al, 1991). In the Survival and Left Ventricular Enlargement (SAVE) Trial, 3 to 16 days postinfarction those patients with ejection fraction less than 40% were randomized to receive either captopril or placebo and were followed up for two to five years. Early, prolonged treatment with captopril 50 mg twice daily reduced mortality from all causes by 17% compared with placebo. However, the mortality rate was not affected in either group during the first ten months of the trial. (See index entry Myocardial Infarction.)

RENAL DISORDERS. Chronic renal disease, including polycystic renal disease, diabetic nephropathy, focal segmental sclerosis, and chronic pyelonephritis, often progresses to end-stage renal failure, possibly as a result of activation of the renin angiotensin system (Asher and Murray, 1991; Brouhard et al, 1991; Kelleher, 1990).

Systemic scleroderma is a complex generalized connective tissue disease marked by inflammatory immunologic reactivity, vascular lesions, and widespread fibrosis of multiple organ systems. Renal insufficiency may develop gradually and be manifested by mild to moderately severe vascular lesions or it may appear abruptly in the form of renal scleroderma manifested by the sudden development of malignant arterial hypertension and subsequent accelerated decline of renal function. Renal scleroderma may cause death within one month.

The observation of elevated peripheral renin levels and severe hypertension in patients with systemic scleroderma are the basis for the use of ACE inhibitors for this condition. Captopril and enalapril appear to be highly effective in controlling elevated arterial pressure and stabilizing renal function in patients with renal scleroderma (Beckett et al, 1985; Lopez-Ovejero et al, 1979; Milsom and Nicholls, 1986). They also may relieve associated peripheral vasospastic manifestations (Lopez-Ovejero et al, 1979) but do not benefit patients with occlusive arterial disease (Beckett et al, 1985).

Diabetic nephropathy, which is characterized by persistent proteinuria and an excessive glomerular filtration rate, is a potentially fatal complication of insulin-dependent and non-insulin-dependent diabetes. It occurs in up to 40% of insulin-dependent patients and peaks after 16 years (Kelleher, 1990). Hypertension is an important risk factor in the development of nephropathy, and all patients with renal disease tend to have higher than average blood pressure levels. Abnormalities in renal function that develop early in diabetic patients include increased glomerular filtration rate, increased renal plasma flow, and impaired autoregulation of renal blood flow. Hyporeninemic hypoaldosteronism occurs in many diabetic patients with severe renal disease. Even at this stage, the renin-angiotensin system may play a crucial role in regulating the filtration rate, which is largely mediated by angiotensin II.

In addition to controlling blood pressure, ACE inhibitors reduce albuminuria without worsening azotemia, probably by reducing glomerular capillary hydraulic pressure through efferent as well as afferent glomerular arteriolar dilation (Björck et al, 1986; Hommel et al, 1986; Marre et al, 1988; Taguma et al, 1985) and by improving the filtering function of the basement membrane (Morelli et al, 1990).

There is some evidence that long-term therapy with ACE inhibitors may decrease the severity of proteinuria (Mathiesen et al, 1991) and slow the progression of diabetic nephropathy (Abraham et al, 1988; Marre et al, 1988); however, beneficial effects are limited if therapy is initiated during the advanced stage (Valvo et al, 1988). Three patients with diabetic nephropathy were observed for an average of 41 months before and 59 months after treatment with ACE inhibitors was begun (Brouhard et al, 1991). Although renal function declined much more rapidly before than during treatment, both mean protein excretion and creatinine clearance decreased after the administration of ACE inhibitors. The renal disease continued to progress.

Enalapril was effective in reducing fluid intake and thus preventing volume overload in a group of patients with end-stage renal disease undergoing dialysis (Oldenburg et al, 1988).

In patients with hypertension associated with renal dysfunction, control of blood pressure with ACE inhibitors may slow progression of chronic renal failure (Bauer and Gaddy, 1985; Opsahl et al, 1987; Ruilope et al, 1989).

Drug Selection

The ACE inhibitors can be classified on the basis of the zinc ion ligand of angiotensin-converting enzyme into three main chemical classes containing sulfhydryl, carboxyl, or phospho-

TABLE 1.
PHARMACOKINETICS OF ACE INHIBITORS

Drug	Bioavailability (%)	Half-life (hours)	Protein Binding (%)	Excretion of Unchanged Drug (%)	Active Metabolite
Benazepril	37	10-11	95-97	1	benazeprilat
Captopril	60-75	1.5-2	25-30	40-50	none
Enalapril	36-44	11	50	60-75	enalaprilat
Fosinopril	36	4	95	1	fosinoprilat
Lisinopril	25-50	12	negligible	~100	none
Quinapril	60	1	97	3	quinaprilat
Ramipril	56	1.1-4.5	56	56	ramiprilat

ryl groups (Salvetti, 1990). Captopril is the only currently marketed ACE inhibitor that contains a sulfhydryl group. Benazepril, enalapril, quinapril, and ramipril contain a carboxyl group and fosinopril contains a phosphoryl group. Captopril and lisinopril are active compounds. Like enalapril, benazepril, fosinopril, quinapril, and ramipril are prodrugs that are converted in vivo to active diacids.

Enalapril and lisinopril have a slower onset and longer duration of action than captopril. Compared with enalapril, benazepril, ramipril, and quinapril reach peak plasma concentrations earlier after oral administration. Both benazepril and quinapril have a shorter half-life than enalapril; in contrast, ramipril and lisinopril have a longer terminal half-life. When the differences in potency between these drugs are compensated by dosage adjustment, the systemic hemodynamic actions of the newer ACE inhibitors are similar to those of enalapril or captopril in the control of hypertension.

The new ACE inhibitors offer a wide choice in terms of pharmacokinetics. It is unclear what pharmacodynamic or clinical benefit these differences may confer. However, the frequency of administration (once daily versus two or three times daily) may be a factor in patient compliance.

Pharmacokinetics

The active metabolites of most ACE inhibitors are primarily eliminated by the kidney; biliary excretion plays a minor role. Hence, except for fosinopril, dosages of ACE inhibitors must be reduced in patients with renal impairment. Fosinoprilat, the prodrug of fosinopril, is eliminated in approximately equal proportions by the renal and hepatic routes in healthy volunteers (Hui et al, 1991; Sica et al, 1991); in patients with renal impairment, total clearance of fosinoprilat is not decreased because of more pronounced biliary excretion.

See also Table 1.

Adverse Reactions and Precautions

Cardiovascular/Renal/Metabolic Reactions: The initial dose of an ACE inhibitor may cause a precipitous, symptomatic fall in blood pressure (which may be accompanied by bradycardia), particularly in patients receiving diuretics, in those on sodium-restricted diets or dialysis, or in hyponatremic individuals. It is advisable to withhold diuretics, if possible, for 24 to 72 hours when treatment with an ACE inhibitor is begun. Occasionally, severe symptomatic hypotension may develop later in the course of therapy, especially in sodium-depleted patients and those undergoing dialysis. Symptomatic hypotension usually responds to sodium repletion.

ACE inhibition may cause a reversible elevation of BUN and serum creatinine levels as a result of reduced renal perfusion pressure and failure of the intrarenal angiotensin-generating mechanism. Acute reversible renal failure may develop in patients with markedly reduced renal perfusion pressure due to bilateral renal artery stenosis or stenosis in a solitary functioning or transplanted kidney. ACE inhibitors should be used with caution in these patients. Functional renal insufficiency also may occur during treatment of severe chronic heart failure, especially in the presence of sodium depletion, hyponatremia, and elevated plasma renin activity (Packer et al, 1987). Azotemia in these patients usually can be managed by reducing the dose of the diuretic, liberalizing salt intake, or reducing the dosage of the ACE inhibitor.

Proteinuria and, less commonly, nephrotic syndrome and membranous glomerulonephritis have been associated with high-dose captopril therapy. However, in general ACE inhibitors tend to decrease proteinuria in patients with diabetic nephropathy, chronic renal failure, and other renal disorders.

ACE inhibitors may occasionally cause hyperkalemia (particularly in elderly patients or those with impaired renal function) even when a potassium-wasting diuretic is given concomitantly. The risk of hyperkalemia is increased if potassium supplements or a potassium-sparing agent is given concurrently.

Dermatologic Reactions: Patients treated with captopril occasionally develop a dose-related erythematous maculopapular or morbilliform rash, sometimes accompanied by fever and/or pruritus. Pruritus also occurs without rash. Lichenoid eruptions, pemphigus-like reactions, cutaneous vasculitis, exacerbation of psoriasis, exfoliative dermatitis, onycholysis, and alopecia have been reported rarely in patients treated with captopril. A severe, scaling erythematous rash, with histologic features resembling the early stages of cutaneous T-cell lymphoma, has been reported in a few patients treated with captopril or enalapril. This rash is not dose-related and appears to have an immunologic pathogenesis; it will not clear unless the drug is discontinued (Furness et al, 1986).

Angioedema and urticaria are occasional complications of therapy with all ACE inhibitors and appear to be caused by activation of kinin (Wood, 1987). If angioedema develops, the drug should be discontinued; when the tongue, glottis, or larynx is involved, subcutaneous epinephrine should be given promptly. Since ACE inhibitors as a class are associated with angioedema, another type of drug should be employed for subsequent therapy (Slater et al, 1988).

Gastrointestinal Reactions: ACE inhibitors may cause gastrointestinal disturbances (nausea, vomiting, dyspepsia, diarrhea). Rarely, both captopril and enalapril have caused hyperesthesia of the oral mucosa, and oral ulcerations have been associated with captopril therapy. Loss or disturbance of taste occurs in approximately 3% to 7% of patients treated with captopril and is dose related and reversible, but it may be necessary to discontinue therapy if anorexia and weight loss develop. Taste disturbances are rare in patients treated with other ACE inhibitors.

Respiratory Reactions: A chronic, nonproductive cough is a common side effect of all ACE inhibitors. It occurs more frequently in women than in men, is especially bothersome when the patient is supine, and may necessitate drug withdrawal. Kinins and prostaglandins have been suggested as possible mediators (Coulter and Edwards, 1987; Semple and Herd, 1986). Some investigators reported that the cough induced by ACE inhibitors occurred in patients with underlying bronchial hyperreactivity (Bucknall et al, 1988; Kaufman et al, 1989), while others found no relationship (Boulet et al, 1989). Only rarely have ACE inhibitors been reported to aggravate respiratory symptoms in asthmatics.

Hematologic Reactions: Neutropenia, the most serious adverse effect of captopril, has occurred in about 0.02% of patients with normal renal function and in 0.3% of those with renal failure or autoimmune disorders or receiving immunosuppressive therapy. Fatal agranulocytosis has occurred occasionally. If detected early, the neutropenia is reversible. In high-risk patients, white blood cell counts should be performed at two-week intervals for the first three months of therapy and periodically thereafter.

Miscellaneous Reactions: ACE inhibitors may cause headache, fatigue, and dizziness. Reversible deafness has been reported in a few patients treated with enalapril (Inman and Rawson, 1987). Rarely, captopril therapy has been associated with cholestatic or mixed cholestatic-hepatocellular jaundice, and there is one published report of hepatitis induced by both captopril and enalapril. Several patients taking enalapril have developed pancreatitis. One case of acute small bowel mucosal edema has been associated with enalapril therapy. Reversible lymphadenopathy has occurred rarely in patients treated with captopril.

Use in Pregnancy: ACE inhibitors should not be given during pregnancy, especially in the second and third trimesters. The cerebral and renal circulations in premature hypertensive infants are especially vulnerable to hypotension, and the marked and persistent reduction in blood pressure induced by ACE inhibitors has led to neurologic complications (eg, seizures) and anuria in these infants (Perlman and Volpe, 1989). Neonatal hypotension, renal failure, limb contracture, craniofacial malformation, hypoplastic lung development, and death have been reported. In addition, ACE inhibitors have been associated with fetal growth retardation and persistent patent ductus arteriosus. Alternative antihypertensive therapy should be prescribed for women who become pregnant while receiving an ACE inhibitor. All seven ACE inhibitors are classified in FDA Pregnancy Category D.

Interactions

See Table 2.

TABLE 2.
INTERACTIONS OF ACE INHIBITORS

Drug(s)	Reaction
Allopurinol	Hypersensitivity reactions (eg, skin eruptions, fever, arthralgia*)
Anesthetics	Enhanced hypotensive effect
Cimetidine	Neurologic disturbances*
Digoxin	Reduced digoxin clearance
Insulin and oral hypoglycemic drugs	Hypoglycemia*
Lithium	Lithium intoxication
Nonsteroidal anti-inflammatory drugs (aspirin, indomethacin)	Reduced antihypertensive effect
Potassium supplements or potassium-sparing diuretics	Hyperkalemia
Thiazides and loop diuretics	Enhanced hypotensive effect

** To date reported only with captopril*

Drug Evaluations

BENAZEPRIL HYDROCHLORIDE
[Lotensin]

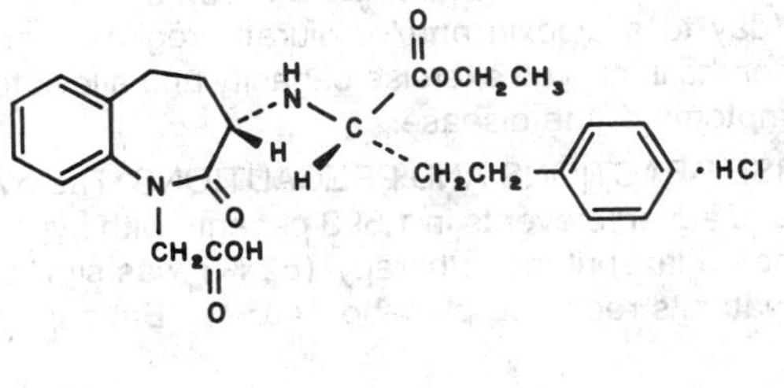

$$\cdot HCl$$

ACTIONS. This potent carboxyl inhibitor of the angiotensin-converting enzyme (ACE) is an ester prodrug that is rapidly absorbed and converted to the active diacid, benazeprilat.

Oral administration of benazepril in healthy human subjects has decreased plasma ACE activity, plasma angiotensin II levels, and plasma aldosterone concentration or urinary aldosterone excretion and has increased plasma angiotensin I levels and plasma renin activity or concentration. More than 90% of plasma ACE activity was inhibited 24 hours after administration of benazepril 5 to 20 mg in healthy volunteers, even though plasma concentrations of angiotensin II and aldosterone generally returned to baseline levels within 24 hours of drug administration, presumably as a result of increased renin secretion and angiotensin I production.

In hypertensive patients, a significant reduction in plasma ACE activity is evident four weeks after treatment with benazepril 5 to 40 mg/day. In patients with congestive heart failure, plasma renin activity increases and ACE activity and aldosterone levels decrease.

USES. Benazepril is given alone or with a diuretic in the management of mild to moderate hypertension. In short-term placebo-controlled trials (≤8 weeks), oral administration of benazepril 10 to 40 mg/day decreased the diastolic and systolic blood pressure in patients with mild to moderate hypertension by 10 to 15 mm Hg and 5 to 10 mm Hg, respectively. A dose of 10 mg once daily controlled blood pressure in approximately 50% of patients; efficacy was increased with higher dosages. The antihypertensive effect was maintained during long-term treatment (one to two years).

In several randomized multicenter studies on mild to moderate hypertensive patients, benazepril 10 mg once daily was as effective as enalapril 20 mg once daily and captopril 50 mg once daily or in divided doses. The efficacy of benazepril 20 mg/day was similar to that of hydrochlorothiazide 25 mg/day, nifedipine 40 mg/day, and propranolol 80 mg/day. Benazepril also is effective in hypertensive patients with renal insufficiency and has not been reported to aggravate the renal condition. It lowers blood pressure in black patients, but it is less effective in these individuals than in nonblacks.

The addition of other drugs to benazepril therapy enhances the antihypertensive effect. The combination of hydrochlorothiazide 25 to 50 mg/day and benazepril 20 to 80 mg/day decreased the diastolic blood pressure by 13 to 17 mm Hg compared with a reduction of 8 to 12 mm Hg with benazepril monotherapy. Systolic blood pressure was reduced by 22 mm Hg after combination therapy compared with decreases of 10 to 12 mm Hg following treatment with benazepril or hydrochlorothiazide alone. Blood pressure reduction following administration of benazepril and nifedipine also was greater than with either drug alone.

In patients with heart failure, the addition of benazepril 2 to 20 mg/day to a digoxin and/or diuretic regimen for one to three months improved exercise capacity and alleviated signs and symptoms of the disease.

ADVERSE REACTIONS AND PRECAUTIONS. The overall incidence of adverse events in 1,693 patients with hypertension receiving benazepril monotherapy (52%) was similar to that in 458 patients receiving placebo (48%) (Balfour and Goa, 1991). Headache was the most common adverse effect and occurred in about 5% of benazepril and placebo recipients. Dizziness, fatigue, cough, nausea, orthostatic hypotension, somnolence, and vertigo were reported in ≤3% of the patients. Dizziness occurred more often in the patients who received benazepril plus hydrochlorothiazide than in those who received benazepril alone, presumably because of the additive hypotensive effect of the two agents. Lip swelling and/or facial swelling occurred rarely.

Neutrophil counts decreased to <1,500/mm^3 in some patients following administration of benazepril, but no signs or symptoms of infection or agranulocytosis were observed. Small decreases in hemoglobin concentration were detected. Hyperkalemia developed in 5% of patients treated with benazepril.

PHARMACOKINETICS. See Table 1.

DOSAGE AND PREPARATIONS.

Oral: For hypertension, *adults*, initially, 10 mg once daily for patients who are not taking a diuretic or 5 mg once daily for those who are also receiving a diuretic. The usual maintenance dose is 20 to 40 mg once daily or in two equally divided doses (maximum, 40 mg daily). For *patients with renal dysfunction* (creatinine clearance, <30 ml/min), initially, 5 mg once daily; the maximum maintenance dose is 10 mg daily.

Lotensin (Ciba). Tablets 5, 10, 20, and 40 mg.

CAPTOPRIL

[Capoten]

ACTIONS. Captopril is the only ACE inhibitor that contains a sulfhydryl group, which may be a factor in the development of rash, taste disturbances, and neutropenia with use of this drug (Brogden et al, 1988). Captopril and lisinopril are the only two ACE inhibitors that are not prodrugs.

The acute effects of oral administration of captopril in healthy subjects and in patients with hypertension and heart failure include inhibition of plasma ACE activity; decreased and increased plasma concentrations of angiotensin II and angiotensin I, respectively; increased plasma renin activity or renin concentration; and decreased aldosterone concentration or urinary aldosterone excretion. Maximal hormonal responses are apparent after one hour and return to control levels after about six to eight hours; however, recovery of ACE activity can take up to 12 to 14 hours. Captopril counteracts the pressor response to infusion of exogenous angiotensin I but not angiotensin II.

USES. Captopril has been widely used in the treatment of essential hypertension and heart failure.

A dose of ≤200 mg daily lowers blood pressure in patients with mild to moderate hypertension when administered alone or in combination with other agents (Brogden et al, 1988). Captopril usually is administered with a diuretic (most often hydrochlorothiazide), which enhances antihypertensive efficacy. The effect of captopril 75 to 300 mg daily in three divided doses is comparable to that of enalapril 10 to 40 mg daily in two divided doses, ramipril 10 mg once daily, propranolol 60 to 120 mg daily, and nifedipine 40 to 80 mg daily as monotherapy or in conjunction with other therapeutic agents. The addition of either captopril 50 to 100 mg or nifedipine 40 to 80 mg daily to atenolol 100 mg plus chlorthalidone 25 mg produced a similar reduction in supine systolic and diastolic blood pressure in patients with mild to moderate hypertension. Captopril 75 mg daily and nifedipine 40 mg daily decreased diastolic blood pressure by 13 mm Hg when both drugs were given alone. A further decrease of 7 to 10 mm Hg in diastolic blood pressure and of 13 to 15 mm Hg in systolic blood pressure was achieved with their combined administration. Long-term trials of captopril alone or with a diuretic indicate that the antihypertensive effect of optimal doses is maintained and that tolerance does not develop.

Treatment of hypertension with captopril alone or with hydrochlorothiazide resulted in significantly higher scores on measures of general well-being, work performance, visual-motor functioning, and life satisfaction than in patients treated with methyldopa (Croog et al, 1986). In addition, captopril plus a diuretic did not alter scores for sexual dysfunction relative to baseline, whereas these total scores worsened in patients receiving diuretics plus methyldopa or propranolol (Croog et al, 1988).

In patients over 55 years with mild to moderate hypertension, captopril $\leq$150 mg daily alone or with a diuretic lowered elevated blood pressure without adversely affecting renal function. Captopril 0.5 to 5.6 mg/kg/day, usually in conjunction with other drugs (eg, beta-adrenergic antagonists), reduced blood pressure in children 0.7 to 16 years with renal hypertension, including hypertension refractory to treatment with other antihypertensive drugs, and in patients with chronic renal failure who were undergoing hemodialysis. Captopril 50 to 100 mg daily alone or with a diuretic also was effective in hypertensive patients with insulin-dependent and noninsulin-dependent diabetes and did not adversely affect carbohydrate metabolism (Brogden et al, 1988).

Results of several trials in patients with chronic heart failure revealed that captopril 37.5 to 150 mg daily given for three to nine months was more effective than placebo in reducing the NYHA functional class by one grade or more and in alleviating dyspnea, breathlessness, fatigue, orthopnea, and edema and improving exercise capacity (Captopril Multicenter Research Group, 1985). Retrospective analysis of the data showed a significant reduction in mortality with captopril compared with placebo over a 90-day period in patients receiving an optimal regimen of digitalis and diuretics (Newman et al, 1988).

In a few patients with heart failure, captopril did not alleviate angina pectoris (Cleland et al, 1991). The reduction in coronary perfusion pressure during exercise may lead to earlier onset of ischemia and exacerbation of angina at rest or during exercise in patients with both angina pectoris and heart failure.

ADVERSE REACTIONS AND PRECAUTIONS. See the Introduction.

PHARMACOKINETICS. Gastrointestinal absorption of captopril may be decreased by food. See also Table 1.

DOSAGE AND PREPARATIONS.

Oral: For hypertension, *adults*, initially, 25 to 50 mg daily in two divided doses one hour before meals. Dosage may be increased at intervals of one to two weeks to 100 or 150 mg daily in two or three divided doses (maximum, 300 mg daily). A diuretic (eg, hydrochlorothiazide 12.5 to 25 mg) should be added before the dose is increased further. *Children over 6 months*, 0.5 to 2 mg/kg daily in three doses (maximum, 6 mg/kg daily). *Infants less than 6 months*, 0.05 to 0.5 mg/kg daily in three doses.

For heart failure, *adults*, initially 6.25 to 12.5 mg three times daily. The dosage may be increased to a maximum of 150 mg/day.

Capoten (Squibb). Tablets 12.5, 25, 50, and 100 mg.

ENALAPRIL MALEATE

[Vasotec, Vasotec I.V.]

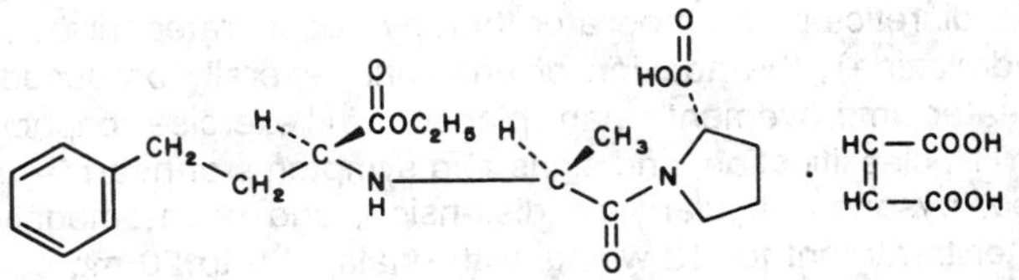

ACTIONS. Enalapril, a carboxyl derivative of captopril, is a prodrug that is converted to form the active ACE inhibitor, enalaprilat. In vitro studies measuring serum, pulmonary, renal, adrenal, and brain ACE from different species showed that enalapril was about three times less potent than enalaprilat and about two times less potent than captopril (Todd and Heel, 1986). The acute effects of enalapril following oral administration in healthy subjects and in patients with hypertension or heart failure include a decrease in the plasma concentration of angiotensin II and an increase in the concentration of angiotensin I, an increase in plasma renin activity or renin concentration, and a decrease in the plasma aldosterone concentration or urinary aldosterone excretion. These effects are usually maintained during long-term treatment. Single oral doses of enalapril higher than 5 mg provide maximal inhibition of the pressor response to exogenous angiotensin I in healthy subjects.

USES. Enalapril is effective in the treatment of essential hypertension and congestive heart failure (Todd and Goa, 1989).

In open and placebo-controlled studies, enalapril 10 to 40 mg daily reduced systolic and diastolic blood pressure by 15% to 20% in patients with mild to severe essential and renovascular hypertension. Adequate blood pressure control was achieved in about 50% to 75% of patients receiving enalapril alone, and the addition of hydrochlorothiazide usually provided adequate control in the remainder. Following daily administration, the efficacy of enalapril was maintained for 24 hours and did not alter the normal diurnal variation in blood pressure. The effect of optimal doses of enalapril on blood pressure is maintained for at least two years.

Enalapril 20 to 40 mg/day or hydrochlorothiazide 50 to 100 mg/day decreases diastolic blood pressure by about 15% when given alone and by about 20% when the two drugs are given concomitantly in patients with mild to moderate hypertension. Black patients have been less responsive to enalapril alone than to hydrochlorothiazide alone. Blacks and nonblacks respond similarly when the drugs are given in combination.

Enalapril ≥20 mg twice daily was at least as effective as captopril 25 mg three times daily, propranolol ≥120 mg twice daily, metoprolol ≥200 mg twice daily, and atenolol ≥100 mg once daily in patients with moderate to severe hypertension. Although the effect of enalapril and beta-adrenergic blocking drugs in lowering diastolic blood pressure was similar, enalapril's effect in lowering systolic blood pressure was consistently greater.

The intravenous form, enalaprilat, may be used to treat severe or sudden elevations in blood pressure that require prompt treatment.

In patients with heart failure who were receiving digitalis and diuretics plus vasodilator therapy (eg, nitrates, prazosin, hydralazine), the addition of enalapril generally produced a greater improvement than placebo in exercise capacity, NYHA classification, and signs and symptoms of heart failure (eg, dyspnea, jugular vein distension, and hepatomegaly). After treatment for 12 weeks with enalapril 5 to 20 mg daily, the NYHA classification improved in 46% of the patients; in comparison, improvement was noted in 10% of those in the placebo group (Enalapril Congestive Heart Failure Investigators, 1987). The enalapril-treated group also experienced fewer episodes of diastolic ventricular gallop, rales, dyspnea, and fatigue. The mean body weight, heart size, and cardiothoracic ratio were decreased and the maximum exercise duration was increased in these patients.

In addition to the beneficial hemodynamic effects, enalapril 5 to 20 mg daily decreased the mortality rate of patients with severe congestive heart failure (NYHA Class IV). In the CONSENSUS trial, after a mean follow-up period of 188 days, mortality was reduced by 40% in the enalapril-treated patients at six months, by 31% at one year, and by 27% at the end of the study (CONSENSUS Trial Study Group, 1987). The survival rate also increased in patients with less severe congestive heart failure (ejection fraction ≤0.35; NYHA Class II and III) following administration of enalapril with conventional treatment (The SOLVD Investigators, 1991). Cumulatively, over a period of 48 months, 510 of 1,284 patients died in the placebo group compared with 452 of 1,285 patients in the enalapril group. The difference in mortality appeared to be most marked in the first 24 months; a similar number of deaths occurred in each group thereafter. A high proportion of deaths in the placebo and enalapril-treated groups (approximately 50%) was due to the progression of heart failure; another 8% to 10% of the deaths were attributed to myocardial infarction. In the VHeFT-II trial, enalapril was more effective in improving the survival rate in patients with heart failure (NYHA Class I and II) than the combination of hydralazine and isosorbide dinitrate (Cohn et al, 1991). The mortality rate was 18% in the enalapril group and 25% in the hydralazine/isosorbide dinitrate group. In the VHeFT-II trial, the reduction in the mortality rate was due to a lower incidence of sudden death.

ADVERSE REACTIONS AND PRECAUTIONS. See the Introduction.

PHARMACOKINETICS. See Table 1.

DOSAGE AND PREPARATIONS.

Oral: For hypertension, *adults*, initially, 2.5 to 5 mg/day in one or two doses. The amount may be doubled at one- or two-week intervals to a maximum of 40 mg daily. For *patients with renal impairment* (creatinine clearance ≤30 ml/min), initially, 2.5 mg/day. A diuretic (eg, hydrochlorothiazide) may be added to enhance the effect; a lower dose of enalapril should be used with the diuretic.

For congestive heart failure, initially, 2.5 mg/day in one or two doses. The dosage can be increased gradually to a maximum of 20 mg/day.

Vasotec (Merck Sharp & Dohme). Tablets 2.5, 5, 10, and 20 mg.

Intravenous: For hypertension, *adults,* initially, 1.25 mg administered over a five-minute period. This dose may be repeated at six-hour intervals. Up to 5 mg every six hours for a maximal duration of 48 hours may be required in some patients. For patients on diuretic therapy and for those with creatinine clearance <30 ml/min, initially, 0.625 mg over a five-minute period. If the response is not adequate, this dose may be repeated in one hour. Additional doses of 1.25 mg may be given at six-hour intervals.

Vasotec I.V. (Merck Sharp & Dohme). Solution (injection) 1.25 mg/ml in 1 and 2 ml containers.

FOSINOPRIL SODIUM
[Monopril]

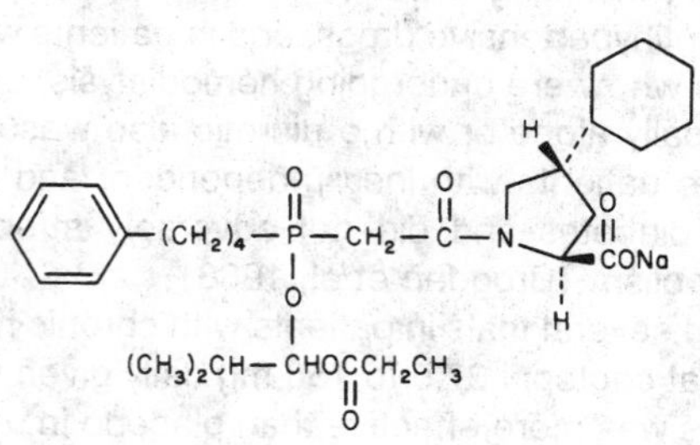

ACTIONS. The prodrug, fosinopril, is a member of a new class of phosphorus-containing ACE inhibitors (DeForrest et al, 1989). It is hydrolyzed completely by intestinal and liver esterases to yield the active diacid, fosinoprilat. Single oral doses of 10 mg or more produced profound and long-lasting inhibition of serum ACE in healthy human subjects and patients with hypertension (Pool, 1990). Oral doses of 10 to 40 mg reduced the pressor response to angiotensin I by 87% or more three to six hours after administration.

USES. Fosinopril given once daily alone or with a diuretic controls blood pressure in patients with mild to moderate essential hypertension. In a double-blind study lasting three months

(Anderson et al, 1991; Fosinopril Study Group II, 1990), fosinopril 40 to 80 mg/day reduced the supine diastolic blood pressure to $\leq$90 mm Hg in 60% of patients after four weeks of therapy and the effect was maintained at eight weeks. The addition of chlorthalidone in patients who did not respond adequately to fosinopril alone further reduced the blood pressure. During long-term treatment (10 to 13 months), the blood pressure continued to be well controlled and there was no evidence of tolerance or tachycardia.

ADVERSE REACTIONS AND PRECAUTIONS. Adverse reactions are generally mild, transient, and not dose-related. Dizziness/lightheadedness is the predominant reaction to fosinopril, especially in patients with renin-dependent hypertension or those maintained on a low-salt diet. Serum potassium concentrations decreased slightly in patients treated with fosinopril and chlorthalidone; fosinopril may have had a mild blunting effect on the kaliuresis induced by chlorthalidone. During long-term studies, moderate elevations in liver function test values were observed in a small number of patients.

PHARMACOKINETICS. See the Introduction and Table 1.

DOSAGE AND PREPARATIONS.

Oral: For hypertension, *adults,* initially, 10 mg once daily. The usual dosage range is 10 to 40 mg/day. The dosage does not have to be reduced in patients with impaired renal function.

Monopril (Mead Johnson). Tablets 10 and 20 mg.

LISINOPRIL

[Prinivil, Zestril]

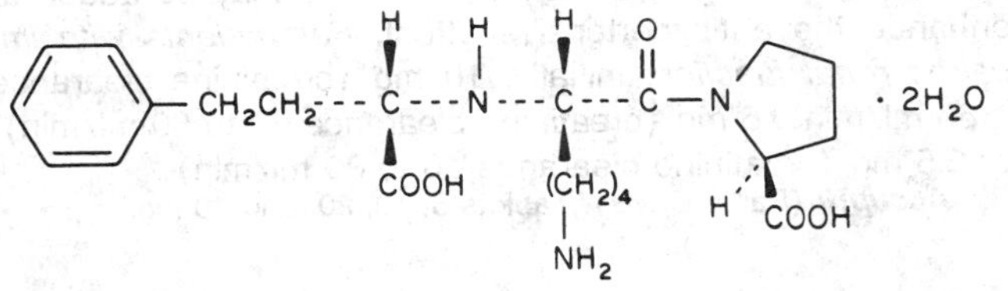

ACTIONS. Lisinopril is a lysine derivative of enalaprilat, the active metabolite of enalapril. In healthy volunteers and patients with hypertension or heart failure, single oral doses of 10 mg reduced plasma angiotensin II, aldosterone, and plasma ACE activity and increased plasma renin activity six hours after administration (Lancaster and Todd, 1988). The effects on the renin-angiotensin-aldosterone system were maintained for up to three weeks during treatment. ACE activity appears to be inhibited more slowly with lisinopril than with captopril or enalapril. In healthy subjects, lisinopril 2.5, 10, and 20 mg inhibited the response to exogenous angiotensin I by 40% to 80%.

USES. Lisinopril is effective in the treatment of hypertension when given alone or with other antihypertensive drugs (Lancaster and Todd, 1988). In several double-blind, placebo-controlled studies, daily oral doses of lisinopril ranging from 1.25 to 80 mg were administered for six weeks to 208 patients with mild to moderate hypertension. Lisinopril 20 mg once daily reduced both systolic and diastolic blood pressure by about 10% to 20% for up to 24 hours compared with placebo. Larger doses did not enhance the hypertensive effect.

Lisinopril 20 to 80 mg once daily was more effective in reducing the mean diastolic pressure (14%) than hydrochlorothiazide 12.5 to 50 mg once daily (8%), and the combination of both drugs was more effective than either drug alone (19%). Nonblack patients were more responsive, both to lisinopril alone and in combination with hydrochlorothiazide, than black patients. The efficacy of lisinopril with or without hydrochlorothiazide was similar in elderly and younger patients.

Lisinopril 20 to 80 mg once daily was at least as effective as atenolol 50 to 200 mg once daily, metoprolol 100 to 200 mg once daily, or nifedipine 40 to 80 mg once daily in patients with mild, moderate, and severe hypertension. In these dosage ranges, the incidence of adverse effects was lowest in the lisinopril-treated patients; beta-adrenergic blocking drugs caused a marked decrease in heart rate, and nifedipine produced peripheral edema, flushing, and headache.

Preliminary data from a placebo-controlled study showed that lisinopril 5 to 20 mg daily for 12 weeks increased left ventricular ejection fraction and the dyspnea/fatigue index in patients with heart failure. Exercise tolerance time was increased significantly with lisinopril compared with baseline and placebo controls, especially in patients over 65 years. Lisinopril produced a greater improvement than placebo in rales, orthopnea, third heart sound, and jugular vein distension but not in paroxysmal nocturnal dyspnea or edema. In one 12-week, randomized, multicenter, double-blind parallel study in patients with NYHA Class II to IV heart failure, lisinopril 5 to 20 mg once daily was more effective than captopril $\leq$150 mg/day in improving mean treadmill exercise time and reduction in rales and jugular vein distension (Powers et al, 1987). Mean ejection fraction was increased in the lisinopril-treated group but not in those treated with captopril.

ADVERSE REACTIONS AND PRECAUTIONS. The most frequent side effects in patients with hypertension include headache, dizziness, cough, and diarrhea. The incidence of dizziness in patients treated with lisinopril plus hydrochlorothiazide was nearly twice that reported with lisinopril alone. In addition, some patients with hypertension developed symptoms suggestive of angioedema, including swelling of the face, lips, mouth, or eyelids. The incidence of the most common side effects to lisinopril monotherapy was similar in elderly and younger hypertensive patients. The most frequent side effects in patients with heart failure were dizziness, diarrhea, and hypotension.

As with other ACE inhibitors, lisinopril has caused a reduction in hemoglobin, an increase in serum potassium, and a reversible increase in serum creatinine.

PHARMACOKINETICS. See Table 1.

DOSAGE AND PREPARATIONS.

Oral: For hypertension, *adults,* initially, 5 to 10 mg once daily. The usual dosage for maintenance is 20 to 40 mg once daily (maximum, 80 mg/day). A diuretic (eg, hydrochlorothiazide) may be added to enhance the antihypertensive effect. For *patients with severe renal impairment,* initially, 5 or 2.5 mg once daily for patients with glomerular filtration rates of 10 to 30 ml/min and <10 ml/min, respectively. The dosage may be increased to a maximum of 40 mg daily.

Prinivil (Merck Sharp & Dohme), ***Zestril*** (Stuart). Tablets 5, 10, 20, and 40 mg.

QUINAPRIL HYDROCHLORIDE
[Accupril]

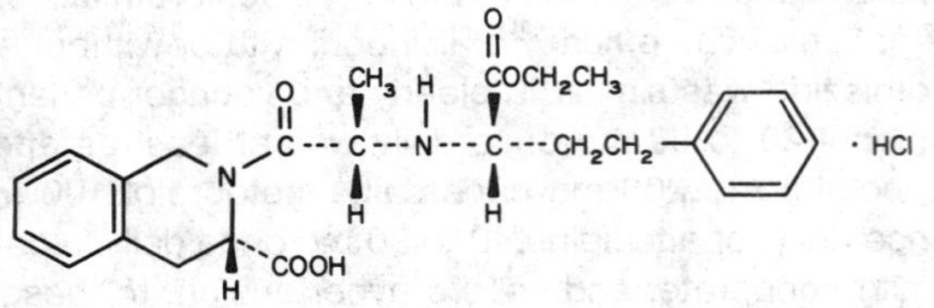

ACTIONS. This carboxyl monoethyl ester is hydrolyzed to form the more active diacid, quinaprilat (Wadsworth and Brogden, 1991). Both quinapril and quinaprilat inhibit ACE activity in a dose-dependent manner, but quinaprilat is approximately three times more potent than quinapril in guinea pig serum. Quinaprilat's inhibitory effect on ACE activity is similar to that of ramiprilat and is more potent than that of enalapril, captopril, and quinapril in human plasma. In healthy volunteers and patients with hypertension, single doses of quinapril decrease plasma ACE activity, increase plasma renin activity or renin concentrations, decrease pressor responses to angiotensin I, and decrease aldosterone concentrations. Marked dose-related decreases in plasma ACE activity are observed within 30 minutes, and the level of inhibition persists for at least eight hours.

USES. Quinapril is effective in the treatment of hypertension when given alone or with other antihypertensive drugs (Wadsworth and Brogden, 1991). In several placebo-controlled trials in patients with mild, moderate, or severe hypertension, administration of quinapril 20 to 80 mg once or twice daily for 12 weeks reduced the systolic blood pressure by 17 to 33 mm Hg and the diastolic blood pressure by 11 to 15 mm Hg more than with placebo. Efficacy was maintained with quinapril 20 to 40 mg/day when the trial was continued in some patients for another nine months.

In randomized, double-blind trials comparing its antihypertensive effects with that of other ACE inhibitors in patients with mild, moderate, and severe hypertension, quinapril 10 to 40 mg/day was as effective in reducing systolic and diastolic pressure as enalapril 10 to 40 mg/day and captopril 50 to 150 mg/day in two or three divided doses. Addition of a diuretic (hydrochlorothiazide 25 mg) to the quinapril, enalapril, or captopril regimen in nonresponsive patients increased the efficacy of all three ACE inhibitors. The addition of atenolol to either quinapril or captopril plus hydrochlorothiazide further reduced the diastolic blood pressure (Goldstein, 1990).

In patients with heart failure, preliminary data demonstrated that quinapril 5 to 30 mg/day produced hemodynamic changes indicative of improved cardiac performance (reduction in systemic vascular resistance, pulmonary capillary wedge pressure, and mean arterial pressure and in increase in cardiac output). The time to onset of these effects was less than one hour and was similar to that observed with captopril (1 to 1.5 hours) and shorter than that with enalapril (four to six hours) (Wadsworth and Brogden, 1991). Quinapril ≤40 mg/day improved the NYHA classification in at least 60% of patients with heart failure. The improvement was maintained for up to one year and was greatest in those with more severe disease (Riegger, 1990). Quinapril 10 to 40 mg/day increased exercise tolerance more than diuretic therapy alone (Kromer and Riegger, 1988).

ADVERSE REACTIONS AND PRECAUTIONS. Quinapril was well tolerated by most patients in clinical trials, including 1,195 patients treated during open studies for up to three years. Adverse effects are generally mild and transient and rarely require withdrawal of treatment. The frequency of adverse effects was similar to that with enalapril and captopril. Dizziness and headache were the most common adverse reactions associated with quinapril monotherapy. Cough, hypotension, abdominal pain, and peripheral edema also were reported in patients with hypertension and heart failure. The incidence of orthostatic and first-dose hypotension has been reported to be lower in quinapril-treated patients than in those treated with captopril.

Quinapril has been associated with increases in plasma creatinine and blood urea nitrogen and with fluctuations in plasma potassium concentrations. White blood cell and neutrophil counts were reduced in some patients.

PHARMACOKINETICS. See Table 1.

DOSAGE AND PREPARATIONS.

Oral: For hypertension, *adults*, initially, 5 to 10 mg once daily. Dosage may be increased after four weeks. The usual range is 10 to 40 mg once daily or in two equally divided doses (maximum, 80 mg once daily). A diuretic may be added to enhance the antihypertensive effect. *For patients with impaired renal function,* initially, 10 mg (creatinine clearance >60 ml/min), 5 mg (creatinine clearance 30 to 60 ml/min), or 2.5 mg (creatinine clearance 10 to 30 ml/min).

Accupril (Parke-Davis). Tablets 5, 10, 20, and 40 mg.

RAMIPRIL
[Altace]

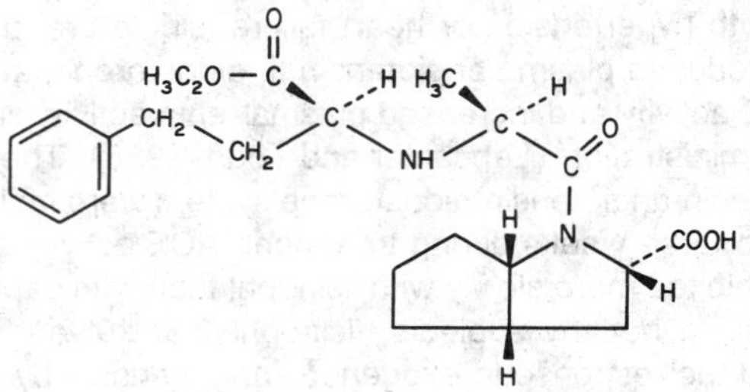

ACTIONS. Ramipril, a structural derivative of enalapril, is a carboxyl prodrug that is hydrolyzed to form the active ACE inhibitor, ramiprilat. Oral administration of ramipril in healthy subjects and in patients with hypertension or congestive heart failure reduced plasma ACE, angiotensin II, and aldosterone levels and increased plasma angiotensin I and renin activity (Todd and Benfield, 1990). The maximum inhibitory effect on the plasma ACE activity was observed one to four hours after oral administration; peak effects on plasma angiotensin I and angiotensin II levels, plasma renin activity, and aldosterone concentration occurred in four to eight hours. These effects were maintained when ramipril was administered for weeks, even though the aldosterone concentration rapidly returned to the pretreatment level after a few days. Arterial infusion of ramipril reversed constriction in the forearm vascular bed induced by infusion of exogenous angiotensin I but not of angiotensin II.

USES. Ramipril is effective in the management of mild, moderate, and severe hypertension when given alone and with a diuretic. In patients with mild to moderate hypertension, oral administration of ramipril 2.5 to 10 mg once daily reduced the systolic and diastolic blood pressure by 2 to 13 mm Hg and 4 to 9 mm Hg, respectively. Once-daily administration regulates blood pressure for 24 hours. Ramipril is equally effective in elderly and younger patients with hypertension and in patients with mild renal impairment. In double-blind, randomized studies lasting six to eight weeks in patients with mild to moderate hypertension, the efficacy of ramipril 5 to 10 mg once daily was comparable to that of atenolol 100 mg once daily, captopril 50 mg twice daily, and enalapril 10 to 20 mg once daily. The efficacy of ramipril is enhanced with the addition of a diuretic (eg, hydrochlorothiazide).

In several studies on a small number of patients with heart failure (NYHA Class III and IV), doses of up to 5 mg once daily reduced pulmonary wedge pressure, mean arterial pressure, and cardiac index and improved exercise duration and NYHA functional class.

ADVERSE REACTIONS AND PRECAUTIONS. The nature and frequency of adverse effects associated with administration of ramipril are similar to those with captopril and enalapril. Dizziness/vertigo and headache were the most frequent side effects; their incidence was lower than that observed with placebo. Fatigue/weakness and nausea also occurred in patients with hypertension. The cough, rash, gastrointestinal pain, and diarrhea observed in patients treated with other ACE inhibitors also occurred in those receiving ramipril. Angioedema was reported in 1 of 2,211 patients receiving this drug. As with other ACE inhibitors, serum potassium, blood urea nitrogen, and serum creatinine levels changed only rarely.

PHARMACOKINETICS. See Table 1.

DOSAGE AND PREPARATIONS.

Oral: For hypertension, *adults*, initially, 1.25 to 2.5 mg once daily. Dosage may be increased at intervals of one to two weeks to a maximum of 10 mg daily. A diuretic may be added to enhance the antihypertensive effect. For *patients with renal impairment* (creatinine clearance <30 ml/min), initially, 1.25 mg once daily. Maximum dosages are 5 and 2.5 mg once daily for patients with creatinine clearance of 10 to 30 ml/min and ≤10 ml/min, respectively.

Altace (Hoechst-Roussel). Capsules 1.25, 2.5, 5, and 10 mg.

Cited References

Abraham PA, et al: Efficacy and renal effects of enalapril therapy for hypertensive patients with chronic renal insufficiency. *Arch Intern Med* 148:2358-2362, 1988.

Alderman MH, et al: Association of the renin-sodium profile with the risk of myocardial infarction in patients with hypertension. *N Engl J Med* 324:1098-1104, 1991.

Anderson RJ, et al: Once-daily fosinopril in the treatment of hypertension. *Hypertension* 17:636-642, 1991.

Ando K, et al: Role of renal hemodynamics in antihypertensive effect of captopril. *Am Heart J* 111:347-352, 1986.

Asher JP, Murray KM: Use of angiotensin-converting-enzyme inhibitors in the management of renal disease. *Clin Pharm* 10:25-31, 1991.

Balfour JA, Goa KL: Benazepril: A review of its pharmacodynamic and pharmacokinetic properties, and therapeutic efficacy in hypertension and congestive heart failure. *Drugs* 42:511-539, 1991.

Bauer JH, Gaddy P: Effects of enalapril alone, and in combination with hydrochlorothiazide, on renin-angiotensin-aldosterone, renal function, salt and water excretion, and body fluid composition. *Am J Kidney Dis* 6:222-232, 1985.

Beckett VL, et al: Use of captopril as early therapy for renal scleroderma: Prospective study. *Mayo Clin Proc* 60:763-771, 1985.

Björck S, et al: Beneficial effects of angiotensin converting enzyme inhibition on renal function in patients with diabetic nephropathy. *BMJ* 293:471-474, 1986.

Boulet L-P, et al: Pulmonary function and airway responsiveness during long-term therapy with captopril. *JAMA* 261:413-416, 1989.

Brogden RN, et al: Captopril: An update of its pharmacodynamic and pharmacokinetic properties, and therapeutic use in hypertension and congestive heart failure. *Drugs* 36:540-600, 1988.

Brouhard BH, et al: Use of angiotensin-converting enzyme inhibitors in chronic progressive renal disease. *Cleve Clin J Med* 58:184-190, 1991.

Bucknall CE, et al: Bronchial hyperreactivity in patients who cough after receiving angiotensin converting enzyme inhibitors. *BMJ* 296:86-88, 1988.

Campbell DJ: Circulating and tissue angiotensin systems. *J Clin Invest* 79:1-6, 1987.

Captopril Multicenter Research Group: A cooperative multicenter study of captopril in congestive heart failure: Hemodynamic effects and long-term response. *Am Heart J* 110:439-447, 1985.

Cleland JGF, et al: Effects of enalapril in heart failure: Double blind study of effects on exercise performance, renal function, hormones, and metabolic state. *Br Heart J* 54:305-312, 1985.

Cleland JGF, et al: Effect of captopril and angiotensin-converting enzyme inhibitor, in patients with angina pectoris and heart failure. *J Am Coll Cardiol* 17:733-739, 1991.

Cohn JN: Current therapy of the failing heart. *Circulation* 78:1099-1107, 1988.

Cohn JN, et al: A comparison of enalapril with hydralazine-isosorbide dinitrate in the treatment of chronic congestive heart failure. *N Engl J Med* 325:303-310, 1991.

CONSENSUS Trial Study Group: Effects of enalapril on mortality in severe congestive heart failure: Results of the Cooperative North Scandinavian Enalapril Survival Study (CONSENSUS). *N Engl J Med* 316:1429-1435, 1987.

Coulter DM, Edwards IR: Cough associated with captopril and enalapril. *BMJ* 294:1521-1523, 1987.

Croog SH, et al: The effects of antihypertensive therapy on the quality of life. *N Engl J Med* 26:1657-1664, 1986.

Croog SH, et al: Sexual symptoms in hypertensive patients. *Arch Intern Med* 148:788-794, 1988.

DeForrest JM, et al: Fosinopril, a phosphinicacid inhibitor of angiotensin I converting enzyme: In vitro and pre-clinical in vivo pharmacology. *J Cardiovasc Pharmacol* 14:730-736, 1989.

Dzau VJ: Circulating versus local renin-angiotensin system in cardiovascular homeostasis. *Circulation* 77(suppl I):I4-I13, 1988.

Dzau VJ: Renin and myocardial infarction in hypertension. *N Engl J Med* 324:1128-1130, 1991.

Enalapril Congestive Heart Failure Investigators: Long-term effects of enalapril in patients with congestive heart failure: A multicenter, placebo-controlled trial. *Heart Failure* 3:102-107, 1987.

Erdös EG: Angiotensin I converting enzyme and the changes in our concepts through the years. *Hypertension* 16:363-370, 1990.

Fosinopril Study Group II: Antihypertensive effect of fosinopril, a new angiotensin converting enzyme inhibitor. *Clin Ther* 12:520-533, 1990.

Furness PN, et al: Severe cutaneous reactions to captopril and enalapril; histological study and comparison with early mycosis fungoides. *J Clin Pathol* 39:902-907, 1986.

Gavras H, et al: Antihypertensive effect of oral angiotensin-converting-enzyme inhibitor SQ 14225 in man. *N Engl J Med* 298:991-995, 1978.

Goldstein RJ: The treatment of moderate to severe hypertension with ACE inhibitors. *J Cardiovasc Pharmacol* 15(suppl 2):S29-S35, 1990.

Hommel E, et al: Effect of captopril on kidney function in insulin-dependent diabetic patients with nephropathy. *BMJ* 293:467-470, 1986.

Hui KK, et al: Pharmacokinetics of fosinopril in patients with various degrees of renal function. *Clin Pharmacol Ther* 49:457-467, 1991.

Inman WHW, Rawson NSB: Deafness with enalapril and prescription event monitoring, letter. *Lancet* 1:872, 1987.

Johnston CI, et al: Long-term effects of captopril (SQ 14 225) on blood-pressure and hormone levels in essential hypertension. *Lancet* 2:493-496, 1979.

Joint National Committee: The 1988 report of the Joint National Committee on Detection, Evaluation, and Treatment of High Blood Pressure. *Arch Intern Med* 148:1023-1038, 1988.

Jungmann E, et al: Aldosterone and prolactin responsiveness after prolonged treatment of congestive heart failure. *Eur J Clin Pharmacol* 28:1-4, 1985.

Kaufman J, et al: Bronchial hyperreactivity and cough due to angiotensin-converting enzyme inhibitors. *Chest* 95:544-548, 1989.

Kelleher CC: ACE inhibitors in the prevention and therapy of diabetic nephropathy. *Drugs* 39:639-645, 1990.

Kromer EP, Riegger AJG: Effects of the ACE-inhibitor quinapril on monotherapy in patients with congestive heart failure (CHF) NYHA class II-III. *Eur Heart J* 9(suppl 1):2, 1988.

Lancaster SG, Todd PA: Lisinopril: A preliminary review of its pharmacodynamic and pharmacokinetic properties, and therapeutic use in hypertension and congestive heart failure. *Drugs* 35:646-669, 1988.

Leslie BR, et al: Absence of blood pressure lowering effect of captopril in anephric patients. *BMJ* 280:1067-1068, 1980.

Levenson DJ, Dzau VJ: Effects on angiotensin-converting enzyme inhibition on renal hemodynamics in renal artery stenosis. *Kidney Int* 31(suppl 20):S173-S179, 1987.

Lijnen P, et al: Increase in plasma aldosterone during prolonged captopril treatment. *Am J Cardiol* 49:1561-1563, 1982.

Lopez-Ovejero JA, et al: Reversal of vascular and renal crises of scleroderma by oral angiotensin-converting-enzyme blockade. *N Engl J Med* 300:1417-1419, 1979.

Marre M, et al: Prevention of diabetic nephropathy with enalapril in normotensive diabetics with microalbuminuria. *BMJ* 297:1092-1095, 1988.

Mathiesen ER, et al: Efficacy of captopril in postponing nephropathy in normotensive insulin dependent diabetic patients with microalbuminuria. *BMJ* 303:81-87, 1991.

Milsom SR, Nicholls MG: Successful treatment of scleroderma renal crisis with enalapril. *Postgrad Med J* 62:1059-1060, 1986.

Morelli E, et al: Effects of converting-enzyme inhibition on barrier function in diabetic glomerulopathy. *Diabetes* 39:76-82, 1990.

Nabel EG, et al: A randomized placebo-controlled trial of combined early intravenous captopril and recombinant tissue-type plasminogen activator therapy in acute myocardial infarction. *J Am Coll Cardiol* 17:467-473, 1991.

Newman TJ, et al: Effects of captopril on survival in patients with heart failure. *Am J Med* 84(suppl 3A):140-144, 1988.

Oldenburg B, et al: Controlled trial of enalapril in patients with chronic fluid overload undergoing dialysis. *BMJ* 296:1089-1091, 1988.

Opsahl JA, et al: Enalapril therapy in chronic renal failure (CRF) patients with hypertension maintains renal function and decreases proteinuria, abstract. *Kidney Int* 31:212, 1987.

Packer M, et al: Preservation of glomerular filtration rate in human heart failure by activation of renin-angiotensin system. *Circulation* 74:766-774, 1986.

Packer M, et al: Functional renal insufficiency during long-term therapy with captopril and enalapril in severe chronic heart failure. *Ann Intern Med* 106:346-354, 1987.

Paulson OB, et al: Role of angiotensin in autoregulation of cerebral blood flow. *Circulation* 77(suppl I):I55-I58, 1988.

Perlman JM, Volpe JJ: Neurologic complications of captopril treatment of neonatal hypertension. *Pediatrics* 83:47-52, 1989.

Pool JL: Antihypertensive effect of fosinopril, a new angiotensin converting enzyme inhibitor: Findings of the Fosinopril Study Group II. *Clin Ther* 12:520-533, 1990.

Powers ER, et al: A double-blind comparison of lisinopril with captopril in patients with symptomatic congestive heart failure. *J Cardiovasc Pharmacol* 9(suppl 3):S82-S88, 1987.

Riegger GAJ: The effects of ACE inhibitors on exercise capacity in the treatment of congestive heart failure. *J Cardiovasc Pharmacol* 15(suppl 2):S41-S46, 1990.

Ruilope LM, et al: Converting enzyme inhibition in chronic renal failure. *Am J Kidney Dis* 13:120-126, 1989.

Salvetti A: Newer ACE inhibitors: A look at the future. *Drugs* 40:800-828, 1990.

Semple PF, Herd GW: Cough and wheeze caused by inhibitors of angiotensin-converting enzyme, letter. *N Engl J Med* 314:61, 1986.

Sica DA, et al: Comparison of the steady-state pharmacokinetics of fosinopril, lisinopril and enalapril in patients with chronic renal insufficiency. *Clin Pharmacokinet* 20:420-427, 1991.

Slater EE, et al: Clinical profile of angioedema associated with angiotensin converting-enzyme inhibition. *JAMA* 260:967-970, 1988.

The SOLVD Investigators: Effect of enalapril on survival in patients with reduced left ventricular ejection fractions and congestive heart failure. *N Engl J Med* 325:293-302, 1991.

Taguma Y, et al: Effect of captopril on heavy proteinuria in azotemic diabetics. *N Engl J Med* 313:1617-1620, 1985.

Todd PA, Benfield P: Ramipril: A review of its pharmacological properties and therapeutic efficacy in cardiovascular disorders. *Drugs* 39:110-135, 1990.

Todd PA, Goa KL: Enalapril: An update of its pharmacological properties and therapeutic use in congestive heart failure. *Drugs* 37:141-161, 1989.

Todd PA, Heel RC: Enalapril: A review of its pharmacodynamic and pharmacokinetic properties, and therapeutic use in hypertension and congestive heart failure. *Drugs* 31:198-248, 1986.

Unger T, et al: Brain angiotensin: Pathways and pharmacology. *Circulation* 77(suppl I):I40-I54, 1988.

Valvo E, et al: Captopril in patients with type II diabetes and renal insufficiency: Systemic and renal hemodynamic alterations. *Am J Med* 85:344-348, 1988.

Wadsworth AN, Brogden RN: Quinapril: A review of its pharmacological properties, and therapeutic efficacy in cardiovascular disorders. *Drugs* 41:378-399, 1991.

Wood SM: Angio-oedema and urticaria associated with angiotensin converting enzyme inhibitors. *BMJ* 294:91-92, 1987.

Drugs Used for Hypertension 25

In the United States, almost 50 million adults aged 25 to 74 years have blood pressure above normal and are considered to be at increased risk of damage to the heart, kidney, brain, and eye that result in premature morbidity and mortality. In general, young men have higher blood pressures than young women; however, older men have lower blood pressures than older women.

CLASSIFICATION OF HYPERTENSION

Individuals may be subdivided according to their blood pressure levels into categories of normal, high normal, and hypertension stages 1, 2, 3, and 4 (Joint National Committee on Detection, Evaluation, and Treatment of High Blood Pressure, 1993) (Table 1). Both systolic and diastolic blood pressures are significant in the diagnosis and treatment of hypertension, since either one is independently capable of precipitating cardiovascular diseases and other complications.

Results of the Tecumseh Blood Pressure Study showed that young individuals who have systolic and diastolic blood pressures of 131 and 94 mm Hg, respectively, already exhibit early signs of cardiovascular disorders (eg, higher heart rates, lower cardiac stroke volume, impaired left ventricular filling) compared to those with corresponding blood pressures of 112 and 75 mm Hg (Julius et al, 1990). If untreated, the blood pressure of these individuals probably will increase progressively, as will the likelihood of developing congestive heart failure, stroke, coronary artery disease, and/or progressive renal failure. Furthermore, the risk of developing hypertension is approximately twofold higher for men and women with an initial diastolic blood pressure of 85 to 89 mm Hg than for those with a value less than 85 mm Hg (Leitschuh et al, 1991).

GUIDELINES FOR TREATMENT

Individuals with high normal blood pressure should be monitored frequently and encouraged to reduce blood pressure by nondrug measures; they do not require pharmacologic therapy.

The goals in treating patients with more pronounced high blood pressure are to achieve and maintain systolic blood pressure below 140 mm Hg and diastolic blood pressure below 90 mm Hg while simultaneously controlling other recognizable cardiovascular risk factors (National High Blood Pressure Education Program Working Group, 1993). The blood pressure may be reduced by pharmacologic and/or nonpharmacologic measures. Nondrug management should be stressed regardless of whether treatment with drugs is also needed. Generally, the prognosis is improved when pharmacologic and nonpharmacologic methods are combined (Collins et al, 1990). Treatment reduces the risk of death from acute left ventricular failure and other cardiac complications. There is strong evidence that drug therapy for mild hypertension reduces the risk of stroke by 40% and of fatal or nonfatal myocardial infarction by 14% (Collins et al, 1990). The benefits are more pronounced in the elderly (Joint National Committee on Detection, Evaluation, and Treatment of High Blood Pressure, 1993).

Nondrug Management

Nonpharmacologic measures to control blood pressure usually necessitate a change of habits and/or lifestyle, and counseling may be required to achieve the intended goals. Nondrug management includes weight control, restriction of sodium and alcohol, and participation in an exercise program (Joint National Committee on Detection, Evaluation, and

TABLE 1.
CLASSIFICATION OF HYPERTENSION*

Category	Systolic BP (mm Hg)	Diastolic BP (mm Hg)	Recommendation
Normal	<130	<85	Recheck in 2 years
High Normal	130-139	85-89	Recheck in 1 year
Hypertension			
Stage 1 (mild)	140-159	90-99	Confirm and treat within 2 months
Stage 2 (moderate)	160-179	100-109	Treat within 1 month
Stage 3 (severe)	180-209	110-119	Treat within 1 week
Stage 4 (very severe)	≥210	≥120	Treat immediately

** Adapted from Joint National Committee on Detection, Evaluation, and Treatment of High Blood Pressure (1993).*

Treatment of High Blood Pressure, 1993). After reduction of sodium and caloric intake, a slight lowering of blood pressure was demonstrable even in healthy men and women with a diastolic blood pressure of 78 to 89 mm Hg (Hypertension Prevention Trial Research Group, 1990).

Excessive weight is common in the United States and varies from less than 20% in younger white men to more than 60% in older black women. A strong correlation between excess weight and development of hypertension has been observed in adults and children of both sexes and in a wide variety of ethnic groups. The risk of developing hypertension is increased two- to sixfold in overweight individuals. Caloric reduction in individuals with high normal blood pressure produced an average weight loss of 3.8 kg at 18 months, with concomitant reduction in systolic and diastolic blood pressures of 2.9 and 2.3 mm Hg, respectively (The Trials of Hypertension Prevention Collaborative Research Group, 1992). Weight loss also has been associated with a 51% reduction in the incidence of hypertension. However, it is emphasized that long-term maintenance of an ideal weight is desirable to achieve the benefits derived from the reduction in blood pressure, since highly variable body weight as a result of repeated episodes of weight loss and gain has been associated with increased mortality and morbidity from coronary heart disease for both men and women (Lissner et al, 1991).

Even though diets varying in total fat and proportions of saturated to unsaturated fats have little effect on blood pressure, dyslipidemia is a major independent risk factor for coronary artery disease (Neaton et al, 1992). Thus, in addition to caloric reduction for weight control, limiting the intake of saturated fat also is desirable (Samuelsson et al, 1987).

The importance of the level of sodium intake is illustrated in a series of stratified analyses in the INTERSALT study (Stamler, 1991). This study showed that the average prevalence of hypertension in individuals with a low body mass index was 1.7% among those with a low sodium intake and 11.9% for those whose diet was high in sodium; a high-sodium intake with light alcohol consumption increased the prevalence rate to 13.4%. Reduced sodium intake had a blood pressure-lowering effect in both normotensive and hypertensive individuals (Law et al, 1991). The average reductions in systolic and diastolic blood pressures for individuals who followed a low-sodium diet were 5 and 3 mm Hg, respectively, for hypertensive patients and 2 and 1 mm Hg, respectively, for those who were normotensive (Cutler et al, 1991). It is recommended that sodium intake not exceed 2.4 g/day (National High Blood Pressure Education Program Working Group, 1993).

Excessive intake of alcohol (eg, three drinks or more per day) leads to elevated blood pressure in some patients and may cause resistance to antihypertensive therapy. On the other hand, light drinkers (less than one ounce of alcohol daily) have a lower mortality risk than either abstainers or heavy drinkers, for the most part due to a lower risk of death from coronary heart disease (Klatsky et al, 1992). Hence, in patients with hypertension, intake of alcohol should be limited to one ounce or less daily.

Sedentary normotensive individuals have an increased risk of developing hypertension compared with more active peers. Increased physical exercise, either alone or as part of a weight loss program, has been associated with an average reduction of 6 to 7 mm Hg for both systolic and diastolic blood pressures; the mechanism is unknown (Arroll and Beaglehole, 1992). The blood pressure reduction was observed in normotensive as well as hypertensive participants and was independent of weight loss. All types of increased physical activity lowered blood pressure. Low- to moderate-intensity endurance exercise requiring 40% to 60% of maximum oxygen consumption (walking, jogging, cycling, dancing, swimming, and gardening) was as effective as high-intensity exercise in reducing blood pressure in patients with stages 1 and 2 hypertension.

Other nonpharmacologic measures (eg, stress management; potassium, calcium, magnesium, fiber, and fish oil supplementation; macronutrient alteration) have limited or unproved efficacy for the management of normotensive individuals and hypertensive patients (National High Blood Pressure Education Program Working Group, 1993).

If the desired blood pressure is not achieved with nonpharmacologic measures within three to six months in patients with borderline or mild hypertension, drug therapy should be instituted.

Drug Therapy

GENERAL POPULATION. Prior to beginning treatment, the patient with mildly or moderately elevated blood pressure (stages 1 and 2) should be seen on at least three separate visits to determine whether the elevation persists, but treatment should not be delayed in those with severe hypertension (stages 3 and 4). The extent of target organ changes, particularly those affecting the optic fundi, brain, heart, and kidneys, should be assessed. Baseline measurements of blood chemistry (serum potassium, creatinine, fasting glucose, and a lipid profile), a complete blood count, urinalysis (protein, blood, and glucose), and an electrocardiogram should be obtained. Measurements of plasma renin activity (PRA) and plasma aldosterone, assessment of renal blood flow, arteriography, and tests for pheochromocytoma or other special examinations should be performed only when specific indications are present.

The initial goal of therapy should be to maintain an arterial pressure of ≤140/90 mm Hg and concurrently control other modifiable cardiovascular risk factors. Further reduction to levels of 130/85 mm Hg may be pursued provided that cardiovascular function, especially for older individuals, is not compromised.

The classes of drugs used for the treatment of hypertensive patients include (1) diuretics, (2) beta-adrenergic blocking agents, (3) alpha- and alpha-beta adrenergic blocking agents, (4) angiotensin-converting enzyme (ACE) inhibitors, (5) calcium channel blocking drugs, and (6) supplemental agents such as centrally acting alpha agonists, rauwolfia alkaloids, and direct vasodilators. Drugs in the first five categories are equally effective (Materson et al, 1993; Neaton et al, 1993) and can be used initially for monotherapy.

Initially, a single drug at the lowest dosage should be used to treat stages 1 and 2 hypertension. If the response is not adequate after one to three months, the dosage can be increased toward maximal levels (if the patient is not experiencing significant side effects), a drug from another class can be substituted, or a second agent from a different class can be added. If it is not used as initial monotherapy, a diuretic often is chosen as a second drug, since it has the potential to enhance the effect of all other antihypertensive agents. After the blood pressure is reduced to the desired level and maintenance doses are established, substitution of an appropriate combination product, especially one containing a diuretic(s), may simplify the patient's regimen and promote compliance.

For patients with stage 3 hypertension, a second or third agent can be added to the initial regimen if control of blood pressure is not achieved within a short time. In these patients, the interval between changes in the drug regimen should be decreased and the maximum dose of some drugs may be prescribed.

Immediate therapy is recommended for patients with stage 4 hypertension and, if significant target organ disease is present, hospitalization may be required.

Because of differences in responsiveness, a regimen should be individualized, and it may be necessary to try various drugs or combinations until the optimal regimen is determined. Effective doses vary considerably from patient to patient. A slow, gradual reduction in blood pressure is better tolerated than an abrupt reduction.

After blood pressure has been maintained at normal levels for at least one year, it may be possible to "step down" therapy slowly and progressively in some patients by first reducing the dose and then discontinuing one or more of the antihypertensive agents (Finnerty, 1984; Levinson et al, 1982). Dose reduction may maintain therapeutic control more effectively than drug withdrawal (Freis et al, 1989). Step-down therapy is especially successful in patients who are diligent in adhering to modifications in lifestyle, but periodic monitoring for any necessary dosage adjustment should continue.

Drug Selection: The selection of an appropriate drug or combination depends on the severity of the disease and the patient's initial response to the therapeutic trial. The choice may be more appropriately individualized by considering the patient's characteristics and the presence of complications caused by hypertension or other medical conditions (see Table 2).

If a diuretic is selected as initial therapy, a thiazide is usually preferred for patients with normal renal function (Table 3). The lowest effective dose should be employed to reduce the risk of metabolic disturbances. Current practice is to add or substitute a drug from another class if the patient does not respond to the equivalent of 25 mg of hydrochlorothiazide. Concurrent treatment with a potassium-sparing agent may prevent hypokalemia. Loop diuretics can be used in combination therapy in patients with impaired renal function or in those who cannot tolerate thiazides.

Diuretics are well tolerated and inexpensive. They control both supine and standing blood pressure in approximately 50% of patients without additional therapy, and, if ineffective alone, are useful to counteract sodium retention and enhance the response to other antihypertensive drugs. Diuretics are more effective than beta blockers in blacks and elderly patients and also are preferred to beta blockers in patients with congestive heart failure, asthma, chronic bronchitis, or peripheral vascular disorders. The possible development of hypokalemia is a concern with use of large doses of diuretics.

A beta blocker is a suitable alternative for initial therapy, particularly in whites, patients with symptomatic coronary artery disease (especially after acute myocardial infarction) or supraventricular arrhythmia, and young patients with hyperdynamic circulation (Table 4). In patients who have survived an acute myocardial infarction, beta blockers reduce the risk of reinfarction and decrease mortality. However, these agents may precipitate heart failure in patients with borderline cardiac reserve, AV block in patients with conduction distur-

TABLE 2.
PROFILED-CARE APPROACH TO DRUG SELECTION IN CHRONIC HYPERTENSION

Patient Characteristics/ Coexisting Conditions	Drug Selection
Advanced age	Thiazides, calcium channel blockers, ACE inhibitors, and beta blockers are usually effective. Avoid drugs causing marked orthostatic hypotension (alpha blockers).
Young age	Calcium channel blockers, alpha blockers, or ACE inhibitors may be better tolerated in physically active patients. A beta blocker may be particularly useful in young patients with hyperdynamic circulation.
Black race	Diuretics are especially useful. Calcium channel blockers also are effective. Beta blockers and ACE inhibitors may be less effective unless given with diuretic.
Races other than black	Beta blockers, diuretics, ACE inhibitors, calcium channel blockers, and alpha blockers have approximately equal antihypertensive efficacy in nonblacks.
Pregnancy	Methyldopa and hydralazine are usually effective. Beta blockers and the alpha-beta blocker, labetalol, also appear to be safe and effective. ACE inhibitors are contraindicated.
Left ventricular hypertrophy	Although the clinical importance is uncertain, all antihypertensive agents except direct-acting vasodilators reduce left ventricular mass and wall thickness.
Dyslipidemia	Diuretics and beta blockers may adversely affect blood lipid levels (although the effect of diuretics may be temporary and the clinical importance of these drug-induced changes is not known). Alpha blockers, alpha agonists, and hydralazine may have beneficial effects on lipid levels. Calcium channel blockers and ACE inhibitors have no effect on lipid levels.
Congestive heart failure	Diuretics, ACE inhibitors, and vasodilators have beneficial hemodynamic effects.
Angina pectoris	Beta blockers or calcium channel blockers are preferred. Avoid drugs that cause reflex tachycardia (eg, arterial vasodilators) unless given with a beta blocker or another antiadrenergic drug.
Postmyocardial infarction	Beta blockers and ACE inhibitors are agents of choice because of their established cardioprotective effects.
Supraventricular tachyarrhythmias	Beta blockers, verapamil, and diltiazem are drugs of choice.
Mitral valve prolapse syndrome	Beta blockers are preferred because they control associated arrhythmias and chest discomfort.
Bradycardia	Beta blockers, verapamil, and diltiazem may further reduce heart rate and should be avoided.
Diabetes mellitus	ACE Inhibitors and some calcium channel blockers may have beneficial renal hemodynamic effects. Central alpha agonists, vasodilators, and alpha blockers usually are well tolerated. Thiazides, loop diuretics, and beta blockers may increase blood glucose levels in a few patients. Beta blockers also may mask hypoglycemic symptoms. Potassium-sparing agents may cause hyperkalemia and should be avoided in patients with moderate to severe diabetes.
Cerebrovascular insufficiency	Avoid drugs that cause orthostatic hypotension (alpha blockers).
Asthma and chronic obstructive pulmonary disease	Calcium channel blockers may protect against exercise-induced asthma. Vasodilators and alpha blockers are potentially beneficial. Avoid beta blockers. ACE inhibitors may produce cough in 5% to 15% of patients.
Raynaud's phenomenon	Calcium channel blockers, alpha blockers, and ACE inhibitors may be useful. Avoid beta blockers.
Migraine	A beta blocker is drug of choice. Calcium channel blockers may be effective.
Hyperthyroidism	Beta blockers are agents of choice for rapid control of signs and symptoms of thyrotoxicosis.
Gout	Thiazides and loop diuretics may precipitate acute attack in predisposed patients and in those with chronic renal failure.
Depression	ACE inhibitors, calcium channel blockers, vasodilators, diuretics, and alpha blockers do not worsen or precipitate depression. Central alpha agonists and beta blockers occasionally may cause or exacerbate depression.

(table continued on next page)

TABLE 2 (continued)

Patient Characteristics/ Coexisting Conditions	Drug Selection
Sexual dysfunction with prior therapy	Any agent that causes a rapid and marked decrease in blood pressure may induce erectile dysfunction. Graded lowering of blood pressure with a class of drugs that has a less pronounced effect should be tried.
Benign prostatic hyperplasia	Alpha blockers are effective.
Stress incontinence	Avoid alpha blockers.
Osteoporosis	Calcium-sparing diuretics (eg, thiazides) are drugs of choice. Loop diuretics, which are calcium wasting, should be avoided.
Renal calculi	Thiazides may prevent recurrence of calcium-containing renal calculi in patients with idiopathic calcium urolithiasis. Loop diuretics should not be used.
Azotemia	Loop diuretics and direct vasodilators (especially minoxidil) are particularly useful; beta blockers, central alpha agonists, and alpha blockers also are usually well tolerated. Thiazides are usually ineffective; potassium-sparing agents should be avoided. ACE inhibitors may cause hyperkalemia and, in volume-depleted patients, may worsen azotemia.
Open-angle glaucoma	Beta blockers reduce intraocular pressure when given topically or systemically.
Essential tremor	Noncardioselective beta blockers may be beneficial.

bances, and bronchospasm in asthmatic patients, and they may mask symptoms of hypoglycemia in insulin-dependent diabetics.

Both diuretics and beta blockers have reduced cardiovascular morbidity and mortality in long-term controlled studies on hypertensive patients. Studies comparing these two drug classes have yielded equivocal results (Medical Research Council Working Party, 1985; Wikstrand et al, 1988; Wilhelmsen et al, 1987).

Calcium channel blockers are effective for initial therapy in both blacks and whites and are well tolerated in the elderly and in physically active patients (Table 5). They are useful in hypertensive patients with coexisting angina and can be used in those who cannot tolerate the pulmonary side effects of beta blockers. These agents, especially verapamil and diltiazem, should be avoided in patients with heart failure. Other adverse effects include AV block (verapamil and diltiazem), tachycardia (nifedipine), ankle edema (nifedipine and other dihydropyridines), constipation (verapamil), headache, and gingival hyperplasia.

Angiotensin-converting enzyme (ACE) inhibitors are useful for initial therapy in whites and are well tolerated by young, physically active patients and the elderly (Table 6). They are preferred drugs in those with coexisting heart failure. Cough, rash, and taste disturbances may occur with ACE inhibitors.

Alpha blocking agents also may be used as initial therapy (Table 7). Alpha$_1$ blockers (doxazosin, prazosin, and terazosin) have added advantage in treating patients with coexisting hypertension and hyperlipidemia because of their beneficial effects on lipids. Phenoxybenzamine and phentolamine, which inhibit both α_1 and α_2 receptors, are useful for patients with pheochromocytoma in the pre- and intraoperative periods but usually are not prescribed for those with uncomplicated hypertension. The alpha-beta blocker, labetalol, can be used for patients with coexisting angina. However, all of these agents may cause orthostatic hypotension; routine monitoring of blood pressure is recommended.

Supplemental antihypertensive drugs include the centrally acting alpha agonists, rauwolfia alkaloids (usually reserpine), and direct vasodilators (Table 8). Most of these agents are less commonly prescribed because of their significant side effect profiles. These agents are usually administered as a second or third drug in the antihypertensive regimen for patients refractory to maximum tolerated doses of standard drugs. However, methyldopa is often used for hypertension associated with pregnancy, and clonidine, sodium nitroprusside, and nitroglycerin are useful in the management of hypertensive emergencies and urgencies.

In addition to lowering the blood pressure, most antihypertensive drugs also reduce left ventricular hypertrophy (Pfeffer and Pfeffer, 1990; Neaton et al, 1993). In a large cohort of the Framingham Heart Study, left ventricular hypertrophy was detected by echocardiography in 20% to 25% of hypertensive patients. In these patients, the number of premature ventricular contractions and episodes of ventricular tachycardia were increased during a 24-hour period, the absolute and reserve arterial blood supply to the myocardium was inadequate, and sudden and ischemic heart-related deaths were more prevalent (Frohlich, 1989 A). Calcium-channel blockers, ACE inhibitors, alpha blockers, centrally acting sympatholytic agents, some beta blockers, and diuretics usually are effective in reducing left ventricular hypertrophy.

Antihypertensive drugs may adversely affect some diseases while they may improve others. They also may interact with medications used to treat other conditions. For example, beta blockers may worsen asthma and peripheral arterial disease, but they may have a beneficial effect on angina pectoris, certain arrhythmias, and migraine headache. In addition, short-term adverse effects on serum triglycerides and cholesterol levels have been reported in hypertensive patients treated with diuretics and nonselective beta blockers (Amery and Lijnen, 1988). The beta blockers also may reduce exercise tolerance. Several antihypertensive drugs may affect sexual function, and centrally acting drugs may impair mental acuity. Thus, awareness of the more common side effects of the various agents is necessary to select drugs that may improve coexisting diseases or symptoms and to avoid those that may adversely affect them. (See also Table 2.)

SYSTOLIC HYPERTENSION IN THE ELDERLY. Isolated systolic hypertension in the elderly (systolic pressure >160 mm Hg, diastolic pressure <90 mm Hg), which may affect up to two-thirds of all individuals with hypertension aged 65 to 89 years (Wilking et al, 1988), is associated with increased morbidity and mortality. This disorder is caused by loss of elasticity in the larger arteries due to atherosclerosis and is associated with reduced cardiac output, elevated total peripheral vascular resistance, and reduced plasma volume (Gifford, 1986; Working Group on Hypertension in the Elderly, 1986). Results of several studies demonstrated that drug therapy for hypertension in elderly patients reduces the risk of cardiovascular complications (Joint National Committee on Detection, Evaluation, and Treatment of High Blood Pressure, 1993).

Diuretics, ACE inhibitors, and calcium channel blockers are used for initial therapy of isolated systolic hypertension in the elderly. If required, any of the drugs from other major classes can be added. Diuretics are especially effective in controlling blood pressure in the elderly, as confirmed by three double-blind studies by the Veterans Administration Cooperative Study Group (Freis, 1991). In the SHEP Cooperative Research Group (1991) trial, administration of chlorthalidone (12.5 mg/day) for an average of 4.5 years substantially lowered the mean systolic blood pressure by 11 to 14 mm Hg in hypertensive patients aged 60 to ≥80 years with isolated systolic hypertension. Treatment was as effective in those ≥80 years as in younger patients in this age group. The incidence of stroke was reduced by 35%, and the number of nonfatal cardiovascular events and deaths from all causes also decreased. Similar reductions in stroke occurrence and mortality from isolated systolic hypertension was reported by the Swedish Trial in Old Patients with Hypertension (STOP-Hypertension) following treatment with a thiazide diuretic or beta blocker in patients aged 70 to 84 years (Dahlof et al, 1991). Reduction in the incidence of stroke also was observed following treatment with hydrochlorothiazide in patients aged 65 to 74 years with mean systolic blood pressures of 160 to 209 mm Hg and mean diastolic blood pressures of <115 mm Hg (Medical Research Council Working Party, 1992).

HYPERTENSIVE URGENCIES AND EMERGENCIES. A severe or sudden elevation in blood pressure without impending complications that requires prompt, but not immediate, treatment is defined as a *hypertensive urgency* (Joint National Committee on Detection, Evaluation, and Treatment of High Blood Pressure, 1993). Possible causes of the elevation in blood pressure include accelerated or malignant hypertension, atherothrombotic brain infarction with severe hypertension, or rebound hypertension after abrupt cessation of antihypertensive drugs. Blood pressure usually can be reduced safely in less than 24 hours by oral antihypertensive drugs, such as clonidine, ACE inhibitors, or calcium channel blockers.

A *hypertensive emergency* presents an immediate risk of cardiovascular complications or death and requires hospitalization and rapid reduction of blood pressure with parenteral antihypertensive drugs. Hypertensive emergencies include hypertensive encephalopathy; eclampsia; pheochromocytoma; hypertension complicated by acute pulmonary edema, acute dissecting aneurysm, acute coronary insufficiency, or subarachnoid or intracranial hemorrhage; and hypertension associated with severe burns, head trauma, unstable angina, or acute myocardial infarction.

In treating hypertensive emergencies, an excessively rapid or marked reduction in blood pressure should be avoided because of the risk of cerebral and myocardial ischemia, particularly in elderly patients and in those with long-standing, severe hypertension. Most hypertensive emergencies are characterized by vasoconstriction with normal or reduced plasma volume. Administration of labetalol, nitroprusside, or nitroglycerin is preferred. The initial reduction in diastolic blood pressure should be approximately 20%; further reductions of 10% every two to four hours until the diastolic pressure reaches 90 to 100 mm Hg are desirable (Calhoun and Oparil, 1990). Patients should be monitored continuously when these potent drugs are used.

The alpha-beta blocker, labetalol, given intravenously, has become a first-line drug for managing many hypertensive emergencies (Cressman et al, 1984; Wilson et al, 1983). This drug usually reduces blood pressure in 5 to 10 minutes without producing reflex tachycardia. During use of intravenous labetalol, the contribution of the postural component should be considered when positioning the patient, and the patient should not be permitted to stand unaided until the ability to do so has been established.

Sodium nitroprusside reduces both peripheral vascular resistance and venous tone. It is the most potent and consistently effective parenteral antihypertensive drug available. It can be used for most hypertensive emergencies, including hypertensive encephalopathy and hypertension complicated by intracranial or subarachnoid hemorrhage. Because of its favorable hemodynamic effect on left ventricular function, nitroprusside is useful in hypertensive or normotensive patients with heart failure and in selected patients with marked pump dysfunction, elevated left ventricular filling pressure, increased peripheral vascular resistance, and decreased cardiac output after acute myocardial infarction. However, to avoid cyanide toxicity, nitroprusside should only be used for short-term treatment and should be infused at a rate <10 mcg/kg/min. (See index entry Heart Failure.)

Intravenous nitroglycerin acts predominantly to reduce venous tone. At high infusion rates, it also reduces total peripheral resistance. Nitroglycerin dilates epicardial coronary arteries and collaterals and improves the regional distribution of myocardial blood flow in patients with coronary artery disease. It relieves refractory chest pain in patients with unstable angina and reduces myocardial ischemia and relieves pulmonary edema in those with severe left ventricular dysfunction following acute myocardial infarction (see index entries Angina; Heart Failure). Nitroglycerin is particularly useful in hypertensive emergencies that occur during and after cardiac surgery. Constant monitoring of blood pressure and regulation of the infusion rate are essential when nitroprusside and nitroglycerin are used.

Certain hypertensive emergencies require the use of other agents. The alpha-adrenergic blocking agents, phentolamine and phenoxybenzamine, and labetalol are used in hypertensive crises caused by pheochromocytoma, drug interaction between monoamine oxidase inhibitors and sympathomimetic amines, and clonidine withdrawal syndrome. Phentolamine and labetalol are used for intravenous therapy; phenoxybenzamine is given orally. Other alpha blockers (prazosin, terazosin, and doxazosin) also are effective.

When given prophylactically, propranolol prevents severe paradoxical hypertension that often develops after repair of coarctation of the aorta. Labetalol is used for postoperative hypertension.

HYPERTENSION DURING PREGNANCY. Hypertension during pregnancy may result in life-threatening consequences for both mother and fetus (National High Blood Pressure Education Program Working Group on High Blood Pressure in Pregnancy, 1990). This condition is diagnosed as increases ≥30 mm Hg of systolic and/or ≥15 mm Hg of diastolic blood pressures compared with the average of values before 20 weeks' gestation.

Chronic Hypertension: Antihypertensive drug treatment is indicated in pregnant patients with diastolic blood pressure ≥100 mm Hg. The goal of treatment is to reduce short-term risks of elevated blood pressure for the mother without compromising the well-being of the fetus. Diuretics and other antihypertensive drugs with the exception of ACE inhibitors may be initiated or continued if they were being taken before pregnancy. ACE inhibitors should not be used, for they may cause neonatal hypotension, renal failure, limb contracture, craniofacial malformation, hypoplastic lung development, and death in the fetus (Perlman and Volpe, 1989).

Methyldopa has been used for treating chronic hypertension during pregnancy. Controlled studies also have documented the efficacy and apparent fetal safety of beta blockers and labetalol. However, atenolol has been associated with intrauterine growth retardation when given after the third month of gestation to patients with mild hypertension (Butters et al, 1990). Hydralazine is safe and effective during pregnancy and may be added when additional control is needed.

Pre-eclampsia, Eclampsia: Pre-eclampsia is a pregnancy-specific condition in which the blood pressure is increased with concomitant proteinuria, edema, or both, and occasionally with abnormalities in coagulation and liver function. Pre-eclampsia primarily occurs in primigravidas and after the 20th week of pregnancy and may progress rapidly to eclampsia, the convulsive phase.

Therapy for pre-eclampsia requires bed rest, control of blood pressure, and seizure prophylaxis when signs of impending eclampsia (eg, headache, visual disturbance, and hyperreflexia) are present. Induction of labor is indicated, regardless of gestational age, when there are signs of fetal distress or of uncontrollable hypertension, deteriorating renal or hepatic function, epigastric pain, or of impending eclampsia in the mother. Antihypertensive treatment should begin if diastolic blood pressure is ≥100 mm Hg. If delivery is not anticipated within 24 hours, an oral agent is preferred (eg, methyldopa, calcium channel blocking drugs, labetalol, beta-adrenergic blocking drugs). When delivery is imminent, a parenteral antihypertensive agent is preferable. Diuretics (eg, furosemide) should be avoided because an acute reduction in intravascular volume may impair uteroplacental perfusion.

Magnesium sulfate is the most commonly used drug in the United States to prevent or control eclamptic convulsions (see index entry Magnesium Sulfate).

HYPERTENSION IN DIABETIC PATIENTS. Diabetes mellitus and hypertension are two of the most common diseases that increase in tandem with aging (Epstein and Sowers, 1992). In the United States, an estimated 2.5 to 3 million people have both diabetes and hypertension; the combination increases morbidity and mortality. The prevalence of hypertension in diabetic patients is approximately twofold that in the nondiabetic population. Chronic hyperglycemia and hyperinsulinemia associated with insulin resistance may contribute to the elevation of blood pressure in diabetic patients.

Since insulin resistance is especially pronounced in hypertensive patients who are obese, nondrug therapy can play an important role in lowering blood pressure in these individuals. Weight reduction and regular aerobic exercise improve sensitivity to insulin, leading to progressive lowering of plasma insulin levels to glucose challenge. The resultant fall in blood pressure probably is associated with the fall in plasma insulin level. Other nondrug measures that modulate hyperinsulinemia and insulin resistance include sodium restriction and moderation in alcohol intake.

Despite adherence to nondrug measures, diabetic patients with hypertension also may require drug therapy. ACE inhibitors, calcium channel blocking agents, and alpha blockers are effective; alpha blockers and ACE inhibitors also may improve insulin sensitivity. Diuretics and beta-adrenergic blocking agents are not recommended as first-line agents (Kaplan, 1992).

Drug Evaluations

DIURETICS

Thiazides and Related Compounds

ACTIONS. The thiazides and related compounds (see Table 3) inhibit sodium and chloride reabsorption in the cortical thick ascending limb of Henle's loop and the early distal tubules. Initially their antihypertensive effect is associated with a reduction in plasma and extracellular fluid (ECF) volume (Freis, 1983); cardiac output and total peripheral resistance are unchanged. With prolonged therapy, cardiac output returns to control levels, total peripheral vascular resistance is reduced, and intravascular (plasma) volume is restored (Frohlich, 1987).

USES. A thiazide often serves as the basis of the antihypertensive regimen: as sole therapy in patients with mild or moderate hypertension or in combination with other antihypertensive drugs in patients not controlled by the diuretic alone (Joint National Committee on Detection, Evaluation, and Treatment of High Blood Pressure, 1993). These drugs are particularly useful in black patients and the elderly; age appears to increase the therapeutic response (Freis et al, 1988). Thiazides are well tolerated and inexpensive. They reduce both supine and standing blood pressures, and their antihypertensive effect is maintained during long-term administration. When used with other antihypertensive drugs, thiazides prevent secondary volume expansion and thus encourage continued responsiveness. Such combined therapy also may permit a decrease in the dosage of other drugs, which reduces the number and severity of adverse reactions.

The various thiazides and related drugs differ primarily in their duration of action. When given in equipotent doses, no clear-cut differences in antihypertensive efficacy or toxicity have been demonstrated.

ADVERSE REACTIONS AND PRECAUTIONS. The thiazides may cause hypokalemia, hypomagnesemia, hyperuricemia, hyperglycemia, hyponatremia, azotemia, hypercalcemia, hypertriglyceridemia, and hypercholesterolemia.

Mild hypokalemia seems to be well tolerated by most ambulatory patients with hypertension. Increased ventricular ectopic activity has been noted in some, but opinion is divided on the role of diuretic therapy or hypokalemia in these disturbances (see index entry Diuretics). Corrective measures (eg, moderate sodium restriction, use of potassium-sparing agents or potassium supplements) are indicated if the serum potassium level falls below 3.5 mEq/L, if the electrocardiogram is abnormal, or if the patient is receiving digitalis.

Dermatologic reactions and blood dyscrasias also have been reported. For further information on adverse reactions, see the chapter, Diuretics.

DOSAGE AND PREPARATIONS. See Table 3. Since the antihypertensive effect of thiazides is not clearly dose related, therapy should be initiated with small daily doses (eg, 12.5 mg of hydrochlorothiazide, chlorthalidone, or the equivalent of other thiazides, with the amount increased if necessary up to 50 mg of hydrochlorothiazide or equivalent). Mild or moderate hypertension often can be controlled with doses that induce minimal biochemical changes (as low as 12.5 mg of hydrochlorothiazide) (Carlsen et al, 1990), but the desire to avoid side effects should not lead to prescription of ineffective doses (Freis and Papademetriou, 1985). Elderly patients may be particularly likely to develop orthostatic hypotension with diuretics, and initiation of therapy with small doses is especially important in this age group (Materson et al, 1993).

Loop Diuretics

BUMETANIDE
[Bumex]

ETHACRYNATE SODIUM
[Sodium Edecrin]

ETHACRYNIC ACID
[Edecrin]

FUROSEMIDE
[Lasix]

TORSEMIDE
[Demadex]

ACTIONS AND USES. The loop diuretics are so named because they block active sodium transport in the medullary and cortical thick ascending limb of Henle's loop. They have a more rapid onset of action and a greater diuretic effect than the thiazides. When given intravenously, loop diuretics act rapidly and are useful adjunctively in the treatment of hypertensive crises. Their oral use in chronic hypertension is usually reserved for patients with impaired renal function (creatinine clearance <30 ml/minute) or in patients who cannot tolerate thiazide diuretics; however, their short duration of action necessitates administration at least twice and occasionally three times daily. In addition, the acute diuresis that occurs in the first few hours after administration can be troublesome.

Furosemide has been used more commonly in antihypertensive therapy than the other loop diuretics because it has a broader dose-response curve, produces fewer gastrointestinal disturbances, and is more convenient for intravenous use. Ethacrynic acid may be useful in patients sensitive to sulfonamides. There has been limited experience with bumetanide and torsemide in antihypertensive therapy.

ADVERSE REACTIONS AND PRECAUTIONS. Proper use of the loop diuretics requires an understanding of their ability to induce electrolyte and fluid derangements. Overzealous therapy can cause dehydration, hypotension, and marked hypokalemia and hypochloremic alkalosis. Like the thiazides, the loop diuretics can cause prerenal azotemia, hyperuricemia, and hyperglycemia. Transient deafness has been reported following rapid parenteral administration of loop diuretics to azotemic or uremic patients. Permanent deafness rarely occurs. Ethacrynic acid appears to be more ototoxic than furosemide. Bumetanide is the least ototoxic loop diuretic. For other adverse effects, see the chapter, Diuretics.

DOSAGE AND PREPARATIONS.
BUMETANIDE:
Intravenous: For hypertensive crises (in conjunction with other antihypertensive drugs), *adults*, initially, 0.5 to 1 mg (maximum, 10 mg/day).

Bumex (Roche). Solution 0.25 mg/ml in 2, 4, and 10 ml containers.

Oral: See Table 3.

ETHACRYNATE SODIUM:

Intravenous: For hypertensive crises (in conjunction with other antihypertensive drugs), *adults,* 50 mg or 0.5 to 1 mg/kg as a single dose; if a second dose is required, it should be injected at another site to avoid thrombophlebitis.

Sodium Edecrin (Merck). Powder equivalent to 50 mg ethacrynic acid.

ETHACRYNIC ACID:

Oral: See Table 3.

FUROSEMIDE:

Intravenous: For hypertensive crises (in conjunction with other antihypertensive drugs), *adults* with normal renal function, 40 to 80 mg administered slowly at a rate not exceeding 4 mg/min. When the glomerular filtration rate is markedly reduced, larger doses may be required.

Lasix (Hoechst-Roussel), ***Generic.*** Solution (sterile) 10 mg/ml in 2, 4, and 10 ml containers.

Oral: See Table 3.

TORSEMIDE:

Intravenous, Oral: See the manufacturer's package insert.

TABLE 3.
ORAL DIURETICS

Drug	Usual Oral Dosage	Preparations
THIAZIDES		
Chlorothiazide	*Adults,* initially, 125 to 250 mg daily. May be increased to 500 mg daily. *Children,* 10 to 20 mg/kg daily in 2 divided doses. Higher doses may be required.	*Diuril* (Merck). Tablets 250 and 500 mg; suspension 250 mg/5 ml (alcohol 0.5%). *Generic.* Tablets 250 and 500 mg.
Hydrochlorothiazide	*Adults,* initially, 12.5 to 25 mg daily. May be increased to 50 mg daily. *Children,* 1 to 2 mg/kg daily in 2 divided doses.	*Esidrix* (CIBA), *HydroDIURIL* (Merck), *Generic.* Tablets 25, 50, and 100 mg. *Oretic* (Abbott). Tablets 25 and 50 mg.
Bendroflumethiazide	*Adults,* initially, 1.25 mg daily. May be increased to 2.5 mg daily. *Children,* initially, 0.1 mg/kg daily in 1 or 2 doses; for maintenance, 0.05 to 0.3 mg/kg daily in 1 or 2 doses.	*Naturetin* (Apothecon). Tablets 5 and 10 mg.
Benzthiazide	*Adults,* initially, 25 mg daily. May be increased to 50 mg daily. *Children,* 1 to 4 mg/kg daily in 3 doses.	*Exna* (Robins) Tablets 50 mg.
Hydroflumethiazide	*Adults,* initially, 25 mg daily. May be increased to 50 mg daily. *Children,* 1 mg/kg daily.	*Diucardin* (Wyeth-Ayerst), *Saluron* (Apothecon), *Generic.* Tablets 50 mg.
Methyclothiazide	*Adults,* initially, 2.5 mg daily. May be increased to 5 mg daily. *Children,* 0.05 to 0.2 mg/kg daily.	*Aquatensen* (Wallace). Tablets 5 mg. *Enduron* (Abbott), *Generic.* Tablets 2.5 and 5 mg.
Polythiazide	*Adults,* initially, 2 mg daily. May be increased to 4 mg daily. *Children,* 0.02 to 0.08 mg/kg daily.	*Renese* (Pfizer). Tablets 1, 2, and 4 mg.
Trichlormethiazide	*Adults,* initially, 1 to 2 mg daily. May be increased to 4 mg once daily. *Children,* 0.07 mg/kg once daily or in divided doses.	*Metahydrin* (Marion Merrell Dow), *Naqua* (Schering), *Generic.* Tablets 2 and 4 mg.
AGENTS RELATED TO THIAZIDES		
Chlorthalidone	*Adults,* initially, 12.5 to 25 mg daily. May be increased to 50 mg.daily. *Children,* 0.5 to 2 mg/kg daily.	*Hygroton* (Rhone-Poulenc Rorer), *Generic.* Tablets 25, 50, and 100 mg. *Thalitone* (Horus). Tablets 15 and 25 mg.
Indapamide	*Adults,* initially, 1.25 mg daily. May be increased to 2.5 to 5 mg daily.	*Lozol* (Rhone-Poulenc Rorer). Tablets 1.25 and 2.5 mg.

(table continued on next page)

TABLE 3 (continued)

Drug	Usual Oral Dosage	Preparations
Metolazone	*Adults,* (*Mykrox*) Initially, 0.5 mg daily; may be increased to 1 mg daily; (*Zaroxolyn*) Initially, 2.5 to 5 mg daily; may be increased to 10 mg daily.	*Mykrox* (Fisons). Tablets 0.5 mg. *Zaroxolyn* (Fisons). Tablets 2.5, 5, and 10 mg.
Quinethazone	*Adults,* initially, 25 mg daily. May be increased to 100 mg daily.	*Hydromox* (Lederle). Tablets 50 mg.
LOOP DIURETICS		
Bumetanide	*Adults,* initially, 0.5 mg daily. May be increased to 5 mg daily in 2 divided doses.	*Bumex* (Roche). Tablets 0.5, 1, and 2 mg.
Ethacrynic Acid	*Adults,* initially, 25 mg twice daily. May be increased to 200 mg daily in 2 divided doses.	*Edecrin* (Merck). Tablets 25 and 50 mg.
Furosemide	*Adults,* initially, 20 to 40 mg daily. If an adequate response is not obtained, dosage may be increased gradually to 320 mg daily in 2 doses. *Children,* 0.5 to 2 mg/kg daily in two doses.	*Lasix* (Hoechst-Roussel), *Generic.* Solution (oral) 10 mg/ml; tablets 20, 40, and 80 mg.
Torsemide	See manufacturer's package insert.	*Demadex* (Boehringer Mannheim). Tablets 5, 10, 20, and 100 mg.
POTASSIUM-SPARING AGENTS		
Amiloride	*Adults,* initially, 5 mg daily. Dosage should be adjusted in accordance with blood pressure and serum potassium level. Dosage should usually not exceed 10 mg daily.	*Midamor* (Merck), *Generic.* Tablets 5 mg.
Amiloride and Hydrochlorothiazide	*Adults,* initially, ½ tablet daily. Dosage should be adjusted in accordance with blood pressure and serum potassium level.	*Moduretic* (Merck), *Generic.* Each tablet contains amiloride hydrochloride 5 mg and hydrochlorothiazide 50 mg.
Spironolactone	*Adults,* initially, 25 mg daily. May be increased to 100 mg daily in a single dose or 2 divided doses. *Children,* 1 to 2 mg/kg daily in 2 doses. The dosage should be adjusted in accordance with blood pressure and serum potassium level.	*Aldactone* (Searle). Tablets 25, 50, and 100 mg. *Generic.* Tablets 25 mg.
Spironolactone and Hydrochlorothiazide	Initially, 1 tablet containing 25 mg of each component daily. May be increased to 50 mg of each component daily in a single dose or in divided doses. The dosage should be adjusted in accordance with blood pressure and serum potassium level.	*Aldactazide* (Searle), *Generic.* Each tablet contains spironolactone 25 mg and hydrochlorothiazide 25 mg (*Aldactazide 25/25*) or spironolactone 50 mg and hydrochlorothiazide 50 mg (*Aldactazide 50/50*).
Triamterene	*Adults,* initially, 50 mg daily. May be increased to 150 mg daily in a single dose or 2 divided doses given after meals. Maximum daily dose is 300 mg. *Children,* 1 to 2 mg/kg daily in 2 doses. The dosage should be adjusted in accordance with blood pressure and serum potassium level.	*Dyrenium* (SmithKline Beecham). Capsules 50 and 100 mg.
Triamterene and Hydrochlorothiazide	*Adults,* initially, 1 capsule daily (may be increased to 2 capsules daily in single or divided doses) or, initially, 1/2 to 1 tablet of *Maxzide-25* daily (may be increased to 2 tablets of *Maxzide-25* or 1 tablet of *Maxzide* daily). The dosage should be adjusted in accordance with blood pressure and serum potassium level.	*Dyazide* (SmithKline Beecham), *Generic.* Each capsule contains triamterene 50 mg and hydrochlorothiazide 25 mg. *Maxzide* (Lederle), *Generic.* Each tablet contains triamterene 37.5 mg and hydrochlorothiazide 25 mg (*Maxzide-25* only) or triamterene 75 mg and hydrochlorothiazide 50 mg (*Maxzide*).

Potassium-Sparing Agents

AMILORIDE HYDROCHLORIDE
[Midamor]

SPIRONOLACTONE
[Aldactone]

TRIAMTERENE
[Dyrenium]

ACTIONS AND USES. Spironolactone, triamterene, and amiloride interfere with sodium reabsorption at the distal sites in the renal tubule where sodium reabsorption is related to the secretion of potassium and hydrogen ions. Spironolactone is an aldosterone antagonist; triamterene and amiloride act directly at the distal exchange sites in the renal tubules.

The potassium-sparing agents are usually employed as adjuncts to a thiazide or loop diuretic to prevent hypokalemia.

ADVERSE REACTIONS AND PRECAUTIONS. Careful monitoring of the serum potassium level is necessary during therapy with potassium-sparing agents because hyperkalemia may occur despite concomitant thiazide therapy. Precipitating factors are impaired renal function, advanced age, moderate to severe diabetes, concomitant use of ACE inhibitors or nonsteroidal anti-inflammatory agents, and a high potassium intake (dietary, supplements, salt substitutes). Renal calculi also may develop with the use of triamterene.

For a more detailed discussion of actions, uses, and other adverse effects, see the chapter, Diuretics.

DOSAGE AND PREPARATIONS. See Table 3.

AVAILABLE MIXTURES.

Potassium-Sparing Diuretic and a Thiazide Diuretic: Since a potassium-sparing diuretic is most useful when given with a thiazide, these combination products are convenient, but occasionally it may be necessary to give the drugs separately for optimal potassium conservation.

For dosage and preparations, see Table 3.

BETA-ADRENERGIC BLOCKING AGENTS

ACTIONS. The nature of beta-adrenergic receptors and the actions, ancillary properties (cardioselectivity, partial agonist [intrinsic sympathomimetic] activity, membrane stabilizing properties, alpha-blocking actions), chemical formulas, and pharmacokinetics of beta blockers are discussed in detail in the chapter, Beta-Adrenergic Blocking Drugs. The beta blockers used in the United States to treat hypertension include the cardioselective agents (acebutolol, atenolol, betaxolol, bisoprolol, and metoprolol) and the nonselective agents (carteolol, nadolol, penbutolol, propranolol, pindolol, and timolol) (Table 4). Acebutolol, carteolol, and pindolol also possess partial agonist activity.

Beta blockers reduce heart rate, myocardial contractility, and cardiac output. The mechanism of their antihypertensive effect remains unresolved (see the chapter, Beta-Adrenergic Blocking Drugs).

USES. Beta blockers may be used as the initial drug in the antihypertensive regimen, and are agents of choice in patients with symptomatic coronary artery disease (particularly after acute myocardial infarction) or supraventricular arrhythmia and in young patients with hyperdynamic circulation (see also Table 2). Beta blockers are more effective in lowering blood pressure in whites than in blacks, in younger patients than in the elderly (Bannon et al, 1986; Greenberg et al, 1984; Veterans Administration Cooperative Study Group on Antihypertensive Agents, 1982), and in nonsmokers than in smokers (Materson et al, 1988; Medical Research Council Working Party, 1988).

Diuretics enhance the antihypertensive effect of beta blockers. A diuretic-beta blocker-hydralazine regimen is useful in moderate to severe hypertension and is usually well tolerated by patients who have experienced disabling side effects with other regimens.

Beta blockers that are available in parenteral formulations (propranolol, atenolol, metoprolol, and the short-acting esmolol) may be used to treat arrhythmias and hypertension in surgical patients. A beta blocker may be given with an alpha-adrenergic blocking agent to prevent tachycardia and ventricular arrhythmias during the preoperative management of patients with pheochromocytoma and for prolonged treatment of patients who are not suitable candidates for surgery. The dosage varies widely and must be individualized. A beta blocker should not be used in pheochromocytoma without first administering adequate doses of an alpha-blocking drug, because it may increase blood pressure if used alone.

Propranolol also prevents the severe systolic hypertension that often occurs after repair of coarctation of the aorta (Gidding et al, 1985; Leenen et al, 1987), but it may initially potentiate the rise in diastolic blood pressure (Leenen et al, 1987). Propranolol is given orally for two days or more before surgery, intravenously during the immediate postoperative period, and orally for the first postoperative week.

ADVERSE REACTIONS AND PRECAUTIONS. Beta blockers may precipitate heart failure in patients with inadequate cardiac reserve, worsen AV conduction disturbances, and provoke bronchospasm in patients with asthma or severe chronic obstructive lung disease. These and other adverse reactions and interactions are discussed in detail in the chapter, Beta-Adrenergic Blocking Drugs.

DOSAGE AND PREPARATIONS. See Table 4.

CALCIUM CHANNEL BLOCKING AGENTS

The properties of these drugs are discussed in detail in the chapter, Calcium Channel Blocking Drugs.

ACTIONS. Calcium channel blocking drugs (calcium antagonists) inhibit the entry of calcium into cardiac cells and smooth muscle cells of the coronary and systemic vasculature. All calcium channel blocking agents increase coronary blood flow, but nifedipine and other dihydropyridines are more potent as peripheral vasodilators than verapamil and diltiazem. Only verapamil and diltiazem depress atrioventricular nodal conduction in vivo. Dihydropyridines cause reflex tachycardia. Although dihydropyridines exert a negative inotropic effect on isolated myocardial tissue, myocardial depression is rarely seen in vivo because of the reflex response to the va-

TABLE 4.
BETA-ADRENERGIC BLOCKING AGENTS

Drug	Usual Oral Dosage	Preparations
Acebutolol	Initially, 200 mg as a single dose. For maintenance, 200 to 800 mg daily. Some patients may require up to 1.2 g daily in two divided doses.	*Sectral* (Wyeth-Ayerst). Capsules 200 and 400 mg.
Atenolol	*Adults,* initially, 25 mg once daily. If the desired response is not obtained, dosage may be increased to 50 mg daily and then to 100 mg daily. The usual daily maximum dose is 100 mg. A further increase is unlikely to produce additional benefit. The following maximal doses are recommended for patients with renal impairment: creatinine clearance 15 to 35 ml/min/1.73 M^2, 50 mg daily; creatinine clearance $<$15 ml/min/1.73 M^2, 50 mg on alternate days. *Children,* 1 to 2 mg/kg daily.	*Tenormin* (ZENECA), *Generic.* Tablets 25, 50, and 100 mg.
Atenolol and Chlorthalidone	Dosage should be individualized.	*Tenoretic 50, 100* (ZENECA), *Generic.* Each tablet contains atenolol 50 or 100 mg and chlorthalidone 25 mg.
Betaxolol	*Adults,* initially, 10 mg once daily. Dosage may be increased within one or two weeks to 20 mg daily. For the elderly and patients on dialysis, the initial dose is 5 mg.	*Kerlone* (Searle). Tablets 10 and 20 mg.
Bisoprolol	*Adults,* initially, 5 mg once daily. Dosage may be increased to 10 mg and then, if necessary, to 20 mg once daily. For patients with renal or hepatic impairment, initially, 2.5 mg daily; caution should be used in titration.	*Zebeta* (Lederle). Tablets 5 and 10 mg.
Bisoprolol and Hydrochlorothiazide	Dosage should be individualized.	*Ziac* (Lederle). Each tablet contains bisoprolol 2.5, 5, or 10 mg and hydrochlorothiazide 6.25 mg.
Carteolol	*Adults,* initially, 2.5 mg daily. For maintenance, 2.5 to 5 mg daily. The usual maximum daily dose is 10 mg.	*Cartrol* (Abbott). Tablets 2.5 and 5 mg.
Metoprolol	The effective dose varies widely and must be titrated on the basis of the therapeutic response. *Adults,* initially, 50 mg daily. If the desired response is not obtained, the dosage may be increased gradually. The maximum maintenance dose is 200 mg daily, most commonly given in one or two doses. If control is not adequate, the drug should be given three times daily. *Children,* 1 to 4 mg/kg daily in two doses.	*Lopressor* (Geigy). Tablets 50 and 100 mg. *Toprol XL* (Astra). Tablets (prolonged-release) 50, 100, and 200 mg.
Metoprolol and Hydrochlorothiazide	Dosage should be individualized.	*Lopressor HCT* (Geigy). Each tablet contains metoprolol tartrate 50 mg and hydrochlorothiazide 25 mg (*Lopressor HCT-50/25*) or metoprolol tartrate 100 mg and hydrochlorothiazide 25 or 50 mg (*Lopressor HCT-100/25* and *Lopressor HCT-100/50,* respectively).

(table continued on next page)

TABLE 4 (continued)

Drug	Usual Oral Dosage	Preparations
Nadolol	The effective dose varies widely and must be titrated on the basis of the therapeutic response. *Adults,* initially, 40 mg once daily. Dosage may be increased gradually to a usual maintenance dose of 40 to 80 mg. Up to 320 mg daily may be required rarely. The dosage interval should be increased as follows in patients with renal impairment: creatinine clearance (ml/min/1.73 M^2) >50, 24 hours; 31 to 50, 24 to 36 hours; 10 to 30, 24 to 48 hours; <10, 40 to 60 hours.	*Corgard* (Bristol). Tablets 20, 40, 80, 120, and 160 mg.
Nadolol and Bendroflumethiazide	Dosage should be individualized.	*Corzide* (Bristol). Each tablet contains nadolol 40 or 80 mg and bendroflumethiazide 5 mg (*Corzide 40/5* and *Corzide 80/5*, respectively).
Penbutolol	Initially, 20 mg daily. The usual maximum dose is 80 mg daily.	*Levatol* (Reed & Carnrick). Tablets 20 mg.
Pindolol	*Adults,* initially, 10 mg twice daily or 5 mg three times daily. If a satisfactory response is not obtained in two to three weeks, the dosage may be increased by 10 mg/day at two- to three-week intervals to 60 mg daily.	*Visken* (Sandoz), *Generic.* Tablets 5 and 10 mg.
Propranolol	Dosage must be titrated on the basis of the therapeutic response because the effective dose varies widely. Maximal effects may not be evident for several weeks. *Regular preparation*: *Adults*, initially, 40 mg twice daily. If the desired response is not obtained, the dosage should be increased to 80 mg twice daily. Further 80-mg increments may be added, if needed. If control is not adequate, the drug should be given three times daily. The daily dose usually need not exceed 320 mg when propranolol is given with a diuretic and hydralazine. *Children,* 1 to 3 mg/kg daily in three doses. *Prolonged-release preparation: Adults*, initially, 60 mg once daily. For maintenance, 120 to 160 mg once daily. Occasionally, a daily dose of 320 mg may be required.	*Generic.* Tablets 10, 20, 40, 60, 80, and 90 mg; solution 20 and 40 mg/5 ml and 80 mg/ml. *Inderal* (Wyeth-Ayerst). Tablets 10, 20, 40, 60, and 80 mg. *Inderal LA* (Wyeth-Ayerst), *Generic.* Capsules (prolonged-release) 60, 80, 120, and 160 mg.
Propranolol and Hydrochlorothiazide	Dosage should be individualized.	*Inderide* (Wyeth-Ayerst), *Generic.* Each tablet contains propranolol hydrochloride 40 or 80 mg and hydrochlorothiazide 25 mg (*Inderide-40/25* and *Inderide-80/25*, respectively). *Inderide LA* (Wyeth-Ayerst). Each capsule (prolonged-release) contains propranolol hydrochloride 80, 120, or 160 mg and hydrochlorothiazide 50 mg (*Inderide LA-80/50, Inderide LA-120/50*, and *Inderide LA-160/50*, respectively).
Timolol	Initially, 10 mg twice daily. For maintenance, 20 to 40 mg daily. Some patients may require 60 mg daily.	*Blocadren* (Merck), *Generic.* Tablets 5, 10, and 20 mg.
Timolol and Hydrochlorothiazide	Dosage should be individualized.	*Timolide* (Merck). Each tablet contains timolol maleate 10 mg and hydrochlorothiazide 25 mg.

sodilating effect. Myocardial depression may be evident, however, in patients with severe heart failure or in those receiving other myocardial depressant drugs.

USES. Although calcium channel blocking drugs differ in their electrophysiologic and hemodynamic effects, all are effective antihypertensive agents. Concurrent diuretic therapy may be less important than with other antihypertensive drugs (Kaplan, 1989). Calcium channel blockers are suitable for initial antihypertensive therapy (Joint National Committee on Detection, Evaluation, and Treatment of High Blood Pressure, 1993). They are effective in both black and white patients and usually are well tolerated in young, physically active patients and in the elderly. (See also Table 2.)

Calcium channel blocking agents also have been used in hypertensive urgencies.

ADVERSE REACTIONS AND PRECAUTIONS. Nifedipine and other dihydropyridines may cause headache and tachycardia. Constipation and headache are the most common side effects of verapamil. Diltiazem is usually well tolerated but may produce headache and dizziness.

Calcium channel blockers may produce congestive heart failure in patients with compromised left ventricular function or in those receiving other myocardial depressant drugs. Their use also has been associated with development of peripheral edema; this is more common with dihydropyridines than with diltiazem or verapamil. Gingival hyperplasia is a common side effect for all calcium channel blockers. For other adverse reactions, precautions, and interactions, see the chapter, Calcium Channel Blocking Drugs.

PHARMACOKINETICS. See the chapter, Calcium Channel Blocking Drugs.

DOSAGE AND PREPARATIONS. See Table 5.

TABLE 5.
CALCIUM CHANNEL BLOCKING AGENTS

Drug	Usual Oral Dosage	Preparations
Amlodipine	*Adults,* initially, 5 mg once daily. After two weeks, the dosage may be increased to 10 mg once daily. For the elderly and patients with hepatic dysfunction, initially, 2.5 mg once daily.	*Norvasc* (Pfizer). Tablets 2.5, 5, and 10 mg.
Diltiazem	*Adults,* initially, 30 to 60 mg three or four times daily (regular preparation); 60 to 120 mg twice daily (prolonged-release preparation); or 180 to 240 mg once daily (extended-release preparation). The usual maintenance dose is 240 to 360 mg daily.	*Cardizem* (Marion Merrell Dow). Tablets 30, 60, 90, and 120 mg; capsules (prolonged-release) 60, 90, or 120 mg *(Cardizem SR)*; capsules (extended-release) 120, 180, 240, and 300 mg (*Cardizem CD*). *Dilacor XR* (Rhone-Poulenc Rorer). Capsules (prolonged-release) 120, 180, and 240 mg. *Generic.* Tablets 30, 60, 90, and 120 mg.
Felodipine	*Adults,* initially, 5 mg once daily. After two weeks, the dosage may be increased to 10 mg once daily (maximum, 20 mg once daily or, for the elderly and patients with hepatic dysfunction, 10 mg daily).	*Plendil* (Merck). Tablets (prolonged-release) 5 and 10 mg.
Isradipine	*Adults,* initially, 5 mg daily. The maximum daily dose is 20 mg.	*DynaCirc* (Sandoz). Capsules 2.5 and 5 mg.
Nicardipine	*Adults* (regular preparation), initially, 20 mg three times daily; for maintenance, 20 to 40 mg three times daily (prolonged-release preparation). Initially, 30 mg two times daily; for maintenance, 30 to 60 mg two times daily.	*Cardene* (Syntex). Capsules 20 and 30 mg; capsules (prolonged-release) 30, 45, and 60 mg (*Cardene SR*).
Nifedipine	*Adults* (regular preparation), initially, 10 mg three times daily; this may be followed by doses of 20 mg three times daily. The usual maximum dose is 180 mg daily (prolonged-release preparation). Initially, 30 or 60 mg once daily (maximum daily dose, 120 mg).	*Adalat* (Miles), *Procardia* (Pratt). Capsules 10 and 20 mg; tablets (prolonged-release) 30, 60, and 90 mg (*Adalat CC, Procardia XL*). *Generic.* Capsules and tablets 10 and 20 mg.
Verapamil	*Adults,* 120 mg daily in three divided doses (regular preparation) or 120 mg once daily in the morning (prolonged-release preparation). The maximum daily dose is 480 mg.	*Calan* (Searle), *Isoptin* (Knoll). Tablets 40, 80, and 120 mg; tablets (prolonged-release) 120, 180, and 240 mg *(Calan SR, Isoptin SR)*. *Verelan* (Lederle, Wyeth-Ayerst). Capsules (prolonged-release) 120, 180, and 240 mg. *Generic.* Tablets 40, 80, and 120 mg; tablets (prolonged-release) 240 mg.

ANGIOTENSIN-CONVERTING ENZYME INHIBITORS

ACTIONS. The function of the renin-angiotensin-aldosterone system and the actions of the ACE inhibitors are discussed in detail in the chapter, Angiotensin-Converting Enzyme Inhibitors. ACE inhibitors block the conversion of angiotensin I to the active angiotensin II by inhibiting the converting enzyme. They also inhibit degradation of the vasodilator, bradykinin. ACE inhibitors are presumed to exert their action on the tissue angiotensin systems in the vasculature and myocardium (Frohlich, 1989 B). These drugs reduce total peripheral resistance, lower systemic blood pressure, and do not cause reflex tachycardia.

USES. ACE inhibitors are useful when given orally to treat mild to severe hypertension and are recommended for initial therapy (Joint National Committee on the Detection, Evaluation and Treatment of High Blood Pressure, 1993). Diuretics enhance their antihypertensive effect. During combined therapy, ACE inhibitors reduce diuretic-induced hyperaldosteronism and lessen hypokalemia.

ACE inhibitors are particularly useful in patients with coexisting hypertension and congestive heart failure. They are well tolerated in young, physically active patients and appear to be effective in the elderly (Schnaper, 1990) (see also Table 2). ACE inhibitors are more effective in white than in black patients when used as sole therapy, but the addition of a diuretic abolishes this difference (Gavras, 1986; Veterans Administration Cooperative Study Group on Antihypertensive Agents, 1984).

Oral ACE inhibitors also may be used for hypertensive urgencies when immediate reduction of blood pressure with parenteral drugs is not required. The intravenous preparation, enalaprilat, is used in hypertensive emergencies.

ADVERSE REACTIONS, PRECAUTIONS, AND INTERACTIONS. Rash, taste disturbances, and cough are frequent side effects of ACE inhibitors; cough is most common. The initial dose of an ACE inhibitor may cause a precipitous, symptomatic fall in blood pressure, especially in volume-depleted patients and in those with high-grade bilateral renal artery stenosis. The hypotensive reaction to lisinopril and enalapril may be prolonged. ACE inhibitors should not be used for the treatment of hypertension during pregnancy (Perlman and Volpe, 1989). These and other adverse reactions, precautions, and interactions are discussed in detail in the chapter, Angiotensin-Converting Enzyme Inhibitors.

PHARMACOKINETICS. See the chapter, Angiotensin-Converting Enzyme Inhibitors.

DOSAGE AND PREPARATIONS. See Table 6.

TABLE 6.
ANGIOTENSIN-CONVERTING ENZYME INHIBITORS

Drug	Usual Dosage	Preparations
Benazepril	*Oral: Adults,* 10 mg once daily for patients who are not taking a diuretic or 5 mg once daily for those who are receiving a diuretic. The usual maintenance dose is 20 to 40 mg once daily or in two equally divided doses (maximum, 80 mg daily). For *patients with impaired renal function* (creatinine clearance <30 ml/min), initially, 5 mg once daily; the maximum maintenance dose is 40 mg daily.	*Lotensin* (CIBA). Tablets 5, 10, 20, and 40 mg.
Captopril	*Oral:* Captopril should be taken one hour before meals. *Adults,* for mild to moderate hypertension, initially, 12.5 mg two times daily. For severe hypertension, initially, 25 mg two times daily, which may be increased to 50 mg two times daily after one or two weeks. If required, the dosage may be increased further at one- to two-week intervals to a maximum of 150 mg twice daily. Volume-depleted patients and those with severe hypertension should be observed carefully for several hours after the initial dose. Dosage should be reduced in patients with impaired renal function. Diuretics enhance the therapeutic response. *Infants under 6 months,* 0.05 to 0.5 mg/kg daily in three doses: *children over 6 months,* 0.5 to 2 mg/kg daily in three doses.	*Capoten* (Squibb). Tablets 12.5, 25, 50, and 100 mg.
Captopril and Hydrochlorothiazide	Dosage should be individualized.	*Capozide 25/15, 25/25, 50/15, 50/25* (Squibb). Each tablet contains captopril 25 or 50 mg and hydrochlorothiazide 15 or 25 mg.

(table continued on next page)

TABLE 6 (continued)

Drug	Usual Dosage	Preparations
Enalapril	*Oral: Adults,* initially, 2.5 mg daily for patients who are receiving a diuretic and those whose renal function is moderately to severely impaired (creatinine clearance ≤30 ml/min). An initial dose of 5 mg daily may be given to those who are not taking a diuretic and to those with normal or mildly impaired renal function. For maintenance, 10 to 40 mg daily in one or two doses.	*Vasotec* (Merck). Tablets 2.5, 5, 10, and 20 mg.
Enalapril and Hydrochlorothiazide	Dosage should be individualized.	*Vaseretic* (DuPont). Each tablet contains enalapril 10 mg and hydrochlorothiazide 25 mg.
Enalaprilat	*Intravenous: Adults,* initially, 1.25 mg administered over a five-minute period. This dose may be repeated at six-hour intervals. Doses up to 5 mg every six hours may be required in some patients. The maximal duration of therapy in controlled trials on hypertensive patients was 48 hours. The recommended starting dose for patients on diuretic therapy and for those with creatinine clearance <30 ml/min is 0.625 mg over a five-minute period. If the response is not adequate, this dose may be repeated in one hour. Additional doses of 1.25 mg may be given at six-hour intervals.	*Vasotec IV* (Merck). Solution 1.25 mg/ml in 1 and 2 ml containers.
Fosinopril	*Oral: Adults,* initially, 10 mg once daily. The usual dosage range is 20 to 40 mg once daily or in two divided doses (maximum, 80 mg daily). No dose adjustment is needed for patients with renal impairment.	*Monopril* (Mead Johnson). Tablets 10 and 20 mg.
Lisinopril	*Oral: Adults,* initially, 10 mg once daily for patients who are not taking a diuretic or 5 mg once daily for those who are receiving a diuretic. The usual maintenance dose is 20 to 40 mg daily. The initial dose should be reduced to 5 mg in patients with a creatinine clearance of 10 to 30 ml/min and to 2.5 mg for those with a creatinine clearance of <10 ml/min.	*Prinivil* (Merck), *Zestril* (Stuart). Tablets 5, 10, 20, and 40 mg.
Lisinopril and Hydrochlorothiazide	Dosage should be individualized.	*Prinzide* (Merck), *Zestoretic* (Stuart). Each tablet contains lisinopril 20 mg and hydrochlorothiazide 12.5 (*Prinzide 12.5, Zestoretic 20/12.5*) or 25 mg (*Prinzide 25, Zestoretic 20/25*).
Quinapril	*Oral: Adults,* initially, 10 mg once daily. Dosage may be increased after two weeks. The usual range is 20 to 80 mg once daily or in two equally divided doses (maximum, 80 mg once daily). A diuretic may be added. For *patients with renal impairment*, initially, 10 mg (creatinine clearance >60 ml/min), 5 mg (creatinine clearance 30 to 60 mg/ml), or 2.5 mg (creatinine clearance 10 to 30 ml/min).	*Accupril* (Parke-Davis). Tablets 5, 10, 20, and 40 mg.

(table continued on next page)

TABLE 6 (continued)

Drug	Usual Dosage	Preparations
Ramipril	*Oral: Adults,* initially, 1.25 to 2.5 mg once daily. Dosage may be increased at intervals of one to two weeks to a maximum of 10 mg daily. A diuretic may be added. For *patients with renal impairment,* initially, 1.25 mg once daily. Maximum dosage is 5 mg once daily (creatinine clearance 10 to 30 ml/min) or 2.5 mg once daily (creatinine clearance ≤10 ml/min).	*Altace* (Hoechst). Capsules 1.25, 2.5, 5, and 10 mg.

ALPHA-ADRENERGIC BLOCKING AGENTS

Alpha-adrenergic receptors are found in most blood vessels but are most abundant in the resistance vessels of the skin, mucosa, intestine, and kidney. Two subtypes have been identified pharmacologically: $alpha_1$ and $alpha_2$. Both types are found at postsynaptic sites on vascular smooth muscle where they mediate vasoconstriction. The postsynaptic $alpha_1$ receptor is under neural control and responds to nerve stimulation, whereas the postsynaptic $alpha_2$ receptor is thought to be a hormonal receptor that responds to circulating catecholamines (Van Zwieten, 1988). $Alpha_2$ receptors also may be present in endothelial cells where they may be involved in release of endothelium-derived relaxing and constricting factors (Langer and Schoemaker, 1989) and in the presynaptic membrane where they regulate the release of norepinephrine from sympathetic nerve terminals. Stimulation of these receptors by high concentrations of norepinephrine in the synaptic cleft inhibits the subsequent release of norepinephrine by a negative feedback mechanism (Van Zwieten et al, 1984). Presynaptic $alpha_1$ receptors regulate the release of acetylcholine from cardiac parasympathetic nerve endings, and this mechanism may contribute to the interaction between the sympathetic and parasympathetic nervous systems in controlling heart rate (McGrattan et al, 1987; McDonough et al, 1986). $Alpha_2$ receptors in the central nervous system are involved in the central regulation of blood pressure.

Phentolamine and phenoxybenzamine block both $alpha_1$ and $alpha_2$ receptors, whereas prazosin, doxazosin, terazosin, and related drugs selectively block $alpha_1$ receptors. The blockade of presynaptic $alpha_2$ receptors by phentolamine and phenoxybenzamine inhibits the normal feedback inhibition of norepinephrine release. For this reason, the prolonged use of these agents is associated with marked tachycardia and loss of antihypertensive efficacy (except in patients with pheochromocytoma). The selective blockade of postsynaptic $alpha_1$ receptors by prazosin, terazosin, doxazosin, and related drugs reduces peripheral vascular resistance and hence systemic blood pressure, but the normal feedback inhibition of norepinephrine is maintained.

In addition to lowering blood pressures, all $alpha_1$ blockers relieve symptoms of benign prostatic hyperplasia.

For dosage and preparations, see Table 7.

DOXAZOSIN MESYLATE

[Cardura]

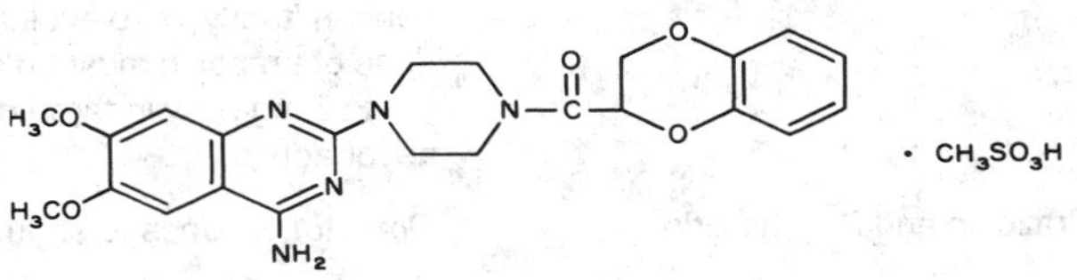

H_3CO, H_3CO, N, N, NH_2, N, N, O, C, O, O, · CH_3SO_3H

ACTIONS. This water-soluble quinazoline analogue of prazosin has selective $alpha_1$-receptor inhibitory action but exerts no direct effect on the vascular smooth muscle. It relaxes arteriolar resistance vessels and the venous capacitance system, thereby reducing peripheral vascular resistance. Doxazosin reduces levels of low-density lipoproteins (LDL), total cholesterol, and triglycerides and increases the high-density lipoprotein (HDL)/total cholesterol ratio (Pool et al, 1990).

USES. Doxazosin is effective in the treatment of mild to moderate hypertension when used alone or in combination with other antihypertensive drugs (Taylor, 1989); single daily dose is adequate. The efficacy of doxazosin is comparable to that of other commonly used antihypertensive drugs in patients of both sexes aged 45 to 69 years (Neaton et al, 1993). It is effective in patients who do not respond adequately to other antihypertensive drugs (eg, nifedipine, captopril, enalapril). Doxazosin controls blood pressure in hypertensive patients who have elevated cholesterol levels (Taylor, 1991), renal insufficiency (Bartels et al, 1988), intermittent claudication (Catalano and Libretti, 1991), asthma and chronic obstructive lung disease (Biernachi and Flenley, 1989), and noninsulin-dependent diabetes mellitus (Castrignano et al, 1988). No loss of effectiveness has been observed with three years of continuous use (Young and Brogden, 1988).

ADVERSE REACTIONS AND PRECAUTIONS. Approximately 31% of patients experience one or more adverse reactions after taking doxazosin (Rosenthal, 1987). In a postmarketing surveillance study, the adverse reaction rate was 17.5% (Langdon, 1991). Most of the side effects are mild or moderate and may disappear with continued therapy. Dizziness is most prevalent, but syncope has occurred rarely with recommended initial doses. Lethargy, fatigue, fluid retention, blurred vision, and dry mouth may be attributable to $alpha_1$-receptor inhibition in susceptible patients.

TABLE 7.
ALPHA- AND ALPHA-BETA ADRENERGIC BLOCKING AGENTS

Drug	Usual Dosage	Preparations
Alpha-Adrenergic Blocking Agents		
Doxazosin	*Oral: Adults,* initially, 1 mg once daily, increased sequentially as needed to 2, 4, and 8 mg once daily. In some patients, 16 mg once daily is needed. The mean optimal dose is 2 to 4 mg once daily.	*Cardura* (Roerig). Tablets 1, 2, 4, and 8 mg.
Prazosin	*Oral: Adults,* initially, 1 mg at bedtime. Subsequently, 1 mg may be given two times daily, then increased to three times daily. For maintenance, the dose may be increased gradually to 20 mg daily in divided doses. Diuretic and beta-adrenergic blocking agents may be administered concomitantly (see evaluation), but the optimal dose of prazosin must be redetermined. *Children,* 0.5 to 7 mg daily in three doses with initial titration as for adults.	*Minipress* (Pfizer), *Generic.* Capsules 1, 2, and 5 mg.
Prazosin and Polythiazide	*Oral: Adults,* dosage should be individualized.	*Minizide 1, 2, 5* (Pfizer). Each capsule contains prazosin 1, 2, or 5 mg and polythiazide 0.5 mg.
Terazosin	*Oral: Adults,* initially, 1 mg given at bedtime. Subsequent doses, 1 mg two times daily, then increased to 1 mg three times daily. Dosage may be gradually titrated upward to a maximum of 20 mg daily.	*Hytrin* (Abbott). Tablets 1, 2, 5, and 10 mg.
Phenoxybenzamine	*Oral: Adults,* for hypertension in pheochromocytoma, dosage varies widely and must be individualized; initially 10 mg twice daily. Dosage should be increased every other day to 20 to 40 mg two or three times a day until optimal dosage is obtained.	*Dibenzyline* (SmithKline Beecham). Capsules 10 mg.
Phentolamine	*Intravenous: Adults,* for hypertension in pheochromocytoma, 5 mg intravenously or intramuscularly one or two hours before surgery, repeated if necessary; 5 mg is given intravenously during surgery as indicated. For hypertensive crises due to interaction of a monoamine oxidase inhibitor with sympathomimetic amines, 5 to 10 mg. For clonidine withdrawal syndrome, 5 to 10 mg at 5-minute intervals to a total dose of 20 to 30 mg.	*Regitine* (CIBA). Powder (lyophilized) 5 mg with diluent.
Alpha-Beta Adrenergic Blocking Agent		
Labetalol	*Oral: Adults,* initially, 100 mg twice daily. Usual maintenance dose is 400 to 800 mg daily in one or two doses. For patients with severe hypertension, up to 1.2 g daily.	*Normodyne* (Schering), *Trandate* (Allen & Hanburys). Tablets 100, 200, and 300 mg.
	Intravenous: Adults, initially, 20 mg infused over two minutes. An additional 40 to 80 mg can be given at 10-minute intervals to a total of 300 mg. Alternatively, a diluted solution containing 1 mg/ml or 2 mg/3 ml is infused at a rate of 0.25 to 0.5 mg/min until desired supine blood pressure is reached.	*Normodyne* (Schering). Solution 5 mg/ml in 20 and 40 ml containers, 20 mg/ml in 4 ml containers, and 40 mg/ml in 8 ml containers. *Trandate* (Allen & Hanburys). Solution 5 mg/ml in 20 and 40 ml containers.

The following adverse reactions were reported in less than 0.5% of the 3,960 patients treated with doxazosin in controlled clinical trials: angina pectoris, myocardial infarction, hypotension, bradycardia, drowsiness, sexual dysfunction. Rarely, rhinitis, polyuria, and urinary incontinence also have occurred.

This drug is classified in FDA Pregnancy Category C.

PHARMACOKINETICS. Doxazosin is metabolized extensively in the liver by oxygen demethylation of the quinazoline substituent or carbon hydroxylation of the benzodioxan moiety to inert byproducts (Young and Brogden, 1988). Approximately 5% of an oral dose is eliminated unchanged in the feces and 9% is excreted unchanged in the urine. Approximately 65% of a dose is eliminated as metabolites in the feces.

Doxazosin is well absorbed orally; bioavailability is 65% in young and elderly patients. Peak plasma concentrations are usually reached two to three hours after oral ingestion and depend on the dose administered and the length of treatment. A peak plasma concentration of approximately 8 mcg/L occurs after ingestion of 1 mg. During prolonged therapy, a mean plasma concentration of 150 mcg/L is observed with a daily dose of 16 mg. The plasma half-life of doxazosin is approximately 19 to 22 hours in all age groups because of low hepatic clearance, allowing for sustained antihypertensive efficacy. The drug is mostly bound to plasma proteins regardless of the dose administered, which explains its retention in the plasma during hemodialysis.

DOSAGE AND PREPARATIONS. See Table 7.

PRAZOSIN HYDROCHLORIDE
[Minipress]

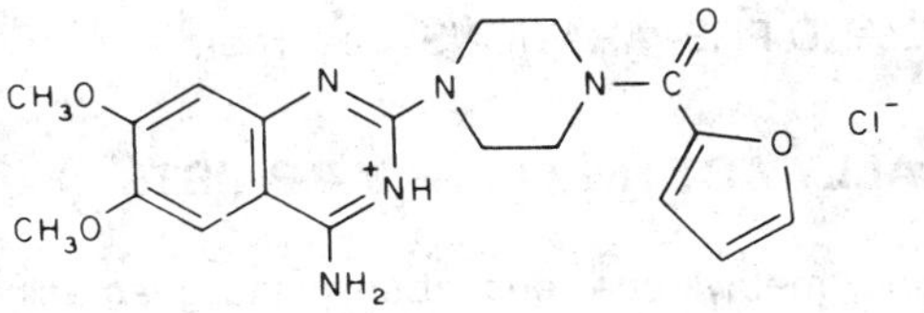

ACTIONS. Prazosin is a quinazoline derivative that reduces total peripheral resistance by blocking $alpha_1$ adrenergic receptors. Its antihypertensive action is similar to that of doxazosin, but prazosin has a shorter duration. This drug does not adversely affect blood lipids and may reduce total cholesterol and triglyceride concentrations (Amery and Lijnen, 1988; Stamler et al, 1988) and counteract the effect of thiazides on blood lipids (Stamler et al, 1988).

USES. Prazosin is used to treat chronic hypertension, usually with a diuretic. When compared as components of a three-drug regimen, prazosin and hydralazine were equally effective, but side effects (dizziness, nightmares, sexual dysfunction) were more common in the regimen containing prazosin (Veterans Administration Cooperative Study Group on Antihypertensive Agents, 1981). Prazosin also may be used for preoperative control of blood pressure in patients with pheochromocytoma.

ADVERSE REACTIONS, PRECAUTIONS, AND INTERACTIONS. Marked orthostatic hypotension, rarely leading to collapse or loss of consciousness, may occur at the onset of treatment ("first dose phenomenon"), especially when the initial dose exceeds 1 mg or when dosage is increased. An associated tachycardia has been noted in some patients and chest pain has occurred rarely. Patients taking diuretics, beta blockers, calcium channel blockers, and/or ingesting a low-sodium diet concomitantly may be particularly susceptible to the first dose phenomenon.

Prazosin may cause fluid retention and edema if a diuretic is not given concomitantly. Dryness of the mouth, nasal congestion, headache, nightmares, sexual dysfunction, and lethargy also may occur. Adverse effects rarely associated with prazosin therapy include urinary frequency, urinary incontinence, priapism, febrile polyarthritis, hypothermia, and dermatologic reactions (including urticaria and angioedema). Psychotic disturbances have been reported in patients with impaired renal function. In one study, antinuclear antibodies (ANA) were noted in one-third of patients taking prazosin; other investigators have found no relationship between prazosin therapy and ANA formation.

This drug is classified in FDA Pregnancy Category C.

PHARMACOKINETICS. The bioavailability of prazosin ranges from 44% to 69%. Its absorption is not influenced by the presence of food in the gastrointestinal tract. The drug is 92% to 97% protein bound, and its volume of distribution is 0.5 L/kg in hypertensive patients. Prazosin is extensively metabolized, and less than 10% is excreted in the urine as unchanged drug. Clearance is 3 ± 0.3 ml/min/kg. The half-life of prazosin is approximately 2.5 hours and is prolonged in elderly patients and those with congestive heart failure.

DOSAGE AND PREPARATIONS. See Table 7.

TERAZOSIN HYDROCHLORIDE
[Hytrin]

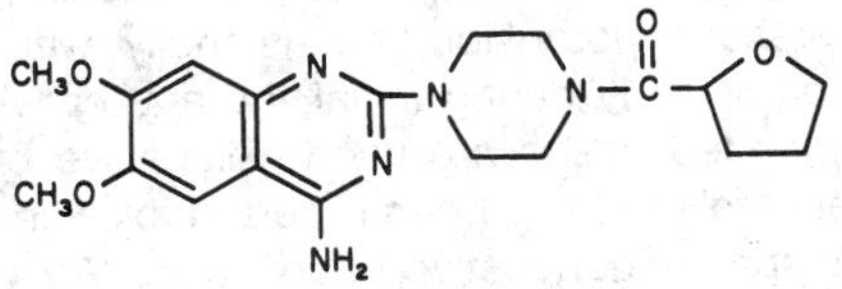

ACTIONS AND USES. Terazosin is a long-acting selective $alpha_1$-blocking agent that reduces total peripheral resistance and has little effect on heart rate. It does not adversely affect blood lipid levels. Terazosin has been used alone or with a diuretic in patients with mild to moderate hypertension. Its antihypertensive efficacy is comparable to that of prazosin, but terazosin is longer acting (Titmarsh and Monk, 1987).

ADVERSE REACTIONS AND PRECAUTIONS. The adverse effects of terazosin resemble those of prazosin. Those reported include dizziness, weakness, sedation, headache, nasal congestion, peripheral edema, nausea, and palpitations.

Terazosin is classified in FDA Pregnancy Category C.

PHARMACOKINETICS. The bioavailability of terazosin is approximately 90%. It is extensively metabolized and its half-life is 12 hours.

DOSAGE AND PREPARATIONS. See Table 7.

ALPHA-BETA ADRENERGIC BLOCKING AGENT

LABETALOL HYDROCHLORIDE
[Normodyne, Trandate]

For chemical formula, see chapter, Beta-Adrenergic Blocking Drugs.

ACTIONS. Labetalol is a competitive antagonist at both alpha- and beta-adrenergic receptor sites. It selectively blocks $alpha_1$ receptors and is nonselective in its action on beta receptors. Labetalol reduces heart rate and myocardial contractility, slows AV conduction, decreases total peripheral resistance, and lowers blood pressure. Following short-term administration, its antihypertensive effect is largely due to vasodilation; during prolonged oral therapy, both peripheral resistance and heart rate are reduced.

USES. Oral labetalol is used to treat mild to severe hypertension and is a preferred drug for patients with coexisting angina and hypertension (Goa et al, 1989). It has been widely employed as a second drug to enhance the antihypertensive effect of a diuretic.

Intravenous labetalol is used to treat various hypertensive emergencies, including hypertensive encephalopathy, hypertension associated with extensive burns, and hypertension in patients with coronary artery disease or acute myocardial infarction. It also has been used in states of catecholamine excess, such as severe tetanus, monoamine oxidase inhibitor-tyramine interaction, pheochromocytoma, and clonidine withdrawal syndrome.

ADVERSE REACTIONS, PRECAUTIONS, AND INTERACTIONS. Labetalol may cause gastrointestinal disturbances (nausea, dyspepsia, abdominal pain, diarrhea), dryness of the mouth, tingling of the scalp, and fluid retention. Symptomatic orthostatic hypotension, occasionally with syncope, may occur, particularly during initial therapy or when larger than recommended doses are used. Excessive bradycardia and acute renal failure have been reported following overdosage. Bronchospasm, congestive heart failure, AV conduction disturbances, and peripheral vascular reactions are less likely to occur with labetalol than with a pure beta-blocking drug but have been reported occasionally.

Elevated hepatic transaminase levels and, rarely, jaundice (usually cholestatic) have been reported. Hepatocellular damage has been observed in some patients treated with labetalol; some fatalities have occurred (Clark et al, 1990). Liver function tests should be performed before and periodically during labetalol therapy. Other adverse reactions include lethargy, nervousness, urinary retention, nasal congestion, facial flushing, palpitations, sexual dysfunction (impotence, failure of ejaculation, decreased libido), paresthesias, muscle cramps or weakness, depression, nightmares, reversible alopecia, and fever. Labetalol has occasionally produced a paradoxical increase in blood pressure in patients with pheochromocytoma or clonidine withdrawal syndrome.

An increased titer of antinuclear antibodies has developed in some patients during long-term therapy, but a systemic lupus syndrome has been reported only rarely. Some patients also developed antimitochondrial antibodies. Various types of rashes have occurred occasionally, including lichenoid skin eruptions, sometimes associated with increased antinuclear antibodies. Labetalol does not alter blood lipid levels.

All of the precautions and contraindications relating to use of beta blockers also pertain to labetalol. (See chapter, Beta-Adrenergic Blocking Drugs.)

Labetalol crosses the placenta (FDA Pregnancy Category C) and is excreted in breast milk.

EFFECT ON LABORATORY TESTS. A specific catecholamine radioenzymatic or high performance liquid chromatographic technique should be used to determine levels of catecholamines or their metabolites, since labetalol interferes with fluorometric and spectrophotometric methods of measuring catecholamines and gives erroneously high readings.

PHARMACOKINETICS. The bioavailability of labetalol is approximately 25% due to extensive first-pass metabolism. Food increases its bioavailability. Bioavailability also is increased in the elderly, in patients with liver disease, or in those taking cimetidine. Labetalol is widely distributed; during prolonged therapy, the volume of distribution at steady state is 9.4 L/kg and protein binding is 50%. This drug is moderately lipophilic. Labetalol is metabolized mainly by conjugation with glucuronic acid.

Less than 5% of a dose is excreted unchanged. The total body clearance is 33 ml/kg/min. The elimination half-life of oral labetalol is six to eight hours and is not affected by impaired renal function.

DOSAGE AND PREPARATIONS. See Table 7.

CENTRALLY ACTING ALPHA AGONISTS

Clonidine, methyldopa, guanabenz, and guanfacine lower blood pressure by activating inhibitory $alpha_2$ receptors in the central nervous system, thus reducing sympathetic outflow. They lower supine and standing blood pressure by reducing total peripheral resistance. Centrally acting antiadrenergic drugs are used less commonly today than in the past because of the availability of alternative drugs with fewer side effects (ie, beta blockers, calcium channel blockers, ACE inhibitors).

For dosage and preparations, see Table 8.

CLONIDINE
[Catapres-TTS]

CLONIDINE HYDROCHLORIDE
[Catapres]

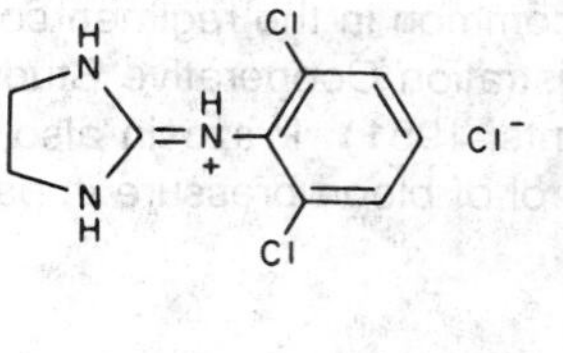

TABLE 8.
SUPPLEMENTAL ANTIHYPERTENSIVE AGENTS

Drug	Usual Dosage	Preparations
Centrally Acting Alpha-Agonists		
Clonidine	*Oral: Adults,* initially, 0.1 mg twice daily for several weeks. Dosage may be increased gradually by increments of 0.1 mg/day. Usual maintenance dose, 0.2 to 0.6 mg daily in divided amounts (maximum dose, 1.2 mg daily). *Children,* 0.05 to 0.4 mg daily in two doses.	*Catapres* (Boehringer), *Generic.* Tablets 0.1, 0.2, and 0.3 mg.
	Transdermal: Adults, initially, *Catapres-TTS-1* is applied once weekly. After one to two weeks, dosage may be increased by adding another *Catapres-TTS-1* or changing to a larger system. Maximum dose is two *Catapres-TTS-3* patches.	*Catapres-TTS-1, -2, -3* (Boehringer). Each patch delivers clonidine 0.1, 0.2, or 0.3 mg/day.
Clonidine and Chlorthalidone	*Oral: Adults,* dosage should be individualized.	*Combipres* (Boehringer), *Generic.* Each tablet contains clonidine 0.1, 0.2, or 0.3 mg and chlorthalidone 15 mg (*Combipres 0.1, Combipres 0.2,* and *Combipres 0.3,* respectively).
Guanabenz	*Oral: Adults,* initially, 4 mg twice daily. Dosage may be increased gradually up to 32 mg twice daily.	*Wytensin* (Wyeth-Ayerst). Tablets 4 and 8 mg.
Guanfacine	*Oral: Adults,* initially, 1 mg daily at bedtime. Dosage may be increased gradually up to 3 mg daily.	*Tenex* (Robins). Tablets 1 and 2 mg.
Methyldopa	*Oral: Adults,* initially, 250 mg at bedtime. Dosage may be increased to 250 mg twice daily after one week. Maximum dose is 1 or 1.5 g daily for most patients. *Children,* initially, 5 to 10 g/kg daily in two doses. Dosage may be titrated at two-day or longer intervals. Maximum dose, 65 mg/kg daily.	*Aldomet* (Merck), *Generic.* Suspension 250 mg/5 ml; tablets 125, 250, and 500 mg.
Methyldopate	*Intravenous:* For postoperative hypertension, *adults,* 250 to 500 mg every six to eight hours. *Children,* 20 to 40 mg/kg daily in four doses.	*Generic.* Solution 50 mg/ml in 10 ml containers. *Aldomet* (Merck). Solution 50 mg/ml in 5 ml containers.
Methyldopa and a Thiazide	*Oral: Adults,* dosage should be individualized.	*Aldoclor-150, -250* (Merck), *Generic.* Each tablet contains methyldopa 250 mg and chlorothiazide 150 or 250 mg. *Aldoril-15, -25* (Merck), *Generic.* Each tablet contains methyldopa 250 mg and hydrochlorothiazide 15 or 25 mg. *Aldoril D30, D50* (Merck), *Generic.* Each tablet contains methyldopa 500 mg and hydrochlorothiazide 30 or 50 mg.
Peripherally Acting Adrenergic Antagonist		
Reserpine	*Oral: Adults and children,* initially and for maintenance, 0.05 to 0.1 mg daily. Maximum dose, 0.25 mg.	*Generic.* Tablets 0.1, 0.25, and 1 mg. *Serpalan* (Lannett). Tablets 0.1 and 0.25 mg.
Reserpine and a Diuretic	*Oral: Adults,* dosage should be individualized.	*Diupres-250, -500* (Merck), *Generic.* Each tablet contains reserpine 0.125 mg and chlorothiazide 250 or 500 mg. *Diutensen-R* (Wallace). Each tablet contains reserpine 0.1 mg and methyclothiazide 2.5 mg.

(table continued on next page)

TABLE 8 (continued)

Drug	Usual Dosage	Preparations
		Hydropres-25, -50 (Merck). Each tablet contains reserpine 0.125 mg and hydrochlorothiazide 25 or 50 mg. *Metatensin #2, #4* (Marion Merrell Dow), *Generic.* Each tablet contains reserpine 0.1 mg and trichlormethiazide 2 or 4 mg. *Regroton* (Rhone-Poulenc Rorer), *Generic.* Each tablet contains reserpine 0.125 mg and chlorthalidone 25 mg (*Demi-Regroton*) or reserpine 0.25 mg and chlorthalidone 50 mg. *Renese-R* (Pfizer). Each tablet contains reserpine 0.25 mg and polythiazide 2 mg. *Salutensin* (Apothecon), *Generic.* Each tablet contains reserpine 0.125 mg and hydroflumethiazide 25 mg (*Salutensin-Demi*) or 50 mg.
Direct Vasodilators		
Hydralazine	*Oral: Adults,* initially, 50 mg in two or three divided doses. Dosage may be increased by 10 to 25 mg increments (maximum dose, 300 mg). *Children,* 1 to 5 mg/kg daily in two or three divided doses.	*Apresoline* (CIBA), *Generic.* Tablets 10, 25, and 50 mg.
Hydralazine with Other Antihypertensive Agents	*Oral: Adults,* dosage should be individualized.	*Apresazide* (CIBA), *Generic.* Each capsule contains hydralazine 25 mg and hydrochlorothiazide 25 mg or hydralazine 50 or 100 mg and hydrochlorothiazide 50 mg. *Ser-Ap-Es* (CIBA), *Tri-Hydroserpine* (Rugby), *Unipres* (Solvay), *Generic.* Each tablet contains hydralazine 25 mg, hydrochlorothiazide 15 mg, and reserpine 0.1 mg.
Minoxidil	*Oral: Adults and children over 12 years,* initially, 5 mg once daily. Dosage may be increased gradually at intervals of three days or longer to 10, 20, and 40 mg daily in single or divided doses. Usual maintenance dose, 10 to 40 mg daily. Maximum dose, 100 mg daily. *Children under 12 years,* initially, 0.2 mg/kg daily. Dosage may be increased in 0.1 or 0.2 mg/kg increments. Maintenance dose, 0.25 to 1 mg/kg daily. Maximum dose, 50 mg/day.	*Loniten* (Upjohn), *Generic.* Tablets 2.5 and 10 mg.
Nitroglycerin	*Intravenous:* For hypertensive emergencies, *adults,* 5 to 100 mcg/min.	*Generic.* Solution 5 mg/ml in 5, 10, and 20 ml containers and 10 mg/ml in 5 and 10 ml containers. *Nitro-Bid IV* (Marion Merrell Dow). Solution 5 mg/ml in 1, 5, and 10 ml containers. *Nitrostat IV* (Parke-Davis). Solution 0.8, 5, and 10 mg/ml in 10 ml containers with or without delivery set. *Tridil* (Du Pont). Solution 0.5 mg/ml in 10 ml containers and 5 mg/ml in 5, 10, and 20 ml containers with or without delivery set (*Tridilset*).
Sodium Nitroprusside	*Intravenous:* For hypertensive emergencies, *adults and children,* 0.3 to 10 mcg/kg/min.	*Nitropress* (Abbott), *Generic.* Powder 50 mg; solution 25 mg/ml in 2 ml containers.

USES. Oral or transdermal clonidine is used to treat chronic hypertension in combination with other antihypertensive agents. Concomitant diuretic therapy enhances the antihypertensive effect. The transdermal preparation, which delivers clonidine uniformly through a rate-controlling membrane during the seven-day wearing period, appears to be as effective as oral clonidine in mild to moderate hypertension (Lowenthal et al, 1986).

Oral clonidine also may be useful in some hypertensive urgencies when an immediate reduction in blood pressure with parenteral drugs is not required. In asymptomatic patients with severe hypertension, only a single oral loading dose followed by maintenance therapy should be administered, since multiple loading doses do not control blood pressure more promptly and may produce severe adverse effects (Zeller et al, 1989).

ADVERSE REACTIONS, PRECAUTIONS, AND INTERACTIONS. The most common side effects of clonidine are drowsiness, dryness of the mouth, and constipation. Rashes, central nervous system disturbances (depression, drowsiness, hallucinations), sexual dysfunction, and gynecomastia also have been reported. Orthostatic symptoms occur occasionally. These reactions may decrease in severity during long-term therapy. Sodium and water retention may be avoided with concurrent use of a diuretic. Localized skin reactions at the site of application are relatively common with use of the transdermal preparation.

A pronounced withdrawal reaction with a rebound increase in blood pressure and symptoms suggesting sympathetic overactivity may develop in 12 to 48 hours if clonidine is discontinued abruptly, especially in patients receiving oral doses exceeding 1.2 mg daily. For a planned withdrawal, dosage should be decreased gradually over one week or more. Psychosis has occurred rarely after abrupt withdrawal of clonidine in patients with pre-existing schizophrenia or manic-depressive illness.

Clonidine may increase bradycardia in patients with sinus node dysfunction, renal insufficiency, or a history of bradycardia. It also has been reported to potentiate the effect of digitalis on AV conduction.

Overdosage usually leads to hypotension and bradycardia but occasionally the blood pressure may increase because of activation of alpha receptors in the peripheral circulation. Atropine has been effective in treating the bradycardia, and volume replacement and vasopressors have been used to manage hypotensive reactions. Other manifestations of toxicity include apnea, drowsiness, miosis, hypothermia, coma, and seizures.

Rarely, a paradoxical hypertensive response has developed during combined therapy with clonidine and a beta-blocking drug. Beta blockers also may exaggerate the rebound hypertension accompanying abrupt withdrawal of clonidine. Therefore, it is recommended that beta blockers be discontinued several days before clonidine is withdrawn. Imipramine, desipramine, and probably other tricyclic antidepressants antagonize the antihypertensive effect of clonidine, resulting in loss of blood pressure control and possibly life-threatening elevations in blood pressure.

Clonidine is classified in FDA Pregnancy Category C.

PHARMACOKINETICS. Clonidine is readily absorbed after oral administration, and its bioavailability is 75% to 95%. The volume of distribution is 2.1 L/kg, and the half-life is approximately 12 to 16 hours. Clonidine is eliminated largely as unchanged drug (40% to 60%); clearance is 3.1 ± 1.2 ml/min/kg.

DOSAGE AND PREPARATIONS. See Table 8. Dosage must be titrated carefully to provide an optimal therapeutic response with minimal side effects.

GUANABENZ ACETATE
[Wytensin]

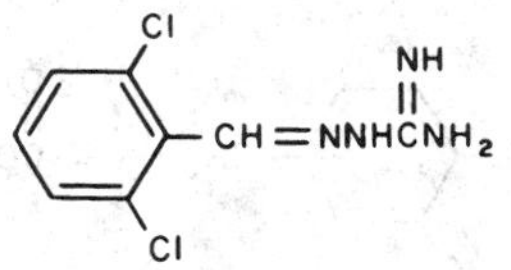

Guanabenz is used to treat chronic hypertension. Concomitant administration of a diuretic enhances the antihypertensive effect.

ADVERSE REACTIONS AND PRECAUTIONS. The adverse effects of guanabenz resemble those of clonidine (see the evaluation on Clonidine Hydrochloride). This drug is classified in FDA Pregnancy Category C.

PHARMACOKINETICS. The bioavailability of guanabenz is 75%. The drug is 90% protein bound and is extensively metabolized. Less than 1% of unchanged drug is recovered in the urine. The half-life is 7 to 10 hours.

DOSAGE AND PREPARATIONS. See Table 8. Dosage should be titrated gradually to provide the optimal therapeutic response with minimal side effects.

GUANFACINE HYDROCHLORIDE
[Tenex]

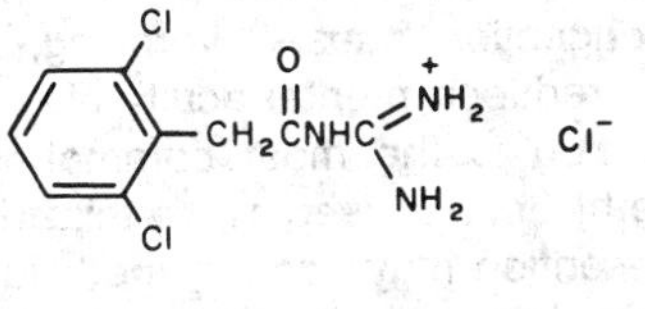

Guanfacine is used to treat chronic hypertension. Concomitant diuretic therapy enhances the antihypertensive effect.

ADVERSE REACTIONS, PRECAUTIONS, AND INTERACTIONS. The adverse effects of guanfacine resemble those of clonidine; however, rebound hypertension associated with drug withdrawal occurs less frequently with guanfacine than with clonidine (Wilson et al, 1986). (See the evaluation on Clonidine Hydrochloride.)

Guanfacine is classified in FDA Pregnancy Category B.

PHARMACOKINETICS. Guanfacine is rapidly and almost completely absorbed (90%) from the gastrointestinal tract. It has a large volume of distribution (276 to 456 L) and, at therapeutic plasma concentrations, is 64% protein bound. Guanfacine enters and leaves the central nervous system more slowly than clonidine. It has a half-life of 16 to 20 hours in patients with normal renal function. Phenobarbital shortens its half-life. Guanfacine is eliminated both by renal excretion of unchanged drug and by hepatic metabolism. Plasma concentrations and the hypotensive effect are not increased in uremic patients.

DOSAGE AND PREPARATIONS. See Table 8. Dosage must be titrated carefully to provide an optimal therapeutic response with minimal side effects.

METHYLDOPA
[Aldomet]

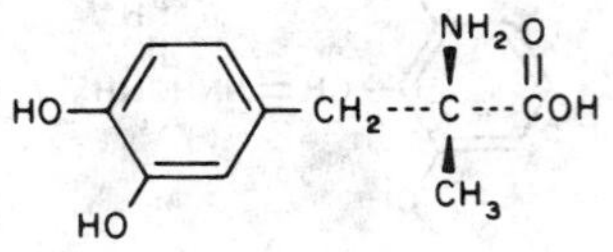

METHYLDOPATE HYDROCHLORIDE
[Aldomet]

USES. Methyldopa is used to treat chronic hypertension. Concomitant diuretic therapy enhances the antihypertensive effect. Although methyldopa crosses the placenta and may slightly reduce blood pressure in newborn infants of treated mothers, it has been used for treating chronic hypertension and pre-eclampsia during pregnancy without serious adverse effects on the fetus.

The intravenous preparation, methyldopate hydrochloride, is administered only rarely to treat hypertensive emergencies because of its delayed onset of action and sedative effect. It is used mainly to treat postoperative hypertension.

ADVERSE REACTIONS, PRECAUTIONS, AND INTERACTIONS. Drowsiness and dryness of the mouth are common. Fatigue may be a problem in the elderly (Materson et al, 1990). Nasal congestion, nausea, vomiting, diarrhea, sexual dysfunction, and reduced mental acuity also may occur. Excessive hypotension is the most common side effect observed when methyldopa is used with a thiazide diuretic. Sodium and water retention may occur if methyldopa is administered without a diuretic.

A positive Coombs' test has been noted in 10% to 20% of patients who received prolonged treatment. Hemolytic anemia occurs only rarely and is generally reversible. Since most patients having a positive Coombs' test do not develop hemolytic anemia, a positive test is not a contraindication to continued use of methyldopa.

Drug-induced hepatitis, sometimes accompanied by fever and malaise, may develop during the first 6 to 12 weeks of treatment. It is usually reversible, but, in a few instances, reexposure to methyldopa caused fatal hepatic necrosis. Liver function tests probably should be performed at monthly intervals during the first four months of treatment or whenever an unexplained fever develops. Drug fever occurs in some patients without hepatic involvement.

Uncommon effects observed with methyldopa therapy include gynecomastia, reversible leukopenia, thrombocytopenia, lichenoid reactions, hypersensitivity myocarditis, acute colitis, pancreatitis, a reversible malabsorption syndrome, and extrapyramidal symptoms. Methyldopa may adversely affect sinus node function in patients with sinus node disorders. Confusion, disorientation, and tremor may result from an interaction between methyldopa and lithium. Oral iron preparations reduce the therapeutic effect of methyldopa.

Hypertensive reactions have been reported rarely after withdrawal of methyldopa or due to interaction with intravenous propranolol or with phenylpropanolamine and a beta blocker. Methyldopa may interfere with determination of urinary catecholamines (fluorescent technique), serum creatinine (alkaline picrate method), uric acid (phosphotungstate method), and AST (colorimetric methods).

Methyldopa is classified in FDA Pregnancy Category B. It crosses the placenta and is excreted in breast milk, but no significant adverse effects have been reported in the fetus or nursing infant.

PHARMACOKINETICS. The bioavailability of methyldopa is 50%, and its volume of distribution is 0.37 ± 0.1 L/kg. It is eliminated by renal excretion of active drug (63%) or conjugates, and its clearance is 3.1 ± 0.9 ml/min/kg. In the presence of renal insufficiency, delayed excretion may result in accumulation of drug and metabolites. The half-life of methyldopa is 1.8 hours and is increased in patients with uremia.

DOSAGE AND PREPARATIONS. See Table 8. Dosage must be titrated carefully to provide an optimal therapeutic response with minimal side effects.

RAUWOLFIA ALKALOIDS

RESERPINE

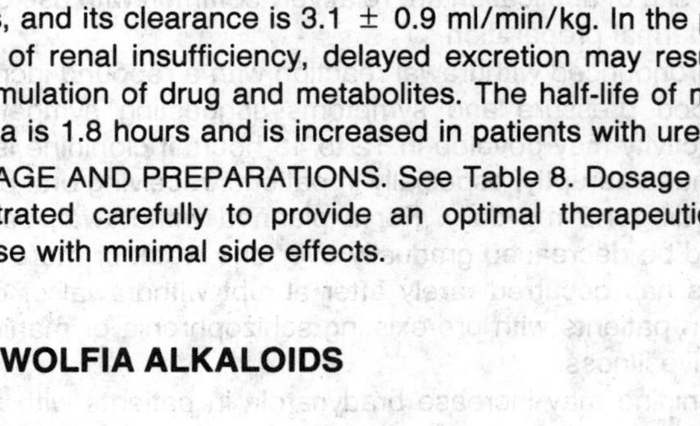

ACTIONS AND USES. Reserpine is the prototype of the rauwolfia alkaloids and is the most commonly used drug in this group. Its antihypertensive effect has been attributed to depletion of catecholamine stores in peripheral sympathetic nerve terminals and the central nervous system. Reserpine decreases total peripheral resistance, heart rate, and cardiac output.

A thiazide-reserpine regimen provides a simple, inexpensive, and reliable means for long-term control of mild to moderate hypertension and compares favorably with other two-drug regimens (Materson et al, 1990; Goldstein et al, 1990). Nevertheless, reserpine is used less commonly today because of the availability of newer drugs with fewer side effects. Small doses (as low as 0.1 mg daily), combined with a diuretic, often are effective and are better tolerated than larger doses (Participating Veterans Administration Medical Centers, 1982).

ADVERSE REACTIONS AND PRECAUTIONS. Lethargy, dryness of the mouth, nasal congestion, and bradycardia may occur with therapeutic doses of rauwolfia alkaloids; fluid retention may develop if a diuretic is not given concomitantly. Other adverse effects include diarrhea, nausea, vomiting, anorexia, sexual dysfunction, stress incontinence, and nightmares.

Reserpine is classified in FDA Pregnancy Category C.

DOSAGE AND PREPARATIONS. See Table 8. The rauwolfia alkaloids have a slow onset and prolonged duration of action. Dosage should be adjusted no more frequently than every five to seven days.

DIRECT-ACTING VASODILATORS

HYDRALAZINE HYDROCHLORIDE

[Apresoline]

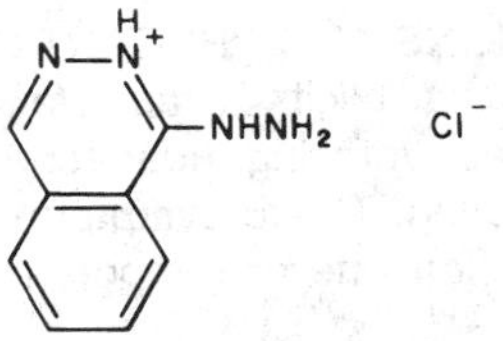

H+ N—N NHNH₂ Cl⁻

ACTIONS AND USES. Hydralazine reduces blood pressure by directly relaxing arteriolar smooth muscle; it has little effect on veins. Heart rate and cardiac output are increased. This drug does not adversely affect lipid levels.

Hydralazine is given orally for the management of chronic hypertension, usually with a diuretic and beta blocker (or other antiadrenergic drug). Since it does not cause sedation or orthostatic hypotension, small doses may be useful in elderly patients, who often have blunted baroreceptor reflexes and do not usually experience tachycardia with hydralazine; a diuretic should be given concomitantly (Goldstein et al, 1990).

ADVERSE REACTIONS, PRECAUTIONS, AND INTERACTIONS. Like other vasodilators, hydralazine causes sodium and water retention if a diuretic is not given concomitantly. Headache and tachycardia are common when hydralazine is given alone and can be minimized by increasing the dose gradually. Tachycardia usually can be prevented by prior and concomitant administration of an antiadrenergic drug, particularly a beta blocker. Coadministration of a beta-blocking drug prevents the tendency of hydralazine to precipitate myocardial ischemia in patients with coronary artery disease. Because it increases the velocity of left ventricular ejection, hydralazine is contraindicated in patients with dissecting aortic aneurysm. Gastrointestinal disturbances, flushing, and rash also may occur.

Hydralazine may produce an acute syndrome simulating systemic lupus erythematosus (SLE); symptoms include fever, myalgia, arthralgia, splenomegaly, edema, and LE cells in the peripheral blood. This syndrome is most common in slow acetylators (most often whites) receiving 200 mg daily or more (rarely below this dose) and occurs more frequently in women than in men. Symptoms of SLE diminish when the drug is withdrawn. In contrast to spontaneously occurring SLE, renal disease is very rare in hydralazine-induced SLE. Hydralazine need not be withdrawn solely on the basis of a positive antinuclear antibody test for SLE, because test results frequently become positive during prolonged therapy in asymptomatic patients (Mansilla-Tinoco et al, 1982).

Rarely, hydralazine causes peripheral neuropathy, blood dyscrasias (including neonatal thrombocytopenia), hepatotoxicity, and acute cholangitis. The neuropathy appears to result from pyridoxine deficiency and can be corrected by administration of pyridoxine. The tartrazine in some brands of hydralazine tablets may cause allergic reactions.

Nonsteroidal anti-inflammatory drugs, beta-adrenergic blocking drugs, and diazoxide attenuate the antihypertensive effect of hydralazine.

Hydralazine crosses the placenta; negligible amounts are excreted in breast milk. This drug is classified in FDA Pregnancy Category C.

PHARMACOKINETICS. The bioavailability of hydralazine is 30% to 50%. It is 87% protein bound, and the volume of distribution is 1.6 L/kg. The drug has a relatively short half-life (2.2 to 2.6 hours) and is eliminated by the kidney as active drug (12% to 14%) and metabolites. Its clearance rate is 8 to 10 ml/min/kg. Metabolic acetylation inactivates the drug. Fast acetylators have lower plasma levels than slow acetylators; however, the rate of elimination from plasma does not differ greatly between the two groups, and other metabolic pathways also may be important.

DOSAGE AND PREPARATIONS. See Table 8.

MINOXIDIL

[Loniten]

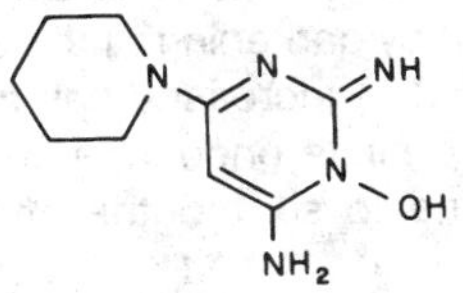

N N NH N OH NH₂

ACTIONS AND USES. Minoxidil acts directly on arterioles to reduce total peripheral resistance. It has little or no effect on the venous system. When given alone, the hypotensive effect of minoxidil is accompanied by a marked increase in heart rate and cardiac output.

Minoxidil is more potent and longer acting than hydralazine and is useful for long-term therapy in patients with severe hypertension refractory to maximum tolerated doses of standard antihypertensive drugs given in combination (Limas and

Freis, 1973). It is often effective in patients with malignant or accelerated hypertension and advanced renal disease and thus provides an alternative to bilateral nephrectomy. Both a diuretic and a beta blocker or other sympathetic depressant drug should be given concomitantly to enhance the therapeutic response by minimizing fluid retention, cardiac workload, and tachycardia. Other antihypertensive drugs also may be continued or added as necessary (Campese, 1981).

ADVERSE REACTIONS AND PRECAUTIONS. Fluid retention, manifested by weight gain and edema, is common but does not result in loss of blood pressure control. Significant volume overload may precipitate or worsen heart failure. If fluid retention occurs, patients who are receiving a thiazide should be given a loop diuretic instead. Combined therapy with a thiazide (especially metolazone) and furosemide may be effective in refractory cases, but close supervision is warranted because this combination can cause marked diuresis, severe hypokalemia, and an increase in the serum creatinine level. Dialysis should be instituted or minoxidil discontinued if excessive fluid retention persists.

Approximately 3% of patients, most commonly those with severely impaired renal function who are not receiving dialysis, have developed pericardial effusion, occasionally with cardiac tamponade, as a result of fluid retention. This condition often persists despite vigorous diuretic therapy. Echocardiography should be performed if pericardial effusion is suspected. The effusion usually abates when minoxidil is withdrawn. Cardiac tamponade should be treated by pericardiocentesis or surgical drainage.

Reflex cardiac stimulation combined with reduced coronary perfusion occasionally may precipitate anginal attacks in patients receiving minoxidil, particularly if beta blockade is inadequate. Myocardial infarction has occurred rarely. Rebound hypertension may sometimes develop when minoxidil is withdrawn abruptly, due in part to the high levels of angiotensin II that are frequently associated with minoxidil therapy.

Electrocardiographic abnormalities (flattening or inversion of T waves, sometimes accompanied by increased QRS voltage) are frequently observed and are usually asymptomatic and reversible.

Hypertrichosis develops in about 80% of patients after one or two months of therapy. The abnormal hair growth usually appears first on the face and later extends to other areas; it may be accompanied by darkening of the skin and coarsening of the facial features. The increased hair growth has not been associated with any definite endocrine abnormalities and disappears gradually one to six months after the drug is withdrawn.

Other side effects occasionally reported are nausea and/or vomiting, headache, fatigue, dermatologic reactions (including Stevens-Johnson syndrome), SLE syndrome, and breast tenderness.

Hypertrichosis and multiple congenital abnormalities have occurred in the offspring of mothers treated with minoxidil. This drug is classified in FDA Pregnancy Category C.

PHARMACOKINETICS. The bioavailability of minoxidil is approximately 90%. The plasma half-life is about 4.2 hours, but therapeutic activity lasts considerably longer (about 75 hours). The drug is extensively metabolized, mainly to the inactive metabolite, minoxidil glucuronide. Parent drug (12%) and metabolites (88%) are eliminated primarily in the urine. Plasma levels do not correlate with the therapeutic response.

DOSAGE AND PREPARATIONS. See Table 8.

SODIUM NITROPRUSSIDE
[Nitropress]

$$Na_2\left[Fe(CN)_5NO\right] \cdot 2H_2O$$

ACTIONS AND USES. This potent vasodilator acts directly to relax both resistance and capacitance vessels. Heart rate is usually increased by reflex mechanisms. Cardiac output generally is not increased because of reduction in venous return following venodilation.

Nitroprusside is used to treat hypertensive emergencies. It reduces blood pressure immediately, but continuous infusion is necessary to maintain the hypotensive response. Because of its beneficial hemodynamic effects, nitroprusside often is the drug of choice in the management of hypertensive emergencies associated with left ventricular failure. In hypertensive patients with cerebral or subarachnoid hemorrhage, nitroprusside infusion permits titration of the blood pressure to any desired level and restoration of a higher level in the event of neurologic deterioration.

ADVERSE REACTIONS AND PRECAUTIONS. A dose of sodium nitroprusside that elicits a rapid fall in blood pressure may produce nausea, vomiting, headache, palpitations, restlessness, and sweating. These symptoms often are relieved by slowing the infusion rate or temporarily discontinuing the infusion.

Prolonged infusion or infusion at rates of 30 to 120 mcg/kg/min may cause muscle twitching, disorientation, delirium, psychotic behavior, hypothyroidism, or death. These adverse effects are usually caused by the accumulation of cyanide and/or thiocyanate, particularly in patients with inadequate endogenous thiosulfate, hepatic disease, or renal disorders. Cyanide is a metabolic product of nitroprusside and is usually converted into thiocyanate for elimination in the urine. Increased blood thiocyanate levels induce metabolic acidosis and occasionally may cause tachyphylaxis. If nitroprusside is infused for more than 72 hours (or less if renal failure is present), blood thiocyanate levels should be determined daily; if levels do not exceed 10 mg/dL, it probably is safe to continue administration. The blood thiocyanate level can be reduced by infusing sodium thiosulfate or hydroxocobalamin.

Drug resistance has been associated with an increase in cardiac output; if volume overload occurs, administration of furosemide is indicated. A beta blocker may be useful if volume overload is not present (Rouby et al, 1982).

A rebound increase in blood pressure has occurred when nitroprusside was discontinued following its use to induce hypotension during anesthesia. Pretreatment with propranolol prevents this response. Nitroprusside may increase intracranial pressure in patients with brain tumors or metabolic encephalopathy. It decreases the platelet count and should be given cautiously to patients with bleeding tendencies or thrombocytopenia. Acute phlebitis has occurred rarely.

Nitroprusside should be avoided during pregnancy because of the risk of fetal cyanide poisoning. It is classified in FDA Pregnancy Category C.

PHARMACOKINETICS. Nitroprusside has a very brief half-life. It is converted by erythrocytes to cyanide, which is then transformed to the final metabolite, thiocyanate, by the hepatic enzyme, rhodanese. This reaction requires thiosulfate (which is derived endogenously from the amino acid, cysteine). Thiocyanate is eliminated by renal excretion. Its half-life is four to seven days in patients with normal renal function.

DOSAGE AND PREPARATIONS. See Table 8. Before using sodium nitroprusside, the manufacturer's prescribing information should be reviewed. Intravenous administration of furosemide will usually prevent fluid overload and ensure a continuing hypotensive response.

NITROGLYCERIN (INTRAVENOUS)
[Nitro-Bid IV, Nitrostat IV, Tridil]

ACTIONS AND USES. This direct-acting vasodilator has a greater effect on the venous than the arterial circulation. It acts predominantly to reduce venous tone but, at high infusion rates, reduces peripheral vascular resistance. Nitroglycerin dilates the large epicardial (conductance) arteries but has little effect on intramyocardial (resistance) vessels. In patients with coronary artery disease, this vasodilator improves the regional distribution of myocardial blood flow and oxygen supply. It is particularly useful in hypertensive emergencies occurring during cardiac surgery.

ADVERSE REACTIONS AND PRECAUTIONS. Nitroglycerin may cause headache, flushing, dizziness, hypotension, and tachycardia. Severe hypotension associated with sinus bradycardia has occurred in some patients. Intravenous preparations contain alcohol and a considerable amount may be administered during prolonged infusion.

Tolerance develops rapidly (within 24 hours) to intravenous nitroglycerin. (See index entry Nitroglycerin, In Heart Failure.)

Intravenous nitroglycerin is classified in FDA Pregnancy Category C.

DOSAGE AND PREPARATIONS. See Table 8.

Cited References

Amery A, Lijnen P: Alterations in lipid metabolism induced by antihypertensive therapy. *Drugs* 36(suppl 2):1-5, 1988.

Arroll B, Beaglehole R: Does physical activity lower blood pressure: A critical review of the clinical trials. *J Clin Epidemiol* 45:439-447, 1992.

Bannon JA, et al: Clinical experience with timolol maleate monotherapy of hypertension. *Arch Intern Med* 146:653-657, 1986.

Bartels ACC, et al: Doxazosin in the treatment of patients with mild or moderate hypertension and mild or moderate renal insufficiency. *Am Heart J* 116:1772-1777, 1988.

Biernachi W, Flenley WC: Doxazosin, a new alpha$_1$-antagonist drug, controls hypertension without causing airway obstruction in asthma and COPD. *J Hum Hypertens* 3:419-425, 1989.

Butters L, et al: Atenolol in essential hypertension during pregnancy. *BMJ* 301:587-589, 1990.

Calhoun DA, Oparil S: Treatment of hypertensive crisis. *N Engl J Med* 323:1177-1183, 1990.

Campese VM: Minoxidil: Review of pharmacological properties and therapeutic use. *Drugs* 22:257-278, 1981.

Carlsen JE, et al: Relation between dose of bendrofluazide, antihypertensive effect, and adverse biochemical effects. *BMJ* 300:975-978, 1990.

Castrignano R, et al: A single-blind study of doxazosin in the treatment of mild-to-moderate essential hypertensive patients with concomitant noninsulin-dependent diabetes mellitus. *Am Heart J* 116:1778-1784, 1988.

Catalano M, Libretti A: A multicenter study of doxazosin in the treatment of patients with mild or moderate essential hypertension and concomitant intermittent claudication. *Am Heart J* 121:367-371, 1991.

Clark JA, et al: Labetalol hepatotoxicity. *Ann Intern Med* 113:210-213, 1990.

Collins R, et al: Blood pressure, stroke, and coronary heart disease: Part 2, short-term reductions in blood pressure: Overview of randomised drug trials in their epidemiological context. *Lancet* 335:827-838, 1990.

Cressman MD, et al: Intravenous labetalol in management of severe hypertension and hypertensive emergencies. *Am Heart J* 107:980-985, 1984.

Cutler JA, et al: An overview of randomized trials of sodium reduction and blood pressure. *Hypertension* 17(suppl I):I-27-I-33, 1991.

Dahlof B, et al: Morbidity and mortality in the Swedish Trial in Old Patients with Hypertension (STOP-Hypertension). *Lancet* 338:1281-1285, 1991.

Epstein M, Sowers JR: Diabetes mellitus and hypertension. *Hypertension* 19:403-418, 1992.

Finnerty FA Jr: Step-down treatment of mild systemic hypertension. *Am J Cardiol* 53:1304-1307, 1984.

Freis ED: How diuretics lower blood pressure. *Am Heart J* 106:185-187, 1983.

Freis ED: Veterans Administration Cooperative Study Group on Hypertensive Agents: Effects of age on treatment results. *Am J Med* 90(suppl 3A):20S-23S, 1991.

Freis ED, Papademetriou V: How dangerous are diuretics? *Drugs* 30:469-474, 1985.

Freis ED, et al: Age and antihypertensive drugs (hydrochlorothiazide, bendroflumethiazide, nadolol and captopril). *Am J Cardiol* 61:117-121, 1988.

Freis ED, et al: Effects of reduction in drugs or dosage after long-term control of systemic hypertension. *Am J Cardiol* 63:702-708, 1989.

Frohlich ED: Diuretics in hypertension. *J Hypertens* 5(suppl 3):43-49, 1987.

Frohlich ED: Left ventricular hypertrophy, cardiac diseases and hypertension: Recent experiences. *J Am Coll Cardiol* 14:1587-1594, 1989 A.

Frohlich ED: Clinical and physiologic significance of local tissue renin-angiotensin systems. *Am J Med* 87(suppl 6B):19-23, 1989 B.

Gavras H: Multicenter trial of enalapril in treatment of essential hypertension. *Clin Ther* 9:24-38, 1986.

Gidding SS, et al: Therapeutic effect of propranolol on paradoxical hypertension after repair of coarctation of aorta. *N Engl J Med* 312:1224-1228, 1985.

Gifford RW Jr: Management of isolated systolic hypertension in the elderly. *J Am Geriatr Soc* 34:106-111, 1986.

Goa KL, et al: Labetalol: A reappraisal of its pharmacology, pharmacokinetics and therapeutic use in hypertension and ischaemic heart disease. *Drugs* 37:583-627, 1989.

Goldstein G, et al: Treatment of hypertension in the elderly, II: Cognitive and behavioral function: Results of a Department of Veterans Affairs Cooperative Study. *Hypertension* 15:361-369, 1990.

Greenberg G, et al: Effects of diuretic and beta-blocker therapy in Medical Research Council trial. *Am J Med* 76:45-51, 1984.

Hypertension Prevention Trial Research Group: The Hypertension Prevention Trial: Three-year effects of dietary changes on blood pressure. *Arch Intern Med* 150:153-162, 1990.

Joint National Committee on Detection, Evaluation, and Treatment of High Blood Pressure: The fifth report of the Joint National Committee on Detection, Evaluation, and Treatment of High Blood Pressure (JNC V). *Arch Intern Med* 153:154-183, 1993.

Julius S, et al: The association of borderline hypertension with target organ changes and higher coronary risk: Tecumseh Blood Pressure Study. *JAMA* 264:354-358, 1990.

Kaplan NM: Calcium entry blockers in the treatment of hypertension: Current status and future prospects. *JAMA* 262:817-823, 1989.

Kaplan NM: Effects of antihypertensive therapy on insulin resistance. *Hypertension* 19 (suppl I):I-116-I-118, 1992.

Klatsky AL, et al: Alcohol and mortality. *Ann Intern Med* 117:646-654, 1992.

Langdon CG: Doxazosin: A study in a cohort of patients with hypertension in general practice: An interim report. *Am Heart J* 121:268-273, 1991.

Langer SZ, Schoemaker H: Alpha-adrenoceptor subtypes in blood vessels: Physiology and pharmacology. *Clin Exp Theory Pract* (suppl 1):21-30, 1989.

Law MR, et al: By how much does dietary salt reduction lower blood pressure? III: Analysis of data from trials of salt reduction. *BMJ* 302:819-824, 1991.

Leenen FHH, et al: Postoperative hypertension after repair of coarctation of aorta in children: Protective effect of propranolol? *Am Heart J* 113:1164-1173, 1987.

Leitschuh M, et al: A high-normal blood pressure progression to hypertension in the Framingham Heart Study. *Hypertension* 17:22-27, 1991.

Levinson PD, et al: Persistence of normal BP after withdrawal of drug treatment in mild hypertension. *Arch Intern Med* 142:2265-2268, 1982.

Limas CJ, Freis ED: Minoxidil in severe hypertension with renal failure: Effect of its addition to conventional antihypertensive drugs. *Am J Cardiol* 31:355-361, 1973.

Lissner L, et al: Variability of body weight and health outcomes in the Framingham population. *N Engl J Med* 324:1839-1844, 1991.

Lowenthal DT, et al: Efficacy of clonidine as transdermal therapeutic system: International clinical trial experience. *Am Heart J* 112:893-900, 1986.

Mansilla-Tinoco R, et al: Hydralazine, antinuclear antibodies, and lupus syndrome. *BMJ* 284:936-939, 1982.

Materson BJ, et al: Cigarette smoking interferes with treatment of hypertension. *Arch Intern Med* 148:2116-2119, 1988.

Materson BJ, et al: Treatment of hypertension in the elderly, I: Blood pressure and clinical changes: Results of a Department of Veterans Affairs Cooperative Study. *Hypertension* 15:348-360, 1990.

Materson BJ, et al: Single-drug therapy for hypertension in men: A comparison of six antihypertensive agents with placebo. *N Engl J Med* 328:914-921, 1993.

McDonough PM, et al: Further characterization of presynaptic alpha-1 receptor modulating ^{3}H ACh release from rat atria. *J Pharmacol Exp Ther* 238:612-617, 1986.

McGrattan PA, et al: Parasympathetic effects on in vivo rat heart can be regulated through an alpha-1 adrenergic receptor. *Circ Res* 60:465-471, 1987.

Medical Research Council Working Party: MRC trial of treatment of mild hypertension: Principal results. *BMJ* 291:97-104, 1985.

Medical Research Council Working Party: Stroke and coronary heart disease in mild hypertension: Risk factors and the value of treatment. *BMJ* 296:1565-1570, 1988.

Medical Research Council Working Party: Medical Research Council trial of treatment of hypertension in older adults: Principal results. *BMJ* 304:405-412, 1992.

National High Blood Pressure Education Program Working Group: National High Blood Education Program Working Group report on primary prevention of hypertension. *Arch Intern Med* 153:186-208, 1993.

National High Blood Pressure Education Program Working Group on High Blood Pressure in Pregnancy: Working group report on high blood pressure in pregnancy. *Am J Obstet Gynecol* 163:1689-1712, 1990.

Neaton JD, et al: Serum cholesterol level and mortality findings for men screened in the Multiple Risk Factor Intervention Trial. *Arch Intern Med* 152:1490-1500, 1992.

Neaton JD, et al: Treatment of Mild Hypertension Study: Final results. *JAMA* 270:713-724, 1993.

Participating Veterans Administration Medical Centers: Low doses v standard dose of reserpine: Randomized, double-blind, multiclinic trial in patients taking chlorthalidone. *JAMA* 248:2471-2477, 1982.

Perlman JM, Volpe JJ: Neurologic complications of captopril treatment of neonatal hypertension. *Pediatrics* 83:47-52, 1989.

Pfeffer MA, Pfeffer JM: Reversing cardiac hypertrophy in hypertension. *N Engl J Med* 322:1388-1390, 1990.

Pool JL, et al: Alpha$_1$-adrenoreceptor blockade and the molecular basis of lipid metabolism alterations. *J Hum Hypertens* 4 (suppl 3):23-33, 1990.

Rosenthal J: A multicenter trial of doxazosin in West Germany. *Am J Cardiol* 59:40G-45G, 1987.

Rouby J-J, et al: Resistance to sodium nitroprusside in hypertensive patients. *Crit Care Med* 10:301-304, 1982.

Samuelsson O, et al: Cardiovascular morbidity in relation to change in blood pressure and serum cholesterol levels in treated hypertension: Results from primary prevention trial in Göteborg, Sweden. *JAMA* 258:1768-1776, 1987.

Schnaper HW: The management of hypertension in older patients. *J Cardiovasc Pharmacol* 15 (suppl 2):S56-S61, 1990.

SHEP Cooperative Research Group: Prevention of stroke by antihypertensive drug treatment in older persons with isolated systolic hypertension: Final results of the Systolic Hypertension in the Elderly Program (SHEP). *JAMA* 265:3255-3264, 1991.

Stamler R: Implications of the INTERSALT study. *Hypertension* 179 (suppl I): I-16-I-20, 1991.

Stamler R, et al: Initial antihypertensive drug therapy: Final report of a randomized, controlled trial comparing alpha-blocker and diuretic. *Hypertension* 12:574-581, 1988.

Taylor SH: Clinical pharmacotherapeutics of doxazosin. *Am J Med* 87 (suppl 2A):2S-11S, 1989.

Taylor SH: Efficacy and safety of doxazosin in the treatment of patients with mild and moderate essential hypertension and elevated levels of cholesterol. *Am Heart J* 121:362-366, 1991.

Titmarsh S, Monk JP: Terazosin: Review of its pharmacodynamic and pharmacokinetic properties, and therapeutic efficacy in essential hypertension. *Drugs* 33:461-477, 1987.

The Trials of Hypertension Prevention Collaborative Research Group: The effects of nonpharmacologic interventions on blood pressure of persons with high normal levels: Results of the Trials of Hypertension Prevention, Phase I. *JAMA* 267:1213-1220, 1992.

Van Zwieten PA: Antihypertensive drugs interacting with alpha- and beta-adrenoceptors: A review of basic pharmacology. *Drugs* 35 (suppl 6):6-19, 1988.

Van Zwieten PA, et al: Role of alpha adrenoceptors in hypertension and in antihypertensive drug treatment. *Am J Med* 77:17-25, 1984.

Veterans Administration Cooperative Study Group on Antihypertensive Agents: Comparison of prazosin with hydralazine in patients receiving hydrochlorothiazide: Randomized, double-blind clinical trial. *Circulation* 64:772-779, 1981.

Veterans Administration Cooperative Study Group on Antihypertensive Agents: Comparison of propranolol and hydrochlorothiazide for initial treatment of hypertension: I. Results of short-term titration with emphasis on racial differences in response. II. Results of long-term therapy. *JAMA* 248:1996-2003, 2004-2011, 1982.

Veterans Administration Cooperative Study Group on Antihypertensive Agents: Low-dose captopril for treatment of mild to moderate hypertension: I. Results of 14-week trial. *Arch Intern Med* 144:1947-1953, 1984.

Wikstrand J, et al: Primary prevention with metoprolol in patients with hypertension: Mortality results from the MAPHY Study. *JAMA* 259:1976-1982, 1988.

Wilhelmsen L, et al: Beta-blockers versus diuretics in hypertensive men: Main results from the HAPPHY trial. *J Hypertens* 5:561-572, 1987.

Wilking SVB, et al: Determinants of isolated systolic hypertension. *JAMA* 260:3451-3455, 1988.

Wilson DJ, et al: Intravenous labetalol in treatment of severe hypertension and hypertensive emergencies. *Am J Med* 75(suppl 4A):95-102, 1983.

Wilson MF, et al: Comparison of guanfacine versus clonidine for efficacy, safety and occurrence of withdrawal syndrome in step-2 treatment of mild to moderate essential hypertension. *Am J Cardiol* 57:43E-49E, 1986.

Working Group on Hypertension in the Elderly: Statement on hypertension in the elderly. *JAMA* 256:70-74, 1986.

Young RA, Brogden RN: Doxazosin: A review of its pharmacodynamic and pharmacokinetic properties, and therapeutic efficacy in mild or moderate hypertension. *Drugs* 35:525-541, 1988.

Zeller KR, et al: Rapid reduction of severe asymptomatic hypertension: A prospective, controlled trial. *Arch Intern Med* 149:2186-2189, 1989.

Antianginal Drugs 26

ANGINA PECTORIS

ETIOLOGY. Angina pectoris develops when the supply of oxygen is insufficient to meet the demands of the heart (Brown and Kloner, 1990; Betriu et al, 1992; Wallace et al, 1990). This occurs when coronary blood flow is reduced and/or does not increase sufficiently at times of elevated myocardial oxygen requirement due to physical exertion (eg, exercise, manual labor, sexual intercourse) or emotion (eg, stress, anger, frustration). The ensuing ischemic episode usually lasts 15 seconds to 15 minutes. Symptoms include substernal discomfort; sensations of pressure, heaviness, or squeezing; and pain that may radiate to the shoulders, arms, neck, jaw, and epigastrium. Angina pectoris is exacerbated by exertion but is relieved within a few minutes by resting in a standing or sitting position or by sublingual nitroglycerin.

Age over 60 years; cigarette smoking; a family history of early heart disease; or the presence of diabetes mellitus, hyperlipidemia, or hypertension increase the likelihood that a patient with chest pain is suffering from angina pectoris. The risk of development of ischemic heart disease is further increased in premenopausal women who have any of these risk factors and are also using oral contraceptives.

Angina pectoris is categorized as stable or unstable (Brown and Kloner, 1990; Betriu et al, 1992).

Stable Angina: Patients in whom chest pain has remained unchanged in severity, frequency, and duration over a period of several weeks to several months have chronic stable angina. Mild ischemic episodes typically occur only after unusual physical exertion or emotional stress and do not require the patient to alter lifestyle to prevent the pain. In severe stable angina, attacks occur frequently and require modification of daily routines to exclude strenuous activities.

Unstable Angina: In unstable angina, transient myocardial ischemia is triggered by a wide range of conditions. Unstable angina includes new-onset angina; angina occurring at rest or with minimal exertion; progressive angina with more severe, prolonged, or frequent episodes superimposed on chronic stable angina; and angina after myocardial infarction.

Two other conditions that are difficult to differentiate initially from unstable angina with fixed coronary obstruction(s) are Prinzmetal's variant angina, which is not related to physical activity but is accompanied by transient ST-segment elevation, and microvascular angina (syndrome X), which is characterized by chest pain with ST-segment depression during exercise and reduced coronary blood flow reserve in normal coronary arteries.

PATHOGENESIS. Myocardial ischemia in patients with angina is usually caused by narrowing of coronary artery lumina with or without superimposed vasomotor constriction (spasm). Fixed narrowing of the coronary arteries is due to atherosclerotic plaque. Increased coronary obstruction caused by rupture of atherosclerotic plaque and thrombus formation are the principal mechanisms for unstable angina (Ambrose, 1992). The variable obstruction of the coronary arteries with increased coronary artery tone and vasospasm is caused by abnormalities in the release of the endothelial-relaxing factor (nitric oxide); endothelin; catecholamines; and various platelet-derived factors, including thromboxane and serotonin (Golino et al, 1991; McFadden et al, 1991). Patients with effort- or exercise-induced angina associated with ST-segment depression usually have fixed atherosclerotic narrowing, while those with Prinzmetal's variant angina suffer from pure coronary artery vasospasm. Patients with emotion-induced, cold-induced, or exercise-induced angina with variable threshold have both fixed atherosclerotic narrowing and vasospasm.

MANAGEMENT. Treatment of angina pectoris should be directed toward restoring sufficient myocardial oxygen supply while minimizing oxygen demand. The goals are to eradicate episodes of myocardial ischemia during routine activities, decrease progression of disease, and prevent cardiac events. Modification of cardiovascular risk factors (eg, hypercholesterolemia, decreased high-density lipoprotein [HDL] levels, increased low-density lipoprotein [LDL] levels, smoking), correction of concurrent disorders (eg, hypertension, arrhythmias, myocardial infarction, heart failure, aortic stenosis, anemia, hyperthyroidism), appropriate exercise, and antianginal drug therapy are all important measures in reducing ischemic episodes. When coronary artery disease is severe and both nonpharmacologic and pharmacologic measures fail, invasive procedures to improve coronary blood flow (percutaneous transluminal coronary angioplasty [PTCA] or coronary artery bypass graft [CABG]) may be considered.

In patients with elevated serum lipids, adherence to a diet low in cholesterol and saturated fat may prevent cardiac events and cause regression of atherosclerotic lesions. In obese patients, symptomatic improvement may follow weight reduction.

Cessation of smoking is particularly important, both to avoid the adverse effects of nicotine and carbon monoxide on the cardiovascular system and anginal symptoms and to eliminate one major factor that may accelerate atherosclerosis and precipitate thrombosis.

Activities or events that precipitate anginal attacks should be recognized and avoided when possible; precipitating factors include the consumption of heavy meals, recreational substance abuse (eg, cocaine) or heavy alcohol intake, undue emotional stress, exposure to cold air, and strenuous, unaccustomed exercise (particularly after meals). Many patients with angina benefit both physically and psychologically from an individualized, graduated exercise program (Franklin et al, 1992).

Patients with angina due to coronary artery disease generally are candidates for further risk assessment (stratification). Those with evidence of life-threatening conditions (eg, left main coronary artery obstruction) should be considered for invasive procedures (ie, CABG, PTCA), even if symptoms can be controlled with medication.

Drug Therapy: Three major classes of drugs, nitrates, beta-adrenergic blocking agents (propranolol, acebutolol, atenolol, betaxolol, carteolol, metoprolol, nadolol, penbutolol, pindolol, timolol), and calcium channel blocking drugs (diltiazem, nicardipine, nifedipine, verapamil, amlodipine, bepridil, felodipine, isradipine, nimodipine, nisoldipine [investigational drug]) are used alone or in combination to treat angina.

In *stable angina*, these drugs are used to increase blood flow to the ischemic myocardium and/or reduce myocardial oxygen requirements. Sublingual nitrates are given as needed to prevent or relieve acute attacks; beta-adrenergic blocking agents, calcium channel blocking agents, and oral, buccal, and topical nitrates are administered for long-term prophylaxis. When monotherapy is ineffective, addition of an agent from another class may enhance the antianginal effect of the first drug. For example, when nitrates are used with beta blockers, the preload-lowering effect of nitrates offsets the tendency of beta blockers to increase left ventricular volume and filling pressure, and the reflex tachycardia occasionally induced by nitrates can be blunted by the bradycardiac effect of beta blockers. However, the combined action of certain drug classes may cause adverse effects. For example, when nitrates and certain calcium channel blocking drugs are given together, reflex tachycardia, hypotension, and headaches may develop. Likewise, addition of a calcium channel blocking agent to a beta blocker regimen can further reduce myocardial oxygen consumption (Strauss and Parisi, 1988): Diltiazem or verapamil in combination with propranolol further attenuates the heart rate response during exercise; adding nifedipine to propranolol further lowers the systolic and diastolic blood pressure response to cold pressor and mental arithmetic stresses, whereas adding verapamil has been shown to blunt the blood pressure response to bicycle exercise. The major adverse effects of concomitant beta blockade and calcium channel blockade (eg, with verapamil or diltiazem) are electrophysiologic disorders (bradycardia, conduction disturbances) and hemodynamic disturbances (left ventricular failure, hypotension). With combination therapy, it is recommended that dosages, especially of beta blockers, be reduced to minimize adverse reactions.

Therapeutic goals in the treatment of *unstable angina* are to decrease myocardial ischemia promptly, preserve left ventricular function, and prevent myocardial infarction and death. Patients with unstable angina should be hospitalized for observation and restricted to bed rest. Those with transient ST-segment alterations associated with angina are easily diagnosed; those without ST-segment alterations frequently require further diagnostic evaluation. Any factor that may aggravate ischemia should be corrected.

Antianginal drug therapy (nitrates, beta-adrenergic blocking drugs, calcium channel blocking drugs, antiplatelet drugs, heparin) should be instituted. Intravenous nitroglycerin is often the drug of first choice but requires careful monitoring of blood pressure and heart rate. The dose of nitroglycerin can be increased until ischemic signs and symptoms are eliminated or until hemodynamic changes (eg, systolic pressure below 90 mm Hg) preclude further increases. Calcium channel blocking drugs help control anginal symptoms but do not prevent the development of myocardial infarction (Held et al, 1989). They should be used with caution in postinfarction patients with residual left ventricular dysfunction (see the chapter on Therapeutic Management of Myocardial Infarction). Calcium channel blocking drugs and nitrates are the most effective drugs for the treatment of variant angina.

Another goal in the treatment of angina is to block the development of thrombi and halt progression from stable angina to unstable angina to myocardial infarction (Brown and Kloner, 1990; Théroux, 1991; Chesebro and Fuster, 1992). This is partially achievable with conventional antithrombotic therapy using aspirin, heparin, or both. Aspirin protects against myocardial infarction and death during all phases of myocardial ischemia. Heparin is beneficial during the acute phase and reduces the incidence of myocardial infarction or recurrent refractory angina (Théroux, 1991). For patients with unstable angina, heparin therapy (partial thromboplastin time, 1.5 to 2 times control) should be administered continuously during the first few days. Before heparin is discontinued, aspirin (75 to 325 mg daily) should be given and continued indefinitely to prevent recurrence of ischemia (Théroux et al, 1992).

The specific role of thrombolytic therapy (eg, streptokinase, urokinase, tissue-type plasminogen activator) in the treatment of unstable angina has not been resolved (Ambrose and Alexopoulos, 1989).

Revascularization: Coronary artery bypass graft (CABG) and percutaneous transluminal coronary angioplasty (PTCA) also can relieve symptoms of angina (Wallace et al, 1990; Wong et al, 1990). The Veterans Administration Cooperative Study compared drug and CABG therapy in patients with unstable angina and found that CABG improved survival among those with lower ejection fractions (between 0.3 and 0.49) (Luchi et al, 1987). There was no difference in survival in patients with ejection fractions between 0.5 and 0.69, and drug therapy improved survival in patients with ejection fractions ≥0.7. CABG did not prevent myocardial infarction.

The use of PTCA in patients with mild angina and single-vessel coronary disease was compared with that of drug therapy in the ACME (Angioplasty Compared to Medicine) trial (Parisi et al, 1992). Both therapies relieved symptoms, but greater relief was observed in patients who had PTCA than in those receiving drugs. Twice as many of those in the PTCA group were free of ischemic discomfort one month after treatment; at six months, 64% of the PTCA group and 46% of the drug group were free of symptoms. In addition, patients in the PTCA group had a greater decrease in the frequency of angina attacks and a greater improvement in psychological well-being. The total exercise time, the maximal heart rate-blood pressure response, and the maximal duration of angina-free exercise were significantly greater in patients treated with PTCA. However, even though results of this trial showed certain short-term benefits with the use of PTCA in patients with single-vessel disease, inherent risks in the procedure include acute myocardial infarction, acute coronary occlusion requiring bypass surgery, and a later need for redilation to treat restenosis. Since survival is not improved by revascularization in patients with single-vessel disease, the value of PTCA to relieve symptoms, improve exercise tolerance, and reduce the need for antianginal medication must be weighed against the small but inherent risks and greater initial costs of the procedure.

PTCA also can be performed in patients with multivessel coronary artery disease, but complete revascularization occurs less frequently than in those with single-vessel disease (Bourassa et al, 1992).

Drug Evaluations

NITRATES

ACTIONS. Organic nitrates are direct-acting vasodilators. They are metabolized by vascular smooth muscle cells to form nitric oxide. The nitric oxide then interacts with endogenous thiols to form S-nitrosothiols, and both nitric oxide and S-nitrosothiols can activate guanylate cyclase to produce cyclic guanosine monophosphate (cGMP), which causes smooth muscle relaxation.

Nitrates reduce myocardial oxygen requirements by decreasing the venous tone of the systemic circulation, resulting in a pooling of blood in peripheral veins and in the splanchnic and mesenteric circulation; this leads to decreased venous return and reduced ventricular volume and myocardial tension (preload). At higher doses, nitrates also cause a moderate decrease in peripheral vascular resistance, which reduces arterial blood pressure and ventricular outflow resistance (afterload).

Nitrates increase myocardial oxygen supply by improving regional myocardial blood flow to ischemic areas. They dilate the large epicardial (conductance) arteries but have little effect on intramyocardial (resistance) vessels. In the normal nonischemic myocardium, coronary blood flow may increase temporarily and then decrease because of the fall in left ventricular wall tension and reduction in myocardial oxygen demand. In patients with coronary artery disease, nitrates relieve coronary artery spasm and dilate those epicardial coronary arteries and collateral vessels that are still capable of responding to vasodilation. These actions improve the regional distribution of myocardial blood flow, even though overall coronary blood flow may decrease (Abrams, 1988; Badger et al, 1985; Brown, 1985).

The beneficial effect of nitrates in stable angina is associated with a reduction in myocardial oxygen requirements. The increase in regional myocardial blood flow may contribute to the therapeutic response. In addition, nitrates dilate susceptible portions of the stenotic lesion itself, which may be a very important mechanism for alleviating ischemia in atherosclerotic anginal syndromes. It has been shown that stenotic constriction occurs during physical exertion in patients with stable angina, and this can be alleviated or prevented by nitroglycerin (Gage et al, 1986).

The beneficial effects of nitrates in unstable angina probably involve both coronary arterial dilation and reduced myocardial oxygen consumption. They also may include increased antiplatelet activity associated with nitrate-induced release of prostacyclin and stimulation of platelet guanylate cyclase (Stamler and Loscalzo, 1991). Nitrates relieve variant angina primarily through their vasodilator effect on the epicardial coronary arteries and also by reducing preload and afterload, thus reducing myocardial oxygen demand.

USES. Sublingual, oral, buccal, chewable, topical, and intravenous nitrates and a lingual aerosol spray are currently used in antianginal therapy.

Sublingual nitrates are given as needed to prevent or relieve acute attacks. Patients whose anginal pain is not relieved by adequate doses of sublingual nitrates are unlikely to benefit from long-acting formulations. Because of its more rapid action, long-established efficacy, and low cost, nitroglycerin (usual dose, 0.3 to 0.4 mg) is the drug of choice among sublingual preparations. When taken at the onset of ischemic discomfort in patients with stable or variant angina, pain is usually relieved within one to three minutes. Since chronic stable angina frequently subsides spontaneously with cessation of activity, nitroglycerin may be useful when taken prophylactically before beginning activities that are known to precipitate an attack. When exercise is not too strenuous, prophylaxis is effective for 20 to 30 minutes and occasionally for up to one hour. Sublingual isosorbide dinitrate may have a longer action (up to two hours).

Nitroglycerin lingual aerosol [Nitrolingual] appears to be as effective as sublingual nitroglycerin and has a comparable onset and duration of action. It may be particularly useful in patients with dry mucous membranes who have problems with dissolution of sublingual preparations (Parker et al, 1986). In contrast to nitroglycerin tablets, which deteriorate over three months, this product has a three-year shelf life.

The *oral nitrates* and *nitroglycerin ointment* have a longer duration of action than sublingual preparations. They are used for long-term prophylaxis of both effort-induced and rest angina. Tolerance to the antianginal action may develop to these preparations if a daily nitrate-free interval is not provided (Erhardt, 1987; Silber et al, 1987).

Buccal nitroglycerin [Nitrogard] may be as long acting as oral formulations, and its onset of action is comparable to that of sublingual nitrates. It is used both for acute relief of symptoms and for prophylaxis.

Transdermal nitroglycerin patches appear to be less effective when used continuously (eg, for 24 hours) because of the eventual development of tolerance (Crean et al, 1984; Leier, 1985; Thadani et al, 1986). Intermittent therapy (12 to 14 hours of wear) is recommended to reduce the risk of tolerance, and other antianginal drugs (beta blockers, calcium channel blockers) should be given concurrently to prevent ischemic episodes (Abrams, 1989).

Intravenous nitroglycerin relieves refractory ischemic chest pain (Mikolich et al, 1980) and is useful in hospitalized patients with severe unstable angina. Intravenous therapy provides more consistent control than oral or topical drugs during the first 24 hours of treatment (Curfman et al, 1983). Intravenous nitroglycerin also is given by the intracoronary route to identify or control vasospasm during coronary angiography, angioplasty, thrombolysis, and bypass surgery. Intracoronary nitroglycerin also can reverse coronary vasospasm induced by provocative testing with ergonovine.

ADVERSE REACTIONS. ***Hypotension and Tachycardia:*** Headache, flushing, and dizziness often are noted early during treatment but can be minimized by using small initial doses. Because of the pronounced action of nitrates on capacitance vessels, their therapeutic effect is enhanced (but adverse effects are increased) when the patient is in the upright position. Marked orthostatic hypotension and, rarely, syncope may occur, particularly if doses are repeated at short intervals; however, the risk of a hypotensive episode can often be diminished by reducing the dosage. The patient should be instructed to sit down before taking a tablet with a rapid onset of action in order to minimize the occurrence of syncope. Rarely, generalized vasodilation may cause profound hypotension and reflex tachycardia, and the fall in perfusion pressure may worsen the symptoms of angina. Excessive hypotension and reflex tachycardia can be avoided, especially during intravenous administration, by avoiding hypovolemia and titrating the dose carefully. Syncope and sweating may simulate symptoms of acute myocardial infarction. Hypovolemic effects can be relieved by immediate assumption of the supine position with elevation of the legs.

Bradycardia: In acute ischemic states, especially myocardial infarction, severe bradycardia occasionally may be associated with hypotension following administration of sublingual nitrates. Since the bradycardia is, at least in part, vagally mediated, it can be reversed by atropine as well as by raising the legs and tilting the head down (to increase central blood volume).

Cerebral Ischemia: Rarely, nitrate-induced hypotension can cause transient cerebral ischemia.

Alcohol Complications: The alcohol diluent (up to 70%) in intravenous preparations has occasionally caused intoxication in patients receiving large doses. Alcohol also may have a depressant effect on the heart and may alter serum uric acid levels and precipitate an acute attack of gout (Shergy et al, 1988). Concomitant intake of alcohol and nitrates may cause excessive hypotension and tachycardia.

Miscellaneous: Allergic contact dermatitis has occasionally been associated with nitroglycerin ointment or patches both in response to the nitroglycerin itself and to the adhesive material on the patches; anaphylactoid reactions have occurred rarely. Precipitation or aggravation of peripheral edema occasionally has been reported with both oral and topical therapy.

PRECAUTIONS. ***Tolerance:*** A steady high level of nitrates leads to a loss in blood vessel responsiveness that may be accompanied by attenuation of the therapeutic response. Loss of responsiveness may occur because sustained drug delivery saturates receptors and depletes intracellular reduced sulfhydryl groups, resulting in a decrease in the conversion of the nitrate molecule into the active vasodilating molecule, nitric oxide (Leier, 1985; Parker, 1992). Activation of neurohormonal systems and plasma volume expansion also may play a role (Abrams, 1989). Tolerance is not caused by increased hepatic metabolism, since plasma nitrate levels actually increase during long-term therapy.

Because sublingual nitrates have a short duration of action, continuous exposure of vascular smooth muscle to the drug is avoided and neither hemodynamic nor clinical tolerance has been a problem. However, their beneficial effect may be reduced transiently when cross-tolerance is caused by concomitant administration of topical or oral nitrate products.

Continuous intravenous infusion of nitroglycerin for 24 to 48 hours leads to attenuation of the drug's effect on the peripheral and coronary circulation (Elkayam et al, 1987; May et al, 1987) and loss of response to sublingual nitroglycerin (Zimrin et al, 1988). In emergency situations (eg, ongoing unstable angina), an adequate therapeutic response to intravenous nitroglycerin sometimes can be achieved by further escalations of dose. Tolerance does not develop during intermittent intravenous therapy (Packer et al, 1987).

Tolerance to the peripheral arterial effect of oral nitrates develops rapidly (within 48 hours when isosorbide dinitrate is given four times daily) and is associated with reduction in the hypotensive response to sublingual nitrates. When the oral nitrate is discontinued, the circulatory response to the sublingual drug is restored within 21 hours (Parker, 1992). Tolerance to the effect of oral nitrates on the venous capacitance vessels also has been described (Manyari et al, 1985). Attenuation of the response appears to be related to sustained plasma levels that are achieved with frequent administration or use of a prolonged-release preparation. To avoid the development of tolerance, the smallest effective dose should be administered and a drug-free interval (10 to 12 hours) should be provided, usually at night (Silber et al, 1987). Buccal nitroglycerin does not induce tolerance, presumably because the tablets are removed at bedtime (Parker et al, 1985).

When applied in doses that improve angina initially, transdermal nitroglycerin patches also are prone to produce tolerance (Crean et al, 1984; Thadani et al, 1986). Loss of responsiveness is apparently associated with sustained nitrate release over 24 hours. Intermittent therapy (ie, 12 hours of continuous use beginning in the morning with removal of the patch for 12 hours overnight) may prevent or reverse tolerance (Transdermal Nitroglycerin Cooperative Study Steering Committee, 1991; Thadani, 1987).

Acetylcysteine (Horowitz et al, 1988; May et al, 1987) or captopril (Metelitsa et al, 1992) may prevent or reverse tolerance by providing more sulfhydryl groups and hence potentiating the vasodilator effect of nitrates.

Dependence: Munitions workers exposed to high levels of nitroglycerin over prolonged periods have developed nitrate dependence. Anginal attacks and, rarely, myocardial infarction and sudden death occurred in some of these workers during withdrawal; these reactions appear to be caused by coronary artery spasm. Nitrate dependence is not common clinically, but rebound vasoconstriction has been documented, and a few fatalities have been reported after the drugs were discontinued abruptly. If nitrates are to be discontinued in patients who have been receiving large doses for prolonged periods, the dosage should be reduced gradually.

The possibility has been raised that withdrawal reactions may develop during drug-free intervals in patients receiving long-acting nitrates. In the Transderm-Nitro Trial, exercise performance of the placebo group was superior to that of the drug groups 12 hours after the patches were removed. In addition, nine patients experienced an exacerbation of angina and one died during a drug-free interval (DeMots and Glasser, 1989). To reduce the risk of aggravating myocardial ischemia during the drug-free intervals, other antianginal drugs (beta blockers, calcium channel blockers) should be prescribed (Abrams, 1989).

Cardioversion: Nitroglycerin patches should be removed before cardioversion to avoid formation of electrical arcs. Nitroglycerin ointment alters electrical resistance of the skin and should not be applied on areas where defibrillation paddles or ECG electrodes are placed.

Hypertrophic Cardiomyopathy: Nitrates should be avoided in patients with hypertrophic cardiomyopathy because they may increase outflow gradients (see index entry Cardiomyopathy).

Methemoglobinemia: Patients with NADH-methemoglobin reductase deficiency may develop methemoglobinemia when exposed to oxidant drugs such as nitrates. Asymptomatic methemoglobinemia also has occurred in patients without this enzyme deficiency who received very large doses of intravenous nitroglycerin.

Miscellaneous: The patient should be cautioned that nitroglycerin ointment or patches can be transferred to the skin of other individuals by direct contact.

DRUG INTERACTIONS. The hypotensive effect of nitrates may be enhanced by alcohol, beta blockers, calcium channel blocking agents, and tricyclic antidepressants. Delayed dissolution of sublingual nitrates due to dry mouth may occur in patients taking drugs with anticholinergic properties.

PHARMACOKINETICS. Organic nitrates are absorbed from the gut, the buccal or sublingual mucosa, and skin. The hepatic enzyme, glutathione-organic nitrate reductase, rapidly converts nitroglycerin to inorganic nitrite and denitrated metabolites, which have little or no vasodilator activity. Nitroglycerin also undergoes significant vascular clearance, and decreased vascular uptake may be more important than hepatic metabolism in attenuation of the therapeutic response. This would explain the observation that plasma nitrate levels increase during long-term administration.

After sublingual administration, peak plasma levels of nitroglycerin are attained in one to two minutes and the half-life is seven minutes. Peak plasma concentrations of 4 to 6 ng/ml are achieved after application of one to four inches of the 2% ointment to a three-by-three inch area on the arm, chest, or thigh. Concentrations achieved with nitroglycerin patches are considerably lower than those attained after use of the ointment (which covers a larger surface area).

Isosorbide dinitrate is metabolized by glutathione-organic nitrate reductase into 2-isosorbide mononitrate and 5-isosorbide mononitrate. The latter compound, which has vasodilator activity, is now approved for treatment of angina. The bioavailability of oral isosorbide dinitrate is approximately 30% and its half-life is brief; 5-isosorbide mononitrate is 100% bioavailable and has a half-life of five hours. Chronic administration of isosorbide dinitrate results in prolonged high plasma levels of both parent drug and metabolites.

DOSAGE AND PREPARATIONS.

SUBLINGUAL NITRATES

NITROGLYCERIN:

Sublingual: Individual sensitivity varies, and the dose must be individualized to relieve symptoms with minimal adverse effects. It is usually preferable to initiate therapy with the lowest dose. *Adults,* 0.15 to 0.6 mg; usual dose, 0.3 to 0.4 mg. If symptoms are not relieved by a single dose, additional or larger doses may be taken at five-minute intervals, but no more than three tablets should be used within a 15-minute period.

Conventional sublingual nitroglycerin tablets gradually lose potency through volatilization; therefore, the drug must be packaged in glass containers with tightly fitting metal screw caps and with no more than 100-dose units in each container. The tablets should be dispensed in the original unopened container, which should be closed tightly after each use. They should not be exposed to heat, and the bulk of the supply should be refrigerated. Stabilized tablets retain potency for a longer period than conventional tablets.

Nitrostat (Parke-Davis). Tablets (stabilized) 0.15, 0.3, 0.4, and 0.6 mg.

ISOSORBIDE DINITRATE:

Sublingual: *Adults,* 2.5 to 5 mg.

Isordil (Wyeth-Ayerst), ***Sorbitrate*** (ICI Pharma), ***Generic***. Tablets 2.5, 5, and 10 mg.

ERYTHRITYL TETRANITRATE:

Sublingual: *Adults,* 5 to 10 mg.

Cardilate (Burroughs Wellcome). Tablets 10 mg.

NITROGLYCERIN LINGUAL AEROSOL:

Lingual: *Adults,* one or two doses are sprayed into the mouth, preferably onto or under the tongue. Administration may be repeated every three to five minutes, but no more than three doses should be given in a 15-minute period.

Nitrolingual (Rhone-Poulenc Rorer). Aerosol 0.4 mg/metered dose.

BUCCAL NITROGLYCERIN

Buccal: *Adults,* initially, 1 mg three times daily every five hours during waking hours. If angina occurs while the tablet is in place, the dosage should be increased to the next tablet strength. The tablet should be placed between the lip and gum above the incisors or between the cheek and gum.

Nitrogard (Forest). Tablets (prolonged-release) 1, 2, 2.5, 3, and 5 mg.

TOPICAL NITRATES

NITROGLYCERIN OINTMENT 2%:

Topical: The 2% ointment contains 15 mg/inch. Initially, 1/2 inch is spread in a thin uniform layer over a 1 × 3 inch area of the skin, usually the chest or back. (It should not be applied on areas of the chest where defibrillation paddles or ECG electrodes are normally placed.) Plasma levels increase when the surface area of application is larger. Dosage and the area of application may be increased if necessary (eg, 1 inch on a 2 × 3 inch area, 2 inches on a 3 × 4 inch area, 3 inches on a 4 × 5 inch area). The frequency of administration recommended in the manufacturers' prescribing literature is every eight hours initially, increased if necessary to every six hours. It should be kept in mind, however, that more frequent application increases the risk of tolerance; therefore, administration three times daily with removal of remaining ointment at bedtime may be preferable.

Generic. Ointment 2% in 30 and 60 g containers.

Nitro-Bid (Marion Merrell Dow). Ointment 2% in 20 and 60 g containers and 1 g unit-dose pouches.

Nitrol (Adria). Ointment 2% in 3, 30, and 60 g containers.

TRANSDERMAL NITROGLYCERIN PREPARATIONS:

Topical: These products consist of a nitroglycerin-impregnated polymer bonded to an adhesive bandage or a liquid nitroglycerin reservoir with dose delivery regulated by a semipermeable membrane opposed to the skin. The delivery of nitroglycerin from the transdermal patches approaches zero-order kinetics and is similar to that with constant intravenous infusion. The amount of nitroglycerin delivered is directly proportional to the size of the patch. The unit is applied to the skin on a site free of hair and should not be placed on the distal parts of the extremities. A new unit should be applied once daily and replaced after bathing or if the product loosens. The application site should be changed each time a new unit is applied to avoid irritation. A nighttime treatment-free interval of 10 to 12 hours may reduce the risk of tolerance. See following table for preparations.

TRANSDERMAL PREPARATIONS

Tradename	Release Rate (mg/hr)	Surface Area (cm^2)	Nitroglycerin Content (mg/unit)
Generic	0.2	10	62.5
	0.4	20	125
Deponit (Schwarz)	0.2	16	16
	0.4	32	32
Minitran (3M Pharmaceuticals)	0.1	3.3	9
	0.2	6.7	18
	0.4	13.3	36
	0.6	20	54
Nitrodisc (Searle)	0.2	8	16
	0.3	12	24
	0.4	16	32
Nitro-Dur (Key)	0.1	5	20
	0.2	10	40
	0.3	15	60
	0.4	20	80
	0.6	30	120
Transderm-Nitro (Summit)	0.1	5	12.5
	0.2	10	25
	0.4	20	50
	0.6	30	75

ORAL NITRATES

ERYTHRITYL TETRANITRATE:

Oral: *Adults,* 10 mg before each meal, as well as at midmorning and midafternoon if needed, and at bedtime for patients subject to nocturnal attacks.

Cardilate (Burroughs Wellcome). Tablets 10 mg.

ISOSORBIDE DINITRATE:

Oral: *Adults,* the recommended maintenance dosage is 10 to 40 mg every six hours (regular preparation) or 40 to 80 mg every 8 to 12 hours (prolonged-release preparation). The risk of tolerance can be reduced by providing a nitrate-free interval, ie, the regular preparation may be taken two or three times daily during waking hours or the prolonged-release preparation may be taken once daily or twice daily at 8 AM and 2 PM (Silber et al, 1987).

Generic. Capsules (plain, prolonged-release) 40 mg; tablets (plain) 5, 10, 20, 30, and 40 mg; tablets (prolonged-release) 40 mg.

Dilatrate-SR (Reed & Carnrick), ***Iso-Bid*** (Geriatric). Capsules (prolonged-release) 40 mg.

Isordil (Wyeth-Ayerst). Tablets 5, 10, 20, 30, and 40 mg; capsules and tablets (prolonged-release) 40 mg.

Sorbitrate (ICI Pharma). Tablets 5, 10, 20, 30, and 40 mg; tablets (prolonged-release) 40 mg.

ISOSORBIDE MONONITRATE:

Oral: *Adults,* for maintenance, 20 mg twice daily; the first dose is taken on awakening and the second dose seven hours later.

ISMO (Wyeth-Ayerst). Tablets 20 mg.

NITROGLYCERIN:

Oral: *Adults,* the manufacturers recommend administration of the lowest effective dose at 8- to 12-hour intervals. The risk of tolerance is increased by frequent administration, and experience with other nitrate preparations suggests that a drug-free interval should be provided.

Generic. Capsules (prolonged-release) 2.5, 6.5, and 9 mg; tablets (prolonged-release) 6.5 and 9 mg.
Nitroglyn (Kenwood). Capsules (prolonged-release) 2.5, 6.5, 9, and 13 mg.
Nitrospan (Rhone-Poulenc Rorer). Capsules (prolonged-release) 2.5 and 6.5 mg.

PENTAERYTHRITOL TETRANITRATE:

Oral: *Adults,* initially, 10 to 20 mg four times daily, one-half hour before or one hour after meals and at bedtime. The dosage may be increased to a maximum of 40 mg four times daily. Alternative maximum dose, 80 mg on rising and 80 mg 12 hours later.

Generic. Capsules (plain, prolonged-release) 80 mg; tablets (plain) 10, 20, 40, and 80 mg; tablets (prolonged-release) 80 mg.
Duotrate (Jones Medical). Capsules (prolonged-release) 30 and 45 mg.
Peritrate (Parke-Davis). Tablets 10, 20, and 40 mg; tablets (prolonged-release) 80 mg (***Peritrate SA***).

INTRAVENOUS NITROGLYCERIN

Caution: Intravenous products of different manufacturers may differ in concentration and/or volume per vial, as well as the diluent to be employed. The manufacturers' literature should be consulted for dilution instructions, and care should be taken when substituting one preparation for another. Nitroglycerin should be diluted with dextrose 5% injection or sodium chloride injection 0.9% and should not be mixed with other drugs. *Glass* containers should be employed for dilution and storage. A solution containing 100 mcg/ml may be used for initial dosage titration; a more concentrated solution (≤400 mcg/ml) may be substituted if it is necessary to limit fluids.

Intravenous: *Adults,* initially, 5 to 10 mcg/min of dilute solution (0.5 to 1 mg/ml) is infused. Dosage may be increased gradually by 5 to 10 mcg/min every three to five minutes until a response is noted. If no response is observed with a dose of 20 mcg/min, increments of 10 and later 20 mcg/min may be employed. On occasion, it may be necessary to increase the infusion rate to 200 mcg/min or more to relieve chest pain, reduce pulmonary artery wedge pressure, and maintain near normal arterial perfusion pressure. Blood pressure and heart rate should be monitored continuously. To minimize tolerance, the infusion should be discontinued as soon as possible; for patients who require intravenous nitroglycerin for more than 24 hours, an intermittent infusion regimen should be established.

Generic. Solution (sterile) 5 mg/ml in 5, 10, and 20 ml containers.
Nitro-Bid IV (Marion Merrell Dow). Solution (sterile) 5 mg/ml in 1, 5, and 10 ml containers (alcohol 70%).
Tridil (DuPont). Solution (sterile) 0.5 mg/ml in 10 ml containers (alcohol 10%) and 5 mg/ml in 5, 10, and 20 ml containers (alcohol 30%) with or without delivery set (***Tridilset***).

BETA-ADRENERGIC BLOCKING DRUGS

The nature of beta adrenergic receptors and the actions, ancillary properties (cardioselectivity, partial agonist activity [PAA], membrane stabilizing properties, alpha blocking actions), chemical formulas, and pharmacokinetics of beta-adrenergic blocking drugs are discussed in detail in the chapter, Beta-Adrenergic Blocking Drugs.

Actions: The beta blockers used in the United States to treat angina are the beta$_1$-selective agents (acebutolol, atenolol, bisoprolol, and metoprolol) and the nonselective agents (carteolol, nadolol, penbutolol, propranolol, pindolol, and timolol). Acebutolol, carteolol, penbutolol, and pindolol have PAA. The beta$_1$ selective agent, betaxolol, is used primarily in antihypertensive therapy and there is little information on its use in angina. Esmolol, a short-acting beta$_1$-selective beta blocker available only for parenteral administration, has been used occasionally to treat unstable angina but generally is not given as sole therapy. Beta$_1$ selectivity, membrane-stabilizing properties, and lipid solubility are not required for the antianginal efficacy of beta blockers. However, beta$_1$ selectivity may lessen some side effects (eg, bronchospasm, peripheral vasospasm). In patients with stable angina, agents with PAA are as effective as those lacking this property (Thadani et al, 1980), but PAA may be associated with reduced efficacy in patients who have angina at rest or severe angina of effort (Quyyumi et al, 1984).

In chronic stable angina, beta blockers reduce the frequency of attacks, decrease nitrate requirements, and improve exercise tolerance. The beneficial effect of beta-blocking drugs derives from their ability to decrease heart rate and myocardial contractility, particularly during exercise. By attenuating the cardiac response to sympathetic stimulation, beta blockade reduces myocardial oxygen requirements and thereby delays the onset of ischemic pain. Blood pressure may be reduced by beta blockade to further decrease myocardial oxygen requirements. These drugs enhance the distribution of limited coronary blood flow; this is especially important for myocardial regions perfused by occluded coronary arteries. The oxygen-sparing effect of beta blockers usually compensates for the tendency of these drugs to increase left ventricular volume and prolong the systolic ejection period. Although administration of beta blockers theoretically might result in coronary vasoconstriction, quantitative coronary angiography performed on patients with stable angina revealed no significant constriction of normal or stenotic epicardial coronary arteries during beta blockade (Prida et al, 1987). In another angiographic study, beta blockade prevented the narrowing of stenotic coronary arteries induced by exercise (Gaglione et al, 1987).

Uses: In the absence of specific contraindications, a beta blocker should be considered for trial in all patients with frequent attacks of stable angina, particularly those who have had a myocardial infarction. This recommendation reflects the favorable effect of beta blockers on postinfarction mortality and reinfarction in addition to their antianginal efficacy. Beta blockers also are effective in suppressing silent ischemic episodes (DePing et al, 1989) and are useful in unstable angina (Lubsen and Tijssen, 1987). Nitrates should be continued, as needed, during beta blocker therapy. Nitrates and beta blockers reduce cardiac work by different mechanisms and thus have an additive effect in reducing myocardial oxygen demand. Beta blockers attenuate the reflex tachycardia induced by nitrates, while nitrates decrease preload and afterload, which may offset the negative inotropic effect of beta blockade.

The use of beta-blocking drugs in variant angina is controversial, and both beneficial and detrimental effects have been reported. Beta blockers generally are avoided but, if used, are seldom given as sole therapy for patients with documented vasospasm.

Transient myocardial ischemia in patients with microvascular angina is thought to be associated with heightened sympathetic nervous system activity, leading to an increase in myocardial oxygen demand. Beta blockers reduce spontaneous ST-segment depression in patients with this disorder (Bugiardini et al, 1989).

In normal volunteers, both selective and nonselective beta blockers attenuate the cardiovascular response to exercise and may diminish exercise performance, particularly during strenuous exercise, but beta blockade does not interfere with skeletal muscle metabolic adaptations (Wolfel et al, 1986). The beneficial effects of training in patients with coronary artery disease are not reduced by beta blockers (Froelicher et al, 1985). In patients with initially low levels of HDL cholesterol, beta blockade does not prevent the increase in this lipoprotein that is induced by exercise (Arvan and Rueda, 1988). Because an increase in parasympathetic tone contributes to training-induced bradycardia, heart rate remains a useful guide for evaluating the effects of physical training in patients receiving beta blockers.

Adequate beta blockade is achieved when the heart rate is 50 to 60 beats/min at rest and does not increase by more than 20 beats/min with moderate exercise (eg, climbing one flight of stairs). Once these rates are established, further increases in the dose of beta blockers can increase the likelihood of adverse effects while producing little clinical benefit. For dosage and preparations, see Table 1.

TABLE 1.
BETA-ADRENERGIC BLOCKING AGENTS

Drug*	Usual Dosage for Angina	Preparations
Acebutolol	***Oral:*** *Adults,* initially, 400 mg daily in two divided doses. Dosage may be increased gradually as needed to control symptoms.	***Sectral*** (Wyeth-Ayerst). Capsules 200 and 400 mg.
Atenolol	***Oral:*** *Adults,* 50, 100, or 200 mg once daily. The dosage interval should be increased in patients with impaired renal function.	***Tenormin*** (ICI Pharma), ***Generic.*** Tablets 25, 50, and 100 mg.
Betaxolol	***Oral:*** *Adults,* 20 to 40 mg once daily (Narahara et al, 1990).	***Kerlone*** (Searle). Tablets 10 and 20 mg.
Bisoprolol	***Oral:*** *Adults,* initially, 10 mg once daily. Dosage may be increased to 20 mg once daily. For patients with renal impairment, maximum daily dose is 10 mg.	***Zebeta*** (Lederle). Tablets 5 and 10 mg.
Carteolol	***Oral:*** *Adults,* information is not sufficient to recommend dosage; 20 to 40 mg once daily has been given.	***Cartrol*** (Abbott). Tablets 2.5 and 5 mg.
Metoprolol	***Oral:*** *Adults,* 50 mg three or four times daily. Twice-daily administration may be effective in some patients with stable angina.	***Lopressor*** (Geigy). Tablets 50 and 100 mg.
Nadolol	***Oral:*** *Adults,* initially, 40 mg once daily; the amount may be increased gradually by 40- to 80-mg increments at three- to seven-day intervals until the desired response is obtained. The usual maintenance dose is 40 or 80 mg once daily. Doses up to 240 mg once daily sometimes may be required. The dosage interval should be increased in patients with renal impairment. The following intervals are suggested: creatinine clearance >50: 24 hours; 31-50: 24-36 hours; 10-30: 24-48 hours; <10: 40-60 hours.	***Corgard*** (Bristol). Tablets 20, 40, 80, 120, and 160 mg.
Penbutolol	***Oral:*** *Adults,* initially, 20 mg once daily. The dose may be increased to 80 mg daily if response is not optimal (Heel et al, 1981).	***Levatol*** (Reed & Carnrick). Tablets 20 mg.
Pindolol	***Oral:*** *Adults,* 10 mg four times daily (Kostis et al, 1982).	***Visken*** (Sandoz). Tablets 5 and 10 mg.
Propranolol	***Oral:*** *Adults, regular preparation,* initially, 10 to 20 mg three or four times daily. The dosage may be increased gradually, as needed, to control symptoms. For maintenance, most patients require at least 160 to 240 mg daily, usually given in four divided doses. Some patients require up to 400 mg daily. Twice-daily administration may be effective in some patients with stable angina.	***Inderal*** (Wyeth-Ayerst), ***Generic.*** Tablets 10, 20, 40, 60, and 80 mg (***Generic*** only).
	Long-acting preparation, initially, 80 mg once daily. The dosage may be increased gradually at three- to seven-day intervals until the optimal response is obtained. The average maintenance dose is 160 mg once daily.	***Inderal LA*** (Wyeth-Ayerst), ***Generic.*** Capsules (prolonged-release) 60, 80, 120, and 160 mg.
Timolol	***Oral:*** *Adults,* 10 to 30 mg twice daily.	***Blocadren*** (Merck Sharp & Dohme), ***Generic.*** Tablets 5, 10, and 20 mg.

* *Sublingual and long-acting nitrates should be continued as needed.*

Adverse Reactions and Precautions: Beta blockers may precipitate heart failure in patients with inadequate cardiac reserve, worsen AV conduction disturbances, increase hypertriglyceridemia, provoke bronchospasm in asthmatic patients, exacerbate peripheral vascular disorders, impair defenses against insulin-induced hypoglycemia in patients with diabetes, and induce depression or other central nervous system disorders. Sudden withdrawal of a beta blocker in patients with severe angina may be followed by recurrence of unstable angina, ventricular tachycardia, myocardial infarction, and sudden death. For a more detailed discussion of these and other adverse reactions and interactions, see index entry Beta-Adrenergic Blocking Agents.

CALCIUM CHANNEL BLOCKING DRUGS

The role of calcium ions in cardiac and vascular smooth muscle function and the actions and pharmacokinetics of the calcium channel blocking drugs (calcium antagonists) are discussed in detail in the chapter, Calcium Channel Blocking Drugs.

The calcium antagonists available in the United States are the benzothiazepine, diltiazem; the diphenyalkylamine, verapamil; the pyrrolidineethanamine, bepridil; and the dihydropyridines, amlodipine, felodipine, isradipine, nifedipine, nicardipine, and nimodipine. (The latter drug has not been used widely as an antianginal agent.) Diltiazem and verapamil reduce heart rate, slow AV conduction, and reduce vascular resistance. Nifedipine is a potent vasodilator that triggers tachycardia with a reflex action and nullifies primary depression of the SA and AV nodes. The other dihydropyridines have actions similar to nifedipine. Calcium antagonists have a depressant effect on myocardial contractility, which is usually offset by the decrease in left ventricular afterload and reflex increase in sympathetic tone, especially with use of the dihydropyridines.

Calcium channel blockers alleviate symptoms of variant angina by relieving coronary artery spasm, thus increasing myocardial oxygen supply, as well as by reducing myocardial oxygen consumption. They prevent increases in coronary artery tone but have less effect than nitroglycerin on basal tone (Brown, 1985; Chew et al, 1983; Feldman et al, 1983; Hossack et al, 1984). Calcium antagonists probably are as effective as nitrates in variant angina. The effects of nifedipine, diltiazem, and verapamil in variant angina have been reported to be comparable (Johnson et al, 1981; Prida et al, 1987; Winniford et al, 1982).

In stable angina, calcium channel blockers reduce the frequency of attacks, decrease nitrate requirements, and improve exercise performance. Their beneficial effect appears to be due primarily to reduced myocardial oxygen demand (De Servi et al, 1986; Joyal et al, 1986). Studies comparing the relative efficacy of the calcium antagonists in patients with stable angina have yielded conflicting results (Dawson et al, 1981; Douard et al, 1989; Frishman et al, 1988; Gill et al, 1987; Klinke et al, 1988; Rodrigues et al, 1988; Johnston et al, 1985; Subramanian et al, 1982; Winniford et al, 1985).

A calcium antagonist may be indicated in stable angina when nitrates are ineffective or poorly tolerated or when beta blockers are contraindicated or produce intolerable side effects. Calcium channel blockers (and diltiazem in particular) also may be used as first-line therapy. Since these agents do not adversely affect airway resistance, they are preferred to beta blockers in patients with bronchospastic disorders. They also may be better tolerated in those with peripheral vascular disease, severe hypertriglyceridemia, or unstable insulin-dependent diabetes mellitus. These drugs may be used for angina after myocardial infarction, although in contrast to beta blockers, they do not appear to prevent recurrent infarction or death (Held et al, 1989).

Clinically important differences among the calcium channel blockers in their effects on myocardial contractility, cardiac conduction, and the peripheral circulation may influence drug selection. Reflex tachycardia occasionally leads to exacerbation of anginal symptoms in patients taking nifedipine or nicardipine. Verapamil and diltiazem usually cause mild bradycardia, which is beneficial in patients with angina. Verapamil has the most pronounced effect on AV nodal conduction and is the calcium antagonist of choice in patients with a coexisting supraventricular tachyarrhythmia. Diltiazem also may be useful in this setting.

Because the direct inhibitory influence of nifedipine and, presumably, other dihydropyridines on the SA and AV nodes is counteracted by reflex sympathetic activity, these calcium antagonists are less likely to precipitate conduction block than verapamil or diltiazem in patients receiving beta blockers and in those with AV conduction disturbances or sinus bradycardia. Diltiazem is less likely to produce severe bradycardia and conduction block than verapamil in patients receiving beta blockers (Strauss and Parisi, 1988).

Data directly comparing the effects of different calcium channel blockers are limited. Nifedipine and diltiazem appear to cause hypotension and congestive heart failure less frequently than other calcium channel blockers in patients with left ventricular dysfunction; however, the ability of calcium channel blockers to aggravate left ventricular dysfunction is well documented in individual patients. Furthermore, diltiazem has significantly increased the occurrence of late-onset congestive heart failure in postinfarction patients with reduced left ventricular ejection fractions (Goldstein et al, 1991). Nicardipine has the least cardiodepressant effect among the dihydropyridines (Visser et al, 1986), but even this agent may worsen heart failure in patients with severe left ventricular dysfunction.

Bepridil depresses the sodium channel current and prolongs cardiac repolarization, which may significantly increase QT-intervals, resulting in torsades de pointes. This drug is not appropriate for patients with hypotension and severe left ventricular dysfunction.

For dosages and preparations used in angina, see Table 2; for information on actions, adverse reactions, precautions, and interactions of individual drugs, see the chapter on Calcium Channel Blocking Drugs.

TABLE 2.
CALCIUM CHANNEL BLOCKING AGENTS

Drug[1]	Usual Dosage For Angina	Preparations
Amlodipine	***Oral:*** *Adults,* initially, 5 mg once daily. After two weeks, the dosage may be increased to 10 mg once daily. For the elderly and patients with hepatic dysfunction, initially, 2.5 mg once daily.	***Norvasc*** (Pfizer). Tablets 2.5, 5, and 10 mg.
Bepridil	***Oral:*** *Adults,* initially, 200 mg once daily. After ten days, the dosage may be increased. The long interval for dosage adjustment is needed because steady-state blood levels are not achieved until after eight days of therapy. Usual maintenance dose, 300 mg once daily (maximum, 400 mg once daily).	***Vascor*** (McNeil). Tablets 200, 300, and 400 mg.
Diltiazem	***Oral:*** *Adults, regular preparation,* initially, 30 mg four times daily before meals; the dose may be increased gradually to a maximum of 360 mg daily. *Prolonged-release preparation,* initially, 120 mg once daily.	***Cardizem*** (Marion Merrell Dow). Tablets 30, 60, 90, and 120 mg. ***Cardizem CD*** (Marion Merrell Dow). Capsules (prolonged-release) 120, 180, 240, and 300 mg.
Felodipine	***Oral:*** *Adults,* 10 mg once daily.	***Plendil*** (Merck Sharp & Dohme). Tablets (prolonged-release) 5 and 10 mg.
Isradipine	***Oral:*** *Adults,* initially, 2.5 mg once daily for two to four weeks. The dosage may be increased in 5-mg increments every two to four weeks until the optimal response is achieved. The maximum dose is 20 mg once daily.	***DynaCirc*** (Sandoz). Capsules 2.5 and 5 mg.
Nicardipine	***Oral:*** *Adults,* initially, 20 mg three times daily. After three days, dose may be increased. Maintenance dose, 20 to 40 mg three times daily.	***Cardene*** (Syntex). Capsules 20 and 30 mg.
Nifedipine	***Oral:*** *Adults, regular preparation,* initially, 10 mg three times daily. The usual effective dose range is 10 to 20 mg three times daily. Some patients, particularly those with variant angina, may require larger doses and/or more frequent administration, eg, 20 to 30 mg three or four times daily. Doses exceeding 180 mg daily are not recommended by the manufacturers. Dosage usually should be titrated over a 7- to 14-day period but may be adjusted more rapidly (eg, over a three-day period) if indicated. In hospitalized patients under close observation, the dose may be increased in 10-mg increments over four- to six-hour periods, but a single dose should rarely exceed 30 mg. *Prolonged-release preparation,* initially, 30 or 60 mg once daily.	***Adalat*** (Miles), ***Procardia*** (Pfizer), ***Generic.*** Capsules 10 and 20 mg. ***Procardia XL*** (Pfizer). Tablets (prolonged-release) 30, 60, or 90 mg.
Nisoldipine[2]	***Oral:*** *Adults,* 20 to 40 mg once daily.	***Syscor*** (Miles).
Verapamil	***Oral:*** *Adults,* 240 to 480 mg daily in three or four divided doses. Patients with severely impaired hepatic function should receive approximately 30% of this dose.	***Calan*** (Searle), ***Isoptin*** (Knoll), ***Verelan*** (Lederle, Wyeth-Ayerst), ***Generic.*** Tablets 40, 80, 120, and 240 mg.

[1] Sublingual and long-acting nitrates should be continued as needed.
[2] Investigational agent.

ANTIPLATELET DRUGS

ASPIRIN. Aspirin has reduced the incidence of myocardial infarction and cardiac death in patients with pre-existing chronic stable or unstable angina (Willard et al, 1992). In patients with stable angina, aspirin (325 mg on alternate days) reduced the incidence of first myocardial infarction by 87% over a five-year period. However, it did not reduce the frequency or severity of ischemic episodes (Ridker et al, 1991). Furthermore, results of the Physicians' Health Study demonstrated that aspirin did not prevent the development of angina in previously healthy subjects (Manson et al, 1990). Since anginal symptoms are not affected, aspirin probably acts by inhibiting the aggregation of platelets and the formation of thrombi at possible sites of plaque rupture rather than by modifying coronary atherosclerosis. In contrast, in patients with unstable angina, the antiplatelet effect of aspirin did reduce the frequency and severity of anginal attacks. Results of randomized, controlled trials showed that low doses of aspirin (75 mg daily) reduce the incidence of myocardial infarction and death from cardiac causes by 50% to 70% in patients with unstable angina (The RISC Group, 1990; Théroux, 1991; Wallentin and Research Group on Instability in Coronary Artery Disease in Southeast Sweden, 1991).

The most common adverse effects of aspirin are gastrointestinal intolerance and hemorrhagic events. Gastrointestinal intolerance may be minimized if the dose of aspirin does not exceed 300 mg daily or 325 mg every other day (The RISC Group, 1990; Willard et al, 1992). Hemorrhagic events, including easy bruising, melena, and epistaxes, are slightly more frequent in patients receiving aspirin than in those receiving placebo, but these effects are rare and mild when the dose is limited to approximately 75 mg daily (The RISC Group, 1990). See also index entry Aspirin, Uses.

OTHER ANTIPLATELET AGENTS. Several other antiplatelet agents have been evaluated alone or in combination with aspirin in patients with ischemic heart disease. Sulfinpyrazone and dipyridamole are less efficacious than aspirin (Willard et al, 1992). In contrast, ticlopidine (250 mg twice daily), which has a different mechanism of action, reduced the incidence of fatal and nonfatal myocardial infarction by approximately 50% following its administration for six months in patients with stable angina (Balsano et al, 1990).

HEPARIN

When administered by continuous intravenous infusion during the acute stage in patients with unstable refractory angina, heparin decreased the number of anginal attacks and silent ischemic episodes and reduced the overall daily duration of ischemia (Neri Serneri et al, 1990). The incidence of myocardial infarction or death also was significantly reduced (Théroux et al, 1988; Théroux, 1991). Bolus injection had no significant effect on these parameters (Neri Serneri et al, 1990; The RISC Group, 1990).

More than 10% of patients with unstable angina who received heparin alone experienced more severe reactivation of the disease process within a short period of time (median, 9.5 hours) following discontinuation of heparin (Théroux et al, 1992). The reactivation was manifested clinically as recurrent unstable angina, myocardial infarction, or both. Concomitant therapy with aspirin prevented this withdrawal phenomenon.

Cited References

Abrams J: Nitrates. *Med Clin North Am* 72:1-35, 1988.

Abrams J: Interval therapy to avoid nitrate tolerance: Paradise regained? *Am J Cardiol* 64:931-934, 1989.

Ambrose JA: Plaque disruption and the acute coronary syndromes of unstable angina and myocardial infarction: If the substrate is similar, why is the clinical presentation different? *J Am Coll Cardiol* 19:1653-1658, 1992.

Ambrose JA, Alexopoulos D: Thrombolysis in unstable angina: Will the beneficial effects of thrombolytic therapy in myocardial infarction apply to patients with unstable angina? editorial. *J Am Coll Cardiol* 13:1666-1671, 1989.

Arvan S, Rueda BG: Nonselective beta-receptor blocker effect on high density lipoprotein cholesterol after chronic exercise. *J Am Coll Cardiol* 12:662-668, 1988.

Badger RS, et al: Coronary artery dilation and hemodynamic responses after isosorbide dinitrate therapy in patients with coronary artery disease. *Am J Cardiol* 56:390-395, 1985.

Balsano F, et al: Antiplatelet treatment with ticlopidine in unstable angina: A controlled multicenter clinical trial. *Circulation* 82:17-26, 1990.

Betriu A, et al: Unstable angina: Outcome according to clinical presentation. *J Am Coll Cardiol* 19:1659-1663, 1992.

Bourassa MG, et al: Strategy of complete revascularization in patients with multivessel coronary artery disease (a report from the 1985-1986 NHLBI PTCA Registry). *Am J Cardiol* 70:174-178, 1992.

Brown BG: Response of normal and diseased epicardial coronary arteries to vasoactive drugs: Quantitative arteriographic studies. *Am J Cardiol* 56:23E-29E, 1985.

Brown E, Kloner RA: Angina pectoris. *Cardiovasc Rev Rep* 11:21-51, 1990.

Bugiardini R, et al: Comparison of verapamil versus propranolol therapy in syndrome X. *Am J Cardiol* 63:286-290, 1989.

Chesebro JH, Fuster V: Thrombosis in unstable angina, editorial. *N Engl J Med* 327:192-194, 1992.

Chew CYC, et al: Effects of verapamil on coronary hemodynamic function and vasomobility relative to its mechanism of antianginal action. *Am J Cardiol* 51:699-705, 1983.

Crean PA, et al: Failure of transdermal nitroglycerin to improve chronic stable angina: Randomized, placebo-controlled, double-blind, double-crossover trial. *Am Heart J* 108:1494-1500, 1984.

Curfman GD, et al: Intravenous nitroglycerin in treatment of spontaneous angina pectoris: Prospective, randomized trial. *Circulation* 67:276-282, 1983.

Dawson JR, et al: Calcium antagonist drugs in chronic stable angina: Comparison of verapamil and nifedipine. *Br Heart J* 46:508-512, 1981.

DeMots H, Glasser SP: Intermittent transdermal nitroglycerin therapy in the treatment of chronic stable angina. *J Am Coll Cardiol* 13:786-793, 1989.

DePing LD, et al: Noradrenergic activity and silent ischaemia in hypertensive patients with stable angina: Effect of metoprolol. *Lancet* 1:403-406, 1989.

De Servi S, et al: Effects of diltiazem on regional coronary hemodynamics during atrial pacing in patients with stable exertional angina: Implications for mechanism of action. *Circulation* 73:1248-1253, 1986.

Douard H, et al: Comparison of the anti-anginal efficacy of nicardipine and nifedipine in patients receiving atenolol: Randomized, double-blind, crossover study. *Int J Cardiol* 22:357-363, 1989.

Elkayam U, et al: Incidence of early tolerance to hemodynamic effects of continuous infusion of nitroglycerin in patients with coronary artery disease and heart failure. *Circulation* 76:577-584, 1987.

Erhardt L: Haemodynamic aspects of nitrate tolerance. *Drugs* 33(suppl 4):55-62, 1987.

Feldman RL, et al: Analysis of coronary responses to nifedipine alone and in combination with intracoronary nitroglycerin in patients with coronary artery disease. *Am Heart J* 105:651-658, 1983.

Franklin BA, et al: Amount of exercise necessary for the patient with coronary artery disease. *Am J Cardiol* 69:1426-1432, 1992.

Frishman W, et al: Diltiazem, nifedipine, and their combination in patients with stable angina pectoris: Effects on angina, exercise tolerance, and the ambulatory electrocardiographic ST segment. *Circulation* 77:774-786, 1988.

Froelicher V, et al: Can patients with coronary artery disease receiving beta blockers obtain training effect? *Am J Cardiol* 55:155D-161D, 1985.

Gage JE, et al: Vasoconstriction of stenotic coronary arteries during dynamic exercise in patients with classic angina pectoris: Reversibility by nitroglycerin. *Circulation* 73:865-876, 1986.

Gaglione A, et al: Is there coronary vasoconstriction after intracoronary beta-adrenergic blockade in patients with coronary artery disease? *J Am Coll Cardiol* 10:299-310, 1987.

Gill JB, et al: Improved left ventricular performance during exercise with verapamil or nifedipine in patients with chronic stable angina. *Am Heart J* 113:700-706, 1987.

Goldstein RE, et al: Diltiazem increases late-onset congestive heart failure in postinfarction patients with early reduction in ejection fraction. *Circulation* 83:52-60, 1991.

Golino P, et al: Divergent effects of serotonin on coronary-artery dimensions and blood flow in patients with coronary atherosclerosis and control patients. *N Engl J Med* 324:641-648, 1991.

Heel RC, et al: Penbutolol: Preliminary review of its pharmacological properties and therapeutic efficacy in hypertension and angina pectoris. *Drugs* 22:1-25, 1981.

Held PH, et al: Calcium channel blockers in acute myocardial infarction and unstable angina: An overview. *BMJ* 299:1187-1192, 1989.

Horowitz JD, et al: Combined use of nitroglycerin and *N*-acetylcysteine in the management of unstable angina pectoris. *Circulation* 77:787-794, 1988.

Hossack KF, et al: Diltiazem-induced blockade of sympathetically mediated constriction of normal and diseased coronary arteries: Lack of epicardial coronary dilatory effect in humans. *Circulation* 70:465-471, 1984.

Johnson SM, et al: Comparison of verapamil and nifedipine in treatment of variant angina pectoris: Preliminary observations in 10 patients. *Am J Cardiol* 47:1295-1300, 1981.

Johnston DL, et al: Clinical and hemodynamic evaluation of propranolol in combination with verapamil, nifedipine, and diltiazem in exertional angina pectoris: Placebo-controlled double-blind, randomized, crossover study. *Am J Cardiol* 55:680-687, 1985.

Joyal M, et al: Effects of diltiazem during tachycardia-induced angina pectoris. *Am J Cardiol* 57:10-14, 1986.

Klinke WP, et al: Randomized double-blind comparison of diltiazem and nifedipine in stable angina. *J Am Coll Cardiol* 12:1562-1567, 1988.

Kostis JB, et al: Treatment of angina pectoris with pindolol: Significance of intrinsic sympathomimetic activity of beta blockers. *Am Heart J* 104:496-503, 1982.

Leier CV: Nitrate tolerance. *Am Heart J* 110:224-232, 1985.

Lubsen J, Tijssen JEP: Efficacy of nifedipine and metoprolol in the early treatment of unstable angina in the coronary care unit: Findings from the Holland Interuniversity Nifedipine/Metoprolol Trial (HINT). *Am J Cardiol* 60:18A-25A, 1987.

Luchi RJ, et al: Comparison of medical and surgical treatment for unstable angina pectoris: Results of a Veterans Administration Cooperative Study. *N Engl J Med* 316:977-984, 1987.

Manson JE, et al: Aspirin in the primary prevention of angina pectoris in a randomized trial of United States physicians. *Am J Med* 89:772-776, 1990.

Manyari DE, et al: Isosorbide dinitrate and glyceryl trinitrate: Demonstration of cross tolerance in capacitance vessels. *Am J Cardiol* 55:927-931, 1985.

May DC, et al: In vivo induction and reversal of nitroglycerin tolerance in human coronary arteries. *N Engl J Med* 317:805-809, 1987.

McFadden EP, et al: Effect of intracoronary serotonin on coronary vessels in patients with stable angina and patients with variant angina. *N Engl J Med* 324:648-654, 1991.

Metelitsa VI, et al: Enhancement of the efficacy of isosorbide dinitrate by captopril in stable angina pectoris. *Am J Cardiol* 69:291-296, 1992.

Mikolich JR, et al: Relief of refractory angina with continuous intravenous infusion of nitroglycerin. *Chest* 77:375-379, 1980.

Narahara KA, et al: Double-blind comparison of once daily betaxolol versus propranolol four times daily in stable angina pectoris. *Am J Cardiol* 65:577-582, 1990.

Neri Serneri GG, et al: Effect of heparin, aspirin, or alteplase in reduction of myocardial ischaemia in refractory unstable angina. *Lancet* 335:615-618, 1990.

Packer M, et al: Prevention and reversal of nitrate tolerance in patients with congestive heart failure. *N Engl J Med* 317:799-804, 1987.

Parisi AF, et al: A comparison of angioplasty with medical therapy in the treatment of single-vessel coronary artery disease. *N Engl J Med* 326:10-16, 1992.

Parker JO: Update on nitrate tolerance. *Br J Clin Pharmacol* 34:11S-14S, 1992.

Parker JO, et al: Comparison of buccal nitroglycerin and oral isosorbide dinitrate for nitrate tolerance in stable angina pectoris. *Am J Cardiol* 56:724-728, 1985.

Parker JO, et al: Nitroglycerin lingual spray: Clinical efficacy and dose-response relation. *Am J Cardiol* 57:1-5, 1986.

Prida XE, et al: Comparison of diltiazem and nifedipine alone and in combination in patients with coronary artery spasm. *J Am Coll Cardiol* 9:412-419, 1987.

Quyyumi AA, et al: Effect of partial agonist activity in β blockers in severe angina pectoris: Double blind comparison of pindolol and atenolol. *BMJ* 289:951-953, 1984.

Ridker PM, et al: Low-dose aspirin therapy for chronic stable angina: A randomized, placebo-controlled clinical trial. *Ann Intern Med* 114:835-839, 1991.

The RISC Group: Risk of myocardial infarction and death during treatment with low dose aspirin and intravenous heparin in men with unstable coronary artery disease. *Lancet* 336:827-830, 1990.

Rodrigues EA, et al: Comparison of nicardipine and verapamil in the management of chronic stable angina. *Int J Cardiol* 18:357-369, 1988.

Shergy WJ, et al: Acute gouty arthritis and intravenous nitroglycerin. *Arch Intern Med* 148:2505-2506, 1988.

Silber S, et al: Induction and circumvention of nitrate tolerance applying different dosage intervals. *Am J Med* 83:860-870, 1987.

Stamler JS, Loscalzo J: The antiplatelet effects of organic nitrates and related nitroso compounds in vitro and in vivo and their relevance to cardiovascular disease. *J Am Coll Cardiol* 18:1529-1536, 1991.

Strauss WE, Parisi AF: Combined use of calcium-channel and beta-adrenergic blockers for the treatment of chronic stable angina: Rationale, efficacy, and adverse effects. *Ann Intern Med* 109:570-581, 1988.

Subramanian VB, et al: Randomized double-blind comparison of verapamil and nifedipine in chronic stable angina. *Am J Cardiol* 50:696-703, 1982.

Thadani U: Effectiveness of transcutaneous nitrate preparations for angina pectoris. *Int J Cardiol* 14:9-14, 1987.

Thadani U, et al: Comparison of five beta-adrenoreceptor antagonists with different ancillary properties during sustained twice daily therapy in angina pectoris. *Am J Med* 68:243-250, 1980.

Thadani U, et al: Transdermal nitroglycerin patches in angina pectoris: Dose titration, duration of effect, and rapid tolerance. *Ann Intern Med* 105:485-492, 1986.

Théroux P: Antiplatelet and antithrombotic therapy in unstable angina. *Am J Cardiol* 68:92B-98B, 1991.

Théroux P, et al: Aspirin, heparin, or both to treat acute unstable angina. *N Engl J Med* 319:1105-1111, 1988.

Théroux P, et al: Reactivation of unstable angina after the discontinuation of heparin. *N Engl J Med* 327:141-145, 1992.

Transdermal Nitroglycerin Cooperative Study Steering Committee: Acute and chronic antianginal efficacy of continuous twenty-four hour application of transdermal nitroglycerin. *Am J Cardiol* 68:1263-1273, 1991.

Visser CA, et al: Effects of intracoronary nicardipine and nifedipine on left ventricular function and coronary sinus blood flow. *Br J Clin Pharmacol* 22 (suppl 3):313S-318S, 1986.

Wallace WA, et al: Unstable angina pectoris. *Clin Cardiol* 13:679-686, 1990.

Wallentin LC, Research Group on Instability in Coronary Artery Disease in Southeast Sweden: Aspirin (75 mg/day) after an episode of unstable coronary artery disease: Long-term effects on the risk of myocardial infarction, occurrence of severe angina and the need for revascularization. *J Am Coll Cardiol* 18:1587-1593, 1991.

Willard JE, et al: The use of aspirin in ischemic heart disease. *N Engl J Med* 327:175-181, 1992.

Winniford MD, et al: Verapamil therapy for Prinzmetal's variant angina: Comparison with placebo and nifedipine. *Am J Cardiol* 50:913-918, 1982.

Winniford MD, et al: Propranolol-verapamil versus propranolol-nifedipine in severe angina pectoris of effort: Randomized double-blind, crossover study. *Am J Coll Cardiol* 55:281-285, 1985.

Wolfel EE, et al: Effects of selective and nonselective β–adrenergic blockade on mechanisms of exercise conditioning. *Circulation* 74:664-674, 1986.

Wong JB, et al: Myocardial revascularization for chronic stable angina: Analysis of the role of percutaneous transluminal coronary angioplasty based on data available in 1989. *Ann Intern Med* 113:852-871, 1990.

Zimrin D, et al: Antianginal effects of intravenous nitroglycerin over 24 hours. *Circulation* 77:1376-1384, 1988.

Antiarrhythmic Drugs

27

Arrhythmias are the leading cause of death from diseases involving the coronary artery.

MECHANISMS OF ARRHYTHMIAS

The performance of the myocardium depends on an ordered sequence of mechanical events involving the four chambers of the heart. Atrial and ventricular systoles are guided by a normally functioning cardiac conduction system in which pacemaker impulses from the sinus node first depolarize the atrial tissues, then propagate slowly through the atrioventricular (AV) node, and finally are distributed rapidly via the His-Purkinje network to the ventricles (Friedman, 1991). Arrhythmias are caused by disorders of electrical impulse formation and/or conduction.

Disorders of Impulse Formation: Automaticity is defined as spontaneous electrical activity arising from a specific focus in the myocardium. Abnormal automaticity is observed when the dominant pacemaker function of the sinus node is taken over by automatic cells in the atria, AV junction, His-Purkinje system, or ventricles. Pacemaker discharge from these ectopic sites may be initiated because the normal automaticity of the sinus node is depressed, as in some bradyarrhythmias, or because automaticity in other cells is enhanced, as in various types of premature ectopy and some tachyarrhythmias. Abnormal rhythms caused by altered automaticity also may occur when the sinus node is the dominant pacemaker but its rate of discharge is inappropriate (eg, sinus bradycardia).

Triggered activity, another cause of abnormal impulse formation, is precipitated by afterdepolarizations or transient oscillations in membrane potential that occur following the upstroke of the action potential (Zipes, 1991; Janse, 1992). Afterdepolarizations may be initiated by a variety of mechanisms, including a calcium current through L-type calcium channels, the sodium "window" or slowly inactivating current, a transient inward current activated by elevated intracellular calcium, intracellular potassium accumulation, the I_{X1} current, and the sodium calcium exchanger.

Afterdepolarizations may occur during repolarization (early afterdepolarization [EAD]) or may be delayed until repolarization is complete or nearly complete (delayed afterdepolarization [DAD]). When these depolarizations are strong enough to reach threshold, the action potential thus initiated is said to be triggered. EADs develop when the heart rate is slow, after long pauses, or when action potentials are otherwise prolonged (eg, by low levels of extracellular potassium, by use of drugs that prolong the action potential). The primary cause of DADs is intracellular calcium overload that results in repetitive release of calcium from the sarcoplasmic reticulum. Calcium overload may be associated with digitalis toxicity, enhanced adrenergic activity, and ischemia and reperfusion. Thus, arrhythmias induced by DADs are dependent on tachycardia, whereas those induced by EADs are dependent on bradycardia. In addition to arrhythmia, both EADs and DADs can cause premature ventricular complexes or contractions (Janse, 1992).

Disorders of Impulse Conduction: Clinically significant arrhythmias also arise from a disturbance of impulse conduction leading to reentry. When a propagating impulse cannot be conducted in the forward direction after encountering a blockage, it may proceed through an alternative and possibly slower pathway. This slowed impulse may be able to proceed in the retrograde direction over the site of orthograde blockage and reenter the initial impulse pathway, thereby completing a circuit. Hence, the primary requirements for reentry are slow conduction and unidirectional block; the pathway for reentry need not be circular. Functional, longitudinal conduction in parallel fiber bundles also may lead to reentry. More complex pathways, such as the figure of eight of El-Sherif, have been observed. The regions of slow conduction and unidirectional block often function without the presence of fixed anatomic structures. Functional abnormalities, including elevation of extracellular potassium concentration and intracellular and extracellular acidosis, may be caused by partial or complete occlusion of the coronary artery resulting in the formation of ischemic or infarct zones.

The initial phase of arrhythmia during acute myocardial infarction usually is due to reentry from the ischemic tissue. Conduction through this area worsens progressively and eventually most of the ischemic tissue becomes inexcitable, at which point the early-phase reentrant ventricular arrhythmias disappear. After six to eight hours, however, surviving subendocardial Purkinje fibers underlying the infarcted myocardium develop abnormal automaticity. Premature ventricular complexes arising from these fibers may trigger reentry (or triggered automaticity) in the border zone of the infarct, where depressed excitability and slow conduction continue. The early-phase ventricular arrhythmias that occur after coronary occlusion are the most likely cause of the 300,000 deaths annually in patients with acute myocardial infarction who die before reaching the hospital. The occurrence of late-phase ventricular arrhythmias necessitates cardiac monitoring for at least 72 hours in patients hospitalized with acute myocardial infarction.

DIAGNOSIS

Management of patients with rhythm disorders requires judgment, experience, and proper evaluation and integration of the results of electrocardiography (ECG) and must be individualized on the basis of the patient's clinical status (Friedman, 1991; Graboys, 1991). The differential diagnosis is facilitated by a classification of arrhythmias based on the width of the QRS interval and the uniformity of the RR cycle. When a tachycardia is observed, a logical progression in the differentiation of the rhythm is to determine if the QRS is wide or narrow and if the cycling is regular or irregular.

The major differential diagnoses include the following:

Regular tachycardia with a wide QRS interval	ventricular tachycardia (VT) supraventricular tachycardia (SVT) with aberration or preexcitation with antegrade accessory tract conduction
Irregular tachycardia with a wide QRS interval	atrial fibrillation with either aberration or fixed or rate-related bundle branch block
Regular tachycardia with a narrow QRS interval	sinus tachycardia paroxysmal tachycardia junctional tachycardia atrial flutter
Irregular tachycardia with a narrow QRS interval	atrial fibrillation multifocal atrial tachycardia (MAT)

In addition to data from the surface electrocardiogram, simultaneously recorded intracardiac (or esophageal) bipolar electrocardiograms from the high atrium (near the sinus node), left atrium, and His bundle region may be needed to diagnose AV conduction disorders.

GENERAL GUIDELINES FOR DRUG SELECTION

Antiarrhythmic agents may be grouped into four categories on the basis of microelectrode studies in isolated cardiac cells. Such classifications describe the drug's predominant electrophysiologic properties in normal tissue, usually Purkinje fibers. Some drugs exhibit characteristics of more than one class, have important indirect actions, have different effects in abnormal tissue, or have active metabolites with electrophysiologic properties different from those of the parent drug.

The drugs used to treat tachyarrhythmias and premature complexes reduce automaticity in ectopic foci and/or affect reentrant excitation by altering conduction velocity and the duration of the refractory period. Agents that increase sinus rate and enhance AV conduction are used occasionally in bradyarrhythmias. The actions and uses of these drugs are summarized in Tables 1 and 2.

Ambulatory electrocardiography (Holter monitoring) and invasive electrophysiologic testing are widely used to assess the response to antiarrhythmic drugs, especially following myocardial infarction (Zipes, 1985). Holter monitoring continuously records the electrocardiogram of an individual patient performing normal daily activities. A drug is considered effective by Holter monitoring when spontaneous ventricular arrhythmia (usually frequent or brief runs of premature ventricular contractions) is largely suppressed. Electrophysiologic testing involves programmed electrical stimulation (PES) to induce arrhythmia. A drug tested by electrophysiologic stimulation is considered effective if previously inducible ventricular tachycardia or fibrillation is no longer inducible by premature ventricular stimulation.

Drug selection often depends as much on tolerance of side effects and ease of administration as on efficacy. Most antiarrhythmic drugs have significant negative inotropic effects, and all should be used cautiously in patients with impaired left ventricular function (Gottlieb et al, 1990). Most antiarrhythmic drugs also have the potential to aggravate the arrhythmia that they are intended to suppress (proarrhythmia) (Kennedy, 1990). Proarrhythmia is more likely to occur in patients

TABLE 1.
AGENTS USED TO TREAT TACHYARRHYTHMIAS

Class/Drug	Actions	Major Uses
CLASS 1		
These drugs are subdivided into 3 categories	Interfere with fast inward depolarizing sodium current.	
CLASS 1A		
Quinidine	Depresses automaticity, particularly at ectopic sites; slows conduction and increases refractoriness of atria, His-Purkinje system, accessory pathways, and ventricles. Has both direct and indirect (anticholinergic) actions.	Maintenance of sinus rhythm after conversion of atrial fibrillation and flutter; maintenance therapy in patients with AV nodal reentrant tachycardia, automatic atrial tachycardia, and arrhythmias associated with the preexcitation syndrome; prevention of ventricular arrhythmias.
Procainamide	Similar to quinidine	Acute termination of supraventricular and ventricular arrhythmias, particularly those associated with the preexcitation syndrome, and maintenance therapy.
Disopyramide	Similar to quinidine	Similar to quinidine
CLASS 1B		
Lidocaine	Depresses automaticity and reduces duration of refractory period in the His-Purkinje system and ventricles. In therapeutic doses, does not slow AV nodal or intraventricular conduction, except in diseased myocardium.	Acute control of ventricular arrhythmias during acute myocardial infarction.
Mexiletine	Similar to lidocaine	Ventricular arrhythmias
Tocainide	Similar to lidocaine	Life-threatening ventricular arrhythmias
CLASS 1C		
Flecainide	Slows conduction in atria, AV node, ventricles, accessory pathways, and particularly in His-Purkinje system; to a lesser extent, increases atrial and ventricular refractoriness; suppresses sinus node automaticity.	Prevention and acute control of supraventricular tachycardia, including AV nodal and AV reentrant tachycardia and atrial fibrillation in patients with normal or near-normal left ventricular function. Refractory life-threatening ventricular arrhythmias.
Moricizine	Prolongs both AH and HV atrioventricular conduction times and PR and QRS intervals.	Life-threatening, sustained ventricular arrhythmias
Propafenone	Similar to flecainide. Also may possess weak beta-blocking and calcium-blocking properties.	Life-threatening ventricular arrhythmias, such as sustained ventricular tachycardia; arrhythmias associated with the preexcitation syndrome
CLASS 2		
Beta-adrenergic blocking agents (eg, propranolol)	Block cardiac beta receptors, thereby reducing sinus rate and myocardial contractility, lengthening AV nodal conduction time and refractoriness, and depressing sinus node automaticity.	Atrial fibrillation and flutter, primarily for rate control; AV nodal reentrant tachycardia; reciprocating tachycardia associated with the preexcitation syndrome; supraventricular and ventricular arrhythmias caused by increased sympathetic tone or circulating catecholamines and those associated with mitral valve prolapse syndrome; supraventricular arrhythmias in hypertrophic cardiomyopathy. Used for both acute control and maintenance therapy.

(table continued on next page)

TABLE 1 (continued)

Drug/Class	Actions	Major Uses
CLASS 2, 3		
Sotalol	Blocks cardiac beta receptors, prolongs atrial and ventricular refractoriness.	Life-threatening ventricular arrhythmias
CLASS 3		
Amiodarone	Increases refractoriness of sinus node, atria, AV node, ventricles, His-Purkinje system, and accessory pathways; depresses sinus node automaticity; slows conduction in atria, AV node, His-Purkinje system, and ventricles.	Prevention of severe, refractory arrhythmias, particularly ventricular tachycardia and fibrillation, atrial flutter and fibrillation in preexcitation syndrome.
Bretylium	After initial increase in automaticity (due to release of norepinephrine), increases refractory period of His-Purkinje system and ventricles without slowing conduction or depressing automaticity.	Prevention and acute control of ventricular tachycardia and fibrillation
CLASS 4		
Calcium channel blocking agents (verapamil, diltiazem)	Prolong AV nodal conduction time and refractoriness and decrease sinus node automaticity by interfering with calcium transport.	Supraventricular arrhythmias, particularly acute episodes of AV nodal reentrant tachycardia; atrial fibrillation and flutter, primarily for rate control (avoid in preexcitation syndrome); reciprocating tachycardia in the preexcitation syndrome.
OTHERS		
Adenosine	Depresses sinus node automaticity and AV nodal conduction.	Acute termination of AV nodal and reentrant tachycardia
Digitalis	Prolongs AV nodal conduction time and functional refractory period, mainly by indirect (cholinergic and antiadrenergic) actions. Slows sinus rate when ventricular function is impaired by virtue of its direct positive inotropic effect, which leads to a reduction in sympathetic stimulation.	Atrial fibrillation and flutter, primarily for rate control (avoid in preexcitation syndrome); AV nodal reentrant tachycardia; arrhythmias associated with congestive heart failure. Used for both acute control and maintenance therapy.

who have left ventricular dysfunction, ventricular fibrillation not related to infarction, or sustained ventricular tachycardia. Concomitant diuretic and digitalis therapy enhances the risk of proarrhythmia. The proarrhythmic effect is manifested by a significant increase in the density of single ectopic beats, emergence of nonsustained ventricular tachycardia, conversion of nonsustained to sustained ventricular tachycardia, or provocation of cardiac arrest (Graboys, 1991).

Class 1 antiarrhythmic agents are especially proarrhythmic in myocardial infarction patients. The Cardiac Arrhythmia Suppression Trial (CAST) was conducted to determine whether the suppression of asymptomatic or mildly symptomatic ventricular arrhythmias with antiarrhythmic drug therapy after myocardial infarction would reduce the incidence of deaths due to arrhythmia. Three Class 1C agents, flecainide [Tambocor], encainide [Enkaid], and moricizine [Ethmozine],

TABLE 2. AGENTS USED TO TREAT BRADYARRHYTHMIAS

Drug/Class	Actions	Major Uses
Atropine	Increases sinus rate and decreases AV nodal conduction time and effective refractory period by decreasing vagal tone.	Sinus bradycardia, sinoatrial arrest, sinoatrial block, type 1 second-degree AV block
Isoproterenol	Increases sinus rate and myocardial contractility, enhances automaticity, and shortens AV nodal conduction time and refractoriness by stimulating cardiac beta receptors.	Second- or third-degree AV block prior to pacing

were tested and found to be effective in suppressing premature ventricular contractions. However, the rates of death from all causes and sudden arrhythmic death in the group treated with placebo were lower than those in the group treated with encainide or flecainide (CAST Investigators, 1989). Over an average 10-month follow-up period, total mortality in the encainide- and flecainide-treated patients was 7.7% compared with 3% in the control group (Echt et al, 1991). Similarly, deaths caused by arrhythmia as well as nonfatal cardiac arrests occurred in 4.5% of the encainide- and flecainide-treated patients and in 1.2% of the placebo-treated patients. These findings led to discontinuation of the testing of flecainide and encainide.

Testing of moricizine was continued in the CAST II study with emphasis on postinfarction patients at greater risk of serious arrhythmia (Greene et al, 1992). Excessive mortality during the first and second week of administration of moricizine was noted. Long-term survival also did not improve; the survival rates of patients treated with moricizine were 95%, 90%, and 88% in the first, second, and third year of follow-up; these rates did not differ from those of patients treated with placebo (95%, 89%, and 85%, respectively). In addition, the rate of occurrence of adverse cardiac events was much higher in moricizine-treated patients (15.8%) than in placebo recipients (8.3%).

Beta-adrenergic blocking agents are the only antiarrhythmic drugs that have been shown to have a favorable effect on survival in the postinfarct patient. Although beta blockers are not potent antiarrhythmic drugs, they are usually well tolerated and the risk of organ toxicity is low.

The antiarrhythmic drugs, digitalis, quinidine, procainamide [Pronestyl, Procan], beta blockers, and lidocaine, appear to be relatively safe for treating arrhythmias in pregnant patients (Rotmensch et al, 1987).

A plasma therapeutic range has been delineated for many antiarrhythmic drugs (Table 3). Measurement of the plasma drug concentration may help assess compliance and facilitate dosage adjustment when age, disease states, or drug interactions alter drug absorption or disposition (Brown and Shand, 1982; Woosley, 1988). Determination of plasma drug levels also may be useful for evaluating therapeutic failure; however, many patients will not respond to a particular drug even if its plasma concentration is in the therapeutic range. Because bioequivalency problems have been reported occasionally, it has been recommended that once a drug has been found to control an arrhythmia, the brand should not be altered; if substitution becomes necessary, plasma drug concentrations should be measured to assure bioequivalency (Nolan, 1989).

For further information on pharmacokinetics, see Table 3.

TABLE 3.
PHARMACOKINETICS OF SELECTED ANTIARRHYTHMIC DRUGS

Drug	Bioavailability (%)	Half-life (hrs)	Protein Binding (%)	Excretion of Unchanged Drug (%)	Therapeutic Plasma Level (mcg/ml)
Adenosine	—	1.5 (sec)	—	—	—
Amiodarone	20-80	26-107 (days)	96	<1	0.5-2
Bretylium	<50	8-12	<1	70-80	not established
Disopyramide	83	8	68	50	2-4
Flecainide	90	20	40	27	0.2-1
Lidocaine	—	1.5-2	low	10	1.5-5
Mexiletine	88	8-10	70	8	0.5-2
Moricizine	40	1.5-3.5	95	<1	not established
Procainamide	75	3	15	50	4-10
N-acetylprocainamide	80	6	15	—	10-20
Propafenone	3-40	5-8	95	<1	not established
Quinidine	70-80	5-12	80-90	20	2.3-5
Tocainide	100	15	10-20	30-50	4-10

SUPRAVENTRICULAR TACHYARRHYTHMIAS

Supraventricular tachycardia encompasses a variety of rhythm disorders that originate at or above the AV node. These disorders are sinus tachycardia, paroxysmal supraventricular tachycardia (AV nodal reentrant tachycardia, AV reentrant tachycardia with concealed pathway, and sinus nodal or atrial reentrant tachycardia), atrial flutter, atrial fibrillation, ectopic or automatic atrial tachycardia, and multifocal atrial tachycardia.

Sinus Tachycardia: Sinus tachycardia is common and usually benign. Generally, the underlying cause (eg, increased sympathetic tone, thyrotoxicosis, fever, heart failure) should be determined and corrected rather than treating the sinus tachycardia as a primary disturbance. When therapy is indicated to control symptoms, a beta-adrenergic blocking agent (eg, propranolol [Inderal]) may be useful if heart failure is not present. Beta blockers slow a rapid sinus rate resulting from enhanced sympathetic tone or increased levels of circulating catecholamines. Digitalis may control sinus tachycardia associated with heart failure but is not useful when the increased sinus rate is due to other causes.

Atrial Tachycardia: Atrial tachycardia caused by premature atrial systoles (extrasystoles), parasystoles, or atrial escapes is relatively common and rarely requires therapy. Some of the precipitating factors for extrasystoles are excess caffeine, nicotine, or alcohol. Propranolol, quinidine, procainamide, or disopyramide [Norpace] may be useful if the premature complexes cause intractable symptoms or presage sustained arrhythmias.

Automatic atrial tachycardia is caused by enhanced automaticity and is associated with acute myocardial infarction, cardiomyopathy, chronic lung disease, or metabolic derangements. Digitalis toxicity also can be a cause, particularly if AV block is present. In the absence of correctable precipitating factors (eg, digitalis toxicity), symptomatic patients may be treated with antiarrhythmic drugs that depress automaticity, such as quinidine, procainamide, flecainide, or disopyramide.

Atrial Fibrillation: Atrial fibrillation is a common arrhythmia (prevalence approximately 2% in the general population and 5% in those over 60 years). The importance of treating atrial fibrillation is emphasized by its association with 6% to 24% of ischemic strokes and 50% of cardioembolic strokes. Atrial fibrillation often is associated with rheumatic valvular disease (20% to 30%) and nonvalvular conditions (70%), including coronary artery disease and hypertension (Albers et al, 1991). Coronary artery disease is present in about 50% of patients with this arrhythmia. It is a complication in 10% of those with myocardial infarction.

Therapy for atrial fibrillation includes cardioversion, rate control, and long-term anticoagulation for stroke prevention (Albers et al, 1991; Pritchett, 1992). Cardioversion can be accomplished electrically and pharmacologically. Direct-current (DC) cardioversion is the most rapid method for restoring sinus rhythm in a patient in whom atrial fibrillation causes hypotension, angina, or heart failure and is successful in about 85% to 90% of patients. With this technique, electrical energy is synchronized with the R-wave to depolarize the reentrant pathway and interrupt the circus movement. Pharmacologic cardioversion using quinidine, procainamide, disopyramide, flecainide, propafenone [Rythmol], or amiodarone [Cordarone] has been successful in up to 80% of patients. Since a large proportion of patients cannot maintain a normal sinus rhythm for a prolonged period of time following DC cardioversion, long-term antiarrhythmic drug therapy (with quinidine, procainamide, disopyramide, flecainide, or propafenone) may be needed to prevent recurrences of atrial fibrillation. However, the safety and efficacy of most antiarrhythmic drugs in this disorder have not been well studied and the risk of sudden death may be increased due to their proarrhythmic effects, especially in patients with structural defects (eg, infarction).

Digoxin, beta-adrenergic blocking drugs, and calcium channel blocking drugs have been used to reduce the rate of the ventricular response to atrial fibrillation. Digoxin is very effective in patients at rest, while beta blockers (eg, nadolol [Corgard], esmolol [Brevibloc]) and calcium channel blockers (eg, verapamil [Calan, Isoptin, Verelan], diltiazem [Cardizem]) are useful in reducing the heart rate during exercise and at the onset of atrial fibrillation. These agents do not restore sinus rhythm and hence are not appropriate for cardioversion.

The incidence of stroke associated with nonvalvular atrial fibrillation is about 5% per year and is higher in the elderly and in patients with severe heart failure, ventricular aneurysm, severe cardiomyopathy, cardiac thrombus, or a recent embolic event (Albers et al, 1991). Results of clinical trials conducted in the United States, Denmark, and Canada indicated that low-dose warfarin can reduce the incidence of stroke by 42% to 86% with minimal risk of significant hemorrhage in patients with atrial fibrillation. The dose of warfarin ranged from an international normalized ratio (INR) of 1.5 to 4.0, based on the prothrombin time ratio with the WHO reference thromboplastin as standard. Patients under 60 years with "lone" atrial fibrillation unaccompanied by evidence of coexisting cardiovascular disease appear to have a risk for stroke of less than 0.5% per year (Albers et al, 1991). Aspirin therapy (325 mg/day) may be more appropriate for this subgroup.

Atrial Flutter: DC cardioversion is the treatment of choice for this arrhythmia; rapid atrial pacing also has been used. Verapamil or diltiazem can be administered to slow the ventricular response rapidly prior to cardioversion. Quinidine, procainamide, or disopyramide may be used to decrease the risk of recurrence following restoration of sinus rhythm. Atrial flutter is more difficult to treat with digitalis. This glycoside may reduce the ventricular response to atrial flutter, but the large doses often required precipitate paroxysmal atrial tachycardia with block. Digitalis also may convert the flutter to atrial fibrillation, and only 50% of these patients attain normal sinus rhythm after a brief period.

AV Nodal Reentrant Tachycardia: AV nodal reentry is the most common cause of paroxysmal supraventricular tachycardia. This arrhythmia frequently is caused by the continuous movement of an electrical wave front over a pathway (reentry) involving the AV node or an associated atrial connection. The reentrant loop consists of dual pathways located within or around the AV node; anterograde conduction usually occurs over a pathway with slow conduction but a short refractory period, and retrograde conduction occurs over a pathway with fast conduction but a longer refractory period. The arrhythmia is often triggered by a premature atrial complex. AV nodal reentrant tachycardia is usually not associated with underlying heart disease, but it frequently causes symptoms and hemodynamic changes.

The treatment of this arrhythmia is based on measures that slow conduction and increase refractoriness in the AV node. Carotid sinus massage or other maneuvers that increase vagal tone will often terminate an acute episode. If not effective as the initial approach, vagal maneuvers may be repeated after each pharmacologic intervention. Carotid sinus massage should be employed cautiously in elderly patients because it occasionally causes hypotension, syncope, asystole, ventricular arrhythmias, and stroke.

When vagal maneuvers alone are ineffective, intravenous adenosine [Adenocard] is usually preferred for acute termination of AV nodal reentrant tachycardia in adults if the patient does not have sinus node disease or left ventricular dysfunction. Adenosine slows conduction and increases refractoriness in the anterograde limb of the AV nodal reentry circuit. Verapamil and diltiazem have similar actions and may be used in place of adenosine. Intravenous digitalis or intravenous propranolol also may be tried. Digitalis, the initial drug of choice in patients with impaired left ventricular function, acts by increasing vagal tone. Propranolol acts by decreasing sympathetic tone. Propranolol generally should not be given intravenously in close temporal proximity to intravenous verapamil.

Intravenous procainamide (which slows conduction in the retrogradely conducting pathway) may be required for acute termination of the arrhythmia when other drugs have failed. In some patients, DC cardioversion or (if digitalis has been given) atrial or ventricular pacing may be advisable. AV node modification with radiofrequency catheter ablation also has been used to treat AV nodal reentrant tachycardia.

Once the acute episode has been terminated, attention should be directed toward preventing recurrences if attacks are frequent or severe. This usually can be accomplished by instituting long-term oral therapy with digitalis and adding or substituting propranolol, verapamil, or diltiazem if necessary. In some patients, a drug that depresses conduction in the retrograde fast pathway (eg, flecainide, disopyramide) may be required.

In infants and young children, digitalis is the preferred drug for terminating AV nodal reentrant tachycardia; DC cardioversion is employed in emergencies. Although intravenous verapamil has been used successfully in some infants, it has caused severe bradycardia and hypotension in neonates with myocardial depression secondary to the arrhythmia (Kirk et al, 1987). Since recurrence is most common during the first year of life, digitalis is usually given prophylactically until age 6 to 12 months. Propranolol may be added if additional control is needed.

AV Reentrant Tachycardia With Concealed Pathway: Some cases of paroxysmal supraventricular tachycardia are caused by AV reentry over a concealed bypass tract that conducts only in a retrograde direction. The approach to terminating an acute episode of this form of tachycardia is the same as that used for AV nodal reentry. To prevent recurrences, an agent that depresses conduction and prolongs refractoriness in the accessory pathway may be required (eg, verapamil). The bypass tract can be interrupted surgically or by catheter ablation when symptoms are not controlled by drugs.

Sinus Nodal or Atrial Reentrant Tachycardia: Occasionally, the reentry circuit is confined to the sinus node or atria. Sinus nodal reentrant tachycardia, which may be difficult to distinguish from sinus tachycardia, is probably initiated by a premature atrial complex. It usually is not sustained. If symptomatic, the measures used to terminate AV nodal reentrant tachycardia may be tried. Intra-atrial reentrant tachycardia also has been described but is uncommon.

Multifocal (Chaotic) Atrial Tachycardia: This rhythm disturbance is usually attributed to enhanced automaticity or triggered activity and is encountered most frequently in patients with chronic pulmonary disease, diabetes, or advanced age. It is difficult to treat. Therapy is directed primarily toward the underlying disorder. Modification of bronchodilator therapy (eg, theophylline) may reduce the intensity of the tachycardia in patients with pulmonary disease.

Patients may respond to verapamil and metoprolol [Lopressor], which reduce atrial and ventricular rates and occasionally convert the arrhythmia to sinus rhythm (Hazard and Burnett, 1987; Levine et al, 1985).

PREEXCITATION SYNDROME (WOLFF-PARKINSON-WHITE SYNDROME)

Preexcitation results from accelerated transmission of impulses from the atrium to the ventricle via accessory pathways that bypass the normal physiologic delay at the AV junction. Preexcitation syndromes are common and occur more frequently in men than women. About two-thirds of patients have no evidence of associated organic heart disease; the remaining one-third have associated defects (eg, Ebstein's anomaly of the tricuspid valve).

The Wolff-Parkinson-White syndrome is one of the preexcitation disorders. The recurrent arrhythmias associated with this disorder are caused by a reentrant circuit involving the normal AV conduction system, an accessory pathway (Kent bundle) with a faster conduction velocity than the AV node, and the atria and ventricles. Usually, anterograde conduction occurs over the normal pathway and retrograde conduction over the bypass tract. The arrhythmia may be initiated by a premature atrial complex that blocks the accessory pathway and is conducted to the ventricle over the normal AV conducting system. The impulse then travels up the bypass tract in a retrograde direction to the atrium and reenters the AV node anterogradely. Less commonly, the accessory pathway serves as the anterograde limb and the AV conduction system as the retrograde limb; in approximately 10% of patients, multiple pathways are involved.

A reciprocating tachycardia is the most common arrhythmia in patients with the Wolff-Parkinson-White syndrome, and measures that prolong conduction in the AV node are used to manage an acute attack. Vagal maneuvers may be tried as the initial approach. When vagal maneuvers alone are ineffective and the refractory period of the accessory pathway is known to be long, intravenous adenosine, verapamil, or diltiazem is often the preferred drug for terminating the arrhythmia. If none of these agents are effective, propranolol or procainamide may be tried.

Atrial fibrillation or flutter in patients with the Wolff-Parkinson-White syndrome, is life-threatening because rapid AV conduction over the accessory pathway may precipitate fatal ventricular fibrillation. Catheter ablation of the accessory pathways with radiofrequency electrical energy appears to be the therapy of choice (Ruskin, 1991). The accessory AV pathways can be precisely located by intracardiac mapping. The lesions produced by radiofrequency current are small, homogeneous, less arrhythmogenic, and not associated with acute ventricular dysfunction. Supraventricular tachycardia is eliminated in 92% to 99% of patients with Wolff-Parkinson-White syndrome, and the procedure has an acceptable short-term safety profile (Calkins et al, 1991; Jackman et al, 1991; Kuck and Schluter, 1991). Surgical ablation also is effective but is less desirable because of the need for thoracotomy and cardiopulmonary bypass.

If ablation therapy must be deferred, quinidine, procainamide, disopyramide, flecainide, propafenone, or amiodarone can be given. These agents maintain sinus rhythm and block antegrade conduction over accessory pathways. Digitalis and calcium channel blockers have no effect on conduction over the accessory pathways and may cause rapid clinical deterioration (ie, ventricular fibrillation).

VENTRICULAR TACHYARRHYTHMIAS

Three or more consecutive rapid ventricular beats or premature ventricular complexes constitute an episode of ventricular tachycardia. The tachycardia is considered to be sustained if the rate exceeds 100 beats/minute and lasts longer than 30 seconds. Ventricular tachycardia that lasts less than 30 seconds and terminates spontaneously is considered to be nonsustained. Patients with nonsustained ventricular tachycardia usually are asymptomatic or mildly symptomatic (eg, palpitations, dizziness).

Ventricular tachycardia can be classified as benign, prognostically significant (potentially lethal), and malignant (lethal) (Bigger, 1983; Morganroth, 1984). Patients with premature ventricular complexes and no underlying heart disease have benign arrhythmias; epidemiologic data suggest that they are not at substantially increased risk of sudden death. Drug treatment is indicated only if the symptoms are sufficiently bothersome to justify the adverse reactions produced by antiarrhythmic drugs (eg, proarrhythmia).

In patients with organic heart disease (myocardial infarction, hypertrophic or dilated cardiomyopathy, or valvular disease) and ventricular ectopy characterized by frequent premature ventricular complexes or nonsustained ventricular tachycardia, the risk for subsequent cardiac mortality is significant. These patients (with prognostically significant tachycardia) are difficult to treat (Weiss et al, 1991) because suppression of the premature ventricular complexes with Class 1 agents (flecainide, encainide, or moricizine) has been shown to increase instead of decrease mortality (CAST Investigators, 1989; Greene et al, 1992). It is possible that other Class 1 agents (eg, propafenone, quinidine, procainamide, mexiletine [Mexitil]) may exert similar actions.

Currently, beta-adrenergic blocking agents are the only class of drugs that have proven to be effective as long-term therapy in clinical trials. These drugs are well tolerated and safe provided that no contraindications are present. They are particularly useful to prevent ventricular arrhythmias associated with myocardial ischemia and infarction and those precipitated by exercise. Beta blocking drugs are more effective in preventing ventricular fibrillation than in suppressing ventricular ectopy. In patients who have survived the acute phase of myocardial infarction, beta blockers reduce the risk of reinfarction and sudden death. This cardioprotective action (which is unrelated to suppression of ventricular ectopy) is observed in both $beta_1$ selective (eg, metoprolol) and nonselective (eg, propranolol) agents and for agents with partial agonist properties (eg, acebutolol [Sectral]). The beneficial effect of beta blockers in the postinfarct patient may be due to antiarrhythmic (particularly antifibrillatory), anti-ischemic, or other actions. High-risk patients have shown the greatest benefit (see index entry Beta-Adrenergic Blocking Agents, Uses, Myocardial Infarction).

Some Class 3 agents are effective in patients at risk of sudden death. Preliminary data indicate that amiodarone increased the survival rate of postinfarction patients who had premature ventricular complexes (Burkhart et al, 1990). The mortality rates for the placebo group, the group given conventional antiarrhythmic therapy to produce a defined degree of suppression of premature ventricular complexes, and the group treated with amiodarone were 13%, 12%, and 5%, respectively. In the Electrophysiologic Study Versus Electrocardiographic Monitoring Trial, sotalol was more efficacious than imipramine, pirmenol, mexiletine, quinidine, procainamide, and propafenone for patients with life-threatening ventricular tachycardia.

Patients with malignant or lethal ventricular arrhythmia have sustained ventricular tachycardia with a propensity to degenerate into ventricular fibrillation. Aggressive treatment has been assumed to be necessary because of the high one-year recurrence rate (30% to 40%). Antiarrhythmic agents may avert ventricular fibrillation by slowing the ventricular rate. Class 3 agents (eg, amiodarone, sotalol) appear to be effective in refractory ventricular tachycardia/fibrillation.

Since antiarrhythmic agents do not eliminate the anatomic substrate responsible for an arrhythmia, other therapy (surgery, catheter ablation, defibrillating and cardioversion devices) have been investigated for patients with lethal ventricular arrhythmia. Map-guided surgery (eg, subendocardial resection) can cure 60% to 80% of selected patients by excising or ablating arrhythmogenic tissue (Klein et al, 1987); however, the mortality rate may be greater than 15%. Catheter ablation of ventricular tachycardia has a success rate of 40% or less (Scheinman et al, 1991). Implantable defibrillating and cardioversion devices are the most recently developed therapy for lethal ventricular arrhythmias. Candidates for implantation include those surviving cardiac arrest, those with recurrent ventricular tachycardia/fibrillation, and those at high risk of sudden death in whom other treatment modalities are inappropriate. A two-year cumulative incidence of sudden death and total mortality among patients with the implanted device was 3.5% (historic control: 15% to 40%) and 13.6%, respectively (Akhtar et al, 1991). Although the incidence of sudden death in the implant recipients was comparatively lower than in those treated with pharmacologic suppression of premature ventricular complexes, empiric amiodarone, or with electrophysiologically guided therapy, the risk of death was higher within 30 days following implantation of the device. In addition, there is a possibility of false-positive defibrillator discharges, and some implant recipients experience psychological adjustment problems that result in anxiety and depression.

BRADYARRHYTHMIAS

Sinus Bradycardia: Sinus bradycardia may not require treatment if cardiac output is adequate. A rate of 50 to 60 beats/minute is usually well tolerated. Marked bradycardia (less than 50 beats/minute) associated with acute myocardial infarction may have serious arrhythmogenic or hemodynamic consequences. If the slow sinus rate is accompanied by hypotension or increased ventricular ectopy, atropine is usually indicated to increase the sinus rate; temporary pacing may be required in unresponsive patients. Because atropine occasionally causes myocardial ischemia and may precipitate severe ventricular arrhythmias, it should not be used routinely in asymptomatic patients.

Sinus Node Disorders: Autonomic blockade with propranolol and atropine has been used to differentiate autonomic dysfunction from intrinsic sinus node disorders, such as sinoatrial block and bradycardia-tachycardia syndrome. Drugs are of limited value for increasing the sinus rate long-term in the presence of intrinsic sinus node disease. Atropine or isoproterenol [Isuprel] may improve sinoatrial conduction for brief periods, and theophylline derivatives occasionally are effective in mild cases. Long-term results generally have been disappointing, because no drug reliably increases heart rate on a long-term basis without producing side effects. Permanent demand pacing is usually preferred if severe symptoms are associated with the bradycardia. Digitalis and other antiarrhythmic drugs can then be used to control any associated tachyarrhythmias.

AV Block and Intraventricular Block: *Primary first-degree AV block* with moderate PR prolongation (0.22 to 0.23 seconds) is a benign condition that rarely progresses to higher degrees of heart block; it does not require therapy (Mymin et al, 1986). In more advanced conduction disturbances, treatment is necessary if the heart rate is not sufficient to maintain an adequate cardiac output during rest and exercise or if other arrhythmias are present.

Type I (Wenckebach) second-degree AV block accompanying acute myocardial infarction is usually transient and is caused by increased vagal tone; it does not require pacing. Atropine may improve conduction in symptomatic patients. Rarely, atropine worsens block by increasing the sinus rate without improving AV conduction. It also may precipitate anginal attacks by increasing heart rate.

Type II second-degree AV block usually signifies a serious conduction disturbance in the His-Purkinje system and often requires temporary or permanent pacing. This conduction abnormality can progress rapidly to *third-degree (complete) AV block*, and the resulting sudden reduction in cardiac output may cause syncope and seizures (Stokes-Adams syndrome). Isoproterenol may improve cardiac output initially in symptomatic patients, but beneficial effects are usually transient. Isoproterenol is most commonly used to maintain heart rate and cardiac output prior to insertion of a pacemaker. Some individuals with complete AV block, particularly the congenital form, maintain an adequate ventricular escape rhythm without long-term drug or pacemaker therapy.

Patients with acute anterior myocardial infarction and *bundle branch* or *fascicular block* may require temporary pacing if the block is acute or is associated with more severe conduction disturbances. Chronic intraventricular block does not require permanent pacing unless there is evidence of AV block. Drugs are not useful for long-term treatment.

Drug Evaluations

AGENTS USED TO TREAT TACHYARRHYTHMIAS

ADENOSINE
[Adenocard]

NH_2 N N N N HOCH$_2$ O OH OH

ACTIONS. Adenosine is a naturally occurring purine nucleoside formed as a degradation product of adenosine triphosphate (ATP). This agent is a potent dilator of coronary arteries, and its antiadrenergic and negative chronotropic actions can decrease cardiac oxygen consumption (Camm and Garratt, 1991). Electrically, adenosine depresses the upstroke of the action potential of the 'N' cells of the AV node. Intravenous administration of bolus doses of adenosine suppresses sinus node automaticity and depresses AV nodal conduction

(DiMarco et al, 1990), resulting in a brief sinus bradycardia, followed by sinus tachycardia. A biphasic blood pressure response also is evident: there is an initial increase in both systolic and diastolic blood pressure at the time of the delay in AV conduction, followed by a decrease at the time of the secondary tachycardia.

USES. Adenosine is used as first-line therapy for acute termination of AV nodal reentrant tachycardia and other supraventricular tachycardias in which the reentry loop involves the AV node (DiMarco et al, 1985; Camm and Garratt, 1991). In a randomized trial comparing adenosine and verapamil in patients with spontaneous or induced paroxysmal supraventricular tachycardia, the two drugs were comparable in efficacy (DiMarco et al, 1990).

When administered during sinus rhythm to patients with a history of paroxysmal supraventricular tachycardia, adenosine may reveal latent preexcitation by slowing or blocking conduction to the ventricles through the AV node, thus demonstrating conduction by an accessory pathway (Camm and Garratt, 1991).

ADVERSE REACTIONS, PRECAUTIONS, AND INTERACTIONS. Symptomatic side effects are common and include transient nausea, metallic taste, dyspnea, chest pain, ventricular ectopy, headache, and flushing. The chest pain may radiate toward the ears, shoulders, ulnar aspect of the upper and lower arms, back, or upper abdomen. It may resemble the pain of cardiac ischemia in patients with chronic stable angina or mimic that of duodenal ulcer. However, since the half-life of adenosine is only 1.5 seconds, the duration of these side effects is brief.

Sinus arrest and atrial fibrillation have occurred rarely. Inhaled adenosine may cause bronchoconstriction in patients with asthma. Methylxanthines (eg, theophylline, caffeine) block both the therapeutic and adverse effects of adenosine.

This drug is classified in FDA Pregnancy Category C.

DOSAGE AND PREPARATIONS.
Intravenous: *Adults,* 6 mg given as a rapid intravenous bolus over one to two seconds. If the arrhythmia is not controlled within one to two minutes, 12 mg may be given as a rapid intravenous bolus. The 12-mg dose may be repeated if required. Individual doses larger than 12 mg are not recommended.

Adenocard (Fujisawa). Solution 3 mg/ml in 2 ml containers.

AMIODARONE HYDROCHLORIDE
[Cordarone]

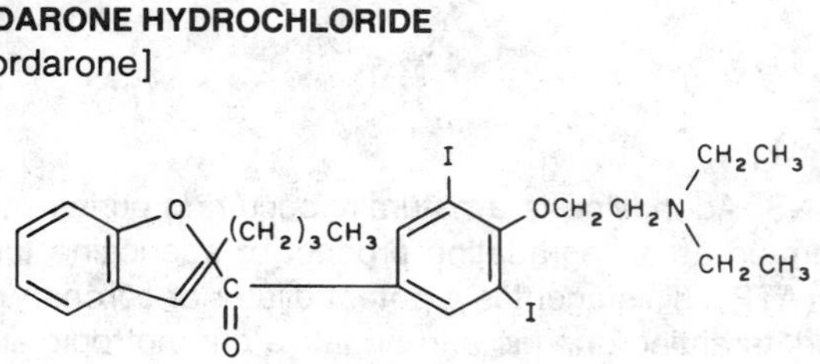

ACTIONS. Amiodarone, an iodine-containing benzofuran derivative, is related structurally to thyroxine. It possesses antiadrenergic and calcium channel blocking properties and exerts both antiarrhythmic and antianginal effects. After prolonged administration, the major electrophysiologic effect of amiodarone is an increase in refractoriness in all cardiac tissue, including the sinus node, atria, AV node, ventricles, His-Purkinje system, and bypass tracts. It also depresses sinus node automaticity and slows conduction in the atria, AV node, His-Purkinje system, and ventricles. After acute intravenous administration, the most prominent electrophysiologic effects of amiodarone are to slow conduction and prolong refractoriness of the AV node.

Amiodarone blocks the peripheral conversion of thyroxine (T_4) to its active metabolite, triiodothyronine (T_3), thereby increasing serum concentrations of reverse T_3. This abnormality in thyroid hormone metabolism may potentiate the direct effect of amiodarone on intraventricular conduction time, but does not explain the drug's long-term effects on ventricular refractoriness (Baerman et al, 1986; Morady et al, 1986).

During prolonged therapy, amiodarone has mild bradycardiac effects and reduces peripheral and coronary vascular resistance. A marked negative inotropic effect may occur following acute administration of intravenous amiodarone.

USES. This Class 3 drug is used to suppress refractory, life-threatening, recurrent ventricular arrhythmias. When given orally, it often is effective in suppressing recurrences of ventricular tachycardia or fibrillation. Amiodarone prevents recurrence of refractory ventricular arrhythmias in 50% to 70% of patients during the first year of treatment (Mason, 1987), but severe side effects or recurrence of the arrhythmia may limit its long-term usefulness.

Amiodarone also prevents recurrences of atrial flutter and fibrillation and AV nodal reentrant tachycardia. In a study on patients who did not respond to or could not tolerate quinidine, approximately two-thirds of those with paroxysmal and one-half of those with chronic atrial fibrillation were successfully maintained on amiodarone for an average of 15 months (Horowitz et al, 1985).

Because it prolongs refractoriness in both the AV node and accessory pathways in addition to slowing AV nodal conduction, amiodarone also has been used in patients with reciprocating tachycardia or atrial flutter and fibrillation associated with the Wolff-Parkinson-White syndrome (Zipes et al, 1984). It appears to be indicated primarily in those with recurrent refractory atrial fibrillation associated with ventricular preexcitation when catheter ablation or surgery is not feasible (Feld et al, 1988).

Amiodarone is employed with increasing frequency to prevent both supraventricular and ventricular arrhythmias in patients with hypertrophic cardiomyopathy. It may control episodes of tachycardia in patients with the bradycardia-tachycardia syndrome; because amiodarone may worsen bradycardia, a permanent pacemaker may be needed.

In a long-term follow-up of 242 patients treated with amiodarone, actuarial survival at 50 months was 66% for the total group, 74% for those with supraventricular arrhythmias, and 52% for those with ventricular arrhythmias (Smith et al, 1986).

Intravenous amiodarone (investigational preparation) is often effective for acute termination of recurrent, refractory life-threatening ventricular arrhythmias (Helmy et al, 1988; Nalos et al, 1991), including those occurring in critically ill patients with coronary artery disease (Ochi et al, 1989). It also has been used to terminate reentrant tachycardias (Holt et al, 1985), to slow the ventricular response to atrial fibrillation or flutter, and to treat multifocal atrial tachycardia.

ADVERSE REACTIONS AND PRECAUTIONS. Adverse effects are common, especially with prolonged therapy; many organ systems are affected. Up to one-third of patients discontinue treatment because of adverse reactions, some of which may be lethal (Mason, 1987).

Amiodarone may cause anorexia, nausea, vomiting, abdominal pain, and constipation (Wilson and Podrid, 1991). When large doses are required, the drug should be given with food to minimize gastrointestinal side effects. Headache, weakness, myalgia, tremor, ataxia, paresthesias, proximal muscle weakness, nystagmus, depression, insomnia, nightmares, and hallucinations also have been reported. Amiodarone-induced peripheral neuropathy is relatively common and is associated with histologic changes in nerve fibers.

Bradycardia, myocardial depression, hypotension, sinoatrial block, atropine-resistant AV block, refractory ventricular arrhythmias, fatal heart failure, cardiogenic shock, and cardiac arrest have occurred in patients taking amiodarone. Hypokalemia may contribute to the development of ventricular arrhythmias in some patients. Amiodarone is less arrhythmogenic than the Class 1 antiarrhythmic drugs, and prolongation of the QT interval during therapy appears to correlate with efficacy rather than toxicity (Torres et al, 1986). Transient ischemic attacks and stroke have been reported, but a cause-and-effect relationship has not been established. This drug should not be used in patients with severe sinus bradycardia or advanced AV block.

Lipofuscin deposits accumulate in the cornea of most patients during long-term therapy. These deposits, which are reported to be reversible, may cause photophobia, the appearance of colored halos around light, and, occasionally, reduced visual acuity. Anterior subcapsular lens opacities; isolated changes in the iris, ciliary body, choroid, and retina; and optic neuropathy also have been reported.

The drug often causes photosensitivity reactions, such as erythema and swelling of areas exposed to sunlight. It also may produce a persistent bluish discoloration of the skin and melanodermatitis due to the development of intracytoplasmic inclusions, which may represent phospholipid membranes associated with amiodarone or its metabolites (Waitzer et al, 1987). Petechiae, erythema nodosum, and other rashes also have been reported.

Amiodarone alters thyroid hormone metabolism and may induce clinical hypothyroidism or, less commonly, hyperthyroidism. Thyroid dysfunction may develop as early as one month or as late as three years after therapy is started and occasionally occurs after the drug is withdrawn. Amiodarone-induced hypothyroidism may require thyroid replacement therapy (which does not abolish the antiarrhythmic effect). Hyperthyroidism may lead to a worsening of arrhythmias and also may require treatment. Thyroid function should be monitored before treatment is begun and frequently during long-term therapy (Albert et al, 1987).

Elevated serum gonadotropin levels have been observed in men receiving amiodarone (Dobs et al, 1991). Although the mean free serum testosterone concentration was maintained, the elevated serum follicle-stimulating hormone and luteinizing hormone levels suggest testicular dysfunction. Amiodarone rarely accumulates in the gonads, and epididymitis causing sterility has been observed in men treated with this drug (Kirkali, 1988).

Pulmonary toxicity is one of the most serious adverse effects of amiodarone and has occurred in approximately 6% to 15% of patients. Common presenting symptoms include dyspnea (particularly with exertion), cough, fever, and malaise, which may mimic infection or heart failure (Kennedy et al, 1987). A reduction in lung diffusion capacity may precede overt clinical toxicity (Gleadhill et al, 1988; Horowitz, 1988). The main pathologic finding is a diffuse interstitial infiltrate of mononuclear cells associated with accumulation of foamy alveolar macrophages, although foamy macrophages also have been identified in patients without symptoms of toxicity (Kennedy et al, 1987).

Serum aminotransferase levels are frequently elevated during amiodarone therapy and may remain so for many months after the drug is discontinued. Elevated serum creatinine levels have been noted in some patients. Hypercholesterolemia, hyperglycemia, and hypertriglyceridemia have been reported. Hematologic reactions (bone marrow depression, thrombocytopenia), epididymitis, vasculitis, polyserositis, alopecia, and Reye's syndrome have occurred rarely.

Amiodarone crosses the placenta and has caused bradycardia in newborn infants of treated mothers. It is secreted in breast milk in concentrations estimated to be equivalent to a low maintenance dose. Amiodarone is classified in FDA Pregnancy Category C.

DRUG INTERACTIONS. Amiodarone enhances the effect of coumarin anticoagulants. The dose of the anticoagulant should be reduced by approximately 50% during concurrent therapy, and prothrombin time should be monitored frequently until a steady state is reached. This interaction is an important consideration when amiodarone is used to treat atrial fibrillation because many patients with this arrhythmia require anticoagulant therapy. The effect may persist for several months after amiodarone is discontinued.

Amiodarone increases serum levels of digoxin, quinidine, procainamide, flecainide, and phenytoin, and the interaction may cause symptoms of toxicity. Ventricular arrhythmias have been attributed to an interaction between amiodarone and Class 1 antiarrhythmic drugs. Hypokalemia also may increase the risk of ventricular arrhythmias. Symptomatic bradycardia or sinus arrest may occur if a beta blocker, digitalis, diltiazem, or verapamil is given to patients treated with amiodarone. Hypotension, bradycardia, and heart block have been reported as a result of an interaction between amiodarone and general anesthetics.

PHARMACOKINETICS. Absorption of amiodarone is slow and variable. During long-term treatment, the active desmethyl metabolite accumulates in plasma and the myocardium, and concentrations may exceed that of the parent compound.

The upper limit of the therapeutic range has not been determined. See also Table 3.

DOSAGE AND PREPARATIONS. Amiodarone has a slow onset of action. The full therapeutic response may not be evident for one week to three months, and effects may persist for 7 to 50 days or more after the drug is discontinued.

Oral: *Adults,* for refractory ventricular arrhythmias, initially, 800 mg to 1.6 g daily for one to three weeks, followed by 600 to 800 mg daily for one month. Thereafter, the usual maintenance dose is 400 mg/day. For supraventricular arrhythmias, 600 mg daily in three divided doses for one week, followed by 200 to 400 mg daily. Thereafter, the lowest effective dose (often 200 mg daily) should be given to minimize side effects. A maintenance dose of 200 mg on alternate days may be effective in some patients. For the bradycardia-tachycardia syndrome (with a pacemaker in place), initially, 200 mg twice daily, followed by 200 to 600 mg daily. *Children,* 3 to 20 mg/kg daily.

Cordarone (Wyeth-Ayerst). Tablets 200 mg.

Intravenous (Investigational): *Adults,* initially, up to 5 mg/kg given over a 5- to 15-minute period; this dose should *not* be repeated within 15 minutes. The drug may then be infused at a dosage of 600 mg to 1.2 g every 12 to 24 hours for several days.

Cordarone (Wyeth-Ayerst).

Beta-Adrenergic Blocking Drugs

The antiarrhythmic effects of these Class 2 drugs (see Table 4) have been attributed to two actions: blockade of postsynaptic cardiac beta-adrenergic receptors and membrane-stabilizing activity. The former action is the most important, because the direct membrane effect (Class 1 antiarrhythmic action) occurs only at concentrations in excess of those usually employed clinically. The cardiac effects of beta blockade include a reduction in heart rate and myocardial contractility, lengthening of AV nodal conduction time and refractoriness, and suppression of automaticity.

TABLE 4.
BETA-ADRENERGIC BLOCKING DRUGS

Drug	Characteristics	Antiarrhythmic Dosage	Preparations
Propranolol	Prototype, nonselective	***Oral:*** *Adults,* effective dose varies widely; 10 to 80 mg three or four times daily. Larger doses (up to 640 mg daily) may be required to suppress chronic ventricular arrhythmias. *Children,* 0.5 to 4 mg/kg daily in four divided doses. As much as 16 mg/kg daily has been used.	*Inderal* (Wyeth-Ayerst), *Generic.* Tablets 10, 20, 40, 60, 80, and 90 (generic only) mg.
		Intravenous: *Adults,* 0.1 to 0.15 mg/kg administered over ten minutes. *Children,* 0.01 to 0.15 mg/kg over ten minutes. The electrocardiogram and blood pressure should be monitored continuously. Smaller doses should be used or the drug avoided if there is a risk of myocardial depression.	*Inderal* (Wyeth-Ayerst), Generic. Solution (for injection) 1 mg/ml in 1 ml containers.
Acebutolol	Cardioselective with partial agonist activity	***Oral:*** *Adults,* initially, 200 mg twice daily, increased gradually as needed. The usual maintenance dose ranges from 400 mg to 1.2 g daily. Doses larger than 800 mg daily should be avoided in elderly patients.	*Sectral* (Wyeth-Ayerst). Capsules 200 and 400 mg.
Atenolol	Cardioselective, long-acting	***Oral:*** *Adults,* initially, 50 mg once daily. The dose may be increased to 100 to 200 mg daily. The dosage interval should be increased in patients with impaired renal function.	*Tenormin* (ICI), *Generic.* Tablets 25 (*Tenormin* only), 50, and 100 mg.
Betaxolol	Cardioselective	***Oral:*** *Adults,* initially, 10 mg once daily. The dose may be increased to 20 to 40 mg once daily.	*Kerlone* (Searle). Tablets 10 and 20 mg.

(table continued on next page)

TABLE 4 (continued)

Drug	Characteristics	Antiarrhythmic Dosage	Preparations
Esmolol	Cardioselective, short-acting	***Intravenous:*** *Adults,* initially, 500 mcg/kg/min for one minute, followed by 50 mcg/kg/min for four minutes. If an adequate response is not obtained within five minutes, initial dose is repeated, followed by maintenance infusion of 100 mcg/kg/min for four minutes. Titration procedure may be continued, repeating loading infusion (500 mcg/kg/min for one minute) and increasing maintenance infusion by increments of 50 mcg/kg/min (for four minutes). As the desired heart rate or a safety end-point (eg, lowered blood pressure) is approached, the loading infusion is omitted and maintenance infusion is reduced to 25 mcg/kg/min or lower. Also, if desired, the interval between titration steps is increased from 5 to 10 minutes.	*Brevibloc* (DuPont). Solution 10 and 250 mg/ml in 10 ml containers.
Metoprolol	Cardioselective	***Oral:*** *Adults,* 50 to 100 mg twice daily. ***Intravenous:*** *Adults,* 0.2 mg/kg.	*Lopressor* (Geigy). Tablets 50 and 100 mg. *Lopressor* (Geigy). Solution 1 mg/ml in 5 ml containers.
Nadolol	Nonselective, long-acting	***Oral:*** *Adults,* initially, 40 mg once daily. The dose may be increased gradually at weekly intervals as needed. The usual maintenance dose is 160 mg daily or less. The dosage interval should be increased in patients with impaired renal function.	*Corgard* (Bristol). Tablets 20, 40, 80, 120, and 160 mg.
Penbutolol	Nonselective	***Oral:*** *Adults,* initially, 20 mg once daily. The dose may be increased to 80 mg daily.	*Levatol* (Reed & Carnrick). Tablets 20 mg.
Pindolol	Nonselective with partial agonist activity	***Oral:*** *Adults,* initially, 5 mg twice daily. The dose may be adjusted in increments of 10 mg/day to a maximum of 60 mg/daily.	*Visken* (Sandoz). Tablets 5 and 10 mg.
Sotalol	Nonselective with Class 3 action	***Oral:*** *Adults,* initially, 80 mg twice daily. The dose may be increased to 240 or 320 mg daily.	*Betapace* (Berlex). Tablets 80, 160, and 240 mg.
Timolol	Nonselective	***Oral:*** *Adults,* 2.5 to 10 mg twice daily.	*Blocadren* (Merck Sharp & Dohme), *Generic.* Tablets 5, 10, and 20 mg.

One beta blocker, sotalol, has additional electrophysiologic properties along with Class 2 actions. Because sotalol prolongs the effective refractory period of Purkinje fibers and atrial and ventricular muscle, it also is classified as a Class 3 drug. It is effective in the treatment of lethal or potentially lethal ventricular arrhythmias (Anastasiou-Nana et al, 1991; Camm and Paul, 1990; Hohnloser et al, 1992).

PROPRANOLOL HYDROCHLORIDE

[Inderal]

For chemical formula, see index entry Beta-Adrenergic Blocking Agents.

USES. The major indications for propranolol as an antiarrhythmic agent are catecholamine-induced arrhythmias, atrial flutter and fibrillation, AV nodal reentrant tachycardia, and selected ventricular arrhythmias.

Propranolol prevents or terminates tachyarrhythmias caused by increased sympathetic tone or an excess of circulating catecholamines, including exercise-induced arrhythmias and those associated with pheochromocytoma. (In the latter, a beta blocker is used only after adequate alpha blockade has been established.) Because the electrophysiologic and therapeutic effects of several antiarrhythmic drugs are reversed by catecholamines, the addition of propranolol may prevent recurrence of arrhythmias.

Because it increases the refractory period of the AV node and prolongs AV nodal conduction time, propranolol often slows the ventricular rate in patients with chronic atrial fibrillation or flutter who are not adequately controlled at rest and during exercise by therapeutic doses of digitalis. This combined therapy represents one of the most important uses of propranolol in the management of arrhythmias. Propranolol also may be useful for short-term control and long-term treatment of AV nodal reentrant tachycardia.

Propranolol is less effective in suppressing ventricular ectopy than the Class 1 antiarrhythmic agents, but it possesses antifibrillatory properties. Plasma concentrations greater than those that produce beta blockade may be required to suppress ventricular arrhythmias. When given in large doses, propranolol is highly effective in preventing exercise-induced ventricular tachycardia; this effect may be associated with a reduction in plasma norepinephrine levels (Sokoloff et al, 1986).

Propranolol is often used as initial therapy for both atrial and ventricular arrhythmias in patients with the mitral valve prolapse syndrome. It is useful for treating ventricular arrhythmias associated with a prolonged QT interval, and appears to reduce the risk of syncope and sudden death when used for long-term therapy in patients with idiopathic long QT syndrome (Moss et al, 1985). Supraventricular arrhythmias associated with hypertrophic cardiomyopathy may respond to beta blockers, but other antiarrhythmic drugs are often needed to control life-threatening ventricular arrhythmias. Lidocaine or phenytoin is preferred to treat digitalis-induced arrhythmias, especially if AV block is present.

Long-term therapy with beta-blocking drugs reduces the risk of reinfarction and sudden death in patients who survive the acute phase of myocardial infarction. It is not known whether this protective effect is due to antifibrillatory, anti-ischemic, or other actions of these drugs (see index entry Beta-Adrenergic Blocking Agents, Uses, Myocardial Infarction).

ADVERSE REACTIONS, PRECAUTIONS, AND INTERACTIONS. The incidence of side effects with beta blockers is low compared with that observed with Class 1 antiarrhythmic drugs. Significant adverse effects include congestive heart failure, worsening of AV conduction disturbances, bradycardia, hypotension, and bronchospasm. Adverse hemodynamic and dromotropic effects may occur when propranolol is given with a calcium channel blocking drug. See index entry Beta-Adrenergic Blocking Agents for a detailed discussion of these and other adverse effects and drug interactions.

PHARMACOKINETICS. See index entry Beta-Adrenergic Blocking Agents.

DOSAGE AND PREPARATIONS. See Table 4.

ESMOLOL HYDROCHLORIDE

[Brevibloc]

For chemical formula, see index entry Beta-Adrenergic Blocking Agents.

This short-acting (half-life, nine minutes) cardioselective beta blocker is used for immediate control of the ventricular response to atrial fibrillation or flutter during and after surgery and in other situations requiring only short-term control. It also has been used for other supraventricular arrhythmias, unstable angina, acute myocardial infarction, and postoperative hypertension. An advantage of esmolol over other intravenous beta blockers is that its action can be terminated rapidly if adverse effects occur (Esmolol Research Group, 1986). Its efficacy is comparable to that of propranolol (Esmolol Multicenter Study Research Group, 1985).

ADVERSE REACTIONS AND PRECAUTIONS. Hypotension, the major adverse effect of esmolol, developed in more than one-third of patients in the multicenter studies and is much more common than with propranolol. In most cases, the hypotension was asymptomatic and rapidly reversible. The drug can cause phlebitis at the infusion site and must be administered in a dilute concentration (10 mg/ml). This can result in a significant fluid load during prolonged infusion. For other adverse effects of beta blockers, see index entry Beta-Adrenergic Blocking Agents.

DOSAGE AND PREPARATIONS. See Table 4.

SOTALOL

[Betapace]

For chemical formula, see index entry Beta-Adrenergic Blocking Agents.

ACTIONS. Sotalol is a nonselective beta-adrenergic blocking agent (Class 2) with no partial agonist or membrane-stabilizing activities (Singh et al, 1987). This drug also possesses Class 3 action, for it increases the duration of the cardiac action potential with a concomitant lengthening of the effective and absolute refractory period.

USES. Intravenous or oral administration of sotalol prevents reinduction of arrhythmias in patients with life-threatening ventricular arrhythmias and recurrence of inducible ventricular tachycardia by programmed electrical stimulation (Singh, 1990). It appears to be as effective as procainamide in suppressing premature ventricular contractions. Sotalol also controls resistant ventricular tachycardia and fibrillation in patients with acute myocardial infarction.

In the Electrophysiologic Study Versus Electrocardiographic Monitoring (ESVEM) Trial conducted to compare the effectiveness of the two procedures in selecting appropriate antiarrhythmic therapy for ventricular tachyarrhythmias, sotalol (320 mg/day) was more effective than imipramine, pirmenol, mexiletine, quinidine, procainamide, or propafenone in reducing the arrhythmia recurrence rate and all-cause mortality.

ADVERSE REACTIONS AND PRECAUTIONS. The adverse reactions of sotalol are due to a combination of its beta-adrenergic blocking action and its ability to lengthen the QT_c interval (Singh et al, 1987).

The frequency of side effects due to beta-blockade (tiredness, lassitude, impotence, depression, headache) is similar to that exhibited by other beta-adrenergic blocking agents. The side effects due to Class 3 action include AV block, bradycardia, hypotension and exacerbation of heart failure. In addition, life-threatening polymorphic ventricular tachycardia or torsades de pointes may occur with overdosage, in patients with renal failure or hypokalemia, or in those receiving concomitant medication that prolongs the QT interval (eg, quinidine, disopyramide, phenothiazines, tricyclic and tetracyclic antidepressants). Torsades de pointes that develops during sotalol administration may be treated by withdrawal of the drug, administration of isoprenaline, ventricular pacing, and correction of serum electrolyte imbalance.

PHARMACOKINETICS. See index entry Beta-Adrenergic Blocking Agents.

DOSAGE AND PREPARATIONS. See Table 4.

BRETYLIUM TOSYLATE
[Bretylol]

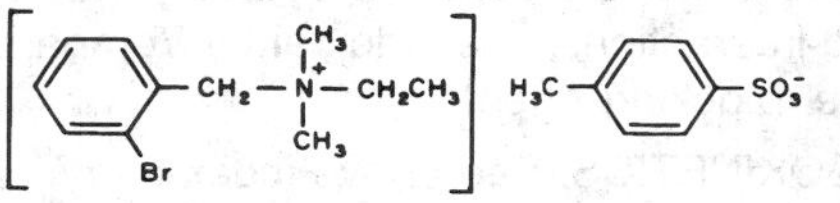

ACTIONS. The major direct effect of bretylium is to prolong action potential duration and refractory period of the His-Purkinje system and ventricles without affecting conduction or automaticity (Class 3). Bretylium also interacts with the sympathetic nervous system. It accumulates in sympathetic ganglia and postganglionic adrenergic neurons where it blocks adrenergic transmission by preventing the release of norepinephrine, thereby inducing a state resembling surgical sympathectomy. It does not antagonize (and may *increase*) sensitivity to circulating catecholamines. A transient increase in automaticity, heart rate, myocardial contractility, and blood pressure occurs prior to the onset of adrenergic neuron blockade; this effect is caused by the initial release of norepinephrine from sympathetic nerve terminals and can be prevented by propranolol. A temporal dissociation between the antiarrhythmic and antiadrenergic effects of bretylium has been noted.

USES. Bretylium is used for the prophylaxis and treatment of ventricular fibrillation and to treat ventricular tachycardia that has failed to respond to lidocaine and other agents. This drug may be more effective in preventing ventricular fibrillation than in suppressing premature ventricular complexes. Its antifibrillatory effects are usually noted within minutes, and it may terminate the arrhythmia, facilitate successful cardioversion, and prevent recurrences.

Bretylium has a delayed onset of action in suppressing ventricular ectopy and tachycardia; the maximal antiarrhythmic action may not be apparent for 20 minutes to 12 hours after injection. (See also Heissenbuttel and Bigger, 1979.)

ADVERSE REACTIONS AND PRECAUTIONS. The initial release of norepinephrine by bretylium may temporarily increase ventricular ectopic activity and elevate blood pressure. These effects may be enhanced if the patient is receiving vasopressor therapy or if the arrhythmia being treated is caused by digitalis toxicity. Bretylium generally should not be administered for digitalis-induced arrhythmias.

The initial pressor effect is followed (usually within one hour) by a fall in supine blood pressure, which is the most common (incidence, up to 66%) and most troublesome adverse reaction. Bretylium is particularly difficult to use in patients who are hypotensive. If the supine systolic pressure falls below 75 mm Hg, placing the patient in an upright position and administering intravenous fluids usually restores blood pressure to an acceptable level. Dopamine or norepinephrine may be infused, but the blood pressure should be monitored closely because bretylium enhances the pressor effect of catecholamines. Patients with severe aortic stenosis or pulmonary hypertension may be unable to increase cardiac output to compensate for a fall in peripheral resistance; if possible, bretylium should be avoided in these patients. It may be given if the arrhythmia is life-threatening, but the patient should be watched closely and vasoconstrictor amines given promptly if hypotension occurs.

Nausea and vomiting may occur, particularly when bretylium is given rapidly. Less common adverse effects include bradycardia, anginal attacks, diarrhea, abdominal pain, hiccups, erythematous macular rash, flushing, fever, sweating, nasal congestion, and mild conjunctivitis.

This drug is classified in FDA Pregnancy Category C.

PHARMACOKINETICS. See Table 3.

DOSAGE AND PREPARATIONS. Bretylium should be used on a short-term basis, and the blood pressure and electrocardiogram should be monitored continuously during therapy. Bretylium is eliminated by the kidneys as unchanged drug, and the dosage should be reduced in patients with impaired renal function.

Intravenous: For immediate control of life-threatening ventricular arrhythmias (particularly ventricular fibrillation), *adults,* 5 mg/kg of undiluted drug is given rapidly. If fibrillation persists, dosage may be increased to 10 mg/kg and repeated as necessary. For immediate control of other ventricular arrhythmias, *adults,* the contents of one ampul should be diluted with at least 50 ml of dextrose injection or sodium chloride injection and 5 to 10 mg/kg infused slowly over eight minutes or more to avoid nausea; the dose may be repeated in one to two hours. For maintenance, *adults,* a dilute solution may be infused continuously at a rate of 1 to 2 mg/min, or 5 to 10 mg/kg may be given by slow intermittent infusion every six hours.

Intramuscular: *Adults,* 5 to 10 mg/kg. Subsequent doses may be given at one- to two-hour intervals if the arrhythmia persists. Thereafter, this dosage is given every six to eight hours.

Bretylol (DuPont), ***Generic***. Solution (sterile) 50 mg/ml in 10 and 20 ml (***Bretylol*** only) containers.

Calcium Channel Blocking Drugs (Calcium Antagonists)

These Class 4 drugs selectively inhibit slow channel calcium ion transport in cardiac tissue. This slow inward current, which contributes to the plateau phase of the cardiac action potential, links myocardial excitation to contraction and controls energy storage and utilization. Action potentials from most specialized cardiac cells depend on both fast (sodium) and slow (calcium) channels, but the pacemaker cells of the SA node and cells in the N zone of the AV node (major site of conduction delay and block) are depolarized primarily by the calcium current. Verapamil and diltiazem have potent antiarrhythmic properties and are useful in treating reentrant tachycardias that incorporate the sinus or AV node. The other available calcium antagonists (amlodipine, felodipine, isradipine, nifedipine, nicardipine, and nimodipine) have minimal or no antiarrhythmic actions.

VERAPAMIL HYDROCHLORIDE

[Calan, Isoptin, Verelan]

For chemical formula, see index entry Verapamil, As Calcium Channel Blocking Agent.

ACTIONS. This synthetic derivative of papaverine blocks the slow (calcium) channel and also has a slight nonspecific sympathetic depressant effect. The antiarrhythmic properties of verapamil derive from its ability to delay impulse transmission through the AV node by a direct action. By increasing AV nodal conduction time and refractoriness, verapamil interrupts reentrant supraventricular tachycardias that incorporate the AV node and slows the ventricular response to rapid atrial rates. It does not significantly affect conduction in accessory pathways. Verapamil also has a direct depressant effect on the sinus node. The negative inotropic effect of verapamil is not prominent with therapeutic doses except in patients with significant heart failure or in those receiving other myocardial depressant drugs.

USES. Verapamil is effective when given intravenously to terminate an acute attack of AV nodal or sinus nodal reentrant tachycardia. It has a rapid onset of action (two to three minutes) and restores sinus rhythm in approximately 80% of patients. A short run of ventricular ectopy may occur during conversion. Intravenous verapamil also slows the ventricular response to atrial fibrillation or flutter. In multifocal atrial tachycardia, intravenous verapamil reduces both the atrial and ventricular rates and may convert the arrhythmia to sinus rhythm (Levine et al, 1985; Salerno et al, 1987).

Large oral doses of verapamil may prevent recurrences of AV nodal reentrant tachycardia; concurrent use of a beta blocker may be beneficial in patients who experience stress-related recurrence (Morady et al, 1989). However, such a combination should be employed cautiously because of potential additive negative inotropic effects.

The use of verapamil with moderate doses of digoxin produces less nighttime bradycardia than large doses of digoxin alone (Channer et al, 1987). The combination also provides better control of exercise-induced tachycardia than digitalis alone but does not improve exercise tolerance (Lewis and McDevitt, 1988). It should be kept in mind that verapamil can significantly increase serum digoxin levels, however.

Verapamil is given intravenously for some arrhythmias associated with the Wolff-Parkinson-White syndrome. Through its action on the AV node, verapamil terminates acute episodes of reciprocating tachycardia but it may be less effective in preventing recurrences. It should be avoided in patients with the Wolff-Parkinson-White syndrome who have or are at risk of developing atrial fibrillation or flutter because the ventricular response may be increased (Rinkenberger et al, 1980; McGovern et al, 1986). Intravenous verapamil is usually contraindicated in any tachycardia manifesting a wide QRS complex (Rankin et al, 1987).

ADVERSE REACTIONS, PRECAUTIONS, AND INTERACTIONS. Significant adverse effects of intravenous verapamil are hypotension, bradycardia, and worsening of AV conduction disturbances and heart failure. Concurrent beta blocker therapy increases the risk of hemodynamic deterioration. Adverse hemodynamic effects have occurred when verapamil was used to treat ventricular tachycardia thought to be of supraventricular origin (Stewart et al, 1986).

Verapamil is classified in FDA Pregnancy Category C.

For a more detailed discussion of these and other adverse effects and interactions, see index entry Verapamil, As Calcium Channel Blocking Agent.

PHARMACOKINETICS. See above index entry.

DOSAGE AND PREPARATIONS. The electrocardiogram and blood pressure should be monitored continuously.

Intravenous: *Adults,* 5 to 10 mg (0.075 to 0.15 mg/kg) given over two minutes (or three minutes in elderly patients). An additional 10 mg may be given if necessary in 30 minutes. For maintenance, infusions of 0.005 mg/kg/min have been employed. *Infants up to 1 year*, 0.1 to 0.2 mg/kg over two minutes, repeated if necessary in 30 minutes. *Children 1 to 15 years*, 0.1 to 0.3 mg/kg, repeated if necessary in 30 minutes. No more than 10 mg should be given as a single dose.

Isoptin (Knoll), ***Generic***. Solution 2.5 mg/ml in 2, 4, and 5 ml (generic only) containers.

Oral: *Adults*, 240 to 480 mg daily in two divided doses (prolonged-release form) or three or four divided doses (standard form).

Calan (Searle), ***Isoptin*** (Knoll), ***Generic***. Tablets 40, 80, and 120 mg; tablets (prolonged-release) 120, 180, and 240 mg (***Calan SR, Isoptin SR***).

Verelan (Lederle). Capsules 120, 180, and 240 mg.

DILTIAZEM HYDROCHLORIDE

[Cardizem]

For chemical formula, see index entry Diltiazem, As Calcium Channel Blocking Agent.

The actions of this calcium channel blocking drug are similar to those of verapamil. Like verapamil, it has been used intravenously for acute control of AV nodal reentrant tachycardia, atrial fibrillation and flutter, and other paroxysmal supraventricular tachycardias (Huycke et al, 1989; Salerno et al, 1989). In patients with the Wolff-Parkinson-White syndrome, it may be useful for acute control of AV reciprocating tachycardia (Shenasa et al, 1987); however, diltiazem is contraindicated in these patients when atrial fibrillation or flutter is associated with an accessory bypass tract.

When given orally with or without digitalis, diltiazem has been used for long-term control of supraventricular tachycardia caused by AV nodal reentry, AV reentrant tachycardia incorporating a concealed accessory pathway, and AV reciprocating tachycardia in the Wolff-Parkinson-White syndrome (Yeh et al, 1983).

For adverse reactions, precautions, interactions, and pharmacokinetics, see index entry Diltiazem, As Calcium Channel Blocking Agent.

DOSAGE AND PREPARATIONS.
Oral: *Adults,* 30 to 90 mg three or four times daily (standard form) or twice daily (prolonged-release form).

Generic. Tablets 30, 60, 90, and 120 mg.

Cardizem (Marion Merrell Dow). Tablets 30, 60, 90, and 120 mg; capsules (prolonged-release) 60, 90, and 120 mg (***Cardizem SR***); capsules (prolonged-release) 120, 180, 240, and 300 mg (***Cardizem CD***).

Intravenous: *Adults,* initially, 0.25 mg/kg (average 20 mg) as a bolus injection over a two-minute period. After 15 minutes, a second bolus dose of 0.35 mg/kg (average 25 mg) over two minutes can be given if needed. For maintenance, 5 to 10 mg/hr is infused for up to 24 hours. The infusion rate may be increased in 5 mg/hr increments to a maximum of 15 mg/hr.

Cardizem Injectable (Marion Merrell Dow). Solution 5 mg/ml in 5 and 10 ml containers.

DIGITALIS GLYCOSIDES

ACTIONS AND USES. The digitalis glycosides have complex direct and indirect effects on the heart. The actions that are of particular importance in antiarrhythmic therapy are lengthening of AV nodal conduction time and functional refractory period, which result from increased vagal tone; an antiadrenergic action; and, to a lesser extent, a direct effect. In addition, the positive inotropic effect of digitalis improves ventricular function and may thereby slow the sinus rate in patients with cardiac failure.

In atrial fibrillation or flutter, digitalis slows the ventricular response in patients at rest. Generally, a larger dose is required to slow the ventricular rate during atrial flutter than during atrial fibrillation, and the ventricular response to atrial flutter is often not easily controllable for prolonged periods (also see the Introduction). Digitalis may terminate AV nodal reentrant tachycardia after vagal maneuvers and other antiarrhythmic drugs have failed.

For the pharmacokinetics, adverse effects, interactions, and dosage and preparations of the digitalis glycosides, see index entry Digitalis, Uses, Heart Failure, Chronic.

DISOPYRAMIDE PHOSPHATE
[Norpace]

O
‖
N CNH_2 $CH(CH_3)_2$
$CCH_2CH_2\overset{+}{N}H$ $H_2PO_4^-$
$CH(CH_3)_2$

ACTIONS AND USES. The electrophysiologic effects of this Class 1A drug are similar to those of quinidine. It also has both direct and anticholinergic actions and local anesthetic properties. Disopyramide has a significant negative inotropic effect, and in contrast to quinidine and procainamide, it causes peripheral vasoconstriction.

Disopyramide is used orally for the same indications as quinidine. It prevents ventricular extrasystoles and ventricular tachycardia and is effective for atrial fibrillation. There is more limited experience with its use in supraventricular tachycardia.

ADVERSE REACTIONS, PRECAUTIONS, AND INTERACTIONS. The most common side effects are related to disopyramide's anticholinergic activity and include dryness of the mouth, blurred vision, constipation, and urinary retention. Efficacy is seldom achieved without mild anticholinergic side effects. Rarely, an attack of acute angle-closure glaucoma has been precipitated. Pyridostigmine was reported to reverse the anticholinergic effects of disopyramide without antagonizing its antiarrhythmic properties (Teichman et al, 1987).

Nausea, vomiting, gastric pain, and diarrhea may occur, but these reactions are less common with disopyramide than with quinidine.

Disopyramide has both a negative inotropic action and a vasoconstrictor effect, and this combination may precipitate heart failure in poorly compensated patients, even those receiving digitalis and diuretics. Heart failure may be more common with disopyramide than with other antiarrhythmic agents (Podrid et al, 1980). Severe myocardial depression may lead to profound hypotension, sometimes associated with increased venous pressure and unexplained abdominal pain. Vasopressor amines (eg, dopamine) can be used to treat this complication. Disopyramide should be used with extreme caution if at all in patients with cardiomegaly, uncompensated or marginally compensated congestive heart failure, and in those receiving beta blockers or other drugs with a negative inotropic effect.

Disopyramide may precipitate or worsen heart block and probably should not be used in patients with second- or third-degree AV block unless a ventricular pacemaker is in place. It also should be avoided in those with sinus node disorders because it may adversely affect sinus node function. Like quinidine, disopyramide may increase the ventricular rate in nondigitalized patients with atrial flutter.

Prolongation of the QT interval, widening of the QRS complex, and a prominent U wave may be present on the electrocardiogram. Occasionally, these electrocardiographic abnormalities may presage ventricular arrhythmias, including torsades de pointes. QT prolongation and ventricular arrhythmias have occurred when erythromycin was added to the regimen of patients receiving disopyramide. The adverse interaction was associated with elevated plasma levels of disopyramide. Conversely, barbiturates, phenytoin, and rifampin lower serum levels of disopyramide. Disopyramide does not increase serum digoxin levels.

Adverse reactions reported rarely include nervousness, dizziness, fatigue, depression, headache, muscle weakness, acute psychosis, severe hypoglycemia, intrahepatic cholestasis, rash, and anaphylactoid reactions.

Disopyramide should not be used for antiarrhythmic therapy during pregnancy because it may initiate uterine contractions. This drug is classified in FDA Pregnancy Category C. Disopyramide and a metabolite are excreted in breast milk.

PHARMACOKINETICS. Protein binding of disopyramide is dose dependent (68% at 0.38 mcg/ml and 28% at 3.8 mcg/

ml); thus, an increase in the dose may result in a more than proportionate increase in free drug concentration. Approximately 20% of a dose is excreted as the mono-N-dealkylated metabolite, which has less antiarrhythmic and atropine-like activity than the parent drug. The half-life of disopyramide is increased in patients with renal insufficiency. See also Table 3.

DOSAGE AND PREPARATIONS.

Oral: *Adults,* (Regular Preparation) initially, 100 to 200 mg every six hours (range, 400 to 800 mg daily). For patients with renal or hepatic insufficiency, the manufacturer recommends a maintenance dose of 100 mg with or without a loading dose of 150 mg at the following intervals: every 8 hours (creatinine clearance 30 to 40 ml/min); every 12 hours (creatinine clearance 15 to 30 ml/min); or every 24 hours (creatinine clearance less than 15 ml/min). Patients of small stature or those with hepatic insufficiency, cardiomyopathy, or cardiac decompensation also may require a smaller dose.

(Prolonged-release Preparation) 300 mg every 12 hours. Dosage should be reduced to 200 mg every 12 hours in patients of small stature or with moderate renal insufficiency. This preparation should not be used in those with severe renal insufficiency, cardiomyopathy, or cardiac decompensation.

For *children,* (Regular Preparation) a 1 to 10 mg/ml suspension can be prepared by adding the entire contents of disopyramide capsules to an appropriate volume of cherry syrup in an amber glass bottle. The suspension is stable for one month when refrigerated and should be thoroughly shaken before use. The suggested daily dosage for *children under 1 year* is 10 to 30 mg/kg; *1 to 4 years,* 10 to 20 mg/kg; *4 to 12 years,* 10 to 15 mg/kg; *12 to 18 years,* 6 to 15 mg/kg.

Norpace (Searle), ***Generic***. Capsules 100 and 150 mg (equivalent to base); capsules (prolonged-release) 100 and 150 mg (equivalent to base) (***Norpace CR, Generic***).

FLECAINIDE ACETATE

[Tambocor]

ACTIONS. This Class 1C agent depresses sinus node automaticity and prolongs conduction in the atria, AV node, ventricles, accessory pathways, and particularly in the His-Purkinje system. To a lesser extent, it increases the refractoriness of atrial and ventricular tissues. Flecainide has a moderate negative inotropic effect.

USES. Flecainide is used for the treatment and prophylaxis of supraventricular tachycardia, including AV nodal and AV reentrant tachycardia and atrial fibrillation in patients with normal or near-normal left ventricular function. Results of short-term (eight weeks), double-blind, placebo-controlled trials showed that oral flecainide increased the time to first episode and the interval between episodes four- to fivefold in patients with paroxysmal supraventricular tachycardia and atrial fibrillation compared with placebo (Anderson et al, 1989; Henthorn et al, 1991). A linear dose-response relationship was observed (Pritchett et al, 1991 A). The number of patients remaining free of paroxysmal supraventricular tachycardia while on flecainide therapy increased with successive increases in dosage (86% of patients receiving 150 mg twice daily compared with 29% of those on placebo). For patients with atrial fibrillation, 18%, 21%, and 54% who received twice-daily doses of 25 mg, 50 mg, and 100 mg of flecainide, respectively, had no episodes compared with 7% of those receiving placebo.

Long-term treatment with oral flecainide in patients with AV reentrant tachycardia, atrial fibrillation, and the Wolff-Parkinson-White syndrome was similarly effective (Wiseman et al, 1990; Cockrell et al, 1991; Hughes et al, 1992).

The estimated one-year mortality rate following treatment with flecainide for supraventricular tachycardia (0.5%) was much lower than that reported for patients with postmyocardial infarction and asymptomatic ventricular arrhythmia (9.2%) in the Cardiac Arrhythmia Suppression Trial (Pritchett and Wilkinson, 1991).

Flecainide should only be used for ventricular tachycardia that is considered to be life-threatening, because it can precipitate more serious arrhythmias and increase mortality in postinfarct patients (CAST Investigators, 1989).

Intravenous flecainide (investigational preparation) has been used to terminate AV nodal reentrant tachycardia and reciprocating tachycardia associated with the Wolff-Parkinson-White syndrome. It also may terminate atrial fibrillation but this route is ineffective in atrial flutter (Camm et al, 1985; Hellestrand, 1988). There is limited information on the use of the intravenous preparation in ventricular arrhythmias.

ADVERSE REACTIONS AND PRECAUTIONS. Blurred vision and dizziness are the most common side effects of flecainide. It also may cause headache, nausea, constipation, dyspnea, chest pain, fatigue, nervousness, insomnia, tremor, paresthesias, tinnitus, rash, difficulty in urination, and sexual dysfunction.

Flecainide may worsen left ventricular function (Greene et al, 1989). It is particularly likely to worsen or precipitate heart failure in patients with an ejection fraction of less than 30% and a history of severe cardiac failure, and it generally should not be used in such patients (de Paola et al, 1987). Flecainide also may precipitate bundle branch block or AV block. It should be avoided in those with advanced conduction disturbances unless a pacemaker is in place. Flecainide increases sinus node recovery time and should be used cautiously in patients with sinus node dysfunction.

Proarrhythmic events (incessant, sustained, monomorphic, wide-complex tachycardia) have been noted in approximately 15% of patients with ventricular arrhythmias treated with flecainide. Aggravation of arrhythmia has occurred most often in those with sustained ventricular tachycardia and/or decreased systolic function (Stanton et al, 1989). The incidence of sudden death increased when flecainide was used to treat asymptomatic or mildly symptomatic ventricular arrhythmias occurring after acute myocardial infarction (CAST Investigators, 1989). Ventricular or supraventricular proarrhythmic events have developed occasionally when flecainide was used to suppress supraventricular arrhythmias or arrhythmias associated with the preexcitation syndrome.

Dysarthria, visual hallucinations, ocular myopathy, neutropenia, and increased antinuclear antibodies have been reported rarely. Flecainide may exacerbate proximal muscle weakness in patients with myopathic disorders.

Activated charcoal reduces the absorption of flecainide and may be useful for treating toxicity.

Flecainide is classified in FDA Pregnancy Category C.

DRUG INTERACTIONS. Flecainide may slightly increase serum digoxin levels. Amiodarone and cimetidine increase serum flecainide levels. During concomitant administration of flecainide and propranolol, plasma levels of both drugs may increase slightly.

PHARMACOKINETICS. See Table 3.

DOSAGE AND PREPARATIONS.

Oral: *Adults,* for supraventricular arrhythmias, initially, 50 mg every 12 hours. The dosage may be increased in 50-mg increments twice daily at four-day intervals until efficacy is achieved (maximum dose, 300 mg/day). For life-threatening ventricular tachycardia, initially, 100 mg every 12 hours. The dose may be increased by 50 mg twice daily every four days until efficacy is achieved or to a maximum of 400 mg daily. The maintenance dose is 100 mg twice daily.

Plasma level monitoring (0.2 to 1 mcg/ml) should guide dosage adjustments in patients with renal failure.

Tambocor (3M Pharmaceuticals). Tablets 50, 100, and 150 mg.

Intravenous (investigational): 1 to 2 mg/kg given as a slow injection or diluted with 5% dextrose and given as a slow infusion.

Tambocor (3M Pharmaceuticals).

LIDOCAINE HYDROCHLORIDE

[Xylocaine Injection for Cardiac Arrhythmias]

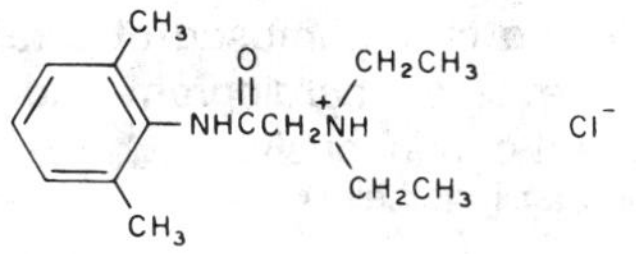

CH_3 O CH_2CH_3 —NHCCH$_2$$\overset{+}{N}$H Cl^- CH_2CH_3 CH_3

ACTIONS AND USES. This Class 1B agent depresses automaticity and reduces refractory period duration in the His-Purkinje system and ventricles but has little effect on atrial tissue. Therapeutic doses do not slow AV nodal or intraventricular conduction velocity except in the ischemic myocardium. Lidocaine can cause hyperpolarization and significant increases in conduction velocity in tissues depolarized by stretch or low extracellular potassium concentrations.

Because it acts rapidly and moderate doses usually do not depress myocardial contractility or AV conduction, intravenous lidocaine has been used for immediate suppression of ventricular ectopy and hemodynamically stable ventricular tachycardia during acute myocardial infarction. However, prophylactic use is no longer recommended, because it does not improve the survival rate (MacMahon et al, 1988).

Lidocaine may control ventricular arrhythmias caused by digitalis toxicity and those that develop during cardiac surgery, cardiac catheterization, or cardioversion. It usually does not correct supraventricular arrhythmias and may increase the ventricular rate.

ADVERSE REACTIONS AND PRECAUTIONS. The major adverse effects of lidocaine are attributable to its action on the central nervous system and include drowsiness, slurred speech, paresthesias, impaired hearing, anxiety (feeling of impending doom), confusion, hallucinations, delusions, muscle twitching, convulsions, coma, and respiratory depression. Large doses may depress myocardial contractility, automaticity, and AV conduction, especially in the presence of conduction system disease. Untoward effects are most common in elderly patients and those with congestive heart failure. The high incidence of side effects in the elderly usually can be avoided if a lower dose is employed.

Lidocaine is classified in FDA Pregnancy Category B.

DRUG INTERACTIONS. Lidocaine clearance is reduced by concomitant administration of either cardioselective or nonselective beta blockers due to decreased cardiac output and hepatic blood flow. Cimetidine also reduces lidocaine clearance and increases its half-life. These interactions may be associated with symptoms of toxicity. When given concomitantly, mexiletine may reduce the threshold of lidocaine toxicity. Hence, the dosage of lidocaine should be decreased when the two drugs are administered together.

TREATMENT OF TOXICITY. Small increments of diazepam or an ultrashort-acting barbiturate are used to control severe convulsions. Vasopressors may be used to treat circulatory depression.

PHARMACOKINETICS. The desethylated metabolites of lidocaine possess antiarrhythmic properties. The half-life of lidocaine may be increased in patients with chronic liver disease. See also Table 3.

DOSAGE AND PREPARATIONS.

Intravenous: *Adults,* for ventricular arrhythmias, a loading dose of 50 to 100 mg given over two to three minutes. This dose may be repeated in five minutes, or one or two supplemental doses of 25 to 50 mg may be given at five- or ten-minute intervals (up to 300 mg in a one-hour period). Following the loading dose, a solution is infused at a rate of 1 to 4 mg/min.

Lidocaine and its active metabolites accumulate in some patients during a constant maintenance infusion over 24 to 36 hours. Monitoring for early evidence of toxicity should be carried out and the dose reduced if toxic effects appear. If symptomatic ventricular arrhythmias occur during the first six hours of infusion, an additional smaller bolus may be given and the infusion rate increased. In patients 70 years and older and those with heart failure, cardiogenic shock, or hepatic disease, the loading dose should be decreased by about one-half and the infusion rate should be reduced to 1 to 2 mg/min.

Children, 0.5 to 1 mg/kg every five minutes for a maximum of three doses, or a solution containing 5 mg/ml infused at a rate of 0.03 mg/kg/min.

Generic. Solution 10 mg/ml in 5, 20, 30, and 50 containers, 20 mg/ml in 5, 10, 20, 30, and 50 ml containers, 40 mg/ml in 5, 25, and 50 ml containers, 100 mg/ml in 10 ml containers, and 200 mg/ml in 5 and 10 ml containers.

Xylocaine Intravenous Injection for Cardiac Arrhythmias (Astra). Solution 10 and 20 mg/ml in 5 ml containers, 40 mg/ml in 25 and 50 ml containers, and 200 mg/ml in 5 and 10 ml containers.

Intramuscular: *Adults,* 300 mg (3 ml of a 10% solution) injected into the deltoid muscle.

Lidocaine Hydrochloride Injection for Cardiac Arrhythmias (Abbott). Solution 100 mg/ml in 10 ml containers.

MEXILETINE HYDROCHLORIDE

[Mexitil]

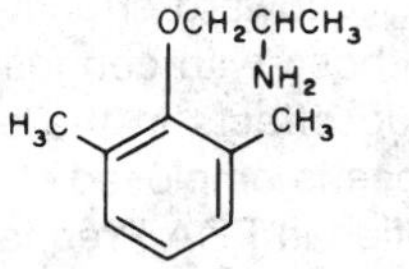

OCH_2CHCH_3 / NH_2 / H_3C / CH_3

ACTIONS. Mexiletine is related structurally to lidocaine and has similar electrophysiologic properties, but, unlike lidocaine, is effective when given both intravenously and orally. It depresses automaticity in the ventricles but has little effect on atrial tissue and does not depress sinus node function except in patients with the sick sinus syndrome. In patients with normal AV conduction, mexiletine does not appear to depress AV nodal function, but AV conduction time may be increased in those with pre-existing conduction disturbances. Mexiletine does not have a clinically important negative inotropic effect.

USES. This Class 1B drug is used to suppress premature ventricular complexes and may be as effective as quinidine or procainamide for this purpose (Morganroth, 1987).

Mexiletine is less effective in patients with recurrent refractory ventricular tachycardia and fibrillation, and extracardiac side effects may limit its long-term usefulness (Poole et al, 1986; Kerin et al, 1990). Concurrent administration of a Class 1A antiarrhythmic drug (eg, quinidine, disopyramide) or propranolol may provide better control of the arrhythmia and permit a reduction in the dose of mexiletine, thus reducing side effects (Duff et al, 1987; Greenspan et al, 1985). Supraventricular arrhythmias are not controlled by mexiletine.

ADVERSE REACTIONS AND PRECAUTIONS. Gastrointestinal and central nervous system side effects are common and include gastric distress, nausea, vomiting, malaise, dizziness, tremor, diplopia, dysarthria, paresthesias, confusion, and ataxia. Most side effects can be minimized by a reduction in dose or administration with food, milk, and/or antacids. Thrombocytopenia, hepatitis, and development of positive antinuclear antibody titers are rare reactions.

Manifestations of cardiovascular toxicity, which are uncommon, include sinus bradycardia or tachycardia, atrial fibrillation, hypotension, dyspnea, and ventricular arrhythmias. Severe bradycardia and prolongation of the sinus node recovery time may occur if mexiletine is given to patients with the sick sinus syndrome. This drug should be avoided in patients with severe bradyarrhythmias. Atropine has controlled mexiletine-induced bradycardia in some patients. In one case of suicidal overdosage, ventricular asystole occurred and the myocardium was refractory to electrical pacing.

Mexiletine is excreted in breast milk. It is classified in FDA Pregnancy Category C.

DRUG INTERACTIONS. Phenytoin, rifampin, and probably other enzyme-inducing drugs decrease the half-life of mexiletine. Opioid analgesics may slow its absorption. Metoclopramide has been reported to accelerate absorption of mexiletine, but the extent of absorption is unchanged. Mexiletine may increase the plasma concentration of theophylline, and combined therapy may lead to proarrhythmic events. Mexiletine lowers the threshold of lidocaine toxicity; hence, the dosage of lidocaine should be decreased when these drugs are administered concomitantly.

PHARMACOKINETICS. The half-life of mexiletine is increased in patients with chronic liver disease. See also Table 3.

DOSAGE AND PREPARATIONS. Mexiletine should be given with food or antacids.

Oral: *Adults,* initially, 200 mg every eight hours. If rapid control is essential, an initial loading dose of 400 mg may be administered, followed by a 200-mg dose in eight hours. Dosage may then be increased or decreased by 50 or 100 mg. A minimum of two or three days between dose adjustments is recommended. The usual maintenance dose is 150 to 200 mg every eight hours. If an adequate response is achieved with a dose of 200 mg or less every eight hours, the same total daily dose may be tried in divided doses every 12 hours while carefully monitoring the patient's response. If a satisfactory response is not achieved and the drug is well tolerated, 400 mg may be given every eight hours or 450 mg every 12 hours. Since the severity of central nervous system side effects increases with total daily dose, the total dose should not exceed 1.2 g/day.

Mexitil (Boehringer Ingelheim). Capsules 150, 200, and 250 mg.

Intravenous (investigational): *Adults,* initially, 200 to 300 mg infused over 30 minutes at a rate of 10 to 15 mg/min. For maintenance, 500 mg to 1 g infused at a rate of 1 mg/min over 24 hours. The electrocardiogram and blood pressure should be monitored continuously.

Mexitil (Boehringer Ingelheim).

MORICIZINE HYDROCHLORIDE

[Ethmozine]

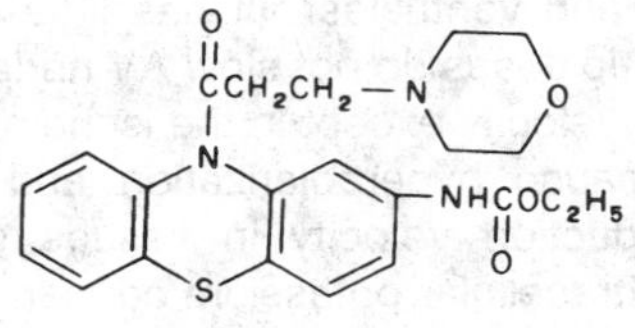

O / CCH_2CH_2-N / O / N / $NHCOC_2H_5$ / O / S

ACTIONS. Moricizine prolongs both AH and HV atrioventricular conduction times and PR and QRS intervals. Although it has some electrophysiologic effects in common with both Class 1A and 1B agents, moricizine probably could be classified as a weak Class 1C agent. In patients with impaired left ventricular function, moricizine has minimal effects on measurements of cardiac performance such as cardiac index, stroke volume index, pulmonary capillary wedge pressure, and systemic or pulmonary vascular resistance or ejection fraction, either at rest or during exercise. A small but consistent increase occurs in resting blood pressure and heart rate. Exercise tolerance in patients with ventricular arrhythmias is not affected. In those with a history of heart failure or angina pectoris, exercise duration and rate-pressure product with maximal exercise are unchanged during administration. Nevertheless, worsened heart failure has been attributed to moricizine in some patients with severe underlying disease.

USES. Moricizine is used to suppress life-threatening ventricular arrhythmias (Morganroth et al, 1987); it was reported to be more effective than disopyramide or low doses of propranolol (Pratt et al, 1987) but less effective than flecainide (CAPS [Cardiac Arrhythmia Pilot Study] Investigators, 1988) in suppressing premature ventricular complexes. Moricizine did not improve the survival rate and increased the incidence of adverse events in patients following myocardial infarction (Greene et al, 1992). It is more effective in preventing recurrences of nonsustained than sustained ventricular tachycardia (Hession et al, 1987); however, moricizine has limited efficacy and carries a considerable risk of inducing life-threatening proarrhythmias in patients with serious ventricular arrhythmias and inducible sustained tachycardia (Damle et al, 1992; Powell et al, 1992).

ADVERSE REACTIONS. Moricizine caused dizziness, nausea, headache, fatigue, dyspnea, and palpitations in more than 5% of the patients in clinical trials (Mann, 1990). The proarrhythmic potential is low in patients with benign arrhythmias but appears to be similar to that of other agents in those with heart disease or serious arrhythmias. Proarrhythmias occurred in 3.7% of 1,072 patients with ventricular arrhythmias who received a wide range of doses under a variety of circumstances; however, in those with malignant ventricular arrhythmia, the incidence of proarrhythmia following treatment with moricizine may approach 15%.

Adverse drug reactions reported in 2% to 5% of patients in clinical trials included sustained ventricular tachycardia, hypoesthesias, abdominal pain, dyspepsia, vomiting, sweating, cardiac chest pain, asthenia, nervousness, paresthesias, congestive heart failure, musculoskeletal pain, diarrhea, dry mouth, sleep disorders, and blurred vision. Thrombocytopenia, hepatitis, and worsening of heart failure have occurred rarely.

Overall mortality was greater in older than in younger patients (9.3% vs 3.9%), but the deaths were not attributed to treatment and the older patients had more serious underlying heart disease.

PRECAUTIONS. Moricizine is contraindicated in patients with pre-existing second- or third-degree AV block.

Hypokalemia, hyperkalemia, or hypomagnesemia should be corrected before moricizine therapy is initiated because these electrolyte disturbances may alter the effects of Class 1 antiarrhythmic drugs.

Patients with hepatic and renal disease should receive lower doses and be closely monitored for excessive pharmacologic effects, including effects on ECG intervals, for dosage adjustment. Moricizine should be used with particular care, if at all, in patients with severe liver disease.

In teratology studies in rats and rabbits, doses up to 6.7 and 4.7 times the maximum recommended daily dose in humans, respectively, were not harmful to the fetus. However, no adequate and well-controlled studies have been performed in pregnant women (FDA Pregnancy Category B).

DRUG INTERACTIONS. The concomitant administration of cimetidine decreased moricizine clearance by 49% and increased plasma levels 1.4 fold in healthy subjects. In patients being treated with cimetidine, initial doses of moricizine should not exceed 600 mg/day.

In patients receiving moricizine and theophylline (conventional or prolonged-release preparations) concomitantly, clearance of theophylline increased 44% to 66% and the plasma half-life decreased 19% to 33% following long-term moricizine therapy. Thus, patients receiving both drugs should be monitored carefully and the doses of moricizine should be adjusted as necessary.

PHARMACOKINETICS. See Table 3.

DOSAGE AND PREPARATIONS.

Oral: *Adults,* for life-threatening ventricular arrhythmias, the usual dosage is 600 to 900 mg/day, given every eight hours in three equally divided doses. Within this range the dosage can be adjusted as tolerated in increments of 150 mg/day at three-day intervals until the desired effect is obtained. Since the antiarrhythmic effect of moricizine persists for more than 12 hours, some responsive patients may be given the same total daily dose every 12 hours to increase convenience and help ensure compliance. However, when higher doses are used, those receiving the drug every 12 hours may experience more dizziness and nausea.

Patients with impaired hepatic or renal function, initially, 600 mg/day or less. These patients should be monitored closely before dosage adjustment.

Ethmozine (DuPont). Tablets 200, 250, and 300 mg.

PROCAINAMIDE HYDROCHLORIDE

[Pronestyl, Pronestyl-SR, Procan SR]

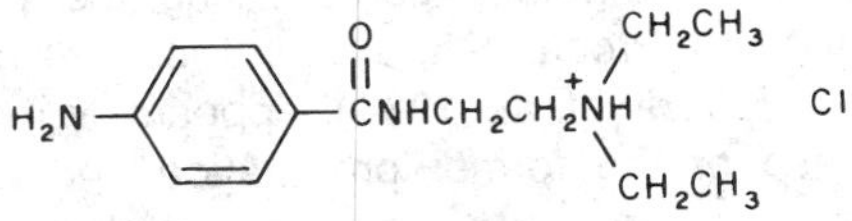

$$H_2N-C_6H_4-C(=O)NHCH_2CH_2\overset{+}{N}H(CH_2CH_3)_2 \quad Cl^-$$

ACTIONS AND USES. The electrophysiologic properties, hemodynamic effects, and antiarrhythmic actions of procainamide are similar to those of quinidine. Although the indications for quinidine and procainamide are the same, they do not always have the same effect in an individual patient. Quinidine is frequently preferred for prolonged oral therapy because of the high incidence of drug-induced lupus associated with long-term administration of procainamide. This Class 1A drug is safer than Class 1C antiarrhythmic drugs in patients with heart failure (Gottlieb et al, 1990).

For intravenous use, procainamide is often preferred to quinidine for terminating supraventricular or ventricular arrhythmias. It is particularly useful in patients with severe ventricular arrhythmias who do not respond to lidocaine. Atrial fibrillation of recent onset may convert to normal sinus rhythm during infusion; however, electrical cardioversion is usually required to convert chronic atrial fibrillation and is preferred in hemodynamically unstable patients. Because it slows conduction and increases the refractory period in accessory pathways, procainamide is useful for acute termination of arrhythmias associated with the Wolff-Parkinson-White syndrome and for slowing the ventricular response during atrial fibrillation or flutter.

ADVERSE REACTIONS, PRECAUTIONS, AND INTERACTIONS. Although procainamide may cause anorexia, nausea, and vomiting, gastrointestinal side effects occur less often than with quinidine. Its adverse cardiovascular effects are similar to those of quinidine (ie, hypotension, myocardial depression, AV block, increased ventricular response to atrial flutter in nondigitalized patients, ventricular arrhythmias [including torsades de pointes]). Excessive QT prolongation and widening of the QRS complex may be early signs of toxicity. Patients with renal insufficiency are particularly at risk due to the accumulation of procainamide and its active metabolite, N-acetylprocainamide, a Class 3 agent.

The usefulness of prolonged therapy is limited because of a reversible lupus erythematosus-like syndrome that develops in more than 12% of patients. Manifestations may include polyarthralgia, arthritis, pleuritic pain, and, less commonly, fever, myalgia, rash, restrictive pericarditis, myocarditis, pleural effusion, thrombocytopenia, and hemolytic anemia. Elevated antinuclear antibody (ANA) titers develop in most patients treated with this drug for more than one year. Patients who develop elevated ANA titers should be monitored closely because such an increase frequently precedes clinical symptoms.

Manifestations of hypersensitivity unrelated to the lupus syndrome (fever, rash, urticaria, neutropenia, agranulocytosis, pancytopenia, and nephrotic syndrome) occur occasionally. A report that severe neutropenia and agranulocytosis may be more common in patients taking the prolonged-release preparation, Procan SR, than in those taking regular procainamide (Ellrodt et al, 1984) appears to reflect the widespread use of the former preparation and its use in patients with more severe disease. When the number of prescriptions for the two preparations is taken into consideration, there is no significant difference in the frequency of these adverse reactions (Meyers et al, 1985).

Rarely, mental disturbances (eg, depression, hallucinations, psychosis), myopathy, tremor, and cerebellar ataxia have occurred in patients taking procainamide.

Procainamide is classified in FDA Pregnancy Category C.

Cimetidine reduces the renal clearance of both procainamide and its active metabolite.

PHARMACOKINETICS. The major metabolic pathway for biotransformation of procainamide is N-acetylation resulting in the formation of N-acetylprocainamide (NAPA). Evaluation of the therapeutic plasma concentrations for procainamide should include measurement of NAPA concentrations. The rate of acetylation shows a bimodal distribution (see index entry Drug Response Variation, Influence of Pharmacogenetics). Renal clearance is decreased in patients with renal insufficiency or when the urine is alkaline. See also Table 3.

DOSAGE AND PREPARATIONS. Dosage should be reduced in patients with impaired renal function.

Oral: (Regular Preparation) *Adults,* initially, 250 to 500 mg every three to six hours around the clock. A loading dose of 1 g produces an effective serum concentration rapidly. *Children,* 50 mg/kg daily in four to six divided doses.

Generic. Capsules 250, 375, and 500 mg; tablets 250 mg.

Pronestyl (Apothecon). Capsules and tablets 250, 375, and 500 mg.

Oral: (Prolonged-release Preparation) *Adults,* for maintenance after initial treatment with the regular preparation, 500 mg to 1 g every six to eight hours or 50 mg/kg daily in divided doses at six-hour intervals.

Pronestyl-SR (Apothecon). Tablets (prolonged-release) 500 mg.

Procan SR (Parke-Davis), ***Generic***. Tablets (prolonged-release) 250, 500, and 750 mg and 1 g (***Procan SR*** only).

Intravenous (slow): *Adults,* 25 to 50 mg/min until the arrhythmia is suppressed (maximum, 1 g). For maintenance, 2 to 4 mg/min. *Children,* 5 to 15 mg/kg given over 30 minutes.

Pronestyl (Apothecon), ***Generic***. Solution (sterile, aqueous) 100 mg/ml in 10 ml containers and 500 mg/ml in 2 ml containers.

PROPAFENONE HYDROCHLORIDE
[Rythmol]

ACTIONS. Propafenone is a Class 1C antiarrhythmic drug that may possess weak beta blocking and calcium channel blocking properties. It slows conduction in the atria, ventricles, AV node, His-Purkinje system, and accessory pathways and, to a lesser extent, increases atrial and ventricular refractoriness. This drug has a negative inotropic effect and may increase peripheral vascular resistance.

USES. Propafenone has been used by the intravenous (investigational) and oral routes for acute termination or long-term suppression of ventricular arrhythmias, particularly recurrent ventricular tachycardia (Chilson et al, 1985; Connolly et al, 1983). It appears to be as effective as quinidine in suppressing frequent premature ventricular complexes, and the frequency of side effects is similar but distinct with the two drugs (Dinh et al, 1985). As a result of the CAST study, propafenone (and other Class 1C antiarrhythmic drugs) is currently labeled only for treatment of life-threatening ventricular arrhythmias. It is not known whether the mild beta blocking properties of propafenone render this drug less likely to precipitate ventricular arrhythmias than other 1C drugs.

Because it depresses both AV nodal and bypass tract conduction, propafenone is useful for immediate termination and long-term prevention of supraventricular reentrant tachycardias involving the AV node or accessory pathways (Ludmer et al, 1987; Shen et al, 1986; Pritchett et al, 1991 B). It also has been used for long-term suppression of refractory, symptomatic atrial fibrillation and flutter (Antman et al, 1988). New atrial flutter with 1:1 AV conduction and QRS prolongation has been reported in a small number of patients treated with propafenone for atrial fibrillation.

ADVERSE REACTIONS AND PRECAUTIONS. Propafenone may substantially increase the PR interval and the duration of the QRS complex. The dose should be reduced if the PR interval exceeds 0.3 seconds and the QRS duration exceeds 0.18 seconds.

Propafenone may worsen congestive heart failure, cause sinus node dysfunction and AV or intraventricular conduction disturbances, and aggravate ventricular arrhythmias. It may cause dizziness, nausea, vomiting, constipation, weakness, fatigue, paresthesias, tremor, taste disturbances, dry mouth, blurred vision, and urinary retention. Rash, bronchospasm, acute pleuritis, and psychotic episodes also have been reported. Abnormal liver function tests, neutropenia, agranulocytosis, lupus-like syndrome, and hyponatremia have been noted rarely.

Propafenone is classified in FDA Pregnancy Category B.

DRUG INTERACTIONS. Propafenone increases serum concentrations of digoxin, warfarin, and propranolol. Cimetidine increases serum levels of propafenone. Small doses of quinidine inhibit the metabolism of propafenone.

PHARMACOKINETICS. The bioavailability of propafenone is reduced by extensive first-pass hepatic metabolism and is dose dependent; the rate of elimination is determined by the debrisoquin hydroxylation (P450IID6) phenotype. Two metabolites, 5-hydroxypropafenone and N-desalkypropafenone, have effects similar to those of the parent compound; the steady-state plasma concentration of each metabolite is approximately 20% that of propafenone. See also Table 3.

DOSAGE AND PREPARATIONS.

Oral: *Adults*, initially, 150 mg every eight hours. If the arrhythmia is not controlled, dosage may be increased at three- to four-day intervals to 225 mg every eight hours and, if necessary, to 300 mg every eight hours.

Rythmol (Knoll). Tablets 150 and 300 mg.

QUINIDINE SULFATE

[Cin-Quin, Quinidex]

QUINIDINE GLUCONATE

[Duraquin, Quinaglute, Quinalan, Quinatime]

QUINIDINE POLYGALACTURONATE

[Cardioquin]

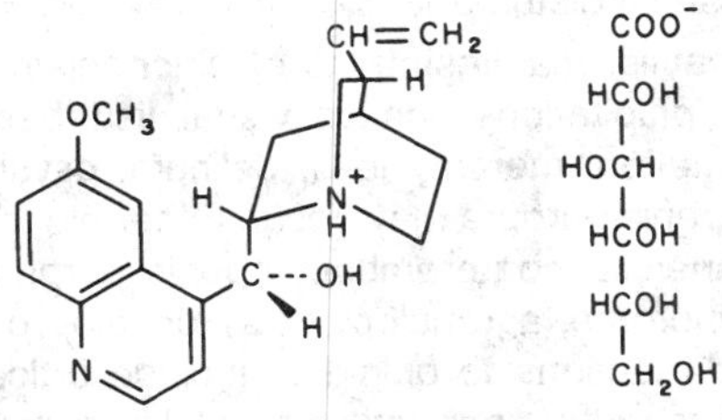

ACTIONS. Quinidine acts directly on the cell membrane to inhibit the sodium channel and has indirect (anticholinergic) effects. It depresses automaticity, particularly in ectopic sites, and slows conduction and increases refractoriness of the atria, His-Purkinje system, accessory pathways, and ventricles. Quinidine usually does not depress sinus node function except in patients with sick sinus syndrome. It dilates resistance and capacitance vessels and has a mild negative inotropic effect.

USES. This Class 1A drug is useful in both supraventricular and ventricular arrhythmias (Coplen et al, 1990; Morganroth and Goin, 1991). Its major uses are to maintain sinus rhythm after conversion of atrial flutter or fibrillation, to prevent ventricular tachycardia, and for long-term prophylaxis in patients with AV nodal reentrant tachycardia and automatic atrial tachycardia. Quinidine also has been used to prevent symptomatic premature supraventricular and ventricular complexes.

Because it slows conduction and prolongs the refractory period of the accessory pathway and suppresses automaticity of ectopic pacemakers, quinidine may prevent recurrences of paroxysmal supraventricular tachycardia caused by reentry over a concealed pathway or AV reciprocating tachycardia associated with the Wolff-Parkinson-White syndrome. It also may slow the ventricular response to atrial flutter or fibrillation in the preexcitation syndrome.

Quinidine is often preferred to procainamide for long-term therapy because elevated antinuclear antibody titers and drug-induced lupus are common during prolonged therapy with procainamide.

ADVERSE REACTIONS AND PRECAUTIONS. The toxic effects of quinidine generally are dose related, but severe reactions may occur after small doses are given to patients who are hypersensitive to the drug. The oral route is preferred because serious cardiovascular reactions (eg, hypotension) are more likely to occur after parenteral administration. Intramuscular injections are painful, increase serum creatine phosphokinase levels, and are erratically and incompletely absorbed.

Diarrhea, nausea, and vomiting are the most common adverse effects of quinidine. Results of largely uncontrolled studies suggested that the gluconate and polygalacturonate salts are better tolerated by some patients, but a controlled trial showed no difference in efficacy or side effects between quinidine gluconate and sulfate preparations (Morganroth and Hunter, 1985). If gastrointestinal reactions become severe, procainamide or disopyramide may be substituted. Aluminum-containing antacids reduce the incidence and degree of gastrointestinal disturbances.

Fever, hepatitis, manifestations of cinchonism (eg, headache, vertigo, palpitations, tinnitus, visual disturbances, confusion, disorientation, memory loss, delirium, psychosis), and thrombocytopenic purpura may occur. Other blood dyscrasias (hemolytic anemia, nonthrombocytopenic purpura, Henoch-Schönlein syndrome, agranulocytosis) develop occasionally. Dermatologic reactions to quinidine include urticaria, photosensitivity, eczematous dermatitis, morbilliform rashes, lichen planus-like eruptions, and abnormal pigmentation. Keratopathy, sicca syndrome, and anterior uveitis are uncommon ocular adverse effects. Rarely, quinidine has induced a lupus erythematosus-like syndrome or isolated polyarthropathy. Reactive lymphadenopathy is another rare complication. Pill-induced esophagitis also has been reported. Quinidine may unmask or exacerbate myasthenia gravis.

In patients with atrial flutter, quinidine may increase the ventricular rate, but this complication generally can be avoided by prior and concomitant treatment with digitalis (with careful monitoring for glycoside toxicity), propranolol, or verapamil. Severe hypotension due to peripheral vasodilation may occur after rapid parenteral administration and should be treated with volume replacement and vasopressor amines. Large doses may depress myocardial contractility and aggravate or induce heart failure in nondigitalized patients. However, because of its vasodilator effect, quinidine may not worsen (and may even improve) hemodynamics in some patients with heart failure.

Quinidine may worsen AV conduction disturbances and should be used cautiously in patients with partial AV block. It probably should not be used in the presence of high-grade second- or third-degree heart block unless a ventricular pacemaker is in place. Quinidine also may adversely affect sinus node function in patients with sinus node disorders.

Other manifestations of cardiac toxicity are excessive prolongation of the QT interval, widening of the QRS complex, and ventricular arrhythmias. Proarrhythmic events may occur at therapeutic or subtherapeutic plasma drug levels, often in association with hypokalemia, and may lead to syncope and sudden death. In a meta-analysis that compared use of quinidine with placebo to maintain sinus rhythm in 800 patients with atrial fibrillation who were treated after cardioversion, 2.9% of patients receiving quinidine died versus 0.8% of those receiving placebo. Similarly, in another study in patients with benign or potentially lethal ventricular arrhythmias, the risk of dying was threefold greater in those receiving quinidine than in those receiving a placebo (Morganroth and Goin, 1991). Most of the patients in these populations died suddenly or experienced lethal ventricular arrhythmias (eg, torsades de pointes).

This drug is classified in FDA Pregnancy Category C.

DRUG INTERACTIONS. Quinidine is a potent inhibitor of cytochrome P450IID6. The concentration of this isozyme is subject to genetic polymorphism. Enzyme activity is lacking or greatly reduced in 5% to 10% of Caucasians resulting in the so-called poor (slow) metabolizer phenotype; less than 1% of Orientals are affected. More than 25 drugs are at least partially eliminated via oxidation by P450IID6. Enzyme inhibition may be an important cause of drug interactions in patients who are extensive metabolizers. Thus, quinidine may impair the metabolism of several drugs, including codeine (reduced formation of action metabolite), tricyclic antidepressants (eg, nortriptyline, desipramine, clomipramine), phenothiazine antipsychotic agents (eg, perphenazine, thioridazine), and other antiarrhythmic drugs (eg, propafenone, flecainide). For further information, see index entry Drug Response Variation, Influence of Pharmacogenetics.

Elevated serum digoxin levels have been noted in patients receiving both quinidine and digoxin (see index entry Heart Failure). Procainamide and disopyramide are alternative antiarrhythmic drugs that do not increase serum digoxin levels. Quinidine also may increase serum digitoxin concentrations, but to a lesser extent. The concomitant administration of quinidine and verapamil may increase the serum quinidine concentration and cause hypotension. Occasionally nifedipine may alter the disposition of quinidine, and the serum quinidine concentration may increase when nifedipine is withdrawn. Bradycardia may occur from an interaction between quinidine and beta blockers (including ophthalmic preparations).

The half-life of quinidine is increased by cimetidine and by drugs that alkalize the urine. The action of coumarin anticoagulants may be enhanced by quinidine. This agent should be used cautiously in patients receiving neuromuscular blocking drugs because the effects may be additive.

In electrophysiologic studies on patients with a history of sustained ventricular tachycardia or reciprocating tachycardia in those with ventricular preexcitation, physiologic doses of epinephrine antagonized the therapeutic effect of quinidine (Morady et al, 1988 A, 1988 B).

TREATMENT OF TOXICITY. There is no specific antidote, and treatment is largely supportive. Rapid volume replacement and administration of sympathomimetic amines may control hypotension and correct some arrhythmias. Charcoal hemoperfusion may enhance quinidine clearance. Cardiovascular assistance with an intra-aortic balloon pump may improve hemodynamics and reverse oliguria. Phenytoin, lidocaine, propranolol, and bretylium have been used to treat quinidine-induced ventricular arrhythmias associated with a prolonged QT interval, but temporary overdrive pacing is the treatment of choice. Molar sodium lactate has been suggested for treating cardiac toxicity but has not been consistently effective.

PHARMACOKINETICS. Food decreases the rate but not the extent of absorption. Bioavailability may differ among the different quinidine preparations, especially the prolonged-release forms. The half-life of quinidine is prolonged in elderly patients and those with impaired hepatic or renal function; dosage reduction may be required in these patients. See also Table 3.

DOSAGE AND PREPARATIONS.

QUINIDINE SULFATE:

Oral: *Adults,* 200 to 400 mg every four to six hours. Loading doses >400 mg significantly increase gastrointestinal irritation. *Children,* 6 mg/kg every four to six hours.

Generic. Capsules 200 mg; tablets 100, 180, 200, and 300 mg.

Cin-Quin (Solvay). Capsules 300 mg; tablets 200 and 300 mg.
Quinidex (Robins). Tablets (prolonged-release) 300 mg.

QUINIDINE GLUCONATE:

Oral: *Adults,* 324 to 972 mg every 8 to 12 hours. As with quinidine sulfate, a loading dose should be given if a rapid antiarrhythmic response is required.

Generic. Tablets 324 mg (prolonged-release).
Duraquin (Warner-Chilcott). Tablets (prolonged-release) 330 mg (equivalent to 248 mg quinidine sulfate).
Quinaglute (Berlex), ***Quinalan*** (Lannett), ***Quinatime*** (CMC). Tablets (prolonged-release) 324 mg (equivalent to 243 mg quinidine sulfate).

Intramuscular: Intramuscular injections are erratically and incompletely absorbed. *Adults,* 400 mg is given initially and may be repeated every four to six hours. In emergencies, administration every two hours (for four or five doses) may be necessary.

Intravenous: This route is rarely used and should be employed only in hospitalized patients. *Adults*, 200 to 400 mg in dilute solution may be given very slowly (approximately 10 mg/min). Normal saline may be administered rapidly simultaneously to counteract the marked reduction in preload produced by quinidine. The electrocardiogram and blood pressure should be monitored continuously.

Generic. Solution 80 mg/ml in 10 ml containers.

QUINIDINE POLYGALACTURONATE:

Oral: The manufacturer's recommended dose for maintenance is: *Adults,* 275 mg two or three times daily.

Cardioquin (Purdue Frederick). Tablets 275 mg (equivalent to 200 mg of quinidine sulfate).

TOCAINIDE HYDROCHLORIDE

[Tonocard]

CH_3 O || + NHC CHNH$_3$ | CH_3 CH_3 Cl^-

ACTIONS. Tocainide is active orally and has electrophysiologic properties similar to those of lidocaine. This Class 1B drug has a moderate myocardial depressant effect and may increase peripheral and pulmonary vascular resistance slightly when given intravenously.

USES. Tocainide is given orally to prevent or treat life-threatening ventricular arrhythmias. Because it may cause blood dyscrasias and severe dermatologic reactions, this drug usually is reserved for patients who have not responded to less toxic agents. Patients who do not respond to lidocaine often do not respond to tocainide. In a controlled study, quinidine was more effective than tocainide in suppressing ventricular ectopy and tachycardia. The usefulness of tocainide in refractory sustained ventricular tachycardia is limited by its low efficacy and frequent adverse effects (Adhar et al, 1988; Morganroth et al, 1985). A combination of tocainide and quinidine, both given in reduced doses, may be more effective and better tolerated than large doses of either drug alone (Kim et al, 1987).

Intravenous tocainide (investigational) has been used to prevent ventricular tachyarrhythmias after acute myocardial infarction. It reduces the incidence of premature ventricular complexes and ventricular tachycardia but has not been particularly effective in preventing primary ventricular fibrillation or improving survival.

Tocainide is not useful in supraventricular arrhythmias.

ADVERSE REACTIONS AND PRECAUTIONS. Tocainide has been discontinued in 20% or more of patients because of adverse reactions, which usually involve the gastrointestinal or central nervous system. Nausea is common; vomiting, abdominal pain, and diarrhea also may occur. Neurologic side effects include dizziness, tremor, paresthesias, blurred vision, and, less commonly, confusion, ataxia, anxiety, and hallucinations. These reactions are dose related and may respond to a reduction in dosage. Dermatologic reactions are relatively common and may be severe, including Stevens-Johnson syndrome, erythema multiforme, and exfoliative dermatitis.

Adverse cardiovascular effects observed only rarely include aggravation of congestive heart failure, conduction disturbances, and ventricular arrhythmias. Tocainide is more likely to worsen heart failure than procainamide (Gottlieb et al, 1990).

Blood dyscrasias (leukopenia, agranulocytosis, hypoplastic anemia, hemolytic anemia, thrombocytopenia) have developed in patients treated with tocainide. Weekly blood counts for the first three or four weeks of therapy have been recommended.

Drug fever, pulmonary fibrosis, interstitial pneumonitis, alveolitis, hepatotoxicity, and elevated ANA titers have been reported rarely.

Tocainide is classified in FDA Pregnancy Category C.

PHARMACOKINETICS. The half-life of tocainide is increased in patients with renal failure. See also Table 3.

DOSAGE AND PREPARATIONS.

Oral: *Adults,* initially, 400 mg every eight hours. The usual maintenance dose is 1.2 to 1.8 g daily in three divided doses. Daily doses exceeding 2.4 g have been given infrequently. In patients who tolerate the drug when it is given three times daily, a twice-daily schedule with careful monitoring may be tried. Smaller doses (less than 1.2 g daily) may be required in patients with renal or hepatic insufficiency.

Tonocard (Merck Sharp & Dohme). Tablets 400 and 600 mg.

AGENTS USED TO TREAT BRADYARRHYTHMIAS

ATROPINE SULFATE

For chemical formula, see index entry Atropine, As Mydriatic-Cycloplegic.

ACTIONS. Atropine increases sinus rate and sinoatrial and AV nodal conduction velocity and decreases the effective refractory period of the AV node by blocking the effects of the parasympathetic neurotransmitter, acetylcholine. Small intravenous doses (less than 0.4 mg) may cause a paradoxical decrease in the sinus rate, which may be followed by an increase. A biphasic response also may be seen immediately after administration of larger doses. The effects of atropine on conduction through the His-Purkinje system are unpredictable (Schweitzer and Mark, 1980), but the drug usually has no effect.

USES. Atropine is used to treat certain reversible bradyarrhythmias that may accompany acute myocardial infarction, particularly marked symptomatic sinus bradycardia. Since a decrease in vagal tone may unmask sympathetic hyperactivity, atropine occasionally may precipitate severe ventricular arrhythmias. For this reason, treatment of asymptomatic sinus bradycardia with atropine is not currently recommended. Pretreatment with atropine may reduce the incidence of ventricular tachyarrhythmias occurring during coronary angiography (Lehmann and Chen, 1989).

Atropine also is used to enhance AV conduction in Wenckebach Type I second-degree AV block. Rarely, a paradoxical worsening of AV block may occur. Atropine is the treatment of choice for bradycardia and hypotension associated with vasovagal episodes. It is sometimes used to increase the heart rate and thereby suppress episodes of drug-induced torsades de pointes prior to temporary pacing (Zipes, 1988).

ADVERSE REACTIONS AND PRECAUTIONS. Therapeutic doses cause dryness of the mouth, cycloplegia, and mydriasis. Large doses may cause hyperpyrexia, urinary retention, and central nervous system effects (eg, confusion, hallucinations). Rarely, systemically administered anticholinergic drugs have induced acute angle-closure glaucoma in predisposed eyes.

Arrhythmias occasionally induced by atropine during acute myocardial infarction include atrial fibrillation and ventricular tachycardia and fibrillation. Rarely, AV block may be worsened because doses that have little direct effect on the AV node may increase the sinus rate, causing more sinus impulses to block.

Atropine is classified in FDA Pregnancy Category B.

DOSAGE AND PREPARATIONS.

Intravenous: *Adults,* initially, 0.4 to 1 mg every one to two hours as needed; larger doses occasionally are required (maximum, 2 mg). *Children,* 0.01 to 0.03 mg/kg.

Generic. Solution 0.05 mg/ml in 5 ml containers; 0.1 mg/ml in 5 and 10 ml containers; 0.3 mg/ml in 1 and 30 ml containers; 0.4 mg/ml in 1 and 20 ml containers; 0.5 mg/ml in 1 and 5 ml containers; 0.8 mg/ml in 1 and 5 ml containers; and 1 and 1.2 mg/ml in 1 and 10 ml containers.

ISOPROTERENOL HYDROCHLORIDE

[Isuprel]

HO–C₆H₃(OH)–CH(OH)CH₂NH₂⁺CH(CH₃)₂ Cl⁻

This adrenergic drug stimulates beta receptors in the heart, blood vessels, and bronchioles, thereby increasing heart rate and myocardial contractility, enhancing automaticity and conduction velocity, dilating resistance vessels (primarily in skeletal muscle), and causing bronchodilation. It has no significant effect on alpha receptors and therefore lacks the marked pressor effect of norepinephrine or epinephrine.

In patients with second- or third-degree AV block, isoproterenol is used to maintain heart rate and cardiac output prior to insertion of a pacemaker. It is particularly useful for the emergency treatment of Stokes-Adams attacks and is indicated for severe myocardial depression induced by beta blockers. Like atropine, isoproterenol is sometimes employed to suppress episodes of drug-induced torsades de pointes prior to temporary pacing (Zipes, 1988). It may precipitate torsades de pointes in patients with congenital long QT syndrome.

Isoproterenol may cause tachycardia, extrasystoles, headache, dizziness, flushing, sweating, and tremors. Because myocardial oxygen demand may be increased, anginal attacks may be precipitated in susceptible individuals. Severe tachyarrhythmias occur occasionally.

DOSAGE AND PREPARATIONS.

Intravenous: *Adults,* 2 mg (10 ml) diluted in 500 ml of 5% dextrose injection is infused at a rate of 0.25 to 1 ml/min (1 to 4 mcg/min) with continuous monitoring of the electrocardiogram. The rate of infusion is determined by the chronotropic response. *Children,* 0.1 to 0.25 mcg/kg/min.

Generic. Solution 1:5,000 (0.2 mg/ml) in 5 ml containers.

Isuprel (Sanofi Winthrop). Solution (sterile) 1:5,000 (0.2 mg/ml) in 1 and 5 ml containers.

Cited References

Adhar GC, et al: Tocainide for drug-resistant sustained ventricular tachyarrhythmias. *J Am Coll Cardiol* 11:124-131, 1988.

Akhtar M, et al: Sudden cardiac death: Management of high-risk patients. *Ann Intern Med* 114:499-512, 1991.

Albers GW, et al: Stroke prevention in nonvalvular atrial fibrillation. *Ann Intern Med* 115:727-736, 1991.

Albert SG, et al: Thyroid dysfunction during chronic amiodarone therapy. *J Am Coll Cardiol* 9:175-183, 1987.

Anastasiou-Nana MI, et al: Usefulness of d, l sotalol for suppression of chronic ventricular arrhythmias. *Am J Cardiol* 67:511-516, 1991.

Anderson JL, et al: Prevention of symptomatic recurrences of paroxysmal atrial fibrillation in patients initially tolerating antiarrhythmic therapy: A multicenter, double-blind, crossover study of flecainide and placebo with transtelephonic monitoring. *Circulation* 80:1557-1570, 1989.

Antman EM, et al: Long-term oral propafenone therapy for suppression of refractory symptomatic atrial fibrillation and atrial flutter. *J Am Coll Cardiol* 12:1005-1011, 1988.

Baerman JM, et al: Interrelationships between serum levels of amiodarone, desethylamiodarone, reverse T_3 and the QT interval during long-term amiodarone therapy. *Am Heart J* 111:644-648, 1986.

Bigger JT: Definition of benign versus malignant ventricular arrhythmias: Targets for treatment. *Am J Cardiol* 52:47C-54C, 1983.

Brown JE, Shand DG: Therapeutic drug monitoring of antiarrhythmic agents. *Clin Pharmacokinet* 7:125-148, 1982.

Burkhart F, et al: Effect of antiarrhythmic therapy on mortality in survivors of myocardial infarction with asymptomatic complex ventricular arrhythmias: Basel Antiarrhythmic Study of Infarct Survival (BASIS). *J Am Coll Cardiol* 16:1711-1718, 1990.

Calkins H, et al: Diagnosis and cure of the Wolff-Parkinson-White syndrome or paroxysmal supraventricular tachycardias during a single electrophysiologic test. *N Engl J Med* 324:1612-1618, 1991.

Camm AJ, Garratt CJ: Adenosine and supraventricular tachycardia. *N Engl J Med* 325:1621-1629, 1991.
Camm AJ, Paul V: Sotalol for paroxysmal supraventricular tachycardias. *Am J Cardiol* 65:67A-73A, 1990.
Camm AJ, et al: Clinical usefulness of flecainide acetate in treatment of paroxysmal supraventricular arrhythmias. *Drugs* 29(suppl 4):7-13, 1985.
CAPS (Cardiac Arrhythmia Pilot Study) Investigators: Effects of encainide, flecainide, imipramine and moricizine on ventricular arrhythmias during the year after acute myocardial infarction. *Am J Cardiol* 61:501-509, 1988.
CAST (Cardiac Arrhythmia Suppression Trial) Investigators: Preliminary report: Effect of encainide and flecainide on mortality in a randomized trial of arrhythmia suppression after acute myocardial infarction. *N Engl J Med* 321:406-412, 1989.
Channer KS, et al: Towards improved control of atrial fibrillation. *Eur Heart J* 8:141-147, 1987.
Chilson DA, et al: Electrophysiologic effects and clinical efficacy of oral propafenone therapy in patients with ventricular tachycardia. *J Am Coll Cardiol* 5:1407-1413, 1985.
Cockrell JL, et al: Safety and efficacy of oral flecainide therapy in patients with atrioventricular re-entrant tachycardia. *Ann Intern Med* 114:189-194, 1991.
Connolly SJ, et al: Clinical efficacy and electrophysiology of oral propafenone for ventricular tachycardia. *Am J Cardiol* 52:1208-1213, 1983.
Coplen SE, et al: Efficacy and safety of quinidine therapy for maintenance of sinus rhythm after cardioversion: A meta-analysis of randomized control trials. *Circulation* 82:1106-1116, 1990.
Damle R, et al: Efficacy and risks of moricizine in inducible sustained ventricular tachycardia. *Ann Intern Med* 116:375-381, 1992.
de Paola AGAV, et al: Influence of left ventricular dysfunction on flecainide therapy. *J Am Coll Cardiol* 9:163-168, 1987.
DiMarco JP, et al: Diagnostic and therapeutic use of adenosine in patients with supraventricular tachyarrhythmias. *J Am Coll Cardiol* 6:417-425, 1985.
DiMarco JP, et al: Adenosine for paroxysmal supraventricular tachycardia: Dose ranging and comparison with verapamil. *Ann Intern Med* 113:104-110, 1990.
Dinh H, et al: Efficacy of propafenone compared with quinidine in chronic ventricular arrhythmias. *Am J Cardiol* 55:1520-1524, 1985.
Dobs AS, et al: Testicular dysfunction with amiodarone use. *J Am Coll Cardiol* 18:1328-1332, 1991.
Duff HJ, et al: Mexiletine-quinidine combination: Electrophysiologic correlates of a favorable antiarrhythmic interaction in humans. *J Am Coll Cardiol* 10:1149-1156, 1987.
Echt DS, et al: Mortality and morbidity in patients receiving encainide, flecainide, or placebo: The Cardiac Arrhythmia Suppression Trial. *N Engl J Med* 324:781-788, 1991.
Ellrodt AG, et al: Severe neutropenia associated with sustained-release procainamide. *Ann Intern Med* 100:197-201, 1984.
Esmolol Multicenter Study Research Group: Efficacy and safety of esmolol vs propranolol in treatment of supraventricular tachyarrhythmias: Multicenter double-blind clinical trial. *Am Heart J* 110:913-922, 1985.
Esmolol Research Group: Intravenous esmolol for treatment of supraventricular tachyarrhythmia: Results of multicenter, baseline-controlled safety and efficacy study in 160 patients. *Am Heart J* 112:498-504, 1986.
Feld GK, et al: Clinical and electrophysiologic effects of amiodarone in patients with atrial fibrillation complicating the Wolf-Parkinson-White syndrome. *Am Heart J* 115:102-107, 1988.
Friedman PL: Atrioventricular conduction disorders. *Cardiovasc Rev Rep* 12:32-45, (April) 1991.
Gleadhill IC, et al: Serial lung function testing in patients treated with amiodarone: Prospective study. *Am J Med* 86:4-10, 1988.
Gottlieb SS, et al: Comparative hemodynamic effects of procainamide, tocainide, and encainide in severe chronic heart failure. *Circulation* 81:860-864, 1990.
Graboys TB: Diagnosis and management of cardiac arrhythmias. *Cardiovasc Rev Rep* 12:35-55, (March) 1991.
Greene HL, et al: Congestive heart failure after acute myocardial infarction in patients receiving antiarrhythmic agents for ventricular premature complexes (Cardiac Arrhythmia Pilot Study). *Am J Cardiol* 63:393-398, 1989.
Greene HL, et al: The Cardiac Arrhythmia Suppression Trial: First CAST. . .then CAST-II. *J Am Coll Cardiol* 19:894-898, 1992.
Greenspan AM, et al: Efficacy of combination therapy with mexiletine and Type IA agent for inducible ventricular tachyarrhythmias secondary to coronary artery disease. *Am J Cardiol* 56:277-284, 1985.
Hazard PB, Burnett CR: Treatment of multifocal atrial tachycardia with metoprolol. *Crit Care Med* 15:20-25, 1987.
Heissenbuttel RH, Bigger JT Jr: Bretylium tosylate: Newly available antiarrhythmic drug for ventricular arrhythmias. *Ann Intern Med* 91:229-238, 1979.
Hellestrand KJ: Intravenous flecainide acetate for supraventricular tachycardias. *Am J Cardiol* 62:16D-22D, 1988.
Helmy I, et al: Use of intravenous amiodarone for emergency treatment of life-threatening ventricular arrhythmias. *J Am Coll Cardiol* 12:1015-1022, 1988.
Henthorn RW, et al: Flecainide acetate prevents recurrence of symptomatic paroxysmal supraventricular tachycardia. *Circulation* 83:119-125, 1991.
Hession MJ, et al: Ethmozine (moricizine HCL) therapy for complex ventricular arrhythmias. *Am J Cardiol* 60:59F-66F, 1987.
Hohnloser SH, et al: Short- and long-term antiarrhythmic and hemodynamic effects of d,l-sotalol in patients with symptomatic ventricular arrhythmias. *Am Heart J* 123:1220-1224, 1992.
Holt P, et al: Intravenous amiodarone in acute termination of supraventricular arrhythmias. *Int J Cardiol* 8:67-76, 1985.
Horowitz LN: Detection of amiodarone pulmonary toxicity: To screen or not to screen, that is the question! Editorial. *J Am Coll Cardiol* 12:789-790, 1988.
Horowitz LN, et al: Use of amiodarone in treatment of persistent and paroxysmal atrial fibrillation resistant to quinidine therapy. *J Am Coll Cardiol* 6:1402-1407, 1985.
Hughes MM, et al: Flecainide therapy in patients treated for supraventricular tachycardia with near normal left ventricular function. *Am Heart J* 123:408-412, 1992.
Huycke EC, at al: Intravenous diltiazem for termination of reentrant supraventricular tachycardia: Placebo-controlled, randomized, double-blind, multicenter study. *J Am Coll Cardiol* 13:538-544, 1989.
Jackman WM, et al: Catheter ablation of accessory atrioventricular pathways (Wolff-Parkinson-White syndrome) by radiofrequency current. *N Engl J Med* 324:1605-1611, 1991.
Janse MJ: The premature beat. *Cardiovasc Res* 26:89-100, 1992.
Kennedy HL: Late proarrhythmia and understanding the time of occurrence of proarrhythmia. *Am J Cardiol* 66:1139-1143, 1990.
Kennedy JI, et al: Amiodarone pulmonary toxicity: Clinical, radiologic, and pathologic correlations. *Arch Intern Med* 147:50-55, 1987.
Kerin NZ, et al: Mexiletine: Long-term efficacy and side effects in patients with chronic drug-resistant potentially lethal ventricular arrhythmias. *Arch Intern Med* 150:381-384, 1990.
Kim SG, et al: Combination of tocainide and quinidine for better tolerance and additive effects in patients with coronary artery disease. *J Am Coll Cardiol* 9:1369-1374, 1987.
Kirk CR, et al: Cardiovascular collapse after verapamil in supraventricular tachycardia. *Arch Dis Child* 62:1265-1282, 1987.
Kirkali Z: Amiodarone-induced sterile epididymitis. *Urol Int* 43:372-373, 1988.
Klein GT, et al: Surgical treatment of tachycardias: Indications and electrophysiologic assessment. *Prog Cardiovasc Dis* 15:139-153, 1987.
Kuck KH, Schluter M: Single-catheter approach to radiofrequency current ablation of left sided accessory pathways in patients with Wolff-Parkinson-White syndrome. *Circulation* 84:2366-2375, 1991.
Lehmann KG, Chen YCJ: Reduction of ventricular arrhythmias by atropine during coronary arteriography. *Am J Cardiol* 63:447-451, 1989.

Levine JH, et al: Treatment of multifocal atrial tachycardia with verapamil. *N Engl J Med* 312:21-25, 1985.

Lewis RV, McDevitt DG: Factors affecting the clinical response to treatment with digoxin and two calcium antagonists in patients with atrial fibrillation. *Br J Clin Pharmacol* 25:603-606, 1988.

Ludmer PL, et al: Efficacy of propafenone in Wolff-Parkinson-White syndrome: Electrophysiologic findings and long-term follow-up. *J Am Coll Cardiol* 9:1357-1363, 1987.

MacMahon S, et al: Effects of prophylactic lidocaine in suspected acute myocardial infarction: Overview of results from the randomized, controlled trials. *JAMA* 260:1910-1916, 1988.

Mann HJ: Moricizine: A new class I antiarrhythmic. *Clin Pharm* 9:842-852, 1990.

Mason JW: Amiodarone. *N Engl J Med* 316:455-466, 1987.

McGovern B, et al: Precipitation of cardiac arrest by verapamil in patients with Wolff-Parkinson-White syndrome. *Ann Intern Med* 104:791-794, 1986.

Meyers DG, et al: Severe neutropenia associated with procainamide: Comparison of sustained release and conventional preparations. *Am Heart J* 109:1393-1395, 1985.

Morady F, et al: Acute and chronic effects of amiodarone on ventricular refractoriness, intraventricular conduction and ventricular tachycardia induction. *J Am Coll Cardiol* 7:148-157, 1986.

Morady F, et al: Antagonism of quinidine's electrophysiologic effects by epinephrine in patients with ventricular tachycardia. *J Am Coll Cardiol* 12:388-394, 1988 A.

Morady F, et al: Effects of epinephrine in patients with an accessory atrioventricular connection treated with quinidine. *Am J Cardiol* 62:580-584, 1988 B.

Morady F, et al: Epinephrine-induced reversal of verapamil's electrophysiologic and therapeutic effects in patients with paroxysmal supraventricular tachycardia. *Circulation* 79:783-790, 1989.

Morganroth J: Premature ventricular complexes: Diagnosis and indications for therapy. *JAMA* 252:673-676, 1984.

Morganroth J: Comparative efficacy and safety of oral mexiletine and quinidine for benign and potentially lethal ventricular arrhythmias. *Am J Cardiol* 60:1276-1281, 1987.

Morganroth J, Goin JE: Quinidine-related mortality in the short-to-medium-term treatment of ventricular arrhythmias: A meta-analysis. *Circulation* 84:1977-1983, 1991.

Morganroth J, Hunter H: Comparative efficacy and safety of short-acting and sustained-release quinidine in treatment of patients with ventricular arrhythmias. *Am Heart J* 110:1176-1180, 1985.

Morganroth J, et al: Comparative efficacy and safety of oral tocainide and quinidine for benign and potentially lethal ventricular arrhythmias. *Am J Cardiol* 56:581-585, 1985.

Morganroth J, et al: Efficacy and tolerance of Ethmozine (moricizine HCL) in placebo-controlled trials. *Am J Cardiol* 60:48F-51F, 1987.

Moss AJ, et al: Long QT syndrome: Prospective international study. *Circulation* 71:17-21, 1985.

Mymin D, et al: Natural history of primary first-degree atrioventricular heart block. *N Engl J Med* 315:1183-1187, 1986.

Nalos PC, et al: Intravenous amiodarone for short-term treatment of refractory ventricular tachycardia or fibrillation. *Am Heart J* 122:1629-1632, 1991.

Nolan PE Jr: Generic substitution of antiarrhythmic drugs, editorial. *Am J Cardiol* 64:1371-1373, 1989.

Ochi RP, et al: Intravenous amiodarone for rapid treatment of life-threatening ventricular arrhythmias in critically ill patients with coronary artery disease. *Am J Cardiol* 64:599-603, 1989.

Podrid PJ, et al: Congestive heart failure caused by oral disopyramide. *N Engl J Med* 302:614-617, 1980.

Poole JE, et al: Intolerance and ineffectiveness of mexiletine in patients with serious ventricular arrhythmias. *Am Heart J* 112:322-326, 1986.

Powell AC, et al: Electrophysiologic response to moricizine in patients with sustained ventricular arrhythmias. *Ann Intern Med* 116:382-387, 1992.

Pratt CM, et al: Antiarrhythmic efficacy of Ethmozine (moricizine HCL) compared with disopyramide and propranolol. *Am J Cardiol* 60:52F-58F, 1987.

Pritchett ELC: Management of atrial fibrillation. *N Engl J Med* 326:1264-1271, 1992.

Pritchett ELC, Wilkinson WE: Mortality in patients with flecainide and encainide for supraventricular arrhythmias. *Am J Cardiol* 67:976-980, 1991.

Pritchett ELC, et al: Flecainide acetate treatment of paroxysmal supraventricular tachycardia and paroxysmal atrial fibrillation: Dose-response studies. *J Am Coll Cardiol* 17:297-303, 1991 A.

Pritchett ELC, et al: Propafenone treatment of symptomatic paroxysmal supraventricular arrhythmias: A randomized, placebo-controlled, crossover trial in patients tolerating oral therapy. *Ann Intern Med* 114:539-544, 1991 B.

Rankin AC, et al: Misuse of intravenous verapamil in patients with ventricular tachycardia. *Lancet* 2:472-473, 1987.

Rinkenberger RL, et al: Effects of intravenous and chronic oral verapamil administration in patients with supraventricular tachyarrhythmias. *Circulation* 62:996-1010, 1980.

Rotmensch HH, et al: Management of cardiac arrhythmias during pregnancy: Current concepts. *Drugs* 33:623-633, 1987.

Ruskin JN: Catheter ablation for supraventricular tachycardia, editorial. *N Engl J Med* 324:1660-1662, 1991.

Salerno DM, et al: Intravenous verapamil for treatment of multifocal atrial tachycardia with and without calcium pretreatment. *Ann Intern Med* 107:623-628, 1987.

Salerno DM, et al: Efficacy and safety of intravenous diltiazem for treatment of atrial fibrillation and atrial flutter. *Am J Cardiol* 63:1046-1051, 1989.

Scheinman MM, et al: Current role of catheter ablative procedures in patients with cardiac arrhythmias: A report for health professionals from the Subcommittee on Electrocardiography and Electrophysiology, American Heart Association. *Circulation* 83:2146-2153, 1991.

Schweitzer P, Mark H: Effect of atropine on cardiac arrhythmias and conduction, parts I and II. *Am Heart J* 100:119-127, 255-261, 1980.

Shen EN, et al: Intravenous propafenone for termination of reentrant supraventricular tachycardia: Placebo-controlled, randomized, double-blind, crossover study. *Ann Intern Med* 105:655-661, 1986.

Shenasa M, et al: Efficacy and safety of intravenous and oral diltiazem for Wolff-Parkinson-White syndrome. *Am J Cardiol* 59:301-306, 1987.

Singh BN: Historical development of the concept of controlling cardiac arrhythmias by lengthening repolarization: Particular reference to sotalol. *Am J Cardiol* 65:3A-11A, 1990.

Singh BN, et al: Sotalol: A review of its pharmacodynamic and pharmacokinetic properties, and therapeutic use. *Drugs* 34:311-349, 1987.

Smith WM, et al: Long-term tolerance of amiodarone treatment for cardiac arrhythmias. *Am J Cardiol* 57:1228-1293, 1986.

Sokoloff NM, et al: Plasma norepinephrine in exercise-induced ventricular tachycardia. *J Am Coll Cardiol* 8:11-17, 1986.

Stanton MS, et al: Arrhythmogenic effects of antiarrhythmic drugs: A study of 506 patients treated for ventricular tachycardia or fibrillation. *J Am Coll Cardiol* 14:209-215, 1989.

Stewart RB, et al: Wide complex tachycardia: Misdiagnosis and outcome after emergent therapy. *Ann Intern Med* 104:766-771, 1986.

Teichman SL, et al: Disopyramide-pyridostigmine interaction: Selective reversal of anticholinergic symptoms with preservation of antiarrhythmic effect. *J Am Coll Cardiol* 10:633-641, 1987.

Torres V, et al: QT prolongation and antiarrhythmic efficacy of amiodarone. *J Am Coll Cardiol* 7:142-147, 1986.

Waitzer S, et al: Cutaneous ultrastructural changes and photosensitivity associated with amiodarone therapy. *J Am Acad Dermatol* 16:779-787, 1987.

Weiss JN, et al: Ventricular arrhythmias in ischemic heart disease. *Ann Intern Med* 114:784-797, 1991.

Wilson JS, Podrid PJ: Side effects from amiodarone. *Am Heart J* 121:158-171, 1991.

Wiseman MN, et al: A study of the use of flecainide acetate in the long-term management of cardiac arrhythmias. *PACE Pacing Clin Electrophysiol* 13:767-775, 1990.

Woosley RL: Role of plasma concentration monitoring in the evaluation of response to antiarrhythmic drugs. *Am J Cardiol* 62:9H-17H, 1988.

Yeh S-J, et al: Effects of oral diltiazem in paroxysmal supraventricular tachycardia. *Am J Cardiol* 52:271-278, 1983.

Zipes DP: Consideration of antiarrhythmic therapy, editorial. *Circulation* 72:949-956, 1985.

Zipes DP: Proarrhythmic events. *Am J Cardiol* 61:70A-76A, 1988.

Zipes DP: Monophasic action potentials in the diagnosis of triggered arrhythmias. *Prog Cardiovasc Dis* 33:385-396, (June) 1991.

Zipes DP, et al: Amiodarone: Electrophysiologic actions, pharmacokinetics and clinical effects. *J Am Coll Cardiol* 3:1059-1071, 1984.

Drugs Used for Heart Failure 28

HEART FAILURE

Heart failure is estimated to develop in 3 to 4 million Americans and is especially common in those ≥65 years of age (American Heart Association, 1992). For those over 75 years, its prevalence is about 10%. The most common underlying causes of heart failure are coronary heart disease, hypertension, idiopathic dilated cardiomyopathy, and valvular heart disease. Approximately 400,000 new cases are diagnosed each year in the United States (Yusef et al, 1989). The total number of cases is likely to grow, because improved therapy has increased the survival rate in patients with underlying acute myocardial infarction and valvular heart disease, even those with significant left ventricular dysfunction.

Although available therapies reduce symptoms and improve exercise capacity, mortality among patients with heart failure remains high; the annual rates range from 15% to 50%, depending on the severity of the condition. The mortality rate increases proportionally with advancing age, and men are at greater risk than women. Data from the National Health and Nutrition Examination Survey-1 Epidemiologic Follow-up Study showed that the 15-year total mortality rate for heart failure in patients ≥55 years was 39% for women and 70% for men (Schocken et al, 1992). Sudden death occurs in about 40% of patients and usually is associated with serious arrhythmias.

Etiology

Heart failure is precipitated by the inability of the myocardium to contract sufficiently during systole, and thus supply an adequate volume of blood for the metabolic needs of the tissues of the body, or to distend sufficiently during diastole, which results in congestion (Kloner, 1991). The syndrome is associated with increased atrial pressure, reduced exercise tolerance, ventricular arrhythmias, and shortened life expectancy. The abnormality in cardiac function may be due to aberrations in the myocardial cells themselves or to some other structural irregularity (eg, valvular stenosis impairing ventricular ejection).

Myocardial failure may be caused by a quantitative loss of functioning myofibrils, as in heart failure associated with a large myocardial infarction, or to a generalized qualitative abnormality in myocyte function, as in idiopathic dilated cardiomyopathy. The precise mechanism for abnormal myocardial function is unknown, but the defects may be due to reduced myofibrillar ATPase content or activity, defective sarcoplasmic reticulum, and/or alterations in mitochondrial function.

In normal individuals, the heart employs several compensatory mechanisms to maintain pumping ability when metabolic demands are increased (eg, exercise, emotional stress). The myocardium can adapt by stretching the cardiac cells to increase the ventricular end-diastolic volume and/or by augmenting the contractile strength of the myofibrils. Factors that alter the end-diastolic volume include total blood volume, body position, intrathoracic and intrapericardial pressure, venous tone, the pumping action of skeletal muscle that returns blood to the heart, and the contribution of the atrium to ventricular filling. Factors that increase the contractile strength of the myocardium include sympathetic nerve stimulation of the myocardial cells and elevation of circulating catecholamines to increase heart rate.

In those with heart failure, compensating mechanisms in response to the decrease in the proportion of functional myocardium include development of myocardial hypertrophy and activation of the neurohumoral systems. The major neurohumoral compensatory mechanisms are an increase in sympathetic tone, activation of the renin-angiotensin-aldosterone system, and release of arginine vasopressin (AVP, antidiuretic hormone, ADH). Sympathetic nervous system activity is consistently increased (Creager et al, 1986; Leimbach et al, 1986). The postsynaptic $alpha_2$ receptor is an important mediator of vasoconstriction in patients with heart failure and, despite high levels of circulating norepinephrine, the $alpha_2$ receptor is not down-regulated (Kubo et al, 1989). The response of the vasopressin and renin-angiotensin systems to hemodynamic stress is independent of that of the sympathetic nervous system (Levine et al, 1986). Plasma norepinephrine concentration and plasma renin activity increase over time (Francis et al, 1988).

The resulting increase in vascular tone and intravascular volume initially is limited by release of atrial natriuretic factor (ANF) and renal prostaglandins, endogenous counter-regulatory substances that promote natriuresis and vasodilation (Creager et al, 1988; Dzau, 1988). As heart failure progresses, these endogenous systems are unable to maintain compensation, and excessive vasoconstriction and volume overload follow. Even though the vasoconstriction occurs throughout the body, the resulting reduction in regional blood flow and capillary perfusion leads to dysfunction in critical organs (eg, decreased glomerular filtration rate and development of azotemia; decreased aerobic/anaerobic metabolism, augmented lactate production, and easy fatigability in skeletal muscle; reduced myocardial oxygen delivery, subendocardial ischemia, and further impairment of cardiac function in the myocardium [Leier, 1992 A]). These regional defects largely produce the symptoms observed in patients, especially in those with low-output heart failure.

Classification

The New York Heart Association (NYHA) has devised a classification system that grades the severity of heart failure according to the amount of exertion required to cause symptoms:

Class I. No limitation of physical activity. No dyspnea, fatigue, or palpitations with ordinary physical activity.

Class II. Slight limitation of physical activity. These patients have fatigue, palpitations, and dyspnea with ordinary physical activity, but are comfortable at rest.

Class III. Marked limitation of activity. Less than ordinary physical activity results in symptoms, but patients are comfortable at rest.

Class IV. Symptoms are present at rest, and any physical exertion exacerbates symptoms.

Anatomically, heart failure can be right- and left-sided. Right-sided ventricular failure, associated with the accumulation of blood in the systemic venous circuit, produces symptoms and signs of edema; congestive hepatomegaly; ascites; and, eventually, weakness and mental confusion. Symptoms and signs of left-sided ventricular failure are caused by blood accumulating behind the left ventricle and pulmonary congestion. Long-standing left-sided ventricular failure may eventually result in signs of right ventricular failure with generalized accumulation of fluid.

Functionally, heart failure can be divided into low- and high-output failure. Heart failure that causes low cardiac output is most common and usually is due to an ischemic, valvular, hypertensive, congenital, or cardiomyopathic process. It is characterized by reduced stroke volume; peripheral vasoconstriction producing cold, pale extremities; reduced pulse pressure; and an increase in arteriovenous oxygen difference. High-output failure is characterized by a widened pulse pressure, peripheral vasodilatation, and warm, flushed extremities and is associated with a decrease in the arteriovenous oxygen gradient. Several conditions rarely may precipitate high-output failure (eg, beriberi, Paget's disease, thyrotoxicosis, arteriovenous fistula, anemia).

Treatment

Precipitating causes of heart failure should be identified and treated (Kloner, 1991; Feldman, 1992). Patients in whom heart failure is due to aortic stenosis may benefit from surgical correction; those with mitral stenosis may benefit from surgical correction or percutaneous balloon valvuloplasty. If severe coronary artery disease with recurrent ischemia is causative, angioplasty or surgical correction may be appropriate. Lowering of blood pressure benefits patients with hypertensive heart disease. Patients with heart failure caused by cardiomyopathy due to alcohol ingestion should abstain from alcohol consumption. Salt restriction, reduction of stressful physical exertion, avoidance of emotional stress, and weight loss by obese patients are important general therapeutic measures.

Exercise testing is an integral part of the assessment of patients with chronic heart failure. Results of several studies indicate that exercise training benefits patients with well-compensated chronic heart failure, even those with considerable left ventricular impairment in whom exercise capacity is reduced because of dyspnea and fatigue (Myers and Froelicher, 1991; Uren and Lipkin, 1992). Such training delays the onset of decreased metabolism in skeletal muscle by reversing the impairment of peripheral vasodilatation and improving blood flow to the exercising muscles. Exercise training is safe and does not induce clinical deterioration as was previously believed.

Patients with Class II, III, or IV heart failure also require drug therapy. Four major categories of drugs are used alone or in combination: diuretics, digitalis glycosides, vasodilators, and nonglycoside inotropic agents (Feldman, 1992).

Diuretics reduce the volume of extracellular fluid and thereby benefit patients with congestive symptoms, pulmonary edema, and systemic edema. However, they may activate neuroendocrine systems, deplete the body of potassium and magnesium, and aggravate arrhythmias. Digitalis glycosides increase cardiac contractility and improve hemodynamics and exercise tolerance. These drugs prevent the worsening of heart failure in patients with systolic dysfunction, even though any improvement in survival has yet to be demonstrated. Vasodilators reduce preload and afterload. Use of angiotensin-converting enzyme (ACE) inhibitors in patients with early symptoms of left ventricular dysfunction reduces left ventricular dilatation. ACE inhibitors also decrease blood pressure and increase serum potassium concentrations. In patients with predominant diastolic abnormalities of the heart (eg, hypertrophic cardiomyopathy), calcium channel blocking agents may improve left ventricular relaxation. Patients with very severe heart failure (Class IV) may require the more potent inotropic agents such as dopamine, dobutamine, or phosphodiesterase inhibitors. Some of these patients may be candidates for special measures, such as cardiac transplantation, left ventricular assist devices, and an artificial heart.

Because of the complex pathophysiology of heart failure and its progressive nature, it is unlikely that one drug can control all signs and symptoms and improve survival. Depending on the patient's condition, a combination of diuretics, digitalis, vasodilators, and inotropic agents may be required. For example, ACE inhibitors or a combination of hydralazine plus isosorbide dinitrate have improved the survival rate in patients with moderate to severe heart failure who are also receiving digoxin and diuretics (Cohn et al, 1991; The SOLVD Investigators, 1991).

DIURETICS

In heart failure, the effective arterial blood volume is reduced and the kidneys, in response to a true volume deficit, retain salt and water. Renin release leads to the formation of angiotensin II, which stimulates aldosterone production by the adrenal cortex. Aldosterone augments renal sodium retention with concomitant potassium loss. Diuretics increase sodium chloride and water excretion and thus reduce preload and relieve symptoms of pulmonary and systemic congestion. By decreasing left ventricular volume and wall tension, they also may reduce myocardial oxygen demand. Their long-term use may reduce peripheral vascular resistance and, thus, aortic impedance. Diuretics are well tolerated and are probably the most commonly used agents for initial therapy in patients with mild chronic heart failure and normal sinus rhythm (Hlatky et al, 1986).

For patients with well-preserved renal function, therapy is usually begun with a thiazide or related diuretic. When the glomerular filtration rate is less than 30 ml/min, thiazides (except metolazone [Diulo, Zaroxolyn] and indapamide [Lozol]) are usually ineffective, but a loop diuretic (furosemide [Lasix], ethacrynic acid [Edecrin], bumetanide [Bumex]) will frequently produce a diuresis. Combinations of diuretics acting at different sites, such as furosemide and a thiazide, are often more effective than larger doses of the loop diuretic in patients with refractory cardiac edema. Potassium-sparing diuretics (spironolactone [Aldactone], triamterene [Dyrenium], amiloride [Midamor]) are given with thiazide or loop diuretics to prevent hypokalemia; they are particularly appropriate for digitalized patients, because hypokalemia may predispose to or accentuate digitalis intoxication. However, potassium-sparing diuretics generally are not used with ACE inhibitors, because the combination may precipitate hyperkalemia.

Diuretics also are useful for treating acute pulmonary edema, but they should not be regarded as substitutes for emergency measures that reduce central blood volume immediately, such as placing the patient in an upright position and administering morphine or venodilators (eg, nitrates). A loop diuretic is usually preferred for the initial management of patients with pulmonary congestion following acute myocardial infarction.

Care should be taken to avoid excessive diuresis, which may cause marked contraction of the plasma volume (often with accompanying hypochloremic alkalosis), reduction in cardiac filling pressure and cardiac output, hypoperfusion of vital organs, renal insufficiency, depletion of potassium and magnesium, and activation of compensatory vasoconstrictor mechanisms. The long-term daily use of diuretics may be inadvisable in some patients. Therefore, the diuretic is continued until the patient's weight has decreased to a stable baseline and is maintained or until an edema-free state is sustained.

For a more detailed discussion of diuretics and dosage information, see index entry Diuretics.

DIGITALIS GLYCOSIDES

ACTIONS. Digitalis has complex direct and indirect cardiovascular actions that are of potential value in the treatment of heart failure. In patients with significant left ventricular systolic dysfunction as evidenced by a reduced ejection fraction <0.4, the direct positive inotropic action of digitalis may increase cardiac output and thereby decrease venous pressure, reduce heart size, and slow compensatory *reflex* tachycardia. Because digitalis decreases ventricular volume, it does not increase myocardial oxygen consumption in the failing heart. Improved renal hemodynamics promote diuresis, thus reducing blood volume and relieving edema. The digitalis glycosides also have a mild direct diuretic action that is independent of changes in the glomerular filtration rate and renal blood flow.

The direct actions of digitalis are believed to result from inhibition of $(Na^+ + K^+)$-ATPase, an enzyme system that provides the energy for active transport of sodium and potassium ions across the myocardial cell membrane. Digitalis combines reversibly with $(Na^+ + K^+)$-ATPase on the cell membrane and thereby prevents the binding of ATP. Inhibition of the sodium-potassium transport system is accompanied by increased cellular uptake of calcium ions due to enhanced sodium-calcium exchange. The increase in cytosolic calcium activates the contractile elements. In addition to its inotropic effects, digitalis may have a beneficial neurohumoral modulating effect by restoring the baroreceptor sensitivity that is decreased in chronic heart failure (Gheorghiade and Ferguson, 1991).

USES. Digitalis is most effective when heart failure is associated with severely depressed systolic function, whether caused by ischemic, hypertensive, valvular, or congenital heart disease. By slowing the ventricular response to atrial fibrillation, glycoside therapy permits adequate time for ventricular filling and emptying. However, digitalis does not usually control the ventricular rate adequately, particularly during exercise, and additional medication may be necessary. To the degree that it decreases the ventricular response in conditions such as mitral stenosis, digitalis can relieve pulmonary congestion, but it is rarely useful in patients with mitral stenosis and normal sinus rhythm.

During long-term therapy, the effect of digitalis on resting hemodynamics is variable, whereas hemodynamic improvement during exercise is sustained (Arnold et al, 1980; Griffiths et al, 1982; Murray et al, 1983). In a multicenter study on patients with mild to moderate heart failure also receiving maintenance diuretic therapy, digitalis increased left ventricular ejection fraction, reduced diuretic requirements, and decreased the frequency of exacerbation of heart failure (Captopril-Digoxin Multicenter Research Group, 1988). Improvement in exercise performance also has been observed in other studies (DiBianco et al, 1989; Enalapril Versus Digoxin French Multicenter Study Group, 1989).

In patients with heart failure due to systolic dysfunction who were treated concurrently with ACE inhibitors, withdrawal of digoxin was associated with clinical and hemodynamic deterioration and decreased exercise capacity (Davies et al, 1991; Packer et al, 1992). Similar deterioration after digoxin withdrawal was observed in patients with heart failure and an ejection fraction of ≤0.35 who were not treated with ACE inhibitors (Young et al, 1992). The National Heart, Lung and Blood Institute and the Department of Veterans Affairs Cooperative Studies Program are currently conducting an international double-blind, randomized, controlled clinical trial (Digitalis Investigation Group, DIG) to assess the effect on mortality of digoxin combined with ACE inhibitors. A total of 7,000 patients with heart failure and ejection fractions <0.45 who are being treated with ACE inhibitors will be randomized to receive either digoxin or placebo.

Approximately 90% of pediatric patients with cardiac failure are infants up to 3 months of age who have severe congenital anomalies that either obstruct ventricular outflow or reroute blood flow. These infants usually respond to digitalis and diuretics.

Glycoside therapy is of limited value in patients with high-output heart failure associated with thyrotoxicosis, chronic anemia, beriberi, or AV fistulas. Effective treatment of these disorders requires correction of the underlying cause. Glycoside therapy often fails to restore compensation when congestive heart failure develops in conjunction with chronic constrictive pericarditis or myocarditis. In patients with hypertrophic cardiomyopathy and other disorders with intact systolic function, the manifestations of heart failure are caused by impaired diastolic function; thus, digitalis usually is not helpful and should be avoided except in those patients with associated atrial fibrillation (see index entry Cardiomyopathy, Hypertrophic).

Digitalis usually does not improve right ventricular function in patients with pulmonary heart disease unless left ventricular function is also impaired (Mathur et al, 1981). Patients with pulmonary heart disease are particularly susceptible to digitalis toxicity; however, digitalis may have a positive inotropic effect on the diaphragm, similar to its effect on the heart, which could be of benefit in patients with chronic obstructive pulmonary disease (Aubier et al, 1987).

FACTORS MODIFYING RESPONSE TO THERAPY. The response to digitalis is influenced by many factors, including the nature and severity of the underlying heart disease, the patient's age, the status of renal function and electrolyte balance, the presence of noncardiac disorders, and the concomitant use of other drugs. Dosage must be individualized, and conditions that predispose to toxicity (eg, hypokalemia, hypercalcemia, hypothyroidism, hypomagnesemia) should be corrected. The dose of digoxin should be reduced and the serum concentration assessed when necessary in patients with renal insufficiency. Even when blood urea nitrogen and creatinine concentrations are within normal limits, the elderly must be assumed to have an age-related reduction in creatinine clearance that necessitates a reduction in dosage, because digoxin is excreted largely unchanged in the urine. Digitoxin, on the other hand, is extensively metabolized before excretion and the dose generally need not be adjusted because of changes in renal function.

A satisfactory response to digitalis is manifested by diuresis, weight loss, reduced pulmonary and systemic venous congestion, decreased heart size and/or rate, and relief of peripheral edema, fatigue, shortness of breath, and orthopnea. If digitalis is the initial and only therapeutic agent employed, these endpoints are useful in titrating dosage. However, sodium restriction, ACE inhibitors, and diuretic therapy also are prescribed for most patients with moderately severe heart failure. Since these measures reduce the load on the heart and relieve edema, the relative contribution of digitalis to the therapeutic response often cannot be assessed. If clinical improvement is not satisfactory and the serum concentration is below or in the lower end of what is considered the usual "therapeutic range," the dose of digitalis may be increased cautiously (Gheorghiade et al, 1992).

MEASUREMENT OF SERUM CONCENTRATIONS. Serum digoxin levels can be measured by radioimmunoassay, which is sensitive to levels of 0.2 to 0.4 ng/ml (Lewis, 1992). Most radioimmunoassays can detect digoxin metabolites, including digoxigenin, bisdigoxiside, and monodigoxiside. However, these assays have relatively low specificity and cross-react with digitalis-like immunoreactive substances, which may be present in patients with renal or hepatic failure, some hypertensive states, or heart failure, as well as during pregnancy. Hence, a baseline serum digoxin concentration should be obtained to determine the presence of these substances before digitalization. In addition, a major error in the use of serum digoxin assays is the failure to allow sufficient time to elapse for equilibration to occur (ie, 12 hours after an oral dose). Five half-lives (10 to 20 days) are usually required to reach steady state after any change in dose. In general, a near-maximal digoxin effect can be expected with a steady-state serum concentration of 1 to 1.5 ng/ml, a range with low risk of toxicity (Lewis, 1992).

Serum digoxin levels are used to validate the dose, monitor patient compliance, evaluate bioavailability, and assess the effects of renal function or of other drugs on elimination. The assay also can be used to evaluate hemodynamic or clinical changes (eg, worsening heart failure), to confirm apparent failure to respond to digoxin, or to diagnose and prevent digoxin toxicity. However, the serum digoxin level should not be considered the definitive measure of clinical condition; other parameters (slowing of heart rate, initiation of diuresis, improvement in dyspnea, disappearance of an S_3 gallop, improvement in chest radiograph) also should be considered.

INTERACTIONS. Hypokalemia predisposes to digitalis toxicity; even a moderate reduction of the serum potassium concentration can precipitate serious arrhythmias. Hypokalemia is encountered most frequently in patients receiving long-term therapy with thiazide or loop diuretics. Since patients with heart failure commonly receive both diuretics and digitalis, hypokalemia may be especially arrhythmogenic and dangerous. These patients should be closely monitored for the development of hypokalemia, and many clinicians routinely prescribe a potassium-sparing diuretic or potassium chloride supplements along with the potassium-wasting diuretic. In children, foods that are high in potassium and low in sodium may be preferable. Supplements and dietary sources are not as reliable as the potassium-sparing diuretics.

Quinidine increases the serum digoxin concentration by reducing its renal and nonrenal clearance and altering its volume of distribution. This interaction has been reported to cause gastrointestinal disturbances and, more important, serious ventricular arrhythmias. It has been recommended that patients receiving both drugs be monitored carefully for signs of digitalis toxicity, particularly during the first five days of combined therapy; that the dose of digoxin be reduced by one-half before starting quinidine (Bigger, 1981); and that patients stabilized on both drugs be evaluated for underdigitalization if quinidine is discontinued.

Several other cardiovascular drugs (verapamil [Calan, Isoptin], flecainide [Tambocor], amiloride [Midamor], amiodarone [Cordarone], propafenone [Rythmol]), as well as quinine, hydroxychloroquine [Plaquenil], and cyclosporine [Sandimmune], increase the serum digoxin concentration. Nifedipine [Procardia] and diltiazem [Cardizem] probably do not cause a clinically important increase in the serum concentration of digoxin, although patients should be monitored for signs of digoxin toxicity when such combinations are used. Symptomatic sinus bradycardia has been reported in patients receiving both digoxin and methyldopa [Aldomet]; however, methyldopa does not alter the disposition of digoxin. Spironolactone has been reported to increase serum digoxin levels, but this apparent interaction now appears to be due to interference with digoxin radioimmunoassay by the spironolactone metabolite, canrenone. The acute administration of certain vasodilator drugs (nitroprusside [Nitropress], hydralazine) reduces serum digoxin levels by increasing renal clearance of the glycoside, and it may be necessary to adjust digoxin dosage during long-term vasodilator therapy. Serum digoxin levels also may be reduced by rifampin [Rifadin, Rimactane] and phenytoin [Dilantin, Diphenylan]. In preterm infants, intravenous indomethacin [Indocin IV] decreases the renal excretion of digoxin.

In approximately 10% of patients, substantial amounts of digoxin are converted to inactive metabolites in the gut, and concurrent antibiotic therapy (erythromycin or tetracycline) markedly increases serum digoxin levels in these individuals. The bioavailability of digoxin is reduced by antacids, dietary bran, kaolin-pectin preparations, cholestyramine resin [Questran], colestipol [Colestid], sulfasalazine [Azulfidine], neomycin, and cytotoxic drugs. Anticholinergic drugs may reduce the gastrointestinal absorption of slowly dissolving brands of digoxin tablets.

ADVERSE REACTIONS AND PRECAUTIONS. The ratio between the full therapeutic and toxic dose of digitalis glycosides is narrow; however, the incidence of digoxin toxicity has diminished from 25% to 2% since radioimmunoassay has been used to determine serum digoxin levels (Lewis, 1992). In part, this also is due to the development of newer classes of drugs for the treatment of both supraventricular arrhythmias and heart failure and to greater recognition of interactions between digoxin and other commonly used cardiovascular agents. The diagnosis of digitalis toxicity is based on the presence of both symptoms and electrocardiographic signs consistent with toxicity, a serum digoxin concentration of at least 1.5 ng/ml, and a close temporal correlation between drug withdrawal or administration of digoxin immune Fab (see Treatment of Toxicity below) and resolution of evidence of toxicity. Digitalis intoxication usually is associated with too rapid loading, accumulation of larger than necessary maintenance doses, the presence of conditions that predispose to toxicity, intentional or accidental overdose, or prescribing digitalis in doses beyond reasonable limits when it is not likely to be effective.

Intoxication usually can be prevented by evaluating therapy frequently, by decreasing the dosage in the presence of factors that tend to cause excessive accumulation (eg, impaired renal function, drug interactions), by correcting conditions that increase toxicity (eg, hypokalemia, alkalosis, hypercalcemia, hypoxia, hypomagnesemia), or by treating underlying diseases (eg, hypothyroidism, anemia, valvular heart disease). When the risk of intoxication is great, a short-acting glycoside should be used.

All digitalis glycosides are classified in FDA Pregnancy Category C.

Extracardiac Reactions: Gastrointestinal and neurologic disturbances may be early signs of digitalis intoxication and serve as a warning that severe cardiotoxicity can result if the drug is not temporarily discontinued or the dosage reduced.

Anorexia, nausea, vomiting, and abdominal pain are the most common gastrointestinal symptoms; diarrhea also may occur. The emetic effect of digitalis is probably of central origin and occurs after either oral or parenteral administration.

Fatigue is the most frequent neurologic manifestation of toxicity. Other symptoms are depression, headache, drowsiness, weakness, lethargy, neuralgia, restlessness, nightmares, personality changes, vertigo, confusion, disorientation, and, rarely, hallucinations and other psychotic reactions. Ocular disturbances include mydriasis, photophobia, modified color perception (particularly yellow vision), visions of flashing or flickering lights, appearance of halos around lights, and reduced visual acuity. The reduction in visual acuity occurs in the form of bilateral central scotomata and appears to be caused by an effect of digitalis on the retinal receptor cells.

Gynecomastia, sexual dysfunction, sweating, and hypersensitivity reactions (urticaria, eosinophilia, thrombocytopenia, vasculitis) occur rarely.

Cardiac Reactions: A disturbance of cardiac rhythm may be the first evidence of digitalis intoxication. Almost any type of arrhythmia may occur; the most common are ventricular bigeminy or trigeminy, multiform premature ventricular complexes, atrial tachycardia with AV block, and nonparoxysmal AV junctional (nodal) tachycardia. The latter arrhythmia is particularly likely to occur in the presence of pre-existing atrial fibrillation. Other digitalis-induced arrhythmias include sinus irregularities (sinus bradycardia, SA block, sinus arrest), unifocal ventricular premature complexes, accelerated ventricular rhythm, fascicular tachycardia, paroxysmal ventricular tachycardia, and ventricular fibrillation. AV dissociation may be induced by a combination of some degree of AV block plus junctional (or ventricular) tachycardia. A bidirectional tachycardia that is of ventricular origin indicates an advanced stage of digitalis intoxication. Digitalis rarely causes atrial fibrillation or flutter.

Treatment of Toxicity: The key to successful treatment is early recognition of an arrhythmia that may be related to digitalis intoxication (Kelly and Smith, 1992). Temporary drug withdrawal usually eliminates symptoms such as ectopic beats or first-degree AV block. Sinus bradycardia, sinoatrial arrest, and AV block are sometimes treated with atropine. Temporary pacing may be necessary.

Digitalis-induced arrhythmias may be exacerbated by both hypokalemia and hyperkalemia. Administration of potassium is most effective in patients with hypokalemia who have atrial tachycardia with AV block, ventricular premature complexes, or ventricular tachycardia as a manifestation of digitalis intoxication. Potassium should be avoided in those with hyperkalemia and severe renal impairment or marked AV conduction disturbances, because hyperkalemia may further impair AV conduction.

Lidocaine [Xylocaine] and phenytoin can be used to treat digitalis-induced ventricular arrhythmias. Although beta-adrenergic blocking drugs may exacerbate AV conduction disturbances caused by digitalis, they decrease catecholamine-induced automaticity and shorten the refractory period of atrial and ventricular muscle while slowing conduction velocity.

Purified digoxin-specific antibody fragments (digoxin immune Fab [ovine] [Digibind]) are used to treat potentially life-threatening digitalis intoxication. These antibody fragments bind with digoxin and digitoxin, and the resulting complexes are excreted rapidly by the kidney. In a multicenter prospective trial of the use of digoxin immune Fab for acute, life-threatening digitalis toxicity, 90% of patients had complete or partial recovery within 88 minutes of infusion (Antman et al, 1990). There were few adverse effects; the most prominent reaction was the rapid development of hypokalemia. Similar results were noted in a subsequent observational surveillance study (Hickey et al, 1991). The median digoxin serum concentration at the time of diagnosis of digitalis intoxication for these patients was 4.2 ng/ml.

Cholestyramine, colestipol, and charcoal can reduce serum digoxin concentrations by binding the drug during transit through the gut lumen via the enteroenteric circulation, but the decrease is not sufficient to alleviate life-threatening toxicity.

Drug Evaluations

DIGOXIN

[Lanoxin]

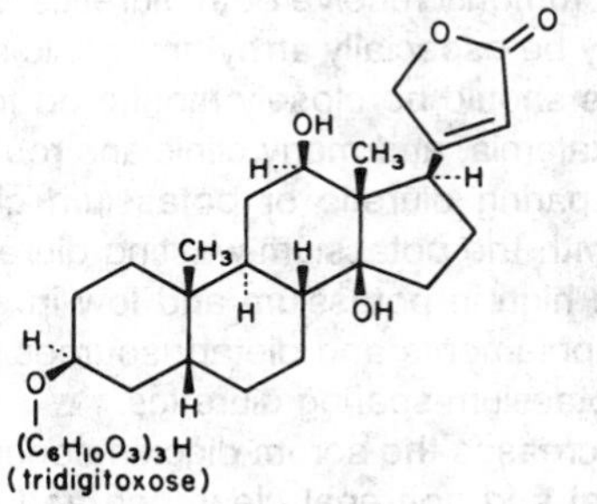

OH, CH_3, H, H, CH_3, H, H, OH, H, O, H, $(C_6H_{10}O_3)_3H$ (tridigitoxose)

Digoxin is a purified digitalis preparation derived from the leaves of *Digitalis lanata.* It is the most widely used digitalis glycoside. Onset of action is within 5 to 30 minutes after an intravenous dose and within one to two hours after oral administration. The maximal effect occurs within one to four hours after intravenous administration and two to six hours after oral administration. Many cardiologists prefer digoxin to other digitalis glycosides for heart failure because its rapid onset of action makes it useful in emergency situations; its relatively short duration of action makes toxic reactions easier to manage; it can be administered both orally and parenterally, making the maintenance dosage easy to establish after emergency intravenous use; and a liquid preparation is available for oral therapy in infants and children.

See the Introduction for a discussion of indications, interactions, and toxicity.

PHARMACOKINETICS. Digoxin is absorbed from the upper small intestine. The bioavailability of Lanoxin tablets is 60% to 80% and that of Lanoxin elixir is 70% to 85%; the capsule-containing solution [Lanoxicaps] is 90% to 100% bioavailable. Food reduces the rate, but not the total amount, absorbed. The absorption of tablets is normal in many patients with limited absorptive surface due to mucosal disease or surgical resection but may be impaired in those with an extremely short length of functioning small intestine.

Digoxin has a high apparent volume of distribution (6 L/kg), which is decreased in elderly patients and in those with impaired renal function. It is widely distributed throughout body tissues; high concentrations appear in skeletal muscle and in the liver, heart, brain, and kidneys. It does not accumulate in adipose tissue. For a given serum level, myocardial accumulation is greater in infants than in adults. Insignificant amounts of digoxin are removed by dialysis. Digoxin is 20% to 25% protein bound.

Digoxin crosses the placenta and, at delivery, the serum concentration in the newborn is similar to that in the mother. Approximately 50% to 75% of a dose is excreted unchanged in the urine of most patients but is more extensively metabolized to both active and inactive metabolites in a small percentage of patients. The half-life of digoxin is 1.5 to 2 days in those with normal renal function. It is prolonged in those with impaired renal function, and dosage should be reduced on the basis of creatinine clearance (Aronson, 1980). The renal clearance of digoxin is lower in patients with heart failure than in those with atrial fibrillation.

Therapeutic serum concentrations of digoxin usually range from 0.8 to 2 ng/ml; however, some patients respond to concentrations as low as 0.5 ng/ml and some can tolerate concentrations as high as 2.5 ng/ml. Sex hormones, bile salts, other digitalis glycosides, and, possibly, spironolactone and its metabolites may interfere with results of digoxin radioimmunoassay (Lewis, 1992). In uremic patients, 6% to 42% of apparent digoxin in the serum may represent metabolites (Gibson and Nelson, 1980).

Baseline serum digoxin levels should be measured prior to initial administration to account for endogenous digitalis-like immunoreactive substances.

DOSAGE AND PREPARATIONS. The following dosages are given to patients who have not received digitalis for at least two weeks. Smaller loading and maintenance doses should be used in small or elderly patients and in those with impaired renal function, electrolyte disturbances (particularly hypokalemia), or metabolic abnormalities (particularly hypothyroidism).

Oral (tablets and elixir): *Adults,* the average digitalizing dose is 0.75 to 1.5 mg. For rapid digitalization, initially, 0.5 to 0.75 mg, followed by 0.25 to 0.5 mg every six to eight hours until full digitalization is achieved. For slow digitalization and maintenance, 0.125 to 0.5 mg daily (0.125 to 0.25 mg in the elderly), depending on lean body weight and renal function as determined by creatinine clearance. The dose should be reduced as renal function decreases. *Institution of maintenance therapy without a loading dose is suitable for many patients with heart failure.* Therapeutic serum levels are achieved after six to seven days of maintenance therapy in patients with normal renal function. Single daily doses are usually satisfactory for maintenance; however, it may be necessary to give two divided doses to some patients with recurrent supraventricular tachyarrhythmias.

For *infants and children,* the following digitalizing doses are given in divided amounts at six-hour intervals. (To ensure adequate absorption, it may be desirable to initiate therapy by the intravenous route and then substitute oral therapy, with the lower dose given first.) *Premature infants,* 0.02 to 0.03 mg/kg; *full-term newborn infants,* 0.025 to 0.035 mg/kg; *1 month to 2 years,* 0.035 to 0.06 mg/kg; *2 to 5 years,* 0.03 to 0.04 mg/kg; *5 to 10 years,* 0.02 to 0.035 mg/kg; *over 10 years,* 0.01 to 0.015 mg/kg. The daily oral maintenance dose is 20% to 30% of the oral loading dose in premature infants and 25% to 35% of the oral loading dose in full-term infants and children. More gradual digitalization can be accomplished by initiating therapy with the appropriate maintenance dose.

Generic. Elixir 0.05 mg/ml; tablets 0.125 and 0.25 mg.
Lanoxin (Burroughs Wellcome). Elixir (pediatric) 0.05 mg/ml; tablets 0.125, 0.25, and 0.5 mg.

Oral (capsules): Dosage recommendations for digoxin solution in capsules are the same as those for intravenous digoxin.

Lanoxicaps (Burroughs Wellcome). Capsules 0.05, 0.1, and 0.2 mg.

Intravenous: *Adults,* the average digitalizing dose is 0.5 to 1 mg. Initially, 0.25 to 0.5 mg, followed by 0.25 mg, is given at four- to six-hour intervals if needed to a total dose of 1 mg. For maintenance, 0.125 to 0.5 mg daily.

For *infants and children,* the following digitalizing doses of the pediatric solution are given in divided amounts at six-hour intervals: *Premature infants,* 0.015 to 0.025 mg/kg; *full-term newborn infants,* 0.02 to 0.03 mg/kg; *1 month to 2 years,* 0.03 to 0.05 mg/kg; *2 to 5 years,* 0.025 to 0.035 mg/kg; *5 to 10 years,* 0.015 to 0.03 mg/kg. The daily intravenous maintenance dose is 20% to 30% of the *oral* loading dose in premature infants and 25% to 30% of the *oral* loading dose in full-term infants and children.

Generic. Solution 0.25 mg/ml in 1 and 2 ml containers.
Lanoxin (Burroughs Wellcome). Solution (pediatric) 0.1 mg/ml in 1 ml containers and 0.25 mg/ml in 2 ml containers (alcohol 10%).

DIGITOXIN

[Crystodigin]

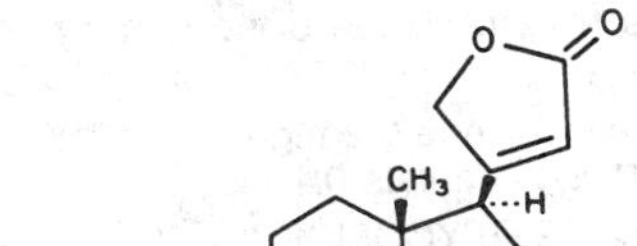

Digitoxin is the chief active glycoside in digitalis leaf; 1 mg of digitoxin is therapeutically equivalent to approximately 1 g of digitalis leaf. Although digitoxin is administered less commonly today than formerly, it is very useful for maintenance therapy because of its long half-life (five to nine days), which provides a sustained therapeutic effect even if a dose is missed. This is a particular advantage in patients with recurrent supraventricular tachyarrhythmias and in those with compliance problems.

See the Introduction for a discussion of indications, adverse reactions and precautions, interactions, and toxicity.

PHARMACOKINETICS. Digitoxin is almost completely absorbed from the gastrointestinal tract. The onset of action is one to four hours, and the maximal effect is attained in 8 to 12 hours. Therapeutic serum concentrations range from 15 to 25 ng/ml, and no variation in bioavailability has been encountered among different preparations. Some methods of measuring serum digitoxin do not differentiate cardioactive glycosides from inactive metabolites.

Digitoxin is 97% bound to plasma protein. Its tissue distribution is similar to that of digoxin. Digitoxin is extensively metabolized in the liver, excreted in the bile, recycled, and eventually excreted in the urine, 80% as inactive metabolites. Since little of the parent compound is eliminated by renal clearance, the half-life of digitoxin is not increased in patients with impaired renal function, and it may be the glycoside of choice in these patients. Insignificant amounts of digitoxin are removed by dialysis. The effect of impaired hepatic function on the pharmacokinetics of digitoxin is not completely understood, but the drug does not appear to accumulate in patients with hepatorenal insufficiency (Kirch et al, 1986).

DOSAGE AND PREPARATIONS. The following dosages are given to patients who have not received digitalis for at least two weeks. Smaller loading and maintenance doses should be used in small or elderly patients or in those with electrolyte disturbances (particularly hypokalemia) or metabolic abnormalities (particularly hypothyroidism).

Oral: *Adults,* for rapid digitalization, initially, 0.8 mg, then 0.2 mg every six to eight hours for two or three doses. For slower digitalization, 0.1 to 0.2 mg one to three times daily to a total of 1.2 to 1.8 mg. For maintenance, 0.1 mg daily (range, 0.05 to 0.2 mg).

For *children,* the following digitalizing doses are given in three or more divided doses at intervals of six hours or more: *Newborn infants,* 0.025 mg/kg; *2 weeks to 1 year,* 0.035 to 0.045 mg/kg; *1 to 2 years,* 0.04 mg/kg; *over 2 years,* 0.02 to 0.03 mg/kg. The maintenance dose is approximately 10% of the digitalizing dose.

Generic. Tablets 0.1 and 0.2 mg.

Crystodigin (Lilly). Tablets 0.1 mg.

OTHER DIGITALIS GLYCOSIDES:

Deslanoside:

Cedilanid-D (Sandoz). Solution 0.2 mg/ml in 2 ml containers (alcohol 9.8%).

Antidote

DIGOXIN IMMUNE FAB (OVINE)
[Digibind]

ACTIONS AND USES. Digoxin immune Fab consists of antigen-binding fragments derived from specific antidigoxin antibodies obtained from immunized sheep. These antibody fragments bind molecules of digoxin or digitoxin and the resulting Fab-glycoside complex is excreted in the urine. Each 40 mg of Fab (one vial) binds approximately 0.6 mg of digoxin or digitoxin.

Digoxin immune antibody fragments are used to treat life-threatening digoxin or digitoxin intoxication manifested by severe tachyarrhythmias or bradyarrhythmias.

ADVERSE REACTIONS AND PRECAUTIONS. Although allergic reactions have been uncommon (0.8%), the possibility of anaphylactic, hypersensitivity, or febrile reactions should be kept in mind, and facilities should be available for treating anaphylaxis. Skin testing may be appropriate for patients previously treated with these antibody fragments or for those allergic to sheep proteins.

The serum potassium level should be monitored closely during treatment because hypokalemia may develop rapidly and require correction. If possible, the serum glycoside concentration should be determined before treatment with digoxin immune Fab. An increase in the serum digitalis concentration may be observed during treatment, but the drug will be bound to the antibody fragments and thus will be unavailable to react with receptors. Standard digoxin assays are not reliable for days to weeks after treatment with digoxin immune Fab.

Because withdrawal of the inotropic or antiarrhythmic action of digitalis may cause the patient's clinical condition to deteriorate, other modalities should be available to treat resulting heart failure or arrhythmias.

Excretion of the Fab-digoxin complex is delayed when renal function is impaired.

Digoxin immune Fab is classified in FDA Pregnancy Category C.

DOSAGE AND PREPARATIONS.

Intravenous: *Adults and children*, see manufacturer's directions.

Digibind (Burroughs Wellcome). Powder (injection) 40 mg.

VASODILATORS

Vasodilator drugs are used to treat chronic heart failure (Class II to IV). Adding vasodilators to digitalis and diuretic therapy results in an increase in survival (Pitt, 1992).

Vasodilators reduce excessive vasoconstriction and are used to relieve the work of the failing heart. They are particularly useful when heart failure is associated with hypertension, ischemic heart disease, idiopathic dilated cardiomyopathy, or mitral or aortic insufficiency. Vasodilators differ in their relative effects on arterial (resistance) and venous (capacitance) vessels. Those that act primarily on resistance vessels reduce aortic impedance and thus increase stroke volume and cardiac output. Venodilators reduce left ventricular filling pressure, improve left ventricular diastolic compliance, and thereby relieve symptoms of pulmonary congestion.

Vasodilators currently used for heart failure include ACE inhibitors and direct-acting agents (nitrates, hydralazine). Most vasodilators modify hemodynamic derangements, but ACE inhibitors have the added advantage of correcting neurohumoral abnormalities.

Vasodilator therapy with ACE inhibitors and, to a lesser extent, with hydralazine and isosorbide dinitrate has been shown to prolong life in patients with heart failure. The first Cooperative Study on Vasodilator Therapy of Heart Failure (V-HeFT I) randomized patients with moderately severe heart failure (Class II and III) who were being treated with digoxin and a diuretic to receive placebo, prazosin, or the combination of hydralazine and isosorbide dinitrate (Cohn et al, 1987). Mortality at two years was decreased 34% in patients receiving the combination of hydralazine and isosorbide dinitrate compared with those receiving placebo. The cumulative two-year mortality rate in the group treated with hydralazine and isosorbide dinitrate was 25.6%, while that in the placebo group was 34.3%. Left ventricular ejection fraction improved with combination therapy, and there was a modest improvement in peak exercise oxygen consumption, but only the former was associated with improved long-term survival. Side effects were common in those treated with hydralazine and isosorbide dinitrate; one or both drugs were discontinued in 19% of patients, and only 55% were taking full doses of both drugs six months after randomization. In this study, prazosin had no effect on survival.

The role of ACE inhibitors was evaluated in the Cooperative North Scandinavian Enalapril Survival Study (CONSENSUS) (Consensus Trial Study Group, 1987). Elderly patients with severe heart failure (Class IV) were randomized to receive enalapril or placebo in addition to digoxin and diuretics. A 40% reduction in one-year mortality was observed in the enalapril-treated group. In addition, improvement in symptoms and signs of left and right ventricular heart failure, reduction of heart size, improvement of NYHA classification category, reduction of concurrent cardiovascular medication, and reduction in the number of hospital admissions and days spent in the hospital were noted in these patients.

The Studies of Left Ventricular Dysfunction (SOLVD) trial assessed the effects of enalapril on mortality, morbidity, and quality of life in two large concurrent clinical trials: a prevention trial, consisting of patients (Class I and II) with low ejection fractions (≤0.35) and no history of overt heart failure, and a treatment trial, consisting of patients (Class II and III) with low ejection fraction (≤0.35) who were receiving diuretics and/or digoxin. In the treatment trial, enalapril reduced the risk of death by 16% in patients with moderately severe heart failure (The SOLVD Investigators, 1991). The largest reduction occurred among those with progressive heart failure. There was no apparent effect of treatment on deaths classified as due to arrhythmia without pump failure. Furthermore, fewer patients died or were hospitalized for worsening heart failure in the enalapril-treated group than in the control group. In the prevention trial, treatment with enalapril significantly delayed the appearance of overt heart failure and the rate of related hospitalizations in patients with heart failure (The SOLVD Investigators, 1992). There also was a tendency toward reduction of mortality from cardiovascular causes. The benefits of enalapril occurred as early as six weeks after initiation of therapy and were greatest among patients with the lowest ejection fraction.

The second cooperative vasodilator trial (V-HeFT II) compared the effects of enalapril with those of hydralazine and isosorbide dinitrate in patients with Class II and III heart failure (Cohn et al, 1991). Mortality after two years was 28% lower in the enalapril arm than in the hydralazine and isosorbide dinitrate arm. In contrast to the results of the SOLVD trial (The SOLVD Investigators, 1991), the lower mortality in enalapril recipients was attributed to a reduction in the incidence of sudden death; mortality or hospitalization due to pump failure was not affected. This finding, which was most prominent in patients with less severe symptoms, suggested that the lower risk of sudden death associated with administration of ACE inhibitors is due to reduction of neurohumoral stimulation. However, exercise tolerance was improved by therapy with hydralazine and isosorbide dinitrate but not with enalapril, even though ACE inhibitors had been shown to increase exercise time in other studies. Left ventricular ejection fraction was increased in both groups, with the patients on hydralazine and isosorbide dinitrate having the greatest increase.

Finally, the Hy-C Trial randomized patients with Class III and IV heart failure to receive either captopril and isosorbide dinitrate or hydralazine and isosorbide dinitrate (Fonarow et al, 1992). Even though the hemodynamic improvement observed in both groups was similar, the survival rate in the captopril group after one year was much higher (81% compared with 51% for the hydralazine group). The decrease in mortality was primarily due to a reduction in sudden death.

All of these trials illustrate the important role of vasodilators in the management of heart failure, especially the ability of the ACE inhibitors to inhibit neurohumoral activity.

ANGIOTENSIN-CONVERTING ENZYME (ACE) INHIBITORS. Captopril [Capoten], enalapril [Vasotec], lisinopril [Prinivil, Zestril], benazepril [Lotensin], fosinopril [Monopril], quinapril [Accupril], and ramipril [Altace] reduce angiotensin II and aldosterone levels by inhibiting the enzyme that converts the inactive angiotensin I to angiotensin II. Inhibition of angiotensin II also reduces circulating catecholamines (norepinephrine). When used to treat refractory heart failure, ACE inhibitors (with most data derived from use of captopril and enalapril) reduce left ventricular volume and filling pressure and decrease total peripheral resistance. ACE inhibitors also increase cardiac output modestly and induce natriuresis. Heart rate may be reduced initially and blood pressure may be reduced markedly after the first few doses. During long-term therapy, renal plasma flow may increase. The combination of captopril and digitalis has an additive beneficial effect on cardiac function at rest and during exercise (Gheorghiade et al, 1989).

Severe but transient hypotension may occur during initiation of therapy with an ACE inhibitor, particularly in patients who are hyponatriuretic. Hypotensive episodes with enalapril or lisinopril may be prolonged. With all ACE inhibitors, therapy should be instituted with a low dose and dosage should be increased carefully, especially in elderly, hypotensive, hyponatremic, or volume-depleted patients. Reduction in dose or the temporary withholding of diuretics may allow these higher-risk patients to tolerate initiation of therapy with ACE inhibitors or other potent vasodilators. (See also index entry Angiotensin-Converting Enzyme Inhibitors.)

The major trials in which ACE inhibitors were shown to reduce mortality in patients with heart failure used relatively high doses of enalapril (escalating doses to achieve a final dose of 10 mg twice daily) and captopril (50 mg three times daily). ACE inhibitors are not indicated or tolerated in all patients with heart failure. In the SOLVD trials, ACE inhibitor therapy was contraindicated in 11% of patients with a left ventricular ejection fraction ≤0.35. In the CONSENSUS trial, SOLVD treatment trial, and V-HeFT-II, 17% to 33.5% of patients randomized to enalapril discontinued therapy prior to the end of the trial, mainly because of symptoms of worsening heart failure or evidence of intolerance, such as hypotension or cough.

DIRECT-ACTING VASODILATORS. Nitrates act predominantly to increase venous capacitance and thus reduce preload and relieve pulmonary congestion. They do not increase cardiac output as effectively as arterial vasodilators. *Sodium nitroprusside* [Nitropress] usually is preferred for short-term intravenous therapy in patients with marked pump dysfunction, elevated left ventricular filling pressure, and a marked increase in peripheral vascular resistance reflected by a normal or increased arterial pressure in the presence of reduced cardiac output. Because it has a balanced vasodilator action on both the arterial and venous beds, nitroprusside reduces left ventricular filling pressure and increases cardiac output in these patients. It is more effective and more rapid-acting than furosemide in acutely decompensated chronic left ventricular failure (Franciosa and Silverstein, 1982). The increase in stroke volume induced by nitroprusside usually counterbalances the fall in peripheral vascular resistance so that arterial blood pressure is not greatly reduced. Heart rate usually is not increased and may decrease because of the improved hemodynamics.

Intravenous nitroglycerin [Nitro-Bid IV, Nitrostat IV, Tridil] may be the drug of choice in patients with coexisting severe coronary artery disease, as well as in those with very high filling pressure and borderline or low arterial pressure. It is particularly useful for lowering elevated left ventricular filling pressure and relieving acute pulmonary edema. It also tends to reduce functional mitral regurgitation resulting from ventricular dilatation. Nitroglycerin reduces preload as effectively as nitroprusside but has less effect on peripheral vascular resistance. It generally does not increase and may reduce cardiac output if left ventricular filling pressure is reduced excessively. This drug dilates epicardial coronary arteries, thereby relieving myocardial ischemia, and it has been used more often after acute myocardial infarction than in chronic heart failure. Adrenergic inotropic agents, such as dopamine [Intropin], may be given with nitroprusside or nitroglycerin when heart failure is complicated by mild or moderate hypotension.

To avoid the development of tolerance to nitrates, the smallest effective dose should be administered and a drug-free interval (intermittent intravenous therapy or 10 to 12 hours overnight for oral dosage forms) should be provided.

Beneficial hemodynamic effects have been observed after administration of oral pentaerythritol tetranitrate [Duotrate, Peritrate], nitroglycerin ointment [Nitro-Bid, Nitrol, Nitrong], and chewable nitrate preparations. Sublingual nitrates are less useful because of their short duration of action, and oral nitroglycerin appears to be relatively ineffective. Although transdermal nitroglycerin patches [Deponit, Minitran, Nitrodisc, Nitro-Dur, Transderm-Nitro] may produce hemodynamic improvement for three to six hours, their effects wane over the next 18 hours and hemodynamic rebound occurs after the patch is removed (Olivari et al, 1983; Roth et al, 1987). (See also index entry Nitrates, Uses, Angina.)

Hydralazine [Apresoline] acts directly on resistance vessels and thus reduces aortic impedance. It improves hemodynamics (Chatterjee et al, 1980) and increases renal and limb blood flow but does not increase exercise capacity. Reflex tachycardia occurs frequently when hydralazine is used to treat hypertension but is less common when the drug is used in patients with heart failure. One group of investigators reported that hydralazine did not retard the development of left ventricular hypertrophy when used to treat aortic regurgitation (Kleaveland et al, 1986); however, in a larger group of patients who were followed for a longer period, a reduction in left ventricular end-diastolic volume and an increase in ejection fraction were observed (Greenberg et al, 1988). Drug-specific tolerance develops in some patients (Packer et al, 1982), and long-term treatment with hydralazine alone has not been shown to be effective (Franciosa et al, 1982).

Combined hydralazine-isosorbide dinitrate therapy reduces left ventricular filling pressure and aortic impedance as effectively as nitroprusside, improves ejection fraction, increases cardiac output, and may increase exercise capacity. Tolerance appears to be uncommon.

The potent direct-acting arteriolar vasodilator, minoxidil [Loniten], improves hemodynamics and left ventricular function during long-term therapy. It does not increase exercise capacity or improve symptomatology, however, and may actually worsen prognosis (Franciosa et al, 1984).

ALPHA-ADRENERGIC BLOCKING AGENTS. Prazosin [Minipress] has a balanced effect on the arteriolar and venous beds. Its hemodynamic effects are more prominent during exercise than at rest. Although orthostatic hypotension may occur during initial therapy for hypertension, it is rare in patients with heart failure, presumably because they have higher filling pressures and are less susceptible to the venodilator actions of the drug. Although prazosin produces short-term hemodynamic improvement, it does not have a favorable effect on symptoms, exercise tolerance, or long-term survival (Markham et al, 1983), possibly because of activation of the renin-angiotensin system (Cohn et al, 1986).

Terazosin [Hytrin], another alpha-adrenergic blocking agent, has been evaluated for use in heart failure in short-term studies. Its effectiveness has not been established (Leier et al, 1986).

CALCIUM CHANNEL BLOCKING AGENTS. Although calcium channel blocking agents (calcium antagonists) have vasodilator properties, the usefulness of these agents in patients with severe systolic dysfunction is limited by their negative inotropic effect, absence of venodilating properties, failure to improve exercise tolerance, and especially their tendency to activate endogenous vasoconstrictor systems (Colucci, 1987; Packer, 1989). Long-term treatment has failed to show beneficial effects (Agostoni et al, 1986).

Drug Evaluations

VASODILATORS

Major vasodilators used orally for long-term therapy of heart failure are listed in the Table. Also see the Introduction.

Angiotensin-Converting Enzyme Inhibitors

Most of the data for the use of ACE inhibitors in the treatment of patients with heart failure are derived from use of captopril and enalapril. For their individual evaluations, see the chapter on Angiotensin-Converting Enzyme Inhibitors. Also see the Table and the Introduction.

Nitrates

NITROGLYCERIN (Intravenous)

[Nitro-Bid IV, Nitrostat IV, Tridil]

$$\begin{array}{l} CH_2-ONO_2 \\ | \\ CH-ONO_2 \\ | \\ CH_2-ONO_2 \end{array}$$

ACTIONS AND USES. Nitroglycerin is a direct-acting vasodilator with a greater effect on the venous than the arterial circulation. Its effect on coronary blood flow depends in part on the status of the coronary circulation. Nitroglycerin dilates the large epicardial (conductance) arteries but has little effect on intramyocardial (resistance) vessels. In the normal nonischemic myocardium, total coronary blood flow may increase temporarily and then may decrease if the central aortic pressure falls substantially or if increased heart rate decreases diastolic filling time. In patients with coronary artery disease, however, nitroglycerin improves the regional distribution of myocardial blood flow and oxygen supply by dilating large atherosclerotic coronary arteries and collateral vessels. Spasm of normal and diseased arteries may be decreased both in angina and in prolonged episodes of ischemia or infarction.

Nitroglycerin is given intravenously to patients with severe, resistant chronic heart failure. It may be the drug of choice in patients with coexisting severe coronary artery disease and in those who have a very high filling pressure and borderline or low arterial pressure. It is less effective than nitroprusside in increasing cardiac output.

ADVERSE REACTIONS AND PRECAUTIONS. Nitroglycerin may cause headache, flushing, dizziness, hypotension, and tachycardia. Severe hypotension associated with sinus bradycardia has occurred in some patients. The bradycardia appears to be, at least in part, vagally mediated because it responds to atropine (Come and Pitt, 1976). Intravenous nitroglycerin preparations contain alcohol, and a considerable amount may be administered during prolonged infusion of large doses. See also the Introduction to this section.

Tolerance develops rapidly (within 24 hours or sooner) to intravenous nitroglycerin, and the dose may have to be increased regularly or therapy interrupted to allow a nitrate-free interval. Nitroprusside may be substituted temporarily. Tolerance also can be reversed by administration of the sulfhydryl-group donor, acetylcysteine (May et al 1987; Packer et al, 1987).

Intravenous nitroglycerin is classified in FDA Pregnancy Category C.

DOSAGE AND PREPARATIONS.

Caution: Several intravenous products are available that differ in concentration and/or volume per vial as well as diluents. The manufacturers' literature should be consulted for dilution instructions, and care should be taken when substituting one preparation for another. Nitroglycerin should be diluted with dextrose 5% injection or sodium chloride 0.9% injection and should not be mixed with other drugs. Only *glass* containers should be used for dilution and storage. (Plastic tubing will absorb considerable amounts of nitroglycerin.) A solution containing 100 mcg/ml may be used for initial dosage titration; a more concentrated solution (200 mcg/ml) may be substituted if it is necessary to limit fluids. Current labeling of some intravenous nitroglycerin products provides dosing guidelines for solutions containing up to 400 mcg/ml.

Intravenous: *Adults,* initially, 5 mcg/min of dilute solution is infused. Dosage may be increased by 5 mcg/min every three to five minutes until a response is noted. Efficacy can be assessed by an adequate fall in pulmonary wedge pressure. Without such measurements, the dose may be increased until a fall in systolic arterial pressure of 5 to 10 mm Hg is noted. If no response is observed with a dose of 20 mcg/min, increments of 10 and later 20 mcg/min may be used. On occasion, it may be necessary to increase the infusion rate to 200 mcg/min or more to relieve chest pain, reduce pulmonary artery wedge pressure, and maintain near normal arterial perfusion pressure. (See precautions above regarding tolerance.) Blood pressure and heart rate should be monitored continuously.

Generic. Solution (sterile) 5 mg/ml in 5, 10, and 20 ml containers; solution in 5% dextrose 25, 50, and 100 mg in 250 ml containers.

Nitro-Bid IV (Marion Merrell Dow). Solution (sterile) 5 mg/ml in 1, 5, and 10 ml containers (alcohol 70%).

Tridil (Dupont). Solution (sterile) 0.5 mg/ml in 10 ml containers (alcohol 10%) and 5 mg/ml in 5, 10, and 20 ml containers (alcohol 30%) with or without delivery set ***(Tridilset).***

SODIUM NITROPRUSSIDE

[Nitropress]

For chemical formula, see index entry Nitroprusside, In Hypertension.

ACTIONS AND USES. This direct-acting vasodilator affects both the venous and arterial beds. It has a more pronounced effect on afterload than does nitroglycerin and therefore is more likely to increase cardiac output. Since the primary action of nitroprusside in the coronary circulation is on resistance rather than conductance vessels, it could precipitate coronary steal. Nitroprusside may increase both myocardial and pulmonary arterial venous shunts; therefore, increases in total blood flow, including coronary blood flow, may not be representative of the portion of the flow that contributes to improved perfusion.

Nitroprusside is preferred for short-term intravenous therapy for severe persistent pump failure in patients with markedly reduced cardiac output and increased peripheral vascular resistance (Cohn and Burke, 1979).

MAJOR VASODILATOR DRUGS USED ORALLY FOR LONG-TERM THERAPY OF HEART FAILURE

Drug	Clinical Considerations	Adverse Reactions	Usual Dosage and Preparations
ANGIOTENSIN-CONVERTING ENZYME INHIBITORS			
Captopril	Improves symptoms and prolongs survival of patients with refractory heart failure receiving digitalis and a diuretic. May prevent development of left ventricular hypertrophy after acute myocardial infarction.	Hypotension, azotemia, hyperkalemia, loss of taste, angioedema, rash, cough, neutropenia	*Oral: Adults,* initially, 25 mg three times daily. Some physicians prefer to administer 6.25 to 12.5 mg three times daily initially to minimize the possibility of a hypotensive effect. Dosage may be titrated upward to 50 mg three times daily. Further increases should be delayed for at least two weeks. Doses larger than 150 mg daily are rarely required (maximal daily dose, 450 mg). In elderly, volume-depleted, or hyponatremic patients and those with moderate to severe impairment of renal function, initial dose should be 6.25 mg three times daily. *Children,* 5 to 10 mg/kg daily in four divided doses. *Capoten* (Bristol-Myers Squibb). Tablets 12.5, 25, 50, and 100 mg.
Enalapril	Improves symptoms and prolongs survival of patients with refractory heart failure receiving digitalis and a diuretic.	Similar to captopril, but hypotensive episodes occur three to four hours after administration and may be more prolonged	*Oral: Adults,* initially, 2.5 mg once or twice daily. The usual maintenance dose is 20 to 40 mg daily given in two divided doses (maximum daily dose, 40 mg). In volume-depleted or hyponatremic patients and in those with moderate to severe impairment in renal function, the initial dose should be reduced to 2.5 mg twice daily, which may be increased to 5 mg twice daily after three or four days. The previous titration plan then may be followed. *Vasotec* (Merck). Tablets 2.5, 5, 10, and 20 mg.
DIRECT-ACTING VASODILATORS			
Hydralazine	A hydralazine-isosorbide dinitrate regimen prolongs survival of patients with refractory heart failure receiving digitalis and a diuretic.	Tachycardia, anginal pain, hypotension, flushing, headache, myocardial ischemia, fluid retention, SLE syndrome, gastrointestinal disturbances	*Oral: Adults,* initially, 40 to 100 mg daily, titrated to 200 to 400 mg daily in two to four doses. Dosage is variable and larger doses may be required in some patients. When given with isosorbide dinitrate, 300 mg daily in four divided doses (Cohn et al, 1986). *Children,* 1 mg/kg every four to six hours. *Apresoline* (CIBA), *Generic.* Tablets, 10, 25, 50, and 100 mg.
Isosorbide dinitrate	See comment under hydralazine	Orthostatic hypotension, headache, flushing, tachycardia, palpitations	*Oral: Adults,* 10 to 80 mg three or four times daily. When given with hydralazine, 160 mg daily in four divided doses (Cohn et al, 1986). For preparations, see index entry Isosorbide Dinitrate, In Angina

ADVERSE REACTIONS AND PRECAUTIONS. As with all vasodilators, hypotension is the major adverse effect of nitroprusside. Tachycardia occurs occasionally. Excess thiocyanate may appear rapidly with overdose or may accumulate during prolonged infusion. If the drug is infused for more than 48 hours, especially in the presence of renal failure, blood thiocyanate levels should be determined daily. High levels of blood cyanide also may appear during infusion of large amounts. Nitroprusside may precipitate coronary steal. (See also index entry Nitroprusside, In Hypertension, for a more detailed discussion of adverse reactions.)

This drug is classified in FDA Pregnancy Category C.

DOSAGE AND PREPARATIONS.

Intravenous: *Adults,* initially, a dilute solution is infused at a rate of 16 mcg/min. The subsequent infusion rate should be determined by hemodynamic monitoring.

Nitropress (Abbott), ***Generic.*** Powder equivalent to sodium nitroprusside dihydrate 50 mg.

NONGLYCOSIDE INOTROPIC AGENTS

The limited therapeutic efficacy of digitalis in severe heart failure led to a search for alternative positive inotropic drugs, including catecholamines and related compounds, dopaminergic agents, and phosphodiesterase inhibitors. These drugs are usually reserved for patients with intractable heart failure refractory to digitalis, diuretics, and vasodilators. In general, these agents are effective for short-term therapy; however, none has been demonstrated to prolong life during long-term treatment and some may increase mortality.

ADRENERGIC AGONISTS. The positive inotropic effect of the adrenergic drugs is due to stimulation of myocardial $beta_1$ receptors. Most of these drugs also have vasodilator properties secondary to activation of $beta_2$ or dopamine receptors. The catecholamine, dopamine [Dopastat, Intropin], acts directly on $beta_1$ receptors and, to a lesser extent, releases norepinephrine from tissue stores. It also acts on alpha receptors. Small doses (0.5 to 2 mcg/kg/min) increase renal and mesenteric blood flow by activating dopaminergic receptors. In standard doses, dopamine can be considered a vasopressor with positive inotropic effects.

Dopamine may be especially effective in patients with heart failure complicated by prerenal azotemia who have become refractory to diuretic therapy. Doses up to 5 mcg/kg/min increase renal and peripheral vasodilation. Higher doses increase myocardial contractility, heart rate, and cardiac output. With doses >10 mcg/kg/min, its alpha-adrenergic vasoconstrictor effect predominates. Dopamine has been used primarily to treat acute circulatory failure in patients with marked hypotension (see index entry Shock), but it also may be useful for short-term therapy in severe refractory chronic heart failure and may be combined with sodium nitroprusside [Nipride, Nitropress] or nitroglycerin.

The synthetic catecholamine, dobutamine [Dobutrex], increases myocardial contractility by stimulating $beta_1$ receptors; the effect on $beta_2$ and alpha receptors is less pronounced and it does not activate dopaminergic receptors. Dobutamine is primarily regarded as a positive inotropic agent. This drug usually is preferred to dopamine in patients with refractory heart failure, especially when the disorder is chronic. Dobutamine tends to lower peripheral resistance and thus augment cardiac output in patients with heart failure and normal blood pressure. Like dopamine, dobutamine is used for short-term treatment (continuous infusion at 1 to 3 mcg/kg/min).

The dopamine precursor, levodopa, which is converted endogenously to dopamine, has beneficial hemodynamic effects in patients with heart failure. Its positive inotropic effect is mediated by $beta_1$ receptors, and a reduction in vascular resistance reflects activation of dopaminergic receptors (Rajfer et al, 1987).

Ibopamine, another dopamine congener, is converted to N-methyldopamine (epinine) after absorption. Long-term administration of this investigational drug improved symptoms and possibly exercise capacity in patients with heart failure (Taylor and Cicchetti, 1990). However, its relatively brief duration of action, the biphasic hemodynamic effect with long-term use, and the impairment of ventricular diastolic function observed in some patients may prevent widespread use of ibopamine (Leier, 1992 B).

The investigational drug, dopexamine [Dopacard], is a selective $beta_2$ agonist that also activates dopaminergic receptors. It has mixed direct and indirect (ie, norepinephrine-releasing) properties. Dopexamine enhances myocardial contractility, stroke volume, and cardiac output; reduces systemic vascular resistance and ventricular afterload; and augments renal and visceral blood flow. In clinical studies in patients with heart failure, dopexamine caused marked vasodilation and increased heart rate, but it had less positive inotropic action than dopamine (Lang et al, 1988). Tachyphylaxis has been observed during prolonged infusion, presumably because of depletion of norepinephrine (Murphy and Hampton, 1988; Port et al, 1990).

Xamoterol [Corwin], a selective $beta_1$ agonist, was developed to mimic the beneficial inotropic effects of catecholamines at rest while antagonizing endogenously released catecholamines during exercise. This investigational drug improved exercise performance and symptoms in patients with mild or moderate heart failure (German and Austrian Xamoterol Study Group, 1988), but it caused marked hemodynamic deterioration in those with severe heart failure (Xamoterol in Severe Heart Failure Study Group, 1990). It also caused bronchospasm in asthmatic patients (Furlong and Brogden, 1988). For these reasons, further testing of xamoterol was discontinued.

PHOSPHODIESTERASE INHIBITORS. Amrinone [Inocor] and milrinone [Primacor] are inotropic agents with substantial vasodilator properties. By inhibiting type III phosphodiesterase, these agents increase intracellular concentrations of cAMP and thus increase the uptake of calcium by myocardial cells. Peripheral arterial and venous vasodilation is largely due to a direct peripheral action rather than to reduction of sympathetic tone.

Short-term intravenous administration of amrinone (Leier, 1992 B) or milrinone (Anderson, 1991) improves hemodynamics, relieves symptoms, and increases exercise capacity in patients with severe refractory heart failure. However, long-term oral therapy with these agents has been disappointing. Numerous serious side effects were associated with long-term use of amrinone, and improvement was limited (Leier, 1992 B). Oral milrinone (40 mg daily given for a median of six months) was associated with a 28% increase in mortality from all causes, a 34% increase in cardiovascular mortality, and no clinical benefit (Packer et al, 1991). The adverse effects of milrinone were greatest in patients with the most severe symptoms. Investigational phosphodiesterase inhibitors, such as enoximone (Vernon et al, 1991), have similar effects. Thus, a pure phosphodiesterase inhibitor may be useful only for short-term or acute therapy in patients with heart failure.

A new group of compounds that inhibits phosphodiesterase and also sensitizes the myofibrillar protein to calcium ions (eg, pimobendan) is being investigated. Short-term (four weeks) oral administration of pimobendan improved resting left ventricular performance and increased exercise duration and peak oxygen uptake in patients with severe heart failure who received digoxin, diuretics, and ACE inhibitors concomitantly (Katz et al, 1992). Similar results were observed in a 12-week study (Kubo et al, 1992). However, studies of longer duration are needed to determine its usefulness in patients with heart failure.

Other myofibrillar calcium sensitizing agents currently under investigation include DPI 201-106 and OPC-8212 [Vesnarinone]. The latter inotropic agent appears to enhance myocardial contractility through phosphodiesterase inhibition, increase levels of intracellular sodium ions, and enhance opening of calcium channels. Results of a randomized, double-blind, placebo-controlled trial in patients with idiopathic dilated cardiomyopathy or ischemic heart disease are encouraging (Feldman et al, 1991).

Drug Evaluations

ADRENERGIC AGONIST

DOBUTAMINE HYDROCHLORIDE

[Dobutrex]

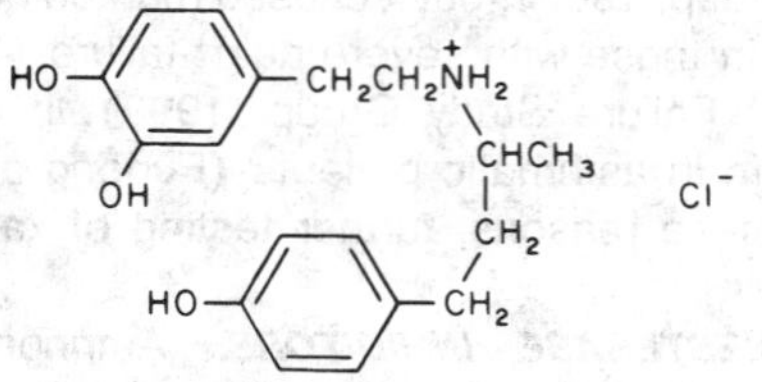

ACTIONS. This synthetic catecholamine was developed in a search for new inotropic agents with minimal chronotropic or vascular activity. Moderate doses increase myocardial contractility without greatly increasing heart rate; large doses may increase heart rate. In animal studies, equivalent inotropic doses of dobutamine had less than one-fourth the chronotropic effect of isoproterenol. This difference appears to be independent of reflex hemodynamic effects and may reflect a relatively selective action on ventricular contractile tissue with a less pronounced effect on the SA node. The hemodynamic effects of dobutamine may be attenuated in the elderly.

USES. Dobutamine is used for short-term therapy to increase cardiac output in patients with severe refractory heart failure. In comparative studies, both dobutamine and dopamine increased cardiac output, but dobutamine was more effective in reducing left ventricular filling pressure (Loeb et al, 1977; Stoner et al, 1977). Combined therapy with the two drugs produced a greater increase in cardiac output, a lower wedge pressure, and a greater reduction in systemic and pulmonary vascular resistance than either drug alone (Mikulic et al, 1977).

Dobutamine also has been used for inotropic support during emergence from cardiac surgery, and it appears to be as effective as isoproterenol in increasing cardiac output. It may cause less tachycardia and fewer arrhythmias than isoproterenol in these patients, although some investigators have found no significant difference between the two drugs.

ADVERSE REACTIONS AND PRECAUTIONS. Tachycardia is the most common adverse effect of dobutamine and usually can be controlled by reducing the dose. Nausea, headache, palpitations, anginal pain, dyspnea, systolic hypertension, hypokalemia, and ventricular arrhythmias also may occur. Proarrhythmic effects may increase mortality in patients with preexisting ventricular tachycardia (Dies et al, 1986). Low doses of dobutamine may cause myocardial ischemia in patients with coronary artery disease who do not have heart failure. Since dobutamine facilitates AV conduction, it may increase the ventricular response to atrial fibrillation. Dobutamine may increase insulin requirements in diabetics.

DOSAGE AND PREPARATIONS. The solution should be further diluted before administration to at least 50 ml (see manufacturer's literature for recommended diluents) and should be used within 24 hours. Dobutamine is incompatible with alkaline solutions and *should not be mixed with sodium bicarbonate injection.*

Intravenous: *Adults,* the rate of infusion required to increase cardiac output usually ranges from 2.5 to 10 mcg/kg/min. Rarely, infusion rates up to 40 mcg/kg/min may be required.

Dobutrex (Lilly). Solution 12.5 mg/ml in 20 ml containers.

DOPAMINE HYDROCHLORIDE

See index entry Dopamine, In Shock.

PHOSPHODIESTERASE INHIBITORS

AMRINONE LACTATE

[Inocor]

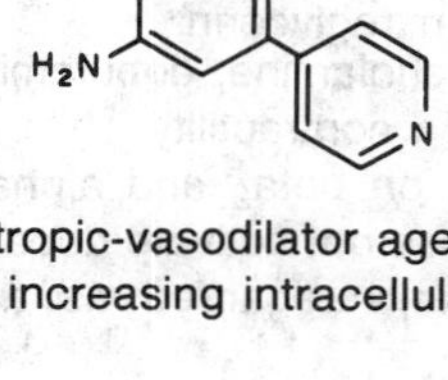

ACTIONS. This inotropic-vasodilator agent inhibits phosphodiesterase, thereby increasing intracellular concentrations of cAMP, which elevates the uptake of calcium by myocardial cells. It reduces peripheral vascular resistance and left ventricular filling pressure, increases myocardial contractility, and enhances cardiac output. Amrinone may cause a modest increase in heart rate, particularly when given in large doses.

The hemodynamic effects of amrinone are similar to those of dobutamine (Benotti et al, 1985), and its positive inotropic effect is less than that of isoproterenol (Firth et al, 1984). Amrinone is most effective in increasing cardiac output in patients with a marked elevation in left ventricular filling pressure. Its inotropic effect depends on adequate stores of cAMP, which may be depleted in patients with severe heart failure (Mancini et al, 1985).

USES. When given intravenously, amrinone acutely improves hemodynamics and exercise performance in many patients with severe chronic heart failure refractory to digitalis, diuretics, and vasodilators (Ward et al, 1983). Its effects are additive to those of digitalis, diuretics, and dobutamine. Long-term oral therapy is not beneficial.

ADVERSE REACTIONS, PRECAUTIONS, AND INTERACTIONS. Hypotension is rare except when ventricular filling pressure is low. Excessive hypotension occurred in one patient treated with amrinone and disopyramide. Dose-dependent, reversible thrombocytopenia also has been reported with oral use but rarely with intravenous use. Hepatotoxicity has been observed rarely. Amrinone may cause discomfort at the infusion site.

This drug is classified in FDA Pregnancy Category C.

PHARMACOKINETICS. Amrinone has a volume of distribution of 1.2 to 1.6 L/kg in patients with chronic heart failure. Protein binding ranges from 10% to 49%. This agent is eliminated by urinary excretion of unchanged drug (30%) and by hepatic metabolism. Clearance ranges from 0.28 to 0.42 L/hr/kg. The terminal elimination half-life of amrinone is 5.8 hours in patients with congestive heart failure.

DOSAGE AND PREPARATIONS. The solution may be administered as supplied or diluted in normal or half normal sodium chloride injection to a concentration of 1 to 3 mg/ml. It should not be diluted with solutions containing dextrose or mixed with furosemide.

Intravenous: *Adults,* initially, 0.75 mg/kg is given as a bolus injection over two to three minutes. If needed, an additional bolus injection of 0.75 mg/kg may be given 30 minutes after initiation of therapy. For maintenance, the drug is infused at a rate of 5 to 10 mcg/kg/min. The total daily dose should not exceed 10 mg/kg. Blood pressure, heart rate, and central venous pressure (if available) should be monitored during therapy with amrinone.

Inocor (Sanofi Winthrop). Solution (lactate) 5 mg/ml in 20 ml containers. Contains sodium metabisulfate.

MILRINONE LACTATE
[Primacor]

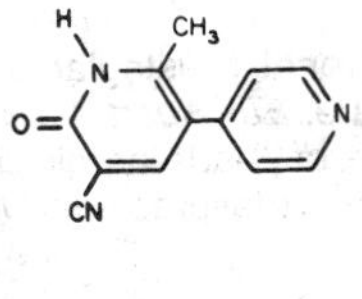

ACTIONS. Milrinone inhibits cAMP phosphodiesterase in both the myocardium and vascular smooth muscle and is 10 to 30 times more potent than amrinone. It possesses vasodilator and positive inotropic properties (Colucci, 1991). Direct infusion of milrinone into the brachial artery was associated with a substantial increase in forearm blood flow and a reduction in forearm vascular resistance, indicating that milrinone exerts a direct vasodilator action. On the other hand, intracoronary administration of milrinone markedly increased left ventricular contractility and stroke work and volume but produced no changes in arterial pressure or systemic vascular resistance; this indicates that milrinone has an inotropic action. These effects are potentiated when dobutamine, a beta-adrenergic agonist, is used with milrinone.

USES. Milrinone is used solely for intravenous therapy in patients with severe refractory heart failure. With acute or short-term administration, milrinone reduced systemic vascular resistance and left ventricular end-systolic wall stress, indicative of vasodilation, and produced a leftward and upward shift of the end-systolic pressure-volume relation, indicative of increased contractility.

ADVERSE REACTIONS AND PRECAUTIONS. The most frequent adverse reaction to milrinone has been ventricular arrhythmias (12%), including ventricular ectopic activity, nonsustained and sustained ventricular tachycardia, and ventricular fibrillation. A few patients experienced more than one type of arrhythmia. Supraventricular arrhythmias have been reported in 3.8% patients receiving milrinone. Other cardiovascular adverse reactions include hypotension and angina.

Headache, hypokalemia, tremor, and thrombocytopenia also have been reported. Diarrhea may occur.

The mortality rate in Class III and IV patients receiving long-term milrinone therapy has been high, ranging from 39% to 66% after six months (Baim et al, 1986; Simonton et al, 1985).

This drug is classified in FDA Pregnancy Category C.

PHARMACOKINETICS. In patients with cardiac failure, the bioavailability of milrinone is 76%. Its volume of distribution is 0.33 to 0.47 L/kg following intravenous administration to patients with severe heart failure. Approximately 80% to 85% of a dose is excreted as unchanged drug. The half-life of milrinone is 1.7 to 2.7 hours in patients with severe heart failure.

DOSAGE AND PREPARATIONS. The solution should be diluted in 0.45% sodium chloride, 0.9% sodium chloride, or 5% dextrose. The final concentration of infusion solutions can be 100 mcg/ml, 150 mcg/ml, or 200 mcg/ml. See the manufacturer's instructions for the rate of infusion.

Intravenous: *Adults,* initially, a loading dose of 50 mcg/kg is given slowly over 10 minutes. For maintenance, the drug is infused at a rate of 0.375 to 0.75 mcg/kg/min. The total daily dose should not exceed 1.13 mg/kg/day. The duration of therapy is determined by the hemodynamic and clinical responses.

Primacor (Sanofi Winthrop). Solution (lactate) 1 mg/ml in 10 and 20 ml single-dose containers and 5 ml sterile cartridge-needle unit [Carpuject] with Interline system cannula.

BETA-ADRENERGIC BLOCKING AGENTS

The use of beta-adrenergic blocking agents in the treatment of heart failure is investigational. The beneficial effects of beta-adrenergic blockade were demonstrated in patients with idiopathic dilated cardiomyopathy (Eichhorn, 1992; Sobotka and Gunnar, 1992), but it is unclear whether this therapy is equally effective in other forms of heart failure (eg, ischemic cardiomyopathy).

In patients with idiopathic dilated cardiomyopathy, beta-adrenergic blocking agents (primarily metoprolol and bucindolol) added to standard therapy with diuretics, digoxin, and vasodilators improved functional status and exercise capacity, increased left ventricular ejection fraction and cardiac index, and improved other hemodynamic measures (eg, pulmonary capillary wedge pressure, systemic vascular resistance, stroke volume) (Engelmeier et al, 1985; Woodley et al, 1991). Very low doses were used initially and the amount was increased in small increments over four to eight weeks (eg, metoprolol tartrate, initially, 6.25 mg daily, increased to a maximum of 100 mg daily in four to eight weeks [Engelmeier et al, 1985]). Further prolongation of the dosage interval may be necessary in some patients. Once the maximal dose was established, beneficial effects were maintained throughout the follow-up periods. Severe decompensation occurred on withdrawal of the beta blocker. Patients receiving beta blockers appeared to have lived much longer than expected compared with historical controls (Swedberg et al, 1980; Waagstein et al, 1989).

The mechanisms proposed for the effects of beta-adrenergic blocking agents include up-regulation of beta receptors, reduction in cardiac energy requirements, protection of the myocardium from norepinephrine toxicity, and antiarrhythmic effects. Further investigation is needed to identify suitable candidates for therapy and the most effective beta-adrenergic blocking agent.

ANTIARRHYTHMIC AGENTS

Life-threatening ventricular arrhythmias are common in patients with heart failure, and about 30% to 40% of these patients die suddenly (Parmley et al, 1991). Symptomatic ventricular arrhythmias should be treated with antiarrhythmic agents, surgery, and/or automatic implantable cardioverter-defibrillators. The role of antiarrhythmic therapy for asymptomatic ventricular arrhythmias in patients with heart failure is unclear, but preliminary studies suggest that amiodarone [Cordarone] may be useful. The Department of Veterans Affairs recently began a randomized, placebo-controlled trial to test the hypothesis that amiodarone may prolong survival in patients with chronic heart failure. However, the use of this drug is limited by pulmonary toxicity and other side effects.

Cited References

American Heart Association 1992 Heart and Stroke Facts. Dallas, American Heart Association, 1992.

Agostoni PG, et al: Afterload reduction: Comparison of captopril and nifedipine in dilated cardiomyopathy. *Br Heart J* 55:391-399, 1986.

Anderson JL: Hemodynamic and clinical benefits with intravenous milrinone in severe chronic heart failure: Results of a multicenter study in the United States. *Am Heart J* 121:1956-1964, 1991.

Antman EM, et al: Treatment of 150 cases of life-threatening digitalis intoxication with digoxin-specific (F(ab) antibody fragments: Final report of a multicenter study. *Circulation* 81:1744-1752, 1990.

Arnold SB, et al: Long-term digitalis therapy improves left ventricular function in heart failure. *N Engl J Med* 303:1443-1448, 1980.

Aronson JK: Clinical pharmacokinetics of digoxin 1980. *Clin Pharmacokinet* 5:137-149, 1980.

Aubier M, et al: Effects of digoxin on diaphragmatic strength generation in patients with chronic obstructive pulmonary disease during acute respiratory failure. *Am Rev Respir Dis* 135:544-548, 1987.

Baim DS, et al: Survival of patients with severe congestive heart failure treated with oral milrinone. *J Am Coll Cardiol* 7:661-670, 1986.

Benotti JR, et al: Comparative vasoactive therapy for heart failure. *Am J Cardiol* 56:19B-24B, 1985.

Bigger JT Jr: Quinidine-digoxin interaction. *Int J Cardiol* 1:109-116, 1981.

Captopril-Digoxin Multicenter Research Group: Comparative effects of therapy with captopril and digoxin in patients with mild to moderate heart failure. *JAMA* 259:539-544, 1988.

Chatterjee K, et al: Oral hydralazine in chronic heart failure: Sustained beneficial hemodynamic effects. *Ann Intern Med* 92:600-604, 1980.

Cohn JN, Burke LP: Nitroprusside. *Ann Intern Med* 91:752-757, 1979.

Cohn JN, et al: Effect of vasodilator therapy on mortality in chronic congestive heart failure: Results of Veterans Administration Cooperative Study. *N Engl J Med* 314:1547-1552, 1986.

Cohn JN, et al: Veterans Administration Cooperative Study on vasodilator therapy of heart failure: Influence of prerandomization variables on reduction of mortality by treatment with hydralazine and isosorbide dinitrate. *Circulation* 75(suppl IV):IV-49-IV-54, 1987.

Cohn JN, et al: A comparison of enalapril with hydralazine-isosorbide dinitrate in the treatment of chronic congestive heart failure. *N Engl J Med* 325:303-310, 1991.

Colucci WS: Usefulness of calcium antagonists for congestive heart failure. *Am J Cardiol* 59:52B-58B, 1987.

Colucci WS: Cardiovascular effects of milrinone. *Am Heart J* 121:1945-1947, 1991.

Come PC, Pitt B: Nitroglycerin-induced severe hypotension and bradycardia in patients with acute myocardial infarction. *Circulation* 54:624-628, 1976.

Consensus Trial Study Group: Effects of enalapril on mortality in severe congestive heart failure: Results of the Cooperative North Scandinavian Enalapril Survival Study (CONSENSUS). *N Engl J Med* 316:1429-1435, 1987.

Creager MA, et al: Contribution of vasopressin to vasoconstriction in patients with congestive heart failure: Comparison with the renin-angiotensin system and the sympathetic nervous system. *J Am Coll Cardiol* 7:758-765, 1986.

Creager MA, et al: Responsiveness of atrial natriuretic factor to reduction in right atrial pressure in patients with chronic congestive heart failure. *J Am Coll Cardiol* 11:1191-1198, 1988.

Davies RJ, et al: Enalapril versus digoxin in patients with congestive heart failure: A multicenter study. *J Am Coll Cardiol* 18:1602-1609, 1991.

DiBianco R, et al: A comparison of oral milrinone, digoxin, and their combination in the treatment of patients with chronic heart failure. *N Engl J Med* 320:677-683, 1989.

Dies F, et al: Intermittent dobutamine in ambulatory outpatients with chronic cardiac failure, abstract. *Circulation* 74(suppl II): II-38, 1986.

Dzau VJ: Vascular and renal prostaglandins as counter-regulatory systems in heart failure. *Eur Heart J* 9(suppl H):H15-H19, 1988.

Eichhorn EJ: The paradox of β-adrenergic blockade for the management of congestive heart failure. *Am J Med* 92:527-538, 1992.

Enalapril Versus Digoxin French Multicenter Study Group: Comparison of enalapril versus digoxin for congestive heart failure. *Am J Cardiol* 63:22D-25D, 1989.

Engelmeier RS, et al: Improvement in symptoms and exercise tolerance by metoprolol in patients with dilated cardiomyopathy: Double-blind, randomized, placebo-controlled trial. *Circulation* 72:536-546, 1985.

Feldman AM: Can we alter survival in patients with congestive heart failure. *JAMA* 267:1956-1961, 1992.

Feldman AM, et al: Usefulness of OPC-8212, a quinolinone derivative, for chronic congestive heart failure in patients with ischemic heart disease or idiopathic dilated cardiomyopathy. *Am J Cardiol* 68:1203-1210, 1991.

Firth BG, et al: Assessment of inotropic and vasodilator effects of amrinone versus isoproterenol. *Am J Cardiol* 54:1331-1336, 1984.

Fonarow GC, et al: Effect of direct vasodilation with hydralazine versus angiotensin-converting enzyme inhibition with captopril on mortality in advanced heart failure: The Hy-C Trial. *J Am Coll Cardiol* 19:842-850, 1992.

Franciosa JA, Silverstein SR: Hemodynamic effects of nitroprusside and furosemide in left ventricular failure. *Clin Pharmacol Ther* 32:62-69, 1982.

Franciosa JA, et al: Hydralazine in long-term treatment of chronic heart failure: Lack of difference from placebo. *Am Heart J* 104:587-594, 1982.

Franciosa JA, et al: Minoxidil in patients with chronic left heart failure: Contrasting hemodynamic and clinical effects in controlled trial. *Circulation* 70:63-68, 1984.

Francis GS, et al: Sequential neurohumoral measurements in patients with congestive heart failure. *Am Heart J* 116:1464, 1988.

Furlong R, Brogden RN: Xamoterol: Preliminary review of its pharmacodynamic and pharmacokinetic properties and therapeutic use. *Drugs* 36:455-474, 1988.

German and Austrian Xamoterol Study Group: Double-blind placebo-controlled comparison of digoxin and xamoterol in chronic heart failure. *Lancet* 1:489-493, 1988.

Gheorghiade M, Ferguson D: Digoxin: A neurohormonal modulator in heart failure? *Circulation* 84:2181-2186, 1991.

Gheorghiade M, et al: Comparative hemodynamic and neurohormonal effects of intravenous captopril and digoxin and their combinations in patients with severe heart failure. *J Am Coll Cardiol* 13:134-142, 1989.

Gheorghiade M, et al: The effects of increasing digoxin dose in rest and exercise ejection fraction, exercise tolerance, and neurohormones in patients with heart failure on maintenance therapy with digoxin. *Circulation* 86 (suppl I):I-1515, 1992.

Gibson TP, Nelson HA: Question of cumulation of digoxin metabolites in renal failure. *Clin Pharmacol Ther* 27:219-223, 1980.

Greenberg B, et al: Long-term vasodilator therapy of chronic aortic insufficiency: Randomized double-blinded, placebo-controlled clinical trial. *Circulation* 78:92-103, 1988.

Griffiths BE, et al: Maintenance of inotropic effect of digoxin on long-term treatment. *BMJ* 284:1819-1822, 1982.

Hickey RA, et al: Digoxin immune F(ab) therapy in the management of digitalis intoxication: Safety and efficacy results of an observational surveillance study. *J Am Coll Cardiol* 17:590-598, 1991.

Hlatky MA, et al: Physician practice in management of congestive heart failure. *J Am Coll Cardiol* 8:966-970, 1986.

Katz SD, et al: A multicenter, randomized, double-blind, placebo-controlled trial of pimobendan, a new cardiotonic and vasodilator agent, in patients with severe congestive heart failure. *Am Heart J* 123:95-103, 1992.

Kelly RA, Smith TW: Recognition and management of digitalis toxicity. *Am J Cardiol* 69:108G-119G, 1992.

Kirch W, et al: Bioavailability and elimination of digitoxin in patients with hepatorenal insufficiency. *Am Heart J* 111:325-329, 1986.

Kleaveland JP, et al: Effects of six-month afterload reduction therapy with hydralazine in chronic aortic regurgitation. *Am J Cardiol* 57:1109-1116, 1986.

Kloner RA: Heart failure. *Cardiovasc Rev Rep* 12:19-59, 1991.

Kubo SH, et al: α_2-Receptor-mediated vasoconstriction in patients with congestive heart failure. *Circulation* 80:1660-1667, 1989.

Kubo SH, et al: Beneficial effects of pimobendan on exercise tolerance and quality of life in patients with heart failure: Results of a multicenter trial. *Circulation* 85:942-949, 1992.

Lang RM, et al: Role of the $beta_2$ adrenoceptor in mediating positive inotropic activity in the failing heart and its relation to the hemodynamic actions of dopexamine hydrochloride. *Am J Cardiol* 62:46C-52C, 1988.

Leier CV: Regional blood flow in human congestive heart failure. *Am Heart J* 124:726-738, 1992 A.

Leier CV: Current status of non-digitalis positive inotropic drugs. *Am J Cardiol* 69:120G-129G, 1992 B.

Leier CV, et al: The hemodynamic and clinical responses to terazosin, a new alpha blocking agent, in congestive heart failure. *Am J Med Sci* 292:128-135, 1986.

Leimbach WN Jr, et al: Direct evidence from intraneural recordings for increased central sympathetic outflow in patients with heart failure. *Circulation* 73:913-919, 1986.

Levine TB, et al: Dissociation of responses of the renin-angiotensin system and sympathetic nervous system to a vasodilator stimulus in congestive heart failure. *Int J Cardiol* 12:165-173, 1986.

Lewis RP: Clinical use of serum digoxin concentrations. *Am J Cardiol* 69:97G-107G, 1992.

Loeb HS, et al: Superiority of dobutamine over dopamine for augmentation of cardiac output in patients with chronic low output cardiac failure. *Circulation* 55:375-381, 1977.

Mancini D, et al: Intravenous use of amrinone for treatment of failing heart. *Am J Cardiol* 56:8B-15B, 1985.

Markham RV Jr, et al: Efficacy of prazosin in management of chronic congestive heart failure: 6-month randomized, double-blind, placebo-controlled study. *Am J Cardiol* 51:1346-1352, 1983.

Mathur PN, et al: Effect of digoxin on right ventricular function in severe chronic airflow obstruction: Controlled clinical trial. *Ann Intern Med* 95:283-288, 1981.

May DC, et al: In vivo induction and reversal of nitroglycerin tolerance in human coronary arteries. *N Engl J Med* 317:805-809, 1987.

Mikulic E, et al: Comparative hemodynamic effects of inotropic and vasodilator drugs in severe heart failure. *Circulation* 56:528-533, 1977.

Murphy JJ, Hampton JR: Failure of dopexamine to maintain haemodynamic improvement in patients with chronic heart failure. *Br Heart J* 60:45-49, 1988.

Murray RG, et al: Evaluation of digitalis in cardiac failure. *BMJ* 284:1526-1528, 1983.

Myers J, Froelicher VF: Hemodynamic determinants of exercise capacity in chronic heart failure. *Ann Intern Med* 115:377-386, 1991.

Olivari MT, et al: Hemodynamic and hormonal response to transdermal nitroglycerin in normal subjects and in patients with congestive heart failure. *J Am Coll Cardiol* 2:872-878, 1983.

Packer M: Pathophysiological mechanisms underlying the adverse effects of calcium channel-blocking drugs in patients with chronic heart failure. *Circulation* 80 (suppl IV):IV-59-IV-67, 1989.

Packer M, et al: Hemodynamic characterization of tolerance to long-term hydralazine therapy in severe chronic heart failure. *N Engl J Med* 306:57-62, 1982.

Packer M, et al: Prevention and reversal of nitrate tolerance in patients with congestive heart failure. *N Engl J Med* 317:799-804, 1987.

Packer M, et al: Effect of oral milrinone on mortality in severe chronic heart failure. *N Engl J Med* 325:1468-1475, 1991.

Packer M, et al: Randomized double-blind placebo-controlled withdrawal study of digoxin in patients with chronic heart failure treated with converting-enzyme inhibitors, abstract. *J Am Coll Cardiol* 19:260A, 1992.

Parmley WM, et al: Congestive heart failure: New frontiers. *West J Med* 154:427-441, 1991.

Pitt B: Congestive heart failure: New therapeutic strategies. *Clin Cardiol* 15 (suppl I):I-2-I-4, 1992.

Port JD, et al: Neurotransmitter depletion compromises the ability of indirect-acting amines to provide inotropic support in the failing human heart. *Circulation* 81:929-938, 1990.

Rajfer SI, et al: Sustained hemodynamic improvement during long-term therapy with levodopa in heart failure: Role of plasma catecholamines. *J Am Coll Cardiol* 10:1286-1293, 1987.

Roth A, et al: Early tolerance to hemodynamic effects of high dose transdermal nitroglycerin in responders with severe chronic heart failure. *J Am Coll Cardiol* 9:858-864, 1987.

Schocken DD, et al: Prevalence and mortality rate of congestive heart failure in the United States. *J Am Coll Cardiol* 20:301-306, 1992.

Simonton CA, et al: Milrinone in congestive heart failure: Acute and chronic hemodynamic and clinical evaluation. *J Am Coll Cardiol* 6:453-459, 1985.

Sobotka PA, Gunnar RM: The use of beta-blockade therapy in treatment of congestive heart failure. *Clin Cardiol* 15:630-635, 1992.

The SOLVD Investigators: Effect of enalapril on survival in patients with reduced left ventricular ejection fractions and congestive heart failure. *N Engl J Med* 325:293-302, 1991.

The SOLVD Investigators: Effect of enalapril on mortality and the development of heart failure in asymptomatic patients with reduced left ventricular ejection fractions. *N Engl J Med* 327:685-691, 1992.

Stoner JD III, et al: Comparison of dobutamine and dopamine in treatment of severe heart failure. *Br Heart J* 39:536-539, 1977.

Swedberg K, et al: Beneficial effects of long-term beta-blockade in congestive cardiomyopathy. *Br Heart J* 44:117-133, 1980.

Taylor SH, Cicchetti V: Efficacy of ibopamine in the treatment of heart failure. *Am Heart J* 120:1583-1590, 1990.

Uren NG, Lipkin DP: Exercise training as therapy for chronic heart failure. *Br Heart J* 67:430-433, 1992.

Vernon MW, et al: Enoximone: A review of its pharmacological properties and therapeutic potential. *Drugs* 42:997-1017, 1991.

Waagstein F, et al: Long-term beta-blockade in dilated cardiomyopathy. *Circulation* 80:551-563, 1989.

Ward A, et al: Amrinone: Preliminary review of its pharmacological properties and therapeutic use. *Drugs* 26:468-502, 1983.

Woodley SL, et al: β-Blockade with bucindolol in heart failure caused by ischemic versus idiopathic dilated cardiomyopathy. *Circulation* 84:2426-2441, 1991.

Xamoterol in Severe Heart Failure Study Group: Xamoterol in severe heart failure. *Lancet* 336:1-6, 1990.

Young JB, et al: Multicenter double-blind placebo-controlled randomized withdrawal trial of the efficacy and safety of digoxin in patients with mild to moderate chronic heart failure not treated with converting enzyme inhibitors, abstract. *J Am Coll Cardiol* 219:259A, 1992.

Yusef S, et al: Changes in hypertension treatment in congestive heart failure mortality in the United States. *Hypertension* 12:174-179, 1989.

Drugs Used for Shock 29

Shock primarily is caused by inadequate supply and consumption of oxygen at vital end organs (Vincent and van der Linden, 1990). Signs and symptoms of shock are complex and include mental obtundation, tachypnea, tachycardia, pallor, cold and clammy skin, oliguria, and metabolic acidosis. Shock may be followed by multiple organ dysfunction, including adult respiratory distress syndrome; acute tubular necrosis; severe left ventricular dysfunction; coagulopathies (hypoprothrombinemia, thrombocytopenia, disseminated intravascular coagulation); hepatic necrosis; and hemorrhagic necrosis of the gut.

Shock is classified according to etiology; types include hypovolemic, septic (distributive), cardiogenic, and extracardiac obstructive shock. This chapter focuses on the treatment of hypovolemic, septic, and cardiogenic shock (see Table for characteristics). For information on anaphylactic shock, see index entry Shock, Anaphylactic.

PRINCIPLES OF THERAPY

Endogenous physiologic compensatory responses strive to maintain overall circulatory function and metabolic integrity after shock but usually are inadequate to meet the demands of tissue oxygenation. Early vigorous therapy reduces morbidity and mortality. The primary initiating event and the major components of the disturbed circulation should be considered in selecting appropriate therapy. The goal of therapy is to ensure a sufficient blood flow for adequate supply of oxygen to vital organs. This requires both adequate intravascular volume and adequate perfusion pressure.

All patients in shock (except cardiogenic shock) should be treated with volume replacement therapy if circulatory volume is low and increased cardiac output is needed (see Table). In addition, the primary initiating event (eg, hemorrhage in hypovolemic shock, bacterial infection in septic shock, myocardial infarction in cardiogenic shock) should be treated. If administration of fluid does not correct tissue hypoxia, the addition of an inotropic agent and, in cardiogenic shock, vasodilators can be considered to increase the cardiac output further. Hypotension is one of the hemodynamic markers for septic and hypovolemic shock, but patients with myocardial infarction who develop cardiogenic shock are not always hypotensive (Shoemaker et al, 1990). If the patient is severely hypotensive, vasopressors are used to maintain sufficient mean arterial pressure for coronary and cerebral perfusion after the maximum effects from fluids and inotropic agents have been achieved.

Hemodynamic, metabolic, and respiratory variables should be monitored to detect potentially reversible disturbances and to assess the effectiveness of therapy. Measurements may include continuous electrocardiographic monitoring of cardiac rate and rhythm, arterial pressure (preferably measured directly by an indwelling catheter), and pulmonary artery occlusive (wedge) pressure using a flow-directed pulmonary artery catheter. The pulmonary wedge pressure provides a reliable estimate of left ventricular filling pressure and is particularly useful for quantitative assessment of the left heart response to fluid challenge.

Arterial blood gases should be measured to assess acid-base status and oxygenation (Adrogué et al, 1989). Serum electrolytes, body temperature, and fluid intake and output also should be monitored. Urine sodium concentration and osmolality should be monitored in selected cases. Measurement of blood lactate may be useful in some instances (Weil et al, 1986).

HYPOVOLEMIC, SEPTIC, AND CARDIOGENIC SHOCK: CHARACTERISTICS AND TREATMENT

	Hypovolemic Shock	Septic Shock	Cardiogenic Shock
CHARACTERISTICS			
Etiology	Hemorrhage or loss of other body fluids	Bacterial, fungal, or viral infection	>40% left ventricular muscle dysfunction; rupture of papillary muscle or free wall; ventricular septal defect
Basic defect	Decreased oxygen supply due to insufficient blood volume	Decreased oxygen extraction by cells	Decreased oxygen supply due to pump failure
Clinical signs			
Cardiac output	Decreased	Normal or elevated, decreased late in sepsis	Decreased
Blood pressure	Hypotension	Hypotension	Hypotension or normal
Heart rate	Tachycardia	Tachycardia	Tachycardia
Pulmonary wedge pressure	Low	Low	Normal or high
Left ventricular function	Normal	Depressed	Depressed due to cell death, muscle rupture or defect
Urinary output	Decreased	Decreased	Decreased
Body temperature	Decreased or normal	Increased or decreased	Normal
TREATMENT			
Volume replacement	Yes	Yes	Usually no
Drug therapy			
Vasopressors (only if severely hypotensive)	Yes	Yes	Yes
Inotropic agents	Possibly	Yes	Yes
Vasodilators	Possibly	No	Possibly
Other therapies			
Surgery	Yes (hemorrhage)	Possibly	Yes (mechanical defect)
Antibacterial therapy	No	Yes	No
Reperfusion therapy	No	No	Yes

Hypovolemic Shock

In hypovolemic shock, tissue perfusion is relatively inadequate due to loss of blood or plasma from the intravascular space. This produces a fall in systolic pressure, which triggers a sympathetic response that results in peripheral vasoconstriction, a rise in pulse rate, and a reduction in pulse pressure. Tachycardia and an increase in cardiac contractility escalate myocardial oxygen requirements.

Therapy for hypovolemic shock should be directed toward improving circulatory function by restoring plasma volume without overloading an already expanded interstitial space. Pulse rate, arterial and central venous pressure, urinary output, temperature, electrocardiographic changes, peripheral oxygen saturation, and mental state should be monitored (Baskett, 1990).

A common characteristic of hypovolemic shock is substantially decreased tissue perfusion throughout the microcirculation. Although resuscitation may restore systemic hemodynamics, volume replacement does not necessarily reverse the impaired microcirculation (eg, in the kidneys and liver) (Wang et al, 1992). Thus, persistent disturbances in the microcirculation may prevent adequate delivery of oxygen and substrate and fail to provide energy needs for several days following resuscitation. However, local damage following ischemia probably is not exclusively due to a lack of oxygen and substrate. Reperfusion of a previously ischemic organ can cause further tissue damage; the primary mechanism appears to be formation of oxygen-free radicals (Haglund and Gerdin, 1991). In addition, tissue damage may stimulate inflammatory cells (eg, macrophages, polymorphonuclear cells, lymphocytes) to release mediators, thus precipitating an intravascular inflammatory response that causes further injury to endothelial cells.

VOLUME REPLACEMENT. Vigorous, rapid volume replacement that maintains pulmonary wedge pressure in the range of 15 to 20 mm Hg is the first and most important measure to employ (Shoemaker et al, 1990). Intravenous fluids should be given to restore an adequate circulating blood volume (Baskett, 1990). Crystalloid, colloid, and albumin solutions; blood in the form of whole blood or red blood cells; or the judicious combination of all of these components may be chosen.

Crystalloid solutions (eg, Ringer's lactate solution) replace both interstitial and intravascular loss, but large volumes are required to restore normal hemodynamic function. It is easier to achieve therapeutic goals with colloid solutions (eg, dextran [Gentran-40, Gentran-75], hetastarch [Hespan], pentastarch [Pentaspan]), which replace intravascular loss and restore hemodynamic values toward normal without overexpansion of interstitial water. These solutions are generally isooncotic, and lost blood volumes can be replaced on a 1:1 basis to normalize hemodynamic values. Crystalloid solutions may be used in patients with mild class I hemorrhage (loss of up to 15% of blood volume). The replacement volume should be three to four times the estimated loss since the electrolyte solution is distributed through the extracellular (intravascular and interstitial) space. The volume should be increased to compensate for urine loss. Administration of fluid should be continued to produce an adequate arterial pressure and a urine flow of 0.5 ml/kg/hr.

SYMPATHOMIMETIC AMINES. After the maximum effect from administration of fluids has been obtained, sympathomimetic amines may be employed to improve tissue perfusion of vital organs. The need for and response to a sympathomimetic amine should be assessed on the basis of cerebral, renal, and myocardial function and possibly the arterial blood lactate level. The rate of infusion must be regulated carefully so that the desired level of blood pressure is not exceeded. Generally, the systolic blood pressure should be maintained between 90 and 100 mm Hg or somewhat higher in previously hypertensive patients.

Sympathomimetic amines used to treat shock include the endogenous catecholamines, norepinephrine [Levophed], epinephrine, and dopamine [Intropin], and the synthetic compound, dobutamine [Dobutrex]. Dobutamine and dopamine are most commonly chosen.

Dobutamine is administered for inotropic support. It acts primarily on $beta_1$ receptors. Moderate doses increase myocardial contractility and cardiac output without substantially increasing heart rate or altering arterial pressure. In contrast to dopamine, dobutamine decreases left ventricular filling pressure. It should produce marked and significant increases in the cardiac output and stroke index, cardiac and stroke work, and oxygen delivery and consumption, as well as decreases in systemic and pulmonary vascular resistance and mean pulmonary artery, central venous, and pulmonary wedge pressures. Blood gases, pH, and the pulmonary venous admixture or shunting are not significantly altered (Shoemaker et al, 1990).

If administration of fluids and dobutamine does not achieve optimal results, dopamine may be given. Small doses activate dopaminergic receptors and thus reduce afterload and increase cardiac output by dilating the renal and mesenteric vascular beds. Moderate doses activate $beta_1$ receptors in the myocardium, resulting in an increase in myocardial contractility, heart rate, and cardiac output. Dopamine should be administered at the lowest dose needed to maintain a mean arterial pressure $>$80 mm Hg and a systolic arterial pressure $>$110 mm Hg. The rate of infusion should be limited to "renal" doses ($\leq$5 mcg/kg/hr) that enhance urine output (Baskett, 1990). Larger doses cause vasoconstriction and tachycardia, which result in increased myocardial oxygen demand that may not be met because of inadequate myocardial blood flow.

Norepinephrine stimulates the myocardium and increases cardiac output by acting on $beta_1$ receptors; it constricts the peripheral vessels by activating alpha receptors. With small doses, the inotropic action is predominant; with larger doses, the vasoconstrictor effect becomes more prominent. Cardiac work and myocardial oxygen consumption are increased. Blood flow to the heart and brain is maintained, while blood flow to other organs, especially abdominal viscera, voluntary muscles, and skin, may be greatly reduced. Norepinephrine is a more potent vasoconstrictor than dopamine. It is used less commonly today than in the past because of the availability of dopamine. However, if hypotension is severe, norepinephrine is the agent of choice to normalize the blood pressure.

Epinephrine acts on $beta_1$ receptors in the heart and on both alpha and $beta_2$ receptors in peripheral blood vessels. Small doses dilate skeletal muscle and mesenteric arterial blood vessels and may decrease blood pressure, but even small amounts constrict cutaneous and renal blood vessels. When administered in large doses, the vasoconstrictor action predominates and blood pressure is increased.

Adverse Reactions and Precautions: Therapeutic doses of sympathomimetic amines may cause headache, restlessness, anxiety, weakness, pallor, dizziness, tremor, precordial pain, palpitations, and respiratory distress. Overdosage can induce hypertension, convulsions, cerebral hemorrhage, and tachyarrhythmias. Excessive cardiac acceleration may reduce cardiac filling time, myocardial efficiency, coronary blood flow, and cardiac output. Fatal ventricular arrhythmias may be precipitated by sympathomimetic amines; therefore, the electrocardiogram should be monitored closely and the drug discontinued or the dosage reduced if an arrhythmia develops. Arrhythmias occur most frequently during administration of large doses, especially in patients with organic heart disease or shock complicated by hypoxia and electrolyte imbalances. Concomitant digitalis therapy may increase the risk of such arrhythmias.

Prolonged administration of vasoconstrictor sympathomimetic amines may reduce plasma volume because constriction of the postcapillary vessels increases capillary pressure and facilitates transcapillary fluid loss. The renal blood flow and glomerular filtration rate, already decreased by hypotension and compensatory vasoconstriction, may be reduced further by amines that constrict the renal vasculature, and acute tubular necrosis may ensue.

Various pathologic changes have been attributed to the prolonged administration of sympathomimetic amines, particularly norepinephrine. These include edema, hemorrhage, and necrosis of the intestine, liver, and kidneys, as well as focal myocarditis, subpericardial hemorrhage, intravascular platelet aggregation, and local slough and gangrene with subsequent loss of fingers or toes, especially in patients with preexisting vascular disease. These changes are most common in patients in severe shock, and it is often difficult to determine whether they are caused by drug therapy or by the shock process alone. Prolonged administration of large doses of norepinephrine produces diffuse necrotic myocardial lesions in experimental animals, and similar lesions have been observed in patients who died after prolonged infusion (Haft, 1974).

Extravasation of norepinephrine may produce local skin necrosis and slough involving subcutaneous and even muscle tissues. These effects can be minimized by prompt infiltration of phentolamine [Regitine] at the site of infusion (Zucker et al, 1960). Local sloughing also has occurred after extravasation of dopamine, but much less commonly than with norepinephrine.

Withdrawal of sympathomimetic amines may result in a fall in arterial blood pressure due to generalized loss of vascular tone or hypovolemia that develops during the infusion. To avoid this complication, discontinuation of therapy should be attempted as soon as possible. It may be advisable to accept a brief episode of hypotension if there is no evidence of tissue hypoperfusion. If there is difficulty in withdrawing the drug, appropriate fluids should be infused and the blood pressure and pulmonary wedge pressure should be monitored. With few exceptions, fluid challenge reverses the hypotensive state. Unless there is a specific indication other than hypotension for resuming sympathomimetic therapy, it is best avoided. The risk of adverse reactions is likely to be greater than the benefit of continued use.

VASODILATORS. These agents occasionally are used to decrease arterial constriction and improve cardiac output. In patients with impaired left ventricular function, vasodilators decrease afterload and thereby improve cardiac output and decrease myocardial oxygen consumption. If the mean arterial pressure is normal or high and the systemic vascular resistance index is high, vasodilation with intravenous nitroglycerin [Nitro-Bid IV, Nitrostat IV, Tridil], sodium nitroprusside [Nitropress], labetalol [Normodyne, Trandate], or alprostadil [Prostin VR] may be considered (Shoemaker and Appel, 1986). Volume replacement always should precede administration of the vasodilator, and fluids should be available in case the drug causes an acute fall in arterial pressure.

SURGICAL TREATMENT. For patients with hemorrhagic shock, surgery may be needed to repair the blood vessel at the site of bleeding.

Septic Shock

Sepsis is defined as a systemic inflammatory response to infection and can be caused by viral, fungal, mycobacterial, rickettsial, or protozoal microorganisms (Billhardt and Rosenbush, 1986; Luce, 1987; Members of the American College of Chest Physicians/Society of Critical Care Medicine Consensus Conference Committee, 1992). However, sepsis and septic shock (sepsis with hypotension) most commonly are associated with aerobic and anaerobic bacterial infections, especially those caused by gram-negative aerobes. The gram-negative aerobes most often responsible are *Escherichia coli, Klebsiella* species, and *Pseudomonas aeruginosa*. The genitourinary and gastrointestinal tracts and the lungs are the primary sites of infection. (For toxic shock syndrome, see index entry on this subject.)

Sepsis and septic shock occur most commonly in patients at the extremes of age who are compromised by coexisting disease or injury (especially malignancies, burns, diabetes, hyposplenism, liver or renal failure), concurrent drug administration (especially corticosteroids and antimetabolites), or procedures (including indwelling urinary bladder catheters and intravascular lines). Sepsis occurs in approximately 10 of 1,000 hospitalized patients, but septic shock develops in only a minority of these individuals (including 40% of those with gram-negative septicemia). However, 60% to 80% of patients with septic shock do not survive. In comparison, only 10% to 20% of hospitalized patients with sepsis die (Perlino and Rimland, 1985).

The series of events leading from sepsis to septic shock probably is initiated by toxins that are liberated by the microorganisms or are bound to their cell walls (Bone, 1991). The endotoxins of gram-negative aerobes, toxic shock syndrome toxin-1, gram-positive aerobe or yeast cell-wall products, and viral or fungal antigens can initiate the sepsis cascade. Once in the circulation, endotoxin mediates the release of tumor necrosis factor α (TNFα); interleukin-1, -6, and -8 (IL-1, IL-6, and IL-8); and platelet activating factor (PAF) from mononuclear phagocytes and endothelial and other cells. TNFα, IL-1, and PAF in turn initiate the metabolism of arachidonic acid to form leukotrienes, thromboxane A_2, and prostaglandins. IL-1 and IL-6 activate the T-cells to produce interferon-γ, IL-2, IL-4, and granulocyte/monocyte colony stimulating factor. Most of these substances and their metabolic products increase endothelial permeability and eventually are injurious. In addition, endotoxin initiates the complement cascade resulting in vascular abnormalities and neutrophil activation. Persistent endothelial damage at one or more sites leads to organ dysfunction, hypoperfusion, and hypotension. Consequences of hypoperfusion include lactic acidosis, oliguria, and acute alteration in mental status. The patient is considered to be in septic shock when hypotension persists despite adequate volume replacement.

In the first stage of septic shock, systemic vascular resistance falls, pulmonary and systemic blood flow increases, and oxygen consumption rises. Although this initial hyperdynamic stage does not progress in some patients, in others the fall in systemic vascular resistance persists and leads to a decline in cardiac output and oxygen consumption. Septic shock also is characterized by impairment of cardiac function. Left ventricular depression appears early and may be directly proportional to the severity of the sepsis and the likelihood of death. Right ventricular depression also can be fatal (Groeneveld et al, 1986; Ognibene et al, 1988; Parrillo et al, 1990). In septic states, the oxygen demand of the cells and the oxygen transport values are typically elevated because of fever and the inflammatory reaction. Decreased ability to extract oxygen limits the capacity of the tissues to increase oxygen uptake. In addition, myocardial depression limits the ability to increase cardiac output to compensate for the oxygen demand.

The reduced cardiac output may be complicated by an increase in pulmonary vascular resistance that occurs relatively late in septic shock and has been attributed to thrombosis, catecholamine excess, hypoxic pulmonary vasoconstriction, and increases in lung volume caused by the mechanical ventilation and positive end-expiratory pressure (PEEP) therapies that are commonly used in septic patients. Other possible explanations for impaired cardiac output in the later stage of septic shock are the presence of circulating anti-inotropic substances (eg, myocardial depressant factor) and the abnormal metabolic state that results from shock. With respect to the latter, lactic acidosis has been shown to alter cardiac performance, presumably by decreasing pH. In addition, venous hypercapnia occurs because of impaired oxygen extraction and may contribute to decreasing pH (Mecher et al, 1990).

Diagnosis and Monitoring: The development of sepsis usually is indicated by temperatures higher than 38.3° C or lower than 36° C, tachycardia (>90 beats/min), tachypnea (>20 breaths/min or hyperventilation), white blood cell count ≥12,000 mm^3 or <4,000 mm^3, and decreased oxygen perfusion (Bone et al, 1992). Hypothermia is observed in a minority of patients, and failure to develop a fever is a poor prognostic sign. Circulating leukocytes increase 30% to 50% in most septic patients. Other significant laboratory findings include hypoglycemia, thrombocytopenia, hypoalbuminemia, hyperbilirubinemia, and an increase in blood urea nitrogen and creatinine concentrations. The most useful test is determination of arterial blood gas levels, which generally indicates respiratory alkalosis and metabolic (lactic) acidosis in the early stages of sepsis. Often the diagnosis is made or confirmed by pulmonary artery catheterization; findings include decreased systemic vascular resistance; increased (or decreased late in sepsis) cardiac output; and narrowed arterial-mixed venous oxygen saturation or content difference that reflects reduced oxygen consumption by the tissues.

Mental obtundation, decreased urine output, and hypotension (systolic blood pressure <90 mm Hg) are cardinal manifestations of septic shock. These patients also may develop hypercapnic respiratory failure due to increased respiratory muscle fatigue in addition to the hypoxemic respiratory failure that results from parenchymal lung disease. PEEP to aid oxygenation and intubation and mechanical ventilation usually are required for these patients.

ANTIBACTERIAL THERAPY. Administration of antibiotics to eliminate the source of infection is essential for survival of patients with sepsis. Selection of an antibiotic should be dictated by epidemiologic data, the site of infection, and results of Gram stains or cultures if available. In most patients, initial therapy for gram-positive and gram-negative bacterial infection is empiric pending culture results because it is difficult to determine the causative microorganism on the basis of clinical symptoms. Antibiotics effective against staphylococci should be given to intravenous drug abusers, and agents effective against anaerobes should be included in the therapeutic regimen for patients with intra-abdominal infections. Combination therapy is recommended for neutropenic patients and for those with infections caused by *Pseudomonas* and *Enterococcus* species; however; serum bactericidal activity appears to be more important than the number of antibiotics. For antimicrobial therapy, see index entry Sepsis.

Despite the use of increasingly potent antibiotics and improved methods for hemodynamic monitoring, the short-term survival rate for patients with septic shock remains poor; slightly more than 50% can be discharged from the intensive care unit. A multivariate analysis indicated that assessment of five variables (left ventricular stroke work index, pulmonary wedge pressure, white blood cell counts, partial pressure of oxygen, and the hematocrit) can predict those patients who are most likely to survive (D'Orio et al, 1990).

IMMUNOTHERAPY. In addition to antibiotics, agents directed at the mediators responsible for sepsis and the immune response are being developed. These investigational agents include the following:

(1) Antiserum against a J5 *E. coli* mutant with an exposed core region, which protects animals against gram-negative infections. Clinical trials of human antiserum compared with control serum demonstrated that passive immunotherapy with anti-J5 antiserum markedly reduced the mortality rate in patients with gram-negative infections (Ziegler et al, 1982) and protected high-risk surgical patients from developing septic shock (Baumgartner et al, 1985).

(2) Two monoclonal IgM antibodies directed against the J5 *E. coli* mutant, E5 and HA-1A, have been produced from mouse hybridoma cells and a primary human cell line, respectively. E5 binds to heterologous smooth lipopolysaccharides, while HA-1A binds only slightly to smooth bacteria that have not been exposed to antibiotics. HA-1A is not as specific as E5, since it also binds to fungi, cardiolipin, and lipoproteins (Baumgartner et al, 1992). In trials comparing E5 and placebo in patients with septic syndrome, survival was improved by E5 only in a small number of patients with gram-negative sepsis who were not in refractory shock (Greenman et al, 1991; Greenberg et al, 1992); E5 did not improve survival in patients with documented gram-negative sepsis (Food and Drug Administration, 1991). Similarly, HA-1A reduced mortality only in a subgroup of patients with gram-negative bacteremia, regardless of whether or not they were in shock (Ziegler et al, 1991), and did not increase survival in the subgroup with gram-negative sepsis. In addition, mortality was slightly higher in HA-1A recipients with nonbacteremic gram-negative infections than in the placebo group 14 and 28 days following treatment (Food and Drug Administration, 1991). Since E5 and HA-1A have not improved survival in those with gram-negative sepsis and since gram-negative bacteremia could not be confirmed until 48 hours or more after culturing the patient's blood, the use of these monoclonal antibodies as a routine adjunctive procedure for the treatment of patients with evidence of sepsis is not yet justified.

(3) Since TNFα plays a key role in the sepsis cascade (Bone, 1991), decreasing its level may lessen the severity of septic syndrome. Administration of a murine anti-TNFα monoclonal antibody (CB0006) to patients with septic syndrome did not decrease the mortality rate (Fisher et al, 1993). However, subgroup analysis showed that in patients with high TNFα levels (>50 pg/ml) initially, survival appeared to improve with large doses of the anti-TNFα monoclonal antibody (10 mg/kg).

(4) A recombinant human IL-1 receptor antagonist (IL-1ra) reduced mortality from endotoxin shock in a rabbit model (Ohlsson et al, 1990). In a multicenter trial conducted by the IL-1ra Phase III Sepsis Syndrome Study Group, patients with septic syndrome were randomized to receive placebo or a regimen consisting of an intravenous loading dose of IL-1ra (100 mg) followed by a continuous 72-hour intravenous infusion (1 or 2 mg/kg/hr). Although no significant difference in the mortality rate between treatment groups was observed, the survival rate in patients treated with IL-1ra increased with increasing severity of the septic syndrome. Patients receiving IL-1ra 2 mg/kg/hr for 72 hours had a mortality rate of 35% compared with 45% in placebo recipients.

VOLUME REPLACEMENT. As with treatment for other forms of shock, an important first step in the management of hypotension is restoration of an adequate intravascular volume, preferably guided by data obtained from pulmonary artery catheterization. Colloid or crystalloid solutions or blood can be used. No one form of fluids has been demonstrated to be superior in enhancing cardiovascular function or decreasing ultimate mortality.

SYMPATHOMIMETIC AMINES. If a patient with septic shock remains hypotensive after volume replacement therapy has raised the pulmonary wedge pressure to 15 to 18 mm Hg, dopamine should be administered to raise the diastolic blood pressure to at least 60 mm Hg. If the dose of dopamine exceeds 15 mcg/kg/min, another vasopressor (usually norepinephrine) can be administered with the dose adjusted to maintain a diastolic blood pressure >60 mm Hg. However, the use of norepinephrine in patients with septic shock who do not respond to dopamine is controversial, since norepinephrine does not improve the peripheral blood flow (Hussain et al, 1988). Nevertheless, more than 200 patients with septic shock have been treated with norepinephrine when volume replacement and dopamine therapy did not increase blood pressure (Parrillo et al, 1990). In many of these patients, shock was reversed and irreversible end-organ damage did not occur. Once blood pressure has been normalized with norepinephrine, the lowest dosage that maintains the diastolic blood pressure at 60 mm Hg should be administered to minimize any potential reduction in organ blood flow. Overall survival in norepinephrine-treated patients is approximately 40%.

Addition of an inotropic agent (eg, dobutamine) can be considered to further increase cardiac output and eliminate tissue hypoxia (Vincent and van der Linden, 1990). Dobutamine also has facilitated fluid administration in septic shock, and the combination of dobutamine and intravenous fluids was particularly effective in enhancing oxygen transport and oxygen consumption in an experimental model of septic shock (Vincent et al, 1987). Dobutamine also has been recommended if myocardial depression becomes evident (Karakusis, 1986). Addition of 5 mcg/kg/min of dobutamine as standard treatment of patients with septic shock may increase cardiac output, oxygen transport, and oxygen consumption without significantly affecting vascular resistance (Vincent et al, 1990).

ADRENAL CORTICOSTEROIDS. Steroids are specifically indicated for shock associated with adrenal insufficiency (addisonian crisis). However, since plasma cortisol concentrations are increased in patients with septic shock (Schein et al, 1990), adrenal insufficiency as judged by absolute plasma cortisol concentrations probably is rare. Corticosteroids may have a supplemental role in anaphylactic shock (see index entry Shock, Anaphylactic), but large doses have not reversed septic shock, prevented the development of adult respiratory distress syndrome, or reduced mortality in large controlled clinical trials (Bone et al, 1987; Veterans Administration Systemic Sepsis Cooperative Study Group, 1987) and may encourage development of secondary infections (Bone et al, 1987). Furthermore, administration of large doses of methylprednisolone increased concentrations of serum bilirubin and blood urea nitrogen in patients with severe sepsis and septic shock compared with those receiving placebo, indicating steroid-induced abnormalities in hepatic and renal function (Slotman et al, 1993). Consequently, the use of steroids should be avoided.

OPIOID ANTAGONISTS. In laboratory animals, endogenous opioids are released in response to stress and may contribute to the pathogenesis of shock (Faden, 1984). The opioid antagonist, naloxone [Narcan], improved cardiovascular function and survival in experimental shock models. Because of its ability to increase the mean arterial pressure, naloxone is effective as a temporizing agent during the treatment of critically ill patients with septic shock (Hackshaw et al, 1990). (For further information on this drug, see index entry Naloxone, In Opioid Overdose.)

SURGICAL TREATMENT. Surgery sometimes is needed in patients with septic shock. For example, drainage of an abscess or excision of necrotic tissue at the septic site is essential. For myometritis accompanying postpartum sepsis, radical hysterectomy may be the treatment of choice.

Cardiogenic Shock

Cardiogenic shock is caused by loss of myocardial contractile function precipitated by myocardial infarction, severe cardiomyopathy, or mechanical obstruction or compression of the heart. It is seen in 7% to 15% of patients with myocardial infarction during the first days after hospitalization. Cardiogenic shock usually results from extension of the initial infarction at its borders and loss of a critical amount of ventricular contractile function, which causes hypotension and inadequate tissue perfusion (Billhardt and Rosenbush, 1986; Hands et al, 1989). Other causes include papillary muscle rupture, free wall rupture, and ventricular septal defect. Regardless of the cause, the physiologic findings are uniform: there is a marked decrease in cardiac output followed by a decrease in coronary blood flow and an increase in peripheral vascular resistance. These changes increase ischemia and lead to continuing necrosis and further worsening of ventricular function in a vicious cycle that is usually fatal. Patients who die from cardiogenic shock have infarction of 40% or more of the left ventricle, and most have severe three-vessel coronary disease. Cardiogenic shock develops more frequently in patients with large infarcts, previous infarction, ejection fractions of <35% on hospitalization, or diabetes and in those of advanced age.

Cardiogenic shock is often indicated by continuing release of MB-creatine kinase and recurring chest pain suggesting infarct extension. Patients have cold and clammy skin (Bolooki, 1989); in addition, tissue perfusion is poor, urine output is <0.5 ml/kg/hr, metabolic acidosis is present, and arterial blood pressure is usually decreased and is associated with tachycardia (heart rate >100 beats/min). Hemodynamically, cardiac output is <2.2 L/min/M^2, pulmonary wedge pressure is >18 mm Hg, and peripheral resistance is >1,800 dyne-sec/cm^{-5}. Treatment is aimed at maintaining cardiac output and perfusion pressure and minimizing ischemia. Cardiac assist techniques, such as intra-aortic balloon counterpulsation, make it possible to sustain the patient pending invasive diagnosis when a surgically treatable complication is suspected.

SYMPATHOMIMETIC AMINES. By increasing arterial blood pressure, sympathomimetic amines may improve coronary perfusion. Some agents also increase blood flow to the renal and mesenteric vascular beds. Those that stimulate the myocardium may increase cardiac output, but sympathomimetic amines should be used with caution because they increase myocardial oxygen consumption by a direct effect on myocardial metabolism and by imposing extra pressure work on the heart. Whether the increased oxygen requirements are met by an adequate increase in coronary blood flow will ultimately depend on the effect of the amine on coronary blood flow.

Dopamine is often the preferred sympathomimetic drug for initial therapy provided that adequate perfusion pressure is maintained and the heart rate does not increase too greatly. Dopamine produces less vasoconstriction than norepinephrine and is less likely to cause skin necrosis if extravasation occurs. It causes less vasodilation and tachycardia than isoproterenol and, in appropriate doses, it may increase blood flow to the kidneys and mesentery (Goldberg, 1972).

Dobutamine is being employed with increasing frequency. Its hemodynamic effects in acute myocardial infarction are comparable to those attained with combined dopamine-nitroprusside therapy (Keung et al, 1981). If marked hypotension is not present, dobutamine may be useful in patients with acute circulatory collapse who have severely impaired pump function, low cardiac output, and elevated left ventricular filling pressure (Francis et al, 1982). A combination of dopamine and dobutamine may be of value in selected patients (Leier and Unverferth, 1983). Intravenous amrinone [Inocor] also may be useful.

Because it acts rapidly and is the most potent pressor agent available, norepinephrine should be reserved for patients with severe hypotension. This drug should not be used for prolonged periods because it may cause ischemia of vital organs and may deplete the plasma volume by constricting small veins, thus increasing capillary (hydrostatic) pressure.

VOLUME REPLACEMENT. In a minority of patients, hypotension accompanying acute myocardial infarction is associated with hypovolemia and a normal or low pulmonary wedge pressure. Hypovolemia may be caused by overuse of diuretics or excessive vasoconstriction due to endogenous or exogenous sympathomimetic amines. These patients may benefit from plasma volume expansion, but pulmonary wedge pressure should be monitored closely (Figueras and Weil, 1979). A subset of patients with right ventricular infarction are often hypotensive with normal or low pulmonary wedge pressure and elevated central venous and right atrial pressures. Fluid administration usually improves their hemodynamic status. If volume replacement alone does not improve cardiac output, dobutamine may be useful (Dell'Italia et al, 1985).

VASODILATORS. A vasodilator may be indicated (most commonly as an adjunct to an inotropic drug) in selected patients with severe pump failure following acute myocardial infarction, especially those with recurrent ischemic pain, increased vascular resistance, normal or reduced cardiac output, or a marked elevation of left ventricular filling pressure. The systolic pressure usually should not be allowed to fall below 110 mm Hg if a vasodilator is used. Vasodilators are of particular value when acute myocardial infarction is complicated by mitral regurgitation or ventricular septal rupture.

Therapy is initiated with intravenous nitroglycerin or sodium nitroprusside. In patients with ongoing ischemia, nitroglycerin is the drug of choice because it improves the regional distribution of myocardial flow and is less likely than nitroprusside to produce coronary steal. When systemic arterial resistance is markedly elevated (>1,500 dyne/sec/cm^{-5}), nitroprusside is preferred. If the systolic pressure falls below 90 mm Hg during vasodilator therapy and volume expansion fails to reverse hypotension promptly, the drug should be discontinued or the dosage reduced. The fall in pressure may be abrupt; therefore, arterial pressure should be monitored carefully. Although the combined hemodynamic effects of a vasodilator and a sympathomimetic amine appear to be beneficial, there is no conclusive evidence that combined therapy improves prognosis.

REPERFUSION THERAPY. The prognosis of patients with cardiogenic shock has not improved appreciably in the past two decades (mortality rate, 65% to 90%) with standard treatment (ie, coronary care unit monitoring; administration of vasopressors, vasodilators, and inotropic agents; intra-aortic balloon counterpulsation) (Bates and Topol, 1991; Goldberg et al, 1991). Although the use of thrombolytic agents would appear to be a logical step in the treatment of patients with cardiogenic shock, only moderate improvement in survival has been observed in isolated trials (Van de Werf, 1988). In other trials (GISSI, 1986; GISSI-2, 1990), neither a decrease in the incidence of cardiogenic shock nor in mortality was observed. However, mechanical revascularization with percutaneous transluminal coronary angioplasty appears to improve the prognosis in patients with cardiogenic shock complicating myocardial infarction (Lee et al, 1988, 1991; Moosvi et al, 1992; Bengtson et al, 1992; Klein, 1992). The mortality rate in patients with successful reperfusion of the infarct artery was 20% to 30% compared with 80% in those whose coronary artery remained occluded even after angioplasty. The 24-month survival rate was significantly better in the former group (54%) than in those who did not respond (11%) (Lee et al, 1991). Improvement in survival is most evident if angioplasty is performed within 24 hours of the onset of cardiogenic shock (Moosvi et al, 1992).

SURGICAL TREATMENT. Prompt surgical intervention is indicated in acute coronary occlusion due to failure of angioplasty, acute papillary muscle rupture, acute ventricular septal defect, acute or false aneurysm of the left ventricle, and persistent postinfarction angina associated with cardiogenic shock. Whenever possible, these patients should receive vasopressors and circulatory assist support (intra-aortic balloon pump, Hemopump, or HeartMate) (Gacioch et al, 1992; Willerson and Frazier, 1991). The coronary anatomy should be defined by coronary arteriography prior to surgery. Mortality associated with surgical revascularization alone is $<10\%$, while the risk with repair of acute mechanical defects with or without surgical revascularization is approximately 50% (Bolooki, 1989).

CARDIAC TRANSPLANTATION. Transplantation is an alternative method of therapy for patients with acute and chronic congestive heart failure that does not respond to drug treatment and/or circulatory assist devices.

Cardiogenic shock occurring in patients following cardiac transplantation poses a special problem in that the normal (donor) heart temporarily is unable to provide adequate cardiac output because of prolonged ischemia or insufficient myocardial function even with use of cold cardioplegic (high potassium) solutions for preservation. Because of myocardial stunning, the cardiac function may not return to normal after restoration of coronary blood flow. Circulatory support (primarily with drugs; rarely, with intra-aortic balloon pump) may be needed for rehabilitation of the donor heart. After transplantation, patients respond well to low-dose isoproterenol infusion, which increases the heart rate to >100/min and maintains low systemic and pulmonary vascular resistance; dobutamine can produce the same effects. Drug therapy may be needed for several days because the denervated donor heart is dependent on the chronotropic response as well as preload to maintain satisfactory cardiac output (Stevenson and Miller, 1991).

Anaphylactic Shock

See index entry Shock, Anaphylactic.

Drug Evaluations

SYMPATHOMIMETIC AMINES

DOPAMINE HYDROCHLORIDE

[Intropin]

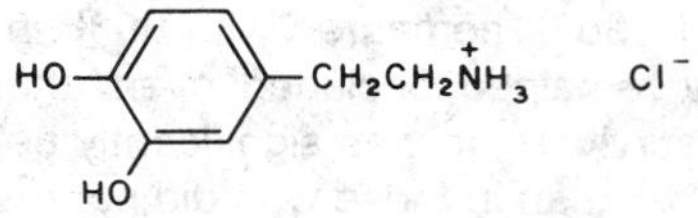

$$HO-C_6H_3(OH)-CH_2CH_2\overset{+}{N}H_3 \quad Cl^-$$

ACTIONS. Dopamine exerts a positive inotropic effect through a direct action on beta-adrenergic receptors and release of norepinephrine from tissue storage sites. Hemodynamic effects vary with dosage. Small doses (<5 mcg/kg/min) activate dopaminergic receptors in the renal and mesenteric vascular beds to produce vasodilation. Slightly larger doses (5 to 10 mcg/kg/min) maintain the effect on dopaminergic receptors and also activate beta receptors; as a result, myocardial contractility, heart rate, and cardiac output are increased. With larger doses (>10 mcg/kg/min), vasoconstriction, which is an alpha-adrenergic effect, predominates and renal blood flow may be reduced; when this occurs, urine output may decrease.

USES. Dopamine is used as an adjunct to volume replacement in patients with shock to increase cardiac output, blood pressure, and urinary flow. It lacks the marked vasoconstrictor properties of norepinephrine but is a more potent pressor agent than dobutamine (which acts predominantly as an inotropic agent). Dopamine is useful in patients with marked hypotension and shock (Vincent et al, 1987; Shoemaker et al, 1989). Because of its unique hemodynamic effects, dopamine often is more beneficial than other sympathomimetic amines in patients with impaired renal function. Small doses (1 mcg/kg/min) may increase renal blood flow and glomerular filtration rate (GFR) and promote diuresis in the early stages of acute oliguric renal failure but may not improve renal function if the baseline GFR is <50 ml/min/1.73 M^2 (Wee et al, 1986).

In selected patients, dopamine may be used with nitroprusside, nitroglycerin, or dobutamine (Shoemaker et al, 1990).

ADVERSE REACTIONS AND PRECAUTIONS. Dopamine may cause nausea, vomiting, headache, nervousness or restlessness, tachyarrhythmias, and anginal pain. Patients with unstable angina may be particularly likely to develop myocardial ischemic episodes during dopamine infusion (Crea et al, 1986). In cardiogenic shock, the improvement in hemodynamic status induced by dopamine may be accompanied by an increase in myocardial oxygen consumption. Small doses occasionally precipitate a fall in blood pressure, which can be corrected by intravenous fluid replacement.

Dopamine is less likely than norepinephrine to cause tissue necrosis following extravasation but, if extravasation occurs, the site should be infiltrated with 10 ml of a solution containing 5 to 10 mg of phentolamine; a fine hypodermic needle should be used. Infusion of dopamine for long periods or in large doses has caused peripheral ischemia and gangrene, necessitating skin grafts and occasionally amputation of an extremity. Bilateral retinal infarction, attributed to dopamine-induced constriction of retinal vessels, has been reported. For further information on the adverse effects of sympathomimetic drugs, see the section on Hypovolemic Shock.

Dopamine is classified in FDA Pregnancy Category C.

DRUG INTERACTIONS. Since dopamine is metabolized by monoamine oxidase, the dose should be reduced to one-tenth the usual amount in patients receiving monoamine oxidase inhibitors.

Cardiac arrest occurred in one patient who was treated with dopamine after receiving a small dose of tolazoline. Dopamine may potentiate the arrhythmogenic effects of other medication, including anesthetics, tricyclic compounds, and digitalis.

DOSAGE AND PREPARATIONS. Dopamine should be administered through a central venous line. Peripheral intravenous administration, even with a large-bore needle, should be avoided.

Intravenous: *Adults,* a solution containing 400 mcg/ml is prepared by diluting the contents of an ampul, vial, or additive syringe with sterile sodium chloride injection or 5% dextrose injection. (This is a more dilute solution than that recommended by the manufacturer.) Initially, the dilute solution is infused at a rate of 2 to 5 mcg/kg/min. In more seriously ill patients, an initial infusion rate of 5 mcg/kg/min may be increased gradually to 5 to 10 mcg/kg/min and, rarely, to 20 to 30 mcg/kg/min. The urine output and electrocardiogram should be monitored closely during the infusion.

Generic. Solution 0.8, 1.6, and 3.2 mg/ml in 5% dextrose in 250 and 500 ml containers, 40 and 80 mg/ml in 5, 10, and 20 ml containers, and 160 mg/ml in 5 ml containers.

Intropin (DuPont). Solution (aqueous) 40, 80, and 160 mg/ml in 5 ml containers.

DOBUTAMINE HYDROCHLORIDE

[Dobutrex]

ACTIONS. Dobutamine acts primarily on myocardial $beta_1$ receptors; it has a less pronounced effect on $beta_2$ and alpha receptors and does not activate dopaminergic receptors. Moderate doses increase myocardial contractility and cardiac output and may reduce peripheral vascular resistance and ventricular filling pressure (Shoemaker et al, 1990); large doses may increase heart rate and blood pressure.

USES. Dobutamine is used for short-term inotropic support in patients with depressed myocardial contractility associated with acute or chronic congestive heart failure or after cardiac surgery (see index entry Heart Failure). It also is useful in *acute* circulatory failure secondary to depressed myocardial contractility (Francis et al, 1982). In patients with acute myocardial infarction complicated by hypotension and severe left ventricular dysfunction, the hemodynamic effects of dobutamine are comparable to those obtained with combined dopamine and nitroprusside therapy (Keung et al, 1981). This drug has also improved cardiac output in patients with right ventricular infarction who do not respond to volume replacement alone (Dell'Italia et al, 1985). If arterial pressure cannot be maintained by dobutamine, dopamine or norepinephrine may be added to the regimen (Leier and Unverferth, 1983; Mueller, 1985).

ADVERSE REACTIONS AND PRECAUTIONS. Dobutamine occasionally causes nausea, headache, palpitations, anginal pain, and shortness of breath. Tachycardia and systolic hypertension, the most common adverse effects, usually can be controlled by reducing the dose or administering antiarrhythmic drugs. Ventricular arrhythmias occur occasionally. Since dobutamine facilitates AV conduction, it may increase the ventricular rate in patients with atrial fibrillation.

DOSAGE AND PREPARATIONS. Dobutamine is incompatible with alkaline solutions and should not be mixed with sodium bicarbonate injection. Before administration, the solution should be further diluted to at least 50 ml (see manufacturer's literature for recommended diluents), and it should be used within 24 hours. The preferred method of administration is by a central venous line.

Intravenous: *Adults,* potentially beneficial hemodynamic effects in patients with acute myocardial infarction have been reported with doses ranging from 8 to 24 mcg/kg/min. The initial rate of infusion is approximately 2 mcg/kg/min; the appropriate dose is determined by titration to achieve the optimal cardiac output, blood pressure, and pulmonary wedge pressure.

Dobutrex (Lilly). Solution 12.5 mg/ml in 20 ml containers.

EPINEPHRINE HYDROCHLORIDE

For chemical formula see index entry Epinephrine, In Asthma.

ACTIONS AND USES. Epinephrine is a highly potent α and β agonist. It is the pressor drug of choice for restoring spontaneous circulation after cardiac arrest caused by asystole, electromechanical dissociation, or ventricular fibrillation. Its beneficial effect in cardiac arrest is due to stimulation of alpha receptors, which increases peripheral vascular resistance, aortic diastolic pressure, and coronary perfusion pressure and blood flow (Otto, 1986; *JAMA*, 1992). Epinephrine also is used after cardiopulmonary bypass surgery when cold cardioplegia is employed, and it is the drug of choice for anaphylactic shock.

ADVERSE REACTIONS AND PRECAUTIONS. See the section on Hypovolemic Shock.

DOSAGE AND PREPARATIONS.

Intravenous: *Adults,* 0.5 to 1 mg (5 to 10 ml of a 1:10,000 solution) is given every three minutes during cardiopulmonary resuscitation. Larger doses have been used in patients who did not respond to standard therapy (Koscove and Paradis, 1988; *JAMA*, 1992).

The endotracheal route is often employed prior to establishing intravenous access, but results of one study indicate that epinephrine is not well absorbed from the tracheobronchial tree (Quinton et al, 1987). Intracardiac administration should be used only if other sites are not accessible.

Generic. Solution 0.1 mg/ml in 10 ml containers.

NOREPINEPHRINE BITARTRATE
[Levophed]

ACTIONS AND USES. Norepinephrine is a potent β_1 agonist and a highly potent α_1 and α_2 agonist. This catecholamine has both inotropic and vasoconstrictor properties. The inotropic effect is evident with small doses; vasoconstrictor effects predominate as the dosage is increased. The marked pressor effect of norepinephrine is primarily due to an increase in peripheral resistance, and, despite its direct positive chronotropic effect, this drug may indirectly reduce the heart rate by reflex mechanisms. Norepinephrine has a prompt and reversible action and is used to treat shock when a potent vasoconstrictor is needed to maintain adequate perfusion of vital organs. Generalized vasoconstriction and the tendency to cause tissue necrosis with prolonged administration limit its usefulness. However, prolonged infusion of norepinephrine may be indicated in patients with shock who have received calcium channel blocking drugs and, especially, in patients who develop hypotension after coronary bypass surgery. Patients receiving antihypertensive agents (eg, ACE inhibitors) who develop hypotension postoperatively also respond well to norepinephrine infusion (Bolooki, 1989).

ADVERSE REACTIONS AND PRECAUTIONS. Norepinephrine can cause tissue necrosis at the site of injection. The risk of ischemic injury is reduced if the drug is infused via a catheter in a deeply seated vein and if a small amount of phentolamine is added to the solution. The infusion site should be changed when prolonged administration is necessary. If extravasation occurs, the site should be infiltrated with 10 ml of a solution containing 5 to 10 mg of phentolamine; a fine hypodermic needle should be used. To reduce the incidence of venous thrombosis, heparin may be added to the infusion solution in amounts that supply 100 to 200 units/hour.

For a general discussion of adverse effects of sympathomimetic amines, see the section on Hypovolemic Shock.

DOSAGE AND PREPARATIONS.

Intravenous: *Adults,* 0.03 to 0.15 mcg/kg/min; for prolonged infusion, the dose range is 1 to 10 mcg/kg/min.

Levophed (Sanofi Winthrop). Solution (sterile, aqueous) equivalent to 1 mg of base/ml in 4 ml containers.

Cited References

Guidelines for cardiopulmonary resuscitation and emergency cardiac care: Part III, adult advanced cardiac life support. *JAMA* 268:2199-2241, 1992.

Transcript of Open Meeting of the Vaccines and Related Biological Products Advisory Committee, September 4, 1991. Bethesda, Md, Food and Drug Administration, 1991, 1-270.

Adrogué HJ, et al: Assessing acid-base status in circulatory failure: Differences between arterial and central venous blood. *N Engl J Med* 320:1312-1316, 1989.

Baskett PJF: Management of hypovolaemic shock. *BMJ* 300:1453-1457, 1990.

Bates ER, Topol EJ: Limitations of thrombolytic therapy for acute myocardial infarction complicated by congestive heart failure and cardiogenic shock. *J Am Coll Cardiol* 18:1077-1084, 1991.

Baumgartner JD, et al: Prevention of gram-negative shock and death in surgical patients by antibody to endotoxin core glycolipid. *Lancet* 2:59-63, 1985.

Baumgartner J-D, et al: The HA-1A monoclonal antibody for Gram-negative sepsis. *N Engl J Med* 523:281-282, 1992.

Bengtson JR, et al: Prognosis in cardiogenic shock after acute myocardial infarction in the interventional era. *J Am Coll Cardiol* 20:1482-1489, 1992.

Billhardt RA, Rosenbush SW: Cardiogenic and hypovolemic shock. *Med Clin North Am* 70:853-876, 1986.

Bolooki H: Emergency cardiac procedures in patients in cardiogenic shock due to complications of coronary artery disease. *Circulation* 79(suppl I):I-137-I-148, 1989.

Bone RC: The pathogenesis of sepsis. *Ann Intern Med* 115:457-469, 1991.

Bone RC, et al: Controlled clinical trial of high-dose methylprednisolone in treatment of severe sepsis and septic shock. *N Engl J Med* 317:653-658, 1987.

Bone RC, et al: Definitions for sepsis and organ failure and guidelines for the use of innovative therapies in sepsis. *Chest* 101:1644-1655, 1992.

Crea F, et al: Provocation of coronary spasm by dopamine in patients with active variant angina pectoris. *Circulation* 74:262-269, 1986.

Dell'Italia LJ, et al: Comparative effects of volume loading, dobutamine, and nitroprusside in patients with predominantly right ventricular infarction. *Circulation* 72:1327-1335, 1985.

D'Orio V, et al: Accuracy in early prediction of prognosis of patients with septic shock by analysis of simple indices: Prospective study. *Crit Care Med* 18:1339-1345, 1990.

Faden AI: Opiate antagonists and thyrotropin-releasing hormone: I, Potential role in treatment of shock. *JAMA* 252:1177-1180, 1984.

Figueras J, Weil MH: Hypovolemia and hypotension complicating management of acute cardiogenic pulmonary edema. *Am J Cardiol* 44:1349-1411, 1979.

Fisher CJ Jr, et al: Influence of an anti-tumor necrosis factor monoclonal antibody on cytokine levels in patients with sepsis. *Crit Care Med* 21:318-327, 1993.

Francis GS, et al: Comparative hemodynamic effects of dopamine and dobutamine in patients with acute cardiogenic circulatory collapse. *Am Heart J* 103:995-1000, 1982.

Gacioch GM, et al: Cardiogenic shock complicating acute myocardial infarction: The use of coronary angioplasty and the integration of the new support devices into patient management. *J Am Coll Cardiol* 19:647-653, 1992.

Goldberg LI: Cardiovascular and renal action of dopamine: Potential clinical applications. *Pharmacol Rev* 24:1-29, 1972.

Goldberg RJ, et al: Cardiogenic shock after acute myocardial infarction: Incidence and mortality from a community-wide perspective, 1975 to 1988. *N Engl J Med* 325:1117-1122, 1991.

Greenberg RN, et al: Observations using antiendotoxin antibody (E5) as adjuvant therapy in humans with suspected, serious, Gram-negative sepsis. *Crit Care Med* 20:730-735, 1992.

Greenman RL, et al: A controlled clinical trial of E5 murine monoclonal IgM antibody to endotoxin in the treatment of Gram-negative sepsis. *JAMA* 266:1097-1102, 1991.

Groeneveld ABJ, et al: Hemodynamic determinants of mortality in human septic shock. *Surgery* 99:140-153, 1986.

Gruppo Italiana per lo Studio della Sopravvivenza nell'Infarto Miocardico (GISSI): GISSI-2: A factorial randomized trial of alteplase versus streptokinase and heparin versus no heparin among 12,490 patients with acute myocardial infarction. *Lancet* 336:65-71, 1990.

Gruppo Italiana per lo Studio della Streptochinasi nell'Infarto Miocardico (GISSI): Effectiveness of intravenous thrombolytic treatment in acute myocardial infarction. *Lancet* 1:349-360, 1986.

Hackshaw KV, et al: Naloxone in septic shock. *Crit Care Med* 18:47-51, 1990.

Haft JI: Cardiovascular injury induced by sympathetic catecholamines. *Prog Cardiovasc Dis* 17:73-86, 1974.

Haglund U, Gerdin B: Oxygen-free radicals (OFR) and circulatory shock. *Circ Shock* 34:405-411, 1991.

Hands ME, et al: The in-hospital development of cardiogenic shock after myocardial infarction: Incidence, predictors of occurrence, outcome and prognostic factors. *J Am Coll Cardiol* 14:40-46, 1989.

Hussain SNA, et al: Effects of norepinephrine and fluid administration on the selective blood flow distribution in endotoxic shock. *J Crit Care* 3:32-42, 1988.

Karakusis PH: Considerations in the therapy of septic shock. *Med Clin North Am* 70:933-960, 1986.

Keung ECH, et al: Dobutamine therapy in acute myocardial infarction. *JAMA* 245:144-146, 1981.

Klein LW: Optimal therapy for cardiogenic shock: The emerging role of coronary angioplasty, editorial comment. *J Am Coll Cardiol* 19:654-656, 1992.

Koscove EM, Paradis NA: Successful resuscitation from cardiac arrest using high-dose epinephrine therapy: Report of two cases. *JAMA* 259:3031-3034, 1988.

Lee L, et al: Percutaneous transluminal coronary angioplasty improves survival in acute myocardial infarction complicated by cardiogenic shock. *Circulation* 78:1345-1351, 1988.

Lee L, et al: Multicenter registry of angioplasty therapy of cardiogenic shock: Initial and long-term survival. *J Am Coll Cardiol* 17:599-603, 1991.

Leier CV, Unverferth DV: Drugs five years later: Dobutamine. *Ann Intern Med* 99:490-496, 1983.

Luce JM: Pathogenesis and management of septic shock. *Chest* 91:883-888, 1987.

Mecher CE, et al: Venous hypercarbia associated with severe sepsis and systemic hypoperfusion. *Crit Care Med* 18:585-589, 1990.

Members of the American College of Chest Physicians/Society of Critical Care Medicine Consensus Conference Committee: American College of Chest Physicians/Society of Critical Care Medicine Consensus Conference: Definitions for sepsis and organ failure and guidelines for the use of innovative therapies in sepsis. *Crit Care Med* 20:864-874, 1992.

Moosvi AR, et al: Early revascularization improves survival in cardiogenic shock complicating acute myocardial infarction. *J Am Coll Cardiol* 19:907-914, 1992.

Mueller HS: Inotropic agents in treatment of cardiogenic shock. *World J Surg* 9:3-10, 1985.

Ohlsson K, et al: Interleukin-1 receptor antagonist reduces mortality from endotoxin shock. *Nature* 348:550-552, 1990.

Ognibene FP, et al: Depressed left ventricular performance: Response to volume infusion in patients with sepsis and septic shock. *Chest* 93:903-915, 1988.

Otto CW: Cardiovascular pharmacology II: Use of catecholamines, pressor agents, digitalis, and corticosteroids in CPR and emergency cardiac care. *Circulation* 74(suppl IV):IV-80-IV-85, 1986.

Parrillo JE, et al: Septic shock in humans: Advances in the understanding of pathogenesis, cardiovascular dysfunction, and therapy. *Ann Intern Med* 113:227-242, 1990.

Perlino CA, Rimland D: Alcoholism, leukopenia, and pneumococcal sepsis. *Am Rev Respir* 132:757-760, 1985.

Quinton DN, et al: Comparison of endotracheal and peripheral intravenous adrenaline in cardiac arrest: Is endotracheal route reliable? *Lancet* 1:828-829, 1987.

Schein RMH, et al: Plasma cortisol levels in patients with septic shock. *Crit Care Med* 18:259-263, 1990.

Shoemaker WC, Appel PL: Effects of prostaglandin E_1 in adult respiratory distress syndrome. *Surgery* 99:275-283, 1986.

Shoemaker WC, et al: Comparison of hemodynamic and oxygen transport effects of dopamine and dobutamine in critically ill surgical patients. *Chest* 96:120-126, 1989.

Shoemaker WC, et al: Therapy of shock based on pathophysiology, monitoring, and outcome prediction. *Crit Care Med* 18:S19-S25, 1990.

Slotman GJ, et al: Detrimental effects of high-dose methylprednisolone sodium succinate on serum concentrations of hepatic and renal function indicators in severe sepsis and septic shock. *Crit Care Med* 21:191-195, 1993.

Stevenson LW, Miller LW: Cardiac transplantation as therapy for heart failure. *Curr Probl Cardiol* 16:219-305, 1991.

Van de Werf F: Lessons from the European Cooperative recombinant tissue-type plasminogen activator (rt-PA) versus placebo trial. *J Am Coll Cardiol* 12:14A-19A, 1988.

Veterans Administration Systemic Sepsis Cooperative Study Group: Effect of high-dose glucocorticoid therapy on mortality in patients with clinical signs of systemic sepsis. *N Engl J Med* 317:659-665, 1987.

Vincent J-L, van der Linden P: Septic shock: Particular type of acute circulatory failure. *Crit Care Med* 18(suppl):S70-S74, 1990.

Vincent J-L, et al: Dopamine compared with dobutamine in experimental septic shock: Relevance to fluid administration. *Anesth Analg* 66:565-571, 1987.

Vincent J-L, et al: Dobutamine administration in septic shock: Addition to a standard protocol. *Crit Care Med* 18:689-693, 1990.

Wang P, et al: Measurement of hepatic blood flow following trauma and severe hemorrhage with different methods: Lack of restoration despite adequate crystalloid resuscitation. *Am J Physiol* 262:G92-G98, 1992.

Wee PM, et al: Effect of intravenous infusion of low-dose dopamine on renal function in normal individuals and in patients with renal disease. *Am J Nephrol* 6:42-46, 1986.

Weil MH, et al: Difference in acid-base state between venous and arterial blood during cardiopulmonary resuscitation. *N Engl J Med* 315:153-156, 1986.

Willerson JT, Frazier OH: Reducing mortality in patients with extensive myocardial infarction. *N Engl J Med* 325:1166-1168, 1991.

Ziegler EJ, et al: Treatment of gram-negative bacteremia and shock with human antiserum to a mutant *Escherichia coli*. *N Engl J Med* 307:1225-1230, 1982.

Ziegler EJ, et al: Treatment of gram-negative bacteremia and septic shock with HA-1A human monoclonal antibody against endotoxin: A randomized, double-blind, placebo-controlled trial. *N Engl J Med* 324:429-436, 1991.

Zucker G, et al: Treatment of shock and prevention of ischemic necrosis with levarterenol-phentolamine mixtures. *Circulation* 22:935-937, 1960.

Drugs Used in Miscellaneous Cardiovascular Disorders

30

PATENT DUCTUS ARTERIOSUS

The ductus arteriosus, a fetal blood vessel connecting the pulmonary artery to the descending aorta, diverts blood away from the lungs to the placenta during fetal life. The ductus begins to constrict within one to two hours after birth and usually closes anatomically within one to several weeks in full-term neonates. Persistent patency of the ductus arteriosus is especially common in infants whose mothers had rubella infection during their first trimester of pregnancy, in premature infants, in infants with lung disease, and in infants born at high altitude. Delay in closure beyond infancy is observed in 5% to 6% of children with congenital heart defects (Liberthson and Waldman, 1991) and is more common in females than in males.

In patients with normal pulmonary arteriolar resistance, blood flows from the aorta to the pulmonary circulation (left to right). Patients with small ductus are asymptomatic. In those with large ductus, excessive pulmonary blood flow causes increased pulmonary artery pressure and left atrial return, left ventricular hypertrophy, and enlargement of the aorta proximal to the ductus. The right atrium and ventricle are normal in size. Virtually all patients with large ductus develop heart failure. In some of these patients, pulmonary vascular resistance may be higher than systemic resistance and blood flow may be reversed to a right-to-left shunting causing cyanosis in the lower extremities and right-sided heart failure. Regardless of the ductus size, infective endocarditis with possible embolization may occur.

Surgical ligation is the most common method of closing a large patent ductus. Emergency surgery is indicated for infants with heart failure; early surgical closure also reduces necrotizing enterocolitis in infants of very low birth weight who require supplemental oxygen (Cassady et al, 1989). Elective ligation is indicated when the diagnosis is confirmed and before symptoms develop. In adults with aneurysmal dilation or calcification of the ductus, precautions to guard against possible dissection and rupture during surgery are essential.

Since ductal patency during fetal life appears to be mediated through prostaglandins of the E type, drugs that inhibit prostaglandin synthesis (eg, indomethacin [Indocin IV]) have been successfully employed as an alternative to surgery in many premature neonates. However, indomethacin is not effective in stimulating closure of the ductus arteriosus in infants more than 4 weeks old, children, or adults.

INDOMETHACIN SODIUM TRIHYDRATE

[Indocin IV]

ACTIONS. This nonsteroidal anti-inflammatory agent is a potent nonselective inhibitor of prostaglandin synthesis. It acts by interfering with formation of endoperoxides, the precursors of all prostaglandins. Its ability to constrict the patent ductus arteriosus in premature infants is believed to be due to this action. Indomethacin may affect the tone of the ductus arteriosus more than that of other blood vessels (Friedman et al, 1978).

USES. Indomethacin is used as a pharmacologic alternative to surgery in premature infants with symptomatic patent ductus arteriosus and respiratory distress syndrome. It also may reduce the incidence of neonatal intraventricular hemorrhage (Bandstra et al, 1988; Ment et al, 1985).

The overall ability of indomethacin to produce constriction depends on the size and number of doses administered and the timing of treatment. Indomethacin appears to be effective when given to infants up to 4 weeks of age of all birth weights and gestational ages within the premature range. In infants with a birth weight <1,000 g, it may be preferable to initiate treatment with indomethacin on confirmation of diagnosis before the infant becomes symptomatic (Mahony et al, 1982; Barst and Gersony, 1989).

ADVERSE REACTIONS, PRECAUTIONS, AND INTERACTIONS. Indomethacin may cause a transient, dose-related decrease in renal function. Although sodium excretion is reduced, severe dilutional hyponatremia has been reported. Indomethacin should not be used in infants with renal impairment. If digoxin is given concomitantly, its dose should be reduced and serum glycoside levels should be monitored because indomethacin reduces digoxin clearance. A similar interaction with aminoglycoside antibiotics suggests that the dosage of these drugs should be reduced as well (Zarfin et al, 1985).

Indomethacin may increase serum concentrations of unconjugated bilirubin by displacing bilirubin from albumin. It interferes with platelet function and has caused gastrointestinal bleeding. Indomethacin may impair the mesenteric circulation and contribute to the development of necrotizing enterocolitis, although this complication also occurs in premature infants who have not received the drug. Indomethacin does not appear to increase the incidence of retinopathy of prematurity or intracranial hemorrhage.

PHARMACOKINETICS. When indomethacin was given intravenously to premature infants with symptomatic patent ductus arteriosus, a twentyfold variation in plasma concentrations was observed. The median half-life was 32 hours, and the clearance was 7 ml/kg/hr. Unsuccessful treatment was associated with lower plasma concentration (<250 ng/ml at 24 hours), shorter half-life, and more rapid clearance (Brash et al, 1981). However, results of other studies indicated that there was no relationship between serum levels and therapeutic effects (Gersony et al, 1983).

DOSAGE AND PREPARATIONS. Indomethacin should be administered in a neonatal intensive care unit. The intravenous route is preferred, although the oral and rectal routes also have been used.

Intravenous: The drug is administered slowly (over 15 to 30 minutes) at 12- to 24-hour intervals for three doses unless closure occurs after the first or second dose or adverse effects develop. The following doses have been recommended:

Age	Dose 1	Doses 2 and 3
<48 hours (or <1 kg wt)	0.2 mg/kg	0.1 mg/kg
2 to 7 days	0.2 mg/kg	0.2 mg/kg
>7 days	0.2 mg/kg	0.25 mg/kg

This regimen may be repeated if the ductus reopens 48 hours or more after initial closure. Surgical ligation should be considered if the ductus does not close after the first course of treatment or if the second course fails and the infant still has cardiorespiratory symptoms.

Indocin IV (Merck). Each vial contains powder (sterile, lyophilized) equivalent to 1 mg of indomethacin.

DUCTAL-DEPENDENT CONGENITAL HEART DISEASE

In infants with certain congenital heart disorders, a patent ductus is needed to provide adequate pulmonary blood flow, prevent systemic hypoperfusion, or, in selected cases, improve pulmonary-systemic arterial mixing prior to surgery. These anomalies include congenital heart disease with (1) decreased pulmonary blood flow due to severe obstruction to right ventricular inflow or outflow (pulmonary atresia or stenosis, tetralogy of Fallot, tricuspid atresia); (2) decreased systemic blood flow due to aortic valve or aortic arch defects (interruption of the aortic arch, coarctation of the aorta, aortic atresia, hypoplastic left heart syndrome); or (3) normal or increased pulmonary blood flow (transposition of the great arteries).

Prostaglandins of the E series dilate isolated rings of the ductus arteriosus and probably play a major role in maintaining ductal patency in the fetus. Persistently elevated serum concentrations of these substances may prevent normal constriction of the ductus in the neonate (Heymann, 1981; Heymann and Rudolph, 1981; Olley and Coceani, 1981). Administration of alprostadil [Prostin VR Pediatric] to maintain ductal patency has been very useful in infants with ductal-dependent congenital heart diseases. Infants can be stabilized prior to undergoing palliative closed-heart procedures or complete open-heart repair.

ALPROSTADIL (Prostaglandin E_1)

[Prostin VR Pediatric]

ACTIONS. Alprostadil is one of a family of naturally occurring compounds derived from arachidonic acid. It has a variety of pharmacologic actions; the most important are vasodilation, inhibition of platelet aggregation, and stimulation of intestinal and uterine smooth muscle. Alprostadil is a potent relaxant of the smooth muscle of the ductus arteriosus and preserves ductal patency in neonates when it is infused before anatomical closure has occurred. It also may dilate the pulmonary vascular bed.

USES. Alprostadil is used in neonates with ductal-dependent congenital heart disorders to maintain the patency of the ductus arteriosus until surgery can be performed. Its efficacy in these disorders is demonstrated by an increase in systemic arterial oxygen tension (PaO_2). In a large-scale collaborative study, the mean PaO_2 of infants increased from 27.5 to 38.9 mm Hg during infusion. Beneficial effects usually were observed within 15 minutes. The greatest clinical improvement occurred in infants less than 4 days old and in those with a low PaO_2 initially (Freed et al, 1981).

Infants with transposition of the great arteries may be managed initially by emergency cardiac catheterization and balloon atrial septostomy to improve mixing of the pulmonary and systemic circulations. At most pediatric cardiac centers, procedures to correct arterial transposition are done within several days after diagnosis; in the majority of cases, surgery is performed within one week. Alprostadil may be useful (1) prior to catheterization and septostomy in critically hypoxemic infants, and (2) as a temporary measure when hypoxemia and acidosis persist despite adequate septostomy. The improvement in systemic oxygen saturation in these infants may be due to both ductal enlargement and decreased pulmonary vascular resistance (Benson et al, 1979). Infants with transposition of the great arteries had a lower PaO_2 before and during infusion than those with other cyanotic congenital heart defects (mean, 22.9 mm Hg before and 31.8 mm Hg during infusion), but the overall increase in oxygenation was similar (Freed et al, 1981).

Alprostadil may improve systemic perfusion in infants with hypoplastic left heart syndrome or aortic arch abnormalities who depend on a patent ductus to supply blood to the aorta. Cyanosis usually is not a prominent feature in these disorders; therefore, measurement of PaO_2 is not useful to determine whether alprostadil has dilated the ductus. Improvement is reflected by the return of palpable femoral pulses, amelioration of metabolic acidosis, increase in urinary output, and decrease in the pressure difference between the main pulmonary artery and the descending aorta (in those with aortic interruption) or between the ascending and descending aorta (in those with coarctation). Clinical improvement was reported in approximately 80% of infants with aortic arch abnormalities during infusion of alprostadil. The maximal response occurred later than in cyanotic infants (up to four hours in those with aortic interruption and up to 11 hours in those with coarctation). The ductus appeared to be closed irreversibly in some unresponsive patients (Freed et al, 1981). The temporary use of alprostadil also has been advocated for infants with critical aortic stenosis to supplement systemic cardiac output.

ADVERSE REACTIONS AND PRECAUTIONS. Apnea has occurred in 10% to 12% of patients. It usually appears during the first hour of infusion and is most common with larger doses and in infants weighing less than 2 kg at birth (Lewis et al, 1981). Bradypnea, wheezing, hypercapnia, respiratory depression, respiratory distress, and tachypnea have been reported rarely. Respiratory status should be monitored throughout treatment, and ventilatory assistance should be available. A distinction between respiratory distress syndrome (RDS) and cyanotic heart disease is essential because alprostadil should not be used in infants with RDS. If full diagnostic facilities are not immediately available, cyanosis and restricted pulmonary blood flow apparent on x-ray are appropriate indicators of congenital heart defects.

Flushing has been reported in about 10% of patients, bradycardia in 7%, hypotension in 4%, and tachycardia in 3%. Edema, conduction disturbances, arrhythmias, cardiac arrest, and heart failure have occurred rarely. Prolonged infusion may increase the fragility of the ductal and juxtaductal structures and may increase the risk of spontaneous or surgically induced rupture of the ductus (Cole et al, 1981).

Seizures have occurred in approximately 4% of patients; hyperpyrexia in 14%; and cerebral bleeding, hyperextension of the neck, hyperirritability, hypothermia, jitteriness, lethargy, or stiffness in less than 1%.

Diarrhea has occurred in 2% of patients and gastric regurgitation and hyperbilirubinemia in less than 1%. Gastric outlet obstruction secondary to antral hyperplasia has been observed.

Infusion of alprostadil rarely has been associated with disseminated intravascular coagulation, anemia, thrombocytopenia, and bleeding. This agent should be used cautiously in infants with bleeding tendencies because it inhibits platelet aggregation.

Anuria and hematuria have been reported rarely.

Long-term use of prostaglandins may cause symmetrical cortical hyperostosis of long bones observable on x-ray. Bone abnormalities generally become apparent within three weeks after the start of therapy and regress within a few weeks or months after treatment is discontinued. Peripheral edema also has been observed with long-term use.

Hypokalemia, hyperkalemia, and hypoglycemia have been reported rarely.

PHARMACOKINETICS. Alprostadil is metabolized rapidly and must be infused continuously. Approximately 80% of circulating alprostadil is metabolized in one pass through the lungs, and the metabolites are excreted by the kidney. Excretion is complete within 24 hours. No unchanged alprostadil has been found in the urine.

MONITORING. In all neonates, arterial pressure should be monitored intermittently by umbilical artery catheter, auscultation, or with a Doppler transducer. If arterial pressure falls significantly, the rate of infusion should be decreased immediately. In infants with restricted pulmonary blood flow, the efficacy of alprostadil is measured by monitoring improvement in blood oxygenation. In infants with restricted systemic blood flow, efficacy is evaluated by monitoring improvement of systemic blood pressure and blood pH.

DOSAGE AND PREPARATIONS. To prepare the infusion solution, 1 ml (500 mcg) should be diluted with sodium chloride or dextrose injection to a volume appropriate for the pump delivery system available. A fresh solution should be prepared every 24 hours.

Intravenous, Intra-arterial: *Infants,* continuous intravenous infusion into a large vein is preferred, but use of a peripheral vein is acceptable. Intra-arterial (umbilical artery) infusion may be considered if venous access is not possible. Prolonged infusion should be avoided; the lowest dose should be infused for the shortest time that will produce the desired effects. The initial infusion rate is 0.05 to 0.1 mcg/kg/min. If the initial dose is inadequate, the amount may be increased gradually to 0.2 mcg/kg/min. After a therapeutic response is obtained, the rate should be reduced to the lowest amount that maintains the response. This may be accomplished by reducing the dosage from 0.1 to 0.05 to 0.025 to 0.01 mcg/kg/min.

The intravenous preparation has been given orally to some infants who are not candidates for surgery and who require prolonged (one to two months) treatment.

Prostin VR Pediatric (Upjohn). Solution (sterile) 500 mcg/ml in dehydrated alcohol in 1 ml containers. The ampuls should be stored in the refrigerator at 2° to 8° C.

PULMONARY HYPERTENSIVE DISORDERS

Primary Pulmonary Hypertension

Primary pulmonary hypertension is an uncommon disorder that is observed predominantly during the third through the fifth decade of life and is more prevalent in women than in men. It is characterized by increased pulmonary artery pressure and pulmonary vascular resistance. Endothelial cell dysfunction and injury contribute to disease progression (Loscalzo, 1992). Inability of the endothelial cells to function leads to decreased production of prostacyclin and endothelium-derived relaxing factor (nitric oxide) and increased release of endothelin, processes that promote pulmonary vasoconstriction and platelet adhesion and activation. The increased afterload to the right ventricle impairs right heart function.

Primary pulmonary hypertension is usually minimally symptomatic until a significant portion of the pulmonary vascular bed is compromised. The impairment of right heart function and reduced cardiac output then cause dyspnea, fatigue, chest pain, and syncope (D'Alonzo et al, 1991). Raynaud's phenomenon is present in about 10% of patients, and the antinuclear antibody test may be positive in some individuals (Rich et al, 1987). Death, which often is sudden, usually occurs about three years after diagnosis; the major cause is right heart failure.

The treatment of primary pulmonary hypertension is directed toward relieving symptoms and preventing progression of the disease (Brown, 1991; Palevsky and Fishman, 1991; Rubin, 1992). There is no definitive cure. Drugs are effective in 30% of patients. For those who are unresponsive to medication, lung transplantation is an option.

OXYGEN SUPPLEMENTATION. Oxygen supplementation to eliminate hypoxic vasoconstriction and secondary erythropoiesis is indicated in any patient who experiences arterial oxygen desaturation either at rest or with physical activity (Palevsky and Fishman, 1991; Rubin, 1992).

DIURETICS. Diuretics alleviate systemic venous congestion, hepatic distention, and peripheral edema in patients with right heart failure. They also reduce pulmonary capillary congestion and extravascular lung fluid and relieve dyspnea and orthopnea. Low doses of furosemide [Lasix] (20 to 40 mg/day) can be given initially, with the amount increased as required (Rubin, 1992). For patients refractory to doses of furosemide that exceed 120 mg/day, metolazone [Diulo, Zaroxolyn] (initially, 2.5 to 5 mg every other day) can be added to the regimen. The serum potassium and magnesium levels should be closely monitored; potassium-sparing diuretics may be given adjunctively.

DIGITALIS. The use of digitalis in patients with right ventricular dysfunction and failure is controversial because digitalis may increase pulmonary vascular resistance, leading to elevation of right ventricular afterload. This adverse effect and the high incidence of digitalis toxicity in patients with severe hypoxemia and lung disease have limited the use of this drug.

VASODILATOR THERAPY. Pulmonary vasoconstriction is an important component of primary pulmonary hypertension in some patients. Vasodilator therapy should reduce pulmonary vascular resistance. Ideally, cardiac output would be increased and pulmonary arterial pressure would be decreased with no change in the systemic arterial blood pressure and oxygenation. However, in practice, the most frequent response after use of vasodilators has been an increase in cardiac output, which often improves exercise tolerance and enhances a sense of well-being but does not produce an appreciable, sustained change in pulmonary arterial pressure or arterial oxygen tension.

A wide variety of oral vasodilators (calcium channel blocking agents, alpha-adrenergic antagonists, beta-adrenergic agonists, angiotensin-converting enzyme (ACE) inhibitors, S_2-serotonergic receptor antagonists, nitrates, and direct-acting vasodilators) have been tested in patients with primary pulmonary hypertension. Only a few have been efficacious in prolonging life expectancy and/or relieving symptoms.

The calcium channel blocking agents, nifedipine [Adalat, Procardia] and diltiazem [Cardizem], appear to be the most effective oral vasodilators for long-term treatment of primary pulmonary hypertension (Rich and Brundage, 1987; Rubin, 1992). Pronounced reductions in pulmonary artery pressure (48%) and pulmonary vascular resistance (60%) were observed in 8 of 13 patients who received much larger than conventional oral doses (nifedipine: up to 240 mg daily; diltiazem: up to 720 mg daily). These effects were sustained after one year in at least five patients and were associated with regression of right ventricular hypertrophy (Rich and Brundage, 1987). In another prospective long-term study, 16 of 17 patients who responded to high-dose therapy with calcium channel blockers were alive after five years compared with 26 of 47 patients who did not respond (Rich et al, 1992). The survival rates of patients in the NIH Primary Pulmonary Hypertension Registry cohort were 68%, 47%, and 38% at one, three, and five years, respectively; in comparison, 94% of patients who responded to high-dose calcium channel blocker therapy were alive at five years. However, only 25% of patients tolerated the high-dose regimen (Rich et al, 1992).

Intravenous epoprostenol (prostacyclin) [Flolan] decreases pulmonary vascular resistance, produces a sustained increase in pulmonary artery oxygen saturation, and increases cardiac output. In a randomized study of 24 patients with primary pulmonary hypertension who did not respond to conventional oral vasodilator therapy, long-term continuous (18 months) administration of epoprostenol by portable infusion pump improved signs and symptoms in 10 of 11 patients (Rubin et al, 1990). Flushing and headache were minor side effects; reversible pulmonary edema occurred in one of these patients. Tolerance may necessitate periodic increases in dose, but the beneficial effect is sustained. Intravenous infusion of iloprost, a stable prostaglandin analogue, produced similar results (Scott et al, 1990). Continuous intravenous infusion of epoprostenol or iloprost in patients with severe primary pulmonary hypertension refractory to oral vasodilator therapy may be useful as a second-line treatment or until lung transplantation can be performed.

Adenosine [Adenocard] is a potent pulmonary vasodilator. In a few patients with primary pulmonary hypertension, doses of adenosine 0.05 to 0.5 mg/kg/min reduced pulmonary artery pressure (8%) and vascular resistance (>35%) without producing systemic side effects (Morgan et al, 1991; Schrader et al, 1992). Cardiac output also was increased by 50%. Adenosine further decreased pulmonary artery pressure and vascular resistance in a small number of patients with primary pulmonary hypertension who had responded to high-dose calcium channel blockers (Inbar et al, 1993).

Inhaled nitric oxide as a substitute for endogenous endothelium-derived relaxing factor also provided potent, selective pulmonary vasodilation as well as antiplatelet activity in patients with primary pulmonary hypertension (Pepke-Zaba et al, 1991).

Since a high proportion of patients with primary pulmonary hypertension do not respond to oral vasodilator therapy, use of short-acting agents like epoprostenol, iloprost, nitric oxide, and adenosine may be feasible and safe for acute screening for pulmonary vasodilatory reserve without subjecting patients to the potential adverse effects associated with prolonged oral vasodilator therapy (Palevsky and Fishman, 1991).

Adverse Reactions and Precautions: Vasodilators may cause adverse hemodynamic effects in patients with advanced pulmonary hypertension whose pulmonary vascular bed is unresponsive. In these individuals, the drug may decrease systemic vascular resistance significantly. Since cardiac output is relatively fixed by the high pulmonary vascular resistance, the fall in systemic resistance may cause profound hypotension. The negative inotropic effects of the calcium channel blockers may become manifest if pulmonary artery pressure is not reduced. Careful monitoring of the hemodynamic effects of any vasodilator is necessary.

Other potential complications of vasodilator drugs are exacerbation of pulmonary hypertension, worsening of right ventricular function, systemic hypoxemia, tachycardia, arrhythmias, anginal pain, heart failure, and cardiac arrest. Vasodilators are particularly hazardous in patients with pulmonary veno-occlusive disease because of the risk of an increase in cardiac output and subsequent elevation of pulmonary capillary wedge pressure. Deaths have occurred when these patients were treated with nifedipine (Rich et al, 1986); however, some patients have been treated successfully (Palevsky and Fishman, 1990).

For other adverse effects, see index entry on the individual drugs.

ANTICOAGULANT THERAPY. As a consequence of endothelial injury and abnormal blood flow, thrombosis in the pulmonary microvasculature has been observed in all forms of primary pulmonary hypertension. The thrombi contribute to the deteriorating course observed in most patients with primary pulmonary hypertension by further decreasing the lumen of the pulmonary blood vessels and causing progressive increases in pulmonary vascular resistance. Peripheral venous thrombosis and pulmonary embolism also can occur as consequences of venous stasis and decreased physical activity in patients with right heart failure. It is not unusual to find fresh intrapulmonary clots at postmortem examination in these individuals.

Results of a retrospective study in a large series of patients with primary pulmonary hypertension showed that anticoagulant therapy appeared to have a beneficial effect on overall survival (Fuster et al, 1984). Treatment with warfarin mildly enhanced survival of those who had not responded to high-dose calcium channel blocking agents (Rich et al, 1992). The one-, three-, and five-year survival rates for this group of patients were 91%, 62%, and 47%; this compared with 52%, 31%, and 31%, respectively, in patients who were not treated with anticoagulants and had not responded to calcium channel blockers.

Warfarin can be administered in amounts sufficient to prolong the prothrombin time to approximately 1.3 to 1.5 times control. Similar doses of subcutaneous heparin can be used in patients at greater risk of hemorrhagic events or who cannot tolerate warfarin. Aspirin and other antiplatelet agents may be useful.

SURGICAL INTERVENTION. Lung transplantation can improve survival and function in patients with end-stage primary pulmonary hypertension. A dramatic decrease in pulmonary artery pressure and resistance associated with an increase in cardiac output occurs within a few hours following surgery. Initially, surgical intervention utilized combined heart-lung transplantation. According to the Registry of the International Society for Heart Transplantation, the one-year survival rate was >60% and the two-year rate was 55% for these patients (Kriett and Kaye, 1990). Recently, single- or double-lung transplantation has been shown to be superior to combined heart-lung transplantation in patients with primary pulmonary hypertension, especially for those who have preserved right ventricular function (Trulock et al, 1991). The procedure is technically less complicated and does not require the use of extracorporeal bypass. Although early mortality is lower, the incidence of obliterative bronchiolitis, a major long-term complication of surgical intervention, is not yet known.

Surgical management can be considered as another option for patients with primary pulmonary hypertension who have not responded to most medical interventions (Palevsky and Fishman, 1991). However, the availability of lungs for transplantation is still limited and there is risk of rejection, infection, and significant perioperative morbidity and mortality.

Secondary Pulmonary Hypertension

Most forms of pulmonary hypertension are secondary to cardiac or lung disorders that increase pulmonary blood flow, pulmonary venous pressure, or pulmonary vascular resistance (Kloner, 1991). Specific disorders that cause secondary pulmonary hypertension include congenital heart diseases, mitral stenosis, collagen-vascular diseases, chronic pulmonary thromboembolism, and chronic obstructive pulmonary disease (COPD). Treatment of secondary pulmonary hypertension is directed toward correction of the underlying cause, if possible.

CONGENITAL HEART DISEASE. The left-to-right shunting of blood increases the pulmonary flow in congenital heart diseases (eg, ventricular septal defect, patent ductus arteriosus, atrial septal defect), and pulmonary hypertension ensues. Prolonged hypertension induces anatomic changes, including medial hypertrophy and intimal cellular proliferation, thereby decreasing the pulmonary arteriolar cross sectional area. Surgical correction of the left-to-right shunt during the initial reversible phase reduces the pulmonary artery pressure. If pulmonary hypertension is not lowered, damage to the pulmonary vascular bed (ie, necrotizing arteritis, plexiform lesions) continues and eventually the shunt is converted to right to left (Eisenmenger's syndrome).

When pulmonary vascular resistance is equal to systemic resistance and the anatomic changes in the vasculature are severe, surgical correction of the intracardiac shunt will not relieve the pulmonary hypertension but will produce severe right ventricular failure; the risk of death is very high. Salt restriction, diuretics, phlebotomy, and chronic oxygen therapy are used to treat these patients. The use of vasodilators is controversial. The overall prognosis for patients with Eisenmenger's syndrome is poor and most do not survive past the fourth decade. Death may be sudden as a result of severe heart failure, ventricular arrhythmias, pulmonary infection, thrombosis, brain abscess, endocarditis, or severe hemoptysis. These patients are candidates for lung transplantation.

MITRAL STENOSIS. Pulmonary hypertension in patients with mitral stenosis is due to impaired pulmonary venous drainage secondary to high left atrial pressure; vasoconstriction with anatomic changes in the vasculature eventually develops. This condition can be treated with mitral valve surgery. The pulmonary artery pressure and resistance fall within the first postoperative week, and many of the anatomic changes (medial hypertrophy, distension of capillaries and lymphatics, swelling of endothelial cells, intimal proliferation) reverse over time.

COLLAGEN-VASCULAR DISEASES. Several collagen-vascular diseases are associated with obliteration of the pulmonary vasculature and lead to pulmonary hypertension. The increase in pulmonary pressure is especially severe in patients with the CREST variant of scleroderma (calcinosis, Raynaud's phenomenon, esophagitis, sclerodactyly, and telangiectasis) and in those with systemic lupus and mixed connective tissue disease. Their response to vasodilators (captopril [Capoten], nifedipine, verapamil [Calan, Isoptin, Verelan], diltiazem, diazoxide [Proglycem], nitroglycerin, hydralazine [Apresoline], and phentolamine [Regitine]) is variable, and long-term effectiveness has not been demonstrated (Brown, 1991).

CHRONIC OBSTRUCTIVE PULMONARY DISEASE (COPD). The cross-sectional area of the pulmonary vascular bed is greatly reduced in patients with COPD due to chronic bronchitis and emphysema (Kloner, 1991). Endothelium-dependent pulmonary artery vasodilation also is compromised (Dinh-Xuan et al, 1991). Most patients with COPD develop cor pulmonale, a heart disease characterized by right ventricular hypertrophy or right heart failure.

COPD is treated with bronchodilators, antibiotics for respiratory infections, supplemental oxygen, postural drainage and chest physical therapy, and smoking cessation. Administration of supplemental oxygen increases the survival rate of patients with cor pulmonale due to COPD. A number of vasodilators have been tried in patients with COPD and/or cor pulmonale, including calcium channel blockers (nifedipine, diltiazem, nitrendipine, verapamil, felodipine [Plendil]), ACE inhibitors (captopril, enalapril [Vasotec]), nitrates (nitroglycerin, isosorbide dinitrate, nitroprusside), hydralazine, phentolamine, diazoxide, and prazosin [Minipress], with varying degrees of success. In general, vasodilators should be used for patients with cor pulmonale only after conventional therapy with bronchodilators and oxygen has been tried. Careful monitoring and blood-gas analysis are appropriate during initial therapy. Diuretics reduce blood volume and improve symptoms of edema in cor pulmonale. The use of digitalis in these patients remains controversial.

HIGH ALTITUDE PULMONARY EDEMA. Hypoxic pulmonary hypertension appears to play a role in the pathogenesis of high-altitude pulmonary edema. Oxygen therapy or transfer of the patient to sea level cures acute cases and ameliorates chronic cases. Nifedipine is useful for the emergency treatment of this life-threatening condition; its effect has been attributed to a reduction in pulmonary artery pressure (Oelz et al, 1989).

PERSISTENT PULMONARY HYPERTENSION OF THE NEWBORN (PPHN, Persistent Fetal Circulation). This syndrome occurs most commonly in full-term or postmature neonates without demonstrable cardiac or pulmonary parenchymal disease. It is characterized by elevated pulmonary vascular resistance and right-to-left shunting of unoxygenated blood through persisting fetal channels (ductus arteriosus and foramen ovale). Affected infants have marked cyanosis, tachypnea, and acidosis. Primary PPHN is believed to be associated with perinatal hypoxemia. Secondary PPHN has been associated with a variety of disorders that predispose to pulmonary vasoconstriction, including sepsis, meconium aspiration, primary pulmonary hypoplasia, and diaphragmatic hernia (Fox and Duara, 1983; Gersony, 1984; Heymann and Hoffman, 1984; Tiefenbrunn and Riemenschneider, 1986).

The goal in the treatment of PPHN is to reduce shunting by decreasing the ratio of pulmonary arterial to systemic pressure. To this end, oxygen, high-frequency mechanical hyperventilation combined with alkalization to produce a marked respiratory and/or metabolic alkalosis, and, in some cases, a vasodilator (usually tolazoline [Priscoline], nitroprusside, epoprostenol, or alprostadil) are employed to reduce pulmonary vascular resistance. Systemic blood pressure is maintained by use of volume expanders and, if necessary, a pressor drug. Epinephrine and dopamine [Intropin] improve cardiac function; the latter is usually the preferred pressor drug. Inhaled nitric oxide also has been beneficial (Kinsella et al, 1992;

Roberts et al, 1992). Metabolic abnormalities should be corrected.

TOLAZOLINE HYDROCHLORIDE
[Priscoline]

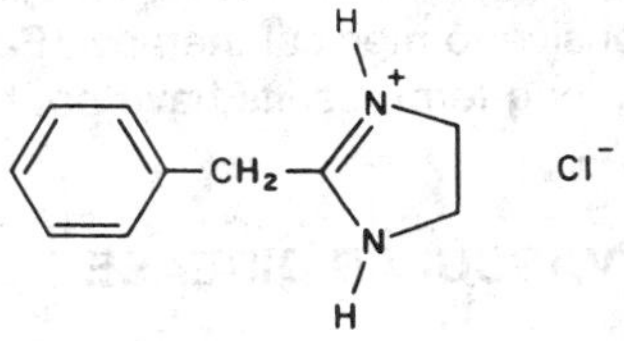

ACTIONS AND USES. Tolazoline is a direct vasodilator with transient alpha blocking actions. It also possesses histamine-like, sympathomimetic, and cholinergic properties. The effect of tolazoline on the pulmonary vasculature has been attributed to its action on histamine receptors, but there is no conclusive evidence that it selectively dilates pulmonary, as opposed to systemic, vessels. Tolazoline also increases cardiac output.

Tolazoline is occasionally used to treat persistent pulmonary hypertension of the newborn when oxygen and mechanical hyperventilation do not relieve hypoxemia or when excessive ventilator settings are required. It initially increases arterial oxygen tension in some infants but does not appear to affect survival (Drummond and Lock, 1984). Published studies have included both full-term and premature infants with PPHN of various etiologies, which may explain the variable degrees of responsiveness to tolazoline (Fox and Duara, 1983).

ADVERSE REACTIONS AND PRECAUTIONS. Adverse effects are common in neonates treated with tolazoline. Hypotension is the most frequent untoward effect, and high concentrations of dopamine and large quantities of colloid infusion may be required to counteract this effect. Oliguria develops in some infants. Thrombocytopenia is relatively common. Other adverse effects include tachycardia, hypochloremic alkalosis, gastrointestinal distension and hemorrhage, and pulmonary hemorrhage. Fatalities have been associated with gastrointestinal, pulmonary, and/or intracranial hemorrhage (Stevenson et al, 1979).

PHARMACOKINETICS. The half-life of tolazoline in neonates ranges from 3 to 10 hours and is longest in infants with poor hemodynamic status.

DOSAGE AND PREPARATIONS.

Intravenous: *Neonates,* initially, 1 to 2 mg/kg via scalp vein, followed by infusion of 1 to 2 mg/kg/hr. If the drug is effective, a response will usually occur within 30 minutes after the initial dose. There is little experience with infusions lasting longer than 36 to 48 hours.

Priscoline (CIBA). Solution 25 mg/ml in 4 ml containers.

HYPERTROPHIC CARDIOMYOPATHY

Hypertrophic cardiomyopathy (idiopathic hypertrophic subaortic stenosis) is a primary myocardial disease that is familial in approximately 60% of cases. This disorder of diastolic function is characterized by myocardial hypertrophy and extensive myofibrillar disarray accompanied by abnormalities of the small intramural coronary arteries (Maron et al, 1987). The increase in myocardial mass is commonly associated with disproportionate involvement of the interventricular septum. Ventricular systolic volume is reduced, contraction is powerful, and ventricular diastolic compliance is markedly impaired. Hemodynamic abnormalities and symptoms have been attributed to dynamic obstruction of left ventricular outflow, impaired diastolic filling, or both. Patients with hypertrophic cardiomyopathy usually develop symptoms during adolescence or middle age, although the disease also has occurred in elderly patients, often in association with hypertension and heavy calcification of the mitral annulus (Lewis and Maron, 1989).

Most adults with hypertrophic cardiomyopathy are asymptomatic or have only mild symptoms that progress slowly if at all. However, the condition of those who are severely affected is prone to deteriorate progressively. Dyspnea, angina, palpitations, and syncope are the most common symptoms. Complications that hasten deterioration are atrial fibrillation, infective endocarditis, mitral regurgitation, left ventricular failure, and myocardial ischemia. The annual mortality rate is 2.5% to 4% and, in many of these patients, death is sudden. The risk factors for sudden death include a family history of sudden death, a young age at diagnosis, syncope, severe symptoms, and nonsustained ventricular tachycardia. The specific cause of sudden death often is not clear, and several mechanisms probably are involved. Ventricular arrhythmias are believed to be the most common cause (Abelmann and Lorell, 1989; Maron et al, 1987); other possible etiologies include supraventricular arrhythmias, complete heart block, asystole, and myocardial infarction.

DRUG THERAPY. Drugs available for the treatment of hypertrophic cardiomyopathy include the beta-adrenergic and calcium channel blocking agents and the antiarrhythmic agents, disopyramide [Norpace] and amiodarone [Cordarone].

The most commonly prescribed beta-adrenergic blocking drug is propranolol [Inderal] (120 to 320 mg daily), which relieves angina, dyspnea, palpitations, and syncope in most patients with hypertrophic cardiomyopathy. It is more effective in relieving symptoms during exercise than at rest. Propranolol reduces the incidence of atrial tachyarrhythmias (McKenna et al, 1980) but may not prevent life-threatening ventricular arrhythmias, which should be managed with additional antiarrhythmic drugs (McKenna et al, 1980).

Other beta-blocking drugs can be effective with the possible exception of those with intrinsic sympathomimetic activity. However, nonselective beta blockers are preferable to cardioselective agents, because the unmasking of peripheral vasoconstrictor inputs can increase ventricular volume (Goodwin, 1988). In addition to symptomatic relief, a rationale for use of beta blockers is to reduce the risk of sudden death. The cardioprotective effect of these drugs in the postinfarct patient is well established, but it is not known whether the risk of sudden death also is reduced in patients with hypertrophic cardiomyopathy (Abelmann and Lorell, 1989).

The calcium channel blocking agent, verapamil, is frequently useful in patients refractory to beta blockers or in those who cannot tolerate beta blockers. Oral verapamil (360 to 480 mg daily) improved exercise tolerance and reduced symptoms in a majority of patients; these improvements were maintained for a long period in more than 50% of patients. However, the electrophysiologic and hemodynamic actions of verapamil may cause particularly severe adverse effects in patients with the obstructive form of hypertrophic cardiomyopathy or with elevated diastolic filling pressure. Adverse reactions include bradycardia, sinus arrest, AV block, myocardial depression, orthostatic hypotension, and pulmonary edema. Fatalities have been reported, usually in patients with symptoms of pulmonary congestion or in those with pulmonary capillary wedge pressures exceeding 22 mm Hg. The concurrent administration of quinidine appeared to contribute to some hypotensive episodes (Epstein and Rosing, 1981; Rosing et al, 1985). There has been limited experience with other calcium antagonists; nifedipine has been shown to improve left ventricular diastolic filling, but its vasodilating effect may cause severe adverse reactions in others.

Antiarrhythmic drugs are often required to control life-threatening arrhythmias in patients with hypertrophic cardiomyopathy (McKenna et al, 1980). Atrial fibrillation is poorly tolerated by these patients. Digitalis may be used to control the ventricular rate if atrial fibrillation develops, but, by increasing myocardial contractility, it may increase left ventricular outflow pressure gradients. Although amiodarone (100 to 600 mg daily) is highly effective in controlling supraventricular and ventricular arrhythmias associated with hypertrophic cardiomyopathy (McKenna et al, 1984), it did not prevent sudden death despite abolition of ventricular tachycardia in patients refractory to beta-adrenergic and calcium channel blockers (Fananapazir et al, 1991). However, significant improvement in the New York Heart Association functional class and exercise tolerance was observed and the survival rate was 80% two years following treatment with amiodarone. This drug also was efficacious in the treatment of new-onset atrial fibrillation in patients with hypertrophic cardiomyopathy (Counihan and McKenna, 1989). Disopyramide (150 mg four times daily), an antiarrhythmic drug with a potent negative inotropic effect, has reduced resting outflow pressure gradients in patients with hypertrophic cardiomyopathy. It may prove to be a useful alternative to propranolol or verapamil in this disorder (Pollick, 1988; Sherrid et al, 1988).

Diuretics may be required to diminish congestive symptoms, but excessive diuresis should be avoided because it will result in higher left ventricular outflow pressure gradients. Nitrates generally should be avoided because they also may increase outflow gradients.

SURGERY. Myotomy-myectomy reduces left ventricular outflow obstruction and relieves symptoms, but it is usually reserved for symptomatic patients who do not respond to aggressive drug therapy. Mitral valve replacement is indicated for severe regurgitation and cardiac transplantation for intractable heart failure and arrhythmias. It is unclear whether surgery improves the long-term survival rate in these patients (Blanchard and Ross, 1991).

PACEMAKER THERAPY. Dual-chamber pacing from the right ventricle may be an effective alternative to surgery in reducing outflow tract gradients and improving functional capacity in patients unresponsive to medical therapy (Fananapazir et al, 1992); however, long-term results have not been reported.

PERIPHERAL VASCULAR DISEASE

Raynaud's Phenomenon

In Raynaud's phenomenon, vasospastic attacks mainly involve the fingers, although toes are also affected in 40% of patients (Coffman, 1991). Idiopathic or primary Raynaud's phenomenon is most common in females aged 11 to 45 years and is characterized by well-demarcated ischemia on one or all digits (excluding the thumb), resulting in pallor or cyanosis. The pallor phase is due to digital artery vasospasm. In the cyanotic phase, the blood flow is slight and slow. Exposure to cold is the most frequent precipitant; in addition, emotional stress has been reported to produce attacks in 9% to 60% of patients.

The etiology of primary Raynaud's phenomenon remains unclear. Low digital artery pressure, thickened vessel walls, increased blood viscosity, persistent vasoconstriction with endothelial abnormalities, and the release of vasoconstrictor agents from platelets could lead to closure of arteries or arterioles during a normal sympathetic stimulus with or without an increase in extravascular pressure. The excessive sensitivity to cold may be produced by the alpha-adrenergic receptors, but serotonergic receptors and low intravascular pressure may be contributing factors. The endothelium, platelet vasoactive factors, neuropeptides, and beta-adrenergic receptors also may be involved.

Causes of secondary Raynaud's phenomenon include connective tissue diseases (scleroderma, systemic lupus erythematosus), drug therapy (methysergide [Sansert], ergot alkaloids, amphetamines, imipramine [Janimine, Tofranil], bromocriptine [Parlodel], combination of vinblastine and bleomycin), carpal tunnel syndrome, and obstructive arterial diseases (thromboangiitis obliterans, arteriosclerosis obliterans, arterial emboli). These secondary causes usually are associated with reduced blood flow or pressure in the digits as a result of vasoconstriction or obstruction. Constant nerve irritation leading to persistent sympathetic vasoconstriction may be the main cause in the carpal tunnel syndrome.

THERAPY. Conservative measures usually provide relief in most patients with primary or secondary Raynaud's phenomenon. The hands and feet must be kept warm and dry (mittens are better than gloves for the hand). All parts of the body (particularly the head and neck) must be protected from exposure to cold to prevent reflex sympathetic vasoconstriction of the digits. Tobacco smoking should cease because of the indirect vasospastic effect of nicotine. Drugs that induce digital vasoconstriction should be discontinued whenever possible.

Drug therapy should be considered if the vasospastic attacks interfere with ability to work or perform daily activities. Several classes of drugs with vasodilatory action have been used to treat Raynaud's phenomenon; these include calcium channel blocking agents, antiadrenergic drugs, direct-acting vasodilators, ACE inhibitors, beta agonists, prostaglandins, thromboxane synthetase inhibitors, and serotonin antagonists.

Calcium channel blockers inhibit contraction of vascular smooth muscle by preventing calcium transport through the slow channel. Nifedipine, verapamil, and diltiazem have been used to relieve vasospasm in primary and secondary Raynaud's phenomenon. Nifedipine (10 to 30 mg three times a day) is the drug of first choice. When given orally, it has potent vasodilator properties and decreases the frequency and severity of attacks in 50% to 60% of patients. Patients with primary Raynaud's phenomenon may experience the most improvement, and digital ulcers have healed in patients with scleroderma. Other dihydropyridines (eg, felodipine, isradipine [DynaCirc]) are as effective as nifedipine. Diltiazem (30 to 120 mg three times a day) also has been reported to benefit patients with primary or secondary Raynaud's phenomenon in small double-blind, placebo-controlled studies. The effects of verapamil (80 mg four times daily) and nicardipine [Cardene] (30 mg three times a day) on these patients are less definitive. The frequent side effects of calcium channel blocking agents (headache, flushing, dizziness, nausea, and edema) may limit their use in many patients.

Reserpine [Serpasil] and guanethidine [Ismelin] have been used for many years in the treatment of Raynaud's phenomenon. Reserpine (0.125 to 1 mg daily) dilates blood vessels by depleting catecholamine stores in sympathetic nerve terminals, and guanethidine (10 to 50 mg daily) acts by interfering with the release of norepinephrine. Both drugs diminish neurogenic vasoconstriction in Raynaud's phenomenon and other peripheral arterial disorders in which episodes of peripheral ischemia are associated with increased sympathetic activity. Reserpine may produce nasal congestion, bradycardia, orthostatic hypotension, dyspepsia, fluid retention, lethargy, and depression. The side effects of guanethidine include orthostatic hypotension, diarrhea, and impotence.

The alpha-adrenergic blocking agents, phenoxybenzamine [Dibenzyline] and phentolamine [Regitine], act at alpha receptor sites to block the response to sympathetic nerve impulses or circulating catecholamines. Even though alpha receptors are abundant in the blood vessels of the skin and skeletal muscles, alpha blockade only increases blood flow to the skin because blood flow to the skeletal muscles is largely controlled by local mechanisms. Intra-arterial administration of phentolamine (50 to 150 mcg/min) is more effective than direct-acting vasodilators in reversing neurogenic digital vasoconstriction (Coffman and Cohen, 1987). Phenoxybenzamine (20 to 60 mg daily) has been given orally to diminish neurogenic vasoconstriction in primary and secondary Raynaud's phenomenon; however, its usefulness may be limited by side effects. The postsynaptic alpha-blocking drug, prazosin (2 to 8 mg daily) has been helpful in some patients with primary or secondary Raynaud's phenomenon. It is better tolerated than phenoxybenzamine, but refractoriness may develop.

Although nitrates have a more pronounced effect on veins than on arterioles, nitroglycerin ointment may be useful as an adjunct to oral antiadrenergic drugs in patients with Raynaud's phenomenon (Franks, 1982). Use of transdermal nitroglycerin alone does not appear to be of benefit (Sovijärvi et al, 1984).

Severe peripheral ischemia caused by ergot poisoning has been treated effectively by continuous infusion of sodium nitroprusside [Nipride, Nitropress] (Carliner et al, 1974) or nitroglycerin or by oral administration of prazosin or the ACE inhibitor, captopril. Captopril (25 mg three times daily) also has relieved vasospastic phenomena when used to control the severe hypertension associated with scleroderma (Lopez-Ovejero et al, 1979).

Other drugs and procedures are being tried abroad or are under investigation in the United States for treating peripheral vascular disorders. In Raynaud's phenomenon, prolonged symptomatic improvement has been reported after plasma exchange (O'Reilly et al, 1979) or intravenous infusion of alprostadil (Clifford et al, 1980), epoprostenol (prostacyclin) (Belch et al, 1983), and iloprost, a stable prostacyclin analogue (Rademaker et al, 1989). Prostaglandins induce vasodilation and inhibit platelet aggregation. However, in one multicenter study, no long-term benefit of alprostadil over placebo was demonstrated (Mohrland et al, 1985). Thromboxane synthase inhibitors are not effective in Raynaud's phenomenon (Ettinger et al, 1984; Malamet et al, 1985).

Ketanserin, a serotonin (5-HT) antagonist that also possesses alpha-blocking properties, was reported to promote healing of digital ulcers in patients with Raynaud's phenomenon (Roald and Seem, 1984), but it did not significantly improve digital circulation in another group of patients with traumatic vasospastic disease (Larsen et al, 1986). In a large multicenter study, ketanserin reduced the frequency of ischemic episodes in patients with primary or secondary Raynaud's phenomenon but had no significant effect on the severity of attacks (Coffman et al, 1989).

Peripheral Obstructive Vascular Disease

Peripheral obstructive vascular disease in the lower extremities is progressively more common in the elderly; the prevalence is 1.8%, 3.7%, and 5.2% in patients under 60 years, 60 to 70 years, and over 70 years, respectively (McDaniel and Cronenwett, 1989). The presence of atherosclerotic lesions is the main cause of progression of this disorder (Hertzer, 1991; Vogt et al, 1992). Plaques are distributed in a segmental pattern and involve the terminal aorta and its major branches, especially the distal portions of the femoral and popliteal arteries. Lesions also are found in the aortic bifurcation, the common femoral, the common iliac bifurcation, and the popliteal and proximal portions of the tibial vessels.

Many patients with lower extremity occlusive disease experience no symptoms. The absence of popliteal or pedal pulses caused by segmental lesions in the superficial femoral artery or in isolated tibial arteries is often an incidental finding in those who either have developed compensatory collateral circulation or have sedentary life-styles. Intermittent claudication, the initial clinical symptom, is characterized by cramping pain in the lower extremities during walking and is relieved by rest. Arterial narrowing in the aorta-iliac region causes ischemic pain in the buttocks, hips, and thighs, while femoral-popliteal lesions produce pain in the calf. As stenosis extends more proximally, longer segments are affected, perfusion is further compromised, vessels become occluded, and pain occurs at rest. The leg may feel cold to the touch, the posterior tibial and dorsalis pedis pulses are absent, and the skin is often pale or cyanotic. Superficial skin ulcers may occur spontaneously or following trauma. Ultimately, gangrene may develop.

Patients with peripheral obstructive vascular disease also have a high prevalence of coronary artery disease. Those who require peripheral revascularization are at increased risk for cardiac complications, including silent ischemia, myocardial infarction, arrhythmia, and death from coronary artery disease.

THERAPY. Peripheral obstructive vascular disease has long been managed by endarterectomy and peripheral arterial bypass. However, nonsurgical therapy (nonpharmacologic, pharmacologic, and mechanical) also can play a role in the management of peripheral vascular disease.

Nonpharmacologic measures that attenuate ischemia or reduce risk factors responsible for the development or further progression of atherosclerotic lesions include smoking cessation, physical exercise, and reduction of serum lipid concentrations. Smoking is a primary risk factor in occlusive vascular disease because nicotine may accelerate atherosclerosis and precipitate thrombosis. Its cessation may increase the maximum treadmill walking distance and decrease pain at rest in patients with intermittent claudication (Quick and Cotton, 1982; Jonason and Bergstrom, 1987). Daily physical exercise, especially walking, increases the walking distance (on average, three times the original values) in patients with claudication (Hiatt et al, 1990). The exact mechanisms by which walking distance is increased are not clear, but it is thought that exercise confers better coordination among leg muscles or induces some beneficial metabolic changes. Adherence to a diet low in cholesterol and saturated fat plays a role in reducing the rate of progression of atherosclerosis in arteries of the lower extremities.

Drugs used for the treatment of peripheral obstructive vascular disease include antiplatelet agents, thrombolytics, pentoxifylline [Trental], and vasodilators (De Felice et al, 1990).

Antiplatelet therapy improves general prognosis and prevents local progression of peripheral arterial disease (Verhaeghe, 1991). Meta-analysis of 28 small trials involving patients with peripheral vascular disease showed that the effect of antiplatelet agents in reducing the risk of serious vascular events was similar to that in cardiovascular and cerebrovascular diseases (Antiplatelet Trialists' Collaboration, 1988). Low-dose aspirin (325 mg on alternate days) also has reduced the need for peripheral arterial surgery in apparently healthy men in the Physicians' Health Study (Goldhaber et al, 1992).

Several trials have been conducted using ticlopidine [Ticlid] in patients with peripheral vascular disease. A meta-analysis of four randomized, double-blind, placebo-controlled trials indicated that treatment with this agent for 6 to 12 months reduced the incidence of fatal and nonfatal cardiovascular events (Boissel et al, 1989). Similar results were noted in the Swedish Ticlopidine Multicenter Study (STIMS) following use of this antiplatelet drug for five years (Janzon et al, 1990). The mechanism by which ticlopidine inhibits platelet aggregation is unclear. This drug was reported to cause hematologic reactions, including pancytopenia, agranulocytosis, and thrombocytopenia (*Lancet*, 1991).

Thrombolytic therapy using low-dose streptokinase [Kabikinase, Streptase], urokinase [Abbokinase], or alteplase [Activase] was reported to be effective in establishing revascularization in recent arterial occlusion in patients with peripheral obstructive vascular disease (De Felice et al, 1990). The initial recanalization rate was 70% to 80%, with a higher success rate when the thrombi were recent or when the duration of the occlusion was less than 6 to 11 months.

Modification of blood rheology can be achieved with pentoxifylline or hemodilution using a starch solution. Pentoxifylline acts by reducing the rigidity of the red and white blood cell membranes and the aggregation of thrombocytes. This drug has been extensively studied, and results of double-blind, placebo-controlled trials showed that pain-free and maximum treadmill walking distance increased significantly in patients with peripheral artery disease (Lindgärde et al, 1989; De Felice et al, 1990). Use of hydroxyethyl starch solution for three weeks reduced hematocrit from 48.5 to 40.5 and increased pain-free walking distance and resting blood flow (Ernst et al, 1987).

The effectiveness of vasodilators has not been proved. The investigational agent, buflomedil, increased pain-free and total walking distance in patients with intermittent claudication in two placebo-controlled trials (Clissold et al, 1987). This agent appears to act by inhibiting alpha adrenoreceptors and improving erythrocyte deformability and oxygen-sparing activity. However, the long-term effectiveness of buflomedil has not been demonstrated.

The efficacy of ketanserin also has been assessed, and reports of its effect on walking distance in patients with intermittent claudication are conflicting and inconclusive (Bounameux et al, 1985; DeCree et al, 1984; PACK Claudication Substudy Investigators, 1989). In a study designed to determine whether ketanserin would improve morbidity and mortality in patients with intermittent claudication, an adverse effect on mortality was noted in patients taking potassium-sparing diuretics concurrently (Prevention of Atherosclerotic Complications with Ketanserin Trial Group, 1989).

When claudication is severe in patients with peripheral obstructive vascular disease, invasive procedures (percutaneous transluminal angioplasty and bypass grafting) may be needed to revascularize the lower limb.

PENTOXIFYLLINE
[Trental]

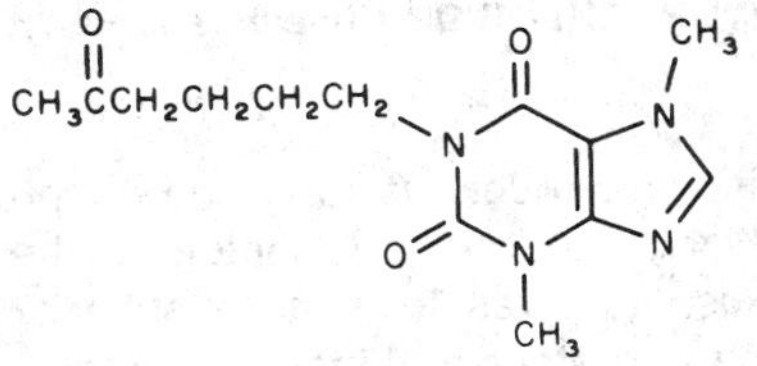

ACTIONS. Pentoxifylline is a trisubstituted xanthine derivative that is classified as a hemorheologic agent. It is claimed to improve oxygenation of ischemic tissues by decreasing blood viscosity. Postulated mechanisms include an increase in erythrocyte and leukocyte flexibility, inhibition of platelet aggregation and granulocyte function, and a reduction in plasma fibrinogen. At the cellular level, pentoxifylline increases the concentration of cyclic adenosine monophosphate (cAMP) in erythrocytes. This agent also has mild vasodilator properties when given intravenously. In microelectrode studies, partial oxygen pressure was increased in calf muscle of patients with chronic occlusive peripheral vascular disease who were treated with pentoxifylline.

USES. Pentoxifylline is used for the treatment of intermittent claudication associated with peripheral obstructive vascular disease. In placebo-controlled trials, doses of 600 mg to 1.2 g/day for at least six weeks improved symptoms (walking distance, rest pain, paresthesia, cramps, ulcer healing, edema, and cyanosis) in 59% to 74% of patients; in contrast, 5% to 29% of patients treated with placebo improved (De Felice et al, 1990; Lindgärde et al, 1989; Ward and Clissold, 1987). In studies that stratified patients according to initial severity of disease, pentoxifylline appeared to produce better results in more severely affected limbs.

After administration for two to three months, pentoxifylline 1.2 g/day significantly increased mean walking distance and improved plethysmographic measurements in patients with chronic peripheral vascular disorder to a greater extent than in those treated with nylidrin 9 mg/day or adenosine 7.2 mg/day. At a lower dosage (300 to 600 mg/day), pentoxifylline was as effective as pyridinolcarbamate 1.5 g/day.

Pentoxifylline also improved symptoms in diabetic patients with lower-limb peripheral vascular disease and in those with cerebrovascular disease.

ADVERSE REACTIONS. The adverse effects of pentoxifylline are dose related and usually involve the gastrointestinal tract. Nausea and dyspepsia are the most common side effects; their incidence can be reduced by giving the drug with food. Flatulence, anorexia, and vomiting are less common.

Adverse effects involving the central nervous system or the cardiovascular system have been observed less frequently. Dizziness, headache, and flushing were noted most often. Nervousness, insomnia, drowsiness, anxiety, and confusion occurred occasionally, and palpitations, angina, arrhythmias, hypotension, dyspnea, and edema were reported rarely. Loss of consciousness, fever, agitation, and convulsions may occur with overdosage.

Blurred vision, rash, pruritus, urticaria, dry mouth, and nasal congestion have occurred occasionally in patients receiving pentoxifylline. Cholecystitis, hepatitis, jaundice, pancytopenia, thrombocytopenia, and purpura have been reported rarely but a cause-and-effect relationship has not been established. Fatal aplastic anemia has occurred rarely.

PRECAUTIONS. Patients who are allergic to xanthines should not be treated with pentoxifylline. Blood pressure should be monitored periodically in those receiving concurrent antihypertensive therapy. Pentoxifylline may reduce plasma fibrinogen levels.

This drug is classified in FDA Pregnancy Category C.

PHARMACOKINETICS. Pentoxifylline is almost completely absorbed after oral administration but undergoes extensive first-pass metabolism. Food delays absorption from an immediate-release capsule (not marketed) but not the total amount absorbed. Plasma levels of metabolites exceed those of the parent drug. The plasma half-life of pentoxifylline is 0.4 to 0.8 hours; the half-lives of its metabolites range from 1 to 1.6 hours. Essentially no parent drug is excreted unchanged.

DOSAGE AND PREPARATIONS.

Oral: *Adults*, 400 mg three times daily with meals. If there is no improvement within 8 to 12 weeks as measured by treadmill exercise performance, the drug should be discontinued. If gastrointestinal or central nervous system side effects develop, the dosage should be reduced to 400 mg twice daily. If adverse effects persist, pentoxifylline should be discontinued.

Trental (Hoechst-Roussel). Tablets (prolonged-release) 400 mg.

ORTHOSTATIC HYPOTENSION

Orthostatic hypotension is characterized by inadequate cerebral perfusion while in the standing position, either immediately on assuming an erect position or after a period of standing upright. Under normal conditions, the transient reduction in venous return to the heart due to redistribution of blood to the capacitance vessels of the legs and splanchnic circulation on standing is compensated for by activation of the baroreflex, resulting in an increase in sympathetic and a decrease in vagal activities. Consequently, heart rate, cardiac contractility, and arteriolar constriction and venoconstriction increase.

In patients with orthostatic hypotension, the reduction in venous return is prolonged, most probably caused by aging, certain drugs (alpha-adrenergic blocking agents, diuretics, centrally acting antihypertensives, nitrates, tricyclic antidepressants, and phenothiazines), or autonomic neuropathy. Secondary causes of orthostatic hypotension include diabetes mellitus, pernicious anemia, amyloidosis, alcoholism, and paraneoplastic syndromes, as well as various genetic disorders including dopamine-beta-hydroxylase deficiency. It may exist alone (Bradbury-Eggleston syndrome) or may accompany central nervous system disorders such as Shy-Drager syndrome, Parkinson's disease, and brain stem lesions, particularly in older persons. The Bradbury-Eggleston syndrome (idiopathic orthostatic hypotension) appears to be precipitated by neuronal cell loss, and it is usually associated with denervation supersensitivity. Orthostatic symptoms are generally most prominent on arising in the morning, during hot weather, and after meals, and many patients have supine hypertension.

The initial approach to treating chronic orthostatic hypotension is nonpharmacologic (Robertson, 1992). The patient can be instructed to perform exercises with dorsiflexion of the feet prior to arising; to arise slowly; to sleep with the head of the bed elevated (which minimizes nocturnal diuresis and supine hypertension); and to avoid heavy lifting and straining, excessive activity after meals, and medications that may adversely affect blood pressure. Use of support garments also may minimize venous pooling and augment venous return to the heart. If these measures are inadequate, pharmacologic therapy is indicated. The salt-retaining steroid, fludrocortisone acetate [Florinef], has been used extensively to treat this condition (Onrot et al, 1986). Midodrine [Amatine], an alpha-adrenergic agonist with a relatively long half-life, is efficacious in the treatment of idiopathic orthostatic hypotension (McTavish and Goa, 1989).

A number of drugs have been used either alone or adjunctively with fludrocortisone to treat orthostatic hypotension. Dihydroergotamine is a relatively selective constrictor of venous capacitance vessels and may control orthostatic symptoms when given parenterally, but bioavailability is low after oral administration and it does not counteract postprandial hypotension (Hoeldtke et al, 1986). Caffeine (250 mg daily) blocks vasodilatory adenosine receptors and may be particularly useful in patients with postprandial hypotension (Hoeldtke et al, 1986; Onrot et al, 1985). Other pharmacologic approaches include use of various sympathomimetic amines, sometimes given with a monoamine oxidase inhibitor; vasopressin analogues; serotonin antagonists; and indomethacin. Orthostatic hypotension associated with dopamine-beta-hydroxylase deficiency has been treated experimentally with DL-dihydroxyphenylserine with the goal of bypassing the enzymatic defect and thus providing endogenous norepinephrine (Biaggioni and Robertson, 1987; Man in'T Veld et al, 1987).

FLUDROCORTISONE ACETATE
[Florinef Acetate]

For chemical formula, see index entry Fludrocortisone, In Adrenal Dysfunction.

This salt-retaining synthetic mineralocorticoid is used to treat orthostatic hypotension in patients who do not have heart failure. Fludrocortisone increases intravascular volume, and large doses may sensitize blood vessels to pressor amines (Onrot et al, 1986; Lipsitz, 1989; Schatz, 1986).

Complications of therapy include fluid retention, hypokalemia, supine hypertension, and heart failure. See also index entry Fludrocortisone, In Adrenal Dysfunction.

DOSAGE AND PREPARATIONS.
Oral: *Adults,* 0.1 to 1 mg daily (Lipsitz, 1989). Dosage should be increased slowly in increments of 0.1 mg until mild peripheral edema develops or symptoms disappear.

Florinef Acetate (Apothecon). Tablets 0.1 mg.

MIDODRINE HYDROCHLORIDE (Investigational drug)
[Amatine]

Midodrine increases venous tone and peripheral vascular resistance by activating alpha receptors in the venous and arterial systems. As a result of these actions, this drug increases supine and standing blood pressure and lowers supine and standing heart rates (McTavish and Goa, 1989).

Midodrine has been used to treat idiopathic orthostatic hypotension (eg, Bradbury-Eggleston syndrome, Shy-Drager syndrome) and the orthostatic hypotension associated with diabetes mellitus and Parkinson's disease. Results of clinical studies in more than 3,000 patients with hypotensive disorders have demonstrated that midodrine increased mean supine and standing blood pressures and improved subjective symptoms of orthostatic hypotension in most patients (McTavish and Goa, 1989; Schirger et al, 1981; Zachariah et al, 1986). Midodrine has been given orphan drug status by the FDA for the treatment of idiopathic orthostatic hypotension. It has been marketed in Europe since 1974 and in Canada since 1991. Midodrine also is being used for the treatment of urinary stress incontinence due to its action on alpha receptors in the urethral sphincter.

ADVERSE REACTIONS. Supine hypertension is the most serious adverse effect of midodrine. Other side effects include pruritus (mainly of the scalp), paresthesias, piloerection, headache, nausea, and a feeling of urinary retention/urgency. Central nervous system stimulation is not associated with use of midodrine.

PHARMACOKINETICS. Midodrine is a prodrug that is rapidly and almost completely absorbed after oral administration and undergoes enzymatic hydrolysis to form the pharmacologically active metabolite, desglymidodrine. After oral administration, peak plasma concentrations of midodrine and desglymidodrine are reached in 30 and 60 minutes, respectively, and elimination half-lives are 30 minutes and two to three hours, respectively. Only 2% to 4% of the parent drug is excreted unchanged.

DOSAGE AND PREPARATIONS.
Oral: *Adults,* 2.5 mg three or four times daily. Dosage may be adjusted at weekly intervals until an optimal response is obtained. Most patients respond to $\leq$30 mg daily given in three or four divided doses. The maximum recommended dose is 40 mg daily.

Amatine (Roberts).

Cited References

Ticlopidine, editorial. *Lancet* 337:459-460, 1991.

Abelmann WH, Lorell BH: Challenge of cardiomyopathy. *J Am Coll Cardiol* 13:1219-1239, 1989.

Antiplatelet Trialists' Collaboration: Secondary prevention of vascular disease by prolonged antiplatelet treatment. *BMJ* 296:320-333, 1988.

Bandstra ES, et al: Prophylactic indomethacin for prevention of intraventricular hemorrhage in premature infants. *Pediatrics* 82:533-542, 1988.

Barst RJ, Gersony WM: Pharmacological treatment of patent ductus arteriosus: Review of the evidence. *Drugs* 38:249-266, 1989.

Belch JJF, et al: Intermittent epoprostenol (prostacyclin) infusion in patients with Raynaud's syndrome: Double-blind controlled trial. *Lancet* 1:313-315, 1983.

Benson LN, et al: Role of prostaglandin E_1 infusion in management of transposition of great arteries. *Am J Cardiol* 44:691-696, 1979.

Biaggioni I, Robertson D: Endogenous restoration of noradrenaline by precursor therapy in dopamine-beta-hydroxylase deficiency. *Lancet* 2:1170-1172, 1987.

Blanchard DG, Ross J Jr: Hypertrophic cardiomyopathy: Prognosis with medical or surgical therapy. *Clin Cardiol* 14:11-19, 1991.

Boissel JP, et al: Is it possible to reduce the risk of cardiovascular events in subjects suffering from intermittent claudication of the lower limbs? *Thromb Haemost* 62:681-685, 1989.

Bounameaux H, et al: Placebo-controlled, double-blind, two-centre trial of ketanserin in intermittent claudication. *Lancet* 2:1268-1271, 1985.

Brash AR, et al: Pharmacokinetics of indomethacin in neonate: Relation of plasma indomethacin levels to response of ductus arteriosus. *N Engl J Med* 305:67-72, 1981.

Brown G: Pharmacologic treatment of primary and secondary pulmonary hypertension. *Pharmacotherapy* 11:137-156, 1991.

Carliner NH, et al: Sodium nitroprusside treatment of ergotamine induced peripheral ischemia. *JAMA* 227:308-309, 1974.

Cassady G, et al: A randomized, controlled trial of very early prophylactic ligation of the ductus arteriosus in babies who weighed 1000 g or less at birth. *N Engl J Med* 320:1511-1516, 1989.

Clifford PC, et al: Treatment of vasospastic disease with prostaglandin E_1. *BMJ* 281:1031-1034, 1980.

Clissold SP, et al: Buflomedil: Review of its pharmacodynamic and pharmacokinetic properties, and therapeutic efficacy in peripheral and cerebral vascular diseases. *Drugs* 33:430-460, 1987.

Coffman JD: Raynaud's phenomenon: An update. *Hypertension* 17:593-602, 1991.

Coffman JD, Cohen RA: Intra-arterial vasodilator agents to reverse human finger vasoconstriction. *Clin Pharmacol Ther* 41:574-579, 1987.

Coffman JD, et al: International study of ketanserin in Raynaud's phenomenon. *Am J Med* 87:264-268, 1989.

Cole RB, et al: Prolonged prostaglandin E_1 infusion: Histologic effects on patent ductus arteriosus. *Pediatrics* 67:816-819, 1981.

Counihan PJ, McKenna WJ: Low-dose amiodarone for the treatment of arrhythmias in hypertrophic cardiomyopathy. *J Clin Pharmacol* 29:436-438, 1989.

D'Alonzo GE, et al: Survival in patients with primary pulmonary hypertension: Results from a national prospective registry. *Ann Intern Med* 115:343-349, 1991.

DeCree J, et al: Placebo-controlled double-blind trial of ketanserin in treatment of intermittent claudication. *Lancet* 2:775-778, 1984.

De Felice M, et al: Current therapy of peripheral obstructive arterial disease: The non-surgical approach. *Angiology* 41:1-11, 1990.

Dinh-Xuan AT, et al: Impairment of endothelium-dependent pulmonary artery relaxation in chronic obstructive lung disease. *N Engl J Med* 324:1539-1547, 1991.

Drummond WH, Lock JE: Neonatal 'pulmonary vasodilator' drugs. *Dev Pharmacol Ther* 7:1-20, 1984.

Epstein SE, Rosing DR: Verapamil: Potential for causing serious complications in patients with hypertrophic cardiomyopathy. *Circulation* 64:437-441, 1981.

Ernst E, et al: Placebo-controlled, double-blind study of haemodilution in peripheral arterial disease. *Lancet* 1:1449-1451, 1987.

Ettinger WH, et al: Controlled double-blind trial of dazoxiben and nifedipine in treatment of Raynaud's phenomenon. *Am J Med* 77:451-456, 1984.

Fananapazir L, et al: Sudden death during empiric amiodarone therapy in symptomatic hypertrophic cardiomyopathy. *Am J Cardiol* 67:169-174, 1991.

Fananapazir L, et al: Impact of dual-chamber permanent pacing in patients with obstructive hypertrophic cardiomyopathy with symptoms refractory to verapamil and β-adrenergic blocker therapy. *Circulation* 85:2149-2161, 1992.

Fox WW, Duara S: Persistent pulmonary hypertension in neonates: Diagnosis and treatment. *Pediatrics* 103:505-514, 1983.

Franks AG Jr: Topical glyceryl trinitrate as adjunctive treatment in Raynaud's disease. *Lancet* 1:76-77, 1982.

Freed MD, et al: Prostaglandin E_1 in infants with ductus arteriosus-dependent congenital heart disease. *Circulation* 64:899-905, 1981.

Friedman WF, et al: Prostaglandins: Physiologic and clinical correlations. *Adv Pediatr* 25:151-204, 1978.

Fuster V, et al: Primary pulmonary hypertension: Natural history and importance of thrombosis. *Circulation* 70:580-587, 1984.

Gersony WM: Neonatal pulmonary hypertension: Pathophysiology, classification, and etiology. *Clin Perinatol* 11:517-524, 1984.

Gersony WM, et al: Effects of indomethacin in premature infants with patent ductus arteriosus: Results of national collaborative study. *J Pediatr* 102:895-906, 1983.

Goldhaber SZ, et al: Low-dose aspirin and subsequent peripheral arterial surgery in the Physicians' Health Study. *Lancet* 340:143-145, 1992.

Goodwin JF: Pharmacologic treatment of hypertrophic cardiomyopathy. *Cardiovasc Drugs Ther* 1:665-668, 1988.

Hertzer NR: The natural history of peripheral vascular disease: Implications for its management. *Circulation* 83(suppl I):I-12-I-19, 1991.

Heymann MA: Pharmacologic use of prostaglandin E_1 in infants with congenital heart disease. *Am Heart J* 101:837-843, 1981.

Heymann MA, Hoffman JIE: Persistent pulmonary hypertension syndromes in the newborn, in Weir EK, Reeves JT (eds): *Pulmonary Hypertension*. Mt Kisco, NY, Futura, 1984, 45-71.

Heymann MA, Rudolph AM: Neonatal manipulation: Patent ductus arteriosus, in Engle MA (ed): *Pediatric Cardiovascular Disease*. Philadelphia, FA Davis, 1981, 301-310.

Hiatt WR, et al: Benefit of exercise conditioning for patients with peripheral arterial disease. *Circulation* 81:602-609, 1990.

Hoeldtke RD, et al: Treatment of orthostatic hypotension with dihydroergotamine and caffeine. *Ann Intern Med* 105:168-173, 1986.

Inbar S, et al: Effects of adenosine in combination with calcium channel blockers in patients with primary pulmonary hypertension. *J Am Coll Cardiol* 21:413-418, 1993.

Janzon L, et al: Prevention of myocardial infarction and stroke in patients with intermittent claudication: Effects of ticlopidine: Results from STIMS, the Swedish Ticlopidine Multicentre Study. *J Intern Med* 227:301-308, 1990.

Jonason T, Bergstrom R: Cessation of smoking in patients with intermittent claudication. *Acta Med Scand* 221:253-260, 1987.

Kinsella JP, et al: Low-dose inhalation nitric oxide in persistent pulmonary hypertension of the newborn. *Lancet* 340:819-820, 1992.

Kloner RA: Pulmonary hypertension and cor pulmonale. *Cardiovasc Rev Rep* 12:27-45, 1991.

Kriett JM, Kaye MP: The Registry of the International Society for Heart Transplantation: Seventh official report—1990. *J Heart Transplant* 9:323-330, 1990.

Larsen VH, et al: Ketanserin in treatment of traumatic vasospastic disease. *BMJ* 293:650-652, 1986.

Lewis AB, et al: Side effects of therapy with prostaglandin E_1 in infants with critical congenital heart disease. *Circulation* 64:893-898, 1981.

Lewis JF, Maron BJ: Elderly patients with hypertrophic cardiomyopathy: A subset with distinctive left ventricular morphology and progressive clinical course late in life. *J Am Coll Cardiol* 13:36-45, 1989.

Liberthson RR, Waldman H: Congenital heart disease in the adult. *Cardiovasc Rev Rep* 12:24-47, 1991.

Lindgärde F, et al: Conservative drug treatment in patients with moderately severe chronic occlusive peripheral arterial disease. *Circulation* 80:1549-1556, 1989.

Lipsitz LA: Orthostatic hypotension in the elderly. *N Engl J Med* 321:952-957, 1989.

Lopez-Ovejero JA, et al: Reversal of vascular and renal crises of scleroderma by oral angiotensin-converting-enzyme blockade. *N Engl J Med* 300:1417-1419, 1979.

Loscalzo J: Endothelial dysfunction in pulmonary hypertension, editorial. *N Engl J Med* 327:117-119, 1992.

Mahony L, et al: Long-term results after atrial repair of transposition of great arteries in early infancy. *Circulation* 66:253-258, 1982.

Malamet R, et al: Nifedipine in treatment of Raynaud's phenomenon: Evidence for inhibition of platelet activation. *Am J Med* 78:602-608, 1985.

Man in'T Veld AJ, et al: Effect of unnatural noradrenaline precursor on sympathetic control and orthostatic hypotension in dopamine-beta-hydroxylase deficiency. *Lancet* 2:1172-1175, 1987.

Maron BJ, et al: Hypertrophic cardiomyopathy: Interrelations of clinical manifestations, pathophysiology, and therapy, parts 1 and 2. *N Engl J Med* 316:780-789; 844-852, 1987.

McDaniel MD, Cronenwett JL: Basic data related to the natural history of intermittent claudication. *Ann Vasc Surg* 3:272-277, 1989.

McKenna WJ, et al: Arrhythmia in hypertrophic cardiomyopathy: Exercise and 48 hour ambulatory electrocardiographic assessment with and without beta adrenergic blocking therapy. *Am J Cardiol* 45:1-5, 1980.

McKenna WJ, et al: Amiodarone for long-term management of patients with hypertrophic cardiomyopathy. *Am J Cardiol* 54:802-810, 1984.

McTavish D, Goa KL: Midodrine: A review of its pharmacological properties and therapeutic use in orthostatic hypotension and secondary hypotensive disorders. *Drugs* 38:757-777, 1989.

Ment LR, et al: Randomized indomethacin trial for prevention of intraventricular hemorrhage in very low birth weight infants. *J Pediatr* 107:937-943, 1985.

Mohrland JS, et al: Multiclinic, placebo-controlled, double-blind study of prostaglandin E_1 in Raynaud's syndrome. *Ann Rheum Dis* 44:754-760, 1985.

Morgan JM, et al: Adenosine as a vasodilator in primary pulmonary hypertension. *Circulation* 84:1145-1149, 1991.

Oelz O, et al: Nifedipine for high altitude pulmonary oedema. *Lancet* 2:1241-1244, 1989.

Olley PM, Coceani F: Prostaglandins and ductus arteriosus. *Annu Rev Med* 32:375-385, 1981.

Onrot J, et al: Hemodynamic and humoral effects of caffeine in autonomic failure: Therapeutic implications for postprandial hypotension. *N Engl J Med* 313:549-554, 1985.

Onrot J, et al: Management of chronic orthostatic hypotension. *Am J Med* 80:454-464, 1986.

O'Reilly MJG, et al: Controlled trial of plasma exchange in treatment of Raynaud's syndrome. *BMJ* 2:1113-1115, 1979.

PACK Claudication Substudy Investigators: Randomized placebo-controlled, double-blind trial of ketanserin in claudicants. *Circulation* 80:1544-1548, 1989.

Palevsky HI, Fishman AP: Pulmonary veno-occlusive disease-response to vasodilator agents. *Am Rev Respir Dis* 142:426-429, 1990.

Palevsky HI, Fishman AP: The management of primary pulmonary hypertension. *JAMA* 265:1014-1020, 1991.

Pepke-Zaba J, et al: Inhaled nitric oxide as a cause of selective pulmonary vasodilatation in pulmonary hypertension. *Lancet* 338:1173-1174, 1991.

Pollick C: Disopyramide in hypertrophic cardiomyopathy: II. Noninvasive assessment after oral administration. *Am J Cardiol* 62:1252-1255, 1988.

Prevention of Atherosclerotic Complications with Ketanserin Trial Group: Prevention of atherosclerotic complications: Controlled trial of ketanserin. *BMJ* 298:424-430, 1989.

Quick CRG, Cotton LT: The measured effect of stopping smoking on intermittent claudication. *Br J Surg* 69 (suppl):524-526, 1982.

Rademaker M, et al: Comparison of intravenous infusions of iloprost and oral nifedipine in treatment of Raynaud's phenomenon in patients with systemic sclerosis: A double blind randomised study. *BMJ* 298:561-564, 1989.

Rich S, Brundage BH: High-dose calcium channel-blocking therapy for primary pulmonary hypertension: Evidence for long-term reduction in pulmonary arterial pressure and regression of right ventricular hypertrophy. *Circulation* 76:135-141, 1987.

Rich S, et al: Primary pulmonary hypertension: Radiographic and scintigraphic patterns of histologic subtypes. *Ann Intern Med* 105:499-502, 1986.

Rich S, et al: Primary pulmonary hypertension: National prospective study. *Ann Intern Med* 107:216-223, 1987.

Rich S, et al: The effect of high doses of calcium-channel blockers on survival in primary pulmonary hypertension. *N Engl J Med* 327:76-81, 1992.

Roald OK, Seem E: Treatment of Raynaud's phenomenon with ketanserin in patients with connective tissue disorders. *BMJ* 289:577-579, 1984.

Roberts JD, et al: Inhaled nitric oxide in persistent pulmonary hypertension of the newborn. *Lancet* 340:818-819, 1992.

Robertson D: Orthostatic hypotension, in Melmon KL, et al (eds): *Clinical Pharmacology*. New York, McGraw-Hill, 1992, 84-103.

Rosing DR, et al: Use of calcium-channel blocking drugs in hypertrophic cardiomyopathy. *Am J Cardiol* 55:185B-195B, 1985.

Rubin LJ: Primary pulmonary hypertension: Practical therapeutic recommendations. *Drugs* 43:37-43, 1992.

Rubin LJ, et al: Treatment of primary pulmonary hypertension with continuous intravenous prostacyclin (epoprostenol): Results of a randomized trial. *Ann Intern Med* 112:485-491, 1990.

Schatz IJ: *Orthostatic Hypotension*. Philadelphia, FA Davis Co, 1986.

Schirger A, et al: Midodrine: New agent in management of idiopathic orthostatic hypotension and Shy-Drager syndrome. *Mayo Clin Proc* 56:429-433, 1981.

Schrader BJ, et al: Comparison of the effects of adenosine and nifedipine in pulmonary hypertension. *J Am Coll Cardiol* 19:1060-1064, 1992.

Scott JP, et al: The acute effect of the synthetic prostacyclin analogue iloprost in primary pulmonary hypertension. *Br J Clin Pharmacol* 44:231-234, 1990.

Sherrid M, et al: Oral disopyramide therapy for obstructive hypertrophic cardiomyopathy. *Am J Cardiol* 62:1085-1088, 1988.

Sovijärvi ARA, et al: Transdermal nitroglycerin in treatment of Raynaud's phenomenon: Analysis of digital blood pressure changes after cold provocation. *Curr Ther Res* 35:832-839, 1984.

Stevenson DK, et al: Refractory hypoxemia associated with neonatal pulmonary disease: Use and limitations of tolazoline. *J Pediatr* 95:595-599, 1979.

Tiefenbrunn LJ, Riemenschneider TA: Persistent pulmonary hypertension of the newborn. *Am Heart J* 111:564-571, 1986.

Trulock EP, et al: The Washington University-Barnes Hospital experience with lung transplantation. *JAMA* 266:1943-1946, 1991.

Verhaeghe R: Prophylactic antiplatelet therapy in peripheral arterial disease. *Drugs* 42 (suppl 5):51-57, 1991.

Vogt MT, et al: Lower extremity arterial disease and the aging process: A review. *J Clin Epidemiol* 45:529-542, 1992.

Ward A, Clissold SP: Pentoxifylline: Review of its pharmacodynamic and pharmacokinetic properties, and its therapeutic efficacy. *Drugs* 34:50-97, 1987.

Zachariah PK, et al: Pharmacodynamics of midodrine, antihypotensive agent. *Clin Pharmacol Ther* 39:586-591, 1986.

Zarfin Y, et al: Possible indomethacin-aminoglycoside interaction in preterm infants. *J Pediatr* 106:511-513, 1985.

Therapeutic Management of Myocardial Infarction

31

In the United States, approximately 1.5 million people develop myocardial infarction annually, and approximately 500,000 die within the first month (25% of all deaths in this country) (American Heart Association, 1988). A large percentage of infarction-related deaths occur in the first hour before medical attention is sought. Of patients who reach the hospital alive, approximately 16% die in the hospital. Of those who survive the acute phase, more than 90% eventually die from coronary artery disease (10% within the first year).

Of the 700,000 patients hospitalized annually because of myocardial infarction, more than 600,000 were completely free of cardiac symptoms or had only mildly symptomatic, stable angina pectoris before the onset. Major risk factors for development of the disease include advanced age, family history of myocardial infarction, lack of exercise, obesity, high serum cholesterol levels, hypertension, smoking, diabetes, psychosocial factors leading to stress, and high circulating levels of factor VII and fibrinogen.

ETIOLOGY

Myocardial infarction is primarily caused by occlusive thrombosis following the rupture of vulnerable atherosclerotic plaques in the coronary artery. Onset is at least three times more likely in the morning (the first few hours after awakening) than in late evening (Cohen and Muller, 1992; Tofler et al, 1992). Some mechanisms responsible for the increased prevalence in the morning include the surge of arterial blood pressure after arising, which may increase the risk of plaque rupture; enhanced platelet aggregability and decreased fibrinolytic activity on standing or sitting; and a possible increase in coronary vasomotor tone that may reduce coronary blood flow in response to morning activities. It is hypothesized that the plaque rupture occurs at a critical time in the morning when a threshold combination of hemodynamic, prothrombotic, and vasoconstrictive forces is rapidly generated by external stresses (eg, moderate to heavy exercise, emotional stress).

Occlusive thrombosis causes acute reduction of blood flow and myocardial ischemia. When the ischemia is sufficiently severe and prolonged, infarction results. There are two phases during the course of acute myocardial infarction: evolving and convalescent (Hagar, 1990; Jennings and Reimer, 1989; Pepine, 1989 A).

The evolving phase generally occurs during the first six hours after the appearance of overt symptoms. Intervention during this time has the best likelihood of reducing mortality. During this phase, hydrogen ion rapidly accumulates in the myocardium. Calcium ion is displaced from contractile proteins in the endoplasmic reticulum and ultimately migrates to the mitochondria, usually with toxic effects. The resulting acidosis and the displaced calcium ion alter the distensibility of the cardiac muscle. Concomitantly, sodium migrates into the cell and sets the stage for swelling and edema. Migration of potassium ion outside the cell may lead to potentially lethal arrhythmias. In addition, cellular metabolism shifts to anaerobic glycolysis within seconds after coronary artery occlusion. Contraction ceases in the area of involvement, and high energy stores of creatine phosphate and then adenosine triphosphate become depleted. Eventually, injury becomes irreversible as it proceeds as a wavefront of cell death from the subendocardium toward the subepicardium and culminates in a transmural infarct.

In experimental studies, the duration of ischemia necessary for completion of cell death has averaged two to six hours. In the absence of reperfusion, evidence of cellular injury can be detected by light microscopy within six to eight hours. Mild infiltration of the white cells begins at the edge of the infarct within 12 hours; by 24 hours, myocyte disruption and coagulative necrosis are evident. By the fourth day, mononuclear cell infiltration and myocyte removal begin to make the infarct even more susceptible to expansion or rupture. Collagen deposition begins at the periphery after 10 to 12 days, and healing with dense scar formation is essentially complete in four to six weeks in all but very large infarcts.

Globally, the onset of severe ischemia initially leads to increased diastolic stiffness that results in elevation of end-diastolic pressure. The systolic function of the involved wall is compromised and the muscle becomes akinetic or dyskinetic, although compensatory hyperkinesis of the remaining nonischemic myocardium may preserve global function in patients with smaller infarcts. Greater loss of functioning myocardium leads to abnormal diastolic and systolic demand on the nonischemic area of the ventricle resulting in subsequent dilatation and remodeling of the heart. In general, infarction of $>10\%$ of left ventricular mass leads to reduction in ejection fraction, of $\geq 25\%$ to dilatation and congestive failure, and of $\geq 40\%$ to cardiogenic shock or death. The loss may be due to single or multiple insults.

If reperfusion occurs early in the course of infarction, a different sequence of events may ensue (Jennings and Reimer, 1989). Restoration of the flow of oxygenated blood leads to substantial increases in tissue water, sodium, and calcium and to explosive disruption of some injured myocytes, which are unable to regulate their cell volume. Salvage of ischemic but viable myocardial cells occurs in the midmyocardial and subepicardial layers of the ventricular wall and commonly results in non-Q-wave infarction. Ventricular arrhythmias often increase, cell infiltration is accelerated, and intramural hemorrhage occurs within the infarct zone. Drug intervention aimed at blunting such effects during re-establishment of coronary blood flow may enhance the myocardial salvage that occurs with reperfusion.

During the convalescent phase, myocardial changes occur from after the first six hours until just before the patient is ready to be discharged from the hospital (usually 3 to 14 days). During the first few days, a large infarction may increase in size (expansion). Extensive geometric remodeling occurs in the remaining myocardium as a result of acute stretching, thinning, and dilatation of the ventricle. This remodeling plays an important role in the pathogenesis of persistent cardiac dilatation, formation of aneurysms, and ventricular septal and even free-wall ruptures. Infarct expansion and rupture occur more often in patients with first infarctions, Q-wave infarctions, and hypertension.

The terms extension and reinfarction generally are used interchangeably to signify additional damage primarily due to further necrosis across the ventricular wall. Extension usually is documented by an increase in the serum level of the MB isozyme of creatine kinase. Recurrent ischemia, ST-segment depression, and a history of previous infarction are risk factors for extension. The mortality rate is many times greater than in those without extension.

Under some conditions, pronounced ischemic injury may produce severe myocardial dysfunction (stunning and hibernating) without evidence of necrosis that persists long after the imbalance between oxygen supply and demand has been corrected. Despite restoration of perfusion, functional, ultrastructural, and biochemical abnormalities in the myocardium may persist, and it may be days or even weeks before function is fully restored. Myocardial stunning may occur when there is acute occlusion of a vessel, which then is reopened or bypassed to reperfuse the affected myocardial region (Braunwald and Kloner, 1982). The myocardium is described as hibernating when a more chronic reduction in blood flow or increase in oxygen demand that causes ischemia occurs (Braunwald and Rutherford, 1986). The myocardium then down-regulates or depresses its function to match its oxygen supply, and a new equilibrium is established between oxygen supply and demand at a level that does not result in necrosis. However, any additional impairment in oxygen supply or increase in oxygen demand can disturb this equilibrium and quickly progress to necrosis.

DIAGNOSIS

The existence of chest pain, abnormalities in the electrocardiogram, and alterations in serum enzyme levels are the current criteria for diagnosis of myocardial infarction.

Chest Pain: A patient with acute myocardial infarction typically complains of severe substernal chest pressure that is described as an intolerable crushing or constricting pain (Hagar, 1990; Kloner, 1989). The sensation of myocardial ischemia, which is transmitted via visceral sympathetic nerves, is often difficult for the patient to describe precisely. The pain often radiates down the arms and occasionally up into the jaws. The pain of myocardial infarction is distinguished from that of angina pectoris by a duration of longer than 20 to 30 minutes and lack of relief with rest and the administration of nitroglycerin. Frequently associated symptoms are caused by activation of the parasympathetic nervous system and include diaphoresis, weakness, or a feeling of impending doom. Nausea, vomiting, and abdominal pain also are common, particularly during inferior wall infarction. When heart failure supervenes, dyspnea and cough with pink frothy sputum may be prominent; when cardiac output starts to decrease due to extensive right or left ventricular infarction, weakness and altered mentation associated with a shock-like state may be noted.

Some patients experience only nonspecific symptoms and believe that they have indigestion. In ≥20% of cases, particularly the elderly and patients with diabetes or hypertension, myocardial infarction is clinically silent and is diagnosed by evolving electrocardiographic changes, by regional wall motion abnormalities, or when complications (heart failure, arrhythmias) develop (Kannel et al, 1984; Grimm et al, 1987; Yano and MacLean, 1989).

Electrocardiographic Recordings: The electrocardiogram (ECG) is of central importance in the diagnosis of acute myocardial infarction (Hagar, 1990; Spodick, 1989). In a large majority of patients, a Q-wave preceded by a period of ST-segment elevation is observed in the ECG tracing. In non-Q-wave infarctions, there is persistent ST-depression or T-wave inversion without Q-wave changes. Evolutionary changes indicative of myocardial infarction are seen on serial tracings in approximately two-thirds of patients with acute myocardial infarction; the remainder have only minor ST-segment alteration and/or T-wave inversion. However, the initial ECG shows only mild or nonspecific abnormalities in as many as 50% of the patients and is normal in about 20% (Kannel et al, 1984; Grimm et al, 1987; Yano and MacLean, 1989). Thus, a single normal or mildly abnormal ECG does not exclude the diagnosis in the appropriate clinical setting.

In the classic pattern, initial hyperacute T-wave peaking followed by elevation of the ST-segment develops promptly after onset of ischemia in the leads facing the area of injury. As cell death occurs, R-wave height is lost in the same leads and a pathologic Q-wave (defined as >0.04 seconds in duration) develops over hours to days. The ST-segment elevation then decreases toward baseline; it returns to normal simultaneously with the development of T-wave inversion during subsequent days. Posterior wall infarction produces an inverted pattern with ST-depression, T-wave peaking, and development of tall and broad R-waves in V_1 and V_2. Right ventricular infarction is manifested electrocardiographically as ST-segment elevation in the right precordial lead, V_{4R} (Zehender et al, 1993). Hence, the V_{4R} lead should always be recorded in patients who arrive at the hospital with ST-segment elevations in the precordial leads, V_2, V_3, and aVF. Frequently, the ST-segment changes in precordial leads V_3-V_2 and sometimes in V_1 also are associated with inferior infarction.

T-wave inversions may persist for weeks or months. Q-waves may diminish in size or disappear over a period of years, particularly with inferior infarction. ST-segment depression, especially anterior ST-depression with inferior infarctions, may be observed in leads remote from the area of infarction. Following early reperfusion after thrombolytic therapy or other measures, ST-elevation may resolve rapidly, development of Q-waves is accelerated, and transient arrhythmias (eg, accelerated idioventricular rhythm) may occur.

Laboratory Tests: The serum level of the MB isozyme of creatine kinase is the assay of choice for the diagnosis of myocardial infarction (Hagar, 1990). It is used in addition to total creatine kinase because MB isozyme levels rise 3 to 12 hours after infarction, peak slightly earlier than the total creatine kinase (20 to 24 hours), and normalize in 36 to 72 hours. The subset of patients (10% to 20%) with elevated creatine kinase-MB isozyme but normal total creatine kinase should be considered to have myocardial infarction if a typical rise and fall in total creatine kinase levels is observed and if the clinical findings are compatible with this diagnosis. Measurement of the isoforms of the MB isozyme (MB1 and MB2) also can be used in the early detection of myocardial infarction. MB2 activity >1 U/L and an MB2:MB1 ratio >1.5 has a 59% sensitivity for diagnosis of myocardial infarction at two to four hours and a 92% sensitivity at four to six hours after onset of symptoms (Puleo et al, 1990).

Reopening of any occluded coronary vessel can be detected by measurement of MB isozyme. An early increase and a shorter time to peak in levels of MB isozyme have been associated with reperfusion following thrombolytic therapy (Ohman et al, 1993). A 2.2-fold increase in MB isozyme levels in patients with inferior myocardial infarction and a 2.5-fold increase in those with anterior myocardial infarction during the initial two hours of treatment are 85% sensitive and 100% specific for detection of recanalization (Garabedian et al, 1988).

Lactate dehydrogenase (LDH) and its five isozymes are useful indicators when the creatine kinase-MB isozyme level is normal and infarction is believed to have occurred at least two to four days earlier. These isozymes rise within 24 to 48 hours of infarction, peak in three to five days, and persist for seven to ten days. Even though LDH is elevated in muscle, the liver, and in those with hematologic disorders, a ratio of LDH_1:LDH_2 of >1.0 is relatively specific for myocardial necrosis. However, a false-positive reading may be observed with hemolysis, which also raises LDH_1.

Since myocardial cell death due to any cause (eg, cardiac contusion after chest wall trauma, electrical injury, pericarditis with concomitant myocardial involvement) will result in a similar rise-and-fall pattern of MB isozyme levels, this marker has drawbacks for early detection of myocardial infarction (Adams et al, 1993 A). In addition, most skeletal muscle contains small amounts (1% to 3%) of MB isozyme that can be released due to any type of skeletal muscle injury, including extremely rigorous exercise, chronic myopathies due to renal failure, and hypothyroidism. In contrast, cardiac troponin I, one of the myofibrillar proteins, is not expressed in skeletal muscle. Since cardiac troponin I is tightly complexed to the contractile apparatus, plasma circulating levels are usually low. In patients with chest pain, elevation of cardiac troponin I levels above the reference range occurs a few hours later than those of MB isozyme (Cummins et al, 1987; Bodor et al, 1992). The increased levels persist for up to one to two weeks after acute myocardial infarction. Because it has a short half-life in plasma and low circulating levels occur in normal volunteers, in patients with skeletal muscle injury or renal failure, and in marathon runners (Adams et al, 1993 B), cardiac troponin I also may serve as a sensitive marker for early detection of myocardial infarction.

Other Diagnostic Methods: Other tests also can be used to assist in the diagnosis of myocardial infarction. ^{99m}Technetium-pyrophosphate scanning is useful because the tracer binds to accumulated calcium within irreversibly damaged myocardium; the sensitivity of this technique is greatest when scanning is performed 24 to 72 hours after Q-wave (transmural) infarction and is significantly lower in non-

Q-wave (nontransmural) infarction. Thallium-201 imaging combined with intracoronary ^{99m}technetium-pyrophosphate scanning can be used to predict myocardial salvage after thrombolysis.

Two-dimensional and Doppler echocardiography also is of considerable value in assessing patients with acute myocardial infarction. Regional wall motion abnormality, location and extent of infarction, and left and right ventricular dysfunction can be characterized. Echocardiography is an aid in the diagnosis of mechanical complications, including papillary muscle rupture, ventricular septal rupture, ventricular aneurysm, ventricular mural thrombus, pericardial effusion, and infarct expansion. Newer applications include tissue characterization and detection of viable myocardial cells following reperfusion.

CLASSIFICATION

Q-wave Infarction: The term Q-wave infarction has replaced transmural infarction because morphologic studies have shown that Q-waves may be seen when necrosis extends partially across the ventricular wall (Pepine, 1989 A; Hagar, 1990).

Coronary angiography has demostrated that acute thrombotic occlusion occurs in 80% to 90% of individuals with Q-wave infarction who were diagnosed within four to six hours of onset. Coronary occlusion is usually caused by the rupture of a vulnerable atherosclerotic plaque and its dynamic interaction with mediators of vascular tone, platelets, and the clotting cascade. Fissuring, rupture, or hemorrhage into an atheromatous plaque often appears to be the initiating event and exposes collagen, atheroma, and tissue thromboplastins to circulating platelets and clotting factors. Platelet aggregation further promotes thrombosis and leads to vasoconstriction and the release of thromboxane A_2, thus overwhelming endogenous vasodilators such as prostacyclin and endothelial-derived relaxation factor. Luminal obstruction results from the combination of atheromatous plaque, platelet-rich thrombus, and variable degrees of spasm.

Non-Q-wave Infarction: Spontaneous thrombolysis occurs in one-third to one-half of infarct-related arteries over hours to days following infarction. Non-Q-wave infarction may result from such spontaneous lysis before the onset of the infarction but also may result from an initially subtotal occlusion or a transmural infarction that fails to produce a Q-wave. Clot lysis results in a fixed stenosis of varying severity and unstable morphology, which may be prone to reocclusion or may heal with incorporation of thrombus and progression of stenosis.

The number of patients with non-Q-wave infarction appears to be increasing. This may be due to improved sensitivity and wider application of the creatine kinase-MB isozyme assay or to better prior medical management (including use of aspirin), which converts probable Q-wave infarctions into non-Q-wave infarctions. The clinical course of patients with non-Q-wave infarction suggests that they may have had partial reperfusion resulting in smaller infarctions with reduced early mortality. However, they also appear to be at a much higher risk for early reinfarction and angina, possibly leading to death. Those with anterior ECG changes, spontaneous or inducible ischemia, a history of prior infarction, or persistent ST-segment depression appear to have an unfavorable prognosis; stable patients under age 70 without prior infarct may fare better.

Atypical Myocardial Infarction: Myocardial infarction may be atypical and lack the classic triad of chest pain, ECG changes, and elevated serum enzymes. These individuals, especially those $\geq$75 years of age, have symptoms of confusion, vomiting, syncope, and shortness of breath (Nadelmann et al, 1990). A number of theories have been proposed to explain why silent or painless myocardial infarction occurs in the elderly. Some investigators suggest the presence of a sensory neuropathy and an increased pain threshold (Glazier et al, 1986) that eliminates the "warning system" (Cohn, 1980). Atypical myocardial infarction also occurs in patients with diabetes.

There is no difference in the incidence of mortality and morbidity in individuals with recognized or atypical myocardial infarctions (Kannel et al, 1984; Grimm et al, 1987; Yano and MacLean, 1989). Since a history of myocardial infarction in the elderly also is associated with an increased risk of future infarcts, there is a need to identify prognostic markers for myocardial ischemia in these individuals.

MANAGEMENT

Since the 1960s, early prehospital supportive care and coronary care unit monitoring have been the standards for the management of the patient with myocardial infarction and have reduced mortality. However, most sudden deaths, primarily caused by ventricular arrhythmias, still occur before medical attention is sought. Most in-hospital deaths are due to cardiogenic shock, which is related to infarct size. With recognition of the importance of thrombosis in the pathogenesis of myocardial infarction and the availability of thrombolytic drugs, early revascularization to salvage the myocardium and minimize infarct size can be achieved (Pepine, 1989 B; Chesebro et al, 1990; Gersh and Anderson, 1993).

Standard treatment of hospitalized patients consists of bed rest during the first days after infarction, supplemental oxygen for hypoxemia, and administration of opioids and antianxiety agents to relieve chest pain or anxiety, low-dose subcutaneous or intravenous heparin to prevent peripheral thromboembolism, and aspirin to inhibit platelet aggregation. Further treatment is individualized and is based on the patient's history. Management of symptoms and/or complications (Hagar, 1990; Lavie and Gersh, 1990), revascularization, and long-term treatment are considered. The optimal strategy is to limit the infarct size through early reperfusion and maintenance of coronary patency. Complications, such as cardiogenic shock, ventricular arrhythmias, and congestive heart failure, are especially life-threatening (see Table 1). After discharge from the hospital, the long-term goals of therapy are to reduce reinfarction and mortality.

TABLE 1.
MANAGEMENT OF COMPLICATIONS OF MYOCARDIAL INFARCTION

Complication	Prognosis	Treatment
Cardiogenic shock	This complicates 7% of left ventricular infarctions in the first days and develops more frequently in those with large infarcts, previous infarction, admission ejection fractions of <35%, diabetes, and advanced age. Ultimate mortality rate from cardiogenic shock is 65% to 90%.	Primary angioplasty greatly reduces mortality. Inotropic drugs (eg, dopamine, dobutamine, amrinone, milrinone) alone or in combination improve contractility. Vasodilators often further improve cardiac output but may worsen coronary perfusion pressure. Intra-aortic balloon counterpulsation improves the hemodynamic profile.
Cardiac rupture	Although rare (≤1% to 2%), rupture is most common several days following a large anterior Q-wave infarction. Shock develops suddenly and circulatory collapse with electromechanical dissociation and signs of tamponade occur. Death is often immediate.	Beta blockade and possibly early vasodilator therapy appear to decrease incidence of cardiac rupture. If stabilized, operative repair (eg, coronary artery bypass) is lifesaving.
Ventricular arrhythmias	These are major causes of death during and after myocardial infarction. Sudden arrhythmia-induced death occurs in the first hour in approximately 15% of patients with acute myocardial infarction and accounts for about 60% of all infarction-related deaths. Most arrhythmias occur before hospital admission but develop in 3% to 9% of patients after admission, usually within 12 hours of infarction.	Prophylactic doses of lidocaine decrease arrhythmias but do not reduce mortality. Amiodarone and beta-adrenergic blockers may be more efficacious than Class 1 antiarrhythmic agents.
Congestive heart failure	Patients have an elevated pulmonary capillary wedge pressure (≥ 15 mm Hg). Pulmonary rales, dyspnea, and radiographic vascular congestion may occur later. About 15% of patients present with frank pulmonary edema. Those with severely depressed cardiac output and pulmonary congestion have the highest mortality rate.	The principal drugs used are diuretics, which reduce preload; inotropic drugs (dobutamine), which increase myocardial contractility; and vasodilators (IV nitrates), which reduce aortic impedance and/or increase venous capacitance. ACE inhibitors may be particularly beneficial both for symptoms and reduction of mortality. Digoxin and ACE inhibitors also may restore baroreceptor sensitivity that results in a decrease in sympathetic outflow and renin production.
Postinfarction angina and/or ischemia	These are associated with higher rates of reinfarction and death.	Complications may be decreased with beta-blockade or angioplasty.
Right ventricular infarction	The right ventricle is involved in roughly one-third of patients with inferior wall infarction and one-tenth of those with anterior wall infarction. Manifestations of right ventricular infarction range from mild jugular venous distention to frank shock.	Initially, hypotensive patients with right ventricular infarction and mild symptoms are treated with volume expansion. After equalization of left- and right-sided pressures, treatment with dobutamine may be necessary when diminished perfusion persists.
Deep venous thrombosis	The incidence of deep venous thrombosis in the lower limbs ranges from 17% to 38%. Deep venous thrombosis forms early after the myocardial infarction (≥50% within 3 days). The incidence is increased after massive or recurrent infarction with heart failure or cardiogenic shock, after prolonged immobilization, and in association with certain characteristics, especially age >70 years.	Heparin (subcutaneous or intravenous) started within 12 to 18 hours after onset of symptoms and continued for 10 days has reduced the incidence of deep venous thrombosis.

(table continued on next page)

TABLE 1 (continued)

Complication	Prognosis	Treatment
Pericarditis	This appears in ≤ 10% of infarctions, most commonly 2 or 4 days after infarction, and is due to inflammation associated with transmural necrosis. It occurs more frequently in those with Q-wave infarctions and with larger and more complicated infarctions.	Usually treated with aspirin. Other nonsteroidal anti-inflammatory agents may precipitate myocardial rupture in patients with large infarcts.
Infarct extension	This occurs in approximately 30% of patients (particularly those with anterior infarction) within 3 to 7 days. It may lead to cardiogenic shock and is associated with a fourfold increase in mortality.	Early revascularization (percutaneous transluminal coronary angioplasty or coronary artery bypass grafting) may be helpful to prevent extension in selected patients.
Ventricular aneurysm	Ventricular aneurysm develops most often in the first 3 months following anterior infarction with poor collateral blood flow. The presence of an aneurysm, especially early after infarction, is associated with a markedly increased risk of heart failure, angina, ventricular arrhythmias, embolization, and death.	Surgical resection may be indicated for patients with intractable heart failure, angina, or arrhythmias if the function of the remaining myocardium is adequate.
Arterial embolism	The overall incidence of mural thrombi is approximately 20% in acute myocardial infarction, 40% in anterior myocardial infarction, and 60% in large anterior myocardial infarction. However, the incidence of systemic embolism is only about 2%, 4%, and 6%, respectively.	Arterial emboli can be prevented by administering subcutaneous or intravenous heparin in a dosage sufficient to prolong APTT to 1.5 to 2 times the control value. Heparin is advocated for patients with a large anteroseptal infarction; it should be administered immediately after the onset of infarct and continued for about 10 days. For patients with chronic left ventricular aneurysm but preserved wall motion outside the zone of infarction, oral anticoagulant therapy should be continued for at least 3 months.

Primary Therapy for Acute Myocardial Infarction

Immediate revascularization utilizing thrombolytic therapy or mechanical means to reperfuse the infarcting myocardium has decreased infarct size, wall motion abnormalities, complications, and the number of fatalities. Concomitant therapy with other drugs may be needed to maintain vessel patency in the reopened coronary arteries.

REPERFUSION THERAPY. Reperfusion therapy consists of the use of thrombolytic agents, percutaneous transluminal coronary angioplasty (PTCA), and coronary artery bypass grafting (CABG). Thrombolytic therapy should be considered first. If it is contraindicated, patients may be candidates for direct PTCA. However, immediate PTCA has been shown to be as effective as thrombolytic therapy in medical centers with appropriate facilities. CABG may be appropriate under certain circumstances (eg, left mainstem subtotal or multivessel occlusion) but is not performed during the acute stage.

Because of delay in seeking medical attention, a nondiagnostic initial ECG, or contraindications to thrombolysis, only approximately 30% to 50% of patients with acute myocardial infarction are candidates for acute revascularization (Murray et al, 1987; GISSI-1, 1986; GISSI-2, 1990).

Thrombolytic Therapy: Four to six hours after the onset of symptoms, an occlusive thrombus in the infarct-related coronary artery is present in nearly 90% of patients with acute myocardial infarction. If patients are treated early enough with thrombolytic agents, eg, streptokinase [Kabikinase, Streptase], urokinase [Abbokinase], tissue-type plasminogen activator (t-PA) that is produced by recombinant DNA technology (rt-PA, alteplase [Activase]), anistreplase (anisoylated plasminogen-streptokinase activator complex, APSAC [Eminase]), reperfusion is possible in most. Thrombolytic agents convert plasminogen to plasmin, a proteolytic enzyme that causes fibrinolysis. (For detailed information on individual agents, see the chapter on Thrombolytics.) Table 2 summarizes pertinent findings from numerous international clinical trials.

Mortality. Results of well-controlled clinical trials demonstrate that mortality was significantly reduced in patients who received thrombolytic therapy within four to six hours after the onset of acute myocardial infarction (Granger et al, 1992). This positive effect is consistent for different myocardial infarction locations and in several major subgroups of patients, including the elderly and those with ST-segment elevation or bundle branch block. However, those with ST-segment depression or a normal ECG do not benefit.

GISSI-2 (1990), the International t-PA/Streptokinase Mortality Trial (1990), and ISIS-3 (1992) compared the effect of different thrombolytic agents with or without subcutaneous heparin. All patients received aspirin. The use of streptokinase or rt-PA (GISSI-2 and International t-PA/Streptokinase

TABLE 2.
INTERNATIONAL TRIALS ON THROMBOLYTIC THERAPY

Trials*	Pertinent Findings
GISSI-1	Streptokinase, administered within 4 to 6 hours after onset of pain, lowered mortality in myocardial infarction.
ASSET, AIMS	rt-PA and anistreplase reduced early mortality in acute myocardial infarction.
TIMI-1, TAMI-1	Angiography showed patent artery in majority of patients following thrombolytic therapy.
TIMI-2, TAMI-1	After rt-PA, angioplasty was needed only for patients with recurrent ischemia.
ISIS-2	Aspirin enhanced reduction of early mortality and reinfarction following streptokinase therapy.
HART	IV heparin prevented reocclusion following rt-PA therapy.
TIMI-1, ECSG-1, PAIMS	Patency was greater following rt-PA than streptokinase.
GISSI-2/Int, ISIS-3	With SC heparin (4 or 12 hours after thrombolytic agent), streptokinase, rt-PA, and anistreplase were equally effective in lowering mortality in myocardial infarction.
TAPS, TAMI-7, RAAMI	Accelerated dose regimen of rt-PA (100 mg/90 min: 15 mg bolus, 50 mg/30 min, and 35 mg/60 min) provided optimal patency within 90 min in occluded coronary arteries.
GUSTO	Mortality at 30 days was significantly lowered with accelerated dose regimen of rt-PA plus IV heparin than with streptokinase plus IV or SC heparin. At 90 minutes, the patency rate was higher with rt-PA than streptokinase.

**AIMS: APSAC Intervention Mortality Study (AIMS Trial Study Group, 1988, 1990)*
ASSET: Anglo-Scandinavian Study of Early Thrombolysis (Wilcox et al, 1988, 1990)
ECSG: European Cooperative Study Group (Van de Werf and the European Cooperative Study Group [ECSG], 1988; Arnold et al, 1992)
GISSI-1: Gruppo Italiana per lo Studio della Streptochinasi nell'Infarto Miocardico (1986)
GISSI-2: Gruppo Italiana per lo Studio della Sopravvivenza nell'Infarto Miocardico (1990)
GUSTO: Global Utilization of Streptokinase and TPA for Occluded Coronary Arteries Trial (1993)
HART: Heparin-Aspirin Reperfusion Trial (Hsia et al, 1990)
Int: International t-PA/Streptokinase Mortality Trial (International Study Group, 1990)
ISIS: First, Second, and Third International Study of Infarct Survival Collaborative Group (ISIS-1, 1986; ISIS-2, 1988; ISIS-3, 1992)
PAIMS: Plasminogen Activator Italian Multicenter Study (Magnani et al, 1989)
RAAMI: Randomized Angiographic Trial of rt-PA in Myocardial Infarction (Carney et al, 1992)
TAMI: Thrombolysis and Angioplasty in Myocardial Infarction (Topol et al, 1987; Bates et al, 1989; Muller et al, 1990; Wall et al, 1992)
TAPS: rt-PA-APSAC Patency Study (Neuhaus et al, 1992)
TIMI Study Group: Thrombolysis in Acute Myocardial Infarction (Chesebro et al, 1987; TIMI Study Group, 1988, 1989)

Mortality Trial) and streptokinase, duteplase (a double chain rt-PA), or anistreplase (ISIS-3) reduced mortality to the same extent. Inclusion of subcutaneous heparin in the regimen had no significant effect on mortality. In contrast, in the GUSTO trial (The GUSTO Investigators, 1993), use of rt-PA saved 10 more lives per 1,000 patients than streptokinase. In this trial, patients were randomly assigned to one of four treatment strategies: (1) streptokinase plus subcutaneous heparin, (2) streptokinase plus intravenous heparin, (3) rt-PA given in accelerated doses plus intravenous heparin, and (4) the combination of rt-PA and streptokinase with intravenous heparin. At 30 days, the mortality rates were 7.2% and 7.4% in patients treated with streptokinase plus subcutaneous or intravenous heparin, respectively, and 6.3% and 7% with the accelerated dose regimen of rt-PA plus intravenous heparin or streptokinase and rt-PA plus intravenous heparin, respectively, four to six hours following onset of symptoms. However, there was an excess of one disabling stroke per 1,000 patients treated with the accelerated dose rt-PA regimen. The majority (70%) of the hemorrhagic strokes were fatal and were included in the mortality data.

Administration of thrombolytic therapy also is beneficial to patients presenting 6 to 12 hours after onset of acute myocardial infarction. The Estudio Multicentrico Estreptoquinasa Republicas de America del Sur (EMERAS) trial revealed a favorable trend in the mortality rate in patients treated with streptokinase 6 to 12 hours after infarction, whereas there was little difference in patients treated with streptokinase or placebo after 13 to 24 hours (EMERAS Collaborative Group, 1993). In the Late Assessment of Thrombolytic Efficacy (LATE) study (LATE Study Group, 1993), patients were randomized to receive rt-PA or placebo 6 to 24 hours after symptom onset. The mortality rate was significantly lower in patients who received rt-PA within 6 to 12 hours than in those who received placebo. However, mortality rates in the placebo and thrombolytic treatment groups were similar when therapy was instituted 12 to 24 hours after the first sign of infarction.

Although patients would still benefit from thrombolytic therapy administered within 12 hours, mortality rates are much lower if thrombolytic therapy is administered at the earliest opportunity. For example, in the GUSTO trial, mortality rates were 4.35% and 5.4% for patients treated with rt-PA and streptokinase, respectively, within two hours of symptom onset, compared with 8.9% and 9.3%, respectively, for those treated within four to six hours (The GUSTO Investigators, 1993). Attempts have been made to reduce the time to initiation of thrombolytic therapy either by treating patients while en route to the hospital or soon after admission. Prehospital thrombolytic therapy administered by paramedics (rt-PA with aspirin and heparin or anistreplase alone) was compared with in-hospital administration (Weaver et al, 1993; The European Myocardial Infarction Project Group, 1993). Although the prehospital group received thrombolytic therapy a median of 33 to 55 minutes earlier than the hospitalized group, no improvement in the mortality rate was associated with initiating treatment before hospital arrival, most probably because most patients in the two groups were treated within two hours of symptom onset. However, patients admitted to other hospitals not participating in thrombolytic trials frequently experienced delays of 50 to 130 minutes (in addition to transit time) before a thrombolytic agent was administered (Sharkey et al, 1989). A "fast track" system in the hospital emergency department could minimize this potentially harmful and avoidable delay (Pell et al, 1992).

The risk of complications, especially bleeding and ischemic stroke, increased with advancing age for those treated with thrombolytic therapy. However, these risks were outweighed by potential benefits. A significantly lower mortality rate was observed in older patients receiving thrombolytic therapy (17.9% compared with 22.1% in those treated with other measures) (Grines and DeMaria, 1990). Similarly, in patients with inferior wall myocardial infarction, the mortality rate was 6.8% with thrombolytics versus 8.7% with placebo.

Patency. The patency rate is a measure of the percentage of patients with open arteries following thrombolytic therapy, as determined by angiography. There appears to be a direct correlation between artery patency and survival. The TIMI classification of reperfusion (grades 0 to 3) in infarct-related arteries is used to define patency (Chesebro et al, 1987): Grade 0 perfusion, no anterograde flow of contrast medium beyond the point of occlusion; grade 1 (minimal perfusion), incomplete around the clot; grade 2 (partial perfusion), complete but delayed perfusion of the distal coronary bed; and grade 3 (complete perfusion), anterograde flow to the entire distal bed at a normal rate.

The ability of the available thrombolytic agents to restore blood flow to infarct-related arteries varies. The early patency rate is lowest with streptokinase and highest with rt-PA given in an accelerated dose regimen (Granger et al, 1992). Using the criteria of TIMI 2 and 3 flows as denoting open arteries and TIMI 0 and 1 as closed ones, the patency rates at 90 minutes for patients treated with streptokinase, anistreplase, urokinase, rt-PA (conventional regimen), and rt-PA (accelerated regimen) were 51%, 70%, 60%, 70%, and 84%, respectively. However, after two to three hours, there was no difference in patency rates (70% to 80%) among the various agents.

The assumption that establishment of TIMI grade 2 flow represents effective recanalization has been challenged, since grade 2 flow may not be sufficient to salvage myocardium and maintain myocardial viability (Lincoff and Topol, 1993). In an analysis of data from the Second Multicenter Thrombolysis Trial of Eminase in Acute Myocardial Infarction (TEAM-2) comparing anistreplase with streptokinase, indexes of infarct size (release of serum enzymes and evolution observed on electrocardiograms) in patients with grade 2 flow 90 to 240 minutes after thrombolysis were comparable to those in patients with grade 0 or 1 flow but were significantly inferior to indexes in patients with grade 3 flow (Karagounis et al, 1992). Similarly, improved outcome, as indicated by ventriculographic, enzymatic, and electrocardiographic indexes, was associated with grade 3 but not grade 2 flow in the TEAM-3 trial in patients treated with anistreplase or rt-PA (Anderson et al, 1993). Direct comparison of rt-PA and streptokinase in the GUSTO trial showed that the percentages of patients with grade 3 flow at 30 minutes were 54%, 29%, and 32% following administration of accelerated rt-PA with intravenous heparin and streptokinase with subcutaneous or intravenous heparin, respectively (The GUSTO Angiographic Investigators, 1993). In addition, in the large cohort of patients prospectively enrolled in four German multicenter randomized thrombolytic trials, the mortality rate among patients with grade 2 flow was essentially the same as that in patients with occluded (grade 0 or 1) arteries and greater than in those with grade 3 flow (Vogt et al, 1993). In the GUSTO trial, the mortality rates at 30 days for patients with grade 0 or 1, grade 2, and grade 3 flows at 90 minutes were 8.9%, 7.4%, and 4.4%, respectively, regardless of thrombolytic treatment (The GUSTO Angiographic Investigators, 1993). Left ventricular function at 90 minutes in those who died within 30 days was consistently worse than in those who were alive after 30 or more days. Thus, TIMI grade 2 and 3 flows are not equivalent and only grade 3 flow should be considered optimal in predicting the survival rate and salvage of myocardial tissues.

Even without thrombolytic therapy, endogenous thrombolysis occurred spontaneously and patency was observed in 20% of patients 90 minutes after symptom onset. After 3 to 21 days, 60% of control or heparin-treated patients exhibited patency in the infarcted vessels. This phenomenon correlates with the observation that t-PA antigen concentrations increase in patients with previous myocardial infarction (Olofssen et al, 1989) and in apparently healthy men who later develop the disease (Ridker et al, 1993). However, the benefit derived from such late occurring and spontaneous reperfusion appears to be limited.

Survival and Patency Enhancement with Anticoagulant and Antiplatelet Agents. Aspirin reduces mortality in patients with acute myocardial infarction. The ISIS-2 trial (1988) studied the effects of administration of streptokinase intravenously for one hour or enteric-coated aspirin orally for one month or both forms of therapy. Combined therapy lowered mortality by 42% compared with 25% for streptokinase alone and 23% for aspirin alone. The effect on survival attributable to aspirin therapy was similar when aspirin was started 0 to 4, 5 to 12, or 13 to 24 hours after symptom onset. Occurrence of nonfatal reinfarction and stroke also was significantly reduced by streptokinase plus aspirin compared with streptokinase alone. This suggests that the effects of streptokinase and aspirin in reducing vascular mortality are additive. In view of these data, aspirin has been recommended as an early adjunctive agent in all patients receiving thrombolytic therapy.

The adjunctive administration of intravenous *heparin* with rt-PA is essential to maintain optimal patency (Prins and Hirsh, 1991). In the Heparin-Aspirin Reperfusion Trial (HART), all patients received rt-PA within four to six hours after onset of myocardial infarction (Hsia et al, 1990). One group received aspirin 80 mg/day and the other group received heparin given intravenously as a 5,000-unit bolus followed by 1,000 units to maintain the activated partial thromboplastin time (APTT) at 1.5 to 2 times normal. Patients underwent cardiac catheterization at 18 hours and again at six to eight days. The patency rate at 18 hours was 82% in patients who received rt-PA with heparin and 52% in those who received rt-PA with aspirin. Similarly, at 55 hours the patency rate was 71% in patients treated with rt-PA and heparin versus 41% in those who received rt-PA and aspirin (Bleich et al, 1990, Hsia et al, 1992). In another study, the patency rate was significantly higher with intravenous heparin (83%) than with placebo (75%) in patients treated with rt-PA and aspirin (de Bono et al, 1992).

The data from these three trials suggest that heparin is needed to sustain the high early patency rates achieved with rt-PA. Since the results of the TAMI-3 study showed that immediate administration of heparin with rt-PA did not result in higher patency rates at 60 to 90 minutes than were achieved with rt-PA alone, it appears that heparin prevents early reocclusion rather than helps rt-PA open vessels (Topol et al, 1989).

Brief versus prolonged heparin therapy was studied in 50 patients receiving rt-PA (Kander et al, 1990). One group received heparin for 24 hours and the other for 72 hours. Patency rates were the same in both groups, but the bleeding rate was 8% in the group receiving heparin for 24 hours versus 24% in those who received it for 72 hours. In the larger (241 patients) National Heart Foundation of Australia Coronary Thrombolysis Group study (1989), all patients received rt-PA followed by intravenous heparin for 24 hours. The patency rate was 80% whether heparin was given for 24 hours or 72 hours. This corresponds to the observation that about one-half of patients who experience reocclusion or reinfarction do so within the first 24 hours. These data suggest that administration of heparin with rt-PA is essential in the first 24 hours to maintain patency rates of 80% and that after 24 to 48 hours, aspirin, but not necessarily heparin, is needed.

It appears to be more important to administer heparin with rt-PA than with streptokinase (Roberts, 1990). Streptokinase is not fibrin-specific, ie, it activates circulating plasminogen as well as plasminogen bound to the clot. As a result, fibrinogen is depleted, and the accompanying increase in fibrin degradation products in turn inhibits platelet aggregation. In contrast, rt-PA, a relatively fibrin-specific agent, activates bound plasminogen but leaves most circulating plasminogen intact. Therefore, the level of fibrin degradation products is much lower and there is a relative lack of inhibitory effect on the platelets. Thus, for the first 2 to 24 hours, heparin may not be as necessary for the prevention of reocclusion in patients receiving streptokinase or other nonspecific thrombolytic agents as it is for those receiving rt-PA.

When used with rt-PA, heparin appears to be more effective when given intravenously than subcutaneously. The GISSI-2 trial (1990) and the International t-PA/Streptokinase Mortality Trial (International Study Group, 1990) compared the efficacy of t-PA and streptokinase with and without heparin, which was administered subcutaneously 12 hours after the start of thrombolytic therapy. These two large-scale trials did not demonstrate any difference in the mortality rates in patients receiving either thrombolytic agent. Similar results were observed in the ISIS-3 trial (1992), even though heparin was administered earlier (four hours after therapy with streptokinase, rt-PA, or anistreplase). In contrast, the mortality rate for patients treated with rt-PA plus intravenous heparin was significantly lower than that with streptokinase plus subcutaneous heparin in the GUSTO trial (The GUSTO Investigators, 1993). If streptokinase plus subcutaneous heparin can be considered the control regimen in all these trials, the combined results suggest that intravenous rather than subcutaneous heparin is essential for rt-PA therapy. However, since rt-PA was administered in an accelerated dose regimen in the GUSTO but not in the ISIS-3 and GISSI-2/International t-PA/Streptokinase Mortality Trial, rt-PA's superiority in reducing the mortality rate could be due to the manner in which rt-PA was delivered, the route of administration of heparin, or both.

A minimum of 12 to 18 hours may be required to produce adequate anticoagulation when heparin is administered subcutaneously (Hull et al, 1986). If heparin is started 4 (ISIS-3) to 12 hours (GISSI-2/International t-PA/Streptokinase Mortality Trial) after initiation of thrombolytic therapy, there are theoretical lag times of 16 to 22 and 24 to 30 hours, respectively, before therapeutic levels are reached. Hence, this route would be expected to have dubious efficacy in patients whose survival may depend on effective lytic therapy followed by maintenance of a patent infarct-vessel.

In the TIMI-5 trial, patients treated with an accelerated dose regimen of rt-PA and aspirin were randomized to receive either *hirudin,* a direct thrombin inhibitor, or heparin, both given in a five-day infusion regimen (Ferguson, 1993). Hirudin appeared to be more effective than heparin in promoting early and sustained grade 3 flow in infarct-related arteries and in reducing the incidence of reocclusion, reinfarction, and mortality up to six weeks following treatment. In addition, bleeding complications were not increased with hirudin. In the TIMI-6 trial, hirudin was compared with heparin in a five-day regimen in patients treated with streptokinase. The mortality and reinfarction rate was 7.7% in hirudin-treated patients compared with 12.5% in those receiving heparin. Thus, hirudin and/or other newer antithrombotic agents may be more efficacious than heparin.

Inhibition of platelet aggregation also can be achieved by a mechanism of receptor blockade that is different from that produced by heparin. On platelet activation, glycoprotein IIb/IIIa, a platelet integrin receptor, binds soluble fibrinogen, von Willebrand factor, and other adhesive proteins that mediate platelet aggregation. The *monoclonal antibody 7E3 Fab* (m7E3 Fab) binds specifically to glycoprotein IIb/IIIa and inhibits platelet aggregation in a dose-dependent manner. In the TAMI 8 Pilot Study, patients presenting within six hours of the onset of myocardial infarction received m7E3 Fab or placebo 3, 6, or 15 hours after administration of rt-PA, intravenous heparin, and aspirin (Kleiman et al, 1993). However, the bolus dose of heparin administered to patients receiving m7E3 Fab at three and six hours after rt-PA was reduced by 50%. Patency rate (grade 2 and 3 flow) at a median range of 121 to 129 hours after administration of m7E3 Fab was substantially increased from 56% (placebo) to 92%. Recurrent ischemic events decreased from 20% (placebo) to 13%. In addition, major bleeding events decreased from 50% (placebo) to 25% because of the decreased dose of heparin used in patients treated with 7E3 Fab.

Administration of heparin in doses sufficient to prolong the APTT to 1.5 to 2 times control also is recommended for acute myocardial infarction in patients not receiving thrombolytic therapy (ACC/AHA Task Force Report, 1990). Heparin infusion is begun on hospital admission and is continued for at least 48 hours. In patients with chronic left ventricular aneurysm, oral anticoagulant (warfarin) therapy should be continued for three months.

Left Ventricular Function. Patients treated with thrombolytic therapy generally have a 3% to 6% increase in ejection fraction compared with placebo recipients (Anderson et al, 1992; Bassand et al, 1991; Voth et al, 1991). Those who are treated within three hours after symptom onset demonstrate a higher left ventricular ejection fraction than those treated later (Kennedy, 1993). The importance of the timing of administration of thrombolytic therapy is reflected in the findings of the Myocardial Infarction, Triage and Intervention (MITI) Prehospital Trial (Weaver et al, 1993). One-half of these patients were treated with rt-PA within 70 minutes of chest pain onset, and their infarct size averaged 5% of left ventricular mass with a corresponding ejection fraction of 53% and a mortality rate of 1.2%. Three-quarters of patients treated within three hours had an infarct size of 10% or less. No infarct zone in the myocardium was detected by thallium SPECT imaging in 40% of these patients at 30 days, even though cardiac enzyme levels had increased. Apparently, the infarct process was aborted with early treatment.

Results of recent trials have shown that rt-PA is more effective in improving left ventricular ejection fraction than anistreplase (Neuhaus et al, 1992) or streptokinase (The GUSTO Angiographic Investigators, 1993), presumably because of the more efficient early thrombolysis and greater myocardial salvage with the accelerated dose regimen of rt-PA.

Reocclusion and Reinfarction. The mortality rate of patients with reocclusion after successful revascularization was twice as high as in those without reocclusion (Ohman et al, 1990). Approximately one-half of the former also had clinical reinfarction. The reocclusion rate generally is higher with rt-PA (13.5%) than with nonfibrin-specific plasminogen activators (8%) (Granger et al, 1992). However, the reinfarction rate with streptokinase and with the accelerated dose regimen of rt-PA was the same (4%) in the GUSTO trial (The GUSTO Investigators, 1993).

Patients with reinfarction after thrombolytic therapy may be treated with supportive care, repeat thrombolytic therapy, or mechanical intervention to re-establish coronary blood flow (Granger et al, 1992). Repeat thrombolytic therapy for threatened reinfarction is frequently effective. Because neutralizing antibodies develop within five days after administration of streptokinase or anistreplase, repeated administration of these agents may be ineffective after that period (White, 1991).

Bleeding and Ischemic Stroke. The most significant side effect of thrombolytic therapy is bleeding, the risk of which is further increased by the concomitant use of aspirin and heparin (Califf et al, 1992). Bleeding may be caused by lysis of a protective hemostatic plug, depletion of clotting factors, and/or loss of vascular integrity. Therapy for life-threatening hemorrhage associated with thrombolytic therapy should include discontinuation of heparin and administration of protamine, cryoprecipitate, and fresh frozen plasma. Platelet transfusion should be considered if bleeding time is prolonged.

Stroke occurs in 1% to 3% of patients with myocardial infarction (Granger et al, 1992). Mortality rates for patients with stroke or intracerebral hemorrhage are 41% and 63%, respectively (Granger et al, 1992). Severe disability occurs in an additional 25% of survivors with intracerebral hemorrhage (Gore et al, 1991). The risk factors for stroke and intracerebral hemorrhage in patients with myocardial infarction are advanced age, hypertension, body weight <65 kg, previous central nervous system dysfunction, and use of an oral anticoagulant. Thrombolytic therapy further increases the risk of intracerebral hemorrhage by 0.3% to 0.9%. In the GISSI-2 (1990), ISIS-3 (1992), and GUSTO (The GUSTO Investigators, 1993) trials, both total stroke and "presumed" intracerebral hemorrhage were more common in patients treated with rt-PA than in those receiving streptokinase. Intracerebral hemorrhage also was more common in patients who received subcutaneous heparin than in those who did not receive heparin (GISSI-2, ISIS-3).

Percutaneous Transluminal Coronary Angioplasty: Percutaneous transluminal coronary angioplasty (PTCA) can restore coronary patency (Oesterle, 1990). In a review of ten studies on its use in patients with acute myocardial infarction without preceding thrombolytic therapy, the average mortality rate in hospitalized patients was 8.3% (Eckman et al, 1992). Poor long-term survival correlated most strongly with a history of previous myocardial infarction, an ejection fraction of <0.4 at discharge, infarct artery occlusion at discharge, and multivessel coronary artery disease.

PTCA, used as primary therapy, was compared with thrombolytic therapy in several randomized trials in patients with evolving myocardial infarction within 6 to 12 hours after the onset of chest pain (Gibbons et al, 1993; Grines et al, 1993; Zijlstra et al, 1993). Immediate angioplasty restored antegrade coronary perfusion in 93% to 98% of patients, and hence was more effective in restoring patency and preventing reocclusion of the infarct-related artery than either rt-PA or streptokinase. Patients who had immediate angioplasty also were more likely to have a patent artery several weeks after infarction and had a lower incidence of recurrent ischemia, reinfarction, and death. There was no difference in myocardial salvage between the two therapies. However, additional data comparing immediate PTCA and thrombolytic therapy are needed to determine whether these observations are valid in larger populations or with the more aggressive accelerated dose rt-PA regimen.

Cardiogenic shock, a condition precipitated by necrosis in >40% of the left ventricular myocardium and caused by ischemia and reinfarction, occurs in 7% of patients with left ventricular myocardial infarction. Standard treatment (coronary care unit monitoring; treatment with vasopressor agents, vasodilators, or inotropic agents; intra-aortic balloon counterpulsation) and thrombolytic therapy have not significantly altered mortality rates in these individuals (Bates and Topol, 1991). However, immediate PTCA can greatly enhance survival in patients with cardiogenic shock and single-vessel disease; restoration of patency appears to be the crucial factor. The mortality rate was reduced from 65% to 80% (historic control) to approximately 40% in these patients. However, no improvement in the mortality rate was observed in patients with multivessel disease and in the elderly (Bates and Topol, 1991; O'Neill, 1992).

Angioplasty performed one to two hours after successful thrombolytic therapy does not further enhance the prognosis of patients with myocardial infarction (Muller and Topol, 1992). It has not improved left ventricular global or regional functional recovery during the early convalescent period following the administration of rt-PA (Topol et al, 1987; TIMI Study Group, 1988; Van de Werf and the European Cooperative Study Group [ECSG], 1988) or streptokinase (Erbel et al, 1989). Furthermore, such treatment is associated with an increase in the incidence of bleeding complications, reocclusion, reinfarction, and the need for emergency coronary artery bypass surgery.

However, "rescue angioplasty" may be useful in selected patients who did not benefit from thrombolytic therapy. In a meta-analysis of 12 studies of rescue angioplasty, overall success rates in achieving artery patency ranged from 71% to 92%, even though there was no detectable improvement in left ventricular function at the time of hospital discharge (Ellis et al, 1992). Reocclusion rates after rescue angioplasty were 14% in patients who did not respond to streptokinase, urokinase, or combination therapy and 24% in patients who did not respond to rt-PA therapy; in comparison, the reocclusion rate was 8% and 13.5% for those who did respond to therapy with streptokinase/urokinase and rt-PA, respectively, without immediate or rescue angioplasty (Ellis et al, 1992; Granger et al, 1992). The high reocclusion rate in patients in whom thrombolytic therapy was unsuccessful may be the result of more extensive fissuring and disruption at the site of acute occlusion and the presence of an intramural, platelet-rich thrombus that is relatively resistant to systemic fibrinolysis. In these individuals, balloon dilation may simply extend the intimal fissure and aggravate an already highly thrombogenic focus.

Even though PTCA is an alternative to thrombolytic therapy in revascularization of patients with myocardial infarction, especially those with cardiogenic shock, the procedure has disadvantages. It can be performed only in hospitals (12% to 18%) where facilities for catheterization and bypass surgery are immediately available. PTCA is contraindicated in patients with multivessel disease, and it may increase the risks in those with severe peripheral vascular disease or diabetic nephropathy.

Coronary Artery Bypass Grafts: Coronary artery bypass grafts (CABG) are sometimes required in patients with acute or recurrent myocardial infarction (Hagar, 1990). Patients with early recurrence of ischemia at rest in spite of medical therapy are candidates for early surgical intervention if they have three-vessel or left main coronary artery disease or other anatomical contraindications to PTCA. Those who did not benefit from PTCA and have large areas of jeopardized myocardium or hemodynamic instability also are candidates. Patients stabilized medically or with inducible ischemia may undergo bypass surgery electively. Including both emergency and elective bypass surgery, 21% of patients in the TAMI trials had the procedure; in the TIMI trials, 10% to 13% of patients, with or without delayed angioplasty, required CABG after thrombolysis; the percentage was higher if PTCA was performed immediately. Operative mortality is increased in patients with poor ventricular function, congestive heart failure, shock, or of advanced age who undergo emergency surgery in the acute phase (Naunheim et al, 1988).

Primary revascularization by CABG in the first hours of infarction also has been performed; mortality rates are acceptable, and long-term results may be better than those obtained when reperfusion does not occur (DeWood et al, 1989); however, no controlled trials have been conducted. The use of CABG for definitive revascularization is impractical for widespread application.

DRUG THERAPY. Beta-Adrenergic Blocking Drugs: During acute myocardial infarction, there is intense stimulation from the central and sympathetic nervous systems. Shortly after coronary occlusion, beta receptors become more numerous and are capable of producing unwanted physiologic responses. All of these adverse effects of high levels of circulating catecholamines can be counteracted by beta blockade, which decreases heart rate, blood pressure, and contractility (Cruickshank, 1990). Beta-adrenergic blocking drugs augment coronary blood flow by lengthening diastolic filling time and increasing collateral blood flow. Some or all of these factors may account for the efficacy of these drugs in acute myocardial infarction.

Results of numerous clinical trials show that the intravenous administration of beta blockers in the absence of thrombolytic therapy and within 12 hours after the onset of myocardial infarction decreases infarct size and controls ventricular arrhythmias (Popma and Topol, 1991).

In ISIS-1 (1986), patients received intravenous atenolol 5 to 10 mg immediately after the infarction, followed by 100 mg/day orally for seven days. Vascular mortality was significantly lower with atenolol than with placebo after seven days and after one year of treatment. Similar findings had been observed with use of intravenous metoprolol 15 mg in the MIAMI (Metoprolol in Acute Myocardial Infarction) research group trial (Miami Trial Research Group, 1985). Analysis of the data from these two trials demonstrated that most of the beneficial effects of atenolol and metoprolol occurred on the first day. A significant proportion of early deaths in patients with myocardial infarction involve cardiac rupture. Early beta blockade may reduce left ventricular wall stress in the noninfarct zone and improve infarct zone motion, thereby decreasing the likelihood of cardiac rupture (Grines et al, 1991).

The TIMI-2B study (TIMI Study Group, 1989; Roberts et al, 1991) assessed the effects of immediate versus deferred beta blocker therapy in patients treated with rt-PA. In the immediate group, metoprolol was given intravenously within two hours after initiating rt-PA and was followed by oral therapy. The patients assigned to the deferred group received oral metoprolol on day 6 following thrombolytic therapy. Immediate and deferred metoprolol therapies were equally effective in improving global and regional left ventricular function and in decreasing the rates of myocardial ischemia and reinfarction. However, intracerebral hemorrhage was reduced in those given immediate metoprolol. The total mortality rate was not altered by immediate beta blocker therapy, but mortality was significantly reduced (from 12% to 5%) in patients who received thrombolytic therapy <2 hours after onset of symptoms. The incidence of recurrent ischemia and reinfarction was reduced as well. The risk of death also may be related to the clinical condition of the patient. Beta blockers significantly reduced mortality during the follow-up period in those who had a high-risk clinical course after infarction (Viscoli et al, 1993).

Thus, beta blockade is useful as adjunctive medical therapy during the process of revascularization. However, because of contraindications (eg, hypotension, bradycardia, reactive airway disease, pulmonary congestion), less than 50% of patients receiving thrombolytic therapy were eligible for beta blockade in the International t-PA/Streptokinase Mortality Trial (International Study Group, 1990).

For a detailed description of individual beta blockers, see the chapter on Beta-Adrenergic Blocking Drugs.

Nitrates: Nitrates also are useful in the treatment of acute myocardial infarction (Jugdutt and Warnica, 1988; Yusuf et al, 1988 A). These agents improve left ventricular function, reduce myocardial oxygen demand, and improve collateral blood flow in patients with acute ischemic injury. Pooled data from ten trials conducted before the advent of thrombolytic therapy showed that the mortality rate among postinfarction patients who received nitroglycerin or nitroprusside was 13% versus 19% in those who received placebo (Yusuf et al, 1988 A). Nitroglycerin is probably more beneficial. This analysis also indicated that intravenous administration of nitroglycerin with careful hemodynamic monitoring for dose adjustment can modify infarct size and reduce early and late mortality. However, recent findings from the GISSI-3 and ISIS-4 trials indicated that nitrates alone given within 35 days to six weeks after acute myocardial infarction did not increase survival. Thus, their use in these patients may require re-evaluation.

Magnesium: Magnesium lowers systemic vascular resistance, dilates coronary arteries, decreases platelet aggregation, improves myocardial metabolism, protects against catecholamine-induced myocardial necrosis, and stabilizes cell membranes (Arsenian, 1993). Magnesium deficiency is associated with intracellular hypokalemia and hypernatremia and augmentation of cell excitability. Autopsy studies on patients who died of myocardial infarction revealed that the intracellular magnesium concentration was lower in both infarcted and noninfarcted myocardial tissues compared with the concentration in those who died of trauma (Speich et al, 1980). In addition, a time-dependent fluctuation of the serum magnesium concentration has been observed during the course of acute myocardial infarction (Giesecke et al, 1986). The serum magnesium concentration increased during the earliest stage of infarction but subsequently declined to a nadir before the creatine kinase enzyme activity peaked. Serum magnesium levels normalized over 24 to 48 hours.

Ventricular arrhythmias occurred more frequently in myocardial infarction patients with low magnesium concentrations. Since administration of magnesium was effective in the treatment of torsades de pointes and some other arrhythmias that are refractory to conventional antiarrhythmic therapy, this agent was tested in patients with myocardial infarction. Pooled data from eight controlled trials showed that intravenous magnesium (30 to 90 mmol) administered within 24 to 48 hours after onset of symptoms decreased ventricular tachycardia and fibrillation by 49% and the incidence of cardiac arrest by 58% in patients who had not been treated with thrombolytics (Horner, 1992). Overall, mortality was reduced by 54% compared with placebo (Horner, 1992). Intravenous magnesium also reduced the mortality rate in patients with suspected myocardial infarction in the second Leicester Intravenous Magnesium Intervention Trial (LIMIT-2) (Woods et al, 1992). Its efficacy was comparable to, but independent of, that of thrombolytic or antiplatelet therapy. In this study, the administration of magnesium was associated with a reduction in the occurrence of heart failure but not of arrhythmias. The efficacy of magnesium in reducing the mortality rate in myocardial infarction patients was challenged by findings from the ISIS-4 trial, which showed that the survival rate was not altered in those treated with magnesium or placebo over a six-month period.

Adverse effects of magnesium include transient flushing and an increase in the incidence of sinus bradycardia.

GUIDELINES FOR PRIMARY THERAPY. The American College of Cardiology/American Heart Association Task Force has issued comprehensive guidelines for management of acute myocardial infarction (ACC/AHA Task Force Report, 1990). In addition, findings from recent trials (eg, GUSTO [1993], LATE [1993]) have provided further refinement.

Criteria for administration of thrombolytic agents are: (1) patients of all ages if no contraindications exist; (2) ST-segment elevation ≥0.1 mV in two of three inferior leads, two contiguous precordial leads, or leads I and aVL or bundle branch block; (3) 20 to 30 minutes of myocardial ischemic pain (not reversed by nitroglycerin); and (4) optimally, less than four to six hours elapsed time from the onset of ischemic pain to thrombolytic therapy, although treatment within 12 hours also is beneficial. Among patients to whom criteria 2 and 3 apply, 99% will have acute myocardial infarction. Thrombolytic therapy may be less effective in patients with

ST-segment depression and in those with unstable angina, since coronary occlusion is more often incomplete in these cases. Heparin and aspirin are recommended in these patients.

No definitive regimen for the administration of any thrombolytic agent was recommended by the ACC/AHA Task Force (1990) (see Table 3 for dosages). However, the accelerated dose regimen is recommended for rt-PA (Neuhaus et al, 1992; The GUSTO Investigators, 1993). For therapy after thrombolysis, the Task Force recommended the administration of intravenous heparin (5,000 units bolus) on initiation of rt-PA therapy with continuation for five days at a dosage sufficient to achieve APTT 1.5 to 2 times the upper limit of normal. It may not be necessary to administer heparin with streptokinase or anistreplase (The GUSTO Investigators, 1993; ISIS-3 Collaborative Group, 1992). Aspirin 160 mg daily should be given immediately and continued thereafter. Early intravenous beta blocker therapy, followed by oral administration, should be considered.

In patients given nitrates, titration of intravenous nitroglycerin should begin with a 15-mcg bolus injection at a pump-controlled infusion rate of 5 to 10 mcg/min (ACC/AHA Task Force Report, 1990). Dosage should be increased by 5 to 10 mcg/min every 5 to 10 minutes, and hemodynamic and clinical responses should be carefully monitored. Doses >200 mcg/min are associated with an increase in the risk of hypotension, and alternative therapy should be considered. The dosage of nitroglycerin should be carefully titrated in patients with inferior wall myocardial infarction (Jugdutt and Warnica, 1988), and this agent should be used with extreme caution, if at all, in patients with suspected right ventricular infarction because of the increased risk of hypotension. Long-acting oral nitrate preparations should not be employed because their effects cannot be terminated rapidly. Topical preparations of nitrates are acceptable. Nitroglycerin should be avoided if marked bradycardia or tachycardia occurs, especially if hypotension is present.

Patients who are stabilized by this initial regimen can be safely monitored in coronary care and step-down units and, if they remain asymptomatic, can undergo limited exercise testing on hospital days 5 to 8 (Hagar, 1990). If the exercise test is negative for ischemia, the patient can be discharged; administration of aspirin and a beta blocker should be continued. Smoking should be avoided. Cardiac catheterization is not obligatory, and patients can receive follow-up exercise testing six weeks after infarction.

If chest pain continues or if the pain initially abates but there is subsequent evidence of severe, spontaneous, recurrent ischemia or if ischemia occurs during the predischarge exercise test, the patient should undergo early coronary arteriography, followed by coronary revascularization with either PTCA or bypass surgery, if feasible, in the hope of reducing the incidence of recurrent ischemic events in the following year.

Secondary Therapy for Myocardial Infarction

Discharge of the patient who survives uncomplicated myocardial infarction typically takes place after six to ten hospital days, and the safety of this practice has been demonstrated repeatedly (Hagar, 1990). Earlier discharge after thrombolysis may be possible in highly selected patients. However, death and/or reinfarction occurs in 5% to 15% of patients in the first year after infarction. Individuals at high risk for recurrent infarction and death, especially those with three-vessel or left main coronary artery disease, must be identified for early intervention. Many factors have been associated with a poor prognosis, but left ventricular dysfunction, severity of coronary artery disease, a large amount of jeopardized myocardium, and early recurrence of ischemia are the most powerful predictors of subsequent cardiac events.

One common strategy for stratifying patients for future therapy is the use of clinical criteria coupled with low-level treadmill exercise data before discharge and symptom-limited maximal exercise data in four to six weeks. However, it should be noted that in a recent study on stabilized patients one to six months after myocardial infarction, noninvasive testing employing electrocardiography during rest, ambulation, and exercise and stress thallium-201 scintigraphy did not consistently identify patients at increased risk for subsequent coronary events (Moss et al, 1993). Patients with complicated infarcts, early recurrence of spontaneous ischemia, previous infarction, or abnormal low-level exercise tests are considered at high risk and are referred for angiography. Inability to complete a low-level exercise test or abnormal hemodynamic response is a better predictor of reinfarction and death than ST-segment depression. Subsequent maximal exercise testing identifies additional patients at increased risk.

In individuals with no abnormalities and normal functional capacity, the one-year mortality rate is approximately 1%; in those with an abnormal test result, the rate is 13%. This prognostic information has additive value beyond clinical assessment alone. With such an approach, coronary angiography is judged appropriate for only about one-half of infarction patients, and those at moderately high risk and extremely low risk are identified. Other strategies and combinations of tests also can be used to stratify patients, depending on clinical signs and the expertise of the physician.

Secondary preventive therapy for postinfarction patients includes nondrug and drug therapy (Goldstein, 1989; Sharpe et al, 1988; Singh, 1990; Yusuf et al, 1988 B).

NONDRUG THERAPY. In the postinfarction patient, intensive efforts should be made to modify coronary risk factors with nondrug treatment (Sytkowski et al, 1990). Progression of the disease and death after infarction are more common among smokers, women, and those with elevated cholesterol levels. Cessation of smoking has reduced mortality in patients after infarction (Rossouw et al, 1990). A decrease in the rate of progression, and in some cases, regression of atherosclerosis also have been observed following ileal bypass surgery (Buchwald et al, 1990). Diabetes and hypertension contribute to increased late mortality as well, and optimal control should be sought. Intensive intervention to reduce risk factors will improve long-term prognosis.

Exercise training of the stable postinfarction patient is intended mainly to avoid the complications of prolonged bed rest and to return the individual to a maximum level of functional capacity following hospital discharge. It hastens the spontaneous improvement in functional capacity that occurs during convalescence and produces further improvement, which is especially beneficial in patients with marked impairment of exercise capacity on predischarge exercise testing. Exercise training programs are clearly safe for the majority of patients, but concern still exists about deleterious effects of early exercise on infarct healing and ventricular remodeling in those with large infarctions. However, in one nonrandomized retrospective study, low levels of physical activity were found to reduce cardiac deaths in a five-year follow-up of 80 men who had survived an infarct (Kitajima et al, 1990).

Education of the postinfarction patient is of great importance. Life-style and dietary changes must be reinforced and guidelines concerning return to work given. Return to work is recommended for patients without marked ischemia or functional impairment. The postdischarge treadmill test is useful to assess disability. Patients may exhibit either excessive anxiety or excessive denial that can hinder their recovery. The physician should be alert for symptoms of depression and social and sexual dysfunction, which are common even after uncomplicated infarction. In addition, compliance is important to ensure the effectiveness of medical treatment. In the Beta Blocker Heart Attack Trial (Horwitz et al, 1990), patients who took ≤75% of prescribed medication were 2.6 times more likely to die within one year than those with a good compliance record, regardless of the severity of the infarct and the presence of risk factors such as smoking and stress. Hence, patient cooperation is imperative.

DRUG THERAPY. Beta-Adrenergic Blocking Agents: Both cardioselective and nonselective beta blockers are effective and safe for long-term secondary prevention after acute myocardial infarction. Analysis of pooled results from 25 trials involving approximately 52,000 patients indicated that the mortality rate was reduced from 9.5% (placebo) to 7.5% (Teo et al, 1993). Results of both the Beta-Blocker Heart Attack (BHAT) Research Group (1982) and the Norwegian timolol study (Norwegian Multicenter Study Group, 1981) indicate that beta blockers (propranolol and timolol) decreased mortality when administered up to six years after an acute myocardial infarction. Mortality also was reduced by long-term beta blockade with propranolol, metoprolol, atenolol, timolol, or nadolol in survivors of acute myocardial infarction without anterograde flow in the infarct artery (Glamann et al, 1991). Beta blockers are especially effective in patients categorized as being at high risk on the basis of recurrent ischemic events, arrhythmias, heart failure, or severe comorbidity during the first year after infarction (Viscoli et al, 1993).

Anticoagulant and Antiplatelet Drugs: Results of ISIS-2 (1988) showed that decreases in mortality (21%) and nonfatal reinfarction (44%) were observed when aspirin was given on the day of myocardial infarction and continued for five weeks thereafter. In patients also treated with streptokinase or rt-PA, the mechanism of action is probably related to aspirin's ability to prevent coronary reocclusion and recurrent ischemia (Roux et al, 1992). A review by the Antiplatelet Trialists' Collaborative Group of all long-term trials of antiplatelet agents for secondary prevention showed that aspirin alone was as effective as aspirin plus another antiplatelet agent (eg, dipyridamole, sulfinpyrazone) (Acheson et al, 1988). In addition, aspirin alone caused fewer side effects. Thus, it appears that aspirin alone may be very effective during the earliest phase of myocardial infarction, during the hyperacute phase, or in those with unstable angina.

The Warfarin Re-infarction Study (Smith et al, 1990) showed that long-term treatment with warfarin in patients who had recovered from acute myocardial infarction resulted in a significant reduction in mortality and reinfarction. The total number of cerebrovascular accidents also was reduced. This finding agrees with pooled results from previous trials (Yusuf et al, 1988 B). A post hoc analysis of the Warfarin Re-Infarction Study indicated that warfarin reduced mortality and reinfarction in patients experiencing their first myocardial infarction but not in those with repeated episodes of infarction (Smith et al, 1992).

Angiotensin-Converting Enzyme (ACE) Inhibitors: ACE inhibitors may play a role in the secondary treatment of myocardial infarction by reducing ventricular enlargement and filling pressures and improving exercise tolerance (Ambrosioni and Borghi, 1989; Jeremy et al, 1989; Sharpe et al, 1988; Pfeffer et al, 1992). In a small number of patients, captopril therapy initiated one to three weeks after the infarct decreased left ventricular end-diastolic volume, prevented further ventricular dilatation, and increased exercise capacity (Pfeffer et al, 1988; Sharpe et al, 1991). Results of the Studies of Left Ventricular Dysfunction (SOLVD) Prevention trial indicated that, compared with placebo, administration of enalapril (initially, 2.5 mg twice daily, titrated to 10 mg twice daily) significantly delayed overt heart failure and reduced the rate of related hospitalizations in patients with ejection fraction ≤0.35 who were not receiving diuretics, digoxin, or vasodilators (The SOLVD Investigators, 1992). The tendency toward mortality from other cardiovascular causes also was reduced in the enalapril group, nearly 80% of whom had a history of myocardial infarction. The beneficial effects occurred as early as six weeks after initiation of therapy and were greatest among patients with the lowest ejection fraction. The incidence of reinfarction or unstable angina in patients who received enalapril for at least six months also was reduced (Yusuf et al, 1992).

In the Survival and Ventricular Enlargement (SAVE) Trial, patients with ejection fraction ≤0.4 but without overt heart failure or symptoms of myocardial ischemia received captopril (initially, 12.5 mg daily, titrated to 25 to 50 mg three times daily) 3 to 16 days after myocardial infarction and were followed for an average of 42 months (Pfeffer et al, 1992). Mortality from all causes was significantly reduced in the captopril group compared with placebo recipients. The incidence of both fatal and nonfatal major cardiovascular events also was consistently reduced. These benefits were observed in patients who did and did not also receive thrombolytics, aspirin, or beta blockers.

In the Cooperative North Scandinavian Enalapril Survival Study II (CONSENSUS II), however, parenteral ACE inhibitor therapy (enalapril) started within 24 hours after the onset of chest pain and followed by oral administration did not improve survival during the 180 days after infarction (Swedberg et al, 1992), even though early treatment (captopril) did attenuate infarct expansion and favorably influence early left ventricular remodeling (Nabel et al, 1991; Oldroyd et al, 1991). The inability of early administration of ACE inhibitors to prolong survival may be related to the increased incidence of hypotension that led to death in some patients following the first dose of the drug (Swedberg et al, 1992).

In the Acute Infarction Ramipril Efficacy (AIRE) Study (1993), survivors of myocardial infarction with clinical evidence of heart failure were randomized to receive ramipril (initially, 2.5 mg twice daily, titrated to 5 mg twice daily) or placebo on day 3 or day 10 after onset of symptoms and were followed for an average of 18 months. Mortality from all causes was significantly lower for patients receiving ramipril (17%) than for those receiving placebo (23%). The incidence of severe or resistant heart failure, reinfarction, and stroke also was reduced. Beneficial effects became apparent as early as 30 days after initiation of drug therapy.

Calcium Channel Blocking Agents: Theoretically, calcium channel blocking agents should protect the myocardium from ischemic injury during acute myocardial infarction because they reduce myocardial oxygen demand by reducing afterload and promote coronary flow to the ischemic area by reducing vasomotor tone and dilating collateral vessels. Ischemia-induced myocardial necrosis may be prevented by reduction of intracellular calcium accumulation. However, results from clinical trials using calcium channel blocking agents have generally been disappointing (Gheorghiade and Goldstein, 1991; Yusuf et al, 1991). In several placebo-controlled trials, including the TRENT study (Wilcox et al, 1986) and the SPRINT I and II trials (Israeli SPRINT Study Group, 1988; Goldbourt et al, 1993), early administration of nifedipine (30 to 60 mg/day) had no effect on the occurrence of sudden death or reinfarction in patients with suspected or confirmed myocardial infarction who had not been treated with thrombolytic therapy. In the TRENT and SPRINT II trials, the mortality rate increased in the nifedipine group at one to six months (Wilcox et al, 1986; Goldbourt et al, 1993). No significant improvement in global left ventricular function, regional wall motion, or infarct size or reduction in the early mortality rate was observed in myocardial infarction patients receiving both thrombolytic and nifedipine therapy (Erbel et al, 1988).

In a multicenter reinfarction study, administration of diltiazem prevented recurrent ischemia and reinfarction but did not improve survival during the first two weeks when given to patients following non-Q-wave myocardial infarction (Gibson et al, 1986). In another double-blind trial on patients who survived either Q-wave or non-Q-wave acute myocardial infarction (Multicenter Diltiazem Postinfarction Trial Research Group, 1988), diltiazem had no significant effect on mortality in either group. Retrospective analysis suggested that mortality was increased in patients with evidence of pulmonary congestion and might have been reduced significantly in those without pulmonary congestion. The effect of diltiazem is in marked contrast to that of beta blockers in which the benefit was evident at all levels of function and appeared to be greater in individuals with cardiomegaly and pulmonary congestion.

The Danish Study Group found no difference in 12-month mortality or 6-month reinfarction rate in 1,436 patients given verapamil or placebo (Danish Study Group on Verapamil in Myocardial Infarction, 1990); however, a subset of patients with incomplete occlusion and/or good collateral circulation and no signs or symptoms of heart failure appeared to benefit from this drug.

In summary, no study to date has conclusively demonstrated that administration of any calcium channel blocking agent reduces mortality after acute myocardial infarction. Morbidity (eg, reinfarction, postinfarction angina) may be reduced with diltiazem or verapamil in a small subset of patients at low risk (eg, with no signs of heart failure). Results of several studies suggest that there is an increase in the risk of mortality when nifedipine is used or when either diltiazem or verapamil is given to high-risk patients. It remains unclear why calcium channel blocking agents do not reduce this risk. One explanation is that they lower blood pressure and cause reflex activation of the sympathetic nervous system and the angiotensin-renin system.

Antiarrhythmic Agents: A number of drugs have been tested for the prevention of ventricular fibrillation, which is common in the hours immediately following myocardial infarction. Class 1 antiarrhythmic agents (Class 1A, 1B, and 1C) increased the risk of death in patients treated with these agents prophylactically after myocardial infarction (Teo et al, 1993). A meta-analysis of 808 patients participating in six trials of quinidine (Class 1A) for control of atrial fibrillation showed that there was a threefold increase in total mortality in those receiving quinidine versus placebo (Morganroth and Goin, 1991). Lidocaine (Class 1B) is clearly effective in the treatment of almost all life-threatening arrhythmias that occur with acute myocardial infarctions (Antman and Berlin, 1992), but the survival rate has not been improved (Teo et al, 1993). An increased mortality rate also was observed in postinfarction patients treated with mexiletine (Class 1B) compared with placebo, and this agent has modest potential for suppressing ventricular premature contractions and causes many noncardiac side effects.

It has been widely believed that the occurrence of high-density or complex premature ventricular contractions following acute myocardial infarction is an independent predictor of sudden cardiac death. A logical corollary is the presumption that the suppression of such arrhythmias will eliminate the trigger mechanisms of ventricular tachycardia and fibrillation. In the Cardiac Arrhythmia Suppression Trial (CAST) Investigation (1989), three Class 1C agents, flecainide, encainide, and moricizine, were found to suppress premature ventricular contractions. However, mortality rates from all causes and from arrhythmia in the group treated with placebo were lower than those in the group treated with encainide or flecainide (Echt et al, 1991). Administration of moricizine also was associated with an excessive number of deaths during the first and second week of administration and with an increase in the long-term rate of occurrence of adverse cardiac events (The Cardiac Arrhythmia Suppression Trial II Investigators, 1992). One possible explanation for the increase in mortality associated with use of these Class 1C antiarrhythmic agents is the interaction between drug treatment and ischemia or autonomic nervous activity (Morganroth and Bigger, 1990). (For detailed information on these agents, see the chapter on Antiarrhythmic Drugs.)

Thus, Class 1 antiarrhythmic drugs should not be prescribed for prophylaxis in asymptomatic patients with potentially malignant ventricular arrhythmias. In patients whose symptoms must be alleviated because of lifestyle-limiting effects, beta blocker therapy should be initiated if these drugs are not already being used. The advisability of the use of antiarrhythmic agents other than beta blockers is unclear at this time. However, results from eight randomized trials of amiodarone showed that the overall mortality rate was reduced from 13% (placebo) to 9.9% (amiodarone) in patients with ventricular arrhythmias during and after myocardial infarction (Teo et al, 1993). Further trials are needed to confirm the beneficial effects of amiodarone.

GUIDELINES FOR SECONDARY THERAPY. Beta blockers should be given intravenously to ensure rapid onset of action as early as possible after the appearance of symptoms. Use of an oral preparation for maintenance therapy should begin within the first few days after infarction and continue for at least two years (ACC/AHA Task Force Report, 1990). ACE inhibitors also should be considered, especially in patients with low ejection fractions (<0.35 to 0.4).

To prevent reocclusion after thrombolysis and to avert early and late reinfarction, long-term aspirin therapy to inhibit platelet aggregation should be given to all patients who can tolerate it. Aspirin should be given as soon after admission as possible and continued for at least several years in doses of 160 to 325 mg/day. In the subgroup of patients with a large anterior myocardial infarction, warfarin may be needed to prevent systemic emboli and is beneficial for the prevention of early and late reinfarction. In this group, it may be reasonable to postpone the use of aspirin until anticoagulants are discontinued after the risk of emboli has ceased.

Drug Evaluations

THROMBOLYTIC AGENTS

Currently available thrombolytic agents include rt-PA (alteplase [Activase]), streptokinase [Kabikinase, Streptase], anistreplase (APSAC [Eminase]), and urokinase [Abbokinase]. These agents act at different points in the fibrinolytic system. The mechanism of action of rt-PA is the same as that of endogenous tissue plasminogen activator. Streptokinase, a bacterial protease, combines with both fibrin-bound and circulating plasminogen to form an active complex that activates other plasminogen and leads to degradation of both fibrin and fibrinogen. Anistreplase is initially inactive, binds to fibrin, and is then deacylated to the active complex. Urokinase activates plasminogen directly. It is not antigenic and produces a slightly less severe lytic state than does streptokinase. Its inactive precursor, scu-PA, is converted to urokinase by plasmin.

Results of the GUSTO trial demonstrated that the accelerated dose regimen of rt-PA (administered within six hours of symptom onset) was more effective than streptokinase in reducing mortality and improving ventricular function (The GUSTO Investigators, 1993; The GUSTO Angiographic Investigators, 1993). The different characteristics of thrombolytic agents are compared in Table 3.

TABLE 3.
COMPARISON OF THROMBOLYTIC AGENTS*

	SK	APSAC	UK	rt-PA
Alpha phase half-life (min)	23	90	16	5
IV dose	1.5 × 10⁶ IU over 0.5-1 hr	30 units bolus over 2-5 min	3 × 10⁶ IU total: 1.5 × 10⁶ IU bolus over 2-5 min, followed by 1.5 × 10⁶ IU over 1 hr	100 mg total: 15 mg bolus, 50 mg/30 min, then 35 mg/hr
Reperfusion rate in 90 min (%)	50-60	60-70	60	70-80
Reocclusion rate (%)	5-10	5-10	10	10-20
Antigenicity	yes	yes	no	no
With IV heparin therapy	no	no	no	yes
Cost (US$) †	313	1,700	2,200	2,200

* *SK: streptokinase; APSAC: anistreplase; UK: urokinase; rt-PA: alteplase (recombinant human tissue plasminogen activator)*

† *as of September 1993.*

ADVERSE REACTIONS AND PRECAUTIONS. Streptokinase and anistreplase induce hypotension with rapid infusion and occasionally cause allergic phenomena and some level of antibody-mediated resistance if administered a second time within one to three years. Systemic fibrinogenolysis is severe and lasts 12 to 48 hours with streptokinase, anistreplase, and urokinase; it is mild with rt-PA.

Major bleeding, especially cerebral, is the most serious complication of thrombolytic therapy. While fibrin-specific agents produce little systemic lytic effect, major bleeding complications caused by disruption of hemostatic plugs can develop at the sites of invasive procedures, in the central nervous system, and elsewhere. In studies in which invasive procedures were employed in the protocol, bleeding episodes occurred in most patients and transfusion was required in 11% to 30% of those receiving thrombolytic therapy (TAMI, TIMI-1). Administration of heparin simultaneously with infusion of the thrombolytic agent also predisposes to an increase in bleeding. When invasive procedures are minimized, bleeding episodes are uncommon; the incidence of any bleeding episode can be expected to be 3.5% to 5% (GISSI-1, 1986; ISIS-2, 1988), and transfusion will be required in 0.3% to 0.5% of patients.

The incidence of intracerebral bleeding varied from 0.1% and 0.2% in the ISIS-2 (1988) and GISSI-1 (1986) trials, respectively, to 0.5% in the TIMI-2 trial (1989) in patients receiving rt-PA 100 mg and 1.9% in the subset of patients treated with rt-PA 150 mg. In the GUSTO trial, the rates of severe or life-threatening bleeding in patients treated with the accelerated dose regimen of rt-PA plus intravenous heparin or with streptokinase plus intravenous or subcutaneous heparin were 0.4%, 0.5%, and 0.3%, respectively (The GUSTO Investigators, 1993). Hypertension, advanced age, and previous cerebrovascular disease are risk factors for intracerebral hemorrhage, which is usually catastrophic. In ISIS-2 (1988) and other trials, the incidence of stroke in control and treated patients was equal because, although intracranial hemorrhage increased with treatment, the incidence of thrombotic and embolic stroke was reduced.

Thrombolytic therapy is contraindicated in any condition that predisposes to major bleeding (Hagar, 1990). Hypotension usually can be controlled rapidly; if not, thrombolytic therapy is contraindicated. Cardiopulmonary resuscitation does not increase bleeding risk if it is brief (<1 minute) and without significant trauma.

Reocclusion, reinfarction, and recurrent ischemia after thrombolytic therapy are significant complications (see Table 1). The incidence of reocclusion after thrombolysis is approximately 3% to 8% within the first 24 hours and 8% to 20% overall during hospitalization. Rethrombosis appears to be related to the adequacy of thrombolysis and the residual minimal diameter of the infarct-related artery at 90 minutes. In rethrombosis due to anchored residual thrombus, most of the residual thrombus produces a persistent stenosis that alters the rheology of blood flow. This tends to produce a thrombogenic substrate that may be even more thrombogenic than the deeply injured arterial wall. Vasoconstriction of the artery also contributes to the severity of residual stenosis after acute arterial injury. In experimental studies, vasodilation produced by nifedipine or verapamil did not decrease platelet deposition. Vasodilation with other drugs, such as receptor blockers for serotonin or thromboxane A_2, significantly reduced vasoconstriction but did not affect platelet deposition in the presence of deep arterial injury.

At 90 minutes after reperfusion of an affected artery, residual thrombus is frequently observed trailing distally beyond the area of stenosis. This resolves within the following 24 hours in about 50% of patients, but it may persist throughout most of the hospitalization period in others. In addition, anticoagulant therapy further reduces residual stenosis and increases the luminal diameter of the artery between the time of lysis and hospital discharge. Most investigators employ both heparin and aspirin during and after thrombolysis (Acheson et al, 1988; ACC/AHA Task Force Report, 1990). (For detailed information on individual thrombolytic agents, see the chapter on Thrombolytics.)

DOSAGE. See Table 3.

BETA-ADRENERGIC BLOCKING AGENTS

Beta blockers reduce the risk of short- and long-term mortality after acute myocardial infarction and can abort threatened infarction. They decrease myocardial oxygen demand by reducing cardiac work and counteract the myocardial effects of high levels of circulating catecholamines and increased number of beta-adrenergic receptors. They also may improve oxygenation of ischemic tissue. Their early intravenous use with continuing oral administration is more likely to decrease mortality than either regimen alone (Goldstein, 1989). Agents without intrinsic sympathomimetic activity are probably more effective for relief of ischemia and prevention of arrhythmias.

For detailed information on individual beta-adrenergic blocking agents, see the chapter on Beta-Adrenergic Blocking Drugs.

ADVERSE REACTIONS AND PRECAUTIONS. Adverse reactions to beta blockade include heart failure, heart block, hypotension, cardiogenic shock, severe bradycardia, and bronchospasm; therefore, these drugs are contraindicated in patients with congestive heart failure or AV block.

DOSAGE.
Oral: Currently recommended regimens after initial intravenous administration include timolol 20 mg, propranolol 180 to 240 mg, and metoprolol 200 mg daily in divided doses and atenolol 100 mg daily. However, the dosage should be individualized, especially in elderly patients and those with other complications.

PREPARATIONS. See the chapter on Beta-Adrenergic Blocking Drugs.

ANGIOTENSIN-CONVERTING ENZYME INHIBITORS

ACE inhibitors are used in the secondary prevention of myocardial infarction. These drugs block the conversion of angiotensin I to angiotensin II by inhibiting angiotensin-converting enzyme. They also inhibit degradation of the vasodilator, bradykinin. ACE inhibitors are presumed to exert their action on the tissue angiotensin systems in the vasculature and myocardium (Frohlich, 1989).

The functions of the renin-angiotensin-aldosterone system and the actions of the individual ACE inhibitors are discussed in detail in the chapter, Angiotensin-Converting Enzyme Inhibitors.

ADVERSE REACTIONS AND PRECAUTIONS. Rash, taste disturbances, and cough (most common) are frequent side effects of ACE inhibitors. The initial dose may cause a precipitous, symptomatic fall in blood pressure, especially in volume-depleted patients and in those with high-grade bilateral renal artery stenosis. The hypotensive effect of lisinopril and enalapril may be prolonged.

DOSAGE.
Oral: Currently recommended regimens include captopril, initially, 12.5 mg daily titrated to 25 to 50 mg three times daily; enalapril, initially, 2.5 mg twice daily titrated to 10 mg twice

daily; and ramipril, initially, 2.5 mg twice daily titrated to 5 mg twice daily.

PREPARATIONS. See the chapter on Angiotensin-Converting Enzyme Inhibitors.

Cited References

ACC/AHA Task Force Report: Guidelines for the early management of patients with acute myocardial infarction. *J Am Coll Cardiol* 16:249-292, 1990.

Acheson J, et al: Secondary prevention of vascular disease by prolonged antiplatelet treatment: Antiplatelet trialists' collaboration. *BMJ* 296:320-321, 1988.

The Acute Infarction Ramipril Efficacy (AIRE) Study Investigators: Effect of ramipril on mortality and morbidity of survivors of acute myocardial infarction with clinical evidence of heart failure. *Lancet* 342:821-828, 1993.

Adams JE III, et al: Biochemical markers of myocardial injury: Is MB creatine kinase the choice for the 1990s? *Circulation* 88:750-763, 1993 A.

Adams JE III, et al: Cardiac troponin I: A marker with high specificity for cardiac injury. *Circulation* 88:101-106, 1993 B.

AIMS Trial Study Group: Effect of intravenous APSAC on mortality after acute myocardial infarction: Primary report of a placebo-controlled clinical trial. *Lancet* 1:545-549, 1988.

AIMS Trial Study Group: Long-term effects of intravenous anistreplase in acute myocardial infarction: Final report of the AIMS study. *Lancet* 335:427-431, 1990.

Ambrosioni E, Borghi C: Potential use of ACE-inhibitors after acute myocardial infarction. *J Cardiovasc Pharmacol* 14 (suppl 1):S92-S94, 1989.

American Heart Association: *1989 Heart Facts*. Dallas, American Heart Association National Center, 1988.

Anderson JL, et al: Anistreplase versus alteplase in acute myocardial infarction: Comparative effects on left ventricular function, morbidity, and 1-day coronary artery patency. *J Am Coll Cardiol* 20:753-766, 1992.

Anderson JL, et al: TIMI perfusion grade 3 but not grade 2 results in improved outcome after thrombolysis for myocardial infarction: Ventriculographic, enzymatic, and electrocardiographic evidence from the TEAM-3 study. *Circulation* 87:1829-1839, 1993.

Antman EM, Berlin JA: Declining incidence of ventricular fibrillation in myocardial infarction: Implications for the prophylactic use of lidocaine. *Circulation* 86:764-773, 1992.

Arnold AER, et al: Recombinant tissue-type plasminogen activator and immediate angioplasty in acute myocardial infarction: One-year follow-up. *Circulation* 86:111-120, 1992.

Arsenian MA: Magnesium and cardiovascular disease. *Prog Cardiovasc Dis* 35:271-310, 1993.

Bassand J-P, et al: Comparative effects of APSAC and rt-PA on infarct size and left ventricular function in acute myocardial infarction: A multicenter randomized study. *Circulation* 84:1107-1117, 1991.

Bates ER, Topol EJ: Limitations of thrombolytic therapy for acute myocardial infarction complicated by congestive heart failure and cardiogenic shock. *J Am Coll Cardiol* 18:1077-1084, 1991.

Bates ER, et al: Thrombolysis and Angioplasty in Myocardial Infarction (TAMI-I) Trial: Influence of infarct location on arterial patency, left ventricular function and mortality. *J Am Coll Cardiol* 13:12-18, 1989.

Beta-Blocker Heart Attack Trial (BHAT) Research Group: Randomized trial of propranolol in patients with acute myocardial infarction. *JAMA* 247:1707-1714, 1982.

Bleich SD, et al: Effect of heparin on coronary arterial patency after thrombolysis with tissue plasminogen activator in acute myocardial infarction. *Am J Cardiol* 66:1412-1417, 1990.

Bodor GS, et al: The development of monoclonal antibodies and an assay for cardiac troponin-I with preliminary results in suspected myocardial infarction. *Clin Chem* 11:2203-2214, 1992.

Braunwald E, Kloner RA: The stunned myocardium: Prolonged postischemic ventricular dysfunction. *Circulation* 66:1146-1149, 1982.

Braunwald E, Rutherford JD: Reversible ischemic left ventricular dysfunction: Evidence for the "hibernating myocardium." *J Am Coll Cardiol* 81:1467-1470, 1986.

Buchwald H, et al: Effect of partial ileal bypass surgery on mortality and morbidity from coronary heart disease in patients with hypercholesterolemia. *N Engl J Med* 323:946-955, 1990.

Califf RM, et al: Clinical risks of thrombolytic therapy. *Am J Cardiol* 69:12A-20A, 1992.

Cardiac Arrhythmia Suppression Trial (CAST) Investigation: Preliminary report: Effect of encainide and flecainide on mortality in randomized trial of arrhythmia suppression after myocardial infarction. *N Engl J Med* 321:406-412, 1989.

Cardiac Arrhythmia Suppression Trial II Investigators: Effect of the antiarrhythmic agent moricizine on survival after myocardial infarction. *N Engl J Med* 327:227-233, 1992.

Carney RJ, et al: Randomized angiographic trial of recombinant tissue-type plasminogen activator (alteplase) in myocardial infarction. *J Am Coll Cardiol* 20:17-23, 1992.

Chesebro JH, et al: Thrombolysis in Acute Myocardial Infarction (TIMI) Trial, Phase I: A comparison between intravenous tissue plasminogen activator and intravenous streptokinase: Clinical findings through hospital discharge. *Circulation* 76:142-154, 1987.

Chesebro JH, et al: New approaches to treatment of myocardial infarction. *Am J Cardiol* 65:12C-19C, 1990.

Cohen MC, Muller JE: Onset of acute myocardial infarction–circadian variation and triggers. *Cardiovasc Res* 26:831-838, 1992.

Cohn PF: Silent myocardial infarction in patients with a defective anginal warning system. *Am J Cardiol* 45:697-702, 1980.

Cruickshank JM: The role of beta blockers in preventing heart attacks and catecholamine-induced cardiovascular damage. *Cardiovasc Rev Rep* 11:10-13, 1990.

Cummins B, et al: Cardiac-specific troponin-I radioimmunoassay in the diagnosis of acute myocardial infarction. *Am Heart J* 113:1333-1344, 1987.

Danish Study Group on Verapamil in Myocardial Infarction: Effect of verapamil on mortality and major events after acute myocardial infarction (The Danish Verapamil Infarction Trial II-DAVIT II). *Am J Cardiol* 66:779-785, 1990.

de Bono DP, et al: Effect of early intravenous heparin on coronary patency, infarct size, and bleeding complications after alteplase thrombolysis: Results of a randomized double blind European Cooperative Study Group trial. *Br Heart J* 67:122-128, 1992.

DeWood MA, et al: Medical and surgical management of early Q wave myocardial infarction, I: Effect of surgical revascularization on survival, recurrent myocardial infarction, sudden death and functional class at 10 or more years of follow-up. II: Effects on mortality and global and regional left ventricular function at 10 or more years of follow-up. *J Am Coll Cardiol* 14:65-77, 1989.

Echt DS, et al: Mortality and morbidity in patients receiving encainide, flecainide, or placebo: The Cardiac Arrhythmia Suppression Trial. *N Engl J Med* 324:781-788, 1991.

Eckman MH, et al: Direct angioplasty for acute myocardial infarction: A review of outcomes in clinical subsets. *Ann Intern Med* 117:667-676, 1992.

Ellis SG, et al: Present status of rescue coronary angioplasty: Current polarization of opinion and randomized trials. *J Am Coll Cardiol* 19:681-686, 1992.

EMERAS (Estudio Multicéntrico Estreptoquinasa Repúblicas de América del Sur) Collaborative Group: Randomised trial of late thrombolysis in patients with suspected acute myocardial infarction. *Lancet* 342:767-772, 1993.

Erbel R, et al: Combination of calcium channel blocker and thrombolytic therapy in acute myocardial infarction. *Am Heart J* 115:529-538, 1988.

Erbel R, et al: Long-term results of thrombolytic therapy with and without percutaneous transluminal coronary angioplasty. *J Am Coll Cardiol* 14:276-285, 1989.

The European Myocardial Infarction Project Group: Prehospital thrombolytic therapy in patients with suspected acute myocardial infarction. *N Engl J Med* 329:383-389, 1993.

Ferguson JJ III: Meeting highlights. *Circulation* 88:6-10, 1993.

Frohlich ED: Clinical and physiologic significance of local tissue renin-angiotensin systems. *Am J Med* 87 (suppl 6B):19-23, 1989.

Garabedian HD, et al: Detection of coronary artery reperfusion with creatine kinase-MB determination during thrombolytic therapy: Correlation with acute angiography. *J Am Coll Cardiol* 11:729-734, 1988.

Gersh BJ, Anderson JL: Thrombolysis and myocardial salvage: Results of clinical trials and the animal paradigm—paradoxic or predictable? *Circulation* 88:296-306, 1993.

Gheorghiade M, Goldstein S: Calcium-channel blockers in postmyocardial infarction patients with special notation to the Danish Verapamil Infarction Trial II. *Prog Cardiovasc Dis* 34:37-43, 1991.

Gibbons RJ, et al: Immediate angioplasty compared with the administration of a thrombolytic agent followed by conservative treatment for myocardial infarction. *N Engl J Med* 328:685-691, 1993.

Gibson RS, et al: Diltiazem and reinfarction in patients with non-Q-wave myocardial infarction: Results of a double-blind, randomized, multicenter trial. *N Engl J Med* 315:423-429, 1986.

Giesecke D, et al: Serum-magnesium konzentration bei myocardinfarct. *Klin Wochenschr* 64:1003-1012, 1986.

Glamann DB, et al: Beneficial effect of long-term beta blockade after acute myocardial infarction in patients without anterograde flow in the infarct artery. *Am J Cardiol* 68:150-154, 1991.

Glazier JJ, et al: Importance of generalized defective perception of painful stimuli as a cause of silent myocardial ischemia in chronic stable angina pectoris. *Am J Cardiol* 58:667-672, 1986.

Goldbourt U, et al: Early administration of nifedipine in suspected acute myocardial infarction: The Second Prevention Reinfarction Israel Nifedipine Trial 2 Study. *Arch Intern Med* 153:345-353, 1993.

Goldstein S: Drug therapy for practical cardioprotection after acute myocardial infarction. *Cardiovasc Rev Rep* 10:21-24, 1989.

Gore JM, et al: Intracerebral hemorrhage, cerebral infarction, and subdural hematoma after acute myocardial infarction and thrombolytic therapy in the thrombolysis in myocardial infarction study. *Circulation* 83:448-459, 1991.

Granger CB, et al: Thrombolytic therapy for acute myocardial infarction: A review. *Drugs* 44:293-325, 1992.

Grimm R, et al: Unrecognized myocardial infarction: Experience in the Multiple Risk Factor Intervention Trial (MRFIT). *Circulation* 75 (suppl II):II-6-II-8, 1987.

Grines CL, DeMaria AN: Optimal utilization of thrombolytic therapy for acute myocardial infarction: Concepts and controversies. *J Am Coll Cardiol* 16:223-231, 1990.

Grines CL, et al: Acute effects of parenteral beta-blockade on regional ventricular function of infarct and noninfarct zones after reperfusion therapy in humans. *J Am Coll Cardiol* 17:1382-1387, 1991.

Grines CL, et al: A comparison of immediate angioplasty with thrombolytic therapy for acute myocardial infarction. *N Engl J Med* 328:673-679, 1993.

Gruppo Italiana per lo Studio della Sopravvivenza nell'Infarto Miocardico: GISSI-2: A factorial randomized trial of alteplase versus streptokinase and heparin versus no heparin among 12,490 patients with acute myocardial infarction. *Lancet* 336:65-71, 1990.

Gruppo Italiana per lo Studio della Streptochinasi nell'Infarto Miocardico (GISSI-1): Effectiveness of intravenous thrombolytic treatment in acute myocardial infarction. *Lancet* 1:349-360, 1986.

The GUSTO Angiographic Investigators: The effects of tissue plasminogen activator, streptokinase, or both on coronary-artery patency, ventricular function, and survival after acute myocardial infarction. *N Engl J Med* 329:1615-1622, 1993.

The GUSTO Investigators: An international randomized trial comparing four thrombolytic strategies for acute myocardial infarction. *N Engl J Med* 329:673-682, 1993.

Hagar JM: The guide to cardiology: Acute myocardial infarction. *Cardiovasc Rev Rep* 11:39-67, 1990.

Horner SM: Efficacy of intravenous magnesium in acute myocardial infarction in reducing arrhythmias and mortality: Meta-analysis of magnesium in acute myocardial infarction. *Circulation* 86:774-779, 1992.

Horwitz RI, et al: Treatment adherence and risk of death after a myocardial infarction. *Lancet* 336:542-545, 1990.

Hsia J, et al: A comparison between heparin and low-dose aspirin as adjunctive therapy with tissue plasminogen activator for acute myocardial infarction. *N Engl J Med* 323:1433-1437, 1990.

Hsia J, et al: Heparin-induced prolongation of partial thromboplastin time after thrombolysis: Relation to coronary artery patency. *J Am Coll Cardiol* 20:31-35, 1992.

Hull RD, et al: Continuous intravenous heparin compared with intermittent subcutaneous heparin in the initial treatment of proximal vein thrombosis. *N Engl J Med* 315:1109-1119, 1986.

International Study Group: In-hospital mortality and clinical course of 20,891 patients with suspected acute myocardial infarction randomized between alteplase and streptokinase with or without heparin. *Lancet* 336:71-75, 1990.

ISIS-1 (First International Study of Infarct Survival) Collaborative Group: Randomized trial of intravenous atenolol among 16,027 cases of suspected acute myocardial infarction: ISIS-1. *Lancet* 2:57-66, 1986.

ISIS-2 (Second International Study of Infarct Survival) Collaborative Group: Randomized trial of intravenous streptokinase, oral aspirin, both, or neither among 17,187 cases of suspected acute myocardial infarction: ISIS-2. *Lancet* 2:349-360, 1988.

ISIS-3 (Third International Study of Infarct Survival) Collaborative Group: ISIS-3: A randomised comparison of streptokinase *vs* tissue plasminogen activator *vs* anistreplase and of aspirin plus heparin *vs* aspirin alone among 41,299 cases of suspected acute myocardial infarction. *Lancet* 339:753-770, 1992.

Israeli SPRINT Study Group: Secondary Prevention Reinfarction Israeli Nifedipine Trial (SPRINT): A randomized intervention trial of nifedipine in patients with acute myocardial infarction. *Eur Heart J* 9:354-364, 1988.

Jennings RB, Reimer KA: Pathobiology of acute myocardial ischemia. *Hosp Pract* 24 (No 1):89-107, 1989.

Jeremy RW, et al: Patterns of left ventricular dilatation during the six months after myocardial infarction. *J Am Coll Cardiol* 13:304-310, 1989.

Jugdutt BI, Warnica JW: Intravenous nitroglycerin therapy to limit myocardial infarct size, expansion, and complications: Effect of timing, dosage, and infarct location. *Circulation* 78:906-919, 1988.

Kander NH, et al: A randomized pilot trial of brief versus prolonged heparin after successful reperfusion in acute myocardial infarction. *Am J Cardiol* 65:139-142, 1990.

Kannel WB, et al: Incidence and prognosis of unrecognized myocardial infarction: An update on the Framingham Study. *N Engl J Med* 311:1144-1147, 1984.

Karagounis L, et al: Does thrombolysis in myocardial infarction (TIMI) perfusion grade 2 represent a mostly patent artery or a mostly occluded artery? Enzymatic and electrocardiographic evidence from the TEAM-2 study. *J Am Coll Cardiol* 19:1-10, 1992.

Kennedy JW: Limiting the size of myocardial infarction by early coronary artery reperfusion. *Heart Dis Stroke* 2:93-97, 1993.

Kitajima K, et al: Prognostic significance of daily physical activity after first acute myocardial infarction. *Am Heart J* 119:1193-1194, 1990.

Kleiman NS, et al: Profound inhibition of platelet aggregation with monoclonal antibody 7E3 Fab after thrombolytic therapy: Results of the Thrombolysis and Angioplasty in Myocardial Infarction (TAMI) 8 Pilot Study. *J Am Coll Cardiol* 22:381-389, 1993.

Kloner RA: The cardiac history. *Cardiovasc Rev Rep* 10:20-23, 1989.

LATE Study Group: Late Assessment of Thrombolytic Efficacy (LATE) study with alteplase 6-24 hours after onset of acute myocardial infarction. *Lancet* 342:759-766, 1993.

Lavie CJ, Gersh BJ: Mechanical and electrical complications of acute myocardial infarction. *Mayo Clin Proc* 65:709-730, 1990.

Lincoff AM, Topol EJ: Illusion of reperfusion: Does anyone achieve optimal reperfusion during acute myocardial infar*tion* 87:1792-1805, 1993.

Magnani B, et al: Plasminogen Activator Italian Multicenter Study (PAIMS): Comparison of intravenous recombinant single-chain human tissue-type plasminogen activator (rt-PA) with intravenous streptokinase in acute myocardial infarction. *J Am Coll Cardiol* 13:19-26, 1989.

MIAMI Trial Research Group: A randomized placebo-controlled international trial. *Eur Heart J* 6:199-226, 1985.

Morganroth J, Bigger JT Jr: Pharmacologic management of ventricular arrhythmias after the Cardiac Arrhythmia Suppression Trial, editorial. *Am J Cardiol* 65:1497-1503, 1990.

Morganroth J, Goin JE: Quinidine-related mortality in the short-to-medium-term treatment of ventricular arrhythmias: A meta-analysis. *Circulation* 84:1977-1983, 1991.

Moss AJ, et al: Detection and significance of myocardial ischemia in stable patients after recovery from an acute coronary event. *JAMA* 269:2379-2385, 1993.

Muller DWM, Topol EJ: Thrombolytic therapy: Adjuvant mechanical intervention for acute myocardial infarction. *Am J Cardiol* 69:60A-70A, 1992.

Muller DWM, et al (TAMI): Two-year outcome after angiographically documented myocardial reperfusion for acute coronary occlusion. *Am J Cardiol* 66:796-801, 1990.

Multicenter Diltiazem Postinfarction Trial Research Group: The effect of diltiazem on mortality and reinfarction after myocardial infarction. *N Engl J Med* 319:385-392, 1988.

Murray N, et al: What proportion of patients with myocardial infarction are suitable for thrombolysis? *Br Heart J* 57:144-147, 1987.

Nabel EG, et al: A randomized placebo-controlled trial of combined early intravenous captopril and recombinant tissue-type plasminogen activator therapy in acute myocardial infarction. *J Am Coll Cardiol* 17:467-473, 1991.

Nadelmann J, et al: Prevalence, incidence and prognosis of recognized and unrecognized myocardial infarction in persons aged 75 years or older: The Bronx Aging Study. *Am J Cardiol* 66:533-537, 1990.

National Heart Foundation of Australia Coronary Thrombolysis Group: A randomized comparison of oral aspirin/dipyridamole versus intravenous heparin after rt-PA for acute myocardial infarction. *Circulation* 80 (suppl II):II-114, 1989.

Naunheim KS, et al: Coronary artery bypass for recent infarction: Predictors of mortality. *Circulation* 78:1-122, 1988.

Neuhaus K-L, et al: Improved thrombolysis in acute myocardial infarction with front-loaded administration of alteplase: Results of the rt-PA-APSAC Patency Study (TAPS). *J Am Coll Cardiol* 19:885-891, 1992.

Norwegian Multicenter Study Group: Timolol-induced reduction in mortality and reinfarction in patients surviving acute myocardial infarction. *N Engl J Med* 304:801-807, 1981.

Oesterle S: Interventional cardiology: Percutaneous transluminal coronary angioplasty. *Cardiovasc Rev Rep* 12:9-27, 1990.

Ohman EM, et al: Consequences of reocclusion after successful reperfusion therapy in acute myocardial infarction. *Circulation* 82:781-791, 1990.

Ohman EM, et al: Noninvasive detection of reperfusion after thrombolysis based on serum creatine kinase MB changes and clinical variables. *Am Heart J* 126:819-826, 1993.

Oldroyd KG, et al: Effects of early captopril administration on infarct expansion, left ventricular remodeling and exercise capacity after acute myocardial infarction. *Am J Cardiol* 68:713-718, 1991.

Olofssen BO, et al: Evidence for increased levels of plasminogen activator inhibitor and tissue plasminogen activator in plasma of patients with angiographically verified coronary artery disease. *Eur Heart J* 10:77-82, 1989.

O'Neill WM: Angioplasty therapy of cardiogenic shock: Are randomized trials necessary? *J Am Coll Cardiol* 19:915-917, 1992.

Pell ACH, et al: Effect of 'fast track' admission for acute myocardial infarction on delay to thrombolysis. *BMJ* 304:83-87, 1992.

Pepine CJ: New concept in the pathophysiology of acute myocardial infarction. *Am J Cardiol* 64:2B-8B, 1989 A.

Pepine CJ: Appropriate therapy of acute myocardial infarction. *Cardiovasc Rev Rep* 10:51-58, 1989 B.

Pfeffer MA, et al: Effects of captopril on progressive ventricular dilatation after anterior myocardial infarction. *N Engl J Med* 319:80-86, 1988.

Pfeffer MA, et al: Effect of captopril on mortality and morbidity in patients with left ventricular dysfunction after myocardial infarction: Results of the Survival and Ventricular Enlargement Trial. *N Engl J Med* 327:669-677, 1992.

Popma JJ, Topol EJ: Adjuncts to thrombolysis for myocardial reperfusion. *Ann Intern Med* 115:34-44, 1991.

Prins MH, Hirsh J: Heparin as an adjunctive treatment after thrombolytic therapy for acute myocardial infarction. *Am J Cardiol* 67:3A-11A, 1991.

Puleo PR, et al: Early diagnosis of acute myocardial infarction based on assay for subforms of creatine kinase-MB. *Circulation* 82:759-764, 1990.

Ridker PM, et al: Endogenous tissue-type plasminogen activator and risk of myocardial infarction. *Lancet* 341:1165-1168, 1993.

Roberts R: Recent clinical findings impact results of GISSI-II. *Hosp Formul* 25 (suppl D):9-12, 1990.

Roberts R, et al: Immediate versus deferred beta-blockade following thrombolytic therapy in patients with acute myocardial infarction: Results of the Thrombolysis in Myocardial Infarction (TIMI) II-B Study. *Circulation* 83:422-437, 1991.

Rossouw JE, et al: The value of lowering cholesterol after myocardial infarction. *N Engl J Med* 323:1112-1118, 1990.

Roux S, et al: Effects of aspirin on coronary reocclusion and recurrent ischemia after thrombolysis: A meta-analysis. *J Am Coll Cardiol* 19:671-677, 1992.

Sharkey SW, et al: An analysis of time delays preceding thrombolysis for acute myocardial infarction. *JAMA* 262:3173-3174, 1989.

Sharpe N, et al: Treatment of patients with symptomless left ventricular dysfunction after myocardial infarction. *Lancet* 1:255-259, 1988.

Sharpe N, et al: Early prevention of left ventricular dysfunction after myocardial infarction with angiotensin-converting-enzyme inhibition. *Lancet* 337:872-876, 1991.

Singh BN: Advantages of beta blockers versus antiarrhythmic agents and calcium antagonists in secondary prevention after myocardial infarction. *Am J Cardiol* 66:9C-20C, 1990.

Smith P, et al: The effect of warfarin on mortality and reinfarction after myocardial infarction. *N Engl J Med* 323:147-152, 1990.

Smith P, et al: Effects of long-term anticoagulant therapy in subgroups after acute myocardial infarction. *Arch Intern Med* 152:993-997, 1992.

The SOLVD Investigators: Effect of enalapril on mortality and the development of heart failure in asymptomatic patients with reduced left ventricular ejection fractions. *N Engl J Med* 327:685-691, 1992.

Speich M, et al: Concentrations of magnesium, calcium, potassium and sodium in human heart muscle after acute myocardial infarction. *Clin Chem* 26:1662-1665, 1980.

Spodick DH: Electrocardiographic responses in acute myocardial infarction: Framework for clinical application and clinicopathologic investigation. *Cardiovasc Rev Rep* 10:55-57, 1989.

Swedberg K, et al: Effects of the early administration of enalapril on mortality in patients with acute myocardial infarction: Results of the Cooperative New Scandinavian Enalapril Survival Study II (CONSENSUS II). *N Engl J Med* 327:678-684, 1992.

Sytkowski PA, et al: Changes in risk factors and the decline in mortality from cardiovascular disease: The Framingham Heart Study. *N Engl J Med* 322:1635-1641, 1990.

Teo KK, et al: Effects of prophylactic antiarrhythmic drug therapy in acute myocardial infarction: An overview of results from randomized controlled trials. *JAMA* 270:1589-1595, 1993.

TIMI Study Group: Immediate versus delayed catheterization angioplasty following thrombolytic therapy for acute myocardial infarction: TIMI IIA results. *JAMA* 260:2849-2858, 1988.

TIMI Study Group: Comparison of invasive and conservative strategies after treatment with intravenous tissue plasminogen activator in acute myocardial infarction: Results of the Thrombolysis in Myocardial Infarction (TIMI) Phase II Trial. *N Engl J Med* 320:618-627, 1989.

Tofler GH, et al: Modifiers of timing and possible triggers of acute myocardial infarction in the thrombolysis in Myocardial Infarction Phase II (TIMI II) Study Group. *J Am Coll Cardiol* 20:1049-1055, 1992.

Topol EJ, et al: A randomized trial of immediate versus delayed elective angioplasty after intravenous tissue plasminogen activator in acute myocardial infarction. *N Engl J Med* 317:581-588, 1987.

Topol EJ, et al: A multicenter, randomized, controlled trial of intravenous tissue plasminogen activator and early intravenous heparin in acute myocardial infarction. *Circulation* 79:281-286, 1989.

Van de Werf F, European Cooperative Study Group (ECSG): Effect of intravenous tissue plasminogen activator on infarct size, left ventricular function and survival in patients with acute myocardial infarction. *BMJ* 297:1374-1379, 1988.

Viscoli CM, et al: Beta-blockers after myocardial infarction: Influence of first-year clinical course on long-term effectiveness. *Ann Intern Med* 118:99-105, 1993.

Vogt A, et al: Impact of early perfusion status of the infarct-related artery on short-term mortality after thrombolysis for acute myocardial infarction: Retrospective analysis of four German multicenter studies. *J Am Coll Cardiol* 21:1391-1395, 1993.

Voth E, et al: Intravenous streptokinase in acute myocardial infarction (I.S.A.M.) trial: Serial evaluation of left ventricular function up to 3 years after infarction estimated by radionuclide ventriculography. *J Am Coll Cardiol* 18:1610-1616, 1991.

Wall TC, et al: Accelerated plasminogen activator dose regimens for coronary thrombolysis. *J Am Coll Cardiol* 19:482-489, 1992.

Weaver WD, et al: Prehospital-initiated vs hospital-initiated thrombolytic therapy: The Myocardial Infarction Triage and Intervention Trial. *JAMA* 270:1211-1216, 1993.

White H: Thrombolytic treatment for recurrent myocardial infarction: Avoid repeating streptokinase or anistreplase. *BMJ* 302:429-430, 1991.

Wilcox RG, et al: Trial of early nifedipine in acute myocardial infarction: The Trent study. *BMJ* 293:1204-1208, 1986.

Wilcox RG, et al: Trial of tissue plasminogen activator for mortality reduction in acute myocardial infarction. *Lancet* 2:525-530, 1988.

Wilcox RG, et al: Effects of alteplase in acute myocardial infarction: 6-month results from the ASSET study. *Lancet* 335:1175-1178, 1990.

Woods KL, et al: Intravenous magnesium sulphate in suspected acute myocardial infarction: Results of the second Leicester Intravenous Magnesium Intervention Trial (LIMIT-2). *Lancet* 339:1553-1558, 1992.

Yano K, MacLean C: The incidence and prognosis of unrecognized myocardial infarction in the Honolulu, Hawaii Heart Program. *Arch Intern Med* 149:1528-1532, 1989.

Yusuf S, et al: Effect of intravenous nitrates on mortality in acute myocardial infarction: An overview of the randomized trials. *Lancet* 1:1088-1092, 1988 A.

Yusuf S, et al: Overview of results of randomized clinical trials in heart disease, I: Treatments following myocardial infarction. *JAMA* 260:2088-2093, 1988 B.

Yusuf S, et al: Update of effects of calcium antagonists in myocardial infarction or angina in light of the Second Danish Verapamil Infarction Trial (DAVIT-II) and other recent studies, editorial. *Am J Cardiol* 67:1295-1297, 1991.

Yusuf S, et al: Effect of enalapril on myocardial infarction and unstable angina in patients with low ejection fractions. *Lancet* 340:1173-1178, 1992.

Zehender M, et al: Right ventricular infarction as an independent predictor of prognosis after acute inferior myocardial infarction. *N Engl J Med* 328:981-988, 1993.

Zijlstra F, et al: A comparison of immediate coronary angioplasty with intravenous streptokinase in acute myocardial infarction. *N Engl J Med* 328:680-684, 1993.

Mechanisms of Blood Coagulation, Thrombus Formation, and Fibrinolysis

32

A system of integrated actions and reactions maintains the normal fluidity of blood and simultaneously promotes a prompt, appropriate response to protect the body from traumatic blood loss (Mosher, 1990; Guyton, 1991; Rapaport, 1991 A). In response to injury, local blood vessels constrict under the influence of humoral factors released by platelets and damaged tissues and as a consequence of smooth muscle spasm and nervous reflexes. Platelets adhere to damaged vascular endothelium and are activated, thus stimulating the aggregation of additional platelets to form a hemostatic plug. The sequential reactions of the coagulation pathways result in the formation of a fibrin clot, which reinforces the initial platelet plug. Natural anticoagulant and fibrinolytic systems restrain the coagulation cascade and maintain blood fluidity distant from the site of injury. The factors involved in coagulation and its regulation appear in the Table, and the reaction sequences of the coagulation cascade and their regulation by limiting factors appear in Figure 1.

Systems of Blood Coagulation

Prothrombin is converted to thrombin by a complex that requires activated factor X (Xa) in addition to other components. Factor X can be activated by either of two pathways, the extrinsic or intrinsic systems (Nemerson, 1990; Guyton, 1991; Rapaport, 1991 A). In the extrinsic system, coagulation is initiated by a substance that normally is extraneous to the blood (tissue factor) but that comes into contact with blood after tissue injury. In the intrinsic system, all the factors necessary for coagulation are present in the blood; the process is initiated in vitro by activation of factor XII.

Extrinsic System: The extrinsic system is activated in vivo when tissue factor, a transmembrane protein present in many tissues, is exposed to blood at sites of tissue damage and forms a calcium-dependent complex with factor VII or with one of the molecules of factor VIIa presumed to be present in the circulation. In vitro assays of clotting by the extrinsic system are performed by adding thromboplastins (lipoprotein complexes extracted from various tissues that contain tissue factor) to anticoagulated blood. The tissue factor/factor VIIa complex converts factor X to its enzymatic form, factor Xa, which then accelerates the process by selectively activating tissue factor-bound factor VII in a feedback reaction. Prothrombin is then converted to thrombin by a complex of factor Xa, factor Va, and calcium ions adsorbed onto phospholipid micelles in vitro or onto the surface of platelets or other cells in vivo. Although activation of factor V is catalyzed by throm-

COAGULATION FACTORS

Factor	Synonym	Clinical Consequences of Hereditary Deficiency†
I	Fibrinogen	Variable bleeding (mild, moderate, or severe)
II*	Prothrombin (thrombin is inhibited by heparin/AT-III)	Moderate to severe bleeding for homozygotes; mild or no bleeding for heterozygotes
V	Labile factor, proaccelerin	Mild to moderate bleeding
VII*	Proconvertin	Severe bleeding if activity $<1\%$ to 2% of normal
VIII	Antihemophilic factor, AHF (circulates in a noncovalent complex with vWf)	Severe bleeding (hemophilia A)
IX*	Christmas factor, plasma thromboplastin component, PTC	Severe bleeding (hemophilia B)
X*	Stuart factor (activated factor X is inhibited by heparin/AT-III)	Moderate to severe bleeding
XI	Plasma thromboplastin antecedent, PTA	Excessive bleeding after surgery; musculoskeletal bleeding is rare
XII	Hageman factor	Increased risk for thromboembolism; clotting times are prolonged
XIII	Fibrin stabilizing factor, FSF	Prolonged bleeding after trauma or surgery; spontaneous bleeding if activity $<1\%$ of normal; impaired wound healing
Tissue factor	Tissue thromboplastin	None reported
HMW-K	High-molecular-weight kininogen, Fitzgerald factor	None (but clotting times are prolonged in PTT test)
Pre-K	Prekallikrein, Fletcher factor	None (but clotting times are prolonged in PTT test)
vWf	von Willebrand factor	Mild to severe bleeding, especially after surgery or trauma (von Willebrand disease)
Antithrombin-III	Heparin cofactor	Increased risk of thrombosis
Protein C*	—	Catastrophic thrombosis in homozygotes; increased risk of thrombosis in heterozygotes
Protein S*	—	Increased risk of thrombosis in heterozygotes

** Vitamin K-dependent and coumarin-sensitive*

† If replacement with exogenous proteins is not provided

bin, factor Xa, or both (Figure 1), it is secreted in a partially activated form during platelet activation. Thrombin initiates coagulation by removing a peptide from each of the alpha and beta chains of fibrinogen. The cleaved fibrinogen is spontaneously polymerized into a gel of fibrin monomer (Mosesson, 1990). Subsequently, the gel is stabilized by covalent crosslinks formed by factor XIIIa (generated from factor XIII in a calcium ion-dependent reaction catalyzed by thrombin) to produce a crosslinked and, thus, stabilized fibrin clot. The extrinsic system of coagulation is measured in the laboratory by the prothrombin time (PT) test.

The importance of the extrinsic pathway for maintaining hemostasis in vivo is demonstrated by the severe, often fatal bleeding diathesis that accompanies hereditary factor VII deficiency when plasma levels of factor VII activity are undetectable. In contrast, patients with levels of factor VII activity between 5% and 20% of normal rarely experience severe bleeding (Rapaport, 1991 A). On the other hand, bleeding in patients with hemophilia A (ie, factor VIII deficiency) or B (ie, factor IX deficiency) shows that activation of factor X by the tissue factor/factor VIIa complex is not sufficient to maintain hemostasis.

Intrinsic System: The intrinsic pathway is activated in vitro when factor XII (Hageman factor) binds to a negatively charged surface (eg, glass, silica). This reaction is facilitated by the formation of complexes between factor XII, high-molecular-weight (HMW) kininogen (Fitzgerald factor), and prekallikrein (Fletcher factor). Complexed factor XIIa then activates factor XI. In the presence of calcium ions, factor XIa transforms factor IX to factor IXa. Factor X is then activated

FIGURE 1. INTRINSIC AND EXTRINSIC SYSTEMS OF BLOOD COAGULATION*

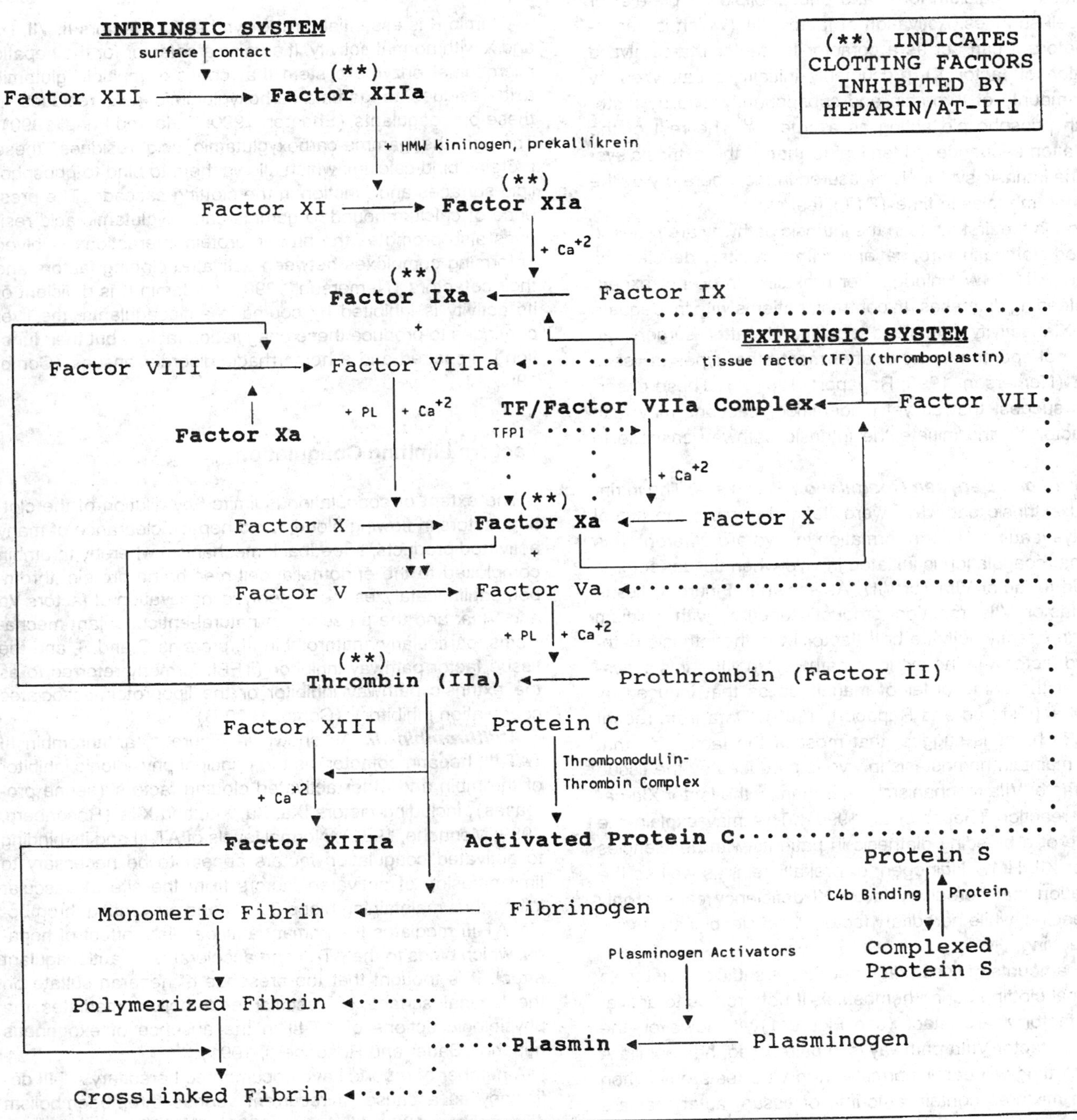

**Precursor/product relationships are indicated by solid arrows that connect procoagulant proteins with their respective activated factors. Activated clotting factors that act as enzymes to activate other factors are indicated in bold type, and those that serve as cofactors in noncovalent complexes with enzymes are indicated in light type. Catalysis of reactions in the clotting pathways is indicated by solid arrows that extend from clotting factors to the centers of other arrows, and additional cofactors (eg, calcium ion=Ca+2) required for optimal reaction rates are shown adjacent to the arrows corresponding to those reactions. Inhibition of reactions, inactivation of factors, or degradation of macromolecular substrates is indicated by dotted arrows, or, for heparin/AT-III, by (**).*
HMW=high molecular weight; PL=phospholipid; TFPI=tissue factor pathway inhibitor

by a complex of factor IXa, activated factor VIII (antihemophilic factor), calcium ions, and phospholipid on platelet or other cell surfaces. Activation of factor VIII (which is necessary before it can act as a cofactor for factor IXa-catalyzed activation of factor X) presumably initially is catalyzed by trace amounts of thrombin and subsequently also by factor Xa with phospholipid acting as a cofactor. The rest of the coagulation sequence is identical to that of the extrinsic system. The intrinsic system is measured in the laboratory by the partial thromboplastin time (PTT) test.

Although the first steps in the intrinsic pathway are required for blood clotting in vitro, patients with hereditary deficiencies of factor XII, HMW kininogen, or prekallikrein do not experience bleeding diatheses. In contrast, patients with inadequate factor XIa activity will bleed significantly after surgery, although not spontaneously or after most other types of tissue trauma (Nemerson, 1990; Rapaport, 1991 A). These observations suggest that as yet unidentified reactions may activate factor XI and initiate the intrinsic pathway cascade in vivo.

Interactions Between Coagulation Pathways: The intrinsic and extrinsic pathways were defined in vitro; the actual pathways leading to fibrin formation in vivo are different. It is likely that coagulation is initiated in vivo when tissue factor is exposed to factor VIIa (or VII). As shown in Figure 1, tissue factor/factor VIIa reaction product, together with calcium ions, can directly activate both factor IX in the intrinsic pathway and factor X in the extrinsic pathway. In vitro, this activation is of the same order of magnitude as that induced by factor XIa (Østerud and Rapaport, 1980). Data from recent studies in humans suggest that most of the factor IXa that acts to maintain hemostasis in vivo is produced by the tissue factor/factor VIIa mechanism rather than by the factor XIa-catalyzed reaction (Bauer et al, 1990). This may explain the absence of a bleeding diathesis in patients with deficiencies of factor XII, HMW kininogen, or prekallikrein, as well as the observation that hereditary factor XI deficiency causes only mild bleeding, while hereditary factor IX deficiency causes severe bleeding.

Small amounts of tissue factor generate sufficient factor Xa for normal clotting during hemostasis if both routes to activation of factor X are intact (see Figure 1). If, however, the factor IXa/factor VIIIa pathway is impaired (eg, hemophilia A or B), clotting will occur normally in in vitro tests only when reaction mixtures contain amounts of tissue factor that are large enough to allow sufficient factor X to be activated by the tissue factor/factor VIIa complex in order to bypass the need for the second route. This explains why plasma from hemophilic patients exhibits normal prothrombin times when measured in vitro. It also suggests that hemophilic patients bleed because blood is exposed to limited amounts of tissue factor after tissue injury, and thus sufficient factor Xa cannot be generated without active participation by the factor IXa/factor VIIIa complex.

Role of Vitamin K

Vitamin K is essential for the synthesis of factors II, VII, IX, and X with normal activity. It acts as a cofactor for the hepatic microsomal enzyme system that converts multiple glutamic acid residues to gamma-carboxyglutamic acid residues in these procoagulants (Shearer, 1990; Furie and Furie, 1990). Through the gamma-carboxyglutamic acid residues, these proteins bind calcium, which allows them to bind to phospholipid surfaces and function in the clotting cascade. The presence of calcium bound to gamma-carboxyglutamic acid residues also promotes the protein-protein interactions involved in forming complexes between activated clotting factors and their cofactors (Nemerson, 1990). If vitamin K is deficient or its activity is inhibited by coumarin anticoagulants, the liver continues to produce these coagulation factors but their function is impaired and a hemorrhagic disorder ensues (Comp, 1990 A).

Factors Limiting Coagulation

The extent of coagulation is limited by dilution of the clotting factors in flowing blood; rapid hepatic clearance of many activated products; a feedback mechanism whereby thrombin complexed to the endothelial cell membrane protein, thrombomodulin, catalyzes the proteolytic inactivation of factors Va and VIIIa; and the presence of natural anticoagulant mechanisms, particularly antithrombin III, proteins C and S, and the tissue factor pathway inhibitor (TFPI; formerly referred to as the extrinsic pathway inhibitor or the lipoprotein-associated coagulation inhibitor) (Comp, 1990 B).

Antithrombin III: As shown in Figure 1, antithrombin III (AT-III, heparin cofactor) is the principal physiologic inhibitor of thrombin and other activated clotting factors (serine proteases), including factors IXa, Xa, XIa, and XIIa (Rosenberg, 1989; Menache, 1991). Normal levels of AT-III and its binding to activated coagulation factors appear to be necessary to limit diffusion of activated factors from the site of vascular injury, thus maintaining blood fluidity and preventing thrombosis. AT-III mediates the primary anticoagulant effect of heparin, which binds to the AT-III and accelerates its anticoagulant effect. It is thought that the presence of heparan sulfate on the luminal surface of vascular endothelium mediates the physiologic actions of AT-III in the absence of exogenous heparin (Bauer and Rosenberg, 1991).

A number of reports have documented hereditary AT-III deficiency as a cause of recurrent venous thromboembolism (Rosenberg, 1989; Menache, 1991). AT-III levels also may be decreased following surgery or in the presence of disseminated intravascular coagulation (DIC), hepatic cirrhosis, nephrotic syndrome, and, infrequently, acute thrombosis. Purified preparations of AT-III are now available for treatment of hereditary AT-III deficiency (see index entry Antithrombin III, As Anticoagulant).

A second heparin-dependent serine protease inhibitor, heparin cofactor II (Comp, 1990 B), inhibits thrombin but not factor Xa. Levels of this protein are reduced in patients with cirrhosis or DIC, and low levels have been reported in some patients with thrombotic diseases.

Protein C and Protein S: Two other coagulation inhibitors, protein C and protein S, depend on vitamin K-dependent gamma-carboxylation of glutamic acid residues for their activity (Kwaan, 1989; Comp 1990 B; Furie and Furie, 1990). Deficiency of either of these proteins in patients receiving warfarin has been associated with skin necrosis (see index entry Necrosis, Drug-induced, Warfarin). Circulating protein C binds to a complex of thrombin with thrombomodulin, which is principally found on the endothelial cell surface where protein C is activated in a calcium ion-dependent reaction (Dittman and Majerus, 1990). As shown in Figure 1, activated protein C exerts its anticoagulant effect by inactivating factors Va and VIIIa. It also enhances fibrinolysis (Sakata et al, 1986). The protein C system thus limits and localizes the clotting process to the vicinity of vascular injury.

Protein C deficiency is inherited as an autosomal codominant trait (Melissari and Kakkar, 1989; Rick, 1990). Heterozygous deficiency is associated with an increased risk of thrombosis in some families but not in others. The reason for this discrepancy has not been determined. Infants with homozygous protein C deficiency develop catastrophic thrombosis and do not survive the neonatal period without protein C replacement (Marlar et al, 1989; Manco-Johnson et al, 1991). Acquired deficiency may occur in conjunction with deficiencies of procoagulant clotting factors in patients with vitamin K deficiency, liver disease, or DIC and in those taking oral anticoagulants. Acquired deficiencies do not pose the same risk for thrombosis as an isolated hereditary deficiency of protein C occurring with normal levels of procoagulant factors.

Protein S acts as a cofactor to accelerate the anticoagulant activity of activated protein C (Kwaan, 1989; Comp, 1990 B). It is present in the circulation both as a free protein and in a noncovalent complex with C4b-binding protein, one of the regulatory proteins of the complement system (Dahlbäck, 1991). Only free protein S is active as a cofactor for activated protein C. Recurrent thrombotic episodes have been associated with heterozygous hereditary protein S deficiency (Engesser et al, 1987; Graves-Hoagland and Walker, 1989).

Two forms of hereditary protein S deficiency have been identified: in about 70% of these patients, the amount of total protein S is one-half or less of normal; the remaining 30% have normal or nearly normal levels of total protein S but no or only very small amounts of free protein S. Acquired protein S deficiency has been observed in patients with the nephrotic syndrome (Vigano-D'Angelo et al, 1987; Allon et al, 1989), liver disease or DIC (D'Angelo et al, 1988), and cerebrovascular occlusion (Sacco et al, 1989). An increased risk of thrombosis has not been demonstrated in those with acquired protein S deficiency.

Tissue Factor Pathway Inhibitor (TFPI): Neither AT-III nor the activated protein C/protein S complex inhibit the catalytic activity of the tissue factor/factor VIIa complex. TFPI, formerly referred to as extrinsic pathway inhibitor or lipoprotein-associated coagulation inhibitor, is a Kunitz-type plasma protease inhibitor that is thought to be the major physiologic regulator of the extrinsic pathway. It forms a quaternary complex with tissue factor, factor VIIa, and factor Xa that lacks catalytic activity (Rapaport, 1991 B). The resulting inhibition may explain bleeding in patients with hemophilia A or B. If production of factor Xa rapidly decreases further activation of factor X by the tissue factor/factor VIIa pathway through formation of this quaternary complex, hemostasis in vivo would depend on continued activation of factor X by factor IXa/factor VIIIa.

Three vascular pools of TFPI have been identified: (1) a plasma pool that circulates in association with plasma lipoproteins, (2) a pool on the luminal surface of the vascular endothelium that can be released by heparin, and (3) a platelet pool that can be released by activation of platelets with thrombin. Limited data are available on the effects of disease on plasma levels of TFPI. Most notably, no reduction was observed in patients experiencing the typical clinical course of active DIC, and serial measurements have not demonstrated that falling levels of TFPI accompany worsening of DIC (Rapaport, 1991 B). However, the TFPI level was markedly reduced in a single patient with sudden, massive DIC (an unusual circumstance). Thus far, screening studies of patients with spontaneous deep vein thrombosis also have not identified any individuals with reduced plasma levels of TFPI.

Thrombus Formation

Thrombus formation represents exaggerated or inappropriate hemostasis (Harker, 1990). The site, composition, and size of thrombi are determined by interactions among three circumstances known as Virchow's triad: restricted or abnormally turbulent blood flow, abnormalities of the blood vessel wall, and abnormalities of the plasma proteins or blood cells involved in clotting. Thrombi are composed of platelets, fibrin, and, where blood flow is impeded, entrapped red cells; the precise composition depends on the conditions of formation and age of the thrombus.

Role of Platelets: Platelets play a major role in thrombus formation and embolization, especially in the arterial system. They adhere to damaged endothelium, form aggregates at the site of vascular damage, and secrete substances that promote further aggregation (eg, adenosine diphosphate [ADP]) or vascular constriction (eg, serotonin) (Bennett and Shattil, 1990). Adhesion to subendothelium involves binding of von Willebrand factor (vWF) to glycoprotein Ib (GPIb) on the platelet surface and to collagen exposed by the vascular damage. Activation of platelets changes the conformation of the platelet surface GPIIb/IIIa complex to promote binding of fibrinogen (Cahill et al, 1992). Because fibrinogen is a symmetrical dimeric molecule, it can bridge activated platelets and mediate their aggregation. Other adhesive proteins (eg, fibronectin, vitronectin, thrombospondin) also are thought to participate in platelet adhesion and/or aggregation.

Along with platelet aggregation, platelet membrane-phospholipases are activated with resultant hydrolysis of membrane phospholipids to release arachidonic acid, which then is converted by fatty acid cyclooxygenase to the cyclic endoperoxides (PGG_2 and PGH_2) (Vane et al, 1990). The endoperoxides are, in turn, converted to thromboxane A_2 (TXA_2) in the platelets and to prostacyclin (PGI_2) in the vessel wall. TXA_2 causes platelet aggregation and vasoconstriction, while PGI_2 dilates coronary, systemic, and pulmonary vascular beds and inhibits platelet aggregation (see Figure 2). The balance between the generation of TXA_2 and PGI_2 may be important in regulating platelet function.

Venous Thrombosis: Venous thrombi frequently occur in the absence of detectable intimal damage and usually develop in regions of slow or disturbed blood flow (eg, valve pockets of deep leg veins). Increased turnover of both platelets and fibrinogen reflects activation of the coagulation mechanism. Small deposits of platelets become interspersed with fibrin and extend in the direction of blood flow. As the thrombus grows, a red tail (mainly fibrin interspersed with red cells) forms and occludes the vein or separates and migrates as an embolus.

Arterial Thrombosis: In contrast, arterial thrombi have a greater platelet component, which may sometimes give them the appearance of white thrombi. They develop at sites of vascular narrowing or irregularity in areas of rapid blood flow, and symptoms are determined by the location rather than by the size of the thrombus. Arterial thrombi may not cause occlusion (unless an artery is markedly stenotic) as readily as venous thrombi. Instead, they tend to remain fixed, acting as a focus for further accumulation. The resulting mass can interfere with blood flow and cause infarctions or it may break loose to form an embolus.

Fibrinolysis

The fibrinolytic system consists of three main components: (1) The circulating proenzyme, plasminogen, and its activated form, plasmin (Francis and Marder, 1990; Henkin et al, 1991). (2) Plasminogen activators, which are enzymes present in blood, vascular endothelium, and numerous tissues that are released in response to local trauma, thrombi, or neurohumoral factors (Francis and Marder, 1990; Vassalli et al, 1991); the most important of these are tissue-type plasminogen activator [tPA], which originates in the endothelial wall,

FIGURE 2. PROSTAGLANDINS AND PLATELET FUNCTION

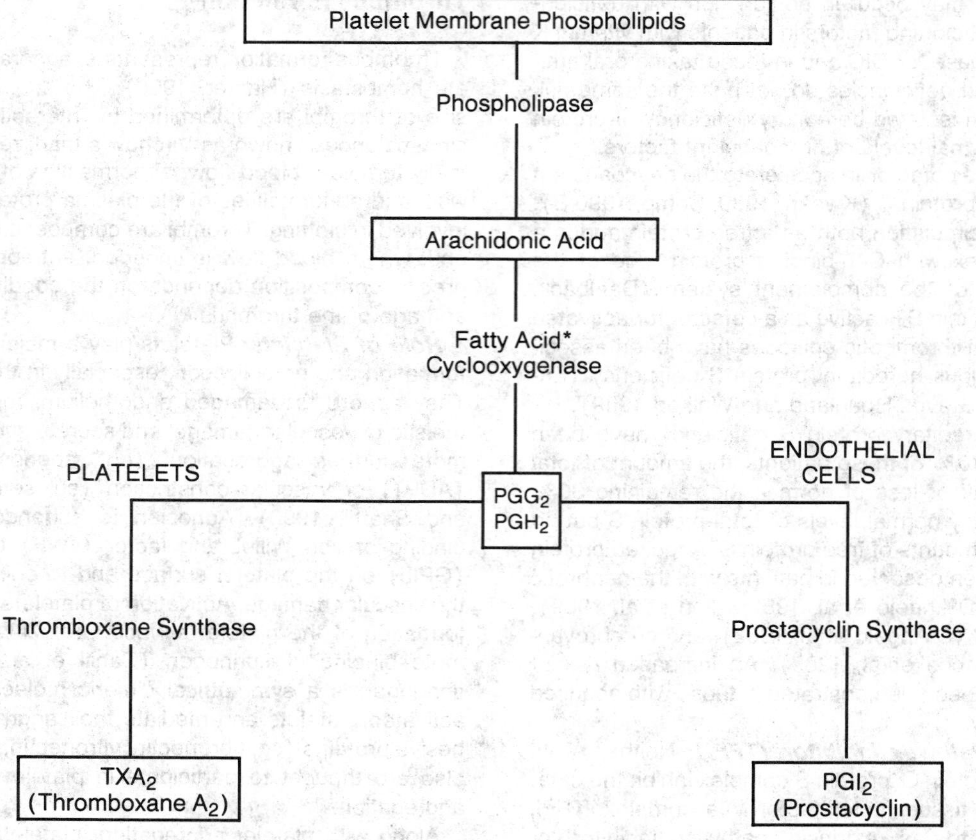

* *Inhibited by aspirin*

and urokinase-type plasminogen activator (uPA), which is secreted by endothelial and epithelial cells as well as by monocytes, fibroblasts, and decidual cells. (3) Specific inhibitors such as α_2-antiplasmin, which rapidly neutralizes plasmin (Saito, 1988; Cucuianu et al, 1991), and plasminogen activator inhibitors (especially PAI-1, which inhibits the activity of both uPA and tPA) (Kruithof et al, 1988; Loskutoff et al, 1989; Andreasen et al, 1990).

Plasminogen binds avidly to lysine residues of fibrin. Only fibrin-bound plasminogen is a substrate for the circulating single-chain form of uPA, while activation by tPA is much more efficient for fibrin-bound than for unbound (circulating) plasminogen. In its two-chain form, uPA activates free as well as fibrin-bound plasminogen. It is postulated that small amounts of α_2-antiplasmin are covalently bound to fibrin by factor XIIIa soon after clotting begins; this neutralizes the plasmin generated initially to maintain the seal provided by the clot. Once these bound molecules of α_2-antiplasmin have been consumed, conversion of additional plasminogen to plasmin initiates fibrinolysis and clot dissolution.

Plasmin also can hydrolyze other proteins, including fibrinogen; factors II, V, VIII, and XII; the first component of complement; and prekallikrein. As fibrin is lysed, both activator and plasmin are released into blood where they are bound by their inhibitors to suppress fibrinogenolysis in circulating blood. PAI-1 and α_2-antiplasmin belong to the serine protease inhibitor (serpin) family, and each rapidly inactivates its target protease(s) (uPA and tPA and plasmin, respectively). Thus, the selective fibrinolysis of thrombi without proteolysis of circulating proteins is regulated both by localization of plasminogen activator-plasminogen complex on the surface of forming fibrin and by enhanced activator- and plasmin-catalyzed proteolytic activity on clot-bound substrate molecules.

Recent reports suggest that dysfunction of the fibrinolytic system may be associated with an increased risk of thrombosis in some patients and that abnormally elevated fibrinolytic activity is an uncommon but important cause of congenital and acquired hemorrhagic disorders (Francis, 1989). Recent analyses support the view that impaired fibrinolysis, usually secondary to increased levels of PAI-1, is associated with an increased risk of postoperative thrombosis (Prins and Hirsh, 1991 A; Wiman and Hamsten, 1991). Inconclusive data suggest that there may be a similar association between impaired fibrinolysis and familial, idiopathic, or recurrent venous thrombosis. In addition, impaired fibrinolysis is more frequent in patients who have experienced a myocardial infarction than in healthy controls, and elevated levels of PAI-1 and reduced levels of tPA are associated with an increased risk of reinfarction in these individuals (Prins and Hirsh, 1991 B; Wiman and Hamsten, 1991). However, understanding of these possible associations is complicated by the fact that PAI-1 is an acute-phase protein and its concentration in plasma is significantly elevated by inflammation and tissue damage.

Cited References

Allon M, et al: Protein S and C antigen levels in proteinuric patients: Dependence on type of glomerular pathology. *Am J Hematol* 31:96-101, 1989.

Andreasen PA, et al: Plasminogen activator inhibitors: Hormonally regulated serpins. *Mol Cell Endocrinol* 68:1-19, 1990.

Bauer KA, Rosenberg RD: Role of antithrombin III as a regulator of in vivo coagulation. *Semin Hematol* 28:10-18, 1991.

Bauer KA, et al: Factor IX is activated in vivo by the tissue factor mechanism. *Blood* 78:731-736, 1990.

Bennett JS, Shattil SJ: Platelet function, in Williams WJ, et al (eds): *Hematology*, ed 4. New York, McGraw-Hill, 1990, 1233-1250.

Cahill M, et al: The human platelet fibrinogen receptor: Clinical and therapeutic significance. *Br J Clin Pharmacol* 33:3-9, 1992.

Comp PC: Production of plasma coagulation factors, in Williams WJ, et al (eds): *Hematology*, ed 4. New York, McGraw-Hill, 1990 A, 1285-1290.

Comp PC: Control of coagulation reactions, in Williams WJ, et al (eds): *Hematology*, ed 4. New York, McGraw-Hill, 1990 B, 1304-1312.

Cucuianu M, et al: α_2-Antiplasmin, plasminogen activator inhibitor (PAI) and dilute blood clot lysis time in selected disease states. *Thromb Haemost* 66:586-591, 1991.

Dahlbäck B: Protein S and C4b-binding protein: Components involved in the regulation of the protein C anticoagulant system. *Thromb Haemost* 66:49-61, 1991.

D'Angelo A, et al: Acquired deficiencies of protein S: Protein S activity during oral anticoagulation, in liver disease, and in disseminated intravascular coagulation. *J Clin Invest* 81:1445-1454, 1988.

Dittman WA, Majerus PW: Structure and function of thrombomodulin: A natural anticoagulant. *Blood* 75:329-336, 1990.

Engesser L, et al: Hereditary protein S deficiency: Clinical manifestations. *Ann Intern Med* 106:677-682, 1987.

Francis RB Jr: Clinical disorders of fibrinolysis: A critical review. *Blut* 59:1-14, 1989.

Francis CW, Marder VJ: Mechanisms of fibrinolysis, in Williams WJ, et al (eds): *Hematology*, ed 4. New York, McGraw-Hill, 1990, 1313-1321.

Furie B, Furie BC: Molecular basis of vitamin K-dependent γ-carboxylation. *Blood* 75:1753-1762, 1990.

Graves-Hoagland RL, Walker FJ: Protein S and thrombosis. *Ann Clin Lab Sci* 19:208-215, 1989.

Guyton AC: Hemostasis and blood coagulation, in: *Textbook of Medical Physiology*, ed 8. Philadelphia, W.B. Saunders, 1991, 390-399.

Harker LA: Pathogenesis of thrombosis, in Williams WJ, et al (eds): *Hematology*, ed 4. New York, McGraw-Hill, 1990, 1559-1569.

Henkin J, et al: The plasminogen-plasmin system. *Prog Cardiovasc Dis* 34:135-164, 1991.

Kruithof EKO, et al: Plasminogen activator inhibitor 1 and plasminogen activator inhibitor 2 in various disease states. *Thromb Haemost* 59:7-12, 1988.

Kwaan HC: Protein C and protein S. *Semin Thromb Hemost* 15:353-355, 1989.

Loskutoff DJ, et al: Type 1 plasminogen activator inhibitor, in Coller BS (ed): *Progress in Hemostasis and Thrombosis.* Philadelphia, W.B. Saunders, 1989, vol 9, 87-115.

Manco-Johnson MJ, et al: Severe neonatal protein C deficiency: Prevalence and thrombotic risk. *J Pediatr* 119:793-798, 1991.

Marlar RA, et al: Diagnosis and treatment of homozygous protein C deficiency: Report of the Working Party on Homozygous Protein C Deficiency of the Subcommittee on Protein C and Protein S, International Committee on Thrombosis and Haemostasis. *J Pediatr* 114:528-534, 1989.

Melissari E, Kakkar VV: Congenital severe protein C deficiency in adults. *Br J Haematol* 72:222-228, 1989.

Menache D (ed): Antithrombin III: Biochemistry, physiology, and management of patients with hereditary deficiency. *Semin Hematol* 28:1-54, 1991.

Mosesson MW: Fibrin polymerization and its regulatory role in hemostasis. *J Lab Clin Med* 116:8-17, 1990.

Mosher DF: Blood coagulation and fibrinolysis: An overview. *Clin Cardiol* 13:VI-5-VI-11, 1990.

Nemerson Y: Sequence of coagulation reactions, in Williams WJ, et al (eds): *Hematology*, ed 4. New York, McGraw-Hill, 1990, 1295-1304.

Østerud B, Rapaport S: Activation of ^{125}I-factor IX and ^{125}I-factor X: Effect of tissue factor and factor VII, factor X_a and thrombin. *Scand J Haematol* 24:213-226, 1980.

Prins MH, Hirsh J: A critical review of the evidence supporting a relationship between impaired fibrinolytic activity and venous thromboembolism. *Arch Intern Med* 151:1721-1731, 1991 A.

Prins MH, Hirsh J: A critical review of the relationship between impaired fibrinolysis and myocardial infarction. *Am Heart J* 122:545-551, 1991 B.

Rapaport SI: Hemostasis, in West JB (ed): *Best and Taylor's Physiological Basis of Medical Practice,* ed 12. Baltimore, Williams & Wilkins, 1991 A, 385-401.

Rapaport SI: The extrinsic pathway inhibitor: A regulator of tissue factor-dependent blood coagulation. *Thromb Haemost* 66:6-15, 1991 B.

Rick ME: Protein C and protein S: Vitamin K-dependent inhibitors of blood coagulation. *JAMA* 263:701-703, 1990.

Rosenberg RD (ed): Role of antithrombin III in coagulation disorders: State-of-the-art review. *Am J Med* 87(3B):1S-67S, 1989.

Sacco RL, et al: Free protein S deficiency: A possible association with cerebrovascular occlusion. *Stroke* 20:1657-1661, 1989.

Saito H: α_2-Plasmin inhibitor and its deficiency states. *J Lab Clin Med* 112:671-678, 1988.

Sakata Y, et al: Mechanism of protein C-dependent clot lysis: Role of plasminogen activator inhibitor. *Blood* 68:1218-1223, 1986.

Shearer MJ: Vitamin K and vitamin K-dependent proteins. *Br J Haematol* 75:156-162, 1990.

Vane JR, et al: Regulatory functions of the vascular endothelium. *N Engl J Med* 323:27-36, 1990.

Vassalli J-D, et al: The plasminogen activator/plasmin system. *J Clin Invest* 88:1067-1072, 1991.

Vigano-D'Angelo S, et al: Protein S deficiency occurs in nephrotic syndrome. *Ann Intern Med* 107:42-47, 1987.

Wiman B, Hamsten A: Impaired fibrinolysis and risk of thromboembolism. *Prog Cardiovasc Dis* 34:179-192, 1991.

Anticoagulants 33

Thromboembolic disorders are a significant cause of morbidity and mortality. Venous thromboembolism occurs as a complication of other disorders, including cancer, diabetes, heart failure, varicose veins, and obesity. Smoking, the postpartum period, oral contraceptive therapy, trauma, surgery, and immobilization, especially following stroke, paraplegia, or myocardial infarction, also are established risk factors. Arterial thromboembolism often accompanies rheumatic heart disease, arrhythmias, the presence of a prosthetic heart valve, or disorders affecting the coronary, cerebral, or peripheral arteries. Acute events in patients with coronary artery disease usually are associated with a ruptured atherosclerotic plaque and platelet clumping leading to intraluminal thrombus formation that is generally resistant to anticoagulant therapy.

ACTIONS

Anticoagulants interfere with fibrin formation and are used to prevent thrombus development and extension. Their major therapeutic application has traditionally been for venous thromboembolic disorders in which stasis, rather than vessel wall damage, plays an important etiologic role. Antiplatelet drugs (antithrombotics) are used to prevent arterial occlusions (see index entry Antiplatelet Drugs). Thrombolytics dissolve existing fresh thrombi and emboli by catalyzing the conversion of plasminogen to plasmin and thereby activating the endogenous fibrinolytic system (see index entry Thrombolytics). The indications for anticoagulants and other antithrombotic drugs were addressed at the American College of Chest Physicians' Second Conference on Antithrombotic Therapy (1989).

The anticoagulants used therapeutically are heparin, the coumarin derivatives (dicumarol and warfarin sodium [Coumadin, Panwarfin]), and the indandione derivative, anisindione [Miradon]. Low-molecular-weight heparins are currently in clinical trial. Direct thrombin inhibitors (eg, hirudin) and fibrinogen depleters, such as ancrod, also are being investigated.

Heparin exerts its anticoagulant effect by binding to antithrombin III. The complex of heparin and antithrombin III rapidly inactivates several activated clotting factors of the intrinsic pathway, including thrombin (IIa), IXa, Xa, XIa, and XIIa. Heparin blocks both the initiation and propagation of thrombi and is the drug of choice when immediate hypocoagulability is required. It also is useful to maintain anticoagulation while therapy with the oral drugs is initiated, for the anticoagulant effect of the oral drugs is delayed until after the first four or five days of administration.

The oral anticoagulants (coumarins and anisindione) lower the plasma activity of the vitamin K-dependent coagulation proteins, factors II, VII, IX, and X and proteins C and S. As a consequence, oral anticoagulants inhibit both the intrinsic and extrinsic pathways of blood coagulation. The coumarins are used for maintenance after the effects of heparin have been established and when long-term therapy is indicated; warfarin is usually the agent of choice (see the section on Coumarin Derivatives). Because of potential toxicity, anisindione is generally reserved for patients who cannot tolerate coumarins.

Hirudin, which is currently being studied in clinical trials, is a naturally occurring anticoagulant protein that was originally isolated from medicinal leeches and is now produced using recombinant DNA technology (Markwardt, 1989, 1991; Walenga et al, 1989; Märki and Wallis, 1990). It forms tightly bound bimolecular complexes with thrombin that block the enzyme's proteolytic activity. This inhibition of thrombin not only prevents further conversion of fibrinogen to fibrin but also blocks thrombin-catalyzed platelet aggregation and activation of clotting factors V, VIII, and XIII. In contrast to heparin, the effects of hirudin on thrombin do not require antithrombin III or other cofactors. In several animal models, hirudin prevented clotting in experimental venous and arterial thrombosis and disseminated intravascular coagulation without significantly prolonging bleeding times in most of these models (Kaiser, 1991). Unlike heparin, hirudin may not induce thrombocytopenia, but trials to confirm this finding have not been completed. These and other properties make hirudin an attractive potential anticoagulant for use in humans.

See also index entry Blood Coagulation, Mechanisms.

USES

Acute Venous Thrombosis and Pulmonary Embolism: For patients who have confirmed acute venous thrombosis of the proximal veins or pulmonary embolism, intrave-nous heparin (to prolong activated partial thromboplastin time [APTT] to 1.5 to 2.5 times control) should be given initially to establish rapid hypocoagulability and should be continued for five to ten days. Subcutaneous heparin does not prolong the APTT into the therapeutic range until at least 12 hours after administration (Hull et al, 1986). Therefore, this route is not recommended for the initial dose administered as acute therapy, but it may be used subsequently to maintain the APTT within the recommended range. (Alternatively, thrombolytic drugs may be considered in appropriate patients; see index entry Thrombolytics, Uses.) Oral anticoagulant therapy (to prolong prothrombin time [PT] to 1.3 to 1.5 times control; equivalent to an international normalized ratio [INR] of 2.0 to 3.0) should be given with heparin for four to five days and continued for at least three months (Hirsh et al, 1989; Hull et al, 1979; Hyers et al, 1989). Comparison of a five-day course of initial intravenous heparin therapy (oral anticoagulation started on day one) with a ten-day course (oral anticoagulation started on day five) demonstrated that both schedules were equally safe and effective for patients with proximal venous thrombosis (Gallus et al, 1986; Hull et al, 1990). The shorter course may reduce the risk of heparin-induced thrombocytopenia (Bell, 1988). Since intravenous heparin must be administered in the hospital, the shorter course also may be more cost effective.

Patients with recurrent venous thromboembolism should be treated with anticoagulants indefinitely (Hyers et al, 1989). If thromboemboli recur despite adequate oral anticoagulant therapy (as documented by measurements of PT time), adjusted-dose subcutaneous heparin (APTT 1.5 times control at the midpoint of the interval between doses) should be substituted or the dosage of the oral anticoagulant should be increased to produce a PT of 1.5 to 2.0 times control (equivalent to an INR of 3.0 to 4.5) (Levine and Hirsh, 1990; British Society for Haematology, 1990). Patients with thromboembolism caused by an inherited or acquired coagulopathy that increases the clotting tendency (sometimes termed thrombophilias [Weston-Smith et al, 1989]) require long-term therapy with anticoagulants. Examples include those with deficiencies of antithrombin III, protein C, or protein S and patients who have the lupus anticoagulant. An antithrombin III concentrate is available for prophylaxis and treatment of thromboembolic episodes in patients with hereditary antithrombin III deficiency (see the evaluation).

In calf vein thrombosis, the risk of embolization is low provided that the thrombi do not extend into the proximal veins (Moser and LeMoine, 1981). After initial treatment with heparin, patients with symptomatic calf vein thrombosis may be treated with oral anticoagulants for six weeks to three months. Alternatively, the patient may be followed up with serial impedance plethysmography while withholding therapy unless extension is documented (Hyers et al, 1989; Lagerstedt et al, 1985; Philbrick and Becker, 1988).

Surgical Prophylaxis: Low-dose subcutaneous heparin (5,000 units two hours prior to surgery, repeated every 8 to 12 hours postoperatively until the patient is discharged or fully ambulatory) prevents venous thromboembolism during surgery in moderate-risk patients, ie, those over age 40 having elective general or abdominal surgery under general anesthesia lasting at least 30 minutes and who have one or more of the following secondary risk factors: prolonged immobilization, paralysis, malignancy, obesity, varicose veins, estrogen use (Hyers et al, 1989; Merli, 1990). An overview of randomized trials in general, orthopedic, and urologic surgery concluded that heparin was especially effective in preventing fatal pulmonary embolism (Collins et al, 1988). Intermittent pneumatic compression is an alternative approach and is preferred by some authorities for patients undergoing neurosurgery, genitourinary surgery, or major knee surgery (Hyers et al, 1989). Other authorities prefer heparin in gynecologic surgery and believe that data are insufficient to determine whether heparin or pneumatic compression is more advantageous in urologic surgery (Merli, 1990).

The optimal prophylactic regimen for patients undergoing hip surgery is not clear. Either adjusted-dose subcutaneous heparin (APTT at the high end of the normal range) or moderate-dose warfarin (PT 1.3 to 1.5 times control) may be effective prophylactically for elective hip surgery; warfarin has been recommended for patients undergoing surgery for a fractured hip or total hip replacement (Hyers et al, 1989; Merli, 1990). Warfarin and pneumatic compression are thought to be of equal efficacy in patients undergoing total knee replacement (Merli, 1990). The combination of antithrombin III and low-dose heparin is being investigated for prophylaxis after total hip or knee replacement (Francis et al, 1991).

Recommendations for management of patients with venous thrombosis or pulmonary embolism at the time of surgery have been published (Merli, 1990). These include use of standard anticoagulant therapy, delay of elective surgery for three to six months, and, for emergency surgery, when possible delay for seven days with constant-infusion heparin therapy. In patients receiving long-term oral anticoagulant therapy (eg, for prosthetic heart valves) who require surgery, intravenous heparin should be substituted three days before the surgery is scheduled, with heparin discontinued six hours before and reinstituted 24 to 36 hours after surgery. The APTT should be measured immediately before surgery; if it is prolonged, it has been suggested that the procedure be delayed for 12 to 24 hours.

The optimal means of preventing thromboembolic complications has not been determined for other high-risk groups, such as those over age 40 with a history of thromboembolism or those undergoing extensive surgery for malignant disease; oral anticoagulants or heparin, along with intermittent pneumatic compression, have been recommended.

Atrial Fibrillation: Atrial fibrillation is a major risk factor for systemic and cerebral embolism, presumably because thrombi that develop as a result of blood stasis in the dilated left atrium are dislodged by sudden changes in cardiac rhythm. Although long-term use of anticoagulants may increase the likelihood of hemorrhage, in subpopulations of patients with atrial fibrillation the benefits of reduced risk of stroke and systemic embolism exceed the risk of life-threatening bleeding if the intensity of the anticoagulant effect is maintained within recommended ranges by regular monitoring of PT (Dunn et al, 1989; Wipf and Lipsky, 1990; Ip et al, 1991). Patients with atrial fibrillation of valvular (rheumatic) origin and a history of systemic embolism within the past two years are at greatest risk, and a PT 1.5 to 2.0 times control (INR 3.0 to 4.5) should be maintained. The risk is slightly lower but still significant in patients with valvular heart disease, mitral stenosis, congestive heart failure, or cardiomyopathy, and long-term warfarin therapy (PT 1.3 to 1.5 times control; INR 2.0 to 3.0) has been recommended for these individuals also. In those with thyrotoxic heart disease, warfarin should be continued for two to four weeks after conversion to sinus rhythm and re-establishment of a euthyroid state.

The risks and benefits of chronic anticoagulation in patients with nonvalvular atrial fibrillation have been evaluated in numerous clinical trials (Petersen et al, 1989; Stroke Prevention in Atrial Fibrillation [SPAF] Study Group Investigators, 1991; Boston Area Anticoagulation Trial for Atrial Fibrillation Investigators, 1990; Connolly et al, 1991). The trials differed in the intensities of anticoagulation used, in some of the endpoints included as negative outcomes, and in other design aspects (eg, unblinded, single-blind, double-blind). Three trials were terminated before completion because interim analyses showed that oral anticoagulants significantly reduced the risk of stroke, thromboembolism, or death in patients with nonvalvular atrial fibrillation, and these results made continued administration of a placebo to patients in a control arm unethical (Laupacis et al, 1991). Because of variations in trial design, reduction in the risks of adverse events ranged from 37% to 86% compared with placebo. No increase in the incidence of major hemorrhage (defined as bleeding that required hospitalization or transfusion) was reported in the patients treated with warfarin.

In some of the trials, aspirin was compared with warfarin for prophylaxis of stroke and thromboembolism in patients with nonvalvular atrial fibrillation. However, the differences between the treatments were not statistically significant and data were insufficient to determine if aspirin was equivalent or superior to warfarin as prophylaxis for stroke in these patients or in certain subgroups. The SPAF II trial is continuing to address this question without the use of a placebo control group. It is currently recommended that oral anticoagulants be used for prophylaxis of stroke and thromboembolism in all patients with nonrheumatic atrial fibrillation except those in whom anticoagulants are contraindicated or who are at low risk of thromboembolic events (Cairns and Connolly, 1991).

Only small numbers of patients with paroxysmal (intermittent) atrial fibrillation were included in these trials, and the lower incidence of strokes and systemic emboli in these patients, compared to patients with chronic atrial fibrillation, may reduce the benefit from anticoagulant therapy below the risk from hemorrhage. Finally, no data suggest that patients under age 60 with idiopathic or "lone" atrial fibrillation (ie, in the absence of other cardiovascular disease or thyrotoxicosis) will benefit from anticoagulant therapy, since the incidence of strokes or systemic emboli in this population is too small to warrant treatment.

When elective cardioversion is planned for patients with atrial fibrillation lasting more than three days, warfarin is often recommended because atrial thrombi may be dislodged when the patient converts. It may be given for three weeks prior to the procedure and continued until sinus rhythm has been maintained for two to four weeks (Dunn et al, 1989; Mancini and Weinberg, 1990). If atrial fibrillation recurs after successful cardioversion, long-term therapy with warfarin is indicated.

Valvular Heart Disease/Prosthetic Heart Valves: In patients with rheumatic mitral valve disease and documented embolism, warfarin should be given for at least one year at a dose sufficient to prolong the PT to 1.5 to 2 times control (INR 3.0 to 4.5), with the dose subsequently reduced (PT 1.3 to 1.5 times control; INR 2.0 to 3.0) for continued therapy. Long-term warfarin therapy (PT 1.3 to 2 times control; INR 2.0 to 3.0) also is recommended for patients with mitral valve disease who have atrial fibrillation, a large left atrium, or severe left ventricular dysfunction (Fuster et al, 1988; Levine et al, 1989).

The risk of thromboemboli in patients with mechanical heart valves is high; these patients should be maintained on warfarin (PT 1.5 to 2 times control; INR 3.0 to 4.5) (Stein et al, 1989; Ip et al, 1991). Dipyridamole (300 to 400 mg daily) may be added if systemic embolism occurs despite warfarin therapy in patients with a history of previous embolism or in those with mechanical valves manufactured before the mid-1970s. Patients with newer, less thrombogenic mechanical valves rarely require the addition of dipyridamole. If bleeding develops or if full-dose anticoagulation is contraindicated, the warfarin dose should be lowered (PT 1.3 to 1.5 times control; INR 2.0 to 3.0) and dipyridamole added. Antiplatelet drugs have not been consistently effective but may be tried if warfarin is contraindicated (Stein and Kantrowitz, 1989).

Bioprosthetic heart valves are less thrombogenic than mechanical valves, particularly when in the aortic position. For patients with valves in the mitral position, warfarin (PT 1.3 to 1.5 times control; INR 2.0 to 3.0) has been recommended for one to three months (Stein et al, 1989; Ip et al, 1991). Long-term warfarin therapy (PT 1.5 to 2.0 times control for the first three months, then 1.3 to 1.5 times control) should be instituted in those with a history of thromboembolism, a large left atrium, or atrial fibrillation (Stein and Kantrowitz, 1989).

Unstable Angina: Results of several well-designed trials demonstrated that aspirin reduces the risk of myocardial infarction and death in patients with unstable angina (see index entry Aspirin, Uses), but data were insufficient to support the routine use of anticoagulants in these patients (Resnekov et al, 1989). Results from the small number of trials comparing aspirin and heparin in those with unstable angina are difficult to pool for a meta-analysis because of differences in doses and routes of administration. In one study, the incidence of myocardial infarction was reduced by both aspirin (325 mg twice daily) and intravenous heparin (APTT 1.5 to 2.0 times control), but only heparin decreased the occurrence of refractory angina. The therapeutic response was not improved by combining the two drugs, although a longer duration of heparin therapy might have increased the efficacy of the combination regimen. Bleeding complications occurred more frequently in patients receiving heparin or the combination (Théroux et al, 1988). A subsequent randomized, placebo-controlled trial used low-dose aspirin (75 mg/day) or bolus intravenous heparin (10,000 units every six hours for the first 24 hours, followed by 7,500 units every six hours for four days), both drugs, or neither drug in patients with unstable angina or non-Q-wave myocardial infarction. Aspirin significantly reduced the risk of myocardial infarction and death at 5, 30, or 90 days after admission; the effect of heparin was not statistically significant either in those taking it alone or combined with aspirin (The RISC Group, 1990). However, as in the above study, the duration of heparin therapy may have been inadequate to enhance the effects of aspirin; thus, longer-term studies on combination therapy are needed.

Some data suggest that in patients with refractory unstable angina (ie, those not responsive to nitrates, calcium channel blockers, and beta-adrenergic blocking drugs), continuous intravenous infusion of heparin for seven days (APTT 1.5 to 2.0 times control) significantly reduces the number and duration of anginal attacks and the number of silent ischemic episodes (Neri Serneri et al, 1990). Intermittent bolus administration of heparin (6,000 units every six hours, with measurement of APTT before each dose to avoid overdose), aspirin (325 mg/day), and alteplase [Activase] (1.75 mg/kg as a 12-hour infusion) were much less effective in reducing symptoms of refractory unstable angina. Data from a retrospective review of percutaneous transluminal coronary angioplasty in patients with unstable angina also suggest that continuous intravenous administration of heparin for at least 24 hours increases the rate of clinical and angiographic success and decreases the incidence of reocclusion within the first 30 minutes after angioplasty (Laskey et al, 1990).

Acute Myocardial Infarction: Anticoagulants are used to achieve several goals in patients with acute myocardial infarction (AMI). In the earliest stage of therapy, heparin is used as an adjunct to thrombolysis. (See the chapters on Therapeutic Management of Myocardial Infarction and Thrombolytics for discussion of results from clinical trials and for current recommendations on dosages and adjunctive regimens.) Anticoagulant therapy also is used in the first several days after AMI to prevent deep venous thrombosis and pulmonary embolism, to prevent arterial embolism from left ventricular mural thrombi, and to reduce early recurrence or extension of myocardial infarction (ACC/AHA Task Force, 1990; Ip et al, 1991). Data are inconclusive on the relative benefits and risks of long-term therapy with oral anticoagulants or antiplatelet drugs for secondary prevention of death, reinfarction, and other cardiac events (eg, unstable angina, pulmonary edema) in patients who survive an AMI. See the chapter on Therapeutic Management of Myocardial Infarction for discussion of results from clinical trials and therapeutic recommendations for these indications.

Coronary Angioplasty and Bypass Grafts: Percutaneous transluminal coronary angioplasty (PTCA) increases the luminal diameter of an occluded vessel, but acute reocclusion and gradual restenosis limit long-term benefits. Acute closure results from both platelet and thrombus deposition at sites of mechanical damage to the blood vessel. Migration and proliferation of smooth muscle cells in response to intimal damage contribute to restenosis after PTCA.

In patients with unstable angina, continuous infusion of heparin for four to seven days before PTCA may be of benefit. For routine PTCA, heparin and antiplatelet therapy during and for 24 hours after the procedure is recommended to increase the success rate and to reduce the incidence of acute closure and mural thrombus (Chesebro et al, 1991). In patients with residual thrombus or stenosis, administration of heparin should continue for several days and should be overlapped with warfarin, which should be continued for an additional three months.

In the only randomized, placebo-controlled trial on use of heparin to decrease the incidence of restenosis in patients with successful, uncomplicated PTCA, heparin had no effect (Ellis et al, 1989); however, pretreatment was omitted and the duration of therapy was only 18 to 24 hours. Additional trials of heparin are in progress, as are studies on low-molecular-weight (fractionated) heparin and heparinoids; the specific thrombin antagonist, hirudin; and combination therapy with heparin and antiplatelet drugs, low-molecular-weight heparin and omega-3 polyunsaturated fatty acids (fish oils), or heparin and glucocorticoids (Chesebro et al, 1991; Berk et al, 1991).

Coronary artery bypass grafts (CABG) are susceptible to reocclusion resulting from thrombosis soon after surgery. Antithrombotic therapy (with anticoagulants or antiplatelet drugs) beginning immediately after CABG surgery has reduced the incidence of early reocclusion. The results of clinical trials to evaluate antithrombotic therapy and compare anticoagulants with antiplatelet drugs for this indication are discussed in the chapter on Antiplatelet Therapy. It has been suggested that anticoagulants will be used less frequently than antiplatelet drugs because of the inconvenience and expense associated with the need to monitor PT times regularly in patients taking oral anticoagulants (Israel et el, 1991). When the risk of occlusion is high (eg, anastomoses to vessels with diameters <1.5 mm, which results in low blood flow through the graft), anticoagulants may be preferred. Whether combination therapy with anticoagulants and antiplatelet drugs may be more efficacious than monotherapy in high-risk patients must be determined in randomized clinical trials.

Cerebral Embolism: The indications for anticoagulants in patients with cerebrovascular disease are limited (Jonas, 1988; Sherman et al, 1989). There is no evidence that anticoagulation reduces the incidence of stroke following single transient ischemic attacks (TIA). There is disagreement on the risk-to-benefit ratio of heparin therapy in patients with multiple (crescendo) TIAs. Although some experts argue that the frequency of cerebral infarction in these patients justifies empiric use of heparin when no contraindications are present (Miller and Hart, 1988), others maintain that use of heparin should be limited to patients with TIA and proven stenosis of a major intracranial artery (eg, middle cerebral or basilar) (Estol and Pessin, 1990). A third view is that the lack of data from randomized, controlled clinical trials and the risk of hemorrhagic complications (including hemorrhagic stroke) suggest that the use of heparin in patients with crescendo TIA be limited to experimental protocols (Phillips, 1989; Scheinberg, 1989). Aspirin has been effective in reducing the risk of TIA recurrence, occlusive stroke, and vascular mortality (see index entry Aspirin, Uses).

Most neurologists agree that patients with acute, partial, stable (thrombotic) stroke do not benefit from heparin therapy. Results of a randomized, placebo-controlled trial in 225 patients found that heparin had no significant effect on stroke progression, neurologic deficits, or functional abilities (Duke et al, 1986). Nevertheless, some advocate its use in patients with partial stroke in the vertebrobasilar system and no contraindications because they are at higher risk of stroke progression (Miller and Hart, 1988); data to support this recommendation are lacking. Heparin may be useful as prophylaxis for thromboembolism after acute stroke, however (McCarthy et al, 1977).

The role of anticoagulants in progressing thrombotic stroke also is in dispute since no data are available from randomized controlled trials to establish their efficacy or safety. For many neurologists, progressing stroke (stroke in evolution) is an accepted indication for heparin in spite of the absence of supporting data (Miller and Hart, 1988; Marsh et al, 1989). Because progressing stroke is often not the result of progressing thrombosis and the risks of hemorrhage after anticoagulant therapy in these patients are substantial, others believe that routine administration of heparin is inadvisable (Philips, 1989; Scheinberg, 1989). A third group believes that patient subgroups should be defined by the vascular mechanism that causes the cerebral ischemia rather than by clinical features such as TIA, acute partial stroke, or progressing stroke (Estol and Pessin, 1990). These authorities maintain that until data from well-designed clinical trials are available, use of heparin in thrombotic stroke should be limited to patients with acute occlusion of a large extracranial or intracranial artery (and mild to moderate neurologic deficits, not major debilitating strokes) and to those with TIA and proven stenosis of a major intracranial artery.

When heparin is used in patients with progressing stroke or crescendo TIA, a constant intravenous infusion adjusted to prolong the APTT to 2.0 to 2.5 times control, with or without an initial bolus of 5,000 to 10,000 units is prescribed most frequently (Miller and Hart, 1988; Marsh et al, 1989). Warfarin (PT to a maximum of 1.5 times control; INR 3.0) may be given after the heparin in some patients with occlusion or stenosis of cerebral arteries (Estol and Pessin, 1990). Aspirin appears to be safer and more effective than anticoagulants in patients with completed thrombotic stroke.

Anticoagulation with heparin followed by warfarin (in a dose sufficient to prolong the PT to 1.5 to 2 times control; INR 3.0 to 4.5) may be considered to prevent recurrence in normotensive patients with small to moderate sized cardiogenic embolic stroke and no hemorrhagic transformation. If there are no recurrences, the dose of warfarin may be reduced (PT 1.3 to 1.5 times control; INR 2.0 to 3.0) after one year. Anticoagulant therapy should be postponed in patients with large embolic strokes, severe hypertension, or hemorrhagic transformation (Sherman et al, 1989; Sherman and Hart, 1986). The use of CT scans within 12 hours of stroke onset to predict the safety of anticoagulation is not recommended, since the scans may not identify infarcts likely to undergo spontaneous hemorrhagic transformation (Cerebral Embolism Study Group, 1987).

Some experts maintain that it is prudent to delay the start of heparin therapy for 24 to 48 hours in patients with cardioembolic stroke to reduce the risk of hemorrhagic transformation (Miller and Hart, 1988), while others believe that anticoagulants should not be given to patients with cardiogenic cerebral emboli because of the magnitude of this risk (Phillips, 1989; Scheinberg, 1989). Although conclusive data are not available, those who favor the use of anticoagulants after cardioembolic stroke estimate that the risk of recurrent cardiogenic emboli (10% to 15% within one month without anticoagulant therapy) exceeds the risk of hemorrhage associated with their use (5%). Thus, well-designed clinical trials also are needed in these patients. Since death after TIA and stroke is more often caused by ischemic heart disease than by recurrent stroke, it may be more beneficial to focus efforts on reducing the incidence of cardiac events.

Peripheral Vascular Disease: Studies on the use of oral anticoagulants in patients with peripheral vascular disease or after bypass surgery of a limb artery have been uncontrolled or limited to small numbers of patients, but the results suggest that the preventive role of anticoagulants is minimal.

Special Situations: Prophylaxis with low-dose heparin or oral anticoagulants should be considered in patients who are immobilized for long periods. Another major use of heparin is to help maintain extracorporeal circulation during open heart surgery or renal hemodialysis.

PRECAUTIONS

Anticoagulation induced by heparin or oral agents must be sufficient to maintain equilibrium between the desired antithrombotic protection and actual bleeding. This requires not only careful calculation of the dose but also repeated sampling and reliable laboratory testing.

Bleeding is a hazard of treatment with any anticoagulant and is the main complication of therapy, but the frequency and severity can be minimized by careful management. The incidence of bleeding depends on the intensity of anticoagulation, the duration of administration, the compliance of the patient, the reliability of laboratory tests, and the occurrence of drug interactions (see Table for interactions with oral anticoagulants). The concurrent use of aspirin with either oral anticoagulants or heparin increases the risk. Hemorrhage also is more likely to occur in patients who have an underlying medical or surgical problem in which anticoagulants are contraindicated or should be given with caution. If gastrointestinal or urinary tract bleeding occurs in the presence of a therapeutic level of anticoagulation, an occult lesion may be present. Cerebral or adrenal hemorrhage, corpus luteum hemorrhage and rupture, subdural hematoma, intestinal submucosal hemorrhage with adynamic ileus or colitis, acute hemorrhagic pancreatitis, and cutaneous hemorrhagic necrosis are possible serious complications.

Anticoagulants should be used with caution in the presence of mild liver or kidney disease, mild hypertension, alcoholism, infective endocarditis, drainage tubes in any orifice, or a history of gastrointestinal ulcers and in those with occupations that are associated with a significant risk of injury resulting in bleeding.

Oral anticoagulants should not be prescribed for outpatient therapy unless the patient is reliable or someone in the household can assume responsibility for competent care. Both verbal and written instructions should be given and the latter carried at all times, and the patient should be encouraged to wear a Medic Alert bracelet. Follow-up visits at weekly intervals are advisable initially.

If major hemorrhagic complications occur, all anticoagulants should be discontinued immediately. Bleeding episodes of any kind indicate the need for immediate reappraisal of the patient's condition.

Pregnancy: If anticoagulation is necessary during pregnancy, heparin should be used instead of oral anticoagulants, because embryopathy has occurred when coumarins were administered during early pregnancy and central nervous system anomalies have been associated with longer and/or later use (Ginsberg and Hirsh, 1989; Hall et al, 1980).

For patients with a history of previous venous thromboembolism, low-dose heparin (5,000 units subcutaneously every 12 hours) has been recommended, with the dosage increased during the last trimester to prolong the APTT at six hours postinjection to 1.5 times control. For those with current venous thromboembolism, full-dose intravenous heparin should be given for seven to ten days, followed by subcutaneous heparin to prolong the APTT to 1.5 times control (Ginsberg and Hirsh, 1988, 1989; Ginsberg et al, 1989 A).

Low-dose heparin may not protect pregnant patients against prosthetic heart valve thrombosis (Iturbe-Alessio et al, 1986), and the optimal dose has not been established. An initial dose of at least 15,000 units subcutaneously every 12 hours has been suggested, with the dose adjusted to maintain the APTT within 1.5 to 2 times control (Fuster et al, 1988).

Use of heparin during pregnancy has been reported to be associated with an increased risk of adverse fetal outcome (Hall et al, 1980), but more recent analyses conclude that coexisting maternal morbidity is primarily responsible and that heparin therapy is safe for the fetus (Ginsberg et al, 1989 A, 1989 B) (see the evaluation).

CONTRAINDICATIONS

Anticoagulants should not be given to patients with cerebral hemorrhage, active ulcerative disease of the gastrointestinal tract, hemorrhagic blood dyscrasias, severe liver or kidney disease, open ulcerative wounds, traumatic surgery resulting in large open surfaces, spinal puncture, or recent surgery of the eye or spinal cord. Other contraindications include dissecting aortic aneurysm, presence of other potential bleeding sites, and moderate to severe hypertension. Anticoagulants also should not be used if adequate laboratory facilities for measurement of coagulation times are unavailable.

Patients receiving anticoagulants should be advised to avoid pregnancy because of the risk of teratogenicity (oral anticoagulants) and intrauterine hemorrhage (both heparin and oral drugs). If pregnancy occurs, the patient should be counseled about the risks to the fetus and options for managing those risks. If anticoagulants must be used, heparin should be employed instead of the oral drugs during the first trimester (and usually thereafter).

Drug Evaluations

HEPARIN CALCIUM
[Calciparine]

HEPARIN SODIUM
[Liquaemin Sodium]

ACTIONS. Heparin, a sulfated mucopolysaccharide, is chemically heterogeneous; it consists of a mixture of molecules that vary in mass from 4,000 to 40,000 daltons (Kessler, 1991). It is synthesized in mast cells and is particularly abundant in the lungs.

Heparin binds to some of the lysine residues of antithrombin III (AT-III) as a consequence of the negative charges borne by the sulfate moieties. A pentasaccharide sequence that is responsible for heparin's binding to AT-III has been identified and synthesized (Hirsh, 1991 A; Kessler, 1991). Binding of heparin induces a conformational change in AT-III, producing a complex with greater affinity for serine proteases than AT-III alone. Therefore, the major effect of heparin is to accelerate AT-III neutralization of activated clotting factors. Heparin:AT-III inactivates factor Xa, thus preventing the conversion of prothrombin to thrombin. The complex also can inactivate thrombin and earlier clotting factors, thus preventing conversion of fibrinogen to fibrin (Kessler, 1991). Heparin also interacts with platelets to inhibit their function and/or induce their aggregation (often resulting in thrombocytopenia; see Adverse Reactions and Precautions below).

Commercial preparations of heparin contain both low- and high-molecular-weight components (mean of 15,000 daltons), which can be further separated. The low-molecular-weight fraction (less than 6,000 daltons) results in a complex with high affinity for factor Xa but lower affinity for thrombin. As a consequence, this fraction has potent anti-Xa activity and moderate antithrombin properties; it also has reduced platelet-activating effects. Small polysaccharides (<18 residues) that contain the critical pentasaccharide sequence bind to AT-III, but the resulting complexes are unable to bind thrombin and thus are specific inhibitors of factor Xa (Hirsh, 1991 A). The high-molecular-weight fraction (more than 25,000 daltons) is active against both factor Xa and thrombin but also can induce platelet aggregation (Kessler, 1991). Heparin prepared from different tissues also appears to vary: More protamine is required to neutralize a unit of beef lung heparin than porcine mucosal heparin (heparin calcium), and the plasma lipolytic activity, antifactor Xa activity, and activated partial thromboplastin time ratio are significantly different.

USES. Heparin is the only anticoagulant used parenterally and is the drug of choice when a rapid effect is desired. Full-dose intravenous or adjusted-dose subcutaneous therapy is employed in patients with established venous thrombosis or pulmonary embolism. The relative effectiveness of the two routes is controversial: Subcutaneous therapy has been reported to be as effective (Doyle et al, 1987; Pini et al, 1990), less effective (Hull et al, 1986), or more effective (Walker et al, 1987) than intravenous therapy. If the dose of heparin is adjusted based on laboratory measurements (see Monitoring Therapy below), the route of administration should not influence its efficacy after the initial intravenous dose establishes hypocoagulability.

For prophylaxis, adjusted-dose subcutaneous heparin should be used in high-risk and low-dose subcutaneous heparin in moderate-risk patients (see the section on Dosage and Preparations for definitions of target APTT ranges). The *routine* use of heparin in general surgical patients younger than 40 years without a thrombotic diathesis is not advocated, because the possibility of hemorrhage and wound complications may exceed the risk of embolism. However, low-dose heparin may be indicated in women under 40 years who are taking oral contraceptives.

Heparin is used after acute myocardial infarction to prevent venous thromboembolism in high-risk patients, to prevent arterial embolism after a large transmural infarction, and to prevent reocclusion after thrombolysis (ACC/AHA Task Force, 1990; Ip et al, 1991; Cairns, 1991). Heparin also may increase the rate of successful reperfusion and decrease the incidence of acute closure and mural thrombus in patients undergoing PTCA (Chesebro et al, 1991).

Heparin should be used instead of oral anticoagulants when therapy is required during pregnancy.

Heparin helps maintain extracorporeal circulation during open heart surgery and renal hemodialysis. It also is used in very small amounts to maintain patency and reduce the incidence of phlebitis in patients with intermittent infusion devices and as a flushing solution to maintain patency in indwelling arterial and venous catheters. A recent review concluded that dilute heparin (10 units/ml) is needed to maintain peripheral venous access devices made of fluoroethylenepropylene when they are used to obtain blood specimens (Weber, 1991); otherwise, normal saline solution is adequate. Data are insufficient to establish the need for heparin in devices constructed of other materials. Although data also are lacking to evaluate the use of dilute heparin in central venous lines, no change in this established procedure is recommended (Weber, 1991).

The use of heparin in the treatment of disseminated intravascular coagulation is controversial (see index entry Disseminated Intravascular Coagulation). Some neurologists advocate its use to treat certain patients with cardioembolic or progressing thrombotic stroke, but this use has not been proved to be efficacious in randomized clinical trials (see the Introduction).

Heparin reduces postprandial lipemia by activating lipoprotein lipase and has a slight antihistaminic effect. Because of these actions, it has been claimed that heparin also may be useful as a hypolipidemic or anti-inflammatory agent, but there is no evidence of its efficacy for such purposes.

Heparin calcium was formulated as an alternative to the sodium salt for subcutaneous administration in low doses to prevent postoperative thromboembolism. The calcium salt has been claimed to produce fewer hematomas or ecchymoses and less pain at the injection site than the sodium salt. However, no substantial difference between the calcium and sodium preparations has been documented with regard to efficacy or side effects.

MONITORING THERAPY. Small doses of heparin (5,000 units every 12 hours) given subcutaneously to prevent venous embolism do not require laboratory monitoring, but monitoring is required to evaluate the response to adjusted-dose intermittent injection or continuous intravenous infusion.

The tests used to monitor heparin therapy are activated clotting time, partial thromboplastin time (PTT), or activated partial thromboplastin time (APTT). The APTT test is the most widely used. The usual therapeutic range varies among laboratories but usually corresponds to an APTT of 1.5 to 2 times control. A nomogram for adjusting the flow rate of intravenous infusions to achieve the target APTT values has been published (Cruickshank et al, 1991).

Patients with elevated pretreatment concentrations of procoagulants may appear to be resistant to heparin because of a poor response measured by the APTT. These patients can be managed by monitoring the circulating heparin concentration. If the heparin level is higher than 0.3 units/ml, dosage need not be increased. True heparin resistance, caused by increased heparin clearance, may occur during initial therapy of pulmonary embolism or severe venous thrombosis and is managed by increasing the dosage. Rarely, resistance is associated with reduced antithrombin III levels.

Frequent monitoring of platelet counts also is necessary (especially after the first five to seven days of therapy) to detect heparin-induced thrombocytopenia (see Adverse Reactions).

ADVERSE REACTIONS AND PRECAUTIONS. Clinically significant bleeding is the most common adverse effect that leads to withdrawal of heparin. Hemorrhage may be less of a problem if dosage is regulated on the basis of the results of clotting tests. Heparin may cause bleeding more often when it is given as intermittent intravenous boluses than when it is administered as a continuous infusion or by subcutaneous injection. Major bleeding is more common in elderly patients, particularly women; those with hypertension, gastrointestinal lesions, renal failure, bleeding disorders, or thrombocytopenia; surgical patients; alcoholics; or those given antiplatelet drugs concomitantly.

Heparin may be the most common cause of drug-related thrombocytopenia in hospitalized patients today. Three forms of thrombocytopenia that vary in severity, time of onset, and incidence have been observed (Cola and Ansell, 1990; Warkentin and Kelton, 1990). The first is an acute and reversible decline in platelet counts that occurs immediately after intravenous administration of a bolus of heparin. This response is common but mild and almost never causes adverse clinical effects; it is thought to result from aggregation and sequestration of platelets through a direct interaction with heparin. A second type of mild thrombocytopenia can develop two to four days after the start of heparin therapy. Platelet counts do not fall below 10^5/microliter and return to normal within five days even if treatment is not terminated; arterial thrombosis does not develop. In the most severe form of heparin-induced thrombocytopenia, which occurs in $<5\%$ of patients, onset is delayed (6 to 14 days after initiation of therapy); platelet counts are reduced below 10^5/microliter but return to normal when heparin therapy is discontinued. The thrombocytopenia can be accompanied by heparin resistance, thromboembolism, and, rarely, disseminated intravascular coagulation. It is thought to result from antiplatelet antibodies, induced in the presence of heparin, that are capable of aggregating platelets.

The delayed-onset form may be more common in patients receiving bovine heparin than in those receiving the porcine preparation (King and Kelton, 1984; Rao et al, 1989), although this finding has been disputed (Ansell et al, 1985). Diagnosis can be difficult because many heparin-treated patients have disorders that could cause the low platelet count. Although most patients have thrombocytopenia only, 10% to 20% have or subsequently develop arterial thrombi or emboli, and morbidity and mortality are high in these patients (Bell, 1988).

A platelet count should be obtained before heparin therapy is initiated and at frequent intervals during treatment. If severe thrombocytopenia develops (platelet counts $\leq 10^5$/microliter), heparin should be discontinued and other measures (thrombolysis, vena caval ligation) instituted to manage the thrombosis. The use of investigational anticoagulants (eg, low-molecular-weight heparins, heparinoids, ancrod) also may be considered. The risk of developing thrombocytopenia can be reduced by introducing warfarin early and discontinuing heparin as soon as the oral anticoagulant becomes effective (Gallus et al, 1986). When thrombocytopenia is complicated by acute arterial thrombosis, other specific treatment may include surgical removal of the thrombus and antiplatelet therapy.

Nausea, vomiting, lacrimation, headache, pruritus, and burning have been reported. Fever, urticaria, bronchospasm, rhinitis, and anaphylaxis occur occasionally after administration of heparin, and myalgia, bone pain, and osteoporosis may be noted with prolonged use. Bone loss has been reported, usually with doses larger than 20,000 units/day given for more than six months; pregnant, menopausal, or elderly patients may be at greatest risk. Heparin can cause elevations in the results of liver function tests. Rare complications include alopecia and a burning sensation in the feet.

Local capillary rupture with subsequent ecchymoses in the area of injection must be anticipated. This has occurred after both subcutaneous and intramuscular injection but is most likely after the latter. Therefore, the intramuscular route should not be used. Subcutaneous injection itself seldom produces serious adverse reactions, although absorption may be irregular and unpredictable and hematoma or cumulative effects may occur after multiple doses. Skin necrosis, which may be severe enough to require grafting, can occur, usually in association with thrombocytopenia. Other adverse reactions to deep subcutaneous injection of heparin include local irritation, erythema, mild pain, or ulceration.

USE DURING PREGNANCY. Heparin should be used if anticoagulation is necessary during pregnancy, but benefits should be weighed against potential risk to the fetus (FDA Pregnancy Category C). The use of heparin during pregnancy has been associated with an increased incidence of maternal hemorrhage, stillbirth, and prematurity (Hall et al, 1980); however, a more recent literature review of heparin therapy in pregnant women suggests that almost all adverse outcomes could be attributed to coexisting conditions in the mother that were themselves associated with adverse fetal or infant outcomes (Ginsberg et al, 1989 A). This conclusion was supported by a retrospective study of 100 pregnancies in 77 women treated with heparin in which rates of prematurity, abortion, stillbirth, neonatal death, and congenital abnormalities were similar to those in the normal population (Ginsberg et al, 1989 B). The bleeding rate with use of heparin was judged acceptably low and safe for the mother and prevented recurrent venous thromboembolism. Concern exists, however, about the potential of increased bleeding during delivery. Although heparin therapy cannot be discontinued at a scheduled time before the onset of natural labor, recent data suggest that it should be discontinued 24 hours before elective induction of labor (Anderson et al, 1991). Heparin also may increase the risk of germinal matrix-intraventricular hemorrhage when used to maintain the patency of vascular catheters in low-birth-weight infants (Lesko et al, 1986).

TREATMENT OF OVERDOSAGE. The action of heparin can be antagonized by the intravenous administration of protamine sulfate, but there are hazards associated with use of this compound (see the evaluation). Data from a recent placebo-controlled study suggest that desmopressin can partially reverse the increase in bleeding time observed in patients with acute venous thromboembolism who are receiving intravenous heparin therapy (Schulman and Johnsson, 1991); however, additional studies are needed to determine if desmopressin will be useful to control hemorrhage in patients treated with excessive doses of heparin (see index entry Desmopressin, As Hemostatic).

DRUG INTERACTIONS. Heparin suppresses aldosterone secretion, even when given in low doses, and it may be prudent to monitor electrolyte balance, particularly in patients with renal insufficiency or diabetes mellitus and in those receiving supplemental potassium, potassium-sparing diuretics, or nonsteroidal anti-inflammatory drugs (Sherman and Ruddy, 1986). Heparin may interact with insulin receptors, altering insulin binding and/or action. Hypoglycemia has been reported during concomitant heparin-glipizide therapy.

There are reports suggesting that the anticoagulant efficacy of heparin is decreased in patients treated simultaneously with intravenous nitroglycerin (Col et al, 1985; Habbab and Haft, 1987). However, these observations were inconclusive since inadequate controls were used and insufficient numbers of patients were tested. Results of more recent controlled studies found that nitroglycerin infusion did not have an acute effect on the ability of heparin to increase the APTT, and the APTT did not increase when nitroglycerin infusion was terminated (Lepor et al, 1989; Bode et al, 1990).

PHARMACOKINETICS. Heparin is rapidly equilibrated throughout the circulation after administration as an intravenous bolus. Absorption after subcutaneous injection is gradual and incomplete and varies considerably among patients. The desired intensity of anticoagulation may not be reached until 12 to 24 hours after administration by this route. Recent data suggest that differences in skinfold thickness may account for much of the variance in absorption after subcutaneous injections (Kroon et al, 1991).

Heparin binds extensively to a variety of plasma proteins, as well as to saturable sites on endothelial cells. It is gradually eliminated by a combination of saturable and first-order mechanisms, resulting in a nonlinear dose-response relationship for its anticoagulant effects within the range of clinically used concentrations (Hirsh, 1991 A). Increasing the intravenous dose from 100 to 400 units/kg lengthens the apparent half-life of heparin activity from 56 to 152 minutes; a half-life of approximately 30 minutes has been measured after an intravenous bolus of 25 units/kg. The apparent volume of distribution is 40 to 60 ml/kg. The mechanisms for elimination of heparin are not fully understood, but a substantial fraction of an intravenous bolus is eliminated in the urine as a partially depolymerized and desulfated metabolite that is about one-half as active as the unmetabolized drug. There are conflicting reports on the effects of liver or kidney disease on heparin pharmacokinetics. Plasma clearance is more rapid in patients with acute pulmonary embolism, although the mechanism for this is not known.

DOSAGE AND PREPARATIONS. Because of its more rapid onset of action, heparin often is given for five to ten days and an oral anticoagulant is overlapped for the last four to five days using stepwise doses until the desired prolongation of PT (or increase in INR) is achieved. Since very large quantities of circulating heparin prolong the PT, this should be measured just before administering bolus doses.

The dosage of heparin is prescribed in units rather than milligrams. One U.S.P. unit is defined as the amount that prevents clotting for one hour after addition of 0.2 ml of 1% calcium chloride to 1 ml of citrated sheep plasma. The U.S.P. standard for minimal potency is 120 units/mg of dry material derived from lung tissue and 140 units/mg of dry material derived from other sources. The potency of commercial preparations ranges from 140 to 190 units/mg. Thus, doses expressed in milligrams have no practical therapeutic meaning, since 100 mg of heparin may represent between 12,000 and 19,000 units of effect. Also, the U.S.P. unit is approximately 10% greater than the international unit (IU) and the difference should be taken into account. The dosage of heparin is identical for the sodium and calcium salts.

Heparin may be administered by intermittent subcutaneous or intravenous injection, by continuous intravenous drip, or by use of a constant infusion pump. Of the intravenous routes, continuous infusion is preferred because it is associated with a more constant intensity of anticoagulation and thus with a lower risk of hemorrhagic complications. The onset of anticoagulant effect is immediate following an intravenous bolus injection of the full therapeutic dose and begins approximately 20 to 30 minutes after subcutaneous injection. With continuous infusion, the two- to three-hour delay in anticoagulant effect may be avoided by injecting 5,000 units of heparin directly into the tubing after the infusion has begun.

Small doses usually are given to prevent thromboembolism. Larger doses are required to prevent propagation of an established thrombus. Still larger doses may be necessary in acute pulmonary embolism.

Intravenous Infusion: *Adults,* initially 5,000 to 10,000 units (alternatively, 100 units/kg) into the tubing after infusion is started, then 20,000 to 40,000 units daily (or occasionally more) at an initial rate of 0.25 unit/kg/min in 5% dextrose injection or isotonic sodium chloride injection. The rate is subsequently adjusted according to the results of the APTT or other clotting time tests performed four hours later. *Children,* 50 units/kg initially, followed by 100 units/kg every four hours or continuous infusion of 20,000 units/M^2/24 hours.

An intravenous drip system or an infusion pump can be used to control the dosage. Although the infusion pump is the most accurate of the two methods, the pump must be monitored carefully since it will continue to force fluid extravascularly if the needle is dislodged, whereas an extravasating intravenous drip will usually stop within a reasonable period.

Intravenous (Intermittent): *Adults,* 10,000 units initially, followed by 5,000 to 10,000 units every four to six hours. Suitable laboratory testing is necessary to regulate the dose. For disseminated intravascular coagulation, one suggested regimen is *adults,* 50 units/kg initially; *children,* 25 units/kg every six hours.

Subcutaneous: *Adults,* for low-dose surgical prophylaxis, 5,000 units two hours before surgery and every 8 to 12 hours thereafter until the patient is discharged or is fully ambulatory. For adjusted-dose prophylaxis or treatment, dosage is guided by the APTT (usually 1.5 to 2 times control). For usual full-dose effects, 8,000 to 10,000 units every eight hours or 15,000 to 20,000 units every 12 hours. The drug should be injected in the smallest volume possible at different sites around the iliac crest, over the lower abdomen, or thigh. A small needle (#27) should be used to prevent massive hematoma.

Intramuscular: This route should not be used because of the likelihood of tissue irritation, local bleeding, or hematoma. Hematoma may not be clinically apparent until 1,000 ml of blood or more has accumulated. In addition, absorption is unpredictable after intramuscular administration.

HEPARIN CALCIUM:

Calciparine (DuPont Multi-Source). Solution (sterile) 5,000 units (from porcine intestinal mucosa) in 0.2 ml pre-filled disposable syringes.

HEPARIN SODIUM:

Generic. Solution 1,000, 2,500, 5,000, 7,500, 10,000, 15,000, 20,000, and 40,000 units/ml.

Liquaemin Sodium (Organon) Solution 1,000, 5,000, 10,000, 20,000, and 40,000 units/ml.

PROTAMINE SULFATE

ACTIONS AND USES. Protamine sulfate binds and inactivates heparin because of its strong electropositive charge. It combines ionically with heparin to form a stable complex. Paradoxically, it has anticoagulant action of its own and prolongs the clotting time in the absence of heparin.

Protamine is used to reverse the anticoagulant effect of heparin. If hemorrhage is severe, transfusion of blood or plasma also may be required. Each milligram of protamine sulfate neutralizes 90 to 115 U.S.P. units of heparin activity, depending on the source of heparin. The reaction is almost instantaneous and effects persist for approximately two hours. However, since the effect of heparin may last longer than that of protamine, bleeding may recur, particularly in postoperative patients, and another injection of protamine may be needed.

ADVERSE REACTIONS AND PRECAUTIONS. Protamine may cause transient hypotension, particularly when given rapidly. Large intravenous doses (up to 200 mg in two hours) have been administered without untoward effects, but no more than 50 mg should be given as a single bolus. This drug must be used cautiously to prevent thrombotic complications.

Diabetic patients receiving protamine zinc insulin may be sensitized to protamine and experience a severe reaction when this agent is administered intravenously (Weiss et al, 1989). Rarely, anaphylactic reactions have occurred, most commonly after repeated exposure or when the drug was given to patients allergic to fish, since protamine is obtained from fish of the salmon family. Vasectomized and infertile men also have been reported to be at risk. When protamine is used, facilities to treat shock and anaphylaxis should be available. Toxic manifestations include acute hypotension, dyspnea, and bradycardia. Occasionally, a feeling of warmth and flushing of the face may be observed.

Prolonged monitoring is necessary when repeated doses of protamine are used to reverse the effect of large doses of heparin (eg, during cardiopulmonary bypass surgery, dialysis). Suggested tests are the activated clotting time (ACT), activated partial thromboplastin time (APTT), or thrombin time (TT).

Protamine is classified in FDA Pregnancy Category C.

DOSAGE AND PREPARATIONS.

Intravenous: Total dosage is determined by the amount of heparin given over the previous three to four hours (each milligram of protamine sulfate, calculated as dry material, neutralizes 90 U.S.P. units of heparin activity derived from lung tissue and 115 U.S.P. units of heparin activity derived from intestinal mucosa). A solution containing 10 mg/ml is injected slowly over one to three minutes, not to exceed 50 mg in any ten-minute period.

Generic. Powder; solution 10 mg/ml in 5, 10, and 25 ml containers.

LOW-MOLECULAR-WEIGHT HEPARINS AND HEPARINOIDS (Investigational Drugs)

Several low-molecular-weight heparins (LMWH) (eg, enoxaparin, fragmin [Kabi 2165], fraxiparin [CY216], logiparin [LHN-1]) and heparinoids (eg, lomoparin [Org 10172]) have been developed. Although some preparations are available in Europe, their use in the United States is limited to clinical trials.

ACTIONS AND USES. LMWH preparations and heparinoids are produced by partial chemical or enzymatic depolymerization of natural heparin followed by fractionation (Levine and Hirsh, 1988; Hirsh, 1990; Verstraete, 1990). The preparations differ from one another both in their mean molecular weights (from < 3,000 to about 9,000 daltons) and in their biological properties (Mammen, 1990). The complexes formed after binding of AT-III to LMWH have markedly reduced inhibitory activity against thrombin when compared to natural heparin but retain high activity against factor Xa. In contrast, lomoparin and other glycosaminoglycan and dermatan heparinoids do not appear to interact with AT-III; instead, they exert their antithrombotic effects through unknown mechanisms that may involve interactions with endothelial cells in the blood vessels (Walenga et al, 1991). Both heparinoids and LMWH interact with platelets to a lesser degree than does standard heparin (Messmore et al, 1991). It has been suggested that these differences might cause less impairment of hemostasis and reduce the risk of hemorrhage at effective antithrombotic doses.

Results of placebo-controlled trials of LMWH and heparinoids demonstrate that some of these preparations are safe and effective for prophylaxis of venous thrombosis (Turpie et al, 1986, 1987; Ockelford et al, 1989). Randomized trials comparing their safety and efficacy with standard heparin for either treatment or prevention of venous thrombosis have yielded mixed results. Some investigators report greater efficacy for LMWH than for standard heparin, with equivalent (*Thromb Haemost*, 1991), reduced (Green et al, 1990), or slightly increased (Bergqvist et al, 1990) hemorrhagic effects. Others report that LMWH preparations and standard heparin are equally efficacious but that the incidence of hemorrhage is lower with LMWH (Albada et al, 1989; Levine et al, 1991). In other studies, the safety and efficacy of standard heparin and LMWH did not differ significantly (Bratt et al, 1990). Some of these differences can be attributed to the use of different LMWH preparations, dosing regimens, and patient populations. There have been a few reports of heparin-induced thrombocytopenia that resolved when a LMWH product was substituted, but in other cases the thrombocytopenia persisted. A recent randomized study compared enoxaparin with dextran 70 as prophylaxis for venous thrombosis in patients undergoing elective total hip replacement (Danish Enoxaparin Study Group, 1991). Enoxaparin (6.5% incidence of thrombosis) was more effective than dextran 70 (21.6% incidence), and their safety was equivalent.

PHARMACOKINETICS. The pharmacokinetic properties of different LMWH preparations vary somewhat, but they are all cleared from the circulation less rapidly than standard heparin (Verstraete, 1990). This may be partially due to a lower affinity of binding sites on endothelial cells for LMWH than for unfractionated heparin. LMWH also are absorbed more completely than standard heparin after subcutaneous injection (Verstraete, 1990; Mammen, 1990), which results in significantly greater bioavailability. In addition, significant anti-factor Xa activity persists in the circulation long after LMWH concentrations have fallen below the limit of detection. Consequently, effective prophylaxis for venous thrombosis can be achieved with a single daily injection rather than the twice-daily injections required with subcutaneous standard heparin. However, optimal dosing regimens have not been established for many of the LMWH preparations. Heparinoids also appear to be cleared more slowly and have greater bioavailability than standard heparin (Walenga et al, 1991).

MONITORING THERAPY. Biological reference materials adopted for standardizing the measurement of LMWH potency differ from those used as references for standard heparin (Thomas, 1989). The tests used to monitor patients during LMWH therapy also differ from those used to monitor standard heparin (eg, APTT, activated clotting time). Most studies have used assays for anti-factor Xa activity that are based on chromogenic substrates to monitor blood levels of LMWH (Verstraete, 1990, Mammen, 1990).

ANTITHROMBIN III CONCENTRATE

[ATnativ, Thrombate III]

ACTIONS. Antithrombin III (AT-III) is the major physiologic inhibitor of thrombin and other activated clotting factors; it also serves as a receptor and cofactor for heparin (Pratt and Church, 1991; Bauer and Rosenberg, 1991). AT-III binds to and inactivates the serine protease catalytic centers of activated clotting factors. Heparin binds to AT-III and accelerates the rate of this inactivation. Normal levels of AT-III maintain blood fluidity by limiting diffusion of activated factors from the site of vascular injury.

USES. Human antithrombin III concentrate is prepared from pooled human plasma. Its use, alone or with heparin, is indicated in the treatment of thromboembolism in patients with hereditary AT-III deficiency and to prevent thromboemboli in congenitally deficient patients who are undergoing surgery, delivery at term, or spontaneous or induced abortion (Menache et al, 1990; Menache, 1991).

Hereditary AT-III deficiency is a rare autosomal-dominant disorder associated with recurrent thrombotic episodes; these may occur spontaneously or be precipitated by surgery, injury, infection, pregnancy, or use of oral contraceptives (Hathaway, 1991). More than 50% of those with this disorder will have a thrombotic episode by age 35 years and more than 85% by age 50. The goal of replacement therapy is to maintain a plasma AT-III concentration at 80% to 120% of normal, which requires frequent monitoring. Less data are available to confirm AT-III concentrate's benefit when it is administered to pregnant women with hereditary AT-III deficiency as prophylaxis for thrombosis or to reduce fetal growth retardation or death (Owen, 1991).

The use of human antithrombin III concentrate in acquired AT-III deficiencies has not been established; such deficiencies usually reflect increased consumption of AT-III and may occur after surgery or trauma, in association with certain diseases or medical conditions (eg, sepsis, disseminated intravascular coagulation, hepatic disease, nephrotic syndrome, protein-losing enteropathy, pre-eclampsia), or after administration of some drugs (eg, heparin, asparaginase, preparations that include estrogen agonists) (Hathaway, 1991). In many instances, acquired AT-III deficiency is not associated with an increased risk of thrombosis.

The effects of AT-III concentrate plus low-dose heparin are under investigation for prophylaxis of deep vein thrombosis after major orthopedic surgery. In separate trials, patients undergoing either total hip replacement or total knee replacement were randomized to receive prophylactic therapy with either dextran-40 or AT-III plus low-dose heparin (Francis et al, 1991). In both trials, the incidence of venous thrombosis was significantly higher among those who received dextran.

ADVERSE REACTIONS, PRECAUTIONS, AND INTERACTIONS. No adverse reactions to human AT-III concentrate have been reported in patients with hereditary deficiency, even at dosages that increased plasma levels to nearly twice normal. In clinical trials, two patients with disseminated intravascular coagulation who were treated for acquired deficiency experienced diuresis and vasodilation that resulted in hypotension. Rapid administration of the concentrate (1,500 units in five minutes) caused dyspnea and hypertension in one healthy subject.

Concomitant use of very large doses of AT-III concentrate and heparin may increase the risk of bleeding. Therefore, the dose of heparin should be monitored carefully when the two drugs are given concurrently.

In pregnant women receiving AT-III and heparin or oral anticoagulants near term, heparin should be discontinued at least 12 hours before delivery and the oral anticoagulant should be terminated several days before delivery or before a therapeutic or elective abortion.

Since human AT-III concentrate is prepared from pooled human plasma, it is heat-treated in solution at 60° C for at least 10 hours. This treatment inactivated several test viruses and human immunodeficiency virus (HIV) that were intentionally added to AT-III concentrate. Plasma used in the manufacture of AT-III concentrate also must be tested and found nonreactive for the hepatitis B surface antigen and antibody to HIV. Nevertheless, elimination of the risk of transmitting viral diseases (eg, hepatitis B or C) cannot be assured. Hepatitis (non-A, non-B) occurred in two patients who received both AT-III concentrate and whole blood or plasma but in none receiving AT-III concentrate alone. Minor episodes of fever have been reported.

The effects of AT-III concentrate on fertility and fetal development have not been studied in experimental animals. No increase in the occurrence of fetal abnormalities has been reported when AT-III was administered during the third trimester. This drug is classified in FDA Pregnancy Category C.

Data are inadequate to assess the safety and efficacy of AT-III concentrate in pediatric or geriatric patients; however, no differences have been observed in therapeutic responses or adverse reactions in adults and the small numbers of children or elderly patients treated thus far.

PHARMACOKINETICS. Plasma levels of AT-III can be measured using either functional or immunologic assays. In asymptomatic subjects with congenital AT-III deficiency, the relationship between the dose of AT-III and the increase in postinfusion plasma level (measured by either technique and expressed as a percentage of the normal mean) is linear when an increment of 1.4% to 1.6%/unit/kg is administered (Schwartz et al, 1989). Similar increments are observed in congenitally deficient patients treated prophylactically or therapeutically with AT-III, whether or not they also were receiving heparin. The mean biological half-life of AT-III was 3.8 ± 1.8 days when measured using functional AT-III assays and 2.5 ± 0.1 days when using an immunologic assay.

DOSAGE AND PREPARATIONS.

Intravenous: The potency of AT-III concentrate is expressed in International Units (IU), defined as the amount of AT-III in 1 ml of pooled normal human plasma and is measured against a standard calibrated with a reference preparation from the World Health Organization. Dosages are based on the degree of AT-III deficiency, an estimation of the desired fraction of normal plasma levels, and the body mass of the patient. The initial dose should be calculated to achieve 120% of the normal AT-III level, and subsequent doses should be calculated to achieve at least 80% of the normal level. Maintenance doses are given every 24 hours. See the manufacturers' literature for recommendations on dosage calculations, reconstitution, and patient monitoring.

ATnativ (Baxter/Hyland). Powder (lyophilized) 500 IU in single-use 50-ml infusion bottles with 90 mg sodium chloride and 100 mg human albumin. Supplied with 10 ml of sterile water for injection. Store at 2° to 8° C.

Thrombate III (Miles/Cutter Biological). Powder (lyophilized) 500 or 1,000 IU in single-dose containers supplied with 10 or 20 ml of diluent. When reconstituted, each IU of AT-III contains 0.110 to 0.210 moles/L sodium chloride, 0.075 to 0.125 moles/L alanine, and 0.004 units (NMT) of heparin.

Coumarin Derivatives

Actions: The coumarin anticoagulants (warfarin [Coumadin, Panwarfin] and dicumarol) block the post-translational modification of clotting factors II, VII, IX, and X and anticoagulant proteins C and S by impairing vitamin K-dependent gamma-carboxylation of N-terminal glutamic acid residues in these factors. Coumarin derivatives inhibit the enzymatic reactivation (reduction) of vitamin K epoxide, leading to its accumulation and to depletion of the active, reduced form (vitamin KH_2). Because of the lack of gamma-carboxylation, synthesized clotting factors are unable to bind calcium (Suttie, 1990; Hirsh, 1991 B; Kessler, 1991). Therefore, formation of thrombin is reduced and coagulation is retarded.

Although inhibition of vitamin K epoxide reductase is essentially complete after absorption and distribution of the first dose of a coumarin derivative, the onset of anticoagulant action requires clearance of the clotting factors already present in the circulation. Since factor VII has the shortest half-life (six to seven hours), it is the first to disappear from the plasma after coumarin administration and produces a mild anticoagulant effect within the first 24 hours. However, the half-life of protein C is close to that of factor VII, and reduction in the level of this anticoagulant protein may counteract the early decline in factor VII activity. Factors II, IX, and X have long half-lives (50 hours, 24 hours, and 36 hours, respectively); thus, the maximal anticoagulant effect is delayed until 72 to 96 hours after coumarin administration has begun.

Uses: The coumarins are used for prophylaxis of thromboemboli in patients with nonvalvular atrial fibrillation, valvular heart disease, or prosthetic heart valves and in selected surgical patients. These drugs also are used as therapy in patients with confirmed acute venous thrombosis or pulmonary embolism for maintenance of anticoagulation after initial treatment with heparin. The coumarins also are administered to prevent arterial emboli after acute myocardial infarction (AMI) in patients at highest risk (ie, those with evidence of mural thrombus or impaired left ventricular wall motion), for secondary prevention of death or recurrence after AMI in patients who cannot tolerate aspirin, and after percutaneous transluminal coronary angioplasty when there is residual thrombus or stenosis. Finally, coumarins may be administered to some patients to prevent reocclusion of coronary artery bypass grafts or to selected stroke patients with occlusion or stenosis of cerebral arteries. (See the Introduction for a more complete discussion of these indications.)

Data from a randomized trial suggest that very small daily doses of warfarin also may prevent thrombosis in patients with chronic indwelling central venous catheters (Bern et al, 1990). Although the dose of warfarin used in this study usually had no measurable effect on the PT, the value was prolonged in some patients. Nevertheless, warfarin 1 mg administered daily from 3 days before to 90 days after catheter insertion reduced the incidence of venogram-documented thrombosis from 37.5% to 9.5%.

Warfarin also has been investigated as a component of several combination chemotherapy regimens in patients with various solid tumors (Zacharski et al, 1990). Its addition to chemotherapy minimally increased survival time and the disease-free interval in patients with advanced small cell lung cancer but had no effect in patients with advanced carcinoma of the colon, prostate, or head and neck. In those with small cell lung cancer, hemorrhage was fatal in 2% and was life-threatening in 6%.

Drug Selection: Warfarin is the oral anticoagulant of choice because it is rapidly and nearly completely absorbed and it has a relatively short half-life. Although the longer action of dicumarol may be useful for maintenance therapy, this drug is so long acting that it may be hazardous if hemorrhage occurs. In addition, the dosage of dicumarol is difficult to control because it is incompletely absorbed.

Monitoring Therapy: The Quick one-stage prothrombin time (PT) test or a modification is used to regulate the dose of oral anticoagulants (British Society for Haematology, 1990; Hirsh, 1991 B). The PT reflects the depression of vitamin K-dependent factors II, VII, and X. (These factors, factor IX, and proteins C and S are affected by coumarin anticoagulants, but proteins C and S and factor IX are not measured by any one-stage prothrombin test.) Since the depression of each of these factors is not additive and each has a markedly different half-life, the factor depressed most quickly and profoundly (usually factor VII) acts as the determinant of prothrombin time during the first few days of treatment. During prolonged therapy, factor X ultimately shows the lowest activity in the steady state.

The thromboplastins used for the PT test in the United States are derived from rabbit brain or brain and lung and are less sensitive to the reduction in vitamin K-dependent clotting factors than are the thromboplastins used in Europe. Variability in the sensitivity of thromboplastins has led to variations in the intensity of anticoagulation achieved for a given target ratio of PT values in treated to untreated individuals. To encourage standardization of the therapeutic range, an international committee recommended adoption of an International Normalized Ratio (INR) to express prothrombin time. This system has now been accepted by most Western nations, although it is not widely used in U.S. hospitals. It relies on standardization of commercially available thromboplastins against a primary international reference preparation distributed by the World Health Organization. An International Sensitivity Index (ISI) is determined for each thromboplastin preparation and is used as the exponent of the PT ratio to calculate the INR (ie, $INR = [PT\ ratio]^{ISI}$). The reference preparation is assigned an ISI value of 1.0, and thromboplastins with lower sensitivity than the reference have ISI values greater than 1.0. Most thromboplastins used in the United States have ISI values ranging from 2.0 to 2.6. When thromboplastins of this sensitivity are used, an INR of 2.0 to 3.0 corresponds to a PT ratio of approximately 1.3 to 1.5 and an INR of 3.0 to 4.5 corresponds to a PT ratio of approximately 1.5 to 2.0.

To adjust the dose of oral anticoagulants, PT should be determined daily for the first five days of therapy, then twice weekly for the following one or two weeks (Hirsh, 1991 B). Measurement of PT should be repeated once weekly for the next one to two months until the values stabilize and then once or twice monthly for the duration of therapy as long as the PT values remain stable. The frequency of monitoring should be increased each time a change in the dose is necessary until PT values stabilize once again. More frequent monitoring also is needed for the duration of therapy in patients with impaired liver function, congestive heart failure, or frequent diarrhea; when the vitamin K content of the diet is drastically changed; or when new drugs are added to or withdrawn from the regimen.

Heparin has little effect on the one-stage PT in the absence of oral anticoagulation, but as the one-stage PT increases with use of oral anticoagulants, its susceptibility to a heparin effect increases. During concurrent therapy, blood samples for PT determination should be taken immediately prior to the next heparin injection if bolus injections are used. For patients on heparin and oral anticoagulants with a one-stage PT within the desired therapeutic range, the PT may decrease by one to three seconds when heparin is discontinued.

Several studies have evaluated the feasibility of patient self-management using a portable PT monitor and capillary blood obtained by fingerstick at home (White et al, 1989; Ansell et al, 1989). These studies concluded that patients can determine PT times accurately and make appropriate adjustments to dosages based on guidelines provided by their physicians. In one study in which the patients measured PT but physicians determined the dose adjustments, those in the self-monitoring group were within the target therapeutic range of PT values a greater percentage of the time than those in a control group monitored at an anticoagulation clinic (White et al, 1989). However, self-monitoring has not yet gained widespread acceptance.

Measurement of the native, fully gamma-carboxylated prothrombin using a specific antibody is an alternative approach that is being developed. Data from a randomized prospective trial suggest that fewer bleeding or thrombotic complications may occur in patients monitored by the antibody-based assay than in those monitored by PT assay (Furie et al, 1990).

Adverse Reactions and Precautions: Hemorrhage is the most common adverse effect leading to withdrawal of coumarin therapy (Hirsh, 1991 B; Harrington and Ansell, 1991). This complication is less frequent when the PT ratio is within the less intense therapeutic range (1.3 to 1.5 times control; INR 2.0 to 3.0). The risk of bleeding is increased in patients with ischemic cerebrovascular disease or venous thromboembolism. Hypertension is an important risk factor in those with cerebrovascular disease. Ulcer, cancer, recent surgery, and paraplegia predispose to bleeding in patients with venous thromboembolism. Intraocular hemorrhage has occurred in patients with iris-fixated intraocular lenses.

A study of the incidence of bleeding in outpatients given oral anticoagulants identified age >65 years, history of stroke or gastrointestinal bleeding, atrial fibrillation, and other serious coexisting conditions (eg, recent AMI, renal impairment, severe anemia) as independent predictors of hemorrhage that can be identified at the start of therapy (Landefeld and Goldman, 1989). Others believe that the age-related increase in the risk of bleeding does not become clinically significant until patients reach 75 years (Launbjerg et al, 1991). However, there is agreement that the risk of hemorrhage increases in proportion to the increase in PT ratio or prolongation of PT times (Landefeld et al, 1989; Launbjerg et al, 1991). This increased risk can be reduced without loss of the therapeutic response by using a less intense anticoagulant regimen that maintains the PT ratio at 1.3 to 1.5 times control (INR 2.0 to

3.0) (Hull et al, 1982; Hirsh 1991 B; Harrington and Ansell, 1991). The incidence of major hemorrhage in patients with atrial fibrillation who were maintained at this level of anticoagulation is 0.5% to 1% (Boston Area Anticoagulation Trial for Atrial Fibrillation Investigators, 1990; Connolly et al, 1991). When the risk of thromboembolism is high (eg, recurrent systemic embolism, mechanical prosthetic heart valves), a PT ratio of 1.5 to 2 times control (INR 3.0 to 4.5) should be maintained. An intensity of anticoagulation greater than this provides no additional benefit and is associated with a higher risk of bleeding (Hirsh et al, 1989).

If hemorrhage is severe and the effects of the oral anticoagulant must be counteracted quickly, administration of fresh frozen plasma (20 ml/kg) is most desirable; fresh single-donor human plasma and factor IX complex also may be used (see index entries Plasma, In Replacement Therapy, and Factor IX Complex Human, As Hemostatic). However, the use of factor IX complex is associated with a significant risk of transmitting viruses and thus is less desirable than fresh plasma. In patients who metabolize warfarin at a slow rate, secondary prolongation of the prothrombin time may occur (in 10 to 12 hours) after the effects of plasma have worn off.

The decision to use vitamin K should be based on a balance between antithrombotic protection and the severity of bleeding and on whether there is a need to resume anticoagulant therapy after the bleeding episode has ceased. If vitamin K is considered necessary, phytonadione (vitamin K_1) may be given orally (adults, 10 to 25 mg; children, 5 to 10 mg) or intramuscularly (adults, 5 to 10 mg; children, 1 to 5 mg). Menadione (vitamin K_3) is not an effective antidote for warfarin-induced hemorrhage (see index entry Hemostatics, In Vitamin K Deficiency). When anticoagulant therapy is resumed after use of phytonadione, larger than usual doses may be required initially.

Necrotic lesions and/or gangrene, presumably caused by thrombosis in the capillaries and venules within the subcutaneous fat, occur occasionally, usually within the third to eighth day after initiating therapy with large doses of warfarin (more than 10 mg) (Comp et al, 1990; Hirsh, 1991 B; Harrington and Ansell, 1991). This complication, which affects women more often than men, begins as petechiae that coalesce to form painful ecchymoses, hemorrhagic bullae, and necrosis. Lesions occur most commonly in adipose tissue or dependent areas, such as the breast, buttocks, thighs, and distal lower extremities. Debridement or amputation of the affected tissue, limb, breast, or penis has been necessary in severe cases. Some fatalities have been reported.

A deficiency of protein C or, less commonly, protein S has been documented in many patients who develop necrotic lesions (Grimaudo et al, 1989). The short half-life of protein C relative to that of clotting factors II, IX, and X may result in a period of hypercoagulability that lasts until activities of these factors fall. In patients with protein C deficiency, the initial decline after beginning oral anticoagulant therapy may lead to microvascular thrombosis and skin necrosis. However, not all patients with heterozygous protein C deficiency develop this response, and some who do are found to have normal levels of both proteins C and S (Comp et al, 1990; Harrington and Ansell, 1991). Other hypercoagulable states that have been associated with anticoagulant-induced skin necrosis include deficiency of antithrombin III and the presence of the lupus anticoagulant. Almost all instances of skin necrosis have occurred in patients being treated for venous thrombosis or pulmonary embolism. Patients receiving coumarin anticoagulants for atrial fibrillation, cerebrovascular insufficiency, or arterial disease rarely experience this reaction.

If an oral anticoagulant is suspected to be the cause of developing necrosis, it should be discontinued immediately and heparin substituted. Phytonadione and fresh frozen plasma (as a source of antithrombin III and proteins C and S) also should be administered. However, no comparative controlled studies have been performed to determine the most effective therapy for warfarin-induced skin necrosis and no treatment is uniformly effective. The risk of developing necrosis has been reported to be reduced if heparin (APTT > 1.5 times control) is given for four to five days prior to starting warfarin and therapy with both drugs overlaps for several days. Some investigators suggest that oral anticoagulant therapy can be successfully resumed after complete resolution of an episode of skin necrosis if very small doses of warfarin are used with full-dose intravenous heparin (Comp et al, 1990).

Occasional adverse reactions include gastrointestinal disturbances (especially diarrhea with dicumarol), elevated transaminase levels, urticaria, dermatitis, leukopenia, fever, hypersensitivity reactions, "purple toe" syndrome, priapism, and alopecia.

Use During Pregnancy and Lactation: When given during the first trimester of pregnancy (especially the sixth to ninth week), warfarin therapy has been associated with embryopathy characterized by nasal hypoplasia and stippled epiphyses. Other abnormalities, including central nervous system and ocular defects, can result from exposure during the second and third trimesters (Hall et al, 1980). Review of case histories reveals that about one-third of infants exposed to coumarin derivatives are stillborn or abnormal if born alive. Heparin should be used if anticoagulant therapy is required during pregnancy. Oral anticoagulants should not be prescribed for women of childbearing age unless absolutely necessary, and those receiving the drug should be counseled regarding measures to avoid pregnancy. If pregnancy occurs, the woman should be counseled about the risks to the fetus and options for managing those risks. Warfarin is classified in FDA Pregnancy Category X.

Although coumarins appear in the milk of lactating women, they are not contraindicated in nursing mothers since no anticoagulant effect has been observed in the breast-fed infant (Ginsberg and Hirsh, 1988).

Drug Interactions: Although many drugs affect the action of oral anticoagulants in laboratory animals, only a small number have been clearly demonstrated to interact in man. Drugs that prolong or intensify the action of oral anticoagulants or diminish the anticoagulant response are listed in the Table. Inclusion of a drug in this list does not imply that its use is contraindicated in patients taking coumarin anticoagulants or in whom their use is contemplated. Most drugs in this list can be used safely and effectively with a coumarin anticoagulant if

INTERACTIONS AFFECTING RESPONSE TO ORAL ANTICOAGULANTS

AGENTS THAT MAY PROLONG OR INTENSIFY THE RESPONSE TO ORAL ANTICOAGULANTS:

- Allopurinol
- Amiodarone
- Anabolic steroids
- Androgens
- Aspirin and other salicylates
- Oral antimicrobial agents plus reduced dietary vitamin K
- Cephalosporins (2nd and 3rd generation)
- Chloramphenicol
- Cimetidine
- Clofibrate
- Cyclophosphamide
- Diflunisal
- Disulfiram
- Erythromycin
- Ethchlorvynol
- Fluconazole
- Fluoroquinolones
- Flurbiprofen
- Gemfibrozil
- Glucagon
- Heparin
- Ifosfamide
- Indomethacin
- Influenza vaccine
- Isoniazid
- Ketoconazole
- Lovastatin
- Magnesium salts
- Mefenamic acid
- Metronidazole
- Miconazole
- Nalidixic acid
- Omeprazole
- Oxyphenbutazone
- Phenylbutazone
- Phenytoin
- Piroxicam
- Propafenone
- Propoxyphene
- Quinidine
- Sulfinpyrazone
- Sulindac
- Tamoxifen
- Thyroid preparations
- Ticlopidine
- Trimethoprim/Sulfamethoxazole
- Vitamin E (megadose)

AGENTS THAT MAY DIMINISH THE RESPONSE TO ORAL ANTICOAGULANTS:

- Aminoglutethimide
- Antacids
- Azathioprine
- Barbiturates
- Carbamazepine
- Cholestyramine resin and other bile acid sequestrants
- Corticosteroids
- Diuretics
- Glutethimide
- Griseofulvin
- Oral contraceptives
- Penicillins (large doses)
- Rifampin
- Thiazide diuretics
- Thioamides (eg, propylthiouracil)
- Trazodone
- Excessive intake of vitamin K (eg, brussels sprouts, other raw vegetables, green tea)

AGENTS THAT HAVE BEEN REPORTED TO INCREASE OR DECREASE PROTHROMBIN TIME:

- Alcohol
- Chloral hydrate
- Ranitidine

PT ratios or INR values are monitored frequently and the appropriate dose adjustments are made during the initial period of combined drug therapy. The only exceptions may be drugs that inhibit platelet aggregation (eg, salicylates, nonsteroidal anti-inflammatory drugs), which may interact with coumarins to cause clinically significant hemorrhage without increasing the PT ratio or INR value.

Coumarins also may interact with oral antidiabetic drugs (chlorpropamide, tolbutamide) to cause hypoglycemia. Dicumarol may displace protein-bound phenytoin [Dilantin] and enhance its toxicity.

WARFARIN SODIUM
[Coumadin, Panwarfin]

Na^+ ^-O CH CH_2CCH_3 O

Warfarin is the oral anticoagulant of choice. It is no longer available for parenteral use. The specific uses of warfarin are discussed at length in the Introduction and reviewed briefly in the previous section on Coumarin Derivatives.

DOSAGE REQUIREMENTS. The former custom of giving a large loading dose, which then is decreased immediately or gradually to the maintenance dose, is no longer recommended. The initial effect of a loading dose primarily reflects depression of factor VII. The benefits of warfarin in preventing formation or extension of thrombi are related largely to depression of factors IX and X. These factors decrease more slowly than factor VII but at the same rate whether a single large loading dose or smaller doses of 10 to 15 mg/day are administered. Prothrombin time should be determined daily and the dosage adjusted accordingly. Avoiding a loading dose minimizes the danger of hemorrhage in patients with diminished tolerance or unusual sensitivity to the anticoagulant and may reduce the risk of skin necrosis (McGehee et al, 1984). Guidelines (Ansell et al, 1989) and computer programs

(Ryan et al, 1989; White and Mungall, 1991) for adjusting the dosage of warfarin based on PT ratios or INR values are available.

PHARMACOKINETICS. Warfarin is intermediate acting; a peak effect is achieved in 36 to 72 hours and the anticoagulant effect persists for two to five days. The drug is rapidly and completely absorbed from the gastrointestinal tract (Shetty et al, 1989; Hirsh 1991 B). The delay in achieving the peak effect results from the long half-lives of clotting factors II, IX, and X, whose levels must decline before maximal anticoagulation is reached.

Warfarin is highly lipophilic and is 99% bound to albumin. Some tissue binding occurs, particularly in the liver. However, only the unbound drug is active and available for hydroxylation in the liver.

The two optically active isomers present in racemic warfarin are metabolized by different pathways and at different rates (Shetty et al, 1989; Hirsh, 1991 B). The R(+) isomer is reduced to an alcohol that is eliminated in the urine, while the S(−) isomer is hydroxylated and excreted in the bile. The half-life of the R(+) enantiomer is 43 hours while that of the S(−) isomer is only 32 hours, but the S(−) enantiomer is three to five times more potent as an antagonist of vitamin K epoxide reductase. The metabolites of both isomers are relatively inactive as anticoagulants. The rate of degradation is proportional to the plasma concentration but there is wide interpatient variabililty. Protein-losing enteropathy (eg, in uremia) may result in decreased protein binding which can lead to increased hepatic clearance, but other forms of impaired renal function do not appear to affect responses to warfarin. However, chronic liver disease may sensitize patients to the drug's effects by reducing hepatic synthesis of clotting factors.

ADVERSE REACTIONS, PRECAUTIONS, AND INTERACTIONS. See the Introduction and the previous discussion on Coumarin Derivatives.

DOSAGE AND PREPARATIONS.
Oral: Prothrombin time (PT) should be determined before the initial dose is given and every day thereafter until the response is stabilized. After a steady state is achieved, the PT should be determined at regular intervals (see the section on Monitoring Therapy). A commonly used regimen is 10 mg/day for two to four days with daily adjustments based on the results of PT determinations. Usually there is little change in the PT during the first 24 hours, followed by a slow rise to 16 to 20 seconds (assuming control values of between 10 and 12 seconds) by the third day. The usual maintenance dose is 2 to 10 mg daily thereafter.

Coumadin (DuPont), ***Panwarfin*** (Abbott), ***Generic.*** Tablets 1 (***Coumadin*** only), 2, 2.5, 5, 7.5, and 10 mg.

DICUMAROL

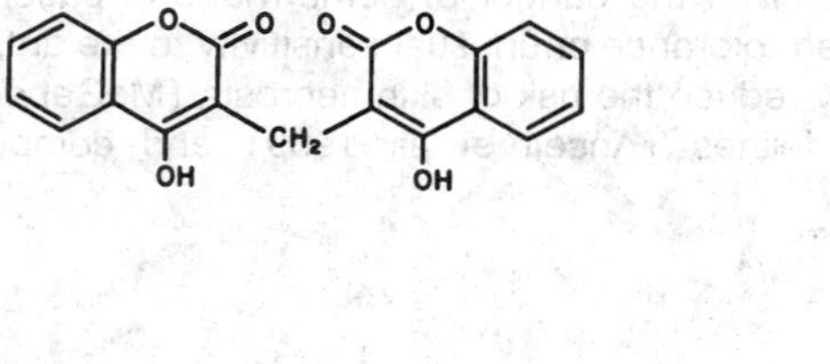

Dicumarol has the same actions and uses as warfarin but is longer acting. In the usual dosage range, the onset of hypocoagulability occurs in 36 to 48 hours while three to five days are required for peak action. Once hypoprothrombinemia is established, the anticoagulant effect usually persists for five to six days (range, two to ten days) following discontinuation of therapy. Dicumarol is incompletely absorbed from the gastrointestinal tract, and maximal plasma concentrations occur in one to nine hours. Dicumarol has a dose-dependent plasma half-life (one to two days); therapy is therefore somewhat difficult to control and frequent monitoring is usually indicated.

Dicumarol frequently causes flatulence and diarrhea. For other adverse reactions, precautions, interactions, and general class characteristics of the coumarin compounds, see the Introduction and the discussion on Coumarin Derivatives.

DOSAGE AND PREPARATIONS.
Oral: *Adults,* 200 to 300 mg on the first day, followed by 25 to 200 mg daily using prothrombin time (PT) determinations as a guide. Frequent dosage adjustments may be necessary during the first 7 to 14 days of therapy (see the discussion on Monitoring Therapy in the section on Coumarin Derivatives). The PT should be determined daily during this period and dosage adjusted to maintain PT ratios or INR values within the therapeutic ranges recommended for each indication (see the Introduction). The maintenance dose varies between 25 and 200 mg daily, depending on the results of these determinations.

Generic. Tablets 25 and 50 mg.

Indandione Derivative

ANISINDIONE
[Miradon]

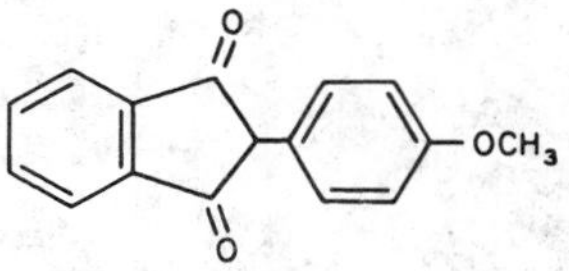

ACTIONS AND USES. This long-acting oral anticoagulant has actions and uses similar to those of the coumarins; however, since anisindione is potentially dangerous, it should be reserved for patients who cannot tolerate the coumarins.

After the initial dose, the peak effect is reached in 48 to 72 hours, and coagulation factors gradually return to normal 24 to 72 hours after the drug is discontinued. As with other oral anticoagulants, both resistance and sensitivity have been reported.

ADVERSE REACTIONS AND PRECAUTIONS. Anisindione may cause dermatitis. Since the related indandione, phenindione (no longer marketed), produced serious and sometimes fatal adverse effects (eg, agranulocytosis, jaundice, nephropathy), anisindione must be assumed to have the potential to cause serious complications. The drug should be discontinued promptly if fever, sore throat, or rash appears, for these symptoms may signal the onset of severe toxicity.

Anisindione occasionally discolors alkaline urine orange; this can be differentiated from hematuria by its disappearance on acidification of the urine. The patient should be advised of this possibility.

See also the Introduction and the discussion on Coumarin Derivatives for hemorrhagic and other complications of oral anticoagulant therapy.

DOSAGE AND PREPARATIONS.

Oral: *Adults,* 300 mg on the first day, 200 mg on the second day, and 100 mg on the third day. For maintenance, the amount that maintains prothrombin time values at 2 to 2.5 times normal should be given; the usual dose ranges from 25 to 250 mg daily.

Miradon (Schering). Tablets 50 mg.

Cited References

A randomised trial of subcutaneous low molecular weight heparin (CY 216) compared with intravenous unfractionated heparin in the treatment of deep vein thrombosis: A collaborative European multicentre study. *Thromb Haemost* 65:251-256, 1991.

ACC/AHA Task Force: ACC/AHA guidelines for the early management of patients with acute myocardial infarction: A report of the American College of Cardiology/American Heart Association Task Force on Assessment of Diagnostic and Therapeutic Cardiovascular Procedures (Subcommittee to Develop Guidelines for the Early Management of Patients With Acute Myocardial Infarction. *Circulation* 82:664-707, 1990.

Albada J, et al: Treatment of acute venous thromboembolism with low molecular weight heparin (Fragmin): Results of a double-blind randomized study. *Circulation* 80:935-940, 1989.

American College of Chest Physicians: Second Conference on Antithrombotic Therapy, symposium. *Chest* 95(suppl):1S-169S, (Feb) 1989.

Anderson DR, et al: Subcutaneous heparin therapy during pregnancy: A need for concern at the time of delivery. *Thromb Haemost* 65:248-250, 1991.

Ansell JE, et al: Heparin-induced thrombocytopenia: What is its real frequency? *Chest* 88:878-882, 1985.

Ansell J, et al: Patient self-management of oral anticoagulation guided by capillary (fingerstick) whole blood prothrombin times. *Arch Intern Med* 149:2509-2511, 1989.

Bauer KA, Rosenberg RD: Role of antithrombin III as a regulator of in vivo coagulation. *Semin Hematol* 28:10-18, (Jan) 1991.

Bell WR: Heparin-associated thrombocytopenia and thrombosis. *J Lab Clin Med* 111:600-605, 1988.

Bergqvist D, et al: Thromboprophylactic effect of low molecular weight heparin started in the evening before elective general abdominal surgery: A comparison with low-dose heparin. *Semin Thromb Hemost* 16(suppl):19-24, 1990.

Berk BC, et al: Pharmacologic roles of heparin and glucocorticoids to prevent restenosis after coronary angioplasty. *J Am Coll Cardiol* 17:111B-117B, 1991.

Bern MM, et al: Very low doses of warfarin can prevent thrombosis in central venous catheters: A randomized prospective trial. *Ann Intern Med* 112:423-428, 1990.

Bode V, et al: Absence of drug interaction between heparin and nitroglycerin: Randomized placebo-controlled crossover study. *Arch Intern Med* 150:2117-2119, 1990.

Boston Area Anticoagulation Trial for Atrial Fibrillation Investigators: The effect of low-dose warfarin on the risk of stroke in patients with nonrheumatic atrial fibrillation. *N Engl J Med* 323:1505-1511, 1990.

Bratt G, et al: Two daily subcutaneous injections of Fragmin as compared with intravenous standard heparin in the treatment of deep venous thrombosis (DVT). *Thromb Haemost* 64:506-510, 1990.

British Society for Haematology, British Committee for Standards in Haematology, Haemostasis and Thrombosis Task Force: Guidelines on oral anticoagulation: Second edition. *J Clin Pathol* 43:177-183, 1990.

Cairns JA: Reperfusion adjunctive therapy. *Chest* 99(suppl):141S-149S, 1991.

Cairns JA, Connolly SJ: Nonrheumatic atrial fibrillation: Risk of stroke and role of antithrombotic therapy. *Circulation* 84:469-481, 1991.

Cerebral Embolism Study Group: Cardioembolic stroke, early anticoagulation, and brain hemorrhage. *Arch Intern Med* 147:636-640, 1987.

Chesebro JH, et al: Importance of antithrombin therapy during coronary angioplasty. *J Am Coll Cardiol* 17:96B-100B, 1991.

Col J, et al: Propylene glycol-induced heparin resistance during nitroglycerin infusion. *Am Heart J* 110:171-173, 1985.

Cola C, Ansell J: Heparin-induced thrombocytopenia and arterial thrombosis: Alternative therapies. *Am Heart J* 119(no. 2, part 1):368-374, 1990.

Collins R, et al: Reduction in fatal pulmonary embolism and venous thrombosis by perioperative administration of subcutaneous heparin: Overview of results of randomized trials in general, orthopedic, and urologic surgery. *N Engl J Med* 318:1162-1173, 1988.

Comp PC, et al: Warfarin-induced skin necrosis. *Semin Thromb Haemost* 16:293-298, 1990.

Connolly SJ, et al: Canadian Atrial Fibrillation Anticoagulation (CAFA) Study. *J Am Coll Cardiol* 18:349-355, 1991.

Cruickshank MK, et al: A standard heparin nomogram for the management of heparin therapy. *Arch Intern Med* 151:333-337, 1991.

Danish Enoxaparin Study Group: Low-molecular-weight heparin (Enoxaparin) vs dextran 70: The prevention of postoperative deep vein thrombosis after total hip replacement. *Arch Intern Med* 151:1621-1624, 1991.

Doyle DJ, et al: Adjusted subcutaneous heparin or continuous intravenous heparin in patients with acute deep vein thrombosis. *Ann Intern Med* 107:441-445, 1987.

Duke RJ, et al: Intravenous heparin for the prevention of stroke progression in acute partial stable stroke: A randomized controlled trial. *Ann Intern Med* 105:825-828, 1986.

Dunn M, et al: Antithrombotic therapy in atrial fibrillation. *Chest* 95(suppl):118S-126S, 1989.

Ellis SG, et al: Effect of 18- to 24-hour heparin administration for prevention of restenosis after uncomplicated coronary angioplasty. *Am Heart J* 117:777-782, 1989.

Estol CJ, Pessin MS: Anticoagulation: Is there still a role in atherothrombotic stroke? *Curr Concepts Cerebrovasc Dis Stroke* 25:1-6, (Jan-Feb) 1990.

Francis CW, et al: Prophylaxis of venous thrombosis following total hip and total knee replacement using antithrombin III and heparin. *Semin Hematol* 28:39-45, (Jan) 1991.

Furie B, et al: Randomized prospective trial comparing the native prothrombin antigen with the prothrombin time for monitoring oral anticoagulant therapy. *Blood* 75:344-349, 1990.

Fuster V, et al: Prevention of thromboembolism induced by prosthetic heart valves. *Semin Thromb Hemost* 14:50-58, 1988.

Gallus A, et al: Safety and efficacy of warfarin started early after submassive venous thrombosis or pulmonary embolism. *Lancet* 2:1293-1296, 1986.

Ginsberg JS, Hirsh J: Optimum use of anticoagulants in pregnancy. *Drugs* 36:505-512, 1988.

Ginsberg JS, Hirsh J: Use of anticoagulants during pregnancy. *Chest* 95(suppl):156S-160S, 1989.

Ginsberg JS, et al: Risks to the fetus of anticoagulant therapy during pregnancy. *Thromb Haemost* 61:197-203, 1989 A.

Ginsberg JS, et al: Heparin therapy during pregnancy: Risks to the fetus and mother. *Arch Intern Med* 149:2233-2236, 1989 B.

Green D, et al: Prevention of thromboembolism after spinal cord injury using low-molecular-weight heparin. *Ann Intern Med* 113:571-574, 1990.

Grimaudo V, et al: Necrosis of skin induced by coumarin in a patient deficient in protein S. *Br Med J* 298:233-234, 1989.
Habbab MA, Haft JI: Heparin resistance induced by intravenous nitroglycerin: Word of caution when both drugs are used concomitantly. *Arch Intern Med* 147:857-860, 1987.
Hall JG, et al: Maternal and fetal sequelae of anticoagulation during pregnancy. *Am J Med* 68:122-140, 1980.
Harrington R, Ansell J: Risk-benefit assessment of anticoagulant therapy. *Drug Saf* 6:54-69, 1991.
Hathaway WE: Clinical aspects of antithrombin III deficiency. *Semin Hematol* 28:19-23, (Jan) 1991.
Hirsh J: From unfractionated heparins to low molecular weight heparins. *Acta Chir Scand Suppl* 556:42-50, 1990.
Hirsh J: Heparin. *N Engl J Med* 324:1565-1574, 1991 A.
Hirsh J: Oral anticoagulant drugs. *N Engl J Med* 324:1865-1875, 1991 B.
Hirsh J, et al: Optimal therapeutic range for oral anticoagulants. *Chest* 95 (suppl):5S-11S, 1989.
Hull RD, et al: Warfarin sodium versus low-dose heparin in the long-term treatment of venous thrombosis. *N Engl J Med* 301:855-858, 1979.
Hull RD, et al: Different intensities of oral anticoagulant therapy in treatment of proximal-vein thrombosis. *N Engl J Med* 307:1676-1681, 1982.
Hull RD, et al: Continuous intravenous heparin compared with intermittent subcutaneous heparin in the initial treatment of proximal-vein thrombosis. *N Engl J Med* 315:1109-1114, 1986.
Hull RD, et al: Heparin for 5 days as compared with 10 days in the initial treatment of proximal venous thrombosis. *N Engl J Med* 322:1260-1264, 1990.
Hyers TM, et al: Antithrombotic therapy for venous thromboembolic disease. *Chest* 95 (suppl):37S-51S, 1989.
Ip JH, et al: Thrombosis and antithrombotic therapy in cardiovascular disease. *Cardiovasc Rev Rep* 12:16-30, 1991.
Israel DH, et al: Antithrombotic therapy in the coronary vein graft patient. *Clin Cardiol* 14:283-295, 1991.
Iturbe-Alessio I, et al: Risks of anticoagulant therapy in pregnant women with artificial heart valves. *N Engl J Med* 315:1390-1393, 1986.
Jonas S: Anticoagulant therapy in cerebrovascular disease: Review and meta-analysis. *Stroke* 19:1043-1048, 1988.
Kaiser B: Anticoagulant and antithrombotic actions of recombinant hirudin. *Semin Thromb Hemost* 17:130-136, 1991.
Kessler CM: The pharmacology of aspirin, heparin, coumarin, and thrombolytic agents: Implications for therapeutic use in cardiopulmonary disease. *Chest* 99 (suppl):97S-112S, 1991.
King DJ, Kelton JG: Heparin-associated thrombocytopenia. *Ann Intern Med* 100:535-540, 1984.
Kroon C, et al: Influence of skinfold thickness on heparin absorption. *Lancet* 337:945-946, 1991.
Lagerstedt CI, et al: Need for long-term anticoagulant treatment in symptomatic calf-vein thrombosis. *Lancet* 2:515-518, 1985.
Landefeld CS, Goldman L: Major bleeding in outpatients treated with warfarin: Incidence and prediction by factors known at the start of outpatient therapy. *Am J Med* 87:144-152, 1989.
Landefeld CS, et al: Bleeding in outpatients treated with warfarin: Relation to the prothrombin time and important remediable lesions. *Am J Med* 87:153-159, 1989.
Laskey MAL, et al: Influence of heparin therapy on percutaneous transluminal coronary angioplasty outcome in unstable angina pectoris. *Am J Cardiol* 65:1425-1429, 1990.
Launbjerg J, et al: Bleeding complications to oral anticoagulant therapy: Multivariate analysis of 1010 treatment years in 551 outpatients. *J Intern Med* 229:351-355, 1991.
Laupacis A, et al: How should results from completed studies influence on-going clinical trials? The CAFA study experience. *Ann Intern Med* 115:818-822, 1991.
Lepor NE, et al: Does nitroglycerin induce heparin resistance? *Clin Cardiol* 12:432-434, 1989.
Lesko SM, et al: Heparin use as risk factor for intraventricular hemorrhage in low-birth-weight infants. *N Engl J Med* 314:1156-1160, 1986.
Levine MN, Hirsh J: Clinical use of low molecular weight heparins and heparinoids. *Semin Thromb Hemost* 14:116-125, 1988.
Levine M, Hirsh J: The diagnosis and treatment of thrombosis in the cancer patient. *Semin Oncol* 17:160-171, 1990.
Levine HJ, et al: Antithrombotic therapy in valvular heart disease. *Chest* 95 (suppl):98S-106S, 1989.
Levine MN, et al: Prevention of deep vein thrombosis after elective hip surgery: A randomized trial comparing low molecular weight heparin with standard unfractionated heparin. *Ann Intern Med* 114:545-551, 1991.
Mammen EF: Why low molecular weight heparin? *Semin Thromb Hemost* 16 (suppl):1-4, 1990.
Mancini GBJ, Weinberg DM: Cardioversion of atrial fibrillation: A retrospective analysis of the safety and value of anticoagulation. *Cardiovasc Rev Rep* 18-23, (Jan) 1990.
Märki WE, Wallis RB: The anticoagulant and antithrombotic properties of hirudins. *Thromb Haemost* 64:344-348, 1990.
Markwardt F: Development of hirudin as an antithrombotic agent. *Semin Thromb Hemost* 15:269-282, 1989.
Markwardt F: The comeback of hirudin as an antithrombotic agent. *Semin Thromb Hemost* 17:79-82, 1991.
Marsh EE III, et al: Use of antithrombotic drugs in the treatment of acute ischemic stroke: A survey of neurologists in practice in the United States. *Neurology* 39:1631-1634, 1989.
McCarthy ST, et al: Low-dose heparin as a prophylaxis against deep-vein thrombosis after acute stroke. *Lancet* 2:800-801, 1977.
McGehee WG, et al: Coumarin necrosis associated with hereditary protein C deficiency. *Ann Intern Med* 100:59-60, 1984.
Menache D: Replacement therapy in patients with hereditary antithrombin III deficiency. *Semin Hematol* 28:31-38, (Jan) 1991.
Menache D, et al: Evaluation of the safety, recovery, half-life, and clinical efficacy of antithrombin III (human) in patients with hereditary antithrombin III deficiency. *Blood* 75:33-39, (Jan) 1990.
Merli GJ: Prophylaxis for deep vein thrombosis and pulmonary embolism in the geriatric patient undergoing surgery. *Clin Geriatr Med* 6:531-542, 1990.
Messmore HL, et al: Interaction of heparinoids with platelets: Comparison with heparin and low molecular weight heparins. *Semin Thromb Hemost* 17 (suppl 1):57-59, 1991.
Miller VT, Hart RG: Heparin anticoagulation in acute brain ischemia. *Stroke* 19:403-406, 1988.
Moser KM, LeMoine JR: Is embolic risk conditioned by location of deep venous thrombosis? *Ann Intern Med* 94 (part 1):439-444, 1981.
Neri Serneri GG, et al: Effect of heparin, aspirin, or alteplase in reduction of myocardial ischaemia in refractory unstable angina. *Lancet* 335:615-618, 1990.
Ockelford PA, et al: A double-blind randomized placebo controlled trial of thromboprophylaxis in major elective general surgery using once daily injections of a low molecular weight heparin fragment (Fragmin). *Thromb Haemost* 62:1046-1049, 1989.
Owen J: Antithrombin III replacement therapy in pregnancy. *Semin Hematol* 28:46-52, (Jan) 1991.
Petersen P, et al: Placebo-controlled, randomised trial of warfarin and aspirin for prevention of thromboembolic complications in chronic atrial fibrillation. *Lancet* 1:175-179, 1989.
Philbrick JT, Becker DM: Calf deep venous thrombosis: A wolf in sheep's clothing? *Arch Intern Med* 148:2131-2138, 1988.
Phillips SJ: An alternative view of heparin anticoagulation in acute focal brain ischemia. *Stroke* 20:295-298, 1989.
Pini M, et al: Subcutaneous vs intravenous heparin in the treatment of deep venous thrombosis: A randomized clinical trial. *Thromb Haemost* 64:222-226, 1990.
Pratt CW, Church FC: Antithrombin: Structure and function. *Semin Hematol* 28:3-9, (Jan) 1991.
Rao AK, et al: Low incidence of thrombocytopenia with porcine mucosal heparin: Prospective multicenter study. *Arch Intern Med* 149:1285-1288, 1989.
Resnekov L, et al: Antithrombotic agents in coronary artery disease. *Chest* 95 (suppl):52S-72S, 1989.

The RISC Group: Risk of myocardial infarction and death during treatment with low dose aspirin and intravenous heparin in men with unstable coronary artery disease. *Lancet* 336:827-830, 1990.

Ryan PJ, et al: Computer control of anticoagulant dose for therapeutic management. *Br Med J* 299:1207-1209, 1989.

Scheinberg P: Heparin anticoagulation. *Stroke* 20:173-174, 1989.

Schulman S, Johnsson H: Heparin, DDAVP and the bleeding time. *Thromb Haemost* 65:242-244, 1991.

Schwartz RS, et al: Clinical experience with antithrombin III concentrate in treatment of congenital and acquired deficiency of antithrombin. *Am J Med* 87 (suppl 3B):3B-53S-3B-60S, 1989.

Sherman DG, Hart RG: Thromboembolism and antithrombotic therapy in cerebrovascular disease. *J Am Coll Cardiol* 8:88B-97B, 1986.

Sherman RA, Ruddy MC: Suppression of aldosterone production by low-dose heparin. *Am J Nephrol* 6:165-168, 1986.

Sherman DG, et al: Antithrombotic therapy for cerebrovascular disorders. *Chest* 95 (suppl):140S-155S, 1989.

Shetty HGM, et al: Clinical pharmacokinetic considerations in the control of oral anticoagulant therapy. *Clin Pharmacokinet* 16:238-253, 1989.

Stein PD, Kantrowitz A: Antithrombotic therapy in mechanical and biological prosthetic heart valves and saphenous vein bypass grafts. *Chest* 95 (suppl):107S-117S, 1989.

Stein B, et al: Antithrombotic therapy in cardiac disease: An emerging approach based on pathogenesis and risk. *Circulation* 80:1501-1513, 1989.

Stroke Prevention in Atrial Fibrillation (SPAF) Study Group Investigators: Stroke Prevention in Atrial Fibrillation Study: Final results. *Circulation* 84:527-539, 1991.

Suttie JW: Warfarin and vitamin K. *Clin Cardiol* 13:VI-16-VI-18, 1990.

Théroux P, et al: Aspirin, heparin, or both to treat acute unstable angina. *N Engl J Med* 319:1105-1111, 1988.

Thomas DP: Biologicals, standards and heparin. *Thromb Haemost* 62:648-650, 1989.

Turpie AGG, et al: Randomized controlled trial of low-molecular-weight heparin (enoxaparin) to prevent deep-vein thrombosis in patients undergoing elective hip surgery. *N Engl J Med* 315:925-929, 1986.

Turpie AGG, et al: Double-blind randomised trial of Org 10172 low-molecular-weight heparinoid in prevention of deep-vein thrombosis in thrombotic stroke. *Lancet* 1:523-526, 1987.

Verstraete M: Pharmacotherapeutic aspects of unfractionated and low molecular weight heparins. *Drugs* 40:498-530, 1990.

Walenga JM, et al: Development of recombinant hirudin as a therapeutic anticoagulant and antithrombotic agent: Some objective considerations. *Semin Thromb Hemost* 15:316-333, 1989.

Walenga JM, et al: Non-heparin glycosaminoglycan-derived drugs: A biochemical and pharmacologic perspective. *Semin Thromb Hemost* 17 (suppl 2):137-142, 1991.

Walker MG, et al: Subcutaneous calcium heparin versus intravenous sodium heparin in treatment of established acute deep vein thrombosis of the legs: A multicentre prospective randomised trial. *Br Med J* 294:1189-1192, 1987.

Warkentin TE, Kelton JG: Heparin and platelets. *Hematol Oncol Clin North Am* 4:243-264, 1990.

Weber DR: Is heparin really necessary in the lock and, if so, how much? *DICP* 25:399-407, 1991.

Weiss ME, et al: Association of protamine IgE and IgG antibodies with life-threatening reactions to intravenous protamine. *N Engl J Med* 320:886-892, 1989.

Weston-Smith S, et al: Thrombophilia. *Br J Hosp Med* 41:368-371, 1989.

White RH, Mungall D: Outpatient management of warfarin therapy: Comparison of computer-predicted dosage adjustment to skilled professional care. *Ther Drug Monit* 13:46-50, 1991.

White RH, et al: Home prothrombin time monitoring after the initiation of warfarin therapy: A randomized, prospective study. *Ann Intern Med* 111:730-737, 1989.

Wipf JE, Lipsky BA: Atrial fibrillation: Thromboembolic risk and indications for anticoagulation. *Arch Intern Med* 150:1598-1603, 1990.

Zacharski LR, et al: Anticoagulants as cancer therapy. *Semin Oncol* 17:217-227, (April) 1990.

Other Selected References

Fuster V, Verstraete M: *Thrombosis in Cardiovascular Disorders.* Philadelphia, WB Saunders, in press.

Halperin JL, Hart RG: Atrial fibrillation and stroke: New ideas, persisting dilemmas. *Stroke* 19:937-941, 1988.

Handin RI, Loscalzo J: Hemostasis, thrombosis fibrinolysis, and cardiovascular disease, in Braunwald E (ed): *Heart Disease: A Textbook of Cardiovascular Medicine,* ed 3. Philadelphia, WB Saunders, 1988.

Harker LA: Antithrombotic therapy, in Williams WJ, et al (eds): *Hematology*, ed 4. New York, McGraw-Hill, 1990, 1569-1581.

Majerus PW, et al: Anticoagulant, thrombolytic, and antiplatelet drugs, in Gilman AG, et al (eds): *Goodman and Gilman's The Pharmacological Basis of Therapeutics*, ed 8. New York, Pergamon Press, 1990, 1311-1331.

Ockelford P: Heparin 1986: Indications and effective use. *Drugs* 31:81-92, 1986.

Wessler S, Gitel SN: Pharmacology of heparin and warfarin. *J Am Coll Cardiol* 8:10B-20B, 1986.

Wessler S, et al (eds): *The New Dimensions of Warfarin Prophylaxis.* New York, Plenum Press, 1987.

New Evaluation 33

ENOXAPARIN
[Lovenox]

ACTIONS. Enoxaparin is a low-molecular-weight heparin (LMWH) prepared from native heparin by a multistep process that includes chemical modification, partial depolymerization, and chromatographic fractionation (Buckley and Sorkin, 1992; Carter et al, 1993). The molecular weight of the sulfated polysaccharides in unfractionated heparin ranges from 2 to 60 kilodaltons. In contrast, the apparent mean molecular weight of enoxaparin is 3.8 kilodaltons when determined by high-performance gel permeation chromatography and 5.6 kilodaltons when measured by refractive index (Buckley and Sorkin, 1992).

Both native heparin and enoxaparin form noncovalent complexes with, and induce a conformational change in, antithrombin III (AT-III) that increase the affinity of the complex for serine protease enzymes (eg, activated coagulation factor X [factor Xa]) (Buckley and Sorkin, 1992; Carter et al, 1993; for additional references, see the evaluation on Heparin). As a result, both anticoagulants accelerate the neutralization of factor Xa, although the activity in units/mg of heparin is slightly higher than the units/mg of enoxaparin. However, enoxaparin is a more selective inhibitor than unfractionated heparin. The heparin/AT-III complex inactivates thrombin at approximately the same rate as it inactivates factor Xa, but the enoxaparin/AT-III complex is three times more active against factor Xa than against thrombin. This apparently is caused by the absence of polysaccharide sequences in enoxaparin (present in native heparin) that mediate formation of a three-way complex with AT-III and thrombin. Furthermore, formation of a three-way complex appears to be necessary for inactivation of thrombin but not for inactivation of factor Xa.

USES. Enoxaparin is indicated to prevent deep vein thrombosis (DVT) and thus reduce the risk of pulmonary embolism in patients undergoing types of orthopedic surgery that have a high risk of thromboembolism (eg, hip replacement). The incidence of DVT confirmed by venography in patients undergoing hip replacement ranged from 6.5% to 12.5% in five clinical trials in which subcutaneous enoxaparin 40 mg was given once daily beginning 8 to 12 hours preoperatively and from 6% to 19.5% in four trials in which 30 mg was given twice daily beginning 12 to 24 hours postoperatively (Buckley and Sorkin, 1992). In contrast, DVT occurred in 51% to 65% of patients who received placebo, in 23% to 25% of those treated with unfractionated heparin, and in 22% of those given dextran 70.

In the trials reviewed (Buckley and Sorkin, 1992), proximal venous thrombosis, which is associated with the greatest risk of pulmonary embolism, occurred in 4% to 7.5% of patients undergoing total hip replacement who received enoxaparin preoperatively, in 5.4% to 6% of those given enoxaparin postoperatively, in 23% of those who received placebo, and in 7% to 19% of those given unfractionated heparin. Thus, data from these and subsequent trials establish that enoxaparin is at least as effective as some of the available alternatives for prophylaxis of DVT and proximal venous thrombosis in patients undergoing total hip replacement and may reduce the mean length of hospitalization and the number of readmissions compared with unfractionated heparin (Menzin et al, 1994). Furthermore, meta-analyses of trials comparing various LMWHs, including enoxaparin, with some of the other agents used for this indication concluded that LMWH may be the most effective anticoagulant (Nurmohamed et al, 1992; Leizorovicz et al, 1992; Mohr et al, 1993; Anderson et al, 1993; Imperiale and Speroff, 1994). However, in trials comparing warfarin with LMWHs other than enoxaparin, the advantages of the latter were less clear. The total incidence of DVT ranged from 12% to 23% and of proximal venous thrombosis from 3.8% to 6% (Green et al, 1994). These data suggest that trials comparing warfarin with enoxaparin might be more clinically relevant than those comparing enoxaparin with heparin.

Few studies have been done on use of enoxaparin in patients undergoing other types of orthopedic surgery. Data from a randomized, double-blind, placebo-controlled trial suggest that enoxaparin inhibited activation of prothrombin and consumption of factor VII in patients undergoing knee arthroplasty or tibial osteotomy (Leclerc et al, 1992; Ofosu et al, 1992). A regimen consisting of enoxaparin 40 mg once daily appeared to be more effective than 20 mg twice daily in elderly patients undergoing surgical repair for fractures of the neck of the femur (Barsotti et al, 1990).

Enoxaparin appears to be comparable to unfractionated heparin for prophylaxis of DVT in patients >40 years with at least one additional predisposing risk factor who undergo general (abdominal, gynecologic, urologic, thoracic) surgery (Combe and Samama, 1991). In a large multicenter trial, there was no difference in efficacy or in hemorrhagic complications among those who received enoxaparin the evening before surgery and those who received it the morning of surgery (Haas and Flosbach, 1993). Data from a nonrandomized trial using a "play-the-winner" design suggest that enoxaparin may be more effective than dextran 70 for prophylaxis of DVT in patients undergoing surgery of the digestive tract and does not cause excessive bleeding (Reiertsen et al, 1993). Results of additional trials suggest that it may be superior to unfractionated heparin in patients undergoing abdominal hysterectomy (Kaaja et al, 1992) but comparable in efficacy and safety in those undergoing aortic surgery and lower limb revascularization (Farkas et al, 1993).

Subcutaneous enoxaparin also has been compared with continuous intravenous infusion of unfractionated heparin as therapy for established DVT in a randomized multicenter trial (Simonneau et al, 1993). Sequential venograms taken during the 10-day treatment period indicated that improvement was significantly greater and there were fewer recurrent thromboembolic events among those treated with enoxaparin. In addition, continuous infusion of heparin is less convenient and may be more costly than a single daily subcutaneous injection of the LMWH. Similarly, five thrombocytopenic patients undergoing bone marrow transplant for malignant disease have been treated successfully with enoxaparin for venous thrombosis induced by the presence of an indwelling Hickman catheter (Drakos et al, 1992). Although additional randomized trials are needed, some LMWHs appear to be at least as effective as and may be superior to unfractionated heparin for established DVT (Cziraky and Spinler, 1993).

Enoxaparin has been studied to prevent clotting in hemodialysis tubing and in cardiopulmonary bypass. A few patients with heparin-induced thrombocytopenia also have been treated successfully for thrombosis with this drug. However, positive cross-reactivity to a different LMWH (Org 10172) occurred in more than 90% of approximately 50 patients with heparin-induced thrombocytopenia (Magnani, 1993). Therefore, enoxaparin should be used with great caution in these patients. Finally, this drug has been used to prevent renal graft thrombosis in several pediatric patients. Data are insufficient to evaluate enoxaparin definitively for any of these uses (for review, see Buckley and Sorkin, 1992).

ADVERSE REACTIONS AND CONTRAINDICATIONS. As with heparin, hemorrhagic complications (wound hematomas, perioperative blood loss, systemic bleeding) are the most serious potential adverse effects of enoxaparin therapy. Limited data from placebo-controlled trials of enoxaparin given postoperatively for prophylaxis of DVT in patients undergoing orthopedic surgery suggest that this drug does not increase the risk of bleeding associated with these procedures (for review, see Buckley and Sorkin, 1992). In dose-ranging studies, the incidence of wound hematomas depended on the dose and schedule of treatment: 2% in those given 20 mg twice daily, 6% in those given 40 mg once daily, 22% in those given 30 mg twice daily, and 12% in those given 60 mg once daily. In trials that compared enoxaparin with unfractionated heparin, the incidence of bleeding was higher in those given heparin 12 to 24 hours postoperatively, and transfusion requirements were somewhat greater after administration of heparin preoperatively (for review, see Buckley and Sorkin, 1992). On the other hand, when compared with warfarin, other LMWHs have been associated with a trend toward increased bleeding and wound hematomas (Hull et al, 1993). Thus, data are needed from trials that compare enoxaparin with warfarin.

Adverse effects of enoxaparin observed infrequently include confusion, fever, and peripheral edema. Although thrombocytopenia appears to occur less frequently than with unfractionated heparin, data are inadequate for definitive comparison. Angioedema, chest pain, dizziness, arrhythmias, shortness of breath, skin necrosis, rash, and urticaria occur rarely.

Enoxaparin is contraindicated in patients with active bleeding, in those with thrombocytopenia and a positive test for antibodies to platelets in the presence of enoxaparin, in those with severe uncontrolled hypertension, and in those with known hypersensitivity to heparin, enoxaparin, or other LMWH. This drug should be used with extreme caution in patients with a history of heparin-induced thrombocytopenia. Enoxaparin also should be used with caution in patients with chronic renal failure because the reduced clearance of the drug (see the section on Pharmacokinetics) may increase the risk of hemorrhage if the dose is not adjusted appropriately.

The carcinogenicity of enoxaparin has not been evaluated. This drug is not mutagenic in vitro or teratogenic in pregnant animals, and it does not appear to cross the placenta (FDA Pregnancy Category B).

PHARMACOKINETICS. Approximately 90% of the dose is absorbed after subcutaneous injection of enoxaparin 20 to 80 mg (Buckley and Sorkin, 1992). Peak plasma levels are achieved three to four hours after injection, and the estimated volume of distribution ranges from 5.2 to 9.3 L. The terminal phase half-life of anti-factor Xa activity is three to six hours. In healthy volunteers, the rate of total body clearance is 0.83 to 1.86 L/hr, primarily by renal elimination. The duration of action for clinically useful doses is approximately 24 hours. In patients with chronic severe renal failure, the rate of clearance appears to be reduced by 50% and the elimination phase half-life is twice that of healthy individuals (Cadroy et al, 1991). This appears to be true of other LMWHs as well. A small portion of the drug is metabolized in the liver by desulfation and depolymerization.

DOSAGE AND PREPARATIONS. Enoxaparin should be injected into the abdominal fat layer, and the injection sites should be rotated. It should not be administered intramuscularly or intravenously.

Subcutaneous: For prophylaxis of DVT and pulmonary embolism in patients undergoing orthopedic surgery, 30 mg twice daily for seven to ten days beginning as soon as possible (but no more than 24 hours) after surgery.

The dosage used in clinical trials for prophylaxis of DVT in patients undergoing general surgery was 20 mg once daily for seven days. In the single study on enoxaparin as therapy for established DVT, 1 mg/kg was given every 12 hours for 10 days.

Lovenox (Rhone-Poulenc Rorer). Solution 30 mg (equivalent to approximately 3,000 IU of anti-factor Xa activity) in 0.3 ml of sterile water for injection in single-use prefilled syringes.

Cited References

Anderson DR, et al: Efficacy and cost of low-molecular-weight heparin compared with standard heparin for the prevention of deep vein thrombosis after total hip arthroplasty. *Ann Intern Med* 119:1105-1112, 1993.

Barsotti J, et al: Comparative double-blind study of two dosage regimens of low-molecular weight heparin in elderly patients with a fracture of the neck of the femur. *J Orthop Trauma* 4:371-375, 1990.

Buckley MM, Sorkin EM: Enoxaparin: A review of its pharmacology and clinical applications in the prevention and treatment of thromboembolic disorders. *Drugs* 44:465-497, 1992.

Cadroy Y, et al: Delayed elimination of enoxaparin in patients with chronic renal insufficiency. *Thromb Res* 63:385-390, 1991.

Carter CA, et al: Enoxaparin: The low-molecular-weight heparin for prevention of postoperative thromboembolic complications. *Ann Pharmacother* 27:1223-1230, 1993.

Combe S, Samama MM: Prevention of thromboembolic disease in general surgery with Clexane (enoxaparin). *Semin Thromb Hemost* 17 (suppl 3):291-295, 1991.

Cziraky MJ, Spinler SA: Low-molecular-weight heparins for the treatment of deep-vein thrombosis. *Clin Pharm* 12:892-899, 1993.

Drakos PE, et al: Low molecular weight heparin for Hickman catheter-induced thrombosis in thrombocytopenic patients undergoing bone marrow transplantation. *Cancer* 70:1895-1898, 1992.

Farkas JC, et al: A randomised controlled trial of a low-molecular-weight heparin (enoxaparin) to prevent deep-vein thrombosis in patients undergoing vascular surgery. *Eur J Vasc Surg* 7:554-560, 1993.

Green D, et al: Low molecular weight heparin: A critical analysis of clinical trials. *Pharmacol Rev* 46:89-109, 1994.

Haas S, Flosbach CW: Prevention of postoperative thromboembolism with enoxaparin in general surgery: A German multicenter trial. *Semin Thromb Hemost* 19 (suppl 1):164-173, 1993.

Hull R, et al: A comparison of subcutaneous low-molecular-weight heparin with warfarin sodium for prophylaxis against deep-vein thrombosis after hip or knee implantation. *N Engl J Med* 329:1370-1376, 1993.

Imperiale TF, Speroff T: A meta-analysis of methods to prevent venous thromboembolism following total hip replacement. *JAMA* 271:1780-1785, 1994.

Kaaja R, et al: Comparison of enoxaparin, a low-molecular-weight heparin, and unfractionated heparin, with or without dihydroergotamine, in abdominal hysterectomy. *Eur J Obstet Gynecol Reprod Biol* 47:141-145, 1992.

Leclerc JR, et al: Prevention of deep vein thrombosis after major knee surgery—A randomized, double-blind trial comparing a low molecular weight heparin fragment (enoxaparin) to placebo. *Thromb Haemost* 67:417-423, 1992.

Leizorovicz A, et al: Low molecular weight heparin in prevention of perioperative thrombosis. *BMJ* 305:913-920, 1992.

Magnani HN: Heparin-induced thrombocytopenia (HIT): An overview of 230 patients treated with Orgaran (Org 10172). *Thromb Haemost* 70:554-561, 1993.

Menzin J, et al: Prevention of deep-vein thrombosis following total hip replacement surgery with enoxaparin versus unfractionated heparin: A pharmacoeconomic evaluation. *Ann Pharmacother* 28:271-275, 1994.

Mohr DN, et al: Prophylactic agents for venous thrombosis in elective hip surgery: Meta-analysis of studies using venographic assessment. *Arch Intern Med* 153:2221-2228, 1993.

Nurmohamed MT, et al: Low-molecular-weight heparin versus standard heparin in general and orthopaedic surgery: A meta-analysis. *Lancet* 340:152-156, 1992.

Ofosu FA, et al: The low molecular weight heparin enoxaparin inhibits the consumption of factor VII and prothrombin activation *in vivo* associated with elective knee replacement surgery. *Br J Haematol* 82:391-399, 1992.

Reiertsen O, et al: Safety of enoxaparin and dextran-70 in the prevention of venous thromboembolism in digestive surgery: A play-the-winner-designed study. *Scand J Gastroenterol* 28:1015-1020, 1993.

Simonneau G, et al: Subcutaneous low-molecular-weight heparin compared with continuous intravenous unfractionated heparin in the treatment of proximal deep vein thrombosis. *Arch Intern Med* 153:1541-1546, 1993.

Antiplatelet Therapy

34

ACTIONS

USES

Angina Pectoris

Acute Myocardial Infarction

Atrial Fibrillation

Cerebrovascular Disease

Secondary Prevention

Primary Prevention

Coronary Artery Bypass Grafts

Coronary Angioplasty

Prosthetic Heart Valves

Peripheral Vascular Disease

Pregnancy-Induced Hypertension and Pre-eclampsia

DRUG EVALUATIONS

Aspirin

Dipyridamole

Sulfinpyrazone

Ticlopidine Hydrochloride

ACTIONS

Aspirin inhibits platelet aggregation by suppressing synthesis of the proaggregatory thromboxane (TXA_2) by platelets (Stein et al, 1989; Webster et al, 1990; Lavie and Genton, 1991). However, it has no effect on platelet adhesion and thus does not prevent deposition of a platelet monolayer at sites of vascular injury. The antithrombotic properties of aspirin are more pronounced on biological surfaces than on synthetic or prosthetic materials. Because aspirin irreversibly acetylates its target enzyme, cyclooxygenase, and the platelet is unable to synthesize new enzyme molecules, the drug's effects persist for the lifetime of the platelet.

Dipyridamole [Persantine] inhibits platelet phosphodiesterase and indirectly activates adenylate cyclase (Stein et al, 1989; Webster et al, 1990; Lavie and Genton, 1991). In addition, uptake of adenosine by vascular endothelium and red blood cells is reduced, and thus plasma levels of adenosine are increased. These responses may combine to increase platelet concentrations of cyclic adenosine monophosphate, which inhibits platelet activation. In contrast to aspirin, dipyridamole blocks platelet adhesion to the vascular subendothelium; however, there is no evidence that these actions contribute to the drug's clinical effects. Dipyridamole also stimulates the release of prostacyclin (PGI_2) from endothelial cells and potentiates its antiaggregating action. Because of the potential for drug synergy that is suggested by their differing mechanisms, dipyridamole is often used with aspirin. Nevertheless, there is little convincing evidence that the combination is more effective clinically or on biological surfaces than aspirin alone (FitzGerald, 1987). However, the combination may result in synergy on prosthetic surfaces.

Sulfinpyrazone [Anturane] is a competitive inhibitor of cyclooxygenase, the enzyme that generates the intermediates required for TXA_2 synthesis. Its inhibitory effects on this enzyme decline when the drug concentration falls below minimally effective levels. However, the precise mechanism responsible for the antithrombotic activity of sulfinpyrazone is not known. It is more effective on prosthetic materials than on biological surfaces.

Nonsteroidal anti-inflammatory drugs, which also inhibit platelet cyclooxygenase to varying degrees, are not used as antiplatelet drugs. They may, however, inhibit platelet function as an adverse reaction when used for other indications.

Ticlopidine [Ticlid] inhibits platelet aggregation in various ex vivo assays of platelet function using platelet-rich plasma isolated from ticlopidine-treated volunteers. Its effects on platelet function persist for the lifetime of the platelet. In contrast, addition of ticlopidine to platelet-rich plasma from untreated subjects inhibits platelet function only at concentrations far in excess of the therapeutic range. The mechanism responsible for this drug's effects on platelets is not understood. Ticlopidine does not inhibit cyclooxygenase or prostaglandin synthase and also does not block elevations of platelet cAMP levels in response to inducers of platelet aggregation. The drug may irreversibly change the platelet membrane to inhibit the binding of fibrinogen and von Willebrand factor, both of which are required for normal platelet function.

Dextran, which is used primarily as a volume expander, also inhibits platelet adhesiveness and decreases vascular stasis by affecting blood flow. A low-molecular-weight dextran [Gentran 40, 10% LMD, Rheomacrodex] has been administered prophylactically to patients undergoing surgery who are at high risk of developing thromboembolic complications. However, dextran has not been shown to be more useful than anticoagulants in these patients and may cause volume overload in those with impaired cardiac or renal function. It appears to be ineffective in patients undergoing coronary angioplasty and is associated with anaphylactoid reactions (incidence 0.6%) (Stein et al, 1989). Nevertheless, dextran may prevent thrombosis on prosthetic surfaces (arterial stents and vascular grafts).

Several other drugs that inhibit platelet aggregation are under investigation. Epoprostenol (prostacyclin, PGI_2) is a naturally occurring arachidonic acid metabolite produced in the vascular endothelium. When administered exogenously, it has vasodilator as well as antiaggregating properties. It is under investigation as a replacement for heparin during hemodialysis as a means of blocking adhesion of platelets to dialyzer membranes and thus may improve the efficiency of hemodialysis (Smith et al, 1982). Epoprostenol also has been used to prevent platelet consumption during cardiopulmonary bypass and charcoal hemoperfusion. Data from pilot studies suggest that this prostaglandin does not affect coronary artery occlusion in patients with acute myocardial infarction (Hackett et al, 1990) or the evolution of unstable angina (Théroux et al, 1990). Clinical use is severely limited by its instability at physiologic pH, its tendency to induce systemic hypotension at effective antiplatelet dosages (especially in anesthetized patients), and its very short duration of action.

Omega-3 polyunsaturated fatty acids (eg, eicosapentaenoic acid), which are found in fatty fish and certain fish oils, alter platelet function after they are incorporated into platelet membranes. Since these acids are alternative substrates for cyclooxygenase, they cause a decline in TXA_2 production with an accompanying increase in production of TXA_3. The latter is much less potent as a vasoconstrictor and stimulator of platelet aggregation than TXA_2. In addition, eicosapentaenoic acid is converted in vascular endothelial cells to PGI_3, which also inhibits platelet aggregation. Epidemiologic and clinical studies suggest a role for these compounds in the treatment and prevention of atherosclerosis (Connor and Connor, 1990). In addition, they possibly may reduce restenosis after coronary angioplasty. However, results from the randomized trials completed thus far are inconclusive (Dehmer et al, 1988; Milner et al, 1989; Reis et al, 1989; Grigg et al, 1989).

Anagrelide decreases platelet count, possibly by inhibiting the budding of new platelets from megakaryocytes. This drug may be of value to reduce the platelet count in disorders such as polycythemia vera and essential thrombocythemia.

Dazoxiben is one of several selective inhibitors of thromboxane synthase that block the formation of TXA_2 and redirect the metabolism of the prostaglandin endoperoxides toward PGI_2 synthesis. Results of studies on the efficacy of these drugs as antiplatelet or anti-ischemic agents have been variable (Mehta and Nichols, 1990). TXA_2 receptor antagonists (eg, sulotroban) also are being investigated (Hall, 1991), and limited data suggest that they may be useful in the treatment of cardiovascular and cerebrovascular ischemia and prevention of thrombosis and reocclusion. In addition, several novel compounds have been synthesized that combine inhibition of thromboxane synthase and TXA_2 receptor antagonism in a single molecule.

Antagonists of the platelet glycoprotein IIB/IIIA complex (GP IIB/IIIA) are a final class of novel antiplatelet drugs being studied (Ellis et al, 1991). GP IIB/IIIA, a receptor present on the outer surface of platelets, binds fibrinogen, von Willebrand factor, or other proteins with the arginine-glycine-aspartic acid (RGD) sequence. Simultaneous binding of an RGD protein to GP IIB/IIIA complexes on two platelets mediates their aggregation. Monoclonal antibodies to this glycoprotein, or the $F(ab')_2$ or Fab fragments generated from such antibodies, can inhibit aggregation. In addition, some natural snake venom RGD peptides and their synthetic analogues are GP IIB/IIIA antagonists and inhibit platelet aggregation. Both classes of antagonists are being investigated as possible inhibitors of acute closure or restenosis after successful angioplasty, to prevent reocclusion in coronary artery bypass grafts or after successful thrombolysis, and in unstable angina. Hirudin, a thrombin inhibitor, is being studied for many of the same indications (see index entry, Hirudin).

USES

Angina Pectoris

Unstable Angina: The significant contribution of intracoronary thrombi to the pathophysiology of unstable angina provides a strong rationale for the use of antiplatelet drugs in these patients (Wallace et al, 1990; Kerins and FitzGerald, 1991). Data from four randomized trials demonstrate that the risk of fatal and nonfatal myocardial infarction (MI) is reduced by ≥50% when aspirin is administered to patients with unstable angina (Lewis et al, 1983; Cairns et al, 1985; Théroux et al, 1988; The RISC Group, 1990). The protective effect of aspirin is apparent in patients hospitalized for unstable angina and during long-term treatment.

The dosages of aspirin used in these studies ranged from 325 mg four times daily (Cairns et al, 1985) to 75 mg once daily (The RISC Group, 1990). The smallest dose appeared to be adequate to protect patients with unstable coronary artery disease (unstable angina or non-Q wave MI) from further coronary events. Furthermore, a randomized, placebo-controlled study used ex vivo measurements of platelet function in men taking 75 mg/day of aspirin for up to two years to show that the ability of this dose to inhibit platelet aggregation does not decrease with time (Berglund and Wallentin, 1991). Because there is a delay of several days before maximal antiplatelet effects are achieved when 75 mg/day is used, a loading dose of 325 mg for the first one or two days may be advisable for optimal protection from the risk of cardiac events early after the onset of symptoms. However, no randomized studies have compared the efficacy of high and low dosages of aspirin for reducing the risk of MI and death in patients with unstable angina, and many cardiologists currently recommend 325 mg once daily (often prescribed in enteric-coated form) as the most appropriate amount.

Sulfinpyrazone therapy was of no benefit when used alone or in combination with aspirin in patients with unstable angina (Cairns et al, 1985). Aspirin also has been compared with intravenous heparin in these patients. (See index entry, Angina, Treatment, Anticoagulants, for a discussion of the results of these clinical trials.)

Stable Angina: Antiplatelet therapy has no measurable effect on chest pain or other symptoms in patients with chronic stable angina (Kerins and FitzGerald, 1991) or in those with coronary artery spasm. However, data from the Physician's Health Study suggest that aspirin (325 mg on alternate days) reduces the risk of MI in patients with chronic stable angina (Ridker et al, 1991), although five years of alternate-day aspirin therapy did not prevent the subsequent development of angina pectoris in individuals with no previous history of MI, stroke, or transient cerebral ischemia (Manson et al, 1990).

Acute Myocardial Infarction

Aspirin is used as an adjunct to thrombolysis in the earliest stage of therapy for acute myocardial infarction (AMI). Other indications for the early use of aspirin in the management of AMI include reducing infarct extension and recurrence and preventing reocclusion of the reperfused artery. Antiplatelet drugs also have been studied as agents for either primary or secondary prevention of AMI. See the chapters on Therapeutic Management of Myocardial Infarction and Thrombolytics for discussion of results from clinical trials and therapeutic recommendations for use of platelet inhibitors for these indications.

Atrial Fibrillation

Patients with atrial fibrillation (AF) are at high risk of developing systemic emboli and stroke (Flegel and Hanley, 1989; Cairns and Connolly, 1991; Wolf et al, 1991). In those with valvular (rheumatic) AF, chronic therapy with oral anticoagulants is preferred for prophylaxis (see index entry Anticoagulants, Uses). In addition, a number of clinical trials demonstrated that the risk of stroke and emboli in patients with nonvalvular AF is reduced by antithrombotic therapy (anticoagulants or antiplatelet drugs) (for review, see Cairns and Connolly, 1991). However, conflicting and inconclusive results regarding the relative efficacy of aspirin and warfarin as prophylactic therapy in these patients were reported in some of these trials (see index entry Atrial Fibrillation). Therefore, randomized trials are continuing to compare aspirin with warfarin for prevention of stroke or systemic emboli in patients with nonvalvular AF. Present recommendations specify that aspirin (325 mg/day) be reserved for patients in whom anticoagulants are contraindicated and in those at low risk of vascular events (young patients with lone AF and possibly those with paroxysmal AF); those at higher risk should receive anticoagulants (Cairns and Connolly, 1991; Cairns, 1991).

Cerebrovascular Disease

Secondary Prevention: Transient ischemic attacks (TIA) carry a high risk of stroke, particularly during the first year after the initial episode. An overview of the secondary prevention trials with antiplatelet drugs showed that long-term aspirin therapy (300 mg to 1.3 g daily) reduced the risk of TIA recurrence, occlusive stroke, and vascular mortality and that antiplatelet regimens other than aspirin alone (eg, aspirin plus dipyridamole, sulfinpyrazone) did not enhance the protective effect (Antiplatelet Trialists' Collaboration, 1988). Aspirin 300 mg/day appears to be as effective as high-dose aspirin (1.2 g/day) (UK-TIA Study Group, 1988).

The European Stroke Prevention Study randomized 2,500 patients who had experienced a TIA, reversible ischemic neurologic deficit, or completed stroke within the preceding three months to receive combination therapy with dipyridamole and aspirin (75 mg and 330 mg, respectively, three times daily) or placebo (ESPS Group, 1990). Treatment with the combination reduced the incidence of death or stroke by 33.5% when an intention-to-treat analysis was used. Similar magnitudes of risk reduction were observed among males (58% of the study population; 34.8% reduction in total endpoint incidence) and females (31.8% reduction of endpoint incidence) (Sivenius et al, 1991 A). Subgroup analyses suggested that patients whose initial cerebral ischemia occurred in the vertebrobasilar artery distribution benefitted more than those whose initial event was in the carotid artery distribution and that patients with TIA were protected from stroke to a greater degree than those who had previously experienced a completed stroke (Sivenius et al, 1991 B). Although many trials have demonstrated that the risk is reduced significantly with aspirin alone (compared with placebo), no data are available from randomized trials that directly compare aspirin plus dipyridamole with either drug alone for secondary prevention of stroke.

Ticlopidine (250 mg twice daily) also has been effective in preventing stroke recurrence, AMI, or death in patients with a recent history of moderate or severe thromboembolic stroke (Gent et al, 1989). Male and female patients were similarly protected. However, adverse effects (eg, neutropenia, rash, diarrhea, bleeding disorders) were reported by 54% of those taking ticlopidine but by only 34% of those in the placebo group. Although the adverse effects were severe in only 8.2% of those given ticlopidine (and in 2.8% of the placebo arm), more than 50% of the patients receiving ticlopidine and 40% of controls dropped out of the study. In a randomized trial comparing ticlopidine (250 mg twice daily) with aspirin (650 mg twice daily), the risk of stroke or death was reduced slightly more in those taking ticlopidine (Hass et al, 1989). However, ticlopidine was also somewhat more likely to produce adverse reactions (diarrhea, rash, and neutropenia).

At present, antiplatelet therapy is recommended for nearly all patients with a recent history of TIA who can tolerate these drugs and for those patients who have had a minor completed stroke with no evidence (eg, by computed tomography) of cerebral hemorrhage (Sandercock, 1991). Since there are no data suggesting that other antiplatelet agents or combination regimens are more effective, aspirin is the drug of choice for secondary prevention of cerebral ischemia. The dosage used most frequently is 160 to 325 mg per day. Ticlopidine is the drug of second choice for those patients who cannot tolerate aspirin. Data from a retrospective study suggest that patients with >75% stenosis of the carotid artery lumen who are receiving aspirin and who develop ischemic neurologic symptoms (aspirin treatment failure) are at high risk of a sudden cerebral infarction not preceded by TIA (Chyatte and Chen, 1990). This may be due to platelet activation by high shear forces caused by flow through the stenosed lumen, a process not inhibited by aspirin. An alternative form of therapy (eg, carotid endarterectomy) may be considered for these patients.

Primary Prevention: When used for primary prevention in healthy men, aspirin (325 mg on alternate days to 500 mg daily) does not appear to reduce the incidence of occlusive fatal or nonfatal stroke and may increase the risk of hemorrhagic stroke (Peto et al, 1988; Steering Committee of the Physicians' Health Study Research Group, 1989). A randomized, placebo-controlled trial is in progress to test the efficacy of aspirin as prophylaxis for TIA, stroke, other vascular events, or death in asymptomatic patients with cervical bruits and carotid stenosis (measured by duplex ultrasonography) of ≥50% of the arterial lumen (The Asymptomatic Cervical Bruit Study Group, 1991).

Coronary Artery Bypass Grafts

Internal mammary artery bypass grafts have a low risk of occlusion, and antiplatelet drugs do not appear to improve the patency rate at one year after surgery (Goldman et al, 1990). In untreated patients with saphenous vein grafts, thrombotic occlusion occurs within the first week after surgery in about 10% and in an additional 5% within six months. Reocclusion after six months is due to intimal hyperplasia and lipid accumulation and thus is much less amenable to antithrombotic therapy. A meta-analysis of 13 randomized, placebo-controlled trials conducted prior to 1988 concluded that protection from early reocclusion was most apparent when antithrombotic therapy with anticoagulants or antiplatelet drugs was begun as soon as possible after surgery was completed (Henderson et al, 1989). The pooled data from these studies demonstrated that the number of patients with one or more grafts occluded was reduced by 30% in those receiving antithrombotic therapy. However, data were insufficient to determine if antiplatelet drugs were more or less effective than anticoagulants or to compare the efficacies of different antiplatelet regimens. In two subsequent trials that compared antiplatelet drugs with oral anticoagulants for preventing CABG reocclusion, efficacy for the two therapies was comparable, but serious complications (death, AMI, severe bleeding) occurred more often in those treated with anticoagulants (Pfisterer et al, 1989; Weber et al, 1990).

An analysis of more recent data also concluded that the two therapies were both efficacious in preventing occlusion of saphenous vein grafts (Israel et al, 1991). However, because of the limited data directly comparing the two therapies, the expense and inconvenience of monitoring prothrombin times, and the increased risk of bleeding in patients receiving oral anticoagulants, antiplatelet therapy is preferred. When the risk of occlusion is high, anticoagulants may be preferred by some cardiologists (see index entry Bypass Grafts, Anticoagulants In), although data to support this opinion are not available. In addition, clinical trials are in progress to determine if combined therapy with low doses of antiplatelet drugs and anticoagulants may be more effective than standard doses of either therapy alone in high-risk patients.

Data comparing different antiplatelet regimens for the prevention of vein graft occlusion are limited. It appears that dipyridamole (75 mg three times daily) may enhance the efficacy of low-dose aspirin (50 mg three times daily) (Sanz et al, 1990) and that a moderate dose of aspirin (325 mg once daily) is equal in efficacy to larger amounts (325 mg three times daily) and to sulfinpyrazone or the combination of aspirin plus dipyridamole (Israel et al, 1991). However, preoperative administration of aspirin increases blood loss during and after surgery (Taggart et al, 1990; Sethi et al, 1990). Furthermore, in a randomized comparison of aspirin therapy started before surgery with aspirin therapy started six hours after surgery, no benefit of the preoperative regimen on early vein graft patency was demonstrable (Goldman et al, 1991). In addition, dipyridamole appears to be more effective than aspirin in inhibiting platelet activation and deposition on prosthetic surfaces (eg, the cardiopulmonary bypass pump used during surgery) (Stein et al, 1989).

Current recommendations specify the use of aspirin beginning as soon as possible after surgery (within six hours by nasogastric tube). Some cardiologists advocate administration of dipyridamole for one or two days before surgery (Israel et al, 1991; Ip et al, 1991 A). Others cite the absence of data demonstrating improved outcome as a result of preoperative therapy and the potential for dipyridamole to cause localized ischemia and exacerbate angina through the "coronary steal" phenomenon as strong arguments against its use before CABG (Rowe and Folts, 1990; Lavie and Genton, 1991). Aspirin therapy should be continued for at least one year (and possibly indefinitely), since data from a randomized comparison show that graft occlusion was more frequent when therapy was discontinued after three months than when it was continued for one year (Pfisterer et al, 1989).

Coronary Angioplasty

Acute closure and gradual restenosis limit the long-term benefits of revascularization using percutaneous transluminal coronary angioplasty (PTCA) (Popma and Topol, 1990; Ip et al, 1991 B). Platelet deposition and thrombosis at the site of mechanical damage to the vessel wall are important contributing factors to acute reocclusion, while migration and proliferation of smooth muscle cells in response to intimal damage contribute to restenosis (Forrester et al, 1991; Hermans et al, 1991). With this understanding of the pathophysiologic responses to PTCA as a rationale, clinical trials showed that antiplatelet drugs can increase patency rates soon after PTCA by reducing the incidence of complications such as AMI and intracoronary thrombi during the procedure. Aspirin, with or without dipyridamole, is effective for this indication. Data suggest that doses of 80 mg and 1.5 g daily may be equally effective and that addition of dipyridamole to aspirin may not reduce the number of periprocedural complications in patients undergoing PTCA (Webster et al, 1990). Current recommendations specify administration of aspirin (150 to 325 mg/day) beginning at least 24 hours before PTCA and continued indefinitely (Webster et al, 1990; Chesebro et al, 1991). The use of heparin before, during, and after the procedure and of oral anticoagulants for patients with residual stenosis or thrombus also is recommended (see index entry Angioplasty, Anticoagulants In). The dose of aspirin should be reduced to 80 mg/day in patients maintained on oral anticoagulants.

Neither antiplatelet drugs nor anticoagulants, alone or in combination, has reduced the incidence (20% to 30%) of gradual restenosis observed after successful PTCA (Forrester et al, 1991; Hermans et al, 1991; Ip et al, 1991 B; Chesebro et al, 1991). Limited data suggest that the combination of aspirin with dipyridamole may lessen the severity of restenosis and the frequency of total or subtotal occlusions (Schwartz et al, 1990). Current clinical trials are investigating the use of thromboxane synthase inhibitors, thromboxane receptor antagonists, omega-3 polyunsaturated fatty acids, or antagonists of the platelet glycoprotein IIB/IIIA complex to reduce gradual stenosis after PTCA (see the Introduction). Pooled data from several studies demonstrate a modest trend toward reduced stenosis in patients treated with fish oils (omega-3 polyunsaturated acids) after PTCA (Milner et al, 1989; Lavie and Genton, 1991). This may result more from blocking responses to growth factors than from a direct antiplatelet action. Local infusion of antimitotic and antiproliferative drugs also is being studied in experimental models and clinical trials (Popma and Topol, 1990). At present, however, no intervention has been reliable in preventing restenosis after PTCA. Some investigators suggest that elevated plasma catecholamines (resulting from stress, smoking, or other mechanisms) may increase the likelihood of restenosis by activating platelets through a mechanism not subject to inhibition by antiplatelet drugs (Folts et al, 1988).

Prosthetic Heart Valves

Anticoagulants are more effective than antiplatelet drugs in preventing formation of thromboemboli in patients with mechanical heart valves. For certain patients, dipyridamole may be used with oral anticoagulants (see index entry Anticoagulants, Uses, for discussion and therapeutic recommendations).

Peripheral Vascular Disease

There is no evidence from randomized, controlled clinical trials that antiplatelet therapy affects the symptoms, need for surgery, or prognosis of patients with atherosclerosis of the peripheral vasculature, but aspirin (150 to 300 mg daily) has been recommended as empiric therapy to prevent MI and stroke in these high-risk patients (Webster et al, 1990). An aspirin-dipyridamole regimen, initiated before surgery and continued for at least six weeks, may improve patency of lower extremity arterial reconstructions, especially when a dacron or polytetrafluoroethylene vascular prosthesis is implanted (Clagett et al, 1989). See index entry Vascular Disease, Peripheral for discussion of other therapies for chronic occlusive vascular disease.

Antiplatelet agents also are being investigated as therapy for intermittent claudication. Although ticlopidine or aspirin plus dipyridamole may relieve some symptoms in these patients (Giansante et al, 1990), there are no data from placebo-controlled trials to establish their efficacy for intermittent claudication.

Pregnancy-Induced Hypertension and Pre-eclampsia

Hypertension occurs in about 10% of pregnancies and increases the maternal risk of abruptio placentae, disseminated intravascular coagulation, cerebral hemorrhage, hepatic failure, or acute renal failure (Working Group on High Blood Pressure in Pregnancy, 1990). Pregnancy-induced hypertension (PIH) is an isolated phenomenon that usually begins after the 20th week of gestation. It may progress to pre-eclampsia in which hypertension is accompanied by proteinuria and/or edema. If untreated, this condition may progress to the seizures that define eclampsia or to microangiopathic hemolytic anemia with liver damage and thrombocytopenia (the HELLP syndrome). The etiology of PIH and pre-eclampsia is not completely understood but is thought to involve inadequate development of the spiral arteries that supply blood to the placenta, leading to endothelial cell damage and then to thrombosis. The inadequate supply of nutrients to the fetus also may result in fetal growth retardation.

Based on the postulated involvement of thrombosis in the etiology of these disorders, clinical trials have been conducted to assess the usefulness of antiplatelet therapy in women at risk. A meta-analysis of six controlled trials of low-dose aspirin (60 to 150 mg/day during the second and third trimesters) in 394 such women found that the risks of PIH, low infant birth weight, and cesarean section were reduced by 65%, 44%, and 66%, respectively, in those receiving aspirin (Imperiale and Petrulis, 1991). No adverse effects on the mother or neonate were associated with the use of low-dose aspirin. Recent data confirm the efficacy and safety of aspirin and failed to demonstrate any added benefit from the combination of dipyridamole with aspirin (Uzan et al, 1991). However, some concerns remain about the potential of aspirin to delay the date of delivery, lengthen labor, increase bleeding during or after delivery, or prematurely close the ductus arteriosus in the fetus (Repke, 1991). Since the number of pregnant women who have been treated is limited, aspirin should not be used routinely in pregnant women who are not at high risk for PIH and pre-eclampsia.

Data suggest that aspirin therapy does not alter the clinical course in women with mild PIH (Schiff et al, 1990). In addition, pre-eclampsia does not respond to aspirin therapy (Repke, 1991). Thus, risk assessment is important so that aspirin therapy may be started before the mother's condition progresses. Various tests have been proposed to predict the risk of PIH and pre-eclampsia, including enhanced sensitivity to elevation of blood pressure by angiotensin II (Wallenburg et al, 1986), an increase in blood pressure on rolling over from the left side onto the back (Schiff et al, 1989), the analysis of Doppler flow-velocity waveforms from the uteroplacental circulation (McParland et al, 1990), and reduced responsiveness of platelet ionized calcium concentrations to stimulation by arginine vasopressin (Zemel et al, 1990). In a retrospective case-control study, multivariate analysis based on the mother's medical history showed that nulliparous women or those with a history of pre-eclampsia were 5.4 and 10.8 times, respectively, more likely to develop pre-eclampsia than those who had previously given birth or those without a history (Eskenazi et al, 1991). However, additional prospective studies are needed to define more fully the risk factors useful for identifying pregnant women who require aspirin therapy to prevent PIH and pre-eclampsia.

Drug Evaluations

ASPIRIN

ACTIONS. Aspirin inactivates the enzyme, cyclooxygenase, thereby suppressing synthesis of proaggregatory thromboxane (TXA_2) by platelets and of antiaggregatory and vasodilator prostacyclin (PGI_2) by endothelial cells that line the blood vessels (Kerins and FitzGerald, 1991; Lavie and Genton, 1991; Weissmann, 1991). Because platelets cannot resynthesize cyclooxygenase, the inhibiting effect of aspirin is irreversible for the life of the platelet. In contrast, endothelial cells can resynthesize the enzyme, and enzymatic activity may be restored following initial inactivation by aspirin. Small doses of aspirin (20 to 40 mg) may suppress TXA_2 formation while sparing PGI_2; nevertheless, the doses prescribed most frequently (160 mg to 1 g daily) are not selective.

USES. Aspirin is used to prevent myocardial infarction in patients with unstable angina; as an adjunct to thrombolysis and to prevent reinfarction and death after acute myocardial infarction; and to prevent transient ischemic attack recurrence, ischemic stroke, and vascular mortality in patients with cerebrovascular disease. Its role in primary prevention remains to be established more definitively. It may reduce the incidence of myocardial infarction in healthy men and women over age 50, but the incidence of hemorrhagic stroke may increase slightly. Aspirin appears to be most beneficial in patients at high risk of arterial thrombotic events (Webster et al, 1990; Ip et al, 1991 A). It also is used to prevent vein graft occlusion after saphenous vein aortocoronary bypass surgery or acute occlusion during angioplasty. Aspirin (with dipyridamole) may improve patency of lower extremity arterial reconstructions, especially when a vascular prosthesis is used. This drug also may prevent pregnancy-induced hypertension and pre-eclampsia in women at high risk for these disorders. Finally, the combination of aspirin and intravenous gamma globulin is the preferred regimen to prevent thrombosis due to coronary aneurysm and coronary artery occlusion in patients with Kawasaki's disease (Shulman, 1989).

For discussions of aspirin use not related to its antiplatelet actions (eg, as an antipyretic, analgesic, antiarthritic, in ocular disorders), see index entry Aspirin, Uses.

Also see the Introduction.

ADVERSE REACTIONS AND PRECAUTIONS. Aspirin may cause abdominal discomfort, heartburn, nausea, and gastrointestinal bleeding. These side effects are dose related and usually can be avoided if the daily dose does not exceed 325 mg. However, overt bleeding from the upper gastrointestinal tract may occur when unbuffered aspirin is administered for long periods even at doses between 75 and 250 mg/day (Naschitz et al, 1990). Concomitant use of an antacid or an H_2 antagonist or substitution of an enteric-coated aspirin product decreases gastrointestinal side effects.

Aspirin may impair surgical hemostasis, and the risk of operative bleeding is increased when it is given with heparin or oral anticoagulants. Severe gastrointestinal bleeding and occasionally intracerebral hemorrhage have occurred when warfarin and aspirin were used concomitantly.

Aspirin is classified in FDA Pregnancy Category D. Although two studies using small patient populations concluded that use of aspirin during the first trimester of pregnancy may increase the risk of congenital cardiac malformations, a larger case-control study found that maternal aspirin use had no effect on fetal heart development (Werler et al, 1989). The FDA recently required aspirin manufacturers to add warnings to the package labeling advising against the use of aspirin during the third trimester of pregnancy (unless specifically prescribed by a physician) because of the risk of impaired hemostasis in the mother, fetus, or neonate.

DOSAGE. A dose of 160 to 325 mg daily is most commonly recommended for antiplatelet therapy, although in most studies on patients with TIA, 1 g or more divided in three or four equal doses was used.

For Kawasaki's disease, 80 to 100 mg/kg/day in four divided doses is administered for 14 days (Shulman, 1989). When the patient becomes afebrile and if no coronary abnormalities are detected by echocardiography, 3 to 5 mg/kg/day is administered for the following six to eight weeks. In patients with coronary abnormalities, aspirin therapy should continue indefinitely.

PREPARATIONS. See index entry Aspirin, Uses, Analgesic.

DIPYRIDAMOLE

[Persantine]

ACTIONS. Dipyridamole inhibits phosphodiesterase, the enzyme that metabolizes cyclic adenosine monophosphate. It also blocks uptake and metabolism of adenosine by erythrocytes and vascular endothelial cells and thus increases its plasma concentration (Webster et al, 1990; Lavie and Genton, 1991). Adenosine inhibits platelet function by stimulating adenylate cyclase and has vasodilator properties. Dipyridamole also potentiates the antiaggregating action of prostacyclin (PGI_2). Because the doses required to affect these functions also cause flushing and headache in about 10% of patients, smaller amounts of dipyridamole are given with aspirin or oral anticoagulants. In doses used clinically, dipyridamole inhibits platelet activation on prosthetic surfaces, but it does not affect platelet adherence to biological surfaces.

USES. The major indication for dipyridamole is as an adjunct to warfarin in patients with artificial heart valves (see the Introduction and index entry Anticoagulants, Uses). It also has been used with aspirin for secondary prevention of acute myocardial infarction, to prevent stroke in patients with transient ischemic attacks, and to maintain patency of coronary artery bypass grafts. The authors of a recent review found no convincing evidence that dipyridamole can prevent myocardial ischemia when used alone (Rowe and Folts, 1990). Furthermore, most studies showing efficacy of the aspirin-dipyridamole regimen did not compare the combination with aspirin alone; when this was done, dipyridamole did not appear to enhance the therapeutic effect (FitzGerald, 1987; Israel et al, 1991; Lavie and Genton, 1991; Rowe and Folts, 1990). Therefore, most experts recommend that aspirin be used alone for these indications. Dipyridamole may be useful to prevent platelet activation by the extracorporeal pump during cardiopulmonary bypass surgery and (with aspirin) to improve patency of lower extremity arterial reconstructions when a vascular prosthesis is implanted.

Also see the Introduction.

ADVERSE REACTIONS AND PRECAUTIONS. Headache, the most common side effect of dipyridamole, is usually dose related and is rarely a problem with the dosage used for antiplatelet therapy. Dizziness, syncope, gastrointestinal disturbances, and rash have been reported.

Dipyridamole, when used in patients with angina pectoris, occasionally causes a worsening of symptoms due to coronary steal (Keltz et al, 1987). This vasodilatory effect of the drug is exploited in a sensitive diagnostic test for coronary artery disease that uses radioisotopes or echocardiography for imaging and intravenous dipyridamole (in place of exercise) to stress the coronary circulation (Scarpa, 1991).

Dipyridamole is classified in FDA Pregnancy Category B.

PHARMACOKINETICS. There is wide interpatient variation in the extent of absorption of dipyridamole. The drug is over 90% protein bound. It undergoes enterohepatic recirculation and is conjugated in the liver and excreted as a glucuronide in the bile. The mean time to peak plasma concentration is 75 minutes after ingestion of a single dose. With prolonged administration, the elimination half-life of dipyridamole is approximately ten hours.

DOSAGE. For long-term prophylaxis in patients with mechanical heart valves, 100 mg four times daily (with warfarin). To prevent platelet activation by the extracorporeal pump during bypass surgery, some experts recommend 100 mg four times daily beginning two days before surgery. In trials that combined dipyridamole with aspirin, 75 mg was given three times daily. However, most experts maintain that there are no advantages to use of the combination compared with aspirin alone.

PREPARATIONS.

Persantine (Boehringer Ingelheim), ***Generic.*** Tablets 25, 50, and 75 mg.

SULFINPYRAZONE

[Anturane]

For chemical formula, see index entry Sulfinpyrazone, In Gout, Hyperuricemia.

ACTIONS AND USES. Sulfinpyrazone has antithrombotic properties, but the mechanism is not known. It appears that competitive inhibition of cyclooxygenase by sulfinpyrazone is not an important factor in the drug's antiplatelet efficacy. When used for secondary prevention of acute myocardial infarction, sulfinpyrazone was reported to reduce the risk of sudden death in one study and to decrease the reinfarction rate in another. It is not effective for prevention of acute myocardial infarction in patients with unstable angina. Sulfinpyrazone may improve bypass graft patency without increasing blood loss, but its tendency to cause transient renal insufficiency limits its usefulness. This drug may be most useful in patients who cannot tolerate aspirin with or without dipyridamole. (See the Introduction.)

ADVERSE REACTIONS, PRECAUTIONS, AND INTERACTIONS. The most common side effects of sulfinpyrazone are gastrointestinal disturbances. Rash has been reported. Blood dyscrasias, acute interstitial nephritis, renal colic, and acute renal failure have occurred occasionally. Sulfinpyrazone may potentiate the anticoagulant effect of warfarin.

PHARMACOKINETICS. See index entry Sulfinpyrazone, In Gout.

DOSAGE AND PREPARATIONS.

Oral: When used for secondary prevention after acute myocardial infarction, a dose of 800 mg daily was employed (Antiplatelet Trialists' Collaboration, 1988).

Anturane (CIBA), ***Generic.*** Capsules 200 mg; tablets 100 mg.

TICLOPIDINE HYDROCHLORIDE

[Ticlid]

Cl S N CH_2 ·HCl

ACTIONS. The mechanism of action of this orally active platelet inhibitor is not completely understood but may involve alteration of the platelet membrane that prevents ADP-induced exposure of the fibrinogen binding site on platelet glycoprotein IIB/IIIA. Ticlopidine (and/or its active metabolites) inhibits ADP-induced platelet aggregation, but it has variable effects on aggregation due to epinephrine, thrombin, platelet-activating factor, arachidonic acid, or collagen. Ticlopidine also may decrease platelet adhesion to some prosthetic surfaces, prolong bleeding time, and decrease blood velocity (McTavish et al, 1990).

USES. Ticlopidine is indicated to reduce the risk of thrombotic stroke in patients who have had a previous thrombotic stroke or precursors to stroke (eg, transient ischemic attack [TIA], reversible cerebral ischemia). However, because of the risk of neutropenia or agranulocytosis associated with use of ticlopidine, current recommendations limit its use to patients who cannot tolerate aspirin.

Two large-scale, long-term clinical trials assessed the efficacy of ticlopidine for stroke prevention in patients with a history of cerebrovascular disease. In the Canadian-American Ticlopidine Study (CATS), ticlopidine reduced the combined incidence of stroke recurrence, myocardial infarction, and vascular death by 30% in patients who had had a recent thromboembolic stroke (Gent et al, 1989).

In the Ticlodipine-Aspirin Stroke Study (TASS), ticlopidine was compared with high-dose aspirin (650 mg twice daily) in patients with a history of TIA, reversible ischemic deficit, or a prior mild stroke. The risk of fatal or nonfatal stroke was marginally lower in patients taking ticlopidine than in those treated with aspirin, but side effects were more frequent with ticlopidine (Hass et al, 1989).

Results of a Swedish multicenter study indicated that long-term prophylaxis with ticlopidine (up to five years) reduced mortality and the incidence of vascular endpoints (eg, stroke, TIA, acute myocardial infarction) in patients with intermittent claudication (Janzon et al, 1990). Ticlopidine also has reduced the risk of myocardial infarction and death in patients with unstable angina, but it has not been directly compared with aspirin therapy for this indication (Balsano et al, 1990). Preliminary data suggest that it may reduce the immediate thrombotic complications of angioplasty (White et al, 1987). This drug appears to be as effective as oral anticoagulants in preventing occlusion of coronary artery bypass grafts during the first three months after surgery (Panak et al, 1983) and reduces the incidence of bypass graft occlusion for up to one year (Limet et al, 1987). However, randomized trials comparing ticlopidine with aspirin for preventing graft occlusion have not been conducted.

Ticlopidine has been used during extracorporal blood circulation in patients undergoing cardiopulmonary bypass surgery or hemodialysis. However, this drug does not prevent platelet deposition on Dacron prosthetic grafts (Stratton and Ritchie, 1984). Other possible uses are in patients with peripheral vascular disease, diabetic retinopathy, and sickle cell crisis. Ticlopidine also has been studied to prevent cerebral vasospasm after subarachnoid hemorrhage.

ADVERSE REACTIONS AND PRECAUTIONS. Gastrointestinal disturbances (nausea, vomiting, cramps, diarrhea) are the most common adverse effects of ticlopidine (McTavish et al, 1990). Hemorrhagic complications also have occurred in patients receiving this drug. Urticaria, rash, and erythema develop occasionally, most commonly during the first month of therapy. Hematologic disorders (leukopenia, agranulocytosis, thrombocytopenia, pancytopenia) are the most serious adverse effects of ticlopidine and may be life threatening. If they are identified early and therapy is discontinued immediately, recovery is the rule; therefore, monitoring of blood counts during the first 12 weeks of therapy is essential. Thrombotic thrombocytopenic purpura (TTP) was reported in four patients after ticlopidine therapy (Page et al, 1991); however, other investigators report that ticlopidine is beneficial in those with TTP (Vianelli et al 1990; De Pasquale et al, 1986; Ishii et al, 1984). The number of patients who have been treated with ticlopidine or who have developed TTP in response to the drug is too small for definitive conclusions to be drawn.

Cholestatic jaundice, hepatitis, icterus, and abnormal liver function tests have been reported rarely. Ticlopidine increases total, HDL, LDL, and VLDL cholesterol levels in some patients.

PHARMACOKINETICS. Ticlopidine is rapidly and extensively (>80%) absorbed after a single oral dose, with peak plasma levels observed approximately two hours after ingestion. Although this drug binds reversibly and nonsaturably to plasma proteins, only 15% or less of the ticlopidine present in plasma after administration of the recommended dose is protein bound. Clearance is reduced with repeated administration; the elimination half-life increased in older volunteers from approximately 12.6 hours to four to five days. Steady state levels are obtained after 14 to 21 days of administration of 250 mg twice daily. Ticlopidine undergoes extensive hepatic metabolism. Approximately 60% of a dose is excreted in the urine (with only trace amounts as intact parent drug), and 23% is eliminated in the feces (33% of which is intact drug). Impaired hepatic function (advanced cirrhosis) appears to only slightly increase plasma levels of the drug, while renal impairment reduces plasma clearance significantly.

DOSAGE AND PREPARATIONS.

Oral: For secondary prevention of stroke, 250 mg twice daily with food.

Ticlid (Syntex). Tablets 250 mg.

Cited References

Antiplatelet Trialists' Collaboration: Secondary prevention of vascular disease by prolonged antiplatelet treatment. *Br Med J* 296:320-331, 1988.

The Asymptomatic Cervical Bruit Study Group: Natural history and effectiveness of aspirin in asymptomatic patients with cervical bruits. *Arch Neurol* 48:683-686, 1991.

Balsano F, et al: Antiplatelet treatment with ticlopidine in unstable angina: A controlled multicenter clinical trial. *Circulation* 82:17-26, 1990.

Berglund U, Wallentin L: Persistent inhibition of platelet function during long-term treatment with 75 mg acetylsalicylic acid daily in men with unstable coronary artery disease. *Eur Heart J* 12:428-433, 1991.

Cairns JA: Stroke prevention in atrial fibrillation trial, editorial. *Circulation* 84:933-935, 1991.

Cairns JA, Connolly SJ: Nonrheumatic atrial fibrillation: Risk of stroke and role of antithrombotic therapy. *Circulation* 84:469-481, 1991.

Cairns JA, et al: Aspirin, sulfinpyrazone, or both in unstable angina: Results of Canadian multicenter trial. *N Engl J Med* 313:1369-1375, 1985.

Chesebro JH, et al: Importance of antithrombin therapy during coronary angioplasty. *J Am Coll Cardiol* 17:96B-100B, 1991.

Chyatte D, Chen TL: Patterns of failure of aspirin treatment in symptomatic atherosclerotic carotid artery disease. *Neurosurgery* 26:565-569, 1990.

Clagett GP, et al: Antithrombotic therapy in peripheral vascular disease. *Chest* 95:S128-S139, 1989.

Connor WE, Connor SL: Diet, atherosclerosis, and fish oil. *Adv Intern Med* 35:139-172, 1990.

Dehmer GJ, et al: Reduction in the rate of early restenosis after coronary angioplasty by a diet supplemented with n-3 fatty acids. *N Engl J Med* 319:733-740, 1988.

De Pasquale A, et al: Possible usefulness of ticlopidine in combined treatment of thrombotic thrombocytopenic purpura: Report of one case. *Haematologica* 71:53-55, 1986.

Ellis SG, et al: Prospects for the use of antagonists to the platelet glycoprotein IIb/IIIa receptor to prevent postangioplasty restenosis and thrombosis. *J Am Coll Cardiol* 17:89B-95B, 1991.

Eskenazi B, et al: A multivariate analysis of risk factors for preeclampsia. *JAMA* 266:237-241, 1991.

ESPS Group: European stroke prevention study. *Stroke* 21:1122-1130, 1990.

FitzGerald GA: Dipyridamole. *N Engl J Med* 316:1247-1257, 1987.

Flegel KM, Hanley J: Risk factors for stroke and other embolic events in patients with nonrheumatic atrial fibrillation. *Stroke* 20:1000-1004, 1989.

Folts JD, et al: Problem with aspirin as antithrombotic agent in coronary artery disease, letter. *Lancet* 1:937-938, 1988.

Forrester JS, et al: A paradigm for restenosis based on cell biology: Clues for the development of new prevention therapies. *J Am Coll Cardiol* 17:758-769, 1991.

Gent M, et al: The Canadian American Ticlopidine Study (CATS) in thromboembolic stroke. *Lancet* 1:1215-1220, 1989.

Giansante C, et al: Treatment of intermittent claudication with antiplatelet agents. *J Int Med Res* 18:400-407, 1990.

Goldman S, et al: Internal mammary artery and saphenous vein graft patency: Effects of aspirin. *Circulation* 82(suppl IV):IV-237-IV-242, 1990.

Goldman S, et al: Starting aspirin therapy after operation: Effects on early graft patency. *Circulation* 84:520-526, 1991.

Grigg LE, et al: Determinants of restenosis and lack of effect of dietary supplementation with eicosapentaenoic acid on the incidence of coronary artery restenosis after angioplasty. *J Am Coll Cardiol* 13:665-672, 1989.

Hackett D, et al: Effect of prostacyclin on coronary occlusion in acute myocardial infarction. *Int J Cardiol* 26:53-57, 1990.

Hall SE: Thromboxane A_2 receptor antagonists. *Med Res Rev* 11:503-579, 1991.

Hass WK et al: Randomized trial comparing ticlopidine hydrochloride with aspirin for prevention of stroke in high-risk patients. *N Engl J Med* 321:501-507, 1989.

Henderson WG, et al: Antiplatelet or anticoagulant therapy after coronary artery bypass surgery: A meta-analysis of clinical trials. *Ann Intern Med* 111:743-750, 1989.

Hermans WRM, et al: Prevention of restenosis after percutaneous transluminal coronary angioplasty: The search for a 'magic bullet.' *Am Heart J* 122:171-187, 1991.

Imperiale TF, Petrulis AS: A meta-analysis of low-dose aspirin for the prevention of pregnancy-induced hypertensive disease. *JAMA* 266:260-264, 1991.

Ip JH, et al: Thrombosis and antithrombotic therapy in cardiovascular disease. *Cardiovasc Rev Rep* 12:16-30, (Mar) 1991 A.

Ip JH, et al: The role of platelets, thrombin and hyperplasia in restenosis after coronary angioplasty. *J Am Coll Cardiol* 17:77B-88B, 1991 B.

Ishii Y, et al: A case of thrombotic thrombocytopenic purpura, successful treatment by ticlopidine. *Clin Hematol* 25:1097-1102, 1984.

Israel DH, et al: Antithrombotic therapy in the coronary vein graft patient. *Clin Cardiol* 14:283-295, 1991.

Janzon L, et al: Prevention of myocardial infarction and stroke in patients with intermittent claudication; effects of ticlopidine: Results from STIMS, the Swedish Ticlopidine Multicentre Study. *J Intern Med* 227:301-308, 1990.

Keltz TN, et al: Dipyridamole-induced myocardial ischemia. *JAMA* 257:1516-1517, 1987.

Kerins DM, FitzGerald GA: The current role of platelet-active drugs in ischaemic heart disease. *Drugs* 41:665-671, 1991.

Lavie CJ, Genton E: Hemostasis, thrombosis, and antiplatelet therapy: Implications for prevention of cardiovascular diseases. *Cardiovasc Rev Rep* 12:24-47 1991.

Lewis HD Jr, et al: Protective effects of aspirin against acute myocardial infarction and death in men with unstable angina: Results of Veterans Administration cooperative study. *N Engl J Med* 309:396-403, 1983.

Limet R, et al: Prevention of aorta-coronary bypass graft occlusion: Beneficial effect of ticlopidine on early and late patency rates of venous coronary bypass grafts: Double-blind study. *J Thorac Cardiovasc Surg* 94:773-783, 1987.

Manson JE, et al: Aspirin in the primary prevention of angina pectoris in a randomized trial of United States physicians. *Am J Med* 89:772-776, 1990.

McParland P, et al: Doppler ultrasound and aspirin in recognition and prevention of pregnancy-induced hypertension. *Lancet* 335:1552-1555, 1990.

McTavish D, et al: Ticlopidine: An updated review of its pharmacology and therapeutic use in platelet-dependent disorders. *Drugs* 40:238-259, 1990.

Mehta JL, Nichols WW: The potential role of thromboxane inhibitors in preventing myocardial ischaemic injury. *Drugs* 40:657-665, 1990.

Milner MR, et al: Usefulness of fish oil supplements in preventing clinical evidence of restenosis after percutaneous transluminal coronary angioplasty. *Am J Cardiol* 64:294-299, 1989.

Naschitz JE, et al: Overt gastrointestinal bleeding in the course of chronic low-dose aspirin administration for secondary prevention of arterial occlusive disease. *Am J Gastroenterol* 85:408-411, 1990.

Page Y, et al: Thrombotic thrombocytopenic purpura related to ticlopidine. *Lancet* 337:774-776, 1991.

Panak E, et al: Ticlopidine: A promise for prevention and treatment of thrombosis and its complications. *Haemostasis* 13:1-54, 1983.

Peto R, et al: Randomised trial of prophylactic daily aspirin in British male doctors. *Br Med J* 296:313-316, 1988.

Pfisterer M, et al: Trial of low-dose aspirin plus dipyridamole versus anticoagulants for prevention of aortocoronary vein graft occlusion. *Lancet* 2:1-7, 1989.

Popma JJ, Topol EJ: Factors influencing restenosis after coronary angioplasty. *Am J Med* 88:1-16N-1-24N, 1990.

Reis GJ, et al: Randomised trial of fish oil for prevention of restenosis after coronary angioplasty. *Lancet* 2:177-181, 1989.

Repke JT: Prevention and treatment of pregnancy-induced hypertension. *Compr Ther* 17:25-31, (May) 1991.

Ridker PM, et al: Low-dose aspirin therapy for chronic stable angina: A randomized, placebo-controlled clinical trial. *Ann Intern Med* 114:835-839, 1991.

The RISC Group: Risk of myocardial infarction and death during treatment with low dose aspirin and intravenous heparin in men with unstable coronary artery disease. *Lancet* 336:827-830, 1990.

Rowe GG, Folts JD: Aspirin and dipyridamole and their limitations in the therapy of coronary artery disease. *Clin Cardiol* 13:165-170, 1990.

Sandercock P: Recent developments in the diagnosis and management of patients with transient ischaemic attacks and minor ischaemic strokes. *Q J Med* 78:101-112, 1991.

Sanz G, et al: Prevention of early aortocoronary bypass occlusion by low-dose aspirin and dipyridamole. *Circulation* 82:765-773, 1990.

Scarpa WJ Jr: New therapy update: Intravenous persantine. *Cardiovasc Rev Rep* 70, (Aug) 1991.

Schiff E, et al: The use of aspirin to prevent pregnancy-induced hypertension and lower the ratio of thromboxane A_2 to prostacyclin in relatively high risk pregnancies. *N Engl J Med* 321:351-356, 1989.

Schiff E, et al: Low-dose aspirin does not influence the clinical course of women with mild pregnancy-induced hypertension. *Obstet Gynecol* 76:742-744, 1990.

Schwartz L, et al: The role of antiplatelet agents in modifying the extent of restenosis following percutaneous transluminal coronary angioplasty. *Am Heart J* 119:232-236, 1990.

Sethi GK, et al: Implications of preoperative administration of aspirin in patients undergoing coronary artery bypass grafting. *J Am Coll Cardiol* 15:15-20, 1990.

Shulman ST (ed): Management of Kawasaki syndrome: A consensus statement prepared by North American participants of the Third International Kawasaki Disease Symposium, Tokyo, Japan, December, 1988. *Pediatr Infect Dis J* 8:663-667, 1989.

Sivenius J, et al: The European Stroke Prevention Study: Results according to sex. *Neurology* 41:1189-1192, 1991 A.

Sivenius J, et al: The European Stroke Prevention Study (ESPS): Results by arterial distribution. *Ann Neurol* 29:596-600, 1991 B.

Smith MC, et al: Prostacyclin substitution for heparin in long-term hemodialysis. *Am J Med* 73:669-678, 1982.

Steering Committee of the Physicians' Health Study Research Group: Final report on the aspirin component of the ongoing physicians' health study. *N Engl J Med* 321:129-135, 1989.

Stein B, et al: Platelet inhibitor agents in cardiovascular disease: An update. *J Am Coll Cardiol* 14:813-836, 1989.

Stratton JR, Ritchie JL: Failure of ticlopidine to inhibit deposition of indium-111-labeled platelets on Dacron prosthetic surfaces in humans. *Circulation* 69:677-683, 1984.

Taggart DP, et al: Low-dose preoperative aspirin therapy, postoperative blood loss, and transfusion requirements. *Ann Thorac Surg* 50:425-428, 1990.

Théroux P, et al: Aspirin, heparin, or both to treat acute unstable angina. *N Engl J Med* 319:1105-1111, 1988.

Théroux P, et al: Hemodynamic, platelet and clinical responses to prostacyclin in unstable angina pectoris. *Am J Cardiol* 65:1084-1089, 1990.

UK-TIA Study Group: United Kingdom transient ischaemic attack (UK-TIA) aspirin trial: Interim results. *Br Med J* 296:316-320, 1988.

Uzan S, et al: Prevention of fetal growth retardation with low-dose aspirin: Findings of the EPREDA trial. *Lancet* 337:1427-1431, 1991.

Vianelli N, et al: Ticlopidine in the treatment of thrombotic thrombocytopenic purpura: Report of two cases. *Haematologica* 75:274-277, 1990.

Wallace WA, et al: Unstable angina pectoris. *Clin Cardiol* 13:679-686, 1990.

Wallenburg HCS, et al: Low-dose aspirin prevents pregnancy-induced hypertension and pre-eclampsia in angiotensin-sensitive primigravidae. *Lancet* 1:1-3, 1986.

Weber MAJ, et al: Low-dose aspirin versus anticoagulants for prevention of coronary graft occlusion. *Am J Cardiol* 66:1464-1468, 1990.

Webster MWI, et al: Platelet inhibitor therapy: Agents and clinical implications. *Hematol Oncol Clin North Am* 4:265-289, 1990.

Weissmann G: Aspirin. *Sci Am* 84-90, (Jan) 1991.

Werler MM, et al: The relation of aspirin use during the first trimester of pregnancy to congenital cardiac defects. *N Engl J Med* 321:1639-1642, 1989.

White CW, et al: Antiplatelet agents are effective in reducing the immediate complications of PTCA: Results from the Ticlopidine Multicenter Trial, abstract. *Circulation* 76 (suppl IV):IV-400, 1987.

Wolf PA, et al: Atrial fibrillation as an independent risk factor for stroke: The Framingham Study. *Stroke* 22:983-988, 1991.

Working Group on High Blood Pressure in Pregnancy: National high blood pressure education program working group report on high blood pressure in pregnancy. *Am J Obstet Gynecol* 163:1689-1712, 1990.

Zemel MB, et al: Altered platelet calcium metabolism as an early predictor of increased peripheral vascular resistance and preeclampsia in urban black women. *N Engl J Med* 323:434-438, 1990.

Other Selected References

Ashby B, et al: Mechanisms of platelet activation and inhibition. *Hematol Oncol Clin North Am* 4:1-26, 1990.

Dutka AJ, Hallenbeck JM: Pharmacologic therapy for ischemic cerebrovascular disease. *Clin Neuropharmacol* 8:161-176, 1990.

Fuster V, Roberts WC (eds): A symposium: Thrombosis and antithrombotic therapy—Direction for the '90s. *Am J Cardiol* 65:1C-50C, 1990.

Fuster V, et al: Antithrombotic therapy in cardiac disease: An approach based on pathogenesis and risk stratification. *Am J Cardiol* 65:38C-44C, 1990.

Hennekens CH: Aspirin in chronic cardiovascular disease and acute myocardial infarction. *Clin Cardiol* 13:V-62-V-72, 1990.

Hirsh J, et al: Aspirin and other platelet active drugs: Relationship among dose, effectiveness, and side effects. *Chest* 95 (suppl): 12S-18S, 1989.

Kroll MH, Schafer AI: Biochemical mechanisms of platelet activation. *Blood* 74:1181-1195, 1989.

Oates JA, et al: Clinical implications of prostaglandin and thromboxane A_2 formation, parts 1 and 2. *N Engl J Med* 319:689-698, 761-767, 1988.

Oczkowski WJ, Turpie AGG: Antithrombotic treatment of cerebrovascular disease. *Baillieres Clin Haematol* 3:781-813, 1990.

Patrono C, FitzGerald GA (eds): *Platelets and Vascular Occlusion.* New York, Raven Press, 1988, vol 54.

Reilly IAG, FitzGerald GA: Aspirin in cardiovascular disease. *Drugs* 35:154-176, 1988.

Schrader BJ, Berk SI: Antiplatelet agents in coronary artery disease. *Clin Pharm* 9:118-124, 1990.

Sila CA, Furlan AJ: Drug treatment of stroke: Current status and future prospects. *Drugs* 35:468-476, 1988.

Thrombolytics

THROMBOLYSIS AND THROMBOLYTIC AGENTS

To maintain the integrity of the vascular system, hemostatic plugs that repair sites of injury are formed through an interdependent series of reactions involving the vessel wall, platelets, and the coagulation system. However, over-responsiveness of the repair mechanism, normal responses in abnormal (atherosclerotic) vascular environments, or failure of the endogenous anticoagulant system to control the activation process can cause a thrombus to form. Obstruction of blood flow by the thrombus contributes to severe dysfunction that may result in myocardial infarction, venous thrombosis, pulmonary embolism, or stroke. To limit the extent of clot formation, the fibrinolytic system is activated simultaneously with hemostasis. Endogenous thrombolysis occurs when the fibrin-bound proenzyme, plasminogen, is converted to the active serine protease, plasmin, which digests the fibrin matrix of the clot. The process is catalyzed by plasminogen activators (tissue-type plasminogen activator [t-PA] and pro-urokinase) that are present in blood, the vascular endothelium, and various tissues. Natural serine protease inhibitors (serpins), especially α_2-antiplasmin, inactivate plasmin in the circulation and thus prevent fibrinogenolysis in circulating blood (see index entry Blood Coagulation, Mechanisms). Fibrin-bound plasmin is partially protected from the effects of α_2-antiplasmin.

Thrombolytics are used when rapid dissolution of a clot is required to preserve organ and limb function (arterial occlusion) or valve function of the veins (venous occlusion). They also may be employed to restore patency to arteriovenous catheters that have been obstructed by blood clots.

Thrombolytic agents are classified as nonfibrin-specific (streptokinase, urokinase, and anistreplase) or fibrin-specific (recombinant t-PA, pro-urokinase, and recombinant plasminogen activator). Streptokinase [Kabikinase, Streptase] is a bacterially derived immunogenic single-chain protein that indirectly activates the fibrinolytic system by combining noncovalently with plasminogen to form an activator complex (Goa et al, 1990; Loscalzo, 1990). Urokinase [Abbokinase], a two-chain serine protease generated by proteolytic cleavage of a proenzyme synthesized in endothelial and mononuclear cells, activates plasminogen directly. Both streptokinase and urokinase catalyze conversion of fibrin-bound and circulating plasminogen to plasmin (Marder and Sherry, 1988; Loscalzo, 1990; Fears, 1990). In addition, both agents may induce a systemic fibrinolytic state characterized by reduced plasma levels of fibrinogen, α_2-antiplasmin, and clotting factors V and VIII; increased levels of fibrin(ogen) degradation products; and activation of plasminogen.

Anistreplase (anisoylated plasminogen-streptokinase activator complex, APSAC [Eminase]) consists of streptokinase complexed noncovalently to a modified form of plasminogen and is catalytically activated by gradual deacylation following binding to fibrin. It has a longer half-life than streptokinase (Fears, 1990; Sherry, 1990). The streptokinase moiety of anistreplase retains its immunogenicity and sensitivity to inhibition by neutralizing antibodies.

Recombinant t-PA (rt-PA, alteplase [Activase]) is produced by recombinant DNA technology and has less potential to induce a systemic effect than the foregoing nonfibrin-specific agents. This agent binds to fibrin and converts the fibrin-bound plasminogen to plasmin. Circulating plasminogen is activated to a lesser extent by rt-PA than by streptokinase. rt-PA is a glycosylated single-chain serine protease that can be cleaved to two chains by plasmin-catalyzed proteolysis (Collen et al, 1989; Becker et al, 1991). A two-chain recombinant preparation of t-PA (duteplase) also has been investigated. Single-chain and two-chain rt-PA have equal enzymatic activities in the presence of fibrin; however, the single-chain form is metabolized 40% more rapidly than the double-chain form and hence a lower dose of duteplase achieves the same level of activity (Mueller et al, 1987).

Recombinant single-chain urokinase-type plasminogen activator (rscu-PA, pro-urokinase, r-proUK [Prolyse]) induces fibrin-specific clot lysis by selectively activating fibrin-bound plasminogen (Collen and Gold, 1989; Bode et al, 1990). Pro-urokinase probably is activated by fibrin-bound plasmin through cleavage of a peptide bond to produce a two-chain protein that is held together by a disulfide bond (high-molecular-weight two-chain urokinase, HMW-tcu-PA). Further proteolysis of HMW-tcu-PA yields urokinase. r-proUK is available for clinical use in the United States only in sponsored clinical trials.

Recombinant plasminogen activator (rPA, BM-06022) is a deletion mutant produced from tissue-type plasminogen activator. It has more potent fibrinolytic activity, similar fibrin specificity, and a longer half-life than rt-PA.

Various approaches to the development of new thrombolytic drugs are being pursued (Lijnen, 1989; Higgins and Bennett, 1990; Collen and Gold, 1990; Fears, 1990; Bode et al, 1990). Among these are mutants and variants of both t-PA (with increased affinity or specificity for fibrin or with decreased clearance rates) and scu-PA (with increased fibrin specificity), chimeric plasminogen activators (eg, recombinant constructs that link the fibrin-binding domain of t-PA with the fibrin-specific catalytic domain of scu-PA), and antibody-targeted thrombolytic agents. The latter group includes (1) plasminogen activators joined by chemical, immunologic, or recombinant DNA techniques to fibrin-specific monoclonal antibodies; (2) bispecific, heteroduplex antibodies that bind both fibrin and a plasminogen activator (ie, chemical conjugates between a monoclonal antibody to a fibrin-specific epitope and a second antibody to t-PA or scu-PA); and (3) constructs in which an antibody to platelet glycoprotein IIb/IIIa (the platelet fibrinogen receptor, which mediates platelet aggregation) is joined to urokinase.

USES

Myocardial Infarction

Almost all patients with myocardial infarction have occlusive thrombi in the infarct-related coronary artery. (See the chapter, Therapeutic Management of Myocardial Infarction.) Decreased oxygen supply to the cardiac muscle cells following the occlusion causes myocardial necrosis, which extends as a wave from the endocardial to the epicardial surface two to six hours after the occlusion. Early in the course of an evolving infarction, recanalization of the infarct-related artery can reperfuse the jeopardized myocardium and thus limit infarct size, preserve left ventricular function, and enhance survival.

Analysis of the results of numerous international clinical trials indicates that thrombolytic agents can restore blood flow to infarct-related arteries, although outcomes vary. rt-PA and streptokinase were directly compared in the Global Utilization of Streptokinase and TPA for Occluded Coronary Arteries (GUSTO) trial. Results showed that the percentage of patients with complete reperfusion (anterograde flow [TIMI grade 3] to the entire distal bed at a normal rate) at 90 minutes was 54%, 29%, and 32% following administration of an accelerated-dose regimen of rt-PA plus intravenous heparin or of streptokinase plus subcutaneous or intravenous heparin, respectively (The GUSTO Angiographic Investigators, 1993); this correlated directly with mortality rates at 30 days of 6.3%, 7.2%, and 7.4%, respectively (The GUSTO Investigators, 1993). The survival rate at one year in patients with open arteries also is higher than in those who did not receive thrombolytic therapy or who had closed arteries at hospital discharge (Kennedy et al, 1985; Chesebro et al, 1987). Other improved outcomes, as indicated by ventriculographic, enzymatic, and electrocardiographic indices, also were associated with TIMI grade 3 flow in the TEAM-3 trial in patients treated with anistreplase or rt-PA (Anderson et al, 1993).

Opening an artery to the infarcted area with thrombolytic therapy reduced the inducibility of ventricular fibrillation or ventricular tachycardia during programmed electrical stimulation and the occurrence of late potentials on signal-averaged ECGs (Vatterott et al, 1991; Zimmermann et al, 1991). Reduction in dispersion, an index of the electrocardiographic QT heterogeneity of myocardial repolarization, also has been associated with successful reperfusion in patients with myocardial infarction. These benefits may be related to the observed reduction in the rate of sudden death in the treated patients (Lange et al, 1990).

Thrombolytic therapy is recommended for patients with chest pain unresponsive to sublingual nitroglycerin for >30 minutes and ST-segment elevation of at least 0.1 mV (1 mm) in at least two contiguous electrocardiographic leads or the I and aVL leads (ACC/AHA Task Force, 1990). Functional and survival benefits are optimal when thrombolytics are administered within six hours of onset of acute myocardial infarction (Granger et al, 1992). Thus, programs have been developed to reduce the time to initiation of therapy by administering these agents either while patients are en route to the hospital or shortly after hospital admission (Weaver et al, 1993; The European Myocardial Infarction Project Group, 1993; Pell et al, 1992). However, patients still benefit when thrombolytic therapy is instituted within 12 hours of symptom onset (EMERAS Collaborative Group, 1993; LATE Study Group, 1993).

When aspirin was given with either rt-PA or streptokinase, the patency rate at 90 minutes was higher and rates of recurrent angina and reocclusion were lower than with placebo (Roux et al, 1992). Thus, aspirin (160 to 324 mg daily) has been recommended as an early adjunctive agent in all patients receiving thrombolytic therapy. Administration of intravenous heparin is essential to achieve lower mortality rates with rt-PA but not with streptokinase or urokinase (Prins and Hirsh, 1991). Even though intravenous heparin is recommended after the administration of anistreplase in patients with myocardial infarction (AIMS Trial Study Group, 1988, 1990), results of the Duke University Clinical Cardiology Study (DUCCS-1) show that the anticoagulant did not enhance the reduction in the incidence of death, reinfarction, recurrent ischemia, or occlusion of the infarct-related artery (O'Connor et al, 1994). Furthermore, withholding heparin resulted in a 46% decrease in bleeding complications after use of anistreplase.

Myocardial infarction in the elderly often is atypical and may lack the classic triad of chest pain, ECG changes, and elevated serum enzymes. These individuals, especially those over 75 years, often have symptoms of confusion, vomiting, syncope, and shortness of breath (Nadelman et al, 1990). As a result, the elderly are more likely to present late for any form of therapy after symptom onset (Williamson et al, 1992). The elderly are at particularly high risk following myocardial infarction: A patient age 75 years with an acute myocardial infarction is seven times more likely to die in the hospital than one age 50 years, and the mortality rate of older patients is twice that of younger patients after discharge (Goldberg et al, 1989). When they were managed conservatively without reperfusion therapy, 31% of patients over age 65 developed heart failure following myocardial infarction compared with 19% of those under age 65 (Weaver et al, 1991). Although older individuals also had a higher overall risk of stroke and reinfarction, thrombolytic therapy increases the overall chance of survival in these patients. In the ISIS-2 trial (1988), the combination of streptokinase and aspirin reduced mortality in those over 80 years from 37% (placebo) to 20%, compared with a reduction of 6% (placebo) to 4% in those under 60 years.

Analysis of the results from nine randomized, controlled trials (GISSI-1, ISAM, AIMS, ISIS-2, ASSET, USIM, ISIS-3, EMERAS, and LATE) indicated that mortality rates were significantly reduced in 55- to 74-year old patients following administration of streptokinase, anistreplase, or rt-PA (Fibrinolytic Therapy Trialists' Collaborative Group, 1994). Recanalization with streptokinase, aspirin, and intravenous heparin was successful in a 110-year-old man during the GUSTO trial (Katz et al, 1993). Thus, there appears to be no upper limit on the age of patients for whom administration of thrombolytics is appropriate, provided that no contraindications exist. Although the incidence of bleeding and intracerebral hemorrhage associated with thrombolytic therapy is higher in the elderly, especially with rt-PA (ISIS-3 Collaborative Group, 1992), the potential reduction in mortality often outweighs this risk.

Absolute contraindications to thrombolytic therapy include active internal bleeding, suspected aortic dissection, prolonged or traumatic cardiopulmonary resuscitation, recent head trauma, intracranial tumor, diabetic hemorrhagic retinopathy or other hemorrhagic ophthalmic condition, pregnancy, previous hypersensitivity reaction to the agent (streptokinase or anistreplase), blood pressure >200/120 mm Hg, or history of hemorrhagic stroke.

See also the chapter on Therapeutic Management of Myocardial Infarction.

Venous Thrombosis and Pulmonary Embolism

Deep vein thrombosis contributes significantly to the morbidity of chronically ill or bedridden patients and is a common complication after surgery (eg, orthopedic surgery of the lower extremity, gynecologic cancer surgery, major abdominal surgery), following trauma, or during pregnancy (Francis and Marder, 1991; Goldhaber, 1993). Deep vein thrombosis may be caused by stasis, endothelial injury, or a hypercoagulable state and can be diagnosed by observing areas of abnormal blood flow on Doppler ultrasonography or absence of venous filling on ascending contrast venography or impedance plethysmography. The outcome of deep venous thrombosis often is development of a pulmonary embolism, which is a contributing factor in at least 50,000 deaths annually in the United States.

Most pulmonary emboli arise from thrombi in the pelvic veins and deep veins of the legs (popliteal, femoral, and iliac). However, pulmonary embolism from thrombi in the upper extremities as a result of effort injury, drug abuse, or anatomic anomalies (eg, cervical ribs, thoracic outlet compression, anomalous musculofascial bands, aberrant arteries), and the long-term use of indwelling central venous catheters appears to be increasing (Monreal et al, 1991).

The goals in treating venous thromboembolism are to reduce mortality from pulmonary emboli; relieve symptoms; alleviate pulmonary and systemic hemodynamic disturbances; prevent permanent damage to the pulmonary vascular bed; and prevent vascular incompetence in the deep veins, which predisposes to persistent venous hypertension and recurrent episodes of deep vein thrombosis (Hirsh and Hull, 1986; Goldhaber, 1990).

Traditional treatment for deep vein thrombosis (eg, anticoagulants) has focused on preventing extension or embolization of the thrombus while leaving it in situ. However, because of the significant risks associated with venous valvular damage and other long-term sequelae (eg, deep venous insufficiency and occlusion), dissolution of the thrombus with thrombolytic agents is an appropriate alternative (Rogers and Lutcher, 1990; Francis and Marder, 1991). In nine randomized trials using pre- and post-treatment venography to verify the results achieved, substantial improvement was observed in 45% of patients treated with streptokinase followed by anticoagulants compared with 5% of patients treated with anticoagulants alone. No change was observed on post-treatment venography in 37% of patients who received thrombolytics and anticoagulants compared with 69% of those treated with anticoagulants alone. Similar results were observed in six randomized studies using phlebography as a diagnostic tool (Goldhaber et al, 1984; Rogers and Lutcher, 1990). Clinical improvement, indicated by decreased incidence of edema, varicosities, pain, discoloration, stasis ulceration, and venous valve damage, has been demonstrated in patients followed for as long as six years after thrombolytic therapy. In a more recent study, three bolus doses of intravenous urokinase administered over a 24-hour period resulted in clot lysis in 50% patients with deep venous thrombosis (Goldhaber et al, 1994). However, streptokinase may be less effective when used to dissolve older thrombi (ie, >3 to 7 days from onset of symptoms compared with ≤3 days) (Rogers and Lutcher, 1990).

Data on the use of rt-PA in patients with deep vein thrombosis are less definitive because of the use of different dosage regimens (35 mg over 4 hours to 185 mg over 35 hours) in various trials. However, more extensive thrombolysis was observed in patients receiving rt-PA and heparin than in those treated with heparin alone (Francis and Marder, 1991).

At present, no one thrombolytic agent is considered therapeutically superior. It is currently suggested that streptokinase or urokinase be infused continuously for up to 27 hours and rt-PA for two hours. Preliminary studies indicate that infusion of thrombolytics via catheter directly into venous clots may be more effective than intravenous infusion (Sherry, 1991), especially for patients with a total obstructive thrombus (Meyerovitz et al, 1992).

About 70% of patients with confirmed pulmonary embolism have thrombosis in deep leg veins and, in about 40% of these patients, the pulmonary embolism is asymptomatic (Kruit et al, 1991; Moser et al 1994). When more than 25% of the pulmonary vascular bed is obstructed, pulmonary arteriolar pressure increases with resultant elevation of right ventricular pressure. The right ventricle ultimately dilates and becomes hypokinetic, leading in turn to tricuspid regurgitation. As the right ventricle fails, right atrial pressure increases and cardiogenic shock ensues. In a multicenter diagnostic trial, the one-year mortality rate of patients with pulmonary embolism was 24%, with cardiac disease, recurrent pulmonary embolism, infection, and cancer causing more than 75% of these deaths (Carson et al, 1992). Thus, pulmonary embolism complicates serious chronic diseases and can be a precursor of death in a substantial proportion of patients.

Anticoagulation with heparin is the mainstay of therapy for pulmonary emboli. However, a thrombolytic agent may be a useful adjunct to heparin in patients with hemodynamic instability, right ventricular dysfunction, massive pulmonary embolism, or extensive deep vein thrombosis. By reestablishing the pulmonary artery blood flow, thrombolysis can quickly reduce the elevated pulmonary artery pressure and reverse right ventricular hypertension, thus preventing right ventricular failure and/or cardiogenic shock.

Clinical benefits from thrombolytic therapy are most evident in those treated for large pulmonary emboli involving more than two lobar arteries (Moran et al, 1989; Marder and Francis, 1990). Streptokinase, rt-PA, and urokinase all improve pulmonary perfusion at 24 hours (Goldhaber, 1993). A randomized controlled trial compared continuous infusion of rt-PA 100 mg over 2 hours with a bolus dose of urokinase 4,400 U/kg followed by 4,400 U/kg/hr infused over 12 hours (Meyer et al, 1992). At two hours, the decrease in total pulmonary resistance was more rapid with rt-PA than with urokinase. However, at 12 hours, the degree of reduction of pulmonary resistance was equivalent with both drugs. The use of angiography to compare the efficacy of these two agents was less sensitive, since improvement assessed two hours after administration of rt-PA and urokinase was similar on the angiogram (Goldhaber et al, 1992).

rt-PA combined with heparin reversed right ventricular dysfunction and restored pulmonary tissue perfusion more rapidly than heparin alone in hemodynamically stable patients with pulmonary emboli (Goldhaber et al, 1993). Although recurrent pulmonary emboli were not observed in the group treated with rt-PA plus heparin, a higher frequency of bleeding was noted. Since low-molecular-weight heparin reduced the risk of major bleeding by 91% during the initial treatment phase in patients with deep vein thrombosis when compared with standard heparin (Hull et al, 1992), this combination may further improve the outcome of patients with pulmonary emboli.

Arterial Thromboembolism

Acute arterial occlusions usually involve vessels of the lower extremities. Prognosis depends on the location of the clot, the presence of collateral circulation, and the extent of irreversible tissue damage at the time of intervention. In patients with limb-threatening ischemia, prompt Fogarty catheter thrombectomy, embolectomy, or arterial reconstructive surgery is indicated. However, the success rate for thrombectomy is low in atherosclerotic arteries or for thrombi distal to the popliteal artery or when it is performed more than 24 hours after onset of the occlusion. Although surgical intervention may be attempted in these patients, infusion of streptokinase, urokinase, or rt-PA offers an alternative or adjunctive approach (Verstraete, 1989). Thrombolytic therapy appears to be most appropriate for patients who can tolerate an additional 24 to 48 hours of occlusion until lysis occurs (eg, those with extensive collateral circulation due to chronic occlusive peripheral vascular disease) or for those whose options are limited because of contraindications to surgery, surgically inaccessible lesions, or lack of suitable vessels for bypass.

The success rate for restoration of blood flow with use of streptokinase or urokinase depends on the time interval between the occlusion and treatment. Recanalization occurred in up to 80% of patients treated within the first 12 hours and in up to 60% of those treated within three days after occlusion, but success rates declined with older thrombi and none older than three months were recanalized. In addition, bleeding was common with the large doses needed for systemic therapy, and fatality rates ranged from 1% to 3%. Intravenous infusion of streptokinase has been successful in a small number of pediatric patients who received the drug for femoral artery thrombosis after cardiac catheterization that did not resolve after 48 hours of heparin infusion (Wessel et al, 1986;

Ino et al, 1988; Brus et al, 1990). However, no controlled trials have been performed in such patients.

Local therapy with smaller doses of thrombolytic drugs can recanalize occluded arteries in most patients, and the incidence of adverse effects is much lower. Two approaches to local thrombolysis of arterial thromboemboli have been used. The first, continuous slow arterial infusion of streptokinase or urokinase in the immediate vicinity of the clot, was successful in clinical trials in 50% to 80% of patients treated at specialized care centers (Verstraete, 1989). Patency of the recanalized artery was maintained in 50% of the patients available for follow-up one year after therapy. In a review of results obtained with this technique in more than 600 patients treated outside of clinical trials by 45 vascular surgeons, the overall recanalization rate was 50%, but the rates of serious complications, major amputations, and mortality were 20%, 16.5%, and 2.3%, respectively (Ricotta et al, 1987). In the second approach, intrathrombotic injection of the thrombolytic drug is repeated every five minutes as the catheter is advanced stepwise between injections until recanalization is achieved. In an overview of 14 clinical trials that used this technique, recanalization was reported in 67% of 474 patients treated with streptokinase and in 81% of 162 patients treated with urokinase (Graor and Olin, 1989). Major complications occurred in 19% of those treated with streptokinase and in 12% of those treated with urokinase. Results of a prospective, randomized trial comparing periodic and slow continuous infusion of urokinase in 25 patients with deep vein thrombosis did not reveal any difference in the speed of lysis, initial success rate, incidence of complication, or 30-day clinical outcome (Kandarpa et al, 1993).

Unstable Angina

Myocardial ischemia in patients with unstable angina is usually caused by atherosclerotic plaque that narrows the coronary artery lumen. Unstable angina usually begins with plaque rupture, followed by platelet aggregation and fibrin-crosslinking at the rupture site. Partial or transient obstruction of the lumen by the resultant thrombus precipitates the symptoms of unstable angina (Ambrose, 1992).

One goal of treatment is to block further enlargement of the thrombus to prevent evolution into myocardial infarction. Because use of aspirin, heparin, or both to reduce the formation of thrombi is only partially effective, trials with thrombolytic agents have been conducted. Although urokinase or rt-PA reduced the incidence of intracoronary filling defect (which reflects the severity of stenosis) in patients with unstable angina, clinical improvement was not observed (Ambrose et al, 1992; Freeman et al, 1992; Karlsson et al, 1992; Bär et al, 1992; The TIMI IIIA Investigators, 1993; The TIMI IIIB Investigators, 1994). Furthermore, these patients were more prone to develop myocardial infarction following thrombolytic therapy than those receiving anticoagulant therapy alone.

The inability of thrombolytic agents to improve clinical outcome may be due to the transient procoagulation effect of thrombolytics in highly stenotic but not occluded coronary vessels, resulting in further extension of thrombosis (Waters and Lam, 1992; Leinbach, 1992). Since thrombin and platelets are activated very early after administration of thrombolytics, reperfusion may be delayed and thus the usefulness of these agents in patients with unstable angina would be negated. It has been suggested that their transient procoagulant effect can be counteracted by administration of more potent anticoagulants (eg, argatroban, hirudin) and by blockade of platelet IIb/IIIa receptors (Waters and Lam, 1992; Leinbach, 1992).

Ischemic Stroke

Ischemic stroke results primarily from occlusion of a cerebral blood vessel that reduces delivery of oxygen and glucose to the affected vascular area (Pulsinelli, 1992). The extent of damage depends on the degree and duration of the impaired blood flow. Most patients benefit from rapid recanalization of the occluded vessel. Following computed tomographic scanning and angiography to exclude intracerebral hemorrhage or hemorrhagic infarction as the cause of symptoms, cerebral arteries were reopened and clinical outcome was improved in 60% of patients with acute ischemic stroke after administration of intra-arterial or intravenous rt-PA, streptokinase, or urokinase in several open trials (Wardlaw and Warlow, 1992; Levine and Brott, 1992). Analysis of the results of four randomized controlled trials on patients treated with thrombolytics indicated that the risk of death was reduced by 37%.

Contrary to the projection that thrombolytic therapy might increase hemorrhagic transformation of cerebral infarcts, the estimated rate of formation of intracerebral hematomas after thrombolysis is 5%, a percentage only slightly higher than that in placebo recipients. In addition, in the Acute Stroke Study Group trial, the rate of cerebral hemorrhage was not higher in patients up to age 80 years than in younger patients (del Zoppo et al, 1992). Furthermore, the incidence of hemorrhagic transformation was directly related to the time of treatment from symptom onset, resting diastolic pressure, and body weight (del Zoppo et al, 1992; Levy et al, 1994). No significant difference in immediate patency rates was observed with rt-PA, streptokinase, or urokinase, even though the cerebral hemorrhage rate may be higher after administration of rt-PA. Thus, thrombolytics may be beneficial in the management of acute ischemic stroke, and the risks involved in their use do not appear to be excessive. However, their routine use should await confirmation from results of large controlled clinical trials.

Occlusion of Surgical Prostheses

DIALYSIS ACCESS SITES. In the absence of renal transplantation, patients with end-stage renal disease require dialysis, with the majority undergoing the procedure three times weekly (Kumpe and Cohen, 1992). These patients require a vascular access site that is easily available and capable of shunting at least 200 ml of blood per minute without interruption. Surgically created hemodialysis access sites can be in the form of external arteriovenous silastic cannula shunts, venous cannulation with one or two catheters, native arteriovenous fistulae, or prosthetic arteriovenous conduits.

The most common complication of long-term internal vascular access is partial or complete obstruction of blood flow due to thrombosis or vascular stenosis. Traditionally, a thrombosed access site is managed with simple thrombectomy. Surgical revision (patch angioplasty, interposition, or venous endarterectomy) also is performed in the presence of a venous anastomosis stenosis. Since the number of access sites that can be created is limited, it is necessary to extend the functional patency of each site with repeated thrombectomies and surgical revision.

Thrombolytic agents can be used as an alternative to surgical intervention. Because recurrent thrombosis necessitates repeated administration of the thrombolytic agent, urokinase is preferred to streptokinase due to its shorter half-life and lack of antigenicity. The success rate of reducing the obstruction is increased with use of a two-catheter technique: Two catheters are placed in a criss-cross pattern directed toward the arterial and venous anastomoses at the site of thrombosis, and urokinase is then infused through both catheters until lysis is complete or near complete. Balloon angioplasty is then performed to remedy any arterial, midgraft, or venous outflow stenoses. The combination of thrombolysis and angioplasty reopened 90% of thrombosed prosthetic conduits in 41 patients (Valji et al, 1991). Advantages of thrombolysis plus angioplasty over thrombectomy or surgical revision are that dialysis can be resumed immediately, placement of a temporary subclavian vein access catheter is unnecessary, and lysis can be performed on outpatients. Long-term secondary patency with the combination of thrombolysis and angioplasty approaches that of surgical therapy.

INDWELLING CATHETERS. Thrombosis of the axillary, subclavian, and central venous circulation occurs in as many as 50% of patients with prolonged subclavian venous access sites and is especially common in children and adult marrow transplant recipients and other cancer patients. Catheter-related subclavian venous thrombosis that obstructs venous circulation in the head and/or upper extremities is manifested by pain in the ipsilateral shoulder and swelling of the ipsilateral arm and hand. Other symptoms may include intrascapular pain, jaw ache, and pain in the opposite shoulder. Catheter function may be preserved by administration of heparin and warfarin (Gould et al, 1993). Because catheter-related venous thrombosis may be complicated by superior vena cava syndrome or pulmonary emboli, catheter removal may be appropriate.

Clot lysis with thrombolytics is an alternative. In the majority of patients with obstructed central venous catheters, instillation of small doses of streptokinase or urokinase followed by incubation for up to one hour has restored patency. One uncontrolled study in a small number of patients suggested that the continuous slow infusion of small doses of urokinase may be safe and effective in children with malignant diseases (Bagnall et al, 1989), and a similar report indicates that prolonged infusion of urokinase can restore catheter patency even after one or more instillations have been unsuccessful (Haire et al, 1990). rt-PA has been used in a few patients to clear occluded central venous catheters that did not open after administration of urokinase (Atkinson et al, 1990).

PROSTHETIC HEART VALVES. Thrombotic occlusion of prosthetic heart valves is a life-threatening event that may be caused by inadequate anticoagulation. The standard therapy, immediate valve replacement, is associated with significant surgical morbidity, especially in elderly patients and those who have severe heart failure; the mortality rate is 4.5% to 25% (McKay, 1993).

Thrombolytic therapy with streptokinase or urokinase has been employed as an alternative to immediate surgical intervention. Use of one of these agents restored the function of thrombosed prosthetic heart valves in 49 of 67 patients (Chen et al, 1992). Partial opening was observed in an additional 10 patients, resulting in stable hemodynamics and reduced surgical risk. In a series of 10 cases of obstructed St. Jude prosthetic valves, treatment with streptokinase or urokinase markedly improved leaflet movement and relieved symptoms within 12 hours in eight patients (Silber et al, 1993). A similar success rate (73%) was observed when streptokinase, urokinase, or rt-PA was utilized to resolve the obstruction in prosthetic valves of 64 patients (Roudaut et al, 1992). In this study, thrombolytic therapy was more efficient for thrombi in aortic prostheses than in mitral valves.

The complications of thrombolytic therapy in patients with thrombosed prosthetic valves vary depending on the thrombolytic agent used and the regimen followed. The major complications reported were systemic embolization, bleeding, and allergic reactions.

ADVERSE REACTIONS AND PRECAUTIONS

Hematologic Reactions: Following a transient procoagulation effect, thrombolytics induce a systemic hypocoagulable state caused by fibrinogenolysis (Loscalzo, 1990). Although this hypocoagulable state is well tolerated by an intact vascular system, the risk of bleeding can be significant and is further increased by the concomitant use of aspirin and heparin (Califf et al, 1992; Granger et al, 1992). Bleeding complications most frequently arise at sites of vascular injury (eg, sites of recent needle puncture, surgery, trauma, or tissue damage [peptic ulceration or cerebral infarction]) and can be minimized by excluding patients with these risk factors. The risk of bleeding also is increased in females, the elderly, and patients with a history of hypertension or who have low body weight (Califf et al, 1992). However, the risk for an individual must be weighed against the likely benefit of thrombolysis and the severity of the thromboembolic condition.

In patients with deep vein thrombosis, the incidence of serious bleeding complications with prolonged systemic thrombolysis followed by anticoagulation is about 9% (Francis and Marder, 1991). The incidence of bleeding severe enough to require transfusion is lower (1%) with the shorter infusion times and smaller dosages used in the treatment of myocardial infarction (ISIS-3 and GISSI-2 trials).

If severe bleeding develops at disturbed sites or internally, the infusion should be discontinued. Major bleeding or impending surgery may necessitate transfusion of whole blood, platelets, red blood cells and cryoprecipitate, or fresh frozen plasma. For rapid reversal of the fibrinolytic state, fibrinolysis inhibitors (eg, aminocaproic acid 100 mg/kg) can be given by slow intravenous injection together with a source of fibrinogen (Sane et al, 1989). (See index entry Aminocaproic Acid.) Protamine sulfate may be useful in treating hemorrhage in patients given heparin as an adjunct to thrombolysis (see index entry Protamine, In Heparin Overdose).

Cardiovascular Reactions: Stroke is a complication of myocardial infarction in 1% to 3% of patients, regardless of treatment with thrombolytics (Granger et al, 1992). In large randomized controlled trials of thrombolytic therapy in patients with myocardial infarction, the risk of intracerebral hemorrhage was increased by 0.3% compared with placebo (ISIS-3 and GISSI-2 trials). Both stroke and "presumed" intracerebral hemorrhage were more common in patients who received rt-PA than streptokinase. In the ISIS-3 trial, the incidence of stroke also was higher with anistreplase than with streptokinase.

The risk of intracerebral hemorrhage increased with the dose of the thrombolytic used: in the TIMI-2 trial, the incidence increased from 0.5% to 1.5% when the dose of rt-PA was raised from 100 to 150 mg in patients with myocardial infarction (Gore et al, 1991).

Transient bradycardia and ventricular arrhythmias are common following thrombolysis for myocardial infarction and are usually regarded as signs of successful reperfusion. If therapy is necessary, the arrhythmias generally respond to conventional antiarrhythmic drugs, such as atropine and lidocaine, respectively. However, these arrhythmias often resolve spontaneously.

Severe hypotension has occurred when large doses of streptokinase were given by rapid intravenous infusion (Lew et al, 1985). Transient, milder, reversible episodes of hypotension also have been reported during or shortly after slower infusions of streptokinase or injections of anistreplase, but they responded to standard measures (eg, change in posture, fluid infusion) and did not recur when temporarily halted infusions of streptokinase were resumed.

Allergic Reactions: Streptokinase may cause allergic reactions, including pruritus, flushing, urticaria and, rarely, angioedema, periorbital swelling, and bronchospasm. A delayed reaction, manifested by fever and arthralgias, is relatively common. A severe serum sickness syndrome, with fever, arthralgias, rash, and renal failure, has occurred rarely. Similar allergic reactions can occur with anistreplase, since it consists of streptokinase complexed with anisoylated plasminogen. The incidence of allergic reactions is higher when readministration of streptokinase is necessary to treat reocclusion of the infarct-related artery soon after successful thrombolysis (White et al, 1990). More important, a high titer of neutralizing antibody will prevent clot lysis if streptokinase or anistreplase is reinfused within five days to two years or more. Antibody-mediated platelet aggregation has been reported after use of streptokinase (Vaughan et al, 1988). Mild reactions may respond to antihistamines and/or corticosteroids. If severe reactions occur, streptokinase should be discontinued and epinephrine, corticosteroids, and antihistamines administered.

Urokinase and rt-PA are not antigenic and hence may be used when thrombolysis is indicated for patients who have been treated with streptokinase or anistreplase within the previous two years (or even longer). However, bronchospasm and angioedema have been reported after alteplase therapy, and allergic reactions characterized by rigor occurred in some patients who received urokinase (Goldhaber et al, 1988; Francis et al, 1991). Other minor allergic reactions have been reported with these agents as well.

Pregnancy: Streptokinase, anistreplase, and rt-PA are classified in FDA Pregnancy Category C, and urokinase is classified in FDA Pregnancy Category B.

Drug Evaluations

ALTEPLASE, RECOMBINANT (rt-PA; Recombinant Human Tissue-Type Plasminogen Activator)
[Activase]

ACTIONS AND USES. Alteplase (rt-PA) is a naturally occurring serine protease that is now produced by recombinant DNA technology. This product has the same characteristics as tissue-type plasminogen activator generated by endothelial cells of the vessel wall as part of the normal but localized physiologic mechanism for digesting fibrin clots.

In the absence of fibrin, rt-PA activates plasminogen at a very slow rate; however, when rt-PA binds to fibrin, the rate of conversion of plasminogen to plasmin increases 1,000-fold (Verstraete, 1989). Thus, when rt-PA is given intravenously in doses that are capable of dissolving clots, plasmin formation in the circulation is more modest than with streptokinase. Streptokinase also causes a more pronounced decrease in plasma concentrations of fibrinogen, α_2-antiplasmin, plasminogen, and factor V and a greater increase in fibrinogen-fibrin degradation products (Collen et al, 1986). When large doses are given for prolonged periods, rt-PA induces systemic fibrinogenolysis. A lytic state is induced in almost all patients receiving therapeutic doses of rt-PA, but it is less pronounced than in those treated with equipotent doses of streptokinase or urokinase.

rt-PA is used to reperfuse occluded coronary arteries after myocardial infarction and as therapy for pulmonary embolism, thromboembolism of the peripheral arteries, and clots in autogenous saphenous vein grafts that bypass occluded peripheral arteries (see the Introduction). Although there is evidence that rt-PA is effective in patients with deep vein thrombosis, additional randomized clinical trials are needed to compare this drug with other therapies for this condition and to determine the optimal dosage regimen.

See the Introduction for information on adverse reactions and precautions.

PHARMACOKINETICS. rt-PA has a plasma half-life for unbound drug of approximately four to five minutes. It is cleared by the liver, and individual variations in hepatic blood flow may explain the variability in plasma concentration. Fibrin-bound rt-PA has a much longer half-life than free drug and thus has a more prolonged duration of action. rt-PA also is inactivated by circulating plasminogen activator inhibitor 1 (PAI-1), whose concentration may vary among patients.

DOSAGE AND PREPARATIONS.

Intravenous: *Adults,* for myocardial infarction the maximum total dose is 100 mg; a bolus of 15 mg is followed by 0.75 mg/kg (maximum, 50 mg) infused over the next 30 minutes and 0.5 mg/kg (maximum, 35 mg) infused over the next hour.

For acute pulmonary embolism confirmed by pulmonary angiography or lung scanning, *adults,* 100 mg infused over two hours. Administration of heparin should be started or reinstituted at the end of the rt-PA infusion when the partial thromboplastin time or thrombin time is twice the normal value or less.

Activase (Genentech). Powder (sterile, lyophilized) 20, 50, and 100 mg (11.6, 29, and 58 million IU) with diluent.

ANISTREPLASE (APSAC, Anisoylated Plasminogen-Streptokinase Activator Complex)

[Eminase]

ACTIONS AND USES. Anistreplase is a noncovalent complex of streptokinase with a modified plasminogen molecule. Native plasminogen contains glutamine as the amino-terminal residue (Glu-plasminogen). Partial proteolysis of Glu-plasminogen yields a slightly smaller molecule with lysine at the amino terminus (Lys-plasminogen), which has a greater affinity for fibrin than Glu-plasminogen. Therefore, anistreplase is somewhat more clot-specific than the activator complex containing endogenous Glu-plasminogen that is formed after administration of streptokinase (Fears, 1990; Sherry, 1990). In addition, the catalytic center of the complex has been blocked reversibly at a serine hydroxyl by acylation (ie, chemical linkage to a *p*-anisoyl group). However, the fibrin-binding sites of its plasminogen moiety, which are located in a different part of the molecule, remain intact. Anisoylation also protects the active site of the complex from inactivation by α_2-antiplasmin and other serpins, significantly lengthens the drug's half-life, allows infusion over a brief (two- to five-minute) period, and reduces the reaction with circulating plasminogen. Deacylation takes place gradually after drug administration and converts anistreplase to an active streptokinase/Lys-plasminogen complex that initiates thrombolysis by converting plasminogen to plasmin in the vicinity of thrombi. At the dosages used clinically, however, anistreplase also has significant systemic effects and induces a prolonged hypocoagulable state (Walker et al, 1984).

Results of clinical trials have demonstrated the efficacy and safety of anistreplase in patients with myocardial infarction. Anistreplase was effective in reducing the mortality rate in patients with myocardial infarction in the GISSI-2 trial (1990), International t-PA/Streptokinase Mortality trial (The International Study Group, 1990), and ISIS-3 trial (1992). In initial studies, the drug was given by the intracoronary route; more recent trials have employed intravenous administration. When given within four hours of onset of symptoms, the reperfusion rate with intravenous anistreplase was similar to that achieved with intracoronary streptokinase; when treatment was delayed beyond four hours, intracoronary streptokinase was more effective. Early reocclusion rates following anistreplase therapy were low (Anderson et al, 1988; Anderson, 1989). However, more recent data show that late reocclusion can occur in approximately 30% of patients with patent arteries after anistreplase therapy, despite adequate therapy with oral anticoagulants (Takens et al, 1990). These patients did not receive aspirin therapy, which may be more effective than anticoagulants for preventing reocclusion. It also was noted that late reocclusion had no effect on survival at one year.

See the Introduction for information on adverse reactions and precautions.

PHARMACOKINETICS. Activation of anistreplase occurs by deacylation, a nonenzymatic first-order reaction with an in vitro half-life in human blood of approximately two hours. The half-life of fibrinolytic activity of circulating anistreplase is 70 to 120 minutes (mean, 94 minutes).

DOSAGE AND PREPARATIONS.

Intravenous: *Adults,* 30 units administered over four to five minutes.

Eminase (SmithKline Beecham). Powder (sterile, lyophilized) 30 units in single-dose containers.

STREPTOKINASE

[Kabikinase, Streptase]

ACTIONS AND USES. Streptokinase, a nonenzymatic protein (molecular weight 47,000 daltons), is a catabolic product secreted by Group C beta-hemolytic streptococci. Streptokinase activates plasminogen in a complex manner: It combines noncovalently with plasminogen in a 1:1 stoichiometric complex to produce a conformational alteration in plasminogen resulting in the uncovering of a catalytic site. The plasminogen thus activated then converts additional plasminogen to the active fibrinolytic and proteolytic enzyme, plasmin. Although the catalytic effect of the streptokinase/plasminogen complex is greatest on fibrin-bound plasminogen, circulating plasminogen also is converted to plasmin and a systemic lytic state is induced.

Most individuals have antibodies to streptokinase as a result of previous streptococcal infections; therefore, a loading dose is given initially. When the resistance level to streptokinase exceeds 1,000,000 IU, this agent is probably inactive and should not be used. Because high antibody titers often are produced beginning five days after therapy, patients treated with streptokinase or anistreplase should not receive streptokinase again for at least six months and probably for as long as two or more years. Preformed antibody titers are otherwise rarely high enough to inhibit streptokinase and do not correlate with coronary artery patency after treatment (Fears et al, 1991).

Streptokinase is used to reperfuse occluded coronary arteries after myocardial infarction. It also is employed as therapy for deep vein thrombosis and pulmonary embolism, peripheral arterial thromboembolism, to lyse clots in autogenous saphenous vein bypass grafts (aortocoronary and peripheral), to open occluded intravenous catheters and arteriovenous cannulae, and to treat the superior vena cava syndrome caused by placement of a central venous catheter. Streptokinase also may be effective to clear occluded prosthetic heart valves. It has been used in patients with unstable angina, thrombosis of renal or retinal arteries or veins, or thrombosis of deep veins of the upper extremities.

See the Introduction for information on adverse reactions and precautions.

PHARMACOKINETICS. The half-life of streptokinase is biphasic: an initial phase of approximately 11 to 13 minutes (due to distribution and to the action of antibodies) and a terminal phase of 23 to 29 minutes (due to disappearance of its catalytic activity). Activity ceases shortly after therapy is discontinued. However, with full-dose therapy, the lytic state persists for several hours.

DOSAGE AND PREPARATIONS.

Intravenous: *Adults,* for myocardial infarction 1.5 million IU infused over a period of up to one hour.

For acute deep vein thrombosis, pulmonary embolism, or acute arterial thrombosis or embolism, a loading dose of 250,000 IU of reconstituted solution is infused over 30 minutes, followed by 100,000 IU/hr (usually for 24 hours in patients with pulmonary embolism, 24 to 72 hours in patients with arterial thrombosis or embolism, and up to 72 hours in patients with deep vein thrombosis). To maintain a systemic lytic state, the dose often must be increased to 200,000 and then to 400,000 IU/hr.

Cannulae Clearance: For local instillation into occluded arteriovenous cannulae after pulling and flushing with heparinized saline have been ineffective, 250,000 IU in 2 ml of intravenous solution may be instilled into each occluded limb of the cannula over a 30-minute period, followed by clamping of the cannula for two hours. Cannula contents then are aspirated and the cannula is flushed with normal saline and reconnected.

Kabikinase (Kabi Pharmacia). Powder (lyophilized) 250,000 and 750,000 IU in 8 ml containers and 1,500,000 IU in 10 ml containers.

Streptase (Astra). Powder (lyophilized) 250,000 and 750,000 IU in 6.5 ml containers and 1,500,000 IU in 6.5 and 50 ml containers.

UROKINASE

[Abbokinase]

ACTIONS AND USES. Urokinase is a serine protease enzyme found in human urine and isolated from tissue cultures of human kidney cells. Two molecular forms exist: S_1, which has a molecular weight of 34,500 ± 2,000 daltons (low-molecular-weight two-chain urokinase), and S_2, which has a molecular weight of 54,000 daltons (high-molecular-weight two-chain urokinase). The S_1 form probably represents a breakdown product of urokinase formed during purification procedures; its amino acid sequence is very similar to the β-chain of thrombin and plasmin. (Abbokinase is primarily the low-molecular-weight form.) Urokinase directly activates plasminogen by proteolytic cleavage to generate plasmin. It is generally thought to be nonantigenic and does not cause the allergic reactions encountered with streptokinase. However, immunologic reactions characterized by rigor have been reported in some patients receiving urokinase for pulmonary embolism (Goldhaber et al, 1988, 1994).

Urokinase is used as therapy for myocardial infarction, pulmonary embolism, and thromboembolic occlusion of peripheral arteries; to clear occluded intravenous catheters; and to treat the superior vena cava syndrome caused by placement of a central venous catheter. It may be effective for occlusions in prosthetic heart valves. Urokinase may be used in patients with cerebral embolism, or with occlusions of renal or retinal blood vessels.

See the Introduction for information on adverse reactions and precautions.

PHARMACOKINETICS. The pharmacokinetic properties of urokinase in humans have not been studied extensively. When administered by intravenous infusion, urokinase is cleared rapidly by the liver. The serum half-life in humans is 20 minutes or less. The half-life would be expected to be prolonged in patients with impaired liver function. As with rt-PA, levels of circulating inhibitors to urokinase may vary among individuals. The presence of circulating complexes between urokinase and a specific inhibitor (identical to the inhibitor of activated protein C) has been demonstrated in plasma obtained from patients undergoing intravenous infusion of urokinase as therapy for myocardial infarction (Geiger et al, 1989). Small fractions of an administered dose are excreted in bile and urine.

DOSAGE AND PREPARATIONS.

Intravenous: *Adults,* for myocardial infarction, a total of 3 million IU is administered, with one-half the dose given as a bolus injection over two to five minutes and the remainder infused over one hour.

For pulmonary embolism, 4,400 IU/kg is infused over ten minutes at a rate of 90 ml/hr, followed by continuous infusion of 4,400 IU/kg/hr at a rate of 15 ml/hr for 12 hours.

Abbokinase (Abbott). Powder (lyophilized) 250,000 IU with mannitol 25 mg, human albumin 250 mg, and sodium chloride 50 mg in 5 ml containers.

Cannulae Clearance: 5,000 IU/ml (in longer lines, 9,000 IU/ml) is gently instilled by tuberculin syringe in amounts equal to the internal volume of the catheter. Aspiration of the clot and urokinase solution is attempted after five to ten minutes. The procedure may be repeated until catheter patency is restored. If the catheter is not open within 30 minutes, it may be clamped to allow the solution to remain within for 30 to 60 minutes before aspiration is again attempted. A second injection may be necessary.

Abbokinase Open-Cath (Abbott). Powder (lyophilized) 5,000 IU in 1 ml containers and 9,000 IU with gelatin, mannitol, sodium chloride, and monobasic sodium phosphate anhydrous in 1.8 ml containers with diluent.

Cited References

ACC/AHA Task Force: ACC/AHA Guidelines for the early management of patients with acute myocardial infarction: A report of the American College of Cardiology/American Heart Association Task Force on Assessment of Diagnostic and Therapeutic Cardiovascular Procedures (Subcommittee to Develop Guidelines for the Early Management of Patients With Acute Myocardial Infarction). *Circulation* 82:664-707, 1990.

AIMS Trial Study Group: Effect of intravenous APSAC on mortality after acute myocardial infarction: Preliminary report of placebo-controlled clinical trial. *Lancet* 1:545-549, 1988.

AIMS Trial Study Group: Long-term effects of intravenous anistreplase in acute myocardial infarction: Final report of the AIMS study. *Lancet* 335:427-431, 1990.

Ambrose JA: Plaque disruption and the acute coronary syndromes of unstable angina and myocardial infarction: If the substrate is similar, why is the clinical presentation different? *J Am Coll Cardiol* 19:1653-1658, 1992.

Ambrose JA, et al: Adjunctive thrombolytic therapy for angioplasty in ischemic rest angina: Results of a double-blind randomized pilot study. *J Am Coll Cardiol* 20:1197-1204, 1992.

Anderson JL: Reperfusion, patency, and reocclusion with anistreplase (APSAC) in acute myocardial infarction. *Am J Cardiol* 64:12A-17A, 1989.

Anderson JL, et al: Multicenter reperfusion trial of intravenous anisoylated plasminogen streptokinase activator complex (APSAC) in acute myocardial infarction: Controlled comparison with intracoronary streptokinase. *J Am Coll Cardiol* 11:1153-1163, 1988.

Anderson JL, et al: TIMI perfusion grade 3 but not grade 2 results in improved outcome after thrombolysis for myocardial infarction: Ventriculographic, enzymatic, and electrocardiographic evidence from the TEAM-3 study. *Circulation* 87:1829-1839, 1993.

Atkinson JB, et al: Investigational use of tissue plasminogen activator (t-PA) for occluded central venous catheters. *J Parenter Enteral Nutr* 14:310-311, 1990.

Bagnall HA, et al: Continuous infusion of low-dose urokinase in the treatment of central venous catheter thrombosis in infants and children. *Pediatrics* 83:963-966, 1989.

Bär FW, et al: Thrombolysis in patients with unstable angina improves the angiographic but not the clinical outcome: Results of UNASEM, a multicenter, randomized placebo-controlled, clinical trial with anistreplase. *Circulation* 86:131-137, 1992.

Becker RC, et al: Recombinant tissue-type plasminogen activator: Current concepts and guidelines for clinical use in acute myocardial infarction, part I. *Am Heart J* 121:220-244, 1991.

Bode C, et al: Future directions in plasminogen activator therapy. *Clin Cardiol* 13:375-381, 1990.

Brus F, et al: Streptokinase treatment for femoral artery thrombosis after arterial cardiac catheterisation in infants and children. *Br Heart J* 63:291-294, 1990.

Califf RM, et al: Clinical risks of thrombolytic therapy. *Am J Cardiol* 69:12A-20A, 1992.

Carson JL, et al: The clinical course of pulmonary embolism. *N Engl J Med* 326:1240-1245, 1992.

Chen HJ, et al: Documentation of successful treatment of prosthetic mitral valve thrombus with intravenous urokinase infusion for twenty-four hours. *Clin Cardiol* 15:127-133, 1992.

Chesebro JH, et al: Thrombolysis in myocardial infarction (TIMI) trial, phase I: Comparison between intravenous tissue plasminogen activator and intravenous streptokinase. *Circulation* 76:142-154, 1987.

Collen D, Gold HK: Fibrin-specific thrombolytic agents and new approaches to coronary artery thrombosis, in Julian DG, et al (eds): *Thrombolysis in Cardiovascular Disease*. New York, Marcel Dekker, 45-68, 1989.

Collen DC, Gold HK: New developments in thrombolytic therapy. *Thromb Res* (suppl X):105-131, 1990.

Collen D, et al: Analysis of coagulation and fibrinolysis during intravenous infusion of recombinant human tissue-type plasminogen activator in patients with acute myocardial infarction. *Circulation* 73:511-517, 1986.

Collen D, et al: Tissue-type plasminogen activator: A review of its pharmacology and therapeutic use as a thrombolytic agent. *Drugs* 38:346-388, 1989.

del Zoppo GJ, et al: Recombinant tissue plasminogen activator in acute thrombotic and embolic stroke. *Ann Neurol* 32:78-86, 1992.

EMERAS (Estudio Multicéntrico Estreptoquinasa Repúblicas de América del Sur) Collaborative Group: Randomised trial of late thrombolysis in patients with suspected acute myocardial infarction. *Lancet* 342:767-772, 1993.

The European Myocardial Infarction Project Group: Prehospital thrombolytic therapy in patients with suspected acute myocardial infarction. *N Engl J Med* 329:383-389, 1993.

Fears R: Biochemical pharmacology and therapeutic aspects of thrombolytic agents. *Pharmacol Rev* 42:201-221, 1990.

Fears R, et al: Pre-treatment anti-streptokinase antibody levels do not influence coronary patency achieved by anistreplase and streptokinase, abstract. *J Am Coll Cardiol* 17:153A, 1991.

Fibrinolytic Therapy Trialists' (FTT) Collaborative Group: Indications for fibrinolytic therapy in suspected acute myocardial infarction: Collaborative overview of early mortality and major morbidity results from all randomised trials of more than 1,000 patients. *Lancet* 343:311-322, 1994.

Francis CW, Marder VJ: Fibrinolytic therapy for venous thrombosis. *Prog Cardiovasc Dis* 34:193-204, (Nov/Dec) 1991.

Francis CW, et al: Angioedema during therapy with recombinant tissue plasminogen activator. *Br J Haematol* 77:562-563, 1991.

Freeman MR, et al: Thrombolysis in unstable angina: Randomized double-blind trial of t-PA and placebo. *Circulation* 85:150-157, 1992.

Geiger M, et al: Complex formation between urokinase and plasma protein C inhibitor in vitro and in vivo. *Blood* 74:722-728, 1989.

Goa KL, et al: Intravenous streptokinase: A reappraisal of its therapeutic use in acute myocardial infarction. *Drugs* 39:693-719, 1990.

Goldberg RJ, et al: The impact of age on the incidence and prognosis of initial acute myocardial infarction—The Worcester Heart Attack Study. *Am Heart J* 117:543-549, 1989.

Goldhaber SZ: Thrombolysis in venous thromboembolism: An international perspective. *Chest* 97(suppl):176S-181S, 1990.

Goldhaber SZ: Recognition and management of pulmonary embolism. *Heart Dis Stroke* 2:142-146, (March/April) 1993.

Goldhaber SZ, et al: Pooled analyses of randomized trials of streptokinase and heparin in phlebographically documented acute deep venous thrombosis. *Am J Med* 76:393-397, 1984.

Goldhaber SZ, et al: Randomised controlled trial of recombinant tissue plasminogen activator versus urokinase in treatment of acute pulmonary embolism. *Lancet* 2:293-298, 1988.

Goldhaber SZ, et al: Recombinant tissue-type plasminogen activator versus a novel dosing regimen of urokinase in acute pulmonary embolism: A randomized controlled multicenter trial. *J Am Coll Cardiol* 20:24-30, 1992.

Goldhaber SZ, et al: Alteplase versus heparin in acute pulmonary embolism: Randomized trial assessing right-ventricular function and pulmonary perfusion. *Lancet* 341:507-511, 1993.

Goldhaber SZ, et al: Efficacy and safety of repeated boluses of urokinase in the treatment of deep venous thrombosis. *Am J Cardiol* 73:75-79, 1994.

Gore JM, et al: Intracerebral hemorrhage, cerebral infarction, and subdural hematoma after acute myocardial infarction and thrombolytic therapy in the Thrombolysis in Myocardial Infarction Study: Thrombolysis in Myocardial Infarction, phase II, pilot and clinical trial. *Circulation* 83:448-459, 1991.

Gould JR, et al: Groshong catheter-associated subclavian venous thrombosis. *Am J Med* 95:419-423, (Oct) 1993.

Granger CB, et al: Thrombolytic therapy for acute myocardial infarction: A review. *Drugs* 44:293-325, 1992.

Graor RA, Olin JW: Regional thrombolysis in peripheral arterial occlusions, in Julian DG, et al (eds): *Thrombolysis in Cardiovascular Disease*. New York, Marcel Dekker, 381-396, 1989.

The GUSTO Angiographic Investigators: The effects of tissue plasminogen activator, streptokinase, or both on coronary artery patency, ventricular function, and survival after acute myocardial infarction. *N Engl J Med* 329:1615-1622, 1993.

The GUSTO Investigators: An international randomized trial comparing four thrombolytic strategies for acute myocardial infarction. *N Engl J Med* 329:673-682, 1993.

Haire WD, et al: Obstructed central venous catheters: Restoring function with a 12-hour infusion of low-dose urokinase. *Cancer* 66:2279-2285, 1990.

Higgins DL, Bennett WF: Tissue plasminogen activator: The biochemistry and pharmacology of variants produced by mutagenesis. *Annu Rev Pharmacol Toxicol* 30:91-121, 1990.

Hirsh J, Hull RD: Treatment of venous thromboembolism. *Chest* 89 (suppl):426S-433S, 1986.

Hull RD, et al: Subcutaneous low-molecular-weight heparin compared with continuous heparin in the treatment of proximal-vein thrombosis. *N Engl J Med* 326:975-982, 1992.

Ino T, et al: Thrombolytic therapy for femoral artery thrombosis after pediatric cardiac catheterization. *Am Heart J* 115:633-639, 1988.

The International Study Group: In-hospital mortality and clinical course of 20,891 patients with suspected acute myocardial infarction randomised between alteplase and streptokinase with or without heparin. *Lancet* 336:71-75, 1990.

ISIS-3 (Third International Study of Infarct Survival) Collaborative Group: ISIS-3: A randomised comparison of streptokinase *vs* tissue plasminogen activator *vs* anistreplase and of aspirin plus heparin *vs* aspirin alone among 41,299 cases of suspected acute myocardial infarction. *Lancet* 339:753-770, 1992.

Kandarpa K, et al: Intraarterial thrombolysis of lower extremity occlusions: Prospective, randomized comparison of forced periodic infusion and conventional slow continuous infusion. *Radiology* 188:861-867, 1993.

Karlsson J-E, et al: Thrombolysis with recombinant human tissue-type plasminogen activator during instability in coronary artery disease: Effect on myocardial ischemia and need for coronary revascularization. *Am Heart J* 124:1419-1426, 1992.

Katz A, et al: Thrombolytic therapy for acute myocardial infarction in a 110-year-old man. *Am J Cardiol* 71:1122-1123, 1993.

Kennedy JW, et al: The Western Washington randomized trial of intracoronary streptokinase in acute myocardial infarction. *N Engl J Med* 312:1073-1078, 1985.

Kruit WHJ, et al: The significance of venography in the management of patients with clinically suspected pulmonary embolism. *J Intern Med* 230:333-339, 1991.

Kumpe DA, Cohen MAH: Angioplasty/thrombolytic treatment of failing and failed hemodialysis access sites: Comparison with surgical treatment. *Prog Cardiovasc Dis* 34:263-278, 1992.

Lange RA, et al: Influence of residual antegrade coronary blood flow on survival after myocardial infarction in patients with multivessel coronary artery disease. *Coronary Artery Dis* 1:59-72, 1990.

LATE Study Group: Late Assessment of Thrombolytic Efficacy (LATE) study with alteplase 6-24 hours after onset of acute myocardial infarction. *Lancet* 342:759-766, 1993.

Leinbach RC: Thrombolysis in unstable angina, editorial. *Circulation* 85:376-377, 1992.

Levine SR, Brott TG: Thrombolytic therapy in cerebrovascular disorders. *Prog Cardiovasc Dis* 34:235-262, (Jan/Feb) 1992.

Levy DE, et al: Factors related to intracranial hematoma formation in patient receiving tissue-type plasminogen activator for acute ischemic stroke. *Stroke* 25:291-297, 1994.

Lew AS, et al: Hypotensive effect of intravenous streptokinase in patients with acute myocardial infarction. *Circulation* 72:1321-1326, 1985.

Lijnen HR: New approaches in the development of thrombolytic agents. *Drugs Today* 25:541-554, 1989.

Loscalzo J: An overview of thrombolytic agents. *Chest* 97 (suppl): 117S-123S, 1990.

Marder VJ, Francis CW: Clinical aspects of fibrinolysis, in Williams WJ, et al (eds): *Hematology,* ed 4. New York, McGraw-Hill, 1543-1558, 1990.

Marder VJ, Sherry S: Thrombolytic therapy: Current status, parts 1 and 2. *N Engl J Med* 318:1512-1520; 1585-1595, 1988.

McKay CR: Prosthetic heart valve thrombosis: 'What can be done with regard to treatment?' Editorial. *Circulation* 87:295-296, 1993.

Meyer G, et al: Effects of intravenous urokinase versus alteplase on total pulmonary resistance in acute massive pulmonary embolism: A European multicenter double-blind trial. *J Am Coll Cardiol* 19:239-245, 1992.

Meyerovitz MF, et al: Short-term response to thrombolytic therapy in deep venous thrombosis: Predictive value of venographic appearance. *Radiology* 184:345-348, 1992.

Monreal M, et al: Upper-extremity deep venous thrombosis and pulmonary embolism: A prospective study. *Chest* 99:280-283, 1991.

Moran KT, et al: The role of thrombolytic therapy in surgical practice. *Br J Surg* 76:298-304, 1989.

Moser KM, et al: Frequent asymptomatic pulmonary embolism in patients with deep venous thrombosis. *JAMA* 271:223-225, 1994.

Mueller HS, et al: Thrombolysis in myocardial infarction (TIMI): Comparative studies of coronary reperfusion and systemic fibrinogenolysis with two forms of recombinant tissue-type plasminogen activator. *J Am Coll Cardiol* 10:479-490, 1987.

Nadelman J, et al: Prevalence, incidence and prognosis of recognized and unrecognized myocardial infarction in persons aged 75 years or older: The Bronx Aging Study. *Am J Cardiol* 66:533-537, 1990.

O'Connor CM, et al: A randomized trial of intravenous heparin in conjunction with anistreplase (anisoylated plasminogen streptokinase activator complex) in acute myocardial infarction: The Duke University Clinical Cardiology Study (DUCCS) 1. *J Am Coll Cardiol* 23:11-18, 1994.

Pell ACH, et al: Effect of "fast track" admission for acute myocardial infarction on delay to thrombolysis. *BMJ* 304:83-87, 1992.

Prins MH, Hirsh J: Heparin as an adjunctive treatment after thrombolytic therapy for acute myocardial infarction. *Am J Cardiol* 67:3A-11A, 1991.

Pulsinelli W: Pathophysiology of acute ischaemic stroke. *Lancet* 339:533-536, 1992.

Ricotta JJ, et al: Use and limitations of thrombolytic therapy in the treatment of peripheral arterial ischemia: Results of a multi-institutional questionnaire. *J Vasc Surg* 6:45-50, (June) 1987.

Rogers LQ, Lutcher CL: Streptokinase therapy for deep vein thrombosis: A comprehensive review of the English literature. *Am J Med* 88:389-395, 1990.

Roudaut R, et al: Mechanical cardiac valve thrombosis: Is fibrinolysis justified? *Circulation* 86 (suppl II):II-8-II-15, 1992.

Roux S, et al: Effects of aspirin on coronary reocclusion and recurrent ischemia after thrombolysis. *J Am Coll Cardiol* 19:671-677, 1992.

Sane DC, et al: Bleeding during thrombolytic therapy for acute myocardial infarction: Mechanisms and management. *Ann Intern Med* 111:1010-1022, 1989.

Sherry S: Pharmacology of anistreplase. *Clin Cardiol* 13 (suppl V):V-3-V-10, 1990.

Sherry S: Thrombolytic therapy for noncoronary disease. *Ann Emerg Med* 20:396-404, 1991.

Silber H, et al: The St. Jude valve: Thrombolysis as the first line of therapy for cardiac valve thrombosis. *Circulation* 87:30-37, 1993.

Takens BH, et al: Reocclusion three months after successful thrombolytic treatment of acute myocardial infarction with anisoylated plasminogen streptokinase activating complex. *Am J Cardiol* 65:1422-1424, 1990.

The TIMI IIIA Investigators: Early effects of tissue-type plasminogen activator added to conventional therapy on the culprit coronary lesion in patients presenting with ischemic cardiac pain at rest: Results of the Thrombolysis in Myocardial Ischemia (TIMI IIIA) Trial. *Circulation* 87:38-52, 1993.

The TIMI IIIB Investigators: Effects of tissue plasminogen activator and a comparison of early invasive and conservative strategies in unstable angina and non-Q-wave myocardial infarction: Results of the TIMI IIIB trial. *Circulation* 89:1545-1556, 1994.

Valji K, et al: Pharmacomechanical thrombolysis and angioplasty in the management of clotted hemodialysis grafts: Early and late clinical results. *Radiology* 178:243-247, 1991.

Vatterott PJ, et al: Late potentials on signal-averaged electrocardiograms and patency of the infarct-related artery in survivors of acute myocardial infarction. *J Am Coll Cardiol* 17:330-337, 1991.

Vaughan DE, et al: Streptokinase-induced, antibody-mediated platelet aggregation: Potential cause of clot propagation in vivo. *J Am Coll Cardiol* 11:1343-1348, 1988.

Verstraete M: Use of thrombolytic drugs in non-coronary disorders. *Drugs* 38:801-821, 1989.

Walker ID, et al: Acylated streptokinase-plasminogen complex in patients with acute myocardial infarction. *Thromb Haemost* 51:204-206, 1984.

Wardlaw JM, Warlow CP: Thrombolysis in acute ischemic stroke: Does it work? *Stroke* 23:1826-1839, 1992.

Waters D, Lam JYT: Is thrombolytic therapy striking out in unstable angina? Editorial. *Circulation* 86:1642-1644, 1992.

Weaver WD, et al: Effect of age on use of thrombolytic therapy and mortality in acute myocardial infarction. *J Am Coll Cardiol* 18:657-662, 1991.

Weaver WD, et al: Prehospital-initiated vs hospital-initiated thrombolytic therapy: The Myocardial Infarction Triage and Intervention Trial. *JAMA* 270:1211-1216, 1993.

Wessel DL, et al: Fibrinolytic therapy for femoral arterial thrombosis after cardiac catheterization in infants and children. *Am J Cardiol* 58:347-351, 1986.

White HD, et al: Safety and efficacy of repeat thrombolytic treatment after acute myocardial infarction. *Br Heart J* 64:177-181, 1990.

Williamson BD, et al: Should older patients with acute myocardial infarction receive thrombolytic therapy? *Drugs Aging* 2:461-468, 1992.

Zimmermann M, et al: Reduction in the frequency of ventricular late potentials after acute myocardial infarction by early thrombolytic therapy. *Am J Cardiol* 67:697-703, 1991.

Hemostatics

36

Excessive bleeding may be caused by defects in the interaction of blood vessels with platelets and circulating clotting factors, abnormal synthesis or activation of clotting factors, or platelet deficiencies. Bleeding disorders may be hereditary or acquired and may be caused by a single or by multiple defects. An understanding of the mechanisms of blood clotting and fibrinolysis is essential to determine the etiology of bleeding and to select appropriate treatment. (See index entry Blood Coagulation, Mechanisms.)

If bleeding results from a specific hereditary clotting factor deficiency, diagnosis may be relatively simple and only replacement therapy may be required. Acquired deficiencies of multiple coagulation factors can be difficult to diagnose and may respond poorly to treatment. Such disorders may result from deficient factor formation or from disseminated intravascular coagulation (DIC).

In addition, both multiple and isolated coagulation deficiencies can be acquired due to development of inhibitors, which are antibodies or paraproteins that interact with clotting factors and alter their function. This is seen most frequently in association with collagen vascular diseases but also has been reported with drug therapy (eg, quinidine, phenothiazines), hematologic malignancies (eg, lymphomas, multiple myeloma), postpartum, and in the elderly. These conditions are much more difficult to diagnose and treat.

Initially, a detailed clinical history must be obtained to identify possible causes of significant mucocutaneous or deep bleeding, particularly following surgery or trauma. A drug history also should be taken, since thrombocytopenia or platelet dysfunction often follows the use of certain drugs. Screening tests that usually are adequate for presumptive diagnosis of a coagulopathy are platelet count, bleeding time, one-stage prothrombin time, activated partial thromboplastin time, and plasma fibrinogen concentration. Any abnormality in these tests indicates the need for referral to a specialist for more detailed diagnostic procedures. A history of significant bleeding also may be sufficient for referral to a coagulation disorder center, even if screening tests are normal.

The ability to diagnose coagulation disorders depends on the quality of the specimen sent to the laboratory. For example, the measures employed in blood collection from intravenous lines to minimize specimen contamination with heparin (used prophylactically to maintain patency) must be adequate to avoid producing spuriously abnormal coagulation times.

HEREDITARY COAGULATION DISORDERS

DESCRIPTION. The most common hereditary bleeding disorders are caused by reduced concentrations or defective activity of factor VIII (antihemophilic factor), von Willebrand factor (vWF), or factor IX (Christmas factor). Hemorrhage requiring specific factor replacement therapy occurs most frequently in inherited factor VIII or IX deficiency.

Hemophilia A (Classic Hemophilia, Factor VIII Deficiency): Factor VIII circulates in a bimolecular complex with vWF; it is dissociable into the procoagulant protein, factor VIII:C, and vWF, which serves as a bridge between platelets and the injured vessel wall and stabilizes factor VIII in the circulation. Factor VIII:C is measured in standard coagulation assays or by its antigenic determinants (VIII:Ag) in immunoassays utilizing human or monoclonal antibodies. It accelerates coagulation through its role as a cofactor in the enzymatic activation of factor X by factor IXa.

Patients with classic hemophilia have factor VIII:C deficiency that is transmitted as an X-linked recessive disorder and thus is manifested almost exclusively in males (Roberts and Jones, 1990). Rarely, females born to a hemophilic father and carrier mother, with Turner's syndrome, or with a high degree of lyonization of the normal X-chromosome resulting in severe carrier status may have symptoms of hemophilia.

The severity of bleeding varies markedly: Frequent, severe, and spontaneous hemorrhages occur in patients with factor VIII activity <1% of normal. A factor activity of 2% to 5% usually is associated with hemarthroses only after trauma, and a concentration >5% usually precludes bleeding except after trauma or surgery. Factor VIII activity >30% of normal is usually adequate to maintain hemostasis during and shortly after surgery. Nevertheless, the target levels for replacement therapy that are recommended by most physicians are >50% of normal prior to minor surgery and 80% to 100% of normal prior to major surgery.

Hemophilia B (Factor IX Deficiency, Christmas Disease): This form of hemophilia also is X-linked but is less common than hemophilia A (Roberts and Jones, 1990). It results from an absence or dysfunction of factor IX, which, in its activated form and together with factor VIIIa, calcium ion, and platelet phospholipids, catalyzes the activation of factor X. The inheritance pattern of hemophilia B is identical to that of hemophilia A, as is the relationship between the frequency and severity of hemorrhage and the percentage of normal factor activity.

von Willebrand Disease: vWF is a multimeric protein that facilitates adhesion of platelets to the injured blood vessel wall, mediates platelet-platelet interactions during aggregation, and serves as a carrier that protects factor VIII:C from rapid degradation in the plasma. The large multimers promote platelet adhesion, and the smaller multimers carry factor VIII:C. vWF is measured by immunologic techniques (vWF:Ag) or by its ability to support ristocetin-induced aggregation of formalin-fixed or washed normal platelets. In addition to plasma vWF, platelet and subendothelial vWF are essential components for primary hemostasis (Bona, 1989; Stel et al, 1985; Turitto et al, 1985).

von Willebrand disease is an autosomal codominant disorder characterized by an alteration in the structure, functions, or concentration of vWF (Montgomery and Hilgartner, 1991). In the most common form, type I or classic von Willebrand disease, the concentration of circulating vWF is reduced. In patients with subtype IA, the size and distribution of vWF multimers (as determined by electrophoretic separation on agarose gels) are the same as in normal individuals; in those with subtype IB, the percentage of the larger multimers is decreased; in those with subtype IC, the satellite bands around each multimer are structurally abnormal. The principal defect in most patients with mild type IA von Willebrand disease is in the secretion of vWF multimers from endothelial cells. In heterozygotes, bleeding from mucous membranes is the principal clinical manifestation, but many affected individuals are asymptomatic. However, severe bleeding may occur with surgery or trauma. Hemorrhagic diathesis is pronounced in the homozygous form (rare) in which no circulating vWF can be detected.

Type II or variant von Willebrand disease is caused by defective vWF. Patients do not assemble large and intermediate multimers (type IIA) or have decreased vWF activity due to the presence of defective larger multimers that bind excessively to platelets (type IIB).

Type III (severe) von Willebrand disease is a recessive disorder characterized by very low levels of both vWF and factor VIII:C. Patients with this form of the disease may have spontaneous major bleeding episodes manifested by both intra-articular and mucosal hemorrhages that begin early in life (Miller, 1990; Bloom, 1991 A).

A condition that may be confused with von Willebrand disease is caused by an intrinsic platelet abnormality (platelet-type von Willebrand disease, pseudo-von Willebrand disease). This is characterized by a heightened affinity of platelets for vWF. Both type IIB and platelet-type von Willebrand disease may be associated with thrombocytopenia. Acquired forms of von Willebrand disease have been described in patients with autoimmune or malignant disorders. The acquired syndrome may be associated with proteolysis or development of a circulating inhibitor.

Other Disorders: Hereditary deficiency of factor XI (plasma thromboplastin antecedent [PTA]) is a less common, usually mild, autosomally inherited disorder that may require transfusion therapy during hemorrhagic episodes and prophylactically prior to and following surgery. The likelihood of excessive bleeding in individuals deficient in factor XI does not appear to correlate with the level of factor XI measured in their plasma.

Other hereditary hemorrhagic disorders associated with clotting factor deficiencies are exceedingly rare, and a specialized text should be consulted for details of treatment.

TREATMENT. Hemophilic patients should exercise regularly to maintain joint flexibility and muscle strength, perform frequent routine dental hygiene measures to minimize the need for extensive restorations and extractions, avoid intramuscular injections, and avoid taking aspirin or other drugs that inhibit platelet function. Patients with hemophilia or other severe bleeding disorders should be referred to a specialized center for hemophilia care when surgery, dental extractions, and treatment of major bleeding episodes are required. They also should be evaluated at least annually at a comprehensive hemophilia center. For routine care, treatment may be administered by the patient or parent, the patient's primary care physician, or performed at the center. Most patients participate in home treatment self-infusion programs, which reduce cost, allow a more normal life, and provide prompt therapy to prevent serious complications when bleeding occurs. Despite home treatment programs, however, new arthropathy may occur or progress, particularly in children 3 to 8 years who do not report hemorrhagic episodes promptly. For this reason, some physicians now recommend routine prophylaxis with factors VIII or IX in hemophiliac children beginning at approximately 2 years of age.

Commercial factor VIII or factor IX concentrates are preferred for home use because they are stable, easy to handle and store, contain a standardized amount of clotting factor, and currently are less likely to transmit viral diseases than cryoprecipitate. These concentrates are prepared from pooled plasma derived from a large number of donors; each unit of plasma has been tested and found to be nonreactive for hepatitis B surface antigen and negative for antibody to HIV. The concentrates also are treated by viral inactivation procedures to reduce the risk of transmission of HIV infection or hepatitis. The inactivation methods currently employed are pasteurization; heating in solvent suspension; use of solvent and detergent with or without heat or vapor treatment; dry heating at 80° C for 72 hours; and immunoaffinity purification. Viral inactivation procedures that use heat during suspension in organic solvents reduce the risk of transmitting HIV but may not attenuate or eliminate hepatitis viruses (The National Hemophilia Foundation Medical and Scientific Advisory Council [MASAC], 1991). Most purified factor VIII concentrates lack the largest vWF multimers, and immunopurified preparations have the lowest level of vWF activity (Fricke and Yu, 1989).

Replacement therapy with clotting factor concentrates is required in most hemophiliacs with active bleeding, whether spontaneous or traumatic, and just prior to surgery. The factor activity in the patient's plasma should be monitored carefully after infusion. The amount of factor needed is determined by the severity and location of bleeding and the baseline activity of the deficient factor. The presence of an inhibitor should be excluded before any intervention is undertaken, even if no inhibitor has been demonstrated previously.

Schedules for administration of clotting factor concentrates are based on the severity of the bleeding diathesis. Hemophilic patients with factor VIII activities 2% to 5% of normal usually do not experience spontaneous bleeding. Bleeding in a confined area (eg, joint) may be controlled with an activity as low as 15% to 20% of normal, but the specific concentration needed to stop bleeding in a given joint has not been determined. A dose calculated to raise the level of factor VIII activity to 25% to 30% of normal generally is recommended. Hemostasis during and after major surgery requires activity >30% of normal, although many physicians prefer levels >50% of normal. See the Table for general guidelines for treatment of bleeding related to factor VIII deficiency. One unit/kg of factor VIII increases the plasma activity of factor VIII by 2% (50 units/kg increase it to 100% of normal activity).

Use of cryoprecipitate is less desirable than an appropriate clotting factor concentrate that has been subjected to adequate viral inactivation techniques (The National Hemophilia Foundation Medical and Scientific Advisory Council [MASAC], 1991). Because several months may elapse between infection with HIV or hepatitis C virus and seroconversion, cryoprecipitate prepared from pooled plasma that was found negative for antibody to these viruses may still be infectious if it included donations from infected individuals who had not yet seroconverted. If special circumstances dictate that cryoprecipitate is the preferred therapy (eg, patient with von Willebrand disease who cannot be treated with desmopressin, see below), it should be prepared from the plasma of one or a few well-screened and frequently tested donor(s) to minimize the risk of disease transmission.

Desmopressin [DDAVP], a synthetic vasopressin analogue, temporarily increases plasma levels of factor VIII:C and vWF. Because of the risks associated with blood products, use of desmopressin in treating mild bleeding disorders has greatly expanded, and it should be employed whenever possible (The National Hemophilia Foundation Medical and Scientific Advisory Council [MASAC], 1991). This agent is injected intravenously prior to dental extractions or minor surgical procedures in patients with mild to moderate hemophilia A or type I von Willebrand disease. The baseline factor VIII activity should be at least 5% of normal for desmopressin to be effective. It may not be adequate for use alone for major surgical procedures or when infusions must be closely spaced because tachyphylaxis is common in these patients. Desmopressin should not be used in type IIB and platelet-type (pseudo) von Willebrand disease, for it may cause thrombocytopenia by promoting binding of vWF multimers to platelets (Mannucci, 1990; Montgomery and Hilgartner, 1991; Aledort, 1991).

Patients with von Willebrand disease who do not respond to desmopressin may be treated with one of the viral-inactivated factor VIII concentrates that is rich in vWF (eg, Humate-P) or with cryoprecipitate prepared as described above. Smaller amounts of cryoprecipitate are needed in patients with von Willebrand disease than in those with hemophilia, because infusion increases endogenous factor VIII activity. Fresh frozen plasma (FFP) may be used if none of the preferred components are available, but hypervolemia and transmission of infectious diseases are additional risks to be considered.

The antifibrinolytic agents, aminocaproic acid [Amicar] and tranexamic acid [Cyklokapron], have specialized applications in hemophilia and von Willebrand disease. They prevent clot lysis by oral secretions and are useful adjuncts to prevent or control bleeding during dental and oral surgery, thus reducing the need for replacement therapy.

For patients with factor IX deficiency, virus-inactivated factor IX complex concentrate [Konȳne-80, Profilnine, Proplex T] is currently recommended (The National Hemophilia Foundation Medical and Scientific Advisory Council [MASAC], 1991). HIV seroconversion has not occurred with use of the current products, but hepatitis may still be a problem with some of them (Pierce et al, 1989). A coagulation factor IX concentrate purified by affinity chromatography [AlphaNine] became available in 1991, and

GENERAL GUIDELINES FOR TREATMENT OF BLEEDING EPISODES IN FACTOR VIII DEFICIENCY*

Condition	Replacement Activity: Prophylaxis	Replacement Activity: Treatment	Comments
MAJOR HEMORRHAGE			
Intracranial trauma			
Without neurologic symptoms		100% (single infusion)	Perform CT scan after factor VIII is administered.
With symptoms	100%	50% for at least five days (infusion repeated at 12-hour intervals), then for prophylaxis every other day for 6 to 12 months.	Perform CT scan after factor VIII is administered.
With persistent neurologic symptoms	100%	>30% for two weeks after bleeding stops, then for prophylaxis every other day for 6 to 12 months.	Perform CT scan, brain scan, and EEG.
Epidural bleeding		100% (prior to lumbar puncture)	
Retroperitoneal bleeding		100% initially, then >50% for five to eight days (or longer if necessary)	Perform ultrasound and CT scan. Administer red cell transfusions as necessary.
Muscle bleeding with nerve compression		70% initially, >30% until tissue is healed, and 50% on the first ambulatory day	Fasciotomy should be performed if necessary. Physical therapy is required after tissues have healed.
Retropharyngeal hemorrhage, airway threatened		100% initially, >30% until bleeding stops (infusion repeated at 12-hour intervals)	Rarely, endotracheal intubation or tracheostomy is required.
Gastrointestinal hemorrhage		70%–100% initially, >30% for several days after bleeding has stopped	Evaluate to determine site of bleeding.
Surgery in patients without inhibitor	70%–100%	30%–50% at completion and in eight hours, then administer factor VIII by continuous infusion or as a bolus every 12 hours for at least two weeks (up to three weeks for major surgery and during physical therapy following joint surgery)	Antifibrinolytic agents (aminocaproic acid [Amicar], tranexamic acid [Cyklokapron]) are *contraindicated* during and after abdominal or orthopedic surgery.
Dental restorations with local anesthesia	30%		Avoid mandibular blocks; administer an antifibrinolytic agent.
Dental extractions	50%–100%	50% if oozing persists	Topical thrombin powder should be applied to the socket. Antibiotics may be required. Antifibrinolytic agents reduce or prevent bleeding episodes during dental procedures, reduce the need for replacement therapy, and decrease recurrent bleeding following oral surgical procedures. One of these agents should be given the evening prior to extraction and for 7 to 10 days thereafter. Aminocaproic acid should *not* be administered in the presence of hematuria. Some physicians believe that aminocaproic acid or tranexamic acid probably should not be administered within eight hours after administration of factor IX concentrate or anti-inhibitor coagulant complex because of a risk of thrombotic complications.

(table continued on next page)

TABLE (continued)

Condition	Replacement Activity: Prophylaxis	Replacement Activity: Treatment	Comments
MINOR HEMORRHAGE†			
Joint hemorrhage			
Early acute		30% (single infusion)	If treated immediately, no other measures necessary.
Late or chronic		30% (two or more infusions)	Use cold compresses and immobilize the joint by sling or splint. Physical therapy should be initiated as soon as bleeding is controlled.
Skin or subcutaneous bleeding		30% (if suturing is required)	
Muscle hemorrhage without nerve compression		30%–50% until bleeding stops (as indicated by softening of muscle mass)	Use cold compresses and immobilize the affected part. Exercises and physical therapy may be necessary. Do *not* administer aminocaproic acid.
Hematuria			
Nontraumatic (spontaneous)		None needed in most cases; 30% if bleeding persists after several days of bedrest	Adequate fluid intake should be maintained. Aminocaproic acid should be avoided.
Traumatic		50% until bleeding stops and injury heals (infusion repeated at 12-hour intervals)	Adequate fluid intake should be maintained. Aminocaproic acid should be avoided.
Epistaxis		30%–50% (single infusion)	Local pressure or nasal packing (without replacement therapy) may suffice.
Mouth bleeding		30%–50% (usually single infusion)	Aminocaproic acid 6 g every six hours should be administered orally. Alternatively, tranexamic acid (25 mg/kg three to four times daily) can be given orally. Topical thrombin powder also may be applied to the site of hemorrhage. Aminocaproic acid should *not* be given in the presence of hematuria.
Tonsil inflammation with bleeding		50% until tonsils heal	

** The presence of an inhibitor should be excluded before treatment of bleeding episode is started. Intermediate-purity factor VIII preparations may contain high titers of anti-A and anti-B agglutinins. If hemolysis occurs (rare), administration of ultrapure factor VIII concentrates is recommended.*

†Desmopressin should be used instead of blood products whenever possible (ie, in persons with mild hemophilia A).

immunoaffinity-purified factor IX preparations currently are being reviewed for marketing approval by the FDA. Coagulation factor IX concentrates are less likely to cause thromboembolic complications than the factor IX complex concentrates (which contain small but clinically significant amounts of activated factors II, VII, IX, and X) (Mannucci et al, 1990; Lusher, 1991; Kim et al, 1991). In the unlikely situation in which factor IX concentrates are not available, FFP from one or a few well-screened and repeatedly tested donor(s) may be used for patients with mild to moderate deficiencies of factor IX. *Antihemophilic Factor (AHF) preparations are not effective.*

Patients with an undefined bleeding disorder or multiple factor deficiencies can be treated with blood group-compatible FFP (15 ml/kg) while diagnostic studies are being performed (Roberts and Jones, 1990). FFP from one or a few well-screened and repeatedly tested donor(s) is the agent of choice in most patients with deficiency of factors II, V, VII, X, or XI if replacement therapy is deemed necessary. For these single-factor deficiencies, the dose of plasma is calculated on the basis of 1 unit of factor IX activity/ml of plasma; 10 to 20 ml/kg usually is given in one to two hours, with administration repeated every 12 hours until bleeding stops. Purified concentrates of factors VII, X, XI, and XIII are being developed but are not generally available at present (Bloom, 1991 B). Factors II, VII, and X (the other vitamin K-dependent factors) also are present in factor IX complex preparations, but the concentration of factor VII is low and quite variable. These preparations have been used to treat deficiency of any of the factors in the complex (eg, congenital deficiency, liver disease, or anticoagulant-induced vitamin K deficiency). However, hepatitis has been reported after use of some factor IX complex concentrates, and the risk of thrombosis is high, especially in patients with severe hepatic dysfunction, following surgery, or in those with inhibitors. Factor IX complex preparations should not be administered to treat the multifactor deficiencies of acquired coagulation disorders such as DIC. These conditions usually are associated with increased fibrinolysis and/or circulating endogenous anticoagulants, as well as with underlying hypercoagulability.

The synthetic androgen, danazol [Danocrine], which has been given to some patients with factor VIII or factor IX deficiency, is not effective and may be harmful.

RESISTANCE. About 10% to 15% of patients with factor VIII deficiency develop inhibitor antibodies that inactivate infused factor VIII, making treatment of subsequent bleeding episodes more difficult (Lusher, 1989). These antibodies develop most commonly in patients with severe deficiency, and they appear before age 20 years in about 65% of hemophilic patients with inhibitors. When inhibitor concentrations remain below 5 Bethesda units, larger amounts of factor VIII may be effective. Patients with inhibitor levels between 5 and 10 Bethesda units may require much larger amounts of factor VIII to overwhelm the inhibitor and treat bleeding. Those with inhibitor levels ≥10 Bethesda units will not respond to even massive quantities of factor VIII, and other replacement products must be given to bypass the inhibitor.

Assay for factor VIII inhibitor should be performed periodically in all hemophiliacs and routinely before surgery. The presence of factor VIII inhibitor should be suspected in patients with a prolonged activated partial thromboplastin time and ecchymoses or bleeding, since inhibitors also develop rarely in healthy individuals, elderly patients, postpartum women, and patients with systemic lupus erythematosus, other autoimmune disorders, drug hypersensitivity, or paraproteinemia.

Purified porcine factor VIII concentrate [Hyate:C], which generally has less cross reactivity with factor VIII antibodies than the human product, has been useful in treating bleeding in hemophiliacs with low- or moderate-titer antibodies. If replacement with porcine factor VIII is being considered, laboratory assays should confirm that the patient's inhibitor has a lower cross reactivity to the porcine factor VIII:C than to human factor VIII:C. As a foreign protein, this product may occasionally be antigenic and rarely can cause thrombocytopenia.

Factor IX complex concentrates also may be useful to treat bleeding in patients with acquired factor VIII inhibitor (see the evaluation on Factor IX Complex). Patients with inhibitors who are bleeding severely or who do not respond to factor IX complex concentrate may be treated with activated anti-inhibitor coagulant complex [Autoplex T, Feiba VH], which has factor VIII inhibitor bypassing activity. The purified coagulation factor IX concentrates (eg, AlphaNine) are not useful in these patients, since the concentration of contaminating clotting factors is suboptimal. Both plasma-derived and recombinant DNA-derived preparations of activated factor VII (VIIa) are being evaluated as therapy for hemophilic patients with inhibitors to factors VIII or IX. When infused, factor VIIa combines with tissue factor to activate factor X directly and is thought by some to be the source of factor VIII-bypassing activity in activated anti-inhibitor coagulant complex. Plasma exchange and pheresis or extracorporeal immunoadsorption columns that remove IgG antibodies are only temporarily effective but may be helpful in life-threatening circumstances.

Although prolonged daily infusions of factor VIII have been reported to suppress inhibitors, the benefits of such regimens must be weighed against cost and the risk of a transient elevation in inhibitor concentrations (Ewing et al, 1988). Some patients (particularly those without hemophilia who acquire inhibitors) have been successfully treated with a combination of immunosuppressive drugs, intravenous IgG, and factor VIII (Lian et al, 1989; Nilsson et al, 1988, 1990).

Circulating inhibitors directed against factor IX occur in 1% to 3% of patients with hereditary factor IX deficiency. A small number of patients with lupus erythematosus appear to have an acquired factor IX inhibitor. Bleeding in the latter patients is frequently due to an inhibitor of factor VIII but may be caused by inhibitors of factor IX or vWF; thus, the presence and identification of an inhibitor must be established prior to treatment. However, lupus-type anticoagulants, antiphospholipid antibodies that prolong the partial thromboplastin time without causing a hemostatic defect, are the most common acquired coagulation inhibitors in these patients. In addition, some patients with lupus develop a non-neutralizing antibody to prothrombin that causes prothrombin deficiency as a result of increased clearance and prolongs prothrombin times.

ADVERSE REACTIONS AND PRECAUTIONS. Type B or C (formerly termed non-A, non-B) hepatitis historically is the most common adverse effect of the concentrated factor VIII and IX clotting factor preparations. Donor screening and viral inactivation procedures have reduced the risk (Epstein and Fricke, 1990) but do not guarantee freedom from hepatitis, which has occurred with products that were heated either dry or in suspension in organic solvent. Available data suggest that pasteurization, solvent/detergent treatment, or dry heating at 80° C for 72 hours may be adequate to inactivate hepatitis viruses (The National Hemophilia Foundation Medical and Scientific Advisory Council [MASAC], 1991); however, only small numbers of patients were included in published studies evaluating these techniques, and additional data documenting the safety of these products are needed.

The hazard with use of cryoprecipitated AHF is the same as with single units of whole blood. Cryoprecipitate prepared from single-donor plasma is a less desirable treatment alternative even for patients who do not require frequent treatment. Immune globulin (gamma globulin) does not attenuate hepatitis B or C viruses, and intramuscular injections are dangerous in any patient with a bleeding disorder. Hepatitis B vaccine should be given to all hemophiliacs who are not already seropositive for hepatitis B surface antigen (see index entry Hepatitis B Vaccine Inactivated).

Approximately 50% to 60% of patients with severe hemophilia are now seropositive for HIV. Use of donor-screened, viral-attenuated clotting factor concentrates has reduced, but has not completely eliminated, the risk of transmitting HIV. Although seroconversion had been associated with dry- and organic solvent-heated products used before 1985, it appears that the newer pasteurized, solvent- and detergent-treated or super dry-heated (80° C for 72 hours) concentrates are much safer (Pierce et al, 1989; Epstein and Fricke, 1990). It is noteworthy that no new instances of HIV seroconversion attributable to clotting factor concentrates have occurred in North America since 1987. Prelicensure clinical trials have been in progress since 1987 to examine the safety and efficacy of recombinant factor VIII preparations (Schwartz et al, 1990; *Semin Hematol*, 1991).

Preparations of factor IX complex have a significant potential to produce thrombotic complications, including DIC (Lusher, 1991). Intravascular thrombosis has occurred most frequently in hemophiliacs undergoing surgery who received large, repeated doses of factor IX complex. It is thought that the high circulating levels of the zymogens produced, prothrombin and factor X, may contribute to the development of thrombosis. These complications have been particularly severe in patients with underlying liver disease; therefore, factor IX complex concentrates or anti-inhibitor coagulant complex (activated prothrombin complex concentrates) should be employed with great caution during the postoperative period in patients with significant liver function abnormalities. Concomitant use of aminocaproic acid is not advocated, as this may increase the risk of thrombosis. The newer preparations of coagulation factor IX concentrate that are purified by affinity chromatography or using immunoaffinity techniques are much less likely to cause thromboembolism since they contain little or no factors II, VII, or X (Mannucci et al, 1990; Kim et al, 1991).

Hemolytic anemia may occur when low or intermediate purity factor VIII preparations are given to individuals with group A, B, or AB red blood cell antigens, because anti-A or anti-B antibodies may be present in the precipitated fraction. The anemia is usually mild and abates after discontinuation of AHF therapy. Spherocytosis of peripheral red blood cells may be the initial sign of hemolysis. Patients who develop hemolysis should be treated with ultrapure factor VIII concentrates. The immunoaffinity-purified products contain little extraneous protein and have not been associated with this complication.

Pulmonary hypertension has developed in some patients receiving heat-dried factor VIII concentrates. This complication may be caused by accumulation of particulate matter in the pulmonary vasculature (Goldsmith et al, 1988).

VITAMIN K DEFICIENCY

Vitamin K is an essential cofactor for the hepatic microsomal enzyme system that converts multiple glutamic acid residues to gamma-carboxyglutamic acid residues in factors II, VII, IX, and X and proteins C and S (Comp, 1990). Through the gamma-carboxyglutamic acid residues, these proteins bind calcium, which allows them to bind to phospholipid surfaces and thus function in the clotting cascade. If vitamin K deficiency occurs, the plasma activity of these procoagulant factors decreases and a hemorrhagic disorder develops.

The vitamin K compounds are fat-soluble naphthoquinones. Vitamin K_1 (phytonadione) occurs in a variety of foods and also is prepared synthetically. Vitamin K_2 is produced by bacteria in the gastrointestinal tract. Like vitamin K_1, vitamin K_3 (menadione) can be prepared synthetically and is used for therapeutic replacement.

ETIOLOGY. Vitamin K_2 accumulates in the liver, spleen, and lungs, but significant amounts are not stored in the body for long periods. The daily requirement of vitamin K is estimated to be 1 to 5 mcg/kg for infants and 0.03 mcg/kg for adults. Dietary sources usually satisfy these requirements, and healthy adults, even those with inadequate diets, are unlikely to develop a deficiency on the basis of an unbalanced diet alone. The major causes of vitamin K deficiency are administration of broad-spectrum antibiotics, impaired absorption, oral anticoagulant therapy, and neonatal deficiency.

Antibiotic Therapy and Malabsorption Syndromes: Vitamin K deficiency may occur during prolonged oral antibiotic therapy, cleansing of the bowel prior to colonic surgery, or when a malabsorption syndrome exists (eg, cystic fibrosis, sprue, short-bowel syndrome, pancreatic insufficiency, dysentery, celiac disease, intestinal fistula, blind loop syndrome). The effects of antibiotics may result from toxicity to the intestinal flora or, with some of the cephalosporins, from inhibition of vitamin K-dependent carboxylation. In young infants, deficiency may result from acute diarrhea, even of short duration. An existing deficiency of vitamin K may be accentuated by alteration of intestinal flora during treatment of infectious diarrhea with antibiotics. Deficiency also can develop rapidly following surgery, particularly if renal failure develops.

Vitamin K supplementation should be routine in patients receiving long-term intravenous feeding and in debilitated patients who may have experienced long periods of inadequate diet. Deficiency develops rapidly during parenteral feeding that is not supplemented with vitamin K, especially if broad spectrum antibiotics are given concomitantly.

The K vitamins, except for the water-soluble salts of menadione (menadione sodium bisulfite, menadiol sodium diphosphate), are absorbed from the gastrointestinal tract only in the presence of adequate quantities of bile salts and pancreatic lipase. Thus, steatorrhea may cause deficiency of vitamin K and consequently of factors II, VII, IX, and X and proteins C and S.

Oral Anticoagulant Therapy: Coumarin derivatives inhibit recycling of oxidized vitamin K (which is inactive as a cofactor for gamma-carboxylation) in the liver, and their use is one of the most common causes of iatrogenic hypocoagulability in humans. Vitamin K-dependent coagulation factor activities often are markedly decreased in patients treated with these drugs.

Vitamin K Deficiency in Neonates: The prothrombin activity in newborn infants is substantially lower than that in adults, but this may not be reflected in prothrombin time determinations. Prothrombin time often is prolonged in infants at birth and may increase during the next two to four days if vitamin K is not given. Spontaneous hemorrhage caused by deficiency of vitamin K-dependent clotting factors is unlikely after the sixth day, particularly if cow's milk (maternal milk contains virtually no vitamin K) is used for feeding. The enzyme systems that synthesize these factors may not be fully developed at birth, and administration of vitamin K usually does not increase levels in infants to the same extent as in adults.

Other conditions that may contribute to defective hepatic synthesis of vitamin K-dependent clotting factors in neonates are a lack of vitamin K-producing bacteria in the gastrointestinal tract (which decreases the amount of vitamin K absorbed), reduced stores of vitamin K, and maternal ingestion of oral anticoagulants or agents that induce cytochrome P-450 (eg, barbiturates, phenytoin).

TREATMENT. Appropriate therapy in cases of apparent vitamin K deficiency requires that true deficiency be differentiated from defective synthesis of vitamin K-dependent clotting factors. For example, in liver disease with severe cellular damage (eg, cirrhosis, hepatitis, hemochromatosis, porphyria cutanea tarda, Wilson's disease), the vitamin K-dependent clotting factors may be reduced significantly despite the presence of adequate vitamin K, and vitamin replacement therapy is ineffective. Although treatment may be unsatisfactory, if bleeding occurs these patients should receive FFP from one or a few well-screened donors who repeatedly test negative for exposure to HIV and the B and C hepatitis viruses. The use of hepatitis B vaccine also should be considered, particularly if repeated transfusions are anticipated. The one-stage prothrombin time (PT) test is used routinely to monitor the efficacy of vitamin K therapy.

Phytonadione, the natural fat-soluble vitamin K_1, is preferred to control severe, acute oral anticoagulant-induced bleeding and for use during the last weeks of pregnancy or in hemorrhagic disease of the newborn. The water-soluble salts of menadione (vitamin K_3) are useful in hypoprothrombinemias caused by conditions that limit the absorption or synthesis of the fat-soluble form of vitamin K (eg, celiac disease, ulcerative colitis). However, because menadione can combine with tissue sulfhydryl groups to produce hemolytic anemia and liver damage, phytonadione is generally preferred when large doses or prolonged therapy is indicated.

In vitamin K deficiency caused by poor nutrition or malabsorption, a single loading dose of phytonadione frequently stops bleeding within a few hours, and additional doses replenish vitamin K stores. If an absorptive defect cannot be localized, small parenteral doses should be given at regular intervals until the defect is corrected. When malabsorption of vitamin K is caused by biliary disease (obstructive jaundice, atresia, fistulas), the PT increases gradually. If hepatic cell damage also is present, hypoprothrombinemia and the associated deficiency of other vitamin K-dependent factors may become even more severe.

The therapeutic strategy for vitamin K deficiency caused by excessive oral anticoagulation depends on the intensity of hypocoagulability, the severity of bleeding, and the need for reinstituting anticoagulant therapy once hemostasis is restored. When the PT is prolonged beyond the desired therapeutic range but no bleeding occurs, a single oral dose of phytonadione often corrects the defect. However, some physicians believe that low-dose parenteral phytonadione (0.5 to 1 mg) is more effective than the orally administered drug. When there is active bleeding, FFP is the therapy of choice. If the hemorrhage is mild to moderate, FFP may be used without concomitant phytonadione. FFP also is preferred when reinstitution of oral anticoagulant therapy is considered after hemostasis is achieved, since phytonadione can increase the difficulty of restoring the PT to the therapeutic range after the mild to moderate bleeding is controlled unless low-dose therapy is used. If severe bleeding occurs, the anticoagulant should be discontinued and intravenous phytonadione [AquaMEPHYTON] therapy initiated. Because the response to vitamin K is delayed for 4 to 24 hours, concomitant transfusion of FFP is essential in life-threatening hemorrhage. The PT should be measured frequently to monitor the effects of the oral anticoagulant and natural decay of the clotting factors in the transfused plasma. Adults usually require two to three units of plasma. When time is critical (eg, central nervous system hemorrhage), use of viral-attenuated factor IX complex may be necessary despite the risk of hepatitis and/or thrombosis.

In pregnant women with vitamin K deficiency or in those who undergo prolonged labor, the administration of phytonadione 12 to 24 hours before delivery may prevent hemorrhagic disease in the neonate. More commonly, a single intramuscular dose of 0.5 to 1 mg is administered to the infant within 24 hours after birth. Because large doses of menadione or its salts may cause kernicterus due to hemolysis or interference with conjugation of bilirubin in the liver, phytonadione is the only acceptable preparation for this purpose. Kernicterus has not been reported with use of this agent, and small doses do not hemolyze red cells deficient in glucose-6-phosphate dehydrogenase (G6PD).

In premature infants with immature liver function or infants with hepatocellular disease, FFP may be required. Phytonadione may not prevent bleeding, and doses exceeding 1 mg may cause hemolytic anemia in these infants.

None of the vitamin K preparations counteract the anticoagulant effects of heparin, and they are often ineffective when hypoprothrombinemia is secondary to liver disease. Patients with hereditary hypoprothrombinemia or hereditary deficiency of factors VII, IX, or X also do not respond to vitamin K therapy.

ADVERSE REACTIONS AND PRECAUTIONS. Adverse reactions are observed only rarely in adults after oral administration of vitamin K. Serious reactions, including fatalities, have occurred in the past during and immediately following intravenous or subcutaneous injection of larger doses. In recent years, no new cases of such reactions have been reported, possibly as a result of dose reductions. The reactions appear to have been caused by hypersensitivity and may have been associated with shock, respiratory arrest, or both. They have occurred in some patients who received vitamin K for the first time. However, some experts suggest that these reactions may have been due to the diluent rather than to vitamin K itself. Other parenteral routes also may be hazardous. One patient developed indurated erythematous plaques with persistent intermittent pruritus at the injection site following intramuscular administration of phytonadione.

When large doses of vitamin K are used to treat hemorrhagic disease in infants, they can increase hemolysis and the plasma levels of unbound bilirubin, resulting in kernicterus, hemolytic anemia, and hemoglobinuria. However, hyperbilirubinemia has been observed only rarely after use of phytonadione, and this drug has not yet been implicated in causing kernicterus. The hemolytic potential of vitamin K is greatest in infants with relatively low activity of G6PD but has also been observed in adults with this deficiency. Plasma concentrations of free bilirubin may increase in premature infants if the mother has received large (more than recommended) doses of menadione sodium bisulfite, although moderate doses are relatively safe and often necessary.

Patients with liver disease should not be given large doses of vitamin K repeatedly if the response to initial administration is unsatisfactory. Those receiving large doses (25 to 50 mg) may be resistant to coumarin drugs given later, making effective anticoagulant therapy difficult until the vitamin is metabolized and excreted. It may be necessary to reinstitute oral anticoagulant therapy with larger doses to overcome resistance or to use heparin.

AFIBRINOGENEMIA AND HYPOFIBRINOGENEMIA

Afibrinogenemia is defined as a complete absence of fibrinogen, while hypofibrinogenemia is manifested by a lower-than-normal concentration of the procoagulant protein. Afibrinogenemia occurs rarely as an autosomal recessive disorder that is manifested clinically in homozygotes. Bleeding is similar to that produced by factor XIII deficiency. Hypofibrinogenemia may represent a heterozygous state. Some patients with low plasma fibrinogen levels are remarkably free of major hemorrhage. More commonly, hypofibrinogenemia is associated with acquired hemorrhagic disorders, particularly liver disease (in which increased destruction and decreased synthesis occur) and DIC. Functional abnormalities of fibrinogen are termed dysfibrinogenemia and may occur in either heterozygous or homozygous forms.

Initial therapy of acquired hypofibrinogenemia should be directed toward control of the underlying disease. If fibrinogen is required, cryoprecipitate is the agent of choice, since fibrinogen is not available as a purified protein concentrate. A dose sufficient to raise the fibrinogen concentration to 50 mg/dL for minor bleeding or to 100 mg/dL for surgery is recommended. ABO-compatible cryoprecipitate should be utilized in children or when large or repeated doses are necessary. If cryoprecipitate is not available, FFP may be substituted. Congenital fibrinogen deficiency in symptomatic patients also is treated with cryoprecipitate or FFP. Most patients with dysfibrinogenemia are asymptomatic and do not require replacement therapy.

Aminocaproic acid or tranexamic acid may be useful adjunctively but should not be used in patients with DIC or in those who are thrombosis-prone. In acute conditions in which hypofibrinogenemia is caused by accelerated consumption mediated by the in vivo generation of excess thrombin, fibrinogen preparations may not only have no effect on hemostasis but, by increasing the available substrate, may increase the level of degradation products and aggravate intravascular clotting.

Tranexamic acid was tested in patients with subarachnoid hemorrhage in a multicenter, double-blind, controlled trial (Vermeulen et al, 1984). Because adequate antifibrinolytic action (rebleeding significantly reduced) was counterbalanced by increases in ischemic complications (eg, cerebral infarction), the drug should not be used in this disorder. Aminocaproic acid also has been used in subarachnoid hemorrhage, but improvement was temporary.

DISSEMINATED INTRAVASCULAR COAGULATION (DIC)

DIC results from excessive activation of both the blood coagulation and the fibrinolytic systems; thus, clinical signs of bleeding and clotting may be observed concurrently. Fibrin deposition occludes small vessels and imperils perfusion of vital organs. The concentrations of some coagulation factors, particularly V, VIII, and fibrinogen, decrease, as do platelets that aggregate on the fibrin masses. Antithrombin III and protein C levels frequently are reduced as well. Fibrin/fibrinogen degradation products are increased due to activation of the fibrinolytic system and further interfere with hemostasis by inhibiting fibrin polymerization to produce unclottable complexes.

Because clotting factors and platelets are consumed, this condition occasionally is termed "consumptive coagulopathy." Hemorrhage can occur spontaneously or after needle puncture, surgery, or other trauma and usually is widespread, but a tendency to bleed may be the only sign. Excessive oozing of blood at multiple sites should be investigated in any patient who has been severely ill for several weeks.

Conditions that precipitate DIC include bacterial septicemia (particularly gram-negative), malignancy, amniotic fluid embolism, abruptio placentae, retention of dead fetus, eclampsia, massive trauma or burn, snakebite, and hemolytic transfusion reaction. Acute DIC is usually characterized by multisite bleeding. In the subacute or chronic form, losses of clotting factors may be compensated by increased synthesis and the patient may present with thrombotic complications.

No single test is specific for DIC, but the combination of prolonged PT, thrombocytopenia, and reduced plasma fibrinogen level is suggestive. In "classic" cases, factors V and VIII are reduced as well. Determination of D-dimer, thrombin time, and serum fibrinogen/fibrin degradation product (FDP) also is useful. Detection of D-dimer indicates that fibrin has been formed intravascularly, has been polymerized and cross-linked, and has been cleaved into D-dimers by plasmin. FDP levels exceeding 80 mcg/ml are strongly suggestive of DIC but are not sufficiently specific when used as an isolated assay.

TREATMENT. Extreme caution is required when treating DIC; continuous laboratory monitoring and the assistance of an experienced hematologist are essential. The primary aims are to determine and treat the underlying disorder and maintain supportive therapy (Marder, 1990). Associated conditions (eg, hypoxemia, hypovolemia, acidosis, anemia, hypotension) also should be treated. If these goals cannot be accomplished, success in elimination of DIC is limited.

When a bleeding diathesis is associated with DIC, treatment includes administration of FFP (2 to 10 units/day for adults or 10 ml/kg every six hours for infants and children) to replace depleted clotting factors. Some hematologists also recommend the use of various plasma serine protease inhibitors, but this is controversial. Platelet concentrates (6 to 10 single-donor or plateletpheresis units given once or twice) also may be administered. Cryoprecipitate may be given to increase the fibrinogen level, particularly if it is less than 100 mg/dL. One bag of cryoprecipitate raises the fibrinogen level by 2 to 5 mg/dL. However, replacement of clotting factors may accelerate DIC, and administration of an excessive amount of platelets or fibrinogen may lead to their rapid consumption and exacerbate microvascular thrombosis. Therefore, many hematologists believe that the consumptive process must end before replacement of the depleted clotting factors and platelets is begun.

Heparin therapy is controversial and is usually reserved for patients with extensive arterial or venous thrombosis, purpura fulminans, neoplastic disease (particularly promyelocytic leukemia), or a retained dead fetus. Many hematologists believe that only small doses of heparin should be administered and the amount titrated as necessary to maintain adequate levels of fibrinogen and platelets when replacement of either is unsuccessful despite administration of large quantities. Some children with purpura fulminans have been treated successfully, with late recovery from thrombocytopenia, using full-dose heparin for two to three weeks. In nearly all other circumstances, full-dose heparin therapy should not be administered unless platelet counts are 80,000/mm^3 or above. Prophylaxis with heparin often is used in acute promyelocytic leukemia before beginning chemotherapy because the incidence of DIC is very high and pretreatment with heparin may have prevented DIC in some patients (Hoyle et al, 1988). However, other retrospective data suggest that heparin prophylaxis may provide no clinical benefit in these patients (Rodeghiero et al, 1990); no data are available from randomized controlled trials.

Antithrombin III infusions have been used investigationally, alone or with heparin, in patients with DIC; results of randomized, controlled clinical studies have shown that AT-III was helpful for treating the rare instances of DIC associated with acute fatty liver of pregnancy.

If bleeding does not respond to heparin and replacement therapy and either hampers care or is life-threatening, fibrinolytic inhibitors such as aminocaproic acid may be used with caution to decrease the concentration of FDPs and stabilize hemostatic plugs.

BLEEDING ASSOCIATED WITH RENAL FAILURE

Bleeding is a common and frequently fatal complication of acute and chronic renal failure that appears to be caused by an acquired defect in platelet function. The anemia of renal failure may play an important role in uremic bleeding. Hemorrhagic complications in renal disease include ecchymoses, purpura, petechiae, epistaxis, bleeding from venipuncture sites, and gingival, gastrointestinal, and cerebral hemorrhage. The most consistent abnormalities are prolonged bleeding time and defective platelet adhesiveness, aggregation, and release.

Dialysis usually improves the hemostatic defect and hemorrhagic complications and is the mainstay of therapy (Couch and Stumpf, 1990). Alternative therapy to decrease bleeding temporarily is infusion of desmopressin or cryoprecipitate. Platelet transfusion has not been consistently effective. When used to correct anemia in uremic patients, recombinant human erythropoietin [Epogen, Procrit] (see index entry Epoetin Alfa) improves hemostatic function (Moia et al, 1987). Conjugated estrogen (intravenous or oral) or estrogen/progesterone therapy has shortened bleeding time over a sustained period and reduced transfusion requirements, thus offering an alternative to desmopressin or cryoprecipitate when an immediate response is not required (Bronner et al, 1986; Livio et al, 1986; Shemin et al, 1990). The mechanism of action of estrogen in renal failure is not known, and its effect is not consistent.

SURGICAL BLOOD LOSS

Hemostatic dysfunction is common after cardiopulmonary bypass for open heart surgery and appears to be caused by multiple factors, including adsorption of platelets and vWF onto artificial surfaces, platelet dysfunction, dilution of coagulation factors, and administration of heparin (Woodman and Harker, 1990). Desmopressin, given intra- or postoperatively, reduces blood loss and transfusion requirements in complex cardiac operations, presumably by increasing the plasma concentration of vWF (Czer et al, 1987; Salzman et al, 1986). This drug also may have a direct effect on the vessel wall that increases platelet adhesion and spreading at sites of injury. However, for uncomplicated primary coronary artery bypass grafts, data suggest that desmopressin does not decrease perioperative blood loss (Hackmann et al, 1989). The serine proteinase inhibitor, aprotinin (not licensed for use in United States), has been reported to be useful for cardiopulmonary bypass surgery (van Oeveren et al, 1990; Havel et al, 1991; Harder et al, 1991). There is only limited information on the use of drugs to prevent postoperative bleeding in noncardiac patients.

Absorbable hemostatics are used to help control surface bleeding and capillary oozing. They include absorbable gelatin sponge [Gelfoam], oxidized cellulose [Oxycel], oxidized regenerated cellulose [Surgicel], microfibrillar collagen hemostat [Avitene], absorbable collagen hemostat [Instat, Helistat, Hemopad, Hemotene], and bovine thrombin [Thrombinar, Thrombogen, Thrombostat]. If significant contamination is present at the site of application, use of these agents is associated with an increased risk of infection. This risk is greatest with particulate hemostatics.

Immunization with the bovine-derived thrombin preparations used for surgical hemostasis may produce prolonged thrombin times if this compound also is used for laboratory testing (Flaherty et al, 1989). However, the antibodies do not cross-react with human thrombin and do not impair clinical hemostasis. A commercially prepared, nonautologous fibrin glue [Tisseel], a human fibrinogen-based material, has been used for some time in Canada and Europe, although it is not licensed as yet in the United States. The investigational use of nonautologous fibrin glue (Kram et al, 1989; Gibble and Ness, 1990) has relied on formulation of the mixture from commercially available and laboratory-generated components.

Caustic agents, such as ferric subsulfate (Monsel's solution) and aluminum chloride solution (eg, 35% in 50% ethanol), also can be used during limited superficial surgery; they produce hemostasis by coagulating skin proteins. Dermal application of ferric subsulfate may result in tattoo marks.

A comparative review of the use of all of these hemostatic agents is available (Larson, 1988).

Drug Evaluations

AGENTS USED FOR CLOTTING FACTOR DEFICIENCIES

DESMOPRESSIN ACETATE

[DDAVP]

ACTIONS. Desmopressin, a synthetic analogue of arginine vasopressin, temporarily increases the concentrations of factor VIII:C and vWF by enhancing their secretion from endothelial cells (Mannucci, 1990; Lusher, 1990). The maximum increase (threefold to fivefold above initial concentrations) occurs in 45 to 90 minutes and persists for up to six hours. Administration of desmopressin more often than every two or three days may lead to a diminished therapeutic response (tachyphylaxis), attributed to depletion of intracellular stores of factor VIII and vWF. The drug also causes release of tissue-type plasminogen activator, but bleeding problems resulting from this are uncommon.

USES. Desmopressin is used for short-term hemostatic control in patients with mild or moderate factor VIII deficiency who have baseline concentrations of at least 5% factor VIII and in those with type I von Willebrand disease (Mannucci, 1990; Czer and Capon, 1990). The drug controls minor bleeding episodes (eg, hemarthroses, mucosal bleeding, bleeding associated with dental extractions) and also has maintained normal coagulation after some types of major surgery. The degree and duration of response should be determined preoperatively before a decision is made to use desmopressin rather than blood products. Desmopressin is not effective in severe factor VIII deficiency or type III von Willebrand disease, for the missing protein cannot be released from intracellular stores, or in factor IX deficiency (Mannucci, 1990; Czer and Capon, 1990). Its effects are variable in type IIA von Willebrand disease. This drug should not be used in type IIB or platelet variants of von Willebrand disease, since it will not be effective and can cause circulating platelet aggregates and thrombocytopenia.

Desmopressin may be employed to reverse uremic bleeding temporarily in patients who require urgent invasive procedures (Mannucci, 1990; Czer and Capon, 1990). Because of an acquired defect in platelet function, uremic patients have an abnormal platelet-vessel wall interaction. The efficacy of desmopressin for uremic bleeding is believed to be associated with release of vWF multimers from endothelial cell storage sites and increased plasma levels of catecholamines, which are mediators of hemostatic function (Escolar et al, 1989). Desmopressin also may temporarily correct the hemostatic defect in patients with chronic liver disease (Cattaneo et al, 1990; Blake et al, 1990) and in those with certain platelet function defects (Kentro et al, 1987; Czer and Capon, 1990; DiMichele and Hathaway, 1990).

When given before cardiopulmonary bypass, desmopressin was reported to reduce intraoperative blood loss (Rocha et al, 1988), and it may reduce total blood loss and transfusion requirements in patients undergoing complex cardiac surgery (Czer et al, 1987; Salzman et al, 1986). These patients have an acquired platelet dysfunction and thus are susceptible to hemorrhage (Mannucci, 1990).

Desmopressin also was reported to reduce operative blood loss and transfusion requirements in hemostatically normal patients undergoing spinal fusion surgery (Kobrinsky et al, 1987). However, it did not decrease perioperative blood loss in patients undergoing initial, uncomplicated coronary artery bypass grafts (Hackmann et al, 1989). A major advantage of desmopressin in all of these disorders is that it avoids the risk of hepatitis and HIV infection associated with blood products.

Desmopressin has been used in Sweden (by intranasal administration 45 minutes before blood donation) to increase factor VIII activity (usually twofold) in the cryoprecipitate or factor VIII concentrate prepared from donated blood.

ADVERSE REACTIONS AND PRECAUTIONS. In patients with type IIB von Willebrand disease, desmopressin may cause release of an abnormal or incomplete vWF protein that has platelet-aggregating properties and can induce thrombocytopenia. In platelet-type (pseudo) von Willebrand disease, normal vWF is released but is bound by the abnormal platelets, which have a heightened affinity for vWF. Therefore, it should not be used to treat these disorders.

Facial flushing is common. Headache, nausea, mild abdominal cramps, and pain and swelling at the site of injection may occur rarely. Slight decreases in blood pressure have been reported sporadically, and thus the drug should be used with caution in patients with coronary artery disease or hypertension. Use of desmopressin has occasionally been followed by cerebral or coronary thrombosis, and it should be used cautiously in elderly patients and those with atherosclerosis. However, the causal relation of desmopressin to these uncommon occurrences remains unclear. Because of the antidiuretic effects of the drug, water intake should be limited, particularly after surgery and in very young and elderly patients, to prevent water intoxication and hyponatremia (Smith et al, 1989; Weinstein et al, 1989).

Desmopressin is classified in FDA Pregnancy Category B.

PHARMACOKINETICS. Desmopressin can be administered by intravenous or subcutaneous injection or intranasally. Bioavailability after subcutaneous injection is nearly equal to that after intravenous infusion; it is approximately 10% when the concentrated intranasal spray is used (Lusher, 1990). The response to desmopressin appears to be saturable, and maximal release of factor VIII/vWF occurs at ≥0.3 mcg/kg (administered parenterally). The maximal response occurs 90 minutes to two hours after infusion. In many patients, the response declines after frequent administration (tachyphylaxis), presumably because of transient depletion of storage pools of the factor VIII/vWF complex in endothelial cells. The mean half-life for clearance of desmopressin from the plasma after intravenous or subcutaneous injection of 0.4 mcg/kg is 3.6 ± 0.4 hours (Lusher, 1990).

DOSAGE AND PREPARATIONS. Desmopressin is almost always given intravenously when used to treat hemostatic disorders. The intranasal preparations of desmopressin currently licensed in the United States (drops, rhinyle) are not used for hemostasis because bioavailability is reduced to approximately 2% with this route of administration. A more concentrated intranasal spray formulation is effective, however (Rose and Aledort, 1991). Once licensed, this formulation should prove useful as home therapy for bleeding (eg, epistaxis, menorrhagia, gum bleeding).

When given intravenously, the dose should be diluted in physiologic sodium chloride solution and infused slowly. In adults and children weighing more than 10 kg, 50 ml of diluent is used; for children under 10 kg, 10 ml of diluent is used. Blood pressure and pulse should be monitored during infusion.

Intravenous: 0.3 mcg/kg infused slowly over a period of 15 to 30 minutes. Dosage should not be repeated within 24 hours.

DDAVP Injection (Rhône-Poulenc Rorer). Solution 4 mcg/ml in 1 and 10 ml containers.

ANTIHEMOPHILIC FACTOR (HUMAN), FACTOR VIII

CRYOPRECIPITATED ANTIHEMOPHILIC FACTOR

COMPOSITION AND STORAGE. Commercially available antihemophilic factor concentrates (factor VIII:C, AHF) are prepared from the pooled plasma of as many as 25,000 donors by a variety of techniques due to the low yields resulting from viral inactivation procedures. Donors are screened for behavior that increases their risk of infection with HIV or hepatitis B virus, and the donated blood is tested for antibodies to HIV, hepatitis B core antigen, and hepatitis C virus and for the hepatitis B surface antigen. Depending on the batch, a vial of concentrate contains 250 to 1,500 IU of factor VIII:C but little fibrinogen or vWF. Although recent regulations have improved standardization of factor VIII preparations, measurement of factor VIII levels in the recipient is still necessary to provide optimal treatment (Epstein and Fricke, 1990; The National Hemophilia Foundation Medical and Scientific Advisory Council [MASAC], 1991).

A single unit of cryoprecipitated antihemophilic factor is made from the plasma of one unit of whole blood centrifuged and frozen within six hours after donation or from one or more units of single-donor fresh frozen plasma. Thawing at 1° to 6° C yields a precipitate rich in factor VIII, vWF, and fibrinogen. Each bag of cryoprecipitate contains 80 to 125 IU of VIII:C, depending on the donor and the efficiency of processing. The percentage of non-AHF plasma factors, including fibronectin 4 mg/ml, vWF, and fibrinogen 250 to 300 mg, is higher than in the lyophilized factor VIII concentrates. Cryoprecipitates must be kept frozen; storage usually should not exceed 12 months at temperatures of −18° C. Cryoprecipitated preparations may represent the most efficient use of community blood resources, since they are inexpensive for community blood banks to prepare, they can be stored in the freezer until needed, and the material remaining in the plasma can be used to process other components such as albumin. However, cryoprecipitate is prepared without the use of viral inactivation procedures. It is less desirable as a treatment alternative than the newer factor VIII concentrates because several months may elapse between infection of a donor with HIV or hepatitis C virus and seroconversion. During this period, it is possible for plasma from an infectious donor to test negative for antibodies to these viruses (The National Hemophilia Foundation Medical and Scientific Advisory Council [MASAC], 1991).

USES. All AHF preparations can be used in patients with hemophilia A (factor VIII deficiency) or in nonhemophiliacs who develop low-responding factor VIII inhibitors. Commercial lyophilized concentrates are most frequently employed to treat severe hemophilia and are preferred for life-threatening hemorrhage, since high activities can be achieved and maintained for long periods. They are preferred for home therapy and during travel because of ease of storage and reconstitution. Since most commercial preparations contain little vWF or fibrinogen, they should not be used to treat hypofibrinogenemia or von Willebrand disease. A few factor VIII concentrates (eg, Humate-P) are effective in von Willebrand disease.

Cryoprecipitate obtained from repeatedly HIV-negative donors is preferred by some physicians, especially to treat factor VIII-deficient patients who are young or have mild to moderate disease, and thus maintenance of high titers of AHF is not required. However, use of this product does carry some risk of hepatitis. Cryoprecipitate from repeatedly HIV-negative donors also may be used to treat hypofibrinogenemia, von Willebrand disease, or factor XIII deficiency and to repair the hemostatic deficit temporarily in patients with renal failure.

ADVERSE REACTIONS AND PRECAUTIONS. Chills, mild fever, and headache may occur shortly after administration of AHF preparations, although these are rare with factor VIII concentrates used currently in the United States. Mild allergic reactions have been reported, and anaphylactic reactions have rarely been associated with use of cryoprecipitate or concentrated factor VIII. Fibrinogen is concentrated in cryoprecipitate and repeated infusion may cause hyperfibrinogenemia.

Cryoprecipitate contains small amounts of groups A and B isohemagglutinins and are usually labeled with the ABO group of the donor. Administration of compatible units is preferred, because large amounts given to patients with blood groups A, B, or AB may cause hemolysis.

The use of donor-screened, dry heat-treated plasma derivatives improved the safety of these blood products, but the risk of viral transmission was not completely eliminated. Newer methods that are safer include pasteurization, solvent/detergent treatment, and use of dry heat at 80° C. Products that are heated while suspended in organic solvent or dry heated at less than 80° C appear to be equally safe with regard to the risk of transmitting HIV but may transmit hepatitis C virus. Factor VIII products made from recombinant DNA, which will pose no risk of contamination from HIV or other blood-borne viruses, have been in prelicensure clinical trials since 1987 (Schwartz et al, 1990; *Semin Hematol*, 1991).

AHF preparations are classified in FDA Pregnancy Category C.

PHARMACOKINETICS. The elimination of factor VIII from plasma is biphasic. The initial phase probably represents equilibration between the vascular compartment and extravascular space. The second phase (half-life, 12 to 15 hours) probably corresponds to the rate of degradation/utilization.

DOSAGE AND PREPARATIONS. Cryoprecipitated AHF should be thawed in a water bath at 37° C (higher temperatures result in loss of factor VIII activity), kept at room temperature after thawing, and used within three hours. The bag should be gently agitated to assure dissolution and the material then administered through a filter.

Lyophilized concentrates should be reconstituted with the sterile diluent supplied.

Intravenous: Various formulas are available to estimate dosage, and details appear in the manufacturers' literature. Based on experimental evidence, approximately 1 unit/kg increases activity about 2%; to maintain the desired level, doses should be repeated every 12 hours. Regardless of the therapeutic guide, if replacement therapy is being used for surgery or to treat a major bleeding episode that threatens life or limb, factor VIII assays should be performed frequently if proper techniques are available to ensure achievement and maintenance of adequate factor VIII activity. These determinations may be imperative when using cryoprecipitated AHF, because there is no uniformity in the concentration of AHF from one plasma donor to the next. A test for factor VIII inhibitors also should be performed prior to infusion. Failure to achieve expected blood levels may be the first indication of the development of an acquired inhibitory antibody.

A circulating AHF activity 20% to 30% of normal usually controls hemarthrosis in hemophiliacs. A single dose of 15 to 20 units/kg given at a rate of 10 to 15 ml/min usually achieves hemostasis and maintains activities sufficient for clotting. For mild bleeding into muscles or soft tissues in noncritical areas, activity should be maintained at 30% to 50% of normal until bleeding stops. For surgery, an activity at least 60% of normal is usually recommended preoperatively for effective hemostasis; postoperatively, it is desirable to maintain a circulating activity 40% to 50% of normal for up to 14 days.

For patients with retroperitoneal, retropharyngeal, or central nervous system bleeding, severe trauma, or spontaneous bleeding into a body cavity, hospitalization is necessary and hemostasis is achieved with initial doses of 40 to 50 units/kg and subsequent doses of 20 to 25 units/kg repeated at 12-hour intervals or, preferably, by continuous infusion of 2 units/kg/hr after the same initial bolus until hemorrhage is controlled or the wound is healed. Bleeding recurs if treatment is discontinued prematurely.

For hypofibrinogenemia, usually four bags of cryoprecipitate/10 kg will raise the fibrinogen concentration by 150 mg/dL.

ANTIHEMOPHILIC FACTOR (HUMAN), FACTOR VIII:

Immunoaffinity Purified and Solvent/Detergent-Treated Products:
Hemofil M (Baxter Healthcare), ***Method M, Monoclonal Purified*** (American Red Cross).

Immunoaffinity Purified and Pasteurized Product:
Monoclate-P (Armour).

Chromatographically Purified and Solvent/Detergent-Treated Product:
MelATE (New York Blood Center).

Products Heated in Aqueous Solution (Pasteurized):
Koate HS (Miles-Cutter), ***Humate P*** (Armour).

Solvent/Detergent-Treated Products:
Factor VIII-SD (New York Blood Center), ***Koate HP*** (Miles-Cutter), ***Profilate OSD*** (Alpha Therapeutic).

Each container is labeled with the number of international units (IU) it contains (200 to 1,700 IU/container). One IU is the AHF activity present in 1 ml of average, normal human plasma pooled from at least ten donors and tested within three hours after collection. These materials must be reconstituted with the diluent supplied to a volume dependent on final container assay of potency and dosage/ml desired.

CRYOPRECIPITATED ANTIHEMOPHILIC FACTOR (HUMAN): This product can be prepared by the hospital blood bank as a byproduct of blood banking. It cannot be standardized, but each bag usually contains 80 to 125 units of factor VIII in a volume of 15 ml.

FACTOR IX COMPLEX (HUMAN)

[Konyne-80, Profilnine Heat-Treated, Proplex T Heat-Treated]

COAGULATION FACTOR IX (HUMAN)

[AlphaNine]

COMPOSITION AND STORAGE. Factor IX complex (prothrombin complex) concentrates are prepared from the supernatants remaining after cryoprecipitation of pooled plasma. These stable, dried, purified plasma fractions contain the vitamin K-dependent coagulation factors (II, VII, IX, and X) and natural coagulation inhibitors (proteins C and S), as well as small amounts of other plasma proteins. Products are alleged to be free of thrombin, thromboplastin-like activity, and anticomplement activity. Konyne-80 and Profilnine Heat-Treated contain no heparin; heparin is added to Proplex T Heat-Treated to help prevent the formation of thrombin after the manufacturing process (eg, with increased temperature during storage). Because amounts of anti-A and anti-B agglutinins are clinically insignificant, factor IX complex (human) may be used without typing or cross-matching. Hypervolemic reactions do not occur because of the concentrated nature of these products and the small amount of fluid needed for administration.

A preparation of human factor IX purified by affinity chromatography [AlphaNine] is now available. Compared with factor IX complex concentrates, this product contains markedly reduced levels of factors II, VII, and X and has a higher specific activity of factor IX. AlphaNine contains very small amounts of heparin (no more than 0.04 units/IU of factor IX activity).

USES. Factor IX complex (human) and affinity-purified coagulation factor IX are used to treat bleeding associated with factor IX deficiency (hemophilia B, Christmas disease). Factor IX complex also may be used to treat deficiency of one or more of the other factors contained in this preparation. However, fresh frozen plasma from repeatedly tested and well-screened donors is preferred when bleeding is not severe. When large amounts of factor IX complex are required, the addition of heparin (5 units/ml of reconstituted product) is recommended by some clinicians to reduce the likelihood of DIC, venous thromboembolism, myocardial infarction, and other thromboembolic complications (Bloom, 1991 B; Lusher, 1991). Addition of heparin is not necessary when affinity-purified coagulation factor IX is used to treat hemophilia B, since the purification procedure removes activated clotting factors and results in a product that is less thrombogenic than factor IX complex (Mannucci et al, 1990; Kim et al, 1991).

Factor IX complex also is used in patients with factor VIII deficiency who develop inhibitor, presumably because it supplies activated factors that participate in the coagulation process beyond the stages where factor VIII is needed. However, if a bleeding episode in these patients does not respond to three or four doses of factor IX complex, additional doses are unlikely to be effective and may increase the risk of acute myocardial infarction or thrombosis (Lusher, 1989). See the section on Resistance in the Introduction for alternative treatment strategies.

Factor IX complex preparations should be used in newborn infants only in those rare situations when life-threatening hemorrhagic disease is caused by proven deficiency of factor II, VII, or X. Infants with congenital deficiency of factor IX who have life-threatening hemorrhage are preferably treated with coagulation factor IX concentrate. Factor IX complex should almost never be given to nonhemophilic patients (ie, those with anticoagulant-induced deficiency of vitamin K-dependent coagulation factors). Such patients should receive fresh frozen plasma if administration of vitamin K alone is inadequate.

Rarely, factor IX complex may be useful in patients with compromised cardiovascular function who are unresponsive to plasma. Also, when rapid reversal of factor IX deficiency is critical in patients with severe hemorrhage, coagulation factor IX may be used to avoid the large volumes of plasma required. If factor IX complex is being considered in these patients, the risk of hepatitis and/or thrombosis must be weighed against the benefits.

ADVERSE REACTIONS AND PRECAUTIONS. Because they are prepared from pooled plasma, there has been a substantial risk of transmitting HIV or hepatitis viruses when factor IX complex concentrates are given. Use of donor-screened, heat-treated factor IX complex has markedly reduced, but not totally eliminated, this risk. However, Konȳne-80, which is dry heat-treated at 80° C, may carry the smallest risk for transmission of blood-borne viruses among the factor IX complex concentrates. Affinity-purified coagulation factor IX is heated while suspended in organic solvent for additional viral attenuation, which is not as effective as pasteurization, solvent/detergent treatment, or heating at 80° C for reducing the risk of transmitting HIV or the hepatitis B and C viruses (The National Hemophilia Foundation Medical and Scientific Advisory Council [MASAC], 1991).

Thromboembolic complications have been reported after administration of factor IX complex, usually in patients undergoing surgery. Increased thrombogenicity appears to result from increased circulating load of procoagulant zymogens, presence of activated factors IX and X and phospholipids in these products, and patient-related factors. Affinity-purified coagulation factor IX is significantly less thrombogenic and should be used for surgery, for severe hemorrhage requiring multiple doses, and for those with a history of thrombotic problems. Factor IX complex concentrates are contraindicated in neonates and in patients with severe liver disease or with milder liver disease when there is any suspicion of DIC or fibrinolysis; these patients have low circulating concentrations of antithrombin III and do not efficiently remove the activated clotting factors due to decreased hepatic clearance.

Transient fever, chills, urticaria, nausea and vomiting, headache, flushing, or tingling can occur shortly after administration of factor IX complex or coagulation factor IX, particularly if the injection is given rapidly. Myocardial infarction has been reported in patients with factor VIII or factor IX inhibitors who received large doses of factor IX complex repeatedly (Lusher, 1991). Rarely, severe hypersensitivity reactions (eg, anaphylactic shock) have been observed.

In bleeding patients with inhibitors, if no response is evident after three or four doses of factor IX complex, other therapy should be tried. Concomitant use of aminocaproic acid or other antifibrinolytic agents is contraindicated.

PHARMACOKINETICS. The immediate recovery of factor IX after infusion of factor IX complex is between 30% and 60% of the infused dose; the mean recovery after administration of affinity-purified coagulation factor IX is approximately 61%. The elimination from plasma is biphasic. The initial phase probably represents equilibration between the vascular compartment and the extravascular space. The second phase (half-life, 22.5 hours) probably corresponds to the rate of degradation or utilization. The mean half-life of affinity-purified coagulation factor IX is 21 hours.

DOSAGE AND PREPARATIONS. Factor IX complex or affinity-purified coagulation factor IX should be given within three hours after reconstitution, and the rate of administration should not exceed 10 ml/min to avoid vasomotor reactions.

Intravenous: The amount of factor IX complex or affinity-purified factor IX required depends on the patient and the nature of the deficiency. Each unit contains the factor IX activity of 1 ml of normal fresh plasma; 1 unit/kg increases factor IX activity 1% and, for maintenance of a desired activity, doses should be repeated every 12 to 24 hours. Overdosage with factor IX complex should be avoided because the long post-infusion half-life of factors II and X can produce unnecessarily high levels of these zymogens. Specific dosage is similar to the lowest dose employed in factor VIII deficiency (see the evaluation on Antihemophilic Factor). Following major surgery, a factor IX activity 40% to 50% of normal should be maintained for four days, with an activity 30% to 40% of normal maintained on days five to eight.

For nonlife-threatening bleeding in patients with hemophilia who have factor VIII inhibitors, initially, 75 units/kg of factor IX complex, repeated once after 6 to 12 hours if necessary. If bleeding persists, alternative therapy, eg, anti-inhibitor coagulant complex (AICC, activated prothrombin complex), porcine factor VIII, or recombinant factor VIIa, may be used. In life-threatening hemorrhage, these patients should receive porcine factor VIII or AICC as the initial therapy.

FACTOR IX COMPLEX (HUMAN):

Konyne-80 (Miles-Cutter). Contains 500 and 1,000 units of factors IX and amounts of factors II, VII, and X approximately proportional to their respective levels in average fresh plasma (heparin-free).

Profilnine Heat-Treated (wet method) (Alpha Therapeutic). Contains factors II, VII, IX, and X; amount of factor IX stated on container (heparin-free).

Proplex T Heat-Treated (Baxter Healthcare). Contains factors II, VII, IX, and X and up to 1.5 units of heparin/ml of reconstituted material; amounts of factor IX stated on container.

COAGULATION FACTOR IX (HUMAN), AFFINITY-PURIFIED:

AlphaNine (Alpha Therapeutic). Heat-treated/solvent suspension in single-dose vials with diluent. The amount of factor IX contained in each vial (in IU) is stated on the label.

ANTI-INHIBITOR COAGULANT COMPLEX

[Autoplex T Heat Treated, FEIBA VH]

Anti-inhibitor coagulant complex (AICC) is prepared from pooled human plasma by a process of controlled activation. It contains variable amounts of activated and precursor clotting factors associated with the prothrombin complex. The two preparations differ in composition. For example, FEIBA VH appears to contain a higher concentration of factor VIIa, while Autoplex T contains more than trace amounts of factors of the kinin-generating system. The active ingredients are unknown except for activated coagulation factor VIIa (and IXa and Xa in Autoplex T). Their duration of effectiveness has not been determined. Although the mechanism of action is not entirely clear, it is postulated that these activated factors exert their effect at a level below factor VIII in the coagulation cascade to achieve fibrin formation and hemostasis.

USES. These AICC concentrates are indicated for active bleeding in patients with factor VIII inhibitors. The experience of many hemophilia centers has shown that these preparations can achieve hemostasis when surgery is essential. However, their effect is not always consistent, and failures have been reported.

ADVERSE REACTIONS, PRECAUTIONS, AND CONTRAINDICATIONS. AICC should be used as initial therapy only in patients who have or have had inhibitor levels exceeding 5 Bethesda units (Abildgaard et al, 1980). It is contraindicated when signs of fibrinolysis or DIC are present. The risks of thrombotic complications and DIC should be kept in mind, particularly following repeated use.

Transient hypofibrinogenemia has been observed in two children; therefore, fibrinogen levels should be monitored in young patients receiving repeated doses (Abildgaard et al, 1980).

Like other blood-derived products, use of AICC is associated with a slight risk of exposure to viral hepatitis or other blood-borne viral diseases. In addition to screening each unit of plasma used in their manufacture, these products are heated either in the presence [FEIBA VH] or absence [Autoplex T] of pressurized water vapor to reduce the risk of viral transmission. The two-step vapor-heating process used for FEIBA VH (10 hours at 60° and 1 hour at 80° C) may be more effective for inactivation of hepatitis viruses. However, neither process completely eliminates the risk of infection with hepatitis virus. The safety and efficacy of the vapor-heated preparation compare favorably with those of an unheated form of the same product (Hilgartner et al, 1990).

The rate of infusion should not exceed 10 ml/min and may have to be decreased if headache, flushing, or changes in pulse rate or blood pressure are noted. If these reactions are severe, the infusion should be stopped until symptoms disappear and then resumed at a rate of approximately 2 ml/min.

AICC is classified in FDA Pregnancy Category C.

DOSAGE AND PREPARATIONS. This complex is standardized by its ability to correct the ellagic acid APTT of factor VIII-deficient plasma. Each vial of Autoplex T is labeled with factor VIII correctional units. (Each unit is that quantity of activated prothrombin complex which, when added to an equal volume of factor VIII-deficient plasma, will correct the ellagic acid-APTT to 35 seconds.) Vials of FEIBA-VH are labeled in units of factor VIII inhibitor bypassing activity. Reconstituted Autoplex T contains a maximum of 2 units/ml of heparin and 0.02 M sodium citrate. The material should be reconstituted with sterile water for injection immediately before injection, and the solution should be given at a rate of no more than 10 ml/min.

Intravenous: 50 to 100 units/kg, depending on the severity of hemorrhage. If minor bleeding problems are treated promptly, lower doses (25 units/kg) may be adequate. If hemostasis is not observed after six hours, the dose should be repeated. Subsequent doses should be adjusted according to the patient's response.

There are no reliable laboratory tests to measure the effect of AICC.

Autoplex T Heat Treated (Baxter Healthcare). Powder in 30 ml containers (each container labeled with factor VIII correctional activity) with sterile diluent (contains up to 2 units heparin/ml).

Feiba VH (Immuno U.S.). Powder (freeze-dried) (each container labeled with factor VIII inhibitor bypassing activity) with sterile diluent (heparin-free).

ANTIHEMOPHILIC FACTOR (PORCINE)

[Hyate:C]

COMPOSITION. This preparation is a freeze-dried concentrate of porcine AHF purified by adsorption and elution from polyelectrolytes. Porcine factor VIII concentrate appears to have a lower immunogenic potential than human factor VIII (Lusher, 1989).

USES. Porcine factor VIII concentrate is used to treat hemophiliacs who have developed antibodies to human factor VIII products (Brettler et al, 1989). One advantage to the use of the porcine product rather than AICC is that the adequacy of treatment can be monitored by measuring factor VIII activity levels. This is not possible in inhibitor patients treated with factor IX complex concentrates or AICC, since the complex bypasses the factor VIII-dependent step in the clotting cascade, thus rendering laboratory monitoring useless. In the past, porcine AHF was reserved for patients with life- or limb-threatening bleeding or those requiring surgery whose antibody titer was greater than 5 Bethesda units/ml (BU/ml) against human factor VIII preparations. However, the routine administration of porcine AHF for uncomplicated bleeding episodes and its use prophylactically in selected patients is becoming much more common as experience increases (Hay and Bolton-Maggs, 1991). Porcine AHF may be ineffective in individuals with antibody titers against human factor VIII greater than 50 BU/ml. Infusion of porcine factor VIII concentrate may lead to an increase in both anti-human and anti-porcine factor VIII antibodies; therefore, inhibitor levels should be determined before and after treatment. During treatment, response to therapy can be monitored by measuring levels of factor VIII activity. In a few carefully chosen patients, therapy with porcine factor VIII induced stable immune tolerance of human factor VIII (Hay et al, 1990).

Porcine AHF also is used in nonhemophiliacs with acquired inhibitory antibodies to factor VIII (Kessler, 1991). Many clinicians regard it as the treatment of choice for bleeding in these patients, since it has never been reported to transmit disease to humans and the response can be monitored with assays of factor VIII activity.

ADVERSE REACTIONS AND PRECAUTIONS. Fever, chills, headache, nausea, vomiting, and rash may occur, particularly during the first infusion. Anaphylactic reactions have developed rarely, and medications to treat such reactions should be readily available. Acute thrombocytopenia has occurred rarely. In Europe, home treatment is used in carefully selected patients and no complications have been reported. A few hemophilia centers in the United States also use home treatment with porcine AHF for patients with inhibitors, but this is recommended only after the patient's tolerance for this preparation is substantiated by the absence of untoward effects during a prehome trial. Porcine factor VIII preparations are not thrombogenic and have not been reported to transmit human blood-borne viruses.

This preparation is classified in FDA Pregnancy Category C.

DOSAGE AND PREPARATIONS.

Intravenous: Initially, 100 to 150 units/kg in patients with human factor VIII antibody levels of less than 50 BU/ml. If the human factor VIII antibody level exceeds 50 BU/ml, the activity of the antibody against the porcine product should be determined. An antiporcine factor VIII antibody level greater than 20 BU/ml suggests that the patient is unlikely to benefit from porcine factor VIII. If the antiporcine factor VIII antibody level is less than 20 BU/ml, an initial dose of 100 to 150 units/kg is recommended.

If recovery of factor VIII:C in the patient's plasma is insufficient after the initial dose, a second larger dose should be given, which may be followed, if necessary, by a third still larger dose.

Hyate:C (Porton). Powder 400 to 700 units to be reconstituted with 20 ml of sterile water for injection.

ANTIFIBRINOLYTIC AGENTS

AMINOCAPROIC ACID

[Amicar]

$$H_2NCH_2(CH_2)_3CH_2\overset{O}{\overset{\|}{C}}OH$$

ACTIONS. Aminocaproic acid may help to control serious hemorrhage associated with excessive fibrinolysis caused by increased activation of plasminogen. Fibrinolysis in the non-pathologic state is regulated by plasminogen activators, which catalyze conversion of fibrin-bound plasminogen to plasmin, and by inhibitors of plasmin (primarily α_2-antiplasmin). Plasminogen and plasmin bind at critical sites of positive charge (ϵ-amino moieties of lysine) in the amino acid sequence of fibrin. Aminocaproic acid is structurally related to lysine and consequently acts as a competitive inhibitor for binding of plasminogen and plasmin to fibrin (Marder and Francis, 1990). As a result, fibrinolysis (and fibrinogenolysis) is inhibited.

QUALIFICATIONS FOR USE. Since this drug inhibits the dissolution of clots, it may interfere with normal mechanisms for maintaining the patency of blood vessels, particularly in thrombosis-prone patients. Before this hemostatic is used, it is important to understand the role of the fibrinolytic system in maintaining the patency and integrity of the vascular system, the laboratory procedures used to determine coagulation defects, and the mechanism of action of aminocaproic acid.

A pathologic fibrinolytic state may be suspected in patients with a predisposing clinical condition when results of laboratory tests suggest increased fibrinolytic activity, prolonged thrombin and prothrombin times, hypofibrinogenemia, or decreased plasminogen levels. However, these conditions and some of the laboratory findings usually are associated with DIC. If aminocaproic acid is given to patients with DIC, it may cause serious or even fatal thrombus formation. For this reason, *most experts do not use aminocaproic acid to treat "fibrinolytic" hemorrhage unless there is definitive proof that DIC is not the underlying cause.* If such proof is lacking, the following criteria may assist in distinguishing between DIC and primary fibrinolysis but they are not diagnostic. In DIC, the platelet count is reduced, the protamine paracoagulation test may be positive, and euglobulin clot lysis (a measure of the fibrinolytic potential of plasma) may be normal or reduced. In primary fibrinolysis (which is rare), the platelet count is normal, the protamine paracoagulation test is negative, and euglobulin clot lysis is reduced. Measurement of D-dimer levels also is useful to distinguish DIC from primary fibrinolysis.

USES. Although cryoprecipitated AHF is preferred for treatment of hypofibrinogenemia, aminocaproic acid may be useful in surgical and nonsurgical hematuria arising from the bladder, prostate, or urethra. In patients undergoing transurethral and suprapubic prostatectomy, postoperative hematuria has been reduced significantly. However, use of aminocaproic acid should be restricted to patients who are seriously threatened by hemorrhage for whom a correctable cause of bleeding from the prostatic bed has been excluded. Isolated case reports suggest that hemorrhagic cystitis may be controlled within 24 hours when aminocaproic acid is given both systemically and intravesically.

Administration of aminocaproic acid as a specific antidote for overdoses of streptokinase or urokinase has been suggested. However, it has produced endocardial hemorrhage and myocardial fat degeneration in animals. Therefore, caution is advocated if this use is considered, because most patients receiving thrombolytic agents have pre-existing cardiac disease.

Aminocaproic acid does not control hemorrhage caused by thrombocytopenia or most other coagulation defects, although it has been very beneficial in hemophiliacs prior to and following tooth extraction and for other traumatic bleeding in the mouth and nasopharynx. Although not yet substantiated by randomized studies, there is some evidence to suggest that aminocaproic acid may be useful for the management of bleeding in patients with immune thrombocytopenia who are refractory to platelet transfusion (Bartholomew et al, 1989). When multiple hemostatic defects exist, other therapeutic measures (eg, fresh frozen plasma, cryoprecipitated AHF, vitamin K) may be required. Since the drug does not control bleeding caused by loss of vascular integrity, valuable time may be wasted if it is used in patients with post-tonsillectomy bleeding, gastrointestinal hemorrhage from ulcers or ruptured esophageal varices, hemoptysis due to bronchiectasis, open surgical wounds, or functional uterine bleeding.

Because aminocaproic acid inhibits C'_1 esterase, it has been used to prevent or control attacks of hereditary angioedema. It has been given following subarachnoid hemorrhage and before and during surgery for ruptured intracranial aneurysms, but it is of questionable value in these conditions.

ADVERSE REACTIONS AND PRECAUTIONS. The most common untoward effects of aminocaproic acid are nausea, diarrhea, and vomiting. Less common are dizziness, pruritus, erythema, rash, hypotension, headache, dyspepsia, inhibition of ejaculation, conjunctival erythema, arrhythmias, fatigue, and nasal congestion. Inflammatory myopathy with myoglobinuria has been reported in a few patients who received doses of 24 to 38 g/day for more than one month (Brodkin, 1980) and in another patient with underlying skeletal muscle disease who received a single dose of 3 g (Morris et al, 1983). Painful urination or urinary frequency has occurred, and one patient developed acute renal failure that required hemodialysis (Biswas et al, 1980). One patient with cirrhosis experienced a grand mal seizure during infusion of aminocaproic acid (Rabinovici et al, 1989). The most serious adverse effect is generalized thrombosis; therefore, hemostatic mechanisms should be monitored. Liver failure has been reported in patients with cirrhosis.

Cardiac and hepatic necroses were found at postmortem examination in one patient who received therapeutic doses of aminocaproic acid. Since subendocardial hemorrhages and myocardial depression have occurred in several animal species, the drug should be used with caution in patients with cardiac disease. It may transiently alter protein metabolism by inhibiting the utilization of lysine.

When aminocaproic acid is given during surgery, care must be taken to free the bladder of blood clots, since the drug accumulates in these clots and inhibits their dissolution. Aminocaproic acid should not be used when renal or ureteral bleeding is suspected, for ureteral clot formation and obstruction may result.

Use of aminocaproic acid in women taking oral contraceptives or estrogens may increase the potential for thromboses.

Teratogenic studies in animals have produced variable results, but no significant abnormalities have been noted clinically. Nevertheless, the drug should not be used during the first and second trimesters unless absolutely essential. It may be given during the last trimester if specifically indicated and if the potential benefit outweighs the possible hazards to the mother and fetus.

PHARMACOKINETICS. Aminocaproic acid is well absorbed orally and also can be given intravenously. It is widely distributed throughout the body. The plasma half-life after intravenous infusion is 77 minutes. This drug is concentrated in the urine and is excreted largely unchanged. Peak plasma levels are obtained about two hours after a single oral dose.

DOSAGE AND PREPARATIONS. Further evidence is needed to determine the safety of prolonged use of aminocaproic acid in the following doses. This drug should not be administered undiluted or injected rapidly.

Intravenous, Oral: *Adults,* initially, 4 to 5 g orally or by *slow* intravenous infusion (in 250 ml of physiologic sodium chloride, sterile water, 5% dextrose, or Ringer's solutions), then 1 g (in 50 ml of diluent if given intravenously) at hourly intervals or 4 to 5 g every four hours if renal function is normal (maximum, 30 g/24 hours). This dosage produces effective plasma concentrations of approximately 13 mg/dL; these concentrations are maintained for slightly less than three hours. The dose should be reduced to 25% in patients with renal disease or oliguria. After prostatic surgery, a dose of 6 g/24 hr is effective because the drug is concentrated in the urine. *Children,* initially, 100 mg/kg followed by 33 mg/kg/hr or 100 mg/kg every six hours (maximum total dose, 18 g/M^2/24 hours). The patient's condition should be re-evaluated after eight hours of continuous therapy.

Generic. Solution (injection) 250 mg/ml in 1, 20, and 96 ml containers.

Amicar (Lederle). Solution (injection) 250 mg/ml in 20 and 96 ml containers; syrup 250 mg/5 ml; tablets 500 mg.

TRANEXAMIC ACID
[Cyklokapron]

ACTIONS AND USES. Tranexamic acid is a synthetic antifibrinolytic agent that acts by competitively inhibiting the activation of plasminogen through a mechanism similar to that of aminocaproic acid. It is indicated for short-term use (two to eight days) in hemophiliacs during and after tooth extraction and oral surgery to reduce or prevent bleeding and to reduce the need for replacement therapy. This drug is also used for hemostasis in patients undergoing oral surgery who are being treated with oral anticoagulants (Sindet-Pedersen et al, 1989). Tranexamic acid has been reported to reduce hemorrhage during and after open heart surgery (Horrow et al, 1990, 1991). In addition, it has been used to reduce gastrointestinal bleeding (Henry and O'Connell, 1989), to control hemorrhage in patients with acute promyelocytic leukemia (Avvisati et al, 1989), and to treat hemothorax in patients with malignant mesothelioma (De Boer et al, 1991).

ADVERSE REACTIONS AND PRECAUTIONS. Tranexamic acid may cause gastrointestinal disturbances (nausea, vomiting, diarrhea), hypotension, and visual disturbances. Although retinal changes have not been reported in humans, retinal degeneration has developed in laboratory animals treated with the drug. Ophthalmologic examination (including visual acuity, color vision, eyeground, and visual fields) is advisable before and during treatment extending over several days. The drug should not be given to patients with acquired defective color vision and should be discontinued if visual disturbances occur. Tranexamic acid is contraindicated in patients with subarachnoid hemorrhage because it may cause cerebral edema and infarction. Its use was associated with thrombotic complications in one patient with idiopathic thrombocytopenic purpura.

This drug is classified in FDA Pregnancy Category B. Tranexamic acid passes through the placenta after administration to pregnant women and achieves concentrations in cord blood that are approximately equal to those in the maternal circulation. The drug is also secreted in the milk of nursing mothers, although at only about 1% of the peak serum concentration.

PHARMACOKINETICS. The oral bioavailability of tranexamic acid is 30% to 50%. It is 3% protein bound (due entirely to binding to plasminogen), and its volume of distribution is 9 to 12 L. Peak plasma levels occur approximately three hours after oral administration of 1 or 2 g. The drug is eliminated mainly by renal excretion (95%). Renal clearance approximates the rate of glomerular filtration. After an intravenous dose of 1 g, the elimination half-life is two hours. Tranexamic acid inhibits fibrinolysis at much lower concentrations than those required for aminocaproic acid. Effective plasma levels persist for six to eight hours after a single dose.

DOSAGE AND PREPARATIONS.

Intravenous: 10 mg/kg before dental surgery; for patients unable to take oral medication, this dose may be repeated three or four times daily for up to eight days. Oral administration is substituted when patients are able to take medication by mouth.

Oral: 25 mg/kg three or four times daily beginning one day prior to dental surgery.

The following dosages are recommended for patients with moderately to severely impaired renal function:

	Dosage	
Serum Creatinine (μmol/L)	**Intravenous**	**Oral**
120-250 (1.36-2.83 mg/dL)	10 mg/kg twice daily	15 mg/kg twice daily
250-500 (2.83-5.66 mg/dL)	10 mg/kg daily	15 mg/kg daily
>500 (>5.66 mg/dL)	10 mg/kg every 48 hours or 5 mg/kg every 24 hours	15 mg/kg every 48 hours or 7.5 mg/kg every 24 hours

Cyklokapron [Kabi Pharmacia]. Tablets 500 mg; solution 100 mg/ml in 10 ml containers.

VITAMIN K PREPARATIONS

PHYTONADIONE (Vitamin K_1)
[AquaMEPHYTON, Konakion, Mephyton]

ACTIONS AND USES. Vitamin K acts as a cofactor for the enzyme system that gamma-carboxylates multiple glutamic acid residues in clotting factors II, VII, IX, and X and in the anticoagulant proteins C and S.

Phytonadione and other vitamin K preparations are used either prophylactically or during bleeding episodes and are the only preparations that reverse the hypoprothrombinemia produced by oral anticoagulants. They do not combat hemorrhage caused by overdosage of heparin.

Phytonadione also is used to prevent or treat hemorrhagic disease in neonates and hypoprothrombinemia caused by inadequate absorption of vitamin K, inadequate synthesis of vitamin K in the gastrointestinal tract, poor nutrition, or the toxic action of certain drugs (eg, trimethoprim/sulfamethoxazole, salicylates) given with anticoagulants.

Phytonadione has a more prompt, potent, and prolonged effect than the other vitamin K analogues and is generally preferred when large doses or long-term therapy is indicated. In contrast to menadione-type drugs, it does not hemolyze red cells in patients who are deficient in G6PD and is generally safe for use in newborn infants if recommended doses are not exceeded.

Phytonadione reverses moderately excessive anticoagulation caused by warfarin overdose. Doses ranging from 0.5 to 10 mg partially correct the prothrombin time in approximately four to six hours, and full correction usually occurs within 24 hours. When further warfarin therapy is not required, up to 10 mg of phytonadione may be used (large doses make the patient resistant to warfarin for several days thereafter); in patients requiring subsequent warfarin maintenance therapy, doses should be limited to 0.5 to 1 mg. The oral and subcutaneous routes are less likely to cause adverse reactions and are preferred for nonemergency situations. Since control of hypoprothrombinemia re-exposes the patient to the same hazards of intravascular clotting that existed prior to anticoagulant therapy, the dose of phytonadione should be as low as possible and prothrombin times should be determined frequently. Heparin's anticoagulant effect is not impaired by large amounts of phytonadione, and it should be readily available if needed to counteract incipient hypercoagulability.

When immediate correction of hypoprothrombinemia is necessary (eg, overdose of oral anticoagulants), transfusion of fresh frozen plasma or factor IX complex concentrates rich in stable vitamin K-dependent clotting factors is indicated. Fresh frozen plasma or blood component therapy also may be needed if bleeding is severe and factors V and VIII are depleted. Concomitant intravenous injection of phytonadione (AquaMEPHYTON only, at a rate that does not exceed 1 mg/min; Konakion is administered intramuscularly only) and plasma (200 to 500 ml) are recommended initially. However, hypervolemia may result and precipitate pulmonary edema in patients with limited cardiac reserve. If rapid reversal of hypoprothrombinemia is necessary in these patients, factor IX complex concentrates may be administered to avoid transfusing large volumes of plasma despite the risk of hepatitis and/or thrombosis.

ADVERSE REACTIONS AND PRECAUTIONS. Intravenous injection of phytonadione can cause flushing of the face, hyperhidrosis, a feeling of chest constriction, cyanosis, acute peripheral vascular failure, shock, and hypersensitivity or anaphylactic-type reactions. Fatalities have occurred (see the Introduction).

The action is more prolonged with subcutaneous and intramuscular administration than with the intravenous route; delayed cutaneous sclerosis and pain may occur at the site of injection.

Parenteral administration in neonates can increase unbound plasma bilirubin significantly and cause hemolytic anemia and hemoglobinuria. These reactions are less likely with phytonadione than with the water-soluble analogues (menadiol sodium diphosphate, menadione sodium bisulfite) and occur rarely if recommended doses are not exceeded. Kernicterus has not yet been reported.

Phytonadione is classified in FDA Pregnancy Category C.

DOSAGE AND PREPARATIONS.

Oral: For anticoagulant overdose and other hypoprothrombinemic states, *adults and children,* 2.5 to 25 mg; rarely, doses as large as 50 mg may be needed.

Mephyton (Merck Sharp & Dohme). Tablets 5 mg.

Parenteral: The preparation may be diluted with 5% dextrose, 0.9% sodium chloride, or 5% dextrose and sodium chloride injection. Other diluents should not be used.

Intramuscular, Subcutaneous: For prophylaxis of hemorrhagic disease in the newborn, 0.5 to 1 mg, given intramuscularly, immediately after birth. For treatment of hemorrhagic disease in the newborn, 1 mg intramuscularly or subcutaneously. If no improvement occurs within six hours, the condition of the infant should be re-evaluated.

Intravenous (slow): The intravenous route should be used only when other routes are not feasible and the risk is justified. The rate of injection should not exceed 1 mg/min. For mild overdose of oral anticoagulants, initially, 0.5 to 5 mg; for moderate to severe hemorrhage, up to 10 mg in divided doses. The frequency of administration and number of additional doses should be determined by the prothrombin time or the patient's condition. If prothrombin time is not satisfactory after six to eight hours, the dose should be repeated. The smallest effective dose should be used to prevent temporary refractoriness to further anticoagulant therapy. If shock occurs or blood loss is excessive, fresh frozen plasma or blood component therapy is essential. For other hypoprothrombinemic states, 2.5 to 25 mg.

AquaMEPHYTON (Merck Sharp & Dohme). Solution 2 mg/ml in 0.5 ml containers and 10 mg/ml in 1, 2.5, and 5 ml containers.

Konakion (Roche). Solution (intramuscular only) 2 mg/ml in 0.5 ml containers and 10 mg/ml in 1 ml containers.

MENADIONE (Vitamin K_3)

O
CH₃
O

Menadione has the same actions and uses as phytonadione, although it is not as active on a weight basis (see the Introduction and the evaluation on Phytonadione). Because it may produce hemolytic anemia and liver damage, menadione should not be given in large doses or for long-term therapy. This preparation is almost insoluble in water and is used orally; the presence of bile salts is required for intestinal absorption.

The incidence of adverse reactions is low when usual therapeutic doses are used, and reactions are similar to those produced by phytonadione. In addition, menadione hemolyzes red blood cells in patients with G6PD deficiency, as well as in newborn (especially premature) infants. Therefore, it probably should not be given to neonates or to women during the last few weeks of pregnancy.

DOSAGE AND PREPARATIONS.
Oral: 2 to 10 mg daily.
Generic. Powder.

MENADIOL SODIUM DIPHOSPHATE
[Synkayvite]

This water-soluble salt of menadione has actions and uses similar to those of phytonadione (see the evaluation); however, it should not be given to prevent or treat hemorrhagic disease in the newborn or to treat hypoprothrombinemia caused by overdosage of oral anticoagulants. Menadiol sodium diphosphate is converted to menadione in the liver. Concomitant administration of bile salts is not necessary for intestinal absorption. Because menadione can produce hemolytic anemia and liver damage, this preparation should not be given when large doses or prolonged therapy is necessary. It is not recommended in patients with obstructive jaundice or biliary fistula.

Adverse reactions are similar to those produced by phytonadione, but the incidence is low when usual therapeutic doses are used. Nevertheless, parenteral forms of menadiol sodium diphosphate should be used only when there is a definite indication for them, since these routes (particularly intramuscular injection) may cause serious toxicity. Like menadione, menadiol sodium diphosphate hemolyzes red blood cells in patients with G6PD deficiency, as well as in newborn (especially premature) infants. Therefore, it probably should not be given to neonates or to women during the last few weeks of pregnancy (FDA Pregnancy Category C).

DOSAGE AND PREPARATIONS.
Oral: *Adults,* for secondary hypoprothrombinemia, 5 to 10 mg daily.
Synkayvite (Roche). Tablets 5 mg.
Subcutaneous, Intramuscular, Intravenous: *Adults,* for secondary hypoprothrombinemia, 5 to 15 mg once or twice daily; *children,* 5 to 10 mg once or twice daily. Doses may be repeated if prothrombin levels do not return to normal.
Synkayvite (Roche). Solution (injection) 5 and 10 mg/ml in 1 ml containers and 37.5 mg/ml in 2 ml containers.

SURGICAL HEMOSTATICS

FIBRIN GLUE

Fibrin glue is used to achieve parenchymal organ hemostasis. It also is effective in patients with disordered coagulation secondary to massive transfusion, chronic disease, or DIC (Kram et al, 1989; Gibble and Ness, 1990). It has been used as well at cannulation sites to attain hemostasis in a variety of surgical procedures, in trauma patients, and in conjunctival surgery in place of sutures. Fibrin glue does not depend on adequate platelet or clotting factor concentrations to be effective. Thrombin interacts with the fibrinogen to produce fibrin monomers, which undergo hydrogen bonding to form strands of fibrin. Calcium catalyzes the chemical reaction. Fibrin glue appears to have good local compatibility and can be used in a wet field.

Fibrin glue is not available commercially in the United States, although clinical trials with one such product [Tisseel] have been conducted (Rousou et al, 1989; Kram et al, 1990, 1991 A). It can be formulated from four components: (1) highly concentrated fibrinogen (total protein approximately 120 mg/ml); (2) aprotinin (3,000 KIU/ml); (3) dried thrombin (500 units/ml); and (4) calcium chloride (400 micromoles/ml). The reconstituted adhesive contains 70 to 100 mg/ml of fibrinogen, 2 to 7 mg/ml of fibronectin (cold-insoluble globulin), 10 units/ml of factor XIII, and 35 mg/L of plasminogen. The fibrinogen is obtained from human donor plasma and, thus, in the absence of viral attenuation procedures, carries the risk of transmitting blood-borne viruses (eg, HIV, hepatitis). (The use of autologous fibrinogen for formulation of fibrin glue has been described [Mandel, 1989; Levinson et al, 1991] and would reduce the risk of viral transmission.) After preheating to 37° C, the fibrinogen is dissolved in aprotinin, and the dried thrombin is reconstituted in calcium chloride. The two solutions are then drawn up into separate syringes that are loaded onto a double-barreled syringe holder designed to mix and apply the components simultaneously. The reconstitution procedure takes 10 to 15 minutes, and the components should be used within four hours. Alternatively, fibrin glue may be applied in aerosol form by the use of an aerosol sprayer (Kram et al, 1991 B).

On application, the components mix to form a clear, viscous solution that firmly adheres to wound surfaces and sets into a white, rubberlike mass within seconds. The adhesive continues to gain in tensile strength, and 70% of the maximum tensile strength is achieved in ten minutes. During the subsequent course of wound healing, the adhesive slowly dissolves by fibrinolysis and eventually is completely removed from the body; aprotinin is added to slow the fibrinolytic process. Because it is completely removed from the body, chronic foreign-body giant-cell inflammatory reactions do not occur. The essential reactions after mixing of the components are proteolysis, fibrin cross-linking, and, finally, lysis and absorption of the clot material during the wound-healing process.

Anaphylaxis was reported in one patient who was deficient in immunoglobulin A with a high titer of IgA antibodies and was treated with fibrin glue made from homologous blood (Milde, 1989). Severe hypotension also has occurred after fibrin glue was applied to deep hepatic wounds or large venous lacerations from separate syringes containing fibrin and thrombin (Berguer et al, 1991); this is hypothesized to result from a systemic reaction to inadvertent intravenous injection of bovine thrombin.

ABSORBABLE GELATIN SPONGE
[Gelfoam]

This sterile, gelatin-base surgical sponge is applied topically as an adjunct to hemostasis when the control of bleeding by conventional procedures is ineffective to reduce capillary ooze or is impractical. Highly vascular areas that are difficult to control by cautery are primary sites of application. Absorbable gelatin sponge is insoluble in water and is usually moistened with sterile sodium chloride before application. Alternatively, it may be moistened with thrombin solution. (A compressed form is available specifically for dry application.)

This preparation is capable of absorbing up to 45 times its weight of blood and other fluids. Only the minimal amount should be used, and it should be held in place at the site until bleeding stops. Absorbable gelatin sponge may be left in place following closure of a surgical wound. When it is packed into cavities or closed tissue spaces, care should be exercised to avoid overpacking, because the material expands to its original size on absorbing fluid and may press on neighboring structures. This is particularly important when nerve tissue is involved. Absorption is complete in four to six weeks without inducing excessive scar tissue formation or cellular reaction. When applied to bleeding nasal, rectal, or vaginal mucosa, it liquifies within two to five days.

Information is insufficient to determine its teratogenic potential, but absorbable gelatin sponge should be used with caution in pregnant women. It should not be employed to control postpartum bleeding or menorrhagia.

Absorbable gelatin sponge cannot be used on graft beds, for it physically separates the graft from the graft site. This material should not be interposed between skin edges in closure of skin incisions (since it may interfere with healing of skin edges) or applied in the presence of infection. It also should not be placed into the vasculature because of the risk of embolization.

ADVERSE REACTIONS AND PRECAUTIONS. Absorbable gelatin sponge or powder may form a nidus for infection or abscess and has been reported to potentiate bacterial growth. Giant-cell granuloma has been reported at the site of absorbable gelatin products implanted in the brain. In one patient, use of absorbable gelatin sponge to reinforce a wrapped cerebral aneurysm resulted in an inflammatory intracranial mass that responded to treatment with intravenous dexamethasone (Guerin and Heffez, 1990). Accumulation of sterile fluid has caused compression of brain and spinal cord. Excessive fibrosis and prolonged fixation of tendons have been reported when absorbable gelatin sponge was used in the repair of severed tendons. The product should not be resterilized by heat or use of ethylene oxide.

DOSAGE AND PREPARATIONS.

Topical (in wound or at operative site): The minimal amount required to control bleeding should be used.

Gelfoam (Upjohn). Blocks 20 × 60 × 3 mm (size 12-3 mm) and 20 × 60 × 7 mm (size 12-7 mm), 80 × 62.5 × 10 mm (size 50) and 80 × 125 × 10 mm (size 100), 80 × 250 × 10 mm (size 200); pleated surgical packs 40 × 2 cm (size 2 cm), 40 × 6 cm (size 6 cm), 10 × 20 × 7 mm (size 2) and 20 × 20 × 7 mm (size 4) (dental packing blocks); compressed blocks 125 × 80 mm (size 100) (dry applications); prostatectomy cones 13 and 18 cm in diameter.

OXIDIZED CELLULOSE
[Oxycel]

OXIDIZED REGENERATED CELLULOSE
[Surgicel]

ACTIONS. These absorbable celluloses are prepared by the controlled oxidation of cellulose or regenerated cellulose. The gauze or fabric apparently does not enter into the normal physiologic clotting mechanism but, when exposed to blood, expands and is converted to a reddish brown or black gelatinous mass whose fibers provide a matrix for clotting. Oxidized cellulose products have a very low pH. Their hemostatic action is not enhanced by other hemostatic agents (thrombin is destroyed by the low pH of this material). Oxidized regenerated cellulose is bactericidal against a wide range of gram-positive and gram-negative organisms, including aerobes and anaerobes.

The rate of absorption depends on the size of the implant, the adequacy of blood supply to the area, and the degree of chemical degradation of the material. The degree of absorption depends on several factors (eg, amount used, degree of saturation with blood tissue bed). Two to seven days are usually required, but the process may take six weeks or longer. Under optimal conditions, absorption from a body cavity occurs without cellular reaction or fibrosis.

USES. Oxidized cellulose or oxidized regenerated cellulose is useful in surgical procedures to assist in the control of moderate bleeding when suturing or ligation is technically impractical or ineffective. Such situations include control of capillary, venous, or small arterial hemorrhage encountered in biliary tract surgery; partial hepatectomy; resections or injuries of the pancreas, spleen, or kidneys; amputations; resection of the bowel, breast, thyroid, or prostate; oral surgery and exodontia; and certain types of gynecologic and otolaryngologic surgery. Oxidized cellulose is not recommended as a wrap in vascular surgery in order to avoid cicatricial contraction.

PRECAUTIONS. Although packing or wadding is sometimes necessary, oxidized regenerated cellulose should not be used in this manner unless it is removed after hemostasis is achieved. It must always be removed when used in, around, or in proximity to foramina in bone, areas of bony confine, the spinal cord, and the optic nerve. Permanent neurologic injury has been reported in a few patients when oxidized regenerated cellulose migrated into the spinal canal after its use during thoracotomy (Short, 1990). These products should not be used for permanent packing or implantation in fractures because they may interfere with bone regeneration and cause cyst formation. Absorbable cellulose products also cannot be used on graft beds, for they physically separate the graft from the graft site. They are less effective on surfaces treated by chemical cautery. The Oxycel brand should not be used as a surface dressing except for immediate control of hemorrhage, since it inhibits epithelialization. Silver nitrate or other corrosive chemicals should not be applied prior to its use.

Information is insufficient to determine the teratogenic potential of these celluloses, and they should be used with caution in pregnant women.

DOSAGE AND PREPARATIONS.

Topical (in wound or at operative site): The minimal amount required to control hemorrhage should be used to facilitate absorption. This material should be placed on the bleeding site and held firmly until hemostasis is obtained.

OXIDIZED CELLULOSE:

Oxycel (Becton-Dickinson). Woven gauze pads 7.6 × 7.6 cm 8 ply; pledgets (cotton type) 5.1 × 2.5 × 2.5 cm; strips (gauze type) 12.7 × 1.3 cm 4 ply, 45.7 × 5.1 cm 4 ply, 91.4 × 1.3 cm 4 ply.

OXIDIZED REGENERATED CELLULOSE:

Surgicel (Johnson & Johnson). Knitted fabric strips 1.3 × 5.1, 5.1 × 7.6, 10.2 × 20.3, and 5.1 × 35.6 cm; 2.5 × 2.5 and 7.6 × 10.2 cm and 15.2 × 22.9 cm ***(Nu-Knit)***.

MICROFIBRILLAR COLLAGEN HEMOSTAT

[Avitene]

ACTIONS AND USES. This water-insoluble fibrous material is prepared from purified bovine corium collagen. The helical structure of this protein, which is preserved during manufacture, is responsible for its inherent hemostatic activity. When applied directly on the bleeding surface, it attracts and entraps platelets to initiate formation of the platelet plug; a natural clot results. Microfibrillar collagen hemostat is assimilated within seven weeks, leaving very little residue.

This material is indicated as an adjunct during surgical procedures when ligature and/or cautery are ineffective or impractical. However, it should not be used instead of ligation or resection to control severe arterial bleeding during surgery.

Microfibrillar collagen hemostat is beneficial in diffuse capillary bleeding (eg, from friable tissues or highly vascular organs). It controls hepatic bleeding, such as that following cholecystectomy, lacerations, biopsy, or resections of hepatic tumors, and capillary bleeding from splenic tears or superficial splenic injuries. This material also is used around vascular anastomoses where only minimal suturing is possible and to control oozing from cancellous bone. However, it should not be used on bone surfaces to which prosthetic materials are to be attached with methylmethacrylate adhesives. This hemostatic appears to retain its effectiveness in heparinized patients and also may be useful in patients with moderate thrombocytopenia but not in those with clinical thrombasthenia. Microfibrillar collagen hemostat is a useful adjunct for patients who are bleeding in the oral cavity, in those with hemophilia, in those receiving coumarin derivatives, and in those with inhibitors to coagulation factors.

ADVERSE REACTIONS AND PRECAUTIONS. Since it is a foreign protein, microfibrillar collagen hemostat may exacerbate infection; abscess formation; dehiscence of cutaneous incisions, where collagen may form a mechanical barrier between opposed skin edges; mediastinitis; and adhesion formation. By sealing the surface, it may conceal deep hemorrhage or hematoma in penetrating wounds. This hemostatic should not be used between skin edges because it interferes with closure of wound edges or between a graft and the graft bed, for it physically separates these sites. However, it does not interfere with epidermal or bone healing.

No systemic allergic reactions or beef antibody responses have been reported. Although weak positive reactions to bovine serum albumin have occurred occasionally, significant IgE antibodies have not developed following use of this product.

Microfibrillar collagen hemostat must be kept dry, since moisture impairs its hemostatic capacity. It is inactivated by autoclaving and should not be resterilized. Sterility is not guaranteed once the container is opened; therefore, the unused portion should be discarded. Care should be taken to avoid spillage on nonbleeding surfaces, particularly in abdominal or thoracic viscera.

Information is insufficient to determine its teratogenic potential, and this preparation should be used with caution in pregnant women.

APPLICATION. Microfibrillar collagen hemostat adheres to tissue surfaces to form a firm flexible film; since it also will adhere to any moist surface (eg, gloves, instruments), dry, smooth, sterile forceps should be used for handling. Surfaces to be treated should first be compressed with dry sponges and then covered with microfibrillar collagen hemostat; moderate pressure with a dry sterile sponge should then be exerted. Pressure for one minute may control superficial capillary bleeding, but five minutes or more may be needed when high-pressure leaks from artery suture holes or other pronounced bleeding is encountered. If oozing is not controlled, additional microfibrillar collagen hemostat may be used. However, only the amount needed to produce hemostasis should be applied and excess material should be removed by teasing or irrigating. This usually can be done without a recurrence of bleeding.

DOSAGE AND PREPARATIONS.

Topical: For capillary bleeding, 1 g is usually sufficient for a 50 cm^2 area. Thicker coverage is required for more pronounced bleeding. To control oozing from cancellous bone, the preparation should be firmly packed into the spongy bone surface and compressed for 5 to 10 minutes.

Avitene (MedChem). Fibrous form (sterile) in 1 and 5 g jars contained in a sealed can; nonwoven web (sterile) 35 x 35 x 1 mm, 70 x 35 x 1 mm, 70 x 70 x 1 mm; and single-use (sterile) endoscopic delivery system 50 x 50 x 1 mm (***Endo-Avitene***).

ABSORBABLE COLLAGEN HEMOSTAT

[Helistat, Hemopad, Hemotene, Instat]

ACTIONS AND USES. Absorbable collagen hemostat is a lyophilized bovine collagen. The material, available as a sponge-like pad product or in noncompressed form, is lightly cross-linked, sterile, nonpyrogenic, and absorbable. Hemostatic activity is an inherent property of collagen and is largely dependent on the basic helical structure of this protein, which is preserved during manufacture. When collagen comes into contact with blood, platelets aggregate on the collagen and release aggregating and activating factors that, together with coagulation factors, result in the formation of fibrin and finally in the formation of a clot.

Absorbable collagen hemostat is indicated in surgical procedures (other than neurologic and ophthalmologic surgery) for use as an adjunct to hemostasis when control of bleeding by ligature or other conventional methods is ineffective or impractical. Pretreatment with anticoagulants does not appear to affect the usefulness of collagen absorbable hemostat. The material is usually absorbed eight to ten weeks after implantation.

Absorbable collagen hemostat is not intended to be used to treat systemic coagulation disorders.

ADVERSE REACTIONS AND PRECAUTIONS. Adverse reactions reported include hematoma, potentiation of infection, wound dehiscence, inflammation, and edema. Other adverse reactions that may be related to the use of absorbable collagen hemostat include adhesion formation, allergic reactions, and foreign body reaction.

This collagen material should not be left in an infected or contaminated space. When placed into cavities or closed spaces, care should be exercised to avoid overpacking, for it may absorb fluid, expand, and press against neighboring structures.

Since this material may interfere with the healing of skin edges, it should not be interposed between them in the closure of skin incisions. Absorbable collagen hemostat should not be applied to a graft site, for the graft will be physically separated from its bed. Absorbable collagen hemostat also should not be applied on bone surfaces to which prosthetic materials are to be attached with methylmethacrylate adhesives because it may reduce their bonding strength. In urologic procedures, the preparation should not be left in the renal pelvis or ureters to eliminate potential foci for calculus formation.

The safety of this product in children and pregnant women has not been established.

Absorbable collagen hemostat is inactivated by autoclaving; it should not be resterilized.

APPLICATION. Absorbable collagen in sponge or noncompressed form is applied directly to the bleeding surface with pressure. Time to hemostasis depends on the type of surgery and degree of bleeding at the surgical site. It usually occurs in two to five minutes. The material maintains its integrity in the presence of blood; it does not stick to instruments, gloves, or sponges, but adheres to bleeding surfaces. Because of its wet strength, it is easily removed after hemostasis has been achieved without reinitiating bleeding.

DOSAGE AND PREPARATIONS.

Topical: Sponges can be cut to the precise size needed to control bleeding at the surgical site. They maintain their shape but can be easily molded when moistened with saline. The noncompressed form can be shaped by hand or instrument.

Helistat (Calgon Vestal). Sponge pads (sterile) 2.5 × 5.0 cm, 7.5 × 10 cm, and 23 × 25 cm.

Hemopad (Astra). Sponge pads (sterile) 2.5 × 5 cm, 5 × 8 cm, and 8 × 10 cm.

Hemotene (Astra). 1 g in noncompressed form in boxes of 5.

Instat (Johnson & Johnson). Sponge pads (sterile) 2.5 x 5.1 cm and 7.6 x 10.2 cm.

THROMBIN

[Thrombinar, Thrombogen, Thrombostat]

ACTIONS AND USES. This sterile plasma protein substance is prepared from bovine prothrombin. It is applied topically to control capillary oozing in operative procedures and also has shortened the duration of bleeding from puncture sites in heparinized patients (eg, after hemodialysis). It also may be used for hemostasis under grafts, for there is no particulate material to separate the graft from its bed. Thrombin may clot whole blood, plasma, or a solution of fibrinogen without the addition of other substances; it also may be combined with gelatin sponge but should not be used to moisten microfibrillar collagen hemostat. Thrombin alone does not control arterial bleeding.

When applied to denuded tissue, thrombin is neutralized rapidly by antithrombins, and its activity is reduced as a result of absorption on fibrin. There is little danger of thrombin being absorbed into the vascular system. It has been used successfully as an adjunct for oral bleeding following dental extractions in patients with hemophilia.

Thrombin has been instilled into the stomach in an effort to hasten hemostasis in ulcerative disease, but activity is limited because of its rapid transit. In addition, thrombin becomes inactive below pH 5.0.

This compound is stable as a dry powder if stored between 2° and 8° C. In solution, it begins to lose activity within eight hours at room temperature or within 48 hours if refrigerated.

PRECAUTIONS. Thrombin should never be injected or allowed to enter large blood vessels, for there is danger of thrombosis and death within a few minutes. Antigenic reactions have occurred in animals, and allergic reactions may develop in persons sensitive to bovine material. Immunization with bovine thrombin may result in prolonged laboratory measurements of thrombin times if bovine thrombin is used in the assay, but hemostasis is not impaired (Flaherty et al, 1989). Hypotension may occur after application of bovine thrombin (Berguer et al, 1991).

Thrombin is classified in FDA Pregnancy Category C.

DOSAGE AND PREPARATIONS.

Topical (in wound or at operative site): Thrombin is dusted on as a powder, applied as a solution by flooding or spraying the site, or combined with a suitable sponge matrix (eg, absorbable gelatin sponge). The usual amount applied is 5,000 units.

Thrombinar (Rhone Poulenc Rorer). Powder (bovine origin) in 1,000, 5,000, 10,000, 20,000, and 50,000-unit containers. The 5,000, 10,000, and 20,000-unit containers are supplied with 5, 10, and 20 ml of isotonic saline as diluent, respectively; spray in 5,000, 10,000, and 20,000 unit containers.

Thrombogen (Jones Medical). Powder (bovine origin) in 1,000, 5,000, 10,000, and 20,000-unit containers. The 5,000, 10,000, and 20,000-unit containers are supplied with 5, 10, and 20 ml of isotonic saline as diluent; spray in 10,000 and 20,000 unit containers with isotonic saline as diluent.

Thrombostat (Parke-Davis). Powder (bovine origin) in 5,000, 10,000, and 20,000-unit containers with 5, 10, and 20 ml, respectively, of isotonic sodium chloride as diluent with phemerol 0.02 mg/ml as preservative.

Cited References

Recombinant factor VIII: Proceedings of the First International Symposium on Recombinant Factor VIII held on August 26, 1989 in Tokyo, Japan. *Semin Hematol* 28 (suppl 1):1-56, 1991.

Abildgaard CF, et al: Anti-inhibitor coagulant complex (Autoplex) for treatment of factor VIII inhibitors in hemophilia. *Blood* 56:978-984, 1980.

Aledort LM: Treatment of von Willebrand's disease. *Mayo Clin Proc* 66:841-846, 1991.

Avvisati G, et al: Tranexamic acid for control of haemorrhage in acute promyelocytic leukaemia. *Lancet* 2:122-124, 1989.

Bartholomew JR, et al: Control of bleeding in patients with immune and nonimmune thrombocytopenia with aminocaproic acid. *Arch Intern Med* 149:1959-1961, 1989.

Berguer R, et al: Warning: Fatal reaction to the use of fibrin glue in deep hepatic wounds: Case reports. *J Trauma* 31:408-411, 1991.

Biswas CK, et al: Acute renal failure and myopathy after treatment with aminocaproic acid. *BMJ* 281:115-116, 1980.

Blake JC, et al: Bleeding time in patients with hepatic cirrhosis. *BMJ* 301:12-15, 1990.

Bloom AL: Von Willebrand factor: Clinical features of inherited and acquired disorders. *Mayo Clin Proc* 66:743-751, 1991 A.

Bloom AL: Progress in the clinical management of haemophilia. *Thromb Haemost* 66:166-177, 1991 B.

Bona RD: von Willebrand factor and von Willebrand's disease: A complex protein and a complex disease. *Ann Clin Lab Sci* 19:184-189, 1989.

Brettler DB, et al: Use of porcine factor VIII concentrate (Hyate:C) in the treatment of patients with inhibitor antibodies to factor VIII: A multicenter US experience. *Arch Intern Med* 149:1381-1385, 1989.

Brodkin HM: Myoglobinuria following epsilon-aminocaproic acid (EACA) therapy: Case report. *J Neurosurg* 53:690-692, 1980.

Bronner MH, et al: Estrogen-progesterone therapy for bleeding gastrointestinal telangiectasias in chronic renal failure: Uncontrolled trial. *Ann Intern Med* 105:371-374, 1986.

Cattaneo M, et al: Subcutaneous desmopressin (DDAVP) shortens the prolonged bleeding time in patients with liver cirrhosis. *Thromb Haemost* 64:358-360, 1990.

Comp PC: Production of plasma coagulation factors, in Williams WJ, et al (eds): *Hematology*, ed 4. New York, McGraw-Hill, 1990, 1285-1290.

Couch P, Stumpf JL: Management of uremic bleeding. *Clin Pharm* 9:673-681, 1990.

Czer LSC, Capon SM: Clinical experience in disorders of haemostasis. *Drug Invest* 2 (suppl 5):32-44, 1990.

Czer LCS, et al: Treatment of severe platelet dysfunction and hemorrhage after cardiopulmonary bypass: Reduction in blood product usage with desmopressin. *J Am Coll Cardiol* 9:1139-1147, 1987.

De Boer WA, et al: Tranexamic acid treatment of hemothorax in two patients with malignant mesothelioma. *Chest* 100:847-848, 1991.

DiMichele DM, Hathaway WE: Use of DDAVP in inherited and acquired platelet dysfunction. *Am J Hematol* 33:39-45, 1990.

Epstein JS, Fricke WA: Current safety of clotting factor concentrates. *Arch Pathol Lab Med* 114:335-340, 1990.

Escolar G, et al: Uremic plasma after infusion of desmopressin (DDAVP) improves the interaction of normal platelets with vessel subendothelium. *J Lab Clin Med* 114:36-42, 1989.

Ewing NP, et al: Induction of immune tolerance to factor VIII in hemophiliacs with inhibitors. *JAMA* 259:65-68, 1988.

Flaherty MJ, et al: Iatrogenic immunization with bovine thrombin: A mechanism for prolonged thrombin times after surgery. *Ann Intern Med* 111:631-634, 1989.

Fricke WA, Yu MW: Characterization of von Willebrand factor in factor VIII concentrates. *Am J Hematol* 31:41-45, 1989.

Gibble JW, Ness PM: Fibrin glue: The perfect operative sealant? *Transfusion* 30:741-747, 1990.

Goldsmith GH Jr, et al: Primary pulmonary hypertension in patients with classic hemophilia. *Ann Intern Med* 108:797-799, 1988.

Guerin C, Heffez DS: Inflammatory intracranial mass lesion: An unusual complication resulting from the use of Gelfoam. *Neurosurgery* 26:856-859, 1990.

Hackmann T, et al: A trial of desmopressin (1-desamino-8-D-arginine vasopressin) to reduce blood loss in uncomplicated cardiac surgery. *N Engl J Med* 321:1437-1443, 1989.

Harder MP, et al: Aprotinin reduces intraoperative and postoperative blood loss in membrane oxygenator cardiopulmonary bypass. *Ann Thorac Surg* 51:936-941, 1991.

Havel M, et al: Effect of intraoperative aprotinin administration on postoperative bleeding in patients undergoing cardiopulmonary bypass operation. *J Thorac Cardiovasc Surg* 101:968-972, 1991.

Hay CRM, Bolton-Maggs P: Porcine factor VIIIC in the management of patients with factor VIII inhibitors. *Transfus Med Rev* 5:145-151, (April) 1991.

Hay CRM, et al: Induction of immune tolerance in patients with hemophilia A and inhibitors treated with porcine VIIIC by home therapy. *Blood* 76:882-886, 1990.

Henry DA, O'Connell DL: Effects of fibrinolytic inhibitors on mortality from upper gastrointestinal haemorrhage. *BMJ* 298:1142-1146, 1989.

Hilgartner M, et al: Efficacy and safety of vapor-heated anti-inhibitor coagulant complex in hemophilia patients. *Transfusion* 30:626-630, 1990.

Horrow JC, et al: Prophylactic tranexamic acid decreases bleeding after cardiac operations. *J Thorac Cardiovasc Surg* 99:70-74, 1990.

Horrow JC, et al: Hemostatic effects of tranexamic acid and desmopressin during cardiac surgery. *Circulation* 84:2063-2070, 1991.

Hoyle CF, et al: Beneficial effect of heparin in the management of patients with APL. *Br J Haematol* 68:283-289, 1988.

Kentro TB, et al: Clinical efficacy of desmopressin acetate for hemostatic control in patients with primary platelet disorders undergoing surgery. *Am J Hematol* 24:215-219, 1987.

Kessler CM (ed): Proceedings of a symposium: Acquired factor VIII inhibitors in the nonhemophiliac: Historical perspectives, current therapies, and future approaches. *Am J Med* 91 (suppl 5A):5A-1S-5A-48S, 1991.

Kim HC, et al: Monoclonal antibody-purified factor IX: Comparative thrombogenicity to prothrombin complex concentrate. *Semin Hematol* 28 (suppl 6):15-19, 1991.

Kobrinsky NL, et al: 1-desamino-8-D-arginine vasopressin (desmopressin) decreases operative blood loss in patients having Harrington rod spinal fusion surgery: Randomized, double-blind, controlled trial. *Ann Intern Med* 107:446-450, 1987.

Kram HB, et al: Fibrin glue achieves hemostasis in patients with coagulation disorders. *Arch Surg* 124:385-387, 1989.

Kram HB, et al: Techniques of splenic preservation using fibrin glue. *J Trauma* 30:97-101, 1990.

Kram HB, et al: Fibrin glue sealing of pancreatic injuries, resections, and anastomoses. *Am J Surg* 161:479-481, 1991 A.

Kram HB, et al: Spraying of aerosolized fibrin glue in the treatment of nonsuturable hemorrhage. *Am Surg* 57:381-384, 1991 B.

Larson PO: Topical hemostatic agents for dermatologic surgery. *J Dermatol Surg Oncol* 14:623-632, 1988.

Levinson AK, et al: Fibrin glue for partial nephrectomy. *Urology* 38:314-316, 1991.

Lian ECY, et al: Combination immunosuppressive therapy after factor infusion for acquired factor VIII inhibitor. *Ann Intern Med* 110:774-778, 1989.

Livio M, et al: Conjugated estrogens for management of bleeding associated with renal failure. *N Engl J Med* 315:731-735, 1986.

Lusher JM: Management of hemophiliacs with inhibitors, in Hilgartner M, Pochedly C (eds): *Hemophilia in the Child and Adult.* New York, Raven Press, 1989, 121-136.

Lusher JM: Pharmacology and pharmacokinetics of desmopressin in haemostatic disorders. *Drug Invest* 2(suppl 5):25-31, 1990.
Lusher JM: Thrombogenicity associated with factor IX complex concentrates. *Semin Hematol* 28(suppl 6):3-5, 1991.
Mandel MA: Autologous fibrin for blepharoplasty incisions, letter. *JAMA* 262:3271-3272, 1989.
Mannucci PM: Desmopressin: A nontransfusional hemostatic agent. *Annu Rev Med* 41:55-64, 1990.
Mannucci PM, et al: Thrombin generation is not increased in the blood of hemophilia B patients after the infusion of a purified factor IX concentrate. *Blood* 76:2540-2545, 1990.
Marder VJ: Consumptive thrombohemorrhagic disorders, in Williams WJ, et al (eds): *Hematology*, ed 4. New York, McGraw-Hill, 1990, 1522-1543.
Marder VJ, Francis CW: Clinical aspects of fibrinolysis, in Williams WJ, et al (eds): *Hematology*, ed 4. New York, McGraw-Hill, 1990, 1543-1558.
Milde LN: An anaphylactic reaction to fibrin glue. *Anesth Analg* 69:684-686, 1989.
Miller JL: von Willebrand disease. *Hematol Oncol Clin North Am* 4:107-128, 1990.
Moia M, et al: Improvement in haemostatic defect of uraemia after treatment with recombinant human erythropoietin. *Lancet* 2:1227-1229, 1987.
Montgomery RR, Hilgartner MW: *Understanding von Willebrand Disease*. New York, The National Hemophilia Foundation, 1991.
Morris CDW, et al: Epsilon-aminocaproic acid-induced myopathy: Case report. *South Afr Med J* 64:363-366, 1983.
The National Hemophilia Foundation Medical and Scientific Advisory Council (MASAC): *Recommendations Concerning HIV Infection, AIDS, Hepatitis and the Treatment of Hemophilia*. New York, The HANDI Information Center, 1991.
Nilsson IM, et al: Induction of immune tolerance in patients with hemophilia and antibodies to factor VIII by combined treatment with intravenous IgG, cyclophosphamide, and factor VIII. *N Engl J Med* 318:947-950, 1988.
Nilsson IM, et al: Noncoagulation inhibitory factor VIII antibodies after induction of tolerance to factor VIII in hemophilia A patients. *Blood* 75:378-383, 1990.
Pierce GF, et al: Use of purified clotting factor concentrates in hemophilia: Influence of viral safety, cost, and supply on therapy. *JAMA* 261:3434-3438, 1989.
Rabinovici R, et al: Convulsions induced by aminocaproic acid infusion. *DICP* 23:780-781, 1989.
Roberts HR, Jones MR: Hemophilia and related conditions: Congenital deficiencies of prothrombin (factor II), factor V, and factors VII to XII, in Williams WJ, et al (eds): *Hematology*, ed 4. New York, McGraw-Hill, 1990, 1453-1473.
Rocha E, et al: Does desmopressin acetate reduce blood loss after surgery in patients on cardiopulmonary bypass? *Circulation* 77:1319-1323, 1988.
Rodeghiero F, et al: Early deaths and anti-hemorrhagic treatments in acute promyelocytic leukemia: A GIMEMA retrospective study in 268 consecutive patients. *Blood* 75:2112-2117, 1990.
Rose EH, Aledort LM: Nasal spray desmopressin (DDAVP) for mild hemophilia A and von Willebrand disease. *Ann Intern Med* 114:563-568, 1991.
Rousou J, et al: Randomized clinical trial of fibrin sealant in patients undergoing resternotomy or reoperation after cardiac operations: A multicenter study. *J Thorac Cardiovasc Surg* 97:194-203, 1989.
Salzman EW, et al: Treatment with desmopressin acetate to reduce blood loss after cardiac surgery: Double-blind randomized trial. *N Engl J Med* 314:1402-1406, 1986.
Schwartz RS, et al: Human recombinant DNA-derived antihemophilic factor (factor VIII) in the treatment of hemophilia A. *N Engl J Med* 323:1800-1805, 1990.
Shemin D, et al: Oral estrogens decrease bleeding time and improve clinical bleeding in patients with renal failure. *Am J Med* 89:436-440, 1990.
Short HD: Paraplegia associated with the use of oxidized cellulose in posterolateral thoracotomy incisions. *Ann Thorac Surg* 50:288-290, 1990.
Sindet-Pedersen S, et al: Hemostatic effect of tranexamic acid mouthwash in anticoagulant-treated patients undergoing oral surgery. *N Engl J Med* 320:840-843, 1989.
Smith TJ, et al: Hyponatremia and seizures in young children given DDAVP. *Am J Hematol* 31:199-202, 1989.
Stel HV, et al: von Willebrand factor in vessel wall mediates platelet adherence. *Blood* 65:85-90, 1985.
Turitto VT, et al: Factor VIII/von Willebrand factor in subendothelium mediates platelet adhesion. *Blood* 65:823-831, 1985.
van Oeveren W, et al: Aprotinin protects platelets against the initial effect of cardiopulmonary bypass. *J Thorac Cardiovasc Surg* 99:788-797, 1990.
Vermeulen M, et al: Antifibrinolytic treatment in subarachnoid hemorrhage. *N Engl J Med* 311:432-437, 1984.
Weinstein RE, et al: Severe hyponatremia after repeated intravenous administration of desmopressin. *Am J Hematol* 32:258-261, 1989.
Woodman RC, Harker LA: Bleeding complications associated with cardiopulmonary bypass. *Blood* 76:1680-1697, 1990.

Other Selected References

Biological products; blood and blood derivatives; implementation of efficacy review, proposed rules. *Federal Register* 50:52602-52723, 1985.
The Other Coagulopathies. New York, The National Hemophilia Foundation, 1989.
Vitamin-K-type coagulants: Proposed bioequivalence requirements. *Federal Register* 45:14063-14067, 1980.
Aledort LM: *Current Management in the Treatment of Hemophilia: A Physician's Manual*. New York, The National Hemophilia Association, 1986.
Aronson DL: The development of the technology and capacity for the production of factor VIII for the treatment of hemophilia A. *Transfusion* 30:748-758, 1990.
Bolan CD, Alving BM: Pharmacologic agents in the management of bleeding disorders. *Transfusion* 30:541-551, 1990.
Bray GL: Recent advances in the preparation of plasma-derived and recombinant coagulation factor VIII. *J Pediatr* 117:503-507, 1990.
Brettler DB, Levine PH: Factor concentrates for treatment of hemophilia: Which one to choose? *Blood* 73:2067-2073, 1989.
Coffin CM: Potentially catastrophic bleeding disorders: Approach to diagnosis and management. *Postgrad Med* 86:217-225, (Sept) 1989.
Dietrich SL: *Comprehensive Care for People With Hemophilia*. New York, The National Hemophilia Association, 1991.
Ey FS, Goodnight SH: Bleeding disorders in cancer. *Semin Oncol* 17:187-197, 1990.
Feinstein DI: Treatment of disseminated intravascular coagulation. *Semin Thromb Hemost* 14:351-362, 1988.
Foster PA, Zimmerman TS: Factor VIII structure and function. *Blood Rev* 3:180-191, 1989.
Jones PK, Ratnoff OD: The changing prognosis of classic hemophilia (factor VIII 'deficiency'). *Ann Intern Med* 114:641-648, 1991.
Kasper CK (ed): *Recent Advances in Hemophilia Care*. New York, Alan R. Liss, 1989, vol 324.
Remuzzi G: Bleeding in renal failure. *Lancet* 1:1205-1207, 1988.

New Evaluation

ANTIHEMOPHILIC FACTOR (RECOMBINANT)
[Bioclate, Helixate, Kogenate, Recombinate]

COMPOSITION AND STORAGE. Recombinant antihemophilic factor (AHF) is a glycoprotein that is synthesized and secreted by cultured hamster (baby kidney or fetal) cells that have been transfected with the cloned human gene for factor VIII (Limentani et al, 1993). The protein is then purified from the cell culture medium using one or more chromatographic steps as well as an immunoaffinity column. The activity of recombinant AHF preparations is expressed in International Units (IU), and it is defined using the same reference standard as for plasma-derived preparations of AHF (human).

USES. Recombinant AHF is indicated in patients with hemophilia A to prevent and control spontaneous and traumatic bleeding episodes and for perioperative management (Schwartz et al, 1990; *Transfus Med Rev*, 1992; Brackmann et al, 1993; Limentani et al, 1993). The recombinant preparations also may be useful to maintain factor VIII activity at recommended levels in patients with inhibitors to factor VIII whose titers are <10 Bethesda units/ml. von Willebrand factor protein is either absent [Helixate, Kogenate] or does not function adequately [Bioclate, Recombinate]; thus, these preparations should not be used to manage patients with von Willebrand disease.

ADVERSE REACTIONS AND PRECAUTIONS. In contrast to plasma-derived factor VIII concentrates and cryoprecipitate, the transmission of blood-borne viruses and other infectious diseases has not been associated with use of recombinant AHF, since this product is not derived from human plasma. The incidence of factor VIII inhibitor antibody development in patients with severe hemophilia A (<1% of normal factor VIII levels) appears to be no greater with recombinant AHF than with plasma-derived preparations. In a prospective study, previously untreated patients with hemophilia A were monitored frequently over a median of 1.5 years while using recombinant AHF for prophylaxis or management of bleeding episodes. Inhibitory alloantibodies to factor VIII protein activity were detected in 16 of 81 individuals tested (Lusher et al, 1993); however, in 9 of the 16 patients, most of the inhibitors were present in low concentrations or disappeared completely with continued episodic treatment. Recent analyses and comparison of these data with those from studies using plasma-derived factor VIII concentrates suggest that alloantibody formation in individuals with severe or moderate hemophilia A may be a part of the natural history of the disease following exposure to replacement products, and their detection appears to depend on the frequency of testing.

Although immunologic reactions to rodent or bovine proteins are theoretically possible because of the origin of the cell lines, culture media, and monoclonal antibodies used in the manufacture and purification of these preparations, no such reactions have been reported. Allergic reactions to the human serum albumin used to stabilize recombinant AHF preparations are possible, but also have never been observed.

During clinical trials, transient, minor adverse reactions occurred after <1% of infusions. Local reactions at the site of infusion included burning, pruritus, or erythema. Systemic reactions included dizziness, nausea, vomiting, diarrhea, chest discomfort, sore throat, cold feet, metallic taste, slight hypotension, facial flushing, rash, and fever. No serious reactions have been reported.

No data are available from long-term studies in animal model systems to evaluate the carcinogenic potential of these preparations. In vitro studies have demonstrated that recombinant AHF is not mutagenic. Its safety in pregnant animals or humans has not been tested (FDA Pregnancy Category C).

PHARMACOKINETICS. Data from a comparative crossover trial in patients with hemophilia A showed that the biologic half-life of factor VIII activity was similar (approximately 14.5 hours) after infusions of Recombinate and a highly purified plasma-derived preparation [Hemofil M] (Morfini et al, 1992). In contrast, the clearance and volume of distribution were slightly smaller and the in vivo recovery of activity was slightly greater for the recombinant protein. Comparison with historical data for intermediate-purity concentrates suggests that the recombinant protein has a slower rate of clearance and a longer biologic half-life. Kogenate appears to be equivalent to plasma-derived factor VIII in the mean recovery of activity in vivo, but it has a slightly longer biologic half-life (15.8 versus 13.9 hours) (Schwartz et al, 1990).

DOSAGE AND PREPARATIONS. The lyophilized powder can be stored refrigerated (2° to 8° C) or at room temperature (<30° C). The diluent should not be frozen. If refrigerated, the powder should be brought to room temperature before reconstitution in the diluent provided and should be administered within three hours.

Intravenous: Directions for estimating the dosage and recommendations for laboratory measurements to assess the efficacy of treatment are included in the manufacturers' literature. For general guidelines, see the evaluation on plasma-derived antihemophilic factor concentrates and the Table.

Bioclate (Armour Pharmaceutical), ***Recombinate*** (Baxter Healthcare). Powder (lyophilized) in single-dose containers of approximately 250, 500, or 1,000 IU, each labeled with the amount measured in vitro and supplied with 10 ml of diluent. The reconstituted solution contains human albumin 12.5 mg/ml, polyethylene glycol 1.5 mg/ml, sodium 180 mEq/L, histidine 55 mM, polysorbate 80 1.5 mcg/IU of AHF activity, and calcium 0.2 mg/ml.

Helixate (Armour Pharmaceutical), ***Kogenate*** (Miles). Powder (lyophilized) in single-dose containers of approximately 250, 500, or 1,000 IU, each labeled with the amount measured in vitro and supplied with 2.5, 5, and 10 ml of diluent, respectively. The reconstituted solution contains glycine 10 to 30 mg/ml, imidazole ≤500 mcg/1,000 IU, polysorbate 80 ≤600 mcg/1,000 IU, calcium chloride 2 to 5 mM, sodium chloride 100 to 130 mEq/L, and human albumin 4 to 10 mg/ml.

Cited References

Proceedings of an international symposium on recombinant factor VIII. *Transfus Med Rev* 6:233-300, 1992.

Brackmann H-H, et al: Two years' experience with two recombinant factor VIII concentrates. *Blood Coagul Fibrinolysis* 4:421-424, 1993.

Limentani SA, et al: Recombinant blood clotting proteins for hemophilia therapy. *Semin Thromb Hemost* 19:62-72, 1993.

Lusher JM, et al: Recombinant factor VIII for the treatment of previously untreated patients with hemophilia A: Safety, efficacy, and development of inhibitors. *N Engl J Med* 328:453-459, 1993.

Morfini M, et al: Pharmacokinetic properties of recombinant factor VIII compared with a monoclonally purified concentrate (Hemofil M). *Thromb Haemost* 68:433-435, (Oct) 1992.

Schwartz RS, et al: Human recombinant DNA-derived antihemophilic factor (factor VIII) in the treatment of hemophilia A. *N Engl J Med* 323:1800-1805, 1990.

New Evaluation 36

APROTININ
[Trasylol]

ACTIONS. Aprotinin, a polypeptide of 58 amino acid residues with a molecular weight of 6,512 daltons, is isolated from bovine lung (Hardy and Desroches, 1992; Westaby, 1993). It is a naturally occurring inhibitor of many serine protease enzymes, including human trypsin, plasmin, and both tissue and plasma kallikrein. The mechanism by which aprotinin blocks catalysis involves reversible (ie, noncovalent) formation of enzyme/aprotinin complexes, and thus the degree of inhibition for each enzyme is a function of the aprotinin concentration and the relative affinities of the enzyme for aprotinin and its natural substrate. The inhibitory activity of aprotinin is expressed in kallikrein inactivator units (KIU). Plasmin is inhibited when the plasma concentration of aprotinin activity is ≥125 KIU/ml and plasma kallikrein is inhibited at concentrations between 250 and 500 KIU/ml (Hardy and Desroches, 1992).

The major hemostatic effect of aprotinin is probably due to its inhibition of plasmin (Hardy and Desroches, 1992; Westaby, 1993), which results in impaired fibrinolysis. Thus, fibrin clots are degraded less rapidly, and platelet dysfunction that might be caused by plasmin-mediated degradation of platelet membrane receptors is prevented.

USES. Aprotinin is used prophylactically to minimize perioperative bleeding and thus reduce exposure to the risks associated with blood transfusions in patients undergoing repeat coronary bypass graft surgery. Data from two randomized, placebo-controlled, double-blind trials on >200 such patients demonstrated that intraoperative use of aprotinin reduced the percentage of patients who required donor blood and decreased the number of units transfused per patient (Cosgrove et al, 1992; Lemmer et al, 1994).

Aprotinin also is used in those undergoing a first bypass, valve, or valve and aortic procedure who are at increased risk of bleeding or for whom transfusion is unavailable or unacceptable. It reduced the use of donor blood and decreased the need for transfusion in 151 patients undergoing a first bypass procedure (Lemmer et al, 1994). However, most surgeons reserve the use of this agent for initial cardiac surgery to patients with acute aortic dissection, systemic infection, suspected preoperative hemorrhagic diathesis, or other factors that elevate the risk of bleeding and thus the likelihood of a requirement for transfusion (Westaby, 1993). In patients without such risk factors before initial surgery, the difference in blood loss between those given aprotinin and placebo (~250 ml) may be insufficient to justify routine use of this hemostatic, since it is costly and potential risks of hypersensitivity and renal dysfunction, however minimal, are associated with its administration (see Adverse Reactions). Aminocaproic acid is a less expensive alternative that has been shown to reduce blood loss after first-time coronary artery bypass grafting in a randomized, prospective, double-blind trial (Daily et al, 1994).

Aprotinin also is used to reduce the risk of bleeding that results from preoperative use of aspirin. Patients undergoing first-time cardiac surgery (45 coronary bypass grafts and 9 valvular operations) who received aspirin within 48 hours of their operations were randomized to receive aprotinin or placebo during the surgery (Murkin et al, 1994). A significantly smaller volume of blood was lost and fewer units of red blood cells were transfused in the group receiving aprotinin.

The effects of aprotinin on perioperative blood loss and/or transfusion requirements also have been investigated in noncardiac surgical patients. Data from a randomized trial on 40 patients undergoing total hip replacement suggest that aprotinin may reduce perioperative blood loss and the need for blood transfusions during this procedure (Janssens et al, 1994). In addition, results from several studies (128 patients total) showed a beneficial effect in those undergoing orthotopic liver transplantation (Suárez et al, 1993; Ickx et al, 1993; Grosse et al, 1993); however, in one placebo-controlled randomized trial on 18 patients, the effect of aprotinin was not statistically significant (Groh et al, 1993).

ADVERSE REACTIONS. Hypersensitivity to this bovine protein is the major adverse effect (Hardy and Desroches, 1992; Westaby, 1993). Symptoms range from skin eruptions, pruritus, dyspnea, nausea, and tachycardia to fatal anaphylactic shock with circulatory failure. Although the overall incidence is only 0.1%, these reactions are more likely to occur on a second exposure to the drug. Since the likelihood of significant blood loss is greater in repeat cardiac surgery than in most first-time operations, the recommendation that aprotinin be reserved for use in repeat surgeries unless the patient is at an increased risk for bleeding during the initial procedure appears reasonable.

Data from a randomized placebo-controlled trial in patients undergoing repeat bypass surgery at a single institution suggested that aprotinin may have increased the incidence of postoperative myocardial infarction (from 9% to 17%; not statistically significant) (Cosgrove et al, 1992). In addition, postmortem examination revealed acute saphenous vein graft thrombosis in 6 of 12 patients who died after receiving aprotinin but in none of five patients in the placebo group who died. However, in a subsequent multicenter trial (Lemmer et al, 1994) and in patients who had received aspirin preoperatively (Murkin et al, 1994), no difference in the incidence of perioperative myocardial infarction was observed between those receiving aprotinin and those given placebo. Furthermore, no significant effect of aprotinin on early vein graft patency was observed in the multicenter trial and in a smaller European trial (Havel et al, 1994).

In the single-institution study, a trend toward impaired renal function (increased serum creatinine, decreased creatinine clearance) was reported among those treated with aprotinin but was not statistically significant (Cosgrove et al, 1992). In animal model studies, reversible obstruction of the proximal tubules resulting from renal drug accumulation was observed (Hardy and Desroches, 1992). In addition, some patients treated with aprotinin during aortic operations that employ deep hypothermic circulatory arrest may develop renal dysfunction and other organ damage that appears to result from disseminated microvascular platelet-fibrin thrombosis (Saffitz et al, 1993). In contrast, aprotinin did not cause a clinically significant increase in renal dysfunction in the large multicenter trial (Lemmer et al, 1994). Similarly, in a small study that specifically evaluated renal function in patients treated with aprotinin, no effect of the drug on serum electrolytes, osmolarity, creatinine concentration, or creatinine clearance was observed (Blauhut et al, 1991). Nevertheless, the potential for development of renal toxicity remains a concern, especially in patients who require moderate to deep hypothermia during cardiopulmonary bypass.

INTERFERENCE WITH LABORATORY TESTS. Because of its inhibitory effect on kallikrein, aprotinin can prolong the activated clotting time (ACT), which is used to monitor heparinization (Hunt et al, 1992; Najman et al, 1993). To avoid underestimating the amount of heparin required to prevent clotting during bypass surgery when aprotinin also is used, patients should be given standard loading doses of heparin and the need for additional amounts of heparin can be monitored using methods that are not affected by aprotinin (ie, protamine titration).

PHARMACOKINETICS. Results from an early study using radiolabeled aprotinin suggested that the plasma concentration declines bi-exponentially after administration of a bolus dose; the distribution phase half-life was 0.7 hours and the elimination phase half-life was seven hours (Kaller et al, 1978). More recent data cited in the manufacturer's literature suggest that aprotinin has a very rapid distribution phase, followed by a second phase with a half-life of 150 minutes and a terminal elimination phase with a half-life of 10 hours that begins >5 hours after administration. Aprotinin is distributed to the total extracellular space. The drug concentration in plasma is a linear function of total dose over the range of 50,000 to 2 million KIU, and the half-lives are independent of dose.

When patients undergoing cardiac surgery are given 2 million KIU each as loading and pump-priming doses, followed by constant infusion of 500,000 KIU/hr, the mean steady-state plasma concentration is 250 KIU/ml. At one-half these doses (1 million KIU each for loading and pump-priming; infusion of 250,000 KIU/hr), the mean steady-state concentration was 137 KIU/ml. Between 25% and 40% of the radioactivity from a single intravenous dose of radiolabeled aprotinin is excreted in the urine over 48 hours. Infusion of 2 million units over 30 minutes results in urinary excretion of 9% of the dose as unmetabolized parent drug; when 1 million units are infused over the same period, 2% appears in the urine as parent drug. Studies in animal models suggest that the drug is filtered by the glomeruli and reabsorbed by the proximal tubules. Aprotinin accumulates and undergoes slow enzymatic degradation in the phagolysosomes of the renal tubular cells.

DOSAGE AND PREPARATIONS. All intravenous doses of aprotinin should be administered through a central line. A 1-ml test dose (10,000 KIU) should be infused at least 10 minutes before administration of the loading dose to assess the potential for hypersensitivity reactions. In patients previously exposed to the drug, an antihistamine should be given before the loading dose.

Intravenous: To prevent excessive bleeding during cardiac surgery, a loading dose of 2 million KIU is infused over 20 to 30 minutes after induction of anesthesia but before sternotomy. An additional 2 million KIU is added to the pump priming fluid of the cardiopulmonary bypass circuit. After infusion of the loading dose, a constant infusion of 500,000 KIU/hr is maintained through a central venous catheter until completion of surgery. No other drugs should be administered through the catheter used for infusion of aprotinin. Total doses >7 million KIU have not been studied in controlled clinical trials.

Trasylol (Miles). Solution (injection) 10,000 KIU/ml (equivalent to 1.4 mg/ml) in isotonic saline in 1 million (100 ml) and 2 million (200 ml) KIU containers.

Cited References

Blauhut B, et al: Effects of high-dose aprotinin on blood loss, platelet function, fibrinolysis, complement, and renal function after cardiopulmonary bypass. *J Thorac Cardiovasc Surg* 101:958-967, 1991.

Cosgrove DM III, et al: Aprotinin therapy for reoperative myocardial revascularization: A placebo-controlled study. *Ann Thorac Surg* 54:1031-1038, 1992.

Daily PO, et al: Effect of prophylactic epsilon-aminocaproic acid on blood loss and transfusion requirements in patients undergoing first-time coronary artery bypass grafting: A randomized, prospective, double-blind study. *J Thorac Cardiovasc Surg* 108:99-108, 1994.

Groh J, et al: Does aprotinin really reduce blood loss in orthotopic liver transplantation? *Semin Thromb Hemost* 19:306-308, 1993.

Grosse H, et al: Influence of high-dose aprotinin on hemostasis and blood requirement in orthotopic liver transplantation. *Semin Thromb Hemost* 19:302-305, 1993.

Hardy J-F, Desroches J: Natural and synthetic antifibrinolytics in cardiac surgery. *Can J Anaesth* 39:353-365, 1992.

Havel M, et al: Aprotinin does not decrease early graft patency after coronary artery bypass grafting despite reducing postoperative bleeding and use of donated blood. *J Thorac Cardiovasc Surg* 107:807-810, 1994.

Hunt BJ, et al: Aprotinin and heparin monitoring during cardiopulmonary bypass. *Circulation* 86 (suppl II):II-410-II-412, 1992.

Ickx B, et al: Effect of two different dosages of aprotinin on perioperative blood loss during liver transplantation. *Semin Thromb Hemost* 19:300-301, 1993.

Janssens M, et al: High-dose aprotinin reduces blood loss in patients undergoing total hip replacement surgery. *Anesthesiology* 80:23-29, 1994.

Kaller H, et al: Pharmacokinetic observations following intravenous administration of radioactive labelled aprotinin in volunteers. *Eur J Drug Metab Pharmacokinet* 2:79-85, 1978.

Lemmer JH Jr, et al: Aprotinin for coronary bypass operations: Efficacy, safety, and influence on early saphenous vein graft patency: A multicenter, randomized, double-blind, placebo-controlled study. *J Thorac Cardiovasc Surg* 107:543-553, 1994.

Murkin JM, et al: Aprotinin significantly decreases bleeding and transfusion requirements in patients receiving aspirin and undergoing cardiac operations. *J Thorac Cardiovasc Surg* 107:554-561, 1994.

Najman DM, et al: Effects of aprotinin on anticoagulant monitoring: Implications in cardiovascular surgery. *Ann Thorac Surg* 55:662-666, 1993.

Saffitz JE, et al: Disseminated intravascular coagulation after administration of aprotinin in combination with deep hypothermic circulatory arrest. *Am J Cardiol* 72:1080-1082, 1993.

Suárez M, et al: Effectiveness of aprotinin in orthotopic liver transplantation. *Semin Thromb Hemost* 19:292-296, 1993.

Westaby S: Aprotinin in perspective. *Ann Thorac Surg* 55:1033-1041, 1993.

Diuretics

Diuretics reduce the volume of extracellular fluid and thereby prevent or alleviate edema. They enhance the urinary excretion of salt and secondarily of water by directly or indirectly impairing sodium chloride reabsorption in the renal tubules. The resulting diuresis is influenced by the drug's site of action in the nephron and, to a lesser extent, by hemodynamic and hormonal regulatory mechanisms that promote the reabsorption of sodium, other ions, and water. The selection and proper use of a diuretic require familiarity with the renal regulation of salt and water balance and with the site and mechanism of action of the different classes of diuretics.

SITE AND MECHANISM OF ACTION OF DIURETICS

All diuretics interfere with sodium chloride reabsorption in the renal tubules but, because they act at different sites, each class has distinctive effects on the pattern of electrolyte excretion, acid-base balance, and the concentrating and diluting capacities of the kidney (see Table 1). Most clinically useful diuretics act from within the renal tubule to inhibit sodium transport mechanisms in the luminal membrane.

Loop Diuretics and Thiazides: The *loop diuretics*, furosemide [Lasix], ethacrynic acid [Edecrin], and bumetanide [Bumex], block sodium chloride reabsorption in both the medullary and cortical portions of the thick ascending limb of Henle's loop by interfering with the chloride binding site of the 1 Na^+, 1 K^+, 2 Cl^- cotransport system. This action reduces the osmotic gradient in the renal medulla and impairs both the concentrating and diluting capacities of the kidney.

Thiazide-type diuretics block the reabsorption of sodium chloride in the cortical thick ascending limb of Henle's loop and the early distal tubule (cortical diluting segment). These diuretics thus interfere with urinary dilution but do not affect the concentrating mechanism.

Thiazides and loop diuretics increase the rate of delivery of tubular fluid and electrolytes to the distal sites of hydrogen and potassium ion secretion, while plasma volume contraction increases the production of aldosterone via the renin-angiotensin-aldosterone system (secondary hyperaldosteronism). The combination of increased delivery and high aldosterone levels promotes sodium reabsorption at the distal sites and thus increases the loss of potassium and hydrogen ions. Loop diuretics also interfere with potassium reabsorption in the thick ascending limb. These changes may be associated with transient hypokalemia and mild hypochloremic alkalosis with or without an effective diuresis. The reduction in extracellular fluid volume activates compensatory mechanisms that increase sodium reabsorption in the proximal tubules, thereby limiting the amount of sodium reaching the distal sites.

Potassium-Sparing Diuretics: Spironolactone [Aldactone] and its related steroids, triamterene [Dyrenium], and amiloride [Midamor] interfere with sodium reabsorption in the cortical collecting duct, thereby promoting sodium excretion while conserving potassium. Spironolactone is a competitive antagonist of aldosterone; triamterene and amiloride interfere directly with electrolyte transport. Amiloride (which also acts in the late distal convoluted tubule) prevents sodium from gaining access to the sodium pump by blocking the sodium channel at the apical membrane. High concentrations of amiloride also interfere with the Na^+/H^+ antiporter in the proximal tubule. The potassium-sparing agents are not potent diuretics when used alone because of the small volume of tubular fluid reaching their sites of action. When given with a more proximally acting diuretic, they reduce potassium loss, enhance sodium excretion, and minimize alkalosis.

Osmotic Diuretics: These agents are believed to produce diuresis by more than one mechanism, and species differences have been noted (Buerkert et al, 1981; Lang, 1987). Mannitol [Osmitrol], the most widely used osmotic diuretic, is freely filtered at the glomerulus and is not reabsorbed or secreted by the renal tubules. Because of its osmotic action, mannitol decreases reabsorption of water in the proximal tu-

TABLE 1.
SITE AND MECHANISM OF ACTION OF DIURETICS

Drug	Major Site of Action	Mechanism of Action
Thiazide	Cortical thick ascending limb of loop of Henle and early distal tubule	Inhibition of sodium chloride reabsorption
Loop	Medullary and cortical thick ascending limb of loop of Henle	Inhibition of luminal cotransport system (1 Na^+, 1 K^+, 2 Cl^-)
Potassium-sparing	Cortical collecting tubule	Inhibition of sodium reabsorption and potassium secretion by competitive antagonism of aldosterone (spironolactone) or by direct action (triamterene and amiloride) on sodium entry across the luminal membrane.
Osmotic	(1) Proximal tubule	Inhibition of sodium and water reabsorption by osmotic action
	(2) Loop of Henle	Inhibition of sodium and water reabsorption by reduction in medullary hypertonicity
	(3) Collecting tubule	Inhibition of sodium and water reabsorption because of papillary washout, high flow rate, or other factors
Carbonic Anhydrase Inhibitor	Early proximal convoluted tubule	Inhibition of sodium bicarbonate reabsorption

bule and descending limb of Henle's loop, which results in a secondary reduction in sodium reabsorption. Mannitol also reduces medullary hypertonicity by increasing medullary blood flow. Sodium and water reabsorption in the collecting tubule is subsequently reduced because of papillary washout (and loss of concentration gradient), high flow rate, or other factors.

Carbonic Anhydrase Inhibitors: Carbonic anhydrase inhibitors (eg, acetazolamide [Diamox]) enhance sodium excretion by reducing sodium bicarbonate reabsorption in the early proximal convoluted tubule. Passive sodium chloride reabsorption in the late proximal convoluted tubule is consequently decreased, but excess chloride (with accompanying sodium) is subsequently reabsorbed in the loop of Henle. Thus, mainly sodium bicarbonate rather than sodium chloride is excreted and the total diuretic effect is minimal. Potassium excretion is increased during initial therapy with carbonic anhydrase inhibitors due to the increased distal tubular flow rate and sodium concentration, the elevated pH of the tubular fluid, and possibly the presence of a nonreabsorbable anion (bicarbonate) in the distal tubular fluid (which increases electronegativity of the tubular lumen). Clinically significant hypokalemia is seldom a problem, because excess hydrogen ions in the extracellular fluid tend to diffuse into the cells and displace potassium ions, which move into the extracellular compartment. After several days of continuous administration, a mild hyperchloremic acidosis develops, which decreases the diuretic effect.

MAJOR USES OF DIURETICS

Chronic Congestive Heart Failure: The kidney plays a central pathophysiologic role in congestive heart failure, and diuretics are a cornerstone of therapy to relieve symptoms (Parmley et al, 1991). By reducing the extracellular fluid volume, diuretics decrease preload and relieve pulmonary congestion and peripheral edema. They also may reduce myocardial oxygen demand by decreasing left ventricular volume and wall tension. With long-term therapy, diuretics reduce peripheral vascular resistance and thus aortic impedance.

Diuretics, digitalis glycosides (eg, digoxin), or vasodilators can be considered first-line therapy for congestive heart failure. Combinations of drugs from these classes produce maximal hemodynamic effects (Cohn et al, 1991; The SOLVD Investigators, 1991). In addition, diuretic therapy is enhanced by concomitant administration of an angiotensin-converting enzyme (ACE) inhibitor (eg, enalapril [Vasotec]), because of the ability of the ACE inhibitors to correct hypokalemia and hyponatremia and attenuate the effects of diuretics on the renin-angiotensin-aldosterone system. The hemodynamics and exercise tolerance of patients with heart failure are improved more when ACE inhibitors are added to diuretics than when a digitalis glycoside is added (Captopril-Digoxin Multicenter Research Group, 1988).

A thiazide is the preferred diuretic if renal function is well preserved. When the glomerular filtration rate (GFR) is less than 30 ml/min, a loop diuretic is preferred.

If cardiac edema is difficult to control with a diuretic and moderate doses of digitalis, the possibility of sodium abuse should be considered. "Refractory" cardiac edema often can be controlled by digitalis and a thiazide if sodium intake is restricted to 50 to 70 mEq daily. Excessive diuretic therapy is another possible cause of "refractory" edema. Intermittent (eg, three days/week) or alternate-day administration may be more effective than continuous daily treatment. The combination of metolazone [Diulo, Zaroxolyn] and a loop diuretic may be useful for initiating diuresis in patients with severe congestive heart failure. These agents act synergistically to block sodium reabsorption in the loop of Henle and early distal tubule simultaneously. If this combination is used, serum electrolyte, blood urea nitrogen (BUN), and creatinine levels should be monitored frequently.

Potassium-sparing agents (amiloride, triamterene, spironolactone) are particularly appropriate when given with a thiazide or loop diuretic to digitalized patients, because hypokalemia may predispose to or accentuate digitalis intoxication. However, in the presence of renal insufficiency, even if it is mild (plasma creatinine level more than 2 mg/dL), potassium-sparing agents should not be given without careful attention to the serum potassium level, because hyperkalemia may occur.

See also index entry Heart Failure.

Acute Pulmonary Edema: Loop diuretics such as furosemide are usually preferred for initial management of patients with pulmonary congestion following acute myocardial infarction and in severe heart failure. The beneficial effect of intravenous loop diuretics is due to rapid reduction in circulatory blood volume combined with vasodilation resulting in a decrease in the amount of venous blood returning to the heart. Although cardiac output tends to decrease transiently, symptoms improve with the reduction in pulmonary arterial pressure. The decrease in pulmonary capillary pressure reduces edema in the perialveolar tissues, thus enhancing oxygenation and lessening systemic arterial hypoxia.

Hypertension: The Joint National Committee on Detection, Evaluation and Treatment of High Blood Pressure (1988) recommended a modified stepped-care approach to treatment of chronic hypertension with the goal of maintaining the arterial blood pressure at or below 140/90 mm Hg. Diuretics are one of the four classes of drugs used in first-line monotherapy for patients with mild to moderate hypertension. In addition, a diuretic is usually the second drug added to a beta-adrenergic blocking agent, calcium channel blocking agent, or ACE inhibitor whenever monotherapy with these agents is not adequate to control blood pressure.

Diuretics initially lower blood pressure by reducing the plasma volume; their long-term effect is associated with a decrease in peripheral vascular resistance. Thiazides are used most commonly. The loop diuretics are usually reserved for patients with markedly impaired renal function unless an immediate action is required (ie, in hypertensive crisis). A potassium-sparing diuretic may be given with the thiazide or loop diuretic when hypokalemia is a problem.

Diuretics are especially effective in controlling blood pressure in the elderly. In the European Working Party on High Blood Pressure in the Elderly (EWPHE) trial (Amery et al, 1985), diuretics (hydrochlorothiazide plus triamterene) controlled blood pressure in 65% of the patients. The death rate from coronary disease also was reduced. The efficacy of diuretics in the older population was confirmed in three double-blind studies of 1,396 hypertensive patients (Freis, 1991). Diuretics are effective both for isolated systolic hypertension, which affects up to two-thirds of all individuals with hypertension aged 65 to 89 years (Wilking et al, 1988), and for diastolic hypertension. In the SHEP Cooperative Research Group (1991) trial, administration of chlorthalidone (12.5 mg/day) for an average of 4.5 years substantially lowered the mean systolic blood pressure by 11 to 14 mm Hg in 2,365 patients aged 60 to ≥80 years with isolated systolic hypertension. Treatment was as effective in those ≥80 years as in the group as a whole. The incidence of stroke was reduced by 35%, and the number of nonfatal cardiovascular events and deaths from all causes also decreased. Similar reductions in stroke occurrence and mortality from isolated systolic hypertension was reported by the Swedish Trial in Old Patients with Hypertension (STOP-Hypertension) following treatment with a thiazide diuretic or a beta blocker in 1,627 patients aged 70 to 84 years with diastolic blood pressure of at least 90 mm Hg (Dahlöf et al, 1991). Diuretics also are particularly effective in blacks.

Because diuretics can worsen hyperglycemia, they should not be prescribed for diabetic patients with hypertension.

See also index entry Hypertension and Table 3 in the chapter on Antihypertensive Drugs.

Nephrotic Syndrome: This condition is characterized by massive edema, pronounced proteinuria, and hypoalbuminemia (Cameron, 1987). Major emphasis should be placed on diagnosis so that the underlying disease process may be treated, if possible. Restriction of dietary sodium is important in managing edema. Diuretics should be considered as ancillary agents, and vigorous diuresis should be avoided. Therapy is often instituted with a thiazide, but nephrotic edema may be more difficult to control than cardiac edema, and a satisfactory diuresis often can be obtained only with a loop diuretic.

Chronic Renal Failure: Chronic renal failure is caused by progressive destruction of the nephrons, resulting in a reduced GFR (Levine, 1989; Risler et al, 1991). The severity of the signs and symptoms of uremia varies according to the number of functioning nephrons remaining in each patient.

Patients with stable chronic renal failure may remain in sodium balance on a normal salt intake but may not readily adapt to a marked deficiency or excess of dietary sodium. Management of these patients requires careful attention to salt and water balance and renal function. If a diuretic is needed to control edema or hypertension, a loop diuretic (usually furosemide or bumetanide) is preferred because thiazides are usually ineffective in patients with a GFR less than 30 ml/min. To avoid excessive sodium depletion, careful dosage adjustment is necessary, and daily diuretic therapy may not be advisable.

Potassium-sparing diuretics should not be used in patients with chronic renal failure because they may cause severe hyperkalemia.

Acute Oliguric Renal Failure: Mannitol and/or furosemide are sometimes employed adjunctively to differentiate prerenal azotemia (hypoperfusion caused by inadequate effective circulating volume) from acute tubular necrosis, but urinalysis and clinical evaluation are safer and probably are more accurate (Levinsky et al, 1981).

During renal hypoperfusion or exposure to potentially nephrotoxic drugs, expansion of the extracellular fluid volume by infusion of sodium chloride may be all that is required to prevent development of acute renal failure. Diuretics are sometimes used prophylactically to increase renal blood flow, prevent tubular obstruction, and limit the development of renal vascular congestion. The most widely used agent, mannitol, may reduce the risk of acute tubular necrosis when administered prior to or immediately after some types of renal insult (eg, during cardiovascular surgery or therapy with nephrotoxic drugs). Furosemide also has been used for prophylaxis but, if administered to volume-depleted patients, it may further reduce the effective blood volume and precipitate rather than prevent acute renal failure. Loop diuretics should not be used without concomitant maintenance of the extracellular fluid volume. If a satisfactory diuresis is achieved (in the absence of cardiopulmonary overload), fluid and solute losses must be replaced carefully to avoid hypovolemia and decreased renal perfusion. When inotropic therapy is required, dopamine [Intropin] is preferred because, when given in small doses, it dilates the renal vascular bed and may promote diuresis in the early stages of acute oliguric renal failure. If larger doses of an inotropic drug are required, it may be more beneficial to add dobutamine [Dobutrex], because large doses of dopamine cause vasoconstriction.

Furosemide may convert established acute oliguric renal failure to the nonoliguric form and, unlike mannitol, it does not cause volume expansion if it fails to produce a diuresis. Although furosemide may reduce the need for dialysis, there is no convincing evidence that this alters the underlying pathology. Although the nonoliguric form of acute renal failure has a better prognosis than the oliguric form, the value of increasing urine volume by use of a diuretic has been questioned (Tiller and Mudge, 1980).

Renal Tubular Acidosis (RTA): Proximal RTA is caused by impaired bicarbonate reabsorption in the proximal tubule leading to hyperchloremic hypokalemic acidosis. Thiazides are given in conjunction with bicarbonate and potassium supplementation to reduce extracellular fluid volume and thus enhance proximal bicarbonate reabsorption (Cogan, 1982).

Diuretics also are used in hyperkalemic hyperchloremic acidosis (Type 4 RTA). Hyporeninemic hypoaldosteronism is an important cause of this disorder in patients with diabetes mellitus, chronic renal disease, or hypertension. Furosemide may be used to lower the serum potassium level and enhance distal hydrogen ion secretion. Furosemide therapy is safer than alternative measures (such as administration of mineralocorticoids, bicarbonate, and potassium-binding resins) in patients with hypertension and/or expanded extracellular fluid volume.

Rarely, mineralocorticoid-resistant hyperkalemia and acidosis with salt retention and hypertension may be caused by enhanced reabsorption of chloride in the distal tubule. This disorder has been successfully treated with salt restriction and/or prolonged therapy with a thiazide or furosemide (Sebastian et al, 1982).

Disorders Characterized by Hypokalemic Alkalosis: Spironolactone normalizes blood pressure and corrects hypokalemia in patients with primary hyperaldosteronism. It is used preoperatively or for long-term therapy (Ganguly and Donohue, 1983).

Hypertension and hypokalemic alkalosis in Liddle's syndrome are corrected by potassium-sparing diuretics that act directly on the renal tubules (triamterene and amiloride). Spironolactone is ineffective in this rare familial disorder, which may be caused by an unidentified mineralocorticoid (Sebastian et al, 1982). Neither potassium-sparing diuretics nor other treatment modalities have been consistently effective in reversing hypokalemia and metabolic alkalosis in Bartter's syndrome, a disorder that may be caused by reduced sodium chloride reabsorption in the thick ascending limb of the loop of Henle.

Chronic Liver Disease: Severe liver disease is frequently complicated by renal dysfunction. Progressive impairment of the kidney's ability to handle sodium may lead to the formation of ascites and peripheral edema. Nausea, anorexia, weakness, discomfort, gastrointestinal bleeding, infection, encephalopathy, and renal failure also may occur independently.

Secondary hyperaldosteronism is common and usually severe in cirrhotic patients. Both the renin-angiotensin and the sympathetic nervous systems appear to be activated by intrahepatic hypertension rather than by volume-dependent mechanisms (Rocco and Ware, 1986). Spironolactone is usually preferred for initial therapy of hyperaldosteronism and is effective in 40% to 75% of patients (Frakes, 1980). If large doses are not effective, a thiazide may be given concurrently. In very resistant cases, a loop diuretic may be substituted for the thiazide, but extreme care must be taken to avoid hypovolemia and electrolyte imbalance.

The development of ascites in a cirrhotic patient marks an important turning point in the quality and length of life. These patients experience discomfort, have impaired mobility, and are at risk of bacterial peritonitis. As more fluid accumulates, respiratory distress, impaired cardiovascular function, and the formation of an umbilical hernia, which may rupture and be potentially fatal, occur.

Ascites is usually treated with bedrest, dietary sodium restriction, and diuretics. Many patients with cirrhosis and ascites retain sodium, but spontaneous diuresis usually occurs in days or weeks when sodium intake is restricted to 10 to 22 mEq daily (Rocco and Ware, 1986). If these measures are ineffective, diuretic therapy may be initiated cautiously. Initially, a diuretic that acts at distal sites (usually spironolactone) is given alone or with a thiazide. If this combination is ineffective, a loop diuretic (furosemide or bumetanide) is administered with spironolactone. Spironolactone 200 to 400 mg and furosemide 40 to 240 mg daily can result in the mobilization and excretion of ascitic fluid (up to 500 ml/day) without adverse consequences. The presence of peripheral edema protects against plasma volume contraction, azotemia, and electrolyte imbalances; therefore, patients with both edema and ascites may undergo a more rapid diuresis than those with ascites only. Once peripheral edema has disappeared, diuretic dosage should be reduced to avoid hypovolemia (Pockros and Reynolds, 1986).

In patients with refractory ascites or those who cannot tolerate diuretics, paracentesis is the next option. Ascites was controlled in all patients treated with daily removal of 4 to 6 liters of serous fluid plus infusion of albumin 40 g (Gines et al, 1988) or a single total paracentesis (6 to 8 L fluid removed) plus intravenous albumin (Tito et al, 1990). When both medical treatment and paracentesis fail, peritoneovenous shunting may be performed (Stanley et al, 1989); however, the survival rate is not altered by this procedure.

Edema of Pregnancy: A pregnant woman may experience various physiologic abnormalities, including edema and hypertension, that regress at the end of the pregnancy. The use of diuretics during pregnancy is controversial, since a reduction of plasma volume may affect the health of the fetus. Results of a meta-analysis of nine randomized trials studying the use of diuretics in more than 7,000 pregnant women indicated that maternal edema or hypertension was reduced without an increase in adverse fetal effects (Collins et al, 1985). Although they are not recommended as first-line drugs in hypertensive pregnant women, diuretics are considered safe and efficacious and can potentiate the response of other antihypertensive drugs (eg, beta-adrenergic blocking agents) in women whose hypertension predated conception or developed before midpregnancy (Working Group on High Blood Pressure in Pregnancy, 1990). (See also index entry Hypertension, Guidelines for Treatment).

Idiopathic Edema: This poorly understood condition occurs primarily in women. Treatment has included avoidance of precipitating causes (eg, prolonged standing), mild salt restriction, periods of recumbency in the afternoon, use of elastic stockings, diuretic therapy (including potassium-sparing agents), and administration of sympathomimetic amines. It must be emphasized that many cases of idiopathic edema are caused or aggravated by diuretic abuse, especially if hypokalemia ensues. Women with this disorder are often overly concerned about their weight and appearance and become habitual users of diuretics, which may be taken surreptitiously. Hypokalemia induced by thiazides or loop diuretics tends to aggravate the edema. Such patients often resist efforts to discontinue the drug because excessive sodium retention, weight gain, and edema develop for a number of days after withdrawal. Successful long-term treatment requires complete abstinence from use of diuretics, which will result in eventual re-establishment of normal sodium and water homeostasis (MacGregor et al, 1979).

Other causes of idiopathic edema that have been considered are psychiatric disturbances (Pelosi et al, 1986), fluctuations in sodium and carbohydrate intake, laxative abuse, self-induced vomiting, capillary leak of albumin, and hormonal disturbances.

Brain Edema: Elevated intracranial pressure is a life-threatening complication of severe head injuries and diseases involving the central nervous system. Acute and transient elevation of intracranial pressure (>15 mm Hg) can be produced by sneezing, coughing, and straining, but because of its short duration, no adverse effect occurs. Spontaneous elevations of intracranial pressure that range from 25 to 60 mm Hg and last 1 to 10 minutes can produce considerable ischemia and serious neurophysiologic complications. Fatalities occur when the intracranial pressure is sustained at >60 mm Hg. Symptoms of elevated intracranial pressure include headache, diplopia, vomiting, decreased vision or episodic blindness, and slowed mentation. Clinical signs include papilledema, bradycardia, bradypnea, fixed pupils unresponsive to light, flaccidity, and hypertension.

In addition to removal of excessive cerebral spinal fluid by means of an intraventricular catheter, osmotic and loop diuretics are the primary pharmacologic agents used to lower elevated intracranial pressure (Woster and LeBlanc, 1990). Since osmotic diuretics (eg, mannitol, urea, glycerin) do not cross the blood-brain barrier, an osmotic gradient is created between the intravascular compartment and the brain, resulting in a net movement of water into the blood. Mannitol is used most commonly; urea and glycerin are less desirable because of their adverse effects. Although loop diuretics (furosemide or ethacrynic acid) have no effect on the intracranial pressure when given alone, their use with mannitol produces a greater and more sustained decrease in the intracranial pressure than mannitol alone. Furosemide (0.5 to 1 mg/kg) is usually given after the osmotic diuretic, and the frequency of administration depends on the response of the patient. Because osmotic and loop diuretics can cause fluid and electrolyte imbalances, the patient should be monitored closely.

Hyponatremic States: Loop diuretics are used as an adjunct to hypertonic sodium chloride to enhance the excretion of free water in patients with acute symptomatic hyponatremia (see index entry Hyponatremia).

Acute Hypercalcemia: Loop diuretics increase the urinary excretion of calcium and are useful (in conjunction with sodium chloride infusion) for the emergency treatment of acute hypercalcemia. Furosemide has been used most commonly for this purpose. Thiazides should not be given because they may increase the serum calcium concentration. (See index entry Hypercalcemia.)

Osteoporosis: Although thiazides were able to delay bone loss and increase bone density, epidemiologic studies showed that these actions did not protect patients from sustaining hip fractures (Framingham Study Cohort [Felson et al, 1991]; Group Health Cooperative of Puget Sound [Heidrich et al, 1991]). (See index entry Osteoporosis.)

Idiopathic Calcium Urolithiasis: Since thiazides decrease urinary calcium excretion, they may prevent recurrence of calcium-containing renal calculi in patients with idiopathic calcium urolithiasis whether or not hypercalciuria is present. Loop diuretics should not be used for this purpose because they increase calcium excretion. (See index entry Urolithiasis.)

Diabetes Insipidus: The thiazides have a paradoxical antidiuretic action in patients with diabetes insipidus and are useful in both the nephrogenic and central forms. The mechanism whereby these agents reduce urine volume appears to involve mild sodium and extracellular volume depletion, which increases sodium and water reabsorption in the proximal tubules and thus reduces delivery of glomerular filtrate to the diluting segment. Amiloride has been used to treat lithium-induced diabetes insipidus. (See index entry Diabetes Insipidus.)

Acute Mountain Sickness: Acute exposure to high altitude (10,000 to 15,000 ft) or reduced oxygen partial pressure induces respiratory alkalosis, which may precipitate symptoms of acute mountain sickness (Johnson and Rock, 1988). Headache, irritability, lassitude, malaise, anorexia, nausea, vomiting, and insomnia usually develop during the first 8 to 24 hours at high altitude. Within one or two days, the body adapts by increasing the renal excretion of bicarbonate; the blood pH then returns to normal and symptoms disappear. Reticulocytosis occurs in approximately five days, and the hematocrit increases in about seven days.

Acute mountain sickness and its severe complications (pulmonary and cerebral edema) usually can be prevented or diminished by "staging" (ie, remaining at an intermediate altitude [7,000 to 10,000 feet] for two to five days before ascending to the altitude of destination) or gradual ascent (less than 1,000 feet/day above 10,000 feet) (Johnson and Rock, 1988). If these measures are not practical, drug therapy can be tried. Acetazolamide [Ak-Zol, Diamox] taken before and during initial exposure to high altitude ameliorates symptoms, presumably by inducing metabolic acidosis (Greene et al, 1981). Pretreatment with acetazolamide mimics the state of acid-base balance that normally takes five days to achieve and has decreased the occurrence of acute mountain sickness by 30% to 50% (Ellsworth et al, 1987). In acclimatized subjects climbing at high altitudes, acetazolamide improves exercise performance and reduces loss of muscle mass and body fat (Bradwell et al, 1986).

Dexamethasone, a synthetic glucocorticoid, appears to be as effective as acetazolamide and has fewer side effects.

In mild cases of acute mountain sickness, a regimen of rest, frequent small meals, avoidance of alcohol, and use of acetaminophen for headache is sufficient. In severe cases, descent is the most successful treatment, because oxygen therapy may not readily reverse the course of the syndrome. Administration of dexamethasone or acetazolamide also is recommended.

Glaucoma Therapy and Intraocular Surgery: Carbonic anhydrase inhibitors reduce intraocular pressure by decreasing the production of aqueous humor. They are used for the long-term treatment of patients with primary open-angle glaucoma and other chronic glaucomas refractory to parasympathomimetic miotics, beta-adrenergic blocking agents, and epinephrine. Carbonic anhydrase inhibitors also are administered for preoperative treatment of acute angle-closure and congenital glaucomas. However, more than 50% of patients treated with oral carbonic anhydrase inhibitors must discontinue therapy because of adverse reactions. Topical preparations, including the investigational agents, MK-417, MK-927, and MK-507, allow use of lower dosages with a corresponding reduction in adverse reactions (Hurvitz et al, 1991).

Osmotic agents are used to reduce intraocular pressure and vitreous volume rapidly prior to iridectomy and other ocular surgical procedures. They also are of temporary benefit in some secondary glaucomas. (See index entry Glaucoma.)

Hirsutism and Acne: Spironolactone has antiandrogen effects and is used in the treatment of hirsutism and acne (see index entries Hirsutism; Acne Vulgaris).

Periodic Paralyses: Acetazolamide is used prophylactically in the management of both hypokalemic and hyperkalemic periodic paralyses. It appears to act by altering muscle membrane function.

Drug Evaluations

Individual and class evaluations are presented in the following order: Thiazides and Related Compounds, Loop Diuretics, Potassium-Sparing Diuretics, Osmotic Diuretics, and Carbonic Anhydrase Inhibitors. The major indications, biochemical side effects, and adverse interactions of diuretics are summarized in Tables 2, 3, and 4.

THIAZIDES AND RELATED COMPOUNDS

The prototype thiazide, chlorothiazide, was introduced in 1958 and was the first reliable, well tolerated, orally effective diuretic. A number of derivatives and four similarly acting nonthiazide agents (chlorthalidone, quinethazone, metolazone, and indapamide) were developed subsequently. The major differences among the various agents involve dosage and duration of action (see Table 5).

ACTIONS AND USES. Thiazide-type diuretics increase the urinary excretion of sodium chloride and water by inhibiting sodium chloride reabsorption in the cortical thick ascending limb of Henle's loop and the early distal tubules (cortical diluting segment). They also increase the urinary excretion of potassium, magnesium, and, to a small extent, bicarbonate ions (the latter effect is due to their slight carbonic anhydrase inhibitory action). During long-term therapy, urinary calcium excretion is reduced.

When renal function is normal, the thiazides are often preferred for initial and maintenance therapy in patients with cardiac edema or essential hypertension. They may be given with a potassium-sparing diuretic to reduce potassium loss and enhance the therapeutic response. In addition, thiazides are used to control edema associated with corticosteroid or estrogen therapy.

Thiazide-type diuretics are usually ineffective in patients with impaired renal function (GFR less than 30 ml/min).

ADVERSE REACTIONS AND PRECAUTIONS. Thiazides may cause dizziness, weakness, fatigue, orthostatic hypotension, and leg cramps, which may reflect electrolyte imbalance. Serum sodium, potassium, chloride, bicarbonate, and magnesium levels should be determined periodically, and the lowest effective dose should be employed to avoid electrolyte disturbances. Short-acting thiazides may cause less severe electrolyte disturbances than the long-acting agents.

The serum potassium frequently falls to a level of 3.3 to 3.8 mEq/L during long-term thiazide therapy and a mild hypochloremic alkalosis also may develop. Since a further decrease in the serum potassium concentration may occur during episodes of diarrhea, vomiting, or anorexia, patients should be instructed to report any such occurrence promptly. In addition, careful consideration should be given to the effect of sodium abuse on the potassium-wasting action of diuretics. Diuretic-induced potassium loss often can be reduced by

TABLE 2.
MAJOR INDICATIONS FOR DIURETICS

Disorder	Drug	Comments
Hypertension	Thiazide-type	Preferred diuretic in patients with normal renal function
	Loop	Used when renal function is impaired or when immediate action is required
	Potassium-sparing	Used in conjunction with thiazide or loop diuretic when hypokalemia is a problem and renal function is normal
Chronic Congestive Heart Failure	Thiazide-type	Used in patients with normal renal function
	Loop	Particularly useful in patients with impaired renal function
	Potassium-sparing	Used in conjunction with thiazide or loop diuretic when hypokalemia is a problem and renal function is normal
Acute Pulmonary Edema	Loop	
Nephrotic Syndrome	Thiazide-type or loop	
Chronic Renal Failure	Loop; metolazone or indapamide may be effective in some patients	The combination of a loop diuretic and metolazone may produce a diuresis when the loop diuretic alone is ineffective. Serum electrolytes should be monitored closely.
Acute Renal Failure	Mannitol and/or furosemide	If diuresis is successful, fluid volume must be replaced carefully.
Renal Tubular Acidosis, Proximal	Thiazide-type	
Renal Tubular Acidosis, Type 4	Furosemide	
Primary Hyperaldosteronism	Spironolactone	
Chronic Liver Disease	Spironolactone alone or with thiazide or loop diuretic	All diuretics, particularly loop diuretics, should be used cautiously. Spironolactone should be avoided if renal function is impaired.
Brain Edema	Osmotic (mannitol) alone or with loop diuretic	Patient should be monitored closely
Hyponatremic States	Loop	Used as adjunct to hypertonic sodium chloride infusion
Hypercalcemia	Furosemide	Used as adjunct to isotonic sodium chloride infusion
Renal Calculi	Thiazide-type	
Diabetes Insipidus	Thiazide-type	Used with low-sodium diet
Acute Mountain Sickness	Acetazolamide	
Open-angle Glaucoma	Carbonic anhydrase inhibitor	Used for long-term therapy
Acute Angle-closure Glaucoma	Osmotic and carbonic anhydrase inhibitor	Used preoperatively
Acne and Hirsutism	Spironolactone	
Periodic Paralyses	Acetazolamide	Effective for prophylaxis of both hypokalemic and hyperkalemic periodic paralysis

TABLE 3. BIOCHEMICAL SIDE EFFECTS OF DIURETICS

Side Effect	Thiazide-type	Furosemide	Ethacrynic acid	Bumetanide	Spironolactone	Triamterene	Amiloride
Hypokalemia and Hypochloremic alkalosis	+	+	+	+	0	0	0
Hyperkalemia	0	0	0	0	+	+	+
Hyperglycemia	+	+	Rare	Rare?	0	Rare	Rare
Azotemia	+	+	+	+	+	+	+
Hyperuricemia	+	+	+	+	+	+	+
Hyponatremia	+	Rare	Rare	Rare	Rare	Rare	+*
Hypercalcemia	+	0	0	0	0	0	0

** Hyponatremia has been a particular problem with the fixed-dose combination of amiloride and hydrochlorothiazide (Bayer et al, 1986; Myers, 1987).*

TABLE 4. CLINICALLY IMPORTANT ADVERSE INTERACTIONS OF DIURETICS

Agent	Diuretic	Effect
Adrenal Corticosteroids	Thiazides Loop	Enhanced hypokalemia
Amantadine	Triamterene with Thiazide	Neurotoxicity
Aminoglycosides	Loop	Increased ototoxicity
Aminoglycosides	Loop Possibly others	Possible increase in nephrotoxicity (due to volume depletion)
Angiotensin-converting Enzyme Inhibitors	Potassium-sparing	Hyperkalemia
Beta blockers	Thiazides Potassium-sparing	Enhanced effect on blood lipid, urate, and glucose levels Hyperkalemia
Chlorpropamide	Thiazides Amiloride with Thiazide	Hyponatremia
Cholestyramine, Colestipol	Thiazides	Decrease in serum thiazide concentration
Diazoxide	Thiazides Furosemide	Hyperglycemia
Digitalis	Thiazides Loop	Increased digitalis toxicity (if hypokalemia occurs)
Hypoglycemic Agents (oral)	Thiazides	Decrease in hypoglycemic effect
Indomethacin	Potassium-sparing (including combination products)	Hyperkalemia
Indomethacin	Triamterene, Amiloride (and combination products)	Acute renal failure

(table continued on next page)

TABLE 4 (continued)

Agent	Diuretic	Effect
Indomethacin and probably other inhibitors of renal prostaglandin synthesis	Loop and, to a lesser extent, Thiazides	Attenuation of natriuretic, antihypertensive, and potassium-wasting effect of the diuretic; acute renal failure (if volume depletion occurs)
Lithium	Thiazides	Increase in serum lithium levels
Phenytoin	Furosemide	Possible decrease in natriuretic response
Potassium supplements	Potassium-sparing	Life-threatening hyperkalemia
Succinylcholine	Loop	Increased neuromuscular blocking effect
Tetracyclines	Probably all	Increased azotemia in patients with pre-existing renal disease
Total parenteral nutrition	Potassium-sparing	Metabolic acidosis
Tubocurarine	Thiazides Loop	Increased neuromuscular blocking effect
Vitamin D, Calcium products	Thiazides	Hypercalcemia

moderate sodium restriction (Ram et al, 1981), as it is accelerated by excessive sodium intake.

Corrective measures should be instituted if symptoms develop, if the serum potassium level falls below 3.5 mEq/L, or if the patient has an irritable myocardium, is receiving digitalis, or has cirrhosis. Thiazide-induced hypokalemia can be minimized by concurrent administration of a potassium-sparing diuretic. Potassium loss also can be reduced by parenteral administration of magnesium; prolonged use of oral magnesium supplements does not affect potassium balance.

The need for routine potassium replacement in healthy, ambulatory patients with hypertension has been questioned (Freis, 1986; Madias et al, 1984; Papademetriou, 1986). Mild hypokalemia is generally well tolerated and is not associated with a clinically important deficiency of total body potassium.

Thiazides increase fasting blood glucose levels and decrease glucose tolerance during long-term therapy. Thiazide-induced glucose intolerance is often attributed to potassium loss; however, concomitant therapy with triamterene does not prevent it (Amery et al, 1978). The effect on glucose tolerance is readily reversed when the drug is discontinued (Murphy et al, 1982) and is not clinically important except in patients with pre-existing or subclinical diabetes who may require an adjustment in dosage of hypoglycemic drugs. In the rare instances in which hyperglycemia is difficult to control, it may be advisable to substitute a diuretic less likely to cause carbohydrate intolerance. Ethacrynic acid appears to be the best choice.

A reversible elevation of the blood urea nitrogen level may occur during thiazide therapy. This prerenal azotemia is caused by a decrease in renal blood flow and glomerular filtration rate secondary to the reduction of blood volume induced by the diuretic. The thiazides also may directly depress renal blood flow.

Thiazides produce an asymptomatic hyperuricemia, which may be caused by decreased secretion of uric acid by the tubular cells into the lumen of the tubule or increased renal tubular reabsorption of uric acid. Diuretic-induced asymptomatic hyperuricemia does not appear to produce any long-term deleterious effects and need not be treated (Langford et al, 1987). The development of acute gouty arthritis is rare, except in patients with chronic renal failure or a hereditary predisposition to gout. Patients with a history of gout may continue to take the thiazide if colchicine or a uricosuric agent (probenecid, sulfinpyrazone) is given concomitantly.

Since thiazides block sodium reabsorption in the diluting segment of the nephron, hyponatremia may occur, especially if water intake is excessive. This complication is most commonly encountered in markedly edematous patients with severe congestive heart failure, cirrhosis, or the nephrotic syndrome who are refractory to diuretics and it is more common in women (especially elderly women) than in men.

Thiazides frequently increase the serum calcium concentration by increasing the protein-bound fraction (hemoconcentration effect). They also increase calcium absorption in the distal convoluted tubule and, by contracting the plasma volume, enhance proximal calcium reabsorption. However, true hypercalcemia (increased ionized calcium) is a rare complication that is usually associated with latent primary hyperparathyroidism. If the serum calcium level does not decrease when the thiazide is discontinued, further evaluation is necessary to rule out the presence of a parathyroid adenoma. Thiazides also may induce transient hypercalcemia in patients who are taking calcium-containing medications (eg, antac-

TABLE 5.
THIAZIDES AND RELATED DIURETICS

Drug and Chemical Structure	Usual Diuretic Dosage*	Duration of Action (hours)	Preparations
THIAZIDES Chlorothiazide	*Oral:* *Adults,* 500 mg to 1 g once or twice daily; *children,* 22 mg/kg daily in 2 doses; *infants under 6 months,* up to 33 mg/kg daily in 2 doses.	6 to 12	*Generic.* Tablets 250 and 500 mg. *Diuril* (Merck Sharp & Dohme). Tablets 250 and 500 mg; suspension 250 mg/5 ml.
Chlorothiazide Sodium	*Intravenous:* *Adults,* 500 mg twice daily.	6 to 12	*Diuril [Sodium]* (Merck Sharp & Dohme). Powder (injection) equivalent to 500 mg chlorothiazide.
Hydrochlorothiazide	*Oral:* *Adults,* initially, 25 to 200 mg once or twice daily for several days; for maintenance, 25 to 100 mg daily or intermittently. *Children,* 2 mg/kg daily in 2 doses; *infants under 6 months,* up to 3 mg/kg daily in 2 doses.	6 to 12	*Generic.* Solution (oral) 10 mg/ml; tablets 25, 50, and 100 mg. *Esidrix* (CIBA), *HydroDIURIL* (Merck Sharp & Dohme). Tablets 25, 50, and 100 mg. *Hydromal* (Hauck). Tablets 50 mg. *Oretic* (Abbott), Tablets 25 and 50 mg.
Bendroflumethiazide	*Oral:* *Adults,* initially, 5 mg daily, preferably in the morning; dose may be increased to 20 mg as a single dose or in 2 doses. For maintenance, 2.5 to 15 mg once daily or intermittently. *Children,* initially, up to 0.4 mg/kg daily in 2 doses. For maintenance, 0.05 to 0.1 mg/kg daily in a single dose.	More than 18	*Naturetin* (Princeton). Tablets 5 and 10 mg.
Benzthiazide	*Oral:* *Adults,* initially, 50 to 200 mg daily for several days, depending on the response. For maintenance, dosage is reduced gradually to minimum effective amount. *Children,* initially, 1 to 4 mg/kg daily in 3 doses. For maintenance, dose is reduced as needed.	12 to 18	*Exna* (Robins), *Generic.* Tablets 50 mg.
Hydroflumethiazide	*Oral:* *Adults,* initially, 50 to 100 mg daily; for maintenance, 25 to 200 mg in divided amounts, depending on response. *Children,* initially, 1 mg/kg daily; for maintenance, dose is adjusted as needed.	18 to 24	*Diucardin* (Wyeth-Ayerst), *Saluron* (Bristol), *Generic.* Tablets 50 mg.
Methyclothiazide	*Oral:* *Adults,* initially, 2.5 to 10 mg once daily; same dose range is used for maintenance. *Children,* 0.05 to 0.2 mg/kg daily.	More than 24	*Aquatensen* (Wallace). Tablets 5 mg. *Enduron* (Abbott), *Generic.* Tablets 2.5 and 5 mg.
Polythiazide	*Oral:* *Adults,* initially, 1 to 4 mg daily, depending on response and severity of the condition; for maintenance, 0.5 to 8 mg daily adjusted for optimal response. *Children,* initially, 0.02 to 0.08 mg/kg daily; for maintenance, dose is adjusted according to response.	24 to 48	*Renese* (Pfizer) Tablets 1, 2, and 4 mg.

(table continued on next page)

TABLE 5 (continued)

Drug and Chemical Structure	Usual Diuretic Dosage*	Duration of Action (hours)	Preparations
Trichlormethiazide	*Oral:* *Adults,* initially, 2 to 4 mg after breakfast daily or twice daily if needed; for maintenance, 1 to 2 mg once daily. *Children,* 0.07 mg/kg daily in single or divided doses.	Up to 24	*Metahydrin* (Marion Merrell Dow), *Naqua* (Schering), *Generic.* Tablets 2 and 4 mg.
RELATED COMPOUNDS			
Chlorthalidone	*Oral:* *Adults,* initially, 50 to 100 mg after breakfast daily or 100 mg on alternate days or 3 times weekly; some patients may require 200 mg. Maintenance doses should be adjusted individually. *Children,* 2 mg/kg 3 times weekly; maintenance dose should be adjusted individually.	24 to 72	*Hygroton* (Rhone-Poulenc Rorer), *Generic.* Tablets 25, 50, and 100 mg. *Thalitone* (Boehringer-Ingelheim). Tablets 25 mg.
Indapamide	*Oral:* *Adults,* initially, 2.5 mg daily. The dose may be increased to 5 mg daily.	24	*Lozol* (Rhone-Poulenc Rorer). Tablets 2.5 mg.
Quinethazone	*Oral:* *Adults,* 50 to 100 mg daily, depending on response and severity of the condition. Some patients may require as much as 150 or 200 mg daily, on alternate days, or 3 times weekly.	18 to 24	*Hydromox* (Lederle). Tablets 50 mg.
Metolazone	*Oral:* *Adults,* 5 to 20 mg daily, depending on response and severity of the condition. Doses as large as 150 mg daily may be required in patients with chronic renal failure.	12 to 24	*Diulo* (Schiapparelli Searle), *Zaroxolyn* (Fisons). Tablets 2.5, 5, and 10 mg.

**For antihypertensive doses, see index entry Thiazides, Uses, Hypertension.*

ids) concurrently and in hypoparathyroid patients taking vitamin D, particularly if renal function is impaired.

Short-term thiazide therapy may increase total cholesterol, triglyceride, and LDL-cholesterol concentrations but probably does not affect HDL levels (Ames, 1986; Ballantyne and Ballantyne, 1983). During long-term therapy, cholesterol and triglycerides tend to return to the pretreatment levels. Factors that may be associated with thiazide-induced changes in serum lipid levels have not been clearly defined, but obesity, glucose intolerance, and hyperuricemia have been mentioned. A lipid-lowering diet may prevent the increase in serum lipid concentrations.

Like other sulfonamides, thiazides may cause rashes, photosensitivity reactions, and fever. Rarely, photosensitivity has persisted after the drug was withdrawn. A dermatologic reaction to one of these drugs generally precludes the use of others, but some patients who experienced rashes with indapamide subsequently tolerated other sulfonamide diuretics (Stricker and Biriell, 1987).

Reactions that have occurred rarely with specific thiazides are idiosyncratic (noncardiac) pulmonary edema (hydrochlorothiazide and chlorothiazide), severe rigor and fever, anaphylactoid reactions (hydrochlorothiazide), and episodes of acute muscle cramps followed by syncope and epileptiform movements (metolazone).

Electrolyte disturbances and thrombocytopenia have been reported in neonates whose mothers were treated with these drugs. Negligible amounts of hydrochlorothiazide and chlorothiazide are excreted in breast milk. These diuretics probably can be given safely to nursing mothers without adverse effects on the infant. Thiazides displace bilirubin from albumin and should be used cautiously in jaundiced infants.

DRUG INTERACTIONS. See Table 4.

PHARMACOKINETICS. Pharmacokinetic data are not available for all thiazide diuretics. Hydrochlorothiazide, metolazone, bendroflumethiazide, and indapamide are absorbed rapidly from the gastrointestinal tract, and their bioavailability ranges from approximately 65% (hydrochlorothiazide and metolazone) to 93% (indapamide) and 100% (bendroflumethiazide). The bioavailability of hydrochlorothiazide is increased to 75% when it is taken with food. Chlorothiazide tablets are absorbed erratically and poorly and bioavailability is not proportional to dose.

The onset of diuretic action occurs within one hour after administration of most thiazides. All are actively secreted in the proximal tubules, and their duration of action appears to be determined by the degree of protein binding and tubular reabsorption (Beermann and Groschinsky-Grind, 1980). Hydrochlorothiazide, hydroflumethiazide, and chlorothiazide are eliminated largely by renal excretion of unchanged drug, whereas bendroflumethiazide and indapamide undergo extensive metabolism. Only 7% of a dose of indapamide is excreted as unchanged drug.

DOSAGE AND PREPARATIONS. See Table 5.

LOOP DIURETICS

The loop diuretics, furosemide [Lasix], ethacrynic acid [Edecrin], and bumetanide [Bumex], block the active transport of sodium, potassium, and chloride in the thick ascending limb of Henle's loop. The loop diuretics have a much greater diuretic effect than the thiazides. Unlike the mercurial diuretics, they remain effective even in the presence of electrolyte and acid-base disturbances. Their proper use requires an understanding of the electrolyte and fluid derangements that they may induce. These potent agents are generally reserved for patients with impaired renal function, refractory edema, acute pulmonary edema, or hypertensive crises.

FUROSEMIDE

[Lasix]

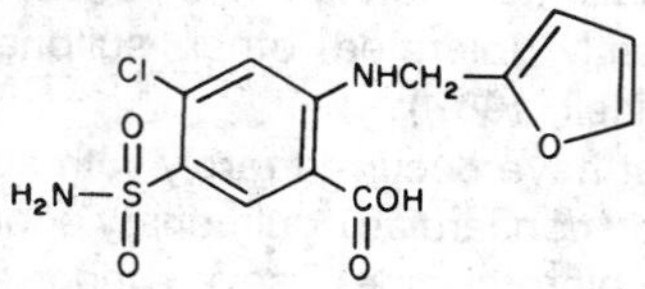

ACTIONS AND USES. Furosemide is a potent, short-acting, sulfonamide diuretic that is chemically similar to the thiazides. When administered orally, the onset of action occurs within 30 to 60 minutes and the diuretic effect lasts two to four hours; with parenteral administration, the diuretic effect is immediate and persists for about two hours. In addition to sodium and chloride, furosemide increases the renal excretion of potassium, magnesium, calcium, and, to a lesser extent, bicarbonate ions.

Furosemide is usually preferred to ethacrynic acid because it (1) is less ototoxic; (2) causes fewer gastrointestinal side effects; (3) is more convenient for intravenous use; (4) may be less likely to cause alkalosis; and (5) is available as an oral solution.

Oral furosemide is usually effective in patients with cardiac edema who do not respond to thiazides. It is of particular value in treating edema associated with impaired renal function because it is effective even when the glomerular filtration rate is greatly reduced. Although some patients with the nephrotic syndrome may respond to less potent diuretics, edema and hypertension in patients with chronic renal failure often can be controlled only with the loop diuretics; large doses may be required, but care should be taken to avoid further depletion of the blood volume. Furosemide should be administered very cautiously if at all to patients with resistant cirrhotic edema and ascites; intensive diuretic therapy may not be desirable in these individuals, especially if plasma volume is borderline.

When fluid retention is refractory to furosemide, the addition of a thiazide-type diuretic may promote diuresis. Serum electrolytes, blood pressure, and renal function should be monitored frequently during such combined therapy because massive fluid and electrolyte losses and fatal circulatory collapse may occur.

Patients with cardiogenic pulmonary edema respond rapidly to intravenous furosemide, and it is often preferred for the initial management of pulmonary congestion following acute myocardial infarction. Since relief of symptoms may precede the diuretic action, a vascular effect (ie, reduced venous tone) has been postulated. Moderate doses reverse acute pulmonary edema without depleting plasma volume (Schuster et al, 1984). Excessive diuresis should be avoided because of the danger of precipitating shock.

Furosemide also is administered intravenously to relieve pulmonary congestion and produce diuresis in patients with severe refractory chronic congestive heart failure. In these patients, clinical improvement may be preceded by a transient worsening of symptoms due to activation of neurohumoral vasoconstrictor mechanisms (Francis et al, 1985).

Intravenous furosemide is sometimes used for diagnosis and prophylaxis of acute renal failure. Administration of a loop diuretic should be preceded by careful restoration of extracellular fluid volume to avoid severe volume depletion and a further decrement in renal function. In patients with established acute tubular necrosis, furosemide may reduce the need for dialysis, but a favorable effect on the mortality rate has not been reported; the value of increasing urine flow in these patients has been questioned. If diuresis is successful, careful fluid replacement is necessary to prevent dehydration and further renal insult.

Furosemide also is given with an osmotic diuretic to relieve elevated intracranial pressure in patients with brain edema (Woster and LeBlanc, 1990).

ADVERSE REACTIONS AND PRECAUTIONS. Because of its potency, therapy with furosemide must be instituted cautiously and dosage should be individualized to avoid excessive diuresis. Overzealous therapy can cause volume depletion, hypotension, azotemia, and marked hypokalemia and hypochloremic alkalosis; therefore, it is advisable to begin therapy with small doses and increase the amount gradually if necessary. During rapid mobilization of edema, serum electrolytes should be monitored carefully and prophylactic measures may be indicated to prevent severe hypokalemia.

Serum electrolyte levels also should be determined periodically in patients receiving long-term therapy. A potassium-sparing diuretic or potassium supplements may be indicated in digitalized or cirrhotic patients. In addition, all those receiving furosemide should be instructed to report promptly any events that might further reduce the serum potassium level (eg, diarrhea, vomiting, anorexia). Like the thiazides, furosemide may cause hyperuricemia and hyperglycemia. Hyponatremia occurs much less frequently, if at all. In patients with latent hypoparathyroidism, furosemide may produce hypocalcemic tetany.

When used to prevent respiratory distress syndrome in premature newborn infants, furosemide may cause excessive volume depletion (Green et al, 1988). Urinary calcium loss induced by furosemide was reported to induce secondary hyperparathyroidism, osteopenia, and renal calcification in these infants (Hufnagle et al, 1982; Venkataraman et al, 1983); the latter complication was prevented by concurrent thiazide therapy (Hufnagle et al, 1982). Other investigators found no relationship between furosemide therapy and osteopenia in preterm neonates (Ryan et al, 1987).

Dermatologic reactions (including urticaria, erythema multiforme, photosensitivity), hematologic disturbances (agranulocytosis, anemia, thrombocytopenia), allergic interstitial nephritis, nonspecific chronic aortitis, and acute pancreatitis have been reported rarely.

Transient deafness has occurred following rapid intravenous administration of large doses and occasionally after administration of small doses and/or during oral therapy. Permanent deafness is rare. Most affected patients had concomitant renal disease or were receiving other ototoxic drugs (aminoglycoside antibiotics or ethacrynic acid). Premature infants also may be at risk.

When furosemide is used for long-term therapy of edematous conditions, rapid withdrawal may be followed by rebound edema. Spironolactone may aid in weaning these patients from furosemide (Chan et al, 1979).

Furosemide is classified in FDA Pregnancy Category C.

DRUG INTERACTIONS. See Table 4. For information on interactions between furosemide and chloral hydrate, see the chapter on Drugs Used for Anxiety and Sleep Disorders.

PHARMACOKINETICS. Food slows the rate of absorption but does not alter the total amount of furosemide absorbed. Absorption is also slowed in patients with decompensated congestive heart failure. Furosemide is 91% to 99% bound to serum albumin, but protein binding is reduced in those with uremia and nephrosis. It is eliminated largely by renal excretion of unchanged drug (50%). The half-life (90 minutes) is prolonged in newborn infants, elderly patients, and those with renal or hepatic impairment (Cutler and Blair, 1979).

DOSAGE AND PREPARATIONS.

Oral: For edema, *adults,* initially, 20 to 80 mg as a single dose, preferably in the morning. If an adequate diuretic response is not achieved, the dose may be increased gradually at intervals of six to eight hours. The effective maintenance dose varies widely and no definite upper limit has been established; however, 600 mg daily is the maximum amount recommended by the manufacturer. The frequency of administration also must be determined individually. Furosemide reaches the site of action within the tubular lumen by glomerular filtration and tubular secretion, and one or two large doses appear to be more effective than small doses administered frequently, especially in patients with renal insufficiency. Furosemide may be administered daily, on alternate days, or for two to four consecutive days per week. In some patients, intermittent therapy may be the most efficient method of mobilizing refractory edema. *Infants and children,* initially, 2 mg/kg given as a single dose. If an adequate response is not obtained, the dose may be increased gradually in increments of 1 or 2 mg/kg/dose no sooner than six to eight hours after the previous dose (maximum, 6 mg/kg).

Lasix (Hoechst-Roussel), ***Generic.*** Solution (oral) 10 mg/ml; tablets 20, 40, and 80 mg.

Intravenous: *Adults,* for acute pulmonary edema, the usual initial dose is 40 mg, which may be repeated in 30 minutes. *Infants and children,* initially, 1 mg/kg given slowly. If an adequate response is not obtained, the amount may be increased in increments of 1 mg/kg no sooner than two hours after the previous dose (maximum, 6 mg/kg). *Premature and full-term newborn infants,* 1 mg/kg given no more frequently than twice daily. (Furosemide also may be administered intramuscularly, but the intravenous route is usually preferred.)

For acute renal failure, *adults,* initially, 80 mg. The amount may then be increased until a diuretic response is obtained, but the total dose should rarely exceed 500 mg in a 24-hour period. *Large intravenous doses should be given at a rate not exceeding 4 mg/min.* If diuresis fails to ensue, the drug should be discontinued. It is important to ascertain that the plasma volume is adequate before furosemide is administered to an oliguric patient. In prerenal azotemia, even large doses may not produce a diuresis without volume replacement. If diuresis is produced, total fluid losses should be replaced every two to four hours (in the absence of edema or cardiopulmonary overload) to maintain adequate plasma volume and renal perfusion.

Lasix (Hoechst-Roussel), ***Generic***. Solution (sterile) 10 mg/ml in 2, 4, and 10 ml containers.

ETHACRYNIC ACID
[Edecrin]

ETHACRYNATE SODIUM
[Sodium Edecrin]

Cl Cl
O O
CH_3CH_2CC — OCH_2COH
CH_2

Ethacrynic acid, a derivative of aryloxyacetic acid, is a potent, short-acting diuretic with an onset and duration of action similar to that of furosemide. The two drugs have the same therapeutic applications, but furosemide is usually preferred.

ADVERSE REACTIONS AND PRECAUTIONS. The electrolyte and fluid derangements induced by ethacrynic acid are identical to those caused by furosemide, and the same precautions should be observed. Ethacrynic acid also may cause azotemia and hyperuricemia. Since hyperglycemia occurs only rarely, this drug may be preferred for use in diabetic patients.

Transient deafness (occasionally accompanied by nystagmus) has been reported, most commonly following rapid intravenous administration of large doses to azotemic or uremic patients or as a result of an interaction with other ototoxic drugs (eg, aminoglycoside antibiotics). Permanent deafness has occurred only rarely but is much more common than with furosemide.

When given orally, ethacrynic acid may cause watery diarrhea and other gastrointestinal disturbances. If these develop, the drug should be discontinued. Gastrointestinal bleeding occurred in some patients during intravenous therapy. Dermatologic reactions, jaundice, abnormal results of liver function tests, agranulocytosis, thrombocytopenia, neutropenia, Henoch-Schonlein purpura, and acute pancreatitis have been reported rarely.

This drug is classified in FDA Pregnancy Category B.

DRUG INTERACTIONS. See Table 4.

DOSAGE AND PREPARATIONS.

Oral: For edema, *adults,* initially, 50 to 100 mg daily. If an adequate response is not obtained, the daily dosage may be increased, usually in increments of 25 or 50 mg. For maintenance, the dose and frequency of administration must be determined individually. Patients with refractory edema may require 400 mg daily (usually in two divided doses); in these patients, intermittent therapy may be the most efficient method of mobilizing edema. *Children,* initially, 25 mg daily. Dosage may be increased gradually by increments of 25 mg.

ETHACRYNIC ACID:

Edecrin (Merck Sharp & Dohme). Tablets 25 and 50 mg.

Intravenous: For acute pulmonary edema, *adults,* initially, 50 mg or 0.5 to 1 mg/kg injected *slowly*; *children,* initially, 1 mg/kg. These doses may be increased if necessary.

ETHACRYNATE SODIUM:

Sodium Edecrin (Merck Sharp & Dohme). Powder equivalent to 50 mg ethacrynic acid.

BUMETANIDE

[Bumex]

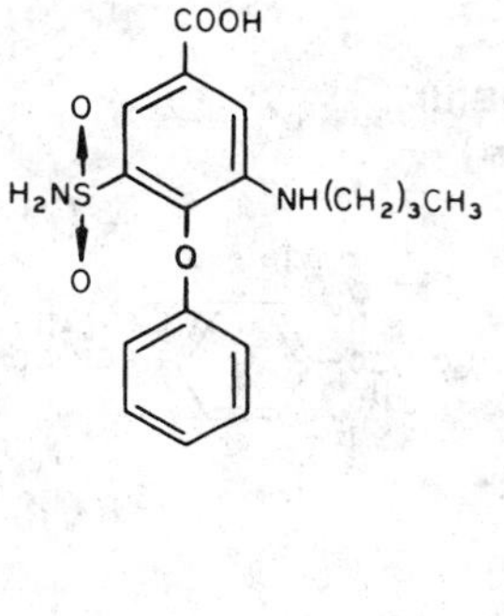

ACTIONS AND USES. Bumetanide is a metanilamide derivative. Its onset and duration of action, diuretic efficacy, and biochemical effects are comparable to those of furosemide, but bumetanide is more active on a weight basis. Given orally, 1 mg of bumetanide is equivalent to approximately 40 mg of furosemide in patients with normal renal function or to 20 mg of furosemide in patients with stable severe chronic renal failure (Voelker et al, 1987).

Oral bumetanide is useful in patients with chronic congestive heart failure, chronic renal failure, cirrhosis with ascites, and the nephrotic syndrome (Ward and Heel, 1984). In most comparative studies, it was as effective as furosemide during both short-term and long-term therapy. Bumetanide also is useful when given intravenously to treat acute pulmonary edema.

ADVERSE REACTIONS AND PRECAUTIONS. The fluid and electrolyte changes induced by bumetanide are similar to those of furosemide, and the same precautions apply (see the evaluation on Furosemide). Bumetanide also may cause azotemia, hyperuricemia, and, rarely, impaired glucose tolerance. In patients with renal failure, large doses may cause myalgia, which may be severe. Nausea, vomiting, abdominal pain, and rashes, including one case of Stevens-Johnson syndrome, have been reported. Blood dyscrasias (granulocytopenia, thrombocytopenia) have occurred rarely.

Audiometric testing has shown that the incidence of drug-related hearing loss is several times higher in patients treated with furosemide than with bumetanide (Tuzel, 1981).

This drug is classified in FDA Pregnancy Category C.

DRUG INTERACTIONS. See Table 4.

PHARMACOKINETICS. The bioavailability of bumetanide is 95%. It is 95% protein bound and the volume of distribution is 12 to 35 L. Approximately 45% of an oral dose is excreted as unchanged drug. The half-life is 1 to 1.5 hours and is prolonged in patients with renal failure.

DOSAGE AND PREPARATIONS.

Oral: *Adults,* for edema, initially, 0.5 to 2 mg as a single dose, preferably in the morning. A second or third dose may be given if required at four- to five-hour intervals. The maximal daily dose recommended by the manufacturer is 10 mg. In some patients, intermittent therapy may be the most efficient method to mobilize refractory edema.

Bumex (Roche). Tablets 0.5, 1, and 2 mg.

Intravenous: *Adults,* for pulmonary edema, initially, 0.5 to 1 mg. A second or third dose may be given at intervals of two to three hours, but the daily dose should not exceed 10 mg.

Bumex (Roche). Solution 0.25 mg/ml in 2, 4, and 10 ml containers.

POTASSIUM-SPARING DIURETICS

The potassium-sparing diuretics promote sodium excretion while conserving potassium by decreasing sodium reabsorption and potassium secretion in the collecting duct. Agents in this group include the aldosterone antagonists, spironolactone [Aldactone] and related investigational steroids (canrenone, canrenoate potassium, and mexrenoate potassium), and the direct-acting agents, triamterene [Dyrenium] and amiloride [Midamor].

Since only a small fraction of filtered sodium normally is reabsorbed at the distal sites, the potassium-sparing agents are not potent diuretics when used alone. Their major use is in conjunction with thiazide or loop diuretics. Such combined therapy reduces potassium excretion, minimizes alkalosis, and may have an additive diuretic effect. Because hypokalemia predisposes to digitalis toxicity, combined therapy is particularly useful in digitalized patients.

During long-term therapy, the potassium-sparing effect of spironolactone is equivalent to or greater than that of triamterene (Jackson et al, 1982); amiloride may be less effective in maintaining normokalemia (Zawada, 1986) but is more effective in correcting metabolic alkalosis (Ramsay et al, 1980). The potassium-sparing diuretics are better tolerated than potassium supplements and, because they block the renal regulatory mechanisms that control potassium excretion, they are more reliable than supplements in preventing diuretic-induced hypokalemia. However, normokalemia is not attained in all patients (Bayer et al, 1986; Papademetriou et al, 1985).

The dosage of potassium-sparing diuretics may be difficult to manipulate in accordance with changes in the serum potassium level, and they are more prone to cause hyperkalemia than potassium supplements, particularly when renal function is impaired. Because renal function decreases with age, potassium-sparing diuretics should be used cautiously if at all in elderly patients. The risk of hyperkalemia is increased with concomitant use of potassium supplements, salt substitutes, angiotensin-converting enzyme inhibitors, or beta blockers (Bailey, 1988).

Potassium-sparing diuretics generally should be avoided in patients with moderate to severe diabetes and mild to moderate renal insufficiency. Such patients have a defect in the renin-angiotensin-aldosterone axis. This defect, in addition to insulin deficiency, makes them particularly prone to life-threatening hyperkalemia. Those with mild diabetes, normal renal function, and a normally responsive renin-angiotensin-aldosterone system do not appear to be at risk.

SPIRONOLACTONE

[Aldactone]

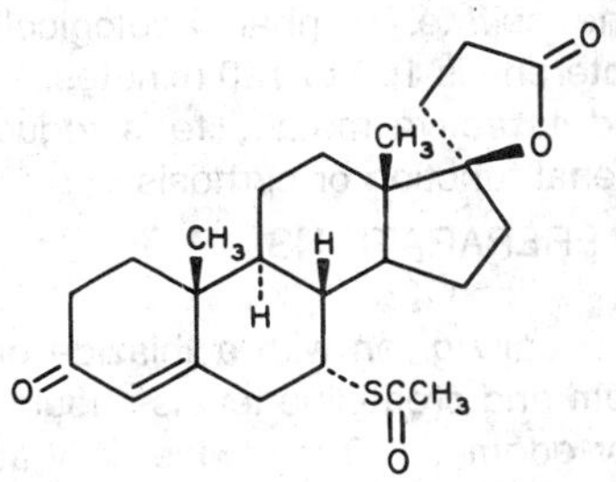

SPIRONOLACTONE AND HYDROCHLOROTHIAZIDE

[Aldactazide, Spirozide]

ACTIONS AND USES. Spironolactone is a steroid that acts as a competitive antagonist of the potent endogenous mineralocorticoid, aldosterone. Although aldosterone must be present for spironolactone to act, it need not be present in large amounts. Spironolactone has a slower onset of action than triamterene or amiloride but its natriuretic and probably its potassium-sparing effects are slightly greater during long-term therapy.

Spironolactone is used to treat edema associated with chronic congestive heart failure, cirrhosis, and the nephrotic syndrome. It is sometimes administered as the sole diuretic agent, particularly in patients with cirrhosis and ascites, but is most commonly used with a thiazide or loop diuretic.

ADVERSE REACTIONS AND PRECAUTIONS. Careful monitoring of the serum potassium level is necessary during therapy with spironolactone because hyperkalemia may occur even when a potassium-wasting diuretic is given concomitantly. Precipitating factors are a high intake of potassium (supplements, salt substitutes, or dietary) and/or impaired renal function. Spironolactone should be used very cautiously, if at all, in patients with a glomerular filtration rate less than 30 ml/min and only if the serum potassium level is monitored closely. Although spironolactone has not been shown to alter carbohydrate metabolism, it generally should be avoided in patients with moderate to severe diabetes. The concurrent use of potassium-sparing diuretics and potassium supplements and/or salt substitutes can be hazardous. Angiotensin-converting enzyme inhibitors and beta blockers also may increase the risk of hyperkalemia.

Spironolactone may increase the blood urea nitrogen level. It has little effect on serum lipid levels. Hyponatremia is rare. The serum bicarbonate concentration should be measured periodically in patients with chronic liver disease because metabolic acidosis may develop.

Daily doses of 100 mg or more often cause gynecomastia in men, which may be related to binding of the active metabolite, canrenone, to tissue androgen receptors. Decreased libido and impotence also have been reported. Menstrual disturbances and breast tenderness may occur in women. Breast cancer has developed in some patients during or after spironolactone therapy, but a cause-and-effect relationship has not been established.

Gastrointestinal disturbances occur occasionally and gastric ulceration rarely. Rashes and neurologic disturbances also have been reported. Agranulocytosis has rarely been associated with spironolactone therapy. Eosinophilia, accompanied by an erythematous macular rash, has occurred in cirrhotic patients treated with spironolactone. A possible association between spironolactone therapy and elevated liver enzyme levels was reported in a patient with primary hyperaldosteronism.

DRUG INTERACTIONS. See Table 4.

EFFECT ON LABORATORY TESTS. Spironolactone interferes with plasma cortisol determinations by the fluorometric method. Spironolactone and its metabolites may interfere with some radioimmunoassay tests for digoxin.

PHARMACOKINETICS. This drug is rapidly and extensively metabolized in the liver, and during prolonged administration approximately 25% of its activity is due to the metabolite, canrenone. Food increases the bioavailability of this active metabolite. Canrenone is 98% bound to plasma proteins and has a half-life of 10 to 35 hours. Canrenone and other metabolites are excreted in the urine and feces.

DOSAGE AND PREPARATIONS.

SPIRONOLACTONE:

The onset of action of spironolactone is relatively slow, and maximal effects usually do not occur until the third day of therapy. When discontinued, effects diminish gradually over two or three days. Spironolactone is usually given with a thiazide or loop diuretic. Serum potassium and creatinine levels should be monitored.

Oral: *Adults,* for edema associated with congestive heart failure, hepatic cirrhosis, or the nephrotic syndrome, initially, 100 mg daily in single or divided doses. Larger doses cause little additional elevation of serum potassium levels and frequently produce side effects. *Children,* 3.3 mg/kg in single or divided doses.

For cirrhotic edema and ascites, *adults,* 300 to 400 mg daily may be required. Occasionally, larger doses (800 mg to 1 g daily) have been used.

For primary hyperaldosteronism, see index entry on this disorder.

Generic. Tablets 25 mg.

Aldactone (Searle). Tablets 25, 50, and 100 mg.

SPIRONOLACTONE AND HYDROCHLOROTHIAZIDE:

The serum potassium response to spironolactone may vary in patients receiving a thiazide; therefore, this combination may not be suitable for some patients. The serum potassium level should be closely monitored.

Oral: *Adults,* for edema, one tablet one to four times daily.

Aldactazide (Searle), ***Spirozide*** (Rugby), ***Generic.*** Each tablet contains spironolactone 25 mg and hydrochlorothiazide 25 mg or spironolactone 50 mg and hydrochlorothiazide 50 mg (***Aldactazide*** only).

TRIAMTERENE

[Dyrenium]

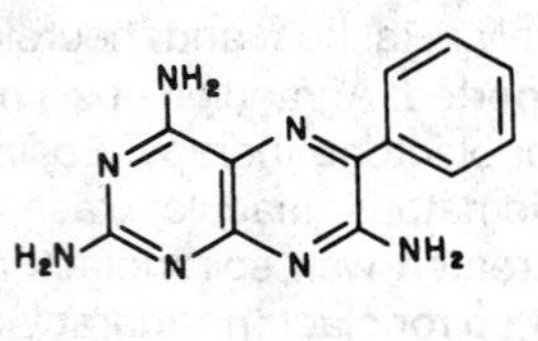

TRIAMTERENE AND HYDROCHLOROTHIAZIDE

[Dyazide, Maxzide]

ACTIONS AND USES. Triamterene is a pteridine derivative that is chemically related to folic acid. It interferes with sodium reabsorption and potassium and hydrogen ion secretion in the cortical collecting tubule by a direct action. Its tubular actions are thought to resemble those of amiloride, but triamterene has not been studied as extensively. Triamterene is given with a thiazide or loop diuretic to treat edema associated with congestive heart failure, cirrhosis, or the nephrotic syndrome. It is used primarily for its potassium-sparing effect.

ADVERSE REACTIONS AND PRECAUTIONS. Like spironolactone, triamterene can cause hyperkalemia, and the same precautions should be observed (see the evaluation on Spironolactone). Glucose intolerance and hyperkalemia may occur in patients with moderate to severe diabetes mellitus and renal insufficiency. Triamterene may increase blood urea nitrogen and serum uric acid levels. Hyponatremia is rare. Gastrointestinal disturbances, rashes, and photosensitivity occur occasionally.

Patients receiving triamterene (usually as Dyazide) have passed urinary stones composed of triamterene and a metabolite, sometimes with other constituents, such as calcium oxalate or uric acid. Although a prior episode of renal lithiasis has not been shown to increase the risk of triamterene calculi, the drug probably should be avoided in patients with such a history. Acute interstitial nephritis also has been associated with triamterene or Dyazide therapy, and nephrogenic diabetes insipidus developed in one patient taking Dyazide. Acute renal failure in patients taking Dyazide may be secondary to crystal deposition, hypovolemia, or acute interstitial nephritis, and the risk is increased by concomitant use of nonsteroidal anti-inflammatory drugs.

Megaloblastic anemia has been reported in cirrhotic patients, but a cause-and-effect relationship has not been definitely established. Anaphylactic reactions have occurred rarely.

Triamterene is classified in FDA Pregnancy Category B.

DRUG INTERACTIONS. See Table 4.

EFFECT ON LABORATORY TESTS. Triamterene interferes with the fluorescent measurement of quinidine.

PHARMACOKINETICS. Triamterene is rapidly absorbed and excreted. Its bioavailability is 52%. The onset of action of a single dose occurs within one hour and reaches a peak in two to three hours. Diuresis usually declines gradually in seven to nine hours. The urinary recovery of triamterene varies among individuals and in the same individual tested on different days. Approximately 20% is excreted unchanged and 80% is recovered as various metabolites. The major metabolite, hydroxytriamterene sulfate, is pharmacologically active. The half-life of triamterene is 100 to 120 minutes. The excretion of triamterene and its active metabolite is reduced in patients with impaired renal function or cirrhosis.

DOSAGE AND PREPARATIONS.

TRIAMTERENE:

Triamterene is usually given with a thiazide or loop diuretic. Serum potassium and creatinine levels should be monitored.

Oral: *Adults,* for edema, 100 mg twice daily after meals; the maximal dose is 300 mg daily. *Children,* 2 to 4 mg/kg daily in divided doses.

Dyrenium (SmithKline Beecham). Capsules 50 and 100 mg.

TRIAMTERENE AND HYDROCHLOROTHIAZIDE:

Combination products containing triamterene and hydrochlorothiazide vary in bioavailability and amount of each component. Both the triamterene and the hydrochlorothiazide components of Maxzide are more bioavailable than those contained in Dyazide. One formulation of Maxzide also contains a larger amount of each drug than does Dyazide (see Preparations).

Oral: *Adults,* for edema, one tablet of Maxzide or one or two tablets of Maxzide-25 MG daily or one or two capsules of Dyazide twice daily after meals. Serum potassium levels should be monitored.

Generic. Each capsule contains triamterene 50 mg and hydrochlorothiazide 25 mg; each tablet contains triamterene 75 mg and hydrochlorothiazide 50 mg.

Dyazide (SmithKline Beecham). Each capsule contains triamterene 50 mg and hydrochlorothiazide 25 mg.

Maxzide (Lederle). Each tablet contains triamterene 37.5 mg and hydrochlorothiazide 25 mg (***Maxide-25 MG***) or triamterene 75 mg and hydrochlorothiazide 50 mg.

AMILORIDE HYDROCHLORIDE
[Midamor]

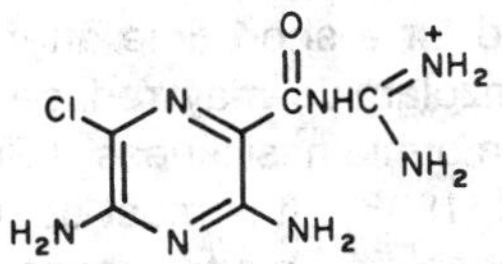

AMILORIDE HYDROCHLORIDE AND HYDROCHLOROTHIAZIDE
[Moduretic]

ACTIONS AND USES. This pyrazine derivative interferes with the epithelial sodium channel in the distal tubule and collecting duct, with a consequent reduction in potassium secretion (Frelin et al, 1987; Howlin et al, 1985; Sonnenberg et al, 1987). Amiloride is given with a thiazide or loop diuretic to treat edema associated with chronic congestive heart failure or cirrhosis. It is used primarily for its antikaliuretic effect.

ADVERSE REACTIONS AND PRECAUTIONS. Like the other potassium-sparing diuretics, amiloride may cause hyperkalemia, and the same precautions apply (see the evaluation on Spironolactone). Patients with moderate to severe diabetes mellitus and renal insufficiency may develop glucose intolerance and hyperkalemia during therapy. Amiloride also may cause azotemia and hyperuricemia. Hyponatremia has been a more common problem with the fixed-dose combination of amiloride and hydrochlorothiazide than with triamterene-hydrochlorothiazide (Bayer et al, 1986) or the thiazide alone (Myers, 1987). This has been attributed to the large amount of thiazide (50 mg) in the combination product (Bayer et al, 1986); however, a relatively high incidence of hyponatremia also occurred with an investigational mixture containing a smaller amount (25 mg) of hydrochlorothiazide (Myers, 1987).

Gastrointestinal disturbances (nausea, vomiting, anorexia, diarrhea) and dizziness also have been reported.

Amiloride is classified in FDA Pregnancy Category B.

DRUG INTERACTIONS. See Table 4.

PHARMACOKINETICS. In fasting subjects, 61% of a 10- to 20-mg dose was recovered in the urine after 48 hours. Bioavailability is decreased when the drug is given with food. Unlike spironolactone and triamterene, amiloride is excreted unchanged by the kidneys. Its half-life is six hours, but is prolonged in patients with impaired renal function.

DOSAGE AND PREPARATIONS.

AMILORIDE HYDROCHLORIDE:

Amiloride is usually given with a thiazide or loop diuretic. Serum potassium and creatinine levels should be monitored.

Oral: *Adults,* 5 to 10 mg daily.

Midamor (Merck Sharp & Dohme), ***Generic.*** Tablets 5 mg.

AMILORIDE HYDROCHLORIDE AND HYDROCHLOROTHIAZIDE:

Some investigators found amiloride to be less effective in preventing hypokalemia when given in a fixed-dose combination with hydrochlorothiazide than when the drugs were given separately in the same dosage ratio (5:50).

Oral: *Adults,* for edema, one or two tablets daily. Serum potassium levels should be monitored.

Moduretic (Merck Sharp & Dohme), ***Generic.*** Each tablet contains amiloride hydrochloride 5 mg and hydrochlorothiazide 50 mg.

OSMOTIC DIURETICS

Osmotic diuretics inhibit sodium and water reabsorption in the proximal tubule, loop of Henle, and collecting duct (Lang, 1987). With the exception of mannitol, which is used for diagnosis and prophylaxis of acute renal failure, osmotic agents are not used as diuretics. Their main clinical applications are to reduce intraocular pressure and vitreous volume prior to ocular surgery and to reduce intracranial pressure pre- and postoperatively in neurosurgical patients.

Mannitol is preferred to urea because it is more convenient to use, less irritating, less likely to cause thrombophlebitis, does not cause tissue necrosis following extravasation, is longer acting, and is safer in patients with renal failure. It is also less likely than urea to cause a rebound increase in intracranial pressure in patients with brain edema.

MANNITOL
[Osmitrol]

For chemical formula, see index entry Mannitol, In Glaucoma.

ACTIONS AND USES. By virtue of its action as a nonreabsorbable solute, mannitol prevents water reabsorption in the water-permeable portions of the nephron, which leads to a reduction in the reabsorption of sodium chloride. It also reduces medullary hypertonicity (Lang, 1987).

This osmotic diuretic is used by some nephrologists for diagnosis and prophylaxis of acute renal failure. It also is used to reduce intraocular pressure and vitreous volume prior to ocular surgery (see index entry Mannitol, In Glaucoma) and to reduce intracranial pressure temporarily in patients with brain edema. Mannitol also can be employed as adjunctive therapy to promote the urinary excretion of toxic substances.

ADVERSE REACTIONS AND PRECAUTIONS. Volume expansion and pseudohyponatremia are predictable side effects of mannitol (Lang, 1987). Headache, nausea, vomiting, chills, dizziness, polydipsia, lethargy, confusion, and sensations of constriction or pain in the chest have been observed. Too rapid administration of large amounts draws intracellular water into the extracellular space, causing cellular dehydration and marked overexpansion of the intravascular space that rarely may precipitate congestive heart failure and pulmonary edema. Fatalities have occurred after large doses. Hyperkalemia may result from movement of potassium from the intracellular to the extracellular space. Rarely, massive infusion of mannitol has caused reversible acute oliguric renal failure. Hence, renal function should be monitored closely when this agent is used in patients with severe renal impairment.

Mannitol may increase cerebral blood flow and thus the risk of postoperative bleeding in neurosurgical patients. Although mannitol crosses the blood-brain barrier less readily than urea, a rebound increase in intracranial pressure has occurred occasionally in patients with Reye's syndrome.

Anaphylactoid reactions have occurred rarely. Hemodialysis is the most effective treatment for mannitol intoxication.

Mannitol is classified in FDA Pregnancy Category C.

DOSAGE AND PREPARATIONS. Hypertonic solutions of mannitol should not be added to whole blood for transfusion because increased osmotic pressure will cause crenation and agglutination of red blood cells. The rate of administration usually should be adjusted to maintain a urine flow of 30 to 50 ml/hr.

Intravenous: To promote diuresis in oliguric patients, after restoration of plasma volume, *adults,* 100 g of a 15% or 20% solution may be given as a single dose (sometimes in conjunction with furosemide). *Children,* 750 mg/kg. If diuresis ensues, fluid losses should be replaced at two- to four-hour intervals to maintain intravascular fluid volume. Doses should not be repeated in patients with persistent oliguria, since this can cause a hyperosmolar state and precipitate congestive heart failure and pulmonary edema due to volume overload.

To prevent acute renal failure during cardiovascular and other surgery, *adults* 50 to 100 g of a 5%, 10%, or 15% solution.

To reduce intracranial pressure, *adults and children,* 1.5 to 2 g/kg of a 15%, 20%, or 25% solution infused over a period of 30 to 60 minutes.

Generic. Solution 5%, 10%, 15%, 20%, and 25%.

Osmitrol (Baxter). Solution (aqueous) 5% in 1,000 ml containers, 10% in 500 and 1,000 ml containers, 15% in 500 ml containers, and 20% in 250 and 500 ml containers.

CARBONIC ANHYDRASE INHIBITORS

Following the observation in 1949 that large doses of sulfanilamide produced diuresis in edematous patients with congestive heart failure and the recognition that the diuresis resulted from inhibition of carbonic anhydrase in the renal tubules, acetazolamide, the first orally administered sulfonamide diuretic, was introduced. Because tolerance develops rapidly, this drug and its analogues proved to be of limited value in diuretic therapy and were soon supplanted by the thiazides. Carbonic anhydrase inhibitors are now used primarily for the prevention and treatment of acute mountain sickness and as adjuncts in glaucoma therapy (see index entry Carbonic Anhydrase Inhibitors, Uses, Glaucoma).

ACETAZOLAMIDE

[Ak-Zol, Diamox]

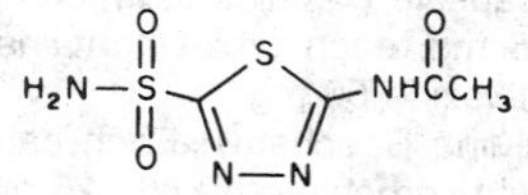

ACTIONS AND USES. Acetazolamide inhibits sodium bicarbonate reabsorption in the proximal tubule. There is no significant increase in chloride excretion and, after several days of continuous administration, a mild hyperchloremic acidosis occurs. Tolerance develops to the diuretic action in the presence of this acid-base disturbance.

Given before and for a short time after acute exposure to high altitude, acetazolamide may reduce the incidence and severity of acute mountain sickness (Greene et al, 1981; Johnson and Rock, 1988). It is most appropriate in individuals who are susceptible to acute mountain sickness and in those who must ascend rapidly. Since acetazolamide does not prevent the life-threatening complications of pulmonary and cerebral edema, it should not be used routinely as a substitute for gradual ascent (Johnson and Rock, 1988). When given to mountain climbers already acclimatized to high altitudes, acetazolamide improves exercise performance and reduces loss of muscle mass and body fat (Bradwell et al, 1986).

Hyperkalemic and hypokalemic periodic paralysis can be managed prophylactically with oral acetazolamide. This drug is postulated to act by altering muscle membrane function (increased uptake of glucose and decreased uptake of potassium). In hypokalemic paralysis, acetazolamide reduces the number of attacks as well as residual muscle weakness. Since periodic paralysis may be precipitated by hypokalemia due to renal or gastrointestinal loss, diuretic or steroid therapy, excessive licorice ingestion, or thyrotoxicosis, overall treatment should be directed toward correcting the causes if possible.

ADVERSE REACTIONS AND PRECAUTIONS. Acetazolamide may cause paresthesias, gastrointestinal disturbances, anorexia, drowsiness, fatigue, and transient myopia. The serum potassium level may fall during the first few weeks of therapy but this decrease is not sustained. No serious problems (eg, enhanced digitalis toxicity) have been associated with the initial hypokalemia.

Carbonic anhydrase inhibitors reduce the excretion of uric acid, and there is one report of exacerbation of gout during acetazolamide therapy. An acute deterioration in renal function may occur when these drugs are used in diabetic patients with nephropathy. Acetazolamide may promote formation of renal calculi by reducing the urinary excretion of citrate. A few patients have died in acute renal failure during acetazolamide therapy; a sulfonamide-like nephropathy may be involved. Urticaria, drug fever, and blood dyscrasias have occurred rarely.

DOSAGE AND PREPARATIONS.

Oral: *Adults,* to prevent acute mountain sickness, 250 mg twice daily (or 500 mg of timed-release preparation once daily) beginning one or two days before arrival at high altitude and continuing for a short time thereafter.

To prevent attacks of familial periodic paralysis, *adults,* 250 to 750 mg daily in two or three divided doses (regular preparation); *children,* 125 mg daily.

Generic. Tablets 125 and 250 mg.

Ak-Zol (Akorn). Tablets 250 mg.

Diamox (Lederle). Capsules (prolonged-release) 500 mg; tablets 125 and 250 mg.

Cited References

Amery A, et al: Glucose intolerance during diuretic therapy. *Lancet* 1:681-683, 1978.

Amery A, et al: Mortality and morbidity results from the European Working Party on High Blood Pressure in the Elderly trial. *Lancet* 1:1349-1354, 1985.

Ames RP: Effects of antihypertensive drugs on serum lipids and lipoproteins: I. Diuretics. *Drugs* 32:260-278, 1986.

Bailey RR: Adverse renal reactions to non-steroidal anti-inflammatory drugs and potassium-sparing diuretics. *Adv Drug React Bull* 131:492-495, 1988.

Ballantyne D, Ballantyne FC: Thiazides, beta blockers and lipoproteins. *Postgrad Med J* 59:483-488, 1983.

Bayer AJ, et al: Plasma electrolytes in elderly patients taking fixed combination diuretics. *Postgrad Med J* 62:159-162, 1986.

Beermann B, Groschinsky-Grind M: Clinical pharmacokinetics of diuretics. *Clin Pharmacokinet* 5:221-245, 1980.

Bradwell AR, et al: Effect of acetazolamide on exercise performance and muscle mass at high altitude. *Lancet* 1:1001-1005, 1986.

Buerkert J, et al: Role of deep nephrons and the terminal collecting duct in mannitol-induced diuresis. *Am J Physiol* 240:411-422, 1981.

Cameron JS: The nephrotic syndrome and its complications. *Am J Kidney Dis* 10:157-171, 1987.

Captopril-Digoxin Multicenter Research Group: Comparative effects of captopril and digoxin in patients with mild to moderate heart failure. *JAMA* 259:539-544, 1988.

Chan MK, et al: Diuretic escape and rebound oedema in renal allograft recipients. *BMJ* 2:1604-1605, 1979.

Cogan MG: Disorders of proximal nephron function. *Am J Med* 72:275-288, 1982.

Cohn JN, et al: A comparison of enalapril with hydralazine-isosorbide dinitrate in the treatment of chronic congestive heart failure. *N Engl J Med* 325:303-310, 1991.

Collins R, et al: Overview of randomised trials of diuretics in pregnancy. *BMJ* 290:17-23, 1985.

Cutler RE, Blair AD: Clinical pharmacokinetics of furosemide. *Clin Pharmacokinet* 4:279-296, 1979.

Dahlöf B, et al: Morbidity and mortality in the Swedish Trial in Old Patients with Hypertension (STOP-Hypertension). *Lancet* 338:1281-1285, 1991.

Ellsworth AJ, et al: Randomized trial of dexamethasone and acetazolamide for acute mountain sickness prophylaxis. *Am J Med* 83:1024-1030, 1987.

Felson DT, et al: Thiazide diuretics and the risk of hip fracture: Results from the Framingham Study. *JAMA* 265:370-373, 1991.

Frakes JT: Physiologic considerations in medical management of ascites. *Arch Intern Med* 140:620-623, 1980.

Francis GS, et al: Acute vasoconstrictor response to intravenous furosemide in patients with chronic congestive heart failure. *Ann Intern Med* 103:1-6, 1985.

Freis ED: Cardiovascular risks of thiazide diuretics. *Clin Pharmacol Ther* 39:239-244, 1986.

Freis ED: Veterans Administration Cooperative Study Group on Hypertensive Agents: Effects of age on treatment results. *Am J Med* 90(suppl 3A):3A-20S-3A-23S, 1991.

Frelin C, et al: Molecular properties of amiloride action and of its Na+ transporting targets. *Kidney Int* 32:785-793, 1987.

Ganguly A, Donohue JP: Primary aldosteronism: Pathophysiology, diagnosis and treatment. *J Urol* 129:241-242, 1983.

Gines P, et al: Randomized comparative study of therapeutic paracentesis with and without intravenous albumin in cirrhosis. *Gastroenterology* 94:1493-1502, 1988.

Green TP, et al: Prophylactic furosemide in severe respiratory distress syndrome: Blinded prospective study. *J Pediatr* 112:605-612, 1988.

Greene MK, et al: Acetazolamide in prevention of acute mountain sickness: Double-blind controlled cross-over study. *BMJ* 283:811-813, 1981.

Heidrich FE, et al: Diuretic drug use and the risk for hip fracture. *Ann Intern Med* 115:1-6, 1991.

Howlin KJ, et al: Amiloride inhibition of proximal tubular acidification. *Am J Physiol* 248:F773-F778, 1985.

Hufnagle KG, et al: Renal calcifications: Complication of long-term furosemide therapy in preterm infants. *Pediatrics* 70:360-363, 1982.

Hurvitz LM, et al: New developments in the drug treatment of glaucoma. *Drugs* 41:514-532, 1991.

Jackson PR, et al: Relative potency of spironolactone, triamterene, and potassium chloride in thiazide-induced hypokalaemia. *Br J Clin Pharmacol* 14:257-263, 1982.

Johnson TS, Rock PB: Acute mountain sickness. *N Engl J Med* 319:841-845, 1988.

Joint National Committee on Detection, Evaluation and Treatment of High Blood Pressure: The 1988 report of the Joint National Committee on Detection, Evaluation and Treatment of High Blood Pressure. *Arch Intern Med* 148:1023-1038, 1988.

Lang F: Osmotic diuresis. *Renal Physiol Basel* 10:160-173, 1987.

Langford HG, et al: Is thiazide-produced uric acid elevation harmful? Analysis of data from the hypertension detection and follow-up program. *Arch Intern Med* 147:645-649, 1987.

Levine SD: Diuretics. *Med Clin North Am* 73:271-282, 1989.

Levinsky NG, et al: Acute renal failure, in Brenner BM, Rector FC Jr: *The Kidney,* ed 2. Philadelphia, WB Saunders, 1981, vol 1, 1181-1236.

MacGregor GA, et al: Is "idiopathic" edema idiopathic? *Lancet* 1:397-400, 1979.

Madias JE, et al: Nonarrhythmogenicity of diuretic-induced hypokalemia: Its evidence in patients with uncomplicated hypertension. *Arch Intern Med* 144:2171-2176, 1984.

Murphy MB, et al: Glucose intolerance in hypertensive patients treated with diuretics; fourteen-year follow-up. *Lancet* 2:1293-1295, 1982.

Myers MG: Hydrochlorothiazide with or without amiloride for hypertension in the elderly: A dose titration study. *Arch Intern Med* 147:1026-1030, 1987.

Papademetriou V: Diuretics, hypokalemia, and cardiac arrhythmias: Critical analysis, editorial. *Am Heart J* 111:1217-1224, 1986.

Papademetriou V, et al: Effectiveness of potassium chloride or triamterene in thiazide hypokalemia. *Arch Intern Med* 145:1986-1990, 1985.

Parmley WW, et al: Congestive heart failure: New frontiers. *West J Med* 154:427-441, 1991.

Pelosi AJ, et al: Psychiatric study of idiopathic oedema. *Lancet* 2:999-1001, 1986.

Pockros PJ, Reynolds TB: Rapid diuresis in patients with ascites from chronic liver disease: Importance of peripheral edema. *Gastroenterology* 90:1827-1833, 1986.

Ram CVS, et al: Moderate sodium restriction and various diuretics in treatment of hypertension: Effects of potassium wastage and blood pressure control. *Arch Intern Med* 141:1015-1019, 1981.

Ramsay LE, et al: Amiloride, spironolactone, and potassium chloride in thiazide-treated hypertensive patients. *Clin Pharm Ther* 27:533-543, 1980.

Risler T, et al: The efficacy of diuretics in acute and chronic renal failure: Focus on torasemide. *Drugs* 41 (suppl 3):69-79, 1991.

Rocco VK, Ware AJ: Cirrhotic ascites: Pathophysiology, diagnosis, and management. *Ann Intern Med* 105:573-585, 1986.

Ryan S, et al: Bone mineral content in bronchopulmonary dysplasia. *Arch Dis Child* 62:889-894, 1987.

Schuster C-J, et al: Blood volume following diuresis induced by furosemide. *Am J Med* 76:585-592, 1984.

Sebastian A, et al: Disorders of distal nephron function. *Am J Med* 72:289-307, 1982.

SHEP Cooperative Research Group: Prevention of stroke by antihypertensive drug treatment in older persons with isolated systolic hypertension: Final results of the Systolic Hypertension in the Elderly Program (SHEP). *JAMA* 265:3255-3264, 1991.

The SOLVD Investigators: Effect of enalapril on survival in patients with reduced left ventricular ejection fractions and congestive heart failure. *N Engl J Med* 325:293-302, 1991.

Sonnenberg H, et al: Effects of amiloride in the medullary collecting duct of rat kidney. *Kidney Int* 31:1121-1125, 1987.

Stanley MM, et al: Peritoneovenous shunting as compared with medical treatment in patients with alcoholic cirrhosis and massive ascites. *N Engl J Med* 321:1632-1638, 1989.

Stricker BHC, Biriell C: Skin reactions and fever with indapamide. *BMJ* 295:1314-1315, 1987.

Tiller DJ, Mudge GH: Pharmacologic agents used in management of acute renal failure. *Kidney Int* 18:700-711, 1980.

Tito L, et al: Total paracentesis associated with intravenous albumin management of patients with cirrhosis and ascites. *Gastroenterology* 98:146-151, 1990.

Tuzel IH: Comparison of adverse reactions to bumetanide and furosemide. *J Clin Pharmacol* 21:615-619, 1981.

Venkataraman PS, et al: Secondary hyperparathyroidism and bone disease in infants receiving long-term furosemide therapy. *Am J Dis Child* 137:1157-1161, 1983.

Voelker JR, et al: Comparison of loop diuretics in patients with chronic renal insufficiency. *Kidney Int* 32:572-578, 1987.

Ward A, Heel RC: Bumetanide: A review of its pharmacodynamic and pharmacokinetic properties and therapeutic use. *Drugs* 28:426-464, 1984.

Wilking SVB, et al: Determinants of isolated systolic hypertension. *JAMA* 260:3451-3455, 1988.

Working Group on High Blood Pressure in Pregnancy: National High Blood Pressure Education Program Working Group Report on high blood pressure in pregnancy. *Am J Obstet Gynecol* 163:1689-1712, 1990.

Woster PS, LeBlanc KL: Management of elevated intracranial pressure. *Clin Pharm* 9:762-772, 1990.

Zawada ET Jr: Antihypertensive therapy with triamterene-hydrochlorothiazide vs amiloride-hydrochlorothiazide: Comparison of effects on urinary prostaglandin E_2 excretion. *Arch Intern Med* 146:1312-1314, 1986.

Drugs Affecting Water Homeostasis

38

Body fluid osmolality is maintained within a narrow range by hypothalamic osmoreceptors that regulate water intake and excretion by controlling thirst and secretion of the antidiuretic hormone, arginine vasopressin (ADH, AVP). Vasopressin and its carrier protein, neurophysin, are synthesized in supraoptic and paraventricular nuclei of the hypothalamus and transported along axons to the median eminence and posterior pituitary where they are stored in the terminal bulbs. Vasopressin is secreted in response to physiologic stimuli processed by the osmoreceptors. An increase in plasma osmolality is the most common stimulus for secretion. Vasopressin also is released by nonosmotic stimuli, including hypotension, decreased plasma volume, pain, and nausea.

The major physiologic action of vasopressin is to increase water reabsorption by the kidney. It interacts with specific receptors in the renal collecting tubules to increase tubular permeability to water and urea, thus permitting an increase in water reabsorption from the lumen. It also enhances the medullary osmotic gradient by stimulating sodium chloride reabsorption in the thick ascending limb of Henle's loop. In addition to its effect on water metabolism, vasopressin increases contractility of vascular smooth muscle and helps maintain blood pressure during hypovolemia in conjunction with the sympathetic nervous system and renin-angiotensin system (Goldsmith, 1987; Rossi and Schrier, 1986).

Two types of vasopressin receptors have been identified: V_1 (subtypes, V_{1a} and V_{1b}) and V_2. V_{1a} receptors located in vascular smooth muscle cells mediate the vasoconstrictor response to the hormone. V_{1b} receptors in the adenohypophysis are involved in release of corticotropin. The actions of V_2 receptors depend on their location. Those in the vascular endothelium increase circulating levels of factor VIII and act on platelets to increase aggregation. V_2 receptors in the renal tubules mediate the vasopressin-induced changes in permeability and transport that concentrate the urine. Dose-dependent regional vasodilation has been observed following vasopressin infusion; this response is thought to involve activation of extrarenal V_2 receptors in selected vascular beds (Hirsch et al, 1989; Suzuki et al, 1989). Vasopressin receptors, particularly those of the V_1 type, also have been described in the central nervous system and these may be important in coordinating autonomic and endocrine responses to homeostatic perturbations (Riphagen and Pittman, 1986). Vasopressin also may affect glycogenolysis through actions on the liver (Thibonnier and Roberts, 1985).

Vasopressin analogues that selectively stimulate V_2 receptors have been developed (eg, desmopressin), and specific V_1 and V_2 antagonists are in the developmental stages of investigation (Laszlo et al, 1991; Thibonnier, 1988). Potential indications for V_1 antagonists are for treatment of heart failure and hypertension. V_2 antagonists may prove to be useful for the treatment of the syndrome of inappropriate secretion of antidiuretic hormone (SIADH), hyponatremia, heart failure, cirrhosis, and nephrotic syndrome.

DIABETES INSIPIDUS

Diabetes insipidus primarily is a disorder of water metabolism characterized by excessive urination, thirst, low urine osmolality, and mild hypernatremia (Moses, 1984). It is caused by partial or complete vasopressin deficiency (central diabetes insipidus) or by inability of the kidney to respond to the hormone (nephrogenic diabetes insipidus). Clinically, diabetes insipidus may resemble primary polydipsia, a disorder in which abnormal regulation or perception of thirst leads to excessive water intake. In contrast to primary polydipsia, increased water intake in patients with diabetes insipidus reflects an appropriate response to osmotic or volume stimuli. Central diabetes insipidus caused by untreated hyponatremia can be fatal (Fraser and Arieff, 1990).

Etiology: Central diabetes insipidus may be idiopathic, familial, or acquired as the result of head trauma, neurosurgery, neoplasms, infection, granulomatous disease, or other conditions that damage the hypothalamus, pituitary stalk, or posterior pituitary. Depending on the location and extent of the lesion, vasopressin deficiency may be partial or complete and, under certain circumstances (eg, postoperatively), it may be transient. In some cases of central diabetes insipidus, particularly those caused by trauma, the thirst center also may be damaged.

Primary nephrogenic (vasopressin-resistant) diabetes insipidus is a rare X-linked disorder in which the renal response to vasopressin is absent although the hormone is secreted in adequate amounts. Resistance to vasopressin may accompany thyrotoxicosis, the nephropathies associated with hypercalcemia and severe potassium depletion, obstructive uropathy, sickle cell anemia, methoxyflurane toxicity, and renal tubular acidosis. Nephrogenic diabetes insipidus also may be induced by certain drugs, particularly lithium and demeclocycline. A form of nephrogenic diabetes insipidus with partial sensitivity to vasopressin has been described in women (Moses et al, 1984), especially during late pregnancy; it is caused by the spontaneous synthesis of vasopressinase, an aminopeptidase that degrades vasopressin, in the placenta (Durr et al, 1987; Shah and Thakur, 1988).

Essential (or adipsic) hypernatremia, a syndrome associated with osmoreceptor dysfunction, is characterized by hypernatremia, hypodipsia, and deficient vasopressin secretion. Polyuria usually does not occur, presumably because of increased renal sensitivity to vasopressin (Dunger et al, 1987).

Diagnosis: A water deprivation test may be employed to establish the etiology of polydipsia/polyuria, especially when vasopressin or one of its analogues is being considered for prolonged therapy.

The first step of the test, water deprivation, establishes an osmotic stimulus for release of endogenous vasopressin. If urinary osmolality rises after water deprivation, vasopressin is present and renal responsiveness is established. If urinary osmolality fails to increase, vasopressin is either absent (complete central diabetes insipidus) or the amount is inadequate to exert an effect (nephrogenic diabetes insipidus). Variable increases in urinary osmolality occur in patients with partial hormone deficiency. In interpreting the water deprivation test, it is important to remember that osmolality can increase from hypotonic to isotonic, even in the absence of vasopressin, if the glomerular filtration rate decreases sufficiently.

The second step is to determine the effect of exogenous vasopressin. When vasopressin is given to patients who failed to concentrate their urine in Step 1, an increase in urine osmolality (60 mOsm/kg) suggests central diabetes insipidus, whereas no change suggests the presence of the nephrogenic variant. When the hormone is given to patients who concentrated their urine in Step 1, a further increase in urine osmolality suggests partial central diabetes insipidus. If urinary osmolality rises no further, primary polydipsia is the presumptive diagnosis. Because urine osmolality may not increase in some patients with partial central diabetes insipidus, measurement of blood or urinary vasopressin by radioimmunoassay may be necessary to confirm the diagnosis.

Therapy: Central diabetes insipidus is treated by hormone replacement with vasopressin, desmopressin, or lypressin. Aqueous vasopressin [Pitressin Synthetic] is a short-acting preparation that is given intramuscularly, subcutaneously, or intravenously when brief antidiuresis is desirable (eg, for initiation of therapy following hypophysectomy, neurosurgery, or head injuries).

Intranasal desmopressin [DDAVP] is long-acting, effective, and has no significant pressor activity. It is generally regarded as the agent of choice for long-term therapy of most patients with central diabetes insipidus. The injectable form of desmopressin acetate [DDAVP Injection, Stimate], which has a longer duration of action than aqueous vasopressin, may be used for short-term replacement therapy or when conditions such as nasal congestion preclude use of the intranasal preparation. A transdermal route was tested in seven healthy volunteers (Svedman et al, 1991) and may prove to be useful for long-term desmopressin therapy after further refinement of the protocol.

Lypressin nasal spray [Diapid] may be used in those with mild to moderate central diabetes insipidus; however, its brief duration of action may result in episodes of abrupt, severe polyuria.

The orally administered nonhormonal agents, chlorpropamide [Diabinese] and clofibrate [Atromid-S], promote release of endogenous vasopressin or enhance its peripheral action (Cobb, 1984). These drugs are useful in mild to moderate partial central diabetes insipidus but may not provide adequate control in patients with severe disease. They may be given singly, in combination, or with a thiazide diuretic. Chlorpropamide and clofibrate are considered secondary therapeutic agents.

By impairing the renal excretion of free water, thiazide diuretics have a paradoxical antidiuretic action in patients with diabetes insipidus. They are rarely effective alone in the central form of the disease but are sometimes useful as sole therapy in nephrogenic diabetes insipidus when employed in conjunction with sodium restriction. Amiloride [Midamor] has been used to treat polyuria associated with lithium therapy, and it may prevent accumulation of lithium in the collecting tubule (Boton et al, 1987). Indomethacin [Indocin] and possibly other nonsteroidal anti-inflammatory agents may reduce free water clearance in the nephrogenic form of the disease (Blachar et al, 1980; Chevalier and Rogol, 1982), particularly when given with a thiazide (Libber et al, 1986). The antiepileptic drug, carbamazepine [Tegretol], has antidiuretic activity, but toxicity limits its usefulness.

Precautions: When the renal excretion of water is impaired and water intake continues, the body fluid volume expands. Water retention or intoxication with resultant hyponatremia has been observed with all forms of antidiuretic therapy. Signs and symptoms of water intoxication (ie, headache, nausea and vomiting, confusion, lethargy, ataxia, coma, convulsions) occur with movement of fluid from the extracellular into the intracellular space, particularly in the central nervous system. Patients with diabetes insipidus who have developed a pattern of excessive water drinking must limit their fluid intake when therapy is initiated. Water intoxication is most likely to be observed in patients with hypothalamic dysfunction and impaired regulation of thirst; in those receiving hypotonic fluids intravenously, especially in the postoperative period; in infants who cannot voluntarily adjust their water intake; or in patients with severe renal dysfunction. Excessive fluid intake can be a major problem in patients who are taking drugs that cause dry mouth (eg, antispasmodics, tricyclic antidepressants).

Water intoxication is managed by water restriction and temporary withdrawal of any antidiuretic agent. Administration of hypertonic sodium chloride with or without furosemide [Lasix] is necessary for symptomatic patients or those with severe hyponatremia.

For adverse drug reactions, see the following evaluations.

Drug Evaluations

ANTIDIURETIC HORMONE AND ANALOGUES

VASOPRESSIN INJECTION

[Pitressin Synthetic]

ACTIONS AND USES. Vasopressin acts on both V_1 and V_2 receptors. The units used to describe antidiuretic activity are defined by a pressor assay in anesthetized animals; vasopressin contains 20 pressor units and not more than 1 oxytocic unit per milliliter (Share, 1988).

The rapid onset of action and brief (two to six hours) antidiuretic effect produced by intramuscular, subcutaneous, or intravenous administration of vasopressin injection (aqueous vasopressin) make this agent useful for diagnosis of diabetes insipidus; for initiating therapy following hypophysectomy, neurosurgery, or head injuries; and for treating acutely ill or unconscious patients.

Antibodies to vasopressin-secreting cells have been identified in the serum of a few patients with central diabetes insipidus (Scherbaum and Bottazzo, 1983). These antibodies appear to develop during treatment with vasopressin (or lypressin) and may result in a reduced antidiuretic response to these drugs (Vokes et al, 1988). A high titer of antibodies to vasopressin without a decrease in response to the hormone also has been observed.

ADVERSE REACTIONS AND PRECAUTIONS. The vasoconstrictor activity of vasopressin is manifested at doses much larger than those usually given to treat diabetes insipidus, but even large doses elevate the blood pressure only slightly (10 to 20 mm Hg) in conscious patients. However, vasopressin may cause significant constriction of the coronary arteries. Angina, electrocardiographic evidence of myocardial ischemia, and myocardial infarction have been reported after injection of 20 units. A latent period of several hours may precede the appearance of chest pain. Ventricular arrhythmias also have occurred when vasopressin was given by the intravenous or intra-arterial route, and cutaneous gangrene has developed after peripheral infusion. Patients with ischemic heart disease should receive the minimal dose needed to control polyuria. If cardiac symptoms occur, desmopressin or an oral antidiuretic agent should be substituted.

Large doses of vasopressin (5 to 20 units) stimulate gastrointestinal smooth muscle and may produce nausea, abdominal cramps, diarrhea, and the urge to defecate. These reactions are more common in women than in men. Uterine cramps also may occur after large doses.

This drug is classified in FDA Pregnancy Category C.

DOSAGE AND PREPARATIONS.

Intramuscular, Intravenous, Subcutaneous: *Adults,* for treatment of central diabetes insipidus, 5 to 10 units (0.25 to 0.5 ml) three or four times daily; for diagnosis of polyuria, 5 units. *Children,* for treatment, 2.5 to 10 units (0.125 to 0.5 ml) three or four times daily.

Pitressin Synthetic (Parke-Davis). Solution (sterile) 10 pressor units in 0.5 ml containers and 20 pressor units in 1 ml containers.

DESMOPRESSIN ACETATE

[DDAVP, DDAVP Injection, Stimate]

ACTIONS AND USES. This vasopressin analogue has a greater affinity for V_2 than V_1 receptors (Richardson and Robinson, 1985). Structural alterations of the naturally occurring human hormone, arginine vasopressin, to desmopressin have increased the antidiuretic/pressor ratio from 0.9 to 2,000 and may prolong the duration of action to 20 hours. In normal individuals and patients with central diabetes insipidus, desmopressin decreases peripheral vascular resistance and blood pressure and increases heart rate, plasma renin activity, and release of factor VIIIc and von Willebrand factor in addition to its antidiuretic action. These changes do not occur in patients with congenital nephrogenic diabetes insipidus (Bichet et al, 1988).

Intranasal desmopressin is generally regarded as the agent of choice for long-term treatment of adults and children with central diabetes insipidus. It is considerably longer acting than lypressin. After a single dose, the antidiuretic effect persists for 8 to 20 hours, whereas the duration of action of lypressin is only three to four hours (Cobb, 1984; Richardson and Robinson, 1985).

Desmopressin usually is not effective in nephrogenic diabetes insipidus, but large doses (20 to 40 mcg) of the nasal spray applied every four hours may be useful in treating women with a variant of the disorder who exhibit partial responsiveness to vasopressin. Combination therapy with indomethacin and desmopressin is effective in some patients with lithium-induced nephrogenic diabetes insipidus (Allen et al, 1989).

The injectable form of desmopressin is a suitable alternative to aqueous vasopressin for use after head trauma or surgery. It also may be substituted for the intranasal preparation when upper respiratory infection, allergy, or changes in the nasal mucosa impair absorption of the latter.

Desmopressin has commonly been used to evaluate renal concentrating capacity.

ADVERSE REACTIONS AND PRECAUTIONS. Desmopressin is well tolerated. Large doses may cause headache and nausea, which disappear upon reduction of the dose. Nasal congestion, mild abdominal cramps, and vulval pain have occurred rarely. Fluid intake should be limited during therapy to avoid hyponatremia and water intoxication, particularly in infants or elderly patients. Although the safety of desmopressin during pregnancy has not been definitely established, no adverse effects were reported in several pregnant women given the drug (FDA Pregnancy Category B).

A transient (one to two day) reduction in the duration of response to intranasal desmopressin has been noted occasionally and may be associated with nasal congestion or with periods of increased physical activity. Rarely, resistance has developed after prolonged therapy (Cobb, 1984). When resistance develops, the addition of an oral antidiuretic agent to the regimen may be beneficial.

DOSAGE AND PREPARATIONS.

Topical (intranasal): Desmopressin is administered as a spray or through a flexible calibrated nasal tube. Therapy should be initiated with a small dose; the amount is then adjusted on the basis of changes in urine volume and osmolality and control of nocturia. For central diabetes insipidus, the usual dose for *adults* is 0.1 ml twice daily (range, 0.1 to 0.4 ml daily as a single dose or divided into two or three doses). For *children 3 months to 12 years,* the usual dosage range is 0.05 to 0.3 ml daily as a single dose or in two divided doses.

DDAVP (Rhone-Poulenc Rorer). Solution (for intranasal administration) 0.1 mg/ml in 2.5 ml containers with two nasal tubes; solution (nasal spray) 50 pressor units/ml (0.1 mg/ml) in 5 ml containers.

Intravenous, Subcutaneous: For central diabetes insipidus, *adults*, 0.5 to 1 ml daily, usually in two divided doses. Morning and evening doses should be adjusted separately on the basis of changes in urine volume and osmolality and control of nocturia. For patients who are switched from intranasal to injectable desmopressin, the dose of the injectable form is approximately one-tenth that of the intranasal dose.

DDAVP Injection (Rhone-Poulenc Rorer). Solution (for injection) 4 mcg/ml in 1 and 10 ml containers.

Stimate (Armour). Solution (for injection) 4 mcg/ml in 10 ml containers.

LYPRESSIN

[Diapid]

ACTIONS AND USES. Lypressin solution contains synthetic lysine-8-vasopressin, a polypeptide found in swine that is similar to arginine-8-vasopressin, the antidiuretic hormone found in the posterior pituitary of humans. It has an activity of 50 posterior pituitary (pressor) units per milliliter (Cobb, 1984).

Lypressin is rapidly absorbed from the nasal mucosa. It is effective as sole therapy in mild to moderate central diabetes insipidus if administered frequently. In more severe disease, treatment may be complicated by episodes of abrupt, severe polyuria that result from the short duration of action of lypressin. Desmopressin is more satisfactory in these patients. Lypressin is not effective in the nephrogenic form of diabetes insipidus.

ADVERSE REACTIONS AND PRECAUTIONS. No significant local or systemic reactions have been reported, although hypersensitivity, manifested by a positive skin test, occurs rarely. Antibody formation with reduced antidiuretic responsiveness may occur more frequently with lypressin than with vasopressin (Vokes et al, 1988). The absorption of lypressin may be impaired in patients with upper respiratory tract infections or allergic rhinitis.

DOSAGE AND PREPARATIONS.

Topical (intranasal): One or more sprays in one or both nostrils. The dose and interval between applications must be determined individually. Each spray delivers approximately 2 pressor units, but the exact amount depends on how vigorously the bottle is squeezed. Four sprays in each nostril provide the maximal amount that can be absorbed at one time without waste. Administration three or four times daily usually is necessary.

Diapid (Sandoz). Solution (nasal spray) 50 pressor units/ml (0.185 mg/ml) in 8 ml containers.

ORALLY ADMINISTERED AGENTS WITH ANTIDIURETIC ACTIVITY

CLOFIBRATE

[Atromid-S]

For chemical formula, see index entry Clofibrate, In Hyperlipidemia.

ACTIONS AND USES. The hypolipidemic agent, clofibrate, has antidiuretic action in patients with mild to moderate central diabetes insipidus (Cobb, 1984). Daily doses of 2 g reduce urine volume by approximately 50%. Clofibrate appears to act by increasing the release of vasopressin from the neurohypophysis; there is no evidence that the peripheral action of vasopressin is enhanced. Clofibrate is less effective as an antidiuretic agent than chlorpropamide. If clofibrate alone does not provide an adequate response, some patients may benefit from the addition of small doses of chlorpropamide or a thiazide to the regimen. Like chlorpropamide, clofibrate is ineffective in patients with complete central diabetes insipidus or the nephrogenic form of the disease.

ADVERSE REACTIONS AND PRECAUTIONS. Gastrointestinal disturbances (nausea, vomiting, diarrhea, dyspepsia, and flatulence) are the most common side effects. Clofibrate increases the risk of cholelithiasis. For other adverse reactions, see index entry Clofibrate, In Hyperlipidemia.

DOSAGE AND PREPARATIONS.
Oral: *Adults,* 1.5 to 2 g daily in divided doses.
Atromid-S (Wyeth-Ayerst), ***Generic.*** Capsules 500 mg.

CHLORPROPAMIDE
[Diabinese]

For chemical formula, see index entry Chlorpropamide, Uses, Diabetes Mellitus.

ACTIONS AND USES. The hypoglycemic agent, chlorpropamide, has an antidiuretic action in many patients with central diabetes insipidus. It is most effective in those with less severe disease; presumably, small amounts of vasopressin are present in the hypothalamus in these patients (Moses, 1984). Chlorpropamide and some of its degradation products reduce free-water clearance by increasing the sensitivity of the renal tubular epithelium to vasopressin or by increasing the renal osmotic gradient for water reabsorption. It also may increase vasopressin release. Urine volume is decreased by approximately 60% with a daily dose of 250 mg. Five to seven days of therapy are often required to achieve a maximal therapeutic effect. If an adequate therapeutic response is not obtained with chlorpropamide alone, better control often can be achieved when clofibrate or a thiazide is given concomitantly. Chlorpropamide is not effective in patients with nephrogenic diabetes insipidus.

ADVERSE REACTIONS AND PRECAUTIONS. Chlorpropamide reduces fasting blood glucose in patients with diabetes insipidus, and significant symptomatic hypoglycemia is not uncommon (Moses, 1984). Hypoglycemic reactions are most common in children, in patients with associated anterior pituitary deficiency, and in those with reduced food intake. Patients should be informed of the importance of not missing meals and warned to avoid alcoholic beverages since disulfiram-like effects may occur. The effects of long-term therapy on the beta cells of the normal pancreas have not been studied (see also index entry Chlorpropamide, Uses, Diabetes Mellitus).

Chlorpropamide is classified in FDA Pregnancy Category C.

DOSAGE AND PREPARATIONS.
Oral: *Adults,* 250 to 500 mg daily; 125 mg daily may be sufficient when another oral antidiuretic agent is given concomitantly.
Diabinese (Pfizer), ***Generic.*** Tablets 100 and 250 mg.

THIAZIDE DIURETICS

ACTIONS AND USES. The thiazide diuretics have a paradoxical antidiuretic action in patients with diabetes insipidus (Cobb, 1984). By producing mild volume depletion, thiazides enhance proximal tubular reabsorption of glomerular filtrate. This action reduces delivery of water to the vasopressin-dependent sites of water reabsorption in the distal nephron. Thiazides are used primarily for nephrogenic diabetes insipidus. Their antidiuretic action in this disorder is enhanced by indomethacin. In central diabetes insipidus, thiazides are rarely useful as sole therapy but may be given with other oral agents, such as chlorpropamide.

ADVERSE REACTIONS AND PRECAUTIONS. Thiazide diuretics are generally well tolerated. Mild symptomatic hypokalemia is common during long-term therapy and can be controlled by addition of a potassium-sparing diuretic to the regimen. Thiazides can increase serum uric acid concentration and may enhance the hyperuricemia observed in some adults with primary nephrogenic diabetes insipidus. For other adverse effects, see index entry Thiazides.

DOSAGE AND PREPARATIONS.
Oral: *Adults,* regimens include chlorothiazide 500 mg to 1 g once or twice daily; hydrochlorothiazide 25 to 50 mg once or twice daily; bendroflumethiazide 5 mg daily; and benzthiazide 50 to 200 mg daily.

For preparations, see index entry Thiazides and Related Diuretics (Table).

AMILORIDE HYDROCHLORIDE
[Midamor]

For chemical formula, see index entry Amiloride, As Diuretic.

This potassium-sparing diuretic has been used to treat lithium-induced nephrogenic diabetes insipidus. Amiloride may help prevent lithium-induced tubular damage by preventing lithium accumulation in the collecting tubule (Boton et al, 1987).

ADVERSE REACTIONS AND PRECAUTIONS. See index entry Amiloride, As Diuretic.

DOSAGE AND PREPARATIONS.
Oral: *Adults,* 5 to 10 mg twice daily.
Midamor (Merck Sharp & Dohme), ***Generic.*** Tablets 5 mg.

SYNDROME OF INAPPROPRIATE SECRETION OF ANTIDIURETIC HORMONE (SIADH)

Etiology: The syndrome of inappropriate secretion of antidiuretic hormone (SIADH) is characterized primarily by ectopic production or sustained pituitary secretion of vasopressin or vasopressin-like substances that elevate plasma levels of vasopressin and lead to water intoxication and hyponatremia. Ectopic production is observed most commonly in patients with neoplasms (particularly oat cell carcinoma of the lung) in which the tumor itself synthesizes vasopressin. SIADH due to sustained pituitary secretion may be associated with central nervous system lesions, nonmalignant pulmonary disease, pain, trauma, emotional stress, surgery, and psychiatric disorders.

The major cause of hyponatremic encephalopathy is an osmotic imbalance between the extracellular fluid and brain cells, leading to net movement of water in the brain with resultant cerebral edema, herniation, and infarction (Fraser and Arieff, 1990). The unrecognized hypotonic state is most common in postoperative patients, especially premenopausal women (Fraser and Arieff, 1990).

Hyponatremia also may occur in response to drug therapy, including many that stimulate vasopressin secretion or enhance its peripheral action (see Table). Thiazides, a frequent cause of hyponatremia, block sodium reabsorption in the diluting segment of the nephron and thus interfere with dilution of the urine but, unlike the loop diuretics, they do not impair the concentrating mechanism. Thiazide-induced hyponatremia is most likely to occur in the elderly and possibly in markedly edematous patients with severe heart failure, cirrhosis, or nephrotic syndrome (see index entry Thiazides).

The diagnosis of SIADH is made by exclusion. All conditions promoting the *appropriate* secretion of vasopressin must be ruled out. The presence of cardiac, renal, hepatic, thyroid, or adrenal disease may make it difficult to establish a diagnosis of SIADH. Hypouricemia also can be present in hyponatremic patients with SIADH (Maesaka et al, 1990). Additional coincidental changes in serum sodium and uric acid concentrations are inversely related to fluid intake. It is hypothesized that the hypouricemia in SIADH is largely due to increased renal urate clearance (Maesaka et al, 1990). Fluid restriction corrects the hyponatremia and the increased urate clearance in these patients; thus, it has been suggested that correction of urate clearance following water restriction can be used to differentiate SIADH from other disorders that produce hyponatremia (Maesaka et al, 1990).

DRUGS CAUSING HYPONATREMIA

DIURETICS
- Primarily Thiazides

HYPOGLYCEMIC AGENTS
- Primarily Chlorpropamide [Diabinese]

PSYCHOPHARMACOLOGIC AND NEUROLOGIC DRUGS
- Amitriptyline [Elavil, Endep]
- Barbiturates
- Carbamazepine [Tegretol]
- Fluoxetine [Prozac]
- Fluphenazine [Permitil, Prolixin]
- Haloperidol [Haldol]
- Opioids
- Thioridazine [Mellaril]
- Thiothixene [Navane]
- Tranylcypromine [Parnate]

ANTINEOPLASTIC AGENTS
- Cyclophosphamide [Cytoxan]
- Vinblastine [Velban]
- Vincristine [Oncovin]

MISCELLANEOUS AGENTS
- Lorcainide (investigational)
- Nicotine
- Oxytocin [Pitocin, Syntocinon]
- Somatostatin Analogues (octreotide [Sandostatin])

Management: The management of hyponatremia depends on whether it is acute or chronic and on its severity (Arieff and Ayus, 1991; Berl, 1990; Cluitmans and Meinders, 1990; Sterns, 1990).

Acute (less than 24 hours) hyponatremia usually responds to water restriction and discontinuation of all medications that cause hyponatremia. When hyponatremia is acute and severe (serum sodium concentration below 115 mmol/L), the risk of neurologic complications is high. Severe neurologic damage or death has occurred in about one-third of patients with severe hyponatremia when treatment was delayed until there was evidence of respiratory insufficiency (Arieff and Ayus, 1991; Fraser and Arieff, 1990).

It is generally accepted that severe acute hyponatremia and chronic hyponatremia associated with severe neurologic symptoms usually require infusion of hypertonic sodium chloride (3% solution). Furosemide [Lasix] (initially 1 mg/kg intravenously with intravenous replacement of excreted electrolytes) is a useful adjunct to enhance the excretion of free water. During the initial two days of treatment, correction of serum sodium >130 mmol/L should be avoided and the absolute increase in serum sodium should not be allowed to exceed 12 mmol/L/day (Arieff and Ayus, 1991; Berl, 1990; Sterns, 1990). In patients with severe chronic hyponatremia, the rate of increase should not exceed 0.5 mmol/L/hr (Cluitmans and Meinders, 1990). Hypertonic sodium chloride is relatively contraindicated for treatment of hyponatremia in patients with heart failure or chronic liver disease.

Mild to moderate chronic hyponatremia is better tolerated and usually can be managed by discontinuing any offending drugs and restricting fluid intake to 500 to 1,500 ml daily. Alternatively, oral furosemide 40 to 80 mg daily can be used. This drug is effective because it prevents excretion of maximally concentrated urine even when vasopressin levels are high. This treatment should be combined with a high salt intake, and appropriate precautions should be taken to avoid hypokalemia.

Demeclocycline [Declomycin] or lithium has been used for the long-term treatment of patients with SIADH who cannot tolerate prolonged fluid restriction or are unable to maintain a serum sodium concentration above 125 to 130 mmol/L. Both drugs interfere with the action of vasopressin on the renal tubules (Moses and Miller, 1974). Demeclocycline (600 mg to 1.2 g daily) is usually preferred because it is more effective and less toxic than lithium (Forrest et al, 1978). It should not be used in young children, however, because of adverse effects on bones and teeth. Demeclocycline also should be used cautiously, if at all, in patients with heart failure or cirrhosis because it may cause azotemia by further reducing the blood volume (Braden et al, 1985). Demeclocycline or lithium should be discontinued periodically to determine whether the syndrome is still present, particularly when the underlying disorder is treatable. See index entries Furosemide and Demeclocycline for evaluations.

Urea corrects hyponatremia in patients with SIADH by producing an osmotic diuresis. Oral administration of urea 30 g daily may be useful for long-term therapy (Decaux et al, 1980, 1985). Several opioids with kappa agonist activity (eg, pentazocine) inhibit the release of vasopressin from the neurohypophysis and may be of value in patients with SIADH of central nervous system origin (Miller, 1980). Hyponatremia associated with head injuries in elderly patients may respond to steroids with mineralocorticoid activity (Ishikawa et al, 1987).

Cited References

Allen HM, et al: Indomethacin in the treatment of lithium-induced nephrogenic diabetes insipidus. *Arch Intern Med* 149:1123-1126, 1989.

Arieff AI, Ayus JC: Treatment of symptomatic hyponatremia: Neither haste or waste. *Crit Care Med* 19:748-751, 1991.

Berl T: Treating hyponatremia: What is all the controversy about? Editorial. *Ann Intern Med* 113:417-419, 1990.

Bichet DG, et al: Hemodynamic and coagulation responses to 1-desamino [8-D-arginine] vasopressin in patients with congenital nephrogenic diabetes insipidus. *N Engl J Med* 318:881-887, 1988.

Blachar Y, et al: Effect of inhibition of prostaglandin synthesis on free water and osmolar clearances in patients with hereditary nephrogenic diabetes insipidus. *Int J Pediatr Nephrol* 1:48-52, 1980.

Boton R, et al: Prevalence, pathogenesis, and treatment of renal dysfunction associated with chronic lithium therapy. *Am J Kidney Dis* 10:329-345, 1987.

Braden GL, et al: Demeclocycline-induced natriuresis and renal insufficiency: In vivo and in vitro studies. *Am J Kidney Dis* 5:270-277, 1985.

Chevalier RL, Rogol AD: Tolmetin sodium in management of nephrogenic diabetes insipidus. *J Pediatr* 101:787-789, 1982.

Cluitmans FH, Meinders AE: Management of severe hyponatremia: Rapid or slow correction? *Am J Med* 88:161-166, 1990.

Cobb WE: Management of neurogenic diabetes insipidus with dDAVP and other agents, in Reichlin S (ed): *The Neurohypophysis*. New York, Plenum Publishing, 1984, 139-163.

Decaux G, et al: Treatment of syndrome of inappropriate secretion of antidiuretic hormone by urea. *Am J Med* 69:99-106, 1980.

Decaux G, et al: Use of urea for treatment of water retention in hyponatraemic cirrhosis with ascites resistant to diuretics. *BMJ* 290:1782-1783, 1985.

Dunger DB, et al: Increased renal sensitivity to vasopressin in two patients with essential hypernatremia. *J Clin Endocrinol Metab* 64:185-189, 1987.

Durr JA, et al: Diabetes insipidus in pregnancy associated with abnormally high circulating vasopressinase activity. *N Engl J Med* 316:1070-1074, 1987.

Forrest JN, et al: Superiority of demeclocycline over lithium in treatment of chronic syndrome of inappropriate secretion of antidiuretic hormone. *N Engl J Med* 298:173-177, 1978.

Fraser CL, Arieff AI: Fatal central diabetes mellitus and insipidus resulting from untreated hyponatremia: A new syndrome. *Ann Intern Med* 112:113-119, 1990.

Goldsmith SR: Vasopressin as vasopressor. *Am J Med* 82:1213-1219, 1987.

Hirsch AT, et al: Vasopressin-mediated forearm vasodilation in normal humans: Evidence for a vascular vasopressin V2 receptor. *J Clin Invest* 84:418-426, 1989.

Ishikawa S, et al: Hyponatremia responsive to fludrocortisone acetate in elderly patients after head injury. *Ann Intern Med* 106:187-191, 1987.

Laszlo FA, et al: Pharmacology and clinical perspectives of vasopressin antagonists. *Pharmacol Rev* 43:73-108, 1991.

Libber S, et al: Treatment of nephrogenic diabetes insipidus with prostaglandin synthesis inhibitors. *J Pediatr* 108:305-311, 1986.

Maesaka JK, et al: Hyponatremia and hypouricemia: Differentiation from SIADH. *Clin Nephrol* 33:174-178, 1990.

Miller M: Role of endogenous opioids in neurohypophyseal function of man. *J Clin Endocrinol Metab* 50:1018-1020, 1980.

Moses AM: Clinical and laboratory features of central and nephrogenic diabetes insipidus and primary polydipsia, in Reichlin S (ed): *The Neurohypophysis*. New York, Plenum Publishing, 1984, 115-138.

Moses AM, Miller M: Drug-induced dilutional hyponatremia. *N Engl J Med* 291:1234-1239, 1974.

Moses AM, et al: Marked hypotonic polyuria resulting from nephrogenic diabetes insipidus with partial sensitivity to vasopressin. *J Clin Endocrinol Metab* 59:1044-1049, 1984.

Richardson DW, Robinson AG: Desmopressin. *Ann Intern Med* 103:228-239, 1985.

Riphagen CL, Pittman QJ: Arginine vasopressin as central neurotransmitter. *Federation Proc* 45:2318-2322, 1986.

Rossi NF, Schrier RW: Role of arginine vasopressin in regulation of systemic arterial pressure. *Ann Rev Med* 37:13-20, 1986.

Scherbaum WA, Bottazzo GF: Autoantibodies to vasopressin cells in idiopathic diabetes insipidus: Evidence for an autoimmune variant. *Lancet* 1:897-901, 1983.

Shah SV, Thakur V: Vasopressinase and diabetes insipidus of pregnancy. *Ann Intern Med* 109:435-436, 1988.

Share L: Role of vasopressin in cardiovascular regulation. *Physiol Rev* 68:1248-1284, 1988.

Sterns RH: The treatment of hyponatremia: First, do no harm, editorial. *Am J Med* 88:557-560, 1990.

Suzuki S, et al: Biphasic forearm vascular responses to intraarterial arginine vasopressin. *J Clin Invest* 84:427-434, 1989.

Svedman P, et al: Administration of antidiuretic peptide (DDAVP) by way of suction de-epithelialised skin. *Lancet* 337:1506-1509, 1991.

Thibonnier M: Use of vasopressin antagonists in human diseases. *Kidney Int* 34 (suppl 26):S48-S51, 1988.

Thibonnier M, Roberts JM: Characterization of human platelet vasopressin receptors. *J Clin Invest* 76:1857-1864, 1985.

Vokes TJ, et al: Antibodies to vasopressin in patients with diabetes insipidus: Implications for diagnosis and therapy. *Ann Intern Med* 108:190-195, 1988.

Fluid, Electrolyte, and Acid-Base Therapy

39

MAINTAINING FLUID AND ELECTROLYTE STATUS

ABNORMAL FLUID STATUS

ACID-BASE DISTURBANCES

POTASSIUM IMBALANCES

MAGNESIUM IMBALANCES

MAINTAINING FLUID AND ELECTROLYTE STATUS

An unstressed adult in a comfortable climate requires approximately 30 to 35 ml/kg/day of fluid to maintain a urine output within the physiologic range. Electrolyte needs generally can be met for short periods by giving sodium 70 to 140 mEq/day and potassium 40 to 80 mEq/day slowly over 24 hours.

Hospitalized patients often have conditions that preclude the oral intake of food or fluids. Various parenteral regimens have been recommended to maintain fluid and electrolyte homeostasis in adults. These include (1) 1,000 ml of dextrose 10% with potassium chloride 20 mEq over 12 hours, followed by 1,000 ml of dextrose 5% and sodium chloride 0.45% with potassium chloride 20 mEq over the next 12 hours (Freitag and Miller, 1980); (2) 1,000 ml of dextrose 5% in Ringer's lactate or sodium chloride 0.9% with potassium chloride or potassium acetate 20 to 40 mEq, followed by 1,500 to 2,000 ml of dextrose 5% with potassium chloride or potassium acetate 30 to 60 mEq over 24 hours (Kopple and Blumenkrantz, 1980); and (3) 1,000 ml of dextrose 5% with potassium chloride 40 mEq over 12 hours, followed by 1,000 ml of sodium chloride 0.9% with potassium chloride 40 mEq over the next 12 hours (Lawson and Henry, 1977). These regimens probably are equally effective for most adults with normally functioning kidneys that are able to maintain the homeostasis of the internal milieu. Volumes should be decreased for infants and children, depending on body weight.

ABNORMAL FLUID STATUS

Isotonic Loss of Sodium and Water (Extracellular Volume Depletion): This may be caused by gastroenteric losses (vomiting, diarrhea, nasogastric suctioning) or renal losses (adrenal disorders). The therapeutic approach depends on the extent of volume depletion and the clinical status of the patient (see Table 1).

Patients of any age who have mild to moderate volume deficits and are capable of consuming fluids, either independently or with assistance, initially should be given oral rehydration solutions (Avery and Snyder, 1990; *WHO Drug Information*, 1990; Mackenzie and Barnes, 1991; Sack, 1991; Santosham and Greenough, 1991). Severely volume-depleted individuals should receive intravenous fluids (preferably Ringer's lactate) until their pulse, blood pressure, and state of consciousness return to normal; thereafter, even these patients should receive oral rehydration therapy until the extracellular volume is restored. Patients who are incapable of consuming fluids orally or by nasogastric intubation, including very young or small infants, must receive intravenous therapy as long as volume depletion persists. Following successful repletion, continuing losses should be replaced (with oral solutions if physically possible) on an equal-volume basis (plus 10 to 12 ml/kg/day to compensate for insensible water loss) until the precipitating cause is controlled.

Oral rehydration solutions are especially recommended for volume-depleted children (American Academy of Pediatrics, Committee on Nutrition, 1985; *WHO Drug Information*, 1990, 1991). Their use has met with some resistance in the United States (Snyder, 1991), partly because they are often associated with "field medicine" in underdeveloped countries (*WHO Drug Information*, 1991). However, oral rehydration of volume-depleted patients in a modern urban setting has been shown to be as effective as intravenous volume repletion (Mackenzie and Barnes, 1991). In addition, oral rehydration is associated with shorter hospitalization, less trauma to the patient, and lower cost.

Oral rehydration solutions (5 to 10 ml every five minutes for children; 10 to 50 ml every five minutes for adults) are absorbed rapidly enough to produce volume repletion in patients who are vomiting intermittently (Sack, 1991; Santosham and Greenough, 1991). If occasional vomiting persists, the solution can be administered via continuous nasogastric intubation. If vomiting worsens, fluids should be given intravenously. In addition, patients with fecal water losses >10 ml/kg/hr

TABLE 1.
EXTRACELLULAR VOLUME DEPLETION: SEVERITY AND THERAPY

Degree of Depletion	Volume Deficit[1]	Clinical Signs	Repletion Therapy[2]
Mild	5%-6%	Increased thirst, slightly dry buccal membranes	Oral rehydration solution (ORS) 50 ml/kg
Moderate	7%-9%	Sunken eyes, sunken fontanelle, loss of skin turgor, dry buccal membranes	ORS 100 ml/kg
Severe	10% +	Above signs, plus rapid thready pulse, cyanosis, lethargy, rapid breathing, orthostatic hypotension, coma	Intravenous fluids 40 ml/kg/hr until pulse and state of consciousness normalize; then ORS 50-100 ml/kg

[1]Volume deficit (%) = (Volume deficit/Normal body water volume) x 100%
Volume deficit = Normal volume − Current volume
[2]Administered within four hours of patient presentation.

require intravenous fluids to supplement oral rehydration solutions.

The international standard for oral rehydration solutions for initial volume repletion is that of the World Health Organization–UNICEF (see Table 2). Use of this formulation has been advocated by the American Academy of Pediatrics (AAP) (American Academy of Pediatrics, Committee on Nutrition, 1985), except that the maximum recommended ratio of carbohydrate to sodium is higher in the AAP guidelines (2.0 versus 1.4). Although several commercial formulations are available for repletion, only Rehydralyte meets the AAP standards and none meet the WHO-UNICEF standards. All of the solutions are within the AAP guidelines for maintenance use after restoration of extracellular fluid volume (see Table 2).

Carbohydrate-based oral rehydration solutions are based on the ability of glucose to act as a transport molecule in carrier-mediated absorption of electrolytes with concurrent movement of water out of the intestinal lumen by osmosis. However, glucose in concentrations >25 g/L may not be absorbed efficiently and increases water movement into the intestinal lumen (osmotic diarrhea); glucose concentrations >50g/L are not recommended. In contrast, starches and glucose polymers contain more glucose moieties/300 milliosmoles/L than does free glucose, providing greater electrolyte transport capability, increased passive water absorption, and more metabolizable energy without imposition of an osmotic penalty. Natural starches are semi-purified and also provide some protein. In addition, the glucose from starches is ab-

TABLE 2.
ORAL REHYDRATION SOLUTIONS

Solution (Manufacturer)	mEq/L Na	K	Cl	Citrate	g/L Dextrose	Rice Syrup Solids	CHO:Na†
WHO–UNICEF	90	20	80	30	20	—	1.2
Pedialyte* (Ross)	45	20	35	30	25	—	3.1
Rehydralyte* (Ross)	75	20	65	30	25	—	1.9
Resol* (Wyeth-Ayerst)	50	20	50	34	20	—	2.2
Ricelyte* (Mead Johnson)	50	25	45	34	—	30	3.3

**Nonprescription*
† Ratio of carbohydrates to sodium. World Health Organization-UNICEF (1986) recommended maximum: 1.4, American Academy of Pediatrics, Committee on Nutrition (1985) recommended maximum: 2.0.

sorbed as rapidly as free glucose (Hirschhorn and Greenough, 1991; Lebenthal and Lu, 1991).

When rice powder (85% to 90% starches, 6% to 9% protein) was used instead of glucose, patients experienced less vomiting, smaller fluid losses with continued diarrhea, more rapid initial water absorption, and a shorter course of disease, and smaller volumes of oral rehydration solution were required (Lebenthal, 1990; Chowdhury et al, 1991; Khin-Maung-U and Greenough, 1991; Lebenthal and Lu, 1991; Gore et al, 1992). Similar results were obtained with rice syrup solids (Pizarro et al, 1991). Corn, wheat, or potato solids may be equally effective (Lebenthal and Lu, 1991). The addition of glycine or alanine also increases electrolyte and water absorption, but because free amino acids increase luminal osmolality, their effectiveness is not superior to that of rice-based oral rehydration therapy (The International Study Group on Improved ORS, 1991; Ribeiro and Lifshitz, 1991; Sazawal et al, 1991).

Food, especially cereals, bananas, and potatoes (and, in infants, breast milk), accelerates recovery when given as soon as possible after initial volume repletion and should be ingested within 24 hours of initiating therapy (American Academy of Pediatrics, Committee on Nutrition, 1985; Khin-Maung-U et al, 1985; Santosham et al, 1985; Casteel and Fiedorek, 1990; Brown, 1991). Cow's milk is not recommended (Lifshitz et al, 1991). Clear liquid beverages also are not recommended because they contain either excessive amounts of sodium and no carbohydrates (broths) or excessive carbohydrates and very little sodium (fruit juices, carbonated beverages, teas, energy replenishment drinks for athletes [eg, Gatorade]).

When intravenous fluid therapy is necessary, Ringer's lactate is preferable to sodium chloride because it provides buffering anions. Once the patient is stabilized, oral rehydration solutions should be substituted if possible. If continued use of parenteral fluids is necessary, serum electrolyte concentrations should be monitored and the composition of the infusion should be tailored to meet the needs of the patient.

For isonatremic volume repletion and maintenance in children and adults, Ringer's lactate is preferred (normal weight infants and children, 100 ml/kg/day; adolescents, 75 to 100 ml/kg/day; adults, 25 to 50 ml/kg/day) (Boineau and Lewy, 1990; El-Dahr and Chevalier, 1990; Kallen, 1990). Care must be taken to avoid overly aggressive therapy in the elderly, who often have limited cardiac reserve and suboptimal renal function and may be at risk for congestive heart failure (Lavizzo-Mourey, 1987). For fluid maintenance in low-birth-weight infants (801 to 2,000 g), 10% dextrose and 0.2% sodium chloride should be given at a rate of 45 to 90 ml/kg/day, depending on body weight (greater volumes) and relative humidity (lower volumes); for those weighing <800 g, 70 to 120 ml/kg/day of 5% or 7.5% dextrose in 0.1% sodium chloride should be given (Baumgart et al, 1982). Dextrose solutions should not be used alone, because the sugar is metabolized rapidly to carbon dioxide and water and its infusion is physiologically equivalent to that of free water and may result in hyponatremia.

Whole blood is the only complete replacement therapy when intravascular volume depletion is caused by hemorrhage (see index entry Blood Whole, In Replacement Therapy). For the treatment of hypovolemic shock, see index entry Shock, Hypovolemic.

Loss of Water in Excess of Sodium (Dehydration): This condition, which causes hypertonic dehydration and hypernatremia (serum sodium concentration >150 mEq/L), may result primarily from inadequate water intake in patients with central nervous system disease who cannot report thirst sensations, in hospitalized elderly patients, in infants given excessively concentrated foods, in water-deprived children, and in very-low-birth-weight infants with excessive losses from evaporation. Hypernatremic dehydration also may result from hyperhidrosis, diabetes insipidus, extensive skin damage caused by burns, and osmotic diuresis (hyperglycemia, high protein tube feeding) or hypotonic diarrhea with inadequate water intake.

The initial volume deficit (in liters) can be estimated by comparing the patient's current body water volume with his or her normal body water volume:

$$\text{Current Body Water Volume} = A \times B \times (BW)$$
$$\text{Normal Body Water Volume} = A \times (BW)$$
$$A = 0.60 \ (\text{Age} < 10 \text{ years})$$
$$0.55 \ (10\text{-}60 \text{ years})$$
$$0.45 \ (> 60 \text{ years})$$
$$B = (140 \text{ mg/dL}) / (\text{serum } [Na])$$
$$BW = \text{body weight in kg}$$

Initially, hypotonic sodium chloride (0.45%) should be given intravenously over several hours until about one-half of the calculated deficit is replaced; the remaining one-half should be given over the next 24 to 48 hours (Feig, 1981). Electrolyte levels should be monitored closely, and potassium chloride should be given if hypokalemia occurs. Idiopathic hypocalcemia commonly accompanies hypernatremia and may require the addition of calcium gluconate to rehydration fluids. Hyperglycemia also may occur in patients with a tendency to develop diabetes and may require treatment with insulin until normal fluid and electrolyte status can be maintained.

Hypertonic dehydration results in efflux of water from within the cells to the extracellular fluid compartment, resulting in intracellular dehydration. However, the brain produces new intracellular solutes (idiogenic osmoles) that protect it from life-threatening dehydration. The rate at which idiogenic osmoles can be removed or inactivated after hypertonicity has been corrected is unknown. Therefore, when administering fluids to treat loss of water in excess of sodium, it is important to monitor the patient for evidence of deteriorating sensorium or for appearance of neurologic signs, because such signs may result from brain cell overhydration and cerebral edema when fluids are infused too rapidly (water intoxication). In general, reduction of the serum sodium concentration to normal within 24 to 48 hours is recommended (Conley, 1990; El-Dahr and Chevalier, 1990).

For the treatment of diabetes insipidus, see index entry Diabetes Insipidus.

Loss of Sodium in Excess of Water: This causes hyponatremia (serum sodium concentration <130 mEq/L). Hypovolemic hyponatremia may be caused by viral gastroenteritis, excessive sweating without fluid replacement, cystic fibrosis, or renal inability to conserve sodium appropriately (diuretic therapy, salt-wasting nephropathies, adrenocortical insufficiency). Euvolemic or hypervolemic hyponatremia occurs when fluid losses (eg, gastrointestinal losses, excessive sweating) are replaced by water without sufficient salt.

When the serum sodium concentration is moderately low and there is clinical evidence of reduced extracellular fluid volume (eg, lethargy, tachycardia, orthostatic hypotension), administration of sodium chloride 0.9% is the treatment of choice and often is all that is required to expand the extracellular fluid volume and normalize the serum concentration of sodium. Maintenance of isonatremia requires successful treatment of the causative condition.

The management of severe symptomatic hyponatremia (ie, plasma sodium concentration <110 to 115 mEq/L; presence of neurologic symptoms such as confusion, stupor, vomiting, or convulsions) has been controversial (Arieff and Ayus, 1991). Because brain cells gradually adapt to hyponatremia by secreting potassium to decrease intracellular osmolarity and reduce water influx, some clinicians have been concerned that increasing serum sodium concentrations rapidly may cause additional efflux of water from brain cells and result in cerebral demyelination. However, rapid reversal of acute hyponatremia (up to 5 mEq/L/hr) apparently is not usually detrimental, possibly because the hyponatremia (and therefore potassium efflux) is limited (Sarnaik et al, 1991). Brain lesions previously attributed to rapid correction of symptomatic hyponatremia (cerebral herniation, diffuse demyelination, infarction, and other signs of hypoxic brain damage) may actually reflect untreated hyponatremia. On the other hand, overcorrection or even restoration of normal serum sodium concentration occasionally can lead to permanent brain damage in patients with severe liver disease or other debilitating primary illnesses. At this time, it appears safe and prudent to infuse hypertonic sodium chloride 3% at a rate calculated to increase the serum sodium concentration by no more than 12.5 mEq/L/day (up to a maximum serum sodium concentration of 125 mEq/L) (Arieff and Ayus, 1991).

Hyponatremia caused by adrenocortical insufficiency should be treated with hormone replacement therapy and sodium chloride 0.9% to support the extracellular and intracellular compartments (see index entry Adrenocortical Insufficiency).

Chronic hyponatremia is often associated with inappropriate secretion of antidiuretic hormone (SIADH). Treatment of SIADH is discussed elsewhere (see index entry Antidiuretic Hormone, Syndrome of Inappropriate Secretion).

Acute Water Intoxication: This occurs in infants who receive water or diluted formula instead of breast milk or full-strength formula (Finberg, 1991). Appropriate therapy is based on the infusion of hypertonic sodium chloride injection (3%) to increase extracellular osmotic forces. When given either as a rapid bolus (Sarnaik et al, 1991) or over 30 to 90 minutes (Keating et al, 1991), this therapy effectively elevates serum sodium concentration and resolves hyponatremic seizures while avoiding the development of central pontine myelinolysis. Mild water intoxication without neurologic dysfunction can be treated with oral sodium chloride when renal function is known to be normal (Finberg, 1991).

Volume Excess: Volume excess with or without edema is observed in adults with congestive heart failure, nephrotic syndrome, or cirrhosis with ascites. Drugs used to treat chronic volume excess in adults are discussed elsewhere (see index entries Heart Failure; Diuretics). Restriction of dietary sodium is important in the management of this imbalance. Water restriction is necessary only when hyponatremia occurs.

TABLE 3.
MULTIPLE ELECTROLYTE INTRAVENOUS SOLUTIONS

		mEq/L							
Tradename (Manufacturer)	**mOsm/L**	**Na^+**	**K^+**	**Ca^{++}**	**Mg^{++}**	**Cl^-**	**HCO_3 Precursor**	**Volume Available (ml)**
Plasma-Lyte 56 (Baxter Healthcare)	111	40	13	—	3	40	Acet 16	1,000
Ringer's Injection (Various)	309	147	4	4	—	156	—	500, 1,000
Normosol-R, Normosol-R pH 7.4 (Abbott)	295	140	5	—	3	98	Acet 27 Gluc* 23	500, 1,000
Isolyte S pH 7.4 (McGaw)	295	141	5	—	3	98	Acet 27 Gluc* 23	500, 1,000
Plasma-Lyte 148, Plasma-Lyte A pH 7.4 (Baxter Healthcare)	294	140	5	—	3	98	Acet 27 Gluc* 23	500, 1,000
Plasma-Lyte R (Baxter Healthcare)	312	140	10	5	3	103	Acet 47 Lac 8	1,000
Ringer's Lactate (Various)	273	130	4	3	—	109	Lac 28	250, 500, 1,000

Gluc = gluconate

TABLE 4. CONCENTRATED MULTIPLE ELECTROLYTE INTRAVENOUS SOLUTIONS[1]

Tradename (Manufacturer)	mOsm/L[2]	mEq/ml Na+	K+	Ca++	Mg++	Cl−	Precursor	Volume Available (ml)
Hyperlyte (McGaw)	6015	1	1.62	0.2	0.32	1.34	Acet 1.624 Gluc[3] 0.2	25 ml in 30 and 50 ml vials
Hyperlyte CR (McGaw)	5500	0.167	0.133	0.013	0.033	0.2	Acet 0.2	250 ml vial
Hyperlyte R (McGaw)	4205	1	0.8	0.2	0.2	1.2	Acet 1	25 ml in 30 ml vial
Lypholyte (LyphoMed)	7562	1.25	2.03	0.25	0.4	1.68	Acet 2.03 Gluc[3] 0.25	20, 40,100, and 200 ml vials
Lypholyte II (LyphoMed)	6200	1.75	1	0.225	0.25	1.75	Acet 1.475	20,40,100, and 200 ml vials
Multilyte-20 (LyphoMed)	4200	1	0.8	0.2	0.2	1.2	Acet 1	25 ml in 50 ml vial
Multilyte-40 (LyphoMed)	6050	1	1.62	0.2	0.32	1.34	Acet 1.62 Gluc[3] 0.2	25 ml in 50 ml vial

[1] *Must be diluted before administration. NOT for direct intravenous administration.*
[2] *Osmolarity of concentrated solution.*
[3] *Gluc=gluconate*

Drug Evaluations

Sodium chloride injection, dextrose injection, or Ringer's lactate may be used to treat most abnormal fluid states. Other solutions have been developed for balanced maintenance or replacement of fluid and electrolytes. In addition to sodium and chloride, these solutions provide potassium; magnesium; and bicarbonate precursors, such as acetate, lactate, and gluconate. In general, it is preferable to individualize therapy. Formulations for oral rehydration solutions appear in Table 2, and partial lists of available parenteral formulations appear in Tables 3, 4, and 5.

SODIUM CHLORIDE

SODIUM CHLORIDE INJECTION

USES. Sodium chloride is used to correct extracellular volume depletion and hyponatremia. It should be administered orally as table salt for replacement therapy whenever possible; oral dosage forms also may be used. A solution containing 3 to 4 g of sodium chloride (1 g of sodium chloride contains 17.1 mEq of sodium) and 1.5 to 3 g of sodium bicarbonate/L (1 g of sodium bicarbonate contains 11.9 mEq of sodium) also is satisfactory for oral use if solid foods cannot be ingested.

Isotonic sodium chloride injection is a 0.9% solution containing 154 mEq of sodium and chloride/L. (In comparison, plasma contains 137 to 147 mEq of sodium and 98 to 106 mEq of chloride/L.) Sodium concentrations of 0.11% to 0.45% are hypotonic, and concentrations of 3% and 5% are hypertonic. The concentration and tonicity of sodium chloride solutions determine their usefulness in different disorders.

Sodium chloride injection 0.9% is infused when sodium and water have been depleted in isotonic proportions. It may be used to maintain effective extracellular fluid volume and a stable circulation during and after surgery in patients with normal cardiovascular and renal function and to maintain plasma volume, thus temporarily postponing the need for blood transfusions in emergencies. Hypertonic sodium chloride injection should be reserved for the treatment of severe symptomatic hyponatremia (serum sodium less than 120 mEq/ml) and should be used only during the critical phase. Hypotonic solutions (usually 0.45% containing 77 mEq sodium and chloride/L) generally are given with dextrose for maintenance therapy in patients who are unable to ingest fluids and nutrients orally for one to three days; they are administered without dextrose in the management of hyperosmolar diabetes mellitus.

PRECAUTIONS. Sodium chloride must be infused with great caution, particularly in patients with congestive heart failure, renal failure, or hypoproteinemia. Signs and symptoms of excessive therapy are peripheral edema and pulmonary congestion (rales, edema). Hypertonic solutions should be given slowly (acutely, up to 5 mEq/L/hr; chronically, up to 12.5 mEq/L/day) and cautiously in small volumes (200 to 400 ml) because of the danger of volume excess, pulmonary ede-

TABLE 5.
DEXTROSE AND MULTIPLE ELECTROLYTE INTRAVENOUS SOLUTIONS

			mEq/L								
Tradename (Manufacturer)	**Calories/L**	**mOsm/L**	**Na^+**	**K^+**	**Ca^{++}**	**Mg^{++}**	**Cl^-**	**$HPO_4^=$**	**HCO_3^- Precursor**	**NH_4^+**	**Volume Supplied**
Ringer's Lactate ½ Strength Dextrose 2.5% (Various)	90	263	65	2	2	—	55	—	Lact 14	—	1,000 ml
Ringer's Lactate Dextrose 10% (Various)	340	775	130	4	3	—	111	—	Lact 28	—	1,000 ml
Ringer's ½ Strength Dextrose 2.5% (Various)	85	280	74	2	2	—	78	—	—	—	500 ml
Ringer's Dextrose 5% (Various)	170	561	147	4	4	—	156	—	—	—	500, 1,000 ml
Electrolyte No. 48 Dextrose 5% (Baxter Healthcare)	180	348	25	20	—	3	24	3	Lact 23	—	250, 500, 1,000 ml
Electrolyte No. 75 Dextrose 5% (Baxter Healthcare)	180	402	40	35	—	—	48	15	Lact 20	—	250, 500, 1,000 ml
Isolyte G Dextrose 5% (McGaw)	170	555	65	17	—	—	149	—	—	70	1,000 ml
Isolyte H Dextrose 5% (McGaw)	170	370	42	13	—	3	39	—	Acet 17	—	1,000 ml
Normosol M Dextrose 5% (Abbott)	170	363	40	13	—	3	40	—	Acet 16	—	500, 1,000 ml
Plasma-Lyte 56 Dextrose 5% (Baxter Healthcare)	170	363	40	13	—	3	40	—	Acet 16	—	500, 1,000 ml
Isolyte M Dextrose 5% (McGaw)	170	400	38	35	—	—	44	15	Acet 20	—	500, 1,000 ml
Isolyte P Dextrose 5% (McGaw)	170	350	25	20	—	3	23	3	Acet 23	—	250, 500, 1,000 ml
Isolyte R Dextrose 5% (McGaw)	170	380	41	16	5	3	40	—	Acet 24	—	1,000 ml
Isolyte S Dextrose 5% (McGaw)	170	555	142	5	—	3	98	—	Acet 30 Gluc* 23	—	1,000 ml
Normosol-R Dextrose 5% (Abbott)	185	547	140	5	—	3	98	—	Acet 27 Gluc* 23	—	500, 1,000 ml
Plasma-Lyte 148 Dextrose 5% (Baxter Healthcare)	190	547	140	5	—	3	98	—	Acet 27 Gluc* 23	—	500, 1,000 ml
Plasma-Lyte R Dextrose 5% (Baxter Healthcare)	181	564	140	10	5	3	103	—	Acet 47 Lact 8	—	1,000 ml
Plasma-Lyte M Dextrose 5% (Baxter Healthcare)	180	377	40	16	5	3	40	—	Acet 12 Lact 12	—	500, 1,000 ml

** Gluc = gluconate*

ma, and hyperosmolarity. The latter may cause confusion, stupor, or coma.

Sodium chloride is classified in FDA Pregnancy Category C.

PREPARATIONS.

ORAL:

Generic. Granules; powder; tablets 650, 1,000, 1,070, and 2,250 mg; tablets (enteric-coated) 1,000 mg.

INTRAVENOUS:

Generic. Solution 0.45%, 0.9%, 3%, and 5%; solution (concentrate) 2.5 and 4 mEq/ml.

ORAL REHYDRATION SOLUTIONS

The World Health Organization has developed a dextrose/electrolyte solution that is useful for managing mild to moderately severe isotonic dehydration (see Tables 1 and 2). Commercial products also are available (see Table 2). Oral rehydration solutions are safe and simple to use, even in patients who are vomiting. They are the oral therapy of choice for isotonic dehydration from any cause in patients of all ages.

Adverse effects are primarily related to electrolyte imbalance and include hypernatremia, hyponatremia, and hypokalemia. A few patients cannot tolerate glucose in the intestine and diarrhea will develop or existing diarrhea will worsen after therapy is initiated.

PREPARATIONS. See Table 2.

BALANCED ELECTROLYTE INJECTION

RINGER'S LACTATE

USES. Ringer's lactate is the preferred treatment for severe volume depletion when oral rehydration is not possible. Although these solutions more closely approximate normal extracellular electrolyte concentrations, additional electrolytes may be necessary to meet the specific needs of the patient (eg, to correct acidosis, alkalosis, or deficits of individual electrolytes). These solutions are not indicated to replace blood or plasma volume expanders when the latter are indicated, except for the temporary maintenance of plasma volume in emergencies.

PREPARATIONS. See Tables 3, 4, and 5.

DEXTROSE INJECTION

DEXTROSE AND SODIUM CHLORIDE INJECTION

USES. Dextrose injection is administered intravenously to provide nutrient and water when oral feeding is not feasible. It usually is administered as a 5% aqueous infusion, which is approximately isotonic compared to blood (277 mOsm/L) and provides about 170 calories/L. Dextrose injection 5% or sodium chloride injection 0.11% to 0.45% with dextrose 5% in water may be used intravenously when there is loss of water in excess of sodium. Solutions containing 10% dextrose provide more nutrient in less volume, but this concentration may be irritating to the veins and, in newborns, may cause hyperglycemia. The immediate intravenous administration of 50 ml (25 g) of 50% dextrose solution is recommended for comatose patients when the cause of the depression is unknown *without waiting for the blood glucose determination* (unless a rapid measurement of blood glucose concentration is possible) in order to prevent brain damage from hypoglycemia. A solution containing 20% to 50% dextrose (often with insulin added) is used to promote the shift of potassium into cells in hyperkalemia associated with arrhythmias or abnormal electrocardiogram patterns. Hypertonic dextrose is infused in a high-flow vein to provide calories in total parenteral nutrition (TPN). (See index entry Nutrition, Enteral, Parenteral.)

The rate of utilization of dextrose varies considerably; however, the average maximal rate is 500 mg/kg/hr (10 ml/kg/hr of dextrose injection 5%) over periods of less than 24 hours. If the patient's capacity to utilize dextrose is exceeded, hyperglycemia, glycosuria, and excessive diuresis will occur.

ADVERSE REACTIONS AND PRECAUTIONS. Dextrose solutions are acidic (pH 3.5 to 5.0) and may produce thrombophlebitis. Subcutaneous administration is very irritating, may distend tissue, and may lead to hypodermaclysis and necrosis. Therefore, this route is never employed. Dextrose injection should not be used as a diluent for blood because it causes clumping of red blood cells and, possibly, hemolysis.

Dextrose injection is classified in FDA Pregnancy Category C.

PREPARATIONS.

DEXTROSE INJECTION:

Generic. Solution 2.5%, 5%, 10%, 20%, 25%, 30%, 38%, 40%, 50%, 60%, and 70%; 5% and 10% with alcohol 5%.

DEXTROSE AND SODIUM CHLORIDE INJECTION:

Generic. Solution containing dextrose 2.5% with sodium chloride 0.45%; dextrose 5% with sodium chloride 0.11%, 0.2%, 0.225%, 0.3%, 0.33%, 0.45%, and 0.9%; dextrose 10% with sodium chloride 0.2%, 0.45%, and 0.9%.

FRUCTOSE INJECTION

INVERT SUGAR INJECTION (containing equal parts of dextrose and fructose)

Fructose offers no advantages over dextrose injection and possesses some disadvantages. It may increase serum concentrations of lactate and urate if given rapidly, and it is considerably more expensive than dextrose. The risk of lactic acidosis is increased in severely ill patients. Fructose infusion has been associated with increased production of uric acid and hyperuricemia and is contraindicated in patients with hereditary fructose intolerance (aldolase deficiency) because it can cause severe reactions (hypoglycemia, nausea, vomiting, tremors, coma, convulsions). Fructose is classified in FDA Pregnancy Category C.

Invert sugar is available in combination with electrolytes for intravenous administration.

PREPARATIONS.

FRUCTOSE INJECTION:

Generic. Solution 10%.

INVERT SUGAR INJECTION (COMBINATION):
Travert (Baxter Healthcare). Solution 5% or 10% with Electrolyte No. 2.

ACID-BASE DISTURBANCES

Acute Metabolic Acidosis: Metabolic acidosis (deficiency of extracellular bicarbonate with pH <7.2) may be caused by excessive production of lactic acid (lactic acidosis) or ketoacids (ketoacidosis), chronic renal failure, a defect in the ability of the kidney to acidify the urine appropriately (renal tubular acidosis), diarrhea, or ingestion of certain drugs or toxins (eg, salicylates, ethylene glycol, methanol, paraldehyde). Identification and correction of the cause of acidosis is preferable to symptomatic treatment and usually corrects the acid-base and fluid derangements. Symptomatic treatment is advisable only when causative factors cannot be identified or corrected.

The role of bicarbonate in the symptomatic treatment of lactic acidosis is controversial. In the past, it was generally accepted that administering alkalizing agents to raise the arterial pH was prudent, and sodium bicarbonate was recommended when the arterial pH dropped below 7.1. However, results of some animal studies suggest that the infusion of bicarbonate in lactic acidosis stimulates excessive production of lactate and actually reduces serum bicarbonate concentration, arterial pH, cardiac output, blood pressure, and tissue perfusion and may produce a "paradoxical" intracellular acidosis (Graf et al, 1985). Nevertheless, some clinicians believe that judicious administration of bicarbonate may raise the arterial pH above a hemodynamically critical level (7.25) and allow the physician additional time to manage the underlying condition (Madias, 1986; Narins and Cohen, 1987). If bicarbonate treatment is chosen, any potassium deficit must first be corrected to avoid bicarbonate-induced hypokalemia (Brewer, 1990).

Chronic Metabolic Acidosis: Patients with chronic renal failure or renal tubular acidosis usually have chronic metabolic acidosis. Mild to moderate acidosis does not require treatment. When the plasma bicarbonate concentration drops below 15 to 20 mEq/L, oral therapy with sodium bicarbonate or sodium citrate should be initiated. The goal is to maintain the plasma bicarbonate concentration at about 20 mEq/L (Quintanilli and Qureshi, 1981). Most patients tolerate oral bicarbonate therapy well, but they must be monitored for evidence of sodium overload, hypertension, and tetany. Sodium bicarbonate is more likely to cause gastrointestinal reactions than sodium citrate. Patients with symptoms of gastric irritation often can be treated with a combination of sodium citrate and citric acid solution (Shohl's solution) [Bicitra].

Metabolic Alkalosis: Metabolic alkalosis (excessive extracellular bicarbonate with pH >7.45) is associated with excessive loss of hydrogen ion (eg, intractable vomiting, gastric suctioning), diuretic-induced hypokalemia, primary hyperaldosteronism, abrupt relief of chronic hypercapnia, or excessive fecal loss of chloride ion (eg, congenital chloridorrhea, villous adenoma of the colon). Treatment of metabolic alkalosis should be aimed at reversing the underlying condition.

Supportive treatment with sodium chloride injection 0.9% and potassium chloride allows the kidneys to excrete bicarbonate and the systemic pH to be normalized. Patients who cannot tolerate volume expansion (eg, those with congestive heart failure) and those who do not respond to more conventional therapy require dialysis. In the past, some clinicians have favored the use of acidifying agents (eg, dilute hydrochloric acid, ammonium chloride, arginine hydrochloride, lysine hydrochloride); however, these agents are dangerous and their use in metabolic alkalosis is not recommended.

The concurrent alkalosis and hypokalemia present in patients with Cushing's syndrome and primary hyperaldosteronism are correctable with potassium chloride given orally or intravenously over several days.

Drug Evaluations

SODIUM BICARBONATE

USES. Sodium bicarbonate is the drug of choice in the treatment of metabolic acidosis secondary to actual loss of bicarbonate from the body. In acute mild to moderate acidosis, oral treatment is preferable to intravenous therapy; tablets (325 and 650 mg), oral solutions (2% to 5%), or a solution containing sodium bicarbonate 0.15% to 0.3% and sodium chloride 0.3% to 0.4% may be used. In severe acute acidosis, sodium bicarbonate may be given intravenously. Commercial solutions are generally hypertonic (4.2%, 5%, 7.5%, and 8.4%) and require dilution. The 7.5% solution, commonly employed in cardiac resuscitation, contains 44.6 mEq/50 ml (892 mEq/L).

ADVERSE REACTIONS AND PRECAUTIONS. Excessive amounts of sodium bicarbonate may cause metabolic alkalosis and hypernatremia. Rapid alkalization may precipitate tetany in hypocalcemic patients and cause cardiotoxicity and paralysis in hypokalemic patients. In addition, too rapid administration produces a transient elevation of PCO_2, and CO_2 diffuses into the cells and cerebrospinal fluid more rapidly than bicarbonate, resulting in intracellular and central nervous system acidosis. If it is administered in excess, sodium bicarbonate increases the production of lactate, worsens cardiac output, and decreases blood pressure in patients with lactic acidosis. Sodium bicarbonate should be given cautiously to patients with congestive heart failure or other edematous or sodium-retaining conditions, oliguria, or anuria.

Sodium bicarbonate injection is classified in FDA Pregnancy Category C.

DRUG INTERACTIONS. Patients receiving corticosteroids may retain excessive sodium if sodium bicarbonate is given. Alkalization of the urine by sodium bicarbonate may decrease the renal clearance of organic bases (eg, amphetamines, ephedrine, flecainide, quinidine, quinine). Conversely, the degree of ionization and renal clearance of organic acids (eg, chlorpropamide, phenobarbital, salicylates) may be increased. The renal clearance of lithium also may be accelerated by the increased renal sodium load.

DOSAGE AND PREPARATIONS. Dosages depend on the severity of acidosis and should be calculated to restore blood pH to the desired range. Dosages range from 1 to 25 mEq/kg of body weight/day (Brewer, 1990).

ORAL:
Generic. Powder; tablets 325 and 650 mg (11.9 mEq/g).

INTRAVENOUS:
Generic. Solution 4.2%, 5%, 7.5%, and 8.4%.

POTASSIUM CITRATE AND CITRIC ACID SOLUTION
[Polycitra-K]

POTASSIUM CITRATE, SODIUM CITRATE, AND CITRIC ACID SOLUTION
[Polycitra]

SODIUM CITRATE AND CITRIC ACID SOLUTION (Shohl's Solution)
[Bicitra]

Shohl's solution contains sodium citrate and citric acid equivalent to 1 mEq sodium and bicarbonate/ml. After absorption, the citrate is metabolized to bicarbonate. This systemic alkalizer is used most frequently in renal tubular acidosis, but it may be employed in chronic metabolic acidosis of other etiologies. For patients on sodium-restricted diets or with conditions requiring sodium restriction, the administration of potassium citrate and citric acid solution may be preferable. Patients who are at risk of hypokalemia after correction of acidosis may be given a solution containing potassium citrate, sodium citrate, and citric acid (Pohlman et al, 1984; Kinkead et al, 1991).

Patients often prefer these preparations to sodium bicarbonate because the former do not cause belching. They may, however, cause diarrhea, and large doses may produce nausea and vomiting.

DOSAGE AND PREPARATIONS.
Oral: *Adults,* for renal tubular acidosis, 0.5 to 2 mEq/kg in four or five divided doses daily. The total dose should be increased until acidosis and hypercalciuria are eliminated. Serum chloride and carbon dioxide content and urinary calcium excretion should be determined approximately twice yearly. The dosage requirement may be increased during intercurrent illness.

POTASSIUM CITRATE AND CITRIC ACID SOLUTION:
Polycitra-K (Willen). Solution containing potassium citrate 1,100 mg and citric acid 334 mg (equivalent to 2 mEq potassium and bicarbonate)/5 ml in 473 ml containers.

POTASSIUM CITRATE, SODIUM CITRATE, AND CITRIC ACID SOLUTION:
Polycitra (Willen). Syrup containing potassium citrate 550 mg, sodium citrate 500 mg, and citric acid 334 mg (equivalent to 1 mEq/ml potassium citrate and 1 mEq/ml sodium citrate or 2 mEq bicarbonate)/5 ml in 473 ml containers.

SODIUM CITRATE AND CITRIC ACID SOLUTION:
Bicitra (Willen). Solution containing sodium citrate dihydrate 500 mg and citric acid monohydrate 334 mg/5 ml in 15, 30, 120, 473, and 3,785 ml containers.

SODIUM LACTATE

Sodium lactate is metabolized to sodium bicarbonate in the liver and has been used to treat metabolic acidosis. However, sodium bicarbonate is preferred for this purpose, because the conversion of lactate to bicarbonate may be impaired in severely ill patients and those with hepatic disease. Its use is contraindicated in those with lactic acidosis.

PREPARATIONS.
Generic. Solution 5 and 167 mEq/L (M1/6).

SODIUM ACETATE

Sodium acetate is often used in total parenteral nutrition as a bicarbonate precursor. Acetate is converted to bicarbonate on an almost equimolar basis. It is readily metabolized outside the liver and its conversion is not impaired in severely ill patients or in those with hepatic disease.

PREPARATIONS.
Generic. Solution 2 mEq/ml in 20, 50, and 100 ml containers and 4 mEq/ml in 50 and 100 ml containers.

POTASSIUM IMBALANCES

Hypokalemia: Hypokalemia is defined as a serum potassium concentration $\leq$3.5 mEq/L; thiazide or loop diuretic therapy is the most common cause of hypokalemia. It also can be caused by decreased intake (eg, anorexia nervosa), increased gastrointestinal losses (eg, diarrhea, vomiting, laxative abuse, villous adenoma), and increased renal losses (eg, increased mineralocorticoid activity; renal tubular acidosis; delivery of large nonabsorbable anions, such as carbenicillin and sodium, to the distal nephron; hypomagnesemia).

Treatment depends on the severity of the condition and its underlying cause. Pharmacologic therapy may not be needed when hypokalemia is mild. Unless hypokalemic patients are receiving digitalis glycosides, have an abnormal electrocardiogram, or are otherwise at risk from hypokalemia, an increase in dietary potassium intake generally is all that is required (Bear and Neil, 1983). Potassium-sparing diuretics (amiloride [Midamor], triamterene [Dyrenium], spironolactone [Aldactone]) may be prescribed for more severe hypokalemia (see index entry Potassium-Sparing Diuretics). Potassium supplements should not be taken in conjunction with these diuretics, except in rare circumstances, because of the risk of hyperkalemia.

Oral replacement therapy is indicated in severe hypokalemia whenever feasible to avoid sudden large increases in serum potassium concentration. Potassium chloride solution is preferred to other salts because, if there is an associated metabolic alkalosis, this salt may correct both the hypokalemia and the metabolic alkalosis. There is little evidence that other salts are tolerated better than potassium chloride, but they are used in rare instances when hypokalemia is associated with acidosis (eg, renal tubular acidosis). Since potassium supplements are not retained well in patients receiving diuretics, large doses may be required. Patients with hypokalemia often have enhanced kaliuresis secondary to hypomagnesemia and require magnesium therapy in conjunction with potassium supplementation to restore potassium homeostasis (Whang et al, 1992). Approximately 60% of those with refractory hypokalemia may have magnesium deficiency concurrently (Whang et al, 1985).

If correction is indicated in patients unable to take potassium orally, potassium chloride is given intravenously. The electrocardiogram should be monitored frequently, because the dangerous effects of hyperkalemia can be detected more rapidly by changes in the electrocardiogram than by measuring serum potassium concentrations; however, the electrocardiogram is *not* a substitute for the determination of serum potassium concentration. An adequate urinary output also must be assured.

Hyperkalemia: Hyperkalemia (serum potassium concentration >5.5 mEq/L) usually is the result of impaired potassium excretion in patients with decreased renal function or impaired secretion of mineralocorticoids (Addison's disease, hypoaldosteronism). It may occur during inappropriate use of potassium supplements by those taking potassium-sparing diuretics or other drugs that either inhibit aldosterone secretion or depress the activity of the Na-K pump in muscle cells. It also may be caused by rapid intravenous administration of potassium-containing solutions, shift of potassium out of the cells (eg, acidosis, tissue breakdown, familial periodic paralysis), metabolic derangements, the effects of a number of drugs, thrombocytosis, or hemolysis (Brem, 1990). Hyperkalemia is more common in the elderly; those with mild to moderate renal failure are especially prone to hyporeninemic and subclinical forms of hypoaldosteronism (Kleinfeld and Corcoran, 1990).

Treatment depends on the degree of hyperkalemia and the severity of its manifestations. In all cases, potassium intake should be discontinued. No further treatment may be needed in those with mild hyperkalemia. When the electrocardiogram is distinctly abnormal (eg, absence of P-wave, widening of QRS complex, S-T segment changes with high peaked T waves) or the serum potassium concentration rises rapidly to more than 6.5 mEq/L, insulin should be administered to increase the cellular uptake of potassium. Concurrent intravenous infusion of dextrose injection 5% or 10% (1 L/10 to 15 units of regular insulin) will prevent iatrogenic hypoglycemia. Although this regimen reduces the serum potassium concentration, total body potassium content will remain elevated unless potassium excretion is stimulated.

An exchange resin (eg, sodium polystyrene sulfonate [Kayexalate]) may be given orally or rectally to promote the gastrointestinal elimination of potassium. The onset of action is slow with oral therapy, but an enema containing 30 to 50 g of the resin suspended in 150 ml of 20% to 70% sorbitol will reduce serum potassium concentration in about one hour. Because cationic exchange resins also bind calcium, calcium infusion may be necessary to avoid hypocalcemia. Loop diuretics also may increase urinary potassium excretion. In nonhypovolemic oliguric patients, hemodialysis or peritoneal dialysis may be indicated to remove large amounts of potassium from the blood, but this treatment is too slow for emergency management.

If cardiotoxicity is severe and the patient is not receiving digitalis, 10 to 30 ml of calcium gluconate 10% may be injected intravenously over a three- to five-minute period to counteract the cardiotoxic effects of potassium; this dose may be repeated once. The electrocardiogram should be monitored continuously. Calcium and sodium bicarbonate must be given separately to avoid calcium ion precipitation.

When the cause of hyperkalemia is not reversible, the serum potassium concentration should be maintained as close to normal as possible. The diet should contain little potassium, and drugs known to predispose to hyperkalemia should be avoided. Thiazide diuretics may be administered, and oral sodium bicarbonate (25 to 100 mEq daily) should be taken routinely (Kleinfeld and Corcoran, 1990).

Drug Evaluations

POTASSIUM CHLORIDE

USES. Since hypokalemia is usually accompanied by metabolic alkalosis, potassium chloride is the agent of choice for treatment. It is used to replace potassium lost by the potassium-wasting effect of thiazide and loop diuretics in those at risk from hypokalemia (eg, digitalized or cirrhotic patients) (see index entry Diuretics). In addition, all potassium-wasting diuretics may cause hypochloremic acidosis, and, if the chloride ion is not replaced, alkalosis and hypokalemia cannot be reversed even if large amounts of potassium are given.

Potassium chloride also may be indicated in those with inadequate dietary intake of potassium, excessive gastrointestinal losses, renal tubular disorders with potassium-wasting primary adrenal disease, or in those receiving corticosteroids. Potassium chloride also is used to treat digitalis intoxication and hypokalemic periodic paralysis.

FORMULATIONS. The liquid form of potassium chloride is the preparation of choice for oral therapy. Most commercial preparations contain 10 to 40 mEq of potassium chloride/15 ml and are flavored to mask the disagreeable taste. Such preparations *must be diluted* before ingestion to minimize gastric irritation, and administration with or after meals is advisable.

For patients who find the liquid unpalatable or intolerable, a prolonged-release preparation may be prescribed. The two primary forms of prolonged-release preparations are a tablet containing potassium chloride in a wax matrix and a capsule containing small microencapsulated particles of potassium chloride. Both forms are designed to release potassium slowly in the gastrointestinal tract; this prevents local exposure to high concentrations of potassium and chloride ions, thus reducing the risk of gastric irritation. Although prolonged-release preparations generally are safer than uncoated products, they occasionally cause small bowel lesions, esophageal ulceration and stricture, and perforation of gastric ulcer. There is no conclusive evidence that the microencapsulated capsule is safer or causes fewer side effects than the wax matrix form (Skoutakis et al, 1984).

The intravenous route is indicated in emergencies or when patients cannot take drugs orally. The electrocardiogram and serum potassium concentration should be monitored frequently, and adequate urinary output must be assured. Concentrated potassium chloride solutions may cause pain when injected into a small vein.

PRECAUTIONS AND DRUG INTERACTIONS. Potassium preparations should be given very cautiously to patients with impaired renal function because severe hyperkalemia may occur. Administering potassium to hypokalemic hypertensive individuals may lower blood pressure excessively. Potassium supplements are particularly dangerous in patients who are also receiving potassium-sparing diuretics. The effectiveness of digitalis is decreased when potassium salts are given concomitantly.

Potassium chloride is classified in FDA Pregnancy Category C.

DOSAGE AND PREPARATIONS. Frequent monitoring of plasma potassium concentrations may be required to avoid iatrogenic hyperkalemia.

Oral: *Adults,* 10 to 20 mEq three or four times daily. Patients receiving thiazide or loop diuretics may require 80 to 100 mEq daily.

For trademark preparations, see Table 6.

TABLE 6.
ORAL POTASSIUM PREPARATIONS

Tradename (Manufacturer)	mEq[1] Potassium	mEq[1] Anion	Formulation
LIQUID POTASSIUM CHLORIDE PRODUCTS			
Generic	10	Cl 10	Liquid
	20	Cl 20	Liquid
	30	Cl 30	Liquid
	40	Cl 40	Liquid
Kaochlor 10% Liquid[2,3] (Adria)	20	Cl 20	Liquid Liquid (sugar-free)
Kaon-Cl 20%[2] (Adria)	40	Cl 40	Liquid (sugar-free)
Kay Ciel[2] (Forest)	20	Cl 20	Liquid (sugar-free)
Klorvess 10%[2] (Sandoz)	20	Cl 20	Liquid
Rum-K (Fleming)	30	Cl 30	Liquid (sugar-free)
POTASSIUM CHLORIDE PRODUCTS FOR RECONSTITUTION			
Generic	20	Cl 20	Powder
Kato (ICN)	20	Cl 20	Powder
Kay Ciel Powder (Forest)	20	Cl 20	Powder (sugar-free)
K-Lor (Abbott)	20	Cl 20	Powder
Klor-Con (Upsher-Smith)	20	Cl 20	Powder (sugar-free)
Klor-Con/25 (Upsher-Smith)	25	Cl 25	Powder (sugar-free)
Klorvess Effervescent (Sandoz)	20	Cl 20	Effervescent powder (sugar-free) Effervescent tablet (sugar-free)
K-Lyte/Cl (Bristol)	25	Cl 25	Effervescent tablet Powder
K-Lyte/Cl 50 (Bristol)	50	Cl 50	Effervescent tablet
PROLONGED-RELEASE POTASSIUM CHLORIDE PRODUCTS			
Generic	1.33	Cl 1.33	Enteric-coated tablet
	8	Cl 8	Enteric-coated tablet
	10	Cl 10	Enteric-coated tablet

(continued on next page)

TABLE 6 (continued)

Tradename (Manufacturer)	mEq[1] Potassium	Anion	Formulation
Kaon Cl[3] (Adria)	6.7	Cl 6.7	Wax-matrix tablet
Kaon Cl-10 (Adria)	10	Cl 10	Wax-matrix tablet
K-Dur 10 (Key)	10	Cl 10	Microencapsulated capsule
K-Dur 20 (Key)	20	Cl 20	Microencapsulated capsule
Klor-Con (Upsher-Smith)	8 10	Cl 10 Cl 10	Wax-matrix tablet Wax-matrix tablet
Klotrix (Bristol)	10	Cl 10	Wax-matrix tablet
K-Tab (Abbott)	10	Cl 10	Wax-matrix tablet
Micro-K (Robins)	8	Cl 8	Microencapsulated capsule
Micro-K 10 (Robins)	10	Cl 10	Microencapsulated capsule
Slow-K (Summit)	8	Cl 8	Wax-matrix tablet
Ten-K (Summit)	10	Cl 10	Microencapsulated capsule
OTHER POTASSIUM PRODUCTS			
Generic	20 2	Gluc[4] 20 Gluc[4] 2	Liquid Tablet
Kaon Tablets (Adria)	5	Gluc[4] 5	Tablet
Klor-Con/EF (Upsher-Smith)	25	Citrate 25	Effervescent tablet (sugar-free)
K-Lyte (Bristol)	25	Bicarbonate and Citrate	Effervescent tablet
K-Lyte DS (Bristol)	50	Bicarbonate and Citrate	Effervescent tablet
Kolyum (Fisons)	20	Cl 3.4 Gluc[4] 16.6	Liquid (sugar-free) Powder (sugar-free)
Tri-K (Century)	45	Acetate, Bicarbonate, and Citrate	Liquid (sugar-free) contains saccharin
Twin-K (Boots)	20	Gluc[4] and Citrate	Liquid

[1] Per 15 ml, packet, or tablet
[2] Contains alcohol
[3] Contains tartrazine
[4] Gluc=Gluconate

Intravenous: Potassium chloride injection must be diluted before infusion. *Adults,* if the serum potassium concentration is greater than 2.5 mEq/L, neuromuscular and cardiac abnormalities are minimal, and renal function is not impaired, potassium is given in concentrations usually no greater than 40 mEq/L at a rate not exceeding 10 to 15 mEq/hr. The total dosage usually should not exceed 100 to 300 mEq/day. If the serum potassium concentration is less than 2 mEq/L in the presence of cardiovascular abnormalities or muscle paralysis, potassium may be given very cautiously in concentrations as high as 60 mEq/L at a rate of up to 40 mEq/hr. When high potassium concentrations are required in the infusate, the volume of fluid in the intravenous lines should be minimized to reduce the potential for harm in the event of an accidental rapid infusion of the complete fluid volume. Total dosage usually should not exceed 400 mEq/day. Infusions must be regulated carefully on the basis of results of continuous electrocardiographic monitoring and repeated serum and urinary potassium determinations.

Generic. Solutions 1.5 mEq/ml in 20 ml containers; 2 mEq/ml in 1, 5, 10, 15, 20, 30, 100, 200, 250, and 500 ml containers; 2.4 mEq/ml in 15 ml containers; 2.5 mEq/ml in 50 and 100 ml containers; 3.3 mEq/ml in 100 ml containers; 5 mEq/ml in 50 and 100 ml containers; and 10 mEq/ml in 100 ml containers. These preparations are extremely concentrated and *must* be diluted prior to use.

AVAILABLE MIXTURES OF DILUTE SOLUTIONS:

Generic. Potassium chloride 10, 20, 30 and 40 mEq/L with dextrose 5% in 1,000 ml containers.

Potassium chloride 20 and 40 mEq/L with sodium chloride 0.9% in 500 and 1,000 ml containers.

Potassium chloride 10, 20, 30, and 40 mEq/L with sodium chloride 0.2%, 0.225%, 0.3%, 0.33%, 0.45%, and 0.9% with dextrose 5% in 250, 500, and 1,000 ml containers.

POTASSIUM BICARBONATE AND CITRATE
[K-Lyte]

POTASSIUM GLUCONATE
[Kaon]

POTASSIUM ACETATE, BICARBONATE, AND CITRATE
[Tri-K]

These preparations are used to treat hypokalemia associated with hyperchloremia (eg, renal tubular acidosis). If they are used in patients with hypokalemic hypochloremic alkalosis, chloride ion also must be provided. There is no convincing evidence that any of these products is better tolerated than potassium chloride.

DOSAGE AND PREPARATIONS.

POTASSIUM BICARBONATE AND CITRATE; POTASSIUM GLUCONATE; POTASSIUM ACETATE, BICARBONATE, AND CITRATE:

Oral: For dosage, see evaluation on Potassium Chloride.

Kaon (Adria), ***K-Lyte*** (Bristol), ***Tri-K*** (Century). See Table 6 for preparations.

POTASSIUM ACETATE, BICARBONATE, AND CITRATE:

Intravenous: These preparations are extremely concentrated and must be diluted prior to use. For dosage, see evaluation on Potassium Chloride.

Generic. Solution 2 mEq/ml in 20 and 50 ml containers and 4 mEq/ml in 50 ml containers.

SODIUM POLYSTYRENE SULFONATE
[Kayexalate]

ACTIONS AND USES. This exchange resin is used occasionally to treat hyperkalemia. It acts by exchanging sodium ion for potassium in the intestine; the potassium-containing resin is then excreted in the feces. In clinical use, much of the exchange capacity is utilized for other cations and, possibly, lipids and proteins; therefore, in vivo exchange of potassium is estimated to be about 0.5 to 1 mEq of potassium/g of resin. Because its action is not evident for hours to days, sodium polystyrene sulfonate is most useful when serum potassium concentrations are not life-threatening or when other measures have reduced the immediate danger.

ADVERSE REACTIONS AND PRECAUTIONS. Adverse reactions usually involve the gastrointestinal tract. The most common are constipation, anorexia, nausea, and vomiting. Fecal impaction may occur in elderly patients when large oral doses are given without concomitant administration of a laxative (eg, sorbitol). Intestinal obstruction due to concretions of aluminum hydroxide coadministered with sodium polystyrene sulfonate have been reported.

Hypokalemia may occur as a result of therapy with sodium polystyrene sulfonate. The risk can be minimized if the serum potassium concentration is monitored at least daily during therapy and the dose is decreased or therapy discontinued when the concentration falls to 4 or 5 mEq/L. Sodium polystyrene sulfonate should be used with caution in patients receiving digitalis, since hypokalemia enhances digitalis toxicity. Hypocalcemia also may occur.

Sodium polystyrene sulfonate exchanges sodium for potassium and, therefore, should be used cautiously in patients who require salt restriction, since volume overload may occur. Because of this problem, calcium and hydrogen ion exchange resins have been used experimentally, but the former may cause hypercalcemia and the latter acidosis.

This drug is classified in FDA Pregnancy Category C.

DRUG INTERACTIONS. Concomitant use of sodium polystyrene sulfonate with antacids containing magnesium or calcium should be undertaken with caution, especially in patients with renal failure (Mangini, 1983). Sodium polystyrene sulfonate is thought to bind to magnesium and calcium, thus preventing these cations from combining with bicarbonate in the small intestine and resulting in systemic alkalosis (Hansten, 1979).

DOSAGE AND PREPARATIONS. Oral administration is generally preferred to rectal use because enemas are not as reliable and often are difficult to recover unless the resin is placed in a dialysis bag. However, patients with impaired coordination during swallowing or with nausea and vomiting because of uremia may aspirate the oral suspension; rectal administration may be preferable for these patients.

Oral: *Adults,* 15 g suspended in 45 to 60 ml of water, syrup, fruit juice, or a soft drink one to four times daily. The preparation may be administered by stomach tube. To prevent constipation, 10 to 20 ml of 70% sorbitol or 30 ml of 50% sorbitol is given every two to three hours until a loose stool is passed, then once or twice daily as needed.

Rectal: *Adults,* 30 to 50 g suspended in 100 ml of aqueous vehicle, such as sorbitol, is given every six hours initially (enemas may be given every one to two hours if the circumstances dictate); the frequency of administration may be decreased on succeeding days. The preparation should be retained as long as possible and should be followed by a cleansing enema. Some authorities prefer placement of the drug in a sealed dialysis bag that is inserted into the rectum.

Kayexalate (Sanofi Winthrop). Powder in 453.6 g containers [sodium content: approximately 100 mg (4.1 mEq)/g].

MAGNESIUM IMBALANCES

Hypomagnesemia: Hypomagnesemia (plasma magnesium concentration <1.8 mg/dL) may accompany inadequate intake, malabsorption (including that secondary to nontopical sprue, bypass surgery for obesity, short-bowel syndrome, laxative abuse, and villous adenoma), prolonged diarrhea, prolonged intravenous feeding without magnesium, pregnancy, lactation, chronic alcoholism, diuretic therapy, renal tubular damage (including nephrotoxicity induced by gentamicin, ticarcillin, carbenicillin, cyclosporine, and cisplatin), hyperaldosteronism, hyperthyroidism, hyperparathyroidism, diabetic ketoacidosis, acute intermittent porphyria, and other disorders often associated with hypocalcemia or hypokalemia. It occurs in approximately 20% of patients receiving digitalis glycoside therapy (Whang et al, 1985).

Magnesium gluconate, magnesium chloride, or magnesium hydroxide (milk of magnesia) may be used orally for supplementation. Magnesium sulfate may be given intramuscularly for treatment of hypomagnesemia. Alternatively, it may be given intravenously in low concentrations alone or as a component of multiple electrolyte solutions to prevent iatrogenic deficiency during routine fluid and electrolyte therapy. Magnesium sulfate should be administered cautiously if renal function is impaired.

Hypermagnesemia: Most patients can tolerate moderately elevated plasma concentrations of magnesium, but toxicity may occur when concentrations exceed 3.6 mg/dL due to oversupplementation, laxative abuse, or prolonged administration of magnesium (eg, in antacid preparations or cathartics) in patients with severe renal impairment. In such patients, hypermagnesemia may cause diarrhea, nausea, vomiting, refractory hypotension, and muscle weakness. Occasionally, third-degree atrioventricular block and respiratory arrest occur. The intravenous administration of 5 to 10 mEq of calcium salts counteracts the depression of the respiratory muscles. As in the treatment of hyperkalemia, dextrose and insulin also may be infused to cause an influx of magnesium into the cells (Parfitt and Kleerekoper, 1980). Dialysis is indicated in severe hypermagnesemia with coexisting renal insufficiency and/or refractory hypotension.

Drug Evaluations

MAGNESIUM CHLORIDE
[Slow-Mag]

MAGNESIUM CITRATE
[Citroma]

MAGNESIUM GLUCONATE
[Magonate]

MAGNESIUM HYDROXIDE (Milk of Magnesia)

MAGNESIUM OXIDE
[Maox, Uro-Mag]

MAGNESIUM SULFATE

USES. Magnesium sulfate is used intravenously or intramuscularly to treat severe hypomagnesemia, to prevent hypomagnesemia during total parenteral nutrition (TPN), and in convulsive states, especially eclampsia. The duration of action of an intramuscular dose of magnesium sulfate is several hours; intravenous doses last only 30 minutes.

Magnesium gluconate is less likely to cause diarrhea and is more rapidly absorbed and bioavailable than the chloride, citrate, oxide, or hydroxide salt (Nicar and Pak, 1982; Lindberg et al, 1990).

PRECAUTIONS AND INTERACTIONS. Magnesium sulfate interacts with succinylcholine and the nondepolarizing neuromuscular blocking agents. It should be given cautiously to patients with impaired renal function and to those receiving digitalis and is contraindicated in patients with heart block. A calcium salt (eg, calcium gluconate) should be available for intravenous injection to counteract the potential hazard of respiratory depression.

Parenteral magnesium sulfate is classified in FDA Pregnancy Category D.

DOSAGE AND PREPARATIONS.
Oral: *Adults and older children,* for magnesium supplementation, 5 mg of magnesium/kg/day. Magnesium gluconate or magnesium hydroxide tablets are generally used and should be taken two hours after a meal to minimize diarrhea and at least one hour before the next meal to maximize absorption (Mansmann, 1991). Intestinal upset can be reduced by ingesting a partial dose initially and gradually increasing intake until stools first begin to soften (Mansmann, 1991). If an oral liquid is preferred, magnesium hydroxide (milk of magnesia) or magnesium gluconate four times/day is recommended (Flink, 1985; Mansmann, 1991).

MAGNESIUM CHLORIDE:
Slow-Mag (Searle). Tablets (enteric-coated, prolonged-release) 64 mg (nonprescription).

MAGNESIUM CITRATE:
Generic. Solution 7% in 300 ml containers (nonprescription).
Citroma (Century). Solution 7% in 296 ml containers (nonprescription).

MAGNESIUM GLUCONATE:
Generic. Tablets 30, 500, and 550 mg.
Magonate (Fleming). Tablets 500 mg (containing magnesium 27 mg); liquid 55 mg/5 ml.

MAGNESIUM HYDROXIDE (MILK OF MAGNESIA):
Generic. Tablets 325 mg; liquid 390 mg/5 ml (nonprescription).

MAGNESIUM OXIDE:
Maox (Kenneth Manne). Tablets 420 mg (contains tartrazine) (nonprescription).
Uro-Mag (Blaine). Capsules 140 mg (nonprescription).

Intramuscular, Intravenous: *Adults and older children,* for severe hypomagnesemia, 2 to 4 g (4 to 8 ml of 50% solution or 16 to 32 mEq) daily intramuscularly in divided doses; administration is repeated daily until serum concentrations return to normal. If the deficiency is not severe, 1 g (2 ml of 50% solution) can be given once or twice daily. Serum magnesium concentrations should serve as a guide to continued treatment. Magnesium sulfate 10% may be infused intravenously at a rate not exceeding 1.5 ml/min. It also may be added to TPN solution (see index entry Nutrition, Parenteral).

For pre-eclampsia and eclampsia, see index entry Magnesium Sulfate.

MAGNESIUM SULFATE:

Generic. Solution 10% in 1, 20, and 50 ml containers, 12.5% in 8 ml containers, and 50% in 2, 5, 10, 20, 30, 50, and 100 ml containers.

Cited References

Essential drugs. *WHO Drug Information* 4:180-182, 1990.

Oral rehydration therapy: Its place in the developed world. *WHO Drug Information* 5:120-121, 1991.

American Academy of Pediatrics, Committee on Nutrition: Use of oral fluid therapy and posttreatment feeding following enteritis in children in a developed country. *Pediatrics* 75:358-361, 1985.

Arieff AI, Ayus JC: Treatment of symptomatic hyponatremia: Neither haste nor waste. *Crit Care Med* 19:748-751, 1991.

Avery ME, Snyder JD: Oral therapy for acute diarrhea: The underused simple solution. *N Engl J Med* 323:891-894, 1990.

Baumgart S, et al: Fluid, electrolyte, and glucose maintenance in the very low birth weight infant. *Clin Pediatr* 21:199-206, (April) 1982.

Bear RA, Neil GA: Clinical approach to common electrolyte problems: 2. Potassium imbalances. *Can Med Assoc J* 129:28-31, 1983.

Boineau FG, Lewy JE: Estimation of parenteral fluid requirements. *Pediatr Clin North Am* 37:257-264, 1990.

Brem AS: Disorders of potassium homeostasis. *Pediatr Clin North Am* 37:419-428, 1990.

Brewer ED: Disorders of acid-base balance. *Pediatr Clin North Am* 37:429-448, 1990.

Brown KH: Dietary management of acute childhood diarrhea: Optimal timing of feeding and appropriate use of milks and mixed diets. *J Pediatr* 118:S92-S98, 1991.

Casteel HB, Fiedorek SC: Oral rehydration therapy. *Pediatr Clin North Am* 37:295-312, 1990.

Chowdhury AMR, et al: Oral rehydration therapy: A community trial comparing the acceptability of homemade sucrose and cereal-based solutions. *Bull WORLD Health Organ* 69:229-234, 1991.

Conley SB: Hypernatremia. *Pediatr Clin North Am* 37:365-372, 1990.

El-Dahr SS, Chevalier RL: Special needs of the newborn infant in fluid therapy. *Pediatr Clin North Am* 37:323-336, 1990.

Feig PU: Hypernatremia and hypertonic syndromes. *Med Clin North Am* 65:271-290, 1981.

Finberg L: Water intoxication: A prevalent problem in the inner city, editorial. *Am J Dis Child* 145:981-982, 1991.

Flink EB: Hypomagnesemia in patient receiving digitalis. *Arch Intern Med* 145:625-626, 1985.

Freitag JJ, Miller LW: *Manual of Medical Therapeutics*, ed 23. Boston, Little Brown, 1980.

Gore SM, et al: Impact of rice based oral rehydration solution on stool output and duration of diarrhoea: Meta-analysis of 13 clinical trials. *Br Med J* 304:287-291, 1992.

Graf H, et al: Evidence for detrimental effect of bicarbonate therapy in hypoxic lactic acidosis. *Science* 227:754-756, 1985.

Hansten PD: *Drug Interactions*, ed 4. Philadelphia, Lea & Febiger, 1979.

Hirschhorn N, Greenough WB III: Progress in oral rehydration therapy. *Sci Am* 264:50-56, (May) 1991.

The International Study Group on Improved ORS: Impact of glycine-containing ORS solutions on stool output and duration of diarrhoea: A meta-analysis of seven clinical trials. *Bull WORLD Health Organ* 69:541-548, 1991.

Kallen RJ: The management of diarrheal dehydration in infants using parenteral fluids. *Pediatr Clin North Am* 37:265-286, 1990.

Keating JP, et al: Oral water intoxication in infants: An American epidemic. *Am J Dis Child* 145:985-990, 1991.

Khin-Maung-U, Greenough WB III: Cereal-based oral rehydration therapy, I: Clinical studies. *J Pediatr* 118:S72-S79, 1991.

Khin-Maung-U, et al: Effect on clinical outcome of breast feeding during acute diarrhoea. *Br Med J* 290:587-589, 1985.

Kinkead TM, et al: The varied forms of RTA and how to treat them. *Contemp Urol* 3:33-54, (April) 1991.

Kleinfeld M, Corcoran AJ: Hyperkalemia in the elderly. *Compr Ther* 16:48-53, (Sept) 1990.

Kopple JD, Blumenkrantz MJ: Total parenteral nutrition and parenteral fluid therapy, in Maxwell MH, Kleeman CR (eds): *Clinical Disorders of Fluid and Electrolyte Metabolism*, ed 3. New York, McGraw-Hill, 1980, 413-498.

Lavizzo-Mourey R: Dehydration. *Drug Ther* 56-61, (Jan) 1987.

Lawson DH, Henry DA: Drug therapy reviews: Intravenous fluid therapy. *Am J Hosp Pharm* 34:1332-1338, 1977.

Lebenthal E: Rice as a carbohydrate substrate in oral rehydration solutions (ORS), editorial. *J Pediatr Gastroenterol Nutr* 11:293-296, 1990.

Lebenthal E, Lu R-B: Glucose polymers as an alternative to glucose in oral rehydration solutions. *J Pediatr* 118:S62-S69, 1991.

Lifshitz F, et al: Refeeding of infants with acute diarrheal disease. *J Pediatr* 118:S99-S108, 1991.

Lindberg JS, et al: Magnesium bioavailability from magnesium citrate and magnesium oxide. *J Am Coll Nutr* 9:48-55 (No. 1), 1990.

Mackenzie A, Barnes G: Randomised controlled trial comparing oral and intravenous rehydration therapy in children with diarrhoea. *Br Med J* 303:393-396, 1991.

Madias NE: Lactic acidosis, forum. *Kidney Int* 29:752-774, 1986.

Mangini RJ (ed): *Drug Interaction Facts*. St Louis, Mo, Facts and Comparisons Division, JB Lippincott, 1983, 430a.

Mansmann HC Jr: Consider magnesium homeostasis point. *Pediatr Asthma Allergy Immunol* 5:273-279, 1991.

Narins RG, Cohen JJ: Bicarbonate therapy for organic acidosis: The case for its continued use. *Ann Intern Med* 106:615-618, 1987.

Nicar MJ, Pak CYC: Oral magnesium load test for the assessment of intestinal magnesium absorption. *Miner Electrolyte Metab* 8:44-51, 1982.

Parfitt AM, Kleerekoper M: Clinical disorders of calcium, phosphorus, and magnesium metabolism, in Maxwell MH, Kleeman CR (eds): *Clinical Disorders of Fluid and Electrolyte Metabolism*, ed 3. New York, McGraw-Hill, 1980, 947-1151.

Pizarro D, et al: Rice-based oral electrolyte solutions for the management of infantile diarrhea. *N Engl J Med* 324:517-521, 1991.

Pohlman T, et al: Renal tubular acidosis. *J Urol* 132:431-436, 1984.

Quintanilli AP, Qureshi N: Renal acidosis. *Comp Ther* 7:51-55, (March) 1981.

Ribeiro HDC Jr, Lifshitz F: Alanine-based oral rehydration therapy for infants with acute diarrhea. *J Pediatr* 118:S86-S90, 1991.

Sack DA: Use of oral rehydration therapy in acute watery diarrhoea: A practical guide. *Drugs* 41:566-573, 1991.

Santosham M, Greenough WB III: Oral rehydration therapy: A global perspective. *J Pediatr* 118:S44-S51, 1991.

Santosham M, et al: Role of soy-based, lactose-free formula during treatment of acute diarrhea. *Pediatrics* 76:292-298, 1985.

Sarnaik AP, et al: Management of hyponatremic seizures in children with hypertonic saline: A safe and effective strategy. *Crit Care Med* 19:758-762, 1991.

Sazawal S, et al: Alanine-based oral rehydration solution: Assessment of efficacy in acute noncholera diarrhea among children. *J Pediatr Gastroenterol* 12:461-468, 1991.

Skoutakis VA, et al: Liquid and solid potassium chloride: Bioavailability and safety. *Pharmacotherapy* 4:392-397, 1984.

Snyder JD: Use and misuse of oral therapy for diarrhea: Comparison of US practices with American Academy of Pediatrics recommendations. *Pediatrics* 87:28-33, 1991.

Whang R, et al: Frequency of hypomagnesemia in hospitalized patients receiving digitalis. *Arch Intern Med* 145:655-656, 1985.

Whang R, et al: Refractory potassium repletion: A consequence of magnesium deficiency. *Arch Intern Med* 152:40-45, 1992.

World Health Organization: Oral rehydration therapy for treatment of diarrhea in the home. *WHO Diarrheal Disease Programme*, 1986.

Drugs Used in Urologic Disorders

40

Lower urinary tract dysfunction (disorders of micturition) may be manifested as recurrent urinary tract infection, recurrent or persistent retention of urine, urinary frequency, or incontinence. It is of paramount importance to examine the patient thoroughly before instituting therapy. Diagnosis of most disorders of urinary function can be suggested by history, physical examination, and simple laboratory tests. Urodynamic tests are indicated in most patients for definitive diagnosis and may be useful to document drug efficacy prior to instituting long-term therapy (Mundy et al, 1984).

Drugs that stimulate or inhibit smooth muscle activity are beneficial in some disorders of the lower urinary tract. The goals of therapy are to improve the storage and/or emptying functions of the urinary bladder and to prevent renal complications.

PHYSIOLOGY

Storage and elimination of urine are accomplished by coordinated activity of (1) the smooth muscle of the bladder wall (detrusor muscle), (2) the smooth muscle of the bladder neck and proximal urethra (the "internal" or "smooth" sphincter), (3) the striated muscle layer of the outer wall of the urethra (the intrinsic rhabdosphincter), and (4) the periurethral striated muscle of the urogenital diaphragm and levator ani (the "external sphincter"). The bladder expands when the volume of urine increases (accommodation or compliance), and continence is maintained by the tonicity of the internal sphincter and activity in the external sphincter. Voluntary contraction of the external sphincter can inhibit micturition indefinitely and terminates micturition in progress promptly. In males, the preprostatic urethra is surrounded by sympathetically innervated smooth muscle that is continuous with the capsule of the prostate. Contraction of this musculature in the bladder neck prevents the retrograde propulsion of seminal fluid into the bladder during ejaculation.

The afferent nerve impulses generated in stretch receptors of the bladder wall are activated by bladder distention (filling). These nerve impulses are relayed to the central nervous system and the efferent arm of the reflex arc, and the pelvic parasympathetic nerves activate the bladder detrusor muscle. At the same time, motor activity in the pudendal nerves is inhibited, which relaxes the periurethral striated muscles of the external sphincter. This "micturition reflex" is integrated in the brain stem rostral pons. Volitional control of the reflex is maintained by excitatory and inhibitory pathways originating in the cerebral cortex. Bladder neck resistance is decreased by inhibition of sympathetic nerve activity resulting in suppression of alpha$_1$-adrenergic receptor activity in the internal sphincter during voiding. Inhibitory neural signals from the frontal cortex prevent uninhibited detrusor contractions (premature contractions of the bladder smooth muscle). In normal micturition, the first urodynamic event is cessation of sphincter activity (which can be measured by electromyography) accompanied by a decrease in outlet resistance. This is followed by contraction of the detrusor muscle; the bladder neck opens concurrently.

Sympathetic tone is presumed to be of minor importance in normal urinary function, but it may be a major element of outlet resistance in some pathologic conditions affecting the lower motor neuron bladder.

The physiology of the lower urinary tract, the influence of certain congenital neuronal anomalies and of central nervous system lesions on function, and the effects of pharmacotherapy have been reviewed (McGuire, 1986 A; Wein, 1992).

UROLOGIC DISORDERS: URINE STORAGE AND EMPTYING

Incontinence in Adults

Incontinence, the involuntary loss of urine, represents a failure in the storage phase of bladder function. Various factors may be responsible, and the specific cause must be determined in order to select the appropriate therapy (Wein, 1992).

Only about 30% of patients with incontinence seek medical assistance. Failure to obtain treatment may be due to embarrassment, fear, or lack of faith in physicians (Fonda, 1990). Incontinence can be eliminated in about one-third of all patients, and leakage can be reduced to a tolerable level in another one-third. For the remaining patients, use of absorbent pads and other methods can allow most to lead normal lives (Resnick, 1990).

Maximal use of nonpharmacologic, nonsurgical measures should be instituted before drugs or surgery are considered; scheduled voiding regimens, pelvic muscle exercises, biofeedback training, or electrical stimulation may be employed prior to or as an adjunct to drug therapy (Weiss, 1991).

Reversible causes of incontinence should be excluded before initiating any therapy. In particular, the patient's current medications should be reviewed to determine if they could be responsible for or contribute to incontinence. Drugs that can potentially weaken bladder contraction include antipsychotic agents (eg, phenothiazines, haloperidol), anticholinergic agents (eg, propantheline, oxybutynin, hyoscyamine), antihistamines, opioids, sedative/hypnotics (eg, benzodiazepines, barbiturates), tricyclic antidepressants (eg, imipramine), and drugs with the potential to affect sympathetic nerve function (eg, antihypertensive agents, alpha-adrenergic receptor agonists and antagonists). For a more extensive list of drugs that adversely affect continence, see Bissada and Finkbeiner, 1988, and Resnick, 1990.

A Consensus Conference (National Institutes of Health, 1989) and various reports (eg, Brandeis and Resnick, 1992; Peggs, 1992) have reviewed management strategies for the incontinent elderly, particularly the institutionalized patient. These should be consulted for assessment of the elderly patient's needs and for information on the efficacy and limitations of various treatment programs for this population.

UNSTABLE BLADDER. The terms unstable bladder, urge incontinence, uninhibited neurogenic bladder, detrusor instability, detrusor hyperreflexia, detrusor overactivity, and detrusor hyperactivity have been used interchangeably when referring to uninhibited, involuntary detrusor contractions. The most accurate terms are detrusor instability or detrusor overactivity. In most incontinent patients, the cause of uninhibited contractions is non-neurogenic and the condition is referred to specifically as detrusor instability. When the contractions are caused by neurologic lesions, the condition is termed detrusor hyperreflexia. The latter is common in patients with lesions superior to the micturition reflex center in the midpons (Parkinson's disease), after stroke, and in individuals with a spinal cord lesion (tumor, multiple sclerosis, or congenital anomalies). In patients with a suprasacral spinal cord lesion (tumor, multiple sclerosis, or congenital anomalies), there also may be dysfunction of the sphincters (Blaivas, 1988 A; McGuire, 1986 B; Wein, 1992).

Urge incontinence refers simply to the condition of a person who cannot always reach the toilet in time; these patients usually have a normal sensorium. Urge incontinence can be mimicked by other conditions, including urinary retention with overflow incontinence. Since frequency and nocturia also may be present in urge as well as overflow incontinence, determination of the postvoid residual volume is essential (McGuire, 1988). Dysuria usually does *not* occur unless there is concurrent infection. In patients with cystitis, the desire to void usually is constant and is unrelieved by urination.

Irritation of the bladder mucosa caused by infection, stones, irradiation, interstitial cystitis, or carcinoma, as well as unstable bladder secondary to outflow obstruction (eg, prostatic hyperplasia, obstruction of the bladder neck) should be ruled out. Acute vaginitis, mucosal atrophy of the urethra and vagina in postmenopausal women, and chronic constipation should be corrected, since these conditions may be associated with unstable bladder. Accessible toilet facilities should be provided for patients with reduced mobility or physical handicaps.

Nondrug Therapy: The following recommendations on the value of behavioral therapy for urinary incontinence are in general accordance with guidelines developed by the Health and Human Services Agency for Health Care Policy and Research (*FDC Reports*, 1992 A; Urinary Incontinence Guideline Panel, 1992).

Detrusor control may improve significantly in patients with non-neurogenic causes of detrusor instability or urge incontinence by instituting a timed voiding schedule with progressively longer intervals between urinations (bladder retraining drill), and this should be the initial treatment of choice (Jarvis, 1982; Weiss, 1983, 1991; Fantl et al, 1991). However, a good initial response may not be sustained (Ferrie et al, 1984). Drug therapy is limited to patients who are unable or unwilling to participate in retraining, for those in whom bladder spasms occur frequently despite retraining, and for those in whom retraining is ineffective or not sustained.

For patients unable to participate in a bladder retraining program but who can urinate on command and retain more than 150 ml of urine in the bladder without eliciting a contraction, a fixed voiding schedule (usually every two hours during the day and every four hours at night) can be instituted. Drugs to suppress or delay detrusor contractions may be useful, but they should be considered only ancillary to the regular schedule of bladder emptying (*Lancet,* 1986).

Drug Therapy: In some patients, anticholinergic agents (eg, propantheline [Pro-Banthine]) or antispasmodics with anticholinergic activity (eg, oxybutynin [Ditropan]) can be used to suppress or at least delay the reflex until intravesical distention is greater (Finkbeiner and Bissada, 1980; Gajewski and Awad, 1986; Lloyd, 1979; Wein, 1986). Some practitioners prefer antispasmodics to the more potent anticholinergic agents (eg, propantheline) (Resnick, 1988); however, these drugs may be less effective in some elderly patients (Brandeis and Resnick, 1992). The side effects of these agents (dryness of the mouth, constipation) are most commonly cited by patients as the reason for lack of compliance.

One-half of the usual dose may control urge incontinence in the elderly as well as in some middle-aged and younger patients and markedly reduces the severity of side effects (Diokno, 1983; Malone-Lee et al, 1992). Results also have been promising in elderly patients, particularly those over 70 years, who are given imipramine [Tofranil] in a single dose at bedtime. Doxepin [Sinequan] may be substituted for imipramine if the latter induces or exacerbates orthostatic hypotension, a particular problem in the elderly (Lose et al, 1989). The effect of tricyclic drugs is additive to that of anticholinergic agents, and care should be exercised to avoid excessive atropine-like side effects when both agents are prescribed. Oxybutynin and other agents with anticholinergic actions can produce overflow incontinence by causing retention in susceptible individuals or when given in large doses. Urinary retention occurs more frequently in patients with coexistent asymptomatic prostatism or other forms of outlet obstruction. These individuals may be managed with intermittent self-catheterization.

To avoid side effects and noncompliance while retaining the effectiveness of anticholinergic agents in patients with urge incontinence, a low dose of medication can be administered continuously. Excellent results were reported with this technique in a small study employing transdermal scopolamine patches [Transderm-Scōp] designed for motion sickness (Wiener et al, 1986). In this study, scopolamine patches containing 1.5 mg were applied to the skin and replaced at three-day intervals. The value of this technique for long-term management of urgency is being assessed.

Because bladder wall activity may be increased by the prostaglandins, inhibitors of prostaglandin synthesis (eg, indomethacin [Indocin]) have been used in patients with detrusor instability (Cardozo and Stanton, 1980), but little objective evidence exists to indicate that they are effective (Wein, 1990). Baclofen [Lioresal] (Taylor and Bates, 1979) and the calcium channel blocking agents (eg, verapamil [Calan, Isoptin, Verelan], nifedipine [Procardia]) have been used investigationally, but data are limited. For patients who do not respond to or are unable to tolerate oral agents, but who are able to perform intermittent self-catheterization, intravesical instillation of some of these agents (eg, oxybutynin, verapamil) has been effective.

Terodiline, an investigational agent with both anticholinergic and calcium channel blocking activity, has been used extensively in Europe for incontinence due to unstable bladder (Langtry and McTavish, 1990; Wein, 1990). In a placebo-controlled study on 98 women in the United States, this agent was effective and safe in reducing urge incontinence (Ouslander et al, 1993). Initially, few adverse reactions were reported, and terodiline appeared to be safer than oxybutynin; moreover, its twice-daily dosing schedule is convenient. However, reports in England of serious cardiotoxicity (eg, heart block, ventricular tachycardia [torsades de pointes] that caused several fatalities) prompted the voluntary withdrawal of this agent worldwide by the manufacturer pending the results of further studies on safety (*Pharmaceut J*, 1991; Veldhuis and Inman, 1991; Ouslander et al, 1993).

STRESS INCONTINENCE. Stress incontinence may be defined as the involuntary loss of small amounts of urine following a sudden increase in intra-abdominal pressure, as may occur during coughing, sneezing, laughing, change to a standing position, or physical exercise (walking, running), usually *without* other urinary symptoms. It usually is caused by sphincter incompetence but sometimes may result from an unstable bladder. It is most often of non-neurogenic origin.

Non-neurogenic stress incontinence (also called genuine stress incontinence) is common in older, particularly multiparous, women. The mechanism of urine loss is controversial but is known to be related to hypermobility of the vesicourethral junction. Elevations in intra-abdominal pressure are transmitted inadequately to the upper urethra where it descends below the pelvic diaphragm (Cantor, 1979). Another form of non-neurogenic stress incontinence is referred to as intrinsic sphincter deficiency and may result from loss of urethral sphincter function. This can be caused by aging, injury, inflammation, denervation, or scarring from instrumentation and surgery, particularly multiple surgical procedures for stress incontinence. It also can be observed in patients with myelodysplasia (Barbalias and Blaivas, 1983; McGuire, 1986 A) and after radical pelvic surgery (eg, hysterectomy, abdominoperineal resection of the rectum) (Blaivas and Barbalias, 1983).

There is now considerable evidence that detrusor instability occurs in many women with stress incontinence; however, whether the two conditions are related is controversial.

Nondrug Therapy: Alternatives to drug therapy that decrease the need for surgery include use of modified Kegel exercises to strengthen pelvic floor muscles; they relieve leakage in 65% to 75% of women with stress incontinence and may cure about 25% (Cammu et al, 1991; Weiss, 1991; Fantl et al, 1991). (These exercises are of less value in men.) A procedure that also strengthens pelvic floor muscles and forces women to use the correct muscles employs weights (Femina cones) that are inserted into the vagina; as pelvic strength improves, heavier weights are used (Cotton, 1990; Olah et al, 1990). In one study, cones used together with Kegel exercises restored muscle tone sooner than the exercises alone (one versus six months). Another promising approach is the use of electrical stimulation devices inserted into the vagina. By strengthening the muscles, electrical stimulation may cure 30% of patients with stress incontinence (Weiss, 1991; Bankhead, 1991). Inhibition of neurologic impulses blocks involuntary detrusor contractions and may cure 60% of individuals with urge incontinence.

Periurethral devices consisting of Teflon or collagen implants inserted around the bladder neck or over the sphincter have controlled incontinence due to intrinsic sphincter dysfunction (Appell, 1990; *FDC Reports*, 1990; Cotton, 1990). Periurethral injection of glutaraldehyde crosslinked collagen appears to be effective and safe in patients with intrinsic sphincter dysfunction, and it may be a suitable alternative to surgery (Herschorn et al, 1992; Stricker and Haylen, 1993). Enthusiasm for suburethral injection of Teflon has waned because the migration of particles to other tissues may cause granulomas, and proper placement is difficult (Stricker and Haylen, 1993). Implantation of an artificial sphincter, which is now approved by the FDA, also may be beneficial (Webster et al, 1992).

Patients with mixed incontinence may respond to a timed voiding pattern at frequent intervals (eg, every two hours), even in the absence of a voiding urge (Godec, 1984). If no benefit is observed within two weeks, drug therapy may be instituted. The effectiveness of surgery for mixed incontinence is controversial.

Drug Therapy: The striated muscle tone of the external sphincter cannot be enhanced by drugs, but proximal urethral resistance can be increased by agents that activate alpha-adrenergic receptors in the smooth muscle of the internal sphincter. For this reason, alpha-adrenergic drugs, such as ephedrine (usually the drug of choice), phenylpropanolamine [Propagest] (the preferred drug if the side effects or potential side effects of ephedrine are unacceptable), and pseudoephedrine [Sudafed, Novafed], sometimes may be used to treat mild stress incontinence; they also have been employed when surgical correction is not appropriate or must be deferred.

Some postmenopausal women with stress incontinence benefit from the administration of an oral or topical vaginal preparation of estrogen (Wein, 1985 A, 1990; Marsh, 1993). There appears to be no correlation between the patient's age, time since menopause, or duration of symptoms and the effectiveness of the therapy. However, a correlation can be demonstrated between the effectiveness of therapy and the appearance during urethral cytologic examination of estrogen-induced maturation from transitional to intermediate squamous epithelium (Bhatia et al, 1989). Pharmacologic doses of estrogen are required for significant effects, and adverse reactions (eg, gallbladder and thromboembolic diseases, hepatic adenomas, endometrial carcinoma) are possible with long-term therapy. The combination of estrogen plus an alpha-adrenergic agent (eg, phenylpropanolamine) appears to have an additive effect (Diokno, 1983; Kinn and Lindskog, 1988).

OVERFLOW INCONTINENCE. Overflow (paradoxical) incontinence is caused by inadequate emptying of the bladder. Continual dribbling occurs when the weight of the urine in the distended bladder overcomes outlet resistance. This condition may result from outflow obstruction (eg, due to prostatic enlargement), hypotonicity of the detrusor muscle (particularly in women), or loss of bladder sensation to filling (sensory neurogenic [paralytic] bladder) that may occur in diabetic visceral neuropathy or tabes dorsalis.

Therapy: Surgery to relieve obstruction or periodic self-catheterization is required. In the absence of obstruction, cholinergic drugs (eg, bethanechol [Duvoid, Myotonachol, Urecholine]) have been administered in an attempt to stimulate bladder contractions, or alpha-adrenergic receptor antagonists (eg, phenoxybenzamine [Dibenzyline], prazosin [Minipress], terazosin [Hytrin]) have been prescribed to relax the smooth muscle of the internal sphincter. However, little or no benefit is obtained with these drugs.

POSTPROSTATECTOMY INCONTINENCE. Mild to moderate incontinence due to injury of smooth and skeletal muscle during prostatectomy, and more commonly when surgery and radiation therapy have been combined, is sometimes improved by drug therapy. Most men recover within a few weeks following resection, but urgency and urge incontinence persist in at least 10% (Jones and Schoenberg, 1985). These can be relieved with anticholinergic drugs (oxybutynin, propantheline, hyoscyamine [Anaspaz, Cystospaz, Levsin]). Adrenergic drugs (phenylpropanolamine) or drugs with multiple actions (imipramine) are used if sphincter incompetence is the primary dysfunction. Ancillary measures, particularly sphincter exercises, also can be beneficial.

Incontinence due to edema or loss of elasticity of the sphincter distal to the verumontanum occasionally improves with time. If drug therapy does not control incontinence after one year, periurethral collagen injection or insertion of an inflatable artificial sphincter should be considered (Gundian et al, 1993). If urodynamic evaluation demonstrates detrusor instability or poor compliance associated with significant stress incontinence, this *must* be corrected before implantation of an artificial sphincter to avoid the potential complications of hydroureteronephrosis and vesicoureteral reflux (Leach et al, 1987).

Neurogenic Urinary Retention in Adults

Neurogenic disorders of the lower urinary tract may result from trauma, surgery, congenital defects, ischemia, tumors, infection (eg, herpes simplex, herpes zoster), neurologic disease, or a defect in corticoregulatory control without a detectable organic lesion. There may be an associated malfunction of the detrusor muscle, internal sphincter, or external sphincter; the disorders may exist alone or with coordinated or uncoordinated bladder-sphincter function (dyssynergia).

After motor and sensory denervation of the urinary bladder, detrusor tone is maintained but reflex contractility is lost. If both the internal and external sphincter are nonfunctional, intravesical pressure remains low because of the resulting incontinence; the bladder will not increase in size and the upper urinary tract remains normal. However, if adequate internal or external sphincter activity, or both, is retained to require an intravesical pressure >40 cm of water to overcome urethral resistance, the bladder wall thickens and becomes trabeculated, the ureters dilate, vesicoureteral reflex may occur, and there is risk of upper urinary tract dysfunction.

Therapy: Patients with high intravesical pressure are maintained with intermittent self-catheterization. If pressure remains high between catheterizations, anticholinergic drugs are employed and catheterization is performed more frequently. Alpha-adrenergic agents and external sphincterotomy can be used in males; striated sphincterotomy can be used in patients with documented dyssynergy (McGuire, 1986 A). High pressure voiding techniques, such as external compression (Credé maneuver), are generally ineffective unless both internal and external sphincter tone are markedly reduced.

The cholinergic drug, bethanechol, has been used to enhance intravesical pressure and thus facilitate bladder emptying in patients with spinal cord lesions above S_2-S_4 (*reflex neurogenic bladder*) during the recovery phase after spinal shock. However, its efficacy remains controversial (Downie, 1984; Finkbeiner, 1985). This drug is not effective during acute spinal shock. Bethanechol also has been used to reduce residual urine volume in patients with lesions involving the afferent limb of the micturition reflex arc (*sensory paralytic bladder*) and in those with incomplete lower motor neuron impairment (*motor paralytic bladder*). It should not be used unless bladder and external sphincter function are coordinated, ie, detrusor contractions occur concomitantly with relaxation of the external sphincter (Diokno and Koppenhoefer, 1976; Sonda et al, 1979). Thus, regardless of the etiology of urine retention, efforts to facilitate bladder emptying with bethanechol have been disappointing (Barrett, 1981; Blaivas, 1985; Wein, 1986). *It is recommended that the drug's effectiveness be documented during a short trial before committing a patient to long-term therapy.*

Results of studies to determine the usefulness of instilling dinoprostone (PGE_2) into the bladder of patients with inactive or hypotonic detrusor function have varied. The patient must be free of organic or functional outlet obstruction and must have an intact sacral reflex arc (absence of complete lower neuron lesion). (It is not possible to induce reflex voiding in patients with complete denervation, in those with spinal cord injuries during the spinal shock phase, or in patients with detrusor-striated sphincter dyssynergia.) Approximately one-half of patients treated with dinoprostone had sustained (months) improvement in mean urine flow rate and decreased residual volume (Desmond et al, 1980). Bethanechol may be continued during therapy with dinoprostone or added to the regimen later. It is possible that dinoprost ($PGF_{2\alpha}$) would be more effective (Tammela et al, 1987).

The alpha-adrenergic blocking agent, phenoxybenzamine, relaxes the internal sphincter and has been used to treat various neurogenic bladder disorders in which residual urine volume is increased because of functional outlet obstruction or internal sphincter dyssynergia. It may be given with bethanechol (Mobley, 1976; Raz and Smith, 1976). In spinal cord injury, only patients with incomplete lesions respond to phenoxybenzamine (Graham, 1981).

Because of the side effects encountered with phenoxybenzamine, particularly reflex tachycardia and orthostatic hypotension, and because phenoxybenzamine is mutagenic and carcinogenic in animals (see the evaluation), agents with selective $alpha_1$ receptor blocking activity are now preferred. Of these, prazosin was beneficial in some adults with lower motor neuron lesions and autonomous bladder. To avoid first-dose phenomenon hypotension, a small dose (1 mg) is given twice daily initially, and the amount is increased gradually at weekly intervals to 3 to 4 mg three times a day (Andersson et al, 1981; Wein, 1984 A; Wein and Barrett, 1988). Suppression of ejaculation appears to be far less of a problem with prazosin than with phenoxybenzamine. Another selective alpha receptor antagonist, terazosin, is structurally similar to prazosin and has similar actions and adverse reactions. Its long half-life (12 hours) permits once-daily dosing, which may improve compliance.

BENIGN PROSTATIC HYPERPLASIA (BPH). Benign hyperplasia of the prostate usually does not develop until after age 40. It is estimated to affect 80% of men by age 80. The mean age of onset of obstructive symptoms is 65 years in white and 60 years in black males. Hyperplasia of the gland occurs predominantly in the periurethral region extending from the verumontanum to the bladder neck. Manifestations include hesitancy; a decrease in the caliber and force of the urinary stream; inability to terminate micturition abruptly, resulting in postvoid dribbling; a sensation of incomplete bladder emptying, which often results in frequency and nocturia; and, occasionally, acute urinary retention. Sustained bladder outlet obstruction may lead to bladder hypertrophy, hydroureteronephrosis, and eventual renal failure (Johnson et al, 1988). The severity of symptoms in most patients varies, often from day to day. Approximately 40% of the total urethral pressure is due to the capsular tone of the enlarged prostate that varies directly with the level of sympathetic activity (Furuya et al, 1982).

It is important to note that, although the symptoms of BPH often are attributed solely to mechanical obstruction, the pathophysiology of this disorder may include impaired detrusor contractility or detrusor instability, sensory abnormalities of the bladder wall, and active contractility of the smooth muscle affecting the prostatic urethra (Blaivas, 1988 B). Sophisticated urodynamic studies may be required to assess these components if the usual treatment is unsuccessful.

Surgery: Transurethral resection of the prostate (TURP) is a common treatment for BPH and is successful in more than 80% of patients (O'Brien, 1991); however, a second surgical procedure may be required in 10% to 15% of patients within eight years. Adverse effects include bleeding, infection, and incontinence; the degree of incontinence is significant in 0.5% to 2% of those undergoing TURP. Impotence may occur in 3% to 35% of patients (Peters and Sorkin, 1993).

Although TURP is often necessary for patients with severe symptoms, many authorities believe that surgery is overused in those with mild to moderate symptoms. Improvement, as measured by quality of life indices, is generally less for patients with moderate symptoms than for those with severe BPH, and those with mild symptoms may experience little benefit (Flood et al, 1992; Riehmann and Bruskewitz, 1993). Because the progression to severe disease may be slow and the ability of individual patients to tolerate mild to moderate symptoms varies widely, "watchful waiting," ie, long-term observation with or without pharmacologic therapy, may postpone or obviate the need for surgery in many individuals.

Surgical alternatives to TURP for symptomatic BPH include open prostatectomy when the prostate is extremely large (80 to 100 g) and transurethral incision of the prostate (TUIP) when the prostate is less than 20 g (Moul, 1993). Alternatives currently being investigated include placement of prostatic stents, microwave therapy, balloon dilation, and laser prostatectomy (Riehmann and Bruskewitz, 1993; Moul, 1993).

Drug Therapy: Symptomatic BPH can be managed medically by reducing the tone of the prostatic smooth muscle in the stroma and capsule with agents that block alpha-adrenergic receptors or by inducing glandular regression with hormones.

Good results had been achieved with the nonselective adrenergic blocking agent, phenoxybenzamine (Caine et al, 1981), but other adrenergic blocking agents now being used are safer. Prazosin, a selective $alpha_1$-adrenergic blocking drug, has been employed in responsive patients and in those who are not suitable candidates for surgery. More recently, a single daily dose of a related $alpha_1$-adrenergic blocking agent, terazosin, has been beneficial. When compared with placebo in controlled clinical trials, terazosin improved symptom scores and increased urinary flow rates to a small but significant extent; adverse reactions did not differ significantly from those of the placebo (Lepor et al, 1992; Brawer et al, 1993; Lowe and Stark, 1993). Symptomatic improvement may occur as early as two weeks after initiation of therapy. Although little data exist on the long-term effects of terazosin, in some studies in patients with BPH, its efficacy and safety was maintained for 24 months (Lepor et al, 1992).

Terazosin and prazosin may be particularly useful in patients with BPH and hypertension (Stein, 1993). Although prazosin must be given three or four times daily compared with once daily for terazosin, the efficacy, actions, and adverse reaction profile of these two drugs are similar; however, terazosin is about ten times more expensive. Some authorities believe that both drugs are appropriate first-line therapy for medical management of symptomatic BPH. Other selective alpha-adrenergic blocking agents that are being investigated for treatment of BPH are doxazosin and alfuzosin. The efficacy of doxazosin is similar to that of terazosin (Christensen et al, 1993).

Castration or hypopituitarism is associated with a decrease in prostate size (Lepor, 1989). Based on the known role of hormones in BPH, various hormonally active substances have been employed to induce androgenic deprivation that could, in time, cause involution of the glandular component of the prostate and reduce the mechanical aspect of bladder outlet obstruction. Greater symptomatic improvement has occurred in men treated with progestins, GnRH analogues, and cyproterone acetate than in those treated with placebo. Gonadotropin and testosterone secretion are inhibited and, in most patients, prostate size diminishes. However, impotence is a common side effect of hormonal therapy, and thus the usefulness of these agents is limited (McConnell, 1990).

Flutamide [Eulexin], a nonsteroidal antiandrogen currently marketed for the treatment of prostate cancer, competes with dihydrotestosterone (DHT) for androgen receptor sites intracellularly. When this drug was administered in doses of 750 mg/day for 12 weeks and six months, prostate volume decreased 18% and 41%, respectively, and urinary flow rate increased 30% and 35%, respectively. Objective improvement was not noted with placebo, but symptomatic improvement was comparable in treated and control patients. Side effects included breast pain or tenderness; gynecomastia; gastrointestinal disorders (incidence, up to 50%), including diarrhea (incidence, up to 14%); and hepatitis (Manyak, 1991; Stone, 1992). Impotence or changes in libido was not reported. Adverse reactions and the drug's modest efficacy limit the value of flutamide for BPH.

Finasteride [Proscar] acts by inhibiting type II 5-α reductase, an enzyme required for the formation of DHT from testosterone (McConnell, 1990; Cotton, 1991; Peters and Sorkin, 1993). The concentration of DHT in the prostate falls markedly and its volume decreases by 20% to 30% following treatment. In two large multicenter trials in patients with BPH treated with this drug, symptoms improved in 30% to 50% of patients and statistically significant but relatively small increases in the urinary flow rate were reported (Gormley et al, 1992; Peters and Sorkin, 1993). Supportive data are lacking, but it is hoped that finasteride will slow progression of BPH and reverse its natural progression in some patients with mild to moderate disease. Preliminary data suggest that the efficacy of a single daily oral dose of finasteride may be maintained for up to three years (*FDC Reports*, 1992 B; Stoner et al, 1994). Decreased libido and impotence occur in 5% to 10% of patients; most patients with sexual dysfunction note a decrease in the volume of ejaculate. Although relief of symptoms and improvement in urinary function are considerably less than the results achieved with TURP, finasteride may allow many patients with moderate symptoms to avoid surgery and may be beneficial for those with severe BPH who cannot tolerate or refuse surgery (Peters and Sorkin, 1993).

Finasteride has no proven prophylactic value. However, the National Cancer Institute is sponsoring a seven-year prospective study in 18,000 men to determine if this drug can prevent prostate cancer.

Finasteride acts on the static or mechanical component of BPH by shrinking the gland, whereas terazosin inhibits the dynamic component of the disorder by blocking smooth muscle sympathetic tone. Some investigators believe that finasteride is preferable to terazosin for patients in whom glandular hyperplasia is predominant, while terazosin is more beneficial than finasteride in patients in whom stromal hyperplasia is predominant (Stone, 1992). Furthermore, the different mechanisms of action of the two drugs may be exploited by using them in combination to obtain greater therapeutic benefit than would be achieved by either agent alone. A major study comparing the effects of finasteride and terazosin as monotherapy and in combination is underway.

Efficacy and safety must be demonstrated for many years before any agent can be regarded as having meaningful long-term value for BPH. Patient characteristics that could help predict which patient subtypes will benefit from drug therapy have not been identified. The symptoms commonly attributed to BPH and assumed to be specific for BPH and obstructive uropathy are unrelated to the degree of obstruction and may be present even if urodynamic evaluation does not reveal any obstruction. Of interest are data suggesting that symptoms previously thought to be relatively specific for BPH and obstructive uropathy are as common in elderly women as in elderly men; presence of symptoms and relief of such symptoms by medication or surgery do not establish conclusively that obstruction is present (Chai et al, 1993).

DETRUSOR-STRIATED SPHINCTER DYSSYNERGIA. This functional obstruction involving the external urethral sphincter develops most often in patients with neurologic damage above the level of the sacral spinal cord. Detrusor-striated sphincter dyssynergia usually is caused by trauma or demyelinating disease, but occasionally may occur after surgery, vascular injury, or radiation (Blaivas et al, 1981; McGuire, 1986 A; Wein, 1992). It also has been reported in patients with no apparent structural or neurologic abnormality, and particularly in young children; this may represent a learned behavior (ie, inappropriate sphincter contractions) and not true dyssynergia.

A substantial number of patients with multiple sclerosis, transverse myelitis, or other upper motor lesions exhibit external sphincter dyssynergia. This condition is related to loss of supraspinal influences on sacral cord function and is usually permanent. The degree of activity of the external sphincter and the detrusor reflex varies greatly and independently in patients with upper motor neuron lesions. Generally, the detrusor reflex occurs at a low volume and sphincter activity is greater than normal. Urine is voided in spurts while the bladder and sphincter contract in a disorganized manner. Treatment is determined after assessment of the relative activity of the sphincter and detrusor (McGuire, 1986 A; Wein, 1992).

Therapy: When no neurologic basis is apparent, diazepam [Valium] has been reported to be effective because of its antianxiety action (Wein, 1986). An alternative is to lessen the uninhibited bladder contractions that may be the real cause of the external sphincter dyssynergia by utilizing timed voiding and anticholinergic agents (Koff et al, 1978).

No drug acts selectively on the external sphincter to relieve spasticity, but dantrolene [Dantrium] and baclofen have been used for this purpose. Dantrolene is presumed to act by inhibiting excitation-contraction coupling in muscle. Urination patterns have improved, but the drug's use is limited by its potential hepatotoxicity. Baclofen acts by enhancing polysynaptic inhibition in the spinal cord. It appears to be more effective than dantrolene in external sphincter spasm and dyssynergias, but its safety and efficacy have not been evaluated fully. Treatment with either drug may result in satisfactory reflex voiding in males, but incontinence will continue to be a major problem in women (McGuire, 1986 A). Diazepam is not effective in detrusor-striated sphincter dyssynergia due to suprasacral lesions.

POSTOPERATIVE URINARY RETENTION. The inability to initiate urination is relatively common after surgery, particularly following genitourinary or anorectal procedures. It is more common in the elderly and in patients who are not ambulatory in the immediate postoperative period. In men over 50 years, an enlarged prostate is often assumed to be responsible for urinary retention after surgery, but this assumption is frequently incorrect (O'Reilly, 1991).

Therapy: If conservative measures (placing the patient in a normal posture for voiding, audibly running water) fail, drug therapy should be undertaken with the understanding that this problem will resolve spontaneously in two to six months in most patients who use intermittent self-catheterization.

A response has been obtained with phenoxybenzamine 10 mg twice a day (Tammela, 1986; Goldman et al, 1988). When phenoxybenzamine or another alpha-adrenergic blocking agent (eg, prazosin, terazosin) is not appropriate or effective or when bladder distention is estimated to be greater than one liter, intermittent catheterization or an indwelling catheter may be required until spontaneous voiding reappears. Patients with pre-existing obstructions or obstruction caused by the surgical procedure (edema, blood clots) are managed more appropriately by an indwelling catheter.

The infusion of dinoprost tromethamine ($PGF_{2\alpha}$) into the bladder has been investigated for the relief of postoperative voiding difficulties in women following periurethral surgery (Tammela et al, 1987). In this study, 10 mg of the drug dissolved in 50 ml of physiologic saline at body temperature was instilled into the drained bladder and retained for two hours. Patients were not permitted fluids for three hours prior to the procedure to prevent dilution of the drug by enhanced urine production. Of 18 patients, 15 were able to urinate after the instillation, but only seven had residual volumes of less than 100 ml. None of the 18 patients receiving a placebo had spontaneous voiding. Few other studies have been performed, and the value of this and other prostaglandins for this purpose is unclear.

The postoperative use of opioids, particularly epidurally, for analgesia causes a significant incidence of postoperative urinary retention. This adverse response usually is not sustained, but one or two catheterizations may be required. If a prolonged course of epidural morphine is anticipated, an indwelling catheter may be placed. The small doses of naloxone [Narcan] that are given to abolish pruritus produced by epidural opioids will not reverse the suppression of the voiding reflex. However, phenoxybenzamine has been reported to reduce the frequency of retention (Evron et al, 1984).

Female Urethral Syndrome

The symptoms of female urethral syndrome are urinary frequency and urgency (sometimes accompanied by hesitancy), dysuria, pressure sensations, abdominal pain, anxiety, and low back pain. Results of urine culture by standard techniques are negative (Testa, 1992); otherwise, findings are similar to those observed in patients with urinary tract infections. However, dysuria generally is less severe than in those with infections, and burning is absent or occurs only at the end of voiding (O'Dowd et al, 1985). Similar symptomatology also occurs in a number of other disorders (acute urethral syndrome, infectious cystitis, urethritis, or vaginitis; carcinoma in situ; early interstitial cystitis; postmenopausal atrophic vulvovaginitis; external sphincter dysfunction; neuropathic bladder) (Gleason, 1978; Graham, 1980; Komaroff and Friedland, 1980; Schmidt, 1985; Bodner, 1988). Patients with acute urethral syndrome who have pyuria and bacteria in their urine respond to antimicrobial therapy (Stamm et al, 1981). See index entry Urethral Syndrome, Treatment. Women with a history of recurrent urinary tract infections may experience symptoms in the absence of infection (Messing, 1986 A).

Female urethral syndrome without bacteriuria or pyuria sometimes requires cystoscopy to rule out carcinoma in situ or interstitial cystitis and/or urodynamic testing to determine the appropriate pharmacologic or surgical intervention. Patients with dysuria not associated with frequency should be evaluated for vaginitis or genital herpes simplex infection.

Female urethral syndrome is a diagnosis of exclusion. Conservative medical, rather than surgical, management is recommended once infection, treatable conditions such as senile dementia, extraneous factors that may induce urethritis or vaginitis (spermicides, tampons, bubble baths, deodorant soap, douches, sexual activity), or a pathologic abnormality have been excluded.

Some authorities believe that the female urethral syndrome is a psychogenic disorder (Testa, 1992). One suggested management protocol includes antimicrobial therapy even though no identifiable bacteria are present; if this does not relieve symptoms, bladder retraining is undertaken with or without one to two weeks of therapy with anticholinergic drugs and/or striated muscle relaxants (eg, alpha-adrenergic blocking agents such as prazosin or terazosin, benzodiazepines such as diazepam). If this therapy is unsuccessful, cystourethroscopy is indicated. If symptoms persist despite the above measures, a psychological evaluation and psychotherapy along with use of antianxiety agents or antidepressants may be beneficial. Physicians may have to spend extra time with patients who are highly anxious due to persistent pain and discomfort (Testa, 1992).

In the postmenopausal patient, the vaginal application of conjugated estrogens 1.25 mg in a cream base nightly for two to three weeks, followed by application one or two times a week thereafter, is adequate for hypoestrogenic urethritis (Scotti and Ostergard, 1985). For contraindications and details of cyclic therapy if long-term application is necessary, see index entry Menopause.

Psychogenic Voiding Disturbances

Chronic *psychogenic urinary retention* is a relatively uncommon condition occurring almost exclusively in women. The urologic component is managed by intermittent self-catheterization and bladder training. Drugs are employed *only* as required for the psychiatric component (Siroky and Krane, 1988).

Male patients with *chronic aseptic prostatitis* (Siroky et al, 1981) or *prostatodynia* (Osborn et al, 1981) who experience hesitancy, weak stream, infrequent voiding, and terminal dribbling but who have no demonstrable neurologic abnormality may benefit from diazepam, baclofen, or phenoxybenzamine. Despite extensive urodynamic studies, the criteria for drug selection have not been established. It is possible that management should be directed primarily at the psychiatric component.

Bashful bladder syndrome is defined as the inability of a male to initiate urination when in the company of others (Beary and Gilbert, 1981). Drugs are inappropriate for this problem. One management technique has been to have the affected individual do silent serial multiplications. This mental activity blocks cortical inhibition and permits the patient to urinate in a public toilet.

An *urgency-frequency syndrome* of psychogenic origin is a diagnosis made by exclusion. It is recognized primarily in women under 60 years and may have some symptoms of urethral syndrome, but is distinguishable by an underlying personality disorder of the somatizing type. Anticholinergic, sedative, and antianxiety drugs rarely are of value. The voiding disorder may respond to a bladder retraining program with timed voidings of gradually increased duration (Frewen, 1984).

Interstitial Cystitis

Interstitial cystitis is a chronic bladder disorder of unknown etiology; more than 90% of those affected are young and middle-aged women. This disorder is characterized by urgency, frequency, nocturia, occasionally dysuria, and suprapubic, pelvic, perineal, or vaginal pain, which is sometimes diminished by voiding. The urine is sterile. Submucosal edema and vasodilation are characteristic histologic findings, and cystoscopic examination after repeated bladder distention with water may reveal glomerulations, mucosal bleeding, reduced bladder capacity, and ulceration (Hunner's ulcers); the latter occurs in $<10\%$ of patients (Messing, 1986 B; Gillenwater and Wein, 1988). Before therapy is initiated, care should be taken to rule out diffuse carcinoma in situ of the bladder. Irritable bowel syndrome and allergies also are common (incidence, 40% and $\geq 50\%$, respectively); symptoms of interstitial cystitis may worsen perimenstrually (Sant and Theoharides, 1994).

Therapy: Symptoms of interstitial cystitis have been reduced by bladder retraining techniques; bladder distention; surgery; and various drugs, including amitriptyline [Elavil, Endep], antihistamines, immunosuppressive agents, and heparin (Hanno and Wein, 1987), as well as oxychlorosene [Chlorpactin WCS-90] and dimethyl sulfoxide (DMSO) [Rimso-50].

Simple bladder distention with water after induction of local or general anesthesia is often the first treatment method employed. It may relieve symptoms in up to 30% of patients, but the effect is short-lived (Sant and Meares, 1990; Levine, 1990). Bladder retraining (increasing the interval between voidings) is effective in patients with little or no pain or in those who can tolerate moderate pain. In one study, increasing the interval by 15 to 30 minutes every month markedly improved symptoms after three months in 71% of patients (Parsons and Koprowski, 1991).

Many physicians prefer to employ intravesical DMSO if patients do not improve substantially with bladder hydrodistention alone. Approximately 60% of patients respond to weekly instillations of DMSO for six weeks but many also require maintenance therapy because of relapses. The anti-inflammatory, analgesic, and muscle relaxing properties of this preparation contribute to relief of symptoms (Sant and Meares, 1990). Other advantages of DMSO include the absence of local or systemic adverse reactions, low cost, lack of need for anesthesia, and ease of administration in the physician's office. Because DMSO is essentially nonirritating, it also can be administered at home by intermittent self-catheterization as needed (Biggers, 1986; Perez-Marrero et al, 1988). Patients who do not respond to the initial course of DMSO may benefit from the addition of 100 mg of hydrocortisone in the usual 50 ml of DMSO (Sant, 1987) or of heparin and bicarbonate.

Intravesical instillation of a 0.4% solution of oxychlorosene has been beneficial in some patients refractory to other therapy. Pain relief can be dramatic and may last for over six months. However, instillation of oxychlorosene is extremely painful and requires general or spinal anesthesia (Messing, 1986 B); severe irritative symptoms may persist for 24 to 48 hours following instillation and may require the use of opioid analgesics (Bowen et al, 1985).

Based on the hypothesis that a deficiency of surface glycosaminoglycans is responsible for the dysfunctional bladder epithelium in patients with interstitial cystitis, the effectiveness of a synthetic sulfated glycosaminoglycan, pentosan polysulfate sodium [Elmiron], is being investigated. Results of most studies indicate that oral administration of this agent is safe and reduces symptoms in 30% to 50% of patients (Parsons, 1987). Pentosan polysulfate sodium may be particularly valuable in patients refractory to DMSO. Beneficial results should be observed within 12 to 16 weeks.

Heparin, another synthetic glycosaminoglycan, has been used intravesically for over 20 years to treat interstitial cystitis (Stone, 1991). In an open pilot study, once monthly instillation for one year prevented recurrence of interstitial cystitis in 20 of 25 patients in whom complete resolution of acute symptoms had been induced by intravesical DMSO alone or DMSO with heparin with or without bladder hydrodistention (Perez-Marrero et al, 1993). In one study, subcutaneous administration of heparin also relieved symptoms (Lose et al, 1985), but this approach is not currently recommended.

In nonblind pilot studies, oral hydroxyzine [Atarax, Vistaril], a histamine$_1$ receptor antagonist, was administered as a single dose of 50 or 75 mg at bedtime for three months to female patients; most reported a 75% decrease in symptoms (Theoharides, 1993, 1994). Double-blind studies are needed to confirm these observations. Amitriptyline also can be considered in patients refractory to other therapy (Hanno et al, 1989). A dose of 25 mg at bedtime, increased gradually during a three-week period to 75 mg, has been employed.

Voiding Dysfunction of Childhood and Adolescence

Enuresis is repeated involuntary urination and is classified as primary if it has persisted since birth. Nocturnal enuresis is the most common form, although some children also suffer from urgency, frequency, and urge incontinence during the day. Numerous causative factors have been proposed (Kass et al, 1979; Nørgaard et al, 1989; Himsl and Hurwitz, 1991). Children who have no daytime urinary symptomatology, neurologic or anatomic abnormalities, or infection usually have normal bladders and do not require urodynamic tests, intravenous pyelography (IVP), or endoscopy. Those with persistent day- and nighttime wetting (with or without recurrent urinary infection) may benefit from more extensive diagnostic evaluation. Enuretic syndromes include unstable bladder (uninhibited bladder), large capacity hypotonic bladder (lazy bladder), and the non-neurogenic neurogenic bladder (Hinman syndrome).

UNSTABLE BLADDER. In this condition, uncontrollable contractions occur in young children who have not developed the ability to voluntarily inhibit the voiding reflex. To keep dry during the involuntary contraction, the child constricts the external sphincter forcefully for its duration, which may be 20 or 30 seconds. This voluntary detrusor external sphincter dyssynergia can lead to high intrabladder pressure, which may damage the bladder and associated structures (Himsl and Hurwitz, 1991). Vesicoureteral reflux may occur in some of these children. Unstable bladder appears to be a common cause of recurrent urinary infection in girls 3 to 8 years. Until the adult pattern of urinary control develops, the goal is elimination of unstable contractions without interfering with normal voiding (Koff, 1984). In many patients, unstable bladder would not be a clinical problem if it were not for the negative social consequences associated with incontinence.

Therapy: Treatment of unstable bladder can improve continence and reduce the incidence of infection in more than 70% of children (Koff et al, 1979). The primary goal is to prevent or eliminate the uninhibited contraction. Some authorities recommend a regimen that includes the use of drugs to eliminate unwanted detrusor contractions or reduce their intensity (Himsl and Hurwitz, 1991); timed voiding to empty the bladder before an uninhibited contraction occurs; and treatment of constipation, if present. Fluid restriction to lengthen the voiding interval also is useful, especially in children with large fluid intakes. The addition of anticholinergic drugs further decreases the rate of urine production and increases functional bladder capacity, leading to a lengthened voiding interval. When the new voiding interval has been established, the child should void voluntarily about 30 minutes before the next uninhibited bladder contraction is expected.

Children with detrusor instability who were treated with oral oxybutynin experienced urodynamic improvement with an increase in total bladder capacity, an increase in bladder volume at first contraction, and a decrease in the frequency and intensity of uninhibited bladder contractions (Fernandes et al, 1991). Propantheline is probably equally effective, but it is not available in a liquid formulation and thus administration is less convenient in children. For short-term management (overnight stays, camping trips), imipramine or another tricyclic antidepressant provides prompt and effective relief in many individuals (Kass et al, 1979; Mikkelsen et al, 1980; Koff, 1986). In addition to inhibition of detrusor contractions, imipramine increases bladder outlet resistance. These actions may result from direct effects on the action potential in bladder smooth muscle cells and from enhanced alpha-adrenergic actions at the bladder outlet. Adverse reactions caused by imipramine can be more problematic than those associated with oxybutynin or propantheline. Drugs with anticholinergic effects can aggravate untreated constipation, which contributes to bladder instability.

Drug therapy without restriction of fluids has little value, and some physicians consider fluid restriction the key element in increasing the length of the voiding interval. Parents should be instructed to limit the child's fluid intake to 24 to 32 ounces per day (which is the usual daily intake in children); this amount can be increased in hot weather and other situations in which more fluids are necessary. However, fluid restriction can worsen constipation. Accumulation of a large hard stool compresses the base of the bladder and trigonal region and exacerbates bladder instability. The fear of a painful bowel movement in constipated children creates a cycle of fecal retention. Children should be given dietary bran in any form they will accept (eg, breads, cereals, muffins). If stronger measures are necessary, bulk-forming laxatives can be beneficial. This approach requires significant motivation on the part of both parents and child.

NOCTURNAL ENURESIS. This term is defined as persistent bed wetting occurring more than twice a month in children over 5 years. The primary problem is the child's lack of subconscious ability to inhibit the detrusor contraction when bladder capacity is exceeded. The etiology of this condition is obscure. Behavioral abnormalities appear to be the result and not the cause of incontinence. The role of heredity is demonstrated by data indicating that a parental history of bed wetting increases the likelihood of the child having the same problem. In severe cases, patients usually have a small functional bladder capacity. Contributing factors for which evidence is weak include sleep disorders, delayed maturation of the nervous system, and food allergies. Recently, increasing attention has been given to an association between decreased levels of antidiuretic hormone (ADH) and nocturnal enuresis in some patients.

Most children who have nocturnal enuresis can be divided into two groups with non-neurogenic disorders: those who have *unstable bladder* and a history of urgency, frequency, dysuria, daytime wetting, or urinary tract infection and those who have *pure nocturnal enuresis*, which can be defined as bed wetting unaccompanied by symptoms of unstable bladder. If the physical findings and urinalysis are normal in these patients, further evaluation (eg, urodynamic studies) has no value. However, parents of children with persistent nighttime wetting may be fearful that an organic cause is responsible for symptoms and that serious damage to the urinary tract and/or general health of the child may occur. An ultrasound examination can allay these concerns and assists the physician when treatment options are discussed with families who need additional reassurance (Rosenfeld and Jerkins, 1991).

Parents should be informed that nocturnal enuresis is not caused by emotional problems and that children should not be disciplined for bedwetting (Miller et al, 1992). Severe and repeated punishment for wetting accidents in young children may lead to involuntary tightening of the external sphincter even during attempts at voiding. When this learned behavior persists into adolescence, external sphincter dyssynergia is associated with high voiding pressure, upper urinary tract dilation, and a large, thick-walled bladder. The external sphincter remains contracted at rest and during filling and the muscle does not relax completely during voiding. Such patients require some degree of psychotherapy and perhaps biofeedback training to complement pharmacologic management (Bauer, 1984).

Therapy: Nocturnal enuresis ceases in 99% of children by age 15 regardless of therapy, if any. If treatment is indicated, motivational conditioning, hypnotherapy, and/or conditioning with a portable waking device that is worn on the body and can detect the first drops of urine (eg, Sleep Dry, Wet-Stop, Potty Pager, Nytone) are usually tried initially. Parents and children must be motivated and follow directions carefully to obtain success with waking devices. For a detailed discussion of the use of these systems, see Himsl and Hurwitz, 1991, and Schmitt, 1990.

Nondrug techniques are superior to drug therapy in carefully selected children with cooperative and understanding parents (Koff, 1986; Fordham and Meadow, 1989; Forsythe and Butler, 1989). Drugs should be considered for use when alarm systems are impractical or have failed after a three-month trial or when rapid control of enuresis is required. Drugs either increase functional bladder capacity (eg, oxybutynin, propantheline, imipramine) or decrease urine production (desmopressin [DDAVP]).

Although oral oxybutynin has been reported to decrease bed wetting in about 40% of children and may eliminate the problem in up to 25%, its value is unproven and the relapse rate is high (Lovering et al, 1988). Imipramine is more useful but has greater toxicity.

Some children with nocturnal enuresis appear to have normal functional bladder capacity that is surpassed at night as a result of decreased secretion of antidiuretic hormone (ADH) (Nørgaard et al, 1989). This suggests that replacement therapy with ADH analogues could be useful for treatment of nocturnal enuresis. Results of a number of studies have demonstrated the effectiveness of desmopressin, a synthetic ADH analogue, in pure nocturnal enuresis (Miller et al, 1989; Klauber, 1989; Hjälmås and Sillén, 1990). In some trials, intranasal desmopressin prevented bed wetting in up to 70% of children (Himsl and Hurwitz, 1991) and decreased it in other children in whom total dryness was not achieved; in other trials, total dryness was achieved in less than 25% of children (Evans and Meadow, 1992; Moffat et al, 1993). Relapses occur in >95% of children after withdrawal of desmopressin (Hjälmås and Sillén, 1990; Rosenfeld and Jerkins, 1991). The drug is well tolerated and produces few adverse reactions (eg, low incidence of hyponatremia and water intoxication).

Desmopressin therapy is effective when it decreases urine production to a level below the bladder trigger capacity. Some authorities do not recommend its use as primary or initial therapy but reserve it for refractory bed wetters or for short-term protection (eg, overnight stays, camping trips). Its use with oxybutynin, propantheline, or another anticholinergic agent may produce additive effects in some patients. No tests are available to predict which children will respond. Combined use of desmopressin and an enuresis alarm may be beneficial in patients resistant to either therapy alone (Sukhai et al, 1989).

LAZY BLADDER SYNDROME. Children with the lazy bladder syndrome, most commonly girls, void infrequently and usually only enough to relieve the pressure of a full bladder. They may experience stress or overflow incontinence secondary to overdistention. This secondary enuresis (occurring after toilet training) requires frequent (every two to three hours) timed voiding. If detrusor activity is inadequate, intermittent catheterization may be required.

NON-NEUROGENIC NEUROGENIC BLADDER. The most serious non-neurogenic voiding dysfunction occurs in children whose bladders resemble true neurogenic bladders both functionally and radiographically. This condition results from inappropriate constriction of the external sphincter during a detrusor contraction and is characterized by infrequent voiding associated with urgency and stress incontinence and often an abnormal voiding pattern. These children experience daytime and nighttime enuresis, urinary tract infections, lower urinary tract damage, constipation, and fecal incontinence; they frequently have severe bladder muscle trabeculation, a large capacity bladder with large volumes of residual urine, upper urinary tract damage, vesicoureteral reflux, and hydronephrosis.

After the urine is sterilized and maintained infection-free, suggestion techniques, voiding retraining, intermittent catheterization, or biofeedback training are instituted to reduce the external sphincter dyssynergia (Hanna et al, 1981; Koff, 1984; Hellström et al, 1987). This management program may be supplemented with diazepam to relax the external sphincter, an alpha-adrenergic receptor antagonist such as prazosin to reduce outflow resistance, and anticholinergic drugs as needed to reduce detrusor contractility (Hinman, 1986). If these measures fail, surgical intervention may be necessary.

GIGGLE INCONTINENCE. This is abrupt, involuntary, uncontrollable, complete emptying of the bladder associated with giggling or laughter. It is distinct from the slight wetting that may occur during laughter in stress incontinence but rarely may be a variant of stress incontinence (Sawczuk and Blaivas, 1984). Giggle incontinence is probably familial, usually begins about age 5 to 7 years, and is more common in girls. Urodynamic and neurologic evaluations generally show no abnormalities. The condition usually resolves gradually, rarely persisting into adulthood. Symptomatic relief was reported in two preadolescent boys following a short course of propantheline (Brocklebank and Meadow, 1981), but no therapy appears to be useful in adolescent girls (Belman, 1988). Giggle incontinence also may be associated with focal seizures; incontinence in these patients responds to antiepileptic therapy (Rogers et al, 1982).

CEREBRAL PALSY. Uninhibited bladder contractions in incontinent children with cerebral palsy usually respond to anticholinergic therapy. Behavior modification and intermittent catheterization for detrusor sphincter dyssynergia or incomplete emptying may be required in some of these children. The incidence of structural changes is high when these patients develop urinary tract infections. Therefore, definitive radiologic tests should be performed when urinary tract infections occur in order to avoid further urologic deterioration (Decter et al, 1987).

CONGENITAL ANOMALIES. In many children over age 3 years with neurogenic bladder caused by spina bifida, meningocele, or traumatic paraplegia, continence may be maintained with intermittent catheterization by either the parent or patient (de la Hunt et al,1989; Joseph et al, 1989). This can be supplemented with a bladder relaxant (eg, propantheline, oxybutynin), particularly if urodynamic assessment indicates uninhibited detrusor contractions or hypertonicity (Mulcahy and James, 1979).

Myelodysplasia may result in voiding dysfunction at any age, and symptoms may be delayed until the growth spurt of early adolescence. Caudal regression syndrome frequently produces similar symptoms. No correlation exists between the level of vertebral defect and the resulting dysfunction. Detrusor hypertonicity and areflexia frequently are present. Either open vesical outlet or detrusor external sphincter dyssynergia also may be present. Urodynamic investigation is necessary to determine treatment (Barrett and Woodside, 1988).

Incontinence, infection, and upper urinary tract deterioration occur in children with sacral agenesis or myelodysplasia. Involvement of the upper urinary tract is related to intravesical pressure. Intermittent catheterization and anticholinergic agents are preferred for initial treatment. Bladder pressure should be measured. If storage occurs when the urodynamic pressure is >40 cm/water, upper tract deterioration will occur. Measures directed at decreasing bladder pressure must be instituted. In about 10% of these patients, true detrusor-sphincter dyssynergia is present; in these individuals, intermittent catheterization and anticholinergic agents should be continued. Continence can be achieved in about 60% to 70% of myelodysplastic patients using these measures. Patients with a tethered spinal cord require early and aggressive neurosurgery to prevent further urologic deterioration (Kaplan et al, 1988; Flanigan et al, 1989).

Retrograde Ejaculation

Reduction of sympathetic tone in the bladder neck may prevent adequate closure of the internal sphincter during ejaculation, which allows retrograde ejection of semen into the urinary bladder. This interruption of normal sympathetic activity may occur after instrumentation or surgery (transurethral resection of the prostate, bilateral lumbar sympathectomy, retroperitoneal lymph node dissection, abdominoperineal resection of the rectum), administration of certain drugs (eg, guanethidine [Ismelin]), or in patients with diabetic visceral neuropathy. Aspermia usually is caused by absence of ejaculation, but if retrograde ejaculation can be demonstrated, alpha-adrenergic agents (eg, ephedrine, phenylpropanolamine) (Proctor and Howards, 1983) or imipramine (Brooks et al, 1980; Nijman et al, 1982) may be beneficial.

In a double-blind controlled study in patients with nondrug-related retrograde ejaculation, no difference in results achieved with the adrenergic agents, dextroamphetamine, ephedrine, pseudoephedrine, and phenylpropanolamine could be discerned (Proctor and Howards, 1983). Although the action of these drugs may be apparent if they are taken one to two hours prior to intercourse, maximal consistent results were achieved after four days of administration. Their value following long-term administration has not been determined, but the beneficial effect of imipramine apparently is maintained with daily dosing.

Autonomic Dysreflexia

The syndrome of autonomic dysreflexia (hyperreflexia) is a medical emergency occurring in quadriplegic or paraplegic patients with complete or incomplete spinal lesions above T-6. It is characterized by symptoms of reflex sympathetic discharge: hypertension, pounding occipital headache, bradycardia, diaphoresis, blotchy flushing of the face and chest, cutis anserina, and nausea. The hypertensive episode may result in retinal or cerebrovascular hemorrhage, seizures, cardiac or renal failure, and death. In approximately 90% of patients, the symptoms are induced by manipulation, irrigation, or distention (infrequent catheterization, obstruction of an indwelling catheter, sphincter dyssynergia) of the bladder. In most of the remaining 10%, symptoms occurred after distention of the bowel or rectal examination.

When this syndrome is caused by bladder distention, it is treated by immediate drainage of the bladder. If the response is inadequate, a prompt-acting vasodilator should be administered. Success has been reported with trimethaphan [Arfonad], nitroprusside [Nipride, Nitropress], hydralazine [Apresoline], phenoxybenzamine, diazoxide [Proglycem], and phentolamine. Nifedipine 10 mg orally was reported to reduce blood pressure within 5 to 10 minutes, with restoration of baseline pressure 30 to 40 minutes following an acute episode of autonomic dysreflexia (Lindan et al, 1985).

The prophylactic use of nifedipine (Dykstra et al, 1987) or a ganglionic blocking agent prior to bladder irrigation or diagnostic procedures on the bladder prevents the autonomic dysreflexia syndrome. Long-term therapy with either calcium channel blockers or alpha-adrenergic antagonists to prevent the syndrome in susceptible patients has not been evaluated extensively.

There are two common predisposing causes for autonomic dysreflexia involving the urinary tract: uninhibited high pressure contractility with detrusor-external sphincter dyssynergia and autonomic dysreflexia that occurs with high bladder volumes in patients on intermittent catheterization. The former can be treated with external sphinterotomy (Barton et al, 1986), sacral rhizotomy, or augmentation cystoplasty, and the latter can be managed by the continued administration of small doses (1 to 3 mg/day) of prazosin or terazosin. Guanethidine appears to be useful (Brown et al, 1979) but may have unacceptable side effects in some patients.

Drug Evaluations

AGENTS USED TO TREAT URINARY INCONTINENCE

Anticholinergic Drugs

Anticholinergic drugs block the action of acetylcholine at postganglionic cholinergic sites, thereby increasing bladder capacity by reducing the number of motor impulses reaching the detrusor muscle. The response of the detrusor muscle to parasympathetic stimulation is relatively resistant to cholinergic blockade; therefore, doses that inhibit the urinary bladder produce the usual anticholinergic side effects (eg, constipation, dryness of the mouth). Anticholinergic drugs are relatively ineffective for sensory urgency without incontinence (McGuire, 1988).

A large number of anticholinergic agents are available commercially. Both the natural belladonna alkaloids (atropine, belladonna tincture, and hyoscyamine) and various synthetic agents (eg, propantheline) have been used in urologic disorders. Because oral quaternary ammonium compounds are absorbed more slowly than the natural belladonna alkaloids, they may have a slightly longer duration of action. There is no evidence that any one is more effective or better tolerated than propantheline.

Other urinary antispasmodics (dicyclomine [Bentyl], flavoxate [Urispas], and oxybutynin) are reported to relax the detrusor and other smooth muscle by cholinergic blockade, as well as by a direct relaxant effect on muscle fibers. They may have less pronounced anticholinergic side effects than the pure anticholinergic agents, and this advantage may be significant, especially in elderly patients.

BELLADONNA TINCTURE

Because this preparation is administered as a liquid, it is used primarily in children with nocturnal enuresis who also experience urgency, frequency, and urge incontinence during the day.

Belladonna produces antimuscarinic effects on the salivary glands, heart, eye, and gastrointestinal tract; large doses may cause flushing, fever, and marked central nervous system effects (eg, excitement, hallucinations, delirium). Belladonna is classified in FDA Pregnancy Category C. See also index entry Anticholinergic Agents.

DOSAGE AND PREPARATIONS.

Oral: *Children over 5 years,* initially, 0.25 to 0.5 ml (10 to 20 drops) three times daily. Dosage may be increased gradually, if necessary, to 1 ml/dose. The dose should be reduced if flushing or other signs of toxicity occur. *Adults* (usually reserved for those who cannot take solid preparations), 0.4 to 1 ml (15 to 40 drops) four times daily.

Generic. Tincture 0.3 mg/ml in 120, 480, 500, and 3,840 ml containers (alcohol 65% to 70%). Available with graduated droppers supplying 40 drops/ml.

DICYCLOMINE HYDROCHLORIDE

[Bentyl]

$\cdot$ HCl

$COOCH_2CH_2N(C_2H_5)_2$

This drug has anticholinergic and antispasmodic properties. It has been reported to increase bladder capacity in adults with detrusor hyperreflexia.

Dicyclomine can produce anticholinergic side effects and is contraindicated in the presence of urinary outflow obstruction (eg, prostatic hypertrophy) or intestinal atony and in patients who cannot tolerate tachycardia.

DOSAGE AND PREPARATIONS.

Oral: *Adults*, 10 to 20 mg four times daily (Wein, 1984 A). As much as 30 mg four times daily is recommended by some urologists (Mundy, 1985).

Generic. Capsules 10 and 20 mg; syrup 10 mg/5 ml; tablets 20 mg.

Bentyl (Marion Merrell Dow). Capsules 10 mg; tablets 20 mg; syrup 10 mg/5 ml.

FLAVOXATE HYDROCHLORIDE

[Urispas]

$^{+}N-CH_2CH_2OC(=O)$ H Cl^- CH_3 O

ACTIONS AND USES. Flavoxate has local anesthetic, analgesic, and anticholinergic properties. It also may have a direct relaxant effect on smooth muscle. Urinary excretion of the drug may contribute to its local effects. The relative contribution of each of these characteristics to the antispasmodic effect is difficult to appraise, however.

Flavoxate has been used to reduce dysuria, nocturia, suprapubic pain, and urinary frequency, urgency, and incontinence associated with cystitis, prostatitis, urethritis, and trigonitis. Despite its various actions, flavoxate has not proved to be more effective in these disorders than other drugs with anticholinergic actions (Benson et al, 1977; Finkbeiner and Bissada, 1980; Chapple et al, 1990), and some clinicians consider it to be no better than a placebo (Briggs et al, 1980; Meyhoff et al, 1983). Flavoxate should not be considered a drug of first choice for incontinence.

ADVERSE REACTIONS AND PRECAUTIONS. Adverse reactions are relatively uncommon; nausea, vomiting, dryness of the mouth, nervousness, vertigo, headache, drowsiness, blurred vision, disturbed visual accommodation, increased intraocular pressure, urticaria and other dermatoses, confusion (especially in the elderly), dysuria, tachycardia, fever, eosinophilia, and reversible leukopenia (one case) have been reported. Some of these reactions resemble anticholinergic effects; therefore, the same precautions and contraindications should apply (see index entry Anticholinergic Agents).

Flavoxate is classified in FDA Pregnancy Category B.

DOSAGE AND PREPARATIONS.

Oral: *Adults,* 100 or 200 mg three or four times daily; the dose may be reduced when symptoms improve. Dosage has not been established for *children under 12 years.*

Urispas (SmithKline Beecham). Tablets 100 mg.

HYOSCYAMINE

[Cystospaz]

HYOSCYAMINE SULFATE

[Anaspaz, Cystospaz-M, Levsin]

H H_3C-N^{+} H $OC-C---H$ O CH_2OH $]_2$ $SO_4^{=} \cdot 2H_2O$

Hyoscyamine has the same actions and side effects as the other belladonna alkaloids. Its most common use in urology has been to treat bladder spasm associated with infection, inflammation, or use of a retention catheter, although these conditions are less responsive to anticholinergic medication than neurogenic bladder disorders.

Adverse effects are similar to those observed with other anticholinergic agents (see index entry Anticholinergic Agents). Hyoscyamine is classified in FDA Pregnancy Category C.

DOSAGE AND PREPARATIONS.

Oral: *Adults,* 0.15 to 0.3 mg of the base three or four times daily or 0.375 mg of the sulfate twice daily.

HYOSCYAMINE:

Cystospaz (Polymedica). Tablets 0.15 mg.

HYOSCYAMINE SULFATE:
Anaspaz (Ascher), ***Generic.*** Tablets 0.125 mg.
Cystospaz-M (Polymedica). Capsules (prolonged-release) 0.375 mg.
Levsin (Schwarz). Capsules (prolonged-release) 0.375 mg (***Levsinex***); drops 0.125 mg/ml (alcohol 5%); elixir 0.125 mg/5 ml (alcohol 20%); tablets 0.125 mg.

OXYBUTYNIN CHLORIDE
[Ditropan]

$C_6H_5-C(OH)(C_6H_{11})-COOCH_2C{\equiv}CCH_2\overset{+}{N}H(CH_2CH_3)_2\ Cl^-$

ACTIONS AND USES. Oxybutynin has both anticholinergic and direct antispasmodic actions and also may possess mild local anesthetic properties. In some clinical trials, this drug increased bladder capacity and improved urinary frequency, urgency, and urge incontinence in adults and children with uninhibited bladder contractions (Koff et al, 1978; Thüroff et al, 1991); it also increased bladder capacity and reduced incontinence in those with reflex neurogenic bladder. Oxybutynin may be less effective in elderly patients with uninhibited bladder contractions (Brandeis and Resnick, 1992). It has not consistently relieved bladder spasm following transurethral surgical procedures.

A solution for intravesical instillation has been prepared by crushing a 5-mg tablet and dissolving it in 10 to 30 ml of sterile sodium chloride solution. Intravesical therapy was effective and safe in adults and children with neurogenic unstable bladder who were refractory to or unable to tolerate oral medication (Weese et al, 1993). In one small study in children, intravesical instillation of oxybutynin produced complete continence in 50% of patients. Daytime continence was achieved in another 30% (Greenfield and Fera, 1991). Adverse reactions were not observed.

The syrup is an acceptable alternative to tincture of belladonna in young children for whom a liquid preparation improves compliance.

ADVERSE REACTIONS AND PRECAUTIONS. Oxybutynin is preferred over other anticholinergic agents (eg, propantheline) because it produces fewer adverse effects; however, adverse reactions do occur. Severe dryness of the mouth is most common; a lingering bad taste, nausea, blurred vision, flushing, and tachycardia also have been observed. The incidence of adverse reactions (eg, hallucinations) is higher in children under 5 years (Jonville et al, 1992). Contraindications are the same as for other drugs with anticholinergic properties (see index entry Anticholinergic Agents).

DOSAGE AND PREPARATIONS.
Oral: *Adults,* 5 mg two or three times daily (maximum, 20 mg daily); up to 10 mg four times a day (maximum, 40 mg/day) has been recommended by some urologists. Doses of 2.5 to 5 mg three times a day are safe in *geriatric patients (older than 80 years).* The lower dose is recommended initially in these patients and may prove sufficient (Ouslander et al, 1988). *Children under 5 years,* 1 mg per year of age given twice daily; *5 years and older,* 5 mg two times daily (maximum, 15 mg daily).
Generic. Tablets 5 mg.
Ditropan (Marion Merrell Dow). Syrup 5 mg/5 ml; tablets 5 mg.
Additional Trademark:
Urotrol (Baker Norton).

PROPANTHELINE BROMIDE
[Pro-Banthīne]

$\text{xanthen-9-yl}-COOCH_2CH_2\overset{+}{N}CH_3(CH(CH_3)_2)_2\ Br^-$

ACTIONS AND USES. This quaternary ammonium compound is a synthetic anticholinergic agent with both antimuscarinic and ganglionic blocking properties. Its therapeutic effects are usually attributed to the antimuscarinic action.

Oral propantheline is used commonly to increase bladder capacity and to reduce urinary frequency, urgency, and urge incontinence associated with uninhibited neurogenic bladder. It may be given with imipramine. In paraplegic patients with lesions above the sacral spinal cord (reflex neurogenic bladder), propantheline also may control reflex detrusor activity and thus preserve continence in the interval between catheterizations.

Many physicians prefer oxybutynin over propantheline because it produces fewer adverse reactions. The lack of a liquid oral formulation is a drawback to the use of propantheline in children.

ADVERSE REACTIONS AND PRECAUTIONS. The adverse reactions produced by propantheline are common to all anticholinergic drugs. Doses that inhibit detrusor contractions also suppress salivation, interfere with ocular accommodation, dilate pupils, increase heart rate, and reduce gastrointestinal motility to cause constipation. Quaternary ammonium compounds do not readily cross the blood-brain barrier; therefore, central nervous system effects are rare. Because of its ganglionic blocking properties, large doses can cause orthostatic hypotension and impotence. Propantheline should be avoided in patients with glaucoma and used with care in those with urinary outlet obstruction. See also index entry Anticholinergic Agents.

DOSAGE AND PREPARATIONS. To improve bioavailability, propantheline should be administered one hour prior to meals.

Oral: To improve bladder capacity in patients with uninhibited neurogenic bladder, *adults,* initially, 15 mg every four to six hours; the amount may be increased by 15 mg/dose at weekly intervals until side effects (particularly visual) become intolerable or to a maximum of 90 mg four times daily (Mundy et al, 1984). *Children 5 years and older*, 7.5 to 15 mg two or three times daily.

To maintain continence between catheterizations in patients with reflex neurogenic bladder, *adults,* 15 to 30 mg every four to six hours; *children,* 7.5 to 15 mg every four to six hours.

Generic. Tablets 15 mg.

Pro-Banthīne (Roberts). Tablets 7.5 and 15 mg.

SCOPOLAMINE

[Transderm-Scōp]

For chemical formula, see index entry Scopolamine, In Motion Sickness.

A small pilot study reported an excellent response to the dermal application of scopolamine for urge incontinence (Wiener et al, 1986). Long-term use of dermal scopolamine in a larger patient population is needed to assess its value for unstable bladder (Baum et al, 1991).

The low systemic concentration of scopolamine was associated with few or no side effects. Application at three-day intervals improves compliance. See also index entry Scopolamine, In Motion Sickness. Scopolamine is classified in FDA Pregnancy Category C.

DOSAGE AND PREPARATIONS.

Topical: *Adults,* one transdermal adhesive unit is applied to clean dry skin in the postauricular area. The unit delivers 0.5 mg over 72 hours. A replacement patch should be applied at three-day intervals. This system may not be suitable for use in *children.*

Transderm-Scōp (CIBA). Adhesive unit 2.5 cm^2 containing 1.5 mg scopolamine.

Tricyclic Drug

IMIPRAMINE HYDROCHLORIDE

[Tofranil]

For chemical formula, see index entry Imipramine, Uses, Depression.

ACTIONS AND USES. Imipramine's mechanism of action in enuresis appears to be related to direct inhibition of bladder muscle (by a mechanism unrelated to anticholinergic effects) and increased outlet resistance (enhanced sympathetic amine activity). It is unclear if the response to imipramine is related to the serum concentrations of the parent drug and its metabolite, desipramine. Estimates of the therapeutic serum concentration of imipramine in enuresis range from 60 to 100 mcg/L (Miller et al, 1992), which is three to four times lower than the effective antidepressant concentration (Jorgensen et al, 1980; Rapoport et al, 1980). However, this drug has a narrow therapeutic window, and serum concentrations >60 mcg/L have been associated with significant adverse reactions (Miller et al, 1992).

Imipramine is used to treat nocturnal enuresis in children 6 years and older. Reported rates of cure range from 10% to more than 50% (Stewart, 1975; McKendry et al, 1975). Those who do not respond within one week usually do not benefit from continued administration of the drug. This drug probably is overused for childhood nocturnal enuresis; it should be employed only after bladder retraining and/or alarm systems have failed (Knapp, 1992).

Tolerance to the antienuretic action of imipramine develops in a few patients within weeks of initiating therapy. It has been recommended that the dose be reduced gradually at three-month intervals to determine the need for continued therapy. Tapering of the dose also may result in a lower incidence of relapse.

Imipramine also is useful in urge incontinence, particularly in elderly patients (over age 70), and may be combined with a pure anticholinergic agent, such as propantheline. It can be tried in the postprostatectomy patient with mild incontinence in whom sphincter weakness appears to be the primary deficit and in patients with demonstrable retrograde ejaculation.

ADVERSE REACTIONS AND PRECAUTIONS. A transient "dull feeling" or drowsiness may be noted for the first one to two weeks of therapy. Dryness of the mouth, constipation, blurred vision, restlessness, sleep disturbances, alterations in appetite, and mood changes are common. Memory loss is a significant side effect in the elderly. See also index entry Imipramine, Uses, Depression.

To avoid misunderstandings, it is recommended that the patient be informed that the drug is *not* being given for its antidepressant action, which requires a much larger dose.

OVERDOSAGE. Overdosage can cause convulsions, coma, and severe cardiovascular reactions, including AV block and marked hypotension. The most common source of imipramine poisoning in children is nonsecured medication belonging to an older, enuretic sibling. The pediatric patient also may increase dosage to dangerous levels in an attempt to secure dryness. Parents should be given adequate warning of this potential danger. Withdrawal reactions (nausea, vomiting, headache, and malaise) have been reported following abrupt discontinuation of long-term therapy (Wein, 1985 B).

PHARMACOKINETICS. See index entry Imipramine, Uses, Depression.

DOSAGE AND PREPARATIONS.

Oral: For nocturnal enuresis, *children 6 to 12 years,* 25 mg daily; if a satisfactory response is not apparent in one week, the dose should be increased to 50 mg daily; *children over 12 years,* up to 75 mg daily. The drug may be administered after the evening meal or up to one hour before bedtime. Some early nighttime bedwetters may benefit from administration in divided doses given at midafternoon and bedtime. When optimal effects are obtained, administration is continued for two to three months; the dose is then reduced gradually over three to four months. Such tapering of the dose may reduce the frequency of relapse and is necessary to prevent withdrawal effects.

For urge incontinence in *adults*, the following dosage has been proposed: Initially, 25 mg is given at bedtime and the amount is increased by 25 mg every third day until the patient is continent or experiences side effects (eg, orthostatic hypotension) to a maximum of 150 mg (Castleden et al, 1981). About 5 to 10 days are required to obtain a maximum effect. This dosage should be reduced by one-half in *elderly patients*

(Wein, 1985 A). In *children* with urge incontinence, smaller doses given every eight hours appear to be more effective than a single bedtime dose.

For postprostatectomy incontinence, up to 75 mg three times daily. For retrograde ejaculation, 25 mg two to four times daily.

Tofranil (Geigy), ***Generic.*** Tablets 10, 25, and 50 mg.

Alpha-Adrenergic Drugs

EPHEDRINE SULFATE

For chemical formula, see index entry Ephedrine, In Asthma.

This adrenergic drug has both alpha- and beta receptor-stimulating properties. It is effective orally, is generally well tolerated, and has a relatively long duration of action. By increasing urethral resistance, ephedrine improves urine storage in patients with mild to moderate stress incontinence of neurogenic or non-neurogenic origin, but it is of little value if the periurethral striated muscle is completely denervated or severely damaged or if there is severe damage to the posterior urethra (Diokno and Taub, 1975).

Since ephedrine increases blood pressure and stimulates the heart, it should be used cautiously in patients with hypertension and other cardiovascular disorders and in those with hyperthyroidism. It also stimulates the central nervous system and may cause insomnia and anxiety.

Ephedrine is classified in FDA Pregnancy Category C.

DOSAGE AND PREPARATIONS.

Oral: For stress incontinence, *adults,* 25 to 50 mg four times daily; *children,* 11 to 20 mg four times daily. For retrograde ejaculation, 50 to 75 mg one to two hours before intercourse; alternatively, 25 mg four times daily may be given.

Generic. Capsules and tablets 25 and 50 mg (nonprescription); syrup 20 mg/5 ml (alcohol 12%) (nonprescription).

PHENYLPROPANOLAMINE HYDROCHLORIDE

[Propagest]

For chemical formula, see index entry Phenylpropanolamine, In Nasal Congestion.

USES. Phenylpropanolamine, marketed for use as an appetite suppressant and nasal decongestant, is effective in mild stress incontinence (Awad et al, 1978). Use of the single-entity agent is preferable to combination products containing this drug.

Any beneficial response that occurs is apparent immediately or within a few days. An excellent response can be expected in mild stress incontinence; good response, but rarely total dryness, is observed in moderate to severe incontinence. Incontinence usually recurs if several doses are omitted or if therapy is discontinued.

ADVERSE REACTIONS AND PRECAUTIONS. The incidence of side effects is low and generally is related to the size of the dose. Reactions include dizziness and headache; central nervous system stimulation is much less marked than with ephedrine, and nervousness and insomnia are rarely a problem. Hypertensive episodes are uncommon. The drug should be used with caution in patients with hypertension, other cardiovascular disease, hyperthyroidism, and diabetes mellitus. Elderly patients may tolerate larger doses poorly.

Phenylpropanolamine is contraindicated in patients receiving monoamine oxidase inhibitors. The antihypertensive effectiveness of guanethidine may be reduced in some individuals.

PHARMACOKINETICS. About 80% to 90% of the dose is eliminated unchanged in the urine within 24 hours. Approximately 10% is metabolized to an active metabolite.

DOSAGE AND PREPARATIONS.

Oral: *Adults*, for incontinence, 50 mg three times a day. The dosage may be increased if required to 75 mg three times a day. Some patients may be able to omit the evening dose without a notable decrease in effectiveness. A single 75-mg prolonged-release preparation each morning may be adequate. For retrograde ejaculation, 75 mg twice daily.

Generic. Capsules (prolonged-release) 75 mg; tablets 25 and 50 mg (both forms nonprescription).

Propagest (Carnrick). Tablets 25 mg (nonprescription).

PHENYLPROPANOLAMINE HYDROCHLORIDE AND CHLORPHENIRAMINE MALEATE

[Drize, Ornade, Triaminic-12]

USES. Women with mild to moderate stress incontinence may respond to this mixture, which contains an alpha-adrenergic stimulant (phenylpropanolamine) and an antihistamine (chlorpheniramine). However, the chlorpheniramine component does not contribute to the urodynamic activity. This preparation is less satisfactory in men with postprostatectomy incontinence, although those with mild symptoms occasionally may improve (Stewart et al, 1976).

ADVERSE REACTIONS AND PRECAUTIONS. Adverse reactions attributable to sympathomimetic, antihistaminic, and anticholinergic effects may occur. Drowsiness, dryness of the mouth and nasal passages, and tachycardia are most common. If these effects are troublesome, the dose should be reduced or a single-entity preparation of phenylpropanolamine should be substituted. This mixture should be used cautiously in patients with hypertension and other cardiovascular disorders and in those with hyperthyroidism.

See also the evaluation on Phenylpropanolamine Hydrochloride.

DOSAGE AND PREPARATIONS.

Oral: For incontinence or retrograde ejaculation, *adults,* one capsule twice daily.

Generic. Capsules (prolonged-release).

Drize (Jones Medical), ***Ornade*** (SmithKline Beecham). Capsules (prolonged-release) containing phenylpropanolamine hydrochloride 75 mg and chlorpheniramine maleate 12 mg.

Triaminic-12 (Sandoz). Tablets (prolonged-release) containing phenylpropanolamine hydrochloride 75 mg and chlorpheniramine maleate 12 mg (nonprescription).

PSEUDOEPHEDRINE HYDROCHLORIDE

[Sudafed, Novafed]

For chemical formula, see index entry Pseudoephedrine, In Nasal Congestion.

Pseudoephedrine hydrochloride, marketed for use as a nasal decongestant, is effective for stress incontinence. It acts similarly to ephedrine but causes less central nervous system stimulation and hypertension. For additional information, see index entry Pseudoephedrine, In Nasal Congestion.

DOSAGE AND PREPARATIONS.

Oral: *Adults*, for stress incontinence, 30 to 60 mg four times daily (Wein, 1984 B) or, prolonged-release form, 20 mg twice daily; for retrograde ejaculation, 60 mg four times a day.

Sudafed (Warner Wellcome), ***Generic.*** Tablets 30 and 60 mg; tablets (prolonged-release) 120 mg (***Sudafed 12 Hour***); liquid 30 mg/5 ml (all forms nonprescription).

Novafed (Marion Merrell Dow). Capsules (prolonged-release) 120 mg.

Hormonal Agent

DESMOPRESSIN ACETATE

[DDAVP]

ACTIONS AND USES. The inadequate secretion of the antidiuretic hormone, vasopressin, may cause the nightly urine volume to exceed bladder capacity in some children. Desmopressin, a synthetic analogue of vasopressin, has potent antidiuretic actions but does not have the pressor activity of the parent compound. In numerous clinical trials, a daily intranasal dose of desmopressin ranging from 5 to 40 mcg has been effective and safe in preventing and treating bed wetting in children with pure nocturnal enuresis (Klauber, 1989; Miller et al, 1989; Himsl and Hurwitz, 1991; Key et al, 1992). Desmopressin appears to have little value in unstable bladder or other forms of enuresis.

Total dryness may occur in up to 70% of children with pure nocturnal enuresis, and the extent of bedwetting is decreased in many others; however, in some trials, total dryness was achieved in less than 25% of children (Evans and Meadow, 1992; Moffat et al, 1993). Increasing the dose from 20 to 40 mcg/day may enhance the response (Terho, 1991; Hjälmås and Sillén, 1990). The duration of action is 10 to 12 hours. Most patients relapse after withdrawal of desmopressin, but gradual tapering of the dose may prevent relapse in some.

The use of this agent for more than six months has not been studied extensively; a few reports indicate that desmopressin retained effectiveness and was safe for up to three years (Belmaker and Belich, 1986; Miller et al, 1989; Hjälmås and Sillén, 1990). It is unclear if this drug should be used for initial or primary therapy (Rosenfeld and Jerkins, 1991); some authorities recommend that it be reserved for patients refractory to other treatment or for specific short-term use (eg, overnight stays, camping trips) (Himsl and Hurwitz, 1991). Its use with oxybutynin, propantheline, or another anticholinergic agent may produce additive effects in some patients. Combined use with an enuresis alarm may be beneficial in children who do not respond to either treatment alone (Sukhai et al, 1989). This drug is expensive; one-month supply (20 mcg/day) costs about $120.00.

ADVERSE REACTIONS AND PRECAUTIONS. This drug is well tolerated. Nasal discomfort has been reported in some patients. Hyponatremia and fluid retention (water intoxication) have been observed rarely; however, hyponatremia-induced convulsions in children have been reported recently (Beach et al, 1992; Hamed et al, 1993; Kallio et al, 1993). Causes have included excessive fluid intake, concomitant therapy with imipramine, and acute illness (eg, diarrhea) affecting water balance. Fluid intake should be limited to no more than 30 ml/kg two to four hours before and 12 hours after administration of desmopressin (Beach et al, 1992).

Rhinorrhea interferes with absorption of desmopressin; administration of an antihistamine or ipratropium nasal spray may be necessary.

For a more detailed discussion of adverse reactions and precautions, see index entry Desmopressin, In Diabetes Insipidus.

DOSAGE AND PREPARATIONS.

Topical (Intranasal): Desmopressin is administered through a flexible calibrated nasal tube or by metered spray. The initial dose is 20 mcg (10 mcg in each nostril) at bedtime. The amount may be increased to a maximum of 40 mcg/day if there is no improvement after two weeks. Patients who do not respond to a four-week trial of therapy (with 40 mcg/day used the last week of therapy) are unlikely to respond to larger doses (Rosenfeld and Jerkins, 1991). After continence is achieved for two or more weeks, the dose may be reduced slowly and the larger amount reinstituted if enuresis reappears.

DDAVP (Rhone-Poulenc Rorer). Solution (intranasal) 100 mcg/ml in 2.5 ml containers with two rhinal tube applicators; solution (spray) 10 mcg/0.1 ml in 5 ml containers.

AGENTS USED TO TREAT URINARY RETENTION

The drugs used to treat urinary retention facilitate bladder emptying by increasing detrusor muscle contractility (cholinergic agents) or by reducing outlet resistance (alpha-adrenergic blocking drugs). Bethanechol, a cholinergic agent, has been used for the management of chronic hypotonic bladder and for short-term treatment of postoperative urinary retention in selected patients; however, its efficacy is limited. The cholinesterase inhibitor, neostigmine methylsulfate [Prostigmin], also has been prescribed for the latter purpose. The alpha-adrenergic blocking drug, phenoxybenzamine, facilitates voiding by relaxing the internal sphincter and is used in certain neurogenic bladder disorders and for outlet obstruction in symptomatic benign prostatic hypertrophy. Because phenoxybenzamine is mutagenic and carcinogenic in rodents, prazosin or terazosin should be used when long-term administration is anticipated. These drugs may be given with bethanechol. Relaxants used primarily to combat spasticity, dantrolene and baclofen, reduce urinary retention secondary to spasm of the external sphincter.

Cholinergic Drug

BETHANECHOL CHLORIDE

[Duvoid, Myotonachol, Urecholine]

$$H_2NCOCH(CH_3)CH_2\overset{+}{N}(CH_3)_3 \quad Cl^-$$

(with C=O on the carbonyl carbon)

ACTIONS AND USES. Bethanechol is a choline ester that acts directly on effector cells. Its muscarinic effects are similar to those of acetylcholine but are more prolonged because bethanechol is relatively resistant to hydrolysis by cholinesterase. Effects on autonomic ganglia are minimal. The action on the urinary bladder and gastrointestinal tract is more pronounced than that on the cardiovascular system. Although response to bethanechol's bladder smooth muscle-stimulating effects is variable and its efficacy for bladder dysfunction has been questioned, it is helpful in an occasional patient and, in the absence of superior agents, this drug is used as discussed below.

Bethanechol has been used in conjunction with intermittent self-catheterization to facilitate emptying of the hypotonic neurogenic bladder. It is sometimes employed during the recovery phase after spinal shock to enhance weak detrusor contractions in patients with coordinated bladder-external sphincter function who have spinal cord lesions above the vesical reflux arc (S_2 to S_4) (Diokno and Koppenhoefer, 1976). If tolerated, bethanechol also may be used for long-term therapy in patients with sensory paralytic bladder or in those with incomplete motor lesions and coordinated sphincter function (Sonda et al, 1979). *Its effectiveness should be documented during a short trial before committing a patient to long-term therapy.*

In neurogenic bladder disorders, bethanechol may be used in conjunction with surgery or other drugs (eg, terazosin) to reduce anatomic or functional outlet obstruction. It also is used to restore normal micturition in selected patients with acute urinary retention associated with surgery or parturition.

ADVERSE REACTIONS AND PRECAUTIONS. Bethanechol may cause flushing, headache, salivation, sweating, nausea, abdominal cramps, diarrhea, asthmatic attacks, and a fall in blood pressure. Some patients cannot tolerate prolonged therapy. Side effects may be counteracted immediately by atropine (children to age 12, 0.01 mg/kg; adults, 0.6 mg); the subcutaneous route is used except in emergencies, and administration may be repeated every two hours if needed. Atropine should be available during the subcutaneous administration of bethanechol.

Bethanechol must not be given intravenously or intramuscularly because acute severe muscarinic effects, including acute circulatory failure and cardiac arrest, may result.

This drug is classified in FDA Pregnancy Category C.

CONTRAINDICATIONS. *Bethanechol is contraindicated in the presence of anatomic or functional urinary tract obstruction. This drug also should be avoided in patients with detrusor-external sphincter dyssynergia* (involuntary detrusor contractions accompanied by contraction of the external sphincter) *unless an effective external sphincter relaxant is given concomitantly,* because prolonged therapy has caused bladder trabeculation, diverticula, and vesicoureteral reflux. Although dyssynergia resulting from internal sphincter overactivity may be less common, the possibility of adverse effects in such cases should be considered.

Bethanechol also is contraindicated in patients with bronchial asthma because it may cause bronchospasm. It may reduce blood pressure and generally should be avoided in patients with hypotension, bradycardia, or coronary artery disease and during therapy with ganglionic blocking agents (eg, mecamylamine, trimethaphan). Additional contraindications include hyperthyroidism, hypertension, and atrioventricular conduction defects.

Because it increases gastrointestinal motility, bethanechol should not be given to patients with peptic ulcer and other gastrointestinal lesions or to those with intestinal obstruction. It should not be employed following recent gastrointestinal resection and anastomosis.

EFFECTS ON LABORATORY TESTS. Serum amylase, lipase, and transaminase (AST) levels may be increased secondary to pancreatic stimulation and contraction of the sphincter of Oddi.

DOSAGE AND PREPARATIONS. The dosage and route of administration must be individualized. The drug should be given before meals to avoid nausea and vomiting. A subcutaneous dose of 5 mg is equivalent to an oral dose of 200 mg.

Subcutaneous: For acute postoperative and postpartum urinary retention in selected *adults,* 5 mg (1 ml). If this dose is ineffective, the patient should be catheterized. Bethanechol should not be used unless the patient is alert and there is no outlet obstruction.

Subcutaneous, Oral: For patients with incomplete spinal cord lesions above the sacral reflex arc and voluntary control of the external sphincter, initially, 2.5 to 5 mg subcutaneously every four to six hours. The patient should be catheterized once or twice daily; when residual urine is less than 50 ml, oral therapy may be substituted (50 mg every six hours) or subcutaneous therapy may be continued (2.5 mg every six hours). This regimen should be continued for at least one week. If the amount of residual urine remains low, the drug may be discontinued following a gradual reduction in dosage. Some patients may require several weeks or months of therapy.

In sensory paralytic bladder and partial motor paralytic bladder with coordinated sphincter function, initially, 5 to 10 mg subcutaneously every four hours around the clock. (An initial dose of 5 mg may be advisable in very frail patients.) The patient should be asked to try to urinate 20 to 30 minutes after the drug is administered. This voiding program may be initiated with an indwelling catheter, which is removed after the first few doses. When the amount of residual urine is less than 50 ml for three days, each dose may be reduced by 2.5 mg. If the response remains satisfactory, dosage may be reduced to a minimum of 5 mg every four hours. Oral therapy (50 mg four times daily) may be substituted when complete bladder emptying is achieved over a three-day period. The drug may be discontinued when the sensory paralytic bladder is rehabilitated, but patients with incomplete motor lesions generally require lifelong treatment.

For *children* with lazy bladder syndrome and inadequate detrusor activity, 0.2 mg/kg or 6.7 mg/M^2 orally three times a day or 0.15 to 0.2 mg/kg or 5 to 6.7 mg/M^2 subcutaneously three times a day. The drug should be discontinued when voiding retraining is accomplished.

Oral: For patients with lesions above the sacral reflex arc and coordinated bladder and sphincter function, initially, 25 mg every six hours. Dosage may be increased or decreased depending on the response (the usual adult dose is 50 to 100 mg four times a day), and the drug should be discontinued if reflex voiding is established.

Generic. Tablets 5, 10, 25, and 50 mg.
Duvoid (Roberts). Tablets 10, 25, and 50 mg.
Myotonachol (Glenwood). Tablets 10 and 25 mg.
Urecholine (Merck). Solution (for injection) 5 mg/ml; tablets 5, 10, 25, and 50 mg.

Alpha-Adrenergic Blocking Agents

PHENOXYBENZAMINE HYDROCHLORIDE

[Dibenzyline]

$$C_6H_5-CH_2\overset{+}{N}H(CH_2CH_2Cl)CH(CH_3)CH_2O-C_6H_5 \quad Cl^-$$

ACTIONS AND USES. By noncompetitively blocking alpha-adrenergic receptors in the smooth muscle of the bladder neck and proximal urethra, phenoxybenzamine relaxes the internal sphincter. It may improve voiding efficiency in patients with functional outlet obstruction and obviate or delay the need for transurethral surgery. Phenoxybenzamine has been effective in some patients with reflex, autonomous, or motor paralytic bladder when urinary retention could not be prevented by other methods, such as reflex voiding, Credé maneuver, or use of bethanechol (Kleeman, 1977; Mobley, 1976; Scott and Morrow, 1978). It is particularly useful in rehabilitating decompensated or atonic bladders when administered with bethanechol (Finkbeiner and Bissada, 1980).

In addition to its use in neurogenic bladder dysfunction, phenoxybenzamine has been employed to treat voiding disturbances in patients with prostatic obstruction who are not suitable candidates for surgery or in those who have only occasional, transient, acute episodes of retention (Caine et al, 1981; Waterfall and Williams, 1980). As an alternative to catheterization of the bladder, phenoxybenzamine can be employed to relieve postoperative retention of urine. A dose of 10 mg orally may be given prophylactically 6 and 18 hours after surgery or if signs of obstruction become evident (Leventhal and Pfau, 1978).

Phenoxybenzamine has no effect on striated muscle and therefore is ineffective in urinary retention caused by excessive or inappropriate activity of the external sphincter.

ADVERSE REACTIONS AND PRECAUTIONS. The major side effects of phenoxybenzamine, orthostatic hypotension and reflex tachycardia, result from blockade of alpha-adrenergic receptors in the peripheral circulation. Elastic stockings may counteract hypotension. Other adverse reactions include nasal congestion, transient lassitude, nausea, diarrhea, miosis, and inhibition of ejaculation.

A two-year study in rats employing large doses showed a proliferation of basal cells in the nonglandular portion of the stomach. For this reason, the manufacturer currently recommends that this drug be reserved for emergency, short-term use, such as the preoperative management of pheochromocytoma.

PHARMACOKINETICS. The gastrointestinal absorption of phenoxybenzamine is erratic; about 20% to 30% of an orally administered dose appears in the systemic circulation. The volume of distribution has not been reported. Phenoxybenzamine has high lipid solubility and accumulates in body fat. About 50% of an intravenous dose is excreted in 12 hours and over 80% in 24 hours.

DOSAGE AND PREPARATIONS.

Oral: *Adults,* initially, 10 mg once daily. If larger amounts are needed, the dosage may be increased by 10-mg increments every four to five days to a maximum of 60 mg daily. Daily doses larger than 10 mg should be divided evenly and given every 8 to 12 hours. The maximum effect usually becomes apparent only after one week following initiation or change in dosage (Wein, 1984 B). *Children,* the dosage is similar to that used in adults, to a maximum of 10 mg three times daily (Diokno and Sonda, 1984).

Dibenzyline (SmithKline Beecham). Capsules 10 mg.

PRAZOSIN HYDROCHLORIDE

[Minipress]

For chemical formula, see index entry Prazosin, Uses, Hypertension.

This antihypertensive agent is a relatively specific alpha$_1$ adrenergic receptor antagonist. In contrast to phenoxybenzamine, prazosin has not demonstrated mutagenic or carcinogenic action in animal studies, and it is preferred to phenoxybenzamine for treatment of symptomatic benign prostatic hyperplasia or functional outlet obstruction. In voiding dysfunction, the efficacy of prazosin is approximately equivalent to that of phenoxybenzamine in most patients (Wein, 1988).

The actions, indications, and adverse reactions of prazosin are similar to those of terazosin, but the dosing schedule (three or four times daily) is less convenient. Prazosin is about ten times less expensive than terazosin, however.

ADVERSE REACTIONS AND PRECAUTIONS. Marked orthostatic hypotension and syncope that occasionally has led to collapse and unconsciousness may occur at the onset of treatment (first-dose phenomenon). An associated tachycardia has been noted occasionally, and chest pain has occurred rarely. Symptomatic orthostatic hypotension appears to be most common when the initial dose exceeds 2 mg and when dosage is increased rapidly; careful dosage titration can prevent this problem. Patients receiving diuretics, a beta blocker, and/or a low-sodium diet may be particularly susceptible. Prazosin may cause edema if a diuretic is not given concomitantly.

Prazosin is classified in FDA Pregnancy Category C.

For additional information on side effects, precautions, and pharmacokinetics, see index entry Prazosin, Uses, Hypertension.

DOSAGE AND PREPARATIONS.

Oral: *Adults*, initially, 1 mg at bedtime, then 1 mg three times daily. This may be increased at weekly intervals by 1 mg/dose until an adequate effect is produced or the side effects become unacceptable. The maximum dose for urologic dysfunction is 3 to 4 mg three times daily (Wein and Barrett, 1988).

Minipress (Pfizer), ***Generic***. Capsules 1, 2, and 5 mg.

TERAZOSIN HYDROCHLORIDE

[Hytrin]

For chemical formula, see index entry Terazosin, In Hypertension.

The actions and indications for this selective alpha-adrenergic receptor blocking agent are similar to those for prazosin. The primary advantage of terazosin over prazosin is its longer half-life, which permits once-daily administration. However, it is considerably more expensive than prazosin.

In several multicenter trials in men with symptomatic benign prostatic hyperplasia (BPH), a single daily oral dose of 10 mg reduced symptom scores by 50% to 70% and urinary flow rates improved significantly (Lepor et al, 1992; Brawer et al, 1993; Lowe and Stark, 1993). Although little data exist on the long-term effects of terazosin, in one study in patients with BPH, its efficacy and safety were maintained for 24 months (Lepor et al, 1992). The value of combined therapy with finasteride is being studied.

ADVERSE REACTIONS AND PRECAUTIONS. Orthostatic hypotension and dizziness have not been significant when the dose is increased gradually up to 10 mg. The patient should be monitored for alterations in blood pressure and especially for the development of orthostatic hypotension. For additional information on side effects, precautions, and pharmacokinetics, see index entry Terazosin, In Hypertension.

DOSAGE AND ADMINISTRATION.

Oral: *Adults,* initially, 1 mg daily at bedtime, increased gradually to 10 mg/day given as a single dose at bedtime for three to seven days. (Because dose-response curves observed in clinical trials indicated that a 10-mg dose was not adequate to produce maximal effects, a 20-mg dose is now being evaluated.)

Hytrin (Abbott). Tablets 1, 2, 5, and 10 mg.

Alpha Reductase Inhibitor

FINASTERIDE

[Proscar]

ACTIONS AND USES. This agent blocks the conversion of testosterone to dihydrotestosterone (DHT) by inhibiting the enzyme, 5-α reductase. Subsequent marked decreases of DHT levels in the prostate in patients with benign prostatic hyperplasia (BPH) are presumed to be responsible for the decrease in prostate size and inhibition of further growth (McConnell, 1990).

Results of a number of investigations, including multicenter studies, indicate that oral administration of 5 mg once daily reduces prostate volume by 20% to 30% and improved symptoms in 30% to 50% of patients; the increase in urinary flow rate over that observed with placebo was small but significant (Gormley et al, 1992; Peters and Sorkin, 1993; McConnell, 1990; Cotton, 1991). A six-month trial is recommended, because this is the length of time required to achieve a beneficial response in some men. It is not possible to identify those who will benefit (*FDC Reports*, 1992 B).

Relief of symptoms and improvement in objective parameters of urinary function are considerably less than the results achieved with TURP; however, use of finasteride may allow patients with moderate symptoms to avoid surgery, and it may be beneficial for those with severe BPH who cannot tolerate or refuse surgery (Peters and Sorkin, 1993). The drug has no prophylactic value.

Preliminary data suggest that the efficacy of finasteride may be maintained for up to two years in responsive patients (*FDC Reports*, 1992 B). Combined use of finasteride and terazosin may have additive effects; a large clinical trial to compare the effect of each drug alone and in combination in patients with symptomatic BPH is underway.

At present, there is no indication for use of this drug in women, and it should not be used in this population.

ADVERSE REACTIONS AND PRECAUTIONS. Finasteride appears to be safe and is well tolerated. A low incidence of impotence as well as decreased ejaculate and diminished libido have been reported (Cotton, 1991; *FDC Reports*, 1992 B). To protect the male fetus, pregnant women or those attempting to become pregnant should avoid contact with the semen of men taking this drug.

DOSAGE AND PREPARATIONS.

Oral: *Men*, 5 mg once daily.

Proscar (Merck). Tablets 5 mg.

External Sphincter Relaxants

BACLOFEN

[Lioresal]

For chemical formula, see index entry Baclofen, In Muscle Spasticity.

ACTIONS AND USES. Baclofen reduces polysynaptic reflex activity in the spinal cord. Its primary indication is spasticity resulting from upper motor neuron lesions (see index entry Baclofen, In Muscle Spasticity). It may be useful in the management of external sphincter hypertonicity or detrusor-external sphincter dyssynergia. Patients with concurrent bladder hypotonicity who demonstrate weak or poorly sustained detrusor contraction on voiding also may require a cholinergic agent, such as bethanechol, to attain the optimal effect. Baclofen apparently is a more potent relaxant of the external sphincter than diazepam or dantrolene.

ADVERSE REACTIONS AND PRECAUTIONS. Baclofen usually is well tolerated. Drowsiness (incidence 10% to 63%), dizziness (incidence 5% to 15%), and muscle weakness may occur but often disappear with continued administration and may be minimized by avoiding abrupt increases in dosage. Occasional reactions include nausea, constipation, insomnia, and headache. Baclofen may increase the frequency of seizures in epileptic patients. Abrupt discontinuation of long-term, high-dose therapy may be associated with visual and auditory hallucinations and agitated behavior. Alcohol and other central nervous system depressants should be avoided.

The safety of baclofen during pregnancy or in children has not been established.

Baclofen may increase blood glucose, serum alkaline phosphatase, and serum AST values.

PHARMACOKINETICS. See index entry Baclofen, In Muscle Spasticity.

DOSAGE AND PREPARATIONS.

Oral: *Adults,* initially, 5 mg three times a day, increased by 15 mg/day every fourth day until the desired effect is achieved. The manufacturer's literature specifies that most patients respond to a total daily dose of 40 to 80 mg and that doses in excess of 80 mg daily should not be used. In one study, however, most patients required an average daily dose of 120 mg to reduce external urethral sphincter spasticity significantly (Leyson et al, 1980). Usually a minimum of five weeks is required to assess the effectiveness of therapy. Baclofen should be discontinued slowly over a one- to two-week period to avoid precipitating hallucinations and/or agitated behavior.

Lioresal (Geigy), ***Generic.*** Tablets 10 and 20 mg.

DANTROLENE SODIUM

[Dantrium]

For chemical formula, see index entry Dantrolene, In Muscle Spasticity.

ACTIONS AND USES. Dantrolene acts directly on skeletal muscle to produce relaxation by interfering with the release of calcium ions from the sarcoplasmic reticulum. It is of some benefit in patients with external sphincter hypertonicity who have excessive residual urine volume and high urethral pressure. Its action may be enhanced by the concomitant administration of diazepam, but the combination may produce significant sedation. In patients with concurrent bladder hypotonicity who demonstrate weak or poorly sustained detrusor contraction on voiding, a cholinergic agent, such as bethanechol, also may be required for an optimal effect. On a theoretical basis, the urethral pressure can be decreased by only 50%. The risks of dantrolene therapy must be weighed against the potential benefit in patients with incomplete neurologic lesions. The drug is not a substitute for external sphincterotomy in male patients with complete spinal cord lesions.

ADVERSE REACTIONS AND PRECAUTIONS. Minor side effects, which usually disappear with continued treatment, are drowsiness, dizziness, nausea, vomiting, and diarrhea. The only adverse reaction that occurs commonly during long-term therapy is an acne-like skin eruption.

The limiting reaction at the dosage levels required to manage external sphincter spasm is generalized muscle weakness. Patients with brain stem or high cervical lesions, amyotrophic lateral sclerosis, or multiple sclerosis may not tolerate large doses of dantrolene because of severe muscle weakness. The drug should be used with caution in patients with impaired pulmonary function, particularly obstructive lung disease or respiratory weakness caused by motor neuron disease. Alcohol should be avoided.

For other adverse reactions, precautions, and pharmacokinetics, see index entry Dantrolene, In Muscle Spasticity.

DOSAGE AND PREPARATIONS. The dosage should be titrated. Usually five to seven weeks are required to assess the value of therapy.

Oral: *Adults,* initially, 25 mg once daily; 25 mg is added every fourth day until the desired effect is attained or until a maximum dose of 400 mg/day is reached. The manufacturer's literature specifies that most patients respond to a total daily dose of 400 mg or less and that only rarely should doses larger than this be given. However, in one study, most patients required 600 mg daily (Hackler et al, 1980). *Children,* a similar schedule should be used, beginning with 0.5 mg/kg twice daily, increased to a maximum of 3 mg/kg four times daily. Doses larger than 400 mg/day should not be given.

Dantrium (Procter & Gamble). Capsules 25, 50, and 100 mg.

DIAZEPAM

[Valium]

For chemical formula, see index entry Diazepam, In Anxiety.

ACTIONS AND USES. Diazepam has an antispastic action in addition to its sedative and antianxiety properties. This effect is believed to be the result of combined presynaptic inhibition in the spinal cord and suppression of the lateral reticular system that is facilitative to the gamma motor neurons. Its beneficial action in voiding, however, is ascribed by many solely to its antianxiety action.

Diazepam is useful as a supplement to voiding retraining or intermittent catheterization in children with external sphincter dyssynergia (non-neurogenic neurogenic bladder of childhood) and as a supplement to anticholinergic agents in women with urethral syndrome due to spasm of the external sphincter. The drug is less effective in spastic external sphincter secondary to upper motor neuron lesions.

For a discussion of adverse reactions, precautions, and pharmacokinetic data, see index entry Diazepam, In Anxiety.

DOSAGE AND PREPARATIONS. The half-life is prolonged in premature infants, elderly patients, and in those with hepatic disease; the latter require a reduction in dosage. Dosage adjustment is not required in those with renal disease.

Oral: The dosage for urologic disorders should not exceed the usual amount given for anxiety. *Children,* 0.2 to 0.4 mg/kg three or four times a day; *adults,* 2 to 5 mg/day in three or four divided doses. This amount is continued for two to six months and then is reduced gradually.

Generic. Solution (oral) 1 and 5 mg/ml; tablets 2, 5, and 10 mg.

Valium (Roche). Tablets 2, 5, and 10 mg.

AGENTS USED TO TREAT INTERSTITIAL CYSTITIS

DIMETHYL SULFOXIDE (DMSO)

[Rimso-50]

$$CH_3-S(=O)-CH_3$$

USES. Dimethyl sulfoxide is available as a 50% solution for direct instillation into the bladder to treat interstitial cystitis. It relieves symptoms for several months in many patients due to its anti-inflammatory, analgesic, and muscle relaxing properties (Sant and Meares, 1990). Although most responsive patients relapse after initial improvement, retreatment is usually successful. In these patients, intermittent self-catheterization in conjunction with administration of DMSO may prove useful. Advantages of DMSO include the absence of significant local or systemic adverse reactions, low cost, lack of need for anesthesia, and ease of administration in the physician's office.

ADVERSE REACTIONS AND PRECAUTIONS. The most common side effect of DMSO, which results from systemic absorption, is a garlic-like taste and odor on the breath and skin that lasts for as long as 72 hours; this is without clinical significance. Other side effects are self-limiting and include suprapubic discomfort, transient chemical cystitis, headache, lethargy, and nausea.

When applied to the skin, DMSO may cause erythema, pruritus, and urticaria. Severe systemic allergic reactions following topical exposure are uncommon, but shortness of breath, angioedema, and other allergic reactions have been reported. Similar reactions probably can occur after intravesical administration. DMSO may be a weak sensitizer. It has been reported to induce a generalized papuloerythematous eruption following multiple intravesical instillations (Nishimura et al, 1988).

Lens opacities have occurred following prolonged administration to animals, but this is species specific and has not been reported in humans.

DMSO is classified in FDA Pregnancy Category C.

PHARMACOKINETICS. The portion of DMSO that is absorbed into the systemic circulation after intravesical instillation is tightly protein bound and can be detected for 36 to 48 hours. A portion is reduced to dimethyl sulfide, which is responsible for the garlic-like taste and odor on the breath. The principal metabolite is an oxidation product, dimethyl sulfone, which may be detected in the serum for longer than two weeks after a single intravesical instillation.

DOSAGE AND PREPARATIONS.

Intravesical Instillation: Following local anesthesia of the urethra, 50 ml of a 50% solution of DMSO is instilled (slowly to avoid bladder spasm) by catheter directly into the bladder. Anticholinergic agents may be given prior to instillation to help prevent bladder spasm. The solution is retained in the bladder for 15 minutes and then eliminated by spontaneous voiding. Approximately 60% of patients respond to weekly instillations of DMSO for six weeks but many also require maintenance therapy because of relapses. Some physicians employ 50 ml of a 25% solution for the initial instillation and the 50% solution thereafter. Instillation may be repeated at one- or two-week intervals in patients with severe symptoms or at three- to six-month intervals in those with milder symptoms (maintenance therapy).

Rimso-50 (Research Industries), ***Generic.*** Solution (sterile) 50% in 50 ml containers.

WARNING: The preparation, ***Cryoserv*** (formerly ***Rimso-100***), which is used for cryogenic preparations, is not intended for human use. The instillation of ***Cryoserv*** into the bladder would cause a tissue-damaging exothermic reaction.

OXYCHLOROSENE SODIUM

[Clorpactin WCS-90]

This topical antiseptic is a mixture of the sodium salt of hypochlorous acid and alkylbenzene sulfonates (see index entry Oxychlorosene, As Antiseptic). A 0.4% solution is instilled to relieve the symptoms of interstitial cystitis. General or spinal anesthesia is required because instillation is extremely painful. An intensification of symptoms (lasting up to 72 hours) may occur immediately following each treatment, and oral opioids may be required for relief. The use of this agent is reserved for patients who do not respond to DMSO and other oral preparations.

Other than extreme pain during instillation, no side effects attributable to this agent or injury to the bladder has been reported. Oxychlorosene may, however, produce ureteral fibrosis in patients with vesicoureteral reflux (Messing and Freiha, 1979). In these patients, the ureteral orifice should be occluded before instillation. Concentrations should not exceed 0.4%.

DOSAGE AND PREPARATIONS.

Intravesical Instillation: A 0.4% solution is prepared immediately prior to use. After the patient is anesthetized, the solution is instilled through a large urethral catheter under low pressure (10 cm water) until the bladder is full. After a five-minute retention period, the bladder is emptied. Instillations are repeated for a total retention time of 15 to 20 minutes. The patient is then observed for four weeks. If symptoms do not subside, up to four additional instillations can be performed at weekly intervals. If improvement is attained during a treatment course, no more is given until symptoms recur. A six-month interval is allowed to elapse prior to a second course of therapy, if this is required (Messing and Stamey, 1978; Messing, 1986 B).

Clorpactin WCS-90 (Guardian). Powder (water-soluble) in 2 g containers (nonprescription).

Cited References

Incontinence implant gains is approvable FDA Advisory Panel concludes; Follow-up data needed. *FDC Reports* 9, (Oct) 1990.

Kabi Pharmacia withdraws its incontinence drug terodiline. *Pharmaceut J* 381, (Sept) 1991.

Urinary incontinence first-line treatment is behavioral therapy; propantheline is effective. *FDC Reports* (March 29) 1992 A.

Merck's *Proscar* requires six-month trial treatment period to determine individual response; Free supplies offered through patient support program. *FDC Reports* 6, (June) 1992 B.

Urinary incontinence in elderly patients. *Lancet* 2:1316-1317, 1986.

Andersson K-E, et al: Effects of prazosin on isolated human urethra and in patients with lower motor neuron lesions. *Invest Urol* 19:39-42, 1981.

Appell RA: New developments: Injectables for urethral incompetence in women. *Int Urogynecol J* 1:117-119, 1990.

Awad SA, et al: Alpha-adrenergic agents in urinary disorders of proximal urethra: Part 1. Sphincteric incontinence. *Br J Urol* 50:332-335, 1978.

Bankhead CD: Pelvic shocks abet continence. *Med World News* 61, (March) 1991.

Barbalias GA, Blaivas JG: Neurologic implications of pathologically open bladder neck. *J Urol* 129:780-782, 1983.

Barrett DM: Effect of oral bethanechol chloride on voiding in female patients with excessive residual urine: Randomized double-blind study. *J Urol* 126:640-642, 1981.

Barrett DM, Woodside JR: Voiding dysfunctions in children: Diagnosis and management, in Yalla SV, et al (eds): *Neurourology and Urodynamics: Principles and Practice,* ed 2. New York, Macmillan, 1988, 237-263.

Barton CH, et al: Effect of modified transurethral sphincterotomy on autonomic dysreflexia. *J Urol* 135:83-85, 1986.

Bauer SB: Genitourinary problems in adolescence. *J Reprod Med* 29:385-390, 1984.

Baum N, et al: Urinary incontinence: Not a 'normal' part of aging. *Postgrad Med* 90:99-109, (Aug) 1991.

Beach PS, et al: Hyponatremic seizures in a child treated with desmopressin to control enuresis. *Clin Pediatr* 31:566-569, 1992.

Beary J III, Gilbert S: Coping with the 'bashful bladder' syndrome, letter. *Lancet* 1:1429-1430, 1981.

Belmaker RH, Belich A: The use of desmopressin in adult enuresis. *Mil Med* 151:660-662, 1986.

Belman AB: Urgency incontinence in children. *West J Med* 149:315, 1988.

Benson GS, et al: Bladder muscle contractility: Comparative effects and mechanisms of action of atropine, propantheline, flavoxate, and imipramine. *Urology* 9:31-35, 1977.

Bhatia NN, et al: Effects of estrogen on urethral function in women with urinary incontinence. *Am J Obstet Gynecol* 160:176-181, 1989.

Biggers RD: Self-administration of dimethyl sulfoxide (DMSO) for interstitial cystitis. *Urology* 28:10-11, 1986.

Bissada NK, Finkbeiner AE: Urologic manifestations of drug therapy. *Urol Clin North Am* 15:725-736, 1988.

Blaivas JG: Pathophysiology of lower urinary tract dysfunction. *Clin Obstet Gynecol* 12:11-25, 1985.

Blaivas JG: Neurologic dysfunctions, in Yalla SV, et al (eds): *Neurourology and Urodynamics: Principles and Practice.* New York, Macmillan, 1988 A, 343-357.

Blaivas JG: Pathophysiology and differential diagnosis of benign prostatic hypertrophy. *Urology* 32 (suppl 6):5-11, 1988 B.

Blaivas JG, Barbalias GA: Characteristics of neural injury after abdomino-perineal resection. *J Urol* 129:84-87, 1983.

Blaivas JG, et al: Detrusor-external sphincter dyssynergia: Detailed electromyographic study. *J Urol* 125:545-548, 1981.

Bodner DR: Urethral syndrome. *Urol Clin North Am* 15:699-704, 1988.

Bowen LW, et al: Interstitial cystitis, in Ostergard DR (ed): *Gynecologic Urology and Urodynamics: Theory and Practice,* ed 2. Baltimore, Williams & Wilkins, 1985, 437-454.

Brandeis GH, Resnick NM: Pharmacotherapy of urinary incontinence in the elderly. *Drug Ther* 93-102, (Feb) 1992.

Brawer MK, et al: Terazosin in the treatment of benign prostatic hyperplasia. *Arch Fam Med* 2:929-935, 1993.

Briggs RS, et al: Effect of flavoxate on uninhibited detrusor contractions and urinary incontinence in the elderly. *J Urol* 123:665-666, 1980.

Brocklebank JT, Meadow SR: Cure of giggle micturition. *Arch Dis Child* 56:232-234, 1981.

Brooks ME, et al: Treatment of retrograde ejaculation with imipramine. *Urology* 15:353-355, 1980.

Brown BT, et al: Guanethidine sulfate in prevention of autonomic hyperreflexia. *J Urol* 122:55-57, 1979.

Caine M, et al: Phenoxybenzamine for benign prostatic obstruction: Review of 200 cases. *Urology* 27:542-546, 1981.

Cammu H, et al: Pelvic physiotherapy in genuine stress incontinence. *Urology* 38:332-337, 1991.

Cantor EB (ed): *Female Urinary Stress Incontinence.* Springfield, Ill, Charles C. Thomas, 1979.

Cardozo LD, Stanton SL: Comparison between bromocriptine and indomethacin in treatment of detrusor instability. *J Urol* 123:399-401, 1980.

Castleden CM, et al: Imipramine: Possible alternative to current therapy for urinary incontinence in the elderly. *J Urol* 125:318-320, 1981.

Chai TC, et al: Specificity of the American Urological Association voiding symptom index: Comparison of unselected and selected samples of both sexes. *J Urol* 150:1710-1713, 1993.

Chapple CR, et al: Double-blind, placebo-controlled, cross-over study of flavoxate in the treatment of idiopathic detrusor instability. *Br J Urol* 66:491-494, 1990.

Christensen MM, et al: Doxazosin treatment in patients with prostatic obstruction: A double-blind placebo-controlled study. *Scand J Urol Nephrol* 27:39-44, 1993.

Cotton P: Physicians hear about incontinence. *JAMA* 264:2361-2362, 1990.

Cotton P: Case for prostate therapy wanes despite more treatment options. *JAMA* 266:459-460, 1991.

Decter RM, et al: Urodynamic assessment of children with cerebral palsy. *J Urol* 138 (part 2):1110-1112, 1987.

de la Hunt MN, et al: Intermittent catheterization for neuropathic urinary incontinence. *Arch Dis Child* 64:821-824, 1989.

Desmond AD, et al: Clinical experience with intravesical prostaglandin E_2: Prospective study of 36 patients. *Br J Urol* 52:357-366, 1980.

Diokno AC: Practical approach to management of urinary incontinence in the elderly. *Compr Ther* 9:67-75, (July) 1983.

Diokno AC, Koppenhoefer R: Bethanechol chloride in neurogenic bladder dysfunction. *Urology* 8:455-458, 1976.

Diokno AC, Sonda LP: Pharmacological management of neuropathic bladder and urethra, in Caine M (ed): *The Pharmacology of the Urinary Tract*. New York, Springer-Verlag, 1984, 77-99.

Diokno AC, Taub M: Ephedrine in treatment of urinary incontinence. *Urology* 5:624-625, 1975.

Downie JW: Bethanechol chloride in urology: Discussion of issues. *Neurourol Urodynam* 3:211-222, 1984.

Dykstra DD, et al: Effect of nifedipine on cystoscopy-induced autonomic hyperreflexia in patients with high spinal cord injuries. *J Urol* 138:1155-1157, 1987.

Evans JHC, Meadow SR: Desmopressin for bed wetting: Length of treatment, vasopressin secretion, and response. *Arch Dis Child* 67:184-188, 1992.

Evron S, et al: Prevention of urinary retention with phenoxybenzamine during epidural morphine. *BMJ* 288:190, 1984.

Fantl JA, et al: Efficacy of bladder training in older women with urinary incontinence. *JAMA* 265:609-613, 1991.

Fernandes E, et al: Medical progress: The unstable bladder in children. *J Pediatr* 118:831-837, 1991.

Ferrie BG, et al: Experience with bladder training in 65 patients. *Br J Urol* 56:482-484, 1984.

Finkbeiner AE: Is bethanechol chloride clinically effective in promoting bladder emptying? Literature review. *J Urol* 134:443-449, 1985.

Finkbeiner AE, Bissada NK: Drug therapy for lower urinary tract dysfunction. *Urol Clin North Am* 7:3-16, 1980.

Flanigan RC, et al: Urologic aspects of tethered cord. *Urology* 33:80-82, 1989.

Flood AB, et al: Assessing symptom improvement after elective prostatectomy for benign prostatic hypertrophy. *Arch Intern Med* 152:1507-1512, 1992.

Fonda D: Taking the 'in' out of incontinence. *Med J Aust* 153:245-247, 1990.

Fordham KE, Meadow SR: Controlled trial of standard pad and bell alarm against mini alarm for nocturnal enuresis. *Arch Dis Child* 64:651-656, 1989.

Forsythe WI, Butler RJ: Fifty years of enuretic alarms. *Arch Dis Child* 64:879-885, 1989.

Frewen WK: Significance of psychosomatic factor in urge incontinence. *Br J Urol* 56:330, 1984.

Furuya S, et al: Alpha-adrenergic activity and urethral pressure in prostatic zone in benign prostatic hypertrophy. *J Urol* 128:836-839, 1982.

Gajewski JB, Awad SA: Oxybutynin versus propantheline in patients with multiple sclerosis and detrusor hyperreflexia. *J Urol* 135:966-968, 1986.

Gillenwater JY, Wein AJ: Summary of the National Institute of Arthritis, Diabetes, Digestive and Kidney Diseases workshop on interstitial cystitis, National Institutes of Health, Bethesda, Maryland, August 28-29, 1987. *J Urol* 140:203-206, 1988.

Gleason DM: Female urologic disorders, in Devine CJ Jr, Stecker JF Jr (eds): *Urology in Practice*. Boston, Little Brown, 1978, 201-230.

Godec CJ: 'Timed voiding': Useful tool in treatment of urinary incontinence. *Urology* 23:97-100, 1984.

Goldman G, et al: α-Adrenergic blocker for posthernioplasty urinary retention: Prevention and treatment. *Arch Surg* 123:35-36, 1988.

Gormley GJ, et al: The effect of finasteride in men with benign prostatic hyperplasia. *N Engl J Med* 327:1185-1191, 1992.

Graham JB: Female urethral syndrome? *Urol Clin North Am* 7:59-62, 1980.

Graham SD: Present urological treatment of spinal cord injury patients. *J Urol* 126:1-4, 1981.

Greenfield SP, Fera M: The use of intravesical oxybutynin chloride in children with neurogenic bladder. *J Urol* 146:532-534, 1991.

Gundian JC, et al: Mayo Clinic experience with the AS800 artificial urinary sphincter for urinary incontinence after transurethral resection of prostate or open prostatectomy. *Urology* 41:318-321, 1993.

Hackler RH, et al: Clinical experience with dantrolene sodium for external urinary sphincter hypertonicity in spinal cord injured patients. *J Urol* 124:78-81, 1980.

Hamed M, et al: Hyponatraemic convulsion associated with desmopressin and imipramine treatment, letter. *BMJ* 306:1169, 1993.

Hanna MK, et al: Urodynamics in children: Part II. Pseudoneurogenic bladder. *J Urol* 125:534-537, 1981.

Hanno PM, Wein AJ: Medical treatment of interstitial cystitis (other than Rimso-50/Elmiron). *Urology* 29(suppl):22-26, (April) 1987.

Hanno PM, et al: Use of amitriptyline in the treatment of interstitial cystitis. *J Urol* 141:846-848, 1989.

Hellström A-L, et al: Rehabilitation of the dysfunctional bladder in children: Method and 3-year followup. *J Urol* 138:847-849, 1987.

Herschorn S, et al: Early experience with intraurethral collagen injections for urinary incontinence. *J Urol* 148:1797-1800, 1992.

Himsl KK, Hurwitz RS: Pediatric urinary incontinence. *Urol Clin North Am* 18:283-293, 1991.

Hinman F Jr: Nonneurogenic neurogenic bladder (Hinman syndrome): 15 years later. *J Urol* 136:769-777, 1986.

Hjälmås K, Sillén U: Pharmacological treatment of bed-wetting. *Drug Invest* 2(suppl 5):17-21, 1990.

Jarvis GJ: Bladder drill for treatment of enuresis in adults. *Br J Urol* 54:118-119, 1982.

Johnson DE, et al: Tumors of the genitourinary tract, in Tanagho EA, McAninch JW (eds): *Smith's General Urology*, ed 12. Norwalk, Conn, Appleton & Lange, 1988, 330-434.

Jones KW, Schoenberg HW: Comparison of incidence of bladder hyperreflexia in patients with benign prostatic hypertrophy and age-matched female controls. *J Urol* 133:425-426, 1985.

Jonville AP, et al: Side-effects of oxybutynine chloride (Ditropan Rm). *Therapie* 47:389-392, (Sept-Oct) 1992.

Jorgensen OS, et al: Plasma concentration and clinical effect in imipramine treatment of childhood enuresis. *Clin Pharmacokinet* 5:386-393, 1980.

Joseph DB, et al: Clean, intermittent catheterization of infants with neurogenic bladder. *Pediatrics* 84:78-82, 1989.

Kallio J, et al: Severe hyponatremia caused by intranasal desmopressin for nocturnal enuresis. *Acta Paediatr* 82:881-882, 1993.

Kaplan WE, et al: Urological manifestations of the tethered cord. *J Urol* 140(part 2):1285-1288, 1988.

Kass EJ, et al: Enuresis: Principles of management and result of treatment. *J Urol* 121:794-796, 1979.

Key DW, et al: Low dose desmopressin in nocturnal enuresis. *Clin Pediatr* 39:299-301, 1992.

Kinn A-C, Lindskog M: Estrogens and phenylpropanolamine in combination for stress urinary incontinence in postmenopausal women. *Urology* 32:273-280, 1988.

Klauber GT: Clinical efficacy and safety of desmopressin in the treatment of nocturnal enuresis. *J Pediatr* 114(suppl):719-722, 1989.

Kleeman FJ: Use of phenoxybenzamine poorly defined. *Urology* 9:708, 1977.

Knapp M: Enuresis and body worn alarms, letter. *Med J Aust* 156:672, 1992.

Koff SA: Non-neuropathic vesico-urethral dysfunction in children, in Mundy AR, et al (eds): *Urodynamics: Principles, Practice and Application*. New York, Churchill Livingstone, 1984, 311-325.

Koff SA: Enuresis, in Walsh PC, et al (eds): *Campbell's Urology*, ed 5. Philadelphia, WB Saunders, 1986, 2179-2192.

Koff SA, et al: Uninhibited bladder in children: Cause for urinary obstruction, infection, and reflux, in Hodson J, Kinkaid-Smith P (eds): *Reflux Nephropathy*. New York, Masson, 1978, 161-170.

Koff SA, et al: Association of urinary tract infection and reflux with uninhibited bladder contractions and voluntary sphincteric obstruction. *J Urol* 122:373, 1979.

Komaroff AL, Friedland G: Dysuria-pyuria syndrome. *N Engl J Med* 303:452-454, 1980.

Langtry HD, McTavish D: Terodiline: A review of its pharmacological properties, and therapeutic use in the treatment of urinary incontinence. *Drugs* 40:748-761, 1990.

Leach GE, et al: Post-prostatectomy incontinence: Influence of bladder dysfunction. *J Urol* 138:574-578, 1987.

Lepor H: Nonoperative management of benign prostatic hypertrophy. *J Urol* 141:1283-1289, 1989.

Lepor H, et al: A randomized, placebo-controlled multicenter study of the efficacy and safety of terazosin in the treatment of benign prostatic hyperplasia. *J Urol* 148:1467-1474, 1992.

Leventhal A, Pfau A: Pharmacologic management of postoperative overdistention of bladder. *Surg Gynecol Obstet* 146:347-348, 1978.

Levine DZ: Interstitial cystitis: An overlooked cause of pelvic pain. *Postgrad Med* 88:101-109, (July) 1990.

Leyson JFJ, et al: Baclofen in treatment of detrusor-sphincter dyssynergia in spinal cord injury patients. *J Urol* 124:82-84, 1980.

Lindan R, et al: Comparison of efficacy of an alpha-1-adrenergic blocker and slow calcium channel blocker in control of autonomic dysreflexia. *Paraplegia* 23:34-38, 1985.

Lloyd LK: Neurogenic bladder dysfunction. *Cont Educat* 11:21-42, 1979.

Lose G, et al: Subcutaneous heparin in the treatment of interstitial cystitis. *Scand J Urol Nephrol* 19:27-29, 1985.

Lose G, et al: Doxepin in the treatment of female detrusor overactivity: Randomized double-blind crossover study. *J Urol* 142:1024-1026, 1989.

Lovering JS, et al: Oxybutynin efficacy in treatment of primary enuresis. *Pediatrics* 82:104-106, 1988.

Lowe FC, Stark E: The use of α-blockers in the management of benign prostatic hyperplasia. *NY State J Med* 93:169-173, 1993.

Malone-Lee J, et al: Low dose oxybutynin for the unstable bladder, letter. *BMJ* 304:1053, 1992.

Manyak MJ: Pharmacologic treatment for benign prostatic hyperplasia. *Drug Ther* 44-52, (Dec) 1991.

Marsh TD: Estrogens for treating urinary incontinence in women. *Am Pharm* NS33:47-48, 90, (Nov) 1993.

McConnell JD: Androgen ablation and blockade in the treatment of benign prostatic hyperplasia. *Urol Clin North Am* 17:661-670, 1990.

McGuire EJ: Innervation and function of lower urinary tract. *J Neurosurg* 65:278-285, 1986 A.

McGuire EJ: Neurogenic bladder problems: Upper motor neuron lesions; Neurogenic bladder problems: Lower motor neuron lesions, in Kaufman JJ (ed): *Current Urologic Therapy,* ed 2. Philadelphia, WB Saunders, 1986 B, 258-265.

McGuire EJ: Adult female urology, in Yalla SV, et al (eds): *Neurourology and Urodynamics: Principles and Practice,* ed 2. New York, Macmillan, 1988, 264-273.

McKendry JBJ, et al: Primary enuresis: Relative success of three methods of treatment. *Can Med Assoc J* 113:953-955, 1975.

Messing EM: Urethral syndrome, in Walsh PC, et al (eds): *Campbell's Urology,* ed 5. Philadelphia, WB Saunders, 1986 A, 1087-1092.

Messing EM: Interstitial cystitis and related syndromes, in Walsh PC, et al (eds): *Campbell's Urology,* ed 5. Philadelphia, WB Saunders, 1986 B, 1070-1086.

Messing EM, Freiha FS: Complication of Clorpactin WCS90 therapy for interstitial cystitis. *Urology* 13:389-392, 1979.

Messing EM, Stamey TA: Interstitial cystitis. *Urology* 12:381-392, 1978.

Meyhoff HH, et al: Placebo: Drug of choice in female motor urge incontinence? *Br J Urol* 55:34-37, 1983.

Mikkelsen EJ, et al: Childhood enuresis: I. Sleep patterns and psychopathology. II. Psychopathology, tricyclic concentration in plasma, and antienuretic effect. *Arch Gen Psychiatry* 37:1139-1145, 1146-1152, 1980.

Miller K, et al: Nocturnal enuresis: Experience with long-term use of internasally administered desmopressin. *J Pediatr* 114 (suppl):723-726, 1989.

Miller K, et al: Drug therapy for nocturnal enuresis: Current treatment recommendations. *Drugs* 44:47-55, 1992.

Mobley DF: Phenoxybenzamine in management of neurogenic vesical dysfunction. *J Urol* 116:737-738, 1976.

Moffat MEK, et al: DDAVP and enuresis. *Pediatrics* 92:420, 1993.

Moul JW: Benign prostatic hyperplasia: New concepts in the 1990s. *Postgrad Med* 94:141-146, 151-152, (Nov) 1993.

Mulcahy JJ, James HE: Management of neurogenic bladder in infancy and childhood. *Urology* 13:235-240, 1979.

Mundy AR: Unstable bladder. *Urol Clin North Am* 12:317-328, 1985.

Mundy AR, et al (eds): *Urodynamics: Principles, Practice and Application.* New York, Churchill Livingston, 1984.

National Institutes of Health, Consensus Conference: Urinary incontinence in adults. *JAMA* 261:2685-2690, 1989.

Nijman JM, et al: Treatment of ejaculation disorders after retroperitoneal lymph node dissection. *Cancer* 50:2967-2971, 1982.

Nishimura M, et al: Systemic contact dermatitis medicamentosa occurring after intravesical dimethyl sulfoxide treatment for interstitial cystitis, letter. *Arch Dermatol* 124:182-183, 1988.

Nørgaard JP, et al: Nocturnal enuresis: An approach to treatment based on pathogenesis. *J Pediatr* 114 (suppl):705-710, 1989.

O'Brien WM: Benign prostatic hypertrophy. *Am Fam Physician* 44:162-171, (July) 1991.

O'Dowd TC, et al: Irritable urethral syndrome: Discussion. *J R Coll Gen Pract* 35:140-141, 1985.

Olah KS, et al: The conservative management of patients with symptoms of stress incontinence: A randomized, prospective study comparing weighted vaginal cones and interferential therapy. *Am J Obstet Gynecol* 162:87-92, 1990.

O'Reilly PH: Postoperative urinary retention in men: Don't automatically blame the prostate. *BMJ* 302:864, 1991.

Osborn DE, et al: Prostatodynia: Physiological characteristics and rational management with muscle relaxants. *Br J Urol* 53:621-623, 1981.

Ouslander JG, et al: Pharmacokinetics and clinical effects of oxybutynin in geriatric patients. *J Urol* 140:47-50, 1988.

Ouslander JG, et al: Terodiline in the Elderly American Multicenter Study Group: Effects of terodiline on urinary incontinence among older non-institutionalized women. *J Am Geriatr Soc* 41:915-922, 1993.

Parsons CL: Sodium pentosanpolysulfate treatment of interstitial cystitis: Update. *Urology* 29 (suppl):14-16, (April) 1987.

Parsons CL, Koprowski PF: Interstitial cystitis: Successful management by increasing urinary voiding intervals. *Urology* 37:207-212, 1991.

Peggs JF: Urinary incontinence in the elderly: Pharmacologic therapies. *Am Fam Physician* 46:1763-1769, 1992.

Perez-Marrero R, et al: Controlled study of dimethyl sulfoxide in interstitial cystitis. *J Urol* 140:36-39, 1988.

Perez-Marrero R, et al: Prolongation of response to DMSO by heparin maintenance. *Suppl Urol* 41:64-66, (Jan) 1993.

Peters DH, Sorkin EM: Finasteride: A review of its potential in the treatment of benign prostatic hyperplasia. *Drugs* 46:177-208, 1993.

Proctor KG, Howards SS: Effect of sympathomimetic drugs on post-lymphadenectomy aspermia. *J Urol* 129:837-838, 1983.

Rapoport JL, et al: Childhood enuresis. II. Psychopathology, tricyclic concentration in plasma, and antienuretic effect. *Arch Gen Psychiatry* 37:1146-1152, 1980.

Raz S, Smith RB: External sphincter spasticity syndrome in female patients. *J Urol* 115:443-446, 1976.

Resnick NM: Voiding dysfunction in the elderly, in Yalla SV, et al (eds): *Neurourology and Urodynamics: Principles and Practice.* New York, Macmillan, 1988, 303-330.

Resnick NM: Urinary incontinence in the older person. *Harvard Med School Health Lett* (suppl):9-12, (Aug) 1990.

Riehmann M, Bruskewitz R: New options in benign prostatic hyperplasia. *Hosp Pract* 17-24, (Feb) 1993.

Rogers MP, et al: Giggle incontinence. *JAMA* 247:1446-1448, 1982.

Rosenfeld J, Jerkins GR: The bed-wetting child: Current management of a frustrating problem. *Postgrad Med* 89:63-70, (Feb) 1991.

Sant GR: Intravesical 50% dimethyl sulfoxide (Rimso-50) in treatment of interstitial cystitis. *Urology* 29 (suppl):17-21, (April) 1987.

Sant GR, Meares EM Jr: Interstitial cystitis: Pathogenesis, diagnosis, and treatment. *Infect Urol* 24-30, (Jan/Feb) 1990.

Sant GR, Theoharides TC: The role of the mast cell in interstitial cystitis. *Urol Clin North Am* 21:41-53, 1994.

Sawczuk I, Blaivas JG: Successful surgical treatment of giggle incontinence: Case report. *Neurourol Urodynam* 3:63-66, 1984.

Schmidt RA: Urethral syndrome. *Urol Clin North Am* 12:349-354, 1985.

Schmitt BD: Efficacy and safety of drugs available for the treatment of nocturnal enuresis. *Drug Invest* 2 (suppl 5):9-16, 1990.

Scott MB, Morrow JW: Phenoxybenzamine in neurogenic bladder dysfunction after spinal cord injury. II. Autonomic dysreflexia. *J Urol* 119:483-484, 1978.

Scotti RJ, Ostergard CR: Urethral syndrome, in Ostergard DR (ed): *Gynecologic Urology and Urodynamics: Theory and Practice,* ed 2. Baltimore, Williams & Wilkins, 1985, 299-321.

Siroky MB, Krane RJ: Psychogenic voiding dysfunction, in Yalla SV, et al (eds): *Neurourology and Urodynamics: Principles and Practice,* ed 2. New York, Macmillan, 1988, 358-370.

Siroky MB, et al: Functional voiding disorders in men. *J Urol* 126:200-204, 1981.

Sonda LP, et al: Further observations on cystometric and uroflowmetric effects of bethanechol chloride on the human bladder. *J Urol* 122:775-777, 1979.

Stamm WE, et al: Treatment of acute urethral syndrome. *N Engl J Med* 304:956-958, 1981.

Stein J: Terazosin: A single drug for hypertension and BPH symptoms. *INPHARMA* 1, (July 17) 1993.

Stewart MA: Treatment of bedwetting. *JAMA* 232:281-283, 1975.

Stewart BH, et al: Stress incontinence: Conservative therapy with sympathomimetic drugs. *J Urol* 115:558-559, 1976.

Stone AR: Treatment of voiding complaints and incontinence in painful bladder syndrome. *Urol Clin North Am* 18:317-325, 1991.

Stone NN: Treatment options in benign prostatic hypertrophy. *Hosp Pract* 85-88, 91-92, (Oct) 1992.
Stoner E, Members of The Finasteride Study Group: Three-year safety and efficacy data on the use of finasteride in the treatment of benign prostatic hyperplasia. *Urology* 43:284-294, 1994.
Stricker P, Haylen B: Injectable collagen for type 3 female stress incontinence: The first 50 Australian patients. *Med J Aust* 158:89-91, 1993.
Sukhai RN, et al: Combined therapy of enuresis alarm and desmopressin in the treatment of nocturnal enuresis. *Eur J Pediatr* 148:465-467, 1989.
Tammela T: Prevention of prolonged voiding problems after unexpected postoperative urinary retention: Comparison of phenoxybenzamine and carbachol. *J Urol* 136:1254-1257, 1986.
Tammela T, et al: Intravesical prostaglandin $F_{2\alpha}$ for promoting bladder emptying after surgery for female stress incontinence. *Br J Urol* 60:43-46, 1987.
Taylor MC, Bates CP: Double-blind crossover trial of baclofen: New treatment for unstable bladder syndrome. *Br J Urol* 51:504-505, 1979.
Terho P: Desmopressin in nocturnal enuresis. *J Urol* 145:818-820, 1991.
Testa GM: The urethral syndrome: Why what we do works, or doesn't. *Med J Aust* 157:549-553, 1992.
Theoharides TC: Hydroxyzine for interstitial cystitis. *J Allergy Clin Immunol* 91:686-687, 1993.
Theoharides TC: Hydroxyzine in the treatment of interstitial cystitis. *Urol Clin North Am* 21:113-119, 1994.
Thüroff JW, et al: Randomized, double-blind, multicenter trial on treatment of frequency, urgency and incontinence related to detrusor hyperactivity oxybutynin versus propantheline versus placebo. *J Urol* 145:813-817, 1991.
Urinary Incontinence Guideline Panel: *Urinary Incontinence in Adults: Clinical Practice Guideline*. AHCPR Pub No. 92-0038, Rockville, Md, Dept of Health and Human Services, 1992.
Veldhuis GJ, Inman WHW: Terodiline and torsades de pointes, letter. *BMJ* 303:519, 1991.
Waterfall NB, Williams G: Effects of phenoxybenzamine on bladder neck opening. *J R Soc Med* 73:345-347, 1980.
Webster GD, et al: Management of type III stress urinary incontinence using artificial urinary sphincter. *Urology* 39:499-503, 1992.
Weese DL, et al: Intravesical oxybutynin chloride: Experience with 42 patients. *Urology* 41:527-530, 1993.
Wein AJ: Pharmacological treatment of non-neurogenic voiding dysfunction, in Caine M (ed): *The Pharmacology of the Urinary Tract*. New York, Springer-Verlag, 1984 A, 100-134.
Wein AJ: Pharmacology of bladder and urethra, in Mundy AR, et al (eds): *Urodynamics: Principles, Practice and Application*. New York, Churchill Livingstone, 1984 B, 26-41.
Wein AJ: Pharmacologic treatment of lower urinary tract dysfunction in the female patient. *Urol Clin North Am* 12:259-269, 1985 A.
Wein AJ: Drug therapy for detrusor hyperactivity: Where are we? *Neurourol Urodynam* 4:337-351, 1985 B.
Wein AJ: Drug therapy for neurogenic and non-neurogenic bladder dysfunction, in Kaufman JJ (ed): *Current Urologic Therapy,* ed 2. Philadelphia, WB Saunders, 1986, 265-272.
Wein AJ: Clinical neuropharmacology of the lower urinary tract, in Yall SV, et al (eds): *Neurourology and Urodynamics: Principles and Practice*. New York, Macmillan, 1988, 377-398.
Wein AJ: Pharmacologic therapy for incontinence. *Suppl Urology* 36:36-42, (Oct) 1990.
Wein AJ: Neurogenic bladder and incontinence, in Walsh PC, et al (eds): *Campbell's Urology*, ed 6. Philadelphia, W.B. Saunders, 1992, 573-613.
Wein AJ, Barrett DM: *Voiding Function and Dysfunction: A Logical and Practical Approach*. Chicago, Year Book Medical Publishers, 1988.
Weiss BD: Unstable bladder in elderly patients. *Am Fam Physician* 28:243-247, (Oct) 1983.
Weiss BD: Nonpharmacologic treatment of urinary incontinence. *Am Fam Physician* 579-586, (Aug) 1991.
Wiener LB, et al: New method for management of detrusor instability: Transdermal scopolamine. *Urology* 28:208-210, 1986.

Drugs Used for Urolithiasis 41

Every year approximately one of every 1,000 Americans experiences the discomfort of renal calculi (Smith, 1989). The likelihood of stone formation in any individual is affected by inherent and environmental factors, including age, race, sex, geographic locale, water intake, diet, occupation, and season (Drach, 1986). Symptomatic urolithiasis occurs four times more often in men than in women, and the incidence is even lower in women taking oral contraceptives containing estrogen (Tawashi et al, 1984). Calculi develop more often in whites than in members of other racial groups. Urolithiasis is most common between age 30 and 60. The rate of spontaneous recurrence among untreated patients averages 50% to 60% within 10 years and is highest among younger individuals (Uribarri et al, 1989).

Although urolithiasis may remain asymptomatic with spontaneous passage of calculi ("silent stones"), patients with symptomatic urolithiasis experience intense renal or ureteral colic. The presence of calculi may be confirmed by urinalysis (which generally shows gross or microscopic hematuria and, sometimes, crystals of the same type as those comprising the stone) and by examination of the kidneys, ureter, and bladder (KUB with tomograms). An intravenous urogram may be needed to determine the degree of obstruction during an acute episode. Ultrasonography of the kidney, ureter, and bladder is useful for localizing large urinary calculi and for detecting radiolucent stones in patients with severe renal colic or in renal failure, and it avoids the hazards associated with radiation or administration of contrast medium (Saita et al, 1988). Periodic KUB with tomograms also may be useful in the early detection of recurrent calculi.

Renal colic results from increased intrapyelic pressure secondary to ureteral obstruction. Acute pain usually has been managed with opioid analgesics (meperidine [Demerol] 50 to 100 mg or morphine 10 to 15 mg, depending on body size, age, coexisting disease, and severity of pain). The administration of belladonna alkaloids with the opioid may increase analgesia, but side effects are common. Continued abnormal intrapyelic pressure induces local prostaglandin production and secretion, which increases diuresis and further exacerbates pressure and pain. Therefore, in patients with less severe discomfort or in those for whom opioids are contraindicated, the following potent inhibitors of prostaglandin synthesis may be as effective as opioids: indomethacin 50 mg in oral or suppository form (Kapoor et al, 1989) or as an aqueous rectal solution (Nissen et al, 1990); diclofenac sodium 50 to 75 mg intramuscularly (Khalifa and Sharkawi, 1986; Sanahuja et al, 1990) or 50 mg orally three times daily (Indudhara et al, 1990); or ketorolac tromethamine [Toradol] 10 mg intramuscularly (Oosterlinck et al, 1990; Litvak and McEvoy, 1990). These agents produce fewer adverse effects than opioids, although the time to maximum analgesia may be slightly longer. Acupuncture also has been successful in alleviating pain associated with urolithiasis (Lee et al, 1992).

Calcium channel blocking agents (eg, nifedipine) have been used to reduce renal colic, but their antispasmodic action generally is inadequate, and their diuretic effect may increase renal colic (Okaniwa et al, 1989).

Most stones smaller than 0.5 cm pass, stones 0.5 to 0.7 cm may pass, and stones larger than 0.7 cm probably will not pass. Extracorporeal shock wave lithotripsy (ESWL), percutaneous nephrostolithotomy, ureteroscopic ultrasonic lithotripsy, and pulsed dye laser lithotripsy are being used increasingly in the management of patients with stones located in the kidney or upper two-thirds of the ureter, and endoscopy is being used for stones in the lower ureter. Major surgery is necessary in less than 5% of patients with acute renal colic (Consensus Conference, National Institutes of Health, 1988; Streem, 1988; Lingeman et al, 1989; Morse and Resnick, 1991; Glowacki et al, 1992).

To improve the effectiveness of preventive therapy, any metabolic abnormality that predisposes a patient to urolithiasis should be identified (Goldwasser et al, 1986; Coe and Parks, 1988; Smith, 1989; Pak, 1989). An effort also should be made to recover the calculus for analysis by both x-ray diffraction and chemical methods. Determination of the composition of recovered calculi may suggest a therapeutic means of minimizing recurrent stone formation. In North America, 70% to 80% of all kidney stones contain calcium salts (as calcium oxalate, calcium phosphate [apatite or brushite], or mixtures of these salts), about 10% are composed of uric acid, about 10% contain "struvite" (magnesium ammonium phosphate mixed with carbonate apatite and hydroxyapatite), and 1% are composed of cystine salts. If infection is present, the stone, stone fragments, or urine should be cultured.

Most clinicians recommend that a serum biochemical profile (calcium, phosphorus, uric acid, and blood urea nitrogen or creatinine) and complete blood count be obtained for all patients. Additional diagnostic information can be obtained from a 24-hour urine specimen analyzed for volume, pH, calcium, magnesium, phosphate, sodium, sulfate, oxalate, citrate, and uric acid (Pak et al, 1985 A; Wilson, 1990). These samples should be obtained one to three months after an acute episode has resolved (Preminger, 1989; Urivetzky et al, 1990 B). Opinions vary on the need for more extensive metabolic evaluations, particularly following an initial episode (Pak, 1989; Uribarri et al, 1989; Seftel and Resnick, 1990). The frequency of recurrent calculus formation will suggest whether the determination of serum parathyroid hormone concentration, creatinine clearance, or urinary excretion of a number of substances in urine specimens after adherence to standard and specific-stress diets is warranted (Kosko and Resnick, 1985; Consensus Conference, National Institutes of Health, 1988; Wilson, 1989).

Patients who have shown radiologic evidence of new stone formation or stone growth or have experienced documented passage of gravel have active urolithiasis and are candidates for long-term prophylactic therapy. *The fundamental principle of preventive therapy is the maintenance of a daily urine volume greater than 2.5 L* (Smith et al, 1978; Pak et al, 1980; Wilson, 1989). Additional fluids should be ingested at meals, at bedtime, and during exercise and episodes of profuse sweating. The ingestion of large volumes of liquids and some basic dietary adjustments usually will prevent recurrent episodes in 50% to 80% of stone formers (Hosking et al, 1983; Ettinger et al, 1986; Wilson, 1990). However, *overhydration should be avoided during an episode of renal or ureteral colic.* Increased diuresis may further elevate intrarenal pressure and produce extravasation of urine, urinoma, or urinary peritonitis (Foster et al, 1990).

If the disease remains active after six months of conservative therapy, medication may be required. Therapeutic approaches appropriate for the variety of metabolic abnormalities associated with urolithiasis appear in the Table. *Many patients with urolithiasis exhibit more than one metabolic abnormality;* therefore, a combination of several agents or forms of therapy in addition to dietary therapy may be necessary.

CALCIUM LITHIASIS. Prophylactic therapy to reduce the recurrence of calcium-containing calculi is based on the management of underlying metabolic defects that result in hypercalciuria, hyperuricosuria, hyperoxaluria, or hypocitruria (see the Table and index entry Calcium, Disorders). Metabolic defects associated with urolithiasis result from hyperparathyroidism, sarcoidosis, multiple myeloma, hypervitaminosis D, primary or enteric hyperoxaluria, hyperthyroidism, metastatic malignant neoplasms, Addison's disease, leukemia, Paget's disease, abrupt or chronic immobilization (casts, traction, quadriplegia), distal renal tubular acidosis, inappropriate nutrition, and poisoning. Hypercalciuria in the absence of any demonstrable metabolic abnormality ("idiopathic") occurs in approximately 50% of all patients who form calcium-containing calculi (Coe and Parks, 1990). In addition, various pharmacologic regimens (such as sulfadiazine for treatment of *Toxoplasma gondii* encephalitis associated with AIDS) can induce urolithiasis (Simon et al, 1990).

Hypercalciurias: Urolithiasis commonly accompanies hypercalciuria, frequently defined as a daily urinary excretion of calcium in excess of 4 mg/kg (Pak, 1988; Lemann and Gray, 1989). However, this definition assumes "average" body size; it will require adjustment for individuals with larger or smaller skeletal frames. Several subcategories of this disorder based on pathogenesis have been identified (Pak et al, 1974; Menon and Koul, 1992).

Resorptive hypercalciuria occurs secondary to a chronic increase in bone resorption and calcium mobilization from the skeleton resulting in fasting hypercalcemia and an increase in the amount of calcium filtered by the kidneys (Silverberg et al, 1990). Most cases are associated with hypersecretion of parathyroid hormone (PTH) in primary hyperparathyroidism or of PTH-like proteins by malignancies that mimic hyperparathyroidism; however, hyperthyroidism, Addison's disease, Paget's disease, or abrupt immobilization also can trigger resorptive hypercalciuria. In addition, PTH stimulation of the production of 1,25-dihydroxyvitamin D_3 with increased absorption of dietary calcium may contribute to renal calcium loading and hypercalciuria in patients with primary hyperparathyroidism (Silverberg et al, 1990). Previously, the presence of hypercalcemia with hypophosphatemia was considered pathognomonic for hyperparathyroidism. However, serum PTH concentration can be measured quite accurately and reliably using radioimmunoassays for the intact molecule; either elevated serum PTH concentration or normal serum PTH concentration in the presence of hypercalcemia are indicative of hyperparathyroidism. Recent evidence suggests that resorptive hypercalciuria also may result from hypersensitivity of bone cell precursors to normal concentrations of PTH (Pacifici et al, 1990) or from parathyroid cell hypersensitivity to calcium ions (Wong et al, 1992).

Absorptive hypercalciuria is characterized by increased intestinal absorption of dietary calcium, increased renal filtered load of calcium, and hypercalciuria (over 200 mg/day), either

MANAGEMENT OF UROLITHIASIS

Type of Stone and Metabolic Abnormality	Therapy
CALCIUM OXALATE/PHOSPHATE	
Calcium urolithiasis (idiopathic)	Dietary manipulation* and high fluid intake
Resorptive hypercalciuria	Correction of endocrine disorder
Absorptive hypercalciuria Types I and II	*Severe† Hypercalciuria:* Cellulose sodium phosphate Magnesium gluconate or magnesium citrate Moderate calcium and oxalate restriction *Mild to Moderate Hypercalciuria:* Thiazide diuretic or neutral orthophosphate Potassium citrate Moderate calcium restriction High fluid intake
Hypophosphatemic hypercalciuria	Neutral orthophosphate
Renal hypercalciuria (idiopathic renal calcium leak)	Thiazide diuretic or indapamide Potassium citrate Restriction of dietary protein and salt
Hyperoxaluria	
Primary (Type I or Type II)	Pyridoxine Neutral orthophosphate Magnesium oxide and potassium citrate Renal/liver transplantation
Enteric	Dietary restriction of fats and oxalate Management of underlying gastrointestinal disorder Calcium salts Potassium citrate or potassium and sodium citrate Magnesium gluconate or magnesium citrate
Distal renal tubular acidosis	Potassium citrate or potassium bicarbonate Restriction of dietary salt and salt substitutes
Hyperuricosuric calcium oxalate lithiasis	Allopurinol and restriction of dietary purines (meat) Potassium citrate
Hypocitruric calcium urolithiasis	Potassium citrate
STRUVITE (magnesium ammonium phosphate)	
Infection with urea-splitting organisms	Antibacterial agents Acetohydroxamic acid Surgical removal of calculi or renal irrigation Restriction of dietary phosphate
URIC ACID	
Hyperuricosuria	Alkalization with potassium citrate Allopurinol Restriction of dietary purines (meat) High fluid intake
CYSTINE	
Cystinuria	Alkalization with potassium citrate Penicillamine or tiopronin and pyridoxine Restriction of dietary protein High fluid intake
XANTHINE/HYPOXANTHINE	
Xanthinuria/Hypoxanthinuria	High fluid intake and restriction of dietary protein Allopurinol (hypoxanthinuria)
SILICATE	
Silicaturia	Reduced antacid ingestion
AMMONIUM URATE	
Hyperuricosuria/ammoniuria	Treatment for chronic diarrhea and reduced laxative use

**Restriction of dietary oxalates, protein, purines, and possibly calcium and sodium. Fiber or magnesium may be added to the diet.*

† > 400 mg/day.

during dietary calcium restriction (Type I) or following an oral calcium load (Type II). Oxalate absorption also often is increased. The increase in fractional calcium absorption may result from varying degrees of idiopathic renal overproduction of 1,25-dihydroxyvitamin D_3 (Coe and Bushinsky, 1984; Lemann and Gray, 1989; Bataille et al, 1991). Plasma calcium concentrations tend to be in the high-normal range and serum immunoreactive PTH activity in the low-normal range.

Hypophosphatemic hypercalciuria (renal phosphate leak, absorptive hypercalciuria Type III) results from increased 1,25-dihydroxyvitamin D_3 production stimulated by chronic hypophosphatemia secondary to inadequate tubular reabsorption of phosphate (Roberts and Knox, 1990).

Renal hypercalciuria (renal calcium leak) is caused by an idiopathic failure of adequate tubular reabsorption of filtered calcium, which results in fasting hypercalciuria (Pak, 1979). Plasma calcium concentrations are in the low-normal range, stimulating PTH secretion, 1,25-dihydroxyvitamin D_3 activation, and bone resorption. Plasma calcium homeostasis is maintained at the expense of bone mineral density (Bataille et al, 1991). Serum osteocalcin concentrations may be elevated. Renal hypercalciuria may be associated with or aggravated by high salt intake, enhanced sensitivity to dietary sodium, or arterial hypertension (McCarron et al, 1980; Wasserstein et al, 1987; Goldfarb, 1988; Cappuccio et al, 1990). It also may account for a substantial portion of the calcium lost after menopause (Nordin et al, 1991).

All hypercalciuric patients should undertake a lifelong effort to increase their fluid intake sufficiently to maintain a daily urine output greater than 2.5 L. If this does not prevent active stone formation or growth, dietary restrictions can be recommended; for many patients, these may be as effective as medications in retarding lithogenesis (Kohri et al, 1990). Patients with absorptive hypercalciuria should reduce their calcium intake to between 400 and 800 mg/day by limiting the ingestion of milk, milk products, calcium-enriched cereals and breads, and calcium supplements; reduction below 400 mg/day significantly increases the risk of osteopenia even in hyperabsorptive individuals and is not recommended (Fuss et al, 1990). *Restriction of dietary calcium is not indicated* in hypercalciuric patients when intestinal calcium absorption is normal; however, even in these patients, calcium intake in excess of 1 g/day should be avoided (Pak et al, 1984).

Most calcium-containing uroliths contain calcium oxalate regardless of their etiology, and oxalate absorption may be increased in stone formers. Oxalate intake should be limited (eg, discontinuation of vitamin C supplements, limited ingestion of tea, nuts, chocolate, cocoa, rhubarb, plums, cranberries, raspberries, asparagus, and spinach). Urinary excretion of calcium and oxalate also may be reduced by restricting the daily intake of animal proteins to no more than 1 g/kg (Robertson et al, 1979; Goldfarb, 1988; Kok et al, 1990; van Beresteijn et al, 1990).

Calciuria also may be reduced by limiting the dietary intake of sodium and refined sugars (Wills et al, 1969; Silver et al, 1983; Holl and Allen, 1987; Goldfarb, 1988). Adding significant amounts of fiber to the diet (eg, 20 g rice bran; 30 g unprocessed wheat bran) also can reduce urinary calcium excretion, probably by chelating calcium in the intestine and decreasing the efficiency of its absorption (Ebisuno et al, 1986; Gleeson et al, 1990). When appropriate, the successful treatment of morbid obesity can improve calcium homeostasis (Andersen et al, 1984), perhaps by the interaction of all of the above dietary interventions.

Moderation of caffeine consumption also may be beneficial; preliminary reports indicate that renal reabsorption of filtered calcium may be decreased and urinary calcium losses may be increased in adults who ingest more than four cups of regular coffee/day, although net calcium balance may be affected only when calcium intakes fall below 600 mg/day (Massey et al, 1987; Barger-Lux et al, 1990). Similarly, alcohol consumption inhibits renal calcium reabsorption (Zechner et al, 1981). Carbonated cola beverages may be hypocitraturic, and their intake should be limited (Weiss et al, 1992).

Renal hypercalciuria not fully corrected by dietary therapy may respond to the long-term administration of a thiazide diuretic (Pak, 1979). Chlorothiazide [Diuril] 500 mg twice daily, hydrochlorothiazide [Esidrix, HydroDIURIL, Oretic] 25 to 50 mg twice daily, trichlormethiazide [Metahydrin, Naqua] 2 mg twice daily or 4 mg once daily, chlorthalidone [Hygroton] 25 mg twice daily or 50 mg once daily, or equivalent doses of other thiazides may be employed. The hypocalciuric effect of thiazides usually begins within two days, becomes maximal within six days, and then is sustained indefinitely (Pak, 1979). Correction of hypercalciuria with thiazides may promote calcium retention in hypercalciuric stone formers and reduce net bone loss. The effectiveness of thiazides is abolished by a high sodium or potassium intake. Because thiazides reduce the renal excretion of citrate, an inhibitor of calculus formation (Kok et al, 1990; McLean et al, 1990), supplementation with potassium citrate [Urocit-K] (10 to 20 mEq three times a day) is recommended to prevent hypocitruria (Pak, 1979).

Unlike the thiazides, loop diuretics (furosemide [Lasix], ethacrynic acid [Edecrin], bumetanide [Bumex]) increase urinary calcium excretion. Such agents should not be used to prevent stone recurrence.

Patients with confirmed severe *absorptive hypercalciuria* may be treated with oral cellulose sodium phosphate (10 to 15 g/day taken with meals). This agent exchanges sodium for calcium in the gut and dramatically reduces calcium absorption and the renal filtered calcium load (Pak, 1981; Lake and Brown, 1985). However, it also binds magnesium (an inhibitor of calculi formation), and the intestinal absorption and renal excretion of magnesium are decreased. In contrast, because less calcium is available to form chelates in the gut, intestinal absorption and urinary excretion of oxalate are increased and calcium oxalate calculi can recur relatively frequently when cellulose sodium phosphate is used alone (Backman et al, 1980). Supplementation with magnesium gluconate (1 to 1.5 g, twice a day) and mild restriction of dietary calcium, oxalate, and ascorbic acid eliminate these complications (Pak, 1981). Alternatively, magnesium citrate (trimagnesium dicitrate 10 mEq taken orally with food four times daily) may be beneficial; its use in patients with absorptive hypercalciuria has been reported to increase urine magnesium and citrate concentrations (Lindberg et al, 1990).

Cellulose sodium phosphate is contraindicated in patients with renal hypercalciuria.

Patients with less severe absorptive hypercalciuria may be treated with a thiazide diuretic and potassium citrate (Pak et al, 1985 B). In addition to their hypocalciuric effects, thiazides may interfere with 1,25-dihydroxyvitamin D_3 production and decrease intestinal calcium absorption by 10% to 20% in some individuals (Coe et al, 1988; Insogna et al, 1989). However, continued administration of thiazides to patients with absorptive hypercalciuria may not reduce intestinal calcium absorption or the rate of new stone formation (Churchill and Taylor, 1985; Uribarri et al, 1989). In many of these patients, the hypocalciuric response becomes attenuated through unknown mechanisms (Preminger and Pak, 1987). Alternatively, the administration of elemental phosphorus as neutral orthophosphate [K-Phos Neutral, Neutra-Phos] (1.5 to 2 g/day of phosphorus in four doses taken after meals) may be as effective as the thiazides in decreasing 1,25-dihydroxyvitamin D_3 production and urinary calcium excretion (Thomas, 1978; Insogna et al, 1989), although increased phosphate intake may induce secondary hyperparathyroidism.

Primary therapy for *resorptive hypercalciuria* associated with urolithiasis consists of identifying and correcting the causative endocrine disorder (see index entries Hypercalcemia; Hyperthyroidism; Adrenocortical Insufficiency, Primary; and Paget's Disease of Bone). The resorptive hypercalciuria triggered by immobilization may be controlled with the use of hydrochlorothiazide 2 to 2.5 mg/kg/day plus amiloride 0.2 to 0.25 mg/kg/day (Bentur et al, 1987), although the patient must be monitored to avoid the risk of inducing potentially fatal hypercalcemia.

Hyperuricosuria: In patients with hyperuricosuria who develop calcium oxalate calculi, uric acid excretion and calculus formation may be decreased by increased fluid intake; decreased calcium, sodium, and purine intake (less than 60 g/day of dietary protein); and potassium citrate therapy (Goldfarb, 1988; Yamamoto et al, 1990). If these measures are inadequate, recurrent calculi can be prevented by inhibiting the conversion of purines to uric acid by the administration of allopurinol [Lopurin, Zyloprim] 200 to 300 mg/day (Ettinger et al, 1986; Coe, 1978). A follow-up 24-hour urine collection should be performed in about eight weeks to assess the effectiveness of the dosages of potassium citrate and allopurinol. This regimen will not be effective in preventing lithogenesis if hypercalciuria is also present and is not treated appropriately (Goldwasser et al, 1984; Fellström et al, 1985; Ettinger et al, 1986).

Primary Hyperoxaluria: In this rare genetic disease, production and excretion of oxalate are increased, resulting in hyperoxaluria (urinary oxalate:creatinine ratios, children <1 year: >0.3 mg/mg; 1 to 5 years: >0.1 mg/mg; >5 years: >0.05 mg/mg [Scheinman, 1991]). Two distinct enzyme deficiencies are involved (Williams and Wandzilak, 1989). In *Type I hyperoxaluria*, there is excessive oxalate synthesis resulting from a deficiency of hepatic peroxisomal pyridoxine-dependent alanine: glyoxylate aminotransferase with an accompanying increase in the hepatic production and urinary excretion of glycolate and oxalate. In *Type II hyperoxaluria*, there is a systemic deficiency of D-glycerate dehydrogenase (glyoxylate reductase) with an increase in the hepatic production and urinary excretion of oxalate and L-glycerate. The two forms can be distinguished by measuring plasma glycolate concentration, which will be elevated at least tenfold in patients with primary hyperoxaluria Type I (Marangella et al, 1992). When severe, primary hyperoxaluria Type I can result in renal failure during infancy; 50% of those less severely affected will develop calcium oxalate stones before age 4 (Leumann, 1985). In some patients, dozens of stones, often large, develop over several years. Calcium oxalate deposition within the kidney (nephrocalcinosis) results in renal failure in about 50% of these patients by age 20 (Steinmuller, 1985).

Large doses of pyridoxine decrease oxalate production in some patients with Type I primary hyperoxaluria (Kasidas and Rose, 1984) by facilitating the conversion of glyoxylate to glycine rather than to oxalate. Initially, 100 mg/day is given for one month. If there is no decrease in urinary oxalate, the dose is doubled at monthly intervals until a response has been produced or until a dose of 800 mg/day has been attained. For children, treatment should begin with 25 mg/day, with the amount increased gradually to a maximum of 250 mg/day (Scheinman, 1991). The arbitrary initial dose in infants is 10 mg/day. Patient compliance should be determined by measuring the amount of 4-pyridoxic acid present in urine collected for oxalate analysis. Only if no significant reduction in oxalate excretion is attained after a six-month trial in a compliant patient should alternative therapy be considered.

Patients with pyridoxine-resistant Type I primary hyperoxaluria or Type II primary hyperoxaluria often benefit from concurrent use of oral orthophosphate (2 g/day elemental phosphorus), magnesium (as magnesium oxide or magnesium hydroxide), and potassium citrate (Smith, 1980; Rose and Samuell, 1987). However, potassium citrate may be hypocalcemic, and its use in hyperoxaluria should be limited to patients with urinary citrate excretion <400 mg/day (Scheinman, 1991). Allopurinol has been used to inhibit endogenous oxalate production, but clinical results are inconclusive; it apparently is not effective in further reducing oxaluria in patients adhering to dietary restrictions (Urivetzky et al, 1990 A). Hydrochlorothiazide does not reduce urinary oxalate excretion (Urivetzky et al, 1991). Pyridoxine-resistant patients with Type I primary hyperoxaluria are candidates for either combined renal and orthoptic liver transplantation (Watts and Mansell, 1990) or renal transplantation followed by long-term daily dialysis (Scheinman, 1991).

Enteric Hyperoxaluria: In this condition, hyperoxaluria (over 40 mg/day) is associated with increased absorption of dietary oxalate secondary to loss of function of the small intestine (eg, ileal resection for Crohn's disease, steatorrhea, jejunoileal bypass, severe chronic bowel disease). Hyperabsorption of dietary oxalate results from increased colonic permeability to oxalate induced by malabsorbed bile acids and dietary fatty acids, from an enlarged absorbable oxalate pool caused by the complexing of calcium with malabsorbed fatty acids accumulating within the intestinal lumen, and from a decrease in oxalate degradation by colonic bacteria (especially *Oxalobacter formigenes*). Increased urinary excretion of oxalate may then contribute to the formation of calcium oxalate uroliths in some patients (Harper and Mansell, 1991; McLeod and Churchill, 1992).

These patients may benefit from a low-fat diet (maximum, 40 g daily) and limited ingestion of oxalate-rich foods. The substitution of medium-chain triglycerides for dietary fat also can be beneficial. The use of ascorbic acid supplements by individuals with intestinal malabsorption and lithiasis should be discontinued because ascorbate may be converted to oxalate prior to its absorption in these patients (Chalmers et al, 1986); urinary oxalate excretion increases 6 to 13 mg/g of supplemental ascorbic acid (Urivetzky et al, 1992). If the urinary excretion of calcium is low (less than 100 mg/24 hours), supplementing the diet with 1 to 3 g of calcium in order to chelate dietary oxalate may help reduce oxalate absorption, but the daily urinary excretion of calcium must be maintained below 4 mg/kg. Because citrate and magnesium absorption often are reduced in patients with intestinal malabsorption, supplementation with oral potassium citrate and intravenous magnesium oxide (Rudman et al, 1980; Johansson et al, 1980) or oral magnesium citrate (Lindberg et al, 1990) may be beneficial. Potassium and sodium citrate [Polycitra] may be given to those patients requiring additional sodium. If malabsorption is not severe, magnesium citrate (10 to 20 mEq, three times daily) also may increase the urinary excretion of citrate and magnesium while decreasing urinary oxalate; however, urinary excretion of calcium also may be increased (Lindberg et al, 1990). In some patients, cholestyramine (4 g four times daily) may bind oxalate and reduce the rate of stone formation, although fat malabsorption may be increased. Patients who have uncorrectable hyperoxaluria and stone formation following intestinal bypass may be candidates for reconstructive surgery.

Renal Hyperoxaluria: Calcium oxalate uroliths can form in mildly hyperoxaluric individuals without producing evidence of hepatic enzyme deficiency or intestinal malabsorption. The observation that the erythrocyte oxalate transport mechanism appears to be abnormal in at least some of these individuals has led to the hypothesis that a similar renal oxalate transport defect results in a renal oxalate leak (Zusman et al, 1991). However, this abnormality is not universal among or limited to stone formers and may not be pathognomonic (Motola et al, 1992). In any case, mild renal ("idiopathic") hyperoxaluria should be managed with dietary oxalate restriction, magnesium citrate supplementation, and high fluid intake.

Secondary Hyperoxaluria: This is an infrequent but potentially lethal complication in the treatment of a number of unrelated diseases (Conyers et al, 1990). The formation of calcium oxalate calculi often accompanies this disorder. A number of agents share minor pathways for oxalate synthesis, including xylitol, sorbitol, sucrose, fructose, lactose, glycerol, methanol, tryptophan, ascorbate, polysorbate, dichloroacetate, and methoxyflurane. Ethylene glycol also is a metabolic precursor of oxalate. The endogenous production of oxalate is proportional to the amount of exogenous substrate provided and may become sufficient to induce hyperoxaluria and calcium oxalate urolithiasis. This complication should be considered when any of these agents is administered. Selection of an alternative therapy or detoxification usually normalizes oxalate production and excretion; the extent of clinical sequelae depends on the severity and duration of oxalosis.

Distal Renal Tubular Acidosis: Calcium nephrolithiasis is common in patients with *incomplete distal renal tubular acidosis*, which is characterized by normal concentrations of serum electrolytes but reduced ability to acidify urine following an acid load. Hypocitruria usually is present, but hypercalciuria may or may not occur. Stone formation ceases following restoration of citrate excretion (Preminger et al, 1985). Potassium citrate (80 mEq/day) is more effective than sodium citrate and is the preferred treatment regardless of the presence of hypercalciuria or the status of systemic acid-base balance (Preminger et al, 1988; Buckalew, 1989). Patients with renal insufficiency must be monitored to prevent hyperkalemia and the development of metabolic alkalosis; in addition to potassium citrate therapy, dietary sodium chloride and salt substitutes should be restricted.

Hypocitruria: Citrate is a potent inhibitor of the crystallization and growth of calcium salts in the urine (Pak, 1987; Achilles et al, 1990), and urinary excretion of citrate is decreased in approximately 50% of all patients with urolithiasis (Pak et al, 1985 C). Chronic diarrhea, malabsorption syndromes, and malnutrition decrease the intestinal absorption of citrate, resulting in hypocitremia, a reduced filtered load of citrate in the kidneys, and hypocitruria (Hamm, 1990). (In the absence of these conditions, citrate absorption is normal in patients with urolithiasis [Fegan et al, 1992].) Strenuous physical exercise without adequate rehydration (Sakhaee et al, 1987) and active urinary tract infection increase citrate metabolism and contribute to hypocitruria. Distal renal tubular acidosis, use of acetazolamide or ethacrynic acid, thiazide-induced hypokalemia, consumption of diets rich in acid ash content, magnesium deficiency, and any other condition that results in urinary pH below 6.0 increase the renal tubular reabsorption of citrate and decrease its excretion in the urine (Simpson, 1983; Pak et al, 1985 C). In addition, patients who form calcium-containing calculi frequently have hypocitruria resulting from idiopathic increased renal tubular reabsorption of filtered citrate (Minisola et al, 1989). Chronic hemodialysis often is accompanied by large reductions in urinary citrate excretion and formation of calcium oxalate uroliths (Daudon et al, 1992). Although there is no direct correlation between the degree of hypocitruria and the rate of stone formation (Hosking et al, 1985; Goldberg et al, 1989), the formation of calcium-containing calculi is more likely if urinary citrate excretion is less than 400 mg/day (Pak et al, 1985 C; Kok et al, 1990).

Oral potassium citrate [Urocit-K] (30 to 100 mEq/day in three doses) elevates urinary citrate concentration and pH and reduces urinary calcium excretion and stone recurrence, regardless of the cause of hypocitruria (Pak, 1987; Sakhaee et al, 1991). Sodium citrate is equally effective in increasing urinary citrate and pH but is not hypocalciuric (Sakhaee et al, 1983). In addition, potassium citrate may be preferable because even mild hypokalemia decreases urinary citrate excretion, and hypernatremia is calciuric (Fourman and Robinson, 1953; Goldfarb, 1988). Magnesium citrate also may be useful. A new formulation, potassium-magnesium citrate [K-Mag], increases urinary citrate and magnesium excretion rates more than either potassium citrate or magnesium citrate alone and inhibits calcium oxalate crystallization more effectively (Koenig et al, 1991; Pak et al, 1992). A dose of supplemental citrate taken late in the evening will decrease the risk of calcium oxalate crystallization during the night, when concentrated urine is formed (Berg et al, 1990), and the effect may be sufficient to allow reliance on a single daily dose (Berg et al, 1992). The urinary citrate excretion rate reaches a maximum two to four hours after citrate ingestion (Koenig et al, 1991; Sakhaee et al, 1992).

STRUVITE LITHIASIS. Struvite calculi are formed in association with urinary tract infection by urea-splitting bacteria (usually *Proteus*), often in conjunction with anatomic abnormalities of the urinary tract. Struvite stone formation is twice as common in women as in men. Calculi that produce obstruction, pain, and bleeding and those associated with active infections must be removed surgically. Traditional open surgery can be performed, but percutaneous lithotripsy or extracorporeal shock wave lithotripsy (ESWL) has become more popular. Use of both lithotripsic methods may be more effective than either alone (Streem and Lammert, 1992). Appropriate bactericidal antibiotic therapy (usually ampicillin for indole-negative *Proteus*) is instituted 48 hours prior to surgery and is continued for 10 to 14 days thereafter. Culture of the stone material, not the urine, is essential to determine appropriate postsurgical antimicrobial therapy (Ohkawa et al, 1992).

The rate of struvite stone formation can be slowed by reducing the availability of phosphate through restriction of dietary phosphate and the administration of aluminum hydroxide gel to further decrease the intestinal absorption of phosphate. However, chronic phosphorus depletion can result in hypercalciuria leading to calcium oxalate urolithiasis. A more modest restriction of dietary phosphate without the antacid may be preferred. In addition, exposure to aluminum can accelerate the development of renal insufficiency, particularly if renal function already is impaired by infection and the presence of calculi. Bacterial urease inhibitors, such as acetohydroxamic acid [Lithostat] 250 mg three or four times daily, can be used to reduce intraluminal ammonia production and pH and may also potentiate the effects of appropriate, culture-specific antimicrobial agents given concurrently (Bagley, 1987; Campbell and Griffith, 1987). Use of acetohydroxamic acid should be restricted to patients (1) with chronic disease due to urease-producing organisms *not* responsive to antimicrobial agents alone, and (2) with adequate renal function (serum creatinine concentration below 3 mg/dL) (Williams et al, 1984). As with other forms of urolithiasis, a large fluid intake should be maintained after calculi are removed.

Various irrigation solutions and procedures are available to dissolve struvite stones in patients who are not candidates for surgery (Drach, 1986) or to remove stone fragments postsurgically or after ESWL (Spirnak et al, 1988). Failure to remove even minute fragments after these procedures may result in recurrent infection and new stone formation. Irrigation of the renal pelvis with a 10% solution of Renacidin (citric acid, gluconolactone, and magnesium carbonate) dissolves all traces of struvite stones (Nemoy, 1980). *Sterile urine and normal kidney function are prerequisites to the use of Renacidin.* Once these are assured, on the fourth or fifth postoperative day, the renal pelvis can be irrigated with saline for 24 to 48 hours at a maximum rate of 120 ml/hr and an infusion pressure not greater than 25 cm water. If no leakage, fever, or flank pain occurs, Renacidin 10% can be instilled at the same rate and pressure. In the absence of visible fragments in plain film tomograms of the kidney, irrigation should be continued for an additional 24 to 48 hours. If visible fragments are present, irrigation should be continued until all stones are dissolved. During irrigation, hypermagnesemia, hyperphosphatemia, and reduced renal function may occur. Because hypermagnesemia is potentially fatal, infusion should be discontinued if the serum magnesium concentration exceeds 5 mEq/L. Urine cultures should be obtained daily and, if positive, the irrigation must be discontinued until the infection is eradicated to avoid fatal sepsis. Because use of Renacidin requires continuous monitoring, hospitalization is required. Additional details of the Renacidin infusion technique are available (Palmer, 1987).

Suby's solution G (32.4 g citric acid monohydrate, 3.8 g anhydrous magnesium oxide, and 4.3 g anhydrous sodium carbonate per liter; pH 4.0) may be substituted for Renacidin. This preparation has been as effective as Renacidin in dissolving struvite calculi (Shortliffe and Spigelman, 1986).

URIC ACID LITHIASIS. Uric acid stones form when the urinary concentration of uric acid (which is sparingly soluble in urine) is increased beyond saturation (ie, when the urine pH is low or the urinary uric acid concentration is high). Low urinary pH (<5.5) with uric acid lithiasis is encountered in patients with primary gout or chronic diarrhea and in those who are dehydrated. Hyperuricosuria with uric acid stone formation results from gout, hemolytic anemia, tumor lysis syndrome, aggressive cytolytic treatment of neoplastic disease, hypercatabolic states, Lesch-Nyhan syndrome (hypoxanthine-guanine phosphoribosyltransferase deficiency), and salicylate or thiazide therapy (Maierhofer, 1987). About one-half of all individuals who excrete more than 800 mg/day of uric acid in their urine form uric acid calculi.

Treatment is aimed at correcting low urinary pH or hyperuricosuria. Maintaining adequate urinary volume and increasing urinary pH to 6.0 to 7.0 increase the solubility of uric acid, reduce new crystal formation, and may promote the dissolution of existing uric acid calculi. If there are no restrictions on sodium intake, urinary alkalization is accomplished most easily by taking sodium bicarbonate 2 to 4 g/day (24 to 48 mEq bicarbonate) or more in divided doses two hours after each meal and at bedtime. Potassium citrate (20 mEq three times daily) also is an excellent alkalizing agent as well as an inhibitor of uric acid crystallization and new uric acid stone formation (Sakhaee et al, 1983; Pak et al, 1986 A; Preminger, 1987; Williams-Larson, 1990). If compliance with daily therapy is a problem, 50 mEq may be given on alternate days (Rodman, 1991).

Sodium citrate [Bicitra, Polycitra] is an alternative alkalizing agent in patients prone to hyperkalemia but is less effective in preventing new stone formation (Sakhaee et al, 1983;

Pak et al, 1986 A). In addition, sodium alkali may cause sparingly soluble sodium urate to form and may enhance calcium stone formation. The patient should attempt to maintain a urinary pH of 6.0 to 7.0 at least 80% of the time, should test urine pH at each voiding, and should adjust alkali intake if necessary. It is particularly important that a sufficient amount of alkali be taken at bedtime to prevent the development of an acid urine on awakening.

If more rapid dissolution is desired, urinary alkalization may be enhanced by direct irrigation with a sodium bicarbonate solution (167 mEq/L in normal saline), utilizing a percutaneous or urethral catheter (Rodman et al, 1984), or by the intravenous administration of 1/6 M sodium lactate (Kursh and Resnick, 1984). However, calcium phosphate may be precipitated at a urinary pH above 7.0, and there is a risk of systemic alkalosis during irrigation with alkali.

Because about one-half of the uric acid derived from dietary purines via xanthine oxidase is excreted in the urine and urinary uric acid excretion decreases with restricted purine intake (Yamamoto et al, 1990), a low-purine diet may be considered. Simply reducing animal protein intake from 100 to 60 g/day can reduce uric acid excretion by 25% (Goldfarb, 1988). Weakly uricosuric drugs (salicylates, thiazides) and drugs that cause systemic acidosis (eg, acetazolamide [Diamox]) should be avoided. It has been reported that ketogenic diets occasionally acidify urine sufficiently to result in uric acid lithiasis (Herzberg et al, 1990). Allopurinol inhibits xanthine oxidase, thereby decreasing uric acid synthesis, serum uric acid concentration, and renal uric acid excretion, and this drug is recommended if hyperuricosuria is present. In the absence of hyperuricosuria, a high fluid intake with urinary alkalization may be adequate. A combination of high fluid intake and urine alkalization with or without allopurinol 150 mg twice daily dissolves existing uric acid calculi and prevents their recurrence (Lingeman et al, 1989). However, a small percentage of patients taking allopurinol develop xanthine calculi (Greene et al, 1969).

CYSTINE LITHIASIS. Hypercystinuria (over 300 mg/day) is inherited as an autosomal recessive trait and causes excessive urinary excretion of the dibasic amino acids, cysteine, ornithine, lysine, and arginine. Only the cysteine disulfide, cystine, forms stones because it is relatively insoluble in urine; the other amino acids are readily soluble. Hypercalciuria, hyperuricosuria, and hypocitruria may accompany cystine nephrolithiasis and contribute to the formation of mixed calcium and cystine stones or noncystine-containing renal calculi (Sakhaee et al, 1989). Cystine stone formers who excrete less than 800 mg of cystine/day usually are managed by measures to achieve a urinary output of 3 to 4 L/day (accomplished by drinking two large glasses of water every two hours during the day and one or more times at night) and by alkalization of the urine to a pH greater than 7.0 with potassium citrate to increase cystine solubility. Oral ascorbic acid has been used to prevent disulfide bonding of cysteine, which reduces cystine formation, but the large dose required (5 g/day) greatly increases the risk of inducing hypercalciuria and hyperoxaluria. Excessive methionine in the diet should be avoided, but low-methionine diets rarely are acceptable to patients. An interesting correlation has been observed between reduction in sodium intake and cystine excretion (Jaeger et al, 1986; Norman and Manette, 1990); however, the effectiveness of sodium restriction in reducing cystine calculus formation has not been demonstrated.

If these measures are inadequate or if increasing the rate of dissolution of cystine calculi is judged to be necessary, the concentration of cystine in urine can be decreased by agents that chelate cysteine and thus prevent cystine formation. Both penicillamine [Cuprimine, Depen] 1 to 2 g/day divided into four doses and tiopronin (alpha-mercaptopropionylglycine) [Thiola] 800 mg to 1.5 g/day decrease urinary cystine, form complexes with cysteine that are much more soluble in urine than is cystine, and reduce the size and formation rate of cystine calculi (Pahira, 1987). These agents should be used cautiously, however, because significant adverse reactions (eg, bone marrow suppression, pruritus, loss of taste, nephrotic syndrome) occur in many patients receiving more than 1 g/day of either drug. However, many patients who cannot tolerate penicillamine may tolerate tiopronin (Pak et al, 1986 B). The dosage of these agents should be adjusted to the smallest amount that will maintain urinary cystine excretion below 300 mg/day. Because these agents also inhibit the conversion of pyridoxine to pyridoxal phosphate, the concurrent administration of oral pyridoxine 50 mg/day is required (Pahira, 1987).

Succimer (*meso*-2,3-dimercaptosuccinic acid, DMSA) [Chemet] may be useful in preventing cystine lithiasis. Preliminary evidence suggests that about 90% of the succimer excreted in the urine of healthy subjects is bound to cysteine (Aposhian et al, 1989; Maiorino et al, 1989). Cysteine appears to bind to succimer in a 2:1 molar ratio; this suggests that succimer may be twice as effective as penicillamine or tiopronin in chelating urinary cysteine. Although experience with short-term use suggests that succimer may produce fewer adverse reactions, the safety of its lifelong use remains to be determined.

The use of percutaneous ultrasonic lithotripsy should be considered an alternative to penicillamine in patients with cystine stones >1.5 cm. ESWL is effective for the fragmentation of cystine stones or fragments <1.5 cm (Kachel et al, 1991).

Penicillamine, tiopronin, tromethamine [Tham-E], and acetylcysteine have been administered to dissolve cystine calculi by pelvicaliceal irrigation. Of these, acetylcysteine in an alkaline solution and tromethamine infusion are most effective (Dretler et al, 1984; Saltzman and Gittes, 1986). Irrigation may be combined with shock wave lithotripsy (Schmeller et al, 1984; Singer and Das, 1989).

XANTHINE LITHIASIS. Xanthine is very poorly soluble in urine, and calculi composed largely of this substance have been reported to occur in patients with hereditary xanthinuria (xanthine oxidase deficiency) and occasionally in patients treated with allopurinol (Greene et al, 1969). Because withdrawal of allopurinol from these individuals is usually not recommended, reduced purine intake and a large fluid intake (at least 3 to 4 L/day) are the only available interventions.

SILICATE LITHIASIS. Silicate calculi are rare and are found only in patients ingesting antacids containing magnesium trisilicate [Magnatril, Bicalma, Algenic Alka Improved, Gaviscon]. About 5% of an ingested dose of silicate appears in the urine and may precipitate as a gel. Treatment consists of reducing the amount of antacid ingested and perhaps substituting alternative therapy (Farrer and Rajfer, 1984).

AMMONIUM URATE LITHIASIS. Calculi containing ammonium urate are extremely rare in developed countries; they appear to occur in conjunction with the abuse of laxatives (Dick et al, 1990). Induced diarrhea results in large losses of water, potassium, and magnesium, which cause intracellular acidosis, excessive ammonium in the urine, and reduced urinary volume and excretion of citrate and magnesium. Urate and ammonium become supersaturated and precipitate. Treatment must focus on removal of the stimulus for excessive laxative use.

ALUMINUM-MAGNESIUM URATE LITHIASIS. As many as 20% of the renal calculi formed by hemodialysis patients are composed of a uric acid salt containing aluminum, magnesium, and potassium (Daudon et al, 1992). These stones are most common in patients receiving oral aluminum salts to bind phosphate.

UROLITHIASIS DURING PREGNANCY. Urolithiasis is the most common nonobstetric diagnosis among pregnant women hospitalized for abdominal pain (Maikranz et al, 1987; Rodriguez and Klein, 1988). Renal colic may trigger premature labor and increases the incidence of spontaneous abortion (Horowitz and Schmidt, 1985; Maikranz et al, 1987). About 10% to 20% of cases of urolithiasis during pregnancy are complicated by urinary tract infections, which can result in stunted fetal growth, premature labor, and increased perinatal mortality (Horowitz and Schmidt, 1985; Maikranz et al, 1987; Marlow, 1989).

The presence of renal calculi is somewhat more common among pregnant women than among nulliparous women (incidence, 0.03% to 0.53% of pregnancies; average, 0.1%) (Gertner et al, 1986; Marlow, 1989). Calculus formation and renal colic are most common during the second and third trimesters (Horowitz and Schmidt, 1985; Rodriguez and Klein, 1988). The causes of gestational calculi are similar to those of calculi formed in nonpregnant patients. However, their prevalence appears to be increased by ureteral abnormalities, pyelonephritis, and multiparity (Horowitz and Schmidt, 1985; Cass et al, 1986). Urinary stasis within the kidney and ureters during pregnancy also may contribute to calculus formation. Gestational hydronephrosis results from the combination of an elevated glomerular filtration rate (GFR) and external compression of the ureters at the pelvic brim by the gravid uterus, while increased progesterone secretion during pregnancy allows relaxation and dilatation of the renal calices, pelves, and ureters (Krieger, 1986; Goldfarb et al, 1989). Calcium oxalate calculi also can form around a ureteral stent inserted to relieve acute hydronephrosis (Rodriguez and Klein, 1988; Goldfarb et al, 1989).

The formation of calcium-containing gestational calculi may be enhanced by metabolic adaptations typical of pregnancy, including hypercalciuria and hyperuricosuria. Increased production of 1,25-dihydroxyvitamin D_3 during gestation causes increased absorption of dietary calcium and decreased secretion of PTH (Heaney and Skillman, 1971; Gertner et al, 1986). The resulting absorptive hypercalciuria occurs independently of changes in the GFR (Gertner et al, 1986; Marya et al, 1987). However, gestational hypercalciuria alone is insufficient to trigger calculus formation; unknown adaptive mechanisms appear to protect most pregnant women from this disorder (Maikranz et al, 1989).

Most patients with gestational calculi can be successfully managed with conservative therapy, ie, hydration, administration of potassium citrate and analgesics, and bed rest (Kroovand, 1992). With such treatment, 50% to 75% of calculi will pass spontaneously. Pharmacologic treatment is not recommended. Thiazides may induce fetal hypoglycemia, hyponatremia, and thrombocytopenia, and penicillamine crosses the placenta and has been associated with birth defects (Ehlers-Danlos syndrome) in humans (Mjølnerød et al, 1971; Maikranz et al, 1987). The safety of allopurinol during pregnancy is unknown and, until ascertained, its use should be avoided.

PEDIATRIC LITHIASIS. Active calculi account for 0.01% to 0.1% of pediatric hospital admissions in the United States, affect boys and girls about equally, and occur predominantly among whites (Polinsky et al, 1987; Stapleton, 1989). Unlike adults, pediatric patients may have diffuse back or abdominal pain in addition to flank pain. Hematuria occurs in more than 90% of children with urolithiasis, and otherwise unexplained hematuria is predictive of hypercalciuria (Hymes and Warshaw, 1984; Stapleton, 1990). Pyuria, bacteriuria, and dysuria commonly accompany pediatric urolithiasis. Urinary calculus formation during childhood is predictive of recurrence (incidence 30% to 40%) (Diamond et al, 1989); identifying effective measures to reduce future morbidity is extremely important.

The causes of uroliths in children are similar to those in adults, although a much lower percentage remain truly "idiopathic" (Polinsky et al, 1987; Gearhart et al, 1991). Many children with calculi also have developmental anomalies of the urinary tract, but these appear to be facilitative rather than causative (Polinsky et al, 1987). In addition, urinary tract infections are more prevalent among children with urolithiasis; often, the infection is secondary to calculi that do not contain struvite, and urease-inhibiting therapies will be inappropriate.

About two-thirds of all very-low-birth-weight (VLBW) infants who receive total parenteral nutrition (TPN) develop calcium oxalate/phosphate calculi (Jacinto et al, 1988). Many cases are associated with calciuric diuretics (eg, furosemide [Lasix]) given for bronchopulmonary dysplasia; however, many VLBW infants who were never treated with diuretics develop urolithiasis (Adams and Rowe, 1992). TPN solutions containing ascorbate and glycine also increase urinary oxalate concentrations in VLBW infants in proportion to the glycine content of the solution (Campfield and Braden, 1989). Many TPN and enteral feeding solutions given these infants are deficient in phosphorus ($<$35 mg/kg/day) and predispose to hypercalciuria (Adams and Rowe, 1992). The combination of furosemide and TPN may be especially lithogenic.

Because of their high rate of bone turnover, chronically immobilized or bedridden children are especially prone to resorptive hypercalciuria (Bentur et al, 1987). About one-third of children with osteogenesis imperfecta are hypercalciuric; the prevalence of urolithiasis in this population is variable (Chines et al, 1991). Primary hyperoxaluria may result in renal failure and death before age 6 months if untreated; in other affected infants, calcium oxalate calculi form early in life and recur along with progressive renal damage (Leumann, 1985; Steinmuller, 1985). In addition to the causes observed in adults, enteric hyperoxaluria in children may be secondary to cystic fibrosis. Children are relatively hyperuricosuric compared to adults, and extreme hyperuricosuria (such as that associated with polycythemia, infantile cyanotic congenital heart disease, and Lesch-Nyhan syndrome) may occur before uric acid calculi are formed. Struvite calculi usually appear in boys before age 5 and recur despite removal and preventive treatment.

Diagnostic evaluation of pediatric patients with calculi is similar to that in adults, but renal and absorptive hypercalciurias are more difficult to distinguish.

Therapeutic interventions are similar to those recommended for adults, with daily doses adjusted as appropriate: potassium citrate 2 to 4 mEq/kg, hydrochlorothiazide 2 mg/kg, pyridoxine 10 to 100 mg/kg, penicillamine 30 mg/kg, and allopurinol 5 to 10 mg/kg. Pediatric resorptive hypercalciuria responds favorably to hydrochlorothiazide 2 mg/kg plus amiloride 0.25 mg/kg daily (Bentur et al, 1987). In patients receiving furosemide, urinary excretion of calcium may be decreased if a thiazide diuretic also is used (Polinsky et al, 1987). The adverse reactions associated with acetohydroxamic acid make this agent unacceptable for use in children. Sodium cellulose phosphate and dietary restriction of calcium or phosphate are not appropriate for use in growing children.

Drug Evaluations

ACETOHYDROXAMIC ACID
[Lithostat]

$$CH_3-\overset{\displaystyle O}{\overset{\|}{C}}-N\begin{matrix}OH\\ H\end{matrix}$$

ACTIONS AND USES. This urease inhibitor is used to prevent the production of ammonia and hydroxide, the alkalization of urine, and the development of struvite stones in the presence of urea-splitting bacteria (usually *Proteus*). It has little antimicrobial activity, and its use should be restricted to patients who continue to form struvite calculi after antibacterial therapy or surgery. An appropriate culture-specific antimicrobial agent should be given concomitantly.

ADVERSE REACTIONS AND PRECAUTIONS. Acetohydroxamic acid should be used only in patients with adequate renal function (serum creatinine concentration less than 3 mg/dL) (Lake and Brown, 1985). It is contraindicated in women who are pregnant or who may become pregnant (FDA Pregnancy Category X). Women of childbearing age who are exposed to this drug should be counseled about its potential teratogenic effects and about the need to avoid conception.

Approximately 15% of patients using this drug develop signs characteristic of a Coombs'-negative hemolytic anemia. Some patients also experience nausea, vomiting, anorexia, and malaise. A greater number exhibit mild reticulocytosis. These responses are reversible with discontinuation of therapy. Since acetohydroxamic acid chelates iron, hypochromic anemia should be managed by administration of iron, which should not coincide with ingestion of acetohydroxamic acid. Large doses of acetohydroxamic acid produce bone marrow depression in animals (leukopenia, thrombocytopenia), but this has not been encountered with clinical doses in humans.

Mild, usually transient, headache responsive to salicylates is common during the first 48 hours of treatment. About 6% of patients experience depression, anxiety, and tremulousness severe enough to warrant interrupting or discontinuing therapy.

Nausea, anorexia, and vomiting not associated with hemolytic anemia are common during initial therapy and usually do not persist. A nonpruritic, maculopapular rash of the upper extremities and face has occurred, particularly with long-term therapy and in patients using alcoholic beverages. Avoidance of alcoholic beverages is recommended.

Superficial phlebitis of the lower extremities, sometimes with secondary pulmonary embolus, has been observed, particularly in patients with poor renal function. A history of thrombophlebitis should be considered a relative contraindication to use of this agent.

DOSAGE AND PREPARATIONS.
Oral: *This drug should be taken on an empty stomach. Adults,* initially, 12 mg/kg/day administered in divided doses at six- to eight-hour intervals. The maximum daily dose should not exceed 1.5 g. A maintenance dose of 250 mg three times a day is usually effective; in unresponsive patients, the amount may be increased to 250 mg four times a day. This agent is unacceptable for use in *children.*

Lithostat (Mission). Tablets 250 mg.

ALLOPURINOL
[Lopurin, Zyloprim]

For chemical formula, see index entry Allopurinol, In Gout.

Allopurinol is employed in the treatment of uric acid lithiasis and idiopathic calcium urolithiasis associated with hyperuricosuria (Lingeman et al, 1989; Ettinger et al, 1986). This drug inhibits xanthine oxidase conversion of purines to uric acid. It does not prevent stone recurrence in the absence of hyperuricosuria.

For a discussion of side effects, toxicity, interactions, and pharmacokinetics, see index entry Allopurinol, In Gout.

DOSAGE AND PREPARATIONS. Dosage should be individualized to obtain the desired serum urate concentrations in hyperuricemic patients; the daily urinary uric acid excretion should be less than 800 mg in men and 750 mg in women. ***Oral:*** The usual *adult* dosage for urolithiasis is 200 to 300 mg once daily; 100 mg daily may be adequate. Allopurinol is better tolerated if taken after a meal. A high urine output (more than 2.5 L/day) must be maintained, and the urine should be kept neutral or slightly alkaline. Dietary intake of animal protein should be less than 120 g/day, but a vegetarian diet should be avoided.

When renal disease is present, the dose or dose interval should be modified and the creatinine clearance and BUN should be evaluated periodically. The following daily doses may be given: creatinine clearance 10 to 20 ml/min, a maximum of 200 mg; 3 to 10 ml/min, a maximum of 100 mg; less than 3 ml/min, dosage interval should be lengthened.

Lopurin (Boots), ***Zyloprim*** (Burroughs Wellcome), ***Generic***. Tablets 100 and 300 mg.

CELLULOSE SODIUM PHOSPHATE
[Calcibind]

ACTIONS AND USES. This agent is taken with meals to reduce the absorption of dietary and secreted calcium from the intestinal tract. It is indicated *only* for severe confirmed absorptive hypercalciuria associated with recurrent calcium oxalate or calcium phosphate urolithiasis. Cellulose sodium phosphate 5 g reduces urinary calcium by approximately 50 mg.

ADVERSE REACTIONS AND PRECAUTIONS. Cellulose sodium phosphate is contraindicated in patients with primary or secondary hyperparathyroidism, including renal hypercalciuria; hypocalcemic disorders (hypoparathyroidism, intestinal malabsorption); bone disease (osteoporosis, osteomalacia, osteitis); hypomagnesemia (serum magnesium less than 1.5 mg/dL); or enteric hyperoxaluria and in patients with seriously impaired renal function (glomerular filtration rate less than 40 ml/min) (Lake and Brown, 1985).

Cellulose sodium phosphate also reduces the intestinal absorption of dietary magnesium. The resulting hypomagnesemia responds to magnesium supplements.

Because less calcium is available to bind oxalate, urinary oxalate increases. This can be managed by a moderate restriction of dietary oxalate. However, the need for every-meal compliance and for magnesium supplementation reduces the usefulness of this preparation in controlling calcium absorption.

Because of their increased dietary calcium requirements, cellulose sodium phosphate should not be used in children younger than 16 years or pregnant or lactating women (FDA Pregnancy Category C).

As the result of the decreased intestinal absorption of calcium, parathyroid function may increase and lead to bone disease. Therefore, parathyroid function, serum calcium, and serum magnesium should be assessed at three- to six-month intervals. If there is an increase in serum parathyroid hormone, the drug should be discontinued or the dosage adjusted. If there is an inadequate response to the drug (a reduction in urinary calcium of less than 30 mg/5 mg cellulose sodium phosphate while patients are on a moderate calcium-restricted diet [400 to 600 mg/day]), therapy should be considered ineffective and the agent discontinued. Therapy also should be reassessed if urinary excretion of oxalate exceeds 55 mg/day. Although the continued use of cellulose sodium phosphate does not seem to affect the levels of copper, zinc, and iron, concentrations of these trace elements should be measured periodically until more experience with this drug has accumulated.

A dose of 15 g contains 23 to 48 mEq of exchangeable sodium, which should be considered before cellulose sodium phosphate is used in patients with congestive heart failure or ascites. Some patients complain of loose bowel movements or diarrhea.

DOSAGE AND PREPARATIONS.

Oral: The drug is suspended in water, a soft drink, or fruit juice and ingested during meals or within 30 minutes after each meal. In patients on a moderate calcium-restricted diet with a 24-hour urinary excretion of calcium greater than 300 mg, the initial dose is 15 g/day. In stone formers who are excreting 200 to 300 mg of calcium daily, the dose is 10 g/day. Dietary restriction of oxalate and reduction of calcium intake should be imposed simultaneously.

Patients taking 15 g/day should receive 1.5 g magnesium gluconate before breakfast and at bedtime at least one hour before or after ingestion of cellulose sodium phosphate. The dose of supplemental magnesium gluconate for patients receiving 10 g/day of cellulose sodium phosphate is 1 g twice daily.

Calcibind (Mission). Powder 2.5 g (sodium approximately 11% and inorganic phosphate approximately 34%).

MAGNESIUM CITRATE
[Citroma, Citro-Nesia]

ACTIONS AND USES. Magnesium citrate decreases the urinary saturation and spontaneous nucleation of calcium oxalate by increasing urinary magnesium excretion and the production and renal clearance of citrate. It is useful in patients with hypocitruria or hypomagnesuria and in those in whom magnesium absorption is inhibited (eg, intestinal malabsorption).

ADVERSE REACTIONS AND PRECAUTIONS. Some patients complain of gastroenteric discomfort, dysgeusia, and a laxative effect. These effects may be minimized by diluting the preparation in water or juice and taking it with meals or snacks.

Magnesium citrate should not be used in patients with urinary tract infection or severe renal impairment. The safety and effectiveness of this preparation in children and pregnant women have not been determined.

PHARMACOKINETICS. More than 90% of an oral dose of magnesium citrate is absorbed. The urinary citrate excretion rate reaches a maximum two to four hours after administration.

DOSAGE AND PREPARATIONS.

Oral: *Adults,* 15 to 30 ml, diluted in water or juice and taken in two to four doses with food.

Citroma (Cumberland-Swan), ***Citro-Nesia*** (Century), ***Generic***. Solution 7% in 300 ml containers (nonprescription). Provides 210 mEq magnesium and citrate per 300-ml container.

ORTHOPHOSPHATES
[K-Phos Neutral, Neutra-Phos, Neutra-Phos-K]

Orthophosphates used in the prevention of urolithiasis consist of monobasic potassium phosphate with or without dibasic potassium phosphate, monobasic sodium phosphate, and dibasic sodium phosphate. The monobasic salts also are known as potassium acid phosphate and sodium acid phosphate, respectively. The combination salts are used to increase urinary pyrophosphate secretion and decrease the tendency of calcium to crystallize in the urine (see the Table and index entry Calcium Metabolism, Drugs Affecting). Acid phosphate salts should not be administered alone, since they may cause hypocitruria and increased stone formation.

ADVERSE REACTIONS AND PRECAUTIONS. The most common adverse effect of phosphate salts is diarrhea. A low initial dosage followed by a gradual increase in the amount given may improve tolerance to the medication but diarrhea-prone patients usually cannot be given an optimal amount. Patients with kidney stones may pass old stones when phosphate therapy is started and should be warned of this possibility. Phosphates are contraindicated in patients with urinary tract infections or infected stones and in those with renal function less than 30% of normal (creatinine clearance less than 30 ml/min). The use of sodium-containing orthophosphates may be contraindicated in patients with congestive heart failure or ascites or in those on sodium-restricted diets.

Phosphate products are classified in FDA Pregnancy Category C.

DOSAGE AND PREPARATIONS.

Oral: An exact dosage does not appear to be critical as long as the patient receives 1.5 to 2 g of elemental phosphorus in divided doses every 24 hours.

K-Phos Neutral (Beach). Tablets containing dibasic sodium phosphate anhydrous 852 mg, monobasic potassium phosphate 155 mg, and monobasic sodium phosphate 130 mg. This supplies 250 mg phosphorus, 298 mg sodium (13.0 mEq), and 45 mg potassium (1.1 mEq) per tablet.

Neutra-Phos (Baker Norton). Capsules and powder containing monobasic and dibasic sodium phosphate 164 mg and monobasic and dibasic potassium phosphate 278 mg (7.125 mEq sodium, 7.125 mEq potassium). This supplies 250 mg phosphorus per capsule or 75 ml of reconstituted solution (nonprescription).

Neutra-Phos-K (Baker Norton). Sodium-free formulation of ***Neutra-Phos,*** except dibasic potassium phosphate 556 mg (14.25 mEq potassium).

PENICILLAMINE (D-penicillamine)
[Cuprimine, Depen]

For chemical formula, see index entry Penicillamine, Uses, Metal Poisoning.

ACTIONS AND USES. This chelating agent prevents the formation of cystine calculi and may facilitate the dissolution of existing calculi by forming a water-soluble mixed disulfide with cysteine, which decreases the availability of cysteine to form the disulfide cystine. Because of its inherent toxicity, penicillamine should be used only if hydration with a urine output greater than 3 L/day and alkalization of the urine have been unsuccessful in preventing stone formation; DL- and L-penicillamine should not be used (Pahira, 1987). A dilute, alkaline urine should be maintained during penicillamine therapy. Oral pyridoxine supplements (50 mg/day) should be taken concurrently to counter the pyridoxine-blocking effect of penicillamine. In addition, iron deficiency may develop, particularly in children and menstruating women. Because preparations containing iron may interfere with the action of penicillamine, at least two hours should elapse between the administration of the drug and iron salts.

ADVERSE REACTIONS AND PRECAUTIONS. The incidence of side effects is high with penicillamine, particularly when daily doses exceed 1 g, and some reactions are potentially fatal. Therefore, medical supervision is essential throughout the period of drug administration. Most reactions occur shortly after therapy is begun (Pahira, 1987).

Various types of rashes with different characteristics may develop. Erythematous maculopapular or morbilliform rashes with pruritus are common and are considered to be hypersensitivity reactions; they often can be alleviated by concomitant administration of antihistamines. This rash usually disappears shortly after discontinuing medication and seldom recurs when therapy is resumed at a lower dosage. Less frequently, rash may occur after six or more months of treatment. This type usually appears on the trunk and is accompanied by intense pruritus. Following discontinuation of penicillamine, the rash may persist for many weeks and usually recurs if therapy is reinstituted.

Drug fever may occur in some patients, usually two or three weeks after initiation of therapy, and it may be accompanied by a macular eruption. Therapy should be discontinued temporarily until this reaction subsides and should be reinstituted at a lower dosage with the amount increased gradually. Systemic steroid therapy is usually helpful if the reaction recurs.

Purpuric or vesicular ecchymoses or rashes accompanied by fever, leukopenia, thrombocytopenia, eosinophilia, arthralgia, and lymphadenopathy may indicate the onset of a penicillamine-induced autoimmune syndrome or bone marrow suppression. Thrombocytopenia and granulocytopenia with occasional eosinophilia are early signs of impending bone marrow aplasia. Thrombocytopenia accompanied by a reduction in megakaryocytes in the marrow is indicative of aplastic anemia; however, if the marrow content of megakaryocytes is normal or increased, the thrombocytopenia is presumed to be an immune reaction. Autoimmune or immune complex disorders that are presumed to be caused by penicillamine include dermatomyositis, polymyositis, lupus erythematosus, diffuse alveolitis, obliterative bronchiolitis, and myasthenia gravis. If any of these disorders appear, therapy must be discontinued and adrenal corticosteroids administered if necessary.

Oral mucosal ulcers resembling aphthae and gastrointestinal upset may occur and usually respond to a reduction in dosage. Oral mucosal ulcers characterized by bullous lesions require discontinuation of penicillamine and treatment with corticosteroids.

Impairment of taste (hypogeusia) develops in some patients and may progress to a total loss of taste. The effect is transient, and normal sensitivity usually returns after two or three months of therapy. The administration of copper salts to overcome this effect is of no benefit.

Anorexia, nausea, vomiting, and epigastric pain may develop. Isolated cases of reactivated peptic ulcer have occurred and cholestatic jaundice and pancreatitis, which presumably were induced by penicillamine, have been reported occasionally.

Nephrotic syndrome may occur after several months of treatment. When proteinuria develops during therapy, the dosage should not be increased further and quantitative urinary protein determinations should be performed periodically. Therapy should be terminated if proteinuria exceeds 2 g/24 hours or if hematuria occurs. Abnormal urinary findings suggestive of Goodpasture's syndrome (glomerulonephritis, hemoptysis, and pulmonary infiltrates) occur rarely and require immediate discontinuation of penicillamine therapy.

Tinnitus, optic neuritis, and peripheral sensory and motor neuropathies, including polyradiculoneuropathy (Guillain-Barré syndrome), have been reported. Muscle weakness may accompany peripheral neuropathies. Visual and psychic disturbances also have been observed. Myasthenic syndrome sometimes occurs and may progress to myasthenia gravis; ptosis and diplopia, with weakness of the extraocular muscles, often are early signs of myasthenia. In the majority of patients, symptoms of myasthenia have receded after withdrawal of penicillamine.

Careful examination of the skin, as well as urinalysis, differential and white blood cell counts, direct platelet counts, and hemoglobin determinations should be performed every three days during the first two weeks of therapy, at least every ten days for three or four months, and monthly thereafter for the duration of treatment. If the white blood count falls below 3,500/microliter and the results are confirmed, discontinuation of penicillamine therapy is mandatory. If the platelet count falls below 100,000/microliter, even in the absence of bleeding, at least temporary cessation of therapy is required. A progressive fall in either platelet count or white blood cell count in three successive determinations also requires at least temporary suspension of the use of penicillamine, even if laboratory values are still within the normal range. When therapy is resumed, the initial dose should be small and the amount increased cautiously.

It is recommended that the drug be withheld from pregnant patients with cystinuria. Infants with generalized connective tissue defects who died following abdominal surgery have been born to cystinuric women who took penicillamine. If calculi continue to form in pregnant patients following withdrawal of penicillamine, the benefits of therapy for the mother must be weighed against the risks to her fetus. If continued therapy with penicillamine is considered necessary, the dosage should be limited to 1 g/day if possible. If cesarean section is planned, the dose should be reduced to 250 mg/day during the last six weeks of pregnancy and during the immediate postoperative period until healing has occurred.

Cross sensitivity between penicillin and penicillamine does not always occur; therefore, penicillamine can be given cautiously to patients who are hypersensitive to penicillin.

DOSAGE AND PREPARATIONS. Penicillamine should be given on an *empty stomach* at least one hour before meals with copious amounts of water, and other medication should not be taken concurrently.

The interruption of therapy for even a few days may cause sensitivity reactions when treatment is reinstituted. *This must be stressed to the patient.* If therapy is interrupted, it should be reinstituted at a lower dosage, which is increased gradually to the full amount.

Oral: For cystinuria, *adults,* initially, 1 g (increasing gradually to 4 g, if necessary) daily in four divided doses at least one hour before or two hours after meals; *young children and infants,* 30 mg/kg/day in four divided doses. If the patient cannot tolerate the full calculated dosage of penicillamine, a daily dose of 250 mg may be given initially and increments added gradually. If equal doses are not possible or if adverse reactions necessitate a reduction in dosage, the largest amount should be given at bedtime. High fluid intake also is required (about 500 ml of water at bedtime and another 500 ml during the night when the urine is more concentrated and more acidic than during the day). Effective therapy is indicated by the urinary excretion of less than 100 to 200 mg of cystine/day.

Because the drug causes the skin to become friable and may inhibit wound healing, the dosage should be reduced to 250 mg/day prior to elective oral or general surgery. Reinstitution of full dosages should be delayed until wound healing is complete.

Cuprimine (Merck Sharp & Dohme). Capsules 125 and 250 mg.
Depen (Wallace). Tablets 250 mg.

POTASSIUM CITRATE
[K-Lyte, Polycitra-K, Urocit-K]

ACTIONS AND USES. Potassium citrate decreases the urinary saturation and spontaneous nucleation of calcium oxalate by increasing the production and renal clearance of citrate. It is useful in all patients with hypocituria and also may be used in those with renal tubular acidosis and enteric hyperoxaluria if a sodium load should be avoided (Pak, 1987; Berg et al, 1990). This preparation can be combined with a thiazide and/or allopurinol to treat hypocitruric or hyperuricosuric calcium oxalate urolithiasis. Potassium citrate also may be used to alkalize the urine in patients with stones composed of cystine or uric acid.

ADVERSE REACTIONS AND PRECAUTIONS. Some patients complain of gastroenteric discomfort, bad taste, and a laxative effect when taking the liquid form [Polycitra-K]. These effects may be minimized by diluting the preparation in water and taking it after meals. These reactions are less common with the tablet [Urocit-K] and crystalline [Polycitra-K] forms. Effervescent tablets containing citrate and bicarbonate [K-Lyte] may be even more acceptable to patients.

Potassium citrate should not be used in patients with urinary tract infection or severe renal impairment. The concurrent administration of other potassium-containing medications or potassium-sparing diuretics, especially in the presence of renal disease, may lead to serious hyperkalemia and systemic alkalosis. The tablet preparation should not be used in patients with active peptic ulcer. In patients who require a potassium-restricted diet, sodium citrate and citric acid solution [Bicitra] should be substituted.

Potassium citrate is classified in FDA Pregnancy Category C.

PHARMACOKINETICS. Potassium citrate is 98% absorbed within three hours in both healthy individuals and stone formers (Fegan et al, 1992).

DOSAGE AND PREPARATIONS.

Oral: (Solution) *Adults,* 15 to 30 ml, diluted in water or juice and taken in two to four divided doses after meals and at bedtime; *children,* 1 ml/kg diluted in water or juice and taken in two to four divided doses after meals and at bedtime. (Tablets) *Adults,* two to four tablets taken two or three times daily within one-half hour after meals. (Crystals) *Adults,* one packet dissolved in at least six ounces of liquid taken two to four times a day after meals and at bedtime. (Effervescent Tablets) *Adults,* one tablet dissolved in at least six ounces of liquid and taken one to five times daily after meals and at bedtime.

K-Lyte (Apothecon). Each effervescent tablet contains 25 mEq (961 mg) potassium as bicarbonate and citrate.

K-Lyte DS (Apothecon). Each effervescent tablet contains 50 mEq (1,922 mg) potassium as carbonate and citrate.

Polycitra-K Oral Solution (Baker Norton). Each 5 ml contains potassium citrate monohydrate 1.1 g and citric acid monohydrate 334 mg. Each 5 ml contains 10 mEq potassium (approximately equivalent to 10 mEq bicarbonate).

Polycitra-K Crystals (Baker Norton). Each packet contains potassium citrate monohydrate 3.3 g and citric acid monohydrate 1 g. When reconstituted, each 15 ml contains 30 mEq potassium (approximately equivalent to 30 mEq bicarbonate).

Urocit-K (Mission). Each tablet contains 5 mEq (540 mg) or 10 mEq (1,080 mg) potassium citrate.

POTASSIUM AND MAGNESIUM CITRATE

[K-Mag]

ACTIONS AND USES. This mixture of potassium and magnesium citrate decreases the urinary saturation and spontaneous nucleation of calcium oxalate by increasing urinary magnesium excretion and the production and renal clearance of citrate. It is useful in patients with hypocitruria or hypomagnesuria and in those with renal tubular acidosis and enteric hyperoxaluria when a sodium load should be avoided. Potassium and magnesium citrate also may be used to alkalize the urine in patients with cystine or uric acid lithiasis. It inhibits calcium oxalate crystallization more effectively than potassium citrate.

ADVERSE REACTIONS AND PRECAUTIONS. The concurrent administration of other potassium-containing medications or potassium-sparing diuretics, especially in the presence of renal disease, may cause severe hyperkalemia and systemic alkalosis. Potassium and magnesium citrate should not be used in patients with urinary tract infection or severe renal impairment.

The safety and effectiveness of this preparation in children and pregnant women have not been determined.

PHARMACOKINETICS. More than 90% of an oral dose of potassium and magnesium citrate is absorbed. The urinary citrate excretion rate reaches a maximum two to four hours after administration.

DOSAGE AND PREPARATIONS.

Oral: *Adults*, three or four tablets twice daily with breakfast and the evening meal.

K-Mag (Bio-Tech Pharmacal). Tablets containing potassium, magnesium, and citrate in a 4:1:2 molar ratio. Each tablet provides 7 mEq potassium, 3.5 mEq magnesium, and 10.5 mEq citrate (nonprescription).

POTASSIUM AND SODIUM CITRATE

[Polycitra]

ACTIONS AND USES. In conditions in which there is loss of both sodium and potassium, a mixture of potassium citrate and sodium citrate is used most commonly to alkalize the urine and increase the production and renal clearance of citrate.

ADVERSE REACTIONS AND PRECAUTIONS. The most common adverse reaction is a laxative effect. This may be minimized if the preparation is taken immediately after meals.

The patient should be instructed to take potassium and sodium citrate with adequate quantities of fluid to avoid the intestinal injury that can be produced by concentrated potassium salts. To avoid hyperkalemia, this preparation should not be used in patients with severe renal impairment or given with potassium-sparing diuretics or other salts containing potassium. Periodic examination of the patient and determination of serum electrolytes are recommended in those with renal disease. The administration of potassium citrate alone may be preferred in patients with congestive heart failure, edema, hypertension, or toxemia of pregnancy.

In patients with distal (type I) tubular acidosis with signs of hypokalemia and systemic acidemia, decreasing serum potassium as the serum pH is corrected can be avoided by initiating therapy with potassium citrate alone. After correction of acidemia and elevation of the potassium concentration into the normal range, the mixture containing potassium citrate and sodium citrate can be used.

Potassium and sodium citrate is classified in FDA Pregnancy Category C.

DOSAGE AND PREPARATIONS.

Oral: *Adults*, 10 to 15 ml two to four times daily within one-half hour after meals and at bedtime. The preparation should be diluted in water and may be taken with additional water. *Children*, 1 ml/kg diluted in water or juice in two to four divided doses.

Polycitra Syrup, Polycitra-LC-Sugar Free Solution (Baker Norton). Each 5 ml of syrup or solution contains potassium citrate monohydrate 550 mg, sodium citrate dihydrate 500 mg, and citric acid monohydrate 334 mg. Each 5 ml contains 5 mEq potassium and 5 mEq sodium and is equivalent to 10 mEq bicarbonate (alcohol free).

RENACIDIN

USES. This renal irrigation solution containing citric acid, gluconolactone, and magnesium carbonate is used to dissolve renal calculi composed of apatite or struvite in patients free of urinary tract infection. It also may be used after lithotripsy or laser treatment to dissolve residual apatite or struvite calculi and fragments after surgery. This preparation does not dissolve calculi composed of calcium oxalate, uric acid, or cysteine. Irrigation of the renal pelvis with Renacidin requires prolonged hospitalization.

ADVERSE REACTIONS AND PRECAUTIONS. Renacidin is contraindicated in the presence of urinary tract infection; deaths from sepsis following such use have been reported. Prolonged irrigation may cause hypermagnesemia with hyporeflexia, dyspnea, apnea, coma, cardiac arrest, and death. Other adverse effects include flank pain, urothelial ulceration or edema, and fever.

DOSAGE AND PREPARATIONS.
Percutaneous: A 10% solution in sterile distilled water is infused for at least 24 to 48 hours at a maximum rate of 120 ml/hr and an infusion pressure less than 25 cm water. For additional details, see Palmer, 1987.

Renacidin Irrigation Solution (Guardian). Solution (sterile) for dilution (1:10) in sterile distilled water in 500 ml containers.

THIAZIDES

The thiazide diuretics are used to reduce urinary calcium excretion in patients with hypercalciuria.

Thiazide-induced hypokalemia should be avoided to prevent hypocitruria because citrate inhibits the crystallization of stone-forming calcium salts. The concomitant administration of potassium citrate in doses of 10 to 25 mEq three times a day is recommended to prevent thiazide-induced hypocitruria (Nicar et al, 1984; Goldberg et al, 1989). For precautions and adverse effects, see index entry Thiazides. These drugs are classified in FDA Pregnancy Category B.

DOSAGE.
Oral: *Adults,* hydrochlorothiazide 25 to 50 mg one or two times daily or the equivalent of other thiazides (eg, chlorthalidone 50 mg/day, trichlormethiazide 4 mg/day). *Children,* hydrochlorothiazide 2 mg/kg/day (Stapleton, 1989). It is important to avoid a dietary intake of sodium greater than 4 g/day because a high sodium intake can negate the hypocalciuric response of the kidneys to the thiazides.

For preparations, see index entry Thiazides.

TIOPRONIN (Alpha-Mercaptopropionylglycine)
[Thiola]

$$CH_3CH(SH)C(=O)NHCH_2C(=O)OH$$

This drug forms a water-soluble mixed disulfide with cysteine and is used to dissolve cystine calculi. The toxicity of tiopronin has been reported to be lower than that of penicillamine, although both drugs produce a dose-related nephrotic syndrome. For this reason, routine monitoring of urinary protein excretion is recommended. Other adverse effects include urticaria, fever, lymphadenopathy, and essentially all of the side effects of penicillamine, although to a lesser degree (Pahira, 1987). Patients who cannot tolerate penicillamine may be able to tolerate tiopronin (Pak et al, 1986 B). Tiopronin is classified in FDA Pregnancy Category C.

DOSAGE AND PREPARATIONS. Tiopronin should be given on an *empty stomach* at least one hour before or two hours after meals, and other medication should not be taken concurrently.

Oral: *Adults,* initially, 800 mg in divided doses three times a day; hydration to maintain a minimum urine output of 3 L/day and alkalization to a urinary pH of 7.0 are essential during therapy.

Thiola (Mission). Tablets 100 mg.

Cited References

Achilles W, et al: The in-vivo effect of sodium-potassium citrate on the crystal growth rate of calcium oxalate and other parameters in human urine. *Urol Res* 18:1-6, 1990.

Adams ND, Rowe JC: Nephrocalcinosis. *Clin Perinatol* 19:179-195, 1992.

Andersen T, et al: Calcium homeostasis in morbid obesity. *Miner Electrolyte Metab* 10:316-318, 1984.

Aposhian HV, et al: Urinary excretion of meso-2,3-dimercaptosuccinic acid in human subjects. *Clin Pharmacol Ther* 45:520-526, 1989.

Backman U, et al: Treatment of recurrent calcium stone formation with cellulose phosphate. *J Urol* 123:9-13, 1980.

Bagley DH: Pharmacologic treatment of infection stones. *Urol Clin North Am* 14:347-352, 1987.

Barger-Lux MJ, et al: Effects of moderate caffeine intake on the calcium economy of premenopausal women. *Am J Clin Nutr* 52:722-725, 1990.

Bataille P, et al: Diet, vitamin D and vertebral mineral density in hypercalciuric calcium stone formers. *Kidney Int* 39:1193-1205, 1991.

Bentur L, et al: Hypercalciuria in chronically institutionalized bedridden children: Frequency, predictive factors and response to treatment with thiazides. *Int J Pediatr Nephrol* 8:29-34, 1987.

Berg C, et al: Effects of different doses of alkaline citrate on urine composition and crystallization of calcium oxalate. *Urol Res* 18:13-16, 1990.

Berg C, et al: The effects of a single evening dose of alkaline citrate on urine composition and calcium stone formation. *J Urol* 148:979-985, 1992.

Buckalew VM Jr: Nephrolithiasis in renal tubular acidosis. *J Urol* 141(part 2):731-737, 1989.

Campbell R, Griffith DP: Infected (struvite) calculi, in Rous SN (ed): *Stone Disease: Diagnosis and Management.* Orlando, Grune & Stratton, 1987, 161-175.

Campfield T, Braden G: Urinary oxalate excretion by very low birth weight infants receiving parenteral nutrition. *Pediatrics* 84:860-863, 1989.

Cappuccio FP, et al: Kidney stones and hypertension: Population based study of an independent clinical association. *BMJ* 300:1234-1236, 1990.

Cass AS, et al: Management of urinary calculi in pregnancy. *Urology* 28:370-372, 1986.

Chalmers AH, et al: A possible etiologic role for ascorbate in calculi formation. *Clin Chem* 32:333-336, 1986.

Chines A, et al: Hypercalciuria in children severely affected with osteogenesis imperfecta. *J Pediatr* 119:51-57, 1991.

Churchill DN, Taylor DW: Thiazides for patients with recurrent calcium stones: Still an open question. *J Urol* 133:749-751, 1985.

Coe FL: Hyperuricosuric calcium oxalate nephrolithiasis. *Kidney Int* 13:418-426, 1978.

Coe FL, Bushinsky DA: Pathophysiology of hypercalciuria, editorial. *Am J Physiol* 247:F1-F13, 1984.
Coe FL, Parks JH: Pathophysiology of kidney stones and strategies for treatment. *Hosp Pract* 23:185-207, (March 15) 1988.
Coe FL, Parks JH: Nephrolithiasis, in Favus MJ (ed): *Primer on the Metabolic Bone Diseases and Disorders of Mineral Metabolism*. Kelseyville, Calif, American Society for Bone and Mineral Research, 1990, 273-276.
Coe FL, et al: Chlorthalidone promotes mineral retention in patients with idiopathic hypercalciuria. *Kidney Int* 33:1140-1146, 1988.
Consensus Conference, National Institutes of Health: Prevention and treatment of kidney stones. *JAMA* 260:977-981, 1988.
Conyers RAJ, et al: The relation of clinical catastrophes, endogenous oxalate production, and urolithiasis. *Clin Chem* 36:1717-1730, 1990.
Daudon M, et al: Urolithiasis in patients with end stage renal failure. *J Urol* 147:977-980, 1992.
Diamond DA, et al: Etiological factors in pediatric stone recurrence. *J Urol* 142 (part 2):606-608, 1989.
Dick WH, et al: Laxative abuse as a cause for ammonium urate renal calculi. *J Urol* 143:244-247, 1990.
Drach GW: Urinary lithiasis, in Walsh PC, et al (eds): *Campbell's Urology*, ed 5. Philadelphia, WB Saunders, 1986, 1094-1190.
Dretler SP, et al: Percutaneous catheter dissolution of cystine calculi. *J Urol* 131:216-219, 1984.
Ebisuno S, et al: Rice-bran treatment for calcium stone formers with idiopathic hypercalciuria. *Br J Urol* 58:592-595, 1986.
Ettinger B, et al: Randomized trial of allopurinol in prevention of calcium oxalate calculi. *N Engl J Med* 315:1386-1389, 1986.
Farrer JH, Rajfer J: Silicate urolithiasis. *J Urol* 132:739-740, 1984.
Fegan J, et al: Gastrointestinal citrate absorption in nephrolithiasis. *J Urol* 147:1212-1214, 1992.
Fellström B, et al: Allopurinol treatment of renal calcium stone disease. *Br J Urol* 57:375-379, 1985.
Foster MC, et al: Urological myths. *BMJ* 301:1421-1423, 1990.
Fourman P, Robinson JR: Diminished urinary excretion of citrate during deficiencies of potassium in man. *Lancet* 2:656-657, 1953.
Fuss M, et al: Involvement of low-calcium diet in the reduced bone mineral content of idiopathic renal stone formers. *Calcif Tissue Int* 46:9-13, 1990.
Gearhart JP, et al: Childhood urolithiasis: Experiences and advances. *Pediatrics* 87:445-450, 1991.
Gertner JM, et al: Pregnancy as state of physiologic absorptive hypercalciuria. *Am J Med* 81:451-456, 1986.
Gleeson MJ, et al: Effect of unprocessed wheat bran on calciuria and oxaluria in patients with urolithiasis. *Urology* 35:231-234, 1990.
Glowacki LS, et al: The natural history of asymptomatic urolithiasis. *J Urol* 147:319-321, 1992.
Goldberg H, et al: Urine citrate and renal stone disease. *Can Med Assoc J* 141:217-221, 1989.
Goldfarb S: Dietary factors in the pathogenesis and prophylaxis of calcium nephrolithiasis. *Kidney Int* 34:544-555, 1988.
Goldfarb RA, et al: Management of acute hydronephrosis of pregnancy by ureteral stenting: Risk of stone formation. *J Urol* 141:921-922, 1989.
Goldwasser B, et al: Change in inhibitory potential in urine of hyperuricosuric calcium oxalate stone formers affected by allopurinol and orthophosphates. *J Urol* 132:1008-1011, 1984.
Goldwasser B, et al: Calcium stone disease: Overview. *J Urol* 135:1-9, 1986.
Greene ML, et al: Urinary xanthine stones: A rare complication of allopurinol therapy. *N Engl J Med* 280:426-427, 1969.
Hamm LL: Renal handling of citrate. *Kidney Int* 38:728-735, 1990.
Harper J, Mansell MA: Treatment of enteric hyperoxaluria. *Postgrad Med J* 67:219-222, 1991.
Heaney RP, Skillman TG: Calcium metabolism in normal human pregnancy. *J Clin Endocrinol* 33:661-670, 1971.
Herzberg GZ, et al: Urolithiasis associated with the ketogenic diet. *J Pediatr* 117:743-745, 1990.
Holl MG, Allen LH: Sucrose ingestion, insulin response and mineral metabolism in humans. *J Nutr* 117:1229-1233, 1987.
Horowitz E, Schmidt JD: Renal calculi in pregnancy. *Clin Obstet Gynecol* 28:324-338, 1985.
Hosking DH, et al: The stone clinic effect in patients with idiopathic calcium urolithiasis. *J Urol* 130:1115-1118, 1983.
Hosking DH, et al: Urinary citrate excretion in normal persons and patients with idiopathic calcium urolithiasis. *J Lab Clin Med* 106:682-689, 1985.
Hymes LC, Warshaw BL: Idiopathic hypercalciuria: Renal and absorptive subtypes in children. *Am J Dis Child* 138:176-180, 1984.
Indudhara R, et al: Oral diclofenac sodium in the treatment of acute renal colic: A prospective randomized study. *Clin Trials J* 27:295-300, 1990.
Insogna KL, et al: Trichlormethiazide and oral phosphate therapy in patients with absorptive hypercalciuria. *J Urol* 141:269-274, 1989.
Jacinto JS, et al: Renal calcification incidence in very low birth weight infants. *Pediatrics* 81:31-35, 1988.
Jaeger P, et al: Anticystinuric effects of glutamine and of dietary sodium restriction. *N Engl J Med* 315:1120-1123, 1986.
Johansson G, et al: Biochemical and clinical effects of prophylactic treatment of renal calcium stones with magnesium hydroxide. *J Urol* 124:770-774, 1980.
Kachel TA, et al: Endourological experience with cystine calculi and a treatment algorithm. *J Urol* 145:25-28, 1991.
Kapoor DA, et al: Use of indomethacin suppositories in the prophylaxis of recurrent ureteral colic. *J Urol* 142:1428-1430, 1989.
Kasidas GP, Rose GA: Metabolic hyperoxaluria and its response to pyridoxine, in Ryall RL, et al (eds): *Urinary Stone*. Melbourne, Churchill Livingstone, 1984, 138-147.
Khalifa MS, Sharkawi MA: Treatment of pain owing to acute ureteral obstruction with prostaglandin-synthetase inhibitor: A prospective randomized study. *J Urol* 136:393-395, 1986.
Koenig K, et al: Bioavailability of potassium and magnesium, and citraturic response from potassium-magnesium citrate. *J Urol* 145:330-334, 1991.
Kohri K, et al: Allopurinol and thiazide effects on new urinary stone formed after discontinued therapy in patients with urinary stones. *Urology* 36:309-314, 1990.
Kok DJ, et al: The effects of dietary excesses in animal protein and in sodium on the composition and the crystallization kinetics of calcium oxalate monohydrate in urines of healthy men. *J Clin Endocrinol Metab* 71:861-867, 1990.
Kosko J, Resnick MI: Urinary calculi: Evaluation and medical management, in Resnick MI (ed): *Current Trends in Urology*. Baltimore, Williams & Wilkins, 1985, vol 3, 59-68.
Krieger JN: Complications and treatment of urinary tract infections during pregnancy. *Urol Clin North Am* 13:685-693, 1986.
Kroovand RL: Stones in pregnancy and in children, editorial. *J Urol* 148:1076-1078, 1992.
Kursh ED, Resnick MI: Dissolution of uric acid calculi with systemic alkalization. *J Urol* 132:286-287, 1984.
Lake KD, Brown DC: New drug therapy for kidney stones: A review of cellulose sodium phosphate, acetohydroxamic acid and potassium citrate. *DICP* 19:530-539, 1985.
Lee Y-H, et al: Acupuncture in the treatment of renal colic. *J Urol* 147:16-18, 1992.
Lemann J Jr, Gray RW: Idiopathic hypercalciuria. *J Urol* 141 (part 2): 715-718, 1989.
Leumann EP: Primary hyperoxaluria: Important cause of renal failure in infancy. *Int J Pediatr Nephrol* 6:13-16, 1985.
Lindberg J, et al: Effect of magnesium citrate and magnesium oxide on the crystallization of calcium salts in urine: Changes produced by food-magnesium interaction. *J Urol* 143:248-251, 1990.
Lingeman JE, et al: *Urinary Calculi: ESWL, Endourology, and Medical Therapy*. Philadelphia, Lea & Febiger, 1989.
Litvak KM, McEvoy GK: Ketorolac, an injectable nonnarcotic analgesic. *Clin Pharm* 9:921-935, 1990.
Maierhofer WJ: Renal disease from excess uric acid. *Postgrad Med* 82:123-129, (Sept) 1987.
Maikranz P, et al: Nephrolithiasis in pregnancy. *Am J Kidney Dis* 9:354-358, 1987.

Maikranz P, et al: Gestational hypercalciuria causes pathological urine calcium oxalate supersaturations. *Kidney Int* 36:108-113, 1989.

Maiorino RM, et al: Determination and metabolism of dithiol chelating agents: VI, Isolation and identification of the mixed disulfides of *meso*-2,3-dimercaptosuccinic acid with L-cysteine in human urine. *Toxicol Appl Pharmacol* 97:338-349, 1989.

Marangella M, et al: Plasma and urine glycolate assays for differentiating the hyperoxaluria syndromes. *J Urol* 148:986-989, 1992.

Marlow RA: Nephrolithiasis in pregnancy. *Am Fam Physician* 40:185-189, 1989.

Marya RK, et al: Urinary calcium excretion in pregnancy. *Gynecol Obstet Invest* 23:141-144, 1987.

Massey LK, et al: Dietary caffeine lowers ultrafiltrable calcium levels in women consuming low dietary calcium. *J Bone Miner Res* 2(suppl 1):abstract 479, 1987.

McCarron DA, et al: Enhanced parathyroid function in essential hypertension: A homeostatic response to a urinary calcium leak. *Hypertension* 2:162-168, 1980.

McLean RJC, et al: Influence of chondroitin sulfate, heparin sulfate, and citrate on proteus mirabilis-induced struvite crystallization in vitro. *J Urol* 144:1267-1271, 1990.

McLeod RS, Churchill DN: Urolithiasis complicating inflammatory bowel disease. *J Urol* 148:974-978, 1992.

Menon M, Koul H: Clinical Review 32: Calcium oxalate nephrolithiasis. *J Clin Endocrinol Metab* 74:703-707, 1992.

Minisola S, et al: Studies on citrate metabolism in normal subjects and kidney stone patients. *Miner Electrolyte Metab* 15:303-308, 1989.

Mjølnerød OK, et al: Congenital connective-tissue defect probably due to D-penicillamine treatment in pregnancy. *Lancet* 1:673-675, 1971.

Morse RM, Resnick MI: Ureteral calculi: Natural history and treatment in an era of advanced technology. *J Urol* 145:263-265, 1991.

Motola JA, et al: Transmembrane oxalate exchange: Its relationship to idiopathic calcium oxalate nephrolithiasis. *J Urol* 147:549-552, 1992.

Nemoy NJ: Renacidin in treatment of infection stones, in Kaufman JJ (ed): *Current Urologic Therapy*. Philadelphia, WB Saunders, 1980, 145-146.

Nicar MJ, et al: Use of potassium citrate as a potassium supplement during thiazide therapy of calcium nephrolithiasis. *J Urol* 131:430-433, 1984.

Nissen I, et al: Treatment of ureteric colic: Intravenous versus rectal administration of indomethacin. *Br J Urol* 65:576-579, 1990.

Nordin BEC, et al: Evidence for a renal calcium leak in postmenopausal women. *J Clin Endocrinol Metab* 72:401-407, 1991.

Norman RW, Manette WA: Dietary restriction of sodium as a means of reducing urinary cystine. *J Urol* 143:1193-1195, 1990.

Ohkawa M, et al: Composition of urinary calculi related to urinary tract infection. *J Urol* 148:995-997, 1992.

Okaniwa T, et al: Effect of nifedipine on urinary concentrating ability: A placebo controlled study. *J Clin Pharmacol* 29:938-945, 1989.

Oosterlinck W, et al: A double-blind single dose comparison of intramuscular ketorolac tromethamine and pethidine in the treatment of renal colic. *J Clin Pharmacol* 30:336-341, 1990.

Pacifici R, et al: Increased monocyte TNFα and GM-CSF secretion in patients with 'resorptive' idiopathic hypercalciuria. *J Bone Miner Res* 5:S100, 1990.

Pahira JJ: Management of the patient with cystinuria. *Urol Clin North Am* 14:339-346, 1987.

Pak CYC: Physiological basis for absorptive and renal hypercalciurias. *Am J Physiol* 237:415-423, 1979.

Pak CYC: A cautious use of sodium cellulose phosphate in the management of calcium nephrolithiasis. *Invest Urol* 19:187-190, 1981.

Pak CYC: Citrate and renal calculi. *Miner Electrolyte Metab* 13:257-266, 1987.

Pak CYC: Medical management of nephrolithiasis in Dallas: Update, 1987. *J Urol* 140:461-467, 1988.

Pak CYC: Role of medical prevention. *J Urol* 141(part 2):798-801, 1989.

Pak CYC, et al: The hypercalciurias: Causes, parathyroid functions and diagnostic criteria. *J Clin Invest* 54:387-400, 1974.

Pak CYC, et al: Evidence justifying high fluid intake in treatment of nephrolithiasis. *Ann Intern Med* 93:36-39, 1980.

Pak CYC, et al: Dietary management of idiopathic nephrolithiasis. *J Urol* 131:850-852, 1984.

Pak CYC, et al: Graphic display of urinary risk factors for renal stone formation. *J Urol* 134:867-870, 1985 A.

Pak CYC, et al: Correction of hypocitraturia and prevention of stone formation by combined thiazide and potassium citrate therapy in thiazide-unresponsive hypercalciuric nephrolithiasis. *Am J Med* 79:284-288, 1985 B.

Pak CYC, et al: Long-term treatment of calcium nephrolithiasis with potassium citrate. *J Urol* 134:11-19, 1985 C.

Pak CYC, et al: Successful management of uric acid nephrolithiasis with potassium citrate. *Kidney Int* 30:422-428, 1986 A.

Pak CYC, et al: Management of cystine nephrolithiasis with alpha-mercaptopropionylglycine. *J Urol* 136:1003-1008, 1986 B.

Pak CYC, et al: Physicochemical action of potassium-magnesium citrate in nephrolithiasis. *J Bone Miner Res* 7:281-285, 1992.

Palmer JM: Administration of 10% Renacidin for renal stones in ambulatory patients, in White RWdeV, Palmer JM (eds): *New Techniques in Urology*. Mount Kisco, NY, Futura, 1987, 73-87.

Polinsky MS, et al: Urolithiasis in childhood. *Pediatr Clin North Am* 34:683-710, 1987.

Preminger GM: Pharmacologic treatment of uric acid calculi. *Urol Clin North Am* 14:335-338, 1987.

Preminger GM: The metabolic evaluation of patients with recurrent nephrolithiasis: A review of comprehensive and simplified approaches. *J Urol* 141(part 2):760-763, 1989.

Preminger GM, Pak CYC: Eventual attenuation of hypocalciuric response to hydrochlorothiazide in absorptive hypercalciuria. *J Urol* 137:1104-1109, 1987.

Preminger GM, et al: Prevention of recurrent calcium stone formation with potassium citrate therapy in patients with distal renal tubular acidosis. *J Urol* 134:20-23, 1985.

Preminger GM, et al: Alkali action on urinary crystallization of calcium salts: Contrasting responses to sodium citrate and potassium citrate. *J Urol* 139:240-242, 1988.

Roberts DH, Knox FG: Renal phosphate handling and calcium nephrolithiasis: Role of dietary phosphate and phosphate leak. *Semin Nephrol* 10:24-30, 1990.

Robertson WG, et al: The effect of high animal protein intake on the risk of calcium stone formation in the urinary tract. *Clin Sci* 57:285-288, 1979.

Rodman JS: Prophylaxis of uric acid stones with alternate day doses of alkaline potassium salts. *J Urol* 145:97-99, 1991.

Rodman JS, et al: Dissolution of uric acid calculi. *J Urol* 131:1039-1044, 1984.

Rodriguez PN, Klein AS: Management of urolithiasis during pregnancy. *Surg Gynecol Obstet* 166:103-106, 1988.

Rose GA, Samuell CT: Hyperoxaluric states, in Rous SN (ed): *Stone Disease: Diagnosis and Management*. Orlando, Grune & Stratton, 1987, 177-205.

Rudman D, et al: Hypocitruria in patients with gastrointestinal malabsorption. *N Engl J Med* 303:657-661, 1980.

Saita H, et al: Ultrasound diagnosis of ureteral stones: Its usefulness with subsequent excretory urography. *J Urol* 140:28-31, 1988.

Sakhaee K, et al: Contrasting effects of potassium citrate and sodium citrate therapies on urinary chemistries and crystallization of stone-forming salts. *Kidney Int* 24:348-352, 1983.

Sakhaee K, et al: Assessment of the pathogenetic role of physical exercise in renal stone formation. *J Clin Endocrinol Metab* 65:974-979, 1987.

Sakhaee K, et al: Spectrum of metabolic abnormalities in patients with cystine nephrolithiasis. *J Urol* 141:819-821, 1989.

Sakhaee K, et al: Contrasting effects of various potassium salts on renal citrate excretion. *J Clin Endocrinol Metab* 72:396-400, 1991.

Sakhaee K, et al: Citraturic response to oral citric acid load. *J Urol* 147:975-976, 1992.

Saltzman N, Gittes RF: Chemolysis of cystine calculi. *J Urol* 136:846-849, 1986.

Sanahuja J, et al: Intramuscular diclofenac sodium versus intravenous Baralgin in the treatment of renal colic. *DICP* 24:361-364, 1990.

Scheinman JI: Primary hyperoxaluria: Therapeutic strategies for the 90's. *Kidney Int* 40:389-399, 1991.

Schmeller NT, et al: Combination of chemolysis and shock wave lithotripsy in treatment of cystine renal calculi. *J Urol* 131:434-438, 1984.

Seftel A, Resnick MI: Metabolic evaluation of urolithiasis. *Urol Clin North Am* 17:159-169, 1990.

Shortliffe LMD, Spigelman SS: Infection stones: Evaluation and management. *Urol Clin North Am* 13:717-726, 1986.

Silver J, et al: Sodium-dependent idiopathic hypercalciuria in renal-stone formers. *Lancet* 2:484-486, 1983.

Silverberg SJ, et al: Nephrolithiasis and bone involvement in primary hyperparathyroidism. *Am J Med* 89:327-334, 1990.

Simon DI, et al: Sulfadiazine crystalluria revisited: The treatment of *Toxoplasma* encephalitis in patients with acquired immunodeficiency syndrome. *Arch Intern Med* 150:2379-2384, 1990.

Simpson DP: Citrate excretion: A window on renal metabolism. *Am J Physiol* 244:F223-F234, 1983.

Singer A, Das S: Cystinuria: Review of the pathophysiology and management. *J Urol* 142:669-673, 1989.

Smith LH: Enteric hyperoxaluria and other hyperoxaluric states, in Coe FL, et al (eds): *Contemporary Issues in Nephrology.* New York, Churchill Livingstone, 1980, vol 5, 136-164.

Smith LH: The medical aspects of urolithiasis: An overview. *J Urol* 141 (part 2):707-710, 1989.

Smith LH, et al: Nutrition and urolithiasis. *N Engl J Med* 298:87-89, 1978.

Spirnak JP, et al: Complex struvite calculi treated by primary extracorporeal shock wave lithotripsy and chemolysis with hemiacidrin irrigation. *J Urol* 140:1356-1359, 1988.

Stapleton FB: Nephrolithiasis in children. *Pediatr Rev* 11:21-30, 1989.

Stapleton FB: Idiopathic hypercalciuria: Association with isolated hematuria and risk for urolithiasis in children. *Kidney Int* 37:807-811, 1990.

Steinmuller DR: Primary hyperoxaluria: Frequently unappreciated cause of chronic renal failure. *Cleve Clin Q* 52:27-30, 1985.

Streem SB: Kidney stones: How new technology has improved management. *Postgrad Med* 84:77-89, (Dec) 1988.

Streem SB, Lammert G: Long-term efficacy of combination therapy for struvite staghorn calculi. *J Urol* 147:563-566, 1992.

Tawashi R, et al: Calcium oxalate crystal growth in normal urine: Role of contraceptive hormones. *Urol Res* 12:7-9, 1984.

Thomas WC Jr: Use of phosphates in patients with calcareous renal calculi. *Kidney Int* 13:390-396, 1978.

Uribarri J, et al: The first kidney stone. *Ann Intern Med* 111:1006-1009, 1989.

Urivetzky M, et al: Absence of effect of allopurinol on oxalate excretion by stone patients on random and controlled diets. *J Urol* 144:97-98, 1990 A.

Urivetzky M, et al: Biochemical evaluation of calcium stone patients: How soon can it be done after stone surgery/passage? *Urology* 36:410-414, 1990 B.

Urivetzky M, et al: Urinary excretion of oxalate by patients with renal hypercalciuric stone disease: Effect of chronic treatment with hydrochlorothiazide. *Urology* 37:327-330, 1991.

Urivetzky M, et al: Ascorbic acid overdosing: A risk factor for calcium oxalate nephrolithiasis. *J Urol* 147:1215-1218, 1992.

van Beresteijn ECH, et al: Relationship between the calcium-to-protein ratio in milk and the urinary calcium excretion in healthy adults: A controlled crossover study. *Am J Clin Nutr* 52:142-146, 1990.

Wasserstein AG, et al: Case-control study of risk factors for idiopathic calcium nephrolithiasis. *Miner Electrolyte Metab* 13:85-95, 1987.

Watts RWE, Mansell MA: Oxalate, livers, and kidneys. *BMJ* 301:772-773, 1990.

Weiss GH, et al: Changes in urinary magnesium, citrate, and oxalate levels due to cola consumption. *Urology* 39:331-333, 1992.

Williams HE, Wandzilak TR: Oxalate synthesis, transport and the hyperoxaluric syndromes. *J Urol* 141 (part 2):742-747, 1989.

Williams JJ, et al: Randomized double-blind study of acetohydroxamic acid in struvite nephrolithiasis. *N Engl J Med* 311:760-764, 1984.

Williams-Larson AW: Urinary calculi associated with purine metabolism: Uric acid nephrolithiasis. *Endocrinol Metab Clin North Am* 19:821-838, 1990.

Wills MR, et al: The interrelationships of calcium and sodium excretion. *Clin Sci* 37:621-630, 1969.

Wilson DM: Clinical and laboratory approaches for evaluation of nephrolithiasis. *J Urol* 141 (part 2):770-774, 1989.

Wilson DM: Clinical and laboratory evaluation of renal stone patients. *Endocrinol Metab Clin North Am* 19:773-803, 1990.

Wong S, et al: Metabolic studies in kidney stone disease. *Q J Med* 82:247-258, (March) 1992.

Yamamoto T, et al: The effect of completely purine-free diet of low sodium content on purine intermediates and end-product. *Eur J Clin Nutr* 44:659-664, 1990.

Zechner D, et al: Nutritional risk factors in urinary stone disease. *J Urol* 125:51-54, 1981.

Zusman CJ, et al (eds): Calcium oxalate nephrolithiasis: Defective oxalate transport, nephrology forum. *Kidney Int* 39:1283-1298, 1991.

Drugs Used in Disorders of the Upper Gastrointestinal Tract

42

PEPTIC ULCER DISEASE

Etiology

Peptic (gastric, duodenal, and esophageal) ulcers occur in areas of the gastrointestinal tract exposed to acid and pepsin and result from an imbalance between the erosive action of acid and pepsin on the one hand and the gastroduodenal mucosal defense system on the other. Although high acid output appears to be an important causative factor in duodenal ulcers, it cannot explain the development of ulcer in every patient (Soll, 1989, 1990 A). Nocturnal acid secretion, rather than total acid output, appears to be of particular importance in the pathogenesis of duodenal ulcers. Furthermore, an individual's ability to neutralize acid delivered to the duodenum may be impaired by inadequate duodenal bicarbonate secretion. In patients with gastric ulcers, however, acid output is normal or reduced, which suggests that altered mucosal resistance is a primary factor in their development. Use of aspirin and other nonsteroidal anti-inflammatory drugs (NSAIDs), smoking, genetic factors, and environmental influences also may contribute to the development of chronic peptic ulcers.

Although antral gastritis is associated with both gastric and duodenal ulcers, the pathogenic relationship has been controversial; the relationship between duodenitis and duodenal ulcer also has not been established. The bacterium, *Helicobacter pylori,* has been isolated in the gastric antrum in a substantial proportion of patients with type B gastritis or with gastric and duodenal ulcers. Colonization of the gastric antrum by *H. pylori* appears to be a major cause of type B antral gastritis and possibly gastric ulcer and may be associated with increased risk of gastric cancer (Taylor and Milne, 1992; Forman, 1991). Similarly, colonization of the duodenum by *H. pylori* (after gastric metaplasia occurs) may contribute to the pathogenesis of duodenal ulcer.

More than 90% of duodenal ulcers and 65% to 70% of gastric ulcers occur in *H. pylori*-positive patients. If gastric ulcers associated with drug therapy (eg, NSAIDs) are excluded, the prevalence of gastric ulcers increases to 90%, which parallels that of duodenal ulcers in these patients (Goodman and Lisowski, 1991). However, since most people infected with this organism do not develop peptic ulcer, it appears that other undetermined risk factors must be present for *H. pylori* to cause ulcers. The organisms can be identified by culture, isolation, and visualization in gastric or duodenal biopsy specimens; by serologic testing; and by the urease breath assay or biochemical assays based on the presence of urease, which catalyzes the conversion of urea to ammonia.

Management

The goals of peptic ulcer therapy are to decrease or abolish symptoms, to hasten healing, to prevent serious complications (hemorrhage, perforation, and obstruction), and to prevent recurrences. These goals usually can be achieved with drug therapy and the avoidance of precipitating or aggravating substances.

DIETARY MEASURES. There is little evidence that any single dietary factor influences the healing of peptic ulcers, and the so-called "ulcer diet" consisting of bland soft foods with milk or cream does not affect the rate of healing or recurrence. However, foods, spices, and liquids that provoke or worsen symptoms should be avoided, and patients should eat three meals a day that comprise a balanced diet of their choosing. Unless an H_2 receptor antagonist or proton pump inhibitor (eg, omeprazole [Prilosec]) is taken concomitantly, a small snack at bedtime may be harmful, since it stimulates nocturnal acid secretion.

Although the ingestion of milk is advocated by some authorities (Lewis, 1983), its value is controversial. It is sometimes recommended that coffee (both caffeinated and decaffeinated), tea, cola drinks, and acidic juices be avoided, but evidence that these beverages are harmful is lacking. Moderate alcohol intake with meals does not aggravate symptoms or delay healing.

AVOIDANCE OF DAMAGING DRUGS. Nonsteroidal Anti-Inflammatory Drugs (NSAIDs): These drugs aggravate mucosal damage, delay healing, and/or predispose to bleeding, and thus they should be avoided in all patients with peptic ulcer. Prolonged ingestion of NSAIDs is one of the primary causes of gastric ulcer and, to a lesser extent, of duodenal ulcer (more than 10% of these patients have an endoscopically verified peptic ulcer) and is a principal reason for lack of healing of these ulcers. Chronic use of NSAIDs has increased significantly in recent years, particularly in the elderly, and the frequency of upper gastrointestinal bleeding and perforated peptic ulcer in these patients, especially elderly women, is disproportionately high. These life-threatening complications often occur without prior warning and may be the first clear indications of the presence of an ulcer (Graham, 1989).

In any patient with a duodenal or gastric ulcer that does not heal after adequate therapy, the ingestion of aspirin or other NSAIDs as well as the presence of a gastrinoma (eg, Zollinger-Ellison syndrome) should be considered as possible causes.

Assessment of the potential that any given NSAID has for producing gastrointestinal damage must take into account the fact that lack of acute damage to the gastrointestinal mucosa does not prove that these agents have no long-term effect on the gastrointestinal tract. Moreover, the higher doses of NSAIDs used for the treatment of arthritis may not provide additional significant therapeutic benefit for some individuals and are associated with a higher percentage of adverse reactions, especially peptic ulcer. Relief of pain in some patients can be achieved at doses lower than those presently used (Graham, 1989).

A systemic effect of absorbed NSAIDs, disruption of mucosal defense mechanisms (eg, disturbance of endogenous prostaglandin synthesis and turnover), is a likely cause of gastric ulcer; direct local mucosal damage produced by unabsorbed drug may not be a critical factor in pathogenesis. This would explain the ability of prostaglandin derivatives (eg, misoprostol [Cytotec]) to prevent NSAID-induced gastric ulcer and the inability of H_2 receptor blocking drugs to do the same (Barrier and Hirschowitz, 1989). Patients who should receive misoprostol prophylaxis include those at high risk for ulcer formation or for the complications of peptic ulcer (eg, the elderly, patients with debilitating disease) (Graham 1989; Jones and Schubert, 1991; Smith, 1991). H_2 receptor blockers are as effective as misoprostol for prophylaxis in patients receiving NSAIDs who have a history of duodenal ulcer.

Once an ulcer has formed following NSAID therapy, H_2 receptor antagonists and other commonly used antiulcer agents (eg, sucralfate [Carafate], antacids) should be used in preference to misoprostol. Any of these agents usually will heal the ulcer if NSAID treatment is withdrawn. In patients who continue to use NSAIDs, omeprazole promotes healing of ulcers more effectively than the H_2 receptor antagonists (Walt, 1992).

The presence of *H. pylori* and NSAID administration may be independent rather than additive risk factors for peptic ulcer formation. When treated with NSAIDs, patients who are positive for *H. pylori* may be at much higher risk of developing gastrointestinal complications than those who are *H. pylori* negative (Ryan, 1991).

Corticosteroids: Corticosteroids appear to enhance peptic ulcer formation in patients receiving NSAIDs concomitantly (Guslandi and Tittobello, 1992). Low doses of corticosteroids may be used with caution in these patients, although it should be borne in mind that corticosteroids may mask symptoms of perforation and other complications (Shearman and Finlayson, 1982).

AVOIDANCE OF SMOKING. The incidence of peptic ulcer is higher in smokers than in nonsmokers. Cigarette smoking also delays healing, may increase the rate of recurrence, increases the need for and risks associated with surgery, and may decrease the effectiveness of cimetidine and other antiulcer medications (McCarthy, 1984; Soll, 1990 A). Thus, patients with peptic ulcers should avoid smoking.

CONTROL OF EMOTIONAL FACTORS. Emotional factors (anxiety, stress) may contribute to the development of peptic ulcers in some patients (Peters and Richardson, 1983; Soll, 1989), but they are not a primary cause. However, anxiety and stress may hasten recurrence of active peptic ulcer disease. The resolution of problems that contribute to emotional distress may reduce the extent and frequency of pain. The physician's reassurance often relieves anxiety and promotes compliance.

Treatment of anxiety disorders should be independent of peptic ulcer treatment. Adjunctive use of diazepam [Valium] or another antianxiety agent occasionally may be useful (Gillespie et al, 1983).

***ERADICATION OF* HELICOBACTER PYLORI.** *H. pylori* appears to be a major cause of chronic type B antral gastritis. Although *H. pylori* has been identified in more than 90% of patients with duodenal ulcer and in 65% to 70% of those with gastric ulcer, investigators who believe that it has a primary role in the development of peptic ulcer disorders could not explain why this organism is also present in more than 50% of asymptomatic individuals with no evidence of peptic ulcer (McKinlay et al, 1990). Nevertheless, it is becoming increasingly apparent that eradication of *H. pylori* prevents relapse of duodenal ulcer and that, in the absence of this organism, the ulcer does not recur (Rauws and Tytgat, 1990; Oderda et al, 1990; Caldwell and Marshall, 1989; Graham et al, 1992 A; Walsh, 1992); this may also be true for gastric ulcer (Graham et al, 1992 A).

Increasing evidence suggests that reinfection with *H. pylori* may be rare and that the relapse of a peptic ulcer results from inadequate eradication. In the absence of NSAID administration or other known ulcerogenic factors, eradication may cure peptic ulcer (Borody et al, 1992).

Drug Therapy

Peptic ulcers usually have a benign prognosis and may be self-limiting. Almost all patients can be treated successfully with drugs and alteration of lifestyle; surgery may be required for those with ulcer complications and those refractory to drug therapy. Most therapeutic failures are due to inadequate therapy, noncompliance, or incorrect diagnosis. The possibility that gastric carcinoma or other serious diseases are present also, must be considered in patients with gastric ulcer.

Drugs that promote healing in acid peptic disorders reduce gastric acidity or enhance mucosal defense systems (Grossman et al, 1981; Soll, 1990 A, 1990 B). Peptic ulcers usually can be healed by single-drug therapy with an H_2 receptor antagonist (cimetidine [Tagamet], ranitidine [Zantac], famotidine [Pepcid], nizatidine [Axid]), omeprazole, or sucralfate. However, when drug therapy is discontinued, peptic ulcers recur within two years in 70% to 95% of patients, and they may recur even during maintenance therapy. H_2 receptor antagonists have been drugs of choice to prevent recurrence of gastric or duodenal ulcer.

For eradication of *H. pylori* in peptic ulcer disorders, oral administration of bismuth salts (eg, colloidal bismuth subcitrate, bismuth subsalicylate [Pepto-Bismol]) with the antimicrobial agent metronidazole and the antibiotics amoxicillin or tetracycline (referred to as triple therapy) is being investigated. This combination has eradicated *H. pylori* and healed chronic type B gastritis and duodenal ulcer in 90% to 95% of affected patients. In clinical trials, combined therapy has been as effective as standard antiulcer therapy (eg, H_2 receptor blockers, antacids, sucralfate) in producing initial healing (Borody et al, 1989) and in preventing relapse of duodenal and gastric ulcer (Graham et al, 1992 A). However, the long-term safety and benefits of combination therapy have not been established, and at present use of this approach for the initial healing of peptic ulcer should be limited to controlled clinical trials.

GUIDELINES FOR THERAPEUTIC MANAGEMENT OF UNCOMPLICATED PEPTIC ULCER. Assessment of the effectiveness of drug therapy is more difficult for gastric than duodenal ulcers. Evidence from many controlled studies suggests that the rate of healing of gastric ulcers equals that of duodenal ulcers when patients follow prescribed regimens (Isenberg et al, 1983; Jadhav and Freston, 1983). The chief differences in therapy involve frequency of administration, dosage, and the endpoint of treatment. The following are guidelines for treatment of patients with uncomplicated gastric and duodenal ulcers:

1. Discontinue all ulcerogenic drugs and cigarette smoking.
2. Prescribe cimetidine, ranitidine, famotidine, nizatidine, sucralfate, antacids, or omeprazole. Results of numerous well-controlled studies have demonstrated endoscopically confirmed healing of duodenal ulcer after four to six weeks of daily treatment with the above agents in most patients; healing of gastric ulcer generally requires 8 to 12 weeks.
3. Therapy can relieve pain rapidly. Patients usually are asymptomatic long before healing occurs. In duodenal ulcer, discontinue drug therapy after six weeks if all symptoms have disappeared, although healing may not be complete in some individuals. For patients with gastric ulcers, confirm healing, preferably by endoscopy, after eight weeks of therapy.

The results of radiologic examinations and the improvement of symptoms do not always reflect the extent of healing of peptic ulcer. Unhealed ulcers can be observed endoscopically in asymptomatic patients, and healed peptic ulcers may be seen in patients still experiencing pain and other symptoms (Isenberg et al, 1983). Unhealed gastric ulcers should be investigated for possible malignancy.

4. Further treatment depends on whether the ulcer produces symptoms, heals completely, or recurs. Patients usually are re-evaluated upon recurrence of symptoms. If the ulcer recurs during the first three or four months, prescribe a full course of drug therapy for four weeks. If the ulcer does not heal, enlarges, or recurs frequently, substitute another drug or combination of drugs or consider *H. pylori* eradication therapy. In therapeutic failures, evaluate compliance, adequacy of dosage, use of NSAIDs, and the possibility of an incorrect diagnosis (eg, gastric cancer). After healing, evaluate the patient at three-month intervals for one year.
5. Bleeding stops spontaneously in approximately 90% of patients with bleeding ulcers. Surgery may be required for intractable bleeding or perforation.

MAINTENANCE THERAPY TO PREVENT RECURRENCE. Whether maintenance therapy should be instituted or drugs withdrawn after peptic ulcer has healed is unclear. Up to one-third of patients may never have a recurrence. Maintenance therapy with H_2 receptor antagonists, sucralfate, or omeprazole usually prevents recurrence of a duodenal ulcer only as long as treatment continues (success rate, 65% to 90%); 5% to 10% of patients may have a relapse despite continued maintenance therapy, and 70% to 95% of untreated patients will relapse within two years (Cave, 1992; Graham et al, 1992 B). Therapy beyond one year is recommended in elderly, debilitated, or other poor-risk patients with duodenal ulcer or in those with prior duodenal ulcer complications such as bleeding or perforation. For gastric ulcer, evidence supporting the value of maintenance therapy with cimetidine or ranitidine beyond one year is not as strong. In one study, the significant prophylactic effect of cimetidine was maintained after one year, but there was little benefit beyond two years (Barr et al, 1983).

For maintenance, one-half the dose used for initial healing is usually sufficient to prevent relapse. However, some patients require the same dose utilized for initial healing, especially those whose ulcer healed slowly and/or who are hypersecretors (Cave, 1992). In two studies in patients with uncomplicated ulcer, a single daily dose of cimetidine 400 mg at bedtime (duodenal ulcer) or two doses daily, one in the morning and one at bedtime (gastric or duodenal ulcer), prevented recurrences in more than 80% of patients for at least one year (Barr et al, 1983; Jadhav and Freston, 1983). For patients experiencing infrequent, uncomplicated recurrences of duodenal ulcer, some practitioners recommend full-dose treatment when symptoms recur, with the drug not given between relapses.

Although it is generally recommended that *H. pylori* eradication therapy be limited to controlled clinical trials, some authorities now endorse consideration of this therapy in the following patients: (1) those with duodenal ulcer who are *H. pylori*-positive (Graham, 1993), (2) those with peptic ulcer who have more than one relapse per year, (3) those who are resistant to H_2 receptor blockers or proton pump inhibitors, (4) those who relapse during therapy with these two classes of antisecretory drugs, (5) those in whom compliance for initial treatment is poor or who refuse long-term maintenance therapy, (6) those with ulcer-associated complications (eg, bleeding, perforation), and (7) those with symptoms severe enough for surgery to be considered (Graham et al, 1992 A; Walsh, 1992).

H. pylori eradication therapy presently being investigated consists of combined use of two or more drugs, one of which is an antibiotic. Such combinations decrease resistance and enhance eradication. H_2 receptor antagonists have no effect on *H. pylori* but are useful in combination with regimens (eg, triple therapy) that eradicate this organism and prevent peptic ulcer recurrence (Graham et al, 1992 A); combined use may shorten the time required for eradication.

In a major long-term study in patients with peptic ulcer, administration of ranitidine (300 mg once daily for up to 16 weeks) healed the ulcers but did not eradicate *H. pylori* in any patient. In contrast, the organism was eradicated in 90% of those who received triple therapy (bismuth subsalicylate, five or eight 262-mg tablets daily; metronidazole, 250 mg three times daily; tetracycline, 500 mg four times daily) plus ranitidine for the first two weeks of therapy. One year after initial healing, recurrence was observed in 95% of duodenal ulcer patients, in 74% of gastric ulcer patients who had received only ranitidine, but in only 12% to 13% of those who had been treated with ranitidine and triple therapy (Graham et al, 1992 A). These data suggest a relationship between the presence of *H. pylori* and ulcer recurrence.

It is unclear if therapy to eradicate *H. pylori* will gain widespread acceptance. The chief drawbacks include compliance with this complicated regimen; adverse reactions (chiefly gastrointestinal disturbances), which also limit compliance; and development of resistance by *H. pylori*, particularly to metronidazole. The use of omeprazole or sucralfate with antibiotics as well as other combinations also are being investigated (Hentschel et al, 1993; Marshall, 1993). To increase the acceptability of eradication therapy, medication with a well-tolerated, simplified dosage regimen must be developed.

REFRACTORY ULCERS AND GASTRIC ACID HYPERSECRETORY DISORDERS. Until the introduction of omeprazole, single-drug therapy was generally unsuccessful for many patients with intractable peptic ulcer, the Zollinger-Ellison syndrome, multiple endocrine adenomas, systemic mastocytosis, or other gastric acid hypersecretory disorders. A single daily dose of omeprazole adequately controls acid output in most of these patients and is regarded as a major therapeutic advance (Decktor and Robinson, 1990; Lindberg et al, 1990). The dose should be titrated for each patient using gastric acid secretion (basal <5 mEq/hour before the next dose) as the endpoint. If the gastrinoma can be resected, cure of the Zollinger-Ellison syndrome can be anticipated in up to 20% to 30% of patients.

The somatostatin analogue, octreotide [Sandostatin], may suppress elevated gastrin levels for prolonged periods and provide significant symptomatic relief in carefully selected patients with the Zollinger-Ellison syndrome (Mozell et al, 1992). Unlike omeprazole, octreotide inhibits both gastric acid and gastrin production; this drug also inhibits secondary peptides released by gastrinomas. However, because it must be given intravenously and is very expensive, use of octreotide may be impractical.

COMBINATION THERAPY. For most patients with uncomplicated gastric or duodenal ulcer, the use of cimetidine, ranitidine, famotidine, nizatidine, or sucralfate in any combination is costly and yields no additional therapeutic advantage while subjecting the recipient to possible additional adverse effects of combination regimens.

In some patients with intractable peptic ulcers, the Zollinger-Ellison syndrome, multiple endocrine adenomas, systemic mastocytosis, or other gastric acid hypersecretory disorders, various drug combinations were investigated prior to the introduction of omeprazole. At present, no combination is recommended since all patients will respond to an adequate dose of omeprazole.

Drug Selection

Factors to consider when selecting a specific drug for ulcer therapy include ease of administration, incidence and severity of adverse effects, availability, and cost. Similar rates of healing (75% to 85%) for peptic ulcer disease are reported for cimetidine, ranitidine, famotidine, nizatidine, sucralfate, antacids, and a number of investigational agents (eg, tripotassium dicitrato bismuthate [colloidal bismuth compound]). Omeprazole is the most efficacious single drug; the rate of healing has been reported to be up to 100% after four weeks of therapy.

HISTAMINE$_2$ RECEPTOR ANTAGONISTS. Cimetidine, ranitidine, famotidine, and nizatidine currently are the drugs of choice for initial treatment and maintenance therapy in most patients with uncomplicated gastric or duodenal ulcer. Studies indicate that a single bedtime dose of cimetidine 800 mg, ranitidine 300 mg, nizatidine 300 mg, or famotidine 40 mg is as efficacious as previously recommended multidose regimens and increases compliance (Gledhill et al, 1983; Gitlin et al, 1987). Ranitidine and cimetidine are currently the most widely used antiulcer medications. However, up to 20% of patients do not respond or respond slowly. In these individuals, use of the H_2 receptor antagonist can be extended an additional six weeks beyond the usual recommended duration of therapy for peptic ulcer; most ulcers heal within 4 to 12 weeks. If patients do not respond to this regimen, another drug (eg, omeprazole) should be tried and the patient evaluated for noncompliance, use of NSAIDs, or presence of gastrinoma (eg, Zollinger-Ellison syndrome). H_2 receptor antagonists have no proven value in terminating hemorrhage in patients with bleeding peptic ulcers.

The overall incidence of adverse reactions to cimetidine is low. Elderly and debilitated individuals, patients with impaired renal function, and those who require prolonged therapy with large doses are the most likely to experience side effects (see the evaluation). Another H_2 receptor antagonist may be preferred for these patients and those who respond poorly.

Ranitidine is about three times more potent than cimetidine, has little antiandrogenic activity (and thus produces gynecomastia only rarely), does not markedly inhibit hepatic drug metabolizing enzymes, and causes fewer drug interactions than cimetidine (Konturek, 1982; Brogden et al, 1982). Larger doses than with cimetidine can be used in refractory patients because of the lower incidence of adverse reactions.

Famotidine is more potent than ranitidine and its duration of action is 30% longer (Friedman, 1987). Like ranitidine, famotidine does not cause antiandrogenic side effects or interfere with hepatic oxidative metabolism. Although reported reactions to famotidine are rare, more experience must be obtained before the effects of long-term use can be assessed.

Nizatidine's potency in inhibiting gastric acid secretion and its efficacy in acid-peptic disorders appear to be similar to those of ranitidine. As with famotidine, few adverse reactions have been reported and drug metabolism has not been affected (Stern, 1988).

If large doses (twice the usual amount) of an H_2 receptor antagonist are required, omeprazole probably should be substituted.

Although some concern has been expressed, the available H_2 receptor blockers are not carcinogenic.

SUCRALFATE. Sucralfate, a sulfated sucrose-aluminum hydroxide complex, is as effective as cimetidine in healing duodenal ulcers. Its value in long-term maintenance therapy to prevent recurrence of duodenal ulcers has been established, but prevention of gastric ulcer recurrence has not been clearly documented. A number of diverse actions contribute to its effects; the exact mechanism of action is not known (Szabo and Hollander, 1989). Sucralfate's chief advantage is lack of significant absorption and, hence, the absence of systemic adverse reactions; constipation and other minor gastrointestinal disturbances are noted infrequently.

PROTON PUMP INHIBITORS. Omeprazole represents a new class of gastric acid inhibitors, the substituted benzimidazoles. It is considerably more potent than the H_2 receptor antagonists and markedly inhibits gastric acid secretion by inhibiting the H^+/K^+ ATPase proton pump in parietal cells. Omeprazole may be particularly effective in healing peptic ulcer or reflux esophagitis that is unresponsive to the H_2 receptor antagonists (Howden, 1991). It also has been highly effective and is the drug of choice for patients with the Zollinger-Ellison syndrome, some of whom had symptoms that were resistant to large doses of H_2 antagonists (Maton et al, 1989; Maton, 1991).

Concern about the long-term use of omeprazole has been raised because of its dramatic effects on gastric acid secretion. Large doses administered lifelong to rats caused gastric carcinoid tumors (Ekman et al, 1985). These tumors appeared to be related to the achlorhydria and resulting hypergastrinemia produced by the drug. This may not be a significant problem in humans (Decktor and Robinson, 1990; Lindberg et al, 1990; Maton et al, 1989, 1990). However, the issue of long-term safety of this drug has been clouded by a report on the development of hyperplastic gastric polyps with no sign of dysplasia or malignancy in three patients treated with omeprazole 20 mg/day for one year (Graham, 1992). Increasing evidence suggests that fear of this and other significant long-term adverse reactions may be groundless (Joelson et al, 1992). See the evaluation.

Lansoprazole [Prevacid], an investigational proton pump inhibitor, has actions, indications, efficacy, and safety similar to those of omeprazole (Barradell et al, 1992; Sekiguchi et al, 1992).

ANTACIDS. Although they are effective and less expensive than other antiulcer drugs, the routine use of antacids in the treatment of peptic ulcer is questionable; many authorities believe that these agents should be used only occasionally for the relief of pain. This should be borne in mind when reading the following discussion.

In several controlled studies, an adequate antacid regimen was as effective as cimetidine in patients with gastric or duodenal ulcer. For uncomplicated duodenal ulcer, an intensive course of liquid antacid (144 mEq of acid neutralizing capacity one and three hours after meals and at bedtime, total 1,008 mEq/day) may be required (Peterson et al, 1977), although considerably smaller amounts are often effective. Tablets appear to be as effective as liquid preparations. In one study, a low-dose regimen of antacid tablets (14 tablets, 280 mEq total daily dose) was as effective as ranitidine in healing duodenal ulcers (Berstad et al, 1982). However, when antacids are used for initial healing, the frequent administration required, lack of palatability, and side effects (diarrhea, constipation) reduce patient compliance significantly, particularly when ulcer symptoms are absent.

Because of the low gastric acidity usually associated with gastric ulcer, relatively low-dose regimens (275 to 375 mEq) of a liquid antacid containing aluminum and magnesium hydroxides heal a significant percentage of gastric ulcers (Romankiewicz and Reidenberg, 1981; Isenberg et al, 1983).

Antacids also may be used with H_2 receptor antagonists or sucralfate in patients with uncomplicated peptic ulcers but only as required to relieve pain in the initial stages of therapy.

Poorly absorbed antacids are preferred in the treatment of peptic ulcer. Certain highly concentrated aluminum and magnesium combinations appear to have a prolonged duration of action and beneficial effects on pH. Mixtures of aluminum oxide-hydroxide and magnesium oxide-hydroxide are used most frequently. Calcium carbonate has a greater neutralizing capacity, but its utilization has decreased because of absorption of calcium, concern regarding possible acid rebound, and the formation of kidney stones.

Sodium bicarbonate, which is an active ingredient of some proprietary preparations, is very soluble and has an immediate and pronounced neutralizing effect, but its duration of action is extremely brief. Because sodium bicarbonate produces metabolic alkalosis when used excessively or in patients with impaired renal function, it must not be taken for long periods. This antacid should not be used routinely in the management of peptic ulcer and is contraindicated in patients requiring a low-sodium diet.

For additional information on the available antacid preparations, see the discussion on Antacids in the evaluations section.

ANTICHOLINERGIC AGENTS. Anticholinergic drugs were important in peptic ulcer management before the introduction of the H_2 receptor antagonists. At present, these drugs have only a minor role and should be used only adjunctively with H_2 receptor antagonists or other agents in peptic ulcer disease if prescribed at all. The antisecretory action of the antimuscarinic anticholinergic drugs is less pronounced than that of the H_2 antagonists and they produce more side effects. (See index entry Antispasmodics.)

PROSTAGLANDINS. Misoprostol has antisecretory and protective effects in gastric and duodenal mucosa. It is the only clinically available prostaglandin analogue that prevents gastric and duodenal ulcer formation in patients receiving long-term therapy with aspirin and other NSAIDs (Dobrilla et al, 1989; Roth, 1990; Walt, 1992). Clinical trials indicate that misoprostol also is effective in healing duodenal and gastric ulcers (Monk and Clissold, 1987), but an H_2 receptor antagonist or sucralfate is preferred. Serious adverse effects are rare. Common minor adverse reactions include diarrhea and abdominal cramping. Because of the abortifacient potential of misoprostol, it is imperative to avoid use of this drug in pregnant women or those of childbearing potential.

INVESTIGATIONAL AGENT. *Tripotassium dicitrato bismuthate* (colloidal bismuth compound) has no significant acid neutralizing activity. At acid pH, it binds protein at the ulcer site and has a demulcent effect that forms a barrier against acid and pepsin. Part of its action appears to be due to its antibacterial effect on *H. pylori* (Lambert, 1990). This compound may be useful in treating gastric and duodenal ulcers (Wilson and Alp, 1982; Richardson and Peterson, 1982). Adverse reactions after short-term use are minimal; the stool is darkened. The adverse effects associated with therapy lasting longer than one year are unknown. Liquid preparations smell of ammonia.

ESOPHAGEAL DISORDERS

REFLUX ESOPHAGITIS. Unlike peptic ulcer, which is characterized by intermittent relapses and symptom-free intervals, chronic reflux esophagitis is an unremitting, essentially incurable disorder that quickly relapses on discontinuation of therapy with all currently available drugs. Many factors are thought to be important in the pathogenesis of reflux esophagitis and heartburn, the most common of which appears to be repeated transient relaxation of the lower esophageal sphincter (LES) not associated with swallowing (Dent, 1981; Holloway et al, 1981; Orr, 1992). Other factors include LES incompetence, impaired ability of the esophagus to clear refluxed material, low intraesophageal pH, delayed gastric emptying, and impaired resistance of the esophageal mucosa to injury.

Initial management should include elevation of the head of the bed; weight reduction in obese patients; elimination of tight garments; avoidance of heavy lifting; avoidance of large meals and of lying down for three to four hours after eating; and elimination of smoking, coffee, alcohol, chocolate, and other foods known to exacerbate symptoms.

Drug Therapy: It is a common misconception that the initial healing and maintenance doses employed in antisecretory regimens for peptic ulcer also are useful for reflux esophagitis. However, larger initial healing doses and much larger maintenance doses are generally required, and treatment must be lifelong.

Antacids or an antacid/alginic acid combination [Gaviscon] provide relief in many patients. Systemic agents are used concomitantly when the response to the above measures is inadequate. In one study, sucralfate was as effective as an antacid/alginic acid combination (Laitinen et al, 1985). However, although this drug appears to protect esophageal mucosa locally and is an attractive choice because of its lack of systemic adverse effects, many authorities believe that sucralfate may be no better than a placebo in patients with reflux esophagitis (Elsborg and Jorgensen, 1991). Others believe that symptomatic relief is possible in many patients but there is little endoscopic evidence of healing (Watson, 1992).

The H_2 antagonists, cimetidine and ranitidine, are often drugs of first choice to relieve symptoms. Although there are less data on famotidine and nizatidine, these drugs also can be effective. H_2 antagonists reduce gastric acid secretion but have no effect on LES pressure or esophageal motility. Antacid consumption is reduced significantly more than with a placebo. The rate of healing, as determined by endoscopy and biopsy, is not increased as much as relief of symptoms. Doses two to three times larger than those used for peptic ulcer healing are often necessary, especially in refractory patients. Such high-dose therapy is costly (up to $3,000/year).

Omeprazole heals esophageal lesions but is indicated only for patients with endoscopically verified esophageal erosions or ulcers that are not healed by H_2 receptor antagonists.

Drugs that improve esophageal motility (eg, bethanechol [Duvoid, Myotonachol, Urecholine], metoclopramide [Maxolon, Octamide PFS, Reglan], domperidone [Motilium] [investigational], cisapride [Propulsid] [investigational]) may provide symptomatic relief of heartburn, but their effects in healing esophageal lesions are marginal and not consistent (Lieberman, 1990). Metoclopramide may have some value in reflux esophagitis with delayed gastric emptying; however, adverse reactions (eg, extrapyramidal effects, drowsiness) may limit the value of this drug. Cisapride is a possible alternative to metoclopramide to enhance gastric emptying. This agent stimulates motility throughout the gastrointestinal tract, elevates LES pressure, and enhances esophageal acid clearance (Johnson, 1992). It may be useful primarily for maintenance therapy in patients with mild reflux esophagitis (Richter, 1992).

Since anticholinergic and calcium channel blocking agents may aggravate reflux and/or reduce saliva, which neutralizes acid, they are contraindicated in patients with this disorder.

Surgery: For patients refractory to drug therapy and young patients with severe disease who will need lifelong drug therapy, surgery is an alternative that often provides prolonged relief (Orr, 1992). Nissen fundoplication and other reflux procedures have yielded excellent results when performed by experienced surgeons.

ACHALASIA AND DIFFUSE ESOPHAGEAL SPASM. Dysphagia is a primary symptom of these disorders of motility. The dysphagia that accompanies motor disorders must be differentiated from that caused by mechanical obstruction of the esophagus due to rings, webs, strictures, and benign or malignant tumors (Meyer and Castell, 1981). Because chest pain is prominent in patients with diffuse esophageal spasm, many patients fear that the pain is cardiac in origin. Accurate diagnosis and patient reassurance are important.

Achalasia is much easier to diagnose and treat than diffuse esophageal spasm. Balloon (pneumatic) dilation or surgery (Heller myotomy) is often required in patients with achalasia (Achem and Kolts, 1992). Although both procedures are successful in most of these individuals, pneumatic dilation is preferred.

Bougie dilation, which may be repeated at intervals, relieves symptoms in many patients with diffuse esophageal spasm. Although it is often recommended that myotomy be avoided in these individuals because it may predispose to severe reflux and esophagitis, this procedure may be useful in selected patients (Ellis, 1992).

Drug Therapy: Drugs generally are not effective in patients with achalasia or diffuse esophageal spasm. The studies described in the following discussion were carried out under highly controlled laboratory conditions and are unlikely to have widespread clinical utility.

The calcium channel blocking agents have been investigated in patients with these disorders of esophageal motility (Achem and Kolts, 1992; Short and Thomas, 1992). Results of open clinical studies demonstrate that nifedipine [Procardia] reduced LES pressure (mean decrease, 58% to 70%), the frequency of spontaneous esophageal contractions, and the amplitude of distal peristaltic esophageal contractions in some patients with achalasia; this drug also decreased LES pressure and the amplitude and frequency of spasm in patients with diffuse esophageal spasm. Gastric emptying was not affected. Verapamil [Calan, Isoptin] and diltiazem [Cardizem] also are being evaluated for use in these disorders (Achem and Kolts, 1992; Short and Thomas, 1992). Although results of a number of studies are conflicting, some investigators believe that sublingual nifedipine (investigational route) may relieve dysphagia and is as effective as pneumatic dilation in patients with stage I and II achalasia (Coccia et al, 1991); they recommend a trial in patients with mild symptoms before pneumatic dilation is considered (Elta and Kochman, 1992; Bortolotti and Coccia, 1992). For additional information on these drugs, see index entry Calcium Channel Blocking Agents.

Isosorbide dinitrate [Isordil, Sorbitrate] has been evaluated in patients with achalasia or diffuse esophageal spasm. An open study (Gelfond et al, 1982) comparing isosorbide dinitrate 5 mg and nifedipine 20 mg in achalasia revealed that both drugs relieved dysphagia subjectively after sublingual administration. Isosorbide dinitrate reduced LES pressure more promptly and eliminated a radionuclide test meal from the esophagus more consistently, but side effects (dizziness, flushing, headache, fainting) were more troublesome.

STRESS ULCERATION AND HEMORRHAGE

The incidence of stress ulcers is high in critically ill patients with hepatic, respiratory, or renal failure; sepsis; burns over more than 35% of the body surface; head injury; or multiple trauma. In addition, some patients develop stress ulcers postoperatively. The major factor underlying the development of stress ulceration appears to be decreased gastric mucosal blood flow that impairs mucosal defenses. Patients with head injury, burns, or sepsis have increased gastric acid output, which also favors the development of ulcers. Although the net gastric acid output may be normal or low in most individuals with altered metabolic states, significant back diffusion of hydrogen ion can occur (Zinner et al, 1981). The inability of compromised or damaged gastric mucosa to tolerate acid appears to be more important than the amount of acid present (Levinson, 1989). In critically ill patients, hemorrhage from stress ulcers is a serious complication, and mortality rates greater than 50% have been reported when gastrointestinal bleeding is severe. Because overt bleeding is difficult to control, emphasis is placed on preventive measures (Zuckerman and Shuman, 1987).

Prophylaxis: *The incidence of upper gastrointestinal tract bleeding in critically ill patients can be greatly decreased by prevention of hypovolemia, systemic acidosis, sepsis, hypoalbuminemia, anemia, and malnutrition.* Patients receiving enteral nutrition are less susceptible to gastrointestinal hemorrhage and may not require prophylactic drug therapy (Pingleton, 1983; Levinson, 1989). The incidence of bleeding in those in intensive care units has decreased markedly with good general management, and bleeding and death in critically ill patients with stress ulcers have become rare (Tryba, 1990).

Pharmacologic prophylaxis is aimed at maintaining the intragastric pH above 4.0, although the evidence is not convincing that this is beneficial in preventing stress ulcer bleeding. Antacid therapy is more effective than placebo in both low-risk and critically ill high-risk patients. However, large doses must be administered by nasogastric intubation every one to two hours, and a high percentage of patients at risk cannot tolerate antacids because of severe diarrhea, hypophosphatemia, metabolic alkalosis, and aspiration (Pingleton, 1983). For these reasons, many physicians feel that prophylactic use of antacids is impractical (Koretz, 1990; Levinson, 1989; Peura, 1990).

Routine use of H_2 receptor antagonists or other drugs in critically ill patients is discouraged (Reusser et al, 1990; Reines, 1990) and may be justified only for a subgroup of critically ill patients with multiorgan failure (Koretz, 1990; Peura, 1990). In low-risk patients, most well-controlled studies indicate that cimetidine is superior to placebo and equivalent to intensive antacid therapy for prophylaxis of bleeding secondary to stress ulcer. Cimetidine has been administered in an intravenous bolus dose every four to six hours (McElwee et al, 1979; Halloran et al, 1980; Peura and Johnson, 1985), but continuous intravenous infusion of an H_2 receptor blocker is more effective than an intermittent bolus in maintaining the intragastric pH above 4.0 (Ostro et al, 1984; Siepler and Trudeau, 1984; Siepler et al, 1989). There have been fewer studies with ranitidine, but results to date are similar to those with cimetidine. Some physicians prefer ranitidine to cimetidine because the former appears to be safer in critically ill patients and produces fewer drug interactions. An H_2 receptor antagonist and an antacid are often combined for prophylactic therapy, but any additional benefit over use of a single agent is unproved and the incidence of adverse reactions may be increased. Neutralization of stomach acid by H_2 receptor antagonists or antacids can potentially cause nosocomial pneumonia.

Sucralfate in suspension form appears to be as effective as antacids and H_2 receptor blockers in preventing stress ulceration and hemorrhage. Its ease of administration, low incidence of adverse effects, and low cost make sucralfate a useful alternative to antacids and H_2 receptor antagonists (Borrero et al, 1985; Bresalier et al, 1987).

If the stomach is functionally normal, sucralfate, an H_2 receptor antagonist, or an antacid can be administered orally or by nasogastric tube. In patients with gastric dysfunction or damage, a parenteral H_2 receptor antagonist is preferable to sucralfate or an antacid (Koretz, 1990; Peura, 1990).

Treatment: It is difficult to assess the efficacy of drugs used to control hemorrhage since mild to moderate bleeding usually is self-limited and severe bleeding generally is refractory to drugs. Most of the evidence suggests that the intermittent or continuous intravenous administration of an H_2 receptor antagonist or oral administration of omeprazole is ineffective in treating acute gastrointestinal bleeding due to stress ulcers (Kandel, 1990; Daneshmend et al, 1992).

Intravenous tranexamic acid [Cyklokapron] blocks fibrinolytic activity and aborts sustained local hemorrhage. Results of a number of clinical trials have indicated that this agent is beneficial in some patients with gastrointestinal bleeding and may be more effective than H_2 receptor blockers. However, it is seldom used for this indication. No serious adverse effects requiring withdrawal of the drug have been reported. Tranexamic acid should be administered as soon as possible after diagnosis. It should be avoided in patients with thrombotic, coagulation, or bleeding disorders (Kandel, 1990).

DISORDERS OF GASTRIC EMPTYING

A variety of conditions are associated with delayed gastric emptying (eg, gastric atony, gastric outlet obstruction). Causes of this disorder include diabetic gastroparesis, vagotomy or partial gastric resection, active duodenal or pyloric ulcer, bile reflux gastritis, collagen diseases, primary anorexia nervosa, and electrolyte imbalance. All of these diseases produce nausea, vomiting, and abdominal distress (flatulence, bloating, epigastric fullness, or pain), which complicate their management.

The pathophysiology of the defect in gastric emptying is unclear. Various abnormalities in gastric muscle function at the cellular level, failure of neurohormonal feedback mechanisms (primarily vagal dysfunction), and psychogenic influences usually are involved (Malagelada, 1982; Heading, 1982; Domstad and Deland, 1982). Delayed emptying of solids due to absent or abnormal gastric antral contractions is characteristic of these disorders. Gastric emptying of liquids often is normal.

In diabetic gastroparesis, which is the most common cause of delayed gastric emptying, vomiting of food can result in insulin overdosage. Gastroparesis is probably due to neural regulatory dysfunction caused by enhanced sympathetic or decreased parasympathetic input to the gastric antrum. Most of these patients have long-standing insulin-dependent diabetes that has been poorly controlled for many years. In some patients, however, gastroparesis may be the only complication of diabetes.

Management: Management of diabetic gastroparesis and other disorders of delayed gastric emptying is similar. Hospitalization may be required if symptoms are frequent or severe. Nonpharmacologic measures include avoidance of anticholinergic drugs and ingestion of a liquid diet or homogenization of solid foods.

In most patients with mild symptoms, metoclopramide enhances gastric emptying and is the drug of choice. It is less useful for relief of severe symptoms. This drug improves gastric motility and acts centrally as an antiemetic (Harrington et al, 1983; Albibi and McCallum, 1983). (See the evaluation.)

Domperidone (investigational), an antidopaminergic drug with actions similar to those of metoclopramide, also has been used in disorders of delayed gastric emptying. It appears to be as efficacious as metoclopramide, although direct comparative studies of the two agents are lacking. Domperidone may have an advantage in long-term maintenance therapy because it causes fewer central nervous system and extrapyramidal side effects. However, a small number of patients experience side effects related to hyperprolactinemia (McCallum, 1985).

In initial studies, cisapride, an investigational prokinetic agent, appeared to be as efficacious as metoclopramide in enhancing gastric emptying and produced fewer side effects; however, in more recent studies, its efficacy has been questioned. Trials of these drugs, as well as dazopride, a substituted benzamide, and naloxone [Narcan], an opioid antagonist, are in progress.

Erythromycin is a specific motilin agonist that, like motilin, stimulates strong contractions of the gastric body and antrum.

Results of a number of investigational studies show that this antibiotic relieves gastroparesis in patients with diabetes or progressive systemic sclerosis (Janssens et al, 1990; Dull et al, 1990), and it may be effective in those who do not respond to metoclopramide.

In the presence of bowel stasis, bacterial overgrowth in the small bowel may aggravate gastrointestinal hypomotility. This can be diagnosed by employing the hydrogen breath test and should be treated with antibiotics. Erythromycin can be used to enhance motility and tetracycline to control bacterial overgrowth.

NONULCER DYSPEPSIA

Although lack of an adequate definition has hampered an understanding of nonulcer dyspepsia, most authorities agree that the term refers to a disorder that produces intermittent upper abdominal complaints, the cause of which cannot be determined by clinical evaluation (Lagarde and Spiro, 1984; Talley and Phillips, 1988). Most patients with nonulcer dyspepsia fall into one of the two large subgroups: those with the classic peptic ulcer symptoms of postprandial epigastric burning pain that is relieved by eating and those with nonperiodic belching, bloating, and indigestion.

By definition, patients in the first group do not have a demonstrable ulcer crater; however, a high proportion have endoscopic evidence of gastritis and/or duodenitis (Greenlaw et al, 1980). It is unclear whether such findings are responsible for the dyspeptic symptoms and whether the gastroduodenitis is part of the spectrum of peptic ulcer disease. Patients with bloating and belching may have a definable disorder of gastroduodenal motility diagnosable by studies of gastric emptying or gastroduodenal motility (Rees et al, 1980). In the future, detailed investigations of patients with nonulcer dyspepsia may reveal that only a small number have no definable cause for symptoms.

Therapy: Most controlled trials suggest that conventional peptic ulcer therapy (eg, H_2 receptor antagonists, omeprazole, sucralfate) is of no therapeutic benefit in the majority of patients with nonulcer dyspepsia (Nyrén et al, 1986). However, their trial is often instituted in patients with classic peptic ulcer symptoms prior to an extensive diagnostic work up. In contrast to results in most studies in which no benefit was demonstrated, in one large controlled study, self-administered on-demand therapy with cimetidine (400 to 800 mg one to three times a day) or another H_2 receptor blocker was reported to relieve dyspepsia in most patients (Johannessen et al, 1992). In those who do not respond to drugs, x-ray and/or endoscopic studies are usually performed.

Most patients with nonclassic symptoms of bloating and belching will have undergone radiologic studies to exclude obvious disorders. When results of these studies are not definitive, a trial of metoclopramide, anticholinergic agents, and/or antianxiety agents can be considered. For most patients in whom the above drugs are not effective and in whom no cause of symptoms can be ascertained, dietary manipulations and attempts at emotional support should be considered. Since there is no clear association between *H. pylori* and nonulcer dyspepsia, *H. pylori* eradication therapy is not warranted (Bernersen et al, 1992).

ASPIRATION PNEUMONITIS

Pulmonary aspiration of gastric contents with subsequent pneumonitis may occur during regurgitation or vomiting when the glottic reflex is obtunded. It is one of the most serious complications in semiconscious or unconscious patients and is a major cause of significant morbidity and occasional mortality in the perioperative period.

Conditions predisposing to high risk of aspiration include reduced level of consciousness, incompetent gastroesophageal sphincter, delayed gastric emptying, and gastric hemorrhage. Surgical patients especially at risk include those undergoing obstetrical procedures, those who require emergency surgery, and those who are morbidly obese (Olsson et al, 1986). Individuals undergoing outpatient surgery, pediatric patients, geriatric patients, and some inpatients undergoing elective surgery also are potentially at risk. Patients with impaired consciousness at risk include those experiencing stroke, convulsions, and alcohol intoxication. Chronic aspiration occurs in children and adults with asthma, seizures, nocturnal cough, or achalasia and in other patients susceptible to reflux.

A patient is thought to be at risk of pulmonary damage in the event of aspiration of at least 25 ml or 0.4 ml/kg of gastric contents with a pH of less than 2.5 (Mendelson, 1946; Teabeaut, 1952; Roberts and Shirley, 1974). The risk of a serious pulmonary reaction increases as the pH of the aspirate decreases below 2.5 (Teabeaut, 1952).

Treatment: Once aspiration has occurred, aggressive measures to restore normal pulmonary function are required promptly because pulmonary damage occurs in seconds. Recommended measures include removal of particulate matter, oxygenation and positive pressure ventilation (usually with positive end expiratory pressure), use of bronchodilators and other procedures to maintain the airway, and replacement of intravascular volume (Cohen, 1982; Kallos et al, 1983; Wynne and Modell, 1977).

Prophylaxis: All of the following measures to decrease the risk of aspiration should be utilized when possible. No oral intake should be permitted immediately before surgery or during labor; patients who are to undergo elective surgery can ingest oral liquids up to three hours before surgery (Sandhar et al, 1989; Scarr et al, 1989). Proper anesthetic technique is essential, including regional anesthesia, adequate preoxygenation, awake intubation or rapid sequence induction with drugs (eg, thiopental, midazolam, etomidate), cricoid pressure, and rapid paralysis with a muscle relaxant to facilitate endotracheal intubation. After general anesthesia has been induced and an endotracheal tube with inflated cuff is in place, evacuation of gastric contents through a nasogastric tube can reduce the risk of aspiration during recovery (Scott, 1981; Cohen, 1982; Kallos et al, 1983; Wynne and Modell, 1977). Removal of gastric contents is necessary only following a recent meal (Brock-Utne et al, 1989). Awake extubation will minimize aspiration on recovery from anesthesia.

Most prophylactic measures have focused on increasing the pH of the gastric contents above 2.5. Some recent investigations also have considered methods of reducing the volume of gastric content and increasing lower esophageal sphincter tone. Drugs used for prophylaxis include clear (nonparticulate) antacids, cimetidine, ranitidine, and metoclopramide. Less data are available on the H_2 receptor blockers, nizatidine and famotidine, and the proton pump inhibitor, omeprazole.

Recent studies indicate that antacids decrease morbidity but have little effect on mortality, which may reflect their inability to raise gastric pH sufficiently, their potential for increasing gastric content volume and acid rebound, and the pulmonary toxicity of particulate antacid-neutralized gastric contents. Because oral antacids act more rapidly than cimetidine or ranitidine, they are more useful for emergency surgery. Antacids raise the gastric pH in 10 to 30 minutes. It is generally not necessary or advisable to administer antacids frequently during labor, especially if clear antacids are used; most practitioners advocate use of a single oral dose prior to anesthesia (Cohen, 1982; Wheatley et al, 1979).

Although almost all particulate antacids studied were reported to produce pathologic changes in the lung parenchyma, magnesium trisilicate has been reported to be safe, efficacious, and reliable when properly administered (Crawford and Potter, 1984). This remains the most commonly used prophylactic antacid in the United Kingdom despite the great interest in nonparticulate antacids and H_2 receptor antagonists (Sweeney, 1986).

The clear, nonparticulate antacid, sodium citrate, is preferred by many physicians for oral prophylaxis. Sodium citrate (0.3 M) has a more rapid effect than particulate antacids, mixes with gastric contents better, and is considered to be safer if aspirated. A single dose administered 10 to 45 minutes prior to anesthesia significantly increases gastric pH (Cohen, 1982; Wrobel et al, 1982; Gibbs et al, 1982; Abboud et al, 1984). Disadvantages of sodium citrate include its lack of palatability, inability to buffer large volumes of gastric fluid, tendency to increase gastric volume, and the need to prepare solutions because commercial single-entity products are not available. One commercial product, Bicitra, contains sodium citrate (0.34 M) with citric acid (0.32 M). Its buffering capacity is less than that of sodium citrate 0.3 M, and results of studies evaluating its efficacy for the prophylaxis of aspiration pneumonitis are conflicting (Gibbs and Banner, 1984; Manchikanti et al, 1985). Another commercial product, Alka-Seltzer, contains sodium and potassium bicarbonates and citric acid in a dry effervescent tablet, and sodium citrate is produced when the tablet is dissolved in water. Results of the only study evaluating the efficacy of Alka-Seltzer for aspiration prophylaxis in emergency surgery were encouraging (Chen et al, 1984); however, the aspirin component of this product may promote bleeding.

Results of a number of controlled studies indicate that cimetidine (Stoelting, 1978; Coombs et al, 1979 A; Manchikanti et al, 1982; Manchikanti and Roush, 1984; Durrant and Strunin, 1982; Morison et al, 1982; Hodgkinson et al, 1983; Kallos et al, 1983) or ranitidine (Durrant and Strunin, 1982; Manchikanti et al, 1984, 1986; McAuley et al, 1983; Morison et al, 1982) raises the pH of the gastric contents significantly more than antacids and decreases gastric content volume. Although little supporting evidence exists, most practitioners believe that, with proper administration, cimetidine, ranitidine, or other H_2 receptor blockers reduce both morbidity and mortality. Use of these drugs in emergency surgery is limited, however, because effects do not occur for 45 to 60 minutes. A single dose of an H_2 receptor blocker given the night prior to surgery may not provide adequate protection against aspiration (Dubin et al, 1989). A double-dose regimen is more effective (Manchikanti et al, 1982); the second dose is given intramuscularly, intravenously, or orally 60 minutes before anesthesia is induced. In some studies, parenteral administration 45 to 90 minutes prior to induction produced a higher gastric pH than oral administration (Williams and Strunin, 1985; Weber and Hirshman, 1979; Coombs et al, 1979 B; Manchikanti et al, 1986; Maile and Francis, 1983). There is no evidence, however, that parenteral administration is more protective (Silverman et al, 1989). Even though cimetidine and ranitidine reliably elevate gastric pH in most patients, usefulness is limited by their inability to neutralize the acid already present in the stomach, the long time interval required following administration for reliable effect, and occasional side effects and drug interactions (Manchikanti et al, 1982; Moir, 1983; Zeldis et al, 1983). Administration of omeprazole the night prior to surgery and the morning of surgery (or with the second dose omitted) appears to be more effective than ranitidine for prophylaxis against aspiration (Ewart et al, 1990; Wingtin et al, 1990).

Combination therapy with an antacid and cimetidine or ranitidine increases acid neutralization of gastric contents in most patients, thus increasing the level of protection in both elective and emergency obstetric surgery (Gillett et al, 1984; Moir, 1983; Okasha et al, 1983). An effervescent cimetidine-sodium citrate formulation (available in England) appears to offer more protection against aspiration than sodium citrate alone (Ormezzano et al, 1990).

The anticholinergic agents, atropine, glycopyrrolate [Robinul], and pirenzipine (investigational), may be useful adjuncts to antacids (Cohen, 1982; Dewan et al, 1982).

It is not clear if metoclopramide decreases gastric volume sufficiently to reduce the risk of pulmonary aspiration or to improve safety significantly when administered alone. When given with antacids (Schmidt and Jørgenson, 1984; Manchikanti et al, 1985) or with H_2 blockers (Cohen, 1982; Manchikanti et al, 1984), results are conflicting. Nevertheless, some investigators believe that it is probably wise to administer this drug adjunctively (especially with H_2 blockers) to patients at high risk from aspiration; an additional benefit of metoclopramide is provided by its ability to increase lower esophageal sphincter tone (Cohen et al, 1984; Manchikanti et al, 1984; Rao et al, 1984; Lerman et al, 1988).

Drug Evaluations

H_2 RECEPTOR ANTAGONISTS

CIMETIDINE
[Tagamet]

CIMETIDINE HYDROCHLORIDE
[Tagamet Hydrochloride]

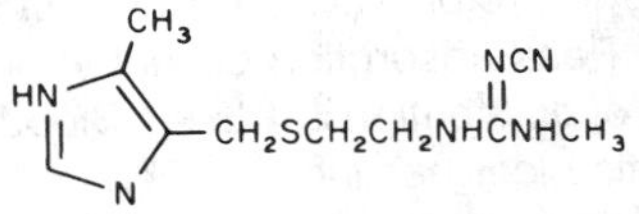

CH_3 HN NCN N $-CH_2SCH_2CH_2NHCNHCH_3$

ACTIONS. Cimetidine promotes healing of peptic ulcer by markedly reducing the volume and concentration of acid secreted both in the resting state and after stimulation by food, histamine, pentagastrin, insulin, and caffeine (Wastell and Lance, 1979). It does not appear to exert a clinically significant effect on gastric motility or emptying, on lower esophageal sphincter pressure, or on secretion by the pancreas or gallbladder.

USES. Cimetidine accelerates the healing of gastric and duodenal ulcer, and it or another H_2 receptor antagonist is the drug of choice for the treatment of an uncomplicated peptic ulcer. A single 400-mg dose at bedtime prevents the recurrence of duodenal ulcer in most patients as long as therapy continues. The value of maintenance therapy in preventing recurrences of gastric ulcer for more than one year is unclear (Barr et al, 1983), although no serious adverse effects of cimetidine have been demonstrated in patients treated for up to ten years.

Like antacids, cimetidine relieves symptoms but conventional doses do not heal lesions in reflux esophagitis.

Gradually decreasing responsiveness after prolonged use has been reported occasionally, but the clinical significance of this phenomenon awaits further study. Basal and postprandial serum gastrin levels increase slightly and progressively during six months of continuous therapy; however, this finding does not appear to have clinical significance, because "acid rebound" is rare in patients with duodenal ulcer after abrupt cessation of cimetidine.

Cimetidine heals some NSAID-induced peptic ulcers but does not prevent their initial occurrence. This drug may prevent recurrence of duodenal but not gastric ulcer in patients taking NSAIDs.

The incidence of adverse effects is increased by the large doses necessary to treat Zollinger-Ellison syndrome and other gastric acid hypersecretory states (eg, systemic mastocytosis); therefore, cimetidine may be less useful than ranitidine in these disorders (Helman and Ou Tim, 1983; Jensen et al, 1983 A, 1983 B). Neither drug is as effective as omeprazole, which is the therapy of choice.

Cimetidine has been used for stress ulcers and bleeding. It is more useful for prophylaxis than for treatment. Cimetidine's value may be enhanced significantly when it is administered by continuous intravenous infusion (Ostro et al, 1984; Siepler and Trudeau, 1984; Siepler et al, 1989).

Cimetidine is a useful alternative to antacids in preventing aspiration pneumonitis during childbirth and elective surgical procedures. It is less useful than antacids during emergency surgery because of its slow onset of action. This drug has been given to prevent alkalosis in patients subjected to prolonged nasogastric aspiration, especially those secreting large amounts of acid, and to decrease ileostomy/jejunostomy output in the short-bowel syndrome.

In patients with pancreatic insufficiency, claims have been made that the reduction in hydrochloric acid secretion induced by cimetidine enhances the efficacy of oral pancreatic enzymes. However, cimetidine is effective only in those with low rates of gastric acid secretion, and such patients rarely require this drug or other adjuvants. Well-controlled studies have demonstrated that cimetidine is ineffective in acute pancreatitis, and it may actually increase and prolong hyperamylasemia.

ADVERSE REACTIONS. The overall incidence of adverse reactions is low. Untoward effects during short-term trials include diarrhea, dizziness, myalgia, or rash (which is usually transient). Confusion and more severe central nervous system reactions have occurred, usually after ingestion of excessive doses, in elderly patients, or in those with renal impairment (Larsson et al, 1982); these symptoms were reversed when the drug was discontinued. Some dementia-like symptoms may reflect interaction between cimetidine and concomitantly administered psychotropic drugs or may be primary side effects because cimetidine crosses the blood-brain barrier.

Drug-related elevations of serum transaminase levels have been noted; no other signs of hepatic dysfunction were observed. Rarely, unexplained elevations in alkaline phosphatase levels have been reported. Slight elevations of creatinine concentrations without evidence of renal dysfunction occur during treatment; appreciable increases associated with interstitial nephritis that cleared on discontinuation of the drug have been documented occasionally (Pitone et al, 1982; Rudnick et al, 1982).

Some questions have been raised about the formation of N-nitroso derivatives of H_2 receptor antagonists and their possible carcinogenicity. Currently available H_2 receptor antagonists do not form such derivatives in humans and are not carcinogenic.

Prolactin levels may be elevated transiently after intravenous administration of cimetidine. Gynecomastia and impotence have developed in patients treated with standard doses for prolonged periods or with larger than usual doses for hypersecretory states or duodenal ulcer (Jensen et al, 1983 B). Swelling and nipple tenderness were usually mild and did not progress after several months of therapy. In one study, a reversible reduction (but within the normal range) in sperm count, complete impotence, and/or gynecomastia were noted in men taking cimetidine for more than two months. The effects were dose dependent in 7 of 19 patients with gastric acid hypersecretion who received large doses of cimetidine (mean, 4.5 g/day; range, 1.2 to 10.8 g/day) for at least 12 months. They did not recur when equieffective doses of ranitidine were given (Allende et al, 1982). The proposed mechanism of these effects is antagonism of androgen receptors or alteration of estrogen metabolism.

A few cases of neutropenia, leukopenia, and thrombocytopenia have been reported, and the incidence of delayed hypersensitivity reactions increased after six weeks of treatment. Fever, bradycardia, and other arrhythmias have occurred, but a direct causal relationship is difficult to verify.

In animals, cimetidine crosses the placenta and is excreted in maternal milk, but toxicity has not been observed. No well-controlled studies have been carried out that assure the safety of this drug during pregnancy (FDA Pregnancy Category B).

Because of the potential for adverse reactions when large doses of cimetidine are required, it is probably advisable to substitute a more potent H_2 receptor antagonist or omeprazole.

DRUG INTERACTIONS. Antacids and metoclopramide reduce the oral bioavailability of cimetidine by 20% to 30% (Gugler et al, 1981; Sorkin and Darvey, 1983). These interactions may not be clinically significant (Hansten, 1985), but an interval of at least one hour should be maintained between the administration of either the antacid or metoclopramide and oral cimetidine.

Because the absorption of ketoconazole is reduced by approximately one-half when this drug is administered with cimetidine, ketoconazole should be given two hours before cimetidine (Sorkin and Darvey, 1983). In addition, ketoconazole requires an acid pH and is less effective at the higher pH produced in patients receiving an H_2 blocker; this interaction also may occur with concomitant use of enoxacin.

Cimetidine inhibits drug metabolizing microsomal enzymes in the liver (Hansten, 1983), which increases the plasma half-life of warfarin and similar anticoagulants, as well as of theophylline and caffeine (Broughton and Rogers, 1981), phenobarbital, phenytoin, carbamazepine, beta-adrenergic blocking agents (eg, propranolol, metoprolol), tricyclic antidepressants (eg, doxepin, imipramine, desipramine, nortriptyline), diazepam, chlordiazepoxide, and probably other benzodiazepines eliminated by oxidation (eg, prazepam, clorazepate). Benzodiazepines that are eliminated almost entirely by glucuronidation (eg, oxazepam, lorazepam) are not affected. Reduced hepatic blood flow has been reported, but the indirect methods used for measurement have been questioned and the significance of this effect is unproven. Cimetidine may inhibit alcohol dehydrogenase in the gastric mucosa. It is unclear if concomitant ingestion of cimetidine with alcoholic beverages increases blood alcohol concentrations (Di Padova et al, 1992; Fraser et al, 1992; Hansten, 1992). Until further data are available, it is probably wise for patients receiving this drug to avoid alcohol. This drug also impairs the disposition and elevates the serum concentrations of antiarrhythmic drugs (eg, procainamide, quinidine), lidocaine, and calcium channel blockers (eg, verapamil, nifedipine, diltiazem) (Hansten and Horn, 1989). Cimetidine may increase the bone marrow toxicity of carmustine and other antineoplastic drugs. It is incompatible with barbiturates in intravenous solutions.

See the manufacturer's literature for further information on drug interactions.

PHARMACOKINETICS. The oral bioavailability of cimetidine is approximately 70%. Bioavailability is essentially 100% after intravenous or intramuscular administration. Plasma binding is limited to about 20%.

Food delays the rate, but not the extent, of absorption; therefore, cimetidine should be administered with or immediately after meals to take advantage of the acid buffering effect of food and to prolong the drug's effect during the postprandial period. Peak absorption occurs in 60 to 90 minutes, and the volume of distribution is 1 L/kg. Blood levels correlate poorly with peptic ulcer healing.

Cimetidine penetrates the central nervous system; the cerebrospinal fluid concentration is 10% to 20% of the serum concentration.

About 50% to 80% of an intravenous dose is excreted as unchanged drug; 40% of an oral dose is excreted unchanged in the urine in patients with peptic ulcer disease. Most of the remainder of the drug appears in the urine as 5-hydroxymethyl or sulfoxide metabolites. The plasma elimination half-life is about two hours; systemic clearance is 8.3 ml/min/kg.

DOSAGE AND PREPARATIONS.

Oral: For gastric or duodenal ulcer, *adults*, 300 mg with or immediately after meals and at bedtime (total, 1.2 g daily). Duodenal ulcer usually heals in four to six weeks with daily treatment; healing of gastric ulcer generally requires 8 to 12 weeks. For duodenal ulcer, alternative schedules include 200 mg with meals and 400 mg at bedtime (Graham et al, 1981), 400 mg in the morning and 400 mg at bedtime (Delattre et al, 1982), or 800 mg at bedtime (Lacerte et al, 1984). Endoscopy is used to verify healing of a gastric ulcer. Some authorities do not recommend repeated endoscopy in patients with duodenal ulcer and consider relief of symptoms after four to six weeks the endpoint of initial therapy.

For maintenance therapy, 400 mg once daily at bedtime for one year prevents recurrence of gastric or duodenal ulcer in about 60% to 80% of patients. Antacids may be taken concurrently but only as needed to control pain, with an interval of at least one hour between the administration of the antacid and cimetidine.

For reflux esophagitis, *adults,* 1.6 g daily in divided doses (800 mg twice daily or 400 mg four times daily). Patients with the Zollinger-Ellison syndrome require treatment indefinitely, and the dosage must be individualized. Most responsive patients have been managed with <2.4 g/day, but up to 10.8 g/day has been used in refractory patients (Jensen et al, 1983 A). Efficacy is usually established by determining that acid output is <5 mEq/hr one hour before the next dose. When the patient has coexisting esophagitis, acid output must be reduced to <2 mEq/hr. The drug is usually administered every six to eight hours. When the total daily dose exceeds 2.4 g, substitution of omeprazole is indicated.

For prevention of aspiration pneumonitis in surgical patients, see the discussion of this disorder in the Introduction.

Children, 20 to 40 mg/kg daily in divided doses has been given; however, clinical experience in children is limited, and the benefit/risk ratio should be considered carefully.

CIMETIDINE:
Tagamet (SmithKline Beecham). Tablets 200, 300, 400, and 800 mg.

CIMETIDINE HYDROCHLORIDE:
Tagamet Hydrochloride (SmithKline Beecham). Liquid 300 mg/5 ml (alcohol 2.8%).

Intravenous, Intramuscular: For short-term use in patients with severe gastric acid hypersecretory disorders (eg, Zollinger-Ellison syndrome) or peptic ulcer disease refractory to oral medication or in those who refuse to take or cannot tolerate oral medication, the following dosages are suggested: *Adults* (intravenous), 1 to 4 mg/kg/hr is infused (continuous administration) or 300 mg is diluted and injected over a five-minute period or infused over a 15- to 20-minute period and repeated at six-hour intervals (intermittent administration). (Intramuscular) 300 mg is given every six to eight hours. When feasible, the dosage should be adjusted to maintain an intragastric pH >4.0. Dosage should be reduced in patients with impaired renal function; if the impairment is severe, 300 mg twice daily is suggested. Oral administration should be substituted as soon as possible (eg, when signs of bleeding have been absent for 48 hours).

For prevention of aspiration pneumonitis in surgical patients, see the discussion of this disorder in the Introduction.

For prophylaxis and treatment of stress ulcers and bleeding (investigational indication), 300 to 400 mg is injected intravenously every six hours or up to 50 to 100 mg/hr (1.2 g/day) is infused (Ostro et al, 1984).

Children, see oral dosage.

CIMETIDINE HYDROCHLORIDE:
Tagamet Hydrochloride (SmithKline Beecham). Solution 150 mg/ml in 2 and 8 ml containers; prefilled syringes containing 300 mg with 2 ml of sterile water.

RANITIDINE HYDROCHLORIDE
[Zantac]

$(CH_3)_2NCH_2$–(furan)–$CH_2SCH_2CH_2NHC(=CHNO_2)NHCH_3$

ACTIONS. This H_2 receptor blocking agent is a competitive antagonist of histamine-induced gastric acid secretion and is about three times more potent than cimetidine (Helman and Ou Tim, 1983; Hirschowitz et al, 1982). Like cimetidine, ranitidine inhibits both the volume and concentration of gastric juice produced nocturnally and by food but does not affect gastric mucus production or lower esophageal sphincter pressure.

USES. Ranitidine is effective for the treatment of duodenal or gastric ulcer and relieves symptoms of reflux esophagitis. It heals some NSAID-induced ulcers but does not appear to prevent their initial occurrence. Ranitidine prevents recurrence of duodenal but not gastric ulcer in patients taking NSAIDs (Barrier and Hirschowitz, 1989). Investigationally, this drug prevented aspiration pneumonitis during surgery, and it appears to be useful for the prophylaxis of bleeding due to stress ulcers.

Many patients with peptic ulcers that did not respond to cimetidine in eight weeks or less have responded to ranitidine (Helman and Ou Tim, 1983; Danilewitz et al, 1982; Zeldis et al, 1983). Because of its greater potency and the lower incidence of adverse effects compared with high-dose cimetidine, ranitidine is often preferred to cimetidine for patients with the Zollinger-Ellison syndrome and other gastric acid hypersecretory states. Efficacy is usually established by determining that acid output is <5 mEq/hr one hour before the next dose. When the patient has coexisting esophagitis, the output must be reduced to <2 mEq/hr. The gynecomastia and impotence that occur during high-dose cimetidine therapy in patients with the Zollinger-Ellison syndrome may disappear when ranitidine is substituted (Zeldis et al, 1983; Jensen et al, 1983 B) but may take 12 to 24 months to regress in some patients. Up to 6 g/day has been used in these patients without untoward effects. However, neither ranitidine nor cimetidine is as effective as omeprazole, which is the drug of choice. If large doses of an H_2 receptor antagonist are required (twice the usual daily dose) in patients with refractory peptic ulcer or reflux esophagitis, substitution of omeprazole is preferred by most authorities.

Ranitidine may be preferred to cimetidine in patients taking multiple drugs (particularly drugs whose metabolism is affected by cimetidine), in those who cannot tolerate cimetidine's adverse effects, and in geriatric patients.

ADVERSE REACTIONS. Minor adverse effects occur infrequently (incidence less than 3%) and include headache and rashes that usually subside with continued therapy, malaise, nausea, constipation, dizziness, and abdominal pain (Zeldis et al, 1983; Helman and Ou Tim, 1983). Usual doses of ranitidine only rarely produce confusion, gynecomastia, hyperprolactinemia, sexual dysfunction, bradycardia, blood dyscrasias, or hepatitis.

In contrast to cimetidine, ranitidine binds minimally to the hepatic mixed-function oxidase system, androgen receptors, or peripheral lymphocytes. Serum transaminase and plasma creatinine levels may increase during therapy but often return to normal with continued treatment. Ranitidine appears in breast milk and should be used with caution in nursing mothers. This drug is classified in FDA Pregnancy Category B.

Some questions have been raised about the formation of N-nitroso derivatives of H_2 receptor antagonists and their possible carcinogenicity. Currently available H_2 receptor antagonists do not form such derivatives in humans and are not carcinogenic.

Hypersensitivity is uncommon, and no cross reaction has occurred when ranitidine was given to a patient who experienced erythema annulare induced by cimetidine.

DRUG INTERACTIONS. Although ranitidine interacts with other medications less frequently than cimetidine, an increasing number of drug interactions are being reported (Tatro, 1992). Interactions with nifedipine, warfarin, theophylline, and metoprolol have been observed. Mechanisms other than inhibition of P450 hepatic drug metabolizing systems may be involved. Ranitidine may decrease the absorption of diazepam and reduce its plasma concentration by 25% (Hansten, 1983); these drugs should be administered at least one hour apart. Ketoconazole requires an acid pH and is less effective at the higher pH produced in patients receiving an H_2 receptor antagonist; this interaction also may occur with concomitant use of enoxacin. It is unclear if concomitant ingestion of ranitidine with alcoholic beverages increases blood alcohol concentrations (Di Padova et al, 1992; Fraser et al, 1992; Hansten, 1992). Until further data are available, it is probably wise for patients receiving this drug to avoid alcohol.

Allowing at least one hour between administration of antacids or anticholinergic drugs and ranitidine is desirable.

PHARMACOKINETICS. The oral bioavailability of ranitidine is about 50% and is increased in patients with liver disease. The plasma half-life is approximately 1.7 to 3 hours in adults and is prolonged in geriatric patients as a result of an age-related decrease in renal function, in those with kidney disease, and, to a much lesser extent, in those with liver disease. Peak plasma concentrations occur within one to three hours after an oral dose of 150 mg. The apparent volume of distribution is 1.2 to 1.9 L/kg. Plasma protein binding is only 15%.

Ranitidine undergoes significant first-pass metabolism after oral administration. It is metabolized in the liver to the pharmacologically inactive desmethylranitidine, ranitidine-N-oxide, and ranitidine-S-oxide.

Less than 10% of an intravenous or oral dose is excreted as metabolites; 68% to 79% of an intravenous dose and 30% of an oral dose appear in the urine as unchanged drug. Ranitidine and its metabolites are excreted principally in the urine; the remainder is recovered in the feces (Helman and Ou Tim, 1983; Zeldis et al, 1983). In healthy individuals, systemic clearance is 10.4 ml/min/kg.

DOSAGE AND PREPARATIONS.

Oral: For gastric or duodenal ulcer, *adults*, 150 mg twice daily. For duodenal ulcer, 300 mg once daily at bedtime is as effective as twice-daily administration (Ireland et al, 1984). Duodenal ulcer usually heals in four to six weeks with daily treatment. Most authorities do not recommend repeated endoscopy in patients with duodenal ulcer and consider relief of symptoms after four to six weeks the endpoint of initial therapy. Healing of gastric ulcer generally requires 8 to 12 weeks; endoscopy is used for verification. For maintenance, 150 mg at bedtime inhibits nocturnal acid secretion and prevents recurrence of gastric or duodenal ulcer (Alstead et al, 1983). Antacids may be taken as needed to control pain if an interval of at least one hour has elapsed between the administration of these agents and ranitidine; however, the need for antacids suggests recurrence of the ulcer.

For reflux esophagitis (unverified lesions), *adults*, 150 mg twice daily for up to six weeks; (endoscopically verified lesions) 150 mg four times daily for up to 12 weeks.

For the Zollinger-Ellison syndrome and other gastric acid hypersecretory disorders, the dose must be titrated for each patient on the basis of acid output and continued indefinitely; 150 mg twice daily or more frequently has been suggested. Up to 6 g/day has been given to those with severe disease, but most authorities now believe that if large doses (twice the usual amount) of an H_2 receptor antagonist are required, omeprazole should be substituted.

For prevention of aspiration pneumonitis in surgical patients, see the discussion of this disorder in the Introduction.

Because ranitidine is excreted primarily by the kidney, adults with impaired renal function (clearance <50 ml/min) generally should not receive more than 150 mg every 24 hours. Dosage may be increased with caution to 150 mg every 12 hours or more frequently if necessary. Hemodialysis slightly reduces the level of circulating ranitidine; therefore, administration of the drug should coincide with the end of hemodialysis.

Zantac (Glaxo). Tablets 150 and 300 mg; syrup 75 mg/5 ml (alcohol 7.5%).

Intramuscular, Intravenous: For temporary use in patients with the Zollinger-Ellison syndrome or other gastric acid hypersecretory disorders, peptic ulcer disease refractory to oral medication, or in patients who refuse to take or cannot tolerate oral medication, dosage is not proportional to the acid output and must be individualized; 50 mg every six to eight hours is commonly used. (No dilution is necessary for intramuscular administration.) When renal clearance is <50 ml/min, the dosing interval should be increased to 18 to 24 hours. Alternatively, 6.25 mg/hr has been administered as a continuous infusion, but this dosage has not been studied in patients with renal impairment.

For prevention of aspiration pneumonitis in surgical patients, see the discussion of this disorder in the Introduction.

Zantac (Glaxo). Solution 25 mg/ml in 2, 6, and 40 ml containers with phenol 0.5% as preservative; solution (premixed) 0.5 mg/ml in 50 ml containers (preservative-free; for intravenous use only).

FAMOTIDINE HYDROCHLORIDE
[Pepcid]

ACTIONS. Famotidine is a competitive H_2 receptor antagonist that inhibits basal, overnight, and pentagastrin-stimulated gastric acid secretion. Pharmacologically, it is three times more potent than ranitidine and 20 times more potent than cimetidine.

USES. Randomized double-blind controlled trials reveal that famotidine effectively heals both active duodenal and gastric ulcers when compared with placebo. Healing rates are comparable to those seen at eight weeks with cimetidine and ranitidine (Friedman, 1987; Berardi et al, 1988). In a six-month controlled trial, the drug also reduced the rate of recurrence of duodenal ulcer. Studies to determine famotidine's efficacy in gastric ulcer prophylaxis and prevention of stress ulceration are being conducted.

Famotidine relieves symptoms and heals lesions in patients with mild to moderate reflux esophagitis (Sabesin et al, 1991; Wesdorp, 1992). It also compares favorably with the other H_2 receptor antagonists in patients with the Zollinger-Ellison syndrome (Howard et al, 1985; Berardi et al, 1988); efficacy is usually established by determining that acid output is <5 mEq/hr one hour before the next dose. When the patient has coexisting esophagitis, acid output must be reduced to <2 mEq/hr. However, omeprazole is the drug of choice in those with severe reflux esophagitis or the Zollinger-Ellison syndrome.

Like ranitidine, famotidine may be preferable to cimetidine in some patients because of its lack of antiandrogenic side effects and drug interactions.

ADVERSE REACTIONS AND PRECAUTIONS. In controlled clinical trials, infrequent minor adverse reactions observed include headache, dizziness, constipation, and diarrhea. No antiandrogenic effects have been reported.

This drug is classified in FDA Pregnancy Category B. Because it is not known whether famotidine is excreted in human breast milk, it should be used with caution in nursing mothers.

Some questions have been raised about the formation of N-nitroso derivatives of H_2 receptor antagonists and their possible carcinogenicity. Currently available H_2 receptor antagonists do not form such derivatives in humans and are not carcinogenic.

DRUG INTERACTIONS.Only a limited number of drugs have been tested with famotidine in humans. No interference with the hepatic oxidative metabolism of diazepam, theophylline, warfarin, or phenytoin has been observed (Friedman, 1987). Ketoconazole requires an acid pH and is less effective at the higher pH produced in patients treated with an H_2 receptor antagonist; this interaction also may occur with concomitant use of enoxacin.

PHARMACOKINETICS. Famotidine is a sulfamoylamidine that differs chemically from cimetidine and ranitidine in that it contains a thiazole ring. The peak plasma concentration occurs approximately two hours after oral administration, and the primary plasma elimination half-life is three to eight hours. The bioavailability of famotidine is 40% to 45%. The only significant metabolite is famotidine-S-oxide. Approximately 25% of the dose is recovered intact in the urine after a single oral dose. In patients with severe renal failure, the elimination half-life of famotidine may exceed 20 hours (Berardi et al, 1988).

DOSAGE AND PREPARATIONS.

Oral: For *adults* with active duodenal or gastric ulcers, 40 mg is given once daily in the morning (Okada et al, 1992). In most studies, more than 90% of ulcers were healed after eight weeks of therapy. The initial dosage in patients with uncomplicated peptic ulcers and creatinine clearance <10 l/min is 20 mg. For maintenance therapy in patients with duodenal ulcers, 20 mg is more effective than placebo. No studies are available to determine the prophylactic dose in those with gastric ulcer.

For reflux esophagitis (unverified lesions), *adults*, 20 mg twice daily for up to six weeks; (endoscopically verified lesions) 20 to 40 mg twice daily for up to 12 weeks.

For patients with the Zollinger-Ellison syndrome and other gastric hypersecretory states, dosage is not proportional to acid output and must be individualized. The suggested initial oral dose is 20 mg every six hours.

Pepcid (Merck). Tablets 20 and 40 mg; suspension (oral) 40 mg/5 ml.

Intravenous: For selected patients with hypersecretory states or in those unable to take oral medications, the dose must be titrated for each patient on the basis of acid output; 20 mg every 12 hours is commonly used but may be insufficient.

Pepcid I.V. (Merck). Solution 10 mg/ml in 2 and 4 ml containers.

NIZATIDINE

[Axid]

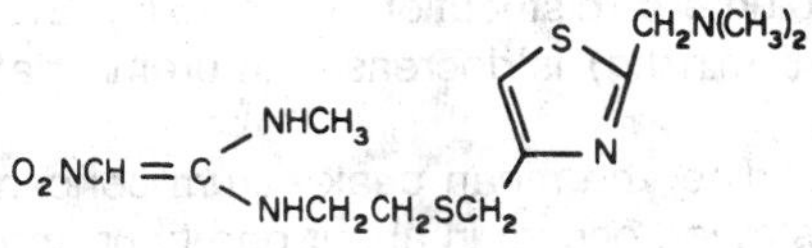

$O_2NCH=C(NHCH_3)NHCH_2CH_2SCH_2$–(thiazole ring, S, N)–$CH_2N(CH_3)_2$

USES. The potency of this H_2 receptor antagonist in inhibiting gastric acid secretion is similar to that of ranitidine. The value of nizatidine in the management of acid-peptic disorders is comparable to that of ranitidine and cimetidine. Once- or twice-daily doses usually heal duodenal ulcer within eight weeks; a single daily dose prevents relapse (Bianchi-Porro and Keohane, 1987; Stern, 1988). The efficacy of nizatidine in the treatment of gastric ulcer appears to be comparable to that of other H_2 receptor blockers, although less data are available.

In the Zollinger-Ellison syndrome and other acid-peptic disorders, the efficacy of nizatidine would be expected to be similar to that of ranitidine, but confirmation in clinical studies is required. Nizatidine relieves symptoms and heals lesions in patients with mild to moderate reflux esophagitis (Cloud et al, 1991, 1992). If large amounts (twice the usual dose) of nizatidine are required in patients with the Zollinger-Ellison syndrome, severe reflux esophagitis, or refractory peptic ulcer, omeprazole should be substituted.

ADVERSE REACTIONS. This agent is well tolerated. Minor gastrointestinal adverse reactions have been noted. During clinical trials, the elevation of serum uric acid as well as transaminase levels observed in a few patients has not appeared to be clinically significant. As with other H_2 receptor antagonists, the potential for hepatotoxicity is low with use of nizatidine. In rats, large doses have produced antiandrogenic effects, but such effects have not been observed with the therapeutic doses used in clinical trials (Stern, 1988).

Some questions have been raised about the formation of N-nitroso derivatives of H_2 receptor antagonists and their possible carcinogenicity. Currently available H_2 receptor antagonists do not form such derivatives in humans and are not carcinogenic.

Nizatidine is classified in FDA Pregnancy Category C.

DRUG INTERACTIONS. Nizatidine may inhibit alcohol dehydrogenase in the gastric mucosa and produce higher serum levels of alcohol, but this does not appear to be clinically significant. With doses comparable to those at which cimetidine inhibits hepatic microsomal drug metabolizing enzymes, nizatidine has produced no effect (Klotz, 1987). In healthy volunteers, no drug interactions were reported when nizatidine and theophylline, lidocaine, warfarin, chlordiazepoxide, diazepam, or lorazepam were used together. Concomitant antacid administration did not significantly decrease absorption of nizatidine. Ketoconazole requires an acid pH and is less effective at the higher pH produced in patients treated with an H_2 blocker; this interaction also may occur with concomitant use of enoxacin.

PHARMACOKINETICS. In one study, the oral bioavailability of nizatidine exceeded 70% and was not affected by food or the anticholinergic drug, propantheline (Knadler et al, 1987). Its apparent volume of distribution is 1.2 L/kg. Systemic clearance (10 ml/min/kg) is decreased in uremic patients and in the elderly.

Like cimetidine, the mean peak serum concentration after oral administration occurs in about one hour and the plasma half-life is about 1.5 hours. Nizatidine has a duration of action of up to 10 hours (Stern, 1988). It is eliminated primarily by the kidneys; 90% of the administered dose (65% as unchanged drug) is recovered in the urine within 16 hours (Knadler et al, 1986).

DOSAGE AND PREPARATIONS

Oral: For *adults* with active duodenal ulcer, 300 mg once daily or 150 mg twice daily. In most studies, ulcers are healed in about 90% of patients after eight weeks of therapy. The initial dosage should be reduced by 50% in patients with uncomplicated peptic ulcers and a creatinine clearance <10 ml/minute. For maintenance therapy in patients with duodenal ulcer, 150 mg at bedtime is more effective than placebo.

For *adults* with active gastric ulcer, the same dosage regimen as for duodenal ulcer was effective in one study, but more data are necessary for confirmation (Naccaratto et al, 1987).

For reflux esophagitis, *adults*, 150 mg twice daily.

Axid (Lilly). Capsules 150 and 300 mg.

ANTACIDS

Actions: The clinically useful antacids are basic aluminum, calcium, and magnesium salts that react with hydrochloric acid to form neutral, less acidic, or poorly soluble salts. Adequate doses increase the pH of the gastric contents to 5.0 or more, thus decreasing pepsin activity and facilitating healing of peptic ulcer.

Tablets with acid neutralizing capacity similar to that of liquid preparations appear to be equally effective for peptic ulcer therapy. The liquid formulation is preferred in patients with duodenal ulcer who would require a large number of tablets daily.

The acid neutralizing effects of different antacids vary widely. Antacids with high neutralizing potency in vitro are generally more efficacious in vivo. The appropriate antacid should be determined individually on the basis of patient response and acceptance. If a generic preparation is prescribed, its neutralizing capacity should be known. The dose should be determined by the milliequivalents of hydrochloric acid neutralized rather than by the total amount of antacid ingested. See Tables 1 and 2 for the acid neutralizing capacities of antacid products.

It has been suggested that antacids may have a cytoprotective action on gastric mucosa mediated by the release of endogenous prostaglandins (Hollander et al, 1984). However, the precise mechanism by which antacids relieve pain has not been explained completely. They do not provide a beneficial coating on or around the ulcer crater.

Uses: For specific indications for antacids, see the discussion of the disorders in the Introduction.

Many authorities now believe that the role of antacids in the treatment of peptic ulcer should be reassessed and suggest that these agents should be used only occasionally for relief of pain rather than for routine, long-term therapy. This should be borne in mind when reading the following discussion on antacids.

Antacids also are commonly taken to treat symptoms such as dyspepsia, heartburn, or so-called acid indigestion. However, hydrochloric acid is not always responsible for these symptoms, which also may occur in patients with achlorhydria. There are no well-controlled studies demonstrating the effectiveness of antacids in these functional disorders.

Aluminum hydroxide, calcium carbonate, and basic aluminum carbonate are used to treat renal calculi and to control hyperphosphatemia encountered early in the course of chronic renal failure (see index entry Osteodystrophy, Renal).

Adverse Reactions and Precautions: The adverse reactions and drug interactions of antacids have been reviewed (Henry and Langman, 1981). The most common reactions associated with prolonged use are diarrhea or constipation. Magnesium salts cause diarrhea, and large, frequently administered doses are not tolerated. Conversely, constipation may occur when large doses of calcium or aluminum preparations are given frequently. Aluminum hydroxide may rarely produce intestinal obstruction in the elderly and in patients with decreased bowel motility, dehydration, or restricted fluid intake, and hemodialysis and renal transplant patients appear to be at high risk for fecal impaction and intestinal obstruction when using aluminum hydroxide preparations (see the evaluation).

Doses of 20 to 40 g of calcium carbonate daily are reported to cause fecal impaction; however, these amounts are well above the manufacturers' maximum recommended daily dose of 8 g. Disruption of normal bowel function can be minimized by teaching the patient how to determine the necessary balance of magnesium salts with calcium or aluminum preparations. However, very few patients achieve perfect regulation of bowel function with high-dose regimens of available fixed-ratio mixtures, and further supplementation with laxative or constipating antacids is often required.

Adverse systemic effects of aluminum and magnesium occur in patients with renal insufficiency; nephrolithiasis has been encountered. Magnesium compounds can produce hypermagnesemia in patients with renal failure. Aluminum intoxication and osteomalacia may also occur. Because aluminum-containing antacids delay gastric emptying, they should not be used to prevent aspiration pneumonitis (Cohen, 1982).

Aluminum encephalopathy may develop in dialysis patients.

All antacids produce a temporary compensatory increase in the secretion of hydrochloric acid, probably because the increased gastric pH induced by antacids enhances the release of antral gastrin (Clayman, 1980; Schrumpf, 1980).

A number of aluminum or magnesium antacid preparations can be used cautiously in patients requiring a low-sodium diet; however, the exact amounts of sodium should be known when antacids are prescribed for these patients (see Tables 1 and 2).

Drug Interactions: Antacids reduce the oral bioavailability of concomitantly administered cimetidine or ranitidine (Hansten, 1985). Although this interaction may not be clinically significant, these drugs probably should be given one hour apart. Because the simultaneous administration of antacids may impair the binding of sucralfate to the ulcerated mucosa, at least 30 minutes should elapse between administration of the antacid and sucralfate.

By altering gastric and renal pH and thus the ionization of drugs, antacids may interfere with the dissolution, absorption, and excretion of concomitantly used medications. Antacids containing calcium, magnesium, or especially aluminum interfere with the absorption of the tetracyclines, the quinolones, and possibly iron, isoniazid, and digoxin. Nonchelating antacids, such as sodium bicarbonate, may decrease tetracycline absorption by decreasing dissolution. If the urine is sufficiently alkalized by the aluminum-magnesium antacids, blood

TABLE 1.
COMPOSITION OF COMMONLY USED NONPRESCRIPTION SINGLE-ENTITY ANTACID PREPARATIONS
(per capsule, tablet, or 5 ml of liquid)

Product (Manufacturer)	Dosage Form	Acid Neutralizing Capacity OTC Method (mEq)	Active Ingredients: Aluminum Hydroxide (mg)	Active Ingredients: Calcium Carbonate (mg)	Active Ingredients: Other (mg)	Sodium Content (mg)	Sodium Content (mEq)
ALternaGEL (Johnson & Johnson/Merck Consumer)	Suspension	16	600	—	—	<2.5	0.109
Amphojel (Wyeth-Ayerst)	Suspension	10	320	—	—	<2.3	0.1
	Tablets (600 mg)	16	600	—	—	2.9	0.13
	(300 mg)	9	300	—	—	1.8	0.08
Basaljel (Wyeth-Ayerst)	Suspension	12	400*	—	—	2.9	0.13
	Capsules	12	500*	—	—	2.8	0.12
	Tablets	13	500*	—	—	2.8	0.12
Dialume (Rhone-Poulenc Rorer)	Capsules	10	500	—	—	<1.2	0.05
Dicarbosil (SmithKline Beecham)	Tablets	10	—	500	—	<2.3	<0.13
Phillips' Milk of Magnesia (Sterling Health)	Suspension	13.9	—	—	Magnesium Hydroxide 400	0.47	0.017
	Tablets	10.9	—	—	Magnesium Hydroxide 311	0.33	0.06
Rolaids (Warner-Lambert)	Tablets	7.5	—	—	Dihydroxy-aluminum Sodium Carbonate 334	53	2.3
Titralac (3M Personal Care)	Tablets	7.5	—	420	Glycine 150	<0.3	0.013
Tums (SmithKline Beecham)	Tablets	10	—	500	—	≤2	0.13
	Extra Strength	15	—	750	—	≤2	<0.2

**Aluminum hydroxide equivalent, present as basic aluminum carbonate*

TABLE 2.
COMPOSITION OF COMMONLY USED NONPRESCRIPTION ANTACID MIXTURES
(per capsule, tablet, or 5 ml of liquid)

Product (Manufacturer)	Dosage Form	Acid Neutralizing Capacity OTC Method (mEq)	Active Ingredients				Sodium Content	
			Aluminum Hydroxide (mg)	Magnesium Hydroxide (mg)	Magnesium Trisilicate (mg)	Other (mg)	(mg)	(mEq)
Aludrox (Wyeth-Ayerst)	Suspension	12	307	103	—	—	2.3	0.1
Chooz (Schering Plough)	Gum	10				Calcium Carbonate	0.99	0.014
	Tablets	10					1.249	0.054
Di-Gel (Schering-Plough)	Tablets (Advance Formula)			128	—	Calcium Carbonate 280 Simethicone 20		
	Suspension	10.5	200[1]	200	—	Simethicone 20	≤5	0.22
Gaviscon (SmithKline Beecham)	Suspension	4	31.7	—	—	Sodium Alginate Magnesium Carbonate 137.3	13	0.5
	Tablets	0.5	80	—	20	Alginic Acid	19	0.8
Gaviscon ESR (SmithKline Beecham)	Suspension	14.2	254			Magnesium Carbonate 237.5	20	0.9
	Tablets	7.5	160			Magnesium Carbonate 105	30	1.3
Gaviscon-2 (SmithKline Beecham)	Tablets	1	160	—	40	Alginic Acid	38	1.6
Gelusil (Warner-Lambert)	Suspension	12	200	200	—	Simethicone 25	0.7	0.03
	Tablets	11	200	200	—	Simethicone 25	0.8	0.035
Kudrox (Schwarz)	Suspension	28	500	450	—	Simethicone 40	<2.5	<0.11
Maalox (Rhone-Poulenc Rorer)	Suspension	13.3	225	200	—	—	1.4	0.06
	Tablets	9.7	200	200	—	—	0.7	0.03
	Tablets (Extra Strength)	23.4	400	400	—	—	1.4	0.06
Maalox Plus (Rhone-Poulenc Rorer)	Suspension (Extra Strength)	29.5	500	450	—	Simethicone 40	1.2	0.05
	Tablets	11.4	200	250	—	Simethicone 25	0.8	0.03
Maalox Therapeutic Concentrate (Rhone-Poulenc Rorer)	Suspension	27.2	600	300	—	—	0.8	0.03
	Tablets	28	600	300	—	—	0.5	0.02
Mylanta (Johnson & Johnson/Merck Consumer)	Suspension	12.7	200	200	—	Simethicone 20	0.68	0.03
	Tablets	11.5	200	200	—	Simethicone 20	0.77	0.03

(Continued on next page)

TABLE 2 (continued)

Product (Manufacturer)	Dosage Form	Acid Neutralizing Capacity OTC Method (mEq)	Active Ingredients: Aluminum Hydroxide (mg)	Active Ingredients: Magnesium Hydroxide (mg)	Active Ingredients: Magnesium Trisilicate (mg)	Active Ingredients: Other (mg)	Sodium Content (mg)	Sodium Content (mEq)
Mylanta II (Johnson & Johnson/Merck Consumer)	Suspension	25.4	400	400	—	Simethicone 40	1.14	0.05
	Tablets	23	400	400	—	Simethicone 40	1.3	0.06
Remegel (American Chicle)	Squares (chewable)	13.2	—	—	—	Aluminum Hydroxide-Magnesium Carbonate Codried Gel 476.4	25	1.1
Riopan (Whitehall)	Tablets	13.5	—	—	—	Magaldrate[2] 480	<0.1	≤0.004
	Suspension	15	—	—	—	540	0.3	0.013
Riopan Plus (Whitehall)	Tablets	13.5	—	—	—	Simethicone 20 Magaldrate[2] 480	<0.1	≤0.004
	Suspension	15	—	—	—	Simethicone 40 Magaldrate[2] 540	0.3	0.013
Riopan Plus 2 Double Strength (Whitehall)	Suspension	30	—	—	—	Magaldrate[2] 1,080 Simethicone 40	≤0.3	0.013
	Tablets	30	—	—	—	Magaldrate[2] 1,080 Simethicone 20	≤0.5	≤0.021
Rolaids Sodium Free (Warner-Lambert)	Tablets	8.5	—	64	—	Calcium Carbonate 317	<0.4	<0.017
Titralac Plus (3M Personal Care)	Liquid	11	—	—	—	Simethicone 20 Calcium Carbonate 500	0.0005	≤0.00002
	Tablets	7.5	—	—	—	Simethicone 21 Calcium Carbonate 420	0.03	≤0.001
WinGel (Sterling Health)	Suspension	11.6	180	160	—	—	2.5	0.11
	Tablets	12.3	180	160	—	—	<2.5	0.11

[1] *Equivalent to dried gel.*

[2] *A complex of aluminum and magnesium hydroxides*

concentrations of quinidine may increase and the concentration of aspirin may decrease because of variations in renal excretion. Ketoconazole requires an acid pH and is less effective at the higher pH produced in patients treated with an antacid. The use of thiazide diuretics with excessive doses of calcium-containing antacids can produce marked hypercalcemia. Concurrent use of magnesium or calcium-containing antacids with sodium polystyrene sulfonate can result in systemic alkalosis (Hansten and Horn, 1991). These interactions can be avoided if the dosing interval between an antacid and the interacting drug is one to two hours.

Aluminum Compounds

ALUMINUM HYDROXIDE GEL

DRIED ALUMINUM HYDROXIDE GEL

ACTIONS AND USES. Aluminum hydroxide is the prototype and most commonly used aluminum compound for acid peptic disorders. The gel is a poorly soluble antacid-buffer that reacts slowly with hydrochloric acid and has low neutralizing capacity. This antacid adsorbs and temporarily inactivates pepsin, which may contribute to healing of peptic ulcer (Sepelyak et al, 1984). Rapid gastric emptying decreases the efficacy of more slowly reactive preparations. Preparations vary in neutralizing potency.

Aluminum hydroxide has demulcent properties that do not contribute to its effect in peptic ulcer. Its astringent action may cause release of prostaglandins. Aluminum hydroxide probably should be reserved for peptic ulcer patients who cannot tolerate magnesium-containing antacids.

ADVERSE REACTIONS AND PRECAUTIONS. The most common adverse reaction is dose-related constipation, and combined therapy with a magnesium compound is almost invariably required. The astringent action or taste of this agent may produce nausea and vomiting. If phosphate intake is low, patients receiving large doses for long periods may develop hypophosphatemia and osteomalacia.

Adverse central nervous system effects ("dialysis dementia") may occur when aluminum hydroxide is given for prolonged periods to dialysis patients. High levels of aluminum in the water of the dialysis bath have been implicated in most cases. Aluminum encephalopathy has not been described in patients taking aluminum antacids who are not being dialyzed, although nondialyzed uremic patients may be at risk for aluminum intoxication if they are given aluminum-containing preparations. The concomitant use of calcium carbonate allows reduction of the dose of aluminum antacid in these patients (Alfrey, 1984). Citrate antacids should not be administered concurrently with aluminum-based antacids used as phosphate binders in patients with renal failure (Kirschbaum and Schoolwerth, 1989).

Neutron activation analysis has demonstrated that the intestinal barrier is permeable to a heavy aluminum load and that aluminum may be deposited in the bones of patients with normal renal function. There is much speculation but no convincing evidence of an association between consumption of aluminum-containing compounds and Alzheimer's disease (Butterworth et al, 1992; Hughes, 1992; Young, 1992).

DRUG INTERACTIONS. See the discussion on drug interactions in the Introduction to this section.

DOSAGE AND PREPARATIONS.
Oral: The dose and frequency of administration depend on the disorder being treated, the frequency and severity of pain, and the degree of relief obtained.

For peptic ulcer, *adults*, 80 and 40 mEq of gel per dose for duodenal and gastric ulcer, respectively, one and three hours after meals and at bedtime.

Generic. Liquid and suspension (gel); tablets 600 and 608 mg (dried gel) (all forms nonprescription).
See Table 1 for trademark preparations.

BASIC ALUMINUM CARBONATE GEL

This gel reacts slowly with hydrochloric acid and is rarely used today as an antacid. It is prescribed primarily in conjunction with a low-phosphate diet to reduce elevated phosphate levels and demineralization of bones in patients with renal insufficiency and to prevent the formation of phosphatic urinary stones.

Patient compliance usually is poor, since the quantities required cause gastrointestinal discomfort, taste intolerance, and constipation. Serum levels of calcium and phosphorus should be monitored periodically in patients with impaired renal function. As with other amphoteric gels, absorption of the tetracyclines is impaired when these drugs are used concomitantly.

DRUG INTERACTIONS. See the discussion on drug interactions in the introduction to this section.

DOSAGE AND PREPARATIONS.
Oral: For peptic ulcer, see the evaluation on Aluminum Hydroxide Gel.
See Table 1 for preparations.

DIHYDROXYALUMINUM SODIUM CARBONATE

This aluminum compound is claimed to have properties of both sodium carbonate and aluminum hydroxide; sodium carbonate reacts rapidly while aluminum hydroxide has a more prolonged effect. Results of a limited number of studies have shown that this agent temporarily neutralizes gastric acid; however, there are no convincing comparative data to demonstrate its superiority to solid dosage forms of other aluminum compounds.

Constipation may occur with large doses.

DRUG INTERACTIONS. See the discussion on drug interactions in the introduction to this section.

DOSAGE AND PREPARATIONS.
Oral: The dose and frequency of administration depend on the disorder being treated and the degree of relief obtained. A suggested dosage for duodenal and gastric ulcer is 80 and 40 mEq per dose, respectively. The traditional dose recommendation in *adults* is one or two tablets four or more times daily.
See Table 1 for preparations.

Calcium Compounds

The calcium compound used most commonly as an antacid is calcium carbonate. Tribasic calcium phosphate has been used occasionally, but its neutralizing action is weak and of brief duration; its principal indication is as a source of calcium and phosphate in deficiency states (see index entry Calcium Metabolism, Drugs Affecting).

CALCIUM CARBONATE

ACTIONS AND USES. Calcium carbonate has a rapid onset of action, very high neutralizing capacity, and a relatively prolonged effect. Its use as an antacid has been abandoned, perhaps prematurely, by many gastroenterologists because of emphasis on the acid rebound and the elevation in serum gastrin level that occur after single doses. However, the calcium specificity of gastrin-stimulated acid rebound has not been proved (Clayman, 1980; Schrumpf, 1980). In the alkaline intestinal milieu, this compound may be reconstituted as insoluble calcium soaps or calcium phosphate resulting in minimal systemic absorption. Significant hypercalcemia occurs in some patients, but usually only when the recommended dosage is exceeded.

ADVERSE REACTIONS AND PRECAUTIONS. Lack of palatability is a frequent complaint of patients using antacids. Dose-related constipation is common when calcium carbonate 20 to 40 g is taken daily, which is well above the manufacturers' maximum recommended daily dose of 8 g. Hemorrhoids, painful and bleeding anal fissures, or fecal impaction also may occur. Acute appendicitis has been produced by impacted calcium carbonate fecoliths. Liberation of carbon dioxide in the stomach may cause eructation and flatulence. Constipation can be minimized by substituting sufficient amounts of a magnesium preparation; a mixture of one part magnesium oxide to five parts calcium carbonate produces relatively normal stools in many patients.

The milk-alkali syndrome may occur after prolonged administration of calcium carbonate with sodium bicarbonate and/or homogenized milk containing vitamin D. This relatively rare syndrome is characterized by hypercalcemic alkalosis with normal or elevated phosphorus levels, azotemia, and normal alkaline phosphatase levels. Renal failure and metastatic calcinosis also occur; the urinary excretion of calcium is generally not increased, but the calcium nephropathy that occurs suggests a relationship between hypercalciuria and calcium carbonate ingestion. Conjunctival and episcleral suffusion accompany the alkalosis, and calcium deposits (manifested by band keratopathy) are noted. Nausea is a common symptom, in part reflecting the hypercalcemia. Symptoms subside gradually following discontinuation of the antacid and/or the milk. Predisposing factors are hypertension, sarcoidosis, dehydration and electrolyte imbalance due to vomiting or aspiration of gastric contents with inadequate intravenous fluid replacement, and renal dysfunction caused by primary renal disease. Magnesium and aluminum salts have not been implicated in this syndrome.

DRUG INTERACTIONS. See the discussion on drug interactions in the introduction to this section.

DOSAGE AND PREPARATIONS.
Oral: The dose and frequency of administration depend on whether an active ulcer or an interval phase is being treated. *Adults,* 1 to 4 g one and three hours after meals and at bedtime; 2 to 4 g every hour may be required to relieve pain. The tablets should be chewed before swallowing.

Generic. Powder; suspension; tablets 500 (chewable), 600, and 650 mg and 1.25 g (all forms nonprescription).

See Table 1 for trademark preparations.

Magnesium Compounds

The carbonate, hydroxide, oxide, phosphate, and trisilicate salts of magnesium are used as antacids, usually in combination with aluminum hydroxide. Magnesium trisilicate reacts slowly in gastric juice, and the stomach may empty before much of the acid is neutralized.

Magnesium salts have a laxative effect; therefore, their correct proportion in combination products will prevent or reduce the constipating effect of aluminum or calcium salts, which reciprocally control the diarrheal effect of magnesium salts. Because large doses must be given frequently to control ulcer pain, most available antacid combinations must be supplemented with aluminum or calcium salts to avoid diarrhea. Magnesium compounds are rarely tolerated as the sole antacid, because the laxative effect occurs at doses only slightly greater than those that produce the antacid effect.

Antacids containing magnesium seldom produce serious toxic effects; however, some compounds may cause hypermagnesemia in patients with severely impaired renal function.

MAGNESIUM HYDROXIDE (Milk of Magnesia)

MAGNESIUM OXIDE

These antacids have the same properties because magnesium oxide is hydrolyzed to the hydroxide in water. They have a high neutralizing capacity with a rapid onset of action.

For adverse reactions, see the preceding discussion on Magnesium Compounds.

DRUG INTERACTIONS. See the discussion on drug interactions in the introduction to this section.

DOSAGE AND PREPARATIONS.
Oral: Like all antacids with laxative properties, the dose and frequency of administration are determined by the number of substitutions for aluminum or calcium salts that result in normal stool consistency.

MAGNESIUM HYDROXIDE (Milk of Magnesia):
Generic. Powder; suspension; tablets (nonprescription).

MAGNESIUM OXIDE:
Generic. Capsules 140 mg; tablets 325, 400, and 420 mg; powder in both heavy and light forms (light form suspends more readily in liquid) (all forms nonprescription).

MAGNESIUM CARBONATE

The effect of magnesium carbonate is similar to that of the hydroxide and oxide salts, but this compound liberates carbon dioxide in the stomach during neutralization. It has a high neutralizing capacity but is rarely used alone for peptic ulcer. See Table 2 for antacid mixtures containing this agent.

For adverse reactions and precautions, see the preceding discussion on Magnesium Compounds.

DRUG INTERACTIONS. See the discussion on drug interactions in the introduction to this section.

Generic. Powder in both heavy and light forms (light form suspends more readily in liquid) (nonprescription).

MAGNESIUM PHOSPHATE

The action of this alkaline powder is similar to that of other magnesium preparations. Its neutralizing capacity is less than that of magnesium carbonate.

For adverse reactions and precautions, see the preceding discussion on Magnesium Compounds.

DRUG INTERACTIONS. See the discussion on drug interactions in the introduction to this section.

Generic. Powder (nonprescription).

Sodium Compound

SODIUM CITRATE

SODIUM CITRATE WITH CITRIC ACID
[Bicitra]

Sodium citrate is the antacid of choice for prophylaxis of aspiration pneumonitis during childbirth (Mendelson's syndrome) and other surgical procedures (Abboud et al, 1984; Gibbs et al, 1982); 30 ml of a 0.3 M solution of this clear nonparticulate antacid is rapid acting and safe for use in emergency surgery. Its chief drawback is lack of palatability. Commercial products containing sodium citrate alone are not available. However, a preparation of Shohl's solution containing sodium citrate with citric acid [Bicitra] has been adapted for this use (Gibbs and Banner, 1984).

Citrate antacids should not be administered with aluminum-based antacids used as phosphate binders in patients with renal failure (Kirschbaum and Schoolwerth, 1989). For other drug interactions, see the discussion in the introduction to this section.

Bicitra (Baker Norton). Solution containing sodium citrate dihydrate 500 mg (0.34 M) and citric acid monohydrate 334 mg (0.32 M)/5 ml in 15, 30, 120, 473, and 3,785 ml containers (sodium 1 mEq/ml, equivalent to 1 mEq bicarbonate).

Mixtures of Antacids

Products containing aluminum and/or calcium compounds with magnesium salts are more commonly used to treat peptic ulcer than single-entity antacids. The antacid effect of these combination products usually is the sum of effects of the individual components, but supplemental amounts of aluminum, calcium, or magnesium often are required to reduce constipation or diarrhea when large doses are employed. Newer formulations have been prepared in an attempt to provide a greater neutralizing action.

PREPARATIONS. See Table 2.

Mixtures of Antacids with Other Ingredients

Several products containing antacid and nonantacid ingredients are claimed to provide additional benefits. The alginic acid in *Gaviscon* forms a foam that acts as a carrier for antacids. The foam purportedly floats on top of the gastric contents and thus brings the antacids in contact with the mucosa, especially during reflux. There is no evidence that the effects of Gaviscon are more beneficial than those of conventional antacids, although some studies demonstrate that Gaviscon is at least as effective as other antacids in relieving heartburn. However, adverse effects may occur less frequently with Gaviscon than with more potent antacids. Alginic acid has no demonstrable effect on reflux esophagitis produced by acid peptic or bile reflux.

The *simethicone* present in some mixtures is claimed to alleviate symptoms of gas; however, its efficacy is doubtful and the rationale for its mechanism of action is dubious (see the evaluation). Simethicone has, however, been designated "safe and effective" by the FDA-OTC Antacid and Antiflatulent Review Panel (*Federal Register*, 1974). There is no convincing evidence that mixtures containing this apparently safe agent have beneficial effects other than those provided by the antacid.

PREPARATIONS. See Table 2.

MISCELLANEOUS AGENTS

METOCLOPRAMIDE HYDROCHLORIDE
[Maxolon, Octamide PFS, Reglan]

Cl, H_2N, OCH_3, $\overset{O}{\|}CNHCH_2CH_2\overset{+}{N}H(CH_2CH_3)_2$

ACTIONS. Metoclopramide is related structurally to procainamide but has a different spectrum of pharmacologic activity; it antagonizes dopamine receptors. This drug stimulates the motility of the upper gastrointestinal tract, increases lower esophageal sphincter (LES) pressure, and increases the rate of gastric emptying. The exact mechanism of action of metoclopramide has not been fully determined. Upper gastrointestinal transit time is accelerated by increased contractions of the esophageal body, increased gastric (especially antral) contractions with coordination of antral and duodenal peristalsis, and enhanced pyloric activity and pressure. Central antiemetic action may contribute to the effectiveness of metoclopramide in gastroparesis (Snape et al, 1982). Effects in the small intestine are similar to those in the esophagus and stomach. Gastric acid secretion is not affected. Gallbladder and bile duct pressure are increased, the sphincter of Oddi is relaxed, and pancreatic secretion is unaffected. No significant effect on colorectal function has been noted.

Therapeutic levels of some drugs that are absorbed primarily in the small intestine are achieved more rapidly, because metoclopramide increases the rate of gastric emptying (Harrington et al, 1983). The clinical significance of this effect has not been determined.

USES. Oral metoclopramide may relieve symptoms of mild diabetic gastroparesis; it may be less useful in patients with severe symptoms. Several studies indicate that this agent may be useful in the treatment of gastric atony occurring after vagotomy and gastric resection for peptic ulcer disease and for idiopathic gastric stasis; it is ineffective after antral resection. Investigationally, metoclopramide has been given adjunctively to improve gastric emptying and prevent aspiration pneumonitis in surgical patients before and during anesthesia (Albibi and McCallum, 1983; Harrington et al, 1983; Cohen et al, 1984).

When long-term therapy is needed, intravenous administration of metoclopramide may be required initially for a few days because inadequate gastric emptying prevents passage of the drug from the stomach to the intestine where it is absorbed.

In one study, metoclopramide was effective in 60% of patients with gastroparesis. Only 25% of those with prior gastric surgery responded to this drug; most of these patients had undergone antrectomy, which suggests that an intact antrum is important to metoclopramide's action (Pellegrini et al, 1983).

The dosage may be increased in unresponsive patients, but the incidence of adverse effects also increases. Lack of response may be due to other factors, such as concomitant treatment with opioids or other analgesics or drugs that impair gastric motility. Metoclopramide is not indicated when mechanical obstruction contributes to delayed emptying (Pellegrini et al, 1983).

Very large doses of metoclopramide have an antiemetic effect but do not prevent motion sickness (see index entry Metoclopramide, In Nausea).

Intravenous metoclopramide facilitates intubation and biopsy of the small intestine, and this route also has been used adjunctively in the radiologic examination of the stomach and small intestine in individuals with delayed gastric emptying. Its value for the latter indication is unproven in clinical trials.

Since metoclopramide increases LES pressure and enhances gastric emptying, it has been used orally as an adjunct to H_2 receptor antagonists to treat reflux esophagitis. It may be particularly valuable in patients with slow gastric emptying. However, no data are available from long-term studies to establish its safety and role when used as an adjunct to the H_2 receptor antagonists in the treatment of this condition. Furthermore, the clear superiority of omeprazole in reflux esophagitis eliminates the need for such combinations.

ADVERSE REACTIONS. Usual doses cause adverse reactions in up to 20% of patients; however, the effects often are mild and are reversible after metoclopramide is withdrawn. Drowsiness and lassitude are common. Constipation, diarrhea, urticarial or maculopapular rash, brief episodes of agitation or anxiety, restlessness, dryness of the mouth, glossal or periorbital edema, hirsutism, and methemoglobinemia have been noted. Hypotension or hypertension can occur occasionally. A hypertensive crisis developed when this drug was given to a patient with pheochromocytoma. Severe depression is a rare but potentially serious adverse effect.

Extrapyramidal reactions occur infrequently but are more common in the elderly, adolescents, and children. They are identical to the reactions produced by phenothiazine and butyrophenone drugs. Parkinsonian symptoms, dystonic movements, and tardive dyskinesia may occur, especially when therapeutic doses are taken daily for many months (Grimes et al, 1982). Unlike parkinsonian symptoms, tardive dyskinesia is not always reversible when the drug is discontinued.

Markedly increased prolactin levels have stimulated lactation, and metoclopramide may be contraindicated in patients with breast cancer who have undergone radiation or chemotherapy.

Particular caution should be employed when metoclopramide is administered to elderly or young patients or to those with hypertension. This drug should not be given to patients with extrapyramidal symptoms or epilepsy, although it has been used safely in those with parkinsonism. The safety of metoclopramide during pregnancy has not been established (FDA Pregnancy Category B), but its short-term use to prevent aspiration pneumonitis during childbirth (investigational indication) is apparently safe.

DRUG INTERACTIONS. The action of metoclopramide on gastrointestinal motility may be impaired by the concomitant administration of atropine or other anticholinergic agents. Metoclopramide should not be given with thioxanthene, phenothiazine, or butyrophenone compounds. Therapy should not be initiated in patients who have received tricyclic antidepressants or monoamine oxidase inhibitors within the previous two weeks. Metoclopramide may impair the vascular effect of dopamine.

Metoclopramide reduces the oral bioavailability of cimetidine by 25% to 30% (Gugler et al, 1981); therefore, at least one hour should elapse between administration of the two drugs. The dose of cimetidine may be increased when the two drugs are administered concomitantly, but this is not preferred.

PHARMACOKINETICS. Metoclopramide is well absorbed orally; the time to peak effect is 30 to 60 minutes. The volume of distribution is 2 to 3 L/kg. The range of plasma half-life is 2.6 to 5 hours. About 85% of an oral dose appears in the urine, one-half as free drug and sulfate and glucuronide conjugates and the remainder as a major and a few minor metabolites.

DOSAGE AND PREPARATIONS.

Oral: To relieve symptoms of diabetic gastroparesis and other disorders of gastric emptying, *adults*, 10 mg given 30 minutes before meals and at bedtime. *Children and young adults*, a maximum of 0.5 mg/kg is given daily in three divided doses. *Children under 6 years* should not receive more than 0.1 mg/kg as a single dose.

Maxolon (SmithKline Beecham). Tablets 10 mg.

Reglan (Robins), ***Generic.*** Syrup 5 mg/5 ml; tablets 5 and 10 mg.

Intravenous, Intramuscular: The following dosages are used for severe symptoms of diabetic gastroparesis when oral administration is not practical. When used intravenously, the injection should be given over one to two minutes. *Adults*, 10 mg is given 30 minutes before meals and at bedtime. *Chil-*

dren over 6 years and young adults, a maximum of 0.5 mg/kg is given daily in three divided doses. *Children under 6 years* should not receive more than 0.1 mg/kg as a single dose.

Intravenous: To facilitate small bowel intubation or when delayed gastric emptying interferes with x-ray examination of the upper gastrointestinal tract or small bowel, the manufacturer's suggested dose for *adults* is 10 mg (2 ml) injected over a one- to two-minute period. For *children 6 to 14 years*, 2.5 to 5 mg; *under 6 years*, 0.1 mg/kg.

Generic. Solution 5 mg/ml.

Octamide PFS (Adria). Solution (preservative-free) 5 mg/ml in 2, 10, and 30 ml containers.

Reglan (Robins). Solution 5 mg/ml in 2, 10, and 30 ml containers.

MISOPROSTOL

[Cytotec]

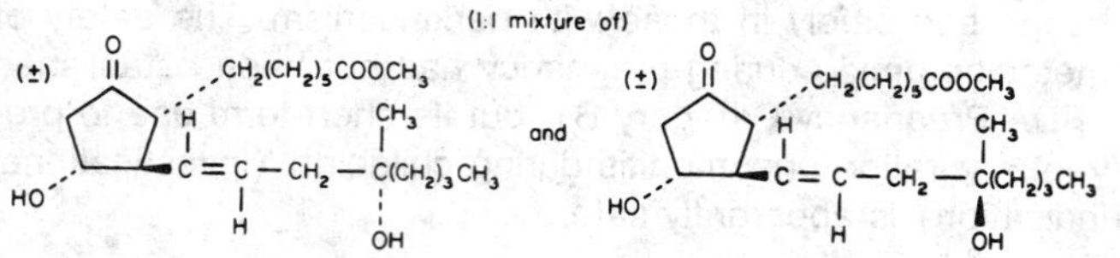

(1:1 mixture of)

(±) and (±)

ACTIONS AND USES. This PGE_1 methyl ester has both antisecretory and protective actions in the gastric mucosa. Misoprostol prevents gastrointestinal damage and peptic ulcer in patients receiving long-term therapy with aspirin or other NSAIDs (Roth, 1990; Bond, 1984, 1985; Henahan, 1985; Walt, 1992). In NSAID-induced peptic ulcer, misoprostol prevents the recurrence of both gastric and duodenal ulcer, whereas H_2 receptor antagonists prevent the relapse of duodenal ulcer but not gastric ulcer (Graham et al, 1991). In clinical trials, misoprostol was as effective as cimetidine for short-term treatment of duodenal ulcer and appeared to be effective for healing gastric ulcer, but H_2 receptor antagonists or sucralfate is preferred for treatment of peptic ulcer not associated with use of NSAIDs.

ADVERSE REACTIONS AND PRECAUTIONS. This drug is generally well tolerated. Minor adverse effects include mild nausea, abdominal discomfort, dizziness, and headache; diarrhea has occurred in 14% to 40% of patients.

Misoprostol should not be used in pregnant women or women of childbearing age. In one clinical trial, bleeding occurred in about 50% of pregnant women in the first trimester, and complete or incomplete abortion was induced in 7%. Misoprostol is classified in FDA Pregnancy Category X.

DOSAGE AND PREPARATIONS.

Oral: For prophylaxis of duodenal or gastric ulcer in high-risk patients receiving long-term therapy with NSAIDs (eg, the elderly, those with a history of gastric ulcer or upper gastrointestinal bleeding), *adults,* 200 mcg four times daily or 400 mcg twice daily. Many practitioners recommend an initial dose of 100 mcg four times daily taken with food to improve gastrointestinal tolerance.

Cytotec (Searle). Tablets 100 and 200 mcg.

OMEPRAZOLE

[Prilosec]

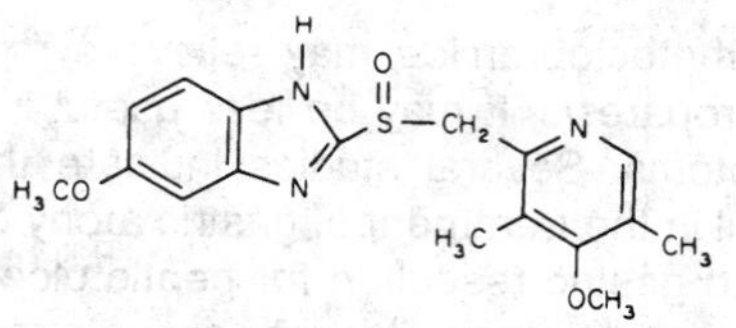

ACTIONS. This substituted benzimidazole inhibits gastric acid secretion by binding to and inactivating the H^+K^+ ATPase pump that exchanges luminal potassium for cellular hydrogen ions. Omeprazole binds irreversibly to this enzyme; the H_2 receptor is unaffected. Oral administration of omeprazole almost completely inhibits basal as well as pentagastrin-stimulated acid secretion.

USES. Omeprazole is effective for the treatment of peptic ulcers when these disorders have not responded to usual doses of the H_2 receptor antagonists (Clissold and Campoli-Richards, 1986; Maton, 1991; Howden, 1991), and the use of this agent for routine treatment of uncomplicated peptic ulcer is increasing. Clinical trials have clearly established that omeprazole heals duodenal ulcers more rapidly than cimetidine or ranitidine. In many studies, after administration of a single daily dose of 40 mg for two weeks, the healing rate achieved by omeprazole is similar to that obtained after four weeks of treatment with H_2 blockers. This agent is as or more efficacious than other drugs in patients with gastric ulcer.

For reflux esophagitis, a single daily dose of 40 mg was more effective than ranitidine 150 mg twice daily (Clissold and Campoli-Richards, 1986). Use of omeprazole in patients with this disorder should be limited to those with lesions refractory to usual doses of H_2 receptor antagonists and/or for those with severe disease (grades 3 and 4).

In some trials lasting as long as five years, a single daily dose has markedly reduced acid hypersecretion and has not produced significant adverse effects in patients with the Zollinger-Ellison syndrome, for which it is the drug of choice, and in other disorders of gastric acid hypersecretion (Maton et al, 1989).

ADVERSE REACTIONS. Few adverse effects were observed in clinical trials. Large doses administered lifelong to rats produced hypertrophy of mucosal enterochromaffin-like cells (ECL cells) leading to carcinoid tumors. The absence of acid secretion and resulting hypergastrinemia are believed to be responsible for stimulation of ECL cell growth. In clinical trials, the safety of long-term administration to patients with the Zollinger-Ellison syndrome suggests that the relative risk to humans is probably very small (Maton et al, 1990). However, in a recent case study, three patients treated with omeprazole 20 mg/day for one year developed hyperplastic gastric polyps with no sign of dysplasia or malignancy (Graham, 1992). Although more data are needed to assess the potential for tumor formation in patients receiving long-term omeprazole therapy, this and fears of other adverse reactions not observed with short-term usage appear to be groundless (Joelson et al, 1992).

Another concern has been raised regarding bacterial overgrowth resulting from the long-term use of omeprazole. In one study, significant increases in bacterial growth and in the nitrite and nitrosamine concentrations were observed in the gastric juice of volunteers given 30 mg for two weeks (Sharma et al, 1984). Illness produced by bacterial overgrowth has not been reported in clinical trials.

Although mild elevations of serum transaminases have been observed, no significant hepatotoxicity has been reported with omeprazole.

Worldwide, gynecomastia and impotence have occurred in 30 patients receiving omeprazole (Lindquist and Edwards, 1992).

Omeprazole is classified in FDA Pregnancy Category C.

DRUG INTERACTIONS. Omeprazole inhibits the drug metabolizing hepatic microsomal P450 mono-oxygenase and can be expected to interfere with the elimination of drugs metabolized in this system. The half-lives of diazepam, warfarin, and phenytoin are prolonged in patients treated with omeprazole (Maton, 1991). Ketoconazole requires an acid pH and is less effective at the higher pH produced in patients treated with omeprazole.

PHARMACOKINETICS. Administration of enteric-coated granules produces mean peak plasma concentrations in 0.5 to 2.5 hours. Increasing the daily dose or continued daily administration increases the bioavailability, probably because inhibition of gastric acid secretion protects omeprazole from rapid breakdown. Plasma protein binding in human plasma is above 95%.

This agent is eliminated rapidly and almost completely by metabolism. Unchanged drug has not been recovered in the urine. The mean elimination half-life in healthy subjects is about one hour.

Omeprazole inhibits acid secretion significantly for days after plasma concentrations have decreased below the limits of detection. This probably reflects the time required for synthesis of new enzyme to replace the irreversibly inhibited ATPase (Clissold and Campoli-Richards, 1986).

DOSAGE AND PREPARATIONS.

Oral: For peptic ulcers, *adults,* 20 or 40 mg once daily for four to six weeks. For reflux esophagitis, *adults*, 20 or 40 mg once daily for up to two months. In some patients, a third month of therapy may be required to achieve complete healing. Thereafter, 20 mg once daily is given. In patients with severe esophagitis, this dosage may be necessary indefinitely (Metz et al, 1992).

For the Zollinger-Ellison syndrome, *adults,* the daily doses required to reduce gastric acid secretion to <5 mEq/hr during the hour before the next dose is to be administered have ranged from 20 to 160 mg. If more than 80 mg/day is required, the drug should be administered twice daily in divided doses. In patients with the Zollinger-Ellison syndrome who also have esophagitis, acid output should be reduced to <2 mEq/hr. After stabilization of disease, the dose can be reduced to 20 mg once or twice daily in 70% of patients (Metz et al, 1992).

Prilosec (Merck). Capsules (prolonged-release) 20 mg.

SUCRALFATE

[Carafate]

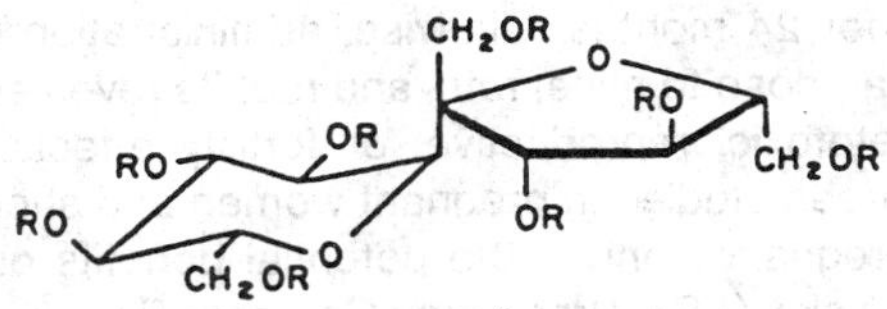

$$R = SO_3[Al_2(OH)_2(H_2O)_y]$$

ACTIONS. Sucralfate is a complex of sulfated sucrose and aluminum hydroxide. It has healing properties in patients with peptic ulcer and other acid-peptic disorders, but the mechanism of action is unclear (Szabo and Hollander, 1989). No gastric acid antisecretory action, acid-neutralizing effect, or direct stimulation of healing at ulcer sites has been demonstrated. Binding to pepsin and bile salts may contribute to acceleration of ulcer healing. Sucralfate also has antibacterial actions but is not active against *Helicobacter pylori* (Tryba and Mantey-Stiers, 1987).

The site of these actions is entirely local; only 2% to 5% of the sulfated disaccharide is absorbed (even in patients with mucosal lesions) and excreted in the urine.

USES. In controlled clinical trials, sucralfate was as effective as cimetidine or antacids in healing duodenal and gastric ulcers. When it was given prophylactically, recurrence of duodenal ulcers was decreased. Unlike H_2 receptor blockers and omeprazole, the efficacy of this drug in those with duodenal ulcer appears to be similar in smokers and nonsmokers (Mathews et al, 1992). Sucralfate's effect in preventing recurrences of gastric ulcers is still unclear.

The usefulness of sucralfate in reflux esophagitis is unresolved; many clinicians believe that its value is limited (Elsborg and Jorgensen, 1991). Others believe that symptomatic relief is possible but there is little endoscopic evidence of healing (Watson, 1992).

In some studies (Borrero et al, 1985; Bresalier et al, 1987), administration of sucralfate by nasogastric tube was as effective as antacids in preventing stress ulcers and bleeding during the first 40 to 48 hours after hospital admission.

ADVERSE REACTIONS. The overall incidence of adverse reactions was 4.7% in studies involving 2,500 patients. The most common side effect was constipation (2.2%). Other untoward effects (no single reaction occurred in more than 0.3% of patients) were similar to those in placebo groups.

Concern has been raised about the presence of aluminum in sucralfate (207 mg of elemental aluminum/g). However, elevated aluminum levels have not been found in patients with normal renal function treated for a prolonged period. Nevertheless, because of its aluminum content, sucralfate should be used with caution in patients with renal failure. There is no association between elevated brain levels of aluminum and Alzheimer's disease (Mathews et al, 1992; Watson, 1992).

No toxicity was reported in animals after the short-term administration of maximum oral doses, and no tumorigenicity was observed after 12 times the human dose was given to animals for 24 months. Likewise, administration of 50 times the human dose to mice, rats, and rabbits revealed no teratogenic, fetotoxic, reproductive, or fertility effects. Sucralfate has not been studied in pregnant women and should be used during pregnancy only if the potential benefits outweigh the possible risks (FDA Pregnancy Category B).

DRUG INTERACTIONS. Various case reports suggest that sucralfate may interfere with the absorption of tetracyclines, warfarin, phenytoin, quinidine, theophylline, or digoxin (*Med Lett Drugs Ther*, 1984; Berardi; et al, 1992). Sucralfate and these drugs should be given two hours apart to minimize this possibility. Sucralfate decreases the bioavailability of ciprofloxacin and norfloxacin (even when doses are taken hours apart). To avoid possible antibiotic failure, these fluoroquinolones should not be administered with sucralfate (Nix et al, 1989; Parpia et al, 1989).

DOSAGE AND PREPARATIONS.

Oral: *Adults,* for treatment of duodenal and gastric ulcer, 1 g four times a day on an empty stomach (one hour before meals and at bedtime). The suggested dose for prophylaxis is 2 g daily. Antacids may be used concurrently as needed for relief of pain, but they should not be taken within one-half hour before or after sucralfate administration.

Carafate (Marion Merrell Dow). Tablets 1 g.

SIMETHICONE

[Gas-X, Mylanta Gas, Mylicon]

This combination of dimethylpolysiloxanes and silica gel is available as a single-entity product and in mixtures containing antacids, belladonna alkaloids, and/or digestive enzymes. Simethicone has an antifoaming action by virtue of its effect on the surface tension of gas bubbles. It is promoted to relieve the symptoms of gaseous distention occurring postoperatively or as a result of aerophagia; however, evidence from controlled studies to prove that symptoms of intestinal gas are relieved by use of this agent, alone or in combination products, is inconclusive. Simethicone eliminates mucus-embedded bubbles that interfere with visualization during gastroscopy. It does not reduce intestinal gas that may interfere with radiologic or ultrasound examination of the abdomen. No adverse reactions have been reported.

Generic. Drops 40 mg/0.6 ml; tablets (chewable) 80 mg.

Gas-X (Sandoz). Tablets 80 and 125 mg.

Mylanta Gas (Johnson & Johnson/Merck Consumer). Tablets 40, 80, and 125 mg.

Mylicon (Johnson & Johnson/Merck Consumer). Drops 40 mg/0.6 ml; tablets (chewable) 40, 80, and 125 mg (all forms nonprescription).

Additional Trademark:

Phazyme (Reed & Carnrick).

Cited References

Antacid and antiflatulent products, part II. *Federal Register* 39:19862-22140, 1974.

Sucralfate for peptic ulcer: Reappraisal. *Med Lett Drugs Ther* 26:43-44, 1984.

Abboud TK, et al: Efficacy of clear antacid prophylaxis in obstetrics. *Acta Anaesthesiol Scand* 28:301-304, 1984.

Achem SR, Kolts BE: Current medical therapy for esophageal motility disorders. *Am J Med* 92(suppl 5A):5A-98S-5A-105S, 1992.

Albibi R, McCallum RW: Metoclopramide: Pharmacology and clinical application. *Ann Intern Med* 98:86-95, 1983.

Alfrey AC: Aluminum intoxication. *N Engl J Med* 310:1113-1115, 1984.

Allende HD, et al: Cimetidine-induced impotence and gynecomastia: Reversal with ranitidine, abstract. *Gastroenterology* 82:1007, 1982.

Alstead EM, et al: Ranitidine in prevention of gastric and duodenal ulcer relapse. *Gut* 24:418-420, 1983.

Barr GD, et al: Two-year prospective controlled study of maintenance cimetidine and gastric ulcer. *Gastroenterology* 85:100-104, 1983.

Barradell LB, et al: Lansoprazole: A review of its pharmacodynamic and pharmacokinetic properties and its therapeutic efficacy in acid-related disorders. *Drugs* 44:225-250, 1992.

Barrier CH, Hirschowitz BI: Controversies in the detection and management of nonsteroidal antiinflammatory drug-induced side effects of the upper gastrointestinal tract. *Arthritis Rheum* 32:926-932, 1989.

Berardi RR, et al: Comparison of famotidine with cimetidine and ranitidine. *Clin Pharm* 7:271-284, 1988.

Berardi RR, et al: Identifying potential interactions of sucralfate with other drugs in hospitalized patients. *Am J Hosp Pharm* 49:1488-1490, 1992.

Bernersen B, et al: Is *Helicobacter pylori* the cause of dyspepsia? *BMJ* 304:1276-1279, 1992.

Berstad A, et al: Controlled clinical trial of duodenal ulcer healing with antacid tablets. *Scand J Gastroenterol* 17:953-959, 1982.

Bianchi-Porro G, Keohane PP (eds): Nizatidine in peptic ulcer disease: Proceedings of First International Symposium on Nizatidine. *Scand J Gastroenterol* 22(suppl 136):1-88, 1987.

Bond WS: Prostaglandins: Next generation of antiulcer agents, part I. *Facts Comparisons Drug Newslett* 3:89-91, 1984.

Bond WS: Prostaglandins: Next generation of antiulcer agents, part II. *Facts Comparisons Drug Newslett* 4:1-3, 1985.

Borody TJ, et al: Recurrence of duodenal ulcer and *Campylobacter pylori* infection after eradication. *Med J Aust* 151:431-435, 1989.

Borody T, et al: *Helicobacter pylori* reinfection 4 years posteradication. *Lancet* 339:1295, 1992.

Borrero E, et al: Comparison of antacid and sucralfate in prevention of gastrointestinal bleeding in patients who are critically ill. *Am J Med* 79(suppl 2C):62-64, 1985.

Bortolotti M, Coccia G: Achalasia treatment: Is nifedipine a viable alternative? Selected summaries. *Gastroenterology* 102:1433-1434, 1992.

Bresalier RS, et al: Sucralfate suspension versus titrated antacid for prevention of acute stress-related gastrointestinal hemorrhage in critically ill patients. *Am J Med* 83(suppl 3B):110-115, 1987.

Brock-Utne JG, et al: Influence of preoperative gastric aspiration on the volume and pH of gastric contents in obstetric patients undergoing caesarean section. *Br J Anaesth* 62:397-401, 1989.

Brogden RN, et al: Ranitidine: Review of its pharmacology and therapeutic use in peptic ulcer disease and other allied diseases. *Drugs* 24:267-303, 1982.

Broughton LJ, Rogers HJ: Decreased systemic clearance of caffeine due to cimetidine. *Br J Clin Pharmacol* 12:155-159, 1981.

Butterworth KR, et al: Bioavailability of aluminum, letter. *Lancet* 339:1489, 1992.

Caldwell SH, Marshall BJ: *Campylobacter pylori* and peptic disease: Therapeutic implications. *Drug Ther* 92-106, (May) 1989.

Cave DR: Therapeutic approaches to recurrent peptic ulcer disease. *Hosp Pract* 33-49, (Sept) 1992.

Chen CT, et al: Evaluation of the efficacy of Alka-Seltzer effervescent in gastric acid neutralization. *Anesth Analg* 63:325-329, 1984.

Clayman CB: The carbonate affair: Chalk one up. *JAMA* 244:2554, 1980.

Clissold SP, Campoli-Richards DM: Omeprazole: Preliminary review of its pharmacodynamic and pharmacokinetic properties, and therapeutic potential in peptic ulcer disease and Zollinger-Ellison syndrome. *Drugs* 32:15-47, 1986.

Cloud ML, et al: Nizatidine *versus* placebo in gastroesophageal reflux disease: A 12-week, multicenter, randomized, double-blind study. *Am J Gastroenterol* 86:1735, 1991.

Cloud ML, et al: Nizatidine *versus* placebo in gastroesophageal reflux disease: A six-week, multicenter, randomized, double-blind comparison. *Dig Dis Sci* 37:865-874, 1992.

Coccia G, et al: Prospective clinical and manometric study comparing pneumatic dilatation and sublingual nifedipine in the treatment of oesophageal achalasia. *Gut* 32:604-606, 1991.

Cohen SE: Aspiration syndrome. *Clin Obstet Gynecol* 9:235-254, 1982.

Cohen SE, et al: Does metoclopramide decrease volume of gastric contents in patients undergoing cesarean section? *Anesthesiology* 61:604-607, 1984.

Coombs DW, et al: Acid-aspiration prophylaxis by preoperative oral administration of cimetidine. *Anesthesiology* 51:352-356, 1979 A.

Coombs DW, et al: Preanesthetic cimetidine: Alteration of gastric fluid volume and pH. *Anesth Analg* 58:183-188, 1979 B.

Crawford JS, Potter SR: Magnesium trisilicate mixture BP: Its physical characteristics and effectiveness as prophylactic. *Anaesthesia* 39:535-539, 1984.

Daneshmend TK, et al: Omeprazole versus placebo for acute upper gastrointestinal bleeding: Randomised double blind controlled trial. *BMJ* 304:143-147, 1992.

Danilewitz M, et al: Ranitidine suppression of gastric hypersecretion resistant to cimetidine. *N Engl J Med* 306:20-22, 1982.

Decktor DL, Robinson MG: Omeprazole. *Drug Ther* 54-60, (April) 1990.

Delattre M, et al: Treatment of duodenal ulceration: Comparative trial of cimetidine (Tagamet) at daily dosages of 800 mg (400 mg b.i.d.) and 1000 mg (250 mg q.i.d.). *Clin Trials J* 19:94-105, 1982.

Dent J: What's new in the esophagus. *Dig Dis Sci* 26:161-169, 1981.

Dewan DM, et al: Antacid anticholinergic regimens in patients undergoing elective caesarean section. *Can Anaesth Soc J* 29:27-30, 1982.

Di Padova C, et al: H_2-receptor antagonists and blood alcohol levels. *Gastroenterology* 103:1102-1104, 1992.

Dobrilla G, et al: An update on the short-term medical treatment of duodenal ulcer. *Curr Ther Res* 45:873-901, 1989.

Domstad PA, Deland FH: Management of gastric outlet obstruction. *Compr Ther* 8:17-20, (Aug) 1982.

Dubin SA, et al: Famotidine: A new H_2 receptor antagonist. *Anesth Analg* 68:S72-S73, 1989.

Dull JS, et al: Successful treatment of gastroparesis with erythromycin in a patient with progressive systemic sclerosis. *Am J Med* 89:528-530, 1990.

Durrant JM, Strunin L: Comparative trial of effect of ranitidine and cimetidine on gastric secretion in fasting patients at induction of anaesthesia. *Can Anaesth Soc J* 29:446-451, 1982.

Ekman L, et al: Toxicological studies on omeprazole. *Am J Gastroenterol* 108:53-69, 1985.

Ellis FH Jr: Esophagomyotomy for noncardiac chest pain resulting from diffuse esophageal spasm and related disorders. *Am J Med* 92(suppl 5A):5A-129S-5A-131S, 1992.

Elsborg L, Jorgensen F: Sucralfate versus cimetidine in reflux oesophagitis: A double-blind clinical study. *Scand J Gastroenterol* 26:146-150, 1991.

Elta GH, Kochman ML: Achalasia treatment: Is nifedipine a viable alternative? Selected summaries. *Gastroenterology* 102:1432-1433, 1992.

Ewart MC, et al: A comparison of the effects of omeprazole and ranitidine on gastric secretion in women undergoing elective caesarian section. *Anaesthesia* 45:527-530, 1990.

Forman D: *Helicobacter pylori* infection: A novel risk factor in the etiology of gastric cancer. *J Natl Cancer Inst* 83:1702-1703, 1991.

Fraser AG, et al: Effects of H_2-receptor antagonists on blood alcohol levels, letter. *JAMA* 267:2469, 1992.

Friedman G: Famotidine. *Am J Gastroenterol* 82:504-506, 1987.

Gelfond M, et al: Isosorbide dinitrate and nifedipine: Treatment of achalasia, clinical, manometric and radionuclide evaluation. *Gastroenterology* 83:963-969, 1982.

Gibbs CP, Banner TC: Effectiveness of Bicitra as preoperative antacid. *Anesthesiology* 61:97-99, 1984.

Gibbs C, et al: Effectiveness of sodium citrate as antacid. *Anesthesiology* 57:44-46, 1982.

Gillespie IE, et al: The stomach, in Gillespie IE, Thompson TJ (eds): *Gastroenterology, An Integrated Course*. New York, Churchill Livingstone, 1983, 46-91.

Gillett GB, et al: Prophylaxis against acid aspiration syndrome in obstetric practice. *Anesthesiology* 60:525, 1984.

Gitlin N, et al: Multicenter, double-blind randomized placebo-controlled comparison of nocturnal and twice-a-day famotidine on treatment of active duodenal ulcer disease. *Gastroenterology* 92:48-53, 1987.

Gledhill T, et al: Single nocturnal dose of H_2 receptor antagonist for treatment of duodenal ulcer. *Gut* 24:904-908, 1983.

Goodman LJ, Lisowski JM: *Helicobacter pylori* and the upper GI tract: A bug for all lesions? *Hosp Formul* 26:792-800, 1991.

Graham DY: Prevention of gastroduodenal injury induced by chronic nonsteroidal antiinflammatory drug therapy. *Gastroenterology* 96:675-681, 1989.

Graham JR: Gastric polyposis: Onset during long-term therapy with omeprazole. *Med J Aust* 157:287-288, 1992.

Graham DY: Treatment of peptic ulcers caused by *Helicobacter pylori*, editorial. *N Engl J Med* 328:349-350, 1993.

Graham DY, et al: Prevention of duodenal ulcer in arthritics who are chronic NSAID users: A multicenter trial of the role of misoprostol. *Gastroenterology* 100(pt 2):A75, 1991.

Graham DY, et al: Effect of treatment of *Helicobacter pylori* infection on the long-term recurrence of gastric or duodenal ulcer: A randomized, controlled study. *Ann Intern Med* 116:705, 1992 A.

Graham DY, et al: Ulcer recurrence following duodenal ulcer healing with omeprazole, ranitidine, or placebo: A double-blind, multicenter, 6-month study. *Gastroenterology* 102:1289-1294, 1992 B.

Greenlaw R, et al: Gastroduodenitis: Broader concept of peptic ulcer disease. *Dig Dis Sci* 25:660-672, 1980.

Grimes JD, et al: Adverse neurologic effects of metoclopramide. *Can Med Assoc J* 126:23-25, 1982.

Grossman MI, et al: Peptic ulcer: New therapies, new diseases. *Ann Intern Med* 95:609-627, 1981.

Gugler R, et al: Impaired cimetidine absorption due to antacids and metoclopramide. *Eur J Clin Pharmacol* 20:225-228, 1981.

Guslandi M, Tittobello A: Steroid ulcers: A myth revisited. Steroids cause peptic ulcers only when given together with non-steroidal anti-inflammatory drugs. *BMJ* 304:655-656, 1992.

Halloran LG, et al: Prevention of acute gastrointestinal complications after severe head injury: Controlled trial of cimetidine prophylaxis. *Am J Surg* 139:44-48, 1980.

Hansten PD: Drug interactions of ranitidine vs cimetidine. *Drug Interact Newslett* 3:31-34, 1983.

Hansten PD: Interactions between antiulcer medications. *Drug Interact Newslett* 5:11-14, 1985.

Hansten PD: Effects of H_2-receptor antagonists on blood alcohol levels, letter. *JAMA* 267:2469, 1992.

Hansten PD, Horn JR: *Drug Interactions,* ed 6. Philadelphia, Lea & Febiger, 1989.

Hansten PD, Horn JR: Antacid drug interactions. *Drug Interact Newslett* 11:519, 1991.

Harrington RA, et al: Metoclopramide: Updated review of its pharmacological properties and clinical use. *Drugs* 25:451-494, 1983.

Heading RC: Gastric emptying: Clinical perspective. *Clin Sci* 63:231-235, 1982.

Helman CA, Ou Tim L: Pharmacology and clinical efficacy of ranitidine, new H_2-receptor antagonist. *Pharmacotherapy* 3:185-192, 1983.

Henahan J: Laboratory devised prostaglandin derivatives offer antiulcer promise. *JAMA* 253:617-620, 1985.

Henry DA, Langman MJS: Adverse effects of anti-ulcer drugs. *Drugs* 21:444-459, 1981.
Hentschel E, et al: Effect of ranitidine and amoxicillin plus metronidazole on the eradication of *Helicobacter pylori* and the recurrence of duodenal ulcer. *N Engl J Med* 328:308-312, 1993.
Hirschowitz BI, et al: Inhibition of basal acid, chloride, and pepsin secretion in duodenal ulcer by graded doses of ranitidine and atropine with studies of pharmacokinetics of ranitidine. *Gastroenterology* 82:1314-1326, 1982.
Hodgkinson R, et al: Comparison of cimetidine (Tagamet) with antacid for safety and effectiveness in reducing gastric acidity before elective cesarean section. *Anesthesiology* 59:86-90, 1983.
Hollander D, et al: Cytoprotective action of antacids against alcohol-induced gastric mucosal injury: Morphologic, ultrastructural and functional time sequence analysis. *Gastroenterology* 86:1114, 1984.
Holloway RH, et al: Upper gastrointestinal motility. I: Pathophysiologic approach to management of reflux esophagitis. *Am J Gastroenterol* 76:280-290, 1981.
Howard JM, et al: Famotidine, a new potent long-acting histamine H_2-receptor antagonist: Comparison with cimetidine and ranitidine in treatment of Zollinger-Ellison syndrome. *Gastroenterology* 88:1026-1033, 1985.
Howden CW: Clinical pharmacology of omeprazole. *Clin Pharmacokinet* 20:38-49, 1991.
Hughes JT: Bioavailability of aluminum, letter. *Lancet* 339:1489, 1992.
Ireland A, et al: Ranitidine 150 mg twice daily vs 300 mg nightly in treatment of duodenal ulcers. *Lancet* 2:274-276, 1984.
Isenberg JI, et al: Healing of benign gastric ulcer with low-dose antacid or cimetidine: Double-blind, randomized, placebo-controlled trial. *N Engl J Med* 308:1319-1324, 1983.
Jadhav GR, Freston JW: Peptic ulcers: Can maintenance therapy prevent relapse? *Drug Ther* 13:183-188, 1983.
Janssens J, et al: Improvement of gastric emptying in diabetic gastroparesis by erythromycin: A preliminary study. *N Engl J Med* 322:1028-1031, 1990.
Jensen RT, et al: Zollinger-Ellison syndrome: NIH combined clinical staff conference. *Ann Intern Med* 98:59-75, 1983 A.
Jensen RT, et al: Cimetidine-induced impotence and breast changes in patients with gastric hypersecreting states. *N Engl J Med* 308:883-887, 1983 B.
Joelson S, et al: Safety experience from long-term treatment with omeprazole. *Digestion* 51 (suppl 1):93-101, 1992.
Johannessen T, et al: Cimetidine on-demand in dyspepsia: Experience with randomized controlled single-subject trials. *Scand J Gastroenterol* 27:189-195, (March) 1992.
Johnson DA: Medical therapy for gastroesophageal reflux disease. *Am J Med* 92 (suppl 5A):5A-88S-5A-97S, 1992.
Jones MP, Schubert ML: What do you recommend for prophylaxis in an elderly woman with arthritis requiring NSAIDs for control? Controversies, dilemmas, and dialogues. *Am J Gastroenterol* 86:264-265, 1991.
Kallos T, et al: Pulmonary aspiration of gastric contents, in Orkin FK, Cooperman LH (eds): *Complications in Anesthesiology*. Philadelphia, JB Lippincott, 1983, 152-164.
Kandel G: Management of nonvariceal upper GI hemorrhage. *Hosp Pract* 171-182, (Jan) 1990.
Kirschbaum BB, Schoolwerth AC: Acute aluminum toxicity associated with oral citrate and aluminum-containing antacids. *Am J Med Sci* 297:9-11, 1989.
Klotz U: Lack of effect of nizatidine on drug metabolism. *Scand J Gastroenterol* 22 (suppl 136):18-23, 1987.
Knadler MP, et al: Nizatidine: An H_2 blocker: Its metabolism and disposition in man. *Drug Metab Dispos* 14:175-182, 1986.
Knadler MP, et al: Absorption studies of H_2-blocker nizatidine. *Clin Pharmacol Ther* 42:514-520, 1987.
Konturek SJ: Pharmacology and clinical use of ranitidine. *Mt Sinai J Med* 49:370-382, 1982.
Koretz RL: Prophylactic therapy of stress-related mucosal damage: Why, which, who, and so what? *Am J Gastroenterol* 85:935-937, 1990.
Lacerte M, et al: Single daily dose of cimetidine for treatment of symptomatic duodenal ulcer. *Curr Ther Res* 35:777-782, 1984.
Lagarde SP, Spiro HM: Non-ulcer dyspepsia. *Clin Gastroenterol* 13:437-446, 1984.
Laitinen S, et al: Sucralfate and alginate/antacid in reflux esophagitis. *Scand J Gastroenterol* 20:229-232, 1985.
Lambert JR: Effect of antiulcer drugs on *Helicobacter pylori*. *Drug Invest* 2 (suppl 1):52-55, 1990.
Larsson R, et al: Pharmacokinetics of cimetidine and sulphoxide metabolite in patients with normal and impaired renal function. *Br J Clin Pharmacol* 13:163-170, 1982.
Lerman J, et al: Effects of metoclopramide and ranitidine on gastric fluid pH and volume in children. *Can J Anaesth* 35:S142-S143, 1988.
Levinson MJ: Gastric stress ulcers. *Hosp Pract* 59-68, (March) 1989.
Lewis JH: Treatment of gastric ulcer. *Arch Intern Med* 143:264-274, 1983.
Lieberman D: Treatment approaches to reflux oesophagitis. *Drugs* 39:674-680, 1990.
Lindberg P, et al: Omeprazole: The first proton pump inhibitor. *Med Res Rev* 10:1-54, 1990.
Lindquist M, Edwards IR: Endocrine adverse effects of omeprazole. *BMJ* 305:451-452, 1992.
Maile CJD, Francis RN: Preoperative ranitidine: Effect of a single intravenous dose on pH and volume of gastric aspirate. *Anaesthesia* 38:324-326, 1983.
Malagelada JR: Gastric emptying disorders: Clinical significance and treatment. *Drugs* 24:353-359, 1982.
Manchikanti L, Roush JR: Effect of preanesthetic glycopyrrolate and cimetidine on gastric fluid pH and volume in outpatients. *Anesth Analg* 63:40-46, 1984.
Manchikanti L, et al: Cimetidine and related drugs in anesthesia. *Anesth Analg* 61:595-608, 1982.
Manchikanti L, et al: Ranitidine and metoclopramide for prophylaxis of aspiration pneumonitis in elective surgery. *Anesth Analg* 63:903-910, 1984.
Manchikanti L, et al: Bicitra (sodium citrate) and metoclopramide in outpatient anesthesia for prophylaxis against aspiration pneumonitis. *Anesthesiology* 63:378-384, 1985.
Manchikanti L, et al: Dose-response effects of intravenous ranitidine on gastric pH and volume in outpatients. *Anesthesiology* 65:180-185, 1986.
Marshall BJ: Treatment strategies for *Helicobacter pylori* infection. *Gastroenterol Clin North Am* 22:183-198, 1993.
Mathews DR, et al: Sucralfate, correspondence. *N Engl J Med* 326:836-837, 1992.
Maton PN: Omeprazole. *N Engl J Med* 324:965-975, 1991.
Maton PN, et al: Long-term efficacy and safety of omeprazole in patients with Zollinger-Ellison syndrome: A prospective study. *Gastroenterology* 97:827-836, 1989.
Maton PN, et al: The effect of Zollinger-Ellison syndrome and omeprazole therapy on gastric oxyntic endocrine cells. *Gastroenterology* 99:943-950, 1990.
McAuley DM, et al: Ranitidine as antacid before elective caesarean section. *Anaesthesia* 38:108-114, 1983.
McCallum RW: Review of current status of prokinetic agents in gastroenterology. *Am J Gastroenterol* 80:1008-1016, 1985.
McCarthy DM: Smoking and ulcers: Time to quit. *N Engl J Med* 311:726-728, 1984.
McElwee HP, et al: Cimetidine affords protection equal to antacids in prevention of stress ulceration following thermal injury. *Surgery* 86:620-626, 1979.
McKinlay AW, et al: *Helicobacter pylori*: Bridging the credibility gap. *Gut* 31:940-945, 1990.
Mendelson CL: Aspiration of stomach contents into lungs during obstetric anesthesia. *Am J Obstet Gynecol* 53:191-205, 1946.
Metz DC, et al: Currently used doses of omeprazole in Zollinger-Ellison syndrome are too high. *Gastroenterology* 103:1498-1508, 1992.
Meyer GW, Castell DO: Evaluation and management of diseases of esophagus. *Am J Otolaryngol* 2:336-344, 1981.

Moir DD: Cimetidine, antacids, and pulmonary aspiration. *Anesthesiology* 59:81-83, 1983.
Monk JP, Clissold SP: Misoprostol: Preliminary review of its pharmacodynamic and pharmacokinetic properties, and therapeutic efficacy in treatment of peptic ulcer disease. *Drugs* 33:1-30, 1987.
Morison DH, et al: Double-blind comparison of cimetidine and ranitidine as prophylaxis against gastric aspiration syndrome. *Anesth Analg* 61:988-992, 1982.
Mozell EJ, et al: Long-term efficacy of octreotide in the treatment of Zollinger-Ellison syndrome. *Arch Surg* 127:1019-1026, 1992.
Naccaratto R, et al: Nizatidine versus ranitidine in gastric ulcer disease: European multicentre trial. *Scand J Gastroenterol* 22 (suppl 136):71-78, 1987.
Nix DE, et al: The effect of sucralfate pretreatment on the pharmacokinetics of ciprofloxacin. *Pharmacotherapy* 9:377-380, 1989.
Nyrén O, et al: Absence of therapeutic benefit from antacids or cimetidine in non-ulcer dyspepsia. *N Engl J Med* 314:339-343, 1986.
Oderda G, et al: Cure of peptic ulcer associated with eradication of *Helicobacter pylori*. *Lancet* 335:1599, 1990.
Okada M, et al: A comparative study of once-a-day morning and once-a-day bedtime administration of 40 mg famotidine in treating gastric ulcers. *Am J Gastroenterol* 87:1009-1013, 1992.
Okasha AS, et al: Cimetidine-antacid combination as premedication for elective caesarean section. *Can Anaesth Soc J* 30:593-597, 1983.
Olsson GL, et al: Aspiration during anaesthesia: A computer aided study of 185,358 anaesthetics. *Acta Anaesthesiol Scand* 30:84-92, 1986.
Ormezzano X, et al: Aspiration pneumonitis prophylaxis in obstetric anaesthesia: Comparison of effervescent cimetidine-sodium citrate mixture and sodium citrate. *Br J Anaesth* 64:503-506, 1990.
Orr WC: Maintenance therapy in gastroesophageal reflux disease. *Hosp Formul* 27:504-508, 1992.
Ostro MJ, et al: Control of gastric pH with cimetidine: Boluses versus primed infusions, abstract. *Gastroenterology* 86:1203, 1984.
Parpia SH, et al: Sucralfate reduces the gastrointestinal absorption of norfloxacin. *Antimicrob Agents Chemother* 33:99-102, 1989.
Pellegrini CA, et al: Diagnosis and treatment of gastric emptying disorders: Clinical usefulness of radionuclide measurements of gastric emptying. *Am J Surg* 145:143-151, 1983.
Peters MN, Richardson CT: Stressful life events, acid hypersecretion, and ulcer disease. *Gastroenterology* 84:114-119, 1983.
Peterson WL, et al: Healing of duodenal ulcer with antacid regimen. *N Engl J Med* 297:341-345, 1977.
Peura DA: Prophylactic therapy of stress-related mucosal damage: Why, which, who, and so what? *Am J Gastroenterol* 85:935-937, 1990.
Peura DA, Johnson LF: Cimetidine for prevention and treatment of gastroduodenal mucosal lesions in patients in intensive care unit. *Ann Intern Med* 103:173-177, 1985.
Pingleton SK: Gastrointestinal hemorrhage. *Med Clin North Am* 67:1215-1231, 1983.
Pitone JM, et al: Cimetidine-induced acute interstitial nephritis. *Am J Gastroenterol* 77:169-171, 1982.
Rao TLK, et al: Metoclopramide and cimetidine to reduce gastric pH and volume. *Anesth Analg* 63:1014-1016, 1984.
Rauws EAJ, Tytgat GNJ: Cure of duodenal ulcer associated with eradication of *Helicobacter pylori*. *Lancet* 335:1233-1235, 1990.
Rees WDW, et al: Dyspepsia, antral motor dysfunction, and gastric stasis of solids. *Gastroenterology* 78:360-365, 1980.
Reines H: Do we need stress ulcer prophylaxis? *Crit Care Med* 18:344, 1990.
Reusser P, et al: Prospective endoscopic study of stress erosions and ulcers in critically ill neurosurgical patients: Current incidence and effect of acid-reducing prophylaxis. *Crit Care Med* 18:270-274, 1990.
Richardson CT, Peterson WL: New agents for peptic ulcer. *Drug Ther* 12:145-151, 1982.
Richter JE: Gastroesophageal reflux: Diagnosis and management. *Hosp Pract* 59-66, (Jan) 1992.
Roberts RB, Shirley MA: Reducing the risk of acid aspiration during cesarean section. *Anesth Analg* 53:859-868, 1974.
Romankiewicz JA, Reidenberg MM: Current status of cimetidine in acid-peptic disorders. *Ration Drug Ther* 15:1-5, (May) 1981.
Roth SH: Misoprostol in the prevention of NSAID-induced gastric ulcer: A multicenter, double-blind, placebo-controlled trial. *J Rheumatol* 17 (suppl 20):20-24, 1990.
Rudnick MR, et al: Cimetidine-induced acute renal failure. *Ann Intern Med* 96:180-182, 1982.
Ryan MF: *Helicobacter pylori* and NSAIDS: More questions than answers. *Am J Gastroenterol* 86:1091-1092, 1991.
Sabesin SM, et al: Famotidine relieves symptoms of gastroesophageal reflux disease and heals erosions and ulcerations: Results of a multicenter, placebo-controlled, dose-ranging study. *Arch Intern Med* 151:2394-2400, 1991.
Sandhar BK, et al: Effect of oral liquids and ranitidine on gastric fluid volume and pH in children undergoing outpatient surgery. *J Anesth* 71:327-330, 1989.
Scarr M, et al: Volume and acidity of residual gastric fluid after oral fluid ingestion before elective ambulatory surgery. *Can Med Assoc J* 141:1151-1154, 1989.
Schmidt JF, Jørgenson BC: Effect of metoclopramide on gastric contents after preoperative ingestion of sodium citrate. *Anesth Analg* 63:841-843, 1984.
Schrumpf E: Effects of antacids on gastrin release. *Scand J Gastroenterol* 15:25-28, 1980.
Scott DB: Mendelson's syndrome, in Rugheimer E, Zindler M (eds): *Anaesthesiology: Proceedings of the 7th World Congress of Anaesthesiologists*. Princeton, Excerpta Medica, 1981, 799-801.
Sekiguchi T, et al: Open study of the clinical effects of lansoprazole in the treatment of reflux oesophagitis. *Drug Invest* 4:422-434, 1992.
Sepelyak RJ, et al: Adsorption of pepsin by aluminum hydroxide, II: Pepsin inactivation. *J Pharmaceut Sci* 73:1517-1521, 1984.
Sharma BK, et al: Intragastric bacterial activity and nitrosation before, during, and after treatment with omeprazole. *BMJ* 289:717-719, 1984.
Shearman DJC, Finlayson NDC: *Peptic Ulceration in Diseases of the Gastrointestinal Tract and Liver*. New York, Churchill Livingstone, 1982, 134-168.
Short TP, Thomas E: An overview of the role of calcium agonists in the treatment of achalasia and diffuse oesophageal spasm. *Drugs* 43:177-184, 1992.
Siepler J, Trudeau W: Treatment of UGIH by constant versus intermittent infusion of cimetidine in intensive care unit. *Gastroenterology* 86:1251, 1984.
Siepler JK, et al: Use of continuous infusion of histamine 2-receptor antagonists in critically ill patients. *DICP* 23:540-543, 1989.
Silverman DG, et al: Oral H2-antagonist prophylaxis in the outpatient setting: Ranitidine vs. famotidine. *Anesth Analg* 68:S263, 1989.
Smith JL: What do you recommend for prophylaxis in an elderly woman with arthritis requiring NSAIDs for control? Controversies, dilemmas, and dialogues. *Am J Gastroenterol* 86:266-267, 1991.
Snape WJ Jr, et al: Metoclopramide to treat gastroparesis due to diabetes mellitus: Double-blind, controlled trial. *Ann Intern Med* 96:444-446, 1982.
Soll A: Duodenal ulcer and drug therapy, in Sleisenger MH, Fordtran JS (eds): *Gastrointestinal Disease: Pathophysiology, Diagnosis, Management*, ed 4. Philadelphia, Saunders, 1989, 814-879.
Soll AH: Pathogenesis of peptic ulcer and implications for therapy. *N Engl J Med* 322:909-916, 1990 A.
Soll AH: Treatment of peptic ulcers. *N Engl J Med* 323:998-999, 1990 B.
Sorkin EM, Darvey DL: Review of cimetidine drug interactions. *Drug Intell Clin Pharm* 17:110-120, 1983.
Stern WR: Summary of 32nd meeting of Food and Drug Administration's gastrointestinal drugs advisory committee. *Am J Gastroenterol* 83:417-419, 1988.
Stoelting RK: Gastric fluid pH in patients receiving cimetidine. *Anesth Analg* 57:675-677, 1978.
Sweeney BL: Use of antacids as a prophylaxis against Mendelson's syndrome in the United Kingdom: Survey. *Anaesthesia* 41:419-422, 1986.

Szabo S, Hollander D: Pathways of gastrointestinal protection and repair: Mechanisms of action of sucralfate. *Am J Med* 86 (suppl 6A):23-31, 1989.

Talley NJ, Phillips SF: Non-ulcer dyspepsia: Potential causes and pathophysiology. *Ann Intern Med* 108:865-879, 1988.

Tatro DS: Update: Ranitidine drug interactions. *Facts Comparisons Drug Newslett* 11:25-27, (April) 1992.

Taylor T, Milne T: New evidence adds weight to the *Helicobacter pylori* story. *Inpharma* 5-7, (May) 1992.

Teabeaut JR II: Aspiration of gastric contents. *Am J Pathol* 28:51-62, 1952.

Tryba M: Stress bleeding prophylaxis with sucralfate: Pathophysiologic basis and clinical use. *Scand J Gastroenterol* 25 (suppl 173):22-33, 1990.

Tryba M, Mantey-Stiers F: Antibacterial activity of sucralfate in human gastric juice. *Am J Med* 83 (suppl 3B):125-127, 1987.

Walsh J: *Helicobacter pylori:* Selection of patients for treatment, editorial. *Ann Intern Med* 116:770-771, 1992.

Walt RP: Misoprostol for the treatment of peptic ulcer and anti-inflamatory-drug—induced gastroduodenal ulceration. *N Engl J Med* 327:1575-1580, 1992.

Wastell C, Lance P: *Cimetidine: The Westminster Hospital Symposium 1978*. London, Churchill Livingstone, 1979.

Watson K: Sucralfate. . .24 years on. *Inpharma* 18, (Feb) 1992.

Weber L, Hirshman CA: Cimetidine for prophylaxis of aspiration pneumonitis: Comparison of intramuscular and oral dosage schedules. *Anesth Analg* 58:426-427, 1979.

Wesdorp ICE: Famotidine in gastroesophageal reflux disease (GERD). *Hepatogastroenterology* 39 (suppl I):24-26, 1992.

Wheatley RG, et al: Milk of magnesia is effective preinduction antacid in obstetric anesthesia. *Anesthesiology* 50:514-519, 1979.

Williams JG, Strunin L: Preoperative intramuscular ranitidine and cimetidine: Double blind comparative trial, effect on gastric pH and volume. *Anaesthesia* 40:242-245, 1985.

Wilson P, Alp MH: Colloidal bismuth subcitrate tablets and placebo in chronic duodenal ulceration: Double-blind randomised trial. *Med J Aust* 1:222-223, 1982.

Wingtin LNG, et al: Omeprazole for prophylaxis of acid aspiration in elective surgery. *Anaesthesia* 45:436-438, 1990.

Wrobel J, et al: Sodium citrate: Alternative antacid for prophylaxis against aspiration pneumonitis. *Anaesth Intensive Care* 10:116-119, 1982.

Wynne JW, Modell JH: Respiratory aspiration of stomach contents. *Ann Intern Med* 87:466-474, 1977.

Young M: Bioavailability of aluminum, letter. *Lancet* 339:1489, 1992.

Zeldis JB, et al: Ranitidine: New H_2-receptor antagonist. *N Engl J Med* 309:1368-1373, 1983.

Zinner MJ, et al: Prevention of upper gastrointestinal tract bleeding in patients in intensive care unit. *Surg Gynecol Obstet* 153:214-220, 1981.

Zuckerman GR, Shuman R: Therapeutic goals and treatment options for prevention of stress ulcer syndrome. *Am J Med* 83 (suppl 6A):29-35, 1987.

THIS EVALUATION WAS PREPARED AFTER COMPLETION OF THIS CHAPTER

New Evaluation 42

CISAPRIDE
[Propulsid]

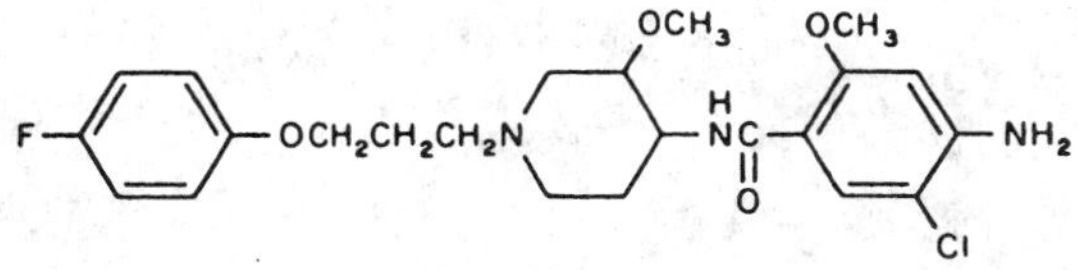

ACTIONS AND USES. This oral serotonin receptor antagonist stimulates motility throughout the gastrointestinal tract, elevates lower esophageal sphincter pressure, and enhances esophageal acid clearance (Johnson, 1992). Cisapride may be beneficial in some patients with mild to moderate reflux esophagitis; its primary value may be for maintenance therapy in patients with mild disease (Richter, 1992; Blum et al, 1993). Some studies suggest that this agent may be as efficacious as metoclopramide and safer for patients with diabetic gastroparesis and other disorders of delayed gastric emptying (Richards et al, 1993).

ADVERSE REACTIONS AND DRUG INTERACTIONS. This drug is usually well tolerated (*FDC Reports*, 1993 A, 1993 B). Seizures and arrhythmogenic effects on the heart have been reported rarely.

Accelerated gastric emptying increases the absorption and serum concentration of cimetidine, ranitidine, and other H_2 antagonists. Likewise, concomitant administration of cimetidine enhances the absorption and increases the serum concentration of cisapride; this does not occur with concomitant use of ranitidine. This serotonin antagonist also may enhance the sedative effects of benzodiazepines and alcohol.

Cisapride is classified in FDA Pregnancy Category C.

DOSAGE AND PREPARATIONS.

Oral: *Adults*, 10 mg four times daily given at least 15 minutes before meals and at bedtime (maximum, 20 mg four times daily).

Propulsid (Janssen). Tablets 10 mg.

Cited References

Janssen's *Propulsid* gastric motility agent is 'approvable.' *FDC Reports* 4-5, (April 19) 1993 A.

Janssen's *Propulsid* approved July 29 for nocturnal heartburn. *FDC Reports* 1-2, (Aug 2) 1993 B.

Blum AL, et al: Effect of cisapride on relapse of esophagitis: A multinational, placebo-controlled trial in patients healed with an antisecretory drug. *Dig Dis Sci* 38:551-560, 1993.

Johnson DA: Medical therapy for gastroesophageal reflux disease. *Am J Med* 92(suppl 5A):5A-88S-5A-97S, 1992.

Richards RD, et al: Objective and subjective results of a randomized, double-blind, placebo-controlled trial using cisapride to treat gastroparesis. *Dig Dis Sci* 38:811-816, 1993.

Richter JE: Gastroesophageal reflux: Diagnosis and management. *Hosp Pract* 59-66, (Jan) 1992.

Drugs Used in Disorders of the Lower Intestinal Tract

43

DIARRHEAL DISORDERS

Diarrhea is characterized by excessive fluidity, altered consistency, and increased volume of stool (more than 250 g/day in adults and 30 g/day in children). It is almost always associated with more frequent defecation (more than three times/day) and may be acute or chronic. Causes include infection, intoxication, ischemia of the bowel, maldigestion, malabsorption, inflammation, functional disorders, tumors of the bowel, allergy, and, rarely, certain extraintestinal hormone-producing neoplasms. The readiness with which diarrhea subsides depends largely on the underlying cause. Appropriate therapy depends on proper diagnosis.

Diarrhea can be classified as acute (<14 days), persistent (>14 days), or chronic (>30 days); the etiology and therapy differ for each.

Chronic diarrhea can be produced by a wide variety of substances, and it is associated with a large number of disorders, ranging from benign, self-limited diseases to life-threatening illnesses (Baldassano and Liacouras, 1991). See Table 1. Drug therapy is a frequent cause of chronic diarrhea; laxative abuse is common in the elderly. For a detailed discussion of drug-induced diarrhea, see Ratnaike and Jones, 1992, and Duncan et al, 1992).

Some authorities classify diarrhea as mild when it does not interfere with daily activities or cause any disturbance in fluid and electrolyte balance. Acute diarrhea causes water and salt depletion that may lead to dehydration and/or electrolyte imbalance, especially hypokalemia and acidosis. Even mild chronic diarrhea may produce hypokalemia with profound weakness and malaise.

Cramping from intermittent spasm and/or distention from gas produced by fermentation can occur. The frequency of defecation may cause unbearable discomfort when the number of bowel movements exceeds ten per day. Perianal irritation is common and hemorrhoids may be irritated.

Infectious Diarrhea

Infectious diarrhea is the most common cause of morbidity and mortality worldwide; as many as five million children under 5 years die annually. The majority of deaths could be prevented with adequate rehydration therapy (Avery and Snyder, 1990). Although acute infectious diarrhea is not as serious a problem in the United States, it accounts for as many as 20% of acute care visits by young children in large urban hospitals and for as many as 10% of potentially preventable deaths in American children.

A variety of organisms cause acute infectious diarrhea, and appropriate therapy depends on identification of the causative organism and the severity of the infection.

TABLE 1. COMMON CAUSES OF CHRONIC DIARRHEA IN ADULTS AND CHILDREN*

Infectious
- Bacterial (*Salmonella, Shigella, Campylobacter, Yersinia, Aeromonas, Plesiomonas*)
- Parasitic (*Giardia, Cryptosporidium, Entamoeba, Cyclospora*)
- *Clostridium difficile*

Postinfectious diarrhea

Drug-induced diarrhea
- Antibiotics
- Laxative abuse
- Chemotherapy

Dietary causes
- Overfeeding
- Intolerance to specific foods
- Sorbitol
- Formulas
- Malnutrition
- Milk-protein/soy allergy

Primary or secondary lactose intolerance

Encopresis

Irritable bowel syndrome

Nonspecific diarrhea of infancy

Inflammatory bowel disease
- Crohn's disease
- Ulcerative colitis

Celiac disease

Bacterial overgrowth

**Adapted from Baldassano and Liacouras, 1991.*

NONDRUG THERAPY. For patients with mild uncomplicated illness, heat applied to the abdomen and food restriction may relieve cramping and diarrhea.

In moderate to severe acute diarrhea, dehydration occurs as fluids are lost in the vomitus and stools and is a major danger. It can be prevented by the judicious administration of oral rehydration liquids (carbohydrate-electrolyte) soon after symptoms appear. Although intake of foods with a high fiber content (unrefined cereals, fruits, and vegetables) may be reduced concurrently, it is more important to establish appropriate rehydration and oral feeding within the first 24 hours to reduce stool frequency, improve nutrition, hasten recovery, and increase survival (Snyder, 1991). In one regimen for infants, all liquids and foods are withdrawn after the onset of diarrhea and oral rehydration solutions are administered for six hours. This is immediately followed by oral refeeding of either full- or half-strength formula (depending on tolerance) or by an unrestricted diet (Bezerra et al, 1992; Kerr, 1992). It is often recommended that lactose-containing products and milk products be avoided in children with acute diarrhea; however, those who have tolerated these products prior to the diarrheal episode are at no risk from their early readministration after oral rehydration. Furthermore, milk may have antidiarrheal properties (Nathavitharana and Booth, 1992).

For oral rehydration, patients require a balanced electrolyte solution containing sodium chloride and dextrose, which provides a favorable osmotic gradient for the increased absorption of water by the small intestine. In those who are vomiting, these solutions must be given in small volumes (5 to 10 ml) every five minutes and the amount increased gradually until the patient can drink normally. Frequent administration of small amounts of oral rehydration fluids also is beneficial for nonvomiting patients. If patients are severely dehydrated, it may be necessary to administer fluids intravenously initially: 50 to 100 ml/kg over four hours, followed by 100 ml/kg every 24 hours for maintenance (Skirrow, 1984). However, even in hospitalized patients, the oral route is preferred to intravenous administration in almost all (>85%) but the most severely dehydrated patients (*WHO Drug Information*, 1991).

Solutions available for oral rehydration in the United States include Pedialyte, Resol, Ricelyte, Rehydralyte, and WHO-UNICEF oral rehydration salts (ORS). The latter two solutions have a higher sodium content (75 to 90 mmol/L) and have been recommended for treatment; however, there is risk of hypernatremia with their use and most patients do not require this amount of sodium. Solutions containing less sodium (40 to 60 mmol/L) have been used primarily to prevent dehydration or for maintenance after rehydration, but they appear to be useful for treatment in most patients (American Academy of Pediatrics Committee on Nutrition, 1985; Santosham and Greenough, 1991). If solutions with a higher sodium content are used for maintenance, they should be alternated with water or low-sodium liquids (eg, low-carbohydrate juices).

Although rice-based or rice-derived solutions (eg, Ricelyte) may deliver more nutrients, provide less osmotic load to the gut lumen, contain less sodium, and reduce stool volume and frequency more effectively than glucose-based solutions (Pizarro et al, 1991 A; *Lancet,* 1992; Nathavitharana and Booth, 1992), their comparative value is controversial (see Pizarro et al, 1991 B; Sloan, 1991; Tochen, 1991; Scanlon and Scanlon, 1992).

Many physicians oppose use of homemade oral rehydration mixtures. However, if commercial oral electrolyte solutions are not available, a mixture of 1 level teaspoonful of table salt and 10 teaspoonsful of sugar in one quart of water can be a temporary substitute. Potassium chloride (1/4 teaspoonful) and sodium bicarbonate (1/2 teaspoonful of baking soda) also may be included (Swedberg and Steiner, 1983; Gaginella, 1983). This home remedy must be used with great caution, particularly in young children, since the amount of sodium in one quart (135 mEq) approaches a dangerous concentration. An equal volume of water should be given after each glassful of this salt solution.

Safer home remedy solutions that are being investigated are cereal based. In one, 1/2 cup of dry, precooked baby rice cereal is mixed with 1/4 teaspoon of salt in two cups of water. The resultant solution is thick but pourable and drinkable; it should not taste salty (50 mEq/L sodium). (However, even a twofold error in the amount of salt does not produce a dangerous sodium concentration.)

Only parents who are capable of following directions should be advised to prepare noncommercial home remedies, and the danger of mixing the components of the solution in the wrong proportions should be stressed. In general, home remedy solutions should be used only when the cost of commercial solutions is prohibitive and when fatalities may result if fluid and electrolyte disturbances are not corrected. For further discussion of this issue, see Meyers et al, 1991 A, 1991 B. See also index entry Rehydration Solution, Oral.

The primary foods recommended for early oral feeding are those containing starch (glucose polymers); useful sources include rice, maize, wheat, and potatoes (Snyder, 1991). Such foods can increase effective absorption of salt and water from the intestine and provide more calories than oral electrolyte solutions (Avery and Snyder, 1990). Overconcern about malabsorption probably has been responsible for the slow reintroduction of oral feeding within the first critical 24 hours (Snyder, 1991).

DRUG THERAPY. The classes of drugs that are useful for treatment of infectious diarrhea include nonspecific agents, which provide symptomatic relief without affecting the underlying cause of the diarrhea, and specific antimicrobial agents, which relieve symptoms by eliminating the causative organism.

For mild infectious diarrhea, if antidiarrheal therapy is used, only nonspecific agents (eg, antimotility agents, bismuth subsalicylate) should be prescribed to prevent the development of asymptomatic carriers or antibiotic-resistant organisms. However, even nonspecific agents are seldom required except in the elderly. Nonspecific agents such as antimotility drugs are contraindicated in infants under 2 years.

Although many physicians and pharmacists worldwide prescribe antibacterial agents for acute diarrhea, less than 10% of individuals affected require treatment with these drugs (Nathavitharana and Booth, 1992; del Costello and Bhutta, 1992). In most patients, antibacterial agents provide little or no benefit and should be reserved for those with diarrhea accompanied by high fever or bloody stools; those with infections caused by culture-proven *C. difficile, Shigella,* or *Campylobacter* and, in infants under 3 months, *Salmonella*; or those with moderate to severe travelers' diarrhea. Because glucose-based solutions (and probably Ricelyte) do not decrease the number of stools, fear by parents that infants and children receiving oral rehydration solutions are not improving leads to the unnecessary and potentially dangerous use of antidiarrheal and/or anti-infectious drugs.

For those relatively few patients with severe acute diarrhea, symptomatic treatment is justified to provide temporary relief until the cause is identified. For a more extensive discussion of criteria for choosing a treatment regimen for acute infectious diarrhea, see Gorbach, 1987, and Ashkenazi and Cleary, 1991.

Rotavirus and Norwalk virus commonly cause brief (24 to 72 hours), self-limited diarrhea, for which antimicrobial drug therapy is *not* effective. Antimicrobial therapy also is not indicated in the treatment of acute food poisoning caused by ingestion of preformed staphylococcal enterotoxins.

Enterotoxigenic strains of *E. coli* and *Vibrio cholerae* are important causes of acute secretory diarrheas; specific antimicrobial therapy (eg, tetracycline) is indicated in the latter infection. Many cases of travelers' diarrhea are due to enterotoxigenic strains of *E. coli.* Treatment with an antimotility agent (eg, loperamide [Imodium, Kaopectate II]) or bismuth subsalicylate [Pepto-Bismol] and an antimicrobial agent (eg, fluoroquinolones, trimethoprim/sulfamethoxazole [Bactrim, Cotrim, Septra]) is preferred to prophylaxis, except in selected individuals for whom infection would pose a high risk of morbidity or disruption of travel (Ericsson et al, 1990; DuPont et al, 1990 A).

In one study, the most rapid relief of travelers' diarrhea was provided by trimethoprim/sulfamethoxazole plus loperamide (Ericsson et al, 1990). The latter is a useful adjunct to antibiotics for patients who have secretory travelers' diarrhea (Ericsson et al, 1990; Taylor et al, 1991). Loperamide is preferable alone for initiation of therapy in patients who have mild diarrhea without fever or dysenteric disease and a history of drug allergy or antimicrobial-induced vaginitis. Many physicians do not recommend its use in children.

When administered orally (investigational route), the antibiotic aztreonam [Azactam] is minimally absorbed from the intestine and produces fewer adverse reactions than trimethoprim/sulfamethoxazole and other antibiotics that are absorbed systemically. These properties make this agent safer for use in pregnant women and children. In one recent study, it was reported that oral aztreonam 100 mg administered three times daily for five days was effective and well tolerated in patients with bacterial travelers' diarrhea (DuPont et al, 1992).

For a more detailed discussion on the antimicrobial treatment of infectious bacterial diarrhea, including diarrhea caused by invasive organisms (eg, *Shigella*, *Salmonella, Campylobacter jejuni, Yersinia enterocolitica*), see index entry Diarrhea, Infectious. For treatment of antibiotic-associated (*Clostridium difficile*) colitis, see index entry Colitis, Pseudomembranous. For treatment guidelines for infectious diarrhea caused by protozoa, see index entries Giardiasis, Amebiasis, and Cryptosporidiosis.

Maldigestion and Malabsorption Syndromes

Patients with disaccharidase deficiencies, gluten-induced enteropathy, and fructose malabsorption require specific dietary therapy. Individuals with symptomatic lactase deficiency often respond to lactase enzyme replacement [LactAid, Lactrase]; these products are taken in or with milk or milk products.

Dietary restriction of fat may ameliorate diarrhea associated with postsurgical vagotomy, hyperthyroidism, or lymphangiectasia and other steatorrheas. Medium-chain triglycerides are a more readily absorbable substitute for fat.

Most patients with maldigestive diarrhea caused by pancreatic insufficiency respond to replacement therapy with pancreatic enzymes (see index entry Pancreatitis).

Patients who have undergone limited ileal resection (<100 cm) may experience diarrhea caused by bile salt malabsorption with increased colonic secretion and reduced colonic absorption of water and electrolytes. These patients often benefit from therapy with cholestyramine resin [Questran], which binds bile acids. Patients with more extensive resection often develop the short bowel syndrome with severe steatorrhea (> 30 g daily). These individuals are not usually helped by cholestyramine but may respond to a low-fat diet with substitution of medium-chain triglycerides.

Hormonal Diarrheas

A number of hormonal or humoral substances produced in excess by certain tumors can cause moderate to severe secretory diarrhea (eg, serotonin in carcinoid syndrome; calcitonin and prostaglandins in medullary carcinoma of the thyroid; calcitonin, gastric inhibitory polypeptide, and/or vasoactive intestinal peptide in the watery diarrhea syndrome [pancreatic nonbeta cell tumors, often referred to as pancreatic cholera]; gastrin in the Zollinger-Ellison syndrome; histamine in mastocytosis). Temporary intravenous parenteral nutrition may be required until surgery and/or cancer chemotherapy is initiated.

Concomitant use of indomethacin [Indocin] and prednisolone has helped control secretory diarrhea produced by pancreatic nonbeta cell tumors in a few patients with tumors secreting vasoactive intestinal peptide (VIPomas, also called pancreatic cholera) (Jaffee et al, 1977). Trifluoperazine [Stelazine] (Donowitz et al, 1980) and lithium carbonate (Pandol et al, 1980) also have been utilized. Other agents that have been effective investigationally in VIPomas include aspirin, clonidine [Catapres], lidamidine hydrochloride (investigational drug), and somatostatin. A synthetic somatostatin analogue, octreotide [Sandostatin], has been effective in treating diarrhea in patients with VIPomas and carcinoid tumors. It also reduces the flushing and wheezing associated with these tumors (Vinik et al, 1986; Rosenberg, 1988). This drug has been used investigationally in diarrhea associated with a number of other conditions and may be beneficial in the management of diarrhea in AIDS patients (see the evaluation).

Drug Evaluations

AGENTS USED TO TREAT DIARRHEAL DISORDERS

Opioids: In adults, the opioids are the most effective and prompt-acting nonspecific antidiarrheal agents. They probably act by slowing gastrointestinal motility and prolonging the transit time of the fecal mass to allow more time for absorption of water and electrolytes from the intestinal lumen. Codeine also interacts with central opioid receptors that regulate intestinal motility. Loperamide may decrease intestinal secretion by inactivating calmodulin, the calcium-dependent regulatory protein (Merritt et al, 1982), and has been reported to increase internal anal sphincter pressure (Read et al, 1979). It is not known if opioids have an antisecretory action that enhances fluid and electrolyte absorption from the intestinal lumen (Gaginella, 1983; Schiller et al, 1984).

Opium tincture and paregoric (camphorated opium tincture) are much more widely used in the United States than the purified alkaloids (eg, codeine), which are equally effective in equivalent doses. Paregoric may be preferable to opium tincture since the dose of the former is measured by teaspoon, while the dose of the latter is in drops. Because usual doses produce neither euphoria nor analgesia, these preparations may be prescribed for acute, self-limited diarrhea with little or no risk of dependence. However, dependence may develop if opioids are used indefinitely to treat chronic diarrhea or diarrhea associated with inflammatory bowel disease.

In a double-blind crossover study in patients with chronic diarrhea, codeine, loperamide, and diphenoxylate with atropine [Lomotil] were equally efficacious in reducing the frequency of bowel movements. However, loperamide and codeine were superior to diphenoxylate with atropine in producing a solid stool and reducing rectal urgency (Palmer et al, 1980).

Because loperamide and diphenoxylate with atropine have little abuse potential, they have become the most widely used nonspecific antidiarrheal preparations. Physical dependence has not been documented clinically with their use in therapeutic doses, and large doses given for long periods did not produce dependence in animals. Nevertheless, these drugs should not be prescribed for long-term, unsupervised use in dependence-prone patients.

Opioids had been combined with other antidiarrheal agents, but such mixtures were judged to be of unproven effectiveness, thus exposing the patient to the adverse effects of the other components at greater expense and with no additional benefit. Such mixtures are no longer available.

The more serious untoward effects of these drugs (see index entry Opioids, Adverse Reactions) are not encountered with usual antidiarrheal doses. Loperamide, diphenoxylate with atropine, and difenoxin may precipitate toxic megacolon in patients with active inflammatory bowel disease or acute colitis caused by bacteria (including *C. difficile*), amebae, schistosomes, or ischemia. Postdiarrheal constipation occurs in some patients after treatment with opioids. Although these agents may alleviate cramping and reduce the number of bowel movements in patients with acute infectious diarrhea, fluid may be sequestered in dilated loops of bowel, especially in children and adolescents. Hepatic coma has developed in patients with severe liver disease, presumably caused by prolonged exposure of colonic contents to urea-splitting bacteria with formation of ammonia and diminished hepatic detoxification.

It is often recommended that opioids be avoided in acute diarrheas caused by antibiotics, poisons, infectious organisms, or exotoxins until mural infection has subsided and/or it can be assumed that most of the toxic material has been eliminated. However, these agents probably are safe when given for brief periods to adults or older children with infectious diarrhea (including travelers' diarrhea) if significant fever and dysentery are absent (DuPont, 1983 A).

Because of their lack of proven benefit and the potential for adverse reactions in infants, opioids and other nonspecific agents (eg, adsorbents) generally are not recommended for use in those under 2 years. Respiratory depression has been reported after overdose of diphenoxylate with atropine in infants and young children. Their safety during pregnancy has not been determined.

Antisecretory Agents: Salicylates and other inhibitors of prostaglandin synthesis often have marked antisecretory effects in experimental animals. Bismuth subsalicylate stimulates absorption of fluid and electrolytes across the intestinal wall and has been effective in secretory diarrhea produced by enterotoxigenic *Escherichia coli*, as well as for nonspecific diarrhea.

Hydrophilic Substances: Polycarbophil, methylcellulose, and various psyllium seed derivatives bind water and bile salts and may be effective in the symptomatic treatment of watery diarrhea. Fewer, bulkier stools may be passed more comfortably, but the amount of stool is not decreased. (See also index entry Laxatives, Cathartics.)

Adsorbent Powders: The use of preparations containing bismuth subcarbonate, subgallate, subnitrate, or subsalicylate to treat diarrhea is empiric. It has been claimed that these salts adsorb intraluminal toxins, bacteria, and viruses or provide a protective coating for the mucosa, but proof of these actions has not been established.

Activated charcoal has been used empirically to treat diarrhea and flatulence, but there are no controlled studies confirming its efficacy for these conditions. This preparation is employed in poisoning caused by certain drugs (see index entry Charcoal, Activated). (It should be noted that activated charcoal contains sorbitol, which may pose problems in patients who cannot tolerate monosaccharides.)

Hydrated aluminum silicate clays such as activated attapulgite can be used alone [Diasorb, Donnagel, Kaopectate, Parepectolin, Rheaban] or in combination (eg, with kaolin, pectin); these ingredients have been claimed to act as adsorbents and protectants. Only a few adequately controlled clinical studies demonstrate their efficacy. Results of animal studies suggest that the fluidity of the stool is decreased, but total water loss appears to be unchanged and sodium and potassium loss may be exacerbated (McClung et al, 1980).

The adsorbents are generally safe, but they may interfere with the absorption of other therapeutic agents; a two- to three-hour interval is recommended between the oral administration of adsorbent powders and other drugs. Adsorbents are contraindicated in patients with suspected obstructive lesions of the bowel and in children less than 3 years.

The anion exchange resin, cholestyramine, binds bile acids and the toxin of *C. difficile*. It relieves diarrhea due to excessive bile salts and may be effective for mild or recurrent cases of antibiotic-induced pseudomembranous colitis. This resin may be especially useful in relapses of pseudomembranous colitis caused by *C. difficile* in which it can be used instead of antibiotics in some patients. Cholestyramine allows the colonic flora to return to normal. It also may be beneficial in the diarrheal form of the irritable bowel syndrome.

Lactobacillus: Viable *Lactobacillus* cultures [Bacid, Lactinex] are promoted for the treatment of diarrhea caused by antibiotics, and they are reported to be useful in the prophylaxis of ampicillin-associated diarrhea (Gotz et al, 1979). Additional well-controlled studies to support their effectiveness are needed. It is suspected that most of the organisms are killed by the normal gastric acidity.

Anticholinergic Antispasmodics: Anticholinergic agents are ineffective in the treatment of acute diarrhea (Reves et al, 1983). They are used most commonly as adjuncts in the treatment of the irritable bowel syndrome. There is no conclusive evidence that any drug in this class exerts a selective effect on the gastrointestinal tract, although dicyclomine has been promoted in such a manner.

Amebicides: Clioquinol (iodochlorhydroxyquin) and iodoquinol (diiodohydroxyquin) [Yodoxin] have been used in the prophylaxis of travelers' diarrhea but proof of their efficacy is lacking, and subacute myelo-optic neuropathy (SMON) has occurred. Since amebae cause only a small percentage of the diarrheas encountered while traveling, the indiscriminate use of such potentially toxic agents is unjustified. Clioquinol is no longer available for systemic use in the United States.

ANTI-INFECTIVE AGENTS

See index entry Diarrhea, Infectious.

BISMUTH SUBSALICYLATE
[Pepto-Bismol]

ACTIONS AND USES. A number of mechanisms of action may be responsible for the antidiarrheal effects of this agent; it is unclear if the actions discussed below or some as yet unknown effects are primary.

Bismuth subsalicylate binds toxins produced by *Vibrio cholerae* and *Escherichia coli*; an antimicrobial action has been demonstrated both in vitro and in vivo. It also has been suggested that the subsalicylate salt is hydrolyzed by coliforms to liberate salicylic acid, which inhibits synthesis of a prostaglandin responsible for intestinal inflammation and hypermotility. Salicylate also may have antisecretory actions and stimulate absorption of fluid and electrolytes across the intestinal wall. Bismuth subsalicylate and the other intestinal bismuth reaction products have antimicrobial effects in vitro (Graham et al, 1983) that are important in the prophylaxis and possibly in the treatment of acute diarrhea (DuPont et al, 1987).

Bismuth subsalicylate is useful for the symptomatic treatment of nonspecific diarrhea. When administered prophylactically as a suspension (DuPont et al, 1977, 1980) or as tablets (Graham et al, 1983; DuPont et al, 1987), bismuth subsalicylate also reduces travelers' diarrhea and other acute infectious diarrhea (Soriano-Brücher et al, 1991). When this agent is taken shortly after the onset of diarrhea caused by enterotoxigenic *E. coli* and viral infections, the frequency of bowel movements is reduced and stomach cramps are relieved. However, the large volume of suspension required (240 ml) and the amount of salicylate ingested (2.1 g) daily (Tolle and Elliot, 1984) may be hazardous if other salicylate-containing compounds also are taken. With a recommended daily dose of 240 ml of the suspension, serum salicylate concentrations equivalent to eight aspirin tablets may result (DuPont, 1983 B). To avoid the large volume, tablets may be used (Graham et al, 1983; DuPont et al, 1987); however, each tablet contains 350 mg of calcium carbonate and up to 2 g of calcium is ingested daily, which occasionally causes hypercalcemia (Levine, 1983).

Bismuth subsalicylate also is being used with antibiotics to eradicate gastrointestinal infection with *Helicobacter pylori* and to treat forms of antral gastritis and peptic ulcer associated with infestation by this pathogen. See index entry Ulcer, Peptic.

ADVERSE REACTIONS, PRECAUTIONS, AND INTERACTIONS. Bismuth may produce constipation or impaction in infants and elderly debilitated patients. Grayish black discoloration of the stool should not be confused with melena. Bismuth is radiopaque and may interfere with radiologic examination of the gastrointestinal tract.

The use of bismuth subsalicylate and other nonacetylsalicylic acid salicylates has not been associated with development of Reye's syndrome, but it is probably wise to avoid ingestion of this and other salicylate-containing agents during outbreaks of varicella or influenza (Soriano-Brücher et al, 1991).

Bismuth subsalicylate decreases the bioavailability of doxycycline and should be given at least two hours after this antibiotic (Ericsson et al, 1982).

DOSAGE AND PREPARATIONS.

Oral: *Adults,* 30 ml of the regular- or maximum-strength suspension or two tablets; *children 3 to 6 years,* 5 ml or one-third tablet; *6 to 9 years,* 10 ml or two-thirds tablet; *9 to 12 years,* 15 ml or one tablet. This dose is repeated every 30 minutes (regular-strength suspension or tablet) or hour (maximum-strength suspension) if needed until eight and four doses are taken, respectively. For prophylaxis, two tablets four times daily (with meals and at bedtime) have been administered for two weeks to young adults (DuPont et al, 1987).

Generic. Powder.

Pepto-Bismol (Procter & Gamble). Suspension 262 mg/15 ml (regular strength) and 525 mg/15 ml (maximum strength) in 120, 240, 360, and 480 (regular-strength only) ml containers; tablets (chewable) 262 mg (all forms nonprescription).

CHOLESTYRAMINE RESIN

[Questran]

USES. Cholestyramine may be useful when diarrhea is caused by increased concentrations of certain bile acids in the colon resulting from defective ileal reabsorption of bile acids or by deconjugation of bile acids by colonic flora in the upper small intestine. In patients with extensive ileal resections (short bowel syndrome) or those with postvagotomy diarrhea who are consuming a normal diet, cholestyramine may reduce the fluidity of diarrhea slightly but may increase steatorrhea due to excessive binding of bile salts (Duncombe et al, 1977). If steatorrhea is a problem, small amounts of cholestyramine given with a diet low in animal fats supplemented with medium-chain triglycerides and a hydrophilic colloid may control diarrhea while permitting caloric balance. Patients with severe steatorrhea (>20 g daily) are unlikely to respond.

Cholestyramine binds the toxin of *Clostridium difficile* and thus may be used to treat mild or recurrent cases of antibiotic-induced pseudomembranous colitis, although metronidazole or vancomycin is preferred in patients with moderate to severe involvement.

Cholestyramine also absorbs dietary oxalate and reduces hyperoxaluria following ileal resection, a cause of calcium oxalate renal stones (Kirsner, 1991).

ADVERSE REACTIONS AND PRECAUTIONS. Cholestyramine resin may cause constipation, heartburn, or perianal irritation. Reduction of serum folate has been reported with long-term administration; folate, vitamin A, and vitamin D supplements may be required. Because of the risk of bowel obstruction, this agent should be used with caution in patients with Crohn's disease if strictures are present. For a more detailed discussion, see index entry Cholestyramine Resin, Uses, Hyperlipidemia.

Because of the sucrose present in the powder preparation, cholestyramine resin may be undesirable for use in patients who cannot tolerate monosaccharides.

DOSAGE AND PREPARATIONS.

Oral: *Adults,* dosage must be individualized. Initially, 2 to 4 g of the bar preparation or powder two or three times daily with adjustments according to the patient's tolerance and response. The powder is suspended in 120 to 180 ml of water or in pulpy juices, mashed banana, applesauce, gelatin, or cooked cereal. Cholestyramine resin should never be swallowed dry because of the hazard of esophageal irritation or blockage.

Cholestyramine resin should be administered at least one hour after or four hours before other oral medications (eg, thyroid hormones, anticoagulants, digitalis glycosides) because the absorption of concurrently administered oral drugs may be decreased or delayed; moreover, when cholestyramine is withdrawn, sudden increased absorption of these drugs can produce toxicity.

Questran (Bristol). Powder 4 g/packet in 5 and 9 g single-dose containers and 210 (***Questran Light***) and 378 g containers.

CODEINE PHOSPHATE

CODEINE SULFATE

For chemical formula, see index entry Codeine, As Analgesic.

Codeine is a purified opium alkaloid used for the short-term symptomatic treatment of mild diarrhea. Indications and contraindications are identical to those of diphenoxylate, loperamide, and the opium extracts. Drug dependence is a small but definite risk with prolonged use. Adverse reactions are similar to those produced by other opioids but are seldom encountered with usual antidiarrheal doses.

Codeine is classified in FDA Pregnancy Category C.

DOSAGE AND PREPARATIONS.

Oral: *Adults,* 15 to 60 mg every four to eight hours as needed. Codeine should not be used in *children under 12 years*.

Intramuscular: 15 to 30 mg every two to four hours as needed.

CODEINE PHOSPHATE:
Generic. Solution 30 mg/ml in 1 and 20 ml containers and 60 mg/ml in 1 ml containers; tablets (soluble) 15, 30, and 60 mg; powder.
CODEINE SULFATE:
Generic. Tablets (oral, soluble) 15, 30, and 60 mg.

DIFENOXIN HYDROCHLORIDE WITH ATROPINE SULFATE
[Motofen]

Difenoxin is the principal active metabolite of diphenoxylate. The uses, actions, adverse reactions and precautions, and drug interactions of this preparation are similar to those of diphenoxylate with atropine. See that evaluation.

Difenoxin with atropine is classified in FDA Pregnancy Category C.

DOSAGE AND PREPARATIONS.
Oral: *Adults,* 2 mg (two tablets) initially, then 1 mg (one tablet) after each loose stool or every three to four hours as needed. The total dosage during any 24-hour period should not exceed 8 mg (eight tablets).

Motofen (Carnrick). Tablets containing 1 mg of difenoxin hydrochloride and 0.025 mg of atropine sulfate.

DIPHENOXYLATE HYDROCHLORIDE WITH ATROPINE SULFATE
[Lomotil]

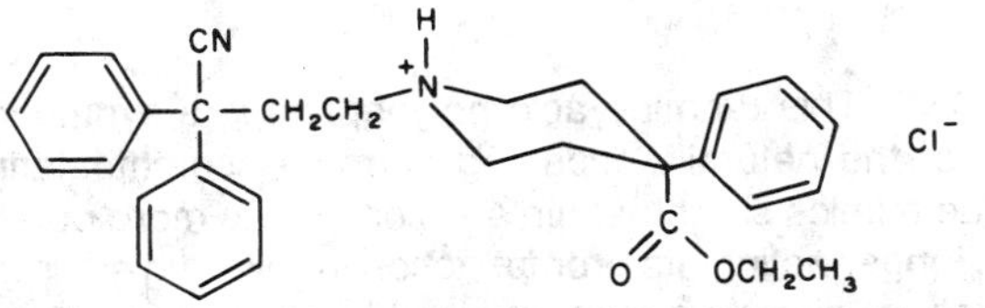

CN, H, $C - CH_2CH_2$, N^+, Cl^-, C, O, OCH_2CH_3

ACTIONS AND USES. This opioid is as effective as the other opium derivatives in relieving diarrhea. It limits peristalsis by inhibiting mucosal receptors, which abolishes the local mucosal peristaltic reflex, and by stimulating segmental contraction. In one controlled study, this preparation decreased frequency of bowel movements and stool volume without affecting sphincter tone or rectal continence in patients with chronic diarrhea and fecal incontinence (Harford et al, 1980).

ADVERSE REACTIONS AND PRECAUTIONS. Diphenoxylate with atropine has minimal dependence liability in recommended doses and is classified as a Schedule V substance under the Controlled Substances Act. The presence of atropine helps prevent abuse but adds the potential for its own unpleasant side effects.

The incidence of adverse reactions is relatively low. Those reported include abdominal distention, intestinal obstruction, dilation of the colon, rash, drowsiness, dizziness, mental depression, restlessness, nausea, headache, and blurred vision.

Toxic megacolon or ileus may occur in patients with idiopathic, infectious (including that caused by *C. difficile*), or ischemic colitis and may be precipitated by anticholinergic and opioid medications; the complication is more likely to occur in severely ill and malnourished patients. Investigationally, large doses (40 to 60 mg) of diphenoxylate have produced a morphine-like euphoria, and toxic doses may cause respiratory depression and coma. Narcotic antagonists are effective antidotes (see index entry Naloxone). Side effects of atropine generally occur after overdosage. This preparation should be used cautiously in patients with liver disease, since delayed intestinal transport has precipitated hepatic coma in patients with cirrhosis.

Diphenoxylate is classified in FDA Pregnancy Category C.

DRUG INTERACTIONS. In large doses, diphenoxylate may potentiate the actions of barbiturates and opioids and other central nervous system depressants.

DOSAGE AND PREPARATIONS.
Oral: *Adults,* initially, 5 mg (two tablets) or 10 ml (two teaspoonsful) of liquid four times daily (20 mg/day). After diarrhea is controlled, the dosage may be reduced. The manufacturer recommends that Lomotil tablets not be used in *children 2 to 12 years*, and neither tablets nor liquid should be used in those *under 2 years*. The total daily dosage suggested for the liquid in children is 0.3 to 0.4 mg/kg (0.6 to 0.8 ml/kg) administered in four divided doses.

Lomotil (Searle), ***Generic.*** Each tablet or 5 ml of liquid contains diphenoxylate hydrochloride 2.5 mg and atropine sulfate 0.025 mg.

LOPERAMIDE HYDROCHLORIDE
[Imodium, Kaopectate II]

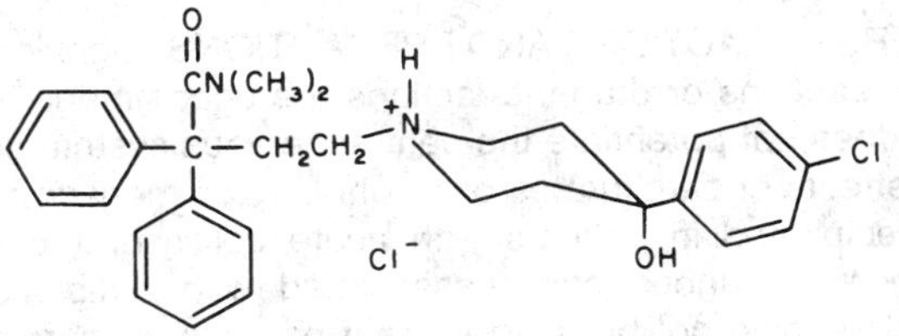

O, $CN(CH_3)_2$, H, $C - CH_2CH_2$, N^+, Cl, Cl^-, OH

ACTIONS. This opioid is a derivative of haloperidol and resembles meperidine structurally. It has much less effect on the central nervous system than haloperidol and meperidine when effective antidiarrheal doses are used. The exact mechanism(s) and site of action have not been determined. In animal studies, loperamide's influence on gastrointestinal contractile activity resembles that of diphenoxylate and other opioids. In addition, loperamide may decrease intestinal secretion by inactivating the calcium-dependent regulatory protein, calmodulin (Merritt et al, 1982), or enhance the rate of absorption of water and electrolytes from the intestinal lumen (Sandhu et al, 1983). In humans, transit time is prolonged, fecal volume is reduced, and loss of water and electrolytes is decreased; this results in decreased frequency of bowel movements and improved consistency of stools. Loperamide also may increase the internal anal sphincter pressure (Read et al, 1979).

USES. In open clinical trials and double-blind crossover comparisons with placebo, diphenoxylate, and other opioids, loperamide was effective and had a prompt and prolonged action in both acute and chronic diarrhea. However, it is more expensive than generic diphenoxylate, codeine, and the opium extracts.

Large doses of loperamide often are effective in acute and chronic infectious diarrhea; abdominal pain is relieved and diarrhea is reduced in patients with infection due to enterotoxigenic *Escherichia coli* and other bacteria. Opioids are not as safe or as effective as antibiotics in severe bacterial diarrhea; their use should be limited to patients with mild to moderate illness who are not dehydrated (DuPont, 1983 A).

For moderate to severe travelers' diarrhea without fever or bloody stools, loperamide is useful in combination with an antimicrobial agent (Ericsson et al, 1990).

The usefulness of loperamide for acute infectious diarrhea in infants is unclear. One report suggests that this drug can be lifesaving in some infants with severe prolonged diarrhea unresponsive to other treatment (Sandhu et al, 1983).

Loperamide may help control chronic diarrhea in patients with the irritable bowel syndrome, colostomy, ileostomy, ileoanal anastomoses, and malabsorption. This drug has been advocated to reduce the volume of ileostomy effluent, decrease the frequency of bowel movements, and improve the consistency of stools in patients with ulcerative colitis and Crohn's disease, but it should not be considered for routine use in these individuals.

In patients who have undergone colectomy for ulcerative colitis (in whom no risk of recurrence exists, unlike those with Crohn's disease), loperamide may be of value when dietary measures alone cannot control the liquidity of the effluent or when renal electrolyte loss is increased and further intestinal loss would be hazardous.

ADVERSE REACTIONS AND PRECAUTIONS. Significant adverse reactions or drug interactions are uncommon. Loperamide does not potentiate the central nervous system depressant effects of barbiturates or alcohol. Toxic megacolon may be precipitated in patients with acute colitis or those with pseudomembranous colitis associated with antibiotic use. Opioids should not be used to treat bacterial or parasitic infection of the bowel wall when significant fever or dysentery is present because they may worsen symptoms, prolong the illness, or cause perforation. This agent should be used with caution in the presence of hepatic insufficiency (since it is metabolized primarily by the liver) or other conditions in which constipation should be avoided.

The safety of loperamide during pregnancy has not been determined; however, no teratogenic effects have been reported (FDA Pregnancy Category B).

Overdose should be treated with naloxone if morphine-like signs and symptoms occur. Administration of activated charcoal can reduce systemic absorption of loperamide ninefold.

PHARMACOKINETICS. About 40% of an oral dose of loperamide is absorbed. Experimentally, a considerable proportion of the remaining drug also is absorbed into the intestinal wall where it is desmethylated and secreted back into the lumen of the intestine (Miyazaki et al, 1982). About one-half of the oral dose is excreted unchanged, primarily in the feces (Heel et al, 1978).

DOSAGE AND PREPARATIONS. Over-the-counter preparations of loperamide are adequate, and it is not necessary to use the prescription product (DuPont et al, 1990 B). The manufacturers' suggested dosages are:

Oral: For acute and chronic diarrhea, *adults,* 4 mg, followed by 2 mg after each diarrheal stool. Subsequent dosage is individualized but is usually 2 to 4 mg once or twice daily (maximum, 8 mg daily OTC product and 16 mg daily prescription product). Loperamide should be discontinued after 48 hours if no improvement is observed in patients with acute diarrhea. Chronic diarrhea is unlikely to be relieved if symptoms are not rapidly alleviated with doses of 16 mg daily.

Children 2 to 12 years, the recommended first-day dosage schedule for acute diarrhea is: (liquid only) *2 to 5 years* (13 to 20 kg), 1 mg three times; *6 to 8 years* (20 to 30 kg), 2 mg twice; *8 to 12 years* (more than 30 kg), 2 mg three times. Subsequently, 1 mg/10 kg should be administered only after a loose stool. The total daily dose should not exceed the recommended first-day dose. The pediatric dosage for chronic diarrhea has not been established. Use of loperamide in *children under 2 years* is not recommended.

Imodium (Janssen). Capsules 2 mg.

Imodium A-D (McNeil Consumer). Liquid 1 mg/5 ml (alcohol 5.25%); tablets 2 mg (both forms nonprescription).

Kaopectate II (Upjohn). Tablets 2 mg (nonprescription).

OCTREOTIDE ACETATE

[Sandostatin]

```
       S ——————————————————————————— S
       |                             |
H — (D)-Phe — Cys — Phe — (D)-Trp — Lys — Thr — Cys — Thr — OL
```

ACTIONS. This 8-amino acid polypeptide is a synthetic analogue of the naturally occurring hormone, somatostatin. Octreotide mimics somatostatin's actions but is more potent and much longer acting. Its prompt action in relieving symptoms in a variety of disorders characterized by severe secretory diarrhea is largely due to inhibition of the release of several gastroenteropancreatic peptide hormones, including gastrin, gastric inhibitory peptide, motilin, neurotensin, secretin, vasoactive intestinal peptide (VIP), insulin, glucagon, and pancreatic polypeptide (Battershill and Clissold, 1989). In addition, octreotide decreases splanchnic blood flow, reduces intestinal motility, and increases water and electrolyte absorption from the gut. The diverse actions of this agent at multiple sites are reflected by the finding that the clinical response does not always parallel the decrease in secretion of marker peptides in various secretory diarrheas (Maton et al, 1989; Rosenberg, 1988).

USES. A number of studies have demonstrated that within 24 hours octreotide can markedly reduce diarrhea and relieve the flushing and wheezing that occur in patients with metastatic carcinoid tumors (the carcinoid syndrome) or VIPomas. This agent is not curative but allows the patient to be ambulatory and to be free of severe chronic diarrhea that is a more immediate threat to life and the quality of life than the slowly growing tumors (Rosenberg, 1988; Maton et al, 1989; Vinik and Moattari, 1989).

Octreotide has been effective investigationally in the treatment of inappropriate secretion of peptide hormones that occurs in patients with acromegaly, pancreatic fistulas, and tumoral hormonal diarrheas; in the treatment of nontumoral secretory diarrhea that may be associated with disorders such as microvillus inclusion disease and diabetes (Cutz et al, 1989; Dudl et al, 1987; Rosenberg, 1988); and in the treatment of the dumping syndrome occurring in patients following gastrectomy (Hopman et al, 1988). It also may be useful in AIDS patients with diarrhea who do not respond to antibacterial or antimotility agents (Cook et al, 1988; Katz et al, 1988). For investigational uses of octreotide in malignant conditions, see index entry Octreotide.

Most patients or their family members can be taught to administer the drug by subcutaneous injection at home. Intravenous bolus injections have been used in emergencies.

ADVERSE REACTIONS AND PRECAUTIONS. Many patients have received the drug for two years or longer and only minor (usually transient) adverse reactions have been reported. Pain at the site of the injection, abdominal cramps, bloating, flatulence, diarrhea, steatorrhea, and nausea are the most frequent complaints. Inhibition of gallbladder emptying may increase the rate of gallstone formation. Patients receiving long-term therapy should be monitored periodically by ultrasound imaging of the gallbladder and bile ducts. Octreotide may exacerbate either hyperglycemia or hypoglycemia in some patients. The dose of insulin may require reduction in diabetics receiving octreotide; little data exist on other possible interactions.

Octreotide is classified in FDA Pregnancy Category B.

PHARMACOKINETICS. After subcutaneous injection, octreotide is rapidly and completely absorbed. Peak plasma concentrations are attained 30 minutes after subcutaneous injection and four minutes after intravenous injection; the half-life of the injected drug is 113 minutes and 45 minutes, respectively. About 30% of the subcutaneous dose is recovered as unchanged drug in the urine; the remainder is excreted in the bile and by proteolysis (Rosenberg, 1988).

DOSAGE AND PREPARATIONS.

Subcutaneous: *Adults,* initially, 50 mcg once or twice daily; subsequent dosage is adjusted on the basis of response. For the carcinoid syndrome, 100 to 600 mcg/day and, for VIPomas, 200 to 300 mcg/day may be given; these amounts are administered in two to four divided doses daily for the initial two weeks of therapy.

Sandostatin (Sandoz). Solution 0.05, 0.1, and 0.5 mg/ml in 1 ml containers.

OPIUM TINCTURE

USES. Opium tincture is prompt-acting and useful for the symptomatic treatment of diarrhea. It is less widely used today than paregoric because the latter, despite an unpleasant taste, is more dilute and teaspoonful doses are more convenient to measure than the dropper quantities of opium tincture. However, the prescription of the tincture may be smaller in volume and the number of drops can be adjusted more precisely to the needs of the patient.

PRECAUTIONS. Opioids should not be used in patients with bacterial or parasitic infection of the bowel wall when significant fever or dysentery is present because they may worsen symptoms, prolong the illness, or cause perforation.

Effective antidiarrheal doses do not relieve pain or produce euphoria or dependence; however, larger doses or prolonged use may cause dependence (see index entry Opioids). Opium tincture is a Schedule II drug under the Controlled Substances Act and is classified in FDA Pregnancy Category C.

DOSAGE AND PREPARATIONS.

Oral: 0.6 ml (range, 0.3 to 1 ml) four times daily. The maximal single dose is 1 ml every two to four hours, and no more than 6 ml should be taken in 24 hours.

Generic. Tincture 10% in 120 and 473 ml containers (alcohol 19%).

PAREGORIC

Paregoric (camphorated opium tincture) is as effective as opium tincture in equivalent doses and provides the convenience of teaspoonful dosage.

ADVERSE REACTIONS AND PRECAUTIONS. Adverse effects are rare, but nausea and other gastrointestinal disturbances occur occasionally. Usual oral doses do not produce euphoria or analgesia, but prolonged use has produced physical dependence despite the drug's unappealing taste. Paregoric is classified as a Schedule III drug under the Controlled Substances Act.

Opioids should not be used to treat patients with bacterial or parasitic infection of the bowel wall when fever or dysentery is present because they may worsen symptoms, prolong the illness, or cause perforation.

This drug is classified in FDA Pregnancy Category C.

DOSAGE AND PREPARATIONS.

Oral: *Adults,* 5 to 10 ml one to a maximum of four times daily until diarrhea is controlled. *Children,* 0.25 to 0.5 ml/kg one to a maximum of four times daily. The amount usually recommended per prescription is 30 or 60 ml.

Generic. Tincture (camphorated) containing morphine 0.4 mg/ml in 5, 60, 480, 1,000, and 3,840 ml containers (alcohol 45%).

INFLAMMATORY BOWEL DISEASE

Ulcerative Colitis and Crohn's Disease

Idiopathic inflammatory bowel disease includes Crohn's disease (ileitis, regional enteritis, granulomatous colitis) and ulcerative colitis. The principal features of Crohn's disease include focal, often transmural, lesions in the small intestine and/or colon with extraintestinal manifestations. Ulcerative colitis is characterized by diffuse superficial colonic mucosal inflammation that extends proximally from the rectum. Although diarrhea is associated with both disorders, bloody diarrhea is more common in ulcerative colitis. Inflammatory bowel disease is characterized by unpredictable relapses, which may be precipitated by stress or upper respiratory infections and other viral diseases. It has been reported that use of nonsteroidal anti-inflammatory drugs (NSAIDs) may correlate with the onset as well as increase the frequency and severity of attacks (Kaufmann and Taubin, 1987).

Individualized medical management often controls ulcerative colitis and Crohn's disease, although recurrence is common. Physicians can fail their patients by exclusive reliance on medication and lack of appreciation of the value of reassurance and emotional support. Individuals with inflammatory bowel disease may have low self-esteem and often are discouraged and disheartened by the prospect of long-term disability, repeated hospitalizations, economic deprivation, social isolation, and an uncertain future (Kirsner, 1991). Continued physician interest and assurance as well as education of patients about their disease should be integral aspects of management.

Inflammatory bowel disease in children may be severe, and many of these patients require surgery. Growth retardation is more frequent and pronounced in children with Crohn's disease than in those with ulcerative colitis and sometimes is permanent. Nutritional intake must be increased 30% to 50% to achieve growth, but compliance may be a problem. Corticosteroid therapy is required in some children with active inflammation but may retard growth if steroid-free intervals are not introduced. Alternate-day corticosteroid therapy may control symptoms and lessen growth retardation. These drugs should not be used for maintenance therapy.

NUTRITIONAL THERAPY. The usefulness of oral (enteral) nutritional therapy (either elemental or polymeric) and total parenteral nutrition (TPN) in patients with inflammatory bowel disease is controversial. Although improved nutrition enhances healing capacity, immune function, and response to drugs or surgery, it is unclear whether oral feeding or TPN can reduce intestinal inflammation and exert a primary therapeutic effect. Furthermore, nutritional therapy may be needed for prolonged periods, is expensive, and may be poorly tolerated.

Any advantage of TPN over oral nutritional therapy is unclear for most patients with inflammatory bowel disease; some patients cannot receive or cannot tolerate oral therapy. Nutritional therapy is more useful for Crohn's disease than for ulcerative colitis. It is beneficial in some patients as an adjunctive measure (Gassull et al, 1986; Silk and Payne-James, 1989) to replace lost protein, calories, and vitamins and may be necessary in some patients with Crohn's disease because anorexia, secondary malnutrition, and weight loss are common. However, although oral elemental feedings, TPN, and bowel rest reduce symptoms and can induce clinical remissions, there is little evidence that the benefits are long lasting and the claim that nutritional therapy should be the primary treatment for Crohn's disease is unproven; most patients who respond also have received corticosteroids (Gray, 1991). In Crohn's disease, continuing weaknesses of studies examining the role of nutritional therapy are failure to include controls to account for the natural history of the disease (occurrence of spontaneous remissions) and a significant placebo effect (Bernstein and Shanahan, 1992).

Evidence for the value of oral nutritional therapy in Crohn's disease is much stronger in children than in adults; when combined with drug therapy or surgery, aggressive nutritional therapy may prevent or reverse growth failure in children and reduce the required dose of corticosteroids (Singleton, 1991; Sutton, 1992). Some investigators have reported that oral feeding can produce remission in many patients with Crohn's disease who are refractory to, dependent on, or cannot tolerate corticosteroids; this may forestall or eliminate the need for surgery (O'Brien et al, 1991; Rigaud et al, 1991). More data are needed to confirm these observations.

In ulcerative colitis, TPN is used mainly in malnourished patients, in those unable to tolerate oral ingestion because of a nonfunctional gut, or as nutritional support prior to surgery.

DRUG THERAPY. Mild to Moderate Inflammatory Bowel Disease: Sulfasalazine [Azulfidine] is effective in acute attacks of mild to moderate ulcerative colitis but probably is less effective in severe disease. It also is useful as maintenance therapy to prevent relapses. Therefore, sulfasalazine should be continued as maintenance therapy for ulcerative colitis, even in patients without signs of active disease.

In the National Cooperative Crohn's Disease study, this drug's usefulness for acute attacks appeared to be limited to patients with colitis or ileocolitis; it did not prevent relapses. However, many physicians prescribe sulfasalazine for ileal disease and continue therapy after remissions are achieved (Sack and Peppercorn, 1983).

Sulfasalazine is metabolized by colonic bacteria to sulfapyridine and 5-aminosalicylic acid (5-ASA). Current evidence suggests that 5-ASA is the active moiety and that most adverse reactions are due to the sulfapyridine metabolite (Azad Khan et al, 1977; Bondesen et al, 1987). Approximately 10% to 15% of patients who are allergic to sulfasalazine also will be allergic to mesalamine, a 5-ASA preparation used orally or rectally in these disorders.

A prodrug for mesalamine, olsalazine sodium (disodium azodisalicylate) [Dipentum], also is available orally for ulcerative colitis. It contains two molecules of 5-ASA linked by an azo bond. The molecules are cleaved by bacteria, and high concentrations of 5-ASA are released in the distal colon. The value of olsalazine for repeated attacks of mild to moderate acute ulcerative colitis is uncertain (Feurle et al, 1989), but its usefulness appears to be similar to that of sulfasalazine for maintenance therapy to prevent relapse (Rao et al, 1989; Ireland et al, 1988). Minimal absorption of the intact diazo compound occurs. Secretory diarrhea, which occurs in up to 15% of patients, may be a limiting side effect of olsalazine and prevent its use for acute attacks of ulcerative colitis (Willoughby et al, 1982; Wadworth and Fitton, 1991).

One oral preparation of mesalamine [Asacol] is a pH-sensitive, polymer-coated tablet that releases 5-ASA in the terminal ileum and colon at or above pH 7.0. It is used in patients with ulcerative colitis for treatment of acute attacks and for maintenance. Both sulfasalazine and 5-ASA preparations reduce the one-year relapse rate of ulcerative colitis from about 70% to 20%.

Unlike sulfasalazine, this oral 5-ASA preparation was effective for maintenance therapy in Crohn's disease in placebo-controlled studies (Prantera et al, 1992; Tremaine, 1992) and is better tolerated than sulfasalazine in doses that would achieve the same concentration of aminosalicylate in the gut lumen that is provided by 5-ASA preparations. It is unclear if aminosalicylates prevent recurrence of Crohn's disease postoperatively.

Adverse reactions with use of oral mesalamine preparations are similar to those of olsalazine, but the incidence of diarrhea may be lower (Sninsky et al, 1991). Delayed-release oral formulations are used because mesalamine is extensively absorbed in the upper gastrointestinal tract when immediate-release forms are used. Delayed-release preparations can deliver larger amounts of the effective agent to specific sites of intestinal inflammation in the ileum or colon than sulfasalazine preparations and are alternatives to sulfasalazine in nonresponsive patients, in those who cannot tolerate sulfasalazine (Sutherland et al, 1987), and in patients with Crohn's disease of the small and large bowel (Bondesen et al, 1987; Jarnerot, 1989).

The oral preparation, Pentasa, which consists of capsules containing ethylcellulose-coated mesalamine beads, has the same indications as Asacol. This formulation permits release of the drug throughout the small and large intestine (Peppercorn 1992 A, 1992 B). An investigational oral preparation of 4-aminosalicylic acid (4-ASA, PAS), an isomer of 5-ASA, was effective in patients with active ulcerative colitis (Ginsberg et al, 1992).

ω-3 fatty acids (investigational) inhibit the formation of leukotriene B4 but do not appear to be effective for maintenance therapy in ulcerative colitis. However, ω-3 fatty acid capsules containing eicosapentaenoic acid and docosahexaenoic acid have reduced the dose of steroids needed in patients with active ulcerative colitis (Aslan and Triadafilopoulos, 1992; Stenson et al, 1992).

Antimicrobial drugs are more useful in Crohn's disease than in ulcerative colitis because intestinal bacterial overgrowth, abscess formation within the abdomen, and perianal and perineal suppuration occur in those with the former disorder (Kirsner, 1991). One antimicrobial drug, metronidazole, may be as effective as sulfasalazine in colonic Crohn's disease and is particularly useful for perianal complications (Frank et al, 1983; Ursing et al, 1982; Sutherland et al, 1991). It should be reserved for patients who do not respond to or cannot tolerate sulfasalazine or 5-ASA preparations. The primary adverse effect is dose-related peripheral neuropathy; the possible occurrence of this disorder necessitates regular re-examination of the patient, even in the absence of symptoms. Change in taste sensation may be the earliest subjective indication of toxicity. Mutagenic, teratogenic, and carcinogenic effects have occurred in animals but not in humans. Antimicrobial agents that may be alternatives to metronidazole in Crohn's disease include trimethoprim/sulfamethoxazole, ciprofloxacin [Cipro], and tetracycline (Kirsner, 1991).

Corticosteroids are the most potent drugs available to treat inflammatory bowel disease. Corticotropin (ACTH) or adrenal corticosteroids are used alone to treat exacerbations of ulcerative colitis or Crohn's disease and are often prescribed for moderate disease refractory to sulfasalazine. Oral or parenteral preparations of hydrocortisone, prednisone, prednisolone, and methylprednisolone are most commonly employed.

Many physicians use corticotropin or a corticosteroid with sulfasalazine for both diseases despite lack of evidence from controlled trials that the addition of sulfasalazine provides an enhanced benefit. In one study, a combination of sulfasalazine and a corticosteroid was reported to produce a more rapid response than either drug alone in patients with Crohn's disease but did not prolong remission (Rijk et al, 1991).

Both sulfasalazine and steroids are safe for use in pregnant or nursing women; the consequences of untreated inflammatory bowel disease are much more dangerous to the fetus than the drugs used to treat these disorders (Baiocco and Korelitz, 1984).

Results of most studies indicate that steroid maintenance therapy has no value and does not prevent relapses of ulcerative colitis or Crohn's disease (Sack and Peppercorn, 1983). Corticosteroids should be withdrawn very gradually when remission has occurred. Patients with Crohn's disease may be more resistant to complete withdrawal than those with ulcerative colitis. Judgment and experience are required to minimize the occurrence of adverse reactions, which are sometimes serious and increase with prolonged systemic use. In some patients with Crohn's disease, the need for steroid therapy can be reduced or eliminated by adhering to a bland diet and using mild antispasmodic-anticholinergic preparations and sedatives (Kirsner, 1991). Crohn's disease of the mouth may respond to mouthwashes containing an antibiotic slurry (Kirsner, 1991) or a paste containing sucralfate or topical hydrocortisone [Orabase HCA] (Peppercorn, 1992 B).

Oral and enema preparations containing steroids that are minimally absorbed and, if absorbed, undergo rapid first-pass hepatic inactivation are being developed. One promising investigational agent, oral budesonide, appears to be as effective as prednisolone for active ileocecal Crohn's disease (Rutgeerts et al, 1993). It is unclear whether any agent currently being investigated lacks adrenocortical suppressive effects or does not cause other serious corticosteroid-related adverse reactions.

Severe ulcerative colitis in hospitalized patients usually requires the use of parenteral steroids, but oral forms can be effective in some individuals. Large oral doses of prednisolone or methylprednisolone (40 to 60 mg/day) are used initially; prednisone or hydrocortisone also can be administered. These drugs are less effective in malnourished hypoproteinemic patients and when courses are repeated after incomplete responses. Patients who do not respond to a five- to seven-day course of intravenous corticosteroids are unlikely to benefit from further corticosteroid therapy (Crotty and Jewel, 1992).

Corticotropin has been used intramuscularly or intravenously in selected patients with ulcerative colitis. Corticosteroids are more effective than corticotropin in patients previously treated with these drugs, while corticotropin is more useful in patients without prior exposure to corticosteroids (Meyers, 1983), perhaps because adrenocortical function has not been suppressed.

Enema preparations containing hydrocortisone [Cortenema] or prednisolone are useful in patients with distal ulcerative colitis or proctitis, who respond poorly to sulfasalazine or oral 5-ASA preparations. A preparation of hydrocortisone acetate foam [Cortifoam] is effective in patients with ulcerative proctitis and allows ambulation immediately after application. Occasionally, such enema preparations obviate the need for oral steroids or, when given with oral steroids, may permit reduction of the oral dose; moreover, because of less extensive absorption, adrenocortical suppression and other systemic adverse effects may be reduced (Sack and Peppercorn, 1983).

In open studies, enema preparations of beclomethasone dipropionate (investigational route) and budesonide (investigational agent) were effective in patients with distal ulcerative colitis, did not suppress hypothalamic-pituitary-adrenal function, and produced no significant adverse reactions (Vignotti et al, 1992; Danish Budesonide Study Group, 1991). In one study, the investigational corticosteroid, fluticasone, was not effective for distal ulcerative colitis (Angus et al, 1992; Kumana et al, 1982; Bansky et al, 1987). A nonsystemic steroid devoid of glucocorticoid or mineralocorticoid actions, tixocortol pivalate, also has been studied. An enema preparation of this investigational agent was as effective as hydrocortisone enemas and did not produce significant adverse effects (Hanauer, 1988).

Rectal forms of mesalamine [ROWASA] are beneficial for distal ulcerative colitis (proctitis, proctosigmoiditis) (Biddle and Miner, 1990; LaRosa et al, 1991). Enemas containing mesalamine 4g are effective in 80% to 90% of patients with active left-sided colitis. Patients who have not responded to sulfasalazine and/or corticosteroids often respond to mesalamine enemas. As with sulfasalazine, the enema also is useful for maintenance. The suppository form of mesalamine is used in the management of active ulcerative proctitis and for maintenance. Some patients with distal colonic Crohn's disease also may respond to mesalamine enema preparations (Klotz et al, 1980).

An enema preparation of 4-aminosalicylic acid [Pamisyl, Rezipas], available as an Orphan Drug, is effective in distal ulcerative colitis and distal Crohn's disease (Ginsberg et al, 1988; Peppercorn, 1992 A).

As in diversion colitis, utilization of energy-providing fatty acids (eg, butyrate) is impaired in the colon of patients with ulcerative colitis; fecal fluid from such patients contains abnormally low concentrations of butyrate and other short-chain fatty acids. In patients with distal ulcerative colitis who were refractory to sulfasalazine, 5-ASA preparations, and low doses of corticosteroids, treatment with an enema solution containing butyrate relieved symptoms significantly compared with placebo (Scheppach et al, 1992; Rowe and Bayless, 1992). These data suggest that butyrate may play a role in the pathogenesis of distal ulcerative colitis.

Antidiarrheal Therapy. Diarrhea in patients with mild ulcerative colitis or Crohn's disease can be relieved by nonspecific antidiarrheal agents (eg, loperamide, diphenoxylate with atropine [Lomotil], bulk-forming agents). Although many patients with mild stable ulcerative colitis or Crohn's disease have used antidiarrheal agents for prolonged periods without adverse effects, in general these drugs should be used only briefly. Nonspecific antidiarrheal agents often are ineffective in acute inflammatory bowel disease and may precipitate ileus or toxic megacolon if prescribed in large amounts for severely ill patients.

Severe Inflammatory Bowel Disease: The role of immunosuppressive agents in the treatment of severe inflammatory bowel disease is now less controversial. Azathioprine [Imuran] and its congener, mercaptopurine [Purinethol], have been effective for treatment and as maintenance therapy in patients with active and chronic Crohn's disease (Present et al, 1980; Sack and Peppercorn, 1983; Korelitz, 1983) and chronic ulcerative colitis unresponsive to other agents (Korelitz, 1983, 1990; Korelitz and Sohn, 1992). These agents also may be effective in some patients with ulcerative colitis who respond poorly to corticosteroids (Present et al, 1980; Adler and Korelitz, 1990; Steinhart et al, 1990; Lobo et al, 1990). In one study, maintenance therapy with azathioprine produced remissions lasting at least two years in patients with ulcerative colitis (Hawthorne et al, 1992). However, when used initially, three to six months may elapse before immunosuppressive agents become effective; subsequent courses produce beneficial effects more rapidly.

These drugs usually are not useful alone in acute active disease. Initial treatment with steroids may be required in more seriously ill patients to allow time for the immunosuppressive drug to exert an effect. Both azathioprine and mercaptopurine have a steroid-sparing effect and allow reduction of steroid dosage. Mercaptopurine may facilitate closure of enteric and perianal fistulas in patients with Crohn's disease. However, up to 5% of patients with Crohn's disease who are treated with azathioprine or mercaptopurine may develop pancreatitis (Singleton et al, 1979).

Cyclosporine [Sandimmune] also is being investigated for use in patients with severe inflammatory bowel disease. In two studies, one of which was placebo-controlled, patients with acute, severe ulcerative colitis that did not respond to ten or more days of intravenous steroid therapy, received intravenous and oral cyclosporine therapy; the drug eliminated the need for colectomy and permitted the withdrawal of steroids in the majority of patients (Lichtiger and Present, 1990; Lichtiger et al, 1993). In both studies, patients were given intravenous cyclosporine initially (mean response time, six to seven days); after improvement was observed, cyclosporine was administered orally. Although cyclosporine was well tolerated in short-term studies, prolonged use has produced paresthesias and hirsutism in a significant number of patients. The risk of development of hypertension and kidney damage also increases with continued treatment (Kirsner, 1991). Cyclosporine should be administered only by experienced investigators under controlled conditions.

Methotrexate [Folex] also is being tested clinically in those with severe inflammatory bowel disease. A single weekly intramuscular injection of low doses (25 mg) for 12 weeks was effective in patients with severe Crohn's disease or ulcerative colitis (Kozarek et al, 1989).

The long-term renal, hepatic, and other adverse effects of therapy with methotrexate or cyclosporine are unknown.

Therefore, it has been recommended that their use be restricted to patients with severe disease refractory to other drugs (including steroids) and to steroid-dependent patients (Sack and Peppercorn, 1983; Peppercorn, 1990). Many physicians do not prescribe immunosuppressive agents because of their potential adverse effects but others believe that the potential benefits outweigh the danger.

For a more extensive discussion of agents under investigation for use in inflammatory bowel disease, see Geier and Miner, 1992; Peppercorn, 1992 A.

SURGERY. Surgery is indicated for ulcerative colitis when complications are severe, the response to maximal medical therapy is poor, or side effects of drug therapy are excessive. Colectomy and ileostomy or ileoanal anastomosis cure ulcerative colitis. Physiologic adjustment after mucosal proctectomy and formation of an ileal reservoir may require many months. However, the majority of patients maintain continence with four to eight liquid stools daily. Bowel movement frequency is reduced in many patients with use of antidiarrheal preparations and/or psyllium fiber supplements. Pouchitis (inflammation within the ileal reservoir) complicates 15% to 40% of cases and usually responds to a course of metronidazole, ciprofloxacin, or possibly rectal 5-aminosalicylic acid (mesalamine [ROWASA]) (Miglioli, 1989).

Surgical resection is indicated for Crohn's disease when persistent intestinal obstruction, abscess, uncontrollable bleeding, or perforation occurs. Total colectomy and ileostomy may be required for severe colonic disease. However, the recurrence rate approaches 100% after intestinal resection and anastomosis. The use of immunosuppressive agents may decrease the need for colectomy in some patients.

Miscellaneous Forms of Colitis

Miscellaneous forms of colitis include diversion, collagenous, lymphocytic (microscopic), ischemic, and that due to enteroinvasive strains of *E. coli* 0157:H7. The latter is being observed more frequently, but identification of *E. coli* requires special laboratory techniques. The hemorrhagic colitis produced by *E. coli* 0157:H7 is similar to that observed in patients with ulcerative colitis; this form of colitis also is characterized by bloody diarrhea, abdominal cramps, and low-grade fever. Antibiotic therapy appears to have little value (Griffen and Tauxe, 1991). Other strains of *E. coli* (eg, *E. coli* 0126:H11), which produce *Shigella*-like cytotoxins, also may cause hemorrhagic colitis and may be associated with the hemolytic uremia syndrome.

Diversion colitis occurs in the colonic segment that is excluded from the fecal stream by a diverting colostomy or ileostomy; this inflammatory disorder resolves after reanastomosis. A nutritional deficiency of the short-chain fatty acids (primarily butyrate) that normally bathe the colonic mucosa may cause diversion colitis (Geraghty and Talbot, 1991). In one uncontrolled study in adults with this disorder, symptoms were relieved by administration of an enema containing short-chain fatty acids (Harig et al, 1989).

In collagenous and lymphocytic colitis, symptoms are mild and usually consist of chronic watery diarrhea (Lazenby et al, 1992). In collagenous colitis, collagen is deposited into a thickened subepithelial layer. This disorder may be related to inflammatory bowel disease, and some cases may result from use of NSAIDs or antibiotics (Kirsner, 1991). Lymphocytic colitis differs from inflammatory bowel disease in the penetration of neutrophils and lymphocytes into the surface epithelium. In ischemic colitis, blood flow to the colon is diminished; this disease may be transient and resemble Crohn's colitis or, less commonly, ulcerative colitis.

Effective therapy for these forms of colitis is lacking. Anecdotal evidence suggests that sulfasalazine or corticosteroids may relieve symptoms of collagenous or lymphocytic colitis.

Drug Evaluations

ADRENAL CORTICOSTEROIDS (SYSTEMIC)

See the Introduction and index entry Adrenal Corticosteroids.

HYDROCORTISONE
[Cortenema]

HYDROCORTISONE ACETATE
[Cortifoam]

USES. The use of retention enemas or rectal preparations containing an adrenal corticosteroid is usually restricted to patients with mild to moderate distal ulcerative colitis, although rectal forms may be useful as an adjunct to other drugs in those with more severe disease. These preparations also may be of value in proctitis caused by radiation. Combined use of oral and enema preparations often permits reduction of the oral steroid dose. See also the discussion on drug therapy for inflammatory bowel disease.

Approximately 30% to 50% of the steroid is absorbed from noninflamed mucosa, but larger amounts may be absorbed if acute inflammation is present. A beneficial effect is usually noted within 48 hours.

ADVERSE REACTIONS AND PRECAUTIONS. All of the serious toxic reactions produced by systemic adrenal corticosteroids may occur with use of these rectal preparations (see index entry Adrenal Corticosteroids); accordingly, the same precautions should be observed. However, the extent of adrenocortical suppression and other systemic adverse effects is much less with rectal preparations (Sack and Peppercorn, 1983).

DOSAGE AND PREPARATIONS.

Rectal: A retention enema containing hydrocortisone 100 mg is instilled once or twice daily. The enema is inserted with the patient in the left Sims's position. Since optimal absorption is achieved with prolonged retention, the patient should lie quietly for at least 30 minutes after instillation. Dosage usually is reduced over a period of weeks as improvement occurs. Alternatively, a foam aerosol preparation (that may reach the distal sigmoid junction) is applied once or twice daily for two to three weeks and then on alternate days. Patients may be ambulatory after application of the foam.

HYDROCORTISONE:
Cortenema (Solvay). Retention enema 100 mg in 60 ml single-dose containers.

HYDROCORTISONE ACETATE:
Cortifoam (Reed & Carnrick). Aerosol 90 mg in 900 mg of foam.

SULFASALAZINE
[Azulfidine]

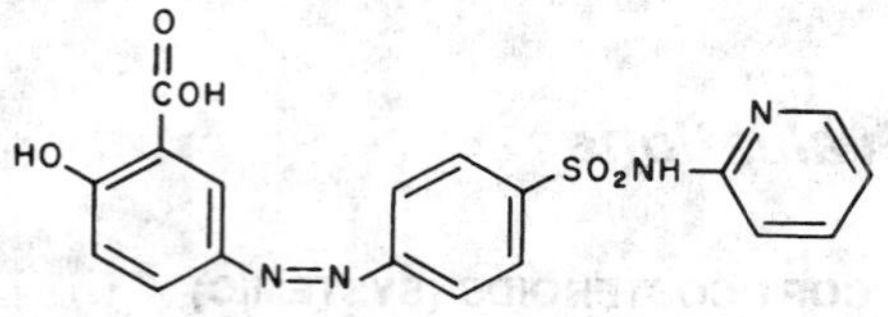

ACTIONS. The actions of sulfasalazine in inflammatory bowel disease are attributed to one of its constituents, 5-aminosalicylic acid (5-ASA). Less than 30% of an oral dose of sulfasalazine is absorbed, almost all of which re-enters the intestine with bile. Thus, the major portion of a dose reaches the colon and is converted to sulfapyridine and 5-ASA by colonic bacteria (Peppercorn and Goldman, 1972; Azad Khan et al, 1977). Sulfapyridine is inactive but is almost completely absorbed and partially metabolized; it accounts for almost all of the adverse reactions produced by sulfasalazine. About 20% to 30% of the 5-ASA formed is absorbed; it is acetylated and eliminated rapidly in the urine. The mechanism of action of 5-ASA has been tentatively ascribed to inhibition of arachidonic acid cascade (cyclooxygenase and lipoxygenase metabolites). Sulfasalazine and 5-ASA block both pathways. However, 5-ASA is a more potent inhibitor of the lipoxygenase pathway and prevents the production of leukotriene B_4 by neutrophils (Bondesen et al, 1987).

USES. Sulfasalazine is most useful in exacerbations of mild to moderate ulcerative colitis. It appears to be less effective in severe disease, but this has not been confirmed by controlled studies. Results of controlled clinical studies indicate that prophylactic use of sulfasalazine decreases the rate of recurrence in patients with chronic, idiopathic ulcerative colitis. Because patients without overt symptoms may still have active disease, its use should not be discontinued prematurely.

This drug also may be useful as an adjunct in about 50% of patients with acute Crohn's disease; the colon appears to be more responsive than the small intestine (Sack and Peppercorn, 1983; Summers et al, 1979; Van Hees et al, 1981). Sulfasalazine used alone is effective in Crohn's colitis and ileocolitis. Results of most studies indicate that sulfasalazine does not prevent relapses of active Crohn's disease or postoperative recurrences.

ADVERSE REACTIONS, PRECAUTIONS, AND INTERACTIONS. Patients in whom sulfapyridine is acetylated slowly may require smaller doses or more gradual initial dosage adjustment and are more likely to develop untoward effects. Generalized adverse reactions, such as nausea and vomiting, headache, abdominal discomfort, malaise, arthralgia, and anorexia, are common, usually dose-related, and often persistent, especially when daily doses exceed 2 g (Singleton et al, 1979; Azad Khan et al, 1980) or the drug is taken on an empty stomach. Gastrointestinal intolerance may be reduced by administering the drug with food or using enteric-coated preparations. Reduction of the dose or discontinuation of therapy may be necessary.

Most patients with mild allergic reactions, such as fever or rash, can be desensitized by increasing the dose gradually (Korelitz et al, 1984; Taffet and Das, 1983). Alternatively, an aminosalicylate can be substituted; however, 10% to 15% of sulfasalazine-sensitive patients will be intolerant of or allergic to an aminosalicylate. Desensitization should not be attempted in those who experience serious adverse reactions.

Idiosyncratic reactions such as hypersensitivity pneumonitis, a lupus-like syndrome, pancreatitis, and toxic hepatitis have been reported.

Agranulocytosis and other blood dyscrasias occur rarely and are sometimes fatal. Both immune and nonimmune hemolytic anemia develop; the latter is more common in G6PD-deficient patients. Complete blood counts should be performed periodically, particularly during the first few weeks of therapy.

Folate deficiency may occur in patients treated with sulfasalazine. Macrocytic anemias may be related to impaired absorption of folic acid. Therefore, adequate intake of folate should be assured (Halsted et al, 1981). Folic acid supplementation (1 mg/day) is recommended since sulfasalazine competitively inhibits folate conjugase and interferes with dietary folate absorption.

A retrospective review of 531 pregnant patients suggests that prospects for normal pregnancies in women with inflammatory bowel disease who take sulfasalazine and/or steroids are better than those for patients with untreated disease and similar to those for the general population (Mogadam et al, 1981). Another study demonstrates that the prognosis for a successful pregnancy improves when the disease is controlled or in remission (Baiocco and Korelitz, 1984). Sulfasalazine is safe for use in nursing mothers. This drug is classified in FDA Pregnancy Category B.

Reversible oligospermia and infertility have been described in men treated with sulfasalazine (Rachmilewitz, 1982). These problems also have been observed in malnourished patients not receiving this agent.

Sulfasalazine can impair the absorption of digoxin. An interval of two to three hours between the oral administration of these drugs is recommended.

DOSAGE AND PREPARATIONS.

Oral: *Adults,* initially, 0.5 g daily, increased by 0.5 g/day until a maximum of 2 to 6 g daily in divided doses is reached. For maintenance, 2 to 4 g daily in divided doses. *Children over 2 years,* initially, 40 to 60 mg/kg daily in four to six divided doses; for maintenance, 30 mg/kg daily in four divided doses. Twice-daily administration is effective in many children. The enteric-coated tablet may be used to reduce gastric irritation.

Generic. Tablets (plain, enteric-coated) 500 mg.
Azulfidine (Kabi Pharmacia). Tablets 500 mg; tablets (enteric-coated) 500 mg (***Azulfidine-EN-tabs***).

MESALAMINE (Rectal) (5-Aminosalicylic Acid, 5-ASA)
[ROWASA]

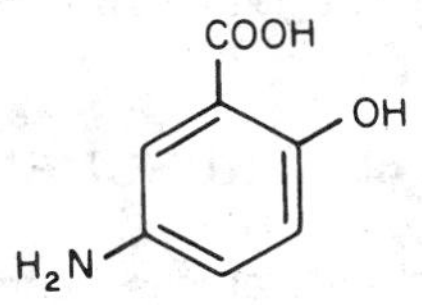

ACTIONS. 5-ASA appears to be the active moiety of sulfasalazine (Azad Khan et al, 1977; Klotz et al, 1980). Its anti-inflammatory properties include inhibition of the arachidonic acid cascade with prevention of leukotriene B_4 production and the ability to scavenge radicals. In contrast to sulfasalazine, 5-ASA scavenges hypochlorite rather than superoxide radicals. When this metabolite is administered alone in enema or suppository form (mesalamine), less than 15% is absorbed from the colon, acetylated, and excreted in the urine. The remainder is excreted in the feces either as free or acetylated 5-ASA.

USES. Rectal suppositories of mesalamine (mesalazine in Europe) are used in the management of active ulcerative proctitis. The enema form is indicated for active ulcerative colitis limited to the left colon (distal to the splenic flexure). Enema preparations reliably spread to the sigmoid colon and often to the splenic flexure (Campieri et al, 1985). Once mucosal healing has occurred, generally after three to six weeks, the number of instillations should be reduced gradually. However, reduction in the number of instillations may induce a relapse of colitis and necessitate resumption of nightly enema therapy and, as with sulfasalazine or steroids, discontinuation of mesalamine enema therapy may precipitate severe relapses necessitating colectomy. The inflammatory reaction rarely may spread more proximally in refractory patients or after discontinuation of treatment. Many patients will require maintenance therapy with an oral form (mesalamine or olsalazine) or with the enema or suppository preparation (administered less frequently) to remain in remission.

Patients with distal ulcerative colitis refractory to therapy with oral sulfasalazine and/or steroids are likely to respond to enema preparations of mesalamine (Biddle and Miner, 1990). Enema preparations also may be useful for the treatment of distal colonic Crohn's disease (Klotz et al, 1980).

ADVERSE REACTIONS AND PRECAUTIONS. This drug usually is well tolerated; the most common adverse effect is mild perianal irritation. Rarely, individuals may develop a fever, rash, or *aggravation* of colitis, probably as a result of sensitivity to salicylates; the drug should be discontinued if the patient reports increased symptoms or rectal bleeding.

Between 10% and 15% of patients who are allergic to sulfasalazine will be intolerant of or allergic to an aminosalicylate; symptoms of hypersensitivity include pancreatitis, alopecia, pneumonitis, and myopericarditis; acute pancreatitis may occur in up to 5% of patients (Fiorentini et al, 1991). Salicylate-related renal damage has been reported in animals with doses of mesalamine above 40 mg/kg (Bondesen et al, 1987). Rarely, renal toxicity with nephritis has been reported in patients treated with Asacol, an oral mesalamine preparation (*Drug Ther Bull*, 1992: Committee on Safety of Medicines, 1990; Daneshmend, 1991).

Sulfasalazine can be used safely during pregnancy and lactation, but mesalamine has not been tested in pregnant or lactating women (FDA Pregnancy Category B). It is probable that mesalamine is as safe as sulfasalazine, since systemic concentrations of 5-ASA and its metabolites are no greater after mesalamine enemas than after ingestion of oral sulfasalazine.

Mesalamine does not induce sperm abnormalities in humans and substituting this drug for sulfasalazine has reversed hypospermia and disturbances of morphology and motility.

DOSAGE AND PREPARATIONS.
Rectal: For ulcerative colitis, patients should be positioned on their left side. A retention enema (4 g) is instilled nightly at bedtime and retained for approximately eight hours if possible. Instillation should continue nightly for four to eight weeks until mucosal healing has occurred. Application then is reduced to every second or third night and gradually reduced further. Nightly enema therapy should resume if flare-ups occur.

For active ulcerative proctitis, *adults*, one suppository (500 mg) twice daily for three to six weeks. Retention for one to three hours or longer produces maximum benefit.
ROWASA (Solvay). Retention enema 4 g in 60 ml single-dose containers; suppositories 500 mg.

MESALAMINE (Oral)
[Asacol, Pentasa]

OLSALAZINE SODIUM
[Dipentum]

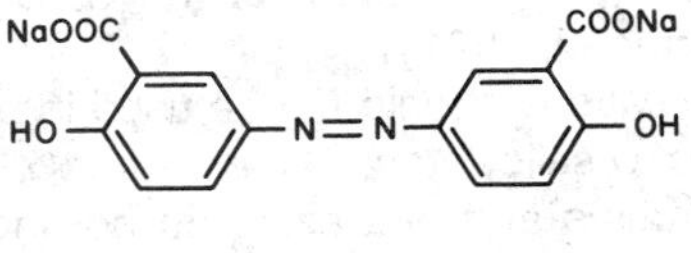

ACTIONS. The linkage of two 5-aminosalicylic acid molecules by an azo bond produces an oral formulation, olsalazine sodium (disodium azodisalicylate), that resists degradation in the upper small intestine. Free 5-ASA is generated in the terminal ileum and colon by the action of bacteria that cleave the azo bond. Oral mesalamine is available as (1) Asacol, a pH-sensitive, polymer-coated tablet that releases active drug in the terminal ileum and colon at or above pH 7.0, and (2) Pentasa, a capsule containing ethylcellulose-coated mesalamine beads that release the drug throughout the small and large intestine. Like rectal mesalamine, the anti-inflammatory properties of these oral forms of 5-ASA include inhibition of the arachidonic acid cascade with prevention of leukotriene B_4 production and the ability to scavenge hypochlorite radicals.

USES. Few trials have compared the available oral 5-ASA preparations. Results of controlled trials indicate that oral mesalamine (mesalazine in Europe) and olsalazine are as effective as sulfasalazine in patients with mild to moderate ulcerative colitis. The oral forms of mesalamine are used for treatment of initial attacks in those with acute disease and as maintenance therapy to prevent relapses. Olsalazine is used to maintain remission; it is not used for treatment of acute attacks (Ireland et al, 1988; Rao et al, 1989; Sninsky et al, 1991; Wadworth and Fitton, 1991). These drugs may be a suitable alternative in patients who cannot tolerate sulfasalazine.

These 5-ASA preparations are being studied as alternatives to sulfasalazine for active Crohn's disease of the small and large bowel (Bondesen et al, 1987; Jarnerot, 1989). Unlike sulfasalazine, in placebo-controlled studies, oral mesalamine was effective for maintenance therapy in Crohn's disease (Prantera et al, 1992; Tremaine, 1992). (In doses that would achieve the same concentration of aminosalicylate in the gut lumen provided by 5-ASA preparations, patients may not tolerate sulfasalazine.) It is unclear if aminosalicylates prevent recurrence of Crohn's disease postoperatively.

Aminosalicylates are considerably more expensive than sulfasalazine.

ADVERSE REACTIONS, PRECAUTIONS, AND INTERACTIONS. Olsalazine causes diarrhea in up to 15% of patients; this can be avoided by using low doses initially, increasing the amount gradually, and taking the drug with meals. Olsalazine should be avoided in patients with active disease; the incidence of diarrhea is greater in patients with more severe or extensive colitis. Oral mesalamine produces diarrhea less frequently than olsalazine (incidence, <5%) (Sninsky et al, 1991). Other reported adverse reactions to oral aminosalicylates include acne, rash, nausea, cramping or abdominal pain, pruritus, transient anxiety attacks, hepatitis, arthralgia, pneumonitis, pericarditis, exacerbation of colitis, and pancreatitis (Wadworth and Fitton, 1991). Rarely, renal toxicity with nephritis has been reported in patients treated with Asacol (*Drug Ther Bull*, 1992; Committee on Safety of Medicines, 1990; Daneshmend, 1991).

These formulations should not be used in patients who are hypersensitive to salicylates.

Oral mesalamine and olsalazine do not induce sperm abnormalities in humans, and substituting these formulations for sulfasalazine has reversed hypospermia and disturbances of morphology and motility. Although sulfasalazine is safe for use during pregnancy and lactation, high-dose aminosalicylate therapy has not been tested in pregnant or lactating women. Olsalazine and the Asacol preparation of mesalamine are classified in FDA Pregnancy Category C. The Pentasa preparation of mesalamine is classified in FDA Pregnancy Category B.

DOSAGE AND PREPARATIONS.

MESALAMINE (Oral):

Oral: For mild to moderate active ulcerative colitis, *adults,* the dosage for Asacol ranges from 2.4 to 4.8 g daily; the dosage for Pentasa ranges from 2 to 4 g daily. For maintenance therapy, dosage is similar but in time may be reduced by one-half.

Asacol (Proctor & Gamble Pharmaceuticals). Tablets (prolonged-release) 400 mg.

Pentasa (Marion-Merrell Dow). Capsules (prolonged-release) 250 mg.

OLSALAZINE SODIUM:

Oral: *Adults,* to maintain remission in ulcerative colitis, 500 mg twice daily taken with food.

Dipentum (Kabi Pharmacia). Capsules 250 mg.

IRRITABLE BOWEL SYNDROME

The irritable bowel syndrome is a common, recurrent, physiologic or functional disorder. At least two forms have been observed: In one, a spastic colon (spastic colitis) produces abdominal pain and constipation or diarrhea. Painless diarrhea also may occur (Shearman and Finlayson, 1982; Langman, 1982). In another form, patients experience alternating episodes of diarrhea and constipation. Mixed forms are common. Gaseous distention of the bowel frequently occurs. Impaired neural coordination of colonic contractions may be responsible for some aspects of this disorder (Snape, 1978); however, generalized neuromuscular abnormalities can occur throughout the gastrointestinal tract (Cann and Read, 1985). There are no objective pathognomonic signs, and a complete history and examination should be performed, since the diagnosis often is made by exclusion.

Emotional stress aggravates this disorder and may precipitate acute episodes in many patients. The alterations in normal motility may be an exaggerated response to stress resulting from a generalized autonomic disturbance. Many investigators consider the etiology to be psychological (Cook et al, 1990; Wald, 1990; Drossman and Thompson, 1992).

TREATMENT. There is no convincing evidence that any therapy is effective in this syndrome; however, several therapeutic approaches make patients more comfortable and allow them to live fairly normal lives. Many physicians do not meet the physical and emotional needs of patients with this disorder, which probably accounts for the fact that up to one-third seek alternatives to standard medical therapy (Drossman and Thompson, 1992). Patient education is essential. Physicians should explain that even in cases associated with stress or other psychological causes, the primary disturbance, a dysfunctional intestinal tract, is not imaginary and symptoms are real. The intestine of patients with the irritable bowel syndrome is overly sensitive to various stimuli (eg, stress, food, menstrual and other hormonal changes). Patients must understand that this chronic disease is not fatal, does not lead to serious disease, and does not shorten life expectancy. For many, treatment that includes simple advice on diet, suggestions for stress avoidance, and temporary drug treatment for exacerbations may be beneficial; these measures, along with adequate patient education, may be the best therapy presently available.

Behavioral Therapy: This form of treatment is only beneficial in motivated patients with moderate to severe symptoms. Some individuals are emotionally disturbed as a result of childhood psychological trauma, including bereavement, physical assault, or sexual abuse; they may have been rewarded in childhood with affection when they complained of intestinal symptoms. As adults, such patients may be conditioned to seek health care for lesser degrees of illness (Almy, 1992). Patients likely to respond to psychotherapy include those with predominant diarrhea and pain, those with overt psychiatric symptoms, and those with intermittent pain exacerbated by stress; those with constant abdominal pain are unlikely to respond (Guthrie et al, 1991). (For a more detailed discussion of behavioral therapy, see Drossman and Thompson, 1992, and Guthrie et al, 1991.)

Less than 5% of patients with severe refractory irritable bowel syndrome insist that they have a serious organic disorder despite negative results of diagnostic tests and physician reassurance. Such patients are strongly resistant to traditional psychotherapy and drugs affecting the intestine. Suggested treatment for these individuals includes specific behavioral therapy and use of psychoactive drugs (Drossman and Thompson, 1992).

Dietary Therapy: The value of dietary fiber is unclear (Guthrie et al, 1991; Everhart and Renault, 1991). Many physicians believe that spastic colon associated with constipation or "pellet" stools may be improved by bulk-forming agents, such as psyllium or bran. In contrast, reduction in unrefined fiber products is often helpful in patients with excess gas or diarrhea, because fiber may aggravate symptoms in these individuals. Causes of specific dietary intolerance (eg, lactose, fructose) should be sought, and aggravating food substances such as sorbitol or caffeine should be avoided.

Drug Therapy: The efficacy of drug therapy in the irritable bowel syndrome is difficult to demonstrate because the placebo response is high, and symptoms often abate without specific treatment. An initial placebo effect may lead patients to take a prescribed medication indefinitely. However, no single drug or combination of drugs should be used chronically, for adverse reactions can occur. At times, a specific exacerbation may cause pain, diarrhea, constipation, or another symptom that is severe enough to impair daily function. A drug targeted at that specific symptom may be useful temporarily.

Anticholinergic drugs frequently are used alone or with an antianxiety agent, but their effectiveness in the irritable bowel syndrome is variable. Antianxiety drugs may block stress-induced increases in colonic motility (Narducci et al, 1982). Although anticholinergic drugs provide only short-term benefits and their adverse effects may outweigh their usefulness, small doses may be helpful. The milder anticholinergic drugs (eg, tincture of belladonna, dicyclomine [Bentyl]) often are useful and produce few side effects. Potent anticholinergic drugs, such as propantheline [Pro-Banthīne], are not recommended. Patients most likely to respond to anticholinergic drugs have postprandial abdominal pain and distention that are relieved when the medication is administered before meals, but these patients constitute only a relatively small proportion of cases (Thompson, 1984). Cisapride, an investigational prokinetic agent, has relieved symptoms of mild idiopathic chronic constipation (Thompson, 1984).

Administration of low doses of tricyclic antidepressants for at least three weeks may be helpful in patients with the irritable bowel syndrome when diarrhea and pain are the predominant symptoms (Camilleri and Prather, 1992); these drugs should be avoided in patients with constipation and pain.

Nonspecific antidiarrheal drugs, such as loperamide, may be effective in patients with loose stools, frequent bowel movements, and urgency. Loperamide also has been useful for episodes of diarrhea in some patients with alternating constipation and diarrhea (Cann et al, 1984; Müller-Lissner et al, 1987) but may aggravate the cyclic pattern in others.

Drug Evaluations

ANTICHOLINERGIC ANTISPASMODICS

ACTIONS. Atropine, the prototype of the *naturally occurring anticholinergic agents*, competitively antagonizes the effect of acetylcholine at muscarinic sites. It does not block transmission either at the neuromuscular junction or at autonomic ganglia unless it is administered in toxic doses. This tertiary amine is readily absorbed from the gastrointestinal tract and crosses the blood-brain barrier.

Atropine reduces both the motility and secretory activity of the gastrointestinal tract. It has much less effect on the smooth muscle of the bile ducts, gallbladder, ureter, urinary bladder, and myometrium. Usual doses have only modest inhibitory action on gastric secretion. Salivary secretions are generally inhibited at doses lower than those required to affect gastrointestinal motility and gastric secretion.

The *quaternary ammonium compounds* are ionized and rarely affect the central nervous system because they do not readily cross the blood-brain barrier. Their ionization is largely responsible for the wide individual variability in absorption noted after oral administration. Most of their actions are attributable to the antimuscarinic effect of usual therapeutic doses. Some antispasmodic actions of quaternary ammonium compounds may be due to their relatively specific ganglionic blocking effects in the gastrointestinal tract.

The *synthetic tertiary amine derivatives* have a more uniform oral bioavailability than the naturally occurring belladonna alkaloids, and central nervous system effects generally are less prominent. Although all of these derivatives have anticholinergic properties, some exhibit an additional or primary noncholinergic gastrointestinal antispasmodic effect experimentally; the mechanism of action is unknown.

Unfortunately, there are no clinically significant, clear-cut differences in efficacy among the anticholinergic antispasmodics to aid in drug selection and, on a practical basis, no available anticholinergic drug has a particular advantage over others.

USES. Anticholinergic antispasmodics are occasionally useful as adjuncts in the treatment of irritable bowel syndrome, usually when postprandial abdominal pain and constipation are prominent (Ivey, 1975; Thompson, 1984). Because of a high placebo effect, it is difficult to assess their value in most patients. (See the Introduction to this section.)

Opinion is divided on the usefulness of anticholinergic antispasmodics in Crohn's disease and acute ulcerative colitis.

The milder antispasmodic preparations are preferable to more potent compounds because of the likelihood of inducing paralysis of colonic musculature and toxic megacolon with the latter (see the section on Inflammatory Bowel Disease). Anticholinergic agents are ineffective for relief of acute diarrhea (Reves et al, 1983).

ADVERSE REACTIONS, PRECAUTIONS, AND INTERACTIONS. Untoward effects associated with therapeutic doses of anticholinergic agents include dryness of the mouth, anhidrosis, mydriasis, cycloplegia, tachycardia, constipation, dysuria, and acute urinary retention. Tolerance to some of these reactions develops with continued use and/or administration of smaller doses, but effectiveness also may be reduced. Hypersensitivity, usually manifested as rash, occurs infrequently.

Toxic doses may produce extreme dryness of the mouth accompanied by a burning sensation, dysphagia, thirst, marked photophobia, flushing in the blush area, fever, leukocytosis, rash, nausea, vomiting, tachycardia, and hypotension or hypertension. Ileus or toxic megacolon has been reported in some patients with severe inflammatory, ischemic, or amebic colitis. Physostigmine may counteract this complication (see index entry Physostigmine, In Anticholinergic Toxicity).

Large doses of the naturally occurring anticholinergic compounds may produce signs of central nervous system excitation (eg, restlessness, tremor, irritability, delirium, hallucinations), which may be followed by respiratory depression and death from medullary paralysis. Children are more susceptible to these toxic effects than adults.

Large doses of the quaternary ammonium compounds may cause ganglionic blockade, as evidenced by orthostatic hypotension and impotence, and toxic doses may cause respiratory arrest as a result of neuromuscular blockade. Since quaternary ammonium compounds do not readily cross the blood-brain barrier, central nervous system effects occur only rarely.

Anticholinergic drugs are contraindicated in patients with reflux esophagitis because they decrease both esophageal and gastric motility and relax the lower esophageal sphincter. They should be used with caution in patients with prostatic hypertrophy, pyloric obstruction, obstruction of the bladder neck, and congestive heart failure with tachycardia. Because of their mydriatic effect, the anticholinergic drugs may precipitate an attack of acute glaucoma in patients predisposed to angle closure. This has occurred occasionally after parenteral administration but only rarely after oral use. Anticholinergic drugs can be given safely to patients with open-angle glaucoma who are being treated with miotics.

Since antacids may interfere with the absorption of anticholinergic agents, these drugs should not be given concomitantly; an interval of at least one hour is suggested.

DOSAGE AND PREPARATIONS. Dosage requirements vary markedly among patients and may differ from those recommended by the manufacturers. The doses suggested in the Table 2 are guidelines for initial therapy. The dose is usually determined by increasing the amount to just below that which causes mild adverse effects (eg, dryness of the mouth, blurred vision). It is not useful to give large doses to maximize the effect; lower doses also improve patient compliance.

Anticholinergic agents usually are administered orally 30 minutes before meals and at bedtime; prolonged-release preparations are given less frequently.

For suggested doses and preparations, see Table 2.

Mixtures Containing Anticholinergic Antispasmodics

Many widely promoted mixtures contain anticholinergic antispasmodics and antianxiety agents (ie, benzodiazepines, hydroxyzine, meprobamate, barbiturates). Combinations containing antispasmodics and antianxiety agents may aid in the relief of the irritable bowel syndrome. If an antianxiety agent is needed, the benzodiazepines appear to be the most efficacious and safest (see index entry Antianxiety Drugs). Some products also contain ergotamine, but controlled studies have not demonstrated that this drug has any special value in gastrointestinal disorders.

Anticholinergic compounds require greater individualization of dosage than most drugs to be effective and to minimize side effects. Since the need for adjustments in the dose of the individual ingredients is seldom parallel, it often is impractical, especially during initial therapy, to utilize combination products.

The following list of commonly used preparations is for information only; inclusion in the list does not indicate approval or recommendation for use.

Generic (Belladonna Alkaloids with Phenobarbital). Each tablet contains hyoscyamine hydrobromide or sulfate 0.1037 mg, atropine sulfate 0.0194 mg, scopolamine hydrobromide 0.0065 mg, and phenobarbital 16.2 mg.

Bellergal-S (Sandoz). Each prolonged-release tablet contains levorotatory alkaloids of belladonna as malates 0.2 mg, ergotamine tartrate 0.6 mg, and phenobarbital 40 mg.

Butibel (Wallace). Each tablet or 5 ml of elixir contains belladonna extract 15 mg, butabarbital sodium 15 mg, and alcohol 7% (elixir).

Chardonna-2 (Schwarz). Each tablet contains belladonna extract 15 mg and phenobarbital 15 mg.

Donnatal (Robins). Each capsule, tablet, or 5 ml of elixir contains hyoscyamine sulfate 0.1037 mg, atropine sulfate 0.0194 mg, scopolamine hydrobromide 0.0065 mg, phenobarbital 16.2 mg, and alcohol 23% (elixir); each No. 2 tablet contains same formulation as ***Donnatal*** except phenobarbital 32.4 mg; each tablet (prolonged-release) contains hyoscyamine sulfate 0.3111 mg, atropine sulfate 0.0582 mg, scopolamine hydrobromide 0.0195 mg, and phenobarbital 48.6 mg ***(Donnatal Extentabs)***.

Kinesed (Stuart). Each tablet (chewable) contains hyoscyamine sulfate 0.12 mg, atropine sulfate 0.012 mg, scopolamine hydrobromide 0.007 mg, and phenobarbital 16 mg.

Levsin w/Phenobarbital (Schwarz). Each tablet contains hyoscyamine sulfate 0.125 mg and phenobarbital 15 mg; each 1 ml of drops (***Levsin-PB Drops***) contains the same formulation as tablets plus alcohol 5%.

Librax (Roche). Each capsule contains clidinium bromide 2.5 mg and chlordiazepoxide hydrochloride 5 mg.

ANORECTAL PREPARATIONS

Hemorrhoids, anal fissures, and cryptitis are common and are often associated with pruritus, bleeding, mucus seepage,

TABLE 2.
ANTICHOLINERGIC ANTISPASMODICS

Drug	Usual Initial Dosage	Preparations
NATURALLY OCCURRING TERTIARY AMINES		
Belladonna Alkaloids		
Atropine Sulfate	*Oral, Subcutaneous: Adults,* 0.3 to 1.2 mg every 4 to 6 hours. *Subcutaneous: Children,* 0.01 mg/kg every 4 to 6 hours.	*Generic.* Solution (for injection) 0.05 mg/ml in 5 ml containers; 0.1 mg/ml in 5 and 10 ml containers; 0.3 mg/ml in 1 ml containers; 0.4 mg/ml in 1 and 20 ml containers; 0.5 mg/ml in 1, 5, and 30 ml containers; 0.8 mg/ml in 0.5 and 1 ml containers; 1 mg/ml in 1 and 10 ml containers; 1.2 mg/ml in 1 ml containers; tablets (oral, soluble) 0.3, 0.4, and 0.6 mg; tablets (plain) 0.4 mg.
l-Hyoscyamine Sulfate	*Oral: Adults,* 0.125 to 0.25 mg every 4 to 6 hours. *Children 2 to 10 years*, one-half above dosage range; *under 2 years*, one-fourth above dosage range. *Intramuscular, Subcutaneous, Intravenous: Adults,* 0.25 to 0.5 mg every 4 to 6 hours. When symptoms are controlled, oral medication is substituted. *Children,* parenteral dosage not established.	*Anaspaz* (Ascher). Tablets 0.125 mg. *Levsin* (Schwarz). Drops 0.125 mg/ml (alcohol 5%); elixir 0.125 mg/5 ml (alcohol 20%); tablets (oral, sublingual [*Levsin/SL*]) 0.125 mg; capsules (prolonged-release) [*Levsinex*] 0.375 mg; solution (for injection) 0.5 mg/ml in 1 and 10 ml containers.
Scopolamine Hydrobromide	*Oral: Adults,* 0.4 to 0.8 mg 3 or 4 times daily. *Intramuscular, Intravenous, Subcutaneous: Adults,* 0.3 to 0.6 mg as a single dose.	*Generic.* Solution (for injection) 0.3, 0.4, and 1 mg/ml in 1 ml containers; and 0.86 mg/ml in 0.5 ml containers.
Belladonna Extract	*Oral: Adults,* 15 mg 3 times daily.	*Generic.* Tablets 15 mg.
Belladonna Leaf	*Oral: Adults,* 30 to 200 mg.	No single-entity dosage form available; compounding necessary for prescription.
Belladonna Leaf, Fluid Extract	*Oral: Adults,* 0.06 ml 3 times daily.	*Generic.* Fluid extract in 500 ml containers.
Belladonna Tincture	*Oral: Adults,* 0.6 to 1 ml 3 or 4 times daily. *Children,* 0.03 ml/kg in 3 or 4 divided doses.	*Generic.* Tincture in 120 ml and pint and gallon containers.
Belladonna (total levorotatory alkaloids of belladonna as malates)	*Oral: Adults,* 0.25 to 0.5 mg 3 times daily. *Children over 6 years*, 0.125 to 0.25 mg 3 times daily.	No single-entity dosage form available; compounding necessary for prescription.
QUATERNARY AMMONIUM DERIVATIVES OF NATURAL OR SEMISYNTHETIC BELLADONNA ALKALOIDS		
Homatropine Methylbromide	*Oral: Adults,* 2.5 to 10 mg 4 times daily. *Children,* 3 to 6 mg 4 times daily. *Infants,* 0.3 mg dissolved in water 5 or 6 times daily.	*Generic.* Powder.
Methscopolamine Bromide	*Oral: Adults,* 2.5 to 5 mg 4 times daily. Total daily dose may be increased to 30 mg, if necessary. *Children,* dosage not established. *Intramuscular, Subcutaneous: Adults,* 0.25 to 1 mg every 6 to 8 hours until acute symptoms are controlled and patient can take oral medication. *Children,* dosage not established.	*Available generically under the name Scopolamine Methylbromide.* Solution; tablets. *Pamine* (Upjohn). Tablets 2.5 mg.

(table continued on next page)

TABLE 2 (continued)

Drug	Usual Initial Dosage	Preparations
OTHER SYNTHETIC QUATERNARY AMMONIUM COMPOUNDS		
Clidinium Bromide	*Oral: Adults,* 2.5 to 5 mg 3 or 4 times daily before meals and at bedtime. For the *aged and debilitated,* 2.5 mg 3 times daily before meals. *Children,* dosage not established.	*Quarzan* (Roche). Capsules 2.5 and 5 mg.
Glycopyrrolate	*Oral: Adults,* initially, 1 or 2 mg 3 times daily; for maintenance, 1 mg 2 times daily. *Children,* dosage not established. *Intramuscular, Intravenous, Subcutaneous: Adults,* 0.1 or 0.2 mg at 4-hour intervals 3 or 4 times daily. *Children,* dosage not established.	*Robinul* (Robins), *Generic.* Tablets 1 and 2 mg (*Robinul Forte*); solution (for injection) 0.2 mg/ml in 1, 2, 5, and 20 ml containers.
Isopropamide Iodide	*Oral: Adults and children over 12 years,* initially, 5 mg every 12 hours; for patients with severe symptoms, 10 mg every 12 hours. Not recommended for *children under 12 years.*	*Darbid* (SmithKline Beecham). Tablets 5 mg.
Mepenzolate Bromide	*Oral: Adults,* 25 or 50 mg 3 times daily, preferably with meals, and 25 or 50 mg at bedtime. Not recommended for *children.*	*Cantil* (Marion Merrell Dow). Tablets 25 mg.
Methantheline Bromide	*Oral: Adults,* initially, 50 to 100 mg every 6 hours; dose is reduced to 25 mg for patients who cannot tolerate larger doses. For maintenance, generally one-half initial dose. *Children,* 5 to 10 mg/kg daily in 4 divided doses.	*Banthine* (Schiaparelli Searle). Tablets 50 mg.
Propantheline Bromide	*Oral: Adults,* 15 mg 3 times daily and 30 mg at bedtime. *Children,* 1.5 mg/kg daily in 4 divided doses.	*Generic.* Tablets 15 mg. *Pro-Banthīne* (Schiaparelli Searle). Tablets 7.5 and 15 mg.
SYNTHETIC TERTIARY AMINE COMPOUNDS		
Dicyclomine Hydrochloride	*Oral, Intramuscular: Adults,* 10 to 20 mg 3 or 4 times daily. Solution should not be given intravenously. *Children,* 10 mg 3 or 4 times daily. *Infants,* 5 mg 3 or 4 times daily. For infants, dose diluted with equal volume of water. Contraindicated in *infants under 6 months.*	*Generic.* Capsules 10 and 20 mg; syrup 10 mg/5 ml; tablets 20 mg; solution (for injection) 10 mg/ml in 2 and 10 ml containers. *Bentyl* (Marion Merrell Dow). Capsules 10 mg; syrup 10 mg/5 ml; tablets 20 mg; solution (for injection) 10 mg/ml in 2 and 10 ml containers.
Oxyphencyclimine Hydrochloride	*Oral: Adults,* 10 mg twice daily, gradually increased to 50 mg if side effects are absent. *Children,* dosage not established.	*Daricon* (SmithKline Beecham). Tablets 10 mg.

and pain, which may become severe, especially during or just after defecation.

Composition: Some topical anorectal preparations afford symptomatic relief, but none are curative (*Federal Register*, 1980). Most of these preparations contain protectants or emollients, often in combination with a local anesthetic and, sometimes, a corticosteroid, which is included for its anti-inflammatory effect. Some preparations also contain ingredients of questionable value, such as belladonna, opium, vitamins, vasoconstrictors, weak antiseptics, and astringents. Convincing data to prove that any one mixture is superior to another are lacking. The more bland, simple formulations probably are safest. None controls bleeding and none is a substitute for personal hygienic measures to keep the affected areas as clean as possible.

The local anesthetics commonly incorporated into these preparations include benzocaine, tetracaine, dibucaine, dyclomine, lidocaine, and pramoxine. The base forms of local anesthetics can be absorbed through unbroken skin, but salt forms are absorbed only through mucosa or abraded surfaces. In some preparations, the concentration of the base is too low to be effective. Benzocaine, one of the most widely used topical anesthetics, is not absorbed through the mucosa in concentrations of less than 5% and is poorly soluble in many aqueous vehicles. (See also index entry Anesthetics, Local.)

The ingredients of all anorectal preparations have been or are being reformulated to comply with FDA guidelines established in a final monograph on OTC anorectal drug products (*Federal Register*, 1990). In this monograph, which delineated the conditions under which OTC anorectal drug products are generally recognized as safe and effective, the FDA determined that the only active ingredients that may be marketed for this indication are *local anesthetics*—benzocaine, benzyl alcohol, dibucaine, dyclonine hydrochloride, lidocaine, pramoxine hydrochloride, tetracaine, and tetracaine hydrochloride; *vasoconstrictors*—ephedrine sulfate, epinephrine, epinephrine hydrochloride, and phenylephrine hydrochloride; *protectants*—aluminum hydroxide gel, calamine, cocoa butter, cod liver oil, glycerin, hard fat, kaolin, lanolin, mineral oil, petroleum, shark liver oil, topical starch, white petrolatum, and zinc oxide; *analgesics, anesthetics, and antipruritics*—camphor, juniper tar, and menthol; *astringents*—calamine, hamamelis water, and zinc oxide; and *keratolytics*—alcloxa and resorcinol. With the exception of hydrocortisone and live yeast cell derivative, all other drugs are considered nonmonograph ingredients (safety and efficacy unproved) and, therefore, must be the subject of an approved New Drug Application (NDA) before OTC marketing (*Federal Register*, 1990).

Dosage Forms: The suppository is the most common dosage form available. Some products may be applied by introduction of a multiple aperture tip into the anal canal, thus avoiding the disadvantage produced when the suppository slips into the rectum to melt and ensuring that the medication is likely to be applied at the site of the lesion. However, the danger of self-inflicted trauma from misdirection of the applicator must be considered. The effectiveness of creams or ointments may be enhanced by intra-anal application up to the distal joint of the rubber-cotted finger.

Adverse Reactions: Untoward systemic effects may result from the absorption of local anesthetics, corticosteroids, or other ingredients from the anal or rectal mucosa or excoriated perianal skin. Hypersensitivity reactions with severe dermatitis may occur after topical application of local anesthetics, antiseptics, and some other drugs present in these preparations. Symptoms of overdosage are uncommon because of the small quantity of the drugs in the formulation. Fatalities have occurred when certain of these products have been ingested by infants.

Preparations: The preparations listed below are those most commonly prescribed or widely used. Those with multiple ingredients are not necessarily preferred to preparations containing topical local anesthetics with or without hydrocortisone.

Americaine Hemorrhoidal Ointment (CIBA). Ointment containing benzocaine 20% and benzethonium chloride 0.1% in a polyethylene glycol base (nonprescription).

Analpram-HC (Ferndale). Cream containing hydrocortisone acetate 1% or 2.5% and pramoxine hydrochloride 1% in a washable, nongreasy base containing stearic acid, cetyl alcohol, propylene glycol, potassium sorbate 0.1%, sorbic acid 0.1%, triethanolamine lauryl sulfate, and water.

Anusol (Warner-Lambert). Ointment containing pramoxine hydrochloride 1%, mineral oil 46.7% and zinc oxide 12.5%; suppositories containing phenylephrine 0.25%, hard fat 88.7%, corn starch, methylparaben, and propylparaben (both forms nonprescription).

Anusol-HC (Parke-Davis). Cream containing hydrocortisone 2.5%; suppositories containing hydrocortisone acetate 25 mg in a hydrogenated cocoglyceride base.

Anusol-HC-1 (Warner Lambert). Ointment containing hydrocortisone acetate 1% with diazolidinyl urea, mineral oil, and white petrolatum (nonprescription).

Medicone Rectal (Medicone). Suppositories containing benzocaine 13%, hydroxyquinoline sulfate 1.6%, menthol 0.9%, zinc oxide 19.5%, and Peruvian balsam 6.5% in cocoa butter-vegetable and petroleum oil base (nonprescription).

Preparation H (Whitehall). Ointment, cream, or suppositories containing shark liver oil 3%, live yeast cell derivative (supplying 2,000 units of skin respiratory factor/30 g of ointment, cream, or suppository base), and phenylmercuric nitrate 1:10,000 (preservative) (all forms nonprescription).

Preparation H Hydrocortisone 1% (Whitehall). Cream containing hydrocortisone 1% with glycerin, lanolin, petrolatum, propylene glycol, simethicone, and sodium benzoate (nonprescription).

Proctocort Cream (Solvay). Cream (buffered) containing hydrocortisone 1%.

Proctocream-HC (Reed & Carnrick). Cream containing hydrocortisone acetate 1% and pramoxine hydrochloride 1%.

Proctofoam-HC (Reed & Carnrick). Aerosol foam containing pramoxine hydrochloride 1% and hydrocortisone acetate 1% in a mucoadhesive base.

Tronolane (Ross). Cream containing pramoxine hydrochloride 1%; suppositories containing zinc oxide 5% (both forms nonprescription).

Tucks (Warner-Lambert). Pads containing witch hazel 50% and glycerin 10% with alcohol 7% and benzalkonium chloride 0.003% (nonprescription).

Wyanoids (Wyeth-Ayerst). Suppositories containing live yeast cell derivative (supplying 2,000 units skin respiratory factor per ounce of cocoa butter base) and shark liver oil 3% (nonprescription).

Cited References

Anorectal drug products for over-the-counter human use; establishment of monograph. *Federal Register* 45:35576-35677, 1980.

Anorectal drug products for over-the-counter human use; final monograph. *Federal Register* 55:31776-31783, (Aug 3) 1990.

Cereal-based oral rehydration solutions: Bridging the gap between fluid and food, editorial. *Lancet* 339:219-220, 1992.

Choosing an oral 5 aminosalicylic acid preparation for ulcerative colitis. *Drug Ther Bull* 30:50-52, 1992.

Oral rehydration therapy: Its place in the developed world. *WHO Drug Information* 5:120-121, 1991.

Adler DJ, Korelitz BI: The therapeutic efficacy of 6-mercaptopurine in refractory ulcerative colitis. *Am J Gastroenterol* 85:717, 1990.

Almy TP: Management of the irritable bowel syndrome: Different views of the same disease. *Ann Intern Med* 116:1027-1028, 1992.

American Academy of Pediatrics Committee on Nutrition: Use of oral fluid therapy and posttreatment feeding following enteritis in children in a developed country. *Pediatrics* 75:358-361, 1985.

Angus P, et al: Oral fluticasone propionate in active distal ulcerative colitis. *Gut* 33:711-714, 1992.

Ashkenazi S, Cleary TG: Antibiotic treatment of bacterial gastroenteritis. *Pediatr Infect Dis J* 10:140-148, 1991.

Aslan A, Triadafilopoulos G: Fish oil fatty acid supplementation in active ulcerative colitis: A double-blind, placebo-controlled, crossover study. *Am J Gastroenterol* 87:432-437, 1992.

Avery ME, Snyder JD: Oral therapy for acute diarrhea: The underused simple solution. *N Engl J Med* 323:891-894, 1990.

Azad Khan AK, et al: An experiment to determine the active therapeutic moiety of sulfasalazine. *Lancet* 2:292-295, 1977.

Azad Khan AK, et al: Optimum dose of sulphasalazine for maintenance treatment in ulcerative colitis. *Gut* 21:232-240, 1980.

Baiocco PJ, Korelitz BI: Influence of inflammatory bowel disease and its treatment on pregnancy and fetal outcome. *J Clin Gastroenterol* 6:211-216, 1984.

Baldassano RN, Liacouras CA: Chronic diarrhea: A practical approach for the pediatrician. *Pediatr Clin North Am* 38:667-686, 1991.

Bansky G, et al: Treatment of distal ulcerative colitis with beclomethasone enemas: High therapeutic efficacy without endocrine side effects: Prospective, randomized, double-blind trial. *Dis Colon Rectum* 30:288-292, 1987.

Battershill PE, Clissold SP: Octreotide: A review of its pharmacodynamic and pharmacokinetic properties, and therapeutic potential in conditions associated with excessive peptide secretion. *Drugs* 38:658-702, 1989.

Bernstein CN, Shanahan F: Braving the elementals in Crohn's disease. *Gastroenterology* 103:1363-1364, 1992.

Bezerra JA, et al: Treatment of infants with acute diarrhea: What's recommended and what's practiced. *Pediatrics* 90:1-4, (July) 1992.

Biddle WL, Miner PB Jr: Long-term use of mesalamine enemas to induce remission of ulcerative colitis. *Gastroenterology* 99:113, 1990.

Bondesen S, et al: 5-aminosalicylic acid in treatment of inflammatory bowel disease. *Acta Med Scand* 221:227-242, 1987.

Camilleri M, Prather CM: The irritable bowel syndrome: Mechanisms and a practical approach to management. *Ann Intern Med* 116:1001-1008, 1992.

Campieri M, et al: 5-aminosalicylic acid for treatment of inflammatory bowel diseases. *Gastroenterology* 89:701-706, 1985.

Cann PA, Read NW: A disease of the whole gut? in Read NW (ed): *Irritable Bowel Syndrome.* New York, Grune & Stratton, 1985, 53-63.

Cann PA, et al: Role of loperamide and placebo in management of irritable bowel syndrome. *Dig Dis Sci* 29:239-247, 1984.

Committee on Safety of Medicines: Nephrotoxicity associated with mesalazine (Asacol). *Curr Probl* 30:2, (Dec) 1990.

Cook DJ, et al: Somatostatin treatment for cryptosporidial diarrhea in a patient with the acquired immunodeficiency syndrome (AIDS). *Ann Intern Med* 108:708-709, 1988.

Cook IJ, et al: Effect of dietary fiber on symptoms and rectosigmoid motility in patients with irritable bowel syndrome: A controlled crossover study. *Gastroenterology* 96:66-72, 1990.

Crotty B, Jewell DP: Drug therapy of ulcerative colitis. *Br J Clin Pharmacol* 34:189-198, 1992.

Cutz E, et al: Microvillus inclusion disease: Inherited defect of brush-border assembly and differentiation. *N Engl J Med* 320:646-651, 1989.

Daneshmend TK: Mesalamine associated thrombocytopenia. *Lancet* 337:1297-1298, 1991.

Danish Budesonide Study Group: Budesonide enema in distal colitis: A randomized dose-response trial with prednisolone enema as positive control. *Scand J Gastroenterol* 26:1225-1230, 1991.

del Costello AM, Bhutta TI: Antidiarrhoeal drugs for acute diarrhoea in children. *BMJ* 304:1-2, 1992.

Donowitz M, et al: Trifluoperazine reversal of secretory diarrhea in pancreatic cholera. *Ann Intern Med* 93:284-285, 1980.

Drossman DA, Thompson WG: The irritable bowel syndrome: Review and a graduated multicomponent treatment approach. *Ann Intern Med* 116:1009-1016, 1992.

Dudl RJ, et al: Treatment of diabetic diarrhea and orthostatic hypotension with somatostatin analogue SMS 201-995. *Am J Med* 83:584-588, 1987.

Duncan A, et al: Laxative induced diarrhoea: A neglected diagnosis. *J R Soc Med* 85:203-205, 1992.

Duncombe VM, et al: Double-blind trial of cholestyramine in post-vagotomy diarrhoea. *Gut* 18:531-535, 1977.

DuPont HL: Using OTC drugs for acute diarrhea. *Drug Ther* 13:127-136, (Feb) 1983 A.

DuPont HL: Traveler's diarrhea, letter response. *N Engl J Med* 308:464, 1983 B.

DuPont HL, et al: Symptomatic treatment of diarrhea with bismuth subsalicylate among students attending Mexican university. *Gastroenterology* 73:715-718, 1977.

DuPont HL, et al: Prevention of traveler's diarrhea (emporiatric enteritis): Prophylactic administration of subsalicylate bismuth. *JAMA* 243:237-241, 1980.

DuPont HL, et al: Prevention of travelers' diarrhea by the tablet formulation of bismuth subsalicylate. *JAMA* 247:1347-1350, 1987.

DuPont HL, et al: Use of bismuth subsalicylate for the prevention of travelers' diarrhea. *Rev Infect Dis* 12 (suppl 1):S64-S67, 1990 A.

DuPont HL, et al: A randomized open-label comparison of prescription loperamide and attapulgite in the symptomatic treatment of acute diarrhea. *Am J Med* 88 (suppl 6A):20s-23s, 1990 B.

DuPont HL, et al: Oral aztreonam, a poorly absorbed yet effective therapy for bacterial diarrhea in US travelers to Mexico. *JAMA* 267:1932-1935, 1992.

Ericsson C, et al: Influence of subsalicylate bismuth on absorption of doxycycline. *JAMA* 247:2266-2267, 1982.

Ericsson CD, et al: Treatment of traveler's diarrhea with sulfamethoxazole and trimethoprim and loperamide. *JAMA* 263:257-261, 1990.

Everhart JE, Renault PF: Irritable bowel syndrome in office-based practice in the United States. *Gastroenterology* 100:998-1005, 1991.

Feurle GE, et al: Olsalazine versus placebo in the treatment of mild to moderate ulcerative colitis: A randomised double blind trial. *Gut* 30:1354, 1989.

Fiorentini MT, et al: Acute pancreatitis during oral 5-aminosalicylic acid therapy. *Ital J Gastroenterol* 23:643-644, 1991.

Frank MS, et al: Pharmacotherapy of inflammatory bowel disease. Part 2: Metronidazole. *Postgrad Med* 74:155-160, (Dec) 1983.

Gaginella TS: Diarrhea: Some new aspects of pharmacotherapy. *Drug Intell Clin Pharm* 17:914-916, 1983.

Gassull MA, et al: Enteral nutrition in inflammatory bowel disease. *Gut* 27 (suppl 1):76, 1986.

Geier DL, Miner PB Jr: New therapeutic agents in the treatment of inflammatory bowel disease. *Am J Med* 93:199-208, 1992.

Geraghty JM, Talbot IC: Diversion colitis: Histological features in the colon and rectum after defunctioning colostomy. *Gut* 32:1020-1023, 1991.

Ginsberg AL, et al: Treatment of left-sided ulcerative colitis with 4-aminosalicylic acid enemas: Double-blind, placebo-controlled trial. *Ann Intern Med* 108:195-199, 1988.

Ginsberg AL, et al: Placebo-controlled trial of ulcerative colitis with oral 4-aminosalicylic acid. *Gastroenterology* 102:448-452, 1992.

Gorbach SL: Bacterial diarrhoea and its treatment. *Lancet* 2:1378-1382, 1987.

Gotz V, et al: Prophylaxis against ampicillin-associated diarrhea with lactobacillus preparation. *Am J Hosp Pharm* 36:754-757, 1979.

Graham DY, et al: Double-blind comparison of bismuth subsalicylate and placebo in prevention and treatment of enterotoxigenic *Escherichia coli*-induced diarrhea in volunteers. *Gastroenterology* 85:1017-1022, 1983.

Gray GM: Gastroenterology: IV, Inflammatory bowel disease, in: *Scientific Medicine.* New York, Scientific American, 1991, 1-16.

Griffin PM, Tauxe RV: The epidemiology of infections caused by *Escherichia coli* 0157:H7, other enterohemorrhagic *E. coli*, and the associated hemolytic uremic syndrome. *Epidemiol Rev* 13:60-98, 1991.

Guthrie E, et al: A controlled trial of psychological treatment for the irritable bowel syndrome. *Gastroenterology* 100:450-457, 1991.

Halsted CH, et al: Sulfasalazine inhibits absorption of folates in ulcerative colitis. *N Engl J Med* 305:1513-1517, 1981.

Hanauer SB: Clinical experience with tixocortol pivalate. *Can J Gastroenterol* 2:156-158, 1988.

Harford WV, et al: Acute effect of diphenoxylate with atropine (Lomotil) in patients with chronic diarrhea and fecal incontinence. *Gastroenterology* 78:440-443, 1980.

Harig JM, et al: Treatment of diversion colitis with short-chain fatty acid irrigation. *N Engl J Med* 320:23-28, 1989.

Hawthorne AB, et al: Randomised controlled trial of azathioprine withdrawal in ulcerative colitis. *BMJ* 305:20-22, 1992.

Heel RC, et al: Loperamide: A review of its pharmacological properties and therapeutic efficacy in diarrhoea. *Drugs* 15:33-52, 1978.

Hopman WPM, et al: Treatment of dumping syndrome with somatostatin analogue SMS 201-995. *Ann Surg* 207:155-159, 1988.

Ireland A, et al: Controlled trial comparing olsalazine and sulphasalazine for the maintenance treatment of ulcerative colitis. *Gut* 29:835, 1988.

Ivey KJ: Are anticholinergics of use in irritable colon syndrome? *Gastroenterology* 68:1300-1307, 1975.

Jaffee BM, et al: Indomethacin-responsive pancreatic cholera. *N Engl J Med* 297:817-821, 1977.

Jarnerot G: Newer 5-aminosalicylic acid based drugs in chronic inflammatory bowel disease. *Drugs* 37:73-86, 1989.

Katz MD, et al: Treatment of severe cryptosporidium-related diarrhea with octreotide in a patient with AIDS. *DICP* 22:134-136, 1988.

Kaufmann NJ, Taubin HL: Nonsteroidal anti-inflammatory drugs activate inflammatory bowel disease. *Ann Intern Med* 107:513-516, 1987.

Kerr CP (ed): The treatment of diarrhea in infants—Is there a right way? *Fam Pract Newslett* 7:33-36, (May) 1992.

Kirsner JB: Inflammatory bowel disease, part II: Clinical and therapeutic aspects. *Dis Mon* 673-746, (Nov) 1991.

Klotz U, et al: Therapeutic efficacy of sulfasalazine and its metabolites in patients with ulcerative colitis and Crohn's disease. *N Engl J Med* 303:1499-1502, 1980.

Korelitz BI: Role of immunosuppressives. *Mt Sinai J Med* 50:144-147, 1983.

Korelitz BI: Immunosuppressives, in Peppercorn MA (ed): *Therapy of Inflammatory Bowel Disease*. New York, Marcel Dekker, 1990, 103-134.

Korelitz BI, Sohn N (eds): Corticosteroids and immunosuppressives in treatment of inflammatory bowel disease, in: *Management of Inflammatory Bowel Disease*. St. Louis, Mosby Yearbook, 1992.

Korelitz BI, et al: Desensitization to sulfasalazine after hypersensitivity reactions in patients with inflammatory bowel disease. *J Clin Gastroenterol* 6:27-31, 1984.

Kozarek RA, et al: Methotrexate induces clinical and histologic remission in patients with refractory inflammatory bowel disease. *Ann Intern Med* 110:353-356, 1989.

Kumana CR, et al: Beclomethasone dipropionate enemas for treating inflammatory bowel disease without producing Cushing's syndrome or hypothalamic pituitary adrenal suppression. *Lancet* 1:579-583, 1982.

Langman MJS: Large bowel disease, in: *A Concise Textbook of Gastroenterology*. New York, Churchill Livingstone, 1982, 84-98.

LaRosa D, et al: Maintenance oral sulfasalazine prolongs remission in ulcerative proctitis and proctosigmoiditis. *Am J Gastroenterol* 86:1456-1460, 1991.

Lazenby AJ, et al: Inflammatory bowel disease, correspondence. *N Engl J Med* 326:574, 1992.

Levine RA: Risk of hypercalcemia from prophylaxis of traveler's diarrhea. *JAMA* 249:1151-1152, 1983.

Lichtiger S, Present DH: Preliminary report: Cyclosporin in treatment of severe active ulcerative colitis. *Lancet* 336:16-19, 1990.

Lichtiger S, et al: Cyclosporin A in the treatment of severe, refractory ulcerative colitis: A double blinded placebo controlled trial, abstract. *Gastroenterology* 104:A372, 1993.

Lobo AJ, et al: The role of azathioprine in the management of ulcerative colitis. *Dis Colon Rectum* 33:374, 1990.

Maton PN, et al: Use of long-acting somatostatin analog SMS 201-995 in patients with pancreatic islet cell tumors. *Dig Dis Sci* 34 (suppl):28S-39S, 1989.

McClung HJ, et al: Effect of kaolin-pectin adsorbent on stool losses of sodium, potassium and fat during lactose-intolerance diarrhea in rats. *J Pediatr* 96:769-771, 1980.

Merritt JE, et al: Loperamide and calmodulin, letter. *Lancet* 1:283, 1982.

Meyers S: Role of corticosteroids. *Mt Sinai J Med* 50:141-143, 1983.

Meyers A, et al: Economic barriers to the use of oral rehydration therapy: A case report. *JAMA* 265:1724-1725, 1991 A.

Meyers A, et al: Oral rehydration for children with diarrhea, letter. *JAMA* 266:517, 1991 B.

Miglioli M: Topical administration of 5-ASA: A therapeutic proposal for the treatment of pouchitis. *N Engl J Med* 320:257, 1989.

Miyazaki H, et al: Loperamide in rat intestines: Unique disposition. *Life Sci* 30:2203-2206, 1982.

Mogadam M, et al: Pregnancy in inflammatory bowel disease: Effect of sulfasalazine and corticosteroids on fetal outcome. *Gastroenterology* 80:72-76, 1981.

Müller-Lissner SA, et al: Treatment of chronic constipation with cisapride and placebo. *Gut* 28:1033-1038, 1987.

Narducci F, et al: Stimulation of colonic myoelectric activity by emotional stress in healthy subjects and irritable bowel syndrome: Effect of pretreatment with librium. *Gastroenterology* 82:1137, 1982.

Nathavitharana KA, Booth IW: Pharmacoeconomics of the therapy of diarrhoeal disease. *PharmacoEconomics* 2:305-323, 1992.

O'Brien CJ, et al: Elemental diet in steroid-dependent and steroid-refractory Crohn's disease. *Am J Gastroenterol* 86:1614-1618, 1991.

Palmer KR, et al: Double-blind cross-over study comparing loperamide, codeine and diphenoxylate in treatment of chronic diarrhea. *Gastroenterology* 79:1272-1275, 1980.

Pandol SJ, et al: Beneficial effect of oral lithium carbonate in treatment of pancreatic cholera syndrome. *N Engl J Med* 302:1403-1404, 1980.

Peppercorn MA: Advances in drug therapy for inflammatory bowel disease. *Ann Intern Med* 112:50-60, 1990.

Peppercorn MA: Drug therapy of inflammatory bowel disease, part I: Newer therapeutic agents. *Drug Ther* 23-42, (Sept) 1992 A.

Peppercorn MA: Drug therapy of inflammatory bowel disease, part II: Patient management recommendations. *Drug Ther* 43-53, (Sept) 1992 B.

Peppercorn MA, Goldman P: The role of intestinal bacteria in the metabolism of salicylazosulfapyridine. *J Pharmacol Exp Ther* 181:555-562, 1972.

Pizarro D, et al: Rice-based oral electrolyte solutions for the management of infantile diarrhea. *N Engl J Med* 324:517-521, 1991 A.

Pizzaro D, et al: Rice-based oral electrolyte solutions in infantile diarrhea, letter. *Lancet* 325:283-284, 1991 B.

Prantera C, et al: Oral 5-aminosalicylic acid (Asacol) in the maintenance treatment of Crohn's disease. *Gastroenterology* 103:363-368, 1992.

Present DH, et al: Treatment of Crohn's disease with 6-mercaptopurine. *N Engl J Med* 302:981-987, 1980.

Rachmilewitz D: Sulphasalazine-induced infertility. *Gastroenterology* 82:996-997, 1982.

Rao SS, et al: Olsalazine or sulphasalazine in first attacks of ulcerative colitis? A double blind study. *Gut* 30:675, 1989.

Ratnaike RN, Jones T: Prescribing for the elderly II: Drug-associated diarrhoea. *Curr Ther* 33:43-46, (Sept) 1992.

Read MG, et al: Effect of loperamide in anal sphincter function in patients with diarrhea, abstract. *Gut* 20:A942, 1979.

Reves RR, et al: Failure to demonstrate effectiveness of an anticholinergic drug in the symptomatic treatment of acute travelers' diarrhea. *J Clin Gastroenterol* 5:223-227, 1983.

Rigaud D, et al: Controlled trial comparing two types of enteral nutrition in treatment of active Crohn's disease: Elemental *v* polymeric diet. *Gut* 32:1492-1497, 1991.

Rijk MC, et al: Sulphasalazine and prednisone compared with sulphasalazine for treating active Crohn disease. *Ann Intern Med* 15:445-450, 1991.

Rosenberg JM: Octreotide: Synthetic analog of somatostatin. *DICP* 22:748-754, 1988.

Rowe WA, Bayless TM: Colonic short-chain fatty acids: Fuel from the lumen? *Gastroenterology* 103:336-339, 1992.

Rutgeerts P, et al: Budesonide versus prednisolone for the treatment of active ileocecal Crohn's disease: A European multicenter trial, abstract. *Gastroenterology* 104:A772, 1993.

Sack DM, Peppercorn MA: Drug therapy of inflammatory bowel disease. *Pharmacotherapy* 3:158-176, 1983.

Sandhu BK, et al: Loperamide in severe protracted diarrhoea. *Arch Dis Child* 58:39-43, 1983.

Santosham M, Greenough WB III: Oral rehydration therapy: A global perspective. *J Pediatr* 118:S44-S51, 1991.

Scanlon T, Scanlon F: Cereal-based oral rehydration solutions, letter. *Lancet* 339:676, 1992.

Scheppach W, et al: Effect of butyrate enemas on the colonic mucosa in distal ulcerative colitis. *Gastroenterology* 103:51-56, 1992.

Schiller LR, et al: Mechanism of antidiarrheal effect of loperamide. *Gastroenterology* 86:1475-1480, 1984.

Shearman DJC, Finlayson NDC: Structure and function of the large intestine: Irritable bowel syndrome, in Shearman DJC, Finlayson NDC (eds): *Diseases of the Gastrointestinal Tract and Liver*. New York, Churchill Livingstone, 1982, 807-815.

Silk DB, Payne-James J: Inflammatory bowel disease: Nutritional implications and treatment. *Proc Nutr Soc* 48:355, 1989.

Singleton JW: Enteral feeding versus drug therapy in Crohn's disease: A continuing story. *Gastroenterology* 101:1127-1128, 1991.

Singleton JW, et al: National Cooperative Crohn's Disease Study: Adverse reactions to study drugs. *Gastroenterology* 77:870-882, 1979.

Skirrow MB: Three Rx steps to calming acute diarrhea. *Mod Med* 235-238, (March) 1984.

Sloan HR: Rice-based oral electrolyte solutions in infantile diarrhea, letter. *Lancet* 325:283, 1991.

Snape WS Jr: Disorders of colonic motility, in Brooks FP (ed): *Gastrointestinal Pathophysiology,* ed 2. New York, Oxford University Press, 1978, 317-326.

Sninsky CA, et al: Oral mesalamine (Asacol) for mildly to moderately active ulcerative colitis: A multicenter study. *Ann Intern Med* 115:350-355, 1991.

Snyder JD: Use and misuse of oral therapy for diarrhea: Comparison of US practices with American Academy of Pediatrics recommendations. *Pediatrics* 87:28-33, 1991.

Soriano-Brücher H, et al: Bismuth subsalicylate in the treatment of acute diarrhea in children: A clinical study. *Pediatrics* 87:18-27, 1991.

Steinhart AH, et al: Azathioprine therapy in chronic ulcerative colitis. *J Clin Gastroenterol* 12:271, 1990.

Stenson WF, et al: Dietary supplementation with fish oil in ulcerative colitis. *Ann Intern Med* 116:609-614, 1992.

Summers RW, et al: National Cooperative Crohn's Disease Study: Results of drug treatment. *Gastroenterology* 77:847-869, 1979.

Sutherland LR, et al: 5-aminosalicylic acid enema in treatment of distal ulcerative colitis, proctosigmoiditis, and proctitis. *Gastroenterology* 92:1894-1898, 1987.

Sutherland L, et al: Double blind, placebo controlled trial of metronidazole in Crohn's disease. *Gut* 32:1071-1075, 1991.

Sutton MM: Nutritional needs of children with inflammatory bowel disease. *Compr Ther* 18:21-25, (Oct) 1992.

Swedberg J, Steiner FJ: Oral rehydration therapy in diarrhea. *Postgrad Med* 74:335-354, (Nov) 1983.

Taffet SL, Das KM: Sulfasalazine: Adverse effects and desensitization. *Dig Dis Sci* 28:833-842, 1983.

Taylor DN, et al: Treatment of travelers' diarrhea: Ciprofloxacin plus loperamide compared with ciprofloxacin alone: A placebo-controlled, randomized trial. *Ann Intern Med* 114:731-734, 1991.

Thompson WG: Irritable bowel. *Gut* 25:305-320, 1984.

Tochen ML: Rice-based oral electrolyte solutions in infantile diarrhea, letter. *Lancet* 325:283, 1991.

Tolle SW, Elliot DL: Evaluation and management of acute diarrhea. *West J Med* 140:293-297, 1984.

Tremaine WJ: Maintenance of remission in Crohn's disease: Is 5'-aminosalicylic acid the answer? Editorial. *Gastroenterology* 103:694-696, 1992.

Ursing B, et al: A comparative study of metronidazole and sulfasalazine for active Crohn's disease: The cooperative Crohn's disease study in Sweden. *Gastroenterology* 83:550-562, 1982.

Van Hees PAM, et al: Effect of sulphasalazine in patients with active Crohn's disease: Controlled double-blind study. *Gut* 22:404-409, 1981.

Vignotti D, et al: Topical treatment of active distal ulcerative colitis with beclomethasone dipropionate. *Curr Ther Res* 52:659-665, 1992.

Vinik A, Moattari AR: Use of somatostatin analog in management of carcinoid syndrome. *Dig Dis Sci* 34 (suppl):14S-27S, 1989.

Vinik AI, et al: Somatostatin analogue (SMS 201-995) in management of gastroenteropancreatic tumors and diarrhea syndromes. *Am J Med* 81 (suppl 6B):23-40, 1986.

Wadworth AN, Fitton A: Olsalazine: A review of its pharmacodynamic and pharmacokinetic properties, and therapeutic potential in inflammatory bowel disease. *Drugs* 41:647-664, 1991.

Wald A: Fiber supplements for irritable bowel syndrome: Do they really make a difference? *Am J Gastroenterol* 85:1652-1653, 1990.

Willoughby CP, et al: Distribution and metabolism in healthy volunteers of disodium azodisalicylate, potential therapeutic agent for ulcerative colitis. *Gut* 23:1081-1087, 1982.

Laxatives and Cathartics 44

Most active, healthy people eating a balanced diet have no problem with bowel function and usually have at least three bowel movements per week. Normal consistency, frequency, and quantity of stool can be maintained by eating adequate amounts of high-residue, natural foods (fruit, vegetables, high-fiber cereals, whole grains) and drinking an ample amount of liquid. Proper toilet habits and regular exercise also contribute to normal bowel function.

The normal stool is neither hard nor loose and can be passed with minimal straining. The consistency of the stool as well as the frequency of elimination determines the extent of constipation. For instance, once daily elimination of a small, hard, "rabbit-like" stool is considered to be constipation (Devroede, 1989; Marshall, 1990). In constipated patients, the slow transit of the fecal bolus allows increased time for the colonic mucosa to absorb water and electrolytes from fecal material.

The most common causes of simple constipation are poor dietary habits, inadequate dietary fiber, and ignoring the defecatory urge. The latter diminishes the rectal response to distention and leads to continued reabsorption of water and electrolytes from the feces; in children with encopresis, rectal distention is massive. Increasing the amount of dietary fiber and obedience to normal defecatory urges often relieve simple constipation. In many patients, bowel retraining procedures improve function in one to two weeks (Stratton and Mackeigan, 1982; Wald, 1990).

When constipation does not abate after six to eight weeks, it is considered to be chronic. Two types of disorders predominate in chronic constipation: colonic atony and abnormal colonic motility. In some patients, propulsive activity is absent; in others, colonic contractions are normal or even increased but coordination of contractions is abnormal. There is increasing evidence to suggest that neuronal dysfunction and disruption of neural modulation of colonic motility (myenteric plexus, autonomic innervation of colon and rectum) are responsible for the development of chronic constipation in some patients (Johanson et al, 1992). In others, colonic transit is normal, but anorectal dysfunction causes retention of feces in the rectum.

In as many as one-third of patients with severe chronic constipation, normal transit of ingested markers suggests that a stress-related disorder may be causative (Wald et al, 1989). Patients with severe idiopathic constipation and a colon of normal diameter are almost exclusively women and are usually of reproductive age; this condition has no known cause. In one study, the serum concentrations of many steroid hormones were consistently reduced in many women with severe idiopathic constipation; it is unclear if this reduction results from or is caused by the disorder (Kamm et al, 1991). This condition generally does not respond to medical therapy (Tremaine, 1990).

For a listing of some factors associated with constipation, see Table 1.

It has been assumed that constipation occurs more frequently in the elderly and this may be true for bedridden patients or those in long-term care facilities (Williams and DiPalma, 1990). Little data support this contention in ambulatory, healthy older individuals; however, some physicians believe that anal dysfunction increases with age (Wald, 1990, 1993). Because of anxiety or depression, many elderly individuals may believe that they are constipated when they are not. This contributes to the greater consumption of laxatives by people over 60 years than by the younger population (Sonnenberg and Koch, 1989). Furthermore, physicians often define constipation primarily as infrequency whereas many elderly indi-

TABLE 1.
SOME CAUSES OF SIMPLE AND CHRONIC CONSTIPATION*

NONSTRUCTURAL PREDISPOSING CONDITIONS	NEUROGENIC CONDITIONS
Age	Amyotrophic lateral sclerosis
Anismus	Cerebral palsy
Dehydration	Cerebrovascular accident
Depression	Chronic idiopathic intestinal pseudo-obstruction (neuropathic or myopathic)
Eating disorders	Hirschsprung's disease (anganglionosis)
Idiopathic slow transit	Multiple sclerosis
Inadequate dietary fiber	Parkinson's disease
Insufficient fluid intake	Spinal cord injuries including myelomeningocele
Irritable bowel syndrome	
Physical inactivity	**METABOLIC-ENDOCRINE ABNORMALITIES**
Poor toilet habits	Diabetes mellitus or insipidus
Pregnancy	Hyperparathyroidism
Stress	Hypokalemia
	Hypothyroidism
DRUG EFFECTS	Uremia
Antacids (with aluminum or calcium)	
Anticholinergic agents	**OTHER SYSTEMIC CONDITIONS**
Antidepressants	Amyloidosis
Barium sulfate	Scleroderma
Bismuth	
Calcium channel blockers	**STRUCTURAL ABNORMALITIES**
Cholestyramine	Anal fissure or stricture
Clonidine	Colorectal neoplasm
Colestipol	Colorectal stricture
Contact laxatives	Descending perineum syndrome
Disopyramide	
Diuretics	
Iron	
Nonsteroidal anti-inflammatory agents	
Opioids	
Phenothiazines	
Phenytoin	
Sucralfate	
Sympathomimetic agents	

* *Adapted from Marshall, 1990, and Tremaine, 1990.*

viduals define it as straining during defecation (Whitehead et al, 1989).

Indications

Laxative-cathartics are used (1) to ease the pain of elimination in patients with episiotomy wounds, painful thrombosed hemorrhoids, anal fissures, or perianal abscesses; (2) to ease elimination and thereby reduce excessive straining and intra-abdominal pressure in those with body wall and diaphragmatic hernias, anorectal stenosis, aneurysm, or other diseases of the cerebral or coronary arteries; (3) to relieve constipation during pregnancy or the puerperium; (4) in geriatric patients with inadequate fiber intake whose abdominal and perineal muscles have lost their tone; (5) in patients with severe neuromuscular diseases; (6) in children with encopresis and congenital or acquired megacolon; (7) when bowel motility has been altered by drugs (eg, anticholinergic agents, opioids); (8) to prevent or decrease colonic absorption of ammonia and other neurotoxins in patients with hepatic encephalopathy; (9) to prepare the bowel prior to surgery or radiologic, proctoscopic, or colonoscopic procedures; (10) to provide a fresh stool for parasitologic examination; (11) to accelerate excretion of various parasites, including nematodes, after anthelmintic therapy; (12) to hasten excretion of poisonous substances; and (13) to modify the effluent in patients with an ileostomy or colostomy.

Enemas may be indicated (1) to relieve impaction; (2) to empty the rectum and colon prior to radiographic or endoscopic procedures; (3) to cleanse the large bowel prior to surgery or childbirth; (4) for patients with fecal incontinence or colostomies; and (5) occasionally, as substitutes for glycerin suppositories and other laxatives to re-establish the rectal reflex in constipated patients.

Constipation can be prevented or alleviated in most patients who are at risk, including women during pregnancy or the puerperium, chronically bedridden or immobilized patients, individuals taking constipating drugs, and those with painful perianal conditions such as inflamed hemorrhoids or fissures. Ingestion of foods high in fiber, as well as use of psyllium or another bulk-forming agent, small doses of senna pod preparations, phenolphthalein, and/or mineral oil taken daily are usually safe and effective (Godding, 1984 A; Klein, 1982; Godding, 1988).

Laxative or cathartic agents promote and/or ease defecation by accelerating the passage of feces through the large intestine, by influencing the consistency and amount of stool, and by facilitating the elimination of feces from the rectum. The terms, laxative and cathartic, reflect the typical intensity and latency of effect. A cathartic usually produces prompt fluid evacuation, while a laxative usually produces a soft formed stool over a protracted period; the same drug may act as a laxative or a cathartic depending on the dose administered or individual patient sensitivity. Enemas cause fragmentation, liquefaction, or lubrication of the feces and fluid distention of the bowel wall with resultant reflex elimination.

The traditional concept that the primary mechanism of action of the stimulant cathartics is to enhance intestinal motility is not accurate. Many laxative-cathartics promote net fluid accumulation within the bowel lumen by a hydrophilic effect, an osmotic action, or a direct action on mucosal cells to decrease absorption and/or enhance secretion of water and electrolytes. These secretory effects are mediated by alterations in the synthesis of sodium-potassium ATPase, adenylate cyclase, prostaglandins, and possibly intracellular calcium. The complex effects of fluid accumulation and the influence of the laxative-cathartics on intestinal motility are not completely understood. See also Drug Selection.

Patients with colonic atony generally respond poorly to laxatives or enemas. Colectomy with ileorectal anastomosis rarely may be required in patients with colonic inertia (Wexner et al, 1991). For a discussion of surgical procedures used to treat severe intractable constipation, see Schouten, 1991, and Pemberton et al, 1991.

Fecal Impaction: Impaction occurs when the fecal mass becomes too large to pass through the anal sphincter. It results from prolonged incomplete evacuation due to prolonged immobility, debility, and the use of constipating drugs. Fecal incontinence can occur in patients with severe constipation and fecal impaction. A variety of treatment regimens are employed. The softening and lubricating effects of mineral oil and minimal manual disimpaction often relieve impaction (see the evaluation on Mineral Oil). In one study, pulsed irrigation of the rectum was used to rehydrate and break up impacted stool (Puet et al, 1991). In this procedure, warm water is forced into the rectum using a programmable pump; an inflatable cuff prevents backwash of water and stool. Four- to six-second pulses of water are followed by a drainage cycle that removes pieces of stool and fluid. It usually requires 15 to 20 minutes to obtain a clear return fluid. Although promising, this procedure may promote infection; more data are needed to establish its efficacy and safety.

Encopresis (Primary Fecal Retention): Volitional withholding of stool by children is thought to be the cause of idiopathic constipation and encopresis (Gleghorn et al, 1991). Social pressures or episodes of painful defecation may prompt withholding. Repetitive episodes can result in colonic dilation, loss of normal defecatory urge, and colorectal dysfunction. Therapy, which is successful in most patients, includes removal of impacted stool, use of laxatives, and behavioral modification. Although the value of adding laxatives to a behavioral modification program aimed at promoting regular bowel movements has never been proved, in one well-controlled study, children who did not respond well to behavioral modification alone improved significantly when laxatives were added (Nolan et al, 1991). When laxatives are used, large initial doses are usually required. Most physicians who advocate the administration of enemas for encopresis recommend their use only when bowel movements do not occur within two or three days. Although enemas are widely used, some authorities believe that they are unnecessary and counterproductive (Gleghorn et al, 1991).

Laxative Habit: In most instances, laxatives should be used only temporarily. Except when employed to prepare the colon for examination or surgery, the agent chosen should not empty the bowel completely. With few exceptions, there is no justification for prescribing or self-administering drugs that perpetuate and intensify the condition for which they are used initially.

Some laxatives may cause evacuation from the ascending colon in addition to the usual site, the distal descending or sigmoid colon. After such overemptying, two to five days usually elapse before the normal fecal mass can be re-established. Worry regarding the lack of bowel movement during this period may lead to repeated use of the laxative, and a vicious cycle can be established: Spontaneous bowel function is reduced, laxatives are used in larger doses, and the laxative habit becomes fixed. Laxative abuse can be responsible for some otherwise unexplained cases of diarrhea (Bytzer et al, 1989). Unfortunately, many people have misconceptions concerning the necessity for daily bowel movements and do not realize that two or three bowel movements a week may be normal. This perception is a major cause of laxative abuse and misuse as is the availability of a variety of laxative preparations that are advertised aggressively.

In general, laxatives should be avoided in children. Some parents give laxatives to their children in the mistaken belief that a daily bowel movement is essential; laxative-dependent constipation may be created in this manner.

Laxatives are sometimes used inappropriately (occasionally in very large doses) for weight reduction (Killen et al, 1986).

Drug Selection

A single appropriate laxative produces the best results in most patients. Ideally, selection should be based on mechanism and site of action. Although data are insufficient for precise classification, laxative-cathartics can be divided into three groups on the basis of the intensity and latency of their effect (Fingl, 1980): agents that usually produce a soft formed stool within one to three days, a soft semifluid stool within 6 to 12 hours, or a watery stool within two to six hours (see Table 2). Although the traditional pharmacologic classification (ie, bulk-forming agents, stimulants, saline cathartics, wetting agents, lubricants) no longer adequately reflects current knowledge, it is well-entrenched in the medical literature and is widely used by physicians.

The choice of the most appropriate drug is based on the indication, the desired effect, the idiosyncrasies of the individual patient, and the differences among the types of laxative-cathartics. A laxative should never be given to patients with undiagnosed abdominal pain or intestinal obstruction. Laxatives other than mineral oil should be avoided in the initial management of fecal impaction. Constipation that reflects a change in bowel habits must be investigated thoroughly because it may be a symptom of colon cancer or other serious diseases.

Laxatives have been reviewed by an Advisory Panel of the FDA as part of the Drug Efficacy Study Implementation project, and a tentative monograph on these agents was published (*Federal Register*, 1985). The Committee on FDA-related Matters of the American College of Gastroenterology also has reviewed the use of laxatives (Tedesco et al, 1985).

Dietary Fiber: Dietary fiber is the portion of plant food that escapes digestion and is composed of lignin and polysaccharides (ie, cellulose, hemicelluloses, pectins, gums, mucilages, alginates). Two distinct mechanisms are proposed for the laxative effect of dietary fiber (Ornstein and Baird, 1987; Anderson, 1986): (1) Cereal fibers generally possess small cells with highly lignified cell walls that resist digestion and

TABLE 2.
CLASSIFICATION AND COMPARISON OF REPRESENTATIVE LAXATIVES*

TYPE OF LAXATIVE-CATHARTIC EFFECT AND LATENCY		
Softening of Formed Stool (1 to 3 days)	**Soft-Semifluid Stool (6 to 12 hours)**	**Watery Stool (2 to 6 hours)**
Bulk-Forming Agents Dietary Fiber Karaya Gum Methylcellulose Psyllium preparations Calcium Polycarbophil	Saline Laxatives (low dose) Milk of Magnesia Magnesium Sulfate	Saline Laxatives (high dose) Milk of Magnesia Magnesium Carbonate Magnesium Citrate Magnesium Oxide Magnesium Sulfate Sodium Phosphate Sodium Sulfate
Docusate Sodium, Potassium, or Calcium Salts	Diphenylmethane Derivatives Phenolphthalein Bisacodyl (oral)	
Lactulose Sorbitol Mineral Oil Malt Soup Extract	Anthraquinone Derivatives Senna (oral) Cascara Sagrada	Bisacodyl (rectal) Senna (rectal) Castor Oil Polyethylene Glycol (PEG)-Electrolyte preparations

**Adapted from Fingl, 1980.*

retain water within their cellular structure. (2) Other types of dietary fiber (eg, apple, carrot, guar, pectin) are digested extensively by and stimulate the growth of colonic flora, which increases fecal mass. Osmotically active metabolites also may contribute to the laxative effect.

Patients with poor dietary habits may add raw bran (2 to 6 tablespoons with each meal) to soft or liquid foods, followed by a glass of water or another beverage. Raw bran changes the texture but not the flavor of food, requires no refrigeration, and is unaffected by heat. A significant laxative effect is not observed for three to five days, and several weeks may be required to relieve chronic constipation. Raw vegetables and fruits have a low fiber content and are not adequate substitutes for raw bran. Many patients take too much bran with too little fluid. Furthermore, ingestion of large amounts of bran can cause nausea, abdominal bloating, or flatulence and can interfere with the absorption of magnesium, calcium, iron, zinc, and other minerals; similar symptoms also can occur in the first few weeks after bran supplementation is initiated. These effects can be decreased by using a very small amount initially and slowly increasing the number of tablespoonsful ingested daily.

Bulk-Forming Drugs: Calcium polycarbophil [Fiberall, FiberCon, Mitrolan], psyllium [Effer-Syllium, Konsyl, Metamucil, Perdiem Fiber, Syllact], methylcellulose [Citrucel], and other bulk-forming laxatives are more refined and concentrated than bran and generally are more effective, but they also are considerably more expensive. The bulk-forming drugs should be well diluted to ensure adequate mixing with the food bolus and, preferably, should be ingested shortly after a meal. These agents also can be taken before meals or at bedtime. When consumed with adequate amounts of liquid, it is generally believed that these drugs increase the water content and bulk volume of the stool by binding to stool contents and/or absorbing water; these actions decrease intestinal transit time. Ingestion of plastic flakes milled to the same dimensions as coarse bran produces similar laxative actions, which may indicate that mechanical stimulation of nerves in the bowel wall is a primary action of dietary fiber and bulk-forming agents (Goldfinger, 1991; Tomlin and Read, 1988).

The response to ingestion of bulk-forming laxatives usually begins in 12 to 24 hours, but up to three days may be required for the fecal mass to reach the rectum in patients who use laxatives chronically. Bulk-forming agents generally are not absorbed and are safe when adequate quantities of liquids are ingested concomitantly. They are used most commonly by patients with diverticulosis or the irritable bowel syndrome. Some bulk-forming agents have been used to improve fecal consistency in patients with disease of the terminal ileum or to modify the effluent in patients with ileostomy or colostomy in order to relieve maceration or discomfort and to reduce the number of evacuations.

Claims that the bulk-forming preparations are effective in the treatment of obesity have not been substantiated.

Psyllium has reduced serum cholesterol in males with mild to moderate hypercholesterolemia (Anderson et al, 1988). (See also index entry Hyperlipidemia.)

Impaction or obstruction may occur if the bulk-forming laxatives are arrested in their passage through the alimentary canal; water is absorbed, and the bolus can become inspissated within the bowel lumen. Thus, abnormal narrowing of the lumen at any level represents a hazard. Inspissation does not occur in the normal bowel if one or more glasses of water are taken with the laxative.

Bloating and flatulence are observed less frequently with psyllium and other commercial bulk-forming agents than with bran. Allergic reactions (urticaria, nonseasonal rhinitis, dermatitis, bronchial asthma) may be a serious consequence of the use of karaya and other plant gums, as well as other bulk-forming agents; this is less likely to occur with the synthetic agents, carboxymethylcellulose sodium and calcium polycarbophil. Digitalis, salicylates, and nitrofurantoin are bound by cellulose, but this interaction is not usually clinically significant. The sugar added to some psyllium preparations to improve palatability can complicate the management of diabetic patients, but sugar-free preparations are available (see the evaluation).

Sodium intake is increased substantially with use of carboxymethylcellulose sodium, which contains 2.7 to 4 mEq/g. Marked fluid retention has been reported when carboxymethylcellulose sodium was used as an anorexiant.

Contact Laxatives: The term contact laxatives is still used even though the primary mechanism of action of these agents is no longer considered to be their irritant effect on gastrointestinal mucosa. Another classification categorizes these agents as *stimulant laxatives* (cascara; senna; bisacodyl; phenolphthalein; castor oil; docusate calcium, potassium, and sodium; and bile acids) (Brunton, 1990). Many practitioners believe that contact laxatives should be used only when milder laxatives or tap water enemas have been ineffective. Since contact laxatives are the agents most often abused, some clinicians recommend that they should be taken for no longer than one week.

The precise mechanism(s) of action for each drug in this group has not been established, but, in general, they produce a net accumulation of fluid and electrolytes in the lumen. Direct stimulation of intramural nerve plexuses has not been proved. There is no conclusive evidence that contact laxatives have a direct mucosal stimulant or irritant effect, but morphologic changes of the surface epithelium occur and water and electrolyte transport is altered.

The continuous use of contact laxatives infrequently produces diarrhea that is severe or prolonged enough to cause hyponatremia, hypokalemia, dehydration, hyperaldosteronism, protein-losing gastroenteropathy with hypoalbuminemia, steatorrhea, and osteomalacia. Changes in the radiologic appearance of the colon can simulate megacolon or ulcerative colitis.

Elderly patients who are being prepared for diagnostic procedures must be monitored closely because weakness, incoordination, and even orthostatic hypotension (often resulting in falls) can be exacerbated by electrolyte loss.

When contact laxatives are used in suppository form or as enemas, the same problems of dependence, habituation, and tolerance observed with oral use occur.

Castor oil is hydrolyzed in the upper small intestine to ricinoleic acid, a long-chain fatty acid that markedly affects the mucosal transport systems to cause a net luminal accumulation of water and electrolytes resulting in watery stools. Its use is limited principally to preparation of the bowel before radiologic procedures when prompt, complete evacuation is desired. The stimulation of anion secretion probably is ricinoleic acid's most important action to alter fluid movement. However, some studies indicate that this agent may erode villous tips, disorganize the microvillous surface of the small intestine, and increase mucosal permeability to molecules with molecular weights as large as 16,000 daltons (eg, dextran).

The anthraquinone-containing laxatives (eg, senna preparations, cascara sagrada) are widely used and abused. These agents usually act within 6 to 12 hours. Cascara has the mildest action and produces a soft or formed stool, usually without causing abdominal cramps. Standardized senna (senna pod) may be particularly helpful in patients with severe constipation and is apparently safe (at least for short-term use) even in large doses. When combined with psyllium or other bulk-forming agents, smaller amounts of senna pod may be employed (Godding, 1984 B). Neither senna pod nor cascara is absorbed significantly when recommended doses are administered. Crude senna also produces a soft or formed stool, but usually causes more muscle contraction with cramping. Rhubarb and aloe preparations are the most potent anthraquinone-containing laxatives and should not be used because they almost always produce colic. All products containing the potent anthraquinone, danthron, were removed from the market because this agent produced tumors in experimental animals.

It should be noted that although most anthraquinone-containing laxatives may discolor the urine and colonic mucosa (melanosis coli), this effect is presumed to be innocuous and is reversible. When melanosis coli is observed in patients with unexplained diarrhea, laxative abuse is a possible cause. Anthraquinones are excreted in the milk of lactating mothers but, at recommended doses, the concentration is rarely sufficient to exert a laxative effect in the infant. If there is concern, a laxative from a different class should be prescribed.

Reflex peristalsis following stimulation of sensory nerves only partly explains the effect of the diphenylmethane laxatives, bisacodyl [Carter's Little Pill, Dulcolax, Fleet Bisacodyl] and phenolphthalein. Both agents alter active electrolyte transport and thus affect fluid movement. Although bisacodyl produces a soft to formed stool usually with little or no colic, an enteric coating is required to minimize gastric irritation; the suppository preparation may cause stinging, tenesmus, and mild proctitis in a few patients. Phenolphthalein is more likely to produce a semifluid stool with little or no colic. Because of significant enterohepatic circulation, its action may be prolonged (three to four days) in sensitive patients.

Docusate sodium [Colace, Correctol Extra Gentle, Dialose, DOS, Doxinate, Modane Soft], docusate potassium [Kasof], and docusate calcium [Surfak] are presumed to soften the feces by an emollient action that reduces surface tension, thus permitting penetration of the fecal mass by intestinal fluids. There also is evidence that these agents increase mucosal permeability, inhibit water absorption in the jejunum and colon, and/or increase accumulation of intraluminal water and electrolytes (Gullikson et al, 1977; Moriarity et al, 1982). In these respects, the docusate drugs act like bile salts, which are anionic detergents and also may be considered contact laxatives. Docusate salts usually produce a soft formed stool.

The calcium and sodium salts of docusate (and probably the potassium salt) are absorbed to some extent in the duodenum and proximal jejunum. Their metabolic fate, the bioavailability of drugs taken with them, and the significance of their absorption are unknown and require further study. Morphologic changes and increased mucosal permeability have been noted in vitro. These contact laxatives should be prescribed in the smallest effective amounts.

Dihydroxy bile acids induce colonic secretion of water and electrolytes, which results in a net accumulation of luminal fluid that produces a mild laxative action. Dehydrocholic acid [Decholin], a synthetic derivative of cholic acid, also has a hydrocholeretic action, but controlled studies to prove that this effect is beneficial are lacking.

Saline Laxatives: Each of these agents is a salt, one or both ions of which are poorly and slowly absorbed. Commonly used preparations are magnesium carbonate, oxide, citrate, hydroxide, or sulfate; sodium sulfate or phosphate; and mixed sodium and potassium tartrate (see Table 3). A hypertonic solution may draw a substantial volume of fluid into the intestinal lumen by osmosis and stimulate stretch receptors to increase propulsive movements. Release of cholecystokinin (CCK) or prostaglandin E from the intestinal wall, which enhances intestinal secretory and motor activity, has been proposed as an additional mechanism of action for the magnesium salts.

Large doses of saline laxatives are used as cathartics to hasten the evacuation of worms or toxic materials. They provide a liquid stool for examination of parasites without rupture of trophozoites. These agents also are given to empty the bowel before various diagnostic and surgical procedures. In one study, it was reported that oral sodium phosphate was more effective and better tolerated than the polyethylene glycol (PEG) electrolyte solutions for bowel evacuation to prepare patients for colonoscopy (Vanner et al, 1990); however, significant alterations in electrolyte levels (particularly phosphate) occurred. In larger doses, saline laxatives usually act within two to six hours. Smaller doses usually produce a soft semifluid stool in 6 to 12 hours.

Congestive heart failure has been precipitated through indiscriminate use of saline laxatives, and coma or death from hyperkalemia and hypermagnesemia has been observed in patients with renal insufficiency who used these drugs. Oral sodium phosphate salts administered to normal volunteers significantly decreased serum calcium levels and increased serum phosphate levels. Therefore, phosphate salts should be used with caution in individuals with cardiac disease, convulsive disorders, or hypocalcemia. Tetany (resulting from hypocalcemia) and hyperphosphatemia may develop when phosphate salts are used by patients with impaired renal function or in children with impaction. Sodium phosphate-biphosphate preparations (eg, Phospho-Soda) may cause sloughing of the surface epithelium of the rectum.

Lubricant: Mineral oil (liquid petrolatum), which is indigestible, is used orally to prevent injury to hemorrhoidal tissue or further irritation of anal fissures and to lessen the strain of evacuation (eg, in patients with hernia or cardiovascular disease) by virtue of its emollient action. It is particularly effective in relieving fecal impaction. Lipid pneumonia caused by aspiration as well as deposition of mineral oil in the liver has been reported. Anal seepage may occur.

Bowel Cleansing Agents: Electrolyte preparations containing polyethylene glycol (PEG) [CoLyte, GoLYTELY, NuLytely, OCL Solution] produce a liquid stool within hours and are useful to cleanse the bowel prior to colonoscopy or colorectal operations. However, when administered on the same day as a barium enema, PEG preparations can interfere with the examination by preventing barium coating of the bowel wall and possibly by causing fluid to be retained. This problem can be eliminated by the administration of four bisacodyl tablets immediately after ingestion of the electrolyte solution (Girard et al, 1984; DiPalma and Brady, 1989). These solutions also have been recommended for gastrointestinal decontamination after acute drug overdose (Tenenbein et al, 1987). In one study, ingestion of a PEG electrolyte preparation (500 ml daily for five days) was effective and well tolerated by patients with chronic constipation (Andorsky and Goldner, 1990).

Net electrolyte excretion in the bowel is minimal, even when the large volumes (four liters) needed to cleanse the bowel are administered. Thus, these solutions are generally safe for use in elderly patients, in those with cardiovascular or renal disorders, and in those who are poorly hydrated. These preparations are more convenient and are equally or more effective than the usual regimen of diet combined with oral laxatives, suppositories, or enemas used for cleansing the bowel. The PEG solutions generally are more effective for bowel cleansing if they are ingested over three to four hours rather than over a much longer time period. Adverse effects are generally infrequent; nausea, vomiting, abdominal bloating or fullness, or cramps occur occasionally but usually subside rapidly.

Kits for cleansing the gastrointestinal tract prior to diagnostic examination also are available (eg, Dulcolax Bowel Prep Kit, Evac-Q-Kwik, Fleet Prep Kit, X-Prep). The solutions, tablets, and suppositories present in these kits are administered sequentially on the afternoon, evening, and/or morning prior to the examination.

Miscellaneous Agents: Because of its hyperosmolarity, administration of glycerin in enema or suppository form [Fleet Babylax, Fleet Glycerin Suppositories] promotes defecation by producing tissue dehydration and reflex rectal contraction; it also lubricates and softens inspissated fecal material. The suppository is safe for temporary use to re-establish proper bowel habits in patients who have lost the rectal reflex. Rectal instillation of hypertonic sorbitol also stimulates defecation but appears to have no advantage over glycerin. Senna and glycerin suppositories are believed to act locally in the rectum and probably the sigmoid colon.

Sorbitol and lactulose are poorly absorbed sugars that are not digested by intestinal enzymes. They are, however, hydrolyzed in part to lactic, acetic, and formic acids by coliforms. Accumulation of fluid in the colon is stimulated by the mild osmotic effect of these acid metabolites, and this usually produces soft formed stools. Large amounts of gas and an acid pH also result; the latter may have an additional effect on colonic transport of water and electrolytes.

Sorbitol and lactulose [Chronulac, Constilac, Duphalac] may be useful in patients with chronic constipation who do not respond to dietary fiber or bulk-forming agents. Sorbitol may be better tolerated, particularly in the elderly (Lederle et al, 1990; Richter, 1991). In one well-controlled study in elderly patients with chronic constipation, 30 to 60 ml of sorbitol 70% administered at bedtime was as effective as lactulose and was well tolerated (Lederle et al, 1990). Sorbitol, which is considerably less expensive than lactulose, may serve as a low-cost alternative to that agent in most constipated patients (Richter, 1991).

For the use of lactulose in portal systemic encephalopathy, see index entry Lactulose.

For information on malt soup extract [Maltsupex], see the evaluation.

The oral benzamide derivative, cisapride, has a prokinetic effect on the cecum and ascending colon and accelerates colonic transit in adults with severe idiopathic chronic constipation (Krevsky et al, 1989); however, its effectiveness has not been demonstrated. This agent also has been used in children with chronic constipation (Staiano et al, 1991). Cisapride may be beneficial in patients with colonic inertia. In one study, the use of cisapride reduced the consumption of laxatives in patients who chronically abused these agents (Müller-Lissner and the Bavarian Constipation Study Group, 1987); more data are needed to confirm this finding.

In investigational studies, oral naloxone reversed opioid-induced constipation and did not affect the analgesic action of morphine in dependent patients (Culpepper-Morgan et al, 1992).

Enemas: Most enemas act by increasing volume. Because they act locally in the rectum and probably the sigmoid colon and have little effect on the more proximal colon and small bowel, enemas may be preferred to contact laxatives. An enema containing only warm tap water relieves constipation in most adults. (Tap water enemas should not be used in infants or children.) Adults who do not respond to oral laxatives and who have no spontaneous bowel movements can self-administer tap water enemas every three to four days. The addition of laxatives or other substances to an enema solution may have little therapeutic value and is potentially harmful. However, the small-volume prepackaged lubricant (mineral oil), hypertonic (sorbitol, sodium phosphate-biphosphate), surfactant (docusate potassium), or contact laxative (bisacodyl) enema kits are convenient and fairly safe for self-administration. Some elderly patients may require a commercial small-volume enema occasionally (Sparberg, 1984), particularly when the stool is not excessively hard.

Isotonic sodium chloride solution (one level teaspoonful/pint of water) is commonly employed in infants, children, and the elderly but should be used cautiously in patients with sodium and fluid retention (eg, those with congestive heart failure, cirrhosis, or nephrosis). Although significant absorption of sodium does not occur when small amounts of sodium phosphate-biphosphate are employed in patients who must restrict sodium intake (Zumoff and Hellman, 1978), small-volume disposable kits containing sorbitol or a detergent (wetting agent) (eg, docusate potassium) may be preferable in these individuals.

Numerous complications are associated with either the solution employed or the mode of administration. Most enema solutions irritate the mucosa, sometimes producing excessive mucus in the stool. Early changes of ulcerative proctosigmoiditis are simulated. Hot water, peroxide, household detergents, and strong hypertonic salt solutions are most irritating. If the rectum must be cleansed before proctoscopy, a saline enema is least likely to alter the appearance of the mucosa. If a question regarding the mucosa remains, the examination should be repeated without prior use of an enema.

Weakness, excessive perspiration, shock, convulsions, and/or coma may result from water intoxication and dilutional hyponatremia after the use of enemas. Children and the elderly are most vulnerable. This syndrome also can occur in patients with megacolon given a tap water enema even in the customary volume (500 ml). Tap water or soapsuds enemas have caused weakness and incoordination in elderly patients. Severe hypokalemia may follow the use of a tap water enema, especially in patients also receiving thiazides or more potent congeners as antihypertensive agents or diuretics. Convulsions with hypocalcemia and hyperphosphatemia have occurred in healthy children or adults with renal dysfunction who absorbed large amounts of the phosphate present in recommended doses of sodium phosphate-biphosphate enemas (Haskell, 1985). Some physicians recommend that phosphate enemas be avoided in children under 3 years and used in reduced doses and with caution in older children (McCabe et al, 1991).

Methemoglobinemia, colitis with toxic megacolon, severe serosanguineous fluid loss, anaphylaxis, and rectal gangrene have followed the use of concentrated soap solutions. Alkaline soapsuds enemas should be avoided; they are particularly hazardous in the presence of portal systemic encephalopathy, since they increase diffusion of ammonia into the portal circulation. Therefore, only pure castile soap should be used (20 ml of soap solution/1 or 1.5 liters of water).

Rectal abrasion and laceration have been produced by aggressive insertion of a hard enema tip, and bleeding or draining pus may result. Perforation may cause ischiorectal abscess. The rectal wall is insensitive above the pectinate line, and the patient may be unaware of the injury. Free perforation with fecal peritonitis occurs when the transmural tear is above the peritoneal reflection. Inflamed sigmoidal diverticula are vulnerable to rupture if water pressure is increased even slightly. Syringes should be avoided to prevent high intraluminal pressure. The enema fluid level should be no higher than 18 to 20 inches above the anus, and no more than 750 ml of fluid should be instilled over a ten-minute period. Only soft plastic or rubber tubes with side openings should be inserted and only gentle pressure should be applied. The anus should be well lubricated with petroleum jelly or similar preparations to avoid injury.

In view of the risks, some authorities believe that enemas should be administered only when there is a clear indication for their use and when no adequate substitute can be provided.

BULK-FORMING DRUGS

CARBOXYMETHYLCELLULOSE SODIUM

R=H or $CH_2CO^-\ Na^+$

METHYLCELLULOSE

[Citrucel]

These synthetic cellulose derivatives are indigestible and nonabsorbable. When mixed with water, a bulky hydrophilic colloid is formed. Softening of the formed stool usually occurs within one to three days. These agents have been used to decrease the fluidity of stools in patients with chronic watery diarrhea. In one study, methylcellulose was reported to be more effective than psyllium in relieving chronic constipation (Hamilton et al, 1988).

For adverse reactions and precautions, see the Introduction. Allergic reactions to these synthetic agents are rare. Fluid retention caused by the substantial amounts of sodium in carboxymethylcellulose has occurred after use of this preparation as an anorexiant; caution should be exercised when it is used for long-term routine therapy of patients with heart or renal disease.

DOSAGE AND PREPARATIONS.

CARBOXYMETHYLCELLULOSE SODIUM:

Oral: *Adults,* 4 to 6 g daily; *children over 6 years*, 1 to 1.5 g daily. The drug should be taken in divided doses with one or two glasses of liquid and ingested rapidly.

Generic. Bulk.

METHYLCELLULOSE:

Oral: *Adults and children over 12 years,* 2 g (one level tablespoonful) in 240 ml (8 oz) of water one to three times daily; one rounded or heaping tablespoonful is recommended by the manufacturer. *Children 6 to 12 years,* 1 g (one rounded teaspoonful) in 120 ml (4 oz) of water three to four times daily.

Generic. Bulk (powder); capsules 500 mg (nonprescription).
Citrucel (SmithKline Beecham). Powder 2 g/tablespoonful in 480 and 900 g containers (nonprescription).

KARAYA GUM (Sterculia Gum)

This indigestible, nonabsorbable vegetable gum contains hydrophilic polysaccharides that act like other bulk-forming laxatives. Allergic reactions and urticaria have been reported rarely. For general indications, adverse reactions, and precautions, see the discussion on bulk-forming agents in the Introduction.

DOSAGE AND PREPARATIONS.

Oral: 5 to 10 g daily taken with an adequate amount of fluid.

Generic. Bulk (powder, nonprescription).

PSYLLIUM HYDROPHILIC COLLOID

[Effer-Syllium, Konsyl, Metamucil, Perdiem Fiber, Syllact]

The whole or powdered seeds of the three species of *Plantago* or the refined colloid obtained from psyllium seed husks are rich in mucilage (a hemicellulose). These preparations increase bulk by absorbing water and are indigestible and nonabsorbable.

Psyllium preparations are commonly used in patients with diverticulosis or the irritable bowel syndrome and may relieve painful defecation in patients with hemorrhoids. Choleretic diarrhea caused by small bowel resection or disease of the terminal ileum may be alleviated by psyllium hydrophilic colloid, but cholestyramine resin is more effective. Psyllium also is useful when combined with senna pod, with or without mineral oil, to prevent constipation in patients at risk or in those who cannot tolerate constipation (Godding, 1984 A, 1984 B).

Allergic reactions, including anaphylaxis, have occurred rarely; in most instances, nurses, other health care workers, or pharmaceutical workers who came into direct contact with the powder were affected (James et al, 1991).

For general adverse reactions and precautions, see the discussion on bulk-forming agents in the Introduction.

DOSAGE AND PREPARATIONS.

Oral: *Adults,* 7 to 30 g daily; one dose (see preparations) is mixed with a glass of water or other suitable fluid and ingested rapidly one to three times daily. A second glass of water enhances the effect. *Children over 6 years*, one-half the adult dose.

Generic. Powder.
Effer-Syllium (Johnson & Johnson-Merck Consumer). Powder (effervescent) 3 g/dose (sodium <5 mg) (nonprescription).
Konsyl (Konsyl). Powder (sugar-free) 6 g/dose (sodium <4 mg); powder 6.5 g/dose (dextrose, sodium <4 mg) ***(Konsyl-D)*** (both forms nonprescription).
Metamucil (Procter & Gamble). Powder 3.4 g/dose (dextrose 3.5 g, potassium 31 mg, sodium <10 mg); powder (sugar-free) 3.4 g/dose (phenylalanine 30 mg/dose, sodium <10 mg) (***Metamucil Regular SF***); powder (effervescent, sugar-free) 3.4 g/dose (phenylalanine 30 mg, potassium 310 mg [orange] or 290 mg [lemon-lime], sodium <10 mg) (***Metamucil Effervescent Flavored***) (all forms nonprescription).
Perdiem Fiber (Rhone-Poulenc Rorer). Granules 4.03 g/dose (sodium 1.8 mg) (nonprescription).
Syllact (Wallace). Powder 3.3 g/dose (nonprescription).
Additional Trademarks.
Fiberall (Ciba), ***Modane Bulk*** (Savage), ***Siblin*** (Parke-Davis) (all forms nonprescription).

CALCIUM POLYCARBOPHIL

[Fiberall, FiberCon, Mitrolan]

Polycarbophil, a hydrophilic polyacrylic resin, is indigestible, nonabsorbable, and metabolically inert. It has more water-binding activity than the other bulk-forming agents, absorbing 60 to 100 times its weight in water. Because of this property, polycarbophil is an effective laxative; however, its superiority over other bulk-forming agents is unproved. Polycarbophil also can be used to modify the effluent in chronic watery diarrhea. The preparation has a low sodium content (0.02 mEq/tablet) and thus may be useful in patients who must restrict the intake of sodium. No toxicity has been observed in animal studies.

Calcium polycarbophil releases free calcium after ingestion and should not be used with tetracyclines or in patients who must restrict the intake of calcium. For general adverse reactions and precautions, see the discussion on bulk-forming agents in the Introduction.

DOSAGE AND PREPARATIONS.

Oral: *Adults,* 1 g one or two times daily (maximum, 6 g); *children 6 to 12 years,* 500 mg one to four times daily (maximum 3 g); *2 to 6 years,* 500 mg one or two times daily (maximum, 1.5 g). Each dose should be taken with one glass of liquid.

Fiberall (Ciba). Tablets (chewable) equivalent to 1 g of base (nonprescription).
FiberCon (Lederle). Tablets equivalent to 500 mg of base (nonprescription).
Mitrolan (Wyeth-Ayerst). Tablets (chewable) equivalent to 500 mg of base (nonprescription).
Additional Trademark.
Equalactin (Numark).

CONTACT LAXATIVES

BISACODYL

[Carter's Little Pill, Dulcolax, Fleet Bisacodyl]

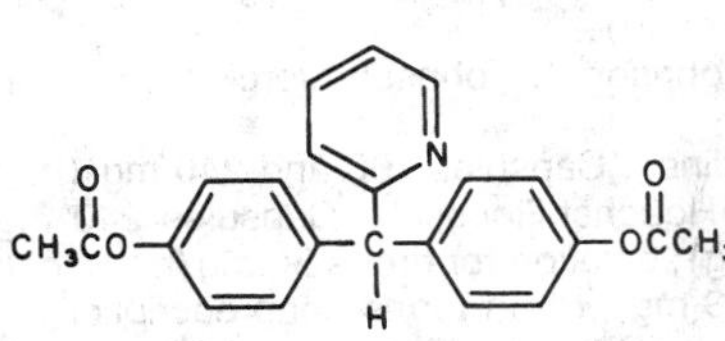

Bisacodyl may produce a soft to formed stool usually within six hours after oral ingestion and 15 to 60 minutes after rectal administration. However, its strong purgative action can be difficult to control. Emptying is sufficient to prepare patients for proctoscopic or colonoscopic procedures. Bisacodyl is useful as an adjunct to improve barium coating of the mucosal wall in patients who receive polyethylene glycol-electrolyte solutions prior to the examination (DiPalma and Brady, 1989).

ADVERSE REACTIONS AND PRECAUTIONS. The tablets must be swallowed whole to avoid gastric irritation. They should not be taken within one hour after ingestion of milk or antacids to prevent premature dissolution of the enteric coating and resultant dyspepsia.

The suppository may produce mild smarting or tenesmus, and continued rectal administration may cause proctitis. Sloughing of the surface epithelium of the rectum also has been observed (Meisel et al, 1977). Inflammatory changes that occur after the short-term use of bisacodyl suppositories may resemble those seen in mild idiopathic ulcerative proctitis. Hence, prolonged use of this dosage form is undesirable.

DOSAGE AND PREPARATIONS.

Oral: *Adults,* 10 mg (range, 5 to 15 mg); up to 30 mg may be given to prepare the lower gastrointestinal tract for special procedures. *Children 6 years and older,* 5 mg.

Generic. Tablets (plain, enteric-coated) 5 mg (nonprescription).
Carter's Little Pill (Carter Products), ***Dulcolax*** (Ciba), ***Fleet Bisacodyl*** (Fleet). Tablets (enteric-coated) 5 mg (nonprescription).

Rectal: *Adults and children over 2 years,* 10 mg (suppository) or 30 ml (enema); *under 2 years,* 5 mg (one-half suppository).

Generic. Suppositories 5 and 10 mg (nonprescription).
Dulcolax (Ciba). Suppositories 10 mg (nonprescription).
Fleet Bisacodyl (Fleet). Suppositories and enema preparation 10 mg (nonprescription).

CASCARA SAGRADA

Cascara is one of the mildest anthraquinone-containing laxatives. Its effect on the small intestine is insignificant or slight, but it stimulates mass peristalsis in the large intestine. A soft or formed stool is produced, usually in six to eight hours, with little or no colic. Casanthranol, a derivative of cascara sagrada, is present in some proprietary mixtures.

Prolonged use of cascara may produce benign pigmentation of the colonic mucosa (melanosis coli) that may regress after therapy is discontinued. This agent imparts a yellowish brown color to acid urine and a reddish color to alkaline urine.

In recommended doses, cascara is safe for use in nursing mothers.

DOSAGE AND PREPARATIONS.

Oral: *Adults,* one tablet (325 mg) at bedtime, 0.5 to 1.5 ml of fluid extract, or 5 ml of aromatic fluid extract. *Infants and children up to 2 years,* 1 to 2 ml of the aromatic fluid extract as one dose only. *Children 2 years and older,* 2.5 ml of the aromatic fluid extract as one dose only; the dose is adjusted for patient size and need.

Generic. Tablets 325 mg; fluid extract (plain, aromatic) (alcohol 18%) (all forms nonprescription).

CASTOR OIL

[Purge]

CASTOR OIL, EMULSIFIED

[Emulsoil, Fleet Castor Oil Emulsion, Neoloid]

ACTIONS AND USES. Castor oil has been classified as a contact cathartic because lipolysis in the small intestine liberates ricinoleic acid. This long-chain fatty acid inhibits the absorption and induces secretion of water and electrolytes, resulting in fluid accumulation in vitro, and these changes are presumed to account for the marked net fluid accumulation in vivo.

Castor oil produces one or more copious, watery evacuations two to six hours after ingestion. The colon is emptied so completely that passage of normal stool may be delayed for two days or more. Since castor oil thoroughly empties gas and feces from the intestine, it is used to prepare patients for radiologic examination. This strong cathartic should not be used to treat common constipation.

Palatability is improved by administering chilled castor oil with fruit juice or by consuming a carbonated beverage immediately after ingestion. A flavored emulsion of castor oil, such as Fleet Castor Oil Emulsion or Neoloid, also may be more palatable.

ADVERSE REACTIONS AND PRECAUTIONS. Castor oil causes morphologic changes in the small intestine and alters mucosal permeability. Colic, dehydration, and electrolyte imbalance may occur.

DOSAGE AND PREPARATIONS.

CASTOR OIL:

Oral: *Adults,* 15 to 60 ml; *children*, 5 to 15 ml; *infants under 2 years*, 1 to 5 ml.

Generic. Liquid (nonprescription).

Purge (Fleming). Liquid 95% (nonprescription).

CASTOR OIL, EMULSIFIED:

Oral: *Adults,* 30 to 60 ml; *children*, 7.5 to 30 ml; *infants*, 2.5 to 7.5 ml.

Emulsoil (Paddock). Emulsion 95% (nonprescription).

Fleet Castor Oil Emulsion (Fleet). Emulsion 67% (nonprescription).

Neoloid (Kenwood). Emulsion 36.4% (nonprescription).

DOCUSATE CALCIUM

[Surfak]

```
 ┌ O       CH2CH3            ┐
 │ ||      |                 │
 │ COCH2CH(CH2)3CH3          │
 │ |                         │
 │ CH2                       │  Ca++
 │ |                         │
 │ CHSO3-                    │
 │ |                         │
 │ COCH2CH(CH2)3CH3          │
 │ ||      |                 │
 └ O       CH2CH3            ┘2
```

DOCUSATE POTASSIUM

[Kasof]

DOCUSATE SODIUM

[Colace, Correctol Extra Gentle, Dialose, DOS, Doxinate, Modane Soft]

ACTIONS AND USES. In vitro studies suggest that these salts of dioctylsulfosuccinic acid lower the surface tension of the stool to permit water and lipids to enter more readily and thus soften the feces. However, more recent evidence indicates that they may stimulate the secretion of water and electrolytes on contact with the mucosa. Water absorption may be inhibited in the small and large bowel. One to two days or more may be required for full effect, since it may be that long before the softened fecal bolus reaches the rectum.

In usual doses, the docusate salts are probably marginally effective (Kallman, 1983). These mild contact laxatives lessen the strain of defecation (eg, in persons with hernia or cardiovascular disease) and relieve constipation caused by delayed rectal emptying. The calcium or potassium salt may be preferred in patients who must restrict sodium intake.

ADVERSE REACTIONS AND PRECAUTIONS. Docusate salts occasionally can cause diarrhea. Morphologic damage to the intestine has been observed in rats. They also may be hepatotoxic (Klein, 1982).

Docusate sodium is classified in FDA Pregnancy Category C.

These agents are often combined with other laxatives with little justification. They may enhance the absorption and, hence, the toxicity of several other laxatives (see the section on Mixtures).

DOSAGE AND PREPARATIONS.

DOCUSATE CALCIUM, DOCUSATE SODIUM:

Oral: *Adults and children over 12 years*, 50 to 360 mg daily; *2 to 12 years*, 50 to 150 mg daily; *less than 2 years,* 25 mg of the sodium salt. It is suggested that 240 to 300 ml of water be taken with each dose.

DOCUSATE CALCIUM:

Generic. Capsules, tablets 240 mg (both forms nonprescription).

Surfak (Upjohn). Capsules 240 mg (alcohol 3%) (nonprescription).

DOCUSATE SODIUM:

Generic. Capsules 50, 100, 240, and 250 mg; liquid 10 mg/ml; syrup 20 mg/5 ml, 60 mg/15 ml, and 100 mg/30 ml; tablets 100 mg (all forms nonprescription).

Colace (Apothecon). Capsules 50 and 100 mg (sodium content 2.65 and 5.3 mg, respectively); solution for drops 10 mg/ml (sodium content 0.73 mg); syrup 60 mg/15 ml (alcohol 1%, sodium content 3.66 mg) (all forms nonprescription).

Correctol Extra Gentle (Schering-Plough). Tablets 100 mg (nonprescription).

Dialose (Johnson & Johnson-Merck Consumer). Tablets 100 mg.

DOS (Goldline). Capsules 100 and 240 mg (nonprescription).

Doxinate (Hoechst-Roussel). Capsules 240 mg (sodium content 12.7 mg); solution for drops 50 mg/ml (alcohol 5%, sodium content 0.73 mg) (both forms nonprescription).

Modane Soft (Savage). Capsules 100 mg (sodium content 5.3 mg) (nonprescription).

DOCUSATE POTASSIUM:

Oral: The manufacturers' recommended dosage is *adults,* 240 mg once daily. Some clinicians believe that administration twice daily is more effective.

Generic. Capsules 100 mg (nonprescription).

Kasof (Roberts). Capsules 240 mg (nonprescription).

PHENOLPHTHALEIN

ACTIONS. Phenolphthalein acts primarily on the large intestine to produce a semifluid stool in four to eight hours with little or no colic. The claim that yellow phenolphthalein is three times more potent than the white form has not been substantiated. The action of a single dose may persist for three to four days as a result of enterohepatic circulation. This drug is the active agent in many over-the-counter laxative preparations.

ADVERSE REACTIONS. Serious adverse effects are rare but can occur with excessive doses. Phenolphthalein should be avoided in the elderly because its prolonged action may severely deplete water and electrolytes.

Dermatitis (fixed eruptions, pruritus, burning, vesiculation, residual pigmentation) may occur in hypersensitive patients. Fatal anaphylactic reactions have been reported, but an absolute causal relationship with phenolphthalein has not been established. Nonthrombocytopenic purpura has been reported occasionally, while dehydration from excessive laxative action or electrolyte imbalance after prolonged use occurs infrequently. Phenolphthalein imparts a pink color to alkaline urine or feces.

DOSAGE AND PREPARATIONS.

Oral: *Adults,* 30 to 270 mg daily; doses >270 mg may be required occasionally. *Children 6 years and older*, 30 to 60 mg daily; *2 to 5 years*, 15 to 20 mg daily in single or divided doses.

Generic. Bulk (powder) (nonprescription).

Available Trademarks.

Alophen (Warner-Lambert), ***Ex-Lax*** (Sandoz), ***Correctol***, ***Feen-a-Mint*** (Schering-Plough), ***Modane*** (Savage), ***Phenolax*** (Upjohn) (all nonprescription).

SENNA WHOLE LEAF PREPARATIONS
[Black Draught]

SENNA POD PREPARATIONS
[Senokot]

CALCIUM SALTS OF SENNOSIDES A AND B
[Gentle Nature]

The actions and uses of this anthraquinone-type contact laxative are similar to those of cascara, but senna is more potent. Senna decreases transit time, softens the stool, and increases stool weight. A soft semifluid stool is produced 6 to 12 hours after ingestion.

Senna is available as the crude drug (senna, senna fluid extract, senna syrup) and as a standardized, purified concentrate [Senokot]. Sennosides A and B are believed to be the active constituents of senna preparations. The purified preparations are used most often and are claimed to produce colic and watery stools only rarely when administered in the recommended dosage.

Low doses of senna are usually effective and are not appreciably absorbed. Senna pod is believed to have the most physiologic action of all the contact laxatives. Colonic bacterial enzymes cleave senna and release the active anthrone metabolite gradually, which may explain the mild action of small doses (Godding, 1984 C). This laxative may inhibit the activity of cyclic sodium-potassium ATPase, and gastrointestinal regulatory peptides may be involved in its action. There is evidence that senna decreases colonic and jejunal water absorption independently of histologic alterations or effects on cyclic adenosine monophosphate; other effects on ion transport also occur (Donowitz et al, 1984).

Senna is particularly useful in patients with severe constipation (Godding, 1984 C). Minimal doses should be used, and the drug should be discontinued as soon as normal bowel function is restored. Large doses of the purified preparations appear to be safe but should not be used for prolonged periods. Senna pod also is useful in combination with a psyllium preparation with or without mineral oil to prevent constipation in patients at risk or in those who cannot tolerate constipation because of debility or disease (Godding, 1984 A, 1984 B). The addition of senna to psyllium results in greater stool moisture than the use of psyllium alone (Marlett et al, 1987). Mixtures containing senna and a docusate salt may be less useful because the latter agent may enhance the absorption of senna (see the section on Mixtures).

Senna is considered safe for use during pregnancy and the puerperium. In recommended doses, significant amounts are not excreted in breast milk. There have been some unconfirmed reports that increased bowel activity occurs in infants whose mothers ingested senna while breast feeding.

Melanosis coli has not been reported with use of senna products. Senna preparations may impart a yellowish brown color to acid urine and a reddish color to alkaline urine; this same effect may occur in breast milk or feces.

DOSAGE AND PREPARATIONS.

SENNA WHOLE LEAF PREPARATIONS:

Oral: *Adults,* 0.5 to 2 g. *Children 6 to 12 years*, one-half adult dose; *2 to 5 years*, one-quarter adult dose; *under 2 years*, one-eighth adult dose.

Generic. Granules; leaves; powder; tablets (all forms nonprescription).

Black Draught (Chattem). Granules; tablets (both forms nonprescription).

SENNA POD PREPARATIONS:

Oral: (Granules) *Adults,* 1 level teaspoonful to a maximum of 2 level teaspoonsful two times daily; *geriatric, obstetric, or gynecologic patients and children over 27 kg*, dosage reduced by one-half. (Syrup) *Adults,* 2 to 3 teaspoonsful one or two times daily; *geriatric, obstetric, or gynecologic patients*, dosage reduced by one-half; *children 5 to 15 years*, 1 to a maximum of 2 teaspoonsful two times daily; *1 to 5 years*, one-half to a maximum of 1 teaspoonful two times daily; *1 month to 1 year*, one-quarter to a maximum of one-half teaspoonful twice daily. (Tablets) *Adults,* two to a maximum of four tablets two times daily; *geriatric, obstetric, or gynecologic patients and children over 27 kg*, dosage reduced by one-half.

Senokot (Purdue Frederick). Granules, syrup, tablets (regular, double-strength) (all forms nonprescription).

Available Mixture.

Perdiem (Rhone-Poulenc Rorer). Granules containing 0.74 g senna and 3.25 g psyllium/15 ml dose in 100 and 250 g containers (sodium 1.8 mg/dose) (nonprescription).

Rectal: *Adults,* one suppository; if necessary, a second suppository may be administered two hours later. *Children over 27 kg*, one-half suppository.

Senokot (Purdue Frederick). Suppositories (nonprescription).
CALCIUM SALTS OF SENNOSIDES A AND B:
Oral: *Adults,* one to three tablets (usually two) at bedtime.
Gentle Nature (Sandoz). Tablets (nonprescription).

SALINE LAXATIVES

MAGNESIUM, POTASSIUM, AND SODIUM SALTS

ACTIONS AND USES. Many salts having essentially the same actions are used as laxatives or cathartics. They usually produce a watery evacuation in two to six hours when doses at the upper range of effectiveness are used and are most effective if taken with substantial amounts (at least 240 ml) of fluid on an empty stomach. Magnesium-containing laxatives cause the release of cholecystokinin from duodenal mucosa, which may contribute to their osmotic action by stimulating colonic motility. Milk of magnesia and magnesium sulfate, in doses at the lower range of effectiveness, usually produce a soft semifluid stool in six to eight hours.

These preparations are given to empty the bowel prior to surgical, radiographic, proctoscopic, or colonoscopic procedures and to remove toxic material in some cases of poisoning. They also are useful to eliminate parasites and toxic vermifuge after anthelmintic therapy. When these preparations are administered orally, the watery diarrhea produced does not destroy the osmotically sensitive trophozoites of *Entamoeba histolytica* or *Giardia lamblia*; thus, they are suitable for the collection of fresh stool specimens for parasite examination. However, the same laxative used as an enema destroys the trophozoites (but not the cyst forms) of *E. histolytica*.

ADVERSE REACTIONS AND PRECAUTIONS. Saline laxatives should be given with large amounts of liquids to prevent dehydration and maximize their effects. Magnesium salts should be avoided in patients with simple constipation. Up to 20% of magnesium may be absorbed and enter the systemic circulation. Magnesium and potassium salts are contraindicated in patients with impaired renal function. The bitter taste of magnesium sulfate may cause nausea. Sodium salts are contraindicated in patients with heart disease who have edema or congestive heart failure or in those on a low-sodium diet. Sodium phosphate should be used cautiously in patients with cardiovascular, renal, or convulsive disorders or with hypocalcemia. The sodium phosphate-biphosphate preparations may cause sloughing of the surface epithelium of the rectum.

DOSAGE AND PREPARATIONS. See Table 3.

TABLE 3.
SALINE CATHARTICS[1]

Preparations	Usual Dose (Adults)[2,3]
Fleet Enema (Fleet) (solution containing 19 g monobasic sodium phosphate and 7 g dibasic sodium phosphate/delivered dose)	118 ml (rectal only)
Magnesium carbonate	8 g
Magnesium citrate solution (1.55 to 1.9 g/100 ml magnesium oxide with citric acid anhydrous and potassium bicarbonate for effervescence)	200 ml
Milk of Magnesia (7% to 8.5% magnesium hydroxide suspension)	15 to 40 ml
Magnesium oxide	4 g
Magnesium sulfate	10 to 15 g
Fleet Phospho-Soda (aqueous solution containing 48 g monobasic sodium phosphate and 18 g dibasic sodium phosphate/100 ml)	20 to 30 ml
Potassium bitartrate	2 g
Potassium phosphate	4 g
Potassium sodium tartrate	5 to 10 g
Dibasic sodium phosphate	3.6 to 7.2 g
Sodium phosphate, effervescent, dried	10 g
Sodium phosphate oral solution	7.5 g

[1]*All nonprescription except potassium phosphate.*
[2]*Dosage is reduced for children.*
[3]*Except where indicated, all doses are administered orally. Flavored preparations of various saline cathartics are marketed but usually are more expensive than the generic preparations.*

LUBRICANT

MINERAL OIL (Liquid Petrolatum)

ACTIONS AND USES. Mineral oil is an indigestible liquid hydrocarbon of limited absorbability. When used in recommended doses, it is safe and is particularly effective when used rectally in the management of fecal impaction. Mineral oil can be used with a psyllium preparation and/or senna pod to prevent constipation in patients at risk or in those who cannot tolerate constipation because of debility or disease. It has been used orally to lessen the strain of evacuation of inspissated stool (eg, patients with hernia or cardiovascular disease). Mineral oil is preferable to contact laxatives because it is safer and tolerance does not occur (Klein, 1982; Sparberg, 1984).

The emulsified preparations are claimed to reduce seepage through the anal sphincter and to be more effective than nonemulsified preparations, but conclusive evidence from controlled studies is not available. Seepage of oil from the rectum can be avoided by reducing the dose.

ADVERSE REACTIONS AND PRECAUTIONS. In recent years, the oral use of mineral oil has not been advocated because of the possibility of interference with the absorption of fat-soluble vitamins and the danger of pulmonary aspiration. The dose required for the former effect exceeds that normally used in clinical practice. Moreover, in one study this was not a significant problem (Clark et al, 1987). Advising the patient to remain upright for at least two hours after administration reduces the danger of lipid pneumonia; some physicians avoid use of this agent in the elderly because of this potential risk. Oral mineral oil should not be given to patients with swallowing abnormalities.

Foreign-body granulomas or paraffinomas in the liver, spleen, or mesenteric lymph nodes have been reported following systemic absorption of mineral oil.

Because concurrent use of the docusate salts may increase the absorption of mineral oil, their concomitant administration is not recommended.

Mineral oil is still prescribed by some surgeons after anorectal surgery despite the fact that it sometimes causes pruritus ani. Laceration of the area from scratching or rubbing can interfere with healing because droplets of the inert material act as a foreign body in the wound.

Mineral oil is classified in FDA Pregnancy Category C.

DOSAGE AND PREPARATIONS.

Oral: *Adults,* 15 to 45 ml two times daily; *children over 6 years*, 10 to 15 ml of plain mineral oil at bedtime or 10 to 15 ml of emulsion two times daily.

For fecal impaction, some authorities recommend that 30 ml be administered hourly while the patient is awake until oil seeps from the rectum (usually within 24 to 48 hours) or the obstruction is relieved. At this point, after most of the softened feces have been removed manually, several tap water enemas are administered followed by an oral cathartic dose of a saline laxative to flush out the rectum (Klein, 1982; Sparberg, 1984; Wrenn, 1989).

Before this regimen is used, the possibility of mechanical bowel obstruction should be eliminated. Large amounts of fluid should be administered to prevent dehydration.

Generic. Liquid (nonprescription).

Available Trademarks.
Kondremul Plain (Ciba), ***Milkinol*** (Schwarz) (both nonprescription).

Rectal: *Adults,* 120 ml; *children over 6 years*, 60 ml.
Fleet Mineral Oil Enema (Fleet) (nonprescription).

BOWEL CLEANSING AGENTS

POLYETHYLENE GLYCOL ELECTROLYTE PREPARATIONS
[CoLyte, GoLYTELY, NuLytely, OCL Solution]

ACTIONS AND USES. Each liter of these isosmotically balanced solutions contains about 60 g of polyethylene glycol (PEG), a nonabsorbable osmotic agent, plus smaller amounts of sodium sulfate, potassium chloride, sodium chloride, sodium bicarbonate, and polysorbate 80 (OCL Solution only). Absorption of sodium is impaired by sulfate, a poorly absorbed anion, and the other electrolytes prevent net absorption or secretion of other ions. PEG solutions cleanse the bowel rapidly by producing a voluminous liquid stool without significantly affecting water and electrolyte balance or mucosal histology (Davis et al, 1980).

When administered four to five hours before a diagnostic procedure, these preparations are equally or more effective than the usual regimen of diet and oral laxatives, suppositories, or enemas for cleansing the bowel. In addition, they act more rapidly and cause less discomfort (*Med Lett Drugs Ther*, 1985). However, some physicians consider these solutions unsatisfactory when taken on the same day as a barium enema because they may interfere with barium coating of the bowel wall using the double-contrast technique. The addition of bisacodyl significantly improves coating with barium by affecting the quality or quantity of colonic mucus (DiPalma and Brady, 1989) and allows evacuation of residual fluid (Girard et al, 1984; MacCollum et al, 1989; Clarkston and Smith, 1991). In one study, the use of an oral senna preparation the night before administration of a PEG solution was more effective in cleansing the bowel than use of the PEG solution alone. Less lavage fluid was needed, and the senna was well tolerated (Ziegenhagen et al, 1991). Many physicians consider PEG electrolyte solutions the preferred cleansing agents to prepare patients for colonic surgery (Beck et al, 1986; DiPalma and Marshall, 1990).

Ingestion of a PEG electrolyte preparation (500 ml daily for five days) was reported to be effective and well tolerated by patients with chronic constipation (Andorsky and Goldner, 1990).

PEG solutions have been used investigationally in infants and children for whole-bowel irrigation for encopresis, severe constipation, preparation for surgery and colonoscopy, and acute iron overdose (Goodale and Noble, 1989; Sondheimer et al, 1991). These solutions were effective and well tolerated; however, large amounts of lavage solution were required.

The results of one small study in patients over 75 years indicated that a PEG solution had no significant advantage over an enema for bowel cleansing, and elderly patients appeared to tolerate the enema better (Lashner et al, 1990).

For information on the treatment of patients with diabetes who require bowel cleansing, see McMahon, 1992.

ADVERSE REACTIONS AND PRECAUTIONS. Nausea, vomiting, abdominal bloating or fullness, and cramps occur occasionally but are transient and usually well tolerated. Metoclopramide does not prevent any of these effects (Brady et al, 1985). Chilling the solution improves the unpleasant salty taste but may cause hypothermia. Compliance may be improved and the taste may be more palatable if the mouth is rinsed with mouthwash after each glassful of the iced preparation (London, 1990). In one study on 87 volunteers, the palatability of CoLyte was improved by addition of Koolaid drink mix sweetened with aspartame; the osmolality of the solution was not affected significantly (Gruber et al, 1991). The use of fermentable sugars with electrocautery must be avoided, for a fatal explosion may occur (Bigard et al, 1979).

A low-sodium sulfate-free preparation [NuLytely] has been developed to reduce the salty taste of the solution and to improve palatability and patient compliance (Fordtran et al, 1990; DiPalma and Marshall, 1990; Beck and DiPalma, 1991). The amount of sodium is reduced by about one-half and the amount of PEG is increased. However, a group of healthy volunteers could not distinguish any difference in taste between the low-salt and standard PEG preparations (Froehlich et al, 1991).

Theoretical problems with PEG solutions include gastrointestinal bleeding and aspiration due to obstruction; however, these adverse effects have not been observed in patients. The same precautions observed with other laxatives apply to use of PEG electrolyte preparations. The solutions should not be used in patients with intestinal obstruction or perforation, ileus, gastric retention, toxic colitis, or megacolon. If the solution is given through a nasogastric tube, the patient should be observed closely to prevent regurgitation and aspiration.

These solutions are generally safe for elderly patients; for those with cardiovascular, hepatic, or renal disorders; or for those who are poorly hydrated. Available data show that these agents also are safe in infants 6 months and older (Goodale and Noble, 1989) and in children; delivery through a nasogastric tube may be required in children. Safety for pregnant women and the fetus has not been established (FDA Pregnancy Category C).

DOSAGE AND PREPARATIONS.

Oral: *Adults,* 200 to 300 ml (7 to 10 oz) orally every 10 to 15 minutes or through a nasogastric tube at a rate of 20 to 30 ml/min. Administration should begin the evening before or four to five hours before the examination and continue until the rectal discharge is clear. This requires 2.5 to 3.5 L in most patients. The first bowel movement usually commences about one hour after administration of the initial dose. Patients should ingest only clear liquids for two to four hours before the examination and until it is complete.

CoLyte (Reed & Carnrick). Powder (plain or with artificial flavor and sweetener ***[Colyte-Flavored]***) containing polyethylene glycol 3350, 240 g in a 4-liter container and 227.1 g in a 3.785-liter container with sodium sulfate, sodium bicarbonate, sodium chloride, and potassium chloride.

GoLYTELY (Braintree). Powder containing polyethylene glycol 3350, 236 g in a 4-liter container with sodium sulfate, sodium bicarbonate, sodium chloride, and potassium chloride.

NuLytely (Braintree). Powder containing polyethylene glycol 3350, 420 g in a 4-liter container with sodium bicarbonate, sodium chloride, and potassium chloride.

OCL Solution (Abbott). Solution containing polyethylene glycol 3350, 6 g in a 1.35-liter container with sodium sulfate, sodium bicarbonate, sodium chloride, potassium chloride, and polysorbate 80 (supplied in 3 containers).

MISCELLANEOUS AGENTS

GLYCERIN

[Fleet Babylax, Fleet Glycerin Suppositories]

Glycerin suppositories promote fecal evacuation in 15 to 30 minutes by stimulating rectal contraction through hyperosmotic and irritant actions. This preparation also may be used to soften and lubricate inspissated fecal material, and it is often employed temporarily to re-establish normal bowel function in laxative-dependent patients. Glycerin suppositories are often useful in bowel retraining regimens and in individuals with intermittent constipation.

Glycerin, given rectally in a liquid form as an enema, is a convenient way to administer a glycerin laxative to children.

DOSAGE AND PREPARATIONS.

Rectal: (Suppository) *Adults*, 2 to 3 g; *children under 6 years*, 1 to 1.7 g. (Enema) *Children 2 to 6 years,* 2 to 5 ml.

Fleet Babylax (Fleet). Solution (enema) 80% v/v in 4 ml containers (nonprescription).

Fleet Glycerin Suppositories (Fleet), ***Generic***. Suppositories (nonprescription).

LACTULOSE

[Chronulac, Constilac, Duphalac]

For chemical formula, see index entry Lactulose, In Portal Systemic Encephalopathy.

ACTIONS AND USES. Lactulose, a synthetic disaccharide, is not hydrolyzed by gastrointestinal enzymes and is not absorbed significantly in the small intestine. As a result, lactulose reaches the colon unchanged where it is metabolized by colonic bacteria to short-chain organic acids (eg, lactic, acetic, and formic acids). The increased osmotic activity of these nonabsorbable acid metabolites results in a modest net accumulation of fluid in the colon. A soft formed stool usually is produced in one to three days but, in some patients, a semifluid stool is produced in 6 to 24 hours.

In several double-blind controlled studies, lactulose was effective in patients with chronic constipation and markedly reduced the incidence of fecal impaction in the elderly. Large doses (30 to 60 ml/day) are usually required, and 24 to 48 hours may elapse before normal bowel function is reestablished. Because of its nonsystemic, colon-specific action, lactulose avoids the potentially harmful effects that result from the absorption of many laxatives. However, many patients receiving lactulose experience cramping and flatulence;

these symptoms are usually transient but may persist in some patients with continued therapy.

Because of its adverse effects, relatively high cost, and lack of proof that it is more efficacious than conventional laxatives, some practitioners recommend that lactulose be reserved for patients who do not respond to other medications (Sparberg, 1984; Bateman and Smith, 1988). It may be useful in elderly patients in whom bulk-forming agents or dietary fiber supplements do not provide relief or are not tolerated; however, these patients may have difficulty swallowing large volumes of the diluted drug (Kallman, 1983).

ADVERSE REACTIONS AND PRECAUTIONS. Initial administration frequently produces flatulence and intestinal cramps. Excessive doses can produce watery stools.

Patients may not tolerate the extremely sweet taste. Because lactulose contains galactose (<2.2 g/15 ml) and lactose (<1.2 g/15 ml), it should be used with caution in diabetic patients and avoided in those requiring a low-galactose diet. Lactulose can produce nausea.

Serum electrolytes should be measured periodically in elderly debilitated patients who receive lactulose for more than six months.

This drug is classified in FDA Pregnancy Category B.

DOSAGE AND PREPARATIONS.

Oral: *Adults,* 15 to 30 ml (10 to 20 g of lactulose) daily, increased to 60 ml daily if necessary. Children, there is insufficient experience to recommend a dose.

Chronulac (Marion Merrell Dow), ***Constilac*** (Alra), ***Duphalac*** (Solvay), ***Generic.*** Each 15 ml of syrup contains lactulose 10 g, galactose less than 2.2 g, lactose less than 1.2 g, and other sugars 1.2 g or less.

SORBITOL (D-glucitol)

```
     H  OH H  OH OH H
     |  |  |  |  |  |
  HO-C--C--C--C--C--C-OH
     |  |  |  |  |  |
     H  H  OH H  H  H
```

ACTIONS AND USES. Following oral administration, this nonabsorbable synthetic disaccharide has actions similar to those of lactulose. It reaches the colon unchanged where it is metabolized to short-chain organic fatty acids that, when present in amounts that exceed the rate of maximal colonic absorption, act osmotically to increase the amount of fluid in the colon. A soft formed stool is usually produced in one to three days. Oral sorbitol may be as effective as lactulose and may be a low-cost alternative to that agent in patients with chronic constipation who do not respond to dietary fiber or bulk-forming agents (Lederle et al, 1990; Richter, 1991). When used rectally, the effects of sorbitol are believed to result from hyperosmotic and local irritant actions.

Oral or rectal sorbitol also is used as an adjunct to sodium polystyrene sulfonate resin in the treatment of hyperkalemia; sorbitol counteracts the constipating effect of the resin and facilitates its passage through the intestine. In addition, it assists in removal of potassium.

ADVERSE REACTIONS AND PRECAUTIONS. This agent is usually well tolerated; adverse reactions after oral administration include bloating, flatulence, and diarrhea. Mild adverse reactions after rectal administration result from a local irritant effect and occur only rarely. Sorbitol may be better tolerated than lactulose, particularly in the elderly.

DOSAGE AND PREPARATIONS.

Oral: *Adults and children over 12 years,* 30 to 60 ml of a 70% solution administered at bedtime; *children 2 to 11 years,* one-quarter to one-half the adult dose has been used.

Rectal (enema): *Adults and children 12 years and older,* 120 ml of a 25% to 30% solution; *children 2 to 11 years,* 30 to 60 ml of a 25% to 30% solution.

For use as an adjunct to sodium polystyrene sulfonate resin, see index entry on this drug.

Generic. Powder; solution (oral, rectal) 70%.

MALT SOUP EXTRACT
[Maltsupex]

Malt soup extract is a concentrated aqueous extract of barley malt; the amylolytic enzymes are removed during processing. Generally, this extract has a mild laxative effect. The exact mechanism of action is unknown. It may act in part as a bulk-forming laxative; however, malt soup extract also lowers fecal pH by forming pyruvic and lactic acids and carbon dioxide.

Malt soup extract is often prescribed for children; however, barley cereal may be more effective and is much less expensive.

DOSAGE AND PREPARATIONS.

Oral: *Adults and children over 12 years*, up to 64 g daily in divided doses. *Children 6 to 12 years*, up to 32 g daily in divided doses; *2 to 6 years*, up to 16 g daily in divided doses.

Maltsupex (Wallace). Powder; liquid; tablets (all forms nonprescription).

MIXTURES

There is no satisfactory evidence that laxative-cathartic mixtures are advantageous. The concomitant use of two or more laxatives to treat constipation does not enhance efficacy sufficiently to justify the additional hazards. With a knowledge of the mechanism of action of the various laxatives and an understanding of the patient's problem, the need for mixtures should be minimized. Too often, constipation caused by delay in passage of fecal material through the colon, delay in evacuating the rectum, or simply insufficient quantity of stool may be converted to a more serious condition by injudicious use of a combination of laxatives. Mixtures containing a docusate salt and another contact laxative are of special concern since the docusate salt may enhance the absorption of the other agent in the mixture.

The following listing of available mixtures is provided for information only; it is not intended to be complete and, in certain instances, represents an unfortunate commentary on the motives that led to the formulation of these products. This listing does not signify a recommendation for use.

Agoral (Parke-Davis). Emulsion (flavored) containing white phenolphthalein 200 mg and mineral oil 4.2 g/15 ml (nonprescription).

Dialose Plus (Johnson & Johnson-Merck Consumer). Each capsule contains casanthranol 30 mg and docusate potassium 100 mg (nonprescription).

Doxidan (Upjohn). Each capsule contains yellow phenolphthalein 65 mg and docusate calcium 60 mg (alcohol 1.5%) (nonprescription).

Haley's M-O (Sterling Health). Emulsion containing magnesium hydroxide 304 mg and mineral oil 1.25 ml/5 ml (nonprescription).

Peri-Colace (Apothecon). Each capsule contains casanthranol 30 mg and docusate sodium 100 mg; each 5 ml of syrup contains casanthranol 10 mg and docusate sodium 20 mg (alcohol 10%) (both forms nonprescription).

Senokot S (Purdue Frederick). Each tablet contains senna concentrate 187 mg and docusate sodium 50 mg (nonprescription).

Cited References

Laxative drug products for over-the-counter human use; tentative final monograph. *Federal Register* 50:2124-2158 (Jan 15), 1985.

Oral electrolyte solutions for colonic lavage before colonoscopy or barium enema. *Med Lett Drugs Ther* 27:39-40, 1985.

Anderson JW: Fiber and health: Overview. *Am J Gastroenterol* 81:892-897, 1986.

Anderson JW, et al: Cholesterol-lowering effects of psyllium hydrophilic mucilloid for hypercholesterolemic males. *Arch Intern Med* 148:292-296, 1988.

Andorsky RI, Goldner F: Colonic lavage solution (polyethylene glycol electrolyte lavage solution) as a treatment for chronic constipation: A double-blind, placebo-controlled study. *Am J Gastroenterol* 85:261-265, 1990.

Bateman DN, Smith JM: A policy for laxatives. *BMJ* 297:1420-1421, 1988.

Beck DE, DiPalma JA: A new oral lavage solution vs cathartics and enema method for preoperative colonic cleansing. *Arch Surg* 126:552-555, 1991.

Beck DE, et al: Comparison of oral lavage methods for preoperative colonic cleansing. *Dis Colon Rectum* 29:699-703, 1986.

Bigard M-A, et al: Fatal colonic explosion during colonscopic polypectomy. *Gastroenterology* 77:1307-1310, 1979.

Brady CE, et al: Golytely lavage—Is metoclopramide necessary? *Am J Gastroenterol* 80:180-184, 1985.

Brunton LL: Agents affecting gastrointestinal water flux and motility, digestants, and bile acids, in Gilman AG, et al (eds): *Goodman and Gilman's The Pharmacological Basis of Therapeutics*, ed 8. New York, Pergamon Press, 1990, 914-932.

Bytzer P, et al: Prevalence of surreptitious laxative abuse in patients with diarrhoea of uncertain origin: A cost benefit analysis of a screening procedure. *Gut* 30:1379-1384, 1989.

Clark JH, et al: Serum beta-carotene, retinol, and alpha-tocopherol levels during mineral oil therapy for constipation. *Am J Dis Child* 141:1210-1212, 1987.

Clarkston WK, Smith OJ: Golytely/Dulcolax combination improves prep for outpatient colonoscopy. *Am J Gastroenterol* 86:1351, 1991.

Culpepper-Morgan JA, et al: Treatment of opioid-induced constipation with oral naloxone: A pilot study. *Clin Pharmacol Ther* 52:90-95, 1992.

Davis GR, et al: Development of a lavage solution associated with minimal water and electrolyte absorption or secretion. *Gastroenterology* 78:991-995, 1980.

Devroede G: Constipation, in: *Gastrointestinal Disease*, ed 4. Philadelphia, WB Saunders, 1989, 331-368.

DiPalma JA, Brady CE III: Colon cleansing for diagnostic and surgical procedures: Polyethylene glycol-electrolyte lavage solution. *Am J Gastroenterol* 84:1008-1016, 1989.

DiPalma JA, Marshall JB: Comparison of a new sulfate-free polyethylene glycol electrolyte lavage solution versus a standard solution for colonoscopy cleansing. *Gastrointest Endosc* 36:285-289, 1990.

Donowitz M, et al: Effects of Senokot on rat intestinal electrolyte transport: Evidence of Ca++ dependence. *Gastroenterology* 87:503-512, 1984.

Fingl E: Laxatives and cathartics, in Gilman AG, et al (eds): *Goodman and Gilman's The Pharmacological Basis of Therapeutics*, ed 6. New York, Macmillan, 1980, 1002-1012.

Fordtran JS, et al: A low-sodium solution for gastrointestinal lavage. *Gastroenterology* 98:11-16, 1990.

Froehlich F, et al: Palatability of a new solution compared with standard polyethylene glycol solution for gastrointestinal lavage. *Gastrointest Endosc* 37:325-328, 1991.

Girard CM, et al: Comparison of Golytely lavage with standard diet/cathartic preparation for double contrast barium enema. *Am J Roentgenol* 142:1147-1149, 1984.

Gleghorn EE, et al: No-enema therapy for idiopathic constipation and encopresis. *Clin Pediatr* 30:669-672, 1991.

Godding EW: Bowel function and dysfunction: Prevention of constipation. *Pharm J* 229-230, (Feb 25) 1984 A.

Godding EW: Bowel function and dysfunction: Rehabilitation of the constipated bowel: Case histories. *Pharm J* 198-200, (Feb 18) 1984 B.

Godding EW: Bowel function and dysfunction: Chemical laxatives. *Pharm J* 168-169, (Feb 11) 1984 C.

Godding EW: Laxatives and the special role of senna. *Pharmacology* 36(suppl 1):230-236, 1988.

Goldfinger SE: Constipation, part 1: The hard facts. *Harvard Health Lett* 16:1-4, (Feb) 1991.

Goodale EP, Noble TA: Pediatric bowel evacuation with a polyethylene glycol and iso-osmolar electrolyte solution. *DICP* 23:1008-1009, 1989.

Gruber M, et al: Palatability of colonic lavage solution is improved by the addition of artificially sweetened flavored drink mixes. *Gastroenterol Nurs* 14:135-137, 1991.

Gullikson GW, et al: Effects of anionic laxatives on hamster small intestinal membrane structure and function: Relationship to surface activity. *Gastroenterology* 73:501-511, 1977.

Hamilton JW, et al: Clinical evaluation of methylcellulose as a bulk laxative. *Dig Dis Sci* 33:993-998, 1988.

Haskell LP: Hypocalcemic tetany induced by hypertonic-phosphate enema. *Lancet* 2:1453, 1985.

James JM, et al: Anaphylactic reactions to a psyllium-containing cereal. *J Allergy Clin Immunol* 88:402-408, 1991.

Johanson JF, et al: Association of constipation with neurologic diseases. *Dig Dis Sci* 37:179-186, (Feb) 1992.

Kallman H: Constipation in the elderly. *Am Fam Physician* 27:179-184, (Jan) 1983.

Kamm MA, et al: Steroid hormone abnormalities in women with severe idiopathic constipation. *Gut* 32:80-84, 1991.

Killen JD, et al: Self-induced vomiting and laxative and diuretic use among teenagers: Precursors of the binge-purge syndrome? *JAMA* 255:1447-1449, 1986.

Klein H: Constipation and fecal impaction. *Med Clin North Am* 66:1135-1141, 1982.

Krevsky B, et al: Cisapride accelerates colonic transit in constipated patients with colonic inertia. *Am J Gastroenterol* 84:882-887, 1989.

Lashner BA, et al: Randomized clinical trial of two colonoscopy preparation methods for elderly patients. *J Clin Gastroenterol* 12:405-408, 1990.

Lederle FA, et al: Cost-effective treatment of constipation in the elderly: A randomized double-blind comparison of sorbitol and lactulose. *Am J Med* 89:597-601, 1990.

London FA: Help the patient comply with the colonic prep, correspondence. *Gastroenterology* 1393, (May) 1990.

MacCollum BJ, et al: Double blind randomized trial to evaluate the effect of a cathartic on a standard colon lavage preparation for colonoscopy. *Am J Gastroenterol* 84:1189, 1989.

Marlett JA, et al: Comparative laxation of psyllium with and without senna in ambulatory constipated population. *Am J Gastroenterol* 82:333-337, 1987.

Marshall JB: Chronic constipation in adults: How far should evaluation and treatment go? *Postgrad Med* 88:49-63, (Sept) 1990.

McCabe M, et al: Phosphate enemas in childhood: Cause for concern. *BMJ* 302:1074, 1991.

McMahon T: Diabetes control during bowel cleansing with PEG-electrolyte solution. *Clin Pharm* 11:751-752, 1992.

Meisel JL, et al: Human rectal mucosa: Proctoscopic and morphological changes caused by laxatives. *Gastroenterology* 72:1274-1279, 1977.

Moriarity KJ, et al: Study on mechanism of action of dioctyl sodium sulphosuccinate in normal human jejunum. *Gastroenterology* 82:1134, 1982.

Müller-Lissner SA, Bavarian Constipation Study Group: Treatment of chronic constipation with cisapride and placebo. *Gut* 28:1033-1038, 1987.

Nolan T, et al: Randomised trial of laxatives in treatment of childhood encopresis. *Lancet* 338:523-527, 1991.

Ornstein MH, Baird IM: Dietary fiber and the colon. *Mol Aspects Med* 9:41-67, 1987.

Pemberton JH, et al: Evaluation and surgical treatment of severe chronic constipation. *Ann Surg* 214:403-411, 1991.

Puet TA, et al: Pulsed irrigation enhanced evacuation: New method for treating fecal impaction. *Arch Phys Med Rehabil* 72:935-936, 1991.

Richter JE: Hurray for brand X, comment. *Gastroenterology* 100:1474-1475, 1991.

Schouten WR: Severe, longstanding constipation in adults: Indications for surgical treatment. *Scand J Gastroenterol Suppl* 188:60-68, 1991.

Sondheimer JM, et al: Safety, efficacy, and tolerance of intestinal lavage in pediatric patients undergoing diagnostic colonoscopy. *J Pediatr* 119:148-152, (July) 1991.

Sonnenberg A, Koch TR: Physician visits in the United States for constipation: 1958 to 1986. *Dig Dis Sci* 34:606-611, 1989.

Sparberg M: Practical pointers for treating constipation. *Drug Ther* 14:97-105, (May) 1984.

Staiano A, et al: Effect of cisapride on chronic idiopathic constipation in children. *Dig Dis Sci* 36:733-736, 1991.

Stratton JW, Mackeigan JM: Treating constipation. *Am Fam Physician* 25:139-142, (June) 1982.

Tedesco FJ, et al: Laxative use in constipation. *Am J Gastroenterol* 80:303-309, 1985.

Tenenbein M, et al: Whole bowel irrigation as decontamination procedure after acute drug overdose. *Arch Intern Med* 147:905-907, 1987.

Tomlin J, Read NW: Laxative properties of indigestible plastic particles. *BMJ* 297:1175-1176, 1988.

Tremaine WJ: Chronic constipation: Causes and management. *Hosp Pract* 89-100, (April) 1990.

Vanner SJ, et al: A randomized prospective trial comparing oral sodium phosphate with standard polyethylene glycol-based lavage solution (Golytely) in the preparation of patients for colonoscopy. *Am J Gastroenterol* 85:422-427, 1990.

Wald A: Constipation and fecal incontinence in the elderly. *Gastroenterol Clin North Am* 19:405-418, 1990.

Wald A: Constipation in elderly patients: Pathogenesis and management. *Drugs Aging* 3:220-231, 1993.

Wald A, et al: Psychological and physiological characteristics of patients with severe idiopathic constipation. *Gastroenterology* 97:932-937, 1989.

Wexner SD, et al: Colectomy for constipation: Physiologic investigation is the key to success. *Dis Colon Rectum* 34:851-856, 1991.

Whitehead WE, et al: Constipation in the elderly living at home: Definition, prevalence and relationship to lifestyle and health status. *J Am Geriatr Soc* 37:423-429, 1989.

Williams SG, DiPalma JA: Constipation in the long-term care facility. *Gastroenterol Nurs* 179-182, (Winter) 1990.

Wrenn K: Fecal impaction. *N Engl J Med* 321:658-662, 1989.

Ziegenhagen DJ, et al: Addition of senna improves colonoscopy preparation with lavage: A prospective randomized trial. *Gastrointest Endosc* 37:547-549, 1991.

Zumoff B, Hellman L: Absorption of sodium from hypertonic sodium phosphate enema solutions. *Dis Colon Rectum* 21:440-443, 1978.

Drugs Used in Disorders of the Liver, Biliary Tract, and Pancreas

45

DISORDERS OF THE LIVER

Chronic Hepatitis

Etiology: Chronic hepatitis should be considered as a possible diagnosis if evidence of inflammation of the liver persists for at least six months regardless of the presence or absence of symptoms. Distinctions have been based on histopathologic criteria but are now based on etiology.

Chronic persistent hepatitis (CPH) is characterized by inflammation around portal spaces without significant architectural distortion of the liver lobule. CPH associated with autoimmune hepatitis is virtually asymptomatic and often nonprogressive, and the prognosis usually is good. In patients with chronic hepatitis B or C, CPH can progress and become symptomatic. Patients with CPH should be examined at 6- to 12-month intervals to ensure that the diagnosis is accurate.

Chronic active hepatitis (CAH) is characterized by inflammation causing erosion of the limiting plate with piecemeal necrosis. This disorder often progresses to cirrhosis and causes premature death from liver failure or the complications associated with portal hypertension. Similar histologic changes and clinical features may be observed in patients with hepatitis B, hepatitis C, and hepatitis D; autoimmune disorders; and even Wilson's disease. They also may be associated with drug therapy. Some patients with CPH associated with hepatitis C eventually develop CAH. Following spontaneous remission or successful therapy, CAH patients can develop CPH.

Approximately 20% to 50% of the estimated three million cases of chronic hepatitis in the United States are due to infection with hepatitis B virus (HBV). In the Far East, infected people acquire HBV most commonly by vertical transmission at birth, whereas those in Western countries become infected most commonly by horizontal transmission during adulthood. Until recently, the response of patients with hepatitis B to antiviral therapy was difficult to predict (Willson, 1990); however, criteria now exist to identify some patients infected with HBV who will respond favorably (Patel et al, 1992). There is a strong association between infection with HBV and development of hepatocellular carcinoma.

Hepatitis C virus (HCV) is the causative agent in most cases of non-A, non-B hepatitis and is an important (but decreasing) cause of post-transfusion chronic hepatitis (Lambiase and Davis, 1992). In patients with acute hepatitis C, the infection becomes chronic in more than 50% and leads to cirrhosis in more than 20% (Hoofnagle and Di Bisceglie, 1989). Moreover, as with HBV, there appears to be a strong association between infection with HCV and the development of hepatocellular carcinoma.

The hepatitis D virus (HDV, delta hepatitis) is a small, defective virus that is not infectious in the absence of coinfection with HBV. Patients with HBV who acquire a superinfection with HDV may develop a much more virulent and severe form of chronic hepatitis that is refractory to treatment and often progresses to cirrhosis and death (Padilla and Schiff, 1991).

Hepatitis A and E are caused by viruses that do not produce chronic hepatitis. The acute hepatitis produced by these two viruses is usually self-limited, but fulminant hepatitis can occur (Schiff, 1992).

Although it is potentially the most virulent form of chronic hepatitis and is usually fatal if not treated, *autoimmune chronic active hepatitis* (AICAH) was, prior to the development of interferon for HBV and HCV, the only type that responded to therapy. AICAH is diagnosed in part by eliminating other possible causes of chronic hepatitis and by confirming the presence in most patients of hypergammaglobulinemia and the ANA, SMA, or anti-actin autoantibodies. Two major types of AICAH exist: Type I, the classic form, is characterized by hypergammaglobulinemia and high titers of ANA. Type II is characterized by the presence of antibody to liver and kidney microsomes (anti-LKM1) and has two subtypes, type IIa and type IIb. Type IIa occurs predominantly in young women and produces antibodies to P450 IID6; type IIb results from infection with HCV and does not produce antibodies to P450 IID6. Types I and IIa are steroid-responsive, whereas type IIb responds to antiviral therapy for HCV but not to steroids (Maddrey, 1993; Yamamoto et al, 1993).

Progression to cirrhosis occurs in up to 30% of patients with AICAH.

Drug Therapy: Depending on etiology, patients with chronic hepatitis may be candidates for treatment, which may be lifesaving. Remission is induced in more than 70% of patients with type I AICAH. Initially, prednisone 30 to 40 mg, with or without azathioprine [Imuran] 1.5 mg/kg, is administered daily for at least one year. When alanine aminotransferase (ALT) and aspartate aminotransferase (AST) concentrations stabilize within normal limits, the dose of prednisone can be reduced gradually. If prednisone is given alone initially, the daily maintenance dose is 10 to 20 mg. Although azathioprine is not needed to induce remission, maintenance therapy with azathioprine permits the withdrawal of prednisone in 50% to 75% of patients in remission (Stellon et al, 1988; Kaplan, 1989). Both short- and long-term toxicity are more common with prednisone than with combination therapy. For this reason, the combined steroid/azathioprine regimen is preferable to corticosteroid monotherapy (Patel et al, 1992; Lambiase and Davis, 1992). Relapses following induction of remission and interruption of treatment are observed frequently, and thus periodic monitoring is required.

Interferon alfa-2b [Intron A] has induced remissions in some patients with chronic hepatitis B or C. Subcutaneous administration of 5 million IU of interferon alfa-2b daily (or 10 million IU three times weekly) for four months has produced long-term remission in 35% to 45% of patients infected with HBV who are positive for hepatitis Be antigen (HBeAg) (Lambiase and Davis, 1992; Patel et al, 1992; Schiff, 1992; Maddrey, 1993; Perrillo et al, 1990). A complete response to interferon alfa-2b is defined as reduction of serum ALT or AST to normal levels, disappearance of viral DNA and HBeAg from serum, and appearance of anti-HBeAg in serum (Schiff, 1992). In one major study, serum hepatitis B surface antigen (HBsAg) disappeared three to seven years after initiation of therapy (Korenman et al, 1991). Relapse is uncommon in patients achieving a complete response. The disappearance of HBsAg and absence of HBV DNA as measured by polymerase chain reaction indicate complete eradication of the infection and probable cure. However, it is possible that some viral DNA integrates into the host genome and the disease could be reactivated. Criteria to identify HBV patients with the greatest likelihood of response to interferon alfa-2b include infection with HBV as an adult, female sex, serum ALT >100 IU, low serum HBV DNA (<100 pg/ml), evidence of active liver inflammation at biopsy, and absence of HIV antibody (Patel et al, 1992; Maddrey, 1993).

The suggestion that a short trial with corticosteroids could enhance the response to interferon has not been confirmed (Lambiase and Davis, 1992); such use of corticosteroids may be dangerous, since their withdrawal may cause hepatic failure in up to 20% of patients with chronic hepatitis B.

Almost 50% of patients with chronic hepatitis C respond to interferon alfa-2b. The subcutaneous administration of 3 million IU three times weekly produces normal ALT concentrations and usually decreases hepatic inflammation markedly (Davis et al, 1989; Di Bisceglie et al, 1989; Patel et al, 1992; Maddrey, 1993). A significant response (indicated by reduction of the ALT concentration to near normal) occurs in an additional 10% of patients. HCV patients who are likely to respond to interferon alfa-2b generally do so within the first 12 weeks of therapy.

Relapses (as indicated by return of elevated ALT levels) occur within six months after withdrawal of interferon alfa-2b therapy in more than 50% of patients with chronic hepatitis C who had a complete or near-complete response (Lambiase and Davis, 1992; Maddrey, 1993). These patients usually respond to another course of therapy.

Interferon alfa-2b may exacerbate or cause autoimmune disease, particularly in patients with chronic hepatitis C, and thus should be avoided in those with underlying autoimmune disease (Papo et al, 1992).

Although patients with advanced cirrhosis or other signs of decompensated liver disease generally have not been viewed as candidates for interferon therapy (Maddrey, 1993), preliminary data indicate that interferon alfa-2b may inhibit the activity of transforming growth factor beta$_1$ (TGF beta$_1$), a cytokine involved in stimulating collagen formation and hepatic fibrosis (Castilla et al, 1991). It is unclear if interferon alfa-2b can reverse or prevent hepatic fibrosis and cirrhosis and improve the prognosis in chronic hepatic diseases (Schiff, 1991).

Liver Transplantation: Liver transplantation should be considered for all patients with progressive hepatic failure or stage 3 or 4 coma regardless of etiology. Reinfection from extrahepatic sources is common in patients with chronic hepatitis B; the course of disease is often virulent and progresses rapidly. In patients with chronic hepatitis C, the rate of reinfection is high after transplantation, but the disease course does not progress rapidly (Martin et al, 1992; Ferrell et al, 1992).

Fulminant Hepatitis

Etiology: HBV (especially when it is associated with HDV) and drug therapy are the causes of massive or submassive hepatic necrosis in the vast majority of patients with fulminant hepatitis. A diagnosis of Wilson's disease should be considered in young patients who have hemolytic anemia in association with fulminant hepatic failure. Mortality rates approach 80% in patients with fulminant hepatitis.

Therapy: Fluid and electrolyte balance should be maintained, and hypoxia, hypotension, hypoglycemia, and clotting defects should be corrected. At present, all therapy is experimental. The only treatment that has reduced the mortality rate is liver transplantation. In contrast to patients with chronic hepatitis B who undergo liver transplantation, recurrent infection following transplantation is unlikely in patients with acute fulminant hepatitis B.

For more detailed information, see index entries Interferons; Hepatitis, Viral; Antiviral Agents.

Primary Biliary Cirrhosis and Primary Sclerosing Cholangitis

The etiology of these inflammatory diseases is unknown, but a disorder of immune function is suspected as the primary cause. In both primary biliary cirrhosis (PBC) and primary sclerosing cholangitis (PSC), the destruction of the bile ducts impairs bile flow (cholestasis) and causes retention of toxic substances, such as bile acids, within the liver.

Signs and Symptoms: PBC is a chronic, progressive, and often fatal cholestatic liver disease that is characterized by the destruction of intrahepatic bile ducts and portal inflammation and scarring. As the disease progresses, signs of chronic cholestasis may develop (eg, pruritus, increasing jaundice, osteoporosis, deficiency of fat-soluble vitamins). It eventually produces cirrhosis and liver failure (Kaplan, 1990 A; Stavinoha and Soloway, 1990).

PBC occurs primarily in middle-aged women, most of whom are asymptomatic when first identified by liver chemistry screening. Asymptomatic individuals have not been treated in the past; however, recent data showing that these patients have shortened life spans and that more than 80% develop active disease suggest the need for earlier treatment (Balasubramaniam et al, 1990; Kaplan, 1990 B).

PSC is a chronic cholestatic disease characterized by inflammation, scarring, and obliteration of both the intrahepatic and extrahepatic biliary ducts (Stavinoha and Soloway, 1990; LaRusso and Wiesner, 1990; Kaplan, 1991). It is twice as common in males as in females. Symptoms do not develop until the disease is advanced, at which time the typical signs of cholestasis (eg, pruritus, increasing jaundice) occur. PSC usually progresses to fibrosis, cirrhosis, and liver failure. More than 70% of patients also have inflammatory bowel disease.

Therapy: In both disorders, treatment is symptomatic. No therapy affects the underlying disease process, provides prolonged relief of symptoms, or prolongs the life of patients with PBC or PSC (Kaplan, 1990 A; LaRusso and Wiesner, 1990). However, results of several studies indicate that ursodiol (ursodeoxycholic acid) [Actigall] and methotrexate may provide substantial symptomatic relief and have the potential to prolong survival.

In several studies involving small numbers of patients, low doses of methotrexate (Kaplan and Knox, 1991; Bergasa et al, 1991; Knox and Kaplan, 1991; Kaplan, 1991) and ursodiol (Beuers et al, 1992; Stavinoha and Soloway, 1990; O'Brien and Senior, 1991; Kaplan, 1991; Poupon et al, 1991) were effective and safe in early-stage PBC or PSC (stages I and II). Both drugs relieved symptoms and improved biochemical markers of liver function and some histologic features of the diseases. The improvement in histology may be less pronounced with ursodiol than with methotrexate and, in some studies, patients with PBC did not respond to ursodiol (Perdigoto and Wiesner, 1992). Long-term use of low doses of methotrexate (average, 15 mg/week [5 mg every 12 hours for three doses]) is well tolerated and has not produced signs of hepatotoxicity, but more data are needed to confirm long-term safety (Hoofnagle and Bergasa, 1991). Methotrexate-associated pneumonitis may occur in up to 8% of patients but is usually reversible on discontinuation of the drug (Kaplan, 1993). Ursodiol 600 mg (300 mg twice daily) or up to 15 mg/kg also is well tolerated and is widely used for treatment of early-stage PBC. More definitive data are needed to determine if methotrexate or ursodiol halts progression of histologic changes or extends the lives of patients.

Cyclosporine [Sandimmune], a potent immunosuppressive agent, also decreased symptoms and improved biochemical markers in patients with early-stage PBC (Wiesner et al, 1990). Its effect on histologic changes has been less evident, and it may not prolong survival (Lombard et al, 1993). A significant number of patients developed hypertension and had kidney damage. Further studies are necessary to determine if long-term therapy halts the histologic progression of PBC and if the benefits justify the risk of toxicity. Controlled studies are being performed to determine the effects of cyclosporine on PSC.

Some practitioners have advocated the use of corticosteroids in patients with PBC (Wiesner et al, 1988). However, because osteoporosis is a major adverse effect of corticosteroids and is also a major complication of PBC, their use is contraindicated in this disorder. Azathioprine has been reported to increase survival time (Christensen et al, 1985), but this observation requires confirmation. Colchicine in doses of 0.6 mg twice daily has produced signs of biochemical improvement, but neither symptoms nor histologic progression of the disease appears to be affected (Kaplan et al, 1986; Zifroni and Schaffner, 1991). Rarely, this drug may cause granulocytopenia (Finklestein et al, 1987). Although penicillamine [Cuprimine, Depen] has relieved symptoms in some patients, its use in PBC is no longer recommended because survival time is not improved significantly and the incidence of side effects is high (Dickson et al, 1985).

Cholestyramine resin [Questran] relieves pruritus, which is often disabling in these patients. Large-volume plasmapheresis relieves pruritus and xanthomatous neuropathy in the rare patient who does not respond to cholestyramine. Ursodiol also has relieved pruritus in those with PBC or PSC. Phenobarbital and antihistamines (eg, hydroxyzine) rarely are useful for pruritus; rifampin [Rifadin, Rimactane] and naloxone [Narcan] are being investigated for this use (Podesta et al, 1991; Bergasa et al, 1992).

Deficiencies of vitamins A, D, E, and K and iron may occur in PBC patients, especially those with severe jaundice, steatorrhea, or malabsorption, and administration of these fat-soluble vitamins or iron to those with iron-deficiency anemia may be necessary. A low-fat diet supplemented with medium-chain triglycerides also is used to treat symptomatic steatorrhea. There is no effective treatment for hepatic osteodystrophy. The administration of vitamin D or its derivatives in a dose of 1,000 to 5,000 units daily rarely may slow progression of the bone disease.

Most patients with end-stage PBC or PSC are candidates for liver transplantation (Wiesner et al, 1992).

Portal Systemic Encephalopathy

Etiology: Portal systemic encephalopathy (PSE) encompasses a spectrum of psychiatric and neurologic abnormalities ranging from subtle impairment of intellectual function to deep coma. This syndrome is the result of a metabolic disorder of the central nervous system that occurs as a complication of hepatic failure or shunting of portal blood into the systemic circulation or as a result of an inherited deficiency of urea cycle enzymes. Four hypotheses concerning the pathogenesis of the derangement of neurotransmission that underlies PSE are being considered (Mullen, 1991; Butterworth, 1992): (1) hyperammonemia caused by defective conversion of ammonia to urea, (2) alterations in gamma-aminobutyric acid ($GABA_A$) receptor complexes in the brain, (3) presence of other neurotoxins (mercaptans and short-chain fatty acids), and (4) presence of false neurotransmitters (eg, octopamine, phenylethanolamine).

Therapy: Current therapy is aimed at improving hepatocellular function and identifying precipitating factors (hypnotic-sedative drugs, gastrointestinal hemorrhage, hypokalemia, sepsis). Therapy to reduce or eliminate sources of excess protein in the gastrointestinal tract is instituted; dietary protein is decreased; and laxatives, enemas, or antibiotics are administered to eliminate ammonia-producing bacteria in the bowel.

The primary drugs used to manage PSE are lactulose [Cephulac], a synthetic disaccharide that may decrease the production of ammonia by bacteria and/or enhance its excretion by producing enteric acidosis, and neomycin [Mycifradin], a poorly absorbed antibiotic that decreases bacterial production of ammonia. Lactulose is effective for acute as well as prolonged maintenance therapy. Neomycin is used rarely as an adjunct for short-term management of severe disease. It may have a more rapid onset of action, but is partially absorbed and can cause significant adverse effects, particularly in patients with impaired renal function. Lactulose is less toxic, especially in older patients and in those with renal impairment or constipation. In one clinical trial, a combination of lactulose and neomycin produced synergistic effects (Weber et al, 1982). In another study, this combination did not appear to be more effective than either drug alone (Crossley and Williams, 1984). Patients who respond poorly to lactulose may respond to nonabsorbable oral antibiotics such as vancomycin [Vancocin] (Tarao et al, 1990) or metronidazole (Morgan et al, 1982).

Investigationally, lactose, a precursor of lactulose, appears to be effective when PSE occurs in association with lactase deficiency. Another investigational disaccharide, lactitol (beta galactoside-sorbitol disaccharide), is more palatable than lactulose and has been effective in clinical trials; it also may be administered by enema (Blanc et al, 1992).

Substantial levels of endogenous substance(s) with benzodiazepine receptor-binding and immunoreactive properties are present in patients with PSE (Mullen et al, 1990; Basile et al, 1991). The benzodiazepine antagonist, flumazenil [Mazicon], has relieved symptoms in some patients (Ferenci et al, 1989; Howard and Seifert, 1993). See index entry Flumazenil, Uses, Portal Systemic Encephalopathy.

Although branched-chain amino acids showed initial promise in those with mild or early PSE (Egberts et al, 1985) and some investigators believe that they may have short-term benefit in reversing coma in acute PSE (Naylor et al, 1989), there is little convincing evidence of their value (Eriksson and Conn, 1989).

Portal Hypertension

Increased resistance to portal blood flow elevates portal pressure. Such increased resistance may be caused by intrahepatic processes resulting in compression of hepatic venules by regenerating nodules in the cirrhotic liver, deposition of collagen in the space of Disse or periportal areas, and/or enlargement of hepatocytes with consequent sinusoidal compression. Other causes of portal hypertension are impaired hepatic venous outflow (eg, Budd-Chiari syndrome, veno-occlusive disease) or obstruction of portal vein flow (eg, portal vein thrombosis).

Bleeding occurs in one-quarter to one-half of patients with esophagogastric varices within one year of diagnosis and, to a large extent, the degree depends on variceal size and portal pressure. The risk of recurrent bleeding is 30% at six weeks and 70% at one year (Graham and Smith, 1981). The mortality rate of patients experiencing variceal bleeding is almost 50%. Because of the great difficulty in treating acute hemorrhage or preventing early recurrent bleeding, prevention of the initial bleeding episode is critical.

Therapy: The intravenous infusion of vasopressin [Pitressin Synthetic] in combination with nitroglycerin is usually employed as the initial therapy for acute variceal bleeding (Conn, 1986). However, vasopressin has not been shown to be effective for acute variceal hemorrhage in controlled trials. Somatostatin analogues (eg, octreotide [Sandostatin]) may be safer than vasopressin (Resnick, 1990), but conflicting conclusions on their value were reported in two major controlled studies (Valenzuela et al, 1989; Burroughs et al, 1990).

For bleeding not controlled by medical therapy, placement of a gastric or esophageal balloon tamponade and endoscopic sclerotherapy are alternative therapies. In the latter procedure, the injection of sclerosing substances (eg, sodium morrhuate, sodium tetradecyl sulfate, ethanolamine oleate) into esophageal varices has stopped acute bleeding in patients with moderate or severe liver disease; success rates have ranged from 75% to 90% (Grace, 1990). Many authorities consider this procedure the treatment of choice for actively bleeding varices. Although the frequency of recurrent bleeding also is decreased, it has not been established whether survival is prolonged (Grace, 1990; Hashizume et al, 1992).

The prophylactic value of sclerotherapy in patients who have never hemorrhaged is unclear and generally it is not recommended in these individuals. Although two meta-analyses of randomized and nonrandomized trials demonstrated benefits for prophylactic sclerotherapy (Van Ruiswyk and Byrd, 1992; Pagliaro et al, 1992), results of two large multicenter studies indicated not only lack of value but a significant increase in mortality (The PROVA Study Group, 1991; The Veterans Affairs Cooperative Variceal Sclerotherapy Group, 1991). Complications, which occur in less than 10% of patients, include severe bleeding, perforation, mediastinitis, esophageal ulcers or strictures, portal vein thrombosis, fistulas, and pulmonary emboli. The administration of propranolol [Inderal] to cirrhotic patients receiving sclerotherapy may be more effective than sclerotherapy alone in reducing the rate of recurrence of bleeding (Vinel et al, 1992).

In patients with alcoholic cirrhosis, propranolol in a dose that reduces the resting pulse by 20% has been reported to reduce the risk of recurrent variceal bleeding by blocking both $beta_1$- and $beta_2$-adrenergic receptors (Lebrec et al, 1981; Pascal et al, 1987); the effectiveness of this drug in these patients has been questioned, however (Burroughs et al, 1983; Dickson et al, 1985; Vorobioff et al, 1987). Beta-blocker therapy may only postpone bleeding episodes rather than eliminate the risk of hemorrhage (Grace, 1990; Conn et al, 1991).

In randomized clinical trials, prophylactic doses of propranolol alone appeared to prevent initial hemorrhage from varices (Pascal et al, 1987), but it is unclear if survival is enhanced (Conn et al, 1991; Poynard et al, 1991). Another beta receptor antagonist, nadolol [Corgard], also has been used (Lebrec et al, 1988). It may have some theoretical advantages over propranolol, but significant differences have not been observed clinically (Poynard et al, 1991). Beta-blocking drugs may be less useful in cirrhotic patients in whom clotting factors are altered significantly because these drugs inhibit platelet aggregation.

In cirrhotic patients with hypertensive portal gastropathy, propranolol reduces the likelihood of recurrent bleeding from gastric lesions (Panés et al, 1993).

Endoscopic ligation or transjugular intrahepatic portasystemic shunt (TIPS) may be effective alternatives to sclerotherapy for bleeding esophageal varices (Stiegmann et al, 1992; *Mayo Clin Update*, 1992). Portasystemic shunt surgery may control recurrent esophageal or gastric bleeding and reduce portal vein pressure in patients with hepatic cirrhosis, but hepatic encephalopathy may occur in up to 30% of patients. Prophylactic shunt surgery is not recommended because it does not prolong survival significantly (Clark, 1982; Grace, 1990).

Drug Evaluations

LACTULOSE
[Cephulac]

OH
CH_2OH
CH_2OH
HO
OH
O
OH HO
CH_2OH

ACTIONS. Lactulose, a poorly absorbed, synthetic disaccharide prepared from lactose, reduces blood ammonia levels by mechanisms that are not fully understood. This drug is not metabolized in the upper intestinal tract and thus is not absorbed. Lactulose is degraded in the colon by intestinal bacteria into low-molecular-weight organic acids that decrease the pH of the colonic contents and have an osmotic laxative action. Acidification inhibits the production of ammonia by bacteria and enhances the transport of blood ammonia to the colonic lumen; there it is converted to ammonium ion, which is poorly absorbed. Colonic transit time is accelerated by the laxative effect of the organic acids and the excretion of ammonium ion is increased (Conn, 1978).

Lactulose also stimulates bacterial growth, enhances protein synthesis, and inhibits protein catabolism. Stimulation of protein synthesis may enhance the incorporation of ammonia from the lumen and tissue stores into bacterial protein. By inhibiting protein breakdown by luminal bacteria, lactulose may block the formation of ammonia, short-chain fatty acids, and other toxic substances (Mortensen et al, 1990).

USES. Lactulose is useful for the treatment of acute episodes and for long-term maintenance therapy in portal systemic encephalopathy (PSE); it also improves protein tolerance in patients with advanced hepatic failure (Conn et al, 1977; Atterbury et al, 1978). Recurrences of encephalopathy are reduced in approximately 75% of patients, and an increase in protein intake and discontinuation of neomycin are usually possible. Improvement may be noted within one to three days, but maximal benefits may not be evident for 10 to 14 days.

The purified crystalline preparation of lactulose (not available in the United States) is equally effective and causes fewer adverse effects.

ADVERSE REACTIONS. Lactulose may cause transient abdominal distention and discomfort, flatulence, nausea, and vomiting. Excessive doses cause diarrhea. Rarely, hyperglycemia may occur.

This drug is classified in FDA Pregnancy Category B.

DOSAGE AND PREPARATIONS.

Oral: Treatment should be initiated with a single cleansing enema (which need not contain lactulose). *Adults,* for acute PSE, initially, 30 to 45 ml (20 to 30 g) every four hours. When laxation occurs, the frequency of administration may be reduced to three or four times daily. For maintenance, 15 to 45 ml (10 to 30 g) is given three or four times daily. Dosage should be adjusted every one or two days to produce two or three soft stools daily. Overdosage of lactulose will produce diarrhea and may create a significant nursing problem and promote bed sores in nonambulatory (especially comatose) patients. *Older children and adolescents,* 30 to 90 ml (20 to 60 g) daily in two or three divided doses. If the initial dose causes diarrhea, subsequent doses should be reduced.

Rectal: *Adults,* 300 ml is mixed with 700 ml of water or saline and given as a retention enema. The enema is retained for 30 to 60 minutes. Administration may be repeated every four to six hours. Coma may be reversed within two hours after the first enema. Enemas should be reserved for adults in impending coma or the coma stage of encephalopathy and when the danger of aspiration exists.

Cephulac (Marion Merrell Dow). Syrup 10 g/15 ml (<2.2 g galactose, <1.2 g lactose, and 1.2 g or less of other sugars).

NEOMYCIN SULFATE

[Mycifradin]

For chemical formula, see index entry Neomycin, As Antibacterial Agent.

ACTIONS AND USES. When given orally, this poorly absorbed aminoglycoside reduces hyperammonemia in patients with portal systemic encephalopathy (PSE), presumably by destroying urea-splitting (urease positive) intestinal bacteria. This mechanism of action has been questioned, however, because neomycin has no effect on anaerobic gut flora, which are the predominant bacteria generating ammonia and other neurotoxins.

Neomycin is used adjunctively for the short-term management of severe PSE and may have a more rapid onset of action than lactulose; however, the latter is less toxic and is preferred for long-term therapy. Neomycin is seldom used now.

ADVERSE REACTIONS AND PRECAUTIONS. Diarrhea and reversible malabsorption are the most common adverse effects; nausea and vomiting also occur. Superinfections may develop after prolonged use. Patients who cannot tolerate or are hypersensitive to other aminoglycosides may respond similarly to neomycin. Contraindications include the presence of inflammatory bowel disorders, which may increase absorption, and intestinal obstruction. Ototoxicity or nephrotoxicity may be observed, especially in patients with inflammatory bowel disease or renal insufficiency or after prolonged use in patients without intestinal or renal disease. The risk of toxicity may be increased when neomycin is used for longer than two weeks.

For additional discussion of adverse reactions and precautions, see index entry Neomycin, As Antibacterial Agent.

DOSAGE AND PREPARATIONS.

Oral: *Adults,* initially, 4 to 8 g daily in divided doses for five to six days; for maintenance, 2 to 4 g daily. The manufacturer's recommended maximum total daily dose is 12 g; however, most authorities limit the dose to 8 g/day.

Generic. Tablets 500 mg.

Mycifradin (Upjohn). Solution (oral) 125 mg/5 ml (equivalent to 87.5 mg of base).

DISORDERS OF THE BILIARY TRACT

Composition of Bile Acids and Salts: The primary bile acids, cholic acid and chenodeoxycholic acid, are formed from cholesterol in the liver. Deoxycholic and lithocholic acids are produced by 7-dehydroxylation of cholic acid and chenodeoxycholic acid, respectively, by anaerobic intestinal bacteria. Ursodeoxycholic acid is present in human bile in trace amounts; it is formed from chenodeoxycholic acid by bacterial action in the large intestine and possibly from the 7-oxo derivative of chenodeoxycholic acid in the liver.

Bile acids do not occur as such in bile, but rather as N-glycine or N-taurine conjugates. Conjugation increases their solubility, makes them more resistant to precipitation by calcium, decreases passive intestinal absorption, and prevents bacterial 7-dehydroxylation. Lithocholic acid is not only conjugated with glycine or taurine but also is sulfated at the 3 position. Sulfation decreases intestinal absorption, thus hastening elimination of this hepatotoxic bile acid.

Endogenous Actions of Bile: In humans, bile serves as the unique excretory pathway for cholesterol, which is transported in bile and dissolved in mixed micelles containing bile acids and phospholipid. Cholesterol is secreted into the intestine during digestion and a mixed micelle with a new composition is formed; this new aggregate contains predominantly fatty acids and monoglycerides formed by the action of lipase and colipase on dietary triglycerides.

Bile acids facilitate absorption by enhancing the diffusion of solubilized fat digestion products through the unstirred layer of water that coats the intestinal mucosa. Micellar solubilization of fat-soluble vitamins is essential for their absorption. The conjugated bile acids are reabsorbed mainly in the ileum by active transport and return to the liver, where they are extracted and re-excreted in bile, thus completing the enterohepatic circulation. The bile acid pool (ie, the mass of bile acids in the enterohepatic circulation) circulates six to ten times a day. The only input of bile acids into the enterohepatic circulation is by synthesis from cholesterol; the only loss is by fecal excretion.

Many conditions interfere with the enterohepatic circulation of bile acids. The major disturbances are biliary obstruction, biliary fistula, ileal disease or resection, and bacterial overgrowth (eg, in the stagnant loop syndrome). These defects impair micelle formation, causing maldigestion of fat and steatorrhea.

Replacement Therapy

At present, no preparation of conjugated bile acids is satisfactory for replacement therapy. Commercial ox bile preparations do not provide an adequate amount of conjugated bile acids (about 4 to 8 g are secreted with each meal) and produce diarrhea (dihydroxy bile acids induce secretion of water and electrolytes by the colon). Thus, they are not useful in conditions in which a deficiency of bile acids in the small intestine causes steatorrhea. However, successful replacement therapy with bile acids was reported in one patient with an ileostomy and significant steatorrhea (Fordtran et al, 1982).

Synthetic dehydrocholic acid [Decholin], an oxidized derivative of cholic acid, is metabolized to cholic acid (and hydroxy-oxo bile acids) in the liver. A hydrocholeretic effect has been reported, but controlled studies demonstrating that such an effect is therapeutically useful are lacking.

Gallstones

Bile acids play an important role in solubilizing cholesterol in bile. When their secretion is decreased or cholesterol secretion is increased, bile cholesterol may precipitate from solution and form cholesterol gallstones. Calcium bilirubinate (pigment) gallstones are formed by deconjugation of bilirubin conjugates after their secretion into bile. The unconjugated bilirubin forms an insoluble salt with calcium ions. The precipitate may polymerize and thus form black pigment stones, usually in the gallbladder. In contrast, brown stones are usually formed in the bile ducts, and bacterial degradation products of bile (ie, calcium bilirubinate, calcium palmitate, small amounts of cholesterol) predominate.

Cholelithiasis affects about 10% of the population of the United States (20% over age 50). Gallstones are three times more common in women than in men. Obesity and/or genetic predisposition are important causative factors. In many patients, the probable mechanism for development is abnormal cholesterol metabolism with decreased synthesis of bile acids in conjunction with increased production of cholesterol. Defects that appear to be present in most patients with cholesterol gallstones include bile that is supersaturated with cholesterol, more rapid cholesterol nucleation, and impaired gallbladder evacuation. The symptoms of active disease include biliary colic and jaundice if bile duct obstruction occurs, but the majority of patients remain asymptomatic. Many practitioners believe that only symptomatic patients require treatment (Hofmann, 1990; Ransohoff et al, 1983; Tangedahl, 1983; Tyor, 1983).

MANAGEMENT OF GALLSTONES. A number of treatment options are available; for reviews, see Strasberg and Clavien, 1992; Johnston and Kaplan, 1993; NIH Consensus Development Panel on Gallstones and Laparoscopic Cholecystectomy, 1993).

Surgery: Surgery is recommended for most patients with symptomatic gallstones, particularly those with complications such as acute cholecystitis, bile duct stones, or pancreatitis. When intervention is required, laparoscopic cholecystectomy (LC) is the therapy of choice (Strasberg and Clavien, 1992; Johnston and Kaplan, 1993; Shaw, 1993). Only about 5% of patients subsequently require conventional cholecystectomy; the percentage varies with the clinical setting and the experience of the surgeon. Acute cholecystitis is no longer considered a contraindication to LC (Wilson et al, 1992).

LC is a rapid, relatively safe, and curative procedure (Reddick and Olsen, 1989; *JAMA,* 1991; Wolfe et al, 1991); compared with conventional cholecystectomy, LC is less painful and less invasive, requires a shorter hospital stay (less than two days), allows the patient to return to full activity more quickly, and produces minimal scarring. Although the incidence of intraoperative bile duct injury has been higher with LC than with conventional cholecystectomy, this has decreased significantly as surgeons have gained greater experience with this procedure (Ratliff et al, 1992). LC requires a larger number of pre- and postoperative endoscopic retrograde cholangiopancreatography procedures and endoscopic sphincterotomy. Therefore, it must be considered a major surgical procedure with risks similar to those of conventional cholecystectomy (Southern Surgeons Club, 1991).

Drug Therapy: With the rapid acceptance of LC as the therapy of choice for symptomatic patients, it is recommended that gallstone dissolution therapy be reserved for patients who require treatment but refuse surgery, for patients in whom surgery or general anesthesia would be hazardous (Johnston and Kaplan, 1993), or for patients in whom complicating illness makes surgery hazardous. Medical therapy can dissolve stones and make surgery unnecessary in many of these individuals. However, delaying surgery may increase operative morbidity and mortality in poor-risk patients (McSherry, 1981).

At present, chenodiol (chenodeoxycholic acid) [Chenix] and ursodiol (ursodeoxycholic acid) [Actigall] are used for gallstone dissolution therapy in carefully selected patients. Some practitioners believe that ursodiol (but not chenodiol) relieves symptoms of biliary distress before dissolution of the gallstones; however, the data are inconclusive. Relief also occurs in some patients given a placebo. Chenodiol and ursodiol decrease cholesterol secretion into bile, thus desaturating bile in most patients and dissolving cholesterol gallstones if the surface is accessible to the desaturated bile and the stones have a very high cholesterol content (Palmer and Carey, 1982).

Results of the National Cooperative Gallstone Study (NCGS) to determine the efficacy of chenodiol were disappointing (Schoenfield et al, 1981). In this controlled, multicenter trial, more than 900 patients received chenodiol 375 or 750 mg/day for two years. The larger dose completely dissolved gallstones in only 14% of patients. A dose of 750 mg/day is equivalent to approximately 11/mg/kg in patients of average body weight and is considered suboptimal. Thus, lean patients received a higher mg/kg dose, and their rate of response was better than that of overweight or obese patients. It is now clear that chenodiol is less effective in doses smaller than 13 mg/kg/day (Tangedahl et al, 1983).

In the NCGS, chenodiol increased serum cholesterol (particularly low density lipoproteins) by 10% and elevated serum AST levels; termination of therapy was required in 3% of those receiving the larger dose (750 mg/day). In several patients, hepatic lesions formed and resembled those induced by lithocholic acid (the major metabolite of chenodiol). Mild diarrhea also occurred.

In a number of studies, the effectiveness of ursodiol in dissolving cholesterol gallstones was similar to that of chenodiol.

Stone dissolution is more rapid in some patients (Ward et al, 1984), and the drug generally is well tolerated. The only significant adverse effect, intolerable diarrhea, is observed in less than 1% of patients. Currently, ursodiol appears to be the drug of choice for gallstone dissolution and is preferred to chenodiol by most physicians (Affronti and Putnam, 1991; Fromm and Albert, 1991; Salen et al, 1990). Although a 1:1 combination of ursodiol and chenodiol has been used and is as effective as ursodiol alone (Sackmann et al, 1991), the possible advantages of this combination have not been established (Podda et al, 1989; Sackmann et al, 1990 A).

Calcification of gallstones acquired during drug therapy has been reported; in the largest study to date, the prevalence of acquired calcification was similar in patients receiving either ursodiol or chenodiol (Frabboni et al, 1985).

Radiopaque cholesterol gallstones containing more than 4% calcium are resistant to complete dissolution by either bile acid. Dissolution often occurs only until a pigment layer, a calcified shell, or an insoluble nidus is reached. Prior to initiating therapy, stone calcium content can best be assessed by CT scanning using 3 to 5 mm slices without contrast. Black pigment gallstones (some of which are radiolucent on conventional x-ray) have greater x-ray attenuation than predominantly cholesterol gallstones and are more radiodense than bile on CT scan (Ell et al, 1991). Oral cholecystography contrast medium may remain in the gallbladder for at least seven to ten days and may be confused with calcium on CT scan.

Overall, some dissolution occurs in 40% to 80% of appropriately selected patients within three months to two years after treatment with adequate doses of either chenodiol or ursodiol; about one-half of these patients experience total dissolution of stones. Complete dissolution occurs more often in those with gallstones less than 15 mm in diameter or with noncalcified radiolucent stones that are "floating" (ie, that float during oral cholecystography) (Malet et al, 1990). Gallstones dissolve completely in over 80% of those with floating radiolucent stones when either bile acid is taken for up to two years (Tangedahl et al, 1983). However, only 10% to 15% of patients have this type of stone. In patients who respond to treatment, the decrease in diameter of the stones is linear, averaging 0.7 mm/month (Senior et al, 1990).

The extent of dissolution is most accurately assessed by oral cholecystography performed at 6- to 12-month intervals. Lack of visualization of the gallbladder is not an indication for discontinuing treatment unless this is observed on two examinations 3 to 6 months apart. Complete dissolution is most accurately verified by ultrasound; two negative examinations are necessary before patients can be considered free of stones. Therapy should be continued for at least three months after apparent complete dissolution. Patients who do not respond to chenodiol or ursodiol after 12 months probably will not achieve complete stone dissolution. Therapy should be discontinued if there is no significant decrease in stone size after 12 to 18 months (Tyor, 1983; Tangedahl, 1983). As long as dissolution is progressing, however, continued treatment may be appropriate.

Following complete dissolution with chenodiol or ursodiol, about 50% of patients with multiple stones experience recurrences within five years; in comparison, the rate of recurrence is 10% to 20% in patients who had a single stone (Villanova et al, 1989). Retreatment is usually successful, but if stones recur, life-long therapy with ursodiol or chenodiol may be necessary. Some authorities believe that x-ray monitoring has no value since asymptomatic patients are not treated.

Patients receiving ursodiol or chenodiol must have a functioning gallbladder (a patent cystic duct) as assessed by oral cholecystography. Chenodiol must not be used in those with evidence of chronic liver disease, hepatobiliary obstruction, or cholestasis. It is generally recommended that pregnant women or those likely to become pregnant should not be treated with chenodiol or ursodiol; however, ursodiol has been used to treat cholestatic syndromes associated with pregnancy and no apparent side effects have been observed.

Extracorporeal Shock Wave Lithotripsy (ESWL): This noninvasive procedure has been introduced into the United States in investigational protocols but is not approved by the Food and Drug Administration (FDA). The technique involves the combination of gallstone fragmentation by focused shockwaves followed by dissolution of the fragments by oral therapy with chenodiol or ursodiol (Albert and Fromm, 1990; Schoenfield et al, 1990; Affronti and Putnam, 1991). Spontaneous passage of gallstone fragments also may occur. The lithotripsy technique is similar in principle to that used for the treatment of renal stones, which has been judged safe and effective by the FDA. At least 12 manufacturers have developed devices utilizing spark gap, piezoelectric, or electromagnetic shock wave generators.

The criteria for selection of eligible patients vary among different investigational protocols but are more restrictive than those used for medical dissolution of gallstones with chenodiol or ursodiol. Typical criteria include the presence of not more than three radiolucent stones, the total diameter of which must be less than 3 cm, and the ability to visualize the gallbladder during oral cholecystography. Patients with evidence of common duct stones have been excluded from most lithotripsy procedures. In addition, it must be possible to localize the stones by ultrasound, and the stones must be positioned in the focal point of the shock wave. In early studies, general anesthesia was used, but intravenous analgesia has been satisfactory (Sackmann et al, 1987). The use of piezoelectric ESWL eliminates the need for analgesia, anesthesia, or sedation in most patients, although more treatment sessions may be required than with use of other shock wave generators (Darzi et al, 1991; Weber et al, 1991).

Experience with ESWL in Germany with several hundred highly selected patients has been satisfactory. Post-treatment pain was mild, and surgical complications or acute pancreatitis occurred in only a small percentage of patients. In 80% of ideal candidates (those with solitary stones less than 20 mm in diameter), all stone fragments dissolved or passed within three to nine months, and the gallbladder appeared to be free of detectable fragments. As with use of chenodiol or ursodiol, gallstones recur in 10% to 20% of patients with a single stone, and the rate of recurrence is higher in those with two or three stones or with defective gallbladder motility (Albert et al, 1990; Sackmann et al, 1990 B, 1991).

In controlled studies, ursodiol used with ESWL was twice as effective in eliminating residual gallstone fragments as ESWL alone (Schoenfield et al, 1990). An advantage of ESWL and ursodiol over dissolution by oral agents alone is most notable in those with a solitary gallstone 1 to 3 cm in diameter; however, only 15% of patients fulfill these criteria (Brink et al, 1990).

Both ESWL and ursodiol are well tolerated. Mild to moderate transient abnormalities in liver tests occur in a small percentage of patients. Mild acute pancreatitis and/or transient cholestasis have been reported in less than 2% of patients, but the risk of biliary colic is substantial in these individuals. Mortality is negligible. If gallstone fragments are not eliminated after oral ursodiol therapy (up to 10% of selected patients), LC or conventional cholecystectomy is required.

The successful use of lithotripters for fragmentation of duct stones also is well established (Becker et al, 1987; Sauerbruch et al, 1989). The combination of ESWL and contact dissolution of gallstones with solvents such as methyl-*tert*-butyl-ether remains investigational (Peine et al, 1989; Holl et al, 1991). Such an approach offers complete dissolution of all gallstone fragments within a few hours after stone fragmentation by ESWL.

Methyl-tert-butyl-ether (MTBE) Dissolution Therapy: MTBE is an alkyl ether that is similar to diethyl ether in physical and chemical properties but, in contrast to diethyl ether, MTBE is liquid at body temperature. MTBE is an excellent solvent for cholesterol (14 g/ml); because of this and its extremely low viscosity, MTBE dissolves cholesterol gallstones at least 50 times more rapidly than monoctanoin [Moctanin]. Limited experience suggests that cholesterol stones in the gallbladder can be dissolved with MTBE in 6 to 12 hours (Allen et al, 1985; Thistle, 1987; Thistle et al, 1989).

A percutaneous transhepatic pigtail catheter of solvent-resistant material is placed in the gallbladder so that its pigtail surrounds the gallstones. The solvent is alternately infused and aspirated using a glass syringe. The infusion volume should be less than the amount that leaks into the cystic duct. Pumps for automated infusion/aspiration of MTBE are being developed (Zakko and Hofmann, 1990; Poterucha et al, 1991). A nasobiliary catheter placed in the gallbladder using endoscopy also has been employed by several investigators.

The advantages of dissolution therapy with MTBE include the lack of need for general anesthesia, absence of abdominal scarring, safety when performed by experienced practitioners, and the relatively low risk for elderly patients and, especially, those with pulmonary or cardiovascular disease (Thistle, 1990; Thistle et al, 1989). Risks of the procedure are those associated with catheter placement and removal or inadvertent overdosage. If an excess of MTBE overflows from the gallbladder, absorption may cause hemolysis and anesthesia. Whether MTBE treatment influences gallbladder function permanently is not known but seems unlikely.

Although MTBE is a remarkably powerful solvent for cholesterol gallstones, at present its use is investigational and is limited in most instances to patients at increased surgical risk. Dissolution therapy with MTBE is a labor-intensive procedure and can be used only by physicians who have obtained approval from the FDA. Other solvents such as ethyl propionate are being tested.

Bile Duct Stones

Bile duct stones are usually cholesterol or black pigment stones from the gallbladder or are primary duct stones composed mainly of a mixture of calcium palmitate and calcium bilirubinate. Primary duct stones form when cholestasis and bacteria are present.

Nonsurgical Therapy: In a patient without a T-tube, bile duct stones usually can be treated by endoscopic retrograde cholangiopancreatography (ERCP) with sphincterotomy, procedures at least as safe as surgery when performed by experienced practitioners (Horton et al, 1991; Johnston and Kaplan, 1993). After ERCP with sphincterotomy, almost 90% of the stones can be removed by balloon, Dormia basket, and/or mechanical lithotripsy. When a T-tube is in place, basket retrieval is usually successful; however, this cannot be done until a tract has formed, which requires at least four or five weeks.

For large bile duct stones, mechanical or extracorporeal shockwave lithotripsy (ESWL) appears to be useful for fragmenting stones (Sauerbruch et al, 1989). MTBE has been used investigationally after ESWL to dissolve the remaining fragments in patients with and without a T-tube. Rarely, a nasobiliary tube is placed and monoctanoin is infused to induce stone dissolution and/or passage (Venu et al, 1982; Vennes, 1983).

For reviews of procedures used for management of bile duct stones, see Johnston and Kaplan, 1993; and the NIH Consensus Development Panel on Gallstones and Laparoscopic Cholecystectomy, 1993.

Drug Evaluations

CHENODIOL (Chenodeoxycholic Acid)
[Chenix]

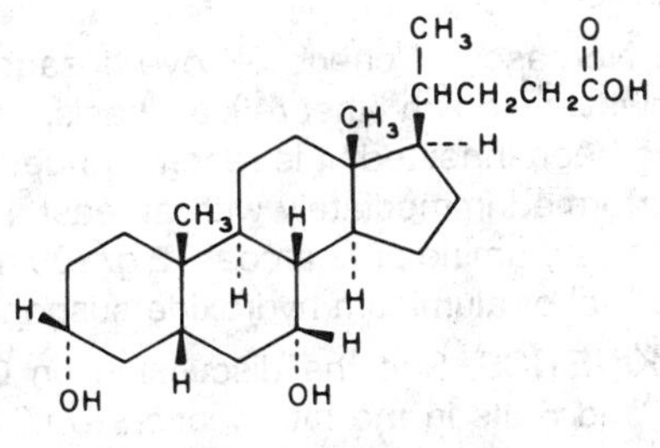

ACTIONS AND USES. Chenodiol, a natural dihydroxy bile acid, decreases cholesterol saturation of bile by decreasing the secretion of cholesterol and, in some patients, by increasing the secretion of bile acids. Thus, it promotes the dissolution of radiolucent cholesterol gallstones in selected patients (Hofmann, 1990). Radiopaque gallstones (containing calcium) and some radiolucent calcium bilirubinate stones (containing pigment) are resistant to dissolution.

Chenodiol has a limited role in gallstone dissolution therapy and has been largely supplanted by ursodiol (Affronti and Putnam, 1991; Salen et al, 1990). Considerable commitment by both the physician and patient is required for successful therapy. Up to one-third of patients do not complete the required duration of therapy (usually 24 months) (Tangedahl et al, 1983). The effectiveness of this agent and guidelines for its use are discussed in the Introduction to this section.

ADVERSE REACTIONS. Intermittent dose-related diarrhea is usually the only side effect. The dose should be reduced by one-half until the diarrhea abates and then increased gradually to the original level; it is only rarely necessary to discontinue treatment. Dyspepsia is uncommon and usually diminishes or disappears two to four weeks after initiation of therapy.

A reversible increase in the serum aspartate aminotransaminase (AST) level develops in some individuals. Therefore, the AST level should be measured before initiating treatment; at one-, three-, and six-month intervals during administration; and at six-month intervals thereafter. If the level is more than twice the upper limit of normal, unrelated viral hepatitis should be excluded. Chenodiol should be discontinued if alkaline phosphatase or bilirubin levels are elevated markedly.

Chenodiol may cause portal tract inflammation in hypersensitive patients (Fisher et al, 1991). This bile acid increases the low density lipoprotein fraction of cholesterol by about 10%, which may be a risk factor for atherosclerosis (Albers et al, 1982). The high density lipoprotein fraction is unaffected.

PRECAUTIONS. Relative contraindications include inflammatory diseases of the bile duct or bowel, obstructive hepatobiliary diseases, acute cholecystitis, and acute or chronic hepatitis. Women of childbearing age should receive chenodiol only in conjunction with effective contraception, because safety during pregnancy has not been documented (FDA Pregnancy Category X). For the same reason, it is not advisable to use this drug in lactating mothers.

DRUG INTERACTIONS. Cholestyramine, colestipol, and aluminum-containing antacids bind chenodiol and may decrease its absorption; therefore, simultaneous administration of these agents is inadvisable.

POISONING. No cases of chenodiol overdosage have been reported; however, on a theoretical basis, if excessive amounts have been ingested, it is recommended that gastric lavage be performed immediately with at least 1 L of a suspension of cholestyramine or charcoal (2 g/100 ml of water), followed by 50 ml of aluminum hydroxide suspension orally.

PHARMACOKINETICS. See the discussion on Composition of Bile Acids and Salts in the Introduction to this section. In patients with normal liver function, the intestinal absorption and hepatic uptake of chenodiol are so rapid that only a slight increase in blood concentration occurs.

DOSAGE AND PREPARATIONS. Chenodiol should be taken with meals or milk since it dissolves more rapidly in intestinal chyme when bile and pancreatic juices are present.

Oral: *Adults,* initially, 500 mg/day; the amount is increased gradually after one or two weeks until an approximate dose of 15 mg/kg/day (1 g/day) in divided amounts is reached. Doses <13 mg/kg/day are less effective.

A single bedtime dose combined with a low-cholesterol diet has been reported to almost double the rate of gallstone dissolution (Kupfer et al, 1982), thus reducing the duration and cost of therapy.

Chenix (Solvay). Tablets 250 mg.

URSODIOL (Ursodeoxycholic Acid)
[Actigall]

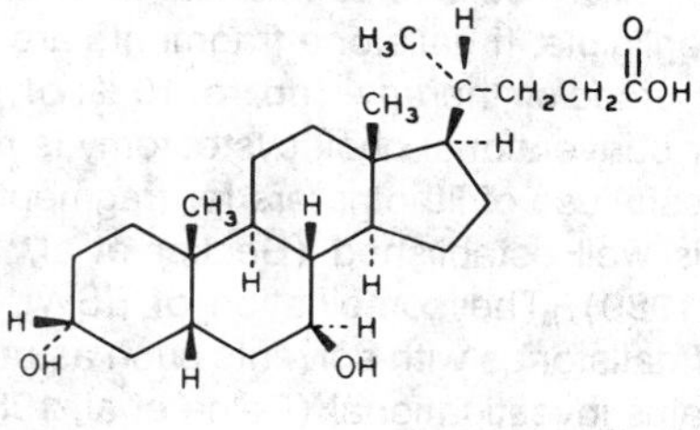

ACTIONS. This natural hydrophilic bile acid is prepared as a drug by chemical modification of chenodeoxycholic or cholic acid. Like chenodiol, ursodiol decreases the saturation index (ie, the bile concentration of cholesterol relative to bile acids), which results in dissolution of cholesterol from the surface of gallstones (Bachrach and Hofmann, 1982; Tint et al, 1986).

Unlike chenodiol, ursodiol does not efficiently solubilize cholesterol in micellar solution or increase the secretion of bile acids into bile. Instead it promotes the formation of a lecithin-cholesterol liquid layer at the surface of the stone (Fromm, 1984). Ursodiol decreases cholesterol secretion into the bile, but apparently not by decreasing cholesterol synthesis. It inhibits the absorption of cholesterol but does not appear to alter serum cholesterol levels in patients with gallstones.

USES. The effectiveness of ursodiol in dissolving radiolucent gallstones in carefully selected patients is similar to that of chenodiol, and ursodiol is preferred to chenodiol by most physicians (Affronti and Putnam, 1991; Shaw, 1993). Symptoms are relieved rapidly in many patients after its use. As with chenodiol, radiopaque gallstones (containing calcium) and some radiolucent calcium bilirubinate stones (containing pigment) are resistant to therapy. Guidelines for use of ursodiol for gallstone dissolution are discussed in the Introduction to this section. In controlled trials, ursodiol enhanced the dissolution of fragments produced by ESWL (Schoenfield et al, 1990).

Ursodiol decreases the proportion of circulating endogenous bile salts (cholic acid, deoxycholic acid). It also has anti-inflammatory actions due to its ability to inhibit the expression of histocompatibility antigens on cell surfaces. Both of these properties may contribute to its value in patients with early-stage primary biliary cirrhosis (PBC) and primary sclerosing cholangitis (PSC). See discussion on PBC and PSC in the Introduction.

ADVERSE REACTIONS AND PRECAUTIONS. Dose-related hypersensitivity-related elevation of serum aspartate aminotransaminase (AST) and alanine aminotransferase (ALT) levels is observed rarely. Intolerable diarrhea has been reported in less than 1% of patients and appears to be dose-related. These side effects occur much less frequently and are less severe than with chenodiol. Hepatic damage has not been reported (Ward et al, 1984; Affronti and Putnam, 1991).

In the largest study to date, the prevalence of acquired calcification of gallstones was similar in patients receiving either ursodiol or chenodiol (Frabboni et al, 1985).

Ursodiol is classified in FDA Pregnancy Category B.

The precautions and drug interactions are similar to those with chenodiol; the treatment of poisoning also is similar (see that evaluation).

PHARMACOKINETICS. Ursodiol is not completely absorbed from the intestine and is rapidly taken up by the liver, from which it is excreted into bile as conjugates with glycine and, to a much less extent, with taurine. Like chenodiol, this agent is converted to lithocholic acid in the distal intestine by colonic bacteria. Some lithocholic acid is absorbed and sulfated in the liver; sulfation prevents enterohepatic cycling and detoxifies this potentially hepatotoxic compound. In patients with normal liver function, oral absorption and hepatic uptake of ursodiol occur so rapidly that only a small increase in blood concentration occurs.

Enterohepatic recirculation of ursodeoxycholyl conjugates of ursodiol is quite efficient. The half-life following oral administration is 3.5 to 5.8 days.

DOSAGE AND PREPARATIONS. This drug should be taken with meals or milk since it dissolves more rapidly in intestinal chyme when bile and pancreatic juices are present.

Oral: *Adults,* 8 to 10 mg/kg/day given twice daily (usually a 300-mg capsule administered in the morning and evening).

Actigall (Summit). Capsules 300 mg.

MONOCTANOIN

[Moctanin]

The major constituents of this semisynthetic vegetable oil are the mono- and diglycerides of octanoic and decanoic acids. The product is predominantly glyceryl 1-mono-octanoate.

Monoctanoin has been effective in up to two-thirds of patients with retained radiolucent biliary duct stones containing more than 40% cholesterol (Palmer and Hofmann, 1986). It is only occasionally effective in recurrent bile duct stones and is ineffective in pigment stones containing little cholesterol.

The availability of endoscopic, percutaneous, and surgical procedures for extracting bile duct stones and the introduction of more effective direct-contact cholesterol solvents have greatly limited the value of monoctanoin and it is used infrequently (Peine, 1992).

Moctanin (Ethitek). Solution (sterile) in 120 ml containers.

DISORDERS OF THE PANCREAS

Optimum digestion of fat, carbohydrate, and protein depends on the exocrine function of the pancreas (ie, secretion of lipase, amylase, trypsin, and chymotrypsin). Pancreatic secretion of bicarbonate also is necessary to raise the pH and protect these enzymes from denaturation by acid and pepsin. Pancreatic enzyme replacement is required when pancreatic secretion is impaired by pancreatectomy, chronic pancreatitis, cystic fibrosis, or pancreatic duct obstruction caused by carcinoma or stricture.

The most common form of chronic pancreatitis is due to alcohol ingestion. In chronic alcoholics, the onset of symptoms with calcification and functional impairment usually occurs between age 40 and 50 years. Abstinence from alcohol is essential for these patients. Other major forms are juvenile and senile idiopathic chronic pancreatitis. The juvenile form is characterized by onset of severe abdominal pain before age 20 and the development of calcification and pancreatic insufficiency before age 30. The senile form occurs in patients 60 to 80 years; it usually is mild and is often asymptomatic (DiMagno and Clain, 1986; Ammann et al, 1987).

The duodenal pH in patients with chronic pancreatitis is often less than 5.0 late in the postprandial period. Glycine-conjugated bile acids may precipitate below pH 5.0, which reduces their bioavailability and further impairs fat absorption. The secretin stimulation test and endoscopic retrograde cholangiopancreatography (ERCP) offer the best sensitivity and specificity for diagnosing chronic pancreatitis (Toskes and Greenberger, 1983). However, simpler indirect tests, such as bentiromide or serum trypsin-like immunoreactivity, also are useful for this assessment (Toskes, 1984; Jacobson et al, 1984).

Replacement Therapy

Drug Selection: The pancreatic enzymes present in pancreatin and pancrelipase (lipase, protease [trypsin or chymotrypsin], and amylase) are extracted from hog pancreata. Pancreatin and pancrelipase are effective for replacement therapy in diseases accompanied by a marked decrease in the secretion of these enzymes (eg, chronic pancreatitis, benign or malignant pancreatic tumors, cystic fibrosis, pancreatectomy). However, these enzymes should be prescribed only after the diagnosis of exocrine pancreatic insufficiency has been confirmed. There is no rationale for their use in gastrointestinal disorders unrelated to pancreatic enzyme deficiency, as remedies for dyspepsia, or as "digestive aids."

Successful enzyme replacement therapy relieves symptoms of steatorrhea (diarrhea, abdominal fullness or bloating, and cramps) and prevents further weight loss or produces weight gain. The effectiveness of therapy can be assessed by comparing the 24-hour fat excretion in stool determined from a baseline measurement with that during therapy (Grendell and Cello, 1983).

The benefits obtained from conventional (plain [uncoated]) preparations and enteric-coated microspheres of pancrelipase or pancreatin usually are similar. Enteric-coated conventional preparations (eg, tablets) also are available but have little clinical value because the coating does not dissolve until the luminal pH is greater than 5.5, which may affect bioavailability in the duodenum and upper jejunum where the enzyme is needed most (Graham, 1986). Furthermore, the particles are too large to empty from the stomach with food.

Patients with severe pancreatic insufficiency manifested by high fecal fat excretion may have either a high or low rate of acid secretion. In those with high rates of acid secretion, much of the enzyme in conventional preparations will be inactivated; thus, a good clinical response often requires the use of enteric-coated microspheres or concomitant administration of conventional preparations with sodium bicarbonate or aluminum hydroxide before or with a meal, which relieves steatorrhea more than the enzymes alone (Graham, 1982). Antacids containing calcium or magnesium should be avoided; they do not reduce steatorrhea and may increase it in some patients (Graham et al, 1982).

Because lipase is irreversibly inactivated below pH 4.0, adjuvants such as histamine$_2$ blockers have been employed to raise the pH of the intragastric contents in an attempt to improve the effectiveness of pancreatic enzymes. Patients with very high rates of gastric acid secretion (eg, those with cystic fibrosis) may have a low intragastric pH even after optimal use of adjuvant H_2 receptor antagonists and may require omeprazole [Prilosec], a more potent inhibitor of gastric acid secretion (Heijerman et al, 1991).

In addition, in some patients with cystic fibrosis, residual lipase activity is inactivated by high levels of gastric acid; administration of omeprazole 20 mg once daily preserves this residual enzyme activity and decreases the dose requirements for pancreatic enzyme replacement therapy (Heijerman et al, 1993).

For children with cystic fibrosis, some physicians recommend mixing the enteric-coated microsphere preparations with applesauce; however, it is unclear whether this enhances or reduces efficacy. Mixing conventional plain pancreatic enzyme preparations with applesauce is inappropriate since the low pH immediately and irreversibly inactivates lipase (Sackman et al, 1982).

Most patients with low rates of gastric acid secretion respond adequately to conventional (plain) preparations of the enzymes alone. The use of adjuvants in these patients will reduce the steatorrhea even further, but the added improvement (although often statistically significant) may not be clinically significant.

Pancreatic enzyme preparations were marketed before 1938 and have not been subject to FDA examination for efficacy and safety. However, because of the problems noted above, the FDA has categorized microsphere preparations as new drugs, and manufacturers are required to submit proof of the efficacy and safety of these formulations (*Federal Register*, 1991).

Pancreatic preparations are not interchangeable and should not be substituted for one another unless proof of efficacy can be demonstrated. New formulations of pancreatic enzyme preparations are now available that contain five to nine times more pancreatic enzymes per capsule or tablet than older preparations. It is unclear if these high-dose preparations will improve compliance and/or therapeutic outcome (Bowler et al, 1993; Miller et al, 1993; Opekun et al, 1993).

Use of generic preparations of enteric-coated pancreatic enzymes has been associated with treatment failures due to inadequate enzyme content or formulation defects that caused premature dissolution of the enteric coating in the stomach where the lipase was destroyed by acid. Furthermore, laboratory analysis of the content of all available microsphere preparations (brand name as well as generic) revealed unacceptable variations in enzyme content, acid stability of the enteric coating, and the pH at which the enzymes are released (Hendeles et al, 1993). The enzyme content of Zymase and Cotazym-S is not released until a pH of 6.0 is exceeded. These products may be less effective in patients with cystic fibrosis than Creon, which releases its enzymes at a pH above 5.5 (Hendeles et al, 1993).

Bile salts or proteolytic enzymes of plant origin are of no benefit in exocrine pancreatic insufficiency.

Adverse Reactions and Precautions: Although allergic reactions to the animal protein in enzyme preparations occur only rarely, allergic rhinitis and bronchospasm have resulted from sensitization induced by repeated inhalation of the powder. These enzymes should be used cautiously in patients who are sensitive to pork. Respiratory symptoms caused by inhalation of pancreatic powder also may develop in the absence of sensitivity to ingested pork.

Large doses of pancreatic enzymes may produce diarrhea, nausea, abdominal cramps, or pain. In children, large doses have been associated with hyperuricemia and hyperuricosuria (Stapleton et al, 1976; Davidson et al, 1978). Whether the pancreatic enzyme formulations have caused these changes or whether the hyperuricemia and hyperuricosuria observed in some cystic fibrosis patients are directly related to the severity of the underlying disease has not been established (Toskes, 1993). A high-fiber diet may decrease the efficacy of oral pancreatic enzymes (Dutta and Hlasko, 1985).

Dosage Requirements: Dosage should be individualized and is based on the activity of the lipase, protease, and amylase in each product rather than on the weight of the extract. Requirements depend on the degree of maldigestion and malabsorption, the degree of acid secretion, the amount of fat in the diet, and the enzyme activity of each preparation. Enzyme preparations should be taken with every meal and snack for maximal effectiveness. Compliance is a problem, particularly in alcoholic patients.

Rarely, it may be necessary to reduce the dietary intake of fat. Usually this is required only in patients with persistent watery diarrhea after steatorrhea has been reduced. In such individuals, medium-chain triglycerides may be necessary to supply additional calories.

Pain Relief in Chronic Pancreatitis

Suppression of pancreatic secretion is induced exclusively by serine proteases (trypsin, chymotrypsin, elastase) delivered into the duodenum. This concept of feedback inhibition of pancreatic secretion by serine proteases is well established as a physiologic mechanism in humans (Owyang et al, 1986; Liener et al, 1988) and has been proposed as the basis for the relief of abdominal pain following oral administration of pancreatic enzymes in patients with chronic pancreatitis. This feedback mechanism may be mediated through inhibition of cholecystokinin by serine proteases (Slaff et al, 1985; Owyang et al, 1986). Large doses of pancreatic enzymes have healed pancreatic fistulae (Boyd et al, 1985) and, in uncontrolled clinical trials, have been reported to decrease the frequency of attacks of acute recurrent pancreatitis.

Results of two double-blind controlled trials that demonstrated that large doses of conventional pancreatic enzyme preparations decrease the chronic abdominal pain observed in patients with chronic pancreatitis (Isaksson and Ihse, 1983; Slaff et al, 1984) have been confirmed by extensive clinical experience. However, some authorities question the feedback concept and the value of pancreatic enzymes to relieve pain in these patients (Pitchumoni, 1991); this may be due to failure to take into account the poor response in patients with dilated ducts (Toskes, 1991).

Patients whose pain responds best to pancreatic enzymes have normal or slightly abnormal ducts and mild to moderate exocrine impairment (abnormal secretin test, normal fat absorption, minimal abnormalities by ERCP). In one study, use of an enteric-coated microsphere preparation [Pancrease] produced modest pain relief (Halgreen et al, 1986).

In one suggested regimen (Toskes, 1992), patients with recurrent or chronic abdominal pain of undetermined origin (after exclusion of other causes) are given a secretin test. If the results are abnormal, a one-month trial of pancreatic enzymes is instituted. Patients whose pain is not significantly relieved by the enzymes undergo ERCP. If duct dilation is observed, ductal decompression surgery is considered. Patients without evidence of duct dilation on ERCP have small duct disease; these individuals continue to receive enzyme therapy with total parenteral nutrition and possibly anticholinergic drugs. If a secretin test is not performed and pain is relieved after a one-month trial of pancreatic enzymes, pancreatitis is the likely diagnosis (Toskes, 1992).

The use of pancreatic enzyme preparations to relieve pain is more complicated than their use as enzyme replacement therapy. Whereas dissolution of the enteric coating in either the duodenum or the jejunum corrects fat malabsorption, pain is not relieved by enteric-coated preparations that do not dissolve in the duodenum, which is the only intestinal site involved in the feedback mechanism that is believed to be responsible for decrease of pancreatic exocrine activity and pain relief (Toskes et al, 1991; Toskes, 1992). For this reason, conventional (uncoated) pancreatic enzyme preparations (eg, Viokase) have been recommended to alleviate pain; however, to achieve a dose sufficient to relieve pain, large numbers of tablets must be ingested (eight before each meal and eight at bedtime). In addition, to protect the enzymes from gastric acid, sodium bicarbonate, an H_2 receptor antagonist, or omeprazole is needed (Toskes, 1992). Claims have been made that the newer enteric-coated microsphere preparations with greater enzyme activity and different formulations (eg, Creon 25; Pancrease-MT 25 and 32; Ultrase MT 20, 24, and 30) are more effective in providing pain relief than conventional uncoated forms; this has not yet been proved in comparative trials.

Octreotide, a somatostatin analogue, suppresses secretion of pancreatic enzymes; increasing evidence suggests that patients with large duct disease who do not respond to pancreatic enzymes may experience significant pain relief from the subcutaneous administration of octreotide 100 to 200 mcg (Lambiase et al, 1993). Duct decompression surgery may be delayed or avoided in those who respond to octreotide.

Anatomic causes of unsuccessful therapy with enzymes include the presence of dilated ducts or pseudocysts. Patients with dilated ducts usually require ductal decompression surgery, after which enzyme therapy may relieve pain. Pseudocysts must be drained and decompressed before enzyme therapy can be resumed.

In patients who do not respond to pancreatic enzymes, a celiac block (produced by injection of a local anesthetic into the nerve plexus) can provide relief of pain for up to six months. The local anesthetic can be injected three or more times and may postpone the need for surgery (Pap et al, 1990).

Considerable relief of pain also can be obtained for fairly long periods by administration of oral nonsteroidal anti-inflammatory agents (Dutta, 1990).

Inflammation of the pancreas and abdominal pain may spontaneously resolve or improve with or without treatment after 5 to 15 years in some patients.

Drug Evaluations

PANCREATIN

[*Conventional:* Pancreatin; *Enteric-coated microspheres:* Creon]

Pancreatin preparations are derived from hog pancreata and contain varying amounts of amylase, proteases, lipases, and other constituents. In the FDA tentative final monograph on exocrine pancreatic insufficiency drug products, pancreatin preparations were classified as safe and effective (*Federal Register*, 1985). Because of problems with standardization of different microsphere preparations, the FDA is requiring proof of efficacy (see the Introduction to this section). Caution is advised when administering pancreatin to patients who are sensitive to pork.

See the Introduction to this section for indications and other precautions. This enzyme is classified in FDA Pregnancy Category C.

DOSAGE AND PREPARATIONS.

Oral: *Adults,* 4 to 18 g of extract (triple U.S.P. strength) daily in divided doses with meals; an extra dose should be taken with any food eaten between meals. Administration at one- or two-hour intervals throughout the day or before and within one hour after meals also has been suggested, but no apparent advantage is gained from taking the enzymes at any time other than when food is ingested, presumably because food acts as a buffer for gastric acidity and the gastric pH is highest during the digestive period. *Children,* initially, 300 to 600 mg with each meal. Dosage or frequency of administration may be increased to reduce steatorrhea further if nausea, vomiting, or diarrhea does not occur.

CONVENTIONAL PREPARATIONS:

Pancreatin (Vitaline). Tablets (4X) containing pancreatin 2.4 g (lipase 12,000 U.S.P. units, protease 60,000 U.S.P. units, and amylase 60,000 U.S.P. units) and tablets (8X) containing pancreatin 7.2 g (lipase 22,500 U.S.P. units, protease 180,000 U.S.P. units, and amylase 180,000 U.S.P. units) (nonprescription).

ENTERIC-COATED MICROSPHERES:

Creon (Solvay). Each capsule contains no less than 8,000 U.S.P. units of lipase, 13,000 U.S.P. units of protease, and 30,000 U.S.P. units of amylase. Only free protease is measured by the U.S.P. method. Total protease activity (free protease and zymogen activity) is approximately 29,000 units (Fatmi et al, 1988).

Creon 10 (Solvay). Each capsule contains 10,000 U.S.P. units of lipase, 37,500 U.S.P. units of protease, and 33,200 U.S.P. units of amylase.

Creon 25 (Solvay). Each capsule contains 25,000 U.S.P. units of lipase, 62,500 U.S.P. units of protease, and 74,700 U.S.P. units of amylase.

PANCRELIPASE

[*Conventional:* Cotazym, Ilozyme, Ku-zyme HP, Viokase; *Enteric-coated microspheres:* Cotazym-S, Pancrease, Pancrease MT, Protilase, Ultrase MT, Zymase]

The action of pancrelipase, which is derived from hog pancreata, is qualitatively similar to that of other pancreatic enzyme preparations. The enteric-coated microspheres may be more useful than conventional products in patients with high rates of acid excretion. Conventional preparations are preferred in other patients.

In the FDA tentative final monograph on exocrine pancreatic insufficiency drug products, pancrelipase preparations were classified as safe and effective (*Federal Register*, 1985). Because of problems with standardization of different microsphere preparations, the FDA is requiring proof of efficacy (see the Introduction to this section). Caution is advised when administering pancrelipase to patients who are sensitive to pork.

See the Introduction to this section for indications and other precautions. Pancrelipase is classified in FDA Pregnancy Category C.

DOSAGE AND PREPARATIONS.

Oral: *Adults,* 300 to 900 mg (one to three tablets or capsules) before each meal, 900 mg with meals, 600 mg within an hour after meals, and 300 mg with any food eaten between meals. *Children,* 300 to 600 mg taken in the same manner outlined for adults. In severe deficiency, 1 g every waking hour has been given.

CONVENTIONAL PREPARATIONS:

Cotazym (Organon). Each capsule contains lipase 8,000 U.S.P. units, protease 30,000 U.S.P. units, amylase 30,000 U.S.P. units, and precipitated calcium carbonate 25 mg.

Ilozyme (Adria). Each tablet contains lipase 11,000 U.S.P. units, protease 30,000 U.S.P. units, and amylase 30,000 U.S.P. units.

Ku-zyme HP (Schwarz). Each capsule contains lipase 8,000 U.S.P. units, protease 30,000 U.S.P. units, and amylase 30,000 U.S.P. units.

Viokase (Robins). Each tablet contains lipase 8,000 U.S.P. units, protease 30,000 U.S.P. units, and amylase 30,000 U.S.P. units; each 700 mg of powder contains lipase 16,800 U.S.P. units, protease 70,000 U.S.P. units, and amylase 70,000 U.S.P. units. (NOTE: The unpleasant taste of the powder reduces compliance.)

ENTERIC-COATED MICROSPHERES:

(NOTE: Capsules should not be crushed or chewed.)

Cotazym-S (Organon). Each capsule contains lipase 5,000 U.S.P. units, protease 20,000 U.S.P. units, and amylase 20,000 U.S.P. units.

Pancrease, Pancrease MT (McNeil). Each capsule contains no less than 4,000 U.S.P. units of lipase, 25,000 U.S.P. units of protease, and 20,000 U.S.P. units of amylase (***Pancrease***); no less than 4,000 U.S.P. units of lipase, 12,000 U.S.P. units of protease, and 12,000 U.S.P. units of amylase (***Pancrease MT 4***); no less than 10,000 U.S.P. units of lipase, 30,000 U.S.P. units of protease, and 30,000 U.S.P. units of amylase (***Pancrease MT 10***); no less than 16,000 U.S.P. units of lipase, 48,000 U.S.P. units of protease, and 48,000 U.S.P. units of amylase (***Pancrease MT 16***); no less than 25,000 U.S.P. units of lipase, 75,000 U.S.P. units of protease, and 75,000 U.S.P. units of amylase (***Pancrease MT 25***); or no less than 32,000 U.S.P. units of lipase, 70,000 U.S.P. units of protease, and 90,000 U.S.P. units of amylase (***Pancrease MT 32***).

Protilase (Rugby). Each capsule contains lipase 4,000 U.S.P. units, protease 25,000 U.S.P. units, and amylase 20,000 U.S.P. units.

Ultrase MT (Scandipharm). Each capsule contains no less than 12,000 U.S.P. units of lipase, 39,000 U.S.P. units of protease, and 39,000 U.S.P. units of amylase (***Ultrase MT12***); no less than 20,000 U.S.P. units of lipase, 65,000 U.S.P. units of protease, and 65,000 U.S.P. units of amylase (***Ultrase MT20***); no less than 24,000 U.S.P. units of lipase, 78,000 U.S.P. units of protease, and no less than 78,000 U.S.P. units of amylase (***Ultrase MT24***); or no less than 30,000 U.S.P. units of lipase, 97,500 U.S.P. units of protease, and no less than 97,500 U.S.P. units of amylase (***Ultrase MT30***).

Zymase (Organon). Each capsule contains no less than 12,000 U.S.P. units of lipase, 24,000 U.S.P. units of protease, and 24,000 U.S.P. units of amylase.

Mixtures

Mixtures containing bile constituents and derivatives, enzymes, sedatives (eg, phenobarbital), antispasmodics, cellulase, and other ingredients have been marketed for the treatment of many ill-defined gastrointestinal syndromes. There is no scientific rationale or evidence of efficacy to support their use, and most are no longer available. Pancreatic enzymes are indicated only when an exocrine pancreatic deficiency has been demonstrated, in which case adequate quantities of the enzymes alone should be prescribed. When the other active ingredients of these mixtures are required, they should be prescribed separately. For these reasons, use of such mixtures cannot be justified. Examples are listed only for information.

Kutrase (Schwarz). Each capsule contains lipase 75 mg, protease 6 mg, amylase 30 mg, hyoscyamine sulfate 0.0625 mg, cellulase 2 mg, and phenyltoloxamine citrate 15 mg.

Ku-zyme (Schwarz). Each capsule contains lipase 75 mg, protease 6 mg, amylase 30 mg, and cellulase 2 mg.

Cited References

Diagnostic and Therapeutic Technology Assessment (DATTA). *JAMA* 265:1585-1587, 1991.

Exocrine pancreatic insufficiency drug products for over-the-counter human use; tentative final monograph. *Federal Register* 50:46594-46600, 1985.

Exocrine pancreatic insufficiency drug products for over-the-counter human use; proposed rulemaking. *Federal Register* 56:32282-32290, 1991.

Transjugular intrahepatic portosystemic shunt (TIPS): A new treatment for recurrent variceal hemorrhage. *Mayo Clin Update* 3-5, 1992.

Affronti J, Putnam WS: New treatment alternatives for gallstone disease. *Hosp Formul* 26:399-414, 1991.

Albers JJ, et al: National Cooperative Gallstone Study: Effect of chenodeoxycholic acid on lipoproteins and apolipoproteins. *Gastroenterology* 82:638-646, 1982.

Albert MB, Fromm H: Extracorporeal shock-wave lithotripsy of gallstones with the adjuvant use of cholelitholytic bile acids. *Semin Liver Dis* 10:197-204, 1990.

Albert MB, et al: Successful outpatient treatment of gallstones with piezoelectric lithotripsy. *Ann Intern Med* 113:164-166, 1990.

Allen MJ, et al: Rapid dissolution of gallstones by methyl tert-butyl ether. *N Engl J Med* 312:217-220, 1985.

Ammann RW, et al: Differences in the natural history of idiopathic (nonalcoholic) and alcoholic chronic pancreatitis: A comparative long-term study of 287 patients. *Pancreas* 2:368-377, 1987.

Atterbury CE, et al: Neomycin-sorbitol and lactulose in treatment of acute portal-systemic encephalopathy: Controlled, double-blind clinical trial. *Am J Dig Dis* 23:398-406, 1978.

Bachrach WH, Hofmann AF: Ursodeoxycholic acid in treatment of cholesterol cholelithiasis, parts I and II. *Dig Dis Sci* 27:737-761, 833-856, 1982.

Balasubramaniam K, et al: Diminished survival in asymptomatic primary biliary cirrhosis: A prospective study. *Gastroenterology* 98:1567-1571, 1990.

Basile AS, et al: Elevated brain concentrations of 1,4-benzodiazepines in fulminant hepatic failure. *N Engl J Med* 325:473-478, 1991.

Becker CD, et al: Treatment of retained cystic duct stones using extracorporeal shockwave lithotripsy. *Am J Roentgenol* 148:1121-1122, 1987.

Bergasa NV, et al: Oral methotrexate (MTX) for primary biliary cirrhosis (PBC): Preliminary report, abstract 51. *Gastroenterology* A-31, 1991.

Bergasa NV, et al: A controlled trial of naloxone infusions for the pruritus of chronic cholestasis. *Gastroenterology* 102:544-549, 1992.

Beuers U, et al: Ursodeoxycholic acid for treatment of primary sclerosing cholangitis: A placebo-controlled trial. *Hepatology* 16:707-714, 1992.

Blanc P, et al: Lactitol or lactulose in the treatment of chronic hepatic encephalopathy: Results of a meta-analysis. *Hepatology* 15:222-228, 1992.

Bowler IM, et al: A double blind lipase for lipase comparison of a high lipase and standard pancreatic enzyme preparation in cystic fibrosis. *Arch Dis Child* 68:227-230, 1993.

Boyd EJ, et al: Aspects of feedback control of pancreatic secretion in man. *Ital J Gastroenterol* 17:18-22, 1985.

Brink JA, et al: Simulation of gallstone fragments by cavitation bubbles during extracorporeal shock wave lithotripsy: Physical basis and in vitro demonstration. *Radiology* 174:787-791, 1990.

Burroughs AK, et al: Controlled trial of propranolol for prevention of recurrent variceal hemorrhage in patients with cirrhosis. *N Engl J Med* 309:1539-1542, 1983.

Burroughs AK, et al: Randomized, double-blind, placebo-controlled trial of somatostatin for variceal bleeding: Emergency control and prevention of early variceal rebleeding: Emergency control and prevention of variceal rebleeding. *Gastroenterology* 99:1388-1395, 1990.

Butterworth RF: Pathogenesis and treatment of portal-systemic encephalopathy: An update. *Dig Dis Sci* 37:321-327, (March) 1992.

Castilla A, et al: Transforming growth factors $\beta1$ and α in chronic liver disease: Effects of interferon alfa therapy. *N Engl J Med* 324:933-940, 1991.

Christensen E, et al: Beneficial effect of azathioprine and prediction of prognosis in primary biliary cirrhosis. *Gastroenterology* 89:1084-1091, 1985.

Clark ML: Portal hypertension, editorial. *J R Soc Med* 75:761-764, 1982.

Conn HO: Lactulose: Drug in search of modus operandi. *Gastroenterology* 74:624-626, 1978.

Conn HO: Vasopressin and nitroglycerin in the treatment of bleeding varices. *Hepatology* 6:523-525, 1986.

Conn HO, et al: Comparison of lactulose and neomycin in treatment of chronic portal-systemic encephalopathy: Double-blind controlled trial. *Gastroenterology* 72:573-583, 1977.

Conn HO, et al: Propranolol in the prevention of the first hemorrhage from esophagogastric varices: A multicenter, randomized clinical trial. *Hepatology* 13:902-912, 1991.

Crossley JR, Williams R: Progress in treatment of chronic portosystemic encephalopathy. *Gut* 25:85-98, 1984.

Darzi A, et al: Combined ultrasound-guided extracorporeal shock-wave lithotripsy and MTBE instillation in the treatment of common bile duct stones. *Hepatogastroenterology* 38:36-38, 1991.

Davidson GP, et al: Iatrogenic hyperuricemia in children with cystic fibrosis. *J Pediatr* 93:976-978, 1978.

Davis GL, et al: Treatment of chronic hepatitis C with recombinant interferon alpha: A multicenter randomized, controlled trial. *N Engl J Med* 321:1501-1506, 1989.

Di Bisceglie AM, et al: Recombinant interferon alpha therapy for chronic hepatitis C: A randomized, double-blind, placebo-controlled trial. *N Engl J Med* 321:1506-1510, 1989.

Dickson ER, et al: Trial of D-penicillamine in advanced primary biliary cirrhosis. *N Engl J Med* 312:1011-1015, 1985.

DiMagno EP, Clain JE: Chronic pancreatitis, in Go VLW, et al (eds): *The Exocrine Pancreas: Biology, Pathobiology and Diseases.* New York, Raven Press, 1986, 541-575.

Dutta SK: Chronic pancreatitis: Exocrine and endocrine insufficiency, in Bayless TM (ed): *Current Therapy in Gastroenterology and Liver Disease-3.* Toronto, BC Decker, 1990, 553-558.

Dutta S, Hlasko J: Dietary fiber in pancreatic disease: Effect of high fiber diet on fat malabsorption in pancreatic insufficiency and in vitro study of interaction of dietary fiber with pancreatic enzymes. *Am J Clin Nutr* 41:517-525, 1985.

Egberts E-H, et al: Branched chain amino acids in treatment of latent portosystemic encephalopathy: Double-blind placebo-controlled crossover study. *Gastroenterology* 88:887-895, 1985.

Ell C, et al: Significance of computed tomography for shock-wave therapy of radiolucent gallbladder stones. *Gastroenterology* 101:1409-1416, 1991.

Eriksson LS, Conn HO: Branched chain amino acids in the management of hepatic encephalopathy: Analysis of variants. *Hepatology* 10:228-246, 1989.

Fatmi AA, et al: An in vitro comparative evaluation of pancreatic enzyme preparations. *Drug Devel Indust Pharm* 14:1429-1438, 1988.

Ferenci P, et al: Successful long-term treatment of portal-systemic encephalopathy by the benzodiazepine antagonist flumazenil. *Gastroenterology* 96:240-243, 1989.

Ferrell LD, et al: Hepatitis C viral infection in liver transplant recipients. *Hepatology* 16:865-876, 1992.

Finklestein M, et al: Granulocytopenia complicating colchicine therapy for primary biliary cirrhosis. *Gastroenterology* 93:1231-1235, 1987.

Fisher RL, et al: The lack of relationship between hepatotoxicity and lithocholic-acid sulfation in biliary bile acids during chenodiol therapy in the National Cooperative Gallstone Study. *Hepatology* 14:454-463, 1991.

Fordtran JS, et al: Ox bile treatment of severe steatorrhea in ileectomy patient. *Gastroenterology* 82:564-568, 1982.

Frabboni R, et al: Acquired gallstone calcification during cholelitholytic treatment with chenodeoxycholic, ursodeoxycholic, and tauroursodeoxycholic acids, abstract. *Hepatology* 5:1004, 1985.

Fromm H: Gallstone dissolution and cholesterol-bile acid-lipoprotein axis: Propitious effects of ursodeoxycholic acid. *Gastroenterology* 87:229-233, 1984.

Fromm H, Albert MB: Mechanical and chemical management of gallstones, in Yamada T, et al (eds): *Textbook of Gastroenterology.* Philadelphia, JB Lippincott, 1991, vol 2, 2650-2662.

Grace ND: A hepatologist's view of variceal bleeding. *Am J Surg* 160:26-31, (July) 1990.

Graham DY: Pancreatic enzyme replacement: Effect of antacids or cimetidine. *Dig Dis Sci* 27:485-490, 1982.

Graham DY: Treatment of steatorrhea in chronic pancreatitis. *Hosp Pract* 21:125-129, (Jan 15) 1986.

Graham D, Smith JL: The course of patients after variceal hemorrhage. *Gastroenterology* 80:800-809, 1981.

Graham D, et al: Mechanism of increase in steatorrhea with calcium and magnesium in exocrine pancreatic insufficiency: Animal model. *Gastroenterology* 83:638-644, 1982.

Grendell JH, Cello JP: Chronic pancreatitis, in Sleisenger MH, Fordtran JS (eds): *Gastrointestinal Disease: Pathophysiology, Diagnosis, Management.* Philadelphia, WB Saunders, vol II, 1983, 1503-1505.

Halgreen H, et al: Symptomatic effect of pancreatic enzyme therapy in patients with chronic pancreatitis. *Scand J Gastroenterol* 21:104-108, 1986.

Hashizume M, et al: Endoscopic injection sclerotherapy for 1,000 patients with esophageal varices: A nine-year prospective study. *Hepatology* 15:69-75, 1992.

Heijerman HG, et al: Omeprazole enhances the efficacy of pancreatin (Pancrease) in cystic fibrosis. *Ann Intern Med* 114:200-201, 1991.

Heijerman HGM, et al: Improvement of fecal fat excretion after addition of omeprazole to pancrease in cystic fibrosis is related to residual exocrine function of the pancreas. *Dig Dis Sci* 38:1-6, (Jan) 1993.

Hendeles L, et al: Generic and alternative brand-name pharmaceutical equivalents: Select with caution. *Am J Hosp Pharm* 50:323-329, 1993.

Hofmann AF: Nonsurgical treatment of gallstone disease. *Annu Rev Med* 41:401-415, 1990.

Hoofnagle JH, Bergasa NV: Methotrexate therapy of primary biliary cirrhosis: Promising but worrisome, editorial. *Gastroenterology* 101:1440-1442, 1991.

Hoofnagle JH, Di Bisceglie AM: Treatment of chronic type C hepatitis with alpha interferon. *Semin Liver Dis* 9:259-263, 1989.

Horton RC, et al: Endoscopic removal of common duct stones: Current indications and controversies. *Postgrad Med J* 67:107-111, 1991.

Howard CD, Seifert CF: Flumazenil in the treatment of hepatic encephalopathy. *Ann Pharmacother* 27:46-48, 1993.

Isaksson G, Ihse I: Pain reduction by oral pancreatic enzyme preparation in chronic pancreatitis. *Dig Dis Sci* 28:97-102, 1983.

Jacobson DG, et al: Trypsin-like immunoreactivity as test for pancreatic insufficiency. *N Engl J Med* 310:1307-1309, 1984.

Johnston DE, Kaplan MM: Pathogenesis and treatment of gallstones. *N Engl J Med* 328:412-421, 1993.

Kaplan M: Chronic liver diseases: Current therapeutic options. *Hosp Pract* 24:111-130, (March 15) 1989.

Kaplan MM: Primary biliary cirrhosis, in Bayless TM (ed): *Current Therapy in Gastroenterology and Liver Disease-3.* Toronto, BC Decker, 1990 A, 481-485.

Kaplan MM: Survival in asymptomatic primary biliary cirrhosis: Not as good as previously reported? *Gastroenterology* 98:1707-1709, 1990 B.

Kaplan MM: Medical approaches to primary sclerosing cholangitis. *Semin Liver Dis* 11:56-63, 1991.

Kaplan M: Personal communication, 1993.

Kaplan MM, Knox TA: Treatment of primary biliary cirrhosis with low-dose weekly methotrexate. *Gastroenterology* 101:1332-1338, 1991.

Kaplan MM, et al: Prospective trial of colchicine for primary cirrhosis. *N Engl J Med* 315:1448-1454, 1986.

Knox TA, Kaplan MM: Treatment of primary sclerosing cholangitis with oral methotrexate. *Am J Gastroenterol* 86:546-552, 1991.

Korenman J, et al: Long-term remission of chronic hepatitis B after alpha-interferon therapy. *Ann Intern Med* 114:629-634, 1991.

Kupfer S, et al: Gallstone dissolution rate during chenic acid therapy. *Dig Dis Sci* 27:1025-1029, 1982.

Lambiase L, Davis GL: Treatment of chronic hepatitis. *Gastroenterol Clin North Am* 21:659-677, 1992.

Lambiase LR, et al: Correlation of pain relief and reduction in fasting serum CCK levels in chronic pancreatitis patients treated with octreotide. *Gastroenterology* 104 (suppl):A315, 1993.

LaRusso NF, Wiesner RH: Sclerosing cholangitis, in Bayless TM (ed): *Current Therapy in Gastroenterology and Liver Disease-3.* Toronto, BC Decker, 1990, 489-493.

Lebrec D, et al: Propranolol for prevention of recurrent gastrointestinal bleeding in patients with cirrhosis: Controlled study. *N Engl J Med* 305:1371-1374, 1981.

Lebrec D, et al: Nadolol for prophylaxis of gastrointestinal bleeding in patients with cirrhosis: Randomized trial. *J Hepatol* 7:118-125, 1988.

Liener IE, et al: Effect of trypsin inhibitor from soybeans (Bowman-Birk) on the secretory activity of the human pancreas. *Gastroenterology* 94:419-427, 1988.

Lombard M, et al: Cyclosporin A treatment in primary biliary cirrhosis: Results of a long-term placebo controlled trial. *Gastroenterology* 104:519-526, 1993.

Maddrey WC: Chronic hepatitis. *Dis Mon* 57-125, (Feb) 1993.

Malet PF, et al: Gallstone composition in relation to buoyancy at oral cholecystography. *Radiology* 177:167-169, 1990.

Martin P, et al: Liver transplantation for viral hepatitis: Current status. *Am J Gastroenterol* 87:409-418, 1992.

McSherry CK: National Cooperative Gallstone Study Report: Surgeon's perspective. *Ann Intern Med* 95:379-380, 1981.

Miller C, et al: Safety and efficacy of a new, high potency pancreatic enzyme in the treatment of pancreatic insufficiency associated with cystic fibrosis, abstract. *Gastroenterology* 104:A322, 1993.

Morgan MH, et al: Treatment of hepatic encephalopathy with metronidazole. *Gut* 23:1-7, 1982.

Mortensen PB, et al: The degradation of amino acids, proteins, and blood to short-chain fatty acids in colon is prevented by lactulose. *Gastroenterology* 98:353-360, 1990.

Mullen KD: Benzodiazepine compounds and hepatic encephalopathy, editorial. *N Engl J Med* 325:509-511, 1991.

Mullen KD, et al: 'Endogenous' benzodiazepine activity in body fluids of patients with hepatic encephalopathy. *Lancet* 336:81-83, 1990.

Naylor CD, et al: Parenteral nutrition with branched-chain amino acids in hepatic encephalopathy: A meta-analysis. *Gastroenterology* 97:1033-1042, 1989.

NIH Consensus Development Panel on Gallstones and Laparoscopic Cholecystectomy: Gallstones and laparoscopic cholecystectomy. *JAMA* 269:1018-1024, 1993.

O'Brien CB, Senior JR: Prolonged ursodiol effects in primary sclerosing cholangitis: A pilot study with two-year follow-up, abstract 56. *Gastroenterology* A-14, 1991.

Opekun AR Jr, et al: Pancreatic enzyme enteric coated microspheres are now available with different lipase activities: Does this result in improved therapy? Abstract. *Gastroenterology* 104:A326, 1993.

Owyang C, et al: Feedback regulation of pancreatic enzyme secretion: Suppression of cholecystokinin release by trypsin. *J Clin Invest* 77:2042-2047, 1986.

Padilla VM III, Schiff ER: Current topics in viral hepatitis. *Compr Ther* 17:7-12, (Sept) 1991.

Pagliaro L, et al: Prevention of first bleeding in cirrhosis: A meta-analysis of randomized trials of nonsurgical treatment. *Ann Intern Med* 117:59-70, 1992.

Palmer RH, Carey MC: Optimistic view of National Cooperative Gallstone Study. *N Engl J Med* 306:1171-1174, 1982.

Palmer KR, Hofmann AF: Intraductal mono-octanoin for direct dissolution of bile duct stones: Experience in 343 patients. *Gut* 27:196-202, 1986.

Panés J, et al: Effects of propranolol on gastric mucosal perfusion in cirrhotic patients with portal hypertensive gastropathy. *Hepatology* 17:213-218, 1993.

Pap A, et al: Is percutaneous celiac plexus block (PCPB) associated with pain relief in chronic pancreatitis? A comparison among analgesic, alcohol and steroid PCPB. *Pancreas* 5:725, 1990.

Papo T, et al: Autoimmune chronic hepatitis exacerbated by alpha-interferon. *Ann Intern Med* 116:51-53, 1992.

Pascal JP, et al: Propranolol in the prevention of first upper gastrointestinal tract hemorrhage in patients with cirrhosis of the liver and esophageal varices. *N Engl J Med* 317:856-861, 1987.

Patel SA, et al: Management of chronic active liver disease. *Hosp Formul* 27:1178-1196, 1992.

Peine CJ: Gallstone-dissolving agents. *Gastroenterol Clin North Am* 21:715-741, 1992.

Peine CJ, et al: Extracorporeal shock-wave lithotripsy and methyl tert-butyl ether for partially calcified gallstones. *Gastroenterology* 97:1229-1234, 1989.

Perdigoto R, Wiesner RH: Progression of primary biliary cirrhosis with ursodeoxycholic acid therapy. *Gastroenterology* 102:1389-1391, 1992.

Perrillo R, et al: A randomized, controlled trial of interferon alfa 2b alone and after prednisone withdrawal for the treatment of chronic hepatitis B. *N Engl J Med* 323:337-339, 1990.

Pitchumoni CS: Is there an effective nonsurgical treatment for pain in chronic pancreatitis? Controversies, dilemmas, and dialogues. *Am J Gastroenterol* 86:26-28, 1991.

Podda M, et al: Efficacy and safety of a combination of chenodeoxycholic acid and ursodeoxycholic acid for gallstone dissolution: Comparison with ursodeoxycholic acid alone. *Gastroenterology* 92:222-229, 1989.

Podesta A, et al: Treatment of pruritus of primary biliary cirrhosis with rifampin. *Dig Dis Sci* 36:216-220, (Feb) 1991.

Poterucha JJ, et al: Dissolution of cholesterol gallstones (CGS) with methyl tert-butyl ether (MTBE) using an infusion-aspiration pump: Phase I clinical studies, abstract. *Suppl Gastroenterol* 100:A334, 1991.

Poupon RE, et al: A multicenter, controlled trial of ursodiol for the treatment of primary biliary cirrhosis. *N Engl J Med* 324:1548-1554, 1991.

Poynard T, et al: Beta-adrenergic-antagonist drugs in the prevention of gastrointestinal bleeding in patients with cirrhosis and esophageal varices: An analysis of data and prognostic factors in 589 patients from four randomized clinical trials. *N Engl J Med* 324:1532-1538, 1991.

The PROVA Study Group: Prophylaxis of first hemorrhage from esophageal varices by sclerotherapy, propranolol or both in cirrhotic patients: A randomized multicenter trial. *Hepatology* 14:1016-1024, 1991.

Ransohoff DF, et al: Prophylactic cholecystectomy or expectant management for silent gallstones. *Ann Intern Med* 99:199-204, 1983.

Ratliff DS, et al: Laparoscopic cholecystectomy: A community experience. *South Med J* 85:942-945, 1992.

Reddick EJ, Olsen DO: Laparoscopic laser cholecystectomy: A comparison with mini-lap cholecystectomy. *Surg Endosc* 3:131-133, 1989.

Resnick RH: Somatostatin for variceal bleeders. *Gastroenterology* 99:1524-1526, 1990.

Sackman JW, et al: Does mixing pancreatic enzyme microspheres (Pancrease) with food damage the enteric coating? *J Pediatr Gastroenterol Nutr* 1:333-335, 1982.

Sackmann M, et al: Extracorporeal shock-wave lithotripsy of gallstones without general anesthesia: First clinical experience. *Ann Intern Med* 107:347-348, 1987.

Sackmann M, et al: Monotherapy with ursodeoxycholic acid is as efficient as a combination of urso- and chenodeoxycholic acid for dissolution of gallstone fragments. *Hepatology* 12:869, 1990 A.

Sackmann M, et al: Early gallstone recurrence after successful shock-wave therapy. *Gastroenterology* 9:392-396, 1990 B.

Sackmann M, et al: The Munich gallbladder lithotripsy study: Results of the first 5 years with 711 patients. *Ann Intern Med* 114:290-296, 1991.

Salen G, et al: Oral dissolution treatment of gallstones with bile acids. *Semin Liver Dis* 10:180-186, 1990.

Sauerbruch T, et al: Fragmentation of bile duct stones by extracorporeal shock waves: A new approach to biliary calculi after failure of routine endoscopic measures. *Gastroenterology* 96:146-152, 1989.

Schiff ER: Hepatic fibrosis: New therapeutic approaches. *N Engl J Med* 324:987-989, 1991.

Schiff ER: Viral hepatitis today. *Emerg Med* 115-132, (Nov) 1992.

Schoenfield LJ, et al: Chenodiol (chenodeoxycholic acid) for dissolution of gallstones: National Cooperative Gallstone Study, controlled trial of efficacy. *Ann Intern Med* 95:257-282, 1981.

Schoenfield LJ, et al: The effect of ursodiol on the efficacy and safety of extracorporeal shock-wave lithotripsy of gallstones: The Dornier National Biliary Lithotripsy Study. *N Engl J Med* 323:1239-1245, 1990.

Senior JR, et al: In vivo kinetics of radiolucent gallstone dissolution by oral dihydroxy bile acids. *Gastroenterology* 99:243-251, 1990.

Shaw MJ: Current management of symptomatic gallstones. *Postgrad Med* 93:183-187, (Jan) 1993.

Slaff JI, et al: Protease-specific suppression of pancreatic exocrine secretion. *Gastroenterology* 87:44-52, 1984.

Slaff JI, et al: Elevated fasting cholecystokinin levels in pancreatic exocrine impairment. *J Lab Clin Med* 105:282-285, 1985.

Southern Surgeons Club: A prospective analysis of 1518 laparoscopic cholecystectomies. *N Engl J Med* 324:1073-1078, 1991.

Stapleton F, et al: Hyperuricemia due to high-dose pancreatic extract therapy in cystic fibrosis. *N Engl J Med* 295:246-248, 1976.

Stavinoha MW, Soloway RD: Current therapy of chronic liver disease. *Drugs* 39:814-840, 1990.

Stellon AJ, et al: Maintenance of remission in autoimmune chronic active hepatitis with azathioprine after corticosteroid withdrawal. *Hepatology* 8:781-784, 1988.

Stiegmann GV, et al: Endoscopic sclerotherapy as compared with endoscopic ligation for bleeding esophageal varices. *N Engl J Med* 326:1527-1532, 1992.

Strasberg SM, Clavien P-A: Cholecystolithiasis: Lithotherapy for the 1990s. *Hepatology* 16:820-839, 1992.

Tangedahl TN: Management of gallstones: New option of bile acid therapy. *Postgrad Med* 74:115-121, (Nov) 1983.

Tangedahl T, et al: Drug and treatment efficacy of chenodeoxycholic acid in 97 patients with cholelithiasis and increased surgical risk. *Dig Dis Sci* 28:545-551, 1983.

Tarao K, et al: Successful use of vancomycin hydrochloride in the treatment of lactulose resistant chronic hepatic encephalopathy. *Gut* 31:702-706, 1990.

Thistle JL: Direct contact dissolution of gallstones. *Semin Liver Dis* 7:311-316, 1987.

Thistle JL: Topical dissolution treatment of cholesterol gallstones with methyl tert-butyl ether. *Semin Liver Dis* 10:187-190, 1990.

Thistle JL, et al: Dissolution of cholesterol gallbladder stones by methyl tert-butyl-ether administered by percutaneous transhepatic catheter. *N Engl J Med* 320:633-639, 1989.

Tint GS, et al: Effect of ursodeoxycholic acid and chenodeoxycholic acid on cholesterol and bile acid metabolism. *Gastroenterology* 91:1007-1118, 1986.

Toskes PP: Bentiromide test for pancreatic exocrine insufficiency. *Pharmacotherapy* 4:74-80, 1984.

Toskes PP: Is there an effective nonsurgical treatment for pain in chronic pancreatitis? Controversies, dilemmas, and dialogues. *Am J Gastroenterol* 86:28-29, 1991.

Toskes PP: Recurrent abdominal pain: Is the pancreas responsible? *Emerg Med* 159-174, (Oct) 1992.

Toskes PP: Therapy of pancreatic disease, in Wolfe M (ed): *Gastrointestinal Pharmacotherapy*. Philadelphia, WB Saunders, 1993, 265-273.

Toskes PP, Greenberger NJ: Acute and chronic pancreatitis. *Dis Mon* 26:1-18, 1983.

Toskes PP, et al: Failure of enteric-coated pancreatin to lower CCK levels and relieve pain in chronic pancreatitis. *Pancreas* 6:722, 1991.

Tyor MP: Selecting patients for gallstone-dissolving therapy. *Drug Ther* 13:237-252, (April) 1983.

Valenzuela JE, et al: A multicentre, randomised, double-blind trial of somatostatin in the management of acute haemorrhage from esophageal varices. *Hepatology* 10:958-961, 1989.

Van Ruiswyk J, Byrd JC: Efficacy of prophylactic sclerotherapy for prevention of a first variceal hemorrhage. *Gastroenterology* 102:587-597, 1992.

Vennes JA: Management of calculi in common duct. *Semin Liver Dis* 3:162-171, 1983.

Venu RP, et al: Gallstone dissolution using mono-octanoin infusion through an endoscopically placed nasobiliary catheter. *Am J Gastroenterol* 77:227-230, 1982.

The Veterans Affairs Cooperative Variceal Sclerotherapy Group: Prophylactic sclerotherapy for esophageal varices in men with alcoholic liver disease: A randomized, single-blind, multicenter clinical trial. *N Engl J Med* 324:1779-1784, 1991.

Villanova N, et al: Gallstone recurrence after successful oral bile acid treatment: A 12-year follow-up study and evaluation of long-term postdissolution treatment. *Gastroenterology* 97:726-731, 1989.

Vinel J-P, et al: Propranolol reduces the rebleeding rate during endoscopic sclerotherapy before variceal obliteration. *Gastroenterology* 102:1760-1763, 1992.

Vorobioff J, et al: Acute and chronic hemodynamic effects of propranolol in unselected cirrhotic patients. *Hepatology* 7:648-653, 1987.

Ward A, et al: Ursodeoxycholic acid: Review of its pharmacological properties and therapeutic efficacy. *Drugs* 27:95-131, 1984.

Weber FL Jr, et al: Effects of lactulose and neomycin on urea metabolism in cirrhotic subjects. *Gastroenterology* 82:213-217, 1982.

Weber J, et al: Extracorporeal piezoelectric lithotripsy for complicated bile duct stones. *Am J Gastroenterol* 86:196-200, 1991.

Wiesner RH, et al: Clinical and statistical analyses of new and evolving therapies for primary biliary cirrhosis. *Hepatology* 8:668-676, 1988.

Wiesner RH, et al: A controlled trial of cyclosporine in the treatment of primary biliary cirrhosis. *N Engl J Med* 322:1419-1424, 1990.

Wiesner RH, et al: Selection and timing of liver transplantation in primary biliary cirrhosis and primary sclerosing cholangitis. *Hepatology* 16:1290-1299, 1992.

Willson RA: Hepatitis update: New trends and treatments. *Drug Ther* 33-42, (June) 1990.

Wilson RG, et al: Laparoscopic cholecystectomy as a safe and effective treatment for severe acute cholecystitis. *BMJ* 305:394-396, 1992.

Wolfe BM, et al: Laparoscopic cholecystectomy: A remarkable development. *JAMA* 265:1573-1574, 1991.

Yamamoto AM, et al: Characterization of anti-liver-kidney microsome antibody (anti-LKM1) from hepatitis C virus-positive and -negative sera. *Gastroenterology* 104:1762-1767, 1993.

Zakko SF, Hofmann AF: Microprocessor-assisted solvent-transfer system for gallstone dissolution: In vitro and vivo validation. *Gastroenterology* 99:1807-1813, 1990.

Zifroni A, Schaffner F: Long-term follow-up of patients with primary biliary cirrhosis on colchicine therapy. *Hepatology* 14:990-993, 1991.

Drugs Used in Adrenocortical Dysfunction

46

Regulation of Adrenocortical Hormone Secretion: The adrenal cortex secretes glucocorticoids, mineralocorticoids, androgens, progesterone, and estrogens (see Figure). Healthy adults and children over 8 years secrete 5 to 15 mg of cortisol and 1.5 to 4 mg of corticosterone, the major glucocorticoids in humans, and 30 to 150 mcg of aldosterone, the most important mineralocorticoid, daily (Linder et al, 1990; Esteban et al, 1991; Kerrigan et al, 1993). The principal androgens secreted by the adrenal cortex are dehydroepiandrosterone (DHEA), DHEA sulfate, and androstenedione.

Glucocorticoid steroidogenesis from cholesterol (see Figure) responds rapidly to stimulation by adrenocorticotropin (ACTH), a polypeptide produced in the basophilic cells of the anterior pituitary gland. The steroidogenic and trophic actions of ACTH on the adrenal cortex are mediated by activation of adenylate cyclase with an increase in the production of cyclic adenosine monophosphate (cAMP). The response to acute stimulation by ACTH occurs within two minutes and is complete in less than one hour. Secretion rapidly follows steroid biosynthesis; only small amounts of adrenocortical hormones are stored within the gland.

The secretion of ACTH is stimulated by corticotropin-releasing hormone (CRH), a peptide synthesized in the hypothalamus and transported to the anterior pituitary gland by the hypophyseal portal blood vessels (Vale et al, 1981). Stimulation of CRH and, therefore, of ACTH secretion occurs in the anterior areas of the brain, including the amygdala, in response to extrahypothalamic central nervous system signals. In individuals who maintain a normal sleep-activity cycle, blood CRH and ACTH concentrations peak between 4 AM and 8 AM and are lowest in the late evening or early sleep period. This circadian rhythm is absent or blunted in patients with ACTH-secreting pituitary adenomas and is accentuated in those with partial adrenal insufficiency. Stimuli from both anterior and posterior brain areas stimulate the release of CRH in the hypothalamus in response to stress (eg, trauma, anxiety, severe infection, hypoglycemia, surgery, severe physical exertion). In addition, extrahypothalamic CRH may be released from damaged peripheral tissues and may prolong the release of ACTH in response to trauma (Petrusz et al, 1985).

Pituitary secretion of ACTH is stimulated by interleukin-1-β (IL-1-β) (Besedovsky et at, 1985); this effect is mediated by cytokine stimulation of hypothalamic neurosecretion of CRH (Berkenbosch et al, 1987; Lumpkin, 1987; Sapolsky et al, 1987 A). In humans, IL-1-β is secreted by hypothalamic neurons that innervate key endocrine and autonomic cell groups, which control the central components of the acute phase reaction of the immune response (Breder et al, 1988). Subsequently, glucocorticoids secreted in response to IL-1-β-stimulated ACTH suppress several aspects of immune function, including additional secretion of IL-1-β, potentially limiting the extent of the immune reaction (Besedovsky et al, 1985).

Glucocorticoids exert two types of negative feedback control on ACTH secretion, which differ in the time required for their inhibitory effects. The fast feedback system acts almost immediately and is responsible for normal minute-to-minute physiologic control. This system may be impaired in some elderly patients, in whom episodes of glucocorticoid secretion in response to ACTH stimulation may be prolonged (Sapolsky et al, 1987 B). The delayed feedback system suppresses basal CRH and ACTH secretion when pharmacologic doses of glucocorticoids are administered. However, severe stress overrides exogenous glucocorticoid suppression of ACTH secretion. (See also reviews by Jones and Gillham, 1988; Reisine, 1988; Taylor and Fishman, 1988; Tyrrell et al, 1991.)

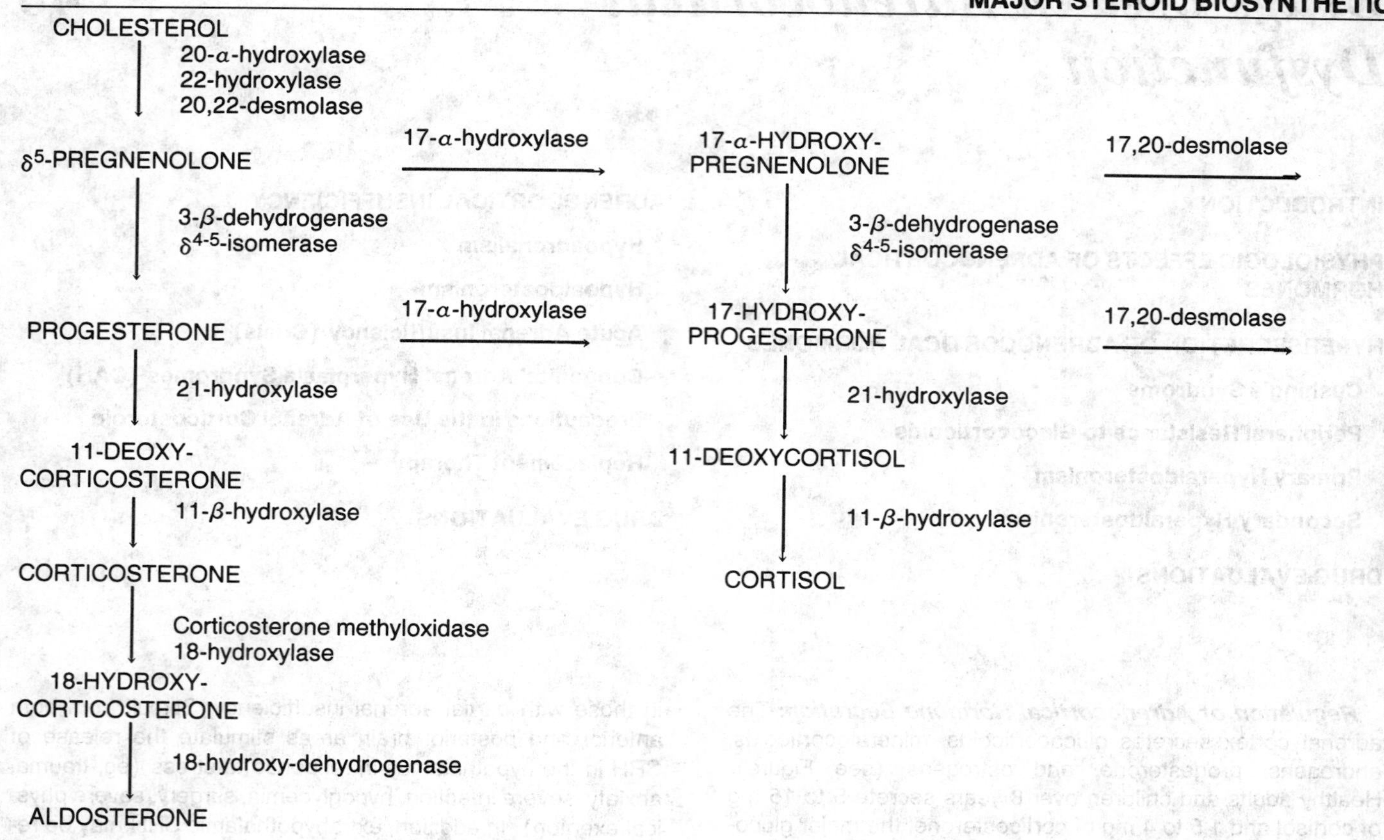

The amount of ACTH secreted at any time is influenced by the integration of CRH stimulation and negative feedback from circulating glucocorticoids. Maximal ACTH secretion in response to stress occurs in the evening, which coincides with the normal nadir of CRH, ACTH, and cortisol secretion. Severe stress is the most potent stimulus for ACTH and cortisol secretion and increases CRH secretion, pituitary sensitivity to CRH, and adrenal sensitivity to ACTH (Naito et al, 1991).

Aldosterone secretion is controlled primarily by the renin-angiotensin system and the serum potassium concentration. When the plasma volume is decreased, secretion of renin by the renal juxtaglomerular apparatus is stimulated. Sympathetic stimulation of the juxtaglomerular apparatus also may increase renin secretion. Renin catalyzes the cleavage of angiotensinogen to angiotensin I; angiotensin-converting enzyme converts angiotensin I to angiotensin II, a potent vasoconstrictor and stimulator of aldosterone synthesis and secretion. Aldosterone secretion also is stimulated directly by increasing plasma potassium concentrations. ACTH also acutely stimulates aldosterone secretion, but the effect is attenuated within 24 hours and there is no significant negative feedback effect on ACTH production. Aldosterone exhibits a slight circadian rhythmicity, and serum concentrations tend to peak in the morning.

ACTH stimulates adrenal androgen as well as cortisol secretion. Another, as yet unidentified, substance secreted by the pituitary may stimulate secretion of adrenal androgens but not other adrenocortical hormones (McKenna and Cunningham, 1991). Pituitary gonadotropins probably stimulate only the secretion of gonadal sex steroids. Adrenal sex steroids do not exert feedback control on ACTH secretion.

Mechanism of Adrenocortical Hormone Action: Like other steroid hormones, corticosteroids exert their cellular effects through interaction with specific receptor proteins in the cytoplasm of responsive cells. The hormone-receptor complex is translocated to the nucleus where it binds to nuclear chromatin, followed by transcription of specific genes into corresponding messenger RNA and by RNA translation into proteins, usually enzymes (Funder, 1993).

Transport and Metabolism of Adrenocortical Hormones: More than 90% of circulating cortisol is reversibly bound to corticosteroid-binding globulin (CBG) and albumin; only the free hormone is biologically active. Only 50% of circulating aldosterone is protein bound, principally to albumin. The synthetic corticosteroids vary in their affinity and capacity for protein binding. Some synthetic corticosteroids (eg, prednisolone) compete for binding to CBG; others (eg, dexamethasone) do not. Most synthetic glucocorticoids are extensively bound to albumin. Variations in plasma protein binding,

PATHWAYS IN THE ADRENAL GLAND

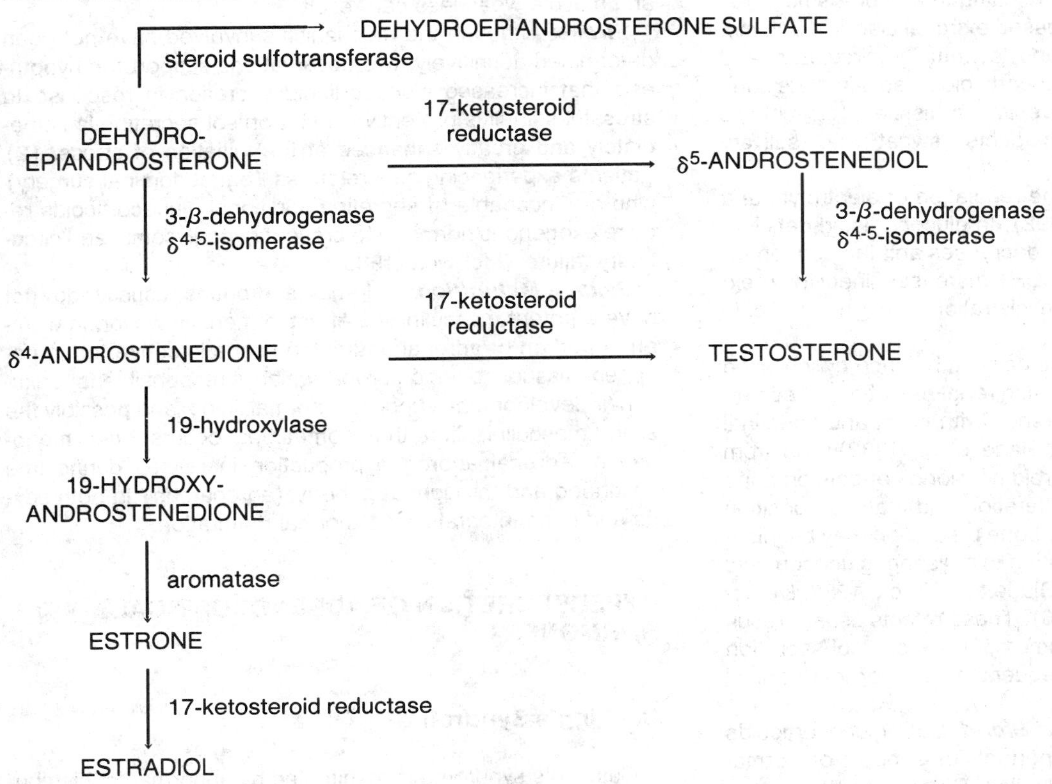

as well as differences in clearance rates, affect the proportion of exogenous steroid available to exert a therapeutic effect and may explain why relatively small doses of some synthetic preparations cause cushingoid effects.

In certain conditions associated with high concentrations of total corticosteroids, the negative feedback mechanism maintains normal free hormone concentrations. For example, during pregnancy, in patients taking estrogens, or in those with diabetes, the concentrations of CBG and total corticosteroid are elevated, but the serum free cortisol concentration remains normal. Conversely, in individuals with hepatic disease, nephrotic syndrome, or hyperthyroidism, the CBG concentration decreases but serum free hormone concentrations are normal. The effect that a disease or drug has on hormone binding to plasma proteins must be taken into account when interpreting the results of some adrenal function tests.

Natural corticosteroids have relatively short plasma half-lives, ranging from 30 minutes for aldosterone to 90 minutes for cortisol. The duration of cortisol's biological effectiveness is approximately 8 to 12 hours. Synthetic glucocorticoids have plasma half-lives varying from 1.5 to 24 hours and exert their effects for 8 to 54 hours.

Most endogenous cortisol is metabolized in the liver and kidneys (Whitworth et al, 1989), where physiologically inactive water-soluble conjugates are formed. These are excreted in the bile, and most are reabsorbed so that 90% of cortisol metabolites are excreted in the urine and the remaining 10% in the feces (Begg et al, 1987).

PHYSIOLOGIC EFFECTS OF ADRENOCORTICAL HORMONES

Intermediary Metabolism: Glucocorticoids affect carbohydrate, protein, and fat metabolism; in contrast, mineralocorticoids have little effect on intermediary metabolism. In general, the glucocorticoids stimulate hepatic gluconeogenesis, proteolysis, and the generation of gluconeogenic precursors. Fatty acid mobilization and hepatic cholesterol synthesis also are enhanced by glucocorticoids. These effects on intermediary metabolism are critical survival responses to starvation and severe stress.

Water and Electrolyte Balance: Although 98% of filtered sodium is reabsorbed by active and passive mechanisms before reaching the distal tubules, mineralocorticoids promote reabsorption of small but significant portions of filtered sodium in these tubules. In exchange, the renal excretion of potassium and hydrogen ions is enhanced. Therefore, severe aldosterone deficiency in the absence of compensatory production of cortisol with its weak mineralocorticoid activity produces excessive sodium loss resulting in a hypo-osmotic extracellular compartment, decreased extracellular fluid volume, hyperkalemia, mild acidosis, and, eventually, circulatory and renal failure and death. Mineralocorticoids also stimulate sodium reabsorption across other epithelial tissues (eg, colonic mucosa, exocrine pancreatic ducts, sweat and salivary glands).

Cortisol also is involved in the regulation of electrolyte and water balance (Clore et al, 1992). In glucocorticoid deficiency, the glomerular filtration rate decreases and the concentration of antidiuretic hormone (ADH) increases; inability to excrete a water load results. Administration of a glucocorticoid restores normal function.

The glucocorticoids decrease calcium balance by inhibiting intestinal absorption and increasing renal excretion. These effects result from direct interference with renal and intestinal cell responses to vitamin D (Glade et al, 1982) and from direct and indirect (via parathyroid hormone) effects on bone cell function. Osteoblastic proliferation and matrix deposition are inhibited, while osteoclastic bone resorption may be inhibited or stimulated, depending on circulating glucocorticoid concentrations (Wong, 1979; Glade and Krook, 1982; Dempster et al, 1983; Reid et al, 1986). These effects usually result in acute net bone loss during times of peak cortisol secretion and are reversed during subsequent periods of low cortisol concentrations.

Cardiovascular System and Blood: Both glucocorticoids and mineralocorticoids are important for support of normal cardiovascular structure and function. Glucocorticoids potentiate the vasoconstrictor action of adrenergic stimuli on small vessels, contributing to the maintenance of capillary integrity. Mineralocorticoids help maintain normal blood volume by stimulating sodium retention.

Glucocorticoids increase plasma hemoglobin concentration and the number of erythrocytes and polymorphonuclear leukocytes (neutrophils) in the blood and elevate the total white blood cell count. In contrast, they decrease the number of circulating eosinophils, basophils, monocytes, and lymphocytes. The observation that daily fluctuations in blood eosinophil levels occur is of historical interest because it suggested the existence of a circadian rhythm of glucocorticoid secretion. For a complete discussion of the immunomodulatory properties of the glucocorticoids, see index entry Adrenal Corticosteroids, Actions.

Central Nervous System: In general, the role of the corticosteroids in central nervous system function is poorly defined. Corticosteroids readily enter the brain and can influence mood, sleep patterns, and EEG activity. Adrenal insufficiency is associated with changes in mood (irritability and depression) and with greater than usual EEG slow wave activity. Both conditions are relieved by the administration of hydrocortisone.

Skeletal Muscle: Corticosteroids are required to maintain normal skeletal muscular strength. The fatigue associated with adrenal insufficiency probably is caused primarily by circulatory incompetence and, to a lesser extent, by disorders of carbohydrate metabolism and electrolyte balance. In contrast, large amounts of glucocorticoids stimulate proteolysis in myocytes and the secretion of glutamine and alanine; pain and muscle weakness can result.

Stress: Although the mechanisms involved have not been determined definitively, two observations support the hypothesis that increased glucocorticoid secretion in response to stressful stimuli is protective: (1) Cortisol secretion is immediately and greatly enhanced at the initiation of stress. (2) Patients experiencing severe stress (eg, abdominal surgery) who are incapable of secreting additional glucocorticoids require exogenous hormone to prevent hypoglycemia and circulatory failure (McEwen, 1988).

Sexual Maturation: Adrenal androgens usually do not have a potent masculinizing effect in men. However, in women, a portion of adrenal androstenedione is converted in peripheral tissues to testosterone, which is responsible for sexual hair development, support of normal libido, and possibly the slight masculinization that sometimes occurs after menopause. Adrenal androgen production increases during late childhood and throughout puberty (adrenarche) in both sexes and is an integral part of normal maturation.

HYPERSECRETION OF ADRENOCORTICAL HORMONES

Cushing's Syndrome

Cushing's syndrome is manifested by abnormal fat distribution and obesity, moon facies, hypertension, hyperpigmentation, skin atrophy and striae, masculinization (acne, hirsutism, menstrual disorders), myopathy, abnormal glucose tolerance, depression (or, less commonly, euphoria and other behavioral abnormalities), osteoporosis, pedal edema, and, in children, growth suppression. Reversible suppression of thyroid-stimulating hormone (TSH) and thyroid hormone secretion mimicking the syndrome of nonthyroidal illness are common (Benker et al, 1990; Bartalena et al, 1991). Central serous chorioretinopathy also may occur (Bouzas et al, 1993). These effects are similar to some side effects of pharmacologic doses of glucocorticoids administered for nonendocrine disorders (see index entry Adrenal Corticosteroids, Adverse Reactions).

Cushing's syndrome results from excessive serum concentrations of glucocorticoids and is either iatrogenic or caused by adrenal hypersecretion (Schteingart, 1989). Primary hypersecretion of glucocorticoids occurs in patients with benign adrenal adenoma, adrenocortical carcinoma, congenital primary pigmented nodular adrenocortical disease (primary adrenal nodular dysplasia [PAND]), or macronodular hyperplasia. Secondary hypersecretion occurs in response to excessive pituitary secretion of ACTH (Cushing's disease [Cushing, 1932]). Cushing's disease is present in about 70% of patients with noniatrogenic hyperglucocorticoidism. Primary pituitary disease has a relatively slow onset and results from hypersecretion of ACTH by a monoclonal pituitary adenoma (Biller et al, 1992; Gicquel et al, 1992). Secondary pituitary corticotropic hyperplasia may result from excessive

CRH secretion by rare, benign, hypothalamic gangliocytomas or by extremely rare, ectopic, CRH-secreting carcinomas (Carey et al, 1984; Trainer and Grossman, 1991).

About 10% to 15% of patients with Cushing's syndrome have bilateral adrenal hyperplasia caused by ectopic nonpituitary ACTH-secreting tumors (ectopic ACTH syndrome) (White and Clark, 1993). In adults, carcinomas of the lung, thyroid, esophagus, islet cell, ovary, breast, or prostate; bronchial adenomas; and carcinoid tumors are the most common ACTH-secreting tumors. In children, ectopic production of ACTH by neural, thymic, and pancreatic tumors is more common. The unregulated ectopic secretion of ACTH may trigger rapidly progressive hypercortisolism, in which the physical signs typical of Cushing's syndrome are minimal but hypertension, hypokalemia, and malaise are common.

Hypersecretion of ACTH from lack of glucocorticoid feedback also can occur when glucocorticoid secretion is inadequate. The skin pigmentation characteristic of Addison's disease or Nelson's syndrome may be caused by ACTH and related peptides, such as β- and γ-melanocyte-stimulating hormone (MSH), which have intrinsic skin-darkening properties.

The pathogenesis of PAND is obscure. Current evidence suggests that it is a familial disease occurring most frequently among females during the first two decades of life. The syndrome may be triggered by circulating adrenal-stimulating ACTH-receptor autoantibodies and might more accurately be termed autoimmune hypercortisolism (Findling, 1989; Young et al, 1989; Wilkin, 1990). Other cases have been attributed to adrenal hypersensitivity to gastric inhibitory peptide (Reznik et al, 1992).

SCREENING. The use of single determinations of plasma cortisol concentrations is of little value for *initial screening* of patients for hypercortisolism (see the Table and the previous discussion on Regulation of Adrenocortical Hormone Secretion). However, plasma cortisol concentrations measured in the morning and evening may be useful; evening concentrations greater than 50% of morning concentrations, even if within a "normal" range, suggest hypercortisolism. Plasma ACTH concentrations >100 pg/ml (22.0 pmol/L) also suggest hypersecretion of ACTH (Cushing's disease or ectopic ACTH syndrome), although there is substantial overlap between unaffected and affected individuals (Kuhn et al, 1989). The 1-mg overnight dexamethasone test is a simple *dynamic screening* technique; nine hours after administration of dexamethasone (1 mg orally at 11 PM), about 70% of unaffected individuals have a plasma total cortisol concentration <140 nmol/L (5 mcg/dL) (Crapo, 1979).

Most endocrinologists prefer to measure urinary free cortisol (UFC) excretion (Sheeler, 1988; Schteingart, 1989; Kaye and Crapo, 1990; Grua and Nelson, 1991). When iatrogenic hypercortisolism is unlikely, 24-hour UFC >70 mcg/M^2 measured by binding assay or >35 mcg/M^2 measured by high-pressure liquid chromatography (HPLC) is diagnostic of Cushing's syndrome (see Table) in 98% of affected adults (Carpenter, 1988) and in 99% to 100% of affected children (Thomas et al, 1984; Jones, 1990; Gomez et al, 1991). Concurrent plasma ACTH concentrations <40 pg/ml (8.8 pmol/L) are indicative of primary adrenal disease (benign adrenal adenoma, adrenal carcinoma, macronodular hyperplasia, or PAND).

DIAGNOSIS. CRH may be used in the differential diagnosis of nonadrenal Cushing's syndrome (Kaye and Crapo, 1990; Loriaux and Nieman, 1991). Increased plasma concentrations of cortisol or ACTH after intravenous administration of CRH suggest Cushing's disease, while lack of response usually indicates an ectopic ACTH source. However, positive responses to CRH stimulation have been reported in patients with ectopic ACTH-producing tumors (Suda et al, 1986; Trainer and Grossman, 1991). In addition, depression, seasonal affective disorder, obesity, anorexia nervosa, alcoholism, and use of opioids inhibit the ACTH response to CRH.

Synthetic ovine and synthetic human CRH have similar effects on pituitary function, and their usefulness in adrenal function testing has been compared (Nieman et al, 1989; Trainer and Grossman, 1991). Many clinicians favor the use of ovine CRH because its effect is three to four times more prolonged, probably because human CRH is cleared from the circulation much faster. However, the antigenic nature of ovine CRH also must be taken into consideration.

The various dexamethasone suppression tests (see Table) determine the ability of exogenous dexamethasone to inhibit ACTH and cortisol secretion (Tyrrell et al, 1986). The high-dose test can be used to differentiate Cushing's disease (suppressible hypersecretion of ACTH) from ectopic ACTH syndrome (nonsuppressible hypersecretion of ACTH), adrenal tumors, or PAND (suppressed secretion of ACTH) (Crapo, 1979). However, this test does not conclusively identify 10% to 15% of patients with pituitary adenomas (Flack et al, 1992). An intravenous dexamethasone suppression test may enhance the ability to detect pituitary adenomas (Biemond et al, 1990). Many obese, depressed, alcoholic, or hospitalized patients and those receiving medications that accelerate hepatic clearance of dexamethasone will be resistant to ACTH suppression by dexamethasone (Schteingart, 1989; Kyriazopoulou and Vagenakis, 1992).

The abilities of the CRH stimulation test and the dexamethasone suppression tests to distinguish a pituitary from an ectopic source of ACTH appear to be comparable (Kaye and Crapo, 1990). When used together, these tests have been reported to result in 100% specificity and sensitivity and 98% to 100% diagnostic accuracy (Hermus et al, 1986; Nieman et al, 1986; Yanovski et al, 1993).

The most accurate and reliable single method for distinguishing pituitary and ectopic ACTH hypersecretion requires sampling of petrosal sinus blood and comparing its ACTH concentration with that of peripheral venous blood following CRH administration (Mampalam et al, 1988; Tabarin et al, 1991 A; Oldfield et al, 1991). Bilateral samples may indicate the location of a pituitary microadenoma in many patients (Loriaux and Nieman, 1991; Oldfield et al, 1991).

Although it is seldom used currently, the ACTH stimulation test also has been employed to test adrenal function and differentiate among adrenal adenoma, adrenal carcinoma, and PAND (Jones, 1990). However, this test is not sufficiently discriminating because of the variability of the response to acute ACTH stimulation. Ultrasound, CT scan, and MRI are

TESTS THAT ASSIST IN THE DIAGNOSIS OF ADRENAL CORTICOSTEROID HYPERSECRETION[1]

Diagnostic Test	Result	Suggested Diagnosis
INITIAL SCREENING:		
Plasma cortisol concentration (8 AM)	275-700 nmol/L (10-25 mcg/dL)	normal
	>700 nmol/L (>25 mcg/dL)	adrenal hypersecretion
Plasma ACTH concentration (8 AM)	2–22 pmol/L (10-100 pg/ml)	normal
	>22 pmol/L (>100 pg/ml)	hypersecretion of ACTH
UFC[2] excretion	>70 mcg/M²/day	adrenal hypersecretion[3]
	>35 mcg/M²/day	adrenal hypersecretion[4]
1-mg overnight dexamethasone suppression test	plasma [cortisol] >140 nmol/L (>5 mcg/dL)	adrenal hypersecretion
IF INITIAL SCREENING SUGGESTS ADRENAL HYPERSECRETION:		
CRH stimulation test	>20% ↑ plasma [cortisol] *and* >50% ↑ plasma [ACTH]	Cushing's disease
	<20% ↑ plasma [cortisol] *and* <50% ↑ plasma [ACTH]	adrenal tumor; ectopic ACTH syndrome
Low-dose dexamethasone suppression test		
48-hour test (6 hr after 8 doses of 0.5 mg every 6 hr)	plasma [cortisol] <140 nmol/L (<5 mcg/dL) *or* UFC <70 mcg/M²/day	normal
	plasma [cortisol] >140 nmol/L (>5 mcg/dL) *or* UFC >70 mcg/M²/day	adrenal hypersecretion
High-dose dexamethasone suppression test		
overnight test (8 hr after 8 mg)	>50% ↓ plasma [cortisol]	Cushing's disease
	<50% ↓ plasma [cortisol]	adrenal tumor; PAND[5]; ectopic ACTH syndrome
48-hr test (6 hr after 8 doses of 2 mg every 6 hr)	>50% ↓ plasma [cortisol] *or* >90% ↓ UFC *and* >64% ↓ 24-hour urinary 17-hydroxysteroid excretion	Cushing's disease
	<50% ↓ plasma [cortisol] *or* <90% ↓ UFC *or* <64% ↓ 24-hour urinary hydroxysteroid excretion	adrenal tumor; PAND[5]; ectopic ACTH syndrome
Bilateral inferior petrosal sinus sampling	ACTH gradient >2	Cushing's disease; lateralization of tumor

[1]See text for details of tests and their interpretations.
[2]Urinary free cortisol
[3]Measured using binding assay.
[4]Measured using high pressure liquid chromatography (HPLC).
[5]Primary adrenal nodular dysplasia

much more useful in the identification of adrenal tumors (Carpenter, 1988).

Metyrapone [Metopirone] has been used to distinguish pituitary causes of Cushing's syndrome from nonpituitary causes. However, metyrapone now is seldom used diagnostically because results are relatively nonspecific and plasma ACTH concentrations can be measured directly.

TREATMENT. Treatment of Cushing's syndrome is directed toward the cause. Transsphenoidal adenomectomy, hypophysectomy, or pituitary irradiation is used to treat the pituitary adenomas associated with Cushing's disease. Disorders of adrenal origin or in which the primary cause cannot be corrected are treated by adrenal surgery. Drugs are most useful as adjuncts to pituitary surgery or irradiation or as palliative treatment for adrenal carcinoma or ectopic ACTH-producing tumors (Miller and Crapo, 1993).

Surgery: Transsphenoidal microadenomectomy is the treatment of choice for most adults when pituitary disorders cause Cushing's syndrome, even in the absence of radiologic evidence of microadenoma (Freidberg, 1989; Grua and Nelson, 1991). Surgical success is indicated by plasma cortisol concentrations <35 nmol/L measured 6 to 12 weeks after surgery; postoperative serum cortisol concentrations >100 nmol/L at 6 to 12 weeks are predictive of clinical relapse (Toms et al, 1991). When surgery is successful, return of normal pituitary-adrenal function usually is not observed for months. During this period, the patient is treated for secondary adrenal insufficiency and appropriate precautions should be observed: increased doses of glucocorticoid should be given during stress (eg, febrile illness, surgical or other trauma), and the patient should wear medical identification and carry an emergency supply of injectable glucocorticoid.

In general, bilateral adrenalectomy is no longer indicated for patients with Cushing's disease. However, adrenalectomy may be employed in patients who do not respond to pituitary surgery, irradiation, or medical therapy and in whom the condition is complicated by hypertension or severe osteoporosis. Bilateral adrenalectomy also may be appropriate in the presence of inoperable ectopic ACTH-producing tumors and in patients with PAND. Following surgery, the incidence of residual cortisol-producing tissue may be relatively high, and subsequent hormone replacement therapy must be individualized (Kemink et al, 1992; McCance et al, 1993).

Unilateral adrenalectomy is the appropriate treatment for benign adenoma or adrenal carcinoma. These patients require glucocorticoid replacement for one year or more until there is recovery of function by the suppressed contralateral adrenal gland.

Women with untreated hypercortisolism who become pregnant and do not spontaneously abort early in gestation should be treated to enhance the likelihood of full-term delivery and to avoid the possibility of neonatal adrenal insufficiency (Buescher et al, 1992). Transsphenoidal surgery and unilateral adrenalectomy are relatively safe for these patients and decrease the incidence of premature labor and fetal loss.

Pituitary Irradiation: High-dose external irradiation of the pituitary with cobalt 60 improves or cures approximately 50% of patients with Cushing's disease. The response is greater in younger individuals; however, hypopituitarism or other neurologic complications resulting from radiation necrosis of the brain may develop years after irradiation in childhood. Pituitary irradiation also may be used in patients at high risk for surgical complications and following unsuccessful pituitary surgery. Remission can be enhanced in some patients with concurrent long-term administration of reserpine 1 to 2 mg daily (Murayama et al, 1992).

Drug Therapy: Use of drugs as the primary treatment for Cushing's syndrome has been only partially successful (Miller and Crapo, 1993). An adrenolytic agent (mitotane [Lysodren]), enzyme inhibitors (metyrapone [Metopirone], aminoglutethimide [Cytadren], trilostane [Modrastane]), ketoconazole [Nizoral], and centrally acting agents (cyproheptadine [Periactin], bromocriptine [Parlodel]) are generally used as adjuncts to prepare patients for adrenal surgery. They also are employed in conjunction with pituitary irradiation to control Cushing's disease, for medical adrenalectomy, or rarely are given alone as primary treatment for Cushing's disease. All drugs used to treat Cushing's syndrome have unpleasant and serious side effects that limit their usefulness. In addition, all patients receiving drugs to control Cushing's syndrome must be monitored to detect iatrogenic adrenal insufficiency, which may develop as therapy becomes effective.

Mitotane destroys adrenocortical cells and is useful when other therapies are ineffective. Lower doses (1.5 to 4 g daily) inhibit steroid synthesis and may control adrenal secretion in Cushing's disease, particularly while awaiting the effects of pituitary irradiation. Larger doses (4 to 12 g daily) are used to destroy metastatic tissue in adrenal carcinoma.

Enzyme inhibitors block the biosynthetic pathway for cortisol production and are less toxic and therefore preferable to mitotane. In pituitary-dependent disease, however, removal of the negative feedback effect of cortisol on the pituitary causes even greater secretion of ACTH, which partially overcomes the metabolic blockade and renders these drugs less effective after several days. Enzyme inhibitors are more useful for treating pituitary-independent forms of Cushing's syndrome such as ectopic ACTH-producing tumors.

Enzyme inhibitors also are used to reduce cortisol secretion temporarily until the effects of pituitary irradiation are realized and in patients being prepared for adrenal surgery who are at high risk due to hypercortisolism. Metyrapone and aminoglutethimide often are used together for their additive effects. They block sex steroid synthesis in the gonads and adrenal glands and may be particularly useful when virilization results from excessive androgen production by an adrenal tumor. Experience with trilostane is inadequate to determine its relative effectiveness.

Ketoconazole, an imidazole with antifungal properties at low dosages, is the agent of choice when decreased cortisol secretion is desired (Jones, 1990; Tabarin et al, 1991 B). Oral administration of 400 mg to 1.2 g/day inhibits steroid production without increasing ACTH secretion (Pont et al, 1982; Sonino, 1987), but disease remission does not occur (Sonino, 1988; Tabarin et al, 1991 B). Patients should be monitored closely for signs of hepatotoxicity (Khanderia, 1991). In addition, ketoconazole can stimulate the secretion of 11-deoxycorticosterone and produce hypokalemia and hypertension (Saadi et al, 1990). Very large doses are sometimes effective in the treatment of ectopic ACTH syndrome (Tabarin et al, 1991 B).

The centrally acting agent, cyproheptadine, a serotonin antagonist, may act directly on pituitary microadenoma cells to inhibit ACTH secretion, but adequate suppression has been sustained in only 10% to 15% of patients receiving up to 24 mg daily and disease recurrence is common (Orth, 1983; Miller and Crapo, 1993). Bromocriptine, a dopamine agonist, decreases ACTH secretion in some patients, but normal cortisol levels are not achieved (Lamberts and Birkenhagr, 1976; Miller and Crapo, 1993). These agents also do not inhibit ACTH secretion when used together (Whitehead et al, 1990). A somatostatin analogue, octreotide [Sandostatin], has suppressed ACTH secretion in a few patients with Cushing's disease at doses >300 mcg/day; lower doses were ineffective (Ambrosi et al, 1990; Invitti et al, 1990; Woodhouse et al, 1993).

An investigational agent, RU486 (mifepristone), 5 to 22 mg/kg/day, may be effective in the treatment of Cushing's syndrome caused by inoperable or hidden ectopic ACTH-secreting tumors (Chrousos et al, 1988). Rather than reducing cortisol secretion, this agent relieves the symptoms of hypercortisolism by preventing glucocorticoid binding to tissue receptors (Svec, 1988). Unfortunately, the drug's effectiveness can only be monitored by observation of the patient's condition, an inexact approach at best.

The safety of metyrapone and aminoglutethimide during pregnancy has not been determined, but both are probably hazardous. Ketoconazole is a known teratogen in animals.

Peripheral Resistance to Glucocorticoids

Primary resistance to cortisol caused by functional abnormalities of the glucocorticoid receptor is characterized by hypercortisolism and elevated UFC and plasma ACTH concentration in the presence of hypertension, hypokalemia, and (in women) hirsutism. Affected individuals have decreased numbers of glucocorticoid receptors on all target tissues, including pituitary corticotropin cells; decreased affinity of glucocorticoid receptors for cortisol; decreased thermal stability of glucocorticoid receptors; and decreased binding of cortisol-receptor complexes to DNA (Iida et al, 1985; Brönnegärd et al, 1986; Nawata et al, 1987). Some patients with AIDS develop acquired hypercortisolism; they have no signs of Cushing's disease but lymphocyte receptor affinity for cortisol is decreased (Norbiato et al, 1992). Long-term administration of dexamethasone normalizes serum cortisol concentration in some of these individuals.

Primary Hyperaldosteronism

Increased plasma aldosterone concentration results in decreased plasma renin activity, hypokalemia (with electrocardiographic changes, muscle weakness, fatigue, paresthesia), metabolic alkalosis, and hypertension (Shenker, 1989; Hambling et al, 1993). Most cases of primary hyperaldosteronism (Conn's syndrome [Conn, 1955]) are caused by aldosterone-producing adrenal adenomas or by bilateral zona glomerulosa hyperplasia (Hambling et al, 1993). Rarely, this syndrome is associated with adrenal carcinoma.

DIAGNOSIS. Primary hyperaldosteronism should be suspected in all hypertensive patients with spontaneous hypokalemia. The diagnosis is confirmed when the ratio of plasma aldosterone concentration to plasma renin activity at 8 AM is greater than 30- or 24-hour urinary 18-hydroxycortisol excretion is greater than 300 mcg and when a high salt diet and administration of fludrocortisone [Florinef]), saline infusion, or oral captopril [Capoten] 25 mg fails to normalize the plasma aldosterone concentration (Melby, 1991; Miyamori et al, 1992; Hambling et al, 1993; Weinberger and Fineberg, 1993). Appropriate treatment requires determination of the cause of hyperaldosteronism. Diagnostic techniques to differentiate adrenal adenoma from bilateral adrenal hyperplasia include postural response tests, measurement of aldosterone precursors in serum (see Figure), determination of adrenal sensitivity to infusion of angiotensin and its blockade by saralasin, adrenal radioiodocholesterol scan, CT or MRI of the adrenal glands, and simultaneous catheterization of the adrenal veins (Melby, 1991; Hambling et al, 1993; Weinberger and Fineberg, 1993).

TREATMENT. When disease is caused by adrenal adenoma or carcinoma, simple resection of the adenoma or removal of the entire adrenal is curative. Plasma potassium concentrations should be normalized before surgery with large doses of spironolactone [Aldactone], a potassium-sparing diuretic and aldosterone antagonist, given for several weeks before surgery in conjunction with a low-sodium diet. If hypokalemia remains uncorrected, some physicians add oral potassium chloride to this regimen for one week prior to surgery. Postoperative mineralocorticoid replacement therapy (see discussion on Adrenocortical Insufficiency) has significantly increased survival (Shenker, 1989).

Hypertension caused by hyperaldosteronism in association with bilateral adrenal hyperplasia is usually not cured by partial resection or bilateral adrenalectomy. Spironolactone is the agent of choice to treat this form of the disease. The plasma potassium concentration may normalize within two weeks after initiation of spironolactone therapy, but several months are required to increase the renin concentration. In addition to antagonizing the effect of aldosterone, spironolactone also may inhibit its synthesis directly, allowing an eventual reduction in dose. Spironolactone has antiandrogenic side effects that may limit long-term use in some individuals, particularly males. In these patients, triamterene [Dyrenium] (100 to 300 mg/day), amiloride [Midamor] (5 to 40 mg/day), or trilostane (120 to 360 mg/day) may be used. Normalization of blood pressure may require the addition of another diuretic, a calcium channel antagonist, or an ACE inhibitor.

In rare familial glucocorticoid-suppressible hyperaldosteronism, fusion of the genes encoding 11-β-hydroxylase and 18-hydroxy-dehydrogenase results in unusually large numbers of "transitional" ACTH-responsive, angiotensin II-unresponsive aldosterone-secreting cells (Lifton et al, 1992). Diagnosis can be confirmed by 24-hour urinary excretion of 18-oxotetrahydrocortisol >100 nmol and of 18-hydroxycortisol >500 nmol (Rich et al, 1992). Treatment with a glucocorticoid (eg, dexamethasone 0.25 to 1 mg/day [Fraser et al, 1989; Shenker, 1989]) suppresses ACTH and aldosterone secretion and usually will correct hypertension and other aberrations caused by hyperaldosteronism (Shenker, 1989).

Secondary Hyperaldosteronism

Several primary disorders of renin physiology can result in secondary hypersecretion of aldosterone. Renovascular hypertension caused by atherosclerosis, renal cortical nephrosclerosis, fibromuscular hyperplasia, renal infarction, solitary renal cysts, or hydronephrosis may be associated with hypersecretion of renin and secondary renin-induced hyperaldosteronism. Severe chronic renal insufficiency with sodium wasting, Bartter's syndrome, estrogen therapy, and practices such as diuretic or laxative abuse or surreptitious vomiting also increase renal sodium excretion and trigger hyperreninism and hyperaldosteronism. Appropriate management of the primary disorder usually ameliorates symptoms of secondary hyperaldosteronism.

"Pseudohypoaldosteronism" is a syndrome characterized by hyperkalemia, hyperaldosteronemia, and hyperreninemia (Holland, 1991). The type I syndrome is associated with salt wasting and reduced blood pressure and is caused by aldosterone receptor deficiency (Armanini et al, 1985), prematurity (Abramson et al, 1992), or aldosterone insensitivity secondary to distal nephron disorders (systemic lupus erythematosus, obstructive uropathy, sickle cell anemia, analgesic nephropathy, chronic pyelonephritis). The severity of the signs depends on the degree of aldosterone insensitivity. Sodium supplementation and administration of oral polystyrene sulfonate resin [Kayexalate] can alleviate clinical signs (Smith and Kemp, 1991). The type II syndrome is associated with salt retention and can be completely reversed with a strict low-salt diet and diuretic therapy.

Drug Evaluations

AMINOGLUTETHIMIDE
[Cytadren]

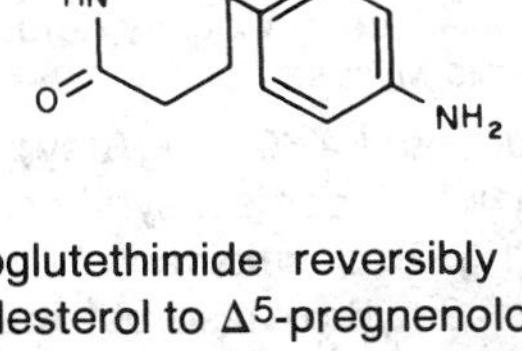

ACTIONS. Aminoglutethimide reversibly inhibits enzymatic conversion of cholesterol to Δ^5-pregnenolone, decreasing the secretion of glucocorticoids, mineralocorticoids, and sex steroids. In addition, aminoglutethimide inhibits aromatase activity in extra-adrenal tissues, decreasing the conversion of androstenedione to estrone and estradiol.

USES. Aminoglutethimide is used alone or with other agents to control cortisol secretion in Cushing's syndrome as an adjunct to pituitary irradiation, to prepare high-risk patients for adrenalectomy, as palliative treatment for metastatic adrenal carcinoma, and to lessen the effects of ectopic ACTH-producing tumors. When Cushing's syndrome results from hypersecretion of ACTH, this drug's efficacy may decrease as negative feedback of cortisol is reduced and ACTH secretion is thus increased enough to partially overcome the enzyme blockade. Aminoglutethimide is not curative; relapse occurs on cessation of therapy.

For a discussion of adverse reactions, teratogenicity, and pharmacokinetics, see index entry Aminoglutethimide, As Antineoplastic Agent.

PRECAUTIONS. Adrenal and thyroid function should be monitored and replacement therapy provided if necessary. Aminoglutethimide should not be used in patients who are hypersensitive to it or to glutethimide. It is not known whether this drug is excreted in human milk, and its safety and effectiveness in children have not been established (FDA Pregnancy Category D).

DRUG INTERACTIONS. Aminoglutethimide induces the hepatic oxidation of several drugs, including itself. If adrenocortical hormone replacement therapy is required, dexamethasone should not be used because its metabolism is accelerated by aminoglutethimide. Hydrocortisone should be used instead. Aminoglutethimide increases the rate of metabolism of oral anticoagulants and may increase the warfarin requirement by approximately 100%. The dose of warfarin may then have to be reduced considerably if aminoglutethimide is withdrawn. This drug also may decrease the steady-state concentrations of digitoxin. Alcohol may potentiate the effects of aminoglutethimide.

DOSAGE AND PREPARATIONS.
Oral: *Adults*, for Cushing's syndrome, 250 mg every six hours initially, increased by 250 mg daily every one to two weeks if necessary to 2 g daily. Plasma cortisol concentrations are monitored until the desired level of suppression is achieved. Dosage reduction or discontinuation of therapy may be necessary if adverse effects develop.

Cytadren (CIBA). Tablets 250 mg.

CORTICOTROPIN (ACTH)
[Acthar, H.P. Acthar Gel]

CHEMISTRY. Corticotropin is a straight-chain polypeptide consisting of 39 amino acids prepared from animal pituitaries and bioassayed against a standard preparation. The sequence of the first 24 amino acids is common to humans, cattle, pigs, and sheep, and this segment contains the biological activity of the molecule. The arrangement of the remaining amino acids varies among species. These heterologous segments may stimulate production of antibodies and cause allergic reactions when corticotropin of animal origin is used in humans. More importantly, animal preparations contain other antigenic proteins or peptides.

ACTIONS AND USES. Corticotropin stimulates the adrenal cortex to secrete cortisol, deoxycorticosterone, androgens, and other steroids. It can be used diagnostically to determine the competence of the hypophyseal-adrenal axis, although the synthetic analogue, cosyntropin, is preferred because of the lower risk of allergic reactions (see the evaluation on Cosyntropin).

Corticotropin also may be used to treat glucocorticoid-responsive diseases in patients with functional adrenal glands (see index entry Adrenal Corticosteroids, Uses); however, treatment with this agent is less predictable, less convenient, more expensive, and usually possesses no advantages over a glucocorticoid. Some investigators prefer corticotropin to glucocorticoids in patients with ulcerative colitis, but objective evidence of superiority is lacking. It has been reported that corticotropin does not inhibit growth to the same extent as glucocorticoids when given to children with chronic diseases responsive to long-term glucocorticoid therapy, but these results have not been confirmed. For other uses, see index entry Corticotropin.

PRECAUTIONS. Corticotropin is contraindicated after recent surgery and in patients with osteoporosis, systemic fungal infections, ocular herpes simplex, peptic ulcer, congestive heart failure, hypertension, or sensitivity to porcine proteins. Immunizations should be undertaken with caution during therapy with corticotropin because of the risk of neurologic complications and lack of antibody response. The effects of corticotropin may be enhanced in patients with hypothyroidism or cirrhosis.

Although corticotropin causes adrenal hyperplasia rather than atrophy, prolonged therapy impairs the ability of the hypophyseal-pituitary-adrenal axis to respond to stress. Its use during glucocorticoid withdrawal does not hasten, and may even impair, the establishment of hypothalamic-hypophyseal-adrenal responsiveness.

ADVERSE REACTIONS. In addition to the adverse effects caused by increased secretion of glucocorticoids, corticotropin can produce electrolyte disturbances and acne, hirsutism, and amenorrhea in women. Acute allergic reactions have occurred in sensitized patients. Corticotropin has an embryocidal effect (FDA Pregnancy Category C). It is not known whether this drug is excreted in human milk.

DOSAGE AND PREPARATIONS. Because adrenal glands vary in their response to corticotropin, the dosage must be individualized to obtain a satisfactory therapeutic effect with minimal dosage and alteration in metabolism. When dosage reduction is necessary, the amount should be decreased gradually. The gel form delays uptake from tissues, thereby prolonging the hormone's action. Because the activity of corticotropin is destroyed by proteolytic enzymes in the gastrointestinal tract, the drug is administered intramuscularly and, occasionally, subcutaneously or intravenously.

Intramuscular: For therapeutic use, 80 units of aqueous solution daily in four divided doses (20 units every six hours) or 40 to 80 units of gel (repository) every 24 to 72 hours.

For diagnostic use, 40 to 80 units of gel daily for one to three successive days.

Available generically and as ACTH: Gel (repository) 40 and 80 units/ml in 5 ml containers; powder 40 units.

Acthar (Rhone-Poulenc Rorer). Powder (sterile, lyophilized) 25 and 40 units.

H.P. Acthar Gel (Rhone-Poulenc Rorer). Gel (repository) 40 and 80 units/ml in 1 and 5 ml containers.

Intravenous: For diagnostic uses, 25 or 40 units dissolved in 500 ml of 5% dextrose infused over an eight-hour period.

Generic. Powder 40 units.

Acthar (Rhone-Poulenc Rorer). Powder (sterile, lyophilized) 25 and 40 units.

COSYNTROPIN
[Cortrosyn]

CHEMISTRY. Cosyntropin is $\alpha^{1\text{-}24}$-corticotropin, a synthetic subunit of ACTH. It is an open-chain polypeptide containing the first 24 of the 39 amino acids of natural ACTH and exhibits the full corticosteroidogenic activity of natural ACTH. Cosyntropin 0.25 mg stimulates the adrenal cortex to the same extent as 25 units of natural ACTH. It has little antigenicity.

USES. Cosyntropin is used in diagnostic screening of patients for adrenocortical insufficiency. It may be administered intramuscularly or intravenously for prompt determination of adrenal function or as an intravenous infusion over a four- to eight-hour period to provide a greater stimulus to the adrenal glands. A low-dose ACTH stimulation test may distinguish adrenocortical insufficiency from glucocorticoid-induced adrenal suppression (Dickstein et al, 1991).

PRECAUTIONS. Hypersensitivity reactions occur rarely; very few other adverse reactions have been reported. The safety of cosyntropin when given to pregnant or lactating women has not been established (FDA Pregnancy Category C).

DOSAGE AND PREPARATIONS.

Intravenous: For rapid diagnostic use, *adults*, a single injection of 0.25 mg stimulates maximal adrenal response in 30 to 60 minutes. For more pronounced stimulation, 0.25 to 0.75 mg may be infused intravenously over four to eight hours. For low-dose test, 1 to 5 mcg. *Children 2 years or less*, 0.125 mg.

Intramuscular: For diagnostic use, a single injection of 0.25 to 0.75 mg produces maximal adrenal response in 30 to 60 minutes.

Cortrosyn (Organon). Powder (sterile, lyophilized) 0.25 mg with mannitol 10 mg in 1 ml containers with diluent.

KETOCONAZOLE
[Nizoral]

For chemical formula, see index entry Ketoconazole, Uses, Subcutaneous, Systemic Mycoses.

ACTIONS. Large doses (>600 mg/day) of this antifungal imidazole reversibly inhibit cortisol synthesis (Sonino, 1987). The drug inhibits 17, 20-desmolase, 17-α-hydroxylase, 18-hydroxylase, and 11-β-hydroxylase but has no effect on 21-hydroxylase and 3-β-dehydrogenase (Engelhardt et al, 1991). Consequently, cortisol secretion is decreased and 11-

deoxycorticosterone secretion is increased (Saadi et al, 1990).

USES. Ketoconazole is the agent of choice when a decrease in the adrenal secretion of cortisol is desired. Relatively large doses reverse hypercortisolism without triggering an increase in ACTH secretion and "cortisol escape." With continued use, both clinical and biochemical signs of ACTH-independent and ACTH-dependent forms of Cushing's syndrome regress, although remission may not be possible. However, even very large doses may be ineffective in the treatment of ectopic ACTH syndrome.

For information on adverse reactions, precautions, drug interactions, and pharmacokinetics, see index entry Ketoconazole, Uses, Subcutaneous, Systemic Mycoses.

DOSAGE AND PREPARATIONS.

Oral: For Cushing's disease and Cushing's syndrome, 400 mg to 1.2 g/day.

Nizoral (Janssen). Tablets 200 mg.

METYRAPONE

[Metopirone]

ACTIONS AND USES. Metyrapone blocks cortisol production, primarily by reversibly blocking 11-β-hydroxylase activity in the adrenal cortex. Although the drug also inhibits aldosterone secretion, the production of deoxycorticosterone, a mineralocorticoid, is increased and mineralocorticoid deficiency usually does not occur.

Metyrapone is used investigationally alone or with other agents to control cortisol secretion in Cushing's syndrome. Its uses in this disorder are similar to those of aminoglutethimide (see that evaluation). The effectiveness of this drug is decreased by the increased secretion of ACTH in pituitary-dependent disease. However, the elevated level of ACTH generally is insufficient to overcome the enzyme blockade. The drug may induce remission but is not curative. Metyrapone also has been used to assess pituitary function, but the ability to measure plasma ACTH concentrations accurately has rendered this use obsolete (see discussion in section on Cushing's Syndrome).

ADVERSE REACTIONS AND PRECAUTIONS. Side effects of metyrapone include nausea, abdominal distress, drowsiness, headache, dizziness, and skin rash. Metyrapone may cause hypertension and hypokalemic alkalosis as 11-deoxycorticosterone accumulates in the blood. Similarly, the increase in the adrenal secretion of dehydroepiandrosterone may cause hirsutism in women.

Since adrenal insufficiency may occur, especially when metyrapone is given with another adrenal suppressant, such as aminoglutethimide, adrenal function should be monitored. Replacement therapy may be instituted if necessary, or the dose of the drug(s) may be reduced.

PREGNANCY AND LACTATION. When metyrapone is administered to pregnant women during the second and third trimesters, it may cause enzymatic blockade and adrenal insufficiency in the fetus (FDA Pregnancy Category C). It is not known whether this drug is excreted in human milk.

PHARMACOKINETICS. Metyrapone is well absorbed after oral administration. The drug is excreted in the urine, mostly as glucuronides, and has an elimination half-life of 1 to 2.5 hours.

DOSAGE AND PREPARATIONS.

Oral: For selected patients with Cushing's syndrome, 250 to 500 mg four times daily.

Metopirone (CIBA). Capsules 250 mg (available from manufacturer under an Investigational New Drug Application).

MITOTANE

[Lysodren]

For chemical formula, see index entry Mitotane, As Antineoplastic Agent.

ACTIONS AND USES. Mitotane is a relatively specific adrenolytic agent; it destroys adrenal cortical cells of the zona fasciculata and reticularis (but not glomerulosa), which permanently decreases the synthesis of adrenal steroids. Adrenal 11-β-hydroxylase and cholesterol side-chain cleavage enzymes are inhibited in surviving cells, which further reduces the synthesis of cortisol and aldosterone. Peripheral metabolism of steroids also is altered; circulating concentrations of 17- hydroxysteroids are decreased and 6-β-hydroxycortisol is increased.

Mitotane is used as palliative treatment for metastatic adrenal carcinoma (see index entry Mitotane, As Antineoplastic Agent). It has been used investigationally as an adjunct to pituitary irradiation to temporarily inhibit or permanently destroy (depending on dose) adrenal tissue in selected patients with Cushing's syndrome. Because the onset of effectiveness may take several weeks, this agent is not suitable for acute therapy.

ADVERSE REACTIONS AND PRECAUTIONS. Toxicity is dose related, and the most frequent and severe adverse reactions are observed with the larger doses used to treat cancer. Less severe effects occur with the lower doses used to treat Cushing's syndrome. Gastrointestinal disturbances (eg, nausea, vomiting, diarrhea) are the most common adverse reactions; central nervous system effects (eg, lethargy, somnolence, dizziness, vertigo) also are observed. Infrequent reactions include visual problems, genitourinary disturbances (eg, hematuria, cystitis, albuminuria), and cardiovascular effects (eg, flushing, hypertension, orthostatic hypotension).

Because the onset of clinical effectiveness is variable, patients should be monitored and treated for adrenal insufficiency (both glucocorticoid and mineralocorticoid replacement) when appropriate. In those with adrenal carcinoma, tumor tissue should be removed before mitotane is administered in order to prevent infarction and hemorrhage produced by its rapid adrenolytic action.

Prolonged administration of mitotane may cause brain toxicity with behavioral and neurologic impairment. Behavioral and neurologic assessments should be made at regular intervals when mitotane therapy is continued for more than two years.

The safety of mitotane in pregnant and lactating women and in children has not been established (FDA Pregnancy Category C).

PHARMACOKINETICS. See index entry Mitotane, As Antineoplastic Agent.

DOSAGE AND PREPARATIONS.

Oral: *Adults*, for adjunctive therapy with pituitary irradiation in selected patients with Cushing's syndrome, initially, 500 mg to 1 g daily in divided doses with the largest amount given at bedtime to minimize discomfort from side effects. The dose can be increased every two to four weeks (to avoid adrenal insufficiency) to a maximum of 4 g daily. The maintenance dose is 500 mg to 2 g daily.

For use in adrenal carcinoma, see index entry Mitotane, As Antineoplastic Agent.

Lysodren (Bristol-Myers Squibb). Tablets 500 mg.

SPIRONOLACTONE

[Aldactone]

For chemical formula, see index entry Spironolactone, Uses, Diuresis.

ACTIONS AND USES. This steroidal aldosterone antagonist promotes natriuresis and inhibits potassium and magnesium excretion by acting as a competitive antagonist of aldosterone in the cortical collecting duct of the renal tubule. Doses exceeding 100 mg/day may inhibit biosynthesis and block the peripheral action of testosterone by competing for androgen receptor sites.

Spironolactone is used to treat primary hyperaldosteronism and to correct potassium depletion prior to surgery in patients with an aldosterone-producing adrenal adenoma. This drug is the agent of choice for the long-term treatment of hyperaldosteronism due to bilateral adrenal hyperplasia and also is used to treat hirsutism (both idiopathic and that associated with polycystic ovary disease).

ADVERSE REACTIONS. Spironolactone may cause a variety of adverse reactions (see index entry Spironolactone, Uses, Diuresis). Their incidence is related to dosage and length of treatment; adverse effects are much less frequent at doses below 150 mg/day (Skluth and Gums, 1990).

For a discussion of drug interactions, effects on laboratory tests, and pharmacokinetics, see index entry Spironolactone, Uses, Diuresis.

PREGNANCY AND LACTATION. Spironolactone crosses the placenta and may affect the fetus. A metabolite of spironolactone, canrenone, appears in human milk. If use of this drug is essential, an alternative method of infant feeding should be considered.

DOSAGE AND PREPARATIONS. Concomitant food intake enhances the absorption of spironolactone; salicylates increase its metabolism and should be avoided.

Oral: To prepare patients with aldosterone-producing adrenal adenoma for surgery, *adults,* 300 to 600 mg/day in four divided doses for three to four weeks before surgery. For prolonged treatment of hyperaldosteronism due to bilateral adrenal hyperplasia, initially, 200 to 400 mg daily. The dosage subsequently may be reduced to 25 to 100 mg daily.

Generic. Tablets 25 mg.

Aldactone (Searle). Tablets 25, 50, and 100 mg.

TRILOSTANE

[Modrastane]

ACTIONS AND USES. This synthetic steroid has no inherent hormonal activity. Trilostane inhibits adrenal 3-β-hydroxysteroid dehydrogenase activity and decreases the secretion of cortisol and aldosterone. When given alone in therapeutic doses, the drug does not suppress adrenal secretion below normal levels, depress testicular testosterone production significantly, or cure the underlying disease process. Carbohydrate metabolism may improve in some patients.

Trilostane has been used in selected patients with Cushing's syndrome to control hypersecretion of glucocorticoids. It has been used investigationally to treat hyperaldosteronism.

ADVERSE REACTIONS AND PRECAUTIONS. Adverse reactions are reported in about 25% of patients and can be minimized by using small doses initially and increasing the amount gradually. Gastrointestinal reactions (eg, diarrhea, abdominal discomfort, nausea) occur in about 17% of patients. Effects observed in less than 10% of patients include oral or nasal burning sensation, flushing, and headache.

Although trilostane alone does not produce adrenal insufficiency, the adrenal response to severe stress may be impaired. The therapeutic response to the drug should be monitored. Trilostane should not be given to patients with severe renal or liver disease.

DRUG INTERACTIONS. Because trilostane inhibits aldosterone secretion, the potassium-wasting effect of thiazide or loop diuretics is reduced.

PHARMACOKINETICS. Data on the pharmacokinetics of trilostane in humans are limited; however, there is considerable variation in the dose-response to the drug.

PREGNANCY AND LACTATION. Trilostane should not be given to pregnant patients (FDA Pregnancy Category X), because it inhibits fetal steroidogenesis. It has terminated pregnancy in rats, monkeys, and women through an interceptive mechanism. Skeletal teratogenesis was observed in rats.

It is not known whether trilostane is excreted in human milk but, because of the potential for adrenal suppression in the infant, lactating mothers should not take this drug. Its safety and efficacy in children have not been established.

DOSAGE AND PREPARATIONS.

Oral: For selected *adults* with Cushing's syndrome, 30 mg four times a day for at least three days. Thereafter, the dosage may be adjusted at three- to four-day intervals according to the patient's response. The usual range is 120 to 360 mg daily. Similar doses may provide temporary relief of primary hyperaldosteronism (Shenker, 1989). Doses $>$480 mg/day are not recommended.

Modrastane (Sanofi Winthrop). Capsules 30 and 60 mg.

ADRENOCORTICAL INSUFFICIENCY

Hypoadrenalism

Inability to secrete corticosteroids results from defects in the hypothalamic-pituitary-adrenal axis. Lack of adrenal function can result from destruction of the adrenal glands, inadequate secretion of ACTH or CRH, or congenital defects in steroidogenesis.

Adrenal atrophy with loss of function (*primary adrenocortical insufficiency*; Addison's disease) is usually caused by autoimmune disease, although tuberculosis also is a significant etiologic factor. Autoimmune adrenocortical insufficiency is characterized by autoantibodies to adrenal microsomal and plasma membrane antigens and lymphocytic infiltration of degenerative adrenal cortices, with sparing of the adrenal medulla. Autoantibodies to other tissue antigens are commonly found in patients with autoimmune hypoadrenalism; Addison's disease, lymphocytic thyroiditis, and insulin-dependent diabetes mellitus often occur together (Type II autoimmune polyendocrinopathy). In addition, hypoadrenalism has been reported in patients with coagulopathies, thrombotic venous occlusions, hemorrhagic adrenal infarctions, and circulating antiphospholipid antibodies (Asherson and Cervera, 1992). These findings are consistent with the hypothesis that autoimmune hypoadrenalism may be a manifestation of a generalized defect in immunoregulation (see reviews by Muir and Maclaren, 1991; Wick et al, 1993).

Asymptomatic adrenocortical insufficiency is common among HIV-seropositive patients. At autopsy, focal adrenal necrosis and hemorrhage are found in a majority of AIDS patients; because cytomegalovirus inclusions are found in the adrenal glands of virtually all of these individuals, the hypoadrenalism is thought to result from cytomegalovirus adrenalitis (Strauss, 1991). Prolonged drug therapy also may suppress adrenal function in AIDS patients (Etzel et al, 1992).

Neoplastic destruction of both adrenal glands secondary to metastatic carcinoma has been described (Addison, 1855; Otabe et al, 1991). Very rarely, isolated glucocorticoid deficiency or Allgrove syndrome (ACTH insensitivity, alacrima, and achalasia) may result from congenital or acquired ACTH receptor defects (Moore et al, 1991).

Secondary adrenocortical insufficiency is caused by ACTH deficiency resulting from surgical ablation of the pituitary, pituitary disease (including autoimmune hypophysitis), or pituitary suppression after prolonged administration of pharmacologic doses of glucocorticoids (see index entry Adrenal Corticosteroids, Adverse Reactions). *Tertiary adrenocortical insufficiency* is rare and results from inadequate secretion of CRH. This abnormality can be caused by cranial irradiation for brain tumors (Constine et al, 1993). Because aldosterone secretion is primarily regulated through the renin-angiotensin system, which is not impaired in secondary or tertiary adrenocortical insufficiency, mineralocorticoid secretion usually is not affected.

DIAGNOSIS. Signs and symptoms of primary adrenocortical insufficiency include muscular weakness, weight loss, anorexia, nausea, vomiting, diarrhea, hypoglycemia, hypotension, hyponatremia, hyperkalemia, and, frequently, hyperreninemia. Hyperpigmentation often accompanies hypersecretion of ACTH in primary adrenocortical insufficiency.

Symptoms usually are milder in those with secondary adrenocortical insufficiency. Hyperkalemia and hyperreninemia are seldom encountered because the renin-angiotensin-aldosterone system remains fully functional.

If the plasma ACTH concentration is elevated and the plasma cortisol concentration is low in the morning, primary adrenal insufficiency should be suspected. If plasma ACTH concentrations are equivocal, synthetic ACTH (cosyntropin [Cortrosyn]) can be administered to test adrenal responsiveness. In normal individuals, plasma cortisol and aldosterone concentrations peak 30 to 60 minutes after a single intravenous or subcutaneous injection of cosyntropin 250 mcg. A subnormal response confirms the diagnosis of adrenal insufficiency, but more prolonged adrenal stimulation is required to distinguish between primary, secondary, or tertiary causes. If the plasma cortisol concentration increases after more prolonged stimulation, functional adrenal tissue exists and insufficiency is probably caused by pituitary or hypothalamic dysfunction. Continued failure to respond to prolonged stimulation verifies the lack of functional adrenal cortical tissue.

If both plasma ACTH and cortisol concentrations are low, the ability of the pituitary to secrete ACTH upon stimulation can be determined by administration of CRH 1 mcg/kg intravenously. Failure to respond to CRH indicates pituitary insufficiency, while a positive response suggests hypothalamic disease.

TREATMENT. The goals of therapy are to restore strength, weight, normal blood pressure, and electrolyte balance. Replacement therapy for adrenocortical insufficiency should simulate normal glucocorticoid secretory patterns (two-thirds of the daily dose in the morning, one-third in the afternoon). Hydrocortisone and cortisone are preferred for initial treatment because they possess strong glucocorticoid and moderate mineralocorticoid properties. When the dose of hydrocortisone is subsequently reduced to the normal replacement range, a potent mineralocorticoid (fludrocortisone [Florinef], administered once daily) usually must be added. Methylprednisolone, prednisone, or prednisolone may be used, but because these drugs lack significant mineralocorticoid activity in the dosages appropriate for replacement therapy, concurrent administration of fludrocortisone is necessary.

Panhypopituitarism requires replacement of thyroid and gonadal hormones as well as adrenal hormones. The glucocorticoid should be administered alone until normal adrenal function is re-established. If thyroid hormone is administered first, acute adrenal insufficiency may be precipitated. Children require replacement of growth hormone; growth hormone-deficient adults also may benefit from administration of this hormone (Rudman et al, 1990).

Hypoaldosteronism

Hyperkalemia that cannot be attributed to renal insufficiency suggests isolated hypoaldosteronism (Holland, 1991). Primary isolated hypoaldosteronism may result from a congenital deficiency of 18-hydroxylase or 18-hydroxy-dehydrogenase. Renin production is not exaggerated unless sodium wasting is present. These patients require treatment with fludrocortisone.

Secondary isolated hypoaldosteronism without glucocorticoid deficiency has been described in patients with moderate renal impairment associated with diabetic renal disease, interstitial nephropathy, glomerulosclerosis, gout, AIDS, or analgesic nephropathy. In the most commonly encountered form, hyporeninemic hypoaldosteronism, renin concentration is reduced by damage to the juxtaglomerular apparatus or by the use of angiotensin-converting enzyme inhibitors, and decreased aldosterone secretion, hyperkalemia, and hypotension result (Nadler et al, 1986). Furosemide [Lasix] corrects the hyperkalemia, and fludrocortisone provides effective replacement therapy in this disorder. However, if hyporeninemia is an appropriate physiologic response to excessive sodium retention that causes hypertension, diuretics should be used alone to avoid exacerbating the hypertension (Holland, 1991).

Paradoxical hyperkalemia with hyperaldosteronemia and hyperreninemia results from renal insensitivity to aldosterone (see discussion on Pseudohypoaldosteronism under Secondary Hyperaldosteronism).

Acute Adrenal Insufficiency (Crisis)

Adrenal (addisonian) crisis can be caused by acute adrenal or pituitary failure (following neurosurgery, head trauma, or hemorrhagic shock), failure to maintain adrenal replacement therapy, rapid withdrawal of large doses of corticosteroids, failure to provide additional corticosteroids to dependent patients subjected to stress, or treatment of patients with mild or subclinical hypoadrenalism with rifampin [Rifadin, Rimactane] (which stimulates the clearance of adrenocortical steroids) (Kyriazopoulou et al, 1984). Occasionally, patients with borderline adrenal insufficiency are diagnosed after an unusual stress (eg, severe infection, surgery) induces adrenal crisis. Symptoms include fever, hypotension, dehydration, weakness, vomiting, and diarrhea. If untreated, this condition proceeds to shock and death. Crisis of the classic addisonian type results from deficiencies of both cortisol and aldosterone leading to sodium loss, marked dehydration, and vascular collapse.

Rapid replacement of salt, fluids, and glucocorticoids is required; a mineralocorticoid is not needed when large doses of hydrocortisone are used. Initially, hydrocortisone is given intravenously as a bolus. Intramuscular cortisone acetate generally should not be administered because absorption may be slow and inadequate and conversion to cortisol may be erratic. Normal saline with dextrose in amounts sufficient to correct the blood pressure is then given, followed by slow intravenous infusion of hydrocortisone. The amount of saline administered in the first 24 hours depends on the degree of volume depletion. The total dose of hydrocortisone given to adults during the first 24 hours is approximately 200 mg/M^2 and should be reduced gradually to replacement levels during the next several days. Hyperkalemia should be corrected if still present. The underlying condition (eg, infection, hemorrhage) must be treated concurrently.

Congenital Adrenal Hyperplasia Syndromes (CAH)

In these syndromes, reduced synthesis of cortisol and sometimes aldosterone results from inherited adrenal enzyme deficiencies (see review by New and Speiser, 1989). Clinical manifestations depend on the specific enzyme(s) involved but, in all patients, low plasma cortisol concentrations stimulate ACTH secretion and adrenal hyperplasia results, often accompanied by incidentaloma (silent adenoma). If the enzyme deficiency is partial, the increase in ACTH secretion may result in normal cortisol concentrations. In all patients, there is hypersecretion of the steroids synthesized prior to the enzyme block and from alternate pathways. Therefore, symptoms may be related to either hormone deficiency or excess depending on whether synthesis of a particular steroid is stimulated or blocked.

TYPES OF CAH. 21-Hydroxylase Deficiency: In 21-hydroxylase deficiency, a monogenic autosomal recessive trait that is found in up to 95% of patients with CAH, the pathways to cortisol synthesis are blocked and hypersecretion of ACTH causes hyperplasia of the adrenal cortex. Excessive secretion of adrenal androgens by the fetus causes masculinization of the external genitalia in female neonates; in affected infants, sexual ambiguity may result and necessitate surgical correction. However, gonadal formation is essentially normal and in many cases the ovaries are fully functional. Excessive androgen production is not always apparent in male infants, but may be manifested by phallic enlargement and scrotal pigmentation. Elevated androgen concentrations suppress the secretion of gonadotropin and the production of testosterone, which is required in high concentrations within the testis to support normal spermatogenesis. Progesterone and 17-hydroxyprogesterone secretion also are increased, causing hypoaldosteronism and salt loss.

Plasma cortisol concentration may be low in the salt-losing form or normal in the simple virilizing form. However, the cortisol response to stress may be diminished, and these patients may require supplementary doses of corticosteroids to avoid addisonian crisis during stress. A partial deficiency of 21-hydroxylase may not produce symptoms of hypoaldosteronism.

11-β-Hydroxylase Deficiency: Deficiency of 11-β-hydroxylase is the second most common form of CAH, occurring in approximately 5% of cases. This disorder may be diagnosed during gestation by increased maternal urinary excretion of tetrahydro-11-deoxycortisol (THS) or abnormally high amniotic fluid THS and 11-deoxycortisol concentrations (Rösler et al, 1988). Plasma 11-deoxycortisol, deoxycorticosterone, and androgen concentrations are elevated in affected neonates, causing masculinizing effects, salt retention, hypertension, and hypokalemia and predisposing to gynecomastia (Hochberg et al, 1991).

Other Forms: In 3-β-hydroxysteroid dehydrogenase deficiency, the synthesis of cortisol and aldosterone is impaired, resulting in salt loss and virilization. A similar enzyme defect in the testes prevents formation of testosterone, and the genitalia of male infants are incompletely developed. The mortality rate is high during infancy. However, spontaneous signs of puberty may occur in those who survive.

In 17-hydroxylase deficiency, androgen and estrogen synthesis are impaired in the adrenal glands and gonads (Yanase et al, 1991). This may result in male pseudohermaphroditism and female hypogonadism with lack of secondary sexual characteristics. Replacement therapy is required to initiate and maintain puberty in these patients. Excessive secretion of deoxycorticosterone causes hypertension and hypokalemia. Aldosterone secretion may be reduced, normal, or increased.

Complete block of steroid synthesis by the adrenal glands and gonads occurs in cholesterol 20, 22-desmolase deficiency. If the enzymatic deficiency is marked, early death results. In less severe cases, there is salt loss as well as cortisol deficiency. The effect on the development of genitalia is similar to that in 17-hydroxylase and 3-β-hydroxysteroid dehydrogenase deficiencies. Puberty also must be induced in these patients.

Lack of maternal placental aromatase activity results in failure to convert circulating androgens to estrogens during pregnancy (Shozu et al, 1991). Progressive maternal virilization and pseudohermaphroditism of a female fetus will occur even in the absence of adrenal enzyme deficiencies.

Nonclassic Forms of CAH: Nonclassic (previously designated "acquired," "late onset," or "attenuated") mild CAH has been diagnosed in late childhood to adulthood. Deficiencies of 3-β-hydroxysteroid dehydrogenase or 11-β- or 21-hydroxylase are not mutually exclusive (Eldar-Geva et al, 1990) and may be detected at or near the time of puberty or later in females who present with hirsutism, acne, menstrual irregularity, and possibly clitoral enlargement. Polycystic ovarian disease or infertility also may occur. In addition to these characteristics, patients with 11-β-hydroxylase deficiency may develop hypertension and hypokalemia, and those with 21-hydroxylase deficiency are often hyperinsulinemic (Walker and Edwards, 1991; Speiser et al, 1992).

Hirsutism of adrenal origin in young adults can be distinguished from excessive ovarian androgen production by the results of a five-day low-dose (2 mg/day) dexamethasone suppression test, which will suppress adrenal but not ovarian androgen secretion (Ehrmann and Rosenfield, 1990). Subsequently, adrenal hydroxylase deficiency can be confirmed by a markedly elevated plasma DHEAS concentration after ACTH stimulation (Siegel et al, 1990); measurements of basal steroid concentrations generally are not useful (Eldar-Geva et al, 1990; Siegel et al, 1990).

Late onset of an incomplete form of 3-β-hydroxysteroid dehydrogenase deficiency is characterized by precocious pubarche in children and by hirsutism and oligomenorrhea in women. Plasma androgen concentrations vary, but DHEAS appears to be increased more than androstenedione or testosterone (Pang et al, 1985). Increased plasma 17-OH pregnenolone concentrations and 17-OH pregnenolone:17-OH progesterone plasma concentration ratios are diagnostic in individuals of normal weight but not in those who are overweight (Pang et al, 1985; Jabbar et al, 1991).

TREATMENT. The goals of treatment are to correct the hormonal imbalance and allow growth to normal height, prevent virilism in girls or prepubertal sexual development in boys, and allow normal puberty and fertility. As in other types of adrenocortical insufficiency, cortisol is replaced (as hydrocortisone or cortisone). Potent long-acting preparations of adrenal corticosteroids (eg, dexamethasone) are useful in adults, but overdosage is difficult to avoid in children and can cause growth retardation, irritability, hyperactivity, and iatrogenic Cushing's syndrome. The dosage must be individualized on the basis of clinical and laboratory assessments of the patient's condition. Enough glucocorticoid is given to suppress ACTH secretion (and thus excess androgen production) but not enough to cause cushingoid changes or inhibit growth. Usually, hydrocortisone 10 to 25 mg/M^2/day orally is required (Winterer et al, 1985). Division and scheduling of the dose have been attempted to optimize suppression of androgen secretion, but a consensus on optimal therapy remains to be established. Whatever regimen is used, the dose employed should be the lowest amount necessary to suppress the elevated androgen secretion.

Frequent (every three months) monitoring is required to adjust the dose of glucocorticoid to the changing requirements of the growing child. Follow-up examination should include assessment of growth rate (most important single parameter), including bone age; monitoring for signs of virilization or Cushing's syndrome; and testing for hypertension.

In 21-hydroxylase deficiency, increased urinary excretion of 17-ketosteroids and pregnanetriol and plasma 17-hydroxyprogesterone concentrations can be used to guide treatment. Newer assays for salivary 17-hydroxyprogesterone and androstenedione also are used to monitor patients with CAH. However, complete normalization of plasma 17-hydroxyprogesterone concentration usually reflects overtreatment with glucocorticoids. Although biochemical measurements are helpful in detecting undertreatment, they may not distinguish between optimal treatment and progressive overtreatment; therefore, clinical status must be carefully considered.

In patients with salt-losing CAH, the mineralocorticoid, fludrocortisone, is prescribed. Mineralocorticoids also are useful in patients who are not overtly losing salt but are nevertheless sodium-depleted and who have high plasma renin concentrations, which may further stimulate ACTH secretion. Administration of mineralocorticoid normalizes the plasma renin concentration, improves hormonal balance, and may decrease the hydrocortisone requirement (Hochberg et al, 1991). Normalization of plasma renin concentration also is associated with increased linear growth.

In patients with hypertensive forms of CAH, hormone replacement is provided by a glucocorticoid with minimal mineralocorticoid activity (eg, prednisone, dexamethasone), and salt restriction is required only rarely. However, hypertension may not be corrected and may require antihypertensive drugs for control.

In adults with nonclassic forms of CAH, fertility can be restored by glucocorticoid therapy or, in some cases, a glucocorticoid plus clomiphene [Clomid] (Birnbaum and Rose, 1984). Alternatively, 50 mg/day of the antiandrogen, cyproterone, which inhibits peripheral responses to androgens (see index entry Cyproterone), may be preferable to hydrocortisone in the treatment of females (Spritzer et al, 1990). During pregnancy, replacement doses of adrenal corticosteroids are often difficult to adjust because placental CRH may exaggerate ACTH stimulation of adrenal androgens.

The necessity for adrenal hormone replacement is lifelong. If therapy is withdrawn before growth is complete, height may be compromised due to premature epiphyseal closure. Later in life, lack of adrenal suppression causes virilization and menstrual disorders in females and oligospermia in males. CAH patients who discontinue glucocorticoid therapy are at risk of inadequate adrenal response to stress (infections, surgery, or trauma). If the mineralocorticoid is discontinued, there is a greater risk of adrenal insufficiency, especially in the presence of salt deprivation.

SALT-LOSING CRISIS. Infants with diagnosed CAH or those with ambiguous genitalia should be observed closely for signs of salt-losing crisis, which generally occurs between the first and third weeks of life but may develop earlier or later. Affected infants eat poorly, vomit, and are dehydrated; death occurs rapidly in the absence of adequate treatment. Fluids containing normal saline and hydrocortisone should be administered intravenously. Potassium is avoided because hyperkalemia may be present, but it may be needed later in the course of treatment. Serum electrolytes and hematocrit values should be monitored until the infant's condition stabilizes. Following the crisis, maintenance therapy is initiated.

PRENATAL DIAGNOSIS AND TREATMENT. Fetal adrenal androgen secretion that causes masculinization of the female fetus occurs between 10 and 16 weeks' gestation. Administration of dexamethasone to the mother (1.5 mg/day in two or three divided doses) beginning as early as the fifth week of gestation and continuing until birth has prevented or significantly reduced fetal masculinization by suppressing fetal ACTH and adrenal androgen secretion. (Cortisone or prednisone is not a suitable substitute for dexamethasone.) Adverse effects on the mother are significant and include excessive weight gain, severe striae, hypertension, reduced glucose tolerance, gastrointestinal disturbances, and extreme irritability (Pang et al, 1992). Only healthy pregnant women whose fetuses are at risk of CAH and who have no apparent risk of hyperglycemia or hypertension should be treated. Chorionic villus sampling should be performed as early as possible (Rumsby et al, 1993), and treatment should be continued only in cases of female fetuses with CAH (Pang et al, 1990).

Precautions in the Use of Adrenal Corticosteroid Replacement Therapy

All patients receiving glucocorticoid replacement therapy require supplemental doses (two to three times replacement amounts) during physical stress. The dose must be increased in proportion to the severity of the stress. Temporary excessive doses are preferred to inadequate replacement. During mild illness, such as upper respiratory infections, doubling the maintenance dose usually is sufficient. When oral intake of steroids is not possible for any reason, including vomiting, a parenteral preparation (hydrocortisone, cortisone acetate, prednisolone phosphate or succinate, or dexamethasone sodium phosphate) can be given intramuscularly, but intravenous administration is preferred. In patients who require mineralocorticoids, adequate salt replacement must be assured or hyponatremia may result.

Patients receiving glucocorticoid replacement therapy who are undergoing major surgery require replacement doses high enough to maintain plasma glucocorticoid concentrations at about twice the normal range immediately before, during, and after the procedure. Replacement of salt, fluid, and mineralocorticoid is prescribed as necessary. If adequate amounts of steroids are administered, salt and fluid replacement is the same as for any patient undergoing similar surgery. If the postoperative course is uncomplicated, the dose can be reduced gradually over two to five days to the usual replacement amount. The physician and patient should be aware that prolonged overtreatment will result in gradual development of cushingoid symptoms.

Steroid dependence and increased dosage requirement under widely variable conditions of stress are of utmost importance and should be understood by the patient or parents. All such patients should carry an identification card and wear a bracelet and necklace indicating their dependence on steroid medication. In addition, care should be taken to assure that an adequate supply of steroids is available at all times for emergencies. This should include oral medication and a glucocorticoid suitable for intramuscular injection. Older patients should be taught to self-administer injections, and parents should be trained to administer these injections to their children.

Drug Evaluations

CORTISONE ACETATE

[Cortone Acetate]

For chemical formula, see index entry Adrenal Corticosteroids, Chemistry.

USES. Cortisone acetate is readily converted in the body to cortisol, the naturally occurring active form. Like hydrocortisone, it is a preferred drug for replacement therapy in chronic adrenocortical insufficiency and for most patients with salt-losing forms of congenital adrenal hyperplasia because it has both glucocorticoid and mild mineralocorticoid effects.

Potential bioequivalency problems for some generic preparations have been reported by the FDA.

See the Introduction for specific indications and precautions. For a detailed discussion of anti-inflammatory actions, uses, adverse reactions, drug interactions, and precautions see index entry Adrenal Corticosteroids.

DOSAGE AND PREPARATIONS. Dosage requirements are variable and must be individualized on the basis of disease severity and patient response.

Oral: For chronic adrenocortical insufficiency, 12 to 20 mg/M^2 daily, a dose slightly greater than basal daily secretion. The daily dosage may be divided, with two-thirds given in the morning on arising and one-third in the afternoon, to simulate normal adrenocortical secretion.

For congenital adrenal hyperplasia, 10 to 30 mg/M^2 daily. The dosage is divided as for treatment of CAH with hydrocortisone (see the evaluation). The dosage must be carefully individualized.

Generic. Tablets 5, 10, and 25 mg.
Cortone Acetate (Merck). Tablets 25 mg.

Intramuscular: For chronic adrenocortical insufficiency, initially, 20 to 30 mg daily. Larger doses (up to 300 mg) are indicated in shock unresponsive to conventional therapy if adrenocortical insufficiency exists or is suspected. The dose is adjusted until the patient's response is satisfactory within a reasonable period of time. Maintenance dosage is determined by gradually decreasing the initial dose to the lowest amount that maintains adequate clinical response. In infants and young children with congenital adrenal hyperplasia, administration only once every three or four days may be adequate for maintenance. When drug withdrawal is necessary, it should be done gradually.

Cortisone generally should not be given intramuscularly for acute adrenal insufficiency because absorption may be erratic and inadequate.

Generic. Suspension 25 mg/ml in 10 and 20 ml containers and 50 mg/ml in 10 ml containers.
Cortone Acetate (Merck). Suspension 50 mg/ml in 10 ml containers.

DEXAMETHASONE
[Decadron, Hexadrol]

DEXAMETHASONE SODIUM PHOSPHATE
[Decadron Phosphate, Dexasone, Hexadrol Phosphate]

For chemical formula, see index entry Adrenal Corticosteroids, Chemistry.

USES. Dexamethasone, a fluorinated derivative of prednisolone, is a high-potency glucocorticoid that is used primarily to treat inflammatory or allergic conditions. It may be used for replacement therapy in adrenal insufficiency. For dosage equivalents, see index entry Adrenal Corticosteroids: Relative Potencies of Glucocorticoids (Table).

Dexamethasone also is used to diagnose endogenous hypercortisolism (see the discussion on the dexamethasone suppression test in the section on Cushing's Syndrome, Diagnosis).

For a detailed discussion of anti-inflammatory actions, uses, adverse reactions, drug interactions, and precautions, see index entry Adrenal Corticosteroids.

DOSAGE AND PREPARATIONS.

DEXAMETHASONE:

Oral: For dexamethasone suppression tests, see the Table. For mild adrenal insufficiency, 0.5 to 0.75 mg/M^2 daily.

Generic. Tablets 0.25, 0.5, 0.75, 1, 1.5, 2, 4, and 6 mg; elixir 0.5 mg/5 ml; solution (drops) 0.5 mg/0.5 ml.
Decadron (Merck). Tablets 0.25, 0.5, 0.75, 1.5, 4, and 6 mg; elixir 0.5 mg/5 ml.
Hexadrol (Organon). Tablets 0.75, 1.5, and 4 mg; elixir 0.5 mg/5 ml.

DEXAMETHASONE SODIUM PHOSPHATE:

Intravenous: For replacement therapy during cosyntropin test, dexamethasone 1 or 2 mg is given after the baseline serum sample for cortisol determination is drawn and after cosyntropin has been administered.

Generic. Solution 4 and 10 mg/ml.
Decadron Phosphate (Merck). Solution 4 mg/ml in 1, 2.5, 5, and 25 ml containers and 24 mg/ml in 5 and 10 ml containers.
Dexasone (Hauck). Solution 4 mg/ml in 5, 10, and 30 ml containers.
Hexadrol Phosphate (Organon). Solution 4 mg/ml in 1 and 5 ml containers, 10 mg/ml in 1 and 10 ml containers, and 20 mg/ml in 5 ml containers.

FLUDROCORTISONE ACETATE
[Florinef Acetate]

CH_2OCCH_3, C=O, OH, HO, H, CH_3, CH_3, H, F, H, H, O

USES. Fludrocortisone, the only oral mineralocorticoid available, is a halogenated derivative of cortisone. It is not suitable for use as an anti-inflammatory agent. Fludrocortisone has very potent mineralocorticoid and moderate glucocorticoid effects and, therefore, is useful for mineralocorticoid replacement therapy in primary chronic adrenocortical insufficiency, salt-losing forms of congenital adrenal hyperplasia, and in patients with elevated plasma renin activity and hyperkalemia associated with isolated hypoaldosteronism.

ADVERSE REACTIONS. Adverse reactions include hypertension, edema, hypokalemia, cardiac hypertrophy, and gynecomastia in adolescent boys. Salt intake must be adjusted to meet individual requirements. Use in hypertensive individuals is contraindicated.

DOSAGE AND PREPARATIONS.

Oral: For chronic primary adrenocortical insufficiency, initially, 0.05 to 0.1 mg (50 to 100 mcg) daily, increased up to 0.2 mg daily. For salt-losing forms of congenital adrenal hyperplasia, initially, up to 0.2 mg (200 mcg) daily; this can be reduced gradually to 0.05 to 0.1 mg (50 to 100 mcg) daily over several months.

Florinef Acetate (Apothecon). Tablets 0.1 mg.

HYDROCORTISONE
[Cortef, Hydrocortone]

HYDROCORTISONE CYPIONATE
[Cortef]

HYDROCORTISONE SODIUM PHOSPHATE
[Hydrocortone Phosphate]

HYDROCORTISONE SODIUM SUCCINATE
[A-hydroCort, Solu-Cortef]

For chemical formula of hydrocortisone, see index entry Adrenal Corticosteroids, Chemistry.

USES. Hydrocortisone is a preferred drug for replacement therapy in acute or chronic adrenocortical insufficiency and salt-losing forms of congenital adrenal hyperplasia because it has both glucocorticoid and mild mineralocorticoid activities and is chemically identical to cortisol, the endogenous glucocorticoid.

The oral preparations (base and cypionate salt) are often used for replacement therapy. The water-soluble forms (sodium phosphate, sodium succinate) are given intravenously or intramuscularly in emergencies, such as acute adrenocortical insufficiency (addisonian crisis); for salt-losing crisis in congenital adrenal hyperplasia; or to prepare patients who require replacement therapy prior to major surgery.

ADVERSE REACTIONS AND PRECAUTIONS. Peptic ulceration may occur during therapy with large doses of hydrocortisone; concurrent prophylactic antacid therapy may be appropriate. When high-dose therapy must be continued for more than 48 hours, hypernatremia may occur. In these patients, hydrocortisone should be replaced with methylprednisolone, which causes little or no sodium retention.

Some preparations of hydrocortisone (eg, Solu-Cortef Act-O-Vial System) are contraindicated in premature infants because they contain benzyl alcohol, which has been associated with a fatal "gasping syndrome" in infants.

For a detailed discussion of anti-inflammatory actions, uses, adverse reactions, drug interactions, and precautions, see index entry Adrenal Corticosteroids.

DOSAGE AND PREPARATIONS. Dosage requirements are variable and must be individualized on the basis of disease severity and patient response.

Oral: For chronic adrenocortical insufficiency, 12 to 18 mg/M^2 daily. The daily dosage may be divided, with two-thirds given in the morning on arising and one-third in the afternoon, to simulate normal adrenocortical secretion.

For congenital adrenal hyperplasia, the dosage must be carefully individualized and ranges between 10 and 25 mg/M^2 (Winterer et al, 1985).

HYDROCORTISONE:
Cortef (Upjohn). Tablets 5, 10, and 20 mg.
Hydrocortone (Merck), ***Generic.*** Tablets 10 and 20 mg.
HYDROCORTISONE CYPIONATE:
Cortef (Upjohn). Oral suspension equivalent to hydrocortisone 10 mg/5 ml.

Intravenous: The dosage depends on the severity of the condition and the size of the patient; smaller doses (minimum, 25 mg) are appropriate for infants. In emergencies, initially, 100 to 500 mg, delivered over 30 seconds (100 mg) to 10 minutes (500 mg) and repeated if necessary. For salt-losing crisis in congenital adrenal hyperplasia, 50 to 100 mg is given with intravenous fluids for one to two days until the crisis is controlled. Larger doses are indicated in shock unresponsive to conventional therapy if adrenocortical insufficiency exists or is suspected.

Intramuscular: The dosage depends on the severity of the condition and the size of the patient; smaller doses are appropriate for infants. For emergencies when the intravenous route is not feasible, initially, 100 to 500 mg, repeated at intervals of two, four, or six hours as indicated by the patient's response.

HYDROCORTISONE:
Generic. Suspension 25 and 50 mg/ml in 10 ml containers.
HYDROCORTISONE SODIUM PHOSPHATE:
Generic, Hydrocortone Phosphate (Merck). Solution 50 mg/ml in 2 and 10 ml containers.
HYDROCORTISONE SODIUM SUCCINATE:
Generic. Powder 100, 250, and 500 mg and 1 g (with and without diluent).
A-hydroCort (Abbott), ***Solu-Cortef*** (Upjohn). Powder 100 mg; powder and diluent 100, 250, and 500 mg and 1 g.

METHYLPREDNISOLONE
[Medrol]

PREDNISOLONE
[Prelone]

PREDNISONE
[Deltasone, Liquid Pred, Meticorten, Orasone, Sterapred]

For chemical formulas, see index entry Adrenal Corticosteroids, Chemistry.

USES. Prednisolone and methylprednisolone are Δ-1 analogues of hydrocortisone, and prednisone is the analogous derivative of cortisone. All are available as oral and parenteral preparations, although only the oral forms are appropriate for hormone replacement therapy. Prednisone must be converted in the body to the active compound, prednisolone; therefore, it may be unsuitable for patients with liver disease. However, reduced nonrenal clearance of unbound prednisolone may compensate for impaired hepatic conversion of prednisone to prednisolone in these individuals (Frey and Frey, 1990).

Because they have little mineralocorticoid activity, these drugs are not suitable as the sole agent in primary adrenocortical insufficiency. However, they can be used alone for replacement therapy in secondary adrenocortical insufficiency or hypertensive (salt-retaining) forms of congenital adrenal hyperplasia. When given with a mineralocorticoid, methylprednisolone, prednisolone, or prednisone can be used in primary adrenocortical insufficiency or salt-losing forms of congenital adrenal hyperplasia. These agents are sometimes preferred for congenital adrenal hyperplasia because they are somewhat longer acting than hydrocortisone or cortisone and more readily induce adrenocortical suppression throughout the day.

Insufficient data are available to determine the bioequivalence of some generic preparations of prednisolone and prednisone.

For a detailed discussion of anti-inflammatory actions, uses, adverse reactions, drug interactions, and precautions, see index entry Adrenal Corticosteroids.

DOSAGE AND PREPARATIONS. Dosage requirements are similar for all three agents but vary among patients and must be individualized on the basis of disease severity and response. Only the oral forms are appropriate for hormone replacement therapy, including congenital adrenal hyperplasia.

Oral: For replacement therapy, initially, 4 mg/M^2 daily. The daily dosage may be divided, with two-thirds given in the morning on arising and one-third in the afternoon, to simulate normal glucocorticoid secretion. For congenital adrenal hyperplasia, initially, 5 mg/M^2 daily given in two or three divided doses.

METHYLPREDNISOLONE:

Generic. Tablets 4 and 16 mg.

Medrol (Upjohn). Tablets 2, 4, 8, 16, 24, and 32 mg.

PREDNISOLONE:

Generic. Tablets 5 mg.

Prelone (Muro). Syrup 5 and 15 mg/5 ml.

PREDNISONE:

Generic. Tablets 1, 2.5, 5, 10, 20, 25, and 50 mg; solution (oral concentrate) 5 mg/ml; solution (oral) 5 mg/5 ml.

Deltasone (Upjohn). Tablets 2.5, 5, 10, 20, and 50 mg.

Liquid Pred (Muro). Syrup 5 mg/5 ml.

Meticorten (Schering). Tablets 1 mg.

Orasone (Solvay). Tablets 1, 5, 10, 20, and 50 mg.

Sterapred (Mayrand). Tablets 5 and 10 mg (***Sterapred DS***).

Cited References

Abramson O, et al: Pseudohypoaldosteronism in a preterm infant: Intrauterine presentation as hydramnios. *J Pediatr* 120:129-132, 1992.

Addison T: *On the Constitutional and Local Effects of Disease of the Suprarenal Capsules.* London, England, Highley, 1855.

Ambrosi B, et al: Failure of somatostatin and octreotide to acutely affect the hypothalamic-pituitary-adrenal function in patients with corticotropin hypersecretion. *J Endocrinol Invest* 13:257-261, 1990.

Armanini D, et al: Aldosterone-receptor deficiency in pseudohypoaldosteronism. *N Engl J Med* 313:1178-1181, 1985.

Asherson RA, Cervera R: The antiphospholipid syndrome: A syndrome in evolution. *Ann Rheum Dis* 51:147-150, 1992.

Bartalena L, et al: The nocturnal serum thyrotropin surge is abolished in patients with adrenocorticotropin (ACTH)-dependent or ACTH-independent Cushing's syndrome. *J Clin Endocrinol* 72:1195-1199, 1991.

Begg EJ, et al: Pharmacokinetics of corticosteroid agents. *Med J Aust* 146:37-41, 1987.

Benker G, et al: TSH secretion in Cushing's syndrome: Relation to glucocorticoid excess, diabetes, goitre, and the 'sick euthyroid syndrome.' *Clin Endocrinol* 33:777-786, 1990.

Berkenbosch F, et al: Corticotropin-releasing factor-producing neurons in the rat activated by interleukin-1. *Science* 238:524-526, 1987.

Besedovsky HO, et al: Immune-neuroendocrine interactions. *J Immunol* 135:750s-754s, 1985.

Biemond P, et al: Continuous dexamethasone infusion for seven hours in patients with the Cushing syndrome: A superior differential diagnostic test. *Ann Intern Med* 112:738-742, 1990.

Biller BMK, et al: Clonal origins of adrenocorticotropin-secreting pituitary tissue in Cushing's disease. *J Clin Endocrinol Metab* 75:1303-1309, 1992.

Birnbaum MD, Rose LI: Late onset adrenocortical hydroxylase deficiencies associated with menstrual dysfunction. *Obstet Gynecol* 63:445-451, 1984.

Bouzas EA, et al: Central serous chorioretinopathy in endogenous hypercortisolism. *Arch Ophthalmol* 111:1229-1233, 1993.

Breder CD, et al: Interleukin-1 immunoreactive innervation of the human hypothalamus. *Science* 240:321-324, 1988.

Brönnegärd M, et al: Primary cortisol resistance associated with a thermolabile glucocorticoid receptor in a patient with fatigue as the only symptom. *J Clin Invest* 78:1270-1278, 1986.

Buescher MA, et al: Cushing syndrome in pregnancy. *Obstet Gynecol* 79:130-137, 1992.

Carey RM, et al: Ectopic secretion of corticotropin-releasing factor as a cause of Cushing's syndrome: A clinical, morphologic, and biochemical study. *N Engl J Med* 311:13-20, 1984.

Carpenter PC: Diagnostic evaluation of Cushing's syndrome. *Endocrinol Metab Clin North Am* 17:445-472, 1988.

Chrousos GP, et al: Glucocorticoids and glucocorticoid antagonists: Lessons from RU 486. *Kidney Int* 34 (suppl 26):S18-S23, 1988.

Clore J, et al: When is cortisol a mineralocorticoid? *Kidney Int* 42:1297-1308, 1992.

Conn JW: Presidential address: Part I, Painting background; Part II, Primary aldosteronism, a new clinical syndrome. *J Lab Clin Med* 45:3-17, (Jan) 1955.

Constine LS, et al: Hypothalamic-pituitary dysfunction after radiation for brain tumors. *N Engl J Med* 328:87-94, 1993.

Crapo L: Cushing's syndrome: A review of diagnostic tests. *Metabolism* 28:955-977, 1979.

Cushing H: The basophil adenomas of the pituitary body and their clinical manifestations (pituitary basophilism). *Bull Johns Hopkins Hosp* 50:137-195, 1932.

Dempster DW, et al: Mean wall thickness and formation periods of trabecular bone packets in corticosteroid-induced osteoporosis. *Calcif Tissue Int* 35:410-417, 1983.

Dickstein G, et al: Adrenocorticotropin stimulation test: Effects of basal cortisol level, time of day, and suggested new sensitive low dose test. *J Clin Endocrinol Metab* 72:773-778, 1991.

Ehrmann DA, Rosenfield RL: Hirsutism—Beyond the steroidogenic block. *N Engl J Med* 323:909-911, 1990.

Eldar-Geva T, et al: Secondary biosynthetic defects in women with late-onset congenital adrenal hyperplasia. *N Engl J Med* 323:855-863, 1990.

Engelhardt D, et al: The influence of ketoconazole on human adrenal steroidogenesis: Incubation studies with tissue slices. *Clin Endocrinol* 35:163-168, 1991.

Esteban NV, et al: Daily cortisol production rate in man determined by stable isotope dilution/mass spectrometry. *J Clin Endocrinol Metab* 72:39-45, 1991.

Etzel JV, et al: Endocrine complications associated with human immunodeficiency virus infection. *Clin Pharm* 11:705-713, 1992.

Findling JW: The Cushing syndromes: An enlarging clinical spectrum, editorial. *N Engl J Med* 321:1677-1678, 1989.

Flack MR, et al: Urine free cortisol in the high-dose dexamethasone suppression test for the differential diagnosis of the Cushing syndrome. *Ann Intern Med* 116:211-217, 1992.

Freidberg SR: Transsphenoidal pituitary surgery in the treatment of patients with Cushing's disease. *Urol Clin North Am* 16:589-595, 1989.

Frey BM, Frey FJ: Clinical pharmacokinetics of prednisone and prednisolone. *Clin Pharmacokinet* 19:126-146, 1990.

Funder JW: Mineralocorticoids, glucocorticoids, receptors and response elements. *Science* 259:1132-1133, 1993.

Gicquel C, et al: Monoclonality of corticotroph macroadenomas in Cushing's disease. *J Clin Endocrinol Metab* 75:472-475, 1992.

Glade MJ, Krook L: Glucocorticoid-induced inhibition of osteolysis and the development of osteopetrosis, osteonecrosis and osteoporosis. *Cornell Vet* 72:76-91, 1982.

Glade MJ, et al: Calcium metabolism in glucocorticoid-treated pony foals. *J Nutr* 112:77-86, 1982.

Gomez MT, et al: Urinary free cortisol values in normal children and adolescents. *J Pediatr* 118:256-258, 1991.

Grua JR, Nelson DH: ACTH-producing pituitary tumors. *Endocrinol Metab Clin North Am* 20:319-362, 1991.

Hambling C, et al: Primary hyperaldosteronism—Evaluation of procedures for diagnosis and localization. *Q J Med* 86:383-392, 1993.

Hermus AR, et al: Corticotropin-releasing-hormone test versus high-dose dexamethasone test in the differential diagnosis of Cushing's syndrome. *Lancet* 2:540-544, 1986.

Hochberg Z, et al: Mineralocorticoids in the mechanism of gynecomastia in adrenal hyperplasia caused by 11β-hydroxylase deficiency. *J Pediatr* 118:258-260, 1991.

Holland OB, et al: Further evaluation of saline infusion for the diagnosis of primary aldosteronism. *Hypertension* 6:717-723, 1984.

Iida S, et al: Primary cortisol resistance accompanied by a reduction in glucocorticoid receptors in two members of the same family. *J Clin Endocrinol Metab* 60:967-971, 1985.

Invitti C, et al: Treatment of Cushing's syndrome with the long-acting somatostatin analogue SMS 201-995 (Sandostatin). *Clin Endocrinol* 32:275-281, 1990.

Jabbar M, et al: Excess weight and precocious pubarche in children: Alterations of the adrenocortical hormones. *J Am Coll Nutr* 10:289-296, 1991.

Jones KL: The Cushing syndromes. *Pediatr Clin North Am* 37:1313-1329, 1990.

Jones MT, Gillham B: Factors involved in the regulation of adrenocorticotropic hormone/β-lipotropic hormone. *Physiol Rev* 68:743-817, 1988.

Kaye TB, Crapo L: The Cushing syndrome: An update on diagnostic tests. *Ann Intern Med* 112:434-444, 1990.

Kemink L, et al: Residual adrenocortical function after bilateral adrenalectomy for pituitary-dependent Cushing's syndrome. *J Clin Endocrinol Metab* 75:1211-1214, 1992.

Kerrigan JR, et al: Estimation of daily cortisol production and clearance rates in normal pubertal males by deconvolution analysis. *J Clin Endocrinol Metab* 76:1505-1510, 1993.

Khanderia U: Use of ketoconazole in the treatment of Cushing's syndrome. *Clin Pharm* 10:12-13, (Jan) 1991.

Kuhn JM, et al: Comparative assessment of ACTH and lipoprotein plasma levels in the diagnosis and follow-up of patients with Cushing's syndrome: A study of 210 cases. *Am J Med* 86:678-684, 1989.

Kyriazopoulou V, Vagenakis AG: Abnormal overnight dexamethasone suppression test in subjects receiving rifampicin therapy. *J Clin Endocrinol Metab* 75:315-317, 1992.

Kyriazopoulou V, et al: Rifampicin-induced adrenal crisis in addisonian patients receiving corticosteroid replacement therapy. *J Clin Endocrinol Metab* 59:1204-1206, 1984.

Lamberts SWJ, Birkenhagr JC: Effect of bromocriptine in pituitary-dependent Cushing's syndrome. *J Endocrinol* 70:315-316, 1976.

Lifton RP, et al: A chimaeric 11β-hydroxylase/aldosterone synthase gene causes glucocorticoid-remediable aldosteronism and human hypertension. *Nature* 355:262-265, 1992.

Linder BL, et al: Cortisol production rate in childhood and adolescence. *J Pediatr* 117:892-896, 1990.

Loriaux DL, Nieman L: Corticotropin-releasing hormone testing in pituitary disease. *Endocrinol Metab Clin North Am* 20:363-369, 1991.

Lumpkin MD: The regulation of ACTH secretion by IL-1. *Science* 238:452-454, 1987.

Mampalam TJ, et al: Transsphenoidal microsurgery for Cushing disease: A report of 216 cases. *Ann Intern Med* 109:487-493, 1988.

McCance DR, et al: Bilateral adrenalectomy: Low mortality and morbidity in Cushing's disease. *Clin Endocrinol* 39:315-321, 1993.

McEwen BS: Glucocorticoid receptors in the brain. *Hosp Pract* 107-121, (Aug) 1988.

McKenna TJ, Cunningham SK: The control of adrenal androgen secretion, commentary. *J Endocrinol* 129:1-3, 1991.

Melby JC: Diagnosis of hyperaldosteronism. *Endocrinol Metab Clin North Am* 20:247-255, 1991.

Miller JW, Crapo L: The medical treatment of Cushing's syndrome. *Endocr Rev* 14:443-458, 1993.

Miyamori I, et al: Determination of urinary 18-hydroxycortisol in the diagnosis of primary aldosteronism. *J Endocrinol Invest* 15:19-24, 1992.

Moore PSJ, et al: Allgrove syndrome: An autosomal recessive syndrome of ACTH insensitivity, achalasia and alacrima. *Clin Endocrinol* 34:107-114, 1991.

Muir A, Maclaren NK: Autoimmune diseases of the adrenal glands, parathyroid glands, gonads, and hypothalamic-pituitary axis. *Endocrinol Metab Clin North Am* 20:619-643, 1991.

Murayama M, et al: Long term follow-up of Cushing's disease treated with reserpine and pituitary irradiation. *J Clin Endocrinol Metab* 75:935-942, 1992.

Nadler JL, et al: Evidence of prostacyclin deficiency in the syndrome of hyporeninemic hypoaldosteronism. *N Engl J Med* 314:1015-1020, 1986.

Naito Y, et al: Biphasic changes in hypothalamo-pituitary-adrenal function during the early recovery period after major abdominal surgery. *J Clin Endocrinol Metab* 73:111-117, 1991.

Nawata H, et al: Decreased deoxyribonucleic acid binding of glucocorticoid-receptor complex in cultured skin fibroblasts from a patient with the glucocorticoid resistance syndrome. *J Clin Endocrinol Metab* 65:219-226, 1987.

New MI, Speiser PW: Disorders of adrenal steroidogenesis, in Vaughan ED Jr, Carey RM (eds): *Adrenal Disorders.* New York, Thieme Medical Publishers, 1989, 191-217.

Nieman LK, et al: Ovine corticotropin-releasing hormone stimulation test and dexamethasone suppression test in the differential diagnosis of Cushing's syndrome. *Ann Intern Med* 105:862-867, 1986.

Nieman LK, et al: The ovine corticotropin-releasing hormone (CRH) stimulation test is superior to the human CRH stimulation test for the diagnosis of Cushing's disease. *J Clin Endocrinol Metab* 69:165-169, 1989.

Norbiato G, et al: Cortisol resistance in acquired immunodeficiency syndrome. *J Clin Endocrinol Metab* 74:608-613, 1992.

Oldfield EH, et al: Petrosal sinus sampling with and without corticotropin-releasing hormone for the differential diagnosis of Cushing's syndrome. *N Engl J Med* 325:897-905, 1991.

Orth DN: Cushing's syndrome, in Krieger DT, Bardin CW (eds): *Current Therapy in Endocrinology 1983-1984*. St Louis, CV Mosby, 1983.

Otabe S, et al: Hyperreninemic hypoaldosteronism due to hepatocellular carcinoma metastatic to the adrenal gland. *Clin Nephrol* 35:66-71, 1991.

Pang S, et al: Late-onset adrenal steroid 3β-hydroxysteroid dehydrogenase deficiency: I. Cause of hirsutism in pubertal and postpubertal women. *J Clin Endocrinol Metab* 60:428-439, 1985.

Pang S, et al: Prenatal treatment of congenital adrenal hyperplasia due to 21-hydroxylase deficiency. *N Engl J Med* 322:111-115, 1990.

Pang S, et al: Maternal side effects of prenatal dexamethasone therapy for fetal congenital adrenal hyperplasia. *J Clin Endocrinol Metab* 75:249-253, 1992.

Petrusz P, et al: Central and peripheral distribution of corticotropin-releasing factor. *Federation Proc* 44:229-235, 1985.

Pont A, et al: Ketoconazole blocks adrenal steroid synthesis. *Ann Intern Med* 97:370-372, 1982.

Reid IR, et al: The effects of hydrocortisone, parathyroid hormone and the bisphosphonate, APD, on bone resorption in neonatal mouse calvaria. *Calcif Tissue Int* 38:38-43, 1986.

Reisine T: Neurohumoral aspects of ACTH release. *Hosp Pract* 77-96, (March 15) 1988.

Reznik Y, et al: Food-dependent Cushing's syndrome mediated by aberrant adrenal sensitivity to gastric inhibitory polypeptide. *N Engl J Med* 327:981-986, 1992.

Rich GM, et al: Glucocorticoid-remediable aldosteronism in a large kindred: Clinical spectrum and diagnosis using a characteristic biochemical phenotype. *Ann Intern Med* 116:813-820, 1992.

Rösler A, et al: 11β-Hydroxylase deficiency congenital adrenal hyperplasia: Update of prenatal diagnosis. *J Clin Endocrinol Metab* 66:830-838, 1988.

Rudman D, et al: Effects of human growth hormone in men over 60 years old. *N Engl J Med* 323:1-6, 1990.

Rumsby G, et al: Prenatal diagnosis of congenital adrenal hyperplasia by direct detection of mutations in the steroid 21-hydroxylase gene. *Clin Endocrinol* 38:421-425, 1993.

Saadi HF, et al: Feminizing adrenocortical tumor: Steroid hormone response to ketoconazole. *J Clin Endocrinol Metab* 70:540-543, 1990.

Sapolsky R, et al: Interleukin-1 stimulates the secretion of hypothalamic corticotropin-releasing factor. *Science* 238:522-524, 1987 A.

Sapolsky R, et al: Stress and glucocorticoids in aging. *Endocrinol Metab Clin* 16:965-980, 1987 B.

Schteingart DE: Cushing's syndrome. *Endocrinol Metab Clin North Am* 18:311-338, 1989.

Sheeler LR: Cushing's syndrome—1988. *Cleve Clin J Med* 55:329-337, 1988.

Shenker Y: Medical treatment of low-renin aldosteronism. *Endocrinol Metab Clin North Am* 18:415-442, 1989.

Shozu M, et al: A new cause of female pseudohermaphroditism: Placental aromatase deficiency. *J Clin Endocrinol Metab* 72:560-566, 1991.

Siegel SF, et al: ACTH stimulation tests and plasma dehydroepiandrosterone sulfate levels in women with hirsutism. *N Engl J Med* 323:849-854, 1990.

Skluth HA, Gums JG: Spironolactone: A re-examination. *DICP* 24:52-59, 1990.

Smith JK, Kemp SF: Pseudohypoaldosteronism: Successful treatment with home electrolyte monitoring. *Clin Pediatr* 30:600-601, 1991.

Sonino N: Use of ketoconazole as inhibitor of steroid production. *N Engl J Med* 317:812-818, 1987.

Sonino N: Current trends in the endocrine use of ketoconazole. *J Endocrinol Invest* 11:741-744, 1988.

Speiser PW, et al: Insulin insensitivity in adrenal hyperplasia due to nonclassical steroid 21-hydroxylase deficiency. *J Clin Endocrinol Metab* 75:1421-1424, 1992.

Spritzer P, et al: Cyproterone acetate *versus* hydrocortisone treatment in late-onset adrenal hyperplasia. *J Clin Endocrinol Metab* 70:642-646, 1990.

Strauss KW: Endocrine complications of the acquired immunodeficiency syndrome. *Arch Intern Med* 151:1441-1444, 1991.

Suda T, et al: Ectopic adrenocorticotropin syndrome caused by lung cancer that responded to corticotropin-releasing hormone. *J Clin Endocrinol Metab* 63:1047-1051, 1986.

Svec F: Differences in the interaction of RU 486 and ketoconazole with the second binding site of the glucocorticoid receptor. *Endocrinology* 123:1902-1906, 1988.

Tabarin A, et al: Usefulness of the corticotropin-releasing hormone test during bilateral inferior petrosal sinus sampling for the diagnosis of Cushing's disease. *J Clin Endocrinol Metab* 73:53-59, 1991 A.

Tabarin A, et al: Use of ketoconazole in the treatment of Cushing's disease and ectopic ACTH syndrome. *Clin Endocrinol* 34:63-69, 1991 B.

Taylor AL, Fishman LM: Corticotropin-releasing hormone. *N Engl J Med* 319:213-222, 1988.

Thomas CG Jr, et al: Hyperadrenalism in childhood and adolescence. *Ann Surg* 199:538-548, 1984.

Toms GC, et al: Predicting relapse after transsphenoidal surgery for Cushing's disease. *J Clin Endocrinol* 129(suppl):132, 1991.

Trainer PJ, Grossman A: The diagnosis and differential diagnosis of Cushing's syndrome. *Clin Endocrinol* 34:317-330, 1991.

Tyrrell JB, et al: An overnight high-dose dexamethasone suppression test for rapid differential diagnosis of Cushing's syndrome. *Ann Intern Med* 104:180-186, 1986.

Tyrrell JB, et al: Glucocorticoids & adrenal androgens, in Greenspan FS (ed): *Basic and Clinical Endocrinology,* ed 3. Norwalk, Appleton & Lange, 1991, 323-362.

Vale W, et al: Characteristics of 41-residue ovine hypothalamic peptide that stimulates secretion of corticotropin and β-endorphin. *Science* 213:1394-1397, 1981.

Walker BR, Edwards CRW: 11β-Hydroxysteroid dehydrogenase and enzyme-mediated receptor protection: Life after liquorice? *Clin Endocrinol* 35:281-289, 1991.

Weinberger MH, Fineberg NS: The diagnosis of primary aldosteronism and separation of two major subtypes. *Arch Intern Med* 153:2125-2129, 1993.

White A, Clark AJL: The cellular and molecular basis of the ectopic ACTH syndrome. *Clin Endocrinol* 39:131-141, 1993.

Whitehead HM, et al: The effect of cyproheptadine and/or bromocriptine on plasma ACTH levels in patients cured of Cushing's disease by bilateral adrenalectomy. *Clin Endocrinol* 32:193-201, 1990.

Whitworth JA, et al: The kidney is the major site of cortisone production in man. *Clin Endocrinol* 31:355-361, 1989.

Wick G, et al: Immunoendocrine communication via the hypothalamo-pituitary-adrenal axis in autoimmune diseases. *Endocr Rev* 14:539-563, 1993.

Wilkin TJ: Receptor autoimmunity in endocrine disorders. *N Engl J Med* 323:1318-1324, 1990.

Winterer J, et al: Effect of hydrocortisone dose schedule on adrenal steroid secretion in congenital adrenal hyperplasia. *J Pediatr* 106:137-142, 1985.

Wong GL: Basal activities and hormone responsiveness of osteoclast-like and osteoblast-like bone cells are regulated by glucocorticoids. *J Biol Chem* 254:6337-6340, 1979.

Woodhouse NJY, et al: Acute and long-term effects of octreotide in patients with ACTH-dependent Cushing's syndrome. *Am J Med* 95:305-308, (Sept) 1993.

Yanase T, et al: 17 α-Hydroxylase/17, 20-lyase deficiency: From clinical investigation to molecular definition. *Endocr Rev* 12:91-108, 1991.

Yanovski JA, et al: Corticotropin-releasing hormone stimulation following low-dose dexamethasone administration: A new test to distinguish Cushing's syndrome from pseudo-Cushing's states. *JAMA* 269:2232-2238, 1993.

Young WF Jr, et al: Familial Cushing's syndrome due to primary pigmented nodular adrenocortical disease. *N Engl J Med* 321:1659-1664, 1989.

Other Selected Reference

James VHT (ed): *The Adrenal Gland,* ed 2. New York, Raven Press, 1992.

Drugs Used in Thyroid Disease 47

Physiology of Thyroid Hormones

Thyroid hormones affect metabolism, growth, and development. Their major metabolic actions in adults are calorigenic: they accelerate the rate of cellular oxidation and increase energy expenditure and heat production. The resulting metabolic stimulation affects the utilization of vitamins, proteins, carbohydrates, lipids, electrolytes, and water and can alter the activities of hormones and drugs. The thyroid hormones also have important effects on protein anabolism and cellular differentiation during growth and development.

The two clinically important thyroid hormones are L-triiodothyronine (T_3) and L-tetraiodothyronine (T_4, thyroxine). The mechanisms of their synthesis and secretion are well defined. The follicular cells of the thyroid concentrate iodide, the rate-limiting substrate for synthesis of the thyroid hormones, by an active membrane transport process. This "trapping" of iodide by thyroid follicular cells can be blocked by inhibitors of oxidative metabolism, by agents that uncouple oxidative phosphorylation (eg, 2-4-dinitrophenol), by inadequate oxygen, and by certain monovalent anions (eg, perchlorate, thiocyanate). After trapping, the iodide is oxidized ("activated") and incorporated into post-translationally modified thyroglobulin molecules as mono- and diiodotyrosines (MIT and DIT) ("organification"). DIT is then coupled with either MIT or another DIT molecule to form T_3 or T_4, respectively.

Thyroglobulin containing T_3 and T_4 is stored within the follicular lumina of the gland. About 1% of these stores are released into the circulation daily (80 to 100 mcg of T_4 and 5 to 8 mcg of T_3).

About 70% of circulating T_4 is bound to thyroxine-binding globulin (TBG), 15% to 25% to transthyretin (formerly termed thyroxine-binding prealbumin), and 5% to 15% to albumin. T_3 also is bound to TBG (but less firmly than T_4) as well as to albumin. About 0.03% of the T_4 and 0.3% of the T_3 are free or nonprotein bound. The protein-bound hormones serve as hormone reservoirs and the binding proteins may act as buffers to maintain relatively stable free hormone concentrations. Serum concentrations of free T_3 and T_4 appear to determine true clinical status. Although the free T_4 concentration is several times larger than the free T_3 concentration, thyroid hormone receptors within target tissues have 10-fold greater affinity for T_3, and T_3 is several times more potent than T_4 in inducing calorigenesis.

Circulating thyroid hormone concentrations are regulated through a feedback system involving the thyroid, anterior pituitary, and hypothalamus. As circulating concentrations of free thyroid hormones decrease, the secretion of thyroid-stimulating hormone (thyrotropin, TSH) by the pituitary is increased. TSH stimulates iodide trapping by thyroid follicular cells as well as each step of hormone synthesis and secretion, acts as a trophic hormone to maintain the viability of normal follicular cells, and facilitates hypertrophy and hyperplasia of thyroid follicular cells during goitrogenesis. TSH secretion also is stimulated by hypothalamic thyrotropin-releasing hormone (TRH), and the tonic intensity and pulsatile frequency of pituitary TSH secretion and hence of thyroid gland activity appear to be maintained by hypothalamic TRH secretion. Conversely, the thyroid hormones inhibit TRH and TSH synthesis and secretion. Hypothalamic somatostatin and dopamine also appear to inhibit TSH secretion. In addition, an intrathyroidal autoregulatory system exists; increased intracellular iodide concentration transiently inhibits iodine organification. Iodide also directly inhibits TSH-stimulated release of hormones from the thyroid gland.

In certain conditions, TBG concentrations may be altered, changing the total extrathyroidal pool of thyroid hormones. For example, TBG concentrations are physiologically elevated in adults in response to increased serum estrogen concentrations, during pregnancy, and in the newborn. Consequently, the serum concentrations of both protein-bound and total T_4 and T_3 are increased, although the concentrations of free hormones are maintained within normal limits and metabolic status is not affected. Other euthyroid hyperthyroxinemic conditions associated with increased serum TBG concentrations include hereditary X-linked TBG excess, treatment with various drugs (eg, methadone, perphenazine, tamoxifen, fluorouracil), heroin use, acute intermittent porphyria, acute hepatocellular inflammation, and chronic active hepatitis (Safran and Braverman, 1987). Failure to recognize that free hormone concentrations can remain normal despite increased TBG concentrations or binding of thyroxine to abnormal thyroid hormone binders (endogenous antibodies, abnormal serum albumin-like proteins) may lead to misdiagnosis of hyperthyroidism.

Conversely, TBG concentrations may be reduced in patients receiving androgens, anabolic steroids, glucocorticoids, asparaginase, phenytoin, carbamazepine, or combined treatment with colestipol and niacin and in those with cirrhosis, nephrotic syndrome, severe or chronic illness, or hereditary TBG deficiency. Malnutrition, fasting, and anorexia nervosa also decrease TBG synthesis and serum concentrations. In addition, a deficiency in TBG binding capacity may occur because binding sites are occupied by drugs (eg, aspirin, diclofenac, diflunisal, phenytoin, furosemide) or long-chain nonesterified fatty acids (especially arachidonic, linoleic, and linolenic acids) (Lim et al, 1988). Hypothyroidism may be misdiagnosed under these conditions if the diagnosis is based solely on total serum hormone concentrations.

In euthyroid individuals, the half-life of T_4 in blood is about six days and that of T_3 is about one day. The half-life of T_4 is shortened in hyperthyroid patients (to as little as three days) and may be prolonged in hypothyroid patients (up to ten days). Conditions associated with elevated amounts of binding protein (eg, pregnancy, treatment with estrogen) increase the half-life, while those associated with reduced amounts of binding protein (eg, kidney or liver disease) may decrease the half-life. About 10% to 20% of secreted thyroid hormone is excreted in the feces via the hepatobiliary system.

Approximately 85% to 90% of thyroid hormones are deiodinated in peripheral tissues, and the iodine released returns to the circulation and is available for reincorporation into new thyroid hormone. Iodine that is not reutilized is excreted in the urine. In addition to the T_3 secreted by the thyroid gland, adults produce about 22 mcg daily in peripheral tissues by the monodeiodination of T_4 at the 5′ position; this represents about 75% of the daily T_3 production. Some T_4 also is deiodinated at the 5 position to form the inert metabolite, reverse T_3 (rT_3). In the normal fetus and neonate and in adults with certain conditions (eg, starvation, anorexia nervosa, acute or chronic debilitating disease, cachexia, surgery, cirrhosis), 5′-deiodination of T_4 is reduced. Under these conditions, serum T_3 concentrations decrease and serum rT_3 concentrations increase.

Thyroid hormones increase tissue oxygen utilization through mechanisms involving cell nuclei and mitochondria. They bind with high affinity and specificity to nuclear DNA-binding protein receptors in a variety of cells (Lazar, 1993). The hormone-receptor complex interacts with a thyroid hormone response element that is present in the promoter regions of several genes and regulates transcription of mRNA and translation of cellular regulatory and functional proteins. Because of the wide-ranging impact of the thyroid hormones, thyroid dysfunction has profound effects on many body systems. Fortunately, effective treatment is available for most dysfunctional states.

Thyroid Function Tests

Although some thyroid diseases are recognized easily after a careful history and physical examination, diagnostic confirmation and the selection of appropriate therapies usually require determination of the status of thyroid function. However, the results of laboratory procedures should be used selectively and should suggest therapeutic measures consistent with clinical judgment. Detailed reviews on the use of thyroid function tests in the diagnosis of thyroid abnormalities are available (Burrow, 1990; Helfand and Crapo, 1990; Oppenheimer and Volpé, 1990; Surks et al, 1990; Bayer, 1991; Felicetta, 1991).

The most useful laboratory tests for screening purposes are measurements of serum free T_4, total T_4, and TSH concentrations. In the past, determination of the *serum free T_4* concentration was difficult and often unreliable (Wong et al, 1992); however, newly developed labeled antibody radioimmunoassays appear to have overcome these problems (Christofides et al, 1992; Sheehan and Christofides, 1992). Serum free T_4 concentration is elevated in most hyperthyroid patients and is usually decreased in those with hypothyroidism. In many patients with alcoholic liver disease, chronic renal failure, acute myocardial infarction, major surgery or trauma, leukemia, poorly controlled diabetes, malnutrition, birth trauma, prematurity, or hypoxia, the serum free T_4 concentrations are normal despite reduced secretion of T_4 (a clinical syndrome known as nonthyroidal illness [previously termed euthyroid sick syndrome or sick euthyroid syndrome]). During treatment of hyperthyroidism with antithyroid drugs, changes in serum free T_4 concentrations occur rapidly and can be used to monitor the effectiveness of therapy.

Serum total T_4 concentration (including both protein-bound and free T_4) is easily measured by immunometric assays. However, serum total T_4 concentration alone is inadequate for diagnosis because it is affected by the *serum TBG* concentration and binding capacity. Potentially abnormal serum total T_4 concentrations should be compared with *serum TSH* concentrations that were measured using an immunochemiluminometric assay capable of detecting TSH in serum at concentrations as low as 0.001 microunit/ml.

Most patients with untreated overt hyperthyroidism have serum TSH concentrations <0.1 microunit/ml (Ross et al, 1989; Surks et al, 1990). Detectable subnormal concentrations (<0.5 microunits/ml) usually indicate subclinical hyperthyroidism (low TSH, normal free T_4 and free T_3). These patients may require further testing or continued surveillance for accurate assessment of their status. The interpretation of subnormal serum TSH concentrations may be confounded by conditions (eg, Cushing's syndrome, severe nonthyroidal illness, chronic renal failure, cigarette smoking, old age) and agents (eg, T_3 [liothyronine], T_4 [levothyroxine], glucocorticoids, dopamine, somatostatin, endorphins) that suppress TSH secretion (Bartalena et al, 1990; Benker et al, 1990; Ericsson and Lindgärde, 1991; Stott et al, 1991; Sundbeck et al, 1991).

More than 95% of patients with serum TSH concentrations between 0.5 and 5 microunits/ml have normal thyroid function. However, a serum TSH concentration in the normal range (0.5 to 5 microunits/ml) does not always reflect euthyroidism. Clinically apparent hypothyroidism of hypothalamic or pituitary origin is characterized by abnormally low tonic TRH secretion, lack of nocturnal TSH surges, and abnormal glycosylation of TSH (with changes in immunoactivity), all of which will decrease measured serum TSH concentration (Samuels and Ridgway, 1992). Abnormally low serum TSH, serum T_4, and total T_3 concentrations may be present in those with nonthyroidal illness despite the absence of clinical signs of hypothyroidism (Romijn and Wiersinga, 1990; Finucane et al, 1991; Mahoney and Wartofsky, 1993). In addition, because TSH secretion remains suppressed for weeks or months after the restoration of euthyroidism in both adults and children (Sills et al, 1992), serum TSH concentrations are not reliable indicators of the effectiveness of therapy in the treatment of hyperthyroidism.

Serum TSH concentrations >5 microunits/ml are considered abnormal. If serum T_4 concentration is normal and other clinical signs are absent, borderline elevated serum TSH concentrations may indicate subclinical or impending hypothyroidism. Subclinical hypothyroidism may progress to overt hypothyroidism or may continue for years without change (Kabadi, 1993).

Serum TSH concentrations >10 microunits/ml usually indicate primary hypothyroidism or hypothyroidism secondary to isolated adrenocorticotropin (ACTH) deficiency (Shigemasa et al, 1992). In patients with primary hypothyroidism, periodic assessment of serum TSH concentrations provides a sensitive and reliable means of monitoring the effectiveness of thyroid hormone replacement therapy. Serum TSH concentrations >10 microunits/ml also are characteristic of hyperthyroidism resulting from pituitary hypersecretion of TSH (TSH adenoma) and pituitary resistance to the negative feedback effects of thyroid hormones on TSH secretion.

The *free thyroxine index* (FT_4I), sometimes referred to as the corrected T_4, is a unitless number that may be obtained by multiplying the serum total T_4 concentration by the thyroid hormone binding ratio (THBR, also called the T_3 resin uptake test [T_3RU]). Despite the increasing popularity of the sensitive serum TSH assays, the FT_4I is still recommended by some for general screening of thyroid function (DeGroot and Mayor, 1992).

Determination of the *serum total T_3* concentration by radioimmunoassay may be used to detect T_3-toxicosis and to confirm hyperthyroidism when other test results are borderline. Serum T_3:T_4 concentration ratios may be elevated in impending hypothyroidism; however, peripheral conversion of T_4 to T_3 maintains normal serum T_3 concentrations and, therefore, serum total T_3 concentration is not a sensitive indicator of hypothyroidism. In contrast, in conditions in which conversion of T_4 to T_3 in peripheral tissues is reduced (eg, nonthyroidal illness), low serum total T_3 concentrations result even though clinical signs of hypothyroidism are absent (Fisher, 1990; Pearce, 1991).

Measurement of *circulating antithyroid antibodies* also may assist diagnosis by indicating the existence of autoimmune thyroid disease. The most important are antithyroglobulin antibodies, antithyroid peroxidase (anti-TPO) antibodies, thyroid stimulating antibodies, and thyroid stimulating blocking antibodies. The interpretation of assay results depends on the antibodies measured and the methods utilized.

Dynamic tests of thyroid function also can be employed. Administration of *protirelin*, a synthetic preparation of *TRH*, has been used to assess thyroid function when hyperthyroidism was suspected; this test has no diagnostic advantage over a sensitive TSH assay (Spencer et al, 1993). The measurement of serum TSH concentration after injection of protirelin has been used in attempts to differentiate hypothalamic hypothyroidism (TRH-sensitive: tonic low TSH secretion resulting from TRH deficiency) from pituitary hypothyroidism (TRH-insensitive: tonic low TSH secretion caused by pituitary defects). Unfortunately, the complexity of hypothalamic-pituitary interactions often prevents this test from providing definitive results and thus it has limited clinical usefulness (Samuels and Ridgway, 1992; see also the evaluation on Protirelin). Increased *serum free T_3* concentration following injection of protirelin has been suggested as an indicator of disease remission in both hyperthyroid and hypothyroid patients (Notsu et al, 1991); however, current methods for measuring serum free T_3 concentration are unreliable (Price et al, 1992).

In a *thyroid scan*, a small amount of radioactive iodine or technetium is given and the morphology of the areas of radioactive uptake (ie, active thyroid tissue) is outlined. Scanning is used (1) to determine whether hyperthyroidism is caused by Graves' disease, thyroid adenoma, thyroiditis, or multinodular goiter, and (2) to help distinguish between "hot" (active) and "cold" (inactive) nodules in determining the likelihood of malignancy. In the *radioactive iodine uptake test*, the proportion of an oral dose of radioactive iodine that accumulates within the thyroid gland is measured; this test is used to determine the dosage for radioactive iodide ablation therapy, in differentiating Graves' disease from hyperthyroidism caused by thyroiditis or exogenous thyroid hormones, and in confirming thyroid dysgenesis in the newborn. *Fine-needle aspiration* to obtain samples for histocytologic evaluation is the procedure of choice to differentiate between benign and malignant nodules (Gharib and Goellner, 1993). *Ultrasonography* is often used in the evaluation of hypofunctioning nodules to differentiate cystic nodules from solid lesions; to measure the size of the glands, cysts, and adenomas; and to guide needle puncture when draining cysts (*therapeutic fine-needle aspiration*). *Ultrasound, magnetic resonance imaging,* and *computerized tomography* may be used to examine the structure of the thyroid gland and associated tissues.

HYPOTHYROIDISM

SYMPTOMS. Clinical manifestations of hypothyroidism include the classical myxedema facies with its round, puffy, sleepy appearance; dry, rough skin and brittle hair; obesity; bradycardia; and slightly elevated diastolic blood pressure. Myalgias and arthralgias are common. Fatigue, somnolence, irritability or apathy, constipation, nonpitting peripheral edema, hyperprolactinemia, galactorrhea, infertility, and intolerance to cold also may be observed. Patients may or may not have a goiter. In those with mild hypothyroidism, serum HDL-cholesterol concentrations may be decreased and serum total and LDL-cholesterol concentrations, plasma Lp(a) concentrations, and the risk of coronary heart disease may be increased (de Bruin et al, 1993). In its most severe form, hypothyroidism may induce hypothermia, seizures, stupor, or coma. However, the severity of symptoms may not correlate with the reduction in serum hormone concentrations. Depression, learning impairment, and attention deficits may be prominent symptoms of hypothyroidism in the elderly (Osterweil et al, 1992). When hypothyroidism occurs congenitally or during early infancy (ie, cretinism), inadequate development of the brain, bones, teeth, and muscles; mental retardation; and delayed skeletal maturation are inevitable.

ETIOLOGY. Clinical hypothyroidism almost always results from inadequate secretion of thyroid hormones. The disease is usually of thyroidal origin (primary), although hypothyroidism also may result from hypopituitarism (secondary hypothyroidism) or hypothalamic injury (tertiary or central hypothyroidism).

Fetal hypothyroidism usually is caused by failure of the thyroid to develop normally (hypoplasia or aplasia) but may result from TSH deficiency; genetic defects in thyroid hormonogenesis, including reduced production of thyroglobulin or production of defective thyroglobulin; or extreme deficiency of iodine (Gruters, 1992; Medeiros-Neto et al, 1993). Maternal ingestion of antithyroid drugs, inadvertent use of sodium iodide I 131 during pregnancy, or the passive placental transfer of TSH-antagonist immunoglobulins also may produce fetal hypothyroidism. Ultrasound-guided percutaneous umbilical cord blood sampling may allow accurate diagnosis when fetal thyroid dysfunction is suspected. Intra-amniotic injection of T_4 (levothyroxine 250 mcg, once weekly) has been reported to resolve confirmed fetal hypothyroidism secondary to excessive maternal intake of an antithyroid drug (Davidson et al, 1991); unless treated, this condition results in symptomatic neonatal hypothyroidism.

Transient hypothyroidism of prematurity is common in preterm infants (Fisher, 1990); the condition results from immaturity of the hypothalamic-pituitary axis and spontaneously remits as the central nervous system reaches a stage of development appropriate for term birth. Normalization of thyroid function requires 4 to 16 weeks, depending on the degree of prematurity at birth.

The incidence of congenital hypothyroidism in female infants is about twice that in males. Hypothyroid neonates tend to have longer gestations (two to three weeks beyond term) and thus greater birth weights than normal infants. Because only 5% of hypothyroid neonates exhibit clinical manifestations at birth, routine screening programs are now in widespread use to ensure the earliest possible detection. Screening is most effective when samples are obtained two to six days after birth (American Academy of Pediatrics, 1993). At this age, serum TSH concentrations >20 microunits/ml suggest congenital hypothyroidism (Fisher, 1991). Samples obtained earlier will tend to cause overestimation of the incidence of congenital hypothyroidism because a brief physiologic TSH secretory surge normally occurs after birth; however, serum TSH concentrations >40 microunits/ml indicate a need for immediate institution of thyroid hormone replacement therapy (American Academy of Pediatrics, 1993). When samples are obtained when the infant is between two and six weeks of age, congenital hypothyroidism is suggested by serum total T_4 concentrations < 84 nmol/L or serum TSH concentrations >7 microunits/ml (Fisher, 1991).

Juvenile hypothyroidism can develop in children who apparently were normal previously and is usually the result of autoimmune thyroiditis, although those inborn errors in thyroid hormonogenesis that escaped detection in the neonatal period also may be expressed initially during early childhood (LaFranchi, 1992).

Autoimmune thyroiditis is the most common cause of spontaneous hypothyroidism in North America. This disease is four times more common in women than in men (incidence, 1% to 4% of all women), four times more common in whites than in blacks, and increasingly common with advancing age. The prototype, chronic lymphocytic (Hashimoto's) thyroiditis (goitrous chronic lymphocytic thyroiditis, struma lymphomatosa), is characterized by an enlarged thyroid exhibiting diffuse lymphocytic infiltration, atrophy of the parenchymal cells, fibrosis, and oxyphilic change in some of the parenchymal cells. Variants include chronic fibrous thyroiditis, in which fibrosis predominates; lymphocytic thyroiditis of childhood and adolescence, in which fibrosis, oxyphilic cell change, and germinal centers are less obvious; and atrophic thyroiditis (idiopathic myxedema), in which the thyroid gland is atrophied rather than hypertrophied.

Postpartum thyroiditis can develop a few months after delivery and is most common in women who have given birth to females (James, 1992). In some patients, thyroid autoantibodies are produced in an apparent reaction to the immunosuppressive effect of early pregnancy; almost 50% will later develop postpartum thyroiditis (Stagnaro-Green et al, 1992). An initial hyperthyroid phase usually is followed by a hypothyroid phase, during which clinical signs become apparent. This condition usually resolves as postparturient immune function normalizes, but recurrences are common following subsequent pregnancies and may eventually culminate in chronic thyroiditis and permanent hypothyroidism (Hara et al, 1992; Roti and Emerson, 1992; Walfish et al, 1992 A). Women with insulin-dependent diabetes mellitus may be at increased risk of symptomatic postpartum thyroid dysfunction (Gerstein, 1993). In some women, postpartum hypothyroidism may precipitate postpartum depression (Harris et al, 1992; Walfish et al, 1992 A).

Autoimmune thyroid disease appears to be a familial disorder of defective immunoregulation (see DeGroot and Quintans, 1989; Volpé, 1991; Weetman et al, 1992). Immune reactivity to thyroid antigens (thyroglobulin, the TSH membrane receptor, and thyroid microsomal antigen/thyroid peroxidase) by a resident population of autoreactive T-lymphocytes occurs normally but at a level that is physiologically insignificant. Individuals with various inherited abnormalities of immunoregulation or those with thyroid cell damage caused by infection or other disorders may produce increased amounts of thyroid antigens and antithyroid antibodies. In those with a genetically induced partial defect in thyroid-directed suppressor T-lymphocytes, the survival of autoreactive helper T-lymphocytes is enhanced and may trigger clinical autoimmune disease. Autoreactive helper T-lymphocytes secrete interferon gamma (IFN-γ), which induces the expression of major histocompatibility complex class II (HLA-DR) antigens on the surface of normal thyroid follicular cells (Kasuga et al, 1991). These antigens sensitize helper T-lymphocytes to follicular cells and may stimulate further IFN-γ secretion. IFN-γ also stimulates thyrocytes to secrete interleukins 2, 6, and 8; these cytokines are chemoattractants for lymphocytes and may activate both B- and T-lymphocytes within the thyroid gland (Weetman et al, 1992).

Sensitized thyroid-specific helper T-lymphocytes activate a subpopulation of B-lymphocytes that secrete autoantibodies directed against a number of antigens, including thyroglobulin, follicular cell surface and microsomal antigens, T_3, T_4, and the TSH receptor. Some of these antibodies may act alone or in association with macrophages or killer lymphocytes to either damage or lyse thyroid follicular cells, inhibit their growth, or attenuate their response to TSH (Chiovato et al, 1990). Other antibodies may stimulate thyroid function by acting as TSH agonists (see the section on Graves' Disease).

Exogenous cytokines used as novel therapeutic agents (eg, interferon alfa, interleukin 2, sargramostim [GM-CSF], tissue necrosis factor) also may cause thyroiditis by stimulating autoantibody secretion (Kung et al, 1992; Weetman et al, 1992). Whether autoimmune thyroid disease is expressed as hypothyroidism or hyperthyroidism or resolves depends on the relative proportions of thyrotoxic and TSH agonist and antagonist antibodies; clinical status can change with fluctuations in this balance (Takasu et al, 1992; Tamai et al, 1990).

The most sensitive indication of the onset of autoimmune thyroiditis is the presence of circulating anti-TPO antibodies. The earliest sign of decreased thyroid reserve resulting from autoimmune thyroiditis is an elevation in the serum TSH concentration. This response to decreasing thyroid function occurs before a decline in serum T_3 or T_4 concentrations to subnormal levels can be detected (a condition known as compensated or subclinical hypothyroidism). Autoimmune thyroiditis is the most common cause of subclinical hypothyroidism and may be the presumptive diagnosis in middle-aged or older adults with normal T_3 and T_4 concentrations but elevated serum TSH concentrations (Francis and Wartofsky, 1992). Often these patients remain clinically euthyroid, although some become hypothyroid.

Primary hypothyroidism also may follow destruction of the thyroid gland by radioactive iodine therapy, external radiation, or surgical removal. The incidence of central hypothyroidism is high (25% to 65%) in the decade following cranial or craniospinal irradiation for brain tumors (Ogilvy-Stuart et al, 1991; Constine et al, 1993). Transient hypothyroidism may accompany subacute lymphocytic thyroiditis (painless or silent thyroiditis) and subacute granulomatous (DeQuervain's) thyroiditis. Familial resistance to thyroid hormones resulting from defects in receptor structure (Refetoff's syndrome) or lack of thyroid hormone receptors also may cause the symptoms of hypothyroidism even though serum concentrations of T_4, T_3, and TSH are elevated (Refetoff et al, 1983). Mild chronic malnutrition inhibits T_4 conversion to T_3, but severe protein-calorie malnutrition (including that resulting from anorexia nervosa or bulimia) induces thyroid involution and a degree of hypothyroidism (Ingenbleek, 1985; Marshall and Lippmann, 1987; Fonseca et al, 1990). However, decreased thyroid function may be an adaptive mechanism in these patients and not an indication for treatment.

Patients with AIDS often have elevated serum total T_4 and normal total T_3 concentrations until late in disease progression (LoPresti et al, 1989). Maintenance of normal serum total T_3 concentration may account for the inexorable weight loss characteristic of HIV infection (Strauss, 1991). In contrast, end-stage disease is accompanied by the low serum TSH, total T_3, and total T_4 concentrations that are typical of nonthyroidal illness. Patients with AIDS who are treated with aerosolized pentamidine are susceptible to *Pneumocystis carinii* infection of the thyroid gland with clinical features similar to those of subacute granulomatous thyroiditis (Guttler and Singer, 1993).

Hypothyroidism also may be induced by drugs (eg, lithium, excessive doses of antithyroid compounds, preparations with high iodine content such as amiodarone), most commonly in patients with underlying thyroid abnormalities (Roti et al, 1993 A). Withdrawal of the causative agent usually cures the condition. If these agents must be continued, thyroid replacement therapy may be given concomitantly. Some drugs (eg, phenobarbital, phenytoin, carbamazepine, nicardipine, rifampin, imidazole antibiotics), industrial chemicals (polycyclic and polyhalogenated aromatic hydrocarbons, tetrachlorodibenzo-pdioxin [the metabolically active contaminant in Agent Orange]), organochlorine pesticides (DDT), and fungicides (hexachlorobenzene) induce the hepatic enzymes that metabolize thyroid hormones and also increase biliary excretion of thyroid hormone metabolites (Curran and DeGroot, 1991). Acute hypothyroid episodes or chronic subclinical hypothyroidism can result from exposure to these substances. The metabolism of some drugs is reduced in hypothyroid patients (eg, anticoagulants, propranolol, phenytoin, oxazepam, cortisone, digoxin, anesthetics, opioids, all sedating drugs that are metabolized in the liver). Therefore, lower doses of these drugs may be appropriate in patients with uncorrected thyroid deficiency.

Indications for Treatment with Thyroid Hormones

Regardless of the etiology of hypothyroidism, replacement therapy with thyroid hormone is the appropriate therapeutic choice. However, mild transient hypothyroidism may be self-limited and often is not treated. When hypothyroidism is a side effect of drug usage, withdrawal of the offending agent is indicated.

CONGENITAL HYPOTHYROIDISM. Early diagnosis and adequate treatment are mandatory for the management of congenital hypothyroidism. Evidence suggests that untreated affected infants lose three to five IQ points monthly during the first year of life (Fisher, 1991). Most of the permanent sequelae of congenital hypothyroidism can be minimized or avoided when appropriate thyroid hormone replacement therapy is begun early in life. Single daily oral doses of T_4 (levothyroxine, 10 to 15 mcg/kg) can restore normal serum free T_4 and T_3 concentrations (7 to 16 and 4 to 7 pg/ml, respectively) in one to two weeks in most affected infants (Gruters, 1992). Infants with undetectable serum total T_4 concentrations should be given levothyroxine 50 mcg daily (American Academy of Pediatrics, 1993). The dosage then must be monitored by regular measurements of serum free T_4 and, if possible, free T_3 concentrations in order to maintain cerebral euthyroidism (Chiovato et al, 1991). Serum TSH concentrations may remain elevated (between 10 and 20 microunits/ml) because the feedback threshold for T_4 suppression of TSH secretion is reset in infants with congenital hypothyroidism.

When treatment is initiated in the first month of life and maintained thereafter, intellectual ability is only slightly compromised (Chiovato et al, 1991; Heyerdahl et al, 1991). Treatment initiated after the infant is about 1.5 months of age does not reverse all of the intellectual impairment that has already occurred but does reverse the physical effects. Hypothyroidism that develops after age 2 to 3 years is not associated with mental retardation but usually is characterized by growth retardation, delayed epiphyseal maturation, and delayed dentition. Reduced adult stature results when treatment of hypothyroidism is delayed; the degree of impairment is correlated with the length of the delay.

AUTOIMMUNE THYROIDITIS. Thyroid hormones are used to treat chronic lymphocytic (Hashimoto's) thyroiditis and its variants. In frankly hypothyroid individuals, the therapeutic goal is to restore the euthyroid state, as indicated by the return of serum TSH concentrations to normal; when this is accomplished, the serum total T_4 concentration often is 1 to 2 mcg/dL greater than normal. By normalizing TSH secretion, replacement therapy also may reduce the size of any existing goiter. Patients with subclinical hypothyroidism may be monitored periodically for the onset of clinical hypothyroidism or may be given prophylactic thyroid hormone therapy.

HYPOTHYROIDISM DURING PREGNANCY AND POSTPARTUM THYROIDITIS. Rarely, symptomatic hypothyroidism will first appear during pregnancy and may increase the incidence of stillbirth. Affected women should be treated with full replacement doses of thyroid hormone in order to achieve serum hormone concentrations in the normal range for pregnancy. Women with pre-existing hypothyroidism usually require increased amounts of replacement hormones during pregnancy to compensate for increased serum TBG concentrations.

Pregnant women who produce antibodies that inhibit binding of TSH to its receptor may transfer these antibodies transplacentally and induce fetal and neonatal hypothyroidism that may persist for several years. Affected infants require replacement therapy from birth until thyroid function normalizes.

Transient autoimmune thyroiditis with hypothyroidism may occur in women during the first few months postpartum. Clinical symptoms usually are mild and transient; if severe, they respond favorably to thyroid hormone replacement therapy until endogenous thyroid function normalizes spontaneously (Roti and Emerson, 1992; Walfish et al, 1992 A).

MYXEDEMA COMA. Acute severe hypothyroidism can be triggered by infections, surgery, neurologic disorders, trauma, or acute illness and is characterized by bradycardia, ileus, hypothermia, psychosis, and coma (Smallridge, 1992). Relatively large doses of T_3 (liothyronine) should be given intravenously as soon as a definitive diagnosis is made (MacKerrow et al, 1992). Intravenous administration is preferable to the oral route because intestinal absorption can be inefficient during acute hypothyroidism. Although T_4 (levothyroxine) can be used, the conversion of T_4 to T_3 may be compromised in those with myxedema coma. Appropriate supportive measures also must be provided (ventilatory assistance, passive warming, regulation of fluids and electrolytes, and administration of dextrose if hypoglycemia is present). Intravenous corticosteroids also should be given because of the difficulty in excluding adrenal insufficiency from the initial diagnosis.

SUBACUTE THYROIDITIS. Transient hypothyroidism occurs during the course of subacute lymphocytic (painless, silent) thyroiditis and subacute granulomatous (DeQuervain's) thyroiditis. Symptomatic improvement can be achieved with replacement doses of levothyroxine during prolonged hypothyroid phases.

THYROID CARCINOMA. Thyroid hormones may produce a demonstrable regression of metastatic papillary lesions, including those developing after neck irradiation. All patients treated for papillary or follicular carcinoma require pituitary suppressing therapy with levothyroxine to minimize TSH stimulation of tumor regrowth. The goal is to administer the minimum amount of thyroid hormone that will either completely suppress pituitary TSH secretion in response to TRH stimulation or produce serum TSH concentrations <0.01 microunits/ml. If no evidence of tumor regrowth is apparent after several years, the dosage of levothyroxine can be reduced to replacement levels.

INAPPROPRIATE INDICATIONS. Amenorrhea, menorrhagia, dysmenorrhea, premenstrual tension, sterility, habitual abortion, oligospermia, obesity, hypercholesterolemia, and vague symptoms suggesting hypometabolism have been treated empirically with thyroid hormones. There is no evidence that such therapy is beneficial unless the patient is also proven to be hypothyroid; furthermore, such treatment may cause iatrogenic thyrotoxicosis.

Drug Selection

The preferred agent for replacement therapy is the synthetic salt of the pure thyroid hormone, T_4 (levothyroxine sodium [LEVO-T, Levothroid, Levoxine, Synthroid]); this also is the drug of choice for treating congenital hypothyroidism (Committee on Drugs, American Academy of Pediatrics, 1978). More precise assessment of clinical progress is possible with its use (see the section on Monitoring Therapy). Substitution of levothyroxine should be considered for patients who are being maintained on desiccated animal thyroid tablets.

Synthetic T_3 (liothyronine sodium [Cytomel, Triostat]) generally is not preferred for maintenance therapy because of the wide oscillations that result from its absorption into a small plasma pool. However, liothyronine is preferred for acute myxedema coma, when resistance to thyroid hormones is encountered, or when conversion of T_4 to T_3 is defective.

A preparation containing both T_4 and T_3 (liotrix [Thyrolar]) is available. This preparation contains T_3 and T_4 in a ratio of 1:4, five times greater than the physiologic ratio. The administration of relatively large amounts of T_3 bypasses the physiologic regulation of T_3 production and may result in hypertriiodothyroninemia. Furthermore, because most circulating T_3 is formed by peripheral monodeiodination of T_4, the T_3 component is not needed if peripheral regulation of thyroxine metabolism is normal. Therefore, current combination products often offer no therapeutic advantage over levothyroxine alone for the routine treatment of hypothyroidism.

Thyroid preparations usually are administered orally. Parenteral preparations of levothyroxine and liothyronine are used in emergencies and when oral administration is impossible.

DOSAGE. Hypothyroid patients have increased sensitivity to thyroid hormones, and determination of the optimum dosage of levothyroxine must be individualized and should be based on apparent clinical status, age, the results of appropriate laboratory tests (see the following section on Monitoring Therapy), and the duration of hypothyroidism (see Dosage and Preparations in the Drug Evaluations section). Factors favoring conservative dosing include coronary artery disease; a history of myocardial infarction; severe, prolonged thyroid disease; possible adrenal insufficiency masked by the low metabolic rate characteristic of clinical hypothyroidism; and advanced age. Because of its more rapid onset of action, liothyronine should not be used in such patients.

Adolescents, young adults, and those with hypothyroidism of short duration can be treated initially with full replacement doses (about 1.6 mcg/kg). Others may be given one-half to three-quarters of the estimated maintenance dosage, with full replacement amounts given after four to six weeks. In those with myxedema, the low initial dose is increased more gradually because these patients are sensitive to the cardiac effects of thyroid hormones.

Maintenance doses currently recommended for adults are lower than those formerly used. If a patient is receiving larger amounts, the dose may be reduced gradually to the minimum required to normalize the serum TSH concentration (Jennings et al, 1984; Ross, 1988). In children, maintenance requirements are relatively higher than in adults.

The half-life of thyroid hormones is increased in elderly patients. These individuals, particularly those with cardiovascular disease, may require a small initial dose, gradual dosage increments, and a lower maintenance dose than younger adults.

MONITORING THERAPY. Measurement of serum TSH concentration by a highly sensitive test is the most useful method for monitoring thyroid hormone therapy in patients with primary hypothyroidism. TSH concentrations begin to decrease within hours after initiating therapy and correlate inversely with thyroid hormone concentrations. Persistently elevated TSH concentrations indicate inadequate replacement dosage or, more often, patient noncompliance. In most individuals, thyroid hormone should be given in increasing doses until the TSH concentration is within the normal range. However, full TSH normalization may not be appropriate for all patients with cardiac disease.

Patients with congenital hypothyroidism may have elevated serum TSH concentrations for months or years, even when appropriate or even excessive doses of thyroid hormones are given. In these individuals, T_3 feedback control of TSH secretion appears to be abnormal, and serum free T_4 concentrations should be monitored and maintained in the upper half of the normal range for the age of the infant or child (serum FT_4I also may be used). This ensures sufficient hormone for the growing child.

The possibility of disease remission may be determined by temporarily withdrawing therapy and examining changes in serum TSH concentrations. Alternatively, TRH can be administered without withdrawing therapy; patients in whom thyroid function has normalized have significantly elevated serum TSH, T_4, and T_3 concentrations two hours after being given 500 mcg of TRH intramuscularly (Takasu et al, 1990).

ADVERSE REACTIONS. If the appropriate amount of thyroid hormone is provided for replacement, no adverse reactions occur. However, overdosage of any thyroid preparation causes thyrotoxicosis. Signs and symptoms include tachycardia, palpitations, wide variations in pulse pressure, angina pectoris, tremor, nervousness, insomnia, headache, change in appetite, diarrhea, weight loss, hyperhidrosis, heat intolerance, fever, myopathy, psychosis, coma, seizure, and (if prolonged) osteoporosis. Prolonged overtreatment of neonates can result in premature craniosynostosis and brain dysgenesis. The dose of thyroid hormone that produces thyrotoxicosis varies widely from patient to patient; regular monitoring during therapy is essential.

The suggestion that the incidence of breast cancer was increased in women receiving thyroid replacement therapy has been evaluated and it was concluded that there was no increased risk associated with long-term use of thyroid hormone. It is recommended that patients with a documented need for thyroid medication continue their therapeutic program (Education Committee, American Thyroid Association, 1977; Shapiro et al, 1980).

PRECAUTIONS. Because hypothyroid patients may discontinue medication when euthyroidism and relief of clinical symptoms have been attained, it is important to stress (1) that their need for thyroid replacement therapy usually is lifelong, (2) that they must inform any new physician of their condition, and (3) that they should participate in a medical alert identification program.

In adults, it is important that replacement doses not be increased too rapidly when there is underlying arteriosclerosis or myocardial disease. In such patients, the capacity of the heart to handle the increased metabolic demands of the body may be exceeded. If cardiovascular symptoms (tachycardia, atrial fibrillation, pain) appear, the dose must be reduced. However, it should be emphasized that the myocardium performs most efficiently in a euthyroid state. Therefore, full replacement should be the goal, although it should be attained slowly and with caution. On the other hand, for patients with myxedema coma or severe myxedema with bowel obstruction, it may be lifesaving to accept the hazards associated with rapid replacement. In younger patients, the dose may be increased to the full replacement amount more rapidly without undue risk.

Hypothyroidism and adrenal insufficiency may coexist, as in pituitary insufficiency or concomitant primary thyroid and adrenal failure (Schmidt's syndrome). If a medical emergency exists and there is reason to suspect hypoadrenalism, adequate amounts of hydrocortisone should be given with thyroid replacement therapy because thyroid hormones increase the metabolic turnover and degradation of adrenocortical hormones and may precipitate acute adrenocortical insufficiency. Otherwise, the function of the pituitary-adrenal axis should be assessed before therapy is begun (see index entry Adrenal Corticosteroids).

TSH-suppressing doses of levothyroxine can result in subclinical hyperthyroidism, with shortened systolic time intervals, elevations in liver enzymes, and accelerated pre- and postmenopausal bone loss (Lakatos et al, 1987; Ross, 1988; Diamond et al, 1990; Stall et al, 1990; Greenspan et al, 1991; Lehmke et al, 1992; Mudde et al, 1992). Doses that result in very low or undetectable serum TSH concentrations in women increase several indicators of the rate of bone resorption: serum osteocalcin concentration (Ribot et al, 1990; Ross, 1991), urinary hydroxyproline excretion (Krakauer and Kleerekoper, 1992), and urinary pyridinoline and deoxypyridinoline excretion (Harvey et al, 1991). These observations have raised concern that treatment with levothyroxine may accelerate the development of osteoporosis and increase the risk of fracture (Cooper, 1988; Greenspan et al, 1991). Consequently, it has been recommended that the doses of levothyroxine used to treat hypothyroidism and benign thyroid disease be limited to amounts that will reduce serum TSH concentration to the low-normal range (Baran and Braverman, 1991; Ross, 1991; Burmeister et al, 1992).

Subclinical hyperthyroidism (spontaneous or levothyroxine-induced) is associated with decreased serum total and LDL-cholesterol concentrations (Arem and Patsch, 1990; Parle et al, 1992). Thyroid hormones may increase binding of LDL-cholesterol to hepatocyte receptors (Franklyn and Sheppard, 1990).

DRUG INTERACTIONS. Thyroid hormones enhance the effect of coumarin anticoagulants by increasing catabolism of vitamin K-dependent clotting factors. If levothyroxine and a coumarin anticoagulant are given concomitantly, the dose of the latter may have to be decreased.

Amiodarone inhibits the conversion of T_4 to T_3, inhibits cellular entry and receptor binding of T_3 in peripheral tissues, and may stimulate TSH secretion. Patients taking amiodarone may require increased doses of levothyroxine to normalize serum TSH concentrations (Figge and Dluhy, 1990). The required dosage of thyroid hormones also is increased in patients taking phenytoin, lithium, or carbamazepine (Utiger, 1990).

Children and adults receiving recombinant human growth hormone (somatrem [Protropin], somatropin [Humatrope]) have decreased serum total T_4 concentrations and increased serum total T_3 concentrations. The growth hormone appears to inhibit TSH secretion and stimulate T_4 conversion to T_3 (see Massa et al, 1991). Patients receiving both growth hormone and levothyroxine should be monitored to avoid the induction of thyrotoxicosis.

Cholestyramine [Cholybar, Questran] and colestipol [Colestid] bind orally administered thyroid hormone in the intestine, delaying or preventing absorption of ingested hormone and reabsorption of hormone excreted in bile. Because 50 mg of cholestyramine can bind 3 mg of levothyroxine, this interaction can be exploited in the treatment of iatrogenic hyperthyroidism (Shakir et al, 1993). To prevent this interaction, there should be a four- to five-hour interval between administration of bile acid sequestrants and an oral thyroid drug.

Initiation of thyroid therapy in diabetic patients may increase the requirement for insulin or oral hypoglycemic agents. In digitalized patients, the requirement for digoxin may be increased.

Oral ferrous sulfate forms insoluble complexes with levothyroxine, and the absorption of both agents is reduced (Campbell et al, 1992).

Drug Evaluations

LEVOTHYROXINE SODIUM

[LEVO-T, Levothroid, Levoxine, Synthroid]

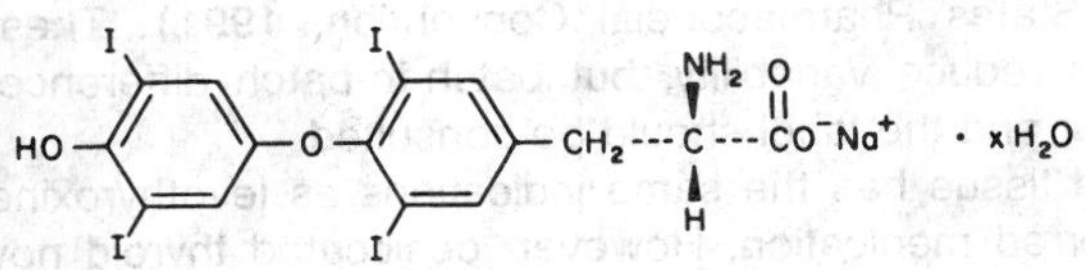

ACTIONS AND USES. *For most indications requiring thyroid replacement, this synthetic sodium salt of the levorotatory isomer of T_4 (thyroxine) is the drug of choice.* It is used most commonly for thyroid hormone replacement therapy in hypothyroidism. In myxedema coma, levothyroxine should be given intravenously with hydrocortisone to forestall adrenal insufficiency (but intravenous liothyronine is preferred). These patients should be treated in the intensive care unit and be monitored with electrocardiography, since this therapy may cause ventricular arrhythmias.

Other uses of levothyroxine include the treatment of simple nonendemic goiter, chronic lymphocytic (Hashimoto's) thyroiditis, thyroid nodules, and differentiated thyroid carcinoma (see the Introduction). It also may prevent the goitrogenic effects of other therapeutic agents (eg, lithium). This agent has not reduced the size of thyroid nodules in a small percentage of affected patients (Edmonds, 1992; Reverter et al, 1992).

ADVERSE REACTIONS. See the Introduction for adverse reactions and precautions with use of levothyroxine. This drug is classified in FDA Pregnancy Category A.

PHARMACOKINETICS. About 80% of an oral dose of levothyroxine is absorbed from the gastrointestinal tract. Its half-life is approximately one week, and a steady-state level is achieved in four to six weeks. Following conjugation in the liver, levothyroxine is excreted in the bile; a portion is released as free hormone and reabsorbed.

DOSAGE AND PREPARATIONS. Levothyroxine usually is administered orally, but the intravenous route is used in myxedema coma or when oral administration is impractical. In general, the intravenous dosage for levothyroxine is about 50% of the oral dosage. Because of small but significant differences in bioavailability and potency, especially with some generic preparations, it is best to use the same brand throughout a patient's treatment.

Oral: *Young and middle-aged adults,* for *mild* hypothyroidism, initially, 100 mcg daily in women and 150 mcg daily in men, increased by 50 mcg or less at four- to six-week intervals until the desired response (normalization of serum TSH concentrations) is maintained. The average maintenance dose is 125 mcg/day in women and 175 mcg/day in men. This dose may need to be increased by up to 50% during pregnancy in hypothyroid women (Mandel et al, 1990; Tamaki et al, 1990). For *severe* hypothyroidism, initially, 50 mcg daily, increased by 25 to 50 mcg at four-week intervals to 100 mcg daily. Further increases by increments of 25 to 50 mcg may be made at four- to six-week intervals until the desired response is maintained. Patients receiving suppressive therapy for thyroid cancer usually require larger doses. *Older adults,* initially, 12.5 to 50 mcg daily for six weeks, increased by 12.5 to 25 mcg every four weeks until the desired response is maintained (usual maintenance dose, 50 to 75 mcg daily). Selected patients with *subclinical* hypothyroidism may be treated with prophylactic doses sufficient to normalize serum TSH concentrations (Kong, 1990).

For otherwise normal *children*, dosage should be carefully adjusted to normalize serum TSH and T_4 concentrations. Common initial dosages are: *premature infants less than 2 kg, infants at risk of cardiac failure, and otherwise normal infants 0 to 2 weeks,* 50 mcg/day until serum total T_4 concentrations are normalized; thereafter, *infants up to 6 months*, 25 mcg/day; *6 to 12 months*, 50 mcg/day; *children 1 to 5 years*, 75 mcg/day; *over 6 years and adolescents*, 100 mcg/day. The dose should be adjusted as necessary to maintain normal serum T_4 and TSH concentrations.

LEVO-T (Lederle), ***Levothroid*** (Forest), ***Generic.*** Tablets 25, 50, 75, 100, 125, 150, 175 (***Levothroid*** only), 200, and 300 mcg.

Levoxine (Daniels), ***Synthroid*** (Boots). Tablets 25, 50, 75, 88, 100, 112, 125, 150, 175, 200, and 300 mcg.

Additional Trademark:

Thysin (Lexis).

Intravenous: For *newborn infants* unable to take oral medication, 50% of the oral dose (see above) is given daily. For myxedema coma, *adults*, 2 to 4 ml of a solution containing 100 mcg/ml infused slowly; 1 to 3 ml may be given on the second day if necessary, then 1 ml/day until oral administration is possible. Hydrocortisone is given concomitantly; 300 mg/day is administered in divided doses, and the amount is decreased gradually over the next four to five days. Hydrocortisone is discontinued when adrenal insufficiency has been excluded from the diagnosis. After the patient's condition has stabilized, levothyroxine is given orally in maintenance doses to prevent recurrence of clinical hypothyroidism. Initial doses should be reduced in patients with heart disease.

Generic. Powder 200 and 500 mcg.

Levothroid (Forest). Powder (lyophilized) 200 and 500 mcg with mannitol 15 mg.

Synthroid (Boots). Powder (lyophilized) 200 and 500 mcg with mannitol 10 mg.

LIOTHYRONINE SODIUM

[Cytomel, Triostat]

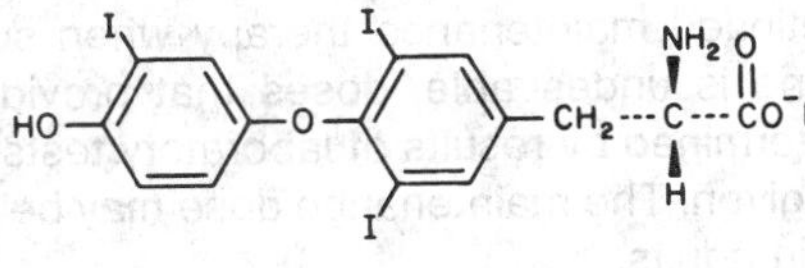

ACTIONS AND USES. This drug is the synthetic sodium salt of the levorotatory isomer of T_3. On a weight basis, liothyronine is about twice as potent as levothyroxine. Its onset and duration of action are short. Monitoring is difficult because blood concentrations fluctuate after each dose. Liothyronine may be preferred to levothyroxine if intestinal absorption of T_4 is impaired and may be necessary in patients resistant to thyroid hormone. Liothyronine also may be used for short-term suppression of thyroid function prior to radioactive iodine scanning or when thyroid therapy must be interrupted periodically, as in patients with thyroid cancer who require ablative radioactive iodine therapy.

Liothyronine alone or with levothyroxine may be given intravenously to treat myxedema coma and precoma (see the Introduction).

ADVERSE REACTIONS. See the Introduction for adverse reactions and precautions. This drug is classified in FDA Pregnancy Category A.

DOSAGE AND PREPARATIONS.

Oral: For the rare individual who is intolerant of levothyroxine and for generalized resistance to thyroid hormones, liothyronine should be given in divided doses two or three times daily. *Young and middle-aged adults,* for mild hypothyroidism, initially, 25 mcg daily increased by 12.5 to 25 mcg at intervals of one to two weeks until the desired response (normalization of serum TSH concentrations) is maintained. For severe hypothyroidism, initially, 5 mcg daily, increased by 5 to 10 mcg at intervals of one to two weeks until a daily dose of 25 mcg is reached; thereafter, this amount is increased by 12.5 to 25 mcg at one- to two-week intervals until the desired response is maintained. The usual maintenance dose is up to 75 mcg/day. *Older adults,* initially, 2.5 to 5 mcg daily for three to six weeks; the amount is then doubled every six weeks until the desired response is maintained.

Generic. Tablets 25 and 50 mcg.

Cytomel (SmithKline Beecham). Tablets 5, 25, and 50 mcg.

Intravenous: For myxedema coma, initial doses in adults range from 10 to 100 mcg. Subsequent doses are determined by the response of the patient.

Triostat (SmithKline Beecham). Solution 10 mcg/ml in 1 ml containers.

LIOTRIX

[Thyrolar]

Liotrix is a mixture of levothyroxine sodium and liothyronine sodium in a ratio of 4:1, respectively. The mixture offers no clinical advantage over administration of levothyroxine and may be disadvantageous (see the Introduction).

This preparation is classified in FDA Pregnancy Category A.

DOSAGE AND PREPARATIONS.

Oral: For continued maintenance therapy when substitution of levothyroxine is undesirable, doses that provide optimal therapy as determined by results of laboratory tests and clinical status are given. The maintenance dose may be greater in children than in adults.

Thyrolar (Forest). Tablets (***Thyrolar-1/4, -1/2, -1, -2,*** and ***-3***) containing, respectively, levothyroxine sodium and liothyronine sodium: 12.5/3.1, 25/6.25, 50/12.5, 100/25, and 150/37.5 mcg.

THYROID, U.S.P.

[Armour Thyroid, S-P-T, Thyrar, Thyroid Strong]

This preparation is the cleaned, dried, powdered thyroid gland of domesticated animals. The U.S.P. standards require that thyroid powder from animal sources contain 38 mcg levothyroxine ±15% and 9 mcg liothyronine ±10% per 65 mg (United States Pharmacopeial Convention, 1991). These standards reduce variability, but batch-to-batch differences may occur and the label should be consulted.

Thyroid tissue has the same indications as levothyroxine, the preferred medication. However, desiccated thyroid now usually is prescribed only for individuals who have been maintained for years on this product, and many of these patients might benefit from a substitution in therapy (see the Introduction). Desiccated thyroid is not recommended for initial therapy in newly diagnosed patients.

This drug is classified in FDA Pregnancy Category A.

DOSAGE AND PREPARATIONS. Desiccated thyroid should be taken on an empty stomach to enhance absorption.

Oral: For continued maintenance therapy, dosages must be individualized. The optimal amount is determined primarily by the clinical response and confirmed by results of laboratory tests (serum TSH concentrations).

Generic. Tablets 15, 30, 60, 120, 180, and 325 mg corresponding to 1/4, 1/2, 1, 2, 3, and 5 grains, respectively; tablets (enteric-coated) 120 and 325 mg, corresponding to 2 and 5 grains, respectively.

Armour Thyroid Tablets (Forest). Tablets (pork extract) 15, 30, 60, 90, 120, 180, 240, and 300 mg, corresponding to 1/4, 1/2, 1, 1 1/2, 2, 3, 4, and 5 grains, respectively.

S-P-T (Fleming). Capsules (liquid, pork extract) 60, 120, 180, and 300 mg, corresponding to 1, 2, 3, and 5 grains, respectively.

Thyrar (Rhone-Poulenc Rorer). Tablets (beef extract) 30, 60, and 120 mg, corresponding to 1/2, 1, and 2 grains, respectively.

Thyroid Strong (Jones). Tablets 30, 60, 120 mg (plain, sugar-coated), and 180 mg (sugar coated), equivalent to 3/4, 1 1/2, 3, and 4 1/2 grains, respectively (50% stronger than Thyroid, U.S.P.).

HYPERTHYROIDISM

Clinical hyperthyroidism (thyrotoxicosis) results from the excessive secretion or ingestion of thyroid hormones and is usually characterized by abnormally high serum concentrations of T_4 and T_3, normal concentrations of TBG, and very low or undetectable concentrations of TSH. Thyrotoxicosis, the development of overt clinical signs associated with hyperthyroidism, is usually caused by Graves' disease (toxic diffuse goiter, autoimmune hyperthyroidism). Other causes include toxic multinodular goiter, thyroiditis, single hyperfunctioning thyroid nodules, exogenous thyroid hormone, metastatic thyroid follicular carcinoma, pituitary hypersecretion of TSH, excess iodide ingestion (Jod-Basedow's syndrome), choriocarcinoma, autonomous struma ovarii, or other rare conditions. Transient thyrotoxicosis of varying severity that resolves spontaneously may occur in some patients after parathyroidectomy, perhaps secondary to intraoperative thyroid gland manipulation (Walfish et al, 1992 B).

In most instances of thyrotoxicosis, thyroidal secretion of T_3 is increased more than that of T_4. In some elderly patients with severe nonthyroidal illness and hypersecretion of T_4, extrathyroidal conversion of T_4 to T_3 may be reduced and serum T_3 concentrations may remain essentially normal, resulting in "T_4 thyrotoxicosis" (Joasoo, 1975). These variations in hyperthyroid function are important only diagnostically; clinical symptoms and effective therapeutic management are similar.

Thyrotoxicosis is characterized by hypermetabolism manifested by effects on temperature regulation (eg, increased heat production with intolerance to heat; warm, moist, flushed skin); cardiovascular effects (eg, rapid, strong heartbeat; in older patients, angina, arrhythmias, heart failure); skeletal muscle weakness and wasting; tremor or choreoathetosis; emotional instability; general overactivity; hypercalcemia, hypercalciuria, increased bone resorption, decreased intestinal absorption of calcium, and osteoporosis; and increased appetite with weight loss if caloric requirements are not met by adequate food intake. The metabolism and clearance of some drugs (eg, propranolol, tolbutamide, theophylline, oxazepam, cortisone, insulin, digoxin, metoprolol, acetaminophen) are increased in those with hyperthyroidism; therefore, larger doses of these drugs may be required in untreated hyperthyroid patients.

Heart disease often complicates hyperthyroidism (Klein and Ojamaa, 1992; Woeber, 1992; Polikar et al, 1993). Atrial arrhythmias are common, and heart failure may occur, especially in the elderly. If congestive heart failure develops, it must be treated conventionally at the same time that control of thyrotoxicosis is initiated. However, higher doses of digitalis preparations are usually needed in these patients until the hyperthyroidism is corrected. Also, in the elderly, hyperthyroidism may exist without the classical signs and often appears as "apathetic" hyperthyroidism in which cardiac abnormalities (eg, heart failure, atrial fibrillation) or cachexia may be the predominant manifestation (Sawin, 1991).

Children with thyrotoxicosis tend to have nontender, diffuse goiter; tachycardia; exophthalmos; and increased pulse pressure (Foley, 1992). Hyperactivity, short attention span, restlessness, and difficulty sleeping adversely affect intellectual performance. Although it has not been studied in children, secretion of growth hormone can increase up to fourfold in those with untreated hyperthyroidism (Iranmanesh et al, 1991).

GRAVES' DISEASE. Evidence suggests that Graves' disease, the most common form of hyperthyroidism, is an autoimmune disorder in which antibodies stimulate the thyroid gland (see the discussion on autoimmune thyroiditis). The Committee on Nomenclature of the American Thyroid Association (1987) has recommended that a single term, *thyroid receptor antibody (TRAb)*, followed by identification of the method of measurement, be used to describe this class of immunoglobulins. However, the *thyroid stimulating antibodies (TSAb)* that bind to the TSH receptor and stimulate cAMP synthesis and thyroid hormone secretion must be distinguished from the *thyroid stimulating blocking antibodies (TSBAb)* that also bind to the TSH receptor but inhibit cAMP synthesis (see the discussion on autoimmune thyroiditis).

TSAb bind to TSH receptors on thyroid follicular cell membranes and stimulate cAMP synthesis, T_4 and T_3 secretion, and glandular hypertrophy (Huber et al, 1991; Laurent et al, 1991). It has been hypothesized that the resulting increases in local concentrations of T_4 and T_3 may further reduce the number and function of suppressor T-lymphocytes and effectively stimulate helper T-lymphocyte activity. Interventions that reduce thyroid hormone secretion may result in disease remission by restoring normal suppression of helper T-lymphocyte activity, thereby decreasing activation of B-lymphocytes and secretion of TSAb. The presence of TSAb in the blood indicates disease activity, and their persistence in high titer after a course of antithyroid therapy may be predictive of relapse. However, the absence of TSAb does not guarantee that relapse will not occur (Volpé, 1991; Ilicki et al, 1992).

Graves' disease is approximately six times more common in women than in men. The disease may develop at any age but most often appears during the third or fourth decade. Stress or other environmental factors (including smoking [Prummel and Wiersinga, 1993]) may precipitate disease expression (Winsa et al, 1991; Ebner et al, 1992). Perhaps because of a genetic interrelationship between autoimmune diseases, other organ-specific autoimmune disorders occur more frequently in patients with Graves' disease, including insulin-dependent diabetes mellitus, pernicious anemia, vitiligo, Addison's disease, myasthenia gravis, idiopathic thrombocytopenic purpura, rheumatoid arthritis, premature menopause, and chronic active hepatitis.

The vast majority of patients with Graves' disease have subclinical ophthalmopathy (Perros and Kendall-Taylor, 1992). Clinical exophthalmos may not be affected when hyperthyroidism is controlled ("malignant exophthalmos") unless therapy is initiated early. It has been suggested that exophthalmos and autoimmune hyperthyroidism are closely related but distinct entities whose clinical appearance is often coincidental (Volpé, 1991; Perros and Kendall-Taylor, 1992). The unpredictability of the ophthalmopathy must be emphasized to the patient. Some patients improve spontaneously, others respond to systemic corticosteroids and immunosuppressive agents alone or in combination, and others require surgical orbital decompression.

Pretibial myxedema is an uncommon manifestation of untreated Graves' disease that may be partially ameliorated by the administration of topical steroids.

TOXIC NODULES (FOLLICULAR ADENOMAS). Toxic thyroid nodules (monoclonal follicular adenomas) arise from autonomous follicular cells that are present from birth and slowly replicate until a sufficient number exist to synthesize and secrete thyroid hormones independent of regulation by TSH (Studer and Ramelli, 1982; Mazzaferri, 1993). The incidence of this disorder increases from late childhood on and is over 50% in the elderly (Hung, 1992; Mazzaferri, 1993). Head and neck irradiation increase the risk of developing thyroid nodules (Mazzaferri, 1993). Single hyperfunctioning nodules are usually benign and may not cause clinical hyperthyroidism for years. Overt signs may be preceded by subclinical thyrotoxicosis (low serum TSH concentrations and increased risk of atrial fibrillation). The diagnosis is often missed because signs and symptoms seen in younger patients (eg, smooth moist skin, nervousness, tachycardia, muscle weakness) occur less frequently or are less severe in older patients. Weight loss occurs in the majority of older hyperthyroid patients, and a compensatory increase in appetite is not common. In contrast, multinodular goiter often is indicative of thyroid carcinoma, particularly in males. Such patients are candidates for surgery.

THYROID STORM. Potentially fatal thyrotoxic crisis may occur in symptomatic hyperthyroid patients spontaneously or following trauma, infection, emotional stress, or inadequate preparation for surgery (Martinelli and Fontana, 1990; Smallridge, 1992). It is manifested by hyperthermia, extreme tachycardia with arrhythmia, profound asthenia, apathy, agitation, delirium, nausea, vomiting, diarrhea, dehydration, high-output heart failure, and, finally, syncope and coma. Without treatment, overall mortality ranges from 10% to 75% (Wartofsky, 1992). Treatment should be started immediately without waiting for laboratory confirmation and includes antithyroid medication, iodine, propranolol or other beta blockers as necessary, hydrocortisone or dexamethasone, and fluids and electrolytes. Ipodate [Oragrafin] also may be given to prevent conversion of T_4 to T_3. Other standard supportive measures (eg, sedation, oxygen, cooling of the patient) should be employed. Although it is almost never required, charcoal hemodialysis may reverse this potentially life-threatening state. Plasmapheresis has been used when conventional therapy has failed.

MATERNAL, FETAL, AND NEONATAL HYPERTHYROIDISM. Serum TBG, free and total T_4, and total T_3 concentrations increase during the first trimester of pregnancy and remain elevated until parturition (Burrow, 1993). In contrast, serum TSH concentrations tend to decrease during the first trimester and slowly increase during the second and third trimesters, but they do not return to preconception levels before parturition. Clinical manifestations of these changes are rare. There is evidence that human chorionic gonadotropin (hCG) acts as a TSH agonist and regulator of thyroid function during the adjustment phase of early pregnancy (Kimura et al, 1993; Lazarus, 1993).

Hyperthyroidism tends to improve during gestation as serum-binding protein concentrations increase and also perhaps as a result of the immunosuppressive nature of pregnancy. However, clinically apparent hyperthyroidism, whether pre-existing or appearing during pregnancy, is associated with morbidity and mortality and can cause growth retardation in utero, premature labor, miscarriage, and stillbirth (Lazarus and Othman, 1991; Mitsuda et al, 1992). Fetal and neonatal thyrotoxicosis can result from placental transfer of TRAb, which will stimulate hyperthyroidism until they are cleared from the infant's circulation in 8 to 12 weeks (Zakarija and McKenzie, 1983; Volpé et al, 1984). Neonatal morbidity (tachycardia, hyperactivity, growth retardation, craniosynostosis) and mortality can be high if treatment is not instituted shortly after birth. Treatment regimens include antithyroid drugs, propranolol, sedatives, and digitalization, as well as appropriate supportive measures. Surgery may be performed in the second trimester if drug therapy is ineffective. Prevention of complications usually can be achieved by treating the pregnant hyperthyroid woman with antithyroid drugs in the lowest doses needed to maintain the fetal heart rate below 160 beats/min. Overtreatment itself poses a danger to the fetus; antithyroid drugs cross the placenta and, in excess, may induce fetal hypothyroidism. Medication can be withdrawn gradually following disease resolution. Radioactive iodine is contraindicated during pregnancy because of the probability of fetal thyroid ablation.

Trophoblastic disease (hydatidiform mole and choriocarcinoma) occur in about one in 2,000 deliveries in the United States, and a small percentage of affected women will develop clinically apparent hyperthyroidism. Symptoms are identical to those of hyperthyroidism from other causes, and cardiac failure or thyroid storm can be fatal. Trophoblastic tumors often secrete hCG in quantities sufficient to directly stimulate the thyroid. Men with hCG-secreting germ cell tumors also can develop hyperthyroidism. Temporary antithyroid treatment (see above) is appropriate when clinical symptoms are apparent.

RESISTANCE TO THYROID HORMONES. Elevated serum concentrations of free T_4, free T_3, rT_3, and TSH can be caused by thyroid hormone receptor deficiencies or defects (Refetoff's syndrome) (Franklyn, 1991; McDermott and Ridgway, 1993). Patients with generalized resistance to thyroid hormones also have normal TSH secretory response to TRH, but negative feedback inhibition of TSH secretion by thyroid hormones is impaired. Although peripheral tissues are less responsive to thyroid hormones, the increased availability of thyroid hormones partially compensates and the usual symptoms of hypothyroidism frequently are absent. The condition should be suspected in any patient with elevated FT_4 I and free T_4 concentrations but normal or elevated TSH concentrations. Indiscriminate measures to reduce elevated thyroid hormone concentrations in resistant patients should be avoided. Some clinicians advocate administering large doses of liothyronine to children with this syndrome in order to flood tissue receptors and prevent irreversible complications produced by hypothyroidism (Refetoff et al, 1983; Franklyn, 1991).

Rarely, patients become hyperthyroid because of selective pituitary resistance to thyroid hormones (PRTH); clinical signs of systemic hyperthyroidism and elevated TSH concentrations are evident (McDermott and Ridgway, 1993). Treatment is problematic; carefully monitored administration of antithyroid drugs may alleviate thyrotoxic symptoms (Franklyn, 1991), but their use is not recommended. Dextrothyroxine (2 mg/day) normalized TSH and thyroid hormone secretion in a single patient (Dorey et al, 1990). A T_3 analogue, 3,5,3′-triiodothyroacetic acid [Triac] (2.1 to 4.2 mg/day), suppressed TSH and T_4 secretion in ten patients with PRTH, but its intrinsic stimulation of peripheral metabolic rate appears to offset its beneficial effects on the pituitary (Kunitake et al, 1989). A somatostatin analogue, octreotide [Sandostatin], has not been effective in suppressing TSH secretion in a few patients with PRTH (Beck-Peccoz et al, 1989).

TSH-SECRETING PITUITARY ADENOMA. Hypersecretion of TSH that is independent of elevated serum thyroid hormone concentrations occurs in patients with rare TSH-secreting pituitary macroadenomas (about 1% of all patients with pituitary tumors). Because these adenomas may metastasize (Mixson et al, 1993), the usual treatment is transsphenoidal adenomectomy. Investigational use of octreotide 50 to 500 mcg three times daily for more than two weeks has normalized TSH and T_4 secretion in most patients, and tumor shrinkage is observed in some (Chanson and Warnet, 1992).

Choice of Therapy

The treatment of hyperthyroidism is directed toward reducing the excessive production of thyroid hormones. This can be accomplished with antithyroid drugs, radioactive iodine, or surgery; the latter two procedures are more definitive. Because many of the signs and symptoms of hyperthyroidism reflect increased cellular sensitivity to adrenergic stimulation, beta-adrenergic blocking drugs such as propranolol [Inderal], esmolol [Brevibloc], or atenolol [Tenormin] may be used adjunctively. In addition, cholestyramine binds thyroxine and prevents the reabsorption of thyroxine excreted in bile, which accelerates the clearance of thyroxine from the body (Solomon et al, 1993). Accurate diagnosis is essential before treatment is started. The choice of therapy depends on careful evaluation of each patient and is influenced by the patient's age, sex, cardiovascular status, degree of hyperthyroidism, and history of previous management of the disease. Opinions vary on which therapeutic modality is best (Glinoer et al, 1987).

Antithyroid drugs of the thioamide type (propylthiouracil and methimazole [Tapazole]) are frequently used for the initial treatment of Graves' disease because spontaneous and possibly permanent remission may occur during their use. The rate of remission appears to be less than 30%. These drugs also are used to stabilize severely symptomatic patients prior to surgery or treatment with radioactive iodine.

Because of the lower rate of remission with thioamides, radioactive iodine is the agent of choice of many endocrinologists in nonpregnant hyperthyroid patients, including children and adolescents (Solomon et al, 1990). In addition, the course and outcome of radioactive iodine treatment are more predictable. In juveniles, therapy has been demonstrated to be without radiation-induced adverse effects for at least 25 years and relapse does not occur (Hamburger, 1985). However, response times to radioactive iodine are slower. In most patients, thyroid function is normalized by antithyroid drugs in four to eight weeks and by radioactive iodine in 12 to 18 weeks.

If radioactive iodine use is undesirable and remission has not occurred after two or more years of antithyroid drug treatment, surgery may be elected. Surgery also may be selected for removal of a large disfiguring goiter. Antithyroid drugs and iodine are employed preoperatively because surgical complications are increased in hyperthyroid patients. However, morbidity is unusual when the surgeon is experienced.

The potential for development of hypothyroidism is more likely after radioactive iodine (Franklyn et al, 1991). Hypothyroidism is especially likely to occur within six months after radioactive iodine treatment in patients with recurrent hyperthyroidism previously treated by subtotal thyroidectomy (Vestergaard and Laurberg, 1992). Patients receiving either form of ablative treatment or antithyroid drugs should be monitored periodically for thyroid status, and the necessity for hormone replacement therapy should be anticipated.

Drug Therapy

THIOAMIDE DERIVATIVES. The principal agents used to inhibit the production of thyroid hormones are thioamide derivatives. The drugs used in this country are propylthiouracil (PTU) and methimazole, which have replaced the more toxic parent compound, thiouracil. Both drugs inhibit the incorporation of iodide into thyroglobulin but do not inactivate or interfere with the release of thyroid hormone previously formed and stored in the gland. They also may be mildly immunosuppressive in patients with autoimmune thyroid disease (Weetman et al, 1984; Burman and Baker, 1985; Hashizume et al, 1991), although this effect may be an indirect result of their inhibition of thyroid cell activity and thus of thyrocyte-immunocyte signaling (Volpé et al, 1986). The effects of thioamide derivatives are reversible. These drugs are used primarily to establish control of hyperthyroidism in preparation for surgery or treatment with radioactive iodine, in the long-term suppression of hyperthyroidism in selected adults and children, and in attempts to achieve disease remission.

Of the two drugs, PTU has been more widely used in the United States. In addition to inhibiting thyroid hormone synthesis, PTU decreases the peripheral conversion of T_4 to T_3. These effects decrease the toxicity of excessive secreted T_4. However, with therapeutically equivalent doses, methimazole is more potent in inhibiting thyroidal hormone synthesis and may have a greater effect in restoring normal immune homeostasis; in addition, the incidence of adverse effects (including bitter aftertaste) is lower (Cooper, 1986). Methimazole also has a longer half-life and accumulates rapidly within the thyroid gland, which make once- or twice-daily administration possible in most patients and facilitates control of the disease. However, many apparent treatment failures with both drugs may have resulted from inadequate frequency of administration. If the patient does not respond to a given dose, a shorter interval (eg, four hours) may be tried before increasing the total dose; this may minimize dose-related side effects.

The effects of these drugs are not apparent until the thyroid hormone reserve has been depleted, which may take several weeks. Patients with severe hyperthyroidism dissipate their stores more rapidly and may respond to therapy more quickly than those with mild hyperthyroidism. As the abnormally high metabolic state of clinical hyperthyroidism is corrected, the half-lives of PTU and methimazole may increase, reducing dosage requirements.

In Graves' disease, the goal of long-term antithyroid drug therapy is to inhibit hormone synthesis and secretion until spontaneous remission occurs. This takes six months to two years in responsive patients. Long-term antithyroid drug therapy is frequently necessary in the treatment of adolescents, for whom the time to remission can be much longer. Decrease in the size of the gland during therapy is correlated with the likelihood of remission. Early remission is much less likely in patients with large goiters, in those who experienced relapse after previous remissions, or in patients with persistently high serum TRAb concentrations. When remission is suspected, the patient's response to slow withdrawal of antithyroid drugs can be monitored. Following remission, relapse is less likely if the intake of iodine-containing drugs and dietary substances is minimized (García-Mayor et al, 1992; Roti et al, 1993 B).

To better manipulate thyroid function, thyroid hormones may be administered when antithyroid drugs have produced mild hypothyroidism. In addition, combining levothyroxine (100 mcg/day) with methimazole (10 mg/day) has been reported to normalize the thyroid function of adults with Graves' disease and also to decrease serum concentrations of antibodies to TSH receptors (presumably TSAb) (Hashizume et al, 1991). Combined therapy was associated with increased rates of disease remission and virtually no incidence of relapse during three years following the withdrawal of methimazole. However, it is more difficult to monitor the effectiveness of antithyroid therapy when thyroid hormones are administered. The implications of combined antithyroid-thyroid therapy during pregnancy are more complex.

Use During Pregnancy and Lactation: Treatment of maternal hyperthyroidism is important to reduce the incidence of premature delivery. PTU is preferred to methimazole in hyperthyroid pregnant women because it crosses the placenta less readily and because methimazole has been associated with aplasia cutis in the newborn (Burrow et al, 1978). However, when pregnant women were maintained on 100 to 200 mg of PTU daily, neonatal thyroxine concentrations were reduced and TSH concentrations were elevated (Cheron et al, 1981). These concentrations returned to normal within five days after birth. In most instances, these effects can be minimized by maintaining mild maternal hyperthyroidism by employing lower doses of PTU during pregnancy.

The administration of an antithyroid-thyroid combination during pregnancy was proposed initially on the basis that exogenous thyroid hormone might cross the placenta and retard the effect of PTU on the fetus. It is now known that minimal amounts of thyroid hormones do cross the placenta, but the clinical importance of this is unknown. Therefore, it is considered prudent to use PTU alone in the lowest effective dosage, erring on the side of slight maternal hyperthyroidism if necessary.

In contrast, there is evidence that when women with hyperthyroidism that is well controlled with antithyroid medications become pregnant, substituting levothyroxine (100 mcg/day) for antithyroid drugs during pregnancy and for at least two years postpartum can inhibit the production of TSAb and prevent the recurrence of hyperthyroidism, even without reinstituting antithyroid medication (Hashizume et al, 1992).

Antithyroid drugs usually are not administered to lactating mothers because of possible detrimental effects on the nursing infant. However, one study demonstrated that the concentration of PTU in milk is only 10% of that in maternal serum. The amount ingested by an infant is minimal (ie, 150 mcg daily when PTU 600 mg/day is taken by the mother) and is thought to be clinically insignificant (Kampmann and Hansen, 1981). However, because methimazole is more lipid soluble than PTU, higher concentrations are found in human milk (Cooper, 1984).

Adverse Reactions and Precautions: If the size of the thyroid gland increases during thioamide treatment, dosage reduction may be required. An elevated serum TSH concentration indicates overtreatment.

In general, the adverse reactions produced by antithyroid drugs are similar (see the evaluation on Propylthiouracil) and cross sensitivity sometimes occurs. Side effects, which include fever, rash, and arthralgias, occur in approximately 5% of patients. Some mild reactions (eg, rash) disappear spontaneously with continued treatment. If a severe reaction necessitates withdrawal of one drug, the other may be tried cautiously, although there is an increased risk of recurrence with administration of the related agent. Agranulocytosis and granulocytopenia are the most serious toxic effects but usually are reversible if detected promptly (Cooper, 1984). Because neutropenia and mild granulocytopenia may be produced by Graves' disease itself, the baseline white blood cell status should be determined before antithyroid drug treatment is initiated and periodically during treatment.

Hypersensitivity reactions can develop after one or more weeks of therapy (Gupta et al, 1992). Symptoms gradually resolve with discontinuation of the drug; however, a small percentage of patients will again become hypothyroid weeks to months after recovery from acute hypersensitivity.

ADRENERGIC BLOCKING AGENTS. Beta-blocking agents, such as propranolol, atenolol, and esmolol (or metoprolol for patients with asthma) are widely prescribed for symptomatic relief in hyperthyroidism and are preferred to reserpine and guanethidine [Ismelin], which produce general sympathetic blockade. Beta blockers rapidly control tachycardia and ameliorate nervousness, hyperactivity, sweating, and tremor, and are useful adjuncts to other appropriate therapy for thyroid storm and neonatal and pediatric thyrotoxicosis (Geffner and Hershman, 1992). Beta blockers are given with antithyroid drugs preoperatively to prevent thyroid storm and to patients with limited tolerance for antithyroid drugs. The duration of therapy may be two to three weeks when beta blockers are used with antithyroid drugs or as long as three months when they are used as adjuncts to radioactive iodine therapy. Dosage depends on the patient's thyroid status. The recommended initial dose of propranolol in neonates is 2 mg/kg in six divided doses; children and adolescents should be given 20 to 30 mg in three to five divided doses (Foley, 1992).

Atenolol may be preferable to propranolol because its effects have a longer duration postoperatively, reducing the need for additional intravenous drug administration during recovery. Alternatively, esmolol may be selected because of its short half-life (9 minutes in adults; 4.5 minutes in children) and duration of action (10 to 20 minutes) (Gray, 1988; Wiest et al, 1991), which allow precise titration of dosage and rapid action (Brunette and Rothong, 1991). Esmolol may be the drug of choice when preparing thyrotoxic patients for emergency surgery (Isley et al, 1990; Helfman et al, 1991).

Beta blockers usually are not used alone in the treatment of thyrotoxicosis. However, monotherapy with propranolol can control signs and symptoms of transient hyperthyroidism (eg, painless subacute thyroiditis) and is effective in the preoperative preparation of hyperthyroid patients and for the long-term control of thyrotoxic symptoms. However, this agent does not decrease thyroid hormone secretion or alter goiter or exophthalmos, although the metabolic effects of hyperthyroidism, including accelerated bone loss, are partially corrected (Wang et al, 1992). Spontaneous remission has been observed after use of propranolol as sole treatment for mild Graves' disease (Codaccioni et al, 1988), but the continued high oxygen demand of incompletely controlled hyperthyroidism during therapy combined with propranolol's negative inotropic effect may produce congestive heart failure. Propranolol may increase uterine irritability during pregnancy. The (R)-enantiomer of propranolol may inhibit the conversion of T_4 to T_3 without adversely affecting cardiac and smooth muscle (Stoschitzky et al, 1992).

IODINE. Iodine, once the only substance available for the management of hyperthyroidism, in sufficient quantities inhibits the synthesis and release of thyroid hormones and may inhibit iodide organification by the thyroid follicular cell membrane (the Wolff-Chaikoff effect). Iodine usually is only partially effective, and control often is not sustained as the thyroid reduces the intrathyroidal iodine concentration by decreasing the active uptake of iodide (iodine escape). In addition, iodine should only be given after antithyroid drug therapy has begun in order to decrease the likelihood that iodine will stimulate thyroid hormone synthesis and secretion (the Jod-Basedow effect). Therefore, its use as an antithyroid drug is now limited to special circumstances: to treat potentially fatal thyrotoxic crisis (thyroid storm) or neonatal thyrotoxicosis, preoperatively to decrease the vascularity of the thyroid gland, and prophylactically following a nuclear accident or weapon detonation. Because the irradiated thyroid is more sensitive to iodine, this agent controls hyperthyroidism more quickly when administered one week after radioactive iodine therapy. It should not be given as monotherapy for long-term control of thyrotoxicosis.

Iodine is not recommended during pregnancy because it crosses the placenta and may block the synthesis of thyroid hormones by the fetal thyroid. High dietary intake and other sources of iodine (eg, iodine douches) also should be avoided by pregnant patients.

LITHIUM. The observation that some patients receiving lithium for psychiatric disorders developed hypothyroidism led to the trial of this drug in the treatment of hyperthyroidism. In a limited number of patients, lithium 300 mg four times daily has ameliorated thyrotoxicosis and decreased circulating thyroid hormone concentrations by rapidly inhibiting thyroid hormone secretion (Wartofsky, 1992). However, TSH secretion and thyroid gland size may be increased (Perrild et al, 1990). Lithium also sensitizes the thyroid to radioactive iodine.

ORAL CHOLECYSTOGRAPHIC AGENTS. Ipodate [Oragrafin] and iopanoic acid [Telepaque] suppress thyroid function in euthyroid and hyperthyroid individuals. Ipodate is more potent in this respect and has been used to treat hyperthyroidism and the acute thyrotoxicosis of thyroid storm; 500 mg once daily inhibits thyroid hormone secretion, increases conversion of T_3 to rT_3, inhibits extrathyroidal conversion of T_4 to T_3, and normalizes serum T_3 and T_4 concentrations (Shen et al, 1991). However, ipodate has no effect on TSAb production and the secretion of thyroid hormones often is stimulated by the slow release of iodine resulting from the metabolism of ipodate, leading to a high relapse rate (Wang et al, 1987; Martino et al, 1991). Recurrent hyperthyroidism after use of ipodate often is resistant to treatment with thioamide derivatives (Martino et al, 1991; Roti et al, 1993 C).

POTASSIUM PERCHLORATE. Potassium perchlorate is a competitive inhibitor of the active transport of iodide by thyroid cells. Daily doses of 120 mg to 1 g have been used in the treatment of iodide- and amiodarone-induced hyperthyroidism (Martino et al, 1986 A) and to normalize thyroid function and reduce TSAb activity (Wenzel and Lente, 1984; Martino et al, 1986 B). However, the risk of inducing aplastic anemia limits the usefulness of this agent.

Radioactive Iodine Therapy

Sodium iodide I 131 [Iodotope] is often the agent of choice in the treatment of hyperthyroidism caused by Graves' disease, multinodular goiter, or a single toxic adenoma. Radioactive iodine also is used to treat metastatic thyroid carcinoma. However, this treatment is beneficial only when the lesions have an affinity for iodine (papillary and follicular carcinoma). Radioactive iodine accumulates in thyroid tissue and destroys adjacent follicular cells, but its radiation cannot penetrate surrounding tissues.

Because radioactive iodine is transported across the placenta and can destroy the fetal thyroid permanently, pregnancy should be ruled out before treatment is begun. Women who elect to receive radiation therapy should be advised to avoid pregnancy during the next year, because retreatment may be required during that time.

A radioactive iodine uptake test should be performed prior to therapy to determine the dosage that will ensure adequate thyroidal accumulation of the radioisotope. A single dose is often sufficient when calculated for the individual patient (Franklyn et al, 1991), but repeated administration may be required, especially in patients with large nodular goiters. In multinodular goiter, the initial dose may be considerably larger than that needed in Graves' disease.

The release of thyroid hormones from the thyroid gland occasionally is increased several days after irradiation as follicular tissue degenerates; this may aggravate the thyrotoxic state. Some physicians recommend that elderly patients or those with severe hyperthyroidism, cardiac disease, diabetes mellitus, or pulmonary disease be treated initially with PTU or methimazole. The antithyroid drug usually is discontinued three to seven days before administration of radioactive iodine to avoid interference with isotope uptake. Some physicians resume drug therapy two to ten days after irradiation to hasten the return to euthyroidism (Solomon et al, 1990).

Although clinical improvement following administration of radioactive iodine may require two to three months to become apparent, serum T_4 and T_3 concentrations are reduced by more than 50% within two weeks (MacLeod et al, 1993). Similarly, biochemical indices of the effects of hyperthyroidism, including indices of bone turnover, begin to normalize within one week. Nevertheless, some clinicians recommend that iodine therapy be started seven to ten days after I 131 treatment to control symptoms of hyperthyroidism until the full clinical effects of radiation become apparent.

Ablation of the thyroid with the intention of eliminating further glandular function and growth is often the goal of radioactive iodine therapy in adults. Even when residual thyroid function is desired, hypothyroidism often develops after radioactive iodine therapy for hyperthyroidism. Reducing the dose of radioisotope decreases the incidence but does not avoid this complication completely. Thyroid insufficiency may become evident years after therapy; 50% to 80% of adults treated with radioactive iodine develop hypothyroidism within 15 years. The need for replacement therapy should be anticipated, and it may be initiated prophylactically if there is a problem in ready access to follow-up care. The possibility that thyroid failure is the natural progression of Graves' disease in some patients may account for some cases of hypothyroidism. Hypothyroidism is seen occasionally after radioactive iodine therapy for toxic nodular goiter in patients with coexisting autoimmune thyroiditis; long-term follow-up is necessary to identify these patients.

Conversely, residual TSH-independent thyroid tissue may survive radioisotope therapy. If such patients are treated with routine doses of replacement hormones, the persistence of non-TSH mediated thyroid function may paradoxically result in hyperthyroidism. Dosages for thyroid hormone replacement therapy after radioisotope therapy should be titrated to achieve normal serum TSH concentrations in order to avoid iatrogenic thyrotoxicosis (Bearcroft et al, 1991).

The goal of I 131 treatment in children is to destroy all thyroid tissue in order to reduce the danger of malignancy later in life. Following ablative doses, life-long thyroid hormone replacement therapy will be necessary.

Radioactive iodine therapy is associated with the onset or exacerbation of exophthalmos in some patients (Tallstedt et al, 1992). I 131 may damage suppressor T-lymphocytes within the thyroid, allowing increased production of thyroid autoantibodies. The relationship between thyroid physiology and exophthalmos remains controversial.

Surgery

Surgery may be performed on a small percentage of patients with large goiters or after relapse of previously treated disease. Preparation for surgery should include administration of PTU or methimazole to induce euthyroidism. A beta-blocking agent also may be given to reduce symptoms. About ten days before surgery, strong iodine solution, U.S.P. (Lugol's solution), potassium iodide, or sodium iodide should be added to the regimen to promote involution and decrease vascularity of the thyroid gland, thus reducing the tendency toward excessive bleeding during surgery.

Subtotal thyroidectomy controls hyperthyroidism in most patients. The principal drawbacks to surgery are cost, operative morbidity, complications (eg, permanent hypothyroidism, hypoparathyroidism, recurrent laryngeal nerve damage with vocal cord paralysis and altered voice quality), and the propensity for recurrence of hyperthyroidism (incidence, 5% to 20%). If there is a recurrence, radioactive iodine therapy or an antithyroid drug is employed because the incidence of complications increases with subsequent surgeries.

Drug Evaluations

PROPYLTHIOURACIL (PTU)

$CH_3CH_2CH_2$ — [structure: pyrimidine ring with H–N, =S, NH, =O]

ACTIONS AND USES. Propylthiouracil is used to manage hyperthyroidism, to prepare hyperthyroid patients for thyroidectomy, and to treat thyrotoxic crisis. It also may be given before or after radioactive iodine (see also the section on Radioactive Iodine Therapy). PTU has a serum half-life of one to two hours and a duration of action of up to 36 hours (Cooper, 1984).

PTU inhibits the synthesis of thyroid hormones by preventing the iodination of tyrosine residues in thyroglobulin. Because it also inhibits the conversion of T_4 to T_3, PTU may be preferred to methimazole in elderly patients, in those with cardiac disease, and in thyrotoxic crisis.

PTU probably crosses the placenta less readily than methimazole and thus also is preferred for pregnant women. However, both drugs are classified in FDA Pregnancy Category D. The concentration of PTU in human milk is low, and a lactating mother may safely breast feed, although it is recommended that PTU ingestion be timed to allow at least three hours before the next nursing session (Momotani et al, 1989) and that the infant's thyroid status be closely monitored. Some clinicians advise women not to breast feed while taking PTU.

ADVERSE REACTIONS AND PRECAUTIONS. Granulocytopenia and agranulocytosis occur rarely and are the most serious adverse reactions of PTU. These effects require immediate cessation of therapy and institution of supportive measures. Most cases are observed during the first two months of treatment, and the incidence gradually declines thereafter. Because neutropenia may be caused by Graves' disease itself, baseline white blood cell status should be determined before an antithyroid drug is administered. Periodic white blood cell counts can assist in the detection of early asymptomatic agranulocytosis (Tajiri et al, 1990) but should not be the sole measure relied on to detect agranulocytosis because of the rapidity with which this complication can develop (Cooper, 1984). Patients should be instructed to report sore throat or fever immediately, for these symptoms may signal the development of agranulocytosis. Milder leukopenias develop when doses exceeding 400 mg/day are used, but discontinuing therapy or reducing the dose is not necessary if blood cell counts are performed periodically and the leukopenia does not become severe.

A lupus erythematosus-like polyserositis syndrome occurs rarely and requires discontinuation of antithyroid drug treatment. Transient asymptomatic increases in serum alanine aminotransferase activities may occur in patients given PTU, but therapy may be continued in the absence of hyperbilirubinemia (Liaw et al, 1993). Toxic hepatitis, which may be fatal, appears to occur only with PTU, whereas cholestatic jaundice is more common with methimazole (Cooper, 1984).

Pruritus is common and may be caused by the drug or by the disease. Rash, usually urticarial or papular, is observed in approximately 3% of patients; it can be severe but usually is mild. Patients occasionally experience nausea, abdominal discomfort, arthralgia, headache, dizziness, paresthesia, and drowsiness. Temporary loss of taste may occur.

DOSAGE AND PREPARATIONS. The plasma half-life of PTU is only about 1.5 hours, but the drug is concentrated within the thyroid gland and has a duration of action of up to 36 hours. Nevertheless, frequent administration is necessary, especially initially, to achieve maximal clinical effectiveness. When large doses are required, a dosing interval of four to six hours may provide more constant suppression of thyroid activity.

Oral: For hyperthyroidism, *adults,* initially, 300 to 600 mg daily in divided doses every six to eight hours. These doses are given until the patient becomes euthyroid. For maintenance thereafter, 100 to 300 mg is given daily in two or three divided doses. *Children 10 years and over,* initially, 150 to 300 mg daily in divided doses every six to eight hours. The usual maintenance dose is 100 to 300 mg daily divided into two doses at 12-hour intervals. *Children 6 to 10 years,* initially, 50 to 150 mg daily in divided doses every six to eight hours; *under 6 years*, initially, 120 to 175 mg/M^2 daily in divided doses every eight hours. Routine evaluation of therapy is advised, with adjustment of dosage as required.

For neonatal thyrotoxicosis, 10 mg/kg daily in divided doses.

For preoperative preparation of the thyroidectomy patient, the drug is given to *adults and children* in the same doses used for hyperthyroidism until the patient becomes euthyroid. Patients with Graves' disease also are given iodine for ten days before surgery (see the evaluation on the iodine salts).

For thyrotoxic crisis, *adults,* 1.2 to 1.5 g daily in divided doses (Wartofsky, 1992); the tablets can be taken orally or crushed and delivered by nasogastric tube. Alternatively, 400 mg can be dissolved in 60 ml of mineral oil and administered rectally (Walter and Bartle, 1990). The initial dose is followed in one hour by administration of iodine (see the evaluation on the iodine salts).

Generic. Tablets 50 mg.

METHIMAZOLE

[Tapazole]

Methimazole has the same actions and indications as PTU (see the section on Hyperthyroidism in the Introduction and the evaluation on Propylthiouracil) but is approximately ten times more potent. The onset of action, degree of response, and incidence of adverse reactions depend on dosage. The plasma half-life of methimazole (three to nine hours) is longer than that of PTU. However, methimazole does not have any effect on peripheral thyroid hormone conversion, and therefore PTU may be preferred for treatment of thyrotoxic crisis. Effective treatment of hyperthyroidism sometimes can be achieved with less frequent administration of methimazole, and a single daily dose may be adequate for initial and maintenance therapy in some patients. Treatment for 18 months has been more effective in promoting stable remission than shorter term therapy (Allannic et al, 1990).

In general, adverse reactions to methimazole are similar to those caused by PTU. Cross sensitivity to PTU may occur in susceptible patients.

Methimazole increases the clearance of prednisolone, and patients receiving glucocorticoids for exophthalmos may require larger doses of steroids when methimazole is given (Legler, 1988).

This drug is classified in FDA Pregnancy Category D.

DOSAGE AND PREPARATIONS.

Oral: *Adults,* initially, 15 to 60 mg daily in divided doses every six to eight hours until the patient becomes euthyroid. A single dose of 10 or 15 mg may be adequate for some (Okamura et al, 1987; Messina et al, 1992), and most patients can be given 30 mg once daily. For maintenance, 5 to 20 mg daily in one to three doses. *Children 6 to 10 years,* initially, 0.4 mg/kg daily in divided doses every six to eight hours; *under 6 years,* 12 to 17.5 mg/M^2 daily in divided doses every eight hours. Routine evaluation of therapy is advised. Dosage is titrated on the basis of serum TSH, T_4, and T_3 concentrations, and the drug is withdrawn after one to two years.

For preoperative preparation of the thyroidectomy patient, the drug is given to *adults and children* in the same doses used for hyperthyroidism until the patient becomes euthyroid. Patients with Graves' disease also are given iodine for ten days before surgery (see the evaluation on the iodine salts).

For thyrotoxic crisis, *adults,* 60 to 120 mg daily in divided doses; the tablets are taken orally or crushed and delivered by nasogastric tube. The initial dose is followed in one hour by administration of iodine (see the evaluation on the iodine salts).

Tapazole (Lilly). Tablets 5 and 10 mg.

POTASSIUM IODIDE

POTASSIUM IODIDE SOLUTION

SODIUM IODIDE

STRONG IODINE SOLUTION (Lugol's Solution)

Iodine is commonly administered as strong iodine solution, U.S.P. (Lugol's solution [5% elemental iodine and 10% potassium iodide]) or potassium iodide solution, U.S.P.; solutions of sodium iodide also are used occasionally. Iodine is given orally with an antithyroid drug to prepare hyperthyroid patients for thyroidectomy or to control hyperthyroidism in the acute period following radioactive iodine therapy and intravenously to treat thyroid storm or neonatal thyrotoxicosis. When used to treat thyrotoxicosis, iodine should be administered with an agent that blocks thyroid hormone synthesis.

If an accident were to occur at a nuclear power reactor, large quantities of radionuclides, including isotopes of radioactive iodine, could be released into the atmosphere. Administration of potassium iodide blocks the accumulation of radioactive iodine by the thyroid gland. The risk of inducing hyperthyroidism associated with short-term use of relatively small doses of potassium iodide in a radiation emergency (projected radiation dose, 25 rem or greater) is judged to be less than that of radioactive iodine-induced thyroid nodules or cancer (Becker, 1987).

ADVERSE REACTIONS AND PRECAUTIONS. The adverse effects of iodine (iodism) usually include the unpleasant (brassy) taste of iodine, burning in the mouth, sore mouth and throat, hypersalivation, painful sialadenitis, acne and other rashes, diarrhea, productive cough, and gynecomastia. In patients with nontoxic nodular goiter, iodide administration may be followed by an increase in serum thyroid hormone concentrations and thyrotoxic symptoms (Jod-Basedow's phenomenon). Conversely, iodide-induced hypothyroidism and goiter may occur in patients who have underlying autoimmune thyroiditis. The use of iodine during pregnancy is not recommended because it is transported across the placenta, and fetal goiter and hypothyroidism may result (FDA Pregnancy Category C).

Acute poisoning is relatively rare but can occur in very sensitive individuals immediately or several hours after administration. Angioedema with swelling of the larynx may lead to dyspnea. Manifestations of serum sickness also may develop.

DOSAGE AND PREPARATIONS.

Oral: *Adults and children,* to prepare hyperthyroid patients for thyroidectomy, a common practice is to administer strong iodine solution, U.S.P. (two to six drops three times daily) or potassium iodide solution, U.S.P. (one or two drops three times daily) for ten days before surgery. For thyroid storm, one hour after antithyroid drugs and as part of the medical emergency treatment, at least two drops of strong iodide solution or 50 to 100 mg of potassium iodide solution, U.S.P., should be administered every 6 to 12 hours. Some clinicians recommend as much as 1 g/day (Wartofsky, 1992).

Individuals likely to receive a projected radioactive iodine dose of 25 rem or greater from radionuclides released into the environment may be given the following amounts of potassium iodide: *adults and children over 1 year*, 130 mg/day; *children under 1 year*, 65 mg/day. This dose is administered for three to ten days.

POTASSIUM IODIDE:
Generic. Tablets 300 mg.
Thyro-Block (Wallace), ***Iostat*** (Anbex). Tablets 130 mg (available only to state and federal agencies).
POTASSIUM IODIDE SOLUTION:
Potassium Iodide (Roxane). Solution 21 mg/drop in 30 ml containers (available only to state and federal agencies).
SODIUM IODIDE:
Generic. Bulk (crystals, granules, powder).
STRONG IODINE SOLUTION:
Generic. Solution containing iodine 5% and potassium iodide 10%. Also marketed under the name Lugol's Solution.

Intravenous: For thyroid storm, 50 to 100 mg of sodium iodide, U.S.P., should be given daily, beginning one hour after initial doses of PTU and propranolol have been administered. Other agents and procedures appropriate for the treatment of thyrotoxicoses are described in the Introduction to this section.

SODIUM IODIDE:
Iodopen (Fujisawa). Solution 118 mcg/ml containing 100 mcg elemental iodide in 10 ml containers.

SODIUM IODIDE I 131
[Iodotope]

ACTIONS AND USES. This radioactive isotope of iodine accumulates in the thyroid gland where its ionizing beta radiation destroys the functional and regenerative capacities of thyroid cells within weeks. It also emits gamma radiation, which contributes relatively little to biological activity but can easily be detected externally to provide an accurate dosage and uptake measurement.

Radioactive iodine is the preferred therapy in the treatment of hyperthyroidism and carcinoma of the thyroid when uptake of the nuclide is sufficient (see also the discussion on Radioactive Iodine Therapy in the Introduction to Hyperthyroidism). Antithyroid drugs should be discontinued three to seven days before administration of radioactive iodine to avoid interfering with the uptake of radioactive iodine by thyroid tissue. Tracer amounts also are used to evaluate thyroid pathology. These diagnostic procedures are believed to be virtually without hazard if test doses are small (eg, infants and small children, 1 microcurie; adults, less than 10 microcuries). However, I 123 has generally replaced I 131 for imaging and dosage estimation procedures because even lower doses of radiation can be used.

ADVERSE REACTIONS AND PRECAUTIONS. Ablative treatment with radioactive iodine following appropriate pretreatment with antithyroid drugs results in few adverse effects. Without effective pretreatment, radioactive iodine can induce transient but potentially serious thyrotoxic reactions during the first few days or weeks following therapy, including the onset or an increase in the severity of exophthalmos. Other complications (hyperpyrexia, tachycardia, dehydration) are of special significance in patients with severe thyrotoxic heart disease. The area over the thyroid gland may become tender and painful as a result of radiation thyroiditis, but this usually is alleviated by analgesics and prednisone. Large cumulative doses of radioactive iodine may cause dryness of the mouth, bone marrow depression, pulmonary fibrosis, and, very rarely, leukemia (Sisson, 1989).

Permanent hypothyroidism is a common consequence of ablative therapy. The incidence is 10% to 50% in the first year and increases by about 2% each successive year. Follow-up studies of patients 10 years or more after ablation indicate that most will eventually develop hypothyroidism and will require thyroid hormone replacement therapy. Life-long monitoring of thyroid status is required to avoid the deleterious effects of unrecognized hypothyroidism. However, because many patients are difficult to follow indefinitely, some clinicians recommend the use of replacement doses of levothyroxine prior to the advent of hypothyroidism in anticipation of this complication.

If 30 millicuries or more are administered as a single dose, Nuclear Regulatory Commission regulations require hospitalization, and appropriate precautions for care of the patient and disposal of body wastes should be observed.

Before treating papillary and follicular carcinomas of the thyroid with large doses of radioactive iodine (100 to 200 millicuries), the residual thyroid should be suppressed either surgically or by pretreatment with lower doses of the radioactive iodine. If significant residual thyroid tissue is present, large doses of radioactive iodine may cause severe laryngitis with necrosis.

There has been concern that radioactive iodine may be carcinogenic or injurious to gametes and therefore should be withheld from patients during their reproductive years (ages 20 to 40). However, review of large numbers of treated patients after two to three decades of follow-up has revealed no increase in the incidence of malignancy and no evidence of gamete injury in offspring (Brill and Becker, 1986; Balan and Critchley, 1992). The incidence of leukemia also is not increased (Hall et al, 1992). Therefore, many physicians use radioactive iodine therapy to treat children and adolescents.

Sodium iodide I 131 crosses the placenta and appears in maternal milk; therefore, it is contraindicated during pregnancy and nursing (FDA Pregnancy Category X).

DOSAGE AND PREPARATIONS.

Oral: For selected patients with Graves' disease and other types of hyperthyroidism, typical therapeutic doses (4 to 10 millicuries) result in the retention of 50 to 160 microcuries/g of gland at 24 hours. If initial treatment is not successful, retreatment after three to four months is usually recommended. Larger doses are required for patients with toxic nodular goiter and for those with high serum concentrations of TRAb.

For thyroid carcinoma, 29.9 millicuries may be used for the ablation of normal thyroid tissue; 100 to 200 millicuries is the usual subsequent therapeutic dose for metastases, although larger doses can be safely administered under certain circumstances (Gershengorn and Robbins, 1987).

Generic. Capsules ranging from 0.75 to 100 millicuries; oral solution ranging from 3.5 to 150 millicuries/ml.

Iodotope (Bristol Myers Squibb). Capsules ranging from 8 to 100 millicuries; oral solution 7.05 millicuries/ml.

DIAGNOSTIC THYROID PREPARATIONS

PROTIRELIN (TRH)

[Relefact TRH, Thypinone]

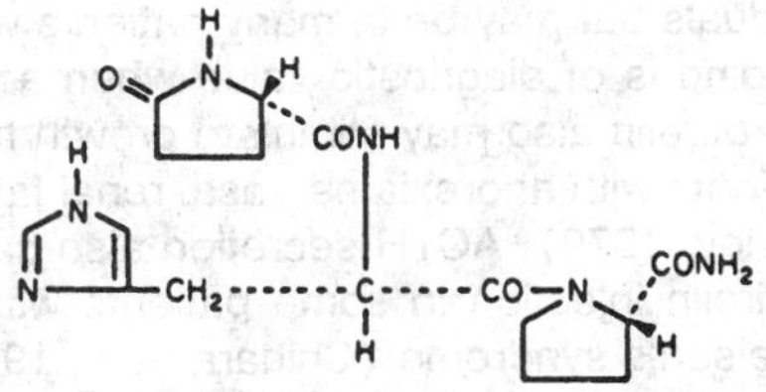

Synthetic thyrotropin-releasing hormone (TRH) (pyroglutamyl-histidyl-proline amide) was the first hypothalamic-releasing hormone to become commercially available in the United States. After intravenous injection, protirelin has a plasma half-life of about five minutes.

ACTIONS AND USES. Protirelin stimulates the release of TSH from the pituitary; measurements of the rate of TSH secretion in response to protirelin can be used to estimate pituitary and, indirectly, hypothalamic and thyroid function. However, use of highly sensitive TSH assays has largely replaced use of the TRH response test.

When pituitary or hypothalamic function is to be tested with protirelin, patients should discontinue taking liothyronine (T_3) at least three weeks before and levothyroxine (T_4) at least six weeks before undergoing diagnostic testing. A normal TSH response to protirelin stimulation will exclude thyrotoxicosis, and a negative response indicates thyrotoxicosis or central hypopituitarism. However, some patients with multinodular goiters or other conditions (eg, renal or liver failure, severe illness, malnutrition, alcoholism, Cushing's syndrome, acromegaly, mania, borderline personality disorder), the elderly, or those taking corticosteroids, dopamine, levodopa, octreotide, growth hormone, calcitonin, aspirin, cocaine, or verapamil may have a suppressed response to protirelin even though they are clinically euthyroid. Suppressed responses also occur in some patients with major depression, and protirelin challenge is employed as an adjunct to clinical observation in the diagnosis of depression. In contrast, adults receiving estrogens, dopamine antagonists, or cimetidine and children with growth hormone deficiency may have an exaggerated response to protirelin (Burrow, 1990).

Protirelin is useful in distinguishing thyrotoxicosis due to TSH-producing tumors (no TSH response to protirelin) from pituitary resistance to thyroid hormone (normal or exaggerated response). Protirelin also may be used to diagnose generalized resistance to thyroid hormone, in which serum concentrations of T_4 and T_3 are elevated but there are no clinical features of hyperthyroidism (patients may appear clinically hypothyroid [Refetoff's syndrome]). Serum TSH concentrations and the TSH response to protirelin are normal or elevated in those with this condition.

Protirelin is a potent stimulator of prolactin secretion by the anterior pituitary gland, especially in women. A prolactin response to protirelin in the absence of a TSH response in hypothyroid patients suggests isolated TSH deficiency; failure of either TSH or prolactin to respond to protirelin is indicative of generalized pituitary insufficiency. The prolactin response to protirelin also is inhibited by high concentrations of thyroid hormones or glucocorticoids and in prolactinomas.

Growth hormone secretion is not stimulated by protirelin in normal individuals but may be in many patients with acromegaly. This finding is of diagnostic value when acromegaly is suspected. Protirelin also may stimulate growth hormone secretion in patients with anorexia nervosa, renal failure, or liver disease (Morley, 1979). ACTH secretion also can be stimulated by protirelin injection in some patients with Cushing's disease or Nelson's syndrome (Chihara et al, 1977).

Because of the wide distribution of TRH in the central nervous system and peripheral tissues, protirelin is being investigated for a variety of uses. Protirelin was reported to reverse hypotension in endotoxic, hemorrhagic, and anaphylactic shock and to aid in neurologic recovery after spinal trauma in animals (Holaday and Bernton, 1984). In one study, protirelin briefly improved motor function of patients with amyotrophic lateral sclerosis (Engel et al, 1983).

ADVERSE REACTIONS. The intravenous injection of protirelin is usually followed by a metallic taste in the mouth, nausea, and flushing. An urge to urinate has been reported in both sexes and, in some women, a vaginal sensation similar to mild sexual arousal may occur. These effects develop almost immediately after injection and last up to several minutes.

Alterations in blood pressure (usually increased) may occur immediately after protirelin administration, and elderly patients or those with hypertension or other cardiovascular disorders should be monitored carefully. Severe hypotensive episodes may be avoided by placing the patient in a supine position during testing.

The safety of protirelin in pregnant women is unknown, and use of this agent during pregnancy should be avoided. In lactating women, breast enlargement and leakage may occur for several days.

DOSAGE AND PREPARATIONS.

Intravenous: For diagnostic testing, a bolus injection of 250 or 500 mcg is administered over 10 to 15 seconds (Burrow, 1990). For *children 6 years and older*, 7 mcg/kg (maximum, 500 mcg) is given. Because thyroid hormones suppress the response to TRH, thyroid replacement therapy must be discontinued three to six weeks before administration unless the purpose of the test is assessment of replacement or suppressive therapy.

Relefact TRH (Hoechst-Roussel), ***Thypinone*** (Abbott). Solution (sterile) 500 mcg/ml in 1 ml containers.

THYROTROPIN (TSH)

[Thytropar]

ACTIONS AND USES. Two forms of thyrotropin (TSH) are produced commercially: Thytropar (isolated from bovine anterior pituitary glands) and Thyrogen (an investigational preparation of recombinant human TSH). TSH stimulates thyroidal iodine uptake, the formation and secretion of thyroid hormones, and growth of the thyroid gland. It may be used to stimulate radioiodine uptake and demonstrate the presence of differentiated thyroid carcinoma or metastases in thyroid carcinoma and to reveal the presence of normal thyroid tissue (using a scan) in patients with toxic nodular or toxic adenomatous goiters. However, the latter use of TSH is now considered obsolete.

This hormone once was used to differentiate primary from secondary hypothyroidism but, because of adverse reactions and the availability of sensitive TSH assays, it is *not* used for this purpose today. Thyrotropin also is inappropriate in the treatment of either secondary or tertiary hypothyroidism.

ADVERSE REACTIONS AND PRECAUTIONS. Thyrotropin can induce hyperthyroidism, especially after repeated injections; thus, it should be used with extreme caution in patients with cardiovascular disease who might not tolerate even mild thyrotoxicosis (eg, those with congestive heart failure or coronary artery disease with or without angina). Thyrotropin also must be administered cautiously to patients with primary (adrenal) or secondary (pituitary) adrenocortical insufficiency because of the danger of precipitating acute adrenocortical crisis. These patients should receive replacement corticosteroid therapy before and during administration of TSH.

Minor untoward effects include nausea, vomiting, headache, and urticaria. Hypotension, arrhythmias, thyroid swelling, and anaphylactic reactions have been reported. Repeated injection can elicit antibody formation with allergic reactions, false elevation of serum TSH concentration, or resistance to subsequent administration of thyrotropin.

To maximize the effect of Thytropar during diagnostic procedures, thyroid hormone replacement may be withdrawn for one to two weeks to allow endogenous TSH secretion to rise and additionally stimulate radioiodine uptake by thyroid tissue or metastases. Withdrawal of Thyrogen is not required.

Thyrotropin is classified in FDA Pregnancy Category C.

DOSAGE AND PREPARATIONS.

Intramuscular, Subcutaneous: To increase the uptake of radioactive iodine, 10 I.U. is given daily for three to five days prior to a tracer or therapeutic dose of I 131.

Thytropar (Rhone-Poulenc Rorer). Powder (sterile, lyophilized) 10 I.U. of thyrotropic activity with diluent.

Cited References

USP Dispensing Information, ed 11. Rockville, Md, United States Pharmacopeial Convention, 1991, vol 3.

Allannic H, et al: Antithyroid drugs and Graves' disease: A prospective randomized evaluation of the efficacy of treatment duration. *J Clin Endocrinol Metab* 70:675-679, 1990.

American Academy of Pediatrics: Newborn screening for congenital hypothyroidism: Recommended guidelines. *Pediatrics* 91:1203-1209, 1993.

Arem R, Patsch W: Lipoprotein and apolipoprotein levels in subclinical hypothyroidism: Effect of levothyroxine therapy. *Arch Intern Med* 150:2097-2100, 1990.

Balan KK, Critchley M: Outcome of pregnancy following treatment of well-differentiated thyroid cancer with ^{131}iodine. *Br J Obstet Gynaecol* 99:1021-1024, 1992.

Baran DT, Braverman LE: Thyroid hormones and bone mass, editorial. *J Clin Endocrinol Metab* 72:1182-1183, 1991.

Bartalena L, et al: Lack of nocturnal serum thyrotropin (TSH) surge in patients with chronic renal failure undergoing regular maintenance hemofiltration: A case of central hypothyroidism. *Clin Nephrol* 34:30-34, 1990.

Bayer MF: Effective laboratory evaluation of thyroid status. *Med Clin North Am* 75:1-26, 1991.

Bearcroft CP, et al: Thyroxine replacement in post-radioiodine hypothyroidism. *Clin Endocrinol* 34:115-118, 1991.

Becker DV: Reactor accidents: Public health strategies and their medical implications. *JAMA* 258:649-654, 1987.

Beck-Peccoz P, et al: Treatment of hyperthyroidism due to inappropriate secretion of thyrotropin with the somatostatin analog SMS 201-995. *J Clin Endocrinol Metab* 68:208-214, 1989.

Benker G, et al: TSH secretion in Cushing's syndrome: Relation to glucocorticoid excess, diabetes, goitre, and the "sick euthyroid syndrome." *Clin Endocrinol* 33:777-786, 1990.

Brill AB, Becker DV: Safety of ^{131}I treatment of hyperthyroidism, in Van Middlesworth L (ed): *The Thyroid Gland: A Practical Clinical Treatise.* Chicago, Year Book Medical Publishers, 1986.

Brunette DD, Rothong C: Emergency department management of thyrotoxic crisis with esmolol. *Am J Emerg Med* 9:232-234, 1991.

Burman KD, Baker JR Jr: Immune mechanisms in Graves' disease. *Endocr Rev* 6:183-232, 1985.

Burmeister LA, et al: Levothyroxine dose requirements for thyrotropin suppression in the treatment of differentiated thyroid cancer. *J Clin Endocrinol Metab* 75:344-350, 1992.

Burrow GN: The hypothalamic-pituitary-thyroid axis, in Burrow GN, et al (eds): *Thyroid Function and Disease.* Philadelphia, WB Saunders, 1990, 41-64.

Burrow GN: Thyroid function and hyperfunction during gestation. *Endocr Rev* 14:194-202, (April) 1993.

Burrow GN, et al: Intellectual development in children whose mothers received propylthiouracil during pregnancy. *Yale J Biol Med* 51:295-296, 1978.

Campbell NRC, et al: Ferrous sulfate reduces thyroxine efficacy in patients with hypothyroidism. *Ann Intern Med* 117:1010-1013, 1992.

Chanson P, Warnet A: Treatment of thyroid-stimulating hormone-secreting adenomas with octreotide. *Metabolism* 41 (suppl 2):62-65, 1992.

Cheron RG, et al: Neonatal thyroid function after propylthiouracil therapy for maternal Graves' disease. *N Engl J Med* 304:525-528, 1981.

Chihara K, et al: Effects of thyrotropin-releasing hormone on sleep and sleep-related growth hormone release in normal subjects. *J Clin Endocrinol Metab* 44:1094-1100, 1977.

Chiovato L, et al: Incidence of antibodies blocking thyrotropin effect *in vitro* in patients with euthyroid or hypothyroid autoimmune thyroiditis. *J Clin Endocrinol Metab* 71:40-45, 1990.

Chiovato L, et al: Evaluation of L-thyroxine replacement therapy in children with congenital hypothyroidism. *J Endocrinol Invest* 14:957-964, 1991.

Christofides ND, et al: One-step, labeled-antibody assay for measuring free thyroxin: I. Assay development and validation. *Clin Chem* 38:11-18, 1992.

Codaccioni JL, et al: Lasting remissions in patients treated for Graves' hyperthyroidism with propranolol alone: A pattern of spontaneous evolution of the disease. *J Clin Endocrinol Metab* 67:656-662, 1988.

Committee on Drugs, American Academy of Pediatrics: Treatment of congenital hypothyroidism. *Pediatrics* 62:413-417, 1978.

Committee on Nomenclature of the American Thyroid Association: Revised nomenclature for tests of thyroid hormones and thyroid-related proteins in serum, letter. *J Clin Endocrinol Metab* 64:1089-1094, 1987.

Constine LS, et al: Hypothalamic-pituitary dysfunction after radiation for brain tumors. *N Engl J Med* 328:87-94, 1993.

Cooper DS: Antithyroid drugs. *N Engl J Med* 311:1353-1362, 1984.

Cooper DS: Which anti-thyroid drug? *Am J Med* 80:1165-1168, 1986.

Cooper DS: Thyroid hormone and the skeleton: A bone of contention, editorial. *JAMA* 259:3175, 1988.

Curran PG, DeGroot LJ: The effect of hepatic enzyme-inducing drugs on thyroid hormones and the thyroid gland. *Endocr Rev* 12:135-150, 1991.

Davidson KM, et al: Successful in utero treatment of fetal goiter and hypothyroidism. *N Engl J Med* 324:543-546, 1991.

de Bruin TWA, et al: Lipoprotein(a) and apolipoprotein B plasma concentrations in hypothyroid, euthyroid, and hyperthyroid subjects. *J Clin Endocrinol Metab* 76:121-126, 1993.

DeGroot LJ, Mayor G: Admission screening by thyroid function tests in an acute general care teaching hospital. *Am J Med* 93:558-564, 1992.

DeGroot LJ, Quintans J: The causes of autoimmune thyroid disease. *Endocr Rev* 10:537-562, 1989.

Diamond T, et al: A therapeutic dilemma: Suppressive doses of thyroxine significantly reduce bone mineral measurements in both premenopausal and postmenopausal women with thyroid carcinoma. *J Clin Endocrinol Metab* 72:1184-1188, 1990.

Dorey F, et al: Thyrotoxicosis due to pituitary resistance to thyroid hormones: Successful control with D thyroxine: A study in three patients. *Clin Endocrinol* 32:221-228, 1990.

Ebner SA, et al: Conjugal Graves disease. *Ann Intern Med* 116:479-481, 1992.

Edmonds C: Treatment of sporadic goitre with thyroxine. *Clin Endocrinol* 36:21-23, 1992.

Education Committee, American Thyroid Association: ATA statement on breast cancer and thyroid hormone therapy. *J Pediatr* 90:683-684, 1977.

Engel WK, et al: Effect on weakness and spasticity in amyotrophic lateral sclerosis of thyrotropin-releasing hormone. *Lancet* 2:73-75, 1983.

Ericsson U-B, Lindgärde F: Effects of cigarette smoking on thyroid function and the prevalence of goitre, thyrotoxicosis and autoimmune thyroiditis. *J Intern Med* 229:67-71, 1991.

Felicetta JV: Thyroid function tests: Interpreting the basic studies. *Consultant* 30-32, (Aug) 1991.

Figge J, Dluhy RG: Amiodarone-induced elevation of thyroid stimulating hormone in patients receiving levothyroxine for primary hypothyroidism. *Ann Intern Med* 113:553-555, 1990.

Finucane P, et al: Thyrotropin response to thyrotropin-releasing hormone in elderly patients with and without acute illness. *Age Ageing* 20:85-89, 1991.

Fisher DA: Euthyroid low thyroxine (T_4) and triiodothyronine (T_3) states in premature and sick neonates. *Pediatr Clin North Am* 37:1297-1312, 1990.

Fisher DA: Management of congenital hypothyroidism. *J Clin Endocrinol Metab* 72:523-529, 1991.

Foley TP Jr: Thyrotoxicosis in childhood. *Pediatr Ann* 21:43-49, 1992.

Fonseca V, et al: Hyperthyroidism and eating disorders. *BMJ* 301:322-323, 1990.

Francis T, Wartofsky L: Common thyroid disorders in the elderly. *Postgrad Med* 92:225-234, (Sept) 1992.

Franklyn JA: Syndromes of thyroid hormone resistance. *Clin Endocrinol* 34:237-245, 1991.

Franklyn JA, Sheppard MC: Thyroxine replacement treatment and osteoporosis: Controversy continues about the optimum dosage. *BMJ* 300:693-694, 1990.

Franklyn JA, et al: Long-term follow-up of treatment of thyrotoxicosis by three different methods. *Clin Endocrinol* 34:74-76, 1991.

García-Mayor RVG, et al: Antithyroid drug and Graves' hyperthyroidism: Significance of treatment duration and TRAb determination on lasting remission. *J Endocrinol Invest* 15:815-820, 1992.

Geffner DL, Hershman JM: β-adrenergic blockade for the treatment of hyperthyroidism. *Am J Med* 93:61-68, 1992.

Gershengorn MC, Robbins J: Thyroid neoplasia, in Green WL (ed): *The Thyroid.* New York, Elsevier, 1987, 293-338.

Gerstein HC: Incidence of postpartum thyroid dysfunction in patients with type I diabetes mellitus. *Ann Intern Med* 118:419-423, 1993.

Gharib H, Goellner JR: Fine-needle aspiration biopsy of the thyroid: An appraisal. *Ann Intern Med* 118:282-289, 1993.

Glinoer D, et al: The management of hyperthyroidism due to Graves' disease in Europe in 1986: Results of an international survey. *Acta Endocrinol* 115 (suppl 285): 1-23, 1987.

Gray RJ: Managing critically ill patients with esmolol: An ultra short-acting β-adrenergic blocker. *Chest* 93:398-403, 1988.

Greenspan SL, et al: Skeletal integrity in premenopausal and postmenopausal women receiving long-term L-thyroxine therapy. *Am J Med* 91:5-14, 1991.

Gruters A: Congenital hypothyroidism. *Pediatr Ann* 21:15-18, 1992.

Gupta A, et al: Drug-induced hypothyroidism: The thyroid as a target organ in hypersensitivity reactions to anticonvulsants and sulfonamides. *Clin Pharmacol Ther* 51:56-67, 1992.

Guttler R, Singer PA: *Pneumocystis carinii* thyroiditis: Report of three cases and review of the literature. *Arch Intern Med* 153:393-396, 1993.

Hall P, et al: Leukaemia incidence after iodine-131 exposure. *Lancet* 340:1-4, 1992.

Hamburger JI: Management of hyperthyroidism in children and adolescents. *J Clin Endocrinol Metab* 60:1019-1024, 1985.

Hara T, et al: The role of thyroid stimulating antibody (TSAb) in the thyroid function of patients with post-partum hypothyroidism. *Clin Endocrinol* 36:69-74, 1992.

Harris B, et al: Association between postpartum thyroid dysfunction and thyroid antibodies and depression. *BMJ* 305:152-156, 1992.

Harvey RD, et al: Measurement of bone collagen degradation in hyperthyroidism and during thyroxine replacement therapy using pyridinium cross-links as specific urinary markers. *J Clin Endocrinol Metab* 72:1189-1194, 1991.

Hashizume K, et al: Administration of thyroxine in treated Graves' disease: Effects on the level of antibodies to thyroid-stimulating hormone receptors and on the risk of recurrence of hyperthyroidism. *N Engl J Med* 324:947-953, 1991.

Hashizume K, et al: Effect of administration of thyroxine on the risk of postpartum recurrence of hyperthyroid Graves' disease. *J Clin Endocrinol Metab* 75:6-10, 1992.

Helfand M, Crapo LM: Testing for suspected thyroid disease, in Sox HC Jr (ed): *Common Diagnostic Tests: Use and Interpretation*, ed 2. Philadelphia, American College of Physicians, 1990, 148-182.

Helfman SM, et al: Which drug prevents tachycardia and hypertension associated with tracheal intubation: Lidocaine, fentanyl, or esmolol? *Anesth Analg* 72:482-486, 1991.

Heyerdahl S, et al: Intellectual development in children with congenital hypothyroidism in relation to recommended thyroxine treatment. *J Pediatr* 118:850-857, 1991.

Holaday JW, Bernton EW: Protirelin (TRH): A potent neuromodulator with therapeutic potential, editorial. *Arch Intern Med* 144:1138-1139, 1984.

Huber GK, et al: Thyrotropin receptor autoantibodies induce human thyroid cell growth and c-*fos* activation. *J Clin Endocrinol Metab* 72:1142-1147, 1991.

Hung W: Nodular thyroid disease and thyroid carcinoma. *Pediatr Ann* 21:50-57, 1992.

Ilicki A, et al: Hyperthyroid Graves' disease without detectable thyrotropin receptor antibodies. *J Clin Endocrinol Metab* 74:1090-1094, 1992.

Ingenbleek Y: Thyroid function in nutritional disorders. *Pediatr Adolesc Endocrinol* 14:345-368, 1985.

Iranmanesh A, et al: Nature of altered growth hormone secretion in hyperthyroidism. *J Clin Endocrinol Metab* 72:108-115, 1991.

Isley WL, et al: Use of esmolol in managing a thyrotoxic patient needing emergency surgery. *Am J Med* 89:122-123, 1990.

James WH: Sex ratio, testosterone and postpartum thyroid dysfunction. *Br J Obstet Gynaecol* 99:698-699, 1992.

Jennings PE, et al: Relevance of increased serum thyroxine concentrations associated with normal serum triiodothyronine values in hypothyroid patients receiving thyroxine: A case for 'tissue thyrotoxicosis.' *BMJ* 289:1645-1647, 1984.

Joasoo A: T_4 thyrotoxicosis with normal or low serum T_3 concentration. *Aust N Z J Med* 5:432-434, 1975.

Kabadi UM: 'Subclinical hypothyroidism': Natural course of the syndrome during a prolonged follow-up study. *Arch Intern Med* 153:957-961, 1993.

Kampmann JP, Hansen JM: Clinical pharmacokinetics of antithyroid drugs. *Clin Pharmacokinet* 6:401-428, 1981.

Kasuga Y, et al: Effects of recombinant human interleukin-2 and tumor necrosis factor-α with or without interferon-γ on human thyroid tissues from patients with Graves' disease and from normal subjects xenografted into nude mice. *J Clin Endocrinol Metab* 72:1296-1301, 1991.

Kimura M, et al: Gestational thyrotoxicosis and hyperemesis gravidarum: Possible role of hCG with higher stimulating activity. *Clin Endocrinol* 38:345-350, 1993.

Klein I, Ojamaa K: Cardiovascular manifestations of endocrine disease. *J Clin Endocrinol Metab* 75:339-342, 1992.

Kong Y-CM: Shared thyroglobulin epitopes in autoimmune thyroiditis, in Bigazzi PE, et al (eds): *Organ-Specific Autoimmunity.* New York, Marcel Dekker, 229-240, 1990.

Krakauer JC, Kleerekoper M: Borderline-low serum thyrotropin level is correlated with increased fasting urinary hydroxyproline excretion. *Arch Intern Med* 152:360-364, 1992.

Kunitake JM, et al: 3,5,3'-Triiodothyroacetic acid therapy for thyroid hormone resistance. *J Clin Endocrinol Metab* 69:461-466, 1989.

Kung AWC, et al: Thyroid functions in patients treated with interleukin-2 and lymphokine-activated killer cells. *Q J Med* 82:33-42, 1992.

LaFranchi S: Thyroiditis and acquired hypothyroidism. *Pediatr Ann* 21:29-39, 1992.

Lakatos P, et al: The effect of thyroid hormone treatment on bone mineral content in patients with hypothyroidism and euthyroid benign adenoma, in Christiansen C, et al (eds): *Osteoporosis 1987.* Copenhagen, Osteopress ApS, 1987, 452-453.

Laurent E, et al: Unlike thyrotropin, thyroid-stimulating antibodies do not activate phospholipase C in human thyroid slices. *J Clin Invest* 87:1634-1642, 1991.

Lazar MA: Thyroid hormone receptors: Multiple forms, multiple possibilities. *Endocr Rev* 14:184-193, (April) 1993.

Lazarus JH: Pregnancy, hCG, thyrotoxicosis and hyperemesis gravidarum, commentary. *Clin Endocrinol* 38:343, 1993.

Lazarus JH, Othman S: Thyroid disease in relation to pregnancy. *Clin Endocrinol* 34:91-98, 1991.

Legler UF: Impairment of prednisolone disposition in patients with Graves' disease taking methimazole. *J Clin Endocrinol Metab* 66:221-223, 1988.

Lehmke J, et al: Determination of bone mineral density by quantitative computed tomography and single photon absorptiometry in subclinical hyperthyroidism: A risk of early osteopaenia in postmenopausal women. *Clin Endocrinol* 36:511-517, 1992.

Liaw Y-F, et al: Hepatic injury during propylthiouracil therapy in patients with hyperthyroidism: A cohort study. *Ann Intern Med* 118:424-428, 1993.

Lim C-F, et al: Drug and fatty acid effects on serum thyroid hormone binding. *J Clin Endocrinol Metab* 67:682-688, 1988.

LoPresti JS, et al: Unique alterations of thyroid hormone indices in the acquired immunodeficiency syndrome (AIDS). *Ann Intern Med* 110:970-975, 1989.

MacKerrow SD, et al: Myxedema-associated cardiogenic shock treated with intravenous triiodothyronine. *Ann Intern Med* 117:1014-1015, 1992.

MacLeod JM, et al: The early effects of radioiodine therapy for hyperthyroidism on biochemical indices of bone turnover. *Clin Endocrinol* 38:49-53, 1993.

Mahoney KM, Wartofsky L: Significance of alterations in thyroid function test results in the critical care setting. *J Intensive Care Med* 7:318-327, 1993.

Mandel SJ, et al: Increased need for thyroxine during pregnancy in women with primary hypothyroidism. *N Engl J Med* 323:91-96, 1990.

Marshall Z, Lippmann S: How do eating disorders affect thyroid function? *Postgrad Med* 82:110-116, (Nov) 1987.

Martinelli AM, Fontana JL: Thyroid storm: Potential perioperative crisis. *AORN J* 52:305-313, 1990.

Martino E, et al: Treatment of amiodarone-associated thyrotoxicosis by simultaneous administration of potassium perchlorate and methimazole. *J Endocrinol Invest* 9:201-207, 1986 A.

Martino E, et al: Short term administration of potassium perchlorate restores euthyroidism in amiodarone iodine-induced hypothyroidism. *J Clin Endocrinol Metab* 63:1233-1236, 1986 B.

Martino E, et al: Therapy of Graves' disease with sodium ipodate is associated with a high recurrence rate of hyperthyroidism. *J Endocrinol Invest* 14:847-851, 1991.

Massa G, et al: Effect of growth hormone therapy on thyroid status of girls with Turner's syndrome. *Clin Endocrinol* 34:205-209, 1991.

Mazzaferri EL: Management of a solitary thyroid nodule. *N Engl J Med* 328:533-559, 1993.

McDermott MT, Ridgway EC: Thyroid hormone resistance syndromes. *Am J Med* 94:424-432, (April) 1993.

Medeiros-Neto G, et al: Defective thyroglobulin synthesis and secretion causing goiter and hypothyroidism. *Endocr Rev* 14:165-183, (April) 1993.

Messina M, et al: Effectiveness of a low fixed dose of methimazole in the initial therapy of hyperthyroidism, independent of the severity of the disease. *Curr Ther Res* 51:792-798, 1992.

Mitsuda N, et al: Risk factors for developmental disorders in infants born to women with Graves disease. *Obstet Gynecol* 80:359-364, 1992.

Mixson AJ, et al: Thyrotropin-secreting pituitary carcinoma. *J Clin Endocrinol Metab* 76:529-533, 1993.

Momotani N, et al: Recovery from foetal hypothyroidism: Evidence for the safety of breast-feeding while taking propylthiouracil. *Clin Endocrinol* 31:591-595, 1989.

Morley JE: Extrahypothalamic thyrotropin releasing hormone (TRH): Its distribution and its functions. *Life Sci* 25:1539-1550, 1979.

Mudde AH, et al: Peripheral bone density in women with untreated multinodular goitre. *Clin Endocrinol* 37:35-39, 1992.

Notsu K, et al: Plasma free triiodothyronine response to thyrotropin-releasing hormone to predict the remission of Graves' disease treated with antithyroid drugs. *J Clin Endocrinol Metab* 73:396-400, 1991.

Ogilvy-Stuart AL, et al: Thyroid function after treatment of brain tumors in children. *J Pediatr* 119:733-737, 1991.

Okamura K, et al: Reevaluation of the effects of methylmercaptoimidazole and propylthiouracil in patients with Graves' hyperthyroidism. *J Clin Endocrinol Metab* 65:719-723, 1987.

Oppenheimer JH, Volpé R: Measurement of thyroid function, in Burrow GN, et al (eds): *Thyroid Function & Disease.* Philadelphia, WB Saunders, 1990, 124-139.

Osterweil D, et al: Cognitive function in non-demented older adults with hypothyroidism. *J Am Geriatr Soc* 40:325-335, 1992.

Parle JV, et al: Circulating lipids and minor abnormalities of thyroid function. *Clin Endocrinol* 37:411-414, 1992.

Pearce CJ: The euthyroid sick syndrome. *Age Aging* 20:157-159, 1991.

Perrild H, et al: Thyroid function and ultrasonically determined thyroid size in patients receiving long-term lithium treatment. *Am J Psychiatry* 147:1518-1521, 1990.

Perros P, Kendall-Taylor P: Pathogenetic mechanisms in thyroid-associated ophthalmopathy. *J Intern Med* 231:205-211, 1992.

Polikar R, et al: The thyroid and the heart. *Circulation* 87:1435-1441, 1993.

Price A, et al: Comparison of methods for the determination of unbound triiodthyronine in pregnancy. *Clin Endocrinol* 37:41-44, 1992.

Prummel MF, Wiersinga WM: Smoking and risk of Grave's disease. *JAMA* 269:479-482, 1993.

Refetoff S, et al: The consequences of inappropriate treatment because of failure to recognize the syndrome of pituitary and peripheral tissue resistance to thyroid hormone. *Metabolism* 32:822-834, 1983.

Reverter JL, et al: Suppressive therapy with levothyroxine for solitary thyroid nodules. *Clin Endocrinol* 36:25-28, 1992.

Ribot C, et al: Bone mineral density and thyroid hormone therapy. *Clin Endocrinol* 33:143-153, 1990.

Romijm JA, Wiersinga WM: Decreased nocturnal surge of thyrotropin in nonthyroidal illness. *J Clin Endocrinol Metab* 70:35-42, 1990.

Ross DS: Subclinical hyperthyroidism: Possible danger of overzealous thyroxine replacement therapy. *Mayo Clin Proc* 63:1223-1229, 1988.

Ross DS: Monitoring L-thyroxine therapy: Lessons from the effects of L-thyroxine on bone density. *Am J Med* 91:1-4, 1991.

Ross DS, et al: Measurement of thyrotropin in clinical and subclinical hyperthyroidism using a new chemiluminescent assay. *J Clin Endocrinol Metab* 69:684-688, 1989.

Roti E, Emerson CH: Postpartum thyroiditis. *J Clin Endocrinol Metab* 74:3-5, 1992.

Roti E, et al: Thyrotoxicosis followed by hypothyroidism in patients treated with amiodarone: A possible consequence of a destructive process in the thyroid. *Arch Intern Med* 153:886-892, 1993 A.

Roti E, et al: Effects of chronic iodine administration on thyroid status in euthyroid subjects previously treated with antithyroid drugs for Graves' hyperthyroidism. *J Clin Endocrinol Metab* 76:928-932, 1993 B.

Roti E, et al: Sodium ipodate and methimazole in the long-term treatment of hyperthyroid Graves' disease. *Metabolism* 42:403-408, 1993 C.

Safran M, Braverman LE: Euthyroid hyperthyroxinemia, in Cohen MP, Foá PP (eds): *Hormone Resistance and Other Endocrine Paradoxes.* New York, Springer-Verlag, 1987, 62-91.

Samuels MH, Ridgway EC: Central hypothyroidism. *Endocrinol Metab Clin North Am* 21:903-919, 1992.

Sawin CT: Thyroid dysfunction in older persons. *Adv Intern Med* 37:223-248, 1991.

Shakir MKM, et al: The use of bile acid sequestrants to lower serum thyroid hormones in iatrogenic hyperthyroidism. *Ann Intern Med* 118:112-113, 1993.

Shapiro S, et al: Use of thyroid supplements in relation to the risk of breast cancer. *JAMA* 244:1685-1687, 1980.

Sheehan CP, Christofides ND: One-step, labeled-antibody assay for measuring free thyroxin: II. Performance in a multicenter trial. *Clin Chem* 38:19-25, 1992.

Shen D-C, et al: Further studies on the long-term treatment of Grave's hyperthyroidism with ipodate: Assessment of a minimal effective dose. *Thyroid* 1:143-146, 1991.

Shigemasa C, et al: Evaluation of thyroid function in patients with isolated adrenocorticotropin deficiency. *Am J Med Sci* 304:279-284, 1992.

Sills IN, et al: Inappropriate suppression of thyrotropin during medical treatment of Graves disease in childhood. *J Pediatr* 121:206-209, 1992.

Sisson JC: Medical treatment of benign and malignant thyroid tumors. *Endocrinol Metab Clin North Am* 18:359-387, 1989.

Smallridge RC: Metabolic and anatomic thyroid emergencies: A review. *Crit Care Med* 20:276-291, 1992.

Solomon B, et al: Current trends in the management of Graves' disease. *J Clin Endocrinol Metab* 70:1518-1524, 1990.

Solomon BL, et al: Adjunctive cholestyramine therapy for thyrotoxicosis. *Clin Endocrinol* 38:39-43, 1993.

Spencer CA, et al: Thyrotropin (TSH)-releasing hormone stimulation test responses employing third and fourth generation TSH assays. *J Clin Endocrinol Metab* 76:494-498, 1993.

Stagnaro-Green A, et al: A prospective study of lymphocyte-initiated immunosuppression in normal pregnancy: Evidence of a T-cell etiology for postpartum thyroid dysfunction. *J Clin Endocrinol Metab* 74:645-653, 1992.

Stall G, et al: Accelerated bone loss in hypothyroid patients overtreated with L-thyroxine. *Ann Intern Med* 113:265-269, 1990.

Stoschitzky K, et al: Racemic (R,S)-propranolol versus half-dosed optically pure (S)-propranolol in humans at steady state: Hemodynamic effects, plasma concentrations, and influence on thyroid hormone levels. *Clin Pharmacol Ther* 51:445-453, 1992.

Stott DJ, et al: Elderly patients with suppressed serum TSH but normal free thyroid hormone levels usually have mild thyroid overactivity and are at increased risk of developing overt hyperthyroidism. *Q J Med* 78:77-84, (Jan) 1991.

Strauss KW: Endocrine complications of the acquired immunodeficiency syndrome. *Arch Intern Med* 151:1441-1444, 1991.

Studer H, Ramelli F: Simple goiter and its variants: Euthyroid and hyperthyroid multinodular goiters. *Endocr Rev* 3:40-61, 1982.

Sundbeck G, et al: Clinical significance of low serum thyrotropin concentration by chemiluminometric assay in 85-year-old women and men. *Arch Intern Med* 151:549-556, 1991.

Surks MI, et al: American Thyroid Association guidelines for use of laboratory tests in thyroid disorders. *JAMA* 263:1529-1532, 1990.

Tajiri J, et al: Antithyroid drug-induced agranulocytosis: The usefulness of routine white blood cell count monitoring. *Arch Intern Med* 150:621-624, 1990.

Takasu N, et al: Test for recovery from hypothyroidism during thyroxine therapy in Hashimoto's thyroiditis. *Lancet* 336:1084-1086, 1990.

Takasu N, et al: Disappearance of thyrotropin-blocking antibodies and spontaneous recovery from hypothyroidism in autoimmune thyroiditis. *N Engl J Med* 326:513-518, 1992.

Tallstedt L, et al: Occurrence of ophthalmopathy after treatment for Graves' hyperthyroidism. *N Engl J Med* 326:1733-1738, 1992.

Tamai H, et al: Follow-up study of thyroid stimulating-blocking antibodies in hypothyroid patients. *Clin Endocrinol* 33:699-707, 1990.

Tamaki H, et al: Thyroxine requirement during pregnancy for replacement therapy of hypothyroidism. *Obstet Gynecol* 76:230-233, 1990.

Utiger RD: Therapy of hypothyroidism: When are changes needed? *N Engl J Med* 323:126-127, 1990.

Vestergaard H, Laurberg P: Radioiodine treatment of recurrent hyperthyroidism in patients previously treated for Graves' disease by subtotal thyroidectomy. *J Intern Med* 231:13-17, 1992.

Volpé R: Autoimmunity causing thyroid dysfunction. *Endocrinol Metab Clin North Am* 20:565-587, 1991.

Volpé R, et al: Graves' disease in pregnancy years after hypothyroidism with recurrent passive-transfer neonatal Graves' disease in offspring. *Am J Med* 77:572-578, 1984.

Volpé R, et al: Evidence that antithyroid drugs induce remissions in Graves' disease by modulating thyroid cellular activity. *Clin Endocrinol* 25:453-462, 1986.

Walfish PG, et al: Prevalence and characteristics of post-partum thyroid dysfunction: Results of a survey from Toronto, Canada. *J Endocrinol Invest* 15:265-272, 1992 A.

Walfish PG, et al: Postparathyroidectomy transient thyrotoxicosis. *J Clin Endocrinol Metab* 75:224-227, 1992 B

Walter RM Jr, Bartle WR: Rectal administration of propylthiouracil in the treatment of Graves' disease. *Am J Med* 88:69-70, 1990.

Wang Y-S, et al: Long term treatment of Graves' disease with iopanoic acid (Telepaque). *J Clin Endocrinol Metab* 65:679-682, 1987.

Wang X, et al: Effect of propranolol on calcium, phosphorus, and magnesium metabolic disorders in Graves' disease. *Metabolism* 41:552-555, 1992.

Wartofsky L: Emergency: Thyrotoxic storm. *Hosp Med* 123-142, (Oct) 1992.

Weetman AP, et al: Evidence for an effect of antithyroid drugs on the natural history of Graves' disease. *Clin Endocrinol* 21:163-172, 1984.

Weetman AP, et al: Thyroid follicular cells produce interleukin-B. *J Clin Endocrinol Metab* 75:328-330, 1992.

Wenzel KW, Lente JR: Similar effects of thionamide drugs and perchlorate on thyroid-stimulating immunoglobulins in Graves' disease: Evidence against an immunosuppressive action of thionamide drugs. *J Clin Endocrinol Metab* 58:62-69, 1984.

Wiest DB, et al: Pharmacokinetics of esmolol in children. *Clin Pharmacol Ther* 49:618-623, 1991.

Winsa B, et al: Stressful life events and Graves' disease. *Lancet* 338:1475-1479, 1991.

Woeber KA: Thyrotoxicosis and the heart. *N Engl J Med* 327:94-98, (July) 1992

Wong TK, et al: Comparison of methods for measuring free thyroxin in nonthyroidal illness. *Clin Chem* 38:720-724, 1992.

Zakarija M, McKenzie JM: Pregnancy-associated changes in the thyroid-stimulating antibody of Graves' disease and the relationship to neonatal hyperthyroidism. *J Clin Endocrinol Metab* 57:1036-1040, 1983.

Agents Used to Regulate Blood Glucose 48

DIABETES MELLITUS

Diabetes mellitus is a chronic disorder with interrelated metabolic and vascular components. A relative or absolute deficiency of insulin secretion and activity is associated with hyperglycemia and altered lipid and protein metabolism. Vascular components consist of accelerated atherosclerosis and microangiopathy primarily affecting the renal and retinal microcirculation. Associated peripheral and autonomic neuropathies are secondary to metabolic abnormalities, especially hyperglycemia, although vascular abnormalities also may be contributory. Subgroups of patients with diabetes have different clinical and genetic characteristics.

Classification

The current classifications and nomenclature for diabetes and other types of glucose intolerance were established by an international workgroup sponsored by the National Diabetes Data Group of the National Institutes of Health (National Diabetes Data Group, 1979). Diabetes mellitus is classified as insulin-dependent diabetes mellitus (IDDM, Type I); non-insulin-dependent diabetes mellitus (NIDDM, Type II); diabetes mellitus associated with other conditions (eg, pancreatic disease, hormonal, drugs), formerly known as secondary diabetes; or gestational diabetes mellitus (GDM, diabetes present only during pregnancy). More recently, the World Health Organization (WHO) has added a fifth subset, malnutrition-related diabetes, which occurs in underdeveloped countries.

IDDM was once termed juvenile onset diabetes (because the age of onset is predominantly before adulthood) or ketosis-prone diabetes. Patients with IDDM require insulin to prevent ketosis and sustain life. NIDDM was previously identified as maturity-onset (MOD), adult-onset (adulthood is the most common time of onset), or ketosis-resistant diabetes. NIDDM is further subdivided into nonobese and obese types. Approximately 60% to 80% of NIDDM patients have the latter type, and the racial or ethnic group of the patient is a significant factor.

Women who experience the *onset* or first recognition of glucose intolerance during pregnancy have GDM. All women should be screened for GDM during pregnancy. Criteria for screening and diagnostic oral glucose tolerance tests have been established (Freinkel, 1985). In those with GDM, the blood glucose must be controlled during pregnancy; insulin is used when dietary management is not successful. The role of exercise during pregnancy is being evaluated, and no firm recommendations are yet available. GDM patients must be rescreened after pregnancy to determine whether glucose intolerance persists.

Patients with glucose values between normal and diabetic are characterized as nondiabetic with impaired glucose tolerance (IGT) and are further subdivided into nonobese, obese, and IGT associated with certain conditions (eg, pancreatic disease, hormonal, drugs). An oral glucose tolerance test is necessary to establish a diagnosis of IGT. Approximately 30% to 50% of patients with IGT will develop diabetes; test results return to normal in approximately 30%. Although atherosclerosis is accelerated in patients with IGT, other complications specific for diabetes (eg, retinopathy, nephropathy) usually do not develop.

Two additional statistical risk categories were established by the National Diabetes Data Group: previous abnormality of glucose tolerance (Prev AGT) and potential abnormality of glucose tolerance (Pot AGT). The former includes patients with normal glucose tolerance who have experienced diabetic hyperglycemia (eg, women with GDM whose glucose tolerance reverted to normal after parturition; formerly obese diabetics whose glucose tolerance became normal after weight loss; patients who were hyperglycemic under stress of infection, myocardial infarction, or surgery). The Pot AGT class includes individuals with no history of glucose intolerance who are at increased risk of developing IDDM (eg, those with islet cell antibodies or autoantibodies to insulin; monozygotic twins, other siblings, or first-degree relatives or offspring of IDDM diabetics) or NIDDM (eg, monozygotic twins or first-degree relatives, mothers of large neonates, members of certain Indian tribes, individuals with acanthosis nigricans). Patients in these risk categories should be monitored for impaired glucose tolerance or frank diabetes mellitus, and the importance of avoiding obesity and being physically active should be stressed.

The diagnostic criteria for diabetes mellitus and related disorders of glucose tolerance are summarized in Table 1. It is emphasized that a glucose tolerance test is not indicated to establish the diagnosis of diabetes mellitus if the fasting plasma glucose repeatedly exceeds 140 mg/dL. In addition, patients with the classic symptoms of uncontrolled diabetes (ie, polyuria, polydipsia) and random blood glucose concentrations >200 mg/dL on repeated determinations have diabetes, and no formal testing is required.

TABLE 1.
CRITERIA FOR THE DIAGNOSIS OF DIABETES MELLITUS[1]

	Plasma Glucose (mg/dL After Oral Glucose Tolerance Test)[2]			
Condition	**Fasting**	**Intervening Sample**	**Two hours**	**Three hours**
Normal				
Adults	<115	<200	<140	
Children	<130	(no criterion for children)		
Impaired glucose tolerance				
Adults	<140	≥200	140-200	
Children	<140	(no criterion for children)	>140	
Diabetes mellitus	≥140	≥200	≥200	
Gestational diabetes mellitus[3]	>105	>190 (one-hour sample)	>165	>145

[1]*Adapted from National Diabetes Data Group: Classification and diagnosis of diabetes mellitus and other categories of glucose intolerance.* Diabetes *28:1039-1057, 1979; American Diabetes Association: Position Statement: Office guide to diagnosis and classification of diabetes mellitus and other categories of glucose intolerance.* Diabetes Care *4:335, 1981; and Moss JM: New diagnostic classification of diabetes mellitus.* Am Fam Physician *23:180, (Feb) 1981 (by permission of the American Academy of Family Physicians).*

[2]*Standard oral glucose load is 75 g in adults, 100 g during pregnancy, and 1.75 g/kg in children. If classic symptoms are not present, at least two specimens on one test must be elevated for diagnosis. The ambulatory patient should receive a high-carbohydrate diet for three days before testing. The test is done in the morning, after a 10- to 16-hour fast. No exercise, smoking, or medication is allowed during testing. The patient should not be experiencing physical or emotional stress or be recovering from recent illness, pregnancy, trauma, or myocardial infarction. For children and nonpregnant adults, blood samples are taken at 0 time (fasting) and at 30-minute intervals for two hours; for pregnant women, blood samples are taken at 0 time (fasting), one, two, and three hours.*

[3]*Two or more of the following values must be equaled or exceeded.*

Etiology and Pathophysiology

IDDM. The presence of islet cell antibodies, autoantibodies against endogenous insulin, and antibodies against a 64K antigen (especially the latter) is common early in IDDM and is predictive of diabetes. The onset of this type of diabetes occasionally follows viral infection. Based on retrospective analysis, it appears that children of IDDM fathers (Warram et al, 1984) and paternal grandparents (McFarland et al, 1988) are at greater risk of developing IDDM than children of IDDM mothers. A strong positive correlation exists between IDDM and the presence of human leukocyte antigens (HLA) DR3 and/or DR4 and DQ genes on the short arm of chromosome 6 (Nepom, 1993). Siblings who are HLA-identical to IDDM patients or share one or more HLA haplotypes have a higher risk of developing the disease. The risk of becoming diabetic by age 25 is 16% if two HLA haplotypes are shared and 9% if one is shared; there is no increased risk if none are shared (Gorsuch et al, 1982; Tarn et al, 1988). When one identical twin has IDDM, the other twin has the disease only 25% to 50% of the time. An additional environmental factor(s) appears to be necessary for expression of IDDM. Ingestion of cow's milk during infancy has been suggested as one such factor. Antibodies to bovine serum albumin (BSA) cross react with a protein on the surface of islet beta cells (Rossini et al, 1993). Newly diagnosed children with IDDM have IgG antibodies to BSA (but not other milk proteins), which disappear within two years. The incidence and concentration of BSA antibodies are lower in normal children (Karjalainen et al, 1992). However, additional evidence is necessary before elimination of cow's milk from the diets of even those children considered at risk for IDDM can be recommended (Maclaren and Atkinson, 1992).

In individuals with IDDM, the islet beta cells are progressively destroyed, production of insulin eventually ceases, and the patient must receive insulin injections to prevent ketoacidosis. These patients usually are lean and may have experienced recent weight loss. Although onset is most common before age 30, IDDM also can occur in the elderly. Onset of symptoms (polyphagia, polydipsia, polyuria) usually is rapid. See also review by Thai and Eisenbarth, 1993.

NIDDM. The inheritance pattern of NIDDM is stronger than that of IDDM (>95% concordance in identical twins); however, the genetic mechanisms are not well understood. NIDDM may occur at an earlier age if parents or other first-degree relatives have diabetes or glucose intolerance (Keen, 1987). Mutations in glucokinase genes have been identified in some families with a high prevalence of maturity-onset diabetes in the young (MODY), an uncommon form of NIDDM. Glucokinase is a critical component in the sensitivity of beta cells to serum glucose concentration; thus, abnormality of the enzyme may be involved in the pathogenesis of some forms of NIDDM (Permutt et al, 1992).

Although treatment with insulin may be necessary to control hyperglycemia, patients with NIDDM are not prone to ketosis. Both dysfunction of beta cell insulin secretion and resistance to insulin are hallmarks of this form of diabetes. Native Americans of the Pima tribe have a high incidence of NIDDM, and children aged 6 to 19 years in this population have higher fasting serum insulin concentrations (indicating insulin resistance) than Caucasian children of similar age (Pettitt et al, 1993).

Hepatic glucose output is elevated in patients with NIDDM; this is reflected by increased fasting blood glucose concentrations. Pulsatile insulin secretion in response to appropriate stimuli is impaired (Kahn and Porte, 1988; Polonsky et al, 1988); later, failure of beta cells to secrete insulin appropriately may be caused by glucotoxicity. Islet cell mass may be decreased. Amyloid deposits are observed frequently in the islet cells, and their role in the pathologic process remains under investigation (Leahy, 1990). Resistance to insulin action occurs at a postreceptor site (Davidson, 1985). Uptake of glucose into skeletal muscle also is decreased and glycogen synthesis is impaired (Shulman et al, 1989). This defect in nonoxidative glucose metabolism in skeletal muscle may be an early abnormality that precedes hyperglycemia or changes in glucose tolerance and can be observed in nondiabetic first-degree relatives of NIDDM patients (Eriksson et al, 1989). Increased hepatic gluconeogenesis also is present in this population of NIDDM relatives (Osei, 1990).

Lipid abnormalities (ie, decreased high-density lipoproteins, elevated triglycerides) together with obesity and hypertension contribute to increased cardiovascular risk. It has been hypothesized that hyperinsulinemia, a manifestation of insulin resistance in both diabetic and nondiabetic subjects, underlies its association with hypertension, obesity, and glucose intolerance (Donahue et al, 1990).

Diet therapy and exercise, alone or in conjunction with oral hypoglycemic agents or insulin, are appropriate to treat NIDDM because they can reduce the severity of insulin resistance.

GDM. This form of diabetes may have phenotypic and genotypic heterogeneity and may include some patients with slowly evolving IDDM (Freinkel et al, 1985) in whom islet cell antibodies are found (McEvoy et al, 1991). There is some evidence that those with GDM are more likely to have diabetic mothers than diabetic fathers (Martin et al, 1985).

MALNUTRITION-RELATED DIABETES. Patients with this form of diabetes are usually between 10 and 40 years old at onset and have marked polyuria, polydipsia, and weight loss. Insulin is usually required to control hyperglycemia, although patients continue to be ketosis-resistant even when insulin is withdrawn. Some individuals experience antecedent abdominal pain radiating to the back, suggesting pancreatitis, and there is evidence of pancreatic destruction, fibrosis, and calcification. However, chronic pancreatitis does not account for the diabetes, since insulin requirements are high; in contrast, patients with diabetes secondary to pancreatitis usually are very sensitive to insulin. Moreover, some patients have no evidence of pancreatitis or pancreatic calcification on x-ray. The role of malnutrition in causing this variant of diabetes is unknown.

Nondrug Management

DIETARY THERAPY. Adherence to an appropriate diet is fundamental in the management of all types of diabetes. A caloric intake that enables achievement and maintenance of desirable body weight consonant with age, sex, height, and build, with reasonable adjustments to fit the individual's living habits and occupation, should be prescribed initially for both symptomatic and asymptomatic patients.

The dietary goals, strategies, and priorities of treatment vary for the different types of diabetes. In those with IDDM and in patients with NIDDM who require insulin, composition and timing of meals and snacks must be planned and relatively constant because of the constraints of the insulin program. Adequate quantities of carbohydrate and protein are needed at each meal to accommodate growth and variable amounts of exercise, particularly in juveniles. In children, three meals a day plus midmorning, midafternoon, and bedtime snacks may facilitate treatment. In adults who are taking insulin, only a bedtime snack usually is required. However, if the patient received intermediate-acting insulin in the morning and there is a long period between the midday and evening meals, a midafternoon snack may be helpful to avoid late afternoon hypoglycemia. In individuals whose diabetes is very closely controlled, hypoglycemia may occur if meals are delayed even 15 to 30 minutes. In overweight patients with NIDDM not treated with insulin, precise timing of meals is unimportant; a more active life-style and caloric restriction to approach desirable body weight are the primary goals.

For adults, American Diabetes Association guidelines recommend distribution of total energy intake as protein 0.8 g/kg of body weight (approximately 15% of total calories; more may be required for the elderly), 55% to 60% as carbohydrates, and less than 30% as fats. Cholesterol should be limited to less than 300 mg per day. Saturated and polyunsaturated fats each should be limited to less than 10% of calories (total of both, 20%); the balance of fat intake should consist of monosaturated fats. Unrefined carbohydrates (eg, those containing more fiber) should be chosen instead of highly refined carbohydrates. These guidelines allow relatively more carbohydrate and less fat than previous diabetic diets (American Diabetes Association, 1987 A). Fiber should include both insoluble and soluble types. Soluble fiber, such as that found in oat bran and dry bean products, has been reported to have a beneficial effect on serum lipids, reducing total cholesterol and LDL (Anderson and Gustafson, 1986). It has been suggested that substitution of monosaturated fats for some dietary carbohydrate may improve the serum lipoprotein profile (increased HDL lipoproteins, decreased triglycerides and VLDL lipoproteins due to decreased carbohydrate intake) in NIDDM patients (Garg, 1991). It also has been suggested that lowering protein intake to approximately 60 g/day may retard the progression of nephropathy and the decline in glomerular filtration rate (Walker et al, 1989).

Previous dietary guidelines stressed avoidance of monosaccharides and disaccharides and preference for complex carbohydrates, such as starch. This was based on the belief that simple sugars were absorbed rapidly and caused postprandial hyperglycemia. However, studies of specific carbohydrate-containing foods have documented numerous exceptions to these rules. Sugars vary in the rapidity with which they affect serum glucose levels: with maltose, the rise is rapid; with sucrose, intermediate; with lactose and fructose, slow. White potatoes, white or whole wheat bread, and corn increase glucose levels markedly, while pasta, legumes, rice, sweet potatoes, and ice cream elevate glucose moderately (Kolata, 1983; American Diabetes Association, 1984). Also, the same carbohydrate source, such as wheat flour, may cause different patterns of glycemic response depending on the type of food in which it is incorporated (Wood and Bierman, 1986). Many of these observations were made when the test food was eaten alone. When eaten as part of a meal, the glycemic effect of specific foods is often blunted. Although further nutritional evaluation of foods consumed at mealtime will be necessary before firm recommendations on specific foods to avoid can be made, considerable evidence is accumulating that avoidance of sucrose by diabetic patients is unnecessary (Bantle et al, 1993). Continuing research may result in further modification of dietary guidelines.

For information on special dietary considerations for diabetic patients with hyperlipidemia, see index entry Lipoproteins, Disorders, Dietary Management.

IMMUNOTHERAPY. Immunosuppressive therapy has been investigated to delay or prevent further islet cell destruction due to immune mechanisms in early IDDM. Temporary remissions have been achieved in some newly diagnosed diabetic patients who were given cyclosporine [Sandimmune] (Stiller et al, 1984); however, these patients eventually relapse when immunosuppressive therapy is withdrawn. Because of the significant risks (eg, kidney damage), this form of therapy cannot be recommended outside of research protocols.

In some studies, treatment with niacinamide, an important metabolic cofactor in the pancreatic islet beta cell, has delayed the development or progression of IDDM, but results have been inconsistent. Niacinamide may impede destruction of the beta cell and stimulate beta cell growth and insulin secretion. Intensive insulin therapy, either in the prediabetic period or at disease onset, also has delayed development of the disease or prolonged beta cell function; however, results are inconsistent and temporary. Insulin is thought to provide "rest" for the beta cells and perhaps protection from immune destruction. See Keller et al, 1993, and reviews by Eisenbarth and Di Mario, 1992, and Skyler and Marks, 1993.

Because the disease process that destroys islet beta cells is not always progressive, diagnostic methods must be developed to identify individuals who would develop IDDM without intervention (Palmer and McCulloch, 1991). If less toxic treatment can be developed and patients identified before significant islet cell destruction occurs, immunotherapy may prevent development of IDDM (Marks and Skyler, 1991; Lernmark at al, 1991). (See also American Diabetes Association, 1990 A.)

TRANSPLANTATION. Research on methods to improve transplantation of pancreatic islet tissue in humans is ongoing. Numerous variations have been performed, from transplanting part or all of a pancreas to transplanting islet cells via injection into various sites. Major obstacles include obtaining an adequate supply of transplantable tissues and graft rejection. Usually, a cadaveric pancreas is used, but part of a pancreas from a living donor also has been employed. Pancreatic exocrine secretions currently are managed by draining secretions into the urinary bladder. At this time, pancreas transplants generally are limited to patients who also require kidney transplants for end-stage renal disease. Although concomitant pancreatic transplantation increases the surgical risk somewhat, a successful pancreas transplant improves quality of life because the need for insulin injections and dietary regimentation is eliminated and hypoglycemic episodes probably are unlikely.

Successful pancreatic transplantation has halted progression of some diabetic complications and improved others. The kidneys of recipients had decreased glomerular mesangial volume compared with control subjects. Effects on retinopathy are less certain, but it appears that stabilization occurs after three years with functioning grafts (Sutherland et al, 1989). In patients with peripheral polyneuropathy, the disorder did not progress and conduction velocity improved slightly after pancreatic transplantation. The degree of improvement may have been limited by previous neural damage (Kennedy et al, 1990). It is probable that successful pancreas transplantation would prevent or delay the long-term complications of diabetes, but more experience is necessary to prove this.

More than 3,000 pancreas transplants have been performed worldwide. Between 1986 and 1990, the average one-year overall patient survival was 89% and functional graft survival was 62%. When bladder drainage was used instead of other duct management techniques and when a kidney was transplanted simultaneously, graft survival rates were higher in North America than Europe (Sutherland, 1991).

Immunosuppressive therapy is a lifelong requirement after pancreas transplantation. Combination immunosuppressive regimens that utilize agents with different mechanisms of action have greater efficacy and lower toxicity. Triple-drug regimens (cyclosporine, azathioprine [Imuran], and prednisone) are commonly used, sometimes with the addition of lymphocyte immune globulin (Cook and Sasaki, 1989).

Transplantation of islet cells by intravenous injection (umbilical vein) instead of a segment or whole pancreas is being investigated in clinical trials. As with pancreas transplantation, islet cells must be protected from immune rejection. One method being studied is to pretreat these cells to prevent rejection. Another approach to islet cell transplantation, which is being investigated in animals, is to first encapsulate the cells in a polymer matrix, which protects them from immunologic destruction and allows secretion of insulin into the system.

See also review by Lacy, 1993.

Research on an implantable artificial pancreas, which would be capable of maintaining glycemic control comparable to that achieved with a normal pancreas, also is in progress. A major problem to overcome is the development of a glucose sensor capable of long-term operation in an implant (Pfeiffer, 1987).

Control of Blood Glucose and Diabetic Complications

The desirability of strict, rather than loose, control of the blood glucose concentration primarily stems from evidence in animals and humans that maintaining near normal levels of blood glucose delays or prevents diabetic complications (Hanssen et al, 1992). Most experts agree that hyperglycemia is a major risk factor in the development of nephropathy, neuropathy, and retinopathy of diabetes. Genetic susceptibility also may play a role in the development of diabetic complications (Raskin and Rosenstock, 1986).

There are well-recognized metabolic differences between IDDM and NIDDM, but the prevalence of microvascular and neuropathic complications is similar for a given duration of disease with one exception: proliferative retinopathy is less prevalent in patients with NIDDM. Lowering the blood glucose level is important in delaying these complications. However, less stringent control may be acceptable in patients who have a tendency toward severe hypoglycemic episodes or in those older than 65 years. Severe hypoglycemia should be avoided in all patients, especially those with autonomic diabetic neuropathy, for symptoms of epinephrine release are absent in these patients (hypoglycemia unawareness).

Observations that support the causal association of hyperglycemia and microvascular and neuronal complications include development of glomerular abnormalities in normal kidneys transplanted into diabetic patients (Maurer et al, 1983); reversal of glomerular pathology in rats and humans after beta cell transplants; and slowing of nerve conduction velocity associated with hyperglycemia that improved after correction of hyperglycemia. During a seven-year observation period, retinopathy developed in more poorly controlled diabetic patients (Howard-Williams et al, 1984).

Retinopathy: Several prospective controlled studies have addressed the issue of progression of microangiopathy with continuous subcutaneous insulin infusion (CSII) versus conventional therapy. Retinopathy worsened in some patients during the first six months of intensive therapy as evidenced by the appearance of more retinal microinfarcts; this is thought to be caused by lowering of the level and possibly the rate of reduction of blood glucose. Although reversal of established retinopathy was not associated with improvement of diabetic control, recent studies suggest that the progression of retinopathy after several years of CSII is less than after less stringent control of blood glucose (Rosenstock et al, 1986). Results of one study of early control and its impact on renal and retinal complications showed that although poor control of blood glucose and duration of disease were associated with increased risk of renal and retinal complications, lack of control was the more important factor associated with renal damage, and duration of disease was more important in producing retinal damage (Chase et al, 1989).

Nephropathy: Nephropathy most commonly develops 10 to 14 years after diagnosis of IDDM. Although results of studies have been inconsistent, it appears that, as with retinopathy, intensive therapy does not alter the course of degeneration once begun (proteinuria in the case of nephropathy) (see references in reviews by Godine, 1988, and Siperstein, 1988). However, microalbuminuria, a predictor of subsequent nephropathy (Mogensen, 1987), is corrected by near euglycemia (Vasquez et al, 1984; Bending et al, 1985; Feldt-Rasmussen et al, 1986; Dahl-Jørgensen et al, 1988).

Neuropathy: Diabetic neuropathy causes demyelination, swelling, and axonal degeneration of peripheral nerves; sympathetic and parasympathetic ganglia also may be affected. A variety of problems may result (eg, sensory loss; increased visceral pain; gastropathy; orthostatic hypotension; anhidrosis; bladder atony; impotence; entrapment neuropathies, such as carpal tunnel syndrome; gustatory sweating). After two years of near normoglycemia, conduction velocity in motor neurons is improved and autonomic function deteriorates less with intensive than conventional insulin therapy (Ward, 1986; Lebovitz, 1987).

One hypothesis suggests that hyperglycemia may cause certain diabetic complications when glucose is diverted to the sorbitol pathway. Intracellular accumulation of sorbitol, which is an intermediate product in the conversion of glucose to fructose, is thought to be responsible for a variety of pathologic manifestations in target tissues. The hyperosmotic effect of sorbitol accumulation in the lens contributes to cellular destruction and eventually cataracts. The elevated sorbitol concentration in neurons caused by the conversion of glucose by aldose reductase may play a role in the pathogenesis of diabetic neuropathy (Brown and Asbury, 1984). Diabetic neuropathy is associated with increased intracellular sorbitol and decreased myo-inositol. Aldolase reductase, the enzyme used to convert glucose to sorbitol, is found in cells of tissues affected by diabetic complications, as well as in other tissues. Aldose reductase inhibitors are being investigated to prevent and treat these complications; beneficial effects have been observed in some studies. It appears that these drugs may be most effective if used early in the disease to prevent complications rather than to treat a well-established problem. Unfortunately, the aldose reductase inhibitors investigated to date cause various adverse reactions (eg, rash, fever, liver toxicity, myalgia, lymphadenopathy, thrombocytopenia, neutropenia), and it is difficult to justify their use for preventive therapy, particularly without clear demonstration of benefit (Kirchain and Rendell, 1990). See also Vinik et al, 1992 and index entry Neuropathy, Diabetic.

Diabetes Control and Complications Trial (DCCT). This large, long-term study should finally eliminate doubts about the beneficial effects of near euglycemia on the microvascular (retinopathy and nephropathy) and neuropathic complications of diabetes. In the DCCT, more than 1,400 IDDM patients were randomly assigned to receive either conventional treatment (ie, one to two insulin injections daily, self-monitoring of blood glucose, quarterly clinic visits, educational materials available) or intensive treatment (ie, maintenance of blood glucose as close to normal as possible by either subcutaneous infusions or three to five injections of insulin daily, self-monitoring of blood glucose, intensive patient education, weekly clinical monitoring). Subjects were followed for an average of seven years. The results showed that regardless of age, sex, or duration of disease, intensive therapy reduced the risk of onset or progression of retinopathy, nephropathy, and neuropathy by approximately 60%. This was apparent even though blood glucose levels averaged 40% above normal (ie, 155 mg/dL; glycated hemoglobin 7.2%). However, intensive therapy had a threefold increased risk of severe hypoglycemic events, greater weight gain, and increased cost of treatment compared with conventional therapy (American Diabetes Association, 1993 A; Diabetes Control and Complications Trial Research Group, 1993).

The results of the DCCT strongly suggest that IDDM patients be treated to achieve the best blood glucose control possible consistent with an acceptable level of risk of adverse events. Intensive therapy is usually appropriate for all willing patients except those with contraindications (eg, very young children or elderly adults, patients with cardiovascular comorbidity or advanced diabetic complications). Although NIDDM patients were not included in the DCCT, close control of blood glucose is probably beneficial in them as well because the mechanisms involved in developing diabetic complications can be expected to be the same as in IDDM.

Macrovascular Complications: A causal association between hyperglycemia and macrovascular complications (ie, myocardial infarction, stroke, peripheral vascular disease) has not been established (University Group Diabetes Program, 1982; American Diabetes Association, 1990 B), but, in epidemiologic studies, hyperglycemia has been associated with an increased prevalence of macrovascular disease. Increased risk of macrovascular complications affects both IDDM and NIDDM patients but appears to be correlated with age and duration of disease only in those with IDDM. The presence of proteinuria is predictive of later development of macrovascular disease (American Diabetes Association, 1989). There is little direct evidence that rigid control of glucose levels will ameliorate the macrovascular complications. However, because poor control of blood glucose is associated with other known or probable risk factors for atherosclerosis (ie, increased total cholesterol, total triglycerides, and LDL in plasma) (Sosenko et al, 1980), achievement of good control seems desirable.

Summary: There is considerable evidence from animal and human studies that hyperglycemia is involved in the pathogenesis of diabetic complications, including nephropathy, retinopathy, and neuropathy. Because there is much evidence to support the causal relationship between hyperglycemia and the severity of microangiopathic complications, it is reasonable to conclude that near normalization of blood glucose levels would prevent and arrest early changes. However, rigid control appears neither to halt progression nor to reverse these complications once they are moderately advanced. One finding of note in several studies, including the DCCT, is the two- to threefold increase in severe hypoglycemic reactions in patients following an intensive compared with a conventional blood glucose control regimen (Godine, 1988).

HYPOGLYCEMIC AGENTS

Choice of Therapy

Patients with IDDM do not respond to oral hypoglycemic agents (OHAs) and require insulin. NIDDM patients taking oral agents or who are controlled adequately by diet and exercise may require insulin if certain complications arise: severely impaired renal or hepatic function, during stress (eg, infection, surgery), when corticosteroid therapy is given concomitantly, and during pregnancy. Insulin also is given to NIDDM patients when the blood glucose concentration is not controlled by maximal doses of OHAs.

Improving insulin action by weight reduction and exercise is the foundation and most important aspect of therapy in obese NIDDM patients. A team approach (patient, physician, nurse, dietitian, person responsible for food preparation) is recommended to achieve and maintain a successful weight control program.

When a hypoglycemic agent is necessary to treat NIDDM, a choice must be made between insulin and an oral sulfonylurea (acetohexamide [Dymelor], chlorpropamide [Diabinese], glipizide [Glucotrol], glyburide [DiaBeta, Micronase, Glynase], tolazamide [Tolinase], tolbutamide [Orinase]). (The only biguanide available in the United States, phenformin, can be obtained only under special circumstances; see the evaluation.)

Drug therapy for NIDDM is often initiated with an OHA when dietary measures have failed (Peters and Davidson, 1990). OHAs are more convenient and easier to administer than insulin. This is particularly important in elderly patients who have poor vision and in whom injection of incorrectly measured doses may cause hypoglycemia. These agents also are sometimes used in the rare NIDDM patient who is allergic to insulin and unwilling or unable to undergo desensitization. However, primary and secondary (after initial control) failures occur routinely with OHAs.

While some physicians prefer insulin if a hypoglycemic agent is needed, most prescribe insulin only when dietary and OHA therapy fail or for certain types of patients (eg, under 40 years, lean). Insulin is sometimes given for initial control if blood glucose levels are very high. Although large doses of OHAs are usually effective in these patients (Davidson, 1992), it will become apparent within one to two weeks of instituting OHA therapy whether insulin is needed. Many patients, particularly those who are obese, will respond. NIDDM patients stabilized on a low daily dose of insulin sometimes may be placed on OHA therapy or diet alone for maintenance. In NIDDM patients in whom insulin was compared with glyburide or glipizide as initial drug therapy or following chlorpropamide failure, slightly more favorable serum lipoprotein patterns (increased HDL cholesterol and decreased LDL:HDL ratio) were observed with insulin, but glycemic control was similar (Schmitt et al, 1987; Nathan et al, 1988).

INSULINS

PREPARATIONS. Insulins available in the United States differ in time of onset and duration of action, purity, and species of origin; most now are available in a U100 (100 units/ml) concentration and are nonprescription. (The production of U80 preparations was discontinued in 1980 and that of U40 preparations and all protamine zinc insulins in 1991.) A U500 preparation, Regular (Concentrated) Iletin II, is available by prescription for patients with severe insulin resistance who require very large total daily doses of insulin.

Insulins may be divided into rapid-, intermediate-, and long-acting groups (see Table 2). Insulin (crystalline zinc insulin, regular insulin) has a rapid onset and short duration of action. Isophane (NPH), an intermediate-acting insulin, is conjugated with protamine, a large protein molecule, which delays absorption and prolongs duration of action. (This preparation has an isoelectric point at physiologic pH, which reduces solubility and contributes to its long action.)

The large particle size and crystalline form of extended insulin zinc suspension (ultralente insulin) also delay absorption and prolong the duration of action. The combination of 70% ultralente and 30% semilente insulin produces insulin zinc suspension (lente insulin), which has an intermediate duration of action and approximates the general characteristics of isophane insulin.

Advances in industrial chemistry continue to improve the stability and purity of insulin. Unbuffered regular insulin with neutral pH (7.4) has been termed Neutral Regular Insulin (NRI). Patients may keep the bottle currently in use (usually a two- to four-week supply) at room temperature but protected from excessive heat, sunlight, or freezing. Additional bottles should be refrigerated until needed.

In 1980, the FDA ordered the purity of insulin products to be designated as "conventional" and "purified." Purified preparations are usually of either bovine or porcine origin and contain less than 10 ppm proinsulin (the most readily quantified protein contaminant); "single component" and "monocomponent" were terms formerly used to distinguish preparations of this purity. In general, since 1980, insulins of much higher purity have become available from several manufacturers. Conventional insulins are single-species insulins or mixtures of bovine-porcine origin. Human insulin, which is purified, is the most frequently used insulin today.

Purified Insulin Preparations: Although purified preparations produce lower antibody titers, the species of origin is more important to immunogenicity than the purity. Pork insulin differs from human insulin by only one amino acid; both preparations are less immunogenic than beef preparations.

Insulin antibodies are minimal in most patients treated solely with purified pork insulin or human insulin. Although lipoatrophy does occur, it is less common in patients treated with purified or human products and generally improves after treatment with these preparations. Lipohypertrophy may occur with use of any insulin preparation.

Human Insulin: The goal of producing the purest insulins possible has led to methods of synthesizing insulin that is identical to that produced by the human pancreas. Several recombinant DNA technologies are used. Synthetic genes for insulin A and B chains are spliced to *Escherichia coli* genes for beta-galactosidase or tryptophan synthetase. The insulin chains are then cleaved from the enzyme and joined with disulfide bonds to form the insulin molecule. Alternatively, the proinsulin gene may be introduced into *E. coli* or yeast and the resulting proinsulin then is converted to insulin.

In some patients, human insulin may have a more rapid onset and shorter duration of action than a comparable pork product, which may increase the number of insulin injections required to maintain the same level of control (Davidson, 1989).

TABLE 2.
INSULIN PREPARATIONS AVAILABLE IN THE UNITED STATES[1]

Preparation (Tradename)	Source	Purified[2]	Concentration[3] (units/ml)	Hours After Subcutaneous Administration[4]: Onset of Action[5]	Maximum Effect	Duration of Action[5]
RAPID-ACTING						
Insulin Injection (Regular, Crystalline Zinc)						
Regular Iletin I (Lilly)	Bovine-porcine	No	100	½–1	2–4	6–8
Regular Insulin (Novo Nordisk)	Porcine	No	100	½	2½–5	8
Pork Regular Iletin II (Lilly)	Porcine	Yes	100	½–1	2–4	6–8
Velosulin Human (Novo Nordisk)	Human	Yes	100	½	1–3	8
Purified Pork Insulin (Novo Nordisk)	Porcine	Yes	100	½	2½–5	8
Humulin R (Lilly)	Human	NA	100	½–1	2–4	6–8
Novolin R (Novo Nordisk)	Human	NA	100	½	2½–5	5–8
Regular (Concentrated) Iletin II,[1] U-500 (Lilly)	Porcine	Yes	500	½	–	24
INTERMEDIATE-ACTING						
Isophane (NPH) 70% Regular Insulin 30%						
Humulin 70/30 (Lilly)	Human	NA	100	½	2–12	24
Humulin 50/50 (Lilly)	Human	NA	100	½	3–5	24
Novolin 70/30 (Novo Nordisk)	Human	NA	100	½	2–12	24
Novolin 70/30 Prefilled (Novo Nordisk)	Human	NA	100	½	2–12	24
Isophane (NPH) Insulin Suspension						
NPH Iletin I (Lilly)	Bovine-porcine	No	100	2	6–12	18–26
NPH Insulin (Novo Nordisk)	Bovine	No	100	1½	4–12	24
Pork NPH Iletin II (Lilly)	Porcine	Yes	100	2	6–12	18–26
NPH Purified Pork Insulin (Novo Nordisk)	Porcine	Yes	100	1½	4–12	24
Humulin N (Lilly)	Human	NA	100	1–2	6–12	18–24
Novolin N (Novo Nordisk)	Human	NA	100	1½	4–12	18–24
Insulin Zinc Suspension (Lente)						
Lente Iletin I (Lilly)	Bovine-porcine	No	100	2–4	6–12	18–26
Lente Insulin (Novo Nordisk)	Bovine	No	100	2½	7–15	24
Pork Lente Iletin II (Lilly)	Porcine	Yes	100	2–4	6–12	18–26
Lente Purified Pork Insulin (Novo Nordisk)	Porcine	Yes	100	2½	7–15	22
Humulin L (Lilly)	Human	NA	100	1–3	6–12	18–24
Novolin L (Novo Nordisk)	Human	NA	100	2½	7–15	18–24
LONG-ACTING						
Extended Insulin Zinc Suspension (Ultralente)						
Ultralente Humulin U (Lilly)	Human	NA	100	4–6	8–20	24–28
Ultralente Insulin (Novo Nordisk)	Bovine	No	100	4	10–30	36
Ultralente Purified Beef Insulin (Novo Nordisk)	Bovine	Yes	100	4	10–30	36

[1] All preparations are nonprescription except Regular (Concentrated) Iletin II, U-500, a concentrated (500 units/ml) purified pork preparation for use in patients with severe insulin resistance. This preparation may be active over a 24-hour period.

[2] Less than 10 ppm proinsulin contamination

[3] In 10 ml containers

[4] The duration of action is for a single injection. With daily injections, the duration of the longer acting insulins is longer than indicated.

[5] Onset and duration of action vary among patients and are influenced by such factors as concentration and volume, site and depth of injection.

Mixing Insulins: Regular insulin may be mixed with other insulins with certain limitations. The action of regular insulin is delayed when it is mixed with lente (Heine et al, 1984; Olsson et al, 1987; Best et al, 1987) or ultralente insulin because the excess zinc in the lente preparations may complex with regular insulin and decrease its solubility. Separate sequential injections of regular and lente insulin through the same needle avoid the retarding effect on regular insulin (Bilo et al, 1987). Insulins with phosphate buffers (eg, Velosulin) should not be mixed with insulin of the lente series. Regular insulin mixed with NPH has the same time-course of action as regular insulin given alone.

The stability of insulin mixtures is affected by the type of insulin, ratio of the components, and species source (Adams et al, 1987). However, purified pork regular (30%) plus NPH mixture (70%), kept refrigerated, was stable at one month (Peters and Davidson, 1987) and three months (Jawadi and Ho, 1986).

Insulins in the lente series can be mixed with each other in any ratio without altering the activity of the components.

Choice of Insulin Preparation: Although human insulin currently is the most frequently used preparation, there appears to be no compelling reason to substitute human insulin for a purified pork or conventional insulin preparation if control of diabetes has been satisfactory. However, theoretically, purified insulin would be preferred to the conventional alternatives. Human insulin is slightly less antigenic than purified pork insulin and is less expensive.

Clinical situations in which purified pork or human insulin is the agent of choice include: (1) Patients with local insulin allergy, immunologic insulin resistance, or lipoatrophy at the injection site. (2) When insulin treatment is temporary (eg, NIDDM patients treated intermittently with insulin during infection or surgery, insulin given as part of total parenteral nutrition). (Patients with systemic insulin allergy or immunologic resistance frequently have a history of interrupted insulin therapy.) (3) Patients with GDM or those who plan to become pregnant. (4) Newly diagnosed patients, especially if they are young, in whom any potential benefits of long-term treatment with low immunogenic insulin might be realized (American Diabetes Association, 1990 B).

Patients should use the same preparation continuously to avoid a change in dosage requirement: *They should not arbitrarily change to insulin of a different degree of purity or of a different species of origin without careful medical supervision.*

DELIVERY SYSTEMS. Insulin Pumps: The importance of strict regulation of blood glucose is now accepted. Portable insulin infusion pumps that provide constant, smoother control of glucose levels have been developed, and several devices that deliver insulin intramuscularly, intraperitoneally, or intravenously are being tested clinically. Devices that deliver insulin subcutaneously are being used by many patients in the United States. However, superiority of pump systems over multiple-injection intensive therapy has not been demonstrated.

The subcutaneous infusion pumps are "open-loop" devices that permit regulation of the infusion rate manually or by preprogrammed control. The patient must be willing and able to monitor blood glucose at home. Models of open-loop implantable insulin pumps also have been successful in achieving control (Point Study Group, 1988). However, technical problems must be solved before these devices are available for widespread clinical use.

More sophisticated "closed-loop" devices contain a built-in glucose sensor that automatically regulates the dose of insulin; these pumps are currently available for bedside use in hospitals and are sometimes used to manage ketoacidosis and to regulate glucose during surgery, labor, and delivery. These devices require constant sampling of blood and are currently used only for acute situations (up to two days). Miniaturization of components and resolution of numerous functional problems (eg, maintenance of the sensing electrode, optimal route of administration, insulin precipitation, power supply, biocompatibility of components) must be accomplished before production and general use of closed-loop pumps become feasible.

Use of continuous subcutaneous insulin infusion (CSII) requires the participation and backup of a skilled professional team, as well as a highly motivated patient. In general, blood glucose control is similar in patients using CSII or multiple insulin injections, and the choice between the two depends on the patient's life-style and preference (American Diabetes Association, 1985).

Patient characteristics and circumstances in which CSII might be utilized are (1) in motivated, disciplined patients who can be expected to derive long-term benefits from close control of blood glucose; (2) in motivated adolescents, particularly those with growth retardation; (3) in patients planning to become pregnant or from the beginning of pregnancy; (4) in patients who have labile control despite adherence to insulin, diet, and exercise regimens or despite conventional intensive insulin therapy; (5) in patients who prefer or may benefit from the increased flexibility in meal scheduling and exercise that may result from CSII; (6) in acute situations, such as surgery, treatment of ketoacidosis, and labor and delivery (however, intravenous infusion may be more appropriate in these instances).

Patients who are not good candidates for CSII and in whom the risk of hypoglycemia may outweigh the benefits include those unable or unwilling to monitor their blood glucose levels; those not expected to derive long-term benefit because of age or life expectancy; those at risk of unrecognized hypoglycemia; and those with renal insufficiency not corrected by a kidney transplant (Bonner, 1985; Felig and Bergman, 1983; Tamborlane and Press, 1984).

Insulin pumps are associated with certain adverse effects. *Infection* at the site of needle insertion is the most common. The incidence may be increased in patients who are nasal carriers of *Staphylococcus aureus* (Mecklenburg et al, 1984); however, another study found no increase in infections at the insertion site among carriers (van Faassen et al, 1989). Proper preparation and care of the infusion site are important, and the infusion set should be changed every other day. *Ketoacidosis* may occur more frequently with CSII than conventional intensive insulin therapy; it may be caused by clogging of the tubing or, rarely, by mechanical malfunction of the pump or battery. Furthermore, ketoacidosis may occur within eight hours of pump failure; the lack of an insulin depot probably contributes to the rapidity of this effect. Unexplained increases in blood glucose should alert the patient to check the integrity of the infusion line. If blood glucose levels remain elevated, the infusion set should be changed (Bonner, 1985). Hypoglycemia also occurs with CSII, but it rarely results from pump malfunction, and the frequency is no greater than with conventional intensive insulin therapy (Mecklenburg et al, 1986). Newer pump models are equipped with alarms and fail-safe devices to detect malfunctions.

Pump systems and other devices designed to improve insulin administration have been reviewed (Selam and Charles, 1990).

Other Recent Developments: New types of injection devices are being developed to decrease discomfort and to increase the efficiency of absorption from the injection site. Sprinkler needles with multiple openings in the needle wall spread insulin over a wider subcutaneous area, and absorption is faster than with a conventional needle (Edsberg et al, 1987). Studies are needed to determine adjustments that may be necessary because of changes in delivery and absorptive patterns (American Diabetes Association Task Force, 1988).

Routes of administration other than by injection would simplify insulin administration and be more convenient and comfortable for the patient. Intranasal application of aerosolized insulin is being studied as a possible adjunct to subcutaneous administration. In one study, five to ten times the usual dose was required. The potential effect on the amount of insulin absorbed if nasal membranes are inflamed or irritated due to viral infections or allergy is not known (Salzman et al, 1985). A transdermal insulin delivery system and the possibility of enclosing insulin within a chemical complex that resists digestion, thus allowing oral administration, also are being investigated.

MANAGEMENT. The initial insulin dosage range for young IDDM patients is 0.5 to 1.5 units/kg. Newly diagnosed patients may experience a partial or, infrequently, a complete but temporary remission and may not require insulin during this period ("honeymoon phase"). This is at least partly due to reversal of "glucose toxicity" and recovery of insulin secretion by surviving beta cells.

An intermediate-acting preparation given twice a day is usually chosen for *initial treatment* of IDDM in adults and NIDDM patients who require insulin. One injection of insulin generally will not control blood glucose satisfactorily throughout a 24-hour period. In lean adults, 8 to 10 units of an intermediate-acting preparation is given 20 to 30 minutes before breakfast and 4 to 5 units before the evening meal (or at bedtime, which shifts the peak action of this dose to before breakfast). For obese patients (>120% of desirable body weight), the amounts are 20 and 10 units, respectively. The doses are increased gradually (4 to 5 units) depending on results of the before-evening meal (for the morning injection) and before-breakfast (for the previous evening injection) blood or urine glucose tests. Thus, increasing the morning dose of intermediate-acting insulin generally corrects hyperglycemia occurring before the evening meal. Prebreakfast hyperglycemia is often controlled by increasing the dose of intermediate-acting insulin the previous evening and/or reducing the size of the bedtime snack.

Other initial dosage recommendations based on patient weight are for IDDM 0.5 to 0.7 units/kg/day and for NIDDM 0.3 to 0.4 units/kg/day (Skyler, 1991). Up to 1.5 to 2 units/kg/day may be required for adolescents (Dunger, 1992).

Regular insulin is often added to control blood glucose prior to lunch and bedtime. Some physicians prefer to wait until the results of the blood tests performed prior to the evening meal and breakfast are <150 mg/dL before adding 2 to 4 units of regular insulin to the intermediate-acting preparation; the dose of the regular insulin is then increased gradually (2 to 4 units) depending on the results of the before-lunch (for the before-breakfast injection) and before-bedtime snack (for the before-evening meal injection) blood tests. Other physicians add regular insulin to the intermediate-acting preparation initially, in which case increases in the amount of regular insulin should be made cautiously because, as the increasing doses of intermediate-acting insulin become effective, less regular insulin will be required. Alternatively, one or two daily injections of long-acting insulin (ultralente) instead of an intermediate-acting preparation are given to provide a basal level of insulin. The final distribution of the total amount of daily insulin varies widely; a common recommendation is two-thirds to three-quarters in the morning and the remainder in the evening.

Most physicians recommend divided doses as the standard regimen to better approximate the physiologic pattern of insulin secretion. Divided doses are especially indicated (1) when diabetes is otherwise difficult to control, (2) when severe prebreakfast hyperglycemia cannot be corrected by one dose daily, and (3) when more than 40 units daily is required. Three or more daily injections of insulin are sometimes used to provide optimum control. Such intensified insulin regimens require the patient to monitor blood glucose at least several times daily (before each meal and the bedtime snack is optimal). In these cases, an intermediate- or long-acting insulin is used in combination with regular insulin, which is added before meals as required (Skyler, 1991). Generally 40% to 60% of the total daily dose is given as intermediate- or long-acting insulin to control the fasting blood glucose, and the balance is administered as regular insulin before meals (Zimmerman, 1986). Almost any multiple-injection regimen (two or more daily injections) combined with frequent blood glucose monitoring (four times per day) and appropriate adjustments of the insulin dosage can provide good control (Hirsch et al, 1990 A). CSII also is utilized in selected patients.

In elderly NIDDM patients receiving insulin, limited expected life span may diminish the long-term benefits achieved with strict control; therefore, higher fasting blood glucose concentrations and less stringent regimens may be acceptable. In addition, strict control in elderly patients with atherosclerosis may increase the risk of neurologic or cardiac damage from hypoglycemia (see reviews on insulin use in NIDDM by Genuth, 1990; Turner and Holman, 1990; Riddle, 1990).

A between-meal snack containing 15 to 25 g of carbohydrate plus additional protein and fat may be necessary in some patients at the time of peak action of the insulin preparation being used; a bedtime snack is necessary for most patients who require insulin. These snacks help to prevent hypoglycemic reactions that occur at night or between meals or that are associated with exercise. In overweight patients, reduction of insulin dosage may be preferable.

Regular exercise may be helpful in diabetic management because it increases uptake and utilization of glucose by muscle and may decrease insulin requirements. It also provides a healthy sense of well-being. Exercise achieves this effect partially by increasing glucose utilization in muscle and, in patients taking insulin, by increasing its absorption from the injection site. The patient may find it helpful to take a small snack before exercise to prevent hypoglycemia. Because of increased absorption of insulin, it may be advisable to avoid exercise immediately after insulin is injected and to inject insulin into a site that does not include the exercising muscles. In patients who use fixed insulin regimens, exercise should be instituted at the same time each day so that it becomes another fixed component of the overall regimen (ie, diet, insulin, exercise).

Every diabetic patient taking insulin should carry some form of readily available carbohydrate, as well as wear a Medic-Alert bracelet or have an identification card containing pertinent information. The availability of glucagon and instruction in its proper use (family members and close friends) are mandatory for all patients who require insulin.

MONITORING. Blood glucose monitoring before meals and at bedtime pinpoints the pattern of hyperglycemia. Capillary glucose determinations using reagent strips are helpful to determine the insulin doses. Many patients can learn to adjust their own insulin doses. Self-monitoring is especially important for those using insulin pumps or receiving multiple injections daily, pregnant (or planning to become pregnant) patients, and those who become hypoglycemic without the usual warning symptoms (American Diabetes Association, 1987 B). Urine testing is essential for detecting ketones in IDDM and GDM patients.

Glycated hemoglobin assays provide information on the average blood glucose levels during the previous several weeks, but they are not helpful for adjusting day-to-day insulin requirements. These assays performed three to four times yearly are an adjunct to the primary method of monitoring blood glucose and validate the patient's home measurements. Because values vary widely, they should always be interpreted with respect to the normal reference range for the analytical method employed. Glycated serum albumin and serum fructosamine also are correlated with glycemic control, although the half-lives are shorter than that of hemoglobin, and therefore they reflect serum glucose levels over a shorter period (approximately one to two weeks). All three measurements are useful to monitor blood glucose in stable patients who require insulin.

USE IN SPECIAL SITUATIONS. Patients who have intercurrent illness, emotional stress, or trauma or those hospitalized for major illness may require, at least temporarily, multiple injections or infusions of a rapid-acting human insulin. Total requirements commonly will increase temporarily. The degree of hyperglycemia and ketonuria that occurs determines the timing, type, and amount of insulin needed.

Pregnancy: Gestational diabetes (GDM) occurs in 2% to 3% of pregnancies and is the most common form of diabetes during pregnancy (90% of diabetic pregnancies). Routine blood glucose screening of all pregnant women by the sixth to seventh month is recommended, and screening should be performed earlier in those with risk factors (eg, GDM in previous pregnancy, family history of diabetes in first-degree relatives, history of high-birth-weight infants) (American Diabetes Association, 1993; Coustan, 1992). GDM is often diagnosed in the third trimester; it is more likely to occur in women who had high-birth-weight infants in past pregnancies and in those in whom weight gain is greater in the present pregnancy compared with a past pregnancy (Philipson and Super, 1989). One-half may develop overt diabetes within 15 years of onset of GDM, and those affected are likely to have had higher fasting serum glucose levels at diagnosis, preterm delivery, and an abnormal glucose tolerance test two months after parturition (Damm et al, 1992).

The diabetogenic effects of the hormones produced during pregnancy (eg, human placental lactogen, estrogen, progesterone) increase insulin requirements, while the placenta simultaneously promotes insulin catabolism. If hyperglycemia does not respond to diet therapy alone, insulin is required. An oral agent should not be used because these agents cross the placenta and may increase fetal insulin levels late in pregnancy. Use of a purified insulin preparation or human insulin may preclude potential insulin sensitization and related problems if overt diabetes develops subsequently (Freinkel et al, 1985).

In pregnant patients with pre-existing diabetes, the risk of many fetal and neonatal complications is increased and some authorities believe it to be related to the severity of the disease. The risk of prematurity, perinatal death, and congenital anomalies is three to four times greater in pregnant IDDM patients with vascular complications. The risk of spontaneous abortion also appears to be higher in those with IDDM (Miodovnik et al, 1984). Poorly controlled diabetes (as determined by hemoglobin A_{1c} levels) in early pregnancy is associated with an increased risk of major structural malformations in neonates (Miller et al, 1981), including an increase in the risk of cardiovascular defects (Becerra et al, 1990). Poor control is associated with delayed lung maturation at any gestational age (Piper and Langer, 1993). Progression of maternal retinopathy also may occur during pregnancy (Klein et al, 1990).

These observations support the advice that diabetic women plan their pregnancies and that close control of blood glucose should be established *before* conception and maintained throughout the critical period of organogenesis, as well as later in pregnancy (Cousins, 1983; Simpson et al, 1983). Many of the complications of diabetic pregnancies (eg, perinatal mortality, macrosomia, neonatal hypoglycemia, neonatal hyperbilirubinemia) have been reduced by meticulous diabetic control during the third and perhaps the second trimester.

Results from the Diabetes in Early Pregnancy Study and other investigations have demonstrated the benefit of early control. Pregnant diabetic women with poor glycemic control in the first trimester were more likely to have a spontaneous abortion than those with good control; the latter had no increased risk (Mills et al, 1988). Another study revealed that pregnant diabetic women who were in fair to good metabolic control before or within three weeks of conception (early entry) had infants with fewer congenital malformations than women who entered the study later in pregnancy (4.9% vs 9%) and were assumed to have been in poor control around the time of conception. In contrast, nondiabetic controls had only 2% fetal anomalies. However, among the early-entry patients, there was no difference in glycemic control between those whose infants had anomalies and those who did not.

Macrosomia is common in newborns of mothers with GDM. It has been assumed that macrosomia is related to maternal hyperglycemia, which causes fetal hyperinsulinemia, and that stricter control of maternal blood glucose would reduce the incidence. However, clinical evidence of a cause-and-effect relationship has been conflicting.

More stringent control of blood glucose levels during pregnancy may require more frequent injections. The usual schedule includes at least two injections (before breakfast and the evening meal) of a combination of short- and intermediate-acting insulins. Commonly, a third or even fourth daily injection may be required for ideal control.

In the pregnant IDDM patient, insulin needs may be quite different than before pregnancy and may vary throughout the course of the pregnancy. Insulin requirements generally are unchanged or even decreased slightly during the first trimester, but they may increase gradually by as much as 100% or more during the second half of gestation. One study showed a disparity between the increased need for insulin in pregnant IDDM and NIDDM patients. Pregnant IDDM patients required 38% more insulin from the second to third trimester (similar to normal pregnant women), while pregnant NIDDM patients required a 98% increase (Rigg et al, 1980). During the last month of pregnancy, insulin needs may decrease slightly. In IDDM patients, it is particularly important to avoid diabetic ketosis and especially ketoacidosis, which tend to occur in the second or third trimester, since these complications may cause fetal death.

Self-monitoring of capillary blood glucose is essential to facilitate accurate dosage adjustments. Urine testing of glucose is not sensitive enough to maintain close control. Maternal blood sugar levels should be regulated so that they are as close as possible to those during normal pregnancy (60 to 120 mg/dL plasma), although this may be very difficult to achieve without causing significant hypoglycemia. Insulin dosage should be adjusted if possible when the fasting plasma glucose exceeds 100 mg/dL or the postprandial glucose exceeds 140 mg/dL. CSII also is used to achieve close blood glucose control during pregnancy. In one study of 22 pregnant diabetic women, both intensive conventional insulin therapy and CSII provided excellent metabolic control, and there were no differences in outcome between the two methods (Coustan et al, 1986).

Close control of blood glucose and fluctuations in insulin requirement during labor can be managed by constant intravenous infusion of dextrose and insulin. The insulin requirement is reduced or may even be absent during labor, as in other forms of strenuous exertion. Euglycemia during labor may reduce but not eliminate the risk of neonatal hypoglycemia, which is caused by endogenous fetal hyperinsulinemia. Frequent monitoring of the infant is important to identify hypoglycemia because it is often asymptomatic. Oral feeding in the first few hours of life is important to avoid severe hypoglycemia.

Delivery of the infant and placenta abruptly ends diabetogenic stress; in the first day postpartum, the insulin requirement may decrease precipitously to one-half to two-thirds of the prepregnancy level. Occasionally, insulin is not required for up to several days postpartum, even in IDDM patients. Thereafter, there is a gradual increase until about three to five days postpartum when the usual prepregnancy level of insulin is needed. In GDM patients, insulin usually is not required postpartum. If premature labor ensues, corticosteroids (to enhance pulmonary maturity) and/or a uterine relaxant, such as ritodrine [Yutopar], to inhibit labor may be used. Supplemental insulin may be necessary to offset the hyperglycemic effects of these agents.

Surgery: Diabetic patients should be prepared for the stress of surgery and maintained intraoperatively with appropriate measures. Patients with long-standing diabetes should be evaluated preoperatively for renal and cardiovascular function, neuropathy and retinopathy, infection, or other conditions that could adversely affect surgical outcome or recovery. Correction of serious problems may necessitate delay of surgery. For example, intraoperative changes in blood pressure or coagulation may cause retinal hemorrhage in a patient with severe retinopathy, which may be better treated before surgery (Gallina et al, 1983). Oral hypoglycemic drugs should not be taken on the day of surgery or from the day before surgery if the long-acting agent, chlorpropamide, is used.

Insulin may be given intravenously during surgery or as an intermediate-acting preparation before and immediately after surgery in the recovery room. Glucose levels must be monitored before, during, and after the procedure, and additional regular insulin may be given intravenously or subcutaneously if required. An infusion pump is preferred to deliver regular insulin in saline.

In IDDM patients, inadequate intraoperative monitoring increases the risk of hyperglycemia, ketoacidosis, and electrolyte imbalance. Those with NIDDM may develop hyperglycemia and hyperosmolarity. If a diabetic patient requires emergency surgery, glycemic control must be established; blood glucose and electrolytes should be monitored. If the patient is severely hyperglycemic, insulin infusion may result in a rapid and dangerous decrease in serum potassium unless appropriate replacement is given.

Postoperatively, the usual insulin regimen or oral hypoglycemic medication and the normal diabetic meal plan may be resumed at the same time. If food intake is restricted, the amount of insulin administered is adjusted proportionately.

Diabetic Ketoacidosis: This potentially life-threatening emergency requires prompt diagnosis, accurate estimation of severity, and recognition and treatment of any precipitating factor, as well as skillful administration of insulin, fluids, and electrolytes (particularly potassium) and prompt treatment of any coexisting condition. Although there usually is intracellular depletion of potassium, serum levels initially may be low, normal, or high. Replacement of potassium should be started as soon as the serum potassium level begins to decline into the normal range or, if the potassium level is not available, when T-wave configuration on the EKG is normal or low. In children with IDDM, potassium replacement is recommended as soon as it is established that the kidneys are functioning. Potassium salts may be given as potassium chloride and potassium phosphate; the latter prevents hypophosphatemia, but it must be administered cautiously to avoid hypocalcemia. Blood levels should be monitored.

Ketoacidosis is now treated with much smaller doses of insulin than were formerly administered. Less than 100 units may be needed using low-dose regimens (see the evaluation on Insulin Injection). The dose should be increased if the blood glucose level is not decreased by 5% to 10%/hr (assuming adequate rehydration). A decrease in serum glucose of approximately 70 mg/dL/hr indicates adequate insulin and hydration therapy (Alberti, 1977; Heber et al, 1977; Kreisberg, 1978). Initially, 0.9% (normal) saline is administered for the first one to two hours to prevent too rapid reduction in osmolality, which may increase the risk of cerebral edema; 0.45% (half-normal) saline then is given.

Although bicarbonate rapidly corrects the pH, its use in ketoacidosis generally is not recommended because the resulting shift of potassium to the intracellular compartment may cause hypokalemia. Some authorities suggest that bicarbonate may be administered in severe acidosis to correct the pH to 7.1 but should not be used beyond that point. However, in one study, its administration to patients with arterial pH 6.9 to 7.14 did not improve outcome variables (eg, rate or time to recovery) compared with controls (Morris et al, 1986). (See also review by Sanson and Levine, 1989, and reviews on diabetic ketoacidosis and hyperosmolar nonketotic coma by Kitabchi and Murphy, 1988; Graves, 1990.)

Hyperosmolar Nonketotic Syndrome (Coma): This condition may be confused initially with stroke or a severe hypoglycemic reaction. It is observed most often in individuals over 60 years and may complicate pre-existing diabetes or it may present as the initial manifestation of diabetes. It rarely occurs in younger diabetic patients. Hyperosmolar nonketotic syndrome represents an incomplete manifestation of the metabolic derangement seen in diabetic ketoacidosis. Although hyperglycemia occurs, lipolysis is not increased and ketosis and ketoacidosis do not result or are present to a slight degree.

Associated illness, physiologic stress, or a history of taking a drug(s) that inhibits insulin secretion or elevates blood glucose is common. The mortality rate is high (10% to 40%), and death is usually caused by the complicating illness rather than the metabolic abnormality. Polydipsia and polyuria are present for several days to several weeks previously. Weight loss, stupor or coma, severe dehydration, and very high levels of glucose (800 to 1,500 mg/dL plasma or more) are observed. Azotemia (often prerenal) and marked hyperosmolarity are present.

Since polyuria and polydipsia occur for a longer period of time in patients with the hyperosmolar nonketotic syndrome than in those with diabetic ketoacidosis, the degree of dehydration is usually greater and more fluid replacement may be needed. There is some disagreement about the most appropriate replacement fluid; 10 or more liters of hypotonic electrolyte solution (eg, 0.45% sodium chloride) may be given during the first 12 to 36 hours to correct hyperosmolarity and dehydration (urine output is monitored). Alternatively, 0.9% saline may be preferred initially if there is severe intravascular volume depletion; hypotonic solution is administered thereafter. Potassium replacement must be monitored carefully, particularly in older patients since cardiac complications may be present. Morbidity and central nervous system complications are common in survivors and are usually due to arterial or venous thrombotic occlusions from the severe dehydration in the early phase of the syndrome. See review by Wachtel, 1990.

Insulin Resistance: Historically, the term, "insulin resistance," has been applied to patients who require more than 200 units daily for several days or longer in the absence of gross obesity, ketoacidosis, or intercurrent infection. It may be caused by unusually high titers of IgG antibodies to insulin, although this has become very rare with the increasing use of purified pork and human insulins. Antibody-mediated insulin resistance should not be confused with the large amounts of insulin often needed to control obese (especially noncompliant) patients.

In immunologic insulin resistance, changing the species source from beef or mixed beef-pork to pork or human insulin may reduce hyperglycemia. If this is tried and the patient still requires more than 200 units daily, corticosteroids may be administered. An increased duration of action is associated with IgG binding of regular insulin, and the corticosteroid may decrease IgG production or reduce the binding of insulin to the antibody. Prednisone 40 to 80 mg daily is given until the insulin requirement decreases or for a maximum of one month. The usual adverse effects of high-dose corticosteroid therapy may occur. Steroid therapy should be initiated in the hospital or with careful outpatient observation because insulin requirements may increase initially due to the hyperglycemic effect of the corticosteroid.

Since immunologic insulin resistance is self-limited, lasting from several months to more than one year, many physicians avoid corticosteroid therapy by using highly concentrated regular insulin (U500) in large enough quantities to avoid ketoacidosis even though the level of control may be unsatisfactory. (U500 regular insulin has a time-course of action similar to that of an intermediate-acting insulin because the high titer of IgG antibodies binds the insulin and releases it slowly.) The patient must be monitored carefully when hypoglycemia signals the gradual (several weeks) return of sensitivity. Both reduction of IgG antibody titers and release of bound insulin contribute to the rapid decrease in insulin requirements (Davidson, 1991).

Rarely, immunologic insulin resistance occurs as a consequence of antibodies directed against the insulin receptor. Extreme insulin resistance can be associated with the development of acanthosis nigricans. Some of these patients have antibodies to the insulin receptor. Others may have genetic syndromes in which the insulin receptor is structurally abnormal (eg, in leprechaunism).

Nonimmunologic insulin resistance is an integral component of diabetic pathophysiology in NIDDM and occurs to some degree even in nonobese patients (Firth et al, 1987; Swislocki et al, 1987). It also is seen in IDDM but only when these patients are in poor control; restoring near euglycemia in IDDM patients improves insulin sensitivity to almost normal. NIDDM patients have a postreceptor defect that impairs both cellular glucose metabolism and glycogen synthesis in target tissues. In contrast to IDDM, restoring near euglycemia in NIDDM improves insulin sensitivity only modestly (Davidson, 1991).

Hypoglycemia: This effect may be observed in any patient receiving insulin or a sulfonylurea hypoglycemic agent. Causes of hypoglycemia are (1) reduction or change in diet (eg, omission or delay of a meal), especially decreased intake of carbohydrate; (2) alleviation of stress; (3) insulin or sulfonylurea overdosage; (4) weight reduction; (5) termination or completion of pregnancy; (6) exercise; (7) correction of disorders associated with hyperglycemia; (8) overindulgence in alcohol without food; or (9) diabetic gastroparesis, which delays food absorption. Hypoglycemia also may be caused by errors in insulin administration (eg, improper measurement, improper injection technique), remission of the diabetic state, or institution of medication (for an unrelated disorder) that may produce hypoglycemia.

Hypoglycemia often occurs near the time of maximal activity of the insulin preparation used. It is more likely to occur with intensified insulin regimens (conventional or pump). Common manifestations are hunger, anxiety, warmth and sweating, tremulousness, weakness, confusion, emotional lability, palpitation, pallor, abnormal behavior, fatigue, paresthesias, and hyperesthesias of the lips, nose, or fingers. The specific cluster of symptoms varies with the individual and tends to recur with hypoglycemic episodes. However, the occurrence of a recent episode of hypoglycemia may lessen the symptomatic response to a second episode (Cryer, 1993).

In severe hypoglycemia, profound cerebrocortical dysfunction may occur, manifested by convulsions, coma, and eventually death. Central nervous system effects are related to the absolute blood glucose concentration. Therefore, if glucose levels decrease slowly, adrenergic signs and symptoms may not precede central nervous system depression.

The symptoms of hypoglycemia are quite variable in children: A child may have a voracious appetite, tremors, and pallor or simply be faint, easily fatigued, or have a headache. Appearance may be apathetic or sleepy, and the parent may mistakenly assume the child wishes to sleep longer.

For treatment of hypoglycemia, see the sections on Oral Hypoglycemic Agents, Interactions; Hyperglycemic Agents. Patient education is an integral part of initiating insulin therapy. Patients and family members should be taught to recognize an insulin reaction and how to treat it. To avoid a severe hypoglycemic reaction, all patients should have glucose readily available and a family member or friend should be knowledgeable about its administration. Glucagon must be prescribed for all patients receiving insulin, and a family member or friend must be instructed on its proper administration.

Dawn Phenomenon, Somogyi Effect: The *dawn phenomenon*, an increase in fasting blood glucose levels and insulin requirements before breakfast, has been observed in IDDM and NIDDM patients. In nondiabetic patients, it is characterized by prebreakfast increased insulin concentrations with no change in glucose levels (Bolli and Gerich, 1984; Bolli et al, 1984 A; Atiea et al, 1987). The principal cause in diabetic patients appears to be an inability to respond to normal nocturnal surges of growth hormone secretion with increased insulin secretion (Campbell et al, 1985).

In both IDDM and NIDDM patients, adjustment of the dosage regimen should control the fasting hyperglycemia. The second dose of intermediate-acting insulin may be given at bedtime instead of before the evening meal so that peak activity occurs closer to the time of expected hyperglycemia. This also may decrease the risk of hypoglycemia during the night by shifting the peak of insulin action to a later time. A programmable insulin pump also may be set to increase insulin delivery at the appropriate time.

The *Somogyi effect* consists of rebound hyperglycemia in response to secretion of counter-regulatory hormones (ie, epinephrine, norepinephrine, growth hormone, cortisol) during unrecognized hypoglycemic episodes. Although the Somogyi effect has been demonstrated in diabetic patients (Bolli et al, 1984 B), its role in causing prebreakfast hyperglycemia is controversial. In one study of IDDM patients on CSII, nocturnal asymptomatic hypoglycemia was followed by slight morning fasting hyperglycemia and a rise in postbreakfast hyperglycemia that was three times higher than the increase in fasting glucose. The effect on postbreakfast glucose levels occurred six to nine hours after the hypoglycemic episode (Perriello et al, 1988). On the other hand, other studies (Havlin and Cryer, 1987; Lerman and Wolfsdorf, 1988; Tordjman et al, 1987; Hirsch et al, 1990 B) have shown that not only does lowering blood glucose in the middle of the night not lead to rebound hyperglycemia, but that fasting hyperglycemia is seldom preceded by nocturnal hypoglycemia. Fasting hyperglycemia is usually due to the waning of insulin effect overnight and requires more, not less, insulin the previous evening.

ADVERSE REACTIONS AND PRECAUTIONS. Allergic Reactions: Although patients treated with insulin have both IgE and IgG antibodies to insulin, serious allergic problems are rare. Allergic reactions to insulin can be either systemic or local; the latter occur about ten times more frequently than the former, and both forms may be observed in some patients.

Local allergy occurred much more commonly with the older, less pure preparations but also has been reported with human insulin (Ganz et al, 1990). It is manifested by an erythematous, indurated area of several centimeters that develops within one to two hours at the site of injection and may persist for several days. The reaction often begins a few weeks after starting insulin treatment. If it commences within the first few days after initiation of therapy, previous sensitization to beef or pork insulin may be causative. Local reactions are thought to be produced by noninsulin or large-molecular-weight materials present in some preparations, and they remit spontaneously after several months.

Local inflammatory responses (which some consider irritant and others allergic) or infection may result from improper cleansing of the skin, contamination of the injection site, use of a sensitizing antiseptic, or accidental intradermal rather than subcutaneous injection. These reactions usually subside spontaneously.

Generalized reactions begin within 10 to 30 minutes after injection and are characterized by a very large lesion at the injection site, often followed by urticarial skin eruptions with or without systemic manifestations that may include angioedema, respiratory symptoms (eg, asthma, dyspnea), and, very rarely, hypotension, shock, and death. These reactions have been ascribed to sensitivity to the insulin molecule itself. Patients with systemic allergy have high titers of IgE antibody to insulin and commonly have a history of (1) intermittent treatment with insulin, in which case allergy is manifested one or two weeks after resumption of therapy; or (2) allergy to other materials (eg, penicillin). Since this IgE-mediated reaction is an allergic response to the insulin molecule itself, switching insulin preparations does not eliminate the reaction. Systemic allergy to human recombinant DNA insulin also has been reported.

Desensitization is indicated in patients with symptoms of systemic allergy who require insulin (a desensitization kit is available from Eli Lilly and Company). The patient may be desensitized to a mixed or single-species preparation. In general, the process involves injection of very small amounts of human or pork insulin initially, gradually increasing the dosage. These small amounts are bound to IgE antibody-mast cell combinations, and degranulation of the mast cells releases histamine and other inflammatory substances. However, the amounts released by small increments of insulin do not cause symptoms, and eventually all IgE antibodies are bound by insulin. The patient can then tolerate therapeutic doses (Davidson, 1991). Since anaphylactic shock can occur occasionally during desensitization, epinephrine, diphenhydramine, and intubation equipment should be readily available.

Lipodystrophies: Some patients may be susceptible to lipodystrophy (atrophy or hypertrophy). In lipoatrophy, a depression in the skin underlying the site of insulin injection is caused by atrophy of fat tissue. This condition may be due to an immune phenomenon and tends to occur more frequently in young female patients and when less pure insulin preparations are used. The injection of a purified pork or human preparation directly into the atrophic area for two to four weeks will cause subcutaneous fat to accumulate. Some authorities advocate injections at the outer margin of the atrophic area and working inward as the depression fills in over time. Unless insulin is injected into affected areas every two to four weeks, atrophy may recur. Return to the use of a less purified preparation also may cause recurrence. Although rare, lipoatrophy also has been reported in patients treated with purified pork or human insulin.

Lipohypertrophy is an accumulation of subcutaneous fat mixed with connective tissue that sometimes develops at sites of repeated insulin injection. Whether this is primarily due to the lipogenic effect of insulin or to an allergic inflammatory response is difficult to determine. Regression occurs gradually if the affected sites are not used for injections.

Vision Changes: In uncontrolled diabetes, a transient loss of accommodation has been attributed to changes in the hydration of the lens secondary to hyperglycemia; this condition is reversed during the early phase of effective management. Since alterations in osmotic equilibrium between the lens and vitreous and aqueous fluids may not stabilize for a few weeks after initiating therapy, evaluation for new corrective lenses should be delayed for three to six weeks. Visual symptoms also may transiently worsen during the period of initial treatment of diabetes.

Interactions: Hormones that tend to counteract the hypoglycemic effect of insulin include growth hormone (somatotropin), glucocorticoids, thyroid hormone, estrogens, progestins, and glucagon. Epinephrine inhibits insulin secretion and stimulates glycogenolysis.

When hypoglycemia occurs in diabetic patients who are also taking beta-adrenergic blocking drugs, the symptomatic response is affected (Hirsch et al, 1991). The tachycardia associated with hypoglycemia may be masked and counter-regulation may be impaired, but sweating is enhanced.

The hypoglycemic effect of insulin also may be potentiated by monoamine oxidase inhibitors, disopyramide [Norpace], alcohol, quinine, high doses of salicylates, and fenfluramine [Pondimin].

Drug Evaluations

RAPID-ACTING PREPARATIONS

INSULIN INJECTION (Crystalline Zinc Insulin, Regular Insulin)
[*Unpurified:* Regular Iletin I, Regular Insulin; *Purified:* Pork Regular Iletin II, Regular (Concentrated) Iletin II]

This rapid-acting agent has a relatively short duration of action. It may be given intravenously and intramuscularly, as well as subcutaneously (see Table 2).

Regular insulin is widely used to supplement intermediate- and long-acting preparations, and, when buffered, it is the insulin used with infusion pumps.

Regular insulin is the preparation of choice in unstable diabetes when complications, such as infection, shock, or surgical trauma, occur. It may be administered intravenously in the presence of ketoacidosis or during surgery. There may be substantial adherence of insulin to in-line intravenous tubing. However, this is not a problem if the infusion tubing is initially flushed with 50 to 100 ml of the insulin solution. A concentrated form (U-500) may be used in patients with severe insulin resistance. This preparation may be active over a 24-hour period.

See the introduction to this section for further information.

DOSAGE AND PREPARATIONS.

Subcutaneous: Dosage must be individualized, and a broad range may be needed. As an adjunct to intermediate-acting preparations, commonly 5 to 10 units of regular insulin are given in the same syringe before breakfast or the evening meal. (When mixing regular insulin with other insulins, NPH preparations are preferred because the effect of the short-acting insulin may be delayed when added to the lente preparations [probably due to the excess zinc].) The dose of regular insulin must be adjusted according to blood glucose measurements at the appropriate times (eg, after breakfast and before lunch for the morning dose of regular insulin; after the evening meal and before the bedtime snack for the before-evening meal dose of regular insulin).

Intravenous: For ketoacidosis, *adults,* 5 to 10 units/hr given by infusion; more may be required in some insulin-resistant patients. *Children,* range, 0.1 unit/kg/hr to the adult dose above given as a continuous infusion.

Intramuscular: For ketoacidosis when facilities for continuous intravenous infusion are limited, 5 to 10 units hourly.

Regular insulin is available from single or mixed species sources and in conventional or purified preparations (see Table 2). Human insulin preparations are also available (see evaluation below).

REGULAR HUMAN INSULIN INJECTION (Biosynthetic)

[Humulin R, Novolin R, Velosulin Human]

This rapid-acting form of human insulin is produced by recombinant DNA techniques. It may be administered subcutaneously, intravenously, intramuscularly, or through an infusion pump.

Therapeutically, this preparation is probably equivalent to purified pork insulin injection. Human regular insulins are absorbed faster than the corresponding purified pork product in some patients. Although the peak serum concentration of human insulin injection after subcutaneous administration is slightly higher than that of purified pork insulin injection, the times to peak concentration and overall bioavailability are similar and control of blood glucose appears to be equivalent. No differences are apparent in binding, actions, metabolism, or potency.

As with purified pork insulin, patients receiving only human insulin subcutaneously rarely have been reported to produce insulin-specific IgG and IgE antibodies and the biological significance, if any, is unknown. When human insulin was substituted for mixed beef-pork insulin, antibody levels and insulin binding to antibodies decreased. When human insulin was substituted for purified pork insulin, insulin binding to antibodies decreased slightly. *Escherichia coli* or *Saccharomyces cerevisiae* peptides have not been found in biosynthetic products, and antibodies to bacterial peptides have not been observed in patients treated with recombinant DNA human insulin. Lipoatrophy has occurred only rarely in patients receiving only human insulin.

There is no evidence that the slight differences between purified pork and human insulin are clinically significant.

These preparations may be mixed with other insulins subject to certain limitations (see the section on Mixing Insulins).

DOSAGE AND PREPARATIONS.

Subcutaneous, Intramuscular, Intravenous: Some patients may require a different dose than with the older, less pure animal-source insulins. The adjustment may be needed with the first dose or over a period of several weeks.

For dosage guidelines, see the evaluation on Insulin Injection.

For preparations, see Table 2.

INTERMEDIATE-ACTING PREPARATIONS

ISOPHANE (NPH) INSULIN SUSPENSION

[*Unpurified:* NPH Iletin I, NPH Insulin; *Purified:* Pork NPH Iletin II, NPH Purified Pork Insulin Mixtures]

Isophane insulin is an intermediate-acting preparation (see Table 2). Absorption is delayed because the insulin is conjugated with protamine in a complex of reduced isoelectric solubility. This preparation is useful in all forms of diabetes except the initial treatment of diabetic ketoacidosis or in emergencies. Isophane insulin (usually in combination with regular insulin) is often used for previously untreated diabetic patients who require insulin. It may be mixed in the same syringe with other insulin preparations subject to certain limitations (see the section on Mixing Insulins in the Introduction).

Hypoglycemic reactions in mid to late afternoon may be less obvious in onset, more prolonged, and more common than with rapid-acting preparations because of the prolonged effect of the dose. See the introduction to this section for additional information.

DOSAGE AND PREPARATIONS.

Subcutaneous (should never be used intravenously): Dosage must be individualized. *Adults,* initially, 10 to 20 units or more (often in combination with regular insulin) 30 to 60 minutes before breakfast. If needed, a combination of this preparation and regular insulin may be given in divided doses to provide approximately one-third of the daily amount 30 minutes before the evening meal. Alternatively, regular insulin is given separately before the evening meal and isophane insulin is given before bedtime.

Isophane insulin suspension is available from single or mixed species sources and in conventional or purified preparations (see Table 2). Human isophane insulin preparations also are available (see evaluation below).

ISOPHANE (NPH) HUMAN INSULIN SUSPENSION

[Humulin N, Novolin N, *Mixtures:* Humulin 70/30, Humulin 50/50, Novolin 70/30 and Novolin 70/30 Prefilled (70% NPH isophane, 30% regular)]

This intermediate-acting form of human insulin is produced by recombinant DNA techniques. It is administered subcutaneously and should not be given intravenously. Absorption is delayed because the insulin is conjugated with protamine in a complex of reduced isoelectric solubility.

Therapeutically, this preparation is probably comparable to purified pork insulin. However, human NPH insulin may have a slightly more rapid onset and shorter duration of action than comparable purified pork products. In patients who receive only one injection of the human preparation daily, glycemic control may be decreased slightly and fasting serum glucose and ketonuria may increase slightly during the night.

There is no evidence that the slight differences between purified pork and human insulin are clinically significant. This insulin may be mixed with other insulins subject to certain limitations (see section on Mixing Insulins).

DOSAGE AND PREPARATIONS.
Subcutaneous: Some patients may require a different dosage than with the older, less pure animal-source insulins. The adjustment may be needed with the first dose or over a period of several weeks.

For dosage guidelines, see the evaluation on Isophane Insulin Suspension.

For preparations, see Table 2.

INSULIN ZINC SUSPENSION (Lente)

[*Unpurified:* Lente Iletin I, Lente Insulin; *Purified:* Pork Lente Iletin II, Lente Purified Pork Insulin]

This intermediate-acting preparation is a mixture of 30% prompt insulin zinc suspension (semilente insulin) and 70% extended insulin zinc suspension (ultralente insulin) (see Table 2). Insulin zinc suspension or isophane insulin (usually in combination with regular insulin) is often used for previously untreated diabetic patients who require insulin. Insulin zinc suspension is not a suitable substitute for regular insulin in emergencies because of its delayed onset of action. Insulins of the lente series can be mixed in any proportion to obtain the desired dose and modified activity.

Hypoglycemic reactions in mid or late afternoon may be less obvious in onset, more prolonged, and more common than with rapid-acting preparations because of the more prolonged effect of the dose. Insulins in the lente series do not contain a modifying protein and can be mixed in any ratio. See the introduction to this section for additional information on adverse reactions.

Pharmacologically, insulin zinc suspension is equivalent to isophane insulin on a unit-for-unit basis. However, responses vary and some patients may have a hypersensitivity reaction to one of these insulins but not the other depending on whether the antigen is zinc (lente series) or protamine (isophane).

DOSAGE AND PREPARATIONS.
Subcutaneous (should never be given intravenously): See the dosage for Isophane Insulin Suspension.

Insulin zinc suspension is available from single or mixed species sources and in conventional or purified preparations (see Table 2). Human insulin preparations also are available (see evaluation below).

HUMAN INSULIN ZINC SUSPENSION (Lente)

[Humulin L, Novolin L]

This intermediate-acting form of human insulin is produced by recombinant DNA techniques. It is administered subcutaneously and should not be given intravenously.

Therapeutically, this preparation is probably comparable to purified pork insulin. No difference in bioavailability has been observed. There is no evidence that the slight differences between purified pork and human insulin are clinically significant.

DOSAGE AND PREPARATIONS.
Subcutaneous: Some patients may require a different dosage than with the older, less pure animal-source insulins. Adjustment may be needed with the first dose or over a period of several weeks. Insulins of the lente series may be mixed without changing the activity of the components.

For dosage guidelines, see the evaluation on Insulin Zinc Suspension.

For preparations, see Table 2.

LONG-ACTING PREPARATIONS

EXTENDED INSULIN ZINC SUSPENSION (Ultralente)

[*Unpurified:* Ultralente Insulin; *Purified:* Ultralente Purified Beef Insulin]

Like prompt insulin zinc suspension (semilente insulin), this long-acting form contains no modifying protein to which patients may be sensitive. Because of its long duration of action, this insulin preparation has limited usefulness when given alone and is not suitable for use in emergencies. It is usually administered in combination with a shorter acting form. In slightly reduced doses, it may be combined with insulin zinc suspension (lente insulin) when blood glucose levels are not adequately controlled during the daytime. Insulins of the lente series can be mixed in any proportion to obtain the desired dose and modified activity.

DOSAGE AND PREPARATIONS.
Subcutaneous (should never be given intravenously): Dosage must be individualized on the basis of patient response.

Extended insulin zinc suspension is available from bovine sources and in conventional or purified preparations (see Table 2). A human insulin preparation also is available (see the evaluation below).

HUMAN EXTENDED INSULIN ZINC SUSPENSION (Ultralente)

[Ultralente Humulin U]

This long-acting form of human insulin is produced by recombinant DNA techniques. It is administered subcutaneously and should not be given intravenously. The time course of this preparation is similar for onset of activity but shorter for maximum activity and duration of action compared with ultralente preparations of animal origin (see Table 2). Insulins of the lente series can be mixed in any proportion to obtain the desired dose and modified activity.

DOSAGE AND PREPARATIONS.
Subcutaneous (should never be given intravenously): Some patients may require a different dosage than with the older,

TABLE 3.
SULFONYLUREA ORAL HYPOGLYCEMIC AGENTS AVAILABLE IN THE UNITED STATES

Drug and Trademark	Daily Dose Range (Usual Dose in Parentheses)	Elimination Half-life (Hours)	Duration of Action (Hours)
FIRST GENERATION			
Acetohexamide Dymelor (Lilly) Generic	500 mg–1.5 g (1 g)	1.3–6 (including metabolite)	12–24
Chlorpropamide Diabinese (Pfizer) Generic	50–750 mg (250 mg)	30–36	1–3 days
Tolazamide Tolinase (Upjohn) Generic	100 mg–1 g (250 mg)	4.7–8	12–24
Tolbutamide Orinase (Upjohn) Generic	500 mg–3 g (2 g)	4–8	6–12
SECOND GENERATION			
Glipizide Glucotrol (Pratt)	2.5–40 mg (5–15 mg)	2–4	10–24
Glyburide			
DiaBeta (Hoechst) Glynase (Upjohn)	1.25–20 mg (2.5–10 mg)	1–12	12–24
Micronase (Upjohn)	0.75–12 mg (1.5–6 mg)	4	12–24

less pure animal-source insulins. The adjustment may be needed with the first dose or over a period of several weeks. Dosage must be individualized on the basis of patient response.

For preparations, see Table 2.

ORAL HYPOGLYCEMIC AGENTS (OHAs)

SULFONYLUREAS. The first-generation sulfonylurea compounds are acetohexamide [Dymelor], chlorpropamide [Diabinese], tolazamide [Tolinase], and tolbutamide [Orinase]. The second-generation compounds are glyburide (glibenclamide in Europe) [DiaBeta, Glynase, Micronase], glipizide [Glucotrol], and the investigational agent, gliclazide (available in some foreign countries). These agents reduce the blood glucose level in selected patients with NIDDM (see the section on Choice of Therapy). The second-generation agents are more potent than the first-generation agents and are as effective as chlorpropamide or tolazamide.

Pharmacokinetics: The absorption of all sulfonylureas is fairly rapid and complete. These agents are weakly acidic and circulate bound to protein (70% to 99%), principally albumin. All are metabolized in the liver to relatively inactive (tolbutamide, tolazamide, glipizide, glyburide) or active compounds (acetohexamide, chlorpropamide) that are excreted in the urine, mainly by tubular secretion (approximately 50% of the metabolites of glyburide are excreted in the bile and 10% of the metabolites of glipizide are excreted in the feces). The primary therapeutic differences among the sulfonylureas are in duration of action, elimination half-life, and relative potencies (see Table 3). However, the maximal hypoglycemic effect is similar for all agents except tolbutamide and acetohexamide, which are less effective. Plasma levels vary widely, and dose-response relationships generally are weak, although responsive patients usually have higher mean plasma levels of drug.

Mechanism of Action: Although the sulfonylureas are sulfonamide derivatives, they have no antibacterial action. Functional beta cells must be present for activity. Sulfonylureas appear to act initially and principally by increasing the sensitivity of the beta cells to glucose and amino acids, which stimulate insulin secretion. These agents potentiate insulin-stimulated glucose transport in adipose tissue and across skeletal muscle membrane. Sulfonylureas probably do not significantly stimulate insulin binding to receptors, but rather act at postreceptor sites (Nelson, 1987; Melander, 1987; Ward, 1987).

The sulfonylureas decrease blood glucose levels in nondiabetic as well as in diabetic individuals. Conversely, usual therapeutic doses of the biguanides, phenformin and metformin, have no hypoglycemic effect in individuals without diabetes.

BIGUANIDES. The biguanide, metformin, which has been in use in Europe and Canada for two decades, recently became available under a Treatment IND in the United States (for further information, contact Lipha Pharmaceuticals, Inc (212/223-1280). This drug reduces fasting blood glucose, glycated hemoglobin, total cholesterol, and triglycerides. Its hypoglycemic action is probably exerted principally by increasing glucose transport across skeletal muscle cell membranes (Klip and Leiter, 1990) and decreasing peripheral resistance to insulin by stimulating nonoxidative glucose metabolism (Widén et al, 1992). Weight gain does not occur as often as with insulin or sulfonylureas, and weight commonly decreases, possibly due to side effects of the drug (ie, nausea, reduced appetite). The incidence of lactic acidosis, which was responsible for withdrawal of phenformin (also a biguanide) from the U.S. market, is reportedly much lower with metformin. Phenformin is available in the United States only under special circumstances (see the evaluation).

α GLUCOSIDASE INHIBITOR. Acarbose, an investigational agent, is one of a class of compounds that inhibit enzymatic degradation of sucrose, maltose, and other oligosaccharides, thus delaying absorption of monosaccharides. Acarbose causes a more gradual and prolonged postprandial rise in blood glucose and a slight decrease in glycated hemoglobin in both NIDDM and IDDM. When acarbose is used as primary therapy for NIDDM, fasting as well as postprandial blood glucose levels decrease. In IDDM, administration of acarbose results in a modest decrease in insulin dosage requirements. Absorption occurs throughout the small intestine. In the large intestine, carbohydrates are metabolized by bacteria to short-chain fatty acids; thus, most common adverse reactions are gastrointestinal (eg, abdominal bloating, flatulence, diarrhea). Acarbose is marketed in several European and South American countries. See also reviews by Marchetti and Navelesi, 1989, and Lebovitz, 1992.

Management

An adequate and documented trial of nonpharmacologic (diet and exercise) therapy alone is essential before any hypoglycemic agent is prescribed in NIDDM (except in certain symptomatic patients or when the patient's history indicates that an appropriate diet is already being followed). If a hypoglycemic agent is then deemed necessary, it should be considered *only a supplement* to continuing caloric restriction and exercise (rather than a substitute for weight reduction). Opinions differ on when hypoglycemic therapy should be instituted in mildly symptomatic or asymptomatic NIDDM patients. Generally, if the fasting blood glucose remains above 140 mg/dL despite dietary compliance, drug therapy should be instituted. Some practitioners utilize drug therapy for patients whose fasting blood sugar is less than 150 mg/dL but whose postprandial levels exceed 200 mg/dL. Since the trend is toward closer control of hyperglycemia, drug therapy may be initiated when glucose levels are less than 140 mg/dL, particularly in younger, lean patients.

Asymptomatic patients in whom blood glucose levels remain elevated despite dietary compliance should be given an OHA. Self-monitoring of blood glucose is recommended before breakfast and after other meals every one to two weeks until the dosage is established and every one to three months thereafter. Alternatively, glycated hemoglobin levels are measured every two to three months with the goal of maintaining the value less than 1.5% above the upper limit of normal for the assay method used. Therapy is continued if the response is satisfactory. If the response is unsatisfactory, the dose is increased gradually to the maximum effective amount. Symptomatic patients should be given an OHA simultaneously with dietary therapy (without prior dietary trial). Dosage adjustments may be required (see the evaluations). In both symptomatic and asymptomatic patients, fasting (or postprandial if fasting values are <140 mg/dL) blood glucose concentrations should be measured one to two weeks after each change in dosage to evaluate effectiveness.

Once control of hyperglycemia is achieved with an oral agent, the importance of continued dietary compliance should be reinforced. In obese patients who lose weight, the dose of the OHA often can be reduced and possibly discontinued. Control can then be maintained with diet and exercise alone.

OHAs do not initially control hyperglycemia in 15% to 30% of patients, depending in part on the degree of compliance with dietary restrictions. Even when initial control is established with an oral agent, secondary failure occurs in 5% of patients/year. It has been suggested that certain HLA typing patterns may identify individuals who are likely to experience secondary failures in the future (Groop et al, 1987). These individuals may have slowly developing IDDM.

If primary or secondary failure occurs, principles of dietary therapy should be re-emphasized. Another oral preparation may be substituted, although the probability of success is markedly reduced when there is a history of failure with a similar agent (unless therapeutic failure was due to bioinequivalence; see the evaluations on Tolazamide and Tolbutamide). The circumstances associated with the change in drug (eg, renewed dietary compliance, increased exercise, weight reduction) may be more important to the success of therapy than the specific preparation substituted. If weight reduction, dietary restriction, exercise, and an oral agent fail to control hyperglycemia, insulin must be substituted or added.

If substitution of an oral agent for insulin is considered, a maximal dose of the OHA should be given and the insulin dose gradually reduced. If ketonuria occurs, the patient probably has IDDM and requires insulin. If hyperglycemia occurs gradually as the dose is lowered, the patient probably has NIDDM and also requires insulin. Approximately one week is necessary for the oral agent to become maximally effective.

When a patient stabilized on any diabetic regimen is exposed to stress (eg, fever, trauma, infection, surgery), a loss of control may occur. Under these circumstances, it may be necessary to discontinue an oral agent and administer insulin.

DRUG SELECTION. Results of studies comparing the effectiveness of sulfonylurea agents demonstrate that chlorpropamide, tolazamide, glyburide, and glipizide are equally effective; tolbutamide and acetohexamide are less effective. If blood glucose is not controlled in a patient receiving the maximal dose of one of the four most effective OHAs, substituting the maximal dose of another of these agents will restore diabetic control in only a small percentage of patients (estimated <10%).

The second-generation drugs are essentially therapeutically equivalent, but some differences exist. Although both glipizide and glyburide often can be administered once daily, glipizide has a shorter serum half-life (Nelson, 1987). Its serum concentration rises higher and more rapidly and is accompanied by greater insulin secretion initially (Groop et al, 1985). Glipizide reduced postprandial blood glucose more effectively, while glyburide was more effective in decreasing fasting blood glucose levels (Frederiksen and Mogensen, 1982) and enhancing basal insulin secretion (Groop et al, 1987); however, there is no universal agreement with this assessment. The recommended time of administration of the two drugs also differs (see the evaluations).

In patients who are well controlled using standard glyburide preparations, there is no need to substitute the newer, micronized preparation (see the evaluation).

Relative potency should not influence drug selection because maximal effectiveness is similar for all agents. A single daily dose of any sulfonylurea (except tolbutamide) is sometimes adequate to control blood glucose in NIDDM patients.

Combination Therapy: The addition of OHAs to the regimen of patients poorly controlled by insulin alone has been suggested to achieve better control. This combination also has been proposed to simplify the regimen for elderly patients who are averse to multiple daily insulin injections or to avoid the hyperinsulinemia that may be required to control blood glucose with OHAs or high doses of insulin. A subset of NIDDM patients characterized by mild obesity, poor glycemic regulation, adequate insulin reserve as demonstrated by high fasting C-peptide serum concentrations, and duration of insulin therapy of less than eight years also may benefit from combined therapy (Lewitt et al, 1989; Lebovitz and Pasmantier, 1990). Fasting serum insulin levels may not decrease even when the dose of exogenous insulin is decreased, probably because the oral agent stimulates secretion of endogenous insulin (Peters and Davidson, 1991; Pugh et al, 1992).

It also has been suggested that the addition of a bedtime dose of NPH insulin in patients not controlled by maximal doses of OHAs may improve diabetic control (Riddle, 1990). The bedtime insulin injection controls fasting glycemia and the OHA controls daytime glycemia. The advantages of this approach include patient acceptance, less disruption of lifestyle, and ease of adjustment of the single insulin dose to achieve acceptable fasting glucose levels (<120 mg/dL). Over a three-month period, the combination regimen was as effective as more traditional insulin regimens in NIDDM patients (Yki-Järvinen et al, 1992). Its effectiveness over longer periods has not been evaluated.

Combined therapy lowers glycated hemoglobin values by approximately 1%. It is currently debated whether this advantage will reduce complications and whether costs and side effects differ substantially between insulin alone and combined therapy.

ADVERSE REACTIONS AND PRECAUTIONS. Side effects are comparable with all of the sulfonylurea agents except chlorpropamide. The alcohol flushing syndrome usually occurs only with chlorpropamide. Dilutional hyponatremia (from water retention secondary to the syndrome of inappropriate secretion of antidiuretic hormone [SIADH]) also has been observed with chlorpropamide and rarely with tolbutamide. Intrahepatic cholestasis develops more frequently with chlorpropamide than with the other agents. See also the evaluations.

Hypoglycemic reactions have been reported after use of all sulfonylureas but are more common with chlorpropamide. Severe reactions are uncommon, but fatalities have occurred. Hypoglycemia also has developed in nondiabetic individuals who received sulfonylureas for other diseases on an investigational basis or who used the agents factitiously. The hypoglycemia may persist for several days and require repeated administration of intravenous dextrose; the severity of this reaction fluctuates during such episodes. Hospitalization usually is required for patients who develop severe hypoglycemia because of the need for prolonged infusions of dextrose to maintain the glucose concentration until the effect of the OHA has abated.

Hypoglycemic reactions have occurred after one dose of a sulfonylurea, after two or three days of therapy, or after many months of previously uneventful treatment. Hypoglycemia may develop after treatment with a single sulfonylurea, after substitution of one oral drug for another, or after an oral drug is substituted for insulin. It may occur in patients who receive an inappropriately large dose, in those who do not eat properly, or in those who do not metabolize or excrete the drug because of impaired renal function. Thus, these agents generally should not be used in patients with renal or hepatic disease, because they are more vulnerable to the hypoglycemic effects. These factors become even more significant in the elderly, who appear to be more sensitive to sulfonylurea agents and, in addition, may be more likely to have insufficient food intake. Hypoglycemia in elderly or debilitated patients may develop insidiously and may be manifested as brain dysfunction and, ultimately, coma. A decreased rate of drug excretion is likely to intensify the hypoglycemia. Thus, because of the potential for hyponatremia and prolonged hypoglycemia, chlorpropamide usually is not recommended for older patients.

Mild hypoglycemia should be treated with oral dextrose and adjustment of drug dosage and/or meal patterns. In severe hypoglycemic episodes with coma, seizure, or other neurologic impairment, the patient should be given dextrose injection intravenously (50% dextrose followed by 10% dextrose to maintain the blood glucose level above 100 mg/dL). If glucagon is available, it should be administered before the paramedics arrive or the patient is transported to the emergency room. Patients should be monitored in the hospital for one or two days thereafter, since hypoglycemia may recur after apparent recovery.

Allergic skin reactions (pruritus, erythema, urticaria, morbilliform or maculopapular rash, lichenoid reactions) have been noted after use of sulfonylureas and biguanides. Most of these effects are transient and may disappear with continued use; if they persist, the drug should be discontinued. Photosensitivity has been reported with all sulfonylureas. Gastrointestinal disturbances (eg, nausea, heartburn, abdominal pain, vomiting, diarrhea, epigastric fullness) are more common with the biguanides but can occur with sulfonylureas. They are alleviated by taking the drug with meals, adjusting the dosage, or dividing the medication into two or three smaller doses each day. If symptoms persist, the drug should be discontinued at least temporarily.

Water retention and subsequent dilutional hyponatremia (SIADH) has been reported after administration of chlorpropamide and rarely with tolbutamide, particularly in patients with a tendency to retain water (eg, those with congestive heart failure or hepatic cirrhosis, those receiving thiazide diuretics). Tolazamide, glipizide, and glyburide are mildly diuretic.

Hyponatremia is a reflection of serum hypo-osmolarity. Sodium excretion persists despite the hyponatremia and is accompanied by impaired ability to dilute urine and to excrete a water load. Chlorpropamide may potentiate endogenous antidiuretic hormone activity at the renal tubular level and augment the hypothalamic-pituitary release of ADH. These abnormalities have been corrected by withdrawing the drugs but have recurred with readministration.

Leukopenia, thrombocytopenia, agranulocytosis, aplastic anemia, hemolytic anemia, pancytopenia, acute intermittent porphyria, and jaundice caused by reversible intrahepatic cholestasis have been reported rarely after use of the sulfonylureas but not the biguanides. Reversible intrahepatic cholestasis is more common with chlorpropamide than with the other sulfonylurea agents.

OHAs have not yet been shown to cause teratogenic effects in humans, but they are not recommended for diabetic women who are pregnant. Insulin is used during pregnancy, principally because the transplacental passage of OHAs may cause neonatal hypoglycemia by stimulating premature maturation of insulin secretion by the fetal pancreas.

The sulfonylureas are contraindicated in *nondiabetic* patients with renal glycosuria, since these agents may cause prolonged or fatal hypoglycemia. They also are contraindicated in patients with known hypersensitivity or allergy to them, as sole therapy for IDDM, and in diabetic ketoacidosis with or without coma.

INTERACTIONS. Agents that aggravate the diabetic state by increasing blood glucose levels include glucocorticoids, estrogens, oral contraceptives, medroxyprogesterone, thyroid hormones, thiazides and other diuretics, sympathomimetics, beta-adrenergic agonists, niacin, isoniazid, and diazoxide. Phenobarbital, rifampin [Rifadin, Rimactane], and other hepatic enzyme inhibitors (eg, alcohol, glutethimide) increase the metabolism of OHAs. Concomitant use may require an increase in the dose of the hypoglycemic agent.

Drugs that may increase the risk of hypoglycemia in patients taking sulfonylureas include insulin, alcohol, biguanides, sulfonamides, ciprofloxacin [Cipro], large doses of salicylates, phenylbutazone [Butazolidin] and other NSAIDs (eg, naproxen [Anaprox], indomethacin [Indocin]), captopril [Capoten] and other ACE inhibitors, methyldopa, dicumarol and other coumarins, chloramphenicol [Chloromycetin], monoamine oxidase inhibitors, beta-adrenergic blocking agents, anabolic steroids, fenfluramine [Pondimin], probenecid, sulfinpyrazone, some azoles (eg, fluconazole [Diflucan], miconazole [Monistat]) and other antifungal agents, cimetidine [Tagamet], magnesium hydroxide, pentamidine, lithium, mebendazole [Vermox], and clofibrate [Atromid-S]. Glipizide and glyburide are less easily displaced from protein binding sites than other oral agents, and the risk of hypoglycemia when they are taken with drugs that are highly protein bound is theoretically lower, although there is as yet no clinical evidence to support this assumption.

Hypoglycemia may be difficult to recognize in patients taking propranolol [Inderal] and other beta blockers because these agents inhibit tachycardia and tremors (but not sweating) induced by hypoglycemia from any cause, including OHAs. Chlorpropamide may decrease tolerance to alcohol; this is manifested by unusual flushing of the skin, particularly of the face and neck, similar to that caused by disulfiram [Antabuse]. Patients taking chlorpropamide may be more likely to develop hyponatremia if thiazide diuretics are taken concomitantly (Kadowaki et al, 1983). The glycemic control of patients taking vitamin E supplements may be falsely exaggerated because this agent suppresses hemoglobin glycation.

Other discussions of adverse effects and interactions with OHAs (Jackson and Bressler, 1981; Paice et al, 1985) and effects of other drugs on glucose tolerance (O'Byrne and Feely, 1990) are available.

Drug Evaluations

SULFONYLUREA COMPOUNDS

ACETOHEXAMIDE

[Dymelor]

$$CH_3\overset{O}{\overset{\|}{C}}-C_6H_4-SO_2NH\overset{O}{\overset{\|}{C}}NH-C_6H_{11}$$

ACTIONS AND USES. Acetohexamide is similar to other OHAs in the sulfonylurea class. Although it is less effective than chlorpropamide, tolazamide, glyburide, and glipizide, some clinicians prefer this agent for diabetic patients with gout because of its uricosuric effect. Acetohexamide is hydroxylated in the liver to hydroxyhexamide, a metabolite with 2.5 times the hypoglycemic effect of the parent compound.

ADVERSE REACTIONS AND PRECAUTIONS. The incidence of untoward effects is low and reactions are reversible when acetohexamide is discontinued. Relatively severe hypoglycemic reactions have been observed occasionally in patients given large doses for prolonged periods without close observation. Since the active metabolite is excreted by the kidney, this drug should be avoided in patients with renal dysfunction. Acetohexamide is classified in FDA Pregnancy Category C.

See also the introduction to the section on Oral Hypoglycemic Agents.

DOSAGE AND PREPARATIONS.
Oral: Dosage should be individualized. The usual range is 500 mg to 1.5 g daily. Doses in excess of this amount will not improve control. Many patients receiving 1 g or less per day can be given the full amount once daily; however, the drug should be given in divided doses before the morning and evening meals if more than 1 g is required.

Dymelor (Lilly), ***Generic.*** Tablets 250 and 500 mg.

CHLORPROPAMIDE
[Diabinese]

$Cl-\bigcirc-SO_2NH\overset{O}{\overset{\|}{C}}NHCH_2CH_2CH_3$

ACTIONS AND USES. Chlorpropamide has essentially the same actions, uses, and limitations as the other sulfonylureas. It has the longest duration of action (one to three days). Primary and secondary failures have been reported less frequently than with tolbutamide. (See also the introduction to this section.)

ADVERSE REACTIONS AND PRECAUTIONS. Untoward reactions have been reported more frequently with chlorpropamide than with other sulfonylureas, and the drug should be used with caution. In a few older patients, hypoglycemic reactions have been severe. Water retention with hyponatremia can be life-threatening in patients with a tendency to retain water (eg, those with congestive heart failure or hepatic cirrhosis). Elderly patients and those taking thiazide diuretics may be more likely to develop this complication. This drug should not be used in patients with renal insufficiency because the duration of action is greatly prolonged and active metabolites are excreted by the kidney. This drug generally is not given to elderly patients.

Facial flushing after ingestion of alcohol occurs in up to one-third of patients taking chlorpropamide. The mechanism, like that of the disulfiram reaction, probably involves inhibition of the oxidation of acetaldehyde, a metabolite of ethanol. The plasma concentration of chlorpropamide may be correlated with chlorpropamide-alcohol flushing (Jerntorp et al, 1983; Groop et al, 1984).

See also the introduction to this section.

This drug is classified in FDA Pregnancy Category C.

PHARMACOKINETICS. Chlorpropamide is metabolized by the liver and unchanged drug and metabolites are excreted by the kidney; 80% to 90% of a single oral dose is excreted within four days.

DOSAGE AND PREPARATIONS.
Oral: Dosage should be individualized; the total amount is given once daily with breakfast. For *middle-aged patients,* initially, up to 250 mg daily, depending on the severity of hyperglycemia. After five to seven days, the blood glucose level reaches a plateau and the dose may be increased or decreased by 50 to 125 mg at weekly intervals. The maintenance dose depends on the response of the patient and the severity of the disease; the usual range is 100 to 750 mg daily. Patients who do not respond adequately to 750 mg daily usually will not respond to larger doses.

Diabinese (Pfizer), ***Generic.*** Tablets 100 and 250 mg.

GLIPIZIDE
[Glucotrol]

$H_3C-(\text{pyrazine})-\overset{O}{\overset{\|}{C}}NHCH_2CH_2-\bigcirc-\underset{O}{\underset{\|}{\overset{O}{\overset{\|}{S}}}}NH\overset{O}{\overset{\|}{C}}NH-(\text{cyclohexyl})$

ACTIONS AND USES. Glipizide is similar to other OHAs in the sulfonylurea class. This second-generation sulfonylurea is at least 100 times as potent as tolbutamide on a weight basis, but the maximal hypoglycemic effect is similar to that produced by the other sulfonylureas.

A single morning dose of glipizide stimulates insulin secretion after three meals over a 12-hour period. Fasting insulin levels are not elevated. Peripheral effects include increased glucose uptake and suppression of hepatic glucose production (Lebovitz, 1985). These effects on insulin secretion persist for more than three years. Long-term control (more than six years) has been reported in more than two-thirds of patients with NIDDM who responded initially. Glipizide has a mild diuretic effect.

ADVERSE REACTIONS. Glipizide is relatively free of serious adverse effects and only approximately 1.5% of patients discontinued this drug because of adverse reactions. Gastrointestinal disturbances are most common (incidence, 1.7% to 3.7%); skin rashes occur in up to 1.4% of patients. This drug is classified in FDA Pregnancy Category C.

See also the introduction to this section.

PHARMACOKINETICS. Glipizide is rapidly and completely absorbed after oral administration, and peak serum concentrations are observed 1 to 3.5 hours after ingestion. Because the presence of food delays absorption, the drug should be taken approximately 30 minutes prior to a meal. Glipizide is 98.4% nonionically bound to plasma albumin. The drug is metabolized in the liver to inactive metabolites. Most of these metabolites, as well as less than 10% of unchanged drug, are excreted in the urine.

DOSAGE AND PREPARATIONS.
Oral: Dosage should be individualized. The drug should be given 30 minutes before a meal for greatest efficacy. The usual initial dose is 5 mg given before breakfast. Elderly patients or those with liver disease may be given 2.5 mg initially. One week should elapse before the dose is increased, and

the amount should be based on the blood glucose level. Increments of 2.5 to 5 mg may be used. Daily doses exceeding 15 mg should be divided and given before meals. Alternatively, the first 20 mg may be given before breakfast and the remaining amount before the evening meal. The maximum recommended daily dose is 40 mg. However, in one placebo-controlled, double-blind crossover study, no further improvement was achieved with dosages >10 mg/day (Stenman et al, 1993).

Glucotrol (Pratt). Tablets 5 and 10 mg.

GLYBURIDE

[*Regular:* DiaBeta, Micronase; *Micronized:* Glynase]

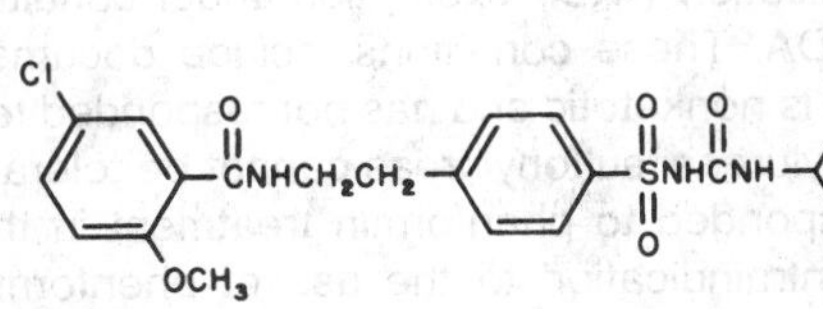

ACTIONS AND USES. Glyburide (glibenclamide in Europe) has actions and uses similar to those of the other sulfonylureas. This drug is 200 times more potent than tolbutamide on a weight basis, but the maximal hypoglycemic effect is similar to that of the other sulfonylureas. Glyburide stimulates secretion of insulin but also increases peripheral sensitivity to insulin by a postreceptor mechanism. Inhibition of hepatic glucose production is an important factor in glycemic control (Simonson et al, 1984). Glyburide has mild diuretic activity.

Primary and secondary therapeutic failures occur, and the overall failure rate after 1.5 years is 10% to 15%.

ADVERSE REACTIONS. The incidence of serious side effects with glyburide is low. Gastrointestinal disturbances develop in 1.8% of patients. Skin rashes occur in 1.5% of patients and may disappear with continued use. This drug is classified in FDA Pregnancy Category B.

PHARMACOKINETICS. Glyburide is absorbed rapidly, and the peak serum concentration occurs 4 to 5.3 hours after ingestion. Bioavailability is greater (90% to 100% versus 60% to 80%) with the micronized preparation, although efficacy is equivalent (5 mg glyburide is equivalent to 3 mg of the micronized preparation). More than 97% of the drug is nonionically bound to serum proteins. Glyburide is metabolized by the liver; about 50% of the metabolites are excreted in the urine, and the rest are excreted in the bile. When patients are switched from other OHAs or from the regular to the micronized form of glyburide, the dosage should be adjusted because equivalence of serum levels among these products are not exact.

See also the introduction to this section. Review articles on glyburide are available (Gavin, 1990).

DOSAGE AND PREPARATIONS. Dosage should be individualized.

REGULAR TABLETS:

Oral: Glyburide should be taken with breakfast or the first main meal. The usual initial dose is 2.5 to 5 mg daily, but 1.25 mg may be adequate in more responsive patients. *Elderly, debilitated, or malnourished patients, or those with liver or renal disease* may be given 1.25 mg daily. The dose may be increased by maximal increments of 2.5 mg at weekly intervals and should be based on the blood glucose level. The usual maintenance dose is 1.25 to 20 mg daily. Amounts larger than 10 mg may be divided into two daily doses.

DiaBeta (Hoechst), ***Micronase*** (Upjohn). Tablets 1.25, 2.5, and 5 mg.

MICRONIZED TABLETS:

Oral: Initially, 1.5 to 3 mg once daily with breakfast or the first main meal (0.75 mg once daily in those at increased risk of hypoglycemia). The dosage may be increased by 1.5 mg increments at weekly intervals until a maintenance dosage (up to 12 mg/day) is reached. Amounts ≥6 mg/day may be administered in two daily doses. Dosage should be adjusted when patients are transferred from regular glyburide or other OHAs.

Glynase (Upjohn). Tablets (micronized) 1.5, 3, 4.5, and 6 mg.

TOLAZAMIDE

[Tolinase]

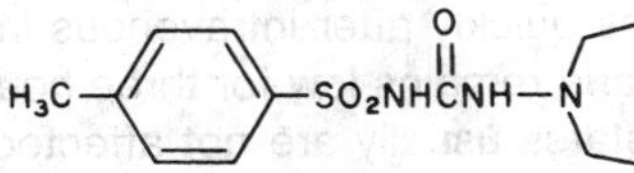

ACTIONS AND USES. Tolazamide has actions and uses similar to those of other sulfonylureas. It is metabolized in the liver to several substances, three of which have weaker hypoglycemic activity. The metabolites are excreted by the kidney. Tolazamide has mild diuretic activity.

ADVERSE REACTIONS. Generally, the untoward effects associated with tolazamide are the same as those noted with the other sulfonylureas; the incidence is low and reactions are reversible when tolazamide is discontinued. Hypoglycemia has been reported occasionally. This drug is classified in FDA Pregnancy Category C.

See also the introduction to this section.

DOSAGE AND PREPARATIONS.

Oral: Dosage should be individualized. Initially, 100 to 250 mg daily is given with breakfast or the first main meal; the amount then is adjusted weekly in increments of 100 to 250 mg. A single daily dose is effective in many patients; if more than 500 mg is required, tolazamide should be given in two daily doses. Amounts larger than 1 g daily probably will not improve control and are not recommended.

Tolinase (Upjohn), ***Generic.*** Tablets 100, 250, and 500 mg.

TOLBUTAMIDE

[Orinase]

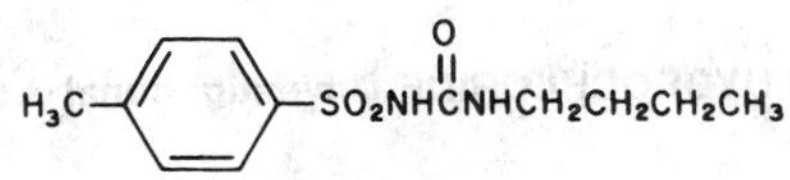

ACTIONS AND USES. Tolbutamide has the same actions, uses, and limitations as other sulfonylurea compounds. It is less effective than chlorpropamide, tolazamide, glyburide, and glipizide. Tolbutamide is metabolized in the liver mainly to two inactive metabolites, which are excreted in the urine.

ADVERSE REACTIONS. The toxicity of tolbutamide appears to be low, and reactions are similar to those observed with other sulfonylureas. This drug is classified in FDA Pregnancy Category C.

See also the introduction to this section.

DOSAGE AND PREPARATIONS.

Oral: Dosage should be individualized. Initially, 500 mg is given twice daily; the dose then is adjusted gradually until the minimal effective amount is established. The maintenance dose is 250 mg to 3 g daily. The total daily dose is given in divided amounts during the day. Doses exceeding 3 g daily are no more effective than smaller amounts and are not recommended; more than 2 g daily is seldom more effective.

Orinase (Upjohn), ***Generic.*** Tablets 250 and 500 mg.

TOLBUTAMIDE SODIUM
[Orinase Diagnostic]

In patients with pancreatic islet cell adenoma, the blood glucose level drops quickly after intravenous injection of tolbutamide sodium and remains low for three hours. Since other hypoglycemic states usually are not affected, tolbutamide sodium may be used in conjunction with estimates of plasma insulin to rule out this condition. The hypoglycemia produced can be severe and may be fatal if not treated. It is reversed with intravenous dextrose.

This agent also has been used during ulcer surgery to verify the completeness of vagus nerve section (by measurement of gastric acid secretion after tolbutamide-stimulated insulin release and subsequent hypoglycemia).

Thrombophlebitis with thrombosis of the injected vein has occurred in 0.8% to 2.4% of patients; no important sequelae have been reported. A burning sensation in the arm along the injected vein may occur. This may be avoided by administering the drug over a two- to three-minute period. Tolbutamide should not be used in patients who have previously had symptoms of allergy to the sulfonylureas.

Tolbutamide sodium is classified in FDA Pregnancy Category C.

DOSAGE AND PREPARATIONS.

Intravenous (diagnostic): 1 g.

Orinase Diagnostic (Upjohn). Powder (sterile, for diagnostic use only) 1 g (present as 1.081 g tolbutamide sodium) with diluent. This preparation must be ordered through a sales representative or distribution center.

BIGUANIDE COMPOUND

PHENFORMIN HYDROCHLORIDE (Investigational drug)

$$C_6H_5-CH_2CH_2NH\underset{\parallel}{\overset{\overset{+}{NH_2}}{C}}NH\underset{\parallel}{\overset{NH}{C}}NH_2 \quad Cl^-$$

STATUS. The FDA removed this drug from general distribution in the United States in 1977 because of the lactic acidosis associated with its use. This complication usually occurs in diabetic patients who have renal insufficiency or are seriously ill with conditions accompanied by hypoxia (eg, cardiac failure, hypotension, liver disease, pulmonary embolism), in those who take the drug with alcohol, or following severe anorexia or vomiting and ketosis; however, lactic acidosis may develop without predisposing conditions. The mortality rate is approximately 50%. Probably very few, if any, patients who cannot be managed by other therapeutic measures require phenformin.

Phenformin is now available only under an Investigational New Drug Application (IND) exemption under conditions set forth by the FDA. These conditions include documentation that the patient is nonketotic and has not responded to diet or diet plus sulfonylureas; sulfonylureas cannot be tolerated; the patient has responded to phenformin treatment in the past; there is no contraindication to the use of phenformin; and insulin cannot be taken. Informed consent must be obtained from the patient or guardian. Physicians may request further information in writing from the Division of Metabolism and Endocrine Drug Products (HFD-510), Room 14B03, Center for Drug Evaluation and Research, Food and Drug Administration, 5600 Fishers Lane, Rockville, MD 20857.

ACTIONS. Phenformin is not related chemically to the insulins or the sulfonylureas. It does not stimulate insulin secretion from the islet cells. Possible mechanisms of action include inhibition of hepatic gluconeogenesis, decreased intestinal absorption of glucose, and increased anaerobic glycolysis, which increases glucose utilization. Large doses appear to inhibit the conversion of alanine and lactate to glucose (gluconeogenesis), whereas small doses enhance glycolysis without inhibiting gluconeogenesis or the conversion of lactate to glucose in vitro. However, it is not known if these effects are responsible for the hypoglycemic action noted with usual doses.

Although some physicians believe that phenformin may cause weight loss in obese, mildly diabetic patients, some double-blind studies have not confirmed this finding. In addition to inducing anorexia, phenformin may retard the absorption of food. This agent inhibits the uptake of glucose by isolated, full-thickness human ileum.

Occasionally, patients in whom normal blood glucose concentrations are maintained by phenformin may experience weight loss, asthenia, and "starvation" ketonuria unless insulin also is administered. Phenformin alone rarely causes hypoglycemia, but this has occurred when it was given with another OHA or after suicide attempts with the drug (Davidson et al, 1966).

HYPERGLYCEMIC AGENTS

Hypoglycemic reactions may follow the use of alcohol and many drugs (eg, large doses of salicylates, propranolol and other beta-adrenergic blocking agents) but are most common after administration of insulin or the sulfonylureas. (See the sections on Hypoglycemia under Insulin Use in Special Situations and Adverse Reactions and Precautions under Oral Hypoglycemic Agents.) The diabetic patient must be aware of the earliest manifestations of hypoglycemia so that a readily available carbohydrate (eg, fruit juice, sugar) can be taken immediately.

For severe hypoglycemia and in unconscious or stuporous patients, intravenous 50% dextrose is preferred, but glucagon may be given intramuscularly (for increased rate of absorption) or subcutaneously before paramedics arrive. Upon rousing, carbohydrate is given orally. Subsequent management of severe hypoglycemia depends on the patient's clinical status and the blood glucose levels; hospitalization usually is required.

Hyperglycemic agents counteract the effects of increased levels of insulin in pathologic states. Diazoxide [Proglycem] blocks insulin secretion and is sometimes given preoperatively for insulinomas. Therapy may be prolonged in patients with small islet cell tumors or when tumors cannot be found at surgery. This agent is sometimes used with streptozocin [Zanosar]. The latter destroys the beta cells of the islet tissue and is used for malignant insulinomas (see also index entry Streptozocin, As Antineoplastic Agent).

Reactive (functional) hypoglycemia is rare. Diagnosis requires documentation of low blood glucose at the time symptoms are experienced, which can be accomplished by examining a sample of capillary blood on filter paper (Palardy et al, 1989). Treatment is primarily dietary. Hyperglycemic agents are not indicated in this condition.

Drug Evaluations

DIAZOXIDE

[Proglycem]

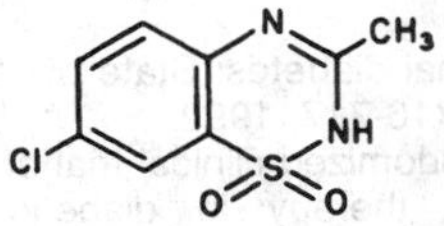

ACTIONS AND USES. This nondiuretic thiazide is used for its hyperglycemic actions when given orally. It produces a prompt, dose-related increase in blood glucose by directly inhibiting insulin secretion and, possibly, by stimulating epinephrine secretion by the adrenal medulla. Diazoxide is used to counteract hyperinsulinism in conditions such as insulinoma. It is not indicated in the treatment of functional hypoglycemia.

ADVERSE REACTIONS, PRECAUTIONS, AND INTERACTIONS. Although diazoxide is a thiazide, it causes sodium and water retention that may necessitate concurrent administration of a diuretic; thiazide diuretics may intensify the drug's hyperglycemic and hyperuricemic effects. Oral diazoxide may potentiate the effects of other antihypertensive drugs, although the effect on blood pressure is not marked when this agent is used alone orally. The hyperglycemic action of diazoxide is antagonized by alpha-adrenergic blocking agents.

Diazoxide also may cause gastrointestinal irritation, thrombocytopenia, eosinophilia, neutropenia, and tachycardia. Excessive hair growth of a lanugo type occurs most frequently in children and is reversible when the drug is withdrawn.

Diazoxide is teratogenic in animals (cardiovascular and skeletal deformities) and causes degeneration of fetal beta islet cells. The safety of this drug in pregnant women has not been established (FDA Pregnancy Category C).

PHARMACOKINETICS. Over 90% of diazoxide is bound to plasma proteins in the blood. The half-life of the oral form is 24 to 36 hours but may be prolonged after overdosage or in individuals with impaired renal function. Because of its long half-life, prolonged observation of patients is necessary. Overdosage can cause marked hyperglycemia sometimes associated with ketoacidosis or nonketotic hyperosmolar coma.

DOSAGE AND PREPARATIONS.

Oral: *Adults and children,* 3 to 8 mg/kg daily; *infants,* 8 to 15 mg/kg daily. The drug is given in two or three equally divided doses.

Proglycem (Baker Norton). Capsules 50 mg; oral suspension 50 mg/ml (alcohol 7.25%).

GLUCAGON

ACTIONS AND USES. Glucagon is a polypeptide produced by the alpha cells of the pancreas. Like insulin, its normal function appears to be to control the homeostasis of glucose, amino acids, and possibly free fatty acids. However, its potent glycogenolytic and gluconeogenic effects are opposite those of insulin and form the basis for glucagon's clinical usefulness. Glucagon also reduces gastric and pancreatic secretions. It increases myocardial contractility but relaxes smooth muscle.

This drug is given principally to treat severe hypoglycemia in diabetic patients. It is often administered by a member of the family at home when a severe hypoglycemic episode occurs and the patient is unable to ingest sugar or simple carbohydrates or is unconscious. An intranasal spray preparation of glucagon is being investigated and may be useful for initial treatment of hypoglycemia (Freychet et al, 1988; Pontiroli et al, 1989).

Glucagon increases the blood glucose concentration by mobilizing hepatic glycogen and thus is effective only when hepatic glycogen is available. Patients with reduced glycogen stores (eg, starvation, adrenal insufficiency, alcoholic hypoglycemia) cannot respond to glucagon.

Glucagon also has been used to diagnose insulinoma and pheochromocytoma. For the former, the rise in plasma insulin concentration following intravenous glucagon may be diagnostic. Other uses (eg, cardiovascular emergencies, meat impaction in the esophagus, beta blocker overdose) have been reviewed (Hall-Boyer et al, 1984).

ADMINISTRATION. Glucagon is effective only when administered parenterally. Its hyperglycemic effect is more gradual than that of dextrose and is of relatively brief duration. However, the blood glucose level often is elevated enough to rouse the unconscious patient to take oral carbohydrate (first simple sugars, then complex carbohydrates for sustained effect), which restores hepatic glycogen and prevents secondary hypoglycemia. If carbohydrate is not ingested, blood glucose levels usually fall to normal or hypoglycemic levels in 60 to 90 minutes. An additional sugar source is especially important in juveniles, since their response is less pronounced than that of adults with stable diabetes. If intravenous dextrose is available, it should be used in comatose patients to avoid the deleterious effects of prolonged cerebral hypoglycemia.

ADVERSE REACTIONS. Nausea and vomiting have occurred occasionally after injection of glucagon; these effects also develop, but less frequently, with hypoglycemia. Hypersensitivity reactions are possible. This drug is classified in FDA Pregnancy Category B.

DOSAGE AND PREPARATIONS.

Intramuscular, Intravenous, Subcutaneous: *Adults and children,* 0.5 to 1 mg (usually subcutaneously, but intramuscularly or intravenously if desired) every 15 to 20 minutes for two or three doses.

The manufacturer's literature also contains instructions for the administration of glucagon by a family member; however, the drug should be used only under the direction of the physician. If it is used in an emergency, the physician should be notified. Any patient receiving insulin therapy should have glucagon available; adult family members or a responsible friend should be instructed on proper administration.

Glucagon (Lilly). Powder (lyophilized) 1 and 10 mg with diluent (see the manufacturer's literature for directions on preparing the solution); solution (for injection) 1 mg with diluent in 1-ml disposable syringe (***Glucagon Emergency Kit***).

Cited References

Adams PS, et al: Stability of insulin mixtures in disposable plastic insulin syringes. *J Pharm Pharmacol* 39:158-163, 1987.

Alberti KGMM: Low-dose insulin in treatment of diabetic ketoacidosis. *Arch Intern Med* 137:1367-1376, 1977.

American Diabetes Association: Position Statement: Office guide to diagnosis and classification of diabetes mellitus and other categories of glucose intolerance. *Diabetes Care* 4:335, 1981.

American Diabetes Association: Policy Statement: Glycemic effects of carbohydrates. *Diabetes Care* 7:607-608, 1984.

American Diabetes Association: Position Statement: Continuous subcutaneous insulin infusion. *Diabetes* 34:946-947, 1985.

American Diabetes Association: Nutritional recommendations and principles for individuals with diabetes mellitus: 1986. *Diabetes Care* 10:126-132, 1987 A.

American Diabetes Association: Consensus Statement: Self-monitoring of blood glucose. *Diabetes Care* 10:95-99, 1987 B.

American Diabetes Association Task Force: Position statement on jet injectors. *Diabetes Care* 11:600-601, 1988.

American Diabetes Association: Consensus Statement: Role of cardiovascular risk factors in prevention and treatment of macrovascular disease in diabetes. *Diabetes Care* 13:573-579, 1989.

American Diabetes Association: Position Statement: Prevention of type I diabetes mellitus. *Diabetes Care* 13:1026-1027, 1990 A.

American Diabetes Association: Position Statement: Insulin administration. *Diabetes Care* 13(suppl 1):28-31, 1990 B.

American Diabetes Association: Position Statement: Gestational diabetes mellitus. *Diabetes Care* 16(suppl 2):5-6, 1993.

American Diabetes Association: Position Statement: Implications of the Diabetes Control and Complications Trial. *Clin Diabetes* 91, 95-96, (July/Aug) 1993 A.

Anderson JW, Gustafson NJ: Type II diabetes: Current nutrition management concepts. *Geriatrics* 41:28-35, 1986.

Atiea JA, et al: Dawn phenomenon: Its frequency in non-insulin-dependent diabetic patients on conventional therapy. *Diabetes Care* 10:461-465, 1987.

Bantle JP, et al: Metabolic effects of dietary sucrose in type II diabetic subjects. *Diabetes Care* 16:1301-1305, 1993.

Becerra JE, et al: Diabetes mellitus during pregnancy and the risks for specific birth defects: A population-based case-control study. *Pediatrics* 85:1-9, 1990.

Bending JJ, et al: Eight-month correction of hyperglycemia in insulin-dependent diabetes mellitus is associated with a significant and sustained reduction of urinary albumin excretion rates in patients with microalbuminuria. *Diabetes* 34(suppl 3):69-73, 1985.

Best JD, et al: Clinical effects of mixing short- and intermediate-acting insulins in treatment of non-insulin-dependent diabetes. *Med J Aust* 146:621-627, 1987.

Bilo HJ, et al: Absorption kinetics and action profiles after sequential subcutaneous administration of human soluble and lente insulin through one needle. *Diabetes Care* 10:466-469, 1987.

Bolli GB, Gerich JE: "Dawn phenomenon": Common occurrence in both non-insulin-dependent and insulin-dependent diabetes mellitus. *N Engl J Med* 310:746-750, 1984.

Bolli GB, et al: Demonstration of dawn phenomenon in normal human volunteers. *Diabetes* 33:1150-1153, 1984 A.

Bolli GB, et al: Glucose counterregulation and waning of insulin in Somogyi phenomenon (posthypoglycemic hyperglycemia). *N Engl J Med* 311:1214-1219, 1984 B.

Bonner RA: Insulin infusion therapy: Potential benefits and risks. *Postgrad Med* 77:153-164, (June) 1985.

Brown MJ, Asbury AK: Diabetic neuropathy. *Ann Neurol* 15:2-12, 1984.

Campbell PJ, et al: Pathogenesis of dawn phenomenon in patients with insulin-dependent diabetes mellitus: Accelerated glucose production and impaired glucose utilization due to nocturnal surges in growth hormone secretion. *N Engl J Med* 312:1473-1479, 1985.

Chase HP, et al: Glucose control and the renal and retinal complications of insulin-dependent diabetes. *JAMA* 261:1155-1160, 1989.

Cook DW, Sasaki T: Current status of pancreas transplantation. *West J Med* 150:309-313, 1989.

Cousins L: Congenital anomalies among infants of diabetic mothers: Etiology, prevention, prenatal diagnosis. *Am J Obstet Gynecol* 147:333-338, 1983.

Coustan DR: Gestational diabetes: State of the union, commentary. *Diabetes Care* 15:716-717, 1992.

Coustan DR, et al: Randomized clinical trial of insulin pump vs intensive conventional therapy in diabetic pregnancies. *JAMA* 255:631-636, 1986.

Cryer PE: Iatrogenic hypoglycaemia in people with type I diabetes: Consequences, risk factors and prevention, in Marshall SM, et al (eds): *The Diabetes Annual*, ed 7. New York, Elsevier Science Publishers, 1993, 317-331.

Dahl-Jørgensen K, et al: Reduction of urinary albumin excretion after 4 years of continuous subcutaneous insulin infusion in insulin-dependent diabetes mellitus: The Oslo Study. *Acta Endocrinol (Copenh)* 117:19-25, 1988.

Damm P, et al: Predictive factors for the development of diabetes in women with previous gestational diabetes mellitus. *Am J Obstet Gynecol* 167:607-616, 1992.

Davidson MB: Pathogenesis of impaired glucose tolerance and type II diabetes mellitus: Current status. *West J Med* 142:219-229, 1985.

Davidson JK: Transferring patients with insulin-dependent diabetes mellitus from animal-source insulins to recombinant DNA human insulin: Clinical experience. *Clin Ther* 11:319-330, 1989.

Davidson MB: *Diabetes Mellitus: Diagnosis and Treatment,* ed 3. New York, Churchill-Livingstone, 1991.

Davidson MB: Successful treatment of markedly symptomatic patients with type II diabetes mellitus using high doses of sulfonylu-

rea agents, correspondence. *West J Med* 157:199-200, (Aug) 1992.
Davidson MB, et al: Phenformin, hypoglycemia and lactic acidosis. *N Engl J Med* 275:886-888, 1966.
Diabetes Control and Complications Trial Research Group: The effect of intensive treatment of diabetes on the development and progression of long-term complications in insulin-dependent diabetes mellitus. *N Engl J Med* 329:977-986, 1993.
Donahue RP, et al: Hyperinsulinemia and elevated blood pressure: Cause, confounder, or coincidence? *Am J Epidemiol* 132:827-836, 1990.
Dunger DB: Diabetes in puberty. *Arch Dis Child* 67:569-570, 1992.
Edsberg B, et al: Sprinkler needle spreads insulin load for diabetic patients. *BMJ* 294:1373-1376, 1987.
Eisenbarth GS, Di Mario U (eds): Immunotherapy of insulin-dependent diabetes mellitus: Practical prevention of IDDM through immunosuppressive therapy. *Diabetes Spectrum* 5:267-306, 1992.
Eriksson J, et al: Early metabolic defects in persons at increased risk for non-insulin-dependent diabetes mellitus. *N Engl J Med* 321:337-343, 1989.
Feldt-Rasmussen B, et al: Effect of two years of strict metabolic control on progression of incipient nephropathy in insulin-dependent diabetes. *Lancet* 2:1300-1304, 1986.
Felig P, Bergman M: Insulin pump treatment of diabetes: Decision-making without definitive data. *JAMA* 250:1045-1047, 1983.
Firth R, et al: Insulin action in non-insulin dependent diabetes mellitus: Relationship between hepatic and extrahepatic insulin resistance and obesity. *Metabolism* 36:1091-1095, 1987.
Frederiksen PK, Mogensen EF: Clinical comparison between glipizide (Glibenese) and glibenclamide (Daonil) in treatment of maturity onset diabetes: Controlled double-blind cross-over study. *Curr Ther Res* 32:1-7, 1982.
Freinkel N (ed): Summary and recommendations of Second International Workshop-Conference on Gestational Diabetes Mellitus. *Diabetes* 34 (suppl 2):123-126, 1985.
Freinkel N, et al: Care of the pregnant woman with insulin-dependent diabetes mellitus. *N Engl J Med* 313:96-101, 1985.
Freychet L, et al: Effect of intranasal glucagon on blood glucose levels in healthy subjects and hypoglycaemic patients with insulin-dependent diabetes. *Lancet* 1:1364-1366, 1988.
Gallina DL, et al: Surgery in the diabetic patient. *Compr Ther* 9:8-16, (Feb) 1983.
Ganz MA, et al: Resistance and allergy to recombinant human insulin. *J Allergy Clin Immunol* 86:45-62, (July) 1990.
Garg A: Dietary recommendations for patients with non-insulin-dependent diabetes mellitus. *Compr Ther* 17:25-31, (Nov) 1991.
Gavin JR III (ed): Glyburide: New insights into its effects on the beta cell and beyond. *Am J Med* 89 (suppl 2A): 2A-1S-2A-53S, 1990.
Genuth S: Insulin use in NIDDM. *Diabetes Care* 13:1240-1264, 1990.
Godine JE: Relationship between metabolic control and vascular complications of diabetes mellitus. *Med Clin North Am* 72:1271-1284, 1988.
Gorsuch AN, et al: Can future type I diabetes be predicted? Study in families of affected children. *Diabetes* 31:862-866, 1982.
Graves L III: Diabetic ketoacidosis and hyperosmolar hyperglycemic nonketotic coma. *Crit Care Nurs Q* 13:50-61, (Nov) 1990.
Groop L, et al: Chlorpropamide-alcohol flush: Significance of body weight, sex and serum chlorpropamide level. *Eur J Clin Pharmacol* 26:723-725, 1984.
Groop L, et al: Pharmacokinetics and metabolic effects of glibenclamide and glipizide in type 2 diabetics. *Eur J Clin Pharmacol* 28:687-704, 1985.
Groop L, et al: Comparison of pharmacokinetics, metabolic effects and mechanisms of action of glyburide and glipizide during long-term treatment. *Diabetes Care* 10:671-678, 1987.
Hall-Boyer K, et al: Glucagon: Hormone or therapeutic agent? *Crit Care Med* 12:584-589, 1984.
Hanssen KF, et al: Blood glucose control and diabetic microvascular complications: Long-term effects of near-normoglycaemia. *Diabetic Med* 9:697-705, 1992.
Havlin CE, Cryer PE: Nocturnal hypoglycemia does not commonly result in major morning hyperglycemia in patients with diabetes mellitus. *Diabetes Care* 10:141-147, 1987.
Heber D, et al: Low-dose continuous insulin therapy for diabetic ketoacidosis: Prospective comparison with "conventional" insulin therapy. *Arch Intern Med* 137:1377-1380, 1977.
Heine RJ, et al: Absorption kinetics and action profiles of mixtures of short- and intermediate-acting insulins. *Diabetologia* 27:558-562, 1984.
Hirsch IB, et al: Intensive insulin therapy for treatment of type I diabetes. *Diabetes Care* 1265-1283, 1990 A.
Hirsch IB, et al: Failure of nocturnal hypoglycemia to cause daytime hyperglycemia in patients with IDDM. *Diabetes Care* 13:133-142, 1990 B.
Hirsch IB, et al: Higher glycemic thresholds for symptoms during β-adrenergic blockade in IDDM. *Diabetes* 40:1177-1186, 1991.
Howard-Williams J, et al: Retinopathy associated with higher glycaemia in maturity-onset type diabetes. *Diabetologia* 27:198-202, 1984.
Jackson JE, Bressler R: Clinical pharmacology of sulphonylurea hypoglycaemic agents, part II. *Drugs* 22:295-320, 1981.
Jawadi MH, Ho LS: Stability and reproducibility of biologic activity of premixed and short-acting and intermediate-acting insulins. *Am J Med* 81:467-471, 1986.
Jerntorp P, et al: Plasma chlorpropamide: Critical factor in chlorpropamide-alcohol flush. *Eur J Clin Pharmacol* 24:237-242, 1983.
Kadowaki T, et al: Chlorpropamide-induced hyponatremia: Incidence and risk factors. *Diabetes Care* 6:468-471, 1983.
Kahn SE, Porte D Jr: Islet dysfunction in non-insulin-dependent diabetes mellitus. *Am J Med* 85 (suppl 5A):4-8, 1988.
Karjalainen J, et al: A bovine albumin peptide as a possible trigger of insulin-dependent diabetes mellitus. *N Engl J Med* 327:302-307, 1992.
Keen H: The genetics of diabetes: From nightmare to headache. *BMJ* 294:917-919, 1987.
Keller RJ, et al: Insulin prophylaxis in individuals at high risk of type I diabetes. *Lancet* 341:927-928, 1993.
Kennedy WR, et al: Effects of pancreatic transplantation on diabetic neuropathy. *N Engl J Med* 322:1031-1037, 1990.
Kirchain WR, Rendell MS: Aldose reductase inhibitors. *Pharmacotherapy* 10:326-336, 1990.
Kitabchi AE, Murphy MB: Diabetic ketoacidosis and hyperosmolar hyperglycemic nonketotic coma. *Med Clin North Am* 72:1545-1563, 1988.
Klein BEK, et al: Effect of pregnancy on progression of diabetic retinopathy. *Diabetes Care* 13:34-40, 1990.
Klip A, Leiter LA: Cellular mechanism of action of metformin. *Diabetes Care* 13:696-704, 1990.
Kolata G: Dietary dogma disproved. *Science* 220:487-488, 1983.
Kreisberg RA: Diabetic ketoacidosis: New concepts and trends in pathogenesis and treatment. *Ann Intern Med* 88:681-695, 1978.
Lacy PE: Status of islet cell transplantation. *Diabetes Rev* 1:76-92, (Spring) 1993.
Leahy JL: Natural history of β-cell dysfunction in NIDDM. *Diabetes Care* 13:992-1010, 1990.
Lebovitz HE: Glipizide: Second-generation sulfonylurea hypoglycemic agent: Pharmacology, pharmacokinetics and clinical use. *Pharmacotherapy* 5:63-77, 1985.
Lebovitz HE: Diabetes management: Case of near-normoglycemic regulation. *Drug Ther* 37-56, (Oct) 1987.
Lebovitz HE: Oral antidiabetic agents: The emergence of α-glucosidase inhibitors. *Drugs* 44 (suppl 3):21-28, 1992.
Lebovitz HE, Pasmantier R: Combination insulin-sulfonylurea therapy. *Diabetes Care* 13:667-675, 1990.
Lerman IG, Wolfsdorf JI: Relationship of nocturnal hypoglycemia to daytime glycemia in IDDM. *Diabetes Care* 11:636-642, 1988.
Lernmark A, et al: Autoimmunity of diabetes. *Endocrinol Metab Clin North Am* 20:589-617, 1991.
Lewitt MS, et al: Effects of combined insulin-sulfonylurea therapy in type II patients. *Diabetes Care* 12:379-383, 1989.
Maclaren N, Atkinson M: Is insulin-dependent diabetes mellitus environmentally induced? Editorial. *N Engl J Med* 327:348-349, 1992.

Marchetti P, Navalesi R: Pharmacokinetic-pharmacodynamic relationships of oral hypoglycemic agents: Update. *Clin Pharmacokinet* 16:100-128, 1989.

Marks JB, Skyler JS: Clinical review 17: Immunotherapy of type I diabetes mellitus. *J Clin Endocrinol Metab* 72:3-9, 1991.

Martin AO, et al: Frequency of diabetes mellitus in mothers of probands with gestational diabetes: Possible maternal influence on the predisposition to gestational diabetes. *Am J Obstet Gynecol* 151:471-475, 1985.

Maurer SM, et al: Development of lesions in glomerular basement membrane and mesangium after transplantation of normal kidneys to diabetic patients. *Diabetes* 32:948-952, 1983.

McEvoy RC, et al: Gestational diabetes mellitus: Evidence for autoimmunity against the pancreatic beta cells. *Diabetologia* 34:507-510, 1991.

McFarland KF, et al: Incidence of diabetes mellitus in parents and grandparents of diabetic children. *Cleve Clin J Med* 55:217-219, 1988.

Mecklenburg RS, et al: Acute complications associated with insulin infusion pump therapy: Report of experience with 161 patients. *JAMA* 252:3265-3269, 1984.

Mecklenburg RS, et al: Malfunction of continuous subcutaneous insulin infusion systems: One-year prospective study of 127 patients. *Diabetes Care* 9:351-355, 1986.

Melander A: Clinical pharmacology of sulfonylureas. *Metabolism* 36(suppl 1):12-16, 1987.

Miller E, et al: Elevated maternal hemoglobin A_{1c} in early pregnancy and major congenital anomalies in infants of diabetic mothers. *N Engl J Med* 304:1331-1334, 1981.

Mills JL, et al: Incidence of spontaneous abortion among normal women and insulin-dependent diabetic women whose pregnancies were identified within 21 days of conception. *N Engl J Med* 319:1617-1623, 1988.

Miodovnik M, et al: Spontaneous abortion among insulin-dependent diabetic women. *Am J Obstet Gynecol* 150:372-376, 1984.

Mogensen CE: Microalbuminuria as a predictor of clinical diabetic nephropathy. *Kidney Int* 31:673-689, 1987.

Morris LR, et al: Bicarbonate therapy in severe diabetic ketoacidosis. *Ann Intern Med* 105:836-840, 1986.

Moss JM: New diagnostic classification of diabetes mellitus. *Am Fam Physician* 23:179-181, (Feb) 1981.

Nathan DM, et al: Glyburide or insulin for metabolic control in non-insulin-dependent diabetes mellitus. *Ann Intern Med* 108:334-340, 1988.

National Diabetes Data Group: Classification and diagnosis of diabetes mellitus and other categories of glucose intolerance. *Diabetes* 28:1039-1057, 1979.

Nelson RL: Non-insulin-dependent diabetes mellitus: Current status of oral hypoglycemic therapy. *Postgrad Med* 81:177-186, (May 1) 1987.

Nepom GT: Immunogenetics and IDDM. *Diabetes Rev* 1:93-103, (Spring) 1993.

O'Byrne S, Feely J: Effects of drugs on glucose tolerance in non-insulin-dependent diabetics, parts I and II. *Drugs* 40:6-18, 203-219, 1990.

Olsson P-O, et al: Miscibility of human semisynthetic regular and lente insulin and human biosynthetic regular and NPH insulin. *Diabetes Care* 10:473-477, 1987.

Osei K: Increased basal glucose production and utilization in nondiabetic first-degree relatives of patients with NIDDM. *Diabetes* 39:597-601, 1990.

Paice BJ, et al: Undesired effects of sulphonylurea drugs. *Adv Drug React Acc Pois Rev* 1:23-36, 1985.

Palardy J, et al: Blood glucose measurements during symptomatic episodes in patients with suspected postprandial hypoglycemia. *N Engl J Med* 321:1421-1425, 1989.

Palmer JP, McCulloch DK: Perspectives in diabetes: Predication and prevention of IDDM—1991. *Diabetes* 40:943-947, 1991.

Permutt MA, et al: Glucokinase and NIDDM: A candidate gene that paid off. *Diabetes* 41:1367-1372, 1992.

Perriello G, et al: Effect of asymptomatic nocturnal hypoglycemia on glycemic control in diabetes mellitus. *N Engl J Med* 319:1233-1239, 1988.

Peters AL, Davidson MB: Effect of storage on action of NPH and regular insulin mixtures. *Diabetes Care* 10:799-800, 1987.

Peters AL, Davidson MB: Use of sulfonylurea agents in older diabetic patients. *Clin Geriatr Med* 6:903-921, 1990.

Peters AL, Davidson MB: Insulin plus a sulfonylurea agent for treating type 2 diabetes. *Ann Intern Med* 115:45-53, 1991.

Pettitt DJ, et al: Insulinemia in children at low and high risk of NIDDM. *Diabetes Care* 16:608-615, 1993.

Pfeiffer EF: On the way to the automated (blood) glucose regulation in diabetes: The dark past, the grey present, the rosy future. *Diabetologia* 30:51-65, 1987.

Philipson EH, Super DM: Gestational diabetes mellitus: Does it recur in subsequent pregnancy? *Am J Obstet Gynecol* 160:1324-1331, 1989.

Piper JM, Langer O: Does maternal diabetes delay fetal pulmonary maturity? *Am J Obstet Gynecol* 168:783-786, 1993.

Point Study Group: One-year trial of a remote-controlled implantable insulin infusion system in type I diabetic patients. *Lancet* 2:866-869, 1988.

Polonsky KS, et al: Abnormal patterns of insulin secretion in non-insulin-dependent diabetes mellitus. *N Engl J Med* 318:1231-1239, 1988.

Pontiroli AE, et al: Intranasal glucagon as a remedy for hypoglycemia: Studies in healthy subjects and type I diabetic patients. *Diabetes Care* 12:604-608, 1989.

Pugh JA, et al: Is combination sulfonylurea and insulin therapy useful in NIDDM patients? A metaanalysis. *Diabetes Care* 15:953-959, (Aug) 1992.

Raskin P, Rosenstock J: Blood glucose control and diabetic complications. *Ann Intern Med* 105:254-263, 1986.

Riddle MC: Evening insulin strategy. *Diabetes Care* 13:676-686, 1990.

Rigg L, et al: Effects of exogenous insulin on excursions and diurnal rhythm of plasma glucose in pregnant diabetic patients with and without residual β-cell function. *Am J Obstet Gynecol* 136:537-544, 1980.

Rosenstock J, et al: Effect of glycemic control on microvascular complications in patients with type I diabetes mellitus. *Am J Med* 81:1012-1018, 1986.

Rossini AA, et al: Immunopathogenesis of diabetes mellitus. *Diabetes Rev* 1:43-75, (Spring) 1993.

Salzman R, et al: Intranasal aerosolized insulin: Mixed-meal studies and long-term use in type I diabetes. *N Engl J Med* 312:1078-1084, 1985.

Sanson TH, Levine SN: Management of diabetic ketoacidosis. *Drugs* 38:289-300, 1989.

Schmitt JK, et al: Modification of therapy from insulin to chlorpropamide decreases HDL cholesterol in patients with non-insulin-dependent diabetes mellitus. *Diabetes Care* 10:692-696, 1987.

Selam J-L, Charles MA: Devices for insulin administration. *Diabetes Care* 13:955-979, 1990.

Shulman GI, et al: Quantitation of muscle glycogen synthesis in normal subjects and subjects with non-insulin-dependent diabetes and ^{13}C nuclear magnetic resonance spectroscopy. *N Engl J Med* 322:223-228, 1989.

Simonson DC, et al: Mechanism of improvement in glucose metabolism after chronic glyburide therapy. *Diabetes* 33:838-845, 1984.

Simpson JL, et al: Diabetes in pregnancy, Northwestern University series (1977-1981): I. Prospective study of anomalies in offspring of mothers with diabetes mellitus. *Am J Obstet Gynecol* 146:263-270, 1983.

Siperstein MD: Diabetic microangiopathy, genetics, environment, and treatment. *Am J Med* 85(suppl 5A):119-130, 1988.

Skyler J: Insulin treatment, in Lebovitz HE (ed): *Therapy for Diabetes and Related Disorders.* Chicago, Ill, American Diabetes Association, 1991.

Skyler JS, Marks JB: Immune intervention in type I diabetes mellitus. *Diabetes Rev* 1:15-42, (Spring) 1993.

Sosenko JM, et al: Hyperglycemia and plasma lipid levels: Prospective study of young insulin-dependent diabetic patients. *N Engl J Med* 302:650-669, 1980.

Stenman S, et al: What is the benefit of increasing sulfonylurea dose? *Ann Intern Med* 118:169-172, 1993.

Stiller CR, et al: Effects of cyclosporine immunosuppression in insulin-dependent diabetes mellitus of recent onset. *Science* 223:1362-1367, 1984.

Sutherland DER: Report from the International Pancreas Transplant Registry. *Diabetologia* 34 (suppl 1):S28-S39, 1991.

Sutherland DER, et al: A 10-year experience with 290 pancreas transplants at a single institution. *Ann Surg* 210:274-288, 1989.

Swislocki ALM, et al: Can insulin resistance exist as primary defect in non-insulin-dependent diabetes mellitus? *J Clin Endocrinol Metab* 64:778-782, 1987.

Tamborlane WV, Press CM: Insulin infusion pump treatment of type I diabetes. *Pediatr Clin North Am* 31:721-733, 1984.

Tarn AC, et al: Predicting insulin-dependent diabetes. *Lancet* 1:845-850, 1988.

Thai A-C, Eisenbarth GS: Natural history of IDDM. *Diabetes Rev* 1:1-14, (Spring) 1993.

Tordjman KM, et al: Failure of nocturnal hypoglycemia to cause fasting hyperglycemia in patients with insulin-dependent diabetes mellitus. *N Engl J Med* 317:1552-1559, 1987.

Turner RC, Holman RR: Insulin use in NIDDM: Rationale based on pathophysiology of disease. *Diabetes Care* 13:1011-1020, 1990.

University Group Diabetes Program: Evaluation of insulin therapy; final report. *Diabetes* 31 (suppl 5):1-18, 1982.

van Faassen I, et al: Carriage of *Staphylococcus aureus* and inflamed infusion sites with insulin-pump therapy. *Diabetes Care* 12:153-155, 1989.

Vasquez B, et al: Sustained reduction of proteinuria in type 2 (non-insulin-dependent) diabetes following diet-induced reduction of hyperglycaemia. *Diabetologia* 26:127-133, 1984.

Vinik AI, et al: Diabetic neuropathies. *Diabetes Care* 15:1926-1975, 1992.

Wachtel TJ: The diabetic hyperosmolar state. *Clin Geriatr Med* 6:797-806, 1990.

Walker JD, et al: Restriction of dietary protein and progression of renal failure in diabetic nephropathy. *Lancet* 2:1411-1414, 1989.

Ward JD: Diabetic neuropathies: Current concepts in prevention and treatment. *Drugs* 32:279-289, 1986.

Ward GM: Insulin receptor concept and its relation to treatment of diabetes. *Drugs* 33:156-170, 1987.

Warram JH, et al: Differences in risk of insulin-dependent diabetes in offspring of diabetic mothers and diabetic fathers. *N Engl J Med* 311:149-152, 1984.

Widén EIM, et al: Metformin normalizes nonoxidative glucose metabolism in insulin-resistant normoglycemic first-degree relatives of patients with NIDDM. *Diabetes* 41:354-358, 1992.

Wood FC Jr, Bierman EL: Is diet the cornerstone in management of diabetes? *N Engl J Med* 315:1224-1227, 1986.

Yki-Järvinen H, et al: Comparison of insulin regimens in patients with non-insulin-dependent diabetes mellitus. *N Engl J Med* 327:1426-1433, 1992.

Zimmerman BR: Practical aspects of intensive insulin therapy. *Mayo Clin Proc* 61:806-812, 1986.

Drugs Used in Disorders of Growth Hormone Secretion

PHYSIOLOGY

The hormones that are particularly important for normal growth and development are growth hormone (GH, somatotropin), thyroid hormones, insulin, insulin-like growth factor (IGF-I), and sex steroids. GH circulates primarily as molecules composed of 176 or 191 amino acids; the former have markedly reduced biological activity. The circulating GH forms appear to be identical to pituitary isomers (Stolar and Baumann, 1986). In normal individuals under physiologic conditions, 50% to 75% of circulating GH is protein bound. When the plasma GH concentration is elevated (ie, >20 ng/ml), measurable protein binding of GH decreases because of partial saturation of the carrier protein (Baumann et al, 1988). See also reviews on GH-binding proteins (Wallis, 1991; Kelly et al, 1991).

Secretion of GH is stimulated by growth hormone-releasing hormone (GHRH) and inhibited by somatostatin, and their interaction regulates the secretion of GH (Hindmarsh et al, 1991 A). In addition, there is evidence that several neurotransmitters, neuropeptides, and other hormones may influence basal growth hormone secretion through their action on GHRH and somatostatin (see Table 1 and Bercu and Diamond, 1986).

The inter-relationships among sex steroid secretion, age, and GH secretion are not completely understood, but results of several studies offer insight into the process. Age and sex affect GH secretion independently. The 24-hour integrated GH secretion is higher during puberty than in childhood or adulthood. The highest peaks are observed during early nocturnal sleep in children who are in the middle to late stages of puberty. In normal adults, GH secretion occurs episodically with a rhythmicity of approximately three to four hours and an overall circadian rhythm that peaks during early slow-wave sleep (Winer et al, 1990). Young adults secrete more GH than older adults. The plasma GH concentration is greater in premenopausal females than in males of the same age (Ho et al, 1987; Lang et al, 1987), and the metabolic clearance of GH is more rapid in men than in women (Rosenbaum and Gertner, 1989).

Testosterone increases GH secretion in males. In one study, when GHRH was administered, the plasma GH response was greater in tall men than in men of average height, but no mean differences in plasma testosterone were observed between the two groups (Batrinos et al, 1989). Observations in pubertal males (Mauras et al, 1987) and adult males with hypogonadotropic hypogonadism who were treated with testosterone (Liu et al, 1987) showed that GH augmentation resulted from increased GH pulse amplitude rather than frequency. Midchildhood and pubertal growth is modulated partly by increased GH pulse amplitude, but the rhythmicity of GH secretion is unchanged at approximately 200 minutes (Hindmarsh et al, 1988).

GH has diverse metabolic effects. It stimulates amino acid uptake by muscle cells and protein synthesis, which increases nitrogen balance and decreases urea production. GH also stimulates lipolysis and fatty acid oxidation and, after an initial stimulation of glucose uptake, decreases the utilization of glucose in tissue (eg, muscle, adipocytes) in spite of increased serum insulin concentrations. GH is a potent antagonist of insulin action, which causes increased blood glucose levels in patients with acromegaly or when exogenous GH is administered in pharmacologic doses.

Growth Hormone-Releasing Hormone (GHRH): GHRH has been found in cells of the ventromedial and arcuate nuclei of the human hypothalamus. It also may be present in the placenta and pancreas and at several loci in the gastrointestinal tract (Vance and Thorner, 1986). Nonhypothalamic secretion may be the source of the small amount of GHRH in the peripheral circulation. Hypothalamic GHRH has been

TABLE 1. SUBSTANCES AFFECTING BASAL GH SECRETION[1]

	Stimulate	Inhibit
NEUROHORMONES		
	Growth hormone-releasing hormone	Somatostatin
NEUROTRANSMITTERS		
	Dopamine Acetylcholine Serotonin GABA α-Adrenergic agonists	Histamine GABA[2] β-Adrenergic agonists
NEUROPEPTIDES		
	Some opioids Some gut hormones Thyrotropin-releasing hormone[3] Galanin[4]	Corticotropin-releasing hormone Some gut hormones
OTHER HORMONES/SUBSTANCES		
	Estrogen Testosterone Thyroxine PGE_2	Calcitonin Glucocorticoids Insulin-like growth factor I

[1] See Bercu and Diamond, 1986, for text and references.
[2] Steardo et al, 1986.
[3] In pathologic states (eg, acromegaly, uncontrolled diabetes, malnutrition).
[4] Bauer et al, 1986.

found to be identical to that originally sequenced from a pancreatic tumor (Guillemin et al, 1982; Spiess et al, 1982; Rivier et al, 1982).

GHRH contains 40 to 44 amino acids and stimulates the secretion of GH but not other pituitary hormones (Gelato et al, 1983; Rosenthal et al, 1983; Thorner et al, 1983; Vance et al, 1984). It has a half-life of 6.8 minutes (Frohman et al, 1986). Primary metabolism of GHRH occurs intravascularly by removal of an amino terminal dipeptide, which renders the molecule biologically inactive (Frohman et al, 1989).

Some data suggest that GHRH may be useful as a diagnostic and therapeutic agent for GH deficiency, but its administration does not appear to be useful for the diagnosis of acromegaly (Gelato et al, 1985). Although a dose-response relationship can be observed when GHRH is administered and GH is measured in the plasma, the same dose does not necessarily produce a quantitatively reproducible response in a given individual. If a hypothalamic defect is responsible for GH deficiency, priming with GHRH may be necessary to achieve a normal GH response. GHRH has been given intravenously, but it also is effective when administered by other routes. The subcutaneous and intranasal routes require larger doses to achieve an effect. The GHRH stimulus to GH secretion does not appear to be down-regulated; therefore, long-acting analogues of GHRH may be potentially useful in some forms of GH deficiency (Vance and Thorner, 1986).

Somatostatin: Somatostatin (growth hormone-inhibiting hormone, somatotropin release-inhibiting hormone [SRIH]) is a tetradecapeptide found in the hypothalamus and other areas of the central and peripheral nervous system, the gastrointestinal tract (stomach antrum, small intestine, D cells of pancreatic islets), the adrenal medulla, and thyroid C cells. It also may exist as a peptide containing 28 amino acids.

Somatostatin inhibits the secretion of GH, thyroid-stimulating hormone (TSH), gastrin, glucagon, insulin, and other hormones, as well as exocrine pancreatic secretion. It does not inhibit the secretion of gonadotropins, prolactin, or ACTH. Somatostatin is involved in the regulation of GH secretion and possibly that of TSH and serves as a neurotransmitter in the central nervous system. Its presence in pancreatic tissue suggests participation in paracrine control of insulin and glucagon secretion (Wass, 1983).

Research is being directed toward the use of long-acting analogues of somatostatin to treat acromegaly (see the discussion in that section) and to control gastrointestinal bleeding in individuals with peptic ulcer. One somatostatin analogue, octreotide [Sandostatin], is used for the treatment of the symptoms associated with carcinoid syndrome and VIPomas that secrete hormones, as well as to decrease GH secretion in patients with acromegaly. Other uses under investigation include treatment of islet cell or gastrointestinal tract tumors (eg, gastrinomas, glucagonomas, insulinomas, pancreatic polypeptide-secreting tumors), diarrhea associated with AIDS, chronic pancreatitis, and some nonendocrine malignancies.

Insulin-Like Growth Factors (IGF, Somatomedin): Many effects of GH on growth are mediated by insulin-like growth factors (Daughaday et al, 1987) elaborated by the liver, kidneys, muscle, bone, and other tissues. The most important member of the group for promoting bone growth is IGF-I (somatomedin C). Normal plasma IGF-I concentrations increase to a maximum at midpuberty; no diurnal variations have been observed. There appears to be a correlation between plasma IGF-I concentration and growth rate during puberty prior to epiphyseal fusion (Cara et al, 1987). However, a low serum IGF-I concentration alone is not a reliable diagnostic indication of GH deficiency (Rosenfeld et al, 1986).

Low IGF-I production is associated with GH deficiency and other conditions that affect GH action (eg, malnutrition, hypothyroidism, liver disease, aging, Laron-type dwarfism, short stature of African pygmies) (Clemmons and Van Wyk, 1984; Hall and Sara, 1984; Merimee et al, 1987). In at least the latter two conditions, an abnormality in the number or structure of GH receptors is the probable cause, and mutations in the gene for GH receptors have been identified in several subjects with Laron dwarfism (Amselem et al, 1989). These individuals have high endogenous blood levels of GH and do not respond to exogenous GH. A classification of GH-insensitive syndromes has been proposed (Laron et al, 1993).

Serum IGF-I levels are high in patients with acromegaly. IGF-II, which is only partially regulated by GH, may play an important role in fetal growth.

GROWTH HORMONE DEFICIENCY

Deficient secretion of GH during childhood may be idiopathic, hereditary, or secondary to a central nervous system lesion, tumor, physical trauma, embryologic defect (eg, septo-optic dysplasia), infection, or cranial irradiation; other tropic hormones also may be impaired. If untreated, dwarfism may result. True GH deficiency as a cause of growth failure must be treated with human GH; animal GH is ineffective because of the formation of heterologous neutralizing antibodies.

Several studies have described short children who may have mild or partial GH deficiency rather than the classic (complete or severe) form (Rudman et al, 1981; Frazer et al, 1982; Van Vliet et al, 1983; Gertner et al, 1984; Spiliotis et al, 1984; Zadik et al, 1985). Some of these patients may have been diagnosed as having constitutional delay of growth. These children have subnormal growth velocities (<5 cm/year) but produced normal quantities of GH after at least one standard pharmacologic stimulus. Their short-term growth rate was accelerated after GH administration; however, a beneficial effect of GH therapy on final height has not been established. One explanation of these observations is that these patients represent a point on the continuum between normal secretory status and classic GH deficiency. In blood samples collected every 20 minutes for 24 hours, total GH secretion, number of secretory pulses, and peak amplitude of GH pulses were lower in the short children subsequently diagnosed with "neurosecretory dysfunction" than in children of normal height (Spiliotis et al, 1984).

Other investigators have divided groups of short children into normal, nonclassic (partial) GH deficiency, or classic GH deficiency on the basis of the total amount of GH secreted over 24 hours; 87% of those with nonclassic GH deficiency responded to GH therapy with an increase in height velocity of more than two standard deviations per year of therapy (Saggese and Cesaretti, 1989). Other studies have found that there is considerable overlap in total GH secreted, as determined by continuous sampling overnight (Lanes, 1989) and over 24 hours (Lin et al, 1989; Costin et al, 1989), among patients who were normal or had partial or classic GH deficiency. These interpretations are controversial, and it is generally thought that any type of testing (ie, standard provocative tests, frequent sampling methods) does not always define a specific GH secretory status. Further, the GH secretory capacity does not necessarily predict the response to GH. Conversely, responsiveness to exogenous GH does not prove that spontaneous GH secretion is deficient or that the GH secreted is not biologically active.

Diagnosis: Factors such as family history of GH deficiency, documentation of subnormal growth rate (see Table 2) over at least six months, elimination of other causes of subnormal growth (eg, hypothyroidism, poor nutrition, psychosocial deprivation), and evidence of delayed bone age all suggest GH deficiency. Serum concentrations of IGF-I also are almost always low in patients with GH deficiency. Laboratory tests of GH secretion are necessary to confirm the diagnosis and determine whether GH deficiency is partial or complete (classic). Criteria for the differential diagnosis of classic GH deficiency appear in Table 2.

TABLE 2.
DEFINITION OF CLASSIC GROWTH HORMONE DEFICIENCY

Poor growth velocity
- <7 cm/yr before age 3 years
- <4-5 cm/yr from age 3 years to onset of puberty

Delayed bone age
- ≥2 SD below mean for chronologic age, generally ≥2 years delayed

Diminished GH response to two or more provocative stimuli
- (levodopa, insulin-induced hypoglycemia, arginine, clonidine, glucagon)

No evidence of other organ system disease

From Bercu, 1987. Reprinted with permission.

Provocative testing of GH deficiency may employ pharmacologic or physiologic stimuli of GH secretion. Pharmacologic stimuli include insulin-induced hypoglycemia, which is probably the most reliable test; levodopa; clonidine; arginine; or glucagon. Two or more provocative stimuli of GH secretion are usually administered to reduce the possibility of an erroneous diagnosis. The physiologic stimulus of 20 minutes of vigorous exercise also is sometimes used.

Integrated measurement of GH secretion over 12 hours (including nocturnal sleep) (Costin and Kaufman, 1987) or 24 hours may reveal subnormal GH secretion that was not detected with provocative testing (Bercu et al, 1986). In one study, the diagnosis of GH deficiency was more accurate after GH sampling over a 24-hour period than after determining the response of GH to pharmacologic stimuli, especially when the deficiency was partial (Zadik et al, 1990). However, other evidence suggests that overnight measurements of physiologic GH secretion vary considerably and that measurement of spontaneous GH secretion over 12 or 24 hours was *less* sensitive than use of stimuli in prepubertal children. Because spontaneous GH secretion increases during puberty, patients and control subjects must be matched carefully for pubertal stage. Failure to do so may account for the disparate results in studies designed to determine the diagnostic significance of measuring stimulated versus spontaneous serum GH levels (Rose et al, 1988).

The concentration and total amount of urinary GH correlate with serum GH measured after administration of insulin and during sleep; this suggests that measurement of urinary GH may have a role in diagnosis of GH deficiency in the future. Demonstration of normal renal clearance excludes the possibility that a high rate of excretion is due to renal tubular impairment (Kida et al, 1992).

Because there is considerable variability among results obtained by different types of commercial GH assays, measurements obtained from different assay systems must be interpreted cautiously (Reiter et al, 1988; Celniker et al, 1989). Patients with classic GH deficiency consistently fail to achieve a peak GH level of 7 to 10 ng/ml during provocative testing as determined by polyclonal antiserum-based radioimmunoassays. However, caution must be exercised in interpreting monoclonal antibody-based immunoradiometric assays, which tend to give values approximately two-thirds those of the polyclonal assays.

Stimulation of GH secretion with GHRH may be useful in the differential diagnosis of GH deficiency (Albini et al, 1988). In a multicenter study, 394 children with subnormal growth were given a single intravenous bolus injection of GHRH (2 mcg/kg), and GH was measured in plasma before and at several intervals after injection. The peak GH values after the single injection reflected the degree of GH deficiency (normal, partial, or complete) as determined previously by conventional testing (Chatelain et al, 1987). However, other investigators who used a different GHRH preparation in one-half the dose given intravenously as a bolus injection found considerable overlap in the response to GHRH between patients with classic deficiency and those with "neurosecretory dysfunction," and they suggested that integrated measurements of unstimulated GH secretion were necessary for the differential diagnosis (Chalew et al, 1986). Others have noted that GH response to GHRH diminishes with the duration of the deficiency and that priming with GHRH may be necessary to induce maximal secretion of GH in patients with long-standing deficiency (Grossman et al, 1986).

The evaluation and treatment of children with short stature and possible GH deficiency have been reviewed (Mahoney, 1987; Raiti, 1989; Jørgensen, 1991; LaFranchi, 1992; Underwood, 1992).

Treatment: Classic GH deficiency has been treated successfully for many years with pituitary GH. Because of the limited supply of human pituitaries, the emphasis in developing treatment regimens was on identifying and treating patients with the most severe GH deficiency and utilizing the lowest dose that would achieve acceptable, but not necessarily optimal, results. The growth rate was highest early in therapy and commonly diminished with continued therapy. The availability of large quantities of recombinant DNA growth hormone (ie, somatrem and somatropin, which appear to have similar clinical effects) has allowed administration of larger doses to overcome this decrease in response. In one study, eight patients with GH deficiency were treated for an average of 4.3 years with GH (somatrem) 0.1 IU/kg three times weekly. After the dose was tripled and administered for an additional eight months, the mean growth rate increased from 5.5 to 8.1 cm/year; this suggests that attenuation of response to GH may be overcome by increasing the dose. It is not known how long this response could be maintained at this or higher dosage levels. No adverse effect on glucose tolerance or serum lipids was observed (Gertner et al, 1987).

Administration of somatrem (methionyl-GH, recombinant DNA derived) [Protropin] accelerates growth in a manner similar to pituitary GH. When somatrem was administered to 36 GH-deficient children for up to four years, growth rates initially increased from 3.2 to 10.5 cm/year, an increase similar to that following pituitary GH therapy (3.8 to 10.1 cm/year) (Kaplan et al, 1986). A second recombinant GH product, somatropin [Humatrope], is chemically identical to endogenous GH, unlike somatrem, which is methionyl-GH. Somatropin was administered to 309 children for periods of up to three years. During the first year of therapy, growth rates increased from 3.8 cm to 8.9 cm in the prepubertal children (Holcombe et al, 1990).

The timing of GH injections may affect outcome. When GH was administered in the evening, metabolic patterns (eg, lipid intermediates, serum alanine and lactate) were more nearly normal than after injections administered in the morning (Jørgensen et al, 1990). Many clinicians prefer to divide the amount of GH given weekly into six or seven daily doses and have observed that daily administration results in greater growth rates than administration three times weekly (Hermanussen et al, 1985; Smith et al, 1988; Zamboni et al, 1991).

Treatment with a recombinant DNA GH preparation is expensive. One year of therapy for a 30-kg child may cost $20,000, and therapy may be required for more than five years (Lantos et al, 1989).

GH therapy may be continued until the patient ceases to respond to treatment and/or the epiphyses fuse (Raiti, 1989). Early withdrawal of therapy may result in lower final height. Generally, final heights are greater in patients who are also deficient in gonadotropins, for pubertal development can be induced later than when puberty is spontaneous. In some GH-deficient children, GH therapy plus gonadal suppression therapy (cyproterone acetate in boys and medroxyprogesterone in girls) delayed completion of puberty and resulted in greater final height compared with similar children who received only GH and experienced spontaneous puberty (Hibi et al, 1989).

In GH-deficient children who also have true precocious puberty, therapy with a combination of GH and a GnRH agonist, which reduces secretion of sex steroids and consequently delays epiphyseal closure, may improve the final height achieved (Cara et al, 1992).

Children with partial GH deficiency also respond to GH therapy with increased growth rates. In one study, the growth rate of 48 children given pituitary GH increased from 3.4 to 6.9 cm/year during the treatment period (Raiti et al, 1987). In other studies of short children who were given somatrem for one year, growth exceeded that in untreated controls (Hindmarsh and Brook, 1987) or resulted in nearly normal adolescent height (Lesage et al, 1991).

Determination of status in nonclassic GH deficiency, and therefore efficacy of therapy, is difficult and is complicated by the lack of standard diagnostic criteria and nomenclature designations. There is probably overlap among some children described as "short normal" or as having "neurosecretory dysfunction." Few patients with partial GH deficiency or short normal children who have been treated with GH preparations have been followed long enough to determine if their temporarily accelerated growth rate will result in enhanced adult height, allow them to achieve height potential earlier, or result in reduced growth rates with no ultimate effect on height when GH therapy is withdrawn.

GH sometimes has been administered with an anabolic steroid to decrease the amount (and expense) of GH required to achieve a therapeutic effect; oxandrolone has frequently been used for this purpose. Theoretically, the anabolic steroid accelerates linear growth. If the bone age is greater than height age before or during therapy, the anabolic steroid should be withheld because of the possibility that final adult height may be limited by early closure of epiphyses. Some practitioners do not favor use of an anabolic steroid with GH except for certain indications (see below).

GHRH or an analogue also has been used to treat subnormal growth conditions that respond to GH therapy. A functional pituitary gland is required to achieve a response. GH-deficient children given GHRH or an analogue by subcutaneous infusion at night or throughout 24 hours or twice-daily by subcutaneous injection (Ross et al, 1987; Smith and Brook, 1987; Thorner et al, 1988; Duck et al, 1992) experienced increased growth rates over the 6 to 30 months of treatment. Similar acceleration of growth was achieved in prepubertal children with partial GH deficiency who received GHRH by continuous subcutaneous infusion (Brain et al, 1990). Desensitization of GH secretory response (down-regulation), was not observed in these studies. Administration of GHRH by continuous infusion for 14 days to normal men also did not cause desensitization of pituitary somatotrophs (Vance et al, 1989). However, in one study, GH therapy was more effective than GHRH in GH-deficient children (Smith and Brook, 1988). Overall, up to 50% of children with GH deficiency respond to therapy with GHRH.

Because clonidine [Catapres] is one of the pharmacologic agents used to stimulate GH secretion when testing for GH deficiency, it has been suggested that clonidine therapy might stimulate GH production in children with partial GH deficiency or constitutional growth delay (CGD). Growth was accelerated in children after two months of treatment with clonidine and remained higher than pretreatment rates after six months of therapy (Loche et al, 1989). However, in other double-blind, placebo-controlled trials, growth velocity was not significantly increased in children with non-GH-deficient short stature after six months of treatment with clonidine (Pescovitz and Tan, 1988; Allen, 1993). Hypotension and drowsiness are associated with clonidine therapy.

Adverse Reactions Associated with Growth Hormone: Overtreatment with GH could induce some degree of the metabolic and structural aberrations associated with endogenous hypersecretion (see the section on Acromegaly below). Since more patients with less severe deficiency are being treated, it becomes even more important to identify adverse effects associated with GH therapy so that the risks and benefits can be weighed appropriately.

In short children who were not GH-deficient, growth was accelerated after one year of GH therapy (Walker et al, 1989). Although serum insulin levels were increased, glucose tolerance was not impaired. Treated children did not develop soft tissue swelling or acromegalic changes and were not more prone to slipped capital femoral epiphyses. Furthermore, GH antibodies did not increase significantly.

A possible association between GH therapy and the occurrence of leukemia has been suggested, but this has not been confirmed (Fisher et al, 1988; Brock et al, 1991).

Patient Selection: GH therapy is clearly indicated for children with classic (severe) GH deficiency. Even though it appears that GH temporarily accelerates growth in patients with only partial deficiency and even in short normal children, there are no firm guidelines to determine who should be treated, when treatment should begin, and how long it should continue. Such use of GH probably should continue to be limited to controlled studies that offer psychological as well as medical evaluation and support (American Academy of Pediatrics, 1983; Underwood, 1992; *Med Lett Drugs Ther,* 1984). Some investigators recommend a six-month trial of GH therapy for carefully selected short children who fulfill all criteria of GH deficiency except subnormal response to GH stimuli and who may have a normal mean 24-hour endogenous GH secretion pattern (Bercu, 1987; Milner, 1986). Others have suggested an arbitrary height (ie, below the first percentile) and evidence of responsiveness to GH treatment, rather than GH deficiency per se, as criteria for patient selection (Allen and Fost, 1990). The decision to treat growth retardation that is not clearly due to classic GH deficiency is complicated by ethical considerations (see below).

Other Indications for Growth Hormone: Growth failure due to conditions other than GH deficiency may respond to GH treatment. Seventy patients with *Turner's syndrome* were given no treatment, somatrem (0.125 mg/kg three times per week), or combined somatrem and oxandrolone (0.0625 mg/kg/day) for a minimum of one year. Treatment with both therapeutic regimens increased the growth rate for up to the six-year duration of the study (Rosenfeld et al, 1992). In another study, 52 patients with Turner's syndrome were given the same dose of GH as in the above study for one year. Growth rates accelerated during treatment but decreased to the baseline rate or, in more than 50% of the patients, to below the baseline rate on withdrawal of therapy (Raiti et al, 1986). In a multicenter study, patients who were treated with GH for three years surpassed their expected adult height, although normal height for age was not reached (Takano et al, 1992). The addition of ethinyl estradiol to the GH regimen did not enhance growth velocity sufficiently to offset the possibility of early breast development or epiphyseal closure (Van der Schueren-Lodeweyckx et al, 1990). The use of GH in Turner's syndrome has been designated an orphan indication by the FDA.

Other indications for GH use are being investigated. There is some clinical evidence to suggest that GH may be useful to increase growth velocity in *children with end-stage renal disease* (Tönshoff et al, 1990; Hokken-Koelega et al, 1991). In children with *Down syndrome* who also had growth retardation and microcephaly, treatment with GH for one year improved linear growth and increased head circumference (Torrado et al, 1991). However, because of the increased risk of leukemia in children with Down syndrome, the possibility of additional risk associated with GH therapy is of concern. Growth rates also were improved in patients with *β thalassemia major* and GH deficiency who were treated with GH (Scacchi et al, 1991).

GH has been administered to *adults with acquired GH deficiency.* Results obtained in these patients were similar to those observed in children who had been treated for GH deficiency. Total body weight did not change, but lean body mass increased and adipose tissue volume decreased. The basal metabolic rate increased, total cholesterol decreased, and isometric strength and exercise capacity were increased in GH-treated patients compared with placebo-treated controls (Jørgensen et al, 1989; Salomon et al, 1989; Whitehead et al, 1992; De Boer et al, 1992).

GH administered to otherwise *normal older males* (61 to 81 years) with plasma IGF-I concentrations 35% of normal also is being investigated. Increased lean body mass, decreased adipose tissue, increased lumbar vertebral density, and increased skin thickness were observed. Small increases in systolic blood pressure and fasting blood glucose also occurred (Rudman et al, 1990). Although the possibility of inhibiting or reversing some age-related changes by administering GH is suggested by results of this study, such use is investigational. More data are necessary to determine the benefits and risks of long-term therapy. Replacement regimens used in adults are similar to those for GH-deficient children and hence are equally costly (Vance, 1990). The addition of GH therapy to a regimen of resistance exercise in young men did not enhance muscle anabolism or function (Yarasheski et al, 1992). For review on use of GH therapy in adults, see Cuneo et al, 1992, and Lamberts et al, 1992.

Use of GH in the treatment of other conditions not involving linear growth is being investigated (eg, certain catabolic states, obesity, osteoporosis, hyperlipidemia, anemia not associated with erythropoietin deficiency, hemophilia, severe sepsis) (Williams and Frohman, 1986; Voerman et al, 1992). GH administered to patients after elective cholecystectomy was associated with improved conservation of nitrogen (Hammarqvist et al, 1992). Administration of GH and insulin to cancer patients reduced whole body and skeletal muscle protein loss (Wolf et al, 1992). Use of GH to enhance nitrogen retention in hospitalized patients suffering from severe burns has been designated an orphan indication by the FDA.

See also review by Hindmarsh et al, 1991 B.

Ethical Considerations: The availability of unlimited supplies of GH underlines the need for guidelines for its use. Long-term use will undoubtedly increase if the current cost of GH is lowered. Already there have been reports of GH abuse by athletes (United States General Accounting Office, 1989) and numerous ethical questions have arisen. GH therapy can be uncomfortable and prolonged (injections three to seven times weekly for six months to several years). Is such treatment justified for trivial medical or psychological indications? Should GH therapy be available for children with genetic short stature in the normal range; for children of those parents who foresee an athletic or business advantage for a taller child; or for any patients who consider short stature a functional handicap? Would the eventual result be an increase in average height or less variability in the height of the population? Since there is no guarantee that GH therapy will be effective, what psychological effect would treatment failure have in a child who has undergone prolonged therapy to correct a perceived defect that otherwise might have been accepted as normal (Benjamin et al, 1984; Underwood, 1992; Lantos et al, 1989)? Answers to these and other questions should be provided by thoughtful and responsible clinical investigations. Because of the adverse effects of excessive endogenous GH (eg, acromegaly including joint disease, cardiovascular problems, glucose intolerance), the use of a potent hormone with potential adverse effects in "normal" children raises serious concern.

Preparations: Somatrem (methionyl-GH [Protropin]) and somatropin (chemically identical to pituitary GH) [Humatrope] are human growth hormone produced by recombinant DNA technology. The pituitary-extracted somatropin preparations [Asellacrin, Crescormon] have been withdrawn from distribution because of the risk of transmitting the virus that causes Creutzfeldt-Jakob disease.

Drug Evaluations

SOMATREM (recombinant DNA produced)
[Protropin]

Somatrem is a preparation of human growth hormone produced by recombinant DNA technology. Because it is not derived from a human source, somatrem carries no risk of transmitting Creutzfeldt-Jakob disease. The product contains 192 amino acid residues, has a molecular weight of approximately 22,000 daltons, and is identical to natural GH except for the addition of methionine on the N-terminus of the molecule. The biological effects appear to be identical to those of GH derived from pituitary glands. One milligram of this preparation is equivalent to 2.6 IU of GH.

USES. Somatrem is indicated for the treatment of GH deficiency in children. Such deficiency should be documented before somatrem is administered. Use in children with various forms of partial GH deficiency or in short normal children is not currently recommended except under investigational protocols. Stimulation of growth in Turner's syndrome and enhancement of nitrogen retention in patients with severe burns have been designated as orphan indications for the use of GH.

Therapy for GH deficiency is usually continued until epiphyseal closure occurs or there is no further response. If therapy is unsuccessful after six months, treatment should be discontinued and the patient re-evaluated.

ADVERSE REACTIONS AND PRECAUTIONS. Antibodies to somatrem were found in approximately 30% of patients (range, 5% of patients previously treated with pituitary GH to 40% in those who received no prior GH therapy). With few exceptions, the antibodies are in low titers and do not interfere with growth stimulation.

GH preparations may be diabetogenic and may cause hyperglycemia and ketosis in patients with insulin deficiency or resistance. However, reports of this effect are rare and cannot be attributed solely to GH administration. Nevertheless, particular caution should be exercised when these agents are administered to diabetic patients. Fasting blood glucose levels should be determined in all patients after several weeks of treatment.

Patients should be evaluated yearly for hypothyroidism, which should be treated with full replacement dosage (Frasier, 1983).

Growth retardation is a side effect of pharmacologic doses of glucocorticoid therapy, and these agents may inhibit the response to somatropin. Daily doses exceeding 10 to 15 mg/M^2 of hydrocortisone or the equivalent will decrease the effectiveness of any GH preparation, and even lower doses may have this effect.

Somatrem is classified in FDA Pregnancy Category C.

DOSAGE AND PREPARATIONS.

Intramuscular, Subcutaneous: Somatrem may be administered intramuscularly or subcutaneously (Russo and Moore, 1982; Wilson et al, 1985). Dosage must be individualized. The usual dosage for GH deficiency is 0.1 mg/kg (0.26 IU/kg) three times per week. The same total dose divided into six or seven injections per week is somewhat more effective. For Turner's syndrome, the maximum dose is 0.125 mg/kg three times per week (0.054 mg/kg daily).

Protropin (Genentech). Powder (sterile, lyophilized) 5 and 10 mg (approximately 13 and 26 IU)/container.

SOMATROPIN (recombinant DNA produced)
[Humatrope]

This preparation is chemically identical to endogenous human pituitary GH but is produced by recombinant DNA techniques. It has a molecular weight of about 22,125 daltons. Because recombinant DNA-produced somatropin is not derived from a human source, it carries no risk of transmitting Creutzfeldt-Jakob disease. This GH preparation differs from somatrem, which is also a recombinant DNA product, in that it lacks the additional methionine on the N-terminus of the molecule. The growth-stimulating properties of somatropin are the same as those of pituitary-extracted human GH and somatrem. One milligram of this preparation is equivalent to 2.6 IU of GH.

USES. Somatropin is indicated for the treatment of GH deficiency in children. Stimulation of growth in Turner's syndrome and enhancement of nitrogen retention in patients with severe burns have been designated as orphan indications for the use of GH. Documentation of deficiency and other considerations concerning administration and monitoring of therapy are similar to those for somatrem (see that evaluation and the Introduction).

ADVERSE REACTIONS AND PRECAUTIONS. In general, these are the same as for somatrem. However, antibodies to somatropin are present in fewer patients than with use of somatrem (about 2% of those treated). With few exceptions, the antibodies do not interfere with growth stimulation.

Somatropin is classified in FDA Pregnancy Category C.

DOSAGE AND PREPARATIONS.

Intramuscular, Subcutaneous: Up to 0.06 mg/kg (0.16 IU/kg) is given three times per week. The same total dose can be injected six or seven times per week. Many endocrinologists use the same dosage regimen for this preparation as for somatrem.

Humatrope (Lilly). Powder (sterile, lyophilized) 5 mg (approximately 13 IU) with 5 ml of diluent.

GROWTH HORMONE EXCESS (ACROMEGALY, GIGANTISM)

Hypersecretion of GH rarely produces gigantism in children and acromegaly in adults. Gigantism usually is caused by a GH-secreting pituitary tumor but also may be caused by hypersecretion of GHRH (Zimmerman et al, 1993). Excessive GH secretion, which is autonomous from tumor tissue in acromegaly, results in an increase in the serum concentration and basal secretion of GH. The excessive secretion also involves increased GH pulse frequency but amplitude is unaffected (Barkan et al, 1989). (This is in contrast to the physiologic increase in GH secretion at puberty in which pulse frequency is relatively constant but amplitude increases.) The increased pulse frequency may be caused by lowered sensitivity of GHRH neurons to negative feedback by IGF-I (Ho et al, 1992). Circulating GH receptor antibodies that have GH activity may contribute to the pathology (Campino et al, 1992).

The physical characteristics of the patient with advanced acromegaly are easily recognized but may have progressed slowly and have been unnoticed for 10 to 20 years. Examination of photographs taken over a number of years may reveal gradual enlargement and coarsening of features. The elevated GH and IGF-I concentrations stimulate bony and cartilaginous overgrowth that result in enlarged and thickened supraorbital ridge, nose, hands, and feet and protruding maxilla and mandible with widely spaced teeth. The patient may have noticed that shoes, hats, and rings or gloves are no longer large enough. Tissue thickening also occurs in the tongue, skin, and other organs (heart, liver, kidneys, lung, brain, and thyroid). The combination of nasal bone and sinus enlargement and laryngeal hypertrophy produces a deep, resonant voice. Acromegalic patients may have visual field impairment, hypertension, and glucose intolerance, and they complain of weakness, fatigue, headache, arthralgias, paresthesias (eg, carpal tunnel syndrome), hyperhidrosis, menstrual irregularities or amenorrhea, and impotence.

Plasma IGF-I concentration is elevated in acromegaly, and failure to suppress serum GH below 3 to 4 ng/ml after a 75-g loading dose of glucose supports the diagnosis (Ezzat and Melmed, 1991). Because of the pulsatile nature of GH secretion, a single plasma sample may be insufficient to exclude a diagnosis. Determination of plasma GH levels after GHRH stimulation is not helpful. In advanced cases, diagnosis is made largely on the basis of history and physical examination.

Acromegaly often is diagnosed at about 40 to 45 years of age, although it may develop any time after closure of the epiphyses. When acromegaly is diagnosed in younger patients, the disease may be more severe (ie, larger tumor) than in older patients, which suggests its more rapid progression in young people (Melmed et al, 1986). There appears to be no sex difference in frequency of the disease.

Acromegaly is caused by a GH-producing adenoma in more than 95% of patients but may result from pituitary hyperplasia or rarely from GHRH- or GH-secreting neoplasms (eg, pancreatic or bronchial tumor) (Melmed, 1991). The plasma IGF-I levels are closely correlated with the logarithm of the mean 24-hour GH concentration (Barkan et al, 1988 A). Measurement of plasma IGF-I is often used to monitor the effects of treatment for acromegaly (Oppizzi et al, 1986).

The diagnosis and treatment of acromegaly have been reviewed (Barkan, 1989; Frohman, 1991; Ezzat and Melmed, 1991).

Surgical and Irradiation Therapy: Acromegaly may be treated surgically, by irradiation, or medically. Transsphenoidal adenomectomy is the initial treatment for small tumors and is the preferred treatment for most tumors. Surgery alone is most effective when tumors are small without extrasellar extension and the plasma GH level is less than 40 ng/ml (Baskin et al, 1982). Surgical correction of large suprasellar tumors may be difficult, particularly if there is lateral extension, and cure rates may be only 25% to 50%. Irradiation and drug therapy may be useful adjuncts in such cases. Adverse effects following surgery may include meningitis, cerebrospinal fluid leakage, hemorrhage, diabetes insipidus, stroke, visual field defects, chronic sinusitis, and destruction of anterior pituitary tissue that requires replacement therapy (Karpf and Braunstein, 1986).

Irradiation is less often used as primary therapy because the full effects take several years to develop, and the otherwise progressive multisystem pathology and disfigurement require more immediate measures. In the past when irradiation was used alone, the GH level was controlled adequately in about 75% of patients after ten years. Radiation therapy is still useful after incomplete excision of large tumors or following surgical failure. Loss of anterior pituitary function will occur in 50% of all patients within 10 years, and, over time, increasing numbers of patients will require pituitary hormone replacement.

Drug Therapy: Acromegaly once was treatable only by surgery or irradiation. Now drugs may be employed as primary treatment of microadenomas if the patient is not a candidate for surgery. More often they are employed as adjuncts to surgery or irradiation. The dopaminergic agent, bromocriptine [Parlodel], sometimes is beneficial. A long-acting analogue of somatostatin, octreotide [Sandostatin], may be more useful but must be given by injection several times a day. Other dopamine receptor agonists (eg, pergolide [Permax]; the investigational agents, lisuride and cabergoline) also have been used.

Bromocriptine is usually employed as an adjunct to an ablative procedure, particularly irradiation. It should not be used as the sole treatment unless the patient is not a candidate for surgery or irradiation. This drug's exact role in acromegaly remains controversial, and a number of investigators consider it only mildly effective.

Bromocriptine is most beneficial in patients with tumors that contain dopamine receptors. Clinical improvement occurs in 70% of these patients, but GH is reduced to ≤10 ng/ml of plasma in only 50% and to 5 ng/ml in 20%. Tumor shrinkage occurs in only 10% to 15% of patients (Frohman, 1991). A good correlation between clinical response to bromocriptine and serum IGF-I has been reported (Wass et al, 1982). Some patients improve clinically (eg, remission of soft tissue swelling) in the presence of decreased IGF-I concentrations, but other patients improve in the absence of changes in either serum GH or IGF-I (Nortier et al, 1985). It has been suggested that the monomeric, most biologically active form of GH is decreased more than less active oligomeric forms, which are nevertheless measured by immunoassay (Wass et al, 1986).

In a randomized, double-blind, placebo-controlled trial on 115 patients, octreotide significantly reduced plasma GH. Integrated mean GH levels were reduced to <5 ng/ml in 53% of patients, and IGF-I levels returned to normal in 68% of patients. Symptoms improved substantially in more than 66% of patients, and tumor size was reduced in 37% after six months of therapy (Ezzat et al, 1992). Results of several additional studies indicate that octreotide may be effective in lowering serum GH levels and normalizing serum IGF-I concentrations, and, in some cases, may lead to reduction in size of the pituitary tumor (Barkan et al, 1988 B, 1988 C; Gorden et al, 1989). The frequency of subcutaneous administration is more important than the total dose (Ho et al, 1990). Octreotide also has been administered by continuous subcutaneous infusion; optimal GH suppression was achieved with doses of 600 mcg/24 hours (James et al, 1989). GH concentration begins to fall within hours of initiating infusion, and it has been suggested that the potential response to octreotide can be determined by continuous infusion for 24 hours (Tauber et al, 1989). Octreotide also was effective when administered in an intranasal preparation, although amounts ten times higher than the usual subcutaneous dose were required to produce equivalent results (Weeke et al, 1992).

About 90% of acromegalic patients respond to octreotide. Results of one study suggested that those with high-density, homogeneous, high-affinity somatostatin receptors are most likely to benefit (Reubi and Landolt, 1989). However, increased GH secretion returns after withdrawal of the drug. Octreotide has reduced both plasma GH and GHRH concentrations in patients with the rare syndrome of ectopic GHRH secretion (Melmed et al, 1988; Moller et al, 1989).

Studies comparing the effectiveness of bromocriptine and octreotide show that octreotide (50 mcg subcutaneously) lowers plasma GH more effectively than bromocriptine (2.5 mg orally). Other investigators found that when octreotide (up to 300 mcg daily) or bromocriptine (up to 22.5 mg daily) was administered in stepwise fashion for 28 days with the final dose maintained for seven weeks, both agents were equally effective. However, the response to bromocriptine depended on the dose, whereas for octreotide frequency of administration was more important than additional dose increments (Halse et al, 1990). Long-term treatment with octreotide also was more effective than bromocriptine in 16 patients, while combined use of these agents in four patients was more effective than either agent alone (Chiodini et al, 1987). Other investigators reported varied responses. A given patient may have been most responsive to bromocriptine, octreotide, or the combination or may not have been responsive to either agent alone or in combination (Lamberts et al, 1986). Since octreotide is a somatostatin analogue and bromocriptine is a dopamine agonist, it is not surprising that the combination may be superior to either drug used alone. The different cellular sites of action of these drugs have been demonstrated (Lamberts et al, 1987).

The role of octreotide in the treatment of acromegaly is not yet definitive. Because it does not compromise pituitary trophic function, it has been suggested as an alternative to radiation therapy when endocrine activity continues after surgery. The drug's drawbacks include the need for lifelong treatment if used as sole therapy (which is true of all drug therapy for acromegaly) rather than as an adjunct to more definitive therapy, the increased risk of gallstones, the high cost (over $6,000/year), and the need for multiple daily injections (Daughaday, 1990).

Drug Evaluations

BROMOCRIPTINE MESYLATE
[Parlodel]

For chemical formula, see index entry Bromocriptine, In Female Hyperprolactinemia.

ACTIONS AND USES. Bromocriptine is a synthetic ergot alkaloid that acts directly on dopaminergic receptors, including those of pituitary cells. It is used in a variety of conditions that respond to dopaminergic therapy (eg, hyperprolactinemia, suppression of postpartum lactation, Parkinson's disease), including acromegaly.

Bromocriptine is indicated as an adjunct to surgery or irradiation in the treatment of acromegaly in about 1% to 20% of patients. In those who are responsive, blood levels of GH decrease within hours and the drug's effectiveness may be assessed within weeks.

Indications of a favorable response include improved glucose tolerance; reduced insulin requirements in diabetic patients; decreased sweating, urinary hydroxyproline levels, and incidence of headaches; and improved libido in men. The latter may be due to concomitant inhibition of prolactin secretion (hyperprolactinemia is associated with acromegaly in one-third of patients). Improvements in phenotypic features include softening of facial features, decreased skin and tongue thickness, and decreased hand and foot size. Regression of early visual defects and evidence of radiologic improvement suggest that bromocriptine may reduce the growth and mass of a minority of GH-producing tumors. However, tumor regression is not as common with GH-secreting tumors as with prolactinoma or mixed prolactin- and GH-producing tumors (Odell, 1984).

In spite of the favorable responses reported, bromocriptine is not curative. If the cause of acromegaly (ie, pituitary tumor, ectopic source) is not eliminated, increased secretion of GH resumes after cessation of treatment.

In summary, the advantage of bromocriptine in acromegaly is that it affects only the secretion of GH and prolactin. It appears to be useful as an adjunct to surgery or irradiation, in the treatment of persistent endocrinopathy after surgery, or to hasten relief of clinical symptoms in the interim between irradiation and realization of its effects. Although some patients appear to benefit, bromocriptine usually suppresses GH only partially and is a temporary noncurative measure.

ADVERSE REACTIONS. Adverse reactions are common when bromocriptine therapy is initiated. Thereafter, their incidence and severity depend on the dosage and its rate of increase. Common untoward effects include nausea, vomiting, dizziness, and orthostatic hypotension. Nausea usually disappears after three to four days and may be minimized by taking the medication with food and at bedtime. Rarely, orthostatic hypotension leads to syncope, even after ingestion of a single dose.

Cerebrospinal fluid rhinorrhea developed during treatment of a pituitary tumor with bromocriptine and may have been due to exposure of a defective sella floor as the tumor tissue retracted (Wilson et al, 1983).

Patients taking larger doses may experience decreased alcohol tolerance, constipation, dyspepsia, dryness of the mouth, nasal congestion, nocturnal leg cramps, depression, nightmares, and peripheral digital vasospasm on exposure to cold.

PHARMACOKINETICS. Bromocriptine is absorbed rapidly after oral administration; peak plasma levels are attained in about one hour. First-pass metabolism occurs with over 90% of the absorbed dose. The plasma half-life is three hours. About 98% is excreted in the feces, and the remaining 2% is eliminated in the urine.

DOSAGE AND PREPARATIONS.

Oral: For acromegaly, initially, 1.25 to 2.5 mg is given in the evening with food for two or three days. This dose may be increased by 2.5 mg on alternate days until tolerance and the maintenance level are reached. The usual therapeutic range is 20 to 30 mg daily in three or four divided doses. Larger doses are unlikely to improve response.

Parlodel (Sandoz). Capsules 5 mg; tablets 2.5 mg.

OCTREOTIDE ACETATE
[Sandostatin]

For chemical formula, see index entry Octreotide, In Diarrhea.

ACTIONS AND USES. Octreotide is an octapeptide with pharmacologic actions similar to those of the endogenous hormone somatostatin. Octreotide suppresses the excessive secretion of serotonin, gastrin, vasoactive intestinal peptide (VIP), glucagon, secretin, motilin, and pancreatic polypeptide in pathologic states. Its usefulness in acromegaly is due to its ability to inhibit GH secretion selectively; the effect is more prolonged than that of the natural hormone. Unlike the effect of somatostatin, GH secretion does not rebound.

Octreotide is rapidly absorbed after subcutaneous injection. The elimination half-life is about two hours, while that of the natural hormone is two to three minutes. Tissue response may extend to 12 hours, however.

ADVERSE REACTIONS AND PRECAUTIONS. The most common adverse effects include headache, hyperhidrosis, fatigue, acne, and joint pain (Ezzat et al, 1992). Nausea, pain at the injection site, diarrhea, abdominal discomfort, and vomiting occur in 3% to 10% of patients. Slight increases in glucosylated hemoglobin and increased excretion of fat in the stool were observed in two patients treated for prolonged periods (Plewe et al, 1986). Like somatostatin, octreotide suppresses cholecystokinin secretion. The lack of cholecystokinin in turn inhibits gallbladder contraction; bile flow also may be inhibited (Daughaday, 1990). Gallstone formation has occurred in up to 25% of patients who received octreotide for acromegaly (McKnight et al, 1989; Daughaday, 1990).

This drug is classified in FDA Pregnancy Category B.

DOSAGE AND PREPARATIONS.

Subcutaneous: For acromegaly, 50 or 100 mcg administered two or three times daily. Doses up to a total of 1.5 mg/day have been used in refractory patients. In several clinical studies, dosages ranged from 75 mcg to 1.5 mg/day (Gorden et al, 1989).

Sandostatin (Sandoz). Solution (for injection) 0.05, 0.1, and 0.5 mg/ml in 1 ml containers.

Cited References

Growth hormone. *Med Lett Drugs Ther* 26:80-81, 1984.

Report to the Chairman, Committee on the Judiciary, US Senate: Drug Misuse: Anabolic Steroids and Human Growth Hormone. Washington, DC, United States General Accounting Office, (Aug) 1989.

Albini CH, et al: Diagnostic value of the growth hormone-releasing factor stimulation test. *Clin Pharmacol Ther* 43:696-700, 1988.

Allen DB: Effects of nightly clonidine administration on growth velocity in short children without growth hormone deficiency: A double-blind, placebo-controlled study. *J Pediatr* 122:32-36, 1993.

Allen DB, Fost NC: Growth hormone therapy for short stature: Panacea or Pandora's box. *J Pediatr* 117:16-21, 1990.

American Academy of Pediatrics: Growth hormone in treatment of children with short stature. *Pediatrics* 72:891-894, 1983.

Amselem S, et al: Laron dwarfism and mutations of the growth hormone-receptor gene. *N Engl J Med* 321:989-995, 1989.

Barkan AL: Acromegaly: Diagnosis and therapy. *Endocrinol Metab Clin North Am* 18:277-310, 1989.

Barkan AL, et al: Plasma insulin-like growth factor-I/somatomedin-C in acromegaly: Correlation with the degree of growth hormone hypersecretion. *J Clin Endocrinol Metab* 67:69-73, 1988 A.

Barkan AL, et al: Treatment of acromegaly with the long-acting somatostatin analog SMS 201-995. *J Clin Endocrinol Metab* 66:16-23, 1988 B.

Barkan AL, et al: Preoperative treatment of acromegaly with long-acting somatostatin analog SMS 201-995: Shrinkage of invasive pituitary macroadenomas and improved surgical remission rate. *J Clin Endocrinol Metab* 67:1040-1048, 1988 C.

Barkan AL, et al: Increased growth hormone pulse frequency in acromegaly. *J Clin Endocrinol Metab* 69:1225-1233, 1989.

Baskin DS, et al: Transsphenoidal microsurgical removal of growth hormone-secreting pituitary adenomas: Review of 137 cases. *J Neurosurg* 56:634, 1982.

Batrinos M, et al: Increased GH response to GHRH in normal tall men. *Clin Endocrinol* 30:13-17, 1989.

Bauer FE, et al: Growth hormone release in man induced by galanin, new hypothalamic peptide. *Lancet* 2:192-195, 1986.

Baumann G, et al: Circulating growth hormone (GH)-binding protein complex: A major constituent of plasma GH in man. *Endocrinology* 122:976-984, 1988.

Benjamin M, et al: Short children, anxious parents: Is growth hormone the answer? *Hastings Cent Rep* 14:5-9, (April) 1984.

Bercu BB: Growth hormone treatment and the short child: To treat or not to treat? *J Pediatr* 110:991-995, 1987.

Bercu BB, Diamond FB Jr: Growth hormone neurosecretory dysfunction. *Clin Endocrinol Metab* 15:537-590, 1986.

Bercu BB, et al: Growth hormone (GH) provocative testing frequently does not reflect endogenous GH secretion. *J Clin Endocrinol Metab* 63:709-716, 1986.

Brain CE, et al: Continuous subcutaneous $GHRH_{(1-29)}$ NH_2 promotes growth over 1 year in short, slowly growing children. *Clin Endocrinol* 32:153-163, 1990.

Brock PR, et al: Malignant disease in Bloom's syndrome children treated with growth hormone, letter. *Lancet* 337:1345-1346, 1991.

Campino C, et al: Growth hormone (GH) receptor antibodies with GH-like activity occur spontaneously in acromegaly. *J Clin Endocrinol Metab* 74:751-756, 1992.

Cara JF, et al: Longitudinal study of relationship of plasma somatomedin-C concentration to pubertal growth spurt. *Am J Dis Child* 141:562-564, 1987.

Cara JF, et al: Height prognosis of children with true precocious puberty and growth hormone deficiency: Effect of combination therapy with gonadotropin releasing hormone agonist and growth hormone. *J Pediatr* 120:709-715, 1992.

Celniker AC, et al: Variability in the quantitation of circulating growth hormone using commercial immunoassays. *J Clin Endocrinol Metab* 68:469-476, 1989.

Chalew SA, et al: Growth hormone (GH) response to GH-releasing hormone in children with subnormal integrated concentrations of GH. *J Clin Endocrinol Metab* 62:1110-1115, 1986.

Chatelain P, et al: Growth hormone (GH) response to single intravenous injection of synthetic GH-releasing hormone in prepubertal children with growth failure. *J Clin Endocrinol Metab* 65:387-394, 1987.

Chiodini PG, et al: Medical treatment of acromegaly with SMS 201-995, a somatostatin analog: Comparison with bromocriptine. *J Clin Endocrinol Metab* 64:447-453, 1987.

Clemmons DR, Van Wyk JJ: Factors controlling blood concentration of somatomedin C. *Clin Endocrinol Metab* 13:113-143, 1984.

Costin G, Kaufman FR: Growth hormone secretory patterns in children with short stature. *J Pediatr* 110:362-368, 1987.

Costin G, et al: Growth hormone secretory dynamics in subjects with normal stature. *J Pediatr* 115:537-544, 1989.

Cuneo RC, et al: The growth hormone deficiency syndrome in adults. *Clin Endocrinol* 37:387-397, 1992.

Daughaday WH: Octreotide is effective in acromegaly but often results in cholelithiasis. *Ann Intern Med* 112:159-160, 1990.

Daughaday WH, et al: On the nomenclature of the somatomedins and insulin-like growth factors, letter. *J Clin Endocrinol Metab* 65:1075-1076, 1987.

De Boer H, et al: Body composition in adult growth hormone-deficient men, assessed by anthropometry and bioimpedance analysis. *J Clin Endocrinol Metab* 75:833-837, 1992.

Duck SC, et al: Subcutaneous growth hormone-releasing hormone therapy in growth hormone-deficient children: First year of therapy. *J Clin Endocrinol Metab* 75:1115-1120, 1992.

Ezzat S, Melmed S: Acromegaly: Etiology, diagnosis and management. *Compr Ther* 17:31-35, (July) 1991.

Ezzat S, et al: Octreotide treatment of acromegaly: A randomized, multicenter study. *Ann Intern Med* 117:711-718, 1992.

Fisher DA, et al: Leukaemia in patients treated with growth hormone. *Lancet* 1:1159-1160, 1988.

Frasier SD: Human pituitary growth hormone (hGH) therapy in growth hormone deficiency. *Endocrinol Rev* 4:155-170, 1983.

Frazer T, et al: Growth hormone-dependent growth failure. *J Pediatr* 101:12-15, 1982.

Frohman LA: Clinical review 22: Therapeutic options in acromegaly. *J Clin Endocrinol Metab* 72:1175-1181, 1991.

Frohman LA, et al: Rapid enzymatic degradation of growth hormone-releasing hormone by plasma in vitro and in vivo to a biologically inactive product cleaved at the NH_2 terminus. *J Clin Invest* 78:906-913, 1986.

Frohman LA, et al: Dipeptidyl-peptidase IV and trypsin-like enzymatic degradation of human growth hormone releasing hormone in plasma. *J Clin Invest* 83:1533-1540, 1989.

Gelato MC, et al: Effects of growth hormone-releasing factor in man. *J Clin Endocrinol Metab* 57:674-676, 1983.

Gelato MC, et al: Effects of growth hormone-releasing factor on growth hormone secretion in acromegaly. *J Clin Endocrinol Metab* 60:251-257, 1985.

Gertner JM, et al: Prospective clinical trial of human growth hormone in short children without growth hormone deficiency. *J Pediatr* 104:172-176, 1984.

Gertner JM, et al: Renewed catch-up growth with increased replacement doses of human growth hormone. *J Pediatr* 110:425-428, 1987.

Gorden P, et al: Somatostatin and somatostatin analogue (SMS 201-995) in treatment of hormone-secreting tumors of the pituitary and gastrointestinal tract and non-neoplastic diseases of the gut. *Ann Intern Med* 110:35-50, 1989.

Grossman A, et al: Growth hormone releasing hormone. *Clin Endocrinol Metab* 15:607-627, 1986.

Guillemin R, et al: Growth hormone-releasing factor from human pancreatic tumor that caused acromegaly. *Science* 218:585-587, 1982.

Hall K, Sara VR: Somatomedin levels in childhood, adolescence and adult life. *Clin Endocrinol Metab* 13:91-111, 1984.

Halse J, et al: A randomized study of SMS 201-995 *versus* bromocriptine treatment in acromegaly: Clinical and biochemical effects. *J Clin Endocrinol Metab* 70:1254-1261, 1990.

Hammarqvist F, et al: Biosynthetic human growth hormone preserves both muscle protein synthesis and the decrease in muscle-free glutamine, and improves whole-body nitrogen economy after operation. *Ann Surg* 216:184-191, 1992.

Hermanussen M, et al: Catch-up growth following transfer from three times weekly im to daily sc administration of hGH in GH deficient patients, monitored by knemometry. *Acta Endocrinol* 109:163-168, 1985.

Hibi I, et al: The influence of gonadal function and the effect of gonadal suppression treatment on final height in growth hormone (GH)-treated GH-deficient children. *J Clin Endocrinol Metab* 69:221-226, 1989.

Hindmarsh PC, Brook CGD: Effect of growth hormone on short normal children. *BMJ* 295:573-577, 1987.

Hindmarsh PC, et al: Growth hormone secretion in children determined by time series analysis. *Clin Endocrinol* 29:35-44, 1988.

Hindmarsh PC, et al: The interaction of growth hormone releasing hormone and somatostatin in the generation of a GH pulse in man. *Clin Endocrinol* 35:353-360, 1991 A.

Hindmarsh PC, et al: Wider indications for treatment with biosynthetic human growth hormone in children. *Clin Endocrinol* 34:417-427, 1991 B.

Ho KY, et al: Effects of sex and age on the 24-hour profile of growth hormone secretion in man: Importance of endogenous estradiol concentrations. *J Clin Endocrinol Metab* 64:51-58, 1987.

Ho KY, et al: Therapeutic efficacy of the somatostatin analog SMS 201-995 (octreotide) in acromegaly: Effects of dose and frequency and long-term safety. *Ann Intern Med* 112:173-181, 1990.

Ho PJ, et al: Regulation of pulsatile growth hormone secretion by fasting in normal subjects and patients with acromegaly. *J Clin Endocrinol Metab* 75:812-819, 1992.

Hokken-Koelega ACS, et al: Placebo-controlled, double-blind, crossover trial of growth hormone treatment in prepubertal children with chronic renal failure. *Lancet* 338:585-590, 1991.

Holcombe JH, et al: Biosynthetic human growth hormone in the treatment of growth hormone deficiency. *Acta Paediatr Scand Suppl* 367:44-48, 1990.

James RA, et al: Continuous infusion of octreotide in acromegaly. *Lancet* 2:1083-1087, 1989.

Jørgensen JOL: Human growth hormone replacement therapy: Pharmacological and clinical aspects. *Endocr Rev* 12:189-207, 1991.

Jørgensen JOL, et al: Beneficial effects of growth hormone treatment in GH-deficient adults. *Lancet* 1:1221-1225, 1989.

Jørgensen JOL, et al: Evening *versus* morning injections of growth hormone (GH) in GH-deficient patients: Effects on 24-hour patterns of circulating hormones and metabolites. *J Clin Endocrinol Metab* 70:207-214, 1990.

Kaplan SL, et al: Clinical studies with recombinant-DNA derived methionyl human growth hormone in growth hormone deficient children. *Lancet* 1:697-700, 1986.

Karpf DB, Braunstein GD: Current concepts in acromegaly: Etiology, diagnosis, and treatment. *Compr Ther* 12:22-30, (Jan) 1986.

Kelly PA, et al: The prolactin/growth hormone receptor family. *Endocr Rev* 12:235-251, 1991.

Kida K, et al: Urinary excretion of human growth hormone in children with short stature: Correlation with pituitary secretion of human growth hormone. *J Pediatr* 120:233-237, 1992.

LaFranchi S: Human growth hormone: Who is a candidate for treatment? *Postgrad Med* 91:367-388, (April) 1992.

Lamberts SWJ, et al: Comparison among the growth hormone-lowering effects in acromegaly of the somatostatin analog SMS 201-995, bromocriptine, and the combination of both drugs. *J Clin Endocrinol Metab* 63:16-19, 1986.

Lamberts SWJ, et al: Comparison between effects of SMS 201-995, bromocriptine, and combination of both drugs on hormone release by cultured pituitary tumour cells of acromegalic patients. *Clin Endocrinol* 27:11-23, 1987.

Lamberts SWJ, et al: The use of growth hormone in adults: A changing scene. *Clin Endocrinol* 37:111-115, 1992.

Lanes R: Diagnostic limitations of spontaneous growth hormone measurements in normally growing prepubertal children. *Am J Dis Child* 143:1284-1286, 1989.

Lang I, et al: Effects of sex and age on growth hormone response to growth hormone-releasing hormone in healthy individuals. *J Clin Endocrinol Metab* 65:535-540, 1987.

Lantos J, et al: Ethical issues in growth hormone therapy. *JAMA* 261:1020-1024, 1989.

Laron Z, et al: Classification of growth hormone insensitivity syndrome. *J Pediatr* 122:241, 1993.

Lesage C, et al: Near normalization of adolescent height with growth hormone therapy in very short children without growth hormone deficiency. *J Pediatr* 119:29-34, 1991.

Lin T-H, et al: Growth hormone testing in short children and their response to growth hormone therapy. *J Pediatr* 115:57-63, 1989.

Liu L, et al: Chronic sex steroid exposure increases mean plasma growth hormone concentration and pulse amplitude in men with isolated hypogonadotropic hypogonadism. *J Clin Endocrinol Metab* 64:651-656, 1987.

Loche S, et al: Augmentation of growth hormone secretion in children with constitutional growth delay by short term clonidine administration: A pulse amplitude-modulated phenomenon. *J Clin Endocrinol Metab* 68:426-430, 1989.

Mahoney CP: Evaluating the child with short stature. *Pediatr Clin North Am* 34:825-849, 1987.

Mauras N, et al: Augmentation of growth hormone secretion during puberty: Evidence for a pulse amplitude-modulated phenomenon. *J Clin Endocrinol Metab* 64:596-601, 1987.

McKnight JA, et al: Changes in glucose tolerance and development of gallstones during high dose treatment with octreotide for acromegaly. *BMJ* 299:604-605, 1989.

Melmed S: Extrapituitary acromegaly. *Endocrinol Metab Clin North Am* 20:507-518, 1991.

Melmed S, et al: Pituitary tumors secreting growth hormone and prolactin. *Ann Intern Med* 105:238-253, 1986.

Melmed S, et al: Medical management of acromegaly due to ectopic production of growth hormone-releasing hormone by a carcinoid tumor. *J Clin Endocrinol Metab* 67:395-399, 1988.

Merimee TJ, et al: Insulin-like growth factors in pygmies: Role of puberty in determining final stature. *N Engl J Med* 316:906-911, 1987.

Milner RDG: Which children should have growth hormone therapy? *Lancet* 1:483-485, 1986.

Moller DE, et al: Octreotide suppresses both growth hormone (GH) and GH-releasing hormone (GHRH) in acromegaly due to ectopic GHRH secretion. *J Clin Endocrinol Metab* 68:499-504, 1989.

Nortier JWR, et al: Bromocriptine therapy in acromegaly: Effects on plasma GH levels, somatomedin-C levels and clinical activity. *Clin Endocrinol* 22:209-217, 1985.

Odell WD: Further considerations of therapy of pituitary tumors, in Odell WD, Nelson DH (eds): *Pituitary Tumors.* New York, Futura, 1984.

Oppizzi G, et al: Relationship between somatomedin-C and growth hormone levels in acromegaly: Basal and dynamic evaluation. *J Clin Endocrinol Metab* 63:1348-1353, 1986.

Pescovitz OH, Tan E: Lack of benefit of clonidine treatment for short stature in a double-blind, placebo-controlled trial. *Lancet* 2:874-877, 1988.

Plewe G, et al: Long-term treatment of acromegaly with somatostatin analogue SMS 201-995, letter. *N Engl J Med* 314:1390-1391, 1986.

Raiti S: Treatment of growth hormone deficiency. *J Endocrinol Invest* 12(suppl 3):21-24, 1989.

Raiti S, et al: Growth-stimulating effects of human growth hormone therapy in patients with Turner syndrome. *J Pediatr* 109:944-949, 1986.

Raiti S, et al: Short-term treatment of short stature and subnormal growth rate with human growth hormone. *J Pediatr* 110:357-361, 1987.

Reiter EO, et al: Variable estimates of serum growth hormone concentrations by different radioassay systems. *J Clin Endocrinol* 66:68-71, 1988.

Reubi JC, Landolt AM: The growth hormone responses to octreotide in acromegaly correlate with adenoma somatostatin receptor status. *J Clin Endocrinol Metab* 68:844-850, 1989.

Rivier J, et al: Characterization of growth hormone-releasing factor from human pancreatic islet tumor. *Nature* 300:276-278, 1982.

Rose SR, et al: The advantage of measuring stimulated as compared with spontaneous growth hormone levels in the diagnosis of growth hormone deficiency. *N Engl J Med* 319:201-207, 1988.

Rosenbaum M, Gertner JM: Metabolic clearance rates of synthetic human growth hormone in children, adult women, and adult men. *J Clin Endocrinol Metab* 69:821-824, 1989.

Rosenfeld RG, et al: Insulin-like growth factors I and II in evaluation of growth retardation. *J Pediatr* 109:428-433, 1986.

Rosenfeld RG, et al: Six-year results of a randomized, prospective trial of human growth hormone and oxandrolone in Turner syndrome. *J Pediatr* 121:49-55, 1992.

Rosenthal SM, et al: Synthetic human pancreas growth hormone-releasing factor (hpGRF, $_{1-44}$NH2) stimulates growth hormone secretion in normal men. *J Clin Endocrinol Metab* 57:677-679, 1983.

Ross RJM, et al: Treatment of growth-hormone deficiency with growth-hormone-releasing hormone. *Lancet* 1:5-8, 1987.

Rudman D, et al: Children with normal-variant short stature: Treatment with human growth hormone for six months. *N Engl J Med* 305:123-131, 1981.

Rudman D, et al: Effects of human growth hormone in men over 60 years old. *N Engl J Med* 323:1-6, 1990.

Russo L, Moore WV: Comparison of subcutaneous and intramuscular administration of human growth hormone in therapy of growth hormone deficiency. *J Clin Endocrinol Metab* 55:1003-1006, 1982.

Saggese G, Cesaretti G: Criteria for recognition of the growth-inefficient child who may respond to treatment with growth hormone. *Am J Dis Child* 143:1287-1293, 1989.

Salomon F, et al: The effects of treatment with recombinant human growth hormone on body composition and metabolism in adults with growth hormone deficiency. *N Engl J Med* 321:1797-1803, 1989.

Scacchi M, et al: Treatment with biosynthetic growth hormone of short thalassaemic patients with impaired growth hormone secretion. *Clin Endocrinol* 35:335-339, 1991.

Smith PJ, Brook CGD: Place of intravenous GHRH 1-40 studies in therapy of growth hormone-deficient children with GHRH. *Clin Endocrinol* 27:97-105, 1987.

Smith PJ, Brook CGD: Growth hormone releasing hormone or growth hormone treatment in growth hormone insufficiency. *Arch Dis Child* 63:629-634, 1988.

Smith PJ, et al: Contribution of dose and frequency of administration to the therapeutic effect of growth hormone. *Arch Dis Child* 63:491-494, 1988.

Spiess J, et al: Sequence analysis of growth hormone releasing factor from human pancreatic islet tumor. *Biochemistry* 21:6037-6040, 1982.

Spiliotis BE, et al: Growth hormone neurosecretory dysfunction: A treatable cause of short stature. *JAMA* 251:2223-2230, 1984.

Steardo L, et al: Pharmacological evidence for dual gabanergic regulation of growth hormone release in humans. *Life Sci* 39:979-985, 1986.

Stolar MW, Baumann G: Big growth hormone forms in human plasma: Immunochemical evidence for their pituitary origin. *Metabolism* 35:75-77, 1986.

Takano K, et al: Treatment of 46 patients with Turner's syndrome with recombinant human growth hormone (YM-17798) for three years: A multicentre study. *Acta Endocrinol* 126:296, 1992.

Tauber JP, et al: Long term effects of continuous subcutaneous infusion of the somatostatin analog octreotide in the treatment of acromegaly. *J Clin Endocrinol Metab* 68:917-924, 1989.

Thorner MO, et al: Human-pancreatic growth-hormone-releasing factor selectively stimulates growth hormone secretion in man. *Lancet* 1:24-28, 1983.

Thorner MO, et al: Acceleration of growth rate in growth hormone-deficient children treated with human growth hormone-releasing hormone. *Pediatr Res* 24:145-151, 1988.

Tönshoff B, et al: Growth-stimulating effects of recombinant human growth hormone in children with end-stage renal disease. *J Pediatr* 116:561-566, 1990.

Torrado C, et al: Treatment of children with Down syndrome and growth retardation with recombinant human growth hormone. *J Pediatr* 119:478-483, 1991.

Underwood LE: Growth hormone therapy for short stature: Yes or no? *Hosp Pract* 192-198, (April) 1992.

Vance ML: Growth hormone for the elderly? Editorial. *N Engl J Med* 323:52-54, 1990.

Vance ML, Thorner MO: Growth-hormone-releasing hormone: Clinical update, editorial. *Ann Intern Med* 105:447-448, 1986.

Vance ML, et al: Human pancreatic tumor growth hormone-releasing factor: Dose-response relationships in normal man. *J Clin Endocrinol Metab* 58:838-844, 1984.

Vance ML, et al: Lack of *in vivo* somatotroph desensitization or depletion after 14 days of continuous growth hormone (GH)-releasing hormone administration in normal men and a GH-deficient boy. *J Clin Endocrinol Metab* 68:22-28, 1989.

Van der Schueren-Lodeweyckx M, et al: Growth-promoting effect of growth hormone and low dose ethinyl estradiol in girls with Turner's syndrome. *J Clin Endocrinol Metab* 70:122-126, 1990.

Van Vliet G, et al: Growth hormone treatment for short stature. *N Engl J Med* 309:1016-1022, 1983.

Voerman HJ, et al: Effects of recombinant human growth hormone in patients with severe sepsis. *Ann Surg* 216:648-655, 1992.

Walker J, et al: Growth hormone treatment of children with short stature increases insulin secretion but does not impair glucose disposal. *J Clin Endocrinol Metab* 69:253-258, 1989.

Wallis M: Growth hormone-binding proteins. *Clin Endocrinol* 35:291-293, 1991.

Wass JAH: Growth hormone neuroregulation and clinical relevance of somatostatin. *Clin Endocrinol Metab* 12:695-724, 1983.

Wass JAH, et al: Changes in circulating somatomedin-C levels in bromocriptine-treated acromegaly. *Clin Endocrinol* 17:369-377, 1982.

Wass JAH, et al: Treatment of acromegaly. *Clin Endocrinol Metab* 15:683-707, 1986.

Weeke J, et al: A randomized comparison of intranasal and injectable octreotide administration in patients with acromegaly. *J Clin Endocrinol Metab* 75:163-169, 1992.

Whitehead HM, et al: Growth hormone treatment of adults with growth hormone deficiency: Results of a 13-month placebo controlled cross-over study. *Clin Endocrinol* 36:45-52, 1992.

Williams TC, Frohman LA: Potential therapeutic indications for growth hormone and growth hormone-releasing hormone in conditions other than growth retardation. *Pharmacotherapy* 6:311-318, 1986.

Wilson JD, et al: Cerebrospinal fluid rhinorrhea during treatment of pituitary tumors with bromocriptine. *Acta Endocrinol* 103:457-460, 1983.

Wilson DM, et al: Subcutaneous versus intramuscular growth hormone therapy: Growth and acute somatomedin response. *Pediatrics* 76:361-364, 1985.

Winer LM, et al: Basal plasma growth hormone levels in man: New evidence for rhythmicity of growth hormone secretion. *J Clin Endocrinol Metab* 70:1678-1686, 1990.

Wolf RF, et al: Growth hormone and insulin reverse net whole body and skeletal muscle protein catabolism in cancer patients. *Ann Surg* 216:280-288, 1992.

Yarasheski KE, et al: Effect of growth hormone and resistance exercise on muscle growth in young men. *Am J Physiol* 262:E261-E267, 1992.

Zadik Z, et al: Do short children secrete insufficient growth hormone? *Pediatrics* 76:355-360, 1985.

Zadik Z, et al: Reproducibility of growth hormone testing procedures: A comparison between 24-hour integrated concentration and pharmacological stimulation. *J Clin Endocrinol Metab* 71:1127-1130, 1990.

Zamboni G, et al: Effects of two different regimens of recombinant human growth hormone therapy on the bone mineral density of patients with growth hormone deficiency. *J Pediatr* 119:483-485, 1991.

Zimmerman D, et al: Congenital gigantism due to growth hormone-releasing hormone excess and pituitary hyperplasia with adenomatous transformation. *J Clin Endocrinol Metab* 76:216-222, 1993.

Drugs Used in Male Reproductive Dysfunction

50

PHYSIOLOGY

INDICATIONS

Constitutional Delay of Growth

Cryptorchidism

Hypogonadism

Micropenis

Impotence

Infertility, General

Infertility Due to Varicocele

Infertility Due to Hypogonadotropic Hypogonadism

Infertility Due to Hyperprolactinemia

Idiopathic Male Infertility

Immunologic Infertility

ANDROGENIC AGENTS

DRUG EVALUATIONS

Anterior Pituitary and Hypothalamic Agents

PHYSIOLOGY

In males, androgens are secreted by the testes and the adrenal cortex. They are responsible for the development and maintenance of primary and secondary sexual characteristics, normal reproductive function, and sexual performance ability, as well as for stimulating the growth and development of the skeleton and skeletal muscle during puberty.

Testosterone is the principal androgen secreted by the steroidogenic Leydig cells, which are located in the interstitial spaces of the testis. Men produce 2.5 to 10 mg of testosterone daily and plasma concentrations are 250 to 1,000 ng/dL. Plasma levels fluctuate in a circadian pattern in young men and are maximal in the early morning. Superimposed on this rhythm are shorter, smaller secretory peaks that follow elevated luteinizing hormone secretion. These variations in plasma hormone levels demonstrate the importance of multiple blood sampling in some experimental and diagnostic situations, although single-point assays are usually sufficient for most clinical situations.

In males, about one-third of the 17-ketosteroids (testosterone precursors) are secreted by the adrenal cortex. However, since the biopotency and rate of conversion to testosterone are low, adrenal androgens are not as important functionally as the smaller amount of testosterone produced by the testis. If Leydig cell function is lost or markedly impaired, the amount of testosterone produced by conversion of the adrenocortical androgens, androstenedione and dehydroepiandrosterone, is inadequate to maintain normal male function.

The anterior pituitary hormone, luteinizing hormone (LH), stimulates steroidogenesis in the Leydig cells. Follicle-stimulating hormone (FSH) is necessary for quantitatively and qualitatively normal spermatogenesis. A negative feedback system involving the hypothalamus, the anterior pituitary, and the testis controls gonadotropic hormone secretion. Testosterone suppresses secretion of LH and, to a lesser extent, FSH.

Estradiol, which is secreted by the testis and produced by the peripheral conversion of testosterone and other androgens, also may participate in the negative feedback control of LH and FSH. Synthetic androgens that cannot be aromatized to estrogen (eg, oxandrolone, mesterolone) are less effective in suppressing gonadotropins than testosterone, which can be aromatized.

Inhibin, a glycoprotein consisting of disulfide-linked α and β subunits secreted by the Sertoli cells of the seminiferous tubules, also inhibits release of FSH. Serum inhibin concentration increases during puberty in both sexes (Burger et al, 1988), and this glycoprotein may play a role in development of FSH target tissues (ie, Sertoli cells, ovarian follicles) at that time (DeJong, 1988).

In men, approximately 98% of circulating testosterone is bound to protein, primarily to sex hormone-binding globulin (SHBG, testosterone-estradiol-binding globulin [TEBG]) and albumin. As with other steroid hormones, the biologically active portion is the free (dialyzable, unbound) fraction. The hepatic synthesis of SHBG is decreased by androgens and elevated by estrogens. Consequently, men have higher levels of free circulating testosterone than women, both proportionately and in total amount. In contrast, because of their high total estradiol secretion, women have higher free estradiol concentrations even though a smaller fraction of plasma estradiol is unbound.

The half-life of endogenous free testosterone in the blood is 10 to 20 minutes. Testosterone is metabolized primarily in the liver and is excreted mainly in the urine as the metabolites, androsterone and etiocholanolone. Small amounts of testosterone glucuronide and sulfate also are excreted. About

6% of the hormone is excreted unaltered in the feces. The plasma half-lives of synthetic androgens are longer because they are metabolized more slowly. Synthetic androgens may be excreted as unaltered hormone or as metabolites.

The steroidogenic activity of LH is mediated through stimulation of cyclic adenosine monophosphate (cAMP) and calmodulin synthesis. The androgenic action of testosterone in some tissues (eg, prostate, seminal vesicle, external genitalia) normally depends on the intracellular reduction of testosterone to 5α-dihydrotestosterone (DHT), which binds to the specific androgen receptor in the cytoplasm of these tissues. The steroid receptor complex is transported to the nucleus where it initiates transcription activity that results in the production of enzymes and other proteins responsible for androgenic expression. In other tissues (eg, skeletal muscle, bone marrow, Sertoli cells), testosterone itself is probably the active intracellular hormone. In the central nervous system, the hormonal effects of testosterone may result in part from its aromatization to estradiol.

Aging: Increasing age in men has been correlated with a decreased number of Leydig cells, reduced sperm production, and elevated serum concentrations of LH and FSH. Elevation of FSH is greater and correlates with lower sperm production (Neaves et al, 1984). In one study, testosterone not bound to SHBG (albumin-bound and free testosterone) was decreased in normal older men (65 to 83 years) but not in younger men (22 to 39 years) (Nankin and Calkins, 1986). In other studies, free plasma testosterone was reported to decline with advancing age, which correlates with reduction of various aspects of sexuality (eg, frequency of activity, erectile and orgasmic function, libido). Hormonal changes are thought to be responsible for only a small part of declining sexual activity with age (Silber, 1991).

There is no male hormonal climacteric analogous to that in women. However, when serum testosterone levels decrease abruptly at any age (eg, following surgical trauma or orchiectomy), vasomotor flushing can occur. This may be alleviated by testosterone replacement therapy.

Behavior: See index entry Sex Offenders, Drug Therapy.

INDICATIONS

CONSTITUTIONAL DELAY OF GROWTH. This condition (height two or more standard deviations below the mean for age and sex) occurs in approximately 2.5% of normal children and more frequently causes concern in boys than in girls. Family history may reveal similar growth retardation in parents, siblings, or other relatives. The diagnosis is made by exclusion and is conclusive after normal but late or prolonged adolescent development. In some instances, boys with idiopathic delayed puberty can be differentiated from those with permanent hypothalamic hypogonadism on the basis of nocturnal LH secretory patterns. Patients with delayed puberty may have elevated, pulsatile patterns of nocturnal LH secretion while those with hypothalamic hypogonadism may not. No differences in baseline testosterone levels or LH response to gonadotropin-releasing hormone (GnRH) injection have been observed (Wagner et al, 1986).

Medical attention frequently is sought because of short stature rather than lack of sexual development, in contrast to patients with primary or hypogonadotropic hypogonadism in whom height is often normal but sexual development is deficient. Characteristics of constitutional delayed growth include normal birth weight, growth curve parallel to normal, low bone age for chronological age but normal for the stage of development (bone age is normal in genetic short stature), and low levels of plasma gonadotropins and adrenal androgens for age but normal for size and stage of sexual development (Rosenfeld et al, 1982; Kelley and Ruvalcaba, 1982; Kulin, 1983).

Bone age is determined at the initial evaluation. Family history of growth development is obtained and nonendocrine causes of growth retardation are considered. Further testing may be postponed during a six-month observation period unless the child is three or more standard deviations below average height or there is no sexual maturation by bone age of 12 to 13 or chronological age of 14 in boys. Extreme anxiety of the patient and parents also may stimulate earlier evaluation. Serum thyroxine and gonadotropins are measured and, if normal, the adequacy of growth hormone secretion may be determined.

Treatment: Drug therapy is not required to achieve normal growth in constitutional delay of growth and puberty; normal development occurs by 18 years, although linear growth may not be complete until after age 20 and final adult height may be slightly below the normal predicted height (LaFranchi et al, 1991). Adult males with a history of constitutional delay of growth have been reported to have decreased bone mineral density (Finkelstein et al, 1992).

When delayed growth and puberty cause significant emotional stress despite reassurance, treatment with androgenic agents may be considered in boys. The goal of therapy is to accelerate initiation of a growth spurt that would otherwise occur later. Patients should be 14 years or older with a bone age at least two years behind the chronological age before treatment is attempted. Care must be taken to avoid doses that produce premature epiphyseal closure, which would compromise adult height. Usually, hormone treatment is employed for three to six months, followed by a drug-free observation period of six months. Bone age should be determined roentgenographically before initiation of therapy and at intervals during and after treatment. The increase in bone age should not exceed the increase in height age. Since stimulation of bone maturation may persist for six months after therapy is discontinued, steroids should be withdrawn well before the skeletal age reaches the norm for the chronological age. Often the pubertal changes initiated by treatment proceed spontaneously after one course of therapy, but a second course may be employed if necessary. However, the need for a second course should prompt reconsideration of the diagnosis of gonadotropin deficiency.

Any anabolic steroid or androgen may be prescribed for constitutional delay of growth. The choice of preparation depends on the balance of growth stimulation and sexual maturation desired; the route of administration preferred also may influence drug selection. For listing, see index entry Anabolic Steroids (Table). Less potent androgens stimulate linear growth but produce relatively less sexual maturation. Oxandrolone [Oxandrin], an anabolic steroid, increased growth velocity in children with constitutional delay of growth compared with untreated controls. However, the effect on growth was short-lived and average adult height either was not increased (Joss et al, 1989) or increased by less than one inch over predicted height (Tse et al, 1990). In another study, oxandrolone was reported to be as effective as growth hormone for treatment of constitutional delay of growth (Loche et al, 1991).

A preparation with greater androgenic activity, usually an intramuscular testosterone ester (eg, testosterone enanthate [Andryl, Delatestryl]), may be chosen if the above guidelines are followed. Low doses (50 mg/month intramuscularly) of testosterone enanthate stimulated height velocity and sexual development in boys with constitutional delay of growth without compromising adult height (Richman and Kirsch, 1988). A sublingual testosterone preparation [AndroTest-SL] has received orphan drug status for this indication and currently is undergoing clinical trials. See also review by Lee and O'Dea, 1990.

CRYPTORCHIDISM. About 5.5% of male infants have cryptorchid testes at birth, and the condition persists in 1.4% at 3 months of age. The incidence is higher in premature infants and in those with certain associated conditions (eg, Kallmann's, Klinefelter's, and Noonan's syndromes). Up to two-thirds of patients with nonscrotal testes have retractile, not cryptorchid, testes. These patients do not develop pathologic testicular changes and do not require therapy (Palmer, 1991).

Little spontaneous testicular descent occurs after 12 months of age, and progressive irreversible tubular damage may begin in cryptorchid testes within the first two years of life; therefore, treatment should begin early to avoid infertility. Initiation of drug therapy usually is recommended by age 2. However, some tubular function may be preserved even when treatment is started in prepubertal boys; delay until puberty usually results in significant impairment of sperm production. Even after testicular descent, normal spermatogenesis may not occur. Among men who underwent orchiopexy for cryptorchidism, the paternity rate was higher in those with unilateral than bilateral cryptorchidism (Elder, 1987). Androgen production is rarely compromised in the cryptorchid testis.

Men with a history of cryptorchidism have an increased relative risk of developing testicular cancer. Although the estimates vary greatly, a relative risk eight times higher than normal for bilateral cryptorchidism and 6.5 times higher than normal for unilateral cryptorchidism seems likely (Depue et al, 1986). A relative risk of testicular cancer 5.9 times higher than that in noncryptorchid subjects was found in another study. In unilateral cryptorchidism, the risk of cancer was higher in the affected testis (Strader et al, 1988). About 10% of men with testicular cancer have a history of cryptorchidism (Chilvers et al, 1986 A). Although questions remain about the relationship between correction of cryptorchidism and testicular cancer (Depue et al, 1986; Pike et al, 1986), a case-control study on 271 patients with testicular cancer provided the first direct, although limited, evidence that the risk increases with age at correction (Pottern et al, 1985). Even though correction of cryptorchidism does not always prevent malignancy, it facilitates detection if malignancy does occur.

Treatment: Correction of cryptorchidism at an early age is currently recommended to preserve fertility and reduce the risk of testicular cancer. However, a therapeutic dilemma exists: early treatment is recommended to reduce future abnormalities, but hormonal therapy is most successful in boys over 7 years of age (Palmer, 1991). If a hernia also is present, surgery should be performed to correct both defects. If not, hormonal therapy probably should be employed before surgery is undertaken. If this is unsuccessful, surgical correction (or removal of the cryptorchid testis if this fails) should be performed.

Chorionic gonadotropin (hCG) has been the standard hormonal therapy for this condition. Gonadorelin (GnRH) has been tried more recently. Success rates for hormonal therapy of cryptorchid testes vary widely; discrepancies may be due to failure to differentiate between retractile and true cryptorchid testes. In a double-blind study in which patients with retractile testes were excluded, neither subcutaneously administered hCG nor intranasally administered gonadorelin stimulated testicular descent; in five boys with retractile testes, hCG induced testicular descent (Rajfer et al, 1986). In a double-blind placebo-controlled study of 252 cryptorchid boys, treatment with gonadorelin nasal spray caused testicular descent in only 18% of subjects. Moreover, the clinical description of the successfully treated subjects suggests that about half had retractile rather than truly cryptorchid testes (de Muinck Keizer-Shrama et al, 1986; Chilvers et al, 1986 B).

HYPOGONADISM. Decreased Leydig cell function can result from abnormality of the testis (primary hypogonadism) or from lack of gonadotropic stimulation (hypogonadotropism) caused by hypothalamic (tertiary) or pituitary (secondary) failure. In one study, almost all patients with idiopathic hypogonadotropic hypogonadism lacked pulsatile LH or FSH secretion. The most severely affected patients had never undergone puberty, and half of these also were anosmic (Kallmann's syndrome). Other patients in whom pulsatile gonadotropin secretion was lacking experienced at least partial spontaneous puberty. Other aberrations in the patterns of gonadotropic secretion include nocturnal pulses similar to those in early puberty and low amplitude pulses (Spratt et al, 1987 A).

Disorders associated with compromised primary Leydig cell function include chromosomal defect (eg, Klinefelter's syndrome), trauma, bilateral torsion, irradiation, or testicular failure associated with disease (eg, myotonic dystrophy, mumps orchitis). Serum gonadotropin levels are high in primary failure (due to lack of negative feedback by androgen) and low in secondary hypogonadism.

The response of Leydig cells to gonadotropin may be tested by administering hCG. If testosterone secretion is stimulated markedly, primary gonadal failure or insensitivity to gonadotropin is ruled out. Human chorionic gonadotropin also can be used to stimulate Leydig cell function, and this agent may produce greater testicular growth than testosterone (Bistritzer et al, 1989).

The time to initiate replacement therapy depends on when clinical manifestations appear, not on whether hypogonadism is primary or secondary. Patients with primary or secondary hypogonadism may seek help because of failure of normal pubertal development or because of impotence, lack of libido, or decreased beard growth after pubertal development was completed. Patients with primary testicular failure may not seek medical attention until adulthood. A patient with Klinefelter's syndrome may have normal height, incomplete virilization, and eunuchoid body proportions but may not consult a physician until infertility becomes apparent in adulthood.

Treatment: Regardless of the cause of hypogonadism, the dose and schedule for replacement therapy depend on age and developmental stage at presentation and the severity of the deficit. Therapy may be directed toward induction of puberty, maintenance of secondary sexual characteristics and sexual behavior, or treatment of infertility. Replacement therapy also increases bone density. Cortical bone increases in all patients, but trabecular bone density increases more in those whose epiphyses are not fused at the time therapy begins (Finkelstein et al, 1989).

When *induction of puberty* is undertaken, a parenteral preparation (eg, testosterone enanthate, testosterone cypionate [Andro-Cyp, Depo-Testosterone, Virilon IM]) achieves the best results. Replacement dosages are generally increased slowly to induce progressive changes of puberty without compromising height. Full sexual development is usually attained in three to four years. Gynecomastia rarely may occur due to aromatization to estrogen. Priapism, which is rarely a problem with appropriate dosage, can be alleviated by adjusting the dose. Although oral therapy with fluoxymesterone [Halotestin] or methyltestosterone [Metandren, Oreton Methyl, Testred, Virilon] may be more convenient for maintenance therapy in patients with hypogonadism, the parenteral testosterone esters are preferred for long-term use because of their greater potency and lack of the hepatotoxicity associated with 17α-alkylated compounds.

An investigational transdermal system consisting of an adhesive film impregnated with testosterone has been successful in providing testosterone in a pattern that mimics normal circadian secretion. A patch is applied daily to the scrotal skin, which is highly permeable because of its vascularity and thin stratum corneum (Korenman et al, 1987). Normal serum testosterone concentrations, as well as satisfactory secondary sexual characteristics, libido, and sexual function, are achieved. However, greatly increased levels of dihydrotestosterone (DHT) are found, probably due to 5α-reductase activity and conversion from testosterone in the scrotal skin. More studies are necessary to determine if long-term risks (eg, prostatic hypertrophy) are associated with the elevated DHT levels (Findlay et al, 1989; Ahmed et al, 1988; Cunningham et al, 1989).

MICROPENIS. This can occur in association with hypospadias, hypogonadotropic or primary hypogonadism, androgen insensitivity, or as an idiopathic condition. Treatment is usually limited to three months to avoid epiphyseal maturation and, ideally, should be undertaken in the neonatal period and repeated once or twice during childhood if necessary. Penile growth may occur after intramuscular administration of testosterone. Alternatively, topical application of testosterone to the penis may be employed, although some authorities feel that the response is better after parenteral administration. Topical application may simplify management and reduce expense, however. It is generally agreed that the action of topical androgen is mediated, at least partly, through systemic absorption of the hormone. Side effects (eg, pubic hair development) can be minimized by using low concentrations (ie, 1.25% and 2.5% testosterone) (Sokol and Swerdloff, 1983). A topical preparation is not available commercially and must be compounded.

IMPOTENCE. Erection involves complex interactions of psychological, hormonal, neural, and vascular functions. Both sympathetic and parasympathetic pathways are utilized. In the flaccid state, α-1-postjunctional adrenoreceptor stimulation of smooth muscle tone in arterioles probably maintains restricted blood flow. Relaxation of smooth muscle in arterioles and sinusoids of the corpora cavernosa and spongiosum reduces peripheral resistance and increases blood flow and engorgement of these tissues. Although acetylcholine may initiate this relaxation, vasoactive intestinal polypeptide (VIP) or nitric oxide (Kim et al, 1991) may be the major neurotransmitters that produce this effect. Compression of venules, probably a passive phenomenon, helps maintain the erection (Lue and Tanagho, 1987; Malloy and Malkowicz, 1987).

Impotence may result from malfunction of one or more of the functional support systems. In the past, it was thought that impotence was of psychogenic origin in more than 90% of the cases. Although there frequently is a psychologic component, organic causes are identified now in about 50% of the cases. Neurologic causes include impotence secondary to a disease (eg, diabetes mellitus, multiple sclerosis) and spinal cord injury or nerve damage caused by surgery (eg, prostatectomy). Decreased blood flow to the penis (eg, arteriosclerosis, vascular damage from injury, bypass procedures, renal transplant), endocrine malfunction (eg, hypogonadism, hyperprolactinemia), or structural abnormality of the penis (eg, Peyronie's disease) also may cause impotence. Numerous drugs can also induce erectile dysfunction (eg, most antihypertensive agents, opioids, antidepressants, antianxiety and antipsychotic agents, ethyl alcohol, chemotherapeutic agents, cimetidine, estrogenic agents) (Buffum, 1986; *Med Lett Drugs Ther,* 1987; McWaine and Procci, 1988). Reviews on impotence (Krane et al, 1989; Morgentaler, 1991) and its occurrence in diabetic patients (Kaiser and Korenman, 1988) and the elderly (Johnson and Morley, 1988) are available.

Diagnosis: Initial diagnostic efforts are directed toward determining whether impotence is psychogenic or organic. A complete physical examination is performed and a history is taken; the latter includes sexual history and questioning about recent emotional upheavals or use of drugs that could affect erectile function. Psychogenic impotence is more likely to be abrupt in onset and of a situational nature (eg, to vary in occurrence or severity with different partners or techniques).

Organic impotence tends to be gradual in onset and occurs more consistently.

Assessment of nocturnal penile tumescence (NPT) can help differentiate psychogenic from organic impotence. Normal men experience one to several erections during nighttime sleep. Men with psychogenic impotence continue to have erections during sleep but are unable to experience or maintain an erection while awake. Several mechanical and electronic devices are available to measure NPT. The former type consists of a band placed around the base of the penis. The band is calibrated so that closures (eg, velcro, plastic) break at various levels of pressure (Bradley, 1987). Further refinement of NPT assessment has taken into account changes in both circumference and rigidity; the latter is determined by the use of microprocessors, servomotors, and loop transducers. A simple but crude mechanical method of NPT assessment is to secure a strip of stamps around the base of the penis; if erection occurs during the night, the strip is broken (Barry et al, 1980).

Intracavernous injection of papaverine also has been used as a screening technique. Patients who fail to have an erection following this procedure probably have vasculogenic impotence; patients who respond positively may be spared angiography (Abber et al, 1986; Buvat et al, 1986). Other diagnostic methods are used to investigate neural (eg, evoked potentials in the pudendal nerve) and vascular (eg, angiography, Doppler pulse-wave analysis) causes of impotence.

Diagnostic methods for vascular (Mueller and Lue, 1988), neural (Padma-Nathan, 1988), and hormonal (McClure, 1988) causes of impotence have been reviewed.

Treatment: The method of treatment for impotence depends on the cause. Psychogenic impotence often can be treated successfully in sex therapy programs, but this approach can be lengthy. Vascular causes may be correctable by surgery (eg, repair of arteries damaged by injury, tying off of leaky veins). Penile prosthetic implants, available as semirigid, inflatable, or articulating devices (Krauss, 1987), are effective for impotence from any cause but should be used only when other methods are unsuitable or fail. A penile implant may preclude the occurrence of a natural erection. External vacuum devices also are available. A discussion of therapeutic options for treatment of impotence is available (Orvis and Lue, 1987).

Pharmacologic treatment is sometimes appropriate. In hypogonadal men, testosterone replacement can restore libido and potency. The effectiveness of androgen therapy in the absence of low serum testosterone is unproven. Some patients helped by empiric therapy may have an underlying gonadal disorder (eg, some diabetic patients have gonadal dysfunction due to diabetes) (Murray et al, 1987). The possibility of stimulating prostate growth in older men should be considered before prescribing testosterone without a clear need for replacement (Meares, 1987). Hyperprolactinemia in men is often accompanied by low serum testosterone and impotence. Bromocriptine lowers or normalizes the serum prolactin concentration, and this is often accompanied by a return of potency (see the discussion on Infertility Due to Hyperprolactinemia). In these instances, administration of testosterone alone generally is ineffective (Malloy and Malkowicz, 1987). Patients with hyperprolactinemia and impotence should be evaluated for pituitary tumor prior to initiation of therapy with bromocriptine.

Yohimbine has long been reputed to be an aphrodisiac, but determination of its effectiveness for the treatment of impotence has been impeded by experimental designs that utilized combination regimens and had other deficiencies. In the study most often cited to date, 23 patients with organic impotence not associated with hypothalamic-pituitary-gonadal deficiency were given yohimbine [Yohimex] 6 mg orally three times daily for ten weeks. This uncontrolled study showed improved quality or complete return of erectile function in 17% and 26% of subjects, respectively (43% positive response) (Morales et al, 1982). Minor side effects, which included nausea, nervousness, and/or dizziness, were reported by three patients. Larger doses caused weakness, elevated blood pressure, and increased heart rate. In later controlled studies by the same group, subjects with organic impotence received the same regimen as above; the response rate for yohimbine was 43.5% versus 27.6% for those who received a placebo, a difference that was not statistically significant (Morales et al, 1987). In other studies, yohimbine was more effective than placebo in men with psychogenic impotence (Reid et al, 1987) and in those with impotence of undetermined origin (Susset et al, 1989). In the latter study, the drug was most effective in younger patients whose impotence was less severe and of shorter duration.

Yohimbine is an α_2 adrenergic antagonist. It purportedly affects erectile function by stimulating presynaptic norepinephrine release (Buffum, 1985). Yohimbine may stimulate erotically induced erection via a sympathetic pathway rather than reflex erection via a parasympathetic pathway as evidenced by failure to produce NPT (*Lancet*, 1986). At this time, documentation of yohimbine's usefulness to treat impotence is sparse and inconclusive. Although the drug may be beneficial in some patients and is probably worthy of further investigation, its efficacy in the treatment of impotence remains unproven.

The most widely used pharmacologic treatment for impotence is the injection of papaverine (Brindley, 1983) or, more commonly, papaverine plus phentolamine, into the corpus cavernosum. Papaverine is a smooth muscle relaxant and phentolamine is an alpha-adrenergic blocking agent. Although papaverine can stimulate an erection when given alone, the addition of phentolamine potentiates the effect (Lue and Tanagho, 1987). Together these agents increase blood flow by promoting smooth muscle relaxation in penile arterioles and sinusoids. In addition, papaverine has been reported to increase venous resistance.

Double-blind placebo crossover studies demonstrate the effectiveness of intracorporal injection of papaverine and phentolamine, and the placebo effect appears to be minimal. In one study of 24 patients, 82.8% had erections after treatment while no patient who received a saline injection had a positive response (Gasser et al, 1987). All 18 patients in another study experienced increased penile length and rigidity immediately after injection with papaverine and phentolamine; although three patients who received saline experienced no immediate effect, they reported improved quality of erection over several weeks (Kiely et al, 1987). In the above studies, most positive responses resulted in erections sufficient for coitus. Improved quality of erection lasted for several weeks in some patients. If sexual activity closely follows treatment, the psychogenic effect of sexual stimulation may enhance the response to the drugs. A less satisfactory response with increasing age of the patient was observed in one study (Strachan and Pryor, 1987).

Patients with venous leakage should *not* be given these injections therapeutically because systemic effects (eg, dizziness, pallor, sweating) have been reported in such individuals after intracavernous papaverine injection (Wespes and Schulman, 1988).

Various regimens were employed in the above studies. A mixture of papaverine and phentolamine was injected with a fine gauge needle into the corpus cavernosum on one side at the base of the penis. Doses ranged from 3 to 30 mg of papaverine plus 0.12 to 1.25 mg of phentolamine administered in a volume of 0.1 to 2 ml (see above references). Generally, injection was recommended no more than twice weekly, with the site of injection alternated. Impotence due to various causes appears to respond to papaverine and phentolamine injection; that due to severe vascular impairment (arterial or venous) is least responsive (Nellans et al, 1987). Neurogenic impotence responds to the lowest doses of papaverine and phentolamine or to papaverine alone (Sidi et al, 1986).

In a preliminary placebo-controlled double-blind crossover study, 8 of 16 impotent men responded positively to oral phentolamine (Gwinup, 1988). Further investigation of this oral preparation, which is no longer marketed in the United States, is likely.

Penile injection of alprostadil (prostaglandin E_1, PGE_1) is an alternative to the use of papaverine/phentolamine. Alprostadil is a potent smooth muscle relaxant that is used to maintain a patent ductus arteriosus in neonates. In controlled studies, this agent was as effective as papaverine/phentolamine and produced erection in some patients with arteriogenic impotence who had not responded to the combination regimen (Lee et al, 1989). Alprostadil was more effective than papaverine in patients with vasculogenic impotence (Kattan et al, 1991) and those with impotence caused by a variety of other disorders (Earle et al, 1990). This prostaglandin also has been used with papaverine, and the combination was more effective than papaverine/phentolamine or alprostadil alone (Floth and Schramek, 1991). As with other regimens, dosage must be individualized but ranged from 5 to 40 mcg of alprostadil per injection in several studies (Artoux and McQueen, 1991). Alprostadil has a shorter duration of action than papaverine, which lessens the likelihood of prolonged erection (Reiss, 1989). Fibrotic plaques do not appear to develop with alprostadil but pain after injection is more likely than with the combination of papaverine and phentolamine (Floth and Schramek, 1991; Bénard and Lue, 1990; Gerber and Levine, 1991). Regimens combining papaverine, phentolamine, and alprostadil in a single injection have been described (Bennett et al, 1991).

Reviews of intracavernous injection therapy for impotence are available (Kursh, 1988; Sidi, 1988; *JAMA*, 1991).

Although variations of the above methods are widely used and appear to be effective, it is emphasized that experience is inadequate to assure safety of long-term therapy. If penile injection of vasoactive agents proves safe and effective, it will probably be used most commonly as an interim measure before implantation of a penile prosthesis rather than for long-term treatment.

Adverse reactions generally are minor and include pain, paresthesia, or bruising or ulcers at the injection site. Prolonged erections are a serious concern, and those lasting more than two to four hours should be treated. If the prolonged erection is painful, indicating ischemia, immediate treatment is indicated. Treatment consists of aspiration of blood or, if that fails, injection of an adrenergic agent. Long-term use of papaverine penile injections may result in Peyronie-like fibrotic plaques at the injection site (Sidi et al, 1986; Malloy and Malkowicz, 1987). One fatality was reported in a paraplegic patient who died from pulmonary thromboembolism presumably caused by papaverine-induced priapism (Hashmat and Abraham, 1987).

INFERTILITY, GENERAL. Almost one-half of cases of infertility are at least partially due to reproductive dysfunction in the male partner. Whatever the etiology, male infertility may be manifested by an alteration in sperm density, motility, or morphology or abnormalities of seminal fluid viscosity or volume. The cause may be an anatomic abnormality (eg, varicocele, cryptorchidism); obstruction of the ductal system due to inflammatory disease (eg, tuberculosis; gonorrhea; iatrogenic, such as following hernia repair); genetic (eg, Klinefelter's syndrome); destruction of the germinal epithelium (eg, mumps orchitis, irradiation); environmental (eg, increased scrotal temperature from hot baths, certain pesticides); immunologic (eg, sperm antibodies); ejaculatory dysfunction (eg, retrograde ejaculation); use of marijuana, which may decrease testosterone levels and cause abnormal spermatogenesis (eg, motility, morphology, sperm count); acute infection as suggested by leukocytes in the semen; or a side effect of drug therapy (see Drife, 1987, and the Table). Only a small proportion of cases of male infertility is caused by a recognized endocrinologic disorder. Reviews that discuss the causes, diagnosis, and management of male infertility include Griffin, 1987; Hirsch and Lipshultz, 1987; Bodner, 1988; and Spark, 1988.

In some cases of male infertility not correctable by drug therapy or surgical intervention, the couple may be suitable candidates for artificial insemination using semen obtained from the husband or a donor. In vitro fertilization (IVF) may be used for certain patients with male infertility involving low sperm count or motility or abnormal morphology, although the couple should be told that the success rate is likely to be low, especially in the presence of poor morphology. Multiple oocyte retrieval may partially offset low fertilization rates (Awadalla et al, 1987) (see also index entry Infertility, Etiology and Treatment in Women).

EFFECTS OF DRUGS ON MALE FERTILITY

Drugs	Reported Effect
Busulfan [Myleran]	Possible sterility, azoospermia, and testicular atrophy
Chlorambucil [Leukeran]	Oligospermia; azoospermia
Cimetidine [Tagamet]	Decreased sperm count
Colchicine	Azoospermia
Cyclophosphamide [Cytoxan, Neosar]	Azoospermia
Diethylstilbestrol (use in pregnancy)	*Sons:* Epididymal cysts; questionable increase in cryptorchidism and infertility
Ethyl Alcohol	Decreased serum testosterone; impaired sperm motility
Marijuana	Decreased serum testosterone; decreased sperm count; impaired sperm motility; abnormal morphology
Methadone [Dolophine]	Decreased serum testosterone
Methotrexate [Folex]	Oligospermia
Phenytoin [Dilantin]	Decreased FSH; oligospermia
Prednisolone	Oligospermia
Spironolactone [Aldactone]	Decreased serum testosterone; increased testosterone clearance
Sulfasalazine [Azulfidine]	Decreased sperm count
Thioridazine [Mellaril]	Slightly decreased serum testosterone

Adapted from Lipman, 1984.

INFERTILITY DUE TO VARICOCELE. About 20% to 40% of infertile males have a varicocele, which may contribute to the infertility. Left varicoceles are most common; bilateral involvement occurs less often, and a right varicocele is rare. Although the exact pathophysiologic mechanisms are not understood, elevated scrotal temperature and reflux of prostaglandins from the left renal and adrenal veins may be involved. In addition, a left varicocele may adversely affect spermatogenesis bilaterally (Takihara et al, 1991). Sperm density and motility decreased over several years of observation in a group of infertile men who had varicoceles (Chehval and Purcell, 1992). When left varicocelectomy fails to improve semen quality, further investigation may reveal a right varicocele; if this is corrected, the quality of semen may improve and pregnancy may be achieved (Amelar and Dubin, 1987). Varicoceles also are common in the fertile male population, and some clinicians have questioned the causal relationship between this condition and infertility (Kursh et al, 1987).

Some men in whom sperm density improved postoperatively also showed normalization of hormonal parameters. An exaggerated response to GnRH and decreased seminal dihydrotestosterone also were altered toward normal after surgery in some patients. However, men who had normal hormonal parameters preoperatively did not experience improvement in sperm density or motility postoperatively, and it was thought that infertility in these men was caused by a factor other than varicocele (Hudson, 1988). This finding was not confirmed by other investigators, who reported improvement in semen quality and fertility in a large series of patients with normal hormonal parameters preoperatively (Dubin and Amelar, 1988).

Adjunctive drug therapy with hCG (Dubin and Amelar, 1977; Mehan and Chehval, 1982) or clomiphene (Check, 1980; Cockett et al, 1984) has been suggested for patients with preoperative sperm counts of less than 10 million/ml. However, the efficacy of such regimens remains unproved.

INFERTILITY DUE TO HYPOGONADOTROPIC HYPOGONADISM. Hypogonadotropic infertility is uncommon. However, spermatogenesis can be initiated and pregnancies achieved in 90% of properly selected patients. Definitive diagnostic tests include those that exclude other causes of infertility in both partners; measurement of serum gonadotropins, prolactin, and testosterone; and testicular biopsy.

Hormonal therapy depends on the severity of the defect. When there is only partial gonadotropin deficiency, hCG alone often increases sperm counts and produces normal ejaculates. In patients with severe deficiency, androgen therapy stimulates virilization during adolescence. Because maximum stimulation of spermatogenesis may require one year of gonadotropin replacement, androgen therapy may be discontinued and administration of gonadotropin begun when the patient reaches his early twenties. Alternatively, gonadotropin therapy may be postponed until the patient desires fertility.

In complete hypogonadotropic hypogonadism, hCG stimulates testicular development only partially despite complete virilization. After normal serum testosterone levels are achieved and there is no further increase in testicular growth or improvement in sperm production, menotropins (hMG) is added to the regimen (see the evaluations). After successful treatment, most patients with complete hypogonadotropic hypogonadism achieve adequate testicular size and produce ejaculates containing 2 to 5 million or more sperm/ml (normal, ≥20 million/ml). Pregnancies have occurred at this low sperm level when the female partner has normal fertility. When maximal stimulation of germinal tissue and sperm output has been achieved, menotropins is withdrawn. Spermatogenesis is maintained by continued administration of hCG (Sherins, 1984), although a study in normal males suggests that FSH activity (present in menotropins but not hCG) is necessary to support production of normal numbers of sperm (Matsumoto et al, 1986).

In men with only partial gonadotropin deficiency, hCG alone stimulated completion of spermiogenesis, and the degree of response correlated with the size of the testis before treatment (ie, the least impaired subjects demonstrated the best response). Pregnancies were achieved with average sperm counts of only 8.7 million/ml (Burris et al, 1988).

Studies have shown that infertile men with hypogonadotropic hypogonadism can be treated successfully by pulsatile subcutaneous administration of GnRH (Shargil, 1987; Aulitzky et al, 1988), but the optimal dose has not been determined. GnRH therapy, which requires the presence of an intact pituitary, offers the appealing possibility of correcting the gonadotropin abnormality with a more physiologic pattern of endogenous gonadotropin secretion than with exogenous administration of gonadotropins. Such therapy, which can be administered using a portable infusion pump, may be preferable to treatment with an hCG-menotropins regimen, which requires several injections weekly. Initiation of spermatogenesis was more rapid with GnRH than with gonadotropin therapy, and gynecomastia was not observed in the group receiving GnRH (Schopohl et al, 1991). However, the need to carry an infusion pump may be a greater inconvenience. The dose, frequency of the pulse, and the total amount of hormone administered can affect the differential pattern of gonadotropin secretion. For example, longer pulse intervals appear to enhance FSH secretion (Gross et al, 1987). Other evidence suggests that pulses every two hours may be optimal for LH secretion (Spratt et al, 1987 B; Whitcomb and Crowley, 1990). GnRH pulse parameters also may affect the biological:immunologic activity ratio of the LH secreted (Veldhuis et al, 1987). Relatively high sperm production (96 million/ml) has been reported when GnRH was used to treat infertility in hypogonadotropic hypogonadism (Crowley, 1988).

Administration of GnRH by the intranasal route also is being investigated. Doses 50 to 100 times greater than those used for intravenous administration are given every two hours except during sleep (Klingmüller and Schweikert, 1985).

INFERTILITY DUE TO HYPERPROLACTINEMIA. Since both men and women require gonadotropic support for gametogenesis, it seems reasonable to expect that the male as well as the female reproductive system may be subject to various inhibitions associated with elevated prolactin levels. Galactorrhea sometimes occurs in males with prolactin-secreting tumors, and impotence is often, but not invariably, present. Hyperprolactinemia may account for refractoriness in some men whose hormonal profiles indicate that they are candidates for clomiphene or hCG therapy. In some men, LH concentration and pulse frequency, sperm counts, and testosterone levels are increased following use of bromocriptine [Parlodel] to normalize serum prolactin levels (Winters and Troen, 1984).

IDIOPATHIC MALE INFERTILITY. Probably 40% to 60% of all infertile males have no identifiable anatomic or endocrine defect. Therapy in these cases is empiric and nonspecific. Clomiphene is commonly employed to treat subfertile males (see the evaluation). However, the lack of controlled studies, standardized patient selection, and treatment regimens makes interpretation of clinical results difficult; consequently, this therapy is not endorsed by all experts, and the use and effectiveness of clomiphene therapy in male infertility remain controversial. Lack of effectiveness was reported in a placebo-controlled study in which clomiphene [Clomid, Serophene] was administered to men with oligospermia and normal hormonal levels. Although gonadotropin and testosterone levels and gonadotropin secretory response to GnRH were increased after clomiphene therapy, no improvement in semen parameters, results of sperm penetration assay, or pregnancy rate was observed (Sokol et al, 1988).

As in women, clomiphene stimulates endogenous gonadotropin secretion. Criteria for patient selection include serum gonadotropin and testosterone levels usually within the normal range. If a testicular biopsy is performed, it may indicate presence of all germinal elements, although decreased in number (hypospermatogenesis). Clomiphene usually increases serum testosterone levels and occasionally may increase the number and motility of sperm. Clomiphene therapy should be withdrawn after six months if there has been no improvement in semen quality, if a marked rise in the FSH or testosterone level occurs, or if there is worsening of the semen quality after earlier improvement.

Successful treatment of some men with idiopathic infertility was reported in an uncontrolled study using tamoxifen [Nolvadex], another antiestrogenic agent (Buvat et al, 1983); however, the initial increase in sperm count may be followed by a decline. In a later report, tamoxifen was found to be no more effective than placebo for this indication (AinMelk et al, 1987). Patients with primary testicular failure (increased serum FSH, hyalinization, or other evidence of permanent epithelial damage) or ductal obstruction are not suitable candidates for gonadotropin or gonadotropin-stimulating therapy (Paulson, 1977).

Gonadotropins (hCG or a combination of hCG and hMG) also have been used to treat idiopathic male infertility, particularly that unresponsive to clomiphene. Although success has been reported in some men (Mehan and Chehval, 1982; Amelar and Dubin, 1988), results generally have been disappointing. The necessity for repeated intramuscular injections is inconvenient, and treatment, particularly when hMG is employed, is expensive. The effectiveness of gonadotropin therapy in males with a normal sperm count is doubtful.

Testosterone rebound has been employed in the past but is no longer recommended. Theoretically, after a period of treatment with exogenous testosterone, withdrawal would stimulate gonadotropin secretion and spermatogenesis. However, improvements in sperm production occurred infrequently and lasted only two to three months, and treatment sometimes was followed by permanent depression of the sperm count (Charny and Gordon, 1978).

In the past, thyroid and adrenal supplements were used empirically; however, more sensitive diagnostic endocrinologic tests are available today, and such treatment cannot be recommended unless thyroid or adrenal hormone deficiency has been documented.

In uncontrolled studies, improved sperm motility with an increase in the number of pregnancies has been reported following administration of low doses of androgen to infertile males with a defect of sperm motility but normal sperm counts, morphology, and serum testosterone levels (Brown, 1975). Prolonged administration may result in decreased sperm counts, and this use of testosterone now is not generally recommended.

Infertile men with poor sperm motility and low seminal zinc concentration responded more favorably to administration of zinc and fluoxymesterone [Halotestin] than to either agent alone. However, pregnancy rates were not reported (Takihara et al, 1983).

The prostaglandin inhibitory effect of some anti-inflammatory drugs is postulated to cause improved sperm quality in oligospermic infertile men (Barkay et al, 1984), but this has not been confirmed. In the presence of infection, appropriate antibiotic therapy may be effective (Megory et al, 1987).

IMMUNOLOGIC INFERTILITY. Antibodies to sperm in the semen or in the female reproductive tract may cause infertility.

Antibodies present on sperm or in the cervical mucus may prevent penetration or progress of sperm in the cervical mucus that results in an abnormal postcoital test. Less frequently, sperm antibodies can directly interfere with fertilization. Antibodies directed at the head or main tailpiece may affect fertility. Antibody testing is suggested for those couples in whom both an abnormal postcoital test and normal semen analysis are found or when there is spontaneous microscopic agglutination of sperm in the semen. Infertility due to sperm antibodies may affect more than one-third of patients who have had vasovasostomy following vasectomy (Bronson, 1988; Tung, 1988).

Attempts to treat infertility caused by sperm antibodies are often unsuccessful, but several options are available. When the female partner is affected, use of a condom reduces exposure to sperm antigens and theoretically may decrease antibody levels. Unprotected coitus at the time of ovulation may then be successful. When the male partner develops autoimmunity to sperm, the semen can be washed to remove antibodies and then used for insemination. However, this technique has not been particularly helpful. Alternatively, artificial insemination of donor semen may be attempted.

Immunosuppressive therapy with large doses of corticosteroids (prednisolone 60 mg/day for 7 or 14 days) has been suggested (Alexander et al, 1983). Pregnancies were achieved within four months in 45% of treated couples compared to 12% of untreated couples. Regimens using larger amounts of corticosteroids have been reported (Shulman and Shulman, 1982). In general, results of corticosteroid immunosuppressive therapy have been inconsistent. The couple must weigh the possibility of adverse effects from this experimental treatment against the importance of a possible pregnancy (see also Bronson, 1988).

ANDROGENIC AGENTS

Unaltered testosterone is not suitable for oral or parenteral administration because absorption and hepatic degradation are rapid. Esterification of testosterone has produced molecules that are less polar and are soluble in oil vehicles and fatty tissue. Generally, the longer the carbon chain of the ester substituent, the more slowly the hormone is released into the circulation. The esters are hydrolyzed to testosterone, which can be assayed in the blood when monitoring therapy. Testosterone esters are administered as the propionate, cypionate [Andro-Cyp, Depo-Testosterone, Virilon IM], and enanthate [Andryl, Delatestryl]. Testosterone propionate is injected two to four times weekly, while the longer-acting cypionate and enanthate are administered every two to four weeks. The latter two preparations are drugs of choice for hypogonadism, which requires long-term therapy.

Methyltestosterone [Android, Oreton Methyl, Testred, Virilon] and fluoxymesterone [Halotestin] are alkylated in the 17α position, which retards hepatic degradation and renders these preparations effective after oral administration. They must be given daily, and their androgenic potency, milligram-for-milligram, is less than that of the parenteral forms of testosterone. Also, 17α-alkylated androgens may be more hepatotoxic (see the discussion on Adverse Reactions and Precautions).

Newer preparations that provide greater ease of administration and effectiveness are being developed. Siloxane capsules containing testosterone are implanted subcutaneously and provide relatively constant blood levels over a long period. An investigational transdermal system consisting of testosterone-impregnated adhesive film also is being tested, and results have been promising (see the section on Hypogonadism above). The undecanoate ester of testosterone (marketed in other countries) and a preparation of microparticulate testosterone that are effective orally also are being investigated.

Certain testosterone derivatives, termed anabolic steroids, are weak androgens designed to provide anabolic activity with less androgenic effect. For indications and preparations, see index entry Anabolic Steroids, Uses.

Adverse Reactions and Precautions: Signs of virilism in prepubertal boys are pubic hair development, phallic enlargement, and increased frequency of erections; a risk of priapism also exists, and any increase in erectile frequency is an indication for reducing the dose or withdrawing the drug temporarily. In aging men, androgens may stimulate prostatic hyperplasia, causing urinary obstruction. Paradoxically, androgens may cause gynecomastia, particularly in boys (eg, when used for constitutional delay of growth), or in men after administration of large doses or in the presence of liver disease. This is probably due to the aromatization of testosterone to estrogen and does not occur with use of steroids that are reduced in the 5α position.

Androgens should not be used to stimulate growth in boys who are small but otherwise normal and healthy, except in selected cases of constitutional delayed growth. When they are used, the rate of skeletal maturation may exceed the rate of linear growth, thereby inducing premature closure of the epiphyses and reducing the attainable adult height. The extent to which this complication occurs depends on the child's bone age, the drug used, dosage, and duration of therapy. The younger the child, the greater the risk of compromising final mature height. The decision to administer anabolic steroids to boys for a specific growth problem should be made only after careful evaluation by an experienced pediatric endocrinologist.

Androgenic and anabolic steroids with an alkyl group substituted in the alpha position on carbon 17 (ie, methyltestosterone, fluoxymesterone, oxymetholone [Anadrol-50], stanozolol [Winstrol]); the impeded androgen, danazol [Danocrine]; and drugs no longer marketed in the United States, including ethylestrenol [Maxibolin] and methandrostenolone, have produced signs of liver dysfunction. Increased sulfobromophthalein (BSP) retention and AST levels appear to be dose-related and are relatively unimportant. Increased serum bilirubin and alkaline phosphatase values indicating excretory dysfunction are rare but important idiosyncratic reactions. Clinical jaundice is unusual and reversible when the drug is discontinued. The histologic findings consist of intrahepatic cholestasis with little or no cellular damage.

Therefore, these drugs should be used with caution in all patients and particularly those with pre-existing liver disease. Long-term administration of 17α-alkylated androgens and anabolic steroids should be avoided.

Rarely, hepatocellular and endothelial malignancies, hepatic adenomas, and intrahepatic hemorrhage associated with peliosis hepatis have developed, particularly in anemic patients treated for long periods with large doses of 17α-alkylated steroids. Hepatocellular adenomas or carcinomas may regress when androgens are discontinued. Patients with Fanconi's syndrome experience more severe liver toxicity from androgen therapy than other patients with anemia; it is not known whether this is due to prolonged androgen therapy or increased susceptibility to liver dysfunction in these patients (Camitta et al, 1982). Patients receiving prolonged androgen therapy should be monitored for functional and structural liver abnormalities.

Abnormal liver function tests are thought to occur less frequently with intramuscular preparations of testosterone and its derivatives and nandrolone phenpropionate and decanoate, which lack the 17α-alkylated group.

Large doses of androgens and anabolic steroids, such as those taken by some athletes for body-building purposes, can cause potentially atherogenic changes in blood lipids, suppress spermatogenesis, and produce other adverse effects. See also index entry Anabolic Steroids, Uses, Athletic Performance. Androgens and anabolic steroids are designated as Schedule III controlled substances under the Anabolic Steroids Control Act of 1990.

Salt and fluid retention are usually not serious but can be undesirable in the elderly, patients with congestive heart failure, or those with a tendency to develop edema from other causes (eg, cirrhosis, hypoproteinemia).

Care should be taken when 17α-alkylated preparations are used in patients on hemodialysis because these drugs may increase blood fibrinolytic activity.

Androgens and anabolic steroids are contraindicated in men with carcinoma of the prostate or breast.

Drug Interactions: When an androgen is administered to patients taking an oral anticoagulant, the activity of the latter is enhanced and severe bleeding episodes may occur. The anticoagulant dose may have to be reduced to 25% of that appropriate for use without androgen. The mechanism of the increased hypoprothrombinemic response is undetermined. The effect occurs rapidly, within several days to a week, and usually reverses in a similar pattern when androgen is discontinued. This interaction is known to occur with 17α-alkylated androgens and with testosterone (Hansten and Horn, 1989). Therefore, when any androgenic steroid is added to or withdrawn from a regimen that also includes an anticoagulant, more frequent prothrombin determinations and adjustments in dose of the anticoagulant should be made.

The requirement for antidiabetic agents may be decreased when anabolic steroids are added to the regimen, because the latter may reduce blood sugar levels directly in diabetics.

Glucocorticoids depress the level of endogenous serum testosterone; the probable mechanism is suppression of hypothalamic GnRH secretion. Conditions such as impotence or osteopenia occurring in men treated for prolonged periods with glucocorticoids may be related to decreased serum testosterone rather than to the illness per se (MacAdams et al, 1986).

Effects on Laboratory Tests: Androgens reduce the level of circulating thyroxine-binding globulin, thereby decreasing thyroid hormone levels and increasing triiodothyronine resin uptake. However, the free T_3 and T_4 are unaffected and there is no evidence of thyroid dysfunction. Androgens enhance blood fibrinolytic activity, increase hematocrit and serum haptoglobin levels, and have variable effects on serum lipids. Administration of testosterone, but not the 17α-alkylated derivatives, elevates urinary 17-ketosteroids.

Drug Evaluations

FLUOXYMESTERONE
[Halotestin]

This short-acting preparation (half-life about nine hours) is used orally. It is less effective for replacement therapy than the long-acting esters of testosterone. Full sexual maturation in patients with prepubertal hypogonadism cannot be achieved easily with fluoxymesterone, but it is sometimes used for replacement therapy when hypogonadism begins in adult life or after secondary sexual characteristics have developed following therapy with a parenteral preparation. However, because of its potential hepatotoxicity, this androgen should not be used for long periods.

See the Introduction and general discussion on Androgens for information on other indications and adverse reactions.

DOSAGE AND PREPARATIONS.

Oral: For androgen deficiency, 10 to 20 mg daily in single or divided doses.

Halotestin (Upjohn), ***Generic.*** Tablets 2, 5, and 10 mg.

METHYLTESTOSTERONE
[Android, Oreton Methyl, Testred, Virilon]

This short-acting preparation (half-life about 2.5 hours) is used orally and buccally. Although absorption is more variable, the bioavailability is greater with buccal administration, probably because the hepatic circulation is bypassed. However, the oral route is used more commonly for convenience.

Methyltestosterone is much less effective for replacement therapy than the long-acting esters of testosterone. Although methyltestosterone does not produce full sexual maturation in patients with prepubertal hypogonadism, it is sometimes used for replacement therapy when hypogonadism begins in adult life or after secondary sexual characteristics have developed following therapy with testosterone. However, because of its potential hepatotoxicity, this androgen should not be used for long periods.

DOSAGE AND PREPARATIONS.

Oral: For androgen deficiency, 10 to 50 mg daily.

Android (ICN), ***Oreton Methyl*** (Schering), ***Generic.*** Tablets 10 and 25 mg.

Testred (ICN), ***Virilon*** (Star). Capsules 10 mg.

Buccal: *Adults,* one-half of oral dosage (rate of absorption is variable).

Oreton Methyl (Schering), ***Generic.*** Tablets (buccal) 10 mg.

TESTOSTERONE CYPIONATE

[Andro-Cyp, Depo-Testosterone, Virilon IM]

TESTOSTERONE ENANTHATE

[Andryl, Delatestryl]

These long-acting, potent esters of testosterone are given intramuscularly to develop or maintain secondary sexual characteristics and other physiologic functions in androgen-deficient males. These agents are preferred to induce full sexual development in eunuchoidal males when testicular disease has interfered with normal pubertal development and to treat postpubertal Leydig cell failure. Peak blood levels are achieved two to three days after administration and decline to baseline levels over several weeks, depending on the dose. Intramuscular administration of these preparations thus results in uneven serum levels of testosterone, and it is recommended that the dosing interval not exceed two to three weeks to avoid long periods without androgen support (Sokol and Swerdloff, 1983).

These preparations also may be given to stimulate growth and initiate puberty in selected boys with constitutional delay of growth.

DOSAGE AND PREPARATIONS.

Intramuscular: For induction of puberty in *boys,* 50 mg/M^2/month closely simulates the first year of puberty; 100 mg/M^2/month simulates normal midpuberty sexual development and growth spurt. The following regimen is suggested: 50 mg is given every four weeks to accomplish growth, followed in the second or third year by 100 mg every four weeks. Dosage is increased gradually thereafter to the following maintenance schedule for adults. For maintenance therapy in androgen deficiency, *adults,* 100 mg/M^2 or 150 to 200 mg every two weeks or 300 mg every three weeks.

TESTOSTERONE CYPIONATE:

Generic. Solution (in oil) 100 and 200 mg/ml in 10 ml containers.

Andro-Cyp (Keene). Solution (in cottonseed oil) 100 and 200 mg/ml in 10 ml containers.

Depo-Testosterone (Upjohn). Solution (in cottonseed oil) 100 mg/ml in 10 ml containers and 200 mg/ml in 1 and 10 ml containers.

Virilon IM (Star). Solution 200 mg/ml in 10 ml containers.

TESTOSTERONE ENANTHATE:

Generic. Solution (in oil) 100 and 200 mg/ml in 5 and 10 ml containers.

Andryl (Keene). Solution (in sesame oil) 200 mg/ml in 10 ml containers.

Delatestryl (Mead Johnson). Solution (in sesame oil) 200 mg/ml in 1 and 5 ml containers.

TESTOSTERONE PROPIONATE

[Testex]

Testosterone propionate can be used to induce or maintain secondary sexual characteristics and other physiologic functions in androgen-deficient males. This relatively short-acting preparation produces a steady response when used parenterally, but this route is not practical for long-term therapy. In older patients, the prostate gland may be sensitive to androgen, and bladder neck obstruction may develop; this complication is more easily corrected if a short-acting preparation is used initially.

DOSAGE AND PREPARATIONS.

Intramuscular: For androgen deficiency, 50 mg three times weekly.

Generic. Solution (in oil) 50 mg/ml in 10 ml containers and 100 mg/ml in 10 and 30 ml containers.

Testex (Pasadena). Solution (in sesame oil) 100 mg/ml in 10 ml containers.

ANTERIOR PITUITARY AND HYPOTHALAMIC AGENTS

BROMOCRIPTINE MESYLATE

[Parlodel]

For chemical formula, see index entry Bromocriptine, In Female Hyperprolactinemia.

ACTIONS AND USES. The usefulness of this semisynthetic ergot alkaloid depends primarily on its dopaminergic activity. Bromocriptine inhibits the secretion of prolactin by the anterior pituitary gland.

Impotence, hypogonadism, or infertility in males associated with elevated prolactin levels sometimes responds to bromocriptine. The drug is not effective in psychogenic impotence or that caused by conditions other than hyperprolactinemia. Symptoms frequently recur upon cessation of therapy.

ADVERSE REACTIONS AND PRECAUTIONS. The doses employed for reproductive dysfunction generally do not cause severe side effects. Nausea is most common, but vomiting, constipation, dizziness, and orthostatic hypotension also occur. These effects can be minimized by taking the medication with food and at bedtime and by initiating therapy with small doses and gradually increasing the amount to effective levels.

DOSAGE AND PREPARATIONS. Bromocriptine should be taken with food.

Oral: In appropriately selected males with elevated plasma prolactin, 2.5 mg twice daily.

Parlodel (Sandoz). Capsules 5 mg; tablets 2.5 mg.

CLOMIPHENE CITRATE

[Clomid, Serophene]

For chemical formula, see index entry Clomiphene, As Ovulatory Stimulant.

USES. This nonsteroidal agent is a mixture of two isomers in approximately a 1:1 ratio and is related chemically to chlorotrianisene. It is sometimes used to stimulate sperm production in selected males with idiopathic infertility. See the discussion in the Introduction.

DOSAGE AND PREPARATIONS.

Oral: For oligospermia in selected males, 25 mg daily is commonly used. Alternatively, 100 mg is given every other day or three times/week (Ross et al, 1980). Medication is continued for 6 to 12 months or until pregnancy is achieved.

Clomid (Marion Merrell Dow), **Serophene** (Serono). Tablets 50 mg.

HUMAN CHORIONIC GONADOTROPIN (hCG)

[A.P.L., Follutein, Pregnyl, Profasi]

ACTIONS AND USES. Human chorionic gonadotropin (hCG) is a placental hormone extracted from the urine of pregnant women. Its biological activity is the same as that of luteinizing hormone and it is used as a substitute for human LH, which is available only in small quantities for investigational studies. Human chorionic gonadotropin has intrinsic thyroid-stimulating properties, which accounts for the thyrotoxic state that occurs in patients with hCG-secreting neoplasms.

This preparation is sometimes used diagnostically in males with delayed puberty or when there is doubt about the steroidogenic ability of the testes to respond to gonadotropin stimulation. Human chorionic gonadotropin also is used to treat cryptorchidism in selected males (see the Introduction) and to treat infertility in males with hypogonadotropic hypogonadism. It stimulates or maintains spermatogenesis depending on the hormonal status of the patient and the regimen used.

The subcutaneous route has been reported to be as effective as intramuscular injection and is more convenient (Saal et al, 1991).

DOSAGE AND PREPARATIONS.

Intramuscular, Subcutaneous: In cryptorchidism, for rapid response and minimal sexual development, 3,000 to 5,000 units every three to four days for four injections; to achieve a greater degree of sexual development, 500 units three times weekly for three weeks, or, for *boys 10 years or older,* 1,000 units twice weekly for three weeks.

In males, for diagnosis of responsiveness to gonadotropin stimulation, 5,000 units given once. Blood levels of testosterone are measured before treatment and three to four days later. An approximate doubling of testosterone levels is normal (Saez and Forest, 1979).

For hypogonadotropic infertility in men, 2,000 units two or three times/week. When normal serum testosterone levels are reached and there is no further testicular growth or improvement in sperm production, menotropins may be added to the regimen. When maximal spermatogenesis is established, sperm production usually continues as long as hCG (2,000 units three times/week) is given.

A.P.L. (Wyeth-Ayerst), ***Generic.*** Powder 5,000, 10,000, and 20,000 U.S.P. units with 10 ml of diluent.

Follutein (Squibb Mark), ***Pregnyl*** (Organon). Powder (lyophilized) 10,000 U.S.P. units with 10 ml of diluent.

Profasi (Serono). Powder (sterile, lyophilized) 5,000 and 10,000 U.S.P. units with 10 ml of diluent.

MENOTROPINS (hMG)

[Pergonal]

ACTIONS AND USES. Menotropins is a preparation of human menopausal gonadotropin (hMG) extracted from the urine of postmenopausal women. FSH and LH activity are present in a 1:1 ratio. The goal of therapy in males is to replace gonadotropins and stimulate spermatogenesis.

Menotropins is sometimes used with hCG to treat hypogonadotropic male infertility, and it has been used investigationally in idiopathic male infertility. Such treatment is prolonged and expensive.

The subcutaneous route has been reported to be as effective as intramuscular injection and is more convenient (Saal et al, 1991).

DOSAGE AND PREPARATIONS.

Intramuscular, Subcutaneous: For hypogonadotropic or idiopathic male infertility (to be given with hCG; see the evaluation on hCG), 75 IU is given three times a week. (One-half of patients respond to 25 IU three times per week. Therefore, lower dosages may be tried.) Effectiveness of therapy is determined after six to nine months at a specific dosage level. When maximal stimulation of the germinal tissue and sperm output has been achieved, menotropins can be discontinued; sperm production continues as long as hCG (2,000 units three times/week) is given.

Pergonal (Serono). Solution containing 75 or 150 IU each of follicle-stimulating hormone (FSH) activity and luteinizing hormone (LH) activity (with 10 mg lyophilized lactose) in 2 ml containers.

Cited References

Diagnostic and Therapeutic Technology Assessment (DATTA). *JAMA* 265:3321-3323, 1991.

Drugs that cause sexual dysfunction. *Med Lett Drugs Ther* 29:65-70, 1987.

Yohimbine: Time for resurrection? *Lancet* 2:1194-1195, 1986.

Abber JC, et al: Diagnostic tests for impotence: Comparison of papaverine injection with the penile-brachial index and nocturnal penile tumescence monitoring. *J Urol* 135:923-925, 1986.

Ahmed SR, et al: Transdermal testosterone therapy in the treatment of male hypogonadism. *J Clin Endocrinol Metab* 66:546-551, 1988.

AinMelk Y, et al: Tamoxifen citrate therapy in male infertility. *Fertil Steril* 48:113-117, 1987.

Alexander NJ, et al: Pregnancy rates in patients treated for antisperm antibodies with prednisone. *Int J Fertil* 28:63-67, 1983.

Amelar RD, Dubin L: Right varicocelectomy in selected infertile patients who have failed to improve after previous left varicocelectomy. *Fertil Steril* 47:833-837, 1987.

Amelar RD, Dubin L: Human chorionic gonadotropin therapy for idiopathic male infertility, in Garcia CR (ed): *Current Therapy of Infertility,* ed 3. Toronto, Decker, 1988, 201.

Artoux MJ, McQueen KD: Alprostadil in impotence. *DICP* 25:363-365, 1991.

Aulitzky W, et al: Pulsatile luteinizing hormone-releasing hormone treatment of male hypogonadotropic hypogonadism. *Fertil Steril* 50:480-487, 1988.

Awadalla SG, et al: In vitro fertilization and embryo transfer as treatment for male factor infertility. *Fertil Steril* 47:807-811, 1987.

Barkay J, et al: Prostaglandin inhibitor effect of antiinflammatory drugs in therapy of male infertility. *Fertil Steril* 42:406-411, 1984.

Barry JM, et al: Nocturnal penile tumescence monitoring with stamps. *Urology* 15:171-172, 1980.

Bénard F, Lue TF: Self-administration in the pharmacological treatment of impotence. *Drugs* 39:394-398, 1990.

Bennett AH, et al: An improved vasoactive drug combination for a pharmacological erection program. *J Urol* 146:1564-1565, 1991.

Bistritzer T, et al: Hormonal therapy and pubertal development in boys with selective hypogonadotropic hypogonadism. *Fertil Steril* 52:302-306, 1989.

Bodner DR: Critical review of pharmacologic therapies. *Semin Reprod Endocrinol* 6:377-384, 1988.

Bradley WE: New techniques in evaluation of impotence. *Urology* 29:383-386, 1987.

Brindley GS: Cavernosal alpha-blockade: New technique for investigating and treating erectile impotence. *Br J Psychiatry* 143:332-337, 1983.

Bronson RA: Current concepts on the relation of antisperm antibodies and infertility. *Semin Reprod Endocrinol* 6:363-368, 1988.

Brown JS: Effect of orally administered androgens on sperm motility. *Fertil Steril* 26:305-308, 1975.

Buffum J: Pharmacosexology update: Yohimbine and sexual function. *J Psychoact Drugs* 17:131-132, 1985.

Buffum J: Pharmacosexology update: Prescription drugs and sexual function. *J Psychoact Drugs* 18:97-106, 1986.

Burger HG, et al: Serum inhibin concentrations rise throughout normal male and female puberty. *J Clin Endocrinol Metab* 67:689-694, 1988.

Burris AS, et al: Gonadotropin therapy in men with isolated hypogonadotropic hypogonadism: Response to human chorionic gonadotropin is predicted by initial testicular size. *J Clin Endocrinol Metab* 66:1144-1151, 1988.

Buvat J, et al: Increased sperm count in 25 cases of idiopathic normogonadotropic oligospermia following treatment with tamoxifen. *Fertil Steril* 39:700-703, 1983.

Buvat J, et al: Is intracavernous injection of papaverine a reliable screening test for vascular impotence? *J Urol* 135:476-482, 1986.

Camitta BM, et al: Aplastic anemia: Pathogenesis, diagnosis, treatment, and prognosis. *N Engl J Med* 306:712-718, 1982.

Charny CW, Gordon JA: Testosterone rebound therapy: Neglected modality. *Fertil Steril* 29:64-68, 1978.

Check JH: Improved semen quality in subfertile males with varicocele-associated oligospermia following treatment with clomiphene citrate. *Fertile Steril* 33:423-426, 1980.

Chehval MJ, Purcell MH: Deterioration of semen parameters over time in men with untreated varicocele: Evidence of progressive testicular damage. *Fertil Steril* 57:174-177, 1992.

Chilvers C, et al: Undescended testis: Effect of treatment on subsequent risk of subfertility and malignancy. *J Pediatr Surg* 21:691-696, 1986 A.

Chilvers C, et al: Luteinizing-hormone-releasing hormone and cryptorchidism, letter. *Lancet* 1:101, 1986 B.

Cockett ATK, et al: Varicocele. *Fertil Steril* 41:5-11, 1984.

Crowley WF Jr: Hypogonadotropic hypogonadism with gonadotropin-releasing hormones, in Garcia CR, et al (eds): *Current Therapy of Infertility,* ed 3. Toronto, Decker, 1988, 192-195.

Cunningham GR, et al: Testosterone replacement with transdermal therapeutic systems: Physiological serum testosterone and elevated dihydrotestosterone levels. *JAMA* 261:2525-2530, 1989.

DeJong FH: Inhibin. *Physiol Rev* 68:555-607, 1988.

de Muinck Keizer-Schrama SMPF, et al: Double-blind, placebo-controlled study of luteinizing hormone-releasing hormone nasal spray in treatment of undescended testes. *Lancet* 1:876-880, 1986.

Depue RH, et al: Cryptorchidism and testicular cancer, letter. *J Natl Cancer Inst* 77:830-833, 1986.

Drife JO: Effects of drugs on sperm. *Drugs* 33:610-622, 1987.

Dubin L, Amelar RD: Varicocelectomy: 986 cases in twelve year study. *Urology* 10:446-449, 1977.

Dubin L, Amelar RD: Varicocelectomy: Twenty-five years of experience. *Int J Fertil* 33:226-235, 1988.

Earle CM, et al: Prostaglandin E1 therapy for impotence, comparison with papaverine. *J Urol* 143:57-59, 1990.

Elder JS: Cryptorchidism: Isolated and associated with other genitourinary defects. *Pediatr Adolesc Endocrinol* 34:1033-1053, 1987.

Findlay JC, et al: Treatment of primary hypogonadism in men by the transdermal administration of testosterone. *J Clin Endocrinol Metab* 68:369-373, 1989.

Finkelstein JS, et al: Increases in bone density during treatment of men with idiopathic hypogonadotropic hypogonadism. *J Clin Endocrinol Metab* 69:776-783, 1989.

Finkelstein JS, et al: Osteopenia in men with a history of delayed puberty. *N Engl J Med* 326:600-604, 1992.

Floth A, Schramek P: Intracavernous injection of prostaglandin E1 in combination with papaverine: Enhanced effectiveness in comparison with papaverine plus phentolamine and prostaglandin E1 alone. *J Urol* 145:56-59, 1991.

Gasser TC, et al: Intracavernous self-injection with phentolamine and papaverine for the treatment of impotence. *J Urol* 137:678-680, 1987.

Gerber GS, Levine LA: Pharmacological erection program using prostaglandin E1. *J Urol* 146:786-789, 1991.

Griffin JE: Diagnosis and management of male infertility. *Adv Intern Med* 32:259-282, 1987.

Gross KM, et al: Differential control of luteinizing hormone and follicle-stimulating hormone secretion by luteinizing hormone-releasing hormone pulse frequency in man. *J Clin Endocrinol Metab* 64:675-680, 1987.

Gwinup G: Oral phentolamine in non-specific erectile insufficiency. *Ann Intern Med* 109:162-163, 1988.

Hansten PD, Horn JR: *Drug Interactions: Clinical Significance of Drug-Drug Interactions,* ed 6. Philadelphia, Lea & Febiger, 1989.

Hashmat AI, Abraham J: Papaverine induced priapism: Lethal complication, abstract. *Urology* 37:201A, 1987.

Hirsch IH, Lipshultz LI: Medical treatment of male infertility. *Urol Clin North Am* 14:307-322, 1987.

Hudson RW: The endocrinology of varicoceles. *Fertil Steril* 49:199-208, 1988.

Johnson LE, Morley JE: Impotence in the elderly. *Am Fam Physician* 38:225-240, (Nov) 1988.

Joss EE, et al: Oxandrolone in constitutionally delayed growth, a longitudinal study up to final height. *J Clin Endocrinol Metab* 69:1109-1115, 1989.

Kaiser FE, Korenman SG: Impotence in diabetic men. *Am J Med* 85(suppl 5A):147-152, 1988.

Kattan S, et al: Double-blind, cross-over study comparing prostaglandin E1 and papaverine in patients with vasculogenic impotence. *Urology* 37:516-518, 1991.

Kelley VC, Ruvalcaba RHA: Use of anabolic agents in treatment of short children. *Clin Endocrinol Metab* 11:25-39, 1982.

Kiely EA, et al: Penile function following intracavernosal injection of vasoactive agents or saline. *Br J Urol* 59:473-476, 1987.

Kim N, et al: A nitric oxide-like factor mediates nonadrenergic-noncholinergic neurogenic relaxation of penile corpus cavernosum smooth muscle. *J Clin Invest* 88:112-118, 1991.

Klingmüller D, Schweikert HU: Maintenance of spermatogenesis by intranasal administration of gonadotropin-releasing hormone in patients with hypothalamic hypogonadism. *J Clin Endocrinol Metab* 61:868-872, 1985.

Korenman SG, et al: Androgen therapy of hypogonadal men with transcrotal testosterone systems. *Am J Med* 83:471-478, 1987.

Krane RJ, et al: Impotence. *N Engl J Med* 321:1648-1659, 1989.

Krauss DJ: Management of impotence. II. Selected surgical procedures: Penile prostheses. *Clin Therapeut* 9:149-156, 1987.

Kulin HE: Delayed puberty in the male, in Krieger DT, Bardin CW (eds): *Current Therapy in Endocrinology 1983-1984*. St Louis, CV Mosby, 1983.

Kursh ED: Injection therapy for impotence. *Urol Clin North Am* 15:625-629, 1988.

Kursh ED, et al: What is the incidence of varicocele in a fertile population? *Fertil Steril* 48:510-511, 1987.

LaFranchi S, et al: Constitutional delay of growth: Expected versus final adult height. *Pediatrics* 87:82-87, 1991.

Lee PA, L St L O'Dea: Primary and secondary testicular insufficiency. *Pediatr Clin North Am* 37:1359-1387, 1990.

Lee LM, et al: Prostaglandin E1 versus phentolamine/papaverine for the treatment of erectile impotence: A double-blind comparison. *J Urol* 141:549-550, 1989.

Lipman AG: Be aware of drugs that may cause infertility. *Mod Med* 231-232, (Sept) 1984.

Loche S, et al: The effect of short-term growth hormone or low-dose oxandrolone treatment in boys with constitutional growth delay. *J Endocrinol Invest* 14:747-750, 1991.

Lue TF, Tanagho EA: Physiology of erection and pharmacological management of impotence. *J Urol* 173:829-836, 1987.

MacAdams MR, et al: Reduction of serum testosterone levels during glucocorticoid therapy. *Ann Intern Med* 104:648-651, 1986.

Malloy TR, Malkowicz B: Pharmacologic treatment of impotence. *Urol Clin North Am* 14:297-305, 1987.

Matsumoto AM, et al: Chronic human chorionic gonadotropin administration in normal men: Evidence that follicle-stimulating hormone is necessary for the maintenance of quantitatively normal spermatogenesis in man. *J Clin Endocrinol Metab* 62:1184-1192, 1986.

McClure RD: Endocrine evaluation and therapy of erectile dysfunction. *Urol Clin North Am* 15:53-64, 1988.

McWaine DE, Procci WR: Drug-induced sexual dysfunction. *Med Toxicol* 3:289-306, 1988.

Meares EM: Testosterone for impotence, letter. *JAMA* 257:3284, 1987.

Megory E, et al: Infections and male fertility. *Obstet Gynecol Surv* 42:283-290, 1987.

Mehan DJ, Chehval MJ: Human chorionic gonadotropin in the treatment of infertile man. *J Urol* 128:60-63, 1982.

Morales A, et al: Nonhormonal pharmacological treatment of organic impotence. *J Urol* 128:45-47, 1982.

Morales A, et al: Is yohimbine effective in treatment of organic impotence? Results of controlled trial. *J Urol* 137:1168-1172, 1987.

Morgentaler A: Current diagnosis and management of impotence. *Compr Ther* 17:25-30, (July) 1991.

Mueller SC, Lue TF: Evaluation of vasculogenic impotence. *Urol Clin North Am* 15:65-76, 1988.

Murray FT, et al: Gonadal dysfunction in diabetic men with organic impotence. *J Clin Endocrinol Metab* 65:127-135, 1987.

Nankin HR, Calkins JH: Decreased bioavailable testosterone in aging normal and impotent men. *J Clin Endocrinol Metab* 63:1418-1420, 1986.

Neaves WB, et al: Leydig cell numbers, daily sperm production, and serum gonadotropin levels in aging men. *J Clin Endocrinol Metab* 59:756-763, 1984.

Nellans RE, et al: Pharmacological erection: Diagnosis and treatment applications in 69 patients. *J Urol* 138:52-54, 1987.

Orvis BR, Lue TF: New therapy for impotence. *Urol Clin North Am* 14:569-581, 1987.

Padma-Nathan H: Neurologic evaluation of erectile dysfunction. *Urol Clin North Am* 15:77-80, 1988.

Palmer JM: The undescended testicle. *Endocrinol Metab Clin North Am* 20:231-240, 1991.

Paulson DF: Clomiphene citrate in management of male hypofertility: Predictors for treatment selection. *Fertil Steril* 28:1226-1229, 1977.

Pike MC, et al: Effect of age at orchidopexy on risk of testicular cancer. *Lancet* 1:1246-1248, 1986.

Pottern LM, et al: Testicular cancer risk among young men: Role of cryptorchidism and inguinal hernia. *J Natl Cancer Inst* 74:377-381, 1985.

Rajfer J, et al: Hormonal therapy of cryptorchidism: Randomized, double-blind study comparing human chorionic gonadotropin and gonadotropin-releasing hormone. *N Engl J Med* 314:466-470, 1986.

Reid K, et al: Double-blind trial of yohimbine in treatment of psychogenic impotence. *Lancet* 2:421-423, 1987.

Reiss H: Use of prostaglandin E_1 for papaverine-failed erections. *Urology* 33:15-16, 1989.

Richman RA, Kirsch LR: Testosterone treatment in adolescent boys with constitutional delay in growth and development. *N Engl J Med* 319:1563-1567, 1988.

Rosenfeld RG, et al: Prospective, randomized study of testosterone treatment of constitutional delay of growth and development in male adolescents. *Pediatrics* 69:681-687, 1982.

Ross LS, et al: Clomiphene treatment of the idiopathic hypofertile male: High-dose, alternate-day therapy. *Fertil Steril* 33:618-623, 1980.

Saal W, et al: Subcutaneous gonadotropin therapy in male patients with hypogonadotropic hypogonadism. *Fertil Steril* 56:319-324, 1991.

Saez JM, Forest MG: Kinetics of human chorionic gonadotropin-induced steroidogenic response of human fetus. I. Plasma testosterone: Implication for human chorionic gonadotropin stimulation test. *J Clin Endocrinol Metab* 49:278-283, 1979.

Schopohl J, et al: Comparison of gonadotropin-releasing hormone and gonadotropin therapy in male patients with idiopathic hypothalamic hypogonadism. *Fertil Steril* 56:1143-1150, 1991.

Shargil AA: Treatment of idiopathic hypogonadotropic hypogonadism in men with luteinizing hormone-releasing hormone: Comparison of treatment with daily injections and with the pulsatile infusion pump. *Fertil Steril* 47:492-501, 1987.

Sherins RJ: Evaluation and management of men with hypogonadotropic hypogonadism, in Garcia C-R, et al (eds): *Current Therapy of Infertility 1984-1985*. Toronto, Decker/Mosby, 1984.

Shulman JF, Shulman S: Methylprednisolone treatment of immunologic infertility in male. *Fertil Steril* 38:591-599, 1982.

Sidi AA: Vasoactive intracavernous pharmacotherapy. *Urol Clin North Am* 15:95-101, 1988.

Sidi AA, et al: Intracavernous drug-induced erections in the management of male erectile dysfunction: Experience with 100 patients. *J Urol* 135:704-706, 1986.

Silber SJ: Effect of age on male fertility. *Semin Reprod Endocrinol* 9:241-248, (Aug) 1991.

Sokol RZ, Swerdloff RS: Hypogonadism: Androgen therapy, in Krieger DT, Bardin CW (eds): *Current Therapy in Endocrinology 1983-1984*. St Louis, Mo, CV Mosby, 1983.

Sokol RZ, et al: A controlled comparison of the efficacy of clomiphene citrate in male infertility. *Fertil Steril* 49:865-870, 1988.

Spark RF: *The Infertile Male: The Clinician's Guide to Diagnosis and Treatment*. New York, Plenum Medical Book, 1988.

Spratt DI, et al: Spectrum of abnormal patterns of gonadotropin-releasing hormone secretion in men with idiopathic hypogonadotropic hypogonadism: Clinical and laboratory correlations. *J Clin Endocrinol Metab* 64:283-291, 1987 A.

Spratt DI, et al: Effects of increasing the frequency of low doses of gonadotropin-releasing hormone (GnRH) on gonadotropin secretion in GnRH-deficient men. *J Clin Endocrinol Metab* 64:1179-1186, 1987 B.

Strachan JR, Pryor JP: Diagnostic intracorporeal papaverine and erectile dysfunction. *Br J Urol* 59:264-266, 1987.

Strader CH, et al: Cryptorchism, orchiopexy, and the risk of testicular cancer. *Am J Epidemiol* 127:1013-1018, 1988.

Susset JG, et al: Effect of yohimbine hydrochloride on erectile impotence: A double-blind study. *J Urol* 141:1360-1363, 1989.

Takihara H, et al: Effect of low-dose androgen and zinc sulfate on sperm motility and seminal zinc levels in infertile men. *Urology* 22:160-164, 1983.

Takihara H, et al: The pathophysiology of varicocele in male infertility. *Fertil Steril* 55:861-868, 1991.

Tse W-y, et al: Long-term outcome of oxandrolone treatment in boys with constitutional delay of growth and puberty. *J Pediatr* 117:588-591, 1990.

Tung K: Immunopathology and male infertility. *Hosp Pract* 191-206, (June 15) 1988.

Veldhuis JD, et al: Preferential release of bioactive luteinizing hormone in response to endogenous and low dose exogenous gonadotropin-releasing hormone pulses in man. *J Clin Endocrinol Metab* 64:1275-1282, 1987.

Wagner IOF, et al: Pulsatile gonadotropin-releasing hormone treatment in idiopathic delayed puberty. *J Clin Endocrinol Metab* 62:95-102, 1986.

Wespes E, Schulman CC: Systemic complication of intracavernous papaverine injection in patients with venous leakage. *Urology* 31:114-115, 1988.

Whitcomb RW, Crowley WF Jr: Clinical Review 4: Diagnosis and treatment of isolated gonadotropin-releasing hormone deficiency in men. *J Clin Endocrinol Metab* 70:3-7, 1990.

Winters SJ, Troen P: Altered pulsatile secretion of luteinizing hormone in hypogonadal men with hyperprolactinaemia. *Clin Endocrinol* 21:257-263, 1984.

Drugs Used for Gynecologic Indications

PHYSIOLOGY. Estradiol 17-β (called estradiol hereafter) is the major estrogen in premenopausal women. A total of 100 to 300 mcg is secreted daily by the ovary. Androstenedione, an androgen precursor, also is secreted by the ovary, where it is converted to testosterone, which then is demethylated and aromatized to estrogen. Androstenedione also may be converted to estrone and then to estradiol. Estradiol and estrone (which is about one-half as potent as estradiol) thus are secreted by the ovary, while estriol (a much weaker estrogen) is formed by the peripheral metabolism of ovarian estrogens. Estradiol and estrone are extensively interconverted in the body.

Estrone also is produced by peripheral conversion of androstenedione in a variety of tissues. In premenopausal women, this conversion accounts for about 25% of the estrone produced; the balance is secreted directly by the ovary. In postmenopausal women, peripheral conversion of androstenedione to estrone is the principal source of this estrogen. Although circulating levels of total estrogens decrease and androstenedione levels are about one-half or less of those in premenopausal women, the daily production of estrone remains similar (about 45 mcg) because of a compensatory increase in the conversion rate of androstenedione. Before menopause, androstenedione is derived almost equally from ovarian and adrenal secretion; after menopause, the principal source of androstenedione is the adrenal cortex.

Progesterone is produced primarily by direct secretion from the ovary (from the corpus luteum after ovulation); a very small amount is secreted by the adrenal cortex. Preovulatory progesterone production is about 1 to 3 mg daily; during the luteal phase, 20 to 30 mg is secreted daily.

A small quantity of testosterone is produced by the ovary in normal women. About one-half of the testosterone present is derived from peripheral conversion of androstenedione and other adrenal androgens, and the balance is secreted directly by the ovary and adrenal cortex.

In the premenopausal years, ovarian estrogen (estradiol) is secreted during the follicular and luteal phase of the cycle, while progesterone is secreted almost entirely during the luteal phase. In the follicular phase, follicle-stimulating hormone (FSH) interacts with receptors on the granulosa cells and luteinizing hormone (LH) interacts with receptors on the thecal cells. The latter results in production of androstenedione and testosterone by the thecal cells. These androgens diffuse into the granulosa cells where aromatizing enzymes (stimulated by FSH) convert them to estrone and estradiol. The combination of FSH and estradiol stimulates growth of new granulosa cells and LH receptors on these cells. During the luteal phase, LH stimulates production of progesterone as well as estrogen in the granulosa cells. Overstimulation of LH receptors may be avoided by down-regulation; that is, the number of receptors may decrease as LH levels increase.

The increasing levels of estrogen before ovulation act as a positive feedback, modulating the effect of luteinizing hormone releasing hormone (LHRH) and enhancing the pituitary response to gonadotropin releasing hormone (GnRH). This results in a midcycle surge of gonadotropin secretion from the anterior pituitary gland. The high level of LH is responsible for ovulation of the mature follicle(s). Estrogen and progesterone produced during the luteal phase exert a negative feedback effect on the hypothalamus and anterior pituitary, and gonadotropin secretion during this time is low.

In the perimenopausal years, ovulatory cycles usually decrease in frequency and the production of ovarian steroids by the follicle and corpora lutea becomes less efficient; this may be due partly to the relative insensitivity of the remaining follicles to the effects of gonadotropin. After menopause, ovarian secretion of estrogen and progesterone essentially ceases, and circulating estrogen (estrone) is produced primarily by peripheral conversion of androstenedione.

The placenta produces enormous quantities of estrogens and progesterone during pregnancy; the resulting high levels of steroids in the maternal circulation rise steadily as pregnancy progresses. Since the placenta does not possess the enzyme systems to accomplish this alone, precursors for progesterone must be supplied from the maternal circulation and precursors for estrogen from the fetal adrenal cortex (the fetoplacental unit for steroid production). The functions of the high levels of estrogen and progesterone during pregnancy are not completely understood, but some are probable: Progesterone may maintain myometrial quiescence and lack of irritability, and it may serve as a precursor for fetal adrenal corticosteroids. Estrogen stimulates uterine growth and uteroplacental blood flow.

In nonpregnant women, estrogen and progesterone support physiologic processes that ultimately result in release of an ovum and preparation of the uterine endometrium to support a conceptus. The interaction of steroid hormones and gonadotropins, the influence of steroids on ovum and sperm transport, and the stimulation by steroids of endometrial growth and glycogen secretion are all directed toward this end.

Estrogen and progesterone stimulate pubertal changes (eg, growth and maturation of uterus, breasts, and other hormone-responsive tissues; stimulation and eventual limitation of linear skeletal growth) and later maintain the integrity of responsive tissues (eg, breast, uterus, vaginal and urethral mucosa). These hormones also have widespread effects on metabolism (eg, transport protein, electrolyte balance). The reduction of circulating estrogen levels following menopause often is associated with symptoms referable to these target tissues (eg, atrophic vagina, urethral irritation, osteoporosis).

The cellular mechanism of action of all steroid hormones is similar. Most evidence has been obtained with estrogen. This hormone crosses cell and nuclear membranes by simple diffusion and binds to intranuclear receptors. In turn, the estrogen-receptor complex is thought to bind to chromatin and activate selective messenger RNA synthesis. As a result of this process, enzymes and other proteins are manufactured and carry out the specific cellular function of the hormone (Press et al, 1986).

Estradiol circulates in the blood 50% to 80% bound to protein transport carriers. Part is bound to sex hormone-binding globulin (SHBG), a beta globulin that is also the carrier protein for testosterone; part is loosely bound to albumin; and a small amount (2%) is unbound. Progesterone is bound largely to corticosteroid-binding globulin (CBG), which is the major binding globulin for cortisol. For all steroid hormones, including estrogen and progesterone, only the relatively small portion that is unbound is biologically active.

The steroids are metabolized to inactive forms in the liver and gastrointestinal tract and then excreted in the urine and bile. Estrogens are converted to sulfates and glucuronides, and progesterone is metabolized to a number of products, including pregnanediol, and then conjugated. Progesterone and other steroids are measured by radioimmunoassays and competitive protein binding assays.

Under normal conditions, the ovaries and adrenal cortex secrete relatively little testosterone in women. Instead, they secrete primarily preandrogens, such as androstenedione and dehydroepiandrosterone, which are metabolized to testosterone in many peripheral tissues. The overall production of testosterone in women averages 0.23 mg daily, and normal plasma concentrations are 20 to 80 ng/dL. About one-half of plasma testosterone is produced by peripheral conversion of androstenedione, and the other one-half is derived equally from other ovarian and adrenal secretory products. Adrenal dehydroepiandrosterone sulfate (DHEAS) is the androgen secreted in greatest quantity after adrenarche, but it is less important functionally because of its low rate of conversion to testosterone.

Secretion of androgen by the adrenal cortex is stimulated principally by corticotropin (ACTH), while ovarian androgens are secreted in response to LH. Probably because 50% of androstenedione is of adrenal origin, the small amplitude circadian periodicity of its secretion coincides with that of cortisol. Also, plasma concentrations of ovarian androgens, including androstenedione and testosterone, increase slightly around midcycle.

Certain pathologic conditions of the adrenal cortex or ovaries (eg, hyperplasia, polycystic ovaries, adenoma, carcinoma) markedly increase the production of testosterone and its precursors. Precocious pubertal development, virilism, or amenorrhea may result if the overproduction is significant and sustained. Hirsutism and/or acne may occur with less severe functional disturbances.

The mechanism of action of androgens in women is the same as that in men. Depending on the target tissue, either testosterone or dihydrotestosterone (DHT) is the active intracellular androgen. Androgen-sensitive hair follicles in women require DHT for stimulation.

THERAPEUTIC PREPARATIONS. Most of the agents used therapeutically are synthetic or natural analogues of endogenous hormones. Therapy may provide hormones to the tissues in unphysiologic patterns, and certain tissues may have relatively greater exposure to exogenous hormone compared with normal secretory patterns. For example, with the commonly used oral preparations, the hepatic-portal circulation carries a greater concentration of the hormone than under conditions of normal physiologic secretion.

Estrogens, progesterone, and progestins (synthetic compounds possessing progestational activity) are available in a variety of preparations for oral, parenteral, transdermal, or topical administration. Natural estrogen and progesterone generally are not useful orally because they are absorbed erratically and are rapidly deactivated by the liver. An exception is the micronized preparation of estradiol [Estrace] in which reduction of particle size greatly increases total surface area with resulting satisfactory absorption. A micronized progesterone preparation is under investigation (Hargrove et al, 1989). Natural estradiol and progesterone are effective when given parenterally. Progesterone also is used as vaginal or rectal suppositories to treat selected patients with infertility (see index entry Progesterone, In Luteal Phase Dysfunction).

All natural estrogen products are steroidal. These include estradiol (see above), estrone compounds, and preparations of conjugated estrogens. Synthetic estrogens may be steroidal or nonsteroidal. The addition of a 17α-ethinyl group to estradiol increases potency and enhances oral activity by impeding hepatic degradation. Quinestrol [Estrovis], which is closely related to ethinyl estradiol [Estinyl, Feminone], is stored in adipose tissue, thus prolonging its action. Esters of estradiol (benzoate, cypionate, valerate) in oily solutions or aqueous suspensions for intramuscular injection have more prolonged activity than oral preparations (see the evaluation).

Most nonsteroidal estrogens are related to stilbene in chemical structure. Diethylstilbestrol (DES), a stilbene, was the first to be synthesized and has potent estrogenic activity. Further modifications in structure yielded other nonsteroidal compounds (eg, dienestrol [DV], chlorotrianisene [TACE]) with varying potency. Clomiphene [Clomid, Serophene], which is related structurally to chlorotrianisene, possesses both estrogenic and antiestrogenic activity and is used to treat infertility (see index entry Clomiphene).

Synthetic progestins are derived from two sources: (1) from modification of the testosterone molecule (norethindrone [Norlutin], norethindrone acetate [Aygestin, Norlutate], and other progestins used only in oral contraceptives), and (2) from 17α-hydroxyprogesterone (hydroxyprogesterone caproate, medroxyprogesterone acetate (MPA) [Amen, Curretab, Cycrin, Depo-Provera, Provera], megestrol acetate [Megace]). Depending on the parent compound and the chemical alterations employed, these agents have varying degrees of progestational or androgenic potency.

The biological activities of the synthetic estrogens and progestins are similar, but not identical, to those of the natural compounds. Potency and side effects vary according to the chemical structure, route of administration, and dose employed.

Indications

Hormones are administered therapeutically to mimic or accentuate the biological effects of endogenous hormones: to supplement inadequate endogenous production (eg, Turner's syndrome, menopause), to correct hormonal imbalance (eg, dysfunctional bleeding), to reverse an abnormal process (eg, hirsutism, endometriosis), and for contraception.

AMENORRHEA. Estrogen and progestins are used both to determine the etiology of amenorrhea and to treat it, if appropriate. Amenorrhea may be primary or secondary, but, if the patient has a uterus in situ, generally the same diagnostic approach is employed in either case. A complete medical history and physical examination are necessary to exclude pregnancy and causes outside the reproductive system. For review of the pathophysiology of amenorrhea, see Doody and Carr, 1990.

Amenorrhea due to hyper- or hypofunction of the adrenal cortex or thyroid or secondary to diabetes mellitus may be corrected by treating the primary disorder. Functional aberrations of neurotransmitters (ie, dopamine, norepinephrine) and/or the endorphin system probably interfere with normal GnRH secretion, causing amenorrhea (Kase, 1983). Other possible etiologies may be referable to dysfunction at any level of the hypothalamic-pituitary-gonadal axis: hypothalamic-pituitary disorders (eg, prolactin-secreting tumors; hypogonadotropism, including craniopharyngioma and Kallmann's syndrome; functional causes); ovarian defects (eg, premature ovarian failure, Turner's syndrome); or uterine-vaginal defects (eg, congenital absence, Asherman's syndrome, imperforate hymen). Amenorrhea also can result from hyperandrogenic disorders (eg, polycystic ovarian disease, ovarian tumor, adrenal hyperfunction or tumor). Hormones and hormone assays are useful to establish the source of the defect (ie, ovary, endometrium, anterior pituitary, hypothalamus, thyroid, adrenal). Progesterone and other steroid concentrations are measured by immunoassays and competitive protein binding assays.

Secondary amenorrhea, particularly in adolescents, may result from inadequate nutrition, excessive exercise, or psychological stress. Amenorrhea also occurs in thin women who engage in regular endurance athletic training (eg, running, dancing, swimming). The cause is unknown but may be related to low body fat or the repeated stress of exercise (Bullen et al, 1985). Another hypothesis suggests that chronic endurance training causes a series of events progressing from increased cardiac output and increased metabolic clearance of gonadal hormones that interferes with normal hypothalamic-pituitary feedback mechanisms to menstrual dysfunction (Casper et al, 1984). When closely matched amenorrheic runners were compared with eumenorrheic runners, no difference was observed in serum LH, FSH, thyroid-stimulating hormone (TSH), or prolactin concentrations. However, gonadotropin response to GnRH was exaggerated in those who were amenorrheic, suggesting an abnormality at the hypothalamic level (Yahiro et al, 1987).

This condition is of concern because of the long-term potential for osteoporosis and the increased risk of cardiovascular disease associated with low levels of estrogen. Vertebral bone was reduced in women with amenorrhea from various causes, including exercise; estrogen levels were in the low-normal range (Cann et al, 1984). Cortical bone loss may be less prevalent when amenorrhea is caused by exercise rather than by other factors (Drinkwater et al, 1984; Jones et al, 1985). Although exercise enhances bone development, the effect may not compensate for low estrogen levels. Amenorrheic athletes should be evaluated for hormonal status after four to six months of missed menses. Bone mineral density increases after resumption of menses, but it is not known if the original bone density is recovered (Drinkwater et al, 1986).

Patients with evidence of anovulation and unopposed estrogen secretion usually are given a progestin only, while hypoestrogenic patients are given estrogen plus progestin (Shangold, 1982). Usual replacement doses of an estrogen and progestin are administered or a low-dose oral contraceptive (OC) may be given; the latter is particularly appropriate if contraception is desired (Shangold et al, 1990). Some form of contraception is advised if the patient is sexually active and a progestin or replacement therapy is prescribed.

Diagnostic Tests: To test for the presence of estrogenic stimulation and ability of the endometrium to respond, oral medroxyprogesterone acetate (MPA) (10 mg daily for five to ten days) or intramuscular progesterone in oil (200 mg) is administered. *Pregnancy must always be ruled out before exogenous hormones are used for diagnosis.* An oral preparation is often preferred for convenience and to avoid the discomfort associated with injection of progesterone. Withdrawal bleeding three to seven days after treatment indicates adequate estrogenic stimulation of the endometrium and anovulation; it suggests inadequate production or abnormal temporal pattern of secretion of gonadotropin (hypothalamic-pituitary-ovarian axis dysfunction). Absence of withdrawal bleeding suggests lack of endogenous estrogen stimulation (including ovulation within the last two weeks), functional causes, ovarian failure (high levels of serum gonadotropins support this diagnosis), or obstruction of outflow from the uterus. If bleeding does not occur, a course of estrogen therapy is given with a progestin added at the end of the cycle (withdrawal bleeding demonstrates the ability of the endometrium to respond to estrogen and progestin).

If the estrogen-progestin challenge fails to produce withdrawal bleeding, a defect in the outflow tract or endometrium is suggested. The latter may result from Asherman's syndrome (uterine synechiae); surgical correction by hysteroscopy and lysis of adhesions is followed by insertion of an IUD, which is left in place for approximately one month. Alternatively, following surgery, a pediatric Foley catheter filled with 3 ml of fluid is placed in the uterus and allowed to remain for seven days. An antibiotic is given concurrently. Estrogen-progestin therapy designed to rebuild a normal endometrium usually follows either of these procedures.

Drug Therapy: Ovarian failure may be congenital (eg, Turner's syndrome, presence of Y chromosome, mosaicism) or caused by premature menopausal changes. Estrogen replacement therapy should be considered to stimulate or maintain secondary sex characteristics and to prevent osteoporosis and premature atherogenic heart disease. A progestin generally is given concurrently when the uterus is intact to prevent unopposed endometrial stimulation. Suggested regimens include conjugated estrogens 0.625 mg daily for 25 days per month with oral MPA 5 to 10 mg daily added during the last 10 to 13 days of estrogen therapy; conjugated estrogens 0.625 mg continuously plus MPA 5 to 10 mg for the first 10 to 12 days of the calendar month; or other dosage-equivalent patterns of other estrogens and progestins. Atypical adenomatous hyperplasia has developed in women taking conjugated estrogens with 10 days or less of MPA therapy. Each cycle can begin on the first of each month for convenience. The adequacy of such therapy is indicated by the relief of symptoms. OCs are generally not used for replacement therapy because they contain pharmacologic, not physiologic, quantities of hormones. However, when contraception is desired, OCs may be used.

Results of one study employing various estrogen regimens to treat *Turner's syndrome* suggested that standard treatment may not be ideal. Estrogen therapy in the form of ethinyl estradiol has a biphasic effect, and linear growth is stimulated by small doses (about 4 mcg daily) and inhibited by standard doses (20 to 50 mcg daily) (Ross et al, 1983). Further utilization of low doses of ethinyl estradiol (100 ng/kg/day or 2 mcg for a 20-kg child) has yielded equivocal results. In a placebo-controlled crossover study of 16 patients with Turner's syndrome treated for six months, there was an increase in predicted adult height with no advancement in bone age compared with those receiving a placebo (Ross et al, 1986). However, in another study of nine patients who received low doses of estrogen for 18 months, peak improvement in growth velocity occurred at six months and declined thereafter. Although this study was uncontrolled, the investigators judged the advancement in bone age relative to linear growth to be unacceptable, and there was no improvement in predicted adult height (Martinez et al, 1987). More evidence is necessary to determine the optimal dose and duration of estrogen therapy that will achieve the greatest adult height in patients with Turner's syndrome. Oxandrolone [Oxandrin], alone or in combination with growth hormone (GH), has enhanced height in those with Turner's syndrome. Although combined treatment with GH is more effective, the cost of oxandrolone therapy is about 10% that of GH. Oxandrolone is available under a treatment IND (investigational new drug) for this indication (see also index entry Growth Hormone and review by Lippe, 1991).

The treatment of amenorrhea caused by *dysfunction of the hypothalamic-pituitary-ovarian (HPO) axis* depends on the goals of the patient. After excluding the presence of a pituitary adenoma, other life-threatening disease, and ovarian failure, induction of ovulation may be attempted if the patient desires pregnancy (see index entry Infertility, Etiology and Treatment in Women). If pregnancy is not desired and the patient has sufficient endogenous estrogen to promote endometrial stimulation, progestin therapy should be administered intermittently (after pregnancy has been excluded) to interrupt this steady-state estrogen effect and prevent endometrial hyperplasia. MPA 10 mg daily for 10 to 13 days monthly will serve this purpose and produce withdrawal bleeding.

Patients with HPO axis dysfunction may unknowingly experience return of spontaneous cyclicity and therefore may be at risk of pregnancy if they are sexually active. Nonhormonal contraceptives are preferred by some practitioners for these patients, but OCs are sometimes administered. There is no evidence that OCs further suppress or alter already abnormal HPO axis function. See also review by Liu, 1990.

Following surgery for *Asherman's syndrome*, conjugated estrogens 1.25 to 2.5 mg daily for three weeks plus MPA 10 mg daily during the last 10 to 12 days of estrogen therapy is given, and the cycle is repeated monthly for three months.

ABNORMAL UTERINE BLEEDING. Abnormal uterine bleeding (ie, excessive in frequency, duration, or amount) may be of organic origin (eg, endometrial cancer, coagulation defects, chronic endometritis, polyps, myomas, complications of pregnancy) or may be dysfunctional, that is, caused by estrogen and progesterone imbalance unassociated with organic pathology. Menorrhagia may be due to a blood dyscrasia. Dysfunctional bleeding is often associated with anovulatory cycles, which are most common during adolescence and the perimenopausal years. This type of cycle produces an estrogen-dominated, fragile, hyperplastic endometrium characterized by periodic profuse bleeding or irregular, possibly chronic, spotting. These abnormalities result from relatively constant, low-level estrogen stimulation uninterrupted by the action of progesterone. Dysfunctional bleeding also may be caused by an atrophic endometrium secondary to progestin dominance. A history of combined OC use with a progressively decreasing volume of withdrawal bleeding or progestin-only (minipill or depot preparation) contraception helps in diagnosing the latter type of bleeding.

Effective management of abnormal uterine bleeding requires determination of etiology. Abnormal bleeding associated with ovulation is only rarely treated with drugs, and polyps, myomas, and similar problems are preferably managed surgically. Endometrial biopsy, hysteroscopy, and medical history assist in determining the rationale of drug therapy. Pregnancy should be excluded before surgical intervention or hormonal therapy is initiated.

Drug Therapy: If the endometrium is proliferative, an oral progestin (MPA 10 mg daily for 10 to 13 days) is useful. Alternatively, norethindrone acetate or norethindrone (2.5 to 5 mg daily) may be given.

If the endometrium is hyperplastic with atypia, an endometrial biopsy or differential dilatation and curettage should be performed before drug treatment is begun. If there is no evidence of an abnormality, a progestin should be administered continuously for two to three months. Patients with endometrial cancer should be referred to a gynecologic oncologist.

The patient with a denuded endometrium may benefit from administration of a high-potency estrogen-progestin combination or estrogen alone to build up a structurally stable endometrium. Conjugated estrogens occasionally are used intravenously to control acute bleeding initially. Suggested oral regimens for initial control or following intravenous estrogen include: (1) three OC pills daily (taken after meals) for seven to ten days; (2) conjugated estrogens 2.5 to 3.75 mg plus MPA 10 mg daily for seven to ten days or conjugated estrogens 5 mg daily for one week with a progestin added the last 5 days (MPA 10 mg or norethindrone acetate 5 mg daily); (3) two OC pills for three days followed by one pill daily for 17 days; (4) one OC pill every six hours for five to seven days, followed by one OC pill daily and cyclically for three months to prevent recurrence. Preparations with the lowest hormone content are likely to be better tolerated. (For a listing of OC preparations, see index entry Contraceptives, Oral.)

In one uncontrolled trial, administration of the GnRH agonist, goserelin [Zoladex], plus cyclic hormone replacement with estrogen and progestin resulted in significant diminution of pain and bleeding (Thomas et al, 1991).

Following treatment, heavy withdrawal bleeding with dysmenorrhea can be expected. Uterine prostaglandin levels normally increase during the luteal phase of the cycle, and dysfunctional bleeding is associated with high levels, particularly of prostacyclin. This substance inhibits platelet aggregation and is a vasodilator, and these actions are consistent with the development of menorrhagia in ovulatory cycles (Strickler, 1985). NSAIDs that are prostaglandin synthetase inhibitors, such as mefenamic acid [Ponstel] or ibuprofen, may reduce excessive menstrual fluid loss and dysmenorrhea when given in usual therapeutic doses (Mishell et al, 1984). The bleeding usually ceases within one to three days; if it continues, curettage may be necessary. Subsequent cycles are regulated by administering OCs for one year or, if contraception is not desired, a progestin alone (MPA 10 mg or norethindrone acetate 2.5 mg daily for ten days preceding expected withdrawal bleeding) can be used during the second six months. Clomiphene may be used to induce ovulation in patients who are infertile and desire pregnancy. If pregnancy does not occur, the ovulatory cycle produced will likely produce normal menses.

Menorrhagia unresponsive to hormonal manipulation or prostaglandin synthetase inhibitors may be alleviated by treatment with the antifibrinolytic agent, tranexamic acid [Cyklokapron] 4 to 6 g daily. An oral iron supplement may be desirable to prevent anemia. Electrosurgical or laser endometrial ablation may be indicated in chronic cases unresponsive to pharmacologic treatment (Andersson, 1991). See also reviews on dysfunctional uterine bleeding by Johnson, 1991 and Hertweck, 1992.

DYSMENORRHEA. Dysmenorrhea secondary to other conditions (eg, endometriosis, leiomyomas) requires treatment of the specific cause. Primary dysmenorrhea probably results from the increased production of prostaglandin (PG) by the secretory endometrium during the luteal phase or to increased sensitivity to PG. Therefore, agents that inhibit ovulation, steroidogenesis, or PG production are often effective. Patients who require contraception as well as relief from primary dysmenorrhea may benefit from treatment with OCs.

Effective and safe PG inhibitors include fenamates (eg, mefenamic acid, flufenamic acid) and phenylpropionic acid derivatives (eg, ibuprofen, naproxen [Naprosyn], naproxen sodium [Anaprox], fenoprofen [Nalfon]). Piroxicam [Feldene], an enolic acid derivative, also is effective. These agents are taken at the onset of menstrual discomfort and are particularly useful when concurrent contraception is unnecessary. Treatment is continued only as long as needed to relieve symptoms, usually two to five days. If a patient does not respond to one agent, another preparation, especially if it is from another chemical group, may be beneficial. Fenamate derivatives theoretically offer an advantage since they inhibit both the synthesis and peripheral action of prostaglandins, but this has not been a consistent finding in controlled clinical trials (Smith, 1988). Indomethacin [Indocin] also is effective, but is probably not the best choice because adverse effects are reported more commonly (Roy, 1983; Wenzloff and Shimp, 1984; Dawood, 1985, 1988; Rawal et al, 1987; Shapiro, 1988). See index entry Anti-inflammatory Agents, Nonsteroidal, for preparations.

If dysmenorrhea is not relieved by OCs or NSAIDs, endometriosis or another organic cause should be considered.

PREMENSTRUAL SYNDROME (PMS). This syndrome may occur in any menstruating woman, but the incidence increases in those over 30 years, and a family history of PMS is common. It is characterized by both psychological (eg, irritability, depression, anxiety) and somatic (eg, abdominal bloating and fluid retention, headache, enlargement and tenderness of breasts) complaints. These symptoms occur premenstrually and not at other times in the cycle. Patterns of symptoms are variable, and there may be several distinct types of PMS with separate etiologies.

Suggested causative factors include change in the concentrations or ratios of estrogen and progesterone, endorphins, prostaglandins, neurotransmitters, angiotensin, or intracellular magnesium, but none of these theories have been proved. It is, therefore, not surprising that none of the wide variety of pharmacologic treatments suggested for PMS has been universally effective. Some treatment regimens have not been proved to be effective by controlled studies, and there are conflicting reports of efficacy among those that are most widely recommended (Havens, 1985). Interpretation of results of studies is difficult because of lack of standard criteria. The same pattern of symptoms tends to recur in a given individual, and therapy usually is individualized to treat specific symptoms. The patient should keep a diary to record symptoms, because timing of symptoms alone may exclude a diagnosis of PMS. Reviews on the diagnosis and management of PMS are available (see Hammarbäck, 1989; Smith and Schiff, 1989; Chihal, 1990; Lurie and Borenstein, 1990).

Drug Therapy: Although numerous approaches have been tried, no specific drug therapy has been proven to be effective in the treatment of PMS. Studies of various therapies for PMS are summarized below. Definitive studies are necessary to determine all etiologic factors more clearly and assist in the development of rational treatment for PMS.

Progesterone has been widely used in severe PMS for many years (Dalton, 1984) and is claimed to be effective for selected patients, although the preponderance of controlled studies do not support this view. Treatment with progesterone is based on the premise that a relative progesterone deficiency or an increased estrogen:progesterone ratio causes PMS. However, the presence of a hormonal abnormality has not been demonstrated in PMS patients (Smith and Schiff, 1989; Freeman et al, 1990). Only one controlled study has shown a beneficial effect from progesterone (micronized) (Dennerstein et al, 1985). Controlled studies on progesterone for the treatment of PMS have been reviewed (Maxson, 1987; Smith and Schiff, 1989; Chihal, 1990). The drug may be administered parenterally, but vaginal or rectal suppositories are more convenient; an intranasal cream is being investigated.

Oral contraceptives, which are effective in dysmenorrhea, have relieved PMS in some patients, but generally they are not considered useful for this indication. A regimen of subcutaneous estradiol implants plus norethindrone tablets, which suppressed ovulation, was more effective than a placebo regimen in relieving symptoms in six symptom clusters (Magos et al, 1986).

An agonist of GnRH suppressed cyclic function, including menses and symptoms of PMS, in some patients (Muse et al, 1984). Use of this type of agent (eg, leuprolide, nafarelin) alone is inappropriate for chronic therapy because of the long-term effects of low estrogen levels (eg, osteoporosis, cardiovascular disease). An estrogen-progestin replacement regimen (0.625 mg conjugated estrogens day 1 to 25; MPA 10 mg day 16 to 25) plus a GnRH agonist maintained relief while providing protection for bone and cardiovascular disease. Conjugated estrogens, MPA, or placebo alone added to the GnRH agonist were less effective in relieving PMS symptoms.

Danazol [Danocrine] has relieved both psychological and somatic complaints of PMS in double-blind placebo-controlled trials. Doses of 200 to 400 mg daily alleviate symptoms, but ovulation usually occurs at the lower dose. In sexually active patients, nonhormonal contraception should be used to prevent pregnancy and avoid possible virilization of a female fetus (Smith and Schiff, 1989; Deeny et al, 1991).

Pyridoxine (vitamin B_6) has alleviated depression associated with high-dose oral contraceptive use. In such instances, contraceptive hormones are believed to cause a relative vitamin B deficiency, alter tryptophan metabolism, and decrease serotonin production, all of which may contribute to depression. The suggestion that a similar hormone-related etiology is responsible for depression during PMS led to the use of pyridoxine for this indication, but results of controlled studies indicate that the vitamin has no specific benefit. Pyridoxine 500 mg daily may cause reversible neuropathy (Berger and Schaumburg, 1984), and it is possible that even lower doses may be toxic in some individuals. The use of pyridoxine in the treatment of PMS has been reviewed (Kleijnen et al, 1990).

Diuretics also are used to treat PMS. They may relieve symptoms related to fluid retention but appear to be ineffective in relieving other symptoms. It was hypothesized that aldosterone levels, which are elevated during the luteal phase of the cycle, may be responsible for fluid retention premenstrually, although aldosterone levels are not increased in women with PMS. Angiotensin, which stimulates secretion of aldosterone, increases capillary permeability and edema. Spironolactone [Aldactone], an aldosterone inhibitor that also interferes with some renal effects of angiotensin in animals

(Hellberg et al, 1991), relieved a variety of premenstrual symptoms (O'Brien et al, 1979) and bloating (Vellacott et al, 1987) in placebo-controlled studies. Spironolactone or MPA was more effective than placebo in improving mood in PMS patients (Hellberg et al, 1991).

Intracellular magnesium concentrations in lymphocytes and polymorphonuclear cells are lower in PMS patients than in unaffected women. Administration of an oral magnesium preparation normalized the intracellular magnesium concentration and improved mood more effectively than placebo (Facchinetti et al, 1991).

Evening primrose oil also has been used to treat PMS. This agent contains *cis*-linoleic acid and gamma-linoleic acid, which are precursors of prostaglandins of the E series. Some patients with PMS may have abnormal levels of these fatty acids, and evening primrose oil may correct the imbalance. Results of a double-blind, placebo-controlled, crossover study showed that this preparation was more effective than placebo in relieving depression associated with PMS (Puolakka et al, 1985).

Alprazolam [Xanax], a benzodiazepine with antianxiety and putative antidepressant effects, also has relieved affective symptoms of PMS in controlled studies. Because of the drug's addictive potential, patients should be carefully selected. Medication should be given only during the luteal phase, and the dosage should be reduced after the onset of menses (Smith and Schiff, 1989). In a double-blind, placebo-controlled crossover study, fluoxetine [Prozac] improved mood and physical symptoms of PMS patients (Wood et al, 1992).

Because prolactin is involved in osmoregulation in some fish and mammals and some symptoms of PMS appear to be related to fluid retention, it has been suggested that this hormone may be a causative factor in PMS. However, no consistent differences in serum prolactin concentrations have been observed in symptomatic and normal women. Bromocriptine [Parlodel], a dopaminergic agent that inhibits prolactin secretion, has been used to treat PMS. No improvement in most premenstrual symptoms has been observed in most trials.

In placebo-controlled trials, a variety of other drugs have shown some success in relieving some PMS symptoms (eg, α-tocopherol, mefenamic acid, naltrexone [Chuong et al, 1988], calcium). Clonidine [Catapres] and verapamil [Calan, Isoptin, Verelan] also were effective in some patients. In one report, thyroid dysfunction was a common finding among patients with PMS, and treatment with levothyroxine relieved PMS symptoms (Brayshaw and Brayshaw, 1986); other investigators have found no association between these disorders (Casper et al, 1989).

HIRSUTISM. Hypersecretion of ovarian androgen due to elevated LH is a common cause of hirsutism; Cushing's syndrome or late-onset congenital adrenal hyperplasia also may cause this condition (Siegel et al, 1990). Hyperinsulinemia, which results from compensatory insulin secretion in response to insulin resistance, also may stimulate secretion of ovarian androgen (Barbieri et al, 1988). Enhanced androgen utilization or sensitivity of the skin to androgen also may be primary or contributing causes of hirsutism (Adashi, 1990).

Plasma androgen levels are elevated in many hirsute women. In one study on 138 hirsute women, the free plasma testosterone level was elevated in 82% and DHEAS was increased in 59% (Wild et al, 1983). Although the total testosterone concentration may be in the normal range, the combination of decreased protein binding of testosterone with elevation of free (biologically active) testosterone may be sufficient to cause hirsutism. In addition, there is great variability in the responsiveness of the pilosebaceous unit to a given level of plasma androgen (Reingold and Rosenfield, 1987). Sensitivity to circulating androgens is probably influenced by androgen receptors and 5α-reductase activity in the skin. Hirsute women have higher levels of 5α-reductase than normal women but similar concentrations of androgen receptors in the skin (Lucky, 1987). It also should be recognized that greater than average hair growth may be a normal characteristic of certain ethnic groups (eg, those of Mediterranean descent). The pathophysiology, diagnosis, and treatment of hirsutism have been reviewed (Rittmaster and Loriaux, 1987).

Diagnostic Tests: Conditions such as Cushing's syndrome, late-onset congenital adrenal hyperplasia, and ovarian or adrenal neoplasms must be considered in the differential diagnosis and treated appropriately if present (Hammond et al, 1986). Diagnostic tests include measurements of serum total testosterone (unbound or free testosterone determination is more expensive and probably not necessary) and DHEAS. The latter yields the same information as the less convenient measurement of 24-hour 17-ketosteroids. Determination of serum prolactin also may be useful because hyperprolactinemia is sometimes associated with hyperandrogenism (Glickman et al, 1982). Androstanediol glucuronide, a measure of peripheral conversion of testosterone to DHT, also is elevated in hirsutism (Greep et al, 1986). Rapidly progressing signs of masculinization and very high serum androgen concentrations (ie, >200 ng/dL testosterone, >700 mcg/dL DHEAS) suggest tumor of the ovary or adrenal gland, respectively. Lower levels usually are associated with ovarian and/or adrenal dysfunction.

Drug Therapy: Various pharmacologic agents have been used to treat hirsutism. A combination OC preparation is frequently selected. The progestin suppresses ovarian steroidogenesis secondary to LH while the estrogen component increases SHBG, which binds to testosterone and decreases the quantity of free hormone. If estrogen is contraindicated, a progestin may be used instead (eg, MPA: oral 10 to 30 mg/day, intramuscular depot 150 mg every three months).

Hirsutism associated with late-onset congenital adrenal hyperplasia can be controlled by a glucocorticoid regimen appropriate for that condition. Since adrenal androgen production is stimulated by ACTH, low doses of glucocorticoid effectively suppress excessive androgen secretion, especially in patients with persistently elevated DHEAS levels. The selection of patients who would benefit from this therapy has been largely empiric. One study suggested a dichotomy of response in hirsute patients. Those who responded to a glucocorticoid with a decrease in serum testosterone greater than 50% also demonstrated lower LH levels with long-term therapy. In patients in whom serum testosterone concentrations decreased less than 50% after glucocorticoid administration, prolonged therapy failed to reduce circulating LH (Karpas et al, 1984). Until it is possible to predict whether a patient is more likely to respond to sex steroids or glucocorticoid therapy, the latter probably should be used as an alternative to sex steroid or other therapy, and the usual precautions associated with glucocorticoid administration should be taken (see index entry Adrenal Corticosteroids, Adverse Reactions).

Spironolactone also appears to be useful for treating hirsutism. It inhibits ovarian androgen synthesis and competes for androgen receptors in susceptible hair follicles (Cumming et al, 1982). Spironolactone therapy causes decreased hair growth rate, decreased hair shaft size, and lighter pigmentation (Tremblay, 1986; Barth et al, 1989). In one study in which 42 of 48 patients reported significant improvement in their condition, spironolactone (100 mg twice daily) was as effective for idiopathic hirsutism as for hirsutism associated with polycystic ovaries (Evans and Burke, 1986). In another study, spironolactone (75 to 100 mg daily) was effective; the most favorable results were reported in women who had regular menses (whether or not OCs were used simultaneously) or who had the most severe hirsutism (Crosby and Rittmaster, 1991). Diuresis may occur for several days after initiating therapy, and menstrual disturbances are common (see the evaluation).

Cyproterone acetate, an agent with antiandrogen and progestin activity, inhibits binding of androgen to intracellular binding protein and also has antigonadotropic activity (Miller and Jacobs, 1986). Successful treatment of hirsutism with a "reverse sequential" regimen (cyclic administration of cyproterone and estrogen followed by estrogen alone) has been reported (Garner and Poznanski, 1984). Cyproterone (2 mg daily) plus an OC was as effective as larger doses of the antiandrogen alone (Barth et al, 1991). In another study, cyproterone and spironolactone were judged to be equally effective (O'Brien et al, 1991). Side effects of cyproterone may include loss of libido and depression. Cyproterone acetate is available as an Orphan Drug for severe hirsutism in the United States and is marketed in some European countries and Canada.

Bromocriptine may be used to treat hirsutism secondary to hyperprolactinemia.

Although cimetidine [Tagamet] also has been suggested to treat hirsutism based on results of an uncontrolled study (Vigersky et al, 1980), a later prospective controlled study showed that it was not effective for this indication (Lissak et al, 1989). A three-month treatment period was used in both investigations.

Ketoconazole [Nizoral] also has been used to treat hirsutism. The drug reduces ovarian and probably adrenal androgen production in a dose-dependent manner. Its usefulness is limited by side effects (eg, dry skin, hair loss, intermenstrual spotting) at the most effective dosages. Adrenal insufficiency and liver enzyme changes are potential problems (Martikainen et al, 1988; Sonino et al, 1990; Pepper et al, 1990). This drug may be considered for treatment of hirsutism if other agents are ineffective.

GnRH agonists have been used to treat hirsutism caused by increased ovarian androgen secretion. These agents decrease gonadotropin secretion and thereby reduce stimulation of ovarian androgen production. Long-term use results in hypoestrogenism with its undesirable consequences (eg, vasomotor flushing, osteoporosis) as well as the desired reduction in androgen levels. Estrogen replacement therapy in addition to the GnRH agonist may provide an approach to treatment that combines therapeutic efficacy with avoidance of hypoestrogenic side effects (Adashi, 1990).

Results of preliminary studies have shown the antiandrogen, flutamide [Eulexin], is effective in the treatment of hirsutism and produces no or minimal alterations in serum androgen and gonadotropin concentrations (Cusan et al, 1990; Motta et al, 1991; Marcondes et al, 1992). Doses ranging from 250 to 750 mg daily have been given. Because flutamide has no contraceptive action, a reliable contraceptive (hormonal or otherwise) should be used in women of childbearing age to prevent pregnancy and possible feminization of a male fetus.

With any type of drug therapy, six months to one year of treatment may be required before effects are apparent. Although hormones suppress new hair growth, normal androgen levels maintain hair that is already present. Electrolysis is useful to hasten the cosmetic results.

ENDOMETRIOSIS. Endometriosis is defined as the presence of endometrial tissue in ectopic sites (probably initiated in most cases by retrograde menstruation). It is found most frequently on the ovaries, the peritoneum of the cul-de-sac, the uterosacral and/or round ligaments, the oviducts, and the serosal surface of the bladder. Endometriosis also may involve the bladder mucosa, ureters, and bowel. Rarely, cells may travel via blood vessels and lymphatics and form implants at distant sites. This disease often is characterized by pelvic or lower back pain that increases prior to menstruation; dysmenorrhea, particularly if it first appears in the late twenties or thirties and becomes progressively worse; and dyspareunia and/or pain on defecation, particularly during menses. The pain of endometriosis probably is related to peritoneal irritation or involvement of other structures that results from scarring, bleeding from the implants during menstruation, or increased production of prostaglandins. The severity of pain is not necessarily related to the extent or location of the disease. Endometriosis occurs predominantly during the childbearing years, because the stimulation of endometrial implants and the associated discomfort depend on cyclic hormonal stimulation, and infertility is common. It also may develop in adolescents as well as in fertile, asymptomatic older women. Like normally located endometrium, the ectopic implants respond to normal cyclic hormonal stimulation, but the response is highly variable.

The pathogenesis and treatment of endometriosis have been reviewed (Metzger and Luciano, 1989; Surrey and Halme, 1989; Barbieri, 1990; Maouris, 1991). Use of standardized staging criteria provides a basis for comparing various therapeutic modalities (American Fertility Society, 1985). The surgical treatment of endometriosis is discussed in the chapter on Drugs Used to Treat Female Infertility.

Drug Therapy: Drugs are employed as the sole treatment or before or after surgery in more severe cases of endometriosis. Like surgical treatment, drugs appear to be most effective in relieving signs and symptoms of endometriosis in severe cases. *Danazol* [Danocrine], an androgen derivative, has been used to treat this disorder. This drug has antigonadotropic (inhibits midcycle surge) and mild anabolic and androgenic activity. Other effects include alteration of ovarian steroidogenesis (Steingold et al, 1986) and, perhaps, a direct effect on the implants. Danazol has been detected in the follicular fluid, and thus it may directly inhibit steroidogenesis at this site (Olsson et al, 1988). Symptoms are somewhat suppressed and some endometrial implants regress. Like surgery, danazol has not been demonstrated to enhance pregnancy rates in patients with mild disease (Seibel et al, 1982; Butler et al, 1984; Bayer et al, 1988).

Many practitioners continue to prescribe *oral contraceptives* for endometriosis, particularly when cost is a limiting factor. These agents are given continuously (not cyclically) for six to nine months and produce a pseudopregnant state in which the uterine endometrium and ectopic implants undergo a decidual reaction, necrosis, and eventual atrophy. Preparations containing less than 50 mcg ethinyl estradiol and a high progestin content are probably best. Symptoms may increase before improvement is noted, and the usual adverse effects of oral contraceptives or estrogens may occur (see index entries Contraceptives, Oral; Estrogens). Oral contraceptives containing ≥50 mcg estrogen should be employed with caution in the presence of myomas, since these agents may stimulate growth.

The newest medical approach to treating endometriosis is the use of *GnRH analogues* (see the review by Erickson and Ory, 1989). These agents inhibit pituitary gonadotropin secretion, suppress normal cyclic ovarian steroid production, and control manifestations of disease; however, like other drug therapy, they are not curative. GnRH analogues induce a hypoestrogenic state but do not have the androgenic side effects of danazol.

The first GnRH analogue to be marketed for the treatment of endometriosis, nafarelin [Synarel], is administered intranasally. In a double-blind placebo-controlled trial, nafarelin (400 or 800 mcg daily) was similar to danazol (800 mg daily) in decreasing the endometriosis laparoscopic score and relieving discomfort. Whereas use of danazol was associated with weight gain and an unfavorable lipoprotein profile (decreased HDL), nafarelin users more frequently reported hot flushes and decreased libido (Henzl et al, 1988; Burry et al, 1989; Välimäki et al, 1989). Biochemical indices of bone turnover increased in patients receiving nafarelin 200 or 400 mcg daily for six months, and bone loss from the forearm and spine occurred in those receiving 400 mcg daily (Johansen et al, 1988). Most bone loss appears to be reversed within one year after treatment is discontinued. The addition of norethindrone to the nafarelin regimen prevented the transient decrease in bone density observed with nafarelin alone (Henzl, 1992). In another study, no decrease in bone mineral density was reported after six months of treatment with danazol or the GnRH analogues, leuprolide and buserelin (Tummon et al, 1988).

An intramuscular depot form of leuprolide acetate [Lupron Depot 3.75 mg] also has been used to treat endometriosis. In a six-month study, danazol and leuprolide similarly decreased the pain and extent of endometriosis, but leuprolide suppressed estrogen secretion more rapidly and effectively (Wheeler et al, 1992). In a prospective randomized trial comparing danazol with an investigational intranasal leuprolide preparation, improvements in endometriosis scores, symptoms, and pregnancy rates were similar with both drugs at the end of one year of treatment (Tummon et al, 1989).

Buserelin (investigational drug) is administered either intranasally or subcutaneously. Both routes were equally effective in causing regression of endometrial implants in one study (Lemay et al, 1988). In another study, subcutaneous implants were more effective in decreasing endometriotic lesions (Donnez et al, 1989). When danazol, gestrinone (an investigational progestin), or buserelin was administered to patients with moderate endometriosis for six months prior to laparotomy, buserelin produced the highest rate of endometriosis regression (73%) and of pregnancy (61%) (Donnez et al, 1990). Loss of trabecular bone (5.9%) and a smaller loss of femoral cortical bone (0.9%) occurred after six months of treatment with buserelin (Matta et al, 1988), but these effects were temporary.

Histrelin [Supprelin] also has been given for this disorder. As with nafarelin, the addition of norethindrone to the regimen largely prevented bone loss during therapy (Surrey et al, 1990). Goserelin also has been reported to relieve symptoms of endometriosis (Reichel et al, 1992; Venturini et al, 1990).

Progestins alone also have been used for endometriosis (eg, MPA 30 mg daily for three months [Moghissi and Boyce, 1976]), particularly when estrogens should be avoided. A depot preparation of MPA is sometimes administered unless pregnancy is desired; its extended duration of action causes prolonged amenorrhea and anovulation (for preparation information, see index entry Medroxyprogesterone). Progestins induce endometrial atrophy, and breakthrough bleeding may be a problem. Use of large doses of MPA or other progestins for an extended period may be associated with an unfavorable change in the serum lipid profile (increased LDL, decreased HDL).

Gestrinone, an investigational 19-nortestosterone derivative, also is being studied for treatment of endometriosis. It suppresses the midcycle gonadotropin surge, weakly binds estrogen receptors, acts as an antiestrogen, and as an agonist and antagonist on progesterone receptors, and demonstrates androgenic activity by its high affinity for SHBG and its effects on serum lipids (ie, increases LDL, decreases HDL). Gestrinone appears to be equivalent to danazol in reducing pain and endometrial implants, but side effects are reportedly fewer and less severe (Fedele et al, 1989; Venturini et al, 1989).

Androgens have been employed to treat endometriosis, but their use is uncommon today and generally not preferred. These hormones may provide temporary relief, but no microscopic changes are observed in ectopic implants. Ovulation is not inhibited, and pregnancy may occur during treatment. Caution must be exercised and the drug discontinued as soon as pregnancy is documented to avoid masculinization of a female fetus.

ABERRANT GROWTH PATTERNS. Puberty may be delayed by associated disorders or *constitutional delay of puberty (CDP)*, a variant of normal, may occur. Short stature is a feature in abnormal states, such as growth hormone deficiency and gonadal dysgenesis. (See index entry Growth Hormone, Deficiency). Girls with CDP may be short but have a height appropriate for the bone age. Differentiation between CDP and hypogonadotropic hypogonadism may be difficult and remain unresolved for years. If there is psychological stress due to lack of development in the interim, brief treatment to stimulate development without advancing bone age is sometimes instituted. Ethinyl estradiol 5 to 10 mcg daily (the smallest tablet currently available is 20 mcg), depot estradiol cypionate (0.5 mg monthly), or conjugated estrogens 0.625 to 1.25 mg daily can be given for three months. The course may be repeated in six months if the condition is unaltered. If short stature is a major concern, therapy can begin with a six-month course of oxandrolone [Anavar] (0.1 mg/kg daily) or a testosterone depot preparation (30 mg monthly). If there is no spontaneous activity by age 17, a gonadotropin deficiency probably exists, and replacement therapy can begin after this has been documented.

The above regimen can induce puberty in girls with sexual infantilism from any cause. Therapy can be initiated at age 12 or, when concomitant growth hormone deficiency exists, it may be delayed until several years after treatment with growth hormone is undertaken. When secondary sexual characteristics appear (the dosage may be doubled if development does not progress), estrogen is given for 25 days per month. When breakthrough bleeding occurs, MPA 5 or 10 mg daily is administered concurrently during the last 10 to 13 days of the cycle. This regimen is repeated monthly. If the uterus has been removed, estrogen alone may be given.

When otherwise normal girls have a predicted adult height (from tables based on present stature and bone age) of greater than six feet and when realization of this growth potential is severely threatening to the child, estrogen therapy is sometimes employed to *suppress the growth rate* and the eventual height attained. Estrogens inhibit production of somatomedin and are effective even though growth hormone levels increase during treatment. Therapy is only effective when begun early, but this principle has limitations. Treatment at age 8 or 9 may be undesirable because of the psychological impact of the long-term regimen (usually one to two years) and the pubertal changes, including induced menses, that result. On the other hand, if therapy is not begun until after the adolescent growth spurt (usually premenarcheal), suppression of growth is often minimal. There is usually an initial acceleration of growth before suppression occurs. If therapy is discontinued before epiphyseal closure, further growth will occur.

When estrogen treatment is initiated by bone age of 11 or 12 years (or early to midpuberty), adult height averages 2 to 3 inches less than the predicted height. Dosages are larger than those used for replacement therapy. Suggested regimens include conjugated estrogens 5 to 10 mg (or the equivalent) daily and continuously, with a progestin (eg, MPA or norethindrone 10 mg daily) added 10 to 13 days each month to induce withdrawal bleeding and thus avoid overstimulation of the endometrium. In a study spanning 15 years, 539 girls received 100 mcg of ethinyl estradiol daily plus MPA 5 mg on day 1 to 10 of the cycle for two years; the average reduction in expected height was approximately 2 inches (Normann et al, 1991). In an earlier study, bromocriptine was suggested as a safe and effective alternative treatment for this indication. This drug reduced the growth hormone response to protirelin and, after 6 to 12 months of therapy, the predicted adult height was reduced in most patients (Evain-Brion et al, 1984).

The potential hazards of estrogen therapy must be considered, and the long-term effects of therapy are unknown. The HPO axis apparently is not suppressed, and almost all patients experience spontaneous regular menses two to six months after cessation of treatment. Decreased antithrombin levels (but not clinical signs of thrombosis) have been observed, and it has been suggested that serum antithrombin levels should be monitored during treatment (Blombäck et al, 1983). Some clinicians feel that the risks of therapy outweigh the benefits of attempting to restrict linear growth.

For a discussion of precocious puberty in both sexes, see index entry Puberty, Precocious.

PREVENTION OF POSTPARTUM LACTATION. Following parturition, prolactin levels usually remain elevated for only one week in the absence of breastfeeding. Lactation ceases in the absence of suckling without drug intervention, but breast engorgement and pain (which can be relieved at least partially by analgesics) are common. Estrogens, alone or with an androgen, often have been used to prevent lactation and the associated discomforts. However, there is an increased risk of thromboembolic phenomena, and rebound lactation often occurs after withdrawal of medication. Androgens are often only partially effective, and masculinizing effects are possible even with brief use.

When bromocriptine is used for 14 days postpartum to prevent lactation, discontinuation of medication does not usually cause rebound prolactin secretion; shorter courses are more likely to be followed by rebound. Once secretion is inhibited and the suckling stimulus is absent, the hormonal conditions necessary to reinitiate lactation are no longer present. Since early ovulation is associated with bromocriptine therapy, there is a risk of unintended pregnancy unless contraception is employed.

Concern has been expressed about the association of certain serious adverse events (eg, stroke, seizure, psychosis) with use of bromocriptine to suppress postpartum lactation. A case-controlled study presented to the FDA by the manufacturer found no association between such use and the occurrence of stroke and seizure; other adverse effects were not addressed (*FDC Rep*, 1988). An FDA Advisory Committee concluded that no drug should be used routinely to suppress postpartum lactation, but that bromocriptine may be appropriate in some cases. Patients should be encouraged to forego pharmacologic therapy for this benign condition, which usually resolves eventually without treatment.

In a multicenter study, the investigational drug, cabergoline (1 mg given once within 27 hours of delivery), was superior to the standard bromocriptine regimen. Complete suppression of lactation occurred more frequently, rebound lactation occurred less frequently, serum prolactin levels were lower, and adverse reactions (ie, hypotension, nausea, dizziness) were less common with cabergoline (European Multicentre Study Group for Cabergoline in Lactation Inhibition, 1991). Cabergoline is available in several European countries.

THREATENED ABORTIONS. Although estrogens have been used to treat *habitual* and *threatened abortions* in the past, such treatment has not been effective. Estrogens now are contraindicated during pregnancy, largely because of the teratogenic effects produced by diethylstilbestrol (DES) and other estrogens in both female and male offspring (see the section on Metabolic Effects, Adverse Reactions, and Precautions and index entry Teratogenicity, Etiology, Oral Contraceptives).

Progestins also have been used to prevent abortion of established pregnancies but are no longer administered for this indication because proof of efficacy is lacking and there is concern about teratogenicity. However, progesterone and hydroxyprogesterone are used for certain indications during pregnancy: Progesterone is employed to treat luteal phase dysfunction from ovulation through early pregnancy (see also index entry Luteal Phase Defect), and hydroxyprogesterone has prevented premature births in some high-risk women when given from the sixteenth week of pregnancy (after organogenesis is complete). No adverse effects have been reported in the offspring (Johnson et al, 1975, 1979 A). Another study in which patients were treated from the twelfth gestational week yielded similar results (Yemini et al, 1985). (See also index entry Infertility, Etiology and Treatment in Women.)

FIBROCYSTIC BREAST CONDITION, MASTALGIA. Breast pain, tenderness, and nodularity are partially or completely relieved in most women with *cyclic fibrocystic breast condition* after administration of danazol, an impeded androgen. Several months of daily treatment may be required. Symptoms may recur within one year after cessation of therapy, and another course may then be initiated. Danazol induces estrogen and progesterone receptors in the breast, and in some women, an increase in the number of progesterone receptors (associated with continued clinical effectiveness) is observed six months after therapy is withdrawn (Panahy et al, 1987).

Bromocriptine also relieves cyclic mastalgia in most patients. In a multicenter randomized, placebo-controlled study conducted by the European Scientific Committee, bromocriptine 2.5 mg twice daily was more effective in relieving symptoms than placebo, and the effect was maintained six months after drug therapy was withdrawn. Clinical improvement was associated with a decline in the serum prolactin concentration, which returned to the original level one month after treatment ceased, even though the clinical improvement continued (Mansel and Dogliotti, 1990).

Other agents that sometimes relieve symptoms include OCs and progestins (Drukker and deMendonca, 1987). Tamoxifen [Nolvadex] is the newest agent to be used investigationally to treat mastalgia; it was more effective than placebo for both cyclic and noncyclic mastalgia (Fentiman et al, 1986; Messinis and Lolis, 1988).

LICHEN SCLEROSUS. Manifestation of this disease includes white patchy appearance of labial skin accompanied by thinning epithelium and presence of subcutaneous collagenization and inflammatory infiltrates. It may occur more frequently within certain families, and it is often found in patients with circulating autoantibodies and autoimmune diseases. Lichen sclerosus occurs most frequently in postmenopausal women; in children, it is more likely to involve nongenital skin sites (Soper and Creasman, 1986). Women with lichen sclerosus may have deficient 5α-reductase activity in the perineal skin, thus limiting tissue conversion of testosterone to dihydrotestosterone (DHT). In affected women, serum testosterone and androstenedione concentrations are elevated and serum DHT is lower than normal.

In women with vulvar disease, topical application of testosterone may induce further enzyme activity, normalizing DHT formation and producing clinical improvement (Friedrich and Kalra, 1984; Ayhan et al, 1989). Treatment with testosterone ointment alleviates pruritus and normalizes the gross and histologic appearance of the skin. (A 2% ointment may be compounded by mixing 30 ml of testosterone propionate [100 mg/ml] with 120 g of petrolatum.) Corticosteroid cream may be used concurrently for prompt relief of pruritus but should not be employed for long periods (Friedrich, 1976). The condition eventually reappears after cessation of treatment.

The classification and treatment of lichen sclerosus and other vulvar dystrophies has been reviewed (*Int J Gynecol Obstet*, 1991).

UTERINE LEIOMYOMAS (FIBROIDS). These benign tumors occur most commonly in women in the late reproductive years but may occur earlier, especially in African American women. They can be asymptomatic or cause menorrhagia, pain, infertility, or inability to support a pregnancy. Leiomyomas are a common indication for hysterectomy. Although surgery is the only curative treatment, drug therapy can suppress tumor size and growth at least temporarily. In many cases, no treatment is required or is needed only to control bleeding patterns.

Several GnRH analogues (eg, leuprolide, nafarelin, histrelin, goserelin, the investigational agents buserelin and triptorelin) have been used to treat this condition. The analogues have been administered daily by subcutaneous injection or intranasally, as well as monthly in a subcutaneous depot preparation (Lemay, 1987). These agents induce down-regulation of pituitary gonadotropin receptors and suppress gonadotropin secretion and ovarian estradiol secretion. The growth of uterine leiomyomas is estrogen-dependent, and uterine volume has decreased an average of 40% to 50% after three to six months of therapy with a GnRH analogue; tumor volume is reduced somewhat less (Friedman et al, 1990). Most of the shrinkage occurs within the first three months. Tumors regress if estrogen is suppressed to the low follicular phase range. When the drug is withdrawn, estrogen secretion resumes and tumor regrowth occurs. The regrowth may be rapid, at least partly because treatment with a GnRH analogue is associated with an increase in the number of estrogen receptors in tumor tissue (Rein et al, 1990). However, longer suppression of tumor regrowth appears to occur with estrogen suppression into the postmenopausal period (Coddington et al, 1986; West et al, 1987; Andreyko et al, 1988). Severe vaginal bleeding rarely is associated with involution of submucosal fibroids (Friedman, 1989).

Treatment of leiomyomas with GnRH agonists is a promising means of reducing tumor size temporarily (eg, prior to surgery, perimenopause), facilitating surgery and possibly allowing a vaginal rather than an abdominal hysterectomy. The amenorrhea induced by GnRH agonists also may correct anemia resulting from tumor-induced bleeding. Large tumors appear to be most responsive to treatment (Vollenhoven et al, 1990 A).

Treatment with GnRH agonists is not suitable for long-term therapy because of the risks associated with a hypoestrogenic state (eg, osteoporosis, cardiovascular disease). Concomitant administration of MPA relieved menopausal symptoms associated with therapy but also impeded the tumor-shrinking activity of leuprolide (Friedman et al, 1988). An estrogen-progestin replacement regimen that is sufficient to prevent hypoestrogenism but insufficient to support tumor growth should be possible. Further clinical experience is necessary to determine appropriate regimens that would allow safe, long-term medical treatment of leiomyomas (Friedman et al, 1990). See also reviews by Vollenhoven et al, 1990 B, and Adamson, 1992.

MENOPAUSE. The menopause is often accompanied by vasomotor symptoms (ie, hot flushes, sweating). Subjective complaints are associated with decreased skin resistance and core temperature, increased skin temperature, perspiration on the upper part of the body, and increased pulse rate. Although the onset of flushing occurs just prior to pulsatile secretion of ACTH, LH, and growth hormone from the pituitary, these secretions are not causative (Meldrum et al, 1984; Tulandi and Lal, 1985); flushes also occur in women who have undergone hypophysectomy and withdrawal from estrogen therapy. Both flushes and pulsatile pituitary secretion are probably due to release of hypothalamic neurotransmitters.

Evidence suggests that decreased endogenous opioids in the hypothalamus and brain stem may trigger increased noradrenergic activity that in turn stimulates neurons involved in thermoregulation and production of releasing hormone (Casper and Yen, 1985). The hypothalamic thermoregulatory set point is lowered, resulting in increased peripheral blood flow and sweating, which facilitate heat loss. Transient changes in plasma catecholamines (increased epinephrine, decreased norepinephrine) have been observed within minutes after a flush and are consistent with increased heart rate and finger blood flow (Kronenberg et al, 1984). Objectively measured hot flushes correlate with waking episodes during sleep, which suggests that menopausal flushes are associated with chronic sleep disturbances. Both the number of flushes and nocturnal waking episodes decrease with estrogen therapy (Erlik et al, 1981).

Manifestations of vaginal and urethral atrophy (eg, vaginitis, dyspareunia, urinary frequency) may occur after menopause and usually respond to estrogen therapy, which may be administered in a topical preparation. The presence of estrogen receptors in the lower urinary tract supports the use of estrogens to treat urinary stress incontinence in postmenopausal women (Iosif et al, 1981). However, larger doses of estrogen may be required than for atrophic indications, and concomitant use of a progestin may attenuate the beneficial effect by decreasing urethral pressure (Miodrag et al, 1988). Changes in vaginal physiology at menopause (ie, increased pH; decreased blood flow, fluid, transvaginal potential difference) also are reversed by estrogen therapy (Semmens and Wagner, 1982).

Emotional complaints (eg, irritability, anxiety, depression), fatigue, and headache sometimes occur and may be secondary to other, particularly vasomotor, disturbances. However, significant improvement in memory and reduction of anxiety have been observed after estrogen therapy in women who did not report vasomotor flushing (Campbell, 1976).

Aging is accompanied by loss of elasticity and wrinkling of the skin. Although a cosmetic benefit from estrogen replacement therapy has not been demonstrated clearly, some observations are of interest. Estrogen receptors in skin increase in number when oophorectomized women are given estrogen. Estrogen reportedly helped to maintain epidermal thickness (Nichols et al, 1984), and postmenopausal women with implants of estrogen and testosterone had higher skin collagen content than untreated women (Brincat et al, 1985).

When estrogen is contraindicated, alternative agents may relieve some menopausal symptoms. However, they are less effective or have unpleasant side effects at effective doses. Progestins, clonidine (available in both tablet and transdermal patch form), or methyldopa [Aldomet] may be tried for vasomotor symptoms. In a placebo-controlled, double-blind, crossover study, MPA 20 mg daily relieved hot flushes and reduced the amplitude and frequency of LH pulses (Albrecht et al, 1981). In addition to relieving vasomotor symptoms, MPA may retard bone resorption (Lobo et al, 1984). Although effectiveness in clinical trials has not been universal, the preponderance of studies has shown that clonidine reduces the number of flushes by at least 50% (Hammar and Berg, 1985). A transdermal preparation may relieve hot flushes at a lower dose than the oral preparation (Nagamani et al, 1987). In another double-blind, placebo-controlled study, propranolol [Inderal] reduced the frequency and severity of vasomotor symptoms (Alcoff et al, 1981). Water-based lubricants may be tried for relief of dyspareunia but are generally not effective. Therapeutic options that do not employ estrogen for treatment of menopausal symptoms have been reviewed (Young et al, 1990).

For further discussion of the menopause, choice of agents and regimen, and the management of related problems, see American College of Obstetricians and Gynecologists, 1992; Grady et al, 1992; American College of Physicians, 1992.

Preparations for Menopausal Estrogen Replacement Therapy: Conjugated estrogens are most commonly used to treat menopausal symptoms in the United States. Other natural and synthetic oral preparations, as well as a transdermal system [Estraderm] that releases estradiol at a constant rate, also are effective.

Currently, the focus is on identifying and developing preparations, routes of administration, and regimens that will, in addition to relieving menopausal symptoms, protect the endometrium and bone; decrease cardiovascular morbidity (including exerting a beneficial effect on serum lipids); and prevent withdrawal bleeding, which may decrease compliance in some patients. An ideal regimen that would provide all the above benefits has not yet been identified, and all benefits may not be achievable by a single regimen. For example, a regimen that most effectively protects bone or inhibits renin substrate production may not exert the most favorable effects on serum lipids and the cardiovascular system.

Effectiveness and side effects may be influenced by the route of administration, pattern of delivery (cyclic or continuous), and dosage, as well as by the inherent properties of the compound or preparation. For example, the hepatic circulation has greater exposure to hormone absorbed orally; thus, the metabolic effects with this route may differ from those exerted with parenteral administration. Relatively more estradiol is converted to estrone when estradiol is given by the oral compared with the parenteral route (Nichols et al, 1984).

Initially, vaginal estrogen preparations are readily absorbed and produce higher blood levels than the same quantity given orally; however, absorption declines when the epithelium becomes cornified. Vaginal preparations are effective for systemic as well as local symptoms. If symptoms of atrophic urogenital changes are the only indication for postmenopausal estrogen therapy, intermittent courses of estrogen in low doses administered intravaginally may be appropriate.

The transdermal preparation [Estraderm] is as effective as conjugated estrogens in relieving hot flushes and other menopausal symptoms (Place et al, 1985). Equivalent doses are conjugated estrogens 0.625 and 1.25 mg and transdermal estradiol 50 and 100 mcg, respectively (Chetkowski et al, 1986). Transdermal estradiol results in a more physiologic hormonal profile as evidenced by the continuous low-level release of estradiol and a normal serum estradiol:estrone ratio rather than the elevated serum estrone level observed with oral estrogen (Powers et al, 1985). This route avoids the first-pass hepatic effect of oral preparations; specifically, no increase in SHBG or other binding globulins or renin substrate occurs with the transdermal patch as it does with oral estrogen. The reduced effect on hepatic metabolism probably also would be reflected by no increased risk of gallbladder disease with the transdermal preparation, although no data are available at present to support this assumption. The beneficial effects on lipoproteins (ie, decreased LDL, increased HDL) observed with oral estrogen are reduced by 50% or more with nonoral preparations. However, the cardioprotective effects of estrogen may be mediated in part by other mechanisms. All of the epidemiologic evidence regarding the cardiovascular benefit of estrogens is derived from use of oral preparations. Widespread use of the transdermal patch is too recent for accrual of enough data to establish clinical endpoints. Bone loss is prevented equally well with use of the oral or transdermal preparation (Stevenson et al, 1990; Ribot et al, 1990). Neither the oral nor the transdermal preparation has elevated clotting factors. With the transdermal estrogen patch, an oral progestin would be taken by women with an intact uterus. Transdermal systems containing estradiol and progesterone are available in Europe.

About 17% of women have skin reactions to the patch; this necessitates discontinuation in 2% of users (the percentage may be higher in very warm climates) (DeLignieres et al, 1986; Chetkowski et al, 1986; Judd, 1987; Utian, 1987; Stanczyk et al, 1988).

In summary, the transdermal patch appears to have advantages and disadvantages compared with oral therapy. Therefore, until further data are available, the choice of preparation may be determined by patient characteristics, preference, and probable compliance with a particular regimen. (See also review on transdermal estrogen by Miller-Bass and Adashi, 1990.)

With injection of long-acting preparations, exposure to the hormone is uninterrupted; injections also are inconvenient and usually expensive. Absorption is inconsistent and blood levels of estrogen are variable. If these preparations are used when the uterus is in place, the addition of a progestin significantly decreases the excess risk of hyperplasia and endometrial cancer. Complete protection of the endometrium under conditions of steady estrogen levels may require progestin therapy for one-half of each month (Gambrell, 1989).

The sublingual and intranasal routes for estrogen delivery are being investigated. Subcutaneous implants provide relatively steady plasma estrogen levels and may be useful after surgical menopause. However, they are difficult to remove if adverse reactions occur. Vaginal rings have similar advantages but are easily removable.

Certain risks, including endometrial cancer (see the section on Metabolic Effects, Adverse Reactions, and Precautions), must be considered in patients receiving estrogen therapy by any route. These women should be re-evaluated at 6- to 12-month intervals to monitor status. Blood pressure, breast, and pelvic examinations should be included. Endometrial biopsy or another method of endometrial sampling should be performed if there is abnormal bleeding and annually if an estrogen alone is administered or if there are other risk factors for endometrial cancer (American College of Obstetricians and Gynecologists, 1992). Papanicolaou smears should include material from the endocervical canal. Any episode of abnormal bleeding should be investigated promptly and thoroughly. If the patient is on a continuous regimen of estrogen and progestin, bleeding that occurs later than the first six months of therapy should be investigated.

The results of dilatation and curettage and vaginal ultrasound were compared in a study of postmenopausal women undergoing diagnostic tests for bleeding. Endometrial tissue $\leq$4 mm (Varner et al, 1991) or 5 mm thick (Nasri et al, 1991; Granberg et al, 1991), as measured by ultrasound, was atrophic, and thicker tissue usually was associated with abnormal histology. Some practioners advocate using transvaginal ultrasound measurement of the endometrium to screen for abnormality, reserving endometrial sampling for patients whose endometrium is thicker than 4 to 5 mm.

Regimens for Menopausal Estrogen Replacement Therapy: Several regimens may be used for hormonal replacement therapy. Those employed when the uterus is intact include (1) cyclic administration of estrogen and a progestin; (2) continuous estrogen and cyclic progestin; and (3) continuous combined estrogen and progestin.

With the cyclic estrogen plus progestin regimen, estrogen is administered daily for 25 days when given orally or twice weekly when transdermal patches are used and a progestin (usually MPA 5 to 10 mg) is administered daily for the last 10 to 13 days of each estrogen cycle to promote maturation of the endometrium and inhibit hyperplastic changes. This regimen is followed by five or six days with no hormonal therapy during which withdrawal bleeding occurs. The hormonal regimen then is resumed whether or not bleeding has ceased. For convenience, each cycle of therapy can be initiated on the first of the month.

In the continuous estrogen and cyclic progestin regimen, oral estrogen is given daily or transdermal patches are applied twice weekly; a progestin (eg, MPA 5 to 10 mg) (Whitehead et al, 1990; Notelovitz, 1989) or MPA 2.5 mg (Lobo, 1992) is added for the first 10 to 13 days of each month. In one study, adequate endometrial secretory transformation was ascertained by endometrial biopsy and was correlated with bleeding on or after day 11 following the start of progestin in the cycle (Padwick et al, 1986).

With continuous combination regimens, both the estrogen and progestin components (eg, conjugated estrogens 0.625 mg plus MPA 2.5 or 5 mg given daily) are administered continuously. Irregular bleeding frequently is a problem, but this decreases in time and amenorrhea is common after six months to a year. Generally, the endometrium is atrophic or exhibits little estrogenic stimulation, even in women who have bleeding episodes. Larger doses of progestin are required to produce a secretory endometrium than to suppress mitotic activity (Gibbons et al, 1986), and it has been suggested that the latter effect is adequate to prevent endometrial hyperplasia while reducing the likelihood of bleeding (Lobo, 1992). The blood lipid profile usually was favorable but may be less so than with sequential therapy (see below) (Prough et al, 1987; Luciano et al, 1988; Notelovitz, 1989; Whitehead et al, 1990; Kable et al, 1990; Weinstein et al, 1990; Yancey et al, 1990). In a pilot study, another regimen (conjugated estrogens 0.625 mg plus MPA 2.5 mg given five days per week) was used to reduce breast tenderness and fluid retention that sometimes occurs with continuous estrogen therapy (Mishell et al, 1991).

In women with no uterus, estrogen is given continuously without a progestin.

A progestin challenge test has been suggested to reduce the risk of endometrial carcinoma in estrogen-treated women and postmenopausal women with high endogenous levels of estrogen (eg, obesity). The test consists of administering a progestin (eg, MPA 10 mg, norethindrone acetate 5 mg) for 10 to 13 days each month as long as withdrawal bleeding occurs. The procedure may be repeated annually after negative results are obtained (Gambrell et al, 1980). Careful monitoring is always required, and abnormal bleeding requires investigation of endometrial status.

In summary, the goal of menopausal estrogen therapy is to relieve specific symptoms and have a favorable effect on other systems (eg, bone, cardiovascular) with the lowest effective dosage. Not all target organs are restored to the normal premenopausal condition, but most symptoms can be controlled by conjugated estrogens 0.625 mg or the equivalent dose of other estrogens given daily and cyclically or continuously. Bone loss and fractures also are prevented by this amount of conjugated estrogens (Hammond, 1984; Lindsay et al, 1984). Eventually, medication may be withdrawn if desired; however, current medical opinion is shifting in favor of prolonged postmenopausal estrogen therapy in the absence of contraindications. When replacement therapy is to be withdrawn, vasomotor symptoms usually diminish when the dose is reduced gradually.

If long-term estrogen therapy is considered in postmenopausal women, the expected benefits must outweigh the risks, and the patient should understand the factors involved and participate in the decision. In one study, an overall decrease in mortality among women who received estrogen replacement therapy was observed, and current users realized greater benefit than past users (Henderson et al, 1991). Initiating therapy in women who are 15 or more years postmenopausal and who have never received estrogen replacement therapy is receiving more support because of the likelihood of beneficial effects on bone (Lindsay and Tohme, 1990; Christiansen and Riis, 1990) and the cardiovascular system. For a discussion of the cardiovascular effects of estrogen replacement therapy, see the section on Metabolic Effects, Adverse Reactions, and Precautions below.

OSTEOPOROSIS. This disorder occurs frequently after menopause and is a more serious problem in women who have earlier loss of ovarian function (eg, surgical menopause, gonadal dysgenesis). Hormone therapy prevents bone loss that occurs after natural or surgical menopause. The most effective use of estrogen in the prevention of osteoporosis is initiation of treatment before significant bone loss has occurred; administration must be continued to maintain the effect. Because of the serious consequences of osteoporosis, long-term estrogen therapy should be considered for high-risk or symptomatic women, for those who have undergone early removal of ovaries (in whom the possibility of endometrial cancer is obviated), and for patients in whom osteopenia has been confirmed by measurement of bone mineral density.

For a discussion of the pathophysiology and diagnosis of osteoporosis and the role estrogens, progestins, and other agents (eg, calcitonin, etidronate, fluoride, calcium, thiazides) play in the treatment of this disorder, see index entry Osteoporosis, Treatment. See also reviews by Tosteson et al, 1990; Duursma et al, 1991; and Prince at al, 1991.

Metabolic Effects, Adverse Reactions, and Precautions with Use of Estrogens and Progestins

In general, some side effects of estrogen and progestin resemble those of hormonal contraceptives (see index entry

Contraceptives, Oral). The dosages prescribed for replacement therapy, the most common noncontraceptive indication for estrogen and progestin, are considerably smaller than those prescribed for contraception and hence the incidence and intensity of effects are lower.

Nausea or vomiting may occur initially when estrogen is administered but can be minimized by taking the medication with food or at bedtime. This reaction usually disappears with continued administration, even when large doses are used to treat cancer. Fullness or tenderness of breasts and edema caused by sodium and water retention may occur with estrogen treatment; if they occur during replacement therapy, these effects may indicate excessive dosage.

METABOLISM. Estrogen replacement therapy usually does not adversely affect glucose tolerance, and transdermal estradiol appears to enhance insulin clearance (Cagnacci et al, 1992). Effects on serum lipids are variable and may be related to the route of administration as well as the preparation (Fahraeus and Wallentin, 1983). Administration of oral estrogens is associated with decreased levels of low density lipoproteins (LDL) and increased levels of high density lipoproteins (HDL), a lipid profile that is associated with a low incidence of coronary heart disease (Wahl et al, 1983; Nichols et al, 1984). Triglyceride levels may increase 30% or more with estrogen or estrogen plus progestin therapy (Egeland et al, 1990).

Progestins that are derivatives of 19-nortestosterone appear to decrease HDL levels in a dose-dependent relationship (larger doses are associated with lower HDL levels), thus possibly neutralizing the beneficial effect of estrogen. Conversely, a low dosage of an androgenic compound may not have an adverse effect. In one study, a postmenopausal replacement regimen of norgestrel 150 mcg (an androgenic progestin) plus conjugated estrogens 0.625 mg did not adversely affect serum lipids overall, whereas an oral contraceptive preparation containing norgestrel 500 mcg and ethinyl estradiol 50 mcg caused increased levels of LDL and total cholesterol and decreased HDL (La Rosa, 1988). Larger doses of MPA (a derivative of hydroxyprogesterone) were required to decrease HDL, and doses used for sequential menopausal therapy (Tikkanen et al, 1986) or MPA 5 mg in a continuous combined regimen (Yancey et al, 1990) did not appear to have this effect. In another study, decreased HDL concentrations were observed when progestin was given with estrogen for replacement therapy, but the effect was more pronounced with levonorgestrel 250 mcg than with MPA 10 mg (Ottosson et al, 1985). Thus, in these studies the effects of progestins on serum lipoproteins range from decreased HDL with androgenic progestins to a smaller or no change in HDL with progesterone or preparations more closely related to progesterone.

Usual replacement doses of conjugated estrogens exert minimal effects on protein synthesis and elevate CBG, SHBG, and renin substrate levels slightly. In postmenopausal women treated with replacement doses of estrogen, changes in hepatic excretory function result in greater cholesterol saturation in the bile, thus predisposing to gallstone formation. The risk of gallbladder surgery is increased 2.5 times in these women. Use of the transdermal estrogen preparation may avoid this adverse effect on the gallbladder, although data are not available to support this assumption. Estrogens should not be given to patients with severe acute (active) liver disease.

CARDIOVASCULAR EFFECTS. Premenopausal women have a lower incidence of coronary heart disease (CHD) than men of comparable age, but this advantage is lost and the risk of CHD increases after bilateral oophorectomy (Centerwall, 1981; Rosenberg et al, 1981); estrogen therapy eliminates the increased risk. Current use of estrogen replacement therapy has been associated with a decrease in the incidence of CHD and cardiovascular mortality (Stampfer et al, 1991). In a meta-analysis of 31 controlled studies, the risk of CHD with postmenopausal estrogen use generally was reduced; in the two best designs (cohort with internal controls and cross-sectional angiography studies), the risk of CHD was estimated to be about one-half that in nonusers (Stampfer and Colditz, 1991).

Among postmenopausal women undergoing coronary angiography, less coronary occlusion was observed in those who received estrogen replacement therapy (Gruchow et al, 1988; Sullivan et al, 1988). The risk of angiographically diagnosed severe CHD was reduced by 50% (McFarland et al, 1989) and 87% (Hong et al, 1992) in postmenopausal women receiving estrogen therapy. A decrease in death from any cause also has been observed in women who received estrogen replacement therapy (Henderson et al, 1991; Stampfer et al, 1991).

Although there are conflicting reports on whether *replacement dosages* of estrogen increase some clotting factors, the risk of clinical thromboembolism is not increased. The risk also is not affected by a combined estrogen-progestin regimen (Notelovitz et al, 1983). Nevertheless, estrogens usually are not administered to menopausal patients with thromboembolic disease or a past history of such disease because these patients are presumably at higher risk. (However, some patients may prefer to assume the risk.) The likelihood of thromboembolic phenomena has been reported to be increased when *pharmacologic doses* of estrogen are used to treat breast or prostatic cancer. Administration of estrogen to suppress postpartum lactation also is associated with a higher incidence of thromboembolism, and this use is no longer recommended (see the section on Indications).

Postmenopausal estrogen therapy is associated with an increase in serum HDL, a change that is consistent with the apparent cardioprotective benefit observed in the above studies (Krauss et al, 1988; Ross et al, 1989). Other cardioprotective benefits of estrogen may be due to its direct effect on the arterial wall or its indirect effects through chemical mediators. Estrogen increases production of prostacyclin, which causes vasodilation, decreases platelet adhesiveness, and decreases production of thromboxane A_2, which has actions that oppose those of prostacyclin (Ylikorkala et al, 1987).

Although the incidence of hypertension generally is not increased, this may occur rarely in sensitive individuals. If hypertension develops or worsens with estrogen therapy, the medication should be discontinued. Results of studies on stroke have not been entirely consistent. The risk of stroke was not elevated in some studies (Judd et al, 1983; Stampfer et al, 1991), while in others the risk of stroke (Finucane et al, 1993) or death due to stroke was reduced (Paganini-Hill et al, 1988; Finucane et al, 1993) in postmenopausal women given estrogen replacement therapy.

In summary, most studies support a favorable role for postmenopausal estrogen replacement in preventing cardiovascular disease and death. The administration of excessive doses of progestins may offset these benefits to some degree.

Mortality from myocardial infarction (MI) was increased in men with a history of MI who were treated with conjugated estrogens 5 mg daily. Cardiovascular deaths also increased in men receiving DES 5 mg daily for prostatic carcinoma but not in those receiving lower dosages. It should be noted that these doses are much higher than those currently used for replacement therapy, treatment was studied in men, and these men had previously documented arteriosclerotic disease. Therefore, these data do not provide an appropriate standard for determination of possible beneficial effects in postmenopausal women.

Estrogens should be administered with caution to patients with migraine and discontinued if attacks increase in number or become more severe.

TERATOGENICITY. Most teratogenic effects of progestins have been observed with agents having high androgenic potency, some of which are no longer marketed. Two studies of progestin (most commonly MPA, which is not androgenic) use during the first trimester of pregnancy showed no increased risk of teratogenicity (Katz et al, 1985; Yovich et al, 1988). However, because of the teratogenic potential, synthetic progestins should not be administered during pregnancy.

Although congenital malformations have occurred rarely with use of 21-carbon compounds (ie, hydroxyprogesterone caproate, progesterone), the incidence is no greater than from chance (Resseguie et al, 1985). It is believed that these agents are safe for specific appropriate indications during pregnancy, including prevention of premature birth (hydroxyprogesterone caproate) and treatment of luteal phase dysfunction (progesterone). See also the section on Indications and index entries Infertility, Etiology and Treatment in Women; Contraceptives.

DES Daughters: The administration of any estrogen is contraindicated during pregnancy. The use of synthetic hormones (estrogens and progestins) to treat threatened abortion is ineffective and carries the risk of teratogenicity. Administration of DES (or other chemically related, nonsteroidal synthetic estrogens, such as dienestrol) for this indication is associated with reproductive tract anomalies, including vaginal adenosis in more than one-third and cervical ectropion in two-thirds of affected patients; rarely, vaginal clear cell carcinoma (adenocarcinoma) has occurred in female offspring and reproductive tract abnormalities in male offspring. In the United States, use of DES during pregnancy probably has ceased.

Young women whose mothers received DES during pregnancy should be examined yearly for early detection of abnormalities. Management of adenosis is conservative; no treatment is generally given, but regular examinations are continued. Recommendations for the identification and management of exposed individuals (male and female) can be found in the 1985 DES Task Force Report (available by contacting DES, Office of Cancer Communication, Building 31, National Cancer Institute, Bethesda, MD 20892; telephone [800]4-CANCER [*JAMA,* 1986]).

Vaginal adenosis and other structural abnormalities may decline or disappear with time (Robboy et al, 1979; Antonioli et al, 1980; Jefferies et al, 1984). This may be due to continuing metaplasia at the junction. The extent of the teratogenic effect is related to the time at which DES was given to the mother: Effects are most severe when the drug was given during embryonal development of müllerian structures. Structural abnormalities (eg, cockscomb, collar, pseudopolyp, hypoplastic cervix) occurred most often when exposure was between weeks 13 to 22 (Jefferies et al, 1984). Steroidal estrogens apparently do not have this effect (Johnson et al, 1979 B). The incidence of urinary tract anomalies is not increased in DES-exposed daughters.

Vaginal adenocarcinoma occurs in 0.1% of exposed female offspring by age 34. Diagnosis was made between the ages of 15 and 27 years in 91% of patients in the Registry for Research on Hormonal Transplacental Carcinogenesis of the University of Chicago (Melnick et al, 1987). This pattern of incidence is temporally related to the declining incidence of abnormally located vaginal tissue with age. Although malignant transformation of vaginal adenosis is thought to be rare, several possible cases have been reported in DES-exposed patients. These patients had been free of malignancy at initial evaluation 1.5 to almost 8 years previously (Veridiano et al, 1981; Kramer et al, 1987). It is not known whether DES-exposed females will be at higher risk for adenocarcinoma later in life when this form of cancer is known to appear most commonly. Risk factors for development of clear cell adenocarcinoma in DES daughters include administration of DES to the mother before the twelfth week of pregnancy and birth of the daughter in the fall (Herbst et al, 1986).

Structural and functional abnormalities of the female reproductive tract also result from in utero exposure to DES. Two-thirds to three-fourths of exposed patients had reproductive tract anomalies demonstrable by hysterosalpingogram. Functional abnormalities include an increased incidence of infertility and early and late complications of pregnancy (Linn et al, 1988). In one study, 36% of DES daughters were unable to conceive for one year or more, but this was unrelated to an abnormal hysterosalpingogram per se. Specific defects (ie, upper uterus constriction, T-shaped uterus) were associated with an approximate doubling of the incidence of infertility (Kaufman et al, 1986). DES daughters displayed a hyperreactive immune response in another study, and the investigators speculated that this may be partly responsible for infertility by an immune mechanism (eg, production of antibodies against sperm or zona pellucida, rejection of the antigenically foreign fetus) (Ways et al, 1987). The incidence of ectopic pregnancy, spontaneous abortion (first and second trimester), incompetent cervix, prematurity, and perinatal deaths also is increased. However, approximately 80% of

DES-exposed daughters who desire children eventually have a live birth (Barnes et al, 1980; Berger and Goldstein, 1980; Herbst et al, 1980).

DES Sons: The reproductive tracts of male offspring exposed to DES were reported to be affected in some studies (Gill et al, 1979; Whitehead and Leiter, 1981). In the latter study, only one-third of DES-exposed patients had normal semen. In general, there was a higher than normal incidence of testicular hypoplasia (often including a history of cryptorchidism), varicocele, and epididymal cyst. DES exposure in males may explain reproductive abnormalities, including infertility. There appears to be no associated risk of cancer (except, possibly, that secondary to cryptorchidism), although testicular cancer has been reported. In contrast to the above reports, one cohort study found no increased risk of urogenital abnormalities in DES-exposed males (Leary et al, 1984).

DES Mothers: The possibility that women who took DES during pregnancy (ie, DES mothers) may have suffered adverse effects has been considered. The risk of developing breast cancer 20 years or more after exposure was increased slightly (relative risk 1.5) (Greenberg et al, 1984), although this may not be a causal relationship. The results of this study of over 3,000 exposed women with more than 85,000 woman-years of follow-up in both exposed and unexposed groups differ from the negative or equivocal results of earlier, smaller studies (Bibbo et al, 1978; Brian et al, 1980). A British study reported no increased risk of breast cancer in 650 DES mothers (Vessey et al, 1983).

CARCINOGENICITY. Women should be examined for breast and genital carcinoma before estrogen therapy is instituted and periodically during administration. Therapy should be withdrawn if estrogen-dependent carcinoma is found or suspected. Most available evidence indicates that menopausal estrogen therapy does not increase the risk of breast cancer (Kaufman et al, 1984; Buring et al, 1987; Wingo et al, 1987; Dupont and Page, 1991). Results of one study showed that there was no overall increased risk of breast cancer associated with past use of replacement estrogen, but the risk was increased slightly in current users (Colditz et al, 1990). Other studies showed no increased risk with current or short-term use but reported an increased risk after five years (Steinberg et al, 1991) or could not rule out additional risk after 15 years of use (Palmer et al, 1991). A meta-analysis of 37 studies showed a slight but statistically significant increase in relative risk for breast cancer (RR = 1.06 overall; RR = 1.3 for natural menopause) associated with postmenopausal hormone replacement therapy (Sillero-Arenas et al, 1992). Greater caution is advised in women with a strong family history or in those who are otherwise at increased risk of the disease.

The possibility that a progestin added to estrogen provides protection against breast cancer was suggested in a study of postmenopausal women in which the incidence of breast cancer was lower in women given a combined regimen than in those receiving estrogen alone (Gambrell, 1986). However, experts feel that there is insufficient evidence to support this claim.

Unopposed estrogen therapy increases the risk of endometrial carcinoma in postmenopausal women. Generally the risk increases with increasing dosage and duration of use and is higher in women who did *not* have conditions previously associated with a higher risk of endometrial cancer (eg, obesity, diabetes, hypertension). The relative risk varied from 4 to 15 times (Stavraky et al, 1981; see references in Hulka, 1980). Endometrial cancer associated with estrogen therapy is usually an early-stage malignancy. The latent period between estrogen administration and development of cancer is relatively short (three to six years), and the risk of cancer is reduced after an estrogen-free interval of two years (Hulka et al, 1980). However, in other studies, the increased risk was reported to persist for at least several years after withdrawal of therapy (Shapiro et al, 1985; Buring et al, 1986). These observations are consistent with the hypothesis that estrogen acts as a tumor promoter rather than as a carcinogen in endometrial carcinoma. However, resolution of this point would not necessarily assist in making therapeutic decisions about estrogen usage.

Addition of a progestin to a cyclic estrogen treatment program or a continuous regimen of daily estrogen and progestin reduces the risk of hyperplasia and endometrial carcinoma to below the rate observed with estrogen only (see the discussion on Menopause and review on endometrial effects of hormones by Creasy et al, 1992).

DRUG INTERACTIONS. Estrogens and progestins presumably have drug interactions that are qualitatively similar to those observed with OCs (see index entry Contraceptives, Oral). However, at the low dosages used for replacement therapy, therapeutic effectiveness might be compromised more easily by drugs that increase metabolism (eg, anticonvulsants, barbiturates, rifampin [Rifadin, Rimactane]) or decrease enterohepatic circulation of hormones (eg, certain antibiotics).

Drug Evaluations

ESTROGENS

Steroidal Estrogens

ESTRADIOL

[Estrace, Estraderm]

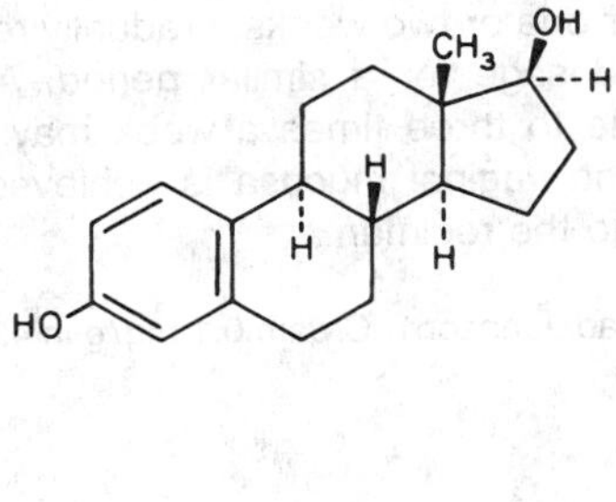

ESTRADIOL BENZOATE

ESTRADIOL CYPIONATE
[Depo-Estradiol]

ESTRADIOL VALERATE
[Delestrogen]

Estradiol is the principal and most biologically potent ovarian estrogen. It is usually injected intramuscularly as esters in oil or aqueous suspension. The onset of action is gradual and the duration is variable (three or four days to three or four weeks).

Oral therapy is generally ineffective because of poor absorption. However, the oral micronized form [Estrace] is effective because the reduced particle size increases surface area, dissolution, and rate of absorption. Orally administered estradiol is metabolized mainly to estrone and its conjugates. A transdermal skin patch also is available.

See the Introduction for specific indications and adverse reactions and information on choice of route of administration. Estrogens used for replacement therapy are frequently given with a progestin.

DOSAGE AND PREPARATIONS.

Intramuscular: For replacement therapy, (estradiol benzoate) 0.5 to 1.5 mg two or three times weekly; (estradiol cypionate) 1 to 5 mg every three to four weeks; (estradiol valerate) 10 to 20 mg every four weeks.

ESTRADIOL BENZOATE:

Generic. Powder 1 and 5 g.

ESTRADIOL CYPIONATE:

Generic. Solution 5 mg/ml (in oil) in 10 ml containers.

Depo-Estradiol (Upjohn). Solution (sterile, in cottonseed oil) 1 mg/ml in 10 ml containers and 5 mg/ml in 5 ml containers.

Additional Trademark.

E-Cypionate (Legere).

ESTRADIOL VALERATE:

Generic. Solution (in oil) 10, 20, and 40 mg/ml in 10 ml containers.

Delestrogen (Mead Johnson). Solution (in sesame oil) 10 mg/ml in 5 ml containers; solution (in castor oil) 20 and 40 mg/ml in 5 ml containers and 20 mg/ml in 1 ml (unit-dose) containers.

Additional Trademarks.

Gynogen L.A. (Forest), ***Menaval*** (Legere).

Oral: For menopausal symptoms, 1 to 2 mg daily for three weeks, then one week without medication; a progestin may be added the last 12 or 13 days. Alternative regimens include the same dose of estrogen given continuously with the addition of a progestin for 12 or 13 days per month or continuously.

ESTRADIOL:

Estrace (Mead Johnson). Tablets (micronized) 1 and 2 mg.

Topical (vaginal): For atrophic vaginitis or kraurosis vulvae, 2 to 4 g daily for one or two weeks, gradually reduced to one-half the initial dosage for a similar period. A maintenance dose of 1 g one to three times a week may be used after restoration of the vaginal mucosa is achieved. A progestin may be added to the regimen.

ESTRADIOL:

Estrace (Mead Johnson). Cream 0.1 mg/g in 42.5 g containers.

Transdermal: For estrogen replacement therapy or menopausal symptoms, a 0.05 or 0.1 mg system is applied to a clean, dry site on the trunk of the body twice weekly to supply medication continuously. The upper portion of the buttocks is preferred and the specific site should be rotated, with an interval of at least one week between applications at a particular site. The patch should not be placed on the breasts, the waistline, or other area subject to rubbing or chafing. A progestin may be added the last 12 or 13 days or taken continuously if the patient has an intact uterus.

ESTRADIOL:

Estraderm (CIBA). Transdermal system 0.05 and 0.1 mg.

ESTRONE

CH_3 O H H H HO

ESTROPIPATE (Piperazine Estrone Sulfate)
[Ogen]

Estrone is an ovarian estrogenic hormone available for oral, vaginal, or intramuscular administration. See the Introduction for specific indications and adverse reactions. Estrogens used for replacement therapy are frequently given with a progestin.

DOSAGE AND PREPARATIONS.

ESTRONE:

Intramuscular: For menopausal symptoms, 0.1 to 2 mg weekly in single or divided doses.

Generic. Suspension (aqueous) 2 mg/ml in 10 and 30 ml containers and 5 mg/ml in 10 ml containers.

ESTROPIPATE:

Oral: For replacement therapy, 0.75 to 1.5 mg daily, cyclically or continuously; a progestin may be added for the last 10 to 13 days or continuously (see also the section on Indications).

Generic. Tablets 1.5 and 3 mg (equivalent to sodium estrone sulfate activity 1.25 and 2.5 mg, respectively).

Ogen (Abbott). Tablets 0.75, 1.5, 3, and 6 mg (equivalent to sodium estrone sulfate activity 0.625, 1.25, 2.5, and 5 mg, respectively).

Topical (vaginal): For atrophic vaginitis or kraurosis vulvae, 2 to 4 g daily and cyclically, depending on the severity of the condition.

Ogen (Abbott). Cream 1.5 mg/g in 42.5 g containers.

CONJUGATED ESTROGENS, U.S.P.
[Premarin]

This is a combination of the sodium salts of the sulfate esters of estrogenic substances, principally estrone and equilin; the esters are similar to the type excreted by pregnant mares. The various preparations contain 50% to 65% estrone sodium sulfate and 20% to 35% equilin sodium sulfate. They are effective orally, parenterally, and vaginally. There is disagreement on whether the parenteral preparation controls spontaneous capillary bleeding rapidly and reduces capillary bleeding during surgery.

Because there have been problems with bioequivalence of generic preparations, new manufacturing specifications to ensure conformity of generic products to Premarin are being developed.

See the Introduction for specific indications and adverse reactions. Estrogens used for replacement therapy are frequently given with a progestin.

DOSAGE AND PREPARATIONS.
Oral: For menopausal symptoms, 0.3 to 1.25 mg daily, cyclically or continuously; a progestin may be added for 10 to 13 days per month or continuously in women with an intact uterus. (See also the section on Indications.)

For replacement therapy in hypogonadism, 0.625 to 1.25 mg daily or a regimen similar to one of the above.

For dysfunctional uterine bleeding due to atrophic endometrium, 5 mg daily in divided doses for one week with a progestin (eg, MPA 10 mg) added to the regimen the last five days; alternatively, 2.5 to 3.75 mg plus MPA 10 mg daily for seven to ten days. See also the section on Indications.

For breast carcinoma, see index entry Estrogens, Conjugated, In Cancer.

Premarin (Wyeth-Ayerst). Tablets 0.3, 0.625, 0.9, 1.25, and 2.5 mg.

Intravenous: For emergency treatment of dysfunctional uterine bleeding when there is a denuded endometrium, 25 mg initially every four hours for three doses; oral treatment with an estrogen-progestin combination is then initiated. See also the section on Indications.

Premarin (Wyeth-Ayerst). Powder (sterile, lyophilized) 25 mg with 5 ml of diluent.

Vaginal: For atrophic vaginitis or kraurosis vulvae, 2 to 4 g daily intravaginally or topically cyclically, depending on the severity of the condition.

Premarin (Wyeth-Ayerst). Cream 0.625 mg/g in 42.5 g containers.

ESTERIFIED ESTROGENS, U.S.P.
[Estratab, Menest]

This is a combination of the sodium salts of the sulfate esters of estrogenic substances, principally estrone; the esters are similar to the type excreted by pregnant mares. Preparations of esterified estrogens contain 75% to 85% sodium estrone sulfate and 6% to 15% sodium equilin sulfate, in such proportion that the total of these two components is not less than 90%. Serum levels of estrone and estradiol are similar after administration of esterified estrogens and conjugated estrogens (Jurgens et al, 1992).

See the Introduction for indications and adverse reactions.
DOSAGE AND PREPARATIONS. For dosage, see the evaluation on Conjugated Estrogens.

Estratab (Solvay), ***Menest*** (SmithKline Beecham). Tablets 0.3, 0.625, 1.25, and 2.5 mg.

ETHINYL ESTRADIOL
[Estinyl]

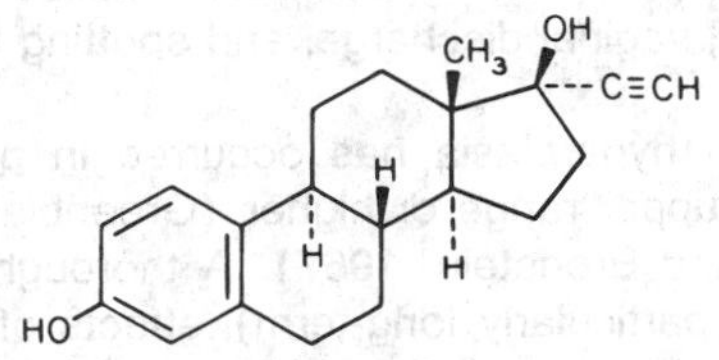

CH_3 OH ---C≡CH H H H HO

This potent, orally effective steroid is related to estradiol, the principal ovarian estrogen. It is used alone and as a component of some estrogen/progestin oral contraceptives (see index entry Contraceptives, Oral). Evidence suggests that ethinyl estradiol 5 mcg may be equivalent to conjugated estrogens 0.625 mg for menopausal replacement therapy, particularly with respect to effects on bone and vaginal epithelium (Mandel et al, 1982). However, this amount is less than that supplied by available preparations.

See the Introduction for specific indications and adverse reactions.

DOSAGE AND PREPARATIONS.
Oral: For menopausal symptoms, 0.02 to 0.05 mg daily or every other day, cyclically or continuously; a progestin may be added for 10 to 13 days per month or continuously in women with an intact uterus (see also the section on Indications).

For dysfunctional uterine bleeding, 0.05 to 0.1 mg given with a progestin for 10 to 13 days (see the section on Indications).

For breast carcinoma, see index entry Ethinyl Estradiol, In Cancer.

Estinyl (Schering). Tablets 0.02, 0.05, and 0.5 mg.

QUINESTROL
[Estrovis]

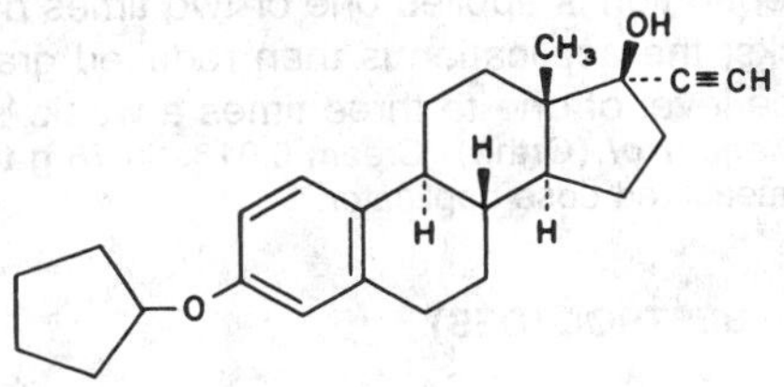

CH_3 OH ---C≡CH H H H O

Quinestrol is the 3-cyclopentyl ether of ethinyl estradiol. After gastrointestinal absorption, it is stored in adipose tissue, released slowly, and metabolized principally to the parent compound. Because of this property, an effective drug level is maintained with once weekly administration after an initial priming regimen.

In one multicenter, double-blind, controlled study, quinestrol was superior to placebo and equivalent to conjugated estrogens in relieving vasomotor flushes in menopausal women (Baumgardner et al, 1978). There is concern because of the depot nature of the drug; the patient is potentially exposed to constant estrogenic stimulation, although hormonal levels are variable. Therefore, the risk of endometrial hyperstimulation may be increased. There are no data on the effect of concurrent progestin therapy with this agent.

ADVERSE REACTIONS. In general, side effects occur infrequently and are similar to those observed with other estrogens. Nausea, breast tenderness, headache, dizziness, blurred vision, vaginal discharge, and spotting have been reported.

Endometrial hyperplasia has occurred in patients taking doses in the upper range or higher (Greenblatt and Zarate, 1967; Ober and Bronstein, 1967). A thorough study of the endometrial (particularly long-term) effects of quinestrol at the recommended dosage has not been published.

DOSAGE AND PREPARATIONS.

Oral: For replacement therapy, 100 mcg once daily for seven days, followed by 100 mcg weekly beginning two weeks after initiating treatment.

Estrovis (Parke-Davis). Tablets 100 mcg.

Nonsteroidal Estrogens

DIENESTROL

[Ortho Dienestrol]

This nonsteroidal estrogen is related chemically to diethylstilbestrol. It is applied topically to relieve symptoms of hypoestrogenic vaginal atrophy. Dienestrol is contraindicated during pregnancy.

See the Introduction and the evaluation on Diethylstilbestrol for adverse reactions.

DOSAGE AND PREPARATIONS.

Topical (vaginal): For atrophic vaginitis and kraurosis vulvae, the preparation is applied one or two times daily for one to two weeks; the application is then reduced gradually to a maintenance level of one to three times a week.

Ortho Dienestrol (Ortho). Cream 0.01% in 78 g tubes with or without measured dose applicator.

DIETHYLSTILBESTROL (DES)

Diethylstilbestrol (DES) is the most potent nonsteroidal estrogen. Since the drug is inactivated slowly, it can be given in single daily doses even when large amounts are required.

DES is generally believed to cause a greater incidence of nausea than some other estrogen preparations and occasionally causes pigmentation (facies, nipples).

This estrogen is contraindicated in pregnant women, especially during the first 16 weeks because vaginal adenosis has occurred in 30% to 90% of postpubertal females whose mothers received DES or a closely related congener during pregnancy. Vaginal adenocarcinoma also has been reported rarely. Yearly examination of patients with this history is recommended. Epididymal cysts, testicular hypoplasia, varicocele, and impaired fertility have been reported in some postpubertal males whose mothers received DES during pregnancy.

See the Introduction for specific indications and adverse reactions. For contraceptive use of DES, see index entry Diethylstilbestrol, As Postcoital Contraceptive.

DOSAGE AND PREPARATIONS.

Oral: For hypogonadism or replacement therapy, 0.2 to 0.5 mg daily and cyclically. A progestin may be added for the last 10 to 13 days.

For use in metastatic breast carcinoma, see index entry Diethylstilbestrol, In Cancer.

Generic. Tablets 1, 2.5, and 5 mg.

Estrogens Combined with Other Drugs

ANDROGEN-ESTROGEN PREPARATIONS

Combined estrogen-androgen therapy has been promoted to restore libido in postmenopausal women and to relieve a variety of symptoms that accompany aging, but there is no evidence that the addition of small amounts of androgen to estrogen retards such symptoms. The use of fixed-dose combinations for any of these indications is not encouraged. Masculinizing effects may occur.

Deladumone (Bristol-Myers Squibb). Each milliliter contains estradiol valerate 4 mg and testosterone enanthate 90 mg in sesame oil.

Depo-Testadiol (Upjohn), ***Duo-Cyp*** (Keene). Each milliliter contains estradiol cypionate 2 mg and testosterone cypionate 50 mg in cottonseed oil.

Estratest (Solvay). Each tablet contains esterified estrogens 1.25 mg and methyltestosterone 2.5 mg or esterified estrogens 0.625 mg and methyltestosterone 1.25 mg [***Estratest H.S.***].

Halodrin (Upjohn). Each tablet contains fluoxymesterone 1 mg and ethinyl estradiol 0.02 mg.

ESTROGENS WITH ANTIANXIETY AGENTS

This type of mixture is used to treat menopausal symptoms. Vasomotor flushes and atrophic vaginitis usually respond readily to estrogen alone. Anxiety may occur secondary to discomfort from these estrogen-responsive complaints. Under these circumstances, when anxiety is not relieved by estrogen therapy, antianxiety agents may be helpful. Therefore, if one of the available combinations contains ingredients appropriate both quantitatively and qualitatively for an individual patient, the use of these mixtures may be acceptable for a *limited* period. Administration of the separate components is preferred, however.

Menrium (Roche). Each tablet contains esterified estrogens 0.2 or 0.4 mg and chlordiazepoxide 5 mg or esterified estrogens 0.4 mg and chlordiazepoxide 10 mg.

PMB (Wyeth-Ayerst). Each tablet contains conjugated estrogens 0.45 mg and meprobamate 200 or 400 mg.

PREPARATIONS CONTAINING ANDROGENS, ESTROGENS, AND OTHER INGREDIENTS

Mixtures containing androgens and estrogens combined with vitamins, minerals, progesterone, sedatives, stimulants, and other drugs are available. They are advocated for use in geriatric patients, but these preparations cannot be considered desirable therapy.

Mediatric (Wyeth-Ayerst). Each capsule contains conjugated estrogens 0.25 mg, methyltestosterone 2.5 mg, methamphetamine hydrochloride 1 mg, vitamin C 100 mg, cyanocobalamin 2.5 mcg, thiamine mononitrate 10 mg, riboflavin 5 mg, niacinamide 50 mg, pyridoxine hydrochloride 3 mg, pantothenate calcium 20 mg, and ferrous sulfate dried 30 mg.

HORMONE COSMETIC PREPARATIONS

Hormones used topically on the skin are marketed principally as quasi-cosmetic rejuvenating creams. Topical preparations containing physiologic amounts of estrogens or natural progesterone have no effect on human sebaceous glands and oil secretion. There is no evidence that hormone creams are any more effective than simple emollients in relieving dryness of the skin, or that they increase the amount of water that the skin can hold or restore fat to the subcutaneous layer. However, there is some evidence that certain topically applied steroid hormones (both active and inactive biologically) may cause slight histologic thickening in some areas of the epidermis of aged skin. Estrogen can increase dermal thickness slightly, but it is unlikely that this alters facial appearance.

Because of the current FDA restrictions on the concentrations of ovarian hormones permitted in such products, there is little likelihood that the amount is sufficient to produce any systemic effects with ordinary use. However, systemic effects have followed *excessive* use of hormone creams.

An FDA Advisory Review Panel concluded that concentrations higher than 1 mg estrone or the equivalent produce systemic effects and should not be available without prescription. Progesterone in concentrations up to 5 mg/30 g is probably safe for daily use when the total amount does not exceed 60 g per month. Higher concentrations of progesterone were not tested (*Federal Register,* 1982).

PROGESTERONE AND PROGESTINS

PROGESTERONE

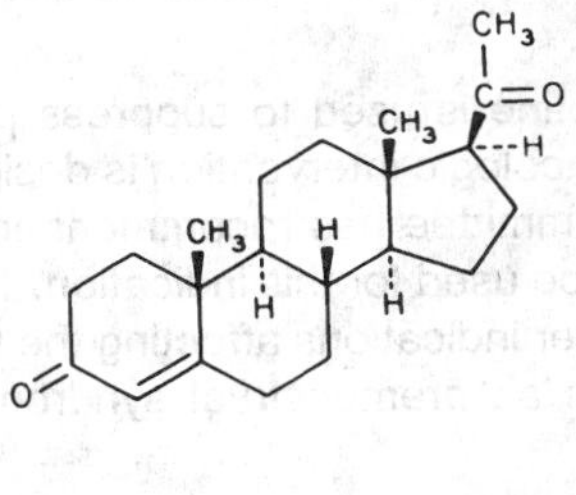

This natural progestational substance acts on target genital tissues and endocrine glands and also has general systemic effects. Parenteral preparations in oil are used primarily to diagnose and treat menstrual disorders; responsiveness of the target organ depends on the priming action of estrogen. The drug is ineffective when given orally.

Progesterone is also available in an IUD [Progestasert] (see index entry Progestasert).

See the Introduction for indications and adverse reactions.

DOSAGE AND PREPARATIONS.

Intramuscular: For diagnostic use in amenorrhea or for dysfunctional uterine bleeding, 200 mg in oil.

Generic. Suspension (in oil) 50 mg/ml in 10 ml containers.

Available Trademark:
Gesterol 50 (Forest).

HYDROXYPROGESTERONE CAPROATE
[Pro-Depo, Prodrox]

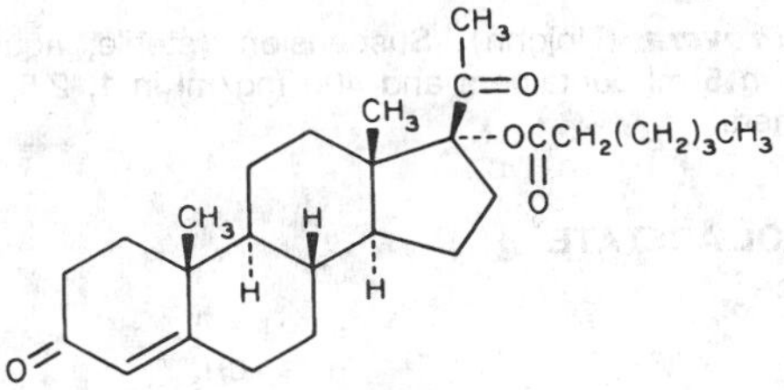

This derivative of progesterone is administered parenterally. Its duration of action is about 9 to 17 days. Since hydroxyprogesterone has no estrogenic activity, priming with estrogen is necessary before a response is noted.

See the Introduction for indications and adverse reactions.

DOSAGE AND PREPARATIONS.

Intramuscular: For menstrual disorders, 125 to 250 mg per cycle.

Generic. Solution 125 mg/ml in 10 ml containers and 250 mg/ml in 5 ml containers.
Pro-Depo (Vortech). Solution 125 mg/ml in 10 ml containers.
Prodrox (Legere). Solution 250 mg/ml in 5 ml containers.

MEDROXYPROGESTERONE ACETATE (MPA)
[Amen, Curretab, Cycrin, Depo-Provera, Provera]

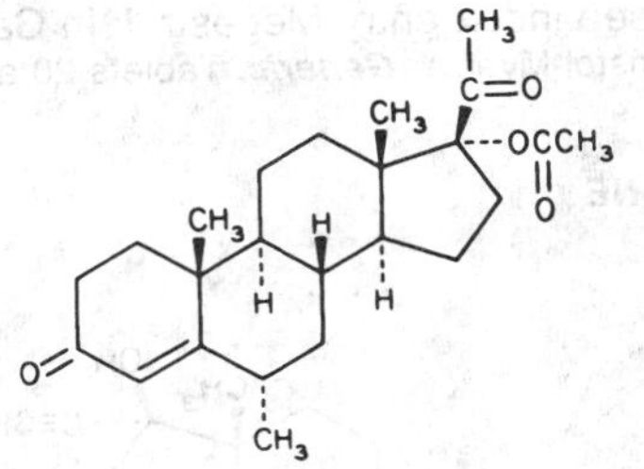

Medroxyprogesterone is effective both orally and parenterally. The duration of action of the depot preparation is variable and occasionally prolonged; therefore, this preparation may be inappropriate in women desiring pregnancy in the imminent future. Since the drug has no inherent estrogenic activity, priming with estrogen is necessary before a response is noted.

See the Introduction for indications and adverse reactions. For use of the parenteral preparation as a contraceptive, see index entry Medroxyprogesterone, As Depot Contraceptive.

DOSAGE AND PREPARATIONS.

Oral: For amenorrhea and dysfunctional uterine bleeding, 5 to 10 mg daily for ten days, depending on the indication.

For endometriosis, 10 to 30 mg daily.

For menopausal replacement therapy, 10 mg for the last 10 to 13 days of estrogen administration or 2.5 mg daily with estrogen for continuous therapy (see the section on Indications).

Amen (Carnrick), ***Curretab*** (Solvay), ***Cycrin*** (Wyeth-Ayerst), ***Generic***. Tablets 10 mg.
Provera (Upjohn). Tablets 2.5, 5, and 10 mg.

Intramuscular: For endometriosis, 150 mg every three months. For endometrial carcinoma, 400 mg to 1 g weekly initially.

Depo-Provera (Upjohn). Suspension (sterile, aqueous) 100 mg/ml in 5 ml containers and 400 mg/ml in 1, 2.5, and 10 ml containers.

MEGESTROL ACETATE
[Megace]

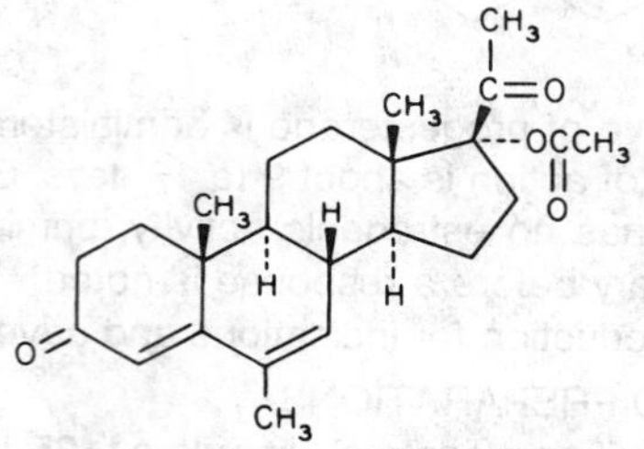

This progestin is used in the palliative treatment of advanced carcinoma of the breast or endometrium. See index entry Progestins, Uses, Cancer.

DOSAGE AND PREPARATIONS.

Oral: In women with recently diagnosed breast carcinoma (in whom estrogen is contraindicated), 40 to 80 mg daily may relieve menopausal symptoms.

For dosages used to treat breast carcinoma and endometrial carcinoma, see index entry Megestrol, In Cancer.

Megace (Bristol-Myers), ***Generic***. Tablets 20 and 40 mg.

NORETHINDRONE
[Norlutin]

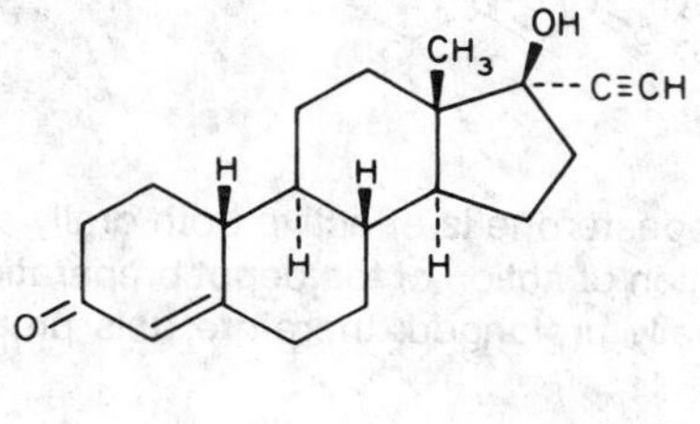

NORETHINDRONE ACETATE
[Aygestin, Norlutate]

This derivative of nortestosterone is a potent oral progestational agent. Its androgenic effects are minor and variable. Norethindrone is given alone or with estrogens for many indications, including contraception (see index entry Contraceptives, Oral). See the Introduction for indications and adverse reactions.

DOSAGE AND PREPARATIONS.

NORETHINDRONE:

Oral: For amenorrhea and dysfunctional uterine bleeding, 5 to 20 mg daily, starting on the fifth day of the cycle and ending on the twenty-fifth day.

For endometriosis, initially, 10 mg daily for two weeks, increased by 5 mg daily every two weeks until a dose of 30 mg daily is reached, then 30 mg daily for maintenance. Maintenance therapy may be continued for six to nine months or until breakthrough bleeding necessitates temporary discontinuation.

For menopausal replacement therapy, 1 to 2.5 mg for 10 to 13 days of each month of estrogen administration in women with an intact uterus.

See also the section on Indications in the Introduction.

Norlutin (Parke-Davis). Tablets 5 mg.

NORETHINDRONE ACETATE:

Oral: For amenorrhea and dysfunctional uterine bleeding, 2.5 to 10 mg, starting on the fifth day of the cycle and ending on the twenty-fifth day.

For endometriosis, initially, 5 mg daily for two weeks, increased by 2.5 mg daily every two weeks until a dose of 15 mg daily is reached, then 15 mg daily for maintenance. Maintenance therapy may be continued for six to nine months or until breakthrough bleeding necessitates temporary discontinuation of therapy.

For menopausal replacement therapy, 1 mg for 10 to 13 days of each month of estrogen administration.

Aygestin (Wyeth-Ayerst), ***Norlutate*** (Parke-Davis). Tablets 5 mg.

OTHER AGENTS

BROMOCRIPTINE MESYLATE
[Parlodel]

For chemical formula, see index entry Bromocriptine, In Female Hyperprolactinemia.

Bromocriptine is a synthetic ergot alkaloid that acts directly on dopaminergic receptors of pituitary cells. It also may exert a central effect on prolactin secretion, but this has not yet been established.

USES. Bromocriptine is used to suppress postpartum lactation when pharmacologic intervention is desired. However, an FDA Advisory Committee has recommended that pharmacologic therapy not be used for this indication. The drug also has been used for other indications affecting the female reproductive system, such as premenstrual syndrome and hirsutism due to hyperprolactinemia. See also the discussion on these disorders in the Introduction.

ADVERSE REACTIONS. Adverse reactions are common when bromocriptine therapy is initiated. Thereafter, their incidence and severity depend on the dosage and its rate of increase. Common untoward effects include headache, nausea, vomiting, dizziness, fatigue, and orthostatic hypotension. Nausea usually disappears after three to four days and may be minimized by taking the medication with food and at bedtime. Rarely, orthostatic hypotension appears to be associated with fainting or collapse in sensitive individuals, even after ingestion of a single dose.

Postpartum hypertension, seizures, stroke, and psychosis have been associated with use of bromocriptine to suppress lactation. Other drugs that may have contributed to the hypertensive effects were taken concomitantly in some cases and causation remains unproven. However, postpartum hypertension or eclampsia has been reported with use of other ergot alkaloids.

The risk of spontaneous abortions or neonatal malformations did not appear to increase when bromocriptine was taken during the first eight weeks of pregnancy (Turkalj et al, 1982).

PHARMACOKINETICS. Bromocriptine is absorbed rapidly after oral administration; peak plasma levels are attained in about one hour. First-pass metabolism occurs with over 90% of the absorbed dose. The plasma half-life is three hours. About 98% is excreted in the feces, and the remaining 2% is eliminated in the urine.

DOSAGE AND PREPARATIONS.

Oral: Patients should be encouraged to forego this or other drugs to prevent postpartum lactation. However, if pharmacologic suppression is still deemed desirable, 2.5 mg one or two times daily is the usual dosage (range, 2.5 to 7.5 mg/day). Therapy is started at least four hours after delivery when vital signs have stabilized and is continued for 14 days. If rebound lactation occurs, 2.5 mg daily may be taken for an additional week.

Parlodel (Sandoz). Capsules 5 mg; tablets 2.5 mg.

DANAZOL

[Danocrine]

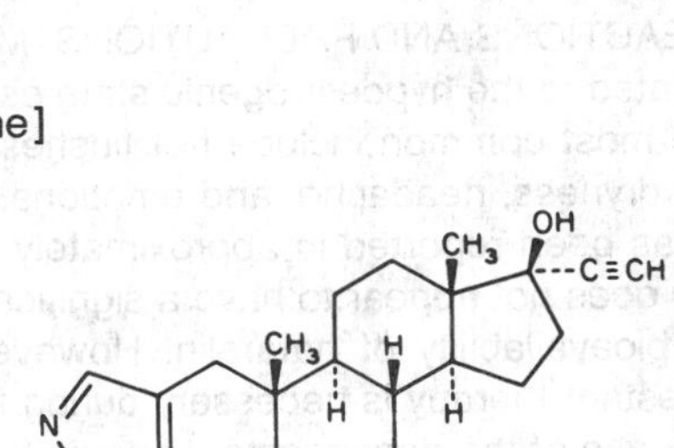

ACTIONS. This synthetic derivative of 17α-ethinyl testosterone (ethisterone) does not exhibit significant estrogenic or progestational properties but acts at several levels of the hypothalamic-pituitary-ovarian axis. It binds to androgen, progesterone, and glucocorticoid (but not estrogen) receptors and to sex hormone-binding and corticosteroid-binding globulins. Danazol inhibits the midcycle gonadotropin surge and multiple enzymes of ovarian steroidogenesis (Barbieri and Ryan, 1981).

USES. Danazol may be useful when suppression of gonadal function is desirable.

Endometriosis: Danazol is indicated for endometriosis amenable to hormonal management; it is thought that this drug is as effective as GnRH analogues. It may be more effective than estrogen-progestin regimens. However, because danazol is considerably more expensive than therapeutically equivalent courses of estrogen-progestin combinations, the latter may be preferred when cost is a consideration and estrogens are not contraindicated. However, this agent is considerably more expensive than therapeutically equivalent courses of oral contraceptives or progestins. A definitive diagnosis of endometriosis should be established before danazol therapy is begun. The drug may be used as sole therapy or preoperatively and/or postoperatively in severe disease. Most patients experience relief of symptoms and exhibit objective improvement upon laparoscopy. Pregnancy rates have not been proven to improve as a result of danazol therapy (see the section on Endometriosis in the Introduction). Endometriosis may recur after discontinuing treatment.

Danazol is not indicated when surgery alone is the treatment of choice and should not be given to women with underlying abnormal genital bleeding.

Fibrocystic Breast Condition: Breast pain and tenderness may be relieved during the first month of danazol therapy, and nodularity may disappear after four to six months of daily administration (Greenblatt et al, 1980) in up to 80% of patients. Irregular menses or amenorrhea is common, especially with larger doses. Symptoms recur in more than one-half of patients within one to two years after cessation of medication, and another course of therapy may then be initiated. Although dosages employed for this indication are probably associated with nonovulatory cycles and an atrophic endometrium, nonhormonal contraception is recommended during danazol therapy.

Miscellaneous Uses: This drug has been used in precocious puberty in both sexes, although GnRH analogues may prove to be preferable for this indication. Regression of secondary sexual characteristics occurs, and girls become amenorrheic. However, the accelerated bone maturation is unaffected, and androgenic side effects may be a problem.

ADVERSE REACTIONS AND PRECAUTIONS. Adverse reactions include weight gain, edema, mood changes, leg cramps, breakthrough bleeding, and androgenic and anabolic effects (acne, mild hirsutism, oily skin or scalp, decreased breast size). Danazol therapy is associated with a decrease in the HDL cholesterol level but no change in triglyceride concentration in the serum. Sequelae of a hypoestrogenic state (vasomotor flushing, sweating, atrophic vaginitis) may occur with lower dosages, but androgenic effects usually are not a problem when less than 600 mg is administered daily.

Danazol should not be administered to pregnant or lactating women (FDA Pregnancy Category X). Masculinization of the external genitalia of female neonates has been reported when this drug was taken inadvertently during the first trimester of pregnancy (Duck and Katayama, 1981; Peress et al,

1982; Kingsbury, 1985). Lower doses of danazol may not inhibit ovulation. The possibility of inadvertent administration during pregnancy may be reduced by initiating therapy after several days of a normal menstrual period and by using a barrier contraceptive during the course of therapy.

Abnormal results of liver function tests and jaundice have been reported. One case report of hepatocellular adenoma associated with danazol use has appeared in the literature (Fermand, 1990). Pseudotumor cerebri has developed in patients during and after withdrawal from danazol treatment (Fanous et al, 1991). This drug should not be taken in the presence of acute liver disease, congestive heart failure, severe hypertension, or renal disease. Danazol may potentiate the action of oral anticoagulants. Lowering of voice pitch, which may return only partially to the pretreatment level, has been reported (Mercaitis et al, 1985).

PHARMACOKINETICS. After administration of danazol 400 mg, peak plasma levels of 80 to 100 ng/ml are attained in one to two hours. The half-life in plasma is about 4.5 hours (Dmowski, 1979). Unaltered steroid appears to be biologically active. Danazol is metabolized to conjugates, sulfates, and glucuronides and is excreted predominantly in the urine but also in feces.

DOSAGE AND PREPARATIONS.

Oral: For endometriosis, dosage is determined on the basis of the severity of disease and is adjusted according to response and the occurrence of adverse reactions. Treatment of moderate to severe disease may be initiated with 800 mg daily in two divided doses. Later, the dose may be reduced to an amount sufficient to maintain amenorrhea; 200 mg daily is adequate in some patients. However, most patients are given 400 to 600 mg daily. Those with more severe disease may require 800 mg daily throughout treatment. The appropriate amount is given daily in two to four divided doses for three to nine months. Serum estradiol is depressed more effectively with the more frequent administration of the same total dose (Dickey et al, 1984). Treatment can be reinstituted if symptoms recur on cessation of therapy.

For fibrocystic breast disease, 50 to 100 mg daily in two divided doses, depending on the severity of symptoms and the patient's response. For pain relief and reduction of nodularity, 100 mg daily for approximately three months is usually effective.

Danocrine (Sanofi Winthrop). Capsules 50, 100, and 200 mg.

LEUPROLIDE ACETATE FOR DEPOT SUSPENSION

[Lupron Depot 3.75 mg]

ACTIONS AND USES. This synthetic analogue of GnRH is administered intramuscularly in a depot form to treat endometriosis. Its actions are similar to those of nafarelin: after initial stimulation of gonadotropin secretion, secretion of pituitary gonadotropins and ovarian steroids is suppressed and menses cease. The pain of endometriosis is usually relieved. Leuprolide is not curative and does not appear to improve fertility. A single monthly injection is as effective as treatment with danazol and does not cause the associated androgenic side effects.

ADVERSE REACTIONS AND PRECAUTIONS. These are similar to reactions associated with nafarelin with the exception of those related to nasal administration of the latter (see the evaluation on Nafarelin Acetate).

DOSAGE AND PREPARATIONS.

Intramuscular: For endometriosis, one injection of 3.75 mg once monthly for six months.

Lupron Depot 3.75 mg (TAP Pharmaceuticals). Powder (sterile, lyophilized microspheres) supplied with diluent.

NAFARELIN ACETATE

[Synarel]

ACTIONS AND USES. Nafarelin, a synthetic analogue of GnRH, is administered intranasally as a spray to treat endometriosis. Paradoxically, it suppresses pituitary gonadotropin secretion (after initially stimulating secretion for several weeks). As a result, production of ovarian steroid decreases and menses cease in most patients but resume in all patients within three months after treatment is discontinued in the absence of pregnancy. Pain caused by endometriosis usually is relieved upon establishment of the hypoestrogenic milieu.

Nafarelin appears to be as effective as danazol in relieving signs and symptoms of endometriosis. Results of clinical trials in the United States and Europe indicated that, after six months of treatment, laparoscopically determined endometriosis scores were similar for the two drugs. Pregnancy rates following treatment also were similar for both agents (approximately 30%). Nafarelin is not curative, however. Of patients who experienced complete relief of symptoms during therapy, 50% remained symptom-free and the remainder did not experience recurrence of severe symptoms six months after treatment ended.

For further information on use of nafarelin for endometriosis, see proceedings of the symposium on Nafarelin in the Management of Endometriosis (*Am J Obstet Gynecol,* 1990).

ADVERSE REACTIONS AND PRECAUTIONS. Most adverse effects are related to the hypoestrogenic state established by nafarelin. The most common include hot flushes, decreased libido, vaginal dryness, headache, and emotional lability. Nasal irritation has been reported in approximately 10% of patients. Rhinitis does not appear to have a significant effect on the systemic bioavailability of nafarelin. However, if topical nasal decongestant therapy is necessary during treatment of endometriosis, use of the decongestant should be delayed at least two hours following administration of nafarelin.

Hypersensitivity reactions have been reported (0.2% of patients).

Although approximately 8% of patients receiving nafarelin in clinical trials experienced weight gain, significant androgenic side effects associated with danazol therapy (eg, decreased HDL and increased LDL lipoprotein concentrations) have not been observed with nafarelin. However, the hypoestrogenic state induced by nafarelin is associated with bone loss of approximately 4% in the lumbar vertebrae after a six-month course of therapy. Most bone loss appears to be reversed within one year after treatment is discontinued. Cortical bone of the distal radius and second metacarpal appeared to be unaffected. Because of concern about cumulative bone loss with long-term therapy, it is recommended that only one six-month course of nafarelin be employed. Patients with existing risk factors (eg, prolonged use of corticosteroids or anticonvulsants, chronic alcohol or tobacco use, strong family history of osteoporosis) theoretically are at higher risk for significant bone loss.

Nafarelin is classified in FDA Pregnancy Category X.

DOSAGE AND PREPARATIONS.
Intranasal: For endometriosis, including reduction in the size and number of endometrial implants and relief of pain and discomfort, 400 mcg daily; one spray (200 mcg) is administered into one nostril in the morning and one spray into the other nostril in the evening. Treatment is begun between days two and four of the menstrual cycle. For the occasional patient in whom regular menses continue after two months of therapy, the dose may be doubled (one spray into each nostril in the morning and evening). The recommended duration of therapy is six months.

Synarel (Syntex). Spray (nasal) 2 mg/ml in 10 ml containers.

SPIRONOLACTONE
[Aldactone]

For chemical formula, see index entry Spironolactone, As Diuretic.

Spironolactone is a steroid that competes for dihydrotestosterone (DHT) receptors in the skin and decreases ovarian microsomal cytochrome P450, which inhibits ovarian androgen production. These properties are responsible for the drug's effectiveness as a treatment for hirsutism. Spironolactone was first used as a diuretic because of its competitive inhibition of aldosterone.

USES. Spironolactone is used to treat hirsutism and appears to be effective regardless of the cause. Clinical improvement may be expected in three to six months. In congenital adrenal hyperplasia, it may be used as an adjunct to glucocorticoid therapy. Oral contraceptive therapy also may be used with spironolactone especially if there is a concurrent need for contraception.

ADVERSE REACTIONS AND PRECAUTIONS. Spironolactone affects the menstrual cycle and the character of menses in the majority of women taking doses in the higher range. Women who previously had normal menstrual periods may develop polymenorrhea, while women who were oligomenorrheic may experience one of a variety of changes (eg, amenorrhea, regular menses, polymenorrhea) (Evans and Burke, 1986). These effects can be prevented by beginning treatment with an oral contraceptive two to three months before initiation of spironolactone therapy.

Since the decrease in androgen secretion may be associated with a return or increase in fertility, contraception should be employed during therapy. Oral contraceptives may be prescribed. Spironolactone should not be taken during pregnancy because of the possibility of feminizing a male fetus.

For discussion of other adverse reactions, pharmacokinetics, and drug interactions, see index entry Spironolactone, As Diuretic.

DOSAGE AND PREPARATIONS.
Oral: For hirsutism, 75 to 200 mg daily taken in divided doses. Doses in the lower range may be effective if spironolactone is being used as an adjunct to another agent (eg, oral contraceptive, glucocorticoid).

Generic. Tablets 25 mg.

Aldactone (Searle). Tablets 25, 50, and 100 mg.

Cited References

Hormone Replacement Therapy, technical bulletin 166. Washington, DC, American College of Obstetricians and Gynecologists, (April) 1992, 1-8.

Lactation suppression indication challenge from HRG. *FDC Rep* Dec 5, 1988, T&G 12.

Nafarelin in the management of endometriosis, symposium. *Am J Obstet Gynecol* 162:565-593, 1990.

Report of recommendations of 1985 DES task force of US Department of Health and Human Services. *JAMA* 255:1849, 1853, 1986.

Topically applied hormone-containing drug products for over-the-counter human use. *Federal Register* 47:429-434, 1982.

Vulvar dystrophies: ACOG Technical Bulletin Number 139—January 1990. *Int J Gynecol Obstet* 35:269-273, 1991.

Adamson GD: Treatment of uterine fibroids: Current findings with gonadotropin-releasing hormone agonists. *Am J Obstet Gynecol* 166:746-751, 1992.

Adashi EY: Potential utility of gonadotropin-releasing hormone agonists in the management of ovarian hyperandrogenism. *Fertil Steril* 53:765-779, 1990.

Albrecht BH, et al: Objective evidence that placebo and oral medroxyprogesterone acetate therapy diminish menopausal vasomotor flushes. *Am J Obstet Gynecol* 139:631-635, 1981.

Alcoff JM, et al: Double-blind, placebo-controlled, crossover trial of propranolol as treatment for menopausal vasomotor symptoms. *Clin Ther* 3:356-364, 1981.

American College of Physicians: Guidelines for counseling postmenopausal women about preventive hormone therapy. *Ann Intern Med* 117:1038-1041, 1992.

American Fertility Society: Revised classification of endometriosis. *Fertil Steril* 43:351-352, 1985. [Copies may be ordered from The American Fertility Society, 2131 Magnolia Avenue, Suite 201, Birmingham, AL 35256.]

Andersson K: Treatment of menorrhagia, in: *Treatment of Gynecological Bleeding Disturbances*. Uppsala, Sweden, Lakemedelsverket, 1991, 85-92.

Andreyko JL, et al: Use of agonistic analog of gonadotropin-releasing hormone (nafarelin) to treat leiomyomas: Assessment by magnetic resonance imaging. *Am J Obstet Gynecol* 158:903-910, 1988.

Antonioli DA, et al: Natural history of diethylstilbestrol-associated genital tract lesions: Cervical ectopy and cervicovaginal hood. *Am J Obstet Gynecol* 137:847-853, 1980.

Ayhan A, et al: Topical testosterone for lichen sclerosus. *Int J Gynecol Obstet* 30:253-255, 1989.

Barbieri RL: Endometriosis 1990: Current treatment approaches. *Drugs* 39:502-510, 1990.

Barbieri RL, Ryan KJ: Danazol: Endocrine pharmacology and therapeutic applications. *Am J Obstet Gynecol* 141:453-463, 1981.

Barbieri RL, et al: Role of hyperinsulinemia in the pathogenesis of ovarian hyperandrogenism. *Fertil Steril* 50:197-212, 1988.

Barnes AB, et al: Fertility and outcome of pregnancy in women exposed in utero to diethylstilbestrol. *N Engl J Med* 302:609-613, 1980.

Barth JH, et al: Spironolactone is an effective and well tolerated systemic antiandrogen therapy for hirsute women. *J Clin Endocrinol Metab* 68:966-970, 1989.

Barth JH, et al: Cyproterone acetate for severe hirsutism: Results of a double-blind dose-ranging study. *Clin Endocrinol* 35:5-10, 1991.

Baumgardner SB, et al: Replacement estrogen therapy for menopausal vasomotor flushes: Comparison of quinestrol and conjugated estrogens. *Obstet Gynecol* 51:445-452, 1978.

Bayer SR, et al: Efficacy of danazol treatment for minimal endometriosis in infertile women: Prospective randomized study. *J Reprod Med* 33:179-183, 1988.

Berger MJ, Goldstein DP: Impaired reproductive performance in DES-exposed women. *Obstet Gynecol* 55:25-27, 1980.

Berger A, Schaumburg HH: More on neuropathy from pyridoxine abuse, letter. *N Engl J Med* 311:986-987, 1984.

Bibbo M, et al: Twenty-five year follow-up study of women exposed to diethylstilbestrol during pregnancy. *N Engl J Med* 298:763-767, 1978.

Blombäck M, et al: Estrogen treatment of tall girls: Risk of thrombosis? *Pediatrics* 72:416-419, 1983.

Brayshaw ND, Brayshaw DD: Thyroid hypofunction in premenstrual syndrome, letter. *N Engl J Med* 315:1486-1487, 1986.

Brian DD, et al: Breast cancer in DES-exposed mothers: Absence of association. *Mayo Clin Proc* 55:89-93, 1980.

Brincat M, et al: Long-term effects of menopause and sex hormones on skin thickness. *Br J Obstet Gynaecol* 92:256-259, 1985.

Bullen BA, et al: Induction of menstrual disorders by strenuous exercise in untrained women. *N Engl J Med* 312:1349-1353, 1985.

Buring JE, et al: Conjugated estrogen use and risk of endometrial cancer. *Am J Epidemiol* 124:434-441, 1986.

Buring JE, et al: Prospective cohort study of postmenopausal hormone use and risk of breast cancer in US women. *Am J Epidemiol* 125:939-945, 1987.

Burry KA, et al: Metabolic changes during medical treatment of endometriosis: Nafarelin acetate versus danazol. *Am J Obstet Gynecol* 160:1454-1461, 1989.

Butler L, et al: Collaborative study of pregnancy rates following danazol therapy of Stage I endometriosis. *Fertil Steril* 41:373-376, 1984.

Cagnacci A, et al: Effects of low doses of transdermal 17β-estradiol on carbohydrate metabolism in postmenopausal women. *J Clin Endocrinol Metab* 74:1396-1400, 1992.

Campbell S: Double blind psychometric studies on effects of natural estrogens on post-menopausal women, in Campbell S (ed): *The Management of the Menopause and Post-Menopausal Years.* Baltimore, University Park Press, 1976, 149-172.

Cann CE, et al: Decreased spinal mineral content in amenorrheic women. *JAMA* 251:626-629, 1984.

Casper RF, Yen SSC: Neuroendocrinology of menopausal flushes: Hypothesis of flush mechanism. *Clin Endocrinol* 22:293-312, 1985.

Casper RF, et al: Effect of increased cardiac output on luteal phase gonadal steroids: Hypothesis for runners' amenorrhea. *Fertil Steril* 41:364-368, 1984.

Casper RF, et al: Thyrotropin and prolactin responses to thyrotropin-releasing hormone in premenstrual syndrome. *J Clin Endocrinol Metab* 68:608-612, 1989.

Centerwall BS: Premenopausal hysterectomy and cardiovascular disease. *Am J Obstet Gynecol* 139:58-61, 1981.

Chetkowski RJ, et al: Biologic effects of transdermal estradiol. *N Engl J Med* 314:1615-1620, 1986.

Chihal HJ: Premenstrual syndrome: An update for the clinician. *Obstet Gynecol Clin North Am* 17:457-479, 1990.

Christiansen C, Riis BJ: 17β-estradiol and continuous norethisterone: A unique treatment for established osteoporosis in elderly women. *J Clin Endocrinol Metab* 71:836-841, 1990.

Chuong CJ, et al: Clinical trial of naltrexone in premenstrual syndrome. *Obstet Gynecol* 72:332-336, 1988.

Coddington CC, et al: Long-acting gonadotropin hormone-releasing hormone analog used to treat uteri. *Fertil Steril* 45:624-629, 1986.

Colditz GA, et al: Prospective study of estrogen replacement therapy and risk of breast cancer in postmenopausal women. *JAMA* 264:2648-2653, 1990.

Creasy GW, et al: Review of the endometrial effects of estrogens and progestins. *Obstet Gynecol Surv* 47 (suppl):654-678, 1992.

Crosby PDA, Rittmaster RS: Predictors of clinical response in hirsute women treated with spironolactone. *Fertil Steril* 55:1076-1081, 1991.

Cumming DC, et al: Treatment of hirsutism with spironolactone. *JAMA* 247:1295-1298, 1982.

Cusan L, et al: Treatment of hirsutism with the pure antiandrogen flutamide. *J Am Acad Dermatol* 23:462-469, 1990.

Dalton K: *The Premenstrual Syndrome and Progesterone Therapy,* ed 2. Chicago, Year Book Medical Publishers, 1984.

Dawood MY: Dysmenorrhea. *J Reprod Med* 30:154-167, 1985.

Dawood MY: Efficacy and safety of suprofen in the treatment of primary dysmenorrhea: Multicenter, randomized, double-blind study. *Curr Ther Res* 44:257-266, 1988.

DeLignieres B, et al: Biological effects of estradiol-17β in postmenopausal women: Oral versus percutaneous administration. *J Clin Endocrinol Metab* 62:536-541, 1986.

Deeny M, et al: Low dose danazol in the treatment of the premenstrual syndrome. *Postgrad Med J* 67:450-454, 1991.

Dennerstein L, et al: Progesterone and premenstrual syndrome: Double blind crossover trial. *BMJ* 290:1617-1618, 1985.

Dickey RP, et al: Serum estradiol and danazol: I. Endometriosis response, side effects, administration interval, concurrent spironolactone and dexamethasone. *Fertil Steril* 42:709-716, 1984.

Dmowski WP: Endocrine properties and clinical application of danazol. *Fertil Steril* 31:237-251, 1979.

Donnez J, et al: Administration of nasal buserelin as compared with subcutaneous buserelin implant for endometriosis. *Fertil Steril* 52:27-30, 1989.

Donnez J, et al: Endometriosis-associated infertility: Evaluation of preoperative use of danazol, gestrinone, and buserelin. *Int J Fertil* 35:297-301, 1990.

Doody KM, Carr BR: Amenorrhea. *Obstet Gynecol Clin North Am* 17:361-387, 1990.

Drinkwater BL, et al: Bone mineral content of amenorrheic and eumenorrheic athletes. *N Engl J Med* 311:277-281, 1984.

Drinkwater BL, et al: Bone mineral density after resumption of menses in amenorrheic athletes. *JAMA* 256:380-382, 1986.

Drukker BH, deMendonca WG: Fibrocystic change and fibrocystic disease of the breast. *Obstet Gynecol Clin North Am* 14:685-701, 1987.

Duck SC, Katayama KP: Danazol may cause female pseudohermaphroditism. *Fertil Steril* 35:230-231, 1981.

Dupont WD, Page DL: Menopausal estrogen replacement therapy and breast cancer. *Arch Intern Med* 151:67-72, 1991.

Duursma SA, et al: Estrogen and bone metabolism. *Obstet Gynecol* 47:38-44, 1991.

Egeland GM, et al: Hormone replacement therapy and lipoprotein changes during early menopause. *Obstet Gynecol* 76:776-782, 1990.

Erickson LD, Ory SJ: GnRH analogues in the treatment of endometriosis. *Obstet Gynecol Clin North Am* 16:123-145, 1989.

Erlik Y, et al: Association of waking episodes with menopausal hot flushes. *JAMA* 245:1741-1744, 1981.

European Multicentre Study Group for Cabergoline in Lactation Inhibition: Single dose cabergoline versus bromocriptine in inhibition of puerperal lactation: Randomised, double blind, multicentre study. *BMJ* 302:1367-1371, 1991.

Evain-Brion D, et al: Studies in constitutionally tall adolescents: II. Effects of bromocriptine on growth hormone secretion and adult height prediction. *J Clin Endocrinol Metab* 58:1022-1026, 1984.

Evans DJ, Burke CW: Spironolactone in treatment of idiopathic hirsutism and the polycystic ovary syndrome. *J R Soc Med* 401-403, (Aug) 1986.

Facchinetti F, et al: Oral magnesium successfully relieves premenstrual mood changes. *Obstet Gynecol* 78:177-181, 1991.

Fahraeus L, Wallentin L: High density lipoprotein subfractions during oral and cutaneous administration of 17α-estradiol to menopausal women. *J Clin Endocrinol Metab* 56:797-801, 1983.

Fanous M, et al: Pseudomotor cerebri associated with danazol withdrawal, letter. *JAMA* 226:1218-1219, 1991.

Fedele L, et al: Gestrinone versus danazol in the treatment of endometriosis. *Fertil Steril* 51:781-785, 1989.

Fentiman IS, et al: Double-blind controlled trial of tamoxifen therapy for mastalgia. *Lancet* 1:287-288, 1986.

Fermand JP: Danazol-induced hepatocellular adenoma. *Am J Med* 88:529-530, 1990.

Finucane FF, et al: Decreased risk of stroke among postmenopausal hormone users: Results from a national cohort. *Arch Intern Med* 153:73-79, 1993.

Freeman E, et al: Ineffectiveness of progesterone suppository treatment for premenstrual syndrome. *JAMA* 264:349-353, 1990.

Friedman AJ: Vaginal hemorrhage associated with degenerating submucous leiomyomata during leuprolide acetate treatment. *Fertil Steril* 52:152-154, 1989.

Friedman AJ, et al: Randomized, double-blind trial of a gonadotropin-releasing hormone agonist (leuprolide) with or without medroxyprogesterone acetate in the treatment of leiomyomata uteri. *Fertil Steril* 49: 404-409, 1988.

Friedman AJ, et al: Efficacy and safety considerations in women with uterine leiomyomas treated with gonadotropin-releasing hormone agonists: The estrogen threshold hypothesis. *Am J Obstet Gynecol* 163:1114-1119, 1990.

Friedrich EG Jr: Lichen sclerosus. *J Reprod Med* 17:147-154, 1976.

Friedrich EG Jr, Kalra PS: Serum levels of sex hormones in vulvar lichen sclerosus, and effect of topical testosterone. *N Engl J Med* 310:488-491, 1984.

Gambrell RD Jr: Role of progestogens in prevention of breast cancer. *Maturitas* 8:169-176, 1986.

Gambrell RD Jr (ed): *Estrogen Replacement Therapy,* ed 2. Dallas, Essential Medical Information Systems, 1989.

Gambrell RD Jr, et al: Use of progestogen challenge test to reduce risk of endometrial cancer. *Obstet Gynecol* 55:732-738, 1980.

Garner PR, Poznanski N: Treatment of severe hirsutism resulting from hyperandrogenism with reverse sequential cyproterone acetate regimen. *J Reprod Med* 29:232-236, 1984.

Gibbons WE, et al: Biochemical and histologic effects of sequential estrogen/progestin therapy on the endometrium of postmenopausal women. *Am J Obstet Gynecol* 154:456-461, 1986.

Gill WB, et al: Association of diethylstilbestrol exposure in utero with cryptorchidism, testicular hypoplasia, and semen abnormalities. *J Urol* 122:36-39, 1979.

Glickman SP, et al: Multiple androgenic abnormalities, including elevated free testosterone, in hyperprolactinemic women. *J Clin Endocrinol Metab* 55:251-257, 1982.

Grady D, et al: Hormone therapy to prevent disease and prolong life in postmenopausal women. *Ann Intern Med* 117:1016-1037, 1992.

Granberg S, et al: Endometrial thickness as measured by endovaginal ultrasonography for identifying endometrial abnormality. *Am J Obstet Gynecol* 164:47-52, 1991.

Greenberg ER, et al: Breast cancer in mothers given diethylstilbestrol in pregnancy. *N Engl J Med* 311:1393-1398, 1984.

Greenblatt RB, Zarate A: Endometrial studies following quinestrol administration. *Int J Fertil* 12:187-202, 1967.

Greenblatt RB, et al: Treatment of benign breast disease with danazol. *Fertil Steril* 34:242-245, 1980.

Greep N, et al: Androstanediol glucuronide plasma clearance and production rates in normal and hirsute women. *J Clin Endocrinol Metab* 62:22-27, 1986.

Gruchow HW, et al: Postmenopausal use of estrogen and occlusion of coronary arteries. *Am Heart J* 115:954-963, 1988.

Hammar M, Berg G: Clonidine in treatment of menopausal flushing. *Acta Obstet Gynecol Scand* 132 (suppl):29-31, 1985.

Hammarbäck S (ed): The premenstrual syndrome: A study of its diagnosis and pathogenesis. *Acta Obstet Gynecol Scand* 151 (suppl):5-48, 1989.

Hammond MG: Managing menopausal signs and symptoms. *Drug Ther* 14:38-45, (Dec) 1984.

Hammond MG, et al: Hyperandrogenism: Tests that simplify evaluation. *Postgrad Med* 79:107-113, (Feb) 1986.

Hargrove JT, et al: Absorption of oral progesterone is influenced by vehicle and particle size. *Am J Obstet Gynecol* 161:948-951, 1989.

Havens C: Premenstrual syndrome: Tactics for intervention. *Postgrad Med* 77:32-37, (May) 1985.

Hellberg D, et al: Premenstrual tension: A placebo-controlled efficacy study with spironolactone and medroxyprogesterone acetate. *Int J Gynecol Obstet* 34:243-248, 1991.

Henderson BE, et al: Decreased mortality in users of estrogen replacement therapy. *Arch Intern Med* 151:75-78, 1991.

Henzl MR: Gonadotropin-releasing hormone analogs: Update on new findings. *Am J Obstet Gynecol* 166:757-761, 1992.

Henzl MR, et al: Administration of nasal nafarelin as compared with oral danazol for endometriosis: Multicenter double-blind comparative clinical trial. *N Engl J Med* 318:485-489, 1988.

Herbst AL, et al: Comparison of pregnancy experience in DES-exposed and DES-unexposed daughters. *J Reprod Med* 24:62-69, 1980.

Herbst AL, et al: Risk factors for development of diethylstilbestrol-associated clear cell adenocarcinoma: Case-control study. *Am J Obstet Gynecol* 154:814-822, 1986.

Hertweck SP: Dysfunctional uterine bleeding. *Pediatr Adolesc Gynecol* 19:129-149, (March) 1992.

Hong MK, et al: Effects of estrogen replacement therapy on serum lipid values and angiographically defined coronary artery disease in postmenopausal women. *Am J Cardiol* 69:176-178, 1992.

Hulka BS: Effect of exogenous estrogen on postmenopausal women: Epidemiologic evidence. *Obstet Gynecol* 35:389-399, 1980.

Hulka BS, et al: Predominance of early endometrial cancers after long-term estrogen use. *JAMA* 244:2419-2422, 1980.

Iosif CS, et al: Estrogen receptors in human female lower urinary tract. *Am J Obstet Gynecol* 141:817-820, 1981.

Jefferies JA, et al: Structural anomalies of cervix and vagina in women enrolled in the Diethylstilbestrol Adenosis (DESAD) Project. *Am J Obstet Gynecol* 148:59-66, 1984.

Johansen JS, et al: The effect of a gonadotropin-releasing hormone agonist analog (nafarelin) on bone metabolism. *J Clin Endocrinol Metab* 67:701-706, 1988.

Johnson CA: Making sense of dysfunctional uterine bleeding. *Am Fam Physician* 44:149-157, 1991.

Johnson JWC, et al: Efficacy of 17 alpha-hydroxyprogesterone caproate in prevention of premature labor. *N Engl J Med* 293:675-680, 1975.

Johnson JWC, et al: High risk prematurity: Progestin treatment and steroid studies. *Obstet Gynecol* 54:412-418, 1979 A.

Johnson LD, et al: Vaginal adenosis in stillborns and neonates exposed to diethylstilbestrol and steroidal estrogens and progestins. *Obstet Gynecol* 53:671-679, 1979 B.

Jones KP, et al: Comparison of bone density in amenorrheic women due to athletics, weight loss, and premature menopause. *Obstet Gynecol* 66:5-8, 1985.

Judd H: Transdermal estradiol bypasses hepatic effects. *Am J Obstet Gynecol* 156:1326-1331, 1987.

Judd HL, et al: Estrogen replacement therapy: Indications and complications. *Ann Intern Med* 98:195-205, 1983.

Jurgens RW Jr, et al: A comparison of circulating hormone levels in postmenopausal women receiving hormone replacement therapy. *Am J Obstet Gynecol* 167:459-460, 1992.

Kable WT, et al: Lipid changes after hormone replacement therapy for menopause. *J Reprod Med* 35:512-518, 1990.

Karpas AE, et al: Effect of acute and chronic androgen suppression by glucocorticoids on gonadotropin levels in hirsute women. *J Clin Endocrinol Metab* 59:780-784, 1984.

Kase NG: Neuroendocrinology of amenorrhea. *J Reprod Med* 28:251-255, 1983.

Katz Z, et al: Teratogenicity of progestogens given during first trimester of pregnancy. *Obstet Gynecol* 65:775-780, 1985.

Kaufman DW, et al: Noncontraceptive estrogen use and risk of breast cancer. *JAMA* 252:63-67, 1984.

Kaufman RH, et al: Upper genital tract changes and infertility in diethylstilbestrol-exposed women. *Am J Obstet Gynecol* 154:1312-1318, 1986.

Kingsbury AC: Danazol and fetal masculinization: Warning. *Med J Aust* 143:410, 1985.

Kleijnen J, et al: Vitamin B6 in the treatment of the premenstrual syndrome: A review. *Br J Obstet Gynaecol* 97:847-852, 1990.

Kramer MS, et al: Diethylstilbestrol-related clear-cell adenocarcinoma in women with initial examinations demonstrating no malignant disease. *Obstet Gynecol* 69:868-871, 1987.

Krauss RM, et al: Effects of estrogen dose and smoking on lipid and lipoprotein levels in postmenopausal women. *Am J Obstet Gynecol* 158:1606-1611, 1988.

Kronenberg F, et al: Menopausal hot flashes: Thermoregulatory, cardiovascular, and circulating catecholamine and LH changes. *Maturitas* 6:31-43, 1984.

La Rosa JC: Varying effects of progestins on lipid levels and cardiovascular disease. *Am J Obstet Gynecol* 158:1619-1621, 1988.

Leary FJ, et al: Males exposed in utero to diethylstilbestrol. *JAMA* 252:2984-2989, 1984.

Lemay A: Monthly implant of luteinizing hormone-releasing hormone agonist: Practical therapeutic approach for sex-steroid dependent gynecologic diseases. *Fertil Steril* 48:10-12, 1987.

Lemay A, et al: Efficacy of intranasal or subcutaneous gonadotropin-releasing-hormone agonist inhibition of ovarian function in the treatment of endometriosis. *Am J Obstet Gynecol* 158:233-236, 1988.

Lindsay R, Tohme JF: Estrogen treatment of patients with established postmenopausal osteoporosis. *Obstet Gynecol* 76:290-295, 1990.

Lindsay R, et al: Minimum effective dose of estrogen for prevention of postmenopausal bone loss. *Obstet Gynecol* 63:759-763, 1984.

Linn S, et al: Adverse outcomes of pregnancy in women exposed to diethylstilbestrol in utero. *J Reprod Med* 33:3-7, 1988.

Lippe B: Turner syndrome. *Endocrinol Metab Clin North Am* 20:121-152, 1991.

Lissak A, et al: Treatment of hirsutism with cimetidine: Prospective randomized controlled trial. *Fertil Steril* 51:247-250, 1989.

Liu JH: Hypothalamic amenorrhea: Clinical perspectives, pathophysiology, and management. *Am J Obstet Gynecol* 163:1732-1736, 1990.

Lobo RA: The role of progestins in hormone replacement therapy. *Am J Obstet Gynecol* 166:1997-2004, 1992.

Lobo RA, et al: Depo-medroxyprogesterone acetate compared with conjugated estrogens for treatment of postmenopausal women. *Obstet Gynecol* 63:1-5, 1984.

Luciano AA, et al: Clinical and metabolic responses of menopausal women to sequential versus continuous estrogen and progestin replacement therapy. *Obstet Gynecol* 71:39-43, 1988.

Lucky AW: Androgens and the skin: Another journey around the circle, editorial. *Arch Dermatol* 123:193-195, 1987.

Lurie S, Borenstein R: The premenstrual syndrome. *Obstet Gynecol Surv* 45:220-228, 1990.

Magos AL, et al: Treatment of premenstrual syndrome by subcutaneous oestradiol implants and cyclical oral norethisterone: Placebo controlled study. *BMJ* 292:1629-1633, 1986.

Mandel FP, et al: Biologic effects of various doses of ethinyl estradiol in postmenopausal women. *Obstet Gynecol* 59:673-679, 1982.

Mansel RE, Dogliotti L: European multicentre trial of bromocriptine in cyclical mastalgia. *Lancet* 335:190-193, 1990.

Maouris P: Asymptomatic mild endometriosis in infertile women: The case for expectant management. *Obstet Gynecol Surv* 46:548-551, 1991.

Marcondes JAM, et al: Treatment of hirsutism in women with flutamide. *Fertil Steril* 57:543-547, 1992.

Martikainen H, et al: Hormonal and clinical effects of ketoconazole in hirsute women. *J Clin Endocrinol Metab* 66:987-991, 1988.

Martinez A, et al: Growth in Turner's syndrome: Long term treatment with low dose ethinyl estradiol. *J Clin Endocrinol Metab* 65:253-257, 1987.

Matta WH, et al: Reversible trabecular bone density loss following induced hypo-oestrogenism with the GnRH analogue buserelin in premenopausal women. *Clin Endocrinol* 29:45-51, 1988.

Maxson WS: Use of progesterone in the treatment of PMS. *Clin Obstet Gynecol* 30:465-477, 1987.

McFarland KF, et al: Risk factors and noncontraceptive estrogen use in women with and without coronary disease. *Am Heart J* 117:1209-1214, 1989.

Meldrum DR, et al: Pituitary hormones during menopausal hot flush. *Obstet Gynecol* 64:752-756, 1984.

Melnick S, et al: Rates and risks of diethylstilbestrol-related clear-cell adenocarcinoma of vagina and cervix: Update. *N Engl J Med* 316:514-516, 1987.

Mercaitis PA, et al: Effect of danazol on vocal pitch: Case study. *Obstet Gynecol* 65:131-135, 1985.

Messinis IE, Lolis D: Treatment of premenstrual mastalgia with tamoxifen. *Acta Obstet Gynecol Scand* 67:307-309, 1988.

Metzger DA, Luciano AA: Hormonal therapy of endometriosis: *Obstet Gynecol Clin North Am* 16:105-122, 1989.

Miller JA, Jacobs HS: Treatment of hirsutism and acne with cyproterone acetate. *Clin Endocrinol Metab* 15:373-389, 1986.

Miller-Bass K, Adashi EY: Current status and future prospects of transdermal estrogen replacement therapy. *Fertil Steril* 53:961-974, 1990.

Miodrag A, et al: Sex hormones and the female urinary tract. *Drugs* 36:491-504, 1988.

Mishell DR Jr, et al: Menorrhagia: Symposium. *J Reprod Med* 29:763-782, 1984.

Mishell DR Jr, et al: Postmenopausal hormone replacement with a combination estrogen-progestin regimen for five days per week. *J Reprod Med* 36:351-355, (May) 1991.

Moghissi KS, Boyce CR: Management of endometriosis with oral medroxyprogesterone acetate. *Obstet Gynecol* 47:265-267, 1976.

Motta T, et al: Flutamide in the treatment of hirsutism. *Int J Gynecol Obstet* 36:155-157, 1991.

Muse KN, et al: Premenstrual syndrome: Effects of "medical ovariectomy." *N Engl J Med* 311:1345-1349, 1984.

Nagamani M, et al: Treatment of menopausal hot flushes with transdermal administration of clonidine. *Am J Obstet Gynecol* 156:561-565, 1987.

Nasri MN, et al: The role of vaginal scan in measurement of endometrial thickness in postmenopausal women. *Br J Obstet Gynecol* 98:470-475, 1991.

Nichols KC, et al: 17β-estradiol for postmenopausal estrogen replacement therapy. *Obstet Gynecol Surv* 39(suppl):230-245, 1984.

Normann EK, et al: Height reduction in 539 tall girls treated with three different dosages of ethinyloestradiol. *Arch Dis Child* 66:1275-1278, 1991.

Notelovitz M: Estrogen replacement therapy: Indications, contraindications, and agent selection. *Am J Obstet Gynecol* 161:8-17, 1989.

Notelovitz M, et al: Combination estrogen and progestogen replacement therapy does not adversely affect coagulation. *Obstet Gynecol* 62:596-600, 1983.

Ober WB, Bronstein SB: Endometrial morphology following oral administration of quinestrol. *Int J Fertil* 12:210-228, 1967.

O'Brien PMS, et al: Treatment of premenstrual syndrome by spironolactone. *Br J Obstet Gynecol* 86:142-147, 1979.

O'Brien RC, et al: Comparison of sequential cyproterone acetate/estrogen versus spironolactone/oral contraceptive in the treatment of hirsutism. *J Clin Endocrinol Metab* 72:1008-1013, 1991.

Olsson J-H, et al: Danazol concentrations in human ovarian follicular fluid and their relationship to simultaneous serum concentrations. *Fertil Steril* 49:42-46, 1988.

Ottosson UB, et al: Subfractions of high-density lipoprotein cholesterol during estrogen replacement therapy: A comparison between progestogens and natural progesterone. *Am J Obstet Gynecol* 151:746-750, 1985.

Padwick ML, et al: Simple method for determining optimal dosage of progestin in postmenopausal women receiving estrogens. *N Engl J Med* 315:930-934, 1986.

Paganini-Hill A, et al: Postmenopausal oestrogen treatment and stroke: Prospective study. *BMJ* 297:519-522, 1988.

Palmer JR, et al: Breast cancer risk after estrogen replacement therapy: Results from the Toronto Breast Cancer Study. *Am J Epidemiol* 134:1386-1395, 1991.

Panahy C, et al: Effects of danazol on incidence of progesterone and oestrogen receptors in benign breast disease. *BMJ* 295:464-466, 1987.

Pepper G, et al: Ketoconazole use in the treatment of ovarian hyperandrogenism. *Fertil Steril* 54:438-444, 1990.

Peress MR, et al: Female pseudohermaphroditism with somatic chromosomal anomaly in association with in utero exposure to danazol. *Am J Obstet Gynecol* 142:708-709, 1982.

Place VA, et al: Double-blind comparative study of Estraderm and Premarin in amelioration of postmenopausal symptoms. *Am J Obstet Gynecol* 152:1092-1099, 1985.

Powers MS, et al: Pharmacokinetics and pharmacodynamics of transdermal dosage forms of 17β-estradiol: Comparison with conventional oral estrogens used for hormone replacement. *Am J Obstet Gynecol* 152:1099-1106, 1985.

Press MF, et al: Estrogen receptor localization in the female genital tract. *Am J Pathol* 123:280-292, 1986.

Prince RL, et al: Prevention of postmenopausal osteoporosis: A comparative study of exercise, calcium supplementation, and hormone-replacement therapy. *N Engl J Med* 325:1189-1195, 1991.

Prough SG, et al: Continuous estrogen/progestin therapy in menopause. *Am J Obstet Gynecol* 157:1449-1453, 1987.

Puolakka J, et al: Biochemical and clinical effects of treating the premenstrual syndrome with prostaglandin synthesis precursors. *J Reprod Med* 30:149-153, 1985.

Rawal MY, et al: Double-blind comparison of efficacy and safety of naproxen and placebo in the treatment of dysmenorrhea. *Curr Ther Res* 42:1073-1080, 1987.

Reichel RP, et al: Goserelin (Zoladex) depot in the treatment of endometriosis. *Fertil Steril* 57:1197-1202, 1992.

Rein MS, et al: Fibroid and myometrial steroid receptors in women treated with gonadotropin-releasing hormone agonist leuprolide acetate. *Fertil Steril* 53:1018-1023, 1990.

Reingold SB, Rosenfield RL: Relationship of mild hirsutism or acne in women to androgens. *Arch Dermatol* 123:209-212, 1987.

Ressegiue LJ, et al: Congenital malformations among offspring exposed in utero to progestins, Olmsted County, Minnesota, 1936-1974. *Fertil Steril* 43:514-519, 1985.

Ribot C, et al: Preventive effects of transdermal administration of 17β-estradiol on postmenopausal bone loss: A 2-year prospective study. *Obstet Gynecol* 75(suppl):42S-46S, (April) 1990.

Rittmaster RS, Loriaux DL: Hirsutism. *Ann Intern Med* 106:95-107, 1987.

Robboy SJ, et al: Pathologic findings in young women enrolled in National Cooperative Diethylstilbestrol Adenosis (DESAD) Project. *Obstet Gynecol* 53:309-317, 1979.

Rosenberg L, et al: Early menopause and risk of myocardial infarction. *Am J Obstet Gynecol* 139:47-51, 1981.

Ross JL, et al: Preliminary study of effect of estrogen dose on growth in Turner's syndrome. *N Engl J Med* 309:1104-1106, 1983.

Ross JL, et al: Effect of low doses of estradiol on 6-month growth rates and predicted height in patients with Turner syndrome. *J Pediatr* 109:950-953, 1986.

Ross RK, et al: Cardiovascular benefits of estrogen replacement therapy. *Am J Obstet Gynecol* 160:1301-1306, 1989.

Roy S: Double-blind comparison of propionic acid derivative (ibuprofen) and fenamate (mefenamic acid) in treatment of dysmenorrhea. *Obstet Gynecol* 61:628-632, 1983.

Seibel MM, et al: Effectiveness of danazol on subsequent fertility in minimal endometriosis. *Fertil Steril* 38:534-537, 1982.

Semmens JP, Wagner G: Estrogen deprivation and vaginal function in postmenopausal women. *JAMA* 248:445-448, 1982.

Shangold MM: Update: Advising patients about exercise. *Fertil News* 16:3-5, (Summer) 1982.

Shangold M, et al: Evaluation and management of menstrual dysfunction in athletes. *JAMA* 263:1665-1669, 1990.

Shapiro SS: Treatment of dysmenorrhoea and premenstrual syndrome with non-steroidal anti-inflammatory drugs. *Drugs* 36:475-490, 1988.

Shapiro S, et al: Risk of localized and widespread endometrial cancer in relation to recent and discontinued use of conjugated estrogens. *N Engl J Med* 313:969-972, 1985.

Siegel SF, et al: ACTH stimulation tests and plasma dehydroepiandrosterone sulfate levels in women with hirsutism. *N Engl J Med* 323:849-854, 1990.

Sillero-Arenas M, et al: Menopausal hormone replacement therapy and breast cancer: A meta-analysis. *Obstet Gynecol* 79:286-294, 1992.

Smith RP: Primary dysmenorrhea and the adolescent patient. *Adolesc Pediatr Gynecol* 1:23-30, 1988.

Smith S, Schiff I: The premenstrual syndrome: Diagnosis and management. *Fertil Steril* 52:527-543, 1989.

Sonino N, et al: Low-dose ketoconazole treatment in hirsute women. *J Endocrinol Invest* 13:35-40, 1990.

Soper JT, Creasman WT: Vulvar dystrophies. *Clin Obstet Gynecol* 29:431-439, 1986.

Stampfer MJ, Colditz GA: Estrogen replacement therapy and coronary heart disease: A quantitative assessment of the epidemiologic evidence. *Prev Med* 20:47-63, 1991.

Stampfer MJ, et al: Postmenopausal estrogen therapy and cardiovascular disease. *N Engl J Med* 325:756-762, 1991.

Stanczyk FZ, et al: Randomized comparison of nonoral estradiol delivery in postmenopausal women. *Am J Obstet Gynecol* 159:1540-1546, 1988.

Stavraky KM, et al: Comparison of estrogen use by women with endometrial cancer, gynecologic disorders, and other illnesses. *Am J Obstet Gynecol* 141:547-555, 1981.

Steinberg KK, et al: A meta-analysis of the effect of estrogen replacement therapy on the risk of breast cancer. *JAMA* 265:1985-1990, 1991.

Steingold KA, et al: Danazol inhibits steroidogenesis by human ovary in vivo. *Fertil Steril* 45:649-654, 1986.

Stevenson JC, et al: Effects of transdermal versus oral hormone replacement therapy on bone density in spine and proximal femur in postmenopausal women. *Lancet* 336:265-269, 1990.

Strickler RC: Dysfunctional uterine bleeding in ovulatory women. *Postgrad Med* 77:235-246, (Jan) 1985.

Sullivan JM, et al: Postmenopausal estrogen use and coronary atherosclerosis. *Ann Intern Med* 108:358-363, 1988.

Surrey ES, Halme J: Endometriosis as a cause of infertility. *Obstet Gynecol Clin North Am* 16:79-91, 1989.

Surrey ES, et al: The effects of combining norethindrone with a gonadotropin-releasing hormone agonist in the treatment of symptomatic endometriosis. *Fertil Steril* 53:620-626, 1990.

Thomas EJ, et al: The combination of a depot gonadotrophin releasing hormone agonist and cyclical hormone replacement therapy for dysfunctional uterine bleeding. *Br J Obstet Gynaecol* 98:1155-1159, 1991.

Tikkanen MJ, et al: Postmenopausal hormone replacement therapy: Effects of progestogens on serum lipids and lipoproteins; review. *Maturitas* 8:7-17, 1986.

Tosteson ANA, et al: Cost effectiveness of screening perimenopausal white women for osteoporosis: Bone densitometry and hormone replacement therapy. *Ann Intern Med* 113:594-603, 1990.

Tremblay RR: Treatment of hirsutism with spironolactone. *Clin Endocrinol Metab* 15:363-371, 1986.

Tulandi T, Lal S: Menopausal hot flush. *Obstet Gynecol Surv* 40:553-563, 1985.

Tummon IS, et al: Bone mineral density in women with endometriosis before and during ovarian suppression with gonadotropin-releasing hormone agonists or danazol. *Fertil Steril* 49:792-796, 1988.

Tummon IS, et al: A randomized, prospective comparison of endocrine changes induced with intranasal leuprolide or danazol for treatment of endometriosis. *Fertil Steril* 51:390-394, 1989.

Turkalj I, et al: Surveillance of bromocriptine in pregnancy. *JAMA* 247:1589-1591, 1982.

Utian WH: Fate of untreated menopause. *Obstet Gynecol Clin North Am* 14:1-11, 1987.

Välimäki M, et al: Comparison between the effects of nafarelin and danazol on serum lipids and lipoproteins in patients with endometriosis. *J Clin Endocrinol Metab* 69:1097-1103, 1989.

Varner RE, et al: Transvaginal sonography of the endometrium in postmenopausal women. *Obstet Gynecol* 78:195-199, 1991.

Vellacott ID, et al: Double-blind placebo-controlled evaluation of spironolactone in premenstrual syndrome. *Curr Med Res Opin* 10:450-456, 1987.

Venturini PL, et al: Endocrine, metabolic, and clinical effects of gestrinone in women with endometriosis. *Fertil Steril* 52:589-595, 1989.

Venturini PL, et al: Treatment of endometriosis with goserelin depot, a long-acting gonadotropin-releasing hormone agonist analog: Endocrine and clinical results. *Fertil Steril* 54:1021-1027, 1990.

Veridiano NP, et al: Delayed onset of clear cell adenocarcinoma of vagina in DES-exposed progeny. *Obstet Gynecol* 57:395-398, 1981.

Vessey MP, et al: Randomized double-blind clinical controlled trial of value of stilbestrol therapy in pregnancy: Long-term follow-up of mothers and their offspring. *Br J Obstet Gynaecol* 90:1007-1017, 1983.

Vigersky RA, et al: Treatment of hirsute women with cimetidine: Preliminary report. *N Engl J Med* 303:1042, 1980.

Vollenhoven BJ, et al: Clinical predictors for buserelin acetate treatment of uterine fibroids: A prospective study of 40 women. *Fertil Steril* 54:1032-1038, 1990 A.

Vollenhoven BJ, et al: Uterine fibroids: A clinical review. *Br J Obstet Gynaecol* 97:285-298, 1990 B.

Wahl P, et al: Effect of estrogen/progestin potency on lipid/lipoprotein cholesterol. *N Engl J Med* 308:862-867, 1983.

Ways SC, et al: Alterations in immune responsiveness in women exposed to diethylstilbestrol in utero. *Fertil Steril* 48:193-197, 1987.

Weinstein L, et al: Evaluation of a continuous combined low-dose regimen of estrogen-progestin for treatment of the menopausal patient. *Am J Obstet Gynecol* 162:1534-1542, 1990.

Wenzloff NJ, Shimp L: Therapeutic management of primary dysmenorrhea. *DICP* 18:22-26, 1984.

West CP, et al: Shrinkage of uterine fibroids during therapy with goserelin (Zoladex): Luteinizing hormone-releasing hormone agonist administered as monthly subcutaneous depot. *Fertil Steril* 48:45-51, 1987.

Wheeler JM, et al: Depot leuprolide versus danazol in treatment of women with symptomatic endometriosis: I. Efficacy results. *Am J Obstet Gynecol* 167:1367-1371, 1992.

Whitehead ED, Leiter E: Genital abnormalities and abnormal semen analyses in male patients exposed to diethylstilbestrol in utero. *J Urol* 125:47-50, 1981.

Whitehead MI, et al: The role and use of progestogens. *Obstet Gynecol* 75 (suppl):59S-76S, (April) 1990.

Wild RA, et al: Androgen parameters and their correlation with body weight in one hundred thirty-eight women thought to have hyperandrogenism. *Am J Obstet Gynecol* 146:602-606, 1983.

Wingo PA, et al: Risk of breast cancer in postmenopausal women who have used estrogen replacement therapy. *JAMA* 257:209-215, 1987.

Wood SH, et al: Treatment of premenstrual syndrome with fluoxetine: A double-blind, placebo-controlled, crossover study. *Obstet Gynecol* 80:339–344, 1992.

Yahiro J, et al: Exaggerated gonadotropin response to luteinizing hormone-releasing hormone in amenorrheic runners. *Am J Obstet Gynecol* 156:586-591, 1987.

Yancey MK, et al: Serum lipids and lipoproteins in continuous or cyclic medroxyprogesterone acetate treatment in postmenopausal women treated with conjugated estrogens. *Fertil Steril* 54:778-782, 1990.

Yemini M, et al: Prevention of premature labor by 17α-hydroxyprogesterone caproate. *Am J Obstet Gynecol* 151:574-577, 1985.

Ylikorkala O, et al: Desogestrel- and levonorgestrel-containing oral contraceptives have different effects on urinary excretion of prostacyclin metabolites and serum high density lipoproteins. *J Clin Endocrinol Metab* 65:1238-1242, 1987.

Young RL, et al: Management of menopause when estrogen cannot be used. *Drugs* 40:220-230, 1990.

Yovich JL, et al: Medroxyprogesterone acetate therapy in early pregnancy has no apparent fetal effects. *Teratology* 38:135-144, 1988.

Drugs Used to Treat Female Infertility

52

Approximately 15% of couples who wish to have a child experience some type of infertility; another 10% have fewer children than desired. Successful pregnancy is achieved in about one-half of the couples who seek medical attention.

Couples who embark on a program of drug treatment for infertility should be counseled carefully and should be fully aware of the potential side effects of this form of therapy and the extended treatment period that may be required. They also should be prepared for the anxiety, frustration, and disappointment that may accompany unsuccessful cycles of treatment and realize that these problems are common to many couples in this circumstance.

Requirements for Fertility: Fertility depends on a complex and integrated hormonal milieu, the anatomic integrity of the reproductive organs, and functional gametes. The responsibility and contribution of the male reproductive system are, in general, the production and delivery of mature, motile sperm in sufficient number and quality to effect fertilization. The role of the female extends beyond gamete production to encompass transport of the male gamete, provision of a hospitable environment for fertilization of the oocyte and implantation of the blastocyst, and maintenance of the sophisticated life support system that nurtures the developing fetus until viability in the external environment is assured.

In both sexes, the physiologic stimulus for gametogenesis is produced by gonadotropins, which are secreted by the anterior pituitary gland. The anterior pituitary releases both follicle stimulating hormone (FSH) and luteinizing hormone (LH) in response to pulsatile production by the hypothalamus of gonadotropin-releasing hormone (GnRH), also called luteinizing hormone-releasing hormone (LHRH). FSH and LH are named for their actions in the female, although they are also necessary for normal reproductive function in the male. In females, FSH stimulates the growth of follicles in the ovary and induces the aromatase enzyme in the granulosa cells. LH stimulates the production of androgens by the thecal cells of the follicle before ovulation; these hormones are aromatized by granulosa cells to estradiol and, to a lesser extent, estrone. LH also stimulates estrogen and progesterone production by the luteinized granulosa and thecal cells of the corpus luteum (CL) after ovulation.

A slight surge in FSH coupled with a pronounced surge in LH secretion occurs at midcycle. The LH surge stimulates ovulation of the mature follicle, and FSH, in the presence of estrogen, induces formation of LH/hCG (human chorionic gonadotropin) receptors on the granulosa cells, thus assuring CL responsiveness to LH or hCG. Estrogen and progesterone produced by the CL prepare the endometrium for nidation. The CL is necessary to support the endometrium during the early weeks of pregnancy before the placenta assumes its steroidogenic function.

Even in the presence of perfectly functioning male and female reproductive systems, coitus must occur during the time when the fertile lives of the sperm (estimated 36 to 72 hours) and the ovum (estimated 12 to 24 hours) overlap. If coitus occurs at least twice weekly, sperm capable of fertilization are almost always present in the woman's reproductive tract, assuming normal receptiveness of her cervical mucus. The pregnancy rate may be improved if intercourse is timed to coincide with ovulation. Timing may be improved by tracking basal body temperature, monitoring cervical mucus, measuring progesterone at midcycle, measuring LH levels in urine or serum, and evaluating follicular growth and endometrial development with ultrasound.

Diagnosis of Infertility: Evaluation of infertility should involve both partners. A detailed description of diagnostic procedures is beyond the scope of this book. The appropriate selection and sequence of tests can maximize the amount of information gained and eventually may spare the couple the time and expense of further testing, the possibility of inappropriate drug therapy, and unwarranted hopefulness. An accurate medical history, including the frequency and timing of coitus, may suggest the need for education rather than infertility tests. A likely cause of infertility deserving early evaluation (eg, mumps orchitis in the male, pelvic inflammatory dis-

SOME EFFECTS OF DRUGS ON FEMALE FERTILITY

Drug	Reported Effect
Busulfan [Myleran]	Amenorrhea, ovarian failure
Chlorambucil [Leukeran]	Amenorrhea, ovarian failure
Cyclophosphamide [Cytoxan, Neosar]	Amenorrhea, ovarian failure
Diethylstilbestrol (use in pregnancy)	*Daughters:* Reduced fertility; increased spontaneous abortions; ectopic pregnancy
DNA-damaging Oncolytic Drugs	See index entry Antineoplastic Agents, DNA Damaging Drugs
Heroin, cocaine ("crack")	Oligomenorrhea; amenorrhea
Levothyroxine [Levothroid, Synthroid]	Anovulation (excessive dose)
Marijuana	Abnormal menstruation; anovulation; decrease of LH
Methyldopa [Aldomet]	Amenorrhea, hyperprolactinemia
Metoclopramide [Reglan]	Amenorrhea, hyperprolactinemia
Nicotine (smoking)	Premature ovarian failure
Spironolactone [Aldactone]	Irregular menses or amenorrhea
Thioridazine [Mellaril]; other antipsychotic drugs	Hyperprolactinemia, amenorrhea

ease or abnormal menstrual function in the female) also may be revealed (see also Jaffe and Jewelewicz, 1991).

A variety of agents also affect fertility in both females and males (see the Table in this chapter and index entry Infertility: Effects of Drugs on Male Fertility [Table]). The effects may be reversible on discontinuation of the drug.

Because the male is the sole partner affected in up to 40% of infertile couples, or because both partners may have impaired reproductive capacity, the couple should be evaluated simultaneously. One or two semen analyses are performed initially. A postcoital test immediately preceding or at ovulation has been used routinely to measure the quality of cervical mucus and evaluate the interaction between sperm and cervical secretions; however, the validity of this procedure as a test to predict the likelihood of pregnancy has been questioned (Griffith and Grimes, 1990). Basal body temperature patterns, measurements of serum progesterone levels at the midluteal phase, and/or endometrial biopsy provide presumptive evidence of ovulatory function. Patency of the fallopian tubes can be demonstrated by hysterosalpingography. Optimal timing of tests allows complete evaluation within two cycles (ie, postcoital tests just before ovulation, endometrial biopsy just before menses, hysterosalpingogram immediately after menses, temperature chart throughout cycle). Care must be taken in interpreting the results of a postcoital test if it is performed following the hysterosalpingogram, for residual contrast media may complicate test interpretation. Measurements of serum prolactin and thyroid stimulating hormone (TSH) are useful to rule out hyperprolactinemia and hypothyroidism, respectively, in patients with ovulatory dysfunction.

When these measures fail to determine the source of infertility, hysterosalpingography is a useful screening procedure that provides important data about the uterine cavity and reveals abnormalities in 10% or more of infertile women. However, its role in infertility investigation is undergoing reanalysis because of higher false-positive and false-negative tubal patency rates compared with laparoscopy (Rice et al, 1986). Laparoscopy may reveal an initially unsuspected cause of infertility (eg, endometriosis, peritubal adhesions) in up to 40% of women tested. Usually this procedure is delayed for up to six months after normal hysterosalpingography because the likelihood of pregnancy is increased during this interval. An alternative is to perform hysteroscopy at the time of laparoscopy.

TREATMENT OF FEMALE INFERTILITY

Female infertility can result from any interference with the necessary delicate hormonal integration that results in failure of ovulation, impairment of the lifespan and function of the CL, or impediment in the access of the sperm to the ovum. The primary causes of female infertility are functional (eg, ovulatory dysfunction) or anatomic (eg, obstruction of the fallopian tubes). Drug therapy has been used to treat infertility due to anovulation, hyperprolactinemia, endometriosis, luteal phase defect, and unfavorable cervical mucus and when the cause is unknown, but clinical studies have failed to support the efficacy of some treatments. See sections below for evaluation of drug therapy for specific diagnoses. See also reviews by Speroff, 1990; Zeevi et al, 1991.

Drug Therapy: Since FSH and LH are necessary to support gametogenesis, clomiphene [Clomid, Serophene], menotropins (hMG) [Pergonal], urofollitropin (FSH) [Metrodin], human chorionic gonadotropin (hCG) [A.P.L., Follutein, Pregnyl, Profasi HP], and gonadorelin (GnRH) [Lutrepulse] can be used to treat anovulation secondary to inadequate secretion or abnormal patterns of secretion of these gonadotropic hormones. Clomiphene stimulates secretion of gonadotropins by the pituitary, while menotropins, urofollitropin, and hCG replace these hormones and directly stimulate the ovary.

Clomiphene requires feedback between the anterior pituitary gland and the hypothalamus to be effective, because endogenous secretion of gonadotropin is stimulated by this agent. Menotropins, a preparation of human menopausal gonadotropins (hMG), contains both FSH and LH activity. It is indicated when the pituitary gland cannot secrete these hormones in response to stimulation or when clomiphene therapy has been unsuccessful in establishing ovulation or pregnancy. Urofollitropin also is used to induce ovulation, and has an advantage in some patients in that it does not contain LH. (Excessive LH levels are thought to be detrimental to the oocyte and to induce premature luteinization.) HCG has the biological activity of LH and stimulates ovulation of follicles that have been stimulated by clomiphene, menotropins, or urofollitropin. In addition to its use as a diagnostic agent, in properly selected patients, pulsatile administration of gonadorelin may induce ovulation by stimulating the gonadotrophs of the anterior pituitary to produce FSH and LH; therefore, an intact anterior pituitary is required.

Danazol, progestins, GnRH agonists, or oral contraceptives are used to treat endometriosis, but evidence increasingly suggests that such therapy does not necessarily enhance fertility in women with mild to moderate disease. Bromocriptine reduces the secretion of abnormally high levels of prolactin and often normalizes cyclic ovulation. When adrenal hyperandrogenism causes ovulatory dysfunction, glucocorticoids suppress excess androgen secretion.

Anovulation and Oligo-ovulation

Clomiphene (alone or with other agents), menotropins, urofollitropin, and hCG are used to treat ovulatory dysfunction. Clomiphene stimulates the endogenous secretion of gonadotropins by an antiestrogenic mechanism, while menotropins and hCG are used to control ovarian hyperstimulation or after clomiphene has failed to induce ovulation, particularly in patients with hypothalamic amenorrhea. In a small number of women, menotropins and hCG replace inadequate quantities of gonadotropins. Gonadorelin, the synthetic form of GnRH, also may be used to induce ovulation; a pulsatile pattern of administration mimics normal endogenous GnRH secretion and stimulates gonadotropin release. There is some evidence that all of these drugs improve cycle fecundity in apparently normally ovulating women (Welner et al, 1988; Aboulghar et al, 1989; Fisch et al, 1989), possibly by stimulating development of multiple follicles. Tamoxifen [Nolvadex], another antiestrogenic compound, has been used investigationally as an alternative to clomiphene.

Clomiphene: The ideal candidates for clomiphene therapy secrete gonadotropins and estrogen but fail to ovulate at all or in a timely fashion because of an abnormality in the feedback mechanisms that control gonadotropin secretion. Menstruation is a demonstration of gonadotropin production, ovarian responsiveness to gonadotropin (ie, secretion of estrogen), and endometrial responsiveness to ovarian steroids. In women with amenorrhea, estrogenic stimulation of the endometrium and a patent outflow tract can be demonstrated by a positive (ie, bleeding within one or two weeks) response to a progesterone withdrawal test (preferably one intramuscular injection of progesterone in oil 100 to 200 mg or oral medroxyprogesterone acetate [Provera] 10 mg daily for five to ten days). Pregnancy should be ruled out with an assay for hCG before a synthetic progestin is administered. Negative results of the test and low concentrations of serum estradiol are predictive of a poor outcome for use of clomiphene. A negative response and a high serum FSH level indicate ovarian failure, which is not responsive to clomiphene or gonadotropin therapy. Women with low or normal gonadotropin levels who do not experience withdrawal bleeding in response to progestins are unlikely to respond to clomiphene, although this agent should be tried in view of its lower cost and lower risk of multiple births compared with menotropins. Women who respond to clomiphene usually have normal FSH and estrogen concentrations and normal to high LH levels.

Before beginning clomiphene therapy, pregnancy should be ruled out and a semen analysis completed. An endometrial biopsy may be performed in patients with long-term anovulation or bleeding of undetermined origin to identify possible endometrial hyperplasia or carcinoma. This is especially important in obese women, who are at greater risk for endometrial carcinoma. Any remaining tests can be performed as needed during the early treatment cycles or as indicated by findings of the initial history and physical examination.

Although the ovulation rate in properly selected patients approaches 75% with use of clomiphene, the pregnancy rate may be only 25% to 45%. Several possibilities may explain this apparent discrepancy: (1) About one-third of clomiphene-treated ovulatory cycles result in either inadequate progesterone production by the CL or an inadequately stimulated endometrium that does not support implantation (luteal phase dysfunction). (2) The antiestrogenic effect of large doses of clomiphene may interfere with production of cervical mucus, thus making sperm penetration unlikely. (3) Luteinization of an unruptured follicle may produce presumptive signs of ovulation, but the ovum is not available for fertilization (luteinized unruptured follicle syndrome). (4) The antiestrogenic component of clomiphene may arrest postfertilization development of the preimplantation embryo through interference with cytoplasmic maturation of the oocyte (Yoshimura and Wallach, 1987).

Menotropins (hMG): Therapy with menotropins is complex and should be undertaken only by a physician experienced in its use and with the patient's full understanding and cooperation. Monitoring of the patient during treatment requires laboratory facilities capable of completing daily serum estradiol assays, including weekends and holidays. Serum estradiol concentration reflects total estrogen production by the ovaries and is not a reliable indication of the number of developing follicles or their stage of maturity (Hull et al, 1986). Utilization of ultrasonography in conjunction with serum estradiol measurements is strongly recommended. If ultrasound examination reveals three or more mature follicles, it has been suggested that administration of hCG be withheld regardless of the serum estradiol level (Adoni et al, 1986). In one study, ovulation occurred in at least 75.2% of patients when follicles measured $\geq$17 mm on the day of hCG administration (Silverberg et al, 1991). If more than one follicle has matured, the couple should be informed about the risk of multiple gestation. A profile of the number and size of all ovarian follicles determined by ultrasound may minimize the risk of ovarian hyperstimulation and multiple gestation; however, visualization of a single mature follicle does not preclude multiple gestation. The occurrence and severity of hyperstimulation increase as the number of follicles and the proportion of small follicles increase. Thus, an unfavorable profile can be identified even if the serum estrogen is within acceptable limits (Blankstein et al, 1987). See also the review on hyperstimulation by Golan et al, 1989.

Induction of ovulation with menotropins usually is reserved for patients who require exogenous supplementation of gonadotropins to achieve pregnancy (Shoham et al, 1991 A). It is the only therapy that can stimulate ovulation in hypophysectomized patients. Anovulatory women with deficient production of gonadotropins and estrogen also are likely to respond to therapy. Some patients who are able to produce estrogen but fail to ovulate with clomiphene may respond to menotropins. Some practitioners recommend a trial of menotropins with or without concomitant intrauterine insemination before resorting to other assisted reproductive technologies (eg, in vitro fertilization [IVF], gamete intrafallopian transfer [GIFT]) in patients with unexplained infertility or who have not responded to other measures. IVF is the more appropriate approach in those with severe tubal pathology.

Patients with ovarian failure, as demonstrated by high levels of serum gonadotropins, are generally not suitable candidates for menotropins. However, pregnancy rarely has been reported in women with premature ovarian failure who received replacement therapy, oral contraceptives, or no treatment (Aiman and Smentek, 1985; Alper et al, 1986).

Patients with polycystic ovaries (PCO) may be hypersensitive to menotropins. Those who do not respond to clomiphene and hCG may be given menotropins with caution (see following discussion on this disorder).

Because of the expense and the potential for complications (eg, multiple births, hyperstimulation syndrome), infertility testing should be performed prior to initiating menotropins treatment to rule out and treat other causes. The cost of the drug may be $500 to $1,500 per cycle, excluding laboratory and physicians' fees. A course of clomiphene combined with hCG may be given before menotropins therapy is begun because, rarely, hypogonadotropic patients will respond to the former agent.

As with clomiphene, there is a discrepancy between the ovulatory and pregnancy rates with menotropins. In properly selected patients, ovulatory rates approach 100%, but only 60% to 80% of treated women become pregnant. Multiple gestations due to ovulation of multiple ova occur in 8% to 30% of pregnancies, and 75% of these result in delivery of twins. Spontaneous abortion is observed in about 25% to 30% of pregnancies and is more likely with multiple gestations. Older patients and/or those who are significantly overweight are at increased risk of spontaneous abortion. In the latter case, an altered hormonal milieu related to excess weight may be contributory. Women whose first menotropins-induced pregnancy aborted spontaneously, especially those who are overweight, also may be at higher risk for spontaneous abortion in subsequent induced pregnancies (Bohrer and Kemmann, 1987; Corsan and Kemmann, 1990). In a study in which ovulation was induced by a variety of regimens, women who had spontaneous abortions had lower serum progesterone:estradiol ratios at the time of implantation compared with those who had successful pregnancies or did not conceive (Maclin et al, 1990). The incidence of congenital abnormalities is not increased with menotropins, FSH, or clomiphene therapy.

Combination Therapy: Selected patients who do not respond to standard ovulation-inducing regimens may benefit from combinations of the above agents. HCG may be added to a clomiphene regimen when patients do not ovulate with clomiphene alone but show evidence of follicular development. These patients may be lacking only the LH surge, which hCG replaces. Other failures with clomiphene may be due to a short luteal phase after ovulation, which also may respond to hCG. (See the evaluation on Clomiphene Citrate for dosages.)

Some candidates for menotropins therapy who retain partial hypothalamic-pituitary-ovarian responsiveness (withdrawal bleeding after administration of progesterone indicating estrogen effect) may benefit from the combined actions of clomiphene, menotropins, and hCG. Partial follicular maturation is induced by clomiphene so that smaller doses of menotropins may be used. HCG is employed as usual to stimulate ovulation. Monitoring is the same as with menotropins-hCG therapy, and the possibility of ovarian hyperstimulation and multiple gestations also is similar. The rationale for this regimen is based on economic, not physiologic, considerations. Preliminary results suggest that the dose of menotropins may be reduced by one-half, thus providing financial relief for this costly therapy (March et al, 1976). (See the evaluation on Menotropins for dosage.)

In a randomized, double-blind, placebo-controlled trial, lower doses of menotropins were needed to stimulate ovulation when human growth hormone was added to the regimen (Homburg et al, 1990).

Gonadorelin (GnRH): This decapeptide hormone may be used to induce ovulation in patients with hypothalamic amenorrhea resulting from disease or traumatic destruction of the hypothalamus or pituitary stalk; weight loss, exercise, or stress; or Kallman's syndrome or other congenital disorders. Gonadorelin must be administered parenterally, and pulsatile administration is required. Ovulation has been induced and pregnancies have been achieved using portable pumps that deliver pulses of gonadorelin intravenously or subcutaneously. Although some authorities may prefer one route of administration over the other, overall results appear comparable (80% to 90% ovulatory cycles; $>$25% cycles achieving pregnancy). However, there are differences that may influence the choice of route for a particular patient.

Intravenous administration produces serum LH concentrations that are sharply peaked and closer to the endogenous pattern, whereas the LH peaks with subcutaneous administration are more blunted and prolonged. Pregnancies are achieved with lower dosages of intravenous gonadorelin (usually 2.5 to 5 mcg versus 5 to 20 mcg for the subcutaneous route), thus reducing the cost per cycle of treatment. Advantages of the subcutaneous route are the low incidence of complications and ease of use. However, infections and pain at the injection site are common, although no major complications have been reported.

In addition to resolving the choice between the subcutaneous and intravenous routes, other issues require further study. These include development of protocols for specific diagnoses and individual patient response and determination of the most beneficial pulse duration, interval, and dose.

Most patients are given hCG or the gonadorelin infusion is continued for luteal support until pregnancy is diagnosed or menses occurs. However, the continued use of gonadorelin increases the inconvenience and expense of therapy and has no demonstrated advantage.

Induction of ovulation with gonadorelin should be monitored carefully in a manner similar to that used for menotropins therapy. Serum estradiol concentrations and ultrasonography should be utilized. See also review by Filicori et al, 1991.

Although hyperstimulation and multiple births may occur, their frequencies appear to be lower than with menotropins therapy. Multiple gestations occur in approximately 7% of pregnancies, and 75% of these gestations result in delivery of twins. The frequency of spontaneous abortions is not increased. Formation of antibodies to GnRH has been reported, but no adverse clinical effect due to antibodies has yet been identified (see reviews by Wong and Asch, 1987; Reid et al, 1988; and Insler, 1988).

Gonadorelin infusion appears to be an effective option for inducing ovulation when conventional methods fail, and it may have advantages over menotropins therapy. The costs of the two methods are approximately equivalent (Sueldo and Swanson, 1986); the higher cost of menotropins is balanced by the expense of the infusion equipment required for gonadorelin therapy. Use of infusion equipment is inconvenient and cumbersome for the patient. The more convenient intranasal route is being investigated.

Polycystic Ovary

Polycystic ovary (PCO) is the most common hyperandrogenic condition associated with female infertility. It is characterized by anovulation and, frequently, by amenorrhea, obesity, and hirsutism. The ovaries may be enlarged with multiple cystic follicles surrounded by a thickened ovarian capsule. Although the etiology varies, pathophysiologic events probably include lack of sufficient follicular stimulation by FSH leading to increased androgen secretion by the follicle; peripheral conversion of the excess androgen (particularly in adipose tissue of obese patients) to estrone; increased intraovarian androgens contributing to accelerated follicular atresia; and increased tonic LH secretion due to slightly elevated estrogen (increased LH:FSH ratio) that stimulates ovarian androgen secretion. Peripherally, the elevated levels of serum androgens decrease sex hormone-binding globulin (SHBG), which may increase the amount of biologically active free serum testosterone in the presence of normal total serum testosterone.

The patient's history often suggests onset of PCO at puberty, perhaps due to excess adrenal androgen production in a disordered adrenarche. Some patients with clinical features of PCO and elevated serum testosterone and 17-hydroxyprogesterone levels may have late-onset congenital adrenal hyperplasia (CAH) (Benjamin et al, 1986; Brodie and Wentz, 1987; New, 1988). Elevated adrenal androgen secretion also occurs in late-onset CAH. In patients with PCO, the aberrations in gonadotropin levels are intermediate between those in normal individuals and those with CAH (Levin et al, 1991). The presence of hyperprolactinemia in some patients with PCO is consistent with an estrogen-induced decrease in hypothalamic dopamine and an increase in LH secretion. Prolactin may stimulate the secretion of adrenal androgen and inhibit ovarian steroidogenesis directly.

Hyperinsulinemia may stimulate androgen secretion by the ovary and is often associated with hyperandrogenism in women; some of these women also may have PCO, particularly those with acanthosis nigricans. Insulin resistance is present to a greater degree than would be attributable to obesity alone (Barbieri and Hornstein, 1988). Hyperandrogenism leads to deposition of abdominal fat (android obesity), the metabolism of which further exacerbates insulin resistance and hyperinsulinemia (Nader, 1991).

The diagnosis of PCO may be apparent from the history and physical findings. Although the serum testosterone level may be normal, elevated testosterone suggests an ovarian source, while increased dehydroepiandrosterone sulfate (DHEAS) suggests an adrenal source. Elevated androstenedione may be of ovarian or adrenal origin. Compared with normal women, in PCO patients the peak FSH secretion is lower and secretion of 17-OH progesterone is elevated (Barnes et al, 1989). If the testosterone or DHEAS level is grossly elevated, ovarian or adrenal tumors, respectively, must be ruled out. Ultrasonography yields diagnostic findings similar to those with laparoscopy; thus, this noninvasive method may be useful to assess ovarian morphology (el Tabbakh et al, 1986). However, endocrine parameters are more sensitive and easier to use in monitoring therapy. The pathophysiology of PCO has been reviewed (Franks, 1989; Gonzalez and Speroff, 1990; Barnes, 1991; McClamrock et al, 1991).

Drug Therapy: Clomiphene is the usual initial choice to induce ovulation in PCO patients (see the section on Anovulation and Oligo-ovulation), although ovulation is not correlated with the gonadotropin secretory response to this agent. If clomiphene alone is unsuccessful, hCG may be added. If ovulation still does not occur, menotropins plus hCG or urofollitropin plus hCG can be substituted. The risks of multiple births and hyperstimulation may be higher in PCO patients, although these effects tend to be idiosyncratic. Estrogen levels should be monitored daily either on initiation of treatment or within several days thereafter. Ultrasound monitoring is especially helpful in these women. Ovulation may occur before administration of hCG (Wang and Gemzell, 1980).

Because the LH:FSH ratio is elevated in most PCO patients, treatment with a purified FSH preparation (instead of menotropins, which contains approximately equal amounts of FSH and LH) seems a reasonable approach to normalize gonadotropic balance. However, overall results of studies using urofollitropin were similar to those obtained with menotropins. Spontaneous LH surges were unpredictable and may have caused luteinization of immature follicles or ovarian hyperstimulation (Flamigni et al, 1985; García et al, 1985). Varying the dose and duration of urofollitropin therapy (with and without hCG) has been tried in an attempt to improve the quantity and quality of ovulatory cycles and reduce hyperstimulation and the incidence of multiple births (Seibel et al, 1985; Claman, 1986; Buvat et al, 1989). It is possible that the LH in menotropins has no added effect because of the high endogenous levels of LH in PCO patients. Thus far, a clear advantage of urofollitropin over menotropins has not been demonstrated.

In one study, urofollitropin was administered to PCO patients in conventional or low-dose regimens. Fewer leading follicles, lower serum estradiol, and no instances of hyperstimulation or multiple births occurred with the low-dose regimen (Shoham et al, 1991 B). In another study, results were similar when low-dose regimens of either urofollitropin or menotropins were administered (Sagle et al, 1991). These studies suggest that the use of lower doses was more important to outcome than the gonadotropin (urofollitropin versus menotropins) preparation employed.

In clomiphene-resistant patients, intravenous infusion of gonadorelin (GnRH) pulses at intervals of 60 to 120 minutes resulted in ovulation in 87% of cycles, but only 30% of patients became pregnant (Burger et al, 1986). A more promising approach is the use of a GnRH analogue, such as leuprolide acetate [Lupron Injection], followed by gonadotropin therapy. Leuprolide suppresses pituitary gonadotropin secretion and decreases the probability of premature luteinization of follicles or other abnormalities when menotropins is administered (Dodson et al, 1987 A; Fleming et al, 1988; Weise et al, 1988). However, when another regimen (suppression with a GnRH analogue followed by gonadotropin) was employed, the ovulatory response, although improved, was still lower in PCO patients than in hypogonadotropic women given gonadotropin alone (Filicori et al, 1988; Surrey et al, 1989).

PCO patients with marginal or slightly elevated DHEAS may benefit from treatment with clomiphene plus dexamethasone (Lobo et al, 1982 A). The glucocorticoid suppresses the secretion of pituitary ACTH and adrenal androgen. This regimen may be successful when clomiphene or clomiphene plus hCG is ineffective, thus obviating the need for gonadotropins. It has been suggested that dexamethasone be used empirically even without evidence of excess adrenal androgen. The rationale is that normalization of the total androgen pool (regardless of the source of excess) may be conducive to induction of ovulation. However, this approach is unproven and generally not favored.

Ovarian wedge resection was used commonly in the past to treat PCO patients. By reducing the volume of ovarian tissue, ovarian androgen production is decreased transiently. However, ovulation does not always result and postoperative adhesions may preclude conception even in the presence of ovulation. Newer approaches include using cautery or a laser beam to ablate a portion of ovarian tissue (Greenblatt and Casper, 1987; Daniell and Miller, 1989). In one study, results of treatment with electrocautery compared favorably with those of hCG administration (Gadir et al, 1990). However, further studies are necessary to determine the risk of postoperative adhesions with these treatment modalities.

See also reviews on ovulation induction in PCO patients (Loy and Seibel, 1988; Blankstein and Quigley, 1988; Filicori et al, 1990; Kelly and Jewelewicz, 1990).

Endometriosis

Endometriosis may be associated with infertility in 25% to 40% of infertile women, although the role of mild endometriosis as a cause of infertility is unclear. Endometriosis is a frequent finding upon laparoscopy in those with previously unexplained infertility. When pregnancy is achieved in women with untreated endometriosis, some investigators have observed an increase in the rate of spontaneous abortions (Wheeler et al, 1983; Groll, 1984), but this association has been questioned (FitzSimmons et al, 1987).

Infertility associated with endometriosis may result from anatomic distortion of pelvic structures, such as ovarian or tubal adhesions that interfere with ovum transport. The prostaglandin concentration and total volume of peritoneal fluid may be increased, but the mechanism by which these conditions influence fertility, if indeed there is a causal connection, is controversial. In patients with endometriosis, a decreased number of ovulatory stigmata was observed at laparoscopy compared with controls. Therefore, it was suggested that unruptured but luteinized follicles may cause infertility in some women (Brosens et al, 1978).

The probability of achieving a second pregnancy after previous infertility caused by endometriosis appears high. Regardless of the prior treatment modality, 76% of patients in one study achieved second pregnancies without treatment. Most of the pregnancies occurred in the first year and the balance in the second year at a rate somewhat lower than that in the normal population (Rosenfeld and Jacob, 1988).

Endometriotic lesions respond to surgery or drug therapy but tend to recur after cessation of drug use. Although the effectiveness of surgery and drug therapy in relieving the pain and discomfort of endometriosis and reducing the size and extent of implants is established, fertility does not appear to be enhanced by either form of treatment.

Drug Therapy: The literature on drug therapy for treatment of mild to moderate endometriosis is voluminous. However, only four studies were randomized, controlled trials that included placebo/no-treatment groups and used pregnancy rate as an endpoint (Evers, 1989). In these studies, pregnancy rates in the placebo/no-treatment groups ranged from 24% to 54% (Seibel et al, 1982; Bayer et al, 1988; Thomas and Cooke, 1987; Telimaa, 1988). In a large nonrandomized study, untreated patients had a 30-month cumulative pregnancy rate of 55% (Hull et al, 1987). Furthermore, newer drug therapies frequently are compared with danazol [Danocrine], the drug most commonly used for endometriosis treatment in the last decade. Although danazol can relieve signs and symptoms of endometriosis, it did not improve fertility in the studies cited above. Other drugs used for the treatment of endometriosis include GnRH analogues (eg, nafarelin [Synarel], leuprolide acetate [Lupron Depot 3.75 mg], buserelin, histrelin, goserelin [Zoladex]), oral contraceptives, and progestins (eg, medroxyprogesterone). For discussion of their use, see index entry Endometriosis, Treatment.

It should be borne in mind (the following discussion notwithstanding) that probably 25% to 50% of endometriosis patients who do not have additional associated factors that preclude pregnancy would become pregnant within 12 to 30 months with no therapy at all.

Surgery: Surgery is usually indicated if the ovaries are greatly enlarged or disease is extensive. Older patients with severe disease who do not wish to become pregnant frequently undergo total hysterectomy and bilateral salpingo-oophorectomy. In patients desiring pregnancy, conservative surgery preserves and enhances reproductive function; pregnancy rates of 40% to 80% have been reported, and response probably reflects the presence or absence of other factors contributing to infertility and, possibly, the severity of the disease. The greatest chance of pregnancy is in the first 18 months after surgery. Surgery may be postponed if pregnancy is desired at a later time.

The role of surgery in enhancing fertility is unproven in mild disease. In a study of 90 patients, those treated with conservative surgery at the time of diagnostic endoscopy had virtually the same pregnancy rate (about 75%) at the end of one year as patients who received endoscopy with no additional treatment (Schenken and Malinak, 1982). In an analysis of 130 infertile patients with endometriosis, conservative surgery was followed by a higher rate of pregnancy only in patients in whom the endometriosis was severe (Olive and Lee, 1986).

Combination Surgical and Drug Treatment: Results with use of danazol before conservative surgery have not been favorable, and many authorities believe that drug therapy during the immediate postoperative period is not beneficial and may actually waste the time in which pregnancy is most likely to succeed. See also reviews by Kettel and Murphy, 1989, and Comite, 1989.

Hyperprolactinemia

Amenorrhea or oligomenorrhea with or without galactorrhea is often associated with elevated levels of plasma prolactin. A hyperprolactinemic state often is associated with impaired fertility, whether it is a normal physiologic condition (postpartum lactation) or is caused by a pathologic disorder (eg, pituitary tumor). The mechanisms underlying the effects of hyperprolactinemia are not completely understood but probably involve central derangement of normal gonadotropin secretion.

Drug Therapy: Bromocriptine [Parlodel], a dopaminergic agonist, has a direct action on the dopamine receptors of prolactin-secreting cells in the anterior pituitary to decrease the secretion of prolactin. When used in women with hyperprolactinemic disorders, the reduction in serum prolactin level is usually followed by normalization of menstrual cycles and return of fertility. Ovulation is induced with bromocriptine in up to 80% of hyperprolactinemic women with either no pituitary pathology or microadenomas and in more than one-third with macroadenomas (Reyniak, 1983). Bromocriptine generally does not restore ovulatory function in amenorrheic women with normal prolactin levels (Coelingh Bennink and van der Steeg, 1983).

During normal pregnancy, rising estrogen levels are associated with anterior pituitary hyperplasia and increased prolactin secretion. Thus, the potential for prolactinoma expansion in the hormonal milieu of pregnancy has been of concern. However, clinical evidence is reassuring, and the presence of a prolactin-secreting tumor is not a contraindication to pregnancy (Ruiz-Velasco and Tolis, 1984). Although up to 40% of untreated patients with macroadenomas may experience complications due to tumor expansion, only 5% of women treated with bromocriptine before pregnancy experience such difficulties (Weil, 1986).

Pergolide [Permax], a long-acting dopaminergic agent, has been used to treat hyperprolactinemia and appears to be as effective as bromocriptine; both drugs have similar adverse effects and produce similar results after cessation of therapy (Blackwell et al, 1983). Although pergolide was associated with greater serum FSH and LH concentrations, clinical effects of pergolide 25 mcg are similar to those achieved with bromocriptine 2.5 mg (Kletsky et al, 1986). It is not known whether patients who are refractory or who develop tolerance to one drug respond to the other. However, response to pergolide has been reported in patients who became resistant to bromocriptine (Ahmed and Shalet, 1986).

Cabergoline, an investigational long-acting oral dopaminergic ergot derivative, is as effective as bromocriptine in reducing prolactin secretion in hyperprolactinemic patients. It also reduces the size of the prolactinomas. Cabergoline is administered only once weekly. After discontinuation of therapy, serum prolactin concentrations remain normal or are reduced for up to two months. Some patients who cannot tolerate either bromocriptine or cabergoline can tolerate the other drug (Ciccarelli et al, 1989).

Luteal Phase Defect

Luteal phase defect (LPD) is a general term describing compromise of CL function, either in the amount of progesterone produced or in the progesterone:estradiol ratio in the luteal phase, which results in an endometrium inadequately prepared for implantation. Most commonly, LPD is manifested as a normal-length luteal phase with inadequate secretion of progesterone. Rarely, it is manifested as a short luteal phase. The function of progesterone in the luteal phase is to induce the synthesis of endometrial peptides and proteins, which are growth promoting and immunosuppressant and have other implantation-promoting effects. About 25% to 40% of patients with recurrent spontaneous abortion and about 35% of clomiphene-treated cycles may be affected, but LPD alone as the primary cause of infertility is uncommon. An abnormal pattern of secretion of FSH and/or LH, causing inadequate follicular stimulation, is one cause of LPD. The abnormal secretion of gonadotropin may be spontaneous or secondary to hyperprolactinemia or clomiphene administration.

LPD can be diagnosed by serial measurements of pregnanediol in urine or progesterone in saliva during the luteal phase (interpretation of results of single measurements are complicated by the pulsatile nature of progesterone secretion). Although the concentration of progesterone is lower in saliva than in serum, the pattern of secretion is qualitatively similar (Riad-Fahmy et al, 1987; Lenton et al, 1988). LPD also may be diagnosed by evidence of an abnormal endometrium as determined by endometrial biopsy (properly dated and taken within two days of the next expected menses). The results of the biopsy must be more than two days out of phase with the normal histologic appearance for the appropriate stage of the cycle (with reference to the onset of the next menses) (Noyes et al, 1950). (A newer method of endometrial dating, which has been claimed to be more accurate than histologic dating, involves taking five morphometric measurements, a procedure requiring about 30 minutes [Li et al, 1988].) Since episodes of luteal dysfunction sometimes occur in women with normal function, the endometrial defect must be present in at least two consecutive cycles in order to establish the diagnosis and initiate drug therapy. Ultrasound may serve as an adjunct to identify those cases associated with an unruptured luteinized follicle.

Endometrial biopsy in the cycle of conception theoretically poses a risk to an early pregnancy, although no increase in associated spontaneous abortions has been reported (Wentz et al, 1986). However, by using a sensitive monoclonal urine test for hCG, early pregnancy can be detected and endometrial sampling can be avoided in the cycle of conception (Herbert et al, 1990).

The etiology, diagnosis, and management of LPD have been reviewed (Brodie and Wentz, 1989; Howe and Wiczyk, 1992).

Drug Therapy: In patients believed to have endometrial inadequacy, it is important to rule out uterine cavity abnormalities using hysterosalpingography (HSG) and to measure serum prolactin and TSH levels. Pharmacotherapy is directed toward treating the cause of the abnormality and should be initiated in the intended cycle of conception rather than after the first missed menses.

Progesterone supplementation is the treatment of choice for women under 35 years with cycles of normal length, a normal HSG, and normal prolactin and TSH levels. Progesterone replacement therapy has generally been the empiric treatment of choice regardless of the etiology of luteal dysfunction. Unlike hCG or clomiphene, efficacy does not depend on a secondary response. Natural progesterone must be used because a synthetic progestin may be luteolytic.

Progesterone 12.5 mg daily may be administered intramuscularly, but this is inconvenient and painful. Vaginal or, less commonly, rectal suppositories (25 mg twice daily) are preferred. Suppositories may be compounded by a pharmacist (see the evaluation). Suppositories are convenient, and the small doses (physiologic) do not delay menses for more than two days if the patient is not pregnant. Intranasal and oral progesterone preparations are being tested clinically.

Administration of progesterone usually is begun after ovulation has occurred (as judged by basal body temperature) in the intended cycle of conception and is continued until placental steroidogenesis is fully functional at about eight to ten weeks of gestation or two weeks after the fetal heart is detected by ultrasonography.

Although clomiphene has been reported to cause luteal phase deficiency in some patients, it also may be effective in the treatment of spontaneous luteal dysfunction resulting from inadequate FSH secretion (eg, short luteal phase, long follicular phase). The efficacy of clomiphene may be due to this drug's ability to stimulate more than one follicle rather than to improve the quality of a single follicle (Guzick and Zeleznik, 1990). Direct replacement of FSH with urofollitropin plus hCG to stimulate ovulation also has been tried. The cumulative pregnancy rate after six cycles approached 50%, and all pregnancies went to term (Minassian et al, 1988). However, this approach is not established, and the expense is much greater than with an equivalent course of clomiphene.

HCG appears to be luteotropic and may be effective when supplementary support of the CL is needed (Blumenfeld and Ruach, 1992). If ovulation is being induced, the initial dose may serve as the trigger and also supports the CL. Rarely, the CL may resist stimulation by hCG and fail to produce adequate progesterone. Menses may be delayed for up to one week if pregnancy does not ensue.

Unfavorable Cervical Mucus

Copious quantities of thin, watery cervical mucus are characteristic of normal estrogenic stimulation around the time of ovulation. If instead the mucus is scant and/or thick, transport of sperm through the cervix may be reduced. Favorable cervical mucus can be demonstrated by the spinnbarkeit test of viscosity, which is performed by drawing out a strand of cervical mucus between two slides. A strand of 10 to 15 cm indicates that conditions are favorable for sperm penetration. Test results are valid only during the pre-ovulatory period when the effect of the estrogen peak on the cervical mucus can be seen. However, sperm survival, as demonstrated by a preovulatory postcoital test, is more important and may occur even when the quality of the cervical mucus does not appear to be ideal.

Formerly, unfavorable cervical mucus was sometimes treated with estrogens, but this approach generally is no longer favored. Intrauterine insemination with washed sperm may be indicated to circumvent the problem.

Assisted Reproductive Technology

The first human birth resulting from in vitro fertilization (IVF) occurred in 1978; since then, several thousand births have been achieved using variations of that initial process. Ethical issues continue to arise as technical advances offer new treatment options and the ramifications are realized. Guidelines have been offered for some of these concerns (American Fertility Society, 1986, 1990; Committee on Ethics, American College of Obstetricians and Gynecologists, 1986; Jones and Schrader, 1987; Bonnicksen, 1988; Ethics Committee, American Fertility Society, 1988; Blackwell et al, 1987). Discussions of relevant legal issues also are available (Quigley and Andrews, 1984; Schenker and Frenkel, 1987; Robertson, 1989). See also general reviews of the current status of IVF technology (Dodson, 1988; Seibel, 1988; Scott and Rosenwaks, 1989; Corsan and Kemmann, 1991; *Int J Gynecol Obstet*, 1991). Guidelines and standards for IVF and gamete intrafallopian transfer (GIFT) programs have been established (American Fertility Society, 1988, 1990, 1991).

The most common indication for IVF is irreparable tubal damage, but some patients have severe endometriosis (Hulme et al, 1990) or other causes of infertility. Male infertility (eg, decreased sperm count or motility) unresponsive to conventional treatment also may be an indication. The procedure is expensive, costing $3,000 to $12,000 per attempt, and often is not covered by medical insurance, although some insurance companies provide at least partial coverage for several treatment cycles and several states have mandated coverage.

The earliest IVF methods utilized a single oocyte retrieved from the patient during a normal ovulatory cycle. Most centers today use regimens that induce superovulation to obtain a larger number of oocytes in a single treatment cycle. Ovulation is induced by regimens consisting of clomiphene alone; clomiphene and hCG; clomiphene, menotropins, and hCG; urofollitropin and hCG; urofollitropin, menotropins, and hCG; or a GnRH analogue plus a menotropins or urofollitropin regimen. Although the agents used are the same as for conventional induction of ovulation, patient selection, treatment schedule, details of monitoring follicular development, and timing of hCG administration may differ. The goal is to develop multiple follicles for IVF; in contrast, only a single mature follicle usually is desired in ovulation induction (see review by Messinis, 1989).

In general, follicular stimulation is initiated earlier in the cycle to achieve development of multiple follicles (Dodson, 1988). When results with menotropins and urofollitropin have been compared, pregnancy rates are similar (Scoccia et al, 1987; Lavy et al, 1988). The technique of first suppressing gonadotropin secretion with a GnRH analogue and then stimulating follicular development with a gonadotropin preparation is claimed to result in fewer premature LH surges, retrieval of more oocytes, and fewer canceled cycles (Palermo et al, 1988; Meldrum et al, 1989; Ron-El et al, 1991; Tummon et al, 1992), but again the use of menotropins or urofollitropin after suppression appears to produce similar results (Bentick et al, 1988; Edelstein et al, 1990). The efficacy of adding a GnRH analogue to the stimulatory regimen has been questioned (Shelton et al, 1991; Corson et al, 1992; Kingsland et al, 1992); discrepancies in the results of various studies may be related to patient selection and differences in the GnRH analogue regimen (eg, timing of initial treatment, dose, and length of treatment) (Benadiva et al, 1990; Thatcher, 1991; Padilla et al, 1991).

Growth hormone (GH) probably plays a role in supporting normal ovulatory function and may act synergistically with hCG to stimulate progesterone secretion (Lanzone et al, 1992). The use of GH as an adjunct to ovulation induction regimens for assisted reproduction is being studied (Christman and Halme, 1992; Bider et al, 1992).

Monitoring for increased serum estradiol levels, measuring follicular size via ultrasound, and identifying other patterns of response to menotropins guide the critical timing of hCG injection. Timing also is critical for oocyte aspiration, in vitro fertilization, and embryo transfer (ET). Oocyte aspiration is accomplished using transvaginal ultrasonography, except that laparoscopic transfer is done 24 hours after transvaginal aspiration with zygote intrafallopian transfer (ZIFT) and tubal embryo transfer.

Although 50% to 90% of recovered oocytes are fertilized, only 75% continue to grow to an appropriate stage for transfer (usually a four- to eight-cell conceptus). The greatest inefficiency in IVF-ET occurs after transfer. Since only a small number of embryos will successfully implant, the clinical pregnancy rate per transfer cycle usually is 15% to 20%. Spontaneous abortion rates for clinical pregnancies may exceed 25% to 30% depending on the age of the patient. In one study in which donor oocytes from women <35 years old were used for IVF, the pregnancy rate was similar in recipients both younger and older than 40 years, which suggests that reduced fertility in older women is specifically due to the age of their oocytes (Sauer et al, 1992).

Transfer of several embryos increases the chance of successful implantation but also the risk of multiple births. Transfer of three or four embryos per attempt is considered an acceptable compromise (Bollen et al, 1991; Penzias et al, 1991). There appears to be no increased risk of congenital abnormalities in successful pregnancies. (See also review by Shoham et al, 1991 C.)

Several variations of the IVF-ET procedure with respect to source of oocyte, sperm, and embryo have been utilized: (1) Wife's oocyte and husband's sperm fertilized in vitro with embryo transfer to the wife. (2) Same as above except that donor sperm is used. (3) "Embryo donation" in which an unused embryo is implanted into another recipient. (4) Donor oocyte is fertilized in vivo using artificial insemination with the husband's sperm. The embryo is flushed from the donor before implantation and transferred to the wife (Bustillo et al, 1984). This procedure allows a woman to be a "gestational mother" of her husband's child if she is the carrier of a genetic disease or is unable to produce oocytes (eg, premature ovarian failure). (5) Oocyte donation (from volunteer or excess from IVF) fertilized in vitro with husband's sperm and transferred to wife's uterus. (6) Embryo cryopreservation for future use. This may be valuable when extra viable embryos are available after an embryo transfer. If the implantation is unsuccessful, an embryo may be thawed and transferred later, and the expense and risks of subsequent follicular recruitment, monitoring, and oocyte retrieval can be avoided. It has been suggested that ET in a later, unstimulated cycle might have a greater chance of success because of the more natural hormonal milieu at the time of implantation. Frozen embryos also may be donated to an unrelated recipient in an "embryo donation" procedure. (7) Gamete intrafallopian transfer (GIFT method), which consists of oocyte stimulation and retrieval followed by injection of ova and motile sperm into the fallopian tube. At least one intact fallopian tube is necessary for this procedure (Asch et al, 1986). (8) Zygote intrafallopian transfer (ZIFT method), in which the zygote is the product of IVF and is transferred into the fallopian tube. (9) Tubal embryo transfer (TET), similar to ZIFT except that an embryo is transferred. (10) Surrogate uterus in which an embryo is implanted into a genetically unrelated recipient.

The success rates of assisted reproduction programs are monitored and recorded in a registry maintained by the Society for Assisted Reproduction Technology (SART). Of cycles stimulated in 1990, records showed that the percentage of oocyte retrievals resulting in a live birth were: for IVF, 14%; for GIFT, 22%; and for ZIFT, 16% (Medical Research International, Society for Assisted Reproductive Technology [SART], 1992).

IVF or GIFT is sometimes used when the fallopian tubes are patent but the patient has not responded to other forms of infertility treatment (unexplained infertility). It has been suggested that controlled trials be performed to compare IVF and GIFT with the technique of superovulation plus intrauterine insemination, a less invasive and less expensive procedure (Dodson et al, 1987 B). The use of intrauterine insemination to treat infertility has been reviewed (Dodson and Haney, 1991).

Drug Evaluations

BROMOCRIPTINE MESYLATE
[Parlodel]

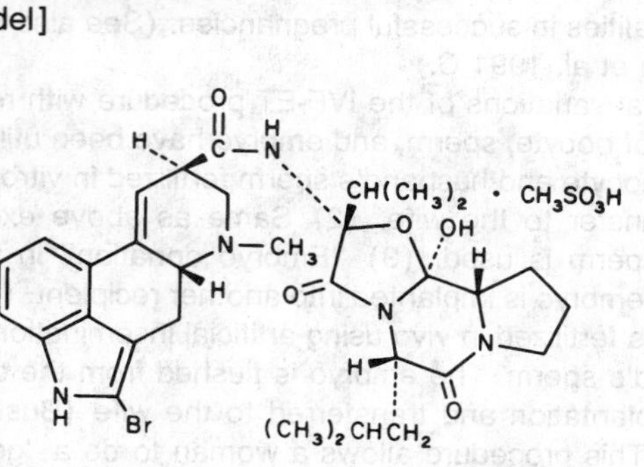

$\cdot\ CH_3SO_3H$

ACTIONS AND USES. The clinical usefulness of this semisynthetic ergot alkaloid to enhance fertility depends primarily on its dopaminergic activity. Bromocriptine inhibits the secretion of prolactin by the anterior pituitary gland and may be used to correct female infertility secondary to hyperprolactinemic states. Recurrence of hyperprolactinemia after cessation of bromocriptine therapy may be expected in virtually all patients within one year. See also the section on Hyperprolactinemia.

Bromocriptine suppresses secretion of prolactin caused by hyperplasia of prolactin-secreting pituitary cells or a pituitary adenoma and may inhibit tumor growth and reduce tumor size. In selected cases, the drug may be used during pregnancy to stop growth of an enlarging prolactinoma. However, bromocriptine is not a substitute for surgery or radiation if either measure is appropriate because of pressure from or growth of the tumor. Otherwise, bromocriptine may be used to induce ovulation in infertile women with hyperprolactinemia.

The natural course of prolactin-secreting microadenomas (less than 1 cm diameter) is not clearly understood, but these neoplasms may prove to be relatively common (asymptomatic microadenomas have been found during routine autopsies) and without threat of morbidity other than that associated with their endocrine function.

ADVERSE REACTIONS AND PRECAUTIONS. The doses employed for reproductive dysfunction generally do not cause severe side effects. Nausea is the most common untoward effect, but vomiting, constipation, dizziness, and orthostatic hypotension also occur. These effects can be minimized by taking the medication with food and at bedtime and by initiating therapy with small doses and gradually increasing the amount to effective levels. Vaginal administration also may reduce the severity of gastrointestinal effects without diminishing drug efficacy (Vermesh et al, 1988).

When ovulation has been induced and pregnancy occurs, bromocriptine usually is withdrawn for the duration of gestation. Although teratogenicity or other adverse effects on mother or fetus are not apparent (Weil, 1986), this drug should not be taken during pregnancy unless indicated. Results from a survey of 29 reproductive endocrinologists indicated that 41% of the patients who had macroadenomas received bromocriptine throughout pregnancy. If the prolactinoma expanded during pregnancy, 90% of respondents favored reinstituting therapy (Blackwell and Chang, 1986).

Visual field impairment or other neurologic symptoms during pregnancy are other indications for resumption of therapy. Bromocriptine reduces prolactin secretion and tumor size and reverses the neurologic effects of suprasellar tumor expansion. If administration is continued or resumed during pregnancy to control symptoms, prolactin secretion is decreased to an amount lower than during normal pregnancy (Ruiz-Velasco and Tolis, 1984). Surgical removal of the adenoma is usually not necessary, but remains an option if bromocriptine therapy fails to control tumor growth.

Following delivery, the patient may nurse if desired. Otherwise bromocriptine may be considered for suppression of lactation, although this use is no longer encouraged. If future pregnancy is desired, administration may be continued. Successful long-term (five to nine years) therapy without tumor progression has been reported (Corenblum and Taylor, 1983).

Cleft lip has occurred in the offspring of rabbits treated with bromocriptine.

DRUG INTERACTIONS. See index entry Bromocriptine, In Parkinsonism.

DOSAGE AND PREPARATIONS. Bromocriptine should be taken with food and preferably at bedtime.

Oral: For amenorrhea-galactorrhea and related conditions, initially, 1.25 to 2.5 mg once daily at the evening meal or bedtime, increased after two or three days to 2.5 mg twice daily. If necessary, dosage may be increased by 2.5 mg every two or three days. Other doses and treatment schedules also have been employed. In one study, 17 of 24 patients (70%) with hyperprolactinemia and serum prolactin levels <100 ng/ml required 2.5 mg or less daily to maintain a normal serum prolactin concentration (Soto-Albors et al, 1987).

Parlodel (Sandoz). Capsules 5 mg; tablets 2.5 mg.

CLOMIPHENE CITRATE

[Clomid, Serophene]

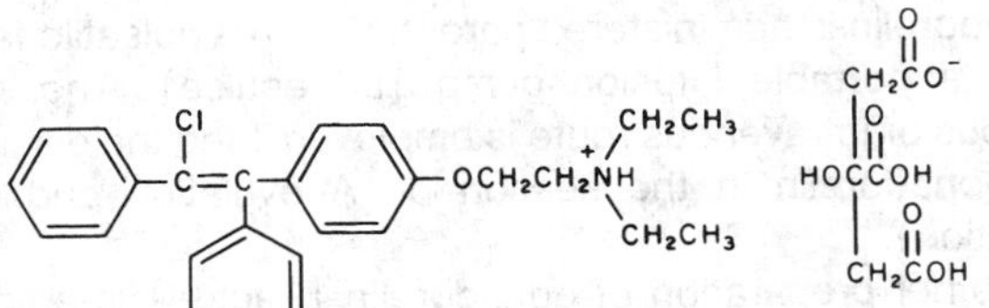

ACTIONS AND USES. This nonsteroidal agent is a mixture of two stereoisomers that depend on the orientation of the side chain; the *cis* conformation is an agonist while the *trans* conformation is an antagonist. These phenolic metabolites isomerize readily to produce a racemic mixture.

In vivo, clomiphene acts as a competitive antagonist of estrogen receptors in the anterior pituitary and anterior hypothalamus to block their activation by endogenous estrogens. In premenopausal women, this produces a low estrogen signal that, in turn, increases the secretion of GnRH and the levels of LH and FSH. Ovarian stimulation results. Clomiphene also may affect the anterior pituitary and ovary directly (Adashi, 1984).

Clomiphene may stimulate ovulation in anovulatory and oligo-ovulatory women with potentially functional hypothalamic-pituitary-ovarian axes and adequate endogenous estrogens. The optimal dose is the lowest amount at which ovulation occurs; incremental dose adjustments are made each treatment cycle until this amount is reached. (The use of 25- to 50-mg increments may be necessary to achieve an ovulatory dose.) If ovulation is achieved but pregnancy does not occur, the ovulatory dose can be repeated cyclically; it should not be exceeded (administering more than the ovulatory dosage may actually decrease the probability of pregnancy). Although 75% of clomiphene-induced pregnancies occur in the first three cycles of treatment (ie, with low doses), a significant number (15%) occur after 150 to 250 mg has been given.

Body weight was positively correlated with the ovulatory dose in one study. Although 85% of women under 50 kg (110 lb) ovulated with 50 mg of clomiphene, only 20% of women over 90 kg (200 lb) did. However, the variability in response related to body weight precluded precise prediction of ovulatory dosage (Lobo et al, 1982 B).

Monitoring is necessary during each treatment cycle to evaluate the dosage in terms of ovulatory response and side effects. Ovulation is assumed to occur if the basal body temperature during the luteal phase is at least 0.5° F higher than during the follicular phase, if an endometrial biopsy during the late luteal phase shows a secretory effect, and/or if the serum progesterone level exceeds 2 ng/ml at any point during the luteal phase. Urinary LH test kits can be used to aid in timing of coitus. When therapy is successful, ovulation usually occurs three to ten days after the last dose. Therefore, patients should have intercourse approximately every other day during this period. Before a subsequent cycle of therapy is begun, the patient should have had confirmed bleeding and basal body temperature should have fallen. Clomiphene therapy should not be resumed if pregnancy has occurred.

ADVERSE REACTIONS AND PRECAUTIONS. Ovarian cysts (persistent ovarian follicles) form in 5% to 10% of patients. The most serious, although very rare, adverse reaction of clomiphene is massive cystic enlargement of the ovaries (hyperstimulation syndrome). Maximal enlargement occurs about one week after ovulation, and regression is usually spontaneous after several days or weeks. Additional therapy should not be given until the ovaries return to pretreatment size (usually within one month). The patient then may be given a lower dose of clomiphene plus hCG when the cervical mucus appears favorable.

When clomiphene induces ovulation, luteal phase defect may occur in up to one-half of the cycles in some patients. This is often treated empirically by adding progesterone or hCG to the regimen. (See the section on Luteal Phase Defect.)

Multiple births are almost always twins; larger multiple gestations have been reported rarely. The incidence of twins is about 8% (six times normal) and the incidence of triplets is 1%; however, these rates are lower than with menotropins. Spontaneous abortions (mostly early miscarriages) have been reported in clomiphene-induced pregnancies; however, the overall incidence does not appear to be significantly different from that in the normal or infertile population.

Blurred vision and scintillating scotomata are dose related and reversible when the drug is discontinued. Objective signs are rarely found, although measurable loss of visual acuity, definable scotomata, and changes in retinal cell function have been reported. Visual abnormalities should be considered a contraindication to further use.

Other adverse reactions include hot flushes resembling menopausal vasomotor symptoms (10% to 20%), depression and mood swings, and, less commonly, nausea, headache, tinnitus, breast engorgement, and abdominal bloating. Symptoms disappear when therapy is stopped. Untoward effects may occur at the lowest dosages in sensitive individuals (see also the Introduction).

TERATOGENICITY. Although there is no evidence that the incidence of fetal anomalies is increased clinically, aberrations have been observed in the offspring of some subprimate animals given clomiphene *during* pregnancy.

In one study, genital tracts from aborted fetuses were implanted under the kidney capsules of immune-deficient mice, and the mice were treated with subcutaneous pellets containing large doses of clomiphene, DES, or tamoxifen for one to two months. In all drug treatment groups, the changes in the implanted tissues were similar to those observed with fetal DES exposure in utero, although changes were not observed in tissues that were less than 16 fetal weeks (Cunha et al, 1987). It is not likely that these changes are relevant to clinical situations in which clomiphene is used to induce ovulation.

Since clomiphene has a circulation half-life of five days and some residual drug may be present in the maternal circulation following implantation of an embryo, there is at least theoretical reason for concern about teratogenicity in humans (March, 1988). However, the teratogenic potential in clinical practice would appear to be low or absent because (1) clomiphene is given prior to ovulation, not during an established pregnancy; and (2) numerous studies since clomiphene has been used to induce ovulation (1967) have failed to identify a teratogenic effect. Nevertheless, there is no indication for clomiphene therapy once conception has been achieved, and this drug should not be administered to pregnant women. The absence of pregnancy should be assured before a subsequent cycle of clomiphene therapy is begun. Theoretically, any potential teratogenic effect would be more likely if the drug were continued inadvertently after pregnancy was established.

PHARMACOKINETICS. Initial metabolism produces long-lived derivatives with antiestrogenic activity; the activity of the *trans* (4-hydroxy) derivative is 100 times greater than that of the parent molecule. About one-half of the ingested dose is excreted in five days; traces appear in the feces up to six weeks after administration. Clomiphene is excreted mainly in the feces; small amounts appear in the urine.

DOSAGE AND PREPARATIONS.

Oral: To induce ovulation, initially, 50 mg daily for five days starting on the third or fifth day of the cycle (spontaneous or induced bleeding) or at any time in patients who have not menstruated recently, provided that pregnancy has been ruled out. Lower doses or a shorter duration of treatment is recommended if unusual sensitivity to pituitary gonadotropin is suspected. If ovulation (monitored by basal body temperature and possibly serum progesterone or endometrial biopsy) without conception occurs, the same dosage is given cyclically (and should not be exceeded) until conception or for three to six cycles. (If conception does not occur after three ovulatory cycles in which cervical mucus is unfavorable prior to ovulation, intrauterine insemination may be attempted.) (See the section on Unfavorable Cervical Mucus.)

If ovulation does not occur, the dosage is increased by 50 mg in each cycle until up to 250 mg/day is given for five days. If doses of 150 to 250 mg daily for five days fail to stimulate ovulation or if there is evidence of ovulatory failure due to lack of an LH surge, hCG may be added to the regimen near the time of anticipated ovulation. A dose of 5,000 to 10,000 USP units is given intramuscularly 12 to 14 days after starting clomiphene if a mature follicle is present or 5,000 USP units is given initially, followed by 5,000 USP units five to seven days later. The optimal day for administering hCG should be determined by awaiting the development of a mature preovulatory follicle as determined by ultrasound. Various protocols for clomiphene regimens appear in the literature (Gysler et al, 1982; García-Flores and Vázquez-Méndez, 1984; Hammond, 1984).

Clomid (Marion Merrell Dow), ***Serophene*** (Serono). Tablets 50 mg.

GONADORELIN HYDROCHLORIDE

[Factrel, Lutrepulse]

USES. Gonadorelin, a synthetic preparation of GnRH that is identical to the endogenous hormone, may be used to induce ovulation in patients refractory to clomiphene or bromocriptine or in lieu of menotropins in those with an intact pituitary. Gonadorelin is administered parenterally in a pulsatile fashion using a portable infusion pump [Lutrepulse]. The subcutaneous or intravenous route is employed (see the discussion on Gonadorelin in the section on Anovulation and Oligo-ovulation).

Another preparation of gonadorelin [Factrel] is employed in the diagnosis of gonadotropin deficiency, but it cannot reliably distinguish pituitary from hypothalamic dysfunction. Repeated administration may improve the specificity of this test.

Gonadorelin also may be used to monitor gonadotropic function in patients who have undergone partial or complete hypophysectomy or pituitary irradiation.

ADVERSE REACTIONS AND PRECAUTIONS. When used to induce ovulation, infections and phlebitis may occur with intravenous administration. Ovarian cyst formation has been reported (Feldberg et al, 1989). Ovarian hyperstimulation may occur, but the frequency is much less than with menotropins. Multiple pregnancies, mostly twins, occur in about 7% of induced pregnancies.

Induction of ovulation with gonadorelin should be monitored in a manner similar to that for menotropins therapy. Treatment of infertility with gonadorelin is very expensive (up to $3,500 per cycle) and should be undertaken only by specialists experienced in its use.

Adverse effects associated with the use of gonadorelin as a diagnostic agent generally are infrequent and not serious. Headache, nausea, abdominal discomfort, lightheadedness, and flushing may occur. Repeated use of large doses may cause luteolysis. Urticaria and an anaphylactic reaction have been reported with use of this agent (Claman et al, 1987; MacLeod et al, 1987).

Drugs that may affect serum levels or pituitary control of gonadotropins (eg, androgens, progestins, estrogens, spironolactone, levodopa, digoxin, phenothiazines) should not be used while performing gonadorelin tests. Although gonadorelin is given to induce ovulation in infertile patients, there are no indications for use of this agent during pregnancy and its safety during pregnancy is unknown (FDA Pregnancy Category B).

DOSAGE AND PREPARATIONS.

For ovulation induction in selected patients:

Subcutaneous: Catheters may be placed in the lower abdominal area (Schriock and Jaffe, 1986). Gonadorelin is then infused as 15- to 20-mcg pulses, or 75 ng/kg, every 90 to 120 minutes for up to 14 days or until adequate follicular development has been demonstrated. Dosages should be adjusted to the patient's weight (300 mcg/kg).

Intravenous: Catheters may be placed in a forearm vein (Schriock and Jaffe, 1986). Gonadorelin is then infused as 1- to 20-mcg pulses every 90 to 120 minutes for up to 14 days or until adequate follicular development has been demonstrated. Dosages should be adjusted to the patient's weight (75 mcg/kg). (See references in Wong and Asch, 1986.)

Lutrepulse (Ferring). Powder (lyophilized) 0.8 or 3.2 mg in 10 ml containers supplied with 10 ml diluent in a kit. The kit also contains sterile catheter tubing, reservoir catheter, intravenous cannula units, syringe, needle, alcohol swabs, elastic belt, and 9-volt battery. For use with Lutrepulse Pump kit.

For diagnostic purposes:

Intravenous, Subcutaneous: *Women,* 100 mcg. The test should be administered between the first and seventh day of the menstrual cycle if that can be established. Venous blood samples are drawn 15 minutes before, immediately before (these two samples are averaged to obtain a baseline value), and 15, 30, 45, 60, and 120 minutes after administration. For interpretation of results, see the manufacturer's literature.

Factrel (Wyeth-Ayerst). Powder (lyophilized) 100 and 500 mcg.

HUMAN CHORIONIC GONADOTROPIN (hCG)

[A.P.L., Follutein, Pregnyl, Profasi HP]

Human chorionic gonadotropin (hCG) is a placental hormone extracted from the urine of pregnant women. It is a glycoprotein with a molecular weight of 30,000. In most radioimmunoassay systems, there is a cross reaction between hCG and LH; however, substantial differences in the sequence of protein and carbohydrate exist. Biologically, hCG mimics the actions of LH. Elimination from plasma is biphasic; the terminal half-life is approximately 24 hours.

USES. HCG serves as a substitute for the LH surge to stimulate ovulation of a prepared follicle when used with clomiphene and/or menotropins. It often is utilized to support production of progesterone by the corpus luteum during the luteal phase. HCG is classified in FDA Pregnancy Category C.

This agent also is used to treat male infertility (see index entry Human Chorionic Gonadotropin, In Male Reproductive Dysfunction).

DOSAGE AND PREPARATIONS.

Intramuscular: To stimulate ovulation, various regimens are employed. In one study, two injections of 5,000 units each given one week apart resulted in a longer luteal phase than a single injection of 10,000 units (Grazi et al, 1991). Also see the evaluations on Clomiphene Citrate and Menotropins.

A.P.L. (Wyeth-Ayerst), ***Generic.*** Powder 5,000, 10,000, and 20,000 U.S.P. units with 10 ml of diluent.

Follutein (Squibb-Mark), ***Pregnyl*** (Organon). Powder (lyophilized) 10,000 U.S.P. units with 10 ml of diluent.

Profasi HP (Serono). Powder (sterile, lyophilized) 5,000 and 10,000 U.S.P. units with 10 ml of diluent.

MENOTROPINS (hMG)

[Pergonal]

ACTIONS AND USES. Menotropins is a preparation of human menopausal gonadotropin (hMG) extracted from the urine of postmenopausal women. FSH and LH activity are present in approximately a 1:1 ratio. The goal of therapy is to replace or supplement gonadotropins and stimulate follicular development. Therapeutic effects are achieved by combination with hCG or clomiphene and hCG.

In anovulatory women judged suitable for gonadotropin therapy (see the Introduction), menotropins is given initially in doses sufficient to induce follicular growth and maturation as determined by serial measurements of serum or urinary estrogens and by ultrasonography of the developing follicle. Following follicular maturation, hCG is given to induce ovulation. Since ovulation of properly prepared follicles usually occurs within 36 to 48 hours after hCG administration, the couple is instructed to have coitus on the evening of the injection and for the next two or three days. Most pregnancies occur within one to five cycles. Therapy beyond five cycles is not likely to increase the success rate except in some women with low endogenous estrogen.

Induction of ovulation with gonadotropins is difficult and expensive and should be carried out only by physicians with specialized training and experience. Proper administration of menotropins requires individualization of dosage based on the patient's response.

Menotropins also is used to treat male infertility (see index entry Menotropins, In Male Infertility).

ADVERSE REACTIONS AND PRECAUTIONS. Symptoms of ovarian overstimulation occur in 10% to 20% of patients and may be observed after any dose but are most common after large doses that result in high serum estradiol levels. Mild overstimulation is manifested by ovarian enlargement and abdominal discomfort, lasts seven to ten days, and requires no treatment. Severe hyperstimulation, which occurs in 0.5% to 1% of patients, is life-threatening and necessitates hospitalization. Ovarian enlargement is accompanied by weight gain, ascites, pleural effusion, oliguria, hypotension, and hypercoagulability. Treatment is largely supportive, although rarely ovarian rupture with intraperitoneal hemorrhage may require surgical intervention. Therapy is directed toward maintenance of adequate intravascular volume; anticoagulation therapy may be necessary. A renin-angiotensin system acting locally in the ovarian follicle may play a role in the manifestation of the hyperstimulation syndrome (Navot et al, 1987).

Multiple gestations occur frequently (incidence, 15% to 30%) in gonadotropin-induced pregnancies and are not predictable solely on the basis of the serum estrogen levels produced; they may be predicted more often by using ultrasound measurements in conjunction with serum estrogen concentration. However, even monitoring by both methods does not ensure detection of all follicles and prevention of multiple gestations (Fedorkow et al, 1988).

Menotropins is classified in FDA Pregnancy Category X.

MONITORING THERAPY. Monitoring patient response is crucial to determine that adequate follicular development occurs without ovarian hyperstimulation and to reduce the likelihood of multiple gestations. Monitoring is required in each cycle of therapy because the patient's response may vary from cycle to cycle.

Ideally, the patient should be examined daily to monitor changes in ovarian size and estrogen production, although this is not necessary during the first several days except in patients with polycystic ovarian disease. Daily examinations and estrogen determinations are recommended beginning on approximately the fifth day of stimulation.

Serum estradiol assays and ultrasonography are used to determine the timing of hCG injection. HCG should be given within 24 hours or up to 36 hours after the last dose of menotropins. When follicular maturation has reached this stage of active estrogen secretion, the rate of estrogen production can be expected to double daily. If estrogen production is lower than optimum, administration of menotropins should be continued. If estrogen production is three to four times greater than the preovulatory level, hCG should not be administered because of the risk of ovarian hyperstimulation unless ultrasound examination of the ovaries suggests that the risk of hyperstimulation is low.

Ultrasonography is indispensable to determine follicle size and to identify multiple follicles. Follicles between 14 and 20 mm after stimulation generally are ready for ovulation induction with hCG. This agent should be withheld if four or more mature follicles are observed with ultrasound or if many small (<10 mm) follicles are detected, even with "safe" levels of serum estradiol.

DOSAGE AND PREPARATIONS.

MENOTROPINS AND hCG:

Intramuscular: For induction of ovulation, the dosage requirement may vary in the same individual and therefore is determined according to the patient's response in each treatment cycle. Usually, patients are initially given one to two ampuls of menotropins (each containing 75 IU FSH and 75 IU LH) daily. The dose should be adjusted and individualized in accordance with the patient's response. Dosage may be continued at this level if there is evidence of estrogen production; if such evidence is lacking, the amount may be increased after the first four to seven days. Up to six ampuls per day may be required to stimulate follicular development.

When the patient has reached the appropriate level of follicular development as judged by serum estrogen measurement and ultrasonography (see the discussion on Monitoring Therapy), a single injection of 5,000 to 10,000 USP units of hCG is administered about 24 hours after the last injection of menotropins. Other variations in the amount and timing of hCG have been employed and are designed not only to provide ovulatory stimulus but also to support corpus luteum function at a critical stage (particularly if there is evidence of luteal phase defect).

MENOTROPINS, CLOMIPHENE, AND hCG:

Oral, Intramuscular: For induction of ovulation, this regimen may be tried in properly selected patients (see the Introduction) to reduce the cost of therapy. Clomiphene is given orally beginning on the third to fifth day of the cycle (spontaneous or induced); 100 mg is given for five to seven days or 200 mg is given for five days. Menotropins is then given and therapy is monitored as above.

Pergonal (Serono). Each 2-ml ampul contains 75 or 150 IU each of follicle-stimulating hormone (FSH) activity and gonadotropin (LH) activity (with 10 mg lyophilized lactose).

PROGESTERONE

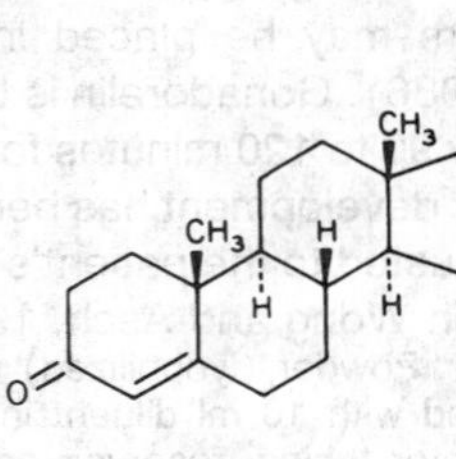

USES. Progesterone is used to treat endometrial inadequacy during the luteal phase that results in infertility or repeated early spontaneous abortion. This disorder should be documented before progesterone therapy is undertaken. Treatment is begun in the intended cycle of conception and generally is continued until placental production of steroids is established (eight to ten weeks after the last menstrual period or six to eight weeks after conception). Treatment may be discontinued two weeks after the fetal heartbeat is detected by vaginal ultrasonography. A synthetic progestin should not be administered for this indication.

Progesterone may be given intramuscularly, which can be painful and inconvenient, or in suppository form. Suppositories may be compounded by a pharmacist using the following formulation: 44 g progesterone powder, 2,096 g polyethylene glycol 400, 1,392 g polyethylene glycol 6,000 (makes 1,760 suppositories containing 25 mg progesterone each). See also the Introduction.

DOSAGE AND PREPARATIONS.

Intramuscular: For support of pregnancy in luteal phase dysfunction, 12.5 mg daily beginning as soon as ovulation can be diagnosed and continuing, if needed, to the eleventh week of gestation.

Generic. Solution (in oil) 25 and 50 mg/ml in 10 and 30 ml containers and 100 mg/ml in 10 ml containers.

Available Trademark:

Gesterol-50 (Forest).

Vaginal, Rectal: For support of pregnancy in luteal phase dysfunction, one 25-mg suppository inserted twice daily beginning as soon as ovulation can be diagnosed and continuing, if needed, up to the eleventh week of gestation.

Generic. Suppositories 25, 50, 100, 200, and 400 mg. Progesterone also is available as a micronized powder for compounding in 5, 10, 25, 50 and 100 g containers. See above for preparation of suppositories.

UROFOLLITROPIN (FSH)

[Metrodin]

Urofollitropin is a preparation of almost pure human FSH (75 IU FSH and less than 1 IU LH per ampul) extracted from the urine of postmenopausal women. This lyophilized preparation stimulates growth of ovarian follicles and may be used with hCG, which simulates the LH surge and causes ovulation of prepared follicles. Urofollitropin is administered in similar doses and produces similar results and adverse reactions as menotropins.

USES. Urofollitropin is indicated as part of a regimen to induce ovulation in PCO patients who have an elevated LH:FSH ratio and who have not responded to clomiphene therapy.

ADVERSE REACTIONS AND PRECAUTIONS. Overstimulation causing ovarian enlargement and abdominal discomfort may occur in 20% of patients who receive urofollitropin-hCG therapy. Symptoms generally regress without treatment within two to three weeks. Hyperstimulation syndrome may occur in 6% of patients so treated and requires hospitalization and appropriate supportive therapy (see the evaluation on Menotropins).

Multiple gestations occur in about 17% of pregnancies; although most are twins, triplet and quintuplet gestations have occurred. The patient should be carefully monitored during each cycle of treatment. Guidelines for monitoring are similar to those employed with menotropins-hCG therapy, including the use of rapid serum estrogen measurements and ultrasound.

Urofollitropin is classified in FDA Pregnancy Category X.

DOSAGE AND PREPARATIONS. Dosage and administration vary depending on the therapeutic indication.

UROFOLLITROPIN AND hCG:

Intramuscular: For induction of ovulation, the dosage is similar to that of menotropins and must be determined individually in each patient and each cycle. Initially, 75 IU urofollitropin is administered daily for 7 to 12 days (or longer) to achieve adequate follicular development as evidenced by serum estrogen and ultrasound evaluation (see above).

One day after the last dose of urofollitropin, 5,000 to 10,000 USP units of hCG is given intramuscularly to stimulate ovulation of the prepared follicle(s).

If ovulation does not occur with this regimen, a similar schedule increasing the dose to 150 IU urofollitropin daily may be tried.

Metrodin (Serono). Each ampul contains 75 IU FSH activity (supplied with 2 ml of sodium chloride injection).

Cited References

New reproductive technologies: ACOG technical bulletin number 140—March 1990. *Int J Gynecol Obstet* 35:274-278, 1991.

Aboulghar MA, et al: Ovarian superstimulation in the treatment of infertility due to peritubal and periovarian adhesions. *Fertil Steril* 51:834-837, 1989.

Adashi EY: Clomiphene citrate: Mechanism(s) and site(s) of action: Hypothesis revisited. *Fertil Steril* 42:331-344, 1984.

Adoni A, et al: Role of ultrasound in ovulation induction by gonadotropins. *Int J Fertil* 31:170-173, 1986.

Ahmed SR, Shalet SM: Discordant responses of prolactinoma to two different dopamine agonists. *Clin Endocrinol* 24:421-426, 1986.

Aiman J, Smentek C: Premature ovarian failure. *Obstet Gynecol* 66:9-14, 1985.

Alper MM, et al: Pregnancies after premature ovarian failure. *Obstet Gynecol* 67(suppl):59S-62S, (March) 1986.

American Fertility Society: Ethical considerations of new reproductive technologies. *Fertil Steril* 46(suppl 1):1S-94S, 1986.

American Fertility Society: Minimal standards for gamete intrafallopian transfer (GIFT). *Fertil Steril* 50:20, 1988.

American Fertility Society: Revised minimum standards for in vitro fertilization, gamete intrafallopian transfer, and related procedures. *Fertil Steril* 53:225-226, 1990.

American Fertility Society: Guidelines for in vitro fertilization, gamete intrafallopian transfer, and related procedures. *Fertil Steril* 56:194-197, 1991.

Asch RH, et al: Preliminary experiences with gamete intrafallopian transfer (GIFT). *Fertil Steril* 45:366-371, 1986.

Barbieri RL, Hornstein MD: Hyperinsulinemia and ovarian hyperandrogenism: Cause and effect. *Endocrinol Metab Clin North Am* 17:685-703, 1988.

Barnes RB: Polycystic ovary syndrome and ovarian steroidogenesis. *Semin Reprod Endocrinol* 9:360-366, 1991.

Barnes RB, et al: Pituitary-ovarian responses to nafarelin testing in the polycystic ovary syndrome. *N Engl J Med* 320:559-565, 1989.

Bayer SR, et al: Efficacy of danazol treatment for minimal endometriosis in infertile women: Prospective randomized study. *J Reprod Med* 33:179-183, 1988.

Benadiva CA, et al: Comparison of different regimens of a gonadotropin-releasing hormone analog during ovarian stimulation for in vitro fertilization. *Fertil Steril* 53:479-485, 1990.

Benjamin F, et al: Prevalence of and markers for attenuated form of congenital adrenal hyperplasia and hyperprolactinemia masquerading as polycystic ovarian disease. *Fertil Steril* 46:215-221, 1986.

Bentick B, et al: Randomized comparative study of purified follicle stimulating hormone and human menopausal gonadotropin after pituitary desensitization with buserelin for superovulation and in vitro fertilization. *Fertil Steril* 50:79-84, 1988.

Bider D, et al: Growth hormone in ovulation induction. *Assist Reprod Rev* 2:23-28, 1992.

Blackwell RE, Chang RJ: Report of national symposium on clinical management of prolactin-related reproductive disorders. *Fertil Steril* 45:607-610, 1986.

Blackwell RE, et al: Comparison of dopamine agonists in treatment of hyperprolactinemic syndromes: Multicenter study. *Fertil Steril* 39:744-748, 1983.

Blackwell RE, et al: Are we exploiting the infertile couple? editorial. *Fertil Steril* 48:735-739, 1987.

Blankstein J, Quigley MM: Induction of ovulation in the patient with polycystic ovarian disease. *Endocrinol Metab Clin North Am* 17:733-749, 1988.

Blankstein J, et al: Ovarian hyperstimulation syndrome: Prediction by number and size of preovulatory ovarian follicles. *Fertil Steril* 47:597-602, 1987.

Blumenfeld Z, Ruach M: Early pregnancy wastage: The role of repetitive human chorionic gonadotropin supplementation during the first 8 weeks of gestation. *Fertil Steril* 58:19-23, 1992.

Bohrer M, Kemmann E: Risk factors for spontaneous abortion in menotropins-treated women. *Fertil Steril* 48:571-575, 1987.

Bollen N, et al: The incidence of multiple pregnancy after in vitro fertilization and embryo transfer, gamete, or zygote intrafallopian transfer. *Fertil Steril* 55:314-318, 1991.

Bonnicksen AL: Embryo freezing: Ethical issues in the clinical setting. *Hastings Cent Rep* 26-30, (Dec) 1988.

Brodie BL, Wentz AC: Late onset congenital adrenal hyperplasia: A gynecologist's perspective. *Fertil Steril* 48:175-188, 1987.

Brodie BL, Wentz AC: Update on the clinical relevance of luteal phase inadequacy. *Semin Reprod Endocrinol* 7:138-154, 1989.

Brosens IA, et al: Study of plasma progesterone, oestradiol-17β, prolactin and LH levels, and of luteal phase appearance of ovaries in patients with endometriosis and infertility. *Br J Obstet Gynaecol* 85:246-250, 1978.

Burger CW, et al: Ovulation induction with pulsatile luteinizing releasing-hormone in women with clomiphene citrate-resistant polycystic ovary-like disease: Clinical results. *Fertil Steril* 46:1045-1054, 1986.

Bustillo M, et al: Nonsurgical ovum transfer as treatment in infertile women. *JAMA* 251:1171-1181, 1984.

Buvat J, et al: Purified follicle-stimulating hormone in polycystic ovary syndrome: Slow administration is safer and more effective. *Fertil Steril* 52:553-559, 1989.

Christman GM, Halme JK: Growth hormone: Revisited. *Fertil Steril* 57:12-14, 1992.

Ciccarelli E, et al: Effectiveness and tolerability of long term treatment with cabergoline, a new long-lasting ergoline derivative, in hyperprolactinemic patients. *J Clin Endocrinol Metab* 69:725-728, 1989.

Claman P: Comparison of intermediate-dose purified urinary follicle-stimulating hormone with and without human chorionic gonadotropin for ovulation induction in polycystic ovarian disease. *Fertil Steril* 46:518-521, 1986.

Claman P, et al: Gonadorelin: Urticaria associated with antigonadorelin antibodies in a woman with Kallman's syndrome: First report. *Obstet Gynecol* 69:503-505, 1987.

Coelingh Bennink HJT, van der Steeg HJ: Failure of bromocriptine to restore menstrual cycle in normoprolactinemic post-pill amenorrhea. *Fertil Steril* 39:238-240, 1983.

Comite F: GnRH analogs and safety. *Obstet Gynecol Surv* 44:319-325, 1989.

Committee on Ethics, American College of Obstetricians and Gynecologists: *Ethical Issues in Human In Vitro Fertilization and Embryo Transfer.* Washington, DC, American College of Obstetricians and Gynecologists, 1986.

Corenblum B, Taylor PJ: Long-term follow-up of hyperprolactinemic women treated with bromocriptine. *Fertil Steril* 40:596-599, 1983.

Corsan GH, Kemmann E: Risk of a second consecutive first-trimester spontaneous abortion in women who conceive with menotropins. *Fertil Steril* 53:817-821, 1990.

Corsan GH, Kemmann E: The role of superovulation with menotropins in ovulatory infertility: A review. *Fertil Steril* 55:468-477, 1991.

Corson SL, et al: Leuprolide acetate-prepared in vitro fertilization-gamete intrafallopian transfer cycles: Efficacy versus controls and cost analysis. *Fertil Steril* 57:601-605, 1992.

Cunha GR, et al: Teratogenic effects of clomiphene, tamoxifen, and diethylstilbestrol on the developing human female genital tract. *Hum Pathol* 18:1132-1143, 1987.

Daniell JF, Miller W: Polycystic ovaries treated by laparoscopic laser vaporization. *Fertil Steril* 51:232-236, 1989.

Dodson WC: In vitro fertilization. *Compr Ther* 14:38-49, (Dec) 1988.

Dodson WC, Haney AF: Controlled ovarian hyperstimulation and intrauterine insemination for treatment of infertility. *Fertil Steril* 55:457-467, 1991.

Dodson WC, et al: Effect of leuprolide acetate on ovulation induction with human menopausal gonadotropins in polycystic ovary syndrome. *J Clin Endocrinol Metab* 65:95-100, 1987 A.

Dodson WC, et al: Superovulation with intrauterine insemination in the treatment of infertility: Possible alternative to gamete intrafallopian transfer and in vitro fertilization. *Fertil Steril* 48:441-445, 1987 B.

Edelstein MC, et al: Equivalency of human menopausal gonadotropin and follicle-stimulating hormone stimulation after gonadotropin-releasing hormone agonist suppression. *Fertil Steril* 53:103-106, 1990.

el Tabbakh GH, et al: Correlation of ultrasonic appearance of ovaries in polycystic ovarian disease and clinical, hormonal, and laparoscopic findings. *Am J Obstet Gynecol* 154:892-895, 1986.

Ethics Committee (1986-1987), American Fertility Society: Ethical considerations of the new reproductive technologies. *Fertil Steril* 49(suppl 1):i-v, 1S-7S, 1988.

Evers JLH: The pregnancy rate of the no-treatment group in randomized clinical trials of endometriosis therapy. *Fertil Steril* 52:906-907, 1989.

Fedorkow DM, et al: Septuplet gestation following the use of human menopausal gonadotropin despite intensive monitoring. *Fertil Steril* 49:364-366, 1988.

Feldberg D, et al: Ovarian cyst formation: A complication of gonadotropin-releasing-hormone agonist therapy. *Fertil Steril* 51:42-45, 1989.

Filicori M, et al: Gonadotropin-releasing hormone (GnRH) analog suppression renders polycystic ovarian disease patients more susceptible to ovulation induction with pulsatile GnRH. *J Clin Endocrinol Metab* 66:327-333, 1988.

Filicori M, et al: Polycystic ovary syndrome: Abnormalities and management with pulsatile gonadotropin-releasing hormone and gonadotropin-releasing hormone analogs. *Am J Obstet Gynecol* 163:1737-1742, 1990.

Filicori M, et al: Ovulation induction with pulsatile gonadotropin-releasing hormone: Technical modalities and clinical perspectives. *Fertil Steril* 56:1-13, 1991.

Fisch P, et al: Unexplained infertility: Evaluation of treatment with clomiphene citrate and human chorionic gonadotropin. *Fertil Steril* 51:828-833, 1989.

FitzSimmons J, et al: Spontaneous abortion and endometriosis. *Fertil Steril* 47:696-698, 1987.

Flamigni C, et al: Use of human urinary follicle-stimulating hormone in infertile women with polycystic ovaries. *J Reprod Med* 30:184-188, 1985.

Fleming R, et al: Combined gonadotropin-releasing hormone analog and exogenous gonadotropins for ovulation induction in infertile women: Efficacy related to ovarian function assessment. *Am J Obstet Gynecol* 159:376-381, 1988.

Franks S: Polycystic ovary syndrome: A changing perspective. *Clin Endocrinol* 31:87-120, 1989.

Gadir AA, et al: Ovarian electrocautery versus human menopausal gonadotrophins and pure follicle stimulating hormone therapy in the treatment of patients with polycystic ovarian disease. *Clin Endocrinol* 33:585-592, 1990.

Garcia N, et al: Induction of ovulation with purified urinary follicle-stimulating hormone in patients with polycystic ovarian syndrome. *Am J Obstet Gynecol* 151:635-640, 1985.

García-Flores RF, Vázquez-Méndez J: Progressive dosages of clomiphene in hypothalamic anovulation. *Fertil Steril* 42:543-547, 1984.

Golan A, et al: Ovarian hyperstimulation syndrome: Update review. *Obstet Gynecol Surv* 44:430-440, 1989.

Gonzalez F, Speroff L: Adrenal morphologic considerations in polycystic ovary syndrome. *Obstet Gynecol Surv* 45:491-508, 1990.

Grazi RV, et al: The luteal phase during gonadotropin therapy: Effects of two human chorionic gonadotropin regimens. *Fertil Steril* 55:1088-1092, 1991.

Greenblatt E, Casper RF: Endocrine changes after laparoscopic ovarian cautery in polycystic ovarian syndrome. *Am J Obstet Gynecol* 156:279-285, 1987.

Griffith CS, Grimes DA: The validity of the postcoital test. *Am J Obstet Gynecol* 162:615-620, 1990.

Groll M: Endometriosis and spontaneous abortion. *Fertil Steril* 41:933-935, 1984.

Guzick DS, Zeleznik A: Efficacy of clomiphene citrate in the treatment of luteal phase deficiency: Quantity versus quality of preovulatory follicles. *Fertil Steril* 54:206-210, 1990.

Gysler M, et al: A decade's experience with an individualized clomiphene treatment regimen including its effect on the postcoital test. *Fertil Steril* 37:161-167, 1982.

Hammond MG: Monitoring techniques for improved pregnancy rates during clomiphene ovulation induction. *Fertil Steril* 42:499-509, 1984.

Herbert CM, et al: Use of a sensitive urine pregnancy test before endometrial biopsies taken in the late luteal phase. *Fertil Steril* 53:162-164, 1990.

Homburg R, et al: Cotreatment with human growth hormone and gonadotropins for induction of ovulation: A controlled clinical trial. *Fertil Steril* 53:254-260, 1990.

Howe RS, Wiczyk HP: The luteal phase and implantation. *Assist Reprod Rev* 2:52-61, 1992.

Hull ME, et al: Correlation of serum estradiol levels and ultrasound monitoring to assess follicular maturation. *Fertil Steril* 46:42-45, 1986.

Hull ME, et al: Comparison of different treatment modalities of endometriosis in infertile women. *Fertil Steril* 47:40-44, 1987.

Hulme VA, et al: Gamete intrafallopian transfer as treatment for infertility associated with endometriosis. *Fertil Steril* 53:1095-1096, 1990.

Insler V: Gonadotropin therapy: New trends and insights. *Int J Fertil* 33:85-97, 1988.

Jaffe SB, Jewelewicz R: The basic infertility investigation. *Fertil Steril* 56:599-613, 1991.

Jones HW Jr, Schrader C: The process of human fertilization: Implications for moral status, editorial. *Fertil Steril* 48:189-192, 1987.

Kelly AC, Jewelewicz R: Alternate regimens for ovulation induction in polycystic ovarian disease. *Fertil Steril* 54:195-202, 1990.

Kettel LM, Murphy AA: Combination medical and surgical therapy for infertile patients with endometriosis. *Obstet Gynecol Clin North Am* 16:167-177, 1989.

Kingsland C, et al: The routine use of gonadotropin-releasing hormone agonists for all patients undergoing in vitro fertilization. Is there any medical advantage? A prospective randomized study. *Fertil Steril* 57:804-809, 1992.

Kletsky OA, et al: Pergolide and bromocriptine for treatment of patients with hyperprolactinemia. *Obstet Gynecol* 154:431-435, 1986.

Lanzone A, et al: Human growth hormone enhances progesterone production by human luteal cells in vitro: Evidence of a synergistic effect with human chorionic gonadotropin. *Fertil Steril* 57:92-96, 1992.

Lavy G, et al: Ovarian stimulation for in vitro fertilization and embryo transfer, human menopausal gonadotropin versus pure human follicle stimulating hormone: A randomized prospective study. *Fertil Steril* 50:74-78, 1988.

Lenton EA, et al: Measurement of progesterone in saliva: Assessment of the normal fertile range using spontaneous conception cycles. *Clin Endocrinol* 28:627-646, 1988.

Levin JH, et al: Is the inappropriate gonadotropin secretion of patients with polycystic ovary syndrome similar to that of patients with adult-onset congenital adrenal hyperplasia? *Fertil Steril* 56:635-640, 1991.

Li T-C, et al: New method of histologic dating of human endometrium in the luteal phase. *Fertil Steril* 50:52-60, 1988.

Lobo RA, et al: Clomiphene and dexamethasone in women unresponsive to clomiphene alone. *Obstet Gynecol* 60:497-501, 1982 A.

Lobo RA, et al: Clinical and laboratory predictors of clomiphene response. *Fertil Steril* 37:168-174, 1982 B.

Loy R, Seibel MM: Evaluation and therapy of polycystic ovarian syndrome. *Endocrinol Metab Clin North Am* 17:785-813, 1988.

MacLeod TL, et al: Anaphylactic reaction to synthetic luteinizing hormone-releasing-hormone. *Fertil Steril* 48:500-502, 1987.

Maclin VM, et al: Progesterone:estradiol ratios at implantation in ongoing pregnancies, abortions, and nonconception cycles resulting from ovulation induction. *Fertil Steril* 54:238-244, 1990.

March CM: Update: Teratogenic effects of ovulatory agents. *Endocr Fertil Forum* 11 (1):1-5, 1988.

March CM, et al: Effect of clomiphene citrate upon amount and duration of human menopausal gonadotropin therapy. *Am J Obstet Gynecol* 125:699-704, 1976.

McClamrock HD, et al: Ovarian hyperandrogenism: The role of and sensitivity to gonadotropins. *Fertil Steril* 55:73-79, 1991.

Medical Research International, Society for Assisted Reproductive Technology (SART): In vitro fertilization-embryo transfer (IVF-ET) in the United States: 1990 results from the IVF-ET registry. *Fertil Steril* 57:15-24, 1992.

Meldrum DR, et al: Routine pituitary suppression with leuprolide before ovarian stimulation for oocyte retrieval. *Fertil Steril* 51:455-459, 1989.

Messinis IE: Drugs used in *in vitro* fertilisation procedures. *Drugs* 38:148-159, 1989.

Minassian SS, et al: Urinary follicle stimulating hormone treatment for luteal phase defect. *J Reprod Med* 33:11-16, 1988.

Nader S: Polycystic ovary syndrome and the androgen-insulin connection. *Am J Obstet Gynecol* 165:346-348, 1991.

Navot D, et al: Direct correlation between plasma renin activity and severity of the ovarian hyperstimulation syndrome. *Fertil Steril* 48:57-61, 1987.

New MI: Polycystic ovarian disease and congenital and late-onset adrenal hyperplasia. *Endocrinol Metab Clin North Am* 17:637-643, 1988.

Noyes RW, et al: Dating the endometrial biopsy. *Fertil Steril* 1:3-25, 1950.

Olive DL, Lee KL: Analysis of sequential treatment protocols for endometriosis-associated infertility. *Obstet Gynecol* 154:613-619, 1986.

Padilla SL, et al: The Lupron screening test: Tailoring the use of leuprolide acetate in ovarian stimulation for in vitro fertilization. *Fertil Steril* 56:79-83, 1991.

Palermo R, et al: Concomitant gonadotropin-releasing-hormone agonist and menotropins treatment for the synchronized induction of multiple follicles. *Fertil Steril* 49:290-295, 1988.

Penzias AS, et al: Gamete intrafallopian transfer: Assessment of the optimal number of oocytes to transfer. *Fertility Steril* 55:311-313, 1991.

Quigley MM, Andrews LB: Human in vitro fertilization and the law. *Fertil Steril* 42:348-355, 1984.

Reid RL, et al: The theory and practice of ovulation induction with gonadotropin-releasing-hormone. *Am J Obstet Gynecol* 158:176-185, 1988.

Reyniak JV: Modern management of prolactinoma. *J Reprod Med* 28:257-263, 1983.

Riad-Fahmy D, et al: Determination of ovarian steroid hormone levels in saliva: Overview. *J Reprod Med* 32:254-272, 1987.

Rice JP, et al: Reevaluation of hysterosalpingography in infertility investigation. *Obstet Gynecol* 67:718-721, 1986.

Robertson JA: Ethical and legal issues in human egg donation. *Fertil Steril* 52:353-364, 1989.

Ron-El R, et al: Gonadotropins and combined gonadotropin-releasing hormone agonist: Gonadotropins protocols in a randomized prospective study. *Fertil Steril* 55:574-578, 1991.

Rosenfeld DL, Jacob J: Subsequent pregnancies in previously infertile women with endometriosis. *Obstet Gynecol* 72:908-910, 1988.

Ruiz-Velasco V, Tolis G: Pregnancy in hyperprolactinemic women. *Fertil Steril* 41:793-805, 1984.

Sagle MA, et al: A comparative, randomized study of low-dose human menopausal gonadotropin and follicle-stimulating hormone in women with polycystic ovarian syndrome. *Fertil Steril* 55:56-60, 1991.

Sauer MV, et al: Reversing the natural decline in human fertility: An extended clinical trial of oocyte donation to women of advanced reproductive age. *JAMA* 268:1275-1279, 1992.

Schenken RS, Malinak LR: Conservative surgery versus expectant management for infertile patient with mild endometriosis. *Fertil Steril* 37:183-186, 1982.

Schenker JG, Frenkel DA: Medico-legal aspects of in vitro fertilization and embryo transfer practice. *Obstet Gynecol Surv* 41:405-413, 1987.

Schriock ED, Jaffe RB: Induction of ovulation with gonadotropin-releasing hormone. *Obstet Gynecol Surv* 41:414-423, 1986.

Scott RT Jr, Rosenwaks Z: Ovulation induction for assisted reproduction. *J Reprod Med* 34 (suppl):108-114, 1989.

Scoccia B, et al: Comparison of urinary human follicle-stimulating hormone and human menopausal gonadotropins for ovarian stimulation in an in vitro fertilization program. *Fertil Steril* 48:446-449, 1987.

Seibel MM: A new era in reproductive technology: In vitro fertilization, gamete intrafallopian transfer, and donated gametes and embryos. *N Engl J Med* 318:828-834, 1988.

Seibel MM, et al: Effectiveness of danazol on subsequent fertility in minimal endometriosis. *Fertil Steril* 38:534-537, 1982.

Seibel MM, et al: Ovulation induction in polycystic ovary syndrome with urinary follicle-stimulating hormone or human menopausal gonadotropin. *Fertil Steril* 43:703-708, 1985.

Shelton K, et al: The use of the GnRH analogue buserelin for IVF—does it improve fertility? *Br J Obstet Gynecol* 98:544-549, 1991.

Shoham Z, et al: Results of ovulation induction using human menopausal gonadotropin or purified follicle-stimulating hormone in hypogonadotropic hypogonadism patients. *Fertil Steril* 56:1048-1053, 1991 A.

Shoham Z, et al: Polycystic ovarian syndrome: Safety and effectiveness of stepwise and low-dose administration of purified follicle-stimulating hormone. *Fertil Steril* 55:1051-1056, 1991 B.

Shoham Z, et al: Early miscarriage and fetal malformations after induction of ovulation (by clomiphene citrate and/or human menotropins), in vitro fertilization, and gamete intrafallopian transfer. *Fertil Steril* 55:1-11, 1991 C.

Silverberg KM, et al: Follicular size at the time of human chorionic gonadotropin administration predicts ovulation outcome in human menopausal gonadotropin-stimulated cycles. *Fertil Steril* 56:296-300, 1991.

Soto-Albors CE, et al: Medical management of hyperprolactinemia: A lower dose of bromocriptine may be effective. *Fertil Steril* 48:213-217, 1987.

Speroff L (ed): New concepts in the induction of ovulation. *Semin Reprod Endocrinol* 8:145-263, (Aug) 1990.

Sueldo CE, Swanson JA: Economics of inducing ovulation with human menopausal gonadotropins versus pulsatile subcutaneous gonadotropin-releasing-hormone. *Fertil Steril* 45:128-129, 1986.

Surrey ES, et al: Effects of gonadotropin-releasing hormone (GnRH) agonist on pituitary and ovarian responses to pulsatile GnRH therapy in polycystic ovarian disease. *Fertil Steril* 52:547-552, 1989.

Telimaa S: Danazol and medroxyprogesterone acetate inefficacious in the treatment of infertility in endometriosis. *Fertil Steril* 50:872-875, 1988.

Thatcher SS: Analogs of gonadotropin-releasing hormone in assisted reproduction. *Assist Reprod Rev* 1:116-131, 1991.

Thomas EJ, Cooke ID: Successful treatment of asymptomatic endometriosis: Does it benefit infertile women? *BMJ* 294:1117, 1987.

Tummon IS, et al: Randomized, prospective comparison of luteal leuprolide acetate and gonadotropins versus clomiphene citrate and gonadotropins in 408 first cycles of in vitro fertilization. *Fertil Steril* 58:563-568, 1992.

Vermesh M, et al: Vaginal bromocriptine: Pharmacology and effect on serum prolactin in normal women. *Obstet Gynecol* 72:693-698, 1988.

Wang CF, Gemzell C: Use of human gonadotropins for induction of ovulation in women with polycystic ovarian disease. *Fertil Steril* 33:479-486, 1980.

Weil C: Safety of bromocriptine in hyperprolactinaemic female infertility: Literature review. *Curr Med Res Opin* 10:172-195, 1986.

Weise HC, et al: Buserelin suppression of endogenous gonadotropin secretion in infertile women with ovarian feedback disorders given human menopausal/human chorionic gonadotropin treatment. *Fertil Steril* 49:399-403, 1988.

Welner S, et al: Human menopausal gonadotropins: A justifiable therapy in ovulatory women with long-standing idiopathic infertility. *Am J Obstet Gynecol* 158:111-117, 1988.

Wentz AC, et al: Cycle of conception endometrial biopsy. *Fertil Steril* 46:196-199, 1986.

Wheeler JM, et al: Relationship of endometriosis to spontaneous abortion. *Fertil Steril* 39:656-660, 1983.

Wong PC, Asch RH: Pulsatile administration of gonadotropin-releasing-hormone (GnRH) for induction of ovulation. *Int J Fertil* 30:11-27, 1986.

Wong PC, Asch RH: Induction of follicular development with gonadotropin-releasing-hormone. *Semin Reprod Endocrinol* 5:399-409, 1987.

Yoshimura Y, Wallach EE: Studies of the mechanism(s) of mammalian ovulation. *Fertil Steril* 47:22-34, 1987.

Zeevi D, et al: Ovulation induction: New approaches. *Assist Reprod Rev* 1:2-8, 1991.

Contraceptives

53

Contraception can be accomplished at any point from gametogenesis in both sexes to endometrial implantation. Combination oral contraceptives (OCs), oral progestins, intramuscular depot progestins, or progestins in subcutaneous capsules prevent ovulation and/or render cervical mucus incompatible to passage of sperm. For males, oral agents that suppress spermatogenesis and sperm maturation are being investigated. Sperm usually can be destroyed by vaginal spermicides, but there is as yet no agent available to destroy released ova. Methods to prevent the union of sperm and ovum utilize timing (eg, natural family planning, ovulation detection, periodic abstinence), surgery (eg, tubal ligation, hysterectomy, vasectomy), mechanical devices (eg, condom, diaphragm, cervical cap, sponge), or chemical agents (eg, spermicidal foams, gels, suppositories, creams; copper intrauterine devices [IUDs]). Even after fertilization has occurred, pregnancy may be prevented with "morning after" methods (eg, high-dose estrogens, some OCs, IUDs, danazol) that alter the uterine environment to prevent nidation.

New Developments in Male and Female Contraception: Mifepristone (RU 486), an antiprogesterone steroid that blocks progesterone-receptor binding, acts as a contraceptive agent by interrupting the luteal phase of the cycle or as an abortifacient when used in early pregnancy. Immunologic approaches are directed toward development of a vaccine against human chorionic gonadotropin or sperm. Analogues of gonadotropin-releasing hormone (GnRH), given by injection or intranasally, may have contraceptive activity by inhibiting ovulation in women (Gudmundsson et al, 1986; Balmaceda et al, 1987) and by interfering with normal gonadotropic stimulation in men (Bhasin and Swerdloff, 1987; Tom et al, 1991). New delivery systems for hormonal contraceptives, such as vaginal rings containing a progestin with or without an estrogen, transdermal contraceptive patches, or monthly injections of depot estrogen-progestin or progestin-only preparations, are in use in other countries or are being tested clinically.

MALE CONTRACEPTION

Only two reliable forms of male contraception currently are available in this country: condoms and vasectomy. When used alone, condoms are quite effective; when used simultaneously with a vaginal spermicide, the contraceptive efficacy is markedly improved (some condoms are coated with a spermicide). Because the condom is a mechanical barrier, it is also thought to prevent transmission of sexually transmitted diseases (STDs) (see Noncontraceptive Benefits of Spermicides/Barrier Methods in the section on Vaginal Spermicides).

Vasectomy is an effective and economical method to achieve permanent sterility. Complications at or soon after surgery may include pain, ecchymosis, infection, and granulomas. No long-term health risks up to 15 years after vasectomy were reported in one study (Rosenberg et al, 1986). However, results of several studies, both prospective and retrospective, have suggested that the relative risk of developing prostate cancer is 1.5 (95% CI, 1.03 to 2.37) to 1.7 (95% CI, 1.25 to 2.21) in vasectomized men, with the higher risk observed approximately 20 years after the procedure (Mettlin et al, 1990; Giovannucci et al, 1993 A, 1993 B). No increased risk of prostate cancer associated with prior vasectomy was found in other studies (*Lancet*, 1991). At this time, it has not been proven that vasectomy increases the risk of prostate cancer, and further studies are required to confirm or deny the association (Howards and Peterson, 1993).

Reversibility has been improved markedly by microsurgical vasovasostomy. However, many men who produce an adequate number of sperm post-anastomosis remain infertile; the development of antisperm antibodies may be responsible.

The pharmacologic approach to male contraception continues to be investigated, but no drugs for this indication are likely to reach the market in the foreseeable future. Pharmacologic agents suppress spermatogenesis through hormonal inhibition of gonadotropin secretion (eg, GnRH analogues, steroids, inhibin), direct inhibition of sperm production without affecting the hormonal milieu (eg, gossypol) (Waites, 1986), or interference with epididymal maturation of sperm.

With long-term use, GnRH analogues act by suppressing secretion of luteinizing hormone (LH) and follicle-stimulating hormone (FSH), which are essential for spermatogenesis. Because LH also is required to stimulate testosterone secretion, libido and potency decrease and secondary sexual characteristics (eg, beard growth) may be affected adversely. To avoid these adverse effects, GnRH analogues must be used with testosterone replacement therapy (initially or after azoospermia is achieved). Various steroid agents, including progestins, testosterone, and other androgens, have been used alone or in combination to suppress gonadotropins and hence spermatogenesis. Combinations used in earlier studies did not produce azoospermia consistently, but results achieved with those employed in recent investigations are more positive. Use of androgens, of course, eliminates the adverse effects on secondary sexual characteristics.

Inhibin, a peptide consisting of an alpha and beta chain linked by disulfide bonds, is secreted in the seminiferous tubules by the Sertoli cells (Ray et al, 1991). This peptide appears to selectively inhibit FSH secretion by the pituitary, which in turn probably inhibits spermatogenesis. Inhibin does not influence LH or testosterone secretion. A male contraceptive that selectively inhibits FSH is an attractive concept, but clinical application awaits development of a suitable preparation.

The main problem with most male contraceptive methods that employ hormonal suppression of spermatogenesis is that the onset and degree of efficacy are inconsistent. Either the dose required for azoospermia is too variable or the decrease in sperm count is inadequate to prevent fertilization. However, it is possible that low sperm counts combined with altered sperm function sufficient to provide contraceptive efficacy may be attainable with regimens currently under investigation.

Gossypol, a pigment extracted from cottonseed oil, directly interferes with spermatogenesis when taken orally and has been investigated in China. Although dramatic reductions in sperm count were obtained (Liu et al, 1987), the high efficacy rates required for marketing a contraceptive agent in the United States may not be achievable. Prolonged use of gossypol is associated with hypokalemia, which may not be reversible with potassium supplementation (Liu and Lyle, 1987). Persistent oligospermia and damage to the spermatogenic epithelium, which may be permanent, have been reported (Wu, 1989). Analogues of gossypol are currently being studied.

Two types of contraceptive vaccines for use in men are being developed. One immunizes against FSH, while the other immunizes against LHRH and would be used with androgen replacement therapy.

FEMALE CONTRACEPTION

Choice of Contraceptive

The best contraceptive for an individual depends on its use-effectiveness for that individual, its relative safety, and the patient's age, parity, and sexual and medical history. For example, patients with menorrhagia or dysmenorrhea may benefit from the endometrial suppression and inhibition of ovulation produced by combination OCs.

EFFECTIVENESS. The effectiveness of contraceptive techniques usually is measured by life table methods, which determine the probability of pregnancy with use of a specific contraceptive method within a given time interval. Failure rates also are expressed by the Pearl index, which is defined as the number of pregnancies/100 woman-years of use.

It is important to distinguish between method-effectiveness (efficacy after consistent correct usage) and use-effectiveness (efficacy after actual conditions of use). The higher failure rates revealed by the use-effectiveness index may be due to improper technique (barrier methods), forgetting to take pills (OCs), and failure to limit coitus to nonfertile times of the cycle (periodic abstinence). Generally, the method- and use-effectiveness rates for IUDs, implants, and medroxyprogesterone acetate (DMPA) are similar because, once inserted or injected, further participation by the patient is required only to ensure timely replacement. However, the use-effectiveness rate for IUDs may be decreased if the device is inserted improperly, is too small for the uterus, or has been expelled spontaneously without the patient's knowledge.

Estimates of effectiveness for the various contraceptive methods as reported in several sources appear in Table 1. For barrier methods (ie, diaphragm, cervical cap, condom), simultaneous use of a vaginal spermicide enhances efficacy. Failure rates for IUDs and diaphragms decline after the first year of use and with increasing age of the user. However, even when contraceptives with low rates of failure are used, the long-term risk of an unwanted pregnancy may appear to be high because the rates are cumulative (see review by Trussell et al, 1990).

SAFETY. In general, OCs probably are associated with a wider variety of adverse effects than other methods of contraception, but complications associated with STDs in IUD users may result in hospitalization and may be more likely to decrease future fertility. Mortality rates are lower with OCs (except in smokers over age 35), IUDs, or elective abortion than with term pregnancy that results from failure to use contraception.

The risk of pelvic inflammatory disease (PID) is increased in the following three groups: (1) nulliparous IUD users less than 25 years old with multiple sexual partners, (2) those with a history of STDs, especially infections caused by *Chlamydia trachomatis* or *Neisseria gonorrhoeae*, and (3) younger women. STDs are the most common cause of PID. Highly effective contraceptives that provide some protective effect against STDs therefore are preferred in these patients. The risk of severe PID may be *decreased* in women who use OCs or barrier methods compared with those using no contraception. However, in one study (Washington et al, 1985), it was hypothesized that OCs may afford no protection and may even increase the risk of *C. trachomatis* cervical infections, which have a milder course but are associated with subsequent infertility in many patients. In another study, OC use was associated with increased risk of both gonococcal and chlamydial infections even after adjusting for the number of sexual partners (Louv et al, 1989).

Because PID may cause infertility, most physicians do not recommend IUDs for nulliparous women who eventually wish to bear children. Older patients whose families are complete are good candidates for barrier methods, levonorgestrel implant [Norplant System], or (if the relationship is mutually monogamous) IUDs, especially if sterilization is not desired.

PATIENT VARIABLES. Other conditions affect the choice of contraceptive. These include the patient's age, knowledge about and attitude toward various methods, frequency of coitus, extent of male participation in contraception, level of protection desired (ie, absolute versus spacing children), benefits in addition to contraception (eg, menstrual regularity, decreased dysmenorrhea and risk of ovarian and endometrial cancer with OCs), attitude toward contraceptive failure (ie, would response to failure be abortion or completion of unwanted pregnancy), cost of contraceptive method, and compliance (eg, unreliability in taking OCs or in utilizing coitus-related methods favors use of an IUD, levonorgestrel implant, or DMPA).

Low-dose OCs are often used by adolescents who have a continuing need for contraception and are willing to comply with the regimen. Some patients in whom OC use is contrain-

TABLE 1.
ESTIMATES OF CONTRACEPTIVE EFFICACY

Method	Approximate Pregnancy Rate First Year of Use*		
	Method-Effectiveness	**Use-Effectiveness**	**Adjusted for Unreported Abortion†**
Oral Contraceptives (combined regimen)	0.1%	2%–3%	6.2%
"Minipill" (progestin only)	0.5%–1%	2.5%–4%	Not available
Intrauterine Devices	<1%	<1%	Not available
Vaginal Spermicides‡	3%	2%–30%	26.3%
Condoms	2%	3%–20%	14.2%
Diaphragms, Cervical Caps	6%	18%	15.6% (Diaphragm)
Rhythm	5%	25%–30%	16.2%
Contraceptive Sponge	3%–9%	6%–27.7%	Not available
Levonorgestrel Implant [Norplant System]	0.04%	0.04%	Not available
Depot Medroxyprogesterone Injection	0.3%	0.3%	Not available
Female Condom	26%	26%	Not available

* *In the absence of contraceptive use by couples, pregnancy would occur in 80% to 85% of the women.*
† *Jones and Forrest, 1989.*
‡ *Gels, creams, foams, suppositories*

dicated may be suitable candidates for IUDs or may choose a barrier method. For women who engage in sporadic sexual activity, a condom, diaphragm or cervical cap, and/or spermicide might be more appropriate than OCs because compliance with an OC regimen may be lax during periods of abstinence and contraceptive protection would be unreliable. Barrier contraceptive methods with spermicides offer partial protection against some STDs and are particularly useful in individuals who have multiple sex partners. The combined use of OCs and condoms may be selected by individuals who have a continuing need for contraception and may be exposed to STDs (eg, those with multiple sexual partners or one nonmonogamous partner).

Use of OCs is no longer discouraged on the basis of age alone; OCs may be the preferred form of contraception for women over age 40 if they are in good health, do not smoke, and other contraindications are not present (Mishell, 1990). Because hormone replacement therapy does not reliably prevent ovulation, low-dose OCs may provide both contraception and relief from menopausal symptoms in the perimenopausal period. (The serum FSH level can be measured annually to determine when menopause has occurred in OC users.) Patients who have completed their families may prefer sterilization (for either the male or female partner) or IUDs to continuing use of other methods of contraception.

In women who are breast-feeding, combination OCs may diminish lactation but may be used after lactation is established. Progestin-only "minipills" and DMPA do not decrease and may increase the volume of milk and, therefore, are preferable. Levonorgestrel implant, which also contains only a progestin, is an alternative. Breast-feeding provides limited contraceptive protection for the first six months depending on the extent of nursing, but return of fertility is more likely when menses resume, which is not predictable in a given patient (Lewis et al, 1991; Dunson et al, 1993).

Proper instruction in contraceptive use is of utmost importance; methods with a potentially high failure rate (eg, diaphragm) may be very effective (failure rate, 3%) if used with a spermicidal agent by highly motivated, properly instructed patients.

Patient preference is paramount when selecting a contraceptive method. A difference in effectiveness of 1% between two methods may be significant on a population basis, but unimportant to a given patient. OCs, IUDs, levonorgestrel implant, DMPA, and barrier methods are all effective, and the best choice among them may be the one that the patient feels most comfortable with and that the couple will use consistently, even though its method-effectiveness is not the highest.

Diaphragms and Cervical Caps

Diaphragms and cervical caps are dome-shaped latex cups that cover the cervix and are inserted before coitus. They should be used with a spermicidal agent that is applied inside and around the edges of the cup.

Diaphragms are larger than cervical caps and are available in several sizes. The circular edge of the diaphragm contains a spring that is flexible, holds the device in place, and aids in insertion and removal. Diaphragms should be left in place for six to eight hours after coitus. Cervical caps are available in a limited number of sizes, which may preclude their use in some women. These devices are held in place by suction and generally are more difficult to insert and remove correctly than diaphragms but may be left in place for 48 hours; however, this length of use may cause malodor. Both types of cervical covers may be dislodged during intercourse, but this appears to be more common with the cervical cap. See also review on cervical caps (Weiss et al, 1991).

Toxic shock syndrome (TSS) has rarely occurred in diaphragm users, although causality has not been established. Most cases occurred in women who wore the device continuously for more than 24 hours; therefore, continuous use should not exceed this period. An association between diaphragm use and urinary tract infections has been suggested but not proved.

The female condom or vaginal pouch, a barrier contraceptive, has been approved by the FDA. The polyurethane sheath is held in place by two flexible rings, one of which covers the labia and one that is placed intravaginally. The device is designed to prevent STDs as well as pregnancy.

Vaginal Spermicides

FORMULATIONS. Spermicidal agents for topical vaginal application are available as creams, gels, foams, films, and suppositories (plain, effervescent) and in a sponge preparation (see Table 2). All can be obtained without prescription, are easily applied, and, when used correctly (particularly in combination with a diaphragm or condom), provide contraceptive protection. Some creams, gels, and foams are designed for use only with a diaphragm. When vaginal spermicides are used alone, agents with the highest concentrations and total amount of active ingredients probably are most effective.

Formulations differ in amount of active ingredient in the preparation, speed of distribution, and degree of surface coverage, and some require special applicators. Suppositories and films are inserted high into the vagina and require a melting and/or effervescence time of 10 to 15 minutes for maximum coverage. In general, aerosol foams are easy to apply, cover the cervix almost immediately, and are distributed over a larger surface area. Effervescent vaginal suppositories are designed to provide similar coverage without the need for a special applicator.

Most vaginal spermicides marketed in the United States contain nonoxynol-9 or octoxynol-9 as the active ingredient. These nonionic surfactants are effective and generally safe, but local irritation (which may be due to the active and/or inactive ingredients, such as perfume in some preparations) may affect either partner. Selection of another product with different components may alleviate irritation.

Proper use of these agents enhances their effectiveness. They should be applied before coitus (from minutes to one hour, as directed) and must be reapplied before each ejaculation. Douching should be avoided for six to eight hours following coitus, since this may dilute the spermicide. Douching itself is *not* effective for contraception.

TABLE 2.
VAGINAL SPERMICIDES (NONPRESCRIPTION)

Product and Manufacturer	Active Ingredient	Other Ingredients
CREAMS		
Koromex Cream* (Schmid)	octoxynol, 3%	propylene glycol, stearic acid, sorbitan stearate, polysorbate 60, boric acid, fragrance
Ortho-Creme* (Ortho)	nonoxynol-9, 2%	benzoic acid, castor oil, cetyl alcohol, fragrance, glacial acetic acid, methylparaben, potassium hydroxide, propylene glycol, propylparaben, purified water, sodium carboxymethylcellulose, sodium lauryl sulfate, sorbic acid, stearic acid, trolamine
GELS		
Conceptrol Disposable Gel (Ortho)	nonoxynol-9, 4%	lactic acid, methylparaben, povidone, propylene glycol, purified water, sodium carboxymethylcellulose, sorbic acid, and sorbital solution
Gynol II* (Ortho)	nonoxynol-9, 2%	same as Conceptrol Disposable Gel
Gynol II Extra Strength (Ortho)	nonoxynol-9, 3%	same as Gynol II
Koromex Gel* (Schmid)	nonoxynol-9, 2%	propylene glycol, cellulose gum, boric acid, sorbitol, simethicone, fragrance
Koromex Jelly* (Schmid)	nonoxynol-9, 3%	same as Koromex Gel
Ortho-Gynol* (Ortho)	octoxynol-9, 1%	benzoic acid, castor oil, fragrance, glacial acetic acid, methylparaben, potassium hydroxide, propylene glycol, purified water, sodium carboxymethylcellulose, sorbic acid
Ramses Vaginal Jelly (Schmid)	nonoxynol-9, 5%	boric acid 1%, ethyl alcohol 5%, jelly base
Shur-Seal Gel* (Milex)	nonoxynol-9, 2%	†
FOAMS		
Delfen Foam (Ortho)	nonoxynol-9, 12.5%	benzoic acid, cetyl alcohol, diethylaminoethyl stearamide, glacial acetic acid, methylparaben, perfume, phosphoric acid, polyvinyl alcohol, propellant 12, propellant 114, propylene glycol, purified water, sodium carboxymethylcellulose, stearic acid
Emko (Schering-Plough)	nonoxynol-9, 8%	benzethonium chloride 0.2%, stearic acid, triethanolamine, glyceryl monostearate, poloxamer 188, polyethylene glycol 600, substituted adamantane
Emko Pre-Fil (Schering-Plough)	nonoxynol-9, 8%	same as Emko
Koromex (Schmid)	nonoxynol-9, 12.5%	propylene glycol, isopropyl alcohol, laureth 4, cetyl alcohol, polyethylene glycol stearate, fragrance, dichlorodifluoromethane, dichlorotetrafluoroethane
SUPPOSITORIES		
Conceptrol (Ortho)	nonoxynol-9, 8.3%	lauroamphodiacetate, sodium trideceth sulfate, polyethylene glycol 1000, polyethylene glycol 1450, povidone
Encare (Thompson)	nonoxynol-9, 3%	polyethylene glycols, sodium bicarbonate, sodium tartrate, tartaric acid, sodium citrate
Semicid (Whitehall)	nonoxynol-9, 100 mg	polyethylene glycol, benzethonium chloride, citric acid, D&C red # 21, D&C red # 33, methylparaben, water

(continued on next page)

TABLE 2 (continued)

Product and Manufacturer	Active Ingredient	Other Ingredients
SPONGE		
Today (Whitehall)	nonoxynol-9, 1 g	benzoic acid, citric acid, sodium dihydrogen citrate, sodium metabisulfite, sorbic acid, water in a polyurethane foam sponge
FILM		
VCF (Apothecus)	nonoxynol-9, 28%	glycerin, polyvinyl alcohol

** Used with diaphragm*

† No further information available from manufacturer

SAFETY. Although the results of several studies have suggested that use of vaginal spermicides may be associated with increased risk of chromosomal or other abnormalities (Strobino et al, 1980; Rothman, 1982; Jick et al, 1981; Polednak et al, 1982; Huggins et al, 1982), the preponderance of evidence strongly supports the safety of these agents (Shapiro et al, 1982; Bracken and Vita, 1983; Cordero and Layde, 1983; Bracken, 1985; Mills et al, 1982, 1985; Linn et al, 1983; Louik et al, 1987; Warburton et al, 1987). In a meta-analysis of maternal spermicide use approximately at or within three months after conception, there was no association with adverse effects on the fetus, including chromosomal aberrations, malformations, neoplasms, and undescended testes (Einarson et al, 1990). Results of studies in which rats were exposed to nonoxynol-9 and octoxynol-9 did not indicate any teratogenic effects and support the above observations (*Popul Rep [H]*, 1984).

CONTRACEPTIVE SPONGE. Another delivery system for spermicide is a disposable polyurethane sponge containing nonoxynol-9 [Today]. The sponge has a concave surface that is designed to be placed over the cervix. It acts as a mechanical barrier to sperm, absorbs seminal fluid, and releases the spermicide that is incorporated into the sponge. A wide range of effectiveness has been reported. In one study, the pregnancy rate among parous women who used the sponge was higher than in those who used a diaphragm (Edelman et al, 1984). The sponge offers potential advantages: It requires no fitting, it is not messy, the spermicide is immediately available, and it may be left in place and is effective for multiple coital encounters over a 24-hour period.

Adverse effects include vaginal irritation and dryness. Insertion and/or removal may be difficult. Although the sponge was left in place for up to 48 hours in early studies, it was found to be much less effective; current instructions recommend that use not exceed 24 hours. Toxic shock syndrome has been reported in a few contraceptive sponge users. Some cases have been associated with predisposing conditions such as menstruation, prolonged use, or use postpartum. The relative risk of TSS on nonmenstrual days is estimated to be 7.8 to 40 times greater for contraceptive sponge users. The actual incidence is rare and is estimated to be 0.015 to 0.28 cases per one million nonmenstrual days (Faich et al, 1986).

NONCONTRACEPTIVE BENEFITS OF SPERMICIDES/BARRIER METHODS. Vaginal contraception may reduce the risk of STDs. In vitro and in vivo studies suggest that spermicides kill the causative microorganisms and offer some protection from gonorrhea, genital herpes, trichomoniasis, and other STDs. PID resulting from such infections also was reduced after use of barrier contraceptives (Kelaghan et al, 1982). The risk of tubal infertility is decreased with use of barrier contraception, particularly if both a mechanical barrier and a spermicide are employed (Cramer et al, 1987). A randomized cross-over study of women at high risk of contracting STDs showed that some protection against *Chlamydia*, but not against yeast infections, may be offered by the contraceptive sponge (Rosenberg et al, 1987). In another study, the incidence of gonorrhea decreased but the rate of HIV seroconversion increased in prostitutes who used the contraceptive sponge (Kreiss et al, 1992). The mechanical barrier provided by diaphragms, cervical caps, sponges, and condoms may contribute to the anti-infective action and also may protect against organisms that initiate or promote cervical cancer (*Popul Rep [H]*, 1984; Coker et al, 1992). Thus, vaginal contraception may be particularly useful for women with multiple sexual partners or for those who are otherwise at increased risk of contracting an STD. On the other hand, these findings should *not* be interpreted to mean that spermicides and/or barrier methods provide reliable protection from STDs, although regular use appears to reduce the risk somewhat.

Intrauterine Devices

In 1985 and 1986, the manufacturers of the Lippes Loop, Saf-T-Coil, and copper-containing devices [Cu-7, Tatum-T] voluntarily discontinued production in the United States. These actions were based on economic rather than medical considerations. Existing supplies of discontinued IUDs continued to be used for some time. Consequently, if any of the formerly available copper-containing products are still in utero, their period of efficacy (three years for the Cu-7 and four years for the Tatum-T) has probably expired and the devices should be replaced.

The World Health Organization has published a series of papers as part of an effort to reassure the international community of the continued safety and efficacy of IUDs for properly selected patients (WHO, 1987 A, 1987 B, 1987 C, 1988).

The only two IUDs currently available in the United States are the intrauterine progesterone contraceptive [Progestasert] system, which requires yearly replacement, and the CuT380A (copper IUD) [ParaGard], which can be worn continuously for eight years without replacement. The CuT380A has almost twice the area of exposed copper as models previously available in this country. This enhances its efficacy, and the use-effectiveness with this model is greater than with OCs. Pregnancy rates were less than 1% during the first year and 1.4% (cumulative rate) after six years of use (*Popul Rep [B]*, 1988; Tatum and Connell, 1986).

Several IUDs are under development in the United States and other countries. One contains levonorgestrel, and others contain copper and silver and differ from the CuT380A in design and the quantity of copper.

An IUD is usually inserted during menses when the absence of pregnancy can be presumed, but it may be inserted at any time during the cycle if a nonpregnant state is assured. Ovulation may be the optimal time for IUD insertion since, contrary to popular belief, the cervix is most patent at that time. In addition, insertion during ovulation has been reported to decrease the expulsion rate (Jovanovic et al, 1988). After a term pregnancy, insertion generally is delayed until involution is complete (approximately four weeks) to decrease the risk of uterine perforation or spontaneous expulsion; a barrier method of contraception may be used in the interim. In one study, women who breastfed were reported to be at substantially greater risk of perforation (Heartwell and Schlesselman, 1983). In another study, immediate postpartum insertion of IUDs designed for such use did not increase infection or uterine perforation, but expulsion rates were higher than after insertion at other times (Cole et al, 1984). Insertion usually can take place immediately after abortion induced during the first trimester. Perforation is less likely, and involution occurs sooner than after full-term delivery.

IUDs have been used as postcoital contraceptives by insertion within three days after unprotected midcycle intercourse. (See also the section on Postcoital Contraception.)

MECHANISM OF ACTION. IUDs alter the biochemical milieu of the endometrium. Leukocytic infiltration occurs soon after insertion, and a sterile inflammatory reaction in the endometrial cavity releases substances toxic to sperm and ova. An increased number of mast cells were observed in the wall of the fallopian tubes in women wearing copper IUDs, and this may be related to local inflammatory reactions (Sandvei et al, 1986). The serum immunoglobulin level is elevated and may interfere with the normal immunologic tolerance that allows successful nidation. Sperm transport to the oviducts also is inhibited.

It was formerly thought that the biochemical changes in the intrauterine environment prevented implantation or caused abortion of the blastocyst and that this was the major mechanism of action of IUDs. Newer evidence suggests that IUD-related changes may develop in the sperm and ovum before fertilization occurs (Alvarez et al, 1988). Therefore, IUDs affect the ovum and sperm separately and before fertilization can take place.

Nonmedicated IUDs are much less effective than medicated IUDs, which have the additional effects of the active agent. The addition of copper increases leukocytic infiltration, which enhances efficacy. Prostaglandin production is greater with copper than with a nonmedicated device, and this probably stimulates the inflammatory reaction. Copper also may decrease sperm motility directly. In addition to enhancing contraceptive efficacy, copper inhibits the growth of gonococci in vitro, but the clinical usefulness of this effect has not been demonstrated. Blood copper levels are not altered. However, copper IUDs should not be used in patients with Wilson's disease.

The Progestasert system continuously releases small quantities (65 mcg daily) of progesterone into the endometrial cavity; glandular atrophy and a chronic decidual reaction that are unfavorable for implantation result. Progesterone also may directly inhibit metabolism, capacitation, and swimming speed of sperm. Results of studies suggest that the risk of ectopic pregnancy is increased compared with other types of IUDs (see section on Adverse Reactions and Contraindications). The progesterone device requires yearly replacement. Normal cyclic function, including ovulation, continues as it does with other IUDs. The amount of progesterone absorbed systemically does not affect carbohydrate or lipid metabolism.

CHOICE OF IUD. In most situations in which an IUD is the desired form of contraception, the CuT380A will be preferred because of its greater efficacy and the need for replacement only every eight years (especially in view of the discomfort and potential cost associated with that procedure). Also, since infections that occur with IUDs are almost entirely associated with insertion, less frequent insertion should reduce this risk. The Progestasert may be selected for patients with a history of heavy menstrual bleeding. The volume of menstrual blood loss (compared with preinsertion cycles or cycles in which a copper device was used) is decreased, and dysmenorrhea may be reduced compared with non-IUD cycles; however, spotting may occur throughout the cycle.

PRECAUTIONS. High fundal placement maximizes efficacy; low placement may be followed by partial expulsion and is associated with decreased effectiveness and increased risk of infection. Spontaneous expulsion may be undetected and usually occurs within six months (highest incidence is in the first month at the time of menses). Factors associated with expulsion of copper IUDs include younger age, increased menstrual blood loss and length of flow, and dysmenorrhea prior to insertion (Zhang et al, 1992). Insertion of another device is usually successful.

The uterus should be sounded carefully before insertion, and a device of appropriate size should be used. Insertion into a uterus of less than 6.5 cm may cause discomfort, bleeding, and expulsion. The presence of the IUD string should be confirmed at least after each menses. Missing strings require prompt investigation: The possibility of pregnancy should first be ruled out (the string can be drawn into the enlarging uterine cavity) and then the presence and location of the device should be confirmed by ultrasound (the string may be coiled in the endocervical canal or perforation into the abdominal cavity may have occurred).

Perforation of the uterine wall and translocation of the device may occur or begin at insertion. IUDs also can become embedded in the endometrium without perforation. Surgical removal, usually by laparoscopy, is common if the IUD is in the peritoneal cavity, particularly when the device contains copper, because tenacious adhesions to the omentum may develop.

If pregnancy occurs with an IUD in situ and the patient elects to complete the pregnancy, the risk of spontaneous first trimester abortion is increased (up to 50%). The risk of prematurity or midtrimester septic abortions also is increased (see below). If the device can be removed without undue resistance, this should be done whether the pregnancy is to be continued or not. There is no evidence that teratogenic effects are produced by IUDs, whether nonmedicated, copper, or medicated.

Fatal septic midtrimester abortions in patients wearing Dalkon Shields led to the withdrawal of this device from the U.S. market. Evidence suggests that the multifilament tail acted as a wick to carry pathogens into the uterine cavity, which normally is separated from the vaginal flora by the cervical mucus. Other noncopper devices also have been associated with sepsis during pregnancy, and it is theoretically possible that any IUD with a string appendage (this includes all IUDs in use in the United States) may present some degree of risk. Patients wearing IUDs who become pregnant should be informed of the risk if the device is not removed and instructed to report symptoms of infection promptly. (See the discussion of pelvic inflammatory disease under Adverse Reactions and Contraindications.)

ADVERSE REACTIONS AND CONTRAINDICATIONS. Insertion of an IUD usually causes temporary discomfort, which may be prevented by administration of an NSAID just prior to insertion. A transient vasovagal response (ie, syncope, bradycardia) may occur. Cramps and bleeding (similar to menstrual cramps and flow) are common for up to 24 hours following insertion. With the Progestasert device, spotting may occur throughout the cycle.

IUDs should not be used during pregnancy, in the presence of genital bleeding of unknown etiology, or in patients with suspected or diagnosed uterine carcinoma. Their use generally is not recommended when the uterine cavity is distorted from any cause, when the uterus is less than 6.5 cm, or when the cervical canal is severely stenotic. See the manufacturers' guidelines for a complete list of contraindications.

Pelvic Inflammatory Disease: With the older devices, the frequency of pelvic inflammatory disease (PID) was reported to be increased two to ten times (Ory, 1978; Kaufman et al, 1980 A, 1983; Vessey et al, 1981; Burkman, 1981; Lee et al, 1983). The noncopper IUD did not provide any protection against PID. The Dalkon Shield was associated with a higher risk of PID than other IUDs (Kaufman et al, 1983; Lee et al, 1983), and these devices should be removed even in asymptomatic women who are still wearing them.

Results of two studies demonstrated increased risk of primary tubal infertility with IUD use in nulliparous women with more than one sex partner; copper-containing IUDs had the lowest risk, followed by nonmedicated devices; the Dalkon Shield had the highest risk (Cramer et al, 1985; Daling et al, 1985). In the former study and a case-controlled study of 657 women hospitalized with PID (Lee et al, 1988), there was no increased risk in women who reported only one sex partner. In a prospective study that compared women who had IUDs removed to allow conception with those who had the device removed because of complications, no difference in subsequent fertility was observed among women in the two groups (Wilson, 1989).

Age appears to be inversely related to risk of PID, but there is no consensus on the influence of parity.

In summary, in certain populations IUDs have a higher relative risk of PID than non-IUD contraception, and the Dalkon Shield repeatedly has had the highest associated risk. However, study results are inconsistent regarding the comparative risk of other types of devices.

If abdominal pain or tenderness, abnormal vaginal discharge, and fever occur in an IUD user, PID should be considered. If the infection is mild and responds to antibiotic therapy within one or two days, some practitioners leave the IUD in place. Severe infection requires removal of the device, hospitalization, and prompt antibiotic therapy. An IUD should not be inserted in the presence of pelvic infection from any cause. Furthermore, women at high risk for PID (eg, history of PID, multiple sex partners) are not good candidates for initial or continuing IUD use. Other contraceptive methods should be considered first for nulliparous women; however, the IUD may be appropriate for some nulliparous women if they are aware that future fertility may be impaired. Nulliparous women with one mutually monogamous sex partner and for whom OCs are contraindicated and who do not wish to use barrier methods may be candidates. (See also reviews on PID and IUDs by Grimes, 1987, and Kessel, 1989.)

Bacterial Infection: *Actinomyces* organisms may be a normal part of the flora in the lower genital tract of healthy women (Persson and Holmberg, 1984). Colonization of these organisms in the upper genital tract appears to be related to long-term IUD use and may cause problems ranging from mild symptoms of infection to endometritis, tubo-ovarian abscess, and, rarely, death. In asymptomatic patients, routine Papanicolaou smears can be tested for *Actinomyces*; if positive, the IUD probably should be removed (Mishell, 1984).

Ectopic Pregnancy: Ectopic pregnancy is less likely to occur in women using any contraceptive method, including IUDs, than in women not using a contraceptive. A case-control study of 274 patients who had an ectopic pregnancy identified current IUD use, history of infertility, history of PID, and prior tubal surgery as independent risk factors for ectopic pregnancy (relative risks of 13.7, 2.6, 3.3, and 4.5, respectively) (Marchbanks et al, 1988). More ectopic pregnancies result from failure of barrier methods and IUDs than from failure with combination OCs (Ory, 1981), perhaps because IUDs prevent intrauterine rather than extrauterine (tubal and ovarian) pregnancy more effectively.

The risk of ectopic pregnancy associated with medicated IUDs appears to be inversely related to the quantity of active ingredient. Thus, IUDs containing ≥ 350 mm^2 of copper are associated with fewer ectopic pregnancies than those containing 200 mm^2. IUDs containing copper or levonorgestrel (investigational product) or nonmedicated devices are associated with fewer ectopic pregnancies than those containing progesterone (Sivin, 1991).

If a patient conceives while using an IUD, the possibility of an ectopic pregnancy (3% to 9%) should be considered

(Mishell, 1984). Women with a history of ectopic pregnancy should not use IUDs thereafter.

Insulin-Dependent Diabetes: In one study, a high failure rate with copper or nonmedicated IUDs was reported in insulin-dependent diabetic women (Gosden et al, 1982), but this has not been confirmed by other investigators. No difference in the pattern of copper corrosion or contraceptive efficacy was observed in insulin-dependent diabetic women compared with nondiabetic controls (Skouby et al, 1984).

PREPARATIONS.

Progestasert System (ALZA). 36 mm tubular vertical stem containing progesterone 38 mg initially (32 mm horizontal crossarms). Replacement required yearly.

ParaGard (GynoPharma). 36 mm stem by 32 mm crossarms; 380 mm^2 exposed copper wire wrapped around stem and crossbars. Replacement required every eight years. (For information on a program that provides free IUDs to women of established economic need who are appropriate candidates for this method of contraception, contact the company at 908/725-3100.)

Oral Contraceptives

Oral contraceptives (OCs) are highly effective in preventing pregnancy. Preparations usually are mixtures containing a synthetic estrogen (ethinyl estradiol or mestranol) and a progestin (norethindrone, norethindrone acetate, ethynodiol diacetate, norgestrel, levonorgestrel, norgestimate, or desogestrel). (Norgestimate and desogestrel were approved as OC components in the United States recently; they have been used in other countries for several years. Another progestin, gestodene, is being evaluated in clinical trials.) Other preparations contain a progestin alone. For the chemical structures of the steroids and the composition of OCs, see the Figure and Table 3. Ethinyl estradiol, norethindrone, and norethindrone acetate also are available as single-entity drugs for noncontraceptive indications. Natural steroids are not used because very large oral doses are required to achieve the desired pharmacologic effect. The addition of a 17α-ethinyl group enhances the oral activity of the steroids used in OCs by inhibiting hepatic degradation.

The steroids present in OCs generally are well absorbed, but their bioavailability is variable (range, approximately 40% for ethinyl estradiol to 65% for norethindrone). These agents are widely distributed with apparent Vds of 1.5 to 4.3 L/kg. They are primarily metabolized in the liver and are excreted in the urine and feces, principally as glucuronide and sulfate conjugates of both the parent compound and metabolites. The glucuronide and sulfate conjugates of ethinyl estradiol (half-life 6 to 14 hours) undergo extensive enterohepatic recycling and may be hydrolyzed by bacterial enzymes, thus regenerating the parent compound. Levonorgestrel (half-life, 5 to 14 hours) and norethindrone (half-life, 7.5 to 9 hours) are metabolized by reduction and conjugation; these conjugates are not cycled appreciably through the enterohepatic circulation.

Discussions on selection, management of patients, and overall benefits and risks of OCs are available (Mishell, 1990; Guillebaud, 1990; Burkman, 1991; Speroff and DeCherney, 1992).

PREPARATIONS. Combination products are available in "low-dose" (less than 50 mcg estrogen) and "high-dose" preparations (50 mcg estrogen). "Low-dose" pills may contain constant doses of estrogen and progestin ("monophasic") or variable doses ("multiphasic"). Variable-dose combination products are either "biphasic" or "triphasic" depending on the number of different dosage regimens in a cycle.

Four biphasic products [GenCept 10/11, Jenest-28, Nelova 10/11, Ortho-Novum 10/11] are marketed in the United States. A constant dose of estrogen is administered for 21 days while the progestin content is increased halfway through the treatment cycle. Triphasic preparations are of two types: In one type, the estrogen content is constant while the progestin changes; in the other, the doses of both estrogen and progestin change during the cycle. There are two preparations of the first type: Ortho-Novum 7/7/7, in which the progestin dose increases throughout the cycle, and Tri-Norinyl, in which the progestin dose first increases then decreases at the end of the treatment cycle. Two preparations of the second type [Tri-Levlen, Triphasil] are available in the United States; the dose of estrogen first increases and then decreases while the dose of progestin increases throughout the cycle.

All combination OCs have similar high efficacy, and although advantages in cycle control may be claimed, all preparations probably provide equivalent contraception.

"Minipills" contain a progestin only (norethindrone [Micronor, Nor-QD], norgestrel [Ovrette]). See Table 3 for information on OC preparations.

ADMINISTRATION. Combination OCs are taken for 21 days of the cycle, followed by one week without medication during which withdrawal bleeding occurs. Most preparations are available in "memory packets" containing 21 active pills and 7 inert pills. Some preparations contain iron in the nonhormonal pills. Minipills are taken daily and continuously.

Administration of combination OCs may be started two to four weeks after full-term pregnancy if the patient is not lactating. Ovulation usually does not occur before this time, and the theoretical danger of associated thromboembolism following delivery probably is reduced by waiting at least two weeks. If bromocriptine [Parlodel] is taken to suppress postpartum lactation, ovulation may occur early and OCs can be resumed two weeks after delivery. The risk of thromboembolic phenomena following abortion is not great, but the chance of early ovulation is high; therefore, OC use may be initiated 24 to 48 hours after a first-trimester spontaneous or induced abortion and within one week after a second-trimester abortion. Minipills may be started immediately after full-term pregnancy or abortion, and are preferred in lactating women.

In general, combination OCs are effective within the first cycle of use if started by the fifth day of the cycle. However, some physicians recommend concomitant utilization of a barrier method during the first month of OC use or until compliance is established. The manufacturer's recommendation should be consulted. Substituting one combination formulation for another may be accomplished easily at the initiation of a new cycle or immediately after the last pill of the previous regimen. Contraceptive effectiveness is not interrupted.

ESTROGENS AND PROGESTINS IN ORAL CONTRACEPTIVES

ESTROGENS

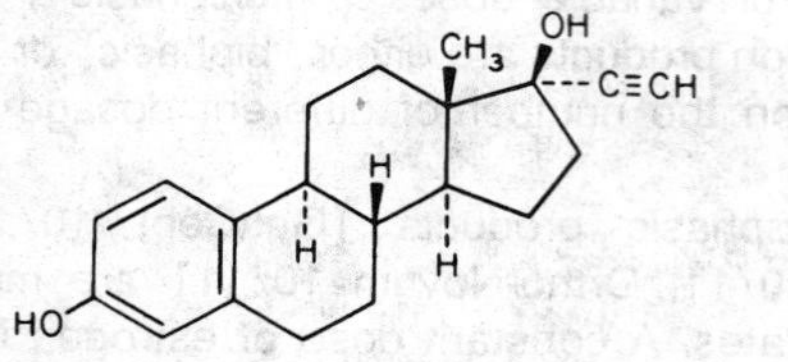

Ethinyl Estradiol

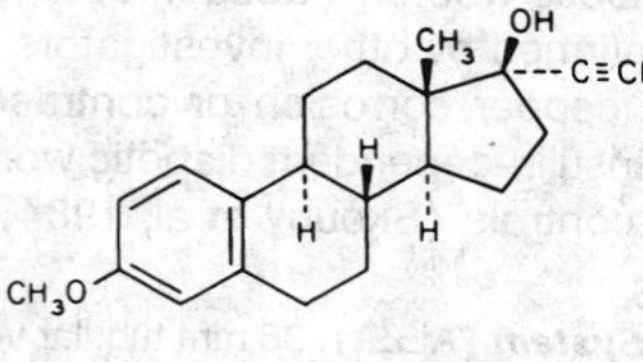

Mestranol

PROGESTINS

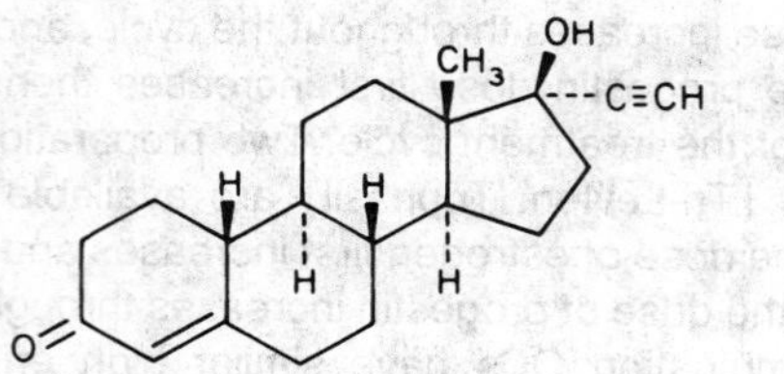

Norethindrone

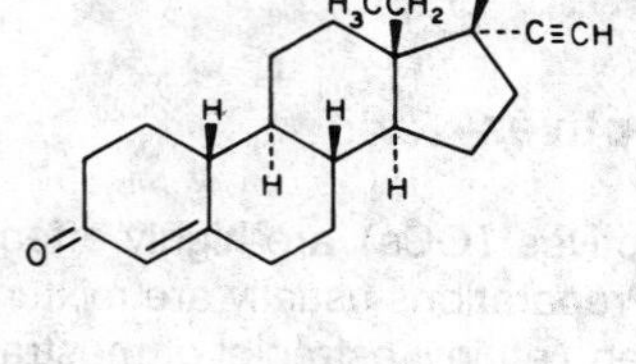

Norgestrel (racemic mixture)
Levonorgestrel (levorotatory isomer)

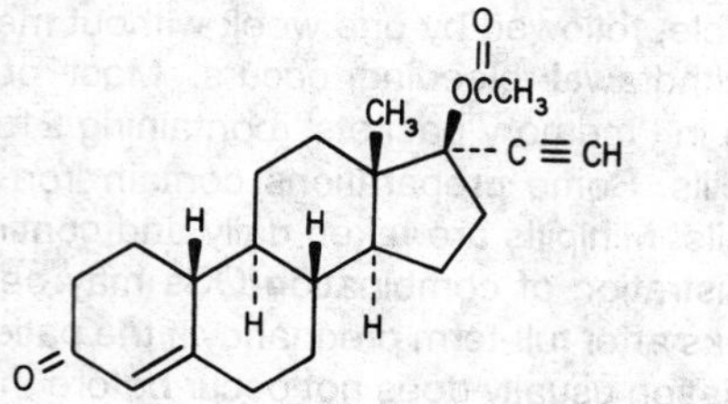

Norethindrone Acetate

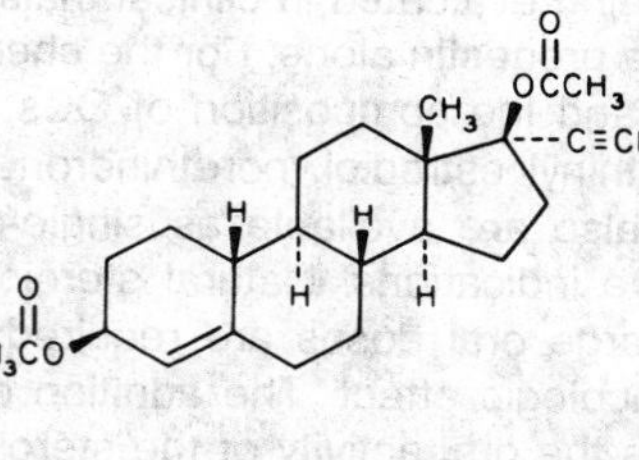

Ethynodiol Diacetate

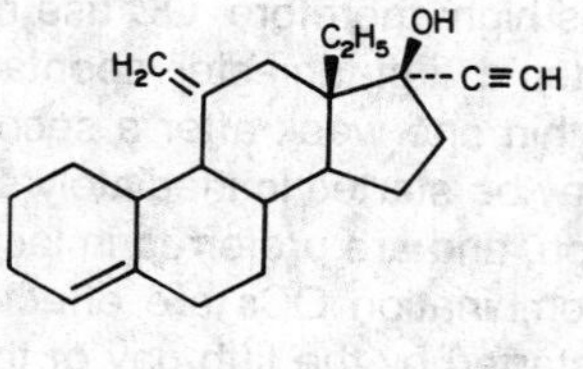

Desogestrel

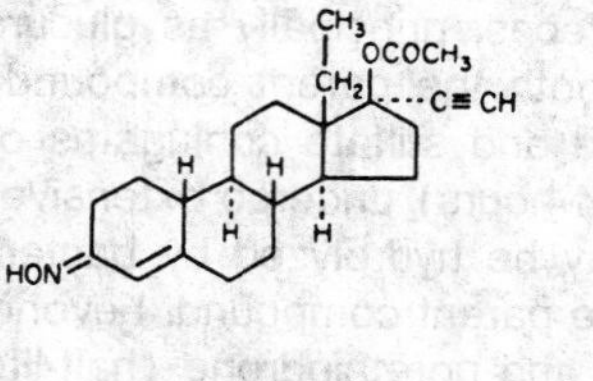

Norgestimate

TABLE 3.
ORAL CONTRACEPTIVES AVAILABLE IN THE UNITED STATES
(Listed within classes according to decreasing estrogen content)

Progestin	Mg	Estrogen	Mcg	Trademarks and Manufacturers	Number of Tablets (Active and Inert) *
PRODUCTS CONTAINING LESS THAN 50 MCG ESTROGEN					
Monophasic Preparations					
Norethindrone	0.4	Ethinyl estradiol	35	Ovcon 35 (Mead Johnson)	21, 28
Norethindrone	0.5	Ethinyl estradiol	35	Brevicon (Syntex) GenCept (Gencon) Genora 0.5/35 (Rugby) Modicon (Ortho) Nelova 0.5/35E (Warner Chilcott) Norminest Fe (Syntex) †	21, 28 Fe (Norminest Fe)
Norethindrone	1	Ethinyl estradiol	35	Genora 1/35 (Rugby) GenCept 1/35 (Gencon) N.E.E. 1/35 (Lexis) Nelova 1/35E (Warner Chilcott) Norcept-E 1/35 (GynoPharma) Norethin 1/35E (Schiapparelli Searle) Norinyl 1 + 35 (Syntex) Norquest Fe (Syntex) † Ortho-Novum 1/35 (Ortho)	21, 28 21, 28 Fe (Norquest Fe)
Norethindrone Acetate	1	Ethinyl estradiol	20	Loestrin 1/20 (Parke-Davis)	21, 28 Fe
Norethindrone Acetate	1.5	Ethinyl estradiol	30	Loestrin 1.5/30 (Parke-Davis)	21, 28 Fe
Desogestrel	0.15	Ethinyl estradiol	35	Desogen (Organon) Ortho-Cept (Ortho)	28 21, 28
Ethynodiol Diacetate	1	Ethinyl estradiol	35	Demulen 1/35 (Searle) Nelulen 1/35 E (Watson)	21, 28
Levonorgestrel	0.15	Ethinyl estradiol	30	Levlen (Berlex) Nordette (Wyeth-Ayerst)	21, 28
Norgestimate	0.25	Ethinyl estradiol	35	Ortho-Cyclen 21, 28 (Ortho)	21, 28
Norgestrel	0.3	Ethinyl estradiol	30	Lo/Ovral (Wyeth-Ayerst)	21, 28
Biphasic Preparations					
Norethindrone	0.5 (7 days); 1 (14 days)	Ethinyl estradiol	35	Jenest-28 (Organon)	28
Norethindrone	0.5 (10 days); 1 (11 days)	Ethinyl estradiol	35; 35	GenCept 10/11 (Gencon) Nelova 10/11 (Warner Chilcott) Ortho-Novum 10/11 (Ortho)	21, 28

(continued on next page)

TABLE 3 (continued)

Progestin	Mg	Estrogen	Mcg	Trademarks and Manufacturers	Number of Tablets (Active and Inert)†
Triphasic Preparations					
Norethindrone	0.5 (7 days); 0.75 (7 days); 1 (7 days)	Ethinyl estradiol	35; 35; 35	Ortho-Novum 7/7/7 (Ortho)	21, 28
Norethindrone	0.5 (7 days); 1 (9 days); 0.5 (5 days)	Ethinyl estradiol	35; 35; 35	Tri-Norinyl (Syntex)	21, 28
Levonorgestrel	0.05 (6 days); 0.075 (5 days); 0.125 (10 days)	Ethinyl estradiol	30; 40; 30	Tri-Levlen (Berlex) Triphasil (Wyeth-Ayerst)	21, 28
Norgestimate	0.18 (7 days) 0.21 (7 days) 0.25 (7 days)	Ethinyl estradiol	35; 35; 35	Ortho Tri-Cyclen 21, 28	21, 28
PRODUCTS CONTAINING 50 MCG ESTROGEN					
Norethindrone	1	Ethinyl estradiol	50	Norethin 1/50M (Schiapparelli Searle) Ovcon-50 (Mead Johnson)	21, 28
Norethindrone	1	Mestranol	50	Genora 1/50 (Rugby) Nelova 1/50M (Warner Chilcott) Noriday 1 + 50 Fe (Syntex) Norinyl 1 + 50 (Syntex) Ortho-Novum 1/50 (Ortho)	21, 28 Fe (Noriday 1 + 50 Fe)
Ethynodiol Diacetate	1	Ethinyl estradiol	50	Demulen 1/50 (Searle) Nelulen 1/50 E (Watson)	21, 28
Norgestrel	0.5	Ethinyl estradiol	50	Ovral (Wyeth-Ayerst)	21, 28
PRODUCTS CONTAINING PROGESTIN ONLY (MINIPILLS) (for continuous administration; all tablets active)					
Norethindrone	0.35			Micronor (Ortho) Nor-QD (Syntex)	28 (Micronor) 42 (Nor-QD)
Norgestrel	0.075			Ovrette (Wyeth-Ayerst)	28

** 20, 21, 42, and 50, all active; 28 (21 active, 7 inert); 28 Fe (21 active, 7 ferrous fumarate 75 mg)*
† Available only to the Agency for International Development (AID).

NONCONTRACEPTIVE BENEFITS OF ORAL CONTRACEPTIVES. The following discussion is based on epidemiologic data from studies that primarily used OC formulations containing estrogen in doses exceeding ethinyl estradiol 35 mcg or mestranol 50 mcg. Oral contraceptives provide highly effective nonsurgical contraception. Although numerous adverse effects have been described, the risks of benign fibrocystic breast disease, menorrhagia, endometrial and ovarian cancer, endometriosis, and iron deficiency anemia are reduced (Mishell, 1982; Dickey, 1987 A, 1987 B). The incidence and severity of dysmenorrhea also are reduced (Milsom and Andersch, 1984). Some women experience improved cycle regularity and decreased premenstrual symptoms.

In contrast to the high-dose estrogen preparations formerly used, the low-dose OCs do not appear to protect against development of functional ovarian cysts, although tricyclic OCs do not appear to increase risk of these cysts (Lanes et al, 1992; Holt et al, 1992).

Both beneficial effects and possible risks related to STDs and PID have been reported in OC users. The severity of the first episode of salpingitis was reduced in women using OCs compared with those using IUDs or neither contraceptive (Svensson et al, 1984). The risk of severe PID associated with gonococcal infections also is reduced with OC use. In patients who have PID, use of OCs appears to be associated with a lower risk of fallopian tube involvement (Wølner-Hanssen et al, 1985); not all data support this finding however.

Available data both refute (del Junco et al, 1985) and support (Vandenbroucke et al, 1986; Hazes et al, 1990) the suggestion that OCs protect against rheumatoid arthritis.

MECHANISM OF ACTION. Combination OCs inhibit ovulation through a negative feedback effect on the hypothalamus. This alters the normal pattern of gonadotropin secretion by the anterior pituitary; both follicular phase FSH and the midcycle surge of gonadotropins are inhibited. The cervical mucus thickens (except with the most estrogenic preparations), which renders it unfavorable to penetration by sperm even if ovulation occurs.

Progestin-only minipills may directly inhibit ovulation, or they may act by causing formation of a thick cervical mucus that is relatively impenetrable to sperm. They also may increase tubal transport time and cause endometrial involution.

CHOICE OF ORAL CONTRACEPTIVE. The numerous combination OC preparations on the market (see Table 3) differ in the type and quantity of estrogen and progestin present in the formulation. Their effectiveness is equivalent with certain exceptions. Conditions that contribute to lower steady-state plasma levels (eg, induction of hepatic drug metabolism) may decrease the efficacy of preparations containing smaller amounts of estrogen (≤35 mcg).

As a general rule, preparations containing the smallest quantity of steroid consistent with efficacy and tolerable side effects are preferred. This means selection of a product containing less than 50 mcg of estrogen for a first-time user. Changing to lower dose preparations is recommended even for patients successfully maintained on older, higher dose estrogen products.

The multiphasic preparations are designed to reduce the total steroid content in the treatment cycle and to provide contraceptive effectiveness comparable to higher dose regimens. It appears that both monophasic and multiphasic preparations are highly effective, but there may be some differences in metabolic effects among the preparations; these are discussed below under the respective sections.

The progestin-only minipill frequently causes menstrual irregularities and is not as widely used (see the section on Metabolic Effects, Adverse Reactions, and Contraindications). Although minipills are slightly less effective than combination OCs, they may be suitable for patients who accept the inconvenience of menstrual irregularities, do not require the most effective protection, and should avoid estrogen-containing medications (eg, those with a history of migraine headaches, patients who experienced estrogen-related side effects from combination OCs). They also may be chosen for lactating women. These considerations also may influence choice of the progestin-only implantable system, levonorgestrel implant [Norplant System], and depot DMPA (also see those evaluations). The following discussion is primarily devoted to combination products.

Relative Potency: The estrogen component of combination OCs marketed in the United States is either ethinyl estradiol or mestranol (ethinyl estradiol 3-methylether). In animal assays, ethinyl estradiol is 50% more potent than mestranol (which must be demethylated to ethinyl estradiol before it is biologically active). Comparison of the two steroids in doses of 50 mcg or more reveals little difference in their effects on the reproductive system, including endometrial histology, inhibition of ovulation, and gonadotropin secretion (Goldzieher et al, 1975). Equivalent blood levels of ethinyl estradiol are achieved following administration of either ethinyl estradiol 35 mcg or mestranol 50 mcg (Brody et al, 1989; Goldzieher, 1990).

The progestin component of an OC may be one of the derivatives of 19-nortestosterone (norethindrone, norethindrone acetate, ethynodiol diacetate) or of gonane (norgestrel, levonorgestrel, norgestimate, desogestrel). Norgestrel is a racemic mixture of levonorgestrel and an inactive isomer and has one-half the potency of levonorgestrel. These two progestins have the most potent androgenic, antiestrogenic, and progestational activity (Dorflinger, 1985; King and Whitehead, 1986). Norethindrone and ethynodiol diacetate possess slight estrogenic activity, and norethindrone has some androgenic activity. Norgestimate and desogestrel are antiestrogenic and have very low androgenicity.

There is disagreement about whether the various formulations available provide real therapeutic alternatives. Attempts have been made to assess the biological activities of the ingredients in order to tailor the OC to the patient's unique hormonal balance. However, numerous considerations complicate interpretation of available data. These include interaction between the estrogen and progestin components and the complex activities of some synthetic progestins, which possess varying degrees of progestational, estrogenic, and androgenic activities. Furthermore, results of the variety of assays available to measure each activity differ, and animal models are not completely analogous to humans. Although different assay systems may show significant differences in potency, they may be unimportant at the dosage ranges employed clinically.

Because of these differences, comparison of OC formulations on the basis of weight of components alone is insufficient. Comparison of commercial products on the basis of their estimated relative hormonal activities provides a rational but theoretical approach for selection of an OC preparation (Dickey, 1987 A). This method probably has less application with low-dose preparations than with the higher dose preparations used formerly.

PRECAUTIONS. Patients should be warned that the risk of pregnancy is increased if pills are missed during the cycle. Pills missed during the first or third weeks of the cycle probably place the patient at higher risk than those missed at other times. If one or two are omitted in the first two weeks, an extra pill should be taken for one or two days, respectively, following the lapse. If two pills are missed, a barrier method of contraception should be used in addition to OCs for the rest of the cycle. A pregnancy test should be performed if menstruation does not occur on time. If two pills are missed in the third week, the remaining pills should be discarded and a new cycle started. If three or more pills are omitted at any time in the cycle, another cycle should be initiated and a barrier contraceptive used for the first two weeks of the new cycle. Detailed recommendations for management when one or more pills are missed are provided with the OC labeling.

The progestin-only minipill is less effective than combination OCs, and pregnancies are more likely to occur during the first six months of use. Therefore, a barrier method should be used around the time of expected ovulation, particularly during the first month of minipill use.

All patients taking OCs should be encouraged to take the pills at the same time every day to enhance compliance and to avoid wide fluctuations in levels of circulating steroids.

Patients taking OCs should be monitored regularly. Annual physical examination, including blood pressure measurement, urinalysis, liver palpation, and breast and pelvic examinations with Papanicolaou smear should be performed. Other laboratory tests, such as measurement of serum glucose and lipid levels, also should be performed when appropriate (women at risk of diabetes or cardiovascular disease on the basis of personal or family history). Patients should be encouraged to examine their breasts monthly.

A periodic pill-free "rest period" is not recommended, since it appears to provide no therapeutic advantage and does not enhance the resumption of ovulatory cycles after cessation of OC therapy. Such intervals may result in noncompliance with the substituted contraceptive and unwanted pregnancies.

METABOLIC EFFECTS, ADVERSE REACTIONS, AND CONTRAINDICATIONS. In reviewing the literature on both adverse effects and noncontraceptive benefits associated with OC use, it should be borne in mind that early preparations contained higher amounts of steroid and that "low-dose" OCs, which became available in the mid-1970s, were established as the agents of choice in the early 1980s. Therefore, some findings reported in earlier studies on high-dose preparations are not relevant to the low-dose preparations currently in use.

The pharmacologic quantities of synthetic steroids present in OC preparations have numerous metabolic effects, some of which resemble those experienced during pregnancy. Effects may be minor, tolerable, or temporary but can be serious and even life-threatening. The patient's medical history must be examined carefully to identify contraindications. This is even more compelling with use of OCs than with other drugs, because patients are healthy before therapy is initiated and alternative contraceptive methods are available.

Some adverse effects associated with OCs are believed to be related to the estrogen component, but cardiovascular changes may be associated with either component. Low-dose estrogen and progestin preparations are associated with fewer cardiovascular complications than products containing larger amounts of steroid, and it is reasonable to expect that other adverse effects attributable to steroid might be influenced similarly.

Common complaints associated with use of combination OCs include nausea sometimes accompanied by vomiting, breast tenderness, and water retention. The nausea is similar to that experienced by some women during early pregnancy and is more common if medication is taken in the early morning or without food. These effects usually occur during the first two or three months of therapy and diminish thereafter.

Although it appears that the progestin-only minipill is devoid of the most deleterious effects of the combination preparations, more experience is necessary for confirmation. The use of progestin-only products has been limited by lack of patient acceptance. The endometrium lacks the structural stability imparted by estrogen, and menstrual irregularities, ranging from intermenstrual spotting to amenorrhea, may result. Anxiety about possible pregnancy also is common. When pregnancy occurs during minipill use, the ectopic/intrauterine ratio is higher than when other agents are employed.

See also reviews by Grimes, 1992 A, and Godsland et al, 1992.

Effects on Reproductive System: Ovarian size is reduced because large follicles and corpora lutea are absent when OCs are being taken. Some growth of follicles occurs, but is followed by early atresia. Gonadotropic stimulation is diminished and resembles that occurring in the early follicular phase of a normal cycle. Likewise, endogenous steroid production is low. Storage of ova and reproductive life span are not increased. The endometrium rapidly progresses from a proliferative to a secretory phase, and glandular atrophy and possibly stromal decidualization then occur, which accounts for decreased or even absent withdrawal bleeding. Regression of the endometrium after a few cycles may be a factor in short-term amenorrhea.

Breakthrough bleeding (BTB) and spotting are common during the first few cycles of use (particularly with low-dose preparations) (Edgren et al, 1989). For example, BTB was most common in the first cycle of triphasic OC use than after these preparations were used for more than six months. If BTB persisted after three cycles, substitution of a monophasic product with a higher progestin content alleviated the problem (Casper and Powell, 1991). Intervention with therapeutic doses of estrogen and/or progestin may be necessary if BTB is heavy or prolonged (see index entry Uterus, Dysfunctional Bleeding) or another contraceptive method may be appropriate.

Cyclic menses usually resume one month after cessation of low-dose OC therapy, although the interval from contraception to conception has been reported to be longer in OC users than in women who used other contraceptive methods (Linn et al, 1982). Occasionally, failure of cyclicity persists for 6 to 12 months and may be due to a pre-existing oligo-ovulatory problem. If pregnancy is desired, the condition should be treated in the same manner as other cases of secondary amenorrhea; usually clomiphene [Clomid] or bromocriptine (if hyperprolactinemia is present) is prescribed (see index entry Infertility, Etiology and Treatment in Women). Results of ovulation induction are similar regardless of contraceptive history (Hull et al, 1981).

It is generally believed that there is no causal relationship between use of OCs and subsequent amenorrhea (postpill amenorrhea). In most studies, this effect was reported in less than 1% of patients who take OCs, which is similar to the incidence in women who do not take OCs. Amenorrhea does not appear to be related to dosage of either component or to duration of use. It may represent progression of an unidentified prior condition with manifestations masked by the regular cycle imposed by OCs. The cause also may be unrelated to contraception (eg, stringent dieting, excessive exercise, underweight, overweight).

Several patients taking phasic (mostly triphasic) OC preparations developed functional ovarian cysts (including corpus luteum cysts) after initial use (within one month to three years), which suggests an association between ovarian cyst formation and use of triphasic OCs (Caillouette and Koehler, 1987). Results of subsequent studies in which the incidence of cyst formation in women who used various OC formulations or did not use OCs was compared indicated that suppression of ovarian cysts was related to the intensity of ovarian suppression (Lanes et al, 1992; Holt et al, 1992). Therefore, the likelihood of suppressing ovarian cyst formation is least likely with triphasic preparations, greater with monophasic low-dose OCs, and greatest with high-dose OCs.

The relative risk of developing uterine leiomyomas has been reported to be lower in OC users with reduction in risk enhanced with increasing duration of OC use (Ross et al, 1986). However, in another study, OC use had no effect on development of leiomyomas, and it was suggested that the earlier finding was the result of indication bias (patients with leiomyomas often are not given OCs) (Parazzini et al, 1992).

The risk of hyperprolactinemia was increased in users of older, high-dose OCs, especially women who began use before age 25 (Badawy et al, 1981). Abnormally high serum prolactin levels (defined in one study as more than 20 ng/ml of serum) were observed in 30% of patients taking high-dose OCs (Reyniak et al, 1980). The risk of galactorrhea, usually associated with elevated prolactin levels, was increased in women who discontinued OCs, particularly for the first year after cessation (Taler et al, 1985). Amenorrhea and menstrual irregularities are common in the presence of hyperprolactinemia and galactorrhea. In one study, the risk of prolactinoma was higher in women who had used OCs for menstrual regulation than in nonusers or those who had used OCs for birth control (Shy et al, 1983). This evidence supports the possibility that OCs may exacerbate underlying pathologic conditions.

The quality and quantity of milk produced during lactation may be adversely affected by some OC preparations. The steroids are secreted in the milk with even low-dose preparations, and, although no adverse effects have been described with use of current formulations, their long-range effects on the nursing infant are not known. The amount of estrogen ingested by the suckling infant is similar whether the source is endogenous production by the lactating mother or estrogen from a combination OC. The progestin component of OCs also is secreted in milk, whereas natural progesterone is not (Committee on Drugs, American Academy of Pediatrics, 1981). Nonhormonal contraception is preferable for nursing mothers but, when steroid contraception is elected, a progestin-only minipill (which contains less progestin than combination pills and may enhance milk production) or a low-dose combination formulation is preferred.

Hepatic Effects: The incidence of *gallbladder disease* and gallstones is thought to be increased when OCs are used; this is probably related to increased cholesterol concentrations in bile. Women who developed jaundice during pregnancy or nulliparous women with a genetic predisposition are at risk of developing *cholestatic jaundice* during therapy. These women are more likely to be affected shortly after hormone exposure (eg, OCs, pregnancy) (Wingrave and Kay, 1982; Scragg et al, 1984). Biopsies reveal cholestasis and, sometimes, minimal hepatocellular degeneration and necrosis. Upon cessation of OC use, jaundice and pruritus disappear and liver function tests return to normal without residual effects. Patients with this history and those with active liver disease should not take OCs; those who have recovered from liver disease (eg, hepatitis, mononucleosis) may receive this medication if hepatic function studies have been normal for one year. In a clinical study using an OC containing 35 mcg ethinyl estradiol, the incidence of abnormal liver function tests was lower than previously reported for products containing 50 to 100 mcg estrogen (Dickerson et al, 1980).

In most reports of hepatic neoplasia associated with OC use, the older, high-dose preparations had been prescribed.

Benign *hepatic adenomas* occur rarely with OC use (Sturtevant, 1979). The relative risk increases greatly after three years of OC use (Rooks et al, 1979), but the absolute (attributable) risk remains extremely low, probably 1 to 5/million OC users (Zucker and Huggins, 1989). The association of OC use with *focal nodular hyperplasia* is not established (Rosenberg, 1991). Adenomas are potentially serious because of the danger of rupture. About one-half of patients present with abdominal pain (sometimes associated with a liver mass) but almost one-third are asymptomatic at the time of diagnosis. Cessation of OC use is mandatory, and spontaneous regression usually occurs.

The relative risk of developing *hepatocellular carcinoma* also is increased in those taking OCs, particularly among long-term users. Case-control studies have estimated that the relative risk increases 3.8 times for ever-users and 20.1 times for those who used OCs for eight or more years (Forman et al, 1986); in another study, the risk increased 7.2 times for those with no evidence of hepatitis B exposure and eight or more years of OC use, but there was no increased risk for ever-users (Neuberger et al, 1986). In a study involving geographic areas where hepatitis B is endemic and the prevalence of hepatic cancer is high, there was no evidence that short-term OC use increased the risk of developing this cancer (WHO Collaborative Study of Neoplasia and Steroid Contraceptives, 1989). These tumors are rarer among OC users than benign hepatic adenomas, so the actual risk is extremely small. The possible evolution of hepatic adenomas into carcinoma has been reported (Gordon et al, 1986). Studies on the association between benign and malignant hepatic tumors and OC use have been reviewed (Rosenberg, 1991).

Carbohydrate, Lipid, and Protein Metabolism: The effect of combination OCs on *carbohydrate metabolism* is complex. Utilization of glucose may be retarded and compensatory insulin secretion increased. A peripheral anti-insulin effect of growth hormone may be involved during the first year of use, since OCs increase the pituitary secretion of growth hormone in some patients. After one year, growth hormone secretion appears to return to normal in some individuals. If alterations in glucose tolerance continue, other diabetogenic factors may be responsible.

Effects of OCs on carbohydrate metabolism are believed to be due to the progestin component. Studies of selected combination OC preparations containing different progestins and progestins alone have shown that all of these agents may elevate blood glucose and insulin levels. Norethindrone, ethynodiol diacetate, norgestimate, and desogestrel appear to be the weakest and levonorgestrel and norgestrel the strongest in this respect. The decreased numbers and affinity of insulin receptors observed in women using low-dose OCs containing norgestrel are consistent with these effects on carbohydrate metabolism (Spellacy, 1982). Progestin-only products containing norethindrone or norgestrel were associated with only minor changes in carbohydrate metabolism (Godsland et al, 1990). In a study comparing users of triphasic OC preparations with those employing nonhormonal contraception, small but statistically significant increases in serum glucose at six months and serum insulin at three months were observed in the OC users. No adverse effect on glucose tolerance was noted, and no differences among the three types of triphasic preparations were reported. Patients with a history of gestational diabetes were excluded from the study (Bowes et al, 1989).

Women who had gestational diabetes and had received low-dose OCs for up to 12 months postpartum did not develop diabetes more frequently than control subjects who used other means of contraception (Kjos et al, 1990). However, even low-dose (including multiphasic) OC preparations slightly decrease glucose tolerance (Luyckx et al, 1986) and/or decrease insulin sensitivity in women with gestational diabetes (Kung et al, 1987; Skouby et al, 1987). There are no data to support the earlier supposition that patients who eventually develop diabetes mellitus (eg, those with a strong family history) may become clinically diabetic earlier with use of OCs. In women with a history of glucose intolerance who are using OCs, deterioration can be detected early by periodic monitoring.

Although increased blood glucose levels can be controlled by adjusting the dose of hypoglycemic agent, some physicians do not recommend OC use in diabetic patients who require hypoglycemic medication. However, the decision must be made on an individual basis. Consideration should be given to the possible increased risk of atherosclerosis in young diabetic patients taking OCs, the risks associated with pregnancy, and the acceptability of other contraceptive methods. Many physicians prescribe low-dose or triphasic OCs for diabetic patients.

Serum lipids also are affected by OCs. In general, estrogen causes elevation of triglycerides and high-density lipoproteins (HDL) and a decrease of low-density lipoproteins (LDL). Progestins derived from testosterone (all such agents used in OC preparations in the United States) have the opposite effects, with the most androgenic progestins having the greatest effect. In clinical studies comparing OC preparations, those containing levonorgestrel and norgestrel had a greater adverse effect on serum lipids than those containing ethynodiol diacetate, norethindrone, or norethindrone acetate. The latter three have lower androgenic potency (Burkman et al, 1988; LaRosa, 1988). However, the effect of progestin on HDL appears to depend on both dose and potency (higher dose associated with lower HDL levels); thus, low doses of an androgenic preparation may have fewer adverse effects on lipids than high doses of a less androgenic preparation.

In a randomized trial that examined the effect of three types of triphasic OC preparations on serum lipid fractions, subjects using these preparations had increased serum triglycerides and decreased HDL_2 compared with those using nonhormonal contraception. No differences were observed among users of the triphasic preparations. Although the direction of the changes was unfavorable, the concentrations of lipid fractions were not abnormal (Patsch et al, 1989).

In a cross-sectional study comparing the effects of nine OC formulations on carbohydrate and lipid metabolism, fasting serum triglyceride concentrations increased with use of combination OC preparations, including triphasic formulations. Combinations containing desogestrel or low-dose norethindrone were associated with decreased LDL and increased HDL concentrations. Serum HDL decreased with use of combinations containing levonorgestrel (Godsland et al, 1990). OCs containing norgestimate are associated with elevated HDL levels and a decreased LDL:HDL ratio (Kafrissen, 1992). Progesterone-derived progestins have little effect on lipid fractions, at least at low doses (Wynn and Niththyananthan, 1982; Lipson et al, 1986; Tikkanen and Nikkilä, 1986; Ellis, 1987). Changes in lipid metabolism do not appear to progress with continued OC use (Fotherby, 1984).

Increased levels of HDL are associated with a lower risk of coronary artery disease, and increased levels of LDL are associated with a higher risk. A serum lipid profile should be obtained in women at higher risk of cardiovascular disease before prescribing OCs and periodically thereafter. If very high levels are found, use of another form of contraception should be encouraged.

Changes in *serum protein* levels during OC use are qualitatively similar to those that occur during pregnancy, but they are generally of less magnitude. Alterations in clotting factors occur (see the discussion on Cardiovascular and Hematologic Effects); $alpha_2$ globulins (including angiotensinogen) and beta globulins are increased and serum albumin levels are decreased.

OCs also increase circulating corticosteroid-binding globulin (CBG, transcortin), which elevates the amount of protein-bound cortisol in peripheral blood. The slight rise in the free (biologically active) cortisol level is probably partly due to the reduced rate of cortisol metabolism. The effect of prolonged elevation of bound cortisol concentrations is unknown. Pituitary-adrenal response to stress remains normal. The level of thyroxine-binding globulin (TBG) also is greater but, since the concentration of free thyroxine is unchanged, thyroid function is not altered. Sex hormone-binding globulin (SHBG) increases with the estrogen level of OCs. Other binding proteins, such as transferrin and ceruloplasmin, also are increased.

Cardiovascular and Hematologic Effects: The preponderance of data from both prospective and retrospective studies reveals that the relative risk of developing idiopathic *thromboembolic phenomena* (including deep vein thrombosis and pulmonary embolism) is approximately 4 to 11 times greater and the relative risk of superficial thrombosis is 2 to 3 times greater among women who use high-dose OCs compared with nonusers. Presumably, the risk was greater in women with conditions that predisposed to thromboembolic disease.

The relative risk of thromboembolic phenomena in OC users increases rapidly during the first month of use and declines at the same rate after discontinuation of treatment. The increased risk, therefore, applies only to current or recent users and is not associated with duration of use. Available data suggest both a reduction (Vessey et al, 1986) or no reduction (Helmrich et al, 1987; Russell and Ramcharan, 1987) in risk associated with use of low-dose OCs. In a cohort study of OC users, the effect of estrogen on venous thromboembolism was dose-dependent with higher risk associated with OC preparations containing ≥50 mcg estrogen (Gerstman et al, 1991).

The relative risk of postoperative venous thrombosis was doubled in OC users, resulting in an absolute risk of 61/10,000 surgical procedures (Stadel, 1981, part 1). The major risk factor is a history of thromboembolic disease. Thromboembolism causing mesenteric vascular ischemia also has occurred rarely in association with OC use (Schneiderman and Cello, 1986).

Intravascular clot formation may be enhanced by increased numbers of platelets or platelet adhesiveness, higher levels of blood clotting factors, decreased fibrinolysis, or inflammatory changes in the blood vessel wall. OCs may alter the concentration of various clotting factors (increased prothrombin and factors VII, VIII, IX, and X; decreased antithrombin III). Larger numbers of platelets and increased adhesiveness are sometimes observed, although decreased or unchanged adhesiveness also has been reported. The hematocrit and plasma fibrinogen levels are elevated, which increases blood viscosity (Lowe et al, 1980).

The increased risk of deep vein thrombosis is believed to be related to the estrogen content of OCs, although occlusion of superficial veins may be related to the progestin component (Dalen and Hickler, 1981). Preparations containing the least amount of estrogen (usually ≤35 mcg) that provides reliable contraception with a minimum of untoward effects (eg, breakthrough bleeding, spotting) should be utilized.

Women with a history of or those with active thromboembolic disease, thrombophlebitis, or hypercoagulable state should not take OCs. In addition, OCs should not be employed within one month before or after major elective surgery or immediately postpartum because of the greater risk of thromboembolism at these times. When OCs cannot be discontinued prior to surgery, as in acute trauma, prophylactic low-dose heparin therapy may be considered.

Most studies showing an increased risk of cardiovascular disease among current OC users were based on use of the older, high-dose preparations. Epidemiologic data on currently used preparations are sparse but suggest that there is little or no increase in disease among nonsmokers (Rosenberg et al, 1990) except when preparations containing 50 mcg estrogen are used (Thorogood et al, 1991). About one-half of all *myocardial infarctions* in young to middle-aged women are attributable to smoking (Willett et al, 1987). This risk is markedly amplified in OC users, with the relative risk twentyfold or more, depending on the number of cigarettes smoked per day, higher than in nonsmoking OC users. A substantial proportion of myocardial infarctions associated with OC use could probably be prevented by not prescribing these agents for women who smoke. The presence of other risk factors (ie, age, hypertension, diabetes, obesity, hyperlipidemia) also increases the risk associated with OC use, but the risk does not appear to increase synergistically as is observed with cigarette smoking.

Nearly all studies, both case-control and cohort, have found that the risk of myocardial infarction was unaffected by past use of OCs, and there is no trend toward increased risk with increasing duration of use (Croft and Hannaford, 1989; Rosenberg et al, 1990; Stampfer et al, 1990 [meta-analysis]).

The relative risk of fatal and nonfatal *stroke* may be increased in OC users. In current users of older high-dose preparations, the risk of thrombotic stroke was increased about tenfold and that of hemorrhagic stroke almost twofold (Collaborative Group for the Study of Stroke in Young Women, 1973). An increased risk of subarachnoid hemorrhage in past OC users also has been suggested. In one study, thrombotic stroke was related to OC dosage in that no strokes were reported in women using low-dose (<50 mcg estrogen) pills (Vessey et al, 1984).

Of the small percentage of fatal strokes among OC users, most are caused by subarachnoid hemorrhages. In addition to OC use, risk factors include hypertension, cigarette smoking, age over 35 years (Longstreth and Swanson, 1984), and alcohol intake (Stampfer et al, 1988). The combination of OC use and hypertension increases the risk of both thrombotic and hemorrhagic stroke; smoking plus use of OCs also has been suggested to increase the risk of subarachnoid hemorrhage.

The pathogenesis of both myocardial infarction (Engel et al, 1983) and stroke associated with current OC use usually is not atheromatous in nature. Myocardial infarctions in young women, whether or not associated with OCs, are usually caused by obstructive coronary artery disease (the left anterior descending coronary artery is a frequent site of the lesion). OCs may contribute to the progression of subclinical thrombosis and to coronary occlusion by their effects on clotting mechanisms. Autopsies on women who died from stroke associated with OC use reveal a common pattern: Thrombi are found at sites of endothelial proliferation and subendothelial fibrosis. These structural characteristics and the increased tendency for clotting may account for occlusion of cerebral arteries (with or without hemorrhage) in affected women. These pathologic patterns, plus the findings that increased risk of myocardial infarction begins at initiation of OC use, ends upon cessation, and is unassociated with duration, strongly suggest that the mechanism is not atherogenesis.

Both the estrogen and progestin components of OCs may contribute to the increased risk of cardiovascular disease. Increases in clotting factors usually are attributed to estrogens. However, in one study, increasing the dose of progestins elevated the relative risk of ischemic heart disease (norethindrone acetate) and strokes (norethindrone acetate and levonorgestrel) (Meade et al, 1980).

It is now considered acceptable to prescribe low-dose OCs for healthy women 40 years or older who are nonsmokers and who are not otherwise at increased risk for cardiovascular disease. These patients should be appropriately screened (eg, blood pressure, serum lipids, glucose tolerance) and monitored (Mishell, 1988).

The risk associated with cigarette smoking and OC use increases synergistically with age. Women over 35 years who smoke should not take OCs, and it is preferable that smoking and OC use not be combined at any age. All women, but especially OC users, should be strongly counseled to stop smoking.

Slight increases in both systolic and diastolic *blood pressure* have been reported, but are usually within the normal range. However, women who use OCs are about three to six times more likely to develop hypertension than nonusers (see references in Dalen and Hickler, 1981). Other evidence suggests that the probability of hypertension increases with duration of OC use and age and is most prominent in women over 35 years. The increase in blood pressure that normally occurs after age 40 apparently is accelerated in current OC users, and women who are already hypertensive may experience a further rise. Changes in blood pressure are usually reversible within one to six months after cessation of therapy.

The mechanism of the OC effect on blood pressure probably involves the renin-angiotensin system. Angiotensinogen (renin substrate) levels increase and the negative feedback control of renin production is impaired; elevated levels of angiotensin, a potent vasoconstrictor, and aldosterone result. Since these changes occur with low-dose OCs (Malatino et al, 1988) and in OC users whether or not they become hypertensive, it appears that individual sensitivity or predisposition is important in the blood pressure response to OCs.

The blood pressure should be monitored after three months of OC therapy and every 6 to 12 months thereafter. If hypertension develops, another form of contraception should be utilized. Other contraceptives are preferred in women who are already hypertensive or who are being treated with antihypertensive agents; if OCs are employed, careful monitoring of blood pressure is necessary.

Several cases of pulmonary hypertension have been reported in women using OCs, although most of these individuals had predisposing conditions.

OCs have been associated with changes in the pattern of *migraine headache*. Attacks that occur frequently during the interval when OCs are not taken may be due to fluid retention and are not dangerous. However, if migraine is first experienced after beginning OC medication or the frequency or intensity increases during treatment, therapy should be discontinued since these may be prodromal symptoms of stroke.

Teratogenicity: Among women who discontinue use of OCs prior to conception, the risk of spontaneous abortion; congenital abnormalities, including any of the so-called VACTERL anomalies (vertebral, anal, cardiac, tracheal, esophageal, renal, or limb); or Down's syndrome in liveborn infants is not increased. In a prospective study of women who were questioned during pregnancy about prior contraceptive use, there was no increased risk of malformation associated with OC use that was discontinued up to one month before conception (Harlap et al, 1985). Some studies have found a higher risk of nongenital malformations among infants exposed to sex steroids, including inadvertent continuation of OCs during susceptible periods in embryogenesis. Cardiovascular and other defects in the VACTERL group have been described (Nora et al, 1978; Heinonen et al, 1977; Janerich et al, 1980), mostly in male infants.

In general, the increased risk of nongenital congenital malformations associated with OC use is small, and the likelihood of a causal association has been questioned (Wilson and Brent, 1981) and refuted (Nora et al, 1982). However, because OCs rarely may cause congenital abnormalities, therapy should be discontinued as soon as pregnancy is confirmed.

Fibrocystic Breast Disease: Women with fibrocystic breast disease who have proliferative lesions on biopsy (especially those with atypia) have an increased risk of breast cancer (Dupont and Page, 1985). Several studies have shown that the risk of *benign breast disease* in women who use combination OCs is not increased (Franceschi et al, 1984) or is decreased (Hislop and Threlfall, 1984). The low-dose formulations currently in use may have no effect (McGonigle and Huggins, 1991). The fact that OCs often are not prescribed for women with a history of benign breast disease may account for the higher prevalence among control subjects. Other studies show no increased risk for OC users with prior benign breast disease (Cancer and Steroid Hormone Study, 1983 A; Rosenberg et al, 1985).

Breast Cancer: Numerous retrospective and prospective studies of a possible association with or causal role of OCs in the development of breast cancer have been conducted and others are ongoing. Most investigators agree that there is no overall increase in the incidence of breast cancer with OC use. Studies to date have been reviewed critically (Thomas, 1991; Staffa et al, 1992; Grimes, 1992 B), and it has been noted that most suffer from potential bias and possible confounding factors and that results are inconsistent (Harlap, 1991). Some studies have suggested that the risk of premenopausal breast cancer is higher in women who used OCs for longer durations before their mid-twenties or prior to first full-term pregnancy, and a meta-analysis of completed studies supported this observation (Romieu et al, 1990). (See the reviews cited for original citations.) Reanalysis of data from the Cancer and Steroid Hormone study showed a relative risk of 1.4 for breast cancer diagnosis between ages 20 to 34 years among ever-users of OCs and a slightly decreased risk among ever-users aged 45 to 54 years (Wingo et al, 1991).

Since estrogen can stimulate growth of pre-existing cancerous breast lesions, OCs are contraindicated in women with known or suspected breast carcinoma, and caution must be exercised if they are prescribed for patients at high risk of breast cancer. Epidemiologic studies continue to monitor this issue, particularly since some carcinogens have very long latencies before they are expressed.

Other Carcinogenicity: The risk of *endometrial carcinoma* among women who have used combined OCs appears to be about one-half that of nonusers overall; the protective effect increases with duration of use and persists for at least 10 to 15 years after discontinuation of OCs. There was no difference in risk associated with use of specific combination OC preparations (Weiss and Sayvetz, 1980; Kaufman et al, 1980 B; Hulka et al, 1982; Cancer and Steroid Hormone Study, 1983 B, 1987 A). However, since estrogen may stimulate the growth of existing endometrial cancer, OCs should not be prescribed for women with undiagnosed abnormal genital bleeding.

The incidence of cervical dysplasia, carcinoma in situ, and invasive *cervical cancer* has been reported to increase with OC use. However, differences between OC users and nonusers with respect to age at commencement of regular intercourse, total number of sexual partners, and use of barrier contraceptives by control subjects appear to explain at least some of this increase. In one study, the incidence of cervical dysplasia and neoplasia was higher in OC users than in IUD users, and there was a trend toward increased risk with increasing duration of OC use. Lack of data on sexual exposure precluded consideration of this confounding variable (Vessey et al, 1983). Later studies support the association of cervical cancer with OC use, however. OC use for seven or more years and first use at 24 years or younger were independent risk factors associated with increased relative risks for invasive cervical cancer of 1.8 and 3.0, respectively (Ebeling et al, 1987). Results of a prospective study of 47,000 women followed for almost 20 years showed an increased risk of cervical cancer with OC use; the incidence quadrupled when the duration of use exceeded 10 years (Beral et al, 1988). It is widely believed that cervical cancer may be caused by a sexually transmitted virus.

Women taking OCs appear to have a reduced risk of *ovarian cancer,* and the risk decreases further with duration of use (Casagrande et al, 1979; Rosenberg et al, 1982). Results of a collaborative reanalysis of data from 12 case-control studies of invasive epithelial ovarian cancer affirmed that the protective effect of OCs occurs within several cycles of treatment, continues to increase for up to six years of use, and lasts 15 years after cessation (Whittemore et al, 1992). The same study indicated that OC use provides less protection from epithelial tumors of low malignancy (borderline tumors) (Harris et al, 1992). The relative risk of epithelial ovarian cancer is 0.6 in OC users. No difference among preparations was found. No assessment of risk for nonepithelial ovarian cancer was possible because of insufficient data (Cancer and Steroid Hormone Study, 1987 B).

OCs do not appear to be causally related to development of benign nevi or melanoma (Green, 1991).

Firm conclusions about the carcinogenicity of OCs are not yet possible because of the potentially long latent period (up to 15 years) between the administration of a carcinogen and the development of cancer and because of the reduction in steroid hormone content of OCs over the last two decades. A comprehensive review of the status of OCs related to various types of neoplasia is available (Zucker and Huggins, 1989).

Miscellaneous Reactions: *Melasma* similar to that observed during pregnancy sometimes develops in women who use OCs. Those with dark complexions or a history of melasma of pregnancy or those exposed to excessive amounts of sunlight are most susceptible. Decreasing the quantity of estrogen may reduce pigmentation. However, even after cessation of medication, pigmentation may be permanent or take a long time to disappear.

Hair loss and changes in hair growth and texture may be related to either the androgenic potency of the progestin component or a decrease in estrogen activity relative to previous endogenous levels. Rarely, a male pattern of hair growth may appear on the face and body or recession of temporal hair may occur. Other manifestations of androgenicity include oily skin and scalp and acne. Use of a preparation containing a progestin with lower androgenicity or a higher estrogen/progestin potency ratio may be considered. Androgen-producing ovarian or adrenal pathologic changes should be ruled out. The effects of changes in drug regimen on hair growth may not be apparent for several months.

Rarely, *chorea* is associated with oral contraceptives, particularly in women with disorders of the basal ganglia. One-half of affected patients have a history of chorea, often associated with rheumatic fever. Symptoms generally resolve upon discontinuation of OCs (Nausieda et al, 1979).

Some women (most commonly those with a history of a psychological disorder) may experience mood changes or develop *depression* while taking OCs. Administration of pyridoxine (vitamin B_6) is sometimes effective in lessening depression in women with a deficiency of this vitamin.

Although the majority of OC users are unaffected, alterations in *libido* sometimes occur. These changes may be in either direction and may be unrelated to steroidal effects (eg, libido may increase because of lack of fear of pregnancy). If decreased libido is a problem, a preparation containing a small amount of estrogen and an androgenic progestin may be helpful.

Changes in blood levels of *vitamins and minerals* have been observed. Plasma pyridoxine, vitamin B_{12}, carotene, calcium, magnesium, manganese, zinc, and phosphorus levels may decrease, while ascorbic acid, vitamin A, iron, and copper levels increase. The clinical significance of these changes is not apparent, and decreased levels do not result in deficiency. Vitamin supplementation is unnecessary in women with adequate diets. Serum folate levels may be depressed by OCs, which may be of clinical significance if a woman becomes pregnant shortly after discontinuing their use.

Ocular abnormalities (eg, retinal vascular occlusion, retinal edema, optic neuropathy, retinal vasculitis) have been associated rarely with use of OCs. Symptoms may appear during therapy, disappear on withdrawal, and reappear on resumption of the drugs. OCs should be discontinued if there is an unexplained decrease in vision or color vision or other serious symptoms, and appropriate diagnostic and therapeutic measures should be taken. Some ophthalmologists recommend discontinuing OCs in women with retinitis pigmentosa because of the impression that pregnancy accelerates peripheral field loss and the similarity between the hormonal milieu of pregnancy and OC therapy (Petursson et al, 1981). Results of controlled studies indicate that OCs probably do not affect *contact lens* tolerance as was thought earlier.

DRUG INTERACTIONS. Two types of drug interactions may occur: those that influence the effectiveness of OCs and those that affect the activity of the second drug. Each type of interaction may either enhance or inhibit the activity of the drug in question. Reviews of OC drug interactions are available (Szoka and Edgren, 1988; Back and Orme, 1990).

Interactions That Decrease the Efficacy of the Second Drug: OCs may decrease the hypoprothrombinemic response to coumarin anticoagulants, and larger doses of the latter may be required. The metabolic clearance of acetaminophen may be accelerated in women taking OCs, and larger doses may be required to achieve the desired response (Baciewicz, 1985). Because estrogen increases the synthesis of thyroxine-binding globulin (TBG), an increase in the dosage of exogenous thyroid hormone may be required when OCs are taken concurrently. OCs may cause an increase in blood glucose concentration that requires adjustment of the dose of the hypoglycemic agent in diabetic patients.

Interactions That Increase the Efficacy or Toxicity of the Second Drug: The plasma concentration of cyclosporine may increase into the toxic range if OCs or androgens are added to the regimen. The probable mechanism is inhibition of cyclosporine metabolism by the liver (Hansten and Horn, 1987). An increased absolute bioavailability of imipramine, consistent with inhibition of hepatic imipramine oxidation, was observed in regular OC users. It was suggested that the dose of imipramine be reduced to achieve desired steady-state plasma concentrations in these individuals (Abernethy et al, 1984). OCs may reduce the metabolism of theophylline, and patients taking this combination should be monitored for theophylline toxicity (Baciewicz, 1985).

When OCs and pharmacologic amounts of corticosteroids are administered concurrently, the metabolism of the latter is reduced and may allow reduction of the corticosteroid dosage. In one study, women taking OCs or postmenopausal estrogen therapy were given prednisolone concurrently. Alterations in metabolism of prednisolone, including increased half-life, were consistent with a potential for enhanced pharmacologic effect or toxicity when prednisolone was added to an estrogen regimen (Gustavson et al, 1986).

Interactions That Decrease the Efficacy of OCs: There have been reports of pregnancies and breakthrough bleeding when OCs were taken with barbiturates, antiepileptic drugs (eg, phenytoin, carbamazepine), griseofulvin, and particularly rifampin. This is probably due to the increased metabolism of estrogen by mixed-function oxidases when these drugs are taken with OCs.

A few case reports of possible interactions with antibiotics, including ampicillin and tetracycline, appear to indicate that contraceptive effectiveness (eg, breakthrough bleeding, pregnancy) may decrease with concomitant use. The suggested mechanism is decreased enterohepatic circulation of hormones due to destruction of bacterial flora in the gut (Hansten and Horn, 1985). Normally, bacterial enzymes hydrolyze hormone conjugates, freeing the steroid for reabsorption by the gut (Back et al, 1981). A study of the effect of gut flora on digoxin metabolism suggested that these organisms may be suppressed for weeks by antibiotics (Lindenbaum et al, 1981).

Although there are studies in which concurrent use of OCs and doxycycline or tetracycline did not decrease serum hormone levels significantly (Neely et al, 1991; Murphy et al, 1991), the wide range of steady-state plasma concentrations of OC steroids observed may partly explain why a few individuals (those with low plasma concentrations) experience decreased contraceptive efficacy with fairly common drug combinations (Back and Orme, 1984). Because of the limited number of reports, an accurate assessment of the frequency of clinically significant interactions is not possible. However, some physicians advise patients to take an OC containing 50 mcg of estrogen during the period of antibiotic therapy, watch for signs of decreased OC efficacy (eg, breakthrough bleeding), and use an additional form of contraception or another contraceptive method during long-term antibiotic treatment.

Interactions That Increase the Efficacy of OCs: Ingestion of ascorbic acid 1 g daily elevates plasma levels of ethinyl estradiol. This implies that patients who initiate OC therapy while taking regular megadoses of vitamin C could experience reduction of estrogen levels in the blood on withdrawal of the vitamin. Conversely, initiating vitamin C administration while taking OCs may elevate the effective estrogen levels. In either case, clinical manifestations are theoretically possible (ie, reduced contraceptive efficacy, estrogen excess). Further verification of this effect and its clinical significance is required.

Miscellaneous Interactions: The blood levels of unbound chlordiazepoxide may be increased in OC users, but differences in clinical effect have not been observed. Low-dose OCs may have a differential effect on benzodiazepine metabolism: metabolism of some agents that undergo conjugation may be accelerated and that of some agents that undergo oxidation may be inhibited (Stoehr et al, 1984).

The combination of aminocaproic acid and oral contraceptives may produce a hypercoagulable state.

EFFECTS ON LABORATORY TESTS. Reversible sulfobromophthalein (BSP) retention may occur during administration of OCs. The defect is in the transfer of BSP from liver cells to bile; storage is not affected.

Estrogens raise the level of thyroxine-binding globulin, which increases values for total thyroxine (T_4) and decreases values for the T_3 resin uptake test. The free thyroxine index (FTI) and direct measurements of T_3 or T_4 by radioimmunoassay remain unchanged. Thyroid function test results return to pretreatment levels within two months after discontinuing therapy. Serum levels of other binding proteins may be elevated.

Serum iron and copper levels may increase because of higher concentrations of their respective transport proteins, transferrin and ceruloplasmin. OCs may cause a false-positive test for LE cells and/or antinuclear antibodies. Urinary 17-hydroxycorticosteroids may be decreased. See also the section on Metabolic Effects, Adverse Reactions, and Contraindications.

Postcoital Contraception

When coitus has occurred without contraceptive protection or a barrier contraceptive method fails and pregnancy is not desired, additional measures may prevent unwanted pregnancy and avoid abortion. Postcoital techniques are often referred to as "morning after" contraception. Various estrogen regimens (see Table 4) or IUDs may be used for this purpose.

The patient who seeks postcoital contraception should understand that high-dose estrogen regimens should be used only infrequently or in emergencies (eg, rape, incest), for the presumed risk of serious side effects after frequently repeated large doses is unacceptable. Breast tenderness is common. Nausea and vomiting occur routinely, and the postcoital regimen may be ineffective in the presence of vomiting.

Estrogen may change the sequence of hormonal influences on the fallopian tubes, thereby disturbing the passage of the ovum. Estrogen also may alter the endometrial milieu and interfere with nidation. Extensive clinical experience and documentation of effectiveness have been obtained with large doses of diethylstilbestrol (DES) administered within 72 hours after unprotected midcycle sexual exposure or ethinyl estradiol or conjugated estrogens administered within 24 (preferably) to 72 hours after coitus (Dixon et al, 1980). See Table 4 for doses.

The preferred postcoital hormonal method (Yuzpe regimen) limits OC use to a 12-hour period, which decreases the total amount of hormone ingested and reduces the frequency and severity of adverse effects. A regimen of ethinyl estradiol 100 mcg and norgestrel 1 mg (two Ovral tablets) taken twice 12 hours apart within 72 hours of a single midcycle coital exposure resulted in 0.6% to 1.9% failures per cycle (Yuzpe, 1984). The failure rate observed over a period of six years utilizing this regimen for 867 postcoital contraceptive treatments was similar (about 2%) (Percival-Smith and Abercrombie, 1987). This regimen compared favorably with the standard ethinyl estradiol-only regimen in a comparative study (Van Santen and Haspels, 1985), and the lowest failure rate was observed when treatment began within 24 hours of unprotected midcycle intercourse (Kane and Sparrow, 1989).

In a comparison with the Yuzpe regimen, two doses of danazol 600 mg were administered 12 hours apart or mifepristone 600 mg was given as a single dose, both regimens within 72 hours of unprotected coitus. Mifepristone was most effective (no pregnancies), the Yuzpe regimen was slightly less effective (2.62% pregnancies), and danazol was least effective (Webb et al, 1992).

As in other situations, the possibility of a previously existing pregnancy should be excluded before hormonal therapy is administered. Administration of DES during the first trimester of pregnancy is associated with a high incidence of vaginal adenosis and other gynecologic abnormalities and, rarely, adenocarcinoma in female offspring, as well as effects on the male urogenital tract (see index entry Diethylstilbestrol, Teratogenicity). Adenosis also has been reported following the use of estrogens other than DES. However, there is no information on the effects of any estrogen given as a postcoital contraceptive on a pregnancy that may ensue in the event of contraceptive failure. If this therapy fails and pregnancy results, some women will elect abortion simply because the pregnancy is unwanted. However, abortion need not be recommended solely on the basis of the teratogenic effects of the estrogen. The patient should be given a realistic assessment of the potential, but uncertain, risks involved before determining the fate of the pregnancy.

IUDs also have been employed for postcoital contraception. The IUD preferably is inserted within one day but may be inserted within five days after unprotected intercourse and left in place, if appropriate, for continuing contraception. Most experience has been with the copper-containing devices. In a

TABLE 4.
POSTCOITAL CONTRACEPTIVE REGIMENS

Estrogen	Dosage
Ethinyl Estradiol and Norgestrel (combination available as Ovral)	100 mcg ethinyl estradiol and 1 mg norgestrel (two Ovral tablets) taken twice 12 hours apart (Yuzpe regimen)
Ethinyl Estradiol	2.5 mg twice daily for five days
Conjugated Estrogens	10 mg three times daily for five days
Estrone	5 mg three times daily for five days
Diethylstilbestrol	25 mg twice daily for five days

survey of studies of various postcoital contraceptive methods, copper IUDs were found to be more effective than a variety of hormonal methods (Fasoli et al, 1989).

Depot Preparations

Several long-lasting depot preparations are available worldwide or are under clinical investigation for use as contraceptives (*Popul Rep [K]*, 1987). These products may contain both an estrogen and a progestin, but a progestin is usually used alone. The depot form of medroxyprogesterone acetate (DMPA) [Depo-Provera Contraceptive Injection] has received the most attention. It is widely used throughout the world and is now approved for this use in the United States. Another preparation available in the United States, levonorgestrel implant [Norplant System], is implanted in Silastic capsules in the upper arm and maintains contraceptive efficacy for five years. A vaginal ring that gradually releases levonorgestrel over several months may be available in some countries in the near future. Norethisterone enanthate, administered by injection or intravaginal ring, also is being investigated in several countries.

Drug Evaluations

MEDROXYPROGESTERONE ACETATE (DMPA)
[Depo-Provera Contraceptive Injection]

For chemical formula, see index entry Medroxyprogesterone, In Gynecologic Disorders.

ACTIONS AND USES. The depot preparation of medroxyprogesterone acetate may be used as a contraceptive. A dose of 150 mg is injected intramuscularly every three months, although the effect usually extends beyond this period. Following a single 150 mg-intramuscular dose, the blood concentration of DMPA increases over a period of three weeks to a peak concentration of 1 to 7 ng/ml. Levels thereafter decline exponentially to less than 100 pg/ml 120 to 200 days after injection. DMPA has the same method-effectiveness as OCs but use-effectiveness is higher.

In a multicenter, multinational study involving 1,216 women, a dose of 100 mg DMPA every 90 days provided contraceptive protection similar to that obtained with a 150-mg dose (WHO, 1987 B), but the data were not considered adequate to recommend changing the current 150-mg contraceptive dose. Intramuscular injection of 400 mg every six months also has been used with only a slight decrease in efficacy.

DMPA inhibits ovulation by suppressing the midcycle surge of LH secretion and also causes thickening of cervical mucus and development of an atrophic endometrium that may not be conducive to nidation. Gonadotropin suppression is not complete, and there is some follicular development; estrogen production is slightly less than in a normal follicular phase.

Resumption of fertility is delayed following discontinuation of DMPA. For this reason, the drug is not recommended for young women who wish to conceive soon after discontinuing use of contraceptives. Average time to conception after the last injection is about one year but may be as long as two and one-half years. This is unrelated to duration of use but may be caused by continuing pituitary suppression after clearance of the progestin or by coincidental pathologic changes. There is considerable variation in the rate of absorption and metabolism of DMPA, which could account for the prolonged contraceptive effect.

ADVERSE REACTIONS AND PRECAUTIONS. Side effects of DMPA include weight gain, depression, headache (1% to 5% of patients), abdominal pain or discomfort, nervousness, dizziness, and asthenia (>5% of patients). The most common problems are irregular menstrual cycles and spotting or amenorrhea, which occur more frequently with a 150-mg than with a 100-mg dose (WHO, 1987 B). Most patients who discontinue therapy do so because of these complaints. Many women tolerate the irregular bleeding if they are informed of the likelihood before therapy begins. If irregular bleeding persists and requires correction, steroidal therapy may be attempted (see index entry Uterus, Dysfunctional Bleeding); however, the routine use of estrogens to "normalize" the menstrual cycle is not advocated in patients using DMPA. An atrophic endometrium develops progressively, and total amenorrhea occurs in 57% of patients after one year and in 68% after two years.

Studies of DMPA's effect on blood pressure have yielded equivocal results but most often no change or a decrease in blood pressure has been reported. In glucose tolerance tests, an exaggerated insulin response to glucose has been observed but is milder than that seen with OCs. No major changes in serum lipid profiles are observed with contraceptive use of DMPA (Garza-Flores et al, 1991).

Seizures have been reported in women taking DMPA, but the possible contributory role of the drug or pre-existing conditions is unclear. The rate of bone loss is increased in DMPA recipients during the early years of use. Progestational agents may cause edema and affect conditions influenced by fluid retention (eg, migraine, cardiac or renal dysfunction). If papilledema or retinal vascular lesions occur while the patient is using this drug, a subsequent dose should not be administered.

Women who complain of severe abdominal pain while using DMPA should be examined for possible ectopic pregnancy.

DMPA has glucocorticoid properties, particularly when given in large doses (eg, to treat endometrial carcinoma). In contraceptive doses, plasma cortisol levels are sometimes decreased and the response to metyrapone may be diminished, but there is no clinical evidence of adrenal insufficiency.

Large doses of DMPA are teratogenic in rabbits; this effect is probably related to the glucocorticoid properties of this agent. DMPA does not appear to have a teratogenic effect in humans. One study of 987 teenage children who had been exposed in utero to DMPA used as a contraceptive revealed no impairment of intellectual development (Jaffe et al, 1988). In another study on children who were exposed to DMPA during pregnancy or lactation, growth and pubertal development were normal (Pardthaisong et al, 1992).

In women treated during pregnancy with large doses of DMPA for threatened abortion or recurrent fetal losses (the treatment apparently was ineffective), there was no statistically significant increase in congenital abnormalities compared with untreated controls (Yovich et al, 1988). However, administration of progestins during pregnancy is generally not recommended, and fetal exposure may be prolonged if a depot preparation is administered during an existing pregnancy or if contraceptive failure occurs. DMPA is classified in FDA Pregnancy Category X.

Results of studies had shown that the risk of breast cancer in women was not increased with contraceptive use of DMPA. However, a case-control study identified a relative risk of 2.0 for development of breast cancer in women aged 25 to 34 years who have used DMPA, and the risk increased with use for six or more years. There was no overall increase in the risk of breast cancer in the study, however (Paul et al, 1989). In a large collaborative international case-control study, the relative risk of breast cancer doubled in women under 35 years whose first exposure to DMPA occurred within the previous four years; however, the overall relative risk for ever-users was low (WHO Collaborative Study of Neoplasia and Steroid Contraceptives, 1991). There was no evidence that DMPA use increased the risk of invasive squamous cell cervical cancer in short- or long-term users (WHO Collaborative Study of Neoplasia and Steroid Contraceptives, 1992).

The main advantages of DMPA as a contraceptive lie in its safety, great effectiveness, and the need for infrequent administration. The latter property is a drawback in the event of side effects, however.

DOSAGE AND PREPARATIONS.

Intramuscular: For contraception, 150 mg is injected deep into the gluteal or deltoid muscle once every three months. To reduce the possibility that the patient is pregnant at the time of first injection, the initial injection should be given within the first five days after the onset of a normal menstrual period, within five days postpartum if not breast feeding, or the sixth week postpartum if breast feeding.

Depo-Provera Contraceptive Injection (Upjohn). Suspension (sterile, aqueous) 150 mg/ml in 1 ml containers. The vial should be shaken vigorously just before use.

LEVONORGESTREL IMPLANT

[Norplant System]

For chemical formula, see Figure.

ACTIONS AND USES. Norplant System consists of the progestin, levonorgestrel, in six Silastic capsules that are implanted subdermally in the upper arm. The levonorgestrel in the capsules is released gradually over the duration of use. Contraceptive efficacy is greater than that of OCs and lasts for five years.

The mechanism of action is the same as that of other progestin-only contraceptives. Ovulation is inhibited in more than 50% of cycles; in addition, levonorgestrel thickens cervical mucus, which interferes with sperm penetration. Alteration of tubal transport and endometrial atrophy also may contribute to contraceptive efficacy (see review by Shoupe and Mishell, 1989).

Norplant System may be an appropriate contraceptive choice for women who want long-term but reversible contraception, for those who cannot or do not wish to use other forms of contraception, or as an alternative to sterilization. It also may be preferable for lactating women. The capsules are implanted immediately postpartum or during the first week of the menstrual cycle, when there is reasonable assurance that the patient is not pregnant. Within 24 hours of implantation, the serum concentration of levonorgestrel is adequate to ensure contraceptive efficacy. Norplant System can be removed any time after insertion, and the contraceptive effects are completely reversible. Eighty-six percent of women who desire pregnancy become pregnant within one year after removal of the system. If continued contraceptive protection is desired after five years, a new Norplant System may be implanted immediately after removal of the old system.

If calculated for the entire five-year period, the cost of Norplant System is comparable to that of OCs. However, early removal of the device would concentrate the same total cost over a shorter period of time.

ADVERSE REACTIONS AND PRECAUTIONS. About 60% to 70% of patients experience irregular menstrual cycles (eg, spotting, breakthrough bleeding, prolonged bleeding, amenorrhea), especially during the first year after implantation. Twenty percent of women discontinue use of Norplant System during the first year, about one-half because of irregular bleeding patterns. Insertion and removal are minor surgical procedures, but the latter is more difficult and time-consuming. Infection at the implantation site with or without expulsion of capsules has been reported (Klavon and Grubb, 1990).

Although the number of days of bleeding may increase during the first year after implantation, hemoglobin levels remain normal or may increase. Occasionally, heavy bleeding may necessitate removal of Norplant System. Thrombocytopenia was reported in 2% of users in one study (Du et al, 1990).

It has been suggested that women whose menstrual cycles are regular while using Norplant System are at highest risk of pregnancy (Shoupe et al, 1991). Ectopic pregnancies occur in 0.15% of users, a rate similar to that associated with other progestin-only contraceptives or IUDs.

Norplant System may cause delay of follicular atresia, continuation of follicle growth, and ovarian cysts. These effects are usually transient and asymptomatic but may require removal of the capsules or, in rare instances, surgical correction.

Headache occurs in 5% to 20% of patients; acne (5%), breast discharge (20%), and weight gain (5%) also may be associated with use of Norplant System. Alterations in carbohydrate metabolism have not been reported. Overall, changes in the lipid profile appear to be beneficial. Total cholesterol, LDL cholesterol, and triglycerides decrease, and HDL cholesterol may decrease or increase.

Norplant System should not be implanted in women who are or may be pregnant (FDA Pregnancy Category X) or in those with undiagnosed genital bleeding, liver tumors (benign or malignant), or known or suspected breast carcinoma. If pregnancy occurs, the implant should be removed. However, no teratogenic effects have been reported in infants born to the small number of women in whom the capsules were retained. No data are available on infants who were breastfed for the first six weeks postpartum and whose mothers had an implant. In infants followed for three years, no adverse effects were observed with use after six weeks postpartum.

PHARMACOKINETICS. Levonorgestrel released from the implant is almost completely bioavailable. Initially, 85 mcg is released daily. Over 1.5 years, the amount gradually decreases to a steady-state release rate of 30 to 35 mcg daily and this continues for 3.5 years.

Maximum serum concentrations of 1,600 pg/ml are achieved within 24 hours of implantation. Over time, these concentrations decrease to an average of 400 pg/ml at three months; 327 pg/ml at 12 months; and 258 pg/ml at five years, at which time the capsules are removed. In women weighing more than 60 kg, serum concentrations decrease about 3 pg/ml/kg. Serum concentrations decrease to 50 pg/ml (the sensitivity level of the assay) within 5 to 14 days after removal of the capsules. Lower concentrations of levonorgestrel are associated with a slight increase in the contraceptive failure rate. Serum FSH and LH decrease when the Norplant system is in place, but the serum estradiol concentration remains normal.

DOSAGE AND PREPARATIONS. A trocar is used to implant the capsules subdermally on the inner surface of the upper arm; training sessions on proper technique for insertion and removal are available for health care providers.

Subdermal: For contraception, the capsules are inserted in a fan-like pattern in the mid-upper arm (8 to 10 mm above the elbow crease) within the first seven days of the menstrual cycle. To maintain efficacy, a new Norplant System must be implanted after five years.

Norplant System (Wyeth-Ayerst). Kit consisting of six flexible closed Silastic capsules, each containing levonorgestrel 36 mg, and implantation instruments (trocar, scalpel, forceps, syringe and needles, skin closures, sponges, bandage, and drapes).

Cited References

New developments in vaginal contraception. *Popul Rep [H]* 12:H159-H190, (Jan-Feb) 1984.

Hormonal contraception: New long-acting methods. *Popul Rep [K]* 15:K57-K87, 1987.

IUDS: A new tool. *Popul Rep [B]* 16:1-12, (March) 1988.

Vasectomy and prostate cancer, editorial. *Lancet* 337:1445–1446, 1991.

Abernethy DR, et al: Imipramine disposition in users of oral contraceptive steroids. *Clin Pharmacol Ther* 35:792-797, 1984.

Alvarez F, et al: New insights on the mode of action of intrauterine contraceptive devices in women. *Fertil Steril* 49:768-773, 1988.

Baciewicz AM: Oral contraceptive drug interactions. *Ther Drug Monit* 7:26-35, 1985.

Back DJ, Orme ML'E: Interindividual variability in oral contraceptive disposition. *TIPS* 480-483, (Nov) 1984.

Back DJ, Orme ML'E: Pharmacokinetic drug interactions with oral contraceptives. *Clin Pharmacokinet* 18:472-484, 1990.

Back DJ, et al: Interindividual variation and drug interactions with hormonal steroid contraceptives. *Drugs* 21:46-61, 1981.

Badawy SZA, et al: Relation between oral contraceptive use and subsequent development of hyperprolactinemia. *Fertil Steril* 36:464-467, 1981.

Balmaceda JP, et al: Luteinizing hormone-releasing hormone analogs: Female contraception. *Semin Reprod Endocrinol* 5:371-380, 1987.

Beral V, et al: Oral contraceptive use and malignancies of the genital tract: Results from the Royal College of General Practitioners' oral contraception study. *Lancet* 2:1331-1335, 1988.

Bhasin S, Swerdloff RS: Contraceptive studies with luteinizing hormone-releasing hormone agonists. *Semin Reprod Endocrinol* 5:381-387, 1987.

Bowes WA Jr, et al: Triphasic randomized clinical trial: Comparison of effects on carbohydrate metabolism. *Am J Obstet Gynecol* 161:1402-1407, 1989.

Bracken MB: Spermicidal contraceptives and poor reproductive outcomes: Epidemiologic evidence against association. *Am J Obstet Gynecol* 157:552-556, 1985.

Bracken MB, Vita K: Frequency of nonhormonal contraception around conception and association with congenital malformations in offspring. *Am J Epidemiol* 117:281-291, 1983.

Brody SA, et al: Pharmacokinetics of three bioequivalent norethindrone/mestranol-50μg and three norethindrone/ethinyl estradiol-35μg OC formulations: Are 'low-dose' pills really lower? *Contraception* 40:269-284, 1989.

Burkman RT: Association between intrauterine device and pelvic inflammatory disease. *Obstet Gynecol* 57:269-276, 1981.

Burkman RT Jr (ed): Benefits and risk of oral contraceptives: A reassessment. *J Reprod Med* 36(suppl):217-252, 1991.

Burkman RT, et al: Lipid and lipoprotein changes associated with oral contraceptive use: Randomized clinical trial. *Obstet Gynecol* 71:33-38, 1988.

Caillouette JC, Koehler AL: Phasic contraceptive pills and functional ovarian cysts. *Am J Obstet Gynecol* 156:1538-1542, 1987.

Cancer and Steroid Hormone Study: Long-term oral contraceptive use and risk of breast cancer. *JAMA* 249:1591-1595, 1983 A.

Cancer and Steroid Hormone Study: Oral contraceptive use and risk of endometrial cancer. *JAMA* 249:1600-1604, 1983 B.

Cancer and Steroid Hormone Study: Combination oral contraceptive use and risk of endometrial cancer. *JAMA* 257:796-800, 1987 A.

Cancer and Steroid Hormone Study: Reduction in risk of ovarian cancer associated with oral-contraceptive use. *N Engl J Med* 316:650-655, 1987 B.

Casagrande JT, et al: "Incessant ovulation" and ovarian cancer. *Lancet* 2:170-173, 1979.

Casper RF, Powell AM: Evaluation and therapy of breakthrough bleeding in women using a triphasic oral contraceptive. *Fertil Steril* 55:292-296, 1991.

Coker AL, et al: Barrier methods of contraception and cervical intraepithelial neoplasia. *Contraception* 45:1-9, 1992.

Cole LP, et al: Postpartum insertion of modified intrauterine devices. *J Reprod Med* 29:677-682, 1984.

Collaborative Group for the Study of Stroke in Young Women: Oral contraception and increased risk of cerebral ischemia or thrombosis. *N Engl J Med* 288:871-878, 1973.

Committee on Drugs, American Academy of Pediatrics: Breast feeding and contraception. *Pediatrics* 68:138-140, 1981.

Cordero JF, Layde PM: Vaginal spermicides, chromosomal abnormalities and limb reduction defects. *Fam Plann Perspect* 15:16-18, 1983.

Cramer DW, et al: Tubal infertility and intrauterine device. *N Engl J Med* 312:941-947, 1985.

Cramer DW, et al: Relationship of tubal infertility to barrier method and oral contraceptive use. *JAMA* 257:2446-2450, 1987.

Croft P, Hannaford PC: Risk factors for acute myocardial infarction in women: Evidence from the Royal College of General Practitioners' oral contraception study. *BMJ* 298:165-168, 1989.

Dalen JE, Hickler RB: Oral contraceptives and cardiovascular disease. *Am Heart J* 101:626-639, 1981.

Daling JR, et al: Primary tubal infertility in relation to use of intrauterine device. *N Engl J Med* 312:937-941, 1985.

del Junco DJ, et al: Do oral contraceptives prevent rheumatoid arthritis? *JAMA* 254:1938-1941, 1985.

Dickerson J, et al: Liver function tests and low-dose estrogen oral contraceptives. *Contraception* 22:597-603, 1980.

Dickey RP: *Managing Contraceptive Pill Patients,* ed 5. Minneapolis, Creative Infomatics, 1987 A.

Dickey RP: *Oral Contraceptive User Guide.* Durant, Okla, Infomatic Guides, Inc, 1987 B.

Dixon GW, et al: Ethinyl estradiol and conjugated estrogens as postcoital contraceptives. *JAMA* 244:1336-1339, 1980.

Dorflinger LJ: Relative potency of progestins used in oral contraceptives. *Contraception* 31:557-570, 1985.

Du MK, et al: Study of Norplant[R] implants in Shanghai: Three-year experience. *Int J Gynecol Obstet* 33:345-357, 1990.

Dunson TR, et al: A multicenter clinical trial of a progestin-only oral contraceptive in lactating women. *Contraception* 47:23-35, 1993.

Dupont WD, Page DL: Risk factors for breast cancer in women with proliferative breast disease. *N Engl J Med* 312:146-151, 1985.

Ebeling K, et al: Use of oral contraceptives and risk of invasive cervical cancer in previously screened women. *Int J Cancer* 39:427-430, 1987.

Edelman DA, et al: Comparative trial of Today contraceptive sponge and diaphragm. *Am J Obstet Gynecol* 150:869-876, 1984.

Edgren RA, et al: Bleeding patterns with low-dose monophasic oral contraceptives. *Contraception* 40:285-297, 1989.

Einarson TR, et al: Maternal spermicide use and adverse reproductive outcome: A meta-analysis. *Am J Obstet Gynecol* 162:655-660, 1990.

Ellis JW: Multiphasic oral contraceptives: Efficacy and metabolic impact. *J Reprod Med* 32:28-36, 1987.

Engel H-J, et al: Coronary atherosclerosis and myocardial infarction in young women: Role of oral contraceptives. *Eur Heart J* 4:1-8, 1983.

Faich G, et al: Toxic shock syndrome and the vaginal contraceptive sponge. *JAMA* 255:216-218, 1986.

Fasoli M, et al: Post-coital contraception: Overview of published studies. *Contraception* 39:459-468, 1989.

Forman D, et al: Cancer of the liver and use of oral contraceptives. *BMJ* 292:1357-1361, 1986.

Fotherby K: New look at progestogens. *Clin Obstet Gynaecol* 11:701-722, 1984.

Franceschi S, et al: Oral contraceptives and benign breast disease: Case-control study. *Am J Obstet Gynecol* 149:602-606, 1984.

Garza-Flores J, et al: Long-term effects of depot-medroxyprogesterone acetate on lipoprotein metabolism. *Contraception* 44:61-71, 1991.

Gerstman BB, et al: Oral contraceptive estrogen dose and the risk of deep venous thromboembolic disease. *Am J Epidemiol* 133:32-37, 1991.

Giovannucci E, et al: A retrospective cohort study of vasectomy and prostate cancer in US men. *JAMA* 269:878-882, 1993 A.

Giovannucci E, et al: A prospective cohort study of vasectomy and prostate cancer in US men. *JAMA* 269:873-877, 1993 B.

Godsland IF, et al: The effects of different formulations of oral contraceptive agents on lipid and carbohydrate metabolism. *N Engl J Med* 323:1375-1381, 1990.

Godsland IF, et al: Clinical and metabolic considerations of long-term oral contraceptive use. *Am J Obstet Gynecol* 166:1955-1963, 1992.

Goldzieher JW: Selected aspects of the pharmacokinetics and metabolism of ethinyl estrogens and their clinical implications. *Am J Obstet Gynecol* 163:318-322, 1990.

Goldzieher JW, et al: Comparative studies of ethinyl estrogens used in oral contraceptives. I. Endometrial response. II. Antiovulatory potency. III. Effect on plasma gonadotropins. *Am J Obstet Gynecol* 122:615-636, 1975.

Gordon SC, et al: Resolution of contraceptive-steroid-induced hepatic adenoma with subsequent evolution into hepatocellular carcinoma. *Ann Intern Med* 105:547-549, 1986.

Gosden C, et al: Intrauterine contraceptive devices in diabetic women. *Lancet* 1:530-534, 1982.

Green A: Oral contraceptives and skin neoplasia. *Contraception* 43:653-666, 1991.

Grimes DA: Intrauterine devices and pelvic inflammatory disease: Recent developments. *Contraception* 36:97-109, 1987.

Grimes DA: The safety of oral contraceptives: Epidemiologic insights from the first 30 years. *Am J Obstet Gynecol* 166:1950-1954, 1992 A.

Grimes DA: Progestins, breast cancer, and the limitations of epidemiology. *Fertil Steril* 57:492-494, 1992 B.

Gudmundsson JA, et al: Intranasal peptide contraception by inhibition of ovulation with gonadotropin-releasing hormone superagonist nafarelin: Six months' clinical results. *Fertil Steril* 45:617-623, 1986.

Guillebaud J: Oral contraceptives in risk groups: Exclusion or monitoring? *Am J Obstet Gynecol* 163:443-446, 1990.

Gustavson LE, et al: Impairment of prednisolone disposition in women taking oral contraceptives or conjugated estrogens. *J Clin Endocrinol Metab* 62:234-237, 1986.

Hansten PD, Horn JR: Inhibition of oral contraceptive efficacy. *Drug Interact Newslett* 5:7-10, 1985.

Hansten PD, Horn JR: Cyclosporine and sex hormones. *Drug Interact Newslett* 7:35-37, 1987.

Harlap S: Oral contraceptives and breast cancer: Cause and effect? *J Reprod Med* 36:374-395, 1991.

Harlap S, et al: Congenital abnormalities in the offspring of women who used oral and other contraceptives around the time of conception. *Int J Fertil* 30:39-47, 1985.

Harris R, et al: Characteristics relating to ovarian cancer risk: Collaborative analysis of 12 US case-control studies: III. Epithelial tumors of low malignant potential in white women. *Am J Epidemiol* 136:1204-1211, 1992.

Hazes JMW, et al: Reduction of the risk of rheumatoid arthritis among women who take oral contraceptives. *Arthritis Rheum* 33:173-179, 1990.

Heartwell SF, Schlesselman S: Risk of uterine perforation among users of intrauterine devices. *Obstet Gynecol* 61:31-36, 1983.

Heinonen OP, et al: Cardiovascular birth defects and antenatal exposure to female sex hormones. *N Engl J Med* 296:67-70, 1977.

Helmrich SP, et al: Venous thromboembolism in relation to oral contraceptive use. *Obstet Gynecol* 69:91-95, 1987.

Hislop TG, Threlfall WJ: Oral contraceptives and benign breast disease. *Am J Epidemiol* 120:273-280, 1984.

Holt VL, et al: Functional ovarian cysts in relation to the use of monophasic and triphasic oral contraceptives. *Obstet Gynecol* 79:529-533, 1992.

Howards SS, Peterson HB: Vasectomy and prostate cancer: Chance, bias, or a causal relationship? Editorial. *JAMA* 269:913-914, 1993.

Huggins G, et al: Vaginal spermicides and outcome of pregnancy: Findings in large cohort study. *Contraception* 25:219-230, 1982.

Hulka BS, et al: Protection against endometrial carcinoma by combination-product oral contraceptives. *JAMA* 247:475-477, 1982.

Hull MGR, et al: Normal fertility in women with post-pill amenorrhoea. *Lancet* 1:1329-1332, 1981.

Jaffe B, et al: Long-term effects of MPA on human progeny: Intellectual development. *Contraception* 37:607-619, 1988.

Janerich DT, et al: Oral contraceptives and birth defects. *Am J Epidemiol* 112:73-79, 1980.

Jick H, et al: Vaginal spermicides and congenital disorders. *JAMA* 245:1329-1332, 1981.

Jones EF, Forrest JD: Contraceptive failure in the United States: Revised estimates from the 1982 National Survey of Family Growth. *Fam Plann Perspect* 21:103-109, (May, June) 1989.

Jovanovic R, et al: Preventing infection related to insertion of an intrauterine device. *J Reprod Med* 33:347-352, 1988.

Kafrissen ME: A norgestimate-containing oral contraceptive: Review of clinical studies. *Am J Obstet Gynecol* 167:1196-1202, 1992.

Kane LA, Sparrow MJ: Postcoital contraception: A family planning study. *N Z Med J* 102:151-153, 1989.

Kaufman DW, et al: Intrauterine contraceptive device use and pelvic inflammatory disease. *Am J Obstet Gynecol* 136:159-162, 1980 A.

Kaufman DW, et al: Decreased risk of endometrial cancer among oral-contraceptive users. *N Engl J Med* 303:1045-1047, 1980 B.
Kaufman DW, et al: Effect of different types of intrauterine devices on risk of pelvic inflammatory disease. *JAMA* 250:759-762, 1983.
Kelaghan J, et al: Barrier-method contraceptives and pelvic inflammatory disease. *JAMA* 248:184-187, 1982.
Kessel E: Pelvic inflammatory disease with intrauterine device use: A reassessment. *Fertil Steril* 51:1-11, 1989.
King RJB, Whitehead MI: Assessment of the potency of orally administered progestins in women. *Fertil Steril* 46:1062-1066, 1986.
Kjos SL, et al: Effect of low-dose oral contraceptives on carbohydrate and lipid metabolism in women with recent gestational diabetes: Results of a controlled, randomized, prospective study. *Am J Obstet Gynecol* 163:1822-1827, 1990.
Klavon SL, Grubb GS: Insertion site complications during the first year of Norplant[R] use. *Contraception* 41:27-37, 1990.
Kreiss J, et al: Efficacy of nonoxynol 9 contraceptive sponge use in preventing heterosexual acquisition of HIV in Nairobi prostitutes. *JAMA* 268:477-482, 1992.
Kung AWC, et al: Glucose and lipid metabolism with triphasic oral contraceptives in women with history of gestational diabetes. *Contraception* 35:257-269, 1987.
Lanes SF, et al: Oral contraceptive type and functional ovarian cysts. *Am J Obstet Gynecol* 166:956-961, 1992.
LaRosa JC: Varying effects of progestins on lipid levels and cardiovascular disease. *Am J Obstet Gynecol* 158:1621-1629, 1988.
Lee NC, et al: Type of intrauterine device and risk of pelvic inflammatory disease. *Obstet Gynecol* 62:1-6, 1983.
Lee NC, et al: The intrauterine device and pelvic inflammatory disease revisited: New results from the Women's Health Study. *Obstet Gynecol* 72:1-6, 1988.
Lewis PR, et al: The resumption of ovulation and menstruation in a well-nourished population of women breastfeeding for an extended period of time. *Fertil Steril* 55:529-536, 1991.
Lindenbaum J, et al: Inactivation of digoxin by gut flora: Reversal by antibiotic therapy. *N Engl J Med* 305:789-794, 1981.
Linn S, et al: Delay in conception for former "pill" users. *JAMA* 247:629-632, 1982.
Linn S, et al: Lack of association between contraceptive usage and congenital malformations in offspring. *Am J Obstet Gynecol* 147:923-928, 1983.
Lipson A, et al: Progestins and oral contraceptive-induced lipoprotein changes: Prospective study. *Contraception* 34:121-135, 1986.
Liu G-z, Lyle KC: Clinical trial of gossypol as male contraceptive drug. Part II. Hypokalemia study. *Fertil Steril* 48:462-465, 1987.
Liu G-z, et al: Clinical trial of gossypol as male contraceptive drug: Part I. Efficacy. *Fertil Steril* 48:459-461, 1987.
Longstreth WT Jr, Swanson PD: Oral contraceptives and stroke. *Stroke* 15:747-750, 1984.
Louik C, et al: Maternal exposure to spermicides in relation to certain birth defects. *N Engl J Med* 317:474-478, 1987.
Louv WC, et al: Oral contraceptive use and risk of chlamydial and gonococcal infections. *Am J Obstet Gynecol* 160:396-402, 1989.
Lowe GDO, et al: Increased blood viscosity in young women using oral contraceptives. *Am J Obstet Gynecol* 137:840-842, 1980.
Luyckx AS, et al: Carbohydrate metabolism in women who used oral contraceptives containing levonorgestrel or desogestrel: 6-month prospective study. *Fertil Steril* 45:635-642, 1986.
Malatino LS, et al: Effects of low-dose estrogen-progestogen oral contraceptives on blood pressure and the renin-angiotensin system. *Curr Ther Res* 43:743-749, 1988.
Marchbanks PA, et al: Risk factors for ectopic pregnancy: A population-based study. *JAMA* 259:1823-1827, 1988.
McGonigle KF, Huggins GR: Oral contraceptives and breast disease. *Fertil Steril* 56:799-819, 1991.
Meade TW, et al: Progestogens and cardiovascular reactions associated with oral contraceptives and comparison of safety of 50- and 30-mcg oestrogen preparations. *BMJ* 280:1157-1161, 1980.
Mettlin C, et al: Vasectomy and prostate cancer risk. *Am J Epidemiol* 132:1056-1061, 1990.
Mills JL, et al: Are spermicides teratogenic? *JAMA* 248:2148-2151, 1982.
Mills JL, et al: Are there adverse effects of periconceptional spermicide use? *Fertil Steril* 43:442-446, 1985.
Milsom I, Andersch B: Effect of various oral contraceptive combinations on dysmenorrhea. *Gynecol Obstet Invest* 17:284-292, 1984.
Mishell DR Jr: Noncontraceptive health benefits of oral steroid contraceptives. *Am J Obstet Gynecol* 142:809-816, 1982.
Mishell DR Jr: Intrauterine devices. *Clin Obstet Gynaecol* 11:679-699, 1984.
Mishell DR Jr: Use of oral contraceptives in women of older reproductive age. *Am J Obstet Gynecol* 158:1652-1657, 1988.
Mishell DR Jr: Oral contraception for women in their 40s. *J Reprod Med* 35 (suppl):447-481, 1990.
Murphy AA, et al: The effect of tetracycline on levels of oral contraceptives. *Am J Obstet Gynecol* 164:28-33, 1991.
Nausieda PA, et al: Chorea induced by oral contraceptives. *Neurology* 29:1605-1609, 1979.
Neely JL, et al: The effect of doxycycline on serum levels of ethinyl estradiol, norethindrone, and endogenous progesterone. *Obstet Gynecol* 77:416-420, 1991.
Neuberger J, et al: Oral contraceptives and hepatocellular carcinoma. *BMJ* 292:1355-1357, 1986.
Nora JJ, et al: Exogenous progestogen and estrogen implicated in birth defects. *JAMA* 240:837-843, 1978.
Nora JJ, et al: Exogenous sex hormones and birth defects: Continuing the dialogue, letter. *Am J Obstet Gynecol* 144:860-862, 1982.
Ory HW: Review of association between intrauterine devices and acute pelvic inflammatory disease. *J Reprod Med* 20:200-204, 1978.
Ory HW: Ectopic pregnancy and intrauterine contraceptive devices: New perspectives. *Obstet Gynecol* 57:137-144, 1981.
Parazzini F, et al: Oral contraceptive use and risk of uterine fibroids. *Obstet Gynecol* 79:430-433, 1992.
Pardthaisong T, et al: The long-term growth and development of children exposed to Depo-Provera during pregnancy or lactation. *Contraception* 45:313-324, 1992.
Patsch W, et al: The effect of triphasic oral contraceptives on plasma lipids and lipoproteins. *Am J Obstet Gynecol* 161:1396-1401, 1989.
Paul C, et al: Depot medroxyprogesterone (Depo-Provera) and risk of breast cancer. *BMJ* 299:759-762, 1989.
Percival-Smith RKL, Abercrombie B: Postcoital contraception with DL-norgestrel/ethinyl estradiol combination: Six years experience in a student medical clinic. *Contraception* 36:287-293, 1987.
Persson E, Holmberg K: Longitudinal study of *Actinomyces israelii* in female genital tract. *Acta Obstet Gynecol Scand* 63:207, 1984.
Petursson GJ, et al: Pharmacology of ocular drugs: 6. Oral contraceptives. *Ophthalmology* 88:368-371, 1981.
Polednak AP, et al: Birth weight and birth defects in relation to maternal spermicide use. *Teratology* 26:27-38, 1982.
Ray S, et al: Development of male-fertility-regulating agents. *Med Res Rev* 11:437-472, 1991.
Reyniak JV, et al: Incidence of hyperprolactinemia during oral contraceptive therapy. *Obstet Gynecol* 55:8-11, 1980.
Romieu I, et al: Oral contraceptives and breast cancer: Review and meta-analysis. *Cancer* 66:2253-2263, 1990.
Rooks JB, et al: Epidemiology of hepatocellular adenoma: Role of oral contraceptive use. *JAMA* 242:644-648, 1979.
Rosenberg L: The risk of liver neoplasia in relation to combined oral contraceptive use. *Contraception* 43:643-652, 1991.
Rosenberg L, et al: Epithelial ovarian cancer and combination oral contraceptives. *JAMA* 247:3210-3212, 1982.
Rosenberg L, et al: Breast cancer and oral contraceptive use. *Am J Epidemiol* 119:167-176, 1985.
Rosenberg L, et al: Risk of myocardial infarction 10 or more years after vasectomy in men under 55 years of age. *Am J Epidemiol* 123:1049-1056, 1986.
Rosenberg MJ, et al: Effect of contraceptive sponge on chlamydial infection, gonorrhea, and candidiasis: Comparative clinical trial. *JAMA* 257:2308-2312, 1987.
Rosenberg L, et al: Oral contraceptive use and the risk of myocardial infarction. *Am J Epidemiol* 131:1009-1016, 1990.

Ross RK, et al: Risk factors for uterine fibroids: Reduced risk associated with oral contraceptives. *BMJ* 293:359-362, 1986.

Rothman KJ: Spermicide use and Down's syndrome. *Am J Public Health* 72:399-401, 1982.

Russell M, Ramcharan S: Oral contraceptive estrogen content and adverse effects: Has a dose-response relationship been established? *Can Fam Physician* 33:445-460, 1987.

Sandvei R, et al: Mast cells in tubal wall in women using intrauterine contraceptive device. *Br J Obstet Gynecol* 93:758-764, 1986.

Schneiderman DJ, Cello JP: Intestinal ischemia and infarction associated with oral contraceptives. *West J Med* 145:350-355, 1986.

Scragg RKR, et al: Oral contraceptives, pregnancy, and endogenous oestrogen in gall stone disease: Case control study. *BMJ* 288:1795-1799, 1984.

Shapiro S, et al: Birth defects and vaginal spermicides. *JAMA* 247:2381-2384, 1982.

Shoupe D, Mishell DR: Norplant: Subdermal implant system for long-term contraception. *Am J Obstet Gynecol* 160:1286-1292, 1989.

Shoupe D, et al: The significance of bleeding patterns in Norplant implant users. *Obstet Gynecol* 77:256-260, 1991.

Shy KK, et al: Oral contraceptive use and occurrence of pituitary prolactinoma. *JAMA* 249:2204-2207, 1983.

Sivin I: Dose- and age-dependent ectopic pregnancy risks with intrauterine contraception. *Obstet Gynecol* 78:291-298, 1991.

Skouby SO, et al: Consequences of intrauterine contraception in diabetic women. *Fertil Steril* 42:568-572, 1984.

Skouby SO, et al: Oral contraception and insulin sensitivity: In vivo assessment in normal women and women with previous gestational diabetes. *J Clin Endocrinol Metab* 64:519-523, 1987.

Spellacy WN: Carbohydrate metabolism during treatment with estrogen, progestogen, and low-dose oral contraceptives. *Am J Obstet Gynecol* 142:732-734, 1982.

Speroff L, DeCherney AH (eds): Next generation of contraception: Oral contraceptives in the 1990s. *Am J Obstet Gynecol* 167 (part 2):1159-1202, 1992.

Stadel BV: Oral contraceptives and cardiovascular disease, part 1. *N Engl J Med* 305:612-618, 1981.

Staffa JA, et al: Progestins and breast cancer: An epidemiologic review. *Fertil Steril* 57:473-491, 1992.

Stampfer MJ, et al: Prospective study of moderate alcohol consumption and the risk of coronary disease and stroke in women. *N Engl J Med* 319:267-273, 1988.

Stampfer MJ, et al: Past use of oral contraceptives and cardiovascular disease: A meta-analysis in the context of the Nurses' Health Study. *Am J Obstet Gynecol* 163:285-291, 1990.

Stoehr GP, et al: Effect of oral contraceptives on triazolam, temazepam, alprazolam, and lorazepam kinetics. *Clin Pharmacol Ther* 36:683-690, 1984.

Strobino B, et al: Exposure to contraceptive creams, jellies, and douches and their effect on zygote, abstract. *Am J Epidemiol* 112:434, (Sept) 1980.

Sturtevant FM: Oral contraceptives and liver tumors, in Moghissi KS (ed): *Controversies in Contraception.* Baltimore, Williams & Wilkins, 1979, 93-150.

Svensson L, et al: Contraceptives and acute salpingitis. *JAMA* 251:2553-2555, 1984.

Szoka PR, Edgren RA: Drug interactions with oral contraceptives: Compilation and analysis of an adverse experience report database. *Fertil Steril* 49 (suppl):31S-38S, 1988.

Taler SJ, et al: Case-control study of galactorrhea and its relationship to use of oral contraceptives. *Obstet Gynecol* 65:665-668, 1985.

Tatum HJ, Connell EB: Decade of intrauterine contraception: 1976 to 1986. *Fertil Steril* 46:173-192, 1986.

Thomas DB: Oral contraceptives and breast cancer: Review of the epidemiologic literature. *Contraception* 43:597-642, 1991.

Thorogood M, et al: Is oral contraceptive use still associated with an increased risk of fatal myocardial infarction? Report of a case-control study. *Br J Obstet Gynaecol* 98:1245, 1991.

Tikkanen MJ, Nikkilä EA: Oral contraceptives and lipoprotein metabolism. *J Reprod Med* 31 (suppl):898-904, 1986.

Tom L, et al: Male contraception: Combined gonadotropin releasing hormone antagonist and testosterone enanthate. *Clin Res* 39:91A, 1991.

Trussell J, et al: Contraceptive failure in the United States: An update. *Stud Fam Plann* 21:51-54, 1990.

Vandenbroucke JP, et al: Noncontraceptive hormones and rheumatoid arthritis in perimenopausal and postmenopausal women. *JAMA* 255:1299-1303, 1986.

Van Santen MR, Haspels AA: Comparison of high-dose estrogens versus low-dose ethinyl estradiol and norgestrel combination in postcoital interception: Study in 493 women. *Fertil Steril* 43:206-213, 1985.

Vessey MP, et al: Pelvic inflammatory disease and intrauterine device: Findings in large cohort study. *BMJ* 282:855-857, 1981.

Vessey MP, et al: Neoplasia of cervix uteri and contraception: Possible adverse effect of the pill. *Lancet* 2:930-934, 1983.

Vessey MP, et al: Oral contraceptives and stroke: Findings in large prospective study. *BMJ* 289:530-531, 1984.

Vessey M, et al: Oral contraceptives and venous thromboembolism: Findings in a large prospective study. *BMJ* 292:526, 1986.

Waites GMH: Male fertility regulation: Recent advances. *Bull WHO* 64:151-158, 1986.

Warburton D, et al: Lack of association between spermicide use and trisomy. *N Engl J Med* 317:478-482, 1987.

Washington AE, et al: Oral contraceptives, *Chlamydia trachomatis* infection, and pelvic inflammatory disease: Word of caution about protection. *JAMA* 253:2246-2250, 1985.

Webb AMC, et al: Comparison of Yuzpe regimen, danazol, and mifepristone (RU486) in oral postcoital contraception. *BMJ* 305:927-931, 1992.

Weiss NS, Sayvetz TA: Incidence of endometrial cancer in relation to use of oral contraceptives. *N Engl J Med* 302:551-554, 1980.

Weiss BD, et al: The cervical cap. *Am Fam Physician* 43:517-523, 1991.

Whittemore AS, et al: Characteristics relating to ovarian cancer risk: Collaborative analysis of 12 US case-control studies: II. Invasive epithelial ovarian cancers in white women. *Am J Epidemiol* 136:1184-1203, 1992.

WHO, Scientific Group on Mechanism of Action, Safety, and Efficacy of Intrauterine Devices. *Contraception* 36:1-167, (July) 1987 A.

WHO: Multicentered Phase-III comparative clinical trial of depot-medroxyprogesterone acetate given three-monthly at doses of 100 mg or 150 mg: I. Contraceptive efficacy and side effects; II. Comparison of bleeding patterns. *Contraception* 34:224-235, 1986; 35:591-610, 1987 B.

WHO: A multicentered pharmacokinetic, pharmacodynamic study of once-a-month injectable contraceptives. I. Different doses of HRP112 and of Depo-Provera. *Contraception* 36:441-457, 1987 C.

WHO: A multicentered Phase III comparative study of two hormonal contraceptive preparations given once-a-month by intramuscular injection: I. Contraceptive efficacy and side effects. *Contraception* 37:1-20, 1988.

WHO Collaborative Study of Neoplasia and Steroid Contraceptives: Combined oral contraceptives and liver cancer. *Int J Cancer* 43:254-259, 1989.

WHO Collaborative Study of Neoplasia and Steroid Contraceptives: Breast cancer and depot-medroxyprogesterone acetate: A multinational study. *Lancet* 338:833-838, 1991.

WHO Collaborative Study of Neoplasia and Steroid Contraceptives: Depot-medroxyprogesterone acetate (DMPA) and risk of invasive squamous cell cervical cancer. *Contraception* 45:299-312, 1992.

Willett WC, et al: Relative and absolute excess risks of coronary heart disease among women who smoke cigarettes. *N Engl J Med* 317:1303-1309, 1987.

Wilson JC: A prospective New Zealand study of fertility after removal of copper intrauterine contraceptive devices for conception and because of complications: A four-year study. *Am J Obstet Gynecol* 160:391-396, 1989.

Wilson JG, Brent RL: Are female sex hormones teratogenic? *Am J Obstet Gynecol* 141:567-580, 1981.

Wingo PA, et al: Age-specific differences in the relationship between oral contraceptive use and breast cancer. *Obstet Gynecol* 78:161-170, 1991.

Wingrave SJ, Kay CR: Oral contraceptives and gallbladder disease: Royal College of General Practitioners' Oral Contraception Study. *Lancet* 2:957-959, 1982.

Wølner-Hanssen P, et al: Laparoscopic findings and contraceptive use in women with signs and symptoms suggestive of acute salpingitis. *Obstet Gynecol* 66:233-238, 1985.

Wu D: An overview of the clinical pharmacology and therapeutic potential of gossypol as a male contraceptive agent and in gynaecological disease. *Drugs* 38:333-341, 1989.

Wynn V, Niththyananthan R: Effect of progestins in combined oral contraceptives on serum lipids with special reference to high-density lipoproteins. *Am J Obstet Gynecol* 142:766-772, 1982.

Yovich JL, et al: Medroxyprogesterone acetate therapy in early pregnancy has no apparent fetal effects. *Teratology* 38:135-144, 1988.

Yuzpe AA: Postcoital contraception. *Clin Obstet Gynaecol* 11:787-797, 1984.

Zhang J, et al: Risk factors for copper T IUD expulsion: An epidemiologic analysis. *Contraception* 46:427-433, 1992.

Zucker PK, Huggins GR: Oral contraceptives and neoplasia: 1989 Update. *Semin Reprod Endocrinol* 7:255-281, 1989.

Uterine Stimulants and Tocolytics

54

UTERINE STIMULANTS

Oxytocic agents stimulate contraction of the myometrium and are used to induce labor at term, to prevent or control postpartum or postabortion hemorrhage, to assess fetal status in high-risk pregnancies, and to induce abortion. Drugs used clinically include the neurohypophyseal hormone, oxytocin [Pitocin, Syntocinon]; the prostaglandins, carboprost tromethamine [Hemabate] and dinoprostone [Prostin E2]; hypertonic saline or urea [Ureaphil]; and the ergot alkaloids, ergonovine [Ergotrate] and methylergonovine [Methergine]. The choice of drug for a specific use is based on its oxytocic and other pharmacologic properties.

Physiology of Labor

The myometrium is capable of contraction at any time; however, the integrated effects of factors involved in the physiologic status of uterine smooth muscle result in a state of relative quiescence throughout most of pregnancy. As pregnancy advances, the myometrium becomes more sensitive to contractile stimulation. Like other smooth muscle, it exhibits spontaneous, repetitive action potentials, but tension is generated only in the presence of synchronized electrical discharge. Contractions are evident weeks before labor begins but initially are weak, uncoordinated, and involve few muscle fibers. Eventually, the strong, synchronous, propagating contractions characteristic of full-term labor begin.

Early in labor, the cervix softens (ripens) and begins to dilate. Prior to and during this process, reconstruction of connective tissue occurs in the cervix and the myometrium; the stretching of the latter may play a functional role in progression of labor (Granström et al, 1989).

Physiologic and pharmacologic factors favoring contraction include production of estrogen, prostaglandins ($PGF_{2\alpha}$ and PGE_2), and oxytocin, as well as stretching of muscle fibers. Factors favoring quiescence include production of progesterone and possibly prostacyclin and beta-adrenergic stimulation.

Progesterone production increases throughout most of pregnancy and generally maintains the uterus in a nonexcitable state. During pregnancy, the resting membrane potential of the muscle fibers of the uterus is hyperpolarized (−60 mv) relative to the nonpregnant uterus (−40 mv). Myometrial cells underlying the placenta may be even more hyperpolarized, possibly caused by the relatively high local concentrations of progesterone produced by the placenta. Hyperpolarization reduces excitability of the muscle cell membrane. Other mechanisms that may contribute to uterine stability include limitation of impulse conduction among cells and sequestration of calcium within the sarcoplasmic reticulum. As pregnancy progresses, the myometrial area under the placenta becomes proportionately smaller and factors enhancing excitability become dominant.

Changes in the hormonal milieu occurring in weeks 34 to 36 of pregnancy probably play a major role in the timing and initiation of labor. A decrease in the progesterone:estrogen ratio in the myometrium occurs at full-term (Batra, 1985). A critical increase in fetal estrogen production probably stimulates synthesis of prostaglandins. The importance of fetal estrogen in this process is suggested by the observation that pregnancy is prolonged when fetal estrogen secretion is impaired in conditions such as anencephaly; fetal adrenal hypoplasia (the fetal adrenal gland is the source of estrogen precursors); or placental deficiency of sulfatase, the enzyme responsible for converting fetal androgenic precursors to estrogen. Estrogen also may increase serum progesterone binding to protein, resulting in less biologically active free progesterone available to myometrial tissue. The stretching of myometrial muscle fibers that occurs with uterine enlargement also is associated with prostaglandin synthesis.

Existing evidence supports the importance of endogenous prostaglandins in labor. Prostaglandin concentration in maternal serum and amniotic fluid increases with the progression of labor. Events or procedures associated with increased prostaglandin synthesis (eg, infection, rupture, or stripping of the fetal membranes; nipple stimulation) also stimulate uterine contractions and labor. At the cellular level, hormonal changes and increased availability of prostaglandins probably promote formation of gap junctions in the myometrial muscle fibers. These low resistance pathways help synchronize electrical activity in the myometrium, allowing an orderly progression of muscle contraction in labor.

Concentrations of beta-endorphins in plasma decrease throughout pregnancy but rise during labor when cervical effacement exceeds 5 cm. Whether these changes contribute to or result from the labor process is unknown (Weissberg et al, 1990).

Although gradual increases in maternal serum oxytocin and myometrial oxytocin receptors occur during pregnancy, oxytocin may play only a permissive role in early labor. Its major contribution may be in strengthening contractions during the second and third stages of labor, when myometrial oxytocin receptor concentration is at its peak. Serum oxytocin increases during the second stage, and fetal oxytocin constitutes a significant portion of the total amount secreted. (See also Speroff et al, 1989; Baxi and Petrie, 1987.)

During the second trimester, uterine muscle is resistant to stimulation. Large doses of prostaglandins can overcome this resistance and are useful to induce labor at this time. The myometrium is relatively resistant to the effects of oxytocin at this stage of pregnancy, and large doses are required to induce labor at this stage.

Although the autonomic nervous system probably is not involved in the initiation of labor, uterine contractions can be influenced by autonomic drugs. Beta-adrenergic drugs inhibit uterine contractions and have been used to delay preterm labor (see the section on Tocolytics). The effect is mediated by increased production of cyclic adenosine monophosphate (cAMP) and effects on intracellular calcium that result in uterine relaxation. The physiology of uterine contraction has been reviewed (Carsten and Miller, 1987).

Indications

INDUCTION OF TERM LABOR. Labor should be induced whenever a medical or obstetrical indication exists. Premature rupture of the membranes and prolonged (post-term) pregnancy probably are the most common indications. Other indications include some instances of antepartum bleeding; intrauterine growth retardation; erythroblastosis fetalis; and placental insufficiency, which may result from diabetes mellitus, pre-eclampsia, or eclampsia. In these situations, induction of labor may reduce maternal and neonatal morbidity and mortality. Because of the increased risk of perinatal morbidity and mortality associated with post-term pregnancies, labor may be induced in some patients, although the criteria for selection are controversial (Dyson, 1988). See relevant texts for management of obstetrical emergencies.

Intravenous infusion of oxytocin is preferred to induce or augment labor. Small doses stimulate uterine contractility at term, and the pattern of contractions approximates that of natural labor. Oxytocin also is used to augment primary or secondary dysfunctional labor (eg, hypotonic myometrial contractions) without increasing fetal distress or the number of cesarean deliveries (Cardozo and Pearce, 1990).

Several prostaglandins are being evaluated for labor induction. These agents stimulate the uterus and may enhance cervical ripening; unlike oxytocin, they do not cause water retention, which may be dangerous in certain patients (eg, those with pre-eclampsia, hypertension, or kidney disease). However, although clinical studies have demonstrated that their efficacy is equivalent to that of oxytocin, the prostaglandins, like oxytocin, can cause hyperstimulation of the uterus, which compromises uteroplacental blood flow; they also have a longer duration of action than oxytocin. Because these effects are difficult to predict and control, enthusiasm for the use of prostaglandins to induce labor has decreased among many specialists. The augmentation and induction of labor with prostaglandins and oxytocin has been reviewed (Brindley and Sokol, 1989).

Dinoprostone is preferred by some investigators and is the prostaglandin most frequently employed in recent clinical studies on labor induction. Since the myometrium is extremely sensitive to prostaglandins at term, small doses should be given to avoid tetanic contractions. Lower doses greatly reduce the gastrointestinal side effects and hyperpyrexia that often develop with the larger doses used for abortion. Adjustment of the dose depending on the degree of cervical dilation (ie, lower dose with higher Bishop's score) has resulted in successful induction, use of lower average doses, and fewer cases of uterine hyperstimulation than when a standard dose is given (Grunstein et al, 1990). Intravaginal forms (eg, gel, suppository) or intracervical administration of gel (not commercially available) show the most promise of effectiveness with diminished side effects (Neher, 1988). (See also the section on Cervical Ripening below.)

When oxytocin is given after dinoprostone, the contractile response is enhanced; therefore, prostaglandins and oxytocin should never be given simultaneously to induce term labor because of the increased risk of uterine hypercontractility and rupture (Claman et al, 1984). A "washout" period (until regular contractions have dissipated; 12 hours is used in some studies) should elapse before oxytocin is administered, and the lowest pump setting should be used initially.

In general, induction of labor with uterine stimulants should not be attempted in cases of cephalopelvic disproportion, malpresentation, complete placenta previa, or vertical uterine scar from previous cesarean section, hysterotomy, or myomectomy. In patients with previous low transverse section delivery, oxytocin has not increased the risk of uterine rupture. Extreme caution should be observed in patients with abruptio placentae, partial placenta previa, and uterine overdistention. In women of high parity (≥5), labor should be induced only with great caution because of the risk of uterine rupture.

During induced labor, the mother and fetus should be monitored carefully to determine fetal and maternal heart rate, maternal blood pressure, and strength of uterine contractions. If uterine hyperstimulation occurs (hypertonus and abnormally frequent contractions), the uterine stimulant should be withdrawn immediately. Although oxytocin (intravenous) and prostaglandins have very short plasma half-lives, the uterine contractions induced by the latter may be prolonged because of their slower absorption. To diminish tetanic contractions produced by prostaglandins, an intravenous bolus of terbutaline [Brethine, Bricanyl] 250 mcg or magnesium sulfate 3 to 4 g may be used if there are no contraindications. Short-term administration of a tocolytic agent is not contraindicated in diabetic patients.

Other oxytocic agents are not suitable for induction or augmentation of labor. Quinine and quinidine are unreliable in safe doses, and there is considerable danger of eighth nerve damage in the infant. The ergot alkaloids and sparteine, a plant alkaloid with stimulant properties, are too long acting and produce excessive, unphysiologic uterine contractions with the potential to cause fetal bradycardia; sparteine is no longer available in the United States.

CERVICAL RIPENING. The state of the cervix is a critical factor in successful induction (Lange et al, 1982), and failure of induction of labor can be attributed partly to an unfavorable cervical condition. Various agents (eg, prostaglandins, relaxin, estrogen, oxytocin, laminaria or other osmotic dilators) are used or are being investigated to ripen the cervix before induction of term labor or dilation and evacuation (D and E) abortion.

Prostaglandins are currently the most widely used pharmacologic agents for softening and dilating unfavorable cervices before labor is induced. Small doses of dinoprostone in a viscous gel (not commercially available in the United States) administered extra-amniotically, intracervically, or intravaginally have been used. Because experimental designs and endpoints for efficacy vary considerably among studies, results are difficult to compare. However, a review of 59 prospective studies of intracervical or intravaginal administration of dinoprostone gel showed that, compared with placebo or no treatment, cervical scores improved, need for oxytocin was decreased, duration of labor was reduced, and fewer cesarean sections were performed (Rayburn, 1989). In a multicenter placebo-controlled trial, a single intracervical dose of dinoprostone (0.5 mg) in a gel preparation was administered. More of the treated women went into labor spontaneously within 12 hours, and the interval between treatment and delivery was shorter in those receiving dinoprostone, even when women who required additional treatment were included (Bernstein, 1991).

Laminaria sticks or Dilapan or Lamicel dilators slowly absorb moisture and expand after placement in the intracervical canal; therefore, they sometimes are used to enhance cervical ripening prior to induction of labor (see the section on Elective Abortion for further information on cervical dilating devices). In one study, time to complete dilation and possibly time to delivery was shorter with Dilapan than with laminaria sticks. With both devices, a standard oxytocin regimen was employed to induce labor following cervical dilation (Blumenthal and Ramanauskas, 1990).

OTHER INDICATIONS FOR INDUCTION OF LABOR. A *hydatidiform mole* increases the risk of pre-eclampsia, uterine hemorrhage, and choriocarcinoma and should be removed promptly on diagnosis. Oxytocin or dinoprostone have been used to stimulate expulsion, but evacuation of the uterine cavity by suction curettage is preferred. The large doses of oxytocin required for this indication increase the risk of water intoxication, especially if the drug is administered in a salt-free solution. It should be noted that there is an increased risk of trophoblastic embolization with any oxytocic agent.

Fetal death in utero often is followed by spontaneous labor within two to three weeks, but labor may be delayed. Prolonging such pregnancies increases the risk of disseminated intravascular coagulation (DIC). All methods employed to induce delivery of the dead fetus, including surgical evacuation, may cause excessive bleeding.

Previously, a conservative approach was to wait for spontaneous delivery for one to two weeks after fetal death if this did not represent an extreme emotional burden on the patient. However, this approach is not usually employed today because improved methods of diagnosing fetal death and safe and effective means of inducing labor are available. Dinoprostone suppositories are used for this purpose through the second trimester. Because of increased uterine sensitivity in the third trimester, oxytocin may stimulate labor when fetal death occurs at this time; if dinoprostone is used, much lower doses are required. Oxytocin and prostaglandins should not be given simultaneously. Carboprost is also administered for this indication, and success rates of 90% to 100% have been reported. Most experience is with its use in the second trimester (Kochenour, 1987).

Reports of induction of preterm labor for *anencephalic fetus* have indicated that dinoprostone is effective, but a long time is usually required to ripen the cervix because of lack of estrogen priming. For this reason, some clinicians recommend slow serial induction with dinoprostone suppositories. Induction of labor avoids the continuing emotional strain on the patient once the diagnosis has been made, particularly in view of the possibility of prolonged gestation in these cases.

CONTRACTION STRESS TEST. A test of fetal well-being is used in certain high-risk obstetrical patients (eg, those with diabetes mellitus, prolonged pregnancy, hypertension, or pre-eclampsia) to assess the clinical condition. The oxytocin challenge test is usually performed in these patients in a hospital at weekly intervals during late pregnancy. The method is similar to that employed for induction of labor at term (see the evaluation on Oxytocin). Chronic fetal distress (fetal hypoxia, placental insufficiency) may be present if late decelerations of fetal heart rate occur after uterine contractions. A negative finding is usually accurate, but one-third of positive test results may be false. Therefore, optimal management requires more detailed assessment of the fetus before the decision to terminate pregnancy is made. Theoretically, this test may increase the risk of preterm labor, but results of one prospective study that followed patients for up to five days indicated that the risk was not increased over that reported with a nonstress test (ie, fetal monitoring of spontaneous contractions) or that expected in the general population (Braly et al, 1981).

Nipple stimulation is frequently used instead of the oxytocin challenge test. The procedure is simpler and less expensive, and although contractions were achieved sooner with nipple stimulation, overall results have been similar to the oxytocin challenge test (Lipitz et al, 1987; Oki et al, 1987; Rosenzweig et al, 1989). However, it has been suggested that the character of uterine activity may differ with the two methods, that nipple stimulation may yield more false-negative results, and that the two tests may require different criteria for correct interpretation (Mashini et al, 1987).

POSTPARTUM USES. Oxytocin may be used to produce firm uterine contractions and decrease uterine bleeding after term delivery or following abortion. The need for oxytocic stimulation is increased if general anesthesia is employed, since this usually decreases spontaneous uterine contractility. It may be most convenient to administer oxytocin by slow intravenous infusion during the immediate postpartum period. Rapid intravenous infusion should be avoided because transient hypotension and increased heart rate may occur and could be life-threatening, particularly in patients with fixed cardiac output or hypotension resulting from hemorrhage.

Ergot alkaloids (ergonovine [Ergotrate], methylergonovine [Methergine]) also can be used postpartum to control uterine hemorrhage and usually are administered intramuscularly. These drugs are preferred when sustained action is required, since they are effective for several hours. Oral tablets are sometimes given prophylactically for one or two days to patients who have undergone abortion. Ergot alkaloids generally should not be given intravenously because of the danger of increasing blood pressure, particularly in hypertensive patients. Methylergonovine has less hypertensive activity than ergonovine.

Prostaglandins are administered by intramyometrial or intramuscular injection to treat postpartum hemorrhage refractory to usual measures and to correct uterine atony (see the evaluation on Carboprost Tromethamine).

Patients who have received a prolonged course of oxytocin are at increased risk of uterine atony after delivery of the infant. These patients may not respond further to oxytocin, and other oxytocic agents may be required during the postpartum period.

STIMULATION OF MILK LET-DOWN REFLEX. The suckling infant stimulates sensory receptors around the nipple, which initiate separate neuroendocrine reflexes that release prolactin from the anterior pituitary and oxytocin from the posterior pituitary. Prolactin is important in initiating and maintaining milk production, and oxytocin stimulates myoepithelial cells in the mammary gland, which causes milk ejection, commonly termed the milk let-down reflex. Oxytocin is not galactopoietic. Milk ejection also can be initiated by psychic stimuli (eg, seeing the infant, hearing the infant cry). When failure of the neuroendocrine reflex is responsible for insufficient breast milk, intranasal oxytocin may be useful.

ELECTIVE ABORTION. In general, abortions performed during the *first trimester* utilize a suction procedure (menstrual extraction or minisuction) and, if done four to six weeks after the last menstrual period (LMP), require little or no cervical dilation.

Suction abortion is relatively rapid and eliminates the necessity of undergoing labor. In addition, it can be performed earlier than instillation techniques that require amniocentesis, thereby reducing the complications associated with abortion as pregnancy progresses. Prostaglandin analogues have been investigated for use during early pregnancy, but suction appears to be superior to prostaglandins during the first trimester.

As pregnancy progresses in the first trimester, *cervical dilation* becomes necessary. When cervical dilation (with or without concomitant administration of uterine stimulants) is required, one of the cervical dilating products may be useful. Laminaria tents are sticks of seaweed that are placed in the cervical canal 4 to 12 hours before the anticipated procedure. As the sticks absorb fluid and expand, the cervix is dilated gradually, usually with less damage than from other methods of mechanical dilation, although cramping and pain may accompany the process. The dose of uterine stimulant drugs required is often reduced and the drug-to-abortion time is sometimes decreased.

Other synthetic products for dilating the cervix are also available or under investigation. One product [Lamicel] is a polyvinyl alcohol sponge impregnated with magnesium sulfate. Its minimum diameter is larger than that of a laminaria stick, but Lamicel appears to cause less pain after insertion. In a double-blind randomized trial comparing Lamicel to laminaria, the two products were equally effective. Because Lamicel is more convenient and less expensive, it may be considered an alternative to multiple laminaria for cervical dilation for abortion (Grimes et al, 1987).

Dilapan is a dilator made of hypan, a hydro-gel polymer with a hard core to resist fragmentation. In a controlled trial of primigravid women seeking first trimester abortion, use of Dilapan resulted in greater cervical dilation within several hours than with meteneprost (an investigational PGE_2 analogue) suppositories or laminaria (Darney and Dorward, 1987).

Dilation and evacuation (D and E) is the most common method used in *second-trimester elective abortions.* Prostaglandins and combinations of agents for intra-amniotic instillation also are used. If an instillation method is employed, a choice must be made between hypertonic saline and urea.

D and E appears to be preferred for early second-trimester abortions, while instillation methods are used more often as pregnancy progresses (Robins and Surrago, 1980; Grimes et al, 1980; Rayburn and Laferla, 1986; Stubblefield, 1986). Advantages of D and E include greater safety in pregnancies through 16 weeks after the LMP, rapidity of the procedure compared to a method that involves undergoing labor, less psychological hardship for the patient (although probably more for the medical personnel), and lower incidence of infections than with an instillation method (Rayburn and Laferla, 1986).

Hypertonic Solutions: When instilled intra-amniotically, hypertonic solutions (usually urea 40% to 50% or saline 20%) act as chemical poisons on the placenta and fetus. Instillation requires amniocentesis and is usually limited to pregnancies of 16 weeks from the LMP or longer when the amniotic cavity is adequate in size.

Hypertonic urea appears to be less effective but safer than hypertonic saline. Inadvertent intravascular injection does not cause serious complications as may occur with saline. The mean abortion time is about 43 hours. Urea can produce dehydration, and coagulation defects have been reported. It should not be used in patients with impaired renal or hepatic function.

Hypertonic saline is effective in more than 90% of cases, and the mean abortion time is about 36 hours. However, major complications result from inadvertent myometrial or intravascular injection. The former causes uterine damage and the latter produces hypernatremia, which may cause DIC that can be fatal. Intravascular injection may be avoided by not injecting saline into bloody amniotic fluid. When general anesthetics and analgesics are withheld, the patient can report symptoms of hypernatremia promptly. Hypertonic saline should not be used in patients whose ability to handle a sodium load is compromised (eg, those with impaired renal or cardiac function, hypertension).

Oxytocin: A dilute solution of oxytocin is not preferred for second trimester abortion because of uterine refractoriness and the risk of water intoxication. However, when concentrated oxytocin solutions (100 to 600 units/L) were administered to patients at 17 to 24 weeks' gestation, effective concentrations were attained in relatively small fluid volumes. The mean time to delivery of the fetus was shorter, and fewer side effects were reported than with dinoprostone suppositories. None of the 22 patients developed water intoxication (Winkler et al, 1991).

Prostaglandins: These agents stimulate labor at any time during gestation and are preferred to a dilute solution of oxytocin for second-trimester induction of labor.

Prostaglandins may be administered as a vaginal suppository (dinoprostone) or by intramuscular injection (15-methyl $PGF_{2\alpha}$, carboprost [Hemabate]) to induce second-trimester abortions. Extraovular administration, sometimes employed in Europe, involves instilling the medication between the fetal membranes and the uterine wall. The intra-amniotic route is preferred to the extraovular route because systemic absorption is reduced, thus decreasing the incidence of adverse effects.

Dinoprostone vaginal suppositories are useful over a wide range of gestational ages, are more convenient than intra-amniotic methods, and have a high success rate. Suppositories also can be used when other abortion methods fail. However, dinoprostone is not useful when there is vaginal hemorrhage and is not recommended in the presence of previous uterine scar. Also, unpleasant side effects and greater length of time to achieve abortion compared to D and E may limit the desirability of this method (Rakhshani and Grimes, 1988).

Carboprost is longer acting than dinoprostone, is easily administered intramuscularly, and can be used over a wide range of gestational ages. It is particularly useful when other methods of abortion have failed and is preferred to dinoprostone when vaginal bleeding is present. Gastrointestinal side effects are more prominent with systemic administration, however.

The incidence of adverse effects (nausea, vomiting, diarrhea) is high with all methods of abortion using prostaglandins. There is also the possibility of delivering a live fetus, which generally is a disadvantage. Carboprost is more likely to cause bronchospasm in asthmatic patients than dinoprostone, but the incidence of febrile reactions is significant with the latter agent.

Combination Regimens: Oxytocin is sometimes used as an *adjunct* to other abortifacients to stimulate contractions and shorten the abortion time. Combination methods have the potential to maximize effectiveness and minimize side effects. *However, caution must be exercised because effects are often additive and the incidence of adverse effects (DIC, cervical detachment, uterine rupture, water intoxication) is increased* (Cederqvist and Birnbaum, 1980).

Investigational Agents: Mifepristone (RU 486), an abortifacient available in France, China, and Great Britain, is an antiprogestin, and its efficacy is based on its ability to competitively inhibit the binding of progesterone to its receptor. This effectively eliminates the availability of progesterone, which is required to support nidation and maintenance of the pregnancy (Nieman et al, 1987; Couzinet and Schaison, 1988; Avrech et al, 1991).

In a study of 100 women with very early pregnancies who were seeking abortions, mifepristone administered within ten days of expected menses induced bleeding in all within four days and complete abortion in 85%. Prolonged bleeding occurred in 18% (Couzinet et al, 1986). In a study of pregnancies up to the eighth week of gestation, administration of oral mifepristone followed by a vaginal pessary containing gemeprost, an investigational prostaglandin analogue, induced complete abortion in 95% of patients (Rodger and Baird, 1987). The effectiveness of mifepristone in inducing early abortion was inversely related to the concentration of the β-subunit of hCG in serum before the drug was administered (Grimes et al, 1988).

To be eligible for mifepristone treatment in France, patients must be amenorrheic for no more than seven weeks after the LMP and have no contraindications (eg, ectopic pregnancy). The regimens currently used are a single oral dose of mifepristone 600 mg plus a prostaglandin, either gemeprost (vaginal) or one of several alternative doses of sulprostone, given by injection two days later. Abortion occurs 4 to 24 hours after administration of the prostaglandin. Uterine bleeding lasts an average of nine days. Abortion occurs most rapidly when a higher dose of sulprostone (0.5 mg) is employed, but pain and the duration of bleeding also are greatest with this regimen. Patients return 8 to 12 days after receiving mifepristone for verification that the abortion is complete. About 2% require further treatment for incomplete abortion and 1% for severe bleeding (Klitsch, 1990). The combination of mifepristone and the oral agent misoprostol [Cytotec] for abortion induction is being evaluated in clinical trials and appears promising (Aubeny and Baulieu, 1991).

Although mifepristone appears to be effective and safe in early clinical studies, bleeding has been a problem and the long-term safety of repeated use is unknown. No adverse effects of mifepristone on embryos surviving failed abortion attempts have been observed, but continued monitoring is necessary.

Other potential clinical applications of mifepristone (contraception, cervical ripening, breast cancer, Cushing's syndrome) have been reviewed (Baulieu, 1989; Heikinheimo et al, 1990).

Epostane, a 3β-hydroxysteroid dehydrogenase inhibitor that blocks synthesis of progesterone, also is being investigated to induce early abortion. When it was administered orally for seven days beginning the fifth through eighth week of gestation, 84% of pregnancies were terminated. Nausea was a common side effect (Crooij et al, 1988).

Adverse Reactions

All uterine stimulants are potentially dangerous, and patients receiving these drugs must be monitored closely. Their injudicious use may cause injury or death of the mother or infant. Hyperstimulation during labor may progress to uterine tetany with marked impairment of uteroplacental blood flow, uterine rupture, cervical laceration, amniotic fluid embolism, or trauma to the infant (eg, hypoxia, intracranial hemorrhage). See also the discussion on Elective Abortion and evaluations.

Drug Evaluations

OXYTOCIN

[Pitocin, Syntocinon]

```
NH2
|
Cys — Tyr — Ile
|              |
S              |
|              |
S              |
|              |
Cys — Asn — Gln
|
Pro — Leu — Gly — NH2
```

Oxytocin is a cyclic octapeptide synthesized in the paraventricular nucleus of the hypothalamus. It is weakly bound to neurophysin within granules and is transported in this form down the axons of the hypothalamic neurons to the posterior pituitary gland where it is stored. Oxytocin circulates in the blood as the free peptide and has a plasma half-life of approximately 10 minutes. Inactivation occurs principally in the liver and kidneys. All available commercial preparations are synthetic.

USES. Oxytocin is the drug of choice to induce labor at term and may be given to augment labor in selected patients with uterine dysfunction (see review by Blakemore and Petrie, 1988, for use of oxytocin to induce labor). This agent also may be used in inevitable or incomplete abortion after 20 weeks of gestation, although prostaglandins are preferred because they are more effective during the second trimester. Oxytocin may be given after term delivery or abortion to prevent or control hemorrhage and to correct uterine hypotonicity. It also is administered to test fetal-placental function in high-risk obstetric patients (oxytocin challenge test). For more information, see the section on Indications in the Introduction.

Depending on the indication, oxytocin is administered intravenously, intramuscularly, or intranasally. For induction of labor, intravenous infusion with an electric pump is preferred because the dosage can be controlled precisely and increased gradually while the patient's response is observed. Intramuscular injections or intravenous infusions may be employed to control postpartum bleeding and uterine hypotonus. Nasal application has been employed to stimulate the milk let-down reflex.

ADVERSE REACTIONS AND PRECAUTIONS. Hypofibrinogenemia and postpartum bleeding have been observed following use of oxytocin during labor, but these disorders are probably related to the underlying problem rather than to the drug. Administration over prolonged periods may result in uterine atony, which is relatively unresponsive to additional oxytocin. Water intoxication with convulsions caused by the inherent antidiuretic effect of oxytocin may occur if large doses (40 to 50 milliunits/min) are infused for long periods. However, this complication should not be a problem at the low concentrations employed to induce labor at term. The risk of water intoxication can be minimized by infusing the drug intravenously in an electrolyte solution (0.9% sodium chloride injection or Ringer's solution) or in a combination of dextrose 5% and a physiologic electrolyte solution instead of dextrose 5% alone. Increasing the concentration of oxytocin rather than the volume of solution infused also minimizes the risk of water intoxication.

Injudicious use of oxytocin may provoke uterine rupture, anaphylactoid and other allergic reactions, and maternal death. Induced uterine contractions of long duration may cause persistent uteroplacental insufficiency, sinus bradycardia, premature ventricular contractions, and other arrhythmias in the fetus, as well as fetal deaths.

Oxytocin should not be used simultaneously by more than one route or with another oxytocic. *If it is given with another oxytocic agent (after a "washout" period), caution must be exercised to prevent additive myometrial hypertonia* (Claman et al, 1984; Cederqvist and Birnbaum, 1980). During induction of labor, uterine contractility, maternal pulse and blood pressure, and fetal heart rate should be monitored, the latter by an external or internal fetal monitor. Administration should be discontinued immediately if tetany occurs.

Contraindications for induction of labor are cephalopelvic disproportion, malpresentation, and complete placenta previa. Except in unusual circumstances, labor should not be induced in the presence of a vertical uterine scar from previous cesarean section, hysterotomy, or myomectomy. With the increasing acceptance of a trial of labor in second pregnancies with previous cesarean deliveries, the benefits and risks of administering oxytocin to augment labor must be weighed. Results of two large studies have shown that, in women with a previous low transverse section, oxytocin did not increase the incidence of dehiscence, hemorrhage, uterine atony, hysterectomy (Horenstein and Phelan, 1985), uterine rupture, maternal or fetal morbidity, or fetal mortality when used according to appropriate guidelines and when the patient was monitored carefully (Flamm et al, 1987).

Oxytocin nasal solution is classified in FDA Pregnancy Category X.

DOSAGE AND PREPARATIONS.

Intravenous Infusion: For induction of labor, a dilute solution (10 milliunits/ml) is administered, preferably with a constant rate infusion pump (counting drops is less reliable). The initial infusion rate is 0.5 milliunits/min, increased by 1 to 2 milliunits/min every 30 to 60 minutes. Studies indicate that approximately 40 minutes are required to reach a steady-state plasma concentration (Seitchik, 1987). The dosage is increased until an optimal uterine response is obtained (three or four contractions similar to normal labor in ten minutes) without evidence of fetal distress. Approximately 75% of patients respond to a final infusion rate of ≤ 5 milliunits/min (Seitchik, 1987). Physiologic saline, Ringer's solution, or a combination of dextrose 5% and a physiologic electrolyte solution should be used as the diluent, especially if a faster rate of infusion is used. As labor progresses, the dose required to maintain contractions often decreases or the drug may be withdrawn altogether.

For the oxytocin challenge test, a dilute solution is infused intravenously starting at the lowest pump setting (approximately 0.5 milliunits/min), and the dose is doubled every 20 to 30 minutes until three contractions are observed every ten minutes (maximum rate, 20 milliunits/min) unless repetitive late deceleration or fetal bradycardia occurs earlier. If either develops, oxytocin should be discontinued immediately.

For prevention of postpartum uterine atony and hemorrhage, 20 to 40 milliunits/ml in an electrolyte solution is given at the rate of 40 milliunits/min or more at a rate sufficient to control uterine atony. The higher concentration assures adequate dosage without excessive fluid. Bolus injection should be avoided because untoward cardiovascular effects (eg, hypotension, tachycardia) may occur even in young healthy patients.

Intramuscular: To control postpartum bleeding, 3 to 10 units (0.3 to 1 ml).

Generic. Solution 10 units/ml in 1 and 10 ml containers.
Pitocin (Parke-Davis). Solution (sterile, aqueous) 5 units/ml in 0.5 ml containers and 10 units/ml in 1 and 10 ml containers.
Syntocinon (Sandoz). Solution (sterile, aqueous) 10 units/ml in 1 ml containers.

Topical (nasal spray): To promote milk ejection, one spray into one or both nostrils two or three minutes before nursing.

Syntocinon (Sandoz). Nasal spray 40 units/ml (40,000 milliunits/ml) in 2 and 5 ml containers.

ERGOT ALKALOIDS

ERGONOVINE MALEATE
[Ergotrate Maleate]

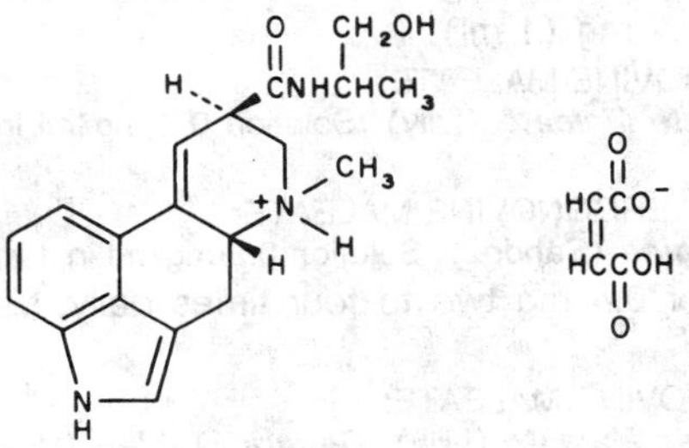

METHYLERGONOVINE MALEATE
[Methergine]

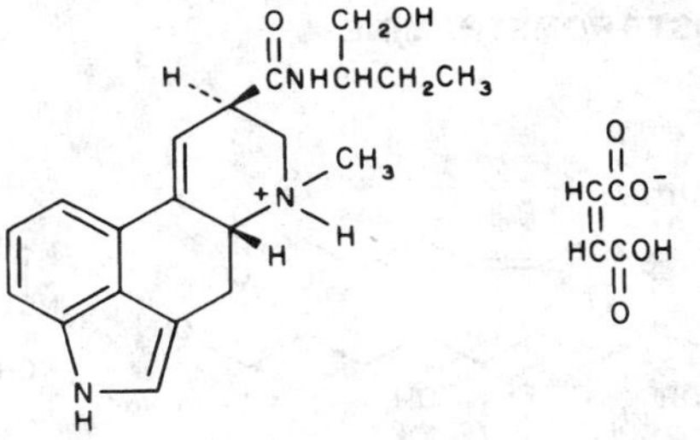

USES. These drugs are used after delivery of the placenta and following suction curettage or instillation abortion to produce firm uterine contractions and decrease uterine bleeding. Both drugs have a rapid onset of action, which varies according to the route of administration (intravenous, 40 seconds; intramuscular, 7 to 8 minutes; oral, 10 minutes). Their usefulness is further enhanced by their prolonged duration of action (several hours).

ADVERSE REACTIONS AND PRECAUTIONS. The adverse effects produced by ergonovine and methylergonovine are similar; because they are more severe after intravenous administration, the intramuscular and oral routes are preferred. Intravenous injection often produces transient hypertension, which is more prominent in patients with chronic hypertension or pre-eclampsia. Hypertensive episodes may be asymptomatic or associated with nausea, vomiting, blurred vision, headaches, and possibly convulsions and death. The intravenous administration of methylergonovine has less tendency to cause hypertension than ergonovine, but preferably neither agent should be given to hypertensive patients.

Ergot alkaloids should not be used in pregnant patients or to induce labor, because of their long duration of action and the unphysiologic uterine contractions that they induce (FDA Pregnancy Category C). They also should not be given to those with a history of hypersensitivity to ergot alkaloids. Both drugs should be administered cautiously to patients with cardiac, hepatic, renal, or obliterative vascular disease.

DOSAGE AND PREPARATIONS.

Intramuscular: To control uterine hemorrhage, 0.2 mg (1 ml); the dose may be repeated in two to four hours if bleeding is severe.

Intravenous: In emergencies to control excessive uterine bleeding, 0.2 mg (1 ml).

ERGONOVINE MALEATE:

Ergotrate Maleate (Lilly). Solution 0.2 mg/ml in 1 ml containers.

METHYLERGONOVINE MALEATE:

Methergine (Sandoz). Solution 0.2 mg/ml in 1 ml containers.

Oral: 0.2 or 0.4 mg two to four times daily, usually for two days.

ERGONOVINE MALEATE:

Ergotrate Maleate (Lilly), ***Generic***. Tablets 0.2 mg.

METHYLERGONOVINE MALEATE:

Methergine (Sandoz). Tablets 0.2 mg.

PROSTAGLANDINS

CARBOPROST TROMETHAMINE

[Hemabate]

ACTIONS AND USES. Carboprost tromethamine (15-methyl $PGF_{2\alpha}$) is a synthetic analogue of the naturally occurring $PGF_{2\alpha}$. Addition of a methyl group at C-15 produces a compound with a longer duration of action. This agent stimulates uterine contractions that are similar to those observed during term labor and is used to induce abortion between 13 and 20 weeks after the LMP.

Abortion is successful in 96% of cases; in 78%, the abortion is complete (ie, complete passage of fetal products without surgical intervention). Time to abortion and total dose increase with greater gestational age but decrease with greater gravidity or parity. Incomplete or failed abortions usually can be completed by D and C or suction curettage.

Carboprost can be used when the membranes have ruptured. An advantage of intramuscular carboprost over intravaginal dinoprostone is that the intramuscular route can be employed in the presence of profuse vaginal bleeding that could lead to expulsion of a vaginal suppository.

Carboprost has controlled persistent postpartum hemorrhage secondary to uterine atony unresponsive to oxytocin and ergonovine or methylergonovine (Herbert and Cefalo, 1984; Nelson, 1980) or manipulative techniques.The need for surgery may be eliminated. In one study, most patients responded to one dose and the average time to increased uterine tone and decreased bleeding was 45 minutes (Hayashi et al, 1984). The intramuscular route is usually employed, but the intramyometrial route also can be utilized. See also the Introduction.

ADVERSE REACTIONS AND PRECAUTIONS. Adverse effects are common but usually not serious and are reversible when administration is discontinued. Because nausea, vomiting, and diarrhea occur in two-thirds of patients, the concurrent administration of antiemetic and antidiarrheal agents is recommended. Transient fever (more than 2° F) occurs in 12% of patients, and care must be taken to differentiate drug-induced pyrexia, which is transient, from that due to endometritis. When carboprost is used to induce abortion, retained placental fragments, excessive bleeding, and endometritis may occur. When used for postpartum hemorrhage, blood pressure may increase.

Carboprost should not be administered to patients who are hypersensitive to the drug or to those with acute pelvic inflammatory disease or active cardiac, pulmonary, renal, or hepatic disease. Patients with a history of asthma; hypertension; cardiovascular, renal, or hepatic disease; anemia; jaundice; diabetes; or epilepsy and those who have undergone uterine surgery, including previous cesarean section, should receive this drug only with caution. Abortion may be incomplete in about 20% of patients, and measures should be taken to ensure completion. Although cervical trauma is unusual, the cervix should be examined after abortion.

As with other prostaglandins, abortion induced by carboprost may result in delivery of a live fetus. Because of the teratogenic potential of certain prostaglandins in animals, pregnancy should be terminated by another method if abortion cannot be induced by carboprost. This drug is classified in FDA Pregnancy Category C.

Carboprost should be administered only by qualified medical personnel in hospitals with obstetric intensive care and surgical facilities.

DOSAGE AND PREPARATIONS.

Intramuscular: A test dose of 100 mcg (0.4 ml) may be administered initially. To induce abortion, 250 mcg deep in the muscle, repeated at intervals of 1.5 to 3.5 hours, depending on the response. Dosage may be increased to 500 mcg if contractility is inadequate after several 250-mcg doses.

To induce labor in instances of fetal death, 250 mcg every two hours. The total dose for this indication should not exceed 12 mg.

For refractory postpartum bleeding, 250 mcg deep in the muscle. Additional doses may be given at intervals of 15 to 90 minutes as determined by the clinical course. If the patient has already received another oxytocic agent, one-half of the dose may be given and the patient observed for systemic effects (eg, decrease in blood pressure, bronchial irritation). The total dose for this indication should not exceed 2 mg.

Hemabate (Upjohn). Solution (sterile) equivalent to 250 mcg carboprost and 83 mcg tromethamine/ml in 1 ml containers. Refrigerate at 36° to 39° F.

DINOPROSTONE
[Prostin E2]

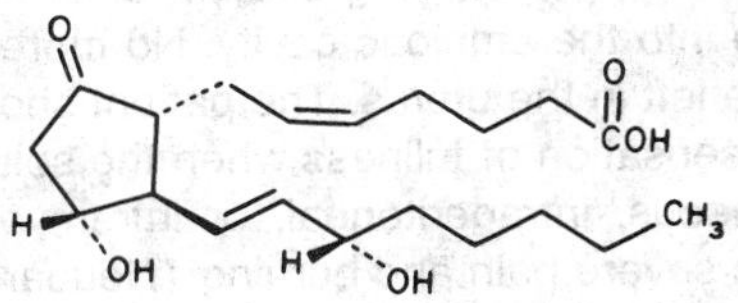

ACTIONS AND USES. Dinoprostone (PGE_2) occurs naturally in mammalian tissues, human seminal plasma, and menstrual fluid. This prostaglandin stimulates smooth muscle contraction and, at the doses used for termination of pregnancy, stimulates gastrointestinal smooth muscle as well as uterine muscle.

Termination of Pregnancy: Dinoprostone is used in suppository form to induce labor in intrauterine fetal death (less than 28 weeks' gestation), missed abortion, benign hydatidiform mole, anencephalic fetus, or elective abortion. Uterine contractions are qualitatively similar to those that occur during term labor.

This prostaglandin also is used to terminate pregnancy from week 12 through 20 of gestation and has been used investigationally for abortions of earlier gestation. Vaginal administration concentrates drug action at the target tissue and is noninvasive. Vaginal application of dinoprostone induces myometrial contractions that usually empty the uterus. It also enhances cervical softening, which facilitates cervical dilatation. Generally, the total dose required to induce delivery declines with advancing gestation so that only a fraction of the 20-mg suppository is needed (Macer et al, 1984).

Dinoprostone can induce uterine contractions when administered orally, intramuscularly, intravenously, or intra- and extra-amniotically, but these routes are still investigational in this country. The effective half-life of prostaglandin action on the uterus is approximately 30 to 60 minutes.

When dinoprostone is used for expulsion of benign hydatidiform mole, blood loss is high and nearly 50% of patients require transfusion. Suction curettage is preferred to evacuate the uterine cavity.

Uses in Term Labor: There are a number of favorable reports on the use of dinoprostone as a cervical ripening agent before induction of labor with oxytocin or as an alternative to oxytocin. Dinoprostone-induced cervical ripening seems to be associated with increased collagenolysis (Ekman et al, 1983) that is similar to the normal ripening process (Uldbjerg et al, 1983), and ripening is not dependent on uterine contractions (Goeschen et al, 1985).

Dinoprostone is preferred to carboprost when induction of labor is necessary but the cervix is unfavorable (eg, following spontaneous rupture of membranes). Intravaginal or intracervical administration of small doses of dinoprostone suppository or gel produces significant cervical softening (increased Bishop scores) and reduces the number of failed inductions. Although the optimal dose has not been determined, dinoprostone gel 0.4 to 0.5 mg extra-amniotically or intracervically (Gordon and Calder, 1983; Ulmsten et al, 1983) and intravaginal suppositories 1 mg were effective (Jagani et al, 1984). The incidence of gastrointestinal adverse reactions is greatly reduced with these doses.

As an alternative to oxytocin for induction of labor, dinoprostone has the advantage of inducing both cervical ripening and uterine contractions. Dinoprostone suppositories or pessaries are used routinely in some countries to induce labor and have been reported to be most useful when the cervix is unfavorable, especially in primigravida patients (Hunter et al, 1984). The incidence of hypertonicity is dose related (Graves et al, 1985), and patients receiving 3 mg or more should be monitored closely. Subsequent augmentation with oxytocin is required in most patients to maintain the established pattern of contractions, but the two uterine stimulants should not be given simultaneously.

ADVERSE REACTIONS AND PRECAUTIONS. Adverse reactions are common with abortive doses of dinoprostone but generally are not serious. Gastrointestinal disturbances are reported most frequently and are related to contractile effects on smooth muscle. Nausea occurs in approximately one-third, vomiting in approximately two-thirds, and diarrhea in 40% of patients. These symptoms can be alleviated by antiemetics and antidiarrheal agents and by increasing the interval between doses.

Transient fever (more than 2° F), frequently with chills, occurs in up to 50% of patients. Drug-induced fever must be differentiated from pyrexia due to endometritis, particularly in intrauterine fetal death when there is a greater risk of sepsis. Also, when the combination of fever and hypotension suggests sepsis, the possibility of drug-induced fever and hypotension due to blood loss associated with uterine rupture should be considered. Myocardial infarction following use of dinoprostone rarely has been reported in patients with a history of cardiovascular disease.

Headache and decreased diastolic blood pressure (by more than 20 mm Hg) occur in 10% of patients. Blood loss resulting from the procedure may contribute to reduced blood pressure. Unlike abortion induced by hypertonic saline, there is no risk of hypernatremia and the incidence of DIC is not increased; however, there is a higher risk of hemorrhage from retained placentas.

Uterine hypertonicity and rupture have been reported (Claman et al, 1984). Rupture of the amniotic and chorionic membranes is not a contraindication to continued use of dinoprostone, but washout of the suppository can occur. Profuse vaginal bleeding also may cause expulsion of the suppository.

Unlike abortion induced by hypertonic saline or urea, that induced by prostaglandins may result in delivery of a live fetus, particularly with increasing gestational age. This agent is not labeled for use beyond 28 weeks and should be employed cautiously in fetal death in utero during the third trimester because of the increased risk of uterine rupture.

In animal studies, certain prostaglandins had teratogenic potential. Therefore, if treatment with dinoprostone fails to abort the fetus, the pregnancy should be terminated by appropriate measures (eg, suction curettage).

Dinoprostone should be used cautiously in patients with cervicitis, infected endocervical lesions, or acute vaginitis, as well as in those with a history of asthma, hypertension or hypotension or other cardiovascular diseases, renal or hepatic disease, anemia, jaundice, diabetes, epilepsy, or uterine scars. It should not be given to patients with acute pelvic inflammatory disease; hypersensitivity to the drug; or active cardiac, pulmonary, renal, or hepatic disease. The concomitant use of oxytocin or other oxytocics to induce abortion is generally not advised because of the increased risk of uterine rupture.

Dinoprostone should be administered only by qualified medical personnel in hospitals with obstetric intensive care and surgical facilities.

This drug is classified in FDA Pregnancy Category C.

DOSAGE AND PREPARATIONS. Suppositories must be stored at or below -20° C (-4° F) and brought to room temperature just before use.

Vaginal: To induce abortion, one 20-mg suppository is inserted high in the vagina; the patient should remain supine for ten minutes following insertion. Subsequently, suppositories are inserted at intervals of three to five hours until abortion occurs. Within this interval, administration time is determined by abortifacient progress, uterine contractility, and patient tolerance. If abortion is incomplete, administration may be continued to completion if blood loss is not excessive and adverse reactions are not severe.

For doses used for cervical ripening and to induce labor (investigational indications), see Actions and Uses.

Prostin E2 (Upjohn). Vaginal suppositories 20 mg.

HYPERTONIC SOLUTIONS

SALINE

USES. Hypertonic saline is used to induce second trimester abortion. It was once the most commonly used agent for this indication but has been replaced to some extent by urea. Some practitioners prefer saline, and the choice among agents depends on several factors (see the discussion on Elective Abortion in the Introduction).

Hypertonic saline is usually administered by transabdominal amniocentesis. It is effective in about 90% of patients; the mean abortion time is approximately 36 hours. Saline may be administered with oxytocin to reduce abortion time. However, care must be taken when more than one uterine stimulant is used because the effects are additive.

PRECAUTIONS. Saline abortion should not be attempted in patients whose ability to handle a sodium load is compromised (eg, those with renal or cardiac failure, hypertension). Inadvertent intravascular injection causes hypernatremia and possibly DIC. Accidental instillation into the uterine wall destroys uterine tissue.

DOSAGE AND PREPARATIONS.

Intra-amniotic Instillation: Following the establishment of an intravenous line and amniocentesis with a properly placed needle for aspiration of amniotic fluid, 200 ml of a 20% or 23% salt solution (40 to 46 g sodium chloride) is instilled with a needle into the amniotic cavity. No more than 40 g of salt should be left in the uterus. The patient should feel nothing or only a sensation of fullness when the solution is injected. Subcutaneous, intraperitoneal, or intramyometrial injection produces severe pain and burning (Neubardt and Schulman, 1977).

Sodium Chloride 20%, 23%. Not available commercially but may be prepared in a hospital pharmacy.

UREA

[Ureaphil]

USES. A hypertonic solution of urea is used as an alternative to hypertonic saline, dinoprostone, or carboprost to induce second trimester abortions. Like saline, urea is administered by transabdominal amniocentesis. The abortion time is longer (43 versus 36 hours) than with saline but urea is theoretically safer.

Oxytocin is sometimes administered after instillation of urea to shorten the abortion time, but care must be taken when more than one uterine stimulant is used because the effects are additive. See also the section on Indications in the Introduction.

ADVERSE REACTIONS AND PRECAUTIONS. Urea may cause hyponatremia, hypokalemia, or hyperkalemia. It should not be used in patients with severely impaired renal or hepatic function, intracranial bleeding, or dehydration. Patients should be encouraged to drink fluids and should receive intravenous fluid during the procedure to enhance excretion of urea. Nausea, vomiting, and headaches also may occur. Inadvertent intravascular spill can cause headache, nausea, uterine cramps, and a feeling of warmth.

Urea is classified in FDA Pregnancy Category C.

DOSAGE AND PREPARATIONS.

Intra-amniotic Instillation: 80 g is reconstituted to a volume of 135 to 200 ml with 5% dextrose solution to make a 40% to 50% solution. It is recommended that a peripheral intravenous line be established initially and then, following amniocentesis with a properly placed needle for aspiration of amniotic fluid, the solution is instilled by gravity via a suitably attached administration set connected to the needle.

Ureaphil (Abbott). Powder (nonpyrogenic) 40 g in 150 ml single-dose containers. The desired diluent can be added directly to the contents.

TOCOLYTICS

Preterm labor (rhythmic uterine contractions less than 10 minutes apart before the end of week 37 of gestation) may occur spontaneously or following premature rupture of the fetal membranes. Many risk factors have been identified and include previous history of preterm labor, low socioeconomic status of the mother, maternal smoking or drug abuse, coital activity, maternal stress, multiple gestation, hydramnios, placental abnormalities, infection of the fetal membranes, and cervical incompetence (Gazaway and Mullins, 1986). Genetic collagen abnormalities may lead to weakening of the fetal membranes, premature rupture, and labor (Schwartz, 1986).

Uterine relaxants (tocolytics) are used in selected patients to inhibit preterm labor in pregnancies that would benefit from longer intrauterine life (ie, until the fetus has matured sufficiently for survival, usually the 32nd week of gestation). Use of selective beta$_2$-adrenergic agents (to relax uterine smooth muscle) has replaced older, less specific approaches, such as infusion of alcohol. Magnesium sulfate is an alternative. These agents also may be employed briefly to delay delivery while treatment with corticosteroids is initiated to stimulate production of fetal lung surfactant. However, theoretically there may be a greater risk of maternal pulmonary edema when corticosteroids are administered with beta-adrenergic agents (see also index entry Adrenal Corticosteroids, Adverse Reactions). The use of a combination of tocolytic agents is increasing, but controlled studies are needed to determine efficacy, maternal tolerance, and neonatal outcome compared with beta-adrenergic therapy alone.

See Besinger and Niebyl, 1990, for an extensive discussion of drugs used to treat preterm labor.

CHOICE OF THERAPY. Uterine contractions may cease spontaneously after conservative treatment with hydration, bed rest, or sedation or may progress to preterm labor. Tocolytic agents are more likely to inhibit labor before it is far advanced.

A national survey of American physicians showed wide variability in the definition and management of preterm labor. The tocolytic agents used most commonly were ritodrine [Yutopar], terbutaline [Brethine, Bricanyl], and magnesium sulfate (in that order); specific protocols differed. Any of these drugs can serve as first-line therapy. Perinatologists appeared more likely than obstetricians to utilize more aggressive therapeutic interventions such as administration of more than one agent, use of amniocentesis and amniotic fluid culture, and initiation of tocolytic therapy when cervical dilation was at a more advanced stage. The majority of physicians reported having observed serious complications with use of tocolytic drugs, which emphasizes that there is significant risk for both the mother and fetus (Taslimi et al, 1989).

When the diagnosis of preterm labor is established, the benefits of therapy may outweigh the risks if the lungs of the fetus are immature (generally when gestation is less than 34 weeks), if the cervix is dilated less than 4 cm, and if there are no contraindications to the drugs. Contraindications include any condition in which treatment and continuation of the pregnancy represent the greater hazard (eg, eclampsia, severe pre-eclampsia, hemorrhage, intrauterine fetal death, chorioamnionitis, maternal cardiovascular disease).

Beta-Adrenergic Agents: These drugs prevent contraction of the myometrium by reducing availability of intracellular calcium. The stimulatory action of oxytocin is inhibited by these agents. *Ritodrine* is the only agent currently labeled for tocolysis in the United States. It has been used extensively throughout the world. *Terbutaline*, commonly used as a bronchodilator, has not been employed as widely, but extensive data indicate that it is therapeutically equivalent to ritodrine and is less expensive. Maternal serum glucose concentrations may be higher with oral (Main et al, 1987) or intravenous (Caritis et al, 1984) terbutaline, but other maternal side effects appear to be similar with these two drugs. They are usually administered intravenously or subcutaneously (0.25 mg every 20 to 60 minutes) until contractions are inhibited. Intramuscular ritodrine (5 to 10 mg every two to four hours) is an alternative route of administration. The alternate routes have similar efficacy and eliminate the possibility of intravenous fluid overload.

After discharge from the hospital, the patient may be maintained on oral medication until delivery of a mature infant is assured. However, tachyphylaxis occurs with long-term therapy and some authorities believe a shorter course of treatment (eg, five days) is equally effective and avoids prolonged exposure of mother and fetus to the drug. If preterm labor recurs, parenteral therapy may be resumed.

Because *isoxsuprine* [Vasodilan], which is promoted for treatment of peripheral vascular disorders, has relatively less specific beta$_2$-adrenergic effects, the incidence and severity of undesirable maternal cardiovascular effects (ie, tachycardia, hypotension) (Caritis, 1983) and neonatal hypocalcemia and hypotension are greater with its use. Other beta$_2$-adrenergic drugs administered to arrest preterm labor are *albuterol* (salbutamol) [Proventil, Ventolin] (available in the United States for treatment of asthma as an oral preparation only) *fenoterol, hexoprenaline,* and *metaproterenol* (orciprenaline).

Maternal hyperglycemia, hypokalemia, angina, tachycardia, hypotension, palpitations, headache, nausea and vomiting, restlessness, tremor, and anxiety have occurred after use of beta-adrenergic agents (Rayburn et al, 1986). Adult respiratory distress syndrome and pulmonary edema, which occur in up to 5% of patients treated with intravenous beta-adrenergic agents, also have developed. These complications may be observed with or without concurrent corticosteroid therapy for fetal lung maturation and usually are observed prior to delivery. Beta-adrenergic agents may exert an antidiuretic effect, and intravenous fluids containing sodium should be avoided. Administration of corticosteroids with mineralocorticoid activity, concurrent infection, and a history of cardiac disease or pulmonary hypertension may contribute to development of pulmonary edema (Besinger and Niebyl, 1990). Although it has been recommended that potent general anesthetics that depress the myocardium be avoided when beta-adrenergic agents are used, clinical data to support this view are lacking.

Magnesium Sulfate: This agent prevents convulsions in pre-eclampsia and inhibits uterine contractions by a direct inhibition of action potentials in the myometrial muscle cells. Excitation and contraction are uncoupled, which decreases the frequency and force of contractions. Magnesium sulfate is administered intravenously and may be as effective as ritodrine (Hollander et al, 1987). However, as with other drugs, it has not been universally effective as a tocolytic agent (Cox et al, 1990). Tocolysis occurs when the serum magnesium concentration is 4 to 8 mEq/L. Within this nontoxic range, only a few side effects are observed in the mother (eg, transient hypotension after administration of a loading dose, sensation of heat, flushing). Serious adverse effects can be avoided by monitoring serum concentration (see the evaluation). Hypotonia, drowsiness, and decreased bowel peristalsis may occur in the infant, because renal excretion of magnesium is delayed in the neonate (Besinger and Niebyl, 1990).

Magnesium sulfate may be used sequentially after failure of a beta-adrenergic agent or as the primary agent, particularly if the cardiovascular side effects of beta-adrenergic agents are of concern. An oral preparation of magnesium oxide was reported to be as effective as oral terbutaline when employed after successful use of parenteral tocolytic therapy (Ridgway et al, 1990). (See the Table for suggested regimen.) However, results of another study suggest that oral therapy may be no more effective than placebo (Ricci et al, 1991).

Magnesium sulfate should not be used in patients with heart block or myocardial damage, severely impaired renal function, or myasthenia gravis; it may be preferred to beta-adrenergic agonists for diabetic, hyperthyroid, or hypertensive patients.

Magnesium sulfate also has been used as an adjunct to ritodrine; the combination may be more effective than ritodrine alone, and the dose of ritodrine required to produce a therapeutic effect may be reduced (Hatjis et al, 1987). Repeated administration of the combination may inhibit preterm labor for one week or longer. However, cardiac side effects may limit the usefulness of this combination (see the evaluation on Ritodrine, Drug Interactions).

Other Agents: Prostaglandins probably play a role in stimulating uterine contractions during normal labor, and their concentrations increase in amniotic fluid and serum during active labor. *Prostaglandin synthetase inhibitors*, particularly indomethacin [Indocin], have been used to delay preterm labor. In controlled clinical trials, indomethacin was more effective than placebo in preventing preterm labor and delivery for periods up to two days (Niebyl et al, 1980; Zuckerman et al, 1984). Indomethacin and ritodrine were similarly effective in preventing delivery for more than 48 hours (Morales et al, 1989) or more than seven days (Besinger et al, 1991). Furthermore, the combination of ritodrine plus indomethacin was more effective than ritodrine alone in prolonging pregnancy (Gamissans et al, 1978; Katz et al, 1983).

Prostaglandins are necessary to maintain a patent ductus arteriosus in the fetus, and prostaglandin synthetase inhibitors may cause premature closure. However, in a large retrospective study using combined suppository and oral indomethacin for 24 to 48 hours to delay preterm labor, premature closure of the ductus arteriosus did not occur (Dudley and Hardie, 1985). In another study, a transient constriction of the ductus arteriosus was observed with administration of indomethacin, but the effect was corrected within 24 hours (Moise et al, 1988). Impaired fetal renal function with oligohydramnios also has been reported and appears to be revers-

SUGGESTED DOSAGE REGIMENS FOR TOCOLYTIC DRUGS*

Drug	Preparation	Loading Dose	Maintenance Dose	
			Short-term	Long-term
Ritodrine [Yutopar]	0.03% solution (150 mg/500 ml) in 5% dextrose and 0.9% normal saline	None	0.05-0.35 mg/min intravenously for 12 hr or longer	10 mg orally every 2 hr for first 24 hr after intravenous therapy and 10-20 mg orally every 4-6 hr thereafter
Terbutaline [Brethine, Bricanyl]	0.001% solution (10 mg/L) in 5% dextrose and 0.45% normal saline	250 mcg intravenously over 1-2 min	10-25 mcg/min intravenously for 12 hr (60-150 ml/hr) or longer	250 mcg subcutaneously every 4 hr; 2.5-5 mg orally every 4-6 hr
Magnesium sulfate	4% solution (40 g/L) in 5% dextrose in water and 0.45% normal saline	4-6 g in 100 ml over 20 min	1-4 g intravenously/hr for 8-12 hr (25-100 ml/hr)	Usually not administered orally (use oral beta-adrenergic drug)
Magnesium oxide† [Mag-Ox, Uro-Mag]	tablets 400 mg capsules 140 mg	----	----	200 mg orally every 3-4 hr

* *Adapted from Rayburn WF, Zuspan FP (eds):* Drug Therapy in Obstetrics and Gynecology, *ed 2. Old Tappin, NJ, Appleton-Century-Crofts, 1986. Reprinted with permission.*

† *Ridgway et al, 1990.*

ible when the drug is withdrawn (Hendricks et al, 1990). Maternal side effects are not serious; nausea and heartburn are commonly reported. Although indomethacin appears to be an effective tocolytic agent, is easy to administer, and causes few maternal side effects, further clinical trials are necessary to resolve questions about fetal safety before its routine use for preterm labor can be recommended.

The calcium channel blocker, *nifedipine*, is the newest drug to be investigated as a tocolytic agent. By inhibiting entry of calcium into the myometrial muscle cells, contractility is reduced, even in the presence of oxytocin or prostaglandins. In one study, nifedipine, administered orally, suppressed uterine contractions more effectively than intravenous ritodrine or no treatment. Adverse effects, which were less numerous and severe than with ritodrine, included flushing, nausea, and increased fetal heart rate but only a transient increase in maternal heart rate (Read and Wellby, 1986). In subsequent studies, ritodrine and nifedipine were equally effective in delaying preterm labor for 48 hours (Meyer et al, 1990) and one week (Ferguson et al, 1990; Janky et al, 1990). Although nifedipine appears to be a useful tocolytic agent, additional data are necessary before assessing its role in therapy for preterm labor.

Diazoxide [Hyperstat IV], a potent antihypertensive agent, occasionally is used to control hypertensive emergencies during labor. This agent also inhibits uterine contractions and has been employed to arrest preterm labor. However, it is not as effective as beta agonists and may cause severe hypotension, marked maternal hyperglycemia, and neonatal hyperglycemia. Therefore, its use generally is not favored.

The use of *intravenous alcohol,* once widely administered to inhibit preterm labor, is now obsolete.

In women at high risk of premature delivery (ie, history of premature deliveries or spontaneous abortions), *hydroxyprogesterone caproate* has been reported to be more effective than placebo in maintaining pregnancy and reducing preterm birth (Johnson et al, 1975; Yemini et al, 1985; Keirse, 1990). The drug was given prophylactically from the 12th to the 37th weeks of pregnancy or until delivery. Although no teratogenic effects have been reported in humans or animals, the possibility of late teratogenic effects must be determined and more experience is necessary before hydroxyprogesterone can be recommended routinely (see also the discussion on alternative therapies for preterm labor in Rayburn et al, 1986).

Drug Evaluations

MAGNESIUM SULFATE

ACTIONS AND USES. This agent decreases muscle contractility in the myometrial cells by uncoupling excitation and contraction. As a result, the frequency and force of contractions are decreased. Because of the inhibitory effect on contraction, magnesium sulfate is used to inhibit preterm labor. When the drug is administered intravenously, onset of action is almost immediate, and the duration is 30 minutes. (See also index entry Magnesium Sulfate, In Eclampsia, Preeclampsia.)

ADVERSE REACTIONS AND PRECAUTIONS. The serum magnesium concentration should be monitored to avoid overdosage. Blood pressure, respiratory rate, and deep tendon reflexes also should be determined to detect signs of toxicity. Tocolysis occurs when the serum magnesium concentration is 4 to 8 mEq/L. Within this nontoxic range, only a few side effects are observed in the mother (eg, transient hypotension after administration of a loading dose, sensation of heat, flushing). Loss of deep tendon reflexes and respiratory depression may occur when serum magnesium exceeds 8 to 10 mEq/L, and conduction abnormalities and cardiac arrest may be observed with concentrations of 15 to 20 mEq/L (Hueston, 1989). Magnesium sulfate is excreted through the kidney, and toxic serum levels may be reached in patients with impaired renal function. Urine output should be at least 30 ml/hr.

Magnesium sulfate crosses the placenta and rapidly equilibrates with the maternal concentration. Hypotonia, drowsiness, and decreased bowel peristalsis may occur in the infant, because renal excretion of magnesium is delayed in the neonate (Besinger and Niebyl, 1990). If possible, administration should be discontinued several hours prior to delivery.

This agent should not be administered to patients with heart block, heart damage from myocardial infarction, renal failure, or myasthenia gravis.

DOSAGE AND PREPARATIONS.

Intravenous: A loading dose of 4 to 6 g is followed by continuous infusion of 2 g/hr; the dose is increased to 3 to 4 g/hr if contractions continue after one hour. The infusion may be given for 24 hours. Serum levels should be monitored every four to six hours.

Generic. Solution 10% in 20 and 50 ml containers and 50% in 2, 5, 10, 20, and 30 ml containers.

RITODRINE HYDROCHLORIDE

[Yutopar]

HO–C_6H_4–CH(OH)–CH(CH_3)NHCH_2CH_2–C_6H_4–OH

ACTIONS. Ritodrine decreases the frequency, intensity, and duration of uterine contractions by direct stimulation of beta$_2$ receptors through activation of adenyl cyclase. Although ritodrine stimulates beta$_2$ receptors principally, it also has some beta$_1$ activity, which is responsible for cardiovascular side effects. Its effect is antagonized by beta blockers, such as propranolol.

USES. This beta$_2$-adrenergic agonist is used to prevent the progress of preterm labor in selected patients (eg, gestation of 20 weeks or more, labor that is not far advanced, intact or ruptured membranes, absence of contraindications). Therapy may be initiated as soon as the diagnosis is established and contraindications are ruled out. Delivery has been delayed for several days to enhance fetal lung maturity with corticosteroid therapy or for weeks to achieve a near normal gestation period. Intravenous administration stops contractions initially; oral therapy is given for maintenance. Intravenous therapy may be repeated if further episodes of preterm labor occur.

Although results of studies have been variable, ritodrine is superior to placebo when preterm labor begins before 33 weeks. However, if gestation exceeds 33 weeks when preterm labor begins, overall advantages have not been demonstrated statistically due to small numbers (Finkelstein, 1981). Ritodrine is less likely to be effective in advanced labor when the cervix is effaced more than 80% and dilated more than 4 cm. In premature rupture of membranes and preterm labor, the addition of ritodrine to expectant management of patients did not prolong pregnancy (Garite et al, 1987). Ritodrine also is used in combination with other tocolytic agents (see the discussion above).

ADVERSE REACTIONS. A diagnosis of preterm labor, as well as absence of contraindications to ritodrine, should be established before this drug is used. Tocolytic therapy with ritodrine should be undertaken only in a hospital equipped to handle potential medical and obstetric complications (Graber, 1989). Cardiovascular and metabolic effects are observed in both mother and fetus. Adverse effects are most severe after intravenous administration and usually are controlled by reducing the dose, although discontinuation of therapy may be required. Theoretically, overdosage can be managed with a beta blocker (Feely et al, 1983), but there is little clinical evidence that this is necessary.

Intravenous infusion has caused tachycardia in almost all patients (maximum increase averages 40 beats/min), increased systolic blood pressure (mean, 12 mm Hg), and decreased diastolic blood pressure (mean, 23 mm Hg). Hemodilution occurs in some patients. Blood glucose and insulin concentrations increase temporarily and return toward normal within 48 to 72 hours, even with continued infusion. Ketoacidosis has been reported in diabetic patients. Serum potassium levels decrease and free fatty acid levels may increase. About one-third of patients experience palpitations, and up to 15% have chest pain, shortness of breath, tremor, nausea and vomiting, headache, or erythema. Less common reactions include nervousness, anxiety, malaise, and cardiovascular effects. Maternal deaths, usually associated with unrecognized cardiopulmonary disease, have been reported (Barden et al, 1980). Rarely, pulmonary edema occurs even after the drug is withdrawn. Ritodrine unmasked latent myotonic muscular dystrophy in one patient (Sholl et al, 1985).

Intravenous administration also may cause tachycardia in the fetus. The concentration of insulin in cord blood may be elevated, resulting in neonatal hypoglycemia. Neonatal hypocalcemia has been reported. Before delivery, the fetus may be affected by maternal ketoacidosis. Infusion should be discontinued as soon as labor appears to be irreversible in order to allow metabolic recovery before delivery.

Fewer and less severe side effects have been reported after *oral* administration. The maternal heart rate may increase, but the blood pressure is not affected significantly. Carbohydrate and electrolyte balance do not appear to be affected. Tremors, palpitations, nausea, nightmares, arrhythmias, and nervousness occur infrequently and are dose related.

Animal studies have shown no teratogenic effects and no impairment of reproductive function. Follow-up studies for two years revealed no deleterious effects on growth, development, or maturation in 7- to 9-year-old children exposed to ritodrine prenatally (Polowczyk et al, 1984).

PRECAUTIONS AND CONTRAINDICATIONS. Fluid balance and serum glucose and potassium levels should be monitored during infusion, particularly in diabetic patients or those taking diuretics that may deplete body potassium. Because cardiovascular effects are most pronounced during intravenous infusion, maternal blood pressure and maternal and fetal heart rate should be monitored. Intravenous solutions containing saline should be avoided to prevent excess fluid load. Cerebral ischemia has been reported during beta-adrenergic therapy in two women with a history of migraine, and caution probably should be observed when ritodrine is used in such patients (Benedetti, 1983). If pulmonary edema develops, infusion should be discontinued and appropriate therapy instituted.

Ritodrine should not be used when continuation of the pregnancy is hazardous to the mother or fetus, as in eclampsia, severe pre-eclampsia, antepartum hemorrhage, chorioamnionitis, maternal cardiovascular disease, or pulmonary hypertension. There are no well-controlled studies on the use of ritodrine prior to 20 weeks' gestation. Caution should be observed in patients with hyperthyroidism or diabetes. This drug is classified in FDA Pregnancy Category B.

DRUG INTERACTIONS. Ritodrine and corticosteroids have additive diabetogenic effects. Insulin requirements may increase greatly during intravenous administration of ritodrine. Pulmonary edema also occurs rarely when ritodrine and corticosteroids are given concurrently, but the contribution of the corticosteroid has not been determined (Benedetti, 1983). The combination of ritodrine and magnesium sulfate has been reported to cause cardiac disturbances that necessitated withdrawal of tocolytic therapy (Ferguson et al, 1984). No additional metabolic changes occur when magnesium sulfate is added to a ritodrine regimen (Ferguson et al, 1987).

Ritodrine may potentiate the effects of other sympathomimetic amines and may have an additive hypotensive effect with drugs such as anesthetics. The possibility of an additive effect on serum potassium with potassium-depleting diuretics also should be considered.

PHARMACOKINETICS. After intravenous infusion in pregnant women, ritodrine exhibited half-lives of six to nine minutes in the distribution phase and two to three hours in the elimination phase.

Oral bioavailability of ritodrine is about 30%, and peak concentrations occur within 40 minutes. Approximately 32% circulates bound to albumin. Up to 90% is excreted in the urine within 24 hours. Ritodrine crosses the placenta, and the cord blood concentration may equal that in the maternal circulation (Finkelstein, 1981).

DOSAGE AND PREPARATIONS. Treatment is individualized, and the optimal dosage is determined by the balance between desired uterine response and undesirable effects. The patient should remain in the left lateral recumbent position to minimize hypotension. Three ampuls or one vial (150 mg) in 500 ml of diluent (eg, 5% dextrose) yield a final concentration of 300 mcg/ml (0.3 mg/ml). Because of the increased risk of pulmonary edema, saline diluents should not be used unless dextrose solution is less desirable (eg, diabetes mellitus) (Philipsen et al, 1981). The solution should be used promptly and discarded after 48 hours or if discoloration or particulate matter is observed.

Intravenous: Initially, 50 mcg/min (0.05 mg/min), increased by the same amount every 20 minutes until contractions are controlled, and maintained for approximately one hour thereafter. This regimen maintains effective blood levels but decreases the amount of drug given and may reduce side effects (Caritis et al, 1990). Repeated intravenous administration may be employed if there are subsequent episodes of preterm labor.

Alternatively, 100 mcg/min (0.1 mg/min), increased by 50 mcg/min (0.05 mg/min) every ten minutes until contractions stop or a rate of 350 mcg/min (0.35 mg/min) is reached.

The lowest dose that maintains uterine quiescence is continued for 12 hours after contractions are controlled. At the recommended rate of infusion, a maximum of approximately 840 ml of fluid would be administered in 12 hours.

Yutopar (Astra), ***Generic.*** Solution (sterile, aqueous) 10 mg/ml in 5 ml containers and 15 mg/ml in 10 ml containers.

Oral: After preterm labor is controlled by intravenous administration, oral therapy is initiated and continued as long as it is desirable to prolong pregnancy or until intravenous therapy is required again. One tablet (10 mg) is taken 30 minutes before intravenous administration is terminated and every two hours thereafter for the first 24 hours; alternatively, two tablets (20 mg) may be given every two to four hours for the first 24 hours; subsequently, one to two tablets (10 to 20 mg) are taken every four to six hours to a maximum total daily dose of 120 mg. Treatment may be continued as long as it is desirable to prolong pregnancy.

Yutopar (Astra). Tablets 10 mg.

TERBUTALINE SULFATE

[Brethine, Bricanyl]

For chemical formula, see index entry Terbutaline, In Asthma.

ACTIONS AND USES. Like ritodrine, this drug is predominantly a $beta_2$-receptor agonist with some $beta_1$ activity, which causes cardiovascular side effects. Terbutaline was employed for preterm labor by a number of physicians before ritodrine was introduced and is still preferred by some. The effectiveness of terbutaline and ritodrine is equivalent, and side effects are similar with intravenous administration. However, in patients with intact membranes, the incidence of tachycardia (more than 130 beats/min) was reported to be greater with ritodrine and the incidence of hyperglycemia (with oral therapy) was greater with terbutaline (Caritis et al, 1984; Main et al, 1987). Oral maintenance therapy with terbutaline 30 mg/day prolonged pregnancy by 40 ± 25 days compared to 22 ± 24 days for oral ritodrine 120 mg/day (Caritis et al, 1984). Labor recurred in fewer women given oral terbutaline for maintenance than with ritodrine.

See the evaluation on Ritodrine Hydrochloride for uses, adverse reactions, interactions, precautions, and contraindications associated with beta-adrenergic therapy.

DOSAGE AND PREPARATIONS.

Intravenous: Initially, 2.5 mcg/min, increased by 2.5 mcg/min every 20 minutes until contractions stop or a rate of 17.5 mcg/min is reached. After contractions are controlled, the rate is reduced by 2.5 mcg/min every 20 minutes until the minimum effective infusion rate is established. This rate is then maintained for 12 hours. If labor recurs during this time, the rate can again be increased by 2.5 mcg/min every 20 minutes to re-establish control. Also see the table for suggested regimens.

Brethine (Geigy), ***Bricanyl*** (Marion Merrell Dow). Solution 1 mg/ml in 1 ml containers.

Oral: For maintenance therapy, 5 mg is given 30 minutes before discontinuing intravenous infusion; subsequently, 5 mg is given every four hours (maximum, 30 mg daily).

Brethine (Geigy), ***Bricanyl*** (Marion Merrell Dow). Tablets 2.5 and 5 mg.

Cited References

Aubeny E, Baulieu EE: Contraceptive activity of RU486 and oral active prostaglandin combination. *C R Acad Sci* 312:539-545, 1991.

Avrech OM, et al: Mifepristone (RU 486) alone or in combination with a prostaglandin analogue for termination of early pregnancy: A review. *Fertil Steril* 56:385-393, 1991.

Barden TP, et al: Ritodrine hydrochloride: Betamimetic agent for use in preterm labor; I. Pharmacology, clinical history, administration, side effects, and safety. *Obstet Gynecol* 56:1-6, 1980.

Batra S: On the role of estradiol and progesterone in parturition: Updated proposal. *Acta Obstet Gynecol Scand* 64:671-672, 1985.

Baulieu E-E: RU-486 as an antiprogesterone steroid: From receptor to contragestion and beyond. *JAMA* 262:1808-1814, 1989.

Baxi LV, Petrie RH: Pharmacologic effects on labor: Effects of drugs on dystocia, labor, and uterine activity. *Clin Obstet Gynecol* 30:19-32, 1987.

Benedetti TJ: Maternal complications of parenteral β-sympathomimetic therapy for preterm labor. *Am J Obstet Gynecol* 145:1-6, 1983.

Bernstein P: Prostaglandin E_2 gel for cervical ripening and labour induction: A multicentre placebo-controlled trial. *Can Med Assoc J* 145:1249-1254, 1991.

Besinger RE, Niebyl JR: The safety and efficacy of tocolytic agents for the treatment of preterm labor. *Obstet Gynecol Surv* 45:415-440, 1990.

Besinger RE, et al: Randomized comparative trial of indomethacin and ritodrine for the long-term treatment of preterm labor. *Am J Obstet Gynecol* 164:981-988, 1991.

Blakemore KJ, Petrie RH: Oxytocin for the induction of labor. *Obstet Gynecol Clin North Am* 15:339-353, 1988.

Blumenthal PD, Ramanauskas R: Randomized trial of dilapan and laminaria as cervical ripening agents before induction of labor. *Obstet Gynecol* 75:365-368, 1990.

Braly P, et al: Incidence of premature delivery following oxytocin challenge test. *Am J Obstet Gynecol* 141:5-8, 1981.

Brindley BA, Sokol RJ: Induction and augmentation of labor: Basis and methods for current practice. *Obstet Gynecol Surv* 43:730-743, 1989.

Cardozo L, Pearce JM: Oxytocin in active-phase abnormalities of labor: A randomized study. *Obstet Gynecol* 75:152-157, 1990.

Caritis SN: Treatment of preterm labor: Review of therapeutic options. *Drugs* 26:243-261, 1983.

Caritis SN, et al: Double-blind study comparing ritodrine and terbutaline in the treatment of preterm labor. *Am J Obstet Gynecol* 150:7-14, 1984.

Caritis SN, et al: Pharmacokinetics of ritodrine administered intravenously: Recommendations for changes in the current regimen. *Am J Obstet Gynecol* 162:420-437, 1990.

Carsten ME, Miller JD: New look at uterine muscle. *Am J Obstet Gynecol* 157:1303-1315, 1987.

Cederqvist LL, Birnbaum SJ: Rupture of uterus after midtrimester prostaglandin abortion. *J Reprod Med* 25:136-138, 1980.

Claman P, et al: Uterine rupture with use of vaginal prostaglandin E_2 for induction of labor. *Am J Obstet Gynecol* 150:889-890, 1984.

Couzinet B, Schaison G: Mifegyne (mifepristone), new antiprogestagen with potential therapeutic use in human fertility control. *Drugs* 35:187-191, 1988.

Couzinet B, et al: Termination of early pregnancy by the progesterone antagonist RU 486 (mifepristone). *N Engl J Med* 315:1565-1570, 1986.

Cox SM, et al: Randomized investigation of magnesium sulfate for prevention of preterm birth. *Am J Obstet Gynecol* 163:767-772, 1990.

Crooij MJ, et al: Termination of early pregnancy by the 3β-hydroxysteroid dehydrogenase inhibitor epostane. *N Engl J Med* 319:813-817, 1988.

Darney PD, Dorward K: Cervical dilation before first trimester elective abortion: Controlled comparison of meteneprost, laminaria, and hypan. *Obstet Gynecol* 70:397-400, 1987.

Dudley DKL, Hardie MJ: Fetal and neonatal effects of indomethacin used as tocolytic agent. *Am J Obstet Gynecol* 151:181-184, 1985.

Dyson DC: Fetal surveillance vs. labor induction at 42 weeks in postterm gestation. *J Reprod Med* 33:262-270, 1988.

Ekman G, et al: Increased postpartum collagenolytic activity in cervical connective tissue from women treated with prostaglandin E_2. *Gynecol Obstet Invest* 16:292-298, 1983.

Feely J, et al: Beta-blockers and sympathomimetics. *Br Med J* 286:1043-1047, 1983.

Ferguson JE II, et al: Adjunctive use of magnesium sulfate with ritodrine for preterm labor tocolysis. *Am J Obstet Gynecol* 148:166-171, 1984.

Ferguson JE II, et al: Adjunctive magnesium sulfate infusion does not alter metabolic changes associated with ritodrine tocolysis. *Am J Obstet Gynecol* 156:103-107, 1987.

Ferguson JE II, et al: A comparison of tocolysis with nifedipine or ritodrine: Analysis of efficacy and maternal, fetal, and neonatal outcome. *Am J Obstet Gynecol* 163:105-111, 1990.

Finkelstein BW: Ritodrine. *Drug Intell Clin Pharm* 15:425-433, 1981.

Flamm BL, et al: Oxytocin during labor after previous cesarean section: Results of multicenter study. *Obstet Gynecol* 70:709-712, 1987.

Gamissans O, et al: A study of indomethacin combined with ritodrine in threatened preterm labor. *Eur J Obstet Gynecol Reprod Biol* 123-128, (Aug) 1978.

Garite TJ, et al: Randomized trial of ritodrine tocolysis versus expectant management in patients with premature rupture of membranes at 25 to 30 weeks of gestation. *Am J Obstet Gynecol* 157:388-393, 1987.

Gazaway P, Mullins CL: Prevention of preterm labor and premature rupture of the membranes. *Clin Obstet Gynecol* 29:835-849, 1986.

Goeschen K, et al: Effect of β-mimetic tocolysis on cervical ripening and plasma prostaglandin $F_{2\alpha}$ metabolite after endocervical application of prostaglandin E_2. *Obstet Gynecol* 65:166-171, 1985.

Gordon AJ, Calder AA: Cervical ripening. *Br J Hosp Med* 30:52-58, 1983.

Graber EA: Dilemmas in the pharmacological management of preterm labor. *Obstet Gynecol Surv* 44:512-517, 1989.

Granström L, et al: Changes in the connective tissue of corpus and cervix uteri during ripening and labour in term pregnancy. *Br J Obstet Gynaecol* 96:1198-1202, 1989.

Graves GR, et al: Effect of vaginal administration of various doses of prostaglandin E_2 gel on cervical ripening and induction of labor. *Am J Obstet Gynecol* 151:178-181, 1985.

Grimes DA, et al: Midtrimester abortion by dilatation and evacuation versus intra-amniotic instillation of prostaglandin $F_{2\alpha}$: Randomized clinical trial. *Am J Obstet Gynecol* 137:785-790, 1980.

Grimes DA, et al: Lamicel versus laminaria for cervical dilation before early second-trimester abortion: Randomized clinical trial. *Obstet Gynecol* 69:887-890, 1987.

Grimes DA, et al: Early abortion with a single dose of the antiprogestin RU-486. *Am J Obstet Gynecol* 158:1307-1312, 1988.

Grunstein S, et al: A scoring system for induction of labor using prostaglandin E_2 vaginal tablets. *Int J Gynecol Obstet* 31:131-134, 1990.

Hatjis CG, et al: Efficacy of combined administration of magnesium sulfate and ritodrine in treatment of premature labor. *Obstet Gynecol* 69:317-322, 1987.

Hayashi RH, et al: Management of severe postpartum hemorrhage with prostaglandin $F_{2\alpha}$ analogue. *Obstet Gynecol* 63:806-808, 1984.

Heikinheimo O, et al: Antiprogesterone RU 486: A drug for non-surgical abortion. *Ann Med* 22:75-84, 1990.

Hendricks SK, et al: Oligohydramnios associated with prostaglandin synthetase inhibitors in preterm labour. *Br J Obstet Gynaecol* 97:312-316, 1990.

Herbert WNP, Cefalo RC: Management of postpartum hemorrhage. *Clin Obstet Gynecol* 27:139-147, 1984.

Hollander DI, et al: Magnesium sulfate and ritodrine hydrochloride: Randomized comparison. *Am J Obstet Gynecol* 156:631-637, 1987.

Horenstein JM, Phelan JP: Previous cesarean section: Risks and benefits of oxytocin usage in trial of labor. *Am J Obstet Gynecol* 151:564-569, 1985.

Hueston WJ: Prevention and treatment of preterm labor. *Am Fam Physician* 40:139-146, (Nov) 1989.

Hunter IWE, et al: Induction of labor using high-dose or low-dose prostaglandin vaginal pessaries. *Obstet Gynecol* 63:418-420, 1984.

Jagani N, et al: Role of prostaglandin-induced cervical changes in labor induction. *Obstet Gynecol* 63:225-229, 1984.

Janky E, et al: A randomised study of treatment of threatened premature labor: Nifedipine as against ritodrine. *J Gynecol Obstet Biol Reprod* 19:478-482, 1990.

Johnson JWC, et al: Efficacy of 17-hydroxy-progesterone caproate in the prevention of premature labor. *N Engl J Med* 293:675-680, 1975.

Katz Z, et al: Treatment of premature labor contractions with combined ritodrine and indomethacin. *Int J Gynaecol Obstet* 21:337-342, 1983.

Keirse MJNC: Progestogen administration in pregnancy may prevent preterm delivery. *Br J Obstet Gynaecol* 97:149-154, 1990.

Klitsch M: French trials of RU 486 find 96 percent abortion rate in pregnancies of less than seven weeks. *Fam Plann Perspect* 22:134-135, (May/June) 1990.

Kochenour NK: Management of fetal demise. *Clin Obstet Gynecol* 30:322-330, 1987.

Lange AP, et al: Prelabor evaluation of inducibility. *Obstet Gynecol* 60:137-147, 1982.

Lipitz S, et al: Breast stimulation test and oxytocin challenge test in fetal surveillance: Prospective randomized study. *Am J Obstet Gynecol* 157:1178-1181, 1987.

Macer J, et al: Induction of labor with prostaglandin E_2 vaginal suppositories. *Obstet Gynecol* 63:664-668, 1984.

Main EK, et al: Chronic oral terbutaline tocolytic therapy is associated with maternal glucose intolerance. *Am J Obstet Gynecol* 157:644-647, 1987.

Mashini IS, et al: Comparison of uterine activity induced by nipple stimulation and oxytocin. *Obstet Gynecol* 69:74-78, 1987.

Meyer WR, et al: Nifedipine versus ritodrine for suppressing preterm labor. *J Reprod Med* 35:649-653, 1990.

Moise KJ Jr, et al: Indomethacin in the treatment of premature labor: Effects on fetal ductus arteriosus. *N Engl J Med* 319:327-331, 1988.

Morales WJ, et al: Efficacy and safety of indomethacin versus ritodrine in the management of preterm labor: A randomized study. *Obstet Gynecol* 74:567-572, 1989.

Neher JO: Prostaglandin E_2 induction of labor. *Am Fam Physician* 38:223-225, (Aug) 1988.

Neibyl JR, et al: The inhibition of premature labor with indomethacin. *Am J Obstet Gynecol* 136:1014-1019, 1980.

Nelson GH: Prostaglandins and reproduction, in Goldstein DP, et al (eds): *Current Problems in Obstetrics and Gynecology*. Chicago, Year Book Medical Publishers, 1980.

Neubardt S, Schulman H: *Techniques of Abortion,* ed 2. Boston, Little Brown, 1977.

Nieman LK, et al: Progesterone antagonist RU 486: Potential new contraceptive agent. *N Engl J Med* 316:187-191, 1987.

Oki EY, et al: Breast-stimulated contraction stress test. *J Reprod Med* 32:919-923, 1987.

Philipsen T, et al: Pulmonary edema following ritodrine-saline infusion in premature labor. *Obstet Gynecol* 58:304-308, 1981.

Polowczyk D, et al: Evaluation of seven- to nine-year-old children exposed to ritodrine in utero. *Obstet Gynecol* 64:485-488, 1984.

Rakhshani R, Grimes DA: Prostaglandin E_2 suppositories as a second-trimester abortifacient. *J Reprod Med* 33:817-820, 1988.

Rayburn WF: Prostaglandin E_2 gel for cervical ripening and induction of labor: A critical analysis. *Am J Obstet Gynecol* 160:529-534, 1989.

Rayburn WF, Laferla JJ: Midgestational abortion for medical or genetic indications. *Clin Obstet Gynecol* 13:71-82, 1986.

Rayburn WF, et al: Drugs to inhibit premature labor, in Rayburn WF, Zuspan FP (eds): *Drug Therapy in Obstetrics and Gynecology,* ed 2. New York, Appleton-Century-Crofts, 1986, 172-190.

Read MD, Wellby DE: Use of calcium antagonist (nifedipine) to suppress preterm labor. *Br J Obstet Gynaecol* 93:933-937, 1986.

Ricci JM, et al: Oral tocolysis with magnesium chloride: A randomized controlled prospective clinical trial. *Am J Obstet Gynecol* 165:603-610, 1991.

Ridgway LE, et al: A prospective randomized comparison of oral terbutaline and magnesium oxide for the maintenance of tocolysis. *Am J Obstet Gynecol* 163:879-882, 1990.

Robins J, Surrago EJ: Alternatives in midtrimester abortion induction. *Obstet Gynecol* 56:716-722, 1980.

Rodger MW, Baird DT: Induction of therapeutic abortion in early pregnancy with mifepristone in combination with prostaglandin pessary. *Lancet* 2:1415-1418, 1987.

Rosenzweig BA, et al: Comparison of the nipple stimulation and exogenous oxytocin contraction stress tests: A randomized, prospective study. *J Reprod Med* 34:950-954, 1989.

Schwartz MF: Genetic aspects of premature rupture of the membranes. *Clin Obstet Gynecol* 29:771-778, 1986.

Seitchik J: Management of functional dystocia in the first stage of labor. *Clin Obstet Gynecol* 30:42-49, 1987.

Sholl JS, et al: Myotonic muscular dystrophy associated with ritodrine tocolysis. *Am J Obstet Gynecol* 151:83-86, 1985.

Speroff L, et al: Prostaglandins, in *Clinical Gynecologic Endocrinology and Infertility,* ed 4. Baltimore, Williams & Wilkins, 1989, 365.

Stubblefield PG: Surgical techniques of uterine evacuation in first- and second-trimester abortion. *Clin Obstet Gynecol* 13:53-70, 1986.

Taslimi MM, et al: A national survey on preterm delivery. *Am J Obstet Gynecol* 160:1352-1360, 1989.

Uldbjerg N, et al: Ripening of human uterine cervix related to changes in collagen, glycosaminoglycans, and collagenolytic activity. *Am J Obstet Gynecol* 147:662-666, 1983.

Ulmsten U, et al: Local application of prostaglandin E_2 for cervical ripening or induction of term labor. *Clin Obstet Gynecol* 26:95-105, 1983.

Weissberg N, et al: The relationship between beta-endorphin levels and uterine muscle contractions during labor. *Int J Gynecol Obstet* 33:313-316, 1990.

Winkler CL, et al: Mid-second-trimester labor induction: Concentrated oxytocin compared with prostaglandin E_2 vaginal suppositories. *Obstet Gynecol* 77:297-300, 1991.

Yemini M, et al: Prevention of premature labor by 17 α-hydroxyprogesterone caproate. *Am J Obstet Gynecol* 151:574-577, 1985.

Zuckerman H, et al: Further study of the inhibition of premature labor by indomethacin: Part II double-blind study. *J Perinat Med* 12:25-29, 1984.

Miscellaneous Endocrine Therapy

55

PRECOCIOUS PUBERTY

Drug Evaluations

ANABOLIC THERAPY

DRUG THERAPY FOR SEX OFFENDERS

HEREDITARY ANGIOEDEMA

Drug Evaluation

Precocious Puberty

Puberty that occurs before the age of 9 years in boys or 8 years in girls is considered precocious. In gonadotropin-releasing hormone (GnRH)-dependent central precocious puberty (CPP), early maturation of the hypothalamic-pituitary axis occurs. CPP may be caused by lesions (eg, hypothalamic hamartomas, gliomas, astrocytomas, traumatic brain injury) or it may be idiopathic; the latter is more common in girls than boys. Peripheral precocious puberty occurs when elevated sex steroid secretion is independent of gonadotropin secretion (eg, adrenal or gonadal tumor, congenital adrenal hyperplasia, hCG-secreting tumor, McCune-Albright syndrome). In familial male precocious puberty, in contrast to GnRH-dependent CPP, testicular activation occurs without the normal pubertal increase in gonadotropin secretion (Pescovitz et al, 1986; Laue et al, 1989) and may be caused by a testicular-stimulating factor in the plasma (Manasco et al, 1991).

In addition to the undesirable physical and emotional effects of early sexual maturation, skeletal maturation also is accelerated resulting in premature epiphyseal fusion and final adult height that is shorter than the genetic potential.

Treatment of both central and peripheral precocious puberty may be either surgical or medical. For example, tumor excision, irradiation, or cyst drainage may be followed by decreased gonadotropin production (Root and Shulman, 1986), or removal of a testicular tumor may be curative for that form of peripheral precocity. In other cases, drug therapy may be attempted.

The long-acting GnRH agonists (ie, histrelin [Supprelin], nafarelin [Synarel], leuprolide [Lupron Injection, Lupron Depot], deslorelin [Somagard] (in Phase III clinical trials), and buserelin are effective in the treatment of GnRH-dependent CPP. Initially, these agents stimulate gonadotropin secretion. Regression of sexual characteristics will not occur until suppression of sex steroids is maintained. With continued treatment, the GnRH agonist induces down-regulation of GnRH receptors, an effect that is then sustained throughout continuous treatment. In responsive patients, nocturnal and GnRH-stimulated gonadotropin secretion is suppressed and growth velocity is decreased in both boys and girls. Serum estradiol decreases once pubertal levels are attained, menstruation ceases, and breast size may regress in girls, while serum testosterone levels and testicular volume decrease in boys. The decrease in the rate of skeletal maturation that occurs results in an increase in the predicted and final adult height.

The dosages of GnRH agonists given for CPP include leuprolide administered subcutaneously (30 to 50 mcg/kg/day) (Kaplan and Grumbach, 1990; Lee et al, 1989) or as the depot preparation monthly (330 mcg/kg/month) (Parker et al, 1991); nafarelin administered intranasally (up to 1.6 mg/day) (Lin et al, 1986) or subcutaneously (4 mcg/kg/day; a preparation for subcutaneous administration is not available commercially) (Kreiter et al, 1990); deslorelin administered subcutaneously (4 mcg/kg/day) (Pescovitz et al, 1991; Manasco et al, 1988, 1989; Oerter et al, 1991); buserelin administered subcutaneously (10 to 20 mcg/kg/day) or intranasally (20 to 40 mcg/kg/day) (Root et al, 1991); and histrelin (see evaluation).

GnRH analogues have been ineffective in the treatment of the peripheral form of precocious puberty.

In familial male precocious puberty, spironolactone [Aldactone] (an antiandrogen) and testolactone [Teslac] (which blocks conversion of androgen to estrogen), given together for up to 18 months, were more effective than either agent alone. Manifestations of precocious puberty and the rate of growth and skeletal maturation were controlled, and no significant adverse effects were observed (Laue et al, 1989). In preliminary studies, ketoconazole [Nizoral] has been effective in treating familial male precocious puberty unresponsive to the GnRH agonist, buserelin (Holland et al, 1985). Combination treatment with a GnRH analogue plus ketoconazole or spironolactone plus testolactone is effective in suppressing puberty in boys in whom central activation of the hypothalamic-pituitary axis has occurred (Holland et al, 1987; Laue et al, in press). However, use of ketoconazole is associated with serious side effects (eg, liver dysfunction, adrenal insufficiency). (See index entry Ketoconazole, Uses, Subcutaneous and Systemic Mycoses.)

In the past in this country, medroxyprogesterone acetate (MPA) was most commonly used to treat precocious puberty. Although this drug may successfully suppress sexual maturation, it is not effective in suppressing the accelerated process of bone maturation and premature epiphyseal closure and may be associated with certain undesirable effects, such as weight gain and development of cushingoid features. Cyproterone acetate, an investigational antiandrogenic progestin, is commonly used to treat precocious puberty in other countries, but its limitations are similar to those of MPA.

Drug Evaluations

HISTRELIN ACETATE
[Supprelin]

ACTIONS AND USES. Histrelin acetate, a synthetic nonapeptide agonist of GnRH, has greater potency than the natural hormone. This agent initially stimulates gonadotropin secretion; long-term administration results in down-regulation of GnRH receptors, inhibition of gonadotropin secretion, and decreased secretion of sex steroids from the gonads in both sexes. When used continuously for central idiopathic precocious puberty, the decrease in secretion of sex steroids is evident within three months, and this results in regression of secondary sex characteristics in the child. The rate of skeletal maturation is slowed, which allows more complete expression of genetic height potential.

Histrelin is administered subcutaneously for the treatment of central (idiopathic or neurogenic) precocious puberty occurring in boys before 9.5 years and in girls before 8 years. Patients should be monitored after the first three months of therapy and every 6 to 12 months thereafter. Treatment is withdrawn when the child reaches the normal age of puberty (approximately age 11).

ADVERSE REACTIONS AND PRECAUTIONS. Skin irritation at the injection site occurs in 45% of patients. Vaginal bleeding may occur in girls during the first three weeks of treatment. Reactions reported infrequently include nausea, vomiting, urticaria, and headache.

Histrelin should not be administered to patients with known hypersensitivity to any of its components.

Histrelin is classified in FDA Pregnancy Category X.

DOSAGE AND PREPARATIONS.

Subcutaneous: For central precocious puberty, 8 to 10 mcg/kg daily given at the same time each day. The site is varied with each injection. Suppression may be incomplete if histrelin is not administered daily. Any unused solution should be discarded.

Supprelin (Roberts). Solution (sterile, hypertonic) 200, 500, or 1,000 mcg/ml in a peptide base with sodium chloride and mannitol (preservative-free) supplied in a kit containing single-dose vials that deliver 0.6-ml. Store between 2° and 8° C and protect from light.

NAFARELIN ACETATE
[Synarel]

ACTIONS AND USES. Nafarelin acetate is a synthetic agonist of GnRH with greater potency than the natural hormone. This agent is administered intranasally to treat central idiopathic precocious puberty in both boys and girls. Its mechanism of action is similar to that of histrelin. Repeated administration of nafarelin suppresses pituitary gonadotropin secretion and hence inhibits gonadal steroid secretion.

ADVERSE REACTIONS AND PRECAUTIONS. Nafarelin initially stimulates the pituitary, so signs of precocious puberty may be exacerbated until the suppressive action becomes effective (several weeks). Estrogen withdrawal bleeding may occur in girls about six weeks after therapy begins but ceases thereafter. There is no evidence that rhinitis affects drug absorption, but if a topical decongestant is used, instillation should be delayed until two hours after nafarelin administration. Hot flushes are reported by 3% of treated children.

DOSAGE AND ADMINISTRATION.

Intranasal: For central precocious puberty, 1.6 mg daily. The dose can be increased to 1.8 mg per day if adequate suppression is not achieved with the lower dose. The 1.6-mg dose is administered as two sprays into each nostril in the morning and evening (eight sprays daily) allowing 30 seconds between successive sprays. The 1.8-mg dose is administered as three sprays three times a day (nine sprays daily) with each set of sprays applied in alternating nostrils.

Synarel (Syntex). Spray (nasal) 2 mg/ml in 10 ml containers. Supplied with a metered spray pump that delivers 200 mcg nafarelin per spray.

Anabolic Therapy

Testosterone and its derivatives have anabolic and somatic growth effects. Attempts to separate the anabolic from the androgenic effects by modifying the testosterone molecule have been only partially successful and have resulted in the development of a number of synthetic analogues, termed anabolic (or anabolic androgenic) steroids. These include the oral preparations, methandrostenolone, oxymetholone [Anadrol-50], oxandrolone [Oxandrin], and stanozolol [Winstrol]. All are 17α-alkylated compounds. Parenteral preparations for intramuscular administration include nandrolone phenpropionate [Androlone, Durabolin, Nandrobolic] and nandrolone decanoate [Androlone-D, Deca-Durabolin], which are not alkylated at the 17α-position (Kochakian, 1990).

All anabolic steroids have androgenic activity, and masculinizing effects occur if sufficient doses are given for a prolonged period. All of these steroids are designated as Schedule III controlled substancs under the Anabolic Steroids Control Act of 1990 (see also index entry Controlled Substance Act).

PROTEIN ANABOLISM. Anabolic steroids reverse the negative nitrogen and calcium balance associated with high-dose glucocorticoid therapy. Although this use of anabolic steroids is a rational approach to prevent some side effects of corticosteroids (eg, muscle wasting and weakness, demineralization of bone), their long-term efficacy has not been established.

Defective protein metabolism with loss of tissue protein may occur in patients with chronic debilitating illnesses and in those convalescing from severe infections, surgery, burns, trauma, irradiation, or cytotoxic drug therapy. Testosterone or related anabolic steroids decrease or reverse negative nitrogen balance, seem to provide a feeling of well-being, and sometimes stimulate appetite; however, there is no evidence that they shorten the period of recovery. Their effectiveness depends on sufficient protein and caloric intake. Although there are no adequate clinical trials proving efficacy, use of anabolic agents as adjunctive or supportive therapy in such conditions, particularly in terminal patients, may be helpful.

Anabolic steroids do not alleviate the symptoms or alter the progress of muscular dystrophy. Masculinizing effects and acceleration of bone age occurred when these agents were used in children with this disorder.

See Table 1 for preparations and dosage of steroids used for anabolic therapy.

TABLE 1.
STEROIDS USED FOR ANABOLIC THERAPY

Drug and Chemical Structure	Usual Dosage	Preparations
TESTOSTERONE ESTERS Testosterone Cypionate 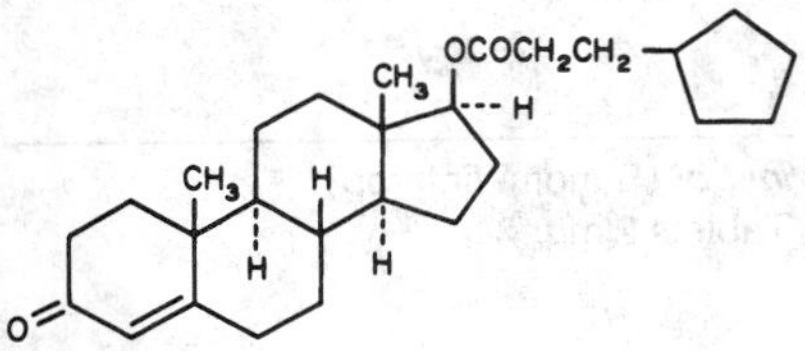 $OCOCH_2CH_2$, CH_3, H, CH_3, H, H, H, O	*Intramuscular: Adults,* 200 mg every 2 weeks or 400 mg every 4 weeks.	*Generic.* Solution (in oil) 100 and 200 mg/ml in 10 ml containers. *Andro-Cyp* (Keene), *Depo-Testosterone* (Upjohn). Solution (in cottonseed oil) 100 and 200 mg/ml in 10 ml containers. *Virilon-IM* (Star). Solution (in cottonseed oil) 200 mg/ml in 10 ml containers.
Testosterone Enanthate	*Intramuscular: Adults,* 200 mg every 2 weeks or 400 mg every 4 weeks.	*Generic.* Solution (in oil) 100 and 200 mg/ml in 5 and 10 ml containers. *Delatestryl* (Gynex). Solution (in sesame oil) 200 mg/ml in 1 and 5 ml containers.
Testosterone Propionate	*Intramuscular: Adults,* 10 to 25 mg daily.	*Generic.* Solution (in oil) 25 mg/ml in 10 ml containers and 50 and 100 mg/ml in 10 and 30 ml containers. *Testex* (Pasadena). Solution (in sesame oil) 100 mg/ml in 10 ml containers.
17α-ALKYLATED COMPOUNDS Fluoxymesterone 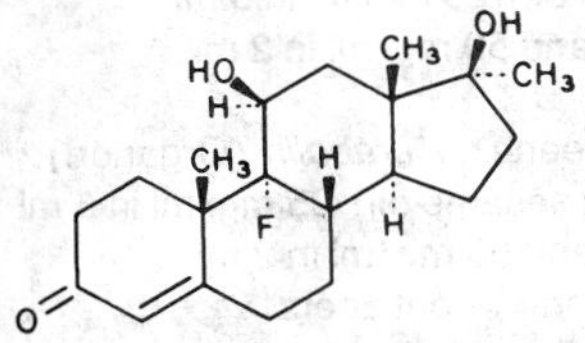 OH, CH_3, HO, H, CH_3, CH_3, H, F, H, O	*Oral: Adults,* 4 to 10 mg daily; for growth stimulation in boys, 2.5 to 10 mg daily; to stimulate erythropoiesis, 0.4 to 1 mg/kg daily.	*Halotestin* (Upjohn), *Generic.* Tablets 2, 5, and 10 mg.

(table continued on next page)

TABLE 1 (Continued)

Drug and Chemical Structure	Usual Dosage	Preparations
Methyltestosterone	*Oral: Adults,* 10 to 20 mg daily; for growth stimulation in boys, 10 to 20 mg daily. *Buccal: Adults,* one-half oral dosage; absorption variable.	*Android* (ICN), *Oreton Methyl* (Schering), *Generic.* Tablets 10 (*Android* only) and 25 mg; tablets (buccal) 5 mg *(Android)* and 10 mg *(Oreton Methyl, Generic).* *Testred* (ICN), *Virilon* (Star). Capsules 10 mg.
Oxandrolone	*Oral: Adults,* 2.5 mg 2 to 4 times daily (range, 2.5 to 20 mg/day). *Children,* total daily dosage should not exceed 0.1 mg/kg.	*Oxandrin* (Gynex). Tablets 2.5 mg.
Oxymetholone	*Oral:* Dose should be individualized. For erythropoiesis, *adults and children,* 1 to 5 mg/kg daily.	*Anadrol-50* (Syntex). Tablets 50 mg.
Stanozolol	*Oral: Adults,* 6 mg daily. *Children 6 to 12 years,* 2 to 6 mg daily; *under 6 years,* 2 mg daily.	*Winstrol* (Sanofi Winthrop). Tablets 2 mg.
OTHER COMPOUNDS		
Nandrolone Decanoate	*Intramuscular* (deep): *Adults,* 50 to 100 mg every 3 to 4 weeks. *Children 2 to 13 years,* 25 to 50 mg every 3 to 4 weeks. For anemia of renal disease, *women,* 50 to 100 mg/week; *men,* 100 to 200 mg/week; *children 2 to 13 years,* 25 to 50 mg every 3 to 4 weeks.	*Generic.* Solution (in oil) 50 and 100 mg/ml in 2 ml containers and 200 mg/ml in 1 ml containers. *Androlone-D* (Keene). Solution (in sesame oil) 200 mg/ml in 1 ml containers. *Deca-Durabolin* (Organon). Solution (in sesame oil) 50 and 100 mg/ml in 1 and 2 ml containers and 200 mg/ml in 1 ml containers.
Nandrolone Phenpropionate	*Intramuscular* (deep): *Adults,* 25 to 50 mg weekly. *Children 2 to 13 years,* 12.5 to 25 mg every 2 to 4 weeks. For erythropoiesis, up to 100 mg weekly.	*Generic.* Solution (in oil) 25 mg/ml in 5 ml containers and 50 mg/ml in 2 ml containers. *Androlone* (Keene), *Durabolin* (Organon). Solution (in sesame oil) 25 mg/ml in 5 ml containers and 50 mg/ml in 2 ml (*Durabolin* only) containers. *Nandrobolic* (Forest). Solution (in sesame oil) 25 mg/ml in 5 ml containers.

ATHLETIC PERFORMANCE. The use of anabolic steroids to improve athletic performance is universally deplored in the medical community (American College of Sports Medicine, 1987; Committee on Sports Medicine, American Academy of Pediatrics, 1989). (See Table 2 for examples of anabolic steroids reported to be used as ergogenic aids.) It was once thought that steroids do not significantly increase muscle mass in healthy young men beyond that due to physical conditioning. However, results of some studies suggest that anabolic steroids increase lean muscle mass, although the tissue may be phosphate-poor and have ultrastructural abnormalities (Mellion, 1984). Body weight increases, but some of the gain is due to fluid retention. Studies designed to identify changes in strength in athletes who have taken steroids have yielded equivocal results (Ryan, 1981; American College of Sports Medicine, 1987; Haupt and Rovere, 1984), but it is now acknowledged that muscular size and strength can be increased in some individuals with the use of anabolic steroids in combination with appropriate diet and exercise intense enough to result in negative nitrogen balance (Yesalis, 1992 A). In a review of placebo-controlled studies in which changes in muscular strength were measured after administration of anabolic steroids, it was concluded that previously trained athletes showed slight improvement in strength, whereas no improvement in strength was observed in untrained volunteers (Elashoff et al, 1991). However, even slight differences in physiologic measurements can have a profound impact on the outcome of athletic competition. Because the doses of steroids used in these studies were in the therapeutic range, the conclusions cannot be extended to situations in which athletes self-administer very large doses (American College of Sports Medicine, 1987) nor can the conclusions be generalized to the population of elite athletes whose training regimens, diet, and psychological state related to training and performance may differ significantly from those of study participants (Yesalis, 1992 A).

TABLE 2.
ANABOLIC STEROIDS USED BY ATHLETES

Generic Name	Trademark(s)	Source*
ORAL PREPARATIONS		
Bolasterone	Tes-10	Foreign
Fluoxymesterone	Halotestin	US
Formebolone (also parenteral)	Esiclene	Foreign
	Hubernol	Foreign
Mesterolone	Mestoranum	Foreign
	Pro-Viron	Foreign
Methandrostenolone (methandienone)	Generic	Foreign
	Dianabol	Foreign
	Nerobol	Foreign
	Danabol	Foreign
	Metanabol	Foreign
Methenolone	Primobolan	Foreign
Methyltestosterone	Android	US
	Oreton Methyl	US
	Testred	US
	Virilon	US
Norethandrolone	Nilevar	Foreign
Oxandrolone	Anavar, Oxandrin	US, Foreign
Oxymesterone	Oranabol	Foreign
Oxymetholone	Anadrol-50	US
Stanozolol	Winstrol	US

(table continued on next page)

TABLE 2 (Continued)

Generic Name	Trademark(s)	Source*
PARENTERAL PREPARATIONS		
Clostebol	Steranabol	Foreign
Nandrolone esters	Androlone, Androlone-D	US
	Durabolin, Deca-Durabolin	US
	Nandrobolic	US
	Turinabol	Foreign
Norethandrolone	Nilevar Injection	Foreign
Testosterone esters	Andro-Cyp	US
	Delatestryl	US
	Depo-Testosterone	US
	Virilon-IM	US
VETERINARY PREPARATIONS		
Boldenone undecylenate	Equipoise	Foreign
Stanozolol	Winstrol-V	US
Trenbolone	Parabolan	Foreign

**Anabolic steroids manufactured in the United States also may be available from foreign sources.*

Regardless of objective evidence supporting or refuting the claim that anabolic steroids enhance athletic performance, many athletes feel that they benefit from the use of large quantities of these agents (Yesalis et al, 1990). Perceived effects include increased muscular strength, heightened aggressive tendencies, more energy, and the ability to train more intensively and shorten the recovery period, thereby allowing more frequent training.

The use of anabolic steroids by athletes is apparently widespread, particularly among weight lifters, shot-putters, discus throwers, and football players, although their use is common in almost all sports requiring strength. Most recently, anabolic steroid use has increased in endurance sports (eg, Nordic skiing, cycling, distance running) and in sprinters. On a written survey of weightlifters who competed in a national championship, 33% admitted having taken steroids; in surveys by telephone, 55% admitted steroid use (Yesalis et al, 1988). In surveys of college students, up to 5% of males participating in some sports (eg, baseball, basketball, tennis) and up to 10% of football players reported using anabolic steroids during the previous 12 months; approximately 1% of women swimmers reported similar usage (Yesalis, 1992 B). Male twelfth grade students from 46 private and public high schools across the United States completed a questionnaire administered by their homeroom teachers. Results showed that 6.6% admitted using anabolic steroids currently or in the past, with more than two-thirds starting steroid use at or before 16 years of age (Buckley et al, 1988). Similar findings have been reported in other surveys: 5% to 12% of male and 1% to 2% of female high school students acknowledge use of anabolic steroids at some time (Yesalis, 1992 B).

ADVERSE EFFECTS OF ANABOLIC STEROIDS. Not only is the use of anabolic steroids to improve physique or athletic performance a medically trivial indication, but adverse effects, some serious, are associated with their use. The potential for adverse effects is presumably greatest in athletes who consume quantities far in excess of therapeutic doses, in those who "stack" drugs (ie, ingest large doses of several steroids simultaneously), or in those who follow repetitive cycles of taking large doses of drugs followed by withdrawal or use of lower doses.

The 17α-alkylated compounds are most commonly used and may alter liver function tests and cause other abnormalities. Because intensive training alone can raise AST and ALT levels, liver-specific indicators, such as LDH_5 and alkaline phosphatase, should be measured to determine the effects of anabolic steroids. Death from liver cancer has been reported in one athlete (Overly et al, 1984).

Endocrinologic effects include decreased glucose tolerance and apparent increased insulin resistance (Cohen and Hickman, 1987), decreased production of thyroid hormones and thyroid binding globulin (TBG), and decreased serum gonadotropin and testosterone concentrations; in one study, the latter remained suppressed for nine weeks after withdrawal of medication (Alen et al, 1987). Depressed spermatogenesis and decreased testicular size also occur (Knuth et al, 1989). Pharmacologic quantities of anabolic steroids may completely suppress secretion of testosterone. Gynecomastia may be observed with use of some preparations.

Retention of salt and fluid may cause hypertension. Although the HDL serum concentration is increased in intensively trained athletes, the opposite effect occurs with anabolic steroid use. Blood lipid patterns show potentially atherogenic changes; HDL levels may decrease by 50% or more and the LDL/HDL ratio increases three times. The effect has persisted for up to seven months after drug administration ceased (Kibble and Ross, 1987). The effects on serum lipoprotein concentrations appear to be significantly greater with an orally administered 17α-alkylated steroid (stanozolol) than with parenterally administered testosterone (Thompson et al, 1989). In male athletes, the unfavorable changes in the serum lipid profile may increase the risk of coronary heart disease three to six times (Glazer, 1991).

Psychological effects also occur with anabolic steroid use in some athletes. Increased aggressiveness, euphoria, and lack of fatigue have been reported (Kibble and Ross, 1987; Lubell, 1989; Bahrke et al, 1990). In one survey of 31 body builders, 15 reported having experienced hallucinations, delusions, manic episodes, or depression at some time; none had such symptoms unassociated with steroid use (Pope and Katz, 1988). Symptoms of depression, including fatigue, anhedonia, and suicidal ideation, have been reported when anabolic steroids were withdrawn (Pope and Katz, 1992).

Anabolic steroids probably stimulate skeletal muscle in female athletes more than in males. In a study of women competitors in strength sports, subjects reported lowering of voice pitch, facial hair, clitoral enlargement, increased aggressiveness, and menstrual irregularities (Strauss et al, 1985). In some women weight lifters who ingested large doses of anabolic steroids, masculinizing effects occurred, levels of serum testosterone exceeding those in normal males were produced, and HDL cholesterol was reduced by 39%, which suggests that use of steroids may increase the risk of cardiovascular disease (Malarkey et al, 1991) and further emphasizes the undesirability of use of these agents in women athletes.

Use of anabolic steroids in juvenile athletes is of particular concern. Puberty may be induced in sexually immature boys, and final adult height may be compromised by premature epiphyseal closure. The possibility of other effects on the maturing hypothalamic-pituitary-gonadal axis also must be considered. See also reviews by Hough, 1990; Lombardo and Sickles, 1992.

The effects on health after long-term anabolic steroid use have not been established.

Drug Therapy for Sex Offenders

Intramuscular injection of medroxyprogesterone acetate (MPA) in large doses (average, 300 mg weekly) or oral administration (average, 100 to 200 mg/day) has been used as an adjunct to psychiatric or psychological counseling in men with a variety of paraphilias. Treatment has decreased serum testosterone, LH, and FSH levels as well as libido and sexual arousal and has helped some men to control deviant behavior, although their sexual orientation was unchanged. Sperm count is appreciably depressed. The repeat-offense rate of untreated male sex offenders is $\geq 60\%$; this rate was reduced to 18% in one group of offenders who were treated with MPA (Meyer et al, in press). The antiandrogen, cyproterone acetate, also has been used for this purpose (Meyer et al, 1985; Cooper, 1986).

Adverse effects observed in some patients treated with MPA include weight gain, leg cramps, fatigue, increased need for sleep, migraine headaches, weakness, decreased glucose tolerance, elevated blood pressure, and gallbladder disease.

Hereditary Angioedema

In this disorder, a deficiency of C1 esterase inhibitor (C1 INH [Type I]) or reduced function caused by abnormal production (C1 INH [Type II]) leads to uncontrolled activation of the complement system, production of vasoactive substances, and angioedema. Edema of the respiratory and gastrointestinal tracts is more common in the hereditary form of angioedema.

Androgens are useful for prophylaxis in this potentially fatal condition. Remission of symptoms and increased hepatic production of the deficient serum α-globulin, C1 INH, are noted after treatment (Gelfand et al, 1976; Gadek et al, 1979). Attenuated androgens, such as danazol [Danocrine] and stanozolol [Winstrol] are preferred, especially in women, because of their effectiveness and low androgenic activity. (For the dose of danazol, see the evaluation.) The dose of stanozolol is 2 mg three times a day; after a favorable response, the amount is reduced gradually to 2 mg daily or on alternate days.

Androgens, as well as antihistamines, corticosteroids, or adrenergic drugs, are ineffective in the treatment of acute attacks. An airway must be established by intubation or tracheostomy when laryngeal edema is severe. C1 INH concentrate from plasma (an investigational drug with orphan drug status in the United States) is available in some European countries for prophylaxis and for treatment of acute attacks (Greaves and Lawlor, 1991; Sim and Grant, 1990; Waytes et al, 1992).

Drug Evaluation

DANAZOL

[Danocrine]

For chemical formula, see index entry Danazol, Uses, Endometriosis.

ACTIONS AND USES. This synthetic derivative of 17α-ethinyl testosterone (ethisterone) has mild androgenic activity. Danazol does not exhibit estrogenic or progestational properties and suppresses the midcycle surge of LH and FSH.

Danazol is a drug of choice in the long-term prophylaxis of hereditary angioedema but is not effective for acute attacks. For other uses, see index entry Danazol.

ADVERSE REACTIONS AND PRECAUTIONS. Most adverse reactions caused by danazol are related to its weak androgenic and anabolic activity. They include weight gain, edema, acne, oily skin, decreased breast size, and hirsutism. Other hypoestrogenic symptoms (flushing, sweating, vaginitis) also occur in women.

In women, therapy should begin during menstruation, or a pregnancy test should be performed to rule out that possibility. Pseudohermaphroditism may occur in female infants whose mothers received danazol during early pregnancy.

As with other 17α-alkylated steroids, danazol has been associated with abnormal liver function tests and jaundice. This drug should not be used in patients with markedly impaired hepatic, renal, or cardiac function or in women with abnormal genital bleeding.

PHARMACOKINETICS. After administration of danazol 400 mg, peak plasma levels of 80 to 100 ng/ml are attained in one to two hours. The half-life in plasma is about 4.5 hours (Dmowski, 1979). Unaltered steroid appears to be biologically active. Danazol is metabolized to conjugates, sulfates, and glucuronides and is excreted predominantly in the urine but also in feces.

DOSAGE AND PREPARATIONS.

Oral: For hereditary angioedema, the initial dose is 400 to 600 mg daily given in divided amounts with step-down titration to determine the lowest effective amount. Treatment can be reinstituted if symptoms recur on cessation of therapy. In one series of 56 patients, 80% responded to a minimal prophylactic dose of $\leq$200 mg/day (Cicardi et al, 1991).

Danocrine (Sanofi Winthrop). Capsules 50, 100, and 200 mg.

Cited References

Alen M, et al: Androgenic-anabolic steroid effects on serum thyroid, pituitary and steroid hormones in athletes. *Am J Sports Med* 15:357-361, 1987.

American College of Sports Medicine: Position stand on the use anabolic-androgenic steroids in sports. *Am J Sports Med* 19:534-539, 1987.

Bahrke MS, et al: Psychological and behavioural effects of endogenous testosterone levels and anabolic-androgenic steroids among males: A review. *Sports Med* 10:303-337, 1990.

Buckley WE, et al: Estimated prevalence of anabolic steroid use among male high school seniors. *JAMA* 260:3441-3445, 1988.

Cicardi M, et al: Long-term treatment of hereditary angioedema with attenuated androgens: A survey of a 13-year experience. *J Allergy Clin Immunol* 87:768-773, 1991.

Cohen JC, Hickman R: Insulin resistance and diminished glucose tolerance in powerlifters ingesting anabolic steroids. *J Clin Endocrinol Metab* 64:960-963, 1987.

Committee on Sports Medicine, American Academy of Pediatrics: Anabolic steroids and the adolescent athlete. *Pediatrics* 83:127-128, 1989.

Cooper AJ: Progestogens in the treatment of male sex offenders: Review. *Can J Psychiatry* 31:73-79, 1986.

Dmowski WP: Endocrine properties and clinical application of danazol. *Fertil Steril* 31:237-251, 1979.

Elashoff JD, et al: Effects of anabolic-androgenic steroids on muscular strength. *Ann Intern Med* 115:387-393, 1991.

Gadek JE, et al: Response of variant hereditary angioedema phenotypes to danazol therapy: Genetic implications. *J Clin Invest* 64:280-286, 1979.

Gelfand JA, et al: Treatment of hereditary angioedema with danazol: Reversal of clinical and biochemical abnormalities. *N Engl J Med* 295:1444-1448, 1976.

Glazer G: Atherogenic effects of anabolic steroids on serum lipid levels: A literature review. *Arch Intern Med* 151:1925-1933, 1991.

Greaves M, Lawlor F: Angioedema: Manifestations and management. *J Am Acad Dermatol* 25:155-165, 1991.

Haupt HA, Rovere GD: Anabolic steroids: Review of literature. *Am J Sports Med* 12:469-484, 1984.

Holland FJ, et al: Ketoconazole in the management of precocious puberty not responsive to LHRH-analogue therapy. *N Engl J Med* 312:1023-1028, 1985.

Holland FJ, et al: Gonadotropin-independent precocious puberty ("testotoxicosis"): Influence of maturational status on response to ketoconazole. *J Clin Endocrinol Metab* 64:328-333, 1987.

Hough DO: Anabolic steroids and ergogenic aids. *Am Fam Physician* 1157-1164, (April) 1990.

Kaplan SL, Grumbach MM: Pathophysiology and treatment of sexual precocity. *J Clin Endocrinol Metab* 71:785-789, 1990.

Kibble MW, Ross MB: Adverse effects of anabolic steroids in athletes. *Clin Pharm* 6:686-692, 1987.

Knuth UA, et al: Anabolic steroids and semen parameters in bodybuilders. *Fertil Steril* 52:1041-1047, 1989.

Kochakian CD: History of anabolic-androgenic steroids, in Linn G, Erinoff L (eds): *Anabolic Steroid Abuse.* Rockville, Md, National Institute on Drug Abuse, 1990, NIDA research monograph 102.

Kreiter M, et al: Preserving adult height potential in girls with idiopathic true precocious puberty. *J Pediatr* 117:364-370, 1990.

Laue L, et al: Treatment of familial male precocious puberty with spironolactone and testolactone. *N Engl J Med* 320:496-502, 1989.

Laue L, et al: Treatment of familial male precocious puberty with spironolactone, testolactone, and deslorelin. *J Clin Endocrinol Metab* In press.

Lee PA, et al: Effects of leuprolide in the treatment of central precocious puberty. *J Pediatr* 114:321-324, 1989.

Lin T-H, et al: Intranasal nafarelin: An LH-RH analogue treatment of gonadotropin-dependent precocious puberty. *J. Pediatr* 109:954-958, 1986.

Lombardo JA, Sickles RT: Medical and performance-enhancing effects of anabolic steroids. *Psychiatric Ann* 22:19-23, (Jan) 1992.

Lubell A: Does steroid abuse cause—or excuse—violence? *Physician Sport Med* 17:176-185, 1989.

Malarkey WB, et al: Endocrine effects in female weight lifters who self-administer testosterone and anabolic steroids. *Am J Obstet Gynecol* 165:1385-1390, 1991.

Manasco PK, et al: Resumption of puberty after long term luteinizing hormone-releasing hormone agonist treatment of central precocious puberty. *J Clin Endocrinol Metab* 67:368-372, 1988.

Manasco PK, et al: Six-year results of luteinizing hormone releasing hormone (LHRH) agonist treatment in children with LHRH-dependent precocious puberty. *J Pediatr* 115:105-108, (July) 1989.

Manasco PK, et al: A novel testis-stimulating factor in familial male precocious puberty. *N Engl J Med* 324:227-231, 1991.

Mellion MB: Anabolic steroids in athletics. *Am Fam Physician* 30:113-119, (July) 1984.

Meyer WJ III, et al: Physical, metabolic, and hormonal effects on men of long-term therapy with medroxyprogesterone acetate. *Fertil Steril* 43:102-109, 1985.

Meyer WJ III, et al: Depo Provera treatment for sex offending behavior: An evaluation of outcome. *Bull Am Acad Psychiatry Law* In press.

Oerter KE, et al: Adult height in precocious puberty after long-term treatment with deslorelin. *J Clin Endocrinol Metab* 73:1235-1240, 1991.

Overly WL, et al: Androgens and hepatocellular carcinoma in the athlete, letter. *Ann Intern Med* 100:158-159, 1984.

Parker KL, et al: Depot leuprolide acetate dosage for sexual precocity. *J Clin Endocrinol Metab* 73:50-52, 1991.

Pescovitz OH, et al: The NIH experience with precocious puberty: Diagnostic subgroups and response to short-term luteinizing hormone releasing hormone analogue therapy. *J Pediatr* 108:47-54, 1986.

Pescovitz OH, et al: Effect of deslorelin dose in the treatment of central precocious puberty. *J Clin Endocrinol Metab* 72:60-64, 1991.

Pope HG Jr, Katz DL: Affective and psychotic symptoms associated with anabolic steroid use. *Am J Psychiatry* 145:487-490, 1988.

Pope HG Jr, Katz DL: Psychiatric effects of anabolic steroids. *Psychiatric Ann* 22:24-29, (Jan) 1992.

Root AW, Shulman DI: Isosexual precocity: Current concepts and recent advances. *Fertil Steril* 45:749-766, 1986.

Root AW, et al: Effectiveness of the gonadotropin-releasing hormone agonist buserelin in the treatment of children with true and complete, central isosexual precocity. *Adolesc Pediatr Gynecol* 4:129-135, 1991.

Ryan AJ: Anabolic steroids are fool's gold. *Fed Proc* 40:2682-2688, 1981.

Sim TC, Grant JA: Hereditary angioedema: Its diagnostic and management perspectives. *Am J Med* 88:656-664, 1990.

Strauss RH, et al: Anabolic steroid use and perceived effects in ten weight-trained women athletes. *JAMA* 253:2871-2874, 1985.

Thompson MD, et al: Contrasting effects of testosterone and stanozolol on serum lipoprotein levels. *JAMA* 261:1165-1168, 1989.

Waytes AT, et al: Use of a vapor-heated C1 inhibitor preparation in hereditary angioedema, abstract. *J Allergy Clin Immunol* 89:247, 1992.

Yesalis CE (ed): *Anabolic Steroids in Sport and Exercise.* Champaign, Ill, Human Kinetics Publishers, 1992 A.

Yesalis CE: Epidemiology and patterns of anabolic-androgenic steroid use. *Psychiatric Ann* 22:7-18, (Jan) 1992 B.

Yesalis CE III, et al: Self-reported use of anabolic-androgenic steroids by elite power lifters. *Physician Sports Med* 16:91-100, 1988.

Yesalis CE, et al: Athletes' projections of anabolic steroid use. *Clin Sports Med* 2:155-171, 1990.

Index

Primary headings appear in boldface type and may be drug names (generic and trademark), indications, or adverse reactions. Drug names followed by (M) are mixtures. Boldface page numbers denote major discussion or individual evaluations.

Dermatologic Therapy: Therapeutic Agents

56

CORTICOSTEROID-RESPONSIVE DERMATOSES

PSORIASIS

DANDRUFF AND SEBORRHEIC DERMATITIS

ACNE

PIGMENTATION DISORDERS

ACTINIC DAMAGE

DRUGS USED FOR MISCELLANEOUS CONDITIONS

- Antipruritics and Topical Anesthetics
- Protectant
- Drugs Used for Dermatitis Herpetiformis
- Debriding Agents
- Drug Used to Stimulate Hair Growth
- Drugs Used for Hyperhidrosis

Topical dermatologic preparations are divided into three main categories: (1) agents used therapeutically, (2) agents used prophylactically, and (3) vehicles. Therapeutic agents are discussed in this chapter. Information on prophylactic agents and vehicles appears in the following chapter.

Preparations: When a topical rather than a systemic preparation is selected to treat a cutaneous disorder, both the active ingredient(s) and the vehicle should be considered. The choice of active ingredient depends on an accurate diagnosis; the choice of vehicle depends on the site of the lesion and the physiologic or pathologic character of the affected skin. In general, concentration or dose, vehicle, and container size are listed in this chapter for prescription drugs but not for all over-the-counter (OTC) preparations. General guidelines for determining the amount of topical medication to apply once the concentration of active ingredient(s) and vehicle have been selected appear in Table 1. Adherence to the guidelines would provide an amount of medication that would be economical but would not lead to overtreatment or inappropriate use by another family member. Information on adverse reactions, contraindications, and precautions appears in the introduction for the therapeutic use or in the individual evaluations.

TABLE 1.
AMOUNT OF TOPICAL MEDICATION FOR TREATMENT*

Area Treated	Single Application (g)	Application Once Daily for 1 week	2 weeks (g)	4 weeks
Hands, head, face, anogenital area	2	15	30	60
One arm, anterior or posterior trunk	3	20	40	80
One leg	4	30	60	120

* *The amounts recommended apply whether a lotion, cream, or ointment is prescribed.*

CORTICOSTEROID-RESPONSIVE DERMATOSES

Topical application of corticosteroids is indicated for corticosteroid-responsive dermatoses (Maibach and Surber, 1992). Response often depends on the disorder and its severity, as well as on the potency of the corticosteroid. Atopic dermatitis, nummular dermatitis, recalcitrant seborrheic dermatitis, mild dyshidrotic dermatitis (hand and foot dermatitis, pompholyx), stasis dermatitis, pityriasis rosea, sunburn, and insect or arthropod bite dermatoses generally respond to topical corticosteroids of low to medium potency. Contact dermatitis associated with irritant or phototoxic chemicals (irritant dermatitis), dryness (inflammatory dermatitis or xerosis), and heat and moisture (noninfectious intertrigo) also may respond, particularly in the later, nonweeping phases. Low to medium potency preparations also are useful in mild psoriasis affecting the face, body folds, palms, soles, elbows, and knees.

Medium to high potency topical corticosteroids are generally required for contact dermatitis caused by allergens; oral corticosteroids may be indicated in more severe cases (eg, poison ivy dermatitis). Medium potency topical corticosteroids may be satisfactory for discoid lupus erythematosus and lichen planus that involve the face and intertriginous areas as well as for alopecia areata and mycosis fungoides; however, high potency preparations will usually be required to treat other areas or more serious forms of these diseases. Necrobiosis lipoidica diabeticorum, lichen simplex chronicus, hypertrophic lichen planus, lichen striatus, and pretibial myxedema also require high potency corticosteroids. If higher concentrations are ineffective, even under occlusion, for hypertrophic lichen planus or necrobiosis lipoidica diabeticorum, intralesional injection of corticosteroids may be necessary. The intralesional route also is recommended for hypertrophic scars early in their development, keloids, granuloma annulare, some acne cysts, sarcoidosis, patchy alopecia areata, and prurigo nodularis. More severe forms of dyshidrotic dermatitis usually require high or occasionally very high potency corticosteroids or, in some cases, short-term oral corticosteroids.

Systemic corticosteroids are required for most patients with the bullous diseases, pemphigus vulgaris and bullous pemphigoid. Rarely, patients with very localized disease will respond to high potency topical preparations. Short-term use of systemic corticosteroids has been successful in patients with polymorphous light eruption.

Oral pastes containing hydrocortisone [Orabase HCA] or triamcinolone may be useful adjunctively in nonherpetic oral inflammatory and ulcerative lesions (eg, oral lichen planus, aphthous stomatitis).

Corticosteroid Preparations

Actions: Actions that probably are responsible for the clinical efficacy of corticosteroids in psoriasis and other keratinizing disorders include the following: inhibition of polyamine synthesis that is involved in cellular growth and proliferation processes; suppression of the immune system that limits release and migration of immune-effector substances to the site of inflammation (ie, induction of lipocortin activity that down-regulates phospholipase A2 and may lower leukotriene production, interruption of lymphokine production by activated T-lymphocytes, suppression of interleukin 1 production by keratinocytes and Langerhans cells); and inhibition of DNA synthesis in fibroblasts, T-lymphocytes, and mast cells (Maibach and Surber, 1992). Neither action is believed to be the sole mechanism by which corticosteroids improve the condition of the skin in psoriasis (Trozak, 1990). Topical corticosteroids suppress keratinocyte DNA synthesis and mitosis and produce vasoconstriction in the upper layer of the dermis. Vasoconstriction limits the entry of circulating inflammatory mediators into the area of involvement and decreases extravasation of serum into the skin, thus inhibiting swelling and discomfort. Tachyphylaxis develops to both keratinocyte suppression and vasoconstriction after repeated application.

The lysosomal membrane-stabilizing effect of corticosteroids inhibits the release of cytotoxic chemicals that cause pain and pruritus. Suppression of mitotic activity diminishes epidermal hyperplasia, but undesirable epidermal and dermal atrophy may result from excessive interference with these synthetic pathways.

Drug Selection: In addition to the disorder and its severity, selection of a corticosteroid depends primarily on the drug's inherent potency, concentration, formulation, and method of application; the site of disease; the patient's age; the amount of skin surface involved; the state of the skin barrier that is affected by the disease; the degree of skin hydration; and the expense.

The formulation and method of application affect the degree of absorption; an occlusive wrap applied for 96 hours can increase absorption as much as tenfold. However, the benefit often is not commensurate. Absorption of corticosteroids also is increased when the skin is hydrated or the skin barrier is altered by disease (eg, increased absorption in atopic dermatitis and exfoliative or erythrodermic psoriasis; decreased absorption in heavily crusted lesions). Selection also is influenced by the character of the lesions (wet or dry). See index entry Vehicles for a more detailed discussion.

Selected topical corticosteroids are grouped on the basis of potency in Table 2 (Cornell and Stoughton, 1993). The most potent topical corticosteroids are generally esterified and/or fluorinated compounds and/or are formulated for delivery in an optimized vehicle. They may be required initially for more recalcitrant disorders. A low-potency steroid may be adequate in permeable areas (eg, scalp, axilla, face, eyelids, neck, perineum, genitals) and should be considered for use only for a few weeks to a month after the acute inflammation subsides, particularly for chronic skin diseases. The prolonged use of fluorinated or medium and high potency steroids on the face should be avoided.

Expense also can be a significant factor in drug selection. Hydrocortisone is a steroid of choice in responsive conditions because it is inexpensive and its application to extensive areas for prolonged periods is relatively safe. Although the risk of adverse reactions generally is increased with agents in the very high and high potency groups and these preparations are generally more expensive, aggressive, short-term therapy with the higher potency agents may lessen the duration of illness, the number of work days lost, and the incidence of noncompliance. Therefore, relative expense is best determined by the physician for the individual patient.

Even when generic and pioneer (innovator) brand products are chemically (ie, same concentration of active agent) and biologically (eg, pharmacologic surrogate endpoint of vasoconstriction in assays of potency) equivalent, clinical efficacy may vary because of differences in formulation, vehicle, and manufacturing processes. For this reason, the definitive bioequivalance (bioavailability) of generic topical corticosteroids has not been determined (Stoughton, 1987; Jackson et al, 1989; Maibach, 1992). Thus, it is important to monitor the patient carefully for the desired therapeutic effect when generic products are substituted for the pioneer product or the reverse.

Adverse Reactions and Precautions: Because of their larger surface area-to-body weight ratio, pediatric patients, especially infants, may be more susceptible to topical corticosteroid-induced suppression of the hypothalamic-pituitary-adrenal (HPA) axis and development of Cushing's syndrome than adults. Elderly patients with atrophic skin may be more susceptible to the systemic as well as cutaneous adverse effects of topical corticosteroids. Careful monitoring for systemic effects and use of less potent agents usually are indicated in these patients.

Predictable adverse reactions to topical corticosteroids are related directly to inherent potency, concentration of drug dispersed, volume applied, skin condition, duration of use, site and area of application, and use of occlusive vehicles or wraps (Bickers et al, 1984; Trozak, 1990). Epidermal and dermal atrophy resulting in thinning of the skin, striae, telangiectases, and purpura are most commonly seen in highly absorptive areas (ie, face, neck, axilla, perineum, genitals), especially in the elderly.

Less common local effects include rosacea-like dermatoses, perioral dermatitis, acne, folliculitis, and miliaria. Hypopigmentation occurs, especially in blacks. Hypertrichosis is a rare side effect of the more potent corticosteroids. Ocular hypertension has been reported when corticosteroids are applied to the eyelids for prolonged periods. Allergic contact dermatitis occurs in about 3% to 5% of all patients in whom patch tests are performed and may be caused by the vehicle components rather than the steroid (Sasaki, 1990). For a comparison of the vehicles used in topical corticosteroid preparations, see Tan et al, 1986. Superficial epidermal fissures that resemble erythema craquele rarely follow termination of prolonged occlusive therapy.

When the more potent steroids are discontinued, patients with generalized or exfoliative erythroderma or erythrodermic or pustular psoriasis may develop severe rebound psoriatic dermatitis on all body surfaces. Rebound local effects include rosacea-like dermatoses and perioral dermatitis on the face or genitalia.

Corticosteroids can mask or aggravate dermatophytoses, impetigo, or scabies (see the section on Corticosteroid-Antibiotic Mixtures).

Pregnancy and Lactation: If prolonged use of occlusive dressings and/or application on extensive areas are avoided to prevent systemic absorption, adverse effects should not be a problem during pregnancy or lactation. Absorption of the more potent topical corticosteroids causes fetal abnormalities in animals but no well-controlled, adequate studies have been performed in pregnant women (FDA Pregnancy Category C).

Toxicity: Systemic toxicity generally is not a major concern except (1) in children (especially when occlusive dressings are applied), who may experience growth suppression even when relatively small amounts of the steroid are absorbed systemically; (2) when high-potency corticosteroids are applied to extensive areas of inflamed skin or under occlusive dressings for prolonged periods, especially in diseases that alter cutaneous permeability (eg, exfoliative erythroderma); miliaria and bacterial and candidal infections may occur with use of occlusive dressings; and (3) with excessive and/or prolonged use of the very high potency steroids (even without occlusion).

When using the latter preparations, assessment of HPA function may be indicated if (1) the weekly dose exceeds 50 g in adults or 30 g in children, (2) daily treatment is required for more than two weeks, or (3) liver function is impaired and it is not possible to reduce the dose or dosage schedule (eg, alternate-day therapy) or substitute a less potent steroid (Parish et al, 1985). If surgery is necessary in individuals receiving large total doses of higher potency corticosteroids, with or without occlusive dressings, a supplemental systemic corticosteroid should be prescribed. For the signs and symptoms of systemic toxicity, see index entry Adrenal Corticosteroids, Adverse Reactions.

Dosage: Lotion, cream, or ointment formulations should be applied sparingly on involved areas. Initially, application of a thin film one or two times daily may be required. Once control is established, the frequency of application should be reduced to the minimum to avoid relapse. Application once a day is usually sufficient, especially for higher potency corticosteroids (Parish et al, 1988; Cornell and Stoughton, 1993). Substitution of a less potent corticosteroid may be desirable to minimize adverse reactions after the acute condition is under control or for maintenance.

Corticosteroid-Antibiotic Mixtures

When secondary pyoderma is superimposed on preexisting dermatitis or when allergic inflammatory dermatitis (eg, eczema) develops in response to primary pyoderma, the concomitant use of a topical corticosteroid and a topical antibiotic may be indicated. The criteria for selection of topical antibiotics and antifungal agents are presented elsewhere; see index entries Antibiotics; Antifungal Agents, In Superficial Mycoses. Criteria for selection of topical corticosteroids are presented in the preceding section on Corticosteroids.

The use of combination products containing a topical corticosteroid and a topical antibiotic or antifungal agent is controversial (Leyden and Kligman, 1978; Hodge, 1980). Those opposed argue that there is insufficient evidence that these

TABLE 2. POTENCY RANKING AND RECOMMENDATIONS FOR USE OF REPRESENTATIVE TOPICAL CORTICOSTEROID PREPARATIONS[1,2]

Drug	Trademark(s) and Preparations	Comments
VERY HIGH POTENCY (SUPER-POTENT)		
Group I		
Betamethasone dipropionate gel 0.05%[3], ointment 0.05%[3]	Diprolene (Schering). Gel and ointment in 15 and 45 g containers.	Preparations in Group I may be used as an alternative to systemic corticosteroid therapy in severe conditions when local areas are involved. There is a high likelihood of skin atrophy. Duration of therapy should be limited to two weeks or less and the dosage to 45 or 50 g/week if possible. After two weeks, if possible, substitute intermittent or pulse therapy or consider use of a less potent corticosteroid. With prolonged intermittent use, periodic assessment of hypothalamic-pituitary-adrenal axis function may be desirable (see discussion under Toxicity). Administration of any preparation in this group that is used with occlusion should be undertaken cautiously in regions of especially high skin permeability.
Clobetasol propionate cream 0.05%, ointment 0.05%[3]	Temovate (Glaxo). Cream and ointment in 15, 30, and 45 g containers. [Also available: Lotion 0.05% in 25 and 50 ml containers]	
Diflorasone diacetate ointment 0.05%	Psorcon (Dermik). Ointment in 15, 30, and 60 g containers.	
Halobetasol propionate ointment 0.05%[3]	Ultravate (Westwood-Squibb). Ointment in 15 and 50 g containers. [Also available: Cream 0.05% in 15 and 50 g containers]	
HIGH POTENCY		
Group II		
Amcinonide cream 0.1%, lotion 0.1%, ointment 0.1%	Cyclocort (Fujisawa). Cream and ointment in 15, 30, and 60 g containers; lotion in 20 and 60 ml containers.	Preparations in Groups II-III may be used for severe eczematous dermatoses, lichen simplex chronicus, and psoriasis for an intermediate duration (except in thickened areas of skin and chronic conditions). They may be used on the face or intertriginous areas for short periods of time.
Betamethasone dipropionate ointment 0.05%	Alphatrex (Savage), Diprosone (Schering), Maxivate (Westwood-Squibb). Ointment in 15 and 45 g containers.	
Desoximetasone cream 0.25%, ointment 0.25%, gel 0.05%	Topicort (Hoechst-Roussel). Cream and ointment in 15, 60, and 120 g (cream only) containers; gel in 15 and 60 g containers.	
Diflorasone diacetate ointment 0.05%	Florone (Dermik), Maxiflor (Allergan Herbert). Ointment in 15, 30, and 60 g containers.	
Fluocinonide gel 0.05%, ointment 0.05%	Lidex (Syntex). Gel and ointment in 15, 30, 60, and 120 g containers. [Also available: Solution 0.05% in 20 and 60 ml containers]	
Halcinonide cream 0.1%	Halog (Westwood-Squibb). Cream in 15, 30, 60, and 240 g containers. [Also available: Cream 0.025% in 15 and 60 g containers; solution 0.1% in 20 and 60 ml containers]	
Mometasone furoate ointment 0.1%	Elocon (Schering). Ointment in 15 and 45 g containers.	

TABLE 2 (continued)

Drug	Trademark(s) and Preparations	Comments
Group III		
Betamethasone dipropionate cream 0.05%	Alphatrex (Savage), Diprolene AF, Diprosone (Schering), Maxivate (Westwood-Squibb). Cream in 15 and 45 g containers. [Also available: Aerosol 0.1% in 85 g containers (Diprosone); lotion 0.05% in 20 (Diprosone), 30 (Diprolene), and 60 ml containers (Alphatrex, Maxivate, Diprolene, Diprosone)]	
Betamethasone valerate ointment 0.1%	Betatrex (Savage), Beta-Val (Lemmon), Valisone (Schering). Ointment in 15 and 45 g containers.	
Diflorasone diacetate cream 0.05%	Florone, Florone E (Dermik), Maxiflor (Allergan Herbert), Psorcon (Dermik). Cream in 15, 30, and 60 g containers. [Also available: Lotion 0.05% in 20 and 60 ml containers (Florone)]	
Fluocinonide cream 0.05%	Generic, Lidex, Lidex E (Syntex). Cream in 15, 30, 60, and 120 g containers. [Also available: Solution 0.5% in 20 and 60 ml containers (Lidex)]	
Fluticasone propionate ointment 0.005%	Cutivate (Glaxo). Ointment in 15, 30, and 60 g containers.	
Halcinonide ointment 0.1%	Halog (Westwood-Squibb). Ointment in 15, 30, 60, and 240 g containers.	
Triamcinolone acetonide cream 0.5%, ointment 0.5%	Generic, Aristocort, Aristocort A (Fujisawa), Kenalog (Westwood-Squibb). Cream in 15 (Generic, Aristocort), 20 (Aristocort A, Kenalog), and 240 g containers (Aristocort); ointment in 15 (Generic, Aristocort) and 240 g containers (Aristocort).	
MEDIUM POTENCY		
Group IV		
Clocortolone pivalate cream 0.1%	Cloderm (Hermal). Cream in 15 and 45 g containers.	Preparations in Groups IV-VI may be used for chronic eczematous dermatoses, hand eczema, and atopic eczema and for a limited period of time on the face and in intertriginous areas.
Desoximetasone cream 0.05%	Topicort LP (Hoechst-Roussel). Cream in 15 and 60 g containers.	
Fluocinolone acetonide ointment 0.025%	Generic, Synalar (Syntex). Ointment in 15, 30, 60, and 425 g containers.	
Flurandrenolide ointment 0.05%	Cordran (Oclassen). Ointment in 15, 30, and 60 g containers. [Also available: Lotion 0.05% in 15 and 60 ml containers (Generic, Cordran); ointment 0.025% in 30 and 60 ml containers, and tape in rolls (Cordran)]	
Hydrocortisone valerate ointment 0.2%[4]	Westcort (Westwood-Squibb). Ointment in 15, 45 and 60 g containers.	
Mometasone Furoate cream 0.1%	Elocon (Schering). Cream in 15 and 45 g containers. [Also available: Lotion 0.1% in 30 and 60 ml containers]	

TABLE 2 (continued)

Drug	Trademark(s) and Preparations	Comments
Trimacinolone acetonide ointment 0.1%	Generic, Aristocort, Aristocort A (Fujisawa), Kenalog, Kenalog-H (Westwood-Squibb), Triacet (Lemmon). Ointment in 15, 60 (Aristocort, Aristocort A, Kenalog), 80 (Generic, Kenalog), 240 (Aristocort, Kenalog), and 454 g (Generic) containers.	
Group V		
Betamethasone benzoate cream 0.025%	Uticort (Parke-Davis). Cream in 15 and 60 g containers. [Also available: Gel and lotion 0.025% in 15 and 60 g containers)	
Betamethasone dipropionate lotion 0.5%	Diprosone (Schering). Lotion in 20 and 60 ml containers.	
Betamethasone valerate cream 0.1%	Betatrex (Savage), Beta-Val (Lemmon), Valisone (Schering). Cream in 15, 45, and 110 and 430 g (Valisone only) containers. [Also available: Cream 0.01% in 15 and 60 g containers]	
Fluocinolone acetonide cream 0.02%	Generic, Synalar, Synemol (Syntex). Cream in 15, 30, 60, and 425 g (Generic, Synalar) containers.	
Fluticasone propionate cream 0.05%	Cutivate (Glaxo). Cream in 15, 30, and 60 g containers.	
Flurandrenolide cream 0.05%	Cordran SP (Oclassen). Cream in 15, 30, and 60 g containers.	
Hydrocortisone butyrate cream 0.1%	Locoid (Ferndale). Cream in 15, 45, and 60 g containers. [Also available: Ointment 0.1% in 15 and 45 g containers; solution 0.1% in 20 and 60 ml containers]	
Hydrocortisone valerate cream 0.2%	Westcort (Westwood-Squibb). Cream in 15, 45, 60, and 120 g containers.	
Triamcinolone acetonide lotion 0.1%	Generic, Kenalog (Westwood-Squibb). Lotion in 15 and 60 g containers.	
LOW POTENCY		
Group VI		
Alclometasone dipropionate cream 0.05%[4], ointment 0.05%[4]	Aclovate (Glaxo). Cream and ointment in 15, 45, and 60 g containers.	
Betamethasone valerate lotion 0.1%	Betatrex (Savage), Beta-Val (Lemmon), Valisone (Schering). Lotion in 20 (Valisone only) and 60 ml containers.	
Desonide cream 0.05%[4]	DesOwen (Owen/Galderma), Tridesilon (Miles). Cream in 15 and 60 g containers. [Also available: Lotion 0.05% (DesOwen) in 60 and 120 ml containers and ointment 0.05% in 15 and 60 g containers]	
Fluocinolone acetonide solution 0.01%	Generic, Fluonid (Allergan Herbert), Synalar (Syntex). Solution in 20 (Generic, Synalar) and 60 g containers. [Also available: Cream 0.01% in 15, 30, 60, and 425 g containers (Generic, Synalar)]	

TABLE 2 (continued)

Drug	Trademark(s) and Preparations	Comments
Triamcinolone acetonide cream 0.1%	Generic, Aristocort, Aristocort A (Fujisawa), Kenalog, Kenalog-H (Westwood-Squibb), Triacet (Lemmon). Cream in 15, 60 (Aristocort, Aristocort A, Kenalog), 80 (Generic, Kenalog, Kenalog-H, Triacet), 240 (Aristocort, Aristocort A, Kenalog), and 454 g (Generic) containers. [Also available: Cream 0.025% in 15 and 60 g containers (Generic, Aristocort, Aristocort A, Kenalog); lotion 0.025% in 60 ml containers (Generic, Kenalog); ointment 0.025% in 15, 80, 240 (Kenalog), and 454 g (Generic) containers; aerosol in 23 and 63 g containers (Kenalog); oral paste 0.1% in 5 g containers (Generic)]	
Group VII		
Topical preparations of Dexamethasone Hydrocortisone[4,5]	DEXAMETHASONE: Aerosol 0.01%: Aeroseb-Dex (Allergan Herbert) Aerosol 0.04%: Decaspray (Merck) DEXAMETHASONE SODIUM PHOSPHATE: Cream 0.1%: Decadron Phosphate (Merck) HYDROCORTISONE: Aerosol 0.5%: Aeroseb-HC (Allergan Herbert) Cream 0.5%: Cort-Dome (Miles), Dermolate[5] (Schering Plough) Cream 1%: Cort-Dome (Miles), Dermacort (Solvay), Hytone (Dermik), Nutracort (Owen/Galderma), Penecort (Allergan Herbert), Synacort (Syntex) Cream 2.5%: Hytone (Dermik), Synacort (Syntex) Lotion 0.25% and 0.5%: Cetacort (Owen/Galderma) Lotion 1%: Cetacort (Owen/Galderma), Dermacort (Solvay), Hytone (Dermik), Nutracort (Owen/Galderma), Texacort (GenDerm) Lotion 2.5%: Hytone (Dermik), Nutracort (Owen/Galderma) Ointment 1% and 2.5%: Hytone (Dermik) HYDROCORTISONE ACETATE: Cream 0.5% and 1%: Cortaid[5] (Upjohn) Lotion 0.5%: Cortaid (Upjohn) Ointment 0.5% and 1%: Cortaid[5] (Upjohn) Oral paste 0.5%: Orabase HCA (Colgate Hoyt/Gel-Kam) Spray 0.5% and 1%: Cortaid[5] (Upjohn)	Safe for long-term application and for use on the face and intertriginous ares and under occlusion. May be used in young children, infants, and the elderly.

1 Adapted from Cornell and Stoughton, 1993 and Maibach and Surber, 1992. Potency is based on vasoconstrictor assay (Stoughton, 1992), which correlates well with clinical efficacy for psoriasis (Cornell, 1992).

2 Potency of steroid preparations descends from Groups I to VII. The generic names of the compounds are listed alphabetically, not by potency, within each group.

3 Package insert specifies no more than 45 g [Diprolene ointment] and 50 g [Diprolene gel, Temovate, Ultravate] weekly for two weeks followed by a rest period; not used under occlusive dressings. No limitation of dose is specified for Psorcon; however, the package insert recommends that patients receiving a large dose applied to a large area or under an occlusive dressing should be evaluated periodically for HPA axis suppression.

4 Nonfluorinated steroids.

5 Available OTC.

mixtures are more effective than the steroid alone in secondary pyodermas and that such therapy may increase the risk of development of resistant organisms and allergic contact dermatitis (especially with neomycin). Furthermore, use of the agents separately allows more flexibility and control over therapy, and the cost to the patient is often reduced (Arndt, 1989). Those in favor of combined therapy point out that such therapy significantly improves results when (1) skin cultures are obtained, if feasible; (2) therapy is initiated early and is limited to one or two weeks' duration; and (3) the combination is chosen on the basis of the area and probable organism involved (eg, neomycin for glabrous skin infections predominantly caused by *Staphylococcus aureus*). Combination therapy should be avoided in patients with intertrigo, diaper dermatitis, and stasis dermatitis or skin ulcers in order to decrease the incidence of antibiotic sensitivity.

A listing of representative mixtures follows.

BETAMETHASONE AND CLOTRIMAZOLE:
Lotrisone (Schering). Cream containing betamethasone dipropionate 0.5% and clotrimazole 1% in 15 and 45 g containers.

DEXAMETHASONE AND NEOMYCIN:
NeoDecadron (Merck). Cream containing dexamethasone sodium phosphate 0.1% and neomycin sulfate 0.5% in 15 and 30 g containers.

FLUOCINOLONE AND NEOMYCIN:
Neo-Synalar (Syntex). Cream containing fluocinolone acetonide 0.025% and neomycin sulfate 0.5% in 15, 30, and 60 g containers.

HYDROCORTISONE AND NEOMYCIN:
Neo-Cortef (Upjohn), ***Generic.*** Ointment containing hydrocortisone acetate 1% and neomycin sulfate 0.5% in 20 g containers.

HYDROCORTISONE, NEOMYCIN, AND POLYMYXIN B:
Cortisporin (Burroughs Wellcome). Cream containing hydrocortisone acetate 0.5%, neomycin sulfate 0.5%, and polymyxin B 10,000 units in 7.5 g containers.
LazerSporin-C (Pedinol). Solution containing hydrocortisone 1%, neomycin sulfate 0.5%, and polymyxin B sulfate 10,000 units in 10 ml containers.

HYDROCORTISONE, NEOMYCIN, POLYMYXIN B, AND BACITRACIN ZINC:
Cortisporin (Burroughs Wellcome). Ointment containing hydrocortisone 1%, neomycin sulfate 0.5%, polymyxin B sulfate 5,000 units, and bacitracin zinc 400 units in 15 g containers.

METHYLPREDNISOLONE AND NEOMYCIN:
Neo-Medrol Acetate (Upjohn). Topical containing methylprednisolone acetate 0.25% and neomycin sulfate 0.5% in 30 g containers.

TRIAMCINOLONE AND NYSTATIN:
Generic. Cream and ointment.
Mycolog II (Westwood-Squibb), ***Mytrex*** (Savage). Cream and ointment containing triamcinolone acetonide 0.1% and nystatin 100,000 units in 15, 30, 60, and 120 (***Mycolog II*** only) g containers.
Myco-Triacet II (Lemmon). Cream and ointment containing triamcinolone acetonide 0.1% and nystatin 100,000 units in 15, 30, and 60 (cream only) g containers.

PSORIASIS

Clinical variants of psoriasis include the following entities: *Psoriasis vulgaris* (chronic plaque psoriasis) is a common chronic papulosquamous inflammatory disease characterized by dry, thick, silver-white, adherent or flaky scale on red papules and sharply demarcated, erythematous, slightly raised plaques. Epidermal proliferation is intense, resulting in parakeratosis and acanthosis. Nails and the skin of the scalp, elbows, knees, and the sacral area are the primary sites of involvement. Intertriginous and anogenital areas are involved secondarily. Eczematous or hyperkeratotic marginated plaques may be present on the palms and soles; nails are often pitted and dystrophic. Epidemiologic, family, twin, and HLA studies have documented the importance of genetic factors in the development of this disease in up to one-third of patients.

Psoriatic arthritis, a seronegative arthritis associated with psoriatic lesions typical of psoriasis vulgaris, occurs in 5% to 15% of patients.

Guttate psoriasis is characterized by spotty oval lesions 1 to 2 cm in diameter and is common in children and young adults following upper respiratory tract infection due to beta-hemolytic streptococci. This form of psoriasis may resolve spontaneously after appropriate treatment of the streptococcal infection. *Flexural (inverse) psoriasis* involves the intertriginous folds of the axillae and the inguinal, inframammary, intergluteal, and perianal skin and is characterized by isolated or confluent lesions. It commonly occurs in obese patients. *Elephantine psoriasis* occurs principally on the lumbosacral skin and legs, especially in patients with long-standing disease; plaques measure 15 cm or more. Less severe cases of these clinical variants usually respond well to conventional drug therapy.

Pustular psoriasis is a severe, highly inflammatory, and often disabling form of the disease that is characterized by sterile superficial pustules associated with the typical lesions of psoriasis vulgaris, psoriatic nail changes, and very painful fissuring of the skin. In its most severe form, acute generalized pustular psoriasis, the mucous membranes also are involved and leukocytosis, high fever, and prostration are present. In *palmoplantar psoriasis*, a variant of pustular psoriasis, the lesions are limited to the palms and soles.

Both generalized pustular psoriasis and *erythrodermic psoriasis*, an exfoliative disorder involving the entire skin surface, may be life-threatening and occur as rebound phenomena after withdrawal of systemic and topical very high or high potency corticosteroids. Unlike palmoplantar psoriasis, these forms are resistant to conventional drug therapy (ie, corticosteroids, tar or anthralin with or without UVB light therapy).

For reviews of variants of psoriasis and their treatment, see Lowe, 1985; Roenigk, 1990; Maibach and Roenigk, 1992 A; Maibach and Roenigk, 1992 B; Moschella and Hurley, 1992.

Pathogenesis: The prime defect of psoriasis is believed but not proven to be in the skin; epidermal hyperproliferation of keratinocytes may be present. The hyperproliferation occurs in the erythematous plaques; it also is observed in normal adjoining skin but there is no inflammation. Hyperproliferation of keratinocytes is not apparent in tissue culture. Experiments suggest that diffusible factors released from dermal fibroblasts may be partially responsible for the hyperproliferation (Rowland Payne, 1987).

Considerable circumstantial evidence and the fact that the disorder responds to immunosuppressive agents suggest that psoriasis may be an immunologic (but not autoimmune) disorder of the skin (Bos, 1988; Barker, 1991; Griffiths, 1992; Baker and Fry, 1992). Altered neutrophils, mast cells, monocytes, macrophages, and T-cell lymphocytes are present in early psoriatic lesions; it is well established that these inflammatory cells respond to soluble mediators (eg, interleukins, interferons) and transmembranous signal transducing systems that can modulate noninflammatory cellular proliferation and differentiation (Martin and Resch, 1988; Smith, 1988). These mediators and other seemingly innocuous systemic substances may augment the hyperproliferation of keratinocytes and produce the characteristic inflammatory signs of psoriasis.

Certain factors often trigger new lesions or exacerbate existing lesions. The most well-recognized factor is skin trauma, whether induced by physical, chemical, mechanical, or thermal means (Koebner's phenomenon). Certain drugs (eg, beta blockers, lithium, indomethacin and possibly other nonsteroidal anti-inflammatory agents, chloroquine and related antimalarials) or emotional stress, pregnancy, obesity, and streptococcal throat infections also may be trigger factors. Abrupt withdrawal of topical or systemic corticosteroid therapy can produce severe rebound psoriasis.

Drug Therapy: The main elements of a management program for psoriasis include (1) patient counseling, (2) avoidance of trigger factors, (3) topical therapy, (4) ultraviolet radiation with or without systemic therapy, and (5) systemic drug therapy. No treatments are curative, but considerable relief and control of the disorder can be achieved.

Counseling to improve understanding promotes compliance and helps patients avoid fraudulent therapy and trigger factors. Such counseling can and usually does markedly augment any positive effects of the drug and/or phototherapeutic regimen selected. The National Psoriasis Foundation, 6600 SW 92nd Ave., Suite 300, Portland, OR 97223 (503/244-7404) can assist the physician in providing information for the patient.

The management of psoriasis depends principally on its severity (Farber and Nall, 1984; Anderson, 1986; Murphy and Greaves, 1988; Menter and Barker, 1991).

Mild Psoriasis. Many patients with mild involvement can be managed with lubricating agents alone. If the thick hyperkeratotic scale and crusts cannot be removed by moist occlusive dressings or long immersion in water, nonprescription formulations (ointment, gel, and shampoo) containing petrolatum alone, salicylic acid 5% to 6% alone or with propylene glycol, alcohol, sulfur, or urea (in 10% to 20% ointment or cream) are used for their keratolytic action. Patients may require medium or high potency topical corticosteroids used with or without occlusive dressings or very high potency steroids generally without occlusive dressings. Some dermatologists recommend intralesional corticosteroids for limited disease or the concomitant use of phototherapy (erythemogenic doses of UVB radiation) if therapy with topical corticosteroids and occlusion is not adequate. Other dermatologists prefer to apply coal tar and measured erythemogenic doses of UVB radiation (Goeckerman regimen) or anthralin [Anthra-Derm, Drithocreme, Lasan].

Moderate Psoriasis. Periodic use of UVB radiation alone or with high concentrations of coal tar or anthralin applied traditionally (Ingram regimen) (Ashton et al, 1983) or preferably in a short-contact, high-concentration regimen (Farber and Nall, 1984; Lowe et al, 1984; Kingston et al, 1987) may be used for moderate psoriasis.

The benefits of sunlight and UVB radiation in the treatment of psoriasis are attributed to increased production of the natural antiproliferative agent, cholecalciferol (vitamin D_3). Although administration of exogenous cholecalciferol is effective in psoriasis, the doses required increase the risk of hypercalcemia and calciuria. Recent studies on an analogue of cholecalciferol, calcipotriol, have shown that it is safe and effective in psoriasis when administered topically, thus obviating concern about development of hypercalcemia and calciuria. Results of a controlled study demonstrated that calcipotriol cream is superior to topical betamethasone valerate in patients with psoriasis vulgaris (Kragballe et al, 1991; Kragballe, 1992; Dubertret et al, 1992). Although calcipotriol is well tolerated, it causes irritation that increases with time and should not be used on the face. It appears to be a promising alternative to topical corticosteroids, tar, anthralin, and UVB radiation (Newbold, 1992).

Severe Psoriasis. When severe disabling psoriasis does not respond adequately to the above regimens, alternative drug therapies are often beneficial but may be associated with greater risk. One employs the cytotoxic drug, methotrexate [Folex PFS]. Another utilizes the psoralen, methoxsalen [Oxsoralen], with UVA radiation, which is termed photochemotherapy (originally termed PUVA therapy) (see the evaluation for a discussion of photochemotherapy). A third regimen utilizes the retinoid, etretinate [Tegison]. Relapses are common after discontinuation of therapy whether methotrexate, photochemotherapy, or retinoids are used. Combination regimens consisting of photochemotherapy and etretinate or methotrexate are now being used extensively. These combinations often permit a reduction in dosage of one or both agents, and they can reduce the time required to control severe disabling psoriasis.

The immunosuppressants, azathioprine [Imuran] and thioguanine [Tabloid], occasionally are used to treat severe psoriasis; however, methotrexate is more effective (Younger et al, 1991; Auerbach, 1992).

Cyclosporine [Sandimmune] is used rarely and only in severe recalcitrant psoriasis that cannot be brought under control rapidly with methotrexate, photochemotherapy, or etretinate (Ellis et al, 1991; Christophers et al, 1992; Menter, 1992). Its action is only suppressive and relapses occur on withdrawal. Because data on long-term safety are limited, especially in patients previously exposed to photochemotherapy, ionizing radiation, and UVB radiation, cyclosporine should be administered only by experts (Mihatsch and Wolff, 1992) and for no longer than three months (Menter, 1992).

Although the antineoplastic agent, hydroxyurea [Hydrea], is well tolerated, it is only variably effective in the treatment of moderate to severe psoriasis; therefore, current guidelines reserve use of this drug alone or in combination with photochemotherapy for patients with psoriasis unresponsive to conventional therapy who are not suitable candidates for more extensive or toxic treatments (eg, methotrexate, etretinate, cyclosporine).

When systemic drug therapy with methotrexate, cyclosporine, or hydroxyurea is indicated for a patient with severe psoriasis, the most critical issues to be weighed are likelihood of teratogenicity; induction of malignancy; hepatic, hematologic, pulmonary, and renal toxicity; and coexistence of hypertension (Wolverton, 1991).

ANTHRALIN

[Anthra-Derm, Drithocreme, Lasan]

OH OH OH

ACTIONS AND USES. Anthralin was developed as a synthetic substitute for chrysarobin in the treatment of psoriasis. It reduces epidermal cell DNA synthesis and mitotic activity of hyperplastic epidermis, thus restoring a normal rate of proliferation and keratinization in patients with moderately severe psoriasis. Anthralin is more effective than topical corticosteroids for psoriasis vulgaris (Ashton et al, 1983; Lowe et al, 1984). If necessary, it may be used with periodic UVB phototherapy. The need for specialized care in a supervised setting has limited the use of this therapy to dermatologists.

A relatively high patient dropout rate is common with conventional regimens of anthralin therapy because of staining and irritation. (Anthralin may stain fabrics permanently and the hair and skin temporarily.) Compared with the conventional overnight 8- or 12-hour Ingram regimens, short-contact high-concentration regimens of anthralin therapy suitable for outpatient or daycare centers cause less staining and irritation and are less expensive (Ashton et al, 1983; Lowe et al, 1984; Farber and Nall, 1984; Schaefer, 1985; Kingston et al, 1987). Thus, these regimens are preferred by dermatologists in the United States.

ADVERSE REACTIONS AND PRECAUTIONS. Significant percutaneous absorption of anthralin has not been observed. Irritation occurs frequently, especially in body folds (eg, groin, axilla) and with concentrations above 0.1%. However, many patients tolerate even the 1% concentration if the dose is increased gradually. Excessive erythema may occur on adjacent normal skin and may require reducing the frequency of application. Sensitivity reactions are rare.

Anthralin should be applied only to quiescent or chronic patches of psoriasis; it should not be used on acute eruptions or excessively inflamed areas and should be used cautiously, if at all, on the face or intertriginous areas. Contact with the eyes may cause conjunctivitis.

It has been suggested that anthralin may be contraindicated in patients with impaired renal function because of possible renal toxicity after percutaneous absorption; however, short-term toxicologic studies using paste and ointment forms indicate that concentrations up to 0.4% do not impair kidney or liver function.

Anthralin is classified in FDA Pregnancy Category C.

DOSAGE AND PREPARATIONS.

Topical: When the response to anthralin has not been previously established, the 0.1% strength should be used initially; if necessary, the concentration is then increased through the range of 0.25%, 0.5%, and 1% at minimum intervals of three to four days. Anthralin may be used in two ways: the conventional overnight (Ingram) regimen and the short-contact regimen. In the overnight regimen, the cream or ointment is applied at bedtime and should remain on the lesions for 8 to 12 hours. To avoid staining of clothing and bed linens, either old clothing should be worn or the treated areas should be covered with suitable dressings. The next morning, the application is removed with soap and water or rubbing alcohol.

In the modified short-contact regimen, 0.1% anthralin cream or ointment is applied initially, left on for 30 minutes, then washed off with soap and hot water. The concentration is increased at three-day intervals as indicated above to a maximum of 1% for 30 minutes providing no burning or irritation is observed (Lowe et al, 1984; Schaefer, 1985).

Dritho-Scalp cream is specially formulated for use on hairy areas. Salicylic acid 3% may be incorporated into anthralin ointments for a keratolytic action on thickened lesions on the soles.

Generic. Powder.

Anthra-Derm (Dermik). Ointment in petrolatum 0.1%, 0.25%, 0.5%, and 1% in 42.5 g containers.

Drithocreme (Dermik). Cream 0.1%, 0.25%, 0.5%, and 1% (***Drithocreme HP***) in 50 g containers and 0.25% and 0.5% ***(Dritho-Scalp)*** in 50 g containers.

Lasan (Stiefel). Ointment 0.4% with salicylic acid in 60 g containers.

CYCLOSPORINE

[Sandimmune]

For chemical formula, see index entry Cyclosporine, Uses, Organ Transplant Rejection.

ACTIONS AND USES. The immunosuppressant, cyclosporine, may be regarded as an alternative to methotrexate, photochemotherapy, and retinoids when recalcitrant severe psoriasis cannot be brought under control with these forms of therapy (Ellis et al, 1991; Christophers et al, 1992).

Cyclosporine blocks the synthesis and/or release of interleukin 1 from monocytes and interleukin 2 from T-helper cells; therefore, it blocks the amplification of T-helper lymphocyte cells. These actions probably account in part for the effectiveness of cyclosporine in patients with psoriasis (Ellis et al, 1991; Christophers, et al, 1992); however, a direct antiproliferative action on keratinocytes may be more relevant. The actions of this agent are quite variable. Relapses occur on withdrawal.

ADVERSE REACTIONS AND PRECAUTIONS. See index entry Cyclosporine, Uses, Organ Transplant Rejection. Because data on long-term safety are limited, only physicians knowledgeable in the treatment of recalcitrant severe psoriasis should use this drug (Mihatsch and Wolff, 1992).

Relative contraindications to the use of cyclosporine include hypertension, active infection, malignancy, extensive ultraviolet damage to the skin, and nephropathy. Since the serum creatinine concentration is a poor predictor of cyclosporine nephrotoxicity, glomerular flow rate and other renal function studies should be conducted before initiation of therapy.

DOSAGE AND PREPARATIONS.

Oral: For severe recalcitrant psoriasis, *adults,* initially, 2.5 to 3 mg/kg/day is administered as a single dose or divided into two doses (Christophers et al, 1992; Menter, 1992; Mihatsch and Wolff, 1992). About two-thirds of patients will respond to this dose; in most of the remaining patients, after about one month it will be necessary to increase the amount gradually to as much as 5 mg/kg/day (recommended maximum) to control the disease. Treatment should not be continued for longer than 12 weeks if cyclosporine is not effective or adverse reactions are intolerable (Menter, 1992). When the disease is under control, the dose should be reduced by 0.5 mg/kg/day until the most effective maintenance dose is determined. Long-term data on safety are incomplete. However, therapy other than cyclosporine is recommended for maintenance to minimize cumulative toxicity (Lowe, 1991). Treatment for longer than two years increases the risk of squamous cell carcinoma of the skin (Bavinck et al, 1991).

Sandimmune (Sandoz). Capsules 25 and 50 mg; solution (oral) 100 mg/ml (alcohol 12.5%).

ETRETINATE

[Tegison]

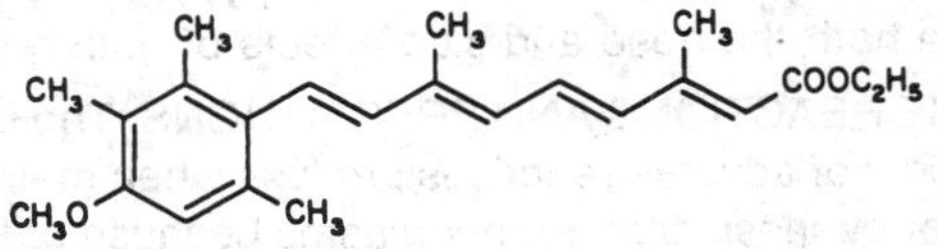

ACTIONS AND USES. Etretinate inhibits keratinization, proliferation, and differentiation of epithelial tissues and inhibits ornithine decarboxylase, which is essential for polyamine synthesis. These actions are responsible in part for its efficacy in proliferative and hyperkeratotic skin disorders. The anti-inflammatory and immunomodulator actions are less defined, but etretinate inhibits the motility and migration of neutrophils and eosinophils into the epidermis, which reduces the antibody-dependent cell-mediated cytotoxicity of polymorphonuclear leukocytes (Ellis et al, 1985); stimulates cell-mediated cytotoxicity and T-killer cells; and suppresses the mitogenic response of lymphocytes.

This retinoid is especially effective in patients with severe forms of psoriasis, such as generalized pustular, palmoplantar pustular, and erythrodermic psoriasis (Ward et al, 1986; Orfanos et al, 1987). It is recommended that only physicians knowledgeable in the treatment of recalcitrant severe psoriasis utilize this drug (Lowe et al, 1988; Shalita and Fritsch, 1992).

Combination therapy consisting of etretinate with tars or anthralin (with or without UVB radiation) or etretinate with photochemotherapy allows use of lower doses and hence reduces the severity of adverse reactions.

Open studies demonstrate that some patients with other disorders of keratinization (eg, lichen planus, pityriasis rubra pilaris, Darier's disease, ichthyosis) also respond satisfactorily to etretinate.

Because of its teratogenic potential and long storage in the body, etretinate should not be used for any dermatologic disorder in women of reproductive potential unless other treatment choices have been exhausted. (See the section on Pregnancy.)

ADVERSE REACTIONS AND PRECAUTIONS. Excessive thirst; sore mouth; thinning and desquamation of the skin, especially the eyelids; dry skin; pruritic rash; red scaly facial skin; fatigue; and irritation of the eyes occur in 50% to 75% of patients. Bruising of the skin, increased susceptibility to sunburn, muscle cramps, and headache develop in 25% to 50% of patients. The following side effects occur in at least 25% of patients: dryness of the nose, lips (cheilitis), and mouth, which may result in sore tongue; epistaxis; peeling of the fingers, palms, and soles; and loss of hair, which has accounted for the majority of withdrawals from therapy. Dryness of the mucosa can be a significant problem in patients with chronic respiratory disease. Nail dystrophies, widespread exfoliation of the skin, conjunctivitis, and nausea are observed in 10% to 25% of patients. Reversible elevations of AST and ALT have been noted in 15% to 25% of patients. Acute severe hepatitis with eosinophilia has been reported rarely within one month of initiation of therapy in some patients. Side effects reported but not documented as causally related to therapy and that develop in less than 10% of patients are usually extensions or complications of the above side effects or represent new organ involvement (eg, earache, external otitis, cardiovascular thrombotic or obstructive events, edema, dyspnea). Pseudotumor cerebri (intracranial hypertension) has been reported in less than 1% of patients. Headache, nausea and vomiting, and visual disturbances should be considered as possible warning signs of papilledema.

Adverse reactions commonly associated with long-term treatment (>2 years) that have been causally related to etretinate include skeletal hyperostosis (usually of the ankles, knees, spine, and pelvis), as well as extraspinal tendon and ligament calcifications (most commonly of the ankles, pelvis, and knees).

The most significant changes in laboratory values include elevations of triglycerides and LDH and decreases of HDL, which are observed in 15% to 50% of the patients. Whether the drug should be discontinued or a lipid-reduction program or period of watchful waiting should be initiated will depend on the degree of change and the presence of cardiovascular risk factors (eg, obesity, diabetes, family history, high pretreatment concentrations of serum triglycerides, alcohol consumption).

Most of the above side effects are a manifestation of the hypervitaminosis A syndrome. The differences and similarities among the clinically useful retinoids have been correlated with that syndrome (Silverman et al, 1987).

PREGNANCY. Like vitamin A and isotretinoin, etretinate is a potent teratogen (FDA Pregnancy Category X). It is imperative that women of reproductive potential not be given etretinate until pregnancy is excluded. Counseling of the patient about the potentially teratogenic effects of etretinate must be conducted and documented. Contraception *must* be practiced for one and preferably two months before and throughout therapy. The drug persists in the body for an extended period; it has been found in the blood of some patients two to three years after discontinuation of therapy. Therefore, it is recommended that pregnancy be avoided for at least two years and probably three years following cessation of therapy (DiGiovanna et al, 1989).

PHARMACOKINETICS. Etretinate is administered orally; bioavailability is approximately 40%. Milk or a diet high in fat enhances absorption. The time to peak absorption varies from two to six hours. This drug is converted to the active, more water-soluble, free acid form (ie, acitretin). Numerous inactive metabolites are found in the urine; however, about 75% of the dose is recovered from the feces.

Etretinate is 99% bound to plasma proteins, principally lipoproteins; its active metabolite, acitretin, is bound to albumin. The volumes of distribution of etretinate and acitretin far exceed total body water due to extravascular sequestration. Steady-state concentrations range from 100 to 500 ng/ml.

Etretinate has a much longer elimination half-life (about 120 days, but the range is variable) than acitretin (50 hours) and isotretinoin (8 to 10 hours). This slow terminal elimination phase results from accumulation in fatty tissue from which it is slowly released. Accumulation may be a factor responsible for the prolonged remissions achieved with etretinate therapy; however, many patients have a rapid recurrence of disease after therapy is discontinued. The lengthening of the elimination half-life with multiple dosing is probably due to lack of assay sensitivity at drug concentrations obtained after single-dose administration rather than to alterations in etretinate's pharmacokinetics (Lucek and Colburn, 1985).

DOSAGE AND PREPARATIONS. *See the warning in the Pregnancy section of this evaluation.*

Oral: *Adults*, for severe psoriasis, 0.75 mg to 1 mg/kg daily in divided amounts, depending on the patient's response (maximum, 1.5 mg/kg daily). The dose may have to be reduced to 0.3 to 0.5 mg/kg daily in patients who are sensitive to the drug. Erythrodermic psoriasis may respond to lower initial doses (0.25 mg/kg daily, gradually increased if necessary by increments of 0.25 mg/kg/day until an optimal initial response is obtained). Although many patients will respond within two to four weeks, treatment may need to be continued for as long as six months before a response is evident in some individuals. Some patients will require prolonged maintenance therapy. Etretinate should be administered with food.

Tegison (Roche). Capsules 10 and 25 mg.

METHOTREXATE

METHOTREXATE SODIUM

[Folex PFS]

For chemical formula, see index entry Methotrexate, Uses, Cancer.

ACTIONS AND USES. Methotrexate, a cytotoxic and immunosuppressant agent, controls severe, recalcitrant, disabling psoriasis that does not respond adequately to topical corticosteroids, tars, or anthralin with or without UVB radiation (Tung and Maibach, 1990; Olsen, 1991).

Actively proliferating tissues (eg, epidermal hyperplasia associated with psoriasis and other disorders of keratinization) are sensitive to this dihydrofolate reductase and thymidylate synthesis inhibitor. Methotrexate also has been used with varying success to treat other dermatologic proliferative and autoimmune disorders (eg, systemic lupus erythematosus, severe epidermolytic ichthyosis or keratoderma, pityriasis rubra pilaris, dermatomyositis, mycosis fungoides, Reiter's disease, bullous pemphigoid, pemphigus vulgaris).

Considerable expertise is required for patient selection and pretreatment evaluation. Dosage schedules must be individualized, and drug interactions and risk factors must be considered. Risk factors that may exclude a patient from receiving methotrexate include abnormal renal or liver function, pregnancy or nursing, immunosuppression, excessive alcohol consumption, infection, diabetes mellitus, obesity, arsenic exposure, peptic ulcer, and probable noncompliance (Tung and Maibach, 1990).

Guidelines for the use of methotrexate in refractory psoriasis have been formulated by an Ad Hoc Committee on Methotrexate of the Psoriasis Task Force of the American Academy of Dermatology (Maibach and Roenigk, 1992 B), and the guidelines should be reviewed prior to use of the drug for this indication. The combination of methotrexate with another agent (eg, etretinate, photochemotherapy) may be desirable to reduce both the dose and side effects of both regimens.

ADVERSE REACTIONS AND PRECAUTIONS. The incidence and severity of adverse reactions are less when methotrexate is used for psoriasis than for neoplasms because of the lower doses required. However, hepatotoxicity is of concern when methotrexate is used for prolonged periods, even at lower doses.

The most common adverse reactions are nausea, malaise, and leukopenia. Chills, fever, fatigue, and dizziness occur less frequently. The most common reason for discontinuing therapy is gastrointestinal side effects.

Methotrexate may cause hepatotoxicity and bone marrow depression, especially during prolonged therapy. Liver function tests should be performed at intervals of approximately three months. This drug also may cause thrombocytopenia, interstitial pneumonitis, immunosuppression, hemorrhagic enteritis, seizures (rare), renal failure, and impaired fertility.

Because methotrexate has caused congenital abnormalities and fetal death, it is not recommended for women of reproductive potential (FDA Pregnancy Category D).

Methotrexate must be used cautiously and only by physicians experienced in the treatment of severe psoriasis. The patient should be fully informed of the risks involved and should remain under the close supervision of a physician.

Nonsteroidal anti-inflammatory agents reduce the rate of excretion of methotrexate and may result in more frequent or severe reactions (Frenia and Long, 1992). Oral antibiotics that alter bacterial flora in the gut suppress the metabolism of methotrexate.

For a more detailed discussion of adverse reactions, precautions, and drug interactions, see index entry Methotrexate, Uses, Cancer.

PHARMACOKINETICS. Conventional oral doses are readily absorbed in most patients; peak serum levels are reached in one to two hours. One-half of the drug is reversibly bound to plasma proteins; aspirin, sulfonamides, phenytoin, chloramphenicol, and tetracyclines can displace methotrexate from these sites.

The disappearance of methotrexate from plasma is triphasic. In patients receiving treatment for psoriasis, the terminal half-life is 3 to 10 hours.

About 10% of an administered dose is metabolized to 7-hydroxymethotrexate and is eliminated by the kidney. About 50% to 90% of methotrexate is excreted by the kidney within 24 hours. Renal clearance (range, 0.63 to 2.62 ml/min/kg) occurs by filtration and active secretion (Chen et al, 1984). Dose-dependent elimination has been observed, presumably due to saturation of renal tubular reabsorption at higher doses.

DOSAGE AND PREPARATIONS. Leucovorin is a specific antidote that can be life-saving in serious methotrexate overdosage. A recommended management program is available (Auerbach, 1992).

Two effective commonly used schedules are based on knowledge of cell proliferation kinetics: (1) a large oral, intravenous, or intramuscular dose is given once weekly; or (2) three oral doses are given weekly over a 24-hour period.

Oral, Intramuscular, Intravenous: The dosage schedules cited below are for a *70-kg adult*. A test dose of 2.5 mg is given in the first week to detect any idiosyncratic reaction followed by 5 mg in the second week. Depending on the patient's response and the desire of the physician, either the weekly single oral or divided oral dose schedule is used.

(1) *Weekly single oral or intramuscular dose:* (a) The usual range for oral administration is 7.5 to 25 mg/week; occasional patients require a maximum of 37.5 mg/week. It is recommended that the total be increased gradually (2.5 to 5 mg/week) with appropriate monitoring of the blood counts. (b) The usual range for intramuscular dosage is 7.5 to 25 mg/week; occasional patients require 30 to a maximum of 50 mg/week. As the total dose is gradually increased, blood counts should be monitored more carefully.

(2) *Divided oral dose schedule:* 5 to 7.5 mg is given at 12-hour intervals for three doses each week. Dosage may be increased gradually by 2.5 mg/week. Blood counts should be monitored.

All schedules should be continually individualized. As the patient improves, the dosage should be reduced and the time interval between the doses can be gradually increased to 14 or more days. The goal is not necessarily to achieve complete clearing of psoriasis, but rather to achieve adequate control with the minimum dosage and the longest rest period. The use of methotrexate may permit the return to conventional topical therapy, which is encouraged.

METHOTREXATE:
Generic. Tablets 2.5 mg.

METHOTREXATE SODIUM:
(Strengths expressed in terms of the base)
Folex PFS (Adria). Solution (preservative-free) 25 mg/ml in 2, 4, 8, and 10 ml containers.
Methotrexate (Lederle). Powder (lyophilized, preservative-free) in 20 and 50 mg and 1 g containers; solution (injection) 25 mg/ml in 2 and 10 ml containers (alcohol 0.9%) and in 2, 4, 8, and 10 ml containers (preservative-free) ***(Methotrexate LPF).***

PHOTOCHEMOTHERAPY

Long-wave ultraviolet radiation in the range of 320 to 400 nm (UVA) produces mild erythema or pigmentation with long exposures, but concomitant use of a circulating photosensitizer (eg, a psoralen) markedly enhances the effect and decreases the time to response. The development of oral psoralen with UVA photochemotherapy as a therapeutic tool has been reviewed (Bickers et al, 1984; Fitzpatrick and Pathak, 1984; Gupta and Anderson, 1987; Helm et al, 1991).

Photochemotherapy, originally termed PUVA therapy (*P*soralen with *UVA* light), is used to treat psoriasis in patients with extensive, active disease who have not responded to conventional regimens (topical steroids; tars or anthralin with or without UVB radiation). Patient selection is complex; however, improvement can be anticipated in about 90% of properly selected patients who have chronic psoriasis vulgaris (Gupta and Anderson, 1987). When used in combination regimens (especially with retinoids or methotrexate) for the treatment of more severe psoriatic disease, effectiveness of therapy is enhanced and the dosage and time required for control of the disease often may be reduced.

Photochemotherapy acts primarily by forming psoralen-DNA photo adducts that interfere with the hyperproliferative epidermal cell turnover characteristic of psoriasis. The psoralen, methoxsalen, is used orally and topically with controlled exposures to UVA light to enhance inhibition of epidermal cell proliferation and minimize burns by decreasing the amount of UVA radiation required. Most lesions usually clear after 12 to 18 therapy sessions, which are commonly spread over a period of 6 to 18 weeks.

Suppression of selected immunologic elements of the skin also provides a beneficial action in some other dermatologic disorders. Photochemotherapy is established clinically for the early stages of mycosis fungoides. Modest improvement in vitiligo may occur, but long-term treatment and careful patient selection, especially in children, is required. Uncontrolled studies support its use in some patients with atopic and dyshidrotic eczema, alopecia areata, parapsoriasis, chronic graft-versus-host reaction, generalized granuloma annulare, lichen planus, pityriasis lichenoides, pityriasis rubra pilaris, persistent palmoplantar pustulosis, urticaria pigmentosa, and polymorphous light eruption. Clinical data are more limited for other disorders (eg, ichthyosis linearis circumflexa, hypereosinophilic syndrome, solar urticaria, scleromyxedema, actinic reticuloid, prurigo nodularis, keratosis lichenoides chronica, lymphomatoid papulosis, hypopigmented sarcoidosis, transient acantholytic dermatosis, generalized granuloma annulare).

ADVERSE REACTIONS. Acute adverse reactions reported with use of photochemotherapy are nausea, pruritus, and erythema, which occur in 15% to 20% of patients; however, these reactions are quite well tolerated except for nausea, which can be quite bothersome and persistent. Scrotal skin is especially sensitive and should be covered during PUVA treatments. Potential chronic major effects include atypical cutaneous pigmentation, accelerated skin aging, and an increased risk of squamous cell skin cancer, especially in fair-skinned individuals with skin types I to III. The risk is increased 12-fold for squamous cell carcinomas of the skin (Lindelof et al, 1991). Patients previously exposed to carcinogens (eg, prior irradiation, chemical carcinogens) or subsequently exposed to immunosuppressive agents may be more at risk. Occasionally, the stimulation of melanogenesis may lead to mottling and lentigenes, but no increase in malignant melanoma has been confirmed. Hypopigmentation has been reported.

Although a cataractogenic action has not been established conclusively, use of proper eye protection (ie, UVA sunblocking sunglasses) is essential during and is strongly recommended for 36 to 48 hours after therapy sessions (especially if the patient goes outside in bright sunlight).

PRECAUTIONS. Criteria for patient selection and dosing regimens are complex. Photochemotherapy should be performed only by dermatologists experienced in its use. The Committee on Drugs of the American Academy of Pediatrics recommends that under no circumstances should children with psoriasis receive such therapy unless it is administered by qualified specialists. The manufacturer of methoxsalen (ICN Pharmaceuticals) distributes information for physicians and patients. The manufacturer's recommendations on the use of any psoralen should be read carefully prior to use for photochemotherapy.

For preparations of methoxsalen, see evaluation in section on Agents Affecting Pigmentation.

TARS

ACTIONS AND USES. Tar presumably suppresses epidermal cell DNA synthesis and mitotic activity (Lowe et al, 1982) and restores a normal rate of proliferation.

Tars, most commonly coal tar, are now used infrequently to treat chronic lichenified and papulosquamous eruptions (Hjorth and Jacobsen, 1983). Although topical corticosteroids are now more commonly used in mild to moderate psoriasis, recalcitrant seborrheic dermatitis, atopic dermatitis, and lichen simplex chronicus, tars are often beneficial in these disorders; they may be less expensive and are useful if patient compliance can be assured in spite of their messiness and ability to stain clothing and towels. Phototherapy with suberythemogenic or erythemogenic doses of UVB radiation following removal of tar has been purported to enhance the suppression of hyperplastic skin in proliferative disorders, but few dermatologists presently use this combination (Goeckerman regimen) for psoriasis (Muller and Perry, 1984).

Tars incorporated into lotions, creams, or ointments containing hydrocortisone 0.25% to 1% and iodoquinol (diiodohydroxyquin) 1% are promoted for the treatment of infected eczemas and atopic dermatitis. Controlled studies comparing this regimen with hydrocortisone or iodoquinol alone are not available.

ADVERSE REACTIONS. An important disadvantage of all tar preparations is their lack of uniformity. Tar formulations cause smarting and burning. They may be photosensitizing, have an unpleasant odor, and frequently stain the skin, hair, and clothes. The irritation caused by usual concentrations of coal tar is minimal and appears to be negligible in patients with psoriasis. However, occlusive therapy or excessive use may aggravate lesions (particularly in guttate or pustular psoriasis) or cause folliculitis. Tars rarely cause allergic sensitization. Juniper tar, birch tar, and pine tar cause sensitization more often and have no advantage over coal tar. Systemic toxicity is not observed following topical administration.

Crude coal tar and its derivatives contain aromatic hydrocarbons and may have carcinogenic potential when used for prolonged periods; however, in an OTC Final Monograph, the FDA classified coal tar preparations as Category I (safe and effective) for psoriasis (*Federal Register*, 1991 A). Considerable experience with the Goeckerman regimen reveals that the incidence of skin cancer is not appreciably increased in patients with psoriasis who have had limited exposure; the risk with long-term exposure is unknown (Muller and Perry, 1984).

Coal tar is classified in FDA Pregnancy Category C.

PREPARATIONS.

COAL TAR (liquor carbonis detergens), U.S.P.:

Generic. Solution 20%. This solution may contain an emulsifier, polysorbate 80 [Tween 80], which forms a fine dispersion when 60 ml is added to the bath. The solution can be incorporated into creams or ointments (2% to 10%) or into tincture of green soap for a shampoo (10%) (nonprescription).

Body Oil:

Balnetar (Westwood-Squibb) 2.5%, ***Doak Oil*** (Doak) 2%, ***Lavatar*** (Doak) 25%, ***Neutrogena T/Derm*** (Neutrogena) 5% (nonprescription), ***Polytar Bath*** (Stiefel) 25% (nonprescription), ***Zetar Emulsion*** (Dermik) 30%.

Cream:

Fototar (ICN) 2%.

Gel:

Estar (Westwood-Squibb) 5%, ***PsoriGel*** (Owen/Galderma) 7.5% (nonprescription).

Lotion:

Doak Tar (Doak) 5% (nonprescription).

Ointment:

Medotar (Medco) 1.5% (nonprescription), ***Unguentum Bossi*** (Doak) 5%.

Paste:

Tarpaste (Doak) 5% (nonprescription).

Shampoo:

Doak Tar Shampoo (Doak) 3%, ***Ionil T 5%, Ionil T Plus 1%*** (Owen/Galderma), ***Pentrax Tar*** (GenDerm) 4.3%, ***Polytar*** (Stiefel) 1%, ***Neutrogena T/Gel*** (Neutrogena) 2%, ***Zetar*** (Dermik) 1% (all forms nonprescription).

Soap:

Packer's Pine Tar (Rydelle) 5.87%, ***Polytar*** (Stiefel) 1% (nonprescription).

DANDRUFF AND SEBORRHEIC DERMATITIS

Dandruff and seborrheic dermatitis are associated with increased rates of maturation and proliferation of epidermal cells, although other characteristics of these disorders, such as type of scale, sebum retention, epidermal hyperplasia, dermal capillary proliferation, areas of involvement, and presence of inflammation, differ considerably.

Some investigators suggest that dandruff affects individuals who are at the upper limit of normal variation with respect to rate of turnover of epidermal cells. The excessive scaling is most obvious on the scalp (and on dark clothing), and it usually is not accompanied by visible inflammation, alteration of sebum kinetics, pathologic change, or epidermal hyperplasia.

Seborrheic dermatitis is an inflammatory scaling disease of the scalp and face and may involve the margins of the eyelids; the area over the sternum, mid-back, nasolabial folds, and intertriginous areas also are involved in the most severe cases. When sebum is retained, the scales become oily; epidermal hyperplasia and an abnormal number of parakeratotic cells are present. Mild pruritus is common.

Agents that are effective in seborrheic disorders are presumed to have a cytostatic action. Some evidence based on the oral and topical use of the antifungal agent, ketoconazole, strongly suggests that the yeasts, *Pityrosporum ovale* and *P. orbicularis* (closely related if not identical organisms), are involved in the pathogenesis of both dandruff and seborrhea (McGrath and Murphy, 1991). However, consensus has not been reached on whether *P. ovale* is a primary cause of seborrheic dermatitis (Jacobs, 1988) because the organism is present on the skin of some individuals who do not have this disorder. It is presumed that other physical factors (eg, moisture, heat, pH and water content of the skin) are necessary to produce symptoms.

Drug Selection: The treatment of choice in seborrheic dermatitis or blepharitis is daily application of a shampoo containing pyrithione zinc [DHS Zinc, Head and Shoulders, Sebulon, Zincon, Zinctex] or selenium sulfide [Exsel, Selsun RX, Selsun Blue, Selsun Gold]. Their modest antifungal action may be as relevant as their cytostatic action in mild to moderately severe seborrheic capitis and dermatitis. Although shampoos containing salicylic acid are beneficial, pyrithione zinc and selenium sulfide are more effective. Salicylic acid has only a weak antifungal action, and its efficacy may depend only on its keratolytic action. It may be necessary to add low potency topical corticosteroids, which decrease mitotic activity and epidermal cell proliferation, to the regimen in those with moderate to severe seborrhea. Topical ketoconazole [Nizoral] may be effective in severe or resistant cases.

Although mild dandruff can be controlled by daily application of non-oily shampoos, most individuals with moderate to severe disease require medicated shampoos. Shampoos containing tar, salicylic acid, zinc pyrithione, or selenium sulfide are moderately effective. Coal tar products may stain hair that is blond, bleached, or gray, and they may produce photosensitivity. Sulfur is only minimally effective in seborrheic disorders to loosen and lyse aggregates of keratin. An FDA final monograph recommends that sulfur be approved for Category I status (safe and effective) for dandruff but not for seborrhea (*Federal Register,* 1991 A).

Chloroxine [Capitrol], a dichlorohydroxy quinoline, is used in the treatment of dandruff and mild to moderately severe seborrhea. When applied topically as a shampoo, chloroxine has antibacterial and antifungal activities against staphylococcal and *Pityrosporum* species. Topical pharmacokinetic data in humans are not available. The preparation should not be used on acutely inflamed (exudative) lesions. Discoloration of light-colored hair (eg, blond, gray, bleached) may occur.

SELENIUM SULFIDE

[Exsel, Selsun RX, Selsun Blue, Selsun Gold]

ACTIONS AND USES. Selenium sulfide shampoos 1% and 2.5% are moderately effective in the treatment of dandruff and seborrhea. The antidandruff and antiseborrheic effects are purported to result from cytostatic activity (*Federal Register*, 1986; Jacobs, 1988) and substantivity (ie, residual adherence to the skin after shampoo and rinse), although an antifungal action may contribute to this agent's usefulness as well.

ADVERSE REACTIONS AND PRECAUTIONS. Little or no toxicity has been observed when selenium sulfide is applied as directed to normal skin and hair. However, it should not be applied to large areas of skin with severe dermatitic lesions because it or the detergent in the formulation may act as an irritant. The product should not be used when acute inflammation or exudation is present, because absorption may be increased. Allergic contact dermatitis has not been documented. The drug irritates conjunctival mucosa on contact.

Selenium sulfide is classified in FDA Pregnancy Category C.

DOSAGE AND PREPARATIONS. For seborrheic dermatitis and dandruff, one or two teaspoonsful of the shampoo are applied and allowed to remain on the scalp and other affected areas for *five to ten minutes* before being rinsed off thoroughly. Alternatively, some physicians prefer two consecutive applications of shampoo and omission of the retention time. Twice-weekly use of the preparation initially may control the condition in mild cases; selenium then should be used no more frequently than required to maintain control. Contact with the conjunctiva should be avoided.

Generic. Lotion shampoo 1% (nonprescription) and 2.5%.

Exsel (Allergan Herbert), ***Selsun RX*** (Ross). Lotion shampoo 2.5% in 120 ml containers.

Selsun Blue, Selsun Gold (Ross Consumer). Lotion 1% in 120, 210, and 330 ml containers (nonprescription).

PYRITHIONE ZINC

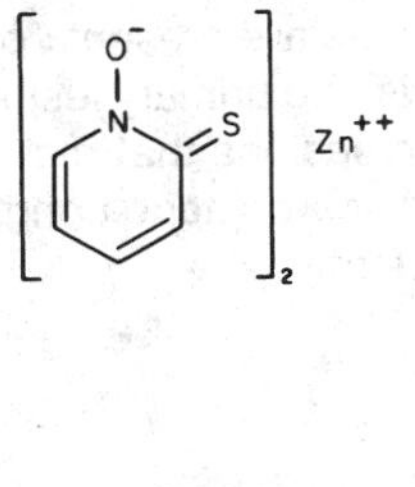

Pyrithione zinc shampoos are widely used nonprescription formulations that are effective in the treatment of dandruff and seborrhea.

Pyrithione zinc possesses cytostatic (*Federal Register*, 1986) and antifungal actions. Its effectiveness in dandruff and seborrhea is purported to result from both these actions and substantivity (ie, residual adherence to the skin after shampoo and rinse).

These shampoos have no apparent toxicity when applied as directed to normal skin and hair.

DOSAGE AND PREPARATIONS. For dandruff and seborrhea, one or two teaspoonsful of shampoo are applied with sufficient water to produce a foam that is allowed to remain on the scalp and other affected areas for up to five minutes before being rinsed off thoroughly; the application is then repeated. Application once or twice weekly controls dandruff in many individuals. Contact with the conjunctiva should be avoided.

Available Trademarks.
DHS Zinc (Person & Covey) 2%, ***Head and Shoulders*** (Procter & Gamble) 1%, ***Sebulon*** (Westwood-Squibb) 2%, ***Zincon*** (Lederle) 1%, ***Zinctex*** (Syosset) 2% (all forms nonprescription).

ACNE

Acne vulgaris principally affects adolescents and young adults, who often are genetically predisposed. The pathogenesis of acne is related to three major events (Leyden and Shalita, 1986): (1) An unexplained exaggerated response to androgenic steroids occurs that results in an increase in sebum production. (2) A proliferation of *Propionibacterium acnes*, a component of the normal flora of the follicle, occurs. *P. acnes* utilizes sebum as a substrate and converts it in part to irritant free fatty acids (FFA). *P. acnes* also activates complement pathways to produce at least two chemotactic factors that promote inflammation. (3) An increase in the number of follicular epithelial cells occurs; the cells are cohesive and produce follicular retention hyperkeratosis. The cause of ductal hyperkeratosis is unknown, but the FFAs produced by *P. acnes* may be the primary comedogenic factor responsible. A deficiency in linoleic acid in the sebum may be the cause of the retention hyperkeratosis (Pochi, 1990).

Retention hyperkeratosis, increased amount of sebum, and proliferation of *P. acnes* cause swelling of the follicle and a keratinized plug (comedo) forms. Inflammation occurs when the comedo ruptures into the dermis; a papule, pustule, nodule, or cyst may then develop. The pilosebaceous follicles on the face, neck, chest, shoulders, and back are most commonly involved (Wilson, 1985; Leyden and Shalita, 1986).

Mild acne lesions are characterized by closed and open comedones (comedonal acne); in moderate acne, inflammatory papules and pustules are present (papulopustular acne). In severe acne vulgaris, the primary lesions are pustules, nodules, and inflammatory lesions that may result in subsequent pitting or hypertrophic scars (acne conglobata). Purulent abscesses occur infrequently.

Nondrug Therapy: Some acneiform eruptions are induced by industrial chemicals or drugs, especially corticosteroids, androgens, iodides, bromides, lithium, and androgenic progestins that are components of some oral contraceptives. If oral contraception is required, preparations containing a nonandrogenic progestin should be used (eg, norgestimate, desogestrel). Efforts to limit or avoid these chemicals and drugs, as well as humid environments, may be as important as drug therapy in the treatment of mild to moderate acne.

Although avoiding use of occlusive cosmetic oils and greases is helpful, prolonged and vigorous washing of the affected skin surface does not remove oils or keratinized plugs and will not resolve lesions. Gentle cleansing of affected areas one or two times daily minimizes surface oiliness, but *scrubbing* with or without abrasives creates friction that may damage the delicate hair follicle openings through which sebum must flow.

Dietary factors do not appear to be relevant in acne management.

Comedo extraction and chemosurgery or cryotherapy may be useful in selected patients.

Drug Selection: The objectives in acne therapy include reducing sebum output and follicular retention hyperkeratosis and decreasing the number of *P. acnes* organisms. The extent of follicular hyperkeratosis, occlusion, and inflammation determines therapy.

Mild to Moderate Acne. Numerous nonprescription products of diverse formulation are available for mild acne, including bar soaps, soap-free cakes, liquid cleansers, lotions, gels, and creams. Keratolytics promote peeling and comedolysis; they include sulfur, resorcinol, and salicylic acid. Benzoyl peroxide is useful because of its antibacterial action on *P. acnes* and its mild comedolytic action. Abrasive particles (pumice, aluminum oxide, sodium tetraborate, polyethylene) are often included in the formulation to remove surface debris; however, excessive washing and vigorous scrubbing should be avoided because the condition may be aggravated by shredding the hair shafts (Leyden and Shalita, 1986). Alcohol or acetone also may be present to promote drying, but the efficacy of this drying action has not been determined conclusively, and the effect may be additive to that of other agents that are also drying.

In the FDA's final monograph on topical acne drug products for OTC use (*Federal Register*, 1991 B), the active ingredients included in Category I (safe and effective) are salicylic acid 0.5% to 2%, sulfur 3% to 10%, and a combination of sulfur 3% to 8% with resorcinol 2% or resorcinol monoacetate 3%. In the FDA's published amendment to the tentative final monograph (*Federal Register*, 1991 C), benzoyl peroxide was reclassified from Category I to Category III (more data needed). The efficacy of benzoyl peroxide is not questioned by the FDA, but because benzoyl peroxide was reported to promote skin tumors in mice, additional studies are needed to determine the relevance of this finding for humans.

Moderate to Severe Acne. Useful topical drugs include benzoyl peroxide, tretinoin, and antibiotics.

Some 5% to 10% strengths of benzoyl peroxide lotions and creams are nonprescription products, but most gels are available only by prescription. Tretinoin also is available only by prescription. The gel formulation of this drug is preferred by some dermatologists for inflammatory acne. Benzoyl peroxide and tretinoin have additive drying and irritating actions; therefore, some dermatologists prefer not to use these drugs in combination. However, because benzoyl peroxide and tretinoin have different mechanisms of action, and because acne is a multifactorial disorder, combination therapy with both agents is considered a rational therapeutic approach by other dermatologists. Tretinoin may potentiate the absorption of other topical medications.

Topical clindamycin [Cleocin T], erythromycin [Aknemycin, A/T/S, Emgel, Erycette, EryDerm, Erygel, Erymax, Staticin, T-Stat], and meclocycline sulfosalicylate [Meclan] are employed in the treatment of inflammatory acne, but controlled comparative studies are limited. Topical clindamycin solution was reported to be more effective than topical tetracycline cream in mild to moderate inflammatory facial acne, and the incidence and severity of adverse effects, such as burning, pruritus, erythema, or peeling, were similar (Padilla et al, 1981). Initial controlled short-term studies comparing 2% erythromycin gel with 1% clindamycin solution in moderate acne revealed no difference in efficacy and adverse reactions (Leyden et al, 1987). There is some concern that antibiotic-resistant strains of bacteria may emerge more rapidly with widespread topical antibiotic therapy (Eady et al, 1982), but this does not appear to be a significant problem at present.

Based on the systemic side effects produced and pharmacokinetic data, the amount of clindamycin absorbed topically appears to be relatively small (Rietschel and Duncan, 1983); however, because pseudomembranous colitis has been reported rarely after use of this route, it is recommended that patients with regional enteritis or ulcerative colitis not use topical preparations of clindamycin.

No adequate, well-controlled, teratogenic studies in humans are available; however, in reproductive studies in animals, clindamycin had no adverse effects. It is present in human milk after systemic administration, but its presence after topical administration is unknown.

If inflammation is severe enough to warrant systemic antibiotic therapy, tetracycline is the drug of choice because of its effectiveness, low toxicity, and low cost (Stern et al, 1984). Oral doses of 250 mg two to four times daily may be required initially for severe inflammation. Optimum response generally requires about 12 weeks, and 250 mg twice daily may be necessary for prolonged maintenance therapy. Erythromycin is an acceptable alternative. Oral clindamycin 150 to 450 mg/day is equally effective; however, because pseudomembranous colitis occurs on occasion after oral administration, this drug should only rarely be used systemically for acne.

Bacterial cross resistance between topical clindamycin and erythromycin (but not oral tetracycline) is usually present. Minocycline 50 to 200 mg or doxycycline 100 to 200 mg once daily orally is suggested if clinical resistance develops to topical clindamycin or erythromycin or if the patient complains of gastric irritation after use of tetracycline. A lack of interaction with food and more rapid alleviation of inflammation (Hubbell et al, 1982) are advantages of minocycline and doxycycline compared with tetracycline; however, the latter is much less expensive.

In women, the systemic use of hormonal drugs (antiandrogenic agents or oral contraceptives) should be reserved for those unresponsive to conventional therapy (Cunliffe, 1987).

Severe Acne. The treatment of severe, nodular inflammatory acne usually requires dermatologic consultation and more aggressive therapy. The treatment of choice of recalcitrant acne is isotretinoin [Accutane]; however, *it is contraindicated during pregnancy.* Larger doses of oral tetracycline (2 g/day) can be given to avoid the long-term complications associated with isotretinoin (eg, altered bowel flora; hepatotoxicity; depressed renal function, especially in those with diabetes mellitus; diabetes insipidus; pseudotumor cerebri). Tetracyclines also are contraindicated during pregnancy and may decrease the effectiveness of oral contraceptives used concurrently. Oral or intralesional injection of corticosteroids is another alternative.

BENZOYL PEROXIDE

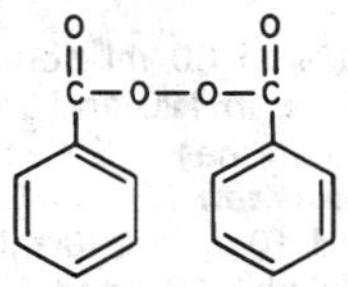

ACTIONS AND USES. Benzoyl peroxide is effective, alone or combined with other appropriate agents (eg, tretinoin, topical antibiotics), in acne vulgaris because of its antibacterial effect. Its bacteriostatic activity against *Propionibacterium acnes* decreases the production of irritant free fatty acids in the follicle. It also has slight keratolytic and mildly comedolytic actions. Benzoyl peroxide is available in untinted or tinted vehicles in concentrations of 2.5% to 10%. Cream, lotion, and gel formulations are available. Gel formulations may be preferable when excessive oiliness is a problem or in warm humid climates where dry skin is less common.

ADVERSE REACTIONS AND PRECAUTIONS. After topical application to the forearm of primates, benzoyl peroxide is absorbed to some extent. Benzoic acid is a major metabolite; however, it is cleared rapidly via the kidney and cumulation does not occur with therapeutic doses (Yeung et al, 1983). Systemic toxicity has not been reported in humans. Some irritation must be accepted, since a dose-response relationship may exist between efficacy and irritation. Contact urticaria and irritation may be severe. Contact hypersensitivity is observed in 1% to 3% of patients under conditions of recommended use. If symptoms are not readily reversible by reducing the frequency of use and dose, the drug should be discontinued.

Benzoyl peroxide should not be applied under an occlusive dressing, because it is a potent experimental contact sensitizer (delayed hypersensitivity), and, in one study in volunteers, a reaction occurred in 70% of subjects after use of occlusive patches containing a 5% or 10% concentration. When hypersensitivity is suspected, patch tests may be performed with a freshly prepared 5% concentration in petrolatum or diluted commercial product.

The potential carcinogenicity of benzoyl peroxide has been questioned by the FDA and the Health Protection Branch in Canada. After initiation with potent aromatic hydrocarbon carcinogens, application of benzoyl peroxide in an acetone vehicle promoted skin tumors in mice. This test is not a routine toxicologic screen, and no correlation between the findings of this short-term test and carcinogenesis in humans has been documented. (For further information, see previous discussion under Drug Selection.)

Benzoyl peroxide is classified in FDA Pregnancy Category C.

DOSAGE AND PREPARATIONS. To avoid severe irritation, the patient should be instructed to limit the volume of material and the frequency of application initially and to increase the amount and duration of contact gradually as tolerance permits. Gels containing acetone or alcohol tend to be more drying.

Topical: The cream or gel is applied twice daily to the affected area.

Liquid Cleanser:
Generic 5% and 10% in 30 ml containers; ***Ben-Aqua Wash*** (Syosset) 5% and 10% in 120 and 240 ml containers; ***Benzac AC Wash*** (Owen/Galderma) 2.5%, 5%, and 10% in 240 ml containers; ***Benzac W Wash*** (Owen/Galderma) 5% in 120 and 240 ml containers and 10% in 240 ml containers; ***Desquam-X Wash*** (Westwood-Squibb) 5% and 10% in 150 ml containers; ***Fostex Benzoyl Peroxide*** (Westwood-Squibb) 10% in 150 ml containers (nonprescription).

Gel (alcohol vehicle):
Generic 5% and 10% in 45 and 120 g containers; ***Benzac 5, 10*** (Galderma) in 60 g containers; ***5-, 10-Benzagel*** (Dermik) in 42 and 85 g containers; ***PanOxyl 5, 10*** (Stiefel) in 60 and 120 g containers.

Gel (without alcohol):
Generic 5% and 10% in 45 g containers; ***Ben-Aqua Gel*** (Syosset) 5% and 10% in 45 and 120 g containers; ***Benzac AC*** (Owen/Galderma) 2.5%, 5%, and 10% in 60 g containers; ***Benzac W 2.5, 5, 10*** (Galderma) in 60 and 90 g containers; ***Desquam-E, Desquam-X 2.5, 5, 10*** (Westwood-Squibb); ***Fostex 5%, 10% BPO*** (Westwood-Squibb) in 45 g containers (nonprescription); ***Neutrogena Acne Mask*** (Neutrogena) 5% in 60 ml containers; ***PanOxyl AQ 2.5%, 5%, 10%*** (Stiefel) in 60 and 120 g containers; ***Persa-Gel W 5%, 10%*** (Ortho) in 45 and 90 g containers; ***Xerac BP 5, 10*** (Person & Covey) in 45 and 90 g containers.

Cleansing Bar:
Fostex Cleansing Bar (Westwood-Squibb) 10% (nonprescription); ***PanOxyl Bar 5, 10*** (Stiefel) (nonprescription).

Cream:
Clearasil (Richardson-Vicks) 10% in 30 g containers; ***Cuticura Acne*** (DEP) 5% in 30 g containers (nonprescription).

Lotion:
Generic 5% and 10% in 30 and 60 ml containers; ***Acne-10*** (Goldline); ***Ben-Aqua 10*** (Syosset) 10% in 30 ml containers; ***Benoxyl 5, 10*** (Stiefel) in 30 and 60 ml containers; ***Clearasil 10%*** (Richardson-Vicks) in 30 ml containers; ***Loroxide*** (Dermik) 5.5% in 25 ml containers; ***Oxy 5, 10*** (SmithKline Beecham) in 30 ml containers; ***Vanoxide*** (Dermik) 5% in 25 and 50 g containers (nonprescription).

Available Mixtures.
Sulfoxyl (Stiefel). Lotion containing benzoyl peroxide 5% and sulfur 2% (Regular) or benzoyl peroxide 10% and sulfur 5% (Strong) in 30 ml containers.
Vanoxide-HC (Dermik). Lotion containing benzoyl peroxide 5% and hydrocortisone 0.5% in 25 g containers.

CLINDAMYCIN PHOSPHATE
[Cleocin T]

ERYTHROMYCIN
[Akne-mycin, A/T/S, Emgel, Erycette, EryDerm, Erygel, Erymax, Staticin, T-Stat]

MECLOCYCLINE SULFOSALICYLATE
[Meclan]

Topical antibiotic therapy is effective in the management of inflammatory acne vulgaris. For further discussion of topical, as well as systemic, antibiotic therapy for acne, see the introduction to this section.

DOSAGE AND PREPARATIONS.

Topical: The preparation is applied twice daily, morning and evening.

CLINDAMYCIN PHOSPHATE:
Cleocin T (Upjohn). Gel 1% in an aqueous vehicle in 30 g containers; lotion 1% in 60 ml containers; solution 1% in a 50% isopropyl alcohol, water, and propylene glycol vehicle in 30 and 60 ml containers.

ERYTHROMYCIN:
Generic. Solution 1.5% and 2% in 60 ml containers.
Akne-mycin (Hermal). Ointment 2% in 25 g containers; solution 2% in a 66% alcohol vehicle in 60 ml containers.
A/T/S (Hoechst Roussel). Gel 2% in a 92% alcohol vehicle in 30 g containers; solution 2% in a 66% alcohol vehicle in 60 ml containers.
Emgel (Glaxo). Gel 2% in 27 and 50 g containers.
Erycette (Ortho). Pledgets 2% in a 66% alcohol vehicle.
EryDerm (Abbott). Solution 2% in a 77% alcohol vehicle in 60 ml containers.
Erygel (Allergan Herbert). Gel 2% in a 92% alcohol vehicle in 30 and 60 g containers.
Erymax (Allergan Herbert). Solution 2% in a 66% alcohol vehicle in 60 and 120 ml containers.
Staticin (Westwood-Squibb). Solution 1.5% in a 55% alcohol vehicle in 60 ml containers.
T-Stat (Westwood-Squibb). Solution 2% in a 71% alcohol vehicle in 60 ml containers; premoistened pads 60/container.

Available Mixture.
Benzamycin (Dermik). Gel containing erythromycin 30 mg and benzoyl peroxide 50 mg/g (after reconstitution) in 23.3 g containers.

MECLOCYCLINE SULFOSALICYLATE:
Meclan (Ortho). Cream 1% in an aqueous (nonalcohol) vehicle in 20 and 45 g containers.

ISOTRETINOIN
[Accutane]

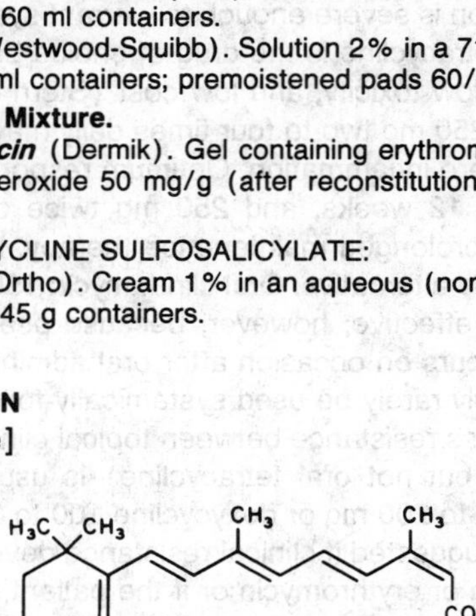

ACTIONS AND USES. ***Nodular or Cystic Inflammatory Acne*** (Acne Conglobata): This *cis* configuration of retinoic (vitamin A) acid is very effective in nodular inflammatory acne. However, because of its potential side effects, use of isotretinoin should be reserved for patients with severe acne who do not respond to or cannot tolerate other therapy (benzoyl peroxide, tretinoin, and topical and systemic antibiotics) (Ward et al, 1984; Millan et al, 1987).

Isotretinoin reduces sebaceous gland cell size, increases separation of pilosebaceous follicular cells, and decreases sebum production. Like other retinoids, isotretinoin also is known to stimulate T-lymphocyte killer cells, enhance tumoricidal effects of macrophages, and inhibit tumor promotion and oncogene expression. These additional actions probably account in part for the wide range of disorders in which the effectiveness of isotretinoin has been explored and validated.

Intensive clinical studies of isotretinoin continue. Data are available for some of the following uses.

Disorders of Keratinization: Prolonged therapy and/or doses larger than those used in acne may be required in some of the following disorders; relapse and retreatment are common (DiGiovanna and Peck, 1983; Ward et al, 1984; Cristofolini et al, 1985): Darier's disease, lamellar ichthyosis, keratosis palmaris et plantaris, erythrokeratodermia variabilis, keratoacanthoma, acantholytic dermatosis (Grover's disease), pityriasis rubra pilaris, and premature sebaceous gland hyperplasia. Less than satisfactory responses were observed in patients with nevus comedonicus, X-linked ichthyosis, and Netherton's syndrome; the latter has worsened following therapy.

Gram-negative Folliculitis: Isotretinoin 0.5 to 1 mg/kg/day for five months is effective in this condition and remissions are often sustained, especially with larger doses (James and Leyden, 1985). An antibacterial action presumably is not responsible. *Staphylococcus aureus* nasal carriage develops in most patients receiving isotretinoin, but colonization has not been a source of significant infection and can be minimized by applying antibiotic ointment (eg, mupirocin) to the anterior inner nares.

Precancerous and Cancerous Disorders: See index entry Isotretinoin, As Antineoplastic Agent.

ADVERSE REACTIONS AND PRECAUTIONS. A status report on all adverse reactions reported to the American Academy of Dermatology has been published (Bigby and Stern, 1988).

Almost all patients experience some of the following reactions: Reversible cheilitis; dry mouth, nose, and skin; skin fragility; epistaxis; conjunctivitis; and pruritus. However, discontinuation of therapy is seldom required. Palmoplantar desquamation and thinning of hair are less common at usual doses (0.5 to 1 mg/kg/day). Inflammation of the urethral meatus may be observed.

Headaches are observed frequently (incidence, 6% to 25%). Because pseudotumor cerebri is infrequently associated with the use of isotretinoin, patients with persistent severe headaches should be examined for papilledema and queried about nausea, vomiting, and visual disturbances. Other less frequent central nervous system signs and symptoms include depression, insomnia, and lethargy. Corneal opacities may be related to long-term use of isotretinoin, especially with large doses (Fraunfelder et al, 1985). Isotretinoin has been associated temporally with inflammatory bowel disease, including regional enteritis, but it has not been shown to be causally related.

Transient elevations in the sedimentation rate and serum levels of ALT and AST have been observed in 40% and 5% to 10% of patients, respectively.

Triglyceride levels are slightly to moderately elevated in approximately 25% of patients treated with 1 mg/kg/day; HDL levels decrease slightly in approximately 15% and cholesterol levels increase slightly in about 7% of patients. Individuals who have diabetes mellitus, are obese, or have a history of excessive alcohol intake and/or a family history of lipid disorders are more susceptible to these effects. The changes are reversible. Monitoring for hyperlipidemia is recommended just before treatment is begun and monthly or bimonthly thereafter, particularly if a known risk factor is present, until the lipid response is established. Peak lipid responses usually are evident after four weeks in men, but may not be observed for 12 weeks in women (Bershad et al, 1985). These elevations are related to the isotretinoin blood concentration rather than the dose, and individuals with high or borderline high serum lipids (eg, triglycerides) >700 mg) or those with pre-existing hypertriglyceridemia are most susceptible.

Onset of arthralgias or muscular pain has been observed in 15% to 20% of patients.

Less than 10% of patients may have hyperuricemia, elevated serum glucose, increased creatine phosphokinase, proteinuria or microscopic or gross hematuria, and a macular erythematous rash.

Skeletal hyperostosis has occurred 4 to 24 months after isotretinoin (mean dose equal to 2.24 mg/kg/day) was administered for chronic disorders of keratinization other than severe acne. Premature closure of the epiphyses has been noted rarely in children receiving long-term high-dose therapy.

One instance of thrombocytopenia verified by rechallenge has been reported (Johnson and Rapini, 1987).

PREGNANCY. Isotretinoin is teratogenic; its placement in FDA Pregnancy Category X signifies that the risk of using this drug during pregnancy clearly outweighs the benefits. Congenital abnormalities include hydrocephalus, microcephaly, microtia, agenesis of the ear canals, conotruncal malformations of the heart, aortic arch atresia, ventricular septal defects, facial dysmorphism, microphthalmos, micrognathia, and cleft palate (*MMWR*, 1984; Lammer et al, 1985). Individuals receiving isotretinoin should not donate blood during treatment and for 30 days after treatment ends to avoid a possible teratogenic effect in pregnant recipients.

Isotretinoin must not be used by females who are pregnant, and women of childbearing potential should not receive isotretinoin until pregnancy is excluded by negative results of a sensitive urine or serum pregnancy test within two weeks prior to initiating therapy and abstinence is practiced or two reliable forms of contraception are used for at least one month before, during, and one month after discontinuation of therapy. The one-month period following termination of therapy appears adequate based on the following study. In 88 women who subsequently became pregnant within 3 to 60 days following their last dose of isotretinoin, the incidence rates of spontaneous abortion or congenital malformations were not significantly different from the rates reported for women of reproductive age in the general population (Dai et al, 1992).

Isotretinoin therapy should begin on the second or third day of a normal menstrual period. Patients should be counseled on the risk to the fetus if pregnancy occurs during treatment and on the desirability of continuing any such pregnancy.

Great concern exists about the numbers of deformed infants who have been born to mothers exposed to isotretinoin during pregnancy (Rosa, 1987; Hogan et al, 1988; Committee on Drugs, 1992). The reasons attributed to the occurrence of this phenomenon are especially disconcerting. Although the teratogenic effect of isotretinoin is entirely preventable, survey data disclosed that 33% of women reported using no method of contraception during isotretinoin therapy. Which cause(s) is primary (ie, patient acquisition of another's medication, physician or pharmacist unwillingness to inform patients about this serious side effect of the drug, inappropriate prescribing by the physician, contraceptive failure) is largely unknown.

To minimize this problem, the FDA has established the following measures: Isotretinoin is to be dispensed only in blister packs with the patient warning included as a part of the package itself along with a representative illustration of an infant with the characteristic visible external deformities caused by the teratogenic action of isotretinoin. In addition, the nonpregnancy pictograph is to be displayed prominently on the package. Furthermore, labeling for physicians states that isotretinoin should be prescribed only by physicians who have special competence in the diagnosis and treatment of severe, recalcitrant acne and who understand the risk of teratogenicity. It also states that isotretinoin is contraindicated in women of childbearing potential unless all of the following conditions apply: (1) the patient has severe, scarring nodular inflammatory acne that is recalcitrant to standard therapies; (2) the patient is reliable in understanding and carrying out instructions; (3) the patient is capable of complying with the mandatory contraceptive measures; (4) the patient has received both oral and written warnings of the hazards of pregnancy and the risks of contraceptive failure and has acknowledged these in writing; and (5) the patient has had a urine or serum pregnancy test with a negative result within two weeks of initiating therapy. The manufacturer recommends monthly pregnancy tests as well during drug treatment.

Physicians are urged to report exposures in pregnant women to the manufacturer by calling 800/526-6367. Arrangements for analyses of abortuses can be made by contacting the Epidemiology Development Branch, Division of Drugs and Biologics Experience, FDA, Rockville, MD. 20852 or the Department of Environmental and Drug-Induced Pathology, Armed Forces Institute of Pathology, Washington, DC, 20306; telephone (202) 576-2434.

PHARMACOKINETICS. The maximum blood concentration occurs one to four hours after oral administration; the presence of food may double the amount absorbed. Isotretinoin is nearly 100% bound to plasma albumin at all therapeutic concentrations.

A major metabolite, 4-oxo-isotretinoin, is formed and then is glucuronidated and excreted via the biliary tract. Enterohepatic circulation occurs in some individuals.

Isotretinoin has a mean elimination half-life of 10 hours in patients with nodular inflammatory acne, and this value did not change significantly following use of 40 mg twice daily for 25 days. The mean half-life of isotretinoin in patients with keratinizing disorders was about 16 hours, while that of its metabolite, 4-oxo-isotretinoin, was 29 hours (Brazzell et al, 1983). The manufacturer reports that the terminal elimination half-life ranged from 10 to 20 hours in volunteers and patients. Negligible amounts of the parent compound are excreted in the urine. Approximately equal amounts of radioactivity are recovered in urine and feces.

DOSAGE AND PREPARATIONS. *See the warning in the Pregnancy section of this evaluation.* Topical agents, such as benzoyl peroxide, sulfur, and tretinoin, should be discontinued before starting isotretinoin therapy because they potentiate the drying effect of isotretinoin. Oral tetracycline and minocycline also should be discontinued because of an increased risk for the development of pseudotumor cerebri. Vitamin A supplements should not be taken concomitantly.

Oral: For most *adults,* the initial dose for nodular inflammatory acne should be 0.5 to 1 mg/kg given in two divided doses daily for 15 to 20 weeks. Patients whose disease is very severe or is manifested primarily on the trunk instead of the face may require the maximum recommended dose of 2 mg/kg/day. Although lower doses (0.1 up to 0.5 mg/kg) may be effective and side effects are not markedly different in frequency or severity than with larger doses, relapses are reported to be more common and occur sooner.

If the total nodule or cyst count has been reduced by more than 70% before 15 to 20 weeks have elapsed, the drug may be discontinued. Improvement usually continues for six months after the first course is terminated. Occasionally an exaggerated healing response manifested by profuse granulation tissue with crusting is noted. A second course may be initiated if warranted by significant recurrence or persistent severe nodular inflammatory acne.

Accutane (Roche). Capsules 10, 20, and 40 mg.

TRETINOIN

[Retin-A]

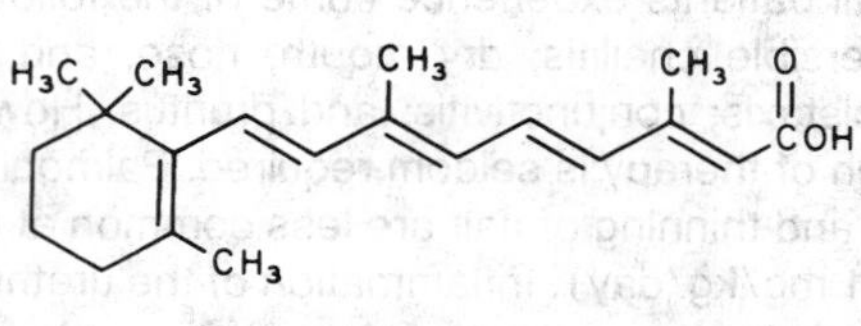

ACTIONS AND USES. ***Acne:*** This retinoid is an all *trans* configuration of retinoic acid (vitamin A acid) used topically to treat acne vulgaris. Tretinoin decreases cohesiveness of the follicular epithelial cells and increases epidermal cell mitosis and cell turnover. It has been suggested that increased turnover of follicular epithelium prevents blockage by keratinous plugs and extrudes existing microcomedones. Acne may be aggravated during the first six weeks of therapy, but good results are noted after three or four months in most patients. Tretinoin also thins the stratum corneum, which enhances the penetration of other topical agents.

Topical tretinoin has been evaluated in more than 40 specific dermatologic disorders, diseases, or conditions. It has varying effectiveness in disorders of altered keratinization (eg, acneiform, ichthyosiform, psoriasiform, infectious, and other inflammatory disorders; keloids and hypertrophic scars; mucocutaneous pigmentation; and premalignant and malignant disorders) (Haas and Arndt, 1986).

Topical tretinoin has reversed some of the clinical and histologic signs of photoaging. Although its topical application does not affect natural aging of the skin, it can improve the appearance of the skin during the period of its use when premature aging is caused primarily by excessive exposure to the sun, especially in those with extensive damage (helicodermatitis). Epidermal thickness and vascularity and compaction of the stratum corneum increase, melanocyte hypertrophy and hyperplasia diminish, and fading of hyperpigmentation (mottling) is enhanced (Weiss et al, 1988; Rafal et al, 1992; Kligman, 1992 A, 1992 B). This drug is not a substitute for a face lift, chemical peel, or dermabrasion nor does it decrease the risk of sun-induced skin cancer. Education by the physician and understanding and acceptance by the patient of the therapeutic program are essential. Cosmetic benefit depends on the patient's compliance; realistic expectations; acceptance of side effects such as irritation (especially in those with Type I skin); avoidance of irritants such as toners, astringents, fragrances and perfumes, harsh soaps, peelers, and cleansers; avoidance of excessive intake of vitamin A; proper use of moisturizing creams or petroleum jelly preparations that do not contain additives; and use of sunscreens to prevent further actinic damage. Treatment may be initiated with low concentrations or alternate-day dosing; the amount of drug is then increased or the dosage interval is reduced, as tolerated. Three to four months of therapy are required for noticeable improvement in the skin, and 8 to 12 months are required for maximum benefit. When therapy is discontinued after one year, histologic benefit may continue, but cosmetic improvement will diminish.

The usefulness of topical tretinoin to reverse photoaging remains controversial (Green et al, 1993). Results obtained in unblinded, open label, and short-term controlled studies require confirmation by long-term controlled studies. Both improvement and adverse reactions appear to be dose dependent. Only a few dermatologic authorities conclude that tretinoin is an adequate treatment for photoaging and the FDA has not approved the drug for this indication. Prevention of photoaging by ensuring proper skin protection is the most desirable approach.

ADVERSE REACTIONS AND PRECAUTIONS. Tretinoin is irritating, even if it is used correctly. Patient sensitivity varies. Initially, once-nightly application or alternate-day therapy and minimizing exposure to the sun or sunlamps will help to reduce irritation. Within 24 to 48 hours, the skin may become red and begin to peel. If this occurs, therapy should be discontinued and resumed only at lower doses and with less frequent applications.

Tretinoin should not be used on eczematous skin. Contact with the corners of the mouth, nose, eyes, or mucous membranes and the number of face washings (which should be gentle) should be limited to minimize skin irritation.

Commercially available formulations of tretinoin penetrate the skin but do not cause systemic toxicity. Contact sensitization has been noted only rarely. An appropriate patch test concentration (0.1% in cream) can be obtained from the manufacturer.

Tretinoin is classified in FDA Pregnancy Category C. No documented cases of human teratogenicity due to tretinoin have occurred, but some authorities recommend its avoidance during pregnancy.

DOSAGE AND PREPARATIONS.
Topical: *Acne.* Use of sunscreens after treatment is recommended. The patient should be instructed to avoid concomitant use of keratolytic preparations (eg, sulfur, resorcinol, salicylic acid) and abrasive soaps except as directed by the physician. Initially, a small section of the involved area may be chosen for treatment. Thereafter, one application nightly or on alternate days to the entire area involved is usually sufficient. The preparation should be applied to dry skin, preferably 15 to 30 minutes after washing. The amount, frequency of application, and dosage form should be individualized to minimize irritation while maintaining effective comedolytic action. The liquid preparation generally is more irritating.

Photoaging. One hour before bedtime, the face should be washed with a mild cleanser (eg, Purpose, Dove, Neutrogena) and patted dry. Initially, a pea-sized amount of the 0.025% cream formulation is applied to the forehead and then gently rubbed over the entire face. No moisturizing agents should be applied for at least one hour after use of tretinoin. If tolerance develops, a stronger concentration may be used. After one year of therapy, two or three applications weekly are adequate for maintenance. Other areas of involvement are treated similarly.

Retin-A (Ortho). Cream 0.025%, 0.05%, and 0.1% in 20 and 45 g containers; gel 0.01% and 0.025% in 15 and 45 g containers (alcohol 90%); liquid 0.05% in 28 ml containers (alcohol 55%).

PIGMENTATION DISORDERS

Hydroquinone [Eldoquin, Melanex], a skin bleaching agent, is applied topically to treat localized macules of *hyperpigmentation,* such as freckles, lentigines, postinflammatory states, and melasma due to pregnancy or oral contraceptives.

Acquired localized disorders of *hypopigmentation* include pityriasis alba and vitiligo, which are characterized by loss of melanocytes, or depigmentation, which is caused by infection or inflammation following bullae, burns, atrophy, or scarring of the skin. Congenital diffuse hypopigmentation or depigmentation (ie, albinism) is distinguished by the presence of melanocytes that lack tyrosinase, the enzyme that produces melanin.

Oral or topical use of the psoralen compounds, trioxsalen or methoxsalen, with subsequent exposure to UVA radiation (photochemotherapy), stimulates melanin synthesis and repigmentation in about one-third of patients; those with albinism are unaffected. If a large proportion of the body surface is affected, it may be easier to lessen or irreversibly destroy the pigmentation of nonvitiliginous areas with monobenzone [Benoquin] provided the patient agrees. If the vitiliginous area is less than 60 cm^2, topical rather than oral administration of the psoralens can be considered.

5-Methoxypsoralen (5-MOP), available for use in Austria and France, has been investigated in open studies as an alternative to methoxsalen (8-methoxypsoralen, 8-MOP). Compared with methoxsalen, this agent is reported to be well tolerated and causes fewer gastrointestinal side effects and pronounced phototoxic reactions without apparent loss of efficacy (Tanew et al, 1988).

HYDROQUINONE

[Eldoquin, Melanex]

ACTIONS AND USES. The skin bleaching agent, hydroquinone, acts by decreasing the proliferative and melanin synthesizing activity of melanocytes. It inhibits tyrosinase in melanocytes, which depresses melanin synthesis, melanin granule formation, and melanocyte growth.

Hydroquinone may decrease cutaneous hyperpigmentation when applied topically in various localized conditions, such as freckles, lentigines, postinflammatory states, and melasma due to pregnancy or oral contraceptives. The decrease in hyperpigmentation is often slow. It is best achieved with a 3% to 4% concentration of hydroquinone in combination with 0.01% to 0.05% tretinoin. Since sunlight darkens the lesions and offsets the bleaching action of hydroquinone, the regular use of a sunscreen with a sun protective factor of at least 15 is recommended during the day. For convenience, sunscreens are present in the formulation of some hydroquinone preparations.

ADVERSE REACTIONS AND PRECAUTIONS. High concentrations of hydroquinone may cause exogenous ochronosis (pseudo-ochronosis) with continuous use and even the 2% preparation has been associated with the development of this adverse reaction (Williams, 1992). No other serious untoward effects have been reported. Tingling or burning on application with subsequent erythema and inflammation was reported in 8% of patients when a 2% concentration of hydroquinone was used and in 32% when a 5% concentration was used. Topical hydrocortisone may be applied to alleviate inflammation. Severe inflammation may result in marked pigmentation.

Allergic contact dermatitis occurs far less frequently than irritation; a 1% concentration of hydroquinone in petrolatum can be obtained from the manufacturer and is suitable for patch testing. Contact with the eyes should be avoided. Some clinicians prefer to limit the extent of the initial application of hydroquinone to minimize liability in case of a severe allergic reaction.

Hydroquinone is classified in FDA Pregnancy Category C.

DOSAGE AND PREPARATIONS.

Topical: *Adults and adolescents over 12 years,* the preparation is applied to the involved areas twice daily for six to eight weeks. A longer duration is required for the treatment of melasma. A sunscreen also should be applied during the day on areas that cannot easily be protected from exposure to the sun to prevent recurrence of hyperpigmentation.

For especially resistant cases, a formula composed of hydroquinone 2% and tretinoin 0.05% to 0.1% in hydrophilic ointment or equal parts of alcohol and propylene glycol can be compounded and is applied twice daily for 6 to 12 weeks (Pathak et al, 1984; Arndt, 1989).

Generic. Powder.

Eldoquin (ICN). Cream 2% (nonprescription) or 4% (***Forte***) in 15 and 30 g containers; lotion 2% (nonprescription) in 15 ml containers.

Melanex (Neutrogena). Solution 3% in 30 ml containers.

Available Mixtures.

HYDROQUINONE AND SUNSCREENS:

Eldopaque (ICN). Cream containing hydroquinone 2% (nonprescription) or 4% ***(Forte)*** in a talc opaque base in 15 and 30 g containers.

Porcelana with Sunscreen (DEP). Cream containing hydroquinone 2% with octyl dimethyl PABA 2.5% in 120 g containers (nonprescription).

Solaquin (ICN). Cream containing hydroquinone 2% (nonprescription) or 4% ***(Forte)*** with ethyl dihydroxypropyl PABA 5%, dioxybenzone 3%, and oxybenzone 2% in 15 (4% only) and 30 g containers; gel containing hydroquinone 4% ***(Forte)*** with ethyl dihydroxypropyl PABA 5% and dioxybenzone 3% in 15 and 30 g containers.

MONOBENZONE

[Benoquin]

Monobenzone is the monobenzyl ether of hydroquinone. Its action is similar to that of hydroquinone except that extensive selective destruction of melanocytes also occurs. Monobenzone causes irreversible depigmentation and is used to remove the few remaining areas of normal pigmentation in patients with vitiligo covering a large portion of the body. Patient consent should be obtained for achieving total depigmentation.

ADVERSE REACTIONS AND PRECAUTIONS. The adverse effects are similar to those caused by hydroquinone, except that the incidence of sensitization is higher.

Monobenzone therapy is often difficult to manage and requires supervision by a physician knowledgeable in its use and careful patient follow-up; bizarre patterns of hypopigmentation may occur at sites distant from the area of application. Alternative management programs should be considered before monobenzone is tried in the treatment of vitiligo, ie, continuous sunscreen protection, psoralen compounds, masking preparations (eg, Covermark Cream), staining-type cosmetics (eg, Vitadye).

Monobenzone is classified in FDA Pregnancy Category C.

DOSAGE AND PREPARATIONS.

Topical: *Adults and adolescents over 12 years,* the preparation is applied to the involved areas twice daily for three to nine months. A sunscreen also should be applied during the day on areas that cannot easily be protected from exposure to the sun.

Benoquin (ICN). Cream 20% in 37.5 g containers.

METHOXSALEN

[Oxsoralen, Oxsoralen-Ultra]

USES. Methoxsalen is administered topically to treat small vitiliginous lesions. A 0.1% concentration of the drug is applied to small macules ranging from 6 to 60 cm^2; the area is subsequently exposed to sunlight or UVA radiation (320 to 400 nm) (photochemotherapy). Oral administration may be considered for larger areas of involvement. Otherwise, it may be easier to lessen or destroy the pigmentation of nonvitiliginous areas with monobenzone. Both topical and oral methoxsalen therapy should be supervised closely by the physician.

ADVERSE REACTIONS AND PRECAUTIONS. Methoxsalen usually is contraindicated in patients with diseases associated with photosensitivity (eg, porphyria, acute systemic lupus erythematosus, hydroa). Other photosensitizing drugs (eg, phenothiazines, tar) should be administered with caution. If overdose occurs, an emetic should be considered, and the patient should remain in a darkened room for eight hours or until cutaneous reactions subside.

Topical: High concentrations of topical methoxsalen and overexposure to UVA radiation can cause toxic reactions (severe erythema and blistering). Therefore, methoxsalen must be diluted to 1:10,000 or 1:1,000 and the exposure dose of UVA radiation carefully controlled.

Oral: Gastric discomfort occasionally follows oral administration of psoralens and is minimized by giving the drug with milk or meals. To protect the eyes and lips, blue-grey sunglasses (with side shields to prevent reflected radiation) opaque to UVA radiation and a light-screening lip balm should be used for 24 or preferably 48 hours after drug ingestion. A cataractogenic action has been established, but this hazard may be avoided if appropriate sunglasses are used. See the discussion on Photochemotherapy in the section on Psoriasis for discussion of the potential cataractogenic and carcinogenic actions of the psoralens.

Both forms of methoxsalen are classified in FDA Pregnancy Category C.

PHARMACOKINETICS. In normal individuals, an oral dose of methoxsalen is variably absorbed (65% to 95%). Time to peak plasma concentration is one to four hours. The duration of photosensitizing action is about ten hours. The terminal elimination half-life is about two hours. Methoxsalen is metabolized in the liver, and more than 90% of a single dose is excreted in the urine within 12 hours. Accumulation has not been observed in those with normal renal function.

Oral methoxsalen has been reformulated from a crystalline [Oxsoralen] to a liquid preparation in a soft gelatin capsule [Oxsoralen-Ultra]. A greater proportion of patients have achieved a good clinical result with the new formulation because it is more rapidly and reliably absorbed; however, an increase in the frequency of nausea and other gastrointestinal complaints has been observed (Lowe et al, 1987).

DOSAGE AND PREPARATIONS. This treatment should be given under the supervision of physicians experienced in photochemotherapy.

Topical: For vitiliginous lesions 6 to 60 cm^2, low concentrations are applied to the affected area (50 to 200 mcg/in^2) on alternate days. Most physicians begin with a 0.1% concentration because of the strong potential for blister formation. The surrounding normal skin is protected by a sunscreen. After 30 to 45 minutes, the treated area is exposed to a UVA radiation source with careful measurement of the dosage and length of UVA exposure. The lesions are then washed with soap and water, and a sunscreen is applied. Direct sunlight should be avoided. The duration of exposure is increased gradually but should not exceed one-half the minimal erythemal dose. Oxsoralen lotion should never be dispensed directly to the patient for home application without adequate instructions for use and information on precautions.

Oxsoralen (ICN). Lotion 1% in 30 ml containers.

Oral: *Adults and children over 12 years,* for repigmentation of idiopathic vitiligo, 0.4 to 0.5 mg/kg as a single dose 75 minutes before exposure to UVA radiation. Patients with brown or black skin can receive 40 mg/day (0.6 mg/kg). UVA exposure should be calculated carefully and phototoxicity testing performed periodically; exposure time is based on the number of joules required. The risk of severe burn to the vitiliginous skin is considerable with methoxsalen. Sunlight exposure also must be limited (see the manufacturer's literature for suggested time limitations), and sunscreens, appropriate sunglasses, and light-screening lip balm must be employed for 24 to 48 hours after exposure to UVA radiation (see Precautions). Oxsoralen capsules should never be dispensed directly to the patient for home use without adequate instructions for use and information on precautions.

Oxsoralen-Ultra (ICN). Capsules 10 mg.

TRIOXSALEN

[Trisoralen]

USES. Trioxsalen, a psoralen derivative, is used for repigmentation of vitiliginous areas and to increase tolerance to sunlight in sun-sensitive individuals (see Table 1 in the following chapter on Dermatologic Therapy: Prophylactic Agents and Vehicles). Tolerance of the skin to ultraviolet radiation is enhanced by increasing pigmentation and, possibly, by thickening of the stratum corneum; therefore, administration of trioxsalen must be followed in approximately two hours by exposure to sunlight or, in expert hands, to long-wave ultraviolet radiation (320 to 400 nm [UVA]). This regimen of trioxsalen and radiation exposure is potentially dangerous to patients with fair skin, for they are more likely to develop keratoses, keratoacanthoma, and basal and squamous cell carcinomas.

ADVERSE REACTIONS. Extensive clinical experience with short-term administration indicates that trioxsalen has minimal toxicity. Gastric discomfort occurs occasionally but can be minimized by taking the medication with food.

See the discussion on Photochemotherapy in the section on Psoriasis for discussion of the potential cataractogenic and carcinogenic actions of the psoralens.

PRECAUTIONS. Since photoprotection develops gradually during multiple treatment sessions, patients are most susceptible to sunburn during initial treatment. Therefore, the dosage and length of exposure to the sun must be controlled closely to prevent injury to the skin. To protect eyes and lips, blue-gray plastic sunglasses (with side shields) opaque to UVA radiation and a visible light-screening lip balm should be used during exposure and for at least 24 and preferably 48 hours following administration. If overdosage occurs, the patient should remain in a darkened room for eight hours or until cutaneous reactions subside.

Trioxsalen is contraindicated in patients with diseases associated with photosensitivity, such as porphyria (porphyria cutanea tarda and erythropoietic porphyria), discoid or systemic lupus erythematosus, and xeroderma pigmentosum. Other photosensitizing drugs (eg, phenothiazines) should be employed cautiously when concomitant use is necessary.

DOSAGE AND PREPARATIONS.

Oral: *Adults and children over 12 years,* to increase tolerance to sunlight, the daily dose usually should not exceed 10 mg (2 tablets), and the total dosage should not exceed 28 tablets on a continuous or interrupted regimen. Trioxsalen is a potent sun-sensitizing agent, and the physician should carefully instruct the patient to adhere to the prescribed dosage schedule and procedure. Graduated, measured, daily exposures to sunlight or UVA radiation should occur two to three hours after ingestion of the tablets. See the manufacturer's literature for suggested time limitations of sun exposure and the section on Precautions for eye and lip protection.

For large lesions of vitiligo (the potential for producing a severe burn is considerable; caution and consultation are advised), 0.6 mg/kg daily is given two or three times a week two hours before exposure to 10 to 15 minutes of mid-day sunlight or UVA radiation. Exposure is increased by 5 to 10 minutes per treatment until a mild erythema develops 24 to 36 hours after exposure that becomes maximal at 48 hours. During exposure to solar radiation, the patient should be in the prone or supine position and should change position at the midpoint of the exposure time. If the desired result is not obtained after a total of 60 minutes of exposure, the dose of trioxsalen is increased by 10-mg increments to a maximum of 80 mg daily. When it occurs, repigmentation, especially on the face and neck, is usually evident after three to four months of treatment. Since few patients benefit from longer use, therapy should be discontinued if results are not significant after four months.

Trioxsalen tablets should never be dispensed without adequate instructions for use and information on precautions; the potential for producing a severe burn is considerable.

See the Precautions section for eye and lip protection.

Trisoralen (ICN). Tablets 5 mg.

ACTINIC DAMAGE

The cytotoxic agents, fluorouracil [Efudex, Fluoroplex] and masoprocol [Actinex], are used to treat actinic (solar) keratoses. For discussion on use of sunscreen preparations, see that section in the following chapter. For use of tretinoin to treat photoaging, see index entry, Tretinoin.

FLUOROURACIL

[Efudex, Fluoroplex]

For chemical formula, see index entry Fluorouracil, As Antineoplastic Agent.

ACTIONS AND USES. This cytotoxic drug is used topically to remove multiple premalignant actinic keratoses; curettage or cryotherapy is preferred for isolated lesions (Bennett et al, 1985). A 1% concentration often is adequate for the face and forehead; higher concentrations may produce severe inflammation in these areas. Lesions on the hands and arms may require higher concentrations and longer treatment periods. Although the inflammatory response may be lessened by limiting the area of initial application, the ultimate effectiveness of treatment is related to the inflammatory response and duration of therapy.

The healing process may continue for one to two months after therapy ceases; restoration of skin color and texture is usually satisfactory.

Fluorouracil acts selectively against atypical rapidly proliferating epidermal cells by inhibiting DNA and RNA synthesis. Even lesions that are not grossly visible respond; for this reason, fluorouracil should be applied to the entire affected area. The drug has less effect on normal epidermis unless occlusive dressings are used.

For other uses of fluorouracil, see index entry Fluorouracil.

ADVERSE REACTIONS AND PRECAUTIONS. Systemic reactions are uncommon after topical use. Pruritus and irritation are the most common adverse reactions. Intense burning pain is reported occasionally. The frequency of severe discomfort can be reduced by careful determination of dosage and instruction of patients. Before therapy is initiated, the patient should be informed that inflammation will develop and is a necessary part of therapy. Discoloration of skin may develop.

If there is excessive inflammation of normal skin, treatment should be discontinued. Fluorouracil should be applied with care to sensitive areas (eg, around the eyes, nasolabial folds). Exposure to sunlight during and for one or two months following treatment should be avoided or minimized by use of sunscreens.

Based on systemic administration, fluorouracil is classified in FDA Pregnancy Category X.

DOSAGE AND PREPARATIONS. Commercial preparations are available in a variety of concentrations and vehicles. Solutions in propylene glycol are more active than creams containing equivalent concentrations of the drug. Fluorouracil should only be prescribed by physicians qualified by training and experience in its use. Patch test kits to determine hypersensitivity can be obtained from the manufacturer.

Topical: Fluorouracil is applied twice daily for two to four weeks. When the inflammatory response reaches the stage of erosion, necrosis, and ulceration, treatment may be terminated or the frequency of application may be reduced in accordance with the intensity of the response. If allergic reactions are not severe, the drug can be applied every three to seven days to maintain the therapeutic effect.

If indicated, post-treatment irritation may be treated with topical corticosteroids.

Efudex (Roche). Cream 5% in 25 g containers; solution 2% and 5% with propylene glycol in 10 ml containers.

Fluoroplex (Allergan Herbert). Cream 1% in 30 g containers; solution 1% with propylene glycol in 30 ml containers.

MASOPROCOL
[Actinex]

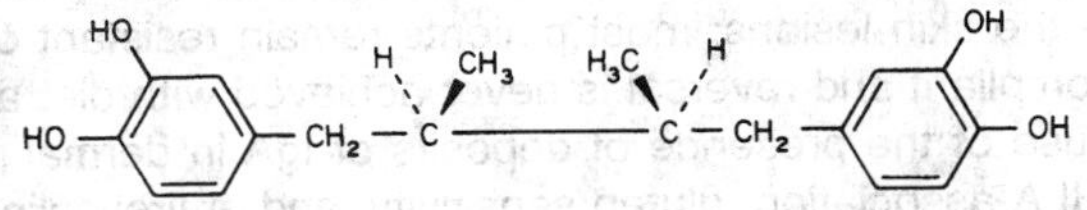

ACTIONS AND USES. Masoprocol, a 5-lipoxygenase inhibitor with antimicrobial and antineoplastic actions, is used topically for premalignant actinic (solar) keratoses. Its antineoplastic actions are probably not responsible for its efficacy in actinic keratoses; however, this has not been definitely established. In one controlled study in 154 patients, a significant mean decrease in lesions from 9.6 ± 5.6 was reported for masoprocol and 2.3 ± 3.7 for the vehicle after application for 28 days; the median percentage of reduction was 71.4% for masoprocol and 4.3% for the vehicle (Olsen et al, 1991). Unlike fluorouracil, the irritation produced by masoprocol does not correlate with efficacy.

ADVERSE REACTIONS AND PRECAUTIONS. The most common adverse reaction is irritation manifested by erythema (46%) and flaking (46%). Pruritus (32%), dryness (27%), edema (14%), burning (12%), and soreness (5%) also occur. Most of these reactions resolve within two weeks after the drug is discontinued.

Masoprocol-induced sensitization (ie, allergic contact dermatitis) developed in 9% of individuals tested; the drug should be discontinued if sensitivity is noted. Cross sensitivity does not occur between masoprocol and fluorouracil; thus, if sensitivity develops to one drug, the other can be tried.

Masoprocol should never be used under occlusive dressings. When the drug is applied with the fingers, the hands should be washed after application. If the cream inadvertently comes into contact with the eye, the eye should immediately be washed out with water. Masoprocol may stain fabrics.

PREGNANCY. In rabbits and rats, topical doses 6 and 16 times the human dose did not produce teratogenic effects. No adequate controlled studies in women are available (FDA Pregnancy Category B). No data are available on whether the drug is excreted in breast milk.

PHARMACOKINETICS. Based on studies of carbon 14-labeled drug in humans, skin absorption was limited to no more than 1% to 2%.

DOSAGE AND PREPARATIONS.

Topical: The skin is washed and dried, and the cream is gently and evenly massaged into affected areas; the eyes and mucous membranes of the nose and mouth should be avoided. The application is repeated morning and evening for 28 days. Occlusive dressings should not be used.

Actinex (Reed & Carnrick). Cream 10% in 30 g containers.

DRUGS USED FOR MISCELLANEOUS CONDITIONS

Antipruritics and Topical Anesthetics

For moderately extensive dermatitic eruptions, application of an agent with anti-inflammatory activity in an appropriate vehicle or a local antipruritic agent in a lotion or cream formulation (eg, menthol 0.25% to 2%, phenol 0.5% to 1.5%, camphor 1% to 3%) usually relieves pruritus and/or pain and avoids the use of topical anesthetics.

The central sedating actions of the first-generation H_1 histamine antagonists or benzodiazepines may be beneficial for more common pruritic dermatoses (eg, dermatitis, psoriasis, lichen planus) in which pruritus is unrelated to peripheral histamine release. Oral nonsedating second-generation H_1 antihistamines, such as astemizole [Hismanal] and terfenadine [Seldane], are effective only when pruritus is due to peripheral release of histamine (eg, wheal reactions of urticaria and dermographism). See also index entry Antihistamines.

Certain antihistamines have local anesthetic activity when applied to mucocutaneous and abraded cutaneous areas, but, because of the risk of allergic contact dermatitis, systemic rather than topical administration is advisable for pruritus.

Topical local anesthetics may be useful in selected disorders affecting mucous membranes, mucocutaneous junctions, and abraded inflamed skin (eg, aphthous stomatitis, oral or anogenital herpes simplex lesions) and for pain caused by cytotoxic therapy for anal and genital warts. They are rarely useful in nonspecific pruritus ani and vulvae and may be sensitizing.

Numerous nonprescription topical mixtures containing a local anesthetic (most commonly, benzocaine) and usually an antiseptic are available for sunburn but they often are ineffective, probably because the concentration of anesthetic is too low and penetration is poor even on sunburned skin. At least a 10% concentration of benzocaine, and probably 20%, usually is necessary on burned skin.

The selection of a topical local anesthetic is based on its availability in a suitable vehicle (ie, solution, viscous solution, jelly, cream, ointment), the patient's prior history of sensitization, and the desired duration of action. Dibucaine may have the longest duration of action (two to four hours). Most topical local anesthetics are available without prescription. In the listing below, they are divided into amide, ester, and miscellaneous (nonamide and nonester) categories for selection in cases of known sensitivity.

Erythema, urticaria, edema, or other manifestations of allergy may develop during use of a topical local anesthetic. These reactions are common even during short-term therapy, especially when used for leg ulcers in elderly patients. These drugs should be used cautiously in patients with allergies or a strong family history of allergy. See also index entry Anesthetics, Local.

Rectal formulations containing local anesthetics are available for relief of symptoms associated with anorectal disorders (see index entry Anorectal Preparations).

AMIDE LOCAL ANESTHETICS.

DIBUCAINE:
Generic. Cream and ointment 1% (nonprescription).
Nupercainal (CIBA). Cream 0.5% in 45 g containers; ointment 1% in 30 and 60 g containers (both forms nonprescription).

LIDOCAINE:
Generic. Ointment 5%; solution 2% (viscous) and 4%.
Xylocaine (Astra). Liquid 5% in 30 ml containers; ointment 2.5% (nonprescription) and 5% in 35 g containers; solution 2% (viscous) in 100 and 450 ml containers and 4% in 50 ml containers; jelly 2% in 30 g containers; oral spray 10% in 60 ml containers.

AMINOBENZOATE ESTER LOCAL ANESTHETICS.

BENZOCAINE:
Generic. Cream 5% (nonprescription).
Americaine (Ciba). Aerosol 20% in 20, 60, and 120 g containers (nonprescription); ointment 20% in 22.5 g containers (nonprescription).
Americaine Anesthetic (Fisons). Gel lubricant 20% in 30 g containers.
Orabase-B (Colgate Hoyt/Gel-Kam). Oral gel 20% in 5 and 15 g containers.

BUTAMBEN PICRATE:
Butesin Picrate (Abbott). Ointment 1% in 30 g containers (nonprescription).

TETRACAINE:
Pontocaine (Sanofi Winthrop). Cream (as hydrochloride) 1% and ointment 0.5% in 30 g containers (both forms nonprescription); solution 0.5% in 15 ml containers and 2% in 30 and 120 ml containers.

NONAMIDE AND NONAMINOBENZOATE ESTER LOCAL ANESTHETICS.

BENZYL ALCOHOL:
Topic (Syntex). Gel 5% in 60 g containers (nonprescription).

DYCLONINE HYDROCHLORIDE:
Dyclone (Astra). Solution 0.5% and 1% in 30 ml containers.

PRAMOXINE HYDROCHLORIDE:
PrameGel (GenDerm). Gel 1% in 120 ml containers (nonprescription).
Tronolane (Ross Consumer). Cream 1% in 30 and 60 g containers (nonprescription).
Tronothane (Abbott). Cream 1% in 30 g containers (nonprescription).

Protectant

COLLODION

This mixture of pyroxylin, ether, and alcohol forms a sticky, tenacious film that adheres to the skin upon drying. Collodion may be used as a protectant from the irritating effects of tar in the treatment of psoriasis or salicylic acid in the treatment of corns, calluses, and warts. This mixture also is employed as a vehicle for salicylic and lactic acids. Flexible collodion also contains camphor 0.2% and castor oil 0.3% and is used as a protectant for fissures.

COLLODION, U.S.P.:
Generic. Liquid in 120, 480, and 3,840 ml containers.

FLEXIBLE COLLODION, U.S.P.:
Generic. Liquid in 120, 480, and 3,840 ml containers.

Drugs Used for Dermatitis Herpetiformis

Dermatitis herpetiformis is a chronic disease characterized by clusters of intensely pruritic papules, urticaria-like lesions, vesicles, and bullae on the extensor surfaces (Hall, 1987; Faure, 1988). A gluten-sensitive jejunopathy similar to that found in celiac disease is observed in so many of these patients that the jejunopathy and dermatitis are considered components of the same disease complex. A gluten-free diet often reverses the generally asymptomatic jejunal abnormality, but strict adherence to the diet is required for months to reverse the skin lesions; most patients remain resistant or are noncompliant and reversal is never achieved with diet alone. Because of the presence of deposits of IgA in dermal papillae, HLA association, gluten sensitivity, and antireticulin antibodies, the disease is classified as an immunologic disorder. An immunosuppressive action of dapsone characterized by inhibition of cytotoxicity induced by the myeloperoxidase-peroxide-halide system supports that concept (Stendahl et al, 1978).

DAPSONE

H_2N — SO_2 — NH_2

USES. Dapsone often controls the skin lesions associated with dermatitis herpetiformis within a few days, and strict adherence to a gluten-free diet usually allows dosage reduction or eventual discontinuation of drug therapy.

In six patients with dermatitis herpetiformis, concurrent administration of cimetidine 400 mg three times daily reduced the level of methemoglobinemia produced by dapsone by 25%. The efficacy of dapsone was not affected, and no adverse reactions to cimetidine were noted. The mechanism of action probably is related to cimetidine's inhibition of cytochrome P450 3A4, which metabolizes dapsone to a hydroxylamine derivative that is responsible for the formation of methemoglobin (Coleman et al, 1992).

Dapsone has been tried in a small number of patients with the bullous form of systemic lupus erythematosus. In one open study, the response was rapid and satisfactory (Hall et al, 1982). It occasionally is used in dermatologic disorders characterized by excessive polymorphonuclear leukocyte activity (eg, bullous pemphigoid, pyoderma gangrenosum, hypereosinophilic syndrome, linear IgA disease) (Venning et al, 1989).

ADVERSE REACTIONS AND PRECAUTIONS. Agranulocytosis is a rare complication of dapsone therapy. Complete blood counts are recommended at weekly intervals during the first month of therapy and every three to four months thereafter.

Less common side effects include dose-related hepatitis and peripheral motor neuropathy that may be idiosyncratic and is usually manifested by weakness or severe neuropathic pain that is not always reversible on drug withdrawal. Reversible, severe hypoalbuminemia has been reported in two patients after 3 and 11 years of dapsone therapy for dermatitis herpetiformis. Toxic epidermal necrolysis can be a serious complication of dapsone therapy.

Larger doses (150 to 300 mg daily) can produce hemolysis, methemoglobinemia, or leukopenia in less than two weeks. Adverse reactions generally diminish following discontinuation of therapy.

For information on pharmacokinetics and additional information on adverse reactions and precautions, see index entry Dapsone, In Leprosy.

DOSAGE AND PREPARATIONS.

Oral: *Adults,* 25 to 50 mg three or four times daily. Alternatively, to minimize toxicity, dosage can be initiated at 50 mg daily and increased by 25 mg every ten days to two weeks until a therapeutic response is achieved.

Generic. Tablets 25 and 100 mg.

SULFAPYRIDINE

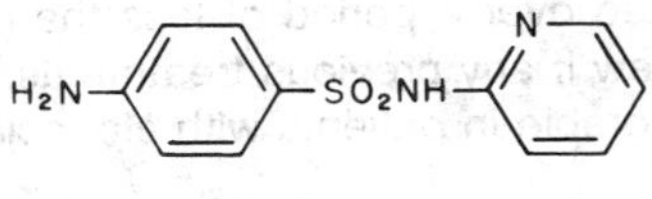

H_2N–(benzene ring)–SO_2NH–(pyridine ring, N)

The sulfonamide, sulfapyridine, was once the treatment of choice for dermatitis herpetiformis but in large part has been replaced by dapsone. Sulfapyridine would be considered obsolete except for its use as an alternative to dapsone for dermatitis herpetiformis.

Sulfapyridine is relatively insoluble and is absorbed slowly following oral administration. The risk of crystalluria with sulfapyridine, unlike many of the newer sulfonamides, is high; oral administration of a sufficient amount of sodium bicarbonate to alkalize the urine and intake of adequate fluid are essential.

DOSAGE AND PREPARATIONS.

Oral: *Adults,* 500 mg to 1 g four times daily; up to 6 g daily has been used.

Generic. Capsules 500 mg.

Debriding Agents

Occlusive Synthetic Dressings: These are available as adjuncts in the management of wound healing. Occlusion prevents loss of drug from the skin, promotes skin hydration, and increases skin temperature. These actions also enhance penetration of certain medications used in the treatment of psoriasis, leg ulcers, some dermatitides, and keratodermas.

The advantages and disadvantages of moist wound healing by use of occlusive biosynthetic dressings have been reviewed (Eaglstein, 1985; Neldner, 1987; Arndt, 1989). Proposed advantages are that a wet wound environment promotes faster healing than a dry one with a better cosmetic result; an environment of relative anoxia is as good or better than one of normal or increased oxygen tension; accumulation of wound exudate and detritus beneath occlusive dressing is not necessarily harmful; bacteria are excluded; and pain and healing time are significantly reduced in such an environment. The major disadvantages include the concerns that occlusive dressings may increase the number of silent and/or visible infections and that patient compliance is reduced because considerable amounts of serous or purulent foul-smelling exudate can accumulate under the dressing or seep from the wound. All occlusive dressings can cause overgrowth of bacteria and *Candida*; therefore, these dressings must be drained or changed frequently.

A variety of synthetic dressings with variable occlusive properties are now available and used for promoting topical drug absorption and for wound healing. Polyurethane transparent occlusive semipermeable dressings are permeable to oxygen and water vapor, but they are impermeable to liquids and bacteria (Pinski, 1986). They will not stick to the wound but do adhere to intact skin and are hypoallergenic. The hydrocolloids are not permeable to oxygen but do have absorptive capacity. The hydrogels have the permeability and nonadherent properties of the polyurethanes, but, like the hydrocolloids, they are absorptive and must be changed daily. The dimethylpolysiloxanes attach to the wound by physical entrapment of fibrin in the nylon mesh; crust formation is minimized and the dressing separates from the wound in five to seven days followed by complete re-epithelization in seven to ten days.

Absorbing beads or granules are not dressings, but cleansing agents that absorb wound secretions and detritus so that they will not interfere with wound healing. Examples include dextran polymers (eg, Debrisan Beads [Johnson & Johnson], DuoDerm Granules [Convatech Division of Squibb]), and graft copolymer starch (eg, Bard Absorption Dressing [Bard]). They can be used only during the wet exudative phase of healing; they are not effective in dry wounds.

Topical Debriding Agents: The value of the adjunctive use of the topical debriding enzymes, collagenase [Santyl], fibrinolysin with desoxyribonuclease [Elase], and sutilains [Travase], is controversial. Although extensively advertised and shown to be efficacious in degrading protein in vitro, the effectiveness of these enzymes in vivo in removing necrotic tissue, clotted blood, purulent exudates, or fibrinous accumulations resulting from burns, trauma, inflammation, infected wounds, or leg ulcers has been questioned by many dermatologists. Because alternative methods for debridement are available (eg, wet dressings, hydrodebridement, surgery), their use is only adjunctive and is not essential for the management of most skin ulcers. They appear to be of value only when the ulcer base has yellowish necrotic connective tissue (mainly collagen) that must be removed before epithelization can proceed. Once the ulcer base is clean, debriding enzymes should no longer be used and in fact may inhibit healing. Only limited controlled data are available. One controlled study found that fibrinolysin with desoxyribonuclease was more effective than saline whether debridement, granulation, or success rate of autologous skin grafts was used to determine outcome (Westerhof et al, 1987).

Effective enzymatic action depends on proper wound preparation prior to application (ie, adequate cleansing of the site to remove detritus, providing for subsequent drainage when necessary). Cross hatching of eschar may be necessary to ensure the enzyme's adequate contact with the wound. Insufficient action may result from improper storage of the enzyme, use of an inappropriate vehicle, or concomitant administration of agents that destroy or inhibit the enzyme (eg, heavy metals, some antiseptics, hexachlorophene). Failure also may result from drying of the substrate, persistence of foreign material or sequestra, and inaccessible location of pus, as in osteomyelitis of cancellous bone.

Drug Used to Stimulate Hair Growth

Normal terminal scalp hair growth (anagen phase) is relatively steady over a mean period of three years (range, two to six years), at which time the follicle enters a resting stage (telogen phase) for about three months. New growth then ensues and the old hair is pushed out of the follicle. Most follicles continue this cycle throughout life, but, in patients with pattern baldness, follicles in the areas of hair loss become progressively smaller, produce thinner and less pigmented indeterminate hair, then nonpigmented, short, soft and fine vellus hair, and finally no hair.

Minoxidil is a potent direct vasodilator that is used orally to treat hypertension. Topical use of this agent has been approved only to stimulate hair growth. In a minority of patients, this agent improves hereditary androgen-dependent alopecia and female androgenetic baldness (diffuse hair loss or thinning of hair in the frontoparietal areas). Minoxidil's degree of efficacy and definitive role in patchy alopecia areata, alopecia totalis (total scalp baldness), and alopecia universalis (total body baldness) have not been established (Clissold and Heel, 1987). These variants of alopecia areata, which is hypothesized to have an autoimmune pathogenesis (Mitchell and Krull, 1984; DeVillez, 1988), have shown some response to high concentrations of topical minoxidil, oral minoxidil, topical or intralesional corticosteroids, topical anthralin, photochemotherapy, oral cyclosporine, and topical allergens (eg, diphencyprone).

MINOXIDIL

[Rogaine]

For chemical formula, see index entry Minoxidil, In Hypertension.

ACTIONS AND USES. Minoxidil causes elongation and normalization of follicles in the area of alopecia; new follicles are not formed. It has no endocrine action. Topical application causes a dose-dependent increase in dermal blood flow as measured by laser doppler velocimetry. In androgenetic alopecia, minoxidil converts vellus hairs to terminal hairs, possibly by stimulating the enlargement and turnover of vellus follicles in early anagen phases (Rumsfield et al, 1987).

The effectiveness of minoxidil in androgenetic alopecia is highly dependent on patient selection and the parameter used to evaluate outcome (Fransway and Muller, 1988). Efficacy is diminished if outcome is based on the patient's perception of a cosmetically acceptable result compared to an objective assessment of the increased number of vellus, indeterminate, and terminal hairs in a predetermined area following treatment. In most trials, when patient satisfaction was the endpoint, a good to excellent response to topical minoxidil 2% was reported in about one-third of the patients with androgenetic alopecia.

A sufficient number of clinical trials have now been done to identify characteristics for patient selection, which should improve the percentage of cosmetically acceptable results obtained (Price, 1987; Fiedler, 1987; Roenigk et al, 1987; Savin and Atton, 1993). In androgenetic alopecia, younger individuals with less hair loss (Hamilton grades II to V) over a shorter period of time (less than five years) will respond best. Older individuals with more than a five-year history of hair loss and with Hamilton grade VI or VII hair loss or with markedly diminished terminal hair density would not be expected to respond in most cases.

Depending on the clinical trial, the efficacy of topical minoxidil 2% in patients with alopecia areata has ranged from less than 33% to 0% (De Groot et al, 1987; Kvedar and Baden, 1987), and the response did not appear to correlate with etiology, ie, whether it is atopic, autoimmune, or idiopathic. Those who are most likely to respond have less than 50% of the scalp affected over a period of less than two years and have received few if any previous treatments. The prognosis is even less favorable in patients with alopecia universalis or alopecia totalis.

The beneficial effect of topical minoxidil ceases when therapy is discontinued; therefore, lifelong treatment is recommended. Generally, at least four months of continuous treatment are required before evidence of hair growth can be expected, and one year of treatment may be necessary before a cosmetically acceptable result occurs (Rietschel and Duncan, 1987). With long-term use, most of the regrown hair is preserved, and the rate of further loss is decreased (Olsen et al, 1990).

ADVERSE REACTIONS AND PRECAUTIONS. A few cases of allergic contact dermatitis and folliculitis have been reported, but local reactions are minimal and treatment is well tolerated. Absorption is poor, averaging about 1.4% (range, 0.3% to 4.5%) from normal intact scalp. The few cardiovascular signs or symptoms reported during clinical trials were not thought to be drug related. However, because of variations in concentration and formulation of extemporaneous preparations, adverse events may not be predictable (Stern, 1987). The FDA strongly recommends that topical formulations not be compounded from available oral tablets for this use.

Adequate controlled studies on use during pregnancy have not been conducted in humans (FDA Pregnancy Category C).

DOSAGE AND PREPARATIONS.

Topical: *Adults,* 1 ml of solution is applied to the total affected scalp (which should be dry) twice a day. The total daily dose should not exceed 2 ml.

Rogaine (Upjohn). Solution 2% in alcohol 60%, propylene glycol, and water in 60 ml containers supplied with either metered spray, extender spray, or rub-on applicator tip.

Drugs Used for Hyperhidrosis

ALUMINUM CHLORIDE HEXAHYDRATE
[Drysol, Xerac AC]

GLUTARAL
[Cidex]

Prescription products containing aluminum chloride hexahydrate 6.25% [Xerac AC] or 20% [Drysol] in absolute ethyl alcohol appear to be effective in some patients with severe hyperhidrosis of the palms, soles, and axillae. They may be applied without occlusion but, for greater effectiveness, the preparation is applied under plastic occlusive dressing to *dry* axillae at bedtime and is washed off in the morning. The number of treatments required depends on the individual. Severe irritation occurs frequently.

Glutaral 2% in a buffered solution (pH 7.5) [Cidex] is available without prescription and has an anhidrotic effect when applied to the palms and soles but not the axillae. It appears to act by occluding the sweat ducts.

Aluminum-containing antiperspirants are classified as Category III substances by the FDA. Iontophoresis with tap water or anticholinergic drugs may be required for patients resistant to these aluminum compounds; the effect may persist for four to six weeks after a few exposures (Simpson, 1988).

The most common adverse effects of antiperspirants are stinging, burning, itching, and irritation. Less common reactions include dermatitis and open ulceration. These preparations should be discontinued at the first sign of irritation, which usually disappears without further complications. Contact sensitization is rare; if patch testing is desirable, the manufacturer should be contacted for appropriate materials, because the final formulation may be inadequate for this purpose.

PREPARATIONS.

ALUMINUM CHLORIDE HEXAHYDRATE:

Drysol (Person & Covey). Solution 20% in 37.5 ml containers.

Xerac AC (Person & Covey). Solution 6.25% in 35 and 60 ml containers.

GLUTARAL:

Cidex (H.L. Moore). Solution (nonprescription).

Cited References

Dandruff, seborrheic dermatitis, and psoriasis drug products for over-the-counter human use; final rule. *Federal Register* 56:63555-63569, (Dec 4) 1991 A.

Topical acne drug products for over-the-counter human use; final monograph; rule. *Federal Register* 56:41008-41020, (Aug 16) 1991 B.

Topical acne drug products for over-the-counter human use; amendment of tentative final monograph; notice of proposed rulemaking. *Federal Register* 56:37622-37635, (Aug 7) 1991 C.

External analgesic drug products for over-the-counter human use: Amendment to tentative final monograph and dandruff, seborrheic dermatitis, and psoriasis drug products for over-the-counter human use; tentative final monograph; further notice of proposed rulemaking and notice of proposed rule making. *Federal Register* 51:27346-27363, 1986.

Isotretinoin: Newly recognized human teratogen. *MMWR* 33:171-173, (April 6) 1984.

Anderson PC: Psoriasis: How to keep mild disease from becoming severe. *Postgrad Med* 79:185-190, (April) 1986.

Arndt KA: *Manual of Dermatologic Therapeutics with Essentials of Diagnosis,* ed 4. Boston, Little Brown, 1989.

Ashton RE, et al: Anthralin: Historical and current perspectives. *J Am Acad Dermatol* 9:173-192, 1983.

Auerbach R: Methotrexate. *Semin Dermatol* 11 (suppl 1):23-29, 1992.

Baker, BS, Fry L: The immunology of psoriasis. *Br J Dermatol* 126:1-9, 1992.

Barker JNWN: The pathophysiology of psoriasis. *Lancet* 338:227-230, 1991.

Bavinck JNB, et al: Cyclosporine for treatment of psoriasis, letter. *N Engl J Med* 324:1894, 1991.

Bennett R, et al: Current management using 5-fluorouracil: 1985. *Cutis* 36:218-236, 1985.

Bershad S, et al: Changes in plasma lipids and lipoproteins during isotretinoin therapy for acne. *N Engl J Med* 313:981-985, 1985.

Bickers DR, et al: Phototherapy and photochemotherapy, in Bickers DR, et al: *Clinical Pharmacology of Skin Disease.* New York, Churchill Livingstone, 1984, 200-216.

Bigby M, Stern RS: Adverse reactions to isotretinoin. *J Am Acad Dermatol* 18:543-552, 1988.

Bos JD: Pathomechanisms of psoriasis; skin immune system and cyclosporin. *Br J Dermatol* 118:141-155, 1988.

Brazzell RK, et al: Pharmacokinetics of isotretinoin during repetitive dosing to patients. *Eur J Clin Pharmacol* 24:695-702, 1983.

Chen ML, et al: Specific HPLC assay to determine pharmacokinetics of methotrexate in patients. *Int J Clin Pharmacol Ther Toxicol* 22:1-6, 1984.

Christophers E, et al: Cyclosporine in psoriasis: A multicenter dose-finding study in severe plaque psoriasis. *J Am Acad Dermatol* 26:86-90, 1992.

Clissold SP, Heel RC: Topical minoxidil: Preliminary review of its pharmacodynamic properties and therapeutic efficacy in alopecia areata and alopecia androgenetica. *Drugs* 33:107-122, 1987.

Coleman MD, et al: The use of cimetidine to reduce dapsone-dependent methaemoglobinaemia in dermatitis herpetiformis patients. *Br J Clin Pharmacol* 34:244-249, 1992.

Committee on Drugs: Retinoid therapy for severe dermatological disorders. *Pediatrics* 90:119-120, 1992.

Cornell RC: Clinical trials of topical corticosteroids in psoriasis: Correlations with the vasoconstrictor assay. *Int J Dermatol* 31 (suppl 1):38-40, 1992.

Cornell RC, Stoughton RB: Topical steroids, in Lowe NJ (ed): *Practical Psoriasis Therapy,* ed 2. St. Louis, Mosby Year Book, 1993, 33-43.

Cristofolini M, et al: The role of etretinate (Tegison, Tigason) in the management of keratoacanthoma. *J Am Acad Dermatol* 12:633, 1985.

Cunliffe WJ: Evolution of strategy for treatment of acne. *J Am Acad Dermatol* 16:591-599, 1987.

Dai WS, et al: Epidemiology of isotretinoin exposure during pregnancy. *J Am Acad Dermatol* 26:599-606, 1992.

De Groot AC, et al: Minoxidil: Hope for the bald? *Lancet* 1:1019-1021, 1987.

DeVillez RL (ed): Androgenetic alopecia: From empiricism to knowledge. *Clin Dermatol* 6:1-235, 1988.

DiGiovanna JJ, Peck GL: Oral synthetic retinoid treatment in children. *Pediatr Dermatol* 1:77-88, 1983.

DiGiovanna JJ, et al: Etretinate: Persistent serum levels after long-term therapy. *Arch Dermatol* 125:246-251, 1989.

Dubertret L, et al: Efficacy and safety of calcipotriol (MC 903) ointment in psoriasis vulgaris: A randomized, double-blind, right/left comparative, vehicle-controlled study. *J Am Acad Dermatol* 27:983-988, 1992.

Eady EA, et al: Use of antibiotics in acne therapy: Oral or topical administration? *J Antimicrob Chemother* 10:89-115, 1982.

Eaglstein WH: Experiences with biosynthetic dressings. *J Am Acad Dermatol* 12:434-440, 1985.

Ellis CN, et al: Etretinate therapy for psoriasis: Reduction of antibody-dependent cell-mediated cytotoxicity of polymorphonuclear leukocytes. *Arch Dermatol* 121:877-880, 1985.

Ellis CN, et al: Cyclosporine for plaque-type psoriasis: Results of a multidose, double-blind trial. *N Engl J Med* 324:277-284, 1991.

Farber EM, Nall L: Appraisal of measures to prevent and control psoriasis. *J Am Acad Dermatol* 10:511-517, 1984.

Faure M: Dermatitis herpetiformis. *Semin Dermatol* 7:123-129, 1988.

Fiedler VC: Minoxidil: Clinical and basic research in perspective. *Semin Dermatol* 6:101-107, 1987.

Fitzpatrick TB, Pathak MA: Research and development of oral psoralen and longwave radiation photochemotherapy: 2000 BC-1982 AD, in Pathak MA, Dunnick JK (eds): *Photobiologic, Toxicologic, and Pharmacologic Aspects of Psoralens*, (monograph 66). Bethesda, Md, USPHS, NIH, NCI, 1984, 3-11.

Fransway AF, Muller SA: 3 percent topical minoxidil compared with placebo for the treatment of chronic severe alopecia areata. *Cutis* 41:431-435, 1988

Fraunfelder FT, et al: Adverse ocular reactions possibly associated with isotretinoin. *Am J Ophthalmol* 100:534-537, 1985.

Frenia ML, Long KS: Methotrexate and nonsteroidal antiinflammatory drug interactions. *Ann Pharmacother* 26:234-237, 1992.

Green LJ, et al: Photoaging and the skin: The effects of tretinoin. *Dermatol Clin* 11:97-105, 1993.

Griffiths CEM: Psoriasis: I. Pathogenesis. *J Am Acad Dermatol* 1:98-101, 1992.

Gupta AK, Anderson TF: Psoralen photochemotherapy. *J Am Acad Dermatol* 17:703-734, 1987.

Haas AA, Arndt KA: Selected therapeutic applications of topical tretinoin. *J Am Acad Dermatol* 15:870-877, 1986.

Hall RP: Pathogenesis of dermatitis herpetiformis: Recent advances. *J Am Acad Dermatol* 16:1129-1144, 1987.

Hall RP, et al: Bullous eruption of systemic lupus erythematosus: Dramatic response to dapsone therapy. *Ann Intern Med* 97:165-170, 1982.

Helm, TN, et al: PUVA therapy. *Am Fam Physician* 43:908-912, 1991.

Hjorth N, Jacobsen M: Coal tar. *Semin Dermatol* 2:281-286, 1983.

Hodge L: Corticosteroid/antibiotic combinations: When should they be used? *Drugs* 19:380-382, 1980.

Hogan DJ, et al: Isotretinoin therapy for acne: Population-based study. *Can Med Assoc J* 138:47-50, 1988.

Hubbell CG, et al: Efficacy of minocycline compared with tetracycline in treatment of acne vulgaris. *Arch Dermatol* 118:989-992, 1982.

Jacobs PH: Seborrheic dermatitis: Causes and management. *Cutis* 41:182-186, 1988.

Jackson DB, et al: Bioequivalence (bioavailability) of generic topical corticosteroids. *J Am Acad Dermatol* 20:791-796, 1989.

James WD, Leyden JJ: Treatment of gram-negative folliculitis with isotretinoin: Positive clinical and microbiologic response. *J Am Acad Dermatol* 12:319-324, 1985.

Johnson TM, Rapini RP: Isotretinoin-induced thrombocytopenia, letter. *J Am Acad Dermatol* 17:838-839, 1987.

Kingston TP, et al: Short-contact anthralin therapy for psoriasis using an aqueous cream formulation. *Cutis* 39:155-157, 1987.

Kligman AM: Current status of topical tretinoin in the treatment of photoaged skin. *Drugs Aging* 2:7-13, 1992 A.

Kligman AM: Tretinoin (Retin-A) therapy of photoaged skin. *Compr Ther* 18:10-13, (Sept) 1992 B.

Kragballe K: Treatment of psoriasis with calcipotriol and other vitamin D analogues. *J Am Acad Dermatol* 27:1001-1008, 1992.

Kragballe K, et al: Double-blind, right/left comparison of calcipotriol and betamethasone valerate in treatment of psoriasis vulgaris. *Lancet* 337:193-196, 1991.

Kvedar JC, Baden HP: Topical minoxidil in treatment of male pattern alopecia. *Pharmacotherapy* 7:191-197, 1987.

Lammer EJ, et al: Retinoic acid embryopathy. *N Engl J Med* 313:837-841, 1985.

Leyden JJ, Kligman AM: Efficacy of steroid-antibiotic combinations. *Drug Ther* 8:114-120, (Feb) 1978.

Leyden JJ, Shalita AR: Rational therapy for acne vulgaris: Update on topical treatment. *J Am Acad Dermatol* 15:907-915, 1986.

Leyden JJ, et al: Erythromycin 2% gel in comparison with clindamycin phosphate 1% solution in acne vulgaris. *J Am Acad Dermatol* 16:822-827, 1987.

Lindelof B, et al: PUVA and cancer: A large-scale epidemiological study. *Lancet* 338:91-93, 1991.

Lowe NJ: *Practical Psoriasis Therapy*. Chicago, Year Book Medical Publishers, 1985.

Lowe NJ: Systemic treatment of severe psoriasis: The role of cyclosporine, editorial. *N Engl J Med* 324:333-334, 1991.

Lowe NJ, et al: New coal tar extract and coal tar shampoos: Evaluation by epidermal cell DNA synthesis suppression assay. *Arch Dermatol* 118:487-489, 1982.

Lowe NJ, et al: Anthralin for psoriasis: Short-contact anthralin therapy compared with topical steroid and conventional anthralin. *J Am Acad Dermatol* 10:69-72, 1984.

Lowe NJ, et al: Comparative efficacy of two dosage forms of oral methoxsalen in psoralens plus ultraviolet A therapy of psoriasis. *J Am Acad Dermatol* 16:994-998, 1987.

Lowe NJ, et al: Etretinate: Appropriate use in severe psoriasis. *Arch Dermatol* 124:527-528, 1988.

Lucek RW, Colburn WA: Clinical pharmacokinetics of retinoids. *Clin Pharmacokinet* 10:38-62, 1985.

Maibach HI (ed): Bioequivalence of topical corticosteroids: A scientific roundtable. *Int J Dermatol* 31 (suppl 1):1-41, 1992.

Maibach HI, Roenigk HH Jr (eds): Psoriasis. *Semin Dermatol* 11:261-324, 1992 A.

Maibach HI, Roenigk HH Jr (eds): Psoriasis symposium. *Semin Dermatol* 11 (suppl 1):1-34, 1992 B.

Maibach HI, Surber C (eds): *Topical Corticosteroids.* Basel, Switzerland, Karger, 1992.

Martin M, Resch K: Interleukin 1: More than a mediator between leukocytes. *TIPS* 9:171-177, 1988.

McGrath, J, Murphy GM: The control of seborrhoeic dermatitis and dandruff by antipityrosporal drugs. *Drugs* 41:178-184, 1991.

Menter A: Cyclosporine. *Semin Dermatol* 11 (suppl 1):30-34, 1992.

Menter A, Barker JNWN: Psoriasis in practice. *Lancet* 338:231-234, 1991.

Mihatsch MJ, Wolff K: Report of a meeting: Consensus conference on cyclosporin A for psoriasis February 1992. *Br J Dermatol* 126:621-623, 1992.

Millan SB, et al: Isotretinoin. *South Med J* 80:494-499, 1987.

Mitchell AJ, Krull EA: Alopecia areata: Pathogenesis and treatment. *J Am Acad Dermatol* 11:763-775, 1984.

Moschella SL, Hurley HJ: *Dermatology*, ed 3. Philadelphia, WB Saunders, 1992, vols 1 and 2.

Muller SA, Perry HO: Goeckerman treatment in psoriasis: Six decades of experience at Mayo Clinic. *Cutis* 34:265-269, 1984.

Murphy GM, Greaves MW: Acne and psoriasis. *BMJ* 296:546-548, 1988.

Neldner KH: Management of leg ulcers, editorial. *J Dermatol Surg Oncol* 13:1297-1298, 1987.

Newbold PCH: Treating psoriasis with calcipotriol: Early studies are promising. *BMJ* 305:847, 1992.

Olsen EA: The pharmacology of methotrexate. *J Am Acad Dermatol* 25:306-318, 1991.

Olsen EA, et al: Five-year follow-up of men with androgenetic alopecia treated with topical minoxidil. *J Am Acad Dermatol* 22:643-646, 1990.

Olsen EA, et al: A double-blind, vehicle-controlled study evaluating masoprocol cream in the treatment of actinic keratoses on the head and neck. *J Am Acad Dermatol* 24:738-743, 1991.

Orfanos CE, et al: Retinoids: Review of their clinical pharmacology and therapeutic use. *Drugs* 34:459-503, 1987.

Padilla RS, et al: Topical tetracycline hydrochloride vs topical clindamycin phosphate in treatment of acne: Comparative study. *Int J Dermatol* 20:445-448, 1981.

Parish LC, et al: Topical corticosteroids. *Int J Dermatol* 24:435-436, 1985.

Parish LC, et al: Topical steroids: What is the optimum application frequency? *Int J Dermatol* 27:19-20, 1988.

Pathak MA, et al: Safety and effectiveness of 8-methoxypsoralen, 4,5′,8-trimethylpsoralen, and psoralen in vitiligo, in Pathak MA,

Dunnick JK (eds): *Photobiologic, Toxicologic and Pharmacologic Aspects of Psoralens*, monograph 66. Bethesda, Md, USPHS, NIH, NCI, 1984, 165-174.

Pinski JB: Dressings for dermabrasion: Occlusive dressings and wound healing. *Cutis* 37:471-476, 1986.

Pochi PE: The pathogenesis and treatment of acne. *Annu Rev Med* 41:187-198, 1990.

Price VH (ed): Rogaine (topical minoxidil, 2%) in management of male pattern baldness and alopecia areata, symposium. *Am J Acad Dermatol* 16(suppl):647-750, (March) 1987.

Rafal ES, et al: Topical tretinoin (retinoic acid) treatment for liver spots associated with photodamage. *N Engl J Med* 326:368-374, 1992.

Rietschel RL, Duncan SH: Clindamycin phosphate used in combination with tretinoin in the treatment of acne. *Int J Dermatol* 22:41-43, 1983.

Rietschel RL, Duncan SH: Safety and efficacy of topical minoxidil in the management of androgenetic alopecia, *J Am Acad Dermatol* 16:677-685, 1987.

Roenigk HH Jr: *Psoriasis.* New York, Marcel Dekker, 1990.

Roenigk HH Jr, et al: Topical minoxidil therapy for hereditary male pattern alopecia. *Cutis* 39:337-342, 1987.

Rowland Payne CME: Psoriatic science. *BMJ* 295:1158-1159, 1987.

Rosa FW: Isotretinoin dose and teratogenicity, letter. *Lancet* 2:1154, 1987.

Rumsfield JA, et al: Topical minoxidil therapy for hair regrowth. *Clin Pharm* 6:386-392, 1987.

Sasaki E: Corticosteroid sensitivity and cross-sensitivity: A review of 18 cases 1967-1988. *Contact Dermatitis* 23:306-315, 1990.

Savin RC, Atton AV: Minoxidil: Update on its clinical role. *Dermatol Clin* 11:55-64, 1993.

Schaefer H: Short-contact therapy, editorial. *Arch Dermatol* 121:1505-1509, 1985.

Shalita AR, Fritsch PO (eds): Retinoids: Present and future: Proceedings of a symposium held at the 18th World Congress of Dermatology. *J Am Acad Dermatol* 27(suppl):S1-S46, (Dec) 1992.

Silverman AK, et al: Hypervitaminosis A syndrome: Paradigm of retinoid side effects. *J Am Acad Dermatol* 16:1027-1039, 1987.

Simpson N: Treating hyperhidrosis, editorial. *BMJ* 296:1345, 1988.

Smith KA: Interleukin-2: Inception, impact, and implications. *Science* 240:1169-1176, 1988.

Stendahl O, et al: Inhibition of polymorphonuclear leukocyte cytotoxicity by dapsone: Possible mechanism in treatment of dermatitis herpetiformis. *J Clin Invest* 61:214-220, 1978.

Stern RS: Topical minoxidil: Survey of use and complications. *Arch Dermatol* 123:62-65, 1987.

Stern RS, et al: Topical versus systemic agent treatment for papulopustular acne: Cost-effectiveness analysis. *Arch Dermatol* 120:1571-1578, 1984.

Stoughton RB: Are generic formulations equivalent to trade name topical glucocorticoids? *Arch Dermatol* 123:1312-1314, 1987.

Stoughton RB: The vasoconstrictor assay in bioequivalence testing: Practical concerns and recent developments. *Int J Dermatol* 31(suppl 1):26-28, 1992.

Tan PL, et al: Current topical corticosteroid preparations. *J Am Acad Dermatol* 14:79-93, 1986.

Tanew A, et al: 5-methoxypsoralen (bergapten) for photochemotherapy: Bioavailability, phototoxicity, and clinical efficacy in psoriasis of new drug preparation. *J Am Acad Dermatol* 18:333-338, 1988.

Trozak DJ: Topical corticosteroid therapy in psoriasis vulgaris. *Cutis* 46:341-350, (Oct) 1990.

Tung JP, Maibach HI: The practical use of methotrexate in psoriasis. *Drugs* 40:697-712, 1990.

Venning VA, et al: Dapsone as first line therapy for bullous pemphigoid *Br J Dermatol* 120:83-92, 1989.

Ward A, et al: Isotretinoin: Review of its pharmacological properties and therapeutic efficacy in acne and other skin disorders. *Drugs* 28:6-37, 1984.

Ward A, et al: Etretinate: Review of its pharmacological properties and therapeutic efficacy in psoriasis and other skin disorders. *Drugs* 26:9-43, 1986.

Weiss JS, et al: Topical tretinoin improves photoaged skin: Double-blind vehicle-controlled study. *JAMA* 259:527-532, 1988.

Westerhof W, et al: Controlled double-blind trial of fibrinolysin-desoxyribonuclease (Elase) solution in patients with chronic leg ulcers who are treated before autologous skin grafting. *J Am Acad Dermatol* 17:32-39, 1987.

Williams H: Skin lightening creams containing hydroquinone: The case for a temporary ban. *BMJ* 305:903-904, 1992.

Wilson DG (ed): Advances in management of acne in general practice and in hospital. *J R Soc Med* 78(suppl 10):1-31, 1985.

Wolverton SE: Systemic drug therapy for psoriasis: The most critical issues, editorial. *Arch Dermatol* 127:565-568, 1991.

Yeung D, et al: Benzoyl peroxide: Percutaneous penetration and metabolic disposition: II. Effect of concentration. *J Am Acad Dermatol* 9:920-924, 1983.

Younger IR, et al: Azathioprine in dermatology. *J Am Acad Dermatol* 25:281-286, 1991.

57

Dermatologic Therapy: Prophylactic Agents and Vehicles

PROPHYLACTIC AGENTS

Chemical Sunscreens and Opaque Sunblocks

Sunlight is necessary for synthesis of vitamin D_3 by the skin and is used therapeutically (phototherapy) in neonatal jaundice, psoriasis, vitiligo, and related papulosquamous disorders. However, sunlight also can produce acute adverse effects on skin, such as sunburn; in addition, exposure to sunlight in association with some drugs and chemicals can result in phototoxicity, which produces a variety of reaction patterns resembling sunburn, or in photoallergy, which usually is manifested as an eczematous rash. Moreover, there is serious concern about adverse effects on the skin when exposure to sunlight is chronic: photoaging or actinic elastosis, premalignant actinic keratoses, basal and squamous cell carcinoma, melanoma, alteration of the immune system causing selective immune incompetence of the skin (Pathak, 1987; Council on Scientific Affairs, 1989; Morison et al, 1991). Although the skin has natural defenses against ultraviolet radiation (UVR) (ie, the presence of keratin, melanin, beta carotene, urocanic acid, the reactive oxygen-scavenging enzymes, superoxide dismutase and glutathione peroxidase reductase), prophylactic measures are recommended for all age groups, particularly infants and children, in order to limit UVR exposure and thus minimize its long-term impact (Pathak, 1987). Such measures include regular use of chemical sunscreens and opaque sunblocks.

Solar Radiation: Solar radiation consists of ultraviolet (6%), visible (48%), and infrared (46%) light. UVR is further subdivided into three categories: (1) UVA or near ultraviolet, 320 to 400 nm; (2) UVB, 290 to 320 nm; and (3) UVC, 200 to 290 nm.

At sea level during the summer months, the solar ultraviolet irradiance of UVB is about 0.5% and that of UVA is about 6.3%. Approximately 90% of the total amount of UVR is UVA because the atmosphere, especially the ozone layer, absorbs UVB radiation below 300 nm and UVC radiation (DeLeo and Maso, 1992). The portion of UVB that is transmitted is 500 to 1,000 times more erythemogenic (sunburn) and melanogenic than UVA radiation. Although seasonal variations in the intensity of UVA (twofold) and UVB (tenfold) radiation occur between June and December, it is generally accepted that UVA radiation accounts for, at most, about one-sixth of the total erythemogenic and melanogenic potential of UVR. However, UVA also can cause chronic adverse effects of radiation; it is known that UVA radiation enhances UVB-induced skin carcinogenesis and aging and is the main spectrum of light responsible for phototoxic drug reactions. Although no appreciable tanning occurs with UVC solar radiation, UVC radiation can be emitted by artificial sources and its erythemogenic potential is greater than that of UVB radiation.

The biologic effects of ionizing radiation are due to photochemical actions and, to a lesser extent, to heat. Causes of thermal effects are nonspecific. Photochemical effects are caused by absorption of specific wavelengths within the ultraviolet and visible spectral regions by particular molecules called chromophores, which are present in DNA, RNA, proteins, and lipids of cells in various compartments of the epidermis, dermis, and subcutis. The mechanisms by which affected chromophores cause cutaneous adverse photobiologic effects are poorly defined (DeLeo and Maso, 1992).

Sun Sensitivity: Because sun sensitivity and the ability to produce pigment vary among individuals, skin has been classified into six types (Table 1). This classification is based on effects observed with the first 45 to 60 minutes of midday summer sun exposure after the winter season or after no sun exposure. The susceptibility of human skin to UVR-induced acute and chronic damage is related to skin type, UVR intensity and duration of exposure, individual habits of sun exposure, and inherent ability to tan and to repair photodamaged DNA. Fair-skinned individuals with normal skin require only 10 to 20 minutes of exposure to sunlight initially after the winter season to develop perceptible sunburn.

Premature aging of the skin caused by excessive exposure to the sun is a distinct process very different from normal chronologic or intrinsic aging of the skin. Although sunscreens have no effect on the latter process, the regular use of sunscreen products over a period of years may lead to a decrease in premature aging of the skin and skin cancer due to sun exposure.

Since adequate studies are unavailable, most sunscreens are not approved for infants less than 6 months; however, protection is particularly important for infants and children (Stern, et al, 1986; Hurwitz, 1988). Since they have more sensitive skin than adults and since the damage done by excessive sun exposure is cumulative, sunscreens with an SPF of at least 15 and/or opaque sunblocks should be applied to the exposed skin of infants and children who are in the sun during peak hours of UVR intensity.

Individuals with certain photosensitivity disorders may require protection with a sunscreen and/or an opaque sunblock depending on the severity of their condition. Common examples include patients with xeroderma pigmentosum, erythropoietic porphyria, systemic lupus erythematosus, extensive vitiligo, polymorphic photodermatitis, or solar urticaria and individuals who are undergoing phototherapy following oral administration of psoralens. Sunscreens are less protective in those who have had a phototoxic (acute) or photosensitivity (delayed allergic) reaction following ingestion of certain drugs (eg, thiazides, phenothiazines, oral or topical retinoids, sulfonamides, sulfonylureas, demeclocycline).

Sunscreen Products: Only topical sunscreens currently are available. A few systemic agents (eg, beta carotene, pso-

TABLE 1.
SKIN TYPES BASED ON SUN SENSITIVITY[1]

Skin Type	Ultraviolet Radiation Sensitivity	Sunburn and Tanning History	Skin Color of Unexposed Buttocks	Recommended SPF to Prevent Sunburn[2]	Sunscreen Product Category Designation
I	Very sensitive	Always burns easily; rarely tans	White	20-30	Ultra High
II	Very sensitive	Always burns easily; tans minimally	White	12[3]-20	Very High
III	Sensitive	Burns moderately; tans gradually and uniformly to a light brown color	White	8-12[3]	High
IV	Moderately sensitive	Burns minimally; always tans well to moderate brown color	White or light Brown	4 to 8[3]	Moderate
V	Minimally sensitive	Rarely burns; tans profusely to dark brown color	Brown	2 to 4[3]	Minimal
VI	Insensitive	Rarely burns; deeply pigmented black color	Chocolate, brown, or black	None Indicated[3]	—

[1] *Adapted from Pathak, 1987;* Federal Register, *1993.*

[2] Sun Protective Factor (SPF) *is the ratio of the amount of ultraviolet energy required to produce a minimal erythema dose (MED) through the applied sunscreen product to the amount required to produce the same reaction without the sunscreen. An MED is the smallest dose of ultraviolet (UV) radiation (expressed as Joules per meter squared) that produces redness reaching the borders of the exposure site. MED (PS) is the minimal erythema dose for protected skin after application of 2 mg/cm^2 of the final formulation of the sunscreen product, and MED (US) is the minimal erythema dose for unprotected skin. Thus, the SPF value is the reciprocal of the effective transmission of the product viewed as a UV radiation filter. Sunscreen products are labeled with SPFs that range from 2 to 45. The SPF test is based on simulated solar radiation, primarily UVB (Lowe et al, 1988).*

[3] *Most dermatologists recommend an SPF of at least 15 in these less-sensitive categories of patients, even including individuals with skin type VI who are chronically exposed.*

ralens, chloroquine) have been used investigationally for specific photosensitivity problems.

The FDA has approved a number of chemicals for use as Category I sunscreen active ingredients (*Federal Register*, 1993). These are listed in Table 2 and are divided into groups on the basis of their ability to block UVB and UVA radiation. Sunscreen active ingredients in group I block only UVB radiation and those in group II partially block UVA radiation, especially in the shorter (320 to 360 nm) wavelengths (Gange et al, 1986; Luftman et al, 1991; DeLeo, 1992). In commercial products, one or more of the agents in group I usually are combined with one of the agents in group II.

TABLE 2.
TYPES OF CHEMICAL SUNSCREENS AND OPAQUE SUNBLOCKS[1]

I. Chemicals effective against UVB radiation only:

Cinnamic acid derivatives
- 2-ethoxyethyl *p*-methoxycinnamate (Cinoxate)
- diethylanolamine *p*-methoxycinnamate (diethanolamine methoxycinnamate)

Para-amino benzoic acid (PABA) and PABA esters
- *p*-amino benzoic acid
- 4-amyldimethyl aminobenzoate (Padimate A)[2]
- 4-octyldimethyl aminobenzoate (Padimate O)
- ethyl 4-[bis (hydroxypropyl)] aminobenzoate
- glyceryl 4-aminobenzoate

Salicylic acid derivatives
- Homosalate
- 2-ethylhexyl salicylate (octyl salicylate)
- triethanolamine salicylate (trolamine salicylate)

Miscellaneous
- digalloyl trioleate
- 2-phenylbenzimidazole-5-sulfonic acid (phenylbenzimidazole sulfonic acid)

II. Chemicals partially effective (shorter > longer wavelengths) against UVA radiation and with variable effectiveness against UVB radiation:

Benzophenone derivatives
- dioxybenzone
- oxybenzone
- sulisobenzone

Cinnamic acid derivative
- ethylhexyl *p*-methoxycinnamate (octyl methoxycinnamate)

Dibenzoylmethane derivatives
- 4-*tert*-butyl methoxydibenzoylmethane (Avobenzone)
- isopropyl dibenzoylmethane (Eusolex 8020)

Miscellaneous
- 2-ethylhexyl 2-cyano 3,3-diphenylacrylate (octocrylene)
- methyl anthranilate

Opaque sunblocks[3]
- Lawsone with dihydroxyacetone
- red petrolatum
- titanium dioxide

[1] *FDA-approved Category I sunscreens* (Federal Register, *1993).*

[2] *At concentrations up to 5%.*

[3] *An opaque sunblock is a sunscreen that reflects, scatters, or absorbs all light in the visible range at wavelengths and some UVA radiation, especially longer wavelengths. Zinc oxide is currently listed as Category III (more data required).*

There is no universally accepted test for determining efficacy against UVA radiation (*Federal Register*, 1993). Some investigators believe that no correlation exists between the results of the SPF test and protection from UVA when sunscreens are compared in a UVA-induced (xenon solar simulator) immediate pigment darkening (IPD) test (Kaidbey and Barnes, 1991). Because approximately 85% of the erythemal action of sunlight results from UVB and 15% from UVA, other investigators question the relevancy of the IPD test and believe that any sunscreen with at least an SPF 10 rating (which by definition blocks over 90% of the total UV damage) must provide UVA protection (Agin, 1992; Agin and Stanfield, 1992; Kaidbey, 1992).

Sunscreen products vary in substantivity, which is usually reflected in the labeling by the terms water-resistant or very water resistant. Part of their substantivity is dependent on the vehicles and other ingredients in the formulations; however, a considerable proportion of substantivity can be inherent in the active agent itself. This is particularly true for PABA. Use of the designation water-resistant or very water-resistant (older, less preferred term is waterproof) requires that the sunscreen product pass a test in which it is shown that photoprotective properties continue to be present after immersion of treated skin in water for periods of 40 and 80 minutes, respectively (*Federal Register*, 1993).

A listing of representative sunscreen products follow; those with an asterisk are available in water-resistant or very water-resistant formulations. See the following sections on Sunscreen Selection and Precautions for additional information on product selection.

Available Trademarks.
Block Out 15*, Clinique 19, Coppertone Moisturizing Sunblock 15*, Elizabeth Arden 15*, Neutrogena Sunblock 15, Photoplex 15*, PreSun 15*, PreSun PABA Free 15*, RVPaque*, Shade UVAGuard 15*, Shiseido 15, SolBar PABA Free 15, Sundown 15*, Total Eclipse 15*.

Sunscreen Selection: Sunscreens are especially indicated for individuals with skin types I, II, and III; those with types IV and V also may derive considerable protection against acute and chronic skin damage (see Table 1). Selection of the SPF of a sunscreen product to prevent sunburn is important. O the basis of concern about all adverse actions of solar r tion, the Skin Cancer Foundation's Seal of Recomme Program and most dermatologists now recomm sunscreen product of at least SPF 15 be u 1992). A generally recommended upper lim

The opaque sunblocks can be useful, especially for selected areas of the body (eg, face, nose, neck, lips, ear helices, hairless scalp) depending on the individual's occupation and length of exposure (eg, outdoor guide, lifeguard, farmer, sailor). However, because many formulations are visible after application and are occlusive, sunblocks often are cosmetically unappealing; they also can discolor clothing and cause folliculitis and acne. Newer sunblocks containing micronized titanium dioxide and other ingredients appear to be more cosmetically acceptable.

Water-resistant or very water-resistant properties, as well as individual preference for cream, lotion, ointment, or gel form, may be important in the selection process. Prior history of allergic reactions to agents related to components of sunscreens is yet another consideration in product selection.

Nondrug measures can be more effective than sunscreens and can markedly augment the effectiveness of those agents (Rustad, 1992). These include the use of protective clothing such as broad-brimmed hats and tightly woven loose clothing that covers the arms and the legs, polarized sunglasses, sunbrellas at the beach, as well as avoidance or limitation of sun exposure at peak hours of UVR intensity, ie, 10 AM to 2 PM (11 AM to 3 PM daylight savings time). Individuals also should be aware of the enhanced effect of reflective surfaces such as water, snow, concrete, ice, and sand; that protection from sun exposure also is important on cloudy or overcast days; and that extra protection will be needed at high altitudes. It may be prudent to reapply sunscreen after sweating, swimming, or bathing even if the preparation is water-resistant or very water-resistant.

Although a darker skin color affords an additional natural protection from UVR, a sun-induced tan from a combination of UVA and UVB radiation is equivalent to an SPF of only approximately 4. Pigmentation from UVB radiation produces epidermal hyperplasia and movement of melanin upward through the epidermis, whereas pigmentation induced by UVA radiation is mainly limited to an increase in the melanin content of the basal layer and no significant hyperplasia. Therefore, tans induced by tanning salons, which utilize principally UVA radiation, are even less protective than tans induced by solar radiation. Tanning salons or sun lamps should be avoided, particularly when solar keratoses are present, there is a known history of sensitivity to sunlight, a family history of skin cancer, or photosensitizing medications are being used.

Precautions: Contact sensitivity and photosensitivity occur in a few individuals with most chemical agents, but a nonsensitizing preparation usually can be found. Sparing use is recommended initially until lack of sensitization is assured. Individuals sensitive to benzocaine, procaine, *p*-phenylene diamine (hair dyes), and sulfanilamide probably should avoid formulations containing PABA and its ester; those sensitive to thiazides and other sulfonamides should avoid the PABA esters as well. Sensitivity to these agents should be determined definitively by patch and photopatch testing. This permits specific recommendations for individual patients and avoids mandating against all related chemicals. Highly alcoholic vehicles should not be used on eczematous or otherwise inflamed skin.

Since sunscreens may decrease cutaneous vitamin D_3 synthesis, it is recommended that elderly patients, whose nutritional intake may be marginal, be evaluated for vitamin D deficiency if they have been using sunscreens for a long period (Matsuoka et al, 1987).

Adjunctive Preparations: Baby oil or mineral oil (with or without iodine), lubricating creams or lotions, cocoa butter, coconut oil, and tanning butters also are available. These preparations provide no protection against sunburn. Furthermore, they enhance the penetration of UVB radiation that promotes sunburn and may induce miliaria and folliculitis. Their sole virtue is that they minimize skin dryness.

A number of artificial tanning preparations (bronzers, body gels, face colors) are available to give the skin a tanned appearance without exposure to the sun; these preparations provide no protection against sunburn unless a sunscreen is incorporated in the formulation.

VEHICLES

Dermatologic vehicles are designed to deliver topical medication in the most beneficial manner (McKay, 1983; Arndt, 1989; Maddin and Ho, 1992). Vehicles are one of a number of important factors that affect percutaneous absorption of chemical agents (Wester and Maibach, 1992) and are used on occasion to enhance penetration of active agents into skin. They can be therapeutic in their own right when properly used. Their actions include skin cleansing, cooling, drying, lubrication, softening, hydration, and protection.

Criteria for selection of a vehicle include its drying, hydrating, or lubricating activity; the manner in which it holds, releases, or assists in the absorption of the active ingredients; and suitability for use on the area intended. Liquids (eg, lotions, foams, tinctures, solutions, shampoos, sprays) are convenient for application to hairy areas. Emulsified vanishing-type creams or lotions are most appropriate for use in body folds (intertriginous sites); if an ointment is used in such areas, it must be spread thinly to avoid maceration.

The principal constituents of vehicles include liquids (water, alcohol, or organic solvents), powders, oils, and ointment bases; pharmaceutic aids often are present as additives.

Liquids have desirable properties in addition to their usefulness as vehicles. Water acts as a vehicle and as a hydrating agent in wet dressings, lotions, baths, creams, and some ointments. When applied as hot or cold compresses, water alters skin temperature and macerates the superficial layer of the skin. Alcohols are solvents and are used to cool the skin; depending on the concentration, they may be antiseptic or astringent. Glycerin, a solvent and emollient in lotions, creams, and pastes, is miscible with water and alcohol. Propylene glycol is an excellent solvent and preservative; it has replaced glycerin as the vehicle for many topical therapeutic agents, cosmetics, and body and hand lotions. It is hygroscopic and has considerable moistening and softening actions. However, irritation (burning and stinging) may limit its use.

Powders increase evaporation, reduce friction and pruritus, and provide a cooling sensation. They are dusted on the skin or are present as a component of lotions and pastes. Examples of U.S.P. powders include zinc oxide, zinc stearate, magnesium stearate, talc, cornstarch, bentonite, titanium dioxide, and precipitated calcium carbonate.

Zinc oxide and talc (mainly hydrous magnesium silicate) are protective and adsorb some water when applied as a paste in petrolatum. Zinc oxide mixed with a small amount of ferric oxide has a pink color; this mixture, calamine, is used in shake lotions. Although insoluble in water, bentonite (hydrated aluminum silicate) combines with water to form a gel; it improves the dispersion of zinc oxide and sulfur in oil-in-water mixtures. Titanium dioxide and zinc oxide contribute to reflection and scattering of both UVA and UVB radiation and are ingredients of lotions or pastes used as sunscreens. They are nonsensitizing and nonirritant in both adults and children. Precipitated calcium carbonate is a fine white powder that is insoluble in alcohol and water; it imparts a dry sensation and is more adsorbent than talc. Talc alone is a lubricant and quite alkaline; it may cause severe granulomatous reactions when applied to open wounds.

Oils are liquid or semisolid hydrocarbons of mineral, vegetable, or animal origin. Vegetable and mineral oils are most widely used for topical application. Hydrogenated vegetable oil in a nonfragrant form (eg, Crisco) used sparingly after a bath in tepid water is an inexpensive example. Cottonseed, corn, castor, olive, and peanut oils are commonly incorporated in creams and lotions. Their emollient effect is similar, but odor, storage stability, and emulsifying capabilities differ.

Mineral oil is a mixture of high-molecular-weight hydrocarbons obtained from petroleum. It is used alone or as an ingredient in lotions, creams, or ointments and, unlike vegetable or animal oils, does not become rancid. Stabilizers (eg, tocopherol, butylhydroxytoluene) often are added. The *United States Pharmacopeia* requires that the stabilizer be identified on the label. Topically applied mineral oil is relatively free of untoward effects, except in acne-prone patients. It occasionally may cause miliaria and folliculitis.

Ointment bases are used in various creams and ointments. They include semisolid vegetable and animal fats and waxes, petroleum hydrocarbons, and silicones.

Emulsifying agents are *pharmaceutic-aid additives* used in topical dermatologic products to provide stability and homogeneity for immiscible liquids. Glyceryl monostearate, polyethylene glycol derivatives (polyoxyl 40 stearate, polysorbate 80), and sodium lauryl sulfate are used as emulsifying agents in lotions, creams, and ointments that contain oily ingredients and water. Other additives include cetyl palmitate and related esters, which improve the consistency and appearance of creams; stearic acid and stearyl alcohol, which act as lubricants or emollients; silicones, which act as antifoaming agents; and methylcellulose and gum tragacanth, which are inert substances used as suspending agents in lotions, creams, ointments, and pastes. The parabens (methylparaben, propylparaben, and butylparaben), oxyquinoline sulfate, organic quaternary ammonium compounds, quaternium 15 [Dowicil 200], imidazolidinyl urea [Germall], parachlorometaxylenol, sorbic acid, benzyl alcohol, and chlorobutanol frequently are added as antimicrobial preservatives. Sorbic acid is often irritating to the face; however, most of these agents are innocuous at the low concentrations present. Preservatives cause sensitization fairly often. The parabens rarely may produce allergic contact dermatitis and sodium lauryl sulfate has the potential for producing irritation. Some additives increase the stratum corneum's permeability not only to medicaments but to noxious agents and thus may directly or indirectly produce irritation.

Wet Dressings

Open wet dressings are indicated for acute inflammation characterized by vesicular eruptions with exudation, oozing (weeping), and crusting. The soft, saturated, tepid dressings should be changed every 5 to 15 minutes for a period of 30 minutes to two hours, depending on the severity of the inflammation. This process may be repeated three or four times daily.

Water is the most important ingredient in wet dressings. In addition to providing evaporative cooling, it is cleansing and helps to drain exudates; the vasoconstriction that results from cooling combats the first stage of an acute inflammatory response. These effects are lost if the wet dressing is occluded by wrapping or covering with plastic or rubber. Softening and maceration of the skin surface result. Aluminum acetate, potassium permanganate, copper and zinc sulfates, acetic acid, or silver nitrate may be present in the formulation for their presumptive antibacterial or astringent action.

A 5% aluminum acetate solution, U.S.P. (Burow's solution), diluted 1:10 to 1:40, is commonly used as a wet dressing. Potassium permanganate 0.025% to 0.1% has astringent properties but stains the skin and the tub or vessel used. *Tablets should be completely dissolved if placed in a tub of water, because they can produce cutaneous necrosis if the patient sits on them.* Silver nitrate solution 0.1% to 0.5% stains the skin but has more antibacterial activity than the other metal salts listed; however, it also permanently stains clothing and linens.

ALUMINUM ACETATE SOLUTION, U.S.P. (Burow's Solution):
Generic. Solution (nonprescription).

ALUMINUM CHLORIDE HEXAHYDRATE, N.F.:
Generic. Powder (nonprescription).

ALUMINUM SULFATE AND CALCIUM ACETATE:
Bluboro (Allergan Herbert). Powder (nonprescription).
Domeboro (Miles). Powder, tablets (nonprescription).

POTASSIUM PERMANGANATE, U.S.P.:
Generic. Tablets.

SILVER NITRATE, U.S.P..:
Generic. Solution.

Baths and Body Oils

Pruritus that accompanies acute dermatitis or extr anthematous lesions is often alleviated by imme of or the entire body in water for a maximum prevent maceration. Cooling diminishes pruritus safely and effectively. When baths are used to hydrate the skin, subsequent gentle drying is desirable, followed by application of an emollient to retard water evaporation.

Colloidal substances can be added to baths for their soothing and antipruritic activities. A paste made of 2 cups of Linit starch, cornstarch, or oatmeal plus 4 cups of cold water is boiled and then added to a tub half filled with water. Commercial products containing colloidal oatmeal [Aveeno Bath Regular, Aveeno Bath Oilated] also are useful.

Occasionally it is desirable to add an oil to bath water. Since oils are insoluble in water, emulsifiers are often added to enhance dispersion and form a milky mixture of microglobules of oil-in-water. A fine film of oil remains on the skin after the bath; it should not be removed when towel-drying. Since the addition of oils may make tubs slippery, body oils should be applied to wet skin after the bath in the elderly and children.

These products may be helpful in ichthyosis or pruritic and chronic eczematous dermatoses. Since these surfactant-treated oils impart a pleasing sensation to the skin, they are often used as emollients. Solutions of coal tar oils also are available for addition to baths; they are particularly useful for treating psoriasis.

MINERAL OIL AND LANOLIN OIL:
Alpha Keri (Bristol-Myers) (nonprescription).

MINERAL OIL:
Doak Fragrance Free, Doak Formula 405 (Doak), ***Domol*** (Miles), ***Lubath*** (Warner-Lambert), ***Mapo Oil*** (Herald) (all forms nonprescription).

SESAME SEED OIL:
Neutrogena Body Oil (Neutrogena) (nonprescription).

Lotions

The term lotion (sometimes called "shake lotion") historically refers to a suspension of powder in a liquid medium (usually water) that requires shaking before application. The term recently has been extended to include commercial liquid emulsions and foams, but they are usually of thin, uniform consistency.

Lotions are used for subacute inflammatory lesions after the severe exudative phase has ceased. Their protective, drying, cooling effect is especially useful at hairy or intertriginous sites or in areas of widespread eruptions. A basic white shake lotion contains zinc oxide, talc, glycerin, and water. Calamine may be added for a flesh tint. Alcohol may be added (to a concentration of 15%) to assist in solubilizing active ingredients and to enhance the drying effect. Propylene glycol may be added to facilitate removal of hyperkeratotic scales.

Menthol 0.25% to 2%, phenol 0.5% to 1.5%, and camphor 1% to 3% have a weak antipruritic action; the latter two agents alter cutaneous nerve transmission, while menthol imparts a cooling sensation. See index entry Phenol. Salicylic acid 1% to 2% and coal tar solution 3% to 10% may have an antipruritic action.

CALAMINE LOTION, U.S.P.:
Generic. Lotion (nonprescription).

PHENOLATED CALAMINE LOTION, U.S.P.:
Generic. Lotion (nonprescription).

MENTHOL LOTION WITH PHENOL:
Schamberg's Lotion (C & M Pharmacal) (nonprescription).

MENTHOL, CAMPHOR, AND PHENOL LOTION:
Sarna Lotion (Stiefel) (nonprescription).

MENTHOL, CAMPHOR, AND/OR CALAMINE:
Rhulicream, Rhuligel, Rhulispray (Rydelle) (nonprescription).

Gels

Gels used for topical preparations are transparent or opaque colloidal dispersions prepared in a solid or semisolid (jelly-like) state. The gel liquifies on contact with skin and dries to a greaseless nonocclusive film; therefore, it is suitable for use in hairy areas. Aqueous, acetone, alcohol, or propylene glycol gels of organic polymers, such as agar, gelatin, polyoxyethylene lauryl ether, hydroxypropyl cellulose, carbomer methylcellulose, pectin, and polyethylene glycol, are the most common ingredients. Sodium lauryl sulfate, an emulsifying and dispensing agent, also often is present and may act as an irritant, especially in inflamed and denuded areas. Gels lack emollient and protective properties, and they are easily removed by perspiration.

The presence of large amounts of water and other solvents characterizes the subclass of gels known as jellies. Jellies are used as vehicles, particularly for application to mucous membranes, and as lubricants for surgical gloves, finger cots, catheters, and sexual intercourse.

A significant percentage of patients experience irritation (burning, stinging) or drying after using gels.

Creams and Ointments

These semisolid preparations serve as vehicles for many drugs and are used alone for their emollient and protective properties. Creams and ointments are particularly suitable for the chronic inflammatory stage of skin diseases. Dry, scaling, thickened, pruritic, and lichenified lesions respond to their softening and lubricating properties. Creams and certain ointments hold or attract water to promote skin rehydration (moisturizers); other types of ointments repel water. Most ointments are sufficiently occlusive to promote the cutaneous absorption of drugs.

Creams and *emulsion ointment bases* consist of emulsions of oil (hydrophobic hydrocarbons, animal or vegetable fats, organic alcohols) and water. Oil-in-water (O/W) emulsions are less greasy and more easily removed (water-washable or vanishing creams) than water-in-oil (W/O) emulsions; however, the latter provide more lubrication and occlusion.

When the amount of oil exceeds that of water by a certain proportion, the emulsion changes from a pourable cream to a semisolid ointment. Although generally true, neither the official nor the manufacturers' designation of a product as a cream or ointment always correlates with O/W or W/O emulsification type, eg, Cold Cream, U.S.P. (W/O); Hydrophilic Ointment, U.S.P. (O/W).

Hydrophilic ointment contains white petrolatum, stearyl alcohol, sodium lauryl sulfate, and propylene glycol in water with preservatives. It is a good vehicle for water-soluble medicaments, has good esthetic properties, and imparts a pleasing sensation. Irritation has been noted, probably due to the emulsifier, sodium lauryl sulfate.

Cold cream, a water-in-mineral oil emulsion containing white wax, cetyl esters, wax, mineral oil, and sodium borate, is widely used. It lubricates and hydrates the skin and imparts a cooling sensation.

The remaining three classes of ointments contain essentially no water. Some are soluble in water or attract and hold it; others are completely insoluble in water, hold little if any water, or may be water-repellent, depending on the base used.

Water-absorbent ointment bases are mixtures of oleaginous materials and emulsifying agents. They are insoluble in water but absorb it and are difficult to wash off. These substances are water-in-oil emulsion ointment bases when hydrated. Examples include Hydrophilic Petrolatum, U.S.P. and Anhydrous Lanolin, U.S.P. The former is composed of white petrolatum, cholesterol, stearyl alcohol, and white wax; it is less greasy and more acceptable cosmetically than petrolatum. Anhydrous lanolin is an oleaginous substance obtained from sheep's wool; it contains less than 0.25% water but is capable of absorbing a considerable amount. It is an ingredient of commercial ointments and some bath oil preparations.

Oleaginous ointment bases are water-repellent and consist of hydrophobic hydrocarbons, hydrogenated vegetable fats, or siloxanes (silicones); some are synthetic mixtures with waxes. They are anhydrous, insoluble in water, and absorb little or no water. They are difficult to wash off, will not dry out, and generally change little during storage (although some fats may become rancid on aging). Oleaginous ointment bases are suitable for use alone or as a vehicle in patients who are sensitive to other bases and/or their ingredients (emulsifiers, stabilizers). Preservatives may be present in some oleaginous ointment bases.

Petrolatum, the most important agent of this group, is a purified mixture of high-molecular-weight hydrocarbons obtained from petroleum. This ointment is protective and emollient when applied to the skin and is an excellent base or vehicle for topical medicaments. It varies in color (off-white to light amber), composition, and consistency depending on the petroleum source and manner of preparation. White Petrolatum, U.S.P., a bleached form of yellow petrolatum, is more esthetically pleasing and, therefore, is the form most commonly used. Yellow petrolatum is preferable for tar preparations because the bleaching agent in white petrolatum may inactivate tars. White Ointment, U.S.P. is white petrolatum with 5% white wax added. This preparation is firmer at room temperature than petrolatum.

Depending on their degree of polymerization, silicones are available as liquid or semisolid preparations. The latter have the properties of other oleaginous ointment bases, except that they are considerably more water-repellent and have a low surface tension, which increases penetration into skin creases. Silicones are used as aqueous-barrier creams because they repel water and provide intimate coverage; however, they do not act as a barrier for organic compounds that may be contact irritants. The polydimethylsiloxanes (dimethicone) are stable, nonsensitizing, and nonirritating.

Water-soluble ointment bases (eg, polyethylene glycol ointment) are greaseless and anhydrous. They absorb water, are water soluble, and are good vehicles for the topical delivery of water-soluble drugs. The oil-in-water emulsion, Hydrophilic Ointment, U.S.P., is soluble in water and can be used similarly.

OIL-IN-WATER EMULSIONS:
Hydrophilic Ointment, U.S.P.
Generic. Ointment (nonprescription).
Acid Mantle Cream (Sandoz), ***Cetaphil Lotion*** (Owen/Galderma), ***Keri Lotion*** (Westwood-Squibb), ***LactiCare Lotion*** (Stiefel), ***Lubriderm Cream*** (Warner-Lambert), ***Moisturel*** (Westwood-Squibb), ***Neutrogena Emulsion*** (Neutrogena), ***Nivea Cream*** (Beiersdorf), ***Nutraderm Cream*** (Owen/Galderma), ***Purpose Dry Skin Cream*** (Johnson & Johnson/Merck Consumer), ***Shepard's Skin Cream*** (Dermik), ***Sofenol 5 Lotion*** (C & M Pharmacal) (all forms nonprescription).
WATER-IN-OIL EMULSIONS:
Cold Cream, U.S.P.
Generic. Cream (nonprescription).
Lanolin, U.S.P.
Generic. Cream; ointment (nonprescription).
Eucerin (Beiersdorf), ***Polysorb Hydrate*** (Fougera) (nonprescription).
WATER-ABSORBENT OINTMENT BASES:
Hydrophilic Petrolatum, U.S.P.
Generic. Ointment (nonprescription).
Anhydrous Lanolin, U.S.P.
Generic. Cream; ointment (nonprescription).
Aquaphor (Beiersdorf), ***Unibase*** (Warner-Chilcott), ***Velvachol*** (Owen/Galderma) (nonprescription).
OLEAGINOUS (WATER-REPELLENT) OINTMENT BASES:
White Petrolatum, U.S.P.
Generic. Gel; ointment (nonprescription).
Vaseline Petroleum Jelly (Chesebrough Ponds) (nonprescription).
White Ointment, U.S.P.
Dimethicone, U.S.P.
Generic. Ointment (nonprescription).
Hydropel (C & M Pharmacal) (nonprescription).
WATER-SOLUBLE OINTMENT BASE:
Polyethylene Glycol Ointment, U.S.P.
Generic. Ointment (nonprescription).
Solumol (C & M Pharmacal) (nonprescription).

Pastes

Simple pastes are made by incorporating finely divided powder(s) into an ointment base in a 1:1 ratio. (If the powder content is less than 50%, the mixture is designated an ointment.) The resulting mixture protects the skin against external irritants and sunlight. The ointment base is usually petrolatum, and the powder is zinc oxide, talc, starch, bentonite, aluminum oxide, or titanium dioxide. Titanium dioxide has particularly good sunscreen properties. Coloring matter may b[illegible] added to make the mixture cosmetically acceptable. A p[illegible] containing zinc oxide, starch, and white petrolatum, Zin[illegible] Paste, U.S.P. (Lassar's Plain Zinc Paste), is a com[illegible] scribed protective paste. Starch may act as subst[illegible] organisms. Pastes generally are poor vehicl[illegible] active pharmacologic agents and for inhibiting water evaporation, but they adhere well and protect skin from friction caused by clothing and bandages. They are applied in subacute and chronic dermatoses, particularly in infants, but generally should be avoided in weeping lesions and hairy areas. Removal of pastes is facilitated by use of mineral or vegetable oil or soap applied with a soft brush.

Humectants

Moisturizers as a class include occlusives and humectants (Wehr and Krochmal, 1987; Spencer, 1988). Occlusive moisturizers provide a partially permeable barrier that allows the skin to retain its own moisture; examples include petrolatum, lanolin, and heavy mineral oil; these are discussed in the section on Creams and Ointments.

When they are absorbed, humectants help the skin retain moisture; examples include urea, glycolic acid, propylene glycol, and lactic acid.

Urea, in a suitable cream or ointment vehicle, may soften the skin in ichthyotic and other dry, scaly conditions, such as psoriasis or atopic dermatitis. It disrupts the normal hydrogen bonding of keratinic proteins through its hydrating and keratolytic actions; this, in turn, promotes desquamation of the stratum corneum. It has not been established whether the antipruritic effect results from a direct action or from improvement of the skin condition. Urea is used to accelerate cutaneous penetration of active ingredients; it increases hydrocortisone absorption twofold. Irritation (burning and stinging) may be noted often with higher concentrations.

Propylene glycol, a widely used vehicle in dermatologic formulations, is isotonic in 2% concentrations. Concentrations up to 70% alter keratin to hydrate and soften the skin and cause desquamation of scales, particularly when used under occlusive dressings. Initially the preparation is applied nightly to wet skin (an occlusive dressing may be applied at bedtime) and the preparation is washed off in the morning. The frequency of application is reduced when improvement is noted. Irritation (burning and stinging) occurs, particularly if the skin is damaged.

Propylene glycol and other hydroalcoholic gels augment the keratolytic action of salicylic acid; this combination may be effective in ichthyosis. If the formulation contains 6% salicylic acid, no more than 20% of the body surface should be covered at any one time to prevent excessive absorption of salicylate.

Patients who cannot tolerate propylene glycol probably experience a special form of irritation but only rarely develop allergic contact dermatitis (Trancik and Maibach, 1982). Other investigators believe that the incidence of allergic contact dermatitis to propylene glycol may be greater than 2% in patients with eczema (Catanzaro and Smith, 1991). Propylene glycol-free dermatologic preparations are suggested for those who cannot tolerate this agent.

UREA:
Generic. Crystals; powder (bulk).
Aqua Care (Menley & James). Cream and lotion 10%.
Aqua Lacten (Herald). Lotion 10%.
Carmol-10 (Syntex). Lotion 10%.
Carmol-20 (Syntex). Cream 20%.
Nutraplus (Owen/Galderma). Cream, lotion 10%.
(All forms nonprescription)

Available Mixture.
Carmol HC (Syntex). Cream containing urea 10% and hydrocortisone acetate 1% in 30 and 120 g containers.

GLYCOLIC ACID:
Aqua Glycolic (Herald). Lotion 10% in 120 and 240 ml containers.

Available Mixtures.
Hydrisalic (Pedinol), ***Keralyt*** (Westwood-Squibb). Gel containing salicylic acid 6% in a propylene glycol and alcohol vehicle in 30 g containers.
Lac-Hydrin (Westwood-Squibb). Lotion containing ammonium lactate equivalent to lactic acid 12% and propylene glycol in 150 and 360 ml containers.

Soaps, Soap Substitutes, and Shampoos

Ordinary soaps are sodium or potassium salts of fatty acids (Oestreicher, 1988). These anionic and cationic surfactants and cleansers emulsify fats, thereby promoting the removal of foreign particles from the skin. The pH of toilet bars varies in solution; some bar soaps are alkaline (pH 8.8 to 10.5) in solution, and superfatted bar soaps are at the lower end of this range. Superfatted soaps contain unsaponified fat, unreacted fatty acids, or emollients (eg, lanolin, cold cream, polysaturated vegetable oils). Neutral toilet bars or "syndets" contain synthetic detergents (soap substitutes, eg, triethanolamine lauryl sulfate, sodium lauryl sulfate) and usually have a pH of 7.5 or slightly less in solution. Badly irritated skin generally should not be exposed to soaps, detergents, or cleansers other than water.

Medicated soaps are widely available. Some abrasive soaps contain inert aluminum oxide, polyethylene, or sodium tetraborate decahydrate particles. Antimicrobial soaps contain antiseptics in sufficient concentration to be effective deodorants or are useful as handwashes for health care personnel, for preoperative preparation of the skin, or for surgical scrubs.

Shampoos are liquid soaps or detergents used to wash the hair and clean the scalp of scales. Most bar soaps can be used similarly. The detergent properties of special shampoos for use on dry, normal, or oily hair differ. Shampoos also are used as vehicles for applying medication to the scalp for dandruff, seborrheic dermatitis, or psoriasis.

NEUTRAL SOAP SUBSTITUTES (SYNDETS):
Acne-Aid Cleansing Bar (Stiefel), ***Aveenobar*** (Rydelle), ***Caress*** (Lever), ***Dermalab Cleansing Bar*** (Dermalab), ***Dove Bar*** (Lever), ***Drytergent*** (C & M Pharmacal), ***Lowila*** (Westwood-Squibb), ***pHisoDerm*** (Winthrop), ***Vel*** (Colgate) (all forms nonprescription).

ALKALINE AND SUPERFATTED SOAPS:
Camay (Procter & Gamble), ***Dermalab Superfatted Soap*** (Dermalab), ***Nivea Creme Soap*** (Beiersdorf), ***Neutrogena Glycerine Soap*** (Neutrogena), ***Shield*** (Lever) ***Oilatum Soap*** (Stiefel) (all forms nonprescription).

ALKALINE AND ANTIMICROBIAL SOAPS:
Coast (Procter & Gamble), ***Irish Spring*** (Colgate), ***Dial*** (Dial Corp), ***Safeguard*** (Procter & Gamble).

Cited References

Sunscreen drug products for over-the-counter human use; tentative final monograph; proposed rule. *Federal Register* 58:28194-28302, (May 12) 1993.

Agin PP: UVA protection percent: A versatile method for determining UVA efficacy of sunscreens, in Urbach F (ed): *Biological Responses to UVA Radiation*. Overland Park, Kan, Valdenmar Publishing, 1992, 347-361.

Agin PP, Stanfield JW: Screening photoprotective agents against UVA radiation, correspondence. *J Am Acad Dermatol* 27:136-137, 1992.

Arndt KA: *Manual of Dermatologic Therapeutics with Essentials of Diagnosis,* ed 4. Boston, Little Brown, 1989.

Catanzaro JM, Smith JG Jr: Propylene glycol dermatitis. *J Am Acad Dermatol* 24:90-95, 1991.

Council on Scientific Affairs: Harmful effects of ultraviolet radiation. *JAMA* 262:380-384, 1989.

DeLeo VA: Testing and labeling sunscreens. *Pharmacy Times* 34-44, (May) 1992.

DeLeo VA, Maso MJ: Photosensitivity, in Moschella SL, Hurley HJ (eds): *Dermatology,* ed 3. Philadelphia, WB Saunders, 1992, 507-531.

Gange RW, et al: Efficacy of sunscreen containing butyl methoxydibenzoylmethane against ultraviolet A radiation in photosensitized subjects. *J Am Acad Dermatol* 15:494-499, 1986.

Hurwitz S: Sun and sunscreen protection: Recommendations for children. *J Dermatol Surg Oncol* 14:657-660, 1988.

Kaidbey K: Screening photoprotective agents against UVA radiation, correspondence. *J Am Acad Dermatol* 27:137-139, 1992.

Kaidbey KH, Barnes A: Determination of UVA protection factors by means of immediate pigment darkening in normal skin. *J Am Acad Dermatol* 25:262-266, 1991.

Lowe NJ, et al: Sunscreens and phototesting. *Clin Dermatol* 6:40-49, 1988.

Luftman DB, et al: Sunscreens: Update and review. *J Dermatol Surg Oncol* 17:744-746, 1991.

Maddin S, Ho VC: Dermatologic therapy, in Moschella SL, Hurley HJ (eds): *Dermatology,* ed 3. Philadelphia, WB Saunders, 1992, 2187-2215.

Matsuoka LY, et al: Sunscreens suppress cutaneous vitamin D_3 synthesis. *J Clin Endocrinol Metab* 64:1165-1168, 1987.

McKay M: Topical dermatologic therapy. *Primary Care* 10:513-524, 1983.

Morison WL, et al: Photobiology. *J Am Acad Dermatol* 25:327-329, 1991.

Oestreicher MI: Detergents, bath preparations and other skin cleansers. *Clin Dermatol* 6:29-36, 1988.

Pathak MA: Sunscreens and their use in preventive treatment of sunlight-induced skin damage. *J Dermatol Surg Oncol* 13:739-750, 1987.

Rustad OJ: Outdoors and active: Relieving summer's seige on skin. *Physician Sportsmed* 20:163-176, (May) 1992.

Spencer TS: Dry skin and skin moisturizers. *Clin Dermatol* 6:24-28, 1988.

Stern RS, et al: Risk reduction for non-melanoma skin cancer with childhood sunscreen use. *Arch Dermatol* 122:537-545, 1986.

Trancik RJ, Maibach HI: Propylene glycol: Irritation or sensitization? *Contact Dermatitis* 8:185-189, 1982.

Wehr RF, Krochmal L: Considerations in selecting a moisturizer. *Cutis* 39:512-515, 1987.

Wester RC, Maibach HI: Percutaneous absorption of drugs. *Clin Pharmacokinet* 23:253-266, 1992.

Principles of Antimicrobial Drug Selection and Therapy of Infectious Diseases

58

Antimicrobial drugs are used extensively by physicians, and the list of clinically useful agents grows longer. The availability of a large number of antimicrobial drugs offers the patient with an infection a greater chance for cure than ever before with less drug-related toxicity and provides a choice among alternatives despite the continuing emergence of drug-resistant pathogenic organisms. For the prescribing physician, however, appropriate antimicrobial drug selection has become increasingly difficult.

The primary goal of chapters in this Section is to present an overview of antimicrobial drug selection for the treatment of bacterial infections. In addition, principles of infectious disease therapy are briefly reviewed.

PRINCIPLES OF ANTIMICROBIAL DRUG SELECTION

Selection of the most appropriate antimicrobial drug for the treatment of an infection is based on several criteria. First, a determination of the primary focus of infection and the possible organism(s) involved can establish a presumptive or definitive *diagnosis*. The most effective classes of antimicrobial agents then can be identified. The possibility of *resistance of microorganisms* to any of these drugs must be considered in order to determine which drugs will most likely succeed in eradicating the organism. *Variation in patient response*, ie, predicting the response of an individual patient to both the organism and the proposed therapy, also aids the physician in determining the most effective, least toxic agents for treatment. Additional criteria required to identify the actual drug(s) of choice for a particular patient include *outpatient versus inpatient management* and *cost*.

Diagnosis: The most probable organism(s) causing an infection often can be determined on the basis of available clinical evidence. Factors that should be considered in identifying the likely pathogen(s) include the primary site of infection (eg, meninges, skin, cardiovascular system, upper or lower respiratory system, urinary tract, bone, joints, gastrointestinal tract, reproductive system) and whether the patient has had recent trauma, burns, drug addiction, sexual activity, hospitalization, prior infection, or antibiotic use or been exposed to contaminated intimate-contact devices (eg, urethral or intravenous catheter, prosthetic implants).

A Gram stain of an *adequate* specimen is a simple, rapid, and inexpensive method that can be particularly helpful in diagnosis when done by someone skilled in this technique. Bacterial culture and antibiotic susceptibility tests are especially important when the suspected causative organisms are known to vary in susceptibility to first-choice drugs (eg, staphylococci, gram-negative bacilli). It is important to obtain appropriate specimens for cultures of body fluids, exudates, and blood before starting antimicrobial therapy. Anaerobic cultures should ' obtained when anaerobic infections are suspected.

Resistance of Microorganisms: Although som isms continue to be susceptible to selected agents (eg, susceptibility of *Treponema pallidum, Streptococcus pyogenes*, and *Neisseria meningitidis* to penicillin G), the development of clinically important antibiotic resistance is common because of the selective pressures associated with antimicrobial drug usage. Organism resistance may be acquired through plasmid transfer, either by conjugation or transformation, or by mutation. The rate of emergence and extent of resistance can vary among organisms and from drug to drug. Depending on the mechanism and degree of resistance within a bacterial population, larger doses of a drug that do not cause serious adverse reactions may effect a clinical cure. In contrast, combinations of antimicrobial drugs are necessary for the effective treatment of certain infections, such as tuberculosis, to avoid rapid selection of highly resistant strains of *Mycobacterium tuberculosis* that appear readily when single drugs are used.

Antimicrobial susceptibility testing is necessary whenever there is doubt about the activity of a given drug against a particular organism. Susceptibility testing is particularly important for bacteria such as *Staphylococcus aureus*, various facultative and aerobic gram-negative bacilli, and anaerobic bacteria such as the *Bacteroides fragilis* group, in which resistance to standard drug therapy is common. However, it should be noted that in vitro susceptibility to a drug does not always correlate with its clinical efficacy.

Patterns of antimicrobial susceptibility can vary from one geographic area to another, among different hospitals within a given area, between units within a single hospital, and between community-acquired and hospital-acquired infections. A current, locally generated antibiotic susceptibility profile for selected organisms is a good source for establishing the frequency of resistance.

Variation in Patient Response: In addition to the virulence of the organism, the severity of an infection is determined by the genetic constitution, age, and health of the patient. Individuals at the extremes of age, those with inadequate humoral and cellular defense mechanisms or neutropenia, and/or those with associated disorders (especially hypovolemia, hypoxemia, and/or acidosis) are most susceptible. An immunologically compromised (usually leukopenic) patient who is receiving radiation and cytotoxic drugs for treatment of a malignancy is the classic example used to define the high-risk individual with an infection. Using bactericidal rather than bacteriostatic agents when either class may be appropriate or using a combination of antibiotics rather than a single drug may be required in high-risk individuals.

Selection of an appropriate drug requires consideration of pharmacokinetic factors that affect the patient's response to the proposed antimicrobial therapy and thus determine drug concentration at the site of infection. Parenteral rather than oral administration of a drug may be necessary to preclude variability in absorption, which frequently is a problem with the latter route.

Distribution characteristics also may determine the drug of choice. This is of particular importance for infections in the cerebrospinal fluid. Small lipophilic molecules, such as chloramphenicol, isoniazid, metronidazole, rifampin, and trimethoprim, penetrate into cerebrospinal fluid better than highly charged or larger molecular weight molecules, such as aminoglycosides, amphotericin B, first and most second generation cephalosporins, clindamycin, and polymyxins. However, if it is necessary to use an agent that penetrates cerebrospinal fluid poorly, lumbar intrathecal or intraventricular (through a shunt) administration may be required for adequate drug delivery.

The remaining two pharmacokinetic parameters, drug metabolism and elimination, must be considered for patients with impaired hepatic or renal function. For example, dosage adjustments must be made for the aminoglycosides in patients with renal insufficiency to avoid severe toxicity, especially ototoxicity and nephrotoxicity.

Additional factors that may limit the use of a particular agent include (1) a reliable history of an allergic reaction to the antibiotic (eg, morbilliform or maculopapular rash, urticaria, angioedema, wheezing, anaphylaxis); (2) potential adverse interactions (eg, avoiding additive nephrotoxicity, ototoxicity, or hepatotoxicity) when other drugs are being given for associated illnesses; and (3) adverse effects that are predictable in certain patients (eg, use of tetracyclines in pregnant women or young children).

Outpatient Versus Inpatient Drug Treatment: Whether hospitalization is required for antimicrobial drug treatment depends primarily on the severity of the infection and the anticipated compliance with therapy. Among equally efficacious alternatives, low toxicity and ease of administration (usually by the oral route) are the most important factors in selecting a particular drug for outpatients. In addition, using drugs that require less frequent administration may improve compliance. In contrast, drug efficacy and the rapid attainment of inhibitory, preferably bactericidal, concentrations at the site of infection are primary considerations in hospitalized patients with life-threatening infections, even when toxic drugs must be administered. Empiric therapy with parenteral (usually intravenous) antimicrobial agents frequently is required in these patients.

Drug selection is usually more complicated for inpatients than for ambulatory patients because (1) nosocomial infections often are associated with uncommon or resistant organisms; (2) inpatients usually have more severe infections and associated underlying illnesses; and (3) severely ill patients are less tolerant of drug toxicity or adverse reactions.

The following core-group of antibiotics is widely used for systemic antimicrobial therapy in ambulatory patients: the penicillins (especially penicillin V, ampicillin, amoxicillin, and the orally bioavailable penicillinase-resistant penicillins, cloxacillin and dicloxacillin), erythromycin, sulfisoxazole, tetracyclines, oral cephalosporins, fluoroquinolones (eg, ciprofloxacin), trimethoprim, and the drug combinations trimethoprim/sulfamethoxazole [Bactrim, Septra], erythromycin/sulfisoxazole [Pediazole], and amoxicillin/potassium clavulanate [Augmentin]. These drugs are effective when employed appropriately and have a good record of safety. (See the following chapters in this section for specific indications.)

Cost: The impact of drug cost continues to be widely discussed. Although the physician's primary responsibility is to select the antimicrobial agent that is most likely to effect a complete cure in the shortest time, alternative preparations of the same antibiotic (generic substitution) or alternative antibiotics often are available. The selection of an appropriate, equally effective but less expensive preparation may ensure compliance in selected patients. The physician is encouraged to seek unbiased sources of information that compare the cost of equally effective preparations. These include the Pharmacy and Therapeutics Committee in local hospitals and antibiotic audit cost-effectiveness reviews in the literature (providing regional costs are consonant with those listed). Surveying local pharmacies for prescription prices also can be useful because prices may vary significantly among pharmacies. Potentially effective mechanisms to decrease antibiotic drug costs within hospitals include the use of competitive bidding for similar antimicrobials (eg, antipseudomonal penicillins, third generation cephalosporins, aminoglycosides) and the use of equally effective and comparably priced drugs that require less frequent administration.

OTHER PRINCIPLES OF INFECTIOUS DISEASE THERAPY

If the preferred antimicrobial agent has been selected on the basis of the preceding criteria, treatment with that drug in an appropriate dosage should produce a concentration of antimicrobial agent at the site of infection that is adequate to eradicate the causative organism. In addition, optimum therapy also will require that the following general principles be given equal consideration.

Relief of Obstruction, Drainage, Surgery, Debridement, and Foreign Body Removal: Relief of gastrointestinal or ureteral obstruction; incision and adequate drainage of furuncles, abscesses, and wound infections; surgical repair of a ruptured colon or removal of an infected gallbladder; as well as debridement of animal and human bite wounds when indicated are necessary to achieve an optimum effect from any antimicrobial agent. In many cases, mechanical correction is the primary factor for determining a successful clinical outcome.

A foreign body, including intimate-contact medical devices (eg, catheters of all types regardless of location, intrauterine devices, prostheses, pacemakers) that must remain in place, should always be considered a potential source of infection in a diagnostic work-up. Successful antimicrobial treatment of an infection associated with a foreign body usually requires the latter's removal.

Supportive Care: Mild to moderate hypovolemia, electrolyte imbalances, and/or acidosis should be corrected to improve the overall management of the patient. Adequate supportive care may help to prevent therapeutic failure in moderate to severe infections. Life-threatening septic shock and other types of cardiovascular depression may require additional therapy with pressor agents (eg, dopamine). Management of increased intracranial pressure is another vital aspect of the supportive care of a patient with an infectious disease (ie, meningitis). Diphtheria antitoxin and tetanus immune globulin (human) also should be administered when indicated.

Monitoring Patient Response: Monitoring the patient's response to antimicrobial therapy is essential to determine the efficacy of treatment and whether a change in drug therapy is indicated. The frequency of monitoring response to therapy is directly related to the severity of the infection.

Measurements of changes in clinical variables, such as resolution of fever, leukocytosis, and other signs of inflammation, and disappearance of the causative organism from post-treatment cultures, are primary methods of determining response to therapy. When a potentially toxic antimicrobial agent (eg, an aminoglycoside) is administered for a prolonged period, monitoring of serum drug concentrations during therapy usually is desirable. Similarly, when a prolonged serum bactericidal effect is necessary to cure an infection (eg, infective endocarditis), measurement of serum bactericidal titers during therapy frequently is done to assess the adequacy of treatment, although the importance of such monitoring is controversial.

Suboptimal response to therapy may be a function of either therapeutic failure or an adverse event. Therapeutic failures commonly occur because of (1) inadequate concentration and/or duration of the antimicrobial agent at the site of infection; (2) prior or developing organism resistance to the drug(s) selected; (3) subsequent development of an unrelated infection or superinfection that is unresponsive to the drug selected; (4) failure to correct an aggravating factor that limits the effectiveness of the antibiotic (eg, failure to drain an abscess, relieve obstruction of an infected viscus, remove a foreign implant, or correct the cause of compromised humoral or cellular immunity); (5) laboratory error resulting in inadequate therapy; (6) initial misdiagnosis; (7) noncompliance by an ambulatory patient; or (8) circumstances in which antimicrobial therapy simply does not alter the immediate course of disease (eg, early pneumococcal pneumonia).

The appearance of an adverse event most probably is related to an adverse drug reaction or drug interaction.

The following are recommended general references on infectious disease therapy:

Selected References

(A) ***Textbooks***

Feigin RD, Cherry JD (eds): *Textbook of Pediatric Infectious Diseases*, ed 2. Philadelphia, WB Saunders, 1987, vols I and II.

Hoeprich PD (ed): *Infectious Diseases*, ed 4. Philadelphia, Harper & Row, 1989.

Holmes KK, et al (eds): *Sexually Transmitted Diseases*, ed 2. New York, McGraw-Hill, 1990.

Kass EH, Platt R (eds): *Current Therapy in Infectious Disease-3.* Philadelphia, BC Decker, 1989.

Mandell GL, et al (eds): *Principles and Practice of Infectious Diseases*, ed 3. New York, Churchill Livingstone, 1990.

Moellering RC Jr: Principles of anti-infective therapy, in Mandell GL, et al (eds): *Principles and Practice of Infectious Diseases*, ed 3. New York, John Wiley & Sons, 1990, 206-218.

Remington JS, Klein JO (eds): *Infectious Diseases of the Fetus and Newborn*, ed 3. Philadelphia, WB Saunders, 1989.

Sande MA, et al: Antimicrobial agents: General considerations, in Gilman AG, et al (eds): *The Pharmacological Basis of Therapeutics*, ed 8. New York, Macmillan, 1990, 1018-1046.

(B) ***Pocketbooks and Manuals***

Report of the Committee on Infectious Diseases: *American Academy of Pediatrics Redbook*, ed 21. Elk Grove Village, IL, American Academy of Pediatrics, 1988.

Bartlett J: *1989-1990 Pocketbook of Infectious Disease Therapy.* Baltimore, Williams and Wilkins, 1990.

Conte JE Jr, Barriere SL: *Manual of Antibiotics and Infectious Diseases*, ed 6. Philadelphia, Lea & Febiger, 1988.

The Medical Letter: *Handbook of Antimicrobial Therapy*. New Rochelle, NY, The Medical Letter, Inc, 1988.

Nelson JD: *1989-1990 Pocketbook of Pediatric Antimicrobial Therapy*, ed 8. Baltimore, Williams & Wilkins, 1989.

Sanford JP: *Guide to Antimicrobial Therapy, 1990.* West Bethesda, Md, Antimicrobial Therapy, Inc, 1990.

(C) ***Reviews***

The choice of antimicrobial drugs. *Med Lett Drugs Ther* 32:41-48, 1990.

Infectious Disease Clinics of North America, vol 1-3. Philadelphia, WB Saunders, 1987-1989 (four issues per volume).

Neu HC: New antibiotics: Areas of appropriate use. *J Infect Dis* 155:403-417, 1987.

Neu HC (ed): Update on antibiotics I. *Med Clin North Am* 71:1051-1216, 1987 (10 articles).

Neu HC: General concepts on chemotherapy of infectious diseases, *Med Clin North Am* 71:1051-1064, 1987.

Neu HC (ed): Update on antibiotics II. *Med Clin North Am* 72:555-743, 1988 (11 articles).

Wilkowske CJ, Hermans PE: General principles of antimicrobial therapy. *Mayo Clin Proc* 62:789-798, 1987.

Antimicrobial Therapy for Common Infectious Diseases

59

BACTEREMIAS AND SEPSIS

BONE AND JOINT INFECTIONS

CARDIOVASCULAR SYSTEM INFECTIONS

CENTRAL NERVOUS SYSTEM INFECTIONS

EAR INFECTIONS

EYE INFECTIONS

GASTROINTESTINAL AND INTRA-ABDOMINAL INFECTIONS

REPRODUCTIVE TRACT INFECTIONS (FEMALE)

REPRODUCTIVE TRACT INFECTIONS (MALE)

RESPIRATORY TRACT INFECTIONS (LOWER)

RESPIRATORY TRACT INFECTIONS (UPPER)

SKIN AND SOFT-TISSUE INFECTIONS

URINARY TRACT INFECTIONS

MISCELLANEOUS INFECTIONS

The purpose of this chapter is to present synopses of recommended antimicrobial drug therapy for common infectious diseases. These guidelines represent a consensus based on evaluation of the current medical literature and the opinions of expert infectious disease consultants.

Unless stated otherwise, the common causative organisms and appropriate antimicrobial drug therapy are for community-acquired infections in normal (eg, immunocompetent) hosts. Hospital-acquired (nosocomial) infections or infections in immunocompromised (eg, neutropenic, diabetic, alcoholic) hosts are indicated as such.

Depending on the nature and severity of the infection, antimicrobial drug therapy may be (1) specific, following identification and susceptibility testing of the causative organism; (2) based primarily on the results of a Gram stain; and/or (3) initially empiric, pending the results of microbial cultures, antibiotic sensitivity tests, or clinical response.

The content of this chapter is limited by the constraints of space. Therefore, it is not possible to provide a detailed discussion of antimicrobial drug therapy or to include all possible drug regimens for each infectious disease. The reader is encouraged to consult the cited references for additional information. The antimicrobial agents, including dosage information, are discussed in other chapters on anti-infective drugs.

Note: In this chapter, when the preferred drug therapy is a penicillin derivative but the patient is allergic to this class of antibiotics, the first nonpenicillin drug (or combination) listed usually becomes the preferred drug therapy. However, penicillin skin testing and desensitization may be indicated for certain serious infections (eg, infective endocarditis). Cephalosporins should not be administered to patients who have experienced an immediate-type hypersensitivity reaction to penicillins (see the chapters Penicillins and Cephalosporins and Related Agents, respectively, for the names of specific penicillin and cephalosporin analogues).

BACTEREMIAS AND SEPSIS

Sepsis of Unknown Etiology

In many cases of sepsis, the probable causative organism(s) can be determined from a suspected source of primary infection prior to blood culture results (for specific examples, see the other sections of this Chapter). After adequate clinical evaluation, if no primary source of infection responsible for bacteremia can be identified and blood culture results are not yet available, EMPIRIC antimicrobial drug therapy (parenteral) to cover the more likely pathogens should be initiated. In NONCOMPROMISED ADULTS AND CHILDREN (GREATER THAN 5 YEARS), coverage should be directed toward gram-negative bacilli, especially *Escherichia coli* and *Klebsiella pneumoniae*, *Neisseria meningitidis*, and gram-positive cocci, including *Staphylococcus aureus, Streptococcus pneumoniae*, and other streptococci. In NONCOMPROMISED INFANTS AND CHILDREN LESS THAN 5 YEARS (EXCEPT NEWBORNS), coverage should be directed toward *Streptococcus pneumoniae* and other streptococci, *Haemophilus influenzae* type b, and *Neisseria meningitidis*; some experts also recommend coverage against *Staphylococcus aureus*. For treatment of sepsis in NEONATES, see the following section entitled Sepsis, Neonatal.

Selected references: Foltzer and Reese, 1986; Word and Klein, 1988; *Med Lett Drugs Ther*, 1990; Sanford, 1990.

EMPIRIC THERAPY

Noncompromised Adults and Children (greater than 5 years)

Gram-negative bacilli (eg, *Escherichia coli, Klebsiella pneumoniae*); *Staphylococcus aureus; Streptococcus pneumoniae*; other streptococci

ALTERNATIVE THERAPY: **(see Remarks)**
Nafcillin (or Oxacillin) *plus* Aminoglycoside (gentamicin, tobramycin, amikacin, netilmicin)
OR
First Generation Cephalosporin (cefazolin, cephalothin, cephapirin, cephradine) *plus* Aminoglycoside
OR
Third Generation Cephalosporin (cefotaxime, ceftizoxime, ceftriaxone, ceftazidime, cefoperazone) *with or without* Aminoglycoside
OR
Ticarcillin/Potassium Clavulanate [Timentin] *with* Aminoglycoside
OR
Ampicillin/Sulbactam [Unasyn] *with* Aminoglycoside
OR
Imipenem/cilastatin [Primaxin] *with or without* Aminoglycoside
OR
Ciprofloxacin (intravenous) *with* or *without* Clindamycin
REMARKS:
(1) No clear-cut consensus for a particular regimen could be obtained from the literature or from our consultants. For life-threatening septicemia, a number of experts recommend a third generation cephalosporin *plus* an aminoglycoside OR ticarcillin/potassium clavulanate *plus* an aminoglycoside OR imipenem/cilastatin *plus* an aminoglycoside. Many experts use imipenem/cilastatin alone, ie, without an aminoglycoside.
(2) When bacterial endocarditis is suspected, nafcillin (or oxacillin) *plus* gentamicin *plus* penicillin G (or ampicillin) can be used.
(3) If methicillin-resistant *Staphylococcus aureus* is suspected, substitute intravenous vancomycin for the penicillinase-resistant penicillin or the other beta lactam antibiotics.
(4) If anaerobic infection with *Bacteroides fragilis* is possible (eg, suspected intra-abdominal focus), clindamycin, metronidazole, or another anti-*B. fragilis* drug should be added when necessary. Ticarcillin/potassium clavulanate, ampicillin/sulbactam, and imipenem/cilastatin have excellent antimicrobial activity against the *B. fragilis* group.
(5) Selection of the particular aminoglycoside should be based on locally generated antibiotic susceptibility profiles.
(6) Most experts do not recommend methicillin in adults or children because of an increased risk of interstitial nephritis.
(7) Switch to most effective drug regimen after blood culture and susceptibility test results are available.
(8) Fluoroquinolones are contraindicated for use in prepubertal children or pregnant women.

Noncompromised Infants and Children (Less Than 5 Years, Excluding Newborns)

Streptococcus pneumoniae, Haemophilus influenzae type b, *Neisseria meningitidis*, other streptococci; some experts also recommend coverage against *Staphylococcus aureus*

PREFERRED THERAPY:
Cefotaxime or Ceftriaxone (or Ceftizoxime) *with or without* Nafcillin (or Oxacillin)
OR
Nafcillin (or Oxacillin) *plus* Chloramphenicol
OR
Ampicillin *plus* Chloramphenicol
REMARKS:
(1) Each of the above regimens has been recommended by various experts.
(2) Chloramphenicol, cefotaxime, ceftizoxime, ceftriaxone, and cefuroxime are active against beta lactamase-producing *H. influenzae* type b, which are prevalent in most geographical areas.
(3) The regimen of ampicillin *plus* chloramphenicol would be inadequate for infections caused by *S. aureus*.
(4) Most experts do not recommend methicillin because of an increased risk of interstitial nephritis.
(5) Cefuroxime, a second generation cephalosporin, has been widely used for *H. influenzae* type b infections in children. However, on a weight basis, this drug is less active than the third generation cephalosporins (eg, cefotaxime, ceftriaxone) against this organism. More important, cefuroxime occasionally has been associated with delayed sterilization of cerebrospinal fluid and even overt therapeutic failure in patients infected with *H. influenzae* type b. Thus, many pediatric infectious disease consultants prefer a third generation cephalosporin (eg, cefotaxime, ceftriaxone) to cefuroxime for severe *H. influenzae* type b infections.
(6) Cefamandole is NOT recommended as an initial therapy for children less than 5 years because of its poor penetration into the cerebrospinal fluid.
(7) In infants between 1 and 3 months, group B streptococci also may be causative. Many pediatric infectious disease experts recommend ampicillin *plus* cefotaxime (or ceftriaxone) for empiric therapy in this age group.
(8) Switch to most effective drug regimen after blood culture and susceptibility test results are available.

Sepsis, Neonatal

The most common causative organisms are *Escherichia coli* and group B streptococci (*Streptococcus agalactiae*). Other causative organisms include *Listeria monocytogenes, Klebsiella-Enterobacter* species, *Proteus* species, group D streptococci (enterococci and *S. bovis*), and non-group D, alpha-hemolytic streptococci. After 5 days of age, nosocomial infections caused by *Staphylococcus aureus* and coagulase-negative staphylococci and multiply resistant gram-negative enteric bacilli also are a possibility.

Initial antimicrobial drug therapy (parenteral) of neonatal sepsis is EMPIRIC pending the results of blood cultures and susceptibility tests.

Selected references: Steinhoff, 1986; St. Geme and Polin, 1988; Nelson, 1991 A.

EMPIRIC THERAPY (NEONATES LESS THAN 1 MONTH)

Streptococcus agalactiae (group B) and other streptococci, including enterococci; *Escherichia coli* and other gram-negative enteric bacilli; *Listeria monocytogenes*

PREFERRED THERAPY:
Ampicillin *plus* Aminoglycoside (gentamicin, tobramycin, amikacin, netilmicin)
ALTERNATIVE THERAPY:
Ampicillin *plus* Cefotaxime (or Ceftriaxone)
REMARKS:
(1) Selection of the particular aminoglycoside should be based on locally generated antibiotic susceptibility profiles.
(2) If *S. aureus* is a suspected pathogen, a penicillinase-resistant penicillin (oxacillin or methicillin) can be added to the regimen. Vancomycin is required for methicillin-resistant strains.
(3) Switch to most effective drug regimen after blood culture and susceptibility test results are available.
(4) The rapid emergence of resistant strains of certain gram-negative bacilli (eg, *Enterobacter cloacae*) to third generation cephalosporins and the increasing incidence of fungal (especially *Candida*) superinfections have caused concern among some neonatologists about the widespread use of these agents as part of routine, initial empiric regimens in the closed environments of neonatal intensive care units (Bryan et al, 1985; McCracken, 1985).
(5) Some consultants recommended caution with ceftriaxone in jaundiced premature infants because this highly protein bound cephalosporin can displace bilirubin from albumin binding sites.

Fever in the Patient with Neutropenia (<1000 Granulocytes/mm^3)

Fever in the presence of granulocytopenia probably is most often encountered in patients receiving cytotoxic drugs for the treatment of neoplasms. In these patients, a decreased granulocyte count is the primary risk factor for the development of subsequent bacterial infection. Additional risk factors are the duration and degree of the granulocytopenia, alterations in cellular and humoral immune functions, breaches in physical barriers to infection (ie, mucosal or integumentary damage), and the quality of the endogenous microbial flora.

In general, all granulocytopenic patients should be considered at risk for infection and, if fever develops, are candidates for empiric antibiotic therapy. Two or three low-grade temperature elevations >38° C (oral) or a temperature >38° C for at least one hour indicate a febrile state.

The definition of granulocytopenia generally indicates a polymorphonuclear leukocyte (PMN) count of <1000/mm^3. A significant discernible increase in the infection rate occurs as the PMN count falls below this level. The risk of infection further increases in patients with a count <500 PMN/mm^3 and becomes overwhelming in those with a PMN count of <100/mm^3 for prolonged periods. In addition to the degree of granulocytopenia, the rate at which the PMN count declines is related to the risk of subsequent infection, with a faster rate of decline indicating increased risk of infection. Thorough medical evaluation of these patients is critical to their survival but is complicated by diminished ability to mount an inflammatory response, which masks the typical signs and symptoms of infection.

Endogenous microbial flora account for at least 80% of primary infections in the granulocytopenic patient. However, since over 50% of infecting strains are acquired in the hospital, antimicrobial drug selection should reflect this and proceed based on local drug susceptibility patterns. Pathogens commonly associated with high mortality are the Enterobacteriaceae, including *Escherichia coli, Klebsiella pneumoniae,* and *Pseudomonas aeruginosa*, although the frequency of infection with the latter organism has inexplicably declined in many hospitals. In contrast, infections caused by gram-positive bacteria have increased in frequency in recent years, especially in patients with indwelling intravascular lines. These organisms include gram-positive cocci, such as *Staphylococcus aureus*, *S. epidermidis* (coagulase-negative staphylococci), and streptococci (*S. pyogenes* and viridans streptococci). In some hospitals, staphylococci are the most common pathogens, and these are not adequately eradicated by most empiric antimicrobial regimens. A major problem is the increasing frequency of methicillin-resistant *S. aureus*, with virtually all institutions now encountering coagulase-negative staphylococci that are resistant to methicillin. Other gram-positive organisms, including *Streptococcus pneumoniae, Enterococcus faecalis, Corynebacterium CDC* J.K., and *Bacillus* species, are isolated occasionally from granulocytopenic patients. The overall mortality associated with infections caused by gram-positive bacteria is substantially less than that in patients with gram-negative bacillary sepsis. However, invasive fungal infections and superinfections with resistant bacterial strains are common in all patients who remain granulocytopenic for prolonged periods; receive antimicrobial therapy for bacterial infections; are hospitalized for long periods; receive corticosteroids; or undergo invasive procedures, such as placement of an indwelling central venous catheter. These subsequent infections are difficult to diagnose, often are resistant to standard therapy, and represent major causes of morbidity and mortality in the neutropenic patient.

The data on antimicrobial therapy for fever in the neutropenic patient do not unequivocally support one regimen over another. Thus, the factors that should be considered in choosing initial EMPIRIC antibiotic therapy include the physical state of the patient; the degree of neutropenia; hepatic and renal function; the presence of indwelling vascular devices; the presence of underlying disease, such as diabetes mellitus; intolerance to penicillins or sulfonamides; the type, frequency of occurrence, and antibiotic susceptibility of bacterial isolates observed in similar patients; and the institutional spectrum of bacterial strains that are resistant to commonly used antibiotics. Guidelines have been published for the use of antimicrobial agents in neutropenic patients with unexplained fever (Hughes et al, 1990). However, therapy must be determined by the evaluation of the individual patient and may require modification during the course of treatment.

Antimicrobial drug therapy prior to blood culture results is essential and EMPIRIC therapy to cover the most common pathogens is indicated. Current consensus is that optimal doses of parenteral, broad spectrum, bactericidal antibiotics in synergistic combinations should be selected (see Remarks).

Selected references: DeJongh et al, 1986 A; Foltzer and Reese, 1986; Klastersky, 1986; Pizzo, 1986, 1990; Klastersky et al, 1986, 1988; Schimpff, 1986, 1990; Calandra et al, 1987; Hathorn et al, 1987; Young, 1987; Bodey, 1989; Sanford, 1990; Wade, 1989; *Med Lett Drugs Ther*, 1990; Meunier, 1990; Nelson, 1991 B.

EMPIRIC THERAPY

Escherichia coli, Klebsiella species, and *Pseudomonas aeruginosa*; possibly *Staphylococcus aureus* and *S. epidermidis* (see Remarks)

PREFERRED THERAPY:

Antipseudomonal Penicillin (piperacillin, azlocillin, mezlocillin, ticarcillin [with or without potassium clavulanate]) *plus* Aminoglycoside (gentamicin, tobramycin, amikacin) (see Remarks)

OR

Ceftazidime *plus* Aminoglycoside (gentamicin, tobramycin, amikacin)

OR

Ceftazidime *plus* Antipseudomonal Penicillin (azlocillin, mezlocillin, piperacillin) (see Remarks)

OR

Aminoglycoside (gentamicin, tobramycin, amikacin) *plus* Antipseudomonal Penicillin (or Ceftazidime) *plus* Vancomycin (see Remarks)

ALTERNATIVE THERAPY:

Monotherapy (Ceftazidime, Imipenem/Cilastatin, Cefoperazone) (see Remarks)

REMARKS:

(1) Current consensus is that combination regimens containing an antipseudomonal beta lactam and an aminoglycoside are preferred for empiric therapy because they frequently have synergistic activity against aerobic gram-negative bacilli (eg, *P. aeruginosa*). Bacteremias caused by these organisms have been associated with the poorest response rates and highest mortality in neutropenic patients, particularly when the neutropenia is profound (<100 granulocytes/mm^3) and persistent.

(2) Selection of the particular aminoglycoside or antipseudomonal penicillin should be based on locally generated antimicrobial susceptibility profiles. Amikacin should be used when gentamicin- and tobramycin-resistant strains are prevalent. Many infectious disease experts now prefer an extended spectrum penicillin, piperacillin or azlocillin, to ticarcillin or mezlocillin because they have greater activity in vitro against *P. aeruginosa.*

(3) Ceftazidime is preferred to the other third generation cephalosporins (eg, cefotaxime, ceftizoxime, ceftriaxone, cefoperazone) because it has the best activity against *P. aeruginosa.*

(4) Controversy currently exists concerning the routine inclusion of vancomycin in empiric regimens (Rubin et al, 1988; Anaissie et al, 1988; Shenep et al, 1988; Bodey et al, 1990). Some investigators suggest that vancomycin can be added after microbiological cultures indicate the presence of sensitive gram-positive organisms, with little or no deleterious effect on the patient. This approach has the advantages of limiting drug exposure and hence drug-related cost (vancomycin is relatively expensive), toxicity (ototoxicity and nephrotoxicity of vancomycin and aminoglycosides may be additive when they are given together), and emergence of resistant bacterial strains (Schwalbe et al, 1987). Other authorities suggest that the routine initial inclusion of vancomycin will be more effective against gram-positive bacteria, avoids potentially deleterious delays in waiting for microbial culture results, and possibly shortens the total duration of therapy. In view of this controversy, the decision to use vancomycin as part of initial therapy must take into account additional local variables, such as institutional antibiotic susceptibility profiles, local prevalence of gram-positive bacteremia, the identification of susceptible strains, routine hospital practices, and consultation with infectious disease experts. Two exceptions exist: (1) vancomycin should be included in the initial regimen when the presence of methicillin-resistant *S. aureus* is suspected (ie, in patients who have been exposed to colonized persons, when institutional infection rates with such strains are high). (2) Infection at exit or tunnel sites of central venous catheters or other lines or nonpatency of vascular lines dictates the inclusion of vancomycin at the onset of the treatment regimen (Hughes et al, 1990).

(5) Because of the toxicity associated with aminoglycosides, regimens to exclude this class of agents have been designed. A number of these regimens, as listed below, have shown comparable efficacy to aminoglycoside-containing combinations as empiric therapy for febrile neutropenic patients in various clinical trials. However, clinical experience is more limited and concerns about each of these alternatives, especially their efficacy in gram-negative rod bacteremias in patients with profound and persistent neutropenia, has, thus far, prevented any of them from becoming clearly preferred therapy in these patients.

(a) Double beta lactam regimens, consisting of an antipseudomonal penicillin (piperacillin, mezlocillin, azlocillin, ticarcillin) *plus* ceftazidime, have proven clinically effective (DeJongh et al, 1986 B; Bodey et al, 1990). Concerns with double beta lactam regimens include the possibility of antagonism between the drugs for certain pathogens, the potential for rapid emergence of resistant bacterial strains, inadequate coverage against staphylococci, increased frequency of adverse reactions, lack of synergy against gram-negative bacilli, and high cost (see Young, 1985; Cohen, 1987). Such regimens may be most useful in patients at increased risk for aminoglycoside toxicity (eg, elderly patients with pre-existing renal dysfunction).

(b) Ceftazidime alone has been as effective as aminoglycoside-containing regimens in some clinical trials (Pizzo et al, 1986; see also Wade et al, 1986). Concerns with ceftazidime monotherapy include the questionable ability of a single drug to cure *P. aeruginosa* infections in the neutropenic host, the potential for rapid emergence of resistant bacterial strains (Johnson and Ramphal, 1990), and inadequate coverage against staphylococci (Young, 1986; Cohen, 1987). Ceftazidime monotherapy may be useful for patients in hospitals where resistance to this drug is minimal and in whom neutropenia is not severe and infection with *P. aeruginosa* is unlikely.

(c) Vancomycin *plus* ceftazidime increases activity against staphylococci, including methicillin-resistant strains, and, in some clinical trials, has been superior to ceftazidime alone (Kramer et al, 1986). The other concerns noted above for vancomycin and for ceftazidime alone also apply to this regimen.

(d) Monotherapy with imipenem, a very broad spectrum, beta lactamase-stable carbapenem, also appears to be effective

(Bodey et al, 1986; Wade et al, 1987; Falloon et al, 1987; Liang et al, 1990), but experience is very limited. Concerns about the use of this drug alone as empiric therapy in febrile neutropenic patients are similar to those listed above for ceftazidime monotherapy. Also, imipenem, which is administered in a 1:1 fixed-ratio combination with cilastatin, a dehydropeptidase-1 inhibitor, has been associated with seizures in some patients.

(e) The combination of vancomycin *plus* aztreonam, a beta lactamase-stable monobactam with excellent activity against aerobic gram-negative bacilli including *P. aeruginosa*, also shows promise (Jones et al, 1986). However, clinical data are very limited. Concerns with this combination are similar to those for vancomycin plus ceftazidime. Interestingly, patients who exhibit immediate-type hypersensitivity reactions to penicillins and cephalosporins appear to tolerate aztreonam, and this drug may be used with caution in these patients.

(6) The optimal duration of empiric antibiotic therapy in the febrile, neutropenic patient is determined primarily by the PMN count (Hughes et al, 1990). Thus, as the PMN count rises above 500/mm^3, the persistence or recurrence of bacterial infection becomes less likely. However, all febrile, granulocytopenic patients must receive antibiotic therapy for a minimum of seven days. If a particular organism has been cultured and its antibiotic sensitivity profile has been determined, the regimen may be modified to provide optimal, cost-effective coverage. However, it is imperative to continue therapy until the causative organism can no longer be cultured, infectious loci have resolved, and fever has disappeared (minimum duration, seven days). Although a PMN count >500/mm^3 is desirable before antibiotic treatment is discontinued, if the aforementioned criteria for discontinuation have been met, the physician may decide to stop therapy before the granulocyte count rises above 500/mm^3. However, this is acceptable only when the patient will be available for continuous, close follow-up, there is no integumental or mucous membrane damage, and no additional cytotoxic chemotherapy or invasive procedures are imminent.

In patients who become and remain afebrile and from whom no particular organism has been isolated, the initial antibiotic therapy should be continued for at least seven days. In the patient who remains afebrile and has a PMN count <500/mm^3, even if no organism can be isolated, the abovementioned guidelines can be applied to determine when to terminate therapy. If the patient remains febrile with a microbiologically documented infection, antibiotics may need to be added or changed. Persistent fever and neutropenia in the absence of documented bacterial infection (ie, negative culture) suggest possible fungal infection with *Candida* or *Aspergillus*; addition of amphotericin B to the regimen should be considered (see Hughes et al, 1990).

Toxic Shock Syndrome

Toxic shock syndrome is an acute clinical illness caused by certain strains of *Staphylococcus aureus* and is characterized by fever, hypotension, erythematous cutaneous eruption followed by desquamation, and multiple organ involvement. It has been associated epidemiologically with young menstruating females who use tampons, particularly those with high absorbency. However, this syndrome also may occur in male and female patients of any age with other *S. aureus* infections (eg, postoperative wound infection, skin infection), and it has been reported as a complication of influenza and influenza-like illness. The pathogenesis of toxic shock syndrome is not completely understood, but it appears to be toxin-mediated. Most strains of *S. aureus* recovered from women with menstrually related toxic shock syndrome produce a pyrogenic exotoxin, called toxic shock syndrome toxin-1 (TSST-1), to which patients lacked circulating antibodies. However, other toxins (eg, enterotoxin B) also may be involved in producing this syndrome. A similar syndrome due to *Streptococcus pyogenes* has been reported.

Antimicrobial drug therapy does not appear to play an important role in treating the acute phase of toxic shock syndrome, unless blood cultures are positive for *S. aureus*. Supportive measures (eg, maintenance of adequate blood pressure with aggressive volume replacement) and removal of the source of presumed infection (eg, removal of tampon, debridement of wound) are of primary importance. Corticosteroids may be beneficial in patients with severe illness. Antibiotics (parenteral) are useful in preventing recurrences of the syndrome.

Selected references: Berkley et al, 1987; MacDonald et al, 1987; Todd, 1988; Chesney, 1989; Resnick, 1990.

SPECIFIC THERAPY

PREFERRED THERAPY:
Nafcillin OR **Oxacillin**
ALTERNATIVE THERAPY:
First Generation Cephalosporin (eg, cefazolin)
REMARKS:
(1) Most experts do not recommend methicillin in adults because of an increased risk of interstitial nephritis.
(2) Vancomycin (intravenous) can be used in patients allergic to penicillins and cephalosporins.
(3) Women who have had menstrual toxic shock syndrome should be advised not to use tampons.

BONE AND JOINT INFECTIONS

Arthritis, Septic

The most common causative organisms of septic arthritis vary with patient age and are usually subdivided according to the following five age groups:

(1) NEONATES AND INFANTS LESS THAN 2 MONTHS: The predominant organisms are *Staphylococcus aureus*, group B streptococci (*Streptococcus agalactiae*), and gram-negative enteric bacilli (eg, *Escherichia coli*) (Note: *Neisseria gonorrhoeae* from an infected mother also may be causative);

(2) CHILDREN 2 MONTHS TO 5 YEARS: *Haemophilus influenzae* type b (more common under 2 years), *S. aureus*, and streptococci (eg, *S. pyogenes, S. pneumoniae*) are the common causative organisms;

(3) CHILDREN 5 TO 15 YEARS: *S. aureus* and streptococci are the major pathogens;

(4) SEXUALLY ACTIVE ADOLESCENTS AND ADULTS (USUALLY BETWEEN 15 AND 40 YEARS): *Neisseria gonorrhoeae* causes most cases; *S. aureus* and streptococci are less common;

(5) OLDER ADULTS (>40 YEARS): *S. aureus* is the predominant pathogen; streptococci, gram-negative bacilli (often

associated with predisposing conditions), and *N. gonorrhoeae* are less common causative organisms.

Although ultimate antimicrobial drug selection for septic arthritis should be SPECIFIC and based on culture (synovial fluid, blood, other sites as indicated) and susceptibility data, EMPIRIC therapy is indicated initially. As outlined below, initial drug selection is based on the age of the patient and results of synovial fluid Gram stain, when available. Parenteral antibiotics are recommended, but intra-articular injection should be avoided. Adequate removal of purulent joint fluid (eg, needle aspiration, open drainage) also is required.

Selected references: Allman and Abruzzo, 1987; Syriopoulou and Smith, 1987; Conte and Barriere, 1988; *Med Lett Drugs Ther,* 1990; *MMWR,* 1989; Sanford, 1990 A; Smith, 1990; Nelson, 1991 A.

EMPIRIC THERAPY (BASED ON INITIAL GRAM STAIN)

Neonates and Young Infants (Less Than 2 Months)

(A) Gram-positive cocci

Staphylococcus aureus; Streptococcus agalactiae (group B)

PREFERRED THERAPY:
Oxacillin (parenteral) OR **Nafcillin**
ALTERNATIVE THERAPY:
Cephalothin or Cephapirin
REMARKS:
(1) In contrast to older children and adults, nafcillin is not recommended in neonates by some experts because of erratic pharmacokinetics, particularly in jaundiced infants.
(2) Penicillin G should be substituted for antistaphylococcal penicillins if susceptibility of *S. aureus* strain is proven.
(3) For methicillin-resistant strains of *S. aureus*, intravenous vancomycin is the drug of choice.
(4) For infections caused by group B streptococci, penicillin G or ampicillin is preferred. Some experts would add either of these agents to the antistaphylococcal penicillin prior to culture and susceptibility test results to improve coverage against group B streptococci.

(B) Gram-negative bacilli

Escherichia coli and other gram-negative enteric bacilli

PREFERRED THERAPY:
Aminoglycoside (gentamicin, tobramycin, amikacin, netilmicin)
OR
Cefotaxime (or Ceftriaxone or Ceftazidime)
REMARKS:
(1) Switch to most effective drug regimen after susceptibility test results are available.
(2) Cefotaxime and ceftriaxone are NOT recommended if *Pseudomonas aeruginosa* is a likely pathogen. Ceftazidime *plus* an aminoglycoside OR an antipseudomonal penicillin (ticarcillin, piperacillin, azlocillin, mezlocillin) *plus* an aminoglycoside are alternative regimens for *P. aeruginosa* infections.

Infants and Young Children (2 Months to 5 Years)

(A) Gram-positive cocci

Staphylococcus aureus; streptococci (*S. pyogenes; S. pneumoniae*)

PREFERRED THERAPY:
Nafcillin (parenteral) OR **Oxacillin (parenteral)**
ALTERNATIVE THERAPY:
Cefazolin, Cephalothin, or Cephapirin; Vancomycin; Clindamycin
REMARKS:
(1) Most experts do not recommend methicillin because of an increased risk of interstitial nephritis.
(2) Penicillin G should be substituted for antistaphylococcal penicillins if susceptibility of *S. aureus* strain is proven.
(3) For methicillin-resistant strains of *S. aureus*, intravenous vancomycin is the drug of choice.
(4) For infections caused by streptococci, penicillin G is preferred.

(B) Gram-negative coccobacilli

Haemophilus influenzae type b

PREFERRED THERAPY:
Cefotaxime (or Ceftizoxime) or Ceftriaxone (or Ceftazidime)
OR
Ampicillin *plus* Chloramphenicol initially
ALTERNATIVE THERAPY:
Chloramphenicol alone; Trimethoprim/Sulfamethoxazole
REMARKS:
(1) Beta lactamase-producing strains of *H. influenzae* type b are resistant to ampicillin and rare strains are resistant to chloramphenicol. Therefore, combined treatment is recommended until susceptibility is determined. Ampicillin usually is preferred for sensitive strains.
(2) All other regimens should be effective against ampicillin-resistant strains of *H. influenzae* type b. Many infectious disease experts now prefer a third generation cephalosporin for these resistant strains or when susceptibility is unknown to avoid the toxicity and problems associated with administration of chloramphenicol (eg, need to monitor serum concentrations).
(3) Cefuroxime, a second generation cephalosporin, has been widely used for *H. influenzae* type b infections in children. However, on a weight basis, this drug is less active against this organism than the third generation cephalosporins (eg, cefotaxime, ceftriaxone). More important, cefuroxime occasionally has been associated with delayed sterilization of cerebrospinal fluid and even overt therapeutic failures in patients infected with *H. influenzae* type b. Thus, many pediatric infectious disease experts prefer a third generation cephalosporin (eg, cefotaxime, ceftriaxone) to cefuroxime for severe *H. influenzae* type b infections.
(4) Cefamandole is NOT recommended as an initial therapy for children less than 5 years because of its poor penetration into cerebrospinal fluid.
(5) Little data are available on the treatment of serious infections with trimethoprim/sulfamethoxazole; resistant strains have emerged during therapy.

Children (5 To 15 Years)

(A) Gram-positive cocci

Staphylococcus aureus; streptococci (*S. pyogenes; S. pneumoniae*)

REMARK:
(1) See Infants and Young Children (2 Months to 5 Years) above for drug selection recommendations and remarks.

Sexually Active Adolescents and Adults (Usually Between 15 and 40 Years)

(A) Gram-negative cocci
Neisseria gonorrhoeae
REMARKS:
(1) See Chapter 3 in this Section, Treatment of Sexually Transmitted Diseases, for treatment guidelines.

(B) Gram-positive cocci
Staphylococcus aureus; streptococci (*S. pyogenes; S. pneumoniae*)
REMARK:
(1) See Infants and Young Children (2 Months to 5 Years) above for drug selection recommendations and remarks.

Older Adults (Greater Than 40 Years)

(A) Gram-positive cocci
Staphylococcus aureus; streptococci (*S. pyogenes; S. pneumoniae*)
REMARK:
(1) See Infants and Young Children (2 Months to 5 Years) above for drug selection recommendations and remarks.

(B) Gram-negative cocci
Neisseria gonorrhoeae
REMARK:
(1) See Chapter 3 in this Section, Treatment of Sexually Transmitted Diseases, for treatment guidelines.

(C) Gram-negative bacilli
Enterobacteriaceae; *Pseudomonas aeruginosa*

PREFERRED THERAPY:
Antipseudomonal Penicillin (ticarcillin, mezlocillin, piperacillin, azlocillin) *plus* Aminoglycoside (gentamicin, tobramycin, amikacin, netilmicin)
ALTERNATIVE THERAPY:
Third Generation Cephalosporin (ceftazidime, cefoperazone, cefotaxime, ceftizoxime; ceftriaxone) *with or without* Aminoglycoside
REMARKS:
(1) Septic arthritis caused by gram-negative bacilli is more common in patients with predisposing risk factors (eg, prior noninfectious joint disease, immunosuppression, narcotic use, underlying chronic debilitating disease). Most experts recommend that coverage include *P. aeruginosa*.
(2) Most experts recommend combination therapy for systemic infections in which *P. aeruginosa* is a probable causative organism.
(3) Third generation cephalosporins alone are NOT recommended for *P. aeruginosa* infections. Among these agents, ceftazidime is the most active against this pathogen. It is the preferred cephalosporin if *P. aeruginosa* is suspected.
(4) Switch to most effective drug regimen after susceptibility test results are available.
(5) Following initial parenteral therapy, oral ciprofloxacin may prove beneficial for completion of therapy for septic arthritis caused by aerobic gram-negative bacilli.

EMPIRIC THERAPY (NO ORGANISMS SEEN ON GRAM STAIN)

Neonates and Young Infants (Less Than 2 Months)
Staphylococcus aureus; Streptococcus agalactiae (group B); *Escherichia coli* and other gram-negative enteric bacilli

PREFERRED THERAPY:
Oxacillin (or Methicillin) *plus* Aminoglycoside (gentamicin, tobramycin, amikacin, netilmicin)
OR
Oxacillin *plus* Cefotaxime or Ceftriaxone (or Ceftazidime)
ALTERNATIVE THERAPY:
Cefazolin (or Cephalothin or Cephapirin) *plus* Aminoglycoside
REMARKS:
(1) Switch to most effective drug regimen after susceptibility test results are available.
(2) In contrast to older children and adults, nafcillin is not recommended in neonates by some experts because of erratic pharmacokinetics, particularly in jaundiced infants; methicillin rarely is nephrotoxic in neonates (Nelson, 1991 B).
(3) If methicillin-resistant strains of *S. aureus* are suspected, substitute intravenous vancomycin for the antistaphylococcal penicillin.
(4) Some experts add penicillin G or ampicillin to the above regimens to improve coverage against group B streptococci.
(5) Some consultants recommend caution with use of ceftriaxone in jaundiced premature infants because this highly protein bound cephalosporin can displace bilirubin from albumin binding sites.

Infants and Young Children (2 Months To 5 Years)
Haemophilus influenzae type b; *Staphylococcus aureus*; streptococci (*S. pyogenes; S. pneumoniae*)

PREFERRED THERAPY:
Nafcillin (or Oxacillin) *plus* Chloramphenicol
OR
Cefotaxime or Ceftriaxone (or Ceftizoxime) *with or without* Nafcillin (or Oxacillin)
ALTERNATIVE THERAPY:
Cefuroxime
REMARKS:
(1) Switch to most effective drug regimen after susceptibility test results are available.
(2) Because ampicillin-resistant strains of *H. influenzae* type b are common in most geographic areas, alternative agents (eg, third generation cephalosporin, chloramphenicol) are preferred until susceptibility test results are known.
(3) Most experts do not recommend methicillin because of an increased risk of interstitial nephritis.
(4) If methicillin-resistant strains of *S. aureus* are suspected, intravenous vancomycin should be used in combination with agents active against *H. influenzae* type b.
(5) Cefotaxime, ceftizoxime, and ceftriaxone have less antistaphylococcal activity than antistaphylococcal penicillins. Some experts recommend adding a second antibiotic (eg, nafcillin, vancomycin) for optimal antistaphylococcal activity pending results of susceptibility tests.
(6) Cefuroxime, a second generation cephalosporin, has been widely used for *H. influenzae* type b infections in children. However, on a weight basis, this drug is less active than the third generation cephalosporins (eg, cefotaxime, ceftriaxone) against this organism. More important, cefuroxime occasionally has been associated with delayed sterilization of cerebrospinal fluid and even overt therapeutic failures in patients infected with

H. influenzae type b. Thus, many pediatric infectious disease consultants prefer a third generation cephalosporin (eg, cefotaxime, ceftriaxone) to cefuroxime for severe *H. influenzae* type b infections.
(7) Cefamandole is NOT recommended as an initial therapy for children less than 5 years because of its poor penetration into cerebrospinal fluid.
(8) Because septic arthritis caused by *H. influenzae* type b usually occurs in infants between 2 months and 2 years, some experts consider age 2 years, rather than 5 years, as the cutoff for coverage against this pathogen. In contrast, others recommend regimens active against *H. influenzae* type b in children up to 6 years or older.

Children (5 to 15 Years)

Staphylococcus aureus; streptococci (*S. pyogenes, S. pneumoniae*)

PREFERRED THERAPY:
Nafcillin (parenteral) OR **Oxacillin (parenteral)**
ALTERNATIVE THERAPY:
Cefazolin, Cephalothin, or Cephapirin; Vancomycin; Clindamycin
REMARKS:
(1) Switch to most effective drug regimen after susceptibility test results are available. Use penicillin G if organism is susceptible.
(2) Most experts do not recommend methicillin because of an increased risk of interstitial nephritis.
(3) If methicillin-resistant strains of *S. aureus* are suspected, substitute intravenous vancomycin for the antistaphylococcal penicillin.
(4) Many experts recommend the addition of an aminoglycoside (gentamicin, tobramycin, amikacin, netilmicin) or third generation cephalosporin (ceftazidime, cefotaxime, ceftizoxime, ceftriaxone) to include coverage against gram-negative bacilli in patients with predisposing risk factors (eg, prior noninfectious joint disease, immunosuppression, narcotic use, underlying chronic debilitating disease).

Sexually Active Adolescents and Adults (Usually Between 15 and 40 Years)

Unless the clinical presentation suggests alternative etiologies, *Neisseria gonorrhoeae* is the most likely causative organism in young healthy adults.

REMARKS:
(1) See Chapter 3 in this Section, Treatment of Sexually Transmitted Diseases, for treatment guidelines.
(2) Many experts recommend the addition of nafcillin (or oxacillin) to provide adequate coverage against *Staphylococcus aureus*.

Older Adults (Greater Than 40 Years)

Staphylococcus aureus most common; streptococci (*S. pyogenes; S. pneumoniae*); possibly aerobic gram-negative bacilli (see Remarks)

PREFERRED THERAPY:
Nafcillin (or Oxacillin) *with or without* Aminoglycoside (gentamicin, tobramycin, amikacin, netilmicin)
OR
Nafcillin (or Oxacillin) *with or without* Third Generation Cephalosporin (ceftazidime, cefotaxime, ceftizoxime, ceftriaxone, cefoperazone)
ALTERNATIVE THERAPY:
Cefazolin (or Cephalothin or Cephapirin) *with or without* Aminoglycoside
OR
Vancomycin *with or without* Aminoglycoside (or Third Generation Cephalosporin)
OR
Imipenem/cilastatin *with or without* Aminoglycoside
REMARKS:
(1) Most experts recommend the addition of an aminoglycoside or third generation cephalosporin to include coverage against gram-negative bacilli in patients with predisposing risk factors (eg, prior noninfectious joint disease, immunosuppression, narcotic use, underlying chronic debilitating disease). Adults with nongonococcal bacterial arthritis frequently have a predisposing risk factor.
(2) Most experts do not recommend methicillin because of an increased risk of interstitial nephritis.
(3) If methicillin-resistant strains of *S. aureus* are suspected, substitute intravenous vancomycin for the antistaphylococcal penicillin.
(4) Switch to most effective drug regimen after susceptibility test results are available. Use penicillin G if organism is susceptible.

Osteomyelitis, Acute Hematogenous

Acute hematogenous osteomyelitis can occur in all age groups, but is most common in children under 16 years. Microbial etiology is related to age and the presence of associated risk factors. In NEONATES AND INFANTS (<3 MONTHS), group B streptococci (*Streptococcus agalactiae*), *Staphylococcus aureus*, and gram-negative enteric bacilli (eg, *Escherichia coli*) are all important causative organisms. In CHILDREN (>3 MONTHS) AND ADULTS, *Staphylococcus aureus* is, by far, the major causative organism. Streptococci, especially *S. pyogenes*, also cause this infection in children and occasionally in adults. In contrast to septic arthritis (see previous section entitled Septic Arthritis), *Haemophilus influenzae* type b is a relatively uncommon cause of osteomyelitis in infants and children under 6 years. However, most infectious disease experts use empiric antimicrobial regimens that provide coverage against this organism, especially in children less than 3 years. Gram-negative bacilli (eg, Enterobacteriaceae, *Pseudomonas aeruginosa*) are more likely to cause osteomyelitis in high-risk patients, including intravenous drug abusers, hemodialysis patients, diabetics, and patients with underlying debilitating diseases (eg, alcoholism, malignancy). Acute hematogenous osteomyelitis is a particularly common infection in CHILDREN AND ADULTS WITH ASSOCIATED HEMOGLOBINOPATHY (SICKLE CELL DISEASE). In addition to the usual pathogens, *Salmonella* species are major causative organisms in these patients.

Although ultimate antimicrobial drug selection for acute hematogenous osteomyelitis should be specific and based on culture (blood, aspirates of subperiosteal pus or intraosseous lesions) and susceptibility data, EMPIRIC therapy is indicated initially. As outlined below, initial drug selection is based on the age of the patient. High-dose parenteral antibiotics are recommended.

Selected references: Dickie, 1986; Norden, 1987, 1990; Conte and Barriere, 1988; Sanford, 1990 B; Nelson, 1991 A.

EMPIRIC THERAPY

Neonates and Young Infants (Less Than 3 Months)

Streptococcus agalactiae (group B); *Staphylococcus aureus; Escherichia coli* and other gram-negative enteric bacilli

PREFERRED THERAPY:
Oxacillin *plus* Aminoglycoside (gentamicin, tobramycin, amikacin, netilmicin)
OR
Oxacillin (or Methicillin) *plus* Cefotaxime (or Ceftazidime or Ceftriaxone)
ALTERNATIVE THERAPY:
Cefazolin (or Cephalothin) *plus* Aminoglycoside
REMARKS:
(1) Switch to most effective drug regimen after susceptibility test results are available.
(2) In contrast to older children and adults, nafcillin is not recommended in neonates by some experts because of erratic pharmacokinetics, particularly in jaundiced infants.
(3) If methicillin-resistant strains of *S. aureus* are suspected, substitute vancomycin for the antistaphylococcal penicillin.
(4) Cefotaxime and ceftriaxone are NOT recommended if *Pseudomonas aeruginosa* is a likely pathogen. Ceftazidime *with or without* an aminoglycoside OR an antipseudomonal penicillin (carbenicillin, ticarcillin, piperacillin, azlocillin, mezlocillin) *plus* an aminoglycoside are alternative regimens for *P. aeruginosa* infections.
(5) Some experts add penicillin G or ampicillin to the above regimens to improve coverage against group B streptococci.
(6) Some consultants recommend caution with ceftriaxone in jaundiced premature infants because this highly protein bound cephalosporin can displace bilirubin from albumin binding sites.
(7) Duration of therapy is usually four to six weeks.

Children (Greater Than 3 Months) and Adults

Staphylococcus aureus

PREFERRED THERAPY:
Nafcillin OR **Oxacillin**
ALTERNATIVE THERAPY:
Cefazolin, Cephalothin, or Cephapirin; Vancomycin; Clindamycin
REMARKS:
(1) Switch to most effective drug regimen after susceptibility test results are available. Use penicillin G if organism is susceptible.
(2) Most experts do not recommend methicillin because of an increased risk of interstitial nephritis.
(3) If methicillin-resistant strains of *S. aureus* are suspected, substitute vancomycin for the antistaphylococcal penicillin.
(4) Although *H. influenzae* type b is a relatively uncommon pathogen in osteomyelitis, many experts recommend that initial, empiric coverage include this pathogen in children under 6 years. The addition of a third generation cephalosporin (cefotaxime, ceftizoxime, ceftriaxone, ceftazidime), ampicillin (usually not recommended initially because of the prevalence of resistant strains of *H. influenzae* type b), or chloramphenicol to the antistaphylococcal penicillin are alternative regimens for these patients. Cefuroxime alone also may be used but is less desirable because it is less potent on a weight basis.
(5) Many experts recommend the addition of an aminoglycoside (gentamicin, tobramycin, amikacin, netilmicin) or, alternatively, a third generation cephalosporin (ceftazidime, cefoperazone, cefotaxime, ceftizoxime, ceftriaxone) to include coverage against gram-negative bacilli in patients with predisposing risk factors (intravenous drug users, hemodialysis patients, diabetics, and patients with underlying debilitating diseases). Ciprofloxacin, orally, looks particularly promising for osteomyelitis caused by aerobic gram-negative bacilli, including *P. aeruginosa*. However, this fluoroquinolone should not be used in pregnant women or prepubertal children.
(6) Duration of therapy is usually four to six weeks. Traditionally, parenteral antibiotics have been used throughout the course of therapy. To decrease cost and the potential complications associated with long-term parenteral administration, a switch to oral antibiotics during the course of therapy may be indicated in selected patients (eg, children with *S. aureus* or streptococcal osteomyelitis in the absence of complicating risk factors) provided that certain criteria are fulfilled: (1) isolation of a bacterial pathogen that is sensitive to an oral agent; (2) administration of the drug in a fashion that ensures peak serum bactericidal titers greater than 1:8 and trough titers greater than 1:2 (monitoring serum bactericidal titers throughout course of therapy is essential); (3) clinical improvement during the first five to seven days of intravenous antibiotics; and (4) patient compliance must be assured (usually by hospitalization).

Children and Adults with Associated Hemoglobinopathy (Sickle Cell Disease)

Staphylococcus aureus; Salmonella; other coliform bacteria

PREFERRED THERAPY:
Nafcillin (or Oxacillin) *plus* Cefotaxime (or Ceftriaxone)
ALTERNATIVE THERAPY:
Nafcillin (or Oxacillin) *plus* Ampicillin
Nafcillin (or Oxacillin) *plus* Chloramphenicol; Cefazolin (or Cephalothin or Cephapirin) *plus* Chloramphenicol; Ciprofloxacin (oral or intravenous) with or without Nafcillin
REMARKS:
(1) Switch to most effective drug regimen after susceptibility test results are available.
(2) Most experts do not recommend methicillin because of an increased risk of interstitial nephritis.
(3) If methicillin-resistant strains of *S. aureus* are suspected, substitute intravenous vancomycin for the antistaphylococcal penicillin.
(4) Some experts avoid chloramphenicol in patients with sickle cell disease, if possible, because of the risk of marrow suppression in the presence of hemolytic anemia.
(5) Duration of therapy is usually four to six weeks.
(6) Fluoroquinolones are contraindicated for use in prepubertal children or pregnant women.

Osteomyelitis, Secondary to Contiguous Focus of Infection or Vascular Insufficiency, Acute and Chronic

Acute (and chronic) osteomyelitis in adults frequently is secondary to a contiguous focus of infection; postoperative and post-traumatic infections are particularly common. Although *S. aureus* still is the most common causative organism, aerobic gram-negative bacilli (eg, Enterobacteriaceae, *P. aeruginosa*), streptococci, *S. epidermidis*, and anaerobic bacteria also may be isolated. Frequently, these infections are polymicrobial. When osteomyelitis is secondary to a puncture wound to the foot (eg, nail), *P. aeruginosa* usually is the causative organism. Acute (and chronic) osteomyelitis in adults also may occur secondary to vascular insufficiency. Most patients are between 50 and 70 years of age and have diabetes mellitus. Polymicrobial etiology is common; *S. aureus*, aerobic gram-negative bacilli (Enterobacteriaceae, *P. aeruginosa*), and gram-positive and gram-negative anaerobic bacteria are common causative organisms. Antimicrobial drug selection for these infections ultimately should be specific and be based on culture and susceptibility data obtained from bone biopsy specimens because sinus tract cultures frequently are unreliable. However, EMPIRIC therapy, as outlined below, often is indicated initially.

Selected references: Swartz and O'Hanley, 1987; Armstrong, 1989; Peterson et al, 1989; Norden, 1990; Sanford, 1990 B.

EMPIRIC THERAPY

Adults

Staphylococcus aureus; Enterobacteriaceae; *Pseudomonas aeruginosa;* anaerobic bacteria

ALTERNATIVE THERAPY **(see Remarks):**

Nafcillin (or Oxacillin) *plus* Aminoglycoside (gentamicin, tobramycin, amikacin, netilmicin)

OR

Third Generation Cephalosporin (cefotaxime, ceftizoxime, ceftriaxone, ceftazidime, cefoperazone) *with or without* Nafcillin (or Oxacillin)

OR

Ticarcillin/Potassium clavulanate [Timentin] with or without Aminoglycoside

OR

Imipenem/cilastatin

OR

Ciprofloxacin (oral or intravenous)

REMARKS:

(1) A number of therapeutic alternatives are reasonable options, and no clear-cut consensus for a particular regimen could be obtained from the literature or from our consultants.

(2) Switch to most effective drug regimen after susceptibility test results are available.

(3) If methicillin-resistant strains of *S. aureus* are suspected, intravenous vancomycin is the drug of choice.

(4) Duration of therapy usually is for four to six weeks. In chronic osteomyelitis, follow-up therapy with oral antimicrobial agents for an additional two months or longer is common. Adequate surgical debridement is extremely important. Generally, cure rates for chronic osteomyelitis are poorer than for acute osteomyelitis.

CARDIOVASCULAR SYSTEM INFECTIONS

Endocarditis, Infective

Streptococci and staphylococci are the major causes of native valve infective endocarditis in nonaddicts, accounting for approximately 55% to 65% and 15% to 20% of cases, respectively. Bacterial endocarditis caused by streptococci usually occurs in patients with underlying heart disease and follows a subacute course. Viridans streptococci (eg, *S. sanguis, S. mutans, S. milleri, S. mitior*) cause about 35% to 40% of cases; enterococci (eg, *Enterococcus faecalis*) cause about 10% to 15% of cases; and nonhemolytic, microaerophilic, anaerobic, or nonenterococcal group D (eg, *S. bovis*) streptococci cause the remaining 10% to 15%. *Staphylococcus aureus* (coagulase-positive) is the major cause of acute bacterial endocarditis. This pathogen can infect normal as well as diseased heart valves. Fastidious, slow-growing, coccobacillary gram-negative bacilli, including *Haemophilus* species, *Actinobacillus actinomycetemcomitans*, *Cardiobacterium hominis*, *Eikenella corrodens*, and *Kingella kingii* (HACEK group), also may cause native valve endocarditis in nonaddicts (approximately 5% to 10% of cases).

Prosthetic valve endocarditis is an infrequent but serious complication of cardiac valve replacement. *Staphylococcus epidermidis* (coagulase-negative) and *S. aureus* are common pathogens in both early onset (less than two months postsurgery) and late onset (greater than two months post-surgery) prosthetic valve endocarditis. In one large study, *S. epidermidis* caused more than 50% of cases occurring within two months of surgery and between three and twelve months after surgery. Furthermore, 80% of *S. epidermidis* strains were methicillin-resistant (Calderwood et al, 1985). Aerobic gram-negative bacilli (common), diphtheroids, fungi, and streptococci are other causes of early onset disease; streptococci are common causative organisms of late onset disease.

In narcotic addicts, *S. aureus* (50%), streptococci (20%), including enterococci, gram-negative bacilli (20%), particularly *Pseudomonas aeruginosa*, and fungi (10%), primarily *Candida*, are the causative organisms of infective endocarditis.

The causative organism of infective endocarditis usually can be isolated from blood cultures, and antimicrobial drug therapy should be SPECIFIC and bactericidal for the offending pathogen. In patients with acute infective endocarditis, EMPIRIC therapy should be employed until the results of blood cultures are known. EMPIRIC therapy usually is unnecessary for subacute forms of the disease. Surgical removal of the infected valve also may be required; this is common in prosthetic valve endocarditis.

Host defense mechanisms play a minimal role in the control of infective endocarditis, and cure is dependent on the administration of adequate dosages (ie, prolonged, high-dose, parenteral administration) of *bactericidal* antibiotics. The usefulness of monitoring serum bactericidal activity is controversial (Scheld and Sande, 1990; Wolfson and Swartz, 1985). Achieving a peak serum bactericidal titer (ie, the killing activity of the patient's serum obtained at the anticipated peak serum antibiotic concentration) of at least 1:8 has been considered a desirable goal. However, a retrospective review of 17 studies failed to confirm any correlation between serum bactericidal activity and therapeutic success (Coleman et al, 1982). In a multicenter collaborative evaluation of a standardized serum bactericidal test, peak serum bactericidal titers of $\geq$64 and trough titers $\geq$32 were associated with bacteriologic cure; adjustment of antibiotic dosages to achieve these titers was recommended to provide optimal therapy of infective endocarditis (Weinstein et al, 1985). However, limitations of this study have been noted (Mellors et al, 1986; Weinstein et al, 1986).

Selected references: Karchmer, 1985; Wilson, 1986; Caputo et al, 1987; Threlkeld and Cobbs, 1990; Nelson, 1991.

SPECIFIC THERAPY

Penicillin-susceptible streptococci (minimum inhibitory concentration [MIC] ≤0.1 mcg/ml), including most viridans streptococci and *S. bovis* (nonenterococcal group D)

(gram-positive cocci)

PREFERRED THERAPY:
Penicillin G *with or without* Gentamicin
OR
Penicillin G *with or without* Streptomycin
ALTERNATIVE THERAPY:
Cefazolin (or Cephalothin); Vancomycin
REMARKS:

(1) The optimum preferred regimen has not been clearly identified, and some controversy exists among experts. The following three regimens are suggested with advantages and disadvantages:

(a) Aqueous penicillin G (adults, 10 to 20 million U/day IV either continuously or in divided doses every four hours; children, 150,000-200,000 U/kg/day IV [not to exceed 20 million U/day] either continuously or in divided doses every four hours) for two weeks *plus either* gentamicin (adults with normal renal function, 1 mg/kg IM or IV [not to exceed 80 mg] every eight hours; children with normal renal function, 2 to 2.5 mg/kg IV [not to exceed 80 mg] every eight hours) *or* streptomycin (adults with normal renal function, 7.5 mg/kg IM [not to exceed 0.5 g] every 12 hours; children with normal renal function, 15 mg/kg IM [not to exceed 0.5 g] every 12 hours) for two weeks is considered by many to be the most cost-effective regimen for patients with native valve endocarditis who are less than 65 years and do not have renal impairment, eighth nerve defects, or serious complications. However, other experts still prefer to treat penicillin-sensitive streptococcal endocarditis for four weeks. Experience with the two-week regimen in children is limited.

(b) Aqueous penicillin G (adults, 10 to 20 million U/day IV either continuously or in divided doses every four hours; children, 150,000 to 200,000 U/kg/day IV [not to exceed 20 million U/day] either continuously or in divided doses every four hours) for four weeks is preferred in patients with relative contraindications to the use of aminoglycosides, including age greater than 65 years, renal impairment, or eighth nerve deficits. This is the preferred regimen of many experts for the majority of patients.

(c) Aqueous penicillin G (adults, 10 to 20 million U/day IV either continuously or in divided doses every four hours; children, 150,000 to 200,000 U/kg/day IV [not to exceed 20 million U/day] either continuously or in divided doses every four hours) for four weeks *plus either* gentamicin (adults with normal renal function, 1 mg/kg IM or IV [not to exceed 80 mg] every eight hours; children with normal renal function, 2 to 2.5 mg/kg IV [not to exceed 80 mg] every 8 hours) *or* streptomycin (adults with normal renal function, 7.5 mg/kg IM [not to exceed 0.5 g] every 12 hours; children with normal renal function, 15 mg/kg IM [not to exceed 0.5 g] every 12 hours) for the initial two weeks is preferred for patients with complicated disease (eg, central nervous system involvement, shock, prosthetic valve) or in individuals who have been ill for three months or longer prior to therapy. Some experts consider this the preferred regimen for all patients who can tolerate aminoglycosides.

(2) In adults, procaine penicillin G (1.2 million units IM every six hours) has been used as an alternative to aqueous crystalline penicillin G in regimens that also include an aminoglycoside. Procaine penicillin G is not recommended in children.

(3) Ideally, serum aminoglycoside concentrations should be monitored. Peak gentamicin and streptomycin levels of 3 mcg/ml and 20 mcg/ml, respectively, are desirable.

(4) Although most reported clinical experience with two-drug regimens involves penicillin and streptomycin, in vitro and animal model data suggest that penicillin and gentamicin also exert a synergistic effect in the treatment of endocarditis caused by viridans streptococci. Gentamicin currently is used more widely in clinical practice than streptomycin. Determinations of serum gentamicin concentrations are more readily available, and, in contrast to streptomycin, gentamicin can be administered either intravenously or intramuscularly. Consensus is that gentamicin is interchangeable with streptomycin in combination treatment regimens (Bisno et al, 1989).

(5) Rare strains of viridans streptococci are highly resistant to streptomycin (MIC ≥1000 mcg/ml). Such strains are susceptible to gentamicin, however, and this aminoglycoside should be used.

(6) In patients whose infection involves prosthetic valves or other prosthetic materials, a six-week regimen of penicillin G is recommended, with an aminoglycoside added for at least the first two weeks.

(7) Vancomycin is an effective alternative and the drug of choice in patients with immediate-type hypersensitivity to penicillin. Cephalothin and cefazolin are effective. Although these agents may be used in some patients with a history of penicillin allergy, *cephalosporins should be avoided in patients with immediate-type hypersensitivity to penicillin.* Dosages are: vancomycin (adults with normal renal function, 30 mg/kg/day IV in two or four equally divided doses; children with normal renal function, 40 mg/kg/day IV in two or four equally divided doses. Each dose should be infused over one hour, and serum vancomycin concentrations should be obtained one hour after infusion and be in the range of 30 to 45 mcg/ml for twice daily dosing and 20 to 35 mcg/ml for four times daily dosing. If serum levels are not monitored, a dose of 2 g/day should not be exceeded.); cephalothin (adults, 2 g IV every four hours; children, 100 to 150 mg/kg/day IV [not to exceed 12 g/day] in equally divided doses every four to six hours); and cefazolin (adults, 1 g IM or IV every eight hours; children, 80 to 100 mg/kg/day IM or IV [not to exceed 3 g/day] in equally divided doses every eight hours). Duration of therapy with any alternative regimen is four weeks.

Strains of viridans streptococci and *S. bovis* relatively resistant to penicillin G (MIC >0.1 mcg/ml and <0.5 mcg/ml) and nutritionally deficient viridans streptococci

(gram-positive cocci)

PREFERRED THERAPY:
Penicillin G *plus* Gentamicin
OR
Penicillin G *plus* Streptomycin
ALTERNATIVE THERAPY:
Cephalothin (or Cefazolin) *plus* Gentamicin (or Streptomycin); Vancomycin alone
REMARKS:

(1) Combination therapy with penicillin G for four weeks and either gentamicin or streptomycin for the initial two weeks is recommended for these relatively resistant strains. The dosage of penicillin G is: adults, 20 million U/day IV either continuously or in divided doses every four hours; children, 200,000 to 300,000 U/kg/day IV (not to exceed 20 million U/day) either continuously or in divided doses every four hours. Dosages of gentamicin and streptomycin are the same as for penicillin-susceptible streptococci (see Specific Therapy of Penicillin-Susceptible Streptococcal Endocarditis above).

(2) When penicillin cannot be used because of immediate hypersensitivity, vancomycin alone for four weeks is the preferred drug. Cephalothin (or cefazolin) for four weeks may be combined with two weeks of aminoglycoside therapy in patients whose penicillin hypersensitivity is not of the immediate type. Dosages of these alternative regimens are the same as for penicillin-susceptible streptococci (see Specific Therapy, Penicillin-susceptible streptococci above).

(3) When endocarditis is caused by viridans streptococci requiring 0.5 mcg/ml or more of penicillin G for inhibition, therapy should be the same as for enterococci (see Specific Therapy, Enterococci below).

Enterococci (*Enterococcus faecalis, E. faecium, E. durans*) and other penicillin-resistant streptococci (MIC >0.5 mcg/ml)

(gram-positive cocci)

PREFERRED THERAPY:
Penicillin G *plus* Gentamicin
OR
Ampicillin *plus* Gentamicin
OR
Penicillin G *plus* Streptomycin
OR
Ampicillin *plus* Streptomycin
ALTERNATIVE THERAPY:
Vancomycin *plus* Gentamicin
OR
Vancomycin *plus* Streptomycin
REMARKS:

(1) Dosages are: Aqueous crystalline penicillin G (adults, 20 to 30 million U/day IV either continuously or in divided doses every four hours; children, 200,000 to 300,000 U/kg/day IV [not to exceed 30 million U/day] either continuously or in divided doses every four hours); ampicillin (adults, 12 g/day IV either continuously or in divided doses every four hours; children, 300 mg/kg/day IV [not to exceed 12 g/day] in divided doses every four to six hours); gentamicin (adults with normal renal function, 1 mg/kg IM or IV [not to exceed 80 mg] every eight hours; children with normal renal function, 2 to 2.5 mg/kg IM or IV [not to exceed 80 mg] every eight hours. Serum concentrations of gentamicin should be monitored and the dose adjusted to obtain a peak level of approximately 3 mcg/ml.); streptomycin (adults with normal renal function, 7.5 mg/kg IM [not to exceed 0.5 g] every 12 hours; children with normal renal function, 15 mg/kg IM [not to exceed 0.5 g] every 12 hours. Serum concentrations of streptomycin should be monitored if possible and the dose adjusted to obtain a peak level of approximately 20 mcg/ml.); and vancomycin (adults with normal renal function, 30 mg/kg/day IV in two or four equally divided doses; children with normal renal function, 40 mg/kg/day IV in two or four equally divided doses. Each dose should be infused over one hour and serum vancomycin concentrations should be obtained one hour after infusion and be in the range of 30 to 45 mcg/ml for twice daily dosing and 20 to 35 mcg/ml for four times daily dosing. If serum levels are not monitored, a dose of 2 g/day should not be exceeded.).

(2) Duration of therapy is four to six weeks. Patients with symptoms of enterococcal endocarditis for more than three months before initiation of therapy and patients with prosthetic valve endocarditis should be treated with combined antimicrobial therapy for six weeks; patients without these high-risk factors can be treated for four weeks (Bisno et al, 1989). Some consultants treat all patients for six weeks, however.

(3) Synergistic antimicrobial combinations are required for bactericidal activity and cure of enterococcal endocarditis.

(4) Streptomycin or gentamicin can be used for susceptible strains of enterococci. Gentamicin is recommended if the organism is highly resistant (ie, MIC ≥2,000 mcg/ml) to streptomycin. Because 40% of enterococcal strains are highly resistant to streptomycin, gentamicin should be used when susceptibility testing cannot be performed. Other aminoglycosides (eg, tobramycin, amikacin) generally should not be substituted for gentamicin or streptomycin.

(5) Enterococci with high-level resistance to gentamicin (and usually to all other aminoglycosides) have become a significant problem in some hospitals (Zervos et al, 1987). Satisfactory regimens for the treatment of endocarditis caused by these organisms remain to be established (see Hoffmann and Moellering, 1987). However, a proportion of these organisms may be susceptible to streptomycin.

(6) Ampicillin is two- to fourfold more active than penicillin G against enterococci in vitro, but the clinical relevance, if any, is uncertain. Some experts prefer ampicillin over penicillin G, however.

(7) Beta lactamase-producing strains of enterococci have been isolated. Patients with these strains should receive vancomycin *plus* an aminoglycoside. (Note: Animal studies suggest ampicillin/sulbactam [Unasyn] *plus* an aminoglycoside may be useful for these strains.)

(8) For patients who are potentially allergic to penicillin G, appropriate skin testing for penicillin allergy is recommended. Some experts recommend desensitization procedures in patients with positive skin tests. The alternative regimen of vancomycin *plus* an aminoglycoside should be effective, but nephrotoxicity may be additive and careful monitoring of renal function is necessary. Vancomycin should not be used alone because of its lack of bactericidal activity in vitro and poor performance in experimental enterococcal endocarditis and because strains resistant to this drug have been isolated. Enterococci are uniformly resistant to all available cephalosporins, and these agents should not be used.

Methicillin-susceptible *Staphylococcus aureus* (coagulase-positive) and coagulase-negative staphylococci (native valve endocarditis, ie, absence of prosthetic materials)

(gram-positive cocci)

PREFERRED THERAPY:
Nafcillin OR **Oxacillin (with optional addition of gentamicin—see Remarks)**
ALTERNATIVE THERAPY:
Cephalothin or Cefazolin (with optional addition of gentamicin); Vancomycin
REMARKS:

(1) Dosages are: Nafcillin (adults, 2 g IV every four hours; children, 150 to 200 mg/kg/day IV [not to exceed 12 g/day] in divided doses every four to six hours); oxacillin (adults, 2 g IV every four hours; children, 150 to 200 mg/kg/day IV [not to exceed 12 g/day] in divided doses every four to six hours); gentamicin (adults with normal renal function, 1 mg/kg IM or IV [not to exceed 80 mg] every eight hours; children with normal renal function, 2 to 2.5 mg/kg IV [not to exceed 80 mg] every eight hours); cephalothin (adults, 2 g IV every four hours; children, 100 to 150 mg/kg/day IV [not to exceed 12 g/day] in divided doses every four to six hours); cefazolin (adults, 2 g IV every eight hours; children, 80 to 100 mg/kg/day IV [not to exceed 6 g/day] in divided doses every eight hours); and vancomycin (adults with normal renal function, 30 mg/kg/day IV in two or four equally divided doses; children with normal renal function, 40 mg/kg/day IV in two or four equally divided doses. Each dose should be infused over one hour, and serum vancomycin concentrations should be obtained one hour after infusion and be in the range of 30 to 45 mcg/ml for twice daily dosing and 20 to 35 mcg/ml for four times daily dosing. If serum levels are not monitored, a dose of 2 g/day should not be exceeded).

(2) Duration of therapy is four to six weeks. Intravenous drug abusers (IVDAs) with right-sided endocarditis usually have less severe disease, and parenteral therapy for four weeks (possibly less) is adequate. In one open study, two-week combination therapy with nafcillin *plus* tobramycin cured 94% of IVDAs with right-sided *S. aureus* endocarditis (Chambers et al, 1988).
(3) Most experts do not recommend the use of methicillin in adults and children because of an increased risk of interstitial nephritis.
(4) Aqueous crystalline penicillin G (adults, 10 to 20 million U/day IV either continuously or in divided doses every four hours; children, 150,000 to 200,000 U/kg/day IV [not to exceed 20 million U/day] either continuously or in divided doses every four hours) for four to six weeks (with optional gentamicin) should be substituted for antistaphylococcal penicillins if susceptibility is proven.
(5) The role of combination chemotherapy with an antistaphylococcal penicillin *plus* gentamicin in *S. aureus* endocarditis remains controversial. This combination exhibits synergistic activity against *S. aureus* in vitro and has greater bactericidal activity than an antistaphylococcal penicillin alone in a rabbit endocarditis model. In humans, nafcillin *plus* gentamicin accelerated the clearance of bacteremia compared to nafcillin alone, but did not alter the cure rate, morbidity, or mortality (Korzeniowski et al, 1982). These data led to the suggestion that combination therapy could be used for the initial three to five days of therapy; after clearance of bacteremia, the aminoglycoside (and its associated toxicity) could be discontinued. Some experts recommend combination therapy in severely ill patients, patients who respond poorly to single drug therapy, or for endocarditis caused by tolerant strains of *S. aureus* (ie, when the minimum bactericidal concentration [MBC] is much greater than the MIC). Routine use of rifampin is not recommended. However, rifampin has been added to an antistaphylococcal penicillin if bacteremia fails to clear with a single agent, or for possible abscesses, or for secondary staphylococcal meningitis. Its use is investigational.
(6) Patients who are allergic to penicillins may be treated with intravenously administered vancomycin (see dosage suggested above). First generation cephalosporins, cephalothin or cefazolin, may be used in some patients with a history of penicillin allergy, but *cephalosporins should be avoided in patients with immediate-type hypersensitivity to penicillin.*
(7) Coagulase-negative staphylococci (eg, *S. epidermidis*) are uncommon causes of native valve endocarditis. Furthermore, many strains of coagulase-negative staphylococci are methicillin-resistant and require therapy as outlined below. Native valve endocarditis caused by methicillin-susceptible coagulase-negative staphylococci can be treated as discussed above for methicillin-susceptible *S. aureus*. Caution must be exercised in interpreting results of antimicrobial susceptibility testing because some systems fail to detect methicillin resistance.

Methicillin-resistant *Staphylococcus aureus* (coagulase-positive) and coagulase-negative staphylococci (native valve endocarditis, ie, absence of prosthetic materials)

(gram-positive cocci)

PREFERRED THERAPY:
Vancomycin
REMARKS:
(1) For patients with normal renal function: Adults, 30 mg/kg/day IV in two or four equally divided doses; children, 40 mg/kg/day IV in two or four equally divided doses. Each dose should be infused over one hour, and serum vancomycin concentrations should be obtained one hour after infusion and be in the range of 30 to 45 mcg/ml for twice daily dosing and 20 to 35 mcg/ml for four times daily dosing. If serum levels are not monitored, a dose of 2 g/day should not be exceeded.
(2) Whether gentamicin should be added for the initial three to five days is controversial. There is evidence of increased nephrotoxicity with this combination without clinical evidence of enhanced efficacy. Furthermore, many strains of methicillin-resistant *S. aureus* also are resistant to aminoglycosides (see Bisno et al, 1989).
(3) Methicillin-resistant staphylococci should also be considered cephalosporin-resistant, but this may not be reliably demonstrated by routine in vitro susceptibility tests.

Coagulase-negative staphylococci (eg, *S. epidermidis*) and prosthetic valve endocarditis (*S. aureus*)

(gram-positive cocci)

PREFERRED THERAPY:
Vancomycin *plus* Rifampin *plus* Gentamicin
REMARKS:
(1) Dosages are: Vancomycin (adults with normal renal function, 30 mg/kg/day IV in two or four equally divided doses; children with normal renal function, 40 mg/kg/day IV in two or four equally divided doses. Each dose should be infused over one hour, and serum vancomycin concentrations should be obtained one hour after infusion and be in the range of 30 to 45 mcg/ml for twice daily dosing and 20 to 35 mcg/ml for four times daily dosing. If serum levels are not monitored, a dose of 2 g/day should not be exceeded); rifampin (adults, 300 mg orally every eight hours; children, 20 mg/kg/day orally [not to exceed 900 mg/day] in divided doses every 12 hours); gentamicin (adults with normal renal function, 1 mg/kg IM or IV [not to exceed 80 mg] every eight hours; children with normal renal function, 2 to 2.5 mg/kg IV [not to exceed 80 mg] every eight hours. Serum concentrations of gentamicin should be monitored and the dose adjusted to obtain a peak level of approximately 3 mcg/ml).
(2) Duration of therapy with vancomycin and rifampin is for a minimum of six weeks. Gentamicin use is limited to the initial two weeks of therapy.
(3) *S. epidermidis* and other coagulase-negative staphylococci should be considered methicillin-resistant and cephalosporin-resistant until proven otherwise. This is especially true when endocarditis develops within the year after surgery. The preferred therapy listed above appears to be the best based on prospective studies (Karchmer et al, 1984; Bisno et al, 1989). Previously, it was shown that cure rates of patients treated with vancomycin were increased by the addition of rifampin or gentamicin (Karchmer et al, 1983). However, the development of rifampin-resistant *S. epidermidis* with treatment failure has been reported in patients receiving only vancomycin plus rifampin therapy for prosthetic valve endocarditis (Karchmer et al, 1983, 1984; Chamovitz et al, 1985). When gentamicin is added to the regimen, the emergence of rifampin resistance is significantly decreased (Karchmer et al, 1984).
(4) Coagulase-negative staphylococci may become resistant to rifampin during combination therapy of prosthetic valve endocarditis. Any *S. epidermidis* strains isolated after initiation of rifampin-containing regimens should be tested for rifampin susceptibility.
(5) If the coagulase-negative staphylococcus is resistant to gentamicin, another aminoglycoside to which it is susceptible may be substituted. If the organism is resistant to all aminoglycosides, the aminoglycoside should be omitted.
(6) Resistance of *S. epidermidis* and other coagulase-negative staphylococci to methicillin or cephalosporins may not be apparent by routine in vitro susceptibility testing (Karchmer et al, 1983; Thornsberry, 1984). Thus, the use of beta lactam antibiotics to treat *S. epidermidis* prosthetic valve endocarditis has resulted in a high failure rate (Karchmer et al, 1983). In those situations where methicillin-susceptible coagulase-negative staphylococci can be clearly documented, treatment with a penicillinase-resistant penicillin (nafcillin or oxacillin) in combination with rifampin and gentamicin may be instituted (see Bisno et al, 1989).
(7) For coagulase-negative staphylococcal infections of pros-

thetic heart valves, particularly when onset occurs within 12 months of cardiac valve replacement or when an aortic valve prosthesis is involved, surgical removal of the affected valve frequently is necessary.

(8) For prosthetic valve endocarditis caused by *Staphylococcus aureus* (coagulase-positive), combination therapy is recommended. For methicillin-susceptible strains, nafcillin or oxacillin (same dosages as for *S. aureus* native valve endocarditis above) should be given for a minimum of six weeks with gentamicin (dosage as in Remark 1 above) for the initial two weeks. For methicillin-resistant strains of *S. aureus,* vancomycin (dosage as in Remark 1 above) should be given for a minimum of six weeks with gentamicin (dosage as in Remark 1 above) for the initial two weeks. Use of rifampin is controversial (Bisno et al, 1989).

EMPIRIC THERAPY

Empiric antimicrobial drug therapy of acute infective endocarditis is recommended prior to isolation of the causative organism from blood culture.

Acute Infective Endocarditis - Native Valve

Staphylococcus aureus and *Enterococcus faecalis* (enterococcus); also *Streptococcus pyogenes* (group A, β hemolytic), *Streptococcus pneumoniae* (pneumococcus), *Neisseria* species, and, occasionally, *Haemophilus* species

PREFERRED THERAPY:
Nafcillin (or Oxacillin) *plus* Gentamicin *plus* Penicillin G (or Ampicillin)
ALTERNATIVE THERAPY:
Vancomycin *plus* Gentamicin
REMARKS:

(1) Guidelines for therapy are controversial and not all of our consultants agreed with the regimens listed above. When methicillin-resistant staphylococci are potential causative organisms, empiric therapy with vancomycin *plus* gentamicin is preferred.

(2) Dosages are: Nafcillin (adults, 2 g IV every four hours; children, 150 to 200 mg/kg/day IV [not to exceed 12 g/day] in divided doses every four to six hours); oxacillin (adults, 2 g IV every four hours; children, 150 to 200 mg/kg/day IV [not to exceed 12 g/day] in divided doses every four to six hours); gentamicin (adults with normal renal function, 1 mg/kg IM or IV [not to exceed 80 mg] every eight hours; children with normal renal function, 2 to 2.5 mg/kg IV [not to exceed 80 mg] every eight hours. Serum concentrations of gentamicin should be monitored and the dose adjusted to obtain a peak level of approximately 3 mcg/ml); aqueous penicillin G (adults, 20 million U/day IV either continuously or in divided doses every four hours; children, 200,000 U/kg/day IV [not to exceed 20 million U/day] either continuously or in divided doses every four hours); ampicillin (adults, 12 g/day IV either continuously or in divided doses every four hours; children, 300 mg/kg/day IV [not to exceed 12 g/day] in divided doses every four to six hours); and vancomycin (adults with normal renal function, 30 mg/kg/day IV in two or four equally divided doses; children with normal renal function, 40 mg/kg/day IV in two or four equally divided doses. Each dose should be infused over one hour, and serum vancomycin concentrations should be obtained one hour after infusion and be in the range of 30 to 45 mcg/ml for twice daily dosing and 20 to 35 mcg/ml for four times daily dosing. If serum levels are not monitored, a dose of 2 g/day should not be exceeded).

(3) Switch to most effective drug regimen after culture and susceptibility test results are available. (Note: Routine susceptibility testing for methicillin-resistant staphylococci may be unreliable [Thornsberry, 1984].)

Acute Infective Endocarditis, Prosthetic Valve

All organisms that cause native valve endocarditis (eg, streptococci, enterococci, *Staphylococcus aureus)* plus *Staphylococcus epidermidis* (methicillin-resistant strains), diphtheroids (corynebacteria), gram-negative bacilli, and fastidious gram-negative coccobacilli (HACEK organisms)

PREFERRED THERAPY:
Vancomycin *plus* Gentamicin *plus* Ampicillin
OR
Vancomycin *plus* Gentamicin *plus* Third Generation Cephalosporin (eg, ceftazidime, cefotaxime, ceftizoxime, ceftriaxone)
REMARKS:

(1) Guidelines for therapy are controversial and not all of our consultants agreed with the regimen listed above.

(2) For dosages, see section on Empiric Therapy, Acute Infective Endocarditis—Native Valve above. For third generation cephalosporins, usual maximum doses are: cefotaxime, 12 g/day; ceftizoxime, 12 g/day; and ceftriaxone, 4 g/day.

(3) Switch to most effective drug regimen after culture and susceptibility test results are available. (Note: Routine susceptibility testing for methicillin-resistant staphylococci may be unreliable [Thornsberry, 1984].)

CENTRAL NERVOUS SYSTEM INFECTIONS

Meningitis, Bacterial

The most common causative organisms vary with patient age and are usually subdivided according to the following four age groups:

(1) OLDER CHILDREN AND ADULTS: The most frequently encountered pathogens are *Streptococcus pneumoniae* (pneumococcus) and *Neisseria meningitidis* (meningococcus); the incidence of meningitis due to *Escherichia coli* and other Enterobacteriaceae and *Haemophilus influenzae* type b increases in adults over 60 years, particularly those with underlying immunocompromising conditions.

(2) CHILDREN 3 MONTHS TO 10 YEARS: The most common causative organism is *Haemophilus influenzae* type b, particularly in infants and younger children; *N. meningitidis* and *S. pneumoniae* also are important;

(3) INFANTS 1 TO 3 MONTHS: *H. influenzae* type b, *N. meningitidis, S. pneumoniae,* group B streptococci *(Streptococcus agalactiae), E. coli* and other gram-negative enteric bacilli, and *Listeria monocytogenes* (ie, organisms commonly encountered in neonates as well as in those seen beyond the newborn period) may be causative;

(4) NEONATES LESS THAN 1 MONTH: The predominant organisms are group B streptococci *(S. agalactiae)* and *E. coli;* other gram-negative enteric bacilli, *L. monocytogenes*, and streptococci other than group B also may be encountered.

Antimicrobial drug therapy of bacterial meningitis can be either SPECIFIC (ie, when the causative organism is known or highly suspected based on results of a Gram stain or a rapid diagnostic test such as counter-immunoelectrophoresis [CIE] or latex agglutination) or EMPIRIC (ie, when the bacterial etiology is unknown but the institution of effective antimicrobial drug therapy is mandatory). Parenteral, preferably intravenous, antimicrobial drug administration is necessary. Bactericidal agents are preferred over bacteriostatic antimicrobials because of inadequate host defense mechanisms (eg, impaired phagocytosis) in cerebrospinal fluid (CSF). Peak CSF drug concentrations at least ten times the minimum bactericidal concentration (MBC) for the infecting pathogen are desirable.

Selected references: Barson et al, 1985; Bryan et al, 1985; Meade, 1985; Rodriguez et al, 1986; *Med Lett Drugs Ther*, 1990; McGee and Baringer, 1990; Modai, 1990; Sanford, 1990; Todd and Brogden, 1990; Scheld and Wispelwey, 1990; Tunkel et al, 1990.

SPECIFIC THERAPY

Streptococcus pneumoniae
(gram-positive cocci)

PREFERRED THERAPY:
Penicillin G OR **Ampicillin**
ALTERNATIVE THERAPY:
Ceftriaxone; Cefotaxime; Ceftizoxime; Cefuroxime; Chloramphenicol
REMARKS:
(1) Susceptibility testing (via oxacillin disk or MIC) is recommended because strains relatively resistant to penicillin G (MIC, 0.1 to 1 mcg/ml) and highly resistant to penicillin G (MIC, >1 mcg/ml) have been reported (Weingarten et al, 1990). Chloramphenicol and cefotaxime may be effective against relatively resistant strains; vancomycin is active in vitro against both relatively resistant and highly resistant strains (Tweardy et al, 1983).
(2) Chloramphenicol is a bactericidal antibiotic for *S. pneumoniae.*
(3) Dexamethasone adjunctive therapy may be used with antimicrobial treatment (see Remarks following section on *H. influenzae* type b below).

Neisseria meningitidis
(gram-negative cocci)

PREFERRED THERAPY:
Penicillin G OR **Ampicillin (see Remarks)**
ALTERNATIVE THERAPY:
Chloramphenicol; Cefuroxime; Cefotaxime; Ceftizoxime; Ceftriaxone; Ceftazidime
REMARKS:
(1) Strains of *N. meningitidis* that produce beta lactamase and thus are resistant to penicillin have been isolated from patients in Europe (Fontanals et al, 1989). Failure of penicillin therapy in treatment of meningococcal disease should alert the clinician to test the penicillin sensitivity of clinical isolates from those patients.
(2) Chloramphenicol is a bactericidal antibiotic for *N. meningitidis.*
(3) Penicillin G and chloramphenicol are not effective for prophylaxis of the meningococcal carrier state. Rifampin is the drug of choice; ciprofloxacin and sulfonamides (when strain is sensitive) also may be useful for prophylaxis (see Chapter 4 in this Section, Antimicrobial Chemoprophylaxis for Ambulatory Patients).

Haemophilus influenzae type b
(gram-negative bacilli)

PREFERRED THERAPY:
Ceftriaxone or Cefotaxime (or Ceftizoxime or Ceftazidime)
OR
Ampicillin plus Chloramphenicol
ALTERNATIVE THERAPY:
Chloramphenicol alone
REMARKS:
(1) An increasing body of data suggest that dexamethasone, given with or just prior to the first dose of antibiotics and continued for four days, can prevent severe neurologic sequelae in some children with bacterial, primarily *H. influenzae* type b, meningitis (Lebel et al, 1988; Kaplan, 1989; McCracken and Lebel, 1989; Gary et al, 1989; Lebel et al, 1989 A, 1989 B).
(2) For infants 2 months or older and children with *H. influenzae* meningitis, the American Academy of Pediatrics Committee on Infectious Diseases (1990) recommends that dexamethasone be considered for adjunctive administration with antibiotic therapy after the physician has weighed the possible risks and benefits in the individual patient. Dexamethasone 0.6 mg/kg/day should be given intravenously in four divided doses for the first four days of antibiotic therapy (Lebel et al, 1988) regardless of the choice of antimicrobial drug. The recommendations state that steroid should be given only to patients with confirmed or strongly suspected (by CSF examination, Gram stain, or antigen test) bacterial meningitis. Although the efficacy of dexamethasone in the treatment of pneumococcal or meningococcal meningitis is not proven, recent data suggest that steroid therapy is beneficial in these infections and should be considered for use in adults and children (Girgis et al, 1989; Täuber and Sande, 1989). No data are available on this use of dexamethasone in infants younger than 2 months or in those with congenital or acquired CNS abnormalities with or without placement of a prosthetic device. In all patients, stools should be examined for occult blood, and hemoglobin levels should be determined regularly during therapy. If melena or gross blood is observed, administration of dexamethasone should be discontinued and the patient observed closely to determine the need for transfusion therapy.
(3) Beta lactamase-producing strains are resistant to ampicillin, and rare strains are resistant to chloramphenicol (some are resistant to both antibiotics). Therefore, combined treatment is recommended until susceptibility is determined. Ampicillin usually is preferred for sensitive strains.
(4) Chloramphenicol is a bactericidal antibiotic for *H. influenzae.*
(5) Intravenous administration of antibiotics usually is indicated. In selected pediatric patients, oral chloramphenicol may be used to complete a course of therapy for *H. influenzae* type b meningitis, provided that compliance can be assured and serum chloramphenicol concentrations are monitored.
(6) Many infectious disease experts now prefer a third generation cephalosporin (eg, cefotaxime, ceftriaxone) for meningitis caused by *H. influenzae* type b strains that are ampicillin-resistant or of unknown susceptibility in order to avoid the toxicity and problems associated with administration of chloramphenicol (eg, need to monitor serum concentrations). One of these cephalosporins becomes the drug of choice for *H. influenzae* type b strains that are resistant to both ampicillin and chloramphenicol. These multiply resistant strains currently are rare in the United States, but they are common in some countries such as Spain (Campos et al, 1986).
(7) Cefuroxime, a second generation cephalosporin, has been widely used for *H. influenzae* type b infections in children, including meningitis. However, on a weight basis, this drug is less

active than the third generation cephalosporins (eg, cefotaxime, ceftriaxone) against this organism. More important, cefuroxime occasionally has been associated with delayed sterilization of cerebrospinal fluid and even overt therapeutic failures in patients infected with *H. influenzae* type b (Marks et al, 1986; Lebel et al, 1989 A; Schaad et al, 1990). Thus, many pediatric infectious disease consultants prefer a third generation cephalosporin (eg, cefotaxime, ceftriaxone) to cefuroxime for severe *H. influenzae* type b infections, especially meningitis (McCracken et al, 1987).

(8) Ampicillin and chloramphenicol are not effective for prophylaxis of the *H. influenzae* type b carrier state. Rifampin is the drug of choice; ciprofloxacin also may be useful for prophylaxis (see Chapter 4 in this Section, Antimicrobial Chemoprophylaxis for Ambulatory Patients).

Streptococcus agalactiae (group B)
(gram-positive cocci)

PREFERRED THERAPY:
Penicillin G (or Ampicillin) ***with or without*** **Aminoglycoside (gentamicin, tobramycin, amikacin, netilmicin)**
ALTERNATIVE THERAPY:
See Remarks
REMARKS:
(1) Alternative antimicrobial therapy to the penicillins has not been studied.
(2) Combination regimen is synergistic in vitro and usually is given until the MIC and MBC of the group B streptococcal strain are determined and the cerebrospinal fluid (CSF) is sterilized. If the organism is susceptible to penicillin G (or ampicillin), the aminoglycoside usually is discontinued, but some experts continue the combination for the full course of therapy.
(3) Penicillin-tolerant strains (ie, inhibited but not killed by concentrations of penicillin G or ampicillin achieved in CSF) are occasionally encountered. Although controversial, combination therapy with ampicillin (or penicillin G) *plus* an aminoglycoside (eg, gentamicin) frequently is recommended throughout the course of therapy for these organisms (see McCracken, 1983).

Escherichia coli and other aerobic gram-negative enteric bacilli

PREFERRED THERAPY:
Cefotaxime OR **Ceftizoxime** OR **Ceftriaxone** OR **Ceftazidime**
ALTERNATIVE THERAPY:
Aminoglycoside (gentamicin, tobramycin, amikacin, netilmicin) ***with or without*** **Ampicillin; Trimethoprim/Sulfamethoxazole**
REMARKS:
(1) Susceptibility testing is recommended.
(2) Presently, cefotaxime is the only third generation cephalosporin among those listed above that is labeled for this indication. However, most of our consultants recommended the inclusion of ceftizoxime, ceftriaxone, and ceftazidime as suitable alternatives. Although moxalactam is labeled for aerobic gram-negative enteric bacillary meningitis, this third generation cephalosporin is not recommended because of serious bleeding disorders associated with its use in adults. Cefoperazone is NOT indicated for central nervous system infections (see also the chapter, Cephalosporins and Related Agents).
(3) Cefotaxime, ceftizoxime, and ceftriaxone are NOT recommended if *Pseudomonas aeruginosa* is a likely causative organism; only ceftazidime is active against this organism (see below).
(4) Aminoglycoside also may be given cautiously by lumbar intrathecal or intraventricular administration in adults if in vitro susceptibility data indicate that an aminoglycoside may be effective. Some of our consultants questioned the efficacy of these routes in children (data indicate these routes should not be used in neonates).
(5) Intravenous trimethoprim/sulfamethoxazole may be a useful alternative for gram-negative bacilli that are resistant to third generation cephalosporins (eg, *Acinetobacter calcoaceticus, Pseudomonas cepacia*, *Flavobacterium meningosepticum*) (Levitz and Quintiliani, 1984). This combination is not active against *P. aeruginosa*, however.
(6) Chloramphenicol frequently is NOT bactericidal for gram-negative enteric bacilli in the central nervous system and high failure rates have been reported. Generally, it is no longer recommended.
(7) Aztreonam may be a useful alternative for patients who are allergic to penicillins or cephalosporins. However, clinical experience is limited in both adults and children (Tunkel and Scheld, 1990).

Pseudomonas aeruginosa
(gram-negative bacilli)

PREFERRED THERAPY:
Ceftazidime ***plus*** **Aminoglycoside**
OR
Antipseudomonal penicillin (ticarcillin, mezlocillin, piperacillin, azlocillin) ***plus*** **Aminoglycoside (gentamicin, tobramycin, amikacin, netilmicin)**
REMARKS:
(1) Aminoglycoside is administered parenterally and intrathecally, either intralumbarly or intraventricularly through an Ommaya reservoir.
(2) Azlocillin and piperacillin are the most active antipseudomonal penicillins in vitro against *P. aeruginosa*, and they are preferred by some consultants.
(3) Ceftazidime given alone also has been effective in the treatment of *P. aeruginosa* meningitis in a limited number of patients (Fong and Tomkins, 1985; Rodriguez et al, 1990). However, because resistance to ceftazidime may develop, the concomitant parenteral use (perhaps including intrathecal administration) of an aminoglycoside is recommended for the first week of treatment.

Listeria monocytogenes
(gram-positive bacilli)

PREFERRED THERAPY:
Ampicillin ***with or without*** **Aminoglycoside (gentamicin, tobramycin, amikacin, netilmicin)**
ALTERNATIVE THERAPY:
Penicillin G ***with or without*** **Aminoglycoside**
REMARKS:
(1) Combination regimen is synergistic in vitro. Most consultants recommended combination therapy for *L. monocytogenes* meningitis.
(2) Trimethoprim/sulfamethoxazole may be a useful alternative in the penicillin-allergic patient (Levitz and Quintiliani, 1984).

EMPIRIC THERAPY

Empiric therapy of bacterial meningitis is based on the patient's age for reasons presented above. Recommendations of the American Academy of Pediatrics Committee on Infectious Diseases (1990) for the use of adjunctive corticosteroids during antibiotic therapy are given above (see Remarks following section on therapy of *H. influenzae* type b meningitis).

Adults (less than 60 years)

Streptococcus pneumoniae and *Neisseria meningitidis*

PREFERRED THERAPY:
Penicillin G
ALTERNATIVE THERAPY:
Cefotaxime; Ceftriaxone; Ceftizoxime; Chloramphenicol
REMARKS:
(1) Some strains of *S. pneumoniae* that are relatively resistant or highly resistant to penicillin G have been reported (Weingarten et al, 1990).
(2) Because of the increasing incidence of *Haemophilus influenzae* type b meningitis in young adults and in some geographical areas, some experts substitute ampicillin for penicillin G, or use combination therapy with a penicillin plus chloramphenicol, or use a third generation cephalosporin, such as cefotaxime or ceftriaxone, that is active against all three organisms.
(3) In older adults (greater than 60 years), additional causative organisms (eg, *Escherichia coli*) should be considered and antimicrobial therapy directed accordingly (eg, cefotaxime, ceftriaxone).

Infants and Children (3 Months to 10 Years)

Haemophilus influenzae type b, *Neisseria meningitidis*, and *Streptococcus pneumoniae*

PREFERRED THERAPY:
Cefotaxime or Ceftriaxone
OR
Ampicillin *plus* Chloramphenicol
ALTERNATIVE THERAPY:
Chloramphenicol alone; Ceftazidime; Ceftizoxime
REMARKS:
(1) Switch to most effective drug regimen after susceptibility test results are available.
(2) *H. influenzae* type b meningitis is most prevalent in infants and younger children (less than 5 years). The selection of 10 years as the upper age limit for empiric therapy that includes coverage against this organism is based on the American Academy of Pediatrics' *Report of the Task Force on Diagnosis and Management of Meningitis* (Klein et al, 1986). However, some pediatric infectious disease consultants recommend an upper age cutoff of 5 to 7 years while others continue empiric coverage for *H. influenzae* type b in children up to 12 years or older.
(3) The American Academy of Pediatrics' Task Force on Diagnosis and Management of Meningitis considered ampicillin *plus* chloramphenicol to be the regimen of choice for empiric therapy of meningitis in infants and children (3 months to 10 years) because of its proven efficacy and safety over many years of use (Klein et al, 1986). However, more recent recommendations by the Academy's Committee on Infectious Diseases indicate that the new cephalosporins are equally acceptable alternatives for initial therapy (American Academy of Pediatrics Committee on Infectious Diseases, 1988). Many pediatric infectious disease experts now prefer monotherapy with an appropriate third generation cephalosporin, usually cefotaxime or ceftriaxone, both for the convenience of single-drug therapy and to avoid the toxicity and problems associated with the administration of chloramphenicol (eg, need to monitor serum concentrations) (McCracken et al, 1987). In numerous controlled trials, these new cephalosporins have shown comparable (but not superior) clinical efficacy to ampicillin *plus* chloramphenicol. Experience with these agents is more limited, however, and comparisons of long-term outcomes with standard therapy have not been published (see Kaplan, 1986; Stutman and Marks, 1987).
(4) Cefuroxime, a second generation cephalosporin, has been widely used for *H. influenzae* type b infections, including meningitis, in children. However, on a weight basis, this drug is less active than the third generation cephalosporins (eg, cefotaxime, ceftriaxone) against this organism. More important, cefuroxime occasionally has been associated with delayed sterilization of cerebrospinal fluid and even overt therapeutic failures in patients infected with *H. influenzae* type b (Marks et al, 1986; Lebel et al, 1989 A; Schaad et al, 1990). Thus, many pediatric infectious disease consultants prefer a third generation cephalosporin (eg, cefotaxime, ceftriaxone) to cefuroxime for severe *H. influenzae* type b infections, especially meningitis (McCracken et al, 1987).

Infants (1 to 3 Months)

Haemophilus influenzae type b, *Neisseria meningitidis, Streptococcus pneumoniae, Streptococcus agalactiae* (group B), *Escherichia coli* and other gram-negative enteric bacilli, and *Listeria monocytogenes*

PREFERRED THERAPY:
Ampicillin *plus* Cefotaxime (or Ceftriaxone)
REMARKS:
(1) The potential pathogens in this age group include organisms commonly encountered in neonates (see below) as well as those seen beyond the newborn period (see above). For empiric therapy, the above regimen provides optimum coverage (see Kaplan, 1986; Klein et al, 1986; McCracken et al, 1987; Stutman and Marks, 1987; American Academy of Pediatrics Committee on Infectious Diseases, 1988; Word and Klein, 1988; Nelson, 1991).
(2) Switch to most effective drug regimen after susceptibility test results are available.

Neonates (Less Than 1 Month)

Streptococcus agalactiae (group B), *Escherichia coli* and other gram-negative enteric bacilli, *Listeria monocytogenes*, and other streptococci

PREFERRED THERAPY:
Ampicillin *plus* Aminoglycoside (gentamicin, tobramycin, amikacin, netilmicin)
OR
Ampicillin *plus* Cefotaxime (or Ceftriaxone)
REMARKS:
(1) No additional benefit from lumbar intrathecal or intraventricular administration of aminoglycoside has been shown in neonates, and these routes are not recommended (McCracken, 1981).
(2) Many pediatric infectious disease experts now prefer a third generation cephalosporin, usually cefotaxime or ceftriaxone, to an aminoglycoside, either in combination with ampicillin, for the empiric therapy of neonatal meningitis because they have better in vitro and CSF bactericidal activity against gram-negative enteric bacilli, are less toxic, and have more predictable pharmacokinetics. However, no study has yet documented superior clinical outcomes with these new cephalosporins and there is considerably less experience with their use. Cefotaxime (or ceftriaxone) is preferred when aminoglycoside serum concentrations cannot be monitored or when the neonate has abnormal renal function (see Klein et al, 1986; Stutman and Marks, 1987; American Academy of Pediatrics Committee on Infectious Diseases, 1988). Ceftazidime is preferred to cefotaxime (or ceftriaxone) in the hospitalized low-birth-weight premature infant in whom nosocomial *Pseudomonas aeruginosa* infection is a possibility (American Academy of Pediatrics Committee on Infectious Diseases, 1988).
(3) Some consultants recommend caution with the use of cef-

triaxone in jaundiced premature infants because this highly protein bound cephalosporin can displace bilirubin from albumin binding sites. In addition, presumably because of its high biliary excretion, ceftriaxone may cause the accumulation of "sludge" (also referred to as pseudolithiasis) in the gallbladder of young children. Symptoms (nausea, epigastric distress, vomiting, right upper quadrant tenderness) subside after discontinuation of ceftriaxone therapy.

(4) Switch to most effective drug regimen after susceptibility test results are available.

Brain Abscess

Brain abscesses may develop as a result of cranial trauma associated with injury or neurosurgery; spread from contiguous sites of infection, particularly otitis/mastoiditis, sinusitis, or odontogenic infections; or hematogenous (or metastatic) spread from a distant site of infection such as lung abscess or empyema or right to left intracardiac shunts in congenital heart disease; or they may be cryptogenic. The bacterial organisms involved in brain abscess depend on the site of any preceding infection, the location of the abscess within the brain, and any underlying clinical circumstances. Gram-positive aerobic and microaerophilic or anaerobic cocci are the most common organisms (in 60% to 70% of brain abscesses), often occurring in mixed culture. These organisms are associated with cryptogenic abscesses, those arising through spread from contiguous foci of infection such as sinusitis or otitis, and abscesses associated with cyanotic congenital heart disease. *Staphylococcus aureus* (in 10% to 15% of brain abscesses) usually are found in abscesses following trauma or neurosurgery. The Enterobacteriaceae and *Bacteroides* sp. may be found in 20% to 40% of brain abscesses, often in mixed culture. They are common in otogenic abscesses. Other bacteria and fungi also may be found in brain abscesses, often in special settings (eg, immunocompromised host).

Surgical excision or drainage (when possible) combined with a lengthy course of high-dose, parenteral antimicrobial agents that penetrate into brain tissue and abscess pus is the recommended treatment of brain abscess. However, optimal treatment guidelines remain to be established. Antimicrobial drug selection ideally should be based on culture and results of susceptibility tests with fluid (pus) obtained from the abscess cavity. However, initial therapy usually is EMPIRIC and should be effective against the most likely pathogens.

Selected references: Jadavji et al, 1985; Benson and Harris, 1986; Yoshikawa and Quinn, 1988; Sáez-Llorens et al, 1989; Wispelwey and Scheld, 1990.

EMPIRIC THERAPY

Aerobic, microaerophilic, and anaerobic streptococci; *Bacteroides* sp., including *B. fragilis*; other anaerobic bacteria; possibly Enterobacteriaceae and *Staphylococcus aureus*

PREFERRED THERAPY:

Penicillin G *plus* Chloramphenicol OR **Penicillin G *plus* Metronidazole (See Remarks)**

REMARKS:

(1) Although no controlled studies on relative efficacy have been performed, the above regimens have been most frequently used for empiric therapy. However, modifications may be indicated, depending on the site of any preceding infection, the anatomic location of the abscess, and any underlying clinical circumstances.

(2) Enterobacteriaceae frequently are isolated from brain abscesses of otic origin, and many experts add a third generation cephalosporin (eg, cefotaxime) to the regimen pending culture results. When *S. aureus* is a likely pathogen (eg, brain abscess after penetrating cranial trauma or neurosurgery, endocarditis), an antistaphylococcal penicillin (eg, nafcillin) is substituted for penicillin G. If the patient is allergic to penicillin or a methicillin-resistant strain of *S. aureus* is identified in pus, vancomycin may be substituted for penicillin G. For brain abscess secondary to frontoethmoid sinusitis, penicillin G alone may be adequate because *B. fragilis* and Enterobacteriaceae are uncommon. In contrast, therapy for brain abscess complicating otitis media, mastoiditis, or pyogenic lung disease requires metronidazole or chloramphenicol because of the frequent involvement of anaerobes, such as *B. fragilis,* in these processes.

(3) Limited data suggest that antimicrobial therapy alone may be sufficient for selected patients in whom surgical intervention is not feasible because of an inaccessible anatomic location or the presence of multiple abscesses (Boom and Tuazon, 1985). Monitoring response to therapy with serial computerized tomographic (CT) or magnetic resonance imaging (MRI) scans is essential.

EAR INFECTIONS

Otitis Media, Acute

Acute otitis media is a very common infection in infants and children, particularly those under 3 years.

The most common causative organisms in all age groups are *Streptococcus pneumoniae* (pneumococcus) (30%) and *Haemophilus influenzae* (usually nontypeable strains) (21%). Other pathogens include *Moraxella (Branhamella) catarrhalis, Streptococcus pyogenes* (group A, beta hemolytic), and, rarely, *Staphylococcus aureus*. The incidence of *M. catarrhalis* as a pathogen appears to have increased in some geographic areas from approximately 5% to 27% (Bluestone, 1986). In neonates up to 6 weeks, particularly those in nursery intensive care units, gram-negative enteric bacilli (eg, *Escherichia coli*) and *S. aureus* may cause up to 20% of cases.

Antimicrobial drug therapy (oral) in ADULTS, CHILDREN, and INFANTS is usually EMPIRIC and should be effective against the two most likely pathogens, *S. pneumoniae* and *H. influenzae*. In NEONATES, many experts recommend that initial treatment be the same as for neonatal sepsis pending isolation of the causative organism (see section on Sepsis, Neonatal above).

The goals of antimicrobial therapy for acute otitis media are (1) to shorten the duration of symptomatic infection and time to recovery; (2) to eradicate the causative organism in the middle ear to prevent suppurative complications; (3) to shorten the duration of middle ear effusion and reduce the period of hearing impairment; and (4) to reduce the recurrence of infections and thus the number of cases of chronic otitis media. Since no single drug is clearly superior to any of the others in accomplishing these goals, it is now apparent that antimicrobial therapy for acute otitis media should be individualized (see Remarks).

Selected references: Marchant, 1986; Bluestone, 1988; Klein, 1990; Lisby-Sutch et al, 1990; Pichichero et al, 1990.

EMPIRIC THERAPY

Adults, Children, and Infants (Greater Than 6 Weeks)
Primarily *Streptococcus pneumoniae* and *Haemophilus influenzae* (usually nontypeable strains)

ALTERNATIVE THERAPY:
Amoxicillin OR **Amoxicillin/Potassium Clavulanate [Augmentin]** OR **Erythromycin Ethylsuccinate-Sulfisoxazole** OR **Trimethoprim/Sulfamethoxazole** OR **Cefaclor** OR **Cefuroxime Axetil** OR **Cefixime**
REMARKS:
(1) Although ampicillin is more cost-effective than amoxicillin, the latter usually is preferred when beta lactamase–producing strains are not prevalent, because it is better absorbed, requires fewer doses per day, can be taken with meals, and may cause less diarrhea. Other aminopenicillins (eg, bacampicillin, cyclacillin) do not appear to offer any important advantages over amoxicillin unless twice-daily dosing (eg, every 12 hours) is desirable. Oral cephalosporins are generally more expensive and should be reserved for patients who cannot tolerate penicillins or sulfonamides. Cefixime may be useful for noncompliant patients because it can be given once daily.
(2) If beta lactamase-producing strains are prevalent (eg, up to 40% of *H. influenzae* and 75% of *M. catarrhalis*) in some geographic areas, a drug that is resistant to enzymatic inactivation (any of those listed except amoxicillin) should be used.
(3) Trimethoprim/sulfamethoxazole is not effective for group A streptococcal infection. Moveover, a recent study showed that up to 30% of *S. pneumoniae* isolates cultured from the nasopharynxes of children in day-care centers were resistant to this combination (Henderson et al, 1988).
(4) An alternative regimen (except Augmentin) should be used in patients allergic to penicillin. However, cephalosporins should not be used in patients who have experienced an immediate-type hypersensitivity reaction to penicillin.
(5) Some consultants suggest doxycycline as a possible alternative in penicillin-allergic adults. This drug should not be given to pregnant women or children under 8 years.
(6) For guidelines on prophylaxis of recurrent otitis media, see Chapter 4 in this Section, Antimicrobial Chemoprophylaxis for Ambulatory Patients.

External Otitis

External otitis is a common inflammatory condition involving the skin of the external auditory canal. When there is a breakdown in the natural defenses, inflammation and secondary infection may ensue. The most common causative bacteria are *Pseudomonas aeruginosa, Escherichia coli, Staphylococcus aureus,* streptococci, or species of *Proteus*. See also index entry Otitis, External.

EMPIRIC THERAPY

PREFERRED THERAPY:
Topical (otic) acetic acid
OR
Topical (otic) neomycin *plus* polymyxin B (or colistin)
REMARKS:
(1) Cleansing the ear canal is the most important part of therapy.
(2) Topical (otic) chloramphenicol is indicated only if the causative organism is proven to be susceptible.

Malignant External Otitis

Malignant (necrotizing, invasive) external otitis is a slowly progressive necrotizing infection of the ear canal that spreads to the soft tissue, cartilage of the external ear, and bone of the skull. This severe infection occurs primarily in elderly, diabetic, debilitated patients, and it may become life-threatening if it extends to the sigmoid sinus, jugular bulb, base of the skull, meninges, and brain. The causative organism is *Pseudomonas aeruginosa.*

SPECIFIC (systemic) antimicrobial drug therapy directed against *P. aeruginosa* in conjunction with local debridement of granulation tissue and infected cartilage usually is recommended.

Selected references: Pelton and Klein, 1988; Rubin and Yu, 1988; Johnson and Ramphal, 1990; Klein, 1990; Sanford, 1990.

SPECIFIC THERAPY

Pseudomonas aeruginosa
(gram-negative bacilli)

PREFERRED THERAPY:
Antipseudomonal Penicillin (ticarcillin, mezlocillin, piperacillin, azlocillin) *plus* Aminoglycoside (gentamicin, tobramycin, amikacin, netilmicin)
OR
Ceftazidime (or Cefoperazone) *plus* Aminoglycoside
ALTERNATIVE THERAPY:
Imipenem/cilastatin *plus* Aminoglycoside; Aztreonam *plus* Aminoglycoside; Ciprofloxacin (oral) *with or without* Rifampin (oral)
REMARKS:
(1) Most experts recommend combination therapy for systemic infections caused by *P. aeruginosa*.
(2) Usual duration of therapy is four to eight weeks. Serum aminoglycoside concentrations should be monitored.
(3) Aztreonam (*plus* aminoglycoside) may be a useful alternative in patients who are allergic to penicillins and cephalosporins.
(4) Limited clinical studies indicate that oral ciprofloxacin (*with or without* rifampin) is effective for malignant external otitis (Lang et al, 1988; Rubin et al, 1989). This oral regimen was less toxic, more convenient, and less costly than conventional parenteral antipseudomonal therapy. If efficacy and safety are confirmed with additional clinical studies, oral ciprofloxacin would likely be the preferred drug for this condition.

EYE INFECTIONS

Conjunctivitis, Bacterial

The most common causative organisms in purulent bacterial conjunctivitis in adults, children, and infants (excluding neonates) are *Staphylococcus aureus* and *S. epidermidis, Streptococcus pneumoniae, Haemophilus influenzae*, and *Moraxella lacunata* (commonly isolated with *S. aureus*). Nonpurulent conjunctivitis is commonly caused by viruses, allergens, or chemical irritants.

EMPIRIC THERAPY

Adults, Children and Infants (Excluding Neonates)

PREFERRED THERAPY:
Topical (ophthalmic) sulfacetamide
OR
Topical (ophthalmic) neomycin-bacitracin-polymyxin B (Gramicidin may be substituted for bacitracin.)
OR
Topical (ophthalmic) bacitracin-polymyxin B
REMARK:
(1) Topical (ophthalmic) gentamicin, tobramycin, tetracycline, or erythromycin is indicated if the causative organism is proven to be susceptible.

Ophthalmia Neonatorum

The most common causative organisms of infectious conjunctivitis during the first ten to twenty days of life are *Chlamydia trachomatis* (onset, 5 to 20 days), *Neisseria gonorrhoeae* (onset, 2 to 5 days), and *Staphylococcus aureus* (onset, variable). *Haemophilus influenzae* and *Streptococcus pneumoniae* also may be causative. Gram stain and culture of exudate and a diagnostic test for chlamydia (eg, culture, direct fluorescent antibody, Giemsa-stained conjunctival scrapings) are necessary to determine the causative organism.

Inclusion conjunctivitis due to *C. trachomatis* and gonococcal ophthalmia are sexually transmitted diseases and treatment guidelines can be found in Chapter 3 of this Section, Treatment of Sexually Transmitted Diseases. Antimicrobial drug selection for ophthalmia neonatorum caused by *S. aureus* appears below.

Ophthalmology consultation should be obtained promptly for patients with ophthalmia neonatorum.

Selected references: Riley and Baker, 1986; *MMWR*, 1989; Nelson, 1991.

SPECIFIC THERAPY

Chlamydia trachomatis

REMARK:
(1) See Chapter 3 of this Section, Treatment of Sexually Transmitted Diseases, for treatment guidelines.

Neisseria gonorrhoeae
(gram-negative cocci)

REMARK:
(1) See Chapter 3 of this Section, Treatment of Sexually Transmitted Diseases, for treatment guidelines.

Staphylococcus aureus
(gram-positive cocci)

SERIOUS INFECTIONS

PREFERRED THERAPY:
Oxacillin (parenteral) ***with or without*** **Neomycin (topical ophthalmic)**
REMARKS:
(1) Nafcillin is not recommended for neonates by some experts because of its erratic pharmacokinetics, particularly in jaundiced infants.
(2) Penicillin G should be substituted for antistaphylococcal penicillins if susceptibility is proven.
(3) For methicillin-resistant strains of *S. aureus*, intravenous vancomycin is the drug of choice.

MINOR INFECTIONS

PREFERRED THERAPY:
Neomycin (topical ophthalmic) only
ALTERNATIVE THERAPY:
Bacitracin (topical ophthalmic); Erythromycin (topical ophthalmic)
REMARK:
(1) Systemic antimicrobial therapy is not required for minor infections.

GASTROINTESTINAL AND INTRA-ABDOMINAL INFECTIONS

Infectious Gastroenteritis/Infectious Diarrhea

Infectious gastroenteritis/infectious diarrhea can be caused by viruses, bacteria, and protozoa.

Rotavirus and Norwalk virus are the most common viral etiologies of infectious diarrhea. Infants between 6 and 24 months are most frequently affected by rotavirus. Norwalk virus tends to occur in epidemics and usually affects school-age children, adolescents, and adults. Antimicrobial drug therapy is NOT effective for these viral infections. Therapy is primarily supportive and consists of correction of dehydration and electrolyte imbalance.

Infectious gastroenteritis/infectious diarrhea caused by bacteria usually is subdivided into three categories:

(1) Acute food poisoning can be caused by ingestion of a preformed enterotoxin. *Staphylococcus aureus* (gram-positive cocci), *Bacillus cereus* (gram-positive bacilli), and *Clostridium perfringens* (anaerobic gram-positive bacilli) are the common bacterial pathogens. Disease is frequently self-limited. Supportive therapy (replacement of fluids and electrolytes) may be necessary, but antimicrobial drug therapy is not indicated.

Although botulism (*Clostridium botulinum*) is a type of acute food poisoning, it is a life-threatening disease characterized by blockade of neuromuscular transmission that is caused by a preformed neurotoxin. Ventilatory support and specific antitoxin are indicated.

(2) Acute secretory diarrheas, characterized by watery diarrhea without fecal leukocytes, are caused by enterotoxins elaborated by causative bacteria. Enterotoxigenic strains of *Escherichia coli* and *Vibrio cholerae* are the major pathogens. Acute secretory diarrheas are common in underdeveloped

countries; enterotoxigenic *E. coli* is the most common cause of travelers' diarrhea.

Supportive therapy (replacement of fluids and electrolytes) and SPECIFIC antimicrobial drug therapy are indicated in the treatment of cholera. Diarrhea caused by enterotoxigenic *E. coli* frequently is self-limited. However, correction of dehydration and electrolyte imbalance also may be necessary, and clinical studies have shown that antimicrobial drug therapy can decrease the severity and duration of the illness.

(3) Invasive bacteria or those that produce a cytotoxin can cause bloody diarrhea with other constitutional symptoms (eg, fever). Leukocytes usually are present in feces. Major causative bacteria include *Shigella* sp. (eg, *S. flexneri, S. sonnei*), *Salmonella* sp. (eg, *S. enteritidis*), and *Campylobacter jejuni*. Other important pathogens include enteroinvasive strains of *Escherichia coli,* enterohemorrhagic *E. coli* 0157:H7, *Yersinia enterocolitica, Vibrio parahaemolyticus, Aeromonas* species, and *Plesiomonas shigelloides.*

When necessary, supportive therapy (replacement of fluids and electrolytes) is indicated for diarrhea caused by any of these pathogens. SPECIFIC antimicrobial drug therapy is recommended for *Shigella* infections. The role of antimicrobial drug therapy for infections caused by the other pathogens is less clear. Acute diarrheal illnesses are often mild and self-limited, and antimicrobial drugs are unnecessary in these cases. When diarrhea is severe and protracted or there is associated bacteremia, SPECIFIC antimicrobial drug therapy usually is recommended. Before culture results are available, EMPIRIC antimicrobial therapy may be indicated for patients with fever and acute, moderate to severe diarrhea who present with dysentery (presence of gross blood and mucus in stools) and/or have microscopic evidence of polymorphonuclear leukocytes in their stools, because infection with an invasive enteropathogen is likely. EMPIRIC therapy is also indicated when a systemic (bacteremic) illness is suspected.

Giardia intestinalis (giardiasis), *Entamoeba histolytica* (amebiasis), and *Cryptosporidium* are the major protozoal etiologies of infectious diarrhea. For treatment guidelines, see index entries Giardiasis; Amebiasis; and Cryptosporidiosis.

Selected references: DuPont, 1985; George et al, 1985; Guerrant et al, 1986; Holmberg et al, 1986; Williams et al, 1986; Levine, 1987; Bishop and Ulshen, 1988; Brenden et al, 1988; Conte and Barriere, 1988 A; Griffen et al, 1988; Cover and Aber, 1989; *Med Lett Drugs Ther*, 1990 A; Cossar et al, 1990; Asperilla et al, 1990; Goodman et al, 1990. See also index entry Diarrhea, Infectious.

SPECIFIC THERAPY

(A) *Supportive therapy (replacement of fluids and electrolytes) PLUS specific antimicrobial drug therapy is recommended for infectious gastroenteritis/infectious diarrhea caused by the following:*

***Shigella* species**
(gram-negative bacilli)

PREFERRED THERAPY:
Trimethoprim/Sulfamethoxazole

ALTERNATIVE THERAPY:
Ciprofloxacin (or Norfloxacin or Ofloxacin); Ampicillin; Nalidixic Acid; Furazolidone

REMARKS:
(1) Antibiotics are indicated because they shorten the duration of illness and decrease the relapse rate.
(2) The fluoroquinolones (eg, ciprofloxacin, norfloxacin) appear promising. They are highly active in vitro against *Shigella* sp., including strains that are resistant to other antimicrobial agents. Furthermore, other major inflammatory gram-negative bacillary enteropathogens (such as *Campylobacter jejuni*) also are susceptible and plasmid-mediated resistance has not occurred with this class of drugs. Fluoroquinolones should not be given to pregnant women or prepubertal children.
(3) Isolates of *Shigella* acquired during foreign travel or residence (eg, while serving in the armed forces) are likely to exhibit multiple antimicrobial resistance (Tauxe et al, 1990; Oldfield et al, 1991). Thus, foreign travel history should be included among selection criteria for initiation of antibiotic therapy prior to receiving results of a susceptibility profile.
(4) Ampicillin-resistant strains are common; this drug frequently is preferred when susceptibility is proven.
(5) Amoxicillin should not be substituted for ampicillin for *Shigella* infections because it is considerably less effective.
(6) Tetracyclines should not be given to pregnant women or children under 8 years.

***Vibrio cholerae* (cholera)**
(gram-negative bacilli)

PREFERRED THERAPY:
Tetracycline

ALTERNATIVE THERAPY:
Trimethoprim/Sulfamethoxazole; Furazolidone; Chloramphenicol

REMARKS:
(1) Antibiotics are indicated because they reduce the duration and volume of diarrhea.
(2) Tetracyclines should not be given to pregnant women or children under 8 years.
(3) Fluoroquinolones (eg, ciprofloxacin, norfloxacin) are highly active in vitro, but clinical studies are not available. These agents should not be given to pregnant women or prepubertal children.

***Giardia intestinalis* (giardiasis)**
(protozoan)

REMARK:
(1) For treatment guidelines, see index entry Giardiasis.

***Entamoeba histolytica* (amebiasis)**
(protozoan)

REMARK:
(1) For treatment guidelines, see index entry Amebiasis.

(B) Infectious gastroenteritis/infectious diarrhea caused by the following pathogens frequently is self-limiting, and supportive therapy (replacement of fluids and electrolytes) ALONE is adequate. When diarrhea is severe or protracted or there is associated bacteremia, SPECIFIC antimicrobial drug therapy also is recommended.

***Salmonella* species (nontyphoidal)**
(gram-negative bacilli)

REMARKS:
(1) Gastroenteritis/diarrhea is self-limited and requires supportive therapy only. Antibiotics may prolong the carrier state. When systemic illness (eg, bacteremia) is present, treat with antimicrobial agents as for typhoid fever (see Typhoid Fever below).
(2) Some pediatric infectious disease experts consider treatment with antimicrobials appropriate for younger children (eg, under 3 months to 1 year) (see American Academy of Pediatrics, 1988; St. Geme et al, 1988).

Campylobacter jejuni
(gram-negative bacilli)

PREFERRED THERAPY:
Erythromycin
OR
Ciprofloxacin (or Norfloxacin or Ofloxacin)
ALTERNATIVE THERAPY:
Tetracycline; Gentamicin; Chloramphenicol
REMARKS:
(1) Definitive treatment guidelines are lacking. In controlled clinical trials, erythromycin shortened the duration of shedding of *C. jejuni* from feces (Anders et al, 1982; Mandal et al, 1984; Salazar-Lindo et al, 1986). When treatment was initiated early, ie, immediately on presentation to a treatment facility, erythromycin also reduced the duration of diarrhea in affected children (Salazar-Lindo et al, 1986). However, this antibiotic failed to alter the clinical course of gastroenteritis when therapy was begun four or more days after the onset of symptoms (Anders et al, 1982; Mandal et al, 1984). Thus, the impact of erythromycin therapy depends on rapid diagnosis of *C. jejuni* gastroenteritis. It appears that mild cases of *C. jejuni* gastroenteritis are self-limited, and erythromycin should be reserved for severe illness or when prevention of transmission of the organism is desirable. Some strains of *C. jejuni* are resistant to erythromycin.
(2) The fluoroquinolones (eg, ciprofloxacin, norfloxacin) are highly active in vitro against *C. jejuni* and other major inflammatory gram-negative bacillary enteropathogens. Also, plasmid-mediated resistance has not occurred with this class of drugs. Although clinical experience (eg, see Pichler et al, 1987) is more limited than with erythromycin, some consultants now prefer the fluoroquinolones for this indication in adults. Fluoroquinolones should not be used in pregnant women or prepubertal children.
(3) Some experts prefer gentamicin or chloramphenicol for patients with bacteremia and other extraintestinal infections. These agents are not used for diarrhea.
(4) Tetracyclines should not be given to pregnant women or children less than 8 years.
(5) Trimethoprim/sulfamethoxazole is NOT effective against *C. jejuni*.

***Escherichia coli* (enteroinvasive strains)**
(gram-negative bacilli)

REMARK:
(1) The role of antimicrobial drug therapy is unclear. Some experts recommend trimethoprim/sulfamethoxazole (alternatives, ciprofloxacin, norfloxacin, or ofloxacin) as for *Shigella*. Laboratory confirmation of invasive *E. coli* infection is not generally available.

***Escherichia coli* O157:H7 (enterohemorrhagic strain)**
(gram-negative bacilli)

REMARKS:
(1) Therapy usually has been supportive, and the role of antimicrobial drugs is controversial. Ciprofloxacin therapy has been advocated by some clinicians.
(2) This organism has been associated with the hemolytic uremic syndrome and thrombotic thrombocytopenic purpura.

Yersinia enterocolitica
(gram-negative bacilli)

REMARK:
(1) Most cases of diarrhea appear to resolve spontaneously. The role of antimicrobial drug therapy is unknown. Trimethoprim/sulfamethoxazole, aminoglycosides (eg, gentamicin), tetracycline, chloramphenicol, the fluoroquinolones (eg, ciprofloxacin, norfloxacin, ofloxacin), and chloramphenicol are active in vitro.

Vibrio parahaemolyticus
(gram-negative bacilli)

REMARK:
(1) Most cases of diarrhea appear to resolve spontaneously. The role of antimicrobial drug therapy is unknown. Tetracycline and the fluoroquinolones (eg, ciprofloxacin, norfloxacin) are active in vitro.

***Aeromonas* species**
(gram-negative bacilli)

REMARK:
(1) The role of antimicrobial drug therapy is unknown. Trimethoprim/sulfamethoxazole, tetracycline, aminoglycosides (eg, gentamicin), third generation cephalosporins (eg, cefotaxime), chloramphenicol, and the fluoroquinolones (eg, ciprofloxacin, norfloxacin, ofloxacin) are active in vitro.

Plesiomonas shigelloides
(gram-negative bacilli)

REMARK:
(1) Most cases of diarrhea are self-limited. The role of antimicrobial drug therapy is unknown. Trimethoprim/sulfamethoxazole, tetracycline, and the fluoroquinolones (eg, ciprofloxacin, norfloxacin, ofloxacin) are active in vitro.

***Escherichia coli* (enterotoxigenic strains)**
(gram-negative bacilli)

REMARK:
(1) Most cases of diarrhea are mild and resolve spontaneously. Although the role of antimicrobial drug therapy is not totally clear, clinical studies have shown that trimethoprim/sulfamethoxazole (alternative, trimethoprim), ciprofloxacin (or norfloxacin or ofloxacin), doxycycline, and bismuth subsalicylate decrease the severity and duration of illness (see TRAVELERS' DIARRHEA below). Laboratory confirmation of enterotoxigenic *E. coli* infection is not generally available.

EMPIRIC THERAPY

Shigella sp., *Salmonella* sp., and *Campylobacter jejuni* are more common; *Escherichia coli* (enteroinvasive strains), *Vibrio parahaemolyticus, Yersinia enterocolitica, Aeromonas hydrophila,* and *Plesiomonas shigelloides* are less common.

PREFERRED THERAPY:
Ciprofloxacin (or Norfloxacin or Ofloxacin) (Adults, see Remarks)

ALTERNATIVE THERAPY:
Trimethoprim/Sulfamethoxazole *with or without* Erythromycin

REMARKS:
(1) Supportive therapy (replacement of fluids and electrolytes) also is indicated.

(2) The fluoroquinolones (eg, ciprofloxacin, norfloxacin, ofloxacin) have advantages over trimethoprim/sulfamethoxazole because they are active against all major inflammatory gram-negative bacillary enteropathogens, including *Campylobacter jejuni.* Furthermore, plasmid-mediated, transferable resistance has not been observed with this class of drugs. However, late relapses of infection due to *Salmonella* sp. may be a problem (Neill et al, 1991). The fluoroquinolones are not active against viruses or protozoa (eg, *Giardia*). These agents should not be used in pregnant women or prepubertal children.
(3) Trimethoprim/sulfamethoxazole is not active against *C. jejuni.* Erythromycin can be added to expand the coverage to include this organism. Trimethoprim/sulfamethoxazole and erythromycin are not active against viruses or protozoa (eg, *Giardia*).

Travelers' Diarrhea

Infectious diarrhea occurs in as many as 50% of U. S. travelers to underdeveloped regions (eg, Mexico, South America, Africa, Southern and Southeast Asia). Most cases have a bacterial etiology. Enterotoxigenic *Escherichia coli* are the most common causative organisms of travelers' diarrhea in all studies, accounting for 30% to 70% of the cases. *Shigella* (0% to 30%), *Salmonella* (0% to 16%), *Campylobacter*, other bacteria, viruses, and protozoa (eg, *Giardia, Cryptosporidium,* amebae) are other important, but less common, pathogens.

Presently, guidelines for the prevention and treatment of travelers' diarrhea are not definitive. All experts agree that awareness and avoidance of possible sources of contamination are of primary importance. The role of antimicrobial prophylaxis is controversial, but the current consensus is that the risks outweigh the benefits for most (if not all) travelers (National Institutes of Health Consensus Development Conference, 1985; *Med Lett Drugs Ther*, 1990 B; see also Chapter 4 in this Section, Antimicrobial Chemoprophylaxis for Ambulatory Patients).

Treatment of mild cases of travelers' diarrhea is usually unnecessary because most are self-limited. Maintenance of fluid and electrolyte balance is of primary importance, although most individuals do not develop serious dehydration. Bismuth subsalicylate [Pepto-Bismol] or antimotility agents (eg, loperamide, diphenoxylate with atropine [Lomotil]) may help relieve symptoms in milder cases, but antimotility agents should be avoided when there is fever or bloody diarrhea, suggesting an inflammatory enteritis (National Institutes of Health Consensus Development Conference, 1985; see also index entry Diarrhea, Infectious). Results of prospective, randomized, double-blind, placebo-controlled studies suggest that early (within 48 to 72 hours of onset of illness) EMPIRIC antimicrobial drug treatment (as outlined below) of more severe cases of travelers' diarrhea can decrease the severity and duration of the illness in most patients (DuPont et al, 1982; Ericsson et al, 1987). In a subsequent study, the concomitant use of an antimotility agent (ie, loperamide) with an antimicrobial agent (trimethoprim/sulfamethoxazole) hastened relief of diarrhea and enteric symptoms in patients with travelers' diarrhea (Ericsson et al, 1990). Such therapy is indicated when symptoms are moderate to severe (three or more loose stools in an eight-hour period with nausea, vomiting, abdominal cramps, fever, or blood in the stools [National Institutes of Health Consensus Development Conference, 1985]). Travelers who have persistent diarrhea with serious fluid loss, fever, and blood or mucus in the stools should seek medical attention.

It is recommended that travelers to areas of high risk obtain an antimotility drug (or bismuth subsalicylate) and an antimicrobial agent prior to their trip in order to avoid buying over-the-counter drugs abroad with potentially dangerous ingredients (National Institutes of Health Consensus Development Conference, 1985).

Selected references: Gorbach and Edelman, 1986; Johnson et al, 1986; Asperilla et al, 1990; Tauxe et al, 1990.

EMPIRIC THERAPY

Enterotoxigenic *Escherichia coli* and *Shigella* species

PREFERRED THERAPY:
Ciprofloxacin (or Norfloxacin or Ofloxacin)
ALTERNATIVE THERAPY:
Trimethoprim/Sulfamethoxazole; Trimethoprim alone
REMARKS:
(1) Dosages are ciprofloxacin 500 mg, norfloxacin 400 mg (DuPont et al, 1987), ofloxacin 200 mg, trimethoprim 160 mg/sulfamethoxazole 800 mg, or trimethoprim 200 mg, all twice daily for three to five days (DuPont et al, 1982; Ericsson et al, 1987). Treatment for three days appears to be effective and is the duration of therapy recommended by the National Institutes of Health Consensus Development Conference (1985).
(2) All of the above regimens were significantly more effective than placebo for infections caused by culture-proven enterotoxigenic *E. coli* or *Shigella* and when diarrhea was not associated with a detectable pathogen. Only 5% of patients receiving trimethoprim/sulfamethoxazole, 8% of patients receiving trimethoprim, and 7% of patients receiving ciprofloxacin were treatment failures (DuPont et al, 1982; Ericsson et al, 1987).
(3) Clinical experience is greatest with trimethoprim/sulfamethoxazole. Plasmid-mediated, transferable resistance to this drug combination among isolates of *E. coli* is becoming widespread in some developing countries (Murray et al, 1985). Also, this regimen is not active against *C. jejuni* or protozoa (eg, *Giardia)*. Despite the disadvantages, trimethoprim 8 to 10 mg/kg for five days is the only regimen appropriate for prepubertal children.
(4) Ciprofloxacin and other fluoroquinolones (eg, norfloxacin, ofloxacin) have advantages over trimethoprim/sulfamethoxazole because they are active in vitro against essentially all aerobic gram-negative enteropathogens *(E. coli, Shigella* sp., *Salmonella* sp., *Vibrio* sp., *Yersinia enterocolitica, Campylobacter jejuni, Aeromonas hydrophila)* and plasmid-mediated, transferable resistance has not been observed. Fluoroquinolones are especially appropriate for patients with a history of hypersensitivity to trimethoprim/sulfamethoxazole or for use in areas where resistance to this drug combination is common. The fluoroquinolones are not active against protozoa (eg, *Giardia)* and should not be used in pregnant women or prepubertal children.
(5) Evidence suggests that doxycycline (100 mg twice daily) also is effective for the treatment of travelers' diarrhea (National Institutes of Health Consensus Development Conference, 1985).

Antibiotic-Associated Pseudomembranous Colitis

The most important cause of antibiotic-associated pseudomembranous colitis is *Clostridium difficile*, an anaerobic, spore-forming gram-positive bacillus that produces two extracellular toxins: toxin A, an enterotoxin, and toxin B, a cytotoxin.

General treatment measures include discontinuation of the causative antimicrobial agent when possible and supportive therapy (replacement of fluids and electrolytes). When necessary, SPECIFIC antimicrobial therapy directed against *C. difficile* is recommended. See also index entry Colitis, Pseudomembranous.

Selected references: Briceland et al, 1988; Lyerly et al, 1988.

SPECIFIC THERAPY

Clostridium difficile
(gram-positive bacilli)

PREFERRED THERAPY:
Vancomycin (oral) OR **Metronidazole (oral)**
ALTERNATIVE THERAPY:
Bacitracin (oral); Cholestyramine resin
REMARKS:
(1) Vancomycin has excellent in vitro activity against *C. difficile*, is not absorbed when given orally, and has an extensive, favorable clinical experience. This agent usually is preferred for severe cases of *C. difficile* pseudomembranous colitis and in high-risk patients. A major disadvantage of vancomycin is its high cost. Most experts agree that the previously recommended adult dosage of 500 mg four times per day (5 to 10 days) can be reduced to 125 mg four times per day (5 to 10 days) in most patients with no decrease in efficacy; this has been demonstrated in a randomized clinical trial (Fekety et al, 1989). Thus, cost of therapy with this agent can be decreased fourfold, but it is still much more expensive than metronidazole.
(2) Oral metronidazole (adults, 250 mg four times daily) was as effective as vancomycin in a prospective, randomized clinical trial (Teasley et al, 1983), and it appears to be an effective and less expensive alternative to vancomycin for mild to moderate cases. (Note: Alternative dosage schedule, adults, 500 mg three times daily.) Metronidazole has been reported to induce *C. difficile* pseudomembranous colitis in a few patients.
(3) Between 10% and 20% of patients relapse after initial successful treatment with vancomycin or metronidazole. Antimicrobial drug-resistant strains of *C. difficile* are not causative, however, because retreatment of these patients with vancomycin or metronidazole frequently is successful. Persistent fecal carriage of *C. difficile*, most likely as antibiotic-resistant spores, after treatment is an important risk factor for relapse.
(4) Cholestyramine resin acts by neutralizing *C. difficile* toxins. The efficacy of this agent has been variable depending on the institution. It should be used only in mild cases of antibiotic-associated pseudomembranous colitis. However, cholestyramine has the potential to bind *C. difficile* toxins in disease that is unresponsive to antimicrobial agents. It can be used with metronidazole or following vancomycin. Because the resin also binds vancomycin, simultaneous use should be avoided.
(5) Experience with bacitracin is limited. However, in two prospective, randomized clinical trials, bacitracin (adults, 20,000 or 25,000 units four times daily) was significantly less effective than vancomycin (adults, 125 or 500 mg four times daily) in clearing *C. difficile* from the stools, although resolution of symptoms and incidence of relapses were similar in each treatment group (Young et al, 1985; Dudley et al, 1986). Occasional strains of *C. difficile* are highly resistant to bacitracin in vitro.
(6) When oral therapy cannot be used (eg, severe ileus, recent surgery) parenteral metronidazole usually is preferred.

Typhoid Fever

Typhoid fever is caused by *Salmonella typhi*. SPECIFIC antimicrobial drug therapy should be directed against this organism.

Selected references: Conte and Barriere, 1988 B; *Med Lett Drugs Ther*, 1990 A; Asperilla et al, 1990; Hook, 1990.

SPECIFIC THERAPY

Salmonella typhi
(gram-negative bacilli)

PREFERRED THERAPY:
Chloramphenicol (see Remarks)
ALTERNATIVE THERAPY:
Ampicillin (or Amoxicillin); Trimethoprim/Sulfamethoxazole; Ceftriaxone (or Cefotaxime); Ciprofloxacin
REMARKS:
(1) Some consultants prefer ampicillin or trimethoprim/sulfamethoxazole for the treatment of typhoid fever in the United States because these agents are less toxic than chloramphenicol, they are more effective against typhoid intestinal carriage (see below), and, unlike in developing countries, cost is not the determining factor in drug selection.
(2) Although uncommon in the United States, chloramphenicol-resistant strains of *S. typhi* have been reported in Southeast Asia, India, the Middle East, and Mexico.
(3) Chloramphenicol is not effective in eradicating the chronic carrier state. Ampicillin (alternative, amoxicillin) has been effective in carriers without gallbladder disease. Although success with trimethoprim/sulfamethoxazole and rifampin has been reported, cholecystectomy may be required for patients with gallbladder disease.
(4) In limited clinical studies, third generation cephalosporins (Soe and Overturf, 1987) and fluoroquinolones (Asperilla et al, 1990) have been effective in typhoid fever and other systemic (nontyphoid) *Salmonella* infections. These agents may be useful alternatives for salmonelloses caused by organisms that are resistant to the standard regimens. Clinical data also suggest that fluoroquinolones are effective in the treatment of chronic typhoid carriers (Asperilla et al, 1990). Optimal agents and dosages and durations of therapy for various *Salmonella* syndromes must be determined by large, controlled trials.

Helicobacter (formerly *Campylobacter*) *pylori*-associated Gastritis

Helicobacter (formerly *Campylobacter*) *pylori*, spiral-shaped, urease-producing, microaerophilic gram-negative bacilli, are significantly associated with and may cause type B (antral) gastritis, and they also may be involved in the development of peptic ulcers. Various antimicrobial agents (eg, penicillin G, amoxicillin, erythromycin, tetracycline, gentamicin, cefoxitin, ciprofloxacin, metronidazole) are active in vitro against *H. pylori*, and these organisms also are susceptible to bismuth salts. However, complete eradication of *H. pylori* from gastric mucosa is difficult and treatment guidelines remain to be established (Graham and Klein, 1987; Dooley and Cohen, 1988). See also index entry Peptic Ulcer.

Hepatitis, Infectious

The major causes of infectious hepatitis are hepatitis A, hepatitis B, and non-A, non-B hepatitis viruses. Recently, an RNA virus designated as hepatitis C virus was shown to be the predominant cause of transfusion-associated non-A, non-B hepatitis (Alter et al, 1989). Conventional antimicrobial drug therapy is NOT effective for these viral infections. However, results of recent randomized, controlled clinical trials suggest that recombinant alfa interferon may be beneficial in transiently reducing disease activity in some patients with chronic hepatitis C (Davis et al, 1989; DiBisceglie et al, 1989) and that prednisone withdrawal followed by recombinant alfa interferon may be an effective treatment for selected patients with chronic type B hepatitis (Perrillo et al, 1988). Further clinical investigation is necessary.

Cholecystitis, Acute

Acute cholecystitis usually results when the cystic duct becomes obstructed by gallstones; secondary bacterial infection occurs in about 50% to 70% of cases. *Escherichia coli*; other gram-negative enteric bacilli, such as *Klebsiella, Enterobacter*, and *Proteus* species; and nonhemolytic streptococci, including enterococci, are causative organisms. Anaerobic bacteria, including *Bacteroides fragilis* and clostridia, also may be involved, particularly in the elderly. When present, anaerobic bacteria frequently are part of polymicrobial infections containing mixtures of anaerobic bacteria and aerobic gram-negative enteric bacilli.

Surgery is the primary treatment of gallstone-associated cholecystitis, but the timing is controversial. Because most cases of acute cholecystitis resolve spontaneously, some surgeons recommend waiting two to three months after the inflammation has subsided. Others advocate immediate surgery. Lithotripsy combined with medical management may offer noninvasive approaches to the treatment of gallbladder disease. Antimicrobial drug therapy (parenteral) of acute cholecystitis should be regarded as adjunctive to surgery (ie, to prevent spread of infection, to sterilize the bloodstream of any associated bacteremia). Drug selection usually is EMPIRIC pending the results of blood cultures and/or biliary operative culture data. Therapy is directed primarily against common aerobic gram-negative enteric bacilli (eg, *E. coli)*. Routine empiric coverage of anaerobic bacteria and enterococci usually is unnecessary except in the elderly and those with prolonged biliary obstruction, repeated gallbladder surgery, and heart valve abnormalities. Antibiotics usually do not eradicate local infection within the biliary tree because penetration of the drugs into bile is inadequate in the presence of complete obstruction.

Selected references: Gregory, 1986; Conte and Barriere, 1988 B; *Med Lett Drugs Ther*, 1990 A; Levison and Bush, 1990.

EMPIRIC THERAPY

Escherichia coli and other enteric gram-negative bacilli (*Klebsiella, Enterobacter, Proteus* sp.); species of *Enterococcus* (*eg, E. faecalis*) and other group D streptococci; possible anaerobic bacteria (*Bacteroides fragilis*, clostridia)

PREFERRED THERAPY:
Ampicillin *plus* Aminoglycoside (gentamicin, tobramycin, amikacin, netilmicin)

ALTERNATIVE THERAPY:
Ampicillin/Sulbactam [Unasyn]; Ticarcillin/Potassium Clavulanate [Timentin]

REMARKS:
(1) Other suggested alternative regimens include mezlocillin *plus* metronidazole; imipenem/cilastatin; cefoxitin *plus* aminoglycoside (gentamicin, tobramycin, amikacin, netilmicin); and cefoxitin *plus* aztreonam (Sanford, 1990). All of the alternative regimens would provide adequate coverage against enteric gram-negative bacilli and anaerobic bacteria, including *B. fragilis*. However, the cefoxitin-containing regimens may be inadequate against enterococci.
(2) For mild infections, single-agent therapy usually is considered adequate. First generation cephalosporins (eg, cefazolin) and ampicillin have been most frequently recommended. Ampicillin/sulbactam; ticarcillin/potassium clavulanate; and cefoxitin also are reasonable choices, especially in the older patient who may have an anaerobic infection.
(3) For life-threatening situations, including perforation with peritonitis or obstructive suppurative cholangitis, immediate surgery and antibiotic regimens, as recommended for secondary peritonitis, are usually necessary (see Peritonitis Secondary to Bowel Perforation below).

Peritonitis Secondary to Bowel Perforation

These infections are typically polymicrobial and contain a mixture of aerobic and anaerobic bacteria that originate from the microbial flora of the large bowel. Among the aerobic bacteria, *Escherichia coli*, other gram-negative enteric bacilli (eg, *Klebsiella, Proteus*), and group D streptococci, particularly enterococci (*Enterococcus faecalis*), are the major causative organisms. *Bacteroides fragilis* sp. and other members of the *B. fragilis* group (eg, *B. ovatus, B. thetaiotaomicron, B. distasonis)* are very common and particularly important anaerobic pathogens. Other common anaerobic bacteria include gram-positive cocci (*Peptostreptococcus* and *Peptococcus*) and clostridia.

The primary treatment of peritonitis secondary to bowel perforation is prompt surgical intervention to correct the intra-abdominal disease processes or injuries that caused the infection or to provide drainage of purulent materials. Supportive therapy (eg, fluid and electrolyte repletion) also is necessary. Antimicrobial therapy is indicated as an adjunct to control bacteremia, prevent the formation of metastatic foci of infection, reduce suppurative complications after bacterial contamination, and prevent local spread of existing infection.

Antimicrobial drug therapy (parenteral) of peritonitis secondary to bowel perforation initially is EMPIRIC pending results of cultures obtained from blood and peritoneal fluid. Broad spectrum antibacterial coverage against both enteric gram-negative bacilli (the aerobic component) and anaerobic bacteria, especially *B. fragilis*, is necessary. Whether enterococci also should be routinely covered is somewhat controversial; coverage is recommended in patients at increased risk of infective endocarditis (eg, prosthetic heart valve; significant heart murmur).

Selected references: Ho and Barza, 1987; Conte and Barriere, 1988 B; *Med Lett Drugs Ther*, 1990 A; Levison and Bush, 1990.

EMPIRIC THERAPY

Escherichia coli and other gram-negative enteric bacilli (eg, *Klebsiella, Proteus* sp.); *Bacteroides fragilis* group (*B. fragilis* sp., *B. thetaiotaomicron, B. ovatus, B. distasonis,* etc) and other anaerobic bacteria (eg, *Peptococcus, Peptostreptococcus*); optional, *Enterococcus faecalis* and other group D enterococci

ALTERNATIVE THERAPY: **(see Remarks)**
Clindamycin *plus* Aminoglycoside (gentamicin, tobramycin, amikacin, netilmicin) *with or without* Ampicillin (or Penicillin G)
OR
Metronidazole *plus* Aminoglycoside *with or without* Ampicillin (or Penicillin G)
OR
Cefoxitin (or Cefotetan) *with or without* Aminoglycoside
OR
Antipseudomonal Penicillin (ticarcillin, mezlocillin, piperacillin, azlocillin) *plus* Aminoglycoside
OR
Imipenem/cilastatin
OR
Ticarcillin/Potassium Clavulanate [Timentin] *with or without* Aminoglycoside
OR
Ampicillin/Sulbactam [Unasyn] *with or without* Aminoglycoside
OR
Clindamycin (or Metronidazole or Chloramphenicol) *plus* Aztreonam *with or without* Ampicillin (or Penicillin G)
OR
Chloramphenicol *plus* Aminoglycoside

REMARKS:

(1) Switch to most effective drug regimen after susceptibility test results are available.

(2) In intra-abdominal infections, there are many therapeutic options, and the severity of illness and the possible presence of resistant organisms play a role in decisions concerning initial empiric therapy. For severely ill patients, a two-drug regimen containing an aminoglycoside plus an agent with excellent activity against anaerobic bacteria, including *B. fragilis*, usually is indicated. The above list of recommended alternative regimens is based on the current literature and consensus opinion among consultants. Ampicillin (or penicillin G) should be added to some of the regimens, as noted above, to increase coverage against enterococci in patients at risk for infective endocarditis (eg, prosthetic heart valve, significant heart murmur). Whether enterococci should be routinely covered in intra-abdominal infections is controversial, however.

(3) Choice of aminoglycoside depends on local susceptibility patterns. Metronidazole, chloramphenicol, and clindamycin are the most active non-beta lactam agents against *B. fragilis*, but some strains are resistant to clindamycin (Cuchural et al, 1988). Hematologic toxicity is associated with chloramphenicol. The most active beta lactam antibiotics against *B. fragilis* are imipenem, ticarcillin/potassium clavulanate, and ampicillin/sulbactam (Cuchural et al, 1988; Finegold and Wexler, 1988; Styrt and Gorbach, 1989).

(4) Cefoxitin is active against most anaerobic bacteria, including *B. fragilis*, and a number of enteric gram-negative bacilli. When used alone, this agent has been as effective as clindamycin *plus* aminoglycoside for community-acquired intra-abdominal infections in controlled clinical studies (Malangoni et al, 1985). Some experts prefer cefoxitin alone for community-acquired infections in mild to moderately ill patients. Despite less clinical experience, cefotetan appears to have comparable efficacy. It should be noted, however, that up to 20% and 35% of strains within the whole *B. fragilis* group may be resistant to cefoxitin and cefotetan, respectively, in some geographic locations. Resistance is greatest for *B. thetaiotaomicron, B. distasonis,* and *B. ovatus* (Cuchural et al, 1988).

(5) Various third generation cephalosporins, including cefotaxime and ceftizoxime, also have been effective for secondary peritonitis when used alone. Each of these antibiotics has excellent activity against aerobic gram-negative enteric bacilli. Moxalactam has activity in vitro against *B. fragilis* comparable to cefoxitin, but serious bleeding has been associated with its use and, generally, it is not recommended. The other third generation cephalosporins are less active against *B. fragilis* and do not appear to offer any advantages over cefoxitin (or cefotetan) when used alone. Some consultants suggest the combination of a third generation cephalosporin (eg, cefotaxime) *plus* an antianaerobic agent (eg, clindamycin) for patients at increased risk for aminoglycoside toxicity (eg, impaired renal function).

(6) Some consultants prefer the newer, extended spectrum penicillins (eg, piperacillin, mezlocillin) to the carboxypenicillins (ticarcillin, carbenicillin) because they are more active against enterococci and *B. fragilis*. These agents should not be used alone because they are susceptible to beta lactamases and resistant bacterial strains are relatively common; therefore, they should be combined with a beta lactamase inhibitor (see below).

(7) The beta lactam/beta lactamase inhibitor combinations, ticarcillin/potassium clavulanate and ampicillin/sulbactam, have exhibited good activity against most intraperitoneal pathogens, including virtually all strains of *B. fragilis*, and they have been promising in studies of clinical infections. Many consultants prefer these agents to cefoxitin (or cefotetan) as monotherapy for mild to moderate infections.

(8) Imipenem, a beta lactamase stable carbapenem antibiotic, has the broadest antimicrobial spectrum of currently available beta lactam antibiotics that includes aerobic gram-negative bacilli (including *P. aeruginosa*), gram-positive cocci (including enterococci), and anaerobic bacteria (including *B. fragilis*). This agent looks promising for empiric monotherapy of polymicrobial infections such as secondary peritonitis (Solomkin et al, 1985, 1990; Hackford et al, 1988). Imipenem is administered in a 1:1 fixed ratio combination with cilastatin, which is a specific inhibitor of dehydropeptidase-I, a renal enzyme that inactivates imipenem.

(9) Aztreonam, a monobactam, is active against the Enterobacteriaceae and *P. aeruginosa*. It may be useful in patients at increased risk for aminoglycoside toxicity and/or those who are allergic to penicillins and cephalosporins. In intra-abdominal infections, it must be combined with an appropriate anti-*B. fragilis* drug (eg, clindamycin, metronidazole).

REPRODUCTIVE TRACT INFECTIONS (FEMALE)

Vaginitis

The major causative organisms of infectious vaginitis are *Candida albicans* (candidiasis), *Trichomonas vaginalis* (trichomoniasis), several species of vaginal bacteria (including anaerobic bacteria and *Gardnerella vaginale*) that interact to produce the syndrome called bacterial vaginosis (formerly nonspecific vaginitis), and Herpes simplex virus. Sexual transmission is believed to play a limited role in candidiasis. In contrast, trichomoniasis, bacterial vaginosis, and genital herpes are sexually transmitted diseases.

Antimicrobial drug therapy of infectious vaginitis is SPECIFIC for the causative organism. Drug selection for vaginal candidiasis is outlined below. For treatment guidelines for trichomoniasis and bacterial vaginosis, see Chapter 3 in this Section, Treatment of Sexually Transmitted Diseases. For treatment of genital herpes infections, see index entry Antiviral Agents.

Selected references: Penn, 1986; Levin et al, 1987; *MMWR*, 1989; Sanford, 1990.

SPECIFIC THERAPY

Candida albicans **(candidiasis)**
(fungus)

PREFERRED THERAPY:
Miconazole (intravaginal) OR **Clotrimazole (intravaginal)**
ALTERNATIVE THERAPY:
Nystatin (intravaginal); Butoconazole (intravaginal); Terconazole (intravaginal)
REMARKS:
(1) In uncomplicated acute infections, larger intravaginal doses and a shorter duration of therapy for miconazole (200 mg/day for three days) and clotrimazole (200 mg/day for three days or 500 mg as a single dose) appear to be as effective as traditional seven-day (100 mg/day) dosage regimens for these agents. For nystatin, a longer treatment period (14 days) may be required. For a detailed discussion, see index entry Candidiasis, Superficial.
(2) Clotrimazole is now available without prescription for the treatment of vaginal candidiasis. However, a physician's diagnosis of candidiasis should be obtained prior to using this drug to rule out other causes of vaginal symptoms. Pregnant women should use this drug only under physician supervision.

Trichomonas vaginalis **(trichomoniasis)**
(protozoan)

REMARK:
(1) See Chapter 3 in this Section, Treatment of Sexually Transmitted Diseases, for treatment guidelines.

Bacterial vaginosis caused by the interaction of several species of vaginal bacteria (including anaerobic bacteria and *Gardnerella vaginale*)

REMARK:
(1) See Chapter 3 in this Section, Treatment of Sexually Transmitted Diseases, for treatment guidelines.

Herpes simplex virus (genital herpes)

REMARK:
(1) For treatment guidelines, see index entry Antiviral Agents.

Cervicitis

Major causative organisms include *Neisseria gonorrhoeae, Chlamydia trachomatis*, and Herpes simplex virus. These are sexually transmitted infections. For treatment guidelines, see Chapter 3 in this Section, Treatment of Sexually Transmitted Diseases. For treatment guidelines for genital herpes infection, see also index entry Antiviral Agents.

Pelvic Inflammatory Disease (PID)

Important causative organisms include *Neisseria gonorrhoeae, Chlamydia trachomatis*, anaerobic bacteria (eg, *Bacteroides*, gram-positive cocci), facultative gram-negative bacilli (eg, *Escherichia coli*), and *Mycoplasma hominis*. Treatment guidelines for PID are outlined in Chapter 3 in this Section, Treatment of Sexually Transmitted Diseases. See also the review by Cunha, 1990.

REPRODUCTIVE TRACT INFECTIONS (MALE)

Genital Ulcers

Causative organisms include Herpes simplex virus, *Treponema pallidum* (syphilis), *Haemophilus ducreyi* (chancroid), *Calymmatobacterium granulomatis* (granuloma inguinale), and LGV serotypes of *Chlamydia trachomatis* (lymphogranuloma venereum). These are sexually transmitted infections. For treatment guidelines, see Chapter 3 in this Section, Treatment of Sexually Transmitted Diseases. See also index entry Antiviral Agents for treatment guidelines to genital herpes infections.

Epididymo-orchitis, Acute

Acute epididymo-orchitis has two forms. A sexually transmitted form usually occurs in men under 35 years, is associated with urethritis, and is caused by *Chlamydia trachomatis* and/or *Neisseria gonorrhoeae*. Nonsexually transmitted epididymo-orchitis usually occurs in men over 35 years, is associated with midstream pyuria and bacteriuria, and is usually caused by *Escherichia coli*; other Enterobacteriaceae and *Pseudomonas aeruginosa* are occasional pathogens. (Note: Mumps and Coxsackie should be considered in the infectious differential diagnosis of epididymo-orchitis. *Mycobacterium tuberculosis* also may cause epididymitis.)

Antimicrobial drug therapy of nonsexually transmitted acute epididymo-orchitis is initially EMPIRIC pending results of urine cultures and susceptibility tests. For treatment of sexually transmitted acute epididymo-orchitis, see Chapter 3 in this Section, Treatment of Sexually Transmitted Diseases.

Selected references: Chodak, 1986; *MMWR*, 1989; Sanford, 1990.

EMPIRIC THERAPY

Nonsexually Transmitted Epididymo-orchitis

Escherichia coli is most frequent pathogen; other Enterobacteriaceae

PREFERRED THERAPY:
Aminoglycoside (gentamicin, tobramycin, amikacin, netilmicin) *with or without* Ampicillin (parenteral)
OR
Trimethoprim/Sulfamethoxazole (oral) depending on severity
ALTERNATIVE THERAPY:
Third Generation Cephalosporin (cefotaxime, ceftizoxime, ceftriaxone, ceftazidime, cefoperazone) (parenteral)
OR
Ciprofloxacin (oral or intravenous, depending on severity)
REMARKS:
(1) For patients with fever, leukocytosis, severe pain and swelling, and a toxic clinical presentation, initial parenteral therapy with an aminoglycoside *with or without* ampicillin usually is preferred. Third generation cephalosporins (eg, cefotaxime) or intravenous ciprofloxacin are alternatives for the severely ill patient.
(2) Switch to most effective, least toxic, and least expensive drug regimen after susceptibility test results are available.
(3) Urologic evaluation is indicated.
(4) In prepubertal males, epididymitis is usually caused by coliforms or *Staphylococcus aureus*. Preferred empiric therapy: Nafcillin *plus* Aminoglycoside (Votteler, 1986).
(5) In a small group of homosexual men under 35 years, *E. coli* was reported to be the primary cause of acute epididymitis, suggesting that the above regimens may be the most appropriate initial therapy in this population (Berger et al, 1987).

Sexually Transmitted Epididymo-orchitis

Chlamydia trachomatis and/or *Neisseria gonorrhoeae*

REMARK:
(1) See Chapter 3 in this Section, Treatment of Sexually Transmitted Diseases, for treatment guidelines.

RESPIRATORY TRACT INFECTIONS (LOWER)

Bronchitis, Acute and Bronchiolitis

Acute bronchitis is caused primarily by viruses for which antimicrobial drug therapy is NOT effective. *Mycoplasma pneumoniae* is occasionally the causative organism. Drug selection for this organism is listed below. When acute bronchitis is accompanied by purulent sputum or symptoms persist beyond one to two weeks, antimicrobial therapy should be considered. Erythromycin frequently is the preferred drug in an otherwise healthy individual.

Bronchiolitis usually occurs within the first two years of life, particularly in infants between 2 and 10 months. It is caused by viruses, most frequently respiratory syncytial virus (RSV). Antimicrobial drug therapy generally is not effective for viral infections. However, ribavirin, administered as a small particle aerosol, may be indicated specifically for hospitalized infants and young children with severe lower respiratory tract infections caused by RSV (see index entry Ribavirin, As Antiviral Agent).

Selected references: Gwaltney, 1990; Hall and Hall, 1990; *Med Lett Drugs Ther*, 1986, 1990.

SPECIFIC THERAPY

Mycoplasma pneumoniae

Chlamydia pneumoniae

PREFERRED THERAPY:
Erythromycin OR **Tetracycline**
REMARK:
(1) Tetracyclines should not be given to pregnant women or children under 8 years.

Acute Exacerbations of Chronic Bronchitis

Streptococcus pneumoniae (pneumococcus) and *Haemophilus influenzae* (usually nontypeable strains) are the two bacterial species most frequently isolated from the sputum of patients with acute exacerbations of chronic bronchitis. *Moraxella (Branhamella) catarrhalis* also may be found. Respiratory viruses and, to a lesser extent, *Mycoplasma pneumoniae* also have been associated with acute exacerbation. However, an unequivocal causative role of these organisms in acute exacerbations of chronic bronchitis remains to be determined.

The effectiveness of short-term antimicrobial drug therapy for acute exacerbations of chronic bronchitis is difficult to assess based on the available data, and this area remains controversial. Many infectious disease experts recommend antimicrobial drug therapy (usually oral) directed against *S. pneumoniae* and *H. influenzae* (and possibly *M. pneumoniae*) in patients with increased cough and purulent sputum production, but without evidence of pneumonia. Treatment is continued or altered as indicated by patient response and/or results of sputum culture.

Selected references: Nicotra et al, 1986; Reynolds, 1990; Anthonisen et al, 1987; Gleckman, 1987; Brown, 1989; Verghese et al, 1990; Oberlin and Hyslop, 1990.

EMPIRIC THERAPY

Adults

Streptococcus pneumoniae and *Haemophilus influenzae;* possibly *Moraxella (Branhamella) catarrhalis* and *Mycoplasma pneumoniae*

PREFERRED THERAPY:
Amoxicillin OR **Tetracycline (or Doxycycline)**
ALTERNATIVE THERAPY:
Trimethoprim/Sulfamethoxazole; Cefaclor; Cefuroxime Axetil; Cefixime; Amoxicillin/Potassium Clavulanate [Augmentin]; Ciprofloxacin; Erythromycin (see Remarks)
REMARKS:
(1) Although ampicillin is a cost-effective alternative, amoxicillin usually is preferred because it is better absorbed, requires fewer doses per day, can be taken with meals, and may cause less diarrhea. Other aminopenicillins (eg, bacampicillin) do not appear to offer any important advantages over amoxicillin.
(2) Trimethoprim/sulfamethoxazole, cefaclor, cefixime, Augmentin, and ciprofloxacin should be effective for infections

caused by amoxicillin-resistant (beta lactamase-producing) strains of *H. influenzae*. Such strains are prevalent (eg, up to 40%) in some geographic areas. Recent results from a national surveillance study indicate that 84.1% of 378 *M. catarrhalis* respiratory isolates produced beta lactamase enzymes (Jorgensen et al, 1990). Thus, any of the alternative regimens, including erythromycin and the tetracyclines, should be active.
(3) Of the drugs listed, tetracycline (or doxycycline) and erythromycin are the only effective drugs against *M. pneumoniae*. However, tetracycline is the least active drug against *S. pneumoniae* and a number of *H. influenzae* strains also are resistant. One of the alternative drugs may be required for tetracyclineresistant strains of these organisms. (Note: Some consultants prefer doxycycline to tetracycline because it is more active in vitro and exhibits better penetration into bronchial secretions.)
(4) Erythromycin provides coverage against *S. pneumoniae, M. pneumoniae,* and *M. catarrhalis,* but is inadequate for *H. influenzae.*
(5) Ciprofloxacin, a fluoroquinolone, has excellent activity against aerobic gram-negative bacteria, including the Enterobacteriaceae, *H. influenzae*, and *M. catarrhalis*, but it has only moderate activity against *S. pneumoniae.* Some consultants suggest this agent for patients with frequent exacerbations of chronic bronchitis who have received multiple courses of antibiotics. These patients often become colonized with gram-negative bacteria and may require the broader spectrum of coverage provided by ciprofloxacin.
(6) Amoxicillin and Augmentin should not be used in penicillin-allergic patients; cefaclor and cefixime should not be used in patients who have had an immediate-type hypersensitivity reaction to penicillin.
(7) Tetracyclines should not be given to pregnant women or children under 8 years. Fluoroquinolones should not be given to pregnant women or prepubertal children.

Pertussis (Whooping Cough)

Selected references: American Academy of Pediatrics, 1988; Conte and Barriere, 1988; *Med Lett Drugs Ther*, 1990; Hewlett, 1990.

SPECIFIC THERAPY
Bordetella pertussis
(gram-negative bacilli)

PREFERRED THERAPY:
Erythromycin
ALTERNATIVE THERAPY:
Trimethoprim/Sulfamethoxazole; Tetracycline
REMARKS:
(1) Antimicrobial agents are given primarily to reduce infectivity by eliminating *B. pertussis* carriage. Although they may ameliorate the disease when given in the catarrhal (preparoxysmal) stage, antimicrobials usually do not affect the clinical course of the illness when given in the paroxysmal stage when the diagnosis is most often first suspected. Supportive care is essential.
(2) Erythromycin orally (adults, 500 mg four times daily; children, 40 to 50 mg/kg daily in four divided doses) for 14 days appears to be the most effective regimen. (Note: A retrospective analysis of the literature suggests that erythromycin estolate has been more effective than erythromycin ethylsuccinate or erythromycin stearate in eliminating *B. pertussis* carriage, presumably due to better penetration of the estolate into respiratory secretions [Bass, 1985].) Less clinical experience has been obtained with the alternative antimicrobial agents.
(3) Ampicillin is active against *B. pertussis* in vitro, but does not reduce communicability or modify the clinical course. Pertussis Immune Globulin (Human) is of no value.
(4) Tetracyclines should not be given to pregnant women or children under 8 years.

Pneumonia

The most common causative organisms of community-acquired pneumonia in otherwise normal hosts are *Streptococcus pneumoniae* (acute bacterial [typical] pneumonia), viruses (viral pneumonias), and *Mycoplasma pneumoniae* (atypical pneumonia syndrome). Relative incidences are related to patient age as follows:

(1) ADULTS GREATER THAN 40 YEARS, *S. pneumoniae*;

(2) ADULTS LESS THAN 40 YEARS AND CHILDREN GREATER THAN 5 YEARS, *M. pneumoniae*;

(3) INFANTS AND CHILDREN LESS THAN 5 YEARS (EXCEPT NEWBORNS), viruses.

Acute bacterial pneumonias are much more common in debilitated elderly patients and persons with predisposing conditions. Although *S. pneumoniae* is usually the most common causative organism, other bacteria are also important pathogens in these patients. Common predisposing conditions and probable causative bacteria are as follows:

(1) CHRONIC OBSTRUCTIVE PULMONARY DISEASE: *S. pneumoniae, Haemophilus influenzae,* and *Moraxella (Branhamella) catarrhalis*;

(2) CHRONIC ALCOHOLISM: *S. pneumoniae*, anaerobic bacteria (aspiration pneumonia), *H. influenzae, Klebsiella pneumoniae, Staphylococcus aureus*, and *Mycobacterium tuberculosis* (tuberculosis);

(3) POSTINFLUENZA BACTERIAL PNEUMONIA: *S. pneumoniae, S. aureus*, and *H. influenzae*;

(4) ELDERLY NURSING HOME PATIENTS: *S. pneumoniae, S. aureus, K. pneumoniae* (and other gram-negative bacilli), and *H. influenzae*;

(5) PATIENTS WITH MENTAL OBTUNDATION, SWALLOWING PROBLEMS, ESOPHAGEAL DISORDERS, SEIZURE DISORDERS, AND POOR DENTAL HYGIENE: Anaerobic bacteria (aspiration pneumonia);

(6) CYSTIC FIBROSIS: *Pseudomonas aeruginosa* and *S. aureus*;

(7) IMMUNOCOMPROMISED HOSTS: Multiple etiologies, including gram-negative bacilli (eg, *Escherichia coli, K. pneumoniae, P. aeruginosa*), *S. aureus*, and other bacteria, as well as viral (eg, cytomegalovirus), fungal (eg, *Aspergillus*), and protozoal (eg, *Pneumocystis carinii*) pathogens. The likely spectrum of causative organisms will vary, depending on the cause of the immunodeficiency (eg, *S. aureus*, aerobic gram-negative bacilli, and *Aspergillus* are likely pathogens in neutropenic patients; *P. carinii* frequently causes pneumonia in AIDS patients).

Additional causative organisms of atypical pneumonia syndromes include *Legionella pneumophila* and other *Legionella* sp., *Chlamydia trachomatis, C. psittaci*, and *Coxiella burnetii. L. pneumophila*, a gram-negative bacillus, is the etiologic agent in Legionnaires' disease. It can cause pneumonia in normal hosts and is a particularly important pathogen in elderly patients with predisposing conditions. The incidence of nonepidemic community-acquired pneumonia due to *L. pneumophila* has increased and is quite common in some reported series. *C. trachomatis* is a common cause of afebrile pneumonia in infants between 2 and 20 weeks of age who have acquired this sexually transmitted organism from mothers with genital tract colonization. Ornithosis (*C. psittaci*) and Q fever (*C. burnetii*, a rickettsial organism) are relatively rare atypical pneumonias associated with exposure to birds and farm animals, respectively. A new chlamydial organism, designated *Chlamydia pneumoniae* strain TWAR, has been reported to be an important cause of atypical pneumonia in adults. The clinical illness caused by this pathogen is very similar to that caused by *M. pneumoniae.*

Ideally, antimicrobial drug selection for a patient with pneumonia should be based on the isolation of a specific causative organism from a site not usually colonized (eg, blood, pleural fluid, lower respiratory tract). However, this may be impossible or impractical in many cases. Thus, antimicrobial drug therapy of community-acquired pneumonia usually is initiated with varying degrees of empiricism based on a number of factors. These include: (1) an adequate history (eg, age; smoking and drinking habits; underlying diseases and predisposing conditions; immune status; recent exposure to specific pathogens; sexual, occupational, travel, and animal exposure history); (2) the clinical presentation (eg, onset, fever, nature of cough, sputum, pleuritic pain); and the results of (3) physical examination; (4) chest x-ray (eg, location of infiltrates, presence of consolidation, effusion, cavitation); (5) clinical laboratory tests (eg, white blood cell count); and, of particular importance, (6) Gram stain of a reliable sputum specimen (less than 10 squamous epithelial cells and greater than 25 polymorphonuclear leukocytes per low power field).

SPECIFIC THERAPY, as outlined below, can be employed when the causative organism is known or highly suspected based on the results of Gram stain and/or these other factors. When the specific etiologic agent is unknown and other factors make the diagnosis equivocal, the institution of rational EMPIRIC THERAPY usually is necessary.

Selected references: Pennington, 1986; Francke, 1983; Donowitz and Mandell, 1990; Gleckman and Roth, 1984; Teele, 1985; Bartlett, 1987; Cunha, 1987; Hager et al, 1987; Marrie et al, 1987; Neu, 1987; Walzer, 1987; Conte and Barriere, 1988; Crane and Komshian, 1988; Brumfitt and Hamilton-Miller, 1989; *Med Lett Drugs Ther*, 1990; Medina et al, 1990; Sanford, 1990; Nelson, 1991.

SPECIFIC THERAPY (ACUTE BACTERIAL PNEUMONIA)

Streptococcus pneumoniae

(gram-positive cocci)

PREFERRED THERAPY:
Penicillin G (IV) OR **Penicillin G Procaine (IM)** OR **Penicillin V potassium (oral) depending on severity**
ALTERNATIVE THERAPY:
Erythromycin; First Generation Cephalosporin (cefazolin, cephalothin, cephapirin, cephradine)
REMARK:
(1) Rare strains of *S. pneumoniae* are totally resistant to penicillin G; these strains are susceptible to vancomycin.

Haemophilus influenzae

(gram-negative bacilli)

PREFERRED THERAPY:
Cefotaxime (or Ceftizoxime or Ceftriaxone or Ceftazidime)
OR
Ampicillin *plus* Chloramphenicol initially
ALTERNATIVE THERAPY:
Trimethoprim/Sulfamethoxazole; Ampicillin/Sulbactam [Unasyn]; Cefuroxime; Ciprofloxacin (oral); Amoxicillin/Potassium Clavulanate
REMARKS:
(1) Beta lactamase-producing strains are resistant to ampicillin and rare strains are resistant to chloramphenicol. Therefore, combined treatment is recommended until susceptibility is determined. Ampicillin usually is preferred for sensitive strains.
(2) All other regimens should be effective against ampicillin-resistant strains of *H. influenzae*. Many infectious disease experts now prefer a third generation cephalosporin for these resistant strains or when susceptibility is unknown to avoid the toxicity and problems associated with administration of chloramphenicol (eg, need to monitor serum concentrations in children).
(3) Some consultants suggest ampicillin/sulbactam, a beta lactam/beta lactamase inhibitor combination, as an excellent alternative regimen in adults. Presently, this drug lacks labeling for pediatric patients.
(4) For milder cases of *H. influenzae* pneumonia in adults, oral therapy with ciprofloxacin in the outpatient setting is a preferred and cost-effective alternative to parenteral therapy in the hospital. Ciprofloxacin, a fluoroquinolone, should not be used in pregnant women or prepubertal children.
(5) Cefuroxime, a second generation cephalosporin, has been widely used for *H. influenzae* infections in children. However, on a weight basis, this drug is less active than the third generation cephalosporins (eg, cefotaxime, ceftriaxone) against this organism. More important, cefuroxime occasionally has been associated with delayed sterilization of cerebrospinal fluid and even overt therapeutic failures in patients infected with *H. influenzae.* Thus, many pediatric infectious disease experts prefer a third generation cephalosporin to cefuroxime for severe *H. influenzae* infections.
(6) Cefamandole is NOT recommended for pediatric cases. Its activity against beta lactamase-producing *H. influenzae* is unreliable and it exhibits poor penetration into cerebrospinal fluid.

Staphylococcus aureus

(gram-positive cocci)

PREFERRED THERAPY:
Nafcillin OR **Oxacillin**
ALTERNATIVE THERAPY:
First Generation Cephalosporin (cefazolin, cephalothin, cephapirin, cephradine); Vancomycin (intravenous)
REMARKS:
(1) Most experts do not recommend methicillin in adults because of an increased risk of interstitial nephritis.
(2) Penicillin G should be substituted for antistaphylococcal penicillins if susceptibility is proven.
(3) For methicillin-resistant strains of *S. aureus*, vancomycin is the drug of choice.

Klebsiella pneumoniae **and other gram-negative enteric bacilli**

PREFERRED THERAPY:

Third Generation Cephalosporin (cefotaxime, ceftizoxime, ceftriaxone ceftazidime) ***with or without*** **Aminoglycoside (gentamicin, tobramycin, amikacin, netilmicin)**

ALTERNATIVE THERAPY:

Ticarcillin/Potassium Clavulanate ***with or without*** **Aminoglycoside; Aztreonam** ***with or without*** **Aminoglycoside; Ciprofloxacin** ***with*** **or** ***without*** **Aminoglycoside.**

REMARKS:

(1) Susceptibility testing is recommended.
(2) Many infectious disease experts prefer combination therapy for documented gram-negative bacillary pneumonia.
(3) Aztreonam, a monobactam, or ciprofloxacin (with or without an aminoglycoside) may be useful alternatives in patients who are allergic to penicillins and cephalosporins.

Pseudomonas aeruginosa
(gram-negative bacilli)

PREFERRED THERAPY:

Antipseudomonal Penicillin (ticarcillin, mezlocillin, piperacillin, azlocillin) ***plus*** **Aminoglycoside (gentamicin, tobramycin, amikacin, netilmicin)**

ALTERNATIVE THERAPY:

Ceftazidime (or Cefoperazone) ***plus*** **Aminoglycoside; Aztreonam** ***plus*** **Aminoglycoside; Imipenem/cilastatin** ***plus*** **Aminoglycoside; Ciprofloxacin** ***with*** **or** ***without*** **Aminoglycoside**

REMARKS:

(1) Most experts recommend combination therapy for systemic infections caused by *P. aeruginosa*.
(2) Aztreonam (*plus* aminoglycoside) or ciprofloxacin (with or without an aminoglycoside) may be useful alternatives in patients who are allergic to penicillins and cephalosporins.

Anaerobic bacteria from oropharyngeal flora, including ***Peptococcus, Peptostreptococcus, Fusobacterium,*** **and** ***Bacteroides*** **(aspiration pneumonia)**

PREFERRED THERAPY:

Penicillin G

OR

Clindamycin

ALTERNATIVE THERAPY:

Ampicillin/Sulbactam [Unasyn]; Cefoxitin

REMARKS:

(1) Traditionally, penicillin G has been preferred for aspiration pneumonia. However, penicillin G-resistant strains of *Bacteroides* sp. (eg, *B. melaninogenicus*) have been increasing. In geographic areas with known increased resistance to penicillin G, clindamycin is preferred.
(2) In hospitalized patients, aspiration pneumonia may be due to gram-negative bacilli present in the oropharynx. Antibiotic therapy must be effective against these organisms when this type of infection is suspected (see above for regimens effective against gram-negative bacilli).

Mycobacterium tuberculosis
(acid fast bacilli)

REMARK:

(1) See index entry Tuberculosis for treatment guidelines.

SPECIFIC THERAPY (ATYPICAL PNEUMONIA SYNDROMES)

Mycoplasma pneumoniae

PREFERRED THERAPY:

Erythromycin OR **Tetracycline**

REMARK:

(1) Tetracyclines should not be given to pregnant women or children under 8 years.

Legionella pneumophila
(gram-negative bacillus)

PREFERRED THERAPY:

Erythromycin ***with or without*** **Rifampin**

REMARKS:

(1) Initial therapy with erythromycin usually is by the intravenous route. In those patients who fail to respond to erythromycin alone, who are critically ill, or who have severe underlying disease, rifampin can be added. Rifampin should not be used alone, however, due to the rapid emergence of resistant organisms.
(2) Presently, there are no good alternatives to erythromycin. Doxycycline *with or without* rifampin or trimethoprim/sulfamethoxazole with or without rifampin may be effective if erythromycin cannot be given. Anecdotal results with ciprofloxacin suggest it may be useful in *Legionella* pneumonia (Edelstein and Meyer, 1988).

Chlamydia trachomatis **(chlamydial pneumonia in infants)**

REMARK:

(1) See Chapter 3 in this Section, Treatment of Sexually Transmitted Diseases, for treatment guidelines.

Chlamydia pneumoniae, strain TWAR

PREFERRED THERAPY:

Tetracycline

ALTERNATIVE THERAPY:

Erythromycin

REMARKS:

(1) Optimum therapy remains to be established. However, treatment failures were common when short-course (eg, five to seven days) erythromycin regimens, commonly used for *M. pneumoniae* infections, were employed (Grayston et al, 1986).
(2) Tetracyclines should not be given to pregnant women or children under 8 years.

Chlamydia psittaci **(ornithosis; psittacosis)**

PREFERRED THERAPY:

Tetracycline

ALTERNATIVE THERAPY:

Erythromycin

REMARKS:

(1) The minimum duration of therapy is 10 to 14 days, and the maximum is 21 days. Some experts recommend treatment for at least 7 to 10 days after good clinical response.
(2) Clinical experience with erythromycin is limited, and its efficacy has been supported in a number of anecdotal reports. It should be used only if there is compelling reason to avoid the use of tetracyclines. Chloramphenicol also is an alternative therapy for psittacosis.
(3) Tetracyclines should not be given to pregnant women or

children under 8 years.

Coxiella burnetii (rickettsial organism responsible for Q fever)

PREFERRED THERAPY:
Tetracycline
ALTERNATIVE THERAPY:
Chloramphenicol
REMARK:
(1) Tetracyclines should not be given to pregnant women or children under 8 years.

Pneumocystis carinii
(protozoan)

PREFERRED THERAPY:
Trimethoprim/Sulfamethoxazole (oral)
OR
Trimethoprim/Dapsone (oral)
OR
Pentamidine isethionate (intravenous)
ALTERNATIVE THERAPY:
Clindamycin plus Primaquine
REMARKS:
(1) *P. carinii* pneumonia is the most common opportunistic infection in patients with AIDS. For more detailed discussion, see index entry Pneumocystis Pneumonia.
(2) Primaquine must not be used in patients with glucose-6-phosphate dehydrogenase deficiency because it may cause hemolysis. It also is contraindicated in pregnant women.

EMPIRIC THERAPY

Guidelines for empiric therapy of community-acquired pneumonia based on patient age and the presence of certain predisposing conditions (if any) are presented. However, it must be emphasized that no single regimen can cover all possible pathogens, and antimicrobial drug selection for any given patient should take into consideration all relevant factors (see above).

Adults (Usually Young to Middle-aged With no Predisposing Condition)

Streptococcus pneumoniae and *Mycoplasma pneumoniae* are most likely; *Legionella pneumophila* is less common.

PREFERRED THERAPY:
Erythromycin
REMARKS:
(1) If *L. pneumophila* is the likely causative organism, a larger dose of erythromycin is necessary.
(2) If the clinical presentation strongly suggests pneumococcal pneumonia (eg, lobar pneumonia, purulent sputum), initial therapy with penicillin G usually is preferred.
(3) For more severely ill patients, the addition of another antibiotic such as a second (eg, cefuroxime) or third generation (eg, cefotaxime) cephalosporin frequently is recommended to provide broader antibacterial coverage.

Adults (Chronic Lung Disease; Alcoholism; Postinfluenza Pneumonia; Elderly Patients)

Streptococcus pneumoniae, Haemophilus influenzae, Staphylococcus aureus, Klebsiella pneumoniae, oropharyngeal anaerobic bacteria, and *Legionella pneumophila*

PREFERRED THERAPY:
Third Generation Cephalosporin (cefotaxime, ceftizoxime, ceftriaxone, ceftazidime, cefoperazone) *with or without* Aminoglycoside (gentamicin, tobramycin, amikacin, netilmicin)
ALTERNATIVE THERAPY:
Ampicillin/sulbactam [Unasyn] *with or without* Aminoglycoside; Ticarcillin/Potassium Clavulanate *with or without* Aminoglycoside; Imipenem/cilastatin *with or without* Aminoglycoside
REMARKS:
(1) Many experts will include the aminoglycoside in patients with severe illness and/or when the clinical presentation suggests gram-negative bacillary pneumonia (eg, *K. pneumoniae*). For patients with mild-to-moderate disease, monotherapy with a beta lactam agent usually is adequate.
(2) Second generation cephalosporins (eg, cefamandole, cefuroxime, cefoxitin, cefonicid) can be used for mild-to-moderate pneumonia in these patient populations and a number of consultants consider them to be suitable alternatives.
(3) None of the above regimens is effective against *L. pneumophila*. The addition of erythromycin to cover this pathogen is recommended when the clinical presentation suggests possible *Legionella* pneumonia and/or in patients with severe illness.
(4) Switch to most effective drug regimen after susceptibility test results are available.

Children (Greater Than 5 Years)

Mycoplasma pneumoniae is most likely; *Streptococcus pneumoniae* is less common. Viruses also may cause pneumonia in this age group, but conventional antimicrobial drug therapy is NOT effective.

PREFERRED THERAPY:
Erythromycin

Infants and Children (Less Than 5 Years; Except Newborns)

Viruses are the most common causes of pneumonia in this age group and, therefore, conventional antimicrobial drug therapy usually is NOT effective. (See Remarks.) *Streptococcus pneumoniae* and *Haemophilus influenzae* type b are the common bacterial causes, and antimicrobial drug therapy should be directed against these pathogens when they are suspected. *Staphylococcus aureus* also may be causative, especially in children less than 2 years of age.

PREFERRED THERAPY:
Cefotaxime or Ceftriaxone (or Ceftizoxime)
ALTERNATIVE THERAPY:
Cefuroxime; Chloramphenicol alone
REMARKS:
(1) Switch to most effective drug regimen after susceptibility test results are available.
(2) Cefuroxime, a second generation cephalosporin, has been widely used for *H. influenzae* type b infections in children. However, on a weight basis, this drug is less active against this organism than the third generation cephalosporins (eg, cefotax-

ime, ceftriaxone). More important, cefuroxime occasionally has been associated with delayed sterilization of cerebrospinal fluid and even overt therapeutic failures in patients infected with *H. influenzae* type b. Thus, many pediatric infectious disease experts prefer a third generation cephalosporin (eg, cefotaxime, ceftriaxone) to cefuroxime for severe *H. influenzae* type b infections.
(3) Cefamandole is NOT recommended as an initial therapy for children less than 5 years because of its poor penetration into cerebrospinal fluid.
(4) Some consultants recommend nafcillin (or oxacillin) plus chloramphenicol in the severely ill child, especially those under 2 years of age, to increase coverage against *Staphylococcus aureus*.
(5) For children who are well enough to be treated as outpatients, oral amoxicillin (alternatives, erythromycin plus sulfisoxazole, amoxicillin/potassium clavulanate) is preferred.
(6) *Chlamydia trachomatis* may cause up to one-third of cases of pneumonia in infants between 2 and 20 weeks of age. If clinical suspicion of *C. trachomatis* is high, erythromycin should be added to the regimen. Infants in this age group who are treated as outpatients should receive erythromycin plus sulfisoxazole.
(7) Conventional antimicrobial therapy is not effective for viral infections. However, ribavirin, administered as a small particle aerosol, may be indicated specifically for hospitalized infants and young children with severe lower respiratory tract infections caused by respiratory syncytial virus (RSV) (see index entry Ribavirin).

Neonates

REMARKS:
(1) Intrapartum bacterial pneumonia most frequently is caused by *Streptococcus agalactiae* (group B) and gram-negative enteric bacilli (eg, *Escherichia coli*). Initial antimicrobial drug therapy is the same as for neonatal sepsis pending isolation of the causative organism (see Sepsis, Neonatal above).
(2) Afebrile pneumonia due to *Chlamydia trachomatis* is seen in neonates between age 2 and 20 weeks; this sexually transmitted pathogen is acquired from infected mothers. See Chapter 3 in this Section, Treatment of Sexually Transmitted Diseases, for treatment guidelines. See also Infants and Children (Less Than 5 Years; Except Newborns) above for additional remarks.

RESPIRATORY TRACT INFECTIONS (UPPER)

Rhinitis, Acute

Acute rhinitis (common cold) is the most common upper respiratory tract infection. However, the etiology is viral and antimicrobial drug therapy is NOT effective.

Pharyngitis/Tonsillitis, Acute

The majority of these infections are caused by viruses for which antimicrobial drug therapy is NOT effective.

A common cause of acute bacterial pharyngitis is the group A beta hemolytic streptococcus (*Streptococcus pyogenes*). Streptococcal pharyngitis ("strep throat"), including scarlet fever, is most common in children between 5 and 15 years and is diagnosed by throat culture or by newer rapid diagnostic (antigen detection) tests. Prevention of acute rheumatic fever is a primary treatment goal. Although the incidence of rheumatic fever declined in the United States over the past two decades, a resurgence of this serious nonsuppurative complication recently has been reported in various areas of this country (Congeni et al, 1987; Hosier et al, 1987; Veasy et al, 1987; Wald et al, 1987).

In adults, in addition to *S. pyogenes*, *Mycoplasma pneumoniae* and *Chlamydia pneumoniae* strain TWAR are relatively common causes of acute pharyngitis. *Corynebacterium hemolyticum* also may be causative in adolescents and young adults.

Less frequent, but important, causes of acute bacterial pharyngitis include *Neisseria gonorrhoeae* and *Corynebacterium diphtheriae*. Gonococcal pharyngitis is a sexually transmitted disease and treatment guidelines can be found in Chapter 3 of this Section, Treatment of Sexually Transmitted Diseases. Diphtheria is rare in the United States today, but it is a potentially life-threatening disease.

Selected references: Dillon, 1987; American Academy of Pediatrics, 1988; Huovinen et al, 1989; *MMWR,* 1989; *Med Lett Drugs Ther,* 1990; Nelson, 1991.

SPECIFIC THERAPY

Streptococcus pyogenes (group A, beta hemolytic)

(gram-positive cocci)

PREFERRED THERAPY:
Penicillin V potassium (orally, for 10 days) OR **penicillin G benzathine (intramuscularly, single dose)**
ALTERNATIVE THERAPY:
Erythromycin (orally, for 10 days)
REMARKS:
(1) Penicillin V potassium usually is preferred to penicillin G (orally, for 10 days) because it is more acid stable, provides greater and more reliable bioavailability, and can be taken with meals.
(2) Oral penicillin V potassium generally is preferred to intramuscular penicillin G benzathine because it is associated with fewer adverse and allergic reactions. However, the single-dose intramuscular injection is preferred in patients who are unlikely to be compliant with a full 10-day course of oral therapy, for rheumatic patients or those in families in which rheumatic fever has occurred, and for geographic areas or socioeconomic settings in which there is substantial risk for development of rheumatic fever.
(3) Approximately 5% of group A beta hemolytic streptococcal strains are now resistant to erythromycin in the United States.
(4) Oral first generation cephalosporins (cephalexin, cephradine, cefadroxil) and clindamycin are other alternatives for streptococcal pharyngitis in patients who are allergic to penicillin and who cannot tolerate erythromycin. However, cephalosporins should not be used in patients who have had an immediate-type hypersensitivity reaction to penicillin.
(5) Some consultants note that cefadroxil, a long-acting oral cephalosporin, has been as effective as penicillin V potassium when administered once or twice daily for 10 days. Although less frequent administration may improve compliance in some situations (eg, in child of parents who both work), the greater cost of cefadroxil when compared to penicillin V potassium also must be considered.
(6) A number of clinical studies have shown that early treatment of streptococcal pharyngitis with penicillin can shorten the duration of symptoms by about 24 hours in children (Randolph et al, 1985; Pichichero et al, 1987), suggesting that initiation of

drug therapy before the results of throat culture are available may be beneficial. However, this issue is controversial (see Smith, 1984; Pichichero et al, 1987). The availability of new rapid diagnostic tests for group A streptococci that are fairly sensitive and highly specific may make earlier diagnosis and, therefore, immediate initiation of specific therapy possible (*Med Lett Drugs Ther*, 1985; Radetsky et al, 1987). Treatment is indicated if such test results are positive. However, negative test results must be confirmed by throat culture (Dajani et al, 1988).
(7) Tetracyclines and sulfonamides are *not* recommended for treatment of streptococcal pharyngitis. Tetracycline-resistant group A, beta hemolytic streptococci are prevalent, and sulfonamides fail to eradicate the streptococci.

Mycoplasma pneumoniae

PREFERRED THERAPY:
Erythromycin OR **Tetracycline**
REMARK:
(1) Tetracyclines should not be given to pregnant women or children under 8 years.

Chlamydia pneumoniae, strain TWAR

PREFERRED THERAPY:
Tetracycline
ALTERNATIVE THERAPY:
Erythromycin
REMARKS:
(1) Optimum therapy remains to be established.
(2) Tetracyclines should not be given to pregnant women or children under 8 years.

Corynebacterium hemolyticum
(gram-positive bacilli)

PREFERRED THERAPY:
Erythromycin

Neisseria gonorrhoeae
(gram-negative cocci)

REMARK:
(1) See Chapter 3 in this Section, Treatment of Sexually Transmitted Diseases, for treatment guidelines.

Corynebacterium diphtheriae
(gram-positive bacilli)

PREFERRED THERAPY:
Antitoxin *plus* Erythromycin
OR
Antitoxin *plus* Penicillin G
REMARK:
(1) Antitoxin is necessary to neutralize toxin produced by *C. diphtheriae*; antimicrobial therapy eradicates the organism and prevents spread.

Laryngitis, Acute

Acute laryngitis is caused by viruses for which antimicrobial drug therapy is NOT effective.

Laryngotracheitis, Acute

Acute laryngotracheitis (viral croup) usually occurs in children under 3 years. It is caused by viruses for which antimicrobial drug therapy is NOT effective. (Note: Bacterial tracheitis is a relatively rare syndrome that mimics viral croup. Causative organisms include *Staphylococcus aureus*, group A beta hemolytic streptococci, and *Haemophilus influenzae* type b. Empiric therapy with intravenous antibiotics should be rapidly initiated. Nafcillin plus chloramphenicol OR third generation cephalosporin [eg, cefotaxime, ceftriaxone] are possible regimens.)

Epiglottitis, Acute

Acute epiglottitis is seen most frequently in children between 2 and 7 years, but may occur at any age. The causative organism usually is *Haemophilus influenzae* type b.

This rapidly progressive and potentially fatal disease should be considered a medical emergency. MAINTENANCE OF AN ADEQUATE AIRWAY IS OF PRIMARY IMPORTANCE. Antimicrobial drug therapy (parenteral) is initially EMPIRIC pending the results of cultures and susceptibility tests.

Selected references: *Med Lett Drugs Ther*, 1990; Todd, 1988; Nelson, 1991.

EMPIRIC THERAPY
Children
Haemophilus influenzae type b

PREFERRED THERAPY:
Cefotaxime (or Ceftriaxone or Ceftizoxime or Ceftazidime)
OR
Ampicillin *plus* Chloramphenicol
ALTERNATIVE THERAPY:
Chloramphenicol alone; Cefuroxime
REMARKS:
(1) Beta lactamase-producing strains of *H. influenzae* type b are resistant to ampicillin and rare strains are resistant to chloramphenicol. Therefore, combined treatment is recommended until susceptibility is determined. Ampicillin usually is preferred for susceptible strains.
(2) Third generation cephalosporins (eg, cefotaxime, ceftriaxone) are highly active against *H. influenzae* in vitro, including beta lactamase-producing strains. Many infectious disease experts now prefer these agents to avoid the toxicity and other problems associated with administration of chloramphenicol (eg, need to monitor serum concentrations).
(3) Cefuroxime, a second generation cephalosporin, has been widely used for *H. influenzae* type b infections in children. However, on a weight basis, this drug is less active than the third generation cephalosporins (eg, cefotaxime, ceftriaxone) against this organism. More important, cefuroxime occasionally has been associated with delayed sterilization of cerebrospinal fluid and even overt therapeutic failures in patients infected with *H. influenzae* type b. Thus, many pediatric infectious disease consultants prefer a third generation cephalosporin (eg, cefotaxime, ceftriaxone) to cefuroxime for severe *H. influenzae* type b infections.
(4) Antimicrobial drug therapy of adults with acute epiglottitis appears to be the same as for children (see Cohen, 1984).

Sinusitis, Acute

The most common causative organisms in both adults and children are *Streptococcus pneumoniae* (pneumococcus) and *Haemophilus influenzae* (usually nontypeable strains). *Moraxella (Branhamella) catarrhalis* (more common in children), *Streptococcus pyogenes* (group A, beta hemolytic), alpha hemolytic streptococci, and *Staphylococcus aureus* are isolated much less frequently.

Antimicrobial drug therapy (usually oral) in ADULTS AND CHILDREN is usually EMPIRIC and should be effective against the two most likely pathogens, *S. pneumoniae* and *H. influenzae*.

Selected references: Bluestone, 1985; Myer, 1987; Daley and Sande, 1988; Wald, 1988.

EMPIRIC THERAPY

Adults and Children

Streptococcus pneumoniae and *Haemophilus influenzae* (usually nontypeable strains)

PREFERRED THERAPY:
Amoxicillin

ALTERNATIVE THERAPY:
Trimethoprim/Sulfamethoxazole OR **Cefaclor** OR **Erythromycin** ***plus*** **Sulfisoxazole** OR **Amoxicillin/Potassium Clavulanate [Augmentin]** OR **Cefuroxime Axetil** OR **Cefixime**

REMARKS:

(1) Although ampicillin is a cost-effective alternative, amoxicillin usually is preferred because it is better absorbed, requires fewer doses per day, can be taken with meals, and may cause less diarrhea. Other aminopenicillins (eg, bacampicillin) do not appear to offer any important advantages over amoxicillin.

(2) All alternative regimens should be effective for infections caused by amoxicillin-resistant (beta lactamase-producing) strains of *H. influenzae*. Such strains are prevalent (eg, up to 40%) in some geographic areas. The majority of *M. catarrhalis* strains also produce beta-lactamase. In areas where amoxicillin resistance is a problem, an alternative regimen should be elevated to preferred status.

(3) Trimethoprim/sulfamethoxazole is not effective for group A streptococcal infection.

(4) An alternative regimen (except Augmentin) should be used in penicillin-allergic patients. However, cephalosporins should not be used in patients who have had an immediate-type hypersensitivity reaction to penicillin.

(5) Prolonged sinus infection in inadequately treated or untreated patients can lead to chronic sinusitis, which is characterized by irreversible damage to the sinus mucous membrane. Anaerobic bacteria (*Bacteroides*, gram-positive anaerobic cocci, *Fusobacterium*) are the predominant organisms isolated. Patients with chronic sinusitis should be referred to an otorhinolaryngologist. Surgical procedures to facilitate drainage may be necessary. Antimicrobial therapy may be useful for acute exacerbations.

(6) Some cases of sinusitis may be severe and parenteral antimicrobial therapy is required. Nosocomial sinusitis due to nasal intubation is usually caused by gram-negative bacilli and requires treatment with an animoglycoside or third generation cephalosporin.

(7) Natural ostia patency may be re-established by the use of topical and/or systemic decongestants, which promote drainage and aeration of sinuses. These agents should be employed for three to five days only. Topical steroids also are effective for cases that do not respond to initial therapy or are of allergic origin.

Influenza

Influenza is caused by influenza A or B virus. Antibiotics are NOT effective for viral infections. Amantadine, if administered within 48 hours of onset of symptoms, may be useful in ameliorating some of the symptoms of influenza A infection; it also is effective for prophylaxis (see index entry Amantadine).

SKIN AND SOFT-TISSUE INFECTIONS

Acne Vulgaris

Acne vulgaris, a chronic inflammatory disease of the sebaceous glands, is believed to be associated with the bacterium *Propionibacterium (Corynebacterium) acnes*. For treatment guidelines, see index entry Acne Vulgaris.

Bacillary Angiomatosis

Bacillary angiomatosis (BA), also known as epithelioid angiomatosis, was initially described in a patient with acquired immunodeficiency syndrome (AIDS) (Stoler et al, 1983). It has been most common in patients with AIDS but may occur in both immunocompromised and immunocompetent patients. This cutaneous infection is characterized by reddish papules of vascular origin that arise due to proliferation of small blood vessels in the skin and visceral organs (Cockerell and LeBoit, 1990). Lesions may be solitary or multiple dermal or subcutaneous nodules and/or solitary or multiple red-to-purple or skin-colored dome-shaped papules with or without ulceration and crusting. They range from pinpoint size to several centimeters in diameter and may number from one to thousands. Deep soft tissues and mucosa may be involved, and lymph node enlargement and peliosis hepatis have been reported (Cockerell and LeBoit, 1990).

A rickettsia-like, gram-negative bacillus that is very closely related to *Rochalimaea quintana* (formerly *Rickettsia quintana*) (Relman et al, 1990) may be the causative organism. Accurate diagnosis of BA depends on distinguishing it from Kaposi's sarcoma; criteria for differential diagnosis have been outlined (Cockerell and LeBoit, 1990). Clinical diagnosis of BA is confirmed by visualization of the bacillus in tissue samples using the Warthin–Starry staining method. The organism appears as tangled masses, which may be abundant, or as single entities in the interstitium between vessels. Conventional stains (eg, acid–fast, periodic acid–Schiff, the Brown–Brenn modification of the Gram stain) are not adequate for confirmation (Cockerell and LeBoit, 1990).

Therapy for this disease must be started as soon as possible, for visceral and mucosal involvement may be fatal. Because of the difficulty of performing the Warthin–Starry stain, and lack of laboratory experience with this stain, antibiotic therapy of BA will most likely be EMPIRIC.

Selected references: Koehler et al, 1988; Berger et al, 1989.

PREFERRED THERAPY:
Erythromycin (oral)
ALTERNATIVE THERAPY:
Trimethoprim/sulfamethoxazole; Doxycycline; Isoniazid; Rifampin
REMARKS:
(1) Oral erythromycin 250 to 500 mg is given four times daily for two weeks to two months (Cockerell and LeBoit, 1990). Shorter treatment periods may be adequate for immunocompetent patients. In some cases, lesions may recur after therapy is discontinued.
(2) To facilitate further study of this disease, the Centers for Disease Control requests that clinicians report new cases of BA to the CDC at the following address: Division of Bacterial Diseases, Centers for Disease Control, Atlanta, GA 30333. Attn: Robert W. Pinner, M.D.

Bites, Animal (Dog and Cat)

Although many microorganisms have been identified in dog and cat bite wounds, the most frequently isolated pathogens are *Pasteurella multocida* (more common with cat bites), α-hemolytic streptococci, *Staphylococcus aureus* and *S. epidermidis,* and oral anaerobic bacteria (nonfragilis *Bacteroides* sp., *Fusobacterium* sp, gram-positive cocci). Unusual aerobic bacteria such as M-5, EF-4, IIj and species of *Capnocytophaga* (formerly known as DF-2) are often isolated from dog bite wounds. In particular, species of the latter may cause fulminant septicemia in asplenic individuals and in those with alcoholic liver disease (Hicklin et al, 1987).

Adequate cleansing, irrigation, and debridement of animal bite wounds are essential aspects of treatment. Elevation to reduce edema also is necessary. Infected wounds should remain open, but opinions differ on the suturing of early-presenting (less than eight hours), noninfected animal bite wounds. Tetanus and rabies prophylaxis may be required, depending on the patient and animal immunization histories. Antimicrobial drug therapy (usually oral) is necessary for wounds that have an established infection. Initial drug selection is EMPIRIC pending the results of culture and susceptibility tests. The role of antimicrobial drugs in patients who present less than eight hours after injury, ie, before an infection is likely to become established, is controversial. Many experts recommend prophylaxis with antimicrobial drugs (regimens as for established infections) routinely in early-presenting, clinically uninfected cases because all moderate to severe bite wounds are assumed to be contaminated and some will eventually develop frank infections. However, others do not favor antimicrobial prophylaxis.

Selected references: Goldstein, 1986, 1989; Marcy, 1986; Goldstein et al, 1987; Sanford, 1990; *Med Lett Drugs Ther*, 1990; Nelson, 1991.

EMPIRIC THERAPY

Pasteurella multocida; α-hemolytic streptococci; *Staphylococcus aureus;* oral anaerobic bacteria (nonfragilis *Bacteroides* sp, *Fusobacterium* sp, gram-positive cocci)

PREFERRED THERAPY:
Amoxicillin/Potassium clavulanate [Augmentin]
ALTERNATIVE THERAPY:
Penicillin V (or Ampicillin) ***with or without*** **Cloxacillin (or Dicloxacillin)**
OR
Penicillin V (or Ampicillin) ***with or without*** **Cephalexin (or Cephradine or Cefadroxil)**
OR
Tetracycline (or Doxycycline or Minocycline) (see Remarks)
REMARKS:
(1) The combination of amoxicillin with potassium clavulanate, a beta lactamase inhibitor, provides broad spectrum coverage against the common bacteria isolated from dog and cat bite wounds, including activity against beta lactamase-producing strains (eg, most *S. aureus*; most anaerobes).
(2) Penicillin V (or ampicillin) alone is not active against beta lactamase-producing bacteria (eg, *S. aureus*) and penicillinase-resistant penicillins and first generation oral cephalosporins are inadequate for *P. multocida* infections.
(3) Some experts use penicillin V alone when *P. multocida* is very likely (eg, infection within 24 hours after a cat bite, especially if gram-negative bacilli on Gram stain).
(4) Tetracyclines should not be administered to pregnant women or children under 8 years.
(5) Switch to most effective drug regimen after culture and susceptibility test results are available.

Bites, Human

Human bites include occlusional bite wounds and clenched-fist injuries. The latter occur when a person delivers a forceful blow with a clenched fist to another's mouth; they frequently are serious. Wounds from human bites are more prone to infection than animal bites and bites to the hand are particularly prone to complications (eg, osteomyelitis, septic arthritis, tenosynovitis). Common pathogens isolated from human bite wounds are α- and β-hemolytic streptococci, *Staphylococcus aureus* and *S. epidermidis, Eikenella corrodens, Haemophilus* species, and oral anaerobic bacteria (nonfragilis *Bacteroides* sp., *Fusobacterium* sp., gram-positive cocci).

Adequate cleansing, irrigation, and debridement of human bite wounds are essential aspects of treatment. Clenched-fist injuries often require immobilization and elevation. Wounds, except perhaps those to the face, should be left open whether infected or uninfected. Closure by delayed primary or secondary intention is recommended. Tetanus prophylaxis may be required, depending on the patient's immunization history. Antimicrobial drug therapy is indicated for all human bite wounds that break the skin and initially is EMPIRIC, pending the results of culture and susceptibility tests.

Selected references: Goldstein, 1986, 1989; Marcy, 1986; Goldstein et al, 1987; Martin, 1987; Sanford, 1990; Nelson, 1991.

EMPIRIC THERAPY

α- and β-hemolytic streptococci; *Staphylococcus aureus; Eikenella corrodens;* oral anaerobic bacteria (nonfragilis *Bacteroides* sp, *Fusobacterium* sp, gram-positive cocci)

PREFERRED THERAPY:
Amoxicillin/Potassium clavulanate [Augmentin] (oral)
OR
Cefoxitin (intravenous) OR **Ampicillin/Sulbactam [Unasyn] (intravenous) depending on severity**
ALTERNATIVE THERAPY:
Penicillin V (or Ampicillin) *plus* Cloxacillin (or Dicloxacillin) (oral)
OR
Penicillin V (or Ampicillin) *plus* Cephalexin (or Cephradine or Cefadroxil) (oral)
OR
Penicillin G *plus* Nafcillin (or Oxacillin) (intravenous) depending on severity
REMARKS:
(1) Outpatient management with oral antimicrobial drugs is not feasible for most patients with clenched-fist injuries or for patients with osteomyelitis, septic arthritis, advancing cellulitis, or systemic symptoms. Hospitalization and intravenous antimicrobial therapy often are necessary for these patients.
(2) The combination of amoxicillin with clavulanic acid, a beta lactamase inhibitor, or cefoxitin, a beta lactamase-stable cephamycin, alone or the combination of ampicillin with sulbactam, a beta lactamase inhibitor, provides broad spectrum coverage against the common bacteria isolated from human bite wounds, including beta lactamase-producing *S. aureus,* anaerobic bacteria, and *Eikenella corrodens.*
(3) Penicillin G or penicillin V (or ampicillin) alone is not active against beta lactamase-producing bacteria (eg, *S. aureus*) and penicillinase-resistant penicillins and first generation cephalosporins are inadequate for *Eikenella corrodens* infections.
(4) Switch to most effective drug regimens after culture and susceptibility test results are available. Continue broad spectrum, initial empiric therapy if cultures are negative.

Burns

The most common causative organisms are gram-negative bacilli, including *Escherichia coli, Klebsiella, Enterobacter, Proteus, Providencia, Serratia marcescens*, and *Pseudomonas aeruginosa*. Frequently, these are hospital-acquired (nosocomial) pathogens that may be resistant to conventional antibiotics. *Staphylococcus aureus* also is an important cause of infection in burn patients. Methicillin-resistant strains may be prevalent in some hospitals.

Systemic (parenteral) antimicrobial drug therapy is indicated for infected burns and, ultimately, drug selection should be based on culture and susceptibility data. Quantitative bacteriologic analyses of full thickness biopsy specimens are necessary to determine the causative organisms; cultures obtained simply from swabbing the burn wound surface are unreliable. When the causative organism is unknown, EMPIRIC therapy, as outlined below, is indicated initially. Appropriate local (eg, debridement) and supportive (eg, nutritional replenishment) treatment measures also are required. This includes the topical application of antimicrobial agents (silver sulfadiazine, mafenide acetate) to control infection within the essentially avascular burn eschar (see index entry Burns, Treatment). Burns simply colonized with bacteria, ie, when there is no deep tissue invasion, are best treated with topical antimicrobial agents alone, without the addition of parenteral antibiotics, in order to minimize selection of resistant organisms.

Selected references: Demling, 1985; Luterman et al, 1986; Tompkins and Burke, 1986; Conte and Barriere, 1988; Sanford, 1990; Yurt and Shires, 1990.

EMPIRIC THERAPY

Gram-negative bacilli (as listed above)
Staphylococcus aureus

PREFERRED THERAPY (see Remarks):
Nafcillin (or Oxacillin) *plus* Aminoglycoside (gentamicin, tobramycin, amikacin, netilmicin)
OR
Cephalosporin *plus* Aminoglycoside; Vancomycin *plus* Aminoglycoside
OR
Ticarcillin/Potassium Clavulanate [Timentin] *plus* Aminoglycoside
ALTERNATIVE THERAPY:
Antipseudomonal Penicillin (ticarcillin, mezlocillin, piperacillin, azlocillin) *plus* Aminoglycoside
REMARKS:
(1) Definitive guidelines for empiric therapy are not available. Each of the above combination regimens has been suggested by various infectious disease experts. An antistaphylococcal agent (nafcillin or oxacillin; cefazolin, cephalothin, or cephapirin; vancomycin) plus an aminoglycoside provides optimum activity against *S. aureus* and adequate coverage against most gram-negative bacilli. Vancomycin is required for methicillin-resistant *S. aureus* strains. Combining an antipseudomonal penicillin with an aminoglycoside provides optimum activity against *P. aeruginosa* and increased coverage against other gram-negative bacilli but may be inadequate for staphylococcal infections. However, the addition of potassium clavulanate, a beta lactamase inhibitor, to ticarcillin restores antistaphylococcal activity. A second or third generation cephalosporin plus an aminoglycoside also increases coverage against gram-negative bacilli and may be adequate for *S. aureus*. Ceftazidime is the preferred cephalosporin for *P. aeruginosa*. The regimen selected for the individual patient should depend on the particular clinical situation and the likelihood of specific pathogens being involved (eg, organism[s] isolated from recent culture; organism[s] that are currently prevalent in the burn unit). Furthermore, the particular aminoglycoside, cephalosporin, antistaphylococcal agent, and/or antipseudomonal penicillin used for empiric therapy should be selected on the basis of locally generated antibiotic susceptibility profiles.
(2) In treating burn patients with systemic antibiotics, it is important to remember that because many such agents, particularly the aminoglycosides, have a shortened plasma half-life as a result of the patients' increased metabolic rate and fluid losses through wounds, monitoring of antibiotic serum concentrations is necessary.
(3) Switch to most effective drug regimen after culture and susceptibility test results are available.
(4) Superinfection with a resistant bacterial organism or fungi is common and patients should be carefully monitored.

Cellulitis

The vast majority of these infections in noncompromised adults and older children are caused by *Streptococcus pyogenes* (group A, beta hemolytic, gram-positive cocci) and *Staphylococcus aureus*. *Haemophilus influenzae* type b is a common cause of cellulitis in children less than 5 years, but is a rare pathogen in adults. Buccal or facial cellulitis, it most commonly occurs as a unilateral infection of the cheek, may have a blue-red to purple-red color, and often is not associated with a primary portal of entry (eg, cut, laceration, insect bite). Enteric gram-negative bacilli (eg, *Escherichia coli, Klebsiella, Enterobacter*) and anaerobic bacteria (eg, *Bacteroides fragilis, Fusobacterium* species, clostridia) are occasional pathogens, usually in patients with complicating factors (eg, immunosuppression, diabetes mellitus) or in patients with cellulitis involving the lower extremities.

Immediate systemic antimicrobial drug therapy is necessary and usually is EMPIRIC based on the clinical presentation. Oral or parenteral administration may be indicated initially, depending on the severity of the infection. Some experts recommend needle aspiration of the cellulitis to obtain material for Gram stain and culture, but the yield is usually low and the procedure may be painful. Blood cultures may be positive when there is associated bacteremia.

Selected references: Hook et al, 1986; Melish, 1986 B; Yamauchi, 1986; Yoshikawa, 1986; Frenkel and the Multicenter Ceftriaxone Pediatric Study Group, 1988; Odom, 1989; Sanford, 1990; Swartz, 1990; Sachs and Pilgrim, 1990; Nelson, 1991.

EMPIRIC THERAPY

(A) Cellulitis (Majority of Cases)

Streptococcus pyogenes and *Staphylococcus aureus* (penicillinase-producing)

PREFERRED THERAPY:
Cloxacillin (or Dicloxacillin) (oral)
OR
Nafcillin (or Oxacillin) OR Cefonicid (parenteral) OR Ceftriaxone (parenteral) depending on severity
ALTERNATIVE THERAPY:
Ampicillin/sulbactam [Unasyn] (intravenous); Erythromycin (oral); Cephalosporin (oral cephalexin, cephradine, cefadroxil; parenteral cefazolin, cephalothin, cephapirin); Vancomycin (parenteral); Clindamycin (oral or parenteral)
REMARKS:
(1) Cloxacillin and dicloxacillin generally are preferred to oxacillin and nafcillin for oral administration because they are better and more reliably absorbed.
(2) Most experts do not recommend methicillin because of an increased risk of interstitial nephritis.
(3) Penicillin G parenterally or penicillin V potassium orally should be substituted if *Streptococcus pyogenes* is shown to be the causative organism or susceptibility of *S. aureus* strain is proven.
(4) For methicillin-resistant strains of *S. aureus*, intravenous vancomycin is the drug of choice.
(5) The relatively long half-life of cefonicid (4.5 hours) permits once-daily intravenous adminstration on an outpatient basis; efficacy is equal to that of intravenous nafcillin (Daly et al, 1990). However, the in vitro activity of cefonicid is relatively poor, and susceptibility studies are required before it is used. Ceftriaxone also may be effective when administered once daily (Bradsher and Snow, 1984).

(B) Facial Cellulitis in Children Less Than 5 Years

Haemophilus influenzae type b, *Staphylococcus aureus, Streptococcus pyogenes,* and *Streptococcus pneumoniae*

PREFERRED THERAPY:
Cefotaxime or Ceftriaxone or Ceftizoxime
OR
Cefuroxime
ALTERNATIVE THERAPY:
Amoxicillin/Potassium Clavulanate
OR
Nafcillin (or Oxacillin) *plus* Chloramphenicol
REMARKS:
(1) Switch to most effective drug regimen after culture and susceptibility test results are available.
(2) Cefuroxime, a second generation cephalosporin, has been widely used for *H. influenzae* type b infections in children. However, on a weight basis, this drug is less active against this organism than the third generation cephalosporins (eg, cefotaxime, ceftriaxone). More important, cefuroxime occasionally has been associated with delayed sterilization of cerebrospinal fluid and even overt therapeutic failures in patients infected with *H. influenzae* type b. Thus, many pediatric infectious disease experts prefer a third generation cephalosporin (eg, cefotaxime, ceftriaxone) to cefuroxime for severe *H. influenzae* type b infections in which central nervous system involvement may be a possibility. Cefuroxime may be used for infections that do not pose the risk of extension to the central nervous system.
(3) Cefamandole is NOT recommended as an initial therapy for children less than 5 years because of its poor penetration into the cerebrospinal fluid.
(4) The above regimens also are recommended empirically in children less than 5 years with preseptal cellulitis or with cellulitis in other sites when accompanied by high fever or significant toxicity, evidence of infection elsewhere (eg, meningitis), or if the lesion has a blue-red to purple-red discoloration.

Cutaneous Abscesses: Carbuncles, Folliculitis, and Furunculosis

The vast majority of these infections are caused by *Staphylococcus aureus* (gram-positive cocci).

Most cases of folliculitis and mild furunculosis can be controlled by local measures (eg, warm soaks to encourage spontaneous drainage). Carbuncles and furuncles with surrounding cellulitis and/or fever or those located in the midfacial area require systemic (usually oral) antibiotic therapy. Drug selection is usually EMPIRIC (based on the clinical presentation) or based on Gram stain. Drainage of these large, fluctuant cutaneous abscesses (except possibly on lips and nose) also is indicated.

A folliculitis caused by *Pseudomonas aeruginosa* is associated with improperly maintained whirlpools, hot tubs, and swimming pools. The disease is usually self-limited (Jacobson, 1985; see also index entry Antibiotics, Uses, Pyodermas).

Selected references: Maibach et al, 1985; Melish, 1986 B; Yoshikawa, 1986; Conte and Barriere, 1988; Sanford, 1990; Swartz, 1990. See also index entry Antibiotics, Uses, Pyodermas.

EMPIRIC THERAPY

Staphylococcus aureus (penicillinase-producing)

PREFERRED THERAPY:
Cloxacillin OR **Dicloxacillin**

ALTERNATIVE THERAPY:
Erythromycin; Oral cephalosporin (cephalexin; cephradine; cefadroxil); Clindamycin; Amoxicillin/Potassium clavulanate [Augmentin]
REMARKS:
(1) Cloxacillin and dicloxacillin generally are preferred to oxacillin and nafcillin for oral administration because they are better and more reliably absorbed.
(2) Recurrent furunculosis is a problem in certain patients and is associated with persistent colonization of the anterior nares by coagulase-positive *S. aureus*. In addition to careful skin cleansing with antistaphylococcal detergents, care of clothing and dressings and application of topical antibiotics (eg, neomycin, bacitracin) to nasal vestibules may prevent recurrences. Recent studies suggest that topical application of 2% mupirocin to anterior nares is very effective in eliminating nasal carriage of *S. aureus* (Casewell and Hill, 1986; Hill et al, 1988). Rifampin (adults, orally 600 mg daily for 10 days) has eradicated these organisms from most nasal carriers for up to 12 weeks (Wheat et al, 1983). This agent, given with another antistaphylococcal agent to prevent the emergence of rifampin-resistant *S. aureus*, may be useful in managing recurrent furunculosis in those patients in whom other measures have failed. Oral therapy with novobiocin (500 mg twice daily) plus rifampin (300 mg twice daily) for five days also has been efficacious in eradicating the carrier state of methicillin-resistant *S. aureus* (MRSA), an important nosocomial infective organism (Arathoon et al, 1990). Low-dose (150 mg/day) oral clindamycin for three months (Klempner and Styrt, 1988) also may be used to manage recurrent furunculosis.
(3) Quinolones such as ciprofloxacin, norfloxacin, and ofloxacin are active against MRSA; however, these agents should be used cautiously because resistance has rapidly increased to levels >50% in some centers following their clinical introduction (Hooper and Wolfson, 1991; Trucksis et al, 1991).

Decubitus Ulcers (With Sepsis)

Causative organisms include *Staphylococcus aureus* (gram-positive cocci); streptococci (gram-positive cocci), including *S. pyogenes* and enterococci; aerobic gram-negative bacilli, including Enterobacteriaceae and *Pseudomonas aeruginosa*; and anaerobic bacteria, including *Bacteroides fragilis* (gram-negative bacilli), gram-positive cocci, and clostridia (gram-positive bacilli).

Antimicrobial drug therapy (parenteral) initially is EMPIRIC pending results of blood cultures. Broad spectrum antibacterial coverage against both aerobic bacteria (enteric gram-negative bacilli, *S. aureus*, non-group D streptococci) and anaerobic bacteria, especially *B. fragilis*, is necessary. Some experts also recommend coverage against enterococci (*E. faecalis*). Local (eg, pressure relief, debridement of necrotic tissue) and supportive (eg, nutritional replenishment) therapy also are indicated.

Selected references: Conte and Barriere, 1988; Allman, 1989; Sanford, 1990. See also index entry Antibiotics, Uses, Pyodermas.

EMPIRIC THERAPY
Gram-negative enteric bacilli (Enterobacteriaceae); *Pseudo monas aeruginosa*; *Bacteroides fragilis* and other anaerobic bacteria (eg, *Peptococcus, Peptostreptococcus*, clostridia); *Staphylococcus aureus*; non-group D streptococci (eg, *S. pyogenes*); *Enterococcus faecalis* and other group D enterococci

PREFERRED THERAPY:
Clindamycin *plus* Aminoglycoside (gentamicin, tobramycin, amikacin, netilmicin) *with or without* Penicillin G (or Ampicillin)
ALTERNATIVE THERAPY:
See Remarks
REMARKS:
(1) The above regimen was obtained from literature sources. However, many additional regimens were considered reasonable alternatives by our consultants, and a number of these experts preferred regimens that, when possible, avoided an aminoglycoside and its associated ototoxicity and nephrotoxicity. Regimens suggested by consultants include: metronidazole *plus* aminoglycoside *with or without* penicillin G (or ampicillin); cefoxitin (or cefotetan) *with or without* aminoglycoside; mezlocillin (or piperacillin) *plus* aminoglycoside; cefazolin *plus* mezlocillin (or piperacillin); nafcillin (or oxacillin) *plus* mezlocillin (or piperacillin); imipenem/cilastatin alone; ticarcillin/potassium clavulanate [Timentin] alone; ampicillin/sulbactam [Unasyn] *with or without* aminoglycoside; clindamycin *plus* aztreonam; ciprofloxacin (oral) *plus* metronidazole.
(2) Switch to most effective drug regimen after culture and susceptibility test results are available.

Ecthyma

The primary causative organism is *Streptococcus pyogenes* (group A, beta hemolytic, gram-positive cocci), which produce the lesions *de novo* or secondarily infect superficial skin lesions (insect bites, excoriations). (It should be noted that lesions mimicking those caused by streptococci may develop during the course of *Pseudomonas* bacteremia [Swartz, 1990].)

Systemic (usually oral) antimicrobial drug therapy is indicated and usually is EMPIRIC based on the clinical presentation. Debridement and cleansing of lesions also are indicated.

Selected references: Odom, 1989; Swartz, 1990. See also index entry Antibiotics, Uses, Pyodermas.

EMPIRIC THERAPY
Streptococcus pyogenes

PREFERRED THERAPY:
Penicillin V potassium
ALTERNATIVE THERAPY:
Erythromycin
REMARK:
(1) Penicillin V potassium usually is preferred to penicillin G (oral) because it is more acid-stable, provides greater and more reliable bioavailability, and can be taken with meals.

Erysipelas

The primary causative organism is *Streptococcus pyogenes* (group A, beta hemolytic, gram-positive cocci).

Systemic antimicrobial drug therapy is necessary and usually is EMPIRIC based on the clinical presentation. Oral or parenteral administration may be indicated initially, depending on the severity of the infection.

Selected references: Melish, 1986 B; Conte and Barriere, 1988; Odom, 1989; Swartz, 1990; Nelson, 1991.

EMPIRIC THERAPY
Streptococcus pyogenes

PREFERRED THERAPY:
Penicillin V potassium (oral) OR **Penicillin G procaine (IM)** OR **Penicillin G (IV) depending on severity**
ALTERNATIVE THERAPY:
Erythromycin (oral); Cephalosporin (oral cephalexin, cephradine, cefadroxil; parenteral cefazolin, cephalothin, cephapirin)
REMARK:
(1) Penicillin V potassium usually is preferred to penicillin G (oral) because it is more acid-stable, provides greater and more reliable bioavailability, and can be taken with meals.

Erythrasma

The causative organism is *Corynebacterium minutissimum*.

Local treatment may be sufficient for mild cases. Systemic (usually oral) antimicrobial drug therapy is indicated for persistent and/or widespread disease.

Selected references: Duncan, 1983; Swartz, 1990. See also index entry Antibiotics, Uses, Pyodermas.

SPECIFIC THERAPY
Corynebacterium minutissimum
(gram-positive bacilli)

PREFERRED THERAPY:
Erythromycin

Fungal Infections (Superficial)

Dermatophytic infections (tinea capitis, tinea corporis, tinea cruris, tinea pedis, and tinea unguium) are caused by species of *Trichophyton, Epidermophyton*, and *Microsporum*. Mucocutaneous mycotic infections include only candidiasis, which is caused most often by *Candida albicans*. For treatment guidelines, see index entry Dermatophytoses.

Impetigo, Bullous

The causative organism is *Staphylococcus aureus* (usually group II, phage type 71). Bullae represent an exfoliative reaction of the epidermis to an exotoxin (exfoliatin) elaborated by this strain of *S. aureus*.

Systemic (usually oral) antimicrobial drug therapy is indicated and usually is EMPIRIC based on the clinical presentation. Debridement and cleansing of lesions also are indicated.

Selected references: Yoshikawa, 1986; Sanford, 1990; Swartz, 1990; Nelson, 1991. See also index entry Antibiotics, Uses, Pyodermas.

EMPIRIC THERAPY
Staphylococcus aureus (penicillinase-producing)

PREFERRED THERAPY:
Cloxacillin (or Dicloxacillin)
ALTERNATIVE THERAPY:
Erythromycin; Oral cephalosporin (cephalexin, cephradine, cefadroxil); Clindamycin; Amoxicillin/Potassium clavulanate [Augmentin]
REMARKS:
(1) Cloxacillin and dicloxacillin generally are preferred to oxacillin and nafcillin for oral administration because they are better and more reliably absorbed. However, the oral suspensions of cloxacillin and dicloxacillin have a bitter taste and may not be accepted by young children.
(2) Oral cephalosporins are more expensive than oral penicillins and erythromycin. However, they may be better tolerated by some patients and should be considered when intolerance to less expensive drugs causes a lack of compliance.

Impetigo, Nonbullous

The primary causative organisms are *Staphylococcus aureus* (gram-positive cocci) and *Streptococcus pyogenes* (group A, beta hemolytic, gram-positive cocci). Frequently, mixtures of *S. pyogenes* and *S. aureus* are isolated from lesions.

Systemic (usually oral) antimicrobial drug therapy generally is indicated and usually is EMPIRIC based on the clinical presentation. Most experts now recommend antimicrobial drugs that are active against both *S. pyogenes* and penicillinase-producing *S. aureus*. Debridement and cleansing of lesions also are indicated.

Selected references: Yoshikawa, 1986; Odom, 1989; Sanford, 1990; Swartz, 1990; Nelson, 1991. See also index entry Antibiotics, Uses, Pyodermas.

EMPIRIC THERAPY

(A) *Streptococcus pyogenes* only

PREFERRED THERAPY:
Penicillin V potassium
ALTERNATIVE THERAPY:
Erythromycin; Penicillin G benzathine (IM); Mupirocin (topical) (see Remarks)
REMARKS:
(1) Duration of therapy with oral antibiotics is 10 days. A single intramuscular injection of penicillin G benzathine is equally effective and is preferred when patient compliance is a likely problem.
(2) Penicillin V potassium usually is preferred to penicillin G (orally, for 10 days) because it is more acid-stable, provides greater and more reliable bioavailability, and can be taken with meals.
(3) Of the oral and parenteral agents listed, only erythromycin is active against penicillinase-producing strains of *S. aureus*. However, in recent experience, between 5% and 25% of these strains derived from skin infections have been erythromycin-resistant, based on results of in vitro susceptibility tests (Coskey and Coskey, 1987).
(4) Mupirocin [Bactroban] is a topical antibiotic that is active against group A streptococci and *Staphylococcus aureus*. A 2%

ointment has been approved for the treatment of impetigo. Results of three randomized, controlled clinical trials showed topical mupirocin to be comparable in efficacy and safety to orally administered erythromycin for the treatment of impetigo (Goldfarb et al, 1988; McLinn, 1988; Mertz et al, 1989). Thus, this topical agent appears to be an effective alternative to systemic therapy for mild to moderate cases of impetigo. Emergence of resistant staphylococci has been reported with long-term topical therapy (*Med Lett Drugs Ther,* 1988). See also index entry Mupirocin.

(B) ***Streptococcus pyogenes*** **and** ***Staphylococcus aureus*** (penicillinase-producing)

PREFERRED THERAPY:
Cloxacillin (or Dicloxacillin)
ALTERNATIVE THERAPY:
Erythromycin; Oral cephalosporin (cephalexin, cephradine, cefadroxil); Clindamycin; Amoxicillin/Potassium clavulanate [Augmentin]; Mupirocin (topical) (see Remarks above)
REMARKS:
(1) Cloxacillin and dicloxacillin generally are preferred to oxacillin and nafcillin for oral administration because they are better and more reliably absorbed. However, the oral suspensions of cloxacillin and dicloxacillin have a bitter taste and may not be accepted by young children.
(2) Oral cephalosporins are more expensive than oral penicillins and erythromycin. However, they may be better tolerated by some patients and should be considered when intolerance to less expensive drugs causes a lack of patient compliance.

Parasitic Infections: Pediculosis

Pediculosis in man is caused by three types of lice: *Phthirus pubis* (crab louse), *Pediculus humanus* (body louse), and *Pediculus capitis* (head louse). For treatment guidelines, see index entry Pediculosis.

Parasitic Infections: Scabies

The causative organism is the itch mite, *Sarcoptes scabiei*. For treatment guidelines, see index entry Scabies.

Scalded Skin Syndrome (Staphylococcal)

The staphylococcal scalded skin syndrome most commonly occurs in neonates and young children and is a potentially severe disease caused by the exfoliative toxin of *Staphylococcus aureus* (usually phage group II).

Parenteral antimicrobial drug therapy is indicated initially and usually is EMPIRIC based on the clinical presentation and skin biopsy. Supportive therapy (eg, fluid and electrolyte replacement) also is indicated.

Selected references: Melish, 1986 A; Swartz, 1990; Nelson, 1991.

EMPIRIC THERAPY
Staphylococcus aureus (penicillinase-producing)

PREFERRED THERAPY:
Nafcillin (parenteral) OR **Oxacillin (parenteral)**
ALTERNATIVE THERAPY:
Cefazolin, Cephalothin, or Cephapirin; Vancomycin (intravenous); Clindamycin
REMARKS:
(1) Methicillin is not recommended (except in newborns) because it is associated with a higher incidence of interstitial nephritis.
(2) If methicillin-resistant strains of *S. aureus* are suspected, substitute intravenous vancomycin for the antistaphylococcal penicillin.

Viral Infections: Cold Sores (Herpes Simplex)

The causative organism is herpes simplex virus. Topical or systemic antiviral therapy in the nonimmunocompromised host generally has been unsuccessful in reducing the severity of herpes simplex labialis. In one study, prophylactic use of oral acyclovir in skiers at high risk for sun-induced herpes labialis resulted in a decrease in the number of persons who developed lesions when compared with placebo controls (Spruance et al, 1988). However, this currently is investigational and specific recommendations are NOT available. For additional discussion, see index entry, Antiviral Agents.

Viral Infections: Shingles (Varicella-Zoster)

The causative organism is varicella-zoster virus. Recent studies in the nonimmunocompromised host suggest that high-dose oral acyclovir (800 mg five times daily for 7 to 10 days) diminishes the severity and shortens the course of herpes zoster infection (Huff et al, 1988; Wood et al, 1988). However, this currently is investigational and specific recommendations are NOT available. For additional discussion, see index entry, Antiviral Agents.

URINARY TRACT INFECTIONS

Pyelonephritis, Acute

Acute pyelonephritis is a common infection in young children, women of childbearing age, and the elderly. It is characterized by fever, chills, flank pain, and costovertebral angle tenderness with associated dysuria and urinary urgency and frequency. Confirmation of acute pyelonephritis is typically based on the observation of pyuria and the presence of uropathogenic bacteria in the normally sterile urine. In 80% of cases, urine will contain $\geq 10^5$ colony-forming units/ml, but 20% of patients have lower colony counts.

Escherichia coli is responsible for approximately 90% of initial infections that are community acquired. *Proteus mirabilis, Klebsiella pneumoniae, Enterobacter* species, *Staphylococcus saprophyticus,* and enterococci (eg, *Enterococcus faecalis)* are occasional causative organisms. These latter pathogens and other gram-negative bacilli, including indole-positive *Proteus* (*Morganella morganii, Providencia rettgeri, Proteus vulgaris*), *Serratia marcescens*, and *Pseudomonas aeruginosa* are more frequently encountered in patients who have had repeated courses of antimicrobial therapy for recurrent infections, those who have undergone frequent instrumentation because of structural abnormalities of the urinary tract, and individuals with hospital-acquired (nosocomial) infections.

Although ultimate antimicrobial drug selection for acute pyelonephritis should be SPECIFIC and based on urine culture and susceptibility data, EMPIRIC therapy, frequently based on a Gram stain of urine, is indicated initially. Patients with acute symptomatic infection frequently require hospitalization and parenteral antimicrobial drug therapy. This group includes bacteremic patients, patients with symptoms of bacterial toxicity, older patients, and patients with other underlying disease. Those experiencing initial attacks who are mildly ill and nonseptic may be treated with orally administered antimicrobial drugs and do not need hospitalization if adequate follow-up care is available.

Selected references: Sabbaj et al, 1985; Gleckman, 1987 A; Stamm et al, 1987, 1989; Lebel and McCracken, 1988; Madrigal et al, 1988; Safrin et al, 1988; Lipsky, 1989; Angel et al, 1990; Jones, 1990; Sandberg et al, 1990; Sobel and Kaye, 1990.

EMPIRIC THERAPY

If possible, a Gram stain of urine should be obtained to aid in appropriate antimicrobial drug selection.

Inpatient Therapy

Escherichia coli most likely in initial, community-acquired infection; other gram-negative bacilli; *Enterococcus faecalis* and other group D enterococci

PREFERRED THERAPY:
Aminoglycoside (gentamicin, tobramycin, amikacin, netilmicin) *plus* Ampicillin (parenteral)

ALTERNATIVE THERAPY:
Trimethoprim/Sulfamethoxazole (parenteral); Third Generation Cephalosporin (cefotaxime, ceftizoxime, ceftriaxone, ceftazidime, cefoperazone); Aztreonam; Ampicillin/Sulbactam [Unasyn]; Ticarcillin/Potassium Clavulanate [Timentin]; Ciprofloxacin, Norfloxacin, Ofloxacin.

REMARKS:

(1) Parenteral ampicillin should no longer be used alone, even for community-acquired infections in patients without previous episodes, due to organism resistance in 20% to 30% of cases.

(2) If Gram stain of urine shows gram-positive cocci in chains, suggesting enterococci, ampicillin should be used.

(3) Some consultants prefer one of the listed alternative therapies to an aminoglycoside because they are less toxic.

(4) Third generation cephalosporins may be preferred in patients with renal impairment, especially when multiply resistant gram-negative bacilli are possible causative organisms (eg, hospital-acquired infection). However, none of these agents is active against enterococci. Only ceftazidime and cefoperazone have activity against *Pseudomonas aeruginosa*.

(5) Aztreonam, a monobactam, is active against the Enterobacteriaceae and *P. aeruginosa*. It may be useful in patients at increased risk for aminoglycoside toxicity and/or those who are allergic to penicillins and cephalosporins. Caution must be exercised, however, in those with severe reactions to penicillins.

(6) Switch to most effective, least toxic, and least expensive drug regimen after susceptibility test results are available.

(7) Most patients with acute pyelonephritis become afebrile by 48 to 72 hours after initiating therapy with appropriate antimicrobial agents. Continuing fever beyond 48 to 72 hours requires further investigation (eg, for urinary obstruction or intrarenal or perinephric abscess).

(8) Parenteral therapy is usually given for at least 24 to 48 hours after the patient becomes afebrile. Oral therapy is then begun. Oral therapy with ciprofloxacin has been successful in moderately severe cases. Current clinical trial data do not support the routine use of less than 14 days of therapy for patients with acute pyelonephritis. If relapse occurs, therapy for up to six weeks is indicated; evaluation for underlying urinary tract abnormalities also is recommended.

(9) In males with acute pyelonephritis, at least one-half of whom have concurrent prostate infection, antimicrobial therapy for a minimum of six weeks is recommended to prevent recurrences, which are frequent in patients given shorter courses of therapy. Follow-up urine cultures are essential to monitor therapeutic results in these patients.

(10) In infants and children, follow-up urine cultures are particularly important after an episode of acute pyelonephritis to document that urine sterility was achieved. These individuals are potentially at risk of renal scars or failure of normal growth of the infected kidney. All children should have radiologic evaluation of the urinary tract following their first infection to exclude a correctable anatomic abnormality.

(11) Fluoroquinolones (ciprofloxacin, norfloxacin, or ofloxacin) are contraindicated in prepubertal children or pregnant women.

Outpatient Therapy

Escherichia coli most likely in initial, community-acquired infection; other gram-negative bacilli; *Enterococcus faecalis* and other enterococci

PREFERRED THERAPY:
Trimethoprim/Sulfamethoxazole (oral)

ALTERNATIVE THERAPY:
Ciprofloxacin, Norfloxacin, or Ofloxacin; Amoxicillin/Potassium clavulanate [Augmentin]; Cephalosporin (oral)

REMARKS:

(1) If Gram stain of urine shows gram-positive cocci in chains, suggesting enterococci, ampicillin should be used.

(2) In some communities, organism resistance to the oral first generation cephalosporins (eg, cephalexin) has increased. Cefuroxime axetil or cefixime, oral second and third generation cephalosporins, respectively, may be preferred in these communities.

(3) Switch to most effective, least toxic, and least expensive drug regimen after susceptibility test results are available.

(4) Duration of therapy is usually 14 days. If relapse occurs, therapy for up to six weeks is indicated; evaluation for underlying urinary tract abnormalities also is recommended.

(5) Fluoroquinolones (ciprofloxacin, norfloxacin, or ofloxacin) should not be used in pregnant women or prepubertal children. Trimethoprim should not be used in pregnant women.

Cystitis, Acute

Acute cystitis, a lower urinary tract infection, is common in women of childbearing or middle age. Dysuria, urinary frequency and urgency, and suprapubic pain accompanied by pyuria and $>10^5$ bacteria/ml of urine are traditional criteria used to define this superficial bladder infection. However, two important points regarding diagnosis of acute cystitis require emphasis. First, it is now apparent that a significant proportion

(≥30%) of women with symptoms restricted to the lower urinary tract have silent renal infection (subclinical pyelonephritis). Second, a large percentage of women with clinical symptoms of cystitis (eg, dysuria, frequency, urgency accompanied by pyuria) also have "negative" or "low-count" bacteriuria (≤10^5 bacteria/ml). Traditionally, these women have been said to suffer from the "acute urethral syndrome," meaning infection localized to the urethra. However, it now is clear that many of these women have infection of both the urethra and bladder (Johnson and Stamm, 1989). These data suggest that the standard criteria for significant bacteriuria (≥10^5 bacteria/ml) should be lower (ie, ≥10^2 bacteria/ml) in a symptomatic woman. Antimicrobial drug therapy of these patients is considered in the section on the Acute Urethral Syndrome below.

In women with uncomplicated acute cystitis, most community-acquired infections are caused by *Escherichia coli* (80%), *Staphylococcus saprophyticus* (11%), and *Enterococcus faecalis*. In patients with complicated cystitis (ie, those with underlying urinary tract abnormalities, catheters, immunosuppression, diabetes mellitus, a history of childhood urinary tract infections, documented relapse of prior urinary tract infection; the elderly; pregnant women), causative organisms also include species of *Enterobacter, Klebsiella, Proteus,* and *Pseudomonas.*

Antimicrobial drug therapy for community-acquired acute cystitis is initially EMPIRIC. For women with uncomplicated infections whose symptoms are recent (less than seven days) and who are available for follow-up, single-dose oral therapy with an appropriate antimicrobial agent has been advocated. However, an analysis of data from 28 clinical trials showed that single-dose antimicrobial therapy (regardless of the drug) is less effective than treatment for ≥3 days (Norrby, 1990). Furthermore, the optimal duration of therapy is determined by the class of agent, and considerable differences exist among the various drugs presumably due to differences in serum half-lives. Thus, cephalosporins and penicillins had unacceptably low cure rates when used as single-dose therapy; a distinct difference was observed between 1, 3, and ≥5 days of treatment, with the latter of greatest efficacy. In contrast, the duration of treatment for trimethoprim/sulfonamide combinations should not exceed three days, since the risk of adverse reactions to the drugs increases with time. Similarly, although the efficacy of beta lactams is greater when the duration of treatment exceeds five days, adverse effects also become more likely; however, the reactions usually are not severe and do not outweigh the risks of disease recurrence and progression that may follow short-term therapy. Thus, the decision to treat acute lower urinary tract infections with short-course antimicrobial therapy must be based on the presence or absence of complicating factors, the pharmacokinetics of the available drugs for this indication, the possible adverse reactions to each drug regimen, the likelihood of full patient compliance and follow-up, and the cost of the various therapies. Many experts now favor three-day regimens of trimethoprim-sulfamethoxazole or trimethoprim for empiric short-course therapy rather than single-dose therapy.

Conventional, multiple-dose antimicrobial therapy for 7 to 14 days is recommended for all other patients, including women with possible upper urinary tract infection (subclinical pyelonephritis), pregnant women, males, and children. Cystitis in men who have not been catheterized or who have not undergone instrumental examination of the urinary tract frequently is prostatic in origin. In such patients, extended therapy (eg, six weeks with proven prostatitis) is recommended. Urologic evaluation is recommended for men and children because of the increased probability of underlying urinary tract abnormalities in these patients.

Selected references: Carlson and Mulley, 1985; Gleckman, 1987 A, 1987 B; Fihn et al, 1988; Corragio et al, 1989; Sobel and Kaye, 1990.

EMPIRIC THERAPY

Short-course therapy (1 to 3 days)
Recommended only for women who are not pregnant, have no apparent renal parenchymal involvement, have no evidence of subclinical pyelonephritis, have recent symptoms (<7 days), and are available for follow-up. *Escherichia coli* is most likely causative organism; *Staphylococcus saprophyticus*; other gram-negative bacilli

PREFERRED THERAPY:
Trimethoprim/Sulfamethoxazole (320 mg/1600 mg [two "double-strength" tablets]) daily for 3 days
ALTERNATIVE SHORT-COURSE 3-DAY THERAPY:
Trimethoprim (200 mg twice daily); Sulfisoxazole (500 mg four times daily); Nitrofurantoin (100 mg four times daily)
ALTERNATIVE SINGLE-DOSE THERAPY:
Sulfisoxazole (2 g); Trimethoprim (400 mg); Tetracycline (2.5 g); Amoxicillin (3 g); Nitrofurantoin (200 mg)
REMARKS:
(1) Advantages of single-dose therapy are increased compliance, decreased risk of adverse drug reactions, lower cost, and decreased likelihood of emergence of resistant bacterial strains. Three-day therapy may provide a higher cure rate than the single-dose regimen and preserve the reduced rate of side effects compared with seven-day therapy.
(2) Most experts do not obtain a urine culture at the initial visit; urinalysis is sufficient. Traditionally, it has been recommended that a urine culture be obtained one week after single-dose therapy as evidence of cure or to identify relapse, but some experts believe test-of-cure cultures for acute uncomplicated cystitis are unnecessary if symptoms are completely resolved (see Komaroff, 1986; Johnson and Stamm, 1987). Patients who fail to respond to single-dose therapy or who relapse (usually within 36 to 96 hours) are considered to have silent renal infection, although rapid reinfection from the perineum also may occur. (Note: Many experts consider response to single-dose therapy as a localization test to distinguish upper from lower urinary tract infection.) For these patients, the urine is cultured and conventional multiple-dose antimicrobial drug therapy is prescribed for 10 to 14 days (see below). Follow-up is essential. Early relapse requires a more prolonged course of therapy (six weeks); evaluation for underlying urinary tract abnormalities also is recommended.
(3) Amoxicillin or sulfonamides alone should not be used empirically unless resistance to these drugs is known to be low (eg, less than 10%) within a given community.
(4) Parenteral aminoglycosides (eg, kanamycin, 500 mg IM) also have been effective as single-dose therapy. Results with oral cephalosporins have been equivocal.

Conventional (multiple-dose) therapy (7 to 14 days)
Recommended for all patients except women who qualify for single-dose therapy (see above). *Escherichia coli* is most likely causative organism; other gram-negative bacilli; *Staphylococcus saprophyticus; Enterococcus faecalis* and other enterococci.

PREFERRED THERAPY:
Sulfisoxazole (or Sulfamethoxazole) OR **Ampicillin (or Amoxicillin)** OR **Trimethoprim/Sulfamethoxazole** OR **Nitrofurantoin**

ALTERNATIVE THERAPY:
Trimethoprim; Tetracycline; Oral Cephalosporin (cephalexin, cephradine, cefadroxil); Ciprofloxacin, Norfloxacin or Ofloxacin; Amoxicillin/Potassium clavulanate [Augmentin]

REMARKS:

(1) Sulfisoxazole (or sulfamethoxazole) is preferred by many experts because it is the least expensive regimen. However, sulfonamide resistance is prevalent in many communities. Some consultants do not recommend its use empirically unless resistance is known to be low (eg, less than 10% of isolates). Sulfonamides should not be used in pregnant women near term or in newborns.

(2) Because resistance to ampicillin and amoxicillin is prevalent in many communities, some consultants do not recommend their use empirically unless resistance is known to be low (eg, less than 10% of isolates).

(3) Expensive alternatives such as cephalosporins, fluoroquinolones (ciprofloxacin, norfloxacin, or ofloxacin), and amoxicillin/potassium clavulanate [Augmentin] should be used only when conventional antimicrobials are contraindicated because of antibiotic-resistant organisms or medication side effects.

(4) Tetracyclines should not be used in pregnant women or children under 8 years. Trimethoprim should not be used in pregnant women. Fluoroquinolones (ciprofloxacin, norfloxacin) should not be used in pregnant women or prepubertal children. Nitrofurantoin should not be used in pregnant women near term or in newborns.

(5) The urinary tract analgesic, phenazopyridine, may provide symptomatic relief of dysuria and urethral irritation during the initial 24 to 48 hours. It should be discontinued after 48 hours.

(6) If relapse occurs, suggesting silent renal infection, a more prolonged course of therapy for six weeks is indicated; evaluation for underlying urinary tract abnormalities also is recommended.

Asymptomatic Bacteriuria

Patients with asymptomatic bacteriuria have significant bacteriuria (ie, $>10^5$ bacteria/ml of urine on more than one consecutive culture) but do not have clinical symptoms of urinary tract infection. Antimicrobial drug therapy is recommended for pregnant women (40% of whom develop pyelonephritis), diabetic patients, other immunocompromised patients, and children. Because asymptomatic bacteriuria of childhood can be a manifestation of underlying structural abnormality, it is recommended that children receive a urological evaluation. Choice of drugs for asymptomatic bacteriuria is dependent on results of culture and susceptibility tests (see Cystitis, Acute above for specific antimicrobial regimens). Tetracyclines, trimethoprim, fluoroquinolones, sulfonamides (near term only), and nitrofurantoin (near term only) should not be administered to pregnant women. Tetracyclines are contraindicated in children under 8 years; fluoroquinolones should not be used in prepubertal children.

At the present time, it is unclear whether it is beneficial to treat asymptomatic bacteriuria in nonpregnant, otherwise healthy, ambulatory adults. Asymptomatic bacteriuria is particularly common in the elderly, and the current consensus is not to treat these individuals.

Selected references: Boscia and Kaye, 1987; Boscia et al, 1987; Patterson and Andriole, 1987; Pedler and Bint, 1987; Sobel and Kaye, 1990.

Acute Urethral Syndrome

Women with the acute urethral syndrome have symptoms of acute cystitis (ie, dysuria, frequency, urgency), but do not have significant bacteriuria as defined by traditional criteria (ie, $>10^5$ bacteria/ml). Patients with pyuria (≥ 8 leukocytes/mm^3 of unspun urine) and between 10^2 and 10^5 bacteria (primarily *Escherichia coli*; also, *Staphylococcus saprophyticus*) per ml of urine essentially are considered to have acute bacterial urethrocystitis, ie, bacterial infection of both the urethra and bladder. Those with pyuria and sterile urine cultures usually are infected with *Chlamydia trachomatis* and have a sexually transmitted disease. (Note: *Neisseria gonorrhoeae* and Herpes simplex virus also may cause the acute urethral syndrome.) Patients with no pyuria and a sterile urine culture have no demonstrable infection. (Note: Vaginitis must always be considered in the differential diagnosis.)

Antimicrobial drug therapy (oral) is indicated for women with symptoms of dysuria, frequency, or urgency who also have pyuria (ie, patients who have the "dysuria-pyuria" syndrome), but not for women who lack pyuria and bacteria in their urine. Two approaches to treatment currently are recommended. EMPIRIC antimicrobial therapy to cover all potential pathogens (ie, *Escherichia coli, Staphylococcus saprophyticus, Chlamydia trachomatis*, *Neisseria gonorrhoeae*) is recommended by some experts. The other, usually preferred, approach is first to differentiate probable coliform (or staphylococcal) infection from chlamydial (or gonococcal) infection using clinical, epidemiologic, and (rapidly available) laboratory data and then treat the patient with a more SPECIFIC, albeit still EMPIRIC, antimicrobial drug regimen. Criteria that suggest coliform (or staphylococcal) infection include abrupt onset of symptoms (<4 days), hematuria, suprapubic pain, previous urinary tract infection, and no recent change in sexual partner. Criteria that suggest chlamydial (or gonococcal) infection include gradual onset of symptoms, >7-day history of symptoms, no hematuria, no suprapubic pain, and recent change in sexual partners. Cervical Gram stain and culture for *N. gonorrhoeae* and rapid immunologic diagnostic testing for *C. trachomatis* may allow for SPECIFIC therapy directed against either of these sexually transmitted pathogens. Treatment guidelines for gonococcal and chlamydial infections and for the acute urethral syndrome caused by these sexually transmitted pathogens can be found in Chapter 3 in this Section, Treatment of Sexually Transmitted Diseases.

Selected references: Komaroff, 1986; *MMWR*, 1989; Sobel and Kaye, 1990.

EMPIRIC THERAPY

(A) Usually effective against all potential pathogens, including *Escherichia coli, Staphylococcus saprophyticus, Chlamydia trachomatis, Neisseria gonorrhoeae*

PREFERRED THERAPY:
Doxycycline
REMARKS:
(1) Tetracycline may be less expensive than doxycycline and should be an effective alternative.
(2) In vitro, resistance to tetracyclines is not uncommon among *E. coli* (up to 30%) and is increasing among gonococci.
(3) Tetracyclines should not be administered to pregnant women or children under 8 years.

(B) Presumed bacterial infection of bladder/urethra; therapy directed against *Escherichia coli, Staphylococcus saprophyticus*
REMARK:
(1) Treat as for acute cystitis with single-dose therapy (preferred, if appropriate) or conventional (multiple-dose) therapy (7 to 14 days). See section entitled Cystitis, Acute above for specific recommendations.

(C) Presumed sexually transmitted infection; therapy directed against *Chlamydia trachomatis* and/or *Neisseria gonorrhoeae*
REMARK:
(1) See Chapter 3 in this Section, Treatment of Sexually Transmitted Diseases, for treatment guidelines.

Recurrent Urinary Tract Infections

Recurrent episodes of urinary tract infection are classified as either due to *relapse* or *reinfection*.

Relapse signifies a post-treatment infection that is caused by the same organism responsible for the initial infection. When relapses do occur, they usually appear within two weeks after a course of therapy has been completed and usually indicate the presence of renal involvement, structural abnormality of the urinary tract (eg, calculi), or, in males, chronic prostatitis. Patients with relapsing urinary tract infections require thorough urologic evaluation to identify surgically correctable abnormalities. If no urological defect is found and the patient has failed to respond to a conventional two-week course of therapy, it is probable that the patient has a deep-seated renal parenchymal infection that may be eradicated only by a six-week course of therapy (see sections above entitled Pyelonephritis, Acute and Cystitis, Acute for specific antimicrobial regimens). Males with chronic bacterial prostatitis also require prolonged courses of antimicrobial therapy (see section below entitled Prostatitis, Chronic).

Reinfections of the urinary tract occur with the introduction and proliferation of an organism (from the fecal-perineal flora) that is different from the one that caused the previously treated infection. Reinfections account for more than 80% of recurrent urinary tract infections in women and girls and usually involve only the lower urinary tract. Most reinfections will occur within weeks to months of the preceding urinary tract infection. If episodes of reinfection are infrequent, each episode can be treated as a separate infection with single-dose or conventional therapy as outlined in the section above, Cystitis, Acute. If reinfections are frequent (eg, three or more episodes per year), long-term antimicrobial prophylaxis may be indicated. See Chapter 4 in this Section, Antimicrobial Chemoprophylaxis for Ambulatory Patients, for guidelines.

Selected references: Nicolle and Ronald, 1987; Brumfitt and Hamilton-Miller, 1990; Sobel and Kaye, 1990; Stapleton et al, 1990.

Urethritis

Urethritis in sexually active males is usually caused by *Neisseria gonorrhoeae* (uncomplicated gonorrhea) or *Chlamydia trachomatis* (nonspecific [non-gonococcal] urethritis). See Chapter 3 in this Section, Treatment of Sexually Transmitted Diseases, for treatment guidelines for these sexually transmitted infections.

Prostatitis, Acute

Escherichia coli is the causative organism in the majority (≥80%) of cases of acute bacterial prostatitis. Other gram-negative bacilli, including *Klebsiella, Proteus, Enterobacter*, and *Pseudomonas* (rare), and enterococci (eg, *E. faecalis*) are occasional causative organisms.

Antimicrobial drug therapy of acute prostatitis initially is EMPIRIC pending results of urine cultures and susceptibility tests.

Selected references: Pfau, 1986; Meares, 1987; Sobel and Kaye, 1990.

EMPIRIC THERAPY
Escherichia coli most likely; other enteric gram-negative bacilli; *Enterococcus faecalis* and other enterococci

PREFERRED THERAPY:
Trimethoprim/Sulfamethoxazole (oral)
OR
Ciprofloxacin, Norfloxacin, or Ofloxacin (oral)
OR
Aminoglycoside (gentamicin, tobramycin, amikacin, netilmicin) *plus* Ampicillin (parenteral)
ALTERNATIVE THERAPY:
Trimethoprim alone
REMARKS:
(1) Although many antibacterial agents appear to penetrate the inflamed prostate adequately, many experts prefer trimethoprim/sulfamethoxazole because of the good penetration of trimethoprim into prostatic tissue. If the causative organism is susceptible and clinical response is favorable, many experts continue trimethoprim/sulfamethoxazole (160 mg/800 mg twice daily) for 30 days in an attempt to prevent the development of chronic prostatitis.
(2) Parenteral therapy with an aminoglycoside *plus* ampicillin may be preferred initially in patients with pronounced systemic symptoms. When the patient becomes afebrile, appropriate oral therapy, based on urine culture and susceptibility testing, is recommended for 30 days.
(3) The fluoroquinolones (eg, ciprofloxacin, norfloxacin, oflox-

acin) have excellent penetration into prostatic tissue and fluid. Initial clinical experience with these compounds suggests that they are at least equally effective, if not more effective, than trimethoprim/sulfamethoxazole. Some experts now prefer the fluoroquinolones for this indication (Lebel, 1988; Tolkoff-Rubin and Rubin, 1988).

Prostatitis, Chronic

Chronic bacterial prostatitis is the most common cause of relapsing urinary tract infections in males. *Escherichia coli* is the causative organism in the majority of cases. Other gram-negative bacilli, including *Klebsiella, Proteus, Enterobacter*, and *Pseudomonas* (rare), and enterococci (eg, *E. faecalis)* are occasional causative organisms. Nonbacterial prostatitis is quite similar to chronic bacterial prostatitis, but an infectious etiology is presently unclear. *Ureaplasma urealyticum* may be causative in some cases. Current evidence does not support a role for *Chlamydia trachomatis* in prostatitis.

Chronic bacterial prostatitis is diagnosed by the prostatic localization test, which shows significantly higher bacterial counts in fluid expressed by prostatic massage or urine voided after massage when compared to urine cultured prior to prostatic massage. Antimicrobial drug therapy (oral) is initiated if bacteria are cultured. Drug selection is limited, however, because few antimicrobial agents adequately penetrate into prostatic fluid.

Selected references: Pfau, 1986; Meares, 1987; Sobel and Kaye, 1990.

EMPIRIC THERAPY
Escherichia coli most likely; other enteric gram-negative bacilli; *Enterococcus faecalis* and other enterococci

PREFERRED THERAPY:
Trimethoprim/Sulfamethoxazole
OR
Ciprofloxacin or Ofloxacin
ALTERNATIVE THERAPY:
Trimethoprim alone
REMARKS:
(1) Most experts prefer trimethoprim/sulfamethoxazole because of the good penetration of trimethoprim into prostatic fluid. If the causative organism is susceptible, most experts will administer trimethoprim/sulfamethoxazole (160 mg/800 mg twice daily) for 12 weeks and some consultants suggest a course of therapy as long as 24 weeks.
(2) Despite prolonged therapy, a significant number of failures will result. Urologic evaluation and surgical resection may be indicated in these patients. Alternatively, some experts initiate long-term suppressive therapy with trimethoprim/sulfamethoxazole (80 mg/400 mg daily) to control symptoms and protect against recurrent urinary tract infections.
(3) The fluoroquinolones have excellent penetration into prostatic tissue and fluid. Although clinical experience is limited, ciprofloxacin and ofloxacin look promising for this indication (see Lebel, 1988; Tolkoff-Rubin and Rubin, 1988). Some consultants now prefer these agents for chronic bacterial prostatitis.
(4) Doxycycline and erythromycin have been suggested in cases of nonbacterial prostatitis in which *Ureaplasma urealyticum* is a potential causative organism.

MISCELLANEOUS INFECTIONS

SPECIFIC antimicrobial drug therapy for miscellaneous bacterial, actinomycetic, rickettsial, and spirochetal infections is outlined in alphabetical order below. Treatment guidelines for fungal, protozoal, helminthic, and viral infections are discussed elsewhere; see index entries Mycoses Deep, Systemic; Antiprotozoal Agents; Anthelmintics; and Antiviral Agents, respectively.

Actinomycosis

Selected references: Conte and Barriere, 1988; *Med Lett Drugs Ther*, 1990; Sanford, 1990 B, 1990 C; Lerner, 1990 A; Nelson, 1991 A, 1991 B.

Actinomyces israelii
(anaerobic, gram-positive, branching, filamentous bacteria)

PREFERRED THERAPY:
Penicillin G
ALTERNATIVE THERAPY:
Tetracycline; Clindamycin; Erythromycin
REMARKS:
(1) High-dose, intravenous penicillin G (10 to 20 million units daily) for the initial four to six weeks, followed by oral penicillin V for 6 to 12 months often is recommended for deep-seated cervicofacial infections. Surgical debridement and drainage frequently are necessary.
(2) Tetracyclines should not be used in pregnant women or children less than 8 years.

Anthrax

Selected references: Conte and Barriere, 1988; Laforce, 1990; *Med Lett Drugs Ther*, 1990; Nelson, 1991 A.

Bacillus anthracis
(gram-positive, spore-forming bacilli)

PREFERRED THERAPY:
Penicillin G
ALTERNATIVE THERAPY:
Erythromycin; Tetracycline
REMARK:
(1) Tetracyclines should not be used in pregnant women or children less than 8 years.

Brucellosis

Selected references: Conte and Barriere, 1988; Hall, 1990; *Med Lett Drugs Ther*, 1990; Mikolich and Boyce, 1990; Sanford, 1990 A, 1990 B; Nelson, 1991 A, 1991 B.

Brucella
(gram-negative bacilli)

PREFERRED THERAPY:
Tetracycline *with or without* Streptomycin
ALTERNATIVE THERAPY:
Chloramphenicol *with or without* Streptomycin; Trimethoprim/Sulfamethoxazole
REMARKS:
(1) Combination regimens are recommended for severe infections.
(2) Trimethoprim/sulfamethoxazole *plus* rifampin or tetracycline *plus* rifampin are other alternative regimens, but clinical experience is limited.
(3) Tetracyclines should not be used in pregnant women or children less than 8 years.

Cat Scratch Disease

Cat scratch disease is usually a self-limited solitary or regional lymphadenitis that is commonly preceded by a cat scratch. Small, pleomorphic gram-negative bacilli are found in affected lymph nodes and in the skin at the primary site of inoculation. This potential etiologic agent recently has been isolated and cultured from patients with the disease. In almost all immunocompetent patients, the disease is self-limited, runs a benign course for several months, and requires no treatment other than analgesics, local heat, and reassurance. Needle aspiration may be necessary if suppuration of the node occurs.

Occasionally, cat scratch disease may cause severe systemic and focal complications, especially in immunocompromised hosts (eg, AIDS patients). Although the effectiveness of antimicrobial therapy is not established, anecdotal reports suggest gentamicin, oral ciprofloxacin, or trimethoprim/sulfamethoxazole may be useful.

Selected references: Fischer, 1990; Holley, 1991.

Clostridial Myonecrosis (Gas Gangrene)

Selected references: Bornstein, 1986; *Med Lett Drugs Ther*, 1990; Sanford, 1990 A; Nelson, 1991 A, 1991 B.

Clostridium perfringens common; also *C. novyi, C. septicum*
(gram-positive bacilli)

PREFERRED THERAPY:
Penicillin G
ALTERNATIVE THERAPY:
Chloramphenicol; Clindamycin; Metronidazole; Tetracycline
REMARKS:
(1) High-dose, intravenous penicillin G (approximately 20 million units per day) is indicated.
(2) Emergency surgical debridement with excision of infected muscle is of primary importance. Hyperbaric oxygen therapy may be a useful adjunct to surgical debridement in the management of the spreading, necrotic type. Antitoxin is no longer recommended.
(3) Tetracyclines should not be used in pregnant women or children less than 8 years.

Erysipeloid

The predominant form is an acute, localized cellulitis caused by *Erysipelothrix rhusiopathiae*. Infection usually occurs in the finger or hand following an abrasion, scratch, or puncture wound while handling organic material (eg, raw fish or poultry) containing the organism. Erysipeloid is an occupational disease of fishermen, butchers, and others handling raw fish or poultry. Rarely, the organism causes bacteremia and endocarditis.

Selected references: Conte and Barriere, 1988.

Erysipelothrix rhusiopathiae
(gram-positive bacilli)

PREFERRED THERAPY:
Penicillin G
ALTERNATIVE THERAPY:
Erythromycin

Glanders

Selected references: *Med Lett Drugs Ther*, 1990; Nelson, 1991 A.

Pseudomonas mallei
(gram-negative bacilli)

PREFERRED THERAPY:
Tetracycline *plus* Streptomycin
ALTERNATIVE THERAPY:
Chloramphenicol *plus* Streptomycin
REMARK:
(1) Tetracyclines should not be used in pregnant women or children less than 8 years.

Leprosy

The causative organism is *Mycobacterium leprae* (acid fast bacilli). For treatment guidelines, see index entry Leprosy.

Leptospirosis

Selected references: Conte and Barriere, 1988; Farrar, 1990; *Med Lett Drugs Ther*, 1990; Sanford, 1990 A; Nelson, 1991 A, 1991 B.

Leptospira species
(spirochete)

PREFERRED THERAPY:
Penicillin G OR **Doxycycline** OR **Tetracycline**
REMARKS:
(1) Therapy early in the course of illness (within four days of onset) appears to favorably affect the signs and symptoms of leptospirosis.
(2) Tetracyclines should not be used in pregnant women or children less than 8 years.

Listeriosis

Selected references: Conte and Barriere, 1988; Gellin and Broome, 1989; Armstrong, 1990; *Med Lett Drugs Ther*, 1990; Sanford, 1990 B; Nelson, 1991 A.

Listeria monocytogenes
(gram-positive bacilli)

PREFERRED THERAPY:
Ampicillin (or Penicillin G) ***with or without*** **Aminoglycoside (gentamicin, tobramycin, amikacin, netilmicin)**
ALTERNATIVE THERAPY:
Trimethoprim/Sulfamethoxazole; Tetracycline; Erythromycin
REMARKS:
(1) Cephalosporins are not active against *L. monocytogenes.*
(2) Tetracyclines should not be used in pregnant women or children less than 8 years.
(3) Combination regimen is synergistic in vitro. It is recommended for serious infections (sepsis, endocarditis, meningitis).

Lyme Disease

Lyme disease is caused by *Borrelia burgdorferi,* a spirochete that is transmitted by *Ixodes* ticks. The disease has three clinical stages that can overlap or occur alone. Stage one (early disease) is characterized by a distinctive skin lesion, erythema (chronicum) migrans, which appears within a few days to a few weeks at the site of the tick bite in approximately two-thirds of patients. This annular skin eruption is often accompanied by nonspecific constitutional symptoms, including fever, headache, fatigue, stiff neck, myalgias, and arthralgias. The second stage follows 2 to 12 weeks after the tick bite and involves neurologic complications (in 10% to 15% of patients), including aseptic meningitis, cranial nerve palsies (most commonly, Bell's palsy), and peripheral neuropathy, and cardiac conduction abnormalities (less than 10% of patients). Stage three Lyme disease occurs from six weeks to two years after the tick bite and is characterized by oligoarticular arthritis in large joints, especially the knee, in approximately 50% of (previously untreated) patients. Chronic neurologic syndromes also may appear.

Treatment of early (stage one) Lyme disease with appropriate antimicrobial agents shortens the duration of erythema migrans and prevents or ameliorates late complications of the disease. Appropriate antibiotics also can be effective for arthritis, carditis, and neurologic involvement, but optimal treatment guidelines remain to be established.

Selected references: Sanford, 1990 A; Goodwin et al, 1990; Abele et al, 1990; Nelson, 1991 B.

Borrelia burgdorferi
(spirochete)

EARLY DISEASE

PREFERRED THERAPY:
Doxycycline (or Tetracycline) (oral)
ALTERNATIVE THERAPY:
Amoxicillin; Penicillin V; Erythromycin (oral)
REMARKS:
(1) Tetracycline and penicillin V were more effective than erythromycin in resolving erythema migrans and associated symptoms in a prospective, randomized study. Tetracycline appeared to be more effective in preventing the late complications of Lyme disease (Steere et al, 1983 A). Many experts now prefer doxycycline and amoxicillin to tetracycline and penicillin V, respectively. Current (oral) dosage recommendations are: doxycycline, *adults,* 100 mg twice daily; tetracycline, *adults,* 250 to 500 mg four times daily; amoxicillin, *adults,* 250 to 500 mg three times daily, and *children,* 20 to 40 mg/kg/day; penicillin V potassium, *adults,* 250 to 500 mg four times daily, and *children,* 50 mg/kg/day; and erythromycin, *adults,* 250 mg four times daily, and *children,* 30 mg/kg/day. Duration of therapy is 10 to 21 days (*Med Lett Drugs Ther,* 1989).
(2) Tetracyclines should not be used in pregnant women or children less than 8 years.

NEUROLOGIC DISEASE
PREFERRED THERAPY:
Doxycycline (oral) OR **Tetracycline (oral)** OR **Amoxicillin (oral) for mild CNS disease (Bell's palsy)**
OR
Ceftriaxone (IV) OR **Penicillin G (IV) for more serious CNS disease**
REMARKS:
(1) For patients with mild symptoms, such as Bell's palsy, oral doxycycline, tetracycline, or amoxicillin can be used in the same dosages as for Early Disease (see above). However, the recommended duration of therapy is one month (*Med Lett Drugs Ther,* 1989).
(2) Tetracyclines should not be used in pregnant women or children less than 8 years.
(3) Intravenous penicillin G was effective in the treatment of more serious neurologic abnormalities (meningitis, peripheral neuropathy) associated with Lyme disease in a small number of patients (Steere et al, 1983 B). Ceftriaxone (IV) also appears useful and was superior to penicillin G (IV) in a small, randomized controlled trial (Dattwyler et al, 1988). Current (intravenous) dosage recommendations are: penicillin G, *adults,* 20 to 24 million units/day and *children,* 250,000 to 400,000 units/kg/day; and ceftriaxone, *adults,* 2 g/day, and *children,* 50 to 80 mg/kg/day. Duration of therapy is 10 to 14 days (*Med Lett Drugs Ther,* 1989).
(4) Intravenous penicillin G or ceftriaxone also has been used in patients with stage three (late) neurologic complications with variable success (see *Med Lett Drugs Ther,* 1989).

CARDIAC DISEASE

PREFERRED THERAPY:
Doxycycline (oral) OR **Tetracycline (oral)** OR **Amoxicillin (oral) for mild cardiac disease**
OR
Penicillin G (IV) OR **Ceftriaxone (IV) for more serious cardiac disease**
REMARKS:
(1) For patients with mild cardiac conduction involvement (first degree atrioventricular block but PR interval less than 0.30 seconds) and no other significant symptoms, oral doxycycline, tetracycline, or amoxicillin can be used in the same dosages as for Early Disease (see above). However, the recommended duration of therapy is 21 days (*Med Lett Drugs Ther,* 1989).
(2) Tetracycline should not be used in pregnant women or children less than 8 years.
(3) Patients with more severe conduction system disease

should be hospitalized and given intravenous penicillin G or ceftriaxone in the same dosages as for Neurologic Disease (see above). Duration of therapy is 10 to 21 days, depending on the rapidity of response. Although the conduction system abnormalities associated with Lyme disease are not permanent, a temporary pacemaker may be necessary (*Med Lett Drugs Ther*, 1989).

ARTHRITIS
PREFERRED THERAPY:
Penicillin G (IV) OR **Ceftriaxone (IV)**
OR
Doxycycline (oral) OR **Tetracycline (oral)** OR **Amoxicillin (oral)**
REMARKS:
(1) Intravenous penicillin G was effective in 11 of 20 patients with established Lyme arthritis, but the response may be delayed for weeks or months (Steere et al, 1985). In a small, randomized controlled trial, ceftriaxone (IV) was superior to penicillin G (IV) and was effective in some patients who failed to respond to penicillin G (Dattwyler et al, 1988). Suggested dosages are the same as for Neurologic Disease (see above), and the duration of therapy is 14 to 21 days (*Med Lett Drugs Ther*, 1989).
(2) Oral doxycycline, tetracycline, or amoxicillin also may be effective for established Lyme arthritis when given in the same dosages as for Early Disease (see above), but for a duration of one month (*Med Lett Drugs Ther*, 1989).
(3) Tetracyclines should not be used in pregnant women or children less than 8 years.
(4) Recalcitrant arthritis may respond to re-treatment with the same or an alternative antibiotic.

Melioidosis

Selected references: Sanford, 1990 B, 1990 D; Conte and Barriere, 1988; *Med Lett Drugs Ther*, 1990; Leelarasamee and Bovornkitti, 1989; Nelson, 1991 A, 1991 B; White et al, 1989.

Pseudomonas pseudomallei
(gram-negative bacilli)

PREFERRED THERAPY:
Trimethoprim/Sulfamethoxazole *with or without* Ceftazidime
OR
Tetracycline *with or without* Chloramphenicol *with or without* Trimethoprim/Sulfamethoxazole
ALTERNATIVE THERAPY:
Ceftazidime
OR
Chloramphenicol *plus* Kanamycin, Gentamicin, or Tobramycin; Sulfonamide
REMARKS:
(1) Antimicrobial therapy should be based on the results of susceptibility testing. Subacute and chronic forms of melioidosis usually respond to treatment with oral trimethoprim/sulfamethoxazole or tetracycline (alternative, chloramphenicol). Combination regimens, administered parenterally, are recommended for severe infections (eg, acute septicemia, severe pneumonitis).
(2) Treatment of acute and chronic forms of melioidosis should be prolonged for at least a month and often for as long as 6 to 12 months because infections tend to persist.
(3) Tetracyclines should not be used in pregnant women or children less than 8 years.

Mycobacterial Infections, Atypical

Causative organisms include *Mycobacterium kansasii, M. avium-intracellulare-scrofulaceum* complex, *M. fortuitum*, and *M. marinum*. For treatment guidelines, see index entry Mycobacterium Infections, Atypical.

Nocardiosis

Selected references: Conte and Barriere, 1988; *Med Lett Drugs Ther*, 1990; Lerner, 1990 B; Sanford, 1990 B and C; Nelson, 1991 A, 1991 B.

Nocardia asteroides
(aerobic, gram-positive, branching, filamentous bacteria)

PREFERRED THERAPY:
Sulfonamide (trisulfapyrimidines, sulfadiazine, sulfisoxazole)
ALTERNATIVE THERAPY:
Trimethoprim/Sulfamethoxazole; Minocycline; Amikacin; Trisulfapyrimidines *plus* Minocycline (or Ampicillin or Erythromycin); Cycloserine
REMARKS:
(1) Optimum treatment guidelines presently are unclear. Some experts prefer trimethoprim/sulfamethoxazole over a sulfonamide alone (see Smego et al, 1983).
(2) Prolonged therapy for 6 to 12 months usually is recommended. Surgical excision or drainage frequently is necessary.

Plague

Selected references: *Med Lett Drugs Ther*, 1990; Butler, 1990; Sanford, 1990 B; Nelson, 1991 A.

Yersinia pestis
(gram-negative bacilli)

PREFERRED THERAPY:
Streptomycin
ALTERNATIVE THERAPY:
Tetracycline; Chloramphenicol; Gentamicin; Trimethoprim/Sulfamethoxazole
REMARKS:
(1) Some experts recommend a combination regimen containing streptomycin *plus* tetracycline.
(2) Tetracyclines should not be used in pregnant women or children less than 8 years.

Pseudomonas cepacia Infections

Selected references: *Med Lett Drugs Ther*, 1990; Sanford, 1990 B; Nelson, 1991 A.

Pseudomonas cepacia
(gram-negative bacilli)

PREFERRED THERAPY:
Trimethoprim/Sulfamethoxazole
ALTERNATIVE THERAPY:
Chloramphenicol; Ceftazidime

Rat Bite Fever

Causative organisms are *Spirillum minus* and *Streptobacillus moniliformis* (Haverhill fever). Antimicrobial drug selection is the same for either organism.

Selected references: Conte and Barriere, 1988; *Med Lett Drugs Ther*, 1990; Nelson, 1991 A.

Spirillum minus
(gram-negative bacilli)

PREFERRED THERAPY:
Penicillin G
ALTERNATIVE THERAPY:
Tetracycline; Streptomycin
REMARK:
(1) Tetracyclines should not be used in pregnant women or children less than 8 years.

Streptobacillus moniliformis
(gram-negative bacilli)

PREFERRED THERAPY:
Penicillin G
ALTERNATIVE THERAPY:
Tetracycline; Streptomycin
REMARK:
(1) Tetracyclines should not be used in pregnant women or children less than 8 years.

Relapsing Fever

Selected references: *Med Lett Drugs Ther*, 1990; Johnson, 1990; Sanford, 1990 A, 1990 B; Nelson, 1991 A.

***Borrelia recurrentis* and other *Borrelia* species**
(spirochete)

PREFERRED THERAPY:
Tetracycline
ALTERNATIVE THERAPY:
Erythromycin; Penicillin G; Chloramphenicol
REMARK:
(1) Tetracyclines should not be used in pregnant women or children under 8 years.

Rickettsial Infections

This group of diseases is caused by rickettsiae (obligate, intracellular, pleomorphic bacteria). All are characterized by fever, chills, headache, rash (except Q fever), myalgias, and prostration. Diseases with worldwide or at least United States distribution include Q fever (*Coxiella burnetii*), rickettsialpox (*Rickettsia akari*), Rocky Mountain spotted fever (*R. rickettsii*), epidemic or Brill-Zinsser typhus (*R. prowazekii*), and endemic or murine typhus (*R. mooseri*). Antimicrobial drug therapy is the same for all rickettsial infections.

Selected references: Kamper et al, 1986; *Med Lett Drugs Ther*, 1990; Saah, 1990; Sanford, 1990 B; Nelson, 1991 A, 1991 B.

Rickettsia

PREFERRED THERAPY:
Tetracycline
OR
Doxycycline
ALTERNATIVE THERAPY:
Chloramphenicol
REMARK:
(1) Tetracyclines should not be used in pregnant women or children less than 8 years.

Syphilis

Syphilis is caused by *Treponema pallidum* (spirochete). See Chapter 3 in this section, Treatment of Sexually Transmitted Diseases, for treatment guidelines for this sexually transmitted infection.

Tetanus

Tetanus is manifested by tonic muscle spasms and hyperreflexia caused by an exotoxin produced by the sporulated form of *Clostridium tetani*. Treatment includes administration of human tetanus immune globulin (TIG) to neutralize the toxin, adequate debridement of the primary wound, supportive care, and the administration of antimicrobial drug therapy, as outlined below.

Selected references: *Med Lett Drugs Ther*, 1990; Cate, 1990; Nelson, 1991 A, 1991 B. For guidelines for the prevention of tetanus, see index entry Tetanus.

Clostridium tetani
(gram-positive, spore-forming bacilli)

PREFERRED THERAPY:
Penicillin G
ALTERNATIVE THERAPY:
Tetracycline
REMARKS:
(1) Avoid intramuscular injections of antimicrobial agents.
(2) Tetracyclines should not be used in pregnant women or children less than 8 years.

Tularemia

Selected references: Conte and Barriere, 1988; *Med Lett Drugs Ther*, 1990; Boyce, 1990; Sanford, 1990 B; Nelson, 1991 A, 1991 B.

Francisella tularensis
(gram-negative coccobacilli)

PREFERRED THERAPY:
Streptomycin OR **Gentamicin**
ALTERNATIVE THERAPY:
Tetracycline; Chloramphenicol
REMARKS:
(1) Tetracycline and chloramphenicol are less effective alternatives and relapses have occurred due to persistence of *F. tularensis*.
(2) Tetracyclines should not be used in pregnant women or children less than 8 years.

Vincent's Infection

Selected references: Lancaster and Attebery, 1986; *Med Lett Drugs Ther*, 1990; Sanford, 1990 A; Nelson, 1991 A.

Leptotrichia buccalis
(gram-negative bacilli)

PREFERRED THERAPY:
Penicillin G
ALTERNATIVE THERAPY:
Tetracycline; Erythromycin; Clindamycin; Metronidazole
REMARK:
(1) Tetracyclines should not be used in pregnant women or children less than 8 years.

Yaws

Selected references: *Med Lett Drugs Ther*, 1990; Nelson, 1991 A.

Treponema pertenue
(spirochete)

PREFERRED THERAPY:
Penicillin G
ALTERNATIVE THERAPY:
Tetracycline
REMARK:
(1) Tetracyclines should not be used in pregnant women or children less than 8 years.

Cited References

Bacteremias and Sepsis

The choice of antimicrobial drugs. *Med Lett Drugs Ther* 32:41-48, 1990.

Anaissie EJ, et al: Randomized trial of beta-lactam regimens in febrile neutropenic cancer patients. *Am J Med* 84:581-589, 1988.

Berkley SF, et al: Relationship of tampon characteristics to menstrual toxic shock syndrome. *JAMA* 258:917-920, 1987.

Bodey GP: Evolution of antibiotic therapy for infection in neutropenic patients: Studies at M. D. Anderson Hospital. *Rev Infect Dis* 11 (suppl 7):S1582-S1590, 1989.

Bodey GP, et al: Imipenem-cilastatin as initial therapy for febrile cancer patients. *Antimicrob Agents Chemother* 30:211-214, 1986.

Bodey GP, et al: β-Lactam regimens for the febrile neutropenic patient. *Cancer* 65:9-16, 1990.

Bryan CS, et al: Gentamicin vs cefotaxime for therapy of neonatal sepsis: Relationship to drug resistance. *Am J Dis Child* 139:1086-1089, 1985.

Calandra T, et al (EORTC International Antimicrobial Therapy Cooperative Group): Ceftazidime combined with short or long course of amikacin for empirical therapy of gram-negative bacteremia in cancer patients with granulocytopenia. *N Engl J Med* 317:1692-1698, 1987.

Chesney PJ: Clinical aspects and spectrum of illness of toxic shock syndrome: Overview. *Rev Infect Dis* 11 (suppl 1):S1-S7, 1989.

Cohen MS: Empiric antibiotic therapy for leukopenic patient: How many antibiotics are enough? *Infect Med* 4:237-246, 1987.

DeJongh CA, et al: Antibiotic synergism and response in gram-negative bacteremia in granulocytopenic cancer patients. *Am J Med* 80 (suppl 5C):96-100, 1986 A.

DeJongh CA, et al: Double beta-lactam combination versus aminoglycoside-containing regimen as empiric antibiotic therapy for febrile granulocytopenic cancer patients. *Am J Med* 80 (suppl 5C):101-111, 1986 B.

Falloon J, et al: Is carbapenem as effective as 3rd generation cephalosporin when used as monotherapy in empiric treatment of febrile (F+) neutropenic (N+) patient (pt)? abstract 1254. 27th Interscience Conference on Antimicrobial Agents and Chemotherapy. New York, Oct 4-7, 1987.

Foltzer MA, Reese RE: Bacteremias and sepsis, in Reese RE, Douglas RG Jr (eds): *A Practical Approach to Infectious Diseases*, ed 2. Boston, Little Brown, 1986, 47-74.

Hathorn JW, et al: Empirical antibiotic therapy in febrile neutropenic cancer patient: Clinical efficacy and impact of monotherapy. *Antimicrob Agents Chemother* 31:971-977, 1987.

Hughes WT, et al: Guidelines for the use of antimicrobial agents in neutropenic patients with unexplained fever. *J Infect Dis* 161:381-396, 1990.

Johnson MP, Ramphal R: β-Lactam-resistant *Enterobacter* bacteremia in febrile neutropenic patients receiving monotherapy. *J Infect Dis* 162:981-983, 1990.

Jones PG, et al: Aztreonam therapy in neutropenic patients with cancer. *Am J Med* 81:243-248, 1986.

Klastersky J: Concept of empiric therapy with antibiotic combinations: Indications and limits. *Am J Med* 80 (suppl 5C): 2-12, 1986.

Klastersky J, et al: Prospective randomized comparison of three antibiotic regimens for empirical therapy of suspected bacteremic infection in febrile granulocytopenic patients. *Antimicrob Agents Chemother* 29:263-270, 1986.

Klastersky J, et al: Empiric antimicrobial therapy for febrile granulocytopenic cancer patients: Lessons from four EORTC trials. *Eur J Cancer Clin Oncol* 24 (suppl 1):S35-S45, 1988.

Kramer BS, et al: Randomized comparison between two ceftazidime-containing regimens and cephalothin-gentamicin-carbenicillin in febrile granulocytopenic cancer patients. *Antimicrob Agents Chemother* 30:64-68, 1986.

Liang R, et al: Ceftazidime versus imipenem-cilastatin as initial monotherapy for febrile neutropenic patients. *Antimicrob Agents Chemother* 34:1336-1341, 1990.

MacDonald KL, et al: Toxic shock syndrome: Newly recognized complication of influenza and influenza-like illness. *JAMA* 257:1053-1058, 1987.

McCracken GH Jr: Use of third-generation cephalosporins for treatment of neonatal infections, editorial. *Am J Dis Child* 134:1079-1080, 1985.

Meunier F: Infections in patients with acute leukemia and lymphoma, in Mandell GL, et al (eds): *Principles and Practice of Infectious Diseases*, ed 3. New York, Churchill Livingstone, 1990, 2265-2275.

Nelson JD: *1991-1992 Pocketbook of Pediatric Antimicrobial Therapy*, ed 9. Baltimore, Williams & Wilkins, 1991 A, 8-14.

Nelson JD: *1991-1992 Pocketbook of Pediatric Antimicrobial Therapy*, ed 9. Baltimore, Williams & Wilkins, 1991 B, 39.

Pizzo PA: Fever and infection in child with cancer, in Nelson JD (ed): *Current Therapy in Pediatric Infectious Disease.* Philadelphia, BC Decker, 1986, 218-223.

Pizzo PA: Empirical therapy and prevention of infection in the immunocompromised host, in Mandell GL, et al (eds): *Principles and Practice of Infectious Diseases*, ed 3. New York, Churchill Livingstone, 1990, 2303-2312.

Pizzo PA, et al: Randomized trial comparing ceftazidime alone with combination antibiotic therapy in cancer patients with fever and neutropenia. *N Engl J Med* 315:552-558, 1986.

Resnick SD: Toxic shock syndrome: Recent developments in pathogenesis. *J Pediatr* 116:321-328, 1990.

Rubin M, et al: Gram-positive infections and the use of vancomycin in 550 episodes of fever and neutropenia. *Ann Intern Med* 108:30-35, 1988.

Sanford JP: *Guide to Antimicrobial Therapy, 1990.* West Bethesda, Md, Antimicrobial Therapy, Inc, 1990, 31-32.

Schimpff SC: Empiric antibiotic therapy for granulocytopenic cancer patients. *Am J Med* 80 (suppl 5C): 13-20, 1986.

Schimpff SC: Infections in the compromised host: An overview, in Mandell GL, et al (eds): *Principles and Practice of Infectious Diseases,* ed 3. New York, Churchill Livingstone, 1990, 2258-2265.

Schwalbe RS, et al: Emergence of vancomycin resistance in coagulase-negative staphylococci. *N Engl J Med* 316:927-931, 1987.

Shenep JL, et al: Vancomycin, ticarcillin, and amikacin compared with ticarcillin-clavulanate and amikacin in the empirical treatment of febrile neutropenic children with cancer. *N Engl J Med* 319:1053-1058, 1988.

St. Geme JW, Polin RA: Neonatal sepsis: Progress in diagnosis and management. *Drugs* 36:784-800, 1988.

Steinhoff MC: Neonatal sepsis and infections, in Reese RE, Douglas RG Jr (eds): *A Practical Approach to Infectious Diseases*, ed 2. Boston, Little, Brown, 1986, 75-98.

Todd JK: Toxic shock syndrome. *Clin Microbiol Rev* 1:432-446, 1988.

Wade JC: Antibiotic therapy for the febrile granulocytopenic cancer patient: Combination therapy vs. monotherapy. *Rev Infect Dis* 11 (suppl 7):S1572-S1581, 1989.

Wade JC, et al: Monotherapy for empiric treatment of fever in granulocytopenic cancer patients. *Am J Med* 80 (suppl 5C): 85-95, 1986.

Wade J, et al: Imipenem vs. piperacillin plus (+) amikacin, empiric therapy for febrile neutropenic patients: Double-blind trial, abstract 1251. 27th Interscience Conference on Antimicrobial Agents and Chemotherapy. New York, Oct 4-7, 1987.

Word BM, Klein JO: Current therapy of bacterial sepsis and meningitis in infants and children: Poll of directors of programs in pediatric infectious diseases. *Pediatr Infect Dis J* 7:267-270, 1988.

Young LS: Double beta-lactam therapy in immunocompromised host. *J Antimicrob Chemother* 16:4-6, 1985.

Young LS: Empirical antimicrobial therapy in neutropenic host. *N Engl J Med* 315:580-581, 1986.

Young LS: New beta-lactam antimicrobics: Controversies about monotherapy versus combinations. *Antimicrob Newslett* 4:17-24, 1987.

Bone and Joint Infections

The choice of antimicrobial drugs. *Med Lett Drugs Ther* 32:41-48, 1990.

1989 Sexually transmitted diseases treatment guidelines. *MMWR* 38 (suppl 8):1-43, 1989.

Allman RL, Abruzzo JL: Diagnosing bacterial arthritis. *Infect Med* 4: 260-284, 1987.

Armstrong EP: Bone and joint infections, in DiPiro JT, et al (eds): *Pharmacotherapy: A Pathophysiologic Approach.* New York, Elsevier, 1989, 1247-1257.

Conte JE Jr, Barriere SL: *Manual of Antibiotics and Infectious Diseases*, ed 6. Philadelphia, Lea & Febiger, 1988, 98, 113-114.

Dickie AS: Current concepts in management of infections in bones and joints. *Drugs* 32:458-475, 1986.

Nelson JD: *1991-1992 Pocketbook of Pediatric Antimicrobial Therapy*, ed 9. Baltimore, Williams & Wilkins, 1991 A, 11, 20-21.

Nelson JD: *1991-1992 Pocketbook of Pediatric Antimicrobial Therapy*, ed 9. Baltimore, Williams & Wilkins, 1991 B, 4.

Norden CW: Treatment of osteomyelitis, in Peterson PK, Verhoef J (eds): *The Antimicrobial Agents Annual/2.* New York, Elsevier, 1987, 405-413.

Norden CW: Osteomyelitis, in Mandell GL, et al (eds): *Principles and Practice of Infectious Diseases*, ed 3. New York, Churchill Livingstone, 1990, 922-930.

Peterson LR, et al: Therapy of lower extremity infections with ciprofloxacin in patients with diabetes mellitus, peripheral vascular disease, or both. *Am J Med* 86:801-808, 1989.

Sanford JP: *Guide to Antimicrobial Therapy, 1990.* West Bethesda, Md, Antimicrobial Therapy, Inc, 1990 A, 19.

Sanford JP: *Guide to Antimicrobial Therapy, 1990.* West Bethesda, Md, Antimicrobial Therapy, Inc, 1990 B, 3.

Smith JW: Infectious arthritis, in Mandell GL, et al (eds): *Principles and Practice of Infectious Diseases*, ed 3. New York, Churchill Livingstone, 1990, 911-918.

Swartz MN, O'Hanley P: Osteomyelitis, in Rubenstein E, Federmen DD (eds): *Scientific American Medicine.* New York, Scientific American, 1987, 7:XVI:1-10.

Syriopoulou VP, Smith AL: Osteomyelitis and septic arthritis, in Feigin RD, Cherry JD (eds): *Textbook of Pediatric Infectious Diseases ed 2.* Philadelphia, WB Saunders, 1987, vol I, 759-779.

Cardiovascular System Infections

Bisno AL, et al: Antimicrobial treatment of infective endocarditis due to viridans streptococci, enterococci, and staphylococci. *JAMA* 261:1471-1477, 1989.

Calderwood SB, et al: Risk factors for development of prosthetic valve endocarditis. *Circulation* 72:31-37, 1985.

Caputo GM, et al: Native valve endocarditis due to coagulase-negative staphylococci: Clinical and microbiologic features. *Am J Med* 83:619-625, 1987.

Chambers HF, et al: Right-sided *Staphylococcus aureus* endocarditis in intravenous drug abusers: Two-week combination therapy. *Ann Intern Med* 109:619-624, 1988.

Chamovitz B, et al: Prosthetic valve endocarditis caused by *Staphylococcus epidermidis*: Development of rifampin resistance during vancomycin and rifampin therapy. *JAMA* 253:2867-2868, 1985.

Coleman DL, et al: Association between serum inhibitory and bactericidal concentrations and therapeutic outcome in bacterial endocarditis. *Am J Med* 73:260-267, 1982.

Hoffmann SA, Moellering RC: Enterococcus: 'Putting the bug in our ears.' *Ann Intern Med* 106:757-761, 1987.

Karchmer AW: Staphylococcal endocarditis: Laboratory and clinical basis for antibiotic therapy. *Am J Med* 78 (suppl 6B):116-127, 1985.

Karchmer AW, et al: *Staphylococcus epidermidis* causing prosthetic valve endocarditis: Microbiologic and clinical observations as guides to therapy. *Ann Intern Med* 98:447-455, 1983.

Karchmer AW, et al: Methicillin-resistant *Staphylococcus epidermidis* (SE) prosthetic valve (PV) endocarditis (E): Therapeutic trial, abstract 476. 24th Interscience Conference on Antimicrobial Agents and Chemotherapy. Washington, DC, Oct 8-10, 1984.

Korzeniowski O, et al: Combination antimicrobial therapy for *Staphylococcus aureus* endocarditis in patients addicted to parenteral drugs and in nonaddicts: Prospective study. *Ann Intern Med* 97:496-503, 1982.

Mellors JW, et al: Value of serum bactericidal test in management of patients with bacterial endocarditis. *Eur J Clin Microbiol* 5:67-70, 1986.

Nelson JD: *1991-1992 Pocketbook of Pediatric Antimicrobial Therapy*, ed 9. Baltimore, Williams & Wilkins, 1991, 30-31.

Scheld WM, Sande MA: Endocarditis and intravascular infections, in Mandell GL, et al (eds): *Principles and Practice of Infectious Diseases*, ed 3. New York, Churchill Livingstone, 1990, 670-706.

Thornsberry C: Methicillin-resistant (heteroresistant) staphylococci. *Antimicrob Newslett* 1:43-47, 1984.

Threlkeld MG, Cobbs CG: Infectious disorders of prosthetic valves and intravascular devices, in Mandell GL, et al (eds): *Principles and Practice of Infectious Diseases,* ed 3. New York, Churchill Livingstone, 1990, 706-716.

Weinstein MP, et al: Multicenter collaborative evaluation of standardized serum bactericidal test as prognostic indicator in infective endocarditis. *Am J Med* 78:262-269, 1985.

Weinstein MP, et al: Current status of serum bactericidal test as monitor of therapeutic efficacy in serious infections. *Antimicrob Newslett* 3:9-14, 1986.

Wilson WR: Antimicrobial therapy of infective endocarditis, in Peterson PK, Verhoef J (eds): *The Antimicrobial Agents Annual/1.* New York, Elsevier, 1986, 420-435.

Wolfson JS, Swartz MN: Serum bactericidal activity as monitor of antibiotic therapy. *N Engl J Med* 312:968-975, 1985.

Zervos MJ, et al: Nosocomial infection by gentamicin-resistant *Streptococcus faecalis:* Epidemiologic study. *Ann Intern Med* 106:687-691, 1987.

Central Nervous System Infections

The choice of antimicrobial drugs. *Med Lett Drugs Ther* 32:41-48, 1990.

American Academy of Pediatrics Committee on Infectious Diseases: Treatment of bacterial meningitis. *Pediatrics* 81:904-907, 1988.

American Academy of Pediatrics Committee on Infectious Diseases: Dexamethasone therapy for bacterial meningitis in infants and children. *Pediatrics* 86:130-133, 1990.

Barson WJ, et al: Prospective comparative trial of ceftriaxone vs conventional therapy for treatment of bacterial meningitis in children. *Pediatr Infect Dis* 4:362-368, 1985.

Benson CA, Harris AA: Acute neurologic infections. *Med Clin North Am* 70:987-1011, 1986.

Boom WH, Tuazon CU: Successful treatment of multiple brain abscesses with antibiotics alone. *Rev Infect Dis* 7:189-199, 1985.

Bryan JP, et al: Comparison of ceftriaxone and ampicillin plus chloramphenicol for therapy of acute bacterial meningitis. *Antimicrob Agents Chemother* 20:361-368, 1985.

Campos J, et al: Multiply resistant *Haemophilus influenzae* type b causing meningitis: Comparative clinical and laboratory study. *J Pediatr* 108:897-902, 1986.

Fong IW, Tomkins KB: Review of *Pseudomonas aeruginosa* meningitis with special emphasis on treatment with ceftazidime. *Rev Infect Dis* 7:604-612, 1985.

Fontanals D, et al: Penicillin-resistant beta-lactamase producing *Neisseria meningitidis* in Spain. *Eur J Clin Microbiol Infect Dis* 8:90-91, 1989.

Gary N, et al: Clinical identification and comparative prognosis of high-risk patients with *Haemophilus influenzae* meningitis. *Am J Dis Child* 143:307-311, 1989.

Girgis NI, et al: Dexamethasone treatment for bacterial meningitis in children and adults. *Pediatr Infect Dis J* 8:848-851, 1989.

Jadavji T, et al: Brain abscesses in infants and children. *Pediatr Infect Dis* 4:394-398, 1985.

Kaplan SL: Bacterial meningitis, in Nelson JD (ed): *Current Therapy in Pediatric Infectious Disease.* Philadelphia, BC Decker, 1986, 104-110.

Kaplan SL: Dexamethasone for children with bacterial meningitis: Should it be routine therapy? *Am J Dis Child* 143:290-292, 1989.

Klein JO, et al: Report of task force on diagnosis and management of meningitis. *Pediatrics* 78 (suppl):959-982, 1986.

Lebel MH, et al: Dexamethasone therapy for bacterial meningitis: Results of two double-blind, placebo-controlled trials. *N Engl J Med* 319:964-971, 1988.

Lebel MH, et al: Comparative efficacy of ceftriaxone and cefuroxime for treatment of bacterial meningitis. *J Pediatr* 114:1049-1054, 1989 A.

Lebel MH, et al: Magnetic resonance imaging and dexamethasone therapy for bacterial meningitis. *Am J Dis Child* 143:301-306, 1989 B.

Levitz RE, Quintiliani R: Trimethoprim-sulfamethoxazole for bacterial meningitis. *Ann Intern Med* 100:881-890, 1984.

Marks WA, et al: Cefuroxime versus ampicillin plus chloramphenicol in childhood bacterial meningitis: Multicenter randomized controlled trial. *J Pediatr* 109:123-130, 1986.

McCracken GH Jr: Perinatal bacterial diseases, in Feigin RD, Cherry JD (eds): *Textbook of Pediatric Infectious Diseases.* Philadelphia, WB Saunders, 1981, vol I, 747-768.

McCracken GH Jr: New concepts in management of infants and children with meningitis. *Pediatr Infect Dis* 2:S51-S55, 1983.

McCracken GH Jr, Lebel MH: Dexamethasone therapy for bacterial meningitis in infants and children. *Am J Dis Child* 143:287-289, 1989.

McCracken GH Jr, et al: Consensus report: Antimicrobial therapy for bacterial meningitis in infants and children. *Pediatr Infect Dis J* 6:501-505, 1987.

McGee ZA, Baringer JR: Acute meningitis, in Mandell GL, et al (eds): *Principles and Practice of Infectious Diseases*, ed 3. New York, Churchill Livingstone, 1990, 741-755.

Meade RH: Bacterial meningitis in neonatal infant. *Med Clin North Am* 69:257-267, 1985.

Modai J: Empiric therapy of severe infections in adults. *Am J Med* 88 (suppl 4A):4A12S-4A17S, 1990.

Nelson JD: *1991-1992 Pocketbook of Pediatric Antimicrobial Therapy,* ed. 9. Baltimore, Williams & Wilkins, 1991, 10.

Rodriguez WJ, et al: Ceftazidime vs. standard therapy for pediatric meningitis: Therapeutic, pharmacologic and epidemiologic observations. *Pediatr Infect Dis* 5:408-415, 1986.

Rodriguez WJ, et al: Treatment of *Pseudomonas* meningitis with ceftazidime with or without concurrent therapy. *Pediatr Infect Dis J* 9:83-87, 1990.

Sáez-Llorens XJ, et al: Brain abscess in infants and children. *Pediatr Infect Dis J* 8:449-458, 1989.

Sanford JP: *Guide to Antimicrobial Therapy 1990.* West Bethesda, Md, Antimicrobial Therapy, Inc, 1990, 4-5.

Schaad UB, et al: A comparison of ceftriaxone and cefuroxime for the treatment of bacterial meningitis in children. *N Engl J Med* 322:141-147, 1990.

Scheld WM, Wispelwey B (eds): Meningitis. *Infect Dis Clin North Am* 4 (No. 4), 1990.

Stutman HR, Marks MI: Therapy for bacterial meningitis: Which drugs, and for how long? *J Pediatr* 110:812-814, 1987.

Täuber MG, Sande MA: Dexamethasone in bacterial meningitis: Increasing evidence for a beneficial effect. *Pediatr Infect Dis J* 8:842-845, 1989.

Todd PA, Brogden RN: Cefotaxime: An update on its pharmacology and therapeutic use. *Drugs* 40:608-651, 1990.

Tunkel AR, Scheld WM: Aztreonam. *Infect Control Hosp Epidemiol* 11:486-494, 1990.

Tunkel AR, et al: Bacterial meningitis: Recent advances in pathophysiology and treatment. *Ann Intern Med* 112:610-623, 1990.

Tweardy DJ, et al: Susceptibility of penicillin-resistant pneumococci to eighteen antimicrobials: Implications for treatment of meningitis. *J Antimicrob Chemother* 12:133-139, 1983.

Weingarten RD, et al: Meningitis due to penicillin-resistant *Streptococcus pneumoniae* in adults. *Rev Infect Dis* 12:118-124, 1990.

Wispelwey B, Scheld WM: Brain abscess. *Clin Neuropharmacol* 10:483-510, 1987.

Wispelwey B, Scheld WM: Brain abscess, in Mandell GL, et al (eds): *Principles and Practice of Infectious Diseases.* New York, Churchill Livingstone, 1990, 777-788.

Word BM, Klein JO: Current therapy of bacterial sepsis and meningitis in infants and children: Poll of directors of programs in pediatric infectious diseases. *Pediatr Infect Dis J* 7:267-270, 1988.

Yoshikawa TT, Quinn W: Aching head: Intracranial suppuration due to head and neck infections. *Infect Dis Clin North Am* 2:265-277, 1988.

Ear Infections

Bluestone CD: Otitis media and sinusitis in children: Role of *Branhamella catarrhalis. Drugs* 31 (suppl 3):132-141, 1986.

Bluestone CD: Management of otitis media in infants and children: Current role of old and new antimicrobial agents. *Pediatr Infect Dis J* 7:S129-S136, 1988.

Henderson FW, et al: Nasopharyngeal carriage of antibiotic-resistant pneumococci by children in group day care. *J Infect Dis* 157:256-263, 1988.

Johnson MP, Ramphal R: Malignant external otitis: Report on therapy with ceftazidime and review of therapy and prognosis. *Rev Infect Dis* 12:173-180, 1990.

Klein JO: Otitis externa, otitis media, mastoiditis, in Mandell GL, et al (eds): *Principles and Practice of Infectious Diseases,* ed 3. New York, Churchill Livingstone, 1990, 505-510.

Lang R, et al: Ciprofloxacin in malignant otitis externa, abstract 337. 28th Interscience Conference on Antimicrobial Agents and Chemotherapy. Los Angeles, Calif, Oct 23-26, 1988.

Lisby-Sutch SM, et al: Therapy of otitis media. *Clin Pharm* 9:15-34, 1990.

Marchant CD: Otitis media, in Nelson JD (ed): *Current Therapy in Pediatric Infectious Disease.* Philadelphia, BC Decker, 1986, 2-4.

Pelton SI, Klein JO: Draining ear: Otitis media and externa. *Infect Dis Clin North Am* 2:117-129, 1988.

Pichichero M, et al: Comparison of cefuroxime axetil, cefaclor, and amoxicillin-clavulanate potassium suspensions in acute otitis media in infants and children. *South Med J* 83:1174-1177, 1990.

Rubin J, Yu VL: Malignant external otitis: Insights into pathogenesis, clinical manifestations, diagnosis and therapy. *Am J Med* 85:391-398, 1988.

Rubin J, et al: Efficacy of oral ciprofloxacin plus rifampin for treatment of malignant external otitis. *Arch Otolaryngol Head Neck Surg* 115:1063-1069, 1989.

Sanford JP: *Guide to Antimicrobial Therapy 1990.* West Bethesda, Md, Antimicrobial Therapy, Inc, 1990, 6-7.

Eye Infections

1989 Sexually transmitted diseases treatment guidelines. *MMWR* 38 (suppl 8):1-43, 1989.

Nelson JD: *1991-1992 Pocketbook of Pediatric Antimicrobial Therapy,* ed 9. Baltimore, Williams & Wilkins, 1991, 9.

Riley GJ, Baker AS: Eye infections, in Reese RE, Douglas RG Jr (eds): *A Practical Approach to Infectious Diseases,* ed 2. Boston, Little Brown, 1986, 156-173.

Gastrointestinal and Intra-abdominal Infections

Advice for travelers. *Med Lett Drugs Ther* 32:33-36, 1990 B.

The choice of antimicrobial drugs. *Med Lett Drugs Ther* 32:41-48, 1990 A.

Report of the Committee on Infectious Diseases, in: *American Academy of Pediatrics Redbook,* ed 21. Elk Grove Village, Ill, American Academy of Pediatrics, 1988, 370-374.

Alter HJ, et al: Detection of antibody to hepatitis C virus in prospectively followed transfusion recipients with acute and chronic non-A, non-B hepatitis. *N Engl J Med* 321:1494-1500, 1989.

Anders BJ, et al: Double-blind, placebo-controlled trial of erythromycin for treatment of *Campylobacter* enteritis. *Lancet* 1:131-132, 1982.

Asperilla MO, et al: Quinolone antibiotics in the treatment of Salmonella infections. *Rev Infect Dis* 12:873-889, 1990.

Bishop WP, Ulshen MH: Bacterial gastroenteritis. *Pediatr Clin North Am* 35:69-87, 1988.

Brenden RA, et al: Clinical disease spectrum and pathogenic factors associated with *Pleisiomonas shigelloides* infections in humans. *Rev Infect Dis* 10:303-316, 1988.

Briceland LL, et al: Multidisciplinary cost-containment program promoting oral metronidazole for treatment of antibiotic-associated colitis. *Am J Hosp Pharm* 45:122-125, 1988.

Conte JE Jr, Barriere SL: *Manual of Antibiotics and Infectious Diseases,* ed 6. Philadelphia, Lea & Febiger, 1988 A, 118-119.

Conte JE Jr, Barriere SL: *Manual of Antibiotics and Infectious Diseases,* ed 6. Philadelphia, Lea & Febiger, 1988 B, 104, 120-121.

Cossar JH, et al: A cumulative review of studies on travellers, their experience of illness and the implications of these findings. *J Infect* 21:27-42, 1990.

Cover TL, Aber RC: *Yersinia enterocolitica. N Engl J Med* 32:16-24, 1989.

Cuchural GJ, et al: Susceptibility of *Bacteroides fragilis* group in United States: Analysis by site of isolation. *Antimicrob Agents Chemother* 32:717-722, 1988.

Davis GL, et al: Treatment of chronic hepatitis C with recombinant interferon alfa: Multicenter randomized, controlled trial. *N Engl J Med* 321:1501-1506, 1989.

DiBisceglie AM, et al: Recombinant interferon alfa therapy for chronic hepatitis C: Randomized, double-blind, placebo-controlled trial. *N Engl J Med* 321:1506-1510, 1989.

Dooley CP, Cohen H: Clinical significance of *Campylobacter pylori. Ann Intern Med* 108:70-79, 1988.

Dudley MN, et al: Oral bacitracin vs vancomycin therapy for *Clostridium difficile*-induced diarrhea: Randomized double-blind trial. *Arch Intern Med* 146:1101-1104, 1986.

DuPont HL: Nonfluid therapy and selected chemoprophylaxis of acute diarrhea. *Am J Med* 78 (suppl 6B):81-90, 1985.

DuPont HL, et al: Treatment of travelers' diarrhea with trimethoprim/sulfamethoxazole and with trimethoprim alone. *N Engl J Med* 307:841-844, 1982.

DuPont HL, et al: Use of norfloxacin in treatment of acute diarrheal disease. *Am J Med* 82 (suppl 6B):79-83, 1987.

Ericsson CD, et al: Ciprofloxacin or trimethoprim/sulfamethoxazole as initial therapy for travelers' diarrhea: Placebo-controlled, randomized trial. *Ann Intern Med* 106:216-220, 1987.

Ericsson CD, et al: Treatment of traveler's diarrhea with sulfamethoxazole and trimethoprim and loperamide. *JAMA* 263:257-261, 1990.

Fekety R, et al: Treatment of antibiotic-associated *Clostridium difficile* colitis with oral vancomycin: Comparison of two dosage regimens. *Am J Med* 86:15-19, 1989.

Finegold SM, Wexler HM: Therapeutic implications of bacteriologic findings in mixed aerobic-anaerobic infections. *Antimicrob Agents Chemother* 32:611-616, 1988.

George WL, et al: *Aeromonas*-related diarrhea in adults. *Arch Intern Med* 145:2207-2211, 1985.

Goodman LJ, et al: Empiric antimicrobial therapy of domestically acquired acute diarrhea in urban adults. *Arch Intern Med* 150:541-546, 1990.

Gorbach SL, Edelman R (eds): Travelers' diarrhea: National Institutes of Health Consensus Development Conference. *Rev Infect Dis* 8 (suppl 2): S109-S233, 1986.

Graham DY, Klein PD: *Campylobacter pyloridis* gastritis: Past, present, and speculations about future. *Am J Gastroenterol* 82:283-286, 1987.

Gregory PB: Gallstones and biliary tract disease, in Rubenstein E, Federman DD (eds): *Scientific American Medicine.* New York, Scientific American, 1986, 4:VI:1-10.

Griffen PM, et al: Illness associated with *Escherichia coli* O157:H7 infections. Broad clinical spectrum *Ann Intern Med* 109:705-712, 1988.

Guerrant RL, et al: Acute infectious diarrhea, I: Epidemiology, etiology and pathogenesis. *Pediatr Infect Dis* 5:353-359, 1986.

Hackford AW, et al: Prospective study comparing imipenem/cilastatin with clindamycin and gentamicin for treatment of serious surgical infections. *Arch Surg* 123:322-326, 1988.

Ho JL, Barza M: Role of aminoglycoside antibiotics in treatment of intra-abdominal infections. *Antimicrob Agents Chemother* 31:485-491, 1987.

Holmberg SD, et al: *Plesiomonas* enteric infections in United States. *Ann Intern Med* 105:690-694, 1986.

Hook EW: *Salmonella* species (including typhoid fever), in Mandell GL, et al (eds): *Principles and Practice of Infectious Diseases,* ed 3. New York, Churchill Livingstone, 1990, 1700-1716.

Johnson PC, et al: Comparison of loperamide with bismuth subsalicylate for treatment of acute travelers' diarrhea. *JAMA* 255:757-760, 1986.

Levine MM: *Escherichia coli* that cause diarrhea: Enterotoxigenic, enteropathogenic, enteroinvasive, enterohemorrhagic, and enteroadherent. *J Infect Dis* 155:377-389, 1987.

Levison ME, Bush LM: Peritonitis and other intra-abdominal infections, in Mandell GL, et al (eds): *Principles and Practice of Infectious Diseases*, ed 3. New York, Churchill Livingstone, 1990, 636-670.

Lyerly DM, et al: *Clostridium difficile*: Its disease and toxins. *Clin Microbiol Rev* 1:1-18, 1988.

Malangoni MA, et al: Treatment of intra-abdominal infections is appropriate with single agent or combination therapy. *Surgery* 98:648-655, 1985.

Mandal BK, et al: Double-blind placebo-controlled trial of erythromycin in treatment of clinical *Campylobacter* infection. *J Antimicrob Chemother* 13:619-623, 1984.

Murray BE, et al: Increasing resistance to trimethoprim/sulfamethoxazole among isolates of *Escherichia coli* in developing countries. *J Infect Dis* 152:1107-1113, 1985.

National Institutes of Health Consensus Development Conference: Travelers' diarrhea. *JAMA* 253:2700-2704, 1985.

Neill MA, et al: Failure of ciprofloxacin to eradicate convalescent fecal excretion after acute salmonellosis: Experience during an outbreak in health care workers. *Ann Intern Med* 114:195-199, 1991.

Oldfield EC III, et al: Endemic infectious diseases of the Middle East. *Rev Infect Dis* 13 (suppl 3):S199-S217, 1991.

Perrillo RP, et al: Prednisone withdrawal followed by recombinant alpha interferon in treatment of chronic type B hepatitis: Randomized controlled trial. *Ann Intern Med* 109:95-100, 1988.

Pichler HET, et al: Clinical efficacy of ciprofloxacin compared with placebo in bacterial diarrhea. *Am J Med* 82 (suppl 4A):329-332, 1987.

Salazar-Lindo E, et al: Early treatment with erythromycin of *Campylobacter jejuni*-associated dysentery in children. *J Pediatr* 109:355-360, 1986.

Sanford JP: *Guide to Antimicrobial Therapy, 1990*. West Bethesda, Md, Antimicrobial Therapy, 1990, 10.

Soe GB, Overturf GD: Treatment of typhoid fever and other systemic salmonelloses with cefotaxime, ceftriaxone, cefoperazone, and other newer cephalosporins. *Rev Infect Dis* 9:719-736, 1987.

Solomkin JS, et al: Randomized trial of imipenem/cilastatin versus gentamicin and clindamycin in mixed flora infections. *Am J Med* 78 (suppl 6A):85-91, 1985.

Solomkin JS, et al: Results of a multicenter trial comparing imipenem/cilastatin to tobramycin/clindamycin for intra-abdominal infections. *Ann Surg* 212:581-591, 1990.

St. Geme JW, et al: Consensus: Management of *Salmonella* infection in first year of life. *Pediatr Infect Dis J* 7:615-621, 1988.

Styrt B, Gorbach SL: Recent developments in understanding of pathogenesis and treatment of anaerobic infections (Parts 1 and 2). *N Engl J Med* 321:240-246, 298-302, 1989.

Tauxe RV, et al: Antimicrobial resistance of *Shigella* isolates in the USA: The importance of international travelers. *J Infect Dis* 162: 1107-1111, 1990.

Teasley DG, et al: Prospective randomised trial of metronidazole versus vancomycin for *Clostridium difficile*-associated diarrhoea and colitis. *Lancet* 2:1043-1046, 1983.

Williams EK, et al: Acute infectious diarrhea, II: Diagnosis, treatment and prevention. *Pediatr Infect Dis* 5:458-465, 1986.

Young GP, et al: Antibiotic-associated colitis due to *Clostridium difficile*: Double-blind comparison of vancomycin with bacitracin. *Gastroenterology* 89:1038-1045, 1985.

Reproductive Tract Infections (Female)

1989 Sexually transmitted diseases treatment guidelines. *MMWR* 38 (suppl 8):1-43, 1989.

Cunha BA: Treatment of pelvic inflammatory disease. *Clin Pharm* 9:275-285, 1990.

Levin S, et al: Office approach to sexually transmitted diseases: Part I. *Dis Mon* 33:121-179, 1987.

Penn RL: Gynecological and obstetrical infections, in Reese RE, Douglas RG Jr (eds): *A Practical Approach to Infectious Diseases*, ed 2. Boston, Little Brown, 1986, 385-421.

Sanford JP: *Guide to Antimicrobial Therapy, 1990*. West Bethesda, Md, Antimicrobial Therapy, Inc, 1990, 16.

Reproductive Tract Infections (Male)

1989 Sexually transmitted diseases treatment guidelines. *MMWR* 38 (suppl 8):1-43, 1989.

Berger RE, et al: Etiology and manifestations of epididymitis in young men: Correlations with sexual orientation. *J Infect Dis* 155:1341-1343, 1987.

Chodak GW: Prostatitis, epididymitis, and balanoposthitis, in Kass EH, Platt R (eds): *Current Therapy in Infectious Disease-2*. Philadelphia, BC Decker, 1986, 248-251.

Sanford JP: *Guide to Antimicrobial Therapy, 1990*. West Bethesda, Md, Antimicrobial Therapy, Inc, 1990, 13-14.

Votteler TP: Epididymitis and orchitis, in Nelson JD (ed): *Current Therapy in Pediatric Infectious Disease*. Philadelphia, BC Decker, 1986, 124-125.

Respiratory Tract Infections (Lower)

The choice of antimicrobial drugs. *Med Lett Drugs Ther* 32:41-48, 1990.

Report of the Committee on Infectious Diseases, in: *American Academy of Pediatrics Redbook*, ed 21. Elk Grove Village, Ill, American Academy of Pediatrics, 1988, 315-325.

Ribavirin (*Virazole*). *Med Lett Drugs Ther* 28:46-48, 1986.

Anthonisen NR, et al: Antibiotic therapy of chronic obstructive pulmonary disease. *Ann Intern Med* 106:196-204, 1987.

Bartlett JG: Anaerobic bacterial infections of lung. *Chest* 91:901-909, 1987.

Bass JW: Pertussis: Current status of prevention and treatment. *Pediatr Infect Dis* 4:614-619, 1985.

Brown RB: Acute and chronic bronchitis: Practical management strategy. *Postgrad Med* 85:249-254, 1989.

Brumfitt W, Hamilton-Miller J: Methicillin-resistant *Staphylococcus aureus*. *N Engl J Med* 320:1188-1196, 1989.

Conte JE Jr, Barriere SL: *Manual of Antibiotics and Infectious Diseases,* ed 6. Philadelphia, Lea & Febiger, 1988, 106-107, 124-126, 127-134.

Crane LR, Komshian S: Gram-negative bacillary pneumonias, in Pennington JE (ed): *Respiratory Infections: Diagnosis and Management,* ed 2. New York, Raven Press, 1988, 314-340.

Cunha BA: Pneumonias acquired from others: 1. History, examination and laboratory findings; 2. Radiographic findings, treatment. *Postgrad Med* 82:126-140; 149-156, 1987.

Donowitz GR, Mandell GL: Acute pneumonia, in Mandell GL, et al (eds): *Principles and Practice of Infectious Diseases*, ed 3. New York, Churchill Livingstone, 1990, 540-555.

Edelstein PH, Meyer RD: *Legionella* pneumonias, in Pennington JE (ed): *Respiratory Infections: Diagnosis and Management,* ed 2. New York, Raven Press, 1988, 381-402.

Francke E: Legionnaires' disease: Clinical and pathologic features and current management. *Postgrad Med* 73:347-354, (Feb) 1983.

Gleckman RA: Bronchial infections: Acute bronchitis and acute exacerbation of chronic bronchitis. *Compr Ther* 13:44-48, 1987.

Gleckman RA, Roth RM: Community-acquired bacterial pneumonia in the elderly. *Pharmacotherapy* 4:81-88, 1984.

Grayston JT, et al: New *Chlamydia psittaci* strain, TWAR, isolated in acute respiratory tract infections. *N Engl J Med* 315:161-168, 1986.

Gwaltney JM Jr: Acute bronchitis, in Mandell GL, et al (eds): *Principles and Practice of Infectious Diseases*, ed 3. New York, Churchill Livingstone, 1990, 529-531.

Hager H, et al: *Branhamella catarrhalis* respiratory infections. *Rev Infect Dis* 9:1140-1149, 1987.

Hall CB, Hall WJ: Bronchiolitis, in Mandell GL, et al (eds): *Principles and Practice of Infectious Diseases*, ed 3. New York, Churchill Livingstone, 1990, 535-540.

Hewlett EL: *Bordetella* species, in Mandell GL, et al (eds): *Principles and Practice of Infectious Diseases*, ed 3. New York, Churchill Livingstone, 1990, 1756-1762.

Jorgensen JH, et al: Antimicrobial resistance among respiratory isolates of *Haemophilus influenzae, Moraxella catarrhalis*, and *Streptococcus pneumoniae* in the United States. *Antimicrob Agents Chemother* 34:2075-2080, 1990.

Marrie TJ, et al: Pneumonia associated with the TWAR strain of *Chlamydia. Ann Intern Med* 106:507-511, 1987.

Medina I, et al: Oral therapy for *Pneumocystis carinii* pneumonia in the acquired immunodeficiency syndrome: A controlled trial of trimethoprim/sulfamethoxazole versus trimethoprim/dapsone. *N Engl J Med* 323:776-782, 1990.

Nelson JD: *1991-1992 Pocketbook of Pediatric Antimicrobial Therapy*, ed 9. Baltimore, Williams & Wilkins, 1991, 25-30.

Neu HC: New antibiotics: Areas of appropriate use. *J Infect Dis* 155:403-417, 1987.

Nicotra B, et al: *Branhamella catarrhalis* as lower respiratory tract pathogen in patients with chronic lung disease. *Arch Intern Med* 146:890-893, 1986.

Oberlin JA, Hyslop DL: Cefaclor treatment of upper and lower respiratory tract infections caused by *Moraxella catarrhalis. Pediatr Infect Dis J* 9:41-44, 1990.

Pennington JE: Treating respiratory infections in era of cost control. *Am Fam Physician* 33:153-160, 1986.

Reynolds HY: Chronic bronchitis and acute infectious exacerbations, in Mandell GL, et al (eds): *Principles and Practice of Infectious Diseases*, ed 3. New York, Churchill Livingstone, 1990, 531-535.

Sanford JP: *Guide to Antimicrobial Therapy, 1990.* West Bethesda, Md, Antimicrobial Therapy, 1990, 22-23.

Teele D: Pneumonia: Antimicrobial therapy for infants and children. *Pediatr Infect Dis* 4:330-335, 1985.

Verghese A, et al: Randomized comparative study of cefixime versus cephalexin in acute bacterial exacerbations of chronic bronchitis. *Antimicrob Agents Chemother* 34:1041-1044, 1990.

Walzer PD: *Pneumocystis carinii* pneumonia. *Infect Med* 4:110-116, 1987.

Respiratory Tract Infections (Upper)

The choice of antimicrobial drugs. *Med Lett Drugs Ther* 32:41-48, 1990.

Rapid office diagnostic tests for streptococcal pharyngitis. *Med Lett Drugs Ther* 27:49-51, 1985.

Report of the Committee on Infectious Diseases, in: *American Academy of Pediatrics Redbook,* ed 21. Elk Grove Village, Il, American Academy of Pediatrics, 1988, 174-179, 386-395.

1989 Sexually transmitted diseases treatment guidelines. *MMWR* 38(suppl 8):1-43, 1989.

Bluestone CD (ed): Diagnosis and management of sinusitis in children. *Pediatr Infect Dis* 4(suppl):S49-S81, 1985.

Cohen EL: Epiglottitis in adult: Recognizing and treating acute case. *Postgrad Med* 75:309-311, (March) 1984.

Congeni B, et al: Outbreak of acute rheumatic fever in northeast Ohio. *J Pediatr* 111:176-179, 1987.

Dajani AS, et al: Prevention of rheumatic fever: Statement for health professionals by the Committee on Rheumatic Fever, Endocarditis, and Kawasaki Disease of the Council on Cardiovascular Disease in the Young, the American Heart Association. *Circulation* 78:1082-1086, 1988.

Daley CL, Sande M: The runny nose: Infection of paranasal sinuses. *Infect Dis Clin North Am* 2:131-147, 1988.

Dillon HC: Streptococcal pharyngitis in the 1980s. *Pediatr Infect Dis J* 6:123-130, 1987.

Hosier DM, et al: Resurgence of acute rheumatic fever. *Am J Dis Child* 141:730-733, 1987.

Huovinen P, et al: Pharyngitis in adults: Presence and coexistence of viruses and bacterial organisms. *Ann Intern Med* 110:612-616, 1989.

Myer CM: Sinusitis and chronic rhinitis: Otolaryngologist's view. *Infect Med* 4:100-116, 1987.

Nelson JD: *1991-1992 Pocketbook of Pediatric Antimicrobial Therapy*, ed 9. Baltimore, Williams & Wilkins, 1991, 25.

Pichichero ME, et al: Adverse and beneficial effects of immediate treatment of Group A beta-hemolytic streptococcal pharyngitis with penicillin. *Pediatr Infect Dis J* 6:635-643, 1987.

Radetsky M, et al: Identification of streptococcal pharyngitis in office laboratory: Reassessment of new technology. *Pediatr Infect Dis J* 6:556-563, 1987.

Randolph MF, et al: Effect of antibiotic therapy on clinical course of streptococcal pharyngitis. *J Pediatr* 106:870-875, 1985.

Smith AL: Does penicillin improve symptoms of strep throat? *Pediatr Alert* 9:17-18, 1984.

Todd JK: The sore throat: Pharyngitis and epiglottitis. *Infect Dis Clin North Am* 2:149-162, 1988.

Veasy LG, et al: Resurgence of acute rheumatic fever in intermountain area of United States. *N Engl J Med* 316:421-427, 1987.

Wald ER: Sinusitis in children. *Pediatr Infect Dis J* 7:S150-S153, 1988.

Wald ER, et al: Acute rheumatic fever in western Pennsylvania and tristate area. *Pediatrics* 80:371-374, 1987.

Skin and Soft-Tissue Infections

The choice of antimicrobial drugs. *Med Lett Drugs Ther* 32:41-48, 1990.

Mupirocin: New topical antibiotic. *Med Lett Drugs Ther* 30:55-56, 1988.

Allman RM: Pressure ulcers among the elderly. *N Engl J Med* 320: 850-853, 1989.

Arathoon EG, et al: Efficacy of short courses of oral novobiocin-rifampin in eradicating carrier state of methicillin-resistant *Staphylococcus aureus* and in vitro killing studies of clinical isolates. *Antimicrob Agents Chemother* 34:1655-1659, 1990.

Berger TG, et al: Bacillary (epithelioid) angiomatosis and concurrent Kaposi's sarcoma in acquired immunodeficiency syndrome. *Arch Dermatol* 125:1543-1547, 1989.

Bradsher RW Jr, Snow RW: Ceftriaxone treatment of skin and soft tissue infections in a once daily regimen. *Am J Med* 63-67, (Oct 19) 1984.

Casewell MW, Hill RLR: Elimination of nasal carriage ot *Staphylococcus aureus* with mupirocin ('pseudomonic acid')—a controlled trial. *J Antimicrob Chemother* 17:365-372, 1986.

Cockerell CJ, LeBoit PE: Bacillary angiomatosis: A newly characterized, pseudoneoplastic, infectious, cutaneous vascular disorder. *J Am Acad Dermatol* 22:501-512, 1990.

Conte JE Jr, Barriere SL: *Manual of Antibiotics and Infectious Diseases*, ed 6. Philadelphia, Lea & Febiger, 1988, 108.

Coskey RJ, Coskey LA: Diagnosis and treatment of impetigo. *J Am Acad Dermatol* 17:62-63, 1987.

Daly JS, et al: Randomized, double-blind trial of cefonicid and nafcillin in the treatment of skin and skin structure infections. *Antimicrob Agents Chemother* 34:654-656, 1990.

Demling RH: Burns. *N Engl J Med* 313:1389-1398, 1985.

Duncan WC: Erythrasma and trichomycosis axillaris, in Hoeprich PD (ed): *Infectious Diseases*, ed 3. Philadelphia, Harper & Row, 1983, 933-936.

Frenkel LD, the Multicenter Ceftriaxone Pediatric Study Group: Once-daily administration of ceftriaxone for the treatment of selected serious bacterial infections in children. *Pediatrics* 82(part 2):486-491, 1988.

Goldfarb J, et al: Randomized clinical trial of topical mupirocin versus oral erythromycin for impetigo. *Antimicrob Agents Chemother* 32:1780-1783, 1988.

Goldstein EJC: Animal bite infection, in Kass EH, Platt R (eds): *Current Therapy in Infectious Disease-2*. Philadelphia, BC Decker, 1986, 112-121.

Goldstein EJC: Management of human and animal bite wounds. *J Am Acad Dermatol* 21:1275-1279, 1989.

Goldstein EJC, et al: Outpatient therapy of bite wounds: Demographic data, bacteriology, and prospective, randomized trial of amoxicillin/clavulanic acid versus penicillin ± dicloxacillin. *Int J Dermatol* 26:123-127, 1987.

Hicklin H, et al: Dysgonic fermenter 2 septicemia. *Rev Infect Dis* 9:884-890, 1987.

Hill RLR, et al: Elimination of nasal carriage of methicillin-resistant *Staphylococcus aureus* with mupirocin during a hospital outbreak. *J Antimicrob Chemother* 22:377-384, 1988.

Hook EW III, et al: Microbiologic evaluation of cutaneous cellulitis in adults. *Arch Intern Med* 146:295-297, 1986.

Hooper DC, Wolfson JS: Fluoroquinolone antimicrobial agents. *N Engl J Med* 324:384-394, 1991.

Huff JC, et al: Therapy of herpes zoster with oral acyclovir. *Am J Med* 85 (suppl 2A):84-89, 1988.

Jacobson JA: Pool-associated *Pseudomonas aeruginosa* dermatitis and other bathing-associated infections. *Infect Control* 6:398-401, 1985.

Klempner MS, Styrt B: Prevention of recurrent staphylococcal skin infections with low-dose oral clindamycin therapy. *JAMA* 260:2682-2685, 1988.

Koehler JE, et al: Cutaneous vascular lesions and disseminated cat-scratch disease in patients with the acquired immunodeficiency syndrome (AIDS) and AIDS-related complex. *Ann Intern Med* 109:449-455, 1988.

Luterman A, et al: Infections in burn patients. *Am J Med* 81 (suppl 1A):45-52, 1986.

Maibach HI, et al: Bacterial infections of the skin, in Moschella SL, Hurley HJ (eds): *Dermatology*, ed 2. Philadelphia, WB Saunders, 1985, 599-642.

Marcy SM: Infection following bite, in Nelson JD (ed): *Current Therapy in Pediatric Infectious Disease*. Philadelphia, BC Decker, 1986, 81-83.

Martin LT: Human bites: Guidelines for prompt evaluation and treatment. *Postgrad Med* 81:221-224, 1987.

McLinn S: Topical mupirocin *vs.* systemic erythromycin treatment for pyoderma. *Pediatr Infect Dis J* 7:785-790, 1988.

Melish ME: Staphylococcal scalded skin syndrome, in Nelson JD (ed): *Current Therapy in Pediatric Infectious Disease*. Philadelphia, BC Decker, 1986 A, 88-90.

Melish ME: Pyogenic skin infections, in Braude AI, et al (eds): *Infectious Diseases and Medical Microbiology*, ed 2. Philadelphia, WB Saunders, 1986 B, 1321-1324.

Mertz PM, et al: Topical mupirocin treatment of impetigo is equal to oral erythromycin therapy. *Arch Dermatol* 125:1069-1073, 1989.

Nelson JD: *1991-1992 Pocketbook of Pediatric Antimicrobial Therapy*, ed 9. Baltimore, Williams & Wilkins, 1991, 18-21.

Odom R: Effective drug therapy in streptococcal skin infections. *Mod Med* 57:130-139, (May) 1989.

Relman DA, et al: The agent of bacillary angiomatosis: An approach to the identification of uncultured pathogens. *N Engl J Med* 323:1573-1580, 1990.

Sachs MK, Pilgrim C: Ampicillin/sulbactam compared with cefazolin or cefoxitin for the treatment of skin and skin structure infections. *Drug Invest* 2:173-183, 1990.

Sanford JP: *Guide to Antimicrobial Therapy, 1990.* West Bethesda, Md, Antimicrobial Therapy, 1990, 27-30.

Spruance SL, et al: Acyclovir prevents reactivation of herpes simplex labialis in skiers. *JAMA* 260:1597-1599, 1988.

Stoler MH, et al: An atypical subcutaneous infection associated with acquired immune deficiency syndrome. *Am J Clin Pathol* 80:714-718, 1983.

Swartz MN: Cellulitis and superficial infections, in Mandell GL, et al (eds): *Principles and Practice of Infectious Diseases*, ed 3. New York, Churchill Livingstone, 1990, 796-807.

Tompkins RG, Burke JF: Infection following burn injury, in Kass EH, Platt R (eds): *Current Therapy in Infectious Disease-2.* Philadelphia, BC Decker, 1986, 106-108.

Trucksis M, et al: Emerging resistance to fluoroquinolones in staphylococci: An alert. *Ann Intern Med* 114:424-426, 1991.

Wheat LJ, et al: Long-term studies of effect of rifampin on nasal carriage of coagulase-positive staphylococci. *Rev Infect Dis* 5 (suppl 3):S459-S462, (July-Aug) 1983.

Wood MJ, et al: Efficacy of oral acyclovir treatment of acute herpes zoster. *Am J Med* 85 (suppl 2A):79-83, 1988.

Yamauchi T: Cellulitis, in Nelson JD (ed): *Current Therapy in Pediatric Infectious Disease.* Philadelphia, BC Decker, 1986, 75-76.

Yoshikawa TT: Cellulitis and soft tissue infection, in Kass EH, Platt R (eds): *Current Therapy in Infectious Disease-2.* Philadelphia, BC Decker, 1986, 266-268.

Yurt RW, Shires GT: Burns, in Mandell GL, et al (eds): *Principles and Practice of Infectious Diseases.* New York, Churchill Livingstone, 1990, 830-834.

Urinary Tract Infections

1989 Sexually transmitted diseases treatment guidelines. *MMWR* 38 (suppl 8):1-43, 1989.

Angel JL, et al: Acute pyelonephritis in pregnancy: A prospective study of oral versus intravenous antibiotic therapy. *Obstet Gynecol* 76:28-32, 1990.

Boscia JA, Kaye D: Asymptomatic bacteriuria in elderly. *Infect Dis Clin North Am* 1:893-905, 1987.

Boscia JA, et al: Asymptomatic bacteriuria in elderly persons: Treat or do not treat? *Ann Intern Med* 106:764-766, 1987.

Brumfitt W, Hamilton-Miller JMT: Comparative study of cephradine and amoxicillin-clavulanate in the treatment of recurrent urinary tract infections. *Antimicrob Agents Chemother* 34:1803-1805, 1990.

Carlson KJ, Mulley AG: Management of acute dysuria: Decision-analysis model of alternative strategies. *Ann Intern Med* 102:244-249, 1985.

Coraggio MJ, et al: Nitrofurantoin toxicity in children. *Pediatr Infect Dis J* 8:163-166, 1989.

Fihn SD, et al: Trimethoprim/sulfamethoxazole for acute dysuria in women: Single-dose or 10-day course: Double-blind, randomized trial. *Ann Intern Med* 108:350-357, 1988.

Gleckman RA: Infections of female urinary tract: Office treatment of selected types. *Postgrad Med* 82:165-171, (Aug) 1987 A.

Gleckman RA: Treatment duration for urinary tract infections in adults. *Antimicrob Agents Chemother* 31:1-5, 1987 B.

Johnson JR, Stamm WE: Diagnosis and treatment of acute urinary tract infections. *Infect Dis Clin North Am* 1:773-791, 1987.

Johnson JR, Stamm WE: Urinary tract infections in women: Diagnosis and treatment. *Ann Intern Med* 111:906-917, 1989.

Jones KV: Antimicrobial treatment for urinary tract infections. *Arch Dis Child* 65:327-330, 1990.

Komaroff AL: Urinalysis and urine culture in women with dysuria. *Ann Intern Med* 104:212-218, 1986.

Lebel M: Ciprofloxacin: Chemistry, mechanism of action, resistance, antimicrobial spectrum, pharmacokinetics, clinical trials, and adverse reactions. *Pharmacotherapy* 8:3-33, 1988.

Lebel MH, McCracken GH: Aztreonam: Review of the clinical experience and potential uses in pediatrics. *Pediatr Infect Dis J* 7:331-339, 1988.

Lipsky BA: Urinary tract infections in men: Epidemiology, pathophysiology, diagnosis, and treatment. *Ann Intern Med* 110:138-150, 1989

Madrigal G, et al: Single dose antibiotic therapy is not as effective as conventional regimens for management of acute urinary tract infections in children. *Pediatr Infect Dis J* 7:316-319, 1988.

Meares EM Jr: Acute and chronic prostatitis: Diagnosis and treatment. *Infect Dis Clin North Am* 1:855-873, 1987.

Nicolle LE, Ronald AR: Recurrent urinary tract infection in adult women: Diagnosis and treatment. *Infect Dis Clin North Am* 1:793-806, 1987.

Norrby SR: Short-term treatment of uncomplicated lower urinary tract infections in women. *Rev Infect Dis* 12:458-467, 1990.

Patterson TF, Andriole VT: Bacteriuria in pregnancy. *Infect Dis Clin North Am* 1:807-822, 1987.

Pedler SJ, Bint AJ: Management of bacteriuria in pregnancy. *Drugs* 33:413-421, 1987.

Pfau A: Prostatitis: Continuing enigma. *Urol Clin North Am* 13:695-715, 1986.

Sabbaj J, et al: Multiclinic comparative study of norfloxacin and trimethoprim/sulfamethoxazole for treatment of urinary tract infections. *Antimicrob Agents Chemother* 27:297-301, 1985.

Safrin S, et al: Pyelonephritis in adult women: Inpatient versus outpatient therapy. *Am J Med* 85:793-798, 1988.

Sandberg T, et al: Randomised double-blind study of norfloxacin and cefadroxil in the treatment of acute pyelonephritis. *Eur J Clin Microbiol Infect Dis* 9:317-323, 1990.

Sobel JD, Kaye D: Urinary tract infections, in Mandell GL, et al (eds): *Principles and Practice of Infectious Diseases*, ed 3. New York, Churchill Livingstone, 1990, 582-611.

Stamm WE, et al: Acute renal infection in women: Treatment with trimethoprim/sulfamethoxazole or ampicillin for two or six weeks. *Ann Intern Med* 106:341-345, 1987.

Stamm WE, et al: Urinary tract infections: From pathogenesis to treatment. *J Infect Dis* 159:400-406, 1989.

Stapleton A, et al: Postcoital antimicrobial prophylaxis for recurrent urinary tract infection: A randomized, double-blind, placebo-controlled trial. *JAMA* 264:703-706, 1990.

Tolkoff-Rubin NE, Rubin RH: Ciprofloxacin in management of urinary tract infection. *Urology* 31:359-367, 1988.

Miscellaneous Infections

The choice of antimicrobial drugs. *Med Lett Drugs Ther* 32:41-48, 1990.

Treatment of Lyme disease. *Med Lett Drugs Ther* 31:57-59, 1989.

Abele DC, et al: The many faces and phases of borreliosis, I: Lyme disease. *J Am Acad Dermatol* 23:167-186, 1990.

Armstrong D: *Listeria monocytogenes,* in Mandell GL, et al (eds): *Principles and Practice of Infectious Diseases,* ed 3. New York, Churchill Livingstone, 1990, 1587-1593.

Bornstein DL: Clostridial myonecrosis, in Braude AI, et al (eds): *Infectious Diseases and Medical Microbiology,* ed 2. Philadelphia, WB Saunders, 1986, 1490-1495.

Boyce JM: *Francisella tularensis* (tularemia), in Mandell GL, et al (eds): *Principles and Practice of Infectious Diseases,* ed 3. New York, Churchill Livingstone, 1990, 1742-1746.

Butler T: *Yersinia* species (including plague), in Mandell GL, et al (eds): *Principles and Practice of Infectious Diseases,* ed 3. New York, Churchill Livingstone, 1990, 1748-1756.

Cate TR: *Clostridium tetani* (tetanus), in Mandell GL, et al (eds): *Principles and Practice of Infectious Diseases,* ed 3. New York, Churchill Livingstone, 1990, 1842-1846.

Conte JE Jr, Barriere SL: *Manual of Antibiotics and Infectious Diseases,* ed 6. Philadelphia, Lea & Febiger, 1988, 109-134.

Dattwyler RJ, et al: Treatment of late Lyme borreliosis: Randomized comparison of ceftriaxone and penicillin. *Lancet* 1:1191-1194, 1988.

Farrar WE: *Leptospira* species (leptospirosis), in Mandell GL, et al (eds): *Principles and Practice of Infectious Diseases,* ed 3. New York, Churchill Livingstone, 1990, 1813-1816.

Fischer GW: The agent of cat scratch disease, in Mandell GL, et al (eds): *Principles and Practice of Infectious Diseases,* ed 3. New York, Churchill Livingstone, 1990, 1874-1877.

Gellin BG, Broome CV: Listeriosis. *JAMA* 261:1313-1320, 1989.

Goodwin SD, et al: Management of Lyme disease. *Clin Pharm* 9:192-205, 1990.

Hall WH: Modern chemotherapy for brucellosis in humans. *Rev Infect Dis* 12:1060-1099, 1990.

Holley HP Jr: Successful treatment of cat-scratch disease with ciprofloxacin. *JAMA* 265:1563-1565, 1991.

Johnson WD Jr: *Borrelia* species (relapsing fever), in Mandell GL, et al (eds): *Principles and Practice of Infectious Diseases,* ed 3. New York, Churchill Livingstone, 1990, 1816-1819.

Kamper CA, et al: Rocky Mountain spotted fever. *Clin Pharm* 7:109-116, 1988.

Laforce FM: *Bacillus anthracis* (anthrax), in Mandell GL, et al (eds): *Principles and Practice of Infectious Diseases,* ed 3. New York, Churchill Livingstone, 1990, 1593-1595.

Lancaster LA, Attebery HR: Vincent's infection, in Braude AI, et al (eds): *Infectious Diseases and Medical Microbiology,* ed 2. Philadelphia, WB Saunders, 1986, 722-724.

Leelarasamee A, Bovornkitti S: Melioidosis: Review and update. *Rev Infect Dis* 11:413-425, 1989.

Lerner PI: *Actinomyces* and *Arachnia* species, in Mandell GL, et al (eds): *Principles and Practice of Infectious Diseases,* ed 3. New York, Churchill Livingstone, 1990 A, 1932-1942.

Lerner PI: *Nocardia* species, in Mandell GL, et al (eds): *Principles and Practice of Infectious Diseases,* ed 3. New York, Churchill Livingstone, 1990 B, 1926-1932.

Mikolich DJ, Boyce JM: *Brucella* species, in Mandell GL, et al (eds): *Principles and Practice of Infectious Diseases,* ed 3. New York, Churchill Livingstone, 1990, 1735-1742.

Nelson JD: *1991-1992 Pocketbook of Pediatric Antimicrobial Therapy,* ed 9. Baltimore, Williams & Wilkins, 1991 A, 44-53.

Nelson JD: *1991-1992 Pocketbook of Pediatric Antimicrobial Therapy,* ed 9. Baltimore, Williams & Wilkins, 1991 B, 18-42.

Saah AJ: Introduction, Section D. Rickettsiosis, in Mandell GL, et al (eds): *Principles and Practice of Infectious Diseases,* ed 3. New York, Churchill Livingstone, 1990, 1463-1465.

Sanford JP: *Guide to Antimicrobial Therapy, 1990.* West Bethesda, Md, Antimicrobial Therapy, 1990 A, 3-32.

Sanford JP: *Guide to Antimicrobial Therapy, 1990.* West Bethesda, Md, Antimicrobial Therapy, 1990 B, 37-40.

Sanford JP: *Guide to Antimicrobial Therapy, 1990.* West Bethesda, Md, Antimicrobial Therapy, 1990 C, 63-67.

Sanford JP: *Pseudomonas* species (including melioidosis and glanders), in Mandell GL, et al (eds): *Principles and Practice of Infectious Diseases,* ed 3. New York, Churchill Livingstone, 1990 D, 1692-1696.

Smego RA Jr, et al: Trimethoprim-sulfamethoxazole therapy for *Nocardia* infections. *Arch Intern Med* 143:711-718, 1983.

Steere AC, et al: Treatment of early manifestations of Lyme disease. *Ann Intern Med* 99:22-26, 1983 A.

Steere AC, et al: Neurologic abnormalities of Lyme disease: Successful treatment with high-dose intravenous penicillin. *Ann Intern Med* 99:767-772, 1983 B.

Steere AC, et al: Successful parenteral penicillin therapy of established Lyme arthritis. *N Engl J Med* 312:869-874, 1985.

White NJ, et al: Halving of mortality of severe melioidosis by ceftazidime. *Lancet* 2:697-701, 1989.

Treatment of Sexually Transmitted Diseases

60

CHLAMYDIA TRACHOMATIS INFECTIONS

GONOCOCCAL INFECTIONS

COMMON STD-ASSOCIATED SYNDROMES

TRICHOMONIASIS

GENITAL HERPES SIMPLEX VIRUS INFECTIONS

GENITAL AND ANAL WARTS (CONDYLOMA ACUMINATUM)

SYPHILIS

CHANCROID

LYMPHOGRANULOMA VENEREUM

GRANULOMA INGUINALE (DONOVANOSIS)

ENTERIC INFECTIONS

PREVENTION OF OPHTHALMIA NEONATORUM

USE OF CONDOMS TO PREVENT STDS

Sexually transmitted diseases (STDs) are among the more common infections in the United States with over 12 million cases diagnosed annually, and they continue to be a major public health problem (Handsfield, 1991). The well-known venereal diseases, gonorrhea and syphilis, continue to be two of the most common reportable infectious diseases; approximately 500,000 and 35,000 cases, respectively, were reported to the Centers for Disease Control and Prevention (CDC) in 1992 (*MMWR*, 1993 A). Because underreporting is common, the actual incidences of these diseases are undoubtedly higher. Chlamydia is the most common sexually transmitted bacterial pathogen in the United States with more than 4 million cases estimated to develop annually (*MMWR*, 1993 B). Although at least 36 states now require reporting of chlamydia infection, no comprehensive national surveillance system exists for this pathogen (Webster et al, 1993). Comprehensive surveillance data for viral sexually transmitted diseases, pelvic inflammatory disease, and vaginitis are not available. However, it is estimated that 700,000 new cases of genital herpes (Webb and Fife, 1987), and at least 1 million cases each of pelvic inflammatory disease (usually resulting from chlamydial and/or gonococcal infection) (Washington and Katz, 1991), trichomonal infection (Rein and Müller, 1990), and genital warts (Cates, 1987) occur annually in this country. In addition, the spectrum of diseases known to be sexually transmitted, and their complications, has enlarged considerably. This is best exemplified by human immunodeficiency virus (HIV) infection and the acquired immunodeficiency syndrome (AIDS), a fatal disease that has become an epidemic crisis throughout the world (Rapoza, 1989). At present, more than 20 etiologic agents that are largely or exclusively dependent on sexual contact for transmission have been identified (Handsfield, 1991).

Guidelines for the selection of appropriate antimicrobial drugs in the treatment of a number of sexually transmitted diseases, ie, infections in which sexual contact is the primary or an important mechanism of transmission, are presented. Most of the recommendations are consistent with 1993 treatment guidelines proposed by the CDC (*MMWR*, 1993 C). However, some recommendations have been updated to reflect more recently published studies and the views of our consultants.

CHLAMYDIA TRACHOMATIS INFECTIONS

Infections caused by *Chlamydia trachomatis* are the most prevalent bacterial sexually transmitted diseases in the United States today, and they are especially common in adolescents and young adults (ie, <25 years of age). The importance of serious complications (eg, pelvic inflammatory disease, infertility, ectopic pregnancy) related to chlamydial infections in women has been established. In the past, diagnosis and treatment of these infections frequently were based on the clinical syndrome, since cultures were not widely available. Reasonably accurate and economical nonculture chlamydia tests (eg, direct fluorescent antibody, enzyme-linked immunoassay, nucleic acid hybridization tests) are increasingly available. Although nonculture tests are less sensitive and specific than high quality cultures for chlamydia, they are useful to diagnose chlamydial genital infections in groups with high prevalence of these infections (>5%) and also can be used in groups with lower prevalence if confirmatory testing is performed (*MMWR*, 1993 B; Stamm, 1993). The CDC recommend that diagnostic testing for *C. trachomatis* be done when possible on all individuals with compatible clinical syndromes, even if treatment must be initiated and sex partners referred before test results become available (*MMWR*, 1993 B). The following guidelines are for treatment of *laboratory-proven* infections caused by *C. trachomatis* (other than lymphogranuloma venereum [LGV] strains). For approaches to the treatment of common chlamydia-associated syndromes when laboratory confirmation is not yet available, or diagnostic testing cannot be performed, see the section of this chapter entitled, Common STD-Associated Syndromes. See also *MMWR*, 1993 B, 1993 C.

Uncomplicated Urethral, Endocervical, or Rectal Infection in Adults (Confirmed Infection)

RECOMMENDED REGIMENS:
Doxycycline: Orally, 100 mg twice daily for seven days;
OR
Azithromycin: Orally, 1 g as a single dose.
ALTERNATIVE REGIMEN(S):
Ofloxacin: Orally, 300 mg twice daily for seven days;
OR
Erythromycin base: Orally, 500 mg four times daily for seven days;
OR
Erythromycin ethylsuccinate: Orally, 800 mg four times daily for seven days.
REMARKS:
(1) Doxycycline and azithromycin appear to be similar in efficacy and toxicity (Martin et al, 1992). Doxycycline has a longer history of extensive use, safety, and efficacy and the advantage of low cost. Azithromycin has the advantage of single-dose administration. Ofloxacin is similar in efficacy to doxycycline and azithromycin, but it is more expensive than doxycycline, cannot be used during pregnancy or in persons ≤17 years of age, and offers no advantage in dosing. Ofloxacin is the only marketed fluoroquinolone with proven efficacy against chlamydial infection.
(2) **Sulfisoxazole,** orally, 500 mg four times daily for 10 days, also is listed as an alternative regimen for uncomplicated chlamydial infections by the CDC, but its efficacy is inferior to the other regimens.
(3) When taken as directed, the doxycycline, azithromycin, and ofloxacin regimens listed above are highly effective. Also, clinically significant antimicrobial resistance of *C. trachomatis* to recommended regimens has not been observed. Therefore, test-of-cure evaluation is not necessary for patients who complete treatment with one of these regimens unless symptoms persist or reinfection is suspected. Retesting may be considered three weeks after completion of treatment with erythromycin or sulfisoxazole.
(4) Sex partners must be notified (eg, by health department). Sex partners of symptomatic patients with *C. trachomatis* should be evaluated and treated for chlamydia with one of the above regimens if their last sexual contact with the index patient was within 30 days of onset of the index patient's symptoms. If the index patient is asymptomatic, sex partners whose last sexual contact with the index patient was within 60 days of diagnosis should be evaluated and treated. (Note: If last sexual intercourse took place before the foregoing time intervals, then the last sex partner of the index case should be treated as a possible source of infection.) Patients should be instructed to avoid sexual intercourse until patient and partner(s) are cured, ie, until therapy is completed and patient and partner(s) are without symptoms.
(5) Doxycycline and ofloxacin are contraindicated in pregnant women, and the efficacy and safety of azithromycin during pregnancy has not been established. Thus, pregnant women with laboratory-proven *C. trachomatis* infections and/or those whose sexual partners have nongonococcal urethritis should be treated with the above **erythromycin base** regimen. The **erythromycin ethylsuccinate** regimen is an alternative. For women who cannot tolerate these regimens, one-half the daily dose (250 mg base; 400 mg ethylsuccinate) four times daily for 14 days should be used. (Note: Erythromycin estolate should not be used during pregnancy, since drug-related hepatotoxicity can result.) The optimal dose and duration of antibiotic therapy for pregnant women have not been established. Guidance for treatment of pregnant women who are allergic to or cannot tolerate erythromycin is limited. At present, the CDC recommend **amoxicillin,** orally, 500 mg three times daily for seven to ten days as an alternative regimen for pregnant women who are allergic to or cannot tolerate erythromycin. However, limited data exist concerning this regimen (Crombleholme et al, 1990; Magat et al, 1993). Limited data also support the use of **clindamycin**, orally, 450 mg three times daily for 10 days in these patients (see Rein, 1993). One consultant suggested that single-dose azithromycin (FDA Pregnancy Category B) can be recommended for pregnant women who cannot tolerate erythromycin, are late in their pregnancy, and have documented chlamydial infection. Close observation for resolution of symptoms and negative cultures for *C. trachomatis* is recommended in pregnant women. Simultaneous treatment of the male partner(s) is an important component of the therapeutic regimen. Partners should be personally counseled prior to treatment; optimally, all partners should be examined and treated for *C. trachomatis*. To prevent maternal postnatal complications and chlamydial infections among infants, the CDC recommend that pregnant women at increased risk be screened for chlamydia during the third trimester, so that treatment, if needed, will be completed before delivery (*MMWR*, 1993 C). Important risk factors include the following: age <25 years, past history or presence of other sexually transmitted diseases, a new sex partner within the preceding three months, or multiple sex partners. Risk factor analysis alone should not dictate the decision to screen, however; physicians should select a screening strategy compatible with their practice population and setting.
(6) Persons with HIV infection and chlamydial infection should receive the same treatment as patients without HIV infection.

Neonatal Conjunctivitis and Pneumonia (Confirmed Infection)

Conjunctivitis

RECOMMENDED REGIMEN:
Erythromycin syrup: Orally, 50 mg/kg/day divided into four doses for 10 to 14 days.
REMARKS:
(1) Appropriate tests (ie, culture if possible) to rule out *Neisseria gonorrhoeae* as the cause should be done.
(2) The diagnosis of chlamydial conjunctivitis can be established by isolation from tissue culture or by nonculture tests, including direct fluorescent antibody tests or immunoassays,

from ocular exudates containing conjunctival cells. A chlamydial etiology should be considered for all infants ≤30 days with conjunctivitis.
(3) There is no indication that supplemental topical therapy provides additional benefit; topical therapy alone is not effective.
(4) The possibility of chlamydial pneumonia should be considered. The efficacy of erythromycin treatment is approximately 80%; a second course of therapy may be required. Follow-up of infants to determine resolution is recommended.
(5) Mothers of infants with chlamydial conjunctivitis and their sex partner(s) should be examined and treated with one of the regimens recommended for chlamydial infection in adults.

Pneumonia

RECOMMENDED REGIMEN:
Erythromycin syrup: Orally, 50 mg/kg/day divided into four doses for 10 to 14 days.
REMARKS:
(1) Specimens should be collected from the nasopharynx for chlamydial testing. Tissue culture remains the definitive standard for diagnosis of chlamydial pneumonia; nonculture tests of nasopharyngeal specimens can be used with the knowledge that such tests produce lower sensitivity and specificity than nonculture tests of ocular specimens. Because of the delay in obtaining test results for chlamydia, initial treatment should include an agent effective against *C. trachomatis* for all infants one to three months of age with possible pneumonia.
(2) The effectiveness of erythromycin treatment is approximately 80%; a second course of therapy may be required. Follow-up of infants is recommended to determine that the pneumonia has resolved. Some infants with chlamydial pneumonia have had abnormal pulmonary function tests later in childhood.
(3) Mothers of infants with chlamydial pneumonia and their sex partner(s) should be examined and treated with one of the regimens recommended for chlamydial infection in adults.

Chlamydial Infections in Children

Uncomplicated chlamydial infection in children <45 kg

RECOMMENDED REGIMEN:
Erythromycin: Orally, 50 mg/kg/day divided into four doses for 10 to 14 days.
REMARKS:
(1) Children weighing ≥45 kg but who are <8 years of age should receive adult regimens of erythromycin (see Uncomplicated Urethral, Endocervical, or Rectal Infection in Adults). The effectiveness of erythromycin treatment is approximately 80%; a second course of therapy may be required.
(2) Children ≥8 years of age should receive the adult regimen of doxycycline. Adult regimens of azithromycin also may be considered for adolescents.
(3) Follow-up cultures are necessary to ensure that treatment has been effective.
(4) Sexual abuse must be considered a cause of chlamydial infection among preadolescent children, although perinatally transmitted *C. trachomatis* infection of the nasopharynx, urogenital tract, and rectum may persist beyond one year. Because of the potential for a criminal investigation and legal proceedings for sexual abuse, diagnosis of *C. trachomatis* should be made by isolation in cell culture. The cultures should be confirmed by microscopic identification of the characteristic intracytoplasmic inclusions, preferably by fluorescein-conjugated monoclonal antibodies specific for *C. trachomatis*. These children should be evaluated for other sexually transmitted diseases (eg, gonorrhea, syphilis, trichomoniasis, HIV, hepatitis B).

GONOCOCCAL INFECTIONS

These guidelines, as proposed by the CDC (*MMWR*, 1993 C) and with modifications based on the views of consultants, take into account the following observations: (1) the anatomic site of the infection; (2) the increasing incidence of infections due to antibiotic-resistant *Neisseria gonorrhoeae*, including penicillinase-producing *N. gonorrhoeae* (PPNG), high-level tetracycline-resistant gonococci (TRNG), and strains with chromosomally mediated resistance to multiple antibiotics (CMRNG); (3) the high frequency of coexisting chlamydial and gonococcal infections, especially in women and heterosexual men; and (4) the side effects and costs of the various treatment regimens. Regimens have been recommended based on the general criteria of efficacy, safety, ease of administration, patient acceptability, and cost.

Antimicrobial resistance in clinical isolates of *Neisseria gonorrhoeae* is a growing problem. Based on results from the Gonococcal Isolate Surveillance Project (GISP), 32.4% of isolates were resistant to penicillin or tetracycline in the United States during 1991. The percentage distribution of resistant isolates was PPNG, 11%; TRNG, 5.7%; PPNG/TRNG, 2.1%; CMRNG (penicillin only), 1.8%; CMRNG (tetracycline only), 7.2%; and CMRNG (penicillin and tetracycline), 4.6% (Gorwitz et al, 1993). Since resistant organisms are so widespread, the CDC continues to recommend *presumptive* treatment for infections caused by resistant strains (*MMWR*, 1993 C).

Uncomplicated Urethral, Endocervical, or Rectal Infection in Adults

RECOMMENDED REGIMEN(S):
Ceftriaxone: Intramuscularly, 125 mg in a single dose;
OR
Cefixime: Orally, 400 mg in a single dose;
OR
Ofloxacin: Orally, 400 mg in a single dose;
OR
Ciprofloxacin: Orally, 500 mg in a single dose;
Plus
A regimen effective against possible coinfection with *C. trachomatis*, such as doxycycline, orally, 100 mg twice daily for seven days or azithromycin, orally, 1 g in a single dose.
ALTERNATIVE REGIMEN:
Spectinomycin: Intramuscularly, 2 g in a single dose (see REMARKS).
Plus
A regimen effective against possible coinfection with *C. trachomatis*, such as doxycycline, orally, 100 mg twice daily for seven days or azithromycin, orally, 1 g in a single dose.
REMARKS:
(1) Single-dose efficacy is a major consideration in choosing an antibiotic regimen to treat persons infected with *N. gonorrhoeae*. In clinical trials, the recommended regimens cured >95% of anal and genital infections, and any of the regimens may be used for uncomplicated anal or genital infection. Some consultants expressed a preference for an oral regimen to avoid the pain of intramuscular injection of ceftriaxone. Published studies indicate that ceftriaxone 125 mg or ciprofloxacin 500 mg can cure ≥90% of pharyngeal infections. If pharyngeal infection is a concern, either of these two regimens should be used.
(2) Because coinfection with *C. trachomatis* is common (20%

to 30%), persons treated for gonorrhea should be treated presumptively with a regimen that is effective against *C. trachomatis*.

(3) Ceftriaxone is a long-acting ($t_{1/2}$=8 hours) third-generation cephalosporin with excellent in vitro activity against *N. gonorrhoeae*, including PPNG, CMRNG, and TRNG strains. No ceftriaxone-resistant strains of *N. gonorrhoeae* have been reported. A single 125-mg intramuscular dose has been highly effective in uncomplicated gonorrhea in adults, including urethral, endocervical, anorectal, and pharyngeal forms of this infection (Handsfield and Murphy, 1983; Collier et al, 1984; Judson et al, 1985; Handsfield and Hook, 1987; see also index entry Ceftriaxone). In the past, the CDC recommended a 250-mg dose, but the 125-mg dose has a comparable therapeutic margin and is now the recommended dose (*MMWR*, 1993 C). Most of our consultants prefer the 125-mg dose because it is less expensive and can be given in a volume of only 0.5 ml, ie, in the deltoid muscle. The drawbacks of ceftriaxone are that it is expensive, currently unavailable in vials <250 mg, and must be administered by injection. Some practitioners report that mixing 1% lidocaine (without epinephrine) with ceftriaxone reduces the discomfort associated with the injection (see manufacturer's literature). No adverse reactions have been associated with use of lidocaine diluent. Ceftriaxone also may cure incubating syphilis.

(4) Cefixime, given orally in a 400-mg dose, does not provide as high nor as sustained a bactericidal level as does a 125-mg dose of ceftriaxone. Cefixime cures anal and genital gonorrhea and appears to be effective against pharyngeal gonococcal infection, but few patients with pharyngeal infection have been included in studies (Handsfield et al, 1991). No cefixime-resistant *N. gonorrhoeae* strains have been reported. The major advantage of cefixime is oral administration. It is not known whether a single 400-mg dose of cefixime can cure incubating syphilis.

(5) Ciprofloxacin in a dose of 500 mg also provides sustained bactericidal levels in blood and, like ceftriaxone, is effective in uncomplicated gonorrhea at all sites, including the pharynx. Ciprofloxacin can be given orally and it is less expensive than ceftriaxone. Although no resistance has been reported in the United States, strains with decreased susceptibility to some quinolones are becoming common in Asia and have been reported in North America. Ofloxacin is active against *N. gonorrhoeae*, has favorable pharmacokinetics, and a 400-mg dose has been effective for uncomplicated anal and genital gonorrhea. Published data are limited regarding its efficacy in pharyngeal gonococcal infection. In contrast to other recommended agents, ofloxacin, orally, 300 mg twice daily for seven days, is effective against both gonococcal and chlamydial infections (Batteiger et al, 1989; Lutz, 1989; Covino et al, 1990). However, a seven-day course of therapy with this fluoroquinolone is considerably more expensive than combination regimens. Quinolones should be used for gonorrhea in patients who are allergic to or cannot tolerate cephalosporin antibiotics. However, quinolones are contraindicated in pregnant or nursing women and for persons ≤17 years of age. Quinolones are not active against *Treponema pallidum*, the organism that causes syphilis.

(6) Spectinomycin has the disadvantages of being administered only by injection, expensive, inactive against *T. pallidum*, and relatively ineffective in pharyngeal gonorrhea. In addition, resistant strains have been reported in the United States. However, spectinomycin remains useful for the treatment of patients who cannot tolerate cephalosporins or quinolones.

(7) Other cephalosporins and quinolones have demonstrated efficacy against uncomplicated anal or genital gonococcal infections. Effective regimens include: **ceftizoxime**, intramuscularly, 500 mg in a single dose; **cefotaxime**, intramuscularly, 500 mg in a single dose; **cefotetan**, intramuscularly, 1 g in a single dose; **cefoxitin**, intramuscularly, 2 g in a single dose; **cefuroxime axetil**, orally, 1 g in a single dose; **cefpodoxime proxetil**, orally, 200 mg in a single dose; **lomefloxacin**, orally, 400 mg in a single dose; and **norfloxacin**, orally, 800 mg in a single dose. However, none of these alternative regimens offers advantages over the recommended regimens, and there is less clinical experience with them for the treatment of uncomplicated gonorrhea.

(8) For patients with uncomplicated pharyngeal gonococcal infection who cannot tolerate cephalosporins or quinolones, a possible alternative is nine "regular strength" tablets of **trimethoprim/sulfamethoxazole** (80 mg/400 mg) as a single daily dose for five days (Moran and Zenilman, 1990; *MMWR*, 1993 C).

(9) Pregnant women with uncomplicated gonorrhea should be treated with a recommended cephalosporin regimen. Those who cannot tolerate cephalosporins should be treated with spectinomycin. Follow-up therapy with one of the erythromycin regimens is necessary to treat coexisting chlamydial infection. Follow-up cervical and rectal cultures for *N. gonorrhoeae* should be obtained four to seven days after treatment is completed. The fluoroquinolones (eg, ofloxacin, ciprofloxacin) and the tetracyclines (including doxycycline) should not be used in pregnant women because of potential adverse effects on the fetus. The CDC recommend that all pregnant women have endocervical cultures for *N. gonorrhoeae* (and be tested for syphilis) at the first prenatal visit. A second culture for gonococci (and tests for *C. trachomatis* and syphilis) late in the third trimester should be done on women at high risk of sexually transmitted diseases.

(10) All patients with gonorrhea should have a serologic test for syphilis when gonorrhea is first detected. Patients with incubating syphilis (those who are seronegative and have no clinical signs of syphilis) may be cured by gonorrhea treatment regimens that include ceftriaxone or a seven-day course of either doxycycline or erythromycin, but few relevant data are available. Patients with gonorrhea and documented syphilis and gonorrhea patients who are sex partners of syphilis patients should be treated for syphilis (see section entitled Syphilis) as well as for gonorrhea.

(11) Sex partners must be notified (eg, by health department). Sex partners of symptomatic patients who have *N. gonorrhoeae* infection should be evaluated and treated for *N. gonorrhoeae* and *C. trachomatis* infections if their last sexual contact with the patient was within 30 days of onset of the patient's symptoms. If the index patient is asymptomatic, sex partners whose last sexual contact with the patient was within 60 days of diagnosis should be evaluated and treated. (Note: If last sexual intercourse took place before the foregoing time intervals, then the last sex partner of the index case should be treated as a possible source of infection). Patients should be instructed to avoid sexual intercourse until patient and partner(s) are cured, ie, until therapy is completed and patient and partner(s) are without symptoms.

(12) Treatment failure following currently recommended regimens is rare; therefore, a follow-up (test-of-cure) culture is not recommended. Persistent symptoms after treatment should be evaluated by culture for *N. gonorrhoeae*, and any gonococcal isolate should be tested for antimicrobial susceptibility. Infections occurring after treatment with one of the recommended regimens are commonly due to reinfection rather than to treatment failure and indicate a need for improved sex partner referral and patient education. Symptoms of urethritis, cervicitis, or proctitis also may be caused by *C. trachomatis* and other organisms.

(13) Persons with HIV infection and gonococcal infection should receive the same treatment as persons not infected with HIV.

Disseminated Gonococcal Infection in Adults (Arthritis-Dermatitis Syndrome)

RECOMMENDED INITIAL REGIMEN:

Ceftriaxone: Intramuscularly or Intravenously, 1 g every 24 hours.

ALTERNATIVE INITIAL REGIMENS:
Cefotaxime: Intravenously, 1 g every eight hours;
OR
Ceftizoxime: Intravenously, 1 g every eight hours;
OR (for persons allergic to β-lactam drugs)
Spectinomycin: Intramuscularly, 2 g every 12 hours.
OR
Ciprofloxacin: Intravenously, 400 mg every 12 hours;
OR
Ofloxacin: Intravenously, 400 mg every 12 hours (see REMARKS)
All parenteral regimens should be continued for 24 to 48 hours after improvement begins. Then therapy may be switched to one of the regimens that follow to complete one full week of therapy: Cefixime, orally, 400 mg twice daily OR Ciprofloxacin, orally, 500 mg twice daily or Ofloxacin, orally, 400 mg twice daily.
REMARKS:
(1) Strains of *N. gonorrhoeae* that cause disseminated gonococcal infection tend to cause little genital inflammation, and these strains have been uncommon in the United States during the past decade. None of the recommended regimens has been adequately studied in prospective, controlled clinical trials in North America. The recommendations reflect opinions of expert consultants.
(2) Hospitalization is recommended for initial therapy, especially for patients who cannot reliably comply with treatment, have uncertain diagnoses, have purulent joint effusions, or have other complications. Attempts should be made to exclude endocarditis or meningitis.
(3) The CDC recommend that patients who are allergic to β-lactam antibiotics be treated with **spectinomycin**, intramuscularly, 2 g every 12 hours (*MMWR*, 1993 C). However, many of our consultants recommend the use of intravenous **ciprofloxacin** or **ofloxacin**, despite limited data.
(4) Patients treated for disseminated gonococcal infections should be presumptively treated for concurrent *C. trachomatis* infection, as outlined in the previous section.
(5) Quinolones (eg, ciprofloxacin) are contraindicated in pregnant or lactating women and in persons ≤17 years of age.
(6) As for uncomplicated infections, sex partners must be notified and referred for evaluation and treatment (see Uncomplicated Urethral, Endocervical, or Rectal Infection in Adults).
(7) Although open drainage of joints other than the hip is not indicated, repeated aspiration may be necessary. Intra-articular injection of antibiotics is contraindicated.
(8) Meningitis and endocarditis caused by *N. gonorrhoeae* require high-dose intravenous therapy with an agent effective against the strain causing the disease. The recommended initial regimen is **ceftriaxone**, intravenously, 1 to 2 g every 12 hours. Treatment should be undertaken in consultation with an expert. Optimal duration of therapy is unknown, but most authorities treat patients with gonococcal meningitis for 10 to 14 days and with gonococcal endocarditis for at least four weeks.

Gonococcal Conjunctivitis in Adults

RECOMMENDED REGIMEN:
Ceftriaxone: Intramuscularly, 1 g in a single dose.
REMARKS:
(1) The single-dose regimen is for adults and children over 20 kg with nonsepticemic gonococcal conjunctivitis; it is based on limited data. If patient is septicemic, treat as for disseminated gonococcal infection in the preceding section.
(2) The infected eye should be lavaged with saline solution once. This may be useful adjunctive therapy to eliminate discharge. All patients must have careful ophthalmologic assessment, including slit-lamp examination, for ocular complications.
(3) Topical antibiotic preparations alone are not sufficient and are unnecessary when appropriate systemic antibiotic therapy is given.
(4) Simultaneous ophthalmic infection with *C. trachomatis* has been reported and should be considered for patients who do not respond promptly.
(5) As for uncomplicated infections, sex partners must be notified and referred for evaluation and treatment (see Uncomplicated Urethral, Endocervical, or Rectal Infection in Adults).

Neonatal Gonococcal Infections

No apparent illness, but born to mother with gonococcal infection

RECOMMENDED REGIMEN:
Ceftriaxone: Intravenously or Intramuscularly, 25 to 50 mg/kg (not to exceed 125 mg) in a single dose.
REMARKS:
(1) The infant born to a mother with untreated gonorrhea is at high risk of infection and requires treatment.
(2) Ceftriaxone should be given cautiously to hyperbilirubinemic infants, especially premature infants, because this highly protein bound cephalosporin can displace bilirubin from albumin binding sites. Some pediatricians prefer not to use ceftriaxone in neonates. Cefotaxime is an alternative, but multiple doses may be required.
(3) Topical prophylaxis for neonatal gonococcal ophthalmia is not adequate treatment for infections at other sites.
(4) Clinical illness requires additional treatment as outlined below.
(5) Mothers of infants with gonococcal infection and their sex partners should be evaluated and treated following the recommendations for treatment of gonococcal infection in adults.
(6) Simultaneous infection with *C. trachomatis* has been reported. Mother and infant should be tested for chlamydial infection.

Gonococcal ophthalmia

RECOMMENDED REGIMEN:
Ceftriaxone: Intravenously or intramuscularly, 25 to 50 mg/kg (not to exceed 125 mg) in a single dose.
REMARKS:
(1) Infants with documented gonococcal ophthalmia should be admitted to the hospital and evaluated for disseminated gonococcal infection, including meningitis. One dose of ceftriaxone is adequate for gonococcal ophthalmia (Laga et al, 1986), but many pediatricians prefer to maintain infants on antibiotics until cultures are negative at 48 to 72 hours. The decision on duration of therapy should be made after consultation with experienced physicians (*MMWR*, 1993 C).
(2) Ceftriaxone should be given cautiously to hyperbilirubinemic infants, especially premature infants, because this highly protein-bound cephalosporin can displace bilirubin from albumin binding sites. Some pediatricians prefer not to use ceftriaxone in neonates. **Cefotaxime**, intravenously or intramuscularly, 25 mg/kg every 12 hours for seven days, is an effective alternative regimen.
(3) Irrigation of the eyes with saline or buffered ophthalmic solutions should be used as adjunctive therapy to eliminate discharge.
(4) Topical antibiotic therapy alone is inadequate and is unnecessary if systemic treatment is administered.
(5) Mothers of infants with gonococcal infection and their sex partners should be evaluated and treated following the recommendations for treatment of gonococcal infection in adults.

(6) Simultaneous ophthalmic infection with *C. trachomatis* has been reported and should be considered in patients who do not respond satisfactorily. Mother and infant should be tested for chlamydial infection at the same time that gonorrhea testing is done.

Bacteremia and arthritis

RECOMMENDED REGIMEN(S):
Ceftriaxone: Intravenously or Intramuscularly, 25 to 50 mg/kg once daily for seven days;
OR
Cefotaxime: Intravenously or Intramuscularly, 25 mg/kg every 12 hours for seven days.
REMARKS:
(1) Infants with documented gonococcal infection should be evaluated for meningitis (CSF cultures) and for gonococcal ophthalmia.
(2) Ceftriaxone should be given cautiously to hyperbilirubinemic infants, especially premature infants, because this highly protein-bound cephalosporin can displace bilirubin from albumin binding sites. Some pediatricians prefer not to use ceftriaxone in neonates.

Meningitis

RECOMMENDED REGIMEN(S):
Ceftriaxone: Intravenously, 25 to 50 mg/kg once daily for 10 to 14 days;
OR
Cefotaxime: Intravenously, 25 mg/kg every 12 hours for 10 to 14 days.
REMARK:
(1) Ceftriaxone should be given cautiously to hyperbilirubinemic infants, especially premature infants, because this highly protein-bound cephalosporin can displace bilirubin from albumin binding sites. Some pediatricians prefer not to use ceftriaxone in neonates.

Gonococcal Infections in Children

Uncomplicated gonorrhea in children <45 kg

RECOMMENDED REGIMEN:
Ceftriaxone: Intramuscularly, 125 mg in a single dose.
ALTERNATIVE REGIMEN (for patients who cannot take ceftriaxone):
Spectinomycin: Intramuscularly, 40 mg/kg (maximum, 2 g) in a single dose.
REMARKS:
(1) Children weighing ≥45 kg should receive adult regimens (see Uncomplicated Urethral, Endocervical, or Rectal Infection in Adults). However, fluoroquinolones (ofloxacin, ciprofloxacin) should not be used in persons ≤17 years of age.
(2) Only parenteral cephalosporins are recommended for use in children; ceftriaxone is labeled for all gonococcal indications in children. Oral cephalosporins have not been adequately evaluated in children.
(3) Follow-up cultures of specimens from infected sites are necessary to ensure that treatment has been effective.
(4) Because sexual abuse must be considered a cause of gonococcal infection among preadolescent children, diagnosis of *N. gonorrhoeae* should only be by standard culture systems and should be confirmed by at least two tests that involve different principles (eg, biochemical, enzyme substrate, or serologic). Isolates should be preserved to permit additional or repeated analysis. These children should be evaluated for other sexually transmitted diseases (eg, *C. trachomatis*, syphilis, trichomoniasis, HIV, hepatitis B).

Complicated gonorrhea (bacteremia, arthritis, or meningitis)
REMARK:
(1) Patients weighing <45 kg with bacteremia and arthritis should be treated with **ceftriaxone** 50 mg/kg (maximum, 1 g) once daily for seven days. For meningitis, the duration of treatment is increased to 10 to 14 days and the maximum dose is 2 g.

COMMON STD-ASSOCIATED SYNDROMES

Several clinical syndromes are associated with STD. Some are more clearly defined etiologically than others. The following guidelines outline approaches to the initial treatment of these conditions when complete microbiological evaluation is not possible or while awaiting the results of specific laboratory tests.

Nongonococcal Urethritis (NGU)

Among men with urethral symptoms, NGU is diagnosed presumptively by Gram stain of a urethral specimen demonstrating polymorphonuclear leukocytes without intracellular gram-negative diplococci; the diagnosis is confirmed by a negative culture for *N. gonorrhoeae*. The most common causative organism is *Chlamydia trachomatis,* which has been implicated as the cause of NGU in 23% to 55% of cases; however, prevalence varies among age groups with lower prevalence rates found among older men. Other organisms that cause NGU include *Ureaplasma urealyticum* (20% to 40% of cases), *Trichomonas vaginalis* (2% to 5% of cases), and occasionally herpes simplex virus. The cause of other cases is unknown.

RECOMMENDED REGIMEN:
Doxycycline: Orally, 100 mg twice daily for seven days.
ALTERNATIVE REGIMEN:
Azithromycin: Orally, 1 g in a single dose.
REMARKS:
(1) For patients in whom tetracyclines are contraindicated or not tolerated, **erythromycin base,** orally, 500 mg four times daily for seven days or **erythromycin ethylsuccinate,** orally, 800 mg four times daily for seven days is recommended. If these high-dose erythromycin regimens are not tolerated, the dosage can be halved and the duration of therapy increased to 14 days.
(2) In most cases, treatment with the recommended regimen has been demonstrated to result in alleviation of symptoms and in microbiologic cure of infection. If the etiologic organism is susceptible to the antimicrobial agent used, sequelae specific to that organism will be prevented, as will further transmission; this is especially important for cases of NGU caused by *C. trachomatis*.
(3) Patients should be instructed to return for evaluation if symptoms persist or recur after completion of therapy. Patients with persistent or recurrent urethritis should be re-treated with

the initial regimen if they failed to comply with the treatment regimen or if they have been re-exposed to an untreated sex partner. Otherwise, the CDC recommend that a wet mount examination and culture of an intraurethral swab specimen for *Trichomonas vaginalis* be performed; if negative, the patient should be re-treated with an alternative regimen extended to 14 days (eg, erythromycin base, orally, 500 mg four times daily for 14 days). (Note: Some consultants recommend adding a single 2-g dose of oral metronidazole to erythromycin for presumptive coverage of *T. vaginalis* in these patients because wet mounts are insensitive and very few laboratories perform cultures for *T. vaginalis*.) The use of alternative regimens ensures treatment of possible tetracycline-resistant *U. urealyticum*. Persistent symptoms or frequent recurrences following adequate treatment with doxycycline and erythromycin usually suggest a condition that is not sexually transmitted.

(4) Sex partners must be notified. Sex partners of symptomatic patients should be evaluated and treated if their last sexual contact with the index patient was within 30 days of onset of symptoms. If the index patient is asymptomatic, sex partners whose last sexual contact was within 60 days of diagnosis should be evaluated and treated. (Note: If last sexual intercourse took place before the foregoing time intervals, then the last sex partner of the index case should be treated as a possible source of infection.) Patients should be instructed to avoid sexual intercourse until patient and partner(s) are cured, ie, until therapy is completed and the patient and partner(s) are without symptoms.

(5) Persons with HIV infection and NGU should receive the same treatment as patients without HIV infection.

(6) Results of a multicenter, randomized, double-blind, double-dummy clinical trial suggest that **azithromycin**, orally, 1 g as a single dose, is as effective as a seven-day course of doxycycline in the treatment of NGU (Stamm et al, 1993).

Acute Pelvic Inflammatory Disease (PID)

Acute pelvic inflammatory disease (PID) includes endometritis, salpingitis, tubo-ovarian abscess, and pelvic peritonitis and refers to an acute clinical syndrome attributed to the ascending spread of microorganisms, unrelated to pregnancy or surgery, from the vagina and endocervix to the endometrium, fallopian tubes, and/or contiguous structures.

Sexually transmitted organisms, especially *Neisseria gonorrhoeae* and *Chlamydia trachomatis*, are implicated in the majority of cases. Microorganisms that can be part of the vaginal flora, including anaerobic bacteria (eg, *Bacteroides*; gram-positive cocci), *Gardnerella vaginalis, Haemophilus influenzae*, enteric gram-negative bacilli (eg, *Escherichia coli*), and Group B streptococci, also may cause PID. Some experts believe that *Mycoplasma hominis* and *Ureaplasma urealyticum* also may be causative.

Because of a wide variation in many symptoms and signs among women with this condition, a clinical diagnosis of acute PID is difficult and imprecise. Although laparoscopy can be used to obtain a more accurate diagnosis of salpingitis and a more complete bacteriologic diagnosis, this diagnostic tool is often neither readily available for acute cases nor easily justifiable when symptoms are mild or vague. Furthermore, laparoscopy will not detect endometritis and may not detect subtle inflammation of the fallopian tubes. Consequently, despite the difficulties, the diagnosis of PID is usually made on the basis of clinical findings. The CDC recommend empiric treatment of PID on the basis of *all* of the following three *minimum* clinical criteria for pelvic inflammation, in the absence of an established cause other than PID: lower abdominal tenderness, adnexal tenderness, and cervical motion tenderness. Additional criteria may be used to increase the specificity of the diagnosis and are especially warranted for women with severe clinical signs. These *routine* criteria for diagnosing PID include oral temperature >38.3°C, abnormal cervical or vaginal discharge, elevated erythrocyte sedimentation rate, elevated C-reactive protein, and laboratory documentation of cervical infection with *N. gonorrhoeae* or *C. trachomatis*. *Elaborate* criteria for diagnosing PID include histopathologic evidence of endometritis on endometrial biopsy, tubo-ovarian abscess on sonography or other radiologic studies, or laparoscopic abnormalities consistent with PID (*MMWR*, 1993 C).

PID therapeutic regimens must provide empiric, broad-spectrum coverage of likely pathogens. The treatment of choice is not established, and no single agent is active against the entire spectrum of pathogens. Therefore, treatment regimens should include a combination of antimicrobial agents that are active against the range of likely pathogens. Antimicrobial coverage should include *N. gonorrhoeae, C. trachomatis*, gram-negative facultative bacteria, anaerobic bacteria, and streptococci.

The following recommended combination regimens exhibit broad activity against major pathogens in PID. The regimens have been subdivided into those used for inpatient treatment and those employed in ambulatory patients. Hospitalization is indicated when (1) the diagnosis is uncertain; (2) surgical emergencies, such as appendicitis and ectopic pregnancy, cannot be excluded; (3) a pelvic abscess is suspected; (4) severe illness or nausea and vomiting precludes outpatient management; (5) the patient is pregnant; (6) the patient is an adolescent; (7) the patient is unable to follow or tolerate an outpatient regimen; (8) the patient has failed to respond to outpatient therapy; or (9) clinical follow-up within 72 hours following the start of antibiotic treatment cannot be arranged. Many experts recommend hospitalization and intravenous antibiotics for all patients with PID. Special consideration should be given to adolescents because compliance with therapy is unpredictable and the long-term sequelae (eg, infertility) are particularly severe in this group. Finally, HIV-infected women who develop PID should be managed aggressively; these women often have tissue inflammation that is more intense and widespread than that suggested by clinical signs and symptoms. Hospitalization and inpatient therapy with one of the intravenous antimicrobial regimens described below is recommended.

For additional discussion of PID, see *MMWR*, 1991 A, 1993 C; McCormack, 1994.

Inpatient Treatment

RECOMMENDED REGIMEN(S):

(A) Cefoxitin: Intravenously, 2 g every six hours OR **Cefotetan: Intravenously, 2 g every 12 hours;**

Plus

Doxycycline: Intravenously, 100 mg every 12 hours.

Continue drugs intravenously for at least 48 hours after patient demonstrates substantial clinical improvement. Then continue doxycycline 100 mg, orally, twice daily to complete 14 days of total therapy.

(B) Clindamycin: Intravenously, 900 mg every eight hours,

Plus

Gentamicin: Intravenously or intramuscularly, 2 mg/kg initially (loading dose), followed by 1.5 mg/kg every eight hours (maintenance dose) in patients with normal renal function.
Continue drugs intravenously for at least 48 hours after patient demonstrates substantial clinical improvement. Then continue with doxycycline 100 mg, orally, twice daily to complete 14 days of total therapy. Continuation of clindamycin 450 mg, orally, four times daily to complete 14 days of total therapy may be considered as an alternative (see Remark 4).

REMARKS:
(1) There has been extensive experience with each of these combination regimens; each regimen provides broad coverage against polymicrobial infection and has shown excellent efficacy against acute PID in randomized controlled clinical trials (see Walker et al, 1993).
(2) Cefotetan has properties similar to those of cefoxitin and requires less frequent administration. Although clinical data are more limited, many experts believe that some third-generation cephalosporins (ceftizoxime, cefotaxime, ceftriaxone), which provide adequate coverage against gonococcal, other facultative gram-negative aerobic, and many anaerobic organisms, also are effective when used in appropriate doses. Third-generation cephalosporins are less active than cefoxitin and cefotetan against anaerobic bacteria, however. Concurrent doxycycline therapy to cover *C. trachomatis* is necessary with third-generation cephalosporins.
(3) Hospitalized patients receiving intravenous therapy should show substantial clinical improvement (eg, defervescence; reduction in direct or rebound abdominal tenderness; or reduction in uterine, adnexal, and cervical motion tenderness) within three to five days after therapy was initiated. Patients who do not demonstrate improvement within this time period usually require further diagnostic work up (such as laparoscopy) or surgical intervention or both.
(4) Continuation of medication after hospital discharge is important, especially for the treatment of possible *C. trachomatis* infection. Clindamycin has more complete anaerobic coverage than doxycycline, and many experts prefer this agent when tubo-ovarian abscess is present. Clindamycin, administered intravenously, appears to be effective against *C. trachomatis* infection; however, the effectiveness of oral clindamycin against salpingitis caused by this organism has not been determined. Doxycycline remains the treatment of choice for patients with chlamydial disease. When *C. trachomatis* is strongly suspected or confirmed as an etiologic agent, doxycycline is preferred. In such instances, doxycycline therapy may be started during hospitalization if initiation of therapy before hospital discharge is thought likely to improve the patient's compliance. Because of the risk of persistent infection, particularly with *C. trachomatis,* patients should have a microbiological re-examination seven to ten days after completing therapy. Some experts also recommend rescreening for *C. trachomatis* and *N. gonorrhoeae* four to six weeks after completing therapy.
(5) Doxycycline administered orally has bioavailability similar to that of the intravenous formulation and may be given if normal gastrointestinal function is present.
(6) Short courses of aminoglycosides in healthy young women usually do not require monitoring of serum aminoglycoside concentrations; monitoring substantially increases the cost of therapy. However, some practitioners may elect to monitor levels. When serum gentamicin levels are monitored, dose or dose interval should be adjusted to maintain a serum level of 5 to 10 mcg/ml 30 minutes after administration.
(7) The CDC suggest two alternative regimens for inpatient therapy of PID. **Ampicillin/sulbactam** *plus* **doxycycline** has good anaerobic coverage and appears to be effective for patients with tubo-ovarian abscess. **Ofloxacin** *plus* **clindamycin (or metronidazole)** provides broad spectrum coverage (*MMWR*, 1993 C).
(8) See Remarks below under Ambulatory Treatment for management of sex partners and patients with intrauterine devices.

Ambulatory Treatment

RECOMMENDED REGIMEN(S):
(A) Cefoxitin: Intramuscularly, 2 g in a single dose given concurrently with probenecid 1 g orally OR Ceftriaxone: Intramuscularly, 250 mg in a single dose OR Other parenteral third-generation cephalosporin (eg, ceftizoxime, cefotaxime)

Plus

Doxycycline: Orally, 100 mg twice daily for 14 days.

(B) Ofloxacin: Orally, 400 mg twice daily for 14 days

Plus

Clindamycin: Orally, 450 mg four times daily for 14 days OR Metronidazole: Orally, 500 mg twice daily for 14 days.

REMARKS:
(1) The above regimens provide broad-spectrum coverage against the common etiologic agents of PID, but evidence from clinical trials supporting their use in outpatients is limited, especially information regarding intermediate and long-term outcomes. Clinical trials have demonstrated that the cefoxitin regimen is effective in obtaining short-term clinical response. Fewer data support the use of the third-generation cephalosporins, but they also are considered effective. Ofloxacin is active against both *N. gonorrhoeae* and *C. trachomatis,* and results of one clinical trial demonstrated the effectiveness of this drug in obtaining a short-term clinical response in patients with PID. Because ofloxacin has poor anaerobic coverage, the addition of clindamycin or metronidazole is recommended. Clindamycin also enhances the gram-positive coverage of the regimen. The ofloxacin-containing regimen is substantially more expensive than cefoxitin/doxycycline.
(2) Information on alternative outpatient regimens is limited. The CDC note that the combination of **amoxicillin/clavulanic acid** *plus* **doxycycline** was effective in obtaining short-term clinical response in one clinical trial, but many patients had to discontinue the regimen because of gastrointestinal side effects.
(3) Outpatients should be re-evaluated after 72 hours to determine the clinical response (see criteria for clinical improvement under Inpatient Treatment); those who fail to respond should be hospitalized for re-evaluation and parenteral therapy.
(4) Because of the risk of persistent infection, particularly with *C. trachomatis*, patients should have a microbiological re-examination seven to ten days after completing therapy. Some experts also recommend rescreening for *C. trachomatis* and *N. gonorrhoeae* four to six weeks after completing therapy.
(5) Sex partners of women with PID should be examined for STD and treated promptly with a regimen effective against uncomplicated gonococcal and chlamydial infections.
(6) Women with intrauterine devices (IUD) should have the IUD removed soon after antimicrobial therapy is initiated (ie, within one to two hours). When an IUD is removed, contraceptive counseling is necessary.

Acute Epididymitis

Acute epididymitis has two forms. Sexually transmitted epididymitis occurs primarily in young men <35 years of age and is associated with the presence of urethritis (which may be subclinical), absence of underlying genitourinary pathology, and absence of gram-negative rods on Gram stain of urine. It is most often caused by *Chlamydia trachomatis* and/or *Neisseria gonorrhoeae*. A nonsexually transmitted form of epididymitis is more common in men >35 years of age and in men who have recently undergone urinary tract instrumentation or surgery. It is associated with urinary tract infections caused by Enterobacteriaceae or *Pseudomonas*. However, homosexual men who are the insertive partners during anal intercourse can have sexually transmitted *Escherichia coli* epididymitis.

Men with epididymitis typically have unilateral testicular pain and tenderness; palpable swelling of the epididymis is usually present. (Note: Testicular torsion is a surgical emergency that should be considered in all cases, and particularly in younger men.) The evaluation of men for epididymitis should include Gram-stained smear of urethral exudate or intraurethral swab specimen for *N. gonorrhoeae* and for nongonococcal urethritis (≥5 polymorphonuclear leukocytes per oil immersion field); culture of urethral exudate or intraurethral swab specimen for *N. gonorrhoeae*; test of intra-urethral swab specimen for *C. trachomatis*; and culture and Gram-stained smear of uncentrifuged urine for gram-negative bacteria.

Recommended initial treatment for suspected sexually transmitted epididymitis, as outlined below, is empiric before culture results are available. Patients with this form of epididymitis should receive an antimicrobial regimen effective against *C. trachomatis* and *N. gonorrhoeae*. For drug selection for nonsexually transmitted acute epididymo-orchitis, see index entry Epididymo-orchitis.

Sexually transmitted epididymitis

RECOMMENDED REGIMEN:
Ceftriaxone: Intramuscularly, 250 mg in a single dose;

Plus

Doxycycline: Orally, 100 mg twice daily for ten days.
ALTERNATIVE REGIMEN:
Ofloxacin: Orally, 300 mg twice daily for ten days.
REMARKS:
(1) Treatment of epididymitis caused by *C. trachomatis* or *N. gonorrhoeae* with either of the above regimens should result in microbiologic cure, improvement in signs and symptoms, and prevention of transmission to others.
(2) The effect of substituting the 125-mg dose of ceftriaxone recommended for treatment of uncomplicated gonorrhea, or the azithromycin single-dose regimen recommended for treatment of uncomplicated *C. trachomatis* infection, is unknown.
(3) Bed rest and scrotal elevation are recommended until fever and local inflammation subside. Failure to improve within three days requires re-evaluation of both the diagnosis and therapy and consideration of hospitalization. Patients with swelling and tenderness that persist after completing antimicrobial therapy should be evaluated for testicular cancer and tuberculous or fungal epididymitis.
(4) Sex partners of men with sexually transmitted acute epididymitis should be evaluated and treated with a regimen effective against uncomplicated gonococcal and chlamydial infection if their last sexual contact with the patient was within 30 days of onset of symptoms. Patients should be instructed to avoid sexual intercourse until patient and partner(s) are cured, ie, until therapy is completed and patient and partner(s) are without symptoms.
(5) Patients with HIV infection and uncomplicated epididymitis should receive the same treatment as persons not infected with HIV. Fungal and mycobacterial causes of epididymitis are more common among immunocompromised patients, however.

Bacterial Vaginosis

Bacterial vaginosis (formerly called nonspecific vaginitis, *Haemophilus*-associated vaginitis, or *Gardnerella*-associated vaginitis) is a clinical syndrome resulting from replacement of the normal H_2O_2-producing *Lactobacillus* spp in the vagina with high concentrations of anaerobic bacteria (eg, *Bacteroides* spp, *Mobiluncus* spp), *Gardnerella vaginalis,* and *Mycoplasma hominis.* This condition is the most prevalent cause of vaginal discharge or malodor, but half of the women meeting clinical criteria for bacterial vaginosis have no symptoms. Although bacterial vaginosis is associated with sexual activity in women, it is not considered exclusively an STD. Bacterial vaginosis frequently occurs as a secondary condition induced by another STD (eg, gonococcal or chlamydial cervicitis). In these cases, many practitioners treat only the STD (eg, gonorrhea, chlamydia) because the bacterial vaginosis resolves spontaneously after treatment. Also, when bacterial vaginosis is diagnosed (see below), the presence of these other STDs should be considered.

Vaginal discharge associated with bacterial vaginosis is nonirritating, malodorous, thin, homogeneous grey or white, and adheres to the vaginal walls. The vaginal pH is elevated (>4.5), and there is release of malodorous amines (fishy odor) from the discharge fluid after alkalization with 10% potassium hydroxide (whiff test). Microscopic examination of vaginal fluid typically reveals small coccobacillary organisms associated with epithelial cells (clue cells). Presence of three or four of these criteria (ie, characteristic discharge, pH, amine odor, clue cells) is sufficient to make the clinical diagnosis. When Gram stain is used, determining the relative concentration of the bacterial morphotypes characteristic of the altered flora of bacterial vaginosis is an acceptable laboratory method for diagnosing bacterial vaginosis. Culture of *Gardnerella vaginalis* is nonspecific and nondiagnostic of this syndrome.

RECOMMENDED REGIMEN:
Metronidazole: Orally, 500 mg twice daily for seven days.
OR
Metronidazole: Orally, 2 g as a single dose.
ALTERNATIVE REGIMEN(S):
(Note: The following three alternative regimens have been effective in clinical trials, but experience with these regimens is limited.)
Clindamycin 2% cream: Intravaginally, one applicatorful (5 g) at bedtime for seven days.
OR
Metronidazole 0.75% gel: Intravaginally, one applicatorful (5 g) twice daily for five days.
OR
Clindamycin: Orally, 300 mg twice daily for seven days.
REMARKS:
(1) Oral metronidazole has been shown in numerous studies to be effective for the treatment of bacterial vaginosis, resulting in

relief of symptoms and improvement in clinical course and flora disturbances. Based on results of four randomized, controlled trials, the overall cure rates are 95% for the seven-day regimen and 84% for the 2-g single-dose regimen. However, some consultants prefer the single-dose regimen because compliance is likely to be greater. Patients should be advised to avoid consuming alcohol during treatment with metronidazole and for 24 hours thereafter (see also index entry, Metronidazole).
(2) Some health care providers prefer the intravaginal route in order to avoid systemic side effects (eg, gastrointestinal upset, unpleasant taste) associated with oral metronidazole.
(3) Clindamycin cream is preferred in cases of allergy or intolerance to metronidazole. Although metronidazole gel may be considered for patients who do not tolerate systemic metronidazole, this topical formulation is contraindicated in patients allergic to oral metronidazole.
(4) Treatment of asymptomatic infections, which are common, is not required.
(5) Follow-up visits are unnecessary if symptoms resolve. Recurrence of bacterial vaginosis is common; alternative treatment regimens may be used for recurrent disease. No long-term maintenance regimen is available.
(6) Treatment of male sex partners does not appear to reduce the risk of recurrence of bacterial vaginosis in the index case and is not routinely recommended. However, some consultants recommend that sex partners be examined and evaluated for STD.
(7) Oral metronidazole is contraindicated during the first trimester of pregnancy. Clindamycin cream is the preferred regimen for pregnant women during the first trimester. Although oral metronidazole may be used during the second and third trimesters, the topical preparations may be preferable. In pregnancy, some studies suggest that bacterial vaginosis may be a factor in premature rupture of membranes and premature delivery. Also, organisms associated with bacterial vaginosis are commonly present in postpartum or postcesarean endometritis. Whether treatment of bacterial vaginosis in pregnant women would reduce the risk of adverse pregnancy outcomes presently is unknown.
(8) Clindamycin cream can weaken latex condoms. Users should be advised of the risk of condom breakage.
(9) Women with HIV infection and bacterial vaginosis should receive the same treatment as women without HIV.

Mucopurulent Cervicitis

The presence of mucopurulent endocervical exudate often suggests mucopurulent cervicitis. This condition may be due to chlamydial or gonococcal infection, although in many cases neither *C. trachomatis* nor *N. gonorrhoeae* can be isolated. Presumptive diagnosis of mucopurulent cervicitis is made by the finding of mucopurulent secretions from the endocervix, which may appear yellow when viewed against a white background (positive swab test); a dramatically increased number of polymorphonuclear leukocytes on cervical Gram stain also is diagnostic of the condition. Patients with mucopurulent cervicitis should have a Gram stain and culture for *N. gonorrhoeae*, and a test for *C. trachomatis*. (Note: The sensitivity of the Gram stain for *N. gonorrhoeae* in the endocervix is only 50%.) Genital herpes also must be considered in the differential diagnosis. For treatment of mucopurulent cervicitis, see the following remarks.

REMARKS:
(1) Treatment for gonorrhea and/or chlamydial infection in women with mucopurulent cervicitis should be based on test results for *N. gonorrhoeae* and *C. trachomatis*, unless the likelihood of infection with either organism is high or the patient is unlikely to return for treatment. The CDC provide the following guidance for treatment of mucopurulent cervicitis: (a) treat for both gonorrhea and chlamydia in patient populations with high prevalences of both infections, such as patients seen at many STD clinics (for regimens, see section entitled Gonococcal Infections: Uncomplicated Urethral, Endocervical, or Rectal Infection in Adults); (b) treat only for chlamydial infection if the prevalence of *N. gonorrhoeae* is low but the likelihood of chlamydia is substantial (for regimens, see section entitled *Chlamydia trachomatis* Infections: Uncomplicated Urethral, Endocervical, or Rectal Infection in Adults); or (c) await test results if the prevalences of both infections are low and if compliance with a recommendation for a return visit is likely. Some consultants recommend treatment of both gonorrhea and chlamydia when the prevalence of each infection is unknown.
(2) Follow-up should be as recommended for the infections for which the woman is being treated.
(3) Male sex partners of women with mucopurulent cervicitis attributed to gonococcal or chlamydial infection should be evaluated and treated with a regimen appropriate for the STD (*N. gonorrhoeae* or *C. trachomatis*) identified for the woman. Partners should be notified, examined, and treated on the basis of test results when possible. However, sex partners of women treated presumptively should receive the same treatment as the woman.
(4) Patients with HIV infection and mucopurulent cervicitis should receive the same treatment as patients without HIV infection.

Acute Urethral Syndrome (Dysuria-Pyuria Syndrome)

The acute urethral syndrome is a common condition that may be associated with STD in women. For description and treatment of the acute urethral syndrome, see index entry Urethral Syndrome, Treatment. For drug selection when the sexually transmitted pathogens *Chlamydia trachomatis* and/or *Neisseria gonorrhoeae* are the suspected causative organisms, see the following remarks.

REMARKS:
(1) If *N. gonorrhoeae* is found on Gram stain or culture of endocervix, urethra, or urine, treatment should be given as recommended for uncomplicated gonorrhea in adults (see section entitled Gonococcal Infections: Uncomplicated Urethral, Endocervical, or Rectal Infection in Adults).
(2) If *N. gonorrhoeae* is not found, treatment should be given as recommended for chlamydial infection in adults (see section entitled *Chlamydia trachomatis* Infections: Uncomplicated Urethral, Endocervical, or Rectal Infection in Adults).
(3) Male sex partners of women with sexually transmitted acute urethral syndrome attributed to gonococcal or chlamydial infection should be evaluated for STD and treated as recommended for contacts exposed to gonorrhea or chlamydial infection.
(4) When the distinction between sexually transmitted acute urethral syndrome and bacterial urinary tract infection is uncertain, **ofloxacin**, orally, 300 mg twice daily for seven days, provides adequate therapy for gonorrhea, chlamydial infection, and most bacterial urinary pathogens.

Vulvovaginal Candidiasis

REMARK:
(1) This common vaginal infection generally is not considered an STD. For drug selection and treatment guidelines, see Chapter 2 in this Section, Antimicrobial Therapy for Common Infec-

tious Diseases, and index entry Candidiasis, Superficial.

TRICHOMONIASIS

This sexually transmitted vaginal infection is caused by *Trichomonas vaginalis.* Symptomatic women typically have a diffuse, malodorous, yellow-green discharge with vulvar irritation. Diagnosis usually is made by direct microscopic visualization (wet preparation) or by culture. Antimicrobial drug therapy should be active against *T. vaginalis.* Symptomatic and asymptomatic patients should be treated.

RECOMMENDED REGIMEN:
Metronidazole: Orally, 2 g in a single dose.
ALTERNATIVE REGIMEN:
Metronidazole: Orally, 500 mg twice daily for seven days.
REMARKS:
(1) Only metronidazole is available in the United States to treat trichomoniasis. Both regimens cure approximately 95% of cases. Patients should be advised to avoid consuming alcohol during treatment with metronidazole and for 24 hours thereafter.
(2) Male sex partners of women with trichomoniasis are usually asymptomatic and should be treated with metronidazole, orally, 2 g as a single dose (alternative, the seven-day regimen), and examined for coexistent STD. Patients should be instructed to avoid sexual intercourse until patient and sex partner(s) are cured, ie, when therapy has been completed and patient and partners are without symptoms.
(3) For women who become asymptomatic after treatment and for males, follow-up is unnecessary.
(4) Infections by strains of *Trichomonas vaginalis* with reduced susceptibility to metronidazole have been observed but are rare. Patients who fail treatment with either regimen should be retreated with metronidazole 500 mg twice daily for seven days. If repeated failure occurs, the patient should be treated with a single 2-g dose of metronidazole once daily for three to five days. Cases with additional culture-documented treatment failure, in which reinfection has been excluded, should be managed in consultation with an expert. Evaluation of such cases should include determination of the susceptibility of *T. vaginalis* to metronidazole.
(5) Metronidazole is contraindicated during the first trimester of pregnancy, and some experts prefer to avoid administering metronidazole throughout pregnancy. However, no other adequate therapy exists. After the first trimester, patients may be treated with 2 g of metronidazole in a single dose. Results from a recent retrospective cohort study showed no increased risk of overall birth defect occurrence in women who received metronidazole during the first trimester (Piper et al, 1993).
(6) Lactating women may be treated with metronidazole, orally, 2 g, in a single dose. Although no adverse reactions in nursing infants have been reported, breast feeding is not recommended for at least 24 hours after therapy.
(7) Infants with symptomatic trichomoniasis or persistent urogenital trichomonal colonization beyond the fourth week of life can be treated with metronidazole 10 to 30 mg/kg daily for five to eight days *(MMWR,* 1985).
(8) Children (prepubertal) with trichomonal infection should be treated with metronidazole, orally, 15 mg/kg daily divided into three doses for seven to ten days. Child abuse should be carefully considered and evaluated (*MMWR,* 1985).
(9) Persons with HIV infection and trichomoniasis should receive the same treatment as persons without HIV.
(10) Intravaginal metronidazole gel, available for bacterial vaginosis, should not be used for trichomoniasis.

GENITAL HERPES SIMPLEX VIRUS INFECTIONS

Genital herpes infection is an STD caused by Herpes simplex virus (HSV), primarily serotype HSV-2; it may be recurrent, and there is no known cure.

Of the estimated 30 million persons in the United States who have genital HSV infection, most never recognize signs or symptoms of disease. Some individuals will have symptoms shortly after infection, ie, the first clinical episode, and never again. A minority of the total infected population will have recurrent episodes of genital lesions. Some cases of the first clinical episode of genital herpes are manifested by extensive disease that requires hospitalization. Many cases of genital herpes are acquired from persons who do not know that they have a genital HSV infection or who were asymptomatic at the time of sexual contact.

Systemic acyclovir provides partial control of the symptoms and signs of herpes episodes when used to treat the first clinical episode or when used as suppressive therapy. However, acyclovir neither eradicates latent virus nor affects subsequent risk, frequency, or severity of recurrences after administration of the drug is discontinued. Topical acyclovir, although available, is less effective than systemically (usually oral) administered drug and is not recommended.

Episodes of HSV infection among HIV-infected patients may require more aggressive therapy. Immunocompromised persons may have prolonged episodes with extensive disease.

First Clinical Episode of Genital Herpes

RECOMMENDED REGIMEN:
Acyclovir: Orally, 200 mg five times daily (or 400 mg three times daily) for seven to ten days or until clinical resolution is attained (see REMARKS).
REMARKS:
(1) The CDC recommend a dosage of 200 mg five times daily. However, others (*Med Lett Drugs Ther*, 1994), including some consultants, prefer a dosage of 400 mg three times daily because it is more convenient to the patient and has comparable efficacy.
(2) Intravenous therapy should be provided for patients with severe disease or complications necessitating hospitalization (disseminated infection that includes encephalitis, pneumonitis, or hepatitis). The recommended regimen is **acyclovir**, intravenously, 5 to 10 mg/kg every eight hours for five to seven days or until clinical resolution is attained.
(3) Patients should be advised to abstain from sexual activity while lesions are present. Patients also should be counseled about the natural history of genital herpes with emphasis on the potential for recurrent episodes and asymptomatic viral shedding and sexual transmission (ie, HSV transmission can occur during asymptomatic periods). The use of latex condoms should be encouraged during all sexual exposures. The risk of neonatal HSV infection should be explained to all patients; women of childbearing age should be instructed to inform their health-care providers of their history of HSV infection if they become pregnant.
(4) Sex partners of patients who have genital herpes are likely to benefit from evaluation and counseling. Symptomatic sex partners should be managed in the same manner as any patient with genital lesions. Asymptomatic partners should be queried about histories of typical and atypical genital lesions and en-

couraged to examine themselves for lesions in the future.
(5) For patients who are allergic to or cannot tolerate acyclovir, effective alternative therapies are not available.
(6) The safety of systemic acyclovir in pregnant women has not been established. However, Burroughs Wellcome Co, in cooperation with the CDC, maintains a registry to assess the effects of the use of acyclovir during pregnancy. Women who receive acyclovir during pregnancy should be reported to this registry (1-800-722-9292, ext. 58465). Current registry findings do not show an association between acyclovir use during pregnancy and an increased incidence of birth defects. However, current sample size precludes any definitive conclusions regarding the risk of acyclovir to pregnant women and to fetuses (*MMWR*, 1993 D). Currently, the CDC recommend that systemic acyclovir not be used for pregnant women without life-threatening disease. In the presence of life-threatening maternal HSV infection (eg, disseminated infection that includes encephalitis, pneumonitis, or hepatitis), intravenous acyclovir is indicated.
(7) Most mothers of infants who acquire neonatal herpes lack histories of clinically evident genital herpes. The risk of transmission to the neonate from an infected mother appears to be greatest among women with first episodes of genital herpes near the time of delivery and is low (≤3%) among women with recurrent herpes. At the onset of labor, all women should be carefully questioned about symptoms of genital herpes and should be examined. Infants of women without symptoms or signs of genital herpes infection (or prodrome) may be delivered vaginally. Among women who have a history of genital herpes, or who have a sex partner with genital herpes, cultures of the birth canal at delivery may aid in decisions relating to neonatal management. Infants delivered through an infected birth canal (proven by virus isolation or presumed by observation of lesions) should be followed carefully, including virus cultures obtained 24 to 48 hours after birth. Prophylactic acyclovir is not recommended for asymptomatic infants delivered through an infected birth canal. Rather, treatment should be reserved for infants who develop evidence of clinical disease and for those with positive postpartum cultures. For treatment of neonatal herpes infection, see *American Academy of Pediatrics Redbook*, 1991; see also index entry, Herpes Infection.

First Clinical Episode of Herpes Proctitis

RECOMMENDED REGIMEN:
Acyclovir: Orally, 400 mg five times daily (or 800 mg three times daily) for ten days or until clinical resolution is attained (see REMARKS).
REMARKS:
(1) The CDC recommend a dosage of 400 mg five times daily. However, others (*Med Lett Drugs Ther*, 1994), including some consultants, prefer a dosage of 800 mg three times daily because it is more convenient for the patient and has comparable efficacy.
(2) For other management considerations, including the management of sex partners and pregnant women, see the section above entitled First Clinical Episode of Genital Herpes.

Treatment of Recurrent Episodes of Genital Herpes

ALTERNATIVE REGIMENS:
Acyclovir: Orally, 200 mg five times daily for five days;
OR
Acyclovir: Orally, 400 mg three times daily for five days;
OR
Acyclovir: Orally, 800 mg twice daily for five days.
REMARKS:
(1) When treatment is instituted during the prodrome or within two days of onset of lesions, some patients with recurrent disease experience limited benefit from therapy. However, since early treatment can seldom be administered, most immunocompetent patients with recurrent disease do not benefit from acyclovir treatment, and it is *not generally recommended*.
(2) For other management considerations, including management of sex partners and pregnant women, see the section above entitled First Clinical Episode of Genital Herpes.

Daily Suppressive Therapy to Prevent Recurrent Episodes of Genital Herpes

RECOMMENDED REGIMEN:
Acyclovir: Orally, 400 mg twice daily.
ALTERNATIVE REGIMEN:
Acyclovir: Orally, 200 mg three to five times daily.
REMARKS:
(1) Daily suppressive therapy reduces the frequency of HSV recurrences by at least 75% among patients with frequent recurrences (≥six per year). Suppressive treatment with oral acyclovir does not totally eliminate symptomatic or asymptomatic viral shedding or the potential for transmission.
(2) Although safety and efficacy have been documented among persons receiving daily therapy for as long as five years, the CDC recommend that *after one year of continuous suppressive therapy, acyclovir be discontinued to allow assessment of the patient's recurrence rate.*
(3) The goal of the alternative regimen is to identify for each patient the lowest dose that provides relief from frequently recurring symptoms.
(4) Although acyclovir-resistant strains of HSV have been isolated from some persons receiving suppressive therapy, these strains usually have not been associated with treatment failure in immunocompetent patients. However, a recent report describes an immunocompetent patient who has had repeated recurrences of genital herpes due to an acyclovir-resistant HSV-2 strain bearing thymidine kinase mutations (Kost et al, 1993).
(5) For other management considerations, including management of sex partners and pregnant women, see the section above entitled First Clinical Episode of Genital Herpes.

Genital Herpes in HIV-Infected Patients

REMARKS:
(1) Lesions caused by HSV are relatively common in HIV-infected patients. Intermittent or suppressive therapy with oral acyclovir may be needed.
(2) The acyclovir dosage for HIV-infected persons is controversial, but experience strongly suggests that immunocompromised patients benefit from increased dosage. Regimens such as 400 mg orally three to five times a day, as used for other immunocompromised persons, have been found to be useful. Therapy should be continued until clinical resolution is attained.
(3) For severe disease, intravenous acyclovir therapy may be required. If lesions persist in patients receiving acyclovir treatment, resistance to the drug should be suspected. These patients should be managed in consultation with an expert. For severe disease caused by proven or suspected acyclovir-resistant HSV strains, hospitalization should be considered. **Foscarnet**, intravenously, 40 mg/kg every eight hours until clinical resolution is attained, appears to be the best available treatment.

GENITAL AND ANAL WARTS (CONDYLOMA ACUMINATUM)

Exophytic genital and anal warts are caused by certain types (most frequently types 6 and 11) of human papilloma virus (HPV). Other types sometimes present in the anogenital region (most commonly types 16, 18, and 31) have been found to be strongly associated with genital dysplasias and carcinoma. These types usually are associated with subclinical infection, however (see below).

Genital warts are generally benign growths that cause minor or no symptoms aside from cosmetic appearance. Treatment of external genital warts is not likely to influence the development of cervical cancer. Results of numerous randomized, controlled clinical trials have shown that currently available therapeutic modalities are 22% to 94% effective in clearing external exophytic genital warts and that recurrence rates are high (usually at least 25% within three months) with all modalities. Treatment appears to be more successful for genital warts that are small and that have been present <1 year. The effect of treatment on transmission and natural history of HPV is unknown. Untreated genital warts may resolve spontaneously (eg, in 20% to 30% of patients within three months), remain unchanged, or enlarge.

No therapy has been shown to eradicate HPV. *Thus, the goals of treatment are removal of exophytic warts and amelioration of signs and symptoms, not the eradication of HPV. Expensive and toxic therapies and procedures that result in scarring should be avoided.* Treatment is optional and decisions should be guided by the preference of the patient. A specific treatment regimen should be chosen with consideration given to anatomic site, size, and number of warts as well as the expense, efficacy, convenience, and potential for adverse effects. Patients with extensive or refractory disease should be referred to an expert.

In most clinical situations, cryotherapy with liquid nitrogen or cryoprobe is an excellent choice for external genital and perianal warts. Cryotherapy is nontoxic, does not require anesthesia, and, if used properly, does not result in scarring. However, special equipment is required and most patients experience moderate pain during and after the procedure. Self-treatment with 0.5% podofilox solution is a practical alternative for external genital warts. Therapy with this topical medication is relatively inexpensive, simple to use, and safe; the medication does not need to be washed off and can be applied by patients at home. Most patients experience mild to moderate pain or local irritation after treatment. Heavily keratinized warts may not respond as well as those on moist mucosal surfaces. Also, patients must be able to see and reach the warts easily. Podophyllin, trichloroacetic acid (TCA), and electrodesiccation/electrocautery are alternative therapies. Treatment with interferon is NOT recommended because of its relatively low efficacy, high incidence of toxicity, and high cost.

The carbon dioxide laser and conventional surgery are useful in the management of extensive warts, particularly for patients who have not responded to other regimens; these alternatives are not appropriate for limited lesions. Like more cost-effective treatments, these therapies do not eliminate HPV and often are associated with recurrence of clinical cases.

After warts have responded to therapy, follow-up is not necessary. Annual cytologic screening is recommended for women with or without genital warts. Presence of genital warts is not an indication for colposcopy.

Examination of sex partners is not necessary for management of genital warts, since the role of re-infection is probably minimal. Sex partners with obvious exophytic warts may desire treatment; counseling of sex partners may be beneficial. Patients with exophytic anogenital warts should be made aware that they are contagious to uninfected sex partners, although the majority of partners probably are already infected with HPV subclinically. The use of condoms may reduce transmission to partners likely to be uninfected.

HPV can cause laryngeal papillomatosis in infants. However, the perinatal transmission rate appears to be very low and the exact route of transmission is unknown. Laryngeal papillomatosis also has occurred among infants delivered by cesarean section. Because its preventive value is unknown, cesarean delivery for prevention of transmission of HPV infection to the newborn presently is not indicated. In rare instances, however, cesarean delivery may be indicated for women with genital warts if the pelvic outlet is obstructed or if vaginal delivery would result in excessive bleeding. Many experts advocate removal of visible warts during pregnancy, but data on this subject are limited.

Persons infected with HIV may not respond to therapy as well as uninfected persons.

Subclinical genital HPV infection is much more common than exophytic warts among men and women. Subclinical infection often is indirectly diagnosed on the cervix by Papanicolaou smear, colposcopy, or biopsy and on the penis, vulva, and other genital skin by the appearance of white areas after application of 5% acetic acid. In the absence of coexistent dysplasia, treatment is not recommended for subclinical genital HPV infection because diagnosis often is questionable and no therapy has been demonstrated to eradicate infection. In the presence of coexistent dysplasia, management should be based on the grade of dysplasia.

External Genital/Perianal Warts

ALTERNATIVE REGIMENS:

Cryotherapy with liquid nitrogen or cryoprobe.

OR

Podofilox: 0.5% solution for self-treatment (*genital warts only*). Patients may use a cotton swab to apply podofilox to warts twice daily for three days, followed by four days of no therapy. This cycle may be repeated as necessary for a total of four cycles. Total wart area treated should be ≤10 cm² and total volume of podofilox should be ≤0.5 ml per day. The health care provider should demonstrate the proper application technique and identify which warts should be treated. If possible, the health care provider should apply the initial treatment to demonstrate the proper technique and identify which warts should be treated.

OR

Podophyllin: 10% to 25% in compound tincture of benzoin. To avoid the possibility of problems with systemic absorp-

tion and toxicity, some experts limit the total volume of podophyllin solution applied to ≤0.5 ml or treat an area ≤10 cm² per session. Wash off thoroughly in one to four hours. Repeat applications once weekly, if necessary. If warts persist after six applications, other therapeutic methods should be considered. Mucosal warts are more likely to respond than are highly keratinized warts on the penile shaft, buttocks, or pubic areas.

OR

Trichloroacetic acid (80% to 90%): Apply only to warts; powder with talc or sodium bicarbonate (baking soda) to remove unreacted acid. Repeat application at weekly intervals, if necessary. If warts persist after six applications, other therapies should be considered.

OR

Electrodesiccation/electrocautery

REMARKS:

(1) In males, wrapping the penis in gauze soaked in 5% acetic acid solution for five minutes prior to cryotherapy allows better visualization of small lesions, ie, they appear as white areas.

(2) Podofilox and podophyllin should not be used during pregnancy because these agents are absorbed through mucous membranes and are teratogenic.

(3) Electrodesiccation is contraindicated in patients with cardiac pacemakers or for lesions proximal to the anal verge.

(4) Patients with extensive or refractory disease should be referred to an expert.

Cervical Warts

For women with exophytic cervical warts, dysplasia must be excluded before treatment is begun. Therefore, management should be carried out in consultation with an expert.

Vaginal Warts

ALTERNATIVE REGIMENS:

Cryotherapy with liquid nitrogen.

OR

Trichloroacetic acid (80% to 90%): Apply only to warts; powder with talc or sodium bicarbonate (baking soda) to remove unreacted acid. Repeat application at weekly intervals, if necessary. If warts persist after six applications, other therapeutic methods should be considered.

OR

Podophyllin: 10% to 25% in compound tincture of benzoin. Treatment area must be dry before speculum is removed. Treat ≤2 cm² per session. Repeat application at weekly intervals.

REMARKS:

(1) The use of a cryoprobe in the vagina is not recommended because of the risk of vaginal perforation and fistula formation.

(2) Podophyllin should not be used during pregnancy because it is absorbed through mucous membranes and is teratogenic. Many experts avoid use of podophyllin on mucosal surfaces (eg, vagina) whenever possible, preferring cryotherapy or trichloroacetic acid.

(3) Patients with extensive or refractory disease should be referred to an expert.

Urethral Meatus Warts

ALTERNATIVE REGIMENS:

Cryotherapy with liquid nitrogen.

OR

Podophyllin: 10% to 25% in compound tincture of benzoin. Treatment area must be dry before contact with normal mucosa. Podophyllin must be thoroughly washed off after one to two hours. Repeat weekly, if necessary. If warts persist after six applications, other therapeutic methods should be considered.

REMARKS:

(1) Podophyllin should not be used during pregnancy because it is absorbed through mucous membranes and is teratogenic. Many experts avoid use of podophyllin on mucosal surfaces (eg, urethra) whenever possible, preferring cryotherapy.

(2) Patients with extensive or refractory disease should be referred to an expert.

Anal Warts

ALTERNATIVE REGIMENS:

Cryotherapy with liquid nitrogen.

OR

Trichloroacetic acid (80% to 90%): Apply only to warts; powder with talc or sodium bicarbonate (baking soda) to remove unreacted acid. Repeat application at weekly intervals if necessary. If warts persist after six applications, other therapeutic methods should be considered.

OR

Surgical removal.

REMARK:

(1) Patients with extensive or refractory disease or warts on rectal mucosa should be referred to an expert.

Oral Warts

ALTERNATIVE REGIMENS:

Cryotherapy with liquid nitrogen.

OR

Electrodesiccation/electrocautery.

OR

Surgical removal.

REMARK:

(1) Patients with extensive or refractory disease should be referred to an expert.

SYPHILIS

Syphilis is a systemic disease caused by *Treponema pallidum*. Patients with syphilis may seek treatment for signs or symptoms of primary infection (ulcer or chancre at site of infection), secondary infection (manifestations that include rash, mucocutaneous lesions, adenopathy), or tertiary (late) infection (cardiac, neurologic, ophthalmic, or auditory symptoms or gummatous lesions). Infections also may be detected during the latent stage by serologic testing. Patients with latent syphilis who are known to have been infected within the preceding year are considered to have early latent syphilis; others have late latent syphilis or syphilis of unknown duration. Theoretically, treatment of late latent syphilis and tertiary syphilis requires therapy of longer duration because organisms are dividing more slowly; however, the validity of this division and its timing are unproven.

Dark-field examinations and direct fluorescent antibody tests of lesion exudate or tissue are the definitive methods for diagnosing early syphilis. Unfortunately, these tests are not performed by most clinical laboratories. Presumptive diagnosis is possible with the use of two types of serologic tests for syphilis: nontreponemal (eg, venereal disease research laboratory [VDRL], rapid plasma reagin [RPR]), and treponemal (eg, fluorescent treponemal antibody absorbed [FTA-ABS], microhemagglutination assay for antibody to *T. pallidum* [MHA-TP]). The use of one type of test alone is not sufficient for diagnosis. Nontreponemal test antibody titers usually correlate with disease activity, and results should be reported quantitatively; a fourfold change in titer (equal to a change of two dilutions) is necessary to demonstrate a substantial difference between two nontreponemal test results that were obtained with the same serologic test. Sequential serologic tests should be performed using the same testing method by the same laboratory. Treponemal test antibody titers correlate poorly with disease activity and should not be used to assess response to treatment.

No single test can be used to diagnose neurosyphilis in all patients. The diagnosis of neurosyphilis can be made based on various combinations of reactive serologic test results, abnormalities of cerebrospinal fluid (CSF) cell count (eg, leukocyte count >5 WBC/mm^3 when active neurosyphilis is present) or protein, or a reactive VDRL-CSF (RPR is not performed on CSF), with or without clinical manifestations. The VDRL-CSF is the standard serologic test for CSF; when reactive in the absence of substantial contamination of CSF with blood, it is considered diagnostic of neurosyphilis. However, the VDRL-CSF may be nonreactive when neurosyphilis is present. Some experts recommend performing an FTA-ABS on CSF. The CSF FTA-ABS is less specific (ie, yields more false-positive results) for neurosyphilis than VDRL-CSF; however, the test is believed to be highly sensitive.

Antimicrobial therapy should be directed against the causative organism, *T. pallidum*. Parenteral penicillin G is the drug of choice in the nonallergic patient for the treatment of all stages of syphilis. The preparation(s) used (ie, benzathine, aqueous procaine, aqueous crystalline penicillin G), the dose, and length of treatment depend on the stage and clinical manifestations of disease. The efficacy of penicillin is based primarily on lengthy clinical experience (rather than randomized controlled clinical trials).

The available evidence suggests that syphilis may contribute to risk for HIV acquisition and possible transmission. Furthermore, the clinical manifestations, serologic responses, efficacy of treatment, and occurrence of complications of syphilis may be altered in patients coinfected with HIV (*MMWR*, 1988; Hook and Marra, 1992; *MMWR*, 1993 C). Thus, *all syphilis patients should be counseled concerning the risks of HIV and should be tested for HIV antibody.* Coinfected patients should be managed accordingly (see section entitled Syphilis in HIV-Infected Patients below; see also *MMWR*, 1988, 1993 C).

Primary and Secondary Syphilis

RECOMMENDED REGIMEN (ADULTS):

Benzathine Penicillin G: Intramuscularly, 2.4 million units in a single dose.

REMARKS:

(1) Lengthy experience indicates that parenteral penicillin G is effective in achieving local cure and in preventing long-term sequelae. However, the optimal penicillin regimen (dose, duration, preparation) remains unclear. Fewer data on nonpenicillin regimens are available.

(2) Penicillin-allergic patients (nonpregnant adults) should receive **doxycycline**, orally, 100 mg twice daily for two weeks OR, alternatively, **tetracycline hydrochloride**, orally, 500 mg four times daily for two weeks. There is less clinical experience with doxycycline, but compliance is better.

(3) In penicillin-allergic patients (nonpregnant adults) who cannot tolerate doxycycline or tetracycline, two options exist: (a) If follow-up or compliance cannot be assured, the patient should have skin testing for penicillin allergy, be desensitized if necessary (for guidelines, see *MMWR*, 1993 C), and treated with penicillin. (b) If compliance and follow-up are assured, **erythromycin**, orally, 500 mg four times daily for two weeks, can be used. Various **ceftriaxone** regimens also may be considered. Treatment failure is more common with erythromycin than with penicillin or the tetracyclines. Data on ceftriaxone are limited, and optimal dose and duration have not been established. However, a regimen that provides eight to ten days of treponemicidal levels in blood should be used. *Single-dose ceftriaxone is not effective therapy for syphilis.* Because patients who are allergic to penicillin may also be allergic to cephalosporins, caution must be used in treating a penicillin-allergic patient with a cephalosporin.

(4) *Recommended regimen for children:* After the newborn period, children diagnosed with syphilis should have a CSF examination to exclude a diagnosis of neurosyphilis, and birth and maternal medical records should be reviewed to assess whether the child has congenital or acquired syphilis (see the section entitled Congenital Syphilis). Children with acquired primary or secondary syphilis should be evaluated (including consultation with child protection services regarding possible sexual abuse) and treated with **benzathine penicillin G**, intramuscularly, 50,000 units/kg in a single dose (maximum, 2.4 million units).

(5) All patients with syphilis should be tested for HIV. In areas with high HIV prevalence, patients with primary syphilis should be retested for HIV after three months.

(6) Treatment failures can occur with any regimen. However, assessing response to treatment is often difficult, and no definitive criteria for cure or failure exist. Serologic test titers may decline more slowly among patients with a prior syphilis infection. Patients should be re-examined clinically and serologically (quantitative nontreponemal VDRL or RPR test) at three and six months. Patients with signs or symptoms that persist or recur, or who have a sustained fourfold increase in nontreponemal test titer compared either with the baseline titer or to a subsequent result, can be considered to have failed treatment or to be reinfected. These patients should be re-treated after evaluation for HIV infection. Unless reinfection is likely, lumbar puncture also should be performed. Failure of nontreponemal test titers to decline fourfold by three months after therapy for primary or secondary syphilis identifies persons at risk for treatment failure. Those persons should be evaluated for HIV infection. Optimal management of such patients is unclear if they are HIV-negative. At a minimum, these patients should have additional clinical and serologic follow-up. If further follow-up cannot be assured, retreatment is recommended. Some experts recommend CSF examination in such patients. When patients are re-treated, most experts recommend three weekly injections of **benzathine penicillin G**, intramuscularly, 2.4 million units per injection, unless CSF examination indicates neurosyphilis is present.

(7) Invasion of the CSF with *T. pallidum* with accompanying

CSF abnormalities is common in adults with primary or secondary syphilis (see Lukehart et al, 1988). Despite the frequency of these CSF findings, very few patients develop clinically overt neurosyphilis when the treatment regimens described above are used. Therefore, unless clinical signs and symptoms of neurologic involvement exist, such as optic, auditory, cranial nerve, or meningeal symptoms, lumbar puncture is not recommended for routine evaluation of patients with primary or secondary syphilis. Patients with signs or symptoms of neurologic or ophthalmic disease should be evaluated and treated accordingly.

(8) Sexual transmission of *T. pallidum* occurs only when mucocutaneous syphilitic lesions are present; such manifestations are uncommon after the first year of infection. Persons sexually exposed to a patient with primary or secondary syphilis should be evaluated clinically and serologically. If the exposure occurred within the previous 90 days, the person may be infected yet seronegative and, therefore, should be presumptively treated. Presumptive treatment also is recommended for persons exposed more than 90 days previously if serologic test results are not immediately available and follow-up is uncertain. The time periods before treatment that are used for identifying at-risk sex partners are three months plus duration of symptoms for primary syphilis and six months plus duration of symptoms for secondary syphilis.

(9) The Jarisch-Herxheimer reaction, an acute febrile reaction often accompanied by headache, myalgia, hypotension, and other symptoms, may occur within the first 24 hours after any therapy for syphilis, and patients should be so warned. Jarisch-Herxheimer reactions are most common in patients with early syphilis. Antipyretics may be recommended, but no proven methods exist for preventing this reaction. Pregnant patients, in particular, should be warned that early labor or fetal distress may occur in association with the Jarisch-Herxheimer reaction.

Latent Syphilis

Latent syphilis is defined as those periods after infection with *T. pallidum* when patients are seroreactive but show no other evidence of disease. Patients who have latent syphilis and who acquired syphilis within the preceding year are classified as having early latent syphilis. Patients can be demonstrated to have acquired syphilis within the preceding year on the basis of documented seroconversion, a fourfold or greater increase in titer of a nontreponemal serologic test, history of symptoms of primary or secondary syphilis, or if they had a sex partner with primary, secondary, or latent syphilis (documented independently as duration less than one year). Nearly all others have latent syphilis of unknown duration and should be managed as if they had late latent syphilis.

RECOMMENDED REGIMENS (ADULTS):

Early Latent Syphilis

Benzathine Penicillin G: Intramuscularly, 2.4 million units in a single dose.

Late Latent Syphilis or Latent Syphilis of Unknown Duration

Benzathine Penicillin G: Intramuscularly, 2.4 million units weekly for three successive weeks (7.2 million units total).

REMARKS:

(1) Treatment of latent syphilis is intended to prevent occurrence or progression of late complications. Clinical experience indicates that penicillin is effective, but optimal penicillin regimens (dose, duration, preparation) have not been determined. There is very little evidence to support the use of nonpenicillin regimens.

(2) For patients who have latent syphilis and who are allergic to penicillin, nonpenicillin therapy should be used only after CSF examination has excluded neurosyphilis. Nonpregnant penicillin-allergic adults should receive **doxycycline**, orally, 100 mg twice daily OR, alternatively, **tetracycline hydrochloride**, orally, 500 mg four times daily. Duration of therapy is two weeks if infection is known to have been less than one year (early latent syphilis); otherwise, treat for four weeks.

(3) *Recommended regimens for children:* After the newborn period, children diagnosed with syphilis should have a CSF examination to exclude a diagnosis of neurosyphilis, and birth and maternal medical records should be reviewed to assess whether the child has congenital or acquired syphilis (see the section entitled Congenital Syphilis). Children with acquired latent syphilis should be evaluated (including consultation with child protection services regarding possible sexual abuse) and treated as follows: *Early Latent Syphilis*, **benzathine penicillin G**, intramuscularly, 50,000 units/kg in a single dose (maximum, 2.4 million units); *Late Latent Syphilis or Latent Syphilis of Unknown Duration*, **benzathine penicillin G**, intramuscularly, 50,000 units/kg (maximum, 2.4 million units) weekly for three successive weeks (total 150,000 units/kg to maximum total dose of 7.2 million units).

(4) All syphilis patients should be tested for HIV.

(5) Quantitative nontreponemal serologic tests should be repeated at 6 and 12 months. Limited data are available to guide evaluation of the response to therapy for a patient with latent syphilis. If titers increase fourfold, or if an initially high titer ($\geq$1:32) fails to decline at least fourfold (two dilutions) within 12 to 24 months, or if the patient develops signs or symptoms attributable to syphilis, the patient should be evaluated for neurosyphilis and re-treated appropriately.

(6) All patients with latent syphilis should be clinically evaluated for evidence of tertiary disease, such as aortitis, neurosyphilis, gumma, and iritis. Recommended therapy for patients with latent syphilis may not be optimal for those with asymptomatic neurosyphilis. However, the yield from CSF examination, in terms of newly diagnosed cases of neurosyphilis, is low. Patients with any of the following criteria should have a CSF examination before treatment: neurologic or ophthalmic signs or symptoms; other evidence of active syphilis (eg, aortitis, gumma, iritis); treatment failure; HIV infection; serum nontreponemal titer $\geq$1:32, unless duration of infection is known to be less than one year; and nonpenicillin therapy planned, unless duration of infection is known to be less than one year. If dictated by circumstances or patient preferences, CSF examination may be performed for persons who do not meet these criteria. If a CSF examination shows abnormalities consistent with CNS syphilis, the patient should be treated for neurosyphilis (see the section entitled Neurosyphilis).

(7) Sexual transmission of *T. pallidum* occurs only when mucocutaneous syphilitic lesions are present; such manifestations are uncommon after the first year of infection. However, persons sexually exposed to a patient with latent syphilis should be evaluated clinically and serologically according to the following recommendations: (a) persons exposed to a patient with early latent syphilis (duration $<$1 year) within the preceding 90 days might be infected even if seronegative and therefore should be presumptively treated; (b) a person who was sexually exposed to a patient with early latent syphilis (duration $<$1 year) more than 90 days earlier should be presumptively treated when serologic test results are not immediately available and the opportunity for followup is uncertain; and (c) for purposes of partner notification and presumptive treatment of exposed sex partners, patients who have syphilis of unknown duration and who have high nontreponemal serologic test titers ($\geq$1:32) may be considered to be infected with early syphilis. The time period before treatment used for identifying at-risk sex partners is one year for early latent syphilis.

(8) The Jarisch-Herxheimer reaction may occur in patients treated for syphilis (see section entitled Primary and Secondary Syphilis).

Late Syphilis

Late (tertiary) syphilis refers to patients with gumma and patients with cardiovascular syphilis (but not neurosyphilis).

RECOMMENDED REGIMEN (ADULTS):
Benzathine Penicillin G: Intramuscularly, 2.4 million units weekly for three successive weeks (7.2 million units total).
REMARKS:
(1) Penicillin-allergic patients (nonpregnant adults) should receive **doxycycline**, orally, 100 mg twice daily for four weeks OR, alternatively, **tetracycline hydrochloride**, orally, 500 mg four times daily for four weeks. If patients are allergic to penicillin, alternative drugs should be used only after CSF examination has excluded neurosyphilis.
(2) CSF examination is recommended for all patients with symptomatic late syphilis before therapy is initiated. If CSF examination reveals findings consistent with neurosyphilis, patients should be treated for neurosyphilis (see next section). Some experts treat all patients who have cardiovascular syphilis with a neurosyphilis regimen. Patients with cardiovascular or gummatous syphilis should be managed in consultation with experts.
(3) There is minimal evidence regarding follow-up of patients infected with late syphilis. Clinical response depends partly on the nature of the lesions.
(4) Long-term sex partners of patients with late syphilis should be evaluated clinically and serologically for syphilis.
(5) All patients with syphilis should be tested for HIV.

Neurosyphilis

Central nervous system disease may occur during any stage of syphilis. Clinical evidence of neurologic involvement (eg, optic and auditory symptoms, cranial nerve palsies) warrants CSF examination regardless of the apparent clinical stage or duration of syphilis.

Syphilitic eye disease frequently is associated with neurosyphilis, and patients with this disease should be treated as for neurosyphilis. CSF examination should be performed.

RECOMMENDED REGIMEN:
Aqueous Crystalline Penicillin G: Intravenously, 2 to 4 million units every four hours for 10 to 14 days.
ALTERNATIVE REGIMEN (IF COMPLIANCE CAN BE ASSURED):
Aqueous Procaine Penicillin G: Intramuscularly, 2.4 million units daily, plus probenecid 500 mg orally four times daily, both drugs for 10 to 14 days.
REMARKS:
(1) Lengthy experience has confirmed the effectiveness of penicillin for neurosyphilis, but the evidence to guide choice of the best regimen is limited.
(2) The durations of these regimens are shorter than that of the regimen used for late syphilis in the absence of neurosyphilis. Therefore, some experts recommend administration of **benzathine penicillin G**, intramuscularly, 2.4 million units after completion of either of these neurosyphilis treatment regimens, to provide a comparable total duration of therapy.
(3) No systematically collected data have evaluated therapeutic alternatives to penicillin. Patients who report being allergic to penicillin should be skin tested, desensitized if necessary (for guidelines, see *MMWR*, 1993 C), and treated with penicillin, or they should be managed in consultation with an expert.
(4) If an initial CSF pleocytosis was present, CSF examination should be repeated every six months until the cell count is normal. Follow-up CSF examinations also may be used to evaluate changes in the VDRL-CSF or CSF protein in response to therapy, but changes in these two parameters are slower and the importance of persistent abnormalities is less certain. If the cell count has not decreased at six months, or is not normal by two years, retreatment should be strongly considered.
(5) All patients with syphilis should be tested for HIV.
(6) Many experts recommend treating patients with evidence of auditory disease caused by syphilis in the same manner as for neurosyphilis, regardless of the findings on CSF exam.
(7) For management of sex partners, see preceding sections.

Syphilis in Pregnancy

All pregnant women should be screened for syphilis early in pregnancy, preferably at the first prenatal visit. In populations in which prenatal care utilization is not optimal, patients should be screened (RPR-card test) and if the test is reactive, treatment should be provided at the time pregnancy is detected. In areas of high syphilis prevalence, or in patients at high risk, serologic screening should be repeated in the third trimester and again at delivery (some states mandate screening at delivery for all women). Any woman who delivers a stillborn infant after 20 weeks' gestation should be tested for syphilis. No infant should be discharged from the hospital without the serologic status of the infant's mother having been determined at least once during pregnancy.

Seropositive pregnant women should be considered infected unless treatment history is clearly documented and sequential serologic antibody titers are showing an appropriate decline.

RECOMMENDED REGIMEN(S):
Penicillin: Pregnant women should receive the penicillin regimen appropriate for the stage of syphilis, as recommended for nonpregnant patients (see preceding sections entitled Primary and Secondary Syphilis; Latent Syphilis; Late Syphilis; and Neurosyphilis; see also REMARKS).
REMARKS:
(1) Penicillin is effective for preventing transmission to a fetus and for treating established infection in a fetus. Evidence is insufficient, however, to determine whether the specific penicillin regimens that are recommended are optimal. Some experts recommend additional therapy (eg, a second 2.4 million-unit dose of intramuscular benzathine penicillin G) one week after the initial dose, particularly for those women in the third trimester of pregnancy and for women who have secondary syphilis during pregnancy.
(2) There are no proven alternatives to penicillin for penicillin-allergic pregnant women. A pregnant woman with a history of penicillin allergy should have skin testing for penicillin allergy, be desensitized if necessary (for guidelines, see *MMWR*, 1993 C), and treated with penicillin. Tetracycline and doxycycline are contraindicated in pregnant women because of potential adverse effects on the fetus. Erythromycin should not be used for the treatment of syphilis during pregnancy because of the high risk of failure to cure infection in the fetus.
(3) Women who are treated for syphilis during the second half of pregnancy are at risk for premature labor and/or fetal distress if their treatment precipitates a Jarisch-Herxheimer reaction. They should be advised to seek medical attention following treatment if they notice any change in fetal movements or have any contractions. Stillbirth is a rare complication of treatment; however, since therapy is necessary to prevent further fetal

damage, this concern should not delay treatment.
(4) Serologic titers should be determined monthly until adequacy of treatment has been assured. The antibody response should be appropriate for the stage of disease.
(5) All patients with syphilis should be tested for HIV.
(6) For management of sex partners, see preceding sections.

Congenital Syphilis

Congenital syphilis may occur if the mother has syphilis during pregnancy. Infants should be evaluated if they were born to seropositive (nontreponemal test confirmed by treponemal test) women who: (1) have untreated syphilis (a woman [pregnant or otherwise] treated for syphilis with a regimen other than those recommended in the preceding sections should be considered untreated); *or* (2) were treated for syphilis less than one month before delivery; *or* (3) were treated for syphilis during pregnancy with erythromycin; *or* (4) were treated for syphilis during pregnancy with the appropriate penicillin regimen, but did not have the expected decrease in nontreponemal antibody titers after treatment to indicate an adequate response ($\geq$ fourfold decrease); *or* (5) do not have a well-documented history of treatment for syphilis; *or* (6) were treated appropriately before pregnancy but had insufficient serologic follow-up to assure that they responded appropriately to treatment and are not currently infected. *An infant should not be released from the hospital without the serologic status of its mother having been documented at least once during pregnancy. Serologic testing also should be performed at delivery in communities and populations at risk for congenital syphilis. Serologic tests may be nonreactive among infants infected late during their mother's pregnancy.*

The clinical and laboratory evaluation of infants born to women described above should include: (1) a thorough physical examination for evidence of congenital syphilis; (2) a quantitative nontreponemal serologic test for syphilis performed on the infant's serum (not on cord blood); (3) CSF analysis for cells, protein, and VDRL; (4) long bone x-rays; (5) other tests as clinically indicated (eg, chest x-ray); (6) for infants who have no evidence of congenital syphilis on the above evaluation, determination of presence of specific antitreponemal IgM antibody by a testing method recognized by the CDC as having either provisional or standard status; and (7) pathologic examination of the placenta or amniotic cord using specific fluorescent antitreponemal antibody staining.

Infants should be treated for presumed congenital syphilis if they were born to mothers who, at delivery, had untreated syphilis or who had evidence of relapse or reinfection after treatment. Additional criteria for presumptively treating infants with congenital syphilis are as follows: (1) any evidence of active disease by physical examination or x-ray; (2) a reactive VDRL-CSF or, for infants born to seroreactive mothers, an abnormal CSF white blood cell count or protein (see NOTE below), regardless of CSF serology; (3) a serum quantitative nontreponemal serologic titer that is at least fourfold higher than the mother's titer (absence of a fourfold higher titer cannot be used as evidence to exclude congenital syphilis); (4) specific antitreponemal IgM antibody detected by a testing method that has been given provisional or standard status by the CDC; and (5) if the infant meets the criteria to be evaluated but has not been fully evaluated. NOTE: In the immediate newborn period, interpretation of CSF test results may be difficult; normal values vary with gestational age and are higher in preterm infants. Other causes of elevated values should also be considered. Although values as high as 25 WBC/mm^3 and 150 mg protein/dL occur in normal neonates, some experts recommend that lower values (5 WBC/mm^3 and 40 mg protein/dL) be considered the upper limits of normal. An infant being evaluated for congenital syphilis should be treated if test results cannot exclude infection.

RECOMMENDED REGIMENS:
Aqueous Crystalline Penicillin G: Intravenously, 100,000 to 150,000 units/kg daily (administered as 50,000 units/kg every 12 hours during the first seven days of life and every eight hours thereafter) for 10 to 14 days;
OR
Aqueous Procaine Penicillin G: Intramuscularly, 50,000 units/kg once daily for 10 to 14 days.

REMARKS:
(1) If more than one day of therapy is missed, the entire course should be restarted.
(2) All symptomatic neonates should also have an ophthalmologic examination.
(3) An infant whose complete evaluation was normal (see above) and whose mother was: (a) treated for syphilis during pregnancy with erythromycin, *or* (b) treated for syphilis less than one month before delivery, *or* (c) treated with an appropriate regimen before or during pregnancy but did not yet have an adequate serologic response should be treated with **benzathine penicillin G**, intramuscularly, 50,000 units/kg in a single dose. In some cases, infants with a normal complete evaluation for whom follow-up can be assured can be followed closely without treatment.
(4) A seroreactive infant (or an infant whose mother was seroreactive at delivery) who is *not treated* for congenital syphilis in the perinatal period should receive careful follow-up examinations at 1, 2, 3, 6, and 12 months of age. Nontreponemal antibody titers should be decreasing by 3 months of age and should have disappeared by 6 months of age if the infant was not infected and the titers were the result of passive transfer of antibody from the mother. If these titers are found to be stable or increasing, the child should be re-evaluated, including CSF examination, and fully treated. Passively transferred treponemal antibodies may be present for as long as one year. If they are present beyond one year, the infant should be re-evaluated and treated for congenital syphilis.
(5) *Treated* infants should also be evaluated every two to three months to assure that nontreponemal antibody titers decline; these infants should have become nonreactive by 6 months of age. Treponemal tests should not be used to evaluate response, since they may remain positive, despite effective therapy, if the child was infected. Infants with CSF pleocytosis should undergo CSF examination every six months or until the cell count is normal. If the cell count is still abnormal after two years, or if a downward trend is not present at each examination, the infant should be retreated. The VDRL-CSF should also be checked at six months; if it is still reactive, the infant should be re-treated.
(6) *After the newborn period*, children diagnosed with syphilis should have a CSF examination to rule out neurosyphilis, and records should be reviewed to assess whether the child has congenital or acquired syphilis. Any child who is thought to have congenital syphilis (or who has neurologic involvement) should be treated with **aqueous crystalline penicillin G**, intravenously, 50,000 units/kg every four to six hours for 10 to 14 days

(200,000 to 300,000 units/kg/day). Follow-up of children treated for congenital syphilis after the newborn period should be the same as that recommended for congenital syphilis among neonates (see above). Older children with definite acquired syphilis and a normal neurologic examination may be treated with **benzathine penicillin G** regimens appropriate for the stage of syphilis (see sections entitled Primary and Secondary Syphilis, and Latent Syphilis). Children who require treatment for syphilis after the newborn period, but who have a history of penicillin allergy, should be skin tested, desensitized if necessary (for guidelines, see *MMWR*, 1993 C), and treated with penicillin.
(7) In cases of congenital syphilis, the mother should be tested for HIV; if the mother is HIV-positive, the infant should be referred for evaluation and appropriate follow-up.

Syphilis in HIV-Infected Patients

The clinical manifestations, serologic responses, efficacy of treatment, and occurrence of complications of syphilis may be altered in patients coinfected with human immunodeficiency virus (HIV). Thus, the CDC have proposed guidelines for the diagnosis, treatment, and follow-up of syphilis in patients coinfected with HIV (*MMWR*, 1993 C).

REMARKS:
(1) *Diagnostic Considerations*: (a) Unusual serologic responses have been observed in HIV-infected persons who also have syphilis. Most reports involved serologic titers that were higher than expected, but falsely negative serologic test results or delayed appearance of seroreactivity also have been reported. *Nevertheless, both treponemal and nontreponemal serologic tests for syphilis are accurate in the vast majority of patients with syphilis and HIV coinfection.* (b) When clinical findings suggest that syphilis is present but serologic tests are negative or inconclusive, it may be helpful to perform alternative tests, such as biopsy of lesions, dark-field examination, and direct fluorescent antibody staining of lesion material. (c) Neurosyphilis should be considered in the differential diagnosis of neurologic disease in HIV-infected persons.
(2) *General Treatment Considerations*: Although adequate research-based evidence is not available, published case reports and expert opinion suggest that HIV-infected patients with early syphilis are at increased risk for neurologic complications and have higher rates of treatment failure with currently recommended regimens. The magnitude of these risks, although not precisely defined, is probably small. No therapy has been demonstrated to be more effective in preventing development of neurosyphilis than those recommended for patients without HIV infection. Careful follow-up after therapy is essential.
(3) *Treatment and Follow-up Considerations for Primary and Secondary Syphilis Among HIV-infected Patients*: (a) Treatment with **benzathine penicillin G**, intramuscularly, 2.4 million units in a single dose, as for patients without HIV infection, is recommended. Some experts recommend additional treatments, such as multiple doses of benzathine penicillin G, as suggested for late syphilis, or other supplemental antibiotics in addition to benzathine penicillin G, 2.4 million units intramuscularly. (b) CSF abnormalities are common in HIV-infected patients who have primary or secondary syphilis, but these abnormalities are of unknown prognostic significance. Most HIV-infected patients respond appropriately to currently recommended penicillin therapy; however, some experts recommend CSF examination before therapy and modification of treatment accordingly. (c) Penicillin regimens should be used to treat HIV-infected patients in all stages of syphilis. Penicillin-allergic patients may be skin tested to confirm penicillin allergy, but data on the utility of that approach in immunocompromised patients are inadequate. Patients may be desensitized and then treated with penicillin. (d) Patients should be evaluated clinically and serologically for treatment failure at 1, 2, 3, 6, 9, and 12 months after therapy. Although of unproven benefit, some experts recommend performing CSF examination after therapy (eg, at six months). (e) HIV-infected patients who meet the criteria for treatment failure should undergo CSF examination and be re-treated just as for patients without HIV infection. CSF examination and re-treatment also should be strongly considered for patients in whom the suggested fourfold decrease in nontreponemal test titer does not occur within three months for primary or secondary syphilis. Most experts would re-treat patients with benzathine penicillin G, intramuscularly, 2.4 million units weekly for three successive weeks (total of 7.2 million units) if CSF examination results are normal.
(4) *Treatment and Follow-up Considerations for Latent Syphilis Among HIV-infected Patients*: (a) Patients who have both latent syphilis (regardless of apparent duration) and HIV infection should undergo CSF examination before treatment. (b) Patients with latent syphilis, HIV infection, and normal CSF examination results can be treated with **benzathine penicillin G,** intramuscularly, 2.4 million units weekly for three successive weeks (total of 7.2 million units). (c) Penicillin regimens should be used to treat HIV-infected patients in all stages of syphilis. Penicillin-allergic patients may be skin tested to confirm penicillin allergy, but data on the utility of that approach in immunocompromised patients are inadequate. Patients may be desensitized and then treated with penicillin.

CHANCROID

Chancroid is a genital ulcer disease caused by *Haemophilus ducreyi*. It is endemic in many areas of the United States and also occurs in discrete outbreaks. Chancroid is well established as a cofactor for HIV transmission, and a high rate of HIV infection among patients with chancroid has been reported in the United States and other countries. The definitive diagnosis requires isolation of *H. ducreyi* from culture of ulcers and/or lymph node aspirates. However, culture for *H. ducreyi* is difficult (culture media not commercially available) and relatively insensitive (≤80%). The decision to treat for chancroid is usually based on a probable diagnosis as follows: The patient has one or more painful genital ulcer(s) and (1) no evidence of *Treponema pallidum* infection by dark-field examination of ulcer exudate (Note: Dark-field examination is not done by most clinical laboratories) or by serologic test for syphilis performed at least seven days after onset of ulcers, and (2) either the clinical presentation of ulcer(s) is not typical of disease caused by herpes simplex virus (HSV) or HSV testing is negative. The combination of a painful ulcer with tender inguinal adenopathy (which occurs in about one-third of patients) is suggestive of chancroid and, when accompanied by suppurative inguinal adenopathy, is almost pathognomonic.

RECOMMENDED REGIMENS:
Azithromycin: Orally, 1 g in a single dose;
OR
Ceftriaxone: Intramuscularly, 250 mg in a single dose;
OR
Erythromycin base: Orally, 500 mg four times daily for seven days.
ALTERNATIVE REGIMENS:
Amoxicillin (500 mg) plus potassium clavulanate (125 mg) orally three times daily for seven days;
OR

Ciprofloxacin: Orally, 500 mg twice daily for three days.
REMARKS:
(1) All three recommended regimens are effective for the treatment of chancroid in patients without HIV infection. Azithromycin and ceftriaxone offer the advantage of single-dose therapy. Strains of *H. ducreyi* resistant to either azithromycin or ceftriaxone have not been reported. Although two isolates resistant to erythromycin were reported from Asia a decade ago, similar isolates have not been reported in the United States. The safety of azithromycin in pregnant or lactating women has not been established.
(2) The two alternative regimens have not been as extensively evaluated as the recommended regimens; neither has been studied in the United States. Ciprofloxacin is contraindicated in pregnant or nursing women and for persons ≤17 years of age.
(3) Patients should be re-examined three to seven days after initiation of therapy. If treatment is successful, ulcers improve symptomatically within three days and improve objectively within seven days after institution of therapy. If no clinical improvement is evident, the clinician must consider whether (a) the diagnosis is correct; (b) coinfection with another STD agent exists; (c) the patient is infected with HIV; (d) treatment was not taken as instructed; or (e) the *H. ducreyi* strain causing infection is resistant to the prescribed antimicrobial drug. The time required for complete healing is related to the size of the ulcer; large ulcers may require two or more weeks. Clinical resolution of fluctuant lymphadenopathy is slower than that of ulcers and may require needle aspiration through adjacent intact skin, even during successful therapy.
(4) Persons who had sexual contact with a patient who has chancroid within 10 days before onset of the patient's symptoms should be examined and treated. The examination and treatment should be administered even in the absence of symptoms.
(5) Patients should be tested for HIV infection at the time of diagnosis. Patients also should be tested three months later for both syphilis and HIV if initial results are negative.
(6) Patients coinfected with HIV should be closely monitored. These patients may require courses of therapy longer than those recommended above. Healing may be slower among HIV-infected persons, and treatment failures do occur, especially after shorter-course treatment regimens. Since data on therapeutic efficacy with the recommended single-dose ceftriaxone and azithromycin regimens in HIV-infected persons are limited, those regimens should be used in these patients only if follow-up can be assured. Some experts suggest using the erythromycin seven-day regimen for treating chancroid in HIV-infected persons.
(7) One consultant stated that if dark-field examination cannot be done, it is difficult to be certain that the patient does not have primary syphilis. In this situation, presumptive treatment for primary syphilis should be given along with therapy for chancroid (see also index entry Syphilis).

LYMPHOGRANULOMA VENEREUM

A rare disease in the United States, lymphogranuloma venereum (LGV) is caused by serovars L_1, L_2, and L_3 of *Chlamydia trachomatis*. In heterosexual men, LGV typically manifests as tender inguinal lymphadenopathy that is most commonly unilateral; among women and homosexually active men, proctocolitis or inflammatory involvement of perirectal or perianal lymphatic tissues is common, often resulting in fistulas or strictures. Diagnosis usually is made serologically and by exclusion of other causes of inguinal lymphadenopathy or genital ulcers.

RECOMMENDED REGIMEN:
Doxycycline: Orally, 100 mg twice daily for 21 days.
ALTERNATIVE REGIMENS:
Erythromycin: Orally, 500 mg four times daily for 21 days;
OR
Sulfisoxazole: Orally, 500 mg four times daily for 21 days (or equivalent sulfonamide course).
REMARKS:
(1) As for other chlamydial infections, doxycycline is preferred. Treatment cures infection and prevents ongoing tissue damage, but tissue reaction may result in scarring.
(2) Patients should be followed until signs and symptoms have resolved. Fluctuant lymph nodes (buboes) should be aspirated as needed through healthy adjacent normal skin. Incision and drainage or excision of nodes delays healing and is contraindicated. Late sequelae, such as stricture and/or fistula, may require surgical intervention.
(3) Persons who have had sexual contact with a patient who has LGV within 30 days before onset of the patient's symptoms should be examined, tested for urethral or cervical chlamydial infection, and treated.
(4) Pregnant and lactating women should be treated with the erythromycin regimen. Tetracyclines (eg, doxycycline) should not be used in pregnant women or children under 8 years. Sulfonamides should not be used in pregnant women near term or in infants under 2 months.
(5) Persons with HIV infection and LGV should be treated with the same regimens listed above.

GRANULOMA INGUINALE (DONOVANOSIS)

Granuloma inguinale is a genital ulcer disease caused by *Calymmatobacterium granulomatis*, and the antimicrobial drug selected should be active against this organism.

Selected references: Felman and Nikitas, 1981; Lynch, 1982; Hart, 1990.

RECOMMENDED REGIMEN:
Tetracycline: Orally, 500 mg four times daily for three weeks or until there is complete healing of all lesions.
REMARKS:
(1) No technique exists for standardized susceptibility testing of the organism, and tetracycline is recommended solely on the basis of clinical experience. For treatment failures or patients who are allergic to or cannot tolerate tetracyclines, gentamicin and chloramphenicol are alternative antibiotics.
(2) A variant of chancroid mimics granuloma inguinale and has accounted for most cases clinically diagnosed as granuloma inguinale in the Atlanta, GA, area. This infection should be treated following the recommendations for chancroid (see Section on Chancroid).
(3) Tetracyclines should not be used in pregnant women or children under 8 years.

SCABIES

This skin infection is caused by the itch mite, *Sarcoptes scabiei*. For treatment guidelines, see index entry Scabies.

PEDICULOSIS PUBIS

This infection is caused by *Phthirus pubis* (crab louse), which primarily infests the pubic region. For treatment guidelines, see index entry Pediculosis.

ENTERIC INFECTIONS

Enteric infections, including proctitis, proctocolitis, and enteritis, can be sexually transmitted and are frequently observed in homosexual or bisexual men due to receptive anal intercourse and to sexual practices that foster fecal-oral contamination. *Proctitis* is inflammation limited to the rectum (the distal 10 to 12 cm) and is associated with anorectal pain, tenesmus, constipation, and rectal discharge. *Neisseria gonorrhoeae*, *Chlamydia trachomatis* (including LGV serovars), *Treponema pallidum*, and herpes simplex virus (HSV) are the most common sexually transmitted pathogens and result from direct anorectal inoculation. In patients coinfected with HIV, herpes proctitis may be especially severe. *Proctocolitis* is associated with symptoms of proctitis plus diarrhea and/or abdominal cramps, and the colonic mucosa is inflamed proximal to 12 cm. Causative organisms include *Campylobacter* spp, *Shigella* spp, *Entamoeba histolytica* (amebiasis), and, rarely, *C. trachomatis* (LGV serovars). Depending on the etiology, proctocolitis can result from either rectal inoculation or oral exposure. Cytomegalovirus (CMV) and other opportunistic organisms may be involved in immunosuppressed patients coinfected with HIV. *Enteritis* in homosexual men usually results in diarrhea and abdominal cramping without signs of proctitis or proctocolitis. In otherwise healthy patients, *Giardia lamblia* (giardiasis) is most commonly implicated; these infections result from oral exposure. In patients coinfected with HIV, CMV, *Mycobacterium avium-intracellulare*, *Salmonella* spp, *Cryptosporidium, Microsporidium*, and *Isospora* must be considered. Enteritis also may be a direct result of HIV infection.

All patients with sexually transmitted enteric infections should be counseled and tested for HIV infection. Evaluation should include appropriate diagnostic procedures, such as anoscopy or sigmoidoscopy, stool examination, and culture.

Treatment of sexually transmitted enteric infections should be based on etiologic diagnosis when possible. Treatment guidelines for proctitis caused by *N. gonorrhoeae* and *C. trachomatis* can be found in the sections of this chapter entitled Gonococcal Infections and *Chlamydia trachomatis* Infections. For drug selection for infections caused by *Campylobacter* spp, *Shigella* spp, and nontyphoidal *Salmonella* spp, see Chapter 2 in this Section, Antimicrobial Therapy for Common Infectious Diseases. For treatment of amebiasis, giardiasis, cryptosporidiosis, and isosporiasis, see index entries on these infections.

HEPATITIS B

An estimated one-third to two-thirds of the 200,000 to 300,000 new hepatitis B (HBV) infections that occurred annually in the United States during the past decade were sexually transmitted. From 6% to 10% of infected adults become chronic HBV carriers; these individuals are capable of transmitting HBV to others and are at increased risk of long-term sequelae (chronic active hepatitis, cirrhosis of the liver, hepatocellular carcinoma) and death. Moreover, infants born to HBV-infected mothers can be infected perinatally.

Interferon alfa-2b [Intron A] is indicated for treatment of chronic hepatitis B in adults with compensated liver disease and HBV replication, ie, patients must be HBsAg-positive for at least six months, be HBeAg-positive, and have elevated serum alanine aminotransferase (ALT). Therapy with interferon alfa-2b has produced virologic remissions (ie, loss of HBeAG and normal serum aminotransferases) in many of these patients. Remissions have been long-term in 35% to 45% of patients. For more detailed discussion, see index entry Hepatitis, Chronic.

HBV infection in both adults and neonates can be readily prevented with a safe and effective vaccine that has been available in the United States for more than 10 years. For recommendations for protection against hepatitis B, see *MMWR*, 1991 B. See also index entry Hepatitis, Viral.

ACQUIRED IMMUNODEFICIENCY SYNDROME

Acquired immunodeficiency syndrome (AIDS) is a late manifestation of a sexually transmissible infection caused by retroviruses known as human immunodeficiency viruses (HIV-1 and HIV-2). Presently, the control measures are primary prevention of sexually transmitted HIV infection (eg, by avoidance of sexual intercourse with an infected individual, by appropriate use of latex condoms) and screening of blood. No interventions have been demonstrated to eradicate HIV infection (secondary prevention) or to totally rehabilitate persons with overt AIDS (tertiary prevention). Also, there is no established treatment available to completely reverse the immune dysfunction of AIDS. Many experimental studies to evaluate the efficacy of potential vaccines, immunomodulatory agents, and antiretroviral compounds active against HIV are in progress. Currently, the nucleoside reverse transcriptase inhibitors, zidovudine [Retrovir; also called AZT], didanosine [Videx; also called ddI], and zalcitabine [Hivid; also called ddC], are the only approved drugs. Treatment and prophylaxis for many of the opportunistic infections and neoplastic complications of AIDS have been variably successful, but require consultation with specialists in infectious diseases, oncology, or dermatology. See also index entries Immunodeficiency Syndrome, Acquired; Antiviral Agents.

PREVENTION OF OPHTHALMIA NEONATORUM

Instillation of a prophylactic agent into the eyes of all newborn infants is recommended to prevent gonococcal ophthalmia neonatorum and is required by law in most states. Although all regimens listed below effectively prevent gonococcal eye disease, none of the regimens appears to prevent chlamydial conjunctivitis reliably (Hammerschlag et al, 1989). Furthermore, they do not eliminate nasopharyngeal colonization with *C. trachomatis* (see also index entry, Conjunctivitis, Chlamydial). Treatment of gonococcal and chlamydial infections in pregnant women is the best method for preventing neonatal gonococcal and chlamydial disease. However, ocular prophylaxis should continue because it can prevent gonococcal ophthalmia neonatorum and, in some populations, >10% of pregnant women may receive no prenatal care.

RECOMMENDED REGIMEN(S):

Silver nitrate (1%) aqueous solution once OR **erythromycin (0.5%) ophthalmic ointment once** OR **tetracycline (1%) ophthalmic ointment once. Instill immediately postpartum and never later than one hour after birth. Drugs are given in a single application into each conjunctival sac with no rinsing of the eyes. Single-use tubes or ampuls are preferred to multiple-use tubes.**

REMARKS:

(1) Silver nitrate is effective in preventing gonococcal ophthalmia neonatorum, but it frequently causes chemical conjunctivitis.

(2) Erythromycin and tetracycline appear to be as effective as silver nitrate in preventing gonococcal ophthalmia and these antibiotic ointments do not cause chemical conjunctivitis. However, erythromycin or tetracycline prophylaxis is considerably more expensive than silver nitrate prophylaxis. Also, ointments are more difficult to administer than drops.

(3) Efficacy of tetracycline and erythromycin in the prevention of gonococcal ophthalmia due to antibiotic-resistant *N. gonorrhoeae* strains (PPNG, CMRNG, TRNG) is unknown, although both probably are effective because of the high concentrations of drug in these preparations. In one study, tetracycline ointment was effective prophylaxis against gonococcal ophthalmia caused by PPNG and strains for which the MICs for tetracycline were relatively high (Laga et al, 1988).

(4) Bacitracin is not recommended.

(5) All infants should be given ocular prophylaxis, whether delivery is vaginal or cesarean. If prophylaxis is delayed (not administered in the delivery room), the hospital should establish a monitoring system to ensure that all infants receive prophylaxis.

USE OF CONDOMS TO PREVENT STDS

Preventing the spread of STDs requires that persons at risk for transmitting or acquiring infections alter their behavior. The most effective way to prevent sexual transmission of STDs, including HIV infection, is to avoid sexual intercourse with an infected partner. However, if a person chooses to have sexual intercourse with a partner whose infection status is unknown or who is infected with HIV or other STDs, men should use a new latex condom with each act of intercourse. Physicians should instruct their patients regarding correct use. See the following recommendations from the CDC (*MMWR,* 1993 C). For more detailed information on STD prevention strategies, see *MMWR*, 1993 C.

Recommendations for Condom Use

1. Use a new condom with each act of intercourse.
2. Carefully handle the condom to avoid damaging it with fingernails, teeth, or other sharp objects.
3. Put the condom on after the penis is erect and before any genital contact with the partner.
4. Ensure that no air is trapped in the tip of the condom.
5. Ensure that there is adequate lubrication during intercourse, possibly requiring the use of exogenous lubricants.
6. Use only water-based lubricants (eg, K-Y Jelly, glycerine) with latex condoms (oil-based lubricants [eg, petroleum jelly, shortening, mineral oil, massage oils, body lotions, cooking oil] that can weaken latex should never be used).
7. Hold the condom firmly against the base of the penis during withdrawal, and withdraw while the penis is still erect to prevent slippage.

Cited References

Drugs for sexually transmitted diseases. *Med Lett Drugs Ther* 36:1-6, 1994.

Report of the Committee of Infectious Diseases: *American Academy of Pediatrics Redbook*, ed 22. Elk Grove Village, Ill, American Academy of Pediatrics, 1991, 259-269.

1985 Sexually transmitted diseases treatment guidelines. *MMWR* 34(suppl):75S-108S, 1985.

Recommendations for diagnosing and treating syphilis in HIV-infected patients. *MMWR* 37:600-608, 1988.

Pelvic inflammatory disease: Guidelines for prevention and management. *MMWR* 40(No. RR-5):1-25, 1991 A.

Hepatitis B virus: A comprehensive strategy for eliminating transmission in the United States through universal childhood vaccination: Recommendations of the Immunization Practices Advisory Committee (ACIP). *MMWR* 40(No. RR-13):1-25, 1991 B.

Summary—Cases of specified notifiable diseases, United States, cumulative, week ending January 2, 1993 (53rd week). *MMWR* 41:979, 1993 A.

Recommendations for the prevention and management of *Chlamydia trachomatis* infections, 1993. *MMWR* 42(No. RR-12):1-39, 1993 B.

CDC sexually transmitted diseases treatment guidelines, 1993. *MMWR* 42(No. RR-14):1-102, 1993 C.

Pregnancy outcomes following systemic prenatal acyclovir exposure—June 1, 1984-June 30, 1993. *MMWR* 42:806-809, 1993 D.

Batteiger BE, et al: Efficacy and safety of ofloxacin in treatment of nongonococcal sexually transmitted disease. *Am J Med* 87(suppl 6C):75S-77S, 1989.

Cates W Jr: Epidemiology and control of sexually transmitted diseases: Strategic evolution. *Infect Dis Clin North Am* 1:1-23, 1987.

Collier AC, et al: Comparative study of ceftriaxone and spectinomycin in treatment of uncomplicated gonorrhea in women. *Am J Med* 11:68-72, 1984.

Covino JM, et al: Comparison of ofloxacin and ceftriaxone in treatment of uncomplicated gonorrhea caused by penicillinase-producing and non-penicillinase-producing strains. *Antimicrob Agents Chemother* 34:148-149, 1990.

Crombleholme WR, et al: Amoxicillin therapy for *Chlamydia trachomatis* in pregnancy. *Obstet Gynecol* 75:752-756, 1990.

Felman YM, Nikitas JA: Sexually transmitted diseases: 1981 schedules for treatment of sexually transmitted diseases as recommended by New York City Health Department Bureau of Venereal Diseases Control, part II. *Cutis* 28:374-394, 1981.

Gorwitz RJ, et al: Sentinel surveillance for antimicrobial resistance in *Neisseria gonorrhoeae*—United States, 1988-1991. *MMWR* 42 (No. SS-3):29-39, 1993.

Hammerschlag MR, et al: Efficacy of neonatal ocular prophylaxis for prevention of chlamydial and gonococcal conjunctivitis. *N Engl J Med* 320:769-772, 1989.

Handsfield HH: Recent developments in STDs: I. Bacterial diseases. *Hosp Pract* 47-56, (July) 1991.

Handsfield HH, Hook EW: Ceftriaxone for treatment of uncomplicated gonorrhea: Routine use of single 125-mg dose in sexually transmitted disease clinic. *Sex Transm Dis* 14:227-230, 1987.

Handsfield HH, Murphy VL: Comparative study of ceftriaxone and spectinomycin for treatment of uncomplicated gonorrhoea in men. *Lancet* 2:67-70, 1983.

Handsfield HH, et al: A comparison of single-dose cefixime with ceftriaxone as treatment for uncomplicated gonorrhea. *N Engl J Med* 325:1337-1341, 1991.

Hart G: Donovanosis, in Holmes KK, et al (eds): *Sexually Transmitted Diseases,* ed 2. New York, McGraw-Hill, 1990, 273-277.

Hook EW III, Marra CM: Acquired syphilis in adults. *N Engl J Med* 326:1060-1069, 1992.

Judson FN, et al: Comparative study of ceftriaxone and spectinomycin for treatment of pharyngeal and anorectal gonorrhea. *JAMA* 253:1417-1419, 1985.

Kost RG, et al: Brief report: Recurrent acyclovir-resistant genital herpes in an immunocompetent patient. *N Engl J Med* 329:1777-1782, 1993.

Laga M, et al: Single-dose therapy of gonococcal ophthalmia neonatorum with ceftriaxone. *N Engl J Med* 315:1382-1385, 1986.

Laga M, et al: Prophylaxis of gonococcal and chlamydial ophthalmia neonatorum: Comparison of silver nitrate and tetracycline. *N Engl J Med* 318:653-657, 1988.

Lukehart SA, et al: Invasion of central nervous system by *Treponema pallidum*: Implications for diagnosis and treatment. *Ann Intern Med* 109:855-862, 1988.

Lutz: Single-dose efficacy of ofloxacin in uncomplicated gonorrhea. *Am J Med* 87 (suppl 6C):69S-74S, 1989.

Lynch PD: Therapy of sexually transmitted diseases. *Med Clin North Am* 66:915-925, 1982.

Magat AH, et al: Double-blind randomized study comparing amoxicillin and erythromycin for the treatment of *Chlamydia trachomatis* in pregnancy. *Obstet Gynecol* 81:745-749, 1993.

Martin DH, et al: A controlled trial of a single-dose of azithromycin for the treatment of chlamydial urethritis and cervicitis. *N Engl J Med* 327:921-925, 1992.

McCormack WM: Pelvic inflammatory disease. *N Engl J Med* 330:115-119, 1994.

Moran JS, Zenilman JM: Therapy for gonococcal infections: Options in 1989. *Rev Infect Dis* 12 (suppl 6):S633-S644, 1990.

Piper JM, et al: Prenatal use of metronidazole and birth defects: No association. *Obstet Gynecol* 82:348-352, 1993.

Rapoza N (ed): *HIV Infection and Disease: Monographs for Physicians and Other Health Care Workers.* Chicago, American Medical Association, 1989.

Rein MF: Sexually transmitted diseases. *Compr Ther* 19:136-144, 1993.

Rein MF, Müller M: *Trichomonas vaginalis* and trichomoniasis, in Holmes KK, et al (eds): *Sexually Transmitted Diseases*, ed 2. New York, McGraw-Hill, 1990, 481-492.

Stamm WE: Toward control of sexually transmitted chlamydial infections. *Ann Intern Med* 119:432-434, 1993.

Stamm WE, et al: Azithromycin in the treatment of nongonoccocal urethritis: A multicenter, double-blind, double-dummy study employing doxycycline as a comparative agent, abstract 10. *33rd Interscience Conference on Antimicrobial Agents and Chemotherapy*. New Orleans, Oct 17-20, 1993.

Walker CK, et al: Pelvic inflammatory disease: Metaanalysis of antimicrobial regimen efficacy. *J Infect Dis* 168:969-978, 1993.

Washington AE, Katz P: Cost of and payment source for pelvic inflammatory disease: Trends and projections, 1983 through 2000. *JAMA* 266:2565-2569, 1991.

Webb DHF, Fife KH: Genital herpes simplex virus infections. *Infect Dis Clin North Am* 1:97-122, 1987.

Webster LA, et al: An evaluation of surveillance for *Chlamydia trachomatis* infections in the United States, 1987-1991. *MMWR* 42 (No. SS-3):21-27, 1993.

Antimicrobial Chemoprophylaxis for Ambulatory Patients

61

PREVENTION OF BACTERIAL ENDOCARDITIS

PREVENTION OF RECURRENT ATTACKS OF RHEUMATIC FEVER (SECONDARY PREVENTION)

PREVENTION OF MENINGOCOCCAL DISEASE

PREVENTION OF *HAEMOPHILUS INFLUENZAE* TYPE b DISEASE

PREVENTION OF PNEUMOCOCCAL INFECTION IN ASPLENIC PATIENTS

PREVENTION OF RECURRENT BACTERIAL URINARY TRACT INFECTIONS (REINFECTIONS) IN WOMEN

PREVENTION OF PERTUSSIS IN EXPOSED PERSONS

PREVENTION OF RECURRENT ACUTE OTITIS MEDIA

PREVENTION OF TRAVELERS' DIARRHEA

The purpose of antimicrobial chemoprophylaxis is to prevent the development of symptomatic infection or to prevent the spread of disease. This is accomplished by administering an antimicrobial agent before, during, or shortly after exposure to an infectious agent. Whether chemoprophylaxis is justified depends on a number of factors, including: (1) the likelihood that the patient will develop symptomatic infection if chemoprophylaxis is not used; (2) the severity of the disease to be prevented; (3) the effectiveness of nonspecific host defenses; (4) the efficacy of the drug in preventing the infection; (5) the acceptability of the drug, based on its adverse reaction potential; (6) the duration of exposure (and the probability of re-exposure) to the infectious agent; (7) the likelihood and consequences of promoting resistance to the drug(s) used; and (8) the cost and availability of the prophylactic regimen (Flynn and Hoeprich, 1983).

Chemoprophylaxis is most often successful when it is directed against a specific pathogenic microorganism that is highly susceptible to the antimicrobial agent and remains susceptible throughout the period of prophylaxis. The use of penicillin G benzathine to prevent recurrent attacks of rheumatic fever by group A beta hemolytic streptococci is an excellent example of chemoprophylaxis directed against a specific pathogen. Prevention of infections at particular body sites by a range of pathogens is more difficult, but can be successfully achieved if the period of risk is defined and brief, if the expected pathogens have predictable antimicrobial susceptibility, and if the site is accessible to the drug. The use of trimethoprim/sulfamethoxazole to prevent recurrent urinary tract infections is an example of this type of chemoprophylaxis. Chemoprophylaxis to prevent secondary infections by any or all microorganisms in patients who are ill with other diseases generally has been unsuccessful. However, short-term chemoprophylaxis with trimethoprim/sulfamethoxazole or the fluoroquinolones (ciprofloxacin, norfloxacin) has been reported to reduce the frequency of bacterial infection in severely neutropenic patients in some studies (see Walsh and Schimpff, 1983; Dekker et al, 1987; Karp et al, 1987; Rozenberg-Arska and Dekker, 1987; see also index entry Trimethoprim and Sulfamethoxazole).

Situations in which antimicrobial chemoprophylaxis of nonsurgical infections in ambulatory patients is of proven, or probable, benefit are discussed below with guidelines for antimicrobial agents of choice, dosages, and durations of prophylaxis. See also Chapter 5 in this Section, Antimicrobial Chemoprophylaxis for Surgical Patients. Immunoprophylaxis of infectious diseases is discussed elsewhere; see index entry Immunization.

General references: Mills and Jawetz, 1982; Scheifele, 1982; Wilson, 1983; Brachman, 1990; Sande et al, 1990; *American Academy of Pediatrics Redbook*, 1991.

Prevention of Bacterial Endocarditis

Antimicrobial chemoprophylaxis of bacterial endocarditis in patients with (1) prosthetic cardiac valves, including bioprosthetic and homograft valves; (2) previous bacterial endocarditis, even in the absence of heart disease; (3) most congenital cardiac malformations (excluding isolated secundum atrial septal defect); (4) rheumatic and other acquired valvular dysfunction, even after valvular surgery; (5) hypertrophic cardiomyopathy (IHSS); and (6) mitral valve prolapse with valvular regurgitation (see NOTE below) is recommended prior to dental procedures known to induce gingival or mucosal bleeding, including professional cleaning, and various other invasive procedures of the upper respiratory, genitourinary, or lower gastrointestinal tract that may be associated with transient bacteremia. Prophylaxis should be effective against α-hemolytic (viridans) streptococci (from oral or respiratory foci) or enterococci (from genitourinary or lower gastrointestinal foci), the likely causative organisms of infective endocarditis. Although the effectiveness of specific regimens for the prevention of bacterial endocarditis has not been documented in controlled clinical studies, the recommendations of the Committee on Rheumatic Fever, Endocarditis and Kawasaki Disease of the Council on Cardiovascular Disease in the Young, American Heart Association (Dajani et al, 1990) are most widely accepted. These guidelines are outlined below. Similar recommendations have been proposed by others (for example, see Keys, 1982; *Med Lett Drugs Ther*, 1989; Durack, 1990; Simmons, 1993).

NOTE: Mitral valve prolapse is a very common condition. Patients with this disorder have a modest increased risk (five- to eightfold) of endocarditis (Clemens et al, 1982), and the risk appears to be greater for those with a precordial systolic murmur with mitral regurgitation (Baddour and Bisno, 1986; MacMahon et al, 1986). Although decision analyses have raised questions about the risk-benefit ratio of prophylaxis for mitral valve prolapse patients (Bor and Himmelstein, 1984; Clemens and Ransohoff, 1984), the current consensus is that those patients with valvular regurgitation should receive antimicrobial prophylaxis (Dajani et al, 1990). Furthermore, although prophylaxis is not recommended in the absence of valvular regurgitation, individuals who have a mitral valve prolapse associated with thickening and/or redundancy of the valve leaflets may be at increased risk for bacterial endocarditis, particularly men who are 45 years of age or older (Dajani et al, 1990). For additional discussion, see Durack, 1990; Greenman and Bisno, 1992.

A. Prophylaxis for dental (including professional cleaning), oral, or upper respiratory tract procedures (risk of bacteremia with various procedures is discussed in Everett and Hirschmann, 1977; LeFrock and Molavi, 1982; Dajani et al, 1990; and Durack, 1990).

PROPHYLACTIC REGIMEN(S)

STANDARD ORAL PENICILLIN-CONTAINING REGIMEN:

Amoxicillin (*adults*, 3 g; *children*, 50 mg/kg) one hour before procedure, then (*adults*, 1.5 g; *children*, 25 mg/kg) six hours after initial dose.

REMARKS:

(1) This is the recommended standard prophylactic regimen for dental, oral, and upper respiratory tract procedures in patients who are at risk, including those with prosthetic heart valves and other high-risk patients.

(2) Amoxicillin, ampicillin, and penicillin V are equally effective in vitro against α-hemolytic streptococci, but amoxicillin is better absorbed from the gastrointestinal tract and provides higher and more sustained serum levels.

(3) Penicillin V (*adults*, 2 g; *children*, 1 g) one hour before procedure, then (*adults*, 1 g; *children*, 0.5 g) six hours after initial dose is still considered a rational and acceptable alternative oral regimen for dental, oral, and upper respiratory tract procedures.

(4) For patients unable to take oral antibiotics prior to a procedure, the following alternative parenteral penicillin-containing prophylactic regimen may be substituted: Ampicillin (*adults*, 2 g; *children*, 50 mg/kg), IM or IV, one-half hour before procedure, then IV or IM ampicillin (*adults*, 1 g; *children*, 25 mg/kg) *or* oral amoxicillin (*adults*, 1.5 g; *children*, 25 mg/kg) six hours after initial dose.

(5) In unusual circumstances or in the case of delayed healing, it may be necessary to provide additional doses of antibiotics even though bacteremia rarely persists longer than 15 minutes after a procedure.

STANDARD ORAL REGIMEN FOR PATIENTS ALLERGIC TO PENICILLIN/AMOXICILLIN:

Erythromycin ethylsuccinate (*adults*, 800 mg; *children*, 20 mg/kg) or erythromycin stearate (*adults*, 1 g; *children*, 20 mg/kg) two hours before procedure, then one-half the amount six hours after initial dose.

REMARKS:

(1) Recommended for dental, oral, or upper respiratory tract procedures in penicillin/amoxicillin-allergic patients who are at risk, including those with prosthetic heart valves and other high-risk patients.

(2) The American Heart Association guidelines state: "Erythromycin ethylsuccinate and erythromycin stearate are recommended because of more rapid and reliable absorption than other erythromycin formulations, resulting in higher and more sustained serum levels." This statement has drawn some criticism. First, due to pharmacokinetic differences, 1.6 g of erythromycin ethylsuccinate (not 800 mg) produces free serum erythromycin concentrations similar to 1 g of erythromycin stearate. Second, enteric-coated formulations of erythromycin base appear to produce serum concentrations comparable to erythromycin stearate (Stierer and Sterchele, 1991; McMorrow and Nahata, 1991; see also index entry Erythromycin). The Chairman of the American Heart Association Committee responded to these criticisms by stating that both of the recommended regimens should result in adequate serum levels against α-hemolytic streptococci; larger doses of erythromycin ethylsuccinate might result in unacceptable gastrointestinal upset; and by simplifying the choices and timing of drug administration, the Committee believed that more reliable erythromycin serum concentrations would be achieved when these recommendations were widely applied (Dajani and Taubert, 1991).

(3) For individuals who cannot tolerate penicillins, another recommended alternative is clindamycin hydrochloride (*adults*, 300 mg; *children*, 10 mg/kg), orally, one hour before procedure, then (*adults*, 150 mg; *children*, 5 mg/kg) six hours after initial dose.

(4) Antibiotic regimens used to prevent the recurrence of acute rheumatic fever are inadequate for the prevention of bacterial endocarditis. Individuals who take an oral penicillin for secondary prevention of rheumatic fever or for other purposes may have viridans streptococci in their oral cavities that are relatively resistant to penicillins (eg, amoxicillin). In such cases, one of the alternative nonpenicillin-containing regimens should be selected for endocarditis prophylaxis.

(5) Tetracyclines and sulfonamides are *not* recommended for endocarditis prophylaxis.

(6) For penicillin/amoxicillin-allergic patients unable to take oral antibiotics prior to a procedure, the following alternative parenteral prophylactic regimen may be substituted: Clindamycin phosphate (*adults*, 300 mg; *children*, 10 mg/kg), IV, one-half hour before procedure, then IV *or* oral clindamycin (*adults*, 150 mg; *children*, 5 mg/kg) six hours after initial dose.

ALTERNATIVE PARENTERAL PENICILLIN-CONTAINING REGIMEN FOR PATIENTS CONSIDERED AT HIGH RISK AND NOT CANDIDATES FOR STANDARD REGIMEN:

Ampicillin (*adults*, 2 g; *children*, 50 mg/kg) *plus* gentamicin (*adults*, 1.5 mg/kg; *children*, 2 mg/kg [not to exceed 80 mg]) IM one-half hour before procedure or IV immediately before procedure, *followed by* oral amoxicillin (*adults*, 1.5 g; *children*, 25 mg/kg) six hours after initial dose. Alternatively, the parenteral regimen may be repeated once eight

hours after the initial dose. (Note: In *children,* the follow-up doses are one-half the initial pediatric doses.)

REMARKS:

(1) Individuals who have prosthetic heart valves, a previous history of endocarditis, or surgically constructed systemic-pulmonary shunts or conduits are at high risk for developing endocarditis, and endocardial infection in such individuals is associated with substantial morbidity and mortality. Previously, parenteral regimens were recommended in these patients. In practice, however, there are substantial logistic and financial barriers to the use of parenteral regimens. Moreover, oral regimens have now been used in other countries in individuals who have prosthetic heart valves, and failures in prophylaxis have not been evident. Thus, the American Heart Association committee recommends the use of the standard prophylactic regimen for dental, oral, or upper respiratory tract procedures in patients who have prosthetic heart valves and in other high-risk groups. Because some practitioners may prefer to use parenteral prophylaxis in these high-risk patients, this alternative regimen is provided.

(2) Initial gentamicin dose should not exceed 80 mg. In patients with compromised renal function, it may be necessary to modify or omit the second dose of gentamicin.

(3) Intramuscular injections for endocarditis prophylaxis should be avoided in patients who receive heparin. The use of warfarin sodium is a relative contraindication to intramuscular injections. Intravenous or oral regimens should be used whenever possible.

ALTERNATIVE PARENTERAL REGIMEN FOR PATIENTS ALLERGIC TO PENICILLIN/AMOXICILLIN/AMPICILLIN AND CONSIDERED AT HIGH RISK:

Vancomycin (*adults*, 1 g; *children*, 20 mg/kg) IV *slowly* over one hour starting one hour prior to procedure. Because of the long half-life of vancomycin, a repeat dose should not be necessary.

REMARKS:

(1) See previous remark on use of parenteral regimens in patients considered to be at high risk.

B. Prophylaxis for genitourinary or gastrointestinal procedures (risk of bacteremia with various procedures is discussed in Everett and Hirschmann, 1977; LeFrock and Molavi, 1982; Dajani et al, 1990; and Durack, 1990).

PROPHYLACTIC REGIMEN(S)

STANDARD PARENTERAL PENICILLIN-CONTAINING REGIMEN:

Ampicillin (*adults*, 2 g; *children*, 50 mg/kg) *plus* gentamicin (*adults*, 1.5 mg/kg; *children*, 2 mg/kg [not to exceed 80 mg]) IM one-half hour before procedure or IV immediately before procedure, *followed by* amoxicillin (*adults*, 1.5 g; *children*, 25 mg/kg), orally, six hours after the initial dose. Alternatively, the parenteral regimen may be repeated once eight hours after the initial dose. (Note: In *children*, the follow-up doses are one-half the initial pediatric doses.)

REMARKS:

(1) This is usually the preferred regimen, particularly in high-risk patients (eg, those with prosthetic heart valves or a previous history of endocarditis).

(2) Initial gentamicin dose should not exceed 80 mg. In patients with compromised renal function, it may be necessary to modify or omit the second dose of gentamicin.

(3) Intramuscular injections for endocarditis prophylaxis should be avoided in patients who receive heparin. The use of warfarin sodium is a relative contraindication to intramuscular injections. Intravenous or oral regimens should be used whenever possible.

SPECIAL PARENTERAL REGIMEN FOR PATIENTS ALLERGIC TO PENICILLIN:

Vancomycin (*adults*, 1 g; *children*, 20 mg/kg) given IV *slowly* over one hour *plus* gentamicin (*adults*, 1.5 mg/kg; *children*, 2 mg/kg [not to exceed 80 mg]) IM or IV one hour before procedure. This regimen may be repeated once eight hours after initial dose. (Note: In *children*, the follow-up doses are one-half the initial pediatric doses.)

REMARK:

(1) Initial gentamicin dose should not exceed 80 mg. In patients with compromised renal function, it may be necessary to modify or omit the second dose of each drug.

SPECIAL ORAL PENICILLIN-CONTAINING REGIMEN:

Amoxicillin (*adults*, 3 g; *children*, 50 mg/kg) one hour before procedure, then (*adults*, 1.5 g; *children*, 25 mg/kg) six hours after initial dose.

REMARK:

(1) This oral regimen may be substituted for minor procedures in low-risk patients.

Prevention of Recurrent Attacks of Rheumatic Fever (Secondary Prevention)

The recommendations of the American Heart Association's (AHA) Committee on Rheumatic Fever, Endocarditis, and Kawasaki Disease of the Council on Cardiovascular Disease in the Young (Dajani et al, 1988) are generally accepted.

Prevention of recurrent rheumatic fever depends upon *continuous prophylaxis* with antimicrobial agents effective against group A beta-hemolytic streptococci (*Streptococcus pyogenes*). Prophylaxis generally is recommended for patients who have a well-documented history of rheumatic fever or Sydenham's chorea and those who show definite evidence of rheumatic heart disease. Prophylaxis should be initiated as soon as the diagnosis of active rheumatic fever or rheumatic heart disease is made. Recommended regimens are listed below.

The most effective protection from rheumatic fever recurrences is afforded by continuous antimicrobial chemoprophylaxis. Risk of recurrence depends on several factors, however. For example, risk decreases as the time interval since the most recent attack lengthens, while individuals with multiple previous attacks are at higher risk. Furthermore, the patient's risk of acquiring a streptococcal upper respiratory tract infection must be considered. Adults with a high risk of exposure to streptococcal infection include parents of young children, teachers, physicians, nurses, allied medical personnel, military personnel, and other individuals living in crowded situations. Thus, physicians must consider each patient's situation when determining appropriate duration of prophylaxis. The AHA committee suggests the following guidelines, depending on whether patients have had rheumatic carditis: "Patients who have had rheumatic carditis are at a relatively high risk for recurrences of carditis and are likely to sustain serious cardiac involvement with each recurrence. Therefore, patients who have had rheumatic carditis should receive long-term antibiotic prophylaxis well into adulthood and perhaps for life. Prophylaxis should continue even after valve surgery, including prosthetic valve replacement, because these patients remain at risk of recurrence of rheumatic fever.

"In contrast, patients who have not had rheumatic carditis are at considerably less risk of cardiac involvement with a recurrence. Therefore, a physician may wish to discontinue prophylaxis in these patients after several years. In general, prophylaxis should continue until the patient is in his or her early 20s and five years have elapsed since the last rheumatic attack. The decision to continue prophylaxis should be made after discussion with the patient of potential risks and benefits and careful consideration of the epidemiological risk factors enumerated above."

PROPHYLACTIC REGIMEN(S)

PREFERRED REGIMEN:
Penicillin G benzathine, intramuscularly, 1.2 million units every four weeks.
REMARKS:
(1) This is the recommended method of secondary prevention.
(2) In countries where the incidence of acute rheumatic fever is particularly high, use of penicillin G benzathine every three weeks may be warranted.
(3) Long-acting penicillin is of particular value in patients at high risk of recurrence, especially those with rheumatic heart disease.
(4) Disadvantages are inconvenience and the pain of the intramuscular injection. As with all penicillins, anaphylaxis, although rare, may occur.
ALTERNATIVE (ORAL) REGIMENS:
Penicillin V, orally, 250 mg twice daily;
OR
Sulfadiazine, orally, 1 g once daily for patients >60 lbs or 500 mg once daily for patients <60 lbs.
REMARKS:
(1) Oral regimens are slightly less efficacious than intramuscular penicillin G benzathine. Thus, the oral regimens are most appropriate for patients with a lower risk of recurrence (eg, a late adolescent or young adult who has not had rheumatic attack in preceding five years).
(2) Success depends on long-term compliance. Careful and repeated instructions to patients about the importance of maintaining continuous prophylaxis is necessary.
(3) Penicillin V is preferred to penicillin G because it is more acid-stable, and, therefore, better absorbed.
(4) Data comparing sulfadiazine and other sulfonamides are not available. However, sulfadiazine may not be obtainable in the United States for this indication (*MMWR*, 1993). Sulfisoxazole probably is effective, but data comparing sulfadiazine and sulfisoxazole are not available (Dajani et al, 1988; *American Academy of Pediatrics Redbook*, 1991).
(5) Erythromycin, orally, 250 mg twice daily may be used in patients allergic to both penicillins and sulfonamides, but studies have not been done.

Prevention of Tuberculosis

For recommendations for chemoprophylaxis of tuberculosis, see index entry Tuberculosis.

Prevention of Meningococcal Disease

Antimicrobial chemoprophylaxis is recommended for household and other intimate contacts of patients with meningococcal disease. Nasopharyngeal cultures are not helpful in determining who warrants prophylaxis. In addition to household contacts, persons at highest risk include nursery school or day-care center contacts (ie, young children), other very close day-to-day contacts who are exposed to the patient's oral secretions either through kissing or sharing of food or beverages, and medical personnel who have direct contact with respiratory secretions of the patient (eg, such as occurs with mouth-to-mouth resuscitation). These contacts should receive antimicrobial prophylaxis as soon as possible, preferably within 24 hours of diagnosis of the primary case. Nasopharyngeal cultures need not be performed before initiating prophylaxis. Prophylaxis is not indicated for casual school or work contacts or for routine contacts of the hospitalized patient. Prophylactic regimens should eliminate nasopharyngeal carriage of *Neisseria meningitidis*.

Selected references: *Med Lett Drugs Ther*, 1981; Shapiro, 1982; Feder, 1983; *MMWR*, 1985; *American Academy of Pediatrics Redbook*, 1991.

PROPHYLACTIC REGIMEN(S)

PREFERRED REGIMEN:
Rifampin (Oral: *Adults*, 600 mg twice daily; *children 1 month to 12 years*, 10 mg/kg twice daily; *newborns less than 1 month*, 5 mg/kg twice daily) for two days.
REMARKS:
(1) Rifampin has been shown to be 90% effective in eradicating nasopharyngeal carriage of *N. meningitidis.* However, resistant organisms have developed during prophylaxis. No serious adverse reactions have been noted. However, rifampin should not be used in pregnant women. The drug stains soft contact lenses and turns secretions and the urine orange.
(2) Sulfonamides are preferred only if the meningococcal isolate is known to be susceptible. Sulfadiazine (Oral: *Adults*, 1 g twice daily; *children 1 to 12 years,* 500 mg twice daily; *infants 2 months to 1 year,* 500 mg once daily) for two days OR sulfisoxazole (Oral: *Adults*, 1 g twice daily; *children 1 to 12 years*, 500 mg twice daily; *infants 2 months to 1 year*, 500 mg daily) for two days is an effective regimen. (NOTE: Sulfadiazine may not be obtainable for this indication in the United States [*MMWR*, 1993].) Sulfonamides should not be used in pregnant women at term or in newborn infants less than 2 months of age.
(3) Ceftriaxone given in a single intramuscular dose of 250 mg for adults and 125 mg for children younger than 12 years of age has been demonstrated to be more effective than oral rifampin in eradicating the meningococcal group A carrier state (Schwartz et al, 1988). However, ceftriaxone is not routinely recommended for prophylaxis because its efficacy has been confirmed only for group A strains. It has the advantages of possible greater efficacy than rifampin, easier dosage administration and availability, and safety during pregnancy (*American Academy of Pediatrics Redbook*, 1991).
(4) Ciprofloxacin has been very effective for eradication of *N. meningitidis* from nasopharyngeal carriers in clinical trials (Dworzack et al, 1988; Gaunt and Lambert, 1988) and may prove useful for this indication in adults. However, the fluoroquinolones should not be given to pregnant women or to prepubertal children.
(5) Although minocycline (100 mg twice daily for five days) is an effective alternative in adults, it generally is not recommended because it causes frequent vestibular side effects. Tetracyclines should not be used in pregnant women or children less than 8 years of age.
(6) Penicillin G and chloramphenicol, preferred drugs in the treatment of meningococcal meningitis, are not useful for chemoprophylaxis because they fail to eliminate nasopharyngeal carriage of *N. meningitidis.*
(7) Presently available meningococcal polysaccharide vac-

cines are not substitutes for chemoprophylaxis since an antibody response is not seen for five days to two weeks following vaccine administration. However, when an outbreak is caused by a vaccine serogroup, meningococcal vaccine can be considered as a possible adjunct to chemoprophylaxis (*American Academy of Pediatrics Redbook*,1991). Serogroups B, C, and W-135 cause 85% to 95% of the meningococcal disease in the United States; serogroup B strains alone are responsible for 50% to 55% of all cases. However, presently available vaccines are only effective against meningococcal disease caused by serogroups A, C, Y, and W-135. Except for the group A component, children less than 2 years of age respond poorly to the vaccine. For uses of meningococcal vaccines, see *MMWR*, 1985 and index entry Meningococcal Polysaccharide Vaccine.

Prevention of *Haemophilus influenzae* Type b Disease

An increased risk of secondary invasive *Haemophilus influenzae* type b disease exists among household contacts less than 4 years of age, particularly unimmunized individuals. The attack rate varies inversely with age and is greatest for children under 2 years of age (see *MMWR*, 1986). Nursery school and day-care center contacts also may be at increased risk, but the magnitude of this is unclear at the present time. Data from published studies are conflicting and suggest that the risk of secondary disease among day-care contacts may vary widely among centers (see Band et al, 1984; Fleming et al, 1985; *MMWR*, 1986; Broome et al, 1987; Mackintubee et al, 1987; Marks and Dorchester, 1987; Murphy et al, 1987; Osterholm et al, 1987; *American Academy of Pediatrics Redbook*, 1991).

Rifampin (20 mg/kg/day in a single dose for four days) effectively eliminates the oropharyngeal carriage of *H. influenzae* type b in 95% of treated individuals (see *MMWR*, 1986; *American Academy of Pediatrics Redbook*, 1991). Limited data from three studies indicate that it also reduces the risk of secondary invasive illness in exposed contacts. In a controlled clinical trial that included household and day-care contacts, this regimen was shown to prevent secondary *H. influenzae* type b disease (Band et al, 1984). This study was criticized for flaws in design and conclusions, however (Osterholm and Murphy, 1984). In a prospective study among day-care classroom contacts, the incidence of secondary *H. influenzae* type b disease was significantly less for children younger than 24 months of age who received rifampin (Mackintubee et al, 1987). Finally, in a retrospective, multicenter collaborative study of day-care centers, rifampin also was found to be effective in preventing secondary cases of invasive *H. influenzae* type b disease in classroom contacts from 0 to 23 months of age (Fleming et al, 1985).

Based on the above information, both the Committee on Infectious Diseases of the American Academy of Pediatrics and the Immunization Practices Advisory Committee of the Centers for Disease Control and Prevention have issued recommendations for antimicrobial chemoprophylaxis of invasive *H. influenzae* type b disease (*MMWR*, 1986; *American Academy of Pediatrics Redbook*, 1991). The recommendations of the American Academy of Pediatrics are listed below. The CDC concurs on most points, but differs with regard to recommendations for prophylaxis of day-care center contacts (see NOTE in item 4 below).

The recommendations of the American Academy of Pediatrics are as follows:

(1) Careful observation of exposed household, day-care, or nursery contacts is essential. Exposed children who develop a febrile illness should receive prompt medical attention. If indicated, antimicrobial therapy appropriate for invasive *H. influenzae* type b infection should be administered.

(2) Rifampin prophylaxis is recommended for all household contacts (children and adults) in households where there is at least one child (other than the index case) less than 48 months of age who has not been adequately immunized. A household contact is an individual living in the residence of the index patient or a nonresident who spent four or more hours with the index patient for at least five of the seven days preceding hospital admission of the index patient. Prophylaxis should be initiated as soon as possible because 54% of secondary cases occur during the first week after hospitalization of the index patient.

(3) The index case should also receive rifampin prophylaxis, which should be initiated during hospitalization, usually just before discharge. (NOTE: Rifampin prophylaxis, given concurrently with therapeutic antimicrobials, ie, starting on day 6 or 7 of therapy, was shown to be as effective as prophylaxis started after therapy was completed, but concern over potential interactions of rifampin with therapeutic antimicrobials, especially chloramphenicol, must be considered [Li and Wald, 1986].)

(4) Nursery and day-care center contacts also may be at increased risk of secondary *H. influenzae* type b disease, but experts disagree on the magnitude of the risk. Most believe that the risk for children attending day-care centers is probably lower than that observed for age-susceptible household contacts, and that secondary disease in contacts is rare when all day-care contacts are older than 2 years of age. Moreover, the efficacy of rifampin in preventing disease in day-care groups is not well established and the difficulties in delivering prophylaxis are considerable. The advisability of rifampin prophylaxis in day-care groups in which a single case has occurred is controversial, and a definitive recommendation regarding administration of rifampin prophylaxis for all types of day-care groups cannot be made at this time. The following guidelines may be useful: (a) in day-care homes that resemble households, such as those with children less than 2 years old, and contact is 25 hours per week or more, rifampin prophylaxis can be employed in the same regimen as recommended for household contacts; and (b) in day-care facilities where all contacts are more than 2 years old, prophylaxis need not be given. Administering rifampin to all attendees and supervisory personnel is recommended when two or more cases of invasive *H. influenzae* type b disease have occurred among attendees within 60 days. Strict and prompt compliance by attendees and supervisory personnel are required for rifampin prophylaxis to be successful. Children and staff should be excluded from the day-care group until rifampin has been initiated. Children entering the group during the time prophylaxis is being given also should receive prophylaxis. (NOTE: Based primarily on the retrospective, multicenter col-

laborative study of day-care centers by Fleming et al [1985], which showed [1] that there was an increased risk of secondary invasive *H. influenzae* type b disease in classroom contacts aged 0 to 23 months who attended day-care for at least 25 hours per week, and [2] that rifampin prophylaxis was effec-tive in preventing secondary disease in these contacts, the CDC recommendations state: "In a day-care classroom in which a case of systemic Hib [*H. influenzae* type b] disease has occurred, and in which one or more children under 2 years old have been exposed, strong consideration should be given to administering rifampin prophylaxis to all children and staff in the classroom, regardless of age" [*MMWR*, 1986].)

(5) In a cohort (household or day-care) in which prophylaxis is given to limit secondary cases, children vaccinated with any *Haemophilus* b vaccine as well as susceptible, unvaccinated children should receive prophylaxis.

(6) Prophylaxis is not recommended for pregnant women who are contacts of the index patient because the effects of rifampin on the fetus are unknown.

PROPHYLACTIC REGIMEN(S)

PREFERRED REGIMEN:
Rifampin (Oral: *Adults and children*, 20 mg/kg once daily [maximum dose, 600 mg daily] for four days).
REMARKS:
(1) The dose for very young infants is not established. Some authorities reduce the dose of rifampin to 10 mg/kg per dose in infants less than 1 month of age.
(2) Rifampin is not commercially available as an oral suspension. For patients unable to swallow rifampin capsules, preweighed rifampin powder mixed with a small amount of applesauce immediately prior to administration may be given. A rifampin suspension (1% in simple syrup), if used, should be freshly prepared and shaken vigorously prior to each administration. The stability of rifampin in solution more than one week following preparation of the solution is unknown. Rifampin stains soft contact lenses and turns secretions and the urine orange.
(3) Ampicillin and chloramphenicol, preferred drugs in the treatment of *H. influenzae* type b disease, are not useful for chemoprophylaxis because they fail to eliminate oropharyngeal carriage of the organism.
(4) Four *H. influenzae* type b polysaccharide conjugate vaccines (*HibTITER, ProHIBit, PedvaxHIB, ActHIB*) are licensed for use in the United States, and a marked decline in the incidence of invasive *H. influenzae* type b disease has been observed since their licensure (see Shapiro,1993). The conjugated vaccine is preferred to the unconjugated Haemophilus b polysaccharide vaccine because it is more immunogenic in infants and young children. Three conjugated vaccines (*HibTITER, PedvaxHIB, ActHIB*) are recommended for all children beginning at 2 months of age. Vaccination may be initiated as early as 6 weeks of age. Two or three booster doses initially are given at two-month intervals and a final booster is administered at 12 to 15 months of age. Any of the four licensed conjugate vaccines may be given at age 15 months or older. Unimmunized children less than 24 months of age who have had invasive *H. influenzae* type b disease should still receive the vaccine because many in this age group fail to develop adequate immunity following the natural disease. Chemoprophylaxis should be given to both vaccinated and unvaccinated contacts of children with *H. influenzae* type b disease because even immune individuals may carry and transmit the pathogen. Vaccination following exposure should not be relied upon to prevent secondary cases (*MMWR*, 1991). For additional discussion, see index entry Haemophilus b Polysaccharide Vaccines.

Prevention of Pneumococcal Infection in Asplenic Patients

Anatomically or functionally asplenic patients (eg, those with sickle cell disease), particularly children, are susceptible to overwhelming infection with encapsulated bacteria, including *Streptococcus pneumoniae, Haemophilus influenzae* type b, and *Neisseria meningitidis*. *S. pneumoniae* is the most frequent and important cause of septicemia in the asplenic child, and continuous antimicrobial chemoprophylaxis directed against this organism traditionally has been recommended for children and adolescents after splenectomy or diagnosis of chronic splenic dysfunction. Whether to use similar chemoprophylaxis in adult patients is less clear.

Selected references: *Med Lett Drugs Ther*, 1977; *American Academy of Pediatrics Redbook*, 1991; Reese and Betts, 1991; Wong et al, 1992; Sickle Cell Disease Guideline Panel, 1993; Sanford, 1993.

PROPHYLACTIC REGIMEN(S)

PREFERRED REGIMEN:
Penicillin V (Oral: *Children less than 5 years*, 125 mg twice daily; *adults and children 5 years and older*, 250 mg twice daily)
REMARKS:
(1) The efficacy of this regimen in preventing pneumococcal septicemia in infants and young children with sickle cell anemia has been demonstrated in a randomized, double-blind, placebo-controlled trial (Gaston et al, 1986). It is recommended that this regimen be initiated in infants who have sickle cell disease beginning before the age of 4 months (*American Academy of Pediatrics Redbook*, 1991).
(2) Some experts recommend use of amoxicillin (20 mg/kg/day) or trimethoprim/sulfamethoxazole (4 mg/20 mg/kg/day) for children less than 5 years of age to include coverage against *H. influenzae* type b. (Note: This organism is less likely to be a concern in patients immunized with Haemophilus b polysaccharide conjugate vaccines.)
(3) Penicillin G benzathine (intramuscularly, 1.2 million units every four weeks) also has been suggested for this indication (see Mandell et al, 1992). Monthly injections of this long-acting penicillin appeared to be effective in preventing pneumococcal infections in young Jamaican children with sickle cell anemia (John et al, 1984). Pain at the site of intramuscular injection is a disadvantage of this regimen. Also, there is some concern that adequate serum concentrations of penicillin G are not maintained during the latter part of the dosing interval (see John et al, 1984).
(4) The optimum duration of prophylaxis is unknown, but in children it traditionally has ranged from two to four years. An unacceptably high incidence of pneumococcal infections in children with sickle cell anemia after they had terminated penicillin prophylaxis at age 3 years (John et al, 1984) suggests that prophylaxis should continue beyond the age of 3 years and perhaps indefinitely. There also is concern that penicillin prophylaxis may prevent the development of natural immunity against pneumococcal infections in young children and, therefore, increase their susceptibility to infection if the prophylactic regimen is terminated (see John et al, 1984; Buchanan and Smith, 1986; Gaston et al, 1986). The 1991 edition of the *American Academy of Pediatrics Redbook* states: "The age at which prophylaxis

can be discontinued is an empirical decision since no studies of this question have been performed. Some experts continue prophylaxis throughout childhood and into adulthood in particularly high-risk patients."

(5) Suboptimal compliance has been associated with failure of prophylaxis (Buchanan and Smith, 1986). Therefore, the necessity for strict compliance to the prophylactic regimen should be emphasized to the patient and/or parents. It also should be stressed that continuous prophylaxis has limitations. Some bacteria that can cause fulminant bacteremia are not susceptible to the antimicrobial agent selected for prophylaxis. Patients and/or parents should be aware that any febrile illness is potentially serious and that immediate medical attention should be sought. When bacteremia is likely, the physician should obtain blood and other appropriate body fluid (eg, cerebrospinal fluid) specimens for culture and should initiate antimicrobial therapy (eg, intravenous ceftriaxone or cefotaxime in children less than 5 years). Although hospitalization of the patient traditionally has been recommended (see *American Academy of Pediatrics Redbook*, 1991), recent studies indicate that many febrile episodes in children with sickle cell disease can be treated safely on an outpatient basis with intramuscular administration of ceftriaxone (Wilimas et al, 1993).

(6) Anatomically or functionally asplenic patients, including those with sickle cell disease, 2 years of age or older also should receive pneumococcal 23-valent polysaccharide vaccine (*MMWR*, 1989) and quadrivalent (A, C, Y, W-135) meningococcal vaccine (*MMWR*, 1985). Anatomically or functionally asplenic patients, including those with sickle cell disease, also should receive Haemophilus b polysaccharide conjugate vaccine (see *MMWR*, 1991). See also index entries Pneumococcal Polysaccharide Vaccine, Meningococcal Polysaccharide Vaccine, and Haemophilus b Polysaccharide Vaccines.

Prevention of Recurrent Bacterial Urinary Tract Infections (Reinfections) in Women

Young to middle-aged nonpregnant women with two or more recurrent episodes of new infection (reinfections) within six months or three or more episodes per year are candidates for long-term antimicrobial chemoprophylaxis. There should be no history of prior urological surgery, renal calculi, or genitourinary tract abnormality.

Selected references: Stamm, et al, 1980, 1981, 1982, 1991; *Med Lett Drugs Ther*, 1981; Ronald and Harding, 1981; Fowler, 1986; Nicolle and Ronald, 1987; Hooton and Stamm, 1991; Nicolle, 1992.

PROPHYLACTIC REGIMEN(S)

PREFERRED REGIMEN:

Trimethoprim (40 mg)/sulfamethoxazole (200 mg), ie, one-half of a regular strength tablet, orally, either once daily at bedtime or three times per week at bedtime (on Sunday, Wednesday, and Friday).

ALTERNATIVE REGIMENS:

Nitrofurantoin, 50 mg (or nitrofurantoin macrocrystals, 100 mg), orally, once daily at bedtime

OR

Trimethoprim, 50 to 100 mg, orally, once daily at bedtime.

OR

Cephalexin, 250 mg, orally, once daily at bedtime.

REMARKS:

(1) Duration of prophylaxis generally is six months. If recurrence of infection then occurs within three months, prophylaxis frequently is reinstituted for two years. Generally, the recurrence of infections is decreased by 95% with the use of prophylaxis.

(2) Trimethoprim penetrates vaginal secretions very well and effectively eradicates Enterobacteriaceae from the fecal reservoir and prevents perineal colonization. Emergence of resistant bacterial strains has not been a major problem. Serious adverse reactions have been rare.

(3) In one study, serious adverse reactions (eg, pulmonary toxicity) were reported with long-term nitrofurantoin administration (Holmberg et al, 1980).

(4) Whether the use of trimethoprim alone will lead to more rapid emergence of trimethoprim-resistant bacterial strains than with administration of the combination is still unresolved. Many experts prefer to reserve trimethoprim alone for patients who are allergic to sulfonamides.

(5) Long-term, low-dose norfloxacin (200 mg once daily at bedtime) or ciprofloxacin (250 mg once daily at bedtime) also is effective for the prevention of recurrent urinary tract infections (Nicolle et al, 1989). Some consultants prefer these agents because they have not been associated with plasmid-mediated, transferable resistance. However, fluoroquinolones cannot be used during pregnancy or in women who might become pregnant during their use.

(6) Prior to beginning chemoprophylaxis, any acute urinary tract infection should be treated with appropriate antimicrobial agents and sterile urine culture obtained.

(7) A screening intravenous pyelogram (IVP) is no longer considered necessary for the majority of women who are candidates for long-term chemoprophylaxis. An exception is relapsing urinary tract infections due to urease-producing bacteria (eg, *Proteus*), in which infected urinary calculi must be considered.

(8) ALTERNATIVE APPROACHES TO LONG-TERM CONTINUOUS CHEMOPROPHYLAXIS:

A. Postcoital prophylaxis. Recurrences of urinary tract infection in some women appear to correlate temporally with sexual intercourse. For such patients, a single prophylactic dose of an appropriate antimicrobial agent taken immediately after intercourse appears to prevent active infections. In a randomized, double-blind, placebo-controlled trial, postcoital antimicrobial prophylaxis with trimethoprim (40 mg)/sulfamethoxazole (200 mg) was shown to be effective in patients with both low ($\leq$2/week) and high ($\geq$3/week) intercourse frequencies; side effects were few and compliance was excellent (Stapleton et al, 1990). Thus, this approach may be an acceptable alternative to long-term chemoprophylaxis for selected women. Nitrofurantoin, trimethoprim, norfloxacin, and ciprofloxacin in doses outlined above also can be used successfully for postcoital prophylaxis.

B. Intermittent self-treatment. Another strategy for managing recurrent urinary tract infections is to prescribe antimicrobial drugs for susceptible women to keep at home and self-administer when symptoms arise. Intermittent self-therapy with single-dose trimethoprim (320 mg)/sulfamethoxazole (1,600 mg) was shown to be efficacious and economical in selected women (eg, those in whom the symptomatic episode was most likely acute cystitis rather than urethritis or vaginitis; those with the ability to accurately self-diagnose acute cystitis) (Wong et al, 1985). For reliable women who prefer this approach, experts recommend either a single-dose or a three-day regimen at the first symptom of urinary tract infection and that patients call their physician if the symptoms are not completely resolved by 48 hours (Hooton and Stamm, 1991).

Prevention of *Chlamydia trachomatis* Infections, Gonococcal Infections, and Syphilis in Sexual Contacts

Guidelines for the prevention of these infections in sexual contacts can be found in Chapter 3 in this Section, Treatment of Sexually Transmitted Diseases.

Prevention of Ophthalmia Neonatorum

Guidelines for the prevention of ophthalmia neonatorum can be found in Chapter 3 in this Section, Treatment of Sexually Transmitted Diseases.

Prevention of Malaria

For recommendations for chemoprophylaxis of malaria, see index entry Malaria.

Prevention of Influenza A Infection

For chemoprophylaxis of influenza A infection with amantadine, see index entry Amantadine. For immunoprophylaxis with influenza vaccine see index entry Influenza Virus Vaccine.

Prevention of *Pneumocystis carinii* Pneumonia in Persons Infected with Human Immunodeficiency Virus (HIV)

For recommendations for chemoprophylaxis of *Pneumocystis carinii* pneumonia in persons infected with HIV, see index entries Antiprotozoal Agents, Pneumocystis Pneumonia, Trimethoprim and Sulfamethoxazole, and Pentamidine Isethionate.

Prevention of Disseminated *Mycobacterium avium* Complex Infections in Persons Infected with Human Immunodeficiency Virus (HIV)

For recommendations for chemoprophylaxis of disseminated *Mycobacterium avium* complex infections in persons infected with HIV, see index entries Mycobacterium Infections, Atypical.

Prevention of Pertussis in Exposed Persons

Exposure to pertussis can result in clinical disease in both immunized and unimmunized contacts. Infants less than 1 year and unimmunized children less than 7 years are at greatest risk. Both the Immunization Practices Advisory Committee (ACIP) of the Centers for Disease Control and Prevention and the Committee on Infectious Diseases of the American Academy of Pediatrics recommend chemoprophylaxis for all household and other close contacts of persons with pertussis, regardless of age and immunization status. The index case also should receive antimicrobial agents to prevent spread (see index entry Pertussis, Treatment).

Selected references: *American Academy of Pediatrics Redbook,* 1991; *MMWR*, 1991.

PROPHYLACTIC REGIMEN(S)

PREFERRED REGIMEN:
Erythromycin, orally, 40 to 50 mg/kg/day (maximum, 2 g/day), divided into four doses for 14 days.
REMARKS:
(1) Erythromycin has been shown to eliminate carriage of *Bordetella pertussis*. Although data from controlled clinical trials are lacking, prophylaxis with erythromycin may reduce transmission (Steketee et al, 1988; *MMWR,* 1991).
(2) A retrospective analysis of the literature suggests that erythromycin estolate has been more effective than erythromycin ethylsuccinate or erythromycin stearate in eliminating *B. pertussis* carriage, presumably due to better penetration of the estolate into respiratory secretions (Bass, 1985), and some experts recommend the estolate preparation (see *American Academy of Pediatrics Redbook,* 1991).
(3) Trimethoprim/sulfamethoxazole (orally, 8 mg/40 mg/kg/day) is recommended as an alternative for individuals who cannot tolerate erythromycin, but its efficacy is not established.
(4) In addition to chemoprophylaxis, the Committee on Infectious Diseases of the American Academy of Pediatrics also recommends the following: (a) Exposed children, especially those incompletely immunized, should be observed carefully for respiratory symptoms for 14 days after contact is broken; (b) household and other close contacts (such as those in day-care centers or classrooms) less than 7 years who are unimmunized or who have received less than four doses of DTP should have DTP immunization initiated or continued according to the recommended schedule. Children who have received their third dose six months or more before exposure should be given their fourth dose at this time. Those who have had at least four doses of pertussis vaccine should receive a booster dose of DTP, unless they have received a dose within the previous three years or they are more than 6 years old (*American Academy of Pediatrics Redbook,* 1991). For a discussion of pertussis immunization, see index entry Pertussis.

Prevention of Recurrent Acute Otitis Media

Antimicrobial chemoprophylaxis has decreased the number of recurrent episodes of acute otitis media in children. However, the most effective drugs, dosage, and the optimum duration of prophylaxis have not been clearly established. Despite these unanswered questions, most infectious disease experts currently recommend antimicrobial chemoprophylaxis (as outlined below) as a reasonable initial approach in children with at least three episodes of acute otitis media in the previous six months or four episodes in one year.

Selected references: Klein, 1984; Bluestone, 1987; Lisby-Sutch et al, 1990; Kempthorne and Giebink, 1991; Teele, 1991; Paradise, 1992; Williams et al, 1993.

PROPHYLACTIC REGIMEN(S)

PREFERRED REGIMENS:
Amoxicillin, orally, 20 mg/kg once daily at bedtime;
OR
Sulfisoxazole, orally, 50 mg/kg once daily at bedtime.
REMARKS:
(1) Some consultants noted that most studies evaluating antimicrobial prophylaxis for recurrent acute otitis media used twice daily dosing. Thus, the following alternative dosage regimens were recommended; amoxicillin, orally, 20 mg/kg/day divided into two doses *or* sulfisoxazole, orally, 70 mg/kg/day divided

into two doses.
(2) Duration of prophylaxis is about six months or during the winter and spring when the incidence of respiratory tract infections is high.
(3) Amoxicillin or sulfisoxazole generally is preferred because of proven effectiveness, safety, and low cost. Although trimethoprim (4 mg/kg)/sulfamethoxazole (20 mg/kg), orally, once daily at bedtime appears to be an effective alternative, some experts express concern about potential legal liability because the package insert recommends against this use (see Paradise, 1992).
(4) If episodes of acute otitis media occur during prophylaxis, an alternative regimen should be used for treatment.
(5) If episodes of acute otitis media recur after conclusion of prophylaxis, reinstitution of chemoprophylaxis is warranted. Myringotomy and insertion of tympanotomy tubes are alternative management options if breakthroughs occur repeatedly (some suggest more than two times) during chemoprophylaxis.
(6) Hazards of antimicrobial chemoprophylaxis include potential for adverse drug reactions and emergence of resistant bacterial strains, but current studies indicate neither is of sufficient importance to withhold initiating a course of chemoprophylaxis.
(7) Because chemoprophylaxis could alleviate symptoms of acute otitis media without eliminating middle ear effusion, monthly evaluation of patients for middle ear effusion is recommended.

Prevention of Travelers' Diarrhea

Although effective chemoprophylactic regimens (as outlined below) are available, the current consensus is that antimicrobial agents are *not recommended* for the prevention of travelers' diarrhea because the risks associated with widespread administration of these agents outweigh the benefits of preventing an illness that usually is mild and self-limited or easily treated. These risks include the potential for: (1) serious adverse drug reactions; (2) the development of superinfections; and (3) the emergence of widespread bacterial resistance to the antimicrobial agents being used (National Institutes of Health Consensus Development Conference, 1985).

For most travelers, awareness and avoidance of possible sources of microbial contamination through dietary restrictions are of primary importance. If diarrhea develops, supportive therapy (replacement of fluids and electrolytes) is indicated (for discussion, see index entry Diarrhea, Infectious). Early treatment with trimethoprim/sulfamethoxazole or a fluoroquinolone (eg, ciprofloxacin) has been shown to decrease the severity of diarrhea caused by enterotoxigenic *Escherichia coli* and *Shigella*, the most common pathogens in travelers' diarrhea (DuPont et al, 1982; Ericsson et al, 1987). Combining an antimicrobial drug with loperamide, an antimotility agent, early in the course of diarrhea may further reduce the duration of diarrhea (Ericsson et al, 1990); some consider combination therapy the best treatment for patients with travelers' diarrhea (DuPont and Ericsson, 1993). Bismuth subsalicylate or loperamide alone also has been useful for the treatment of mild cases of travelers' diarrhea. However, these drugs should not be used in young children and antimotility agents should be avoided when there is fever or bloody diarrhea, suggesting an inflammatory enteritis. In summary, early treatment of travelers' diarrhea presently is preferable to prophylaxis (National Institutes of Health Consensus Development Conference, 1985). See also Chapter 2 in this Section, Antimicrobial Therapy for Common Infectious Diseases, for more detailed discussion.

Despite the widely disseminated recommendations of the National Institutes of Health Consensus Development Conference, many travelers continue to take an antimicrobial drug or bismuth subsalicylate for prophylaxis (DuPont and Ericsson, 1993). In 1992, an international working group of experts concluded that chemoprophylaxis should be considered a reasonable approach for some travelers with trips of short duration (three weeks or less) to areas of Latin America, Africa, or Southern Asia with high incidences of diarrhea (Farthing et al, 1992). Recommendations adapted from this working group are as follows: (1) for travelers with an important underlying illness, including active inflammatory bowel disease, conditions requiring the use of H^+/K^+ − ATPase inhibitors (such as omeprazole), insulin-dependent diabetes mellitus, heart disease in an elderly person, and acquired immunodeficiency syndrome (AIDS), antimicrobial chemoprophylaxis should be considered; (2) for healthy travelers whose trip will be ruined by a brief illness that might force a change in itinerary, bismuth subsalicylate (preferred) or antimicrobial prophylaxis should be considered; and (3) for other healthy travelers who prefer prophylaxis and who are unwilling to follow careful dietary restrictions, prophylaxis with bismuth subsalicylate should be considered (DuPont and Ericsson, 1993).

Only the traveler can determine the importance of not having diarrhea during a trip and the risk he or she is willing to take for a given degree of protection. The physician helping to make the decision about prophylaxis should make certain that the traveler understands the risks involved (DuPont and Ericsson, 1993).

Selected references: Sack et al, 1978, 1979; DuPont et al, 1980, 1983, 1987; Gorbach, 1982; Satterwhite and DuPont, 1983; Siegel, 1984; National Institutes of Health Consensus Development Conference, 1985; Gorbach and Edelman, 1986; Johnson et al, 1986; Reves et al, 1988; Rademaker et al, 1989; Ericsson et al, 1990; DuPont, 1991; Farthing et al, 1992; *Med Lett Drugs Ther*, 1992; Tellier and Keystone, 1992; DuPont and Ericsson, 1993.

PROPHYLACTIC REGIMEN(S)

Each of the regimens listed below was shown to be significantly more effective than a placebo in the prevention of travelers' diarrhea in at least one prospective, randomized, double-blind clinical trial. Some of the advantages and disadvantages of each regimen are considered in the Remarks.

ALTERNATIVE REGIMENS:
(A) Bismuth subsalicylate [Pepto-Bismol], orally, two tablets (containing 262 mg bismuth subsalicylate per tablet) chewed well four times daily (with meals and at bedtime) beginning on day of travel and continuing until two days after return home.
REMARKS:
(1) A laboratory study by Graham et al (1983) suggested that

bismuth subsalicylate (600-mg doses) in nonliquid form is effective in preventing travelers' diarrhea. This was confirmed in a field trial involving U.S. students in Mexico, in which two bismuth subsalicylate tablets (262 mg/tablet) four times daily for three weeks provided a 65% protection rate against travelers' diarrhea when compared with placebo (diarrhea incidences, 14% [drug] versus 49% [placebo]). The drug was well tolerated; the most common side effects were blackening of tongues and stools (DuPont et al, 1987).
(2) Although less effective than antimicrobial drugs, bismuth subsalicylate appears to provide effective prophylaxis in all high-risk areas and has the fewest side effects (DuPont and Ericsson, 1993).
(3) A comparable protection rate previously was reported with the liquid form of bismuth subsalicylate [Pepto-Bismol] given in a dosage of 60 ml (containing 1.05 g bismuth subsalicylate) four times daily (DuPont et al, 1980). This appears to be a less desirable alternative to the tablet formulation, however, because the large volumes are an inconvenience to most travelers.
(4) The salicylate contained in eight tablets or 240 ml of bismuth subsalicylate [Pepto-Bismol] is equivalent to five or eight 5-grain aspirin tablets, respectively. These regimens should not be used in patients allergic to salicylates, those taking large daily doses of aspirin for arthritis, individuals receiving oral anticoagulants, uricosurics, or methotrexate (*Med Lett Drugs Ther*, 1980), or patients with other contraindications to salicylate therapy. Although not reported, salicylate toxicity also is a potential complication in children receiving large doses of bismuth subsalicylate. Some consultants recommend that this compound not be used for prophylaxis of travelers' diarrhea in prepubertal children.

(B) Norfloxacin, orally, 400 mg once daily beginning on day of travel and continuing until two days after return home.
OR
Ciprofloxacin, orally, 500 mg once daily beginning on day of travel and continuing until two days after return home.
OR
Ofloxacin, orally, 300 mg once daily beginning on day of travel and continuing until two days after return home.

REMARKS:
(1) In a single field trial involving U.S. students in Mexico, norfloxacin provided an 88% protection rate against travelers' diarrhea when compared with placebo (diarrhea incidences, 7% [drug] versus 61% [placebo]), adverse reactions were minimal, and emergence of norfloxacin-resistant gram-negative bacilli in fecal flora did not occur (Johnson et al, 1986). Similarly, ciprofloxacin provided a 94% protection rate against travelers' diarrhea when compared with placebo (diarrhea incidences, 4% [drug] versus 64% [placebo]) in healthy travelers to Tunisia. One ciprofloxacin recipient suffered severe sunburn with blistering (Rademaker et al, 1989). Ofloxacin is comparably effective (DuPont and Ericsson, 1993).
(2) The fluoroquinolones have advantages over trimethoprim/sulfamethoxazole and doxycycline (see below) because they are active in vitro against essentially all aerobic gram-negative enteropathogens (*E. coli, Shigella* sp, *Salmonella* sp, *Vibrio* sp, *Yersinia enterocolitica, Campylobacter jejuni, Aeromonas hydrophila*) and plasmid-mediated, transferable resistance has not been observed. Presently, fluoroquinolones are effective for antimicrobial prophylaxis in all high-risk areas (DuPont and Ericsson, 1993).
(3) Although the fluoroquinolones generally are well tolerated, photosensitivity reactions have been reported. The fluoroquinolones should not be used in pregnant women or prepubertal children. See also index entries Norfloxacin, Ciprofloxacin, and Ofloxacin.

(C) Trimethoprim (160 mg)/sulfamethoxazole (800 mg), ie, one double-strength tablet, orally, once daily beginning on day of travel and continuing until two days after return home.

REMARKS:
(1) Plasmid-mediated, transferable resistance to this drug combination among isolates of *E. coli* is becoming widespread in some developing countries (Murray et al, 1985). Presently, trimethoprim/sulfamethoxazole remains effective for those traveling to the interior of Mexico (eg, Mexico City, Guadalajara, or Monterrey) during the summer (DuPont and Ericsson, 1993).
(2) Generally well tolerated, but skin rashes (3%) have been observed. Although uncommon, sulfonamides can cause severe, including fatal, skin (eg, Stevens-Johnson syndrome) or hematologic (eg, hemolytic and aplastic anemias) adverse reactions. Trimethoprim/sulfamethoxazole should be avoided in individuals who are allergic to sulfonamides.
(3) Suggested pediatric dosage is 4 to 5 mg/kg/day of the trimethoprim component, although prophylaxis in children generally is not advised.

(D) Doxycycline, orally, 200 mg on day of travel, followed by 100 mg once daily, continuing until two days after return home.

REMARKS:
(1) Resistant strains of enterotoxigenic *E. coli* and other enteropathogens are widespread in most developing countries. Currently, the role of doxycycline for prophylaxis of travelers' diarrhea is extremely limited (DuPont and Ericsson, 1993).
(2) Drug-induced gastrointestinal upset, including diarrhea, and photosensitivity reactions are important side effects of tetracyclines. Also tetracyclines should not be administered to pregnant women or children less than 8 years of age.
(3) The bismuth subsalicylate contained in a 60-ml dose of suspension [Pepto-Bismol] significantly decreased the bioavailability of doxycycline, 200 mg orally (Ericsson et al, 1982). Thus, the two agents should not be taken together.

Cited References

Introduction

Report of the Committee on Infectious Diseases: *American Academy of Pediatrics Redbook*, ed 22. Elk Grove Village, Ill, American Academy of Pediatrics, 1991, 527-548.

Brachman PS: Principles of chemoprophylaxis and immunoprophylaxis, in Mandell GL, et al (eds): *Principles and Practice of Infectious Diseases*, ed 3. New York, Churchill Livingstone, 1990, 158-160.

Dekker AW, et al: Infection prophylaxis in acute leukemia: Comparison of ciprofloxacin with trimethoprim/sulfamethoxazole and colistin. *Ann Intern Med* 106:7-12, 1987.

Flynn NM, Hoeprich PD: Chemoprophylaxis of infectious diseases, in Hoeprich PD (ed): *Infectious Diseases*, ed 3. Philadelphia, Harper & Row, 1983, 238-254.

Karp JE, et al: Oral norfloxacin for prevention of gram-negative bacterial infections in patients with acute leukemia and granulocytopenia: Randomized, double-blind, placebo-controlled trial. *Ann Intern Med* 106:1-7, 1987.

Mills J, Jawetz E: Clinical use of antimicrobials, in Katzung BG (ed): *Basic and Clinical Pharmacology*. Los Altos, Calif, Lange Medical Publications, 1982, 538-552.

Rozenberg-Arska M, Dekker AW: Prevention of bacterial and fungal infections in granulocytopenic patients, in Peterson PK, Verhoef J (eds): *The Antimicrobial Agents Annual/2*. New York, Elsevier, 1987, 471-481.

Sande MA, et al: Antimicrobial agents: General considerations, in Gilman AG, et al (eds): *The Pharmacological Basis of Therapeutics*, ed 8. New York, Pergamon Press, 1990, 1018-1046.

Scheifele DW: Prophylactic antibiotics in children. *Pediatr Infect Dis* 1:420-424, 1982.

Walsh TJ, Schimpff SC: Prevention of infection among patients with cancer. *Eur J Cancer Clin Oncol* 19:1333-1344, 1983.

Wilson WR: Antimicrobial chemoprophylaxis. *Med Clin North Am* 67:99-112, 1983.

Prevention of Bacterial Endocarditis

Prevention of bacterial endocarditis. *Med Lett Drugs Ther* 31:112, 1989.
Baddour LM, Bisno AL: Infective endocarditis complicating mitral valve prolapse: Epidemiologic, clinical, and microbiologic aspects. *Rev Infect Dis* 8:117-137, 1986.
Bor DH, Himmelstein DU: Endocarditis prophylaxis for patients with mitral valve prolapse: Quantitative analysis. *Am J Med* 76:711-717, 1984.
Clemens JD, Ransohoff DF: Quantitative assessment of pre-dental antibiotic prophylaxis for patients with mitral valve prolapse. *J Chron Dis* 37:531-544, 1984.
Clemens JD, et al: A controlled evaluation of the risk of bacterial endocarditis in persons with mitral-valve prolapse. *N Engl J Med* 307:776-781, 1982.
Dajani AS, Taubert KA: Prevention of bacterial endocarditis, letter. *JAMA* 265:1688, 1991.
Dajani AS, et al: Prevention of bacterial endocarditis: Recommendations by the American Heart Association. *JAMA* 264:2919-2922, 1990.
Durack DT: Prophylaxis of infective endocarditis, in Mandell GL, et al (eds): *Principles and Practice of Infectious Diseases*, ed 3. New York, Churchill Livingstone, 1990, 716-721.
Everett ED, Hirschmann JV: Transient bacteremia and endocarditis prophylaxis: Review. *Medicine* 56:61-77, 1977.
Greenman RL, Bisno AL: Prevention of bacterial endocarditis, in Kaye D (ed): *Infective Endocarditis,* ed 2. New York, Raven Press, 1992, 465-481.
Keys TF: Antimicrobial prophylaxis for patients with congenital or valvular heart disease. *Mayo Clin Proc* 57:171-175, 1982.
LeFrock JL, Molavi A: Transient bacteremia associated with diagnostic and therapeutic procedures. *Compr Ther* 8:65-71, (Feb) 1982.
MacMahon SW, et al: Risk of infective endocarditis in mitral valve prolapse with and without precordial systolic murmurs. *Am J Cardiol* 58:105-108, 1986.
McMorrow J, Nahata MC: Prevention of bacterial endocarditis, letter. *JAMA* 265:1687-1688, 1991.
Simmons NA: Recommendations for endocarditis prophylaxis, letter. *J Antimicrob Chemother* 31:437-438, 1993.
Stierer RC, Sterchele JA: Prevention of bacterial endocarditis, letter. *JAMA* 265:1687, 1991.

Prevention of Recurrent Attacks of Rheumatic Fever (Secondary Prevention)

Report of the Committee on Infectious Diseases: *American Academy of Pediatrics Redbook*, ed 22. Elk Grove Village, Ill, American Academy of Pediatrics, 1991, 445-446.
Update: Availability of Sulfadiazine—United States. *MMWR* 42:105, 1993.
Dajani AS, et al: Prevention of rheumatic fever: Statement for health professionals by the Committee on Rheumatic Fever, Endocarditis, and Kawasaki Disease of the Council on Cardiovascular Disease in the Young, the American Heart Association. *Circulation* 78:1082-1086, 1988.

Prevention of Meningococcal Disease

Meningococcal vaccines. *MMWR* 34:255-259, 1985.
Update: Availability of Sulfadiazine—United States. *MMWR* 42:105, 1993.
Preventing spread of meningococcal disease. *Med Lett Drugs Ther* 23:37-38, 1981.
Report of the Committee on Infectious Diseases: *American Academy of Pediatrics Redbook*, ed 22. Elk Grove Village, Ill, American Academy of Pediatrics, 1991, 323-326.
Dworzack DL, et al: Evaluation of single-dose ciprofloxacin in eradication of *Neisseria meningitidis* from nasopharyngeal carriers. *Antimicrob Agents Chemother* 32:1740-1741, 1988.
Feder HM Jr: Chemoprophylaxis in ambulatory pediatrics. *Pediatr Infect Dis* 2:251-257, 1983.
Gaunt PM, Lambert BE: Single dose ciprofloxacin for eradication of pharyngeal carriage of *Neisseria meningitidis. J Antimicrob Chemother* 21:489-496, 1988.
Schwartz B, et al: Comparative efficacy of ceftriaxone and rifampicin in eradicating pharyngeal carriage of group A *Neisseria meningitidis. Lancet* 1:1239-1242, 1988.
Shapiro ED: Prophylaxis for contacts of patients with meningococcal or *Haemophilus influenzae* type b disease. *Pediatr Infect Dis* 1:132-138, 1982.

Prevention of Haemophilus influenzae *Type b Disease*

Recommendations of the Immunization Practices Advisory Committee (ACIP): Update: Prevention of *Haemophilus influenzae* type b disease. *MMWR* 35:170-180, 1986.
Recommendations of the Immunization Practices Advisory Committee (ACIP): Haemophilus b conjugate vaccine for prevention of *Haemophilus influenzae* type b disease among infants and children 2 months of age and older. *MMWR* 40(RR-1):1-7, 1991.
Report of the Committee on Infectious Diseases: *American Academy of Pediatrics Redbook*, ed 22. Elk Grove Village, Ill, American Academy of Pediatrics, 1991, 220-229.
Band JD, et al: Prevention of *Haemophilus influenzae* type b disease. *JAMA* 251:2381-2386, 1984.
Broome CV, et al: Use of chemoprophylaxis to prevent spread of *Haemophilus influenzae* B in day-care facilities. *N Engl J Med* 316:1226-1228, 1987.
Fleming DW, et al: Secondary *Haemophilus influenzae* type b in day-care facilities: Risk factors and prevention. *JAMA* 254:509-514, 1985.
Li KI, Wald ER: Use of rifampin in *Haemophilus* influenzae type b infections. *Am J Dis Child* 140:381-385, 1986.
Mackintubee S, et al: Transmission of invasive *Haemophilus influenzae* type b disease in day care settings. *J Pediatr* 111:180-186, 1987.
Marks MI, Dorchester WL: Secondary rates of *Haemophilus influenzae* type b disease among day care contacts, editorial. *J Pediatr* 111:305-306, 1987.
Murphy TV, et al: Risk of subsequent disease among day-care contacts of patients with systemic *Haemophilus influenzae* type b disease. *N Engl J Med* 316:5-10, 1987.
Osterholm MT, Murphy TV: Does rifampin prophylaxis prevent disease caused by *Haemophilus influenzae* type b? *JAMA* 251:2408-2409, 1984.
Osterholm MT, et al: Risk of subsequent transmission of *Haemophilus influenzae* type b disease among children in day care: Results of a two-year statewide prospective surveillance and contact survey. *N Engl J Med* 316:1-5, 1987.
Shapiro ED: Infections caused by *Haemophilus influenzae* type b: The beginning of the end? Editorial. *JAMA* 269:264-266, 1993.

Prevention of Pneumococcal Infection in Asplenic Patients

Meningococcal vaccines. *MMWR* 34:255-259, 1985.
Prevention of serious infections after splenectomy. *Med Lett Drugs Ther* 19:2-4, 1977.
Recommendations of the Immunization Practices Advisory Committee (ACIP): Pneumococcal polysaccharide vaccine. *MMWR* 38:64-76, 1989.
Recommendations of the Immunization Practices Advisory Committee (ACIP): Haemophilus b conjugate vaccine for prevention of *Haemophilus influenzae* type b disease among infants and children 2 months of age and older. *MMWR* 40(RR-1):1-7, 1991.
Report of the Committee on Infectious Diseases: *American Academy of Pediatrics Redbook*, ed 22. Elk Grove Village, Ill, American Academy of Pediatrics, 1991, 52-53, 373-378.
Buchanan GR, Smith SJ: Pneumococcal septicemia despite pneumococcal vaccine and prescription of penicillin prophylaxis in children with sickle cell anemia. *Am J Dis Child* 140:428-432, 1986.

Gaston MA, et al: Prophylaxis with oral penicillin in children with sickle cell anemia: Randomized trial. *N Engl J Med* 314:1593-1599, 1986.

John AB, et al: Prevention of pneumococcal infection in children with homozygous sickle cell disease. *BMJ* 288:1567-1570, 1984.

Mandell GL, et al: *Handbook of Antimicrobial Therapy 1992*. New York, Churchill Livingstone, 1992, 106-107.

Reese RE, Betts RF: Antibiotic use, in Reese RE, Douglas RG Jr (eds): *A Practical Approach to Infectious Diseases*, ed 3. Boston, Little Brown, 1991, 853-854.

Sanford JP: *Guide to Antimicrobial Therapy, 1993.* West Bethesda, Md, Antimicrobial Therapy Inc, 1993, 94-98.

Sickle Cell Disease Guideline Panel: *Sickle Cell Disease: Screening, Diagnosis, Management, and Counseling in Newborns and Infants.* Clinical Practice Guideline No. 6. AHCPR Pub. No. 93-0562. Rockville, Md, Agency for Health Care Policy and Research, Public Health Service, U.S. Department of Health and Human Services. (April) 1993, 39-42.

Wilimas JA, et al: A randomized study of outpatient treatment with ceftriaxone for selected febrile children with sickle cell disease. *N Engl J Med* 329:472-476, 1993.

Wong W-Y, et al: Infection caused by *Streptococcus pneumoniae* in children with sickle cell disease: Epidemiology, immunologic mechanisms, prophylaxis, and vaccination. *Clin Infect Dis* 14:1124-1136, 1992.

Prevention of Recurrent Bacterial Urinary Tract Infections (Reinfections) in Women

Treatment of urinary tract infections. *Med Lett Drugs Ther* 23:69-70, 1981.

Fowler JE: Urinary tract infections in women. *Urol Clin North Am* 13:673-683, 1986.

Holmberg L, et al: Adverse reactions to nitrofurantoin: Analysis of 921 reports. *Am J Med* 69:733-738, 1980.

Hooton TM, Stamm WE: Management of acute uncomplicated urinary tract infection in adults. *Med Clin North Am* 75:339-357, 1991.

Nicolle LE: Prophylaxis: Recurrent urinary tract infection in women. *Infection* 20(suppl 3): S203-S205, 1992.

Nicolle LE, Ronald AR: Recurrent urinary tract infection in adult women: Diagnosis and treatment. *Infect Dis Clin North Am* 1:793-806, 1987.

Nicolle LE, et al: Prospective, randomized, placebo-controlled trial of norfloxacin for prophylaxis of recurrent urinary tract infection in women. *Antimicrob Agents Chemother* 33:1032-1035, 1989.

Ronald AR, Harding GKM: Urinary infection prophylaxis in women. *Ann Intern Med* 94:268-270, 1981.

Stamm WE, et al: Antimicrobial prophylaxis of recurrent urinary tract infections: Double-blind, placebo-controlled trial. *Ann Intern Med* 92:770-775, 1980.

Stamm WE, et al: Is antimicrobial prophylaxis of urinary tract infections cost effective? *Ann Intern Med* 94:251-255, 1981.

Stamm WE, et al: Urinary prophylaxis with trimethoprim and trimethoprim/sulfamethoxazole: Efficacy, influence on natural history of recurrent bacteriuria, and cost control. *Rev Infect Dis* 4:450-455, 1982.

Stamm WE, et al: Natural history of recurrent urinary tract infections in women. *Rev Infect Dis* 13:77-84, 1991.

Stapleton A, et al: Postcoital antimicrobial prophylaxis for recurrent urinary tract infection: A randomized, double-blind, placebo-controlled trial. *JAMA* 264:703-706, 1990.

Wong ES, et al: Management of recurrent urinary tract infections with patient-administered single-dose therapy. *Ann Intern Med* 102:302-307, 1985.

Prevention of Pertussis in Exposed Persons

Recommendations of the Immunization Practices Advisory Committee (ACIP): Diphtheria, tetanus, and pertussis: Recommendations for vaccine use and other preventive measures. *MMWR* 40 (No. RR-10):1-28, 1991.

Report of the Committee on Infectious Diseases: *American Academy of Pediatrics Redbook*, ed 22. Elk Grove Village, Ill, American Academy of Pediatrics, 1991, 358-369.

Bass JW: Pertussis: Current status of prevention and treatment. *Pediatr Infect Dis* 4:614-619, 1985.

Steketee RW, et al: Evidence for high attack rate and efficacy of erythromycin prophylaxis in pertussis outbreak in facility for the developmentally disabled. *J Infect Dis* 157:434-440, 1988.

Prevention of Recurrent Acute Otitis Media

Bluestone CD: Otitis media and sinusitis: Management and when to refer to otolaryngologist. *Pediatr Infect Dis J* 6:100-106, 1987.

Kempthorne J, Giebink GS: Pediatric approach to diagnosis and management of otitis media. *Otolaryngol Clin North Am* 24:905-929, 1991.

Klein JO: Antimicrobial prophylaxis for recurrent acute otitis media. *Pediatr Ann* 13:398-403, 1984.

Lisby-Sutch SM, et al: Therapy of otitis media. *Clin Pharm* 9:15-34, 1990.

Paradise JL: Antimicrobial prophylaxis for recurrent acute otitis media. *Ann Otol Rhinol Laryngol* 101(suppl 155):33-36, 1992.

Teele DW: Strategies to control recurrent acute otitis media in infants and children. *Pediatr Ann* 20:609-616, 1991.

Williams RL, et al: Use of antibiotics in preventing recurrent acute otitis media and in treating otitis media with effusion: A meta-analytic attempt to resolve the brouhaha. *JAMA* 270:1344-1351, 1993.

Prevention of Travelers' Diarrhea

Advice for travelers. *Med Lett Drugs Ther* 34:41-44, 1992.

Salicylate in Pepto-Bismol. *Med Lett Drugs Ther* 22:63, 1980.

DuPont HL: Chemoprophylaxis remains an option in travelers' diarrhea, editorial. *Am J Gastroenterol* 86:402-404, 1991.

DuPont HL, Ericsson CD: Prevention and treatment of travelers' diarrhea. *N Engl J Med* 328:1821-1827, 1993.

DuPont HL, et al: Prevention of travelers' diarrhea (emporiatric enteritis): Prophylactic administration of subsalicylate bismuth. *JAMA* 243:237-241, 1980.

DuPont HL, et al: Treatment of travelers' diarrhea with trimethoprim/sulfamethoxazole and with trimethoprim alone. *N Engl J Med* 307:841-844, 1982.

DuPont HL, et al: Prevention of travelers' diarrhea with trimethoprim/sulfamethoxazole and trimethoprim alone. *Gastroenterology* 84:75-80, 1983.

DuPont HL, et al: Prevention of travelers' diarrhea by the tablet formulation of bismuth subsalicylate. *JAMA* 257:1347-1350, 1987.

Ericsson CD, et al: Influence of subsalicylate bismuth on absorption of doxycycline. *JAMA* 247:2266-2267, 1982.

Ericsson CD, et al: Ciprofloxacin or trimethoprim/sulfamethoxazole as initial therapy for travelers' diarrhea: Placebo-controlled, randomized trial. *Ann Intern Med* 106:216-220, 1987.

Ericsson CD, et al: Treatment of traveler's diarrhea with sulfamethoxazole and trimethoprim and loperamide. *JAMA* 263:257-261, 1990.

Farthing MJG, et al: Treatment and prevention of travelers' diarrhea. *Gastroenterol Int* 5:162-175, 1992.

Gorbach SL: Travelers' diarrhea, editorial. *N Engl J Med* 307:881-883, 1982.

Gorbach SL, Edelman R (eds): Travelers' diarrhea: National Institutes of Health Consensus Development Conference. *Rev Infect Dis* 8(suppl 2): S109-S283, 1986 (12 papers).

Graham DY, et al: Double-blind comparison of bismuth subsalicylate and placebo in prevention and treatment of enterotoxigenic *Escherichia coli*-induced diarrhea in volunteers. *Gastroenterology* 85:1017-1022, 1983.

Johnson PC, et al: Lack of emergence of resistant fecal flora during successful prophylaxis of travelers' diarrhea with norfloxacin. *Antimicrob Agents Chemother* 30:671-674, 1986.

Murray BE, et al: Increasing resistance to trimethoprim/sulfamethoxazole among isolates of *Escherichia coli* in developing countries. *J Infect Dis* 152:1107-1113, 1985.

National Institutes of Health Consensus Development Conference: Travelers' diarrhea. *JAMA* 253:2700-2704, 1985.

Rademaker CMA, et al: Results of double-blind placebo-controlled study using ciprofloxacin for prevention of travelers' diarrhea. *Eur J Clin Microbiol Infect Dis* 8:690-694, 1989.

Reves RR, et al: Cost-effective comparison of use of antimicrobial agents for treatment or prophylaxis of travelers' diarrhea. *Arch Intern Med* 148:2421-2427, 1988.

Sack DA, et al: Prophylactic doxycycline for travelers' diarrhea: Results of prospective double-blind study of Peace Corps volunteers in Kenya. *N Engl J Med* 298:758-763, 1978.

Sack RB, et al: Prophylactic doxycycline for travelers' diarrhea: Results of prospective double-blind study of Peace Corps volunteers in Morocco. *Gastroenterology* 76:1368-1373, 1979.

Satterwhite TK, DuPont HL: Infectious diarrhea in office practice. *Med Clin North Am* 67:203-220, 1983.

Siegel JD: Prophylactic antibiotics. *Pediatr Infect Dis* 3:537-541, 1984.

Tellier R, Keystone JS: Prevention of traveler's diarrhea. *Infect Dis Clin North Am* 6:333-354, 1992.

Antimicrobial Chemoprophylaxis for Surgical Patients

62

ABDOMINAL SURGERY

CARDIOVASCULAR SURGERY

NEUROSURGERY

OBSTETRIC-GYNECOLOGIC SURGERY

ORTHOPEDIC SURGERY

OTOLARYNGOLOGIC SURGERY

THORACIC SURGERY

The purpose of antimicrobial chemoprophylaxis for surgical patients is to reduce the risk of postoperative wound and some other infections. The benefit of prophylaxis for each surgical procedure must be weighed against the potential risks to both the patient and the environment, including adverse drug reactions, superinfections, the emergence of antibiotic-resistant bacterial strains, and the total monetary cost of antimicrobial administration.

Surgical procedures are classified into four categories according to the expected level of bacterial contamination at the operative field: *clean, clean-contaminated, contaminated*, and *dirty*. The risk of postoperative infection increases as the degree of bacterial contamination and the virulence of the contaminating bacteria increase; the presence of foreign material, highly traumatized tissue, or a compromised host immune system potentiates the risk of infection. Furthermore, within a given classification, risk of infection varies with the type of surgical procedure (Kaiser, 1990). Generally, antimicrobial prophylaxis should be limited to patients at high risk of postoperative infection, ie, those undergoing clean-contaminated or contaminated surgery, or those in whom the development of an infection might be associated with a catastrophic end result, such as patients undergoing clean surgical procedures involving the insertion of prostheses. Recent guidelines developed by the Antimicrobial Agents Committee of the Surgical Infection Society suggest extending antimicrobial prophylaxis to other categories of clean wounds but only for patients with two or more risk factors established by criteria in the study of the efficacy of nosocomial infection control (SENIC); the baseline infection rate in these patients is high enough to justify prophylaxis (Page et al, 1993). Dirty surgery implies that infection already exists, and the use of antimicrobial agents in such procedures usually is considered treatment rather than prophylaxis.

The timing and duration of antimicrobial administration are important for effective surgical prophylaxis. An adequate concentration of a drug that is active against the likely pathogens must be present in vulnerable tissues at the time of the initial incision and *throughout the procedure*, which is the time of maximal contamination. Thus, parenteral antimicrobial prophylaxis should begin just prior to the operation (Classen et al, 1992). Usually, a single intravenous dose administered shortly before the first incision, ie, in the operating room immediately prior to induction of anesthesia (preinduction), provides sufficient tissue concentrations of antimicrobial agent throughout the procedure. Administration of the antimicrobial regimen on call to the operating room is not recommended because delays in beginning the surgery can result in inadequate drug concentrations and increased failure of prophylaxis (Galandiuk et al, 1989). When the surgical procedure is prolonged (eg, more than two hours), an additional dose of antimicrobial agent, intraoperatively, often is required to maintain adequate tissue concentrations. This is particularly true when antimicrobial agents with relatively short serum and tissue half-lives are employed. Postoperative doses of prophylactic drugs generally are unnecessary. There are little or no data supporting the need for prophylaxis beyond 24 hours.

Selection of the most appropriate antimicrobial regimen for surgical prophylaxis depends on a number of factors, including antimicrobial activity against the likely infecting organisms for the particular operative site and hospital environment; the toxicity and pharmacokinetics of the drug; evidence of effectiveness in controlled clinical trials; and, other factors being equal, the total cost of the prophylactic regimen (this should include the costs of drug acquisition, drug administration, and any necessary monitoring). For most surgical procedures, cefazolin has been preferred because it is effective, has limited toxicity, has a moderately long plasma half-life, and is relatively inexpensive. When methicillin-resistant staphylococci are prevalent, vancomycin should be used; when anaerobic coverage is required (eg, colorectal surgery), cefoxitin and cefotetan are often preferred (American Society of Hospital Pharmacists [ASHP] Commission on Therapeutics, 1992; *Med Lett Drugs Ther*, 1993; Page et al, 1993).

An important consideration is selection of a prophylactic regimen with the most limited effective antimicrobial spectrum (ie, the regimen should be effective against those organisms that are likely to cause postoperative wound infection, but it need not eradicate every potential pathogen). The intent is to avoid use of unnecessarily broad-spectrum antimicrobial agents that frequently are valuable for empiric therapy. This strategy should minimize the emergence of bacterial resistance to these valuable *therapeutic* agents. Because of this, third-generation cephalosporins are *not* recommended for surgical prophylaxis (ASHP Commission on Therapeutics, 1992; *Med Lett Drugs Ther*, 1993; Page et al, 1993).

Guidelines for antimicrobial chemoprophylaxis of those surgical procedures for which prophylaxis is justified, based on controlled clinical trials, are presented below. However, it should be emphasized that definitive recommendations remain to be established, pending the results of future studies.

Selected references: Hirschmann and Inui, 1980; DiPiro et al, 1981, 1983, 1984, 1986; Hirschmann, 1981; Lennard and Dellinger, 1981; Guglielmo et al, 1983; Polk et al, 1983; Burnakis, 1984; Conte et al, 1984; Kaiser, 1986, 1990; Conte and Barriere, 1988; Nichols, 1988, 1991, 1992; Conte, 1989; Platt and Kaiser, 1991; ASHP Commission on Therapeutics, 1992; Haines, 1992; *Int J Gynecol Obstet*, 1992; Malangoni and Jacobs, 1992; Ulualp and Condon, 1992; Van Scoy and Wilkowske, 1992; Ehrenkranz, 1993; *Med Lett Drugs Ther*, 1993; Page et al, 1993; Sanford, 1993.

ABDOMINAL SURGERY

Elective Biliary Tract Surgery (Clean-Contaminated)

INDICATIONS:
Most postoperative infections occur in patients with positive bile cultures. Traditionally, prophylaxis has been recommended only for patients at high risk for bactibilia, including those over 70 years and those with obstructive jaundice, acute cholecystitis, or common duct stones (*Med Lett Drugs Ther*, 1993). However, series reporting the incidence of positive bile cultures from low-risk patients give wide-ranging values (from 10% to 50%). Furthermore, a meta-analysis of 42 studies indicated that antimicrobial prophylaxis was effective in both low- and high-risk patients undergoing biliary tract surgery (Meijer et al, 1990). Thus, many experts now recommend prophylaxis for all patients undergoing biliary tract surgery (ASHP Commission on Therapeutics, 1992; Page et al, 1993). Appropriate recommendations for laparoscopic cholecystectomy are not yet clear, but prophylactic antibiotics are commonly used (Page et al, 1993).

POTENTIAL PATHOGENS:
Gram-negative enteric bacilli (*Escherichia coli, Klebsiella*), *Staphylococcus aureus, Enterococcus faecalis* and other group D enterococci, and *Clostridium perfringens* (less than 20% of cases)

RECOMMENDED REGIMEN:
Cefazolin[1] (*adults*, 1 to 2 g IV immediately prior to induction of anesthesia)

REMARKS:
(1) Meta-analysis indicates that cefazolin is as effective as second- or third-generation cephalosporins and that single-dose prophylaxis is as effective as multiple doses (Meijer et al, 1990).
(2) Gentamicin, *adults*, 1.5 to 1.7 mg/kg IV at induction of anesthesia and every eight hours for three doses is effective in patients with β-lactam allergy (Kaiser, 1990; Mandell et al, 1992).

Gastroduodenal Surgery (Clean-Contaminated)

INDICATIONS:
Prophylaxis is recommended only for high-risk patients with decreased gastric acidity or motility. This includes patients with gastric ulcer, gastric malignancy, obstructing or bleeding duodenal ulcer, and achlorhydria or those receiving chronic H_2-blocker (eg, cimetidine) or omeprazole therapy. Prophylaxis also is recommended for morbidly obese patients undergoing gastric bypass procedures and for percutaneous endoscopic gastrostomy.

POTENTIAL PATHOGENS:
Mixed oropharyngeal flora (eg, aerobic and anaerobic streptococci); gram-negative bacilli; and *Staphylococcus aureus*

RECOMMENDED REGIMEN:
Cefazolin[1] (*adults*, 1 to 2 g IV immediately prior to induction of anesthesia)

REMARK:
(1) In patients with β-lactam allergy, intravenous clindamycin (600 to 900 mg) *plus* gentamicin (1.7 mg/kg) is a suggested alternative regimen, but data are limited (see Kaiser, 1990).

Elective Colorectal Surgery (Clean-Contaminated)

INDICATIONS:
Three general approaches are used: oral antimicrobial agents; parenteral antimicrobial agents; and a combination of oral and parenteral antimicrobial agents (Gorbach, 1991; Gorbach et al, 1992; *Med Lett Drugs Ther*, 1993; Page et al, 1993). Current consensus in the United States is that patients undergoing elective procedures should receive mechanical bowel preparation, usually with a polyethylene glycol-electrolyte lavage solution, and prophylactic antimicrobial agents orally. European surgeons often prefer systemic prophylaxis with parenteral antibiotics only, and some consultants stated that this is an acceptable approach. Use of parenteral agents is essential for emergency colorectal operations, when there is bowel obstruction, or when surgery involves a site distal to an established colostomy. Whether the addition of a parenteral (systemic) antibiotic to the oral regimen provides better prophylaxis currently is unresolved. However, most colon and rectal surgeons in the United States use both oral and injectable antimicrobial regimens plus bowel cleansing (Solla and Rothenberger, 1990). A combination of oral and parenteral agents should be given (1) when intestinal lavage is incomplete or oral antimicrobials are not administered in a timely fashion or in sufficient dosage; (2) when the onset of surgery has been delayed; (3) when there is intraoperative spillage of intestinal contents; (4) when the operation is prolonged (eg, generally longer than 3.5 hours); and (5) when there is rectal resection (Gorbach, 1991; Gorbach et al, 1992;

Ehrenkranz, 1993).
POTENTIAL PATHOGENS:
Gram-negative enteric bacilli (eg, *Escherichia coli*); anaerobic bacteria (especially *Bacteroides fragilis*); and rarely *Enterococcus faecalis* and other group D enterococci
RECOMMENDED REGIMEN (ORAL):
Neomycin *plus* erythromycin base (orally, 1 g of each at 1 PM, 2 PM, and 11 PM on the day prior to surgery [surgery at 8 AM])
RECOMMENDED REGIMENS (PARENTERAL):
Cefoxitin (*adults*, 2 g IV immediately prior to induction of anesthesia)
OR
Cefotetan (*adults*, 2 g IV immediately prior to induction of anesthesia)
OR
Cefmetazole (*adults*, 2 g IV immediately prior to induction of anesthesia)
REMARKS:
(1) For prolonged operations (eg, longer than two hours), a second intraoperative dose of cefoxitin is indicated because of this drug's short elimination half-life.
(2) For patients allergic to β-lactam antibiotics, the following are alternative regimens: Clindamycin (*adults*, 600 to 900 mg IV immediately prior to induction of anesthesia) (or metronidazole, *adults*, 1 g IV infused over 30 to 60 minutes prior to induction of anesthesia) *plus* gentamicin (*adults*, 1.7 mg/kg IV immediately prior to induction of anesthesia) (Bartlett, 1993); clindamycin (*adults*, 600 to 900 mg IV) *plus* aztreonam (*adults*, 1 g IV) immediately prior to induction of anesthesia (Rodolico et al, 1991).
(3) Various third-generation cephalosporins (eg, ceftizoxime) and β-lactam/β-lactamase inhibitor combinations (eg, ampicillin/sulbactam) have been shown to be effective for prophylaxis of elective colorectal surgery, but whether they offer any advantages over cefoxitin, cefotetan, or cefmetazole remains to be established by comparative, controlled clinical trials.

Appendectomy (Clean-Contaminated)

INDICATIONS:
Current consensus is that all patients undergoing appendectomy should receive prophylactic antimicrobial agents. If the appendix is found to be gangrenous or perforated, then continued therapeutic antibiotic administration for three to five days usually is necessary because these settings represent treatment of active infection rather than prophylaxis (Gorbach, 1991; Gorbach et al, 1992).
POTENTIAL PATHOGENS:
Gram-negative enteric bacilli (eg, *Escherichia coli*); anaerobic bacteria (especially *Bacteroides fragilis*); and rarely *Enterococcus faecalis* and other group D enterococci
RECOMMENDED REGIMENS:
Cefoxitin (*adults*, 2 g IV immediately prior to induction of anesthesia)
OR
Cefotetan (*adults*, 2 g IV immediately prior to induction of anesthesia)
OR
Cefmetazole (*adults*, 2 g IV immediately prior to induction of anesthesia)
ALTERNATIVE REGIMENS:
Clindamycin (*adults*, 600 to 900 mg IV immediately prior to induction of anesthesia) (or metronidazole, *adults*, 1 g IV infused over 30 to 60 minutes prior to induction of anesthesia) *plus* gentamicin (*adults*, 1.7 mg/kg IV immediately prior to induction of anesthesia)
REMARKS:
(1) Some experts consider ceftizoxime (*adults*, 1 to 2 g IV immediately prior to induction of anesthesia) an acceptable alternative to the second-generation cephalosporins listed above (Browder et al, 1989; Gorbach, 1991; ASHP Commission on Therapeutics, 1992).
(2) Because of lack of data supporting use of a single agent for children, pediatric surgeons continue to prefer the combination of ampicillin, gentamicin, and clindamycin (ASHP Commission on Therapeutics, 1992).

Penetrating Abdominal Trauma (Contaminated)

INDICATIONS:
Intra-abdominal infection (eg, peritonitis, abscess) may follow surgery for penetrating abdominal trauma, especially when there is colon perforation. The incidence of these infections can be decreased significantly in patients with bacterial contamination of the abdomen secondary to penetrating abdominal trauma if prompt surgical intervention and administration of appropriate antimicrobial agents are performed. The Antimicrobial Agents Committee of the Surgical Infection Society states that when antibiotics are administered for traumatic enteric perforations that are operated on within 12 hours of injury, the antibiotics should be considered prophylactic (Bohnen et al, 1992). Current consensus is that all patients with penetrating abdominal trauma should receive prophylactic antimicrobial therapy (Dellinger, 1991; Malangoni and Jacobs, 1992; Page et al, 1993).
POTENTIAL PATHOGENS:
Gram-negative enteric bacilli (eg, *Escherichia coli*); anaerobic bacteria (especially *Bacteroides fragilis*); and rarely *Enterococcus faecalis* and other group D enterococci
RECOMMENDED REGIMENS:
Cefoxitin (*adults*, 2 g IV as early as possible [eg, during early resuscitation] and then every six hours for 24 hours) (see REMARKS)
OR
Cefotetan (*adults*, 2 g IV as early as possible [eg, during early resuscitation] and then every 12 hours for 24 hours) (see REMARKS)
ALTERNATIVE REGIMEN:
Clindamycin (*adults*, 900 mg IV as early as possible [eg, during early resuscitation] and then every eight hours for 24 hours) *plus* gentamicin (*adults*, 1.7 mg/kg IM or IV as early as possible [eg, during early resuscitation] and then every eight hours for 24 hours) (see REMARKS)
REMARKS:
(1) For prolonged operations (eg, longer than two hours), a second intra-operative dose of cefoxitin is indicated because of the drug's short elimination half-life.
(2) When antimicrobial agents are given as soon as possible after injury, shorter courses are as effective in preventing infections as traditional five- to seven-day durations of therapy (Stone et al, 1979; Oreskovich et al, 1982; Hofstetter et al, 1984; Jones et al, 1985; Dellinger et al, 1986; Fabian et al, 1992). Current consensus is that if an exploratory laparotomy reveals no injury to the bowel and no other source of endogenous contamination, antibiotic prophylaxis can be discontinued after a single dose. If bowel injury is documented, administration of antibiotics should be continued for 24 hours (Dellinger, 1991; Fabian et al, 1992; Malangoni and Jacobs, 1992; Page et al, 1993).
(3) Single-agent prophylaxis with cefoxitin or cefotetan appears to be as effective as combination regimens containing clindamycin plus an aminoglycoside in preventing infections after penetrating abdominal injuries (Hofstetter et al, 1984; Nichols et al, 1984; Jones et al, 1985; Fabian et al, 1992; see also Dellinger, 1991; Malangoni and Jacobs, 1992; Page et al, 1993). Although results of one randomized, double-blind clinical trial suggested that cefotetan was inferior to cefoxitin for penetrating abdominal trauma (Nichols et al, 1993), greater risk factors among patients in the cefotetan group raise questions

about the conclusions of this study. Other β-lactam antibiotics recommended by some consultants for prophylaxis of penetrating abdominal trauma include ampicillin/sulbactam and ceftizoxime. Clindamycin plus an aminoglycoside is a useful alternative regimen for patients who are allergic to β-lactam antibiotics.
(4) An alternative dosing regimen for intravenous clindamycin is 600 mg every six hours.

CARDIOVASCULAR SURGERY

Cardiac Surgery (Clean)

INDICATIONS:
Prophylaxis is recommended when a prosthetic heart valve is inserted to decrease the risk of prosthetic valve endocarditis, a frequently fatal infection. Patients undergoing other open-heart surgery, including coronary artery bypass graft surgery, also should receive prophylactic antimicrobial agents. Prophylaxis may not be necessary for pacemaker insertion in institutions with a low incidence of infection. Prophylaxis is not routinely recommended for cardiac catheterization (*Med Lett Drugs Ther*, 1993).
POTENTIAL PATHOGENS:
Staphylococcus aureus; S. epidermidis; diphtheroids; gram-negative enteric bacilli; and rarely fungi
RECOMMENDED REGIMENS:
Cefazolin (*adults*, 2 g IV immediately prior to induction of anesthesia)
OR
Cefuroxime *(adults,* 1.5 g IV immediately prior to induction of anesthesia) (see REMARKS)
ALTERNATIVE REGIMENS:
Cefamandole *(adults,* 2 g IV immediately prior to induction of anesthesia)
OR
Vancomycin (*adults*, 1 g IV infused over 60 minutes prior to induction of anesthesia) (see REMARKS)
REMARKS:
(1) For prolonged operations (longer than four hours), a second intraoperative dose of cefazolin or cefuroxime is recommended.
(2) Optimal duration of prophylaxis is unknown. Some surgeons prefer to continue prophylaxis for an additional 48 hours until intravascular monitoring catheters are removed, although there are no data to validate this practice. Most reviews of the subject suggest a maximum duration of 48 hours (eg, cefazolin, *adults*, 1 to 2 g IV every eight hours for 48 hours; cefuroxime, *adults*, 1.5 g IV every 12 hours for 48 hours) (Ariano and Zhanel, 1991; ASHP Commission on Therapeutics, 1992; Kreter and Woods, 1992; Page et al, 1993).
(3) The cephalosporin of choice for prophylaxis of open-heart surgery is controversial. In two prospective, randomized controlled trials, cefuroxime (IV, 1.5 g every 12 hours for 48 hours) or cefamandole (IV, 2 g immediately prior to induction of anesthesia, 1 g every two hours during surgery, and 1 g every four hours after surgery for 72 hours) was significantly more effective than cefazolin (IV, either 1 g every eight hours for 48 hours or 2 g immediately prior to induction of anesthesia, 1 g every four hours during surgery, and 1 g every six hours after surgery for 72 hours) in preventing postoperative wound infections, especially those caused by staphylococci, following open-heart surgery (Slama et al, 1986; Kaiser et al, 1987). However, two other controlled clinical trials did not show differences in efficacy (Gentry et al, 1988; Townsend et al, 1993), and a fifth study showed cefazolin to be more effective than cefuroxime (Doebbeling et al, 1990). A meta-analysis of controlled clinical trials suggests a 1½-fold reduction in total wound infection prevalence with the use of second-generation cephalosporins (cefuroxime or cefamandole) when compared with cefazolin (Kreter and Woods, 1992). (Note: The meta-analysis did not include the study of Townsend et al, 1993.) Some experts continue to recommend cefazolin as the preferred prophylactic agent (Page et al, 1993), but others also consider cefuroxime an appropriate first-choice agent (ASHP Commission on Therapeutics, 1992; Van Scoy and Wilkowske, 1992; *Med Lett Drugs Ther*, 1993). Cefuroxime (or cefamandole) should be considered in institutions in which methicillin-susceptible *S. aureus* wound infections continue to occur despite cefazolin prophylaxis (see Kaiser, 1990).
(4) In hospitals with a high incidence of methicillin-resistant *S. aureus* or *S. epidermidis*, vancomycin is the drug of choice. Patients allergic to β-lactam antibiotics also should receive this agent. Because gram-negative bacilli have become common pathogens in open heart surgery, consideration should be given to adding a cephalosporin or gentamicin to the vancomycin regimen.

Peripheral Vascular Surgery (Clean)

INDICATIONS:
Prophylaxis is recommended for arterial reconstructive surgery on the abdominal aorta and vascular operations on the leg involving a groin incision. Generally, prophylaxis is justified for any vascular procedure in which a prosthesis is implanted, including grafts for vascular access to hemodialysis. It is not recommended for brachial or carotid arterial surgery if a prosthesis is not involved; the incidence of infection is low and there are no data on the effectiveness of prophylaxis. See also REMARKS.
POTENTIAL PATHOGENS:
Staphylococcus aureus; S. epidermidis; diphtheroids; and gram-negative enteric bacilli
RECOMMENDED REGIMEN:
Cefazolin[1] (*adults*, 1 to 2 g IV immediately prior to induction of anesthesia)
REMARKS:
(1) Two postoperative doses (at eight-hour intervals) commonly are employed (ASHP Commission on Therapeutics, 1992; Page et al, 1993).
(2) Vancomycin (dosage as above for Cardiac Surgery) is an alternative agent in patients with β-lactam allergy or in hospitals with a high incidence of methicillin-resistant staphylococci. Because gram-negative bacilli frequently are encountered in infections involving a groin incision, consideration should be given to adding a cephalosporin or gentamicin to vancomycin in procedures involving the groin site.
(3) Antimicrobial prophylaxis is indicated in amputation of the lower extremity for ischemia. Staphylococci, gram-negative enteric bacilli, and clostridia are potential pathogens. Cefazolin (IV, 1 g immediately prior to induction of anesthesia) is recommended by some experts (see *Med Lett Drugs Ther*, 1993); cefoxitin (IV, 2 g immediately prior to induction of anesthesia) is preferred by others because of its better anaerobic coverage (see Kaiser, 1990).

NEUROSURGERY

Elective Neurosurgical Operations (Clean)

INDICATIONS:
Prophylaxis is recommended for craniotomy. Despite limited data, antimicrobial prophylaxis for other clean neurosurgical procedures also is a reasonable option (ASHP Commission on Therapeutics, 1992; Haines, 1992; Page et al, 1993).
POTENTIAL PATHOGENS:
Staphylococcus aureus; S. epidermidis

RECOMMENDED REGIMEN:
Cefazolin *(adults,* 1 g IV immediately prior to induction of anesthesia)

ALTERNATIVE REGIMEN:
Vancomycin (*adults,* 1 g IV infused over 60 minutes prior to induction of anesthesia)

REMARKS:
(1) Because of limited data, the optimal regimen for prophylaxis is unknown. Current consensus is that a single preoperative dose of cefazolin will provide effective prophylaxis (ASHP Commission on Therapeutics, 1992; *Med Lett Drugs Ther,* 1993; Page et al, 1993).
(2) Antibiotics used in clinical trials for prophylaxis during elective neurosurgical operations do not reliably cross the blood-cerebrospinal fluid (CSF) barrier. CSF penetration is not important in the prevention of these postoperative infections, presumably because most are soft-tissue infections (Haines, 1992).
(3) Vancomycin is an alternative agent in patients with β-lactam allergy or in hospitals with a high incidence of methicillin-resistant staphylococci.

OBSTETRIC-GYNECOLOGIC SURGERY

Hysterectomy (Clean-Contaminated)

INDICATIONS:
Prophylaxis is recommended for vaginal hysterectomy. The role of antimicrobial prophylaxis in abdominal hysterectomy has been less clear, although some clinical trials have shown significantly decreased rates of postoperative wound infection. A recent meta-analysis of 25 randomized controlled trials concluded that preoperative antibiotics are highly effective in the prevention of serious infections associated with abdominal hysterectomy (Mittendorf et al, 1993). Thus, prophylaxis for abdominal hysterectomy is a reasonable option.

POTENTIAL PATHOGENS:
Escherichia coli and other Enterobacteriaceae; anaerobic bacteria (eg, gram-positive cocci, *Prevotella, Bacteroides*); *Enterococcus faecalis* and other group D enterococci; and *Streptococcus agalactiae* (group B)

RECOMMENDED REGIMEN:
Cefazolin[1] (*adults,* 1 to 2 g IV immediately prior to induction of anesthesia)

REMARKS:
(1) If surgery lasts more than two to three hours, a second intraoperative dose of cefazolin should be administered (*Int J Gynecol Obstet*, 1992).
(2) Cefoxitin, cefotetan, third-generation cephalosporins, and extended spectrum penicillins have been shown to be effective for prophylaxis of vaginal and abdominal hysterectomy, but whether any of these antimicrobial agents offers any advantages over cefazolin remains to be established by published comparative, controlled clinical trials. Cefazolin currently remains the drug of choice for prophylaxis (*Int J Gynecol Obstet*, 1992; Hemsell, 1991; ASHP Commission on Therapeutics, 1992; *Med Lett Drugs Ther*, 1993; Page et al, 1993). (Note: Two gynecological consultants noted that a prospective, randomized, blinded clinical trial conducted by Hemsell et al and involving over 500 women undergoing abdominal hysterectomy found cefotetan [1 g] to be superior to cefazolin [1 g] for this indication. However, the results of this study have not yet been published.)
(3) In patients with β-lactam allergy, the following regimens have been suggested: (a) doxycycline, *adults*, 100 mg orally at bedtime the night before surgery and 100 mg orally three to four hours before surgery (Hemsell, 1991); or (b) clindamycin, *adults*, 600 to 900 mg IV; (c) metronidazole, *adults*, 500 mg IV; or (d) doxycycline, *adults*, 200 mg IV preoperatively (*Int J Gynecol Obstet*, 1992).

Cesarean Section (Clean-Contaminated)

INDICATIONS:
Prophylaxis is useful in reducing postoperative infectious complications (eg, endometritis) in nonelective cesarean sections in high-risk women. This includes patients in active labor or with premature rupture of membranes and those who require internal fetal monitoring. The usefulness of prophylaxis in uncomplicated elective cesarean sections is controversial. Although some data support the efficacy of prophylaxis in low-risk populations (Ehrenkranz et al, 1990), various experts disagree on whether low-risk populations will benefit from prophylaxis (see Hemsell, 1991; ASHP Commission on Therapeutics, 1992, *Med Lett Drugs Ther*, 1993; Page et al, 1993).

POTENTIAL PATHOGENS:
Escherichia coli and other Enterobacteriaceae; anaerobic bacteria (eg, gram-positive cocci, *Prevotella, Bacteroides*); *Enterococcus faecalis* and other group D enterococci; and *Streptococcus agalactiae* (group B)

RECOMMENDED REGIMEN:
Cefazolin[1] (*adults,* 2 g IV after cord clamping)

REMARKS:
(1) To avoid delivery of the antibiotic to the fetus, the single dose for prophylaxis should be administered after the umbilical cord is clamped.
(2) Cefoxitin, cefotetan, third-generation cephalosporins, and extended spectrum penicillins have been shown to be effective for prophylaxis of cesarean section, but whether any of these antimicrobial agents offers any advantages over cefazolin remains to be established by comparative, controlled clinical trials. (Note: One gynecological consultant now prefers cefoxitin or cefotetan, agents with increased anaerobic coverage, to cefazolin.)
(3) In patients with β-lactam allergy, the following regimens have been suggested: (a) metronidazole, *adults*, 500 mg IV after cord clamping (Kaiser, 1990); (b) doxycycline, *adults*, 200 mg IV after cord clamping; or (c) clindamycin, *adults*, 600 to 900 mg IV after cord clamping (Hemsell, 1991).

ORTHOPEDIC SURGERY

Orthopedic Surgery (Clean)

INDICATIONS:
Prophylaxis decreases the incidence of both early and late postoperative infection following total hip replacement, a potentially disastrous complication, and is recommended. Prophylaxis also appears to be justified for other artificial joint insertions and is recommended for hip or other fracture operations in which internal fixation is achieved with nails, plates, screws, or wires. Other clean orthopedic surgery not involving the insertion of a prosthesis usually does not require prophylactic antimicrobial drugs; the incidence of infection is low and the effectiveness of prophylaxis is unproven.

POTENTIAL PATHOGENS:
Staphylococcus aureus; *S. epidermidis*; and other skin flora

RECOMMENDED REGIMEN:
Cefazolin[1] (*adults,* 1 to 2 g IV immediately prior to induction of anesthesia)

ALTERNATIVE REGIMEN:
Vancomycin (*adults,* 1 g IV infused over 60 minutes prior to induction of anesthesia)

REMARKS:
(1) Data on the efficacy of single-dose cefazolin prophylaxis are lacking. Many orthopedic surgeons recommend a second postoperative dose.
(2) Vancomycin is the preferred agent for patients with β-lactam allergy or in hospitals with a high incidence of methicillin-resistant *S. aureus* or *S. epidermidis*.
(3) Operating rooms with ultraclean air also reduce the frequency of deep wound infection following total joint replacement. Antibiotic-impregnated cement is effective in preventing early infection following total joint replacement. At present, it is not clear whether systemic antibiotics in combination with either ultraclean air or antibiotic-impregnated cement produce additive or cumulative effects (see Norden, 1991, for suggestions for combined use).

Compound (Open) Fracture (Contaminated or Dirty)

INDICATIONS:
Risk of infection correlates with the severity of the fracture and the degree of damage to surrounding soft tissue; Grades 3B and 3C fractures have the highest infection rates (Dellinger, 1991). Antimicrobials are indicated for all open fractures. Traditionally, this has been considered treatment rather than prophylaxis.

POTENTIAL PATHOGENS:
Staphylococcus aureus; *Streptococcus pyogenes* (group A beta hemolytic); and clostridia. Gram-negative bacilli (eg, *Enterobacter* sp. and *Pseudomonas aeruginosa*) frequently are recovered from sites of infection complicating Grade 3 fractures.

RECOMMENDED REGIMEN:
Cefazolin[1] (*adults*, 1 to 2 g IV immediately and then 1 g every eight hours for 24 hours to five days or longer) (see REMARKS)

ALTERNATIVE REGIMENS:
Vancomycin (*adults*, 1 g IV, infused over a 60-minute period immediately and then every 12 hours for 24 hours to five days or longer)
OR
Clindamycin (*adults*, 900 mg IV immediately and then every eight hours for 24 hours to five days or longer)

REMARKS:
(1) Some experts would add penicillin G for better coverage against clostridia.
(2) Some experts have observed an increased incidence of gram-negative bacillary infections in open fractures and, therefore, recommend the addition of an aminoglycoside (or possibly a third-generation cephalosporin) to the regimen (Patzakis et al, 1983 A, 1983 B; Gustilo et al, 1984). However, available data do not permit a conclusion regarding the efficacy of this practice (Dellinger, 1991).
(3) Results of prospective, randomized clinical trials suggest that a brief course (one day) of antibiotic (cefonicid and cefamandole were used) administration, begun within six hours of injury, is not inferior to a prolonged course (five days) of antibiotics for prevention of postoperative open fracture-site infections (Dellinger et al, 1988 A, 1988 B). Some experts believe that contaminated compound fractures that are surgically managed within a few hours (eg, six hours) of the traumatic episode may be effectively treated by as brief as a one-day course of preoperative/postoperative antimicrobials to prevent development of infection (Dellinger, 1991; Ehrenkranz, 1993). A longer course of postoperative antimicrobial therapy (eg, five days or longer) is generally necessary for more established infections.
(4) An alternative dosing regimen for intravenous clindamycin is 600 mg every six hours.
(5) Some trauma surgeons find the local use of aminoglycoside-impregnated polymethyl methacrylate beads effective in open-extremity fractures; such therapy results in high local bone and tissue levels of antibiotic with little systemic absorption (see Calhoun and Mader, 1989; Malangoni and Jacobs, 1992).

OTOLARYNGOLOGIC SURGERY

Head and Neck Surgery (Clean-Contaminated)

INDICATIONS:
Prophylaxis is recommended for surgical procedures requiring an incision that enters the oral cavity or pharynx (eg, as in surgery for laryngeal and pharyngeal carcinomas).

POTENTIAL PATHOGENS:
Mixture of oropharyngeal aerobic bacteria (eg, *Staphylococcus aureus*, streptococci, gram-negative bacilli [eg, *Klebsiella*]), and anaerobic bacteria (eg, peptostreptococci, *Bacteroides* [rarely *B. fragilis*])

RECOMMENDED REGIMENS:
Clindamycin (*adults*, 600 to 900 mg IV immediately prior to induction of anesthesia) *with or without* gentamicin (*adults*, 1.7 mg/kg IV immediately prior to induction of anesthesia) (see REMARKS)
OR
Cefazolin[1] (*adults*, 2 g IV immediately prior to induction of anesthesia) (see REMARKS)

REMARKS:
(1) Each of the above regimens was continued every eight hours postoperatively for 24 hours (Johnson et al, 1984 A, 1986, 1987).
(2) Traditionally, a prophylactic regimen (eg, clindamycin plus aminoglycoside) with broad spectrum coverage against gram-positive and gram-negative aerobic and anaerobic bacteria has been recommended. However, in a randomized, double-blind clinical trial, clindamycin alone was as effective as the combination in preventing postoperative wound infections, suggesting that aerobic gram-negative coverage may be unnecessary, except in selected patients (Johnson et al, 1987). A meta-analysis of studies on prophylactic antimicrobials in head and neck surgery also suggests that a one-day course of clindamycin may be the most effective regimen (Velanovich, 1991). Various experts support the use of clindamycin alone (Shapiro, 1991; *Med Lett Drugs Ther*, 1993); others still prefer the combination regimen (ASHP Commission on Therapeutics, 1992; Mandell et al, 1992).
(3) Cefazolin (2 g IV immediately prior to induction of anesthesia and then every eight hours for 24 hours) also appears to be effective for prophylaxis of head and neck surgery (Johnson et al, 1986); this regimen is recommended by a number of experts (Shapiro, 1991; ASHP Commission on Therapeutics, 1992; *Med Lett Drugs Ther*, 1993; Page et al, 1993).
(4) The third-generation cephalosporins, cefotaxime and cefoperazone, also have been effective for prophylaxis of head and neck surgery (Johnson et al, 1984 B, 1986), but whether they offer any advantages over clindamycin with or without an aminoglycoside or high-dose cefazolin remains to be established by comparative, controlled clinical trials.

THORACIC SURGERY

Elective General Thoracic Operations (Clean)

INDICATIONS:
Controlled clinical trials are limited and have resulted in conflicting data about the efficacy of prophylaxis for pulmonary resections. However, the Antimicrobial Agents Committee of the Surgical Infection Society has stated that the use of prophylactic antibiotics is standard practice and provides recommendations

(Page et al, 1993).
POTENTIAL PATHOGENS:
Oral anaerobic bacteria; *Staphylococcus aureus*; streptococci; gram-negative enteric bacilli
RECOMMENDED REGIMEN:
Cefazolin[1] (*adults*, 1 to 2 g IV immediately prior to induction of anesthesia)

FOOTNOTE
[1]*Cephapirin is an alternative to cefazolin. However, cefazolin is preferred because it has the following advantages: (1) a longer serum half-life; (2) higher tissue levels (for equivalent weight of drug); and (3) less pain with IM injection. Based on current data, there is no advantage to using second- or third-generation cephalosporins in this situation.*

Cited References

Antimicrobial prophylaxis in surgery. *Med Lett Drugs Ther* 35:91-94, 1993.

Antimicrobial therapy for gynecologic infections: ACOG Technical Bulletin Number 153—March 1991. *Int J Gynecol Obstet* 38:131-139, 1992.

Ariano RE, Zhanel GG: Antimicrobial prophylaxis in coronary bypass surgery: A critical appraisal. *DICP Ann Pharmacother* 25:478-484, 1991.

ASHP Commission on Therapeutics: ASHP therapeutic guidelines on antimicrobial prophylaxis in surgery. *Clin Pharm* 11:483-513, 1992.

Bartlett JG: 1993 Pocket Book of Infectious Disease Therapy. Baltimore, Williams & Wilkins, 1993, 98-102.

Bohnen JMA, et al: Guidelines for clinical care: Anti-infective agents for intra-abdominal infection: A Surgical Infection Society policy statement. *Arch Surg* 127:83-89, 1992.

Browder W, et al: Nonperforative appendicitis: A continuing surgical dilemma. *J Infect Dis* 159:1088-1094, 1989.

Burnakis TG: Surgical antimicrobial prophylaxis: Principles and guidelines. *Pharmacotherapy* 4:248-271, 1984.

Calhoun JH, Mader JT: Antibiotic beads in the management of surgical infections. *Am J Surg* 157:443-449, 1989.

Classen DC, et al: The timing of prophylactic administration of antibiotics and risk of surgical-wound infection. *N Engl J Med* 326:281-286, 1992.

Conte JE Jr: Antibiotic prophylaxis: Non-abdominal surgery, in Remington JS, Swartz MN (eds): *Current Clinical Topics in Infectious Diseases-10*. Boston, Blackwell Scientific Publications, 1989, 254-305.

Conte JE Jr, Barriere SL: *Manual of Antibiotics and Infectious Diseases*, ed 6. Philadelphia, Lea & Febiger, 1988, 153-157.

Conte JE Jr, et al: *Antibiotic Prophylaxis in Surgery: Comprehensive Review*. Philadelphia, JB Lippincott, 1984.

Dellinger EP: Antibiotic prophylaxis in trauma: Penetrating abdominal injuries and open fractures. *Rev Infect Dis* 13(suppl 10):S847-S857, 1991.

Dellinger EP, et al: Efficacy of short-course antibiotic prophylaxis after penetrating intestinal injury: Prospective randomized trial. *Arch Surg* 121:23-30, 1986.

Dellinger EP, et al: Duration of preventive antibiotic administration for open extremity fractures. *Arch Surg* 123:333-339, 1988 A.

Dellinger EP, et al: Risk of infection after open fracture of arm or leg. *Arch Surg* 123:1320-1327, 1988 B.

DiPiro JT, et al: Antimicrobial prophylaxis in surgery: Parts I and II. *Am J Hosp Pharm* 38:320-334, 487-494, 1981.

DiPiro JT, et al: Prophylactic use of antimicrobials in surgery. *Curr Probl Surg* 20:69-132, 1983.

DiPiro JT, et al: Prophylactic parenteral cephalosporins in surgery: Are the newer agents better? *JAMA* 252:3277-3279, 1984.

DiPiro JT, et al: Single dose systemic antibiotic prophylaxis of surgical wound infections. *Am J Surg* 152:552-559, 1986.

Doebbeling RN, et al: Cardiovascular surgery prophylaxis: A randomized, controlled comparison of cefazolin and cefuroxime. *J Thorac Cardiovasc Surg* 99:981-989, 1990.

Ehrenkranz NJ: Antimicrobial prophylaxis in surgery: Mechanisms, misconceptions, and mischief. *Infect Control Hosp Epidemiol* 14:99-106, 1993.

Ehrenkranz NJ, et al: Infections complicating low-risk cesarean sections in community hospitals: Efficacy of antimicrobial prophylaxis. *Am J Obstet Gynecol* 162:337-343, 1990.

Fabian TC, et al: Duration of antibiotic therapy for penetrating abdominal trauma: A prospective trial. *Surgery* 112:788-795, 1992.

Galandiuk S, et al: Re-emphasis of priorities in surgical antibiotic prophylaxis. *Surg Gynecol Obstet* 169:219-222, 1989.

Gentry LO, et al: Antibiotic prophylaxis in open-heart surgery: Comparison of cefamandole, cefuroxime, and cefazolin. *Ann Thorac Surg* 46:167-171, 1988.

Gorbach SL: Antimicrobial prophylaxis for appendectomy and colorectal surgery. *Rev Infect Dis* 13(suppl 10):S815-S820, 1991.

Gorbach SL, et al: General guidelines for the evaluation of new anti-infective drugs for prophylaxis of surgical infections. *Clin Infect Dis* 15(suppl 1):S313-S338, 1992.

Guglielmo BJ, et al: Antibiotic prophylaxis in surgical procedures: Critical analysis of the literature. *Arch Surg* 118:943-955, 1983.

Gustilo RB, et al: Problems in management of Type III (severe) open fractures: New classification of Type III open fractures. *J Trauma* 24:742-746, 1984.

Haines SJ: Antibiotic prophylaxis in neurosurgery: The controlled trials. *Neurosurg Clin North Am* 3:355-358, 1992.

Hemsell DL: Prophylactic antibiotics in gynecologic and obstetric surgery. *Rev Infect Dis* 13(suppl 10):S821-S841, 1991.

Hirschmann JV: Rational antibiotic prophylaxis. *Hosp Pract* 16:105-123, (Nov) 1981.

Hirschmann JV, Inui TS: Antimicrobial prophylaxis: Critique of recent trials. *Rev Infect Dis* 2:1-23, 1980.

Hofstetter SR, et al: Prospective comparison of two regimens of prophylactic antibiotics in abdominal trauma: Cefoxitin versus triple drug. *J Trauma* 24:307-310, 1984.

Johnson JT, et al: Antimicrobial prophylaxis for contaminated head and neck surgery. *Laryngoscope* 94:46-51, 1984 A.

Johnson JT, et al: Efficacy of two third-generation cephalosporins in prophylaxis for head and neck surgery. *Arch Otolaryngol* 110:224-227, 1984 B.

Johnson JT, et al: Cefazolin or moxalactam? Double-blind randomized trial of cephalosporins in head and neck surgery. *Arch Otolaryngol Head Neck Surg* 112:151-153, 1986.

Johnson JT, et al: Assessment of need for gram-negative bacterial coverage in antibiotic prophylaxis for oncological head and neck surgery. *J Infect Dis* 155:331-333, 1987.

Jones RC, et al: Evaluation of antibiotic therapy following penetrating abdominal trauma. *Ann Surg* 201:576-585, 1985.

Kaiser AB: Antimicrobial prophylaxis in surgery. *N Engl J Med* 315:1129-1138, 1986.

Kaiser AB: Postoperative infections and antimicrobial prophylaxis, in Mandell GL, et al (eds): *Principles and Practice of Infectious Diseases,* ed 3. New York, Churchill Livingstone, 1990, 2245-2257.

Kaiser AB, et al: Efficacy of cefazolin, cefamandole, and gentamicin as prophylactic agents in cardiac surgery: Results of prospective, randomized, double-blind trial in 1,030 patients. *Ann Surg* 206:791-797, 1987.

Kreter B, Woods M: Antibiotic prophylaxis for cardiothoracic operations: Metaanalysis of thirty years of clinical trials. *J Thorac Cardiovasc Surg* 104:590-599, 1992.

Lennard ES, Dellinger EP: Prophylactic antibiotics in surgery: Rationale for family physician. *J Fam Pract* 12:461-467, 1981.

Malangoni MA, Jacobs DG: Antibiotic prophylaxis for injured patients. *Infect Dis Clin North Am* 6:627-642, 1992.

Mandell GL, et al: *Principles and Practice of Infectious Diseases: Handbook of Antimicrobial Therapy, 1992*. New York, Churchill Livingstone, 1992, 98-100.

Meijer WS, et al: Meta-analysis of randomized, controlled clinical trials of antibiotic prophylaxis in biliary tract surgery. *Br J Surg* 77:283-290, 1990.

Mittendorf R, et al: Avoiding serious infections associated with abdominal hysterectomy: A meta-analysis of antibiotic prophylaxis. *Am J Obstet Gynecol* 169:1119-1124, 1993.

Nichols RL: Prophylaxis in abdominal surgery, in Peterson PK, Verhoef J (eds): *The Antimicrobial Agents Annual/3*. New York, Elsevier, 1988, 477-499.

Nichols RL: Surgical wound infection. *Am J Med* 91 (suppl 3B):3B-54S-3B-64S, 1991.

Nichols RL: Prophylaxis for surgical infections, in Gorbach SL, et al (eds): *Infectious Diseases*. Philadelphia, WB Saunders, 1992, 393-403.

Nichols RL, et al: Risk of infection after penetrating abdominal trauma. *N Engl J Med* 311:1065-1070, 1984.

Nichols RL, et al: Prospective alterations in therapy for penetrating abdominal trauma. *Arch Surg* 128:55-64, 1993.

Norden CW: Antibiotic prophylaxis in orthopedic surgery. *Rev Infect Dis* 13 (suppl 10):S842-S846, 1991.

Oreskovich MR, et al: Duration of preventive antibiotic administration for penetrating abdominal trauma. *Arch Surg* 117:200-205, 1982.

Page CP, et al: Antimicrobial prophylaxis for surgical wounds: Guidelines for clinical care. *Arch Surg* 128:79-88, 1993.

Patzakis MJ, et al: Use of antibiotics in open tibial fractures. *Clin Orthop* 178:31-35, 1983 A.

Patzakis MJ, et al: Considerations in reducing the infection rate in open tibial fractures. *Clin Orthop* 178:36-41, 1983 B.

Platt R, Kaiser AB (eds): International Symposium on Perioperative Antibiotic Prophylaxis. *Rev Infect Dis* 13 (suppl 10):S779-S890, 1991 (15 articles).

Polk HC Jr, et al: Guidelines for prevention of surgical wound infection. *Arch Surg* 118:1213-1217, 1983.

Rodolico G, et al: Colorectal surgery: Short-term prophylaxis with clindamycin plus aztreonam or gentamicin. *Rev Infect Dis* 13 (suppl 7):S612-S615, 1991.

Sanford JP: *Guide to Antimicrobial Therapy 1993*. West Bethesda, Md, Antimicrobial Therapy, Inc, 1993, 94-98.

Shapiro M: Prophylaxis in otolaryngologic surgery and neurosurgery: A critical review. *Rev Infect Dis* 13 (suppl 10):S858-S868, 1991.

Slama TG, et al: Randomized comparison of cefamandole, cefazolin, and cefuroxime prophylaxis in open-heart surgery. *Antimicrob Agents Chemother* 29:744-747, 1986.

Solla JA, Rothenberger DA: Preoperative bowel preparation: Survey of colon and rectal surgeons. *Dis Colon Rectum* 33:154-159, 1990.

Stone HH, et al: Prophylactic and preventive antibiotic therapy: Timing, duration and economics. *Ann Surg* 189:691-699, 1979.

Townsend TR, et al: Clinical trial of cefamandole, cefazolin, and cefuroxime for antibiotic prophylaxis in cardiac operations. *J Thorac Cardiovasc Surg* 106:664-670, 1993.

Ulualp K, Condon RE: Antibiotic prophylaxis for scheduled operative procedures. *Infect Dis Clin North Am* 6:613-625, 1992.

Van Scoy RE, Wilkowske CJ: Prophylactic use of antimicrobial agents in adult patients. *Mayo Clin Proc* 67:288-292, 1992.

Velanovich V: A meta-analysis of prophylactic antibiotics in head and neck surgery. *Plast Reconstr Surg* 87:429-434, 1991.

Other Selected Reference

Dellinger EP, et al: Quality standard for antimicrobial prophylaxis in surgical procedures. *Clin Infect Dis* 18:422-427, 1994.

Penicillins

63

A unique combination of high efficacy and low toxicity makes the penicillins one of the most commonly prescribed and generally useful groups of antimicrobial drugs.

Chemistry, Source, and Classification

All penicillins contain a common nucleus (6-aminopenicillanic acid) composed of a thiazolidine ring (A) and a β-lactam ring (B) connected to a side chain (R_3) (see Figure). An intact β-lactam ring is necessary for biological activity, but the side chain primarily determines antibacterial spectrum, susceptibility to acid and β-lactamases, and pharmacokinetic properties. The natural penicillin, penicillin G, is extracted from cultures of *Penicillium chrysogenum.* Semisynthetic penicillins usually are prepared by adding side chains to 6-aminopenicillanic acid.

Currently, 15 penicillin derivatives are marketed in the United States. These can be divided according to antimicrobial spectrum into the following subclasses: natural penicillins, penicillinase-resistant (antistaphylococcal) penicillins, aminopenicillins, and antipseudomonal penicillins (see Figure). In addition, three penicillin derivatives are marketed in combination preparations that incorporate inhibitors of bacterial β-lactamases. These are ampicillin/sodium sulbactam [Unasyn], amoxicillin/potassium clavulanate [Augmentin], and ticarcillin/potassium clavulanate [Timentin]; for information on these drugs, see the chapter, Other Beta Lactam Antimicrobial Agents.

There may be significant differences among penicillin subclasses, particularly with regard to antimicrobial spectrum and uses. Differences among members of a given subclass frequently are of a pharmacologic nature (eg, pharmacokinetics, adverse effects), although one compound in a group may be more active than another against a particular microorganism.

Mechanism of Action

Penicillins exert their bactericidal effect on actively dividing cells and have little or no effect on intracellular organisms, dormant bacteria, or organisms that lack cell walls (eg, eukaryotic cells). In the presence of a penicillin, the cell walls of susceptible bacteria develop abnormally, which ultimately results in death of the organism.

The rigid structure of the bacterial cell wall is due to peptidoglycan, a mucopeptide made up of linear polysaccharide chains that are cross linked by peptide bonds. Bacterial cell wall synthesis is a complex process that involves at least 30 enzymes; it is usually subdivided into three stages. In the first stage, cell wall precursor (UDP-acetylmuramyl-pentapeptide) is synthesized and accumulates in the cytoplasm of the bacterial cell. In the second stage, the UDP-acetylmuramyl-pentapeptide binds to phospholipid in the cell membrane and is then linked to UDP-N-acetylglucosamine with release of uridine nucleotides. This disaccharide pentapeptide undergoes further modification (eg, the addition of five glycine residues in *Staphylococcus aureus*) and finally is linked to pre-existing portions of the cell wall, resulting in a linear peptidoglycan polymer. The third stage occurs outside the cell membrane and involves cross linking of linear peptidoglycan polymers via peptide bonds, thus completing formation of the tough outer envelope of the bacterial cell.

The β-lactam antibiotics, which include the penicillins, cephalosporins, monobactams, and carbapenems, have been considered to act by inhibition of the terminal cross-linking step (ie, inhibitors of transpeptidation) (Tipper, 1986; see also Pratt and Fekety, 1986). This explanation now appears to be oversimplified, however, and the penicillins' actual mechanism of action is not completely understood. In *S. aureus,* bactericidal concentrations inhibit the transpeptidase enzyme that catalyzes the cross-linking reaction. Although it

CHEMICAL STRUCTURES OF PENICILLINS

Penicillin Nucleus[1]

Generic Name	R_1	R_2	R_3
NATURAL PENICILLINS			
Penicillin G[2]	H	H	O, CH_2C
Penicillin V	H	H	O, OCH_2C
PENICILLINASE-RESISTANT PENICILLINS			
Methicillin	H	H	OCH_3, O, C, OCH_3
Nafcillin	H	H	O, C, OC_2H_5
ISOXAZOLYL PENICILLINS			
Oxacillin	H	H	N, O, C, O, CH_3
Cloxacillin	H	H	Cl, N, O, C, O, CH_3

Generic Name	R_1	R_2	R_3
Dicloxacillin	H	H	[structure: 3-(2,6-dichlorophenyl)-5-methylisoxazol-4-yl C=O; labels Cl, Cl, N, O, C, O, CH_3]
AMINOPENICILLINS			
Ampicillin	H	H	[structure: phenyl–C(H)(NH₂)–C=O; labels H, O, C, C, NH_2]
Amoxicillin	H	H	[structure: HO–phenyl–C(H)(NH₂)–C=O; labels HO, H, O, C, C, NH_2]
Bacampicillin	CH_3 O CHO–COCH$_2$CH$_3$	H	[structure: phenyl–C(H)(NH₂)–C=O; labels H, O, C, C, NH_2]
Cyclacillin	H	H	[structure: cyclohexyl with NH_2 and C=O]
ANTIPSEUDOMONAL PENICILLINS			
CARBOXYPENICILLINS			
Carbenicillin Indanyl	H	H	[structure: phenyl–C(H)(CO–O–indanyl)–C=O; labels H, O, C, C, CO, O]
Ticarcillin	H	H	[structure: 3-thienyl–C(H)(COOH)–C=O; labels S, H, O, C, C, COH, O]

(figure continued on next page)

Generic Name	R_1	R_2	R_3
UREIDOPENICILLINS			
Mezlocillin	H	H	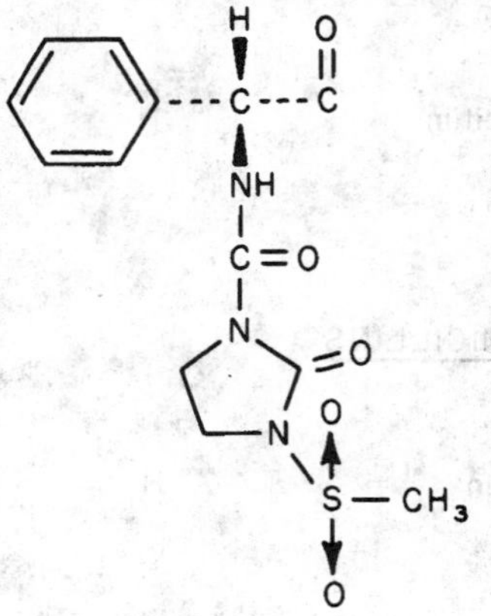 [structure: phenyl–CH(NH–C(=O)–imidazolidinone N-SO2CH3)–C=O]
Piperacillin	H	H	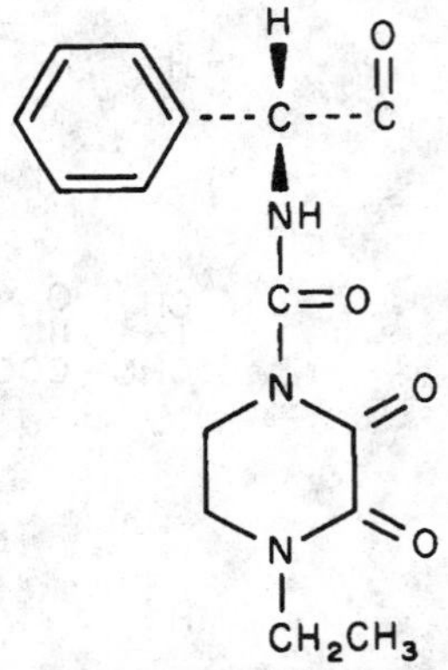 [structure: phenyl–CH(NH–C(=O)–4-ethyl-2,3-dioxopiperazine)–C=O]

[1]*For 6-aminopenicillanic acid,* $R_1 = R_2 = R_3 = H$; *A = thiazolidine ring; B =* β-lactam ring. The arrow is the site of β-lactamase attack.

[2]*Penicillin G procaine (not shown) is a stable aqueous suspension of a poorly water-soluble (0.4%) crystalline salt that contains equimolar amounts of procaine and penicillin G, the active drug. Penicillin G benzathine (not shown) is a stable aqueous suspension of a very poorly water-soluble (0.02%) salt that contains one mole of an ammonium base and two moles of penicillin G, the active drug.*

is believed to be important, this effect probably does not completely explain the bactericidal action of penicillin. In gram-positive species, cell wall lysis also seems to depend on the ability of penicillin to decrease the availability of an inhibitor of bacterial murein hydrolase, a cell wall autolytic enzyme whose normal function is unclear. In the presence of penicillin, this uninhibited autolysin destroys the structural integrity of the cell wall (Pratt and Fekety, 1986). Thus, the penicillins may increase breakdown of the cell wall as well as inhibit its synthesis.

A number of proteins that are associated with bacterial cell membranes have been identified and isolated from both gram-positive and gram-negative bacteria. These proteins (penicillin-binding proteins [PBPs]), which form covalent complexes with penicillin, are enzymes (eg, transpeptidases, transglycosylases, carboxypeptidases) that are involved in bacterial cell wall division, wall elongation, septum formation, and the maintenance of cell shape. Each bacterial species has a unique set of PBPs. The PBPs of gram-negative and gram-positive bacteria differ considerably, but PBPs of different gram-negative bacteria appear to have similarities to each other. However, the selective affinity patterns of β-lactam antibiotics for PBPs of different bacterial species vary and provide the basis for the distinctive structural or microbicidal effects caused by the antimicrobial agent (Neu, 1990; Tomasz, 1986; Tipper, 1986).

The antibacterial activity of β-lactam antibiotics also depends on the concentration of active drug available for binding to essential PBPs. This is primarily determined by the stability of the antibiotic to various β-lactamases produced by gram-positive and gram-negative bacteria and the ability of a drug to penetrate the outer membrane of gram-negative bacteria (see also the section on Resistance).

Antimicrobial Spectrum

NATURAL PENICILLINS. Penicillin G (benzylpenicillin) has excellent in vitro activity against most gram-positive cocci, including *Streptococcus pyogenes* (group A), *S. agalactiae* (group B), nonenterococcal group D streptococci (eg, *S. bovis*), viridans streptococci, anaerobic streptococci (*Peptostreptococcus*), *Peptococcus*, and microaerophilic streptococci. Most strains of *Staphylococcus aureus* produce β-lactamase and are resistant. However, penicillin G is active against *S. aureus* strains that do not produce β-lactamases. The majority of isolates of pneumococci (*S. pneumoniae*) are highly susceptible to penicillin G, but strains that are moderately to highly resistant (minimal inhibitory concentration [MIC] >0.01 mcg/ml) to this drug have been reported in the United States (Weingarten et al, 1990; Spika et al, 1991) and Spain (Viladrich et al, 1988). These strains are considered to be resistant because of reduced binding affinity for penicillin in specific PBPs (Weingarten et al, 1990). Similarly, enterococci (eg, *E. faecalis, E. faecium*) are intrinsically resistant to killing by penicillin alone due to alterations in their PBPs (Grayson et al, 1991); penicillin G must be given with an aminoglycoside or rifampin for bactericidal activity against these species.

Susceptible gram-positive bacilli include *Bacillus anthracis*, most strains of *Corynebacterium diphtheriae*, *Listeria monocytogenes*, *Erysipelothrix rhusiopathiae*, most clostridia (eg, *Cl. perfringens*, *Cl. tetani*), and *Eubacterium*.

Penicillin G is highly active against susceptible gram-negative cocci, including *Neisseria meningitidis* and *N. gonorrhoeae*. Low-level penicillin resistance, presumably due to altered PBPs, has been reported in meningococcal isolates from Spain (Mendelman et al, 1988), but the clinical significance of this observation is unclear, and most meningococci remain highly susceptible to this drug. Penicillin-resistant *N. gonorrhoeae* strains, especially penicillinase-producing *N. gonorrhoeae* (PPNG), have become widespread in the United States. *Veillonella,* anaerobic gram-negative cocci, are susceptible to penicillin G.

Susceptible gram-negative aerobic bacilli include *Streptobacillus moniliformis*, *Pasteurella multocida*, *Leptotrichia buccalis*, *Capnocytophaga* species, and *Spirillum minor*. Although many strains of *Haemophilus influenzae* are susceptible in vitro, β-lactamase-producing *H. influenzae* are resistant. Among gram-negative anaerobic bacilli, most *Fusobacterium* and many oropharyngeal strains of *Bacteroides* are susceptible. However, some strains of *B. melaninogenicus* and *Fusobacterium nucleatum* are resistant. The *B. fragilis* group are usually resistant. Most other gram-negative bacilli are resistant to penicillin G, including important clinical pathogens, such as the Enterobacteriaceae and *Pseudomonas aeruginosa*.

Actinomyces israelii is susceptible to penicillin G, but *Nocardia* species are resistant. Spirochetes, including *Treponema pallidum*, *T. pertenue*, *Leptospira*, and *Borrelia burgdorferi*, the causative organism of Lyme disease, are susceptible. Mycobacteria, mycoplasma, chlamydia, rickettsia, fungi, amebae, plasmodia, and viruses are resistant to all penicillins.

The in vitro activity of penicillin V (phenoxymethyl penicillin) [Ledercillin VK, PenVee K, V-Cillin K, Veetids] against most gram-positive bacteria is comparable to that of penicillin G. However, this derivative is less active than penicillin G against gram-negative bacteria, particularly *Neisseria* and *Haemophilus*.

For additional discussion, see Parry, 1987; Neu, 1990.

PENICILLINASE-RESISTANT PENICILLINS. The penicillinase-resistant penicillins (methicillin [Staphcillin], nafcillin [Nafcil, Unipen]) and the isoxazolyl derivatives, oxacillin [Bactocill, Prostaphlin], cloxacillin [Cloxapen, Tegopen], and dicloxacillin [Dycill, Dynapen, Pathocil]), are active against staphylococci, including β-lactamase-producing strains, and most pneumococci and streptococci, but they are less potent than penicillin G. Enterococci (eg, *E. faecalis*) are resistant.

Although some gram-positive bacilli (eg, *Clostridium perfringens*, *Corynebacterium diphtheriae*, *Listeria monocytogenes*) are susceptible in vitro, antistaphylococcal penicillins are not used clinically for infections caused by these organisms. Gram-negative bacteria generally are resistant.

AMINOPENICILLINS. Another group of semisynthetic penicillins, the aminopenicillins, include ampicillin [Omnipen, Polycillin, Principen], amoxicillin [Amoxil, Larotid, Polymox, Trimox], bacampicillin [Spectrobid], and cyclacillin. With few exceptions, the antibacterial spectra of the aminopenicillins are comparable. The in vitro potencies of amoxicillin and ampicillin, which can be administered as the parent drug or generated from the hydrolysis of the prodrug bacampicillin, are similar. Cyclacillin is less active than the others on a weight basis.

The gram-positive antibacterial spectrum of the aminopenicillins is similar to that of penicillin G, but these drugs are slightly more active against *Enterococcus faecalis* and *Listeria monocytogenes*. Because the aminopenicillins are susceptible to β-lactamases, most staphylococci are resistant. The gram-negative cocci, *Neisseria meningitidis* and *N. gonorrhoeae* (except PPNG and chromosomally mediated resistant *Neisseria gonorrhoeae* [CMRNG]), are susceptible to the aminopenicillins.

Most strains of *Haemophilus influenzae* are susceptible, but resistant β-lactamase-producing strains are prevalent in many areas. In contrast to penicillin G, the aminopenicillins are active against several aerobic gram-negative enteric bacilli, including strains of *Escherichia coli*, *Proteus mirabilis*, *Salmonella*, and *Shigella*. However, resistant β-lactamase-producing strains of these organisms are prevalent in some areas (see also the Uses section). Other Enterobacteriaceae (eg, *Klebsiella*, *Enterobacter*, *Serratia*, indole-positive *Proteus*, *Providencia*), *Pseudomonas aeruginosa*, and most *Acinetobacter* are resistant to the aminopenicillins. Among gram-negative anaerobic bacteria, *Fusobacterium* and oropharyngeal strains of *Bacteroides* are usually susceptible, but the *B. fragilis* group are resistant. Ampicillin is active in vitro against *Gardnerella* (*Haemophilus*) *vaginalis* and *Eikenella corrodens*.

For additional discussion, see Neu, 1990.

ANTIPSEUDOMONAL PENICILLINS. The antipseudomonal penicillins are semisynthetic derivatives that include the carboxypenicillins, carbenicillin [Geopen] (no longer marketed in the United States), carbenicillin indanyl [Geocillin], an ester of carbenicillin for oral administration, and ticarcillin [Ticar]; as well as the ureidopenicillins, azlocillin [Azlin] (no longer marketed in the United States), mezlocillin [Mezlin], and piperacillin [Pipracil]. Many infectious disease experts classify ureidopenicillins separately as fourth generation or extended spectrum penicillins. Like the aminopenicillins, antipseudomonal penicillins are susceptible to destruction by various β-lactamases that are produced by gram-positive and gram-negative bacteria.

Antipseudomonal penicillins have a broader spectrum of activity against gram-negative bacilli than ampicillin. Nonβ-lactamase-producing strains of *Haemophilus influenzae* are susceptible to these drugs. Among the Enterobacteriaceae, many strains of *Escherichia coli*, *Proteus mirabilis*, *Salmonella*, *Shigella*, *Enterobacter*, *Citrobacter*, and indole-positive *Proteus* (*Providencia rettgeri*, *Morganella morganii*, *Proteus vulgaris*) are susceptible to all of these analogues. Generally, mezlocillin and piperacillin are slightly more potent than ticarcillin and carbenicillin for most of these organisms. Furthermore, mezlocillin and piperacillin are active against some *Klebsiella* and *Serratia* strains. Most *Serratia*, essentially all *Klebsiella,* and *Xanthomonas maltophilia* are resistant to carbenicillin and ticarcillin. The number of strains of gram-negative bacilli that are resistant to the antipseudomonal penicillins is quite large, and the emergence of resistant β-lactamase-producing strains is relatively common.

The antipseudomonal penicillins are active against many strains of *Pseudomonas aeruginosa*, which accounts for their major clinical advantage over earlier penicillins (eg, ampicillin, penicillin G). In vitro, the order of decreasing potency (based on minimal inhibitory concentrations) for the various antipseudomonal penicillins against *P. aeruginosa* is piperacillin >mezlocillin = ticarcillin >carbenicillin. However, there appears to be a greater inoculum effect with the newer ureidopenicillins than with the carboxypenicillins. Whether these differences in vitro are of clinical significance is unresolved. Many strains of *Acinetobacter* also are susceptible to the antipseudomonal penicillins.

Among gram-negative anaerobic bacteria, *Fusobacterium* and *Bacteroides*, including many strains of *B. fragilis*, are susceptible.

Mezlocillin and piperacillin are comparable to ampicillin in activity against gram-positive bacteria and gram-negative cocci. Ticarcillin generally is less potent against these organisms and has poor activity against enterococci (eg, *E. faecalis*). β-lactamase-producing strains of staphylococci are resistant to all of the antipseudomonal penicillins.

For additional discussion, see Eliopoulos and Moellering, 1982; Neu, 1982 B, 1983, 1990; Drusano et al, 1984; Parry and Pancoast, 1984; Norris, 1985; and Parry, 1987.

Resistance

Mechanisms by which bacteria resist penicillin activity include: (1) drug inactivation by bacterial β-lactamases; (2) decreased permeability of the bacterial cell to the penicillin, which prevents the antibiotic from reaching the appropriate binding proteins; (3) alterations in PBPs that reduce binding affinity to the penicillin; and (4) tolerance. Clinically, the most important mechanism of acquired resistance is the production of inactivating enzymes (ie, β-lactamases) that cleave the β-lactam ring of the penicillin nucleus, resulting in the formation of inactive penicilloic acid derivatives (see Figure).

Staphylococcal β-lactamases are encoded by plasmids that can be transferred from one bacterium to another by transduction. These enzymes can be induced and are secreted extracellularly. They are considered to be true penicillinases because they inactivate penicillin molecules but not cephalosporins. Methicillin, nafcillin, and the isoxazolyl derivatives (oxacillin, cloxacillin, and dicloxacillin) are resistant to staphylococcal penicillinases. However, methicillin-resistant staphylococci (MRSA) are now frequently encountered in intravenous drug abusers who have community-acquired endocarditis and in acute and long-term care facilities, where they pose significant problems for nosocomial infection control (Boyce, 1990; Kauffman et al, 1990). The mechanism of resistance among MRSA is related to failure of penicillins to bind PBPs (see below).

Genetic information for the various β-lactamases produced by gram-negative bacteria can be encoded in chromosomes or plasmids. These enzymes may be either constitutive or inducible and are located in the periplasmic space between the inner and outer membranes of the bacterial cell. Some β-lactamases of gram-negative bacteria are specific for either penicillins or cephalosporins, but others can hydrolyze both types of these drugs. Differences in their stability to β-lactamases account for some of the differences in the in vitro activities of the various penicillins against some gram-negative bacteria.

The cell walls of gram-negative bacteria are covered by a lipopolysaccharide-containing outer membrane. Some penicillins (eg, the penicillinase-resistant penicillins) are unable to penetrate the porin protein channels of this outer membrane. Therefore, gram-negative bacteria are naturally resistant to these agents. In addition, some gram-negative bacteria, including *Neisseria gonorrhoeae*, *Serratia*, *Enterobacter*, and *Pseudomonas*, develop resistance to ampicillin and/or antipseudomonal penicillins due to changes in their cell envelopes that result in decreased permeability to the antibiotic.

Intrinsic resistance due to altered PBPs is another mechanism of increasing clinical importance for some bacterial pathogens, including methicillin-resistant *Staphylococcus aureus* and *S. epidermidis*, CMRNG, and highly resistant South African strains of *Streptococcus pneumoniae*. This mechanism of resistance also has been demonstrated in *Enterococcus faecalis* and *Haemophilus influenzae.* Intrinsic resistance may result from reduced binding affinities of essential PBP for penicillins, the appearance of a new low affinity PBP that binds poorly to antibiotic, or a combination of both (eg, *S. pneumoniae)* (see Tomasz, 1986).

Tolerance to penicillins has been reported primarily in gram-positive bacteria, such as viridans streptococci (eg, *S. sanguis*), *S. pneumoniae*, *E. faecalis, S. aureus,* and *Listeria*. Penicillin-tolerant strains are resistant to the lethal action of a normally bactericidal penicillin. In vitro, tolerance is suggested initially by large differences between the minimal inhibitory concentration (MIC), which is usually within the normal range, and the minimal bactericidal concentration (MBC), which is much higher. Confirmation of tolerance requires follow-up time-kill studies and more detailed microbiologic studies using genetically and physiologically homogeneous cultures of the isolate. The mechanistic basis of tolerance is not completely understood. The murein hydrolase (autolytic enzyme) of many of these strains appears to be suppressed, thus preventing their lysis, but other mechanisms may be involved as well (see Handwerger and Tomasz, 1985).

For additional discussion, see Neu, 1990.

Uses and Drug Selection

This section describes general concepts applicable to selection of a particular penicillin for clinical use. In addition, information on specific infections for which penicillins are the preferred (or alternative) drugs is summarized according to site of infection. Except in a few instances, alternatives to the penicillins are not discussed in this section. Treatment guidelines outlining therapeutic alternatives to the penicillins can be found in the chapters in the section, Anti-Infective Therapy, or by consulting the index entry on Antimicrobial Drugs or those for specific infections.

Penicillins are bactericidal antibiotics with a high therapeutic to toxic ratio; they are frequently drugs of choice for infections caused by susceptible organisms in nonallergic patients.

NATURAL PENICILLINS. Penicillin G is preferred for infections caused by most frequently encountered gram-positive bacteria (except staphylococci and, in some situations, enterococci) and susceptible gram-negative cocci. It also is the drug of choice for infections caused by certain gram-negative bacilli (eg, *Spirillum minus, Streptobacillus moniliformis, Leptotrichia buccalis*), actinomycetes, and spirochetes.

Procaine penicillin G and benzathine penicillin G are repository forms that provide tissue depots from which drug is absorbed over hours (procaine penicillin G) or days (benzathine penicillin G). When administered intramuscularly, these preparations are indicated for certain infections (eg, early syphilis, late latent syphilis, endocarditis due to penicillin-susceptible streptococci) when prolonged therapeutic blood levels are needed and the frequent dosing requirements of aqueous penicillin G (due to its short half-life) are undesirable. However, when high, sustained concentrations of antibiotic are required, parenteral aqueous penicillin G should be used.

Penicillin V is less labile to gastric acid than penicillin G, and thus blood levels are higher with penicillin V than with penicillin G when equivalent oral doses are given. Furthermore, the absorption of this phenoxymethyl derivative is not affected by the presence of food in the gastrointestinal tract. Thus, penicillin V is frequently preferred to penicillin G when oral administration is indicated, although larger oral doses of buffered penicillin G may be equally effective. (See also the section on Pharmacokinetics.)

PENICILLINASE-RESISTANT PENICILLINS. The penicillinase-resistant penicillins offer no therapeutic advantages over penicillin G except in staphylococcal infections, in which the majority of strains are now resistant to penicillin G. Thus, these agents are drugs of choice only for staphylococcal infections. The penicillinase-resistant penicillins differ mainly in their pharmacologic properties (see the section on Pharmacokinetics). Parenteral nafcillin, oxacillin, and methicillin are alternative choices for serious staphylococcal infections. In adults and children, use of methicillin frequently has been associated with the development of interstitial nephritis, and the other agents are often preferred. Oral dicloxacillin, cloxacillin, and, less frequently, oxacillin are alternative choices for mild to moderate infections. When methicillin-resistant strains of *Staphylococcus aureus* or *S. epidermidis* are known or suspected to be present, vancomycin is the drug of choice (see also index entry Vancomycin).

AMINOPENICILLINS. These agents usually are drugs of choice for infections caused by enterococci (penicillin G often is preferred in enterococcal endocarditis, however) and nonpenicillinase producing strains of *Haemophilus influenzae* and Enterobacteriaceae, particularly *Proteus mirabilis* and community-acquired *Escherichia coli.* Ampicillin, the prototype of this group, is often the agent of choice against susceptible organisms because it is less expensive than the other aminopenicillins and is the only agent of this class available for parenteral administration in the United States. Amoxicillin is preferred for oral use, however, because it is absorbed more rapidly and completely and equivalent doses produce higher serum levels than ampicillin. Furthermore, absorption of amoxicillin is not affected by the presence of food, and diarrhea appears to occur less often, particularly in young children. Higher serum levels with oral administration also may be achieved by using bacampicillin, a proampicillin. Generally, bacampicillin and cyclacillin do not offer significant clinical advantages over amoxicillin, and they are more expensive. (See also the section on Pharmacokinetics.)

ANTIPSEUDOMONAL PENICILLINS. Despite their broad antibacterial spectra, the only preferred use for parenteral antipseudomonal penicillins (ticarcillin, mezlocillin, piperacillin) is treatment of infections caused by or suspected of being caused by *Pseudomonas aeruginosa* or susceptible aerobic gram-negative bacilli that frequently are resistant to other penicillins and cephalosporins. Systemic pseudomonal infections are usually serious and difficult to eradicate. They frequently are of nosocomial origin and thus commonly affect compromised hosts (eg, febrile, neutropenic cancer patients; burn patients; cystic fibrosis patients). A serious problem with these infections is the emergence of resistant bacterial strains, particularly when they are treated with an antipseudomonal penicillin alone. Thus, antipseudomonal penicillins are virtually always given with an aminoglycoside (gentamicin [Garamycin], tobramycin [Nebcin], netilmicin [Netromycin]) for the treatment of these systemic infections. Such combinations often have demonstrated antibacterial synergism against *P. aeruginosa.* Also, the rate of emergence of resistant organisms may be decreased with combination therapy, but this has not been documented clinically. In general, however, if narrower spectrum, less expensive antimicrobials (eg, penicillin G, ampicillin) are appropriate in a given clinical situation, they should be substituted for the antipseudomonal penicillins.

Most physicians preferred ticarcillin over parenteral carbenicillin for infections caused by *P. aeruginosa* because it could be given in lower dosages, resulting in decreased sodium load and other adverse effects (eg, hypokalemia, abnormal coagulation); therefore, the parenteral form of carbenicillin is no longer marketed in the United States. The ureidopenicillins, piperacillin and mezlocillin, have potential clinical advantages over ticarcillin in institutions where ticarcillin-resistant, but ureidopenicillin-susceptible, strains of *P. aeruginosa* (or other gram-negative bacilli) are a problem or when their broader antimicrobial spectrum is desirable. Piperacillin and mezlocillin contain less sodium per gram than ticarcillin, which is an advantage in patients who must severely restrict sodium intake, and their effect on platelet aggregation may be less pronounced. Differences in drug costs may be an important factor in selecting an antipseudomonal penicillin for general use in a given hospital.

Carbenicillin indanyl sodium is used only orally for urinary tract infections, including chronic bacterial prostatitis. The blood levels obtained with this analogue are not high enough to be effective systemically. This drug has largely been replaced by other orally administered agents, such as trimethoprim/sulfamethoxazole or the fluoroquinolones.

For additional information on penicillin uses, see Parry, 1987; *Med Lett Drugs Ther*, 1990; Neu, 1990; Reese and Betts, 1991; Wright and Wilkowske, 1991.

SPECIFIC INFECTIONS. Bacteremia: Parenterally administered penicillins frequently are preferred to treat sepsis caused by susceptible known pathogens (eg, penicillin G for *Streptococcus pneumoniae*; nafcillin, oxacillin, or methicillin for *Staphylococcus aureus*). They also may be used in combination regimens for empiric therapy before the etiologic agent has been identified. For example, a penicillinase-resistant penicillin plus an aminoglycoside sometimes is recommended for sepsis of unknown etiology in nonimmunocompromised adults and older children. Ampicillin plus chloramphenicol, a penicillinase-resistant penicillin (nafcillin or oxacillin) plus chloramphenicol, or a penicillinase-resistant penicillin plus a third-generation cephalosporin (ceftriaxone, cefotaxime, ceftizoxime) is a regimen of choice in immunocompetent infants and children (excluding newborns). Ampicillin plus an aminoglycoside or ampicillin plus cefotaxime may be used for presumptive therapy in nonimmunocompromised neonates. An antipseudomonal penicillin plus either an aminoglycoside or ceftazidime, with or without vancomycin in either regimen, may be used empirically in febrile, neutropenic patients who require broad-spectrum, rapidly bactericidal therapy that is effective against *P. aeruginosa* and gram-positive species (Hughes et al, 1990). For detailed guidelines, see index entry Bacteremias and Sepsis. (See also Bodey, 1989.)

Bone and Joint: *Staphylococcus aureus* and, to a lesser extent, streptococci (eg, *S. pyogenes, S. pneumoniae*) are the most common causes of septic arthritis in adults over 40 years and children under 15 years. A parenteral penicillinase-resistant penicillin (eg, nafcillin, oxacillin) is the drug of choice when the Gram stain reveals that a gram-positive coccus is the causative organism; it also should be given when no organism is seen on Gram stain. *Haemophilus influenzae* type b is an important pathogen for this disease in children between the ages of 2 months and 5 years. In these patients, a combination of parenteral ampicillin plus chloramphenicol may be used initially, especially if β-lactamase producing *H. influenzae* b strains are prevalent or the susceptibility of the isolate to antimicrobial drugs is unknown. If the infecting pathogen proves to be susceptible to ampicillin, this drug may be continued alone. However, many infectious disease experts now prefer a third-generation cephalosporin (eg, cefotaxime, ceftriaxone) for this indication to avoid the toxicity and other problems associated with use of chloramphenicol (eg, the need to monitor serum concentrations). In patients between the ages of 15 and 40, *Neisseria gonorrhoeae* is the most likely cause of septic arthritis. For the role of penicillins in treatment, see also index entry Arthritis, Septic.

In children older than 3 months and adults, the most likely causative organism of acute hematogenous osteomyelitis is *S. aureus,* and a parenteral penicillinase-resistant penicillin (oxacillin or nafcillin) is the initial therapy of choice. Intravenous penicillin G may be substituted for the antistaphylococcal penicillin if the pathogen is proven to be susceptible to this drug. Aerobic gram-negative bacilli also may cause this infection in neonates and young infants, and a penicillinase-resistant penicillin (oxacillin) in combination with either an aminoglycoside or a third-generation cephalosporin (cefotaxime, ceftazidime) is indicated for presumptive therapy.

Cardiovascular: Infective endocarditis is most commonly caused by gram-positive cocci (approximately 90% of all cases), including viridans streptococci (40%); nonhemolytic, microaerophilic, anaerobic, or nonenterococcal group D streptococci (together 20%); enterococci (group D streptococci, 10%); and coagulase-positive (*S. aureus*) and coagulase-negative (*S. epidermidis*) staphylococci (together 20%). The remaining 10% of bacterial endocardial infections may be caused by any of a diverse group of organisms, including *Haemophilus* or other fastidious gram-negative organisms, species of *Pseudomonas*, aerobic gram-negative bacilli, pneumococci, and gonococci. Because gram-positive cocci predominate in causing bacterial endocarditis, presumptive therapy is usually directed against these organisms, although clinical presentation can be valuable in identifying an infecting pathogen. For more information, see index entry Endocarditis, Treatment.

In patients who are not hypersensitive to β-lactam drugs, penicillin G alone is the drug of choice for endocarditis caused by viridans group streptococci or *S. bovis* that is highly susceptible (MIC <0.1 mcg/ml) to this agent. To produce a synergistic effect, streptomycin or gentamicin can be added to this regimen for selected patients (eg, those at low risk for aminoglycoside toxicity) during the first two weeks of therapy; however, the superiority of this combination to penicillin alone has not been established. Vancomycin should be used in penicillin-allergic patients with infection caused by streptococci; if the penicillin allergy is not of the immediate anaphylactic type, cephalothin or cefazolin may be given with streptomycin or gentamicin added as described above (Bisno et al, 1989).

Penicillin-tolerant patients with endocarditis caused by viridans streptococci or *S. bovis* that are relatively resistant to penicillin (MIC >0.1 and <0.5 mcg/ml) should be treated with penicillin G plus streptomycin or gentamicin. Vancomycin is the drug of choice for use against these organisms in patients with immediate-type hypersensitivity to penicillin; those who have non-IgE mediated allergy to penicillin may be cautiously treated with cephalothin or cefazolin, plus an aminoglycoside for the first two weeks (Bisno et al, 1989).

In patients who are not hypersensitive to penicillin, endocarditis caused by enterococci or viridans streptococci with a penicillin MIC >0.5 mcg/ml is optimally treated with penicillin G or ampicillin plus streptomycin or gentamicin. Vancomycin plus streptomycin or gentamicin is the therapy of choice for those who are truly hypersensitive to penicillin. Enterococci that produce β-lactamases have been recognized in patients with endocarditis; these infections should be treated with an aminoglycoside plus either vancomycin or, if tolerated, ampicillin/sodium sulbactam (Bisno et al, 1989).

Nafcillin or oxacillin with or without gentamicin is the regimen of choice for staphylococcal endocarditis caused by methicillin-sensitive strains in penicillin-tolerant patients who do not have intracardiac prosthetic materials in place; patients with these conditions who are allergic to penicillin but do not have immediate-type hypersensitivity may receive a cephalosporin (cephalothin or cefazolin); the addition of gentamicin is optional. Endocarditis due to MRSA in patients without prosthetic material is treated with vancomycin alone. In those who have a prosthetic valve or other prosthetic material, endocarditis caused by MRSA is treated with a combination of vancomycin, rifampin (coagulase-negative isolates only), and gentamicin for the first two weeks (Bisno et al, 1989). Nafcillin or oxacillin plus rifampin (coagulase-negative staphylococci only) plus gentamicin as indicated above are used to treat endocarditis caused by methicillin-susceptible staphylococci in patients who can tolerate penicillins. A first-generation cephalosporin or vancomycin is used in this regimen for penicillin-allergic patients (Bisno et al, 1989); however, cephalosporins should be avoided in patients with immediate-type penicillin hypersensitivity.

Rare cases of endocarditis caused by *P. aeruginosa* (eg, in intravenous drug abusers) may be treated with an antipseudomonal penicillin (ticarcillin) plus an aminoglycoside, although an optimum regimen has not been determined; surgery may be required for cure (see Mandell et al, 1992, for empiric treatment guidelines; see also Brandriss and Lambert, 1991).

Central Nervous System: Antimicrobial therapy of bacterial meningitis may be given presumptively or may be directed toward specific pathogens. Whereas drug selection for presumptive treatment is generally age-specific and should be effective against the most common etiologic organisms for each age group, specific therapy may be tailored to the susceptibility of a known pathogen. The primary role of the penicillins in the treatment of meningitis has decreased in some cases because of the increased resistance of a number of pathogens and the development of newer agents designed to overcome these problems; however, penicillins still have a vital role in this disease and remain drugs of choice for eradicating several pathogens.

In neonates, causative organisms include *Streptococcus agalactiae* (group B) and other streptococci, *E. coli* and other coliforms, and *Listeria monocytogenes*. Intravenous ampicillin plus an aminoglycoside or ampicillin plus cefotaxime are preferred for empiric therapy in this age group; ceftriaxone is not recommended for use in neonates because it displaces bilirubin from albumin binding sites and may cause biliary sludging. For infants aged 1 to 3 months, causative organisms in addition to those listed for neonates include *H. influenzae* type b, *N. meningitidis*, and *S. pneumoniae*; ampicillin plus either cefotaxime or ceftriaxone is preferred for empiric treatment. In infants and children 3 months to 10 years, the pathogen usually is *H. influenzae* type b, *N. meningitidis*, or *S. pneumoniae*; a third-generation cephalosporin (cefotaxime or ceftriaxone) is currently the drug of choice for empiric therapy. Although ampicillin plus chloramphenicol is equally efficacious and is an excellent alternative to the broad-spectrum cephalosporins in this age group, the potential toxicity and hence the need to monitor serum concentrations of chloramphenicol have diminished enthusiasm for this combination among infectious disease specialists. For empiric treatment of meningitis in children older than 10 years and adults up to 50 years, therapy should be effective against *S. pneumoniae* and *N. meningitidis*; a broad-spectrum cephalosporin (cefotaxime or ceftriaxone) or, alternatively, intravenous penicillin G, are recommended. In adults >50 years, gram-negative aerobic bacilli, including *P. aeruginosa*, may be the causative pathogens; a broad-spectrum cephalosporin that is effective against these species (ceftazidime for *P. aeruginosa*; cefotaxime, ceftriaxone, or ceftizoxime for other gram-negative enteric bacilli) with or without an aminoglycoside is preferred for these infections. An antipseudomonal penicillin (piperacillin, ticarcillin, mezlocillin) plus an aminoglycoside is an alternative regimen for *P. aeruginosa* meningitis, and ampicillin plus an aminoglycoside is an alternative for infections presumably caused by *E. coli* or other gram-negative aerobic bacilli in adults.

When a pathogen has been identified, antimicrobial regimens may be adjusted according to the results of susceptibility assays. Intravenous penicillin G or ampicillin is preferred for meningitis caused by susceptible isolates of *S. pneumoniae* or *N. meningitidis*. However, strains of *S. pneumoniae* that are relatively (MIC 0.1 to 1.0 mcg/ml) to highly (MIC ≥2.0 mcg/ml) resistant to penicillins may be encountered; for the former, a third-generation cephalosporin should be substituted for penicillin G or ampicillin and, for the latter, vancomycin is the drug of choice. If a penicillin-resistant pneumococcal infection does not respond quickly to a third-generation cephalosporin, vancomycin or possibly chloramphenicol should be substituted for the latter. Similarly, although their clinical significance is unknown, relatively penicillin-resistant isolates of meningococci with altered PBPs and β-lactamase-producing strains that are absolutely resistant to penicillin have been recognized; vancomycin is indicated for these cases. Intravenous penicillin G (or ampicillin) with or without an aminoglycoside is preferred for treatment of group B streptococcal (*S. agalactiae*) meningitis; alternatives to this regimen have not been established.

Infections due to an isolate of *H. influenzae* type b that produces β-lactamase may be treated with ceftriaxone or cefotaxime (preferred) or ampicillin plus chloramphenicol. However, if the *H. influenzae* isolate is susceptible to ampicillin, this drug may be used alone.

A third-generation cephalosporin (cefotaxime, ceftriaxone, ceftizoxime) is preferred for meningitis caused by *E. coli* or other gram-negative aerobes; intravenous ampicillin with or without an aminoglycoside is a good alternative for these infections. Either ceftazidime or an antipseudomonal penicillin (piperacillin, mezlocillin, ticarcillin) plus an aminoglycoside are preferred for meningitis caused by *P. aeruginosa*.

Intravenous ampicillin with or without an aminoglycoside is preferred for meningeal infections caused by *L. monocytogenes*. Aqueous penicillin G with or without an aminoglycoside is an alternative regimen.

Intravenous penicillin G may be used for anaerobic infections of the central nervous system (eg, brain abscess) if the causative organism is proven to be susceptible. Penicillin G plus metronidazole or chloramphenicol is preferred for presumptive therapy of anaerobic CNS infections pending results of culture because of the possible involvement of penicillin-resistant *B. fragilis*.

Intravenously administered aqueous crystalline penicillin G can be used for gonococcal meningitis caused by susceptible strains of *Neisseria gonorrhoeae*.

For additional information, see American Academy of Pediatrics Committee on Infectious Diseases, 1988; Sáez-Llorens and McCracken, 1990; Tunkel et al, 1990; Wispelwey et al, 1990; see also index entry Meningitis.

Ear: The most common causative organisms of acute otitis media are *Streptococcus pneumoniae* and *Haemophilus influenzae* (usually nontypable strains); *Moraxella (Branhamella) catarrhalis* also are frequent pathogens in some geographic areas (Thoene and Johnson, 1991). Amoxicillin is one of several drugs of choice for initial treatment of this infection. However, the incidence of amoxicillin-resistant *H. influenzae* and *M. catarrhalis* is increasing. Amoxicillin/potassium clavulanate [Augmentin] is an effective alternative for these resistant strains.

Gastrointestinal Tract: Ampicillin in combination with an aminoglycoside is a preferred regimen for empiric therapy of biliary tract infections. Causative organisms of these infections include *Escherichia coli*, other Enterobacteriaceae, and enterococci.

Ampicillin (but not amoxicillin) may be effective in gastroenteritis caused by susceptible *Shigella* strains. However, the number of ampicillin-resistant shigellae is considerable and other drugs may be required for shigellosis caused by resistant strains. No antibiotics are recommended for uncomplicated gastroenteritis due to *Salmonella* in the immunocompetent host. However, ampicillin and amoxicillin are alternatives to chloramphenicol or quinolones for systemic infections (eg, bacteremia, enteric fever syndrome including typhoid fever) caused by *Salmonella* species, including *S. typhi*; these agents often are effective against chloramphenicol-resistant strains. Ampicillin (or amoxicillin) plus probenecid has eliminated the typhoid carrier state in patients without gallstones, although a quinolone is preferred.

Peritonitis following bowel perforation is usually caused by a mixture of pathogens, including aerobic gram-negative bacilli; anaerobic bacteria, particularly the *Bacteroides fragilis* group; and enterococci. The antipseudomonal penicillins (eg, piperacillin, mezlocillin) in combination with an aminoglycoside (to eradicate aerobic gram-negative bacilli) have been effective because these penicillins have significant activity against the *B. fragilis* group. However, clindamycin and metronidazole are current drugs of choice for the *B. fragilis* group and are used with an aminoglycoside to treat these mixed infections; penicillin G or ampicillin also may be added to cover enterococci. Finally, ticarcillin/potassium clavulanate [Timentin] and ampicillin/sulbactam [Unasyn] (ie, penicillins in combination with β-lactamase inhibitors) also are useful for this indication.

Reproductive Tract, Female: Currently, antimicrobial drugs other than penicillins are preferred for acute pelvic inflammatory disease. However, single-dose ampicillin (or amoxicillin) or penicillin G procaine may be used in ambulatory patients (milder cases) when penicillin-susceptible *N. gonorrhoeae* is the causative organism. Follow-up therapy with oral doxycycline [Vibramycin] frequently is recommended to cover potential coexisting *C. trachomatis* infection adequately. (See index entry Pelvic Inflammatory Disease for a detailed discussion.)

For the role of penicillins in the treatment of cervicitis, see the index entry Cervicitis, Mucopurulent.

Reproductive Tract, Male: Epididymo-orchitis caused by *Neisseria gonorrhoeae* and/or *Chlamydia trachomatis* in males under 35 years frequently is sexually transmitted. Ampicillin (or amoxicillin) or penicillin G procaine is effective in acute epididymo-orchitis due to susceptible *N. gonorrhoeae*, but ceftriaxone is the current drug of choice for empiric therapy. Because of the increasing frequency of *C. trachomatis* as the causative organism of epididymo-orchitis, follow-up therapy with doxycycline or tetracycline is recommended by the Centers for Disease Control (see index entry Sexually Transmitted Diseases for a detailed discussion).

Respiratory Tract, Lower: The most common causative bacterial organism of community-acquired, acute pneumonia in a normal host is *Streptococcus pneumoniae*. Intravenous penicillin G is the drug of choice for this infection, and procaine penicillin G or penicillin V may be adequate in uncomplicated cases caused by susceptible strains.

In infants and young children, *Haemophilus influenzae* may be the causative organism of pneumonia. Parenteral ampicillin plus chloramphenicol (initially) is a regimen of choice for susceptible organisms. Amoxicillin/potassium clavulanate and ampicillin/sulbactam [Unasyn] should be effective against penicillin-resistant *H. influenzae*.

Penicillin G has been traditionally preferred for bronchopulmonary infections caused by susceptible anaerobic bacteria (eg, aspiration pneumonia). The major penicillin G-resistant anaerobic pathogen, *Bacteroides fragilis*, is not a frequent cause of infections above the diaphragm. However, the prevalence of penicillin G-resistant (β-lactamase-producing) strains of *B. melaninogenicus*, a common anaerobic pathogen in the respiratory tract, is increasing. In these geographic areas, clindamycin is preferred by many authorities for aspiration pneumonia and lung abscess involving anaerobic bacteria (Gudiol et al, 1990). Penicillin G plus metronidazole or ampicillin/sulbactam are alternative regimens.

Nosocomial pneumonias are frequently caused by gram-negative bacilli (eg, *K. pneumoniae*). When *Pseudomonas aeruginosa* is the infectious agent, an antipseudomonal penicillin (piperacillin, ticarcillin, mezlocillin) in combination with an aminoglycoside is a recommended regimen. When methicillin-sensitive *Staphylococcus aureus* is the documented cause of pneumonia, a penicillinase-resistant penicillin (nafcillin or oxacillin) frequently is preferred.

Penicillins are not active against pneumonia caused by *Mycoplasma pneumoniae, Chlamydia,* or *Legionella pneumophila*. Erythromycin (or tetracycline [except for *Legionella*]) is preferred for these infections.

Respiratory Tract, Upper: Acute sinusitis is caused by the same organisms that cause acute otitis media. Although amoxicillin is a drug of choice for empiric therapy, because penicillin-resistant strains of *H. influenzae* and *M. catarrhalis* may be highly prevalent (>40% in some areas), alternative therapy that is effective against such isolates should be considered.

Oral penicillin V (ten-day course of therapy) or intramuscular benzathine penicillin G (single injection) is the preferred drug for pharyngitis due to *Streptococcus pyogenes* (group A, β hemolytic streptococci [GABHS]). However, because the incidence of acute rheumatic fever and other invasive disease caused by GABHS varies cyclically across the United States (Bisno, 1991), the need for effective alternative treatments for GABHS pharyngitis (and other invasive infections caused by GABHS) has not declined. This pattern of disease resurgence may be a consequence of synergistic infections in which colonizing organisms that produce β-lactamase (eg, *S. aureus, H. influenzae, M. catarrhalis*) protect the GABHS from penicillins that are susceptible to enzymatic inactivation in a process termed copathogenicity (Pichichero, 1990; Pichichero and Margolis, 1991). Although this concept is controversial, this possibility should be suspected in patients with GABHS pharyngitis who do not respond readily to penicillins, and alternative therapy should be considered.

Penicillin G is a drug of choice for Vincent's gingivitis and frequently is preferred for periodontal infections caused by anaerobic bacteria in the oral cavity. Penicillin V may be used in mild infections.

Penicillin G procaine is an alternative to ceftriaxone for gonococcal pharyngitis caused by susceptible strains of *Neisseria gonorrhoeae*. Because resistant strains of this bacteria have become prevalent in recent years, ampicillin or amoxicillin are generally not adequate for this form of gonorrhea. For a detailed discussion of infection caused by penicillin-resistant *N. gonorrhoeae* (eg, PPNG), see index entry Gonococcal Infections.

Specific antitoxin plus antibiotic therapy with penicillin G (or erythromycin) is required to treat diphtheria caused by *Corynebacterium diphtheriae*. Penicillin G can be used to eliminate the carrier state, although many infectious disease experts prefer erythromycin.

Epiglottitis is a life-threatening infection caused by *Haemophilus influenzae* type b. Although either a third-generation cephalosporin (cefotaxime, ceftriaxone, ceftizoxime) or intravenous ampicillin plus chloramphenicol can be used for empiric treatment of this condition, most infectious disease specialists recommend the cephalosporin in this situation. If the pathogen subsequently proves susceptible to ampicillin, treatment may be continued with this drug alone. Maintaining an airway is of critical importance in acute epiglottitis.

Sexually Transmitted Diseases: Penicillin G and its repository forms are drugs of choice for all stages of syphilis in the nonallergic patient. In adults and children with all forms of uncomplicated gonococcal infection or sexual contacts, single-dose ceftriaxone has replaced the penicillins as the drug of choice. Ceftriaxone also is the preferred drug for other forms of gonorrhea (eg, gonococcal arthritis, endocarditis, meningitis, and ophthalmia in adults; all neonatal gonococcal infections). For detailed treatment guidelines, see index entry Sexually Transmitted Diseases.

Skin: Pyodermas caused by *Staphylococcus aureus* (eg, folliculitis, furuncles, carbuncles, bullous impetigo) or *Streptococcus pyogenes* (eg, erysipelas, ecthyma, nonbullous impetigo) frequently require systemic antibiotics. Penicillinase-resistant penicillins (cloxacillin or dicloxacillin) are drugs of choice for staphylococcal pyodermas; amoxicillin/potassium clavulanate is an alternative. Penicillin V is preferred for streptococcal pyodermas.

Amoxicillin/potassium clavulanate is a preferred therapy for infections associated with animal bites; penicillin V (or ampicillin) with or without either cloxacillin (or dicloxacillin) or an oral cephalosporin (cephalexin, cephradine, cefadroxil) are alternative regimens.

For the treatment of infections caused by human bites, oral amoxicillin/potassium clavulanate or intravenous ampicillin/sulbactam are preferred, depending on the severity of infection. Penicillin V (or ampicillin) plus either cloxacillin (or dicloxacillin) or an oral cephalosporin (see above) are alternative regimens for oral therapy; aqueous penicillin G plus nafcillin (or oxacillin) is an alternative parenteral treatment.

Intravenous penicillin G is a drug of choice for gas gangrene due to *Clostridium perfringens,* necrotizing fasciitis due to *S. pyogenes*, or streptococcal myositis. Surgical debridement is essential for these infections.

Infections following burns frequently are caused by gram-negative aerobic bacilli (including *Pseudomonas aeruginosa)* and *S. aureus*. A penicillinase-resistant penicillin (nafcillin or oxacillin) combined with an aminoglycoside is a preferred empiric therapy. Alternative penicillin-containing empiric regimens include either ticarcillin/potassium clavulanate or an antipseudomonal penicillin (piperacillin, mezlocillin, ticarcillin) in combination with an aminoglycoside. For topical antibacterial therapy for burn infections, see index entry Burns.

Urinary Tract: *Escherichia coli* causes more than 90% of initial community-acquired urinary tract infections. Other coliform organisms and enterococci cause these infections less frequently. In addition, *Staphylococcus saprophyticus* is responsible for some cases of acute bacterial cystitis, particularly in younger women.

Resistance to ampicillin or amoxicillin among community-acquired *E. coli* has become a problem in many geographic locations, however, and these drugs should not be used alone for mild (nonbacteremic) acute pyelonephritis in ambulatory patients. Although amoxicillin/potassium clavulanate may be useful in these patients, many authorities prefer an alternative (see index entry Urinary Tract Infections, Treatment). For more severe (inpatient) cases, parenteral ampicillin in combination with an aminoglycoside frequently is recommended until results of cultures and susceptibility tests are available.

Short-course (one to three days) antimicrobial therapy currently is preferred for initial attacks of acute bacterial cystitis in females who are not pregnant, have no renal parenchymal involvement or evidence of subclinical pyelonephritis, are treated soon after onset of symptoms, and are available for follow-up. A single 3-g oral dose of amoxicillin is an alternative to three days of oral trimethoprim/sulfamethoxazole (preferred) for this indication. For pyelonephritis, conventional therapy for 7 to 14 days is recommended. Drugs of choice include ampicillin and amoxicillin. Penicillins are not generally used for prophylaxis of recurrent urinary tract infections or empiric treatment of the acute urethral syndrome.

The causative organisms and treatment of acute prostatitis are similar to those for acute pyelonephritis. However, the aminopenicillins are not indicated for chronic bacterial prostatitis. Oral carbenicillin indanyl sodium may be useful. For additional information, see index entry Prostatitis, Treatment.

For the role of penicillins in the treatment of urethritis, see the chapter on Treatment of Sexually Transmitted Diseases.

Other Infections: The penicillins, particularly penicillin G, play a role in the treatment of certain infectious diseases (eg, Lyme disease, syphilis) that may involve more than one organ system. For treatment guidelines, see index entry Antimicrobial Drugs.

Prophylaxis: See the chapter Antimicrobial Chemoprophylaxis for Ambulatory Patients for guidelines for prophylaxis of rheumatic fever (see also Dajani et al, 1988) and bacterial endocarditis (see also Dajani et al, 1990) and for information on the use of penicillins for the prevention of pneumococcal infection in asplenic patients and those with recurrent otitis media.

For the role of penicillins in the prophylaxis of sexual contacts of syphilis or gonorrhea patients, see index entry Sexually Transmitted Diseases. For detailed discussion of the role of penicillins in surgery, see the chapter Antimicrobial Chemoprophylaxis for Surgical Patients.

Adverse Reactions and Precautions

HYPERSENSITIVITY REACTIONS. The most common adverse effects of the penicillins are hypersensitivity reactions that range in severity from rashes to immediate anaphylaxis. The overall chance of developing a hypersensitivity reaction per course of therapy is approximately 2%. Among the antimicrobials, the penicillins cause the largest number of allergic reactions and are the most common cause of anaphylaxis in the United States. This probably reflects the wide use of these agents as well as their potential for causing allergic sensitization.

Allergic reactions to penicillins can occur during a first course of treatment. However, it is more common for a patient to tolerate penicillins initially and develop an allergic reaction during a subsequent exposure. Nontherapeutic exposures to environmental (eg, food, milk) and occupational sources of penicillin also may sensitize a patient.

Although early reports suggested that allergic reactions to penicillins were more common in atopic patients, more recent studies have shown that these reactions occur no more often in atopic individuals than in the rest of the population. Hypersensitivity reactions to penicillins can occur after exposure by any route of administration: intradermal, parenteral, or oral. However, reactions are less likely when a penicillin is taken orally than when it is administered by the parenteral route. Regardless of the cause of the ostensible sensitization, recent data suggest that patients who report a history of penicillin allergy may not actually be allergic (Surtees et al, 1991). The existence of allergy can be confirmed if necessary. In individuals who report vague or minor prior reactions, negative skin tests to native drug provide sufficient evidence to ensure that an oral penicillin can be given safely (see the section on Skin Testing for Penicillin Hypersensitivity below).

Penicillins (and metabolites thereof) can be viewed as low-molecular-weight haptens that must covalently bind to carrier molecules (eg, host membrane and serum proteins) to be immunogenic. Most of a penicillin bound to protein (about 95%) is in the penicilloyl form, and this is called the major antigenic determinant. Other metabolites (eg, penicilloate, penilloate, penicilloyl-amine) and the native penicillin itself also may be bound to proteins (about 5%) and are collectively called minor antigenic determinants. The terms major and minor refer only to the quantity of hapten and not to their immunologic importance. Both the major and minor antigenic determinants can cause IgE-mediated hypersensitivity reactions. However, minor determinants are considered to be the cause of most systemic anaphylactic reactions. These reactions are the adverse effects most likely to be reported.

Allergic reactions to penicillins and other β-lactam antimicrobial agents can be characterized according to their latency and their mechanism (see Condemi, 1991; Shepherd, 1991).

In susceptible patients, anaphylaxis is the most important and dangerous of the *immediate responses*. Such responses are rare, occurring in only 0.01% to 0.05% of treatment courses. However, anaphylaxis may be fatal in approximately 10% of affected patients (Parry, 1987). It usually begins 2 to 30 minutes after exposure to antibiotic and is mediated by the interaction between protein-bound hapten (eg, penicillin metabolites) and IgE antibodies that are bound to the surface of tissue mast cells or blood basophils. This results in the release of vasoactive compounds (eg, histamine, leukotrienes) as well as the formation of other pharmacologic mediators outside the mast cell. Chemoattractants, which also are released from mast cells during the allergic reaction, induce the migration of other cell types (eg, neutrophils, eosinophils) to the vicinity and their subsequent release of other chemical mediators into the local environment. Manifestations of immediate hypersensitivity include vasodilation, hypotension, laryngeal edema, bronchoconstriction, urticaria, angioedema, wheezing, rhinitis, erythema or pruritus, and, occasionally, severe nausea, vomiting, diarrhea, and abdominal cramps.

A second group of IgE-mediated hypersensitivity responses, classified as *accelerated allergic reactions*, occur 1 to 72 hours following drug treatment. Symptoms include angioedema, erythema or pruritus, urticaria, laryngeal edema, wheezing, and rhinitis. With the exception of laryngeal edema, these reactions are not usually life-threatening. They further differ from immediate IgE-mediated hypersensitivity in that they are tempered by IgG blocking antibodies.

The *late reactions* to penicillins account for 80% to 90% of all allergic responses to these drugs. They may develop 72 hours after initiation of treatment but most commonly appear approximately seven days after exposure. Symptoms include nonurticarial skin rashes, urticaria-angioedema and urticaria-arthralgia syndromes, and serum sickness. The mechanism of rash formation has not been determined. Serum sickness is caused by the deposition of complexes of IgG or IgM antibody and the drug in tissue spaces or on cells of the skin, kidneys, or other organs, thus eliciting further immune responses.

Rare hypersensitivity reactions to penicillins include immune hemolytic anemia, interstitial nephritis, pulmonary infiltration with eosinophilia, drug fever, hypersensitivity vasculitis, erythema multiforme, granulocytopenia, thrombocytopenia, and drug-induced systemic lupus erythematosus. For many of these, an immunologic mechanism has not been confirmed; nevertheless, they do fulfill criteria established for their classification as allergic responses to drug therapy (see Condemi, 1991). It also should be noted that exfoliative dermatitis and the Stevens-Johnson syndrome are uncommon adverse drug reactions that are often confused with allergic responses to penicillins.

Urticarial rashes may occur following the administration of any penicillin but, at least in the case of ampicillin and other aminopenicillins, the vast majority of rashes do not appear to be allergic in nature. These mildly pruritic maculopapular eruptions usually occur within 1 to 28 days following initiation of therapy, are not associated with positive IgE-immediate reacting skin tests, and resolve whether or not penicillin administration is continued. Such rashes are particularly common in patients with viral infections, such as infectious mononucleosis, with lymphatic leukemias, and in those receiving concomitant allopurinol therapy (see the section on Drug Interactions and Interference with Laboratory Tests). They do not preclude the future use of a penicillin.

In order to minimize the risk of penicillin hypersensitivity reactions, a careful history of previous allergic reactions should be taken. For most patients with a positive history, an alternative, noncross-reacting antimicrobial agent usually can be selected. When an effective alternative is not available, skin testing can help identify patients at high risk of developing an IgE-mediated (eg, immediate) reaction (see below).

Once a hypersensitivity reaction to any penicillin occurs, it should be assumed that the patient will react to all other drugs in the class. Thus, other penicillin derivatives should not be used. Although the chemical structures of cephalosporins and penicillins are similar, probably less than 5% of individuals with a history of penicillin allergy, including those with a history of IgE-mediated reactions, also are allergic to cephalosporins (Shepherd, 1991). Therefore, it generally is considered safe to administer a cephalosporin to a patient with a history of a non-IgE-mediated hypersensitivity reaction (eg, maculopapular skin rash) to penicillins. However, cephalosporins should not be used in individuals who experienced immediate hypersensitivity reactions (eg, urticaria, angioedema, bronchospasm, anaphylaxis) to penicillins because the consequences of these adverse reactions could be catastrophic (see also index entry Cephalosporins).

Aztreonam [Azactam], a monobactam, and imipenem [Primaxin], a carbapenem, are structurally related to the penicillins and cephalosporins. Although some cross-reactivity between these drugs would be expected, the available data indicate that clinically relevant cross-reaction between aztreonam and the penicillins is minimal or nonexistent and that aztreonam may be safely, albeit cautiously, administered to patients who are hypersensitive to penicillins and cephalosporins. In contrast, cross-reaction between imipenem and penicillins appears to be substantial, based on clinical trials and results of skin tests. These data indicate that imipenem should be used very cautiously in patients who are allergic to penicillins or cephalosporins (for additional information, see index entries Aztreonam, Imipenem/Cilastatin).

If an allergic reaction to a penicillin does occur, the offending drug should be discontinued. For immediate IgE-mediated reactions, epinephrine (subcutaneous or intramuscular for mild reactions and intravenous for more serious reactions) will usually abort the reaction and can be lifesaving in severe anaphylactic shock (see index entry Shock, Anaphylactic). Accelerated and late urticaria may be treated with antihistamines. Maculopapular rashes are self-limiting, but antihistamines relieve pruritus. Glucocorticoids will suppress the clinical manifestations of most allergic drug reactions and may be used to treat severe urticaria, prolonged systemic anaphylaxis or serum sickness, contact dermatitis, exfoliative and bullous skin reactions, pulmonary and hepatic reactions, and interstitial nephritis.

Skin Testing for Penicillin Hypersensitivity: Skin testing for the presence of IgE-mediated hypersensitivity to a penicillin is indicated for patients who have a history suggesting penicillin allergy and have serious infections for which noncross-reacting alternative antimicrobial agents are either unavailable or undesirable (eg, because of toxicity). Various studies have documented the fact that many patients who purport to have a history of penicillin allergy will have a negative skin test and can tolerate drugs in this class without experiencing a serious reaction. Possible reasons for this discrepancy are that the original reaction was not hypersensitive in nature or was not IgE-mediated and that IgE-antipenicillin antibodies (as detected by skin testing) decline over time.

Skin testing with penicilloyl-polylysine (PPL [Pre-Pen]), penicillin G, and a minor determinant mixture (MDM) of penicilloic and penilloic acids is a highly efficient procedure for detecting IgE-antipenicillin antibodies and, thereby, identifying patients at risk for allergic reactions. Several protocols are used for skin testing. One common approach is to perform prick (scratch) tests with PPL (6×10^{-5} M), penicillin G (10,000 U/ml, 10^{-2} M), and a MDM (10^{-2} M). If no positive reactions are observed, intradermal skin tests are performed using these reagents at the same concentrations used for prick testing. Penicilloyl-polylysine and penicillin G are commercially available, but minor determinants are not. At present, MDM is not commercially available and must be freshly prepared (Levine and Redmond, 1969). In the absence of a MDM reagent, some clinicians will perform skin testing with PPL and penicillin G alone. This will detect approximately 90% of patients at risk for acute allergic reaction to penicillin therapy. Unfortunately, some of the patients missed may be at risk for severe, life-threatening anaphylactic reaction. Thus, including the MDM is highly desirable to preclude this possibility. None of the skin test reagents will predict non-IgE-mediated hypersensitivity reactions, such as serum sickness, hemolytic anemia, contact dermatitis, maculopapular rashes, or interstitial nephritis. Acceptable skin test reagents for assessing cephalosporin, carbapenem, and monobactam hypersensitivity are not commercially available. For more detailed discussion of skin testing for penicillin hypersensitivity, see Condemi, 1991; Shepherd, 1991.

Individuals who have positive results of skin tests are at high risk of developing an acute allergic reaction if given a therapeutic dose of a penicillin. Patients with serious infections who cannot receive alternative noncross-reacting antimicrobials are candidates for acute desensitization. Because of the potential hazards of this procedure (eg, anaphylactic shock), it should be performed under well-controlled conditions (eg, in an intensive care unit, under constant physician supervision, emergency cart at bedside). Oral and parenteral desensitization procedures have been used; for references to various protocols, see Condemi, 1991; Shepherd, 1991.

OTHER ADVERSE REACTIONS. The penicillins have relatively little direct toxicity in humans. Many adverse reactions are caused by the irritant effects of these agents. Pain and sterile inflammation may occur at the site of intramuscular injection, and phlebitis or thrombophlebitis is sometimes seen when these drugs are given intravenously. Pyrosis, anorexia, nausea, vomiting, and mild to severe diarrhea may result from irritation of the gastrointestinal tract, especially with oral administration. Ampicillin has been associated with diarrhea most frequently.

Central Nervous System: The most serious consequences of the irritant properties of the penicillins involve the nervous system. Accidental injection into a peripheral nerve causes pain and dysfunction of that part of the body innervated by the nerve. This effect usually is slowly reversible. If penicillin penetrates and accumulates in high concentrations in the central nervous system (CNS), a variety of neurotoxic reactions ranging from lethargy, confusion, and hallucinations to convulsions, coma, and fatal encephalopathy may occur. Intrathecal administration has produced arachnoiditis and fatal encephalopathy, and this route should be avoided.

Immediate-type toxic reactions to the procaine component of penicillin G procaine may occur in some individuals, particularly when a large single dose is administered in the treatment of gonorrhea (4.8 million units). These reactions probably represent inadvertent intravascular administration and may be manifested by CNS-related disturbances, including anxiety, confusion, agitation, depression, weakness, seizures, hallucinations, combativeness, and expressed fear of impending death. Reactions occur in 1 of 500 patients and are transient, lasting 15 to 30 minutes.

Renal/Electrolyte: Nephropathy, an allergic reaction manifested as interstitial nephritis, has been reported. The fully expressed clinical syndrome is characterized by fever, macular rash, eosinophilia, proteinuria, hematuria, leukocyturia, and eosinophiluria; ultimately, the reaction can progress to acute nonoliguric renal failure. Interstitial nephritis is associated most often with the use of methicillin but may be caused by any of the penicillins. Patients usually recover when the drug is discontinued, but fatalities have been reported. Hemorrhagic cystitis also has been reported rarely in patients treated with methicillin (for additional discussion see the evaluation).

The administration of large intravenous doses of any penicillin, particularly ticarcillin, can produce hypokalemia due to the large amount of nonreabsorbable anion in the distal renal tubules. Excessive sodium intake also can be a problem with disodium salt preparations (eg, ticarcillin) in patients who have impaired sodium excretion mechanisms (eg, those with pre-existing cardiac, renal, or hepatic disease).

Blood: Hematologic toxicity occurs occasionally following administration of the penicillins. Neutropenia has been observed after use of all penicillins, particularly with large doses, and is reversible after discontinuation of therapy. Thrombocytopenia and reticulocytopenia have been reported rarely. The mechanism underlying these penicillin-induced cytopenias generally is considered to be immune-mediated. However, neutropenia resulting from a direct toxic effect on proliferation of myeloid precursor cells also has been reported (Neftel et al, 1985). Coombs'-positive hemolytic anemia is a rare adverse reaction to the penicillins. High concentrations of all penicillins, but particularly carbenicillin and ticarcillin, bind adenosine diphosphate receptors in platelets and prevent their normal aggregation. This can result in prolongation of the bleeding time. Although infrequent, carbenicillin and ticarcillin may be associated with clinically significant hemorrhage when large doses of these drugs are administered to patients who have impaired renal function or underlying disorders of hemostasis or to those receiving other drugs that may contribute to bleeding diatheses (see Fass et al, 1987).

Hepatic: Transient increases in serum concentrations of liver enzymes (eg, ALT, AST) have been reported occasionally with a number of penicillins (eg, nafcillin, isoxazolyl penicillins, aminopenicillins, antipseudomonal penicillins). Symptoms of hepatitis have rarely been associated with these elevated enzyme levels in patients receiving oxacillin and cloxacillin.

Gastrointestinal: Penicillins may alter the bacterial flora in certain areas of the body (eg, intestinal tract, respiratory tract) by eliminating susceptible microorganisms. This usually is of little clinical significance, and re-establishment of the normal microflora occurs after therapy is discontinued. However, serious superinfections with resistant microorganisms (eg, *Klebsiella, Pseudomonas, Candida*) may follow long-term therapy with any penicillin; this may be more likely with broad spectrum analogues.

Diarrhea or antibiotic-associated pseudomembranous colitis (AAPMC) due to *Clostridium difficile* may develop during or after penicillin therapy. Ampicillin has been one of the more frequently implicated antibiotics in this disorder. This potentially life-threatening adverse effect requires prompt discontinuation of the offending antibiotic, maintenance of fluid and electrolyte balance, and possible therapy with oral metronidazole or vancomycin (see also index entry Lincosamides).

Pregnancy: Generally, penicillins have proven to be the safest antibiotics for use during pregnancy. Although less information is available concerning the safety of the newer semisynthetic penicillin derivatives during pregnancy, there is no evidence that these agents are teratogenic (see Chow and Jewesson, 1985). The penicillins are classified in FDA Pregnancy Category B.

For additional discussion of adverse reactions and precautions, see Parry, 1987; Neu, 1990.

Drug Interactions and Interference with Laboratory Tests

The ureidopenicillins (ticarcillin, mezlocillin, piperacillin), which usually are given in large doses, can inactivate aminoglycosides, particularly gentamicin and tobramycin, when mixed together in intravenous solutions, and this practice should be avoided. Furthermore, in patients with renal failure, in vivo antagonism between penicillins and aminoglycosides has been observed and may be clinically significant. Serum aminoglycoside concentrations should be monitored in such patients and the dosage adjusted accordingly to maintain therapeutic levels (Mangini, 1984; Hansten, 1985 A). For a more detailed discussion, see index entry Aminoglycosides.

In theory, bacteriostatic antimicrobial drugs that inhibit protein synthesis (eg, chloramphenicol, tetracyclines, erythromycin, clindamycin) could interfere with the bactericidal effect of penicillins. However, the clinical significance of this interaction is not known and such combinations are recommended under certain circumstances (eg, chloramphenicol plus ampicillin for empiric therapy of *Haemophilus influenzae* type b meningitis). When such combinations are considered necessary, it is recommended that adequate amounts of each drug be administered and, if possible, the penicillin should be given a few hours or more before the bacteriostatic antibiotic (see Hansten, 1985 A).

Oral neomycin decreases the gastrointestinal absorption of penicillin V, presumably due to the production of a malabsorption syndrome. Although this has not been demonstrated for other penicillins, it is recommended that parenteral penicillins be used when patients are receiving oral neomycin (Hansten, 1985 A).

Patients receiving heparin or oral anticoagulants (eg, warfarin) may be at increased risk for bleeding complications when high doses of intravenous penicillins, particularly carboxypenicillins, are administered. Caution should be exercised and coagulation status should be carefully monitored (see Mangini, 1986).

Large doses of some penicillins (eg, penicillin G, nafcillin, mezlocillin) have been associated with false-positive reactions for urinary protein (pseudoproteinuria) when certain assay methods were employed (eg, sulfosalicylic acid and boiling test, acetic acid test, biuret reaction, nitric acid test). This should be distinguished from the true proteinuria that may follow the use of methicillin, oxacillin, and possibly other penicillins.

Pharmacokinetics

Claims that one penicillin is clinically superior to another based on in vitro sensitivity are questionable, because such tests do not take into account factors such as stability in gastric acid, rates of absorption and excretion, degree of protein binding, diffusion into abscesses or body cavities, and minimal effective blood and tissue concentrations.

The pharmacokinetic properties of the penicillins are summarized in the Table.

Absorption: There are marked differences in oral absorption of the penicillins (see Table). Oral preparations of penicillin G are susceptible to destruction by gastric acid and therefore are absorbed erratically and incompletely. To obtain comparable blood concentrations in young, healthy patients, the oral dose of penicillin G must be four to five times greater than the intramuscular dose. However, in elderly or other achlorhydric patients, oral penicillin G will be absorbed more rapidly and completely than in those who produce normal amounts of gastric acid. Because the presence of food also reduces the gastrointestinal absorption of penicillin G, if oral administration is desired, this penicillin must be given one hour before or two hours after meals to ensure adequate blood levels.

Penicillin V potassium is less susceptible than penicillin G to destruction by gastric acid and, when given with meals, produces blood levels almost as high as those obtained when the drug is taken on an empty stomach. In similar patients, comparable doses of penicillin V produce blood levels that are two- to fivefold higher than those obtained with penicillin G. Thus, penicillin V is preferred for oral administration.

Methicillin is not used orally because of its susceptibility to gastric acid. The other penicillinase-resistant penicillins are resistant to gastric acid, but their absorption is incomplete (see Table). Also, because nafcillin and, to a lesser extent, oxacillin are absorbed more erratically than cloxacillin and dicloxacillin, only the latter two drugs are recommended for oral use. The absorption of all penicillinase-resistant penicillins is impeded by food in the gastrointestinal tract.

The aminopenicillins are resistant to destruction by gastric acid. However, amoxicillin and bacampicillin, which is hydrolyzed to ampicillin, are better absorbed than ampicillin, particularly in the presence of food. Amoxicillin is the preferred aminopenicillin for oral use because its bioavailability is superior to that of ampicillin.

The antipseudomonal penicillins (eg, ticarcillin, mezlocillin, piperacillin) are acid-labile and are not absorbed orally. However, carbenicillin indanyl sodium, an ester derivative of car-

CLASSIFICATION OF THE PENICILLINS WITH SOME PHARMACOKINETIC DATA

Class and Generic Name	Trade Name(s)	Route(s) of Administration	Oral Absorption (%)
NATURAL PENICILLINS			
Penicillin G	Many (see evaluation)	Oral Intramuscular Intravenous	20-30
Penicillin V	Many (see evaluation)	Oral	60
PENICILLINASE-RESISTANT (ANTISTAPHYLOCOCCAL) PENICILLINS			
Methicillin	Staphcillin	Intramuscular Intravenous	None
Nafcillin	Nafcil Unipen Nallpen	Oral Intramuscular Intravenous	Erratic (10-20)
Isoxazolyl Penicillins			
Oxacillin	Bactocill Prostaphlin	Oral Intramuscular Intravenous	30
Cloxacillin	Cloxapen Tegopen	Oral	50
Dicloxacillin	Dycill Dynapen Pathocil	Oral	50
AMINOPENICILLINS			
Ampicillin	Many (see evaluation)	Oral Intramuscular Intravenous	40
Amoxicillin	Amoxil Larotid Polymox Trimox	Oral	75-90
Bacampicillin[1]	Spectrobid	Oral	~ 95
Cyclacillin	Cyclapen-W[2]	Oral	~ 95
ANTIPSEUDOMONAL PENICILLINS			
Carboxypenicillins			
Carbenicillin[2]	Geopen[2]	Intramuscular Intravenous	None
Carbenicillin Indanyl[1]	Geocillin	Oral	30
Ticarcillin	Ticar	Intramuscular Intravenous	None
Ureidopenicillins			
Azlocillin[2]	Azlin[2]	Intravenous	None
Mezlocillin	Mezlin	Intramuscular Intravenous	None
Piperacillin	Pipracil	Intramuscular Intravenous	None

Protein Bound (%)	Metabolized (%)	Urinary Recovery (%)	Approximate Half-life (hours)	Volume of Distribution (L/kg)
50-60	20	20 (oral) 60-90 (parenteral)	0.5	0.3-0.42
80	55	29-37	0.5-1	---
35-40	10	80	0.5	0.31
87-90	60	30	0.5	0.31-0.38
90-93	45-50	30-50	0.5	0.12-0.4
93-95	20	30-50	0.5	0.15-0.2
95-97	10	60	0.5-0.7	0.13-0.19
17-20	10	40-45 (oral) 90 (parenteral)	1	0.17-0.31
17-20	10	50-70	1	0.25-0.42
17-20	10	75	1	---
20	15-17	80	0.5-0.75	---
50-60	2	85-95	1.1	0.18
50-60	2	30	1.1	---
50-60	10-15	75-85	1.2	0.22
20-40	<10	50-70	0.8-1.2	~0.2
16-42	<10	45-70	0.8-1.2	~0.2
16-22	---	60-80	0.6-1.3	0.18-0.3

[1] These penicillins are prodrugs; after oral absorption, bacampicillin is hydrolyzed to ampicillin, and carbenicillin indanyl is hydrolyzed to carbenicillin.

[2] No longer marketed in the United States.

benicillin, is adequately absorbed to yield antibacterial concentrations in urine and it should only be used for certain urinary tract infections.

Transient high blood concentrations of penicillin G can be produced by injecting an aqueous solution intravenously or intramuscularly every three to six hours. However, intramuscular administration causes irritation and pain. When large doses (eg, 10 million units or more daily) are required, penicillin G must be given intravenously. High tissue levels can be obtained after continuous or intermittent intravenous infusion. Intrathecal injection should never be used because of the epileptogenic effect that may be produced by even small doses of penicillin given by this route.

When more sustained effects are desired, repository preparations of penicillin G may be given intramuscularly for infections caused by susceptible microorganisms. Penicillin G procaine can be given every 6 to 12 hours or even once daily, depending on the infection and the dose needed. Penicillin G benzathine provides detectable blood levels for as long as four weeks after a single intramuscular injection. However, because low blood levels are produced, this form of penicillin is effective against only very susceptible organisms (see the Uses section).

Penicillin preparations for topical use are no longer marketed in the United States, because hypersensitization is a frequent complication.

Distribution: Plasma protein binding of the penicillins varies widely (see Table). Only the free drug has antibacterial activity. However, the protein-penicillin complex dissociates readily and, as free drug is withdrawn from plasma, additional penicillin is released from protein binding sites.

The penicillins are well distributed to most areas of the body, including lung, liver, kidney, muscle, and bone. High concentrations are achieved in urine. Most of these agents, especially ampicillin, amoxicillin, nafcillin, piperacillin, and mezlocillin, enter the bile in concentrations well above the MIC for most susceptible organisms. In the presence of inflammation, concentrations achieved in synovial, pericardial, pleural, and peritoneal fluids and the middle ear are sufficient to inhibit most susceptible bacteria. Diffusion into cerebrospinal fluid, the eye, and the prostate is poor, even when very large doses are given, unless inflammation is present.

Penicillins cross the placenta. Compounds that exhibit low protein binding may produce fetal serum concentrations equivalent to those in the maternal serum 30 to 60 minutes after injection. Highly protein-bound penicillins achieve only low concentrations in both the fetal serum and the amniotic fluid.

Elimination: Most penicillins are excreted rapidly in the urine, primarily as unchanged drug. Because active renal tubular secretion is the predominant mechanism, probenecid delays excretion of most penicillins. The rate of elimination in newborns is lower than in older children and adults because of their immature renal function. Only nafcillin is excreted primarily by the liver; 60% of a dose is metabolized. Penicillin V and oxacillin also are metabolized significantly. Other penicillins are metabolized to a minor degree. Biliary excretion of penicillins does occur, but probably is important only for nafcillin, mezlocillin, and piperacillin.

The dosage of some penicillins should be adjusted if renal function is impaired. In patients with creatinine clearance rates of 30 to 50 ml/min, modification of carbenicillin and ticarcillin dosage is required. In those with rates of 10 ml/min or less, the dosage of all penicillins, except the isoxazolyl compounds (oxacillin, cloxacillin, dicloxacillin) and nafcillin, must be reduced or the intervals between doses increased (see the evaluations).

Drug Evaluations

NATURAL PENICILLINS

PENICILLIN G

MECHANISM OF ACTION, ANTIMICROBIAL SPECTRUM, AND RESISTANCE. Penicillin G is a naturally derived (from *Penicillium chrysogenum*) antibiotic that inhibits cell wall formation in susceptible bacteria and usually is bactericidal. It is susceptible to hydrolysis by β-lactamases and therefore bacteria that produce these enzymes are resistant to penicillin G. For a detailed discussion of the mechanism of action and antimicrobial spectrum of the penicillins, see the Introduction.

USES. Penicillin G frequently is the drug of choice for a variety of infections caused by susceptible organisms in nonallergic patients. The oral, parenteral, or repository formulations are used for specific indications based on the severity of the infection and the required duration of therapy (see the discussion on Uses in the Introduction).

Oral formulations of penicillin G should be used only for mild or stabilized infections and long-term prophylaxis. Penicillin V generally is preferred for oral administration because it has more reliable bioavailability (see the evaluation on Penicillin V).

Aqueous crystalline penicillin G, available as the potassium (usually preferred) or sodium salt, is administered intramuscularly or intravenously to produce high serum concentrations rapidly. When large doses are indicated for severe infections (eg, pneumococcal meningitis, enterococcal endocarditis, gas gangrene), the intravenous route should be used.

Penicillin G procaine and penicillin G benzathine are repository forms of penicillin G that are administered intramuscularly. They provide tissue depots from which active drug can be absorbed over a period of hours (penicillin G procaine) or days (penicillin G benzathine). Thus, these formulations of penicillin G are useful for certain infections caused by sensitive organisms when prolonged therapeutic blood levels are required and it is desirable to avoid frequent dosing.

ADVERSE REACTIONS AND PRECAUTIONS. Hypersensitivity reactions are the most common adverse effects of penicillin G, and this drug should be avoided in patients known to be allergic to penicillins. If a hypersensitivity reaction occurs, the drug should be discontinued immediately and appropriate ameliorative treatment given if necessary (see the Introduction). In most instances, discontinuation of penicillin G is sufficient. If further treatment of the infection is necessary, an alternative antibacterial agent, selected on the basis of organism susceptibility and the type and severity of infection involved, should be given. For alternative agents, see index entry Antimicrobial Drugs.

Convulsions have followed intravenous dosages of more than 20 million units of penicillin G daily, especially in neonates, patients with renal insufficiency or epilepsy, or other susceptible individuals (eg, those undergoing cardiopulmonary bypass).

Intrathecal administration has produced arachnoiditis and fatal encephalopathy, and this route should be avoided.

Rapid administration of massive intravenous doses of penicillin G potassium (1.7 mEq of potassium/million units) may produce hyperkalemia, arrhythmias, and cardiac arrest, particularly in patients with impaired renal function.

For a detailed discussion of other adverse reactions and precautions, see the Introduction.

In addition to the standard adverse reactions associated with penicillin G, the procaine component of penicillin G procaine has been associated with immediate, but transient, mental disturbances after injection of large single doses (eg, 4.8 million units). The Jarisch-Herxheimer reaction has been reported in patients treated for syphilis with penicillin G benzathine.

DRUG INTERACTIONS AND INTERFERENCE WITH LABORATORY TESTS. See the Introduction.

PHARMACOKINETICS. Comparative pharmacokinetic data on the penicillins appear in the Table.

Following an oral dose of 500 mg (800,000 units) in fasting adults, peak total serum concentrations of drug range between 1.5 and 2.5 mcg/ml after 30 to 60 minutes; peak concentrations of free drug are between 0.6 and 1 mcg/ml. Absorption in neonates and the elderly is greater because gastric pH is higher. The presence of food in the gastrointestinal tract decreases absorption; therefore, penicillin G should be administered either one hour before or two to three hours after a meal.

Peak serum concentrations are attained approximately 15 to 30 minutes after intramuscular injection and immediately after intravenous administration of aqueous crystalline penicillin G, and they usually are about four- to fivefold higher than those following oral administration. For example, a 625-mg (1,000,000 units) intravenous dose of aqueous crystalline penicillin G results in a total peak serum concentration of about 10 mcg/ml.

The drug readily distributes to many tissues (eg, muscle, lung, liver, kidney, bone) and body fluids (eg, interstitial, synovial, pericardial, peritoneal, pleural). High concentrations are achieved in bile and urine. Penetration into cerebrospinal fluid, the aqueous humor, and the prostate is poor in the absence of inflammation, but therapeutic concentrations can be achieved for susceptible organisms in the presence of inflammation. Penicillin G crosses the placenta.

Penicillin G is rapidly eliminated, primarily by renal tubular secretion. Excretion is delayed by probenecid. Additionally, a small percentage of drug is eliminated via the bile. A small proportion (see Table) is metabolized to inactive penicilloic acid derivatives. The half-life is prolonged in patients with renal impairment (eg, 6 to 10 hours in anuric patients) and dosage adjustments are necessary. Because of incompletely developed renal function in young infants and deteriorating renal function in the elderly, the half-life of penicillin G is longer in these patients than in older children and younger adults, respectively.

The elimination of oral penicillin G is the same as for the parenteral form. However, only about 20% of a dose is recovered from urine as unchanged drug because of limited gastrointestinal absorption. Most unabsorbed penicillin G is inactivated by bacteria in the colon; the amount of unchanged drug in feces is low.

Penicillin G Procaine. This repository form of penicillin G slowly releases active drug from the tissue depot at the site of intramuscular injection. A plateau-type of peak serum concentration (eg, approximately 3 mcg/ml after a 750-mg [1.2 million units] dose) is reached after one to three hours and falls slowly over 15 to 20 hours. Usually 60% to 90% of a dose is excreted in the urine within 24 to 36 hours, but drug may be detected in serum five to seven days after injection. Although intramuscular administration of penicillin G procaine does not result in the rapid, high serum concentrations of antibiotic that can be achieved with an equivalent parenteral dose of aqueous crystalline penicillin G, a more prolonged therapeutic serum concentration is attained for certain susceptible microorganisms (see the discussion on Uses in the Introduction). Thus, a longer, more convenient dosing interval can be used.

Penicillin G Benzathine. This repository form of penicillin G releases active drug very slowly from the tissue depot at the site of intramuscular injection. The result is a low peak serum concentration (eg, 0.1 mcg/ml 24 hours after a 750-mg [1.2 million units] dose), but a very flat serum concentration versus time curve. When given in this formulation, penicillin G is detectable in serum for up to 30 days. These prolonged, low serum concentrations are therapeutically effective for certain infections caused by highly susceptible microorganisms and obviate the need for more frequent dosing (see the discussion on Uses in the Introduction).

DOSAGE AND PREPARATIONS. To convert units of penicillin G to milligrams, 1 unit is equivalent to 0.6 mcg (1.6 million units equals 1 g).

PENICILLIN G POTASSIUM:

Oral: A dose is administered one hour before or two hours after meals. *Adults and children over 12 years*, 1.6 to 3.2 million units (1 to 2 g) daily in divided doses four times daily (The Medical Letter, 1990); *children under 12 years*, 40,000 to 80,000 units (25 to 50 mg)/kg daily in divided doses every six to eight hours (Nelson, 1991 A).

Generic. Powder (for oral solution) 250,000 and 400,000 units/5 ml; tablets 200,000, 250,000, 400,000, 500,000, and 800,000 units; tablets (buffered) 200,000, 250,000, and 400,000 units.

Pentids, Pentids 400, Pentids 800 (Apothecon). Powder (for oral solution) 200,000 and 400,000 units/5 ml; tablets 200,000, 400,000, and 800,000 units.

PENICILLIN G SODIUM, POTASSIUM:

Intramuscular, Intravenous: Total daily dosage and route of administration depend on the type and severity of infection. For example, high-dose intravenous penicillin G is used in meningitis (eg, pneumococcal, meningococcal), some forms of endocarditis (eg, enterococcal), and severe clostridial infections.

Adults, 1.2 to 24 million units daily (The Medical Letter, 1990). Daily dosage can be given intermittently in equally divided doses at four (range, two to six)-hour intervals or by constant intravenous infusion. Large doses (10 to 20 million units daily) should be given intravenously.

Children, 100,000 to 250,000 units/kg daily in divided doses every four hours (Nelson, 1991 A).

Infants over 7 days and weighing more than 2 kg, 100,000 units/kg daily in divided doses every six hours; for meningitis, 200,000 units/kg daily in divided doses every six hours; *over 7 days and weighing 1.2 to 2 kg,* 75,000 units/kg daily in divided doses every eight hours; for meningitis, 225,000 units/kg daily in divided doses every eight hours; *under 7 days and weighing more than 2 kg,* 60,000 units/kg daily in divided doses every eight hours; for meningitis, 150,000 units/kg daily in divided doses every eight hours; *under 7 days and weighing 1.2 to 2 kg,* 50,000 units/kg daily in divided doses every 12 hours; for meningitis, 100,000 units/kg daily in divided doses every 12 hours; *0 to 28 days and weighing less than 1.2 kg,* 50,000 units/kg daily in two doses every 12 hours; for meningitis, 100,000 units/kg daily in two doses every 12 hours (Nelson, 1991 B).

For dosage guidelines in syphilis, see index entry on this disease.

PENICILLIN G (AQUEOUS) POTASSIUM:

Generic. Powder (sterile) 1, 5, 10, and 20 million units; solution (premixed, frozen) 1, 2, and 3 million units.

Pfizerpen (Roerig). Powder (buffered) 1, 5, and 20 million units.

PENICILLIN G (AQUEOUS) SODIUM:

Generic. Powder (sterile) 5 and 25 million units.

PROCAINE PENICILLIN G:

Intramuscular: *Adults and children,* 600,000 to 1.2 million units daily in one or two doses depending on the condition being treated. Ten days to two weeks of therapy is usually sufficient. *Newborn infants,* 50,000 units/kg once daily (Nelson, 1991 B).

Certain patients with infective endocarditis caused by penicillin-sensitive streptococci (eg, most viridans streptococci, *S. bovis*) have been successfully treated with procaine penicillin G 1.2 million units four times daily for two weeks plus streptomycin 500 mg twice daily for two weeks (see index entry Endocarditis, Treatment).

For uncomplicated penicillin-susceptible gonococcal infections, a total dose of 4.8 million units, injected at two sites, with probenecid 1 g orally.

For dosage guidelines in the treatment of syphilis, see index entry on this infection.

Generic. Suspension (sterile) 300,000 units/ml in 10 ml containers.

Crysticillin 300 A.S. (Apothecon). Suspension (sterile, aqueous) 300,000 units/ml in 10 ml containers.

Crysticillin 600 A.S. (Apothecon). Suspension (sterile, aqueous) 600,000/1.2 ml in 12 ml containers.

Pfizerpen-AS (Roerig). Suspension (aqueous) 300,000 units/ml in 10 ml containers.

Wycillin (Wyeth-Ayerst). Suspension (sterile, aqueous) 600,000 units/ml in 1, 2, and 4 ml containers.

BENZATHINE PENICILLIN G:

Intramuscular: The following dosages are recommended by the American Heart Association for group A streptococcal upper respiratory tract infections (eg, pharyngitis): *adults and children weighing more than 27 kg,* 1.2 million units as a single dose; *infants and children weighing 27 kg or less,* 600,000 units as a single dose (Dajani et al, 1988). Alternatively, the manufacturers' recommended dosages for group A streptococcal upper respiratory tract infections (eg, pharyngitis) are *adults,* 1.2 million units in a single dose; *older children,* a single injection of 900,000 units; *infants and children weighing less than 27 kg,* a single dose of 300,000 to 600,000 units. For *neonates*, a single dose of 50,000 units/kg has been recommended (Nelson, 1991 B).

For dosage guidelines in the treatment of syphilis, see index entry on this infection.

For dosage guidelines in the prophylaxis of rheumatic fever, see index entry on this disease.

Bicillin L-A (Wyeth-Ayerst). Suspension (sterile) 300,000 units/ml in 10 ml containers and 600,000 units/ml in 1, 2, and 4 ml containers.

Permapen (Roerig). Suspension (aqueous) 600,000 units/ml in 2 ml containers.

COMBINATIONS OF PROCAINE AND BENZATHINE PENICILLIN G: Combinations of procaine penicillin G and benzathine penicillin G are marketed for the convenience of physicians who believe that they may be helpful in situations requiring both immediate and long-term effects when the patient cannot conveniently return for care. In general, however, it is preferable to administer penicillins as single-entity preparations for specific indications. Thus, dosage recommendations generally are not given. However, a single dose of the combination of 900,000 units of benzathine penicillin G and 300,000 units of procaine penicillin G [Bicillin C-R 900/300] may be a satisfactory alternative for smaller patients with group A streptococcal pharyngitis, but this dosage is based on limited data (Dajani et al, 1988).

Bicillin C-R (Wyeth-Ayerst). Suspension (aqueous) containing benzathine penicillin G and procaine penicillin G 150,000 units/ml each in 10 ml containers or 300,000 units/ml each in 1, 2, and 4 ml containers.

Bicillin C-R 900/300 (Wyeth-Ayerst). Suspension (aqueous) containing benzathine penicillin G 900,000 units and procaine penicillin G 300,000 units/ml in 2 ml containers.

PENICILLIN V

POTASSIUM PENICILLIN V

[Ledercillin VK, Pen-Vee K, V-Cillin K, Veetids]

Penicillin V (phenoxymethyl penicillin) is a derivative of penicillin G that is designed for oral use. The activity of penicillin V against most gram-positive bacteria is comparable to that of penicillin G. However, it is less active against gram-negative microorganisms (eg, *Neisseria, Haemophilus*).

Penicillin V is susceptible to hydrolysis by β-lactamases; thus, β-lactamase-producing strains of various bacteria (eg, most staphylococci) are resistant to this drug.

For a detailed discussion of the mechanism of action and antimicrobial spectrum of the penicillins, see the Introduction.

USES. Penicillin V, especially the potassium salt, is preferred to penicillin G when oral administration is indicated because it is more reliably absorbed and can be administered with food (see Pharmacokinetics below).

For a detailed discussion, see the section on Uses in the Introduction; see also index entry Antimicrobial Drugs.

ADVERSE REACTIONS AND PRECAUTIONS. Hypersensitivity reactions are the most common adverse effects. For a discussion of these and other adverse reactions, see the Introduction.

DRUG INTERACTIONS AND INTERFERENCE WITH LABORATORY TESTS. Oral neomycin decreases the gastrointestinal absorption of penicillin V, presumably due to the production of a malabsorption syndrome.

Fatal anaphylactic reactions to oral penicillin V were reported in two patients who also were receiving the nonselective beta-adrenergic blocking agents, nadolol and propranolol, respectively (Berkelman et al, 1986). Although a definite association cannot be made on the basis of this isolated report, beta-adrenergic antagonists may potentiate and increase the severity of penicillin-induced anaphylactic reactions. Furthermore, patients receiving beta-adrenergic blocking agents are less responsive to epinephrine and may be difficult to treat (see Toogood, 1987). Clinicians should be aware of this possible life-threatening interaction. For additional information, see the Introduction.

PHARMACOKINETICS. Comparative pharmacokinetic data on the penicillins appear in the Table.

In contrast to penicillin G, penicillin V is stable in gastric acid. Following a dose of 500 mg (800,000 units), peak serum concentrations of total drug range from 3 to 5 mcg/ml after 30 to 60 minutes; peak concentrations of free drug are about 0.8 mcg/ml. Unlike its effect on penicillin G, the presence of food in the gastrointestinal tract does not appreciably decrease the absorption of penicillin V. The potassium salt of penicillin V is better absorbed than other salts.

Because there is less individual variability in absorption, penicillin V produces total serum concentrations that are two- to fivefold higher than after comparable doses of penicillin G. However, when higher serum concentrations are required (eg, for more serious infections), parenteral penicillin G is indicated.

Like other penicillins, penicillin V primarily distributes into the extracellular fluid volume and is eliminated rapidly by renal tubular secretion. Probenecid delays its elimination. Penicillin V is metabolized to penicilloic acid derivatives. For additional discussion, see the section on Pharmacokinetics in the Introduction.

DOSAGE AND PREPARATIONS.

Oral: *Adults,* 125 to 500 mg four times daily. In the presence of severe renal impairment (creatinine clearance, 10 ml/min or less), the dose probably should not exceed 250 mg every six hours. *Children,* 25 to 50 mg/kg daily in divided doses every six to eight hours. The duration of treatment for streptococcal pharyngitis should be ten days.

For dosage guidelines in the prophylaxis of bacterial endocarditis in high-risk patients prior to dental procedures or surgery or instrumentation of the upper respiratory tract and for the prophylaxis of rheumatic fever, see index entry Antimicrobial Drugs.

PENICILLIN V:
Generic. Powder for oral solution 125 and 250 mg/5 ml; tablets 250 and 500 mg.

POTASSIUM PENICILLIN V:
Generic. Powder for oral solution 125 and 250 mg/5 ml; tablets 125, 250, and 500 mg.
Ledercillin VK (Lederle), ***Pen-Vee K*** (Wyeth-Ayerst), ***Veetids*** (Apothecon). Powder for oral solution 125 and 250 mg/5 ml; tablets 250 and 500 mg.
V-Cillin K (Lilly). Powder for oral solution 125 and 250 mg/5 ml; tablets 125, 250, and 500 mg.

Additional Trademarks.
Beepen-VK (SmithKline Beecham), ***Betapen-VK*** (Apothecon), ***Robicillin VK*** (Robins).

PENICILLINASE-RESISTANT (ANTISTAPHYLOCOCCAL) PENICILLINS

METHICILLIN SODIUM

[Staphcillin]

MECHANISM OF ACTION, ANTIMICROBIAL SPECTRUM, AND RESISTANCE. Methicillin sodium is a water-soluble, penicillinase-resistant semisynthetic salt for parenteral use. It is active against most strains of *Staphylococcus aureus*, including β-lactamase-producing strains. Many strains of *S. epidermidis* also are susceptible. Because most staphylococci produce β-lactamase and are resistant to penicillin G, the penicillinase-resistant penicillins are primary drugs for infections caused by these pathogens. Most streptococci, including *S. pyogenes, S. pneumoniae*, and viridans streptococci, also are susceptible to the antistaphylococcal penicillins. However, penicillin G is more potent against streptococci and is preferred clinically. Enterococci are resistant to methicillin. Gram-negative bacteria generally are resistant.

Over the past decade, methicillin-resistant strains of *Staphylococcus aureus* (MRSA) have become prevalent in the United States (Boyce, 1990). Although initially these strains were found primarily in large acute-care hospitals, they now also occur in the community, especially in abusers of illicit intravenous drugs, and have become a problem in chronic-care facilities (Kauffman et al, 1990). Methicillin resistance also is common among strains of *S. epidermidis*, which is a primary pathogen in infections associated with prosthetic devices and other foreign bodies. Virtually all MRSA strains also are resistant to the other penicillinase-resistant penicillins and to the cephalosporins, although this may not be reliably demonstrated by routine in vitro antimicrobial susceptibility tests. High-level resistance to fluoroquinolones also has been observed in MRSA isolated from patients in the United States and Europe (Blumberg et al, 1991).

For additional discussion of the mechanism of action and antimicrobial spectrum of the penicillins, see the Introduction.

USES. Penicillinase-resistant penicillins are recommended only for infections known or suspected to be caused by penicillinase-producing staphylococci. However, methicillin-resistant strains are common. Thus, an alternative drug such as vancomycin should be selected for empiric therapy of suspected staphylococcal infections pending the availability of accurate susceptibility data (see index entry Antimicrobial Drugs). Nafcillin and oxacillin usually are preferred to methicillin because of the greater association of interstitial nephritis with the latter agent in adults and older children (see Adverse Reactions and Precautions). Methicillin is used in neonates because interstitial nephritis is rare in this age group. Penicillin G is preferred if susceptibility is confirmed. For additional discussion, see the section on Uses in the Introduction to this chapter; index entry Antimicrobial Drugs; and the evaluations on Nafcillin and Oxacillin; see also Neu, 1982 A, 1990; Reese and Betts, 1991.

ADVERSE REACTIONS AND PRECAUTIONS. Methicillin generally is well tolerated; untoward effects are usually mild and most commonly consist of the allergic and other reactions typical of all penicillins (see the Introduction).

Interstitial nephritis has been associated with use of methicillin more frequently than with other antistaphylococcal penicillins. The incidence appears to be greater in males than in females. Methicillin-induced nephrotoxicity may develop at any age (but is uncommon in neonates) and is not dose-related. The disease begins 2 to 37 days (mean, 15 days) after initiation of therapy and is characterized by fever, rash, eosinophilia, hematuria, proteinuria, leukocyturia, and eosinophiluria. Ultimately, the reaction can progress to renal failure. Biopsy of the kidney routinely shows an interstitial infiltrate of mononuclear and eosinophilic cells with tubular damage, but no glomerular lesions. In most cases, renal function returns to normal when the drug is discontinued. The mechanism is unknown, but interstitial nephritis may be a hypersensitivity reaction because of the lack of a dose relationship, the presence of rash and eosinophilia, the renal pathology, and the occurrence of cross-sensitivity in some patients when another penicillin was substituted (Ditlove et al, 1977).

Hemorrhagic cystitis has been reported with methicillin and is most likely to occur in patients with low urine output given large doses. The mechanism is unknown.

DRUG INTERACTIONS AND INTERFERENCE WITH LABORATORY TESTS. See the Introduction.

PHARMACOKINETICS. Comparative pharmacokinetic data on the penicillins appear in the Table.

Methicillin is labile in gastric acid and is not absorbed following oral administration. Thus, it must be administered parenterally. Peak serum concentrations of 12 to 17 mcg/ml are attained 30 to 60 minutes after intramuscular injection of 1 g. After an intravenous dose of 1 g, peak serum concentrations range between 20 and 40 mcg/ml.

Methicillin exhibits the lowest plasma protein binding among the antistaphylococcal penicillins. Like other penicillins, this drug primarily distributes into the extracellular fluid volume.

Methicillin is rapidly eliminated primarily by renal tubular secretion; probenecid delays its excretion. The half-life is prolonged in patients with renal impairment (eg, about four hours in anuric patients) and dosage adjustments are necessary. For additional discussion, see the Introduction.

DOSAGE AND PREPARATIONS. Methicillin can be administered by intramuscular injection (solution containing 500 mg/ml), direct intravenous injection (solution containing 20 mg/ml and given at the rate of 10 ml/min), or by continuous intravenous drip. See the manufacturers' instructions for the appropriate dilution of the drug, a list of compatible diluents and intravenous solutions, and stability of methicillin in these solutions. When used with other drugs, methicillin should not be physically mixed with the other agent(s).

Intramuscular, Intravenous: *Adults*, 4 to 12 g daily in equally divided doses every four to six hours (The Medical Letter, 1990). In those with severe renal impairment (creatinine clearance, 10 ml/min or less), the dose probably should not exceed 2 g every 12 hours (The Medical Letter, 1990).

Children, 100 to 200 mg/kg daily in equally divided doses every four to six hours (The Medical Letter, 1990).

Infants over 7 days and weighing more than 2 kg, 100 mg/kg daily in divided doses every six hours; for meningitis, 200 mg/kg daily in divided doses every six hours; *infants over 7 days and weighing 1.2 to 2 kg*, 75 mg/kg daily in divided doses every eight hours; for meningitis, 150 mg/kg daily in divided doses every eight hours; *infants under 7 days and weighing more than 2 kg*, 75 mg/kg daily in divided doses every eight hours; for meningitis, 150 mg/kg daily in divided doses every eight hours; *infants under 7 days and weighing 1.2 to 2 kg*, 50 mg/kg daily in divided doses every 12 hours; for meningitis, 100 mg/kg daily in divided doses every 12 hours; *infants 0 to 28 days and weighing less than 1.2 kg,* 50 mg/kg daily in two doses every 12 hours; for meningitis, 100 mg/kg daily in two doses every 12 hours (Nelson, 1991 B).

Staphcillin (Apothecon). Powder (buffered) 1, 4, 6, and 10 g (900 mg methicillin base with 3 mEq sodium/g).

NAFCILLIN SODIUM

[Nafcil, Nallpen, Unipen]

MECHANISM OF ACTION, ANTIMICROBIAL SPECTRUM, AND RESISTANCE. Nafcillin sodium is highly resistant to staphylococcal β-lactamases and is usually administered parenterally. The mechanism of action and antimicrobial spectrum are the same as for methicillin (see that evaluation and the Introduction). On a weight basis, nafcillin is more potent than methicillin in vitro against susceptible bacteria.

USES. The indications for parenteral nafcillin are the same as those for methicillin; the primary use is serious infections caused by *Staphylococcus aureus* or other staphylococci (see the evaluation on Methicillin). Nafcillin (or oxacillin) usually is preferred to methicillin in adults and older children because of the association of interstitial nephritis with methicillin. See the discussion on Uses in the Introduction; index entry Antimicrobial Drugs; and the evaluations on Methicillin and Oxacillin. See also Neu, 1982 A, 1990; Reese and Betts, 1991.

ADVERSE REACTIONS AND PRECAUTIONS. Nafcillin generally is well tolerated; untoward effects are usually mild and most commonly consist of the allergic and other reactions typical of all penicillins (see the Introduction). Neutropenia, which is immediately reversible on discontinuation of the drug, has been reported in 10% to 20% of patients receiving 150 to 200 mg/kg daily for 10 to 14 days or longer (Conte and Barriere, 1984). Nafcillin usually is not recommended in neonates or patients with hepatic disease.

DRUG INTERACTIONS AND INTERFERENCE WITH LABORATORY TESTS. Warfarin resistance, demonstrated by decreased prothrombin time, was observed in one patient receiving high-dose intravenous nafcillin therapy. The warfarin half-life was markedly reduced when the patient received nafcillin. Both the prothrombin time and warfarin half-life gradually returned to expected values after discontinuation of nafcillin (Qureshi et al, 1984).

For additional information, see the Introduction.

PHARMACOKINETICS. Comparative pharmacokinetic data on the penicillins appear in the Table.

Although nafcillin is available for oral administration, absorption is usually low (10% to 20% of a dose) and erratic. Thus, this antistaphylococcal penicillin primarily is administered parenterally. Peak serum concentrations of 5 to 8 mcg/ml are attained 60 minutes after intramuscular injection of 500 mg. After an intravenous dose of 15 mg/kg, peak serum concentrations range between 20 and 40 mcg/ml.

Nafcillin exhibits significantly greater plasma protein binding than methicillin but is less protein bound than the isoxazolyl derivatives. Like other penicillins, nafcillin primarily distributes into the extracellular fluid volume. Concentrations achieved in bile in the absence of obstruction are higher than with other antistaphylococcal penicillins. Penetration into cerebrospinal fluid is adequate in the presence of inflammation.

Unlike other penicillins, nafcillin is primarily excreted by the liver and, to a lesser extent, by the kidney. The half-life is increased minimally (to 80 minutes) in anuric patients, and dosage adjustments are not required in these patients. However, dosage adjustments are necessary if there also is coexisting hepatic dysfunction. For additional discussion, see the Introduction. Nafcillin pharmacokinetics in the newborn are erratic, especially in those with jaundice.

DOSAGE AND PREPARATIONS.

Oral: Serum concentrations of nafcillin after oral administration are low and unpredictable, and this route is not recommended. The following dosages are included only for completeness. Nafcillin should be administered at least one hour before or two hours after meals. *Adults,* 2 to 4 g daily in equally divided doses every six hours; *children,* 50 to 100 mg/kg daily in four divided doses every six hours.

Strengths expressed in terms of the base:
Unipen (Wyeth-Ayerst). Capsules (buffered) 250 mg; powder for oral solution 250 mg/5 ml; tablets (buffered) 500 mg.

Intramuscular, Intravenous: Nafcillin can be administered by intramuscular injection (solution containing 250 mg/ml), direct intravenous injection (required amount of drug diluted in 15 to 30 ml and injected over 5 to 10 minutes), or by continuous intravenous drip. See the manufacturers' instructions for the appropriate dilution of the drug, a list of compatible diluents and intravenous solutions, and stability of nafcillin in these solutions. When used with other drugs, nafcillin should not be physically mixed with the other agent(s).

Adults, 2 to 9 g daily in equally divided doses every four to six hours; up to 12 g daily can be given for severe infections (The Medical Letter, 1990). *Children*, 100 to 200 mg/kg daily in equally divided doses every four to six hours (The Medical Letter, 1990). Although nafcillin generally is not recommended for newborn infants, the following dosage guidelines are presented: *infants over 7 days and weighing more than 2 kg*, 150 mg/kg daily in divided doses every six hours; *infants over 7 days and weighing 1.2 to 2 kg*, 75 mg/kg daily in divided doses every eight hours; *infants under 7 days and weighing more than 2 kg*, 60 mg/kg daily in divided doses every eight hours; *infants under 7 days and weighing 1.2 to 2 kg*, 50 mg/kg daily in divided doses every 12 hours; *infants 0 to 28 days and weighing less than 1.2 kg,* 50 mg/kg daily in two doses every 12 hours (Nelson, 1991 B).

Dosage adjustments are not required in patients with impaired renal function.

Strengths expressed in terms of the base:
Nafcil (Apothecon), ***Nallpen*** (SmithKline Beecham), ***Unipen*** (Wyeth-Ayerst), ***Generic.*** Powder (buffered) 500 mg and 1, 2, and 10 g (sodium, 2.9 mEq/g).

OXACILLIN SODIUM
[Bactocill, Prostaphlin]

MECHANISM OF ACTION, ANTIMICROBIAL SPECTRUM, AND RESISTANCE. Oxacillin is a semisynthetic, penicillinase-resistant penicillin for parenteral or oral use. This isoxazolyl derivative is chemically related to cloxacillin and dicloxacillin. Its mechanism of action and antimicrobial spectrum are the same as for methicillin (see that evaluation and the Introduction). On a weight basis, oxacillin is more potent than methicillin in vitro against susceptible bacteria.

USES. The indications for parenteral oxacillin are the same as those for methicillin; the primary use is serious infections caused by *Staphylococcus aureus* or other staphylococci (see the evaluation on Methicillin). Oxacillin (or nafcillin) usually is preferred to methicillin in adults and older children because of the association of interstitial nephritis with the latter agent. Oral oxacillin is an alternative to dicloxacillin and cloxacillin for the treatment of mild to moderate *S. aureus* infections of the skin and soft tissues, respiratory and genitourinary tracts, and joints.

For additional discussion on Uses, see the Introduction; index entry Antimicrobial Drugs; and the evaluations on Methicillin, Nafcillin, Cloxacillin, and Dicloxacillin. See also Neu, 1982 A, 1990; Reese and Betts, 1991.

ADVERSE REACTIONS AND PRECAUTIONS. Oxacillin is generally well tolerated; untoward effects are usually mild and most commonly consist of the allergic and other reactions typical of all penicillins (see the Introduction). Elevations in hepatic enzymes (eg, AST, ALT) have been reported more frequently with oxacillin than other antistaphylococcal penicillins. Reversible cholestatic hepatitis also has occurred. Abnormal results of liver function tests are reversible when the drug is discontinued (see Neu, 1982 A).

DRUG INTERACTIONS AND INTERFERENCE WITH LABORATORY TESTS. See the Introduction.

PHARMACOKINETICS. Comparative pharmacokinetic data on the penicillins appear in the Table.

Oxacillin can be administered orally, intramuscularly, and intravenously. Although it is stable in gastric acid, only a small percentage of an oral dose is absorbed from the gastrointestinal tract. Following administration of 500 mg to fasting individuals, total peak serum concentrations of 4 to 6 mcg/ml are attained in about one hour; peak concentrations of free drug are approximately 0.6 mcg/ml. Although peak serum concentrations of total (ie, bound and unbound) oxacillin are lower than with equivalent doses of cloxacillin and dicloxacillin, free drug concentrations are similar for all three derivatives due to differences in plasma protein binding. Like other penicillins, oxacillin primarily distributes into the extracellular fluid volume. The presence of food in the gastrointestinal tract decreases the absorption of oxacillin, and this drug preferably should be administered one hour before or two hours after meals.

Following intramuscular injection of 500 mg, peak serum concentrations of 14 to 16 mcg/ml are achieved after 30 to 60 minutes. A peak of approximately 30 to 40 mcg/ml is obtained in serum one hour after a 1-g intravenous dose.

Oxacillin is rapidly eliminated, primarily by renal tubular secretion; probenecid delays its excretion. Oxacillin is metabolized to a greater extent than other isoxazolyl penicillins. The half-life is increased minimally (to 30 to 60 minutes) in anuric patients, and dosage adjustments are not required in these patients. For additional discussion, see the Introduction.

DOSAGE AND PREPARATIONS.

Oral: Oxacillin should be taken at least one hour before or two hours after meals. *Adults and children weighing more than 40 kg,* 500 mg to 1 g every six hours; *less than 40 kg,* 50 to 100 mg/kg daily in divided doses every six hours.

Strengths expressed in terms of the base:
Bactocill (SmithKline Beecham). Capsules 250 and 500 mg.
Prostaphlin (Apothecon), ***Generic.*** Capsules 250 and 500 mg; powder (for oral solution) 250 mg/5 ml.

Intramuscular, Intravenous: Oxacillin can be administered by intramuscular injection (solution containing 250 mg/1.5 ml), direct intravenous injection (solution containing ≤100 mg/ml and injected slowly to avoid vein irritation), or by continuous intravenous drip. See the manufacturers' instructions for the appropriate dilution of the drug, a list of compatible diluents and intravenous solutions, and stability of oxacillin in these solutions. When used in conjunction with other drugs, oxacillin should not be physically mixed with the other agent(s).

Adults, 2 to 12 g daily in equally divided doses every six hours (maximum daily dose, 12 g) (The Medical Letter, 1990). *Children*, 100 to 200 mg/kg daily in equally divided doses every six hours (The Medical Letter, 1990). *Infants over 7 days and weighing more than 2 kg*, 150 mg/kg daily in divided doses every six hours; *infants over 7 days and weighing 1.2 to 2 kg*, 90 mg/kg daily in divided doses every eight hours; *infants under 7 days and weighing more than 2 kg*, 75 mg/kg daily in divided doses every eight hours; *infants under 7 days and weighing 1.2 to 2 kg*, 50 mg/kg daily in divided doses every 12 hours; *infants 0 to 28 days and weighing less than 1.2 kg,* 50 mg/kg daily in two doses every 12 hours (Nelson, 1991 B).

Dosage adjustments are not required in patients with renal impairment.

Strengths expressed in terms of the base:
Bactocill (SmithKline Beecham). Powder 500 mg and 1, 2, 4, and 10 g (sodium, 3.1 mEq/g).
Prostaphlin (Apothecon), ***Generic.*** Powder 250 and 500 mg and 1, 2, 4, and 10 g (sodium, 2.8 mEq/g).

CLOXACILLIN SODIUM
[Cloxapen, Tegopen]

MECHANISM OF ACTION, ANTIMICROBIAL SPECTRUM, AND RESISTANCE. Cloxacillin is a semisynthetic, penicillinase-resistant penicillin for oral use. This isoxazolyl derivative is chemically related to oxacillin and dicloxacillin. The mechanism of action and antimicrobial spectrum are the same as for methicillin (see that evaluation and the Introduction). On a weight basis, cloxacillin is more potent than methicillin in vitro against susceptible bacteria.

USES. Orally administered cloxacillin (or dicloxacillin) is a preferred drug for the treatment of mild to moderate *Staphylococcus aureus* (and other staphylococcal) infections of the skin and soft tissue (the most common use), respiratory and genitourinary tracts, and joints. For more severe infections, a parenteral penicillinase-resistant penicillin should be used initially (see evaluations of Methicillin, Nafcillin, and Oxacillin).

For additional discussion on Uses, see the Introduction, index entry Antimicrobial Drugs, and the evaluation on Dicloxacillin. See also Neu, 1982 A, 1990; Reese and Betts, 1991.

ADVERSE REACTIONS AND PRECAUTIONS. Cloxacillin generally is well tolerated; untoward effects are usually mild and most commonly consist of gastrointestinal disturbances or the allergic and other reactions typical of all penicillins (see the Introduction). Symptoms of hepatitis have rarely been associated with elevated serum concentrations of liver enzymes (eg, ALT, AST) in patients given cloxacillin.

The oral suspension has a bitter taste and may not be accepted by young children.

DRUG INTERACTIONS AND INTERFERENCE WITH LABORATORY TESTS. See the Introduction.

PHARMACOKINETICS. Comparative pharmacokinetic data on the penicillins appear in the Table.

Cloxacillin is stable in gastric acid and is absorbed from the gastrointestinal tract. Following administration of 500 mg to fasting individuals, total peak serum concentrations of approximately 10 mcg/ml are attained in about one hour; peak concentrations of free drug are 0.6 mcg/ml. Although peak serum concentrations of total (ie, bound and unbound) cloxacillin are lower than with equivalent doses of dicloxacillin, the levels of free drug are similar due to differences in plasma protein binding. The presence of food in the gastrointestinal tract decreases the absorption of cloxacillin, and this drug preferably should be administered one hour before or two hours after meals.

Among the isoxazolyl penicillins, cloxacillin is less bound to plasma proteins than dicloxacillin but more bound than oxacillin (see the evaluations). Like other penicillins, cloxacillin primarily distributes into the extracellular fluid volume.

Cloxacillin is rapidly eliminated, primarily by renal tubular secretion; probenecid delays its excretion. The half-life is not significantly increased in anuric patients, and dosage adjustments are not required in these patients. For additional discussion, see the Introduction.

DOSAGE AND PREPARATIONS.

Oral: Cloxacillin should be taken at least one hour before or two hours after meals. *Adults and children weighing 20 kg or more*, 500 mg to 1 g every six hours (250 mg every six hours is recommended by the manufacturer for mild to moderate upper respiratory tract infections or localized skin and soft tissue infections). *Children weighing less than 20 kg,* 50 to 100 mg/kg daily in four equal doses every six hours.

A parenteral penicillinase-resistant penicillin (eg, nafcillin, oxacillin) should be used initially for serious staphylococcal infections.

Strengths expressed in terms of the base:
Cloxapen (SmithKline Beecham). Capsules 250 and 500 mg.
Tegopen (Apothecon), ***Generic***. Capsules 250 and 500 mg; powder for oral solution 125 mg/5 ml.

DICLOXACILLIN SODIUM
[Dycill, Dynapen, Pathocil]

MECHANISM OF ACTION, ANTIMICROBIAL SPECTRUM, AND RESISTANCE. Dicloxacillin is a semisynthetic, penicillinase-resistant penicillin for oral use. This isoxazolyl derivative is chemically related to cloxacillin and oxacillin. The mechanism of action and antimicrobial spectrum are the same as for methicillin (see that evaluation and the Introduction). On a weight basis, dicloxacillin is more potent than methicillin in vitro against susceptible bacteria.

USES. Orally administered dicloxacillin (or cloxacillin) is a preferred drug for the treatment of mild to moderate *Staphylococcus aureus* (and other staphylococcal) infections of the skin and soft tissues (the most common use), respiratory and genitourinary tracts, and joints. For more severe infections, a parenteral penicillinase-resistant penicillin should be used initially (see evaluations of Methicillin, Nafcillin, and Oxacillin).

For additional discussion on Uses, see the Introduction; index entry Antimicrobial Drugs; and the evaluation of Cloxacillin. See also Neu, 1982 A, 1990; Reese and Betts, 1991.

ADVERSE REACTIONS AND PRECAUTIONS. Dicloxacillin generally is well tolerated; untoward effects are usually mild and most commonly consist of gastrointestinal disturbances or the allergic and other reactions typical of all penicillins (see the Introduction). Symptoms of hepatitis rarely have been associated with elevated serum concentrations of liver enzymes (eg, ALT, AST) in patients given dicloxacillin.

The oral suspension has a bitter taste and may not be accepted by young children.

DRUG INTERACTIONS AND INTERFERENCE WITH LABORATORY TESTS. Dicloxacillin has been reported to shorten prothrombin times in patients receiving warfarin (Krstenansky et al, 1987). Thus, an altered response to warfarin is a possibility if dicloxacillin therapy is initiated or discontinued (see Hansten, 1984). For additional information, see the Introduction.

PHARMACOKINETICS. Comparative pharmacokinetic data on the penicillins appear in the Table.

Dicloxacillin is stable in gastric acid and is absorbed from the gastrointestinal tract. Following administration of 500 mg to fasting individuals, total peak serum concentrations of approximately 15 mcg/ml are attained in about one hour; peak concentrations of free drug are 0.6 mcg/ml. Although peak serum concentrations of total (ie, bound and unbound) dicloxacillin are higher than with equivalent doses of cloxacillin, those of free drug are similar due to differences in plasma protein binding. The presence of food in the gastrointestinal tract decreases the absorption of dicloxacillin, and this drug preferably should be administered one hour before or two hours after meals.

Dicloxacillin is the most highly protein bound isoxazolyl penicillin (see the evaluations of Oxacillin and Cloxacillin). Like other penicillins, dicloxacillin primarily distributes into the extracellular fluid volume.

Dicloxacillin is rapidly eliminated, primarily by renal tubular secretion; probenecid delays its excretion. The half-life is not significantly increased in anuric patients, and dosage adjustments are not required in these patients. For additional discussion, see the Introduction.

DOSAGE AND PREPARATIONS.

Oral: Dicloxacillin should be taken at least one hour before or two hours after meals. *Adults and children weighing 40 kg or more*, 1 to 2 g daily in equally divided doses every six hours (maximum daily dose, 4 g) (The Medical Letter, 1990) (125 mg every six hours is recommended by the manufacturer for mild to moderate upper respiratory tract infections or localized skin and soft tissue infections.) *Children weighing less than 40 kg*, 12.5 to 25 mg/kg daily in equally divided doses every six hours (The Medical Letter, 1990).

A parenteral penicillinase-resistant penicillin (eg, nafcillin, oxacillin) should be used initially for serious staphylococcal infections.

Strengths expressed in terms of the base:
Dycill (SmithKline Beecham), ***Generic.*** Capsules 250 and 500 mg.
Dynapen (Apothecon). Capsules 125, 250, and 500 mg; powder for oral suspension 62.5 mg/5 ml.
Pathocil (Wyeth-Ayerst). Capsules 250 and 500 mg; powder for oral suspension 62.5 mg/5 ml.

AMINOPENICILLINS

AMPICILLIN
[Omnipen, Polycillin, Principen, Totacillin]

AMPICILLIN SODIUM
[Omnipen-N, Polycillin-N, Totacillin-N]

MECHANISM OF ACTION, ANTIMICROBIAL SPECTRUM, AND RESISTANCE. Ampicillin is a semisynthetic penicillin for oral and parenteral use. It inhibits cell wall formation in susceptible bacteria and usually is bactericidal.

Like penicillin G, ampicillin is active in vitro against most gram-positive bacteria (except β-lactamase-producing staphylococci), gram-negative cocci, and anaerobic bacteria (except the *Bacteroides fragilis* group). However, this aminopenicillin also is active against certain aerobic gram-negative bacilli and thus has a broader antimicrobial spectrum than penicillin G.

Ampicillin is hydrolyzed by β-lactamases produced by various bacteria and is not active against strains that produce these enzymes.

For a detailed discussion of the mechanism of action and antimicrobial spectrum of the penicillins, see the Introduction.

USES. Ampicillin is usually bactericidal, has a high therapeutic index, can be administered parenterally as well as orally, and is relatively inexpensive. Thus, it frequently is a preferred drug for infections caused by susceptible organisms at a wide variety of sites in nonallergic patients, although it usually should not be substituted for penicillin G when the latter drug is equally effective. Many experts prefer amoxicillin over ampicillin for oral administration because gastrointestinal absorption of amoxicillin is intrinsically greater, resulting in higher serum concentrations; the presence of food in the gastrointestinal tract does not interfere with its absorption; and amoxicillin appears to cause diarrhea less frequently. Other aminopenicillins (bacampicillin, cyclacillin) do not appear to offer any significant advantages over these two drugs and they are more expensive (see the evaluations).

Ampicillin also is frequently employed in combination with another antibiotic for empiric therapy when one or more of a number of possible causative organisms may be involved and susceptibility to ampicillin is not known, and for antibacterial synergism.

For a more detailed discussion on Uses, see the Introduction and index entry Antimicrobial Drugs. See also Parry, 1987; Neu, 1990; Reese and Betts, 1991.

ADVERSE REACTIONS AND PRECAUTIONS. Ampicillin is usually well tolerated. Adverse reactions are generally mild and consist most often of skin rashes or diarrhea. The incidence of diarrhea has been reported to be up to 11% in adults and 20% in children. Diarrhea usually is not severe enough to require discontinuing the drug. However, antibiotic-associated pseudomembranous colitis (AAPMC) caused by *Clostridium difficile* may occur during ampicillin therapy. Although this adverse effect is relatively rare, ampicillin has been one of the more frequently implicated antibiotics in this condition. This potentially life-threatening adverse effect requires prompt discontinuation of ampicillin, maintenance of fluid and electrolyte balance, and possible therapy with oral metronidazole or vancomycin (see also index entry Lincosamides).

Other adverse reactions, both allergic and nonallergic, that are typical of all penicillins can occur with ampicillin. For a detailed discussion, see the Introduction.

DRUG INTERACTIONS AND INTERFERENCE WITH LABORATORY TESTS. Isolated cases of breakthrough bleeding and pregnancy have been reported in women receiving oral contraceptives and oral ampicillin. The clinical significance of this observation is unknown, but the addition of other forms of contraception appears warranted when a course of ampicillin therapy is initiated in these women (see Back et al, 1981; Hansten and Horn, 1985; and index entry Contraceptives, Oral).

Either allopurinol or hyperuricemia appears to predispose patients receiving ampicillin to rashes (Jick and Porter, 1981). No special precautions appear to be necessary, however (Hansten, 1985 A).

The bioavailability of atenolol [Tenormin] was reported to be decreased by concurrent administration of oral ampicillin in six healthy volunteers; exercise tachycardia was significantly higher in those given both drugs than in those who received atenolol alone (Schäfer-Korting et al, 1983). Although additional data are required to confirm the clinical significance of this interaction, it should be recognized that an altered response to atenolol may occur if ampicillin therapy is started or stopped (Hansten, 1985 B). For additional information, see the Introduction.

PHARMACOKINETICS. Comparative pharmacokinetic data on the penicillins appear in the Table.

Ampicillin can be administered orally, intramuscularly, and intravenously. It is stable in gastric acid, but is not absorbed well from the gastrointestinal tract. Following a 500-mg dose to fasting individuals, peak serum concentrations of 2.5 to 5 mcg/ml are attained in one to two hours. The presence of food in the gastrointestinal tract decreases absorption. Following intramuscular injection of 500 mg of ampicillin, peak serum concentrations of approximately 8 mcg/ml are achieved within one hour. A peak of approximately 8 to 37 mcg/ml is obtained in serum after a 1-g intravenous dose.

Like other penicillins, ampicillin primarily distributes into the extracellular fluid volume. High concentrations are achieved in bile and urine. Penetration into cerebrospinal fluid is adequate in the presence of inflammation.

Ampicillin is rapidly eliminated, primarily by renal tubular secretion; probenecid delays its excretion. Urinary recovery of unchanged drug is higher after parenteral administration than after oral administration (due to incomplete absorption). The half-life is prolonged in patients with renal impairment (eg, 8 to 12 hours in anuric patients) and dosage adjustments are necessary. For additional discussion, see the Introduction.

DOSAGE AND PREPARATIONS.

AMPICILLIN (TRIHYDRATE OR ANHYDROUS):

Oral: Ampicillin preferably is given one hour before or two hours after meals. *Adults*, 2 to 4 g daily in equally divided doses every six to eight hours; *children,* 50 to 100 mg/kg daily in equally divided doses every six to eight hours (The Medical Letter, 1990).

For dosages for uncomplicated gonococcal infections, see index entry on this subject.

Strengths expressed in terms of the base:

Generic. Capsules 250 and 500 mg; powder for oral suspension 125 and 250 mg/5 ml; solution (oral) 100 mg/ml.

Omnipen (Wyeth-Ayerst). Capsules (anhydrous) 250 and 500 mg; powder for oral suspension (trihydrate) 125 and 250 mg/5 ml.

Polycillin (Apothecon). Capsules (trihydrate) 250 and 500 mg; powder for oral suspension (trihydrate) 125, 250, and 500 mg/5 ml; solution (oral) 100 mg/ml (pediatric).

Principen (Apothecon), ***Totacillin*** (SmithKline Beecham). Capsules (trihydrate) 250 and 500 mg; powder for oral suspension (trihydrate) 125 and 250 mg/5 ml.

Available Mixtures.

NOTE: The following are used for uncomplicated infections (urethral, endocervical, rectal) caused by susceptible *N. gonorrhoeae* in adults.

Polycillin-PRB (Apothecon), ***Generic.*** Powder for oral suspension containing ampicillin (trihydrate) 3.5 g and probenecid 1 g in a single-dose bottle.

Principen W/Probenecid (Apothecon). Capsules containing ampicillin (trihydrate) 389 mg and probenecid 111 mg/nine-capsule package.

AMPICILLIN SODIUM:

Intravenous, Intramuscular: Ampicillin can be administered by intramuscular injection, direct intravenous injection, or intravenous drip. The intravenous route generally is preferred. See the manufacturers' literature for the appropriate dilution of the drug, a list of compatible diluents and intravenous solutions, and stability of ampicillin in those solutions.

Adults, 2 to 12 g daily in equally divided doses every six to eight hours; the maximum daily dose in equally divided doses every four hours should be used for meningitis (The Medical Letter, 1990). *Children*, 100 to 200 mg/kg daily in equally divided doses every six to eight hours; for meningitis caused by ampicillin-sensitive *H. influenzae* type b, up to 400 mg/kg daily in equally divided doses every four hours is recommended (The Medical Letter, 1990).

Infants over 7 days and weighing more than 2 kg, 100 mg/kg daily in divided doses every six hours; for meningitis, 200 mg/kg daily in divided doses every six hours; *infants over 7 days and weighing 1.2 to 2 kg*, 75 mg/kg daily in divided doses every eight hours; for meningitis, 150 mg/kg daily in divided doses every eight hours; *infants under 7 days and weighing more than 2 kg*, 75 mg/kg daily in divided doses every eight hours; for meningitis, 150 mg/kg daily in divided doses every eight hours; *infants under 7 days and weighing 1.2 to 2 kg*, 50 mg/kg daily in divided doses every 12 hours; for meningitis, 100 mg/kg daily in divided doses every 12 hours; *infants 0 to 28 days and weighing less than 1.2 kg*, 50 mg/kg daily in two doses every 12 hours; for meningitis, 100 mg/kg daily in two doses every 12 hours (Nelson, 1991 B).

In the presence of severe renal impairment (creatinine clearance, 10 ml/min or less), the dosage interval should be increased to 12 hours (The Medical Letter, 1990).

For dosage recommendations in the prophylaxis of infective endocarditis, see index entry on this disease.

Strengths expressed in terms of the base:

Omnipen-N (Wyeth-Ayerst), ***Polycillin-N*** (Apothecon), ***Generic.*** Powder 125, 250, and 500 mg and 1, 2, and 10 g.

Totacillin-N (SmithKline Beecham). Powder 250 and 500 mg and 1, 2, and 10 g.

AMOXICILLIN TRIHYDRATE

[Amoxil, Larotid, Polymox, Trimox, Wymox]

MECHANISM OF ACTION, ANTIMICROBIAL SPECTRUM, AND RESISTANCE. Amoxicillin is a semisynthetic aminopenicillin for oral use. The in vitro antimicrobial spectrum of amoxicillin is essentially identical to that of ampicillin (see the evaluation). However, because amoxicillin has somewhat less activity than ampicillin against *Shigella* species and is absorbed from the gastrointestinal tract to a much greater extent than the latter, it is not useful clinically for the gastrointestinal infections caused by this pathogen.

Amoxicillin is hydrolyzed by β-lactamases produced by various bacteria and is not active against these strains. For a detailed discussion of the mechanism of action and antimicrobial spectrum of the penicillins, see the Introduction.

USES. Infections for which amoxicillin is the preferred or alternative drug are discussed in the Introduction. See also index entry Antimicrobial Drugs and Parry, 1987; Neu, 1990; Reese and Betts, 1991.

Many infectious disease experts prefer amoxicillin to ampicillin for infections requiring oral administration (see Pharmacokinetics). Other aminopenicillins (bacampicillin, cyclacillin) do not appear to offer any significant advantage over amoxicillin and they are more expensive (see the evaluations). See also McCracken, 1983.

ADVERSE REACTIONS AND PRECAUTIONS. Adverse reactions to amoxicillin are similar to those seen with ampicillin. However, diarrhea occurs less frequently with amoxicillin, particularly in children (see the evaluation of Ampicillin and the Introduction).

DRUG INTERACTIONS AND INTERFERENCE WITH LABORATORY TESTS. See the Introduction.

PHARMACOKINETICS. Comparative pharmacokinetic data on the penicillins appear in the Table.

Amoxicillin is stable in gastric acid and is well absorbed from the gastrointestinal tract. Following a dose of 500 mg, peak serum concentrations range from 6 to 8 mcg/ml after one to two hours. Because amoxicillin has better bioavailability than ampicillin and, in contrast to the latter drug, absorption is not appreciably affected by the presence of food in the gastrointestinal tract, many experts prefer this aminopenicillin for oral administration.

Like other penicillins, amoxicillin primarily distributes into the extracellular fluid volume. High concentrations are achieved in bile and urine. Amoxicillin is rapidly eliminated, primarily by renal tubular secretion; probenecid delays its excretion. The half-life is prolonged in patients with renal impairment (eg, 8 to 16 hours in anuric patients), and dosage adjustments are necessary. For additional discussion, see the Introduction.

DOSAGE AND PREPARATIONS.

Oral: *Adults and children weighing more than 20 kg*, 750 mg to 1.5 g daily; *less than 20 kg*, 20 to 40 mg/kg daily. These daily doses are administered in divided portions at eight-hour intervals. The larger doses are used in more severe infections. In the presence of severe renal impairment (creatinine clearance, 10 ml/min or less), the adult dose probably should not exceed 500 mg every 12 hours.

For dosage recommendations in gonorrhea, see index entry Gonococcal Infections.

Amoxil (SmithKline Beecham), ***Polymox*** (Apothecon), ***Generic.*** Capsules 250 and 500 mg; powder for oral suspension 50 mg/ml (pediatric) and 125 and 250 mg/5 ml; tablets (chewable) 125 and 250 mg (***Amoxil*** only).

Larotid (SmithKline Beecham), **Trimox** (Apothecon), ***Wymox*** (Wyeth-Ayerst). Capsules 250 and 500 mg; powder for oral suspension 125 and 250 mg/5 ml.

BACAMPICILLIN HYDROCHLORIDE

[Spectrobid]

MECHANISM OF ACTION, ANTIMICROBIAL SPECTRUM, AND RESISTANCE. Bacampicillin is the 1-ethoxycarbonyloxyethyl ester of ampicillin. This prodrug has little antibacterial action itself but is rapidly and completely converted to ampicillin in vivo by hydrolytic cleavage of the ester moiety from the ampicillin base. The antibacterial spectrum of bacampicillin is identical to that of ampicillin (see the Introduction and the evaluation).

USES. The uses of bacampicillin are very similar to those of oral ampicillin or amoxicillin. Bacampicillin does not appear to offer any significant clinical advantages over amoxicillin for routine use and it is more expensive (see the evaluation on Amoxicillin; see also Scheife and Neu, 1982; McCracken, 1983).

ADVERSE REACTIONS AND PRECAUTIONS. Adverse reactions to bacampicillin are similar to those seen with ampicillin. However, diarrhea occurs less frequently with bacampicillin, presumably due to more complete absorption (see the evaluation on Ampicillin and the Introduction; see also Scheife and Neu, 1982).

DRUG INTERACTIONS AND INTERFERENCE WITH LABORATORY TESTS. See the Introduction. The manufacturer recommends that bacampicillin not be given with disulfiram [Antabuse] because products of bacampicillin hydrolysis include acetaldehyde and ethanol.

PHARMACOKINETICS. Comparative pharmacokinetic data on the penicillins appear in the Table.

Bacampicillin is stable in gastric acid. It is rapidly and almost completely absorbed from the gastrointestinal tract following oral administration. During the process of absorption, bacampicillin is hydrolyzed to ampicillin, the active drug; approximately 1.4 mg of bacampicillin is equivalent to 1 mg of ampicillin. Following 400, 800, and 1,600 mg doses of bacampicillin, average peak serum ampicillin concentrations of 7.9, 12.9, and 20.1 mcg/ml, respectively, are attained in 45 to 60 minutes. These are considerably higher than those obtained with equivalent doses of ampicillin because of the superior absorption of the prodrug. In contrast to ampicillin, the presence of food in the gastrointestinal tract does not decrease the absorption of bacampicillin.

Following hydrolysis of the prodrug, the distribution and elimination of bacampicillin-derived ampicillin are the same as for ampicillin. However, concentrations in tissues and body fluids generally are higher after bacampicillin. Approximately 75% of a dose is recovered from urine as active ampicillin within eight hours. (See the evaluation of ampicillin and the Introduction; see also Neu, 1981.)

DOSAGE AND PREPARATIONS. The interval between doses recommended by the manufacturer is longer than that for ampicillin or amoxicillin. This so-called "pulse-dosing" appears to produce equally effective results but offers no clear-cut advantage over more frequent administration of ampicillin or amoxicillin and this drug is considerably more expensive.

Oral: *Adults*, 800 mg to 1.6 g daily in equally divided doses every 12 hours; *children*, 25 to 50 mg/kg daily in equally divided doses every 12 hours. In the presence of severe renal impairment (creatinine clearance, 10 ml/min or less), the adult dose probably should not exceed 800 mg every 24 hours (The Medical Letter, 1990).

Spectrobid (Roerig). Tablets 400 mg (equivalent to 280 mg ampicillin); powder for oral suspension 125 mg/5 ml (equivalent to 87.5 mg ampicillin).

CYCLACILLIN

MECHANISM OF ACTION, ANTIMICROBIAL SPECTRUM, AND RESISTANCE. Cyclacillin is an oral aminopenicillin that is chemically related to ampicillin. The in vitro antimicrobial spectrum of cyclacillin is similar to that of ampicillin and amoxicillin. However, on a weight basis, cyclacillin is less active than these other aminopenicillins. Cyclacillin is inactivated by β-lactamase-producing bacterial strains. See the evaluations of Ampicillin and Amoxicillin and the Introduction.

USES. The uses of cyclacillin are very similar to those of oral ampicillin and amoxicillin. Cyclacillin does not appear to offer any significant clinical advantages over amoxicillin and it is more expensive (see the evaluation of Amoxicillin).

ADVERSE REACTIONS AND PRECAUTIONS. Adverse reactions to cyclacillin are similar to those seen with ampicillin. However, diarrhea occurs less frequently with cyclacillin, presumably due to more complete absorption (see the evaluation of Ampicillin).

DRUG INTERACTIONS AND INTERFERENCE WITH LABORATORY TESTS. See the Introduction.

PHARMACOKINETICS. Comparative pharmacokinetic data on the penicillins appear in the Table.

Cyclacillin is stable in gastric acid, and it is rapidly and almost completely (95%) absorbed from the gastrointestinal tract after oral administration. Following a dose of 500 mg, peak serum concentrations of 11 to 12 mcg/ml are achieved in 40 to 60 minutes. The effect of food on absorption is not known. Although peak serum concentrations of cyclacillin are higher and appear earlier than those obtained with a comparable (ie, 500 mg) dose of ampicillin, cyclacillin is eliminated more rapidly; serum cyclacillin concentrations are lower than those of ampicillin after three hours (see below). Consequently, no differences in clinical efficacy have been reported. See also the evaluation of Ampicillin and the Introduction.

A low percentage of cyclacillin is bound to plasma proteins, and it penetrates into most tissues and body fluids. Cyclacillin is rapidly eliminated, primarily by renal tubular secretion; probenecid delays excretion. The half-life is prolonged in patients with renal impairment, and dosage adjustments are necessary.

DOSAGE AND PREPARATIONS.
Oral: *Adults*, 1 to 2 g daily in equally divided doses every six hours; *children*, 50 to 100 mg/kg daily in equally divided doses every six hours (The Medical Letter, 1990).

For patients with reduced renal function, the dosage interval should be increased to 12 to 24 hours when creatinine clearance is 50 to 10 ml/min and to 24 hours when it is less than 10 ml/min (The Medical Letter, 1990).

Generic. Tablets 250 and 500 mg.

ANTIPSEUDOMONAL PENICILLINS

CARBENICILLIN INDANYL SODIUM
[Geocillin]

Oral carbenicillin indanyl, a semisynthetic carboxypenicillin, is hydrolyzed in the body to carbenicillin, the active metabolite. Although plasma concentrations are low, the active drug is rapidly excreted in the urine and is useful only in the treatment of urinary tract infections caused by susceptible gram-negative bacilli, particularly *Pseudomonas aeruginosa, Enterobacter*, and *Proteus* species. Carbenicillin indanyl also has been used in chronic prostatitis due to susceptible bacteria, but other drugs are now preferred for this indication.

For a more detailed discussion, see index entries Urinary Tract Infections and Prostatitis.

ADVERSE REACTIONS AND PRECAUTIONS. Carbenicillin indanyl sodium is relatively well tolerated, but any of the adverse reactions generally associated with the use of penicillins may occur with this derivative (see the Introduction). See also Neu, 1982 B.

DRUG INTERACTIONS. Elevated serum methotrexate levels have been reported in a patient receiving large doses (30 g daily) of carbenicillin concomitantly. An enhanced methotrexate effect may be observed (see Hansten, 1985 A). For a discussion of other potential drug interactions involving the penicillins, see the Introduction.

PHARMACOKINETICS. Carbenicillin indanyl is stable in gastric acid. After oral administration, the prodrug is absorbed from the gastrointestinal tract and is rapidly hydrolyzed to carbenicillin, the active drug. Peak serum concentrations of about 10 mcg/ml are attained approximately one hour after administration of two tablets (equivalent to 764 mg of carbenicillin). These are inadequate for systemic infections, and this drug is indicated only for urinary tract infections and prostatitis (see Uses and the Table).

For additional discussion, see the Introduction.

DOSAGE AND PREPARATIONS.
Oral: For urinary tract infections in *adults,* one to two tablets four times daily. Clinical data are insufficient to recommend a dose for *children.* (See also the manufacturer's literature.)

This drug should be avoided in patients with severe renal impairment (creatinine clearance, 10 ml/min or less).

Geocillin (Roerig). Tablets equivalent to 382 mg of carbenicillin.

TICARCILLIN DISODIUM
[Ticar]

MECHANISM OF ACTION, ANTIMICROBIAL SPECTRUM, AND RESISTANCE. Ticarcillin disodium is a semisynthetic carboxypenicillin that is not absorbed orally and thus must be given either intravenously or intramuscularly. The antibacterial spectrum of ticarcillin provides wider coverage than the aminopenicillins against gram-negative bacilli and includes *Pseudomonas aeruginosa* and the *Bacteroides fragilis* group.

Ticarcillin is inactivated by various β-lactamases. The number of ticarcillin-resistant strains is quite large for many bacteria, and susceptibility testing is usually necessary before institution of therapy, especially when ticarcillin is used alone.

For a detailed discussion of the mechanism of action and antimicrobial spectrum of the penicillins, see the Introduction.

USES. The primary indications for ticarcillin are suspected or proven infections caused by *P. aeruginosa*. It may be used in bacterial septicemia and skin and soft tissue, respiratory tract, genitourinary tract, and intra-abdominal infections.

The combination of ticarcillin with an aminoglycoside frequently results in antibacterial synergism against *P. aeruginosa*, and combination therapy is recommended for systemic infections caused by this pathogen. Whether the newer ureidopenicillins (piperacillin and mezlocillin) offer significant clinical advantages over ticarcillin is currently unresolved. These newer agents have potential advantages in institutions where ticarcillin-resistant, but ureidopenicillin-susceptible, strains of *P. aeruginosa* (or other gram-negative bacilli) are a problem or when their broader antimicrobial spectrum is desirable. Furthermore, at usual therapeutic doses, piperacillin and mezlocillin contain less sodium per gram than ticarcillin, which is an advantage in patients who must severely restrict sodium intake, and they also may have less effect on platelet aggregation (see the evaluations and the Introduction).

For a more detailed discussion on the uses of antipseudomonal penicillins, see the Introduction and the index entry Antimicrobial Drugs. See also Parry, 1987; Neu, 1990; Reese and Betts, 1991.

ADVERSE REACTIONS AND PRECAUTIONS. Adverse reactions to ticarcillin include various hypersensitivity reactions, dose-related inhibition of platelet aggregation with the potential for bleeding, and hypokalemia. Each gram of ticarcillin disodium contains 5.2 mEq of sodium, and large doses may contribute significantly to the salt load in patients with impaired sodium excretion mechanisms (eg, those with renal, cardiac, or liver disease). Transient increases in serum concentrations of hepatic enzymes (eg, ALT, AST) may occur in patients given ticarcillin. For a more detailed discussion of these and other adverse reactions, see the Introduction and Neu, 1982 B.

DRUG INTERACTIONS AND INTERFERENCE WITH LABORATORY TESTS. Ticarcillin and other antipseudomonal penicillins can inactivate aminoglycosides, particularly gentamicin and tobramycin. Therefore, these antibiotics should not be mixed together prior to administration. Furthermore, in patients with renal failure, in vivo antagonism between ticarcillin and aminoglycosides has been observed. Serum aminoglycoside concentrations should be monitored in such patients and the dosage adjusted accordingly (Mangini, 1984; Hansten, 1985 A; and index entry Aminoglycosides).

Adverse interactions also may occur in patients who are given ticarcillin and heparin or oral anticoagulants, and coagulation status should be monitored regularly (Mangini, 1986).

For a discussion of other drug interactions involving the penicillins, see the Introduction.

PHARMACOKINETICS. Comparative pharmacokinetic data on the penicillins appear in the Table.

Ticarcillin is labile in gastric acid and is not absorbed following oral administration. Thus, it must be administered parenterally. Peak serum concentrations between 20 and 30 mcg/ml are attained about one hour after a 1-g intramuscular injection. Rapid intravenous injection of 5 g produces serum concentrations greater than 300 mcg/ml after 15 minutes.

Like other penicillins, ticarcillin primarily distributes into the extracellular fluid volume. It is rapidly eliminated, primarily by renal tubular secretion; probenecid delays its excretion. The half-life is prolonged in patients with renal impairment (eg, about 15 hours in anuric patients), and dosage adjustments are necessary. For additional discussion, see the Introduction.

DOSAGE AND PREPARATIONS.
Intramuscular: This route is used primarily for uncomplicated urinary tract infections. No more than 2 g should be injected at one time. Intravenous therapy in higher doses should be used for serious urinary tract and systemic infections.

For uncomplicated urinary tract infections, *adults*, 4 g daily in divided doses every six hours; *children weighing less than 40 kg*, 50 to 100 mg/kg daily in divided doses every six to eight hours.
Intravenous: This is the preferred route for serious urinary tract and systemic infections. Ticarcillin disodium can be administered by slow injection or by intermittent or continuous infusion. See the manufacturer's literature for the appropriate dilution of the drug, a list of compatible diluents and intravenous solutions, and stability of ticarcillin in these solutions.

For severe systemic infections (eg, septicemia; respiratory tract, skin and soft tissue, intra-abdominal, and female pelvic and genital tract infections), *adults,* 200 to 300 mg/kg daily in divided doses every four or six hours; *children weighing less than 40 kg*, 200 to 300 mg/kg/day in divided doses every four or six hours (the daily dose should not exceed that used for adults); *infants less than 7 days and weighing more than 2 kg*, 225 mg/kg daily in divided doses every eight hours; *infants over 7 days and weighing more than 2 kg*, 300 mg/kg daily in divided doses every six hours; *infants ≤7 days and weighing 1.2 to 2 kg*, 150 mg/kg daily in divided doses every 12 hours; *infants over 7 days and weighing 1.2 to 2 kg*, 225 mg/kg daily in divided doses every eight hours; *infants 0 to 28 days and weighing less than 1.2 kg,* 150 mg/kg daily in two doses every 12 hours (Nelson, 1991 B).

For uncomplicated urinary tract infections, *adults,* 4 g daily in divided doses every six hours; *children weighing less than 40 kg,* 50 to 100 mg/kg/day in divided doses every six to eight hours.

For urinary tract infections with complications, *adults and children,* 150 to 200 mg/kg/day in divided doses every four to six hours.

The following schedule is used for *adults and children weighing more than 40 kg* with renal insufficiency (see also the manufacturer's literature): An initial loading dose of 3 g followed by:

Creatinine Clearance (ml/min)	Dosage
>60	3 g every 4 hours
60–30	2 g every 4 hours
30–10	2 g every 8 hours
<10	2 g every 12 hours (or 1 g intramuscularly every 6 hours)
<10 (with hepatic dysfunction)	2 g every 24 hours (or 1 g intramuscularly every 12 hours)
Patients on peritoneal dialysis	3 g every 12 hours
Patients on hemodialysis	2 g every 12 hours supplemented with 3 g after each dialysis

Ticar (SmithKline Beecham). Powder 1, 3, 6, 20, and 30 g (equivalent to base) (sodium, 5.2 to 6.5 mEq/g).

MEZLOCILLIN SODIUM
[Mezlin]

MECHANISM OF ACTION, ANTIMICROBIAL SPECTRUM, AND RESISTANCE. Mezlocillin sodium is a broad spectrum, semisynthetic ureidopenicillin for parenteral use; it is not absorbed when given orally. Among the currently available penicillins, mezlocillin exhibits one of the broadest spectrums of activity, including organisms susceptible to both ampicillin and ticarcillin. However, like these other penicillins, mezlocillin also is sensitive to various β-lactamases.

For a detailed discussion of the mechanism of action and antimicrobial spectrum of the penicillins, see the Introduction.

USES. The indications for mezlocillin are similar to those for ticarcillin; the primary use is suspected or proven infections caused by *P. aeruginosa*. It may be used in bacterial septicemia and skin and soft tissue, intra-abdominal, gynecologic, and urinary and lower respiratory tract infections. Although mezlocillin is effective in uncomplicated gonorrhea, other drugs are preferred (see index entry Gonococcal Infections).

In vitro, mezlocillin combined with an aminoglycoside (eg, gentamicin, tobramycin, amikacin) often produced a synergistic effect against a number of susceptible organisms, including *P. aeruginosa* (Neu and Fu, 1978). As with ticarcillin, such a combination is recommended in *P. aeruginosa* infections or in empiric therapy of severe infections.

It is unclear whether mezlocillin provides significant clinical advantages over ticarcillin, at least in terms of improved cure rates. This agent has potential advantages in institutions where ticarcillin-resistant, but mezlocillin-susceptible, strains of *P. aeruginosa* or other gram-negative bacilli are a problem or when mezlocillin's broader antimicrobial spectrum is desirable. Because it is more active against enterococci than ticarcillin, some infectious disease experts now prefer mezlocillin to ticarcillin for intra-abdominal and pelvic infections.

Despite mezlocillin's broad antibacterial spectrum, resistant bacteria are fairly common and resistance has developed during therapy. Thus, this drug usually should not be used alone for empiric therapy of suspected infections. However, mezlocillin alone has been comparable in efficacy and safety to cefoxitin or clindamycin plus gentamicin for treatment of early postpartum endometritis (Faro et al, 1987). Further studies are indicated.

For a more detailed discussion of the uses of antipseudomonal penicillins, see the Introduction and index entry Antimicrobial Drugs. See also Parry, 1987; Neu, 1990; Reese and Betts, 1991.

ADVERSE REACTIONS AND PRECAUTIONS. Mezlocillin is generally well tolerated. The most common side effects are skin rashes and minor gastrointestinal disturbances (incidence, 2% to 3%). Other adverse effects that are typical of the antipseudomonal penicillins either have been reported or are likely to occur with mezlocillin (see the Introduction and Parry and Neu, 1982).

Studies in normal volunteers have shown that the effect of mezlocillin on platelet function was less than that of ticarcillin (Somani et al, 1983). Also, significant clinical bleeding occurred less frequently in a series of hospitalized patients treated with mezlocillin than in those receiving ticarcillin; bleeding was intermediate with piperacillin (Fass et al, 1987). Thus, the risk of a clinical bleeding disorder may be less with mezlocillin than with other antipseudomonal penicillins. Whether other adverse reactions such as hypokalemia will occur less frequently with mezlocillin than with ticarcillin remains to be determined.

Each gram of mezlocillin monosodium contains 1.85 mEq (42.6 mg) of sodium, and large doses may contribute significantly to the sodium load in patients with impaired sodium excretion mechanisms (eg, those with renal, cardiac, or liver disease). However, therapeutic doses of mezlocillin contain less sodium than ticarcillin, which is a possible advantage in these patients (see the evaluation on Ticarcillin).

DRUG INTERACTIONS AND INTERFERENCE WITH LABORATORY TESTS. Mezlocillin and other antipseudomonal penicillins can inactivate aminoglycosides, particularly gentamicin and tobramycin (Pickering and Rutherford, 1981). Therefore, these antibiotics should not be mixed together prior to administration. Furthermore, in patients with renal failure, in vivo antagonism between mezlocillin and aminoglycosides has been observed. Serum aminoglycoside concentrations should be monitored in such patients and dosage adjusted accordingly (Mangini, 1984; Hansten, 1985 A; and index entry Aminoglycosides).

For a discussion of other drug interactions involving the penicillins, see the Introduction.

PHARMACOKINETICS. Comparative pharmacokinetic data on the penicillins appear in the Table.

Mezlocillin is labile in gastric acid and is not absorbed following oral administration. Thus, it must be administered parenterally. After intramuscular injection of 1 g, a peak serum concentration of about 15 mcg/ml is achieved in approximately 45 minutes. Mean serum concentrations observed five minutes after rapid intravenous injection (five minutes) of 2 and 5 g were 253 and 411 mcg/ml, respectively. Immediately after intravenous infusion (30 minutes) of 3 g, an average serum concentration of 263 mcg/ml was measured. Serum concentrations are not proportional to dose.

Like other penicillins, mezlocillin primarily distributes into the extracellular fluid volume. High concentrations are achieved in bile and urine.

Mezlocillin is rapidly eliminated, primarily by renal tubular secretion; probenecid delays excretion. Up to 26% of a dose may be excreted in the bile. The half-life in patients with normal renal function is dose-dependent, ie, it increases somewhat with larger doses, suggesting that saturable extrarenal mechanisms are also involved (Bergan, 1978). The half-life is prolonged in patients with renal impairment and dosage adjustments are necessary in those with moderate to severe insufficiency. For additional discussion, see the Introduction.

DOSAGE AND PREPARATIONS.

Intramuscular: For uncomplicated urinary tract infections, *adults,* 1.5 to 2 g every six hours (100 to 125 mg/kg daily). No more than 2 g should be injected at one time.

Intravenous (direct injection over a three- to five-minute period or by intermittent infusion over a 30-minute period): For uncomplicated urinary tract infections, *adults,* 1.5 to 2 g every six hours (100 to 125 mg/kg daily). For complicated urinary tract infections, *adults,* 3 g every six hours (150 to 200 mg/kg daily).

For severe lower respiratory tract, intra-abdominal, gynecologic, and skin and skin structure infections or septicemia, *adults,* 4 g every six hours or 3 g every four hours (225 to 300 mg/kg daily).

For life-threatening infections, dosage may be increased to 4 g every four hours (maximum, 24 g daily). The usual duration of therapy is 7 to 10 days but may be longer for some infections.

The following schedule is suggested for serious systemic infections in *adults with impaired renal function* (creatinine clearance, ≤30 ml/min): 3 g every eight hours if creatinine clearance is 10 to 30 ml/min and 2 g every eight hours if creatinine clearance is <10 ml/min. For life-threatening infections, the same doses may be administered every six hours. Patients on hemodialysis for renal failure should be given 3 to 4 g after each dialysis and then every 12 hours. Patients on peritoneal dialysis should be given 3 g every 12 hours. (See the manufacturer's literature for additional information.)

The following dosage schedules are recommended for *children and infants*: *infants over 7 days and weighing more than 2 kg,* 225 mg/kg daily in divided doses every eight hours; *infants under 7 days and weighing more than 2 kg,* 150 mg/kg daily in two doses every 12 hours; *infants over 7 days and weighing 1.2 to 2 kg,* 225 mg/kg daily in divided doses every eight hours; *infants under 7 days and weighing 1.2 to 2 kg,* 150 mg/kg daily in two doses every 12 hours; *infants 0 to 28 days and weighing less than 1.2 kg,* 150 mg/kg daily in two doses every 12 hours (Nelson, 1991 B).

Mezlin (Miles). Powder (sterile) 1, 2, 3, 4, and 20 g (equivalent to base) (sodium, 1.85 mEq/g).

PIPERACILLIN SODIUM

[Pipracil]

SPECTRUM OF ACTIVITY. Piperacillin is a broad spectrum, semisynthetic penicillin for parenteral use; it is not absorbed when given orally. Piperacillin and mezlocillin have essentially identical antibacterial spectra and, in vitro, the potencies of these extended spectrum penicillins are comparable for most susceptible bacteria, including *Escherichia coli, Klebsiella, Enterobacter, Proteus mirabilis,* indole-positive *Proteus, Citrobacter, Acinetobacter, Serratia, Providencia, Salmonella, Shigella,* streptococci (including *E. faecalis),* and the *Bacteroides fragilis* group (Fu and Neu, 1978). Piperacillin is more active in vitro than all other penicillins against *Pseudomonas aeruginosa* (Fu and Neu, 1978; Winston et al, 1978). This drug is active against a number of bacterial strains that are resistant to other penicillins (eg, ticarcillin). Piperacillin is sensitive to various β-lactamases, however, and organisms that produce these inactivating enzymes are resistant. Therefore, acquired drug resistance can be expected to be a problem with this antibiotic. Consequently, susceptibility testing is usually necessary before institution of therapy, especially when piperacillin is used alone.

Like mezlocillin, an inoculum effect and large differences between minimal inhibitory concentrations (MIC) and minimal bactericidal concentrations (MBC) have been observed in vitro with *P. aeruginosa.*

For a detailed discussion of the mechanism of action and antimicrobial spectrum of the penicillins, see the Introduction.

USES. The indications for piperacillin are similar to those for ticarcillin and mezlocillin; the primary use is suspected or proven infections caused by *P. aeruginosa*. It may be used in bacterial septicemia and skin and soft tissue, intra-abdominal, gynecologic, bone and joint, and urinary and lower respiratory tract infections (Winston et al, 1980; Pancoast et al, 1981). Although piperacillin is effective in uncomplicated gonorrhea, other drugs are preferred (see index entry Gonococcal Infections).

In vitro, piperacillin combined with an aminoglycoside (eg, gentamicin, tobramycin, amikacin) often produces a synergistic effect against a number of susceptible organisms, including *P. aeruginosa* (Fu and Neu, 1978; Winston et al, 1978). As with ticarcillin and mezlocillin, such a combination is recommended in *P. aeruginosa* infections or in empiric therapy of severe infections, particularly in immunocompromised patients (Hughes et al, 1990). Combination therapy also is recommended to decrease the emergence of piperacillin-resistant organisms, which have appeared when this drug was used alone (Winston et al, 1980; Simon et al, 1980).

It is unclear whether piperacillin provides significant clinical advantages over ticarcillin, at least in terms of improved cure rates. This agent has potential advantages in institutions where ticarcillin-resistant but piperacillin-susceptible strains of *P. aeruginosa* or other gram-negative bacilli are a problem or when piperacillin's broader antimicrobial spectrum is desirable. Some infectious disease experts now prefer piperacillin (or mezlocillin) for empiric combination therapy (with an aminoglycoside) in febrile neutropenic patients or for intra-abdominal and pelvic infections. Because penicillinase-producing strains of bacteria may be present, monotherapy with piperacillin (or any of the antipseudomonal penicillins) generally is not recommended.

Despite piperacillin's broad antibacterial spectrum, resistant bacteria are fairly common and resistance has developed during therapy. Thus, this drug usually should not be used alone for empiric therapy of suspected infections. However, piperacillin alone has been comparable in efficacy and safety to cefoxitin for treatment of early postpartum endometritis (Rosene et al, 1986). Further studies are indicated.

For a more detailed discussion of the uses of antipseudomonal penicillins, see the Introduction and index entry Antimicrobial Drugs. See also Parry, 1987; Neu, 1990; Reese and Betts, 1991.

ADVERSE REACTIONS AND PRECAUTIONS. Piperacillin is generally well tolerated. The most common side effects have been thrombophlebitis (4%), diarrhea (3%), and skin rashes (2%). Other adverse reactions (eg, hypersensitivity reactions, leukopenia and eosinophilia, platelet dysfunction, elevated hepatic enzyme levels, central nervous system irritation, hypokalemia) that are typical of the antipseudomonal penicillins either have been reported or are likely to occur with piperacillin (see the Introduction; see also Fortner et al, 1982; Holmes et al, 1984).

In normal volunteers, the effect of piperacillin on platelet function was less than that of ticarcillin at equivalent dosages (Gentry et al, 1981). Also, significant clinical bleeding occurred less frequently in a series of hospitalized patients treated with piperacillin than in those receiving ticarcillin, but mezlocillin caused fewer bleeding episodes than piperacillin (Fass et al, 1987). Thus, the risk of a clinical bleeding disorder with piperacillin appears to be less than with ticarcillin but greater than with mezlocillin. Whether the incidence of other adverse reactions, such as hypokalemia, will be less with piperacillin than with ticarcillin remains to be determined. A high incidence of fever has been reported in patients with cystic fibrosis who received piperacillin (Stead et al, 1984).

Each gram of piperacillin monosodium contains 1.85 mEq (42.5 mg) of sodium, and large doses may contribute significantly to the sodium load in patients with impaired sodium excretion mechanisms (eg, those with renal, cardiac, or liver disease). However, therapeutic doses of piperacillin contain less sodium than the disodium salt, ticarcillin, a possible advantage in these patients (see the evaluation on Ticarcillin).

DRUG INTERACTIONS AND INTERFERENCE WITH LABORATORY TESTS. Piperacillin and other antipseudomonal penicillins can inactivate aminoglycosides, particularly gentamicin and tobramycin (Pickering and Rutherford, 1981).

Therefore, these antibiotics should not be mixed together prior to administration. Furthermore, in patients with renal failure, in vivo antagonism between piperacillin and aminoglycosides has been observed. Serum aminoglycoside concentrations should be monitored in such patients and dosage adjusted accordingly (Mangini, 1984; Hansten, 1985 A; see also index entry Aminoglycosides).

For a discussion of other drug interactions involving the penicillins, see the Introduction.

PHARMACOKINETICS. Comparative pharmacokinetic data on the penicillins appear in the Table.

Piperacillin is labile in gastric acid and is not absorbed following oral administration. Thus, it must be administered parenterally. After intramuscular injection of 2 g, a peak serum concentration of about 36 mcg/ml is achieved in approximately 30 minutes. Mean serum concentrations observed immediately after rapid intravenous injection (two to three minutes) of 2 and 4 g were 305 and 412 mcg/ml, respectively. Immediately after intravenous infusion (30 minutes) of 4 or 6 g, average serum concentrations of 244 and 353 mcg/ml, respectively, were measured. Serum concentrations are not proportional to dose.

Like other penicillins, piperacillin primarily distributes into the extracellular fluid volume. High concentrations are achieved in bile and urine.

Piperacillin is rapidly eliminated, primarily by renal tubular secretion; probenecid delays its excretion. Up to 25% of an administered dose may be excreted in the bile. The half-life in patients with normal renal function is dose-dependent, ie, it increases somewhat with larger doses. The half-life is prolonged in patients with renal impairment and dosage adjustments are necessary in those with moderate to severe insufficiency. Piperacillin is eliminated more rapidly in patients with cystic fibrosis. For additional discussion, see the Introduction.

DOSAGE AND PREPARATIONS.

Intramuscular: For uncomplicated urinary tract infections and most community-acquired pneumonia, *adults,* 6 to 8 g (100 to 125 mg/kg) daily in equally divided doses every 6 to 12 hours.

No more than 2 g should be injected at one time.

Intravenous (by direct injection over a three- to five-minute period or by intermittent infusion over a 20- to 30-minute period): For uncomplicated urinary tract infections and most community-acquired pneumonia, *adults,* 6 to 8 g (100 to 125 mg/kg) daily in equally divided doses every 6 to 12 hours.

For complicated urinary tract infections, *adults,* 8 to 16 g (125 to 200 mg/kg) daily in equally divided doses every six to eight hours.

For severe lower respiratory tract, intra-abdominal, gynecologic, skin and soft tissue infections or septicemia, *adults,* 12 to 18 g (200 to 300 mg/kg) daily in equally divided doses every four to six hours.

The maximum daily dose for adults is usually 24 g/day. The usual duration of therapy is 7 to 10 days but may be longer for some infections.

The following schedule is suggested for serious systemic infections *in adults with impaired renal function* (creatinine clearance, <40 ml/min): 4 g every eight hours if creatinine clearance is 20 to 40 ml/min and 4 g every 12 hours if creatinine clearance is <20 ml/min. Patients on hemodialysis for renal failure should be given 2 g every eight hours and 1 g after each dialysis. (See the manufacturer's literature for additional information.)

Dosage labeling for piperacillin for *children under 12 years* has not been approved. Most infectious disease experts suggest 200 to 300 mg/kg daily in divided doses every four to six hours for serious systemic infections (The Medical Letter, 1990; Nelson, 1991 A).

Pipracil (Lederle). Powder (sterile) 2, 3, 4, and 40 g (equivalent to base) (sodium 1.85 mEq/g).

Cited References

The choice of antimicrobial drugs. *Med Lett Drugs Ther* 32:41-48, 1990.

American Academy of Pediatrics Committee on Infectious Diseases: Treatment of bacterial meningitis. *Pediatrics* 81:904-907, 1988.

Back DJ, et al: Interindividual variation and drug interactions with hormonal steroid contraceptives. *Drugs* 21:46-61, 1981.

Bergan T: Pharmacokinetics of mezlocillin in healthy volunteers. *Antimicrob Agents Chemother* 14:801-806, 1978.

Berkelman RL, et al: Beta-adrenergic antagonists and fatal anaphylactic reactions to oral penicillin, letter. *Ann Intern Med* 104:134, 1986.

Bisno AL: Group A streptococcal infections and acute rheumatic fever. *N Engl J Med* 325:783-793, 1991.

Bisno AL, et al: Antimicrobial treatment of infective endocarditis due to viridans streptococci, enterococci, and staphylococci. *JAMA* 261:1471-1477, 1989.

Blumberg HM, et al: Rapid development of ciprofloxacin resistance in methicillin-susceptible and -resistant *Staphylococcus aureus. J Infect Dis* 163:1279-1285, 1991.

Bodey GP: Evolution of antibiotic therapy for infection in neutropenic patients: Studies at M. D. Anderson Hospital. *Rev Infect Dis* 11(suppl 7):S1582-S1590, 1989.

Boyce JM: Increasing prevalence of methicillin-resistant *Staphylococcus aureus* in the United States. *Infect Control Hosp Epidemiol* 11:639-642, 1990.

Brandriss MW, Lambert JS: Cardiac infections, in Reese RE, Douglas RG (eds): *A Practical Approach to Infectious Diseases*, ed 3. Boston, Little Brown, 1991, 278-304.

Chow AW, Jewesson PJ: Pharmacokinetics and safety of antimicrobial agents during pregnancy. *Rev Infect Dis* 7:287-313, 1985.

Condemi JJ: Allergy to penicillin and other antibiotics, in Reese RE, Betts RF (eds): *A Practical Approach to Infectious Diseases,* ed 3. Boston, Little Brown, 1991, 801-820.

Conte JE, Barriere SL: *Manual of Antibiotics and Infectious Diseases,* ed 5. Philadelphia, Lea & Febiger, 1984, 63-64.

Dajani AS, et al: Prevention of rheumatic fever: Statement for health professionals by the Committee on Rheumatic Fever, Endocarditis, and Kawasaki Disease of the Council on Cardiovascular Disease in the Young, the American Heart Association. *Circulation* 78:1082-1086, 1988.

Dajani AS, et al: Prevention of bacterial endocarditis: Recommendations by the American Heart Association. *JAMA* 264:2919-2922, 1990.

Ditlove J, et al: Methicillin nephritis. *Medicine* 56:483-491, 1977.

Drusano GL, et al: Acylampicillins: Mezlocillin, piperacillin, and azlocillin. *Rev Infect Dis* 6:13-32, 1984.

Eliopoulos GM, Moellering RC Jr: Azlocillin, mezlocillin, and piperacillin: New broad-spectrum penicillins. *Ann Intern Med* 97:755-760, 1982.

Faro S, et al: Comparative efficacy and safety of mezlocillin, cefoxitin, and clindamycin plus gentamicin in postpartum endometritis. *Obstet Gynecol* 69:760-766, 1987.

Fass RJ, et al: Platelet-mediated bleeding caused by broad-spectrum penicillins. *J Infect Dis* 155:1242-1248, 1987.

Fortner CL, et al: Piperacillin sodium: Antibacterial spectrum, pharmacokinetics, clinical efficacy, and adverse reactions. *Pharmacotherapy* 2:287-299, 1982.

Fu KP, Neu HC: Piperacillin: A new penicillin active against many bacteria resistant to other penicillins. *Antimicrob Agents Chemother* 13:358-367, 1978.

Gentry LO, et al: Effects of sodium piperacillin on platelet function in normal volunteers. *Antimicrob Agents Chemother* 19:532-533, 1981.

Grayson ML, et al: Increasing resistance to β-lactam antibiotics among clinical isolates of *Enterococcus faecium:* A 22-year review at one institution. *Antimicrob Agents Chemother* 35:2180-2184, 1991.

Gudiol F, et al: Clindamycin vs penicillin for anaerobic lung infections: High rate of penicillin failures associated with penicillin-resistant *Bacteroides melaninogenicus. Arch Intern Med* 150:2525-2529, 1990.

Handwerger S, Tomasz A: Antibiotic tolerance among clinical isolates of bacteria. *Rev Infect Dis* 7:368-386, 1985.

Hansten PD: Warfarin and nafcillin. *Drug Interact Newslett* 4:24, 1984.

Hansten PD: *Drug Interactions*, ed 5. Philadelphia, Lea & Febiger, 1985 A, 194-260.

Hansten PD: *Drug Interactions*, ed 5. Philadelphia, Lea & Febiger, 1985 B, 23.

Hansten PD, Horn JR: Inhibition of oral contraceptive efficacy. *Drug Interact Newslett* 5:7-10, 1985.

Holmes B, et al: Piperacillin: Review of its antibacterial activity, pharmacokinetic properties, and therapeutic uses. *Drugs* 28:375-425, 1984.

Hughes WT, et al: Guidelines for the use of antimicrobial agents in neutropenic patients with unexplained fever. *J Infect Dis* 161:381-396, 1990.

Jick H, Porter JB: Potentiation of ampicillin skin reactions by allopurinol or hyperuricemia. *J Clin Pharmacol* 21:456-458, 1981.

Kauffman CA, et al: Methicillin-resistant *Staphylococcus aureus* in long-term care facilities. *Infect Control Hosp Epidemiol* 11:600-603, 1990.

Krstenansky PM, et al: Effect of dicloxacillin sodium on the hypoprothrombinemic response to warfarin sodium. *Clin Pharm* 6:804-806, 1987.

Levine BB, Redmond AP: Minor haptenic determinant-specific reagins of penicillin hypersensitivity in man. *Int Arch Allergy Appl Immunol* 35:445-455, 1969.

Mandell GL, et al: *Principles and Practice of Infectious Diseases: Handbook of Antimicrobial Therapy 1992.* New York, Churchill Livingstone, 1992.

Mangini RJ (ed): *Drug Interaction Facts*. St Louis, Mo, JB Lippincott, 1984, 14.

Mangini RJ (ed): *Drug Interaction Facts*. St Louis, Mo, JB Lippincott, 1986, 66, 277.

McCracken GH Jr: Comparative evaluation of the aminopenicillins for oral use. *Pediatr Infect Dis* 2:317-329, 1983.

The Medical Letter: *Handbook of Antimicrobial Therapy*. New Rochelle, NY, The Medical Letter, Inc, 1990, 42-55.

Mendelman PM, et al: Relative penicillin G resistance in *Neisseria meningitidis* and reduced affinity of penicillin-binding protein 3. *Antimicrob Agents Chemother* 32:706-709, 1988.

Neftel KA, et al: Inhibition of granulopoiesis in vivo and in vitro by β-lactam antibiotics. *J Infect Dis* 152:90-98, 1985.

Nelson JD: *1991-1992 Pocketbook of Pediatric Antimicrobial Therapy*, ed 9. Baltimore, Williams & Wilkins, 1991 A, 66-80.

Nelson JD: *1991-1992 Pocketbook of Pediatric Antimicrobial Therapy*, ed 9. Baltimore, Williams & Wilkins, 1991 B, 16-17.

Neu HC: Pharmacokinetics of bacampicillin. *Rev Infect Dis* 3:110-116, 1981.

Neu HC: Antistaphylococcal penicillins. *Med Clin North Am* 66:51-60, 1982 A.

Neu HC: Carbenicillin and ticarcillin. *Med Clin North Am* 66:61-77, 1982 B.

Neu HC: Structure-activity relations of new β-lactam compounds and in vitro activity against common bacteria. *Rev Infect Dis* 5(suppl 2):S319-S336, 1983.

Neu HC: Penicillins, in Mandell GL, et al (eds): *Principles and Practice of Infectious Diseases*, ed 3. New York, Churchill Livingstone, 1990, 230-246.

Neu HC, Fu KP: Synergy of azlocillin and mezlocillin combined with aminoglycoside antibiotics and cephalosporins. *Antimicrob Agents Chemother* 13:813-819, 1978.

Norris SM: Penicillins with antipseudomonal activity. *Infect Control* 6:165-168, 1985.

Pancoast S, et al: Clinical evaluation of piperacillin therapy for infection. *Arch Intern Med* 141:1447-1450, 1981.

Parry MF: The penicillins. *Med Clin North Am* 71:1093-1112, 1987.

Parry MF, Neu HC: The safety and tolerance of mezlocillin. *J Antimicrob Chemother* 9(suppl A):273-280, 1982.

Parry MF, Pancoast SJ: Antipseudomonal penicillins, in Ristuccia AM, Cunha BA (eds): *Antimicrobial Therapy*. New York, Raven Press, 1984, 197-207.

Pichichero ME: Controversies in the treatment of streptococcal pharyngitis. *Am Fam Physician* 42:1567-1576, 1990.

Pichichero ME, Margolis PA: A comparison of cephalosporins and penicillins in the treatment of group A beta-hemolytic streptococcal pharyngitis: A meta-analysis supporting the concept of microbial copathogenicity. *Pediatr Infect Dis J* 10:275-281, 1991.

Pickering LK, Rutherford I: Effect of concentration and time upon inactivation of tobramycin, gentamicin, netilmicin, and amikacin by azlocillin, carbenicillin, mecillinam, mezlocillin, and piperacillin. *J Pharmacol Exp Ther* 217:345-349, 1981.

Pratt WB, Fekety R: *The Antimicrobial Drugs*. New York, Oxford University Press, 1986, 85-152.

Qureshi GD, et al: Warfarin resistance with nafcillin therapy. *Ann Intern Med* 100:527-529, 1984.

Reese RE, Betts RF: Antibiotic use, in Reese RE, Douglas RG (eds): *A Practical Approach to Infectious Diseases,* ed 3. Boston, Little Brown, 1991, 821-876.

Rosene K, et al: Polymicrobial early postpartum endometritis with facultative and anaerobic bacteria, genital mycoplasmas, and *Chlamydia trachomatis*: Treatment with piperacillin or cefoxitin. *J Infect Dis* 153:1028-1037, 1986.

Sáez-Llorens X, McCracken GH Jr: Bacterial meningitis in neonates and children. *Infect Dis Clin North Am* 4:623-644, 1990.

Schäfer-Korting M, et al: Atenolol interaction with aspirin, allopurinol, and ampicillin. *Clin Pharmacol Ther* 33:283-288, 1983.

Scheife RT, Neu HC: Bacampicillin hydrochloride: Chemistry, pharmacology, and clinical use. *Pharmacotherapy* 2:313-321, 1982.

Shepherd GM: Allergy to β-lactam antibiotics. *Immunol Allergy Clin North Am* 611-633, 1991.

Simon GI, et al: Clinical trial of piperacillin with acquisition of resistance by *Pseudomonas* and clinical relapse. *Antimicrob Agents Chemother* 18:167-170, 1980.

Somani P, et al: The effects of mezlocillin, ticarcillin, and placebo on blood coagulation and bleeding time in normal volunteers. *J Antimicrob Chemother* 11(suppl C):33-41, 1983.

Spika JS, et al: Antimicrobial resistance of *Streptococcus pneumoniae* in the United States, 1979-1987. *J Infect Dis* 163:1273-1278, 1991.

Stead RJ, et al: Adverse reactions to piperacillin in cystic fibrosis. *Lancet* 1:857-858, 1984.

Surtees SJ, et al: Allergy to penicillin: Fable or fact? *BMJ* 302:1051-1052, 1991.

Thoene DE, Johnson CE: Pharmacotherapy of otitis media. *Pharmacotherapy* 11:212-221, 1991.

Tipper DJ: Mode of action of beta-lactam antibiotics, in Queener SF, et al: *Beta-Lactam Antibiotics for Clinical Use.* New York, Marcel Dekker, 1986, 17-48.

Tomasz A: Penicillin-binding proteins and the antibacterial effectiveness of β-lactam antibiotics. *Rev Infect Dis* 8(suppl 3):S260-S278, 1986.

Toogood JH: Beta blocker therapy and the risk of anaphylaxis. *Can Med Assoc J* 136:929-933, 1987.

Tunkel AR, et al: Bacterial meningitis: Recent advances in pathophysiology and treatment. *Ann Intern Med* 112:610-623, 1990.

Viladrich PF, et al: Characteristics and antibiotic therapy of adult meningitis due to penicillin-resistant pneumococci. *Am J Med* 84:839-846, 1988.

Weingarten RD, et al: Meningitis due to penicillin-resistant *Streptococcus pneumoniae* in adults. *Rev Infect Dis* 12:118-124, 1990.

Winston DJ, et al: In vitro studies of piperacillin, a new semisynthetic penicillin. *Antimicrob Agents Chemother* 13:944-960, 1978.

Winston DJ, et al: Piperacillin therapy for serious bacterial infections. *Am J Med* 69:255-261, 1980.

Wispelwey B, et al: Bacterial meningitis in adults. *Infect Dis Clin North Am* 4:645-659, 1990.

Wright AJ, Wilkowske CJ: The penicillins. *Mayo Clin Proc* 66:1047-1063, 1991.

Cephalosporins and Related Agents 64

INTRODUCTION

DRUG EVALUATIONS

Since the introduction of cephalothin [Keflin] for clinical use in the early 1960s, the cephalosporins have become a widely used and rapidly expanding class of antibiotics. Presently, 17 cephalosporins and 4 chemically related antibiotics, cefoxitin [Mefoxin], cefotetan [Cefotan], and cefmetazole [Zefazone], the cephamycins, and moxalactam [Moxam], an oxa-β-lactam, are being marketed in the United States. Additional cephalosporin derivatives undoubtedly will be approved for use in the future. On the other hand, three recently approved parenteral cephalosporins (cefotiam, cefmenoxime, cefpiramide) have not been marketed in this country, presumably because of the intense competition in the cephalosporin marketplace.

CHEMISTRY AND CLASSIFICATION

Like the penicillins, cephalosporins contain a β-lactam ring that is necessary for antimicrobial activity. However, the penicillins are derivatives of 6-aminopenicillanic acid (6-APA) (see index entry Penicillins), whereas the parent nucleus of the cephalosporins is 7-aminocephalosporanic acid (7-ACA) (see Figure). This compound is derived from cephalosporin C, which is a fermentation product of *Cephalosporium acremonium.*

7-Aminocephalosporanic acid is composed of a dihydrothiazine ring (A) and a β-lactam ring (B), and it is resistant to penicillinases, such as those produced by staphylococci. This nucleus has been modified with different side chains to create a whole family of cephalosporin antibiotics (see Figure). Modifications (R_1) at position 7 of the β-lactam ring are associated with changes in antibacterial activity and stability to β-lactamases. Substitutions (R_2) at position 3 of the dihydrothiazine ring affect metabolism and pharmacokinetic properties of the drugs to a greater extent than antibacterial activity.

The cephamycins are related chemically to cephalosporin C, differing primarily in that they possess a 7-α-methoxy group (R_3), which enhances stability to certain β-lactamases. Cefoxitin is derived from cephamycin C, which is elaborated by *Streptomyces lactamdurans.* Cefotetan is a semisynthetic derivative of organomycin G, which is produced by *Streptomyces organonensis.* Cefmetazole is produced synthetically from 7-aminocephalosporanic acid.

Moxalactam has a dihydro-oxazine ring instead of the dihydrothiazine ring common to the cephalosporins and cephamycins. Therefore, technically it is not a penicillin, cephalosporin, or cephamycin but is related to all three. It also is a totally synthetic compound.

For additional discussion of chemistry, see Neu, 1982 A, 1983, 1985; Garzone et al, 1983 A; Barriere and Flaherty,

CHEMICAL STRUCTURES OF CEPHALOSPORINS

Cephalosporin Nucleus[1]

Generic Name (Trade Name)	R_1	R_2	R_3
FIRST GENERATION			
Cephalothin (Keflin)	(2-thienyl)$CH_2C(=O)$	$CH_2OC(=O)CH_3$	H
Cefazolin (Ancef, Kefzol)	(tetrazol-1-yl)$N-CH_2C(=O)$	CH_2-S-(5-methyl-1,3,4-thiadiazol-2-yl) CH_3	H
Cephapirin (Cefadyl)	(4-pyridyl)$SCH_2C(=O)$	$CH_2OC(=O)CH_3$	H
Cephradine (Anspor, Velosef)	(cyclohexadienyl)$C(H)(NH_2)C(=O)$	CH_3	H
Cephalexin (Keflex, Keftab)	(phenyl)$C(H)(NH_2)C(=O)$	CH_3	H
Cefadroxil (Duricef, Ultracef)	HO-(phenyl)$C(H)(NH_2)C(=O)$	CH_3	H
SECOND GENERATION			
Cefamandole Nafate (Mandol)	(phenyl)$C(H)(OCH)C(=O)$	CH_2S-(1-methyltetrazol-5-yl) CH_3	H
Cefuroxime (Zinacef, Kefurox)	(2-furyl)$C(=N-OCH_3)C(=O)$	$CH_2OC(=O)NH_2$	H

(Continued on next page)

FIGURE (continued)

Generic Name (Trade Name)	R_1	R_2	R_3
Cefonicid (Monocid)	Phenyl–CH(OH)–C(=O)	CH_2S–tetrazolyl (N-CH_2SO_3H)	H
Ceforanide (Precef)	2-(CH_2NH_2)phenyl–$CH_2C(=O)$	CH_2S–tetrazolyl (N-CH_2COOH)	H
Cefaclor (Ceclor)	Phenyl–CH(NH_2)–C(=O)	Cl	H
Cephamycins			
Cefoxitin (Mefoxin)	2-thienyl–$CH_2C(=O)$	$CH_2OC(=O)NH_2$	OCH_3
Cefotetan (Cefotan)	$H_2NC(=O)$(HOC(=O))C=(1,3-dithietane)–C(=O)	CH_2S–tetrazolyl (N-CH_3)	OCH_3
Cefmetazole (Zefazone)	$N{\equiv}C-CH_2-S-CH_2-C(=O)$	CH_2S–tetrazolyl (N-CH_3)	OCH_3
THIRD GENERATION			
Cefotaxime (Claforan)	2-amino-4-thiazolyl–C(=N–OCH_3)–C(=O)	$CH_2OC(=O)CH_3$	H
Ceftizoxime (Cefizox)	2-amino-4-thiazolyl–C(=N–OCH_3)–C(=O)	H	H

(continued on next page)

FIGURE (continued)

Generic Name (Trade Name)	R_1	R_2	R_3
Ceftriaxone (Rocephin)	(2-amino-4-thiazolyl)–C(=N–OCH_3)–C(=O)	CH_2S–(triazinone ring: 2-methyl-5-hydroxy-6-oxo-1,2,4-triazin-3-yl; N–CH_3, OH, =O)	H
Ceftazidime (Fortaz, Tazidime, Tazicef)	(2-amino-4-thiazolyl)–C(=N–OC(CH_3)(CH_3)COOH)–C(=O)	CH_2–N^+(pyridinium)	H
Cefoperazone (Cefobid)	CH_3CH_2–N(2,3-dioxopiperazine)N–CNH(=O)–C(H)(p-hydroxyphenyl)–C(=O)	CH_2S–(1-methyltetrazol-5-yl; N–CH_3)	H
Moxalactam[2] (Moxam)	HO–(p-phenylene)–CHC(=O), with –COH(=O)	CH_2S–(1-methyltetrazol-5-yl; N–CH_3)	OCH_3
Cefixime (Suprax)	(2-amino-4-thiazolyl)–C(=N–OCH_2COOH)–C(=O)	$CH=CH_2$	H

[1] For 7-aminocephalosporanic acid (7-ACA), $R_1 = R_3 = H$ and $R_2 = CH_2OCCH_3$ (with =O on C); A = dihydrothiazine ring; B = beta-lactam ring. The arrow is the site of beta-lactamase attack.

[2] Moxalactam is actually an oxy-cephem antimicrobial; it has an oxygen atom instead of sulfur in position one of ring A (see the Cephalosporin Nucleus).

1984; Norris, 1984 A; Quintiliani et al, 1984; Fried and Hinthorn, 1985; Ward and Richards, 1985; and Donowitz and Mandell, 1990.

It is convenient to classify the cephalosporins and related agents as first, second, or third generation compounds based on their activity against gram-negative bacteria. The first generation cephalosporins were the initial agents developed, and they have a narrower gram-negative antibacterial spectrum than the compounds developed later. However, first generation analogues generally are more active against gram-positive bacteria than second and third generation cephalosporins. First generation cephalosporins currently marketed in the United States include cephalothin, cefazolin [Ancef, Kefzol], and cephapirin [Cefadyl] for parenteral use only; cephalexin [Keflex] and cefadroxil [Duricef, Ultracef] for oral use only; and cephradine [Anspor, Velosef], which can be administered orally or parenterally.

The available second generation cephalosporins for parenteral use are cefamandole [Mandol], cefuroxime [Zinacef, Kefurox], cefonicid [Monocid], and ceforanide [Precef] and the cephamycins, cefoxitin, cefmetazole, and cefotetan. However, some experts classify this last agent as a third generation cephalosporin. Cefaclor [Ceclor] and cefuroxime axetil [Ceftin], the acetoxyethyl ester of cefuroxime, are second generation cephalosporins for oral administration. Although there are differences among individual agents, second generation cephalosporins generally are more active against gram-negative bacteria than first generation analogues. Cefoxitin, cefmetazole, cefotetan, and cefuroxime are more resistant to certain gram-negative bacterial β-lactamases than most other compounds.

The third generation cephalosporins are even more active and have a still broader in vitro spectrum of activity against gram-negative bacteria, including organisms resistant to earlier generation cephalosporins. They also show increased stability to β-lactamases produced by many gram-negative bacteria. However, the third generation cephalosporins generally are less active than first generation analogues against gram-positive bacteria. Currently, parenteral cefotaxime [Claforan], ceftizoxime [Cefizox], ceftriaxone [Rocephin], ceftazidime [Fortaz, Tazidime, Tazicef], cefoperazone [Cefobid], and moxalactam are available in the United States. Ceftazidime and cefoperazone are more active against *Pseudomonas aeruginosa* than the other available third generation cephalosporins (see Antimicrobial Spectrum). Cefixime [Suprax] is the first available oral cephalosporin to be classified in the third generation.

For additional discussion, see Neu, 1982 A; Bertino and Speck, 1983; Garzone et al, 1983 A; *Med Lett Drugs Ther*, 1983 A, 1986; Thompson and Wright, 1983; Barriere and Flaherty, 1984; Norris, 1984 A; Quintiliani et al, 1984; Fried and Hinthorn, 1985; Tartaglione and Polk, 1985; Ward and Richards, 1985; Faulkner et al, 1987; Donowitz and Mandell, 1990.

MECHANISM OF ACTION

The cephalosporins are primarily bactericidal antibiotics with a mechanism of action very similar to that of the penicillins. These β-lactam antibiotics inhibit the third and final stage of bacterial cell wall formation by preferentially binding to one or more penicillin binding proteins (PBPs) that are located in the cytoplasmic membrane beneath the cell walls of susceptible bacteria. Thus, the intrinsic activity of a cephalosporin against a particular bacterial strain depends, in part, on its binding affinity to these protein receptor molecules. For example, first generation cephalosporins exhibit greater affinity for essential PBPs of staphylococci than third generation derivatives. Conversely, third generation cephalosporins usually have greater affinity for critical PBPs of the Enterobacteriaceae. Other factors also affect the antibacterial activity of β-lactam antibiotics. These include the stability of the antibiotic to various β-lactamases produced by gram-positive and gram-negative bacteria and the ability of a drug to penetrate the outer membrane of gram-negative bacteria (see also the section on Resistance). For a detailed discussion on the mechanism of action of β-lactam antibiotics, see index entry Penicillins; see also Neu, 1982 B, 1985.

ANTIMICROBIAL SPECTRUM

First Generation Cephalosporins: All of these agents have similar antibacterial spectra that include most gram-positive and some gram-negative bacteria.

The first generation cephalosporins have the highest degree of activity in vitro against gram-positive bacteria. They are active against most staphylococci, including penicillinase-producing *S. aureus*. However, methicillin-resistant staphylococci should be considered resistant to all cephalosporins, although in vitro resistance is not always readily demonstrated. Most streptococci, including *S. pyogenes* (group A, β-hemolytic), *S. agalactiae* (group B), viridans streptococci, anaerobic streptococci, and *S. pneumoniae* are susceptible. However, penicillin-resistant *S. pneumoniae* are resistant to first generation cephalosporins. Enterococci (eg, *E. faecalis*, *E. faecium*) are resistant to all cephalosporins. There do not appear to be major differences in activity between the various parenteral first generation cephalosporins against gram-positive cocci, although cephalothin may be slightly more active against staphylococci than cefazolin. Recent data suggest that some strains of *S. aureus* are less susceptible to cefazolin because of β-lactamase instability (Kernodie et al, 1990). The parenteral agents generally are more active than oral cephalosporins in vitro and in vivo against aerobic gram-positive cocci.

Susceptible gram-positive bacilli include certain *Clostridium* species (eg, *C. perfringens*) and *Corynebacterium diphtheriae*. *Listeria monocytogenes* is resistant to all cephalosporins.

The clinically relevant spectrum of first generation cephalosporins against gram-negative bacteria is limited to *Escherichia coli*, *Klebsiella*, and *Proteus mirabilis*. Cefazolin generally is more active than cephalothin. Variable percentages of strains of these three species are resistant to the first generation cephalosporins, however; resistant strains are more common in hospital-acquired infections. These resistant strains may be susceptible to second and particularly third generation cephalosporins (see below).

Although in vitro susceptibility to first generation cephalosporins has been demonstrated for many strains of *Salmonella*, *Shigella*, *Haemophilus influenzae*, and the gram-negative cocci, *Neisseria gonorrhoeae* and *N. meningitidis*, clinical usefulness has not been demonstrated. Indole-positive *Proteus*, *Providencia*, *Enterobacter*, *Serratia*, *Citrobacter*, *Pseudomonas*, *Acinetobacter*, and the *Bacteroides fragilis* group are resistant. *Legionella pneumophila* should be considered resistant to the cephalosporins.

For additional discussion, see Bertino and Speck, 1983; Garzone et al, 1983 B; Jones and Preston, 1983; *Med Lett Drugs Ther*, 1983 A; Thompson and Wright, 1983; Norris, 1984 B; Quintiliani et al, 1984; Fried and Hinthorn, 1985; Sahm et al, 1985 A; Donowitz and Mandell, 1990.

Second Generation Cephalosporins: These antibiotics have enhanced activity against a greater variety of gram-negative bacteria when compared to first generation cephalosporins. The second generation agents also differ among themselves with regard to their in vitro activities against various bacteria.

Second generation cephalosporins are active in vitro against most staphylococci, including penicillinase-producing *S. aureus*, *Streptococcus pyogenes*, *S. pneumoniae*, *S. agalactiae*, viridans streptococci, and gram-positive anaerobes (eg, *Peptococcus*, *Peptostreptococcus*, clostridia). As with first generation agents, enterococci (eg, *E. faecalis*), methicillin-resistant staphylococci, penicillin-resistant pneumococci, and *Listeria monocytogenes* are resistant.

The in vitro activity of parenteral second generation cephalosporins against most streptococci and pneumococci is comparable to or slightly less than that observed with parenteral first generation agents. Cefamandole and cefuroxime generally are the most potent agents against these organisms. The in vitro activity of the second generation derivatives against staphylococci is variable. The most active agents are cefamandole, cefuroxime, and cefmetazole, which are slightly less potent than first generation agents. Cefoxitin and the newer second generation cephalosporins with longer half-lives, cefonicid, ceforanide, and cefotetan, are less active against staphylococci. Oral cefaclor has comparable activity in vitro to cephalexin against gram-positive cocci. In general, second generation cephalosporins offer no clinical advantages over first generation derivatives for infections caused by gram-positive bacteria.

Neisseria gonorrhoeae and *N. meningitidis*, gram-negative cocci, are susceptible to the second generation cephalosporins. Of particular clinical relevance are (1) the high degree of activity of cefoxitin and cefotetan for *N. gonorrhoeae*, including penicillinase-producing strains (PPNG), and (2) the good activity of cefuroxime against the meningococcus, making it the only second generation cephalosporin that achieves therapeutic concentrations against this organism in cerebrospinal fluid (see Uses and Pharmacokinetics).

The second generation cephalosporins are considerably more active in vitro against *Haemophilus influenzae* than the first generation antibiotics and also are active against many ampicillin-resistant strains. Among the parenteral second generation agents, cefuroxime appears to be the most useful clinically. When compared with cefamandole, it has increased stability to β-lactamases (eg, plasmid-mediated TEM-1) produced by *H. influenzae* and achieves therapeutic concentrations in cerebrospinal fluid (see Uses and Pharmacokinetics). The oral congener of cefuroxime, cefuroxime axetil, may be useful for otitis media. Oral cefaclor is more active in vitro than cephalexin against *H. influenzae* and also is useful in otitis media (see Uses).

Among the Enterobacteriaceae, second generation cephalosporins are more active in vitro than first generation agents against *Escherichia coli*, *Klebsiella*, and *Proteus mirabilis*, including strains resistant to first generation drugs. All have good activity against *Citrobacter diversus*. For other Enterobacteriaceae, the in vitro activity often varies with the second generation agent being considered. Cefamandole, cefuroxime, cefonicid, and ceforanide are most similar and are active against a number of isolates of *C. freundii*, *Enterobacter* species, and the indole-positive *Proteus*; they are not active against *Serratia* species. In contrast, cefoxitin and cefmetazole are less active against *C. freundii* and *Enterobacter* species but are more active against indole-positive *Proteus*, especially *Proteus vulgaris*, and they are active against some *Serratia* species. Strains resistant to these second generation cephalosporins are relatively common among some species of Enterobacteriaceae, however. The third generation cephalosporins clearly have superior activity against most Enterobacteriaceae (see below).

Cefotetan is the most active second generation cephalosporin against the Enterobacteriaceae. Its potency in vitro approaches that of the third generation compounds against *E. coli, Klebsiella* species, *P. mirabilis, C. diversus,* and *P. vulgaris.* Thus, some experts classify this agent as a third generation cephalosporin. Cefotetan has intermediate activity against other *Proteus* species, *Providencia* and *Morganella* species, and *Salmonella* and *Shigella* species. Its activity against *Enterobacter* and *Serratia* species and *C. freundii* is variable and, generally, cefotetan is less active than the third generation cephalosporins against these species.

Cefoxitin is the most active of any currently available cephalosporin against the *Bacteroides fragilis* group because it is not usually hydrolyzed by β-lactamases produced by these gram-negative anaerobic bacilli. Most other anaerobic bacteria, except some *Clostridium* species and a few *Fusobacterium*, also are susceptible to cefoxitin. Thus, this second generation cephalosporin is clinically useful in pelvic and intra-abdominal infections in which *B. fragilis* is a common pathogen (see Uses). In general, cefotetan and cefmetazole are comparable to cefoxitin in vitro against anaerobic bacteria, including the *B. fragilis* species. However, these newer cephamycins are less active against other species within the *B. fragilis* group (eg, *B. ovatus, B. distasonis, B. thetaiotaomicron*). The clinical significance of these in vitro differences is uncertain.

Second generation cephalosporins are not active against *Pseudomonas aeruginosa* or *Acinetobacter*.

For additional discussion, see Barriere and Mills, 1982; Muytjens and van der Ros-van de Repe, 1982; Bertino and

TABLE 1.
COMPARATIVE IN VITRO ACTIVITY OF PARENTERAL THIRD GENERATION CEPHALOSPORINS[1,2]

Organism	Cefotaxime[3]	Ceftizoxime	Ceftriaxone	Ceftazidime	Cefoperazone	Moxalactam
Staphylococcus aureus	++	++	++	+	++	+
Staphylococcus epidermidis	++	+/++	+/++	R/+	++	R/+
Streptococcus, Group A	+++	++++	++++	+++	+++	++
Streptococcus, Group B	++++	++++	++++	+++	+++	++
Streptococcus pneumoniae	+++/++++	+++	+++/++++	+++	+++/++++	++/+++
Haemophilus influenzae[4]	++++	++++	++++	+++/++++	+++	++++
Neisseria gonorrhoeae[4]	++++	++++	++++	+++/++++	++++	++++
Neisseria meningitidis	++++	++++	++++	++++	++++	++++
Escherichia coli	+++/++++	+++	+++/++++	+++	+/++	+++
Klebsiella pneumoniae	+++/++++	+++/++++	+++	+++	+/++	+++
Enterobacter aerogenes	++/+++	++	+++	++/+++	+/++	++/+++
Enterobacter cloacae	+/++	+/++	+/++	+/++	+/++	++/+++
Citrobacter freundii	+/++	++	++	++	+	++
Citrobacter diversus	+++	+++	+++	+++	+++	+++
Serratia marcescens	++	++/+++	++	+++	+/++	++
Proteus mirabilis	++++	++++	++++	++++	+++	+++
Morganella morganii	++	++++	++++	++	++	+++
Providencia stuartii	++/+++	++	++	++	+	++
Pseudomonas aeruginosa[5]	R(64)	R(64)	R(64)	++(8)	+(32)	+(32)

[1]*Adapted from Barriere and Flaherty, 1984. Data for ceftazidime obtained from Bodey et al, 1981; Muytjens and van der Ros-van de Repe, 1982; Fass, 1983; Neu, 1983; Richards and Brogden, 1985; and Thornsberry, 1985. This table was generated from published reports of in vitro susceptibilities from a variety of geographic areas. However, susceptibilities to these drugs may differ markedly from data in the table in a given institution.*

[2]*Legend: ++++ = MIC_{90} ≤ 0.1 mcg/ml (highly susceptible); +++ = MIC_{90} 0.2-1 mcg/ml (very susceptible); ++ = MIC_{90} 2-8 mcg/ml (susceptible); + = MIC_{90} 16-32 mcg/ml (moderately susceptible); R = MIC_{90} > 32 mcg/ml (resistant).*

[3]*In vivo, cefotaxime is partially metabolized to 3-desacetylcefotaxime, an active, beta lactamase-stable metabolite. The antibacterial activity of desacetylcefotaxime (not shown) generally is four- to eightfold less than that of cefotaxime for most bacterial strains, but this metabolite is more active than cefazolin, cefamandole, and cefoxitin against most aerobic gram-negative bacteria. Furthermore, studies in vitro suggest that cefotaxime and desacetylcefotaxime act synergistically against a number of bacterial strains (see Jones et al, 1982; Neu, 1982 E; Chin and Neu, 1984; Jones, 1987).*

[4]*Includes penicillinase-producing strains*

[5]*MIC_{90} in parentheses*

Speck, 1983; Garzone et al, 1983 B; Gold and Rodriguez, 1983; *Med Lett Drugs Ther*, 1983 A, 1986; Smith and LeFrock, 1983; Thompson and Wright, 1983; Dudley et al, 1984; Norris, 1984 B; Pontzer and Kaye, 1984; Quintiliani et al, 1984; Fried and Hinthorn, 1985; Sahm et al, 1985 A; Sanders et al, 1985; Tartaglione and Polk, 1985; Ward and Richards, 1985; Saltiel and Brogden, 1986; Campoli-Richards et al, 1987; Williams and Moosdeen, 1987; Jones, 1989; Donowitz and Mandell, 1988, 1990.

Third Generation Cephalosporins: These antibiotics generally have increased potency and a wider spectrum of activity against clinically important gram-negative bacteria when compared to first and second generation cephalosporins. Comparative in vitro activities of the parenteral third generation cephalosporins are summarized in Table 1.

Although the parenteral third generation cephalosporins are active against most staphylococci, including penicillinase-producing strains, they are considerably less potent than parenteral first generation agents (eg, cephalothin, cefazolin). Moxalactam and ceftazidime are the least active parenteral third generation cephalosporins against *S. aureus* and coagulase-negative staphylococci. Methicillin-resistant staphylococci are resistant to all of these agents. Parenteral cefotaxime, ceftizoxime, and ceftriaxone have excellent activity against *Streptococcus pyogenes*, *S. agalactiae*, and *S. pneumoniae*, including strains that are moderately resistant to penicillin. Ceftazidime, cefoperazone, and, in particular, moxalactam are less active against streptococci and pneumococci. Enterococci (eg, *E. faecalis*) and *Listeria monocytogenes* are resistant to all of these agents. In general, third generation cephalosporins offer no clinical advantages over first generation derivatives for infections (other than meningitis) caused by gram-positive bacteria.

Currently available parenteral third generation cephalosporins are highly active against *Neisseria gonorrhoeae*, including penicillinase-producing strains (PPNG); ceftriaxone, cefotaxime, and ceftizoxime are used clinically for infections caused by these organisms (see Uses). *N. meningitidis* and *Moraxella (Branhamella) catarrhalis* also are very susceptible to these agents.

Parenteral third generation cephalosporins show excellent activity against many aerobic gram-negative bacilli, including *Haemophilus influenzae* and most of the Enterobacteriaceae (eg, *Escherichia coli, Klebsiella, Enterobacter, Proteus, Morganella, Providencia, Citrobacter, Serratia, Salmonella, Shigella*) including strains resistant to earlier generation cephalosporins, penicillins, and aminoglycosides. This activity is related to the agents' excellent β-lactamase stability and high affinity for penicillin binding proteins. Third generation cephalosporins offer distinct clinical advantages over earlier generation cephalosporins against these aerobic gram-negative bacilli. In general, *Enterobacter* species, *Citrobacter freundii*, *Serratia marcescens*, and *Providencia* species are less susceptible to the third generation agents than other Enterobacteriaceae, but there is variability among published reports. Cefoperazone is less active than other third generation cephalosporins against most Enterobacteriaceae. This drug is more susceptible to certain β-lactamases (eg, TEM-1, TEM-2), and β-lactamase-producing strains of *E. coli* and *Klebsiella* that are susceptible to other third generation cephalosporins have been resistant to cefoperazone (see also Resistance).

The activity of parenteral third generation cephalosporins against *Pseudomonas aeruginosa* is variable. Ceftazidime has the greatest activity, including some strains that are resistant to aminoglycosides and antipseudomonal penicillins. Cefoperazone has moderate activity against *P. aeruginosa*; the other agents are considerably less active. Other than ceftaziactive against *Acinetobacter* species.

Although parenteral third generation cephalosporins are active against anaerobic streptococci, some clostridia (not *C. difficile*), fusobacteria, actinomycetes, and most *Bacteroides*, they generally are inferior to the penicillins. Against the *B. fragilis* group, only moxalactam has activity comparable to that of cefoxitin. The other third generation agents generally have less activity against this pathogen.

For additional discussion, see Bodey et al, 1981; Beam, 1982, 1985; Funk and Strausbaugh, 1982; Muytjens and van der Ros-van de Repe, 1982; Neu, 1982 A; Bertino and Speck, 1983; Carmine et al, 1983 A and B; Fass, 1983; Garzone et al, 1983 B; *Med Lett Drugs Ther*, 1983 A; Barriere and Flaherty, 1984; Quintiliani et al, 1984; Richards et al, 1984; Fried and Hinthorn, 1985; Gentry, 1985; Norris, 1985; Richards and Brogden, 1985; Richards and Heel, 1985; Sahm et al, 1985 B; Thornsberry, 1985; Aldridge, 1987; Williams and Moosdeen, 1987; Donowitz and Mandell, 1988, 1990.

Cefixime is the first orally administered cephalosporin that can be classified in the third generation. In vitro, this beta lactamase-stable antibiotic has increased potency and a broader spectrum of activity against most clinically important gram-negative bacteria when compared to other oral cephalosporins. Cefixime has excellent activity against most Enterobacteriaceae (eg, *E. coli, Klebsiella), Haemophilus influenzae, Moraxella (Branhamella) catarrhalis, Neisseria meningitidis,* and *N. gonorrhoeae*, including beta lactamase-producing strains. Against gram-positive cocci, cefixime is more active than other orally administered cephalosporins against *Streptococcus pneumoniae, S. pyogenes,* and *S. agalactiae.* However, *Staphylococcus aureus* and coagulase-negative staphylococci are resistant to cefixime; this represents a major drawback in its antimicrobial spectrum. As with other oral cephalosporins, cefixime is inactive against enterococci (eg, *E. faecalis*), methicillin-resistant staphylococci, penicillin-resistant pneumococci, *Listeria monocytogenes, Pseudomonas, Acinetobacter,* and *Bacteroides fragilis* (see Barry and Jones, 1987; Neu, 1987 A; Brogden and Campoli-Richards, 1989).

RESISTANCE

Mechanisms of resistance to cephalosporins include: (1) inactivation by bacterial β-lactamases (see Figure); (2) decreased permeability of the bacterial cell, which prohibits the cephalosporin from reaching the appropriate binding proteins; and, (3) alterations in penicillin binding protein(s) that prevent binding to the cephalosporin (see Livermore, 1987 A; Donowitz and Mandell, 1990). Clinically, β-lactamase inactivation and, to a lesser extent, altered permeability are most important in gram-negative bacteria. Decreased affinity for penicillin binding proteins occurs with some gram-positive bacteria, but it is not a common cause of clinical resistance to cephalosporins among gram-negative bacteria.

Many β-lactamases have been identified. The enzymes produced by *Staphylococcus aureus* are considered to be true penicillinases because they inactivate penicillin molecules but not cephalosporins. Thus, cephalosporins are active against penicillinase-producing *S. aureus*, although recent data suggest that some strains of *S. aureus* are less susceptible to cefazolin because of β-lactamase instability (Kernodie et al, 1990). The decreased activities of newer generation cephalosporins against staphylococci appear to be due to decreased affinities for penicillin binding proteins rather than increased susceptibilities to β-lactamases. Methicillin-resistant staphylococci are resistant to cephalosporins; this is due to alterations in penicillin binding proteins. The lack of activity of cephalosporins against enterococci also is related to failure to bind critical penicillin binding proteins in these bacteria (see Livermore, 1987 A).

The β-lactamases of gram-negative bacteria fall into five broad enzyme classes (Richmond and Sykes, 1973; Sykes, 1982). These enzymes can be chromosomal- or plasmid-mediated, constitutive or inducible, and are strategically located in the periplasmic space between the inner and outer membranes of the bacterial cell. Some of these enzymes preferentially inactivate either penicillins or cephalosporins, while others work equally well on both classes of drugs. First generation cephalosporins are susceptible to many β-lactamases produced by gram-negative bacteria. This accounts, in part, for their more limited antibacterial spectrum and the development of strains resistant to their antibacterial effect (see Livermore, 1987 A; Donowitz and Mandell, 1990). Second generation cephalosporins, particularly cefoxitin, cefmetazole, cefotetan, and cefuroxime, and most third generation derivatives have been chemically engineered to be considerably more stable to β-lactamase degradation. Thus, in addition to greater intrinsic antibacterial activity, newer generations of cephalosporins are less likely to be inactivated by βlactamases (see Neu, 1982 C; Sykes and Bush, 1983).

Variable susceptibility to different β-lactamases is still evident with the newer cephalosporins, however. For example, some strains of *E. coli* and *Klebsiella* are resistant to cefoperazone because this drug remains susceptible to certain β-lactamases (eg, TEM-1, TEM-2) that may be produced by these bacteria (Sykes and Bush, 1983). Differences in susceptibility of *B. fragilis* and *P. aeruginosa* to the various analogues can be explained in part by differences in susceptibilities of the various drugs to β-lactamases elaborated by these organisms (Sykes and Bush, 1983). With increased use of the newer cephalosporins, it is likely that strains resistant to all of these drugs will emerge to some extent. For example, novel, plasmid-mediated, transferable β-lactamases (eg, TEM-3 [CTX-1], TEM-5 [CAZ-1]) that confer resistance to third generation cephalosporins recently have been isolated from *Klebsiella pneumoniae* and other Enterobacteriaceae in Europe (see Sirot et al, 1988; Philippon et al, 1989). Also, strains of resistant *P. aeruginosa* and *Serratia marcescens* have appeared due to permeability mechanisms (see Sanders and Sanders, 1985).

Of increasing concern is the rapid development of resistance to supposedly β-lactamase stable, third generation cephalosporins by certain nonfastidious gram-negative bacilli, particularly species of *Enterobacter*, *Serratia*, and *Pseudomonas*. Therapeutic failures and relapses, as well as nosocomial spread of these organisms, have been reported. Furthermore, routine antimicrobial susceptibility test procedures may fail to detect these strains. The mechanism of resistance involves the production of large quantities of Type 1 chromosomal β-lactamases, either by the selection of stably derepressed mutant strains or by the reversible induction of enzyme synthesis with inducer β-lactam antibiotics (eg, cefoxitin). Type 1 β-lactamases bind third generation cephalosporins with high affinity and render them inactive. In most cases, slow hydrolysis of the antibiotic also appears to occur. Type 1 β-lactamase-producing bacterial strains also are resistant to other cephalosporins, penicillins (except amdinocillin), and monobactams (eg, aztreonam), but they are susceptible to imipenem. Interestingly, this carbapenem is a potent inducer of these enzymes. It should be emphasized that inducers of Type 1 β-lactamases, such as cefoxitin and imipenem, are potentially antagonistic to other β-lactams if used in combination regimens. Type 1 β-lactamases are not inhibited by clavulanic acid or sulbactam. For additional discussion, see Sanders, 1983, 1984; Sanders and Sanders, 1983, 1985, 1986, 1987; Dworzack et al, 1987; Follath et al, 1987; Livermore, 1987 B. See also index entries Aztreonam; Imipenem/Cilastatin.

The above discussion emphasizes the importance of maintaining locally generated antibiotic susceptibility profiles and of performing appropriate in vitro susceptibility tests when using the cephalosporins (see Amsterdam, 1984; Sanders, 1984; Sahm et al, 1985 A and B).

USES

The cephalosporins are broad spectrum bactericidal antibiotics with a high therapeutic/toxic ratio. They are effective in a wide variety of infections and are used frequently. However, first and second generation analogues usually have not been regarded as antibiotics of first choice for the treatment of most infections because of the availability of equally effective and less expensive alternatives. The third generation cephalosporins are preferred drugs for some infections (eg, enteric gram-negative bacillary meningitis). They will likely become primary drugs for other infections, but additional clinical experience, including comparative trials, is required to demonstrate that they are as reliable as the already proven therapeutic agents. A problem with these newer agents also is their relatively high cost to the patient, but this may be justified by lower toxicity, greater efficacy, or both in comparison with drugs of more reasonable cost. As the number of cephalosporins continues to expand, drug selection among the available agents will become more difficult.

For additional discussion, see index entry, Antimicrobial Drugs: Antimicrobial Drug Selection for Common Infectious Diseases (Table); see also Neu, 1982 A and D, 1987 B; Brooks and Barriere, 1983; Garzone et al, 1983 B; *Med Lett Drugs Ther*, 1983 A, 1988 A; Barriere and Flaherty, 1984; Norris, 1984 B, 1985; Smith, 1984; Eichenwald, 1985; Fried and Hinthorn, 1985; Sanders et al, 1985, 1988; Tartaglione and Polk, 1985; Barriere, 1986; Goldberg, 1987; Thompson, 1987; Donowitz and Mandell, 1988, 1990.

Parenteral First Generation Cephalosporins: Antimicrobial chemoprophylaxis during certain surgical procedures effectively reduces the risk of postoperative wound infection. Parenteral first generation cephalosporins frequently are preferred for prophylaxis during many of these procedures, including prosthetic heart valve insertion and other open-heart surgery (some experts prefer cefuroxime or cefamandole), reconstructive surgery of the abdominal aorta, total hip replacement, gastroduodenal and biliary tract surgery in high-risk patients, vaginal and abdominal hysterectomy, cesarean section in high-risk patients, and head and neck surgery requiring an incision that enters the oral cavity or pharynx (some experts prefer clindamycin with or without an aminoglycoside). Cefazolin usually is preferred over other first generation analogues because it produces higher serum concentrations and has a longer elimination half-life (see Pharmacokinetics). Usually, a single dose administered shortly before the first surgical incision (eg, intravenously at induction of anesthesia) provides sufficient tissue concentrations of cefazolin throughout the procedure. Additional doses given either earlier or later usually are unnecessary; continuation of prophylaxis for more than 24 hours after surgery is not indicated. For a more detailed discussion, see index entry Antimicrobial Drugs: Chemoprophylaxis for Surgical Patients (Table). See also DiPiro et al, 1981, 1983, 1986; Lennard and Dellinger, 1981; Guglielmo et al, 1983; Burnakis, 1984; Conte et al, 1984; Gilbert, 1984; Kaiser, 1986, 1990; *Med Lett Drugs Ther,* 1987, 1989 C. A number of second and third generation cephalosporins have been shown to be effective as prophylactic agents for various surgical procedures (see Tartaglione and Polk, 1985; Barriere and Flaherty, 1984). However, except for cefoxitin in colorectal surgery (see *Med Lett Drugs Ther*, 1989 C) and possibly cefuroxime or cefamandole for open-heart surgery (Slama et al, 1986; Kaiser et al, 1987), there is no evidence, based on controlled, comparative clinical studies, that these newer cephalosporins offer any advantages over first generation cephalosporins. Thus, at present, none are indicated over available therapy (DiPiro et al, 1983, 1984; Rapp and Blue, 1985; *Med Lett Drugs Ther*, 1987).

Parenterally administered first generation cephalosporins (cephalothin, cefazolin, cephapirin, cephradine) are rarely drugs of choice for the treatment of bacterial infections. They may be used in serious infections caused by gram-positive cocci (except enterococci), *Klebsiella pneumoniae, Escherichia coli*, or *Proteus mirabilis*, based on the results of susceptibility tests. These include infections of the lower respiratory tract, skin, soft tissues, bone, joints, heart, and urinary tract and bacteremias. They are not effective in meningitis. First generation cephalosporins may be combined with an aminoglycoside for serious *Klebsiella* infections (eg, pneumonia) or to provide broad spectrum empiric coverage for severe community-acquired infections (eg, pneumonia, septicemia) in nonimmunocompromised patients.

First generation cephalosporins often are the preferred alternatives to antistaphylococcal penicillins or penicillin G for serious staphylococcal and/or streptococcal (except enterococcal) infections (except meningitis) when the patient is allergic to penicillins. These infections include severe pyodermas, staphylococcal pneumonia, pneumococcal pneumonia (erythromycin is often preferred), septic arthritis, osteomyelitis, and endocarditis caused by viridans streptococci and *Staphylococcus aureus* (not methicillin-resistant strains). However, cephalosporins should not be administered to patients who experienced an immediate-type hypersensitivity reaction to a penicillin (see Adverse Reactions and Precautions; see also index entry Penicillins).

When a cephalosporin is used for a gram-positive infection, first generation derivatives are recommended because they have the best activity against gram-positive bacteria and they are less expensive than newer cephalosporins. Cefazolin usually is the preferred parenteral first generation cephalosporin because of its better pharmacokinetic properties (see above and Pharmacokinetics); also, it is less painful than cephalothin and cephapirin when administered intramuscularly. However, some experts prefer cephalothin for severe staphylococcal infections, such as endocarditis, because it is more impervious to attack by some staphylococcal β-lactamases (See Kernodie et al, 1990).

For additional discussion, see index entry Antimicrobial Drugs: Antimicrobial Drug Selection for Common Infectious Diseases (Table); see also Neu, 1982 D; *Med Lett Drugs Ther*, 1983 A; Fried and Hinthorn, 1985; Goldberg, 1987; Donowitz and Mandell, 1988, 1990.

Parenteral Second Generation Cephalosporins: Clinical uses of second generation cephalosporins must differentiate the two patterns of antibacterial activity included in this generation: that of the cephamycins, cefoxitin, cefotetan, and cefmetazole and that of the other second generation derivatives (see Antimicrobial Spectrum).

Cefoxitin is suitable for treating intra-abdominal infections that result from breaches in the intestinal mucosa. Such infections usually are caused by mixtures of aerobic gram-negative enteric bacilli and anaerobic bacteria, including the *Bacteroides fragilis* group. For community-acquired infections, cefoxitin alone has been shown to be as effective as the traditional therapy of clindamycin [Cleocin] plus gentamicin [Garamycin] (Tally et al, 1981; Drusano et al, 1982; Nichols et al, 1984; Malangoni et al, 1985; see also DiPiro and May, 1988). It frequently is a preferred drug in mildly to moderately ill patients with community acquired infections in areas where resistance is not a problem. For more severely ill patients and/or for intra-abdominal infections of nosocomial origin, an aminoglycoside should be included (see index entry Antimicrobial Drugs: Antimicrobial Drug Selection for Common Infectious Diseases [Table]; see also Neu, 1982 D; LeFrock et al, 1984 A; Fried and Hinthorn, 1985; Sanders et al, 1985; DiPiro and May, 1988; Finegold and Wexler, 1988). Other drugs effective against the *B. fragilis* group include clindamycin, metronidazole [Flagyl, Metryl], chloramphenicol [Chloromycetin], the antipseudomonal penicillins, imipenem/cilastatin [Primaxin], ticarcillin/potassium clavulanate [Timentin], and ampicillin/sulbactam [Unasyn].

Gynecologic pelvic infections (eg, acute pelvic inflammatory disease, endometritis, pelvic cellulitis) can be caused by a variety of bacterial pathogens and frequently are caused by more than one organism. Etiologic agents include members of the normal vaginal microflora, such as facultative gram-negative bacilli (eg, *Escherichia coli*) and anaerobic bacteria (eg, *Bacteroides* [*B. bivius, B. disiens*, and, less frequently, *B. fragilis*], gram-positive cocci), and the sexually transmitted pathogens, *Neisseria gonorrhoeae* and *Chlamydia trachomatis.* Depending on the clinical situation and likely causative organisms, cefoxitin, alone or in combination, may be the preferred drug (see Neu, 1982 D; LeFrock et al, 1984 B; Sanders et al, 1985; DiPiro and May, 1988). It is active against *N. gonorrhoeae*, including penicillinase-producing strains (PPNG); many gram-negative bacilli; and most anaerobic bacteria, including *B. fragilis*. Combination with doxycycline [Vibramycin] will expand coverage to include *C. trachomatis*; this combined regimen (alternative, cefotetan combined with doxycycline) is recommended by the Centers for Disease Control for acute pelvic inflammatory diseases likely to be caused by sexually transmitted pathogens (*MMWR*, 1989). Combination of cefoxitin with an aminoglycoside will expand coverage against aerobic gram-negative bacilli, but may not be adequate against *C. trachomatis*. An alternative to cefoxitin-containing regimens is clindamycin plus an aminoglycoside, which provides good coverage against anaerobic bacteria and aerobic gramnegative bacilli, but may not be adequate against *N. gonorrhoeae* or *C. trachomatis*. For additional discussion, see index entry Sexually Transmitted Diseases: Treatment (Table).

Cefoxitin alone also has been effective in mixed aerobic-anaerobic skin and soft tissue infections (Sanders et al, 1985). It is an effective alternative for uncomplicated gonorrhea caused by PPNG, but ceftriaxone is now the preferred cephalosporin (*MMWR*, 1989). Depending on the results of susceptibility tests, cefoxitin may be used in serious lower respiratory tract, urinary tract, bone, joint, skin, and soft tissue infections, or bacteremias, provided that equally effective, less toxic, and less expensive alternatives are not available. Because of its greater activity against the *B. fragilis* group when compared to first generation cephalosporins, cefoxitin is used to prevent infections after appendectomy or colorectal surgery in patients who cannot take the oral neomycin/erythromycin combination (eg, due to emergency operations or intestinal obstruction) (see index entry Antimicrobial Drugs: Chemoprophylaxis for Surgical Patients [Table]).

Cefotetan has been effective in intra-abdominal, obstetric and gynecologic, skin and soft tissue, complicated urinary tract, and lower respiratory tract infections caused by susceptible bacteria (see Ward and Richards, 1985). Although overall clinical experience is less with cefotetan, this cephamycin has been comparable to cefoxitin for the treatment of community-acquired intra-abdominal infections in moderately ill patients (Wilson et al, 1988); obstetric and gynecologic infections (Sweet et al, 1988); and skin and superficial soft tissue infections (Geckler et al, 1988); and for prophylaxis in colorectal surgery (Jagelman et al, 1988) in multicenter, randomized, controlled clinical trials. Thus, cefotetan appears to be an alternative to cefoxitin for these infections that are frequently polymicrobial, involving both aerobic gram-negative bacilli and anaerobic bacteria (including the *B. fragilis* group). When compared to cefoxitin, advantages of cefotetan include an expanded spectrum of activity against aerobic gram-negative bacilli and a longer elimination half-life (about 3.5 hours), which allows it to be administered twice daily. Possible disadvantages include the presence of a methylthiotetrazole side chain that has been associated with hypoprothrombinemia and bleeding as well as somewhat lower activity in vitro against some species of the *B. fragilis* group (eg, *B. ovatus, B. distasonis*). It should be emphasized that up to 20% of *B. fragilis* strains are resistant to both cefoxitin and cefotetan in some institutions and they probably should not be used alone for intra-abdominal infections in severely ill patients or when such infections are nosocomially acquired.

Cefmetazole has been effective in intra-abdominal, skin and skin structure, urinary tract, and lower respiratory tract infections caused by susceptible bacteria (Griffith et al, 1989), and the results of comparative clinical trials suggest that this new cephamycin antibiotic is comparable in efficacy and safety to cefoxitin for the treatment of these infections (Holloway et al, 1989; Frank et al, 1989; Burke et al, 1989; Yangco et al, 1989) as well as for prophylaxis in abdominal surgery (DiPiro et al, 1989). Thus, the place of cefmetazole in infectious disease therapy would appear to be as an alternative to cefoxitin and cefotetan, but clinical experience with this agent is limited. When compared with cefoxitin, the only apparent advantages of cefmetazole are somewhat better activity in vitro against *S. aureus* and other gram-positive cocci and a slightly longer elimination half-life (about 1.2 hours), which allows cefmetazole to be administered three or four times daily. However, cefotetan can be administered twice daily and its activity in vitro against aerobic gram-negative bacilli is superior to that of cefmetazole. Like cefotetan, cefmetazole has the potential disadvantages of a methylthiotetrazole side chain that has been associated with hypoprothrombinemia and disulfiram-like reaction as well as with somewhat lower activity in vitro against some species of the *B. fragilis* group (eg, *B. ovatus, B. thetaiotaomicron*).

Cefamandole and the newer second generation cephalosporins, cefuroxime, ceforanide, and cefonicid, have similar antibacterial spectra (see Antimicrobial Spectrum). Any of these agents may be used to treat infections of the lower respiratory tract, urinary tract, skin and skin structures, bone, and joints or bacteremias caused by susceptible bacteria, provided that equally effective, less toxic, and less expensive alternatives are not available. All of these agents have been approved for perioperative prophylaxis during certain surgical procedures (Tartaglione and Polk, 1985). However, with the possible exception of cefuroxime or cefamandole for open-heart surgery (Slama et al, 1986; Kaiser et al, 1987), none have been shown to offer any advantages over first generation cephalosporins (DiPiro et al, 1984; Rapp and Blue, 1985). Presently, it would appear that only one of these agents needs to be included in the hospital formulary.

Cefuroxime resembles cefamandole, but appears to offer a number of advantages. These include increased stability to certain β-lactamases (eg, TEM-1 of *Haemophilus influenzae*); a longer half life (1.3 hours versus 0.6 to 0.8 hours), which permits a longer dosing interval; and the absence of hypoprothrombinemia and a disulfiram-like reaction as adverse effects (see Antimicrobial Spectrum, Resistance, Pharmacokinetics, and Adverse Reactions and Precautions). Cefuroxime, unlike cefamandole, can achieve adequate concentrations in cerebrospinal fluid and has been effective in meningitis caused by the common meningeal pathogens, *H. influenzae* type b (including β-lactamase-producing strains), *Neisseria meningitidis*, and *Streptococcus pneumoniae* (Pfenninger et al, 1982; Report from a Swedish Study Group, 1982; Marks et al, 1986; see also Pharmacokinetics), although this use is being questioned (see below).

Cefuroxime is effective in community-acquired pneumonia in adults in whom ampicillin-resistant *H. influenzae* is a possible etiologic agent (Donowitz and Mandell, 1988, 1990). This second generation cephalosporin also can be used for single-agent empiric therapy of community-acquired bacterial pneumonia, suppurative bone and joint infections, and buccal and orbital cellulitis in infants and young children between 2 months and 5 years because it provides adequate coverage against the likely causative organisms (ie, *Staphylococcus aureus*, streptococci, pneumococci, *H. influenzae*) (see Gold and Rodriguez, 1983; Nelson, 1983; Smith and LeFrock, 1983; *Med Lett Drugs Ther*, 1984 A; Eichenwald, 1985). Cefuroxime also has been proposed as an effective single-agent alternative to ampicillin plus chloramphenicol for initial therapy of meningitis in infants and young children (see American Academy of Pediatrics Committee on Infectious Diseases, 1988). However, reports of delayed sterilization of cerebrospinal fluid, treatment failure and relapse, and serious sequelae (moderate-to-profound hearing loss) in patients with *H. influenzae* type b infection (Marks et al, 1986; Arditi et al, 1989; LeBel et al, 1989; Schaad et al, 1990) have raised concerns about cefuroxime (see McCracken et al, 1987). Most pediatric infectious disease experts prefer one of the third generation cephalosporins, usually cefotaxime or ceftriaxone, for meningitis (and other bacteremic *H. influenzae* type b infections) in infants and young children (see McCracken et al, 1987). On a weight basis, these third generation agents are considerably more potent than cefuroxime and they achieve much higher bactericidal titers in cerebrospinal fluid (see also discussion below and index entry Antimicrobial Drugs: Antimicrobial Drug Selection for Common Infectious Diseases [Table]).

When compared to cefuroxime or cefamandole, the elimination half-lives of cefonicid ($t_{1/2}$, 4.5 hours) and ceforanide ($t_{1/2}$, 3 hours) are longer, which permit dosage intervals of 24 and 12 hours, respectively (Barriere and Mills, 1982; Dudley et al, 1984; Pontzer and Kaye, 1984; Tartaglione and Polk, 1985; Saltiel and Brogden, 1986; Campoli-Richards et al, 1987; see also Pharmacokinetics). Thus, these agents have the potential to reduce the cost of drug therapy. However, both ceforanide and cefonicid have considerably less activity in vitro than cefuroxime or cefamandole against *Staphylococcus aureus*. Failures with cefonicid in the treatment of serious staphylococcal infections (eg, endocarditis) have been reported (Chambers et al, 1984; see also Dudley et al, 1984; Pontzer and Kaye, 1984; Tartaglione and Polk, 1985; Saltiel and Brogden, 1986). Ceforanide also has inferior activity against *Haemophilus influenzae* (Barriere and Mills, 1982; *Med Lett Drugs Ther*, 1984 B; Tartaglione and Polk, 1985; Campoli-Richards et al, 1987). Unlike cefuroxime, neither cefonicid nor ceforanide adequately penetrates into cerebrospinal fluid to be useful in meningitis (Tartaglione and Polk, 1985). Published clinical studies with cefonicid, particularly in serious infections, are still somewhat limited (Jacob and Layne, 1984; see also Saltiel and Brogden, 1986). However, because of the advantages of once-daily administration, this long-acting second generation cephalosporin is being used to treat a variety of mild-to-moderate infections, including community-acquired pneumonias, urinary tract infections, and skin and soft tissue infections (Donowitz and Mandell, 1988). Cefonicid also is being used to continue parenteral antibiotic therapy in outpatient settings (Kunkel and Iannini, 1984; Nadworny and Markowitz, 1987). Ceforanide does not appear to offer any advantages over cefuroxime or cefonicid and its clinical usefulness probably will remain limited (*Med Lett Drugs Ther*, 1984 B).

Parenteral Third Generation Cephalosporins: In contrast to first and most second generation cephalosporins, the available third generation cephalosporins (except cefoperazone) show considerable usefulness in certain types of meningitis. Cefotaxime and moxalactam have produced excellent results in gram-negative enteric bacillary meningitis, particularly against *Escherichia coli, Klebsiella*, and *Proteus* (Landesman et al, 1981; Cherubin et al, 1982; Rahal, 1982; Rahal and Simberkoff, 1982; Cherubin and Eng, 1986). Although clinical experience is more limited, ceftizoxime, ceftriaxone, and ceftazidime also appear useful for this indication (see Neu, 1987 B; Donowitz and Mandell, 1988, 1990). Because of high failure rates with chloramphenicol and the difficulties associated with intrathecal aminoglycoside administration, these third generation cephalosporins have become drugs of choice for meningitis known to be caused by gram-negative enteric bacilli (see index entry Antimicrobial Drugs: Antimicrobial Drug Selection for Common Infectious Diseases [Table]; see also Corrado et al, 1982; Rahal and Simberkoff, 1982; *Med Lett Drugs Ther*, 1983 A, 1988 A; Barriere and Flaherty, 1984; Fried and Hinthorn, 1985; Neu, 1987 B; Donowitz and Mandell, 1988, 1990). Ceftazidime appears to be the most useful third generation cephalosporin for meningitis caused by *Pseudomonas aeruginosa* (Fong and Tomkins, 1985). Presently, ceftazidime plus an aminoglycoside should be considered a preferred regimen (alternative regimen, an antipseudomonal penicillin plus an aminoglycoside) for this indication; the aminoglycoside is administered intravenously and intrathecally (or intraventricularly) (Neu, 1987 B; *Med Lett Drugs Ther*, 1990). Although ceftazidime alone has been effective in a limited number of cases of *P. aeruginosa* meningitis (Fong and Tomkins, 1985), additional clinical studies are necessary before it can be recommended as monotherapy for this very serious infection.

All of the above third generation cephalosporins also have been very effective against meningitis caused by *Haemophilus influenzae* type b (including β-lactamase-producing strains), a frequent causative organism in young children. Most infectious disease consultants now prefer a third generation cephalosporin (eg, cefotaxime, ceftriaxone) to ampicillin and chloramphenicol for initial treatment of *H. influenzae* type b meningitis. Penicillin G remains the drug of choice for pneumococcal and meningococcal meningitis; chloramphenicol remains an alternative, particularly in patients who are allergic to β-lactam antibiotics. Ceftriaxone and cefotaxime have excellent activity in vitro against all three of these common meningeal pathogens, and they have been shown to be as effective as ampicillin plus chloramphenicol for the empiric therapy of meningitis in infants and young children (Del Rio et al, 1983; Steele and Bradsher, 1983; Congeni, 1984; Barson et al, 1985; Bryan et al, 1985 A; Jacobs et al, 1985; Odio et al, 1986). A twice daily dosage schedule was adequate for the long-acting ceftriaxone; in one study (Bryan et al, 1985 A), once daily administration was effective. Thus, these third generation cephalosporins are now considered to be equally effective single-agent alternatives to ampicillin plus chloramphenicol for initial therapy of pediatric meningitis (American Academy of Pediatrics Committee on Infectious Diseases, 1988; see also index entry Antimicrobial Drugs: Antimicrobial Drug Selection for Common Infectious Diseases [Table]). Most pediatric infectious disease experts prefer monotherapy with an appropriate third generation cephalosporin, usually cefotaxime or ceftriaxone, both for the convenience of single-drug therapy and to avoid the toxicity and problems associated with administration (eg, need to monitor serum concentrations) of chloramphenicol (see McCracken et al, 1987). In addition to meningitis, third generation cephalosporins (eg, cefotaxime, ceftriaxone) also have become preferred empiric therapy of many pediatric infectious disease consultants for other serious infections in infants and young children between 2 months and 5 years where *H. influenzae* type b is a likely pathogen. These infections include facial cellulitis, septic arthritis, osteomyelitis, bacteremia, acute epiglottitis, and pneumonia (see index entry Antimicrobial Drugs: Antimicrobial Drug Selection for Common Infectious Diseases [Table]).

Neonatal meningitis most often is caused by *Streptococcus agalactiae* (group B) and other streptococci, *Escherichia coli* and other gram-negative enteric bacilli, and *Listeria monocytogenes*. The currently recommended empiric therapy for neonatal meningitis is ampicillin plus an aminoglycoside or ampicillin plus a third generation cephalosporin (American Academy of Pediatrics Committee on Infectious Diseases, 1988; see also index entry Antimicrobial Drugs: Antimicrobial Drug Selection for Common Infectious Diseases [Table]). Many pediatric infectious disease experts now prefer a third generation cephalosporin, usually cefotaxime or ceftriaxone, to an aminoglycoside, either in combination with ampicillin, for the empiric therapy of neonatal meningitis because they have better in vitro and CSF bactericidal activity against gram-negative enteric bacilli, are less toxic, and have more predictable pharmacokinetics. However, studies (see McCracken et al, 1984; Naqvi et al, 1985) have not shown superior clinical outcomes with these new cephalosporins and there is considerably less experience with their use. Additionally, the exclusive use of cefotaxime in neonatal intensive care units has led to outbreaks of cefotaxime-resistant *Enterobacter cloacae* (Bryan et al, 1985 B). Cefotaxime (or ceftriaxone) would be preferred when aminoglycoside serum concentrations could not be monitored or when the neonate has abnormal renal function (see Klein et al, 1986; Stutman and Marks, 1987; American Academy of Pediatrics Committee on Infectious Diseases, 1988). Ceftazidime is preferred to cefotaxime (or ceftriaxone) in the hospitalized low-birth-weight premature infant in whom nosocomial *Pseudomonas aeruginosa* infection is a possibility (American Academy of Pediatrics Committee on Infectious Diseases, 1988). Third generation cephalosporins should not be used alone for neonatal meningitis because none are active against *L. monocytogenes* or enterococci and some agents, such as moxalactam, lack adequate activity against group B streptococci (see Neu, 1982 A and D; Barriere and Flaherty, 1984; see also Antimicrobial Spectrum).

All third generation cephalosporins are highly active against *Neisseria gonorrhoeae*, including penicillinase-producing strains (PPNG) (see Antimicrobial Spectrum). In particular, the long-acting ceftriaxone ($t_{1/2}$, 8 hours), administered intramuscularly in a single 250-mg dose, has been shown to be very effective in uncomplicated gonorrhea in adults, including urethral, cervical, anorectal, and pharyngeal forms of this infection (Handsfield and Murphy, 1983; Judson et al, 1983, 1985; Collier et al, 1984). Presently, it is the drug of choice for all uncomplicated gonococcal infections, including PPNG, tetracycline-resistant *N. gonorrhoeae* (TRNG), and chromosomal-mediated resistant *N. gonorrhoeae* (CMRNG) infections (*MMWR*, 1989). Although cephalosporins are likely to cure incubating syphilis, they are not active against *Chlamydia trachomatis* and concomitant therapy with doxycycline (or tetracycline) is recommended for coexisting chlamydial infections (*MMWR*, 1989). Parenteral ceftriaxone (alternative, cefotaxime) also is preferred for disseminated gonococcal infections in adults and children and for neonatal gonococcal infections. A single 250-mg intramuscular dose of ceftriaxone is a treatment of choice (alternative, oral erythromycin for seven days) for chancroid caused by *Haemophilus ducreyi* (*MMWR*, 1989). For a more detailed discussion, see index entry Sexually Transmitted Diseases: Treatment (Table). Ceftriaxone, administered intravenously, has become a preferred drug for the treatment of serious neurologic, cardiovascular, and joint abnormalities associated with Lyme disease (Dattwyler et al, 1988; *Med Lett Drugs Ther*, 1989 A; see also index entry Antimicrobial Drugs: Antimicrobial Drug Selection for Common Infectious Diseases [Table]).

The third generation cephalosporins have been effective, frequently as empiric monotherapy, in a wide variety of serious gram-negative bacillary infections outside the central nervous system. These include lower respiratory tract, uncomplicated and complicated urinary tract, intra-abdominal, gynecologic, skin and skin structure, bone, and joint infections and bacteremias; these infections often are of nosocomial origin (see Neu, 1982 D; Barriere and Flaherty, 1984; Smith, 1984; see also Other Selected References for symposia publications on the individual agents). However, the exact role of third generation cephalosporins in these infections and optimal drug selection among the available third generation derivatives remain to be clarified. The decision to use a third generation cephalosporin should depend, in part, on the particular clinical situation and locally generated antibiotic susceptibility profiles. In general, less expensive, narrower spectrum, first (or second) generation cephalosporins should be used when they are equally effective. First generation cephalosporins clearly are preferable for known gram-positive bacterial infections and for surgical prophylaxis (see Neu, 1982 D; *Med Lett Drugs Ther*, 1983 A; DiPiro et al, 1984; Fried and Hinthorn, 1985; Goldberg, 1987; Donowitz and Mandell, 1988, 1990).

The following represent some of the more likely uses of third generation cephalosporins in serious gram-negative bacillary infections, based on current clinical experience: (1) When bacteria that are known to be multiply resistant to other, less expensive antibiotics (eg, penicillins, older cephalosporins), but are susceptible to a third generation cephalosporin, the latter is indicated. (2) When equally effective, third generation cephalosporins are usually preferred to aminoglycosides because of the ototoxicity and nephrotoxicity and requirement to monitor serum concentrations associated with the latter agents. This is especially important in patients at increased risk for aminoglycoside toxicity (see index entry, Aminoglycosides) or those requiring prolonged therapy (eg, osteomyelitis). (3) The high in vitro activity of third generation cephalosporins against most gram-negative bacilli makes these agents more desirable than less expensive alternatives for certain severe infections, such as pneumonia caused by *Klebsiella pneumoniae* (see Neu, 1982 D, 1987 B; Barriere and Flaherty, 1984; Smith, 1984; Fried and Hinthorn, 1985; Goldberg, 1987; Donowitz and Mandell, 1988, 1990).

The efficacy of monotherapy with a third generation cephalosporin, as an alternative to antimicrobial combination therapy that frequently includes an aminoglycoside, for broad spectrum empiric treatment of serious infections (eg, pneumonia, septicemia) or to treat infections of polymicrobial origin (eg, intra-abdominal, pelvic) has been documented in a number of clinical studies (Oblinger et al, 1982; Mandell et al, 1983, 1987; Stone et al, 1983; Warren et al, 1983; Smith et al, 1984; Mangi et al, 1988 A; see also Neu, 1982 D; Barriere and Flaherty, 1984; Smith, 1984; Moellering, 1985 A; and index entry Antimicrobial Drugs: Antimicrobial Drug Selection for Common Infectious Diseases [Table]). However, rapid development of resistance during therapy with third generation cephalosporins has been observed clinically (see Sanders et al, 1988), and the judicious use of these agents is recommended.

An important consideration for empiric therapy of nosocomial infections is the incidence of *Pseudomonas aeruginosa* in a particular hospital. Of the available third generation cephalosporins, ceftazidime is the most active agent against this organism. When used alone, ceftazidime has been as effective as standard combination therapy (eg, antipseudomonal penicillin plus aminoglycoside) for nosocomial sepsis (Rapp et al, 1984; Cone et al, 1985; Young, 1985), acute pulmonary exacerbations of cystic fibrosis (Mastella et al, 1983; Gold et al, 1985), and for initial therapy of febrile neutropenic patients (Pizzo et al, 1986; see also Wade et al, 1986). However, ceftazidime-resistant strains of *P. aeruginosa* have been isolated and monotherapy with this agent for serious *P. aeruginosa* infections requires further study. Current consensus is that ceftazidime should be used with an aminoglycoside for febrile neutropenic patients because the combination is more effective than ceftazidime alone for patients with gram-negative rod bacteremia (Calandra et al, 1987; see also Young, 1986; Hughes et al, 1990).

Selecting a particular third generation cephalosporin for routine use is somewhat difficult because they infrequently have been compared directly for clinical efficacy and toxicity. However, results of the randomized, prospective clinical trials that have been done suggest no differences among various third generation cephalosporins, except an increased incidence of bleeding with moxalactam (Joshi et al, 1986; Yangco et al, 1987; Mangi et al, 1988 B; Mandell et al, 1989; Smith et al, 1989; see also Neu, 1987 B). Guidelines for drug selection usually are based on noncomparative clinical studies, in vitro antimicrobial activity, pharmacokinetics, adverse reaction profiles, and cost (Barriere, 1986). As discussed above, when *P. aeruginosa* is a probable causative organism, ceftazidime is the preferred third generation cephalosporin. Cefoperazone is an alternative, but it has inferior activity against most strains of this organism. When *P. aeruginosa* is not under consideration, ceftriaxone, ceftizoxime, and cefotaxime have advantages over moxalactam, which has unacceptable hematologic toxicity, and cefoperazone, which also has been associated with hematologic side effects, has poorer activity against many Enterobacteriaceae, is not recommended for meningitis, and is not labeled for use in children, infants, and neonates. Ceftriaxone, ceftizoxime, and cefotaxime have good activity against most gram-positive bacteria (although a few authorities have expressed some concern about the activity of ceftriaxone against *S. aureus*), excellent activity against most gram-negative bacteria, and good adverse reaction profiles that are similar to first and most second generation cephalosporins. These three agents differ primarily in pharmacokinetic properties and in the amount of clinical experience. The primary advantage of cefotaxime is lengthy clinical experience, particularly in gram-negative enteric bacillary meningitis. Cefotaxime has a half-life of only one hour, which suggests that the drug should be administered every six hours for serious infections. However, more recent clinical studies indicate that an eight-hour dosage interval is adequate because of the more prolonged half-life (about 1.6 hours) of desacetylcefotaxime, its active metabolite (see Neu, 1990, and the evaluation). Ceftizoxime is essentially identical to cefotaxime; it has a longer half-life and also can be administered every eight hours for serious infections. However, there are fewer published data on its use in meningitis and it is not labeled for use in infants less than 6 months. Ceftriaxone has the longest half-life ($t_{1/2}$, 8 hours) among third generation cephalosporins and can be administered once daily for most serious infections and twice daily for meningitis. Once-daily therapy with ceftriaxone makes parenteral antibiotic treatment practical on an outpatient basis. See also Antimicrobial Spectrum, Adverse Reactions and Precautions, Pharmacokinetics, and the evaluations.

Oral Cephalosporins: Cephalexin, cephradine, cefadroxil, and cefaclor are rarely drugs of choice for bacterial infections, but these expensive oral antibiotics may be indicated in mild to moderate infections of the respiratory tract, urinary tract, skin and skin structures, and bone caused by susceptible organisms when preferred agents are ineffective or cannot be tolerated. Likely indications for first generation derivatives (cephalexin, cephradine, cefadroxil) include urinary tract infections when the causative organism is resistant to preferred and less expensive drugs (eg, sulfonamides, ampicillin, trimethoprim/sulfamethoxazole [Bactrim, Septra]) and minor staphylococcal pyodermas in patients with non-IgE-mediated (ie, nonimmediate) hypersensitivity reactions to penicillins. Cefaclor, a second generation cephalosporin, is more active than the first generation agents against *Haemophilus influenzae* and is active against many amoxicillin-resistant *H. influenzae* and *Moraxella (Branhamella) catarrhalis* strains. This agent is an alternative to erythromycin/sulfisoxazole [Pediazole], trimethoprim/sulfamethoxazole, and amoxicillin/potassium clavulanate [Augmentin] for acute otitis media and acute sinusitis caused by these amoxicillin-resistant organisms. For additional discussion, see index entry Antimicrobial Drugs: Antimicrobial Drug Selection for Common Infectious Diseases (Table); see also Neu, 1982 D; Rehm and McHenry, 1983; Norris, 1984 B; Eichenwald, 1985; Gordon, 1985; and Reese and Betts, 1986.

Sequential parenteral-oral cephalosporin therapy for suppurative bone and joint infections in infants and children has been successfully employed. However, large doses of oral cephalosporins usually are required, organism susceptibility must be known, and careful monitoring for compliance and serum bactericidal activity is required (see Nelson et al, 1982; Eichenwald, 1985).

Cefuroxime axetil is an ester that is hydrolyzed to cefuroxime after absorption from the gastrointestinal tract. This oral second generation cephalosporin has been effective in treating pharyngitis, acute otitis media, bronchitis, urinary tract infections, skin and skin structure infections, and uncomplicated gonorrhea caused by susceptible pathogens (see *Med Lett Drugs Ther*, 1988 B; Marx and Fant, 1988). Comparative clinical trials are limited, however. Cefuroxime axetil appears clinically to be as effective as cefaclor for acute otitis media (Aronovitz, 1988; McLinn et al, 1988) and lower respiratory tract infections (Schleupner et al, 1988), and it probably will be used to treat acute otitis media, acute sinusitis, and bronchitis. In vitro, it is superior to cefaclor against β-lactamase-producing *H. influenzae* and *M. catarrhalis*, but the lack of an oral suspension currently limits its usefulness in young children (see *Med Lett Drugs Ther*, 1988 B). Cefuroxime axetil has increased activity in vitro against *Escherichia coli* and other Enterobacteriaceae when compared to older cephalosporins, and was reported to be more effective than cefaclor and cephalexin for complicated urinary tract infections (Cox et al, 1987). Thus, cefuroxime axetil may be useful for urinary tract infections that are resistant to less expensive drugs, but there are a number of other antimicrobial agents (eg, trimethoprim/sulfamethoxazole [Bactrim, Septra], amoxicillin/potassium clavulanate [Augmentin], ciprofloxacin [Cipro], cefixime [Suprax]) for this indication. Cefuroxime axetil, 1 g as a single dose, plus probenecid (1 g) is effective for uncomplicated urethral, endocervical, and rectal gonorrhea (Gottlieb and Mills, 1986; Baddour et al, 1989) and is listed as an alternative to ceftriaxone for this indication by the Centers for Disease Control (*MMWR,* 1989). The CDC also recommends this oral cephalosporin to complete the course of therapy for disseminated gonococcal infection after parenteral ceftriaxone is given initially. Cefuroxime axetil offers no apparent advantages to other antimicrobial agents for skin infections or pharyngitis.

Cefixime is the first oral third generation cephalosporin to be approved for use in the United States. It has been effective in treating pharyngitis, acute otitis media, bronchitis, and urinary tract infections caused by susceptible pathogens following once-daily administration (see Brogden and Campoli-Richards, 1989; *Med Lett Drugs Ther,* 1989 B). Comparative clinical trials are very limited, however, and the therapeutic role of cefixime remains to be defined. The suspension formulation, which has better bioavailability than cefixime tablets (see Pharmacokinetics and the evaluation), has been compared to amoxicillin and cefaclor in acute otitis media. Cefixime had similar efficacy to cefaclor (Kenna et al, 1987) and, in one study, to amoxicillin (McLinn, 1987), although more side effects (gastrointestinal upset, rash) were seen in the cefixime group. In another study, however, cefixime was more effective than amoxicillin for acute otitis media caused by β-lactamase-producing *H. influenzae*, but less effective against *S. pneumoniae.* Furthermore, *S. aureus,* an organism that is resistant to cefixime, was isolated from middle ear fluid of nine patients taking this third generation cephalosporin, compared to none in the amoxicillin group (Howie and Owen, 1987). Thus, based on current evidence, cefixime does not appear to offer any clear advantages over older antimicrobial agents for this indication. Cefixime was as effective as amoxicillin for the treatment of acute bacterial bronchitis (Kiani et al, 1988), but any potential advantages over current therapies remain to be determined. Cefixime has excellent activity in vitro against *E. coli* and other Enterobacteriaceae when compared to older oral cephalosporins. It has been comparable to amoxicillin (Iravani et al, 1988) and trimethoprim/sulfamethoxazole (Cox, 1989; see also Brogden and Campoli-Richards, 1989) for uncomplicated urinary tract infections in clinical trials and may be useful for urinary tract infections that are resistant to less expensive drugs. However, there are a number of other effective antimicrobial agents (eg, trimethoprim/sulfamethoxazole, amoxicillin/potassium clavulanate, ciprofloxacin) for this indication. Cefixime offers no advantages to other antimicrobial agents for pharyngitis.

ADVERSE REACTIONS AND PRECAUTIONS

Hypersensitivity Reactions: Cephalosporins generally are well tolerated. Hypersensitivity reactions are the most common systemic adverse effects. The majority of these are maculopapular skin rashes that usually occur after several days of therapy. Rashes frequently are accompanied by fever and eosinophilia. Immediate-type, IgE-mediated reactions, including urticaria, bronchospasm, and anaphylaxis, are uncommon with the cephalosporins. Immune-mediated leukopenia, thrombocytopenia, and anemia have been reported rarely and are reversible with discontinuation of treatment. Direct and indirect positive Coombs' tests are relatively common with large doses, but hemolytic anemia is rare and usually mild. A serum sickness reaction, characterized by skin rash with polyarthritis and, frequently, fever, has been associated most often with cefaclor (Murray et al, 1980; Ackley and Felsher, 1981; Leng and Anderson, 1985; Levine, 1985).

Although the chemical structures of cephalosporins and penicillins are similar (see Chemistry and Classification; see also index entry Penicillins), cross-hypersensitivity between these two groups of antibiotics is low. Clinically, probably fewer than 5% of individuals with a history of penicillin allergy, including those with a history of IgE-mediated reactions, also are allergic to cephalosporins (Saxon, 1983; Quintiliani et al, 1984; Anderson, 1986). Therefore, it generally is considered safe to administer a cephalosporin to a patient with a history of a non-IgE-mediated hypersensitivity reaction (eg, maculopapular skin rash) to penicillins. However, the current consensus is that cephalosporins should not be used in individuals who experienced immediate hypersensitivity reactions (eg, urticaria, angioedema, bronchospasm, anaphylaxis) to penicillins because the consequences of these adverse reactions could be catastrophic (Quintiliani et al, 1984).

Hematologic Reactions: Bleeding has been reported with cefamandole, cefoperazone, cefotetan, cefmetazole, and, particularly, moxalactam. A total of 2.5% of clinical trial patients treated for four or more days with moxalactam experienced a bleeding event, most of which were serious (manufacturer's literature). Each of these cephalosporins contains a methylthiotetrazole side chain that has been associated with hypoprothrombinemia in some patients, particularly elderly debilitated individuals, those with severe renal insufficiency, and malnourished patients receiving total parenteral nutrition. The prolongation of prothrombin time appears to result from interference with hepatic vitamin K metabolism by the methylthiotetrazole side chain of these cephalosporins (Lipsky, 1988; Shearer et al, 1988), but eradication of vitamin K-producing intestinal microorganisms also may be involved (Bang and Kammer, 1983). Administration of vitamin K reverses the hypoprothrombinemia. In some patients, prophylactic vitamin K administration may be desirable when using these five cephalosporins; vitamin K (adults, 10 mg per week) is now recommended in all patients receiving moxalactam (see the evaluation).

Moxalactam also has prolonged the bleeding time and caused bleeding diathesis in some patients because of dose-dependent inhibition of platelet function (Weitekamp and Aber, 1983). This is not reversible by vitamin K. In adults with normal renal function, doses exceeding 4 g per day for more than three days may result in platelet dysfunction. Patients with reduced renal function are particularly susceptible. Bleeding time should be monitored in patients requiring more than 4 g of moxalactam per day for more than three days. All patients with renal dysfunction should have appropriate dosage adjustments and should be monitored periodically with bleeding times. If the bleeding time becomes unduly prolonged, moxalactam should be discontinued (see evaluation). Because of the coagulopathy associated with moxalactam use, third generation cephalosporins usually are preferred (see Uses).

Gastrointestinal Reactions: Gastrointestinal disturbances associated with cephalosporins include pyrosis, anorexia, nausea, vomiting, and diarrhea. Cefoperazone may cause more diarrhea than other cephalosporins, perhaps because of greater biliary excretion (Carlberg et al, 1982; Mulligan et al, 1982). Rarely, antibiotic-associated pseudomembranous colitis (AAPMC) due to *Clostridium difficile* occurs with the cephalosporins. If this potentially life-threatening adverse effect develops, the drug should be discontinued, supportive measures should be initiated to maintain normal fluid and electrolyte balance, and, if necessary, treatment with oral vancomycin (alternative, metronidazole) should be instituted (see index entries Vancomycin; Metronidazole).

Renal and Hepatic Reactions: Cephalosporins may temporarily increase blood urea nitrogen (BUN) levels, but generally they are not considered to be nephrotoxic at usually recommended dosages. However, cephalothin rarely has caused more serious nephrotoxicity (tubular necrosis), especially when given in large dosages or to patients with preexisting renal impairment. Additive nephrotoxicity has been reported when cephalothin and an aminoglycoside were administered concomitantly (see Drug Interactions and Interference with Laboratory Tests). Some signs of hepatic dysfunction, manifested by transient increases in serum transaminase (ALT, AST) and alkaline phosphatase concentrations, also have been noted following administration of the cephalosporins. Reversible cholestatic jaundice has been reported rarely.

Miscellaneous Reactions: Cephalosporins are irritants and can cause pain at the site of intramuscular injection or thrombophlebitis after intravenous administration. Among first generation cephalosporins, cefazolin is less irritating than cephalothin, cephapirin, and cephradine and is preferred for intramuscular use. Phlebitis usually can be prevented by alternating veins or by slow injection of a solution diluted with sodium chloride or dextrose injection. Intrathecal injection of cephalosporins is not recommended, because animal studies and limited clinical observations indicate that this route may be neurotoxic; nystagmus, hallucinations, and convulsions have been observed.

Cephalosporins may cause clinically significant superinfections. *Pseudomonas, Candida*, and enterococci (particularly with third generation derivatives like moxalactam) are likely causative organisms. If superinfection occurs, appropriate measures should be undertaken.

Ceftriaxone has been associated with the formation of biliary sludge in the gallbladder, which may lead to signs and symptoms of cholecystitis. This was reversible after drug discontinuation (Schaad et al, 1988, 1990; Pigrau et al, 1989). This highly protein bound cephalosporin also can displace bilirubin from albumin binding sites (Fink et al, 1987), and some consultants recommended caution in the use of ceftriaxone in jaundiced or premature infants.

The risk to the fetus when the cephalosporins are administered to pregnant women has not been fully assessed but, as with the penicillins, there is no evidence of teratogenicity in man (see Chow and Jewesson, 1985). All cephalosporins except moxalactam are in FDA Pregnancy Category B; moxalactam is in Category C.

For additional discussion of adverse reactions and precautions, see *Med Lett Drugs Ther*, 1983 A; Barriere and Flaherty, 1984; Quintiliani et al, 1984; Smith, 1984; Fried and Hinthorn, 1985; Tartaglione and Polk, 1985; Norrby, 1986; Sattler et al, 1986; Goldberg, 1987; Donowitz and Mandell, 1988, 1990.

DRUG INTERACTIONS AND INTERFERENCE WITH LABORATORY TESTS

An increase in nephrotoxicity has been observed in patients receiving an aminoglycoside plus cephalothin (Wade et al, 1978; see also Luft, 1982; Mangini, 1984 A; and Hansten and Horn, 1989). This appears to be most likely in patients with pre-existing renal disease. Except for cephaloridine (no longer marketed), there is no evidence that other cephalosporins also potentiate aminoglycoside nephrotoxicity (see Mangini, 1984 A). Current recommendations are to administer aminoglycoside-cephalosporin combinations with caution, particularly in patients with pre-existing renal disease (Hansten and Horn, 1989). Avoidance of cephalothin in these patients should be considered.

Cephalothin also may increase the nephrotoxic effects of colistimethate, and renal function should be monitored. The availability of alternative antibiotics probably makes use of this combination unnecessary (Mangini, 1984 B; Hansten and Horn, 1989).

Acute alcohol intolerance, ie, a disulfiram-like reaction, has been attributed to certain cephalosporins containing a methylthiotetrazole side chain. Facial flushing, nausea, headache, sweating, tachycardia, and, infrequently, hypotensive episodes have been reported in patients who imbibed alcohol while receiving cefamandole, cefoperazone, moxalactam, cefotetan, or cefmetazole (Neu and Prince, 1980; Portier et al, 1980; Kannangara et al, 1984; see also Witt and Witt, 1983; Mangini, 1984 C; Stockley, 1985; Kline et al, 1987; Hansten and Horn, 1989; Saito, 1989). Symptoms usually occur within 30 minutes of alcohol ingestion and last for several minutes to several hours. The exact incidence of this reaction is not known. Methylthiotetrazole-containing cephalosporins increased acetaldehyde concentrations in animals when ethanol was administered (Buening et al, 1981), and although not completely understood, acetaldehyde accumulation is presumed to be the cause of this reaction in humans. It is recommended that alcoholic beverages or ethanol-containing pharmaceuticals be avoided in patients receiving cefamandole, cefoperazone, moxalactam, cefotetan, or cefmetazole and for two to three days after antibiotic therapy is discontinued (Hansten and Horn, 1989).

A false-positive reaction for glucose in the urine may occur when Benedict's or Fehling's solution or Clinitest tablets are employed. Cephalosporins apparently do not interfere with results obtained from enzyme-based tests, such as Tes-Tape or Clinistix.

High concentrations of cefoxitin, ceforanide, or cephalothin may interfere with measurement of creatinine levels by the Jaffe reaction and produce false results (see Guay et al, 1983). Serum samples from cefoxitin-treated patients should not be analyzed for creatinine if withdrawn within two hours of drug administration.

PHARMACOKINETICS

Some pharmacokinetic values for the cephalosporins are shown in Table 2.

Oral Cephalosporins: Cephalexin, cephradine, and cefadroxil (first generation cephalosporins), cefaclor and cefuroxime axetil (second generation cephalosporins), and cefixime (third generation cephalosporin) are stable in gastric acid and can be administered orally. The oral first generation cephalosporins and cefaclor are well absorbed from the gastrointestinal tract and similar peak serum concentrations are attained with comparable doses (eg, approximately 15 mcg/ml after a dose of 500 mg). In contrast, cefuroxime axetil and cefixime are incompletely absorbed with bioavailabilities of 36% to 52% and 40% to 50%, respectively (Faulkner et al, 1987; Finn et al, 1987; Marx and Fant, 1988; Brogden and Campoli-Richards, 1989). Except for cefadroxil and cefuroxime axetil, the presence of food decreases the rate of absorption in adults, but the extent of absorption (ie, the area under the serum concentration time curve [AUC]) is unchanged (see Nightingale et al, 1980; Norris, 1984 B; Fried and Hinthorn, 1985; Faulkner et al, 1987). The absorption of cefuroxime axetil is enhanced when taken with food or milk (Finn et al, 1987; Marx and Fant, 1988). In infants and children, the ingestion of milk was reported to decrease the bioavailability of cephalexin and cephradine, but not that of cefadroxil or cefaclor (Ginsburg, 1982).

All of the oral cephalosporins bind poorly to plasma proteins. Although these agents distribute to a wide variety of tissues and body fluids, they do not achieve therapeutic concentrations in the cerebrospinal fluid, even in the presence of inflammation.

Oral cephalosporins are eliminated by the kidneys, primarily by renal tubular secretion, and are recovered as unchanged drugs in the urine. Excretion of most of these agents is delayed by probenecid. The elimination half-lives of cephalexin, cephradine, and cefaclor are similar (about 50 minutes). However, the elimination half-lives of cefadroxil (about 90 minutes), cefuroxime axetil (about 80 minutes), and cefixime (three to four hours) are more prolonged, allowing longer dosing intervals. Dosage reductions are required when cephalexin, cephradine, cefadroxil, cefuroxime axetil, and cefixime are used in patients with impaired renal function. Cefaclor, however, is unstable in biological fluids and does not accumulate in these patients.

See also Table 2 and the evaluations. For additional discussion, see Nightingale et al, 1975, 1980; Rehm and McHenry, 1983; Norris, 1984 B; Quintiliani et al, 1984; Fried and Hinthorn, 1985; Faulkner et al, 1987; Finn et al, 1987; Marx and Fant, 1988; Brogden and Campoli-Richards, 1989.

Parenteral First Generation Cephalosporins: These agents can be administered intravenously or intramuscularly. Cefazolin is preferred to cephalothin, cephapirin, and cephradine for intramuscular administration because it causes less pain at the site of injection. At equivalent doses, cefazolin achieves peak serum concentrations significantly higher than those obtained with other first generation cephalosporins. This is due, in part, to the higher plasma protein binding and lower volume of distribution observed with cefazolin.

Parenteral first generation cephalosporins distribute to a wide variety of tissues (eg, myocardium, bone, gallbladder) and body fluids (eg, pericardial, pleural, synovial, bile, urine). However, they fail to achieve therapeutic concentrations in the cerebrospinal fluid, even in the presence of inflammation.

All parenterally administered first generation cephalosporins are eliminated by the kidneys. However, the mechanisms and rates of elimination differ among the four agents. Both cephalothin and cephapirin are partially metabolized to considerably less active desacetyl metabolites. Parent drugs plus metabolites are rapidly eliminated by renal tubular secretion.

TABLE 2.
PHARMACOKINETIC VALUES FOR THE CEPHALOSPORINS[1]

Generic Name	Trade Name(s)	Route(s) of Administration	Plasma Protein Bound (%)	Volume of Distribution (L/kg)
FIRST GENERATION				
Cephalothin	Keflin	Intravenous Intramuscular	70	0.26 ± 0.11
Cefazolin	Ancef, Kefzol	Intravenous Intramuscular	85	0.12 ± 0.03
Cephapirin	Cefadyl	Intravenous Intramuscular	45-50	0.13 ± 0.05
Cephradine	Anspor, Velosef	Oral Intravenous Intramuscular	10-20	0.25 ± 0.01
Cephalexin	Keflex, Keftab	Oral	10-15	0.26 ± 0.03
Cefadroxil	Duricef, Ultracef	Oral	15-20	0.31
SECOND GENERATION				
Cefamandole	Mandol	Intravenous Intramuscular	70-80	0.16 ± 0.05
Cefuroxime[3]	Zinacef, Kefurox	Intravenous Intramuscular	33	0.19 ± 0.04
Ceforanide	Precef	Intravenous Intramuscular	80	0.16-0.19
Cefonicid	Monocid	Intravenous Intramuscular	95-98	0.11
Cefaclor	Ceclor	Oral	25	0.24-0.36
Cephamycins				
Cefoxitin	Mefoxin	Intravenous Intramuscular	70-80	0.13-0.22
Cefotetan	Cefotan	Intravenous Intramuscular	88	0.12-0.19
Cefmetazole	Zefazone	Intravenous	65	?

Metabolized (%)	Urinary Recovery (%)	Approximate Half-Life (hours)	Effect of Probenecid	References
20-30	70-80 (50)[2]	0.5-0.9	+	Nightingale et al, 1975, 1980; Bennett et al, 1983; Norris, 1984 B; Benet and Sheiner, 1985
None	95	1.8	+	Nightingale et al, 1975, 1980; Quintiliani and Nightingale, 1978; Bennett et al, 1983; Norris, 1984 B; Benet and Sheiner, 1985
40	90 (50)[2]	0.6-0.8	+	Nightingale et al, 1975, 1980; Bennett et al, 1983; Norris, 1984 B; Benet and Sheiner, 1985
None	90	0.8	+	Nightingale et al, 1975, 1980; Bennett et al, 1983; Norris, 1984 B; Benet and Sheiner, 1985
None	90	0.9	+	Nightingale et al, 1975, 1980; Bennett et al, 1983; Rehm and McHenry, 1983; Norris, 1984 B; Benet and Sheiner, 1985
None	90	1.4	−	Nightingale et al, 1980; Bennett et al, 1983; Rehm and McHenry, 1983; Norris, 1984 B
None	80-95	0.6-1	+	Nightingale et al, 1980; Norris, 1984 B; Benet and Sheiner, 1985; Sanders et al, 1985; Tartaglione and Polk, 1985
None	90-95	1.3-1.7	+	Gold and Rodriguez, 1983; Smith and LeFrock, 1983; Norris, 1984 B; Benet and Sheiner, 1985; Tartaglione and Polk, 1985
None	90	2.7-3.0	−	Barriere and Mills, 1982; Bennett et al, 1983; Norris, 1984 B; Tartaglione and Polk, 1985
None	90	3.5-4.5	+	Dudley et al, 1984; Norris, 1984 B; Pontzer and Kaye, 1984; Benet and Sheiner, 1985; Tartaglione and Polk, 1985
None	60-85	0.6-0.9	+	Nightingale et al, 1980; Bennett et al, 1983; Rehm and McHenry. 1983; Norris, 1984 B
<2	80-95	0.7-1	+	Nightingale et al, 1980; Bennett et al, 1983; Norris, 1984 B; Sanders et al, 1985; Tartaglione and Polk, 1985
None	60-80	3-4.6	+	Ward and Richards, 1985; Smith et al, 1986; Bergan, 1987
None	85	1.2	+	Manufacturer's literature

(table continued on next page)

TABLE 2 (Continued)

Generic Name	Trade Name(s)	Route(s) of Administration	Plasma Protein Bound (%)	Volume of Distribution (L/kg)
THIRD GENERATION				
Cefotaxime	Claforan	Intravenous Intramuscular	38	0.25-0.39
Ceftizoxime	Cefizox	Intravenous Intramuscular	30	0.35-0.40
Ceftriaxone	Rocephin	Intravenous Intramuscular	83-96	0.12-0.14
Ceftazidime	Fortaz, Tazicef, Tazidime	Intravenous Intramuscular	<10	0.21-0.28
Cefoperazone	Cefobid	Intravenous Intramuscular	87-93	0.14-0.20
Moxalactam	Moxam	Intravenous Intramuscular	50	0.25-0.40
Cefixime	Suprax	Oral	65-70	0.11-0.22

[1] *The pharmacokinetic values shown in this Table represent average or most frequently reported values from the literature. In some cases, however, there is considerable variation among different laboratories.*

[2] *Number in parentheses represents percentage of dose excreted in the urine as unchanged drug.*

[3] *Cefuroxime axetil [Ceftin], an orally administered product, also is available.*

[4] *The half-life of desacetylcefotaxime is 1.5 to 1.6 hours.*

Cephradine also is rapidly eliminated by renal tubular secretion, but it is not metabolized. The half-lives of cephalothin, cephapirin, and cephradine are under one hour. In contrast, cefazolin is eliminated more slowly ($t_{1/2}$, 1.8 hours) by glomerular filtration and renal tubular secretion. Because of its higher and more prolonged serum concentrations, cefazolin usually can be given in lower doses and less frequently than other parenteral first generation cephalosporins and, thus, often is preferred (see Uses). The half-lives of all of these analogues are prolonged in patients with renal impairment and dosage adjustments are required.

See also Table 2 and the evaluations. For additional discussion, see Nightingale et al, 1975, 1980; Quintiliani and Nightingale, 1978; Norris, 1984 B; Quintiliani et al, 1984; and Fried and Hinthorn, 1985.

Parenteral Second Generation Cephalosporins: These agents can be administered intravenously or intramuscularly. At equivalent dosages, peak serum concentrations vary among the individual agents. In general, cefonicid and cefotetan achieve the highest peak serum concentration followed by ceforanide, cefuroxime, and the older derivatives, cefoxitin and cefamandole. Plasma protein binding also varies; cefonicid is the most highly bound (greater than 95%) and cefuroxime is the least bound (33%) second generation cephalosporin.

Metabolized (%)	Urinary Recovery (%)	Approximate Half-Life (hours)	Effect of Probenecid	References
30-50	85 (50-60)[2]	1-1.1[4]	+	LeFrock et al, 1982; Neu, 1982 A; Carmine et al, 1983 A; Garzone et al, 1983 A; Barriere and Flaherty, 1984; Balant et al, 1985; Benet and Sheiner, 1985
None	80-90	1.4-1.8	+	Neu, 1982 A; Bennett et al, 1983; Garzone et al, 1983 A; Barriere and Flaherty, 1984; Balant et al, 1985; Richards and Heel, 1985
None	40-65[5]	6-9	−	Neu, 1982 A; Bennett et al, 1983; Garzone et al, 1983 A; Barriere and Flaherty, 1984; Patel and Kaplan, 1984; Richards et al, 1984; Balant et al, 1985; Beam, 1985
None	80-90	1.9	−	Neu, 1982 A; Garzone et al, 1983 A; Smith, 1984; Balant et al, 1985; Benet and Sheiner, 1985; Gentry, 1985; Richards and Brogden, 1985
None	25[6]	1.9-2.1	−	Funk and Strausbaugh, 1982; Neu, 1982 A; Bennett et al, 1983; Garzone et al, 1983 A; Barriere and Flaherty, 1984; Balant et al, 1985
None	70-94	2-2.3	−	Fitzpatrick and Standiford, 1982; Neu, 1982 A; Bennett et al, 1983; Carmine et al, 1983 B; Garzone et al, 1983 A: Barriere and Flaherty, 1984; Balant et al 1985
None	50[7]	3-4	?	Faulkner et al, 1987; Brogden and Campoli-Richards, 1989

[5] *Although the primary route of excretion is renal, about 40% of a dose is eliminated unchanged in the bile. Dosage reductions are not necessary in patients with severe renal dysfunction.*

[6] *Unlike other cephalosporins, the primary route of excretion is biliary (70% as unchanged drug). Dosage reductions are not necessary in patients with severe renal dysfunction.*

[7] *Urinary recovery is expressed as percentage of absorbed dose.*

All of these agents distribute to a wide variety of tissues and body fluids, including pleural and synovial fluids, sputum, bone, bile, and urine. However, cefuroxime is the only second generation cephalosporin that achieves therapeutic concentrations in the cerebrospinal fluid of patients with meningitis (see Gold and Rodriguez, 1983; see also Uses).

All parenteral second generation cephalosporins are excreted as unchanged drugs via the kidneys by glomerular filtration and renal tubular secretion. They are not metabolized. These agents differ in their rates of elimination, however. The half-lives of the newer derivatives, particularly cefonicid ($t_{1/2}$, 3.5 to 4.5 hours), cefotetan ($t_{1/2}$, 3 to 4.6 hours), and ceforanide ($t_{1/2}$, 2.7 to 3 hours), are considerably longer than those of cefoxitin and cefamandole ($t_{1/2}$, less than one hour). Cefmetazole has a half-life of 1.2 hours. The half-life of cefuroxime is 1.3 to 1.7 hours. The half-lives of all of these agents are prolonged in patients with renal impairment and dosage adjustments are necessary.

Longer dosing intervals can be employed with cefonicid (24 hours), cefotetan (12 hours), ceforanide (12 hours), cefuroxime (8 hours), and cefmetazole (6 to 8 hours) when compared with cefoxitin and cefamandole (4 to 6 hours). The pharmacokinetics of these newer second generation cephalosporins, particularly cefonicid, have the potential to reduce the cost of cephalosporin therapy. However, equal or improved efficacy (without added toxicity) of these newer agents must be clearly established by comparative clinical trials before they can be recommended over established therapies (see Uses).

See also Table 2 and the evaluations. For additional discussion, see Barriere and Mills, 1982; Gold and Rodriguez, 1983; Smith and LeFrock, 1983; Dudley et al, 1984; Norris, 1984 B; Pontzer and Kaye, 1984; Fried and Hinthorn, 1985; Sanders et al, 1985; Tartaglione and Polk, 1985; Ward and Richards, 1985; Smith et al, 1986; and Bergan, 1987.

Parenteral Third Generation Cephalosporins: Parenteral third generation cephalosporins are poorly absorbed orally and must be administered intravenously or intramuscularly. At equivalent doses, peak serum concentrations vary among the individual agents. In general, ceftriaxone and cefoperazone achieve the highest peak serum concentrations. This is due, in part, to their higher plasma protein binding and lower volumes of distribution.

Third generation cephalosporins distribute to a wide variety of tissues (eg, myocardium, myometrium, bone, gallbladder) and body fluids (eg, synovial, pleural, peritoneal, pericardial). Adequate biliary concentrations are achieved with all of these agents, and very high concentrations are observed with cefoperazone and ceftriaxone. Urinary concentrations achieved with all third generation cephalosporins are far in excess of minimum inhibitory concentrations for susceptible organisms.

In contrast to first and second generation cephalosporins (except cefuroxime), the third generation agents are able to penetrate inflamed meninges to achieve therapeutic cerebrospinal fluid concentrations for a number of pathogens, including *Escherichia coli* and other gram-negative enteric bacilli, *Haemophilus influenzae, Neisseria meningitidis*, and, for some analogues, *Streptococcus pneumoniae*. Except for cefoperazone, for which cerebrospinal fluid penetration has been more variable, the third generation cephalosporins are useful agents for meningitis (see Uses).

The third generation cephalosporins exhibit considerable differences in elimination routes and half-lives. Cefotaxime is the only third generation agent that undergoes metabolism. This compound is partially metabolized by hepatic esterases to desacetylcefotaxime, which is four- to eightfold less active than the parent compound. However, desacetylcefotaxime is more active than cefazolin, cefamandole, and cefoxitin against most aerobic gram-negative bacteria, and studies in vitro suggest that cefotaxime and desacetylcefotaxime act synergistically against a number of bacterial strains (see Jones et al, 1982; Neu, 1982 E; Chin and Neu, 1984). Cefotaxime and its metabolite are eliminated primarily by renal tubular secretion; probenecid delays excretion. Cefotaxime has the shortest half-life (one hour) among third generation cephalosporins and, therefore, has been administered every six hours for serious infections. However, the relatively longer half-life of desacetylcefotaxime ($t_{1/2}$, 1.6 hours) permits less frequent dosing in many situations. Because cefotaxime has an important nonrenal route of elimination, little parent drug accumulates in individuals with renal impairment. However, elimination of the desacetyl metabolite is prolonged and dosage reductions are recommended when the creatinine clearance is less than 20 ml/min.

Ceftizoxime, ceftazidime, and moxalactam are excreted as unchanged drugs by the kidneys. Ceftizoxime ($t_{1/2}$, 1.4 to 1.8 hours) is eliminated by glomerular filtration and renal tubular secretion; probenecid delays excretion. In contrast, ceftazidime ($t_{1/2}$, 1.8 hours) and moxalactam ($t_{1/2}$, 2 to 2.3 hours) are eliminated by glomerular filtration, and probenecid does not affect their rates of excretion. The intermediate elimination half-lives of these three agents allows them to be administered every eight hours for serious infections. The half-lives of ceftizoxime, ceftazidime, and moxalactam are substantially longer in individuals with renal impairment and dosage reductions are necessary to avoid drug accumulation.

Ceftriaxone is eliminated as unchanged drug both via the renal (about 60%, by glomerular filtration) and biliary (about 40%) routes. It has the longest elimination half-life (six to nine hours) of any third generation cephalosporin and can be administered once daily for serious infections outside the central nervous system. Thus, it is a particularly attractive agent because of the potential for cost savings. It also may be useful for home intravenous antibiotic therapy. The elimination half-life of ceftriaxone is only minimally increased in patients with severe renal impairment and dosage reductions are unnecessary. Accumulation does occur in patients with severe combined renal and hepatic failure and dosage modifications are required.

Cefoperazone is the only cephalosporin eliminated primarily unchanged in bile (about 70%); about 25% of a dose is recovered in the urine. This third generation cephalosporin has an intermediate elimination half-life (1.9 to 2.1 hours); most infectious disease experts recommend an eight-hour dosing interval for serious infections. Accumulation of cefoperazone does not occur in patients with end-stage renal disease and the half-life is only increased two- to fourfold in the presence of hepatic disease. However, substantial accumulation occurs in patients with combined renal and hepatic failure and dosage reductions are necessary.

See also Table 2 and the evaluations. For additional discussion, see Neu, 1982 A; Garzone et al, 1983 A; Barriere and Flaherty, 1984; Smith, 1984; Balant et al, 1985; and Noble and Barza, 1985.

Drug Evaluations

PARENTERAL FIRST GENERATION CEPHALOSPORINS

CEPHALOTHIN SODIUM

[Keflin]

MECHANISM OF ACTION, ANTIMICROBIAL SPECTRUM, AND RESISTANCE. The mechanism of action, antimicrobial spectrum, and resistance properties are essentially the same as for cefazolin (see that evaluation and the Introduction). Cephalothin is highly resistant to staphylococcal β-lactamases.

USES. Cephalothin has the same indications as cefazolin, but the latter drug frequently is preferred because it achieves higher serum concentrations, has a longer elimination half-life, and causes less pain on intramuscular injection. However, some experts prefer cephalothin for severe staphylococcal infections, such as endocarditis, because it is more impervious to attack by some staphylococcal β-lactamases (see Kernodie et al, 1990; see also the evaluation on Cefazolin Sodium and the Introduction).

ADVERSE REACTIONS AND PRECAUTIONS. See the Introduction. Nephrotoxicity (renal tubular necrosis) has been reported rarely with cephalothin, usually when large doses were given or after administration to patients with renal impairment.

DRUG INTERACTIONS AND INTERFERENCE WITH LABORATORY TESTS. Cephalothin plus an aminoglycoside can increase nephrotoxicity, particularly in patients with pre-existing renal disease. For additional discussion, see the Introduction.

PHARMACOKINETICS. Because of pain on intramuscular injection, cephalothin usually is administered intravenously. Peak serum concentrations of 30 to 60 mcg/ml are obtained after an intravenous dose of 1 g.

Approximately 70% of circulating cephalothin is bound to plasma protein. The volume of distribution is 0.26 ± 0.11 L/kg. The drug enters many tissues and body fluids, but it fails to achieve therapeutic concentrations in cerebrospinal fluid even in the presence of inflammation. Cephalothin crosses the placenta.

Up to 30% of cephalothin is metabolized to the less active desacetyl metabolite. Parent drug and metabolite are excreted by the kidneys, primarily by renal tubular secretion; probenecid delays excretion. The elimination half-life ranges from 30 to 55 minutes. The half-life is prolonged in patients with renal impairment and dosage adjustments are required.

DOSAGE AND PREPARATIONS. Cephalothin can be administered intravenously (preferred) or by intramuscular injection deep into a large muscle mass to minimize pain and induration. Intravenous administration can be by slow injection or by intermittent or continuous infusion. See the manufacturer's instructions for the appropriate dilution of the drug, compatible diluents and intravenous solutions, and stability of cephalothin in these solutions.

Intravenous, Intramuscular (deep): *Adults*, 2 to 12 g daily in equally divided doses every four to six hours (The Medical Letter, 1988). The usual dosage is 500 mg to 1 g every four to six hours, depending on the severity of the infection and the susceptibility of the causative organism. In severe, life-threatening infections, doses up to 2 g every four hours may be required.

Infants and children, 75 to 125 mg/kg daily in equally divided doses every four to six hours (Nelson, 1989 A). The manufacturer recommends a dosage range of 80 to 160 mg/kg daily in divided doses.

Newborns over 7 days and weighing more than 2 kg, intravenously, 80 mg/kg daily in divided doses every six hours; *newborns over 7 days and weighing less than 2 kg*, intravenously, 60 mg/kg daily in divided doses every eight hours; *newborns 0 to 7 days and weighing more than 2 kg*, intravenously, 60 mg/kg daily in divided doses every eight hours; *newborns 0 to 7 days and weighing less than 2 kg*, intravenously, 40 mg/kg daily in divided doses every 12 hours (Nelson, 1989 B).

Patients with impaired renal function require modification in doses and/or frequency of administration depending on the degree of impairment, severity of the infection, and susceptibility of the causative organism. For *adults with impaired renal function*, the manufacturer of Keflin recommends an intravenous loading dose of 1 to 2 g and maximum maintenance dosages as shown in the following table.

Renal Function	Maximum Adult Maintenance Dosage
Mild Impairment (Ccr = 80-50 ml/min)	2 g every 6 hours
Moderate Impairment (Ccr = 50-25 ml/min)	1.5 g every 6 hours
Severe Impairment (Ccr = 25-10 ml/min)	1 g every 6 hours
Marked Impairment (Ccr = 10-2 ml/min)	0.5 g every 6 hours
Essentially No Function (Ccr < 2 ml/min)	0.5 g every 8 hours when dialysis is not being performed

From manufacturer's literature

A supplemental dose should be given after hemodialysis (Norris et al, 1990).

Generic. Powder 1 and 2 g (sodium, 2.8 mEq/g) in 10, 20 (2 g only), and 100 ml containers; solution 1 and 2 g (equivalent to base) (sodium, 2.4 mEq/g) in 0.9% sodium chloride or 5% dextrose in 50 ml containers.

Keflin (Lilly). Powder 1, 2, 4, and 20 g (equivalent to base) (sodium 2.8 mEq/g).

CEFAZOLIN SODIUM

[Ancef, Kefzol]

MECHANISM OF ACTION, ANTIMICROBIAL SPECTRUM, AND RESISTANCE. The clinically relevant antimicrobial spectra of first generation cephalosporins are the same. These agents have excellent activity against most gram-positive bacteria, including nonpenicillinase- and penicillinase-producing staphylococci, streptococci (except enterococci), and many anaerobic bacteria. In general, they are more active than second or third generation cephalosporins against gram-positive bacteria. Gram-negative activity of first generation cephalosporins essentially is limited to *Escherichia coli, Klebsiella*, and *Proteus mirabilis*. Cefazolin generally is more active than cephalothin. However, all first generation agents are less active than second and, particularly, third generation cephalosporins against these gram-negative species.

For additional discussion of the mechanism of action, antimicrobial spectrum, and resistance properties of the cephalosporins, see the Introduction.

USES. Parenteral first generation cephalosporins frequently are drugs of choice for prophylaxis during certain cardiovascular (some experts prefer cefuroxime or cefamandole), orthopedic, gastroduodenal, biliary tract, obstetric-gynecologic, and head and neck (some experts prefer clindamycin with or without an aminoglycoside) surgical procedures. Cefazolin usually is preferred to other first generation cephalosporins because it has superior pharmacokinetic properties (ie, higher plasma protein binding, lower volume of distribution, slower rate of elimination) that result in higher and more sustained serum concentrations (see the Introduction; see also index entry Antimicrobial Drugs: Chemoprophylaxis for Surgical Patients [Table]).

Parenterally administered first generation cephalosporins are rarely drugs of choice for the treatment of bacterial infections. However, they may be used to treat serious lower respiratory tract, skin, soft tissue, bone, joint, heart, or urinary tract infections and bacteremias, based on the results of susceptibility tests. They are not effective in meningitis. Frequently, they are preferred for serious staphylococcal and/or streptococcal (except enterococcal) infections (eg, pneumonia, septic arthritis, osteomyelitis, endocarditis) in patients who are allergic to penicillins. However, they should not be used in patients who have experienced an immediate-type (IgE-mediated) hypersensitivity reaction to a penicillin. First generation cephalosporins may be given with an aminoglycoside for *Klebsiella* pneumonia (third generation cephalosporin usually preferred) and for severe infections before the results of culture studies are known. Because of its pharmacokinetic advantages, cefazolin often is preferred to other first generation cephalosporins for these indications. However, some experts prefer cephalothin for severe staphylococcal infections, such as endocarditis, because it is more impervious to attack by some staphylococcal β-lactamases than cefazolin (Kernodie et al, 1990; see also the Introduction and index entry Antimicrobial Drugs: Antimicrobial Drug Selection for Common Infectious Diseases [Table]).

ADVERSE REACTIONS AND PRECAUTIONS. See the Introduction. Cefazolin causes less pain on intramuscular injection than other first generation cephalosporins.

DRUG INTERACTIONS AND INTERFERENCE WITH LABORATORY TESTS. See the Introduction.

PHARMACOKINETICS. Cefazolin is administered intramuscularly or intravenously. Peak serum concentrations of approximately 65 mcg/ml and 185 mcg/ml are achieved after intramuscular and intravenous doses of 1 g, respectively. The higher serum concentrations obtained with cefazolin compared to cephalothin, cephapirin, and cephradine are due, in part, to higher plasma protein binding and a smaller volume of distribution (see the Introduction and these evaluations).

Approximately 85% of circulating cefazolin is bound to plasma protein. The volume of distribution is 0.12 ± 0.03 L/kg. The drug enters many tissues (eg, myocardium, bone, gallbladder) and body fluids (eg, pericardial, pleural, synovial). Adequate concentrations are achieved in bile and high concentrations are obtained in urine. However, cefazolin fails to achieve therapeutic concentrations in cerebrospinal fluid even in the presence of inflammation. Cefazolin crosses the placenta.

Up to 95% of a dose is excreted in the urine as unchanged drug by glomerular filtration and renal tubular secretion. Cefazolin is not metabolized. The elimination half-life is approximately 1.8 hours, which is considerably longer than that of cephalothin, cephapirin, and cephradine (see the Introduction and the evaluations). The half-life is prolonged in patients with renal impairment and dosage adjustments are required.

DOSAGE AND PREPARATIONS. Cefazolin can be administered intramuscularly by injection into a large muscle mass or intravenously by direct injection or by intermittent or continuous infusion. Pain is uncommon after intramuscular injection. See the manufacturer's instructions for the appropriate dilution of the drug, compatible diluents and intravenous solutions, and stability of cefazolin in these solutions.

Intramuscular, Intravenous: *Adults*, 1 to 6 g daily in equally divided doses every six to eight hours (The Medical Letter, 1988). The usual dosage for mild infections caused by susceptible gram-positive cocci, 250 to 500 mg every eight hours; for moderate to severe infections, 500 mg to 1 g every six to eight hours; for severe, life-threatening infections (eg, endocarditis, septicemia), 1 to 1.5 g every six hours. For acute uncomplicated urinary tract infections, 1 g every 12 hours is probably adequate. For dosage recommendations in perioperative prophylaxis, see index entry Antimicrobial Drugs: Chemoprophylaxis for Surgical Patients (Table).

Children and infants over 1 month, 25 to 100 mg/kg daily in equally divided doses every six to eight hours (The Medical Letter, 1988). The usual dosage for mild to moderately severe infections is 25 to 50 mg/kg daily in divided doses every six to eight hours. For severe infections, 100 mg/kg daily may be required.

Newborns over 7 days and weighing more than 2 kg, 60 mg/kg daily in divided doses every eight hours; *newborns over 7 days and weighing less than 2 kg*, 40 mg/kg daily in divided doses every 12 hours; *newborns 0 to 7 days*, 40 mg/kg daily in divided doses every 12 hours (Nelson, 1989 B).

Patients with impaired renal function require modification in doses and/or frequency of administration depending on the degree of impairment, severity of the infection, and susceptibility of the causative organism. Various dosage recommendations for these patients have been proposed. For *adults with impaired renal function*, the manufacturers of Ancef and Kefzol recommend an initial loading dose appropriate to the severity of the infection and maintenance dosages as follows:

Creatinine clearance of 55 ml/min or greater or serum creatinine of 1.5 mg/dl or less, full therapeutic doses; creatinine clearance of 35 to 54 ml/min or serum creatinine of 1.6 to 3 mg/dl, full therapeutic doses with dosage interval restricted to at least eight hours; creatinine clearance of 11 to 34 ml/min or serum creatinine of 3.1 to 4.5 mg/dl, one-half the usual dose every 12 hours; creatinine clearance of 10 ml/min or less or serum creatinine of 4.6 mg/dl or greater, one-half the usual dose every 18 to 24 hours (manufacturers' product information brochure).

Alternative dosage recommendations for *adults with impaired renal function* are 0.5 to 1.5 g every eight hours for creatinine clearance of 80 to 50 ml/min; 0.5 to 1 g every 8 to 12 hours for creatinine clearance of 50 to 10 ml/min; 0.5 to 1 g every 24 hours for creatinine clearance less than 10 ml/min (The Medical Letter, 1988). A supplemental dose of 0.25 to 0.5 g should be given after hemodialysis (Norris et al, 1990).

In *children with impaired renal function*, a usual therapeutic dose can be given as a loading dose, followed by maintenance doses according to the following schedule: creatinine clearance 70 to 40 ml/min, 60% of the usual daily dose in equally divided doses every 12 hours; 40 to 20 ml/min, 25% of usual daily dose in equally divided doses every 12 hours; 20 to 5 ml/min, 10% of normal daily dose every 24 hours. See the manufacturers' literature for further information.

Strengths expressed in terms of base.

Generic. Powder (lyophilized, sterile) 250 and 500 mg and 1, 5, 10, and 20 g (sodium 2 mEq/g); solution (sterile) 500 mg and 1 g (sodium 2 mEq/g) in 5% dextrose in 50 ml containers.

Ancef (Smith Kline & French). Powder (lyophilized, sterile) 500 mg and 1 g (sodium 2 mEq/g); solution (sterile) 500 mg and 1 g (sodium 2 mEq/g) in 5% dextrose in 50 ml containers.

Kefzol (Lilly). Powder (sterile) 250 and 500 mg and 1, 10 and 20 g (sodium 2.1 mEq/g); solution 500 mg and 1 g (sodium 2.1 mEq/g) in 10 ml containers.

CEPHAPIRIN SODIUM
[Cefadyl]

MECHANISM OF ACTION, ANTIMICROBIAL SPECTRUM, AND RESISTANCE. The mechanism of action, antimicrobial spectrum, and resistance properties are essentially the same as for cefazolin (see that evaluation and the Introduction).

USES. Cephapirin has the same indications as cefazolin, but the latter drug frequently is preferred because it achieves higher serum concentrations, has a longer elimination half-life, and causes less pain on intramuscular injection (see the evaluation on Cefazolin Sodium and the Introduction).

ADVERSE REACTIONS AND PRECAUTIONS. See the Introduction.

DRUG INTERACTIONS AND INTERFERENCE WITH LABORATORY TESTS. See the Introduction.

PHARMACOKINETICS. The pharmacokinetics of cephapirin are similar to those of cephalothin. Because of pain on intramuscular injection, cephapirin usually is administered intravenously. Peak serum concentrations of 40 to 70 mcg/ml are obtained after an intravenous dose of 1 g.

Between 45% and 50% of circulating cephapirin is bound to plasma proteins. The volume of distribution is 0.13 ± 0.05 L/kg. The drug enters many tissues and body fluids, but it fails to achieve therapeutic concentrations in cerebrospinal fluid even in the presence of inflammation. Cephapirin crosses the placenta.

Up to 40% of cephapirin is metabolized to the less active desacetyl metabolite. Parent drug and metabolite are excreted by the kidneys, primarily by renal tubular secretion; probenecid delays excretion. The elimination half-life ranges from 35 to 50 minutes. The half-life is prolonged in patients with renal impairment and dosage adjustments are required.

DOSAGE AND PREPARATIONS. Cephapirin can be administered intravenously (preferred) or by intramuscular injection deep into a large muscle mass to minimize pain and induration. Intravenous administration can be by slow injection or by intermittent or continuous infusion. See the manufacturer's instructions for the appropriate dilution of the drug, compatible diluents and intravenous solutions, and stability of cephapirin in these solutions.

Intravenous, Intramuscular (deep): *Adults,* 2 to 12 g daily in equally divided doses every four to six hours (The Medical Letter, 1988). The usual dosage is 500 mg to 1 g every four to six hours, depending on the severity of the infection and the susceptibility of the causative organism. In severe, life-threatening infections, doses up to 2 g every four hours may be required.

Children and infants over 3 months, 40 to 80 mg/kg in equally divided doses every six hours (Nelson, 1989 A). Cephapirin has not been extensively studied in infants under 3 months and dosage guidelines are unavailable.

Patients with impaired renal function require modification in dose and/or frequency of administration depending on the degree of impairment, severity of the infection, and susceptibility of the causative organism. Various dosage recommendations for these patients have been proposed. For *adults with reduced renal function* (moderately severe oliguria or serum creatinine greater than 5 mg/dl), the manufacturer recommends a dose of 7.5 to 15 mg/kg every 12 hours. Patients with severely reduced renal function who are undergoing hemodialysis should receive 7.5 to 15 mg/kg just before dialysis and every 12 hours thereafter.

Alternative dosage recommendations for *adults with impaired renal function*, 500 mg to 2 g every six hours for creatinine clearance of 80 to 50 ml/min; every eight hours for creatinine clearance of 50 to 10 ml/min; every 12 hours for creatinine clearance less than 10 ml/min (The Medical Letter, 1988). A supplemental dose of 7.5 to 15 mg/kg should be given just before hemodialysis (Norris et al, 1990).

Generic, Cefadyl (Bristol). Powder (sterile) 500 mg and 1, 2, 4, and 20 g (equivalent to base) (sodium 2.36 mEq/g).

CEPHRADINE
[Anspor, Velosef]

Cephradine can be administered orally and parenterally. The evaluation is included under Oral Cephalosporins (see below).

PARENTERAL SECOND GENERATION CEPHALOSPORINS

CEFAMANDOLE NAFATE
[Mandol]

MECHANISM OF ACTION, ANTIMICROBIAL SPECTRUM, AND RESISTANCE. Cefamandole has a broader antibacterial spectrum against aerobic gram-negative bacilli than the first generation cephalosporins. Among the Enterobacteriaceae, it often has greater activity against *Escherichia coli*, *Klebsiella*, and *Proteus mirabilis*, including cephalothin-resistant strains; its spectrum also includes some indole-positive *Proteus*, *Citrobacter*, and *Enterobacter* strains. Cefamandole-resistant strains of Enterobacteriaceae occur and are relatively common for some species. Third generation cephalosporins clearly have superior activity against most Enterobacteriaceae. Cefamandole is not active against the nonfermenting gram-negative bacilli, *Pseudomonas aeruginosa* and *Acinetobacter* species. Activity against the *Bacteroides fragilis* group, gram-negative anaerobic bacilli, is poor (see the Introduction).

Compared to first generation cephalosporins, cefamandole has enhanced in vitro activity against *Haemophilus influenzae*, including many ampicillin-resistant strains. However, it is less active than ampicillin against ampicillin-sensitive *H. influenzae*. Furthermore, possible tolerance of *H. influenzae* isolates, ineffective killing, and an inoculum effect have been observed with cefamandole (see Sanders et al, 1985). Third generation cephalosporins and cefuroxime are more reliably active against *H. influenzae* when compared to cefamandole (see the evaluations and the Introduction).

Cefamandole is active against most gram-positive bacteria, including nonpenicillinase- and penicillinase-producing staphylococci, streptococci (except enterococci), and anaerobic bacteria. Although its potency against gram-positive bacteria is comparable to or only slightly less than first generation cephalosporins, cefamandole offers no advantages for known gram-positive infections.

Cefamandole is active in vitro against *Neisseria meningitidis* and many *N. gonorrhoeae* strains but is not used clinically in these infections.

For additional discussion of the mechanism of action, antimicrobial spectrum, and resistance properties of the cephalosporins, see the Introduction.

USES. Cefamandole is rarely the drug of choice for the treatment of bacterial infections. It may be used to treat infections of the lower respiratory tract, urinary tract, skin and skin structures, bone, and joints or bacteremias caused by susceptible bacteria, provided that equally effective, less toxic, and less expensive alternatives are unavailable. For example, this second generation cephalosporin may be indicated as a replacement for an aminoglycoside to treat infections caused by gram-negative bacilli (eg, *E. coli, Klebsiella, Proteus*) when susceptibility to cefamandole is known. Although this drug has been used as an alternative to ampicillin or chloramphenicol for serious infections (eg, pneumonia) caused by *H. influenzae*, some failures have been reported (see Sanders et al, 1985). Also, cefamandole is not effective in meningitis. The third generation cephalosporins and cefuroxime are better alternatives for *H. influenzae* infections. They are more reliably active against β-lactamase-producing strains and are useful in meningitis (see the evaluations and the Introduction).

Cefamandole is active against *S. pneumoniae, H. influenzae, S. aureus, K. pneumoniae*, and oropharyngeal anaerobes and has been used empirically, either alone or with an aminoglycoside, to treat community-acquired pneumonia in adults with certain predisposing factors (eg, chronic lung disease, alcoholism, postinfluenza bacterial pneumonia, debilitated elderly patients). Third generation cephalosporins or cefuroxime may be preferred, however. None of the cephalosporins is active against *Legionella pneumophila* or other organisms (eg, *Mycoplasma pneumoniae*) causing atypical pneumonias.

Cefamandole is active against group A, β-hemolytic streptococci, *S. aureus*, pneumococci, and *H. influenzae* and has been used as single-agent empiric therapy in young children (2 months to 5 years) with pneumonia, bone and joint infections, or buccal and orbital cellulitis. However cefamandole does not penetrate adequately into cerebrospinal fluid and "breakthrough" meningitis, especially with *H. influenzae* type b, has been reported (see Nelson, 1983; Eichenwald, 1985; Sanders et al, 1985). A third generation cephalosporin (eg, cefotaxime, ceftriaxone) or cefuroxime is preferred for these pediatric infections (see the evaluation and the Introduction).

Cefamandole does not appear to offer any advantages over first generation cephalosporins against known gram-positive bacterial infections or for surgical prophylaxis, except possibly for open-heart surgery (see the Introduction; see also index entry Antimicrobial Drugs: Chemoprophylaxis for Surgical Patients [Table]).

ADVERSE REACTIONS AND PRECAUTIONS. Hypersensitivity reactions (eg, maculopapular rash, fever, eosinophilia, urticaria) and other adverse effects associated with cephalosporins have been observed with cefamandole (see the Introduction). In addition, this second generation derivative contains a methylthiotetrazole side chain and has been associated with hypoprothrombinemia and, occasionally, bleeding. Elderly debilitated patients, individuals with severe renal insufficiency, and malnourished patients receiving total parenteral nutrition are at highest risk. Vitamin K reverses the hypoprothrombinemia, and prophylactic administration may be desirable in some patients (see the Introduction).

DRUG INTERACTIONS AND INTERFERENCE WITH LABORATORY TESTS. Methylthiotetrazole-containing cephalosporins have been associated with a disulfiram-like reaction. For additional discussion, see the Introduction.

PHARMACOKINETICS. Cefamandole is administered intramuscularly or intravenously. Peak serum concentrations of 20 to 36 mcg/ml (after 30 to 120 minutes) and 88 to 139 mcg/ml (after 10 minutes) are obtained after intramuscular and intravenous doses of 1 g, respectively.

Between 70% and 80% of circulating cefamandole is bound to plasma protein. The volume of distribution is 0.16 ± 0.05 L/kg. This drug enters many tissues (eg, myocardium, bone, gallbladder) and body fluids (eg, pleural, synovial). High concentrations are obtained in bile and urine. However, it fails to achieve therapeutic concentrations in cerebrospinal fluid even in the presence of inflammation. Cefamandole crosses the placenta.

Approximately 85% of a dose is excreted by the kidneys (glomerular filtration and renal tubular secretion) as unchanged drug over an eight-hour period; excretion is delayed by probenecid. Cefamandole is not metabolized. The elimination half-life is 35 to 60 minutes. The half-life is prolonged in

Renal Function	Less Severe Infections (Adult Maintenance Dosage)	Life-threatening Infections (Maximum Adult Maintenance Dosage)
Mild Impairment (Ccr = 80-50 ml/min)	0.75-1.5 g every 6 hours	1.5 g every 4 hours or 2 g every 6 hours
Moderate Impairment (Ccr = 50-25 ml/min)	0.75-1.5 g every 8 hours	1.5 g every 6 hours or 2 g every 8 hours
Severe Impairment (Ccr = 25-10 ml/min)	0.5-1 g every 8 hours	1 g every 6 hours or 1.25 g every 8 hours
Marked Impairment (Ccr = 10-2 ml/min)	0.5-0.75 g every 12 hours	0.67 g every 8 hours or 1 g every 12 hours
Essentially No Function (Ccr < 2 ml/min)	0.25-0.5 g every 12 hours	0.5 g every 8 hours or 0.75 g every 12 hours

From manufacturer's literature

patients with renal impairment and dosage adjustments are required.

DOSAGE AND PREPARATIONS. Cefamandole can be administered by intramuscular injection into a large muscle mass or intravenously by direct injection or intermittent or continuous infusion. See the manufacturer's instructions for the appropriate dilution of the drug, compatible diluents and intravenous solutions, and stability of cefamandole in these solutions.

Intravenous, Intramuscular (deep): *Adults*, 1.5 to 12 g daily in equally divided doses every four to eight hours (The Medical Letter, 1988). The usual dosage range is 500 mg to 1 g every four to eight hours, depending on the severity of the infection and the susceptibility of the causative organism. For severe, life-threatening infections, up to 2 g every four hours may be required. For perioperative prophylaxis in cardiac surgical procedures, see index entry Antimicrobial Drugs: Chemoprophylaxis for Surgical Patients (Table).

Children and infants over 1 month, 50 to 150 mg/kg daily in equally divided doses every four to eight hours (The Medical Letter, 1988). For most infections, 50 to 100 mg/kg daily in equally divided doses every four to eight hours has been effective. In severe infections, up to 150 mg/kg daily (not to exceed the maximum adult dose) may be given.

Patients with impaired renal function require modification in doses and/or frequency of administration depending on the degree of impairment, severity of the infection, and susceptibility of the causative organism. Various dosage recommendations for these patients have been proposed. In *adults with impaired renal function*, the manufacturer recommends an initial loading dose of 1 to 2 g and maintenance dosages as shown in the table.

Alternative dosage recommendations for *adults with impaired renal function* are 1 to 2 g every six hours for creatinine clearance of 80 to 50 ml/min; 1 to 2 g every eight hours for creatinine clearance of 50 to 10 ml min; 0.5 to 1 g every 12 hours for creatinine clearance less than 10 ml/min (The Medical Letter, 1988).

Mandol (Lilly). Powder (sterile) 500 mg and 1, 2, and 10 g (equivalent to base) (sodium 3.3 mEq/g).

CEFUROXIME SODIUM
[Kefurox, Zinacef]

MECHANISM OF ACTION, ANTIMICROBIAL SPECTRUM, AND RESISTANCE. Cefuroxime has good activity against most staphylococci, including β-lactamase-producing strains. However, the antistaphylococcal activity of this second generation cephalosporin is less than that of cephalothin. Cefuroxime has excellent activity against streptococci, including *S. pyogenes* (group A, β-hemolytic), *S. agalactiae* (group B), *S. pneumoniae*, viridans streptococci, and anaerobic streptococci (*Peptostreptococcus*). However, enterococci are resistant. Gram-positive anaerobes, including *Peptococcus* and many clostridia, are usually susceptible. In general, despite its excellent activity against gram-positive bacteria, cefuroxime does not appear to offer any clinical advantages over first generation cephalosporins for infections (other than meningitis) known to be caused by these organisms.

The gram-negative cocci, *Neisseria meningitidis* and *N. gonorrhoeae*, including β-lactamase-producing strains (PPNG), are very susceptible. Cefuroxime is more active than first generation cephalosporins against *Haemophilus influenzae*, including ampicillin-resistant strains. It exhibits excellent stability to β-lactamases produced by this gram-negative bacillus. *Moraxella (Branhamella) catarrhalis*, including β-lactamase-positive strains, also are susceptible.

Among the Enterobacteriaceae, cefuroxime is more active than first generation cephalosporins against *Escherichia coli, Klebsiella*, and *Proteus mirabilis*, including some cephalothin-resistant strains, and its spectrum also includes most *Citrobacter* and some *Enterobacter* and indole-positive *Proteus* strains. However, third generation cephalosporins clearly have superior activity against most Enterobacteriaceae. Cefuroxime is not active against the nonfermenting gram-negative bacilli, *Pseudomonas aeruginosa* and *Acinetobacter* species. The *Bacteroides fragilis* group (gram-negative anaerobic bacilli) usually are resistant.

In summary, the antimicrobial spectrum of cefuroxime is similar to that of cefamandole (see the evaluation). However, cefuroxime has increased resistance to certain β-lactamases (eg, TEM-1) of various gram-negative bacteria (eg, *Haemo-*

philus influenzae, Neisseria gonorrhoeae*), a potential clinical advantage for infections caused by these bacterial strains (see Gold and Rodriguez, 1983; Nelson, 1983; Smith and LeFrock, 1983).

For additional discussion of the mechanism of action, antimicrobial spectrum, and resistance properties of the cephalosporins, see the Introduction.

USES. Cefuroxime has been a widely used drug for single-agent empiric therapy of serious community-acquired bacterial pneumonia, suppurative bone and joint infections, or buccal and orbital cellulitis in infants and young children between 2 months and 5 years. This drug is active against the likely causative organisms, *Haemophilus influenzae* type b (including β-lactamase-producing strains), pneumococci, *Streptococcus pyogenes*, and *Staphylococcus aureus*. Cefuroxime also has been used for bacterial meningitis in this pediatric population (American Academy of Pediatrics Committee on Infectious Diseases, 1988). However, reports of delayed sterilization of cerebrospinal fluid, treatment failure and relapse, and serious sequelae (moderate-to-profound hearing loss) in patients with *H. influenzae* type b infection (Marks et al, 1986; Arditi et al, 1989; LeBel et al, 1989; Schaad et al, 1990) have raised concerns about cefuroxime (see McCracken et al, 1987). Most pediatric infectious disease experts prefer one of the third generation cephalosporins, usually cefotaxime or ceftriaxone, for meningitis, and frequently for other bacteremic *H. influenzae* type b infections as well, in infants and young children (see McCracken et al, 1987). On a weight basis, these third generation agents are considerably more potent than cefuroxime and they achieve much higher bactericidal titers in cerebrospinal fluid (see also the Introduction and index entry Antimicrobial Drugs: Antimicrobial Drug Selection for Common Infectious Diseases [Table]).

Other indications for cefuroxime appear to be similar to those for cefamandole (see the evaluation). However, cefuroxime appears to offer a number of advantages over cefamandole, including increased β-lactamase stability (eg, TEM-1 of *H. influenzae*), a longer elimination half-life, and the absence of hypoprothrombinemia and a disulfiram-like reaction as adverse effects (see the Introduction).

ADVERSE REACTIONS AND PRECAUTIONS. These are the same as for first generation cephalosporins (see the Introduction).

DRUG INTERACTIONS AND INTERFERENCE WITH LABORATORY TESTS. See the Introduction.

PHARMACOKINETICS. Cefuroxime sodium is administered intramuscularly or intravenously. The peak serum concentration obtained after intramuscular injection of 0.75 g was approximately 27 mcg/ml after 45 minutes (range, 15 to 60 minutes). Following intravenous doses of 0.75 and 1.5 g, serum concentrations were approximately 50 and 100 mcg/ml, respectively, at 15 minutes.

Approximately 33% of circulating cefuroxime is bound to plasma protein. The volume of distribution approximates that of the extracellular fluid, ie, 0.2 L/kg. The antibiotic reaches therapeutic levels in a number of tissues (interstitial fluids) and body fluids, including pleural and synovial fluids, sputum, bile, bone, and urine. Unlike first and other second generation cephalosporins, cefuroxime penetrates the inflamed meninges and achieves cerebrospinal fluid concentrations that usually are adequate for the treatment of bacterial meningitis caused by susceptible organisms (eg, *S. pneumoniae, H. influenzae, N. meningitidis*). Cefuroxime crosses the placenta.

More than 90% of a dose of cefuroxime is excreted in the urine as unchanged drug within 24 hours; it is not metabolized. Elimination appears to be by renal tubular secretion and glomerular filtration and is delayed by probenecid. The elimination half-life is approximately 1.3 to 1.7 hours, which is longer than that of cefamandole (0.6 to 1 hour). The half-life is prolonged in patients with renal impairment, and dosage adjustments are required when the creatinine clearance falls below 20 ml/min. The half-life in infants less than 1 week ranges from 3.5 to 5.5 hours.

DOSAGE AND PREPARATIONS. Cefuroxime can be administered by intramuscular injection deep into a large muscle mass or intravenously by direct injection or by intermittent or continuous infusion. See the manufacturer's instructions for the appropriate dilution of the drug, compatible diluents and intravenous solutions, and stability of cefuroxime in these solutions.

Intravenous, Intramuscular (deep): *Adults*, 2.25 to 9 g daily in equally divided doses every eight hours (The Medical Letter, 1988). The usual dosages for uncomplicated urinary tract infections, skin and skin structure infections, disseminated gonococcal infections, and uncomplicated pneumonia are 750 mg every eight hours; for severe or complicated infections, 1.5 g every eight hours. In life-threatening infections or infections due to less susceptible organisms, 1.5 g every six hours may be required. In bacterial meningitis, the dose should not exceed 3 g every eight hours. For uncomplicated gonococcal infections, 1.5 g intramuscularly given as a single dose at two different sites together with probenecid, 1 g orally. For perioperative prophylaxis in cardiac surgical procedures, see index entry Antimicrobial Drugs: Chemoprophylaxis for Surgical Patients (Table).

Infants and children over 3 months, 50 to 100 mg/kg daily in equally divided doses every six to eight hours. The higher dosage (not to exceed the maximum adult dosage) should be used for the more severe or serious infections. For bacterial meningitis, 200 to 240 mg/kg daily in equally divided doses every six to eight hours.

Modification of dosage is unnecessary in patients with creatinine clearances above 20 ml/min. The manufacturer recommends that *adults* with creatinine clearances of 20 to 10 ml/min receive 750 mg every 12 hours and those with creatinine clearances less than 10 ml/min receive 750 mg every 24 hours. In *children* with impaired renal function, the manufacturer recommends that the frequency of administration be modified as for adults. In patients undergoing hemodialysis, a supplemental dose of cefuroxime should be given after each dialysis period.

Kefurox (Lilly). Powder (sterile) 750 mg and 1.5 and 7.5 g (equivalent to base) (sodium 2.4 mEq/g).

Zinacef (Glaxo). Powder (sterile) 750 mg and 1.5 and 7.5 g (equivalent to base) (sodium 2.4 mEq/g); solution 750 mg and

1.5 g (sodium 2.4 mEq/g) in 100 ml containers and frozen premixed minibags (50 ml).

CEFONICID SODIUM
[Monocid]

Cefonicid is a semisynthetic second generation cephalosporin that is structurally similar to cefamandole (see Figure).

MECHANISM OF ACTION, ANTIMICROBIAL SPECTRUM, AND RESISTANCE. The mechanism of action, antimicrobial spectrum, and resistance properties of cefonicid are similar to those of cefamandole. Like cefamandole, the in vitro activity of cefonicid against aerobic gram-negative bacteria generally is superior to that of first generation cephalosporins, but inferior to that of third generation cephalosporins. Cefonicid is usually active against *Escherichia coli, Proteus mirabilis, Klebsiella, Citrobacter diversus*, and *Neisseria meningitidis*. It also has good activity against *N. gonorrhoeae* and *Haemophilus influenzae*, including β-lactamase-producing strains. Its activity against *Enterobacter* species and *C. freundii* is variable. *Serratia marcescens, Providencia, Pseudomonas aeruginosa, Acinetobacter*, and the *Bacteroides fragilis* group (gram-negative anaerobic bacilli) are usually resistant.

Most gram-positive cocci, including nonpenicillinase- and penicillinase-producing *Staphylococcus aureus* and streptococci (except enterococci), are susceptible in vitro. However, the activity of cefonicid against those organisms, especially staphylococci, is less than that of first generation cephalosporins, cefamandole, and cefuroxime. The activity against *S. aureus* is decreased in the presence of serum, which appears to result from the high binding of cefonicid to plasma proteins (see Pharmacokinetics).

For additional discussion, see *Med Lett Drugs Ther*, 1984 C; Dudley et al, 1984; Pontzer and Kaye, 1984; Tartaglione and Polk, 1985; see also the Introduction and the evaluations of Cefamandole Nafate and Cefuroxime Sodium.

USES. Cefonicid has the longest elimination half-life (3.5 to 4.5 hours) among currently available first and second generation cephalosporins. Administered once daily, it is being used to treat a variety of mild-to-moderate infections, including community-acquired pneumonias, urinary tract infections, and skin and soft tissue infections (Donowitz and Mandell, 1988). Cefonicid also is being used to continue parenteral antibiotic therapy in outpatient settings (see Kunkel and Iannini, 1984; Nadworney and Markowitz, 1987). However, published comparative clinical studies with this long-acting second generation cephalosporin, particularly in serious infections, are still somewhat limited (Jacob and Layne, 1984; see also Saltiel and Brogden, 1986).

There is concern over the efficacy of cefonicid in serious *Staphylococcus aureus* infections (eg, endocarditis) because this agent was ineffective in three of four patients with *S. aureus* endocarditis (Chambers et al, 1984). Also, in one study (Lea et al, 1982), cefonicid was shown to be less effective than cefazolin for skin and soft tissue infections caused by this pathogen. Cefonicid is not recommended for the treatment of bacterial meningitis (see *Med Lett Drugs Ther*, 1984 C). When administered as a single 1-g dose, it has been less than adequate for anorectal or pharyngeal gonococcal infections (Handsfield and Murphy, 1985). Although single-dose (1 g) cefonicid has been shown to be effective as perioperative prophylaxis in various surgical procedures, including biliary tract surgery, vaginal and abdominal hysterectomy, cesarean section, colorectal surgery, and prosthetic arthroplasty (see Jacob and Layne, 1984), no advantages over currently recommended cephalosporins (usually cefazolin) have been shown in controlled clinical trials (see DiPiro et al, 1984; *Med Lett Drugs Ther*, 1984 C; Rapp and Blue, 1985; see also index entry Antimicrobial Drugs: Chemoprophylaxis for Surgical Patients [Table]). For additional discussion, see the Introduction.

ADVERSE REACTIONS AND PRECAUTIONS. Cefonicid generally has been well tolerated and most adverse reactions (eg, hypersensitivity reactions, pain on intramuscular injection, gastrointestinal disturbances, mild reversible laboratory abnormalities) are similar to those of first generation cephalosporins (see the Introduction). A "flu-like syndrome" developed in 3 of 15 patients receiving the drug for more than two weeks (Kunkel and Iannini, 1984). Although cefonicid contains a methylthiotetrazole side chain, it has not been associated with hypoprothrombinemia or a disulfiram-like reaction. The absence of these side effects may be related to the presence of a methylsulfonic acid group on the methylthiotetrazole side chain rather than the methyl group present in cefamandole, cefoperazone, and moxalactam (see Pontzer and Kaye, 1984; see also the Introduction and Figure).

DRUG INTERACTIONS AND INTERFERENCE WITH LABORATORY TESTS. See the Introduction. A disulfiram-like reaction has not been reported (see the above discussion).

PHARMACOKINETICS. Cefonicid is administered intramuscularly or intravenously. Peak serum concentrations of 98 mcg/ml (after one to two hours) and 221 mcg/ml (after five minutes) are obtained after intramuscular and intravenous doses of 1 g, respectively.

Greater than 95% of circulating cefonicid is bound to plasma protein. The volume of distribution is approximately 0.11 L/kg. Therapeutic levels are achieved in a number of tissues (eg, bone, gallbladder wall, uterus) and body fluids (eg, sputum, wound fluid, pleural and pericardial fluids, bile). High concentrations are obtained in urine. However, therapeutic concentrations are not achieved in cerebrospinal fluid even in the presence of inflammation. Cefonicid crosses the placenta.

More than 90% of a dose is excreted by the kidneys (renal tubular secretion and glomerular filtration) as unchanged drug within 24 hours. Excretion is delayed by probenecid. Cefonicid is not metabolized. The elimination half-life is approximately 3.5 to 4.5 hours. The half-life is prolonged in patients with renal impairment and dosage adjustments are required.

DOSAGE AND PREPARATIONS. Cefonicid can be administered by intramuscular injection deep into a large muscle mass or intravenously by direct injection or infusion. See the manufacturer's instructions for the appropriate dilution of the drug, compatible diluents and intravenous solutions, and stability of cefonicid in these solutions.

Creatinine Clearance (ml/min/1.73 M²)	Mild to Moderate Infections (Adult Maintenance Dosage)	Severe Infections (Adult Maintenance Dosage)
79-60	10 mg/kg every 24 hours	25 mg/kg every 24 hours
59-40	8 mg/kg every 24 hours	20 mg/kg every 24 hours
39-20	4 mg/kg every 24 hours	15 mg/kg every 24 hours
19-10	4 mg/kg every 48 hours	15 mg/kg every 48 hours
9-5	4 mg/kg every 3-5 days	15 mg/kg every 3-5 days
<5	3 mg/kg every 3-5 days	4 mg/kg every 3-5 days

NOTE: It is not necessary to administer additional dosage following dialysis.
From manufacturer's literature

Intramuscular (deep), Intravenous: *Adults*, 500 mg to 2 g once daily. The usual dosages for uncomplicated urinary tract infections are 500 mg once daily; for mild to moderate infections, 1 g once daily; for severe or life-threatening infections, 2 g once daily. With a dosage of 2 g intramuscularly once daily, one-half of the dose is given in different large muscle masses.

Dosage recommendations for *children* currently are unavailable.

Patients with impaired renal function require modification in doses and/or frequency of administration depending on the degree of impairment, severity of the infection, and susceptibility of the causative organisms. For *adults with impaired renal function*, the manufacturer recommends an initial loading dose of 7.5 mg/kg, intramuscularly or intravenously, followed by maintenance dosages as shown in the table.

Monocid (Smith Kline & French). Powder (sterile) 500 mg and 1 and 10 g (equivalent to base) (sodium 3.7 mEq/g).

CEFORANIDE
[Precef]

Ceforanide is a semisynthetic second generation cephalosporin that is structurally similar to cefamandole (see Figure).

MECHANISM OF ACTION, ANTIMICROBIAL SPECTRUM, AND RESISTANCE. The mechanism of action, antimicrobial spectrum, and resistance properties of ceforanide are similar to those of cefamandole. Like cefamandole, the in vitro activity of ceforanide against members of the Enterobacteriaceae family generally is superior to that of first generation cephalosporins but inferior to that of third generation cephalosporins. Ceforanide is usually active against *Escherichia coli, Klebsiella, Proteus mirabilis*, and *Citrobacter diversus*, including some cephalothin-resistant strains. Activity against indole-positive *Proteus* species and *Enterobacter* species is variable; *Serratia marcescens* are resistant. The nonfermenting gram-negative bacilli, *Pseudomonas aeruginosa* and *Acinetobacter*, are resistant. The *Bacteroides fragilis* group, anaerobic gram-negative bacilli, also are resistant.

Neisseria meningitidis, N. gonorrhoeae, and *Haemophilus influenzae*, including β-lactamase-producing strains, usually are susceptible in vitro. However, ceforanide is considerably less active than cefuroxime, cefamandole, or cefonicid against *H. influenzae*.

Most gram-positive cocci, including nonpenicillinase- and penicillinase-producing *Staphylococcus aureus* and streptococci (except enterococci), are susceptible in vitro. However, the activity of ceforanide against these organisms, particularly staphylococci, is less than that of first generation cephalosporins, cefamandole, and cefuroxime.

For additional discussion, see Barriere and Mills, 1982; Garzone et al, 1983 B; *Med Lett Drugs Ther*, 1984 B; and Tartaglione and Polk, 1985. See also the Introduction and the evaluations on Cefamandole Nafate, Cefuroxime Sodium, and Cefonicid Sodium.

USES. Ceforanide has a longer elimination half-life (2.7 to 3 hours) than currently available first and second generation cephalosporins (except cefonicid) and, administered twice daily, has been shown to be effective in urinary tract, community-acquired lower respiratory tract, skin and skin structure, bone, and joint infections caused by susceptible bacteria (see Barriere and Mills, 1982; LeFrock et al, 1984 C; Tartaglione and Polk, 1985). In one study, ceforanide failed to eradicate *H. influenzae* from the sputum of patients with pneumonia, although clinical outcomes were successful (Wallace et al, 1981); in addition, one infant treated with ceforanide for periorbital cellulitis caused by *H. influenzae* type b relapsed with bacteremia one week after therapy was stopped (Thirumoorthi et al, 1983).

Ceforanide 1 to 2 g every 12 hours intramuscularly also has been shown to be effective for right-sided endocarditis caused by *S. aureus* and nonenterococcal streptococci in intravenous drug abusers. However, serum bactericidal titers for ceforanide against *S. aureus* were inferior to those seen with antistaphylococcal penicillins (eg, nafcillin) or first generation cephalosporins (Cooper et al, 1981; Greenman et al, 1984).

Ceforanide fails to achieve therapeutically effective concentrations in cerebrospinal fluid and is not useful in bacterial meningitis.

Presently, clinical experience with ceforanide is very limited, and randomized, double-blind comparative clinical trials with established therapies generally are unavailable (Barriere and Mills, 1982; *Med Lett Drugs Ther*, 1984 B; Tartaglione and Polk, 1985). Thus, its role in infectious disease therapy is largely undefined. Ceforanide does not appear to offer any advantages over first generation cephalosporins for infections caused by gram-positive bacteria or for perioperative prophylaxis and is inferior to cefuroxime and third generation cephalosporins for *H. influenzae* infections (see *Med Lett Drugs Ther*, 1984 B; Tartaglione and Polk, 1985; see also the Introduction and the evaluations).

ADVERSE REACTIONS AND PRECAUTIONS. Ceforanide generally has been well tolerated, and the majority of adverse reactions (eg, hypersensitivity reactions, gastrointestinal disturbances, mild reversible laboratory abnormalities) are similar to those reported with first generation cephalosporins (see the Introduction). Although ceforanide contains a methylthiotetrazole side chain, it has not been associated with hypoprothrombinemia or a disulfiram-like reaction. The absence of these side effects may be related to the presence of a carboxymethyl group on the methylthiotetrazole side chain rather than the methyl group present in cefamandole, cefoperazone, and moxalactam (see Barriere and Mills, 1982, and Tartaglione and Polk, 1985. See also the Introduction and Figure).

DRUG INTERACTIONS AND INTERFERENCE WITH LABORATORY TESTS. See the Introduction. A disulfiram-like reaction has not been reported (see the above discussion).

PHARMACOKINETICS. Ceforanide is administered intramuscularly or intravenously. Peak serum concentrations of approximately 70 mcg/ml (after one hour) and 125 mcg/ml (after a 30-minute infusion) are obtained after intramuscular and intravenous doses of 1 g, respectively.

About 80% of circulating ceforanide is bound to plasma protein. The volume of distribution ranges from 0.16 to 0.19 L/kg. The antibiotic reaches therapeutic levels in a number of tissues (eg, bone, gallbladder, myocardium) and body fluids (eg, pericardial and synovial fluids, bile). High concentrations are obtained in urine. However, therapeutic concentrations are not achieved in cerebrospinal fluid even in the presence of inflammation. Ceforanide crosses the placenta.

More than 90% of a dose is excreted as unchanged drug via the kidneys, primarily by glomerular filtration. Probenecid does not delay excretion. Ceforanide is not metabolized. The elimination half-life is approximately 2.7 to 3 hours. The half-life is prolonged in patients with renal impairment and dosage adjustments are required.

DOSAGE AND PREPARATIONS. Ceforanide can be administered by intramuscular injection deep into a large muscle mass or intravenously by direct injection or infusion. See the manufacturer's instructions for the appropriate dilution of the drug, compatible diluents and intravenous solutions, and stability of ceforanide in these solutions.

Intramuscular (deep), Intravenous: *Adults*, 1 to 2 g daily in equally divided doses every 12 hours; *children*, 20 to 40 mg/kg daily in equally divided doses every 12 hours.

Patients with impaired renal function require modification in doses and/or frequency of administration depending on the degree of impairment, severity of the infection, and susceptibility of the causative organism. The manufacturer recommends a 12-hour dosing interval when creatinine clearance is 60 ml/min/1.73 M^2 or greater; a 24-hour dosing interval when creatinine clearance is between 59 and 20 ml/min/1.73 M^2; a 48-hour dosing interval when creatinine clearance is between 19 and 5 ml/min/1.73 M^2; and a 48- to 72-hour dosing interval when creatinine clearance is less than 5 ml/min/1.73 M^2. Patients on hemodialysis should receive a supplemental dose (adults, 0.5 to 1 g) after each hemodialysis session (Norris and Mandell, 1985).

Precef (ICN). Powder (sterile) 500 mg and 1 g (equivalent to base).

CEFOXITIN SODIUM
[Mefoxin]

Cefoxitin, a β-lactam antibiotic closely related to the cephalosporins, is technically classified as a cephamycin. It is derived from cephamycin C, which is produced by *Streptomyces lactamdurans*.

MECHANISM OF ACTION, ANTIMICROBIAL SPECTRUM, AND RESISTANCE. The presence of a 7-α-methoxyl group (see Figure) provides cefoxitin with a high degree of resistance to β-lactamases. This antibiotic has a broader antibacterial spectrum against gram-negative bacteria than first generation cephalosporins. Among the Enterobacteriaceae, it is more active against *Escherichia coli*, *Klebsiella*, and *Proteus mirabilis*, including cephalothin-resistant strains; its spectrum also includes indole-positive *Proteus* species, especially *P. vulgaris*; *Providencia* species; and some strains of *Serratia marcescens*. It is less active than cefamandole against *Enterobacter* species, however. The nonfermenting gram-negative bacilli, *Pseudomonas aeruginosa* and *Acinetobacter* species, are resistant.

Cefoxitin is the most active cephalosporin against the *Bacteroides fragilis* group because it is resistant to β-lactamases produced by these anaerobic gram-negative bacilli. Usually between 85% and 95% of *B. fragilis* clinical isolates are susceptible, depending on the institution (*Med Lett Drugs Ther*, 1984 D). Other anaerobic bacteria, except some *Clostridium* species (other than *C. perfringens*) and a few *Fusobacterium* strains, also are susceptible.

Cefoxitin has good activity against *Neisseria gonorrhoeae*, including penicillinase-producing strains (PPNG) and is useful clinically in these infections. Although this antibiotic is active against *N. meningitidis* and *H. influenzae*, including β-lactamase-producing strains, it usually is not used for infections caused by these bacteria.

Although cefoxitin is active against most gram-positive bacteria, including nonpenicillinase- and penicillinase-producing staphylococci and streptococci (except enterococci), it is less potent than first generation cephalosporins, particularly against staphylococci. It offers no advantages over these earlier generation cephalosporins for gram-positive infections.

For additional discussion of the mechanism of action, antimicrobial spectrum, and resistance properties of the cephalosporins, see the Introduction.

USES. Cefoxitin is useful in the treatment of intra-abdominal infections, such as peritonitis secondary to bowel perforation. These are frequently polymicrobial infections caused by mixtures of aerobic gram-negative enteric bacilli (eg, *Escherichia coli*) and anaerobic bacteria, including the *Bacteroides fragilis* group. Initial therapy usually is empiric, and broad spectrum antimicrobial coverage is indicated. Cefoxitin alone appears to be as effective as clindamycin plus an aminoglycoside for mildly to moderately ill patients with community-acquired intra-abdominal infection (Tally et al, 1981; Drusano et al, 1982; Nichols et al, 1984; Malangoni et al, 1985; see also DiPiro and May, 1988) and frequently is a preferred drug in such situations, provided that resistance is not a problem in the particular geographic location. For more severely ill patients and/or for nosocomial infections, combination therapy with an anti-*B. fragilis* agent (eg, metronidazole, clindamycin, chloramphenicol, cefoxitin, cefotetan, imipenem/cilastatin, ticarcillin/potassium clavulanate, ampicillin/sulbactam) plus an aminoglycoside usually is indicated (see the Introduction and index entry Antimicrobial Drugs: Antimicrobial Drug Selection for Common Infectious Diseases [Table]).

Gynecologic pelvic infections (eg, pelvic inflammatory disease, endometritis, pelvic cellulitis) also are typically mixed infections involving aerobic and anaerobic bacteria and cefoxitin has a role in therapy. For pelvic inflammatory disease in sexually active women, cefoxitin plus doxycycline is a preferred regimen of the Centers for Disease Control (*MMWR*, 1989). In such patients, cefoxitin provides antimicrobial coverage against *Neisseria gonorrhoeae*, including PPNG strains; many gram-negative bacilli; and most anaerobic bacteria, including the *B. fragilis* group. Doxycycline expands the spectrum to include *Chlamydia trachomatis* (see the Introduction and index entry Sexually Transmitted Diseases: Treatment (Table).

Cefoxitin has been useful in the treatment of uncomplicated and disseminated gonococcal infections caused by PPNG strains. However, the more highly active third generation agent, ceftriaxone, is now the preferred cephalosporin (*MMWR*, 1989; see also index entry Sexually Transmitted Diseases: Treatment [Table]).

Because of its greater activity against the *B. fragilis* group when compared to first generation cephalosporins, cefoxitin usually is the preferred parenteral antibiotic for prophylaxis in colorectal surgical procedures (see the Introduction and index entry Antimicrobial Drugs: Chemoprophylaxis for Surgical Patients [Table]).

Depending on the results of susceptibility tests, cefoxitin may be used in serious lower respiratory tract, urinary tract, bone, joint, skin, and soft tissue infections or bacteremias, provided that equally effective, less toxic, and less expensive alternatives are unavailable.

ADVERSE REACTIONS AND PRECAUTIONS. These are the same as for first generation cephalosporins (see the Introduction).

DRUG INTERACTIONS AND INTERFERENCE WITH LABORATORY TESTS. See the Introduction. High serum concentrations of cefoxitin may interfere with measurement of creatinine by the Jaffe method. Serum samples withdrawn within two hours of cefoxitin administration should not be assayed for serum creatinine concentrations.

PHARMACOKINETICS. Cefoxitin is administered intramuscularly or intravenously. Peak serum concentrations of 20 to 25 mcg/ml (after 20 to 30 minutes) and 56 to 110 mcg/ml (after five minutes) are obtained after intramuscular and intravenous doses of 1 g, respectively.

Between 70% and 80% of circulating cefoxitin is bound to plasma protein. The volume of distribution ranges from 0.13 to 0.22 L/kg. The antibiotic reaches therapeutic levels in a number of tissues and body fluids, including myometrium; pleural and synovial fluids; bile; and urine. However, it fails to achieve therapeutic concentrations in cerebrospinal fluid even in the presence of inflammation. Cefoxitin crosses the placenta.

Approximately 85% of a dose is excreted by the kidneys (glomerular filtration and renal tubular secretion) as unchanged drug over a six-hour period. Excretion is delayed by probenecid and cefoxitin is minimally metabolized. The elimination half-life is approximately 40 to 60 minutes. The half-life is prolonged in patients with renal impairment and dosage adjustments are required.

DOSAGE AND PREPARATIONS. Cefoxitin can be administered by intramuscular injection deep into a large muscle mass or intravenously by direct injection or by intermittent or continuous infusion. Large doses should be given only by the intravenous route because of the large volumes or high concentrations required. See the manufacturer's instructions for the appropriate dilution of the drug, compatible diluents and intravenous solutions, and stability of cefoxitin in these solutions.

Intravenous, Intramuscular (deep): *Adults,* 3 to 12 g daily in equally divided doses every four to eight hours (The Medical Letter, 1988). The usual dosages for mild uncomplicated infections are 1 g every six to eight hours intravenously or intramuscularly (total daily dosage, 3 to 4 g); for moderate or severe infections, 1 g every four hours or 2 g every six to eight hours intravenously (total daily dosage, 6 to 8 g); for life-threatening infections, 2 g every four hours or 3 g every six hours intravenously (total daily dosage, 12 g). For uncomplicated gonorrhea (including PPNG), 2 g intramuscularly with probenecid, 1 g orally, given at the same time or up to 30 minutes before cefoxitin. For pelvic inflammatory disease, see index entry Sexually Transmitted Diseases: Treatment (Table). For perioperative prophylaxis in colorectal surgical procedures, see index entry Antimicrobial Drugs: Chemoprophylaxis for Surgical Patients (Table).

Infants over 3 months and children, 80 to 160 mg/kg daily divided into four to six equal doses. The maximum daily dosage is 12 g.

Patients with impaired renal function require modification in doses and/or frequency of administration depending on the degree of impairment, severity of the infection, and susceptibility of the causative organism. Various dosage recommendations for these patients have been proposed. For *adults with impaired renal function*, the manufacturer recommends an initial loading dose of 1 to 2 g and maintenance dosages as follows:

Renal Function	Adult Maintenance Dosage
Mild Impairment (Ccr = 50-30 ml/min)	1-2 g every 8-12 hours
Moderate Impairment (Ccr = 29-10 ml/min)	1-2 g every 12-24 hours
Severe Impairment (Ccr = 9-5 ml/min)	0.5-1 g every 12-24 hours
Essentially No Function (Ccr < 5 ml/min)	0-5-1 g every 24-48 hours

From manufacturer's literature

In patients undergoing hemodialysis, a loading dose of 1 to 2 g can be given after each hemodialysis session, followed by a maintenance dose as indicated above.

Alternative dosage recommendations for *adults with impaired renal function* are 1 to 2 g every eight hours for creatinine clearance of 80 to 50 ml/min; 1 to 2 g every 12 hours for creatinine clearance of 50 to 10 ml/min; 0.5 to 1 g every 12 to 24 hours for creatinine clearance less than 10 ml/min (The Medical Letter, 1988). A supplemental dose of 1 to 2 g should be given after hemodialysis (Norris et al, 1990).

Mefoxin (Merck Sharp & Dohme). Powder (sterile) 1, 2, and 10 g (equivalent to base) (sodium 2.3 mEq/g); solution 1 and 2 g (equivalent to base) in 5% dextrose in 50 ml containers.

CEFOTETAN DISODIUM
[Cefotan]

Cefotetan is a cephamycin antibiotic derived semisynthetically from oganomycin G, which is produced by *Streptomyces oganonensis*. Like cefoxitin and moxalactam, it contains a 7α-methoxy substitution on the basic cephalosporin nucleus that enhances its stability to most β-lactamases. Cefotetan generally is classified as a second generation cephalosporin, but some experts would consider it a third generation agent.

MECHANISM OF ACTION, ANTIMICROBIAL SPECTRUM, AND RESISTANCE. The mechanism of action of cefotetan is the same as for other cephalosporins (see the Introduction).

In general, cefotetan has increased potency and a broader antimicrobial spectrum against gram-negative bacteria than first and other second generation cephalosporins. Among the Enterobacteriaceae, it has excellent activity against *Escherichia coli, Klebsiella* species, *Proteus mirabilis*, and *Proteus vulgaris* with most strains susceptible in vitro at concentrations less than 1 mcg/ml. Other *Proteus* species, *Providencia* and *Morganella* species, and *Salmonella* and *Shigella* species are susceptible at concentrations less than 8 mcg/ml. Activity against *Enterobacter*, *Serratia*, and *Citrobacter* species is variable and, generally, cefotetan is less active than third generation cephalosporins against these species.

Cefotetan is active against *Haemophilus influenzae* and *Neisseria gonorrhoeae*, including β-lactamase-producing strains. Its potency (MIC_{90}, 1 to 4 mcg/ml) is comparable to that of cefoxitin and is considerably less than third generation cephalosporins. Cefotetan is active against *Neisseria meningitidis*.

The nonfermenting gram-negative bacilli, *Pseudomonas aeruginosa* and *Acinetobacter* species, are resistant to cefotetan.

Cefotetan has only modest activity against most gram-positive cocci (MIC_{90} = 2 to 16 mcg/ml), including nonpenicillinase- and penicillinase-producing staphylococci and most streptococci. It is similar to cefoxitin in activity against these species and offers no advantages over first generation derivatives (eg, cefazolin) for known gram-positive bacterial infections. None of the cephalosporins are active against enterococci (eg, *Enterococcus faecalis*), methicillin-resistant staphylococci, penicillin G-resistant pneumococci, and *Listeria monocytogenes*.

Cefotetan is active in vitro against anaerobic bacteria. *Bacteroides* (including the *B. fragilis* group), *Clostridium,* and *Fusobacterium* species usually are more susceptible to cefotetan, cefoxitin, and moxalactam than cephalosporins lacking the 7α-methoxy substitution, but activity varies considerably among different institutions. In general, cefotetan is comparable to cefoxitin in vitro against anaerobic bacteria, including the *B. fragilis* species. However, it is less active against other species within the *B. fragilis* group (eg., *B. ovatus, B. distasonis*). The clinical significance of these in vitro differences is uncertain. Like cefoxitin, cefotetan is less active in vitro than clindamycin, metronidazole, chloramphenicol, imipenem, ticarcillin/potassium clavulanate, and ampicillin/sulbactam against the clinically important *Bacteroides* (eg, *B. fragilis*) species. Most anaerobic gram-positive cocci are susceptible to cefotetan.

Like other 7α-methoxy cephalosporins, cefotetan is resistant to most β-lactamases, although it is hydrolyzed by certain β-lactamases from *Pseudomonas aeruginosa* and *Enterobacter cloacae*. Resistant strains of *Bacteroides fragilis*, *Serratia liquifaciens*, and *Citrobacter freundii* also have been reported.

For additional discussion, see Ward and Richards, 1985; Williams and Moosdeen, 1987.

USES. Cefotetan has been shown to be effective in intra-abdominal, obstetric and gynecologic, skin and soft tissue, complicated urinary tract, and lower respiratory tract infections caused by susceptible bacteria (see Ward and Richards, 1985).

Although overall clinical experience is less with cefotetan, this cephamycin has been comparable to cefoxitin for the treatment of community acquired intra-abdominal infections in moderately ill patients (Wilson et al, 1988); obstetric and gynecologic infections (Sweet et al, 1988); skin and superficial soft tissue infections (Geckler et al, 1988); and for prophylaxis in colorectal surgery (Jagelman et al, 1988) in multicenter, randomized, controlled clinical trials. Thus, cefotetan appears to be an alternative to cefoxitin for these infections that are frequently polymicrobial, involving both aerobic gram-negative bacilli and anaerobic bacteria (including the *B. fragilis* group). When compared to cefoxitin, advantages of cefotetan include an expanded spectrum of activity against aerobic gram-negative bacilli and a longer elimination half-life (about 3.5 hours), which allows it to be administered twice daily. Possible disadvantages include the presence of a methylthiotetrazole side chain, which has been associated with hypoprothrombinemia and bleeding, as well as somewhat lower activity in vitro against some species of the *B. fragilis* group (eg, *B. ovatus, B. distasonis*). It should be emphasized that up to 20% of *B. fragilis* strains are resistant to both cefoxitin and cefotetan in some institutions and they probably should not be used alone for intra-abdominal infections in severely ill patients or when such infections are nosocomially acquired (see Antimicrobial Spectrum, Adverse Reactions and Precautions, and Pharmacokinetics, the evaluation on Cefoxitin, and the Introduction; see also index entries Antimicrobial Drugs: Antimicrobial Drug Selection for Common Infectious Diseases [Table]; Sexually Transmitted Diseases: Treatment (Table); and Antimicrobial Drugs: Chemoprophylaxis for Surgical Patients [Table]).

ADVERSE REACTIONS AND PRECAUTIONS. Cefotetan generally has been well tolerated in clinical trial patients and the adverse reaction profile has been similar to other cephalosporins. Hypersensitivity reactions (eg, rash, pruritus, fever), gastrointestinal disturbances (eg, diarrhea, nausea, vomiting), local reactions (eg, phlebitis, local pain), and minor hematologic (eg, eosinophilia, leukopenia) and hepatic (eg, elevated ALT, AST, alkaline phosphatase) laboratory abnormalities have been reported most frequently (Ward and Richards, 1985; manufacturer's literature; see also the Introduction).

Cefotetan contains a methylthiotetrazole side chain and has been associated with hypoprothrombinemia and, occasionally, bleeding. Elderly debilitated patients, individuals with severe renal insufficiency, and malnourished patients receiving total parenteral nutrition are at highest risk. Prothrombin times should be monitored in patients at risk and exogenous vitamin K administered as indicated (see the Introduction).

DRUG INTERACTIONS AND INTERFERENCE WITH LABORATORY TESTS. Methylthiotetrazole-containing cephalosporins have been associated with a disulfiram-like reaction. For additional discussion, see the Introduction.

PHARMACOKINETICS. Cefotetan is not absorbed following oral administration and must be administered intramuscularly or intravenously. Bioavailability after intramuscular injection is 100%. Peak serum concentrations obtained after intramuscular and bolus intravenous injections of 1 g are 50 to 80 mcg/ml (after one to two hours) and 140 to 250 mcg/ml, respectively. Following intravenous infusion of 1 g over a 30-minute period, peak serum levels of approximately 160 mcg/ml are achieved.

Approximately 88% of circulating cefotetan is bound to plasma protein. Apparent volumes of distribution ranging from 8 to 13 L have been reported, indicating distribution to the extracellular water space. Cefotetan has been shown to distribute into a variety of tissues and body fluids, including skin, muscle, fat, myometrium, endometrium, cervix, ovary, kidney, ureter, bladder, maxillary sinus mucosa, tonsil, bile, peritoneal fluid, umbilical cord serum, and amniotic fluid. High concentrations are obtained in urine. Penetration into cerebrospinal fluid appears to be low, but data are very limited.

Cefotetan is eliminated by the renal route. Between 51% and 81% of a dose is recovered as unchanged drug in the urine over a 24-hour period. The drug does not appear to be metabolized. The elimination half-life in adults with normal renal function ranges from 3 to 4.6 hours. In pediatric subjects, a slightly shorter half-life (range, 1.85 to 3.5 hours) usually is observed; in newborn infants with urinary tract infections, a longer half-life of 5.4 hours has been reported. The elimination half-life is prolonged in patients with impaired renal function and dosage adjustments are necessary.

For additional discussion, see Ward and Richards, 1985 and the manufacturer's literature.

DOSAGE AND PREPARATIONS. Cefotetan can be administered by intramuscular injection deep into a large muscle mass or intravenously by direct injection or by intermittent infusion. See the manufacturer's instructions for the appropriate dilution of the drug, compatible diluents and intravenous solutions, and stability of cefotetan in these solutions.

Intramuscular (deep), Intravenous: *Adults*, 1 to 6 g daily in equally divided doses every 12 hours is the dosage range recommended by the manufacturer. The usual adult dosage is 1 or 2 g every 12 hours. The following general guidelines for dosage of cefotetan according to type of infection have been recommended by the manufacturer: urinary tract, 500 mg every 12 hours or 1 to 2 g every 24 hours or 1 to 2 g every 12 hours; other sites, 1 to 2 g every 12 hours; severe, 2 g every 12 hours (intravenous); life-threatening, 3 g every 12 hours (intravenous). The maximum daily dosage should not exceed 6 g. For pelvic inflammatory disease, see index entry Sexually Transmitted Diseases: Treatment (Table). For perioperative prophylaxis in colorectal surgical procedures, see index entry Antimicrobial Drugs: Chemoprophylaxis for Surgical Patients (Table).

Patients with impaired renal function require modification in doses and/or frequency of administration depending on the degree of impairment, severity of the infection, and susceptibility of the causative organism. For *adults with impaired renal function*, the manufacturer recommends: for creatinine clearance of >30 ml/min, the usual recommended dose every 12 hours; for creatinine clearance of 10 to 30 ml/min, the usual recommended dose every 24 hours; for creatinine clearance of <10 ml/min, the usual recommended dose every 48 hours. Alternatively, the dosing interval may remain constant at 12-hour intervals, but the dose reduced to one-half the usual recommended dose for patients with creatinine clearance of 10 to 30 ml/min and one-quarter of the usual recommended dose for patients with creatinine clearance of <10 ml/min. For patients undergoing intermittent hemodialysis, one-quarter of the usual recommended dose should be given every 24 hours on days between dialysis and one-half the usual recommended dose on the day of dialysis.

Pediatric dosage guidelines are presently unavailable.

Cefotan (Stuart). Powder (sterile) 1, 2, and 10 g (equivalent to base) (sodium 3.5 mEq/g).

CEFMETAZOLE SODIUM

[Zefazone]

Cefmetazole is a cephamycin antibiotic that is produced synthetically from 7-aminocephalosporanic acid. Like cefoxitin, cefotetan, and moxalactam, it contains a 7 α-methoxy substitution on the basic cephalosporin nucleus that enhances its stability to most β-lactamases.

MECHANISM OF ACTION, ANTIMICROBIAL SPECTRUM, AND RESISTANCE. The mechanism of action, antimicrobial spectrum, and resistance properties are very similar to those of cefoxitin. In vitro, the minimum inhibitory concentrations (MICs) of cefmetazole were approximately two- to eightfold lower than those of cefoxitin against a number of commonly isolated aerobic bacterial species such as *Escherichia coli, Klebsiella* species, *Proteus mirabilis, Staphylococcus aureus, Streptococcus pyogenes, S. pneumoniae,* and *Haemophilus influenzae.* Cefmetazole was as or slightly less active than cefoxitin against *Neisseria gonorrhoeae* and *N. meningitidis.* Among anaerobic bacteria, the in vitro activity of cefmetazole was superior to that of cefoxitin against *Clostridium* and *Fusobacterium* species, comparable against gram-positive cocci (eg, *Peptostreptococcus* species), slightly less against *Bacteroides fragilis* species, and inferior against other species within the *B. fragilis* group (eg, *B. ovatus, B. thetaiotaomicron*) (Cornick et al, 1987; Jones, 1989; see also the evaluation on Cefoxitin Sodium and the Introduction). The clinical significance of these in vitro differences remains to be determined.

USES. Cefmetazole has been effective in intra-abdominal, skin and skin structure, urinary tract, and lower respiratory tract infections caused by susceptible bacteria (Griffith et al, 1989), and the results of comparative clinical trials suggest that this new cephamycin antibiotic is comparable in efficacy and safety to cefoxitin for the treatment of these infections (Holloway et al, 1989; Frank et al, 1989; Burke et al, 1989; Yangco et al, 1989), as well as for prophylaxis in abdominal surgery (DiPiro et al, 1989). Thus, the place of cefmetazole in infectious disease therapy would appear to be as an alternative to cefoxitin and cefotetan, but clinical experience with this agent is limited. When compared with cefoxitin, the only apparent advantages of cefmetazole are somewhat better activity in vitro against *S. aureus* and other gram-positive cocci and a slightly longer elimination half-life (about 1.2 hours), which allows cefmetazole to be administered three or four times daily. However, cefotetan can be administered twice daily and its activity in vitro against aerobic gram-negative bacilli is superior to that of cefmetazole. Like cefotetan, cefmetazole has the potential disadvantages of a methylthiotetrazole side chain that has been associated with hypoprothrombinemia and a disulfiram-like reaction, as well as somewhat lower activity in vitro against some species of the *B. fragilis* group (eg, *B. ovatus, B. thetaiotaomicron*) (see Antimicrobial Spectrum, Adverse Reactions and Precautions, and Pharmacokinetics; the evaluations on Cefoxitin Sodium and Cefotetan Disodium; and the Introduction).

ADVERSE REACTIONS AND PRECAUTIONS. Cefmetazole generally has been well tolerated in clinical trials in the United States (Griffith et al, 1989) and during postmarketing surveillance in Japan (Saito, 1989). The adverse reaction profile has been similar to that of other cephalosporins. Gastrointestinal disturbances (eg, diarrhea, nausea), hypersensitivity reactions (eg, rash, pruritus, urticaria), local reactions (eg, phlebitis, local pain), and transient hematologic (eg, eosinophilia, leukopenia) and hepatic laboratory abnormalities (eg, elevated ALT and AST) have been reported most frequently (Griffith et al, 1989; Saito, 1989; manufacturer's literature; see also the Introduction).

Cefmetazole contains a methylthiotetrazole side chain that has been associated with hypoprothrombinemia. Elderly debilitated patients, those with severe renal insufficiency, and malnourished patients receiving total parenteral nutrition are at highest risk. Prothrombin times should be monitored in patients at risk, and vitamin K should be administered as indicated (see the Introduction).

DRUG INTERACTIONS AND INTERFERENCE WITH LABORATORY TESTS. Methylthiotetrazole-containing cephalosporins have been associated with a disulfiram-like reaction. For additional discussion, see the Introduction.

PHARMACOKINETICS. Cefmetazole is administered intravenously. Peak serum concentrations obtained following intravenous infusions of 2 g over 5 and 60 minutes were 214 mcg/ml and 143 mcg/ml, respectively.

Approximately 65% of circulating cefmetazole is bound to plasma protein. The antibiotic reaches therapeutic levels in a number of tissues and body fluids, including gallbladder wall; vaginal, uterine, and adnexal tissues, wound muscle, bile, and interstitial fluid. High concentrations are attained in urine. Data on penetration into cerebrospinal fluid are not available.

Approximately 85% of a dose is excreted by the kidneys (renal tubular secretion) as unchanged drug over a 12-hour period. Excretion is delayed by probenecid. The elimination half-life is approximately 1.2 hours. The half-life is prolonged in patients with renal impairment and dosage adjustments are required.

DOSAGE AND PREPARATIONS. Cefmetazole is administered intravenously by injection over three to five minutes or by intermittent infusion over 10 to 60 minutes. See the manufacturer's instructions for the appropriate dilution of the drug, compatible diluents and intravenous solutions, and stability of cefmetazole in these solutions.

Intravenous: *Adults,* 2 g every 6 to 12 hours is the dosage range recommended by the manufacturer. The following general guidelines for dosage of cefmetazole according to type and severity of infection have been recommended by the manufacturer: urinary tract, 2 g every 12 hours; other sites (mild to moderate infections), 2 g every eight hours; other sites (severe to life-threatening infections), 2 g every six hours. Usual duration of therapy is 5 to 14 days. Dosage guidelines for *children* have not been established.

Patients with impaired renal function require a reduction in dosage. For *adults with impaired renal function,* the manufacturer recommends the following: for mild impairment (creatinine clearance 90 to 50 ml/min/1.73 M^2), 1 to 2 g every 12 hours; for moderate impairment (creatinine clearance 49 to 30 ml/min/1.73 M^2), 1 to 2 g every 16 hours; for severe impairment (creatinine clearance 29 to 10 ml/min/1.73 M^2), 1 to 2 g every 24 hours; and for essentially no function (creatinine clearance <10 ml/min/1.73 M^2), 1 to 2 g every 48 hours (administered after hemodialysis).

Zefazone (Upjohn). Powder (sterile) 1 and 2 g (equivalent to base) (sodium 2 mEq/g).

PARENTERAL THIRD GENERATION CEPHALOSPORINS

CEFOTAXIME SODIUM
[Claforan]

Cefotaxime is one of several third generation cephalosporins that contain an aminothiazolyl-acetyl side chain with an α-syn-methoximino group at the 7-position of the β-lactam ring (see Figure). The aminothiazolyl side chain enhances antibacterial activity, particularly against Enterobacteriaceae, and the methoximino group imparts stability against hydrolysis by many β-lactamases (see Neu, 1982 A). Cefotaxime was the first cephalosporin of the third generation to be marketed in the United States.

MECHANISM OF ACTION, ANTIMICROBIAL SPECTRUM, AND RESISTANCE. Cefotaxime has increased potency and a wider spectrum of activity against clinically important gram-negative bacteria when compared to first and second generation cephalosporins. This drug has excellent activity against *Neisseria meningitidis, N. gonorrhoeae, Moraxella (Branhamella) catarrhalis, Haemophilus influenzae*, and most of the Enterobacteriaceae (eg, *Escherichia coli, Klebsiella, Enterobacter, Proteus, Morganella, Providencia, Citrobacter, Serratia, Salmonella, Shigella*), including strains that are resistant to earlier generation cephalosporins, penicillins, and aminoglycosides. This activity is related to cefotaxime's excellent β-lactamase stability and high affinity for penicillin binding proteins in these gram-negative bacteria. The nonfermenting gram-negative bacilli, *Pseudomonas aeruginosa* and *Acinetobacter*, generally are resistant, however. Cefotaxime has only fair activity against the *Bacteroides fragilis* group, anaerobic gram-negative bacilli.

Among gram-positive bacteria, cefotaxime has excellent activity against *Streptococcus pyogenes*, *S. agalactiae*, and *S. pneumoniae* and good activity against nonpenicillinase- and penicillinase-producing staphylococci. However, this agent offers no clinical advantages over first generation cephalosporins for infections (other than meningitis) that are known to be caused by gram-positive bacteria. Enterococci, methicillin-resistant staphylococci, and *Listeria monocytogenes* are resistant to all cephalosporins.

Although cefotaxime is stable to the hydrolytic activity of most β-lactamases, resistance to this third generation cephalosporin can occur among certain nonfastidious gram-negative bacilli, particularly *Enterobacter, Serratia*, and *Pseudomonas* species, via the induction of Type I chromosomal β-lactamases that appear to tightly bind and, therefore, inactivate the drug. In Europe, novel plasmid-mediated transferable β-lactamases (eg, TEM-3 [CTX-1]) that confer resistance to third generation cephalosporins have been isolated from *Klebsiella pneumoniae* and other Enterobacteriaceae (see Sirot et al, 1988; Philippon et al, 1989).

In vivo, cefotaxime is partially metabolized to 3-desacetylcefotaxime, an active, β-lactamase-stable metabolite. The antibacterial activity of desacetylcefotaxime is four- to eight-fold less than that of cefotaxime, but this metabolite is more active than cefazolin, cefamandole, and cefoxitin against most aerobic gram-negative bacteria. Studies in vitro suggest that cefotaxime and desacetylcefotaxime act synergistically against a number of bacterial strains (see Jones et al, 1982; Neu, 1982 E; Chin and Neu, 1984).

For additional discussion of the mechanism of action, antimicrobial spectrum, and resistance properties of the cephalosporins, see the Introduction.

USES. Cefotaxime is useful in the treatment of certain types of bacterial meningitis and, among third generation cephalosporins, clinical experience is probably greatest with this agent. It is a preferred drug for meningitis caused by susceptible gram-negative enteric bacilli (eg, *Escherichia coli, Klebsiella, Proteus*). However, it should not be considered adequate single-drug therapy for meningitis caused by *Pseudomonas aeruginosa*. Cefotaxime (and most third generation cephalosporins) is effective in meningitis caused by *Haemophilus influenzae* type b, including β-lactamase-producing strains. Most infectious disease consultants now prefer a third generation cephalosporin (eg, cefotaxime, ceftriaxone) to ampicillin plus chloramphenicol for this indication. Cefotaxime is active against the common causative organisms (*H. influenzae* type b, *Neisseria meningitidis, Streptococcus pneumoniae*) of meningitis in infants and young children and is an effective single-agent alternative to ampicillin plus chloramphenicol for the empiric therapy of meningitis in this age group (American Academy of Pediatrics Committee on Infectious Diseases, 1988). Most pediatric infectious disease experts prefer monotherapy with an appropriate third-generation cephalosporin, usually cefotaxime or ceftriaxone, both for the convenience of single-drug therapy and to avoid the toxicity and problems associated with administration (eg, need to monitor serum concentrations) of chloramphenical (see McCracken et al, 1987). The combination of ampicillin plus cefotaxime is an alternative to ampicillin plus an aminoglycoside for initial therapy of neonatal meningitis and is the regimen of choice for infants between 1 and 3 months of age (American Academy of Pediatrics Committee on Infectious Diseases, 1988). For additional discussion, see the Introduction; see also index entry Antimicrobial Drugs: Antimicrobial Drug Selection for Common Infectious Diseases (Table).

Cefotaxime has been effective, frequently as empiric monotherapy, in a wide variety of serious gram-negative bacillary infections outside the central nervous system. These include lower respiratory tract, complicated urinary tract, intra-abdominal, gynecologic, skin and skin structure, bone, and joint infections and bacteremias. These frequently are of nosocomial origin and are caused by bacterial strains that are resistant to penicillins, older cephalosporins, and aminoglycosides. However, the exact role of cefotaxime (or other third generation cephalosporins) in the treatment of these infections remains to be determined. It would appear to be particularly useful (1) for infections caused by susceptible gram-negative bacilli that exhibit multiple resistance to other, less expensive antimicrobial agents; (2) as an effective alternative to a more toxic aminoglycoside, particularly in patients at high risk for aminoglycoside toxicity or when prolonged therapy is required (eg, for osteomyelitis); and (3) for certain serious infections, such as *Klebsiella* pneumonia, for which a third generation cephalosporin is the most active agent. Cefotaxime alone may replace combination regimens that contain an aminoglycoside for initial treatment of seriously ill patients with infections of undetermined etiology, but when gram-negative aerobic bacilli are suspected pathogens. However, rapid development of resistance during therapy with third generation cephalosporins has been observed clinically (see Sanders et al, 1988), and the judicious use of these agents is recommended. Cefotaxime should not be used alone when *P. aeruginosa* is a likely causative organism.

Cefotaxime (or other third generation cephalosporins) should not be used when less expensive, narrower spectrum, first generation cephalosporins are equally effective (eg, for known gram-positive infections, perioperative prophylaxis). For additional discussion, see the Introduction and index entry Antimicrobial Drugs: Antimicrobial Drug Selection for Common Infectious Diseases (Table).

Cefotaxime has been useful in the treatment of uncomplicated and disseminated gonococcal infections, including those caused by PPNG strains. However, the more active third generation agent, ceftriaxone, often is the preferred cephalosporin for these infections (*MMWR*, 1989; see also index entry Sexually Transmitted Diseases: Treatment (Table).

ADVERSE REACTIONS AND PRECAUTIONS. Cefotaxime generally is well tolerated, and adverse reactions and precautions are the same as for first generation cephalosporins (see the Introduction).

DRUG INTERACTIONS AND INTERFERENCE WITH LABORATORY TESTS. See the Introduction.

PHARMACOKINETICS. Cefotaxime is administered intramuscularly or intravenously. Peak serum concentrations obtained after intramuscular or intravenous injections of 1 g are 20 mcg/ml (after 30 minutes) and 100 mcg/ml, respectively. Following intravenous infusion of 1 g over a 30-minute period, peak serum levels of 40 to 45 mcg/ml are achieved.

About 38% of circulating cefotaxime is bound to plasma protein. Volumes of distribution ranging from 0.25 to 0.39 L/kg have been reported. Cefotaxime has been shown to distribute into a variety of tissues and body fluids, including synovial, pericardial, pleural, and peritoneal fluids; bile; and urine. It enters cerebrospinal fluid in the presence of inflammation and achieves therapeutic concentrations for a number of pathogens. This antibiotic crosses the placenta.

Up to 50% of a dose is metabolized to desacetylcefotaxime, which has some antimicrobial activity, and other unknown, inactive metabolites. Parent drug and metabolites are excreted via the kidneys by renal tubular secretion and glomerular filtration; probenecid delays excretion. Between 50% and 60% of a dose is recovered as unchanged drug in the urine; 15% to 25% is recovered as desacetylcefotaxime. The elimination half-life of cefotaxime is about one hour; the half-life of desacetylcefotaxime is 1.6 hours. Little parent drug accumulates in patients with impaired renal function. However, elimination of the desacetyl metabolite is prolonged, and dosage reduction is recommended when the creatinine clearance is less than 20 ml/min.

DOSAGE AND PREPARATIONS. Cefotaxime can be administered by intramuscular injection deep into a large muscle mass or intravenously by direct injection or by intermittent or continuous infusion. See the manufacturer's instructions for the appropriate dilution of the drug, compatible diluents and intravenous solutions, and stability of cefotaxime in these solutions.

Intravenous, Intramuscular (deep): *Adults*, 2 to 12 g daily in equally divided doses every four to eight hours (The Medical Letter, 1988). The usual dosage for moderate to severe infections is 1 to 2 g every eight hours; for infections commonly needing antibiotics in higher dosage (eg, septicemia), 2 g intravenously every six to eight hours; for life-threatening infections, 2 g intravenously every four hours. The manufacturer recommends 1 g every 12 hours for uncomplicated urinary tract infections. For uncomplicated gonorrhea (including PPNG), 1 g intramuscularly as a single dose without probenecid. For disseminated and neonatal gonococcal infections, see index entry Sexually Transmitted Diseases: Treatment (Table).

Infants over 1 month and children, 100 to 200 mg/kg daily in equally divided doses every four to eight hours (The Medical Letter, 1988). The larger dosage is recommended for meningitis. *Neonates over 7 days*, 150 mg/kg daily in divided doses every eight hours; *neonates 0 to 7 days*, 100 mg/kg daily in divided doses every 12 hours (The Medical Letter, 1988; Nelson, 1989 B).

Patients with impaired renal function require modification in doses and/or frequency of administration depending on the degree of impairment, severity of the infection, and susceptibility of the causative organism. Various dosage recommendations for these patients have been proposed. The manufacturer recommends that the dose of cefotaxime be halved when creatinine clearance is less than 20 ml/min/1.73 M^2. Alternative dosage recommendations for patients with impaired renal function are to increase the dosage interval to 6 to 12 hours for creatinine clearance of 50 to 10 ml/min and to 12 hours for creatinine clearance less than 10 ml/min (The Medical Letter, 1988). A supplemental dose equal to 50% of the maintenance dose should be given after hemodialysis (Norris et al, 1990).

Claforan (Hoechst-Roussel). Powder (sterile) 1, 2, and 10 g (equivalent to base) (sodium 2.2 mEq/g); solution 1 and 2 g (sodium 2.2 mEq/g) in 50 ml containers.

CEFTIZOXIME SODIUM

[Cefizox]

Ceftizoxime is an aminothiazolyl *syn*-methoximino cephalosporin that is structurally very similar to cefotaxime (see Figure).

MECHANISM OF ACTION, ANTIMICROBIAL SPECTRUM, AND RESISTANCE. The mechanism of action, antimicrobial spectrum, and resistance properties are essentially the same as for cefotaxime (see that evaluation and the Introduction; see also Barriere and Flaherty, 1984; Neu, 1984; Richards and Heel, 1985).

USES. Ceftizoxime has been effective, frequently as empiric monotherapy, in a wide variety of serious gram-negative bacillary infections, including lower respiratory tract, complicated urinary tract, intra-abdominal, gynecologic, skin and skin structure, bone, and joint infections and bacteremias. These frequently are of nosocomial origin and are caused by bacterial strains that are resistant to penicillins, older cephalosporins, and aminoglycosides. This drug is not recommended as sole therapy for *Pseudomonas aeruginosa* infections, however (see Parks et al, 1982; Barriere and Flaherty, 1984; Neu, 1984; Richards and Heel, 1985). The exact role of ceftizoxime in the treatment of these infections remains to be determined, but it appears to have indications very similar to those of cefotaxime (see that evaluation; see also the Introduction and index entry Antimicrobial Drugs: Antimicrobial Drug Selection for Common Infectious Diseases [Table]).

The elimination half-life of ceftizoxime (1.4 to 1.8 hours) is longer than that of cefotaxime (about one hour). Thus, it has the advantage of a more prolonged dosage interval. However, clinical experience with ceftizoxime, particularly for meningitis, is more limited than with cefotaxime. Ceftizoxime has approved labeling for meningitis caused by *Haemophilus influenzae* and looks promising for other forms of bacterial meningitis (Overturf et al, 1984).

ADVERSE REACTIONS AND PRECAUTIONS. These are the same as for first generation cephalosporins (see the Introduction).

DRUG INTERACTIONS AND INTERFERENCE WITH LABORATORY TESTS. See the Introduction.

PHARMACOKINETICS. Ceftizoxime is administered intramuscularly or intravenously. The peak serum concentration obtained after intramuscular injection of 1 g was 39 mcg/ml (after 60 minutes). Following intravenous infusion of 1 g over a 30-minute period, serum levels of 80 to 90 mcg/ml were achieved.

Approximately 30% of circulating ceftizoxime is bound to plasma proteins. Volumes of distribution ranging from 0.35 to 0.40 L/kg have been reported. Ceftizoxime has been shown to distribute into a variety of tissues and body fluids, including pleural, ascitic, prostatic, surgical wound, and peritoneal fluids; bile; urine; saliva; aqueous humor; heart; gallbladder; bone; and biliary, peritoneal, prostatic, and uterine tissues. Ceftizoxime enters cerebrospinal fluid in the presence of inflammation. This antibiotic crosses the placenta and is found in breast milk.

Up to 90% of a dose is excreted in the urine as unchanged drug by renal tubular secretion and glomerular filtration; excretion is delayed by probenecid. Ceftizoxime is not metabolized. The elimination half-life is approximately 1.4 to 1.8 hours. The half-life is prolonged in patients with renal impairment and dosage adjustments are required.

DOSAGE AND PREPARATIONS. Ceftizoxime can be administered by intramuscular injection deep into a large muscle mass or intravenously by direct injection or by intermittent or continuous infusion. See the manufacturer's instructions for the appropriate dilution of the drug, compatible diluents and intravenous solutions, and stability of ceftizoxime in these solutions.

Intravenous, Intramuscular (deep): *Adults*, 2 to 12 g daily in equally divided doses every six to 12 hours (The Medical Letter, 1988). The usual dosages are as follows: for moderate infections outside the urinary tract, 1 g every 8 to 12 hours intramuscularly or intravenously; for severe or refractory infections, 1 g every eight hours or 2 g every 8 to 12 hours intramuscularly or intravenously; for life-threatening infections, 3 to 4 g every eight hours intravenously (up to 2 g every four hours has been given). For uncomplicated urinary tract infections, the manufacturer recommends 500 mg every 12 hours (a higher dosage is recommended for urinary tract infections caused by *Pseudomonas aeruginosa*). For uncomplicated gonorrhea (including PPNG), 1 g intramuscularly as a single dose without probenecid. When 2 g is administered intramuscularly, one-half of the dose is given in different large muscle masses.

Children 6 months or older, 150 to 200 mg/kg daily in equally divided doses every six to eight hours (not to exceed the maximum daily dosage for adults). Dosage guidelines for infants less than 6 months have not been established.

Patients with impaired renal function require modification in doses and/or frequency of administration depending on the degree of impairment, severity of the infection, and susceptibility of the causative organism. In *adults with impaired renal function*, the manufacturer recommends an initial loading dose of 500 mg to 1 g intramuscularly or intravenously and maintenance dosages as shown in the table:

Renal Function	Creatinine Clearance (ml/min)	Less Severe Infections (Adult Maintenance Dosage)	Life-threatening Infections (Adult Maintenance Dosage)
Mild Impairment	79-50	500 mg every 8 hours	0.75-1.5 g every 8 hours
Moderate to Severe Impairment	49-5	250-500 mg every 12 hours	0.5-1 g every 12 hours
Dialysis Patients	4-0	500 mg every 48 hours or 250 mg every 24 hours	0.5-1 g every 48 hours or 0.5 g every 24 hours

From manufacturer's literature

No additional supplemental dosing is required following hemodialysis. However, the dosage schedule should be timed so that the dose (according to the table) is given at the end of the dialysis session.

Cefizox (Smith, Kline & French). Powder (sterile) 1, 2, and 10 g (equivalent to base) (sodium 2.6 mEq/g); solution 1 and 2 g in 5% dextrose (sodium 2.6 mEq/g) in 50 ml containers.

CEFTRIAXONE SODIUM
[Rocephin]

Ceftriaxone is an aminothiazolyl *syn*-methoximino cephalosporin that is structurally similar to cefotaxime and ceftizoxime (see Figure).

MECHANISM OF ACTION, ANTIMICROBIAL SPECTRUM, AND RESISTANCE. The mechanism of action, antimicrobial spectrum, and resistance properties are essentially the same as for cefotaxime (see that evaluation and the Introduction; see also Barriere and Flaherty, 1984; Cleeland and Squires, 1984; Richards et al, 1984; Beam, 1985).

USES. Ceftriaxone has outstanding activity against *Neisseria gonorrhoeae*, including penicillinase-producing strains (PPNG), chromosomal-mediated resistant *N. gonorrhoeae* (CMRNG), and tetracycline-resistant *N. gonorrhoeae* (TRNG). A single intramuscular 250-mg dose of this long-acting third generation cephalosporin has been highly effective in uncomplicated gonorrhea in adults, including urethral, endocervical, anorectal, and pharyngeal forms of this infection (Handsfield and Murphy, 1983; Judson et al, 1983 and 1985; Collier et al, 1984). Presently, it is the drug of choice for all uncomplicated gonococcal infections (*MMWR*, 1989). Because cephalosporins are not active against *Chlamydia trachomatis*, follow-up therapy with doxycycline or tetracycline for seven days is recommended for coexisting chlamydial infections. Parenteral ceftriaxone also is preferred for disseminated gonococcal infections in adults and children and for neonatal gonococcal infections (*MMWR*, 1989). A single intramuscular 250-mg dose of ceftriaxone was highly effective in the treatment of chancroid (Taylor et al, 1985); it is a preferred drug (alternative, erythromycin) for this infection caused by *Haemophilus ducreyi* (*MMWR*, 1989). For additional discussion, see the Introduction and index entry Sexually Transmitted Diseases: Treatment (Table).

Ceftriaxone is highly active against the common causative organisms (*Haemophilus influenzae* type b, *Neisseria meningitidis, Streptococcus pneumoniae*) of meningitis in infants and young children, and it has been shown to be an effective single-agent alternative to ampicillin plus chloramphenicol for the empiric therapy of meningitis in this age group (Del Rio et al, 1983; Steele and Bradsher, 1983; Congeni, 1984; Barson et al, 1985; Bryan et al, 1985 A; American Academy of Pediatrics Committee on Infectious Diseases, 1988). Most pediatric infectious disease experts prefer monotherapy with an appropriate third generation cephalosporin, usually cefotaxime or ceftriaxone, both for the convenience of single-drug therapy and to avoid the toxicity and problems associated with administration (eg, need to monitor serum concentrations) of chloramphenicol (see McCracken et al, 1987). Like cefotaxime, ceftriaxone also is effective for gram-negative enteric bacillary meningitis (eg, *Escherichia coli, Klebsiella*) and, in combination with ampicillin, for neonatal meningitis. It is not active against *Listeria monocytogenes*, enterococci, or *Pseudomonas aeruginosa*. For additional discussion, see the Introduction, the evaluation of Cefotaxime Sodium, and index entry Antimicrobial Drugs: Antimicrobial Drug Selection for Common Infectious Diseases (Table).

Ceftriaxone has been effective, frequently as empiric monotherapy, in a wide variety of serious gram-negative bacillary infections, including lower respiratory tract, complicated urinary tract, intra-abdominal, gynecologic, skin and skin structure, bone, and joint infections and bacteremias. These frequently are of nosocomial origin and are caused by bacterial strains that are resistant to penicillins, older cephalosporins, and aminoglycosides. However, this drug is not recommended as sole therapy of *Pseudomonas aeruginosa* infections (see Barriere and Flaherty, 1984; McClosky, 1984; Richards et al, 1984; Beam, 1985). The exact role of ceftriaxone in the treatment of these infections remains to be determined, but the indications appear to be very similar to those of cefotaxime (see that evaluation; see also the Introduction and index entry Antimicrobial Drugs: Antimicrobial Drug Selection for Common Infectious Diseases [Table]).

Ceftriaxone, administered intravenously, has become a preferred drug for the treatment of serious neurologic, cardiovascular, and joint abnormalities associated with Lyme disease (Dattwyler et al, 1988; *Med Lett Drugs Ther,* 1989 A; see also index entry Antimicrobial Drugs: Antimicrobial Drug Selection for Common Infectious Diseases [Table]. Ceftriaxone and other third generation cephalosporins look promising for systemic salmonellosis, particularly for infections caused by *Salmonella* strains that are resistant to current drugs (eg, ampicillin) (Soe and Overturf, 1987; Islam et al, 1988). Ceftriaxone also may be useful in eradicating pharyngeal carriage of *N. meningitidis* (Schwartz et al, 1988).

The major advantage of ceftriaxone is a long elimination half-life (six to nine hours) that permits administration once daily for most infections. Thus, the potential to reduce the cost of antimicrobial therapy and, for certain infections, to administer parenteral antibiotics in an outpatient setting may be realized with ceftriaxone.

Although single-dose ceftriaxone has been shown to be effective as perioperative prophylaxis for various surgical procedures (see Beam, 1985), no advantages over currently recommended cephalosporins, usually cefazolin, have been shown in controlled clinical trials (see DiPiro et al, 1984; Barriere, 1985; Polk, 1985; see also the Introduction and index entry Antimicrobial Drugs: Chemoprophylaxis for Surgical Patients [Table]).

ADVERSE REACTIONS AND PRECAUTIONS. Ceftriaxone generally has been well tolerated, and most adverse reactions (eg, skin rashes and other hypersensitivity reactions, diarrhea and other gastrointestinal disturbances, mild reversible laboratory abnormalities) are similar to those reported for first generation cephalosporins (see the Introduction). Hypoprothrombinemia is very rare, and bleeding has not been reported. Although ceftriaxone does not possess the methylthiotetrazole side chain that has been associated with coagulopathy, the manufacturer suggests that monitoring of prothrombin time, with supplemental vitamin K, may be reasonable in patients with impaired vitamin K synthesis or low vitamin K stores (eg, chronic hepatic disease, malnutrition). Because of its broad antimicrobial spectrum and high biliary excretion, ceftriaxone markedly alters colonic flora. Diarrhea generally has been reported in only 3% to 6% of patients but has occurred in over 20% of pediatric patients in some studies. The incidence of superinfections with resistant organisms does not appear to be greater than with other third generation cephalosporins (see Barriere and Flaherty, 1984; Moskovitz, 1984; Oakes et al, 1984; Richards et al, 1984; Beam, 1985; Noble and Barza, 1985; Brogden and Ward, 1988).

Ceftriaxone has been associated with the formation of biliary sludge in the gallbladder, which may lead to signs and symptoms of cholecystitis. This was reversible after drug discontinuation (Schaad et al, 1988, 1990; Pigrau et al, 1989). This highly protein bound cephalosporin also can displace bilirubin from albumin binding sites (Fink et al, 1987), and some consultants recommend caution in the use of ceftriaxone in jaundiced or premature infants.

DRUG INTERACTIONS AND INTERFERENCE WITH LABORATORY TESTS. See the Introduction. Although ceftriaxone does not contain a methylthiotetrazole side chain, a disulfiram-like reaction has been reported in one patient (Moskovitz, 1984). It has been suggested by one of our consultants that the methylthiotriazine group at the 3-position of ceftriaxone may have structural similarities to the methylthiotetrazole side chain of cefamandole, cefoperazone, and moxalactam (see Figure).

PHARMACOKINETICS. Ceftriaxone is administered intramuscularly or intravenously. A peak serum concentration of 40 to 45 mcg/ml is obtained between two and three hours after intramuscular injection of 500 mg. Following intravenous infusion of 1 g over a 30-minute period, a serum concentration of approximately 150 mcg/ml is achieved.

Between 83% and 96% of circulating ceftriaxone is bound to plasma protein. Protein binding is concentration-dependent; the free ceftriaxone fraction increases from 4% to 17% over the serum concentration range of 5 mcg/ml to 300 mcg/ml. The apparent volume of distribution of (total) ceftriaxone is 0.12 to 0.14 L/kg. Ceftriaxone distributes to a wide variety of tissues (eg, myometrium, gallbladder wall, bone) and body fluids (eg, synovial, pleural, peritoneal). Large concentrations are present in bile and urine. Ceftriaxone enters the cerebrospinal fluid in the presence of inflammation and achieves therapeutic concentrations for a number of pathogens. This antibiotic crosses the placenta.

Ceftriaxone is eliminated by both renal (glomerular filtration) and biliary routes. It is not metabolized. Between 40% and 65% of a dose is recovered from urine as unchanged drug; the remainder is secreted into bile and ultimately is found in the feces as microbiologically inactive compounds. The elimination half-life is between six and nine hours in healthy volunteers. Elimination is prolonged only slightly in patients with severe renal impairment, and dosage adjustments are unnecessary, provided the total daily dosage does not exceed 2 g. The effect of hepatic dysfunction on elimination also is minimal. However, accumulation occurs in those with combined renal and hepatic impairment and dosage reductions are required.

DOSAGE AND PREPARATIONS. Ceftriaxone can be administered by intramuscular injection deep into a large muscle mass or intravenously by intermittent infusion. See the manufacturer's instructions for the appropriate dilution of the drug, compatible diluents and intravenous solutions, and stability of ceftriaxone in those solutions.

Intramuscular (deep), Intravenous: *Adults*, the usual dosage is 1 to 2 g once daily (or in equally divided doses every 12 hours) depending on the type and severity of the infection (*Med Lett Drugs Ther*, 1985 A; manufacturer's literature). The total daily dose should not exceed 4 g. For uncomplicated gonococcal infections, 250 mg intramuscularly as a single dose. *Infants and children*, for serious infections other than meningitis, 50 to 75 mg/kg daily (maximum of 2 g per day) in equally divided doses every 12 hours; for meningitis, 100 mg/kg daily (maximum of 4 g per day) in divided doses every 12 hours, with or without a loading dose of 75 mg/kg (*Med Lett Drugs Ther*, 1985 A; manufacturer's literature).

For dosage in other gonococcal infections, see index entry Sexually Transmitted Diseases: Treatment (Table); for dosages in Lyme disease, see index entry Antimicrobial Drugs: Antimicrobial Drug Selection for Common Infectious Diseases (Table).

Dosage adjustments are unnecessary in patients with impaired renal or hepatic function. However, the manufacturer recommends monitoring of serum concentrations in patients with severe renal impairment (eg, dialysis patients) and in those with combined renal and hepatic dysfunction.

Rocephin (Roche). Powder (sterile) 250 and 500 mg and 1, 2, and 10 g (equivalent to base) (sodium 3.6 mEq/g); solution 1 and 2 g (sodium 3.6 mEq/g) in 50 ml containers.

CEFTAZIDIME

[Fortaz, Tazicef, Tazidime]

Ceftazidime is an aminothiazolyl cephalosporin similar to cefotaxime, ceftizoxime, and ceftriaxone. However, it differs from these agents because it contains a 2-carboxy-2-oxypropane imino group rather than a methoximino group, which the others have (see Figure). The carboxy side chain of ceftazidime reduces its activity against gram-positive cocci but increases its activity against *Pseudomonas aeruginosa* (see Neu, 1982 A).

Ceftazidime is being marketed by three manufacturers in the United States, which may allow hospital pharmacists to reduce their acquisition cost through competitive bidding.

MECHANISM OF ACTION, ANTIMICROBIAL SPECTRUM, AND RESISTANCE. Ceftazidime is a broad spectrum β-lactamase-stable third generation cephalosporin. Like other aminothiazolyl cephalosporins (eg, cefotaxime) and moxalactam, it has excellent activity against a variety of gram-negative bacteria, including *Neisseria meningitidis, N. gonorrhoeae, Moraxella (Branhamella) catarrhalis, Haemophilus influenzae*, and most Enterobacteriaceae (eg, *Escherichia coli, Klebsiella, Enterobacter, Proteus, Morganella, Providencia, Citrobacter, Serratia, Salmonella, Shigella*). Strains of these gram-negative bacteria that are resistant to earlier generation cephalosporins, penicillins, and aminoglycosides frequently are susceptible.

The primary advantage of ceftazidime when compared to other currently available third generation cephalosporins is its good activity against *Pseudomonas aeruginosa*. It is superior to cefoperazone and, in most instances, is more active in vitro than aminoglycosides, carbenicillin, ticarcillin, azlocillin, and piperacillin against *P. aeruginosa*, including strains that are resistant to these other antibiotics. Ceftazidime also is active against many strains of other nonfermenting gram-negative bacilli, including other *Pseudomonas* species (eg, *P. cepacia*) and *Acinetobacter*.

Among gram-positive bacteria, ceftazidime is generally active in vitro against nonpenicillinase- and penicillinase-producing *Staphylococcus aureus*, but it is somewhat less potent than cefotaxime, ceftizoxime, and ceftriaxone and is considerably less active than parenteral first generation cephalosporins. Activity against coagulase-negative staphylococci (eg, *S. epidermidis*) is marginal and many strains are resistant. As with all cephalosporins, methicillin-resistant staphylococci are resistant. Most streptococci (except enterococci) are susceptible to ceftazidime, but it is less potent than cefotaxime, ceftizoxime, ceftriaxone, and the first generation cephalosporins. *Listeria monocytogenes* are resistant to ceftazidime and all other cephalosporins.

Overall, the activity of ceftazidime against anaerobic bacteria is fair, but it has poor activity against the *Bacteroides fragilis* group. Clostridia (other than *C. perfringens*) usually are resistant.

Although ceftazidime is stable to the hydrolytic activity of most β-lactamases, resistance has emerged during therapy with this antibiotic, particularly among *Pseudomonas* and *Enterobacter* species (see Sanders and Sanders, 1985). In Europe, novel plasmid-mediated, transferable β-lactamases (eg, TEM-5 [CAZ-1]) that confer resistance to ceftazidime have been isolated from *Klebsiella pneumoniae* and other Enterobacteriaceae (see Sirot et al, 1988; Philippon et al, 1989).

For additional discussion of the mechanism of action, antimicrobial spectrum, and resistance properties of ceftazidime, see the Introduction; see also Smith, 1984; Gentry, 1985; and Richards and Brogden, 1985.

USES. Ceftazidime has been effective, frequently as empiric monotherapy, in a wide variety of serious infections caused by *Pseudomonas aeruginosa* and other aerobic gram-negative bacilli. These include lower respiratory tract, complicated urinary tract, skin and soft tissue, bone, and joint infections and bacteremias. These are frequently of nosocomial origin and are caused by bacterial strains that are resistant to penicillins, other cephalosporins, and aminoglycosides (see Smith, 1984; Gentry, 1985; *Med Lett Drugs Ther*, 1985 B; Richards and Brogden, 1985). Thus, ceftazidime appears to be a useful agent for hospital-acquired gram-negative infections and would be preferred to other third generation cephalosporins when *P. aeruginosa* is a potential causative organism. Although this agent has been used to treat intra-abdominal and gynecologic infections (see Smith, 1984), its usefulness as a single agent in these situations must be questioned because of its lack of efficacy against many strains of *Bacteroides fragilis* (see Gleckman, 1985; Moellering, 1985 B; Richards and Brogden, 1985). For additional discussion, see the Introduction.

Ceftazidime is the most useful third generation cephalosporin for meningitis caused by *P. aeruginosa* (Fong and Tomkins, 1985). Presently, it should be considered a preferred alternative to an antipseudomonal penicillin for combination therapy with an aminoglycoside (intravenous and intrathecal administration) (Neu, 1987 B; *Med Lett Drugs Ther,* 1990). Although ceftazidime alone also has been effective in a limited number of cases of *P. aeruginosa* meningitis (Fong and Tompkins, 1985), additional clinical studies are necessary before it can be recommended as monotherapy for this very serious infection. Ceftazidime also is useful for meningitis caused by gram-negative enteric bacilli, such as *Escherichia coli, Klebsiella*, and *Proteus* (see Norrby, 1985), but experience with cefotaxime and moxalactam is greater. In one study, ceftazidime was as effective as ampicillin plus chloramphenicol for meningitis in infants and children from 1 month to 15 years; causative organisms were primarily *Haemophilus influenzae, Neisseria meningitidis*, and *Streptococcus pneumoniae* (Rodriguez et al, 1985). However, cefotaxime and ceftriaxone have been studied more extensively. For additional discussion, see the Introduction and the evaluations; see also index entry Antimicrobial Drugs: Antimicrobial Drug Selection for Common Infectious Diseases (Table).

Ceftazidime is particularly useful in patients whose underlying conditions predispose them to infections with *P. aeruginosa*. Used alone, ceftazidime has produced clinical improvement in some patients with acute pulmonary exacerbations of cystic fibrosis (Mastella et al, 1983; Blumer et al, 1985; Gold et al, 1985) and was as effective as ticarcillin plus tobramycin in a randomized, controlled trial (Gold et al, 1985). Although short-term reductions in sputum colony counts of *P. aeruginosa* were observed, ceftazidime failed to produce long-term *P. aeruginosa* eradication. This is consistent with results obtained with other antipseudomonal antibiotics. The response to ceftazidime was less satisfactory in cystic fibrosis patients with lower respiratory tract infections caused by *P. cepacia* (Gold et al, 1985).

Because of its good activity against *P. aeruginosa*, ceftazidime also has been used alone and in combination with other agents for presumptive and definitive therapy of bacterial infections in neutropenic patients. Some published studies suggest that ceftazidime monotherapy may be as effective as standard combination regimens (eg, antipseudomonal penicillin plus aminoglycoside) for initial therapy of febrile neutropenic patients (de Pauw et al, 1983; Morgan et al, 1983; Reilly et al, 1983; Pizzo et al, 1986; see also Smith, 1984; Pizzo et al, 1985; Wade et al, 1986). However, concerns with ceftazidime monotherapy include the questionable ability of a single drug to cure *P. aeruginosa* infections in the neutropenic host, the potential for rapid emergence of resistant bacterial strains, and inadequate coverage against staphylococci (see Young, 1986). Current consensus is that ceftazidime should be used with an aminoglycoside for febrile neutropenic patients because the combination is more effective than ceftazidime alone for patients with gram-negative rod bacteremia (Calandra et al, 1987; see also Young, 1986; Hughes et al, 1990). Ceftazidime monotherapy may be useful for patients in hospitals where resistance to this drug is minimal and in whom neutropenia is not severe and infection with *P. aerugi-*

nosa is unlikely. In some studies, "breakthrough" infections with gram-positive bacteria (eg, staphylococci) have been frequent when ceftazidime was used alone, prompting some investigators to recommend the addition of an agent (eg, nafcillin, vancomycin) with good gram-positive activity for primary coverage in neutropenic patients (Darbyshire et al, 1983; Fainstein et al, 1983; Ramphal et al, 1983; Kramer et al, 1986). For additional discussion, see index entry Antimicrobial Drugs: Antimicrobial Drug Selection for Common Infectious Diseases [Table]).

As with other third generation cephalosporins, ceftazidime is not indicated for infections that can be effectively treated (or prevented) with less expensive, narrower spectrum, first (or second) generation cephalosporins. In particular, it offers no advantages over first generation cephalosporins for known gram-positive infections or for perioperative prophylaxis (see the Introduction).

ADVERSE REACTIONS AND PRECAUTIONS. These are the same as for first generation cephalosporins (see the Introduction).

DRUG INTERACTIONS AND INTERFERENCE WITH LABORATORY TESTS. See the Introduction.

PHARMACOKINETICS. Ceftazidime is administered intravenously or intramuscularly. Peak serum concentrations obtained after intramuscular and bolus intravenous injections of 1 g are 39 mcg/ml (after 60 minutes) and 107 to 119 mcg/ml, respectively. Following intravenous infusion of 1 g over a 30-minute period, peak serum levels of about 70 mcg/ml are achieved.

Less than 10% of circulating ceftazidime is bound to plasma protein. Apparent volumes of distribution ranging from 0.21 to 0.28 L/kg have been reported. Ceftazidime has been shown to distribute into a variety of tissues (eg, gallbladder wall, myometrium, bone) and body fluids (eg, peritoneal, pleural, and synovial fluids; bile). High concentrations are obtained in urine. Ceftazidime enters the cerebrospinal fluid in the presence of inflammation and achieves therapeutic concentrations for a number of pathogens. This antibiotic crosses the placenta.

Between 80% and 90% of a dose is excreted in the urine as unchanged drug within 24 hours by glomerular filtration without renal tubular secretion. Probenecid has no effect on elimination. Ceftazidime is not metabolized. The elimination half-life is approximately 1.9 hours. The half-life is prolonged in patients with renal impairment and dosage adjustments are required.

DOSAGE AND PREPARATIONS. Ceftazidime can be administered by intramuscular injection deep into a large muscle mass or intravenously by direct injection or by intermittent or continuous infusion. See the manufacturer's instructions for the appropriate dilution of the drug, compatible diluents and intravenous solutions, and stability of ceftazidime in these solutions.

Intramuscular (deep), Intravenous: *Adults*, the usual dosage for moderately severe infections is 1 to 2 g intravenously every 8 to 12 hours; for serious or life-threatening infections such as meningitis or fever in a granulocytopenic patient, the maximum dosage of 2 g every 8 hours should be used (*Med Lett Drugs Ther*, 1985 B).

The following dosages are recommended by the manufacturer for specific indications: uncomplicated urinary tract infections, 250 mg intravenously or intramuscularly every 12 hours; bone and joint infections, 2 g intravenously every 12 hours; complicated urinary tract infections, 500 mg intravenously or intramuscularly every 8 to 12 hours; uncomplicated pneumonia and mild skin and skin structure infections, 500 mg to 1 g intravenously or intramuscularly every 8 hours; serious gynecologic and intra-abdominal infections, 2 g intravenously every 8 hours; meningitis, 2 g intravenously every 8 hours; very severe life-threatening infections, especially in immunocompromised patients, 2 g intravenously every 8 hours; pseudomonal pulmonary infections in patients with cystic fibrosis and normal renal function, 30 to 50 mg/kg intravenously every 8 hours (maximum, 6 g daily).

Infants and children from 1 month to 12 years, 30 to 50 mg/kg intravenously every eight hours (maximum, 6 g daily) (*Med Lett Drugs Ther*, 1985 B; manufacturer's literature). The higher dosage (50 mg/kg every eight hours) is recommended for immunocompromised children or children with cystic fibrosis or meningitis.

Neonates 1 to 4 weeks, 30 mg/kg intravenously every eight hours; *neonates 0 to 7 days*, 30 mg/kg intravenously every 12 hours; the dose should be increased to 50 mg/kg for neonatal meningitis (*Med Lett Drugs Ther*, 1985 B). (NOTE: The manufacturer recommends a dosage of 30 mg/kg intravenously every 12 hours for neonates 0 to 4 weeks).

Patients with impaired renal function require modification in doses and/or frequency of administration depending on the degree of impairment, severity of the infection, and susceptibility of the causative organism. In *adults with impaired renal function*, the manufacturer recommends an initial loading dose of 1 g and maintenance dosages as follows:

Creatinine Clearance (ml/min)	**Adult Maintenance Dosage**
50-31	1 g every 12 hours
30-16	1 g every 24 hours
15-6	500 mg every 24 hours
<5	500 mg every 48 hours

From manufacturer's literature

For patients with severe infections who would normally receive 6 g daily were it not for renal insufficiency, the unit dose given in the table above may be increased 50% or the dosing frequency increased appropriately. In adults undergoing hemodialysis, a loading dose of 1 g is recommended, followed by 1 g after each dialysis period.

Ceftazidime can also be used in patients undergoing intraperitoneal dialysis and continuous ambulatory peritoneal dialysis. In adults, a loading dose of 1 g is given, followed by 500 mg every 24 hours. In addition to intravenous use, ceftazidime can be incorporated in dialysis fluid at a concentration of 250 mg/2 L of dialysis fluid (manufacturer's literature).

Fortaz (Glaxo). Powder (sterile) 500 mg and 1, 2, and 6 g (equivalent to anhydrous ceftazidime) (sodium 2.3 mEq/g); solution 1 g with 2.2 g of dextrose and 2 g with 1.6 g of dextrose in 50 ml containers.

Tazicef (Smith Kline & French). Powder (sterile) 1, 2, and 6 g (equivalent to ceftazidime activity) (sodium 2.3 mEq/g).

Tazidime (Lilly). Powder (sterile) 500 mg and 1, 2, and 6 g (equivalent to ceftazidime activity) (sodium 2.3 mEq/g).

CEFOPERAZONE SODIUM
[Cefobid]

This semisynthetic cephalosporin differs structurally from other third generation cephalosporins (see Figure). Similar to piperacillin, cefoperazone contains a piperazine side chain at position 7 of the cephalosporin nucleus. This enhances its antipseudomonal activity but decreases its stability to certain β-lactamases. Like cefamandole and moxalactam, cefoperazone contains a methylthiotetrazole side chain at position 3 that increases antibacterial activity and helps to prevent metabolism of the drug but also is associated with certain adverse effects (see Neu, 1983).

MECHANISM OF ACTION, ANTIMICROBIAL SPECTRUM, AND RESISTANCE. Similar to other third generation cephalosporins, cefoperazone has increased potency and a wider spectrum of activity against clinically important gram-negative bacteria when compared to first and second generation cephalosporins. This drug has excellent activity against *Neisseria meningitidis, N. gonorrhoeae*, and *Haemophilus influenzae*, including β-lactamase-producing strains of these species. Cefoperazone also is highly active against most Enterobacteriaceae (eg, *Escherichia coli, Klebsiella, Enterobacter, Proteus, Morganella, Providencia, Citrobacter, Serratia, Salmonella, Shigella*), but other third generation cephalosporins generally are superior. Cefoperazone is more susceptible to certain β-lactamases (eg, TEM-1, TEM-2), and β-lactamase-producing organisms, including strains of *E. coli* and *Klebsiella*, that are susceptible to other third generation cephalosporins occasionally will be resistant to cefoperazone (Sykes and Bush, 1983). Cefoperazone has better activity against *Pseudomonas aeruginosa* than other currently available third generation cephalosporins with the exception of ceftazidime. The activity of cefoperazone against *Acinetobacter*, nonfermenting gram-negative bacilli, is poor. Although most anaerobic bacteria are susceptible, many *Bacteroides fragilis* strains are resistant.

Among gram-positive bacteria, cefoperazone has good activity against nonpenicillinase- and penicillinase-producing staphylococci and most streptococci (except enterococci). However, as with other third generation cephalosporins, this agent offers no clinical advantages over first generation cephalosporins for infections that are known to be caused by gram-positive bacteria.

Cefoperazone has been reported to be a poorer inducer of Type I β-lactamases of certain gram-negative bacilli (eg, *Enterobacter cloacae*) when compared to other third generation cephalosporins (Minami et al, 1980; Sykes and Bonner, 1985). Whether this is an advantage clinically is unknown.

For additional discussion on the mechanism of action, antimicrobial spectrum, and resistance properties of cefoperazone, see the Introduction; see also Funk and Strausbaugh, 1982; Barriere and Flaherty, 1984; Smith, 1984.

USES. Cefoperazone has been effective, frequently as empiric monotherapy, in a wide variety of serious gram-negative bacillary infections outside the central nervous system. These include lower respiratory tract, complicated urinary tract, intra-abdominal, gynecologic, skin and skin structure, bone, and joint infections and bacteremias. These infections often are of nosocomial origin and are caused by bacterial strains that are resistant to penicillins, older cephalosporins, and aminoglycosides (see Funk and Strausbaugh, 1982; Warren et al, 1983; Barriere and Flaherty, 1984; Cohen et al, 1984).

The exact role of cefoperazone in the treatment of serious gram-negative bacillary infections remains to be determined, however. This agent has better activity than cefotaxime, ceftizoxime, ceftriaxone, and moxalactam against *Pseudomonas aeruginosa*. However, most infectious disease experts do not recommend cefoperazone as sole therapy for serious systemic *P. aeruginosa* infections (see *Med Lett Drugs Ther*, 1983 B; Barriere and Flaherty, 1984; Quintiliani et al, 1984). Furthermore, ceftazidime has better activity than cefoperazone against this gram-negative organism and is the preferred third generation cephalosporin for infections known or presumed to be caused by *P. aeruginosa* (see the evaluation and the Introduction).

Cefoperazone has inferior activity in vitro against most Enterobacteriaceae and, with the exception of moxalactam, has been associated with more undesirable adverse reactions (eg, hypoprothrombinemia, bleeding) than other third generation cephalosporins. Also, it exhibits variable penetration into cerebrospinal fluid and it is not indicated for meningitis. Thus, the apparent disadvantages of cefoperazone appear to outweigh its advantages when compared to other available third generation cephalosporins. However, well-controlled clinical trials comparing cefoperazone to the other agents are generally unavailable. For additional discussion, see the Introduction.

As with other third generation cephalosporins, cefoperazone is not indicated for infections that can be effectively treated (or prevented) with less expensive, narrower spectrum first (or second) generation cephalosporins. In particular, it offers no advantages over first generation cephalosporins for known gram-positive infections or for perioperative prophylaxis (see the Introduction).

ADVERSE REACTIONS AND PRECAUTIONS. Hypersensitivity reactions (eg, maculopapular rash, fever, eosinophilia) and other adverse effects associated with cephalosporins have been observed with cefoperazone (see the Introduction). Because of its broad antimicrobial spectrum and high biliary excretion, cefoperazone markedly alters colonic flora (Alestig et al, 1983; see also Barriere and Flaherty, 1984; Noble and Barza, 1985). Diarrhea was reported frequently in some studies (Carlberg et al, 1982; Mulligan et al, 1982; Mastella et al, 1983; see also Barriere and Flaherty, 1984) but not in others (Cohen et al, 1984). Superinfections with resistant organisms occur, but the incidence does not appear to be greater than with other third generation cephalosporins (see Barriere and Flaherty, 1984; Noble and Barza, 1985).

Cefoperazone contains a methylthiotetrazole side chain and has been associated with hypoprothrombinemia and, occasionally, bleeding. Elderly debilitated patients, individuals with severe renal insufficiency, and malnourished patients receiving total parenteral nutrition are at highest risk. Vitamin K reverses the hypoprothrombinemia, and prophylactic administration may be desirable in some patients (see the Introduction).

DRUG INTERACTIONS AND INTERFERENCE WITH LABORATORY TESTS. Methylthiotetrazole-containing cephalosporins also have been associated with a disulfiram-like reaction. For additional discussion, see the Introduction.

PHARMACOKINETICS. Cefoperazone is administered intramuscularly or intravenously. Peak serum concentrations obtained after intramuscular and intravenous injections of 1 g are 65 to 74 mcg/ml (after one hour) and 200 mcg/ml (within 15 minutes), respectively. Following intravenous infusion of 1 g over a 15-minute period, a serum level of 153 mcg/ml is achieved.

Between 87% and 93% of circulating cefoperazone is bound to plasma proteins. Volumes of distribution ranging from 0.14 to 0.20 L/kg have been reported. The drug penetrates into most body fluids and tissues; highest concentrations occur in bile. Antibacterial concentrations can be achieved in the cerebrospinal fluid when the meninges are inflamed. However, penetration into cerebrospinal fluid has been variable and cefoperazone is not used to treat meningitis. The drug crosses the placenta.

Approximately 70% of a dose is eliminated in the bile as unchanged drug. About 30% is eliminated in the urine (glomerular filtration). The serum half-life ranges from 1.9 to 2.1 hours and is not prolonged in patients with renal impairment. In patients with hepatic dysfunction, the serum half-life is prolonged two- to fourfold and there is a compensatory increase in urinary excretion. Cefoperazone accumulates in patients with combined renal and hepatic failure and dosage adjustments are necessary.

DOSAGE AND PREPARATIONS. Cefoperazone can be administered by intramuscular injection deep into a large muscle mass or intravenously by intermittent or continuous infusion. See the manufacturer's instructions for the appropriate dilution of the drug, compatible diluents and intravenous solutions, and stability of cefoperazone in these solutions.

Intramuscular (deep), Intravenous: *Adults*, 2 to 4 g daily in equally divided doses every 12 hours is the usual dosage recommended by the manufacturer. In severe infections or infections caused by less sensitive organisms, the manufacturer states that the dose and/or frequency of administration may be increased. Patients have been successfully treated with a total daily dosage of 6 to 12 g divided into two, three, or four administrations ranging from 1.5 to 4 g per dose. Most infectious disease experts recommend a dosing interval of every eight hours (or even every six hours) for serious or life-threatening infections (Garzone et al, 1983 A; Fried and Hinthorn, 1985; Noble and Barza, 1985; The Medical Letter, 1988).

Children, 100 to 150 mg/kg daily in divided doses every 8 to 12 hours has been recommended (Nelson, 1989 A). However there is no approved labeling for use in children.

The dosage usually does not require adjustment in patients with severely impaired renal function. A total daily dosage above 4 g generally is unnecessary in those with hepatic disease and/or biliary obstruction. If higher dosages are used, serum concentrations should be monitored. In patients with both hepatic dysfunction and significant renal disease, dosage should not exceed 1 to 2 g daily and serum concentrations should be monitored.

Cefobid (Roerig). Powder (sterile) in 1 and 2 g containers (equivalent to base) (sodium 1.5 mEq/g); solution 1 and 2 g (sodium 1.5 mEq/g) in 50 ml containers.

MOXALACTAM DISODIUM

[Moxam]

This broad spectrum, β-lactam antibiotic differs from the other third generation cephalosporins in that it is an oxa-β-lactam (1-oxa-cephalosporin) in which the sulfur of the dihydrothiazine ring is replaced by an oxygen to form a dihydro-oxazine ring (see Figure). It is a totally synthetic molecule and it is administered only parenterally.

MECHANISM OF ACTION, ANTIMICROBIAL SPECTRUM, AND RESISTANCE. As with the aminothiazolyl cephalosporins (eg, cefotaxime), moxalactam has increased potency and β-lactamase stability and a wider spectrum of activity against clinically important gram-negative bacteria when compared to first or second generation cephalosporins. This drug has excellent activity against *Neisseria meningitidis, N. gonorrhoeae, Haemophilus influenzae*, and most Enterobacteriaceae (eg, *Escherichia coli, Klebsiella, Enterobacter, Proteus, Morganella, Providencia, Citrobacter, Serratia, Salmonella, Shigella*), including strains that are resistant to earlier generation cephalosporins, penicillins, and aminoglycosides. Moxalactam, unlike other third generation cephalosporins, has reasonably good activity against the *Bacteroides fragilis* group; it is comparable to cefoxitin against these gram-negative anaerobic bacilli. The nonfermenting gram-negative bacilli, *Pseudomonas aeruginosa* and *Acinetobacter*, generally are resistant, however.

Although moxalactam is active against nonpenicillinase- and penicillinase-producing staphylococci and most streptococci (except enterococci), it is inferior to other third generation cephalosporins against these gram-positive bacteria.

For additional discussion of the mechanism of action, antimicrobial spectrum, and resistance properties of moxalactam, see the Introduction; see also Fitzpatrick and Standiford, 1982; Carmine et al, 1983 B; Barriere and Flaherty, 1984.

USES. Substantial clinical experience has been obtained with moxalactam. This drug has been effective in the treatment of meningitis caused by gram-negative enteric bacilli (eg, *E. coli, Klebsiella, Proteus*) and *H. influenzae*. Moxalactam has been effective, frequently as empiric monotherapy, in a wide variety of serious gram-negative bacillary infections outside the central nervous system, including lower respiratory tract, complicated urinary tract, intra-abdominal, gynecologic, skin and skin structure, bone, and joint infections and bacteremias. These frequently are of nosocomial origin and are caused by bacterial strains that are resistant to penicillins, older cephalosporins, and aminoglycosides.

Unfortunately, moxalactam has been associated with serious bleeding episodes, including fatalities, in a number of patients. With the availability of a number of comparably effective and less toxic third generation cephalosporins, the usefulness of moxalactam has diminished greatly. For additional discussion, see the Introduction; see also Barriere and Flaherty, 1984.

ADVERSE REACTIONS AND PRECAUTIONS. All of the adverse reactions common to the cephalosporins (eg, skin rash, other hypersensitivity reactions, gastrointestinal disturbances) may occur with moxalactam (see the Introduction).

Clinically, bleeding has been a particularly common and serious problem with moxalactam. It has been reported that 2.5% of clinical trial patients receiving this antibiotic for four days or longer suffered a bleeding event, most of which were serious (manufacturer's literature). Numerous case reports of moxalactam-associated coagulopathy, including some fatalities, have appeared in the literature (Holt et al, 1981; Pakter et al, 1982; Jones and Kimbrough, 1983; Lee et al, 1983; MacLennan et al, 1983; Panwalker and Rosenfeld, 1983; Slonaker and Luper, 1983; Weitekamp and Aber, 1983; Au and Geiger, 1984; Bach, 1984; Brandstetter et al, 1984; Conly et al, 1984; Meisel, 1984).

Moxalactam affects hemostasis via three mechanisms: hypoprothrombinemia, platelet dysfunction, and, very rarely, immune-mediated thrombocytopenia. Like cefamandole and cefoperazone, moxalactam contains a methylthiotetrazole side chain and has caused hypoprothrombinemia and bleeding in certain patients, particularly elderly, debilitated patients, those individuals with severe renal insufficiency, and malnourished patients receiving total parenteral nutrition. Prothrombin times should be monitored; if they become prolonged, vitamin K should be given. Because vitamin K can prevent the hypoprothrombinemia, it is now recommended that vitamin K (adults, 10 mg per week) be administered prophylactically to all patients receiving moxalactam (manufacturer's literature).

Moxalactam also has caused prolonged bleeding time and bleeding diathesis in some patients by inhibiting platelet function; this is dose dependent and not reversible by vitamin K (Weitekamp and Aber, 1983; Weitekamp et al, 1985). In adults with normal renal function, doses greater than 4 g per day for more than three days may result in platelet dysfunction (manufacturer's literature), although lower dosages also have been implicated (Bach, 1984). Patients with reduced renal function are particularly susceptible. The manufacturer recommends that the bleeding time be monitored in patients requiring more than 4 g of moxalactam per day and who are treated for more than three days. All patients with renal dysfunction should have appropriate dosage adjustments and should be monitored periodically with bleeding times. If the bleeding time becomes unduly prolonged, moxalactam should be discontinued. If hemorrhage should occur by this mechanism, the drug should be discontinued and appropriate supportive measures (eg, administration of fresh frozen plasma, packed red cells, platelet concentrates) should be undertaken. Substitution of moxalactam with another beta lactam antibiotic that also can cause platelet dysfunction (eg, carbenicillin) should be with caution.

Superinfections with enterococci have been reported more frequently with moxalactam than with other third generation cephalosporins. This may be associated with moxalactam's very poor activity against these organisms (see Jones and Thornsberry, 1985).

DRUG INTERACTIONS AND INTERFERENCE WITH LABORATORY TESTS. Similar to other methylthiotetrazole-containing cephalosporins, moxalactam has been associated with a disulfiram-like reaction. For additional discussion, see the Introduction.

Concomitant use of "high-dose" heparin (more than 20,000 units/day), oral anticoagulants, and other drugs that affect hemostasis (eg, aspirin) are factors that may increase the risk of bleeding during therapy with moxalactam.

PHARMACOKINETICS. Moxalactam is administered intramuscularly or intravenously. Peak serum concentrations after intramuscular and intravenous injections of 1 g are 23 to 52 mcg/ml (after one to two hours) and 95 to 120 mcg/ml, respectively. Following intravenous infusion of 1 g over a 30-minute period, a serum level of 60 to 70 mcg/ml is achieved.

Approximately 50% of circulating moxalactam is bound to plasma proteins. Volumes of distribution ranging from 0.25 to 0.40 L/kg have been reported. Moxalactam has been shown to distribute into a variety of tissues and body fluids, including pleural, interstitial, peritoneal, and synovial fluids; bile; urine; aqueous humor; bronchial secretions; bone; prostatic tissue; and atrial appendage. Moxalactam enters the cerebrospinal fluid in the presence of inflammation and achieves therapeutic concentrations for a number of pathogens. This antibiotic crosses the placenta and is found in breast milk.

Up to 90% of a dose of moxalactam is excreted in the urine as unchanged drug within 24 hours; it is not metabolized. The primary mechanism of elimination is by glomerular filtration and probenecid has little effect on excretion. The serum half-life ranges from 2 to 2.3 hours. The half-life is prolonged in patients with renal impairment and dosage adjustments are required.

DOSAGE AND PREPARATIONS. Moxalactam can be administered by intramuscular injection deep into a large muscle mass or intravenously by direct injection or by intermittent or continuous infusion. See the manufacturer's instructions for the appropriate dilution of the drug, compatible diluents and intravenous solutions, and stability of moxalactam in these solutions.

It is recommended that patients who receive moxalactam be given 10 mg of vitamin K per week prophylactically. Bleeding times should be monitored in patients who receive more than 4 g moxalactam per day for more than three days. All patients with significantly reduced renal impairment should have appropriate dosage reduction (see below) and bleeding times should be monitored periodically.

Intramuscular (deep), Intravenous: *Adults*, 2 to 12 g daily in equally divided doses every eight hours (The Medical Letter, 1988). Most infectious disease experts recommend 2 g every eight hours for serious infections (Fitzpatrick and Standiford, 1982; Fried and Hinthorn, 1985; Noble and Barza, 1985; Reese and Betts, 1986). For life-threatening infections (eg, meningitis) or infections caused by less susceptible organisms, up to 4 g every eight hours may be needed. (NOTE: The manufacturer states that the usual daily dosage is 2 to 4 g administered every 8 to 12 hours and that most mild to moderate infections can be expected to respond to 500 mg to 2 g every 12 hours. The manufacturer's recommendations for specific infections are as follows: mild skin and skin structure infections and uncomplicated pneumonia, 500 mg every eight hours; mild, uncomplicated urinary tract infections, 250 mg every 12 hours; urinary tract infections that are more difficult to treat, 500 mg every 12 hours; serious urinary tract infections, 500 mg every eight hours; life-threatening infections or infections caused by less susceptible organisms, up to 4 g every eight hours.)

Children, 150 to 200 mg/kg daily in equally divided doses every six to eight hours; *infants 1 month to 1 year*, 200 mg/kg daily in equally divided doses every six hours; *neonates 1 to 4 weeks*, 150 mg/kg daily in equally divided doses every eight hours; *neonates 0 to 7 days*, 100 mg/kg daily in equally divided doses every 12 hours. In pediatric gram-negative meningitis, an initial loading dose of 100 mg/kg is recommended by the manufacturer. The maximum daily dosage recommended by the manufacturer for serious infections is 200 mg/kg (not to exceed 12 g).

Patients with impaired renal function require modification in doses and/or frequency of administration depending on the degree of impairment, severity of the infection, and susceptibility of the causative organism. In *adults with impaired renal function*, the manufacturer recommends an initial loading dose of 1 to 2 g and maintenance dosages as shown in the table.

The serum half-life of moxalactam during hemodialysis ranges from two to five hours. Maintenance doses should be repeated following regular hemodialysis.

Moxam (Lilly). Powder (sterile) 1, 2, and 10 g (equivalent to base) (sodium 3.8 mEq/g).

ORAL CEPHALOSPORINS

CEPHALEXIN MONOHYDRATE
[Keflex]

CEPHALEXIN HYDROCHLORIDE MONOHYDRATE
[Keftab]

MECHANISM OF ACTION, ANTIMICROBIAL SPECTRUM, AND RESISTANCE. The clinically relevant antibacterial spectrum of cephalexin is similar to that of other first generation cephalosporins. It is active against most gram-positive bacteria, including nonpenicillinase- and penicillinase-producing staphylococci, streptococci (except enterococci), and many anaerobic bacteria. The in vitro potency against gram-positive cocci generally is less than that of parenteral first generation cephalosporins (eg, cephalothin, cefazolin). The gram-negative antibacterial activity of first generation cephalosporins essentially is limited to *Escherichia coli, Klebsiella*, and *Proteus mirabilis*. Cephalexin is not very active against *Haemophilus influenzae*.

For additional discussion of the mechanism of action, antimicrobial spectrum, and resistance properties of the cephalosporins, see the Introduction.

USES. Cephalexin is rarely the drug of choice for bacterial infections. It may be indicated in mild to moderate infections of the respiratory tract, urinary tract, skin and skin structures, and bone caused by susceptible organisms when preferred agents are ineffective or cannot be tolerated. It often is among the alternatives for penicillins in patients who have a history of hypersensitivity reactions (other than the immediate type) to penicillins. For example, cephalexin is a likely alternative to antistaphylococcal penicillins in certain staphylococcal pyodermas. Although it could be used in streptococcal infections (eg, pharyngitis), erythromycin is usually the preferred alternative to penicillin G. Cephalexin usually is not recommended in upper respiratory tract infections or otitis media in which *H. influenzae* is an important pathogen; cefaclor, cefuroxime axetil, and cefixime are oral cephalosporins that may be useful for this organism, however (see the evaluations). Cephalexin may be useful for urinary tract infections when the causative organism is resistant to currently preferred drugs (eg, sulfisoxazole, ampicillin, trimethoprim/sulfamethoxazole) but sensitive to cephalexin.

A consistent problem with the oral cephalosporins has been their relatively high cost to the patient, a factor the physician should take into consideration when alternative, less expensive, but equally effective antibacterial drugs are available.

Creatinine Clearance (ml/min/1.73 M²)	Renal Function	Life-threatening Infections (Maximum Adult Maintenance Dosage)	Less Severe Infections (Adult Maintenance Dosage)
>80	Normal	4 g every 8 hours	0.5-2 g every 8-12 hours
50-80	Mild Impairment	3 g every 8 hours	0.5-1 g every 8 hours
25-50	Moderate Impairment	2 g every 8 hours or 3 g every 12 hours	0.25-1 g every 12 hours
2-25	Severe Impairment	1 g every 8 hours or 1.25 g every 12 hours	0.25-0.5 g every 8 hours
<2	0	1 g every 24 hours	0.25-0.5 g every 12 hours

From manufacturer's literature

For additional discussion, see the Introduction; see also index entry Antimicrobial Drugs: Antimicrobial Drug Selection for Common Infectious Diseases (Table).

ADVERSE REACTIONS AND PRECAUTIONS. Cephalexin generally is well tolerated. Gastrointestinal disturbances (eg, diarrhea) and hypersensitivity reactions (eg, skin rash) are most common. For detailed discussion, see the Introduction.

DRUG INTERACTIONS AND INTERFERENCE WITH LABORATORY TESTS. See the Introduction.

PHARMACOKINETICS. Cephalexin is stable to gastric acid and is well absorbed following oral administration. Following doses of 250 mg, 500 mg, and 1 g, average peak serum concentrations of approximately 9, 18, and 32 mcg/ml, respectively, were obtained at one hour. Although food delays absorption, the total amount of drug absorbed is not affected.

Cephalexin is only 10% to 15% bound to plasma protein. The volume of distribution is 0.26 ± 0.03 L/kg. The drug enters most tissues and body fluids, but fails to achieve therapeutic concentrations in cerebrospinal fluid even in the presence of inflammation. Cephalexin crosses the placenta.

Approximately 90% of a dose is excreted as unchanged drug in the urine within eight hours, primarily by renal tubular secretion. Excretion is delayed by probenecid. The elimination half-life is approximately 50 minutes. The half-life is prolonged in patients with renal impairment and dosage adjustments are required.

DOSAGE AND PREPARATIONS.

Oral: *Adults,* 1 to 4 g daily in equally divided doses every six hours (maximum, 4 g daily in divided doses). If more than 4 g is needed, a parenteral cephalosporin should be substituted. *Children,* 25 to 50 mg/kg daily in equally divided doses every six hours; for severe infections, this dosage may be doubled.

Patients with impaired renal function require modifications in doses and/or frequency of administration depending on the degree of impairment, severity of the infection, and susceptibility of the causative organism. Various dosage recommendations for these patients have been proposed. One recommendation is to increase the dosing interval to 8 to 12 hours when creatinine clearance is between 50 and 10 ml/min and to 24 to 48 hours when creatinine clearance is less than 10 ml/min (The Medical Letter, 1988).

CEPHALEXIN MONOHYDRATE:

Generic. Capsules 250 and 500 mg; suspension 125 and 250 mg/5 ml (after reconstitution); tablets 250 and 500 mg and 1 g.

Keflex (Dista). Capsules 250 and 500 mg; drops (pediatric) 100 mg/ml (after reconstitution); suspension 125 and 250 mg/5 ml (after reconstitution); tablets 250 and 500 mg and 1 g (***Keflet***).

CEPHALEXIN HYDROCHLORIDE MONOHYDRATE:

Keftab (Dista). Tablets 250 and 500 mg.

CEPHRADINE

[Anspor, Velosef]

Cephradine can be administered both orally and parenterally. Structurally, it is a close congener of cephalexin (see Figure).

MECHANISM OF ACTION, ANTIMICROBIAL SPECTRUM, AND RESISTANCE. The mechanism of action, antimicrobial spectrum, and resistance properties are essentially the same as for cephalexin (see that evaluation and the Introduction).

USES. Oral cephradine has the same indications as cephalexin (see that evaluation and the Introduction). Intramuscular or intravenous cephradine has the same indications as cefazolin, but the latter drug frequently is preferred because it achieves higher serum concentrations, has a longer elimination half-life, and causes less pain on intramuscular injection (see the evaluation of Cefazolin Sodium and the Introduction).

ADVERSE REACTIONS AND PRECAUTIONS. Cephradine generally is well tolerated. Gastrointestinal disturbances (eg, diarrhea) and hypersensitivity reactions (eg, skin rash) are most common. For detailed discussion, see the Introduction.

DRUG INTERACTIONS AND INTERFERENCE WITH LABORATORY TESTS. See the Introduction.

PHARMACOKINETICS. Cephradine is stable in gastric acid and is well absorbed when given orally. Following doses of 250 mg, 500 mg, and 1 g, average peak serum concentrations of approximately 9, 17, and 24 mcg/ml, respectively, were obtained within one hour. Although food delays absorption, the total amount of drug absorbed is not affected.

Cephradine also can be administered intramuscularly and intravenously. Peak serum concentrations after intramuscular injection (eg, 5.8 to 6.3 mcg/ml after a 500-mg dose) are actually lower than those obtained by the oral route, but total drug absorbed is the same. Cephradine is absorbed more slowly and serum concentrations are lower in women than in men after injection into the gluteus maximus. A single intravenous dose of 1 g cephradine results in an average peak serum level of 86 mcg/ml after five minutes.

Cephradine is only 10% to 20% bound to plasma protein. The volume of distribution is 0.25 ± 0.01 L/kg. The drug enters most tissues and body fluids, but therapeutic concentrations are not achieved in cerebrospinal fluid even in the presence of inflammation. Cephradine crosses the placenta.

Approximately 90% of a dose is excreted as unchanged drug in the urine within six hours, primarily by renal tubular secretion. Excretion is delayed by probenecid. The serum half-life is approximately 50 minutes. It is prolonged in patients with renal impairment and dosage adjustments are required.

DOSAGE AND PREPARATIONS. Cephradine can be administered orally, intramuscularly deep into a large muscle mass, or intravenously by direct injection or by intermittent or continuous infusion. See the manufacturer's instructions for the appropriate dilution of the drug, compatible diluents and intravenous solutions, and stability of cephradine in these solutions.

Oral: *Adults,* 1 to 4 g daily in equally divided doses every six hours; *children over 9 months,* 25 to 50 mg/kg daily in equally divided doses every six hours (The Medical Letter, 1988). The maximum daily dosage should not exceed 4 g.

Patients with impaired renal function require modification in doses and/or frequency of administration depending on the degree of impairment, severity of the infection, and susceptibility of the causative organism. Various dosage recommendations for these patients have been proposed. For *adults with impaired renal function*, the manufacturers recommend 500 mg every six hours when creatinine clearance is greater than 20 ml/min; 250 mg every six hours when creatinine clearance is between 20 and 5 ml/min; and 250 mg every 12 hours when creatinine clearance is less than 5 ml/min. If the patient is on chronic, intermittent hemodialysis, 250 mg should be given at the start of dialysis and 250 mg at 12 hours and 36 to 48 hours after the start of dialysis. Children may require dosage modification proportional to their weight and the severity of infection.

Generic, Anspor (Smith Kline & French), ***Velosef*** (Squibb-Mark). Capsules 250 and 500 mg; suspension 125 and 250 mg/5 ml.

Intravenous, Intramuscular (deep): *Adults*, 2 to 8 g daily in equally divided doses every four to six hours (The Medical Letter, 1988). The usual daily dosage is 500 mg to 1 g every six hours. In severe infections, up to 8 g daily may be given in divided doses every four to six hours. *Children over 1 year*, 50 to 100 mg/kg daily in equally divided doses every six hours (The Medical Letter, 1988; Nelson, 1989 A).

Patients with impaired renal function require modification in doses and/or frequency of administration depending on the degree of impairment, severity of the infection, and susceptibility of the causative organism. Various dosage recommendations for these patients have been proposed. In *adults with impaired renal function*, the manufacturer recommends 500 mg every six hours when creatinine clearance is greater than 20 ml/min; 250 mg every six hours when creatinine clearance is between 20 and 5 ml/min; and 250 mg every 12 hours when creatinine clearance is less than 5 ml/min. If the patient is on chronic, intermittent hemodialysis, 250 mg should be given at the start of dialysis and 250 mg at 12 hours and 36 to 48 hours after the start of dialysis. Children may require dosage modification proportional to their weight and the severity of infection.

Velosef (Squibb-Mark). Powder (sterile) 250 and 500 mg and 1 and 2 g (intramuscular or intravenous) (sodium 6 mEq/g).

CEFADROXIL

[Duricef, Ultracef]

This orally administered first generation cephalosporin is structurally similar to cephalexin (see Figure).

MECHANISM OF ACTION, ANTIMICROBIAL SPECTRUM, AND RESISTANCE. The mechanism of action, antimicrobial spectrum, and resistance properties of cefadroxil are essentially the same as for cephalexin (see that evaluation and the Introduction).

USES. Cefadroxil has the same indications as cephalexin (see that evaluation and the Introduction). Elimination of cefadroxil is more prolonged, however, and the longer dosing interval may increase patient compliance.

ADVERSE REACTIONS AND PRECAUTIONS. Cefadroxil generally is well tolerated. Gastrointestinal disturbances (eg, diarrhea) and hypersensitivity reactions (eg, skin rash) are most common. For detailed discussion, see the Introduction.

DRUG INTERACTIONS AND INTERFERENCE WITH LABORATORY TESTS. See the Introduction.

PHARMACOKINETICS. Cefadroxil is stable in gastric acid and is well absorbed following oral administration. Following single doses of 500 mg and 1 g, average peak serum concentrations of approximately 16 and 28 mcg/ml, respectively, were obtained at 1.5 to 2 hours. Absorption does not appear to be affected by the presence of food.

Cefadroxil is only 15% to 20% bound to plasma protein. The apparent volume of distribution is 0.31 L/kg. The drug enters most tissues and body fluids, but therapeutic concentrations are not achieved in cerebrospinal fluid even in the presence of inflammation. Cefadroxil crosses the placenta.

More than 90% of a dose is excreted as unchanged drug in the urine within 24 hours by renal tubular secretion and glomerular filtration. The serum half-life of approximately 1.4 hours is somewhat longer than that of cephalexin or cephradine. The half-life is prolonged in patients with renal impairment and dosage adjustments are required.

DOSAGE AND PREPARATIONS.

Oral: *Adults*, 1 to 2 g daily in equally divided doses every 12 hours or once every 24 hours (The Medical Letter, 1988). The usual dosages recommended by the manufacturer are: for uncomplicated lower urinary tract infections, ie, cystitis, 1 to 2 g daily in a single dose or in divided doses every 12 hours; for all other urinary tract infections, 2 g daily in divided doses every 12 hours; for skin and skin structure infections, 1 g daily as a single dose or in divided doses every 12 hours; for group A, β-hemolytic streptococcal pharyngitis or tonsillitis, 1 g daily in a single dose or in divided doses every 12 hours for 10 days.

Children, 30 mg/kg daily in divided doses every 12 hours (The Medical Letter, 1988; Nelson, 1989 A). The manufacturer states that for group A, β-hemolytic streptococcal pharyngitis or tonsillitis, 30 mg/kg daily in a single dose or in divided doses every 12 hours for 10 days should be administered.

In patients with impaired renal function, doses and/or frequency of administration must be modified depending on the degree of renal impairment, severity of the infection, and susceptibility of the causative organism. In *adults with renal impairment*, the manufacturers suggest a loading dose of 1 g followed by administration of 500 mg at the following intervals: Mild to moderate impairment (Ccr 50 to 25 ml/min), every 12 hours; moderate to severe impairment (Ccr 25 to 10 ml/min), every 24 hours; severe impairment to essentially no function (Ccr 10 to 0 ml/min), every 36 hours. Patients with a creatinine clearance value of more than 50 ml/min may be considered to have normal renal function for therapeutic purposes.

Generic, Duricef (Mead Johnson). Capsules 500 mg; tablets 1 g; suspension 125, 250, and 500 mg/5 ml.

Ultracef (Bristol). Capsules 500 mg; tablets 1 g; suspension 125 and 250 mg/5 ml.

CEFACLOR
[Ceclor]

This orally administered second generation cephalosporin is structurally similar to cephalexin (see Figure).

MECHANISM OF ACTION, ANTIMICROBIAL SPECTRUM, AND RESISTANCE. Cefaclor has an in vitro antibacterial spectrum similar to that of the oral first generation cephalosporins, except that it generally is more active against gram-negative bacilli. In particular, it is more active than cephalexin against *Haemophilus influenzae*, including ampicillin-resistant strains; some *H. influenzae* strains are resistant to cefaclor, however (see the evaluation on Cephalexin Monohydrate and the Introduction).

USES. Cefaclor is rarely the drug of choice for the treatment of bacterial infections. It is used primarily in the treatment of acute otitis media and acute sinusitis caused by strains of *H. influenzae* or *Moraxella (Branhamella) catarrhalis* that are resistant to amoxicillin, the usual drug of choice. Cefaclor is an alternative to erythromycin/sulfisoxazole, trimethoprim/sulfamethoxazole, and amoxicillin/potassium clavulanate for infections caused by these resistant strains and usually is preferred in patients who are allergic to sulfonamides. For additional discussion, see the Introduction and index entry Antimicrobial Drugs: Antimicrobial Drug Selection for Common Infectious Diseases (Table).

Similar to oral first generation cephalosporins, cefaclor may be indicated in other mild to moderate infections of the respiratory tract, urinary tract, or skin and skin structures caused by susceptible organisms when preferred agents are ineffective or cannot be tolerated (see the evaluation on Cephalexin Monohydrate and the Introduction).

ADVERSE REACTIONS AND PRECAUTIONS. Cefaclor generally is well tolerated. Gastrointestinal disturbances and hypersensitivity reactions are most common. Serum sickness-like reactions have been reported more frequently with cefaclor than with other cephalosporins (Murray et al, 1980; Ackley and Felsher, 1981; Leng and Anderson, 1985; Levine, 1985). In a large comparative study, the incidences of serum sickness, erythema multiforme, and urticaria were significantly greater in infants and children receiving cefaclor than in those given amoxicillin (Levine, 1985).

For detailed discussion of the adverse reactions and precautions associated with cephalosporin use, see the Introduction.

DRUG INTERACTIONS AND INTERFERENCE WITH LABORATORY TESTS. See the Introduction.

PHARMACOKINETICS. Cefaclor is stable in gastric acid and is well absorbed following oral administration. Following administration of 250 mg, 500 mg, and 1 g doses to fasting subjects, average peak serum levels of approximately 7, 13, and 23 mcg/ml, respectively, were obtained in 30 to 60 minutes. Although the presence of food delays absorption and decreases the peak level by 25% to 50%, the total amount of drug absorbed is not affected.

Cefaclor is only 25% bound to plasma protein. The apparent volume of distribution ranges between 0.24 and 0.36 L/kg. The drug enters most tissues and body fluids, but therapeutic concentrations are not achieved in cerebrospinal fluid even in the presence of inflammation. Cefaclor crosses the placenta.

Between 60% and 85% of a dose is excreted as unchanged drug in the urine within eight hours, primarily by renal tubular secretion. Excretion is delayed by probenecid. The serum half-life ranges from 0.6 to 0.9 hours in patients with normal renal function and is only slightly prolonged in individuals with renal impairment. In those with no renal function, the half-life of cefaclor is 2.3 to 2.8 hours. The drug does not accumulate in such patients because it is unstable in biological fluids.

DOSAGE AND PREPARATIONS.

Oral: *Adults*, 750 mg to 1.5 g daily in equally divided doses every eight hours (The Medical Letter, 1988). The usual dosage is 250 mg every eight hours; for severe infections or those caused by less susceptible organisms, 500 mg every eight hours. The maximum daily dosage recommended by the manufacturer is 4 g.

Children and infants over 1 month, 20 to 40 mg/kg daily in equally divided doses every eight hours (The Medical Letter, 1988). For otitis media, severe infections, or those caused by less susceptible organisms, the larger dosage (40 mg/kg/day) is recommended. The maximum daily dosage is 1 g.

In patients with impaired renal function, cefaclor usually can be administered without modification of the usual dosage. For patients on hemodialysis, a supplemental dose should be administered after each dialysis session (Norris and Mandell, 1985).

Ceclor (Lilly). Capsules 250 and 500 mg; powder (for oral suspension) 125, 187, 250, and 375 mg/5 ml.

CEFUROXIME AXETIL
[Ceftin]

This orally administered second generation cephalosporin is the acetoxyethyl ester of cefuroxime, the active compound.

MECHANISM OF ACTION, ANTIMICROBIAL SPECTRUM, AND RESISTANCE. The mechanism of action, antimicrobial spectrum, and resistance properties are the same as for cefuroxime (see that evaluation and the Introduction). When compared to other oral cephalosporins, cefuroxime has comparable activity against gram-positive cocci, including *Streptococcus pneumoniae, S. pyogenes* (group A, β-hemolytic), and *Staphylococcus aureus.* Cefuroxime has superior activity to cefaclor against gram-negative bacteria, including *Neisseria gonorrhoeae* (including PPNG strains), *Haemophilus influenzae* (including beta lactamase-producing strains), *Moraxella (Branhamella) catarrhalis* (including beta lactamase-producing strains), and the Enterobacteriaceae (eg, *Escherichia coli, Klebsiella, Proteus mirabilis*). In general, cefuroxime is more resistant than cefaclor to beta lactamases produced by gram-negative bacteria.

USES. Cefuroxime axetil has been effective in the treatment of pharyngitis, acute otitis media, bronchitis, urinary tract infections, skin and skin structure infections, and uncomplicated gonorrhea caused by susceptible pathogens (see *Med*

Lett Drugs Ther, 1988 B; Marx and Fant, 1988). Comparative clinical trials are limited, however. Cefuroxime axetil appears clinically to be as effective as cefaclor for acute otitis media (Aronovitz, 1988; McLinn et al, 1988) and lower respiratory tract infections (Schleupner et al, 1988), and it probably will be used to treat acute otitis media, acute sinusitis, and bronchitis. Although the in vitro activity of cefuroxime axetil is superior to cefaclor against beta lactamase-producing *H. influenzae* and *M. catarrhalis*, the lack of an oral suspension currently limits its usefulness in young children; the crushed tablets have a bitter taste and are poorly tolerated (see *Med Lett Drugs Ther,* 1988 B).

Cefuroxime axetil has increased activity in vitro against *Escherichia coli* and other Enterobacteriaceae when compared to older cephalosporins, and it was reported to be more effective than cefaclor and cephalexin for complicated urinary tract infections (Cox et al, 1987). Thus, cefuroxime axetil may be useful for urinary tract infections that are resistant to less expensive drugs, but there are a number of other antimicrobial agents (eg, trimethoprim/sulfamethoxazole, amoxicillin/potassium clavulanate, ciprofloxacin, cefixime) for this indication. Cefuroxime axetil, 1 g as a single dose, plus probenecid (1 g) is effective for uncomplicated urethral, endocervical, and rectal gonorrhea (Gottlieb and Mills, 1986; Baddour et al, 1989), and it is listed as an alternative to ceftriaxone for this indication by the Centers for Disease Control *(MMWR,* 1989). The CDC also recommends this oral cephalosporin to complete the course of therapy for disseminated gonococcal infection after parenteral ceftriaxone is given initially.

Cefuroxime axetil offers no apparent advantages over other antimicrobial agents for skin infections or pharyngitis.

ADVERSE REACTIONS AND PRECAUTIONS. Cefuroxime axetil generally has been well tolerated. The most common side effects have been gastrointestinal and include nausea (2.4%), vomiting (2.0%), diarrhea (3.5%), and loose stools (1.3%). Pseudomembranous colitis has been reported rarely.

As noted above, cefuroxime axetil is available only in a tablet formulation and the crushed tablets have a very bitter taste. Discontinuance of therapy due to taste and/or problems of administering this drug occurred in 13% of children (range 2% to 28% across centers) during clinical trials. The manufacturer recommends that alternative therapy be considered in a child who cannot ingest cefuroxime axetil tablets reliably.

Hypersensitivity reactions have been uncommon and include rash (0.6%), pruritus (0.3%), and urticaria (0.2%). One case of severe bronchospasm has been reported. Headache and dizziness have been reported in 0.7% and 0.2% of patients, respectively. Vaginitis occurred in 1.9% of female patients. Transient elevations in hepatic enzymes (AST, ALT, LDH) have been reported in 1% to 2% of patients. A positive Coombs' test also has been observed (0.4%).

For additional discussion, see Marx and Fant, 1988, and the manufacturer's literature.

DRUG INTERACTIONS AND INTERFERENCE WITH LABORATORY TESTS. See the Introduction.

PHARMACOKINETICS. Cefuroxime axetil is incompletely absorbed from the gastrointestinal tract. The absolute bioavailability of the tablet formulation that is available in the United States varies from 36% when taken while fasting to 52% when taken with food (Finn et al, 1987). Absorption is increased when the drug is taken with food or milk. When cefuroxime axetil was administered immediately after a meal, peak serum concentrations of bioactive cefuroxime occurred at approximately two hours and were 4.1 mcg/ml and 7 mcg/ml for 250 mg and 500 mg doses, respectively.

The distribution and elimination of bioactive cefuroxime is the same as for the injectable product (see the evaluation of Cefuroxime Sodium). Urinary recovery of unchanged cefuroxime ranges from 43% to 52% of an administered dose of the oral ester after 12 hours.

DOSAGE AND PREPARATIONS.

Oral: Cefuroxime axetil may be given without regard to meals, but absorption is enhanced when the drug is administered with food. *Adults and children 12 years of age and older,* 250 mg twice daily; for more severe infections or those caused by less susceptible organisms, 500 mg twice daily; for uncomplicated urinary tract infections, 125 to 250 mg twice daily. *Infants and children up to 12 years of age,* 125 mg twice daily. For otitis media, *children less than 2 years,* 125 mg twice daily; *children 2 years of age or older,* 250 mg twice daily.

Ceftin (Allen & Hanburys). Tablets 125, 250, and 500 mg.

CEFIXIME

[Suprax]

This is the first orally administered third generation cephalosporin to be marketed in the United States. Cefixime is an aminothiazolyl cephalosporin that is structurally similar to cefotaxime (see Figure).

MECHANISM OF ACTION, ANTIMICROBIAL SPECTRUM, AND RESISTANCE. In vitro, this beta lactamase-stable antibiotic has increased potency and a broader spectrum of activity against most clinically important gram-negative bacteria when compared to other oral cephalosporins. Cefixime has excellent activity against most Enterobacteriaceae (eg, *Escherichia coli, Klebsiella*), *Haemophilus influenzae, Moraxella (Branhamella) catarrhalis, Neisseria meningitidis,* and *N. gonorrhoeae,* including beta lactamase-producing strains. Against gram-positive cocci, cefixime is more active than other oral cephalosporins against *Streptococcus pneumoniae, S. pyogenes,* and *S. agalactiae.* However, *Staphylococcus aureus* and coagulase-negative staphylococci are resistant to cefixime, which represents the major drawback in its antimicrobial spectrum. Similar to other oral cephalosporins, enterococci (eg, *E. faecalis*), methicillin-resistant staphylococci, penicillin-resistant pneumococci, *Listeria monocytogenes, Pseudomonas, Acinetobacter,* and *Bacteroides fragilis* are resistant to cefixime (see Barry and Jones, 1987; Neu, 1987 A; Brogden and Campoli-Richards, 1989).

USES. Cefixime has been effective in treating pharyngitis, acute otitis media, bronchitis, and urinary tract infections caused by susceptible pathogens following once-daily administration (see Brogden and Campoli-Richards, 1989; *Med Lett Drugs Ther,* 1989 B). Comparative clinical trials are very limited, however, and the therapeutic role of cefixime remains to be defined.

The suspension formulation, which has better bioavailability than cefixime tablets (see Pharmacokinetics), has been compared to amoxicillin and cefaclor in acute otitis media. Cefixime had similar efficacy to cefaclor (Kenna et al, 1987) and, in one study, to amoxicillin (McLinn, 1987), although more side effects (gastrointestinal upset, rash) were seen in the cefixime group. In another study, however, cefixime was more effective than amoxicillin for acute otitis media caused by beta lactamase-producing *H. influenzae,* but less effective against *S. pneumoniae.* Furthermore, *S. aureus,* an organism that is resistant to cefixime, was isolated from middle ear fluid of nine patients taking this third generation cephalosporin, compared to none in the amoxicillin group (Howie and Owen, 1987). Thus, based on current evidence, cefixime does not appear to offer any clear advantages over older antimicrobial agents for this indication.

Cefixime was as effective as amoxicillin for the treatment of acute bacterial bronchitis (Kiani et al, 1988), but any potential advantages over current therapies remain to be determined. Cefixime offers no advantages over other antimicrobial agents for streptococcal pharyngitis.

Cefixime has excellent activity in vitro against *E. coli* and other Enterobacteriaceae when compared to other oral cephalosporins. It has been comparable to amoxicillin (Iravani et al, 1988) and trimethoprim/sulfamethoxazole (Cox, 1989; see also Brogden and Campoli-Richards, 1989) for uncomplicated urinary tract infections in clinical trials and may be useful for urinary tract infections that are resistant to less expensive antimicrobial agents. However, there are a number of other effective antimicrobial agents (eg, trimethoprim/sulfamethoxazole, amoxicillin/potassium clavulanate, ciprofloxacin) for this indication.

ADVERSE REACTIONS AND PRECAUTIONS. Most adverse reactions observed in clinical trials were of a mild or transient nature, but 5% of patients required discontinuation of cefixime. The most common adverse reactions have been gastrointestinal, particularly diarrhea (16%). Loose or frequent stools (6%), abdominal pain (3%), nausea (7%), dyspepsia (3%), and flatulence (4%) also were reported. Gastrointestinal adverse reactions were classified as severe in 2% of patients, and several patients developed severe diarrhea and/or documented pseudomembranous colitis. In comparative clinical trials, cefixime was more likely to cause diarrhea than amoxicillin (McLinn, 1987; see also Tally et al, 1987).

Other side effects reported for cefixime include dizziness, headache, genital pruritus, and vaginitis. Hypersensitivity reactions were uncommon and included rashes, pruritus, drug fever, and urticaria. Transient elevations in hepatic enzymes (AST, ALT), BUN, and creatinine occurred in less than 1% of patients. Mild and reversible thrombocytopenia, leukopenia, and eosinophilia were reported in less than 1% of patients.

For additional discussion see Tally et al, 1987.

DRUG INTERACTIONS AND INTERFERENCE WITH LABORATORY TESTS. See the Introduction.

PHARMACOKINETICS. Cefixime is slowly and incompletely absorbed from the gastrointestinal tract. The absolute bioavailability is about 40% to 50%. Peak serum concentrations occur between two and six hours following administration of either the tablet or suspension formulation. Single 200 mg or 400 mg doses of cefixime tablets yield average peak serum concentrations of 2 mcg/ml and 3.7 mcg/ml, respectively. The oral suspension, in equivalent doses, produces average peak serum concentrations that are 25% to 50% higher and areas under the time versus concentration curve (AUC) that are 10% to 25% greater. Therefore, the two formulations are not bioequivalent, and the manufacturer recommends that tablets should not be substituted for the oral suspension in the treatment of otitis media. The presence of food does not affect the amount of cefixime that is absorbed, but delays the time to maximal absorption by about 50 minutes.

Approximately 65% to 70% of circulating cefixime is bound to plasma protein. The drug has a steady-state volume of distribution that approximates that of the extracellular fluid. Data on the penetration of cefixime into various tissues and body fluids are limited. High concentrations are achieved in bile and urine (see Brogden and Campoli-Richards, 1989).

Cefixime is eliminated primarily by the renal route. Approximately 50% of an absorbed dose is recovered as unchanged drug in the urine after 24 hours. Greater than 10% of an administered dose is excreted via the bile. Cefixime is not metabolized. The serum half-life in patients with normal renal function is between three and four hours; the half-life is prolonged in patients with renal impairment (11.5 hours for creatinine clearance of 5 to 20 ml/min). Cefixime is not removed significantly from the blood by hemodialysis or peritoneal dialysis.

For additional discussion, see Faulkner et al, 1987; Brogden and Campoli-Richards, 1989.

DOSAGE AND PREPARATIONS.
Oral: *Adults and children older than 12 years or weighing more than 50 kg,* 400 mg once daily or 200 mg every 12 hours; *children 6 months or older,* 8 mg/kg of the suspension once daily or 4 mg/kg of the suspension every 12 hours. For otitis media, the tablet should *not* be substituted for the suspension. The efficacy and safety of cefixime in infants less than 6 months have not been established.

Patients with impaired renal function require modification of dosage depending on the degree of impairment. The manufacturer recommends 75% of the standard dosage (ie, 300 mg daily) when creatinine clearance is between 21 and 60 ml/min or for patients on renal hemodialysis, and 50% of the standard dosage (ie, 200 mg daily) when creatinine clearance is less than 20 ml/min or for patients on continuous ambulatory peritoneal dialysis.

Suprax (Lederle). Tablets 200 and 400 mg; powder for oral suspension 100 mg/5 ml in 50 and 100 ml containers.

Cited References

Choice of cephalosporins. *Med Lett Drugs Ther* 25:57-60, 1983 A.

Cefoperazone sodium (Cefobid). *Med Lett Drugs Ther* 25:29-30, 1983 B.

Cefuroxime sodium (Zinacef). *Med Lett Drugs Ther* 26:15-16, 1984 A.
Ceforanide (Precef). *Med Lett Drugs Ther* 26:91-92, 1984 B.
Cefonicid sodium (Monocid). *Med Lett Drugs Ther* 26:71-72, 1984 C.
Drugs for anaerobic infection. *Med Lett Drugs Ther* 26:87-89, 1984 D.
Ceftriaxone sodium (Rocephin). *Med Lett Drugs Ther* 27:37-39, 1985 A.
Ceftazidime (Fortaz). *Med Lett Drugs Ther* 27:85-87, 1985 B.
Cefotetan disodium (Cefotan). *Med Lett Drugs Ther* 28:70-72, 1986.
Antimicrobial prophylaxis for surgery. *Med Lett Drugs Ther* 29:91-94, 1987; 31:105-108, 1989 C.
Choice of antimicrobial drugs. *Med Lett Drugs Ther* 30:33-40, 1988 A; 32:41-48, 1990.
Cefuroxime axetil. *Med Lett Drugs Ther* 30:57-59, 1988 B.
Treatment of Lyme disease. *Med Lett Drugs Ther* 31:57-59, 1989 A.
Cefixime—New oral cephalosporin. *Med Lett Drugs Ther* 31:73-75, 1989 B.
1989 Sexually transmitted diseases treatment guidelines. *MMWR* 38 (suppl 8):1-43, 1989.
Ackley AM Jr, Felsher J: Adverse reactions to cefaclor. *South Med J* 74:1550, 1981.
Aldridge KE: Controversies in susceptibility testing of anaerobes. *Clin Ther* 10 (suppl A): 2-18, 1987.
Alestig K, et al: Effect of cefoperazone on faecal flora. *J Antimicrob Chemother* 12:163-167, 1983.
American Academy of Pediatrics Committee on Infectious Diseases: Treatment of bacterial meningitis. *Pediatrics* 81:904-907, 1988.
Amsterdam D: Editorial comment. *Antimicrob Newslett* 1:32-33, 1984.
Anderson JA: Cross-sensitivity to cephalosporins in patients allergic to penicillin. *Pediatr Infect Dis J* 5:557-561, 1986.
Arditi M, et al: Cefuroxime treatment failure and *Haemophilus influenzae* meningitis: Case report and review of literature. *Pediatrics* 84:132-135, 1989.
Aronovitz GH: Treatment of otitis media with cefuroxime axetil. *South Med J* 81:978-980, 1988.
Au JP, Geiger GS: Thrombocytopenia associated with moxalactam administration. *Drug Intell Clin Pharm* 18:140-143, 1984.
Bach MC: Prolonged bleeding time associated with 'low-dose' moxalactam therapy, letter. *JAMA* 251:3082, 1984.
Baddour LM, et al: Clinical comparison of single-oral-dose cefuroxime axetil and amoxicillin with probenecid for uncomplicated gonococcal infections in women. *Antimicrob Agents Chemother* 33:801-804, 1989.
Balant L, et al: Clinical pharmacokinetics of third generation cephalosporins. *Clin Pharmacokinet* 10:101-143, 1985.
Bang NU, Kammer RB: Hematologic complications associated with β-lactam antibiotics. *Rev Infect Dis* 5 (suppl 2):S380-S393, 1983.
Barriere SL: Ceftriaxone: Beta-lactamase-stable, broad-spectrum cephalosporin with extended half-life, commentary. *Pharmacotherapy* 5:252-253, 1985.
Barriere SL: Controversies in antimicrobial therapy: Formulary decisions on third-generation cephalosporins. *Am J Hosp Pharm* 43:625-629, 1986.
Barriere SL, Flaherty JF: Third generation cephalosporins: Critical evaluation. *Clin Pharm* 3:351-373, 1984.
Barriere SL, Mills J: Ceforanide: Antibacterial activity, pharmacology, and clinical efficacy. *Pharmacotherapy* 2:322-327, 1982.
Barry AL, Jones RN: Cefixime: Spectrum of antibacterial activity against 16,016 clinical isolates. *Pediatr Infect Dis J* 6:954-957, 1987.
Barson WJ, et al: Prospective comparative trial of ceftriaxone vs conventional therapy for treatment of bacterial meningitis in children. *Pediatr Infect Dis* 4:362-368, 1985.
Beam TR Jr: Third generation cephalosporins, parts I and II. *Ration Drug Ther* 16:1-6 (June), 1-5 (July), 1982.
Beam TR Jr: Ceftriaxone: Beta-lactamase-stable, broad spectrum cephalosporin with extended half-life. *Pharmacotherapy* 5:237-253, 1985.
Benet LZ, Sheiner LB: Design and optimization of dosage regimens. Pharmacokinetic data, in Gilman AG, et al (eds): *The Pharmacological Basis of Therapeutics*, ed 7. New York, MacMillan, 1985, 1663-1733.
Bennett WM, et al: Drug prescribing in renal failure: Dosing guidelines for adults. *Am J Kidney Dis* 3:155-193, 1983.
Bergan T: Pharmacokinetic properties of cephalosporins. *Drugs* 34 (suppl 2):89-104, 1987.
Bertino JS Jr, Speck WT: Cephalosporin antibiotics. *Pediatr Clin North Am* 30:17-26, 1983.
Blumer JL, et al: Ceftazidime therapy in patients with cystic fibrosis and multiply-drug-resistant *Pseudomonas*. *Am J Med* 79 (suppl 2A):37-46, 1985.
Bodey GP, et al: Comparative in vitro study of new cephalosporins. *Antimicrob Agents Chemother* 20:226-230, 1981.
Brandstetter RD, et al: Moxalactam disodium-induced pulmonary hemorrhage. *Chest* 86:644-645, 1984.
Brogden RN, Campoli-Richards DM: Cefixime: Review of its antibacterial activity, pharmacokinetic properties and therapeutic potential. *Drugs* 38:524-550, 1989.
Brogden RN, Ward A: Ceftriaxone: Reappraisal of its antibacterial activity and pharmacokinetic properties, and update on its therapeutic use with particular reference to once-daily administration. *Drugs* 35:604-645, 1988.
Brooks GF, Barriere SL: Clinical use of new beta-lactam drugs: Practical considerations for physicians, microbiology laboratories, pharmacists, and formulary committees. *Ann Intern Med* 98:530-535, 1983.
Bryan JP, et al: Comparison of ceftriaxone and ampicillin plus chloramphenicol for therapy of acute bacterial meningitis. *Antimicrob Agents Chemother* 28:361-368, 1985 A.
Bryan CS, et al: Gentamicin vs cefotaxime for therapy of neonatal sepsis: Relationship to drug resistance. *Am J Dis Child* 139:1086-1089, 1985 B.
Buening MK, et al: Disulfiram-like reaction to β-lactams, (letter). *JAMA* 245:2027-2028, 1981.
Burke BM, et al: Comparison of cefmetazole and cefoxitin for treatment of patients hospitalized with acute urinary tract infections. *J Antimicrob Chemother* 23 (suppl D):35-38, 1989.
Burnakis TG: Surgical antimicrobial prophylaxis: Principles and guidelines. *Pharmacotherapy* 4:248-271, 1984.
Calandra T, et al (EORTC International Antimicrobial Therapy Cooperative Group): Ceftazidime combined with short or long course amikacin for empirical therapy of gram-negative bacteremia in cancer patients with granulocytopenia. *N Engl J Med* 317:1692-1698, 1987.
Campoli-Richards DM, et al: Ceforanide: Review of its antibacterial activity, pharmacokinetic properties and clinical efficacy. *Drugs* 34:411-437, 1987.
Carlberg H, et al: Intestinal side effects of cefoperazone. *J Antimicrob Chemother* 10:483-487, 1982.
Carmine AA, et al: Cefotaxime: Review of its antimicrobial activity, pharmacological properties and therapeutic use. *Drugs* 25:223-289, 1983 A.
Carmine AA, et al: Moxalactam (latamoxef): Review of its antibacterial activity, pharmacokinetic properties, and therapeutic use. *Drugs* 26:279-333, 1983 B.
Chambers HF, et al: Failure of once-daily regimen of cefonicid for treatment of endocarditis due to *Staphylococcus aureus*. *Rev Infect Dis* 6 (suppl 4):S870-S874, 1984.
Cherubin CE, Eng RHK: Experience with use of cefotaxime in treatment of bacterial meningitis. *Am J Med* 80:398-404, 1986.
Cherubin CE, et al: Treatment of gram-negative bacillary meningitis: Role of new cephalosporin antibiotics. *Rev Infect Dis* 4 (suppl):S453-S464, 1982.
Chin N, Neu HC: Cefotaxime and desacetylcefotaxime: Example of advantageous antimicrobial metabolism. *Diagn Microbiol Infect Dis* 2:21S-31S, 1984.
Chow AW, Jewesson PJ: Pharmacokinetics and safety of antimicrobial agents during pregnancy. *Rev Infect Dis* 7:287-313, 1985.
Cleeland R, Squires E: Antimicrobial activity of ceftriaxone: Review. *Am J Med* 77 (suppl 4C):3-11, 1984.
Cohen MS, et al: Multicenter clinical trial of cefoperazone sodium in the United States. *Am J Med* 77 (suppl 1B):35-41, 1984.

Collier AC, et al: Comparative study of ceftriaxone and spectinomycin in the treatment of uncomplicated gonorrhea in women. *Am J Med* 77(suppl 4C):68-72, 1984.

Cone LA, et al: Ceftazidime versus tobramycin-ticarcillin in treatment of pneumonia and bacteremia. *Antimicrob Agents Chemother* 28:33-36, 1985.

Congeni BL: Comparison of ceftriaxone and traditional therapy of bacterial meningitis. *Antimicrob Agents Chemother* 25:40-44, 1984.

Conly JM, et al: Hyperprothrombinemia in febrile, neutropenic patients with cancer: Association with antimicrobial suppression of intestinal microflora. *J Infect Dis* 150:202-212, 1984.

Conte JE Jr, et al: *Antibiotic Prophylaxis in Surgery: Comprehensive Review.* Philadelphia, JB Lippincott, 1984.

Cooper RH, et al: Evaluation of ceforanide as treatment for staphylococcal and streptococcal endocarditis. *Antimicrob Agents Chemother* 19:256-259, 1981.

Cornick NA, et al: Activity of cefmetazole against anaerobic bacteria. *Antimicrob Agents Chemother* 31:2010-2012, 1987.

Corrado ML, et al: Designing appropriate therapy in treatment of gram-negative bacillary meningitis. *JAMA* 248:71-74, 1982.

Cox CE: Cefixime versus trimethoprim/sulfamethoxazole in treatment of patients with acute, uncomplicated lower urinary tract infections. *Urology* 34:322-326, 1989.

Cox CE, et al: Evaluation of cefuroxime axetil, cefaclor, and cephalexin in treatment of urinary tract infections in adults. *Curr Ther Res* 42:124-137, 1987.

Darbyshire PJ, et al: Ceftazidime in treatment of febrile immunosuppressed children. *J Antimicrob Chemother* 12(suppl 2A):357-360, 1983.

Dattwyler RJ, et al: Treatment of late Lyme borreliosis: Randomized comparison of ceftriaxone and penicillin. *Lancet* 1:1191-1194, 1988.

Del Rio M, et al: Ceftriaxone versus ampicillin and chloramphenicol for treatment of bacterial meningitis in children. *Lancet* 1:1241-1244, 1983.

de Pauw BE, et al: Randomized study of ceftazidime versus gentamicin plus cefotaxime for infections in severe granulocytopenic patients. *J Antimicrob Chemother* 12(suppl A):93-99, 1983.

DiPiro JT, May JR: Use of cephalosporins with enhanced antianaerobic activity for treatment and prevention of anaerobic and mixed infections. *Clin Pharm* 7:285-302, 1988.

DiPiro JT, et al: Antimicrobial prophylaxis in surgery, parts 1 and 2. *Am J Hosp Pharm* 38:320-334, 487-494, 1981.

DiPiro JT, et al: Prophylactic use of antimicrobials in surgery. *Curr Probl Surg* 20:69-132, 1983.

DiPiro JT, et al: Prophylactic parenteral cephalosporins in surgery: Are newer agents better? *JAMA* 252:3277-3279, 1984.

DiPiro JT, et al: Single dose systemic antibiotic prophylaxis of surgical wound infections. *Am J Surg* 152:552-559, 1986.

DiPiro JT, et al: Single-dose cefometazole versus multiple dose cefoxitin for prophylaxis in abdominal surgery. *J Antimicrob Chemother* 23(suppl D):71-77, 1989.

Donowitz GR, Mandell GL: Beta-lactam antibiotics (part 2). *N Engl J Med* 318:490-500, 1988.

Donowitz GR, Mandell GL: Cephalosporins, in Mandell GL, et al (eds): *Principles and Practice of Infectious Diseases,* ed 3. New York, Churchill Livingstone, 1990, 246-257.

Drusano GL, et al: Prospective randomized controlled trial of cefoxitin versus clindamycin-aminoglycoside in mixed anaerobic-aerobic infections, *Surg Gynecol Obstet* 154:715-720, 1982.

Dudley MN, et al: Review of cefonicid, long-acting cephalosporin. *Clin Pharm* 3:23-32, 1984.

Dworzack DL, et al: Emergence of resistance in gram-negative bacteria during therapy with expanded-spectrum cephalosporins. *Eur J Clin Microbiol* 6:456-459, 1987.

Eichenwald HF: Antimicrobial therapy in infants and children: Update 1976-1985, part I. *J Pediatr* 107:161-168, 1985.

Fainstein V, et al: Randomized study of ceftazidime compared to ceftazidime and tobramycin for treatment of infections in cancer patients. *J Antimicrob Chemother* 12(suppl A):101-110, 1983.

Fass RJ: Comparative in vitro activities of third-generation cephalosporins. *Arch Intern Med* 143:1743-1745, 1983.

Faulkner RD, et al: Pharmacokinetic profile of cefixime in man. *Pediatr Infect Dis J* 6:963-970, 1987.

Finegold SM, Wexler HM: Therapeutic implications of bacteriologic findings in mixed aerobic-anaerobic infections. *Antimicrob Agents Chemother* 32:611-616, 1988.

Fink S, et al: Ceftriaxone effect on bilirubin-albumin binding. *Pediatrics* 80:873-875, 1987.

Finn A, et al: Effect of dose and food on bioavailability of cefuroxime axetil. *Biopharm Drug Dispos* 8:519-526, 1987.

Fitzpatrick BJ, Standiford HC: Comparative evaluation of moxalactam: Antimicrobial activity, pharmacokinetics, adverse reactions, and clinical efficacy. *Pharmacotherapy* 2:197-212, 1982.

Follath F, et al: Clinical consequences of development of resistance to third generation cephalosporins. *Eur J Clin Microbiol* 6:446-450, 1987.

Fong IW, Tomkins KB: Review of *Pseudomonas aeruginosa* meningitis with special emphasis on treatment with ceftazidime. *Rev Infect Dis* 7:604-612, 1985.

Frank E, et al: Treatment of skin and soft tissue infections: Comparative study of cefmetazole and cefoxitin. *J Antimicrob Chemother* 23(suppl D):55-60, 1989.

Fried JS, Hinthorn DR: Cephalosporins. *DM* 31:1-60, (July) 1985.

Funk EA, Strausbaugh LJ: Antimicrobial activity, pharmacokinetics, adverse reactions, and therapeutic indications of cefoperazone. *Pharmacotherapy* 2:185-196, 1982.

Garzone P, et al: Third-generation and investigational cephalosporins: I. Structure-activity relationships and pharmacokinetic review. *Drug Intell Clin Pharm* 17:507-515, 1983 A.

Garzone P, et al: Third-generation and investigational cephalosporins: II. Microbiologic review and clinical summaries. *Drug Intell Clin Pharm* 17:615-622, 1983 B.

Geckler RW, et al: Multicenter comparative study of cefotetan once daily and cefoxitin thrice daily for treatment of infections of skin and superficial soft tissue. *Am J Surg* 155(suppl 5A):91-95, 1988.

Gentry LO: Antimicrobial activity, pharmacokinetics, therapeutic indications, and adverse reactions of ceftazidime. *Pharmacotherapy* 5:254-267, 1985.

Gilbert DN: Current status of antibiotic prophylaxis in surgical patients. *Bull NY Acad Med* 60:340-357, 1984.

Ginsburg CM: Comparative pharmacokinetics of cefadroxil, cefaclor, cephalexin, and cephradine in infants and children. *J Antimicrob Chemother* 10(suppl B):27-31, 1982.

Gleckman RA: Antimicrobial activity, pharmacokinetics, therapeutic indications, and adverse reactions of ceftazidime, commentary. *Pharmacotherapy* 5:265-266, 1985.

Gold B, Rodriguez WJ: Cefuroxime: Mechanisms of action, antimicrobial activity, pharmacokinetics, clinical applications, adverse reactions and therapeutic indications. *Pharmacotherapy* 3:82-100, 1983.

Gold R, et al: Controlled trial of ceftazidime vs ticarcillin and tobramycin in treatment of acute respiratory exacerbations in patients with cystic fibrosis. *Pediatr Infect Dis* 4:172-177, 1985.

Goldberg DM: Cephalosporins. *Med Clin North Am* 71:1113-1133, 1987.

Gordon RC: Sorting out the cephems: Role of new cephalosporins in pediatric therapeutics. *Pediatr Ann* 14:278-287, 1985.

Gottlieb A, Mills J: Cefuroxime axetil for treatment of uncomplicated gonorrhea. *Antimicrob Agents Chemother* 30:333-334, 1986.

Greenman RL, et al: Twice-daily intramuscular ceforanide therapy of *Staphylococcus aureus* endocarditis in parenteral drug abusers. *Antimicrob Agents Chemother* 25:16-19, 1984.

Griffith DL, et al: Clinical experience with cefmetazole sodium in United States: Overview. *J Antimicrob Chemother* 23(suppl D):21-33, 1989.

Guay DRP, et al: Interference of selected second- and third-generation cephalosporins with creatinine determination. *Am J Hosp Pharm* 40:435-438, 1983.

Guglielmo BJ, et al: Antibiotic prophylaxis in surgical procedures: Critical analysis of the literature. *Arch Surg* 118:943-955, 1983.

Handsfield HH, Murphy VL: Comparative study of ceftriaxone and spectinomycin for treatment of uncomplicated gonorrhoea in men. *Lancet* 2:67-70, 1983.

Handsfield HH, Murphy VL: Treatment of uncomplicated gonorrhea in women with single-dose cefonicid. *Sex Transm Dis* 12:90-92, 1985.

Hansten PD, Horn JR: *Drug Interactions*, ed 6. Philadelphia, Lea & Febiger, 1989, 203-267.

Holloway WJ, et al: Cefmetazole treatment of intra-abdominal infection. *J Antimicrob Chemother* 23 (suppl D):47-54, 1989.

Holt RJ, et al: Hypoprothrombinemia associated with moxalactam treatment of septic sternoclavicular arthritis due to *Citrobacter diversus*. *Drug Intell Clin Pharm* 15:288-289, 1981.

Howie VM, Owen MJ: Bacteriologic and clinical efficacy of cefixime compared with amoxicillin in acute otitis media. *Pediatr Infect Dis J* 6:989-991, 1987.

Hughes WT, et al: Guidelines for use of antimicrobial agents in neutropenic patients with unexplained fever. *J Infect Dis* 161:381-396, 1990.

Iravani A, et al: Double-blind, multicenter, comparative study of safety and efficacy of cefixime versus amoxicillin in treatment of acute urinary tract infections in adult patients. *Am J Med* 85 (suppl 3A):17-23, 1988.

Islam A, et al: Randomized treatment of patients with typhoid fever by using ceftriaxone or chloramphenicol. *J Infect Dis* 158:742-747, 1988.

Jacob LS, Layne P: Cefonicid: Overview of clinical studies in United States. *Rev Infect Dis* 6 (suppl 4):S791-S802, 1984.

Jacobs RF, et al: Prospective randomized comparison of cefotaxime vs ampicillin and chloramphenicol for bacterial meningitis in children. *J Pediatr* 107:129-133, 1985.

Jagelman DG, et al: Single-dose cefotetan versus multiple-dose cefoxitin as prophylaxis in colorectal surgery. *Am J Surg* 155 (suppl 5A):71-76, 1988.

Jones RN: Review of cephalosporin metabolism: Lesson to be learned for future chemotherapy. *Antimicrob Newslett* 4:69-74, 1987.

Jones RN: Review of in-vitro spectrum and characteristics of cefmetazole (cs-1170). *J Antimicrob Chemother* 23 (suppl D):1-12, 1989.

Jones RN, Preston DA: Antimicrobial activity of cephalexin against old and new pathogens. *Postgrad Med J* 59 (suppl 5):9-15, 1983.

Jones RN, Thornsberry C: Gram-positive superinfections: Consequence of modern β-lactam chemotherapy. *Antimicrob Newslett* 2:17-24, 1985.

Jones RN, et al: Antimicrobial activity of desacetylcefotaxime alone and in combination with cefotaxime: Evidence of synergy. *Rev Infect Dis* 4 (suppl):S366-S373, 1982.

Jones SR, Kimbrough RC III: Moxalactam and hemorrhage, letter. *Ann Intern Med* 99:126, 1983.

Joshi M, et al: Double-blind, prospective, multicenter trial comparing ceftazidime with moxalactam in treatment of serious gram-negative infections. *Antimicrob Agents Chemother* 30:90-95, 1986.

Judson FN, et al: Comparative study of ceftriaxone and aqueous procaine penicillin G in treatment of uncomplicated gonorrhea in women. *Antimicrob Agents Chemother* 23:218-220, 1983.

Judson FN, et al: Comparative study of ceftriaxone and spectinomycin for treatment of pharyngeal and anorectal gonorrhea. *JAMA* 253:1417-1419, 1985.

Kaiser AB: Antimicrobial prophylaxis in surgery. *N Engl J Med* 315:1129-1138, 1986.

Kaiser AB: Postoperative infections and antimicrobial prophylaxis, in Mandell GL, et al (eds): *Principles and Practice of Infectious Diseases,* ed 3. New York, Churchill Livingstone, 1990, 2245-2257.

Kaiser AB, et al: Efficacy of cefazolin, cefamandole, and gentamicin as prophylactic agents in cardiac surgery: Results of prospective, randomized, double-blind trial in 1,030 patients. *Ann Surg* 206:791-797, 1987.

Kannangara DW, et al: Disulfiram-like reactions with newer cephalosporins: Cefmenoxime. *Am J Med Sci* 287:45-47, 1984.

Kenna MA, et al: Cefixime vs. cefaclor in treatment of acute otitis media in infants and children. *Pediatr Infect Dis J* 6:992-996, 1987.

Kernodie DS, et al: Failure of cephalosporins to prevent *Staphylococcus aureus* surgical wound infections. *JAMA* 263:961-966, 1990.

Kiani R, et al: Comparative, multicenter studies of cefixime and amoxicillin in treatment of respiratory tract infections. *Am J Med* 85 (suppl 3A):6-13, 1988.

Klein JO, et al: Report of task force on diagnosis and management of meningitis. *Pediatrics* 78 (suppl):959-982, 1986.

Kline SS, et al: Cefotetan-induced disulfiram-type reactions and hypoprothrombinemia. *Antimicrob Agents Chemother* 31:1328-1331, 1987.

Kramer BS, et al: Randomized comparison between two ceftazidime-containing regimens and cephalothin-gentamicin-carbenicillin in febrile granulocytopenic cancer patients. *Antimicrob Agents Chemother* 30:64-68, 1986.

Kunkel MJ, Iannini PB: Cefonicid in once-daily regimen for treatment of osteomyelitis in ambulatory setting. *Rev Infect Dis* 6 (suppl 4):S865-S869, 1984.

Landesman SH, et al: Past and current roles for cephalosporin antibiotics in treatment of meningitis: Emphasis on use in gram-negative bacillary meningitis. *Am J Med* 71:693-703, 1981.

Lea AS, et al: Comparative trial of cefonicid vs cefazolin for treatment of skin and soft tissue infections caused by gram-positive cocci, abstract 794. *23rd Interscience Conference on Antimicrobial Agents and Chemotherapy*. Miami Beach, Oct 4-6, 1982.

LeBel MH, et al: Comparative efficacy of ceftriaxone and cefuroxime for treatment of bacterial meningitis. *J Pediatr* 114:1049-1054, 1989.

Lee S, et al: Coagulopathy associated with moxalactam, letter. *JAMA* 249:2019-2020, 1983.

LeFrock JL, et al: Mechanism of action, antimicrobial activity, pharmacology, adverse effects, and clinical efficacy of cefotaxime. *Pharmacotherapy* 2:174-184, 1982.

LeFrock JL, et al: Nonprophylactic role of cephalosporins in surgery. *Bull NY Acad Med* 60:394-402, 1984 A.

LeFrock JL, et al: Nonprophylactic role of cephalosporins in obstetrics and gynecology. *Bull NY Acad Med* 60:416-425, 1984 B.

LeFrock JL, et al: In vitro and clinical evaluation of ceforanide. *Am J Med Sci* 287:21-25, 1984 C.

Leng M, Anderson PO: Serum sickness with cefaclor. *Drug Intell Clin Pharm* 19:186-187, 1985.

Lennard ES, Dellinger EP: Prophylactic antibiotics in surgery: Rationale for family physician. *J Fam Pract* 12:461-467, 1981.

Levine LR: Quantitative comparison of adverse reactions to cefaclor vs amoxicillin in surveillance study. *Pediatr Infect Dis* 4:358-361, 1985.

Lipsky JJ: Antibiotic-associated hypoprothrombinemia. *J Antimicrob Chemother* 21:281-300, 1988.

Livermore DM: Mechanisms of resistance to cephalosporin antibiotics. *Drugs* 34 (suppl 2):64-88, 1987 A.

Livermore DM: Clinical significance of beta-lactamase induction and stable derepression in gram-negative rods. *Eur J Clin Microbiol* 6:439-445, 1987 B.

Luft FC: Cephalosporin and aminoglycoside interactions: Clinical and toxicologic implications, in Whelton A, Neu HC (eds): *The Aminoglycosides: Microbiology, Clinical Use, and Toxicology*. New York, Marcel Dekker, 1982, 387-399.

MacLennan FM, et al: Severe depletion of vitamin-K-dependent clotting factors during postoperative latamoxef therapy, letter. *Lancet* 1:1215, 1983.

Malangoni MA, et al: Treatment of intra-abdominal infections is appropriate with single agent or combination antibiotic therapy. *Surgery* 98:648-655, 1985.

Mandell LA, et al: Multicentre prospective randomized trial comparing ceftazidime with cefazolin/tobramycin in treatment of hospitalized patients with nonpneumococcal pneumonia. *J Antimicrob Chemother* 12 (suppl A):9-20, 1983.

Mandell LA, et al: Prospective randomized trial of ceftazidime versus cefazolin/tobramycin in treatment of hospitalized patients with pneumonia. *J Antimicrob Chemother* 20:95-107, 1987.

Mandell LA, et al: Once-daily therapy with ceftriaxone compared with daily multiple-dose therapy with cefotaxime for serious bacterial infections: Randomized, double-blind study. *J Infect Dis* 160:433-441, 1989.

Mangi RJ, et al: Cefoperazone versus combination antibiotic therapy of hospital-acquired pneumonia. *Am J Med* 84:68-74, 1988 A.

Mangi RJ, et al: Cefoperazone versus ceftazidime monotherapy of nosocomial pneumonia. *Am J Med* 85(suppl 1A):44-48, 1988 B.

Mangini RJ (ed): *Drug Interaction Facts*. St Louis, JB Lippincott, 1984 A, 12.

Mangini RJ (ed): *Drug Interaction Facts*. St Louis, JB Lippincott, 1984 B, 455.

Mangini RJ (ed): *Drug Interaction Facts*. St Louis, JB Lippincott, 1984 C, 245.

Marks WA, et al: Cefuroxime verus ampicillin plus chloramphenicol in childhood bacterial meningitis: Multicenter randomized controlled trial. *J Pediatr* 109:123-130, 1986.

Marx MA, Fant WK: Cefuroxime axetil. *Drug Intell Clin Pharm* 22:651-658, 1988.

Mastella G, et al: Alternative antibiotics for treatment of pseudomonas infections in cystic fibrosis. *J Antimicrob Chemother* 12(suppl A):297-311, 1983.

McClosky RV: Clinical and bacteriologic efficacy of ceftriaxone in the United States. *Am J Med* 77(suppl 4C):97-103, 1984.

McCracken GH Jr, et al: Moxalactam therapy for neonatal meningitis due to gram-negative enteric bacilli: Prospective controlled evaluation. *JAMA* 252:1427-1432, 1984.

McCracken GH, et al: Consensus report: Antimicrobial therapy for bacterial meningitis in infants and children. *Pediatr Infect Dis J* 6:501-505, 1987.

McLinn SE: Randomized, open label, multicenter trial of cefixime compared with amoxicillin for treatment of acute otitis media with effusion. *Pediatr Infect Dis J* 6:997-1001, 1987.

McLinn SE, et al: Clinical trial of cefuroxime axetil versus cefaclor for acute otitis media with effusion. *Curr Ther Res* 43:1-11, 1988.

The Medical Letter: *Handbook of Antimicrobial Therapy*. New Rochelle, NY, The Medical Letter, Inc, 1988, 38-49.

Meisel S: Severe bleeding diathesis associated with moxalactam administration. *Drug Intell Clin Pharm* 18:721-722, 1984.

Minami S, et al: Induction of β-lactamase by various β-lactam antibiotics in *Enterobacter cloacae*. *Antimicrob Agents Chemother* 18:382-385, 1980.

Moellering RC Jr: Can third-generation cephalosporins eliminate need for antimicrobial combinations? *Am J Med* 79(suppl 2A):104-109, 1985 A.

Moellering RC Jr: Ceftazidime: New broad spectrum cephalosporin. *Pediatr Infect Dis* 4:390-393, 1985 B.

Morgan G, et al: Ceftazidime as single agent in management of children with fever and neutropenia. *J Antimicrob Chemother* 12(suppl A):347-351, 1983.

Moskovitz BL: Clinical adverse effects during ceftriaxone therapy. *Am J Med* 77(suppl 4C):84-88, 1984.

Mulligan ME, et al: Impact of cefoperazone therapy on fecal flora. *Antimicrob Agents Chemother* 22:226-230, 1982.

Murray DL, et al: Cefaclor: Cluster of adverse reactions, letter. *N Engl J Med* 303:1003, 1980.

Muytjens HL, van der Ros-van de Repe J: Comparative activities of 13 β-lactam antibiotics. *Antimicrob Agents Chemother* 21:925-934, 1982.

Nadworny HA, Markowitz A: Parenteral antibiotic therapy at home: Experience with intramuscular cefonicid. *Clin Ther* 10:82-91, 1987.

Naqvi SH, et al: Cefotaxime therapy of neonatal gram-negative bacillary meningitis. *Pediatr Infect Dis* 4:499-502, 1985.

Nelson JD: Cefuroxime: Cephalosporin with unique applicability to pediatric practice. *Pediatr Infect Dis* 2:394-396, 1983.

Nelson JD: *1989-1990 Pocketbook of Pediatric Antimicrobial Therapy*, ed 8. Baltimore, Williams & Wilkins, 1989 A, 64-77.

Nelson JD: *1989-1990 Pocketbook of Pediatric Antimicrobial Therapy*, ed 8. Baltimore, Williams & Wilkins, 1989 B, 20-21.

Nelson JD, et al: Benefits and risks of sequential parenteral-oral cephalosporin therapy for suppurative bone and joint infections. *J Pediatr Orthop* 2:255-262, 1982.

Neu HC: New beta-lactamase-stable cephalosporins. *Ann Intern Med* 97:408-419, 1982 A.

Neu HC: Factors that affect *in vitro* activity of cephalosporin antibiotics. *J Antimicrob Chemother* 10(suppl C):11-23, 1982 B.

Neu HC: In vitro activity, human pharmacology, and clinical effectiveness of new β-lactam antibiotics. *Ann Rev Pharmacol Toxicol* 22:599-642, 1982 C.

Neu HC: Clinical uses of cephalosporins. *Lancet* 2:252-255, 1982 D.

Neu HC: Antibacterial activity of desacetylcefotaxime alone and in combination with cefotaxime. *Rev Infect Dis* 4(suppl):S374-S378, 1982 E.

Neu HC: Structure-activity relations of new β-lactam compounds and in vitro activity against common bacteria. *Rev Infect Dis* 5(suppl 2):S319-S337, 1983.

Neu HC: Ceftizoxime: β-lactamase-stable, broad-spectrum cephalosporin: Pharmacokinetics, adverse effects, and clinical use. *Pharmacotherapy* 4:47-60, 1984.

Neu HC: Relation of structural properties of beta-lactam antibiotics and antibacterial activity. *Am J Med* 79(suppl 2A):2-13, 1985.

Neu HC: In vitro activity of new broad spectrum, beta-lactamase-stable oral cephalosporin, cefixime. *Pediatr Infect Dis J* 6:958-962, 1987 A.

Neu HC: New antibiotics: Areas of appropriate use. *J Infect Dis* 155:403-417, 1987 B.

Neu HC: Pathophysiologic basis for use of third-generation cephalosporins. *Am J Med* 88 (suppl 4A):35-115, 1990.

Neu HC, Prince AS: Interaction between moxalactam and alcohol, letter. *Lancet* 1:1422, 1980.

Nichols RL, et al: Risk of infection after penetrating abdominal trauma. *N Engl J Med* 311:1065-1070, 1984.

Nightingale CH, et al: Pharmacokinetics and clinical use of cephalosporin antibiotics. *J Pharm Sci* 64:1899-1927, 1975.

Nightingale CH, et al: Cephalosporins, in Evans WE, et al (eds): *Applied Pharmacokinetics: Principles of Therapeutic Drug Monitoring*. San Francisco, Applied Therapeutics, 1980, 240-274.

Noble JT, Barza M: Pharmacokinetic properties of newer cephalosporins: Valid basis for drug selection? *Drugs* 30:175-181, 1985.

Norrby SR: Role of cephalosporins in treatment of bacterial meningitis in adults: Overview with special emphasis on ceftazidime. *Am J Med* 79(suppl 2A):56-61, 1985.

Norrby SR: Adverse reactions and interactions with newer cephalosporin and cephamycin antibiotics. *Med Toxicol Adverse Drug Exp* 1:32-46, 1986.

Norris SM: Cephalosporin antibiotic agents, I: Considered as a group. *Infect Control* 5:493-496, 1984 A.

Norris SM: Cephalosporin antibiotic agents, II: First- and second-generation agents. *Infect Control* 5:577-582, 1984 B.

Norris SM: Cephalosporin antibiotic agents, III: Third generation cephalosporins. *Infect Control* 6:78-83, 1985.

Norris SM, Mandell GL: Tables of antimicrobial agent pharmacology, in Mandell GL, et al (eds): *Anti-Infective Therapy*. New York, John Wiley & Sons, 1985, 428-503.

Norris SM, et al: Tables of antimicrobial agent pharmacology, in Mandell GL, et al (eds): *Principles and Practice of Infectious Diseases*, ed 3. New York, Churchill Livingstone, 1990, 434-460.

Oakes M, et al: Abnormal laboratory test values during ceftriaxone therapy. *Am J Med* 77(suppl 4C):89-96, 1984.

Oblinger MJ, et al: Moxalactam therapy vs standard antimicrobial therapy for selected serious infections. *Rev Infect Dis* 4(suppl):S639-S649, 1982.

Odio CM, et al: Cefotaxime vs. conventional therapy for treatment of bacterial meningitis of infants and children. *Pediatr Infect Dis* 5:402-407, 1986.

Overturf GD, et al: Treatment of bacterial meningitis with ceftizoxime. *Antimicrob Agents Chemother* 25:258-262, 1984.

Pakter RL, et al: Coagulopathy associated with use of moxalactam. *JAMA* 248:1100, 1982.

Panwalker AP, Rosenfeld J: Hemorrhage, diarrhea, and superinfection associated with use of moxalactam, letter. *J Infect Dis* 147:171-172, 1983.

Parks D, et al: Ceftizoxime: Clinical evaluation of efficacy and safety in the U.S.A. *J Antimicrob Chemother* 10 (suppl C):327-338, 1982.

Patel IH, Kaplan SA: Pharmacokinetic profile of ceftriaxone in man. *Am J Med* 77 (suppl 4C):17-25, 1984.

Pfenninger J, et al: Cefuroxime in bacterial meningitis. *Arch Dis Child* 57:539-543, 1982.

Philippon A, et al: Extended-spectrum β-lactamases. *Antimicrob Agents Chemother* 33:1131-1136, 1989.

Pigrau C, et al: Ceftriaxone-associated biliary pseudolithiasis in adults. *Lancet* 2:165, 1989.

Pizzo PA, et al: New beta-lactam antibiotics in granulocytopenic patients: New options and new questions. *Am J Med* 79 (suppl 2A):75-82, 1985.

Pizzo PA, et al: Randomized trial comparing ceftazidime alone with combination antibiotic therapy in cancer patients with fever and neutropenia. *N Engl J Med* 315:552-558, 1986.

Polk R: Ceftriaxone: Beta-lactamase-stable, broad-spectrum cephalosporin with an extended half-life, commentary. *Pharmacotherapy* 5:251-252, 1985.

Pontzer RE, Kaye D: Cefonicid: Long-acting, second-generation cephalosporin: Antimicrobial activity, pharmacokinetics, clinical efficacy, and adverse effects. *Pharmacotherapy* 4:325-333, 1984.

Portier H, et al: Interaction between cephalosporins and alcohol, letter. *Lancet* 2:263, 1980.

Quintiliani R, Nightingale CH: Cefazolin. *Ann Intern Med* 89 (part I):650-656, 1978.

Quintiliani R, et al: Cephalosporins: Overview, in Ristuccia AM, Cunha BA (eds): *Antimicrobial Therapy*. New York, Raven Press, 1984, 289-303.

Rahal JJ Jr: Moxalactam therapy for gram-negative bacillary meningitis. *Rev Infect Dis* 4 (suppl):S606-S609, 1982.

Rahal JJ, Simberkoff MS: Host defense and antimicrobial therapy in adult gram-negative bacillary meningitis. *Ann Intern Med* 96:468-474, 1982.

Ramphal R, et al: Early results of comparative trial of ceftazidime versus cephalothin, carbenicillin and gentamicin in treatment of febrile granulocytopenic patients. *J Antimicrob Chemother* 12 (suppl A):81-88, 1983.

Rapp RP, Blue D: Role of extended half-life second generation cephalosporins in surgical prophylaxis. *Drug Intell Clin Pharm* 19:214-215, 1985.

Rapp RP, et al: Ceftazidime versus tobramycin/ticarcillin in treating hospital acquired pneumonia and bacteremia. *Pharmacotherapy* 4:211-215, 1984.

Reese RE, Betts RF: Antibiotic use, in Reese RE, Douglas RG (eds): *A Practical Approach to Infectious Diseases*, ed 2. Boston, Little Brown and Company, 1986, 559-679.

Rehm SJ, McHenry MC: Oral antimicrobial drugs. *Med Clin North Am* 67:57-98, 1983.

Reilly JT, et al: Ceftazidime compared to tobramycin and ticarcillin in immunocompromised haematological patients. *J Antimicrob Chemother* 12 (suppl A):89-92, 1983.

Report from a Swedish Study Group: Cefuroxime versus ampicillin and chloramphenicol for treatment of bacterial meningitis. *Lancet* 1:295-298, 1982.

Richards DM, Brogden RN: Ceftazidime: Review of its antibacterial activity, pharmacokinetic properties, and therapeutic use. *Drugs* 29:105-161, 1985.

Richards DM, Heel RC: Ceftizoxime: Review of its antibacterial activity, pharmacokinetic properties, and therapeutic use. *Drugs* 29:281-329, 1985.

Richards DM, et al: Ceftriaxone: Review of its antibacterial activity, pharmacological properties and therapeutic use. *Drugs* 27:469-527, 1984.

Richmond MH, Sykes RG: β-lactamases of gram-negative bacteria and their possible physiological role. *Rev Microb Physiol* 9:31-88, 1973.

Rodriguez WJ, et al: Ceftazidime in treatment of meningitis in infants and children over one month of age. *Am J Med* 79 (suppl 2A):52-55, 1985.

Sahm DF, et al: β-lactam antibiotics: First- and second-generation cephalosporins. *Antimicrob Newslett* 2:25-28, 1985 A.

Sahm DF, et al: β-lactam antibiotics: Third-generation cephalosporins and other newer β-lactams. *Antimicrob Newslett* 2:33-40, 1985 B.

Saito A: Cefmetazole postmarketing surveillance in Japan. *J Antimicrob Chemother* 23 (suppl D):131-139, 1989.

Saltiel E, Brogden RN: Cefonicid: Review of its antibacterial activity, pharmacological properties and therapeutic use. *Drugs* 32:222-259, 1986.

Sanders CC: Novel resistance selected by new expanded-spectrum cephalosporins: Concern. *J Infect Dis* 147:585-589, 1983.

Sanders CC: Failure to detect resistance in antimicrobial susceptibility tests: "Very major" error of increasing concern. *Antimicrob Newslett* 1:27-31, 1984.

Sanders CC, Sanders WE Jr: Emergence of resistance during therapy with newer β-lactam antibiotics: Role of inducible β-lactamases and implications for the future. *Rev Infect Dis* 5:639-648, 1983.

Sanders CC, Sanders WE Jr: Microbial resistance to newer generation β-lactam antibiotics: Clinical and laboratory implications. *J Infect Dis* 151:399-406, 1985.

Sanders CC, Sanders WE: Type I β-lactamases of gram-negative bacteria: Interactions with β-lactam antibiotics. *J Infect Dis* 154:792-800, 1986.

Sanders CC, Sanders WE: Clinical importance of inducible beta-lactamases in gram-negative bacteria. *Eur J Clin Microbiol* 6:435-437, 1987.

Sanders CV, et al: Cefamandole and cefoxitin. *Ann Intern Med* 103:70-78, 1985.

Sanders CC, et al: Cephalosporins and cephamycins, in Peterson PK, Verhoef J (eds): *The Antimicrobial Agents Annual/3*. New York, Elsevier, 1988, 77-98.

Sattler FR, et al: Potential for bleeding with new beta-lactam antibiotics. *Ann Intern Med* 105:924-931, 1986.

Saxon A: Immediate hypersensitivity reactions to β-lactam antibiotics. *Rev Infect Dis* 5 (suppl 2):S368-S379, 1983.

Schaad UB, et al: Reversible ceftriaxone-associated biliary pseudolithiasis in children. *Lancet* 2:1411-1413, 1988.

Schaad UB, et al: Comparison of ceftriaxone and cefuroxime for treatment of bacterial meningitis in children. *N Engl J Med* 322:141-147, 1990.

Schleupner CJ, et al: Blinded comparison of cefuroxime to cefaclor for lower respiratory tract infections. *Arch Intern Med* 148:343-348, 1988.

Schwartz B, et al: Comparative efficacy of ceftriaxone and rifampicin in eradicating pharyngeal carriage of group A *Neisseria meningitidis*. *Lancet* 1:1239-1242, 1988.

Shearer MJ, et al: Mechanism of cephalosporin-induced hypoprothrombinemia: Relation to cephalosporin side chain, vitamin K metabolism, and vitamin K status. *J Clin Pharmacol* 28:88-95, 1988.

Sirot J, et al: *Klebsiella pneumoniae* and other Enterobacteriaceae producing novel plasmid-mediated β-lactamases markedly active against third-generation cephalosporins: Epidemiologic studies. *Rev Infect Dis* 10:850-859, 1988.

Slama TG, et al: Randomized comparison of cefamandole, cefazolin, and cefuroxime prophylaxis in open-heart surgery. *Antimicrob Agents Chemother* 29:744-747, 1986.

Slonaker CE, Luper WE: Moxalactam-associated platelet dysfunction, letter. *JAMA* 250:729-730, 1983.

Smith BR: Cefsulodin and ceftazidime, two antipseudomonal cephalosporins. *Clin Pharm* 3:373-385, 1984.

Smith BR, LeFrock JL: Cefuroxime: Antimicrobial activity, pharmacology, and clinical efficacy. *Ther Drug Monit* 5:149-160, 1983.

Smith BR, et al: Cefotetan pharmacokinetics in volunteers with various degrees of renal function. *Antimicrob Agents Chemother* 29:887-893, 1986.

Smith CR, et al: Cefotaxime compared with nafcillin plus tobramycin for serious bacterial infections: Randomized, double-blind trial. *Ann Intern Med* 101:469-477, 1984.

Smith CR, et al: Ceftriaxone compared with cefotaxime for serious bacterial infections. *J Infect Dis* 160:442-447, 1989.

Soe GB, Overturf GD: Treatment of typhoid fever and other systemic salmonelloses with cefotaxime, ceftriaxone, cefoperazone, and other newer cephalosporins. *Rev Infect Dis* 9:719-736, 1987.

Steele RW, Bradsher RW: Comparison of ceftriaxone with standard therapy for bacterial meningitis. *J Pediatr* 103:138-141, 1983.

Stockley IH: Disulfiram-type reaction with some cephalosporins. *Pharmaceut J* 234:239-240, 1985.

Stone HH, et al: Third-generation cephalosporins for polymicrobial surgical sepsis. *Arch Surg* 118:193-200, 1983.

Stutman HR, Marks MI: Therapy for bacterial meningitis: Which drugs, and for how long? *J Pediatr* 110:812-814, 1987.

Sweet RL, et al: Multicenter clinical trials comparing cefotetan with moxalactam or cefoxitin as therapy for obstetric and gynecologic infections. *Am J Surg* 155 (suppl 5A):56-60, 1988.

Sykes RB: Classification and terminology of enzymes that hydrolyze β-lactam antibiotics. *J Infect Dis* 145:762-765, 1982.

Sykes RB, Bonner DP: Aztreonam: First monobactam. *Am J Med* 78 (suppl 2A):2-10, 1985.

Sykes RB, Bush K: Interaction of new cephalosporins with β-lactamases and β-lactamase-producing gram-negative bacilli. *Rev Infect Dis* 5 (suppl 2):S356-S367, 1983.

Tally FP, et al: Randomized comparison of cefoxitin with or without amikacin and clindamycin plus amikacin in surgical sepsis. *Ann Surg* 193:318-323, 1981.

Tally FP, et al: Safety profile of cefixime. *Pediatr Infect Dis J* 6:976-980, 1987.

Tartaglione TA, Polk RE: Review of new second-generation cephalosporins: Cefonicid, ceforanide, and cefuroxime. *Drug Intell Clin Pharm* 19:188-198, 1985.

Taylor DN, et al: Comparative study of ceftriaxone and trimethoprim/sulfamethoxazole for treatment of chanchroid in Thailand. *J Infect Dis* 152:1002-1006, 1985.

Thirumoorthi MC, et al: Efficacy and safety of ceforanide in treatment of childhood infections. *Pediatr Infect Dis* 2:377-380, 1983.

Thompson RL: Cephalosporin, carbapenem, and monobactam antibiotics. *Mayo Clin Proc* 62:821-834, 1987.

Thompson RL, Wright AJ: Cephalosporin antibiotics. *Mayo Clin Proc* 58:79-87, 1983.

Thornsberry C: Review of in vitro activity of third-generation cephalosporins and other newer beta-lactam antibiotics against clinically important bacteria. *Am J Med* 79 (suppl 2A):14-20, 1985.

Wade JC, et al: Cephalothin plus aminoglycoside is more nephrotoxic than methicillin plus an aminoglycoside. *Lancet* 2:604-606, 1978.

Wade JC, et al: Monotherapy for empiric treatment of fever in granulocytopenic cancer patients. *Am J Med* 80 (suppl 5C):85-95, 1986.

Wallace RJ, et al: Ceforanide and cefazolin therapy of pneumonia: Comparative clinical trial. *Antimicrob Agents Chemother* 20:648-652, 1981.

Ward A, Richards DM: Cefotetan: Review of its antibacterial activity, pharmacokinetic properties and therapeutic use. *Drugs* 30:382-426, 1985.

Warren JW, et al: Randomized, controlled trial of cefoperazone vs cefamandole-tobramycin in treatment of putative, severe infections with gram-negative bacilli. *Rev Infect Dis* 5 (suppl):S173-S180, 1983.

Weitekamp MR, Aber RC: Prolonged bleeding times and bleeding diathesis associated with moxalactam administration. *JAMA* 249:69-71, 1983.

Weitekamp MR, et al: Effects of latamoxef, cefotaxime, and cefoperazone on platelet function and coagulation in normal volunteers. *J Antimicrob Chemother* 16:95-101, 1985.

Williams JO, Moosdeen F: In vitro antibacterial effects of cephalosporins. *Drugs* 34 (suppl 2):44-63, 1987.

Wilson SE, et al: Cephalosporin therapy in intra-abdominal infections: Multicenter randomized, comparative study of cefotetan, moxalactam, and cefoxitin. *Am J Surg* 155 (suppl 5A):61-66, 1988.

Witt LG, Witt LD: Cephalosporins and ethanol. *Drug Interact Newslett* 3:27-30, 1983.

Yangco BG, et al: Comparative efficacy and safety of ceftizoxime, cefotaxime and latamoxef in treatment of bacterial pneumonia in high risk patients. *J Antimicrob Chemother* 19:239-248, 1987.

Yangco BG, et al: Comparative evaluation of safety and efficacy of cefmetazole and cefoxitin in lower respiratory tract infections. *J Antimicrob Chemother* 23 (suppl D):39-46, 1989.

Young LS: Ceftazidime in treatment of nosocomial sepsis. *Am J Med* 79 (suppl 2A):89-95, 1985.

Young LS: Empirical antimicrobial therapy in neutropenic host, editorial. *N Engl J Med* 315:580-581, 1986.

Other Selected References

Cefamandole and cefoxitin. *Med Lett Drugs Ther* 21:13-15, 1979.

Two new oral cephalosporins. *Med Lett Drugs Ther* 21:85-87, 1979.

Cefotaxime sodium (Claforan). *Med Lett Drugs Ther* 23:61-62, 1981.

Moxalactam disodium (Moxam). *Med Lett Drugs Ther* 24:13-14, 1982.

Ceftizoxime sodium (Cefizox). *Med Lett Drugs Ther* 25:109-110, 1983.

Current and future directions in use of antimicrobial agents. *Bull NY Acad Med* 60:313-446, 1984 (13 papers).

Andriole VT, Kirby WMM (eds): Use of cefoperazone and other injectable antibiotics in patients with altered host defense. *Am J Med* 85 (suppl 1A):1-58 (11 papers).

Barza M, et al (eds): Efficacy and cost implications of new cephalosporins. *Am J Surg* 155 (suppl 5A):1-110, 1988.

Brogden RN, et al: Cefoxitin: Review of its antibacterial activity, pharmacological properties and therapeutic use. *Drugs* 17:1-37, 1979.

Brogden RN, et al: Cefoperazone: Review of in vitro antimicrobial activity, pharmacological properties and therapeutic efficacy. *Drugs* 22:423-460, 1981.

Cherubin CE, et al (eds): Current status of cefotaxime sodium: New cephalosporin. *Rev Infect Dis* 4 (suppl):S281-S488, 1982 (27 papers).

Conte JE Jr (ed): Clinical and economic impact of cefonicid. *Rev Infect Dis* 6 (suppl 4):S777-S937, 1984 (24 papers).

Cunha BA, Ristuccia AM: Third generation cephalosporins. *Med Clin North Am* 66:283-291, 1982.

Farber BF, Moellering RC Jr: New cephalosporins. *Drug Ther* 12:51-59, (May) 1982.

Finch R, et al: Cefmetazole: Clinical appraisal. *J Antimicrob Chemother* 23 (suppl D):1-142, 1989 (18 papers).

Finegold SM, Kirby WMM (eds): Changing patterns of hospital infections: Implications for therapy. *Am J Med* 77 (suppl 1B):1-41, 1984 (6 papers).

Geddes AM, et al (eds): Cefotaxime: New cephalosporin antibiotic. *J Antimicrob Chemother* 6 (suppl A):1-303, 1980 (55 papers).

Gleckman R: Third-generation cephalosporins: Plea for restraint, editorial. *JAMA* 142:1267-1268, 1982.

Hoffbrand BI, Kory M (eds): Cephalexin: Twelve years of clinical and laboratory experience. *Postgrad Med J* 59 (suppl 5):1-56, 1983 (9 papers).

Jones RN, et al (eds): Workshop on five years of clinical experience with cefotaxime (with special references to gram-positive infections). *Infection* 13 (suppl 1):S1-S162, 1985 (32 papers).

Klein JO, Neu HC (eds): Empiric therapy of bacterial infections: Evaluation of cefoperazone. *Rev Infect Dis* 5 (suppl 1):S1-S209, 1983 (22 papers).

Lambert HP, et al (eds): Ceftazidime in clinical practice. *J Antimicrob Chemother* 12 (suppl A):1-414, 1983 (63 papers).

Lyon JA: Cefoperazone (Cefobid, Pfizer). *Drug Intell Clin Pharm* 17:7-11, 1983.

Mandell GL, Sande MA: Cephalosporins, in Gilman AG, et al (eds): *The Pharmacological Basis of Therapeutics,* ed 7. New York, Macmillan, 1985, 1137-1149.

McCracken GH (ed): Cefixime: Clinical overview of new oral third-generation cephalosporin. *Am J Med* 85 (suppl 3A): 1-25, 1988 (5 papers).

Moellering RC Jr (ed): Clinical significance of newer beta-lactam antibiotics: Focus on cefuroxime. *Therapeutics Today Series*. New York, ADIS Press, 1983, vol 3, 1-126 (13 papers).

Moellering RC Jr (ed): Ceftriaxone: Long-acting cephalosporin. *Am J Med* 77 (suppl 4C): 1-118, 1984 (21 papers).

Moellering RC Jr (ed): Symposium on ceftriaxone: Long-acting cephalosporin. *Am J Surg* 148 (suppl 4A): 1-43, 1984 (10 papers).

Moellering RC Jr, Waldvogel FA (eds): Cefaclor. *Clin Ther* 11 (suppl A): 1-96, 1988 (10 papers).

Moellering RC Jr, Young LS (eds): Moxalactam international symposium. *Rev Infect Dis* 4 (suppl): S489-S726, 1982 (38 papers).

Nahata MC, Barson WJ: Ceftriaxone: Third generation cephalosporin. *Drug Intell Clin Pharm* 19:900-906, 1985.

Neu HC (ed): Advances in cephalosporin therapy: Beyond the third generation. *Am J Med* 79 (suppl 2A): 1-118, 1985 (19 papers).

Neu HC, Phillips I (eds): Cefotaxime. *J Antimicrob Chemother* 14 (suppl B): 1-344, 1984 (50 papers).

Neu HC, Barza M (eds): Efficacy and cost implications of new cephalosporins. *Am J Obstet Gynecol* 158:687-746, 1988 (13 papers).

Neu HC, McCracken GH (eds): Proceedings of conference: Clinical pharmacology and efficacy of cefixime *Pediatr Infect Dis J* 6:951-1009, 1987.

Neu HC, et al (eds): Ceftizoxime, broad-spectrum β-lactamase stable cephalosporin. *J Antimicrob Chemother* 10 (suppl C): 1-355, 1982 (46 papers).

Neu HC, et al (eds): Cefotaxime: Proceedings from 15th International Congress of Chemotherapy. *Drugs* 35 (suppl 2): 1-231, 1988 (48 papers).

Neu HC, et al (eds): Third-generation cephalosporins: Decade of progress in treatment of severe infections. *Am J Med* 88 (suppl 4A): 15S:-45S, 1990 (8 papers).

Phillips I, Wise R (eds): Role of cefadroxil in oral antibiotic therapy. *J Antimicrob Chemother* 10 (suppl B): 1-162, 1982 (24 papers).

Phillips I, et al (eds): Cefotetan: New cephamycin. *J Antimicrob Chemother* 11 (suppl A): 1-239, 1983 (32 papers).

Polk RE: Moxalactam (Moxam, Eli Lilly). *Drug Intell Clin Pharm* 16:104-114, 1982.

Quintiliani R (ed): Symposium on cefotetan. *Am J Obstet Gynecol* 154:945-963, 1986 (4 papers).

Quintiliani R, et al: First and second generation cephalosporins. *Med Clin North Am* 66:183-197, 1982.

Smith GH: Oral cephalosporins in perspective. *DICP* 24:45-51, 1990.

Williams JD (ed): Cephalosporin antibiotics. *Drugs* 34 (suppl 2): 1-258, 1987 (17 papers).

Williams JD, Casewell MW (eds): Ceftazidime. *J Antimicrob Chemother* 8 (suppl B): 1-358, 1981 (61 papers).

New Evaluation 64

CEFPODOXIME PROXETIL
[Vantin]

Cefpodoxime proxetil is a semisynthetic prodrug conjugate of cefpodoxime, a broad-spectrum iminomethoxy aminothiazolyl cephalosporin. Following oral administration, cefpodoxime, the active moiety, is released in the gastrointestinal tract by de-esterification of cefpodoxime proxetil. Unless otherwise specified, the following discussion refers only to cefpodoxime.

MECHANISM OF ACTION, ANTIMICROBIAL SPECTRUM, AND RESISTANCE. This bactericidal drug has a mechanism of action similar to that of other β-lactam antibiotics. Its primary target appears to be penicillin-binding protein (PBP) 3, a cell wall component involved in cell division. Binding inhibits growth and causes filamentation of susceptible bacteria (Wise et al, 1990).

The in vitro antimicrobial spectrum of cefpodoxime is similar to that of cefixime, another iminomethoxy aminothiazolyl oral cephalosporin (Chin and Neu, 1988; Jones and Barry, 1988; Wise et al, 1990). At in vitro concentrations of $\leq$2 mcg/ml, cefpodoxime inhibits the growth of many aerobic gram-negative bacteria, including most Enterobacteriaceae (eg, *Escherichia coli, Klebsiella pneumoniae, Citrobacter diversus, Proteus mirabilis*), *Salmonella* species, *Shigella* species, and *Yersinia enterocolitica*. Its in vitro potency against *Morganella morganii* and species of *Enterobacter, Aeromonas*, and *Providencia* is variable. Many isolates of the latter three genera are resistant, as are most isolates of *Acinetobacter, Pseudomonas, Serratia*, and *Bacteroides fragilis* (Fass and Helsel, 1988; Wise et al, 1990; Sheppard et al, 1991). Similarly, *Bordetella pertussis* and *B. parapertussis* are resistant (minimum inhibitory concentration [MIC] for 90% of isolates >16 mcg/ml) (Hoppe and Müller, 1990). In contrast, cefpodoxime is extremely potent in vitro against the common fastidious gram-negative pathogens, *Haemophilus influenzae* and *Moraxella catarrhalis*, and the pathogenic Neisseriaceae, *Neisseria gonorrhoeae* and *N. meningitidis*, including β lactamase-producing isolates. In general, its in vitro potency is equivalent to or slightly less than that of cefixime against most susceptible gram-negative bacteria but is substantially greater than that of other oral cephalosporins (eg, cephalexin, cefaclor, cefuroxime axetil) and amoxicillin.

The majority of penicillin-susceptible hemolytic streptococci (eg, groups A, B, C, F, and G) and *S. pneumoniae* (Chin and Neu, 1988; Fass and Helsel, 1988; Jones and Barry, 1988) are extremely susceptible to cefpodoxime in vitro (MIC <0.06 mcg/ml). When tested against these isolates, it generally is equivalent or slightly superior to amoxicillin (alone or with potassium clavulanate), cefixime, and cefuroxime and usually is substantially more potent than cefaclor and cephalexin. In vitro, the growth of penicillin-resistant pneumococci may be inhibited by cefpodoxime, but this effect is inconsistent (Jones and Barry, 1988). Cefpodoxime generally appears to be as potent or more potent in vitro (MIC 4 mcg/ml or greater) against *Staphylococcus aureus* (methicillin-susceptible, penicillin-susceptible, or resistant) and most coagulase-negative staphylococci than cefaclor, cefixime (Fass and Helsel, 1988; Wise et al, 1990), and cephalexin. Methicillin-resistant staphylococci and enterococci (eg, *Enterococcus faecalis, E. faecium*) are resistant to cefpodoxime. Isolates of *Listeria monocytogenes* and *Corynebacterium* species group JK also are resistant to cefpodoxime, but some clostridia are susceptible (Chin and Neu, 1988).

Like cefuroxime and cefixime, cefpodoxime is not hydrolyzed by most plasmid-coded β lactamases (Chin and Neu, 1988; Wise et al, 1990). Because of this stability, the activity of cefpodoxime is not substantially reduced when the inoculum of bacteria (eg, staphylococci, *H. influenzae, E. coli, Klebsiella*) that produce these enzymes is increased. In contrast, cefpodoxime is degraded by certain chromosomal cephalosporinases (eg, Type I) and thus bacteria that produce these enzymes (eg, *Enterobacter cloacae*) are subject to an inoculum effect with $>10^7$ colony-forming units [cfu]/ml (Jones and Barry, 1988; Wise et al, 1990).

USES. Because of its broad in vitro antimicrobial spectrum of activity and pharmacokinetic properties (see below), oral cefpodoxime proxetil may be effective in the treatment of a wide range of mild to moderate infections caused by common bacterial pathogens. These include infections of the upper (eg, acute otitis media and sinusitis, pharyngitis/tonsillitis) and lower (eg, acute bronchitis, acute exacerbations of chronic bronchitis, community-acquired pneumonia) respiratory tracts, uncomplicated urinary tract infections, infections of the skin and skin structures, and sexually transmitted diseases (eg, gonorrhea).

Cefpodoxime proxetil has been compared with several established antimicrobial agents in randomized clinical trials in adults with infections of the upper respiratory tract (for reviews, see Safran, 1990; Bergogne-Berezin, 1991). Doses of 100 mg twice daily appear to be as effective and well tolerated as standard regimens of potassium penicillin V, cefuroxime axetil, and amoxicillin in adults with acute pharyngitis/tonsillitis. In most of these studies, clinical cure and bacterial eradication rates >95% were observed in patients given cefpodoxime proxetil or the other agents. The results of a small, randomized trial in children aged 2 to 16 years suggest that cefpodoxime proxetil is as effective and well tolerated in this age group as potassium penicillin V in the treatment of pharyngitis/tonsillitis due to group A streptococci (Kline and Kline, 1991). However, cefpodoxime is considerably more expensive than potassium penicillin V, and the efficacy of cefpodoxime in preventing subsequent rheumatic fever in pediatric patients is not established. Thus, it is not recommended for this use.

In a randomized study in adults with acute sinusitis due to common bacterial pathogens (eg, *H. influenzae, S. pneumoniae, M. catarrhalis*), cefpodoxime proxetil 200 mg twice daily was as effective as cefaclor 500 mg three times daily (95% versus 93% clinical cure plus improvement, respectively) (Gehanno et al, 1990). Summary results of clinical trial data on 83 Japanese patients with sinusitis indicated that cefpodoxime proxetil produced lower cure rates (70%) in sinusitis. However, the treatment protocol(s) was not fully described (Kumazawa, 1991).

Data on the efficacy of cefpodoxime proxetil in acute otitis media (AOM) are limited. In a review of clinical trials in children given this drug in suspension form, cure or improvement in six of nine patients with AOM was reported (Fujii, 1991). Similar results were reported in a larger number (169 of 247) of Japanese adults with AOM, but study parameters were not given (Kumazawa, 1991). In a recent comparative trial on patients with AOM, the efficacy of cefpodoxime administered twice daily was similar to that of amoxicillin/potassium clavulanate administered three times daily (Mendelman et al, 1992). Thus, although the in vitro antimicrobial spectrum of cefpodoxime encompasses the predominant pathogens that cause AOM and preliminary data suggest it is clinically effective, more comparative data are needed to fully assess the role of this drug in treating AOM.

The use of cefpodoxime proxetil in lower respiratory tract infections has been studied in a number of double-blind, randomized trials (for reviews, see Safran, 1990; Geddes, 1991). When given at a dosage of 200 mg twice daily for 5 to 10 days, cefpodoxime proxetil was as effective as amoxicillin 500 mg three times daily in adults with community-acquired pneumonia caused primarily by *S. pneumoniae* and *H. influenzae*. In these trials, the clinical response was judged to be satisfactory in 90% and 93% of evaluable patients given cefpodoxime proxetil and amoxicillin, respectively, and the bacteriologic responses were satisfactory in 100% and 94% of patients, respectively. A 10-day trial compared the efficacy of cefpodoxime proxetil 200 mg twice daily with that of intramuscularly administered ceftriaxone 1 g daily in hospitalized, high-risk patients (eg, those with additional risk factors, including age 65 years or more, smoking, diabetes, alcoholism, drug addiction, malnutrition) who had confirmed bacterial pneumonia caused by *S. pneumoniae, H. influenzae, Klebsiella* species, and other gram-negative bacilli (Zuck et al, 1990). An overall favorable response, defined as improvement or cure, was observed in the two groups (98% in the cefpodoxime proxetil group versus 95% in the ceftriaxone group). The bacteriologic response was satisfactory in 94% and 97% of patients given cefpodoxime proxetil and ceftriaxone, respectively. Further study is required to determine whether cefpodoxime proxetil may be useful in outpatients who previously would have required hospitalization for this infection.

Cefpodoxime proxetil also was compared with amoxicillin 250 mg three times daily for seven days in two randomized, double-blind trials in patients with acute bronchitis or acute exacerbations of chronic bronchitis (AECB) caused by *Haemophilus* species, *M. catarrhalis, S. pneumoniae,* or mixed infections with these pathogens (see Geddes, 1991). Dosages of cefpodoxime proxetil 100 or 200 mg twice daily produced results similar to those with standard regimens of amoxicillin in clinical (85% and 86% versus 88% and 86%, respectively) and bacteriologic (94% and 94% versus 85% and 88%, respectively) response. In another randomized trial, cefpodoxime proxetil 200 mg twice daily was comparable to amoxicillin/potassium clavulanate 500/125 mg three times daily in both clinical and bacteriologic efficacy in patients with AECB caused by *H. influenzae, S. aureus, M. catarrhalis,* and *S. pneumoniae* (Periti et al, 1990).

In two seven-day randomized trials in patients with uncomplicated infections of the urinary tract, cefpodoxime proxetil 100 mg twice daily was compared with cefaclor or amoxicillin, each 250 mg three times daily (Cox et al, 1991). The most common pathogens isolated were *E. coli, Klebsiella* species, *P. mirabilis,* and *S. saprophyticus*. Cure rates were 79%, 79%, and 72% in patients who received cefpodoxime proxetil, cefaclor, and amoxicillin, respectively; the corresponding bacteriologic eradication rates were 80%, 82%, and 70%. These results are consistent with data from clinical trials in Japan, which established the efficacy and safety of cefpodoxime proxetil in the treatment of urinary tract infections (Kumazawa, 1991). However, these eradication rates are somewhat lower than those observed with drugs from other classes (eg, fluoroquinolones).

Cefpodoxime proxetil has been evaluated in a single noncomparative trial in adults with mild to moderate skin and skin structure infections, primarily abscesses, cellulitis, and wound infections, most commonly due to *S. aureus, S. epidermidis, S. pyogenes*, and *E. coli* (Tack et al, 1991). Most of the patients received cefpodoxime proxetil 200 mg twice daily; those with severe infections received 400 mg twice daily. Both groups were treated for 7 to 14 days. Clinical cure or improvement occurred in 100% of patients, and overall the bacterial eradication rates were 98% and 100% in the 200-mg and 400-mg recipients, respectively. A favorable clinical response rate of 85% was reported in a summary of Japanese experience with cefpodoxime proxetil in patients with infections of the skin and skin structures, but the complete treatment protocol(s) was not given (Kumazawa, 1991). Because of the relatively weak activity of cefpodoxime against *S. aureus,* more clinical trials comparing this drug with established agents are necessary to confirm these data and determine its role for these indications.

Published data demonstrating the clinical effectiveness of cefpodoxime proxetil in sexually transmitted diseases (eg, gonorrhea) are unavailable at present. However, gonococci are highly susceptible to cefpodoxime and this drug is approved for the treatment of acute uncomplicated urethral and cervical gonorrhea and anorectal infections in women. The role of cefpodoxime in the treatment of chancroid is unknown, and it is not effective against chlamydia.

For additional information on established and alternative drugs for all of the preceding indications, see index entry Antimicrobial Drugs.

ADVERSE REACTIONS AND PRECAUTIONS. Cefpodoxime proxetil is generally well tolerated when given in multiple doses to adults and pediatric patients. However, as with other broad-spectrum antibiotics, administration of cefpodoxime may be associated with the occurrence of antibiotic-associated pseudomembranous colitis. The spectrum and frequency of other adverse reactions are similar to those associated with other oral β-lactam drugs (eg, amoxicillin with or without potassium clavulanate, potassium penicillin V, other cephalosporins).

This agent is classified in FDA Pregnancy Category B.

For a detailed discussion of the adverse reactions and precautions associated with the use of cephalosporins, see the Introduction to this chapter.

DRUG INTERACTIONS. The bioavailability of cefpodoxime proxetil may be reduced by approximately 40% when this drug is administered with the H_2 receptor antagonist, famotidine, or the antacid, aluminum magnesium hydroxide [Maalox] (Saathoff et al, 1992). Corresponding changes were observed in the maximal plasma concentrations, 24-hour urine recovery, and time to maximum concentration of drug in serum. These effects have been attributed to an increase in the gastric pH, which reduces the stability and rate of dissolution of the drug. Therefore, at least two hours should elapse between ingestion of an antacid or histamine H_2 antagonist and cefpodoxime proxetil. No other significant drug interactions have been reported for cefpodoxime proxetil.

PHARMACOKINETICS. Following its absorption by the gastrointestinal epithelial cells, cefpodoxime proxetil is de-esterified by nonspecific esterases, releasing the active moiety, cefpodoxime.

The pharmacokinetics of the tablet and suspension formulations of cefpodoxime proxetil are linear after single or multiple doses of 100 to 400 mg. However, there is evidence that the rate and extent of drug absorption are dose dependent (for review, see Borin, 1991). The absolute bioavailability of this drug is 50%. The extent but not the rate of absorption of the tablet formulation is enhanced by the presence of food; food has no effect on the extent but decreases the rate of absorption of the suspension. Single- and multiple-dose (every 12 hours) administration of 100 to 400 mg of cefpodoxime proxetil produces average peak plasma concentrations ranging from 1 to 4.5 mcg/ml. In general, a peak plasma concentration of approximately 1 mcg/ml can be expected for each 100 mg of cefpodoxime proxetil. The maximal plasma concentration occurs approximately two to three hours after administration of up to 400 mg. Average 12-hour trough plasma concentrations of approximately 0.09 mcg/ml, 0.15 mcg/ml, and 0.28 mcg/ml have been observed following twice-daily administration of 100, 200, or 400 mg, respectively, for 15 days to healthy volunteers.

Cefpodoxime is distributed throughout all body compartments as evidenced by a volume of distribution of approximately 32 L. This large volume of distribution is attributed to cefpodoxime's low plasma protein binding (range, 21% to 29%). After a 100- or 200-mg dose, clinically effective concentrations of cefpodoxime are detected in most tissues and fluids (eg, bile, blister fluid, lung, maxillary sinus mucosa, myometrium, pleural fluid, prostatic tissue, seminal fluid, tonsillar tissue), and these levels are maintained at most sites for up to 12 hours. Very low concentrations of cefpodoxime (<0.08 mcg/ml) have been detected in breast milk.

Cefpodoxime is eliminated from the body primarily by glomerular filtration and tubular secretion. After doses of 100 to 800 mg, approximately 24% to 41% of the dose is recovered in the urine as cefpodoxime, with 90% of this excreted in the first 12 hours. In the urine, concentrations of up to 60 mcg/ml have been observed after a 100-mg dose and up to 196 mcg/ml after an 800-mg dose. Concurrent administration of probenecid decreases urinary excretion of cefpodoxime and can increase maximal serum concentrations by 20%. Renal clearance may be decreased and cefpodoxime may accumulate in patients with impaired renal function; to avoid this, the dosage interval should be increased. Because age has no clinically significant effect on renal clearance of cefpodoxime, dosage adjustment is not necessary in elderly patients with normal age-adjusted creatinine clearance. This drug is removed by hemodialysis, but therapeutic serum concentrations may still be present after a routine dialysis procedure.

Cefpodoxime undergoes minimal hepatic biotransformation. Therefore, it is not necessary to adjust the dose in patients with impaired liver function. The unabsorbed drug is extensively degraded in the gastrointestinal tract and excreted in the feces.

DOSAGE AND PREPARATIONS. The drug should be administered with food to enhance absorption.

Oral: The following doses are given to patients with mild to moderate infections caused by susceptible bacteria: *Adults and children over 13 years* (tablets and suspension), acute community-acquired pneumonia, 200 mg twice daily for 14 days; pharyngitis/tonsillitis, 100 mg twice daily for 10 days; skin and skin structure, 400 mg twice daily for 7 to 14 days; uncomplicated urinary tract, 100 mg twice daily for seven days. For uncomplicated gonorrhea (men and women) and rectal gonococcal infections (women), the manufacturer recommends 200 mg in a single dose. *Children 6 months to 12 years* (suspension), for acute otitis media, 5 mg/kg (maximum, 200 mg/dose) twice daily for 10 days; pharyngitis/tonsillitis, 5 mg/kg (maximum, 100 mg/dose) twice daily for 10 days.

For patients with severe renal impairment (creatinine clearance <30 ml/min), the dosing interval should be increased to 24 hours.

Vantin (Upjohn). Tablets 100 and 200 mg; granules (flavored) 50 and 100 mg/5 ml after suspension in water.

Cited References

Bergogne-Berezin E: Cefpodoxime proxetil in upper respiratory tract infections. *Drugs* 42(suppl 3):25-33, 1991.

Borin MT: A review of the pharmacokinetics of cefpodoxime proxetil. *Drugs* 42(suppl 3):13-21, 1991.

Chin N-X, Neu HC: In vitro activity of an oral iminomethoxy aminothiazolyl cephalosporin, R-3745. *Antimicrob Agents Chemother* 32:671-677, 1988.

Cox CE, et al: Review of clinical experience in the United States with cefpodoxime proxetil in adults with uncomplicated urinary tract infections. *Drugs* 42(suppl 3):41-50, 1991.

Fass RJ, Helsel VL: In vitro activity of U-76,252 (CS-807), a new oral cephalosporin. *Antimicrob Agents Chemother* 32:1082-1085, 1988.

Fujii R: Clinical trials of cefpodoxime proxetil suspension in paediatrics. *Drugs* 42(suppl 3):57-60, 1991.

Geddes AM: Cefpodoxime proxetil in the treatment of lower respiratory tract infections. *Drugs* 42(suppl 3):34-40, 1991.

Gehanno P, et al: Comparison of cefpodoxime proxetil with cefaclor in the treatment of sinusitis. *J Antimicrob Chemother* 26(suppl E):87-91, 1990.

Hoppe JE, Müller J: In vitro susceptibilities of *Bordetella pertussis* and *Bordetella parapertussis* to six new oral cephalosporins. *Antimicrob Agents Chemother* 34:1442-1443, 1990.

Jones RN, Barry AL: Antimicrobial activity and disk diffusion susceptibility testing of U-76,253A (R-3746), the active metabolite of the new cephalosporin ester, U-76,252 (CS-807). *Antimicrob Agents Chemother* 32:443-449, 1988.

Kline NE, Kline MW: Cefpodoxime proxetil versus penicillin V in the treatment of streptococcal pharyngitis in children. *Curr Ther Res* 49:807-813, 1991.

Kumazawa J: Summary of clinical experience with cefpodoxime proxetil in adults in Japan. *Drugs* 42(suppl 3):1-5, 1991.

Mendelman PM, et al: Cefpodoxime proxetil compared with amoxicillin-clavulanate for the treatment of otitis media. *J Pediatr* 121:459-465, 1992.

Periti P, et al: Efficacy and tolerance of cefpodoxime proxetil compared with coamoxiclav in the treatment of exacerbations of chronic bronchitis. *J Antimicrob Chemother* 26(suppl E):63-69, 1990.

Saathoff N, et al: Pharmacokinetics of cefpodoxime proxetil and interactions with an antacid and an H_2 receptor antagonist. *Antimicrob Agents Chemother* 36:796-800, 1992.

Safran C: Cefpodoxime proxetil: Dosage, efficacy and tolerance in adults suffering from respiratory tract infections. *J Antimicrob Chemother* 26(suppl E):93-101, 1990.

Sheppard M, et al: In vitro activity of cefpodoxime, a new oral cephalosporin, compared with that of nine other antimicrobial agents. *Eur J Clin Microbiol Infect Dis* 10:573-581, 1991.

Tack KJ, et al: Cefpodoxime proxetil in the treatment of skin and soft tissue infections. *Drugs* 42(suppl 3):51-56, 1991.

Wise R, et al: The in-vitro activity of cefpodoxime: A comparison with other oral cephalosporins. *J Antimicrob Chemother* 25:541-550, 1990.

Zuck P, et al: Efficacy and tolerance of cefpodoxime proxetil compared with ceftriaxone in vulnerable patients with bronchopneumonia. *J Antimicrob Chemother* 26(suppl E):71-77, 1990.

New Evaluation 64

CEFPROZIL
[Cefzil]

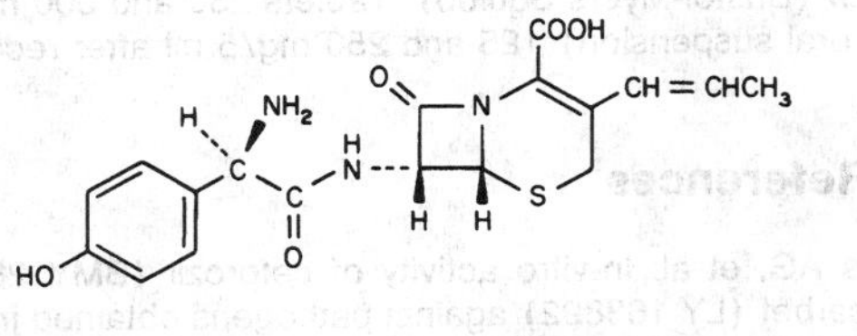

This semisynthetic, orally administered, broad spectrum cephem cephalosporin is structurally similar to cephalexin, cefadroxil, and cefaclor.

MECHANISM OF ACTION, ANTIMICROBIAL SPECTRUM, AND RESISTANCE. Although the mechanism of action, antimicrobial spectrum, and resistance properties of cefprozil are generally similar to those of other oral cephalosporins (cephalexin, cefadroxil, cefaclor, cefuroxime axetil), it is more potent on a weight basis. Thus, this drug has good to excellent bactericidal activity in vitro against most aerobic gram-positive cocci (eg, staphylococci, beta-hemolytic streptococci) with the exception of most species of enterococci, viridans group streptococci, and all methicillin-resistant staphylococcal strains (Eliopoulos et al, 1987; Chin and Neu, 1987). Compared with the older oral analogues (eg, cephalexin, cefadroxil), cefprozil has moderate to good in vitro activity against many aerobic gram-negative bacteria, including *Haemophilus influenzae, Moraxella (Branhamella) catarrhalis, Neisseria gonorrheae, Escherichia coli, Klebsiella pneumoniae, Proteus mirabilis*, and species of *Shigella, Salmonella,* and *Vibrio*. It is inactive in vitro against *Citrobacter freundii, Proteus vulgaris, Serratia marcescens, Morganella morganii, Providencia stuartii*, and most *Pseudomonas* and *Enterobacter* strains (Eliopoulos et al, 1987; Chin and Neu, 1987; Scribner et al, 1987). Cefprozil has good in vitro activity against many anaerobic species, including *Clostridium, Fusobacterium, Peptostreptococcus*, and *Propionibacterium*; it does not inhibit most strains of the *Bacteroides fragilis* group.

Cefprozil is not hydrolyzed by the plasmid-encoded β-lactamases produced by *H. influenzae, M. catarrhalis*, or staphylococci and is more stable than cefaclor in the presence of these enzymes. Its activity is diminished in acidic environments ($\leq$ pH 5) and is adversely affected by large ($>10^7$ CFU/ml) bacterial inocula (Arguedas et al, 1991 A).

USES. Cefprozil has good to excellent activity against bacteria that commonly cause acute otitis media and infections of the upper and lower respiratory tract, urinary tract, and skin. However, because it is given orally, cefprozil is indicated only for mild to moderate illnesses.

In a small, comparative, randomized trial in children with acute otitis media caused by *Streptococcus pneumoniae, H. influenzae*, or *M. catarrhalis*, clinical and bacteriologic cure rates with cefprozil 15 mg/kg twice daily were comparable to those with amoxicillin/potassium clavulanate 40 mg/kg daily in three divided doses (Arguedas et al, 1991 B). In this study, children who received cefprozil had only mild, reversible adverse reactions and none discontinued therapy.

In patients with acute uncomplicated urinary tract infections caused predominantly by *E. coli*, cefprozil 500 mg once daily was comparable to cefaclor 250 mg three times daily; the cure rate was approximately 90% after ten days of therapy (Christenson et al, 1991 A; Iravani, 1991). Although reversible adverse reactions (nausea, leukopenia, vaginal fungal infections) were more common in the patients treated with cefprozil, the differences were not statistically significant. The efficacy of cefprozil after shorter courses of treatment (eg, one to three days) for urinary tract infections is unknown.

Cefprozil given once daily also appears to be promising as an alternative to other established agents for the treatment of acute group A beta-hemolytic streptococcal (GABHS) pharyngitis (Christenson et al, 1991 B). However, once-daily dosing may be appropriate only in the mildest cases, for which antimicrobial intervention may not be required at all. In more severe cases, antibiotic therapy of sufficient potency and duration must be given to prevent the possible development of rheumatic fever as a complication of this infection.

Current data suggest that the efficacy of cefprozil in mild to moderate otitis media, urinary tract infections, and GABHS pharyngitis is comparable to that of established oral agents. Because of this and its favorable pharmacokinetic profile (see below) relative to other oral cephalosporins, cefprozil is a reasonable alternative when oral therapy is indicated. However, additional studies in larger patient samples are required to determine its role in these situations. Similarly, until sufficient data become available on the efficacy and safety of cefprozil in the treatment of infections caused by susceptible bacteria in the lower respiratory tract and skin and skin structures, its role in treating these conditions cannot be adequately evaluated.

ADVERSE REACTIONS AND PRECAUTIONS. The type and frequency of adverse reactions caused by cefprozil are essentially the same as those caused by other oral cephalosporins. This drug is generally well tolerated when given orally in single or multiple doses (Barbhaiya et al, 1990 A, 1990 B). Headache, nausea, diarrhea, dizziness, and rash have been reported; however, only 2% of patients have discontinued treatment because of adverse effects.

Cefprozil is classified in FDA Pregnancy Category B and should be used by pregnant women only if clearly needed.

For a more detailed discussion of the adverse reactions and precautions associated with use of cephalosporins, see the Introduction to this chapter.

DRUG INTERACTIONS AND INTERFERENCE WITH LABORATORY TESTS. See the Introduction to this chapter.

PHARMACOKINETICS. Cefprozil is well absorbed from the gastrointestinal tract; bioavailability is approximately 95%. Plasma protein binding approaches 36% and is independent of concentration in the range of 2 to 20 mcg/ml. Mean peak plasma levels of approximately 6.2, 9.3, and 17.7 mcg/ml occur within 1.5 hours after single oral doses of 250 mg, 500 mg, and 1 g, respectively (Barbhaiya et al, 1990 A). The maximal plasma concentrations do not change significantly after multiple dosing (Barbhaiya et al, 1990 B) and do not appear to be significantly affected by the presence of food in the gastrointestinal tract (Barbhaiya et al, 1990 C).

The elimination half-life is approximately 1.3 hours, and the area under the plasma drug concentration-time curve (AUC) is double that of cefaclor (Barbhaiya et al, 1990 C). Consequently, plasma levels of cefprozil remain above the minimum inhibitory concentration (MIC) for susceptible organisms longer than with similar oral cephalosporins (eg, cefaclor, cefadroxil, cephalexin). As indicated by results obtained in a skin blister fluid model, cefprozil may produce higher tissue concentrations that are maintained for a longer period than with cefaclor (Barbhaiya et al, 1990 D). Results of a small study in pediatric patients (aged 8 months to 8 years) showed that the mean peak plasma concentration and elimination half-life of cefprozil slightly exceed those observed in healthy adult volunteers (Sáez-Llorens et al, 1990). Since accumulation of other cephalosporins has been reported in neonates, cefprozil also may accumulate in these infants.

Cefprozil is eliminated primarily by glomerular filtration and tubular secretion; mean urinary concentrations range from 175 to 658 mcg/ml during the first four hours following single oral doses of 250 mg and 1 g, respectively (Barbhaiya et al, 1990 A). The mean urinary recovery of this drug ranges from 57% to 70% of the dose. The manufacturer has reported that concomitant administration of probenecid doubles the AUC of cefprozil (see manufacturer's literature).

Adjustment of the dosage has been recommended in patients with a creatinine clearance of 30 ml/min or less and in those undergoing hemodialysis (Shyu et al, 1991). The plasma half-life may reach 5.2 hours in patients with severe renal dysfunction; in those with no renal function, it may be as long as 5.9 hours. Hepatic impairment does not necessitate a reduction in dosage.

DOSAGE AND PREPARATIONS.

Oral: *Adults*, 500 mg to 1 g daily in two divided doses for up to 10 days, depending on the severity of the infection and susceptibility of the causative or suspected organism; for infections due to *Streptococcus pyogenes*, cefprozil should be administered for at least 10 days. Mild to moderate urinary tract infections due to susceptible organisms may be treated with a single daily dose of 500 mg to 1 g for 10 days.

Children and infants over 6 months, 30 mg/kg daily in two divided doses for 10 days. Efficacy and safety in *children under 6 months* have not been established.

Cefzil (Bristol-Myers Squibb). Tablets 250 and 500 mg; powder (for oral suspension) 125 and 250 mg/5 ml after reconstitution.

Cited References

Arguedas AG, et al: In-vitro activity of cefprozil (BMY 28100) and loracarbef (LY 163892) against pathogens obtained from middle ear fluid. *J Antimicrob Chemother* 27:311-318, 1991 A.

Arguedas AG, et al: Comparative trial of cefprozil *vs.* amoxicillin clavulanate potassium in the treatment of children with acute otitis media with effusion. *Pediatr Infect Dis J* 10:375-380, 1991 B.

Barbhaiya RH, et al: Phase I study of single-dose BMY-28100, a new oral cephalosporin. *Antimicrob Agents Chemother* 34:202-205, 1990 A.

Barbhaiya RH, et al: Phase I study of multiple-dose cefprozil and comparison with cefaclor. *Antimicrob Agents Chemother* 34:1198-1203, 1990 B.

Barbhaiya RH, et al: Comparison of the effects of food on the pharmacokinetics of cefprozil and cefaclor. *Antimicrob Agents Chemother* 34:1210-1213, 1990 C.

Barbhaiya RH, et al: Comparison of cefprozil and cefaclor pharmacokinetics and tissue penetration. *Antimicrob Agents Chemother* 34:1204-1209, 1990 D.

Chin N-X, Neu HC: Comparative antibacterial activity of a new oral cephalosporin BMY-28100. *Antimicrob Agents Chemother* 31:480-483, 1987.

Christenson JC, et al: Comparative efficacy and safety of cefprozil and cefaclor in the treatment of acute uncomplicated urinary tract infections. *J Antimicrob Chemother* 28:581-586, 1991 A.

Christenson JC, et al: Comparative efficacy and safety of cefprozil (BMY-28100) and cefaclor in the treatment of acute group A beta-hemolytic streptococcal pharyngitis. *Antimicrob Agents Chemother* 35:1127-1130, 1991 B.

Eliopoulos GM, et al: In vitro activity of BMY-28100, a new oral cephalosporin. *Antimicrob Agents Chemother* 31:653-656, 1987.

Iravani A: Comparison of cefprozil and cefaclor for treatment of acute urinary tract infections in women. *Antimicrob Agents Chemother* 35:1940-1942, 1991.

Sáez-Llorens X, et al: Pharmacokinetics of cefprozil in infants and children. *Antimicrob Agents Chemother* 34:2152-2155, 1990.

Scribner RK, et al: In vitro activity of BMY-28100 against common isolates from pediatric infections. *Antimicrob Agents Chemother* 31:630-631, 1987.

Shyu WC, et al: Pharmacokinetics of cefprozil in healthy subjects and patients with renal impairment. *J Clin Pharmacol* 31:362-371, 1991.

New Evaluation

LORACARBEF
[Lorabid]

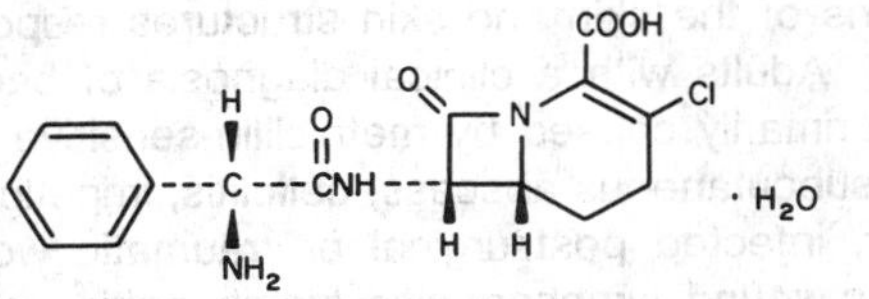

Loracarbef is an orally administered, broad spectrum, semisynthetic carbacephem antimicrobial drug. It is structurally identical to cefaclor except that a methylene group is substituted for sulfur at position 1 of the dihydrothiazine ring, resulting in a tetrahydropyridine ring. As a result of this chemical modification, loracarbef is significantly more stable than other β-lactam antibiotics in solid form and in solutions (eg, plasma, urine). Although loracarbef is not a true cephalosporin, it is closely related to drugs of this class (see Cooper, 1992).

MECHANISM OF ACTION, ANTIMICROBIAL SPECTRUM, AND RESISTANCE. The antibacterial mechanism of loracarbef is similar to that of other β-lactam drugs, including all oral cephalosporins (eg, cephalexin, cephradine, cefadroxil, cefaclor, cefuroxime axetil, cefixime, cefprozil). However, loracarbef may differ somewhat from individual cephalosporins in certain aspects of antimicrobial spectrum, in vitro potency, susceptibility to hydrolysis by bacterial β lactamases, and pharmacokinetics.

Loracarbef is generally bactericidal; the mechanism of action is irreversible interaction with penicillin-binding proteins and subsequent inhibition of cell wall biosynthesis (Sato et al, 1989).

The in vitro antibacterial spectrum of loracarbef is slightly broader than that of earlier oral cephalosporins (eg, cephalexin, cefadroxil) and is comparable to that of cefaclor, cefuroxime, cefixime, and cefprozil (Cao et al, 1988; Knapp and Washington, 1988; Shelton and Nelson, 1988; Pelosi and Fontana, 1988; Howard and Dunkin, 1988; Jones and Barry, 1988; Sato et al, 1989; Arguedas et al, 1991; Doern et al, 1991; for review, see Doern, 1992). When tested in vitro, loracarbef inhibits a majority (>90%) of isolates of methicillin-susceptible, coagulase-positive and -negative staphylococci and streptococci at concentrations attainable in vivo in recommended oral doses (see below). Its in vitro activity against these bacteria generally is comparable or slightly superior to that of cefadroxil, cephalexin, cefaclor, cefixime, cefuroxime (except for *S. pneumoniae*), and cefprozil. Like other cephalosporins, loracarbef does not inhibit enterococci (*Enterococcus faecalis, E. faecium*) or methicillin-resistant staphylococci. It is not active against *Bordetella pertussis* or *B. parapertussis* (Hoppe and Müller, 1990).

Loracarbef inhibits many common gram-negative bacteria, including *Haemophilus influenzae* and *Moraxella catarrhalis* (β lactamase-positive and -negative isolates), *Escherichia coli, Klebsiella pneumoniae, Citrobacter diversus, Proteus mirabilis, Neisseria meningitidis*, and *N. gonorrhoeae* (β lactamase-positive and -negative isolates). Its in vitro activity against these bacteria generally exceeds that of cephalexin, cefadroxil, and cephradine and is comparable to that of cefaclor and cefprozil. Cefuroxime and cefixime are usually more active in vitro than loracarbef against many gram-negative isolates, especially the Enterobacteriaceae that are susceptible to the latter drug (eg, *E. coli, K. pneumoniae*, and *P. mirabilis*). Other genera and species of Enterobacteriaceae and all pseudomonads are resistant to loracarbef.

The anaerobic bacteria susceptible to loracarbef include peptostreptococci, *Propionibacterium acnes, Eubacterium lentum, Clostridium perfringens*, and some *Bacteroides* species; *B. fragilis* are resistant (Cao et al, 1988; Sato et al, 1989). Thus, the antianaerobic activity of loracarbef is similar to that of cefaclor, cephalexin, and amoxicillin.

The in vitro activity of loracarbef is reduced in the presence of large inocula (10^7 CFU/ml) of some beta lactamase-positive isolates of *H. influenzae* and *Staphylococcus aureus*, presumably because it is not stable in the presence of the β lactamases produced by these organisms (Knapp and Washington, 1988). This is consistent with additional in vitro data demonstrating that loracarbef and cefaclor are more susceptible to the actions of many β lactamases than are cephalexin, cefadroxil, and cefuroxime (Jones and Barry, 1987; Pelosi and Fontana, 1988; Cao et al, 1988; Shelton and Nelson, 1988). However, in vitro assays indicate that loracarbef is far less susceptible to hydrolysis by bacterial β lactamases than penicillin, ampicillin, and amoxicillin.

As with similar agents, loracarbef activity in vitro is unaffected by the presence of human serum but is reduced at pH 5.0 (which is similar to that of purulent fluid) but not at pH 6.0 to 8.0 (Arguedas et al, 1991).

USES. Because the in vitro antimicrobial spectrum of loracarbef encompasses the predominant pathogens that cause infections of the upper and lower respiratory tracts, urinary tract, skin, skin structures, and acute otitis media (AOM) in adults and children, it has been evaluated clinically for these indications. However, since it is given orally, this agent should be used only for mild to moderate infections.

The efficacy and safety of 10 days of therapy with loracarbef (30 mg/kg daily in two doses) or amoxicillin/potassium clavulanate (40 mg/kg daily in three doses) were compared in a randomized trial in children with AOM caused by isolates of *H. influenzae, M. catarrhalis*, and *S. pneumoniae*, 37% of which produced β lactamase (Gan et al, 1991). Although the proportion of patients experiencing treatment failure and recurrence of infection was greater in the loracarbef group (27%) than in the amoxicillin/potassium clavulanate group (9%), the difference was not statistically significant. Results of two other randomized trials show that loracarbef (30 mg/kg daily in two doses) is as effective as amoxicillin/potassium clavulanate (40 mg/kg daily in three doses) or amoxicillin alone (40 mg/kg daily in three doses) in the treatment of children with AOM and effusion (Foshee and Qvarnberg, 1992). These results with loracarbef appear comparable to those observed in unrelated studies of cefuroxime axetil and cefaclor in children with AOM (see Pichichero et al, 1990).

In one small randomized study, loracarbef 15 mg/kg daily in two doses for 10 days was equivalent to potassium penicillin V 20 mg/kg daily in four doses in children with pharyngitis caused by group A β-hemolytic streptococci (Nahata and Koranyi, 1992). However, the small number of patients in this study may have biased the outcome so that potassium penicillin V and loracarbef appeared to be equivalent in efficacy. This concern has been alleviated by the results of two subsequent large randomized trials comparing loracarbef (15 mg/kg daily in two doses) and potassium penicillin V (20 mg/kg daily in four doses) in adults (McCarty, 1992) and children (Disney et al, 1992) with pharyngitis and tonsillitis due to group A β hemolytic streptococci (GABHS). In both studies, the highly favorable clinical (90% to 95% resolution of signs and symptoms) and bacteriologic outcomes with loracarbef were comparable to those in patients given potassium penicillin V.

Other mild to moderate infections of the upper and lower respiratory tracts respond well to loracarbef. Loracarbef 400 mg given twice daily for seven to ten days was as effective clinically and bacteriologically as amoxicillin/potassium clavulanate 500 mg (amoxicillin component) three times daily or doxycycline 100 mg daily in patients with acute bacterial maxillary sinusitis caused by *S. pneumoniae, H. influenzae*, and *M. catarrhalis* (Nielsen, 1992). Similar favorable clinical and bacteriologic results were obtained in a series of randomized trials (7 to 14 days in length) comparing loracarbef 400 mg twice daily with amoxicillin/potassium clavulanate or amoxicillin alone (both 500 mg three times daily) in patients with acute exacerbations of chronic bronchitis (Zeckel, 1992) or lobar and bronchial pneumonia (Hyslop, 1992) caused by the same three bacterial pathogens. In all of these studies, short- and long-term clinical and bacteriologic outcomes were nearly identical with the three regimens.

Loracarbef 200 mg once daily was comparable to cefaclor 250 mg three times daily in a randomized seven-day trial in women with acute, uncomplicated urinary tract infections caused primarily by susceptible isolates of *E. coli* and other aerobic gram-negative bacilli (Iravani, 1991; see also Iravani and Bischoff, 1992). Similar results were observed in a large randomized seven-day trial of loracarbef (200 mg once daily) or norfloxacin (400 mg twice daily) in patients with uncomplicated cystitis caused primarily by susceptible isolates of *E. coli* (Iravani and Bischoff, 1992). Loracarbef 400 mg twice daily also was as effective (favorable response in 94% of patients) as cefaclor 500 mg three times daily (favorable response in 96%) or norfloxacin 400 mg twice daily (favorable response in 98%) in two seven-day randomized trials in outpatients with uncomplicated pyelonephritis caused predominantly (85%) by *E. coli* (Hyslop and Bischoff, 1992). In general, the short- and long-term cure rates (>80%) produced by loracarbef in patients with acute, uncomplicated urinary tract infections appear comparable to those observed in unrelated trials in young women treated with other drugs, including oral cephalosporins (Johnson and Stamm, 1989).

Infections of the skin and skin structures respond well to loracarbef. Adults with a clinical diagnosis of bacterial skin infection primarily caused by methicillin-sensitive *S. aureus*, including subcutaneous abscess, cellulitis, impetigo, infected skin ulcer, infected postsurgical or traumatic wound other than a burn wound, lymphadenitis, lymphangitis, or pyoderma, received loracarbef 200 mg twice daily or cefaclor 250 mg three times daily in a randomized trial (McCarty et al, 1992). Both clinical (93% successful) and bacteriologic (92% eradication) responses to loracarbef were comparable to those obtained with cefaclor. Nearly identical outcomes also were observed in a randomized trial in children with similar skin and skin structure infections who were treated with loracarbef 200 mg twice daily or cefaclor 250 mg three times daily (Hanfling et al, 1992). Most of these infections involved methicillin-sensitive *S. aureus*, either alone (42% to 46% of infections) or mixed with group A streptococci (18% to 26%).

Overall, loracarbef does not appear to provide a significant therapeutic advantage over established oral agents of choice or alternatives used to treat mild to moderate susceptible infections. However, because of its relatively long serum half-life and chemical stability in solution (see Pharmacokinetics), twice-daily administration of loracarbef can be effective. This may be a significant advantage for loracarbef when it is necessary to select an agent from among the large number of oral antimicrobial drugs currently available.

ADVERSE REACTIONS AND PRECAUTIONS. Loracarbef is generally well tolerated when given to children and adults in multiple doses, as shown by a compilation of data from 22 clinical trials involving over 9,000 patients (Therasse, 1992). Most adverse events were mild and transient, and only 1.5% of patients discontinued therapy because of a drug-related side effect. Diarrhea was the most commonly reported adverse reaction, but it occurred significantly less frequently in patients given loracarbef than in those who received other drugs (especially amoxicillin/potassium clavulanate). In contrast, headache occurred significantly more often in patients treated with loracarbef than in those given other drugs. No significant alterations in biochemical laboratory parameters or gastrointestinal flora have been reported in patients who received loracarbef.

For a more detailed discussion of the adverse reactions and precautions associated with the use of cephalosporins, see the Introduction to this chapter.

DRUG INTERACTIONS AND INTERFERENCE WITH LABORATORY TESTS. See the Introduction to this chapter.

PHARMACOKINETICS. Loracarbef is rapidly and almost completely absorbed from the gastrointestinal tract under fasting conditions; the presence of food delays oral absorption and reduces the maximal plasma concentration (DeSante and Zeckel, 1992). Thus, this drug should be administered one hour before or two hours after meals. In fasting adults given single oral doses (capsule formulation), the mean serum concentrations after 1.5 and 3 hours were, respectively, 13.2 and 4.3 mcg/ml after a 400-mg dose and 6.9 and 1.7 mcg/ml after a 200-mg dose (Van der Auwera, 1992). Although the extent of oral absorption appeared to vary among subjects in this study, a linear correlation was observed with dosage and serum reciprocal bactericidal titers. The serum half-life is approximately 1.1 hours in adults.

In infants and children given loracarbef (suspension formulation) two hours following a meal, peak plasma concentrations of 12.6 and 18.7 mcg/ml occurred 45 minutes after single doses of 7.5 or 15 mg/kg; the mean half-lives were 51 and 47 minutes, respectively (Nelson et al, 1988). The area under the plasma concentration-versus-time curve (AUC) of loracarbef was 38 mcg/hr/ml after a single dose of 15 mg/kg.

In children, loracarbef penetrates middle ear fluid (MEF) and accumulates at concentrations that range from 42% to 48% of that in plasma approximately two hours after a single oral dose of 7.5 or 15 mg/kg, respectively (Kusmiesz et al, 1990). In this study, the mean concentration of drug in MEF (3.9 mcg/ml) after the larger dose was above the minimum inhibitory concentration (MIC) for 90% of the pathogens that usually cause AOM.

Loracarbef is eliminated primarily by glomerular filtration and tubular secretion. Approximately 90% of a dose is recovered unchanged in the urine within 24 hours. Hepatic transformation of the drug is minimal. Small amounts, which may be unabsorbed drug, can be recovered from the feces. Administration with probenecid decreases renal clearance of loracarbef, causing a 50% increase in the half-life (to 1.5 hr) and doubling the AUC.

Compared with cefaclor, loracarbef has superior bioavailability, penetrates MEF to a greater extent, has a longer plasma half-life, and, because of its chemical structure (ie, a carbacephem), is more stable in plasma.

DOSAGE AND PREPARATIONS. Loracarbef should be taken at least one hour before or two hours after meals.

Oral: For mild to moderate infections caused by susceptible bacteria, *adults*, 200 to 400 mg twice daily; *children and infants over 6 months*, 7.5 to 15 mg/kg twice daily (*Med Lett Drugs Ther*, 1992). See the package insert for dosages for specific indications. *Infants under 6 months,* efficacy and safety have not been established. The dosage should be modified in patients with renal impairment; see the package insert for details.

Lorabid (Lilly). Capsules 200 mg; powder (flavored, for oral suspension) 100 and 200 mg/5 ml after reconstitution. The reconstituted suspension can be stored unrefrigerated at room temperature for 14 days without significant loss of potency.

Cited References

Loracarbef. *Med Lett Drugs Ther* 34:87-88, 1992.

Arguedas AG, et al: In-vitro activity of cefprozil (BMY 28100) and loracarbef (LY 163892) against pathogens obtained from middle ear fluid. *J Antimicrob Chemother* 27:311-318, 1991.

Cao C, et al: In-vitro activity and β-lactamase stability of LY163892. *J Antimicrob Chemother* 22:155-165, 1988.

Cooper RDG: The carbacephems: A new beta-lactam antibiotic class. *Am J Med* 92(suppl 6A):6A-2S-6A-6S, 1992.

DeSante KA, Zeckel ML: Pharmacokinetic profile of loracarbef. *Am J Med* 92(suppl 6A):6A-6S-6A-19S, 1992.

Disney FA, et al: Loracarbef (LY163892) *vs.* penicillin VK in the treatment of streptococcal pharyngitis and tonsillitis. *Pediatr Infect Dis J* 11:S20-S26, 1992.

Doern G: In vitro activity of loracarbef and effects of susceptibility test methods. *Am J Med* 92(suppl 6A):6A-7S-6A-15S, 1992.

Doern GV, et al: In vitro activity of loracarbef (LY163892), a new oral carbacephem antimicrobial agent, against respiratory isolates of *Haemophilus influenzae* and *Moraxella catarrhalis. Antimicrob Agents Chemother* 35:1504-1507, 1991.

Foshee WS, Qvarnberg Y: Comparative United States and European trials of loracarbef in the treatment of acute otitis media. *Pediatr Infect Dis J* 11:S12-S19, 1992.

Gan VN, et al: Comparative evaluation of loracarbef and amoxicillin-clavulanate for acute otitis media. *Antimicrob Agents Chemother* 35:967-971, 1991.

Hanfling MJ, et al: Loracarbef *vs.* cefaclor in pediatric skin and skin structure infections. *Pediatr Infect Dis J* 11:S27-S30, 1992.

Hoppe JE, Müller J: In vitro susceptibilities of *Bordetella pertussis* and *Bordetella parapertussis* to six new oral cephalosporins. *Antimicrob Agents Chemother* 34:1442-1443, 1990.

Howard AJ, Dunkin KT: Comparative in-vitro activity of a new oral carbacephem, LY163892. *J Antimicrob Chemother* 22:445-456, 1988.

Hyslop DL: Efficacy and safety of loracarbef in the treatment of pneumonia. *Am J Med* 92(suppl 6A):6A-65S-6A-69S, 1992.

Hyslop DL, Bischoff W: Loracarbef (LY163892) versus cefaclor and norfloxacin in the treatment of uncomplicated pyelonephritis. *Am J Med* 92(suppl 6A):6A-86S-6A-94S, 1992.

Iravani A: Loracarbef versus cefaclor in the treatment of urinary tract infections in women. *Antimicrob Agents Chemother* 35:750-752, 1991.

Iravani A, Bischoff W: Antibiotic therapy for urinary tract infections. *Am J Med* 92(suppl 6A):6A-95S-6A-100S, 1992.

Johnson JR, Stamm WE: Urinary tract infections in women: Diagnosis and treatment. *Ann Intern Med* 111:906-917, 1989.

Jones RN, Barry AL: Beta-lactamase hydrolysis and inhibition studies of the new 1-carbacephem LY163892. *Eur J Clin Microbiol* 6:570-571, 1987.

Jones RN, Barry AL: Antimicrobial activity of LY163892, an orally administered 1-carbacephem. *J Antimicrob Chemother* 22:315-320, 1988.

Knapp CC, Washington JA II: In vitro activities of LY163892, cefaclor, and cefuroxime. *Antimicrob Agents Chemother* 32:131-133, 1988.

Kusmiesz H, et al: Loracarbef concentrations in middle ear fluid. *Antimicrob Agents Chemother* 34:2030-2031, 1990.

McCarty J: Loracarbef versus penicillin VK in the treatment of streptococcal pharyngitis and tonsillitis in an adult population. *Am J Med* 92(suppl 6A):6A-74S-6A-79S, 1992.

McCarty J, et al: Loracarbef (LY163892) versus cefaclor in the treatment of bacterial and skin-structure infections in an adult population. *Am Med J* 92(suppl 6A):6A-80S-6A-85S, 1992.

Nahata MC, Koranyi KI: Efficacy and safety of loracarbef in children with streptococcal pharyngitis and acute otitis media. *Drug Invest* 4:112-115, 1992.

Nelson JD, et al: Pharmacokinetics of LY163892 in infants and children. *Antimicrob Agents Chemother* 32:1738-1739, 1988.

Nielsen RW: Acute bacterial maxillary sinusitis: Results of U.S. and European comparative therapy trials. *Am J Med* 92(suppl 6A):6A-70S-6A-73S, 1992.

Pelosi E, Fontana R: In vitro activity and beta-lactamase stability of LY163892. *Eur J Clin Microbiol Infect Dis* 7:549-551, 1988.

Pichichero M, et al: Comparison of cefuroxime axetil, cefaclor, and amoxicillin-clavulanate potassium suspensions in acute otitis media in infants and children. *South Med J* 83:1174-1177, 1990.

Sato K, et al: *In vitro* and *in vivo* antibacterial activity of KT3777, a new orally active carbacephem. *J Antibiotics* 42:1844-1853, 1989.

Shelton S, Nelson JD: In vitro susceptibilities of common pediatric pathogens to LY163892. *Antimicrob Agents Chemother* 32:268-270, 1988.

Therasse DG: The safety profile of loracarbef: Clinical trials in respiratory, skin, and urinary tract infections: *Am J Med* 92(suppl 6A):6A-20S-6A-25S, 1992.

Van der Auwera P: Bactericidal titers of loracarbef (LY 163892) in serum and killing rates in volunteers receiving 400 versus 200 milligrams. *Antimicrob Agents Chemother* 36:521-526, 1992.

Zeckel ML: Loracarbef (LY163892) in the treatment of acute exacerbations of chronic bronchitis: Results of U.S. and European comparative clinical trials. *Am J Med* 92(suppl 6A):6A-58S-6A-64S, 1992.

65 Other Beta Lactam Antimicrobial Agents

MONOBACTAM

Aztreonam

BETA LACTAM/BETA LACTAMASE INHIBITOR COMBINATIONS

Amoxicillin/Potassium Clavulanate

Ticarcillin Disodium/Potassium Clavulanate

Ampicillin Sodium/Sulbactam Sodium

CARBAPENEM COMBINATION

Imipenem/Cilastatin Sodium

MONOBACTAM

AZTREONAM

[Azactam]

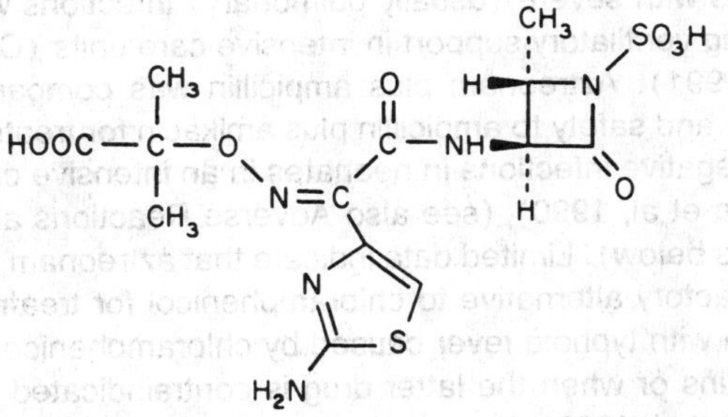

Aztreonam is the first of a new class of β-lactam antimicrobial agents called *monobactams* to be approved for clinical use in the United States. Unlike the penicillins, cephalosporins, and carbapenems, which have fused double-ring nuclei, the monobactams are monocyclic β-lactam agents containing 3-aminomonobactamic acid as the basic nucleus (see following structure).

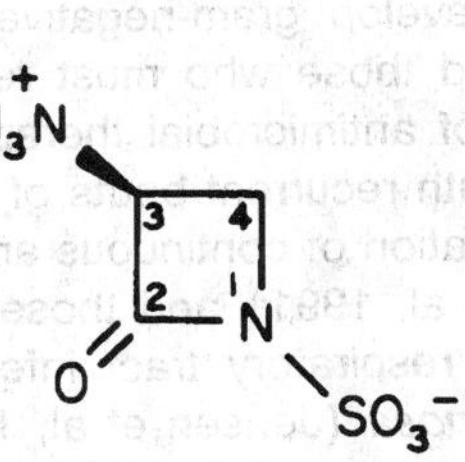

The first monobactams to be discovered were naturally occurring compounds isolated from bacteria (eg, *Gluconobacter, Acetobacter, Chromobacterium*), but they exhibited poor antibacterial properties. In contrast, aztreonam is a totally synthetic monobactam that has been designed (principally by the addition of an aminothiazole oxime side chain with an added carboxylic acid group at the 3-position and an α-methyl group at the 4-position) to have potent activity against aerobic gram-negative bacteria, including *Pseudomonas aeruginosa*, and excellent stability to β-lactamases (Sykes and Bonner, 1985; Neu, 1988; Tunkel and Scheld, 1990).

MECHANISM OF ACTION, ANTIMICROBIAL SPECTRUM, AND RESISTANCE. Like other β-lactam antibiotics, aztreonam inhibits bacterial cell wall formation. This antimicrobial agent readily penetrates the outer membrane and cell wall of aerobic gram-negative bacteria and binds with high affinity to penicillin binding protein 3 (PBP-3). This interaction causes filamentation of bacteria, inhibition of cell division, and, ultimately, cell death. Minimum bactericidal concentrations of aztreonam generally do not differ significantly from the minimum inhibitory concentrations. In contrast to its effect on aerobic gram-negative bacteria, aztreonam does not bind appreciably to essential PBPs of gram-positive or anaerobic bacteria.

Aztreonam is only active against facultative or aerobic gram-negative bacteria, including β-lactamase-producing strains of meningococci, gonococci, and *Haemophilus influenzae*. Its potency is comparable to that of third generation cephalosporins against most Enterobacteriaceae, including isolates that are resistant to penicillins, older cephalosporins, and aminoglycosides. Aztreonam also is active against most strains of *Pseudomonas aeruginosa*, including some that are resistant to other antipseudomonal antibiotics (eg, antipseudomonal penicillins, aminoglycosides). Its potency against this organism is slightly less than that of ceftazidime. Aztreonam has poor activity against other *Pseudomonas* species (eg, *P. cepacia*), however, and is not active against *Acinetobacter* species, *Xanthomonas maltophilia, Achromobacter xylosoxidans, Alcaligenes* species, and *Legionella pneumophila*. Isolates of *Citrobacter freundii, Enterobacter aerogenes*, and *E. cloacae* that are resistant to cefotaxime and ceftazidime frequently are not susceptible to aztreonam (Neu, 1990 B).

Like most third generation cephalosporins, aztreonam possesses a high degree of resistance to enzymatic hydrolysis by most common plasmid and chromosomally mediated β-lactamases. However, it is destroyed by the cefotaxime-ceftazidime hydrolyzing plasmid-coded β-lactamases (eg, TEM 3, 5, 7, 9) and by a chromosomally mediated Richmond-Sykes Type IV enzyme (K-1) produced by some uncommon strains of *Klebsiella oxytoca* (Neu, 1990 B). Aztreonam is a poor inducer of Type I chromosomal β-lactamases of certain gram-negative bacilli (eg, *E. cloacae, Citrobacter, Pseudomonas, Serratia*) when compared with cefoxitin and some third generation cephalosporins (Neu, 1990 B). However, the resistance of some strains of *E. cloacae* and *P. aeruginosa* to aztreonam may be due to stably derepressed Type I β-lactamase in those isolates. Slow hydrolysis of the monobactam is a suggested resistance mechanism; decreased outer membrane permeability to the drug also has been proposed (see also index entry Cephalosporins).

The effect of increasing inoculum concentration (10^4 to 10^6 colony-forming units) on susceptibility to aztreonam generally is slight for most susceptible bacteria. Unlike the aminoglycosides, aztreonam is fully active in an anaerobic or acidic environment.

The in vitro activities of nafcillin, cloxacillin, erythromycin, and vancomycin against gram-positive bacteria and of clindamycin or metronidazole against various anaerobic bacteria were unaffected or were increased additively by combination with aztreonam. The combination of aztreonam with gentamicin, tobramycin, or amikacin was synergistic against a high percentage of strains of *P. aeruginosa* (see Sykes and Bonner, 1985).

USES. Aztreonam is effective when given alone or combined with other antimicrobial drugs in the treatment of serious gram-negative aerobic bacterial infections, many of which are of nosocomial origin or are caused by strains resistant to other agents. These include complicated urinary tract, lower respiratory tract, skin and skin structure, obstetric and gynecologic, intra-abdominal, bone and joint, and central nervous system infections and systemic bacteremias in adults and children (Gentry, 1990; Neu, 1990 A, 1990 B; Bosso and Black, 1991; Clergeot et al, 1991; Conrad et al, 1991; Lentnek and Williams, 1991; Sklavunu-Tsurutsoglu et al, 1991; Stutman, 1991).

The antimicrobial spectrum of aztreonam generally parallels that of the aminoglycosides, with the exception of some aerobic gram-positive cocci (eg, staphylococci, including methicillin-resistant strains; some enterococci), which are susceptible to drugs of the latter class while all gram-positive species typically are resistant to aztreonam. Consequently, aztreonam can replace an aminoglycoside as sole therapy when the pathogen is known or strongly suspected to be susceptible, or it can be substituted for an aminoglycoside in combination regimens used to treat presumed mixed flora infections at a variety of sites. However, its use alone in empiric therapy is not recommended because aztreonam is ineffective against the gram-positive or anaerobic pathogens that may be present.

In various randomized controlled trials, aztreonam was more effective than tobramycin for treatment of nosocomial gram-negative pneumonias, comparable to tobramycin plus azlocillin for acute pulmonary exacerbations of cystic fibrosis, and as effective as gentamicin for serious gram-negative urinary tract infections. The combination of aztreonam plus clindamycin was similar in efficacy to tobramycin plus clindamycin for treatment of serious lower respiratory tract infections caused by aerobic gram-negative bacilli, to tobramycin (or gentamicin) plus clindamycin for intra-abdominal infections, and to gentamicin plus clindamycin for endometritis after caesarean section (see Tunkel and Scheld, 1990; Williams and Hotchkin, 1991).

Aztreonam plus vancomycin with or without amikacin was effective for empiric treatment of febrile, granulocytopenic adults (Rolston et al, 1990). In neutropenic pediatric patients with underlying malignancies, aztreonam plus floxacillin (flucloxacillin) was comparable to piperacillin plus gentamicin in resolving clinically documented and unexplained febrile episodes (Heney et al, 1991). Empiric therapy with aztreonam plus either cloxacillin or oxacillin may be a good alternative to tobramycin plus a cephalosporin (cefuroxime or cefotaxime) in adults with severe (usually pulmonary) infections who are receiving ventilatory support in intensive care units (Colardyn et al, 1991). Aztreonam plus ampicillin was comparable in efficacy and safety to ampicillin plus amikacin for treatment of gram-negative infections in neonates in an intensive care unit (Umaña et al, 1990) (see also Adverse Reactions and Precautions below). Limited data indicate that aztreonam may be a satisfactory alternative to chloramphenicol for treatment of children with typhoid fever caused by chloramphenicol-resistant strains or when the latter drug is contraindicated (Tanaka-Kido et al, 1990); however, these observations require further confirmation.

Thus, aztreonam appears to be a suitable alternative to the aminoglycosides or other potentially toxic drugs for serious gram-negative bacillary infections. Patients who especially may benefit from such substitution include those with renal failure (Sion et al, 1991), in whom ototoxicity and nephrotoxicity are likely to develop with aminoglycoside use; frail, elderly patients who develop gram-negative aerobic infections (Jones, 1990); and those who must receive prolonged or repeated courses of antimicrobial therapy. The latter group includes patients with recurrent bouts of gram-negative peritonitis as a complication of continuous ambulatory peritoneal dialysis (Dratwa et al, 1991) and those with cystic fibrosis who have chronic respiratory tract infections with mucoid strains of *P. aeruginosa* (Jensen et al, 1991). Furthermore, because aztreonam appears to exhibit little cross-allergenicity with penicillins and cephalosporins (see below), it may be useful in patients who are allergic to these agents (see also index entries Cephalosporins; Penicillins).

Despite the positive results discussed above, the ultimate role of aztreonam is still evolving and must be determined in comparison with the aminoglycosides, extended-spectrum cephalosporins (eg, ceftazidime), and penicillins. This is particularly true in patients with gram-negative bacillary meningitis and those who are febrile and neutropenic because of underlying malignancy and its treatment (Rolston et al, 1990). The use of aztreonam as the sole agent directed against gram-negative bacilli in febrile, granulocytopenic cancer patients is controversial and not generally accepted by infectious disease experts (Hughes et al, 1990). However, aztreonam plus a drug that is effective against gram-positive bacteria (eg, vancomycin) may be the only viable alternative for those patients who require broad-spectrum empiric coverage but cannot tolerate aminoglycosides or other β-lactam antibiotics. For patients who are not allergic to β-lactam drugs, it has not been established whether aztreonam has any advantage over the third-generation (antipseudomonal) cephalosporins or imipenem/cilastatin for treatment of infections caused by gram-negative aerobic pathogens.

ADVERSE REACTIONS AND PRECAUTIONS. Aztreonam is generally well tolerated, and its adverse reaction profile resembles that of most other β-lactam antibiotics.

Pain and phlebitis at the intravenous injection site occur in approximately 2% of patients. Mild gastrointestinal upset is observed in less than 2% of patients; nausea (0.8%) and diarrhea (0.7%) are most common. *Clostridium difficile*-associated diarrhea has been reported but is extremely rare.

Although rash has occurred in approximately 2% of patients treated with aztreonam, a possible IgE-mediated urticarial rash was observed in only one of a large number of patients with a history of allergy to penicillin and/or cephalosporins. The potential for immunologic cross-reactivity between aztreonam and the penicillins and cephalosporins has been investigated. In a recent study, patients with documented hypersensitivity to other β-lactam antimicrobials tolerated parenteral administration of aztreonam (Vega et al, 1991). In another study, cystic fibrosis patients with known allergy to β-lactam antibiotics, including anaphylaxis and generalized urticaria, had a negative skin test to aztreonam and were successfully treated with this drug (Jensen et al, 1991). Finally, in a retrospective study of 121 cystic fibrosis patients who received 2,793 courses of various β-lactam antibiotics, the risk for hypersensitivity reactions to aztreonam was very low and appeared to be restricted to those with a high propensity for β-lactam hypersensitivity (Koch et al, 1991). Although caution is warranted, these results indicate that there is very little cross-reactivity between aztreonam and other β-lactam antibiotics. Aztreonam has the same aminothiazoyl oxime side chain as ceftazidime, but possible cross-reactivity between these two drugs has not been evaluated.

Aztreonam has not been associated with nephrotoxicity, neurotoxicity, or coagulopathies (Tartaglione et al, 1986).

Superinfections have been reported in about 10% of patients receiving aztreonam; about 40% of these required specific therapy for this condition. Enterococcal colonization or superinfection in the urinary tract of patients receiving this drug has been observed (Chandrasekar et al, 1984).

Abnormalities in results of laboratory studies appear to be relatively mild and reversible in patients given aztreonam. Transient elevations in serum concentrations of hepatic transaminases (ALT, AST) have been reported in a few patients (see Neu, 1990 B).

The impact of aztreonam on the fecal flora is primarily directed against facultative gram-negative bacilli (eg, Enterobacteriaceae) (see Rolston et al, 1990).

The routine use of aztreonam in neonates is not recommended until data are available to show that the high arginine content of the preparation (780 mg/g of antibiotic) does not cause significant hypoglycemia.

This drug is classified in FDA Pregnancy Category B.

DRUG INTERACTIONS. Concurrent administration of aztreonam with cephradine, clindamycin, gentamicin, metronidazole, or nafcillin in healthy male volunteers resulted in no clinically significant pharmacokinetic drug interactions (Creasey et al, 1984).

PHARMACOKINETICS. Aztreonam is not absorbed following oral administration and must be administered intramuscularly or intravenously. Bioavailability after intramuscular injection is 100%. Peak serum concentrations obtained after intramuscular and bolus intravenous injections of 1 g are 46 mcg/ml (after 60 minutes) and 125 mcg/ml, respectively. Following intravenous infusion of 1 g over a 30-minute period, peak serum levels of 90 to 164 mcg/ml are achieved.

Approximately 56% of circulating aztreonam is bound to plasma protein. Apparent volumes of distribution range from 0.11 to 0.18 L/kg, indicating distribution to the extracellular water space. Aztreonam distributes into a variety of tissues and body fluids, including synovial, pleural, pericardial, peritoneal and blister fluids, bronchial secretions, bone, gallbladder, liver, lungs, kidneys, muscle, endometrium, intestinal tissue, and bile. High concentrations are obtained in urine. Aztreonam penetrates the uninflamed prostate and reaches concentrations (approximately 8 mcg/g of tissue one to three hours after a 1-g intramuscular dose) that are likely to be higher than the minimal inhibitory concentrations for most Enterobacteriaceae (Madsen et al, 1984). Concentrations attained in the cerebrospinal fluid of patients with inflamed meninges were, on the average, fourfold greater than those obtained in the absence of inflammation; however, these concentrations were five- to tenfold higher than necessary to inhibit most Enterobacteriaceae (Duma et al, 1984). Aztreonam crosses the placenta.

About 65% to 70% of a dose of aztreonam is excreted in the urine as unchanged drug by glomerular filtration and tubular secretion; probenecid delays excretion. About 7% of a dose is metabolized, and the metabolite is also eliminated in urine. Only 1% of a dose is recovered as unchanged drug in feces. The average elimination half-life of aztreonam in adults with normal renal function is 1.7 hours (range 1.6 to 2.1 hours). A similar half-life is observed in pediatric patients over 1 month of age; in newborns, the half-life ranges from 2.5 hours in those weighing more than 2.5 kg to 5.7 hours in those weighing less than 2.5 kg (Stutman et al, 1984).

In patients with impaired renal function, the elimination half-life of aztreonam is prolonged (eg, to six hours in renal failure) and dosage adjustments are necessary. About 50% of the drug is removed during hemodialysis, and supplemental dosing is required in patients who undergo this procedure. Total body clearance of aztreonam decreases by 20% to 25% in patients with alcoholic hepatic cirrhosis, and dosage adjustments may be necessary (eg, when therapy is prolonged).

For further discussion of pharmacokinetics, see Swabb, 1985.

DOSAGE AND PREPARATIONS. Aztreonam can be administered by intramuscular injection deep into a large muscle or intravenously by slow bolus injection or by intermittent infusion over a 20- to 60-minute period. See the manufacturer's instructions for the appropriate dilution of the drug, compatible diluents and intravenous solutions, and stability of aztreonam in these solutions.

Intramuscular, Intravenous: *Adults*, 1 to 8 g daily in divided doses every 6 to 12 hours (The Medical Letter, 1990). The manufacturer recommends the following dosages: for urinary tract infections, 500 mg or 1 g every 8 or 12 hours; for moderately severe systemic infections, 1 or 2 g every 8 or 12 hours; and for severe systemic or life-threatening infections, 2 g every six or eight hours. The maximum recommended dose is 8 g per day. The intravenous route is recommended for patients who require single doses greater than 1 g or those with bacterial septicemia, localized parenchymal abscess (eg, intra-abdominal abscess), peritonitis, or other severe systemic or life-threatening infections. For systemic *P. aeruginosa* infections, 2 g every six or eight hours is recommended, at least on initiation of therapy. In elderly patients, the manufacturer suggests estimating creatinine clearance to assess renal function and making appropriate dosage modifications, if necessary. For *infants and children,* dosages have not been established, but 90 to 120 mg/kg/day in divided doses every six to eight hours has been suggested (Nelson, 1991).

For *adults with renal impairment,* the manufacturer recommends the following: for creatinine clearance of 30 to 10 ml/min/1.73 M^2, an initial dose of 1 or 2 g, followed by a maintenance dose that is one-half the usual dose at the usual intervals (6, 8, or 12 hours); for creatinine clearance of less than 10 ml/min/1.73 M^2, an initial dose of 500 mg, 1 g, or 2 g, followed by a maintenance dose that is one-fourth the usual dose at the usual intervals (6, 8, or 12 hours). For serious or life-threatening infections, in addition to the maintenance doses, one-eighth of the initial dose should be given after each hemodialysis session.

Azactam (Squibb). Powder (sterile) 500 mg and 1 and 2 g.

BETA LACTAM/BETA LACTAMASE INHIBITOR COMBINATIONS

Clavulanic acid is a β-lactam derivative that is isolated from *Streptomyces clavuligerus*. Sulbactam is a penicillanic acid sulfone that is derived synthetically from 6-aminopenicillanic acid (see following structures). Both of these compounds have only weak antibacterial properties of their own; however, they are potent inhibitors of many bacterial β-lactamases, the enzymes that hydrolyze penicillins and cephalosporins to inactive compounds.

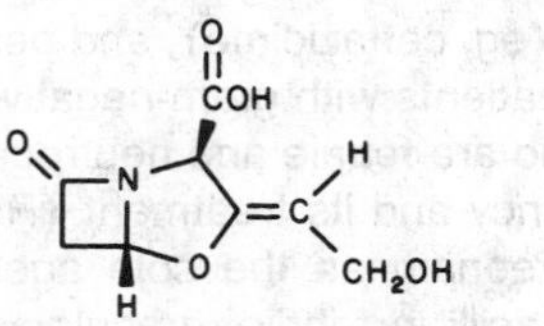

Clavulanic Acid

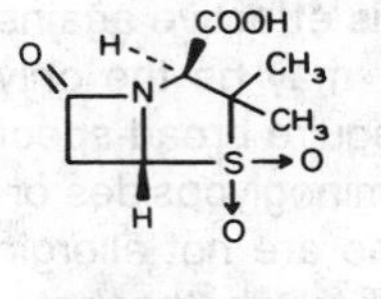

Sulbactam

Clavulanic acid and sulbactam inhibit the plasmid-mediated exoenzymes from staphylococci and the β-lactamases of the Richmond and Sykes Types II, III, IV, V, and VI. These include the common plasmid-mediated TEM-1 enzymes (Type III) that are present in *Haemophilus* (eg, *H. influenzae*), *Neisseria gonorrhoeae, Escherichia coli, Salmonella*, and *Shigella*; other plasmid-mediated β-lactamases produced by certain gram-negative bacteria; and the chromosomally mediated enzymes of *Klebsiella* (Type IV), *Bacteroides fragilis*, and *Legionella*. Inducible, chromosomally mediated Richmond and Sykes Type I β-lactamases that are present in *Enterobacter, Serratia, Morganella, Citrobacter, Pseudomonas,* and *Acinetobacter* generally are not inhibited by clavulanic acid and sulbactam unless these drugs are present in high concentrations that cannot be attained clinically (see Neu, 1985 A, 1990 A; Jacoby and Archer, 1991; Murray, 1991).

The mechanism of inhibition by clavulanic acid or sulbactam depends on the particular β-lactamase. Although in some cases inhibition may be reversible, clavulanic acid or sulbactam frequently acts as a suicide inactivator, which, after forming an acyl enzyme intermediate, irreversibly inactivates the enzyme (Neu, 1990 A; Maddux, 1991; Rolinson, 1991).

Clavulanic acid and sulbactam are used in fixed-ratio combinations with β-lactam antibiotics that are susceptible to β-lactamase inactivation when administered alone. Amoxicillin/potassium clavulanate [Augmentin], ampicillin/sulbactam [Unasyn], and ticarcillin/potassium clavulanate [Timentin] are marketed in the United States. The rationale for these combinations is that the β-lactamase inhibitor protects the β-lactam antibiotic from inactivation by bacterial β-lactamases, thus extending the antibacterial spectrum of the β-lactam agent to include these strains.

AMOXICILLIN/POTASSIUM CLAVULANATE

[Augmentin]

This combination of amoxicillin trihydrate, an aminopenicillin, and potassium clavulanate, a β-lactamase inhibitor, is marketed in 2:1 and 4:1 fixed-ratio dosage forms for oral administration.

MECHANISM OF ACTION, ANTIMICROBIAL SPECTRUM, AND RESISTANCE. Amoxicillin alone is active in vitro against a wide variety of nonβ-lactamase-producing aerobic and anaerobic gram-positive and gram-negative bacteria. The addition of clavulanic acid does not alter the susceptibility of amoxicillin-sensitive strains and extends the in vitro activity of amoxicillin to include, at achievable serum concentrations, β-lactamase-producing strains of intrinsically susceptible species. The combination is not active against methicillin-resistant strains of *S. aureus.* Many strains of *Acinetobacter, Citrobacter, Enterobacter, Morganella, Proteus, Pseudomonas,* and *Serratia* also are resistant, presumably because they produce Richmond and Sykes Type I chromosomal β-lactamases.

For additional discussion of the mechanism of action of clavulanic acid and amoxicillin, see Neu, 1990 A; Todd and Benfield, 1990; and index entry Amoxicillin.

USES. Amoxicillin/potassium clavulanate is effective orally in adults and children with acute otorhinolaryngologic and mild to moderate lower respiratory tract infections (eg, acute exacerbations of chronic bronchitis) caused by penicillinase-producing strains of *H. influenzae* and *M. catarrhalis* (for review, see Lisby-Sutch et al, 1990; Neu, 1990 A; Todd and Benfield, 1990). It is comparable or superior to erythromycin/sulfisoxazole, trimethoprim/sulfamethoxazole, and oral cephalosporins for these indications and is a rational alternative when resistant strains of the causative bacteria are prevalent. If penicillinase-mediated resistance is not a problem, amoxicillin alone is the drug of choice for oral therapy of these infections, especially since cost has become a major consideration in drug selection. In addition, the administration of potassium clavulanate with amoxicillin reduces the gastrointestinal tolerance of amoxicillin (see below), which may limit the usefulness of the combination in children.

Many studies have demonstrated the efficacy of amoxicillin/potassium clavulanate in the treatment of complicated and uncomplicated simple and recurrent urinary tract infections caused by β-lactamase producing strains of *E. coli* and other pathogens in adults and children. However, since other oral agents (eg, trimethoprim/sulfamethoxazole, fluoroquinolones, cephalosporins) are effective, generally well tolerated, and, in some instances, less expensive (eg, cotrimoxazole), amoxicillin/potassium clavulanate should be reserved for patients with recurrent infection caused by resistant species (for reviews, see Johnson and Stamm, 1989; Todd and Benfield, 1990; and index entry Urinary Tract Infections).

Amoxicillin/potassium clavulanate has been effective in the treatment of skin and soft-tissue infections caused by a variety of pathogens, including β-lactamase-producing strains of staphylococci, and is considered an alternative to oral penicillinase-resistant penicillins (eg, dicloxacillin), erythromycin, and oral first-generation cephalosporins (eg, cephalexin) for these indications. It also is effective in infections caused by human (eg, *Eikenella corrodens*, streptococci, *S. aureus*, oral anaerobes) and animal (eg, *Pasteurella multocida*, streptococci, *S. aureus,* oral anaerobes) bite wounds and is considered the drug of choice for these indications by some authorities (Goldstein et al, 1987; see also Todd and Benfield, 1990; and the index entry Bite Wounds).

Amoxicillin/potassium clavulanate is an alternative to erythromycin or ceftriaxone for chancroid caused by β-lactamase-producing strains of *H. ducreyi* (*MMWR*, 1989). Single large doses of amoxicillin (3 g) plus potassium clavulanate (125 to 500 mg) have been effective in some cases of uncomplicated gonorrhea caused by penicillinase-producing *N. gonorrhea* (PPNG). However, failures have occurred with this regimen, and more reliable treatment of PPNG has required multiple doses of the combination or a single large dose with concomitant administration of probenecid (Todd and Benfield, 1990). The Centers for Disease Control recommends oral amoxicillin/potassium clavulanate (alternatives, cefuroxime axetil, ciprofloxacin) to complete the course of therapy for disseminated gonococcal infection after parenteral ceftriaxone is given initially (*MMWR*, 1989).

ADVERSE REACTIONS AND PRECAUTIONS. Amoxicillin/potassium clavulanate generally is well tolerated. With the exception of diarrhea, which appears to occur more frequently with large doses (eg, $\geq$250 mg) of potassium clavulanate, the spectrum of adverse reactions associated with this combination is similar to that of amoxicillin alone. There have been a few reports that amoxicillin/potassium clavulanate may cause liver injury, which is manifested by elevated serum transaminase levels. Hepatic dysfunction causally related to this combination has been reported in 18 patients, of whom six had a syndrome classified as mixed cholestatic-hepatocellular, four had hepatocellular defects, and the remainder were unclassified. All patients recovered without complications when the combination was withdrawn.

Patients allergic to any penicillin should be considered allergic to amoxicillin/potassium clavulanate. (See index entry Amoxicillin; for review, see also Todd and Benfield, 1990.)

This combination is classified in FDA Pregnancy Category B.

DRUG INTERACTIONS AND INTERFERENCE WITH LABORATORY TESTS. See index entry Amoxicillin.

PHARMACOKINETICS. The pharmacokinetic properties of both components are similar and are not affected by administration together (see index entry Amoxicillin and Neu, 1990 A; Todd and Benfield, 1990). Absorption of potassium clavulanate is not affected by food, dairy products, or antacids, and the drug is stable in the gastric environment.

Mean peak serum concentrations of 3.5 to 3.9 mcg/ml of potassium clavulanate are reached one to two hours following a single oral dose of 125 mg in healthy subjects given the drug with 500 mg of amoxicillin (eg, one Augmentin '500' tablet). About 30% of potassium clavulanate is bound to plasma protein, and unbound drug distributes primarily into the extracellular fluid volume. Adequate concentrations of potassium clavulanate appear in bile, pleural and peritoneal fluid, and middle ear effusion. Concentrations in cerebrospinal fluid are low in the absence of inflammation and appear to be inadequate to treat infections caused by β-lactamase-producing pathogens. Studies of the penetration of potassium clavulanate into sputum have yielded variable results, possibly due to differences in assay methodology (Todd and Benfield, 1990). However, large doses of this drug have produced concentrations in sputum that are sufficient to protect amoxicillin from enzymatic inactivation by β-lactamases of common respiratory tract pathogens (Maesen et al, 1987).

Potassium clavulanate crosses the placenta to achieve peak concentrations in amniotic fluid and umbilical cord serum of up to 50% of maternal levels.

Potassium clavulanate is excreted by the kidneys, but probenecid has no effect on renal clearance. About 25% to 40% of this agent is recovered unchanged in the urine after six hours. This compound appears to be extensively metabolized. Its elimination half-life of about one hour is prolonged in patients with impaired renal function; dosage adjustments are made for the amoxicillin component of the combination.

DOSAGE AND PREPARATIONS.

Oral: *Adults and children weighing more than 40 kg,* the usual dose is amoxicillin 250 mg/potassium clavulanate 125 mg (one Augmentin '250' tablet) every eight hours; for more severe infections and infections of the respiratory tract, amoxicillin 500 mg/potassium clavulanate 125 mg (one Augmentin '500' tablet) every eight hours. (*NOTE*: Since both Augmentin '250' and '500' tablets contain the same amount of clavulanic acid, ie, 125 mg as the potassium salt, two Augmentin '250' tablets are not equivalent to one Augmentin '500' tablet.) For chancroid and disseminated gonococcal infections, see index entry Infection, Reproductive Tract.

Children weighing less than 40 kg, the usual dose is 20 mg/kg daily (based on the amoxicillin component) in divided doses every eight hours; for otitis media, sinusitis, lower respiratory infections, and other more severe infections, 40 mg/kg daily (based on the amoxicillin component) in divided doses every eight hours.

Augmentin (SmithKline Beecham). Powder (for oral suspension) containing 125 or 250 mg amoxicillin and 31.25 or 62.5 mg clavulanic acid (as potassium salt)/5 ml (potassium 0.16 or 0.32 mEq/5 ml) (***Augmentin '125', '250' for Oral Suspension***); tablets containing 250 or 500 mg amoxicillin (as trihydrate) and 125 mg clavulanic acid (as potassium salt; potassium 0.63 mEq/tablet) (***Augmentin '250', '500' Tablets***); tablets (chewable) containing 125 or 250 mg amoxicillin (as trihydrate) and 31.25 or 62.5 mg clavulanic acid (as potassium salt; potassium 0.16 or 0.32 mEq/tablet) (***Augmentin '125', '250' Chewable Tablets***).

TICARCILLIN DISODIUM/POTASSIUM CLAVULANATE

[Timentin]

The combination of ticarcillin disodium, a carboxypenicillin, and potassium clavulanate, a β-lactamase inhibitor, is marketed in 30:1 and 15:1 fixed-ratio dosage forms for parenteral administration.

MECHANISM OF ACTION, ANTIMICROBIAL SPECTRUM, AND RESISTANCE. Ticarcillin is a broad spectrum antipseudomonal penicillin that is active in vitro against most gram-positive bacteria (except some enterococci and β-lactamase-producing and methicillin-resistant staphylococci), gram-negative cocci, and, when compared with ampicillin, an expanded spectrum of gram-negative bacilli. However, β-lactamase-producing strains of these gram-negative bacilli can inactivate ticarcillin and are relatively common (for detailed discussion, see index entry Ticarcillin).

Administration of ticarcillin with clavulanic acid does not alter the susceptibility of ticarcillin-sensitive strains and extends the in vitro activity of ticarcillin to include, at achievable serum concentrations, β-lactamase-producing strains of intrinsically susceptible species of gram-positive and gram-negative bacteria, including anaerobes (Itokazu and Danziger, 1991). However, the in vitro susceptibilities of *Pseudomonas aeruginosa, Acinetobacter calcoaceticus*, and a number of *Serratia marcescens* and *Enterobacter* strains are not enhanced by the presence of clavulanic acid at concentrations attainable in serum. Thus, these organisms and methicillin-resistant strains of staphylococci should be considered resistant to ticarcillin/potassium clavulanate if they are resistant to ticarcillin alone (Clarke and Zemcov, 1984; Pulverer et al, 1986). For discussion of the mechanism of action of ticarcillin, see index entry Ticarcillin.

USES. Ticarcillin/potassium clavulanate is indicated for serious lower respiratory tract, urinary tract, bone and joint, and skin and soft tissue infections and septicemia caused by susceptible β-lactamase-producing strains of various gram-negative bacilli and *Staphylococcus aureus* or by ticarcillin-susceptible organisms (Brittain et al, 1985; Gentry et al, 1985; Cox, 1986; Meylan et al, 1986; File and Tan, 1991; Itokazu and Danziger, 1991; Pankey, 1991). Because of its broad antibacterial spectrum, this combination is useful for the treatment of mixed infections such as intra-abdominal and gynecologic infections (Faro, 1990; McGregor, 1990; Neu, 1990 A; Faro, 1991; Faro et al, 1991; Itokazu and Danziger, 1991). It often is used as presumptive therapy prior to the identification of the causative organisms. Because attainable serum concentrations of clavulanic acid do not enhance the susceptibility of *Pseudomonas aeruginosa* to ticarcillin, many authorities recommend that ticarcillin/potassium clavulanate be combined with an aminoglycoside for treatment of systemic infections with this organism.

A combination regimen consisting of ticarcillin/potassium clavulanate plus an aminoglycoside has been effective in the empiric treatment of febrile, neutropenic patients, but its use for this indication is not unanimously recommended (see Hughes et al, 1990). Other antipseudomonal penicillins (eg, piperacillin) or third-generation cephalosporins (eg, ceftazidime) are preferred as the β-lactam element of a combination regimen with an aminoglycoside because their potency against *P. aeruginosa* is greater than that of ticarcillin (see index entries Ticarcillin; Fever, Treatment).

ADVERSE REACTIONS AND PRECAUTIONS. Ticarcillin/potassium clavulanate generally is well tolerated, and adverse reactions are similar to those seen with ticarcillin alone (see index entry Ticarcillin). Patients allergic to any penicillin should be considered allergic to ticarcillin/potassium clavulanate.

This drug is classified in FDA Pregnancy Category B.

DRUG INTERACTIONS AND INTERFERENCE WITH LABORATORY TESTS. As with ticarcillin alone, mixing ticarcillin/potassium clavulanate with an aminoglycoside in parenteral solutions prior to administration can inactivate the aminoglycoside. In vivo antagonism in patients with renal failure also can occur (see index entries Ticarcillin; Aminoglycosides).

For a discussion of other drug interactions involving the penicillins, see index entry Penicillins.

PHARMACOKINETICS. After intravenous infusion (30 minutes) of ticarcillin (3 g)/potassium clavulanate (100 mg) (Timentin 3.1 g formulation), peak serum concentrations of both drugs were attained immediately after completion of the infusion. Ticarcillin serum concentrations were similar to those produced by an equivalent dose of ticarcillin alone (mean peak serum concentration, 330 mcg/ml). The corresponding mean peak serum concentration of clavulanic acid was 8 mcg/ml (manufacturer's literature).

In patients with impaired renal function, dosage adjustments are made for the ticarcillin component.

For additional discussion, see the manufacturer's literature; see also index entry Ticarcillin.

DOSAGE AND PREPARATIONS.

Intravenous: Ticarcillin/potassium clavulanate should be administered by intermittent infusion over 30 minutes. See the manufacturer's literature for the appropriate dilution of the drug, a list of compatible diluents and intravenous solutions, and stability of ticarcillin/potassium clavulanate in these solutions. The manufacturer's dosage recommendations are as follows:

For systemic and urinary tract infections for *average weight (60 kg) adults;* ticarcillin 3 g/potassium clavulanate 100 mg, ie, 3.1 g Timentin, every four to six hours; for *patients weighing less than 60 kg,* 200 to 300 mg/kg daily (based on the ticarcillin component) in divided doses every four to six hours. For *infants and children under 12*, dosages have not been established, but some experts suggest 200 to 300 mg/kg daily (based on the ticarcillin component) in divided doses every four to six hours (The Medical Letter, 1990; Nelson, 1991).

In *adults with renal insufficiency*, an initial loading dose of 3.1 g should be followed by doses based on creatinine clearance and type of dialysis as indicated below:

Creatinine Clearance (ml/min)	Dosage
> 60	3.1 g every 4 hours
60–30	2 g every 4 hours
30–10	2 g every 8 hours
< 10	2 g every 12 hours
< 10 (with hepatic dysfunction)	2 g every 24 hours
Patients on peritoneal dialysis	3.1 g every 12 hours
Patients on hemodialysis	2 g every 12 hours supplemented with 3.1 g after each dialysis

Half-life of ticarcillin in patients with renal failure, about 13 hours

From manufacturer's literature

Timentin (SmithKline Beecham). Powder (sterile) containing 3 g ticarcillin (as disodium salt) and 100 mg clavulanic acid (as potassium salt) in 3.1 g containers (sodium, 4.75 mEq/g) or 3 g ticarcillin (as disodium salt) and 200 mg clavulanic acid (as potassium salt) in 3.2 g containers (sodium, 4.75 m Eq/g).

AMPICILLIN SODIUM/SULBACTAM SODIUM

[Unasyn]

The combination of ampicillin sodium, an aminopenicillin, and sulbactam sodium, a β-lactamase inhibitor, is marketed in a 2:1 fixed-ratio dosage form for parenteral administration.

MECHANISM OF ACTION, ANTIMICROBIAL SPECTRUM, AND RESISTANCE. Ampicillin alone is active in vitro against a wide variety of nonβ-lactamase-producing gram-positive and gram-negative bacteria and various anaerobic bacteria (see index entry, Ampicillin). The addition of sulbactam does not alter the susceptibility of ampicillin-sensitive strains and extends the in vitro activity of ampicillin to include many β-lactamase-producing strains (but not methicillin-resistant staphylococci) and many anaerobic bacteria (including the *Bacteroides fragilis* group). Resistance to ampicillin/sulbactam has been noted for *E. coli* strains that are prevalent in hospital intensive care units. Similarly, strains of Enterobacteriaceae *(Acinetobacter, Citrobacter, Enterobacter, Morganella, Proteus, Providencia, Pseudomonas,* and *Serratia*) that produce inducible chromosomal Richmond and Sykes Type I β-lactamases usually are resistant to ampicillin/sulbactam (Neu, 1985 A, 1990 A; *Med Lett Drugs Ther*, 1987; Kerins, 1991).

For a discussion of the mechanism of action of ampicillin, see index entry Penicillins.

USES. The combination of ampicillin and sulbactam is used parenterally to treat gynecologic, intra-abdominal, and skin and other soft tissue infections in adults and children over 12 years of age. Because of its broad spectrum of activity against β-lactamase-producing gram-positive and gram-negative aerobes and anaerobes, ampicillin/sulbactam may be useful in mixed infections caused by susceptible organisms. In a number of randomized trials in patients with a variety of soft-tissue pelvic infections (eg, endometritis, salpingitis, pelvic peritonitis, tubo-ovarian abscess), the efficacy of ampicillin/sulbactam was comparable to that of metronidazole alone, clindamycin plus gentamicin, cefoxitin plus doxycycline plus metronidazole, cefoxitin alone, and cefotetan. The results of a randomized trial in patients with intra-abdominal infections showed no significant differences between ampicillin/sulbactam and the combination of clindamycin plus gentamicin when clinical or microbiological outcomes were compared (for reviews, see Campoli-Richards and Brogden, 1987; Neu, 1990 A; Kerins, 1991).

Ampicillin/sulbactam also has been effective for the treatment of bone, joint, lower respiratory and urinary tract infections, and uncomplicated gonorrhea (including that caused by PPNG strains), as well as for prophylaxis during gastrointestinal and obstetric/gynecologic surgery.

Ampicillin/sulbactam is effective in the treatment of acute epiglottitis in children (Wald et al, 1986). In a randomized trial comparing this combination with ceftriaxone, the two regimens were clinically and bacteriologically equivalent for soft tissue and bone infections in children (see Kerins, 1991).

Because ampicillin/sulbactam has good to excellent activity against mixed aerobic and anaerobic bacterial infections at a variety of sites, does not produce ototoxicity and nephrotoxicity, is relatively easy to administer, and is relatively inexpensive, it is a reasonable alternative to other more established therapy. However, more clinical trials are required before its therapeutic role is definitively established, especially in life-threatening infections.

ADVERSE REACTIONS AND PRECAUTIONS. Ampicillin/sulbactam generally is well tolerated but has the potential to produce any of the hypersensitivity reactions or other adverse effects associated with ampicillin therapy alone (see index entry Ampicillin and Lees et al, 1986). Patients allergic to any penicillin should be considered allergic to ampicillin/sulbactam.

Ampicillin is classified in FDA Pregnancy Category B.

DRUG INTERACTIONS AND INTERFERENCE WITH LABORATORY TESTS. These are the same as for ampicillin alone (see index entry Ampicillin).

PHARMACOKINETICS. The pharmacokinetics of both components are similar and are not altered when the combination is administered (see index entry Ampicillin). Immediately following a 15-minute infusion of 2 g ampicillin plus 1 g sulbactam, the average peak serum concentrations are 120 mcg/ml and 60 mcg/ml, respectively. About one hour following intramuscular injection of 1 g ampicillin plus 500 mg sulbactam, average peak serum concentrations of 18 mcg/ml and 13 mcg/ml, respectively, are achieved.

About 38% of circulating sulbactam is bound to plasma protein. It primarily distributes into the extracellular fluid volume. High concentrations are achieved in urine. Adequate concentrations of the drug are found in bile, peritoneal fluid, sputum, middle ear fluid, pus, and biliary, female genital tract, and intestinal mucosal tissues. Penetration of sulbactam into cerebrospinal fluid in the presence of bacterial meningitis has been observed (Foulds et al, 1987). Sulbactam crosses the placenta and is found in breast milk.

Sulbactam is eliminated as unchanged drug in the urine by glomerular filtration and renal tubular secretion. Probenecid delays its excretion. Approximately 75% to 85% of the drug is recovered unchanged from urine after eight hours. The elimination half-life of sulbactam is approximately one hour in healthy adult volunteers. It is increased in newborn infants, the elderly, and in patients with impaired renal function. The kinetics of elimination of ampicillin and sulbactam are similar in patients with varying degrees of renal dysfunction. Dosage reductions are necessary in patients with renal impairment.

For additional discussion, see Kerins, 1991; see also index entry Ampicillin.

DOSAGE AND PREPARATIONS. Ampicillin/sulbactam can be administered by intramuscular injection deep into a large muscle mass, intravenously by slow injection (over at least 10 to 15 minutes) or, after dilution with 50 ml to 100 ml of a compatible diluent, by intravenous infusion over 15 to 30 minutes. See the manufacturer's instructions for the appropriate dilution of the drug, compatible diluents and intravenous solutions, and stability of ampicillin/sulbactam in those solutions.

Intravenous, Intramuscular (deep): *Adults,* 1.5 g (1 g ampicillin as the sodium salt plus 0.5 g sulbactam as the sodium salt) to 3 g (2 g ampicillin as the sodium salt plus 1 g sulbactam as the sodium salt) every six hours. The total dose of sulbactam should not exceed 4 g per day. Safety in *children under 12 years of age* has not been established, and dosage recommendations are unavailable.

In patients with impaired renal function, the elimination kinetics of ampicillin and sulbactam are similarly affected, and the ratio of one to the other remains constant regardless of renal function. The manufacturer recommends that in *adults with renal impairment* the dose of ampicillin/sulbactam (expressed in grams of the combination) be administered according to the following schedule:

Creatinine Clearance (ml/min/1.73 M²)	Ampicillin/Sulbactam Half-Life (Hours)	Recommended Dosage
≥30	1	1.5-3 g every 6-8 hours
15-29	5	1.5-3 g every 12 hours
5-14	9	1.5-3 g every 24 hours

When only serum creatinine is available, the following formula (based on sex, weight, and age of the patient) may be used to convert this value into creatinine clearance. The serum creatinine should represent a steady state of renal function.

$$\text{Males} \quad \frac{\text{weight (kg)} \times (140 - \text{age})}{72 \times \text{serum creatinine}}$$

$$\text{Females} \quad 0.85 \times \text{above value}$$

Unasyn (Roerig). Powder (sterile) 1.5 g (1 g ampicillin as the sodium salt plus 0.5 g sulbactam as the sodium salt) and 3 g (2 g of ampicillin as the sodium salt plus 1 g of sulbactam as the sodium salt) (sodium 5 and 10 mEq, respectively).

CARBAPENEM COMBINATION

IMIPENEM/CILASTATIN SODIUM

[Primaxin I.M., Primaxin I.V.]

Imipenem

Cilastatin Sodium

Imipenem is the only carbapenem antimicrobial agent licensed for use in the United States. It is the chemically stable N-formimidoyl derivative of thienamycin, a compound produced by *Streptomyces cattleya.* Like the penicillins and cephalosporins, imipenem contains a β-lactam ring in its structure; unlike that of penicillin, the five-membered ring of imipenem does not contain an endocyclic sulfur atom and is unsaturated (Birnbaum et al, 1985).

Imipenem is metabolized to inactive, potentially nephrotoxic derivatives by dehydropeptidase-1, an enzyme located in the brush border of the proximal renal tubules. As a consequence of this process, only very low concentrations of native drug can be detected in the urine. To counteract this enzymatic breakdown, cilastatin, a bacteriologically inert inhibitor of dehydropeptidase-1, is given in equal amounts with imipenem, thus increasing urinary recovery of active imipenem and avoiding renal toxicity.

MECHANISM OF ACTION, ANTIMICROBIAL SPECTRUM, AND RESISTANCE. Imipenem has the widest spectrum of activity of any currently available antimicrobial drug; most aerobic and anaerobic gram-positive and gram-negative species are susceptible (for review, see Kropp et al, 1985). Its bactericidal potency and broad spectrum probably stem from three basic chemicobiological properties: it readily penetrates the cell wall of gram-positive and gram-negative bacteria; it is highly resistant to the activity of most β-lactamases, whether they are of plasmid or chromosomal origin; and it preferentially binds to a critical penicillin-binding protein, PBP 2 (Neu, 1985 B; see also index entry Penicillins).

Imipenem is highly active in vitro against almost all gram-positive cocci, including staphylococci, streptococci, and pneumococci, and its potency exceeds that of the newer extended-spectrum β-lactam antibiotics. It also is active against most penicillinase-producing strains but does not inhibit true methicillin-resistant *S. aureus* or coagulase-negative species. Among the enterococci (group D streptococci), *E. faecalis* is usually susceptible, but *E. faecium* isolates are usually resistant.

Among gram-negative bacteria, imipenem's spectrum includes most Enterobacteriaceae, against which its activity is comparable to that of aztreonam and the most potent third-generation cephalosporins, and strains that are resistant to antipseudomonal penicillins, aminoglycosides, and some third-generation cephalosporins. Imipenem has excellent activity against meningococci, gonococci, and *Haemophilus influenzae*, including penicillinase-producing strains. It is very active against most *Acinetobacter* strains, and its in vitro potency equals or exceeds that of ceftazidime against *Pseudomonas aeruginosa. P. cepacia* and *Xanthomonas maltophilia* are resistant to this drug.

Except for *Clostridium difficile*, imipenem is highly active against most clinically important anaerobic species; its potency is comparable to that of clindamycin and metronidazole. Although imipenem inhibits a number of less common bacterial species in vitro (eg, *Actinomyces* species, *Aeromonas hydrophila, Campylobacter jejuni, Legionella, Nocardia asteroides, Yersinia enterocolitica*, atypical *Mycobacterium*), the clinical relevance of these findings is unclear.

In a comparison of 30,665 bacterial isolates, 29,220 (95%) and 30,023 (98%) were susceptible to imipenem at 4 mcg/ml and 8 mcg/ml, respectively (Kropp et al, 1985). These concentrations can be sustained in patients receiving the drug for the treatment of moderate and severe infections.

In contrast to many other β-lactam antimicrobial agents, the minimum bactericidal concentration (MBC) of imipenem is generally comparable to the minimum inhibitory concentration (MIC) when tested in vitro over a 10,000-fold inoculum range. The MBC exceeds the MIC for a small number of susceptible isolates, including methicillin-resistant strains of staphylococci and some strains of *P. aeruginosa*. The clinical significance of these observations is uncertain. Imipenem has a marked postantibiotic effect against most susceptible bacteria (see Neu, 1990 A).

Combinations of imipenem with aminoglycosides (gentamicin, tobramycin) appear to act synergistically against many isolates of *P. aeruginosa* and *E. faecalis* and may be useful when rapid and complete bactericidal activity is essential (Neu, 1985 B; Kropp et al, 1985). However, as with some cephamycins and aminothiazolyl cephalosporins, imipenem can induce production of Richmond and Sykes Type I (chromosomal) β-lactamases in certain gram-negative aerobes. In contrast to the inhibitory effect of this enzyme induction on these cephalosporins, phenotypic resistance to imipenem occurs only rarely, presumably because of its excellent penetration of bacterial cell walls and the stability to the β-lactamases it induces. These properties probably account for the general lack of cross-resistance and in vitro antagonism that have been observed between imipenem and other β-lactams (Kropp et al, 1985; Ashby et al, 1987). However, imipenem was reported to be susceptible to hydrolysis by β-lactamases produced by *X. maltophilia* and specific strains of *B. fragilis*.

In addition to inactivation by certain β-lactamases, resistance to imipenem has been postulated to be related to decreased penetration of the bacterial cell by the drug. This mechanism may be responsible for resistance in occasional strains of *S. marcescens* and *E. cloacae* and has been demonstrated for resistant strains of *P. aeruginosa* that have emerged during imipenem therapy (Vurma-Rapp et al, 1990). Cross-resistance with other β-lactams and aminoglycosides does not occur via this mechanism.

USES. Imipenem plus cilastatin has been effective in the treatment of a wide variety of serious nosocomial and community-acquired bacterial infections caused by gram-positive cocci, gram-negative aerobic bacilli, and anaerobes, including strains resistant to other antimicrobial agents. These include lower respiratory tract (Acar, 1985), intra-abdominal (Kager and Nord, 1985), obstetric and gynecologic (Sweet, 1985), complicated urinary tract (Cox and Corrado, 1985) and skin and soft tissue infections (Fass et al, 1985); osteomyelitis (Gentry, 1990); endocarditis primarily caused by *Staphylococcus aureus* (Dickinson et al, 1985); and bacteremias (Eron, 1985). In randomized, comparative clinical trials, the effectiveness of imipenem/cilastatin in serious infections compared favorably with that of moxalactam (Calandra et al, 1984), cefotaxime (Diaz-Mitoma et al, 1985), and the combination of clindamycin plus gentamicin (Guerra et al, 1985). In a multicenter trial, the use of imipenem/cilastatin as initial therapy in patients with mixed flora intra-abdominal infections was associated with significantly fewer treatment failures than tobramycin plus clindamycin (Solomkin et al, 1990). This was ascribed to the greater ability of imipenem/cilastatin to eradicate gram-negative aerobes at the site of infection, thus reducing the incidence of recurrent infection and the need for additional intervention.

The exact role of imipenem/cilastatin has not been completely defined, but this combination is a good choice for cephalosporin-resistant Enterobacteriaceae infections, especially those caused by *Citrobacter freundii* and *Enterobacter* species. Imipenem/cilastatin also is indicated for empiric therapy of serious infections in patients previously treated with multiple antibiotics because there is a high likelihood that organisms resistant to more conventional β-lactam antimicrobial agents will be encountered (see Neu, 1990 A). Imipenem/cilastatin appears to be particularly useful in the treatment of infections caused by mixtures of bacteria for which a combination of antibiotics, often including an aminoglycoside, would otherwise be necessary (Jaresko and Barriere, 1988; Neu, 1990 A). Examples include certain pulmonary, soft tissue, and bone infections. The activity of imipenem/cilastatin against the *Bacteroides fragilis* group and *E. faecalis* when compared with third generation cephalosporins makes it a good choice for the treatment of mixed intra-abdominal infections.

Because resistant strains of *Pseudomonas aeruginosa* have emerged during therapy with imipenem/cilastatin, its use alone for the treatment of serious infections caused by this pathogen probably should be avoided (Neu, 1990 A). Similarly, although imipenem/cilastatin alone has been effective empiric therapy in febrile neutropenic cancer patients (Bodey et al, 1986; Liang et al, 1990; Mortimer et al, 1991; Winston et al, 1991), other antipseudomonal β-lactams (eg, ceftazidime, piperacillin) or imipenem combined with an aminoglycoside are frequently preferred for this indication (see index entries Fever, Treatment). The role of imipenem/cilastatin in the treatment of meningitis and endocarditis caused by susceptible *S. aureus* and streptococci remains to be established.

ADVERSE REACTIONS AND PRECAUTIONS. Imipenem/cilastatin (dosage range, 1 to 4 g of each component daily) generally is well tolerated, and its adverse reaction profile resembles that of most other β-lactam antibiotics (Calandra et al, 1985).

Hypersensitivity reactions have been observed in 2.7% of patients and include drug fever, pruritus, urticaria, and other rashes; anaphylactic reactions have not been reported. However, the incidence of allergic reactions could be higher because all patients with a history of serious allergy to β-lactam antibiotics were excluded from clinical trials. Imipenem/cilastatin produced allergic manifestations in 2 of 12 patients with a history of nonanaphylactic hypersensitivity reactions to penicillins. In another study, 10 of 20 subjects who were positive to one or more penicillin determinants during in vivo skin testing also reacted to imipenem reagents (Saxon et al, 1988). These data indicate that standard precautions should be observed when individuals who are allergic to penicillin receive imipenem. Because lidocaine hydrochloride is used as the diluent in the intramuscular preparation, this product is contraindicated in patients who are hypersensitive to local anesthetics of the amide type and patients in shock or experiencing heart block.

The most common adverse reactions to intravenous and intramuscular administration of imipenem/cilastatin involve the gastrointestinal tract. Drug-related nausea and vomiting have been observed in 1.3% and 0.9% of patients, respectively. In some patients, a syndrome characterized by nausea and vomiting and accompanied by hypotension, dizziness, and sweating has been associated with rapid intravenous infusion of imipenem/cilastatin. If slowing the rate of infusion does not relieve these symptoms, the drug may have to be discontinued.

Diarrhea has occurred in about 3.3% of patients who receive imipenem/cilastatin. *Clostridium difficile* or its toxin was reported in 0.76% of patients and actual pseudomembranous colitis, diagnosed by colonoscopy, has occurred in four (0.16%).

Local adverse reactions at the site of infusion, usually phlebitis/thrombophlebitis, have been considered to be drug related in about 2% of patients. Pain at the site of intramuscular injection has been reported in 1.2% of patients.

Seizures were reported in 3% of 1,754 patients receiving imipenem/cilastatin in Phase III dose-ranging studies in the United States, but they were considered drug-related in only 16 patients (0.9%). Central nervous system lesions (eg, stroke, head injury, intracranial neoplasm), prior history of convulsions, and renal insufficiency were strong risk factors for seizures; the incidence of seizures was highest (12% to 32%) in patients with predisposing risk factors who also had received an excess dosage of drug (see Calandra et al, 1988). Seizures appear to respond to a reduction in dosage or discontinuation of imipenem/cilastatin therapy and to treatment with phenytoin or benzodiazepines. Most authorities believe that imipenem/cilastatin is more epileptogenic than other β-lactam antibiotics in humans; this also was suggested in animal studies (Eng et al, 1989). Thus, this combination should be used with caution in patients at increased risk for seizures, and some clinicians would avoid it in these patients. Dosages of imipenem/cilastatin should be adjusted for low body weight and be reduced in patients with renal impairment, ie, creatinine clearance $\leq$70 ml/min/1.73 M^2 (see Dosage and Preparations below). However, seizures have been reported even when these guidelines are followed (Eng et al, 1989; Leo and Ballow, 1991). Blood level determinations of imipenem are not routinely performed in most hospitals to assist in dosage adjustment.

Imipenem/cilastatin has not been associated with nephrotoxicity or coagulopathies.

Among severely ill patients receiving this combination, the incidences of colonization with resistant bacteria and fungi were 3.2% and 8%, respectively. The incidence of actual superinfections was 2.8% for bacteria, usually *Pseudomonas aeruginosa* or *X. maltophilia,* and 1.5% for *Candida*.

Abnormalities in results of laboratory studies in patients treated with imipenem/cilastatin appear to be relatively mild and reversible. Most common were transient elevations in liver function values, including AST (1.1%), ALT (1.2%), and alkaline phosphatase (0.8%). Eosinophilia and positive direct Coombs' test results have been observed. However, hemolytic anemia has not occurred. Reversible neutropenia, thrombocytopenia, and hypoprothrombinemia have been reported rarely. Thrombocytosis was observed in 15 patients (0.6%).

Despite its broad antimicrobial spectrum, the impact of imipenem/cilastatin on the fecal flora is modest (Nord et al, 1985).

Well-controlled studies of imipenem/cilastatin in pregnant women have not been performed. It is classified in FDA Pregnancy Category C.

DRUG INTERACTIONS. Acute central nervous system disturbances (eg, agitation, confusion, severe tremor) occurred in a renal transplant patient receiving cyclosporine [Sandimmune] and imipenem/cilastatin concomitantly (Zazgornik et al, 1986). Because both agents can cause central nervous system disturbances, patients receiving both drugs should be carefully observed for signs of toxicity and altered cyclosporine serum concentrations pending further information about this possible interaction (Hansten and Horn, 1989).

PHARMACOKINETICS. Neither imipenem nor cilastatin is appreciably absorbed following oral administration and, therefore, must be given parenterally. Mean plasma concentrations after a 30-minute intravenous infusion of 1 g of each drug were 52 and 65 mcg/ml, respectively. Six hours later, these values had fallen to 1 mcg or less per milliliter. Following intramuscular administration of 500 or 750 mg of imipenem/cilastatin, peak plasma levels of imipenem (10 and 12 mcg/ml, respectively) occurred in two hours. Peak plasma levels for cilastatin were 24 and 33 mcg/ml one hour after administration.

Approximately 20% of circulating imipenem is bound to plasma protein, and about 40% of cilastatin is protein bound. The drug is well distributed into most tissues and body fluids. In patients with meningitis, cerebrospinal fluid concentrations ranged between 0.5 and 11 mcg/ml following administration of 1 g every six hours for four doses (Modai et al, 1985). Concentrations of imipenem in bile generally are low. No data are available on drug concentrations in milk, placenta, or fetal tissue.

When administered with cilastatin, about 70% of a dose of imipenem is excreted as unchanged drug in urine within 10 hours of administration; both glomerular filtration and renal tubular secretion are involved. The remainder is eliminated primarily by metabolic inactivation. Approximately 75% of cilastatin also is recovered as unchanged drug in urine. The remainder appears to be metabolized, and 12% of a dose is recovered in urine as N-acetyl cilastatin, the major metabolite. Less than 1% of imipenem or cilastatin is excreted in the feces.

The elimination half-lives of both imipenem and cilastatin are about one hour in patients with normal renal function. In patients with renal failure, the half-life of imipenem increases to 3.5 to 4 hours and that of cilastatin increases to 16 hours; dosage adjustments are necessary. Both drugs are substantially removed by hemodialysis; the half-lives are 2.5 hours for imipenem and 3.8 hours for cilastatin. Supplemental dosing after hemodialysis is necessary.

For additional discussion, see Gibson et al, 1985; Rogers et al, 1985.

DOSAGE AND PREPARATIONS. The dosages listed refer to the amount of imipenem to be administered; an equal amount of cilastatin is present in the solution. See the manufacturer's instructions for the appropriate dilution of the drug, compatible diluents and solutions, and the stability of imipenem/cilastatin in these solutions. The dry powder should be stored below 30° C (86° F) before reconstitution.

Intravenous: For *adults with normal renal function*, the following schedule is recommended. (NOTE: Doses cited are for a 70-kg adult. A proportionate reduction in dose is recommended by the manufacturer for patients weighing less than 70 kg.) The drug is infused intravenously over 20 to 60 minutes, depending on the dose. In patients who develop nausea during the infusion, the rate of infusion may be slowed.

Type or Severity of Infection	Fully susceptible organisms including gram-positive and gram-negative aerobes and anaerobes	Moderately susceptible organisms, primarily some strains of *P. aeruginosa*
Mild	250 mg every 6 hours	500 mg every 6 hours
Moderate	500 mg every 8 hours-500 mg every 6 hours	500 mg every 6 hours-1 g every 8 hours
Severe, life-threatening	500 mg every 6 hours	1 g every 8 hours-1 g every 6 hours
Uncomplicated urinary tract infection	250 mg every 6 hours	250 mg every 6 hours
Complicated urinary tract infection	500 mg every 6 hours	500 mg every 6 hours

Maximum daily dosage not to exceed 50 mg/kg/day or 4 g/day, whichever is lower.

From manufacturer's literature

For *adults with impaired renal function*, the following dosages (based on a body weight of 70 kg) are recommended:

Creatinine Clearance (ml/min/1.73 M²)	Renal Function	Fully susceptible organisms including gram-positive and gram-negative aerobes and anaerobes	Moderately susceptible organisms, primarily some strains of *P. aeruginosa*
31-70	Mild impairment	500 mg every 8 hours	500 mg every 6 hours
21-30	Moderate impairment	500 mg every 12 hours	500 mg every 8 hours
6-20	Severe to marked impairment	250 mg every 12 hours	500 mg every 12 hours[2]
0-5	None, but on hemodialysis[1]	250 mg every 12 hours	500 mg every 12 hours[2]

[1] *Imipenem/cilastatin therapy is not recommended in these patients unless hemodialysis is instituted within 48 hours.*

[2] *There may be an increased risk of seizures at the higher dosages.*

From manufacturer's literature

A supplemental dose of imipenem/cilastatin should be given after each hemodialysis session unless the next dose is scheduled within four hours.

Primaxin I.V. (Merck Sharp & Dohme). Powder (sterile) 250 and 500 mg (equivalent to imipenem component) (sodium 0.8 and 1.6 mEq, respectively).

Intramuscular: Lidocaine hydrochloride 1% (without epinephrine) should be used to prepare the suspension. Dosage should be based on the location and severity of the infection, the susceptibility of the infecting pathogen(s), and renal function. For *adults with normal renal function,* the following schedule is recommended by the manufacturer:

Type/Location of Infection	Severity	Dosage Regimen
Lower respiratory tract, skin and skin structure, gynecologic	Mild/Moderate	500 or 750 mg every 12 hours depending on the severity of infection
Intra-abdominal	Mild/Moderate	750 mg every 12 hours

Total daily dosages greater than 1.5 g are not recommended. The duration of therapy depends upon the type and severity of the infection. Generally, intramuscular imipenem/cilastatin should be administered for at least two days after signs and symptoms of infection have resolved; the safety and efficacy of treatment beyond 14 days have not been established.

The safety and efficacy of this preparation of imipenem/cilastatin have not been established in patients with creatinine clearance of <20 ml/min/1.73 M². Serum creatinine alone may not be a sufficiently accurate measure of renal function. Creatinine clearance (Tcc) may be estimated from the following equation:

Tcc (male) = (wt in kg) (140 - age)/(72) (creatinine in mg/dl).

Tcc (female) = 0.85 X above value.

Primaxin I.M. (Merck Sharp & Dohme). Powder (sterile) 500 mg (sodium 1.4 mEq) and 750 mg (sodium 2.1 mEq) equivalent to imipenem component.

Cited References

Ampicillin/sulbactam (Unasyn). *Med Lett Drugs Ther* 29:79-81, 1987.

1989 Sexually transmitted diseases treatment guidelines. *MMWR* 38(suppl 8):1-43, 1989.

Acar JF: Therapy for lower respiratory tract infection with imipenem/cilastatin: A review of worldwide experience. *Rev Infect Dis* 7(suppl 3):S513-S517, 1985.

Ashby J, et al: Effect of imipenem on strains of Enterobacteriaceae expressing Richmond and Sykes Class I β-lactamases. *J Antimicrob Chemother* 20:15-22, 1987.

Birnbaum J, et al: Carbapenems, a new class of beta-lactam antibiotics: Discovery and development of imipenem/cilastatin. *Am J Med* 78(suppl 6A):3-21, 1985.

Bodey GP, et al: Imipenem-cilastatin as initial therapy for febrile cancer patients. *Antimicrob Agents Chemother* 30:211-214, 1986.

Bosso JA, Black PG: The use of aztreonam in pediatric patients: A review. *Pharmacotherapy* 11:20-25, 1991.

Brittain DC, et al: Ticarcillin plus clavulanic acid in treatment of pneumonia and other serious infections. *Am J Med* 79(suppl 5B):81-83, 1985.

Calandra GB, et al: Multiclinic randomized study of comparative efficacy, safety and tolerance of imipenem/cilastatin and moxalactam. *Eur J Clin Microbiol* 3:478-487, 1984.

Calandra GB, et al: Review of adverse experience and tolerability in first 2,516 patients treated with imipenem/cilastatin. *Am J Med* 78(suppl 6A):73-78, 1985.

Calandra G, et al: Factors predisposing to seizures in seriously ill infected patients receiving antibiotics: Experience with imipenem/cilastatin. *Am J Med* 84:911-918, 1988.

Campoli-Richards DM, Brogden RN: Sulbactam/ampicillin: Review of its antibacterial activity, pharmacokinetic properties, and therapeutic use. *Drugs* 33:577-609, 1987.

Chandrasekar PH, et al: Enterococcal superinfection and colonization with aztreonam therapy. *Antimicrob Agents Chemother* 26:280-282, 1984.

Clarke AM, Zemcov SJV: Clavulanic acid in combination with ticarcillin: *In vitro* comparison with other β-lactams. *J Antimicrob Chemother* 13:121-128, 1984.

Clergeot A, et al: Efficacy and safety of low-dose aztreonam in the treatment of moderate to severe infections due to gram-negative bacilli. *Rev Infect Dis* 13(suppl 7):S648-S651, 1991.

Colardyn F, et al: Infections in patients in intensive care units: Can the combination of a monobactam and a penicillin replace the classic combination of a β-lactam agent and an aminoglycoside? *Rev Infect Dis* 13(suppl 7):S640-S644, 1991.

Conrad DA, et al: Efficacy of aztreonam in the treatment of skeletal infections due to *Pseudomonas aeruginosa*. *Rev Infect Dis* 13(suppl 7):S634-S639, 1991.

Cox CE: Timentin versus piperacillin in treatment of hospitalized patients with urinary tract infections. *J Antimicrob Chemother* 17(suppl C):93-96, 1986.

Cox CE, Corrado ML: Safety and efficacy of imipenem/cilastatin in treatment of complicated urinary tract infections. *Am J Med* 78(suppl 6A):92-94, 1985.

Creasey WA, et al: Pharmacokinetic interaction of aztreonam with other antibiotics. *J Clin Pharmacol* 24:174-180, 1984.

Diaz-Mitoma F, et al: Prospective, randomized comparison of imipenem/cilastatin and cefotaxime for treatment of lung, soft tissue, and renal infections. *Rev Infect Dis* 7 (suppl 3):S452-S457, 1985.

Dickinson G, et al: Efficacy of imipenem/cilastatin in endocarditis. *Am J Med* 78 (suppl 6A):117-121, 1985.

Dratwa M, et al: Treatment of gram-negative peritonitis with aztreonam in patients undergoing continuous ambulatory peritoneal dialysis. *Rev Infect Dis* 13 (suppl 7):S645-S647, 1991.

Duma RJ, et al: Penetration of aztreonam into cerebrospinal fluid of patients with and without inflamed meninges. *Antimicrob Agents Chemother* 26:730-733, 1984.

Eng RHK, et al: Seizure propensity with imipenem. *Arch Intern Med* 149:1881-1883, 1989.

Eron LJ: Imipenem/cilastatin therapy of bacteremia. *Am J Med* 78 (suppl 6A):95-99, 1985.

Faro S: Ticarcillin/clavulanate: An alternative to combination antibiotic therapy for treating soft tissue pelvic infections in women. *J Reprod Med* 35 (suppl):353-358, 1990.

Faro S: The effect of timentin in the treatment of female pelvic soft tissue infections. *Pharmacotherapy* 11 (2, part 2):80S-83S, 1991.

Faro S, et al: Ticarcillin/clavulanate for treatment of postpartum endometritis. *Rev Infect Dis* 13 (suppl 9):S758-S762, 1991.

Fass RJ, et al: Treatment of skin and soft tissue infections with imipenem/cilastatin. *Am J Med* 78 (suppl 6A):110-112, 1985.

File TM Jr, Tan JS: Ticarcillin-clavulanate therapy for bacterial skin and soft tissue infections. *Rev Infect Dis* 13 (suppl 9):S733-S736, 1991.

Foulds G, et al: Penetration of sulbactam and ampicillin into cerebrospinal fluid of infants and young children with meningitis. *Antimicrob Agents Chemother* 31:1703-1705, 1987.

Gentry LO: Antibiotic therapy for osteomyelitis. *Infect Dis Clin North Am* 4:485-499, 1990.

Gentry LO, et al: Ticarcillin plus clavulanic acid (Timentin) therapy for osteomyelitis. *Am J Med* 79 (suppl 5B):116-121, 1985.

Gibson TP, et al: Imipenem/cilastatin: Pharmacokinetic profile in renal insufficiency. *Am J Med* 78 (suppl 6A):54-61, 1985.

Goldstein EJC, et al: Outpatient therapy of bite wounds: Demographic data, bacteriology, and prospective, randomized trial of amoxicillin/clavulanic acid versus penicillin ± dicloxacillin. *Int J Dermatol* 26:123-127, 1987.

Guerra JG, et al: Imipenem/cilastatin vs gentamicin/clindamycin for treatment of moderate to severe infections in hospitalized patients. *Rev Infect Dis* 7 (suppl 3):S463-S470, 1985.

Hansten PD, Horn JR: *Drug Interactions.* Philadelphia, Lea & Febiger, 1989, 224.

Heney D, et al: Aztreonam therapy in children with febrile neutropenia: A randomized trial of aztreonam plus flucloxacillin versus piperacillin plus gentamicin. *J Antimicrob Chemother* 28:117-129, 1991.

Hughes WT, et al: Guidelines for the use of antimicrobial agents in neutropenic patients with unexplained fever. *J Infect Dis* 161:381-396, 1990.

Itokazu GS, Danziger LH: Ampicillin-sulbactam and ticarcillin-clavulanic acid: A comparison of their in vitro activity and review of their clinical efficacy. *Pharmacotherapy* 11:382-414, 1991.

Jacoby GA, Archer GL: New mechanisms of bacterial resistance to antimicrobial agents. *N Engl J Med* 324:601-612, 1991.

Jaresko GS, Barriere SL: Imipenem monotherapy versus combination therapy in management of mixed bacterial infection: Critical appraisal. *Pharmacotherapy* 8:324-333, 1988.

Jensen T, et al: Safety of aztreonam in patients with cystic fibrosis and allergy to β-lactam antibiotics. *Rev Infect Dis* 13 (suppl 7):S594-S597, 1991.

Johnson JR, Stamm WE: Urinary tract infections in women: Diagnosis and treatment. *Ann Intern Med* 111:906-917, 1989.

Jones SR: Infections in frail and vulnerable elderly patients. *Am J Med* 88 (suppl 3C):3C-30S-3C-33S, 1990.

Kager L, Nord CE: Imipenem/cilastatin in treatment of intra-abdominal infections: Review of worldwide experience. *Rev Infect Dis* 7 (suppl 3):S518-S521, 1985.

Kerins DM: Ampicillin/sulbactam: A combination of an old and a new agent in the treatment of infection. *Am J Med Sci* 301:406-411, 1991.

Koch C, et al: Retrospective clinical study of hypersensitivity reactions to aztreonam and six other β-lactam antibiotics in cystic fibrosis patients receiving multiple treatment courses. *Rev Infect Dis* 13 (suppl 7):S608-S611, 1991.

Kropp H, et al: Antibacterial activity of imipenem: First thienamycin antibiotic. *Rev Infect Dis* 7 (suppl 3):S389-S410, 1985.

Lees L, et al: Sulbactam plus ampicillin: Interim review of efficacy and safety for therapeutic and prophylactic use. *Rev Infect Dis* 8 (suppl 5):S644-S650, 1986.

Lentnek AL, Williams RR: Aztreonam in the treatment of gram-negative bacterial meningitis. *Rev Infect Dis* 13 (suppl 7):S586-S590, 1991.

Liang R, et al: Ceftazidime versus imipenem-cilastatin as initial monotherapy for febrile neutropenic patients. *Antimicrob Agents Chemother* 34:1336-1341, 1990.

Leo RJ, Ballow CH: Seizure activity associated with imipenem use: Clinical case reports and review of the literature. *DICP* 25:351-354, 1991.

Lisby-Sutch SM, et al: Therapy of otitis media. *Clin Pharm* 9:15-34, 1990.

Maddux MS: Effects of β-lactamase-mediated antimicrobial resistance: The role of β-lactamase inhibitors. *Pharmacotherapy* 11 (2, part 2):40S-50S, 1991.

Madsen PO, et al: Aztreonam concentrations in human prostatic tissue. *Antimicrob Agents Chemother* 26:20-21, 1984.

Maesen FPV, et al: Amoxycillin/clavulanate in acute purulent exacerbations of chronic bronchitis. *J Antimicrob Chemother* 19:373-383, 1987.

McGregor JA: Ticarcillin/clavulanate for the treatment of female genital tract infections: Efficacy, safety and comparative microbiology. *J Reprod Med* 35:333-338, 1990.

The Medical Letter: *Handbook of Antimicrobial Therapy.* New Rochelle, NY, The Medical Letter, Inc, 1990, 42-55.

Meylan PR, et al: Clinical experience with Timentin in severe hospital infections. *J Antimicrob Chemother* 17 (suppl C):127-139, 1986.

Modai J, et al: Penetration of imipenem and cilastatin into cerebrospinal fluid of patients with bacterial meningitis. *J Antimicrob Chemother* 16:751-755, 1985.

Mortimer JE, et al: Comparison of cefoperazone and mezlocillin with imipenem/cilastatin in febrile neutropenic patients with cancer. *Curr Ther Res* 49:701-710, 1991.

Murray BE: New aspects of antimicrobial resistance and the resulting therapeutic dilemmas. *J Infect Dis* 163:1185-1194, 1991.

Nelson JD: *1991-1992 Pocketbook of Pediatric Antimicrobial Therapy*, ed 8. Baltimore, Williams & Wilkins, 1991, 66-80.

Neu HC: Contribution of beta-lactamases to bacterial resistance and mechanisms to inhibit beta-lactamases. *Am J Med* 79 (suppl 5B): 2-12, 1985 A.

Neu HC: Carbapenems: Special properties contributing to their activity. *Am J Med* 78 (suppl 6A):33-40, 1985 B.

Neu HC: Aztreonam: The first monobactam. *Med Clin North Am* 72:555-566, 1988.

Neu HC: Other beta-lactam antibiotics, in Mandell GL, et al (eds): *Principles and Practice of Infectious Diseases*, ed 3. New York, Churchill Livingstone, 1990 A, 257-263.

Neu HC: Aztreonam activity, pharmacology, and clinical uses. *Am J Med* 88 (suppl 3C):25-65, 1990 B.

Nord CE, et al: Effect of imipenem/cilastatin on colonic microflora. *Rev Infect Dis* 7 (suppl 3):S432-S434, 1985.

Pankey GA: Diagnosis and treatment of skin and soft tissue infections: Clinical experience with ticarcillin disodium-clavulanate potassium. *Pharmacotherapy* 11 (2, part 2):90S-98S, 1991.

Pulverer G, et al: In-vitro activity of ticarcillin with and without clavulanic acid against clinical isolates of gram-positive and gram-negative bacteria. *J Antimicrob Chemother* 17 (suppl C):1-5, 1986.

Rogers JD, et al: Pharmacokinetics of imipenem and cilastatin in volunteers. *Rev Infect Dis* 7 (suppl 3):S435-S446, 1985.

Rolinson GN: Evolution of β-lactamase inhibitors. *Rev Infect Dis* 13 (suppl 9):S727-S732, 1991.

Rolston KVI, et al: Aztreonam in the prevention and treatment of infection in neutropenic cancer patients. *Am J Med* 88 (suppl 3C):3C-24S-3C-29S, 1990.

Saxon A, et al: Imipenem cross-reactivity with penicillin in humans. *J Allergy Clin Immunol* 82:213-217, 1988.

Sion ML, et al: Efficacy and safety of aztreonam in the treatment of patients with renal failure. *Rev Infect Dis* 13 (suppl 7):S652-S654, 1991.

Sklavunu-Tsurutsoglu S, et al: Efficacy of aztreonam in the treatment of neonatal sepsis. *Rev Infect Dis* 13 (suppl 7):S591-S593, 1991.

Solomkin JS, et al: Results of a multicenter trial comparing imipenem/cilastatin to tobramycin/clindamycin for intra-abdominal infections. *Ann Surg* 212:581-591, 1990.

Stutman HR: Clinical experience with aztreonam for treatment of infections in children. *Rev Infect Dis* 13 (suppl 7):S582-S585, 1991.

Stutman HR, et al: Single-dose pharmacokinetics of aztreonam in pediatric patients. *Antimicrob Agents Chemother* 26:196-199, 1984.

Swabb EA: Review of clinical pharmacology of monobactam antibiotic aztreonam. *Am J Med* 78 (suppl 2A):11-18, 1985.

Sweet RL: Imipenem/cilastatin in treatment of obstetric and gynecologic infections: Review of worldwide experience. *Rev Infect Dis* 7 (suppl 3):S522-S527, 1985.

Sykes RB, Bonner DP: Aztreonam: First monobactam. *Am J Med* 78 (suppl 2A):2-10, 1985.

Tanaka-Kido J, et al: Comparative efficacies of aztreonam and chloramphenicol in children with typhoid fever. *Pediatr Infect Dis J* 9:44-48, 1990.

Tartaglione TA, et al: In vitro and in vivo studies of effect of aztreonam on platelet function and coagulation in normal volunteers. *Antimicrob Agents Chemother* 30:73-77, 1986.

Todd PA, Benfield P: Amoxicillin/clavulanic acid: An update of its antibacterial activity, pharmacokinetic properties and therapeutic use. *Drugs* 39:264-307, 1990.

Tunkel AR, Scheld WM: Aztreonam. *Infect Control Hosp Epidemiol* 11:486-494, 1990.

Umaña MA, et al: Evaluation of aztreonam and ampicillin *vs.* amikacin and ampicillin for treatment of neonatal bacterial infections. *Pediatr Infect Dis J* 9:175-180, 1990.

Vega JM, et al: Tolerance to aztreonam in patients allergic to beta lactam antibiotics. *Allergy* 46:196-202, 1991.

Vurma-Rapp U, et al: Mechanism of imipenem resistance acquired by three *Pseudomonas aeruginosa* strains during imipenem therapy. *Eur J Clin Microbiol Infect Dis* 9:580-587, 1990.

Wald E, et al: Sulbactam/ampicillin in treatment of acute epiglottitis in children. *Rev Infect Dis* 8 (suppl 5):S617-S619, 1986.

Williams RR, Hotchkin D: Aztreonam plus clindamycin versus tobramycin plus clindamycin in the treatment of intraabdominal infections. *Rev Infect Dis* 13 (suppl 7):S629-S633, 1991.

Winston DJ, et al: Beta-lactam antibiotic therapy in febrile granulocytopenic patients: A randomized trial comparing cefoperazone plus piperacillin, ceftazidime plus piperacillin, and imipenem alone. *Ann Intern Med* 115:849-859, 1991.

Zazgornik J, et al: Potentiation of neurotoxic side effects by coadministration of imipenem to cyclosporine therapy in a kidney transplant recipient: Synergism of side effects or drug interaction? *Clin Nephrol* 26:265-266, 1986.

New Evaluation

PIPERACILLIN SODIUM/TAZOBACTAM SODIUM
[Zosyn]

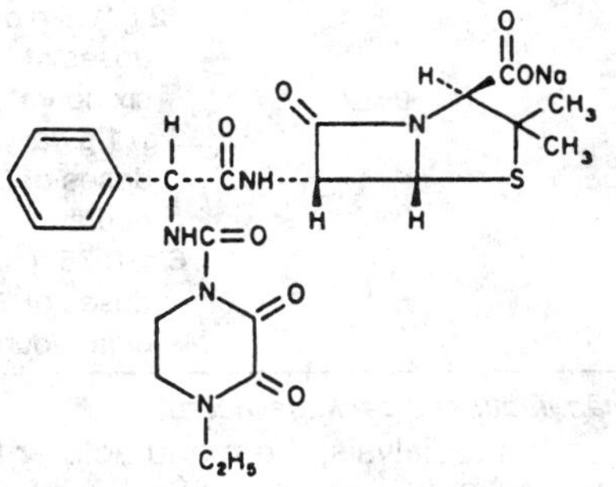

Piperacillin Sodium

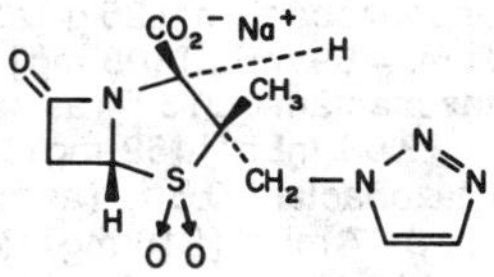

Tazobactam Sodium

The combination of piperacillin sodium, an extended spectrum ureidopenicillin, and tazobactam sodium, a β-lactamase inhibitor of the penicillanic acid sulfone class, is marketed as an 8:1 fixed-ratio dosage form for intravenous administration.

MECHANISM OF ACTION, ANTIMICROBIAL SPECTRUM, AND RESISTANCE. Piperacillin is a broad spectrum antipseudomonal penicillin that is active in vitro against most gram-positive bacteria, gram-negative cocci, and, when compared with ampicillin, an expanded spectrum of gram-negative bacilli including *Pseudomonas aeruginosa*. However, β-lactamase-producing strains of these organisms (eg, β-lactamase-producing strains of staphylococci, *Haemophilus influenzae, Escherichia coli*, and the *Bacteroides fragilis* group) can inactivate piperacillin and are relatively common (for detailed discussion, see index entry Piperacillin).

Like other available β-lactamase inhibitors (clavulanic acid and sulbactam), tazobactam has little intrinsic antibacterial activity, but it irreversibly binds to many β-lactamase enzymes to extend the antibacterial spectrum of piperacillin. Administration of piperacillin with tazobactam does not alter the susceptibility of piperacillin-sensitive strains and extends the in vitro activity of piperacillin to include, at achievable serum concentrations, β-lactamase-producing strains of staphylococci, *H. influenzae*, many Enterobacteriaciae (eg, *E. coli*), and the *B. fragilis* group (Appelbaum et al, 1986; Gutmann et al, 1986; Jacobs et al, 1986; Kuck et al, 1989). Methicillin-resistant staphylococci and highly penicillin-resistant enterococci are resistant to piperacillin/tazobactam. Furthermore, the addition of tazobactam to piperacillin does not increase activity against most strains of *Pseudomonas aeruginosa*, and the majority of piperacillin-resistant *P. aeruginosa* strains also are resistant to the combination (Acar et al, 1993). For discussion of the mechanism of action of piperacillin, see index entry Piperacillin.

USES. Piperacillin/tazobactam is indicated for the following conditions caused by piperacillin-resistant, piperacillin/tazobactam-susceptible, β-lactamase-producing strains of the organisms listed: appendicitis (complicated by rupture or abscess) and peritonitis caused by *E. coli* or the *B. fragilis* group (*B. fragilis, B. ovatus, B. thetaiotaomicron*, or *B. vulgatis*); uncomplicated and complicated skin and skin structure infections, including cellulitis, cutaneous abscess, and ischemic/diabetic foot infections, caused by *S. aureus*; postpartum endometritis or pelvic inflammatory disease caused by *E. coli*; and community-acquired pneumonia (moderate severity only) caused by *H. influenzae*.

Infections caused by piperacillin-susceptible bacteria also are susceptible to piperacillin/tazobactam. Thus, the combination regimen is useful as presumptive therapy of polymicrobial infections prior to identification of causative organisms because of its broad spectrum of activity against gram-positive and gram-negative aerobic and anaerobic bacteria. Results of randomized, prospective clinical trials have shown that piperacillin/tazobactam is comparable to clindamycin plus gentamicin for intra-abdominal (Polk et al, 1993) and pelvic (Sweet et al, 1994) infections and to ticarcillin/clavulanic acid in complicated skin and skin structure infections (Tan et al, 1993). In an open, randomized, European multicenter trial, piperacillin/tazobactam was more effective than imipenem/cilastatin for intra-abdominal infections (Brismar et al, 1992); however, the dosage used for imipenem/cilastatin (500 mg every eight hours) was lower than that usually recommended in the United States (500 mg every six hours to 1 g every eight hours). In summary, the currently available published data suggest that piperacillin/tazobactam will be another useful agent for polymicrobial infections.

Although piperacillin is a useful antibiotic for *Pseudomonas aeruginosa* infections, the manufacturer's literature for piperacillin/tazobactam does not list *P. aeruginosa* as a susceptible pathogen. Moreover, the recommended daily dosage for piperacillin/tazobactam of 12 g (see below) may not be effective for infections caused by this organism (see *Med Lett Drugs Ther*, 1994).

The manufacturer's literature for piperacillin/tazobactam states that clinical trial data showed that this combination was not effective for complicated urinary tract infections at the dosage studied (ie, 3.375 g every eight hours).

ADVERSE REACTIONS AND PRECAUTIONS. Piperacillin/tazobactam generally has been well tolerated in clinical trials. Of 2,621 patients treated in Phase III clinical trials worldwide, only 3.2% discontinued therapy; adverse events involving the skin (1.3%) and gastrointestinal tract (0.9%) were most frequently cited. The most commonly reported adverse events during North American clinical trials also involved the gastrointestinal tract (diarrhea, nausea, vomiting) and skin (rash, pruritus). The most common laboratory abnormalities were related to liver function (see manufacturer's literature; Kuye et al, 1993). Adverse reactions are similar to those seen with piperacillin alone (see index entry Piperacillin). Patients who are allergic to any penicillin should be considered allergic to piperacillin/tazobactam.

Patients over 65 years are not at an increased risk of developing adverse effects solely because of age. However, dosage should be adjusted in the presence of renal insufficiency (see below). Safety and efficacy in children under 12 years have not been established.

This combination product is classified in FDA Pregnancy Category B.

DRUG INTERACTIONS AND INTERFERENCE WITH LABORATORY TESTS. As with piperacillin alone, mixing piperacillin/tazobactam with an aminoglycoside in parenteral solutions prior to administration can inactivate the aminoglycoside. In vivo antagonism also can occur in patients with renal failure (see index entries Piperacillin; Aminoglycosides).

For a discussion of other drug interactions involving the penicillins, see index entry Penicillins.

PHARMACOKINETICS. Peak plasma concentrations of piperacillin and tazobactam are attained immediately after completion of an intravenous infusion; piperacillin concentrations are similar to those produced when the drug is administered alone. Following 30-minute infusions of 2.25, 3.375, and 4.5 g of piperacillin/tazobactam, peak plasma concentrations were 134, 242, and 298 mcg/ml for piperacillin and 15, 24, and 34 mcg/ml for tazobactam, respectively (see manufacturer's literature).

The distribution and elimination of piperacillin and tazobactam are similar. Both drugs are approximately 30% bound to plasma proteins, are widely distributed into tissues and body fluids, are eliminated primarily as unchanged drugs by the kidney (glomerular filtration and renal tubular secretion), and have plasma half-lives between 0.7 and 1.2 hours. Half-lives of both drugs increase in patients with renal impairment, and dosage adjustments are recommended when the creatinine clearance is below 40 ml/min. Hemodialysis removes 30% to 40% of a dose of piperacillin/tazobactam.

For additional discussion, see the manufacturer's literature; see also index entry Piperacillin.

DOSAGE AND PREPARATIONS.

Intravenous: Piperacillin/tazobactam should be administered by intermittent infusion over 30 minutes. See the package insert for the appropriate dilution of the drug, a list of compatible diluents and intravenous solutions, and stability of piperacillin/tazobactam in these solutions.

The manufacturer's recommended total daily dose for *adults* is piperacillin 12 g/tazobactam 1.5 g, given as 3.375 g every six hours. Duration of therapy usually is for 7 to 10 days, but length of therapy depends on the patient's condition and the severity of the infection.

In *adults with renal insufficiency,* the recommended daily doses are as follows:

Creatinine Clearance (ml/min)	Dosage
>40	12 g/1.5 g daily in divided doses of 3.375 g every six hours
20-40	8 g/1 g daily in divided doses of 2.25 g every six hours
<20	6 g/0.75 g daily in divided doses of 2.25 g every eight hours

From manufacturer's package insert

For patients on hemodialysis, the manufacturer recommends a maximum dose of 2.25 g every eight hours plus an additional dose of 0.75 g following each dialysis period.

Zosyn (Lederle). Powder (sterile) containing piperacillin 2 g (as sodium salt) and tazobactam 0.25 g (as sodium salt) in 2.25 g containers (sodium, 4.69 mEq [108 mg]); piperacillin 3 g (as sodium salt) and tazobactam 0.375 g (as sodium salt) in 3.375 g containers (sodium, 7.03 mEq [162 mg]); piperacillin 4 g (as sodium salt) and tazobactam 0.5 g (as sodium salt) in 4.5 g containers (sodium, 9.37 mEq [216 mg]); and piperacillin 36 g (as sodium salt) and tazobactam 4.5 g (as sodium salt) in 40.5 g bulk containers (sodium, 84.36 mEq/container).

Cited References

Piperacillin/tazobactam. *Med Lett Drugs Ther* 36:7-9, 1994.

Acar JF, et al: Susceptibility survey of piperacillin alone and in the presence of tazobactam. *J Antimicrob Chemother* 31(suppl A):23-28, 1993.

Appelbaum PC, et al: Comparative activity of β-lactamase inhibitors YTR 830, clavulanate, and sulbactam combined with β-lactams against β-lactamase-producing anaerobes. *Antimicrob Agents Chemother* 30:789-791, 1986.

Brismar B, et al: Piperacillin-tazobactam versus imipenem-cilastatin for treatment of intra-abdominal infections. *Antimicrob Agents Chemother* 36:2766-2773, 1992.

Gutmann L, et al: Comparative evaluation of a new β-lactamase inhibitor, YTR 830, combined with different β-lactam antibiotics against bacteria harboring known β-lactamases. *Antimicrob Agents Chemother* 29:955-957, 1986.

Jacobs MR, et al: Comparative activities of the β-lactamase inhibitors YTR 830, clavulanate, and sulbactam combined with ampicillin and broad-spectrum penicillins against defined β-lactamase-producing aerobic gram-negative bacilli. *Antimicrob Agents Chemother* 29:980-985, 1986.

Kuck NA, et al: Comparative in vitro and in vivo activities of piperacillin combined with the β-lactamase inhibitors tazobactam, clavulanic acid, and sulbactam. *Antimicrob Agents Chemother* 33:1964-1969, 1989.

Kuye O, et al: Safety profile of piperacillin/tazobactam in Phase I and III clinical studies. *J Antimicrob Chemother* 31(suppl A):113-124, 1993.

Polk HC Jr, et al: Prospective randomized study of piperacillin/tazobactam therapy of surgically treated intra-abdominal infection. *Am Surg* 59:598-605, 1993.

Sweet RL, et al: Piperacillin and tazobactam versus clindamycin and gentamicin in the treatment of hospitalized women with pelvic infection. *Obstet Gynecol* 83:280-286, 1994.

Tan JS, et al: Treatment of hospitalized patients with complicated skin and skin structure infections: Double-blind, randomized, multicenter study of piperacillin-tazobactam versus ticarcillin-clavulanate. *Antimicrob Agents Chemother* 37:1580-1586, 1993.

Macrolides and Lincosamides 66

MACROLIDES

The macrolide antibiotics that are currently used in the United States include the prototype, erythromycin (derived from strains of *Streptomyces erythreus*), and two recently marketed agents, clarithromycin [Biaxin] and azithromycin [Zithromax]. Troleandomycin [Tao], a macrolide derived from strains of *Streptomyces antibioticus*, offers no advantages over erythromycin in the treatment of infectious diseases and is not recommended. It is used occasionally in severe asthma in combination with methylprednisolone (see index entry Troleandomycin, In Asthma).

Chemically, these drugs contain a macrocyclic lactone ring to which sugars are attached (see Figure 1). Clarithromycin is 6-methoxy-erythromycin. Azithromycin has an additional nitrogen group giving it a 15-membered macrolide ring, also referred to as an azalide. These structural changes improve the stability of these compounds in acid, enhance their bioavailability, and may reduce gastrointestinal irritation compared with erythromycin. The microbiologic activity of clarithromycin and azithromycin is similar to that of erythromycin, but there are some important differences (Neu 1991 A, 1991 B) (see the section Antimicrobial Spectrum).

The macrolides are of major clinical importance. These antibiotics have some primary indications and frequently are the preferred alternative to penicillin G for a number of infections in penicillin-allergic individuals. They also are among the safest antibiotics in use today.

Mechanism of Action

Macrolides inhibit bacterial protein synthesis. They reversibly bind to the 50S ribosomal subunit and prevent elongation of the peptide chain, most likely by interfering with the translocation step. These agents do not bind to mammalian 80S ribosomes; this accounts in part for their selective toxicity. The binding sites for the macrolides overlap those for chloramphenicol and the lincosamides; therefore, the binding of one of these antibiotics to the ribosome may inhibit the activity of the other (Pratt and Fekety, 1986). There are no clinical indications for their concurrent use.

Macrolides may be bacteriostatic or bactericidal depending on the concentration of drug, organism susceptibility, growth rate, and size of the inoculum. Bacterial killing is favored by higher antibiotic concentrations, lower bacterial density, and rapid growth. The antibacterial activity of macrolides is pH-dependent, with greater activity demonstrated at neutral or slightly alkaline rather than acidic conditions (Steigbigel, 1990; Washington and Wilson, 1985; Barry et al, 1988; Hardy et al, 1988). Erythromycin is inactivated in an acidic medium (eg, stomach gastric acid, abscess pus).

Antimicrobial Spectrum

Erythromycin has a relatively broad spectrum and is active in vitro against most gram-positive and some gram-negative bacteria, actinomycetes, mycoplasmas, spirochetes, chlamydiae, rickettsiae, and certain mycobacteria other than *M. tuberculosis* (Steigbigel, 1990; Washington and Wilson, 1985; Brittain, 1987).

Among gram-positive cocci, *Streptococcus pyogenes* (group A, beta-hemolytic streptococci) and *S. pneumoniae* are highly susceptible to erythromycin, which exerts a bactericidal action against these organisms; occasional strains (eg, about 5% of group A streptococci) are resistant in the United States (Steigbigel, 1990; Brittain, 1987). However, resistance of *S. pneumoniae* to macrolides and lincosamides has become more common in Europe (eg, 25% in France; 17% in

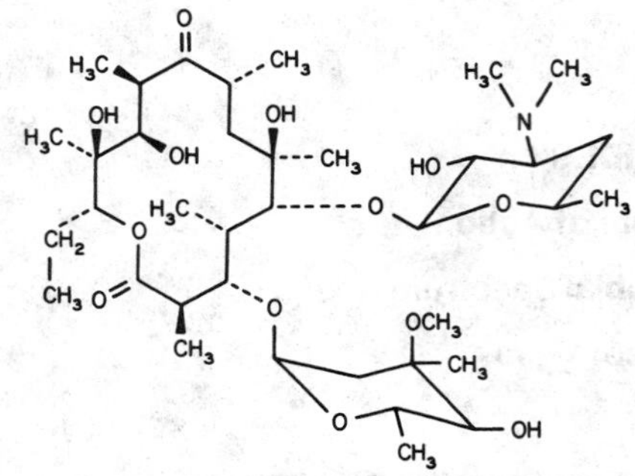

Erythromycin

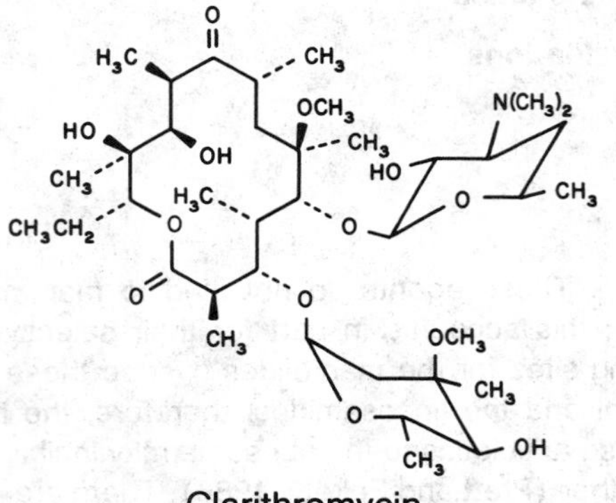

Clarithromycin

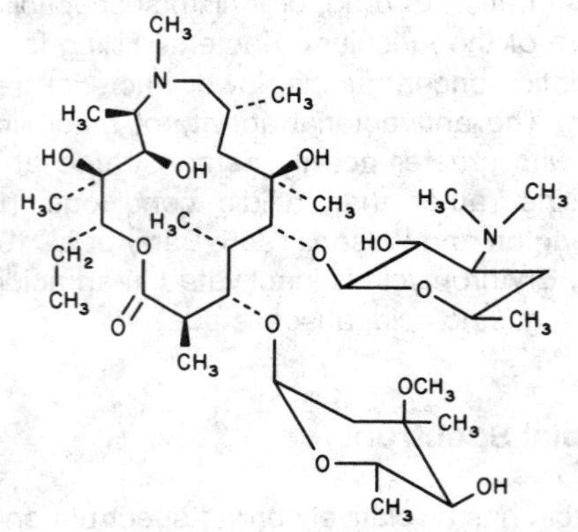

Azithromycin

FIGURE 1. CHEMICAL STRUCTURES OF MACROLIDES

Belgium) (Fremaux et al, 1992; Verhaegen et al, 1988). In general, resistance to erythromycin among groups A, B, C, and G streptococci has reached 14% in Europe (Soussy et al, 1992). These developments may herald increasing problems in the United States.

Erythromycin also is active against most viridans and anaerobic streptococci. It is inhibitory against a small number of strains of *Enterococcus faecalis*. Approximately 50% of *Staphylococcus aureus* and *S. epidermidis* are susceptible; however, many strains of *S. aureus*, particularly nosocomial isolates, are resistant or rapidly develop resistance during therapy. Clarithromycin is two- to fourfold more active and azithromycin two- to fourfold less active than erythromycin against most streptococci and staphylococci (Chin et al, 1987; Barry et al, 1988; Maskell et al, 1990). Streptococci and staphylococci that are resistant to erythromycin are resistant to clarithromycin and azithromycin as well. Depending on the geographic region, 15% to 45% of *S. aureus* strains causing nosocomial infection have the MLS_B phenotype (see Resistance below) and are resistant to macrolides (Duval, 1985). Less than 20% of methicillin-resistant staphylococci are inhibited by macrolides.

Aerobic gram-positive bacilli that are susceptible to macrolides include *Bacillus anthracis, Corynebacterium diphtheriae, C. minutissimum, Erysipelothrix rhusiopathiae,* and *Listeria monocytogenes*. Occasional strains of *C. diphtheriae* are resistant to erythromycin; most are resistant to azithromycin. Erythromycin is active against *Actinomyces israelii. Nocardia asteroides* has variable susceptibility to erythromycin.

Among the anaerobic bacteria, *Clostridium tetani* is susceptible, but many strains of *C. perfringens* are only moderately so. Species of *Bacteroides* isolated in the oropharynx are usually susceptible, but more than one-half of *B. fragilis* strains are resistant. Many *Fusobacterium* strains also are resistant. Concentrations that inhibit some anaerobic species are significantly lower for azithromycin than for erythromycin (Retsema et al, 1987; Neu et al, 1988; Hardy et al, 1988).

Most strains of *Neisseria gonorrhoeae* and *N. meningitidis*, gram-negative cocci, are susceptible to macrolides. *Moraxella (Branhamella) catarrhalis* also are susceptible (Kallings, 1986; Nicotra et al, 1986). Azithromycin is the most active macrolide against these pathogens.

Among gram-negative bacilli, most strains of *Bordetella pertussis, Campylobacter jejuni, Eikenella corrodens, Haemophilus ducreyi* (azithromycin most active), and some *Brucella* species are susceptible to macrolides (Slaney et al, 1990); *Haemophilus influenzae* is only moderately susceptible to erythromycin, but azithromycin is four to eight times more active (Retsema et al, 1987; Hardy et al, 1988; Goldstein et al, 1990). An active metabolite of clarithromycin (14-hydroxy-clarithromycin) acts in an additive or synergistic manner against *Haemophilus* (Hardy et al, 1990; Dabernat et al, 1991; Bergeron et al, 1992). Macrolides also are active against *Helicobacter pylori*.

Azithromycin, unlike erythromycin and clarithromycin, inhibits some aerobic gram-negative bacilli (Retsema et al, 1987; Neu et al, 1988). The majority of these bacilli, including the Enterobacteriaceae, are intrinsically resistant to erythromycin and clarithromycin because the cell envelopes prevent passive diffusion. Organisms that are moderately susceptible to azithromycin include most *Salmonella, Shigella,* and *Aeromonas* species; *Escherichia coli*; and *Yersinia enterocolitica*. Azithromycin has excellent activity against *Vibrio cholerae* and species isolated in patients with vaginitis, such as *Gardnerella vaginalis* and *Mobiluncus*.

Macrolides are active against *Mycoplasma pneumoniae, Ureaplasma urealyticum, Treponema pallidum, Legionella pneumophila, L. micdadei*, and many strains of *Rickettsia* and *Chlamydia*. In vitro, clarithromycin is more active than the other macrolides against *Chlamydia trachomatis* and *C. pneumoniae* (Segreti et al, 1987; Scieux et al, 1990; Ridgway et al, 1991). Clarithromycin inhibits *Mycobacterium avium* complex at concentrations achievable in lung tissue or macrophages, and both new macrolides are more active than erythromycin against other atypical mycobacteria such as *M. chelonae* (clarithromycin most active), *M. chelonae abscessus,* and *M. fortuitum* (Brown et al, 1992).

Both clarithromycin and azithromycin inhibit *Borrelia burgdorferi* at lower concentrations than erythromycin. Azithromycin has excellent activity against *Toxoplasma gondii* and appears to kill cyst forms (Araujo et al, 1988); clarithromycin also is active in vitro and in murine models (Chang et al, 1988). Yeasts, fungi, and viruses are resistant to erythromycin.

Resistance

Various mechanisms of acquired resistance to erythromycin have been reported. Bacteria with such resistance to erythromycin also are resistant to azithromycin and clarithromycin. Decreased binding of macrolides to their target site accounts for nearly all of the resistant strains isolated from patients. This alteration usually results from methylation of adenine in the 23S ribosomal subunit and confers broad resistance to other macrolides (M), lincosamides (L), and some streptogramin (S) type B antibiotics (the so-called MLS_B phenotype). MLS_B resistance has been described for a variety of bacteria, including *Staphylococcus* species, *Streptococcus* species including *S. pneumoniae, Corynebacterium diphtheriae, B. fragilis, C. perfringens, C. difficile, Listeria*, and *Legionella* species, and some Enterobacteriaceae (Leclercq and Courvalin, 1991 A). This resistance is usually mediated by a plasmid that contains a gene for an RNA methylase, and it can be constitutive or inducible; the latter occurs in *S. aureus*. The methylase may be induced when antibiotic concentrations are subinhibitory for protein synthesis; 14- and 15-membered macrolides are the most effective inducers of RNA methylase. MLS_B resistance in *Streptococcus* species also can be expressed constitutively or inducibly; however, unlike in staphylococci, some macrolides or lincosamides may act as inducers.

Another resistance mechanism involves alteration in a protein component of the bacterial 50S ribosomal subunit resulting in decreased binding affinity for erythromycin (and often other macrolides and lincosamides). This one-step, high-level resistance is due to a chromosomal mutation and has been demonstrated in *Bacillus subtilis, S. pyogenes, E. coli*, and probably *S. aureus*.

Two other mechanisms of resistance, decreased permeability of the cell wall to erythromycin and plasmid-mediated esterase or phosphotransferase, are exhibited by the Enterobacteriaceae (Leclercq and Courvalin, 1991 B) (see also Antimicrobial Spectrum).

Uses

A macrolide is the preferred or alternative therapy for a number of indications as outlined below.

Ear: The most common causative organisms of acute otitis media are *S. pneumoniae* and *H. influenzae* (usually nontypeable strains). *M. catarrhalis* is a common pathogen in some geographic areas. Antimicrobial drug therapy is usually empiric and should be effective against the two most likely pathogens. Acute otitis media due to *S. pneumoniae* or *S. pyogenes* usually responds to erythromycin (amoxicillin or ampicillin preferred), but if the infection is caused by *H. influenzae*, the concentration of erythromycin achieved in the middle ear may be inadequate to eradicate the organism. The combination of erythromycin and a sulfonamide usually is more effective than erythromycin alone in children with acute otitis media caused by *H. influenzae*. This combination is useful when the patient is allergic to penicillins or when β lactamase-producing aminopenicillin-resistant strains of *H. influenzae* or *M. catarrhalis* are causative. A fixed-ratio combination product containing erythromycin ethylsuccinate and sulfisoxazole acetyl [Pediazole] is available (see index entry Pediazole). In vitro, azithromycin and the combination of clarithromycin and 14-OH clarithromycin are more active than erythromycin against *H. influenzae* and *M. catarrhalis.* Preliminary results of several clinical trials indicate that clarithromycin suspension (investigational) may be useful in pediatric patients with acute otitis media. For other alternatives in the treatment of acute otitis media caused by amoxicillin-resistant organisms, see index entry Otitis Media, Treatment.

Eye: Conjunctivitis in infants caused by *C. trachomatis* is a primary indication for the use of erythromycin. See index entry Conjunctivitis, Neonatal.

Gastrointestinal and Intra-abdominal: In children, erythromycin is the drug of choice for gastroenteritis caused by *C. jejuni;* ciprofloxacin is an effective alternative in adults. Definitive treatment guidelines are lacking but, in the absence of a rapid diagnostic technique, it appears that mild cases of *C. jejuni* gastroenteritis are self-limited and erythromycin should be reserved for those with severe illness (eg, presence of fever, bloody diarrhea, symptoms unimproved or worsening at the time of diagnosis), infection in immunocompromised hosts (eg, cancer patients), or when transmission of the organism must be prevented. Some strains of *C. jejuni* are resistant to erythromycin. The recommended dosage is adults, 250 mg orally four times daily for five to seven days; children, 30 to 50 mg/kg/day in four divided doses.

Based on preliminary studies, clarithromycin appears to eradicate *H. pylori* from the stomach (Graham et al, 1991).

Because of its effectiveness in animal models, azithromycin is being tested in the treatment of typhoid fever.

Respiratory Tract (Lower): Erythromycin is the drug of choice for the treatment of atypical pneumonia caused by *M. pneumoniae* and *L. pneumophila* (Legionnaires' disease). In the latter, the usual adult daily dose of erythromycin (2 g orally) may be inadequate; thus, the intravenous route is usually used initially (2 to 4 g daily) in all but the mildest cases. *Legionella* may persist despite therapy, and radiographic evidence of resolution often requires many weeks. Rifampin [Rifadin, Rimactane] frequently is added to the regimen for severely ill patients or for those who do not respond satisfactorily to erythromycin alone. The duration of erythromycin therapy for Legionnaires' disease should be three weeks or longer because higher relapse rates have been reported with shorter courses. Erythromycin also is effective for infections caused by *L. micdadei* (Pittsburgh pneumonia agent).

Pneumonia in infants and children due to *C. trachomatis* is a primary indication for the use of erythromycin.

Because erythromycin is an effective alternative to penicillin G for pneumococcal pneumonia and is active against *M. pneumoniae* and *C. pneumoniae*, this antibiotic frequently is preferred for empiric therapy of mild to moderate cases of community-acquired pneumonia in older children and younger adults without predisposing conditions. (*M. pneumoniae* and *S. pneumoniae* are the most common causes of pneumonia in this population.)

The newer macrolides also are effective in pneumonia caused by *S. pneumoniae*. On the basis of animal and in vitro experiments, azithromycin and clarithromycin should be as effective as erythromycin for infections caused by *M. pneumoniae* and *Legionella*. In one multicenter, double-blind, randomized trial, clarithromycin 250 mg twice daily was at least as effective as erythromycin 500 mg four times daily for the treatment of community-acquired pneumonia and was better tolerated (Anderson et al, 1991). Similar results were reported in an open multicenter randomized trial that compared azithromycin with erythromycin in the treatment of atypical pneumonia (Schönwald et al, 1990). See also index entry Pneumonia, Treatment.

In children and college students, lower respiratory tract infections caused by *C. pneumoniae* (TWAR) were very similar to mycoplasma pneumonia. However, the dosage customarily used to treat mycoplasma pneumonia (ie, erythromycin 250 mg four times a day for five to seven days) was ineffective in many patients with *C. pneumoniae* pneumonia (Grayston et al, 1986). It has been suggested that tetracycline (1 to 2 g/day for 14 to 21 days) or a 14-day course of erythromycin be used for *C. pneumoniae* infections, but optimal dosage and duration of treatment remain to be determined (Schachter, 1986; Grayston et al, 1989). The in vitro activity of clarithromycin against *C. pneumoniae* is greater than that of erythromycin and azithromycin (Hammerschlag et al, 1992) and, based on limited data, clarithromycin may be effective in the treatment of this disease.

Many agents are available to treat bacterial exacerbations of bronchitis. Azithromycin and clarithromycin are superior to erythromycin when *H. influenzae* is the causative pathogen. Azithromycin is as effective as cefaclor [Ceclor] (Dark, 1991), erythromycin (Daniel and European Azithromycin Study Group, 1991), ampicillin (Mertens et al, 1992), and amoxicillin (Daniel and European Azithromycin Study Group, 1991) or amoxicillin/clavulanic acid (Balmes et al, 1991); clarithromycin is as effective as ampicillin (Bachand, 1991; Aldons, 1991). Improved patient tolerance due to decreased gastrointestinal upset must be balanced against the increased cost of these new macrolides. See also index entry Bronchitis, Treatment.

A 14-day course of erythromycin is recommended for patients with pertussis. This antibiotic also is administered prophylactically to exposed persons, although proof of efficacy is not fully established (Report of the Committee on Infectious Diseases, 1986). See also index entry Pertussis, Chemoprophylaxis, Treatment.

Patients with acute diphtheria, including some who did not respond to penicillin, have been treated successfully with erythromycin and diphtheria antitoxin. The antibiotic eradicates the causative organism and prevents spread. Erythromycin is preferred for treating carriers of this disease.

Respiratory Tract (Upper): Erythromycin is employed routinely as an alternative to penicillin G (or penicillin V potassium) to treat acute bacterial pharyngitis/tonsillitis and scarlet fever in patients allergic to penicillins. It is the drug of choice to treat other common causes of bacterial pharyngitis in adolescents and adults (eg, *M. pneumoniae, C. pneumoniae, Arcanobacterium* [formerly *Corynebacterium*] *haemolyticum*). See also index entry Pharyngitis.

Erythromycin plus sulfisoxazole is an alternative empiric treatment for acute sinusitis. Clarithromycin and azithromycin are as effective as aminopenicillins in the treatment of acute maxillary sinusitis (Karma et al, 1991 A; Casiano, 1991). Azithromycin penetrates into sinus fluid and tissue, particularly in patients with acute sinusitis, and persists at significant levels for up to four days (Karma et al, 1991 B). Clarithromycin also appears in high concentrations in nasal mucosa and maxillary sinus fluid (Fraschini et al, 1991). For further information, see index entry Sinusitis.

Sexually Transmitted Diseases: Although tetracyclines are the preferred antibiotics for *C. trachomatis* infections (eg, urethritis, cervicitis, proctitis, lymphogranuloma venereum) in nonpregnant adults, erythromycin (2 g/day for at least seven days) is an effective alternative. *C. trachomatis* infections in children (eg, urethritis, cervicitis secondary to sexual abuse) are primary indications for the use of erythromycin. The results of three comparative clinical trials demonstrate that azithromycin 1 g as (1) a single dose, (2) 500 mg twice daily, or (3) 500 mg initially followed by 250 mg for the next two days is as effective as the standard (100 mg) seven-day twice-daily course of doxycycline for uncomplicated genital infections caused by *C. trachomatis* (Johnson, 1991). The convenience and efficacy of single-dose therapy with azithromycin help ensure compliance. Follow-up cultures obtained three to five weeks post-therapy indicated that no relapses had occurred among 112 patients (Martin et al, 1992). Azithromycin also inhibits other organisms that cause sexually transmitted diseases (eg, *N. gonorrhoeae, H. ducreyi*, *T. pallidum*).

Erythromycin may be preferred for urethritis caused by *Ureaplasma urealyticum*. It is a drug of choice in chancroid (alternative, ceftriaxone). This antibiotic may be used as an alternative to penicillin G for early syphilis, but doxycycline (or tetracycline) is the current preferred alternative in penicillin-allergic patients. The use of erythromycin in penicillin-allergic pregnant women with syphilis is now discouraged by the Centers for Disease Control (CDC) (*MMWR*, 1989) because congenital syphilis has occurred in offspring of mothers receiving the macrolide (Fenton and Light, 1976; Fiumara,

1983; *MMWR*, 1986). All patients with syphilis who are treated with erythromycin must be followed carefully to assure eradication of the organism. Although erythromycin also has been used as an alternative drug in gonorrhea, other drugs are more effective against *N. gonorrhoeae* and are preferred. See also index entry Sexually Transmitted Diseases and *MMWR*, 1987, 1988, and 1989 for additional discussion.

Skin and Soft Tissue: Erythromycin is the drug of choice in erythrasma, a superficial skin infection caused by *Corynebacterium minutissimum* and is the preferred therapy for bacillary angiomatosis caused by *Rochalimaea henslei* (see index entry Angiomatosis, Bacillary). Macrolides are used for systemic treatment of impetigo, cellulitis, ecthyma, and erysipelas caused by group A beta hemolytic streptococci (eg, *S. pyogenes*) in patients who are allergic to penicillin. They may be used in patients with relatively minor staphylococcal infections (eg, bullous impetigo, carbuncles). However, they are not drugs of first choice for severe staphylococcal infection because they usually are not bactericidal against this organism. Furthermore, the emergence of appreciable numbers of resistant strains of *S. aureus* limits this use of macrolides. See also index entry Pyoderma.

Oral erythromycin may be useful in the management of pityriasis lichenoides in children (Truhan et al, 1986). The etiology of this cutaneous disorder is obscure.

For use of erythromycin in acne vulgaris, see index entry on this disorder.

Prophylaxis: Prophylactic therapy with erythromycin to prevent bacterial endocarditis is indicated prior to dental procedures or instrumentation of the upper airway in certain penicillin-allergic patients with cardiac abnormalities. Erythromycin also can be used as an alternative to penicillin G in the prophylaxis of recurrences of rheumatic fever in patients who have a history or demonstrable sequelae of rheumatic fever but are allergic to penicillin and sulfadiazine, the preferred alternative (see index entries Endocarditis, Chemoprophylaxis; Rheumatic Fever).

The combination of erythromycin base and neomycin, as an adjunct to mechanical bowel preparation, appears to have reduced the number of infections associated with elective colorectal surgery. This oral combination is a preferred prophylactic regimen for this type of surgery. See also index entry Colorectal Surgery, Elective.

Miscellaneous: Erythromycin has been employed as an alternative to penicillin G in the treatment of anthrax, Vincent's gingivitis, erysipeloid, actinomycosis, and *Listeria monocytogenes* infections (not in the central nervous system). It may be combined with a sulfonamide to treat *Nocardia* infections. Erythromycin is an alternative to ampicillin for *Eikenella corrodens* infections. It may be an alternative to the tetracyclines in *Borrelia* infections, including early Lyme disease or relapsing fever, and in granuloma inguinale due to *Calymmatobacterium granulomatis*. Azithromycin and clarithromycin are more active than erythromycin against *Borrelia burgdorferi*. Studies comparing these two agents with amoxicillin and tetracycline as therapy for Lyme disease are ongoing (Neu, 1992). In one study on patients with early Lyme disease, azithromycin (500 mg on the first day followed by 250 mg once daily for four days) was as effective as a 10-day course of amoxicillin/probenecid or doxycycline (Massarotti et al, 1992). For treatment guidelines, see index entry Lyme Disease, Description, Treatment.

Clarithromycin and azithromycin are being evaluated for the treatment of opportunistic infections due to *Toxoplasma gondii* or *M. avium* complex, and azithromycin is being evaluated for treatment of cryptosporidiosis in patients with AIDS. Both drugs are active against the causative organisms in vitro and in animal models of *T. gondii* infection (Araujo et al, 1988; Chang et al, 1988); azithromycin appears to potentiate the activity of sulfadiazine or pyrimethamine [Daraprim] in this infection (Derouin et al, 1992). In a pilot study, 8 of 13 AIDS patients completed a six-week course of clarithromycin 2 g plus pyrimethamine 75 mg daily; overall, 80% improved clinically, but most patients experienced side effects including liver abnormalities, hearing loss, nausea and vomiting, and skin rash (Fernandez-Martin et al, 1991). Additional trials are in progress to evaluate efficacy and determine the optimal dosing regimen of the newer macrolides in the therapy of toxoplasmic encephalitis.

In short-term trials, clarithromycin (1 g twice daily) alone or in multidrug regimens (with rifampin, isoniazid, ethambutol [Myambutol], and clofazimine [Lamprene] or with ciprofloxacin [Cipro] and amikacin) clears *M. avium* complex from the blood of AIDS patients within two to eight weeks (Dautzenberg et al, 1991; de Lalla et al, 1992). In a multicenter open trial on patients with late-stage AIDS and disseminated *M. avium* complex infection, treatment with clarithromycin 1.5 to 2 g daily eradicated the organism from blood. However, after two to seven months of treatment, relapse occurred in association with acquired resistance (Dautzenberg et al, 1993). Azithromycin 500 mg daily for 30 days has reduced *M. avium* complex bacteremia within two to three weeks in AIDS patients (Young et al, 1991).

Clarithromycin is the most active macrolide against many other atypical mycobacteria and has resolved cutaneous mycobacterial infections due to *M. chelonae* and *M. marinum* (Neu, 1992).

Adverse Reactions and Precautions

The macrolides are among the safest antimicrobial agents and seldom cause serious adverse reactions.

Gastrointestinal irritation, including epigastric distress, abdominal cramps, nausea, vomiting, and diarrhea, is the most common adverse effect produced by erythromycin and usually is associated with oral administration but also may occur after intravenous administration (Bowler et al, 1992). This effect probably is related to the prokinetic action of erythromycin on the gut that is mediated, at least in part, by stimulation of motilin receptors (Catnach and Fairclough, 1992). Symptoms are dose related, and gastrointestinal intolerance is more common and severe with larger doses (eg, ≥ 2 g daily of erythromycin). Some brands of enteric-coated tablets and the ester derivatives (eg, ethylsuccinate, estolate) may be taken with food to minimize these untoward effects. Pseudomembranous colitis caused by *Clostridium difficile* has been reported rarely.

In general, azithromycin and clarithromycin produce less gastrointestinal irritation than erythromycin. In clinical trials involving nearly 4,000 patients, adverse reactions with azithromycin were reported by 12% of patients. The most common were diarrhea (3.6%), nausea (2.6%), and abdominal pain (2.5%) (Hopkins, 1991). The incidence of these reactions with clarithromycin is similar.

When administered to normal subjects, erythromycin has produced myasthenic-like decrements in neuromuscular transmission, as detected by electromyography, but not weakness; however, the condition of one patient with myasthenia gravis worsened after administration of erythromycin (Absher and Bale, 1991).

Hypersensitivity reactions, such as skin rashes, drug fever, and eosinophilia, have occurred occasionally after administration of macrolides; serious reactions (eg, anaphylaxis, interstitial nephritis) are rare. Macrolides should not be used in patients with known hypersensitivity to these antibiotics.

One of the more serious adverse effects of erythromycin is a characteristic syndrome of cholestatic hepatitis. Erythromycin estolate has been associated with hepatotoxicity most often (Nicholas, 1977; Gribble and Chow, 1982; Steigbigel, 1990; Washington and Wilson, 1985; Brittain, 1987; Auckenthaler et al, 1988). Only a few cases of hepatic dysfunction have been associated with other forms of erythromycin, primarily the ethylsuccinate ester (Patel and Schneider, 1984). Patients 12 years of age or older appear to be most susceptible.

Hepatotoxicity typically begins after ten days of therapy, but occurs most frequently and rapidly (within two to three days) in patients who previously received erythromycin estolate. Symptoms consist of nausea, vomiting, and right upper quadrant pain, followed by jaundice, fever, and changes in hepatic function tests suggesting cholestatic hepatitis. These symptoms may be accompanied by rash, leukocytosis, and eosinophilia. The syndrome appears to be a hypersensitivity reaction because it may rapidly return upon rechallenge. It is reversible when the antibiotic is discontinued, and no deaths have been reported.

Despite the relative rarity of this adverse effect, erythromycin estolate should be used with caution, particularly in adults. Other forms of erythromycin or clarithromycin are preferred in patients with a history of liver disease or in those suspected of having impaired liver function. In clinical trials of azithromycin and clarithromycin, hepatic abnormalities were rare; the most common was transient increases of ALT and AST (<2% of patients). One case of cholestatic hepatitis was recorded during clinical trials of azithromycin.

Bilateral flat- or high-frequency sensorineural loss may develop within a few hours to several days after initiating erythromycin therapy. The hearing loss usually reverses gradually after discontinuation of therapy or dosage reduction. The ototoxicity is dose dependent (eg, >2 g daily) and is associated with reduced systemic clearance of erythromycin. In one prospective study, 21% of patients with community-acquired pneumonia receiving erythromycin 4 g/day intravenously developed symptomatic ototoxicity (tinnitus or hearing loss) (Swanson et al, 1992). Mean peak concentration in affected patients was 17.1 mcg/ml. Ototoxicity did not occur when peak concentrations were below 12 mcg/ml. The elderly, patients with renal or hepatic dysfunction, and those receiving other ototoxic drugs (eg, aminoglycosides, loop diuretics) may be most susceptible. Ototoxicity also has occurred with the large doses of clarithromycin and azithromycin used to treat *M. avium* complex infections.

Superinfections (eg, *Candida*) have been reported with erythromycin.

Thrombophlebitis may occur with intravenous administration of erythromycin gluceptate or lactobionate. This can be minimized by slow infusion of more dilute solutions. (Intramuscular administration of erythromycin is not recommended because injection is extremely painful.) Administration of erythromycin also rarely has been associated with the development of ventricular arrhythmias, including ventricular tachycardia and torsades de pointes in individuals with prolonged QT intervals (Nattel et al, 1990; Lindsay et al, 1990; Schoenberger et al, 1990).

Safety during pregnancy is not established, but congenital defects have not been reported despite widespread use of these agents. Erythromycin estolate has been associated with elevated serum AST concentrations in about 10% of pregnant women (McCormack et al, 1977), and this ester probably should not be used during pregnancy. Erythromycin base and azithromycin are classified in FDA Pregnancy Category B, and clarithromycin is classified in FDA Pregnancy Category C.

Drug Interactions

Concomitant use of erythromycin and terfenadine [Seldane] or astemizole [Hismanal] may dangerously elevate the plasma concentration of the antihistamine and cause lethal arrhythmias; therefore, this combination is contraindicated. Concomitant use of other macrolides with terfenadine also should be avoided.

Erythromycin can reduce clearance and increase serum theophylline levels in some patients, particularly those receiving large doses of the methylated xanthine. The mechanism appears to be inhibition of hepatic metabolism of theophylline by erythromycin. Because the potential for theophylline toxicity (eg, nausea, vomiting, cardiovascular instability, seizures) is increased, patients should be carefully monitored. Measurement of theophylline plasma concentrations is recommended (Ludden, 1985), or the dose of theophylline may be decreased by one-third temporarily. Clarithromycin also increases the plasma concentration of theophylline, and monitoring may be required.

Plasma levels of carbamazepine [Tegretol] also can be elevated by erythromycin and clarithromycin, leading to carbamazepine toxicity (eg, nausea, vomiting, drowsiness, nystagmus, ataxia). Close monitoring of patients receiving these two drugs concurrently is recommended; carbamazepine plasma concentrations also should be monitored.

The following drug interactions have not been reported in clinical trials with clarithromycin or azithromycin, but, because they have been observed with erythromycin, similar precautions may apply to their use.

Concomitant administration of erythromycin and warfarin [Coumadin, Panwarfin] can prolong prothrombin time and result in hemorrhage. Monitoring of prothrombin time is necessary when these drugs are given together.

Erythromycin can increase plasma concentrations of cyclosporine [Sandimmune], which may result in nephrotoxicity. This combination should be used with caution; renal function and cyclosporine plasma concentrations should be monitored.

Two patients receiving disopyramide [Norpace] developed QT prolongation, polymorphic ventricular tachycardia, and elevated disopyramide serum concentrations when erythromycin was added to their regimens. Although verification of this potentially fatal drug interaction is necessary, avoidance of erythromycin in patients receiving disopyramide is suggested (Ragosta et al, 1989). If concomitant erythromycin is required, monitoring of disopyramide serum concentrations and the electrocardiogram is recommended.

Erythromycin reduced the clearance and increased plasma concentrations of triazolam [Halcion] in normal volunteers, but the clinical significance is unknown (Phillips et al, 1986). As with troleandomycin, the elimination of methylprednisolone is reduced by erythromycin (LaForce et al, 1983; see Ludden, 1985). Although less well studied than the theophylline-erythromycin interaction, the mechanism for the interaction of erythromycin with each of the above six drugs also appears to be inhibition of hepatic drug metabolism by erythromycin (Ludden, 1985). Antacids that contain aluminum and magnesium reduce the peak serum level (rate) but not the extent of azithromycin absorption.

Approximately 10% of patients convert substantial amounts of digoxin [Lanoxin] to inactive metabolites in the gastrointestinal tract. Certain antimicrobial agents, including erythromycin, alter gut microbial flora and prevent the inactivation of digoxin, which can cause marked increases in serum digoxin levels. The effects of this interaction can persist for several months (Lindenbaum et al, 1981). Careful monitoring of patients receiving these drugs is recommended (Doherty, 1981).

Acute ergot toxicity (eg, peripheral vasospasm) has been reported when erythromycin was administered to patients receiving ergotamine tartrate [Ergomar, Ergostat] (Francis et al, 1984; Tatro, 1989); the mechanism is unknown. Careful monitoring for symptoms of ergot toxicity is recommended when ergot alkaloids and macrolides are given concurrently.

Macrolides, which are primarily bacteriostatic, may interfere with the action of bactericidal agents such as the penicillins. However, the clinical significance is unknown. Such a combination should be used only when it has been demonstrated to be beneficial. Erythromycin may inhibit the activity of other antibiotics that bind to the 50S ribosome (ie, chloramphenicol, clindamycin).

Parenteral dosage forms of erythromycin (gluceptate, lactobionate) may be physically and/or chemically incompatible with solutions containing vitamin B complex, ascorbic acid, cephalothin [Keflin], tetracycline, colistin [Coly-Mycin S], chloramphenicol, heparin, metaraminol [Aramine], and phenytoin [Dilantin].

For a general discussion on drug interactions associated with the macrolides, see Hansten and Horn, 1990.

Interference With Laboratory Tests

Erythromycin may cause false-positive elevations in AST concentrations when determined by colorimetric methods. This must be distinguished from drug-induced hepatotoxicity (see above). Erythromycin also may falsely elevate urinary catecholamine and 17-hydroxycorticosteroid levels.

Pharmacokinetics

The biologically active form of erythromycin is the free base, and it is is absorbed intact. However, erythromycin base is inactivated by gastric acid, and this decreases its gastrointestinal absorption. The structural differences of clarithromycin and azithromycin improve their stability in acid and enhance their gastrointestinal absorption compared with erythromycin. Methods to reduce the acid degradation of erythromycin base include protective coating (eg, film, enteric) on capsules or tablets and chemical modification of the base (ie, stearate salt, ethylsuccinate ester, propionyl ester sulfate salt). These properties and the presence or absence of food in the stomach affect peak serum levels (see the Table); considerable variability exists among subjects from study to study.

When oral erythromycin preparations are administered in the correct dose and with proper timing in relation to food intake, it appears that no one type of preparation offers a significant therapeutic advantage, at least in mild to moderate infections caused by susceptible organisms (Gribble and Chow, 1982; *Federal Register*, 1982; Steigbigel, 1990). Erythromycin estolate usually is not recommended for adults because of the increased risk of reversible cholestatic hepatitis (see Adverse Reactions and Precautions); the estolate ester rarely causes hepatitis in children. Some pediatric infectious disease experts prefer the estolate over the ethylsuccinate because of better bioavailability (Ginsburg et al, 1976, 1982, 1984; *Med Lett Drugs Ther*, 1985); both preparations are tasteless and form stable suspensions in water. When high blood levels are required (eg, for serious infections), the gluceptate and lactobionate salts may be given intravenously.

Distribution: Macrolides are lipid soluble and thus widely distributed, and they penetrate well into most tissues including bronchial, prostatic, middle ear, and bone. Therapeutic concentrations generally are not achievable in the central nervous system. Erythromycin crosses the placenta, but fetal blood concentrations are no higher than 10% (usually closer to 2%) of those in the maternal circulation; higher concentrations accumulate in fetal tissues and amniotic fluid. Erythromycin, clarithromycin, and 14-hydroxyclarithromycin appear in

PEAK SERUM LEVELS OF MACROLIDES IN ADULTS[a]

Preparation	Dose (mg)	Route	Peak Serum Level: Hours After Dose	Peak Serum Level: mcg/ml	Comments
Erythromycin					
Base	250	Oral	4	0.3-1.0[b]	Absorption of enteric-coated erythromycin base may be erratic; administration under fasting conditions increases the peak serum level.
	500			0.3-1.9	
Stearate	250 (fasting)	Oral	3	0.2-1.3	The stearate is acid labile; bioavailability is increased when this derivative is taken with large fluid volumes but is decreased when it is taken with food.
	500 (fasting)		3	0.4-1.8	
	500 (after food)		3	0.1-0.4[c]	
Ethylsuccinate	500[d]	Oral	0.5-2.5	1.5[e] (0.6[e])	Absorbed directly as the inactive ester; food does not decrease absorption and some studies suggest that food can enhance absorption.
Estolate	250	Oral	2-4	1.4-1.7[f]	Acid stable; absorption is not affected by food.
	500		3.5-4	4.2[e] (1.1[e])	
Lactobionate	200	Intravenous	Immediately	3-4	
	500		1	9.9	
Gluceptate	250	Intravenous	Immediately	3.5-10.7	
	1000		1	9.9	
Azithromycin	500	Oral		0.4	Food decreases bioavailability by approximately 50%; the drug should be taken on an empty stomach. Tissue concentrations are substantially higher than those in serum.
	250			0.24[g]	
Clarithromycin	500	Oral	2	2.1	Food delays absorption but does not decrease bioavailability; the drug may be taken without regard to meals.
	250		1-4	1.0[h]	
				0.7-0.8	
				0.6[h]	

[a] *Adapted from Steigbigel NH: Erythromycin, lincomycin, and clindamycin, in Mandell GL, et al (eds):* Principles and Practice of Infectious Diseases, *ed 3. New York, Churchill Livingstone, 1990, 310.*

[b] *Somewhat higher levels reported with some enteric-coated preparations after repeated doses (McDonald et al, 1977; DiSanto and Chodos, 1981). Many physicians administer erythromycin base with meals in the hope of minimizing gastrointestinal upset; peak serum levels will be lower, but therapeutic efficacy may not be significantly affected.*

[c] *Some studies note higher levels (to 2.8 mcg/ml) when dose taken with food (Malmborg, 1979).*

[d] *Erythromycin ethylsuccinate is not available as 500-mg tablets. The 400-mg tablet is equivalent to 250 mg erythromycin base.*

[e] *Free base*

[f] *Total drug (inactive ester and free base)*

[g] *After five days of therapy*

[h] *Concentrations of the active 14-hydroxylated metabolite*

breast milk. Concentrations of the latter are approximately 25% and 75% of the corresponding serum concentrations. Corresponding data for azithromycin are not available.

These agents are concentrated intracellularly by polymorphonuclear leukocytes and alveolar macrophages, which may be important in the treatment of infections caused by intracellular pathogens (eg, *Legionella*). Azithromycin has a unique pharmacokinetic profile that is characterized by low concentrations in the serum but high and persistent concentrations in tissues. It remains in the tissues for up to four days after a dose, and exposure of bacteria to phagocytes containing accumulated azithromycin causes release of the drug; tissue concentrations of azithromycin may exceed those in serum by 10- to 100-fold (Foulds et al, 1990). Thus, regimens for treatment of some infections can be shortened. Depending on the site measured, clarithromycin concentrations in tissues are 2 to 20 times those in the serum (Hardy et al, 1992).

The volume of distribution (Vd) of azithromycin is approximately 31 L/kg compared with 0.75 L/kg for erythromycin; the weight-corrected Vd for clarithromycin is approximately 1.5 to 2 L/kg (Peters and Clissold, 1992). Clarithromycin (65% to 70%) and erythromycin (70% to 75%) are somewhat more protein bound than azithromycin (range, 12% to 50% at concentrations of 0.5 mcg/ml and 0.05 mcg/ml, respectively).

Elimination: Erythromycin and azithromycin are concentrated in the liver, and high concentrations are normally excreted into the bile; some drug is demethylated. A considerable portion of an oral dose of both agents is eliminated in the feces. Only 2% to 5% of an oral dose of erythromycin and 6% of an oral dose of azithromycin is eliminated in the urine; after intravenous administration of erythromycin the percentage may approach 15%.

Clarithromycin is more extensively metabolized in the liver by both oxidative and hydrolytic mechanisms than erythromycin. Approximately 20% of an oral dose is converted to an active metabolite, 14-hydroxyclarithromycin, and approximately 30% of a dose can be recovered in the urine. The elimination half-times of clarithromycin and its active metabolite are dose dependent, averaging three to four hours and five to six hours, respectively, after a 250-mg dose, and five to seven hours and seven hours, respectively, after a 500-mg dose. The half-life is significantly increased in patients with creatinine clearances below 30 ml/min, and a reduction in dosage may be necessary.

The elimination of azithromycin is polyphasic; the terminal half-life associated with release from tissue sites is approximately 68 hours. In contrast, the serum half-life of erythromycin is about 1.6 hours (range, 1.2 and 2.6 hours) in individuals with normal renal function (Bennett et al, 1980; Benet and Sheiner, 1985).

The half-life of erythromycin is increased to approximately five hours in anuric patients. Generally, there is no need to adjust dosage in patients with renal insufficiency. However, erythromycin may be ototoxic in those with renal failure (see Adverse Reactions and Precautions). Erythromycin is not removed by peritoneal dialysis or hemodialysis.

Because erythromycin is excreted primarily by the liver, caution should be exercised in patients with impaired hepatic function. The estolate ester is not recommended in these individuals (see Adverse Reactions and Precautions).

Drug Evaluations

AZITHROMYCIN DIHYDRATE
[Zithromax]

Like clarithromycin, azithromycin is acid stable. Thus, it is better absorbed and causes less gastrointestinal irritation than erythromycin.

ANTIMICROBIAL SPECTRUM. This azalide, a subclass of macrolide antibiotics, is two- to fourfold less active than erythromycin against most staphylococci and streptococci; erythromycin-resistant staphylococci and streptococci also are resistant to this drug. Azithromycin is more active than other macrolides against *Haemophilus influenzae, H. ducreyi,* and certain anaerobic organisms and, unlike other macrolides, is active against certain aerobic and facultative gram-negative bacilli. Like other macrolides, azithromycin is active against respiratory tract pathogens responsible for atypical pneumonia (eg, *Mycoplasma pneumoniae, Chlamydia pneumoniae, Legionella pneumophila*). It also is active against sexually transmitted pathogens (ie, *Chlamydia trachomatis, Ureaplasma urealyticum, Neisseria gonorrhoeae, Treponema pallidum*), the agent responsible for Lyme disease (*Borrelia burgdorferi*), and certain pathogens causing opportunistic infections in AIDS patients (eg, *Toxoplasma gondii, Mycobacterium avium* complex, *Cryptosporidium*).

USES. Azithromycin is an alternative antibiotic for the treatment of mild to moderate pharyngitis/tonsillitis due to streptococcal species. It also is indicated for the treatment of (1) mild to moderate acute bacterial exacerbations of chronic bronchitis due to *H. influenzae, M. catarrhalis*, or *Streptococcus pneumoniae*; (2) pneumonia due to *S. pneumoniae* or *H. influenzae*; (3) uncomplicated skin and skin structure infections due to *S. aureus, Streptococcus pyogenes,* or *Staphylococcus agalactiae,* and; (4) urethritis and cervicitis due to *C. trachomatis*. Azithromycin is being evaluated for the treatment of typhoid fever, Lyme disease, and certain opportunistic infections in AIDS patients (ie, *M. avium* complex, toxoplasmosis [encephalitis], cryptosporidiosis).

PRECAUTIONS. Because azithromycin is principally eliminated by the liver, it should be administered cautiously to patients with impaired hepatic function. Azithromycin should not be used in patients with pneumonia who are not candidates for outpatient oral therapy because of moderate to severe illness or in patients with pneumonia who are elderly or debilitated, have nosocomial infections, have known or suspected bacteremia, or may have an impaired immune response.

For further information on pharmacokinetics, adverse reactions, drug interactions, and other precautions regarding the use of azithromycin, see the Introduction.

PREGNANCY AND LACTATION. No teratogenic effects of azithromycin were evident in animal studies; however, there are no adequate controlled studies in pregnant women.

Therefore, this drug should be used during pregnancy only if it is clearly indicated (FDA Pregnancy Category B). It is not known whether azithromycin is excreted in human milk and therefore caution should be exercised when this drug is administered to nursing women.

DOSAGE AND PREPARATIONS. The safety and effectiveness of azithromycin in individuals under 16 years has not been established. This drug should be given at least one hour before or two hours after meals.

Oral: *Adults*, for mild to moderate pharyngitis/tonsillitis, acute bacterial exacerbations of bronchitis, pneumonia, and uncomplicated skin and skin structure infections, 500 mg as a single dose on the first day followed by 250 mg once daily for four additional days. For nongonococcal urethritis and cervicitis due to *C. trachomatis*, 1 g in a single dose.

Zithromax (Pfizer). Capsules containing azithromycin dihydrate equivalent to 250 mg of base.

CLARITHROMYCIN
[Biaxin]

Clarithromycin is 6-methoxy-erythromycin, a compound that is acid stable. Thus, it is better absorbed and causes less gastrointestinal irritation than erythromycin.

ANTIMICROBIAL SPECTRUM. In general, clarithromycin has an in vitro spectrum of activity that is similar to that of erythromycin, but it is two- to fourfold more active against susceptible streptococci and staphylococci; gram-positive cocci resistant to erythromycin are resistant to clarithromycin as well. The active metabolite (14-OH clarithromycin) acts in an additive or synergistic fashion against *Haemophilus influenzae*. Clarithromycin also is slightly more active in vitro than erythromycin against certain pathogens responsible for atypical pneumonias (ie, *Legionella pneumophila, Mycoplasma pneumoniae, Chlamydia pneumoniae*) (Jones et al, 1990; Logan et al, 1991; Hammerschlag et al, 1992) and Lyme disease (*Borrelia burgdorferi*). This macrolide is somewhat more active than erythromycin against *Chlamydia trachomatis* and is considerably more active against *Ureaplasma urealyticum* (Renaudin and Bébéar, 1990). It also is active against *Toxoplasma gondii*, *Cryptosporidium,* and *Mycobacterium avium* complex; it is the most active macrolide against other atypical mycobacteria (Brown et al, 1992).

USES. Clarithromycin is indicated for the treatment of pneumonia caused by *M. pneumoniae* or *Streptococcus pneumoniae*. Based on limited comparative studies, it appears to be as effective as erythromycin and can be considered an alternative agent for the treatment of atypical pneumonias. Clarithromycin also is indicated for the treatment of (1) acute bacterial exacerbations of chronic bronchitis due to *H. influenzae, M. catarrhalis*, or *S. pneumoniae*; (2) pharyngitis/tonsillitis due to *Streptococcus pyogenes*; (3) acute maxillary sinusitis due to *S. pneumoniae* in penicillin-allergic patients; and, (4) uncomplicated skin and skin structure infections due to *Staphylococcus aureus* or *S. pyogenes*. This drug is an alternative in the treatment of infections due to *U. urealyticum*, early Lyme disease (*Med Lett Drugs Ther*, 1992), and certain opportunistic infections in AIDS or other immunocompromised patients (eg, atypical mycobacteria, *T. gondii* encephalitis). Some experts consider it the drug of choice for treatment or prophylaxis of *M. avium* complex infections (*Med Lett Drugs Ther*, 1992). Clarithromycin is being investigated in the treatment of colonization of the stomach by *Helicobacter pylori*.

PREGNANCY AND LACTATION. Clarithromycin causes teratogenic effects in laboratory animals. Data in pregnant women are lacking; therefore, it should not be used during pregnancy except when no alternative therapy is appropriate (FDA Pregnancy Category C). Since clarithromycin is excreted in human milk, caution should be exercised when this drug is administered to nursing women.

For further information on pharmacokinetics, adverse reactions, drug interactions, and other precautions regarding the use of clarithromycin, see the Introduction.

DOSAGE AND PREPARATIONS. The safety and effectiveness of clarithromycin in children under 12 years have not been established. Clarithromycin may be given with or without food.

Oral: *Adults*, for mild to moderate pharyngitis/tonsillitis due to *S. pyogenes*, 250 mg every 12 hours for 10 days; for uncomplicated skin and skin structure infections and acute exacerbations of chronic bronchitis due to *S. pneumoniae* or *M. catarrhalis* or pneumonia due to *S. pneumoniae* or *M. pneumoniae*, 250 mg every 12 hours for 7 to 14 days; for acute exacerbations of chronic bronchitis due to *H. influenzae*, 500 mg every 12 hours for 7 to 14 days; for acute maxillary sinusitis, 500 mg every 12 hours for 14 days. Dosage reduction may be required in the elderly and in patients with renal impairment.

Biaxin (Abbott). Tablets (film-coated) 250 and 500 mg.

ERYTHROMYCIN
[*film-coated:* Erythromycin Base Filmtabs; *enteric-coated:* E-Mycin, ERYC, Ery-Tab, PCE Dispertab, Robimycin]

ERYTHROMYCIN ESTOLATE
[Ilosone]

ERYTHROMYCIN ETHYLSUCCINATE
[E.E.S., EryPed]

ERYTHROMYCIN GLUCEPTATE
[Ilotycin Gluceptate]

ERYTHROMYCIN LACTOBIONATE
[Erythrocin Lactobionate-IV]

ERYTHROMYCIN STEARATE
[Erythrocin Stearate, Wyamycin S]

All erythromycins (base, salt, esters) have the same spectrum of antibacterial activity and uses; adverse reactions also are similar, except that erythromycin estolate has a greater propensity to cause hepatotoxicity. See the introductory section on Macrolides for a detailed discussion.

DOSAGE AND PREPARATIONS. All doses and strengths are expressed in terms of the base. For group A streptococcal infections, therapy should be continued for at least ten days. ***Oral:*** (Base) *Adults,* 250 to 500 mg every six hours. The manufacturers' recommended alternative schedules for the lower dosage are 333 mg every eight hours (*E-Mycin, Ery-Tab,* and *PCE Dispertab* only) or 500 mg every 12 hours. See the manufacturers' labeling to determine whether a specific preparation should be administered with or without food.

(Estolate) *Adults,* 250 to 500 mg every six hours. The manufacturers' recommended alternative schedule for the lower dosage is 500 mg every 12 hours.

(Ethylsuccinate) *Adults,* 400 to 800 mg four times daily. The manufacturers' recommended alternative schedules for the lower dosage are 600 mg every eight hours or 800 mg every 12 hours.

(Stearate) *Adults,* 250 to 500 mg every six hours. The manufacturers' recommended alternative schedule for the lower dosage is 500 mg every 12 hours. Preferably, the drug is given on an empty stomach. See the manufacturers' recommendations for specific preparations.

(All forms) For severe infections in *adults,* up to 4 g may be given daily in divided doses. These larger doses are necessary for the treatment of known or suspected *Legionella* infections. The duration of therapy for Legionnaires' disease is usually 21 days. *Children,* 30 to 50 mg/kg daily in four divided doses; for severe infections, the dose may be doubled.

For prophylaxis of rheumatic fever or infective endocarditis, see index entries on these infections.

For treatment of sexually transmitted diseases, including chlamydial infections, chancroid, and syphilis, see index entry Sexually Transmitted Diseases.

For prophylaxis prior to elective colorectal surgery, see index entry on this condition.

ERYTHROMYCIN:
Generic. Capsules (enteric-coated pellets) 250 mg; tablets (plain, enteric-coated) 250, 333, and 500 mg.
Erythromycin Base Filmtab (Abbott). Tablets (film-coated) 250 and 500 mg.
E-Mycin (Boots). Tablets (enteric-coated) 250 and 333 mg.
ERYC (Parke-Davis). Capsules (enteric-coated pellets) 250 mg.
Ery-Tab (Abbott). Tablets (enteric-coated) 250, 333, and 500 mg.
PCE Dispertab (Abbott). Tablets (enteric-coated particles in tablet) 333 and 500 mg.
Robimycin (Robins). Tablets (enteric-coated) 250 mg.

ERYTHROMYCIN ESTOLATE:
Generic. Capsules, tablets 250 mg; suspension 125 and 250 mg/5 ml.
Ilosone (Dista). Capsules 250 mg; suspension 125 and 250 mg/5 ml; tablets 500 mg.

ERYTHROMYCIN ETHYLSUCCINATE:
Generic. Suspension 200 and 400 mg/5 ml; tablets (plain, chewable, and film-coated) 400 mg.
E.E.S. (Abbott). Granules for oral suspension 200 mg/5 ml after reconstitution; suspension 200 and 400 mg/5 ml; tablets (film-coated) 400 mg.
EryPed (Abbott). Powder for oral suspension 100 mg/2.5 ml and 200 and 400 mg/5 ml after reconstitution; tablets (chewable) 200 mg.

ERYTHROMYCIN STEARATE:
Erythrocin Stearate Filmtab (Abbott), ***Wyamycin S*** (Wyeth-Ayerst), ***Generic.*** Tablets (film-coated) 250 and 500 mg.

Intravenous: For severe infections, *adults,* 1 to 4 g daily; *children,* 15 to 50 mg/kg daily (maximum, 4 g daily) (The Medical Letter, 1988; Norris and Mandell, 1985). The larger doses (eg, 4 g daily) are necessary for known or suspected *Legionella* infections. (*Note:* The manufacturers state that the usual dosage for adults and children with severe infections is 15 to 20 mg/kg/day and that higher dosages [up to 4 g/day] may be given in very severe infections.)

Administration is by slow intermittent infusion in divided doses at intervals not greater than every six hours or by continuous infusion. Because of the irritating properties of erythromycin, intravenous push is not acceptable. For instructions on the preparation of intravenous solutions and drug administration, consult the manufacturers' literature.

An oral dosage form should be substituted as soon as possible.

ERYTHROMYCIN GLUCEPTATE:
Ilotycin Gluceptate (Dista). Powder 1 g.

ERYTHROMYCIN LACTOBIONATE:
Erythrocin Lactobionate-IV (Abbott), ***Generic.*** Powder (sterile, lyophilized) 500 mg and 1 g.

LINCOSAMIDES

The lincosamides include lincomycin [Lincocin], an antibacterial agent produced by *Streptomyces lincolnensis* var. *lincolnensis*, and its semisynthetic derivative, clindamycin [Cleocin]. These drugs contain an amino acid linked to an amino sugar. Clindamycin (7-chloro-7-deoxylincomycin) differs chemically from lincomycin by the substitution of a chlorine atom for a hydroxyl group on the parent molecule (see Figure 2). With this slight molecular modification, clindamycin has increased antibacterial potency and is better absorbed from the gastrointestinal tract after oral administration (McGehee et al, 1968). Thus, it is the preferred lincosamide for clinical use and the discussion in this section will focus primarily on clindamycin.

FIGURE 2. CHEMICAL STRUCTURES OF LINCOSAMIDES

GENERIC NAME	R
Lincomycin	OH
Clindamycin	Cl

Mechanism of Action

Clindamycin and lincomycin inhibit bacterial protein synthesis by binding to the 50S ribosomal subunit and probably prevent elongation of the peptide chain by interfering with peptidyl transfer (Davis, 1980). The clindamycin ribosomal binding site overlaps those for chloramphenicol and erythromycin, but they are not identical (Pratt and Fekety, 1986). There are no clinical indications for the concurrent use of these antibiotics.

The lincosamides are primarily bacteriostatic. However, depending on the antibiotic concentration, the organism's susceptibility, and the size of the inoculum, bactericidal activity has been demonstrated against some organisms (eg, *Streptococcus pneumoniae, S. pyogenes*, *Bacteroides fragilis*).

Antimicrobial Spectrum

The lincosamides are active against most gram-positive and anaerobic gram-negative bacteria; clindamycin is more potent than lincomycin.

Clindamycin resembles erythromycin in its activity in vitro against various streptococci, including *S. pneumoniae*, *S. pyogenes*, and viridans streptococci. However, enterococci (eg, *E. faecalis*) are resistant. It also is active against penicillinase- and nonpenicillinase-producing *Staphylococcus aureus*, although some resistant strains have been reported. Methicillin-resistant staphylococci frequently are resistant to clindamycin. *Corynebacterium diphtheriae* are susceptible.

Anaerobic organisms susceptible to clindamycin in vitro are *Bacteroides* species, including the *B. fragilis* group, of which 6% to 7% of strains are resistant (Cuchural et al, 1988). Other susceptible anaerobic organisms include *Fusobacterium, Propionibacterium*, *Eubacterium*, *Bifidobacterium*, *Peptostreptococcus, Veillonella* species, and *Peptococcus* (of which about 10% are resistant). Most *Clostridium perfringens* (*welchii*) and *C. tetani* are susceptible, but *C. sporogenes* and *C. tertium* often are resistant, as are several *Actinomyces* species.

Chlamydia trachomatis is moderately susceptible to clindamycin. Most strains of *Mycoplasma pneumoniae* are susceptible, but other antibiotics (eg, erythromycin, tetracycline) are preferred. Most aerobic gram-negative bacteria (eg, the Enterobacteriaceae, *Haemophilus influenzae, Neisseria meningitidis*) and most *Nocardia* species are resistant. Yeasts, fungi, and viruses also are resistant. Lincosamides have activity against certain protozoa (ie, *Toxoplasma gondii, Plasmodium falciparum*) and *Pneumocystis carinii* (Pfefferkorn et al, 1992).

Resistance

Acquired resistance to clindamycin has been observed for gram-positive cocci and the *B. fragilis* group.

Occasional clinical isolates of clindamycin-resistant *S. pneumoniae, S. pyogenes*, and viridans streptococci have been reported; these strains also are resistant to lincomycin and usually to erythromycin.

Strains of *S. aureus* also may become resistant to clindamycin. In vitro, staphylococcal resistance usually develops in a slow, stepwise manner, but can occur more rapidly in strains that are already resistant to erythromycin. Clinical isolates of clindamycin-resistant staphylococci frequently are resistant to erythromycin. Cross resistance between clindamycin and lincomycin is complete for staphylococci; mechanisms appear to involve alterations in the 50S ribosomal binding site or in the 23S RNA component of the 50S subunit. A few isolates of staphylococci, including *S. aureus*, may inactivate clindamycin by enzymatic nucleotidylation (see Steigbigel, 1990; see also the section on Macrolides).

Resistance of the *B. fragilis* group to clindamycin in the United States during the years 1981 to 1985 was assessed in a multicenter study. The average rate of resistance per year varied between 3% and 9%, but this ranged from 0 to 17% among various institutions (Cuchural et al, 1988). High-level, plasmid-mediated, transferable clindamycin resistance has been demonstrated; resistance to erythromycin also is carried on these genes (Tally et al, 1979, 1983). Clinically, *B. fragilis* strains resistant to clindamycin have caused severe infections (Yee et al, 1982). Because antimicrobial resistance can be a problem with this organism, antimicrobial susceptibility testing should be performed.

Uses

Clindamycin is preferred to lincomycin for all indications because it has greater antibacterial potency and is better absorbed after oral administration (see Antimicrobial Spectrum and Pharmacokinetics).

Clindamycin often is effective in the treatment of anaerobic infections outside of the central nervous system that may be caused by the *B. fragilis* group (except anaerobic bacterial endocarditis) or other penicillin-resistant anaerobic bacteria. (Metronidazole is preferred in the treatment of anaerobic bacterial endocarditis caused by *B. fragilis* because of its consistent bactericidal activity against this organism.)

Bacteremias and Sepsis: Certain serious soft tissue infections, such as infected decubitus ulcers with sepsis, frequently are associated with anaerobic bacteria, including the *B. fragilis* group, as well as coliforms. Clindamycin, usually in combination regimens, is a preferred drug for the anaerobic pathogens.

Bone and Joint: Clindamycin may be an alternative drug for the treatment of septic arthritis and osteomyelitis (including acute hematogenous osteomyelitis) caused by susceptible gram-positive cocci, usually *S. aureus*, in patients over 3 years who are allergic to both penicillins and cephalosporins. Although high concentrations of clindamycin are attained in bone, an advantage of this drug for the treatment of osteomyelitis has not been established; some experts prefer vancomycin [Vancocin], a bactericidal drug, in patients who are allergic to β-lactam antibiotics. Clindamycin also may be useful, as a component of a combination regimen, in the treatment of mixed-flora bone infections, such as osteomyelitis affecting the foot in diabetic patients.

Gastrointestinal, Intra-abdominal, and Pelvic: There are many therapeutic options in intra-abdominal infections (eg, peritonitis, abscesses) and in gynecologic infections (eg, endometritis, nongonococcal tubo-ovarian abscess, pelvic cellulitis). The severity of illness and possible presence of resistant organisms are important factors in determining therapy. Clindamycin plus an aminoglycoside is a commonly used therapeutic option. For treatment of infections likely to involve anaerobes, see index entries Gastrointestinal Tract Infections; Pelvic Inflammatory Disease.

Respiratory Tract (Lower): For anaerobic infections above the diaphragm, including aspiration pneumonia and lung abscess, penicillin G traditionally has been the preferred antibiotic. Clindamycin is an effective alternative in penicillin-allergic patients and for anaerobic bronchopulmonary infections that do not respond to penicillin G. The role of clindamycin in serious anaerobic bronchopulmonary infections has become more prominent. Penicillin G-resistant strains of *Prevotella melaninogenica*, a common anaerobic pathogen in the respiratory tract, are increasing and, although relatively uncommon, members of the *B. fragilis* group cause some bronchopulmonary infections (Tally, 1981; Bartlett, 1982; *Med Lett Drugs Ther*, 1984). In two prospective, randomized, controlled, clinical trials comparing clindamycin with penicillin G for the treatment of community-acquired lung abscess and necrotizing pneumonia, clindamycin was superior (Levison et al, 1983; Gudiol et al, 1990). Most infectious disease experts now prefer clindamycin to penicillin G for the initial treatment of serious anaerobic bronchopulmonary infections.

Sexually Transmitted Diseases: In one randomized comparative trial, clindamycin was as effective as erythromycin in the treatment of *C. trachomatis* infections in sexually active women (Campbell and Dodson, 1990) and caused fewer reactions. In a randomized, placebo-controlled trial involving pregnant women with *C. trachomatis* infections, the same findings were reported (Alger and Lovchik, 1991). These preliminary studies suggest that clindamycin can be considered an alternative to standard treatment regimens in these patient populations.

Skin and Soft Tissue: Clindamycin may be an alternative antibiotic for mild to moderate skin and soft tissue infections caused by susceptible gram-positive cocci, usually *S. aureus*, or anaerobes in patients who are allergic to both penicillins and cephalosporins. Because clindamycin is not reliably bactericidal against *S. aureus* and because of the potential emergence of resistant strains, it is not recommended for deep-seated or life-threatening *S. aureus* infections. Also, clindamycin should not be used to treat methicillin-resistant staphylococcal infections. Clindamycin has been used as an alternative to penicillin G in infections caused by *Clostridium perfringens* and *Actinomyces israelii*.

Prophylaxis: Clindamycin has been effective in certain surgical prophylactic regimens, particularly in combination with an aminoglycoside in 'dirty' colorectal surgical procedures (see index entry Antimicrobial Drugs: Chemoprophylaxis for Surgical Patients).

Miscellaneous: The combination of clindamycin plus quinine appears to be useful for the treatment of babesiosis, a malaria-like infection caused by *Babesia microti*. This intraerythrocytic protozoan parasite is transmitted by *Ixodes dammini* ticks (*Med Lett Drugs Ther*, 1988).

Clindamycin, in combination with pyrimethamine, is potentially useful for the treatment of central nervous system toxoplasmosis, particularly in AIDS patients who cannot tolerate sulfonamides (Rolston and Hoy, 1987; Dannemann et al, 1988). In a randomized, unblinded, multicenter trial that allowed crossover in cases of treatment failure or intolerance, the efficacy of clindamycin plus pyrimethamine was approximately equal to that of sulfadiazine plus pyrimethamine for toxoplasmic encephalitis in AIDS patients (Dannemann et al, 1992). Initially, the dosage of clindamycin was 1.2 g intravenously every six hours for three weeks, followed by 300 mg every six hours or 450 mg every eight hours for three weeks. In another study employing clindamycin 300 mg twice daily as prophylaxis for AIDS-associated toxoplasmic encephalitis, dose-limiting toxicity occurred in more than 40% of patients (Jacobson et al, 1992). Similarly, in another large trial of clindamycin plus pyrimethamine versus pyrimethamine alone for prophylaxis of toxoplasmosis, dose-limiting toxicity (ie, diarrhea) forced early discontinuation of clindamycin therapy. Thus, clindamycin does not appear to be useful for prophylaxis; its role for treatment of this infection is still under investigation.

For information on the use of clindamycin in the treatment of pneumonia due to *Pneumocystis carinii* and malaria, see index entries on these infections.

Adverse Reactions and Precautions

Antibiotic-Associated Pseudomembranous Colitis: Lincomycin and clindamycin are usually well tolerated. A common adverse effect is diarrhea; the incidence associated with clindamycin therapy has been reported to be as low as 2% and as high as 21% (mean, about 8%). The lincosamides also can cause antibiotic-associated pseudomembranous colitis (AAPMC) that can be fatal. AAPMC has been estimated to occur in less than 0.01% to more than 10% of patients (Tedesco, 1977; Swartzberg et al, 1977; Gurwith et al, 1977; Lusk et al, 1977; Neu et al, 1977); this disparity may reflect different diagnostic methods and the variable epidemiology of *Clostridium difficile*. However, essentially all antibiotics can cause diarrhea, including AAPMC. Those most frequently associated with AAPMC are ampicillin, the lincosamides, and the cephalosporins (Fekety, 1978; Bartlett, 1981; Chang, 1981; Aronsson et al, 1985); lincosamides (ie, clindamycin) probably have the highest incidence when utilization rates are considered. Thus, the following discussion of AAPMC applies to other antibiotics in addition to the lincosamides.

Older individuals, particularly those with chronic, debilitating diseases, are at greater risk of developing AAPMC. The incidence is unrelated to the route of administration, total dosage, duration of therapy, or underlying disease.

The most frequently observed clinical features of AAPMC are watery diarrhea, crampy abdominal pain, fever, and leukocytosis, although the frequency of fecal leukocytosis is variable. Mucus and blood in the stools also may be observed. Sigmoidoscopic examination often reveals plaque-like lesions (pseudomembranes) on the colonic or rectal mucosa. Histologically, the pseudomembrane is composed of polymorphonuclear leukocytes, chronic inflammatory cells, fibrin, and epithelial debris (Tedesco, 1982).

The majority of patients present with watery diarrhea between the fourth and ninth days of therapy. However, 25% develop diarrhea and AAPMC from two to as long as ten weeks after completion of therapy. Diarrhea that develops during antibiotic administration usually is self-limiting and ceases 4 to 14 days after the medication is discontinued. The disorder is usually more protracted (two to four weeks' duration) and debilitating in patients who continue to receive antibiotic therapy in spite of diarrhea or in those who initially develop diarrhea after the course of antibiotic therapy has been completed (Tedesco, 1982).

It is now known that *C. difficile* produces two extracellular toxins: toxin A, a potent enterotoxin with slight cytotoxic activity, and toxin B, a very potent cytotoxin. Toxin A and toxin B have been purified, and both are lethal when injected into animals. Currently, it is believed that toxin A is primarily responsible for the pathogenesis of AAPMC in humans.

Although sigmoidoscopy may be sufficient to visualize colonic changes in the majority of cases, colonoscopy is necessary to detect pseudomembranous lesions in the cecum or transverse colon. The etiologic diagnosis of *C. difficile*-induced pseudomembranous colitis requires demonstration of the *C. difficile* toxin (primarily toxin B) by tissue culture assay. Other immunologic methods (eg, latex agglutination, enzyme immunoassay) to detect toxin are commercially available. These assays are not as sensitive as the tissue culture toxin assay, but they provide more rapid results (two to three hours versus 24 to 48 hours) and can be performed by laboratories that do not have tissue culture facilities. *C. difficile* also can be isolated from stool using anaerobic cultures and a selective medium. However, isolation of *C. difficile* from stool is a relatively nonspecific finding, since asymptomatic carriage of the organism occurs in about 3% of healthy adults, 10% to 20% of hospitalized patients, and 20% to 80% of patients receiving selected antibiotics (McFarland et al, 1989; Chachaty et al, 1992).

Once AAPMC has been diagnosed, the offending antibiotic should be discontinued (if possible) and procedures initiated to restore and maintain normal fluid and electrolyte balance. These measures may be sufficient in the mildly ill patient, and diarrhea frequently will subside in seven to ten days. Additional treatment is necessary in patients with more severe colitis (eg, high temperature, marked abdominal pain, leukocytosis), in those who are elderly or debilitated (regardless of severity), in those who require continued administration of the inducing antibiotic, or in those who are unresponsive to supportive therapy alone (Kaatz and Fekety, 1986).

Specific therapy aimed at either eradication of the *C. difficile* organism or removal of the toxin is available. See index entry Colitis, Pseudomembranous, Treatment, and Tedesco, 1982; Gotz and Rand, 1982; Bartlett, 1985; Kaatz and Fekety, 1986; Lyerly et al, 1988; Fekety et al, 1989. Oral vancomycin (125 to 500 mg every six hours for seven to ten days in adults with normal renal function) has been a drug of choice, especially in more severe cases of AAPMC and in high-risk patients (see index entry Vancomycin). However, some authorities recommend that the use of oral vancomycin be reduced to lessen the possible development of vancomycin-resistant enterococci. Response to vancomycin usually is prompt and impressive; diarrhea, fever, and abdominal cramps often subside in two to four days and toxin levels in stool samples decline gradually over three to seven days. In a randomized clinical trial, the 125-mg dose was as effective as the 500-mg dose and resulted in considerable cost savings (Fekety et al, 1989).

Oral metronidazole [Flagyl, Metryl, Protostat, Satric] (adults, 250 mg four times daily or 500 mg three times daily), bacitracin (adults, 25,000 units four times daily), and cholestyramine resin [Questran] (or colestipol [Colestid]) adults, 4 g of either resin three times daily) also have been useful in treating AAPMC. Like vancomycin, metronidazole and bacitracin eradicate the *C. difficile* organism. Metronidazole was as effective as vancomycin in a prospective, randomized trial (Teasley et al, 1983), and it appears to be an effective and less costly alternative to vancomycin in mildly to moderately ill patients (Bartlett, 1985; Kaatz and Fekety, 1986). Many infectious disease experts now recommend metronidazole as first-line therapy in mildly to moderately ill patients with AAPMC because of cost considerations. However, metronidazole has occasionally caused AAPMC. Clinical experience with bacitracin is limited. Cholestyramine (or colestipol) binds and neutralizes the toxin. Because the resin also binds vancomycin, simultaneous use should be avoided. Success rates have been variable with cholestyramine, and it appears to be more effective for mild AAPMC.

Occasionally, more aggressive supportive treatment may be necessary, particularly in the elderly. In all hospitalized patients with AAPMC, enteric isolation precautions are recommended to prevent nosocomial spread of *C. difficile*.

Relapses of AAPMC have been observed in 10% to 20% of patients after initial successful treatment. Persistent fecal carriage of *C. difficile*, most likely as antibiotic-resistant spores, after treatment is an important risk factor. Most patients respond to a second course of vancomycin or metronidazole and experience only one relapse. However, some individuals suffer multiple relapses. Optimum treatment guidelines for recurrent AAPMC have not been established, but a low dose of vancomycin (125 mg every other day) or vancomycin plus rifampin has been used successfully in some patients (Tedesco et al, 1985; see also Bartlett, 1985; Kaatz and Fekety, 1986).

Although steroids have been used systemically, there is little evidence that they are beneficial in AAPMC, and their use should be avoided. Antiperistaltic drugs, such as loperamide [Imodium], and the antidiarrheal mixture, diphenoxylate with atropine [Lomotil], are contraindicated; their effectiveness is questionable, they may prevent clearance of the toxin from the stool, and toxic megacolon has been associated with their use in AAPMC.

In summary, AAPMC is not unique to the lincosamides, is relatively uncommon, and is treatable. As with any antimicrobial agent, physicians should prescribe lincosamides when clearly indicated and should be alert to the potential for this adverse reaction.

Other Adverse Reactions and Precautions: Other reported adverse gastrointestinal effects of the lincosamides include nausea, vomiting, and abdominal pain.

Hypersensitivity reactions have occurred with both clindamycin and lincomycin. Generalized mild to moderate morbilliform skin rashes are relatively common. Pruritus, maculopapular rash, and urticaria also have been observed. Severe hypersensitivity reactions, such as erythema multiforme and anaphylactoid reactions, have been reported rarely. Lincosamides should not be used in patients with known hypersensitivity to these antibiotics.

Transient leukopenia and eosinophilia have been reported. Agranulocytosis and thrombocytopenia rarely have been associated with use of the lincosamides, but no direct etiologic relationship has been established.

Transitory changes in liver function tests have occurred after administration of lincomycin and clindamycin. More serious hepatotoxicity, including jaundice, has been reported rarely.

An unpleasant or metallic taste experienced during infusions of 600 mg or more of clindamycin phosphate is probably due to the high concentration of drug in saliva.

Hypotension, electrocardiographic changes, and, rarely, cardiac arrest have been associated with too rapid administration of large intravenous doses of lincomycin and clindamycin. Cardiac arrest also has been reported in one patient after 600 mg of undiluted clindamycin was injected over several minutes into a central intravenous line (Aucoin et al, 1982).

The safety of these drugs during pregnancy has not been established, although no harmful effects have been observed in several hundred pregnant women who received lincomycin or clindamycin during all stages of pregnancy. At dosages of 150 mg orally to 600 mg intravenously, the amount of clindamycin that has been reported to appear in breast milk ranges from 0.7 to 3.8 mcg/ml. The decision to discontinue the drug should take into consideration the importance of the drug to the mother.

Although pain, induration, and sterile abscesses after intramuscular administration and thrombophlebitis after intravenous administration have been reported, local irritative reactions are uncommon and these drugs are generally well tolerated after parenteral administration. Local reactions can be minimized or avoided by giving deep intramuscular injections. Parenteral formulations of lincosamides contain benzyl alcohol as a preservative, which has been associated with a fatal "gasping syndrome" in premature infants.

Drug Interactions

Clindamycin and lincomycin have a slight neuromuscular blocking effect and may enhance the action of other neuromuscular blocking drugs. This combination should be used with caution and only when necessary (Tatro, 1988). Lincosamides may inhibit the activity of macrolides and chloramphenicol. A solution of clindamycin phosphate is physically incompatible with ampicillin, phenytoin, barbiturates, aminophylline, calcium gluconate, and magnesium sulfate (Steigbigel, 1990).

Pharmacokinetics

Essentially all (90%) of an oral dose of clindamycin hydrochloride is absorbed, and mean peak serum concentrations of 2.5 and 3.6 mcg/ml have been attained 45 to 60 minutes after ingestion of 150 and 300 mg, respectively, in adults. Clindamycin palmitate, which is rapidly hydrolyzed in vivo to clindamycin, also is absorbed rapidly and efficiently after oral administration, but serum levels are slightly lower than those achieved with comparable doses of clindamycin hydrochloride. Food interferes with the absorption of oral lincomycin, but the absorption of clindamycin preparations does not appear to be appreciably retarded.

After intravenous administration, biologically inactive clindamycin phosphate is rapidly converted to active clindamycin. In healthy adults, peak serum concentrations of active drug were 7, 10, 11, and 14 mcg/ml after infusions of 300 mg (over 10 minutes), 600 mg (over 20 minutes), 900 mg (over 30 minutes), and 1.2 g (over 45 minutes), respectively. After intramuscular administration, peak concentrations of clindamycin are reached after three hours in adults and one hour in children. With both oral and parenteral preparations of clindamycin, peak serum concentrations increase linearly with increasing dose.

Clindamycin is approximately 90% protein bound. The volume of distribution is 0.66 ± 0.1 L/kg (Benet and Sheiner, 1985). It is widely distributed throughout the body and penetrates well into various tissues and body fluids, including saliva, sputum, respiratory tissue, pleural fluid, bile, liver, gallbladder, appendix, soft tissues, prostate, semen, and bones and joints (see LeFrock et al, 1982). However, effective concentrations are not attained in the cerebrospinal fluid, even when meninges are inflamed. Clindamycin readily crosses the placenta and it is found in breast milk. This drug is actively transported into polymorphonuclear leukocytes and macrophages and achieves relatively high concentrations in experimental abscesses (see Steigbigel, 1990).

Clindamycin is primarily metabolized in the liver to bioactive and inactive metabolites. N-demethyl clindamycin (more active than parent drug) and clindamycin sulfoxide (less active than parent drug) are the major bioactive metabolites. Metabolites are excreted in the urine and bile. Within 24 hours, approximately 10% of an administered dose is excreted in the urine and 3.6% in the feces as active drug and metabolites.

The elimination half-life of clindamycin ranges from 2.4 to 3 hours in adults and children with normal renal function. Half-lives of 8.7 and 3.6 hours have been reported in premature and term neonates, respectively (Bell et al, 1984). The half-life is increased slightly in patients with markedly reduced renal function, and little or no dosage modification is needed when hepatic function is normal in these patients. Dosage reduction is necessary in patients with combined severe renal and hepatic disease. Hemodialysis and peritoneal dialysis do not remove clindamycin from the serum.

For a description of the clinical pharmacology of lincomycin, see Fass, 1980.

Drug Evaluations

CLINDAMYCIN HYDROCHLORIDE
[Cleocin Hydrochloride]

CLINDAMYCIN PALMITATE HYDROCHLORIDE
[Cleocin Pediatric]

CLINDAMYCIN PHOSPHATE
[Cleocin Phosphate]

Clindamycin is a semisynthetic derivative of lincomycin that is more potent and better absorbed than the parent compound. Thus, it is the preferred lincosamide for all indications. For antimicrobial spectrum, uses, pharmacokinetics, adverse reactions and precautions, and interactions, see the section on Lincosamides.

DOSAGE AND PREPARATIONS. For group A streptococcal infections, treatment should be continued for at least ten days.

Oral: (Hydrochloride) *Adults,* for serious infections, 150 to 300 mg every six hours; for more severe infections, 300 to 450 mg every six hours. *Children,* for serious infections, 8 to 16 mg/kg daily in three or four divided doses; for more severe infections, 16 to 20 mg/kg daily in three or four divided doses. To avoid the possibility of esophageal irritation, clindamycin hydrochloride should be taken with a full glass of water.

(Palmitate Hydrochloride) *Adults and children weighing more than 10 kg*, for serious infections, 8 to 12 mg/kg daily in three or four divided doses; for severe infections, 13 to 16 mg/kg daily in three or four divided doses; for more severe infections, 17 to 25 mg/kg daily in three or four divided doses. *Children weighing 10 kg or less*, 37.5 mg three times daily is the minimum recommended dose.

Food does not adversely affect the absorption of clindamycin hydrochloride or clindamycin palmitate.

CLINDAMYCIN HYDROCHLORIDE:
Generic. Capsules 75 and 150 mg (equivalent to base).
Cleocin Hydrochloride (Upjohn). Capsules 75, 150, and 300 mg (equivalent to base). The 75- and 150-mg capsules contain tartrazine.

CLINDAMYCIN PALMITATE HYDROCHLORIDE:
Cleocin Pediatric (Upjohn). Granules for suspension 75 mg/5 ml (equivalent to base).

Intramuscular: This route of administration is rarely indicated; oral therapy should be substituted as soon as possible. Intramuscular injection of more than 600 mg at a single site is frequently painful and is not recommended. *Adults*, for serious infections with aerobic gram-positive cocci and more sensitive anaerobes, 600 mg to 1.2 g daily in two, three, or four equally divided doses. For more severe infections, particularly those suspected or caused by *Bacteroides fragilis, Peptococcus*, or *Clostridium* (other than *C. perfringens*), 1.2 to 2.7 g daily in two, three, or four equally divided doses. *Children over 1 month*, for serious infections, 15 to 25 mg/kg (alternative, 350 mg/M^2) daily in three or four equally divided doses; for more severe infections, 25 to 40 mg/kg (alternative, 450 mg/M^2) daily in three or four equally divided doses. *Neonates less than 1 month*, 15 to 20 mg/kg daily in three or four equal doses. The smaller amount may be adequate for small premature infants.

Intravenous: Oral therapy should be substituted as soon as possible. *Adults,* for serious infections with aerobic gram-positive cocci and more sensitive anaerobes, 600 mg to 1.2 g daily in two, three, or four equally divided doses; for more severe infections, particularly those suspected or caused by *B. fragilis, Peptococcus,* or *Clostridium* (other than *C. perfringens*), 1.2 to 2.7 g daily in two, three, or four equally divided doses; for life-threatening infections, as much as 4.8 g daily has been given. As an alternative to intermittent infusion, the initial dose may be administered as a single rapid infusion, followed by continuous infusion (see manufacturer's recommendations). *Children over 1 month*, for serious infections, 15 to 25 mg/kg (alternative, 350 mg/M^2) daily in three or four equally divided doses; for more severe infections, 25 to 40 mg/kg (alternative, 450 mg/M^2) daily. *Neonates less than 1 month*, 15 to 20 mg/kg daily in three or four equal doses. The smaller amount may be adequate for small premature infants.

Clindamycin phosphate should *not* be injected intravenously undiluted as a bolus. It should be diluted with an appropriate solution for injection to a concentration of not more than 18 mg/ml and infused at a rate of not more than 30 mg/min. See manufacturer's recommendations for appropriate infusion rates. Administration of more than 1.2 g in a single one-hour infusion is not recommended.

CLINDAMYCIN PHOSPHATE:
Generic. Solution 150 mg/ml (equivalent to base).
Cleocin Phosphate (Upjohn). Solution (sterile, for intramuscular, intravenous use) 150 mg/ml in 2, 4, 6, and 60 ml containers (equivalent to base); and 600 mg/4 ml with 50 ml diluent and 900 mg/6 ml with 100 ml diluent *(ADD-Vantage vials; for intravenous use only)*.
Cleocin Phosphate IV (Upjohn). Solution (sterile) 6, 12, and 18 mg/ml with dextrose 5% in 50 ml containers.

LINCOMYCIN HYDROCHLORIDE MONOHYDRATE
[Lincocin]

Lincomycin offers no therapeutic advantages over clindamycin. Consequently, it has become obsolete and no dosage is cited.

For antimicrobial spectrum, adverse reactions, and precautions, see the section on Lincosamides.

Lincocin (Upjohn).

Cited References

The choice of antibacterial drugs. *Med Lett Drugs Ther* 34:49-56, (May) 1992.

Drugs for anaerobic infections. *Med Lett Drugs Ther* 26:87-89, 1984.

Drugs for parasitic infections. *Med Lett Drugs Ther* 30:15-24, 1988.
Erythromycin estolate: Withdrawal of proposal to revoke provisions for certification of tablets and capsules; response to petition; labeling. *Federal Register* 47:22547-22568, (May 25) 1982.
Oral erythromycins. *Med Lett Drugs Ther* 27:1-3, 1985.
Congenital syphilis—United States, 1983-1985. *MMWR* 35:625-628, 1986.
Antibiotic-resistant strains of *Neisseria gonorrhoeae*: Policy guidelines for detection, management, and control. *MMWR* 36:1S-18S, 1987.
Guidelines for prevention and control of congenital syphilis. *MMWR* 37:S1-S13, 1988.
1989 Sexually transmitted diseases treatment guidelines. *MMWR* 38(suppl 8):1-43, 1989.
Absher JR, Bale JF Jr: Aggravation of myasthenia gravis by erythromycin. *J Pediatr* 119:155-156, 1991.
Aldons PM: A comparison of clarithromycin with ampicillin in the treatment of outpatients with acute bacterial exacerbation of chronic bronchitis. *J Antimicrob Chemother* 27(suppl A): 101-108, 1991.
Alger LS, Lovchik JC: Comparative efficacy of clindamycin versus erythromycin in eradication of antenatal *Chlamydia trachomatis. Am J Obstet Gynecol* 165:375-381, 1991.
Anderson G, et al: A comparative safety and efficacy study of clarithromycin and erythromycin stearate in community-acquired pneumonia. *J Antimicrob Chemother* 27(suppl A):117-124, 1991.
Araujo FG, et al: Azithromycin: A macrolide antibiotic with potent activity against *Toxoplasma gondii. Antimicrob Agents Chemother* 32:755-757, 1988.
Aronsson B, et al: Antimicrobial agents and *Clostridium difficile* in acute enteric disease: Epidemiological data from Sweden, 1980-1982. *J Infect Dis* 151:476-481, 1985.
Auckenthaler RW, et al: Macrolides, in Peterson PK, Verhoef J (eds): *The Antimicrobial Agents Annual/3.* New York, Elsevier, 1988, 122-137.
Aucoin P, et al: Clindamycin-induced cardiac arrest. *South Med J* 75:768, 1982.
Bachand RT Jr: Comparative study of clarithromycin and ampicillin in the treatment of patients with acute bacterial exacerbations of chronic bronchitis. *J Antimicrob Chemother* 27(suppl A):91-100, 1991.
Balmes P, et al: Comparative study of azithromycin and amoxicillin/clavulanic acid in the treatment of lower respiratory tract infections. *Eur J Clin Microbiol Infect Dis* 10:437-439, 1991.
Barry AL, et al: In vitro activities of azithromycin (CP 62,993), clarithromycin (A-56268; TE-031), erythromycin, roxithromycin, and clindamycin. *Antimicrob Agents Chemother* 32:752-754, 1988.
Bartlett JG: Antibiotic-associated pseudomembranous colitis. *Hosp Pract* 16:85-95, (Dec) 1981.
Bartlett JG: Anti-anaerobic antibacterial agents. *Lancet* 2:478-481, 1982.
Bartlett JG: Treatment of *Clostridium difficile* colitis, editorial. *Gastroenterology* 89:1192-1195, 1985.
Bell MJ, et al: Pharmacokinetics of clindamycin phosphate in first year of life. *J Pediatr* 105:482-486, 1984.
Benet LZ, Sheiner LB: Design and optimization of dosage regimens: Pharmacokinetic data, in Gilman AG, et al (eds): *The Pharmacological Basis of Therapeutics*, ed 7. New York, Macmillan, 1985, 1663-1733.
Bennett WM, et al: Drug therapy in renal failure: Dosing guidelines for adults. I. Antimicrobial agents, analgesics. *Ann Intern Med* 93:62-89, 1980.
Bergeron MG, et al: In vitro activity of clarithromycin and its 14-hydroxy-metabolite against 203 strains of *Haemophilus influenzae. Infection* 20:164-167, 1992.
Bowler WA, et al: Gastrointestinal side effects of intravenous erythromycin: Incidence and reduction with prolonged infusion time and glycopyrrolate pretreatment. *Am J Med* 92:249-253, 1992.
Brittain DC: Erythromycin. *Med Clin North Am* 71:1147-1154, 1987.
Brown BA, et al: Activities of four macrolides, including clarithromycin, against *Mycobacterium fortuitum, Mycobacterium chelonae*, and *M. chelonae*-like organisms. *Antimicrob Agents Chemother* 36:180-184, 1992.
Campbell WF, Dodson MG: Clindamycin therapy for *Chlamydia trachomatis* in women. *Am J Obstet Gynecol* 162:343-347, 1990.
Casiano RR: Azithromycin and amoxicillin in the treatment of acute maxillary sinusitis. *Am J Med* 91(suppl 3A):3A-27S-3A-30S, 1991.
Catnach SM, Fairclough PD: Erythromycin and the gut. *Gut* 33:397-401, 1992.
Chachaty E, et al: Presence of *Clostridium difficile* and antibiotic and β-lactamase activities in feces of volunteers treated with oral cefixime, oral cefpodoxime proxetil, or placebo. *Antimicrob Agents Chemother* 36:2009-2013, 1992.
Chang T-W: Antimicrobial-associated diarrhea and enterocolitis. *Drug Ther (Hosp)* 6:71-78, (May) 1981.
Chang HR, et al: In vitro effects of four macrolides (roxithromycin, spiramycin, azithromycin [CP-62, 993], and a-56268) on *Toxoplasma gondii. Antimicrob Agents Chemother* 32:524-529, 1988.
Chin N-X, et al: Activity of A-56268 compared with that of erythromycin and other oral agents against aerobic and anaerobic bacteria. *Antimicrob Agents Chemother* 31:463-466, 1987.
Cuchural GJ, et al: Susceptibility of *Bacteroides fragilis* group in United States: Analysis by site of infection. *Antimicrob Agents Chemother* 32:717-722, 1988.
Dabernat H, et al: The activity of clarithromycin and its 14-hydroxy metabolite against *Haemophilus influenzae,* determined by in-vitro and serum bactericidal tests. *J Antimicrob Chemother* 27(suppl A):19-30, 1991.
Daniel R, European Azithromycin Study Group: Simplified treatment of acute lower respiratory tract infection with azithromycin: A comparison with erythromycin and amoxycillin. *J Int Med Res* 19:373-383, 1991.
Dannemann BR, et al: Treatment of toxoplasmic encephalitis with intravenous clindamycin. *Arch Intern Med* 148:2477-2482, 1988.
Dannemann B, et al: Treatment of toxoplasmic encephalitis in patients with AIDS: A randomized trial comparing pyrimethamine plus clindamycin to pyrimethamine plus sulfadiazine. *Ann Intern Med* 116:33-43, 1992.
Dark D: Multicenter evaluation of azithromycin and cefaclor in acute lower respiratory tract infections. *Am J Med* 91(suppl 3A):3A-31S-3A-35S, 1991.
Dautzenberg B, et al: Activity of clarithromycin against *Mycobacterium avium* infection in patients with acquired immune deficiency syndrome. *Am Rev Respir Dis* 144:564-569, 1991.
Dautzenberg B, et al: Clarithromycin and other antimicrobial agents in the treatment of disseminated *Mycobacterium avium* infections in patients with acquired immunodeficiency syndrome. *Arch Intern Med* 153:368-372, 1993.
Davis BD: Protein synthesis, in Davis BD, et al (eds): *Microbiology,* ed 3. Hagerstown, Md, Harper & Row, 1980, 229-255.
de Lalla F, et al: Clarithromycin-ciprofloxacin-amikacin for therapy of *Mycobacterium avium-Mycobacterium intracellulare* bacteremia in patients with AIDS. *Antimicrob Agents Chemother* 36:1567-1569, 1992.
Derouin F, et al: Synergistic activity of azithromycin and pyrimethamine or sulfadiazine in acute experimental toxoplasmosis. *Antimicrob Agents Chemother* 36:997-1001, 1992.
DiSanto AR, Chodos DJ: Influence of study design in assessing food effects on absorption of erythromycin base and erythromycin stearate. *Antimicrob Agents Chemother* 20:190-196, 1981.
Doherty JE: Digoxin-antibiotic drug interaction, editorial. *N Engl J Med* 305:827-828, 1981.
Duval J: Evolution and epidemiology of MLS resistance. *J Antimicrob Chemother* 16(suppl A):137-149, 1985.
Fass RJ: Lincomycin and clindamycin, in Kagan BM (ed): *Antimicrobial Therapy,* ed 3. Philadelphia, WB Saunders, 1980, 97-116.
Fekety R: Antibiotic-associated pseudomembranous colitis. *Clin Microbiol Newslett* (preview issue) Oct 1978.
Fekety R, et al: Treatment of antibiotic-associated *Clostridium difficile* colitis with oral vancomycin: Comparison of two dosage regimens. *Am J Med* 86:15-19, 1989.

Fenton LJ, Light IJ: Congenital syphilis after maternal treatment with erythromycin. *Obstet Gynecol* 47:492-494, 1976.

Fernandez-Martin J, et al: Pyrimethamine-clarithromycin combination for therapy of acute *Toxoplasma* encephalitis in patients with AIDS. *Antimicrob Agents Chemother* 35:2049-2052, 1991.

Fiumara NJ: Therapy guidelines for sexually transmitted diseases, letter. *J Am Acad Dermatol* 9:600-601, 1983.

Foulds G, et al: The pharmacokinetics of azithromycin in human serum and tissues. *J Antimicrob Chemother* 25 (suppl A):73-82, 1990.

Francis H, et al: Severe vascular spasm due to erythromycin-ergotamine interaction. *Clin Rheumatol* 3:243-246, 1984.

Fraschini F, et al: The diffusion of clarithromycin and roxithromycin into nasal mucosa, tonsil and lung in humans. *J Antimicrob Chemother* 27 (suppl A):61-65, 1991.

Fremaux A, et al: In-vitro antibacterial activity of RP 59500, a semisynthetic streptogramin, against *Streptococcus pneumoniae. J Antimicrob Chemother* 30 (suppl A):19-23, 1992.

Ginsburg CM, et al: Concentrations of erythromycin in serum and tonsil: Comparison of estolate and ethylsuccinate suspensions. *J Pediatr* 89:1011-1013, 1976.

Ginsburg CM, et al: Management of group A streptococcal pharyngitis: Randomized controlled study of twice-daily erythromycin ethylsuccinate versus erythromycin estolate. *Pediatr Infect Dis* 1:384-387, 1982.

Ginsburg CM, et al: Erythromycin therapy for group A streptococcal pharyngitis: Results of comparative study of estolate and ethylsuccinate formulations. *Am J Dis Child* 138:536-539, 1984.

Goldstein FW, et al: Bacteriostatic and bactericidal activity of azithromycin against *Haemophilus influenzae. J Antimicrob Chemother* 25 (suppl A):25-28, 1990.

Gotz VP, Rand KH: Medical management of antimicrobial-associated diarrhea and colitis. *Pharmacotherapy* 2:100-109, 1982.

Graham DY, et al: Clarithromycin for the eradication of *H. pylori*, in: *Program and Abstracts of the 31st Interscience Conference on Antimicrobial Agents and Chemotherapy.* Washington, DC, American Society for Microbiology, 1991, 25B.

Grayston JT, et al: New *Chlamydia psittaci* strain, TWAR, isolated in acute respiratory tract infections. *N Engl J Med* 315:161-168, 1986.

Grayston JT, et al: Current knowledge of *Chlamydia pneumoniae,* strain TWAR, an important cause of pneumonia and other acute respiratory diseases. *Eur J Clin Microbiol Infect Dis* 8:191-202, 1989.

Gribble MJ, Chow AW: Erythromycin. *Med Clin North Am* 66:79-89, 1982.

Gudiol F, et al: Clindamycin vs penicillin for anaerobic lung infections: High rate of penicillin failures associated with penicillin-resistant *Bacteroides melaninogenicus. Arch Intern Med* 150:2525-2529, 1990.

Gurwith MJ, et al: Diarrhea associated with clindamycin and ampicillin therapy: Preliminary results of cooperative study. *J Infect Dis* 135 (suppl):104-110, 1977.

Hammerschlag MR, et al: In vitro activities of azithromycin, clarithromycin, L-ofloxacin, and other antibiotics against *Chlamydia pneumoniae, Antimicrob Agents Chemother* 36:1573-1574, 1992.

Hansten PD, Horn JR. *Drug Interactions and Updates*, ed 6. Malvern, Penn, Lea & Febiger, 1990, 263-267.

Hardy DJ, et al: Comparative in vitro activities of new 14-, 15-, and 16-membered macrolides. *Antimicrob Agents Chemother* 32:1710-1719, 1988.

Hardy DJ, et al: Enhancement of the in vitro and in vivo activities of clarithromycin against *Haemophilus influenzae* by 14-hydroxy-clarithromycin, its major metabolite in humans. *Antimicrob Agents Chemother* 34:1407-1413, 1990.

Hardy DJ, et al: Clarithromycin, a unique macrolide: A pharmacokinetic, microbiologic, and clinical perspective. *Diagn Microbiol Infect Dis* 15:39-53, 1992.

Hopkins S: Clinical toleration and safety of azithromycin. *Am J Med* 91 (suppl 3A):3A-40S-3A-45S, 1991.

Jacobson MA, et al: Toxicity of clindamycin as prophylaxis for AIDS-associated toxoplasmic encephalitis. *Lancet* 339:333-334, 1992.

Johnson RB: The role of azalide antibiotics in the treatment of chlamydia. *Am J Obstet Gynecol* 164:1794-1796, 1991.

Jones RN, et al: In vitro activity of clarithromycin (TE-031, A-67268) and 14OH-clarithromycin alone and in combination against *Legionella* species. *Eur J Clin Microbiol Infect Dis* 9:846-848, 1990.

Kaatz GW, Fekety R: Combating colonization of *Clostridium difficile. Consultant* 26:45-58, (Sept) 1986.

Kallings I: Sensitivity of *Branhamella catarrhalis* to oral antibiotics. *Drugs* 31 (suppl 3):17-22, 1986.

Karma P, et al: The comparative efficacy and safety of clarithromycin and amoxycillin in the treatment of outpatients with acute maxillary sinusitis. *J Antimicrob Chemother* 27 (suppl A):83-90, 1991 A.

Karma P, et al: Azithromycin concentrations in sinus fluid and mucosa after oral administration. *Eur J Clin Microbiol Infect Dis* 10:856-859, 1991 B.

LaForce CF, et al: Inhibition of methylprednisolone elimination in presence of erythromycin therapy. *J Allergy Clin Immunol* 72:34-39, 1983.

Leclercq R, Courvalin P: Bacterial resistance to macrolide, lincosamide, and streptogramin antibiotics by target modification. *Antimicrob Agents Chemother* 35:1267-1272, 1991 A.

Leclercq R, Courvalin P: Intrinsic and unusual resistance to macrolide, lincosamide, and streptogramin antibiotics in bacteria. *Antimicrob Agents Chemother* 35:1273-1276, 1991 B.

LeFrock JL, et al: Clindamycin. *Med Clin North Am* 66:103-120, 1982.

Levison ME, et al: Clindamycin compared with penicillin for treatment of anaerobic lung abscess. *Ann Intern Med* 98:466-471, 1983.

Lindenbaum J, et al: Inactivation of digoxin by gut flora: Reversal by antibiotic therapy. *N Engl J Med* 305:789-794, 1981.

Lindsay J, et al: Torsades de pointes associated with antimicrobial therapy for pneumonia. *Chest* 98:222-223, 1990.

Logan MN, et al: The in-vitro activity and disc susceptibility testing of clarithromycin and its 14-hydroxy metabolite. *J Antimicrob Chemother* 27:161-170, 1991.

Ludden TM: Pharmacokinetic interactions of macrolide antibiotics. *Clin Pharmacokinet* 10:63-79, 1985.

Lusk RH, et al: Gastrointestinal side effects of clindamycin and ampicillin therapy. *J Infect Dis* 135 (suppl):111-119, 1977.

Lyerly DM, et al: *Clostridium difficile:* Its disease and toxins. *Clin Microbiol Rev* 1:1-18, 1988.

Malmborg AS: Effect of food on absorption of erythromycin: Study of two derivatives, the stearate and the base. *J Antimicrob Chemother* 5:591-599, 1979.

Martin DH, et al: A controlled trial of a single dose of azithromycin for the treatment of chlamydial urethritis and cervicitis. *N Engl J Med* 327:921-925, 1992.

Maskell JP, et al: Comparative in-vitro activity of azithromycin and erythromycin against gram-positive cocci, *Haemophilus influenzae* and anaerobes. *J Antimicrob Chemother* 25 (suppl A):19-24, 1990.

Massarotti EM, et al: Treatment of early Lyme disease. *Am J Med* 92:396-403, (April) 1992.

McCormack WM, et al: Hepatotoxicity of erythromycin estolate during pregnancy. *Antimicrob Agents Chemother* 12:630-635, 1977.

McDonald PJ, et al: Studies on absorption of newly developed enteric-coated erythromycin base. *J Clin Pharmacol* 17:601-606, 1977.

McFarland LV, et al: Nosocomial acquisition of *Clostridium difficile* infection. *N Engl J Med* 320:204-210, 1989.

McGehee RF Jr, et al: Comparative studies of antibacterial activity in vitro and absorption and excretion of lincomycin and clindamycin. *Am J Med Sci* 256:279-292, 1968.

The Medical Letter: *Handbook of Antimicrobial Therapy.* New Rochell, NY, The Medical Letter, 1988, 38-49.

Mertens JCC, et al: Double-blind randomized study comparing the efficacies and safeties of a short (3-day) course of azithromycin and a 5-day course of amoxicillin in patients with acute exacerbations of chronic bronchitis. *Antimicrob Agents Chemother* 36:1456-1459, 1992.

Nattel MD, et al: Erythromycin-induced long QT syndrome: Concordance with quinidine and underlying cellular electrophysiologic mechanism. *Am J Med* 89:235-238, 1990.

Neu HC: The development of macrolides: Clarithromycin in perspective. *J Antimicrob Chemother* 27 (suppl A):1-9, 1991 A.

Neu HC: Clinical microbiology of azithromycin. *Am J Med* 91 (suppl 3A):3A-12S-3A-18S, 1991 B.

Neu HC: New macrolide antibiotics: Azithromycin and clarithromycin. *Ann Intern Med* 116:515-517, 1992.

Neu HC, et al: Incidence of diarrhea and colitis associated with clindamycin therapy. *J Infect Dis* 135 (suppl):120-125, 1977.

Neu HC, et al: Comparative in vitro activity of the new oral macrolide azithromycin. *Eur J Clin Microbiol Infect Dis* 7:541-544, 1988.

Nicholas P: Erythromycin: Clinical review. I. Clinical pharmacology. *NY State J Med* 77:2088-2094, 1977.

Nicotra B, et al: *Branhamella catarrhalis* as lower respiratory tract pathogen in patients with chronic lung disease. *Arch Intern Med* 146:890-893, 1986.

Norris SM, Mandell GL: Tables of antimicrobial agent pharmacology, in Mandell GL, et al (eds): *Anti-Infective Therapy*. New York, John Wiley & Sons, 1985, 470-471.

Patel J, Schneider R: Hepatotoxic reaction to erythromycin ethylsuccinate. *South Med J* 77:1343-1349, 1984.

Peters DH, Clissold SP: Clarithromycin: A review of its antimicrobial activity, pharmacokinetic properties and therapeutic potential. *Drugs* 44:117-164, 1992.

Pfefferkorn ER, et al: Parasiticidal effect of clindamycin on *Toxoplasma gondii* grown in cultured cells and selection of a drug-resistant mutant. *Antimicrob Agents Chemother* 36:1091-1096, 1992.

Phillips JP, et al: Pharmacokinetic drug interaction between erythromycin and triazolam. *J Clin Psychopharmacol* 6:297-299, 1986.

Pratt WB, Fekety R: *The Antimicrobial Drugs*. New York, Oxford University Press, 1986, 184-228.

Ragosta M, et al: Potentially fatal interaction between erythromycin and disopyramide. *Am J Med* 86:465-466, 1989.

Renaudin H, Bébéar C: Comparative in vitro activity of azithromycin, clarithromycin, erythromycin and lomefloxacin against *Mycoplasma pneumoniae, Mycoplasma hominis* and *Ureaplasma urealyticum*. *Eur J Clin Microbiol Infect Dis* 9:838-841, 1990.

Report of the Committee on Infectious Diseases: *American Academy of Pediatrics Redbook*, ed 20. Elk Grove Village, Ill, American Academy of Pediatrics, 1986, 266-275.

Retsema J, et al: Spectrum and mode of action of azithromycin (CP-62,993), a new 15-membered-ring macrolide with improved potency against gram-negative organisms. *Antimicrob Agents Chemother* 31:1937-1947, 1987.

Ridgway GL, et al: The in-vitro activity of clarithromycin and other macrolides against the type strain of *Chlamydia pneumoniae* (TWAR). *J Antimicrob Chemother* 27 (suppl A):43-45, 1991.

Rolston KV, Hoy J: Role of clindamycin in treatment of central nervous system toxoplasmosis. *Am J Med* 83:551-554, 1987.

Schachter J: *Chlamydia psittaci:* "Reemergence" of forgotten pathogen, editorial. *N Engl J Med* 315:189-191, 1986.

Schoenberger RA, et al: Association of intravenous erythromycin and potentially fatal ventricular tachycardia with Q-T prolongation (torsades de pointes). *BMJ* 300:1375-1376, 1990.

Schönwald S, et al: Comparison of azithromycin and erythromycin in the treatment of atypical pneumonias. *J Antimicrob Chemother* 25 (suppl A):123-126, 1990.

Scieux C, et al: In-vitro activity of azithromycin against *Chlamydia trachomatis*. *J Antimicrob Chemother* 25 (suppl A): 7-10, 1990.

Segreti J, et al: In vitro activity of A-56268 (TE-031) and four other antimicrobial agents against *Chlamydia trachomatis*. *Antimicrob Agents Chemother* 31:100-101, 1987.

Slaney L, et al: In-vitro activity of azithromycin, erythromycin, ciprofloxacin and norfloxacin against *Neisseria gonorrhoeae, Haemophilus ducreyi,* and *Chlamydia trachomatis*. *J Antimicrob Chemother* 25 (suppl A):1-5, 1990.

Soussy CJ, et al: A collaborative study of the in-vitro sensitivity to RP 59500 of bacteria isolated in seven hospitals in France. *J Antimicrob Chemother* 30 (suppl A):53-58, 1992.

Steigbigel NH: Erythromycin, lincomycin, and clindamycin, in Mandell GL, et al (eds): *Principles and Practice of Infectious Diseases,* ed 3. New York, John Wiley & Sons, 1990, 308-317.

Swanson DJ, et al: Erythromycin ototoxicity: Prospective assessment with serum concentrations and audiograms in a study of patients with pneumonia. *Am J Med* 92:61-68, 1992.

Swartzberg JE, et al: Clinical study of gastrointestinal complications associated with clindamycin therapy. *J Infect Dis* 135 (suppl):99-103, 1977.

Tally FP: Therapeutic approaches to anaerobic infections. *Hosp Pract* 16:117-132 (Dec) 1981.

Tally FP, et al: Plasmid-mediated, transferable resistance to clindamycin and erythromycin in *Bacteroides fragilis*. *J Infect Dis* 139:83-88, 1979.

Tally FP, et al: Susceptibility of *Bacteroides fragilis* group in United States in 1981. *Antimicrob Agents Chemother* 23:536-540, 1983.

Tatro DS (ed): *Drug Interaction Facts*. St. Louis, JB Lippincott, 1988, 175 and 530.

Tatro DS (ed): *Drug Interaction Facts*. St. Louis, JB Lippincott, 1989, 315.

Teasley DG, et al: Prospective randomized trial of metronidazole versus vancomycin for *Clostridium difficile*-associated diarrhoea and colitis. *Lancet* 2:1043-1046, 1983.

Tedesco FJ: Clindamycin and colitis: Review. *J Infect Dis* 135 (suppl):95-98, 1977.

Tedesco FJ: Pseudomembranous colitis: Pathogenesis and therapy. *Med Clin North Am* 66:655-664, 1982.

Tedesco FJ, et al: Approach to patients with multiple relapses of antibiotic-associated pseudomembranous colitis. *Am J Gastroenterol* 80:867-868, 1985.

Truhan AP, et al: Pityriasis lichenoides in children: Therapeutic response to erythromycin. *J Am Acad Dermatol* 15:66-70, 1986.

Verhaegen J, et al: Erythromycin-resistant *Streptococcus pneumoniae*. *Lancet* 2:1432-1433, 1988.

Washington JA II, Wilson WR: Erythromycin: Microbial and clinical perspective after 30 years of clinical use, parts 1 and 2. *Mayo Clin Proc* 60:189-203, 271-278, 1985.

Yee MH, et al: Clinical significance of clindamycin-resistant *Bacteroides fragilis*. *JAMA* 248:1860-1863, 1982.

Young LS, et al: Azithromycin reduces M. avium complex (MAC) bacteremia and relieves its symptoms in patients with AIDS, in: *Program and Abstracts of the 31st Conference on Antimicrobial Agents and Chemotherapy*. Washington, DC, American Society for Microbiology, 1991, 148.

Other Selected References

Erythromycin symposium. *Scott Med J* 22 (suppl 1):349-407, 1977.

Derrick CW Jr, Reilly KM: Erythromycin, lincomycin, and clindamycin. *Pediatr Clin North Am* 30:63-69, 1983.

Ginsburg CM: Macrolides: Erythromycin, troleandomycin, and josamycin, in Kagan BM (ed): *Antimicrobial Therapy*, ed 3. Philadelphia, WB Saunders, 1980, 84-97.

Hermans PE: Lincosamides, in Peterson PK, Verhoef J (eds): *The Antimicrobial Agents Annual/3*. New York, Elsevier, 1988, 113-121.

Klainer AS: Clindamycin. *Med Clin North Am* 71:1169-1175, 1987.

Kucers A: Chloramphenicol, erythromycin, vancomycin, tetracycline. *Lancet* 2:425-429, 1982.

Nelson JD (chairman): Evolving role of erythromycin in medicine: Proceedings of symposium. *Pediatr Infect Dis* 5:118-176, 1986.

Nicholas P: Erythromycin: Clinical review. II. Therapeutic uses. *NY State J Med* 77:2243-2246, 1977.

Phillips I, et al (eds): Roxithromycin: New macrolide. *J Antimicrob Chemother* 20 (suppl B): 1-187, 1987.

Wilson WR, Cockerill FR: Tetracyclines, chloramphenicol, erythromycin, and clindamycin. *Mayo Clin Proc* 62:906-915, 1987.

Young RA, et al: Roxithromycin: Review of its antibacterial activity, pharmacokinetic properties and clinical efficacy *Drugs* 37:8-41, 1989.

Tetracyclines and Chloramphenicol

67

TETRACYCLINES

Source, Chemistry, and Classification

The tetracycline antibiotics were discovered as the result of a systematic screening of soil samples collected from many parts of the world for antibiotic-producing microorganisms. The first tetracycline to be introduced was chlortetracycline in 1948. Presently, five tetracycline analogues are marketed in the United States. Tetracycline, oxytetracycline [Terramycin], and demeclocycline [Declomycin] are naturally derived compounds from various species of *Streptomyces*. Doxycycline [Vibramycin] is derived semisynthetically from oxytetracycline, and minocycline [Minocin] is prepared by chemical modification of tetracycline.

All tetracyclines contain a hydronaphthacene nucleus consisting of four fused rings. Differences among the various analogues are determined by different substitutions on the basic structure (Figure).

The tetracyclines are broad spectrum antimicrobial agents. In general, patterns of microbial susceptibility and resistance to the tetracyclines are similar, but there are some differences in the degree of activity among the various analogues. The newer tetracyclines, minocycline and doxycycline, are more active than the parent compound against some organisms. The tetracyclines differ considerably in their pharmacology, and these antibiotics are usually subdivided into short- (tetracycline, oxytetracycline), intermediate- (demeclocycline), and long-acting (doxycycline, minocycline) analogues.

CHEMICAL STRUCTURES OF TETRACYCLINES

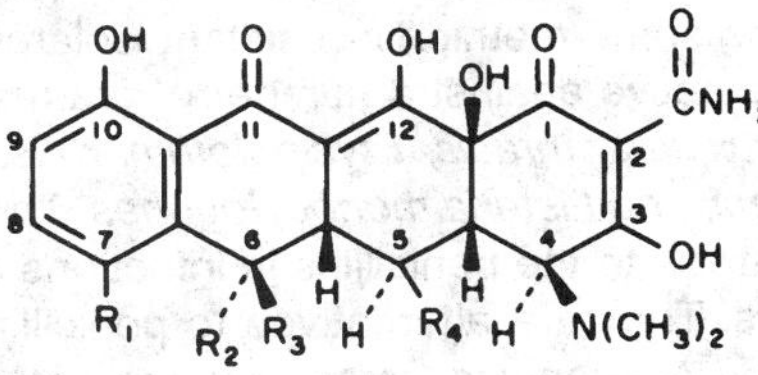

Generic Name	R_1	R_2	R_3	R_4
SHORT-ACTING				
Tetracycline	H	OH	CH_3	H
Oxytetracycline	H	OH	CH_3	OH
INTERMEDIATE-ACTING				
Demeclocycline	Cl	OH	H	H
LONG-ACTING				
Doxycycline	H	H	CH_3	OH
Minocycline	$N(CH_3)_2$	H	H	H

Mechanism of Action

Tetracyclines interfere with protein synthesis by blocking the attachment of aminoacyl transfer RNA to the acceptor site on the messenger RNA-ribosome complex (see Pratt and Fekety, 1986). Binding of antibiotic occurs primarily at the bacterial 30S ribosomal subunit. Tetracyclines also can inhibit mammalian protein synthesis in cell-free systems. Their selective toxicity for bacteria appears to depend, in part, on energy-dependent uptake of antibiotic by bacterial, but not mammalian, cells. This results in a greater accumulation of tetracyclines by bacterial cells. However, since active transport does not occur in various intracellular microorganisms (eg, rickettsiae, chlamydiae) that are highly susceptible to tetracyclines, other factors also appear to be involved.

Tetracyclines are usually bacteriostatic at blood levels achieved clinically.

Antimicrobial Spectrum

Tetracyclines are active in vitro against a great variety of bacteria, including gram-positive, gram-negative, aerobic, and anaerobic organisms. In addition, they are active against spirochetes, mycoplasmas, rickettsiae, chlamydiae, and some protozoa (Siegel, 1978, part II; Ory, 1980; Cunha et al, 1982; Francke and Neu, 1987; Williams, 1988; Standiford, 1990).

Among gram-positive cocci, a number of strains of *Streptococcus pyogenes* (group A), *S. agalactiae* (group B), viridans streptococci, and anaerobic streptococci are susceptible. However, the tetracyclines usually are not used to treat streptococcal infections because many strains are resistant and more effective drugs (eg, penicillin G, erythromycin, cephalosporins) are available. Many strains of *S. pneumoniae* are now resistant to the tetracyclines. Essentially all strains of enterococci (eg, *E. faecalis)* are resistant. Many strains of *Staphylococcus aureus* also are resistant to the tetracyclines. Minocycline has greater antistaphylococcal activity than other analogues, including some methicillin-resistant isolates.

Tetracyclines are active against a number of gram-positive bacilli including *Bacillus anthracis, Erysipelothrix rhusiopathiae, Clostridium tetani,* and *Listeria monocytogenes.* These antibiotics are alternatives to the penicillins in infections caused by these organisms. They are alternatives to penicillin G for infections caused by *Actinomyces israelii*, and minocycline is active against *Nocardia asteroides.*

Many *Neisseria gonorrhoeae* (gram-negative cocci) are susceptible, but there has been an increasing emergence of tetracycline-resistant strains in the United States *(MMWR* 1985, 1986, 1987; Knapp et al, 1987; Schwarcz et al, 1990; Reichart et al, 1992). The Centers for Disease Control no longer recommends tetracyclines as sole therapy for gonococcal infections (*MMWR*, 1989; Moran and Zenilman, 1990; see also Uses). *N. meningitidis* are susceptible to the tetracyclines, particularly minocycline. However, tetracyclines are inadequate therapy for meningococcal infections because they are only bacteriostatic. Furthermore, the usefulness of minocycline in meningococcal prophylaxis is limited by an unacceptably high incidence of vestibular side effects. *Moraxella (Branhamella) catarrhalis* are susceptible to the tetracyclines, particularly doxycycline (Kallings, 1986; Nicotra et al, 1986).

Tetracyclines are active against and are among the preferred antibiotics in infections caused by a number of gram-negative bacilli, including *Brucella, Helicobacter pylori, Pseudomonas mallei, P. pseudomallei, Vibrio cholerae,* and *Calymmatobacterium granulomatis.* They also are active against *Francisella tularensis, Campylobacter jejuni, Haemophilus ducreyi* (a number of strains have become resistant), *Vibrio parahaemolyticus, V. vulnificus, Yersinia pestis, Y. enterocolitica, Pasteurella multocida, Spirillum minor, Streptobacillus moniliformis, Leptotrichia buccalis, Bordetella pertussis,* and *Eikenella corrodens.* Many strains of *Haemophilus influenzae* are susceptible. Doxycycline is active against *Legionella pneumophila,* although erythromycin (with or without rifampin [Rifadin, Rimactane]) is the drug of choice.

Tetracyclines are active against many strains of community-acquired *Escherichia coli* at concentrations achieved in the urine. Some strains of *Shigella* are susceptible. However, many strains of Enterobacteriaceae (eg, *E. coli, Klebsiella, Enterobacter, Proteus mirabilis,* indole-positive *Proteus, Serratia*) are resistant. *Pseudomonas aeruginosa* are almost uniformly resistant; many *Acinetobacter* strains also are resistant.

Among gram-negative anaerobic bacteria, *Fusobacterium* and a number of *Bacteroides* strains are susceptible. However, resistance to most tetracycline analogues is common among members of the *B. fragilis* group. Doxycycline is the most active analogue against the *B. fragilis* group, but other drugs (eg, clindamycin [Cleocin], metronidazole [Flagyl, Metryl]) generally are preferred for infections caused by these pathogens.

Tetracyclines are among the agents of choice in infections caused by *Mycoplasma pneumoniae* and *Ureaplasma urealyticum.* They are the drugs of choice for chlamydial (eg, *C. trachomatis, C. psittaci, C. pneumoniae*), and rickettsial (eg, *R. akari, R. rickettsii, R. prowazekii, R. mooseri, Coxiella burnetii, Ehrlichia chaffeensis*) infections. Among the spirochetes, tetracyclines are active against *Borrelia recurrentis, B. burgdorferi* (cause of Lyme disease), *Leptospira, Treponema pallidum,* and *T. pertenue.* The atypical mycobacteria, *M. fortuitum* and *M. marinum,* are susceptible to doxycycline and minocycline, respectively.

High concentrations of tetracyclines are active against the protozoans, *Entamoeba histolytica, Dientamoeba fragilis, Balantidium coli*, and certain strains of *Plasmodium falciparum.*

Resistance

Several species of bacteria have become increasingly resistant to the tetracyclines (see Siegel, 1978, part I; Pratt and Fekety, 1986; Williams, 1988). Many Enterobacteriaceae (eg, *Shigella, E. coli*) and most *P. aeruginosa* are resistant. Many strains of staphylococci, streptococci, pneumococci, and *Bacteroides* are no longer susceptible. Emergence of high-level tetracycline-resistant *N. gonorrhoeae* (TRNG) strains is common in some geographic areas. Bacterial resistance to clinically useful tetracyclines is primarily acquired, as resistant strains have emerged due to the selective pressure exerted on bacteria by widespread use of these antibiotics in humans and animals.

Resistance may occur through several mechanisms (Jacoby and Archer, 1991; Chopra et al, 1992). A primary mechanism of resistance is decreased accumulation of tetracyclines by the bacterial cell. This is due to alterations in bacterial cytoplasmic membrane-located proteins that result in an energy-dependent increased efflux of antibiotic from the bacterial cell. This type of resistance is common for the Enterobacteriaceae. Clinically, resistance to tetracyclines also may occur by ribosomal protection whereby tetracyclines can no longer bind effectively to the bacterial ribosome. Various gram-positive and gram-negative bacteria, including *Neisseria*, exhibit this form of resistance to tetracycline. Although there is laboratory evidence that some bacteria may be induced to synthesize enzymes that inactivate tetracyclines, the clinical significance is unknown. Resistance to one tetracycline usually implies resistance to all, but there are exceptions (eg, doxycycline's activity against *B. fragilis*).

The genes determining resistance to tetracyclines usually reside in plasmids and/or transposons. Thus, tetracycline resistance usually can be passed readily from one organism to another.

Uses

Tetracyclines are the preferred or alternative drugs for a number of infectious diseases as outlined below. However, they should not be administered to pregnant women or children less than 8 years (see Adverse Reactions and Precautions). Doxycycline or tetracycline generally is preferred, and these antibiotics are administered orally when possible.

Tetracyclines are drugs of choice in brucellosis (often combined with streptomycin or rifampin), cholera, *Vibrio vulnificus* infections, relapsing fever, melioidosis (combined with chloramphenicol and/or trimethoprim/sulfamethoxazole [Bactrim, Septra] in seriously ill patients; some physicians prefer trimethoprim/sulfamethoxazole with or without ceftazidime), glanders (combined with streptomycin), leptospirosis (some physicians prefer penicillin G), *Mycoplasma pneumoniae* infections (erythromycin is preferred by some physicians), and rickettsial infections (ie, Rocky Mountain spotted fever, typhus fever, Q fever, rickettsialpox). Some physicians prefer chloramphenicol for rickettsial infections. Tetracyclines also are preferred antibiotics for the treatment of ehrlichiosis, a tick-borne rickettsial infection caused by *Ehrlichia chaffeensis* (Eng et al, 1990; Schutz, 1992).

A 10- to 21-day course of oral doxycycline or tetracycline is preferred for adults (nonpregnant) and children older than 8 years with Stage I (early) Lyme disease (Steere et al, 1983; *Med Lett Drugs Ther,* 1989; Dattwyler et al, 1990). These agents, given for 30 days, also may be useful in patients with Stage II Lyme disease who have mild neurologic (eg, Bell's palsy alone) or cardiac (eg, minor conduction system involvement) disorders or in patients with Stage III Lyme disease who have arthritis (*Med Lett Drugs Ther,* 1989).

Tetracyclines are preferred drugs for chlamydial infections, including those caused by *Chlamydia trachomatis* (nongonococcal urethritis, mucopurulent cervicitis, proctitis, pelvic inflammatory disease, epididymo-orchitis, lymphogranuloma venereum, trachoma, inclusion conjunctivitis [should not be used in neonates]), *C. psittaci* (psittacosis, ornithosis), and *C. pneumoniae* strain TWAR (a cause of atypical pneumonia) (Grayston et al, 1986, 1989; Schachter, 1986). They are drugs of choice for various other venereal diseases, including granuloma inguinale and urethritis due to *Ureaplasma urealyticum* (some physicians prefer erythromycin). Although penicillin G is still the drug of choice for syphilis, tetracycline is an alternative. Tetracyclines may be effective against chancroid, but a number of strains of *H. ducreyi* are now resistant and other agents (eg, ceftriaxone [Rocephin], erythromycin) are preferred. Because of the increasing emergence of resistant *Neisseria gonorrhoeae* strains (see Antimicrobial Spectrum), tetracyclines are no longer recommended as sole therapy for gonorrhea. However, a seven-day course of doxycycline (or tetracycline) after single-dose antigonococcal therapy (eg, with ceftriaxone) is recommended for coverage of frequently coexisting *C. trachomatis* infection (*MMWR*, 1989). See index entry Sexually Transmitted Diseases for detailed discussions on the treatment of these diseases.

Other diseases for which tetracyclines provide effective therapy and may be suitable alternatives include actinomycosis, tularemia, anthrax, yaws, plague, *Pasteurella multocida* infections, gastroenteritis caused by *Yersinia enterocolitica* and *Campylobacter jejuni,* Vincent's angina, Whipple's disease, tetanus, rat bite fever, tropical sprue, small bowel overgrowth, sinusitis, and certain *Listeria monocytogenes* infections. Tetracyclines can be effective in the treatment of acute, uncomplicated lower urinary tract infections (cystitis), although other antimicrobial agents generally are used for these infections (see index entry Urinary Tract Infections, Treatment).

Atypical pneumonias caused by *Chlamydia, Coxiella, Francisella, Mycoplasma,* and *Legionella* have become difficult diagnostic and therapeutic problems. If *Legionella pneumophila* is the most likely causative organism, erythromycin is the drug of choice. However, for other cases of atypical pneumonia in which the diagnosis is uncertain, tetracyclines are active against most of the potential causative organisms.

Although the precise role of bacterial infection in the pathogenesis of acute exacerbations of chronic bronchitis has yet to be clarified, it has been customary to prescribe antibiotics. The tetracyclines are one class of antibiotics that have been used for this indication. For other alternatives, see index entry Bronchitis, Treatment.

The efficacy of oral tetracyclines in acne is well documented (Ad Hoc Committee on Use of Antibiotics in Dermatology, American Academy of Dermatology, 1975). Tetracyclines are the drugs of first choice when systemic therapy is required for chronic, severe, inflammatory lesions refractory to topical therapy alone. See index entry Acne Vulgaris for a more detailed discussion.

Tetracycline is considered the drug of choice for balantidiasis and is a preferred drug in dientamoebiasis (some physicians prefer iodoquinol). Tetracyclines (preferred alternative, combined use of a sulfonamide with pyrimethamine) are used in combination with quinine for malaria caused by chloroquine-resistant strains of *Plasmodium falciparum*; doxycycline is an alternative to mefloquine for prophylaxis of malaria in chloroquine-resistant areas. Tetracyclines occasionally are useful in acute intestinal amebiasis (*Entamoeba histolytica*). See index entry Antiprotozoal Agents for additional discussion.

The addition of "triple therapy" consisting of tetracycline (500 mg four times daily), metronidazole (250 mg three times daily), and bismuth subsalicylate [Pepto-Bismol] (five to eight tablets daily, each tablet containing 151 mg bismuth) to standard ranitidine [Zantac] (300 mg daily) therapy is regarded by some as the preferred treatment of peptic ulcer disease associated with *H. pylori* in patients with resistant ulcers, those with ulcer-associated complications, and those with symptoms severe enough to be candidates for surgery (Graham et al, 1992).

Doxycycline is the preferred tetracycline for certain infections. Despite some resistant isolates, doxycycline has good activity against pneumococci, *Haemophilus influenzae*, and *Moraxella (Branhamella) catarrhalis* and it has excellent penetration into respiratory secretions. Thus, some consider this agent to be the tetracycline of choice for acute exacerbations of chronic bronchitis (Cunha et al, 1982).

Organisms that cause acute pelvic inflammatory disease include *N. gonorrhoeae, C. trachomatis*, anaerobic bacteria (eg, *Bacteroides*, gram-positive cocci), facultative gram-negative bacilli (eg, *E. coli*), streptococci (eg, Group B), and mycoplasmas (eg, *Mycoplasma hominis*), and regimens, consisting of more than one antimicrobial agent, are employed to cover a broad range of pathogens. A tetracycline usually is included in these combination regimens, and doxycycline is the recommended analogue (*MMWR* 1989, 1991; see also index entry Pelvic Inflammatory Disease, Treatment). It is a preferred drug for *C. trachomatis* infections. Also, doxycycline has better activity against most anaerobes, including *B. fragilis*, than conventional tetracycline and certain pharmacokinetic advantages (see Pharmacokinetics). When intravenous administration is necessary, doxycycline is better tolerated than tetracycline.

Doxycycline is often the drug of choice for the empiric treatment of the acute urethral syndrome (symptoms characteristic of cystitis, but less than 100,000 organisms/ml of urine) because the most likely causative organisms (*E. coli, Staphylococcus saprophyticus*, and chlamydia) are usually susceptible (Stamm et al, 1981). Conventional tetracycline also should be effective for this indication.

Doxycycline has been shown to prevent travelers' diarrhea caused by enterotoxigenic *E. coli* (Sack et al, 1978, 1979). Prophylaxis generally is not recommended, however, because of the potential for adverse drug reactions (eg, photosensitivity), superinfections, and the emergence of resistant bacterial strains (National Institutes of Health Consensus Development Conference, 1985; see also index entry Diarrhea, Travelers'). Despite limited clinical experience, doxycycline has been suggested as an alternative to trimethoprim/sulfamethoxazole or ciprofloxacin in the treatment of more severe cases of travelers' diarrhea (National Institutes of Health Consensus Development Conference, 1985). However, in some geographic areas up to 60% of enterotoxigenic *E. coli* and *Shigella* strains are now resistant to doxycycline (Hyams et al, 1991).

Doxycycline (combined with amikacin) is a preferred regimen for *Mycobacterium fortuitum* infections.

In general, doxycycline offers a number of pharmacologic advantages over conventional tetracycline, including better gastrointestinal absorption resulting in the need for smaller doses, a longer half-life that permits longer intervals between doses, increased lipid solubility leading to higher tissue concentrations, and a mechanism of elimination that is independent of renal function and causes less diarrhea (see Pharmacokinetics). In the past, doxycycline was considerably more expensive than tetracycline, an important consideration in drug selection for those infections in which the two analogues are equally effective. However, the cost of therapy with some generic doxycycline preparations that are now available is similar to that of tetracycline, and many infectious disease experts prefer this long-acting analogue. Doxycycline is the only recommended tetracycline derivative for patients with impaired renal function.

Minocycline is more active than the other tetracyclines against *Nocardia asteroides* and is an alternative drug in nocardiosis. This antibiotic also is effective in *Mycobacterium marinum* infections. The good activity of minocycline against *Neisseria meningitidis* has led to its use in the prophylaxis of the meningococcal carrier state. However, the high incidence of vestibular toxicity has limited its usefulness in this and other infections (see Adverse Reactions and Precautions).

Adverse Reactions and Precautions

Gastrointestinal: The tetracyclines produce varying degrees of gastrointestinal irritation in some patients. These effects are more common after oral administration. Anorexia, pyrosis, nausea, vomiting, flatulence, and diarrhea are most common. They are usually dose related and occur in about 10% of patients receiving 2 g or more of tetracycline or its equivalent daily, and their incidence increases after prolonged administration. These reactions usually are not disabling but may become severe enough to require discontinuation or interruption of therapy. The presence of food may ameliorate the irritating effects of oral tetracyclines on the upper gastrointestinal tract. However, food decreases the absorption of some analogues (eg, tetracycline) more than others (eg, doxycycline) (see Pharmacokinetics).

When diarrhea is severe or persistent, it is important to determine whether it is due to nonspecific irritation or pseudomembranous colitis caused by overgrowth of *Clostridium difficile.* The latter condition can be life-threatening and is more likely to occur in elderly, debilitated patients. Management must be prompt and requires immediate cessation of tetracycline administration. Fluid and electrolyte replacement, other supportive therapy, and treatment with oral vancomycin [Vancocin] or metronidazole may be necessary. Poorly absorbed tetracyclines (eg, tetracycline hydrochloride) are more likely to cause diarrhea and alter the enteric flora than well absorbed analogues (eg, doxycycline).

Tetracyclines are very acidic in solution (doxycycline hyclate in water has a pH of 3.0). Esophageal ulceration with retrosternal pain that is intensified by swallowing has been reported after ingestion of tetracycline hydrochloride and doxycycline hyclate, usually when capsules (or tablets) were taken without water at bedtime. Individuals with esophageal obstruction or hiatal hernia are at increased risk. Having the patient remain upright for at least 90 seconds after taking any tetracycline (and especially doxycycline hyclate) and taking the medication with a full glass of water (240 ml) at least one hour before bedtime may minimize this problem.

Other undesirable gastrointestinal reactions include dryness of the mouth, stomatitis sometimes associated with vesiculopapular oral lesions, glossitis and black hairy tongue, pharyngitis, hoarseness, dysphagia, and proctitis. Inflammatory lesions caused by candidal overgrowth of the oral, vulvovaginal, and perianal regions are not uncommon complications of tetracycline therapy.

Acute pancreatitis has been observed rarely in patients without liver dysfunction who are receiving tetracycline therapy (Nicolau et al, 1991).

Renal: Tetracyclines can produce negative nitrogen balance and increase blood urea nitrogen (BUN) levels, presumably by inhibiting protein synthesis in host cells. This is generally of no clinical importance when usual doses are given to patients with normal renal function, but tetracyclines (except doxycycline) may exacerbate renal dysfunction (eg, increase azotemia, hyperphosphatemia, acidosis) in patients with impaired renal function.

Tetracyclines other than doxycycline should not be used in patients with renal dysfunction. Unlike the other analogues, doxycycline is excreted by the gastrointestinal tract under these circumstances; its half-life remains unchanged and it does not accumulate in the serum of patients with renal insufficiency (see also Pharmacokinetics).

Demeclocycline causes nephrogenic diabetes insipidus characterized by polyuria, polydipsia, and weakness in some patients. The syndrome is reversible upon discontinuation of the antibiotic. This effect has been utilized therapeutically to reverse the chronic syndrome of inappropriate secretion of antidiuretic hormone (SIADH) (Forrest et al, 1978).

Epianhydrotetracycline, a degradation product in outdated tetracycline preparations containing citric acid, has produced a Fanconi-like syndrome. Albuminuria, glycosuria, aminoaciduria, hypophosphatemia, hypokalemia, and renal tubular acidosis are manifestations of this condition. Such formulations are no longer available, and it is unlikely that this complication will recur. The use of outdated tetracyclines also has been associated with a systemic lupus erythematosus-like syndrome. As with any drug, outdated preparations should not be used.

Hepatic: The tetracyclines may cause liver damage that is sometimes associated with pancreatitis, particularly when large doses (2 g or more of tetracycline daily) are administered intravenously. The damage is detectable by liver function studies. Diffuse, fine, vacuolar, fatty metamorphosis of the liver has been demonstrated histologically (Timbrell, 1983). Patients with pre-existing hepatic or renal insufficiency, those suffering from malnutrition, or individuals receiving other hepatotoxic drugs are at increased risk. Hepatotoxicity is a particular hazard to pregnant or postpartum women with pyelonephritis or other renal dysfunction. A number of deaths have been reported, most of them occurring when doses of tetracycline greater than 1 g daily were given intravenously. Therefore, tetracyclines should not be administered to pregnant women unless there are no therapeutic alternatives.

Bones and Teeth: Tetracyclines are deposited in developing bones and teeth where they can chelate with calcium to form a tetracycline-calcium orthophosphate complex. Bone growth is depressed temporarily in the fetus and in young children. The danger is greatest from midpregnancy to 3 years of age, but it may continue to age 7 and possibly longer. The incidence is influenced more by the total quantity of tetracycline ingested by mother or child than by the duration of treatment.

Tetracyclines can interfere with the development of deciduous teeth when administered antepartum or in children up to 4 to 6 months and of permanent teeth when administered to children between age 4 to 6 months and 6 years or older. Permanent discoloration of teeth ranging from gray-brown to yellow can result, and enamel hypoplasia has been reported. The degree of discoloration correlates with the total quantity of antibiotic administered and increases with repeated courses.

Because of these adverse effects, tetracyclines should not be used during the last half of pregnancy or in children under 8 years (see statement of Committee on Drugs, American Academy of Pediatrics, 1975) unless there are compelling reasons to do so. Some infectious disease experts consider it reasonable to administer a single course of tetracycline to a young child with a known serious infection (eg, Rocky Mountain spotted fever) when alternative therapy (eg, chloramphenicol) is potentially more toxic. Doxycycline and oxytetracycline may produce less tooth discoloration than other analogues.

Nervous System: Vestibular toxicity is unique to minocycline. This very lipid-soluble tetracycline analogue appears to concentrate in lipid-laden cells of the vestibular apparatus to produce vertigo. Symptoms of lightheadedness, loss of balance, dizziness, nausea, and tinnitus usually begin two to three days after therapy is initiated and occur in a high percentage of patients (eg, up to 70% receiving the drug for meningococcal prophylaxis). This adverse effect is more common in women than in men. Although vestibular toxicity is reversible after discontinuation of the drug, it has limited the use of minocycline. Patients receiving this analogue should be advised of this adverse effect and cautioned about driving a motor vehicle or operating machinery if they experience central nervous system side effects.

The tetracyclines can cause a rare condition known as pseudotumor cerebri. Tense bulging of the fontanelles caused by increased intracranial pressure occurs in infants, and meningeal irritation with papilledema is observed in adults. Except for the elevated pressure, the spinal fluid is normal and the diagnosis, chiefly one of exclusion, may require careful neurologic appraisal. When the antibiotic is discontinued, spinal fluid pressure returns to normal over a period of days or weeks.

Photosensitivity: Reactions on exposure to the sun or other sources of ultraviolet light have been observed. These occur most frequently and are most severe with demeclocycline, but other analogues, most notably doxycycline, also can cause photosensitivity reactions (*Med Lett Drugs Ther,* 1986). Usual manifestations are exaggerated sunburn and marked erythema on exposed areas of the body; rarely, bullae develop. Paresthesias, primarily tingling of the hands, feet, and nose, may be early indicators of abnormal sunburn reactions. Photosensitivity is reversible over a period of days or weeks. A few cases of papular eruption have been reported, and onycholysis occurs in about 25% of those affected. In most cases, photosensitivity reactions to tetracyclines are phototoxic rather than photoallergic in nature and appear to result from accumulation of the drugs in the skin (Epstein and Wintroub, 1985). Patients likely to be exposed to direct sunlight or ultraviolet light should be advised that an exaggerated sunburn reaction can occur with tetracyclines. Treatment should be discontinued at the first evidence of skin erythema.

Hypersensitivity: Hypersensitivity reactions most often involve the skin (eg, morbilliform rashes), although they are generally rare. Urticaria, angioedema, exfoliative dermatitis, idiopathic nonthrombocytopenic purpura, and exacerbations of systemic lupus erythematosus have been reported. Anaphylaxis has been reported rarely. Patients who are allergic to any of the tetracyclines should not receive these drugs.

Hematologic: Tetracyclines have been shown to depress plasma prothrombin activity. Patients receiving anticoagulant therapy may require a reduction in the dosage of anticoagulant.

Hemolytic anemia, thrombocytopenia, thrombocytopenic purpura, neutropenia, and eosinophilia have occurred rarely with tetracyclines.

Miscellaneous: Tetracyclines can cause thrombophlebitis after intravenous administration. This is more likely to occur with short-acting analogues (tetracycline, oxytetracycline) than long-acting derivatives (doxycycline, minocycline). Intramuscular injection of tetracycline or oxytetracycline is extremely painful, and this route of administration is not recommended.

Tetracyclines may result in overgrowth of nonsusceptible organisms, including fungi. Vaginitis due to overgrowth of *Candida* is one of the more common side effects of tetracycline therapy in women.

When given for prolonged periods, tetracyclines have been reported to produce brown-black discoloration of the thyroid gland. However, no abnormalities in thyroid function are known to occur.

Pigmentation of the skin, nails, and mucous membranes has been reported, most frequently after use of minocycline. This analogue also has been associated with tooth discoloration in young adults treated for acne (Poliak et al, 1985).

The Jarisch-Herxheimer reaction has occurred occasionally when tetracyclines were used to treat brucellosis or spirochetal infections.

Tetracyclines are classified in FDA Pregnancy Category D (see above).

Drug Interactions

Divalent or trivalent cations (eg, Ca++, Mg++, Fe++, Zn++, Al+++) can chelate tetracyclines. Thus, tetracyclines should not be administered with milk or milk products (doxycycline and minocycline are minimally affected), antacids, vitamin and mineral preparations, or cathartics containing divalent or trivalent cations because insoluble complexes form, resulting in decreased and erratic absorption of the antibiotic (see also Pharmacokinetics).

Tetracyclines are primarily bacteriostatic and may interfere with the bactericidal action of penicillins. When such combinations are considered necessary, it is recommended that adequate amounts of each drug be administered and, if possible, the penicillin should be given a few hours or longer before the tetracycline.

Concomitant administration of tetracyclines and methoxyflurane [Penthrane] has caused serious renal toxicity and deaths have been reported. These drugs should not be used together.

The half-life of doxycycline may be decreased by concurrent administration of carbamazepine [Tegretol], phenytoin [Dilantin], or barbiturates, which increase the hepatic metabolism of this antibiotic. Chronic ethanol ingestion also may reduce the doxycycline half-life by this mechanism.

The bismuth subsalicylate contained in a 60-ml dose of Pepto-Bismol significantly decreased the bioavailability of oral doxycycline 200 mg (Ericsson et al, 1982). Thus, the two agents should not be taken together to prevent travelers' diarrhea. This drug interaction also occurs with other tetracycline analogues (see Hansten and Horn, 1992 A).

Tetracyclines can increase plasma prothrombin time and, despite minimal clinical evidence, could potentiate the effects of coumarin-type anticoagulants. Patients should be monitored for an enhanced anticoagulant effect when these drugs are used concurrently.

It has been reported that concurrent administration of tetracyclines and diuretics can increase blood urea nitrogen (BUN) concentrations. However, no special precautions appear to be necessary; one or both drugs should be discontinued if uremia occurs (see Tatro, 1992).

Sodium bicarbonate has been reported to decrease serum concentrations of the tetracyclines. The mechanism is not established, and no special precautions appear to be necessary (see Hansten and Horn, 1992 A).

Approximately 10% of patients convert substantial amounts of digoxin to inactive metabolites in the gastrointestinal tract. Certain antimicrobial agents, including tetracycline, have been shown to alter gut microbial flora and prevent this inactivation of digoxin from occurring. Thus, marked increases in serum digoxin levels result in these individuals. The effects of this interaction can persist for several months (Lindenbaum et al, 1981). Careful clinical monitoring of patients is recommended (Doherty, 1981).

Isolated cases of breakthrough bleeding and pregnancy have been reported in women receiving oral contraceptives and antibiotics, including tetracyclines. The addition of other forms of contraception appears warranted when a course of tetracycline therapy is initiated in a woman receiving oral contraceptives (see Back et al, 1981; Hansten and Horn, 1985; see also index entry Contraceptives, Oral).

Oxytetracycline has been reported to enhance the hypoglycemic effects of insulin or tolbutamide in a few patients, and antidiabetic drug dosage requirements may be reduced (Hansten and Horn, 1992 B).

Single case reports suggest that tetracycline may elevate lithium or theophylline plasma concentrations. The mechanism(s) is not established. Patients receiving either of these drugs concomitantly with tetracycline should be observed for lithium or theophylline toxicity (Hansten and Horn, 1992 C).

Pharmacokinetics

Some pharmacokinetic properties of the tetracyclines are compared in the Table.

Routes of Administration: Tetracyclines usually are given orally, the preferred route of administration. Doxycycline hyclate and minocycline hydrochloride also can be administered intravenously. This route is employed initially in those with severe infections or malabsorption syndromes and in critically ill or comatose patients. Rapid intravenous injection (less than five minutes) should be avoided. These long-acting analogues (doxycycline, minocycline) are less irritating to the vein than tetracycline, and they are less likely to cause thrombophlebitis. The parenteral formulation of tetracycline is no longer marketed.

Intramuscular injection of oxytetracycline also can be employed but is extremely painful, even when the preparation contains a local anesthetic and is injected into a large muscle mass. Furthermore, the serum concentrations attained tend to be low, even with maximum doses. Thus, intramuscular administration is not recommended.

Absorption: The short-acting (tetracycline and oxytetracycline) and intermediate-acting (demeclocycline) tetracyclines are adequately but incompletely absorbed from the gastrointestinal tract; absorption is decreased in the presence of food. The long-acting analogues, doxycycline and minocycline, are more completely absorbed, and absorption appears to be affected only slightly by the presence of food.

Tetracyclines form insoluble complexes in the gut with calcium, magnesium, zinc, iron, aluminum, and other bivalent and trivalent cations. Therefore, the presence of milk and milk products, vitamin and mineral preparations, or cathartics and antacids containing metal salts may result in decreased and erratic absorption. An exception is that milk and milk products appear to minimally affect the absorption of doxycycline and minocycline. Achlorhydria does not appear to interfere with the gastrointestinal absorption of the tetracyclines (see Cunha et al, 1982).

Peak serum concentrations generally are attained one to three hours after oral administration and correlate with the degree of absorption of the various analogues. A 500-mg dose of tetracycline hydrochloride results in a peak serum concentration of 4 mcg/ml, highest of the short- (or intermediate-) acting analogues. Doxycycline and minocycline, given in single 200-mg doses, achieve serum concentrations of approximately 2.5 mcg/ml.

Intravenous injection of the usual 200-mg loading dose of doxycycline or minocycline produces serum concentrations of approximately 4 mcg/ml after 30 minutes. Once tissue distribution of the long-acting analogues occurs, levels are similar to the concentrations achieved orally.

Distribution: The tetracyclines are bound to plasma proteins to varying degrees. Although values reported in the literature are quite variable, the intermediate- and long-acting analogues usually exhibit greater plasma protein binding.

The apparent volume of distribution for most tetracyclines is greater than that of extracellular body water, which indicates sequestration in tissues, most likely the liver. Minocycline and doxycycline have the smallest volumes of distribution.

As a group, tetracyclines penetrate variably into many different body fluids and tissues including bile, liver, lung, kidney, prostate, urine, cerebrospinal fluid, brain, sputum, and bone. The highest concentrations are found in bile and are 5 to 20 times those in the serum. Concentrations of conventional tetracycline in the cerebrospinal fluid are approximately 10% to 20% of those in the serum. Tetracyclines have an affinity for rapidly growing or metabolizing tissue and tend to localize in the liver and new bone and teeth, particularly before birth and during the first three years of life. The tetracyclines cross the placenta and appear in the milk of lactating women.

The tetracyclines differ markedly in their lipid solubility, which correlates directly with tissue penetration. Since doxycycline and minocycline are considerably more lipid soluble than the shorter acting tetracyclines, they penetrate into tissues and secretions more efficiently. For example, doxycycline has excellent penetration into endometrial, myometrial, prostatic, and renal tissues. This may explain, in part, its efficacy in the treatment of pelvic inflammatory disease and chronic pyelonephritis. Similarly, therapeutic concentrations of minocycline are achieved in saliva and tears to eradicate the meningococcal carrier state. Unfortunately, the high lipid solubility of minocycline also appears to result in its concentration in the lipid-laden cells of the vestibular apparatus leading to the vestibular toxicity that is unique to this analogue.

Elimination: The tetracyclines usually are classified on the basis of their duration of action (see the Table). Although these drugs undergo enterohepatic circulation and are, in part, recoverable in the feces, their half-lives are determined primarily by the rates of renal excretion. Tetracycline and oxytetracycline are eliminated rapidly by glomerular filtration as unchanged drugs and thus have the shortest half-lives. Demeclocycline is intermediate. The half-lives of these three drugs are prolonged significantly in patients with renal insufficiency.

Minocycline has a low renal clearance, and less than 10% of a dose is recovered unchanged in urine. The drug undergoes enterohepatic circulation and may be metabolized to a considerable extent. Its high lipid solubility causes it to be retained in fatty tissues. Data are conflicting as to whether the half-life of this drug is prolonged in patients with renal insufficiency.

The elimination of doxycycline, the longest acting tetracycline, differs from the other analogues and is independent of both renal and hepatic function. This drug is excreted in the feces, largely as an inactive chelated product. Thus, the dose does not require modification in patients with renal or hepatic insufficiency. Furthermore, the inactive product has relatively

PHARMACOKINETIC VALUES FOR THE TETRACYCLINES[1]

Antibiotic	Oral Dose Absorbed (%)	Half-life (hours)	Renal Clearance[2] (ml/min/1.73m²)	Urinary Recovery (%)	Apparent Volume of Distribution[2] (liters)	Protein Binding[3] (%)
SHORT-ACTING						
Oxytetracycline	58	9	99	70	128	35
Tetracycline	77	8	74	60	108	65
INTERMEDIATE-ACTING						
Demeclocycline	66	12	35	39	121	91
LONG-ACTING						
Doxycycline	93	18	20	42	50	93
Minocycline	95	16	9	6	60	76

[1]*Adapted from Standiford HC: Tetracyclines and chloramphenicol, in Mandell GL, et al (eds)*: Principles and Practice of Infectious Diseases, *ed 3. New York, Churchill Livingston, 1990, 287.*
[2]*Following single-dose intravenous administration.*
[3]*Ultrafiltration technique.*

less impact on the intestinal microflora resulting in a lower incidence of irritative diarrhea and candidial overgrowth.

Doxycycline offers a number of pharmacologic advantages over conventional tetracycline, including better gastrointestinal absorption resulting in the need for smaller doses, a longer half-life that permits longer intervals between doses, increased lipid solubility leading to higher tissue levels, and a mechanism of elimination that is independent of renal function and causes less diarrhea.

Drug Evaluations

SHORT-ACTING TETRACYCLINES

TETRACYCLINE

[Sumycin]

TETRACYCLINE HYDROCHLORIDE

[Achromycin V, Panmycin, Robitet, Sumycin]

Tetracycline has been the most widely used drug in its class, in part, because it is inexpensive. With the availability of comparably priced generic doxycycline products, many infectious disease experts prefer this latter agent (see the Introduction).

See the Introduction for a complete discussion of the actions, antimicrobial spectrum, uses, pharmacokinetics, adverse reactions and precautions, and drug interactions of tetracycline.

DOSAGE AND PREPARATIONS. Tetracyclines should not be used in pregnant or nursing women or children under 8 years unless there are compelling reasons to do so. This agent should not be given to patients with impaired renal function. ***Oral:*** Therapy should be continued for at least 24 to 48 hours after signs and symptoms have subsided. Tetracycline should be given one hour before or two hours after meals (see Pharmacokinetics). It should be administered with a full glass of water (240 ml) to minimize esophageal irritation. *Adults,* 250 to 500 mg every six hours; the larger dose should be reserved for severe infections. *Children over 8 years*, 25 to 50 mg/kg daily in four divided doses.

For the treatment of brucellosis, 500 mg four times daily for three weeks with streptomycin, intramuscularly, 1 g twice daily the first week and once daily the second week. Alternatively, tetracycline 500 mg four times daily plus rifampin, orally, 600 mg daily for six weeks.

For treatment of sexually transmitted diseases, including chlamydial infections and syphilis, see index entry Sexually Transmitted Diseases.

For treatment of acne, see index entry Acne Vulgaris.

TETRACYCLINE:
(Strengths expressed in terms of the hydrochloride salt.)
Generic. Suspension 125 mg/5 ml.
Sumycin (Apothecon). Syrup (buffered with potassium metaphosphate) 125 mg/5 ml.

TETRACYCLINE HYDROCHLORIDE:
Generic. Capsules 100, 250, and 500 mg.
Achromycin V (Lederle), ***Robitet*** (Robins). Capsules 250 and 500 mg.
Panmycin (Upjohn). Capsules 250 mg (contains tartrazine).
Sumycin (Apothecon). Capsules, tablets 250 and 500 mg.

OXYTETRACYCLINE

[Terramycin IM]

OXYTETRACYCLINE HYDROCHLORIDE

[Terramycin]

The actions, antimicrobial spectrum, indications, pharmacokinetics, adverse reactions and precautions, and interactions of oxytetracycline are similar to those of tetracycline (see the Introduction).

DOSAGE AND PREPARATIONS. Tetracyclines should not be used in pregnant or nursing women or children under 8 years unless there are compelling reasons to do so. Oxytetracycline should not be given to patients with impaired renal function.
Oral: Therapy should be continued for at least 24 to 48 hours after signs and symptoms have subsided. Oxytetracycline should be given one hour before or two hours after meals (see Pharmacokinetics). It should be administered with a full glass of water (240 ml) to minimize esophageal irritation. *Adults,* 1 to 2 g daily in four equally divided doses, depending on the severity of the infection. *Children over 8 years*, 25 to 50 mg/kg daily in four equally divided doses.

OXYTETRACYCLINE HYDROCHLORIDE:

Generic. Capsules 250 mg.

Terramycin (Pfizer). Capsules equivalent to 250 mg of base.

Intramuscular: This route is not recommended because injection can be extremely painful and, at usual dosages, serum concentrations are lower than after oral administration. Thus, no dosage recommendations are given.

OXYTETRACYCLINE:

Terramycin IM (Roerig). Solution 50 mg/ml with 2% lidocaine in 2 and 10 ml containers and 125 mg/ml with 2% lidocaine in 2 ml containers.

INTERMEDIATE-ACTING TETRACYCLINE

DEMECLOCYCLINE HYDROCHLORIDE
[Declomycin]

The actions, antimicrobial spectrum, indications, and adverse effects of demeclocycline are comparable to those of tetracycline, but its half-life (12 hours) is somewhat longer (see the Introduction). Therefore, longer intervals between doses may be employed. The cost of demeclocycline is considerably greater than that of tetracycline, however.

Demeclocycline is the tetracycline most frequently associated with photosensitivity reactions at therapeutic dosage levels. Also, this analogue has been implicated in a few cases of nephrogenic diabetes insipidus, all of which were reversible within four weeks after medication was discontinued. This side effect has been utilized therapeutically to reverse the chronic syndrome of inappropriate secretion of antidiuretic hormone (SIADH).

DOSAGE AND PREPARATIONS. Tetracyclines should not be used in pregnant or nursing women or children under 8 years unless there are compelling reasons to do so. Demeclocycline should not be given to patients with impaired renal function.
Oral: Therapy should be continued for at least 24 to 48 hours after signs and symptoms have subsided. Demeclocycline should be given one hour before or two hours after meals (see Pharmacokinetics). It should be administered with a full glass of water (240 ml) to minimize esophageal irritation. *Adults,* 600 mg daily in two or four divided doses; *children over 8 years*, 6 to 12 mg/kg daily, depending on the severity of the infection, in two or four divided doses.

Declomycin (Lederle). Capsules 150 mg; tablets 150 and 300 mg.

LONG-ACTING TETRACYCLINES

DOXYCYCLINE CALCIUM
[Vibramycin]

DOXYCYCLINE HYCLATE
[Doryx, Doxy-Caps, Doxychel, Doxy-Tabs, Vibramycin, Vibra-Tabs]

DOXYCYCLINE MONOHYDRATE
[Monodox, Vibramycin]

Doxycycline, a synthetic analogue of oxytetracycline, provides certain pharmacokinetic advantages over tetracycline and is more active against some organisms. Thus, it is the analogue of choice for certain indications (eg, pelvic inflammatory disease) and in patients with impaired renal function (see the Introduction). For those indications in which any member of this class of antibiotics would be equally effective, tetracycline usually was preferred because of its lower cost. However, the cost of therapy with some generic doxycycline preparations that are now available is similar to that of tetracycline, and many infectious disease experts prefer this long-acting analogue.

See the Introduction for a complete discussion of the actions, antimicrobial spectrum, uses, pharmacokinetics, adverse reactions and precautions, and drug interactions of doxycycline.

DOSAGE AND PREPARATIONS. Tetracyclines should not be used in pregnant or nursing women or children under 8 years unless there are compelling reasons to do so.
Oral: Therapy should be continued for at least 24 to 48 hours after signs and symptoms have subsided. If gastric irritation occurs, doxycycline can be administered with food, including milk. The absorption of this agent is not markedly affected by the presence of food or milk. It should be administered with a full glass of water (240 ml) to minimize esophageal irritation. The manufacturer recommends that doxycycline not be given just prior to bedtime; an upright position should be maintained after administration.

Adults and children over 8 years weighing 45 kg or more, 200 mg on the first day of treatment divided into two doses at 12-hour intervals, followed by 100 mg daily as a single dose or in two doses every 12 hours or, for more severe infections, 100 mg every 12 hours. *Children over 8 years weighing less than 45 kg,* 4.4 mg/kg on the first day of treatment divided into two doses at 12-hour intervals, followed by 2.2 mg/kg daily as a single dose or in two doses every 12 hours; for more severe infections, 2.2 mg/kg is given every 12 hours. In *patients with renal impairment*, doxycycline in recommended doses does not accumulate excessively.

For the treatment of sexually transmitted diseases, including pelvic inflammatory disease (PID), chlamydial infections, and syphilis, see index entry Sexually Transmitted Diseases.

For the prophylaxis of travelers' diarrhea, 200 mg on the day of travel, followed by 100 mg once daily, continuing until two days after return home (Sack et al, 1978, 1979; Satterwhite and DuPont, 1983); prophylaxis generally is not recommended, however (see Uses). For the treatment of travelers' diarrhea, 100 mg every 12 hours for three to five days (National Institutes of Health Consensus Development Conference, 1985).

For the treatment of brucellosis, doxycycline 100 mg twice daily plus rifampin, orally, 600 to 900 mg daily for six weeks (Mikolich and Boyce, 1990; Ariza et al, 1992).

DOXYCYCLINE CALCIUM:

Vibramycin (Pfizer). Syrup equivalent to 50 mg of base/5 ml.

DOXYCYCLINE HYCLATE:

Generic. Capsules 50 and 100 mg; tablets 100 mg.

Doryx (Parke-Davis). Capsules (coated pellets) equivalent to 100 mg of base.

Doxychel (Rachelle). Capsules and tablets equivalent to 50 and 100 mg of base.

Doxy-Caps (Barr), ***Vibramycin*** (Pfizer). Capsules equivalent to 50 and 100 mg of base.

Doxy-Tabs (Barr), ***Vibra-Tabs*** (Pfizer). Tablets equivalent to 100 mg of base.

DOXYCYCLINE MONOHYDRATE:

Monodox (Oclassen). Capsules equivalent to 50 and 100 mg of base.

Vibramycin (Pfizer). Powder for oral suspension equivalent to 25 mg of base/5 ml after reconstitution.

Intravenous: Intravenous therapy is indicated only when oral therapy is inadequate or not tolerated. Oral therapy should be substituted as soon as possible. The duration of intravenous infusion may vary with the dose (100 to 200 mg/day), but is usually one to four hours. A recommended minimum infusion time for 100 mg of a 0.5 mg/ml solution is one hour. The therapeutic antibacterial serum activity usually persists for 24 hours following use of the recommended dosage. See the manufacturer's literature for instructions on the preparation of solution for intravenous administration.

Adults and children over 8 years weighing 45 kg or more, 200 mg on the first day of treatment given in one or two infusions, followed by 100 to 200 mg daily (depending on the severity of infection) in one or two infusions. *Children over 8 years weighing less than 45 kg*, 4.4 mg/kg on the first day of treatment given in one or two infusions, followed by 2.2 mg/kg to 4.4 mg/kg daily (depending on the severity of infection) in one or two infusions. In *patients with renal impairment*, doxycycline in recommended doses does not accumulate excessively.

For the treatment of pelvic inflammatory disease (PID), see index entry Sexually Transmitted Diseases.

DOXYCYCLINE HYCLATE:

Generic. Powder (sterile) 100 and 200 mg.

Doxy (Lyphomed), ***Doxychel*** (Rachelle). Powder (sterile) equivalent to 100 or 200 mg of base.

Vibramycin IV (Roerig). Powder (sterile) equivalent to 100 or 200 mg of base with ascorbic acid 480 or 960 mg, respectively.

MINOCYCLINE HYDROCHLORIDE

[Minocin]

The clinical use of minocycline is limited by the vestibular toxicity that is unique to this tetracycline analogue. Also, it is considerably more expensive than tetracycline. See the Introduction for a complete discussion of the actions, antimicrobial spectrum, uses, pharmacokinetics, adverse reactions and precautions, and drug interactions of minocycline.

DOSAGE AND PREPARATIONS. Tetracyclines should not be used in pregnant or nursing women or children under 8 years unless there are compelling reasons to do so. Minocycline should not be used in patients with impaired renal function.

Oral: Therapy should be continued for at least 24 to 48 hours after signs and symptoms have subsided. If gastric irritation occurs, minocycline can be administered with food, including milk. The absorption of this agent is not markedly affected by the presence of food or milk. It should be administered with a full glass of water (240 ml) to minimize esophageal irritation. *Adults*, 200 mg initially, followed by 100 mg every 12 hours (alternatively, 50 mg every six hours). *Children over 8 years*, 4 mg/kg initially, followed by 2 mg/kg every 12 hours.

For prophylaxis of meningococcal infections, *adults*, 100 mg every 12 hours for five days. However, this regimen is associated with a high incidence of vestibular toxicity (see index entry, Meningococcal Infection, Chemoprophylaxis).

For *Mycobacterium marinum* infections, optimal dosage has not been established; 100 mg twice daily for six to eight weeks has been effective in a limited number of patients.

MINOCYCLINE HYDROCHLORIDE:

Generic. Capsules and tablets equivalent to 50 and 100 mg of base.

Minocin (Lederle). Capsules (pellet-filled) equivalent to 50 and 100 mg of base; oral suspension equivalent to 50 mg of base/5 ml (alcohol 5%).

Intravenous: Intravenous therapy is indicated only when oral therapy is inadequate or not tolerated. Oral therapy should be substituted as soon as possible. The drug should be diluted before administration (see the manufacturer's literature). *Adults,* 200 mg initially, followed by 100 mg every 12 hours (maximum, 400 mg daily). *Children over 8 years*, 4 mg/kg initially, followed by 2 mg/kg every 12 hours.

MINOCYCLINE HYDROCHLORIDE:

Minocin IV (Lederle). Powder (sterile) 100 mg.

MIXTURE

UROBIOTIC

This product contains a tetracycline, a sulfonamide, and a urinary analgesic and is promoted for the treatment of urinary tract infections, although tetracyclines are not primary drugs for this indication. Since there is no recognized advantage for the fixed-ratio combination (eg, no synergism has been demonstrated between tetracyclines and sulfonamides), the use of either agent alone is preferred.

Because proof of efficacy is lacking, no dosage recommendation is made.

Urobiotic-250 (Roerig). Each capsule contains oxytetracycline hydrochloride equivalent to oxytetracycline 250 mg, sulfamethizole 250 mg, and phenazopyridine hydrochloride 50 mg.

CHLORAMPHENICOL

CHLORAMPHENICOL
[Chloromycetin]

CHLORAMPHENICOL PALMITATE
[Chloromycetin Palmitate]

CHLORAMPHENICOL SODIUM SUCCINATE
[Chloromycetin Sodium Succinate]

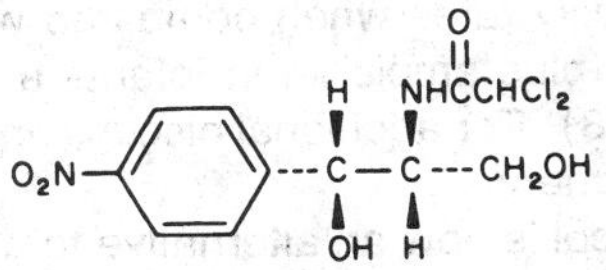

O
‖
H NHCCHCl$_2$
O_2N–⟨benzene ring⟩---C—C---CH_2OH
OH H

Chloramphenicol is a broad spectrum antibiotic that was originally derived from *Streptomyces venezuelae* but is now prepared synthetically. The potential of this drug to cause fatal aplastic anemia has limited its usefulness to the treatment of serious infections in which the anatomic location of the infection, the susceptibility of the causative organism, or individual patient characteristics limits or prevents the use of less toxic agents (see Uses).

MECHANISM OF ACTION. Chloramphenicol acts by inhibiting bacterial protein synthesis. This antibiotic reversibly binds to the 50S subunit of the bacterial 70S ribosome and prevents the attachment of the amino acid-containing end of the aminoacyl-tRNA to the acceptor site on the ribosome. Thus, the amino acid substrate cannot interact with the enzyme, peptidyl transferase, and peptide bond formation does not occur (see Pratt and Fekety, 1986). Chloramphenicol usually is bacteriostatic but can be bactericidal against common meningeal pathogens (*Hemophilus influenzae, Neisseria meningitidis, Streptococcus pneumoniae*) at therapeutic concentrations (Rahal and Simberkoff, 1979).

Mammalian mitochondria contain 70S ribosomes with physical and chemical characteristics similar to those found in bacterial cells. Many of the adverse effects of chloramphenicol, including dose-dependent bone marrow depression and the gray syndrome, appear to result from inhibition of protein synthesis in host mitochondria (see also Adverse Reactions and Precautions).

ANTIMICROBIAL SPECTRUM. Chloramphenicol is active in vitro against a great variety of bacteria, including gram-positive, gram-negative, aerobic, and anaerobic organisms. In addition, this antibiotic is effective against rickettsiae, chlamydiae, spirochetes, and mycoplasmas (Standiford, 1990).

Among gram-positive cocci, *Streptococcus pneumoniae, S. pyogenes, S. agalactiae*, and viridans streptococci are usually susceptible. Enterococci (eg, *E. faecalis*) are variably susceptible. Many strains of *Staphylococcus aureus* are susceptible, but this varies with local utilization patterns. Methicillin-resistant *S. aureus* usually are resistant. *Peptococcus* and *Peptostreptococcus*, anaerobic gram-positive cocci, are susceptible.

Susceptible gram-positive bacilli include *Bacillus* species, *Listeria monocytogenes, Corynebacterium diphtheriae*, clostridia (including *C. perfringens*), and *Eubacterium*.

Most strains of *Neisseria meningitidis* and *N. gonorrhoeae*, gram-negative cocci, are susceptible. *Veillonella* species, obligate anaerobes, also are susceptible.

Among gram-negative bacilli, *H. influenzae* are usually susceptible. Chloramphenicol also is active against *Brucella* species, *Bordetella pertussis, Pasteurella multocida, Pseudomonas pseudomallei, P. mallei, P. cepacia, Yersinia pestis, Vibrio cholerae, Francisella tularensis, Campylobacter jejuni*, and anaerobic gram-negative rods, including virtually all strains of the *Bacteroides fragilis* group, other *Bacteroides* species, and *Fusobacterium*. Response of the Enterobacteriaceae is variable; many organisms that were originally susceptible are now resistant. Salmonellae, including *S. typhi*, are generally susceptible in the United States, although imported strains (eg, from India, Southeast Asia, the Middle East) may be highly resistant. Although an epidemic of typhoid fever caused by chloramphenicol-resistant *S. typhi* occurred in Mexico in the early 1970s, most strains from that country are now susceptible (see Bartlett, 1988). Chloramphenicol is active against most strains of *Shigella, Escherichia coli, Klebsiella pneumoniae*, and *Proteus mirabilis*. However, most strains of *Serratia, Enterobacter, Providencia*, and *Proteus rettgeri* are resistant. *Pseudomonas aeruginosa* are resistant.

Rickettsiae (*R. akari, R. rickettsii, R. prowazekii, R. mooseri, Coxiella burnetii*), chlamydiae (*C. trachomatis, C. psittaci*), mycoplasmas, and treponemes are usually susceptible. Fungi, yeasts, viruses, and protozoa are resistant to chloramphenicol.

RESISTANCE. Chloramphenicol resistance among most gram-negative bacilli is due to drug inactivation by an acetyltransferase that is R-factor mediated. Resistance in gram-positive bacteria appears to develop by a similar mechanism, but is less well understood. *P. aeruginosa* and some strains of *Proteus* and *Klebsiella* become resistant through a nonenzymatic mechanism involving an inducible change in permeability that blocks the entry of chloramphenicol into the bacterial cell.

USES. Chloramphenicol has a relatively low therapeutic:toxic ratio. Also, this antibiotic rarely has caused fatal aplastic anemia (see Adverse Reactions and Precautions). It should not be used to treat trivial infections, for indications for which there are equally effective and less toxic alternatives, or as a prophylactic agent. However, chloramphenicol has unusual properties of lipid solubility with good penetration into cerebrospinal fluid and brain tissue (see Pharmacokinetics), and it is active against a number of important microbial pathogens, including some for which alternative drug therapies are limited (see Antimicrobial Spectrum). Thus, chloramphenicol is recommended for well-defined indications in seriously ill patients, as outlined below, when the location of the infection, the susceptibility of the causative organism, or individual patient characteristics limits or prevents the use of less toxic agents.

Chloramphenicol traditionally has been regarded as the preferred drug for the treatment of acute typhoid fever. Resistant strains of *S. typhi* have not become a serious problem in the United States, although they have appeared in other areas of the world (eg, Mexico, India, Southeast Asia, the Middle East). However, because of the toxicity associated with chloramphenicol and its lack of efficacy in eradicating the chronic typhoid carrier state, many infectious disease experts now prefer alternative antimicrobial agents for treatment of acute typhoid fever in the United States. These alternatives include ampicillin, amoxicillin, trimethoprim/sulfamethoxazole, third generation cephalosporins (eg, cefotaxime [Claforan], ceftriaxone [Rocephin]) (Soe and Overturf, 1987; The Medical Letter, 1990) or a fluoroquinolone (eg, ciprofloxacin [Cipro]) (Asperilla et al, 1990; Hooper and Wolfson, 1991). For additional discussion, see index entry Typhoid Fever, Treatment.

Relapses of typhoid fever respond to retreatment with chloramphenicol, but this compound is not effective in typhoid carriers, who should be treated with ampicillin or amoxicillin (if the strain is susceptible to either of these drugs), trimethoprim/sulfamethoxazole, or, if cholecystitis or cholelithiasis is present, by cholecystectomy. Approximately 10% of patients become postinfective carriers following administration of chloramphenicol, whereas ampicillin or amoxicillin may essentially eliminate the carrier state. Available data also suggest that the fluoroquinolones (eg, ciprofloxacin) are effective in the treatment of chronic typhoid carriers (Asperilla et al, 1990; Hooper and Wolfson, 1991).

For severe salmonellosis (eg, bacteremia, invasive disease) caused by nontyphoidal *Salmonella* species, chloramphenicol is an alternative to other antimicrobial agents, including ampicillin, amoxicillin, trimethoprim/sulfamethoxazole, third generation cephalosporins (eg, cefotaxime, ceftriaxone) (Soe and Overturf, 1987; The Medical Letter, 1990), or the fluoroquinolones (eg, ciprofloxacin) (Asperilla et al, 1990; Hooper and Wolfson, 1991). Drug selection often depends on antimicrobial resistance patterns in a particular geographic location. It is emphasized that antimicrobial drugs generally are not recommended for mild gastroenteritis caused by *Salmonella*, which is usually self-limited. Antimicrobial therapy may not shorten the duration of illness and may prolong the convalescent carrier state.

Chloramphenicol readily penetrates the blood-brain barrier (see Pharmacokinetics) and has been widely used for infections of the central nervous system caused by susceptible organisms. However, it rarely is used in bacterial meningitis today because various third generation cephalosporins are equally effective or, in the case of gram-negative enteric bacillary meningitis, more effective than chloramphenicol.

Chloramphenicol is bactericidal in vitro against most strains of the common meningeal pathogens, *H. influenzae* (usually type b), *N. meningitidis*, and *S. pneumoniae*. Because of the prevalence of ampicillin-resistant (beta lactamase-producing) strains of *H. influenzae*, chloramphenicol, usually in combination with ampicillin, has been widely used in the past for the initial empiric treatment of bacterial meningitis in infants and young children (see Klein et al, 1986). However, recommendations by the Committee on Infectious Diseases of the American Academy of Pediatrics state that certain third generation cephalosporins (cefotaxime, ceftriaxone) are equally acceptable first-line drugs for the therapy of bacterial meningitis in infants and children (Plotkin et al, 1988; American Academy of Pediatrics, 1991). Most pediatric infectious disease experts now prefer monotherapy with an appropriate third generation cephalosporin, usually ceftriaxone or cefotaxime, for this indication, primarily to avoid the problems associated with chloramphenicol administration (eg, need to monitor serum concentrations) (see McCracken et al, 1987). Although the third generation cephalosporins have superior in vitro activity against common meningeal pathogens and greater bactericidal activity in cerebrospinal fluid, they have not sterilized cerebrospinal fluid cultures more rapidly or improved case fatality rates when compared with conventional chloramphenicol plus ampicillin in infants and children (see Plotkin et al, 1988). For additional discussion, see index entry Meningitis, Treatment.

Chloramphenicol is now an alternative to a third generation cephalosporin for documented ampicillin-resistant *H. influenzae* meningitis. It is primary therapy in patients who are allergic to cephalosporins. Meningitis caused by *N. meningitidis* or *S. pneumoniae* (including strains relatively resistant to penicillin) usually responds to chloramphenicol, and this antibiotic frequently is the preferred treatment in patients who are allergic to penicillin G. However, some infectious disease experts now prefer cefotaxime or ceftriaxone in patients whose hypersensitivity to penicillin is not of the immediate (IgE-mediated) type. Although chloramphenicol-resistant strains of *H. influenzae, N. meningitidis*, and *S. pneumoniae* have been reported in the United States, their incidence remains rare.

Most authorities now consider chloramphenicol to be an inappropriate drug for gram-negative enteric bacillary meningitis involving susceptible strains of Enterobacteriaceae, presumably because of its lack of bactericidal activity; third generation cephalosporins (eg, cefotaxime) are preferred (Rahal and Simberkoff, 1982; Barriere and Flaherty, 1984; see also index entry Meningitis, Treatment).

Chloramphenicol frequently is used for anaerobic infections in the central nervous system (eg, brain abscess). Penicillin G and metronidazole are alternatives. When *Bacteroides fragilis* is the likely causative organism, either metronidazole (often preferred because it is bactericidal) or chloramphenicol should be used because this gram-negative anaerobic bacillus usually is resistant to penicillin G. For empiric therapy of pyogenic brain abscesses, combination therapy with penicillin G plus metronidazole (or chloramphenicol) frequently is employed; some experts also would add a third generation cephalosporin (eg, cefotaxime, ceftriaxone). For additional discussion, see index entry Brain Abscess, Treatment.

In addition to meningitis, *H. influenzae* (usually type b) frequently causes other serious infections, particularly in infants and young children. These include acute epiglottitis, pneumonia, facial cellulitis, septic arthritis, and bacteremia. Because of the prevalence of ampicillin-resistant strains of *H. influenzae* in most geographic locations, it has become necessary to use alternative antimicrobial agents for these infections, at least for empiric therapy (ie, before culture and susceptibility test results are available). Most infectious disease experts currently prefer a third generation cephalosporin. Chloramphenicol, often in combination with ampicillin, is alternative therapy for these infections (see index entry Antimicrobial Drugs).

Most anaerobic bacteria are susceptible to chloramphenicol, including virtually all strains of the *B. fragilis* group, an important pathogen in serious infections below the diaphragm (eg, intra-abdominal abscess, peritonitis secondary to bowel perforation). Chloramphenicol combined with an aminoglycoside (to cover aerobic gram-negative bacilli) is still effective therapy for these mixed anaerobic/aerobic infections. However, with the availability of many less toxic anti-*B. fragilis* antibiotics (eg, metronidazole, clindamycin, cefoxitin [Mefoxin], cefotetan [Cefotan], the antipseudomonal penicillins (eg, mezlocillin, piperacillin), imipenem/cilastatin [Primaxin], ticarcillin/potassium clavulanate [Timentin], and ampicillin/sulbactam [Unasyn]), there is seldom the need to use chloramphenicol except possibly in a patient with multiple drug allergies that prevent the use of these other agents (see index entry Peritonitis, Treatment).

Chloramphenicol is as effective as the tetracyclines in Rocky Mountain spotted fever, Q fever, and other rickettsial infections. It can be used when the tetracyclines are contraindicated (eg, in pregnant women, infants and children under 8 years; in hypersensitive patients; when parenteral antibiotics are necessary because of severe illness). Chloramphenicol also is an alternative to tetracyclines for treatment of ehrlichiosis, a tick-borne rickettsial infection caused by *Ehrlichia chaffeensis* (Eng et al, 1990; Schutz, 1992).

Chloramphenicol frequently is combined with a tetracycline for the treatment of severe melioidosis. This antibiotic is an effective alternative in glanders (with streptomycin), brucellosis (with or without streptomycin), plague, certain chlamydial infections (eg, psittacosis), relapsing fever, *Pseudomonas cepacia* infections, tularemia, and gas gangrene.

Chloramphenicol is effective in certain ocular and otic infections (see index entries Conjunctivitis; Otitis).

ADVERSE REACTIONS AND PRECAUTIONS. ***Hematologic:*** The most important adverse effects of chloramphenicol are on the hematopoietic system and can be subdivided into two types of bone marrow depression. The first type is characterized by anemia (with or without thrombocytopenia and leukopenia), reticulocytopenia, and increased levels of serum iron. There is increased cellularity of bone marrow with cytoplasmic vacuolization and maturation arrest of erythroid and myeloid precursors. This form of bone marrow depression is common, occurs during therapy, and is dose related. It is more likely to occur in patients receiving large doses (eg, 4 g or more per day) or prolonged therapy and in those with impaired hepatic function. It frequently is associated with serum levels greater than 25 mcg/ml. This type of bone marrow depression is not a prodrome to aplastic anemia (see below) and is reversible within one to three weeks after the drug is discontinued. The mechanism appears to be related to inhibition of host mitochondrial protein synthesis.

The second, more serious type of bone marrow depression is aplastic anemia. This is not dose related and typically occurs weeks to months after the drug has been discontinued. It is characterized by peripheral pancytopenia and hypoplastic or aplastic bone marrow. The prognosis is very poor, since the anemia usually is irreversible. The incidence of aplastic anemia has been estimated to be 1 in 25,000 to 1 in 40,000 courses of therapy. It is believed to be an idiosyncratic reaction of unknown mechanism. It has been suggested that the nitrated benzene radical of chloramphenicol, or one of its metabolites, may cause irreversible marrow toxicity in genetically predisposed individuals (Yunis et al, 1980). Interestingly, thiamphenicol, an analogue of chloramphenicol used in Europe and Japan, has the nitro group on the benzene ring replaced by a methysulfone and it has not been associated with aplastic anemia (see Standiford, 1990).

There is debate as to whether chloramphenicol given orally is more likely to cause aplastic anemia than when administered by other routes. Although the incidence following intravenous administration is extremely low, some cases have been reported (Domart et al, 1961; Grilliat et al, 1966; Restrepo and Zambrano, 1968; Wallerstein et al, 1969; Daum et al, 1979; Plaut and Best, 1982; Alavi, 1983; West et al, 1988). It also has been observed after topical ophthalmic administration (Rosenthal and Blackman, 1965; Carpenter, 1975; Abrams et al, 1980; Fraunfelder et al, 1982; Fraunfelder and Bagby, 1983). Thus, it must be assumed that this serious adverse effect can occur when chloramphenicol is administered by *any* route.

Chloramphenicol also may precipitate hemolytic anemia in patients with the Mediterranean form of glucose-6-phosphate dehydrogenase (G6PD) deficiency; individuals with milder type A G6PD deficiency (usually blacks) usually are not affected.

Since dose-related bone marrow depression can occur in any patient and is reversible, serial blood monitoring should be conducted in all patients receiving chloramphenicol. Complete blood counts and differential reticulocyte counts should be measured frequently (eg, every two to three days) to permit early detection of bone marrow depression. Serum iron levels also may be monitored. The drug should be discontinued or, at the least, the dosage should be reduced when there is evidence of bone marrow depression (eg, white blood cell count less than 3,000/mm^3 [Bartlett, 1982]). Unfortunately, routine hemograms cannot predict the occurrence of aplastic anemia.

When possible, prolonged or repeated courses of chloramphenicol or concomitant administration with other drugs that depress the bone marrow should be avoided.

Gray Syndrome: The "gray syndrome" refers to a potentially fatal adverse effect that has occurred with excessive dosage. This syndrome generally is associated with serum chloramphenicol concentrations greater than 40 mcg/ml, which can inhibit host mitochondrial electron transport in the liver, myocardium, and skeletal muscle (see Bartlett, 1982; Ambrose, 1984; Shalit and Marks, 1984). It usually begins two to nine (average, four) days after treatment with chloramphenicol is started and is manifested by vomiting, tachypnea, abdominal distention, cyanosis, green stools, lethargy, refractory metabolic acidosis, hypothermia, and an ashen color. It can progress to vasomotor collapse and death (40% of cases), which commonly occurs within two days of initial symptoms. The gray syndrome is most common in neonates (usually less than 2 weeks), particularly premature infants, who receive excessive amounts of the drug. This is because such patients have inadequate glucuronyl transferase activity combined with decreased renal excretion of unconjugated chloramphenicol. If chloramphenicol must be administered to premature infants and neonates, the dosage should be reduced (see Dosage and Preparations) and antibiotic serum concentrations should be monitored. Although this syndrome has been termed the "gray baby syndrome," it can also occur in older children and adults with excessive serum levels of the drug (eg, from overdosage, in patients with hepatic dysfunction).

Methods used to accelerate the removal of chloramphenicol in infants with the gray syndrome have included charcoal-column hemoperfusion (Mauer et al, 1980; Freundlich et al, 1983) and multiple exchange transfusions (Kessler et al, 1980; Stevens et al, 1981; Freundlich et al, 1983). Although the data are very limited, the former method appears to be more effective.

Chloramphenicol crosses the placenta and is excreted in breast milk. Therefore, it should be avoided, if possible, in pregnant women, particularly those near term or in labor, or in breast-feeding mothers.

Neurologic: Neurologic complications are usually associated with prolonged chloramphenicol therapy, particularly in cystic fibrosis patients, and include optic neuritis, peripheral neuritis, confusion, and delirium. Visual loss associated with optic neuritis may not be completely reversible. Vision should be monitored in selected patients (eg, those on long-term therapy, those with cystic fibrosis) because of the risk of optic neuritis. Patients should be requested to report any visual loss promptly.

Gastrointestinal: Nausea, vomiting, glossitis, unpleasant taste, stomatitis, and diarrhea have been reported. Although bacterial or fungal superinfections can occur, antibiotic-associated pseudomembranous colitis due to *Clostridium difficile* is uncommon.

Hypersensitivity: Rashes, fever, urticaria, angioedema, and anaphylaxis have been observed but are uncommon. Herxheimer-like reactions have been reported during treatment of typhoid fever.

Other: A population-based case-control interview study of 309 childhood leukemia cases and 618 age- and sex-matched controls suggests a correlation between chloramphenicol and the risk of acute lymphocytic and nonlymphocytic leukemias, especially in children treated for more than 10 days (Shu et al, 1987). Until this is more clearly understood, it seems prudent to change, whenever possible, from chloramphenicol to an alternative agent if clinical and susceptibility data allow (see Standiford, 1990).

DRUG INTERACTIONS. Chloramphenicol can prolong the half-lives and increase the serum concentrations of phenytoin, tolbutamide, chlorpropamide, dicumarol, and possibly other drugs by inhibiting their metabolism by hepatic microsomal enzymes. Increased toxicity and deaths have been reported. Conversely, phenobarbital, phenytoin, and rifampin (Prober, 1985) have been reported to decrease the serum concentration of chloramphenicol, presumably because of hepatic enzyme induction. Monitoring of chloramphenicol serum concentrations is recommended during concomitant administration with other drugs that may affect its pharmacokinetics.

Chloramphenicol may delay the response of anemias to iron, folic acid, or vitamin B_{12}. This antibiotic may interfere with the anamnestic response to tetanus toxoid. Concomitant administration of chloramphenicol and active immunizing agents probably should be avoided.

Antagonism of penicillin's bactericidal effect by chloramphenicol has been demonstrated in vitro and in animal studies. However, the clinical significance is unclear. This combination should be used only when such treatment has been demonstrated to be beneficial.

PHARMACOKINETICS. Three preparations of chloramphenicol are available for systemic use: chloramphenicol base in capsules for oral use; chloramphenicol palmitate, a tasteless ester, in suspension for oral use; and chloramphenicol succinate, a soluble ester, for intravenous administration. The palmitate and succinate esters are prodrugs that require hydrolysis to liberate biologically active chloramphenicol.

Absorption: Chloramphenicol base is readily absorbed from the gastrointestinal tract; bioavailability ranging from 76% to 93% has been reported. Peak plasma concentrations have been observed between 0.5 and 6 hours, and occur between 0.5 and 2 hours with products having fast dissolution and deaggregation rates (see Ambrose, 1984). After a single 1-g dose, a mean peak plasma concentration of 11.2 mcg/ml was reported at one hour. Multiple dosing at six-hour intervals resulted in somewhat higher plasma concentrations on the second day (18.4 mcg/ml after the fifth dose) with no subsequent increases (see manufacturer's literature).

Chloramphenicol palmitate must be hydrolyzed by pancreatic esterases in the small intestine to active chloramphenicol base, which is subsequently absorbed. Bioavailability of chloramphenicol is approximately 80% when it is administered as the palmitate ester and peak plasma concentrations usually occur two to three hours after administration (see Ambrose, 1984). The absorption of chloramphenicol after oral administration of the palmitate ester has been reported to be incomplete, prolonged, and erratic in premature and term newborns (Shankaran and Kauffman, 1984).

After intravenous administration, circulating chloramphenicol succinate must be hydrolyzed to free chloramphenicol, the active drug; this probably occurs in the liver, kidney, and lung. Initially, it was believed that metabolic conversion of the succinate ester to free chloramphenicol was rapid and complete, but this is not the case. The rate and extent of hydrolysis of chloramphenicol succinate are variable and incomplete and, on the average, about 30% of a dose is eliminated as unhydrolyzed ester in the urine in both adults and children. In addition, there is wide interpatient variability in the amount of succinate ester that is excreted in urine. Thus, the mean 70% bioavailability of free chloramphenicol following intravenous administration of chloramphenicol succinate is actually lower than that obtained following oral administration. More importantly, bioavailability after intravenous administration is quite variable among patients, especially in newborns, infants, and young children (see Kauffman et al, 1981 A, 1981 B; Smith and Weber, 1983; Ambrose, 1984; Kramer et al, 1984; Shalit and Marks, 1984). In newborns (eg, less than 1 month), both the hydrolysis and renal excretion of chloramphenicol succinate appear to be considerably reduced when compared to other age groups (see Ambrose, 1984; Shalit and Marks, 1984).

Distribution: Between 50% and 60% of circulating chloramphenicol is bound to plasma protein. Reported mean values for the apparent volume of distribution range from 0.6 to 1 L/kg (see Ambrose, 1984). The drug has good lipid solubility and readily penetrates most tissues and body fluids. This includes the cerebrospinal fluid where concentrations approximately one-half the corresponding plasma concentration can be achieved with or without meningitis. Concentrations in brain tissue are higher than those in plasma. Therapeutic concentrations are achieved in synovial, pleural, and ascitic fluid. Chloramphenicol penetrates intracellularly, which facilitates efficacy against phagocytized organisms. Good penetration into the aqueous and vitreous humors is also observed. Chloramphenicol readily crosses the placenta and can be found in breast milk. Only small amounts of active chloramphenicol are recovered from bile (see Ambrose, 1984; Standiford, 1990).

Metabolism and Excretion: Chloramphenicol is eliminated primarily by metabolism to inactive products. In patients with normal hepatic function, approximately 90% of chloramphenicol is conjugated to the glucuronide in the liver. The inactive conjugate subsequently is excreted by the kidneys. Minor metabolites also have been identified. Only about 5% to 15% is excreted by glomerular filtration as active, unchanged chloramphenicol in urine. The mean elimination half-life is approximately four hours in adults and children (see Ambrose, 1984).

The metabolism and excretion of chloramphenicol are diminished in neonates and premature infants in whom hepatic (eg, glucuronyl transferase system) and renal function are not fully developed. Mean elimination half-lives of chloramphenicol have been reported to be about nine hours in neonates from 1 week to 2 months and 12 hours in those less than 1 week of age; there is substantial individual variation (see Smith and Weber, 1983; Ambrose, 1984).

Patients with hepatic dysfunction (eg, cirrhosis) conjugate active chloramphenicol at a slower rate, resulting in a prolonged elimination half-life and accumulation in serum. Dosage reductions are necessary.

With impaired renal function, there is a delay in the excretion of the glucuronide conjugate, but this metabolite is biologically inactive and apparently nontoxic. After oral administration, the elimination half-life of chloramphenicol is unchanged and serum accumulation of the active and potentially toxic free drug does not occur. Chloramphenicol bioavailability in patients with renal dysfunction may be greater after intravenous infusion, however, because less succinate ester will be excreted in urine (see Ambrose, 1984). Neither peritoneal nor hemodialysis alters serum levels sufficiently to require dosage alterations.

Monitoring Chloramphenicol Serum Concentrations: In general, peak serum chloramphenicol concentrations of 10 to 20 mcg/ml and trough concentrations of 5 to 10 mcg/ml are thought to be desirable for most infections. This drug has a low therapeutic:toxic ratio, and dose-dependent bone marrow depression has been associated with peak serum concentrations greater than 25 mcg/ml and trough concentrations greater than 10 mcg/ml (see Ambrose, 1984; see also the section on Adverse Reactions and Precautions). Therefore, sequential monitoring of peak and trough serum chloramphenicol concentrations is indicated to ensure efficacy and prevent toxicity (see Bartlett, 1982; Smith and Weber, 1983; Ambrose, 1984; Shalit and Marks, 1984). This is particularly important for pediatric patients in whom wide variations in chloramphenicol metabolism and excretion have been reported. Dosage requirements may vary threefold in children of the same age. Even greater variation is observed in newborn and young infants, making serum monitoring imperative in this age group (Friedman et al, 1979; Kauffman et al, 1981 A; Tuomanen et al, 1981; Yogev et al, 1981). Monitoring of serum chloramphenicol concentrations also is very important in individuals with hepatic dysfunction, those with renal impairment who are given the succinate ester intravenously, and patients receiving concomitant therapy with other drugs (eg, phenytoin, phenobarbital, rifampin) that can alter chloramphenicol pharmacokinetics (see Drug Interactions) (see Bartlett, 1982; Smith and Weber, 1983; Ambrose, 1984; Shalit and Marks, 1984).

DOSAGE AND PREPARATIONS. Current dosage recommendations for oral chloramphenicol base or palmitate or for intravenous chloramphenicol sodium succinate are the same, despite some differences in bioavailability among these preparations (see Pharmacokinetics). The intravenous route is recommended initially in the treatment of most serious infections. Oral therapy may be substituted when conditions warrant. With appropriate monitoring (eg, continued hospitalization, measurement of serum chloramphenicol concentrations), the oral route has been shown to be as effective as the intravenous route for completion of chloramphenicol therapy in children with *H. influenzae* type b meningitis (Tuomanen et al, 1981).

Intramuscular administration of chloramphenicol generally is not recommended because delayed absorption results in substantially lower serum concentrations and therapeutic failures have been reported. However, this has been disputed in a study (Shann et al, 1985) that showed peak serum chloramphenicol concentrations and areas under the serum concentration-time curves to be similar after intramuscular and intravenous administration of chloramphenicol sodium succinate to children with pneumonias or other serious infections.

In general, peak chloramphenicol serum concentrations of 10 to 20 mcg/ml and trough concentrations of 5 to 10 mcg/ml are thought to be desirable for most infections. Sequential monitoring of peak and trough chloramphenicol serum concentrations is recommended because of the low therapeutic:toxic ratio of this antibiotic and the wide interpatient variation in chloramphenicol pharmacokinetics that has been observed. This is of particular importance in pediatric patients, especially newborns and premature infants, patients with hepatic dysfunction, and those receiving concomitant therapy with other drugs that can alter chloramphenicol pharmacokinetics (see Pharmacokinetics and Drug Interactions).

Oral, Intravenous: *Adults*, 50 mg/kg daily in divided doses every six hours for most indications (eg, typhoid fever, rickettsial infections); 100 mg/kg daily in divided doses every six hours for meningitis and brain abscess (see Standiford, 1990). Ideally, serum concentrations of chloramphenicol should be monitored periodically (see above).

Children, 50 to 75 mg/kg daily in divided doses every six hours for most indications; 75 to 100 mg/kg daily in divided doses every six hours for meningitis (Nelson, 1991 A). Ideally, serum concentrations of chloramphenicol should be monitored periodically (see above).

Neonates over 7 days weighing more than 2 kg, 50 mg/kg daily in divided doses every 12 hours; *neonates from birth to 7 days weighing more than 2 kg*, 25 mg/kg once daily; *neonates weighing between 1.2 and 2 kg*, 25 mg/kg once daily; *neonates under 1.2 kg*, 22 mg/kg once daily (Nelson, 1991 B). Serum concentrations of chloramphenicol should be monitored periodically (see above).

In *patients with impaired hepatic function*, dosage reductions may be necessary. Clear guidelines are not available and, ideally, serum concentrations should be monitored. In *adults*, an initial loading dose of 1 g followed by 500 mg every six hours has been suggested (see Standiford, 1990).

CHLORAMPHENICOL:
Chloromycetin (Parke-Davis), ***Generic.*** Capsules 250 mg.
CHLORAMPHENICOL PALMITATE:
Chloromycetin Palmitate (Parke-Davis). Suspension (oral) equivalent to chloramphenicol 150 mg/5 ml.
CHLORAMPHENICOL SODIUM SUCCINATE:
Generic. Powder (for injection) 1 g.
Chloromycetin Sodium Succinate (Parke-Davis). Powder (for injection) 1 g (equivalent to 100 mg of chloramphenicol/ml when reconstituted [see manufacturer's instructions]).

Cited References

Report of the Committee on Infectious Diseases, in: *American Academy of Pediatrics Redbook*, ed 22. Elk Grove Village, Ill, American Academy of Pediatrics, 1991, 220-229, 323-326, 373-378.

Drugs that cause photosensitivity. *Med Lett Drugs Ther* 28:51-52, 1986.

Treatment of Lyme disease. *Med Lett Drugs Ther* 31:57-59, 1989.

Tetracycline-resistant *Neisseria gonorrhoeae*--Georgia, Pennsylvania, New Hampshire. *MMWR* 34:563-570, 1985.

Plasmid-mediated tetracycline-resistant *Neisseria gonorrhoeae*—Georgia, Massachusetts, Oregon. *MMWR* 35:304-306, 1986.

Sentinel surveillance system for antimicrobial resistance in clinical isolates of *Neisseria gonorrhoeae. MMWR* 36:585-593, 1987.

1989 Sexually transmitted diseases treatment guidelines. *MMWR* 38 (suppl 8):1-43, 1989.

Pelvic inflammatory disease: Guidelines for prevention and management. *MMWR* 40(No. RR-5):1-25, 1991.

Abrams SM, et al: Marrow aplasia following topical application of chloramphenicol eye ointment. *Arch Intern Med* 140:576-577, 1980.

Ad Hoc Committee on Use of Antibiotics in Dermatology, American Academy of Dermatology: Systemic antibiotics for treatment of acne vulgaris: Efficacy and safety. *Arch Dermatol* 111:1630-1636, 1975.

Alavi JB: Aplastic anemia associated with intravenous chloramphenicol. *Am J Hematol* 15:375-379, 1983.

Ambrose PJ: Clinical pharmacokinetics of chloramphenicol and chloramphenicol succinate. *Clin Pharmacokinet* 9:222-238, 1984.

Ariza J, et al: Treatment of human brucellosis with doxycycline plus rifampin or doxycycline plus streptomycin: Randomized, double-blind study. *Ann Intern Med* 117:25-30, 1992.

Asperilla MO, et al: Quinolone antibiotics in the treatment of *Salmonella* infections. *Rev Infect Dis* 12:873-889, 1990.

Back DJ, et al: Interindividual variation and drug interactions with hormonal steroid contraceptives. *Drugs* 21:46-61, 1981.

Barriere SL, Flaherty JF: Third generation cephalosporins: Critical evaluation. *Clin Pharm* 3:351-373, 1984.

Bartlett JG: Chloramphenicol. *Med Clin North Am* 66:91-102, 1982.

Bartlett JG: Chloramphenicol, in Peterson PK, Verhoef J (eds): *The Antimicrobial Agents Annual/3*. New York, Elsevier, 1988, 99-105.

Carpenter G: Chloramphenicol eye-drops and marrow aplasia. *Lancet* 2:326-327, 1975.

Chopra I, et al: Review: Tetracyclines, molecular and clinical aspects. *J Antimicrob Chemother* 29:245-277, 1992.

Committee on Drugs, American Academy of Pediatrics: Requiem for tetracyclines. *Pediatrics* 55:142-143, 1975.

Cunha BA, et al: Tetracyclines. *Med Clin North Am* 66:293-302, 1982.

Dattwyler RJ, et al: Amoxycillin plus probenecid versus doxycycline for treatment of erythema migrans borreliosis. *Lancet* 336:1404-1406, 1990.

Daum RS, et al: Fatal aplastic anemia following apparent dose-related chloramphenicol toxicity. *J Pediatr* 94:403-406, 1979.

Doherty JE: Digoxin-antibiotic drug interaction. *N Engl J Med* 305:827-828, 1981.

Domart A, et al: Aplasie medullaire mortelle aprés administration de chloramphénicol par voie intra-musculaire chez duex adultes. *Sem Hop Paris* 37:2256-2258, 1961.

Eng TR, et al: Epidemiologic, clinical, and laboratory findings of human ehrlichiosis in the United States, 1988. *JAMA* 264:2251-2258, 1990.

Epstein JH, Wintroub BU: Photosensitivity due to drugs. *Drugs* 30:42-57, 1985.

Ericsson CD, et al: Influence of subsalicylate bismuth on absorption of doxycycline. *JAMA* 247:2266-2267, 1982.

Forrest JN Jr, et al: Superiority of demeclocycline over lithium in treatment of chronic syndrome of inappropriate secretion of antidiuretic hormone. *N Engl J Med* 298:173-177, 1978.

Francke EL, Neu HC: Chloramphenicol and tetracyclines. *Med Clin North Am* 71:1155-1168, 1987.

Fraunfelder FT, Bagby GC Jr: Ocular chloramphenicol and aplastic anemia, letter. *N Engl J Med* 307:1536, 1983.

Fraunfelder FT, et al: Fatal aplastic anemia following topical administration of ophthalmic chloramphenicol. *Am J Ophthalmol* 93:356-360, 1982.

Freundlich M, et al: Management of chloramphenicol intoxication in infancy by charcoal hemoperfusion. *J Pediatr* 103:485-487, 1983.

Friedman CA, et al: Chloramphenicol disposition in infants and children. *J Pediatr* 95:1071-1077, 1979.

Graham DY, et al: Effect of treatment of *Helicobacter pylori* infection on long-term recurrence of gastric or duodenal ulcer: Randomized, controlled study. *Ann Intern Med* 116:705-708, 1992.

Grayston JT, et al: New *Chlamydia psittaci* strain, TWAR, isolated in acute respiratory tract infections. *N Engl J Med* 315:161-168, 1986.

Grayston JT, et al: Current knowledge on *Chlamydia pneumoniae*, strain TWAR, an important cause of pneumonia and other acute respiratory diseases. *Eur J Clin Microbiol Infect Dis* 8:191-202, 1989.

Grilliat JP, et al: Cytopenié mortelle aprés therapeutique par hemisuccinate de chloramphenicol. *Ann Med Nancy* 5:754-762, 1966.

Hansten PD, Horn JR: Inhibition of oral contraceptive efficacy. *Drug Interact Newslett* 5:7-10, 1985.

Hansten PD, Horn JR: Anti-infective drug interactions, in: *Drug Interactions and Updates.* Vancouver, Wash, Applied Therapeutics, 1992 A, 300-305.

Hansten PD, Horn JR: Antidiabetic drug interactions, in: *Drug Interactions and Updates.* Vancouver, Wash, Applied Therapeutics, 1992 B, 216.

Hansten PD, Horn JR: *Drug Interactions and Updates.* Vancouver, Wash, Applied Therapeutics, 1992 C, 304, 499-500.

Hooper DC, Wolfson JS: Fluoroquinolone antimicrobial agents. *N Engl J Med* 324:384-394, 1991.

Hyams KC, et al: Diarrheal disease during Operation Desert Shield. *N Engl J Med* 325:1423-1428, 1991.

Jacoby GA, Archer GL: New mechanisms of bacterial resistance to antimicrobial agents. *N Engl J Med* 324:601-612, 1991.

Kallings I: Sensitivity of *Branhamella catarrhalis* to oral antibiotics. *Drugs* 31 (suppl 3):17-22, 1986.

Kauffman RE, et al: Pharmacokinetics of chloramphenicol and chloramphenicol succinate in infants and children. *J Pediatr* 98:315-320, 1981 A.

Kauffman RE, et al: Relative bioavailability of intravenous chloramphenicol succinate and oral chloramphenicol palmitate in infants and children. *J Pediatr* 99:963-967, 1981 B.

Kessler DL Jr, et al: Chloramphenicol toxicity in neonate treated with exchange transfusion. *J Pediatr* 96:140-141, 1980.

Klein JO, et al: Report of task force on diagnosis and management of meningitis. *Pediatrics* 78 (suppl):959-982, 1986.

Knapp JS, et al: Frequency and distribution in United States of *Neisseria gonorrhoeae* with plasmid-mediated, high-level resistance to tetracycline. *J Infect Dis* 155:819-822, 1987.

Kramer WG, et al: Comparative bioavailability of intravenous and oral chloramphenicol in adults. *J Clin Pharmacol* 24:181-186, 1984.

Lindenbaum J, et al: Inactivation of digoxin by gut flora: Reversal by antibiotic therapy. *N Engl J Med* 305:789-794, 1981.

Mauer SM, et al: Treatment of infant with severe chloramphenicol intoxication using charcoal-column hemoperfusion. *J Pediatr* 96:136-139, 1980.

McCracken GH Jr, et al: Consensus report: Antimicrobial therapy for bacterial meningitis in infants and children. *Pediatr Infect Dis J* 6:501-505, 1987.

The Medical Letter: *Handbook of Antimicrobial Therapy.* New Rochelle, NY, The Medical Letter, Inc, 1990, 27-41.

Mikolich DJ, Boyce JM: Brucella species, in Mandell GL, et al (eds): *Principles and Practice of Infectious Diseases*, ed 3. New York, Churchill Livingstone, 1990, 1735-1742.

Moran JS, Zenilman JM: Therapy for gonococcal infections: Options in 1989. *Rev Infect Dis* 12 (suppl 6):S633-S644, 1990.

National Institutes of Health Consensus Development Conference: Travelers' diarrhea. *JAMA* 253:2700-2704, 1985.

Nelson JD: *1991-1992 Pocketbook of Pediatric Antimicrobial Therapy*, ed 9. Baltimore, Williams & Wilkins, 1991 A, 66-80.

Nelson JD: *1991-1992 Pocketbook of Pediatric Antimicrobial Therapy*, ed 9. Baltimore, Williams & Wilkins, 1991 B, 16-17.

Nicolau DP, et al: Tetracycline-induced pancreatitis. *Am J Gastroenterol* 86:1669-1671, 1991.

Nicotra B, et al: *Branhamella catarrhalis* as lower respiratory tract pathogen in patients with chronic lung disease. *Arch Intern Med* 146:890-893, 1986.

Ory EM: Tetracyclines, in Kagan BM (ed): *Antimicrobial Therapy*, ed 3. Philadelphia, WB Saunders, 1980, 117-126.

Plaut ME, Best WR: Aplastic anemia after parenteral chloramphenicol: Warning renewed, letter. *N Engl J Med* 306:1486, 1982.

Plotkin SA, et al: Treatment of bacterial meningitis. *Pediatrics* 81:904-907, 1988.

Poliak SC, et al: Minocycline-associated tooth discoloration in young adults. *JAMA* 254:2930-2932, 1985.

Pratt WB, Fekety R: *The Antimicrobial Drugs.* New York, Oxford University Press, 1986, 184-228.

Prober CG: Effect of rifampin on chloramphenicol levels, letter. *N Engl J Med* 312:788-789, 1985.

Rahal JJ Jr, Simberkoff MS: Bactericidal and bacteriostatic action of chloramphenicol against meningeal pathogens. *Antimicrob Agents Chemother* 16:13-18, 1979.

Rahal JJ Jr, Simberkoff MS: Host defense and antimicrobial therapy in adult gram-negative bacillary meningitis. *Ann Intern Med* 96:468-474, 1982.

Reichart CA, et al: Temporal trends in gonococcal antibiotic resistance in Baltimore. *Sex Transm Dis* 19:213-218, 1992.

Restrepo A, Zambrano F: Anemia aplastica tardia secundaria a cloranfenicol. Descripcion de diez casos. *Antioquia Medica* 18:593-606, 1968.

Rosenthal RL, Blackman A: Bone-marrow hypoplasia following use of chloramphenicol eyedrops. *JAMA* 191:148-149, 1965.

Sack DA, et al: Prophylactic doxycycline for travelers' diarrhea: Results of prospective double-blind study of Peace Corps volunteers in Kenya. *N Engl J Med* 298:758-763, 1978.

Sack RB, et al: Prophylactic doxycycline for travelers' diarrhea: Results of prospective double-blind study of Peace Corps volunteers in Morocco. *Gastroenterology* 76:1368-1373, 1979.

Satterwhite TK, DuPont HL: Infectious diarrhea in office practice. *Med Clin North Am* 67:203-220, 1983.

Schachter J: *Chlamydia psittaci*: "Reemergence of forgotten pathogen," editorial. *N Engl J Med* 315:189-191, 1986.

Schutz GE: *Ehrlichia chaffeensis. Infect Dis Newslett* 11:17-19, (March) 1992.

Schwarcz SK, et al: National surveillance of antimicrobial resistance in *Neisseria gonorrhoeae. JAMA* 264:1413-1417, 1990.

Shalit I, Marks MI: Chloramphenicol in the 1980s. *Drugs* 28:281-291, 1984.

Shankaran S, Kauffman RE: Use of chloramphenicol palmitate in neonates. *J Pediatr* 105:113-116, 1984.

Shann F, et al: Absorption of chloramphenicol sodium succinate after intramuscular administration in children. *N Engl J Med* 313:410-414, 1985.

Shu XO, et al: Chloramphenicol use and childhood leukaemia in Shanghai. *Lancet* 2:934-937, 1987.

Siegel D: Tetracyclines: New look at old antibiotic: I. Clinical pharmacology, mechanism of action, and untoward effects. II. Clinical use. *NY State J Med* 78:950-956, 1115-1120, 1978.

Smith AL, Weber A: Pharmacology of chloramphenicol. *Pediatr Clin North Am* 30:209-236, 1983.

Soe GB, Overturf GD: Treatment of typhoid fever and other systemic salmonelloses with cefotaxime, ceftriaxone, cefoperazone, and other newer cephalosporins. *Rev Infect Dis* 9:719-736, 1987.

Stamm WE, et al: Treatment of acute urethral syndrome. *N Engl J Med* 304:956-958, 1981.

Standiford HC: Tetracyclines and chloramphenicol, in Mandell GL, et al (eds): *Principles and Practice of Infectious Diseases*, ed 3. New York, Churchill Livingstone, 1990, 284-295.

Steere AC, et al: Treatment of early manifestations of Lyme disease. *Ann Intern Med* 99:22-26, 1983.

Stevens DC, et al: Exchange transfusion in acute chloramphenicol toxicity. *J Pediatr* 99:651-653, 1981.

Tatro DS (ed): *Drug Interaction Facts.* St. Louis, Mo, Facts and Comparisons, 1992, 694.

Timbrell JA: Drug hepatotoxicity. *Br J Clin Pharmacol* 15:3-14, 1983.

Tuomanen EI, et al: Oral chloramphenicol in treatment of *Haemophilus influenzae* meningitis. *J Pediatr* 99:968-974, 1981.

Wallerstein RO, et al: Statewide study of chloramphenicol therapy and fatal aplastic anemia. *JAMA* 208:2045-2050, 1969.

West BC, et al: Aplastic anemia associated with parenteral chloramphenicol: Review of 10 cases, including second case of possible increased risk with cimetidine. *Rev Infect Dis* 10:1048-1051, 1988.

Williams DN: Tetracyclines, in Peterson PK, Verhoef J (eds): *The Antimicrobial Agents Annual/3.* New York, Elsevier, 1988, 218-228.

Yogev R, et al: Pharmacokinetic comparison of intravenous and oral chloramphenicol in patients with *Haemophilus influenzae* meningitis. *Pediatrics* 67:656-660, 1981.

Yunis AA, et al: Nitroso-chloramphenicol: Possible mediator in chloramphenicol-induced aplastic anemia. *J Lab Clin Med* 96:36-46, 1980.

Other Selected References

Barza M, Schiefe RT: Antimicrobial spectrum, pharmacology and therapeutic use of antibiotics: Part 1. Tetracyclines. *Am J Hosp Pharm* 34:49-57, 1977.

Feder HM Jr: Chloramphenicol: What we have learned in the last decade. *South Med J* 79:1129-1134, 1986.

Kucers A: Chloramphenicol, erythromycin, vancomycin, tetracyclines. *Lancet* 2:425-429, 1982.

Meissner HC, Smith AL: Current status of chloramphenicol. *Pediatrics* 64:348-356, 1979.

Nahata MC: Chloramphenicol, in Evans WE, et al (eds): *Applied Pharmacokinetics: Principles of Therapeutic Drug Monitoring,* ed 2. Spokane, Wash, Applied Therapeutics, Inc, 1986, 437-462.

Reese RE, Betts RF: Antibiotic use: Chloramphenicol; tetracyclines, in Reese RE, Betts RF (eds): *A Practical Approach to Infectious Diseases*, ed 3. Boston, Little Brown, 1991, 949-954, 968-974.

Ristuccia AM: Chloramphenicol: Clinical pharmacology in pediatrics. *Ther Drug Monit* 7:159-167, 1985.

Smilack JD, et al: Tetracyclines, chloramphenicol, erythromycin, clindamycin and metronidazole. *Mayo Clin Proc* 66:1270-1280, 1991.

Aminoglycosides 68

The aminoglycoside antibiotics were discovered as the result of a systematic screening of soil actinomycetes for the elaboration of antimicrobial substances. Streptomycin, the first clinically useful aminoglycoside, was isolated in 1944.

Nine aminoglycoside antibiotics are approved for use in the United States. Streptomycin, neomycin [Mycifradin], kanamycin [Kantrex], tobramycin [Nebcin], and paromomycin [Humatin] are natural compounds derived from various species of *Streptomyces*; gentamicin [Garamycin] and sisomicin [Siseptin] are obtained from species of *Micromonospora*. Amikacin [Amikin] and netilmicin [Netromycin] are semisynthetic aminoglycosides produced by chemical modification of kanamycin and sisomicin, respectively. Sisomicin is not currently marketed in the United States. Paromomycin is used as a luminal amebicide or anthelmintic in certain cestode infections; see index entry Paromomycin.

Aminoglycosides have similar antibacterial spectra and pharmacokinetic properties, and their potential toxicities affect the same organ systems; however, subtle and important differences exist.

Chemistry

The aminoglycosides are more appropriately designated aminoglycosidic aminocyclitols. These agents all contain a six-membered aminocyclitol ring (aglycone) to which are attached by glycosidic linkages a variety of amino- and nonamino-containing sugars. The aminocyclitol ring of streptomycin is streptidine. The other aminoglycosides have 2-deoxystreptamine as the aglycone in a centrally located position.

The 2-deoxystreptamine subclass can be further subdivided into aminoglycoside families based on the number and types of sugars attached to the aminocyclitol ring. The neomycin family, which includes neomycin and paromomycin, has three sugars (two amino hexoses and one nonamino pentose) attached to 2-deoxystreptamine. The kanamycin (kanamycin, tobramycin, amikacin) and gentamicin (gentamicin, sisomicin, netilmicin) families have only two amino hexoses attached to this central aglycone. These latter two families differ in the type of 3-amino hexose found in the C ring position; for the kanamycin family it is kanosamine and for the gentamicin family it is garosamine. Variations within families of aminoglycosides result from differences in side chains on the amino sugars and, in the case of amikacin and netilmicin, on the aglycone. The chemical structures of the aminoglycosides are shown in the Figure.

Mechanism of Action

Under aerobic conditions, the aminoglycosides are bactericidal, but their exact mechanism of action is unknown. Based on studies done primarily with streptomycin, the bacterial ribosome is considered to be the principal target of these agents. Streptomycin blocks bacterial protein synthesis by binding to the bacterial 30S ribosomal subunit to produce a nonfunctional 70S initiation complex. In addition, ribosomally bound streptomycin increases the frequency of misreading of the genetic code due to incorrect codon-anticodon interaction (Moellering, 1983; Pratt and Fekety, 1986; Lietman, 1990). The 2-deoxystreptamine-containing aminoglycosides also bind to the 30S subunit, inhibit protein synthesis, and cause incorrect reading of the genetic code. However, they appear to have different interactions with this subunit than streptomycin and also bind to the 50S subunit. Thus, there is evidence of selective affinities for 30S and 50S binding sites among the 2-deoxystreptamine-containing aminoglycosides (Moellering, 1983; Pratt and Fekety, 1986; Lietman, 1990).

Despite abundant information on the adverse effects of aminoglycosides on bacterial protein synthesis and the fidelity of translation, it is unclear why these agents are rapidly bactericidal while other antimicrobial agents, such as chloramphenicol and the tetracyclines, which are equally effective in inhibiting protein synthesis, usually are bacteriostatic. A number of alternative mechanisms for aminoglycoside activity have been proposed, some of which involve effects on bacterial

STREPTIDINE

STREPTOMYCIN

NEOMYCIN[1]

cytoplasmic membrane integrity, but these remain speculative (Hancock, 1981; Bryan, 1984; Lietman, 1990).

Aminoglycosides must enter bacterial cells to be effective. These drugs penetrate the periplasmic space of gram-negative bacteria by diffusion through the external membrane via aqueous channels formed by porin proteins and subsequently are transported across the cytoplasmic membrane by a two-phase, active process; concentrations then accumulate that greatly exceed the local external concentration. The first phase of active transport of these drugs, termed energy-dependent phase I (EDP I), requires the existence of an electrochemical gradient of protons across the cytoplasmic membrane. This gradient is generated by respiratory processes or the hydrolysis of adenosine 5′-triphosphate. After entering the interior of bacteria, the aminoglycosides bind to polysomes and thus inhibit protein synthesis. This process causes an increase in the rate of transport of the drug, a phase designated energy-dependent phase II (EDP II). EDP II may be linked with progressive disruption of the cytoplasmic membrane, loss of permeability control, and perhaps cell death (Bryan, 1984).

Conditions that reduce or abolish the electrochemical gradient across the bacterial cytoplasmic membrane (by altering either the electrical or chemical component) also attenuate or prevent the transport of aminoglycosides in the EDP I phase. Thus, anaerobiasis, low extracellular pH, and hyperosmolarity of the external environment inhibit aminoglycoside membrane translocation in bacteria. This process also is inhibited by high external concentrations of divalent cations (eg, Ca2+, Mg2+) and polyamines. Therefore, the antibacterial effectiveness of aminoglycosides is markedly reduced in the anaerobic environment of an abscess or in hyperosmolar urine. The effect of divalent cations also is relevant to the selection and use of appropriate, consistent media for in vitro susceptibility testing of aminoglycosides (Lietman, 1990).

The long postantibiotic effect (PAE) of aminoglycosides has particular clinical importance; the PAE refers to the period following the complete removal of an antimicrobial drug from the immediate environment during which no further growth of a susceptible organism occurs (Zhanel et al, 1991). When tested against aerobic gram-negative bacilli, aminoglycosides have PAEs of >3.5 hours, which permit the use of longer intervals between doses than with other antimicrobial drugs (eg, β lactams). These considerations have led some authorities to advocate the use of single-dose regimens to reduce the toxicity, inconvenience to patients, and relatively high nondrug costs associated with standard multiple daily-dose aminoglycoside dosage regimens (see sections on Pharmacokinetics and Dosage Determinations below).

THE AMINOGLYCOSIDES

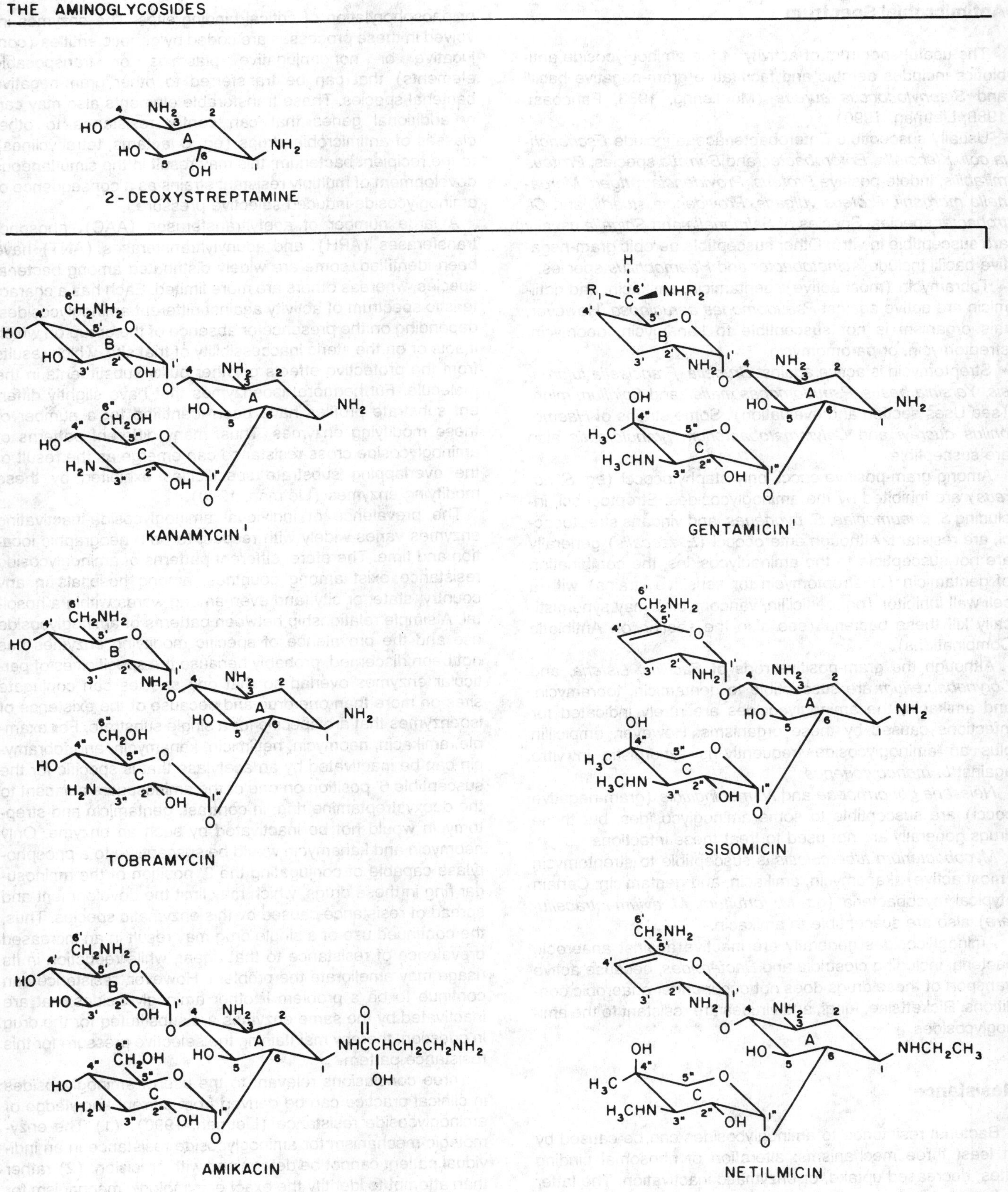

2-DEOXYSTREPTAMINE

KANAMYCIN[1]

GENTAMICIN[1]

TOBRAMYCIN

SISOMICIN

AMIKACIN

NETILMICIN

Antimicrobial Spectrum

The useful spectrum of activity of the aminoglycoside antibiotics includes aerobic and facultative gram-negative bacilli and *Staphylococcus aureus* (Moellering, 1983; Pancoast, 1988; Lietman, 1990).

Usually susceptible Enterobacteriaceae include *Escherichia coli, Klebsiella, Enterobacter,* and *Serratia* species, *Proteus mirabilis*, indole-positive *Proteus, Providencia rettgeri, Morganella morganii, Proteus vulgaris, Providencia stuartii*, and *Citrobacter* species. Species of *Salmonella* and *Shigella* usually are susceptible in vitro. Other susceptible aerobic gram-negative bacilli include *Acinetobacter* and *Haemophilus* species.

Tobramycin (most active), gentamicin, amikacin, and netilmicin are active against *Pseudomonas aeruginosa*. However, this organism is not susceptible to kanamycin, neomycin, streptomycin, or paromomycin.

Streptomycin is active against *Brucella, Francisella tularensis, Yersinia pestis, Pseudomonas mallei*, and *Spirillum minor* (see Uses section and evaluation). Some strains of *Haemophilus ducreyi* and *Calymmatobacterium granulomatis* also are susceptible.

Among gram-positive cocci, only staphylococci (eg, *S. aureus*) are inhibited by the aminoglycosides. Streptococci, including *S. pneumoniae, S. pyogenes,* and viridans streptococci, are resistant. Although enterococci (*E. faecalis*) generally are not susceptible to the aminoglycosides, the combination of gentamicin (or streptomycin for sensitive strains) with a cell wall inhibitor (eg, penicillin, vancomycin) may synergistically kill these bacteria (see also the section on Antibiotic Combinations).

Although the gram-positive rods of *Bacillus, Listeria,* and *Corynebacterium* are susceptible to gentamicin, tobramycin, and amikacin, the aminoglycosides are rarely indicated for infections caused by these organisms. However, ampicillin plus an aminoglycoside frequently is synergistic in vitro against *L. monocytogenes*.

Neisseria gonorrhoeae and *N. meningitidis* (gram-negative cocci) are susceptible to some aminoglycosides, but these drugs generally are not used to treat these infections.

Mycobacterium tuberculosis is susceptible to streptomycin (most active), kanamycin, amikacin, and gentamicin. Certain atypical mycobacteria (eg, *M. fortuitum, M. avium-intracellulare*) also are susceptible to amikacin.

Aminoglycosides generally are inactive against anaerobic bacteria, including clostridia and *Bacteroides*, because active transport of these drugs does not occur under anaerobic conditions. Rickettsiae, fungi, and viruses are resistant to the aminoglycosides.

Resistance

Bacterial resistance to aminoglycosides can be caused by at least three mechanisms: alteration of ribosomal binding sites, decreased uptake, or enzymatic inactivation. The latter is the most common and clinically important mechanism. The aminoglycosides are inactivated by acetylation, adenylation, or phosphorylation of critical binding sites. The enzymes involved in these processes are coded by genetic entities (conjugative or nonconjugative plasmids or transposable elements) that can be transferred to other gram-negative bacterial species. These transferable elements also may carry additional genes that can confer resistance to other classes of antimicrobial drugs (eg, β lactams, tetracyclines) to the recipient bacterium; this may result in the simultaneous development of multiply resistant strains as a consequence of aminoglycoside-induced selective pressure.

A large number of acetyltransferases (AAC), phosphotransferases (APH), and adenylyltransferases (ANT) have been identified; some are widely distributed among bacterial species, whereas others are more limited. Each has a characteristic spectrum of activity against different aminoglycosides, depending on the presence or absence of the group on which it acts or on the steric inaccessibility of that site, which results from the protective effects of other bulky substituents in the molecule. Furthermore, isoenzymes that have slightly different substrate profiles have been identified for a number of these modifying enzymes. Thus, many different patterns of aminoglycoside cross-resistance can emerge as the result of the overlapping substrate specificities exhibited by these modifying enzymes (Lietman, 1990).

The prevalence of individual aminoglycoside-inactivating enzymes varies widely with respect to both geographic location and time. Therefore, different patterns of aminoglycoside resistance exist among countries; among hospitals in any country, state, or city; and even among wards within a hospital. A simple relationship between patterns of aminoglycoside use and the prevalence of specific modifying enzymes has not been discerned, probably because the specificities of particular enzymes overlap so that one species can conjugate sites on more than one drug and because of the existence of isoenzymes that are specific for a single substrate. For example, amikacin, neomycin, netilmicin, kanamycin, and tobramycin can be inactivated by an acetylase that is specific for the susceptible 6′ position on one of the aminosugars adjacent to the deoxystreptamine ring; in contrast, gentamicin and streptomycin would not be inactivated by such an enzyme. Only neomycin and kanamycin would be susceptible to a phosphorylase capable of conjugating the 3′ position of the aminosugar ring in these drugs, which may limit the development and spread of resistance caused by this enzymatic species. Thus, the continued use of a single drug may result in an increased prevalence of resistance to that agent, while reduction in its usage may ameliorate the problem. However, resistance can continue to be a problem if other aminoglycosides that are inactivated by the same enzymes are substituted for the drug in question, thereby maintaining the selective pressure for this resistance pattern.

Three conclusions relevant to the use of aminoglycosides in clinical practice can be derived from current knowledge of aminoglycoside resistance (Lietman, 1990): (1) The enzymologic mechanism for aminoglycoside resistance in an individual patient cannot be determined with precision; (2) rather than attempt to identify the exact enzymologic mechanism for resistance in a patient, the clinician should rely on established tests (eg, MIC, MBC) of susceptibility to a drug; and (3) the current practice of reserving use of a drug (eg, amikacin) to preclude or reduce the emergence of local resistance to that agent may not be rational because the continued use of other aminoglycosides that are inactivated by the same enzyme(s) can exert sufficient selective pressure to cause the emergence of resistance to the reserved drug.

Gram-negative bacilli that are resistant to amikacin frequently are resistant to all aminoglycosides; strains of *E. coli*, *Pseudomonas*, *Enterobacter*, and *Serratia* that are resistant to all aminoglycosides have been isolated. The mechanism of this resistance is thought to be decreased uptake of antibiotic by the bacterial cell (Moellering, 1983; Maloney et al, 1989). Despite increased clinical use, resistance to amikacin does not appear to have become more prevalent in some institutions, and gentamicin/tobramycin resistance frequently has decreased. However, this finding has not been universal, and the possibility of amikacin resistance requires continued surveillance (Cunha, 1988, 1990; Edson and Terrell, 1991).

Among gram-positive species, high-level resistance to all aminoglycosides has emerged in some nosocomial strains of enterococci (*E. faecalis, E. faecium*) and has spread to other isolates of this species by transmission on plasmids and transposons that carry the genetic determinants that code these functions (Murray, 1991). In some of these isolates, concurrent resistance to other antimicrobial drugs (eg, vancomycin, β lactams, erythromycin) has been observed. This presents a significant clinical challenge in that it effectively eliminates the synergy between the aminoglycosides and cell wall-active agents (eg, β lactams, vancomycin) that has been a mainstay of therapy for serious infections caused by these species. This may necessitate a return to single-agent treatment of these conditions and result in reduced efficacy and possibly an increase in morbidity and mortality.

Chromosomal mutations that alter the 30S ribosomal subunit binding site (S12 protein) can result in a rapid, single-step resistance to streptomycin. This mechanism of resistance appears to be clinically important for *Mycobacterium tuberculosis* and enterococci, but not for gram-negative bacilli. Although resistance to 2-deoxystreptamine-containing aminoglycosides has been demonstrated at the ribosomal level, it is generally uncommon and of little clinical importance (see Moellering, 1983; Lietman, 1990).

Uses

Aminoglycosides must be administered parenterally for systemic infections. Amikacin, gentamicin, kanamycin, netilmicin, streptomycin, and tobramycin are the currently available parenteral aminoglycosides. These agents are indicated in severe, complicated infections caused by susceptible organisms. Because of their ototoxic and nephrotoxic potential, these antibiotics should not be used for trivial infections or for those that can be eradicated with less toxic agents.

Parenteral Aminoglycosides for Serious Aerobic Gram-negative Bacillary Infections: The primary use of parenteral aminoglycosides, alone or in combination regimens, is for the treatment of serious infections caused by aerobic gram-negative bacilli, principally the Enterobacteriaceae, *Listeria monocytogenes*, and *Pseudomonas aeruginosa*. These include bacteremias; intra-abdominal infections (eg, acute cholecystitis, peritonitis secondary to bowel perforation, nonvenereal pelvic inflammatory disease); skin and soft tissue infections (eg, infected burns with sepsis, necrotizing fasciitis); lower respiratory tract infections (eg, nosocomial pneumonia); bone and joint infections (eg, osteomyelitis, septic arthritis); malignant external otitis caused by *P. aeruginosa*; complicated urinary tract infections (eg, acute pyelonephritis, acute prostatitis); meningitis (lumbar intrathecal or intraventricular administration may be required except in newborns); and severe nonsexual epididymo-orchitis (Pancoast, 1988; Lietman, 1990; Edson and Terrell, 1991; Reese and Betts, 1991). (See also index entry Antimicrobial Drugs). Amikacin, gentamicin, kanamycin, netilmicin, or tobramycin may be used for these infections when the susceptibility of the causative organism is known.

Empiric therapy with an aminoglycoside frequently is used for a presumed gram-negative bacillary infection before the identification and susceptibility of the causative organism are known. Under these circumstances, drug selection should depend on a number of factors, including the prevalence of aminoglycoside resistance in a given hospital (based on current, locally generated antibiotic susceptibility profiles), the severity and type of infection (community acquired or nosocomial), the ability to monitor aminoglycoside serum concentrations, and the cost of antibiotic therapy (Reese and Betts, 1991). Possible differences in drug toxicity also may be considered, although conflicting results have made it difficult to assess relative differences in risk among the various aminoglycosides. There is considerable controversy about whether one aminoglycoside offers sufficient advantages over other analogues to warrant being considered the drug of choice. The following discussion considers some of the advantages and disadvantages of each agent with regard to the above factors. Ultimately, hospital staff must evaluate the aminoglycosides relative to their institution's requirements before selecting a particular agent for the hospital formulary.

Gentamicin, tobramycin, amikacin, and netilmicin usually are interchangeable for general use. Kanamycin is not active against *P. aeruginosa*, and resistance to this agent among the Enterobacteriaceae is prevalent in many hospitals. Thus, kanamycin has significant disadvantages when compared with the other aminoglycosides in serious gram-negative bacillary infections and is rarely indicated.

At the present time, gentamicin and tobramycin are most frequently selected for general use. Either is an appropriate drug of choice for infections that are likely to be caused by susceptible organisms. Since gentamicin is considerably less expensive than tobramycin, amikacin, or netilmicin, this can be an important consideration when all other factors are equal.

Tobramycin is more potent than gentamicin in vitro against *P. aeruginosa*, including some gentamicin-resistant strains, and frequently is preferred (usually in combination with an antipseudomonal penicillin, a third-generation cephalosporin [eg, ceftazidime], or aztreonam) for infections likely to be caused by this organism (eg, infection in the neutropenic patient). However, there is no conclusive proof that tobramycin is clinically superior to gentamicin against *P. aeruginosa* (Lietman, 1990). Although some infectious disease experts have recommended tobramycin over gentamicin for all infections likely to be caused by susceptible organisms because tobramycin has been reported to be less nephrotoxic (based on serum creatinine determinations) than gentamicin, its use for all patients does not appear to be warranted. Tobramycin may be preferable in patients at increased risk for nephrotoxicity, such as the elderly and those requiring prolonged therapy, particularly when individualized dosing methods are not employed (Moore et al, 1984 A; see also section on Adverse Reactions and Precautions).

Cross-resistance between gentamicin and tobramycin is common, and resistance to these two aminoglycosides is becoming more widespread, particularly in nosocomial infections. Amikacin usually is effective in infections caused by organisms (eg, strains of Enterobacteriaceae, *P. aeruginosa*) that are resistant to gentamicin and tobramycin, because it is less susceptible to aminoglycoside-inactivating enzymes (see section on Resistance). Thus, amikacin should be the drug of choice for empiric therapy of infections caused by aerobic gram-negative bacilli in hospitals where gentamicin- and tobramycin-resistant strains are common. Furthermore, even in hospitals without a major resistance problem, when there is concern about gentamicin- and tobramycin-resistant gram-negative bacilli in a particular clinical situation (eg, severe nosocomial infection in a patient who is immunosuppressed, receiving other antibiotics, or in the intensive care unit), amikacin frequently is recommended for initial therapy before the results of susceptibility tests are known.

The selection of amikacin as the aminoglycoside of choice for general use is controversial. The rationale of reserving this antibiotic for situations in which gentamicin or tobramycin resistance is a problem is that extensive use of amikacin will result in the unnecessary emergence of amikacin-resistant bacterial strains. However, there is no evidence that restriction of amikacin usage will delay the emergence of resistance to this drug (Lietman, 1990; Reese and Betts, 1991). Furthermore, in some hospitals where amikacin was the primary aminoglycoside, resistance to this agent did not increase and gentamicin/tobramycin resistance actually decreased (Berk et al, 1986).

In addition to its lower susceptibility to enzymatic inactivation, some infectious disease experts prefer amikacin over gentamicin (or tobramycin) for general use because it has a better pharmacokinetic profile, including more reliable predictability of adequate, nontoxic, peak serum concentrations, a higher therapeutic ratio, a longer dosing interval, and decreased susceptibility to inactivation by β-lactam antibiotics (Holm et al, 1983; Cunha, 1988; see also the section on Drug Interactions and the evaluations). The clinical significance of these factors is unclear, however, and others have reported wide interpatient variation in amikacin pharmacokinetics similar to that observed with gentamicin and tobramycin (Zaske, 1986; Bauer and Blouin, 1983). Finally, based on current data, it is unclear whether there are any clinically significant differences in toxicity between amikacin and gentamicin (or tobramycin) (see below).

The efficacy of netilmicin is comparable to that of gentamicin, tobramycin, and amikacin in infections caused by susceptible gram-negative bacilli. Netilmicin also is active against some gentamicin- and tobramycin-resistant strains of various Enterobacteriaceae, but it does not appear to offer any advantages in spectrum of activity over amikacin. Clinical experience with this agent is more limited (*Med Lett Drugs Ther*, 1983; Craig et al, 1983; Pancoast, 1988); however, it is less expensive than amikacin. Although data in animals and humans suggest that netilmicin may be less toxic than the other commonly used parenterally administered aminoglycosides, especially in patients who are at high risk of developing ototoxicity, this has not been established clinically (see section on Adverse Reactions and Precautions below).

Specific Uses of Streptomycin: Streptomycin frequently is the preferred drug in the treatment of tularemia, plague, severe brucellosis (in combination with a tetracycline or chloramphenicol), and glanders (in combination with a tetracycline or chloramphenicol). See index entry Streptomycin.

Streptomycin is used in combination regimens to treat tuberculosis. Kanamycin also is used rarely for this disease. For guidelines for the treatment and prophylaxis of tuberculosis, see index entry on this disease.

Streptomycin has been used in granuloma inguinale and chancroid, but other antimicrobial drugs are preferred (see index entry Sexually Transmitted Diseases).

For the use of streptomycin in the treatment of infective endocarditis, see the following section, Antibiotic Combinations, and the evaluation.

Uses of Oral Aminoglycosides: Gastrointestinal absorption of orally administered aminoglycosides is negligible in patients with normal renal function and an intact gastrointestinal tract (see section on Pharmacokinetics). Some analogues have been used by the oral route for their local effects in the gastrointestinal tract.

Neomycin and kanamycin have been used to suppress the bacterial flora of the bowel as a prophylactic measure before elective colorectal surgery. Oral neomycin plus erythromycin base is a regimen of choice for this indication (see index entry Colorectal Surgery).

Neomycin is used as an adjunct in the treatment of hepatic coma because it decreases the number of ammonia-forming bacteria in the intestinal tract. For additional discussion, see index entry Neomycin, In Portal Systemic Encephalopathy.

Neomycin reduces the absorption of cholesterol by precipitating it from micellar solution and has been used in patients with hyperlipoproteinemia. For additional discussion, see index entry Neomycin, In Hypercholesterolemia.

Uses of Topical Aminoglycosides: Neomycin is most commonly used topically for infections of the eye, ear, and skin, frequently as a component of an antibiotic mixture. Topical ophthalmic preparations of gentamicin and tobramycin are used in conjunctivitis caused by susceptible gram-negative bacilli. Although a dermatologic preparation of gentamicin [Garamycin] is available for topical application, such use is *not recommended* because selection of gentamicin-resistant strains occurs very rapidly; widespread resistance has been reported in burn units where topical gentamicin was used. For additional information on the use of the aminoglycosides in infectious diseases of the eye, ear, and skin, see index entry Aminoglycosides, Uses.

The administration of neomycin as a peritoneal or pleural irrigant after surgery is of questionable value and is dangerous, since a sufficient amount of drug can be absorbed to cause serious ototoxicity and nephrotoxicity (Weinstein et al, 1977) or neuromuscular blockade, particularly when used with muscle relaxants. Approval of neomycin for the irrigation of surgical wounds, joints, and various body cavities (other than the intact urinary bladder) has been withdrawn by the U.S. Food and Drug Administration (FDA) (*Federal Register,* 1988 A).

Antibiotic Combinations

Aminoglycosides frequently are combined with another antibiotic to treat certain infections in order to (1) obtain a synergistic antibacterial effect, (2) prevent the emergence of antibiotic-resistant bacteria, and (3) expand the antimicrobial spectrum (see index entry Antimicrobial Drugs, Principles of Drug Selection). The following combinations are often employed clinically.

(1) An antipseudomonal penicillin (ticarcillin [with or without potassium clavulanate], mezlocillin, piperacillin) frequently is combined with an aminoglycoside (gentamicin, tobramycin, amikacin, netilmicin) for serious infections caused by *Pseudomonas aeruginosa* (see index entry Penicillins).

(2) A regimen containing an antipseudomonal aminoglycoside (gentamicin, tobramycin, amikacin, netilmicin) in combination with an antipseudomonal penicillin and/or a cephalosporin (eg, ceftazidime) is often used for initial empiric therapy in febrile neutropenic patients (Hughes et al, 1990). Because of possible gentamicin and tobramycin resistance, amikacin often is the preferred aminoglycoside for this indication.

(3) A regimen containing penicillin G or ampicillin in combination with gentamicin or streptomycin (for susceptible strains) is frequently employed to treat enterococcal endocarditis when rapid bactericidal activity is necessary. Similarly, streptomycin (or gentamicin) and penicillin G are more rapidly bactericidal against viridans streptococci, although penicillin G alone is very active against this organism. The combination of an aminoglycoside with vancomycin also is synergistic against most streptococci, including enterococci. However, because additive ototoxicity and nephrotoxicity may occur in patients who are given this combination (see the section on Drug Interactions), it should be administered only when necessary (eg, for enterococcal endocarditis in patients allergic to penicillin). In some geographic areas, a substantial percentage of enterococcal strains exhibits high-level resistance to gentamicin, streptomycin, and all other aminoglycosides. The optimal drug regimen for the treatment of endocarditis caused by these aminoglycoside-resistant enterococci has not been established (Bisno et al, 1989; Lipman and Silva, 1989).

(4) A penicillinase-resistant penicillin (or vancomycin) plus an aminoglycoside may be synergistic in vitro against *Staphylococcus aureus*; however, the indications for such combination therapy remain to be clarified.

(5) Gentamicin, tobramycin, amikacin, or netilmicin may be combined with a cephalosporin to treat serious *Klebsiella* infections or as empiric therapy for nosocomial pneumonia. Although cephalosporin/aminoglycoside combinations exhibit synergistic activity, some controversy exists concerning their use because increased nephrotoxicity has occurred with cephalothin/aminoglycoside combinations (Wade et al, 1978; see also the section on Drug Interactions).

(6) Gentamicin, tobramycin, amikacin, or netilmicin often is used in combination with a drug effective against the *Bacteroides fragilis* group to treat abdominal or pelvic sepsis or prophylactically prior to "dirty" colorectal surgery. For therapy guidelines, see index entry Antimicrobial Drugs.

(7) Gentamicin, tobramycin, amikacin, or netilmicin may be used with another antibiotic in other empiric therapy when an expanded antimicrobial spectrum is desirable (eg, with ampicillin for neonatal meningitis or biliary tract infections).

(8) Oral neomycin plus erythromycin base is a regimen of choice for prophylaxis of infection after elective colorectal surgery (for details, see index entry Colorectal Surgery).

Some combinations of an aminoglycoside and a nonaminoglycoside antibiotic are antagonistic. In vitro tests and studies in animals indicate that chloramphenicol and tetracycline antagonize the actions of streptomycin in infections caused by streptococci and *Klebsiella*. Similarly, chloramphenicol antagonizes the action of gentamicin in *Proteus mirabilis* infections in neutropenic mice or in mice with meningitis.

Adverse Reactions and Precautions

The aminoglycosides have a low therapeutic index compared with most other antibiotics that are used systemically. In particular, they have the potential to produce irreversible ototoxicity. They also can be nephrotoxic and neurotoxic. Parenteral administration of neomycin is contraindicated in all patients because of the extreme toxicity associated with its use.

Ototoxicity: All aminoglycosides have the potential to produce ototoxicity; both the hearing (cochlear) and equilibrium (vestibular) functions may be affected. These antibiotics are toxic initially to the hair cells and then to the supporting cells of the neuroepithelium and secretory tissues of the vestibular and cochlear apparatuses of the inner ear. Cellular damage appears to be related to the accumulation and slow elimination of aminoglycosides from the perilymph and endolymph that bathe the relevant target cells. Toxicity is frequently irreversible because the cells of the cochlear and vestibular apparatuses cannot regenerate once they have been destroyed (Lietman, 1990).

Clinical manifestations of auditory toxicity include tinnitus, a feeling of "fullness" in the ears, or any degree of hearing loss ranging from temporary inability to detect certain (usually high frequency) tones to total, irreversible deafness. Hearing loss is usually bilateral. Because tinnitus or a feeling of fullness in the ear may be an early sign of ototoxicity, patients should be instructed to report such sensations immediately; however, these symptoms frequently are not reliable premonitors of auditory toxicity (Lietman, 1990). Symptomatic hearing loss usually begins with reduced high-frequency acuity and progresses to loss of lower-frequency hearing (Fausti et al, 1992). By the time hearing loss can be detected by the inability of the patient to react to normal conversational tones, considerable permanent damage will have occurred. Baseline and subsequent serial audiograms are indicated for certain high-risk patients, including those with renal failure and those receiving prolonged therapy (ten days or longer). However, it may not be possible to obtain reliable conventional audiograms in critically ill patients. Because of this and the seriousness of permanent loss of hearing, an abridged five-frequency test encompassing higher frequencies (9 to 20 kHz) has been advocated for early detection of aminoglycoside-induced ototoxicity (Fausti et al, 1992). This test can be performed in 10 minutes and may identify >80% of patients before hearing loss progresses into the conversational range. Auditory testing is not routinely performed in patients without associated risk factors.

Symptoms of vestibular toxicity include nausea, vomiting, vertigo, dizziness, and an unsteady gait with nystagmus. These are difficult to evaluate in critically ill patients. Laboratory measurement of vestibular function by electronystagmography is not performed in most patients receiving aminoglycosides.

Ototoxicity is dose related and may be associated with excessive aminoglycoside serum concentrations. It is more likely to occur with prolonged (more than ten days) or repeated courses of therapy. Ototoxicity also can develop long after discontinuation of treatment. Inappropriately high doses of these drugs in patients with impaired renal function, dehydrated individuals, the elderly, or the obese increase the risk of ototoxicity. Other reported risk factors include bacteremia, fever, liver dysfunction, an elevated ratio of serum urea nitrogen to serum creatinine as a measure of dehydration, and concurrent administration of other ototoxic drugs, such as ethacrynic acid [Edecrin] (Lietman, 1990; Moore et al, 1984 B; see also the section on Drug Interactions). Aminoglycoside serum concentrations should be carefully monitored and adjusted in these high-risk patients (see section on Dosage Determinations).

The incidence of aminoglycoside ototoxicity reported in the literature varies widely, presumably due to differences in patient populations, the criteria used to determine ototoxicity, and whether serum concentrations were optimally controlled (Brummett and Fox, 1989). For example, auditory or vestibular toxicity has been estimated to occur in 3% to 5% of patients receiving gentamicin, tobramycin, or amikacin, based on audiometric or electronystagmographic testing, respectively. However, in other studies, clinically detectable hearing loss or vestibular dysfunction occurred in about 0.5% of patients (see Lietman, 1990). The risk for each patient may be substantially reduced or eliminated by the use of individualized dosing regimens based on pharmacokinetic parameters (see the section on Dosage Determinations below).

The ototoxic potentials of gentamicin, tobramycin, and amikacin do not appear to differ significantly (see Lietman, 1990; Buring et al, 1988), although one report suggests that tobramycin is less vestibulotoxic than gentamicin (Fee, 1983). In animal studies, netilmicin was less ototoxic than gentamicin, tobramycin, and amikacin (Szot and Tabachnick, 1980), but this has not been demonstrated unequivocally in humans. However, a retrospective review of aminoglycoside clinical toxicity (Kahlmeter and Dahlager, 1984) and other comparative studies (Buring et al, 1988; see also Uses) suggests that netilmicin may be less ototoxic than the other aminoglycosides. In one multicenter controlled clinical trial, netilmicin (plus ticarcillin) was reported to be significantly less ototoxic than tobramycin (plus ticarcillin) (Lerner et al, 1983).

Nephrotoxicity: All aminoglycosides have dose- and duration-dependent potential to cause nephrotoxicity at the level of the proximal renal tubular cells. Aminoglycosides are actively reabsorbed by these cells and accumulate over prolonged periods to yield renal cortical levels five- to fiftyfold higher than those observed in plasma. The morphologic effects of aminoglycosides on proximal renal tubular cells consist of swelling and the appearance of cytoplasmic vacuoles and myeloid bodies within lysosomes. Eventually, tubular necrosis can occur. Glomerular filtration subsequently is decreased, but glomerular lesions have not yet been observed in humans. The mechanism for reduced glomerular filtration is unclear (see Lietman and Smith, 1983; Lietman, 1990).

The severity of aminoglycoside nephrotoxicity can range from trivial effects on proximal renal tubules to life-threatening complications of acute tubular necrosis. A syndrome of hypokalemia, hypocalcemia, and hypomagnesemia has been reported rarely. Fortunately, nephrotoxicity usually is mild when aminoglycoside dosage is adjusted carefully for changing glomerular function. Furthermore, it is usually reversible with drug discontinuation because proximal renal tubular cells, unlike the hair cells of the inner ear, readily regenerate. The toxicity usually is nonoliguric (Lietman and Smith, 1983; Lietman, 1990) and should not be a deterrent to the use of these antibiotics in therapeutically effective doses. Aminoglycosides should be given when appropriate in seriously ill patients with routine measurement of serum creatinine and BUN levels.

The earliest effects of aminoglycoside-induced nephrotoxicity begin to appear within one to two days after treatment is begun and include proteinuria caused by increased excretion of β_2-microglobulin and several renal tubular enzymes (alanine aminopeptidase, β-D-glucosaminidase, alkaline phosphatase). Although these early effects are the most sensitive indicators of renal tubular dysfunction, most infectious disease experts consider them to be too nonspecific to be useful in seriously ill patients who also may be receiving other potentially nephrotoxic drugs (eg, amphotericin B, ibuprofen). Urinary casts derived from sloughing of proximal renal tubular cells also appear early. Clinical nephrotoxicity usually is defined by elevations in serum creatinine (alternative, blood urea nitrogen [BUN]) (see Lietman and Smith, 1983; Lietman, 1990). For example, nephrotoxicity can be defined as an increase in serum creatinine levels of ≥0.5 mg/dL if the initial serum creatinine level is <3 mg/dL or an increase of ≥1 mg/dL if the initial serum creatinine level is ≥3 mg/dL (Lietman and Smith, 1983). Elevations in serum creatinine reflect reductions in the glomerular filtration rate. This usually occurs only after five to seven days of aminoglycoside therapy.

Nephrotoxicity is dose related and is more likely to occur with prolonged (more than ten days) or repeated courses of aminoglycoside therapy. It frequently has been associated with elevated serum aminoglycoside trough concentrations (>2 mcg/ml for gentamicin or tobramycin; >4 mcg/ml for netilmicin; >10 mcg/ml for amikacin). However, it is unclear whether this is a true cause-and-effect relationship or simply reflects an already diminished glomerular filtration rate. Inappropriately high doses in patients with impaired renal function, dehydrated individuals, the elderly, and the obese increase the risk of nephrotoxicity. Other reported risk factors for aminoglycoside nephrotoxicity include hypotension, liver dysfunction, obstructive jaundice, female sex, a high initial creatinine clearance, and concurrent administration of other nephrotoxic agents. Potent diuretics (eg, furosemide [Lasix]) can increase the risk of nephrotoxicity if volume depletion is not corrected (Lietman and Smith, 1983; Lietman, 1990; Moore et al, 1984 A). Aminoglycoside serum concentrations should be carefully monitored and adjusted in these high-risk patients (see section on Dosage Determinations).

The incidence of aminoglycoside nephrotoxicity has been reported to range from 1% to 25% or greater in various clinical trials (see Lietman, 1990). The considerable variability among studies is presumably due to differences in the definition of nephrotoxicity, clinical protocols, methodologies, patient populations, the aminoglycoside employed, dosage regimens, and method of determining aminoglycoside dosing (eg, individualized, nomogram).

A number of clinical studies have been undertaken to identify differences in the nephrotoxic potentials of the important parenterally administered aminoglycosides (gentamicin, tobramycin, amikacin, netilmicin). In most cases, data that convincingly show differences in nephrotoxicity are unavailable. Cumulative evidence does suggest that tobramycin and amikacin probably are less nephrotoxic than gentamicin, and this has caused considerable controversy in drug selection (see Uses). Netilmicin was less nephrotoxic than gentamicin, tobramycin, and amikacin in animal studies (Szot and Tabachnak, 1980) and may be less nephrotoxic than tobramycin in humans. However, these differences have not been demonstrated unequivocally (*Med Lett Drugs Ther*, 1983; Craig et al, 1983; Buring et al, 1988; Pancoast, 1988).

Neuromuscular Blockade: The aminoglycosides rarely may cause neuromuscular blockade that can lead to progressive flaccid paralysis and potentially fatal respiratory arrest. This adverse effect is associated with very high concentrations of aminoglycoside at the neuromuscular junction. The risk is greatest with intraperitoneal or intrapleural instillation of large doses or after rapid (bolus) intravenous administration, but a curare-like paralysis also has occurred following intravenous infusion, intramuscular injection, or even oral administration. Blockade is most common in patients already compromised by other drugs (eg, general anesthetics, neuromuscular blocking agents [see section on Drug Interactions]), diseases (eg, myasthenia gravis), or conditions (eg, hypocalcemia) that affect neuromuscular transmission. Blockade usually can be counteracted by the prompt administration of calcium gluconate; response to cholinesterase inhibitors, such as neostigmine [Prostigmin], has been variable.

Hypersensitivity: Hypersensitivity reactions have been observed infrequently following use of aminoglycosides. Rashes, pruritus, urticaria, and, rarely, exfoliative dermatitis have been reported. Drug fever, hypotension, and anaphylactic shock also have been associated with aminoglycoside use. Patients who are allergic to aminoglycosides should not receive these drugs.

Topical application of neomycin frequently has resulted in sensitization to the drug.

Miscellaneous Adverse Reactions: Gastrointestinal side effects are usually mild. Nausea, vomiting, stomatitis, and diarrhea have been reported. Superinfection caused by nonsusceptible organisms has occurred, but pseudomembranous colitis due to *Clostridium difficile* is extremely rare (or does not occur) with aminoglycosides. A malabsorption syndrome may develop after prolonged oral administration.

Blood dyscrasias, including anemia, eosinophilia, neutropenia, thrombocytopenia (including purpura), and agranulocytosis, have been observed, but they are very uncommon.

Headache, lethargy, paresthesias, tremor, peripheral neuritis, visual disturbances, arthralgia, and, rarely, convulsions have been reported.

Increased ALT, AST, LDH, and unbound serum bilirubin levels, possibly drug-related, sometimes develop.

Pain at the site of intramuscular injection also has been noted.

Although there is no conclusive evidence that the aminoglycosides are teratogenic, ototoxic, or nephrotoxic in the fetus, it must be assumed that these effects are possible. Aminoglycosides should be given to pregnant women only when life-threatening infections do not respond to other antibiotics.

Acute Overdose: In patients with normal renal function, maintenance of adequate urine output (3 to 6 ml/kg/hour) with intravenous fluids appears to be the treatment of choice following a single acute overdose with an aminoglycoside (Fuquay et al, 1981; Green et al, 1981). Hemodialysis (preferred) or peritoneal dialysis should be considered in patients with renal failure.

Drug Interactions

Aminoglycosides and various penicillin derivatives chemically interact in a 1:1 molar ratio by forming a covalent bond between an amino group on the aminoglycoside and a carboxyl group from a broken β-lactam ring. However, for this reaction to proceed efficiently, a high molar ratio of penicillin to aminoglycoside is required. Thus, only the aminoglycoside activity is measurably lost (see Lietman, 1990). The antipseudomonal penicillins (ticarcillin, mezlocillin, piperacillin), which usually are given in large doses, inactivate aminoglycosides, particularly gentamicin and tobramycin, when mixed together in intravenous solutions prior to administration, and this practice should be avoided. When these antibiotics are administered separately, loss of aminoglycoside activity is unlikely in patients with normal renal function but has been reported in those with renal failure (see Tatro, 1988; Hansten and Horn, 1990 A); this may be clinically significant. Amikacin and netilmicin appear to be less susceptible than gentamicin or tobramycin to inactivation by antipseudomonal penicillins in vitro (Pickering and Rutherford, 1981). Serum concentrations of any aminoglycoside should be monitored and the dosage adjusted accordingly in patients with renal failure who receive these drugs in combination with antipseudomonal penicillins (Tatro, 1988; Hansten and Horn, 1990 A). Serum specimens containing aminoglycoside-penicillin combinations should be tested immediately or frozen before antibiotic assay (Pickering and Rutherford, 1981). For information on incompatibility between parenteral aminoglycosides and other drugs or substances in intravenous solutions, see Trissel, 1988.

The ototoxicity produced by ethacrynic acid can be additive with that of the aminoglycosides. This combination should be avoided (Hansten and Horn, 1990 A). Whether additive ototoxicity also occurs with the other loop diuretics (furosemide, bumetanide [Bumex]) is unresolved. The combination of furosemide or bumetanide and an aminoglycoside was more toxic to the cochlea than the aminoglycoside alone in animal studies; however, enhanced toxicity of these combinations in humans is not supported by existing data. In a retrospective analysis of three prospective, controlled, randomized, double-blind clinical trials evaluating nephrotoxicity and auditory toxicity of gentamicin, tobramycin, and amikacin, the concurrent administration of furosemide did not increase the incidence of aminoglycoside ototoxicity (or nephrotoxicity) (Smith and Lietman, 1983). Until more information is available, physicians should closely follow aminoglycoside serum concentrations and monitor for signs of nephrotoxicity and ototoxicity in patients receiving furosemide or bumetanide concurrently (Guglielmo, 1984; Hansten and Horn, 1990 A). Also, it should be emphasized that appropriate monitoring of the patient's hydration status is particularly important when potent diuretics are administered with aminoglycosides, because a significant decrease in extracellular fluid volume may cause serum levels of antibiotic to rise to toxic levels.

Although clinical examples are lacking, the possibility that the symptoms of aminoglycoside ototoxicity can be masked by dimenhydrinate [Dramamine] should be considered (Hansten and Horn, 1990 A).

Additive or synergistic nephrotoxicity may occur when aminoglycosides are administered with certain other nephrotoxic agents. This has been documented for methoxyflurane [Penthrane], and aminoglycosides should not be given to patients who recently received this anesthetic unless absolutely necessary (Hansten and Horn, 1990 A). Administration of aminoglycosides with amphotericin B [Fungizone] (Hansten and Horn, 1990 A), vancomycin (Farber and Moellering, 1983; Pauly et al, 1990), cisplatin [Platinol] (Hansten and Horn, 1990 A), cyclosporine [Sandimmune] (Hansten and Horn, 1990 A), or intravenous indomethacin [Indocin IV] (given for closure of patent ductus arteriosus in neonates) (Hansten and Horn, 1990 A) also can result in increased nephrotoxicity. When administration of one of these combination regimens is necessary, close monitoring of renal function is essential.

An increase in nephrotoxicity has been observed in patients receiving an aminoglycoside plus cephalothin [Keflin] (Tatro, 1988; Hansten and Horn, 1990 A). This appears to be most likely in patients with pre-existing renal disease. Except for cephaloridine (no longer marketed), there is no evidence that other cephalosporins potentiate aminoglycoside nephrotoxicity (see Tatro, 1988). However, it is recommended that aminoglycoside-cephalosporin combinations be administered with caution, particularly in patients with pre-existing renal disease (Hansten and Horn, 1990 A). Avoidance of cephalothin in these patients should be considered.

The neuromuscular blockade produced by skeletal muscle relaxants (eg, succinylcholine [Anectine, Quelicin, Sucostrin], tubocurarine) can be potentiated by the aminoglycosides and cause respiratory paralysis. These agents should be given concomitantly only with extreme caution. Calcium or anticholinesterase agents may counteract the blockade (Hansten and Horn, 1990 A; see also the section on Adverse Reactions and Precautions).

Orally administered neomycin or kanamycin may potentiate the action of coumarin anticoagulants by reducing bacterial vitamin K production in the large intestine and/or by decreasing vitamin K absorption. Dietary vitamin K deficiency is an additional predisposing factor for this interaction. Careful monitoring of prothrombin time is recommended in patients receiving oral neomycin or kanamycin and coumarin anticoagulants concomitantly (Hansten and Horn, 1990 B). Oral neomycin also appears to inhibit the gastrointestinal absorption of digoxin. Serum digoxin levels should be monitored when these drugs are given together (Hansten and Horn, 1990 A).

Pharmacokinetics

The pharmacokinetics of individual aminoglycosides are essentially the same in normal, healthy humans. However, considerable interpatient variability in the disposition of aminoglycosides may occur as a function of age, renal capacity, or hydration status or in the presence of underlying pathology (Lietman, 1990). These variables must be considered when determining dosages and dose intervals.

Absorption: The aminoglycosides are highly polar polycations at the pH of the small intestine and are poorly absorbed from the intact gastrointestinal tract. Following oral administration, therapeutic serum concentrations are not attained. Nevertheless, ingestion of quantities sufficient to reduce bacterial flora in the bowel or to treat hepatic coma may produce detectable serum levels, especially in patients with renal failure. Aminoglycosides penetrate poorly through intact skin, but considerable absorption may occur following topical application to large denuded or burned areas. Variable amounts are absorbed during irrigation of closed body cavities or infected wounds.

Aminoglycosides must be given intramuscularly or intravenously (usually by infusion over a period of 30 to 60 minutes) for the treatment of most infections. After intramuscular injection, almost 100% of the dose is absorbed systemically, and peak serum concentrations usually are attained after approximately 60 minutes (range, 30 to 90 minutes). The concentrations attained are similar to those observed 30 minutes after completion of an intravenous infusion of an equal dose over a 30-minute period. Average peak serum concentrations for gentamicin (1.5 mg/kg), tobramycin (1.5 mg/kg), amikacin (7.5 mg/kg), netilmicin (2 mg/kg), and kanamycin (7.5 mg/kg) are 4 to 8, 4 to 8, 15 to 25, 7, and 20 to 25 mcg/ml, respectively.

Distribution: The aminoglycosides are bound weakly to serum proteins; streptomycin is approximately 35% bound and the other aminoglycosides are less than 10% bound. These drugs distribute mainly to extracellular fluids; the volume of distribution using a two-compartment model is between 0.2 and 0.3 L/kg. Various factors can affect the volume of distribution. For example, the presence of edema or ascites increases the volume of distribution and decreases serum levels. The reverse usually is true in obese patients. Because these drugs distribute poorly into adipose tissue, dosage adjustment may be required in obese individuals.

Aminoglycoside concentrations in body tissues and fluids are lower than corresponding serum levels except in the kidney, where these drugs become tightly bound to renal cortical tissue, and in the urine (Lietman, 1990). Penetration of aminoglycosides into cerebrospinal fluid (CSF) is inadequate for antibacterial activity in adults, even in the presence of inflammation; lumbar intrathecal or intraventricular injection is necessary to produce therapeutic CSF levels of these drugs. However, therapeutic levels may be achieved in the CSF of neonates with meningitis after intravenous administration (see McCracken, 1981). Antibacterial concentrations cannot be attained in the vitreous humor of the eye and are not attained consistently in the aqueous humor. Direct instillation by intravitreal or subconjunctival injection, respectively, is necessary to treat infections in these spaces. Biliary concentrations usually are variable and lower than serum levels. Concentrations approximating 25% to 50% of those in the serum are achieved in bronchial, pericardial, peritoneal, pleural, and synovial fluids. These drugs readily enter the perilymph of the inner ear, and high concentrations found in this space correlate with ototoxicity. The aminoglycosides also cross the placenta (Weinstein et al, 1976), and effects on the fetus or newborn infant must be considered if an aminoglycoside is administered during pregnancy. These drugs should be given to pregnant women only when life-threatening infections do not respond to other antibiotics.

Excretion: The aminoglycosides are eliminated from the body almost entirely by glomerular filtration, although some proximal tubular reabsorption may occur (see section on Adverse Reactions and Precautions). These drugs are not metabolized, and more than 90% of a dose is recovered in urine as unchanged drug within 24 hours.

In adults and infants more than 6 months old with normal renal function, the elimination half-life of the aminoglycosides is two to three hours. In infants less than 1 week old, particularly those born prematurely or of low birth weight (less than 2 kg), the half-life may be 8 to 11 hours. The half-life in neonates whose birth weight exceeds 2 kg is approximately five hours. The half-life usually is decreased in febrile patients. Since aminoglycosides are excreted by the kidney, a pronounced increase in elimination half-life is observed with decreases in renal function (eg, up to fortyfold in uremic patients); dosage adjustment is necessary in such patients to avoid serious toxicity (see the sections on Adverse Reactions and Precautions and Dosage Determinations). The aminoglycosides can be removed by hemodialysis and peritoneal dialysis.

During administration of the first three to five doses of an aminoglycoside, the rate of plasma clearance exceeds that of renal excretion by 10% to 20%. Thereafter, an equilibrium is maintained. The initial lag phase represents saturation of binding sites in tissues (eg, renal cortex). The half-life of tissue-bound aminoglycoside is long (eg, 30 to 700 hours), and these drugs can be recovered in the urine for 20 days or longer after discontinuation of therapy.

Dosage Determinations

The following factors apply to parenterally administered aminoglycosides:

(1) The aminoglycosides have a low therapeutic index, ie, there is a narrow range between serum concentrations that are therapeutically effective and those that are toxic.

(2) Results of a number of studies have shown that adequate peak serum aminoglycoside concentrations are associated with desired therapeutic response (Noone et al, 1974; Zaske et al, 1982 A; Moore et al, 1984 C, 1984 D, 1987) and that subinhibitory serum aminoglycoside concentrations can result in treatment failures (Jackson and Riff, 1971; Anderson et al, 1976).

(3) A correlation between excessive serum aminoglycoside concentrations, particularly when they are maintained throughout the course of therapy, and the toxicity (ototoxicity, nephrotoxicity) caused by these agents also is accepted by most infectious disease experts (for reviews, see Zaske, 1986; Wenk et al, 1984). For gentamicin, tobramycin, amikacin, kanamycin, and netilmicin, sustained peak concentrations greater than 12, 12, 35, 35, or 16 mcg/ml, respectively, and trough concentrations greater than 2, 2, 10, 10, or 4 mcg/ml, respectively, have been associated with an increased probability of ototoxicity and nephrotoxicity.

(4) The relationship between standard doses of aminoglycosides and the serum drug concentrations that are attained is generally poor because wide variations in aminoglycoside pharmacokinetics, particularly in volumes of distribution and elimination rates, exist among patients. Thus, standard aminoglycoside dosage regimens may require modification to account for these variables.

Because of the above, serum concentrations of aminoglycosides should be monitored to assure adequate therapeutic levels and to avoid potentially toxic concentrations. This is particularly important in seriously ill or poorly responding patients and for those individuals who are likely to require dosage adjustments. These include (1) patients with pre-existing renal disease; (2) patients with rapidly changing renal function or fluid status; (3) elderly patients; (4) obese patients; (5) patients with sepsis; (6) febrile patients who may have supranormal renal clearance; (7) patients with altered or changing volumes of distribution due to conditions such as cirrhosis (ascites) or heart failure (edema); (8) burn patients; (9) cystic fibrosis patients; (10) patients receiving other drugs that can affect aminoglycoside serum concentrations (eg, antipseudomonal penicillins that can inactivate aminoglycosides in vivo in patients with renal dysfunction; potent diuretics); (11) azotemic patients on dialysis (aminoglycosides are dialyzable molecules); and (12) neonates.

Guidelines have been established to help the clinician obtain peak and trough serum aminoglycoside concentrations that will produce a favorable therapeutic outcome with a minimum risk of toxicity. The desired peak concentrations range from 6 to 10 mcg/ml for gentamicin, tobramycin, and netilmicin and 20 to 30 mcg/ml for amikacin. The desired trough concentrations are 0.5 to 2 mcg/ml for gentamicin, tobramycin, and netilmicin and 1 to 8 mcg/ml for amikacin. Within these guidelines, a dosing protocol may be designed to achieve higher peak concentrations but avoid excessive trough concentrations for patients with more severe infections (eg, gram-negative sepsis or pneumonia) or infections with less susceptible isolates (Zaske, 1986).

Peak concentrations are attained approximately 30 minutes after completion of a 30- to 60-minute intravenous infusion or one hour after an intramuscular injection. Trough concentrations are considered to occur within 15 minutes of the next dose under steady-state conditions (Zaske, 1986). Serum concentration data can be used optimally only if the exact times for beginning and ending an intravenous infusion (or the time of an intramuscular injection) and the exact times for obtaining serum samples are known. A number of fast and reliable assay methods for aminoglycosides are available (see Wenk et al, 1984).

Individualization of aminoglycoside dosage regimens can be accomplished either by utilizing pharmacokinetic principles (Sawchuk and Zaske, 1976; Sawchuk et al, 1977) or by the empiric method. When available, pharmacokinetically based dosing appears to be superior to empiric determinations. In this method, three timed serum concentrations are obtained over two to three half-lives, preferably during the first dosing interval. Assuming a one-compartment model, the serum concentration-time data are then used to determine drug pharmacokinetic parameters, ie, volume of distribution, elimination rate constant. After the desired peak and trough concentrations are determined, the pharmacokinetic parameters are used to calculate the dose and dosage interval. Equations and programs for computers and programmable calculators are available to "fit" the serum concentration-time data, calculate pharmacokinetic parameters, and determine the dosage regimen. Serum concentrations should be monitored periodically throughout the course of therapy and dosage adjustments made to control serum concentrations (see Zaske, 1986).

The Sawchuk-Zaske individualized pharmacokinetic dosing method has been evaluated extensively with gentamicin (Zaske et al, 1982 B) in burn (Zaske et al, 1982 A), surgical (Zaske et al, 1980), gynecologic (Zaske et al, 1981), and elderly (Zaske et al, 1982 C) patients. It also has been tested in a limited number of patients given tobramycin (Cipolle et al, 1980), netilmicin (Rotschafer et al, 1983), or amikacin (Zaske, 1986). In all of these studies, wide interpatient variation in pharmacokinetic parameters was observed and dosages both below and above those used in "standard" regimens were necessary to achieve desired peak and trough serum concentrations. Measured peak and trough serum concentrations obtained with this pharmacokinetic dosing method were in close agreement with predicted values. Furthermore, the incidence of nephrotoxicity was less than 2% and ototoxicity was not observed. In burn patients, survival was significantly increased in patients receiving individualized dosages of gentamicin when compared with those given standard dosage regimens (Zaske et al, 1982 A), and pharmacokinetically based dosing was determined to be cost-beneficial in these patients (Bootman et al, 1979).

When pharmacokinetically based dosing is not available, individualization of aminoglycoside dosage regimens can be done by the empiric method. Peak and trough serum concentrations can be measured, and doses and dosage intervals can then be adjusted using empirical judgments in order to achieve acceptable results. For example, once the initial dosage regimen has been selected, peak and trough serum concentrations should be determined after the steady-state level has been achieved (four to five drug half-lives). In critically ill patients, a peak concentration also should be determined after the loading dose to ensure that it is within the desired therapeutic range. A trough concentration usually is obtained about the fifth to seventh day and intermittently thereafter as an indication of drug accumulation (NOTE: Some experts recommend monitoring peak and trough concentrations beginning on the second or third day). Patients who are likely to need dosage adjustments during therapy (eg, due to changes in volume of distribution or renal function) will require more intensive monitoring.

The empiric method is useful when the patient is at steady state and the clinician is skilled in collecting and using the data. Otherwise, many dosage errors can occur because important parameters, such as the dose, time of infusion, and time of sample collection, frequently are inaccurately known. Also, the empiric method usually requires more time than the pharmacokinetically based dosing method for optimal adjustment of dosage (Zaske, 1986).

A number of nomograms also are available to help determine the appropriate dosage of aminoglycosides in patients with normal renal function and in those with various degrees of renal impairment. Unfortunately, these predictive algorithms generally are based on the invalid assumptions of a constant volume of distribution for all patients and that creatinine clearance (or serum creatinine) has a high degree of correlation with aminoglycoside clearance (Zaske, 1986).

Thus, there can be substantial variation in serum concentrations achieved with the use of these nomograms when compared to predicted values (Lesar et al, 1982). Nomograms do provide acceptable initial dosage guidelines, however, with further dosage adjustment depending on measured peak and trough serum concentrations (Zaske, 1986).

Dosage guidelines based on predictive nomograms also can be used when serum aminoglycoside concentrations cannot be measured. The method of Sarubbi and Hull (1978), which is applicable to gentamicin, tobramycin, amikacin, kanamycin, and netilmicin, generally is preferred. This method uses estimates of renal function, lean body weight, age, and sex to predict required dosage regimens. The method allows the physician to select a different dose or dosing interval for patients who have varying degrees of renal function and severity of infection. The procedure is as follows:

An appropriate loading dose, expressed in mg/kg of ideal body weight, is selected from the dosing chart (see the Table) to attain a peak serum concentration (mcg/ml) in the desired range. Because the aminoglycoside antibiotics are poorly distributed in adipose tissue, the loading dose is calculated using the lean (or ideal) body weight of the patient in order to avoid excessive serum concentrations in obese patients. Ideal (nonobese) body weight is calculated as follows:

Male Ideal Weight = 50 kg + 2.3 kg for every inch over 5 feet

Female Ideal Weight = 45.5 kg + 2.3 kg for every inch over 5 feet

NOTE: Other data have shown that aminoglycosides are partially distributed in adipose tissue and that use of only the ideal body weight for dose determinations may result in unduly low serum concentrations. Thus, many experts recommend that the dose for obese patients be calculated on the basis of a corrected weight that equals the sum of the ideal body weight plus 40% of the excess adipose mass (Schwartz et al, 1978; Bauer et al, 1983).

Maintenance dosage is based on the weight-corrected creatinine clearance [C(c)cr] of the patient. This value can be calculated for males and females as follows:

$$C(c)cr\ male = \frac{140 - age}{serum\ creatinine}$$

$$C(c)cr\ female = 0.85 \times C(c)cr\ male$$

The maintenance dose is then calculated as a percentage of the loading dose according to the corrected clearance determination and can be administered every 8, 12, or 24 hours as shown in the Table. The interval between doses should be extended to 12 or 24 hours as C(c)cr declines (eg, to less than 50% of the loading dose) in order to avoid drug accumulation and elevated trough serum concentrations.

Use of Single Daily-Dose Regimens: The administration of aminoglycosides in multiple daily doses is an established practice for treatment of infections caused by susceptible organisms. However, recent research suggests that these agents may be given to selected patients in single daily doses without loss of efficacy and with a similar (or reduced) risk of toxicity compared with administration of the same amount of drug in a standard divided-dose regimen. This possibility was first suggested by the results of in vitro studies showing that the extent and rate of bacterial killing and the duration of the PAE of aminoglycosides are proportional to the drug concentration (see Gilbert, 1991).

AMINOGLYCOSIDE DOSING CHART

1. Select Loading Dose in mg/kg (IDEAL WEIGHT) to provide peak serum concentrations in range listed below for desired aminoglycoside.

Aminoglycoside	Usual Loading Dose	Expected Peak Serum Concentrations
Tobramycin Gentamicin	1.5 to 2 mg/kg	4 to 10 mcg/ml
Amikacin Kanamycin	5 to 7.5 mg/kg	15 to 30 mcg/ml
Netilmicin	1.3 to 3.25 mg/kg*	4 to 12 mcg/ml*

2. Select Maintenance Dose (as percentage of chosen loading dose) to continue peak serum concentrations indicated above according to desired dosing interval and the patient's corrected creatinine clearance.

Percentage of Loading Dose Required for Dosage Interval Selected

C(c)cr (ml/min)	Half-life** (hours)	8 hours	12 hours	24 hours
90	3.1	84%	—	—
80	3.4	80	91%	—
70	3.9	76	88	—
60	4.5	71	84	—
50	5.3	65	79	—
40	6.5	57	72	92%
30	8.4	48	63	86
25	9.9	—	57	81
20	11.9	—	50	75
17	13.6	—	46	70
15	15.1	—	—	67
12	17.9	—	—	61
10***	20.4	—	—	56
7	25.9	—	—	47
5	31.5	—	—	41
2	46.8	—	—	30
0	69.3	—	—	21

** Values for netilmicin were obtained from the manufacturer's literature.*

*** Alternatively, one-half of the chosen loading dose may be given at an interval approximately equal to the estimated half-life.*

**** Dosing for patients with C(c)cr < 10 ml/min should be assisted by measured serum levels.*

Adapted from Sarubbi and Hull, 1978.

Studies in animal models provide additional support for this concept, indicating that the antibacterial efficacy of aminoglycosides is greater and the occurrence of toxicity is lower with single-dose regimens that produce substantially higher peak serum concentrations and larger AUCs than with intermittent boluses or constant infusions. Furthermore, results of studies in rats, mice, and rabbits suggest that during the interval between single daily doses, the serum aminoglycoside concentrations can fall below the MIC of the infecting pathogen without loss of efficacy because of the substantial PAE of these drugs (Kapusnik and Sande, 1986; Drusano, 1988; Mattie et al, 1989; Gilbert, 1991). These results with aminoglycosides differ from those obtained with β lactams, which, because they have little or no PAE, must be given at intervals that do not allow the serum concentrations to fall below the MIC in order to be effective in humans and neutropenic animals (Drusano, 1988).

Single-dose regimens have been investigated in humans with infections at a variety of sites (Kovarik et al, 1989; Gilbert, 1991; Nordström et al, 1990; Pechère et al, 1991). Although much of the available data are from nonrandomized, noncomparative studies, the results of several recent randomized trials provide strong support for considering their use in selected patients. For example, one study in elderly patients with severe bacterial infections (primarily urinary and respiratory tracts) compared the efficacy and toxicity of netilmicin given at an average daily dose of approximately 4 mg/kg in a single bolus or the same dose in three divided intravenous infusions (in combination with single daily doses of ceftriaxone) (ter Braak et al, 1990). In patients who received netilmicin once daily, the favorable response rate was comparable to that observed in those given the aminoglycoside in the conventional regimen. Although the overall incidence of ototoxicity or nephrotoxicity was similar, nephrotoxicity was significantly delayed in patients who received prolonged treatment with the single-dose regimen. In two additional randomized trials, patients received netilmicin (4.5 or 6 mg/kg daily) plus metronidazole (Hollender et al, 1989) or tinidazole (de Vries et al, 1990) for the treatment of mixed flora intra-abdominal infections. The clinical and bacteriologic responses were equivalent whether the aminoglycoside was given as a single daily dose or the same amount was given in three divided doses. In both studies, the incidence of auditory, vestibular, or renal dysfunction was similar. Finally, in an interim report of an ongoing randomized trial in patients with serious systemic bacterial infections, amikacin 15 mg/kg given once daily with a β-lactam antibiotic (piperacillin or ampicillin) or clindamycin appears to be clinically and bacteriologically equivalent to amikacin 7.5 mg/kg given twice daily and no difference in toxicity has been noted (Maller et al, 1991).

Thus, the evidence at the present time suggests that the administration of standard doses of aminoglycosides in single daily bolus infusions or intramuscular injections produces therapeutic outcomes that are equivalent or superior to those produced by traditional divided-dose regimens in normosthenuric patients with serious systemic bacterial infections. The incidence of auditory, vestibular, or renal toxicity with single-dose therapy does not appear to be significantly different from that associated with traditional dosing schedules, despite the production of significantly higher (but transient) peak serum concentrations. Compared with multiple-dose administration, single bolus dosing also may be less costly and more advantageous for the patient and hospital staff. However, because severely neutropenic (granulocyte count <1000/mm^3) patients have been excluded from most studies and the most effective therapy for bacterial infections in this group is not established (Hughes et al, 1990), the single-dose regimen is not recommended for these patients. Furthermore, it will still be necessary to determine initial peak serum concentrations and regularly monitor trough levels to detect possible accumulation of these drugs and prevent the occurrence of ototoxic and nephrotoxic side effects.

Drug Evaluations

Parenteral Aminoglycosides

AMIKACIN SULFATE

[Amikin]

Amikacin is a semisynthetic, water-soluble acylated derivative of kanamycin A. Acylation of susceptible hydroxyl and amino groups protects them from aminoglycoside-inactivating enzymes, thus making amikacin resistant to most of the enzymes that inactivate kanamycin, gentamicin, tobramycin, and netilmicin.

MECHANISM OF ACTION, ANTIMICROBIAL SPECTRUM, AND RESISTANCE. Amikacin primarily is active against aerobic gram-negative bacilli, including the Enterobacteriaceae and *Pseudomonas aeruginosa*. It also is active against *Staphylococcus aureus, Mycobacterium tuberculosis*, and certain atypical mycobacteria (eg, *M. fortuitum*).

In vitro, amikacin is somewhat less potent on a weight basis than either gentamicin or tobramycin. However, this is not clinically significant because amikacin also is less toxic on a weight basis and larger doses can be administered.

Amikacin is susceptible to only two of the known aminoglycoside-inactivating enzymes (see the Introduction). Therefore, it is active against many gentamicin- and tobramycin-resistant strains of aerobic gram-negative bacilli. Bacterial strains that are resistant to amikacin usually have a defective aminoglycoside transport mechanism. These mutants exhibit cross-resistance to all other aminoglycosides.

See also the Introduction.

USES. Amikacin is used to treat serious infections caused by susceptible aerobic gram-negative bacilli (eg, a number of the Enterobacteriaceae, *P. aeruginosa*). Such infections include bacteremias; intra-abdominal, soft tissue (including burns), bone or joint, lower respiratory tract, and complicated urinary tract infections; and meningitis.

The major advantage of amikacin is its superior resistance profile (see previous section and the Introduction). Thus, it is the aminoglycoside of choice for infections caused by aerobic gram-negative bacilli that are known or suspected to be resistant to other aminoglycosides. It should be the aminoglycoside of choice for general use in hospitals where the prevalence of resistance to gentamicin and tobramycin is known to be high or when there is concern about gentamicin- and tobramycin-resistant gram-negative bacilli in a particular clinical situation.

Because amikacin is the only currently available aminoglycoside effective against many gentamicin- and tobramycin-resistant organisms, many infectious disease experts have felt that its use should be restricted to minimize the emergence of additional resistant strains. However, there is no evidence that such restriction has delayed the emergence of resistance (see Lietman, 1990; Edson and Terrell, 1991; Reese and Betts, 1991). Furthermore, reports from hospitals that rely on amikacin as the primary aminoglycoside suggest that resistance to amikacin does not increase despite widespread use and gentamicin/tobramycin resistance actually may decrease (Berk et al, 1986). Nevertheless, general use of amikacin in hospitals without a gentamicin or tobramycin resistance problem remains controversial. Amikacin is considerably more expensive than gentamicin, an important consideration in a cost-conscious environment. For a detailed discussion of aminoglycoside drug selection, see the Introduction.

ADVERSE REACTIONS AND PRECAUTIONS. Toxicity caused by amikacin in humans does not appear to be significantly different in incidence or severity from that caused by gentamicin or tobramycin. For a detailed discussion, see the Introduction.

Amikacin is classified in FDA Pregnancy Category D.

DRUG INTERACTIONS. When compared with gentamicin and tobramycin, amikacin is less susceptible to inactivation by antipseudomonal penicillins (eg, ticarcillin) both in vitro and in vivo in patients with renal failure. Amikacin may have advantages in patients with renal failure who require concurrent therapy with an antipseudomonal penicillin. For a detailed discussion of this and other drug interactions, see the Introduction.

PHARMACOKINETICS. For a detailed discussion of the pharmacokinetics of the parenterally administered aminoglycosides, see the Introduction.

Although amikacin pharmacokinetics may be more predictable than those of gentamicin and tobramycin (Holm et al, 1983; Cunha, 1988, 1990; see also the Introduction), wide interpatient variation has been reported (Bauer and Blouin, 1983; Zaske, 1986). Theoretically, amikacin may achieve a higher therapeutic ratio against those bacterial strains with minimum inhibitory concentrations that are similar for gentamicin, tobramycin, and amikacin because higher serum concentrations of amikacin can be achieved (Dyas et al, 1983).

DOSAGE AND PREPARATIONS. The following are standard dosages. However, monitoring of aminoglycoside serum concentrations and individualization of dosage regimens, preferably based on pharmacokinetic principles (eg, Sawchuk-Zaske method), is recommended, particularly for seriously ill or poorly responsive patients and for other high-risk individuals in whom dosage adjustments are likely to be necessary (eg, the elderly, neonates, patients with impaired renal function or changing volumes of distribution). Predictive nomograms (eg, Sarubbi-Hull) may provide acceptable dosage guidelines for initiation of treatment. For detailed discussion, see the Introduction.

For amikacin, prolonged peak serum concentrations that exceed 35 mcg/ml and trough serum levels greater than 10 mcg/ml should be avoided (Meyer, 1981; see also the Introduction).

Intramuscular, Intravenous: When given intravenously, amikacin can be diluted in 5% dextrose or isotonic sodium chloride injection and should be infused over a 30- to 60-minute period in adults and children and a one- to two-hour period in infants.

Uncomplicated infections caused by susceptible organisms usually respond in 24 to 48 hours. If a response is not observed in three to five days, bacterial susceptibility should be redetermined and therapy re-evaluated. For both adults and children, the duration of therapy should not exceed ten days except in unusual circumstances.

Patients with normal renal function: Adults, children, and older infants, 15 mg/kg daily in equally divided doses at 12- or 8-hour intervals. The total daily dose for heavier adults should not exceed 1.5 g. When indicated for uncomplicated urinary tract infections in adults, 250 mg twice daily is frequently sufficient. *Neonates* should be given a loading dose of 10 mg/kg, followed by 7.5 mg/kg every 12 hours.

Patients with impaired renal function: Dosage modification is indicated. Amikacin serum concentrations should be monitored to help determine dosage (see above and the Introduction). If these measurements are unavailable or unreliable, amikacin may be given to *adults* according to the dosing chart proposed by Sarubbi and Hull (see the Introduction).

Amikin (Apothecon). Solution (sterile) 50 mg/ml in 2 ml containers, 250 mg/ml in 2 and 4 ml containers, and 500 mg/2 ml syringe for injection.

GENTAMICIN SULFATE
[Garamycin]

Gentamicin is a mixture of three closely related antibacterial substances (gentamicins C_1, C_2, and C_{1A}) obtained from cultures of *Micromonospora purpurea*.

MECHANISM OF ACTION, ANTIMICROBIAL SPECTRUM, AND RESISTANCE. Gentamicin primarily is active against aerobic gram-negative bacilli, including the Enterobacteriaceae and *Pseudomonas aeruginosa*. It also is active against *Staphylococcus aureus*.

In vitro, the potency of gentamicin is similar to that of tobramycin for most bacterial species; it is somewhat more potent on a weight basis than amikacin and kanamycin. Gentamicin generally is more active in vitro than tobramycin against *Serratia*, but it is less active against *P. aeruginosa*.

Gentamicin-resistant strains of Enterobacteriaceae and *P. aeruginosa* are prevalent in some hospitals; cross-resistance with tobramycin is common. Many of these strains are susceptible to amikacin, which is resistant to most aminoglycoside-inactivating enzymes.

See also the Introduction.

USES. This aminoglycoside is used to treat serious infections caused by aerobic gram-negative bacilli (eg, a number of the Enterobacteriaceae, *P. aeruginosa*). These include lower respiratory tract, intra-abdominal, soft tissue, bone or joint, wound, and complicated urinary tract infections; bacteremias; and meningitis (by intrathecal administration; see Dosage and Preparations).

Gentamicin often is the preferred aminoglycoside for general use in hospitals where the prevalence of bacterial resistance to this agent is low (based on locally generated antimicrobial susceptibility profiles). Its major advantage over tobramycin, amikacin, and netilmicin is lower cost. The empiric use of gentamicin or tobramycin is not justified in hospitals where gentamicin resistance is common; amikacin is the aminoglycoside of choice in these locales. For a detailed discussion of aminoglycoside drug selection for aerobic gram-negative bacillary infections, see the Introduction.

The combination of gentamicin plus penicillin G (or ampicillin) exhibits synergistic activity against enterococci (eg, *Enterococcus faecalis*) and viridans streptococci and frequently is the regimen of choice for the treatment of endocarditis caused by these organisms. Streptomycin is an alternative to gentamicin for streptomycin-susceptible strains of enterococci. Enterococcal clinical isolates with high-level resistance to gentamicin and other aminoglycosides (minimum inhibitory concentrations, >2,000 mcg/ml) have been reported. Therapy for endocarditis caused by these gentamicin-resistant enterococci is not established, but some isolates do remain susceptible to streptomycin, which may be given with penicillin to treat this infection (see index entry Cardiovascular Infections; see also the Introduction and the evaluation on Streptomycin Sulfate).

Gentamicin is recommended by the American Heart Association for parenteral prophylactic use with ampicillin or vancomycin in patients who are at high risk of developing bacterial endocarditis but are unable to take the standard oral regimen prior to undergoing invasive procedures involving the oral cavity and upper respiratory, gastrointestinal, or genitourinary tract (Dajani et al, 1990). For additional details and treatment guidelines, see index entry Endocarditis.

For other uses of gentamicin, either alone or in combination, see the Introduction.

ADVERSE REACTIONS AND PRECAUTIONS. For a detailed discussion, see the Introduction. This drug is classified in FDA Pregnancy Category C.

DRUG INTERACTIONS. Gentamicin appears to be more readily inactivated by antipseudomonal penicillins (eg, ticarcillin) than amikacin both in vitro and in vivo in patients with renal failure. For a detailed discussion of this and other drug interactions, see the Introduction.

PHARMACOKINETICS. For a detailed discussion of the pharmacokinetics of the parenterally administered aminoglycosides, see the Introduction.

DOSAGE AND PREPARATIONS. The following are standard dosages for gentamicin. However, monitoring of aminoglycoside serum concentrations and individualization of dosage regimens, preferably based on pharmacokinetic principles (eg, Sawchuk-Zaske method), is recommended, particularly for seriously ill or poorly responding patients and for other high-risk individuals in whom dosage adjustments are likely to be necessary (eg, the elderly, neonates, patients with impaired renal function or changing volumes of distribution). Predictive nomograms (eg, Sarubbi-Hull) may provide acceptable dosage guidelines for initiation of treatment. For detailed discussion, see the Introduction.

For gentamicin, prolonged peak serum concentrations that exceed 12 mcg/ml and trough serum levels greater than 2 mcg/ml should be avoided (see the Introduction).

Intramuscular, Intravenous: When given intravenously, gentamicin can be diluted in 5% dextrose or isotonic sodium chloride injection and administered over 30 to 60 minutes. The total duration of therapy by either route generally should not exceed ten days.

Patients with normal renal function: Adults, 3 to 5 mg/kg daily in three equally divided doses every eight hours. The larger dose is used only for life-threatening infections. *Children,* 6 to 7.5 mg/kg daily in three equally divided doses every eight hours. *Infants 1 week or older,* 7.5 mg/kg daily in three equally divided doses every eight hours. *Premature or full-term neonates less than 1 week,* 5 mg/kg daily in two divided doses every 12 hours.

For dosages for the treatment and prophylaxis of bacterial endocarditis, see index entry Endocarditis.

Patients with impaired renal function: Dosage modification is indicated. Gentamicin serum concentrations should be monitored to help determine dosage (see above and the Introduction). If these measurements are unavailable or unreliable, gentamicin may be given to *adults* according to the dosing chart proposed by Sarubbi and Hull (see the Introduction).

Patients undergoing hemodialysis: Adults, for most infections, 1 to 1.7 mg/kg (depending on the severity of infection) at the end of each six-hour dialysis period. *Children,* 2 mg/kg at the end of each six-hour dialysis period. Gentamicin serum levels must be measured in patients undergoing dialysis.

Garamycin (Schering), ***Generic.*** Solution (sterile) 10 mg/ml (pediatric) in 2 ml containers and 40 mg/ml in 1.5, 2, and 20 ml containers (strengths expressed in terms of the base).

Gentamicin I.V. Piggyback Injection (Lypho-Med). Ready-to-use intravenous piggyback unit containing 1 mg of gentamicin per ml of intravenous solution (0.9% sodium chloride injection) supplied in 60 ml (60-mg dose), 80 ml (80-mg dose), and 100 ml (100-mg dose) units.

Generic. Ready-to-use intravenous solutions containing 60, 80, or 100 mg doses of gentamicin in 60, 80, or 100 ml of 5% dextrose or 40, 60, 70, 80, 90, 100, or 120 mg doses of gentamicin in 50 or 100 ml of 0.9% sodium chloride injection (see manufacturers' literature for specific preparations).

Additional Trademark.
Jenamicin (Hauck).

Intrathecal: Direct administration of a preservative-free gentamicin preparation into the cerebrospinal fluid is intended as adjunctive therapy in patients with central nervous system infections. Although dosage depends on factors such as age and weight of the patient, site of injection, degree of obstruction to cerebrospinal fluid flow, amount of cerebrospinal fluid estimated to be present, and concomitant treatment with intramuscular or intravenous gentamicin, generally recommended dosages are: *adults,* 4 to 8 mg once daily; *children and infants 3 months and older,* 1 to 2 mg once daily.

Garamycin Intrathecal (Schering). Solution (sterile, preservative-free) 2 mg/ml in 2 ml containers.

KANAMYCIN SULFATE
[Kantrex]

Kanamycin is derived from *Streptomyces kanamyceticus*. It is a mixture of kanamycins A (more than 95%) and B (less than 5%).

MECHANISM OF ACTION, ANTIMICROBIAL SPECTRUM, AND RESISTANCE. Kanamycin is active against aerobic gram-negative bacilli, principally members of the Enterobacteriaceae. Unlike gentamicin, tobramycin, amikacin, and netilmicin, it is not active against *Pseudomonas aeruginosa*. Strains of *Mycobacterium tuberculosis* and *Staphylococcus aureus* frequently are sensitive to kanamycin.

Kanamycin is susceptible to a number of aminoglycoside-inactivating enzymes, and kanamycin-resistant bacterial strains are prevalent in many geographic locations.

See also the Introduction.

USES. Bacterial resistance to kanamycin is common and other aminoglycosides (gentamicin, tobramycin, amikacin, netilmicin) are usually preferred for systemic use. Also, kanamycin is not effective against infections caused by *P. aeruginosa*. For a detailed discussion of aminoglycoside drug selection, see the Introduction.

Kanamycin may be used in combination therapy for treatment of active tuberculosis only if susceptibility studies indicate its value over other primary and secondary antituberculous drugs. Since this is relatively uncommon, kanamycin is rarely used in tuberculosis therapy.

Oral kanamycin is an alternative to oral neomycin to suppress the bacterial flora of the bowel as a prophylactic measure before elective colorectal surgery.

ADVERSE REACTIONS AND PRECAUTIONS. Kanamycin may produce irreversible ototoxicity. Both the hearing (cochlear) and equilibrium (vestibular) functions may be affected, but this aminoglycoside usually has been associated with auditory toxicity. For a detailed discussion, see the Introduction.

Although intestinal absorption of kanamycin is poor, caution must be exercised when it is given orally to patients with renal insufficiency, since toxic serum levels may result because of unanticipated absorption through the gastrointestinal epithelium. As with neomycin, a malabsorption syndrome may occur after prolonged oral administration.

Kanamycin is classified in FDA Pregnancy Category D.

DRUG INTERACTIONS AND PHARMACOKINETICS. See the Introduction.

DOSAGE AND PREPARATIONS. The following are standard dosages for kanamycin. However, monitoring of aminoglycoside serum concentrations and individualization of dosage regimens, preferably based on pharmacokinetic principles (eg, Sawchuk-Zaske method), is recommended, particularly for seriously ill or poorly responding patients and for other high-risk individuals in whom dosage adjustments are likely to be necessary (eg, the elderly, neonates, patients with impaired renal function or changing volumes of distribution). Predictive nomograms (eg, Sarubbi-Hull) may provide acceptable dosage guidelines for initiation of treatment. For detailed discussion, see the Introduction.

For kanamycin, prolonged peak serum concentrations that exceed 35 mcg/ml and trough serum levels greater than 10 mcg/ml should be avoided (see the Introduction).

Intramuscular, Intravenous: When the intravenous route must be used, the drug should be diluted to 2.5 to 5 mg/ml in normal sodium chloride injection or 5% dextrose injection and the appropriate dose infused slowly over a 30- to 60-minute period. Duration of therapy with parenteral kanamycin generally should not exceed ten days.

Adults, children, and older infants with normal renal function, 15 mg/kg daily in two equally divided doses every 12 hours (occasionally, an eight-hour interval is used). The maximum daily dose in adults is 1.5 g. *Neonates up to 1 week with normal renal function who weigh 2 kg or less*, 15 mg/kg daily in two equally divided doses every 12 hours. *Neonates up to 1 week with normal renal function who weigh more than 2 kg,* 20 mg/kg daily in two equally divided doses every 12 hours.

Patients with impaired renal function: Dosage modification is indicated and should be determined on the basis of serum concentrations (see above and the Introduction). If this cannot be done, the dosing chart proposed by Sarubbi and Hull can be used for *adults* (see the Introduction).

Kantrex (Apothecon), ***Generic.*** Solution (sterile) 37.5 (pediatric) and 250 mg/ml in 2 ml containers and 333 mg/ml in 3 ml containers (strengths expressed in terms of the base).

Oral (not for systemic effects): *Adults,* as an adjunct in extended therapy of hepatic coma, 8 to 12 g daily in divided doses. *Adults*, as an adjunct in short-term mechanical cleansing of the large bowel, 1 g every hour for four hours, followed by 1 g every six hours for 36 to 72 hours. *Infants and children,* for suppression of bowel flora, 150 to 250 mg/kg daily in divided doses every hour to every six hours (Nelson, 1991).

Kantrex (Apothecon). Capsules equivalent to 500 mg of base.

NETILMICIN SULFATE
[Netromycin]

Netilmicin, a semisynthetic aminoglycoside, is the 1-N-ethyl derivative of sisomicin.

MECHANISM OF ACTION, ANTIMICROBIAL SPECTRUM, AND RESISTANCE. Netilmicin primarily is active against aerobic gram-negative bacilli, including the Enterobacteriaceae and *Pseudomonas aeruginosa*. It also is active against *Staphylococcus aureus*. In general, the in vitro potency of netilmicin is similar to that of gentamicin and tobramycin. However, netilmicin is less active against *P. aeruginosa* than these aminoglycosides. The clinical significance of this difference is unknown (*Med Lett Drugs Ther*, 1983; Craig et al, 1983).

Netilmicin is susceptible to fewer aminoglycoside-inactivating enzymes than gentamicin and tobramycin, and some gram-negative bacilli that are resistant to these latter agents will be susceptible to netilmicin. However, most of these strains are susceptible to amikacin as well, and amikacin also is active against most netilmicin-resistant strains of these bacteria. Thus, netilmicin does not appear to offer any advantages in spectrum of activity over amikacin for the treatment of gentamicin- or tobramycin-resistant organisms (*Med Lett Drugs Ther*, 1983; Craig et al, 1983; Pancoast, 1988).

See also the Introduction.

USES. Netilmicin is administered to treat serious infections caused by aerobic gram-negative bacilli (eg, a number of Enterobacteriaceae, *P. aeruginosa*). These include bacteremias and lower respiratory tract, intra-abdominal, soft tissue, bone or joint, wound, and complicated urinary tract infections.

The clinical role of netilmicin is unresolved. In situations in which gentamicin- or tobramycin-resistant bacterial strains are unlikely, the efficacy of netilmicin appears to be no greater than that of these older analogues. Gentamicin is considerably less expensive than netilmicin. When gentamicin or tobramycin resistance is a problem, the drug of choice for empiric therapy is amikacin because it is least susceptible to enzymatic inactivation. However, netilmicin is an effective alternative for susceptible bacterial isolates and is less expensive than amikacin (see the Introduction). Current evidence suggests that netilmicin is inherently less ototoxic than the other aminoglycosides. Thus, this drug may have advantages in patients at high risk for ototoxicity, particularly when individualized dosing methods are not employed (see the following section and the Introduction).

ADVERSE REACTIONS AND PRECAUTIONS. In animal studies, netilmicin was less ototoxic and nephrotoxic than gentamicin, tobramycin, and amikacin (Szot and Tabachnick, 1980). Although these differences have not been demonstrated unequivocally in humans, results of comparative studies suggest that less ototoxicity is associated with the use of netilmicin than with other aminoglycosides (Buring et al, 1988; Kahlmeter and Dahlager, 1984; Lerner et al, 1983).

For a detailed discussion of aminoglycoside adverse reactions and precautions, see the Introduction. This drug is classified in FDA Pregnancy Category D.

DRUG INTERACTIONS. Netilmicin was reported to be less susceptible to inactivation by antipseudomonal penicillins (eg, ticarcillin) in vitro than gentamicin and tobramycin (Pickering and Rutherford, 1981). For a detailed discussion of this and other drug interactions, see the Introduction.

PHARMACOKINETICS. For a detailed discussion of the pharmacokinetics of the parenterally administered aminoglycosides, see the Introduction.

DOSAGE AND PREPARATIONS. The following are standard dosages for netilmicin cited in the manufacturer's literature. However, monitoring of aminoglycoside serum concentrations and individualization of dosage regimens, preferably based on pharmacokinetic principles (eg, Sawchuk-Zaske method), is recommended, particularly for seriously ill or poorly responding patients and for other high-risk individuals in whom dosage adjustments are likely to be necessary (eg, the elderly, neonates, patients with impaired renal function or changing volumes of distribution). Predictive nomograms (eg, Sarubbi-Hull) may provide acceptable dosage guidelines for initiation of treatment. For detailed discussion, see the Introduction.

For netilmicin, prolonged peak serum concentrations that exceed 16 mcg/ml and trough serum levels greater than 4 mcg/ml should be avoided (manufacturer's literature; see also the Introduction).

Intramuscular, Intravenous: When given intravenously in *adults*, a single dose of netilmicin injection may be diluted in 50 to 200 ml of various parenteral solutions (see manufacturer's literature for a list of compatible parenteral solutions). In infants and children, the volume of diluent is decreased according to the fluid requirements of the patient. The solution may be infused over a period of 30 minutes to two hours.

The duration of therapy with netilmicin usually ranges from 7 to 14 days.

Patients with normal renal function: *Adults with serious systemic infections,* 4 to 6.5 mg/kg daily in equally divided doses every 8 to 12 hours. *Adults with complicated urinary tract infections*, 3 to 4 mg/kg daily in equally divided doses every 12 hours. *Infants and children (6 weeks through 12 years)*, 5.5 to 8 mg/kg daily in equally divided doses every 8 to 12 hours. *Neonates (less than 6 weeks)*, 4 to 6.5 mg/kg daily in equally divided doses every 12 hours.

Patients with impaired renal function: Dosage modification is indicated. Netilmicin serum concentrations should be monitored to help determine dosage (see above and the Introduction). If these measurements are unavailable or unreliable, netilmicin may be given to *adults* according to the dosing chart proposed by Sarubbi and Hull (see the Introduction).

Netromycin (Schering). Solution (sterile) 100 mg/ml in 1.5 ml containers.

STREPTOMYCIN SULFATE

Streptomycin is derived from *Streptomyces griseus*.

MECHANISM OF ACTION, ANTIMICROBIAL SPECTRUM, AND RESISTANCE. Although this drug has a broad spectrum of activity in vitro against common aerobic gram-negative bacilli (eg, Enterobacteriaceae), the widespread emergence of resistant strains has rendered it clinically obsolete for infections caused by these organisms. Naturally resistant organisms include *Pseudomonas aeruginosa*, most gram-positive organisms, anaerobic bacteria, rickettsiae, fungi, and viruses.

See also the Introduction.

USES. Streptomycin frequently is the preferred drug in the treatment of tularemia, plague, severe brucellosis (in combination with a tetracycline or chloramphenicol), and glanders (in combination with a tetracycline or chloramphenicol). It is an alternative agent in rat bite fever. See index entry Streptomycin. It also has been used in granuloma inguinale and chancroid, but other drugs currently are preferred (see index entry Sexually Transmitted Diseases). When used for the treatment of plague, streptomycin may be so rapidly bactericidal that it occasionally precipitates a Herxheimer-like reaction, which can be fatal.

This antibiotic has long been used with large doses of penicillin G (or ampicillin) to treat enterococcal endocarditis because the combination is synergistic against susceptible enterococci (see the Introduction). However, 40% to 50% of enterococcal strains are now almost totally resistant to streptomycin in vitro (eg, minimal inhibitory concentration, >2,000 mcg/ml). The combination of gentamicin and penicillin G (or ampicillin) is usually effective against streptomycin-resistant enterococci. Combinations of streptomycin and penicillin G are still commonly used for endocarditis caused by viridans streptococci, which usually are susceptible both in vitro and in vivo. See index entry Endocarditis.

Streptomycin currently is used in the treatment of tuberculosis in the United States; it is given in combination therapy when organism resistance precludes the use of isoniazid and/or rifampin, and/or parenteral management is desirable. For treatment guidelines, see index entry Tuberculosis.

ADVERSE REACTIONS AND PRECAUTIONS. This aminoglycoside frequently has been associated with vestibular toxicity. Nephrotoxicity appears to occur less commonly with streptomycin than with the other aminoglycosides.

Streptomycin causes hypersensitivity reactions ranging from skin rashes (fairly common) to exfoliative dermatitis and anaphylactic shock. Hematopoietic reactions (leukopenia, thrombocytopenia, pancytopenia, hemolytic anemia) have been reported.

Administration of streptomycin to pregnant women has been reported to affect eighth cranial nerve function in the fetus (Conway and Birt, 1965). Streptomycin should not be given with other ototoxic drugs because effects may be additive.

Streptomycin is usually administered intramuscularly. Injection should be deep into the muscle, because pain and sterile abscesses have developed with more superficial injection. The intrapleural or intrathecal route of administration is rarely, if ever, employed. The latter route has produced radiculitis, transverse myelitis, arachnoiditis, nerve root pain, and even paraplegia.

The topical application of streptomycin is contraindicated because of the high risk of sensitization and rapidly developing bacterial resistance.

For a detailed discussion of aminoglycoside adverse reactions and precautions, see the Introduction.

DRUG INTERACTIONS. See the Introduction.

PHARMACOKINETICS. See index entry Streptomycin, In Mycobacterial Infections.

DOSAGE AND PREPARATIONS. All doses are expressed in terms of the base and are for patients with normal renal function. Dosage for patients with renal impairment must be based on creatinine clearance and decreased in direct proportion to the degree of dysfunction.

Intramuscular: *Adults,* 1 to 2 g daily in divided doses every 12 hours; *children,* 20 to 30 mg/kg daily in divided doses every 12 hours *(The Medical Letter,* 1988).

For tularemia, an accepted dosage for *adults* is 2 g daily in divided doses every 12 hours; for plague, 2 g daily in divided doses every 12 hours; and for brucellosis, 1 g daily in divided doses every 12 hours together with tetracycline (Lietman, 1990).

For tuberculosis, see index entry Streptomycin, In Mycobacterial Infections. For infective endocarditis due to penicillin-sensitive streptococci (eg, viridans streptococci) and enterococcal endocarditis caused by streptomycin-susceptible enterococci, see index entry Endocarditis, Treatment.

Generic. Powder (for solution) 1, 5, 25, and 100 g (strengths expressed in terms of the base); solution 400 mg/ml in 12.5 ml containers.

TOBRAMYCIN SULFATE

[Nebcin]

This water-soluble aminoglycoside is derived from *Streptomyces tenebrarius*.

MECHANISM OF ACTION, ANTIMICROBIAL SPECTRUM, AND RESISTANCE. Tobramycin primarily is active against aerobic gram-negative bacilli, including the Enterobacteriaceae and *Pseudomonas aeruginosa*. On a weight basis, it is two to five times more active in vitro than gentamicin against *P. aeruginosa*. Strains of *P. aeruginosa* that are moderately resistant to gentamicin are usually sensitive to tobramycin. When there is a high degree of resistance to gentamicin, however, the organisms also are frequently resistant to tobramycin. This drug is usually less active in vitro than gentamicin against *Serratia marcescens*.

Cross-resistance between tobramycin and gentamicin is common, and resistant strains of aerobic gram-negative bacilli are prevalent in some hospitals. Many of these strains are susceptible to amikacin, which is resistant to most aminoglycoside-inactivating enzymes.

Most gram-positive organisms except *Staphylococcus aureus* are resistant to tobramycin. In contrast to gentamicin, this drug has poor activity in combination with penicillin G (or ampicillin) against some enterococci (essentially all strains of *Enterococcus faecium* are highly resistant).

See also the Introduction.

USES. Tobramycin is administered to treat serious infections caused by aerobic gram-negative bacilli (eg, a number of the Enterobacteriaceae, *P. aeruginosa*). These include lower respiratory tract, intra-abdominal, soft tissue, bone or joint, wound, and complicated urinary tract infections; bacteremias; and meningitis.

Tobramycin frequently is the aminoglycoside of choice for infections caused by *P. aeruginosa* because of its greater in vitro activity against this organism. However, superior clinical efficacy is unproven. It usually is given in combination with an antipseudomonal penicillin for severe, systemic *P. aeruginosa* infections (see the Introduction).

Some infectious disease experts have preferred the more costly tobramycin to gentamicin for general use in hospitals where resistance is not a problem because it appears to be less nephrotoxic. However, this does not appear to be warranted when all of the available data are evaluated. For a detailed discussion of aminoglycoside drug selection, see the Introduction.

Amikacin is the aminoglycoside of choice in hospitals where gentamicin and tobramycin resistance is a problem (see the Introduction).

ADVERSE REACTIONS AND PRECAUTIONS. For a detailed discussion, see the Introduction. This drug is classified in FDA Pregnancy Category D.

DRUG INTERACTIONS. Tobramycin appears to be more readily inactivated by antipseudomonal penicillins (eg, ticarcillin) than amikacin. For a detailed discussion of this and other drug interactions, see the Introduction.

PHARMACOKINETICS. For a detailed discussion of the pharmacokinetics of the parenterally administered aminoglycosides, see the Introduction.

DOSAGE AND PREPARATIONS. The following are standard dosages for tobramycin. However, monitoring of aminoglycoside serum concentrations and individualization of dosage regimens, preferably based on pharmacokinetic principles (eg, Sawchuk-Zaske method), is recommended, particularly for seriously ill or poorly responding patients and for other high-risk individuals in whom dosage adjustments are likely to be necessary (eg, the elderly, neonates, patients with impaired renal function or changing volumes of distribution). Predictive nomograms (eg, Sarubbi-Hull) may provide acceptable dosage guidelines for initiation of treatment. For detailed discussion, see the Introduction.

For tobramycin, prolonged peak serum concentrations that exceed 12 mcg/ml and trough serum levels greater than 2 mcg/ml should be avoided (see the Introduction).

Intramuscular, Intravenous: When given intravenously, tobramycin can be diluted in 5% dextrose or isotonic sodium chloride injection and administered over 30 to 60 minutes. The total duration of therapy by either route generally should not exceed ten days.

Patients with normal renal function: Adults, 3 to 5 mg/kg daily in three equally divided doses every eight hours. The larger dose is used only for life-threatening infections. *Children*, 6 to 7.5 mg/kg daily in three equally divided doses every eight hours. *Premature or full-term neonates 1 week of age or less*, up to 4 mg/kg daily in two divided doses every 12 hours.

Patients with impaired renal function: Dosage modification is indicated. Tobramycin serum concentrations should be monitored to help determine dosage (see above and the Introduction). If these measurements are unavailable or unreliable, tobramycin may be given to *adults* according to the dosing chart proposed by Sarubbi and Hull (see the Introduction).

Nebcin (Lilly), ***Generic***. Solution (sterile) 10 mg/ml (pediatric) in 2 ml containers and 40 mg/ml in 1.5 and 2 ml containers; powder 1.2 g (strengths expressed in terms of the base) ***(Nebcin*** only).

Nonparenteral Aminoglycoside

NEOMYCIN SULFATE
[Mycifradin Sulfate]

Neomycin, derived from *Streptomyces fradiae*, is the most toxic aminoglycoside antibiotic. It should not be administered parenterally for systemic infections because this route of administration causes serious ototoxicity and nephrotoxicity. Products containing neomycin sulfate for injection were withdrawn from the market by the FDA (*Federal Register,* 1988 B). Therapeutic use is limited to topical and oral administration for local antibacterial effects.

MECHANISM OF ACTION, ANTIMICROBIAL SPECTRUM, AND RESISTANCE. In vitro, neomycin is active against many aerobic gram-negative bacilli, principally members of the Enterobacteriaceae. *Pseudomonas aeruginosa* are resistant, however. Many strains of *Staphylococcus aureus* are susceptible, but most other gram-positive bacteria are resistant. Other resistant organisms include anaerobic bacteria, rickettsiae, fungi, and viruses.

See also the Introduction.

USES. Oral neomycin, in combination with erythromycin base, is frequently a preferred regimen for prophylaxis of postoperative infection in elective colorectal surgery (see the Introduction and index entry Surgery). Neomycin also can be used orally as an adjunct in the treatment of hepatic coma, since the drug reduces the number of ammonia-producing bacteria in the intestinal tract, and in lipoprotein disorders.

Neomycin is most commonly used topically to treat infections of the eye, ear, and skin, frequently as a component of an antibiotic mixture. For these indications, see index entry Neomycin.

The efficacy of this drug as a peritoneal or pleural irrigant is questionable, and absorption may be sufficient to cause serious toxicity. Approval of neomycin for the irrigation of surgical wounds, joints, and various body cavities (other than the intact urinary bladder) has been withdrawn by the FDA (*Federal Register*, 1988 A).

ADVERSE REACTIONS AND PRECAUTIONS. Although only small amounts of neomycin are absorbed following oral administration, this antibiotic may accumulate, particularly in patients with renal impairment, and cause toxicity (Ward and Rounthwaite, 1978). Nausea, vomiting, and diarrhea are the most common adverse reactions following oral administration. Superinfections and a malabsorption syndrome (particularly with prolonged use) also can occur.

Nephrotoxicity, ototoxicity, and neuromuscular blockade have been reported. Therefore, neomycin should not be administered with other drugs that are potentially ototoxic or nephrotoxic, since effects may be additive.

Topical application of neomycin frequently has resulted in sensitization.

This drug is classified in FDA Pregnancy Category D.

DRUG INTERACTIONS. See the Introduction.

PHARMACOKINETICS. Neomycin is poorly absorbed from the intact gastrointestinal tract following oral administration. Unabsorbed neomycin is excreted unchanged in the feces. Any amount that is absorbed will be excreted via the kidneys (glomerular filtration) as unchanged drug.

DOSAGE AND PREPARATIONS.

Oral: For prophylaxis of postoperative infection in patients undergoing elective intestinal or colorectal surgery, *adults*, neomycin plus erythromycin base (1 g of each at 1 PM, 2 PM, and 11 PM on the day prior to surgery [surgery at 8 AM], accompanied by mechanical bowel preparation). No postoperative dose is necessary. For guidelines and alternative regimens, see index entry Antimicrobial Drugs, Chemoprophylaxis for Surgical Patients.

Generic. Tablets 500 mg; solution 125 mg/5 ml.

Mycifradin (Upjohn). Solution 125 mg/5 ml equivalent to 87.5 mg of base.

Topical: For dosages and preparations for topical application, see index entry Neomycin, As Antibacterial Agent.

Cited References

Netilmicin sulfate (Netromycin). *Med Lett Drugs Ther* 25:65-67, 1983.

Oligosaccharide antibiotic drugs; neomycin sulfate for compounding oral products. *Federal Register* 53:12644-12658, 1988 A.

Oligosaccharide antibiotic drugs; neomycin sulfate for injection; withdrawal of approval of abbreviated antibiotic drug applications. *Federal Register* 53:49232-49233, 1988 B.

Anderson ET, et al: Simultaneous antibiotic levels in "breakthrough" gram-negative rod bacteremia. *Am J Med* 61:493-497, 1976.

Bauer LA, Blouin RA: Influence of age on amikacin pharmacokinetics in patients without renal disease: Comparison with gentamicin and tobramycin. *Eur J Clin Pharmacol* 24:639-642, 1983.

Bauer LA, et al: Influence of weight on aminoglycoside pharmacokinetics in normal weight and morbidly obese patients. *Eur J Clin Pharmacol* 24:643-647, 1983.

Berk SL, et al: Clinical and microbiologic consequences of amikacin use during a 42-month period. *Arch Intern Med* 146:538-541, 1986.

Bisno AL, et al: Antimicrobial treatment of infective endocarditis due to viridans streptococci, enterococci, and staphylococci. *JAMA* 261:1471-1477, 1989.

Bootman JL, et al: Individualizing gentamicin dosage regimens in burn patients with gram-negative septicemia: Cost-benefit analysis. *J Pharmaceut Sci* 68:267-272, 1979.

Brummett RE, Fox KE: Aminoglycoside-induced hearing loss in humans. *Antimicrob Agents Chemother* 33:797-800, 1989.

Bryan LE: Mechanisms of action of aminoglycoside antibiotics, in Root RK, Sande MA (eds): *Contemporary Issues in Infectious Diseases (Vol I): New Dimensions in Antimicrobial Therapy.* New York, Churchill Livingstone, 1984, 17-36.

Buring JE, et al: Randomized trials of aminoglycoside antibiotics: Quantitative overview. *Rev Infect Dis* 10:951-957, 1988.

Cipolle RJ, et al: Systematically individualizing tobramycin dosage regimens. *J Clin Pharmacol* 20:570-580, 1980.

Conway N, Birt BD: Streptomycin in pregnancy: Effect on foetal ear. *BMJ* 2:260-263, 1965.

Craig WA, et al: Netilmicin sulfate: Comparative evaluation of antimicrobial activity, pharmacokinetics, adverse reactions, and clinical efficacy. *Pharmacotherapy* 3:305-315, 1983.

Cunha BA: Aminoglycosides: Current role in antimicrobial therapy *Pharmacotherapy* 8:334-350, 1988.

Cunha BA: Aminoglycosides in urology. *Urology* 36:1-14, 1990.

Dajani AS, et al: Prevention of bacterial endocarditis: Recommendations by the American Heart Association. *JAMA* 264:2919-2922, 1990.

de Vries PJ, et al: Prospective randomized study of once-daily versus thrice-daily netilmicin regimens in patients with intraabdominal infections. *Eur J Clin Microbiol Infect Dis* 9:161-168, 1990.

Drusano GL: Role of pharmacokinetics in the outcome of infections. *Antimicrob Agents Chemother* 32:289-297, 1988.

Dyas A, et al: Reproducibility study of pharmacokinetics of amikacin, gentamicin, and tobramycin: Three-way crossover study. *J Antimicrob Chemother* 12:371-376, 1983.

Edson RS, Terrell CL: The aminoglycosides. *Mayo Clin Proc* 66:1158-1164, 1991.

Farber BF, Moellering RC Jr: Retrospective study of toxicity of preparations of vancomycin from 1974 to 1981. *Antimicrob Agents Chemother* 23:138-141, 1983.

Fausti SA, et al: High-frequency audiometric monitoring for early detection of aminoglycoside ototoxicity. *J Infect Dis* 165:1026-1032, 1992.

Fee WE Jr: Gentamicin and tobramycin: Comparison of ototoxicity. *Rev Infect Dis* 5(suppl 2):S304-S313, 1983.

Fuquay D, et al: Management of neonatal gentamicin overdosage. *J Pediatr* 99:473-476, 1981.

Gilbert DN: Once-daily aminoglycoside therapy. *Antimicrob Agents Chemother* 35:399-405, 1991.

Green FJ, et al: Management of amikacin overdose. *Am J Kidney Dis* 1:110-112, 1981.

Guglielmo RB: Furosemide-aminoglycoside interaction. *Drug Interact Newslett* 4:34-35, 1984.

Hancock REW: Aminoglycoside uptake and mode of action—with special reference to streptomycin and gentamicin: I. Antagonists and mutants. II. Effects of aminoglycosides on cells. *J Antimicrob Chemother* 8:249-276, 429-445, 1981.

Hansten PD, Horn JR: *Drug Interactions and Updates,* Malvern, Penn, Lea & Febiger, 1990 A, 243-250.

Hansten PD, Horn JR: *Drug Interactions and Updates,* Malvern, Penn, Lea & Febiger, 1990 B, 117.

Hollender LF, et al: A multicentric study of netilmicin once daily versus thrice daily in patients with appendicitis and other intraabdominal infections. *J Antimicrob Chemother* 23:773-783, 1989.

Holm SE, et al: Prospective, randomized study of amikacin and gentamicin in serious infections with focus on efficacy, toxicity and duration of serum levels above the MIC. *J Antimicrob Chemother* 12:393-402, 1983.

Hughes WT, et al: Guidelines for the use of antimicrobial agents in neutropenic patients with unexplained fever. *J Infect Dis* 161:381-396, 1990.

Jackson GG, Riff LJ: *Pseudomonas* bacteremia: Pharmacologic and other bases for failure of treatment with gentamicin. *J Infect Dis* 124(suppl):S185-S191, 1971.

Kahlmeter G, Dahlager JI: Aminoglycoside toxicity: Review of clinical studies published between 1975 and 1982. *J Antimicrob Chemother* 13(suppl A):9-22, 1984.

Kapusnik JE, Sande MA: Challenging conventional aminoglycoside dosing regimens: Value of experimental models. *Am J Med* 80(suppl 6B):179-181, 1986.

Kovarik JM, et al: Once-daily aminoglycoside administration: New strategies for an old drug. *Eur J Clin Microbiol Infect Dis* 8:761-769, 1989.

Lerner AM, et al: Randomised, controlled trial of comparative efficacy, auditory toxicity, and nephrotoxicity of tobramycin and netilmicin. *Lancet* 1:1123-1126, 1983.

Lesar TS, et al: Gentamicin dosing errors with four commonly used nomograms. *JAMA* 248:1190-1193, 1982.

Lietman PS: Aminoglycosides and spectinomycin: Aminocyclitols, in Mandell GL, et al (eds): *Principles and Practice of Infectious Diseases*, ed 3. New York, Churchill Livingstone, 1990, 269-284.

Lietman PS, Smith CR: Aminoglycoside nephrotoxicity in humans. *Rev Infect Dis* 5(suppl 2):S284-S293, 1983.

Lipman ML, Silva J: Endocarditis due to *Streptococcus faecalis* with high-level resistance to gentamicin. *Rev Infect Dis* 11:325-328, 1989.

Maller R, et al: Efficacy and safety of amikacin in systemic infections when given as a single daily dose or in two divided doses. *J Antimicrob Chemother* 27(suppl C):121-128, 1991.

Maloney J, et al: Analysis of amikacin-resistant *Pseudomonas aeruginosa* developing in patients receiving amikacin. *Arch Intern Med* 149:630-634, 1989.

Mattie H, et al: Determinants of efficacy and toxicity of aminoglycosides. *J Antimicrob Chemother* 24:281-293, 1989.

McCracken GH Jr: Perinatal bacterial diseases, in Feigin RD, Cherry JD (eds): *Textbook of Pediatric Infectious Diseases.* Philadelphia, WB Saunders, 1981, vol 1, 747-768.

The Medical Letter: *Handbook of Antimicrobial Therapy.* New Rochelle, NY, The Medical Letter, 1988, 38-49.

Meyer RD: Amikacin: Drugs five years later. *Ann Intern Med* 95:328-332, 1981.

Moellering RC Jr: In vitro antibacterial activity of aminoglycoside antibiotics. *Rev Infect Dis* 5(suppl 2):S212-S232, 1983.

Moore RD, et al: Risk factors for nephrotoxicity in patients treated with aminoglycosides. *Ann Intern Med* 100:352-357, 1984 A.

Moore RD, et al: Risk factors for development of auditory toxicity in patients receiving aminoglycosides. *J Infect Dis* 149:23-30, 1984 B.

Moore RD, et al: Association of aminoglycoside plasma levels with mortality in patients with gram-negative bacteremia. *J Infect Dis* 149:443-448, 1984 C.

Moore RD, et al: Association of aminoglycoside plasma levels with therapeutic outcome in gram-negative pneumonia. *Am J Med* 77:657-662, 1984 D.

Moore RD, et al: Clinical response to aminoglycoside therapy: Importance of ratio of peak concentration to minimal inhibitory concentration. *J Infect Dis* 155:93-99, 1987.

Murray BE: New aspects of antimicrobial resistance and the resulting therapeutic dilemmas. *J Infect Dis* 163:1185-1194, 1991.

Nelson JD: *1991-1992 Pocketbook of Pediatric Antimicrobial Therapy*, ed 9. Baltimore, Williams & Wilkins, 1991, 71.

Noone P, et al: Experience in monitoring gentamicin therapy during treatment of serious gram-negative sepsis. *BMJ* 1:477-481, 1974.

Nordström L, et al: Does adminstration of an aminoglycoside in a single daily dose affect its efficacy and toxicity? *J Antimicrob Chemother* 25:159-173, 1990.

Pancoast SJ: Aminoglycoside antibiotics in clinical use. *Med Clin North Am* 72:581-612, 1988.

Pauly DJ, et al: Risk of nephrotoxicity with combination vancomycin-aminoglycoside antibiotic therapy. *Pharmacotherapy* 10:378-382, 1990.

Pechère J-C, et al: Once daily dosing of aminoglycoside: One step forward. *J Antimicrob Chemother* 27 (suppl C):149-152, 1991.

Pickering LK, Rutherford I: Effect of concentration and time upon inactivation of tobramycin, gentamicin, netilmicin, and amikacin by azlocillin, carbenicillin, mecillinam, mezlocillin, and piperacillin. *J Pharmacol Exp Ther* 217:345-349, 1981.

Pratt WB, Fekety R: *The Antimicrobial Drugs.* New York, Oxford University Press, 1986, 153-183.

Reese RE, Betts RF: Antibiotic use: Aminoglycosides, in Reese RE, Douglas RG Jr (eds): *A Practical Approach to Infectious Diseases*, ed 3. Boston, Little Brown, 1991, 933-945.

Rotschafer JC, et al: Clinical use of one-compartment model for determining netilmicin pharmacokinetic parameters and dosage recommendations. *Ther Drug Monit* 5:263-267, 1983.

Sarubbi FA Jr, Hull JH: Amikacin serum concentrations: Prediction of levels and dosage guidelines. *Ann Intern Med* 89:612-618, 1978.

Sawchuk RJ, Zaske DE: Pharmacokinetics of dosing regimens which utilize multiple intravenous infusions: Gentamicin in burn patients. *J Pharmacokinet Biopharm* 4:183-195, 1976.

Sawchuk RJ, et al: Kinetic model for gentamicin dosing with use of individual patient parameters. *Clin Pharmacol Ther* 21:362-369, 1977.

Schwartz SN, et al: Controlled investigation of pharmacokinetics of gentamicin and tobramycin in obese subjects. *J Infect Dis* 138:499-505, 1978.

Smith CR, Lietman PS: Effect of furosemide on aminoglycoside-induced nephrotoxicity and auditory toxicity in humans. *Antimicrob Agents Chemother* 23:133-137, 1983.

Szot RJ, Tabachnick IIA: Animal studies with netilmicin. *Clin Trials J* 17:318-337, 1980.

Tatro DS (ed): *Drug Interaction Facts.* St. Louis, JB Lippincott, 1988, 20-23.

ter Braak EW, et al: Once-daily dosing regimen for aminoglycoside plus β-lactam combination therapy of serious bacterial infections: Comparative trial with netilmicin plus ceftriaxone. *Am J Med* 89:58-66, 1990.

Trissel LA: *Handbook on Injectable Drugs*, ed 5. Bethesda, Md, American Society of Hospital Pharmacists, 1988.

Wade JC, et al: Cephalothin plus an aminoglycoside is more nephrotoxic than methicillin plus an aminoglycoside. *Lancet* 2:604-606, 1978.

Ward KM, Rounthwaite FJ: Neomycin ototoxicity. *Ann Otol Rhinol Laryngol* 87:211-215, 1978.

Weinstein AJ, et al: Placental transfer of clindamycin and gentamicin in term pregnancy. *Am J Obstet Gynecol* 124:688-691, 1976.

Weinstein AJ, et al: Systemic absorption of neomycin irrigating solution. *JAMA* 238:152-153, 1977.

Wenk M, et al: Serum level monitoring of antibacterial drugs: Review. *Clin Pharmacokinet* 9:475-492, 1984.

Zaske DE: Aminoglycosides, in Evans WE, et al (eds): *Applied Pharmacokinetics: Principles of Therapeutic Drug Monitoring,* ed 2. Spokane, Wash, Applied Therapeutics, 1986, 331-381.

Zaske DE, et al: Gentamicin dosage requirements: Wide interpatient variations in 242 surgery patients with normal renal function. *Surgery* 87:164-169, 1980.

Zaske DE, et al: Increased gentamicin dosage requirements: Rapid elimination in 249 gynecology patients. *Am J Obstet Gynecol* 139:896-900, 1981.

Zaske DE, et al: Increased burn patient survival with individualized dosages of gentamicin. *Surgery* 91:142-149, 1982 A.

Zaske DE, et al: Gentamicin pharmacokinetics in 1,640 patients: Method for control of serum concentrations. *Antimicrob Agents Chemother* 21:407-411, 1982 B.

Zaske DE, et al: Wide interpatient variations in gentamicin dose requirements for geriatric patients. *JAMA* 248:3122-3126, 1982 C.

Zhanel GG, et al: The postantibiotic effect: A review of in vitro and in vivo data. *DICP* 25:153-162, 1991.

69

Sulfonamides and Trimethoprim

SULFONAMIDES

History, Chemistry, and Scope of Discussion

The modern antimicrobial chemotherapeutic era began in the early 1930s when Prontosil, a chemical developed by the German dye industry, was shown to combat streptococcal infection in mice after metabolism to para-aminobenzene sulfonamide (sulfanilamide), an antibacterial compound.

Sulfanilamide is similar in structure to para-aminobenzoic acid (PABA), a precursor required by bacteria for folic acid synthesis (Figure 1). The clinically useful sulfonamides are synthetically derived from sulfanilamide. Most derivatives contain a free para-amino group, which is necessary for antibacterial activity, and heterocyclic aromatic substitutions on the sulfonamide group (Figure 1). Such modifications of the basic sulfanilamide molecule result in increased antibacterial activity. The nature of these substitutions also determines other pharmacologic properties of the drug, such as absorption, solubility, and gastrointestinal tolerance.

Although many sulfonamides have been tested for clinical usefulness, only four derivatives currently are marketed in the United States as single-entity drugs for systemic use. These include the short-acting sulfonamides, sulfisoxazole [Gantrisin], sulfamethizole [Thiosulfil Forte], and sulfadiazine [Microsulfon], and the intermediate-acting analogue, sulfamethoxazole [Gantanol]. The structures of these derivatives are shown in Figure 1. Long-acting sulfonamides (eg, sulfamethoxypyridazine, sulfameter) are no longer available as single agents because they have been associated with severe hypersensitivity reactions, such as the Stevens-Johnson syndrome.

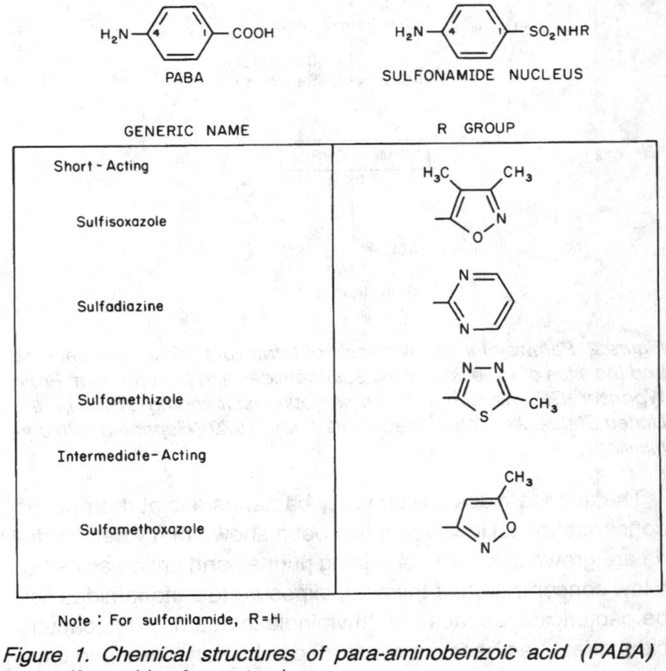

H_2N–C₆H₄–COOH — PABA

H_2N–C₆H₄–SO_2NHR — SULFONAMIDE NUCLEUS

GENERIC NAME	R GROUP
Short-Acting	
Sulfisoxazole	
Sulfadiazine	
Sulfamethizole	
Intermediate-Acting	
Sulfamethoxazole	

Note: For sulfanilamide, R=H

Figure 1. Chemical structures of para-aminobenzoic acid (PABA) and sulfonamides for systemic use.

This section is limited to a discussion of the above single-entity preparations and systemic fixed-ratio mixtures containing more than one sulfonamide or a sulfonamide and another drug (see the discussion on Mixtures).

For information on sulfonamides limited to use in the gastrointestinal tract (sulfasalazine), eye (sulfacetamide), or skin (mafenide, silver sulfadiazine), see index entries on these drugs.

Mechanism of Action

Bacteria require tetrahydrofolic acid, a derivative of folic acid, as a cofactor in the synthesis of thymidine, purines, and, ultimately, DNA. Most bacterial cells are impermeable to folic acid and must synthesize it from para-aminobenzoic acid (PABA). The sulfonamides are structural analogues of PABA and competitively inhibit the synthesis of dihydropteroic acid, the immediate precursor of dihydrofolic acid, from PABA and pteridine (see Figure 2). Mammalian cells are unaffected by this inhibition because they require preformed folic acid and cannot synthesize it.

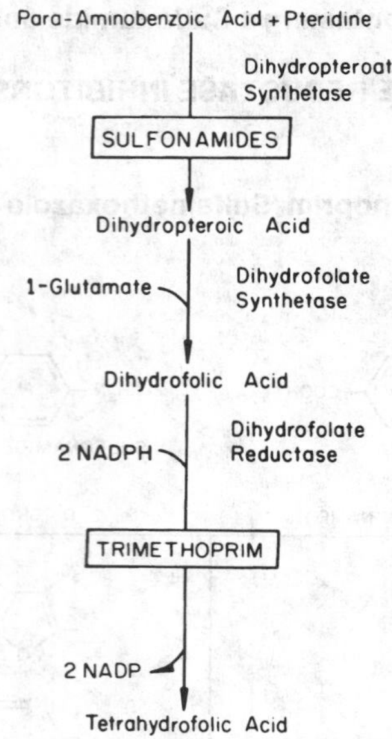

Figure 2. Pathway for the synthesis of tetrahydrofolic acid in bacteria and the sites of inhibition by the sulfonamides and trimethoprim. From Wormser GP, Keusch GT: Trimethoprim-sulfamethoxazole in the United States. Ann Intern Med *91:420-429, 1979 (Reprinted with permission).*

The sulfonamides are primarily bacteriostatic at therapeutic concentrations. However, it has been shown that when bacteria are grown in media containing purines and amino acids but a low concentration of thymine, exposure to sulfonamides can be bactericidal because of "thymineless death." This bactericidal effect has been demonstrated in human blood and urine (Then and Angehrn, 1973 A, 1973 B; see also Pratt and Fekety, 1986).

Sulfonamide-induced inhibition of bacterial cell growth can be reversed in vitro by adding certain agents (eg, thymidine, purines, methionine, serine) to the growth medium. This may be of clinical importance, since pus may contain many of these substances as the result of cell breakdown, and their presence may inhibit the effectiveness of these drugs in purulent infections. Also, when in vitro susceptibility is being determined, it is essential that the culture medium be free of PABA, since trace amounts of this compound may interfere with results.

Antimicrobial Spectrum

The sulfonamides originally were active against a wide range of gram-positive and gram-negative bacteria. However, resistant strains have become common for many bacteria, and the usefulness of the sulfonamides has decreased accordingly. Among microorganisms usually susceptible in vitro to sulfonamides are *Streptococcus pyogenes, S. pneumoniae, Haemophilus influenzae, H. ducreyi, Nocardia* species, *Actinomyces, Calymmatobacterium granulomatis,* and *Chlamydia trachomatis* (Mandell and Sande, 1990). The protozoa, *Plasmodium falciparum* and *Toxoplasma gondii,* also are susceptible (*Med Lett Drugs Ther*, 1992 A).

Neisseria gonorrhoeae and *N. meningitidis* were susceptible in the past, but the majority of strains are now resistant to the sulfonamides. Similarly, most strains of *Shigella sonnei* and *S. flexneri* are now resistant. Although community-acquired *Escherichia coli* frequently have been susceptible to sulfonamides at concentrations achieved in urine, a substantial percentage of strains (25% to 35%) are now resistant (Mandell and Sande, 1990; Sobel and Kaye, 1990). Resistance is common among other Enterobacteriaceae.

Resistance

Many bacteria have become highly resistant to the sulfonamides. Resistance can be chromosomally mediated or transferred by R-factor plasmids. The latter method frequently is seen with Enterobacteriaceae. The mechanisms of resistance include (1) overproduction of PABA; (2) a decreased affinity of dihydropteroate synthetase for the sulfonamide; (3) a decreased permeability of the bacterium to the drug; and (4) increased inactivation of the drug. Cross-resistance between sulfonamides is usual.

Acquired resistance to the sulfonamides is widespread and severely limits their clinical usefulness. For example, significant resistance among gonococci, meningococci, staphylococci, streptococci, and shigellae has rendered the sulfonamides clinically obsolete in treating infections caused by these bacteria. Resistance among community-acquired *E. coli* also is common in most geographic locations. This has raised concern about the continued usefulness of sulfonamides in acute uncomplicated urinary tract infections (see below).

Uses

The sulfonamides were once a mainstay in the treatment of infectious diseases, but their usefulness has been limited as bacterial resistance has increased and safer and more effective antibiotics have been developed.

Urinary Tract Infections: Sulfonamides have been used primarily for acute, uncomplicated urinary tract infections (ie, cystitis). However, because resistance among community-acquired *E. coli* is common in most geographic areas, sulfonamides are no longer recommended for empiric therapy of these infections (see Johnson and Stamm, 1987; Mandell and Sande, 1990; Sobel and Kaye, 1990). The combination of trimethoprim/sulfamethoxazole [Bactrim, Cotrim, Septra] often is preferred for this indication (see the section on Dihydrofolate Reductase Inhibitors).

Single-entity sulfonamides should be effective for acute, uncomplicated urinary tract infections when the causative organism is known to be susceptible. The short-acting sulfonamides, usually sulfisoxazole, are preferred because they are rapidly excreted in high concentrations (largely in the active rather than the acetylated form) and have good solubility in acidic urine.

Sulfonamides should not be used to treat acute pyelonephritis; parenteral antibiotics (eg, an aminoglycoside, β lactam, or fluoroquinolone) frequently are required for this infection. The use of sulfonamides for the prophylaxis of recurrent urinary tract infections also is not recommended. However, trimethoprim/sulfamethoxazole often is used for this indication (see the section on Dihydrofolate Reductase Inhibitors). For a more detailed discussion of antimicrobial drug selection, see index entry Urinary Tract Infections.

Nocardiosis: Sulfonamides, including sulfadiazine, sulfisoxazole, trisulfapyrimidines, and sulfamethoxazole, traditionally have been preferred drugs for nocardiosis. Some clinicians recommend that minocycline, ampicillin, or erythromycin be used with a sulfonamide for this indication, but there are no clinical data to show that combination therapy is better than a sulfonamide alone. Trimethoprim/sulfamethoxazole (preferred therapy of some experts), minocycline [Minocin], and amikacin are alternative therapies for *Nocardia* infections.

Chlamydia trachomatis Infections: Although not the drugs of choice, certain sulfonamides, including sulfisoxazole and sulfamethoxazole, can effectively treat *Chlamydia trachomatis* infections (eg, urethritis, pneumonia, trachoma, inclusion conjunctivitis, lymphogranuloma venereum).

Antibacterial Chemoprophylaxis: Sulfadiazine is recommended for the prophylaxis of rheumatic fever in penicillin-allergic patients. Erythromycin is an alternative. Sulfonamides should *not* be used in the treatment of established streptococcal pharyngitis because they fail to eradicate the causative organism, and late sequelae (eg, rheumatic fever, glomerulonephritis) may develop.

Rifampin [Rifadin, Rimactane] is the drug of choice for prophylaxis of meningococcal meningitis in household or other close contacts. Sulfadiazine (or sulfisoxazole) can be given only if the susceptibility of the organism to this agent is known; its use is rare in the United States. Sulfonamides are no longer used to treat meningococcal meningitis because of the prevalence of resistant strains of *Neisseria meningitidis*.

Sulfisoxazole is an alternative to amoxicillin for the chemoprophylaxis of recurrent acute otitis media (for discussion, see index entry Otitis Media, Chemoprophylaxis).

Based on the results of a randomized, controlled trial comparing long-term (six months) sulfisoxazole therapy to use of ventilation tubes for long-standing otitis media with effusion, antimicrobial therapy may be an effective option before considering ventilation tube placement. One-third of the patients receiving sulfisoxazole avoided surgery (Bernard et al, 1991).

Protozoal Infections: Sulfonamides, usually in combination with other antiprotozoal agents, also are used in various protozoal infections. Sulfadoxine, a long-acting derivative available only with pyrimethamine in a fixed-ratio combination [Fansidar] in the United States, and sulfadiazine may be used adjunctively in combination with pyrimethamine (plus quinine sulfate) in malaria caused by chloroquine-resistant strains of *Plasmodium falciparum*. Sulfadiazine with pyrimethamine is useful in toxoplasmosis due to *Toxoplasma gondii*. *Pneumocystis carinii* infections often are treated with trimethoprim/sulfamethoxazole (see the section on Dihydrofolate Reductase Inhibitors). For additional discussion, see index entries on these infections.

Adverse Reactions and Precautions

The sulfonamides are capable of producing a wide variety of adverse reactions that affect a number of organ systems, including the blood and bone marrow, skin, kidney, liver, and nervous system. As discussed below, many of these adverse effects traditionally have been considered hypersensitivity reactions. However, it has been suggested that some of these actually may be idiosyncratic reactions caused by toxic sulfonamide metabolites that are produced in genetically predisposed individuals (Shear et al, 1986). The incidence of adverse reactions to sulfonamides is higher in HIV-infected patients (see the evaluation of trimethoprim/sulfamethoxazole for discussion).

Cutaneous and Mucocutaneous: Hypersensitivity reactions affecting the skin and mucous membranes include urticaria and maculopapular rashes that are often accompanied by pruritus and fever. More serious dermatologic reactions (eg, exfoliative dermatitis, toxic epidermal necrolysis, erythema nodosum) occur less frequently. The sulfonamides also may provoke erythema multiforme and its severe form, Stevens-Johnson syndrome, especially in children. This syndrome involves both the skin and mucous membranes and is fatal in 5% to 25% of patients (Araujo and Flowers, 1984). Therefore, sulfonamide therapy should be discontinued in patients who develop a skin rash.

Photosensitivity reactions also have occurred with the use of sulfonamides. Patients should be cautioned that an exaggerated sunburn reaction after exposure to the sun is possible during sulfonamide therapy.

Hematologic: The incidence of blood dyscrasias is low, but they can be extremely serious and deaths have occurred. Sulfonamides may cause agranulocytosis, hemolytic or aplastic (rare) anemia, leukopenia, thrombocytopenia, hypoprothrombinemia, eosinophilia, and methemoglobinemia. Hemolytic anemia has been observed in patients with and without deficiency of erythrocytic glucose-6-phosphate dehydrogenase (G6PD). This hazard should be borne in mind if there is a family history of G6PD deficiency, which is most common in blacks and Mediterranean ethnic groups.

Blood studies performed at regular intervals are necessary during prolonged therapy with any sulfonamide, since they detect the milder leukopenias. Clinical signs, such as sore throat, fever, pallor, purpura, or jaundice, may be early indications of serious blood disorders, and blood counts should be performed.

Hypersensitivity Reactions: In addition to hypersensitivity reactions involving the skin and blood, sulfonamides may cause drug fever, a serum sickness-like syndrome, urticaria, anaphylaxis, polyarteritis nodosa, and systemic lupus erythematosus. An allergic reaction to one sulfonamide precludes the later use of another derivative.

Renal: Earlier, less soluble sulfonamides, including sulfadiazine, frequently caused crystalluria in the renal calices and pelvis, ureters, or bladder that resulted in hematuria, irritation, and obstruction. This complication was minimized by maintenance of a high urine flow and alkalization of the urine to increase solubility of the drug. The risk of crystalluria has diminished markedly with the use of more soluble sulfonamides (sulfisoxazole, sulfamethizole, sulfamethoxazole). However, since these agents are excreted primarily by the kidneys, an adequate urine volume must be maintained. Before sulfonamide therapy is begun, urinary output should be 1,000 to 1,500 ml/day for adults with normal renal function and appropriate hydration (eg, maintenance of an adequate fluid intake) should be continued throughout the treatment period. Because the sulfonamides are more soluble in alkaline urine, efforts to alkalize the urine (eg, with sodium bicarbonate) may be desirable in some patients. However, this probably is unnecessary with the newer, more soluble agents (eg, sulfisoxazole).

Sulfonamides infrequently cause toxic nephrosis with oliguria and anuria but without evidence of crystalluria. Tubular necrosis or necrotizing angiitis are the pathologic manifestations of this adverse effect.

Sulfonamides must be used cautiously in patients with impaired renal function. Urinalyses with careful microscopic examination and renal function tests should be performed during therapy, particularly for those patients with impaired renal function.

Hepatic: Hepatitis with focal or diffuse necrosis and cholestatic jaundice may occur. The conjugation of sulfonamides is reduced in patients with impaired liver function, and toxic reactions may follow usual therapeutic doses.

Neurologic: Reactions involving the central nervous system include headache, lethargy, dizziness, and mental depression. Peripheral neuritis, psychoses, ataxia, vertigo, tinnitus, and convulsions have been reported rarely.

Gastrointestinal: Anorexia, nausea, vomiting, and diarrhea are common side effects of sulfonamide therapy.

Miscellaneous Reactions: Sulfonamides are similar chemically to some goitrogens and oral hypoglycemic agents, and they rarely have been reported to produce goiters or hypoglycemia.

Precautions in Pregnancy, Nursing Mothers, and Young Infants: Sulfonamides cross the placenta and are excreted into breast milk. Since they compete with bilirubin for albumin binding, high levels of free bilirubin can cause kernicterus in infants born to mothers who take sulfonamides near term and in nursing neonates whose mothers are taking sulfonamides. Therefore, use of sulfonamides in pregnant women near term or in nursing mothers is inadvisable. In addition, sulfonamides should not be given to infants less than 2 months of age, unless indicated for congenital toxoplasmosis.

Drug Interactions and Interference With Laboratory Tests

Sulfonamides may displace certain drugs from plasma albumin and/or inhibit their biotransformation, thus potentiating their pharmacologic effect. For example, hypoglycemia has been reported after antibacterial sulfonamides were given to a few patients receiving tolbutamide [Orinase] or chlorpropamide [Diabinese]; for this reason, these agents should be given cautiously to patients receiving any oral hypoglycemic agent. Sulfonamides also should be used cautiously with coumarin anticoagulants, methotrexate, phenytoin [Dilantin], and thiopental [Pentothal] since they have been reported to enhance the action of these agents. Conversely, sulfonamides may be displaced from plasma protein binding sites by other drugs (eg, phenylbutazone, salicylates, probenecid [Benemid]), resulting in increased sulfonamide activity.

Sulfamethizole [Thiosulfil Forte] and sulfathiazole have formed insoluble precipitates with formaldehyde in the urine; therefore, concomitant administration of sulfonamides (especially the less soluble analogues) with methenamine compounds (eg, methenamine mandelate [Mandelamine]) should be avoided.

PABA-containing compounds and local anesthetics derived from PABA (eg, procaine [Novocain]) may directly inhibit the activity of sulfonamides.

Sulfonamides have been reported to produce false-positive Benedict's tests for urine glucose and false-positive sulfosalicylic acid tests for urine proteins.

Pharmacokinetics

Single-entity sulfonamides for systemic use are given orally. Parenteral preparations (eg, sulfisoxazole diolamine, sulfadiazine sodium) were rarely used and are no longer marketed.

Absorption: Following oral administration, the systemic sulfonamides are readily absorbed from the gastrointestinal tract, primarily from the small intestine. Approximately 70% to 100% of an oral dose is absorbed. Estimates of therapeutically effective serum concentrations for most infections vary between 60 and 150 mcg/ml of free (ie, unconjugated, unbound) sulfonamide. Because the sulfonamides are concentrated in the urine, however, the serum levels necessary in the treatment of urinary tract infections are lower than those needed for systemic infections. The serum level of sulfamethizole is too low to treat systemic infections outside the urinary tract because of rapid elimination of the drug.

Distribution: All sulfonamides are reversibly bound to plasma proteins in varying degrees. These drugs are widely distributed throughout the body; concentrations approaching 80% of serum levels may be attained in pleural, synovial, and peritoneal fluids. Concentrations of sulfadiazine, sulfisoxazole, and sulfamethoxazole in cerebrospinal fluid have been reported to be 40% to 80%, 30% to 50%, and 25% to 30% of serum levels, respectively (see Zinner and Mayer, 1990). Sulfonamides readily cross the placenta and are present in fetal blood and amniotic fluid. Blood and tissue levels are related to the degrees of protein binding and lipid solubilities of the various analogues.

Metabolism: Sulfonamides are metabolized to varying extents in the liver by N^4-acetylation or conjugation with glucuronic acid. Either process may alter solubility of the drug in urine, the major route of excretion. Acetylated metabolites and glucuronide derivatives lack antimicrobial activity.

Elimination: Both active unchanged sulfonamides and their metabolites are excreted by the kidneys. Excretion is primarily by glomerular filtration, although tubular reabsorption and active tubular secretion may play a role. The half-lives of sulfonamides are dependent on the rates of renal excretion. Generally, urinary excretion is more rapid for sulfonamides with low pKa values (eg, sulfisoxazole). Alkalization of the urine increases solubility and enhances urinary excretion.

The sulfonamides can be classified according to their duration of action in the body as short-, intermediate-, or long-acting. The long-acting sulfonamides are no longer marketed as single agents in the United States, however, because they have been associated with hypersensitivity reactions, such as the Stevens-Johnson syndrome.

Short-acting Sulfonamides. Sulfisoxazole and sulfamethizole are short-acting agents with elimination half-lives of four to seven hours. Sulfamethizole is eliminated primarily as unchanged drug that is readily soluble in urine. Sulfisoxazole is eliminated as acetylated (30%) and free drug; both forms are readily soluble in urine.

Although sulfadiazine also is classified as short-acting, its half-life is 17 hours. It is partially acetylated. In contrast to other systemic sulfonamides, urinary solubility is a problem with sulfadiazine and the patient must be kept well hydrated (maintain urine volume of at least 1,500 ml/day in adults) to avoid crystalluria (see Adverse Reactions and Precautions).

Other short-acting sulfonamides (eg, sulfamerazine, sulfamethazine) are relatively insoluble or weakly anti-infective and are rarely used except in combination with other drugs. Sulfamerazine and sulfamethazine are combined with sulfadiazine in a short-acting mixture known as trisulfapyrimidines (see the section on Mixtures).

Intermediate-acting Sulfonamide. Sulfamethoxazole is an intermediate-acting sulfonamide with a half-life of 10 to 12 hours. It is partially acetylated. Although sulfamethoxazole requires less frequent administration than sulfisoxazole (twice versus four times daily), its acetylated metabolite is less soluble in urine. Thus, the risk of crystalluria is somewhat greater and the patient should be adequately hydrated (maintain urine volume of at least 1,500 ml/day in adults).

Drug Evaluations

Short-acting Sulfonamides

SULFADIAZINE

MECHANISM OF ACTION, ANTIMICROBIAL SPECTRUM, AND RESISTANCE. See the Introduction.

USES. Sulfadiazine is a preferred drug for nocardiosis. Trisulfapyrimidines and sulfisoxazole are other sulfonamides that are used in this disease.

Sulfadiazine in combination with pyrimethamine is the preferred sulfonamide for toxoplasmosis. Sulfadiazine (sulfadoxine usually preferred) also may be used adjunctively with pyrimethamine (plus quinine sulfate) for treatment of malaria caused by chloroquine-resistant strains of *Plasmodium falciparum.*

Sulfadiazine is indicated for the prophylaxis of rheumatic fever in penicillin-allergic patients. Erythromycin is an alternative. The use of sulfadiazine for the prophylaxis of meningococcal meningitis in household or other close contacts should be restricted to cases in which the causative organism is known to be susceptible, and it is rarely used. Rifampin is the current drug of choice for this prophylactic indication.

Sulfadiazine is not recommended for the treatment of urinary tract infections because large doses and alkalization of the urine are necessary. When a sulfonamide is indicated, the more soluble analogues (eg, sulfisoxazole) should be given.

ADVERSE REACTIONS AND PRECAUTIONS. Sulfadiazine is less soluble in the urine than other currently available sulfonamides (eg, sulfisoxazole). Thus, the risk of crystalluria is greater. Patients receiving sulfadiazine must be kept well hydrated in order to maintain an adequate urinary volume (at least 1,500 ml daily in adults). Alkalization of the urine (eg, with sodium bicarbonate) increases urinary solubility.

For other adverse reactions and precautions, see the Introduction.

DRUG INTERACTIONS AND INTERFERENCE WITH LABORATORY TESTS. See the Introduction.

PHARMACOKINETICS. Orally administered sulfadiazine is rapidly absorbed, and peak serum concentrations are attained within three to six hours after a single dose. The blood level should be maintained at 100 to 150 mcg/ml for systemic infections. About 45% of circulating sulfadiazine is bound to plasma proteins. The drug is widely distributed in body fluids and tissues, and therapeutic concentrations are attained in the cerebrospinal fluid. Between 15% and 40% of a dose is acetylated; both acetylated and unchanged drug are excreted by the kidney. The half-life is 17 hours.

DOSAGE AND PREPARATIONS.

Oral: *Adults,* 2 to 4 g initially, then 1 g every four to six hours. *Children and infants over 2 months,* 75 mg/kg initially, then 150 mg/kg daily in four to six divided doses. The total daily dose should not exceed 6 g. Duration of therapy for nocardiosis is four to six months or longer.

For prophylaxis of rheumatic fever, 500 mg once daily for patients under 27 kg and 1 g daily for those over 27 kg.

For prophylaxis of meningococcal disease (only if the *Neisseria meningitidis* isolate is known to be susceptible), *adults*, 1 g twice daily for two days; *children 1 to 12 years*, 500 mg twice daily for two days; *infants 2 months to 1 year*, 500 mg once daily for two days.

For dosages in toxoplasmosis and malaria, see index entries on these infections.

Generic. Tablets 500 mg.

Available Trademark:
Microsulfon (Consolidated Midland).

SULFAMETHIZOLE
[Thiosulfil Forte]

MECHANISM OF ACTION, ANTIMICROBIAL SPECTRUM, AND RESISTANCE. See the Introduction.

USES. Sulfamethizole is used only to treat acute, uncomplicated urinary tract infections caused by susceptible bacteria. However, sulfisoxazole is usually preferred to this sulfonamide. Because of rapid renal excretion, the plasma levels of sulfamethizole are low and the drug is not used for systemic infections outside of the urinary tract.

ADVERSE REACTIONS AND PRECAUTIONS, DRUG INTERACTIONS, AND INTERFERENCE WITH LABORATORY TESTS. See the Introduction.

Sulfamethizole is classified in FDA Pregnancy Category C.

PHARMACOKINETICS. Sulfamethizole is readily absorbed following oral administration and is rapidly eliminated by renal excretion (80% of a dose is recovered in urine within eight hours). Approximately 90% of a dose is excreted in the active unchanged form, which is readily soluble in urine within the normal acidic pH range.

DOSAGE AND PREPARATIONS.

Oral: *Adults,* 500 mg to 1 g three or four times daily. *Children and infants over 2 months,* 30 to 45 mg/kg daily in four divided doses.

Thiosulfil Forte (Wyeth-Ayerst). Tablets 500 mg.

SULFISOXAZOLE
[Gantrisin]

SULFISOXAZOLE ACETYL
[Gantrisin]

MECHANISM OF ACTION, ANTIMICROBIAL SPECTRUM, AND RESISTANCE. See the Introduction.

USES. When a sulfonamide is indicated, sulfisoxazole often is preferred for the treatment of acute, uncomplicated urinary tract infections. However, because of widespread resistance among community-acquired *E. coli,* single-entity sulfonamides are no longer recommended for empiric therapy of these infections (see the Introduction).

Sulfisoxazole frequently is the preferred sulfonamide for susceptible systemic infections. Because of problems with amoxicillin-resistant strains of *Haemophilus influenzae,* sulfisoxazole, in combination with erythromycin, is often used to treat acute otitis media caused by such strains (see the section on Mixtures). This sulfonamide also is used for prophylaxis of recurrent otitis media. It is an alternative to sulfadiazine and trisulfapyrimidines in nocardiosis. Although it is not the drug of choice, sulfisoxazole has been used in *Chlamydia trachomatis* infections (eg, urethritis, pneumonia, trachoma, inclusion conjunctivitis, lymphogranuloma venereum) and for prophylaxis of meningococcal disease.

ADVERSE REACTIONS AND PRECAUTIONS, DRUG INTERACTIONS, AND INTERFERENCE WITH LABORATORY TESTS. See the Introduction.

Sulfisoxazole is classified in FDA Pregnancy Category C.

PHARMACOKINETICS. Sulfisoxazole is absorbed rapidly and completely from the gastrointestinal tract following oral administration. Peak plasma concentrations occur in two to four hours. Sulfisoxazole acetyl is a tasteless soluble derivative for oral use that usually is preferred by children. It is converted to sulfisoxazole in the intestine and, therefore, absorption of active drug is delayed with this preparation.

Sulfisoxazole is 90% bound to plasma proteins. The volume of distribution (0.15 L/kg) approximates that of the extracellular fluid. The drug readily distributes to most tissues and body fluids, including pleural, synovial, peritoneal, and cerebrospinal fluids, and crosses the placenta.

About 30% of a dose of sulfisoxazole is acetylated, and both the free and acetylated drug are rapidly eliminated by the kidneys. The half-life ranges from five to six hours, and about 95% of a dose is recovered from the urine within 24 hours. Both the free and acetylated forms are highly soluble in urine within the normal acidic pH range.

DOSAGE AND PREPARATIONS. All concentrations are expressed in terms of the base.

Oral: *Adults,* 2 to 4 g initially, then 4 to 8 g daily in four to six divided doses. *Children over 2 months,* 75 mg/kg initially, then 150 mg/kg daily in divided doses every four to six hours (maximum, 6 g daily).

For dosages for *Chlamydia trachomatis* (including lymphogranuloma venereum serotype) infections and for prophylaxis of meningococcal disease or recurrent otitis media, see index entries on these infections.

SULFISOXAZOLE:
Gantrisin (Roche), ***Generic***. Tablets 500 mg.

SULFISOXAZOLE ACETYL:
Gantrisin (Roche). Suspension (pediatric) 500 mg/5 ml (0.3% alcohol); syrup 500 mg/5 ml (0.9% alcohol).

Intermediate-acting Sulfonamide

SULFAMETHOXAZOLE
[Gantanol]

MECHANISM OF ACTION, ANTIMICROBIAL SPECTRUM, AND RESISTANCE. See the Introduction.

USES. The indications for this intermediate-acting sulfonamide are the same as for sulfisoxazole and include lower urinary tract and certain systemic infections caused by susceptible organisms. Because sulfamethoxazole is eliminated more slowly than sulfisoxazole, it requires less frequent administration, which may help with compliance. However, the acetylated metabolite of sulfamethoxazole is less soluble in urine and the risk of crystalluria is greater. During therapy, maintenance of an adequate urinary output (at least 1,500 ml daily in adults) by ensuring adequate fluid intake is important, but alkalization of the urine usually is unnecessary. See the evaluation on Sulfisoxazole and the Introduction.

Sulfamethoxazole also is marketed with trimethoprim as a fixed-ratio combination for oral and parenteral use (see the evaluation on this mixture).

ADVERSE REACTIONS AND PRECAUTIONS, DRUG INTERACTIONS, AND INTERFERENCE WITH LABORATORY TESTS. See the Introduction.

Sulfamethoxazole is classified in FDA Pregnancy Category C.

PHARMACOKINETICS. Sulfamethoxazole is completely absorbed following oral administration, although it is absorbed more slowly than sulfisoxazole. It is 70% bound to plasma proteins. The volume of distribution (0.21 L/kg) approximates that of the extracellular fluid. The drug readily distributes to most tissues and body fluids, including pleural, synovial, peritoneal, and cerebrospinal fluids, and crosses the placenta.

Sulfamethoxazole is partially acetylated; both free and acetylated drug are eliminated by the kidneys, primarily by glomerular filtration. The half-life ranges from 10 to 12 hours, which is longer than the half-life of sulfisoxazole. As discussed above, acetylated sulfamethoxazole is less soluble than acetylated sulfisoxazole in the urine.

DOSAGE AND PREPARATIONS.

Oral: *Adults,* 2 g initially, then 1 g two or, for severe infections, three times daily. *Children over 2 months,* initially, 50 to 60 mg/kg then one-half of this amount every 12 hours (maximum, 75 mg/kg/24 hours).

Generic. Tablets 500 mg.

Gantanol (Roche). Suspension 500 mg/5 ml; tablets 500 mg.

MIXTURES

Mixture Containing Only Sulfonamides

The rationale for combining several sulfonamides in a single preparation for systemic use is that the solubilities of the sulfonamides are independent of each other but their therapeutic effects are at least additive. Use of combination therapy thereby decreases the risk of crystalluria. Trisulfapyrimidines is the only such mixture still marketed. The availability of newer single-entity agents (eg, sulfisoxazole) that are more soluble in urine has made combined sulfonamide preparations essentially obsolete for systemic indications.

TRISULFAPYRIMIDINES
[Triple Sulfa No. 2]

This combination contains equal amounts of sulfadiazine, sulfamerazine, and sulfamethazine. It appears to produce somewhat higher total blood levels of sulfonamide than equal doses of sulfadiazine alone, but the effectiveness remains the same. The incidence of crystalluria (but not of other untoward effects) is reduced with trisulfapyrimidines when compared to larger doses of the individual components. However, newer sulfonamides (eg, sulfisoxazole) are considerably more soluble than trisulfapyrimidines and are usually preferred.

For actions, antimicrobial spectrum, indications, adverse reactions and precautions, and drug interactions, see the Introduction.

DOSAGE AND PREPARATIONS.

Oral: *Adults,* 2 to 4 g initially, then 2 to 4 g daily in three to six divided doses. *Children and infants over 2 months,* 75 mg/kg initially, then 150 mg/kg daily in four to six divided doses.

Triple Sulfa No. 2 (Rugby), ***Generic.*** Suspension 500 mg/5 ml; tablets 500 mg.

Mixtures Containing a Sulfonamide and Another Drug

Fixed-ratio combinations containing a sulfonamide and phenazopyridine, a urinary tract analgesic, or a sulfonamide and another antimicrobial agent presently are available for systemic use. See the evaluations for discussions. See the section on Dihydrofolate Reductase Inhibitors for the evaluation on Trimethoprim/Sulfamethoxazole.

SULFONAMIDES AND PHENAZOPYRIDINE

Phenazopyridine, a urinary tract analgesic, is combined with sulfonamides (eg, sulfisoxazole, sulfamethoxazole) in fixed-ratio preparations promoted for the treatment of urinary tract infections. Since phenazopyridine may relieve such symptoms as pain, burning, urgency, and frequency, its concomitant use with a sulfonamide may be beneficial. However, this analgesic preferably should be given separately rather than in a fixed-ratio combination product so that it can be eliminated from the regimen as soon as symptoms are controlled. Phenazopyridine therapy should not be continued beyond the first 48 hours in urinary tract infections because efficacy has not been demonstrated after this time (*Federal Register*, 1983). This drug is an azo dye and colors the urine red or orange (see index entry Phenazopyridine).

DOSAGE AND PREPARATIONS.

Oral: Dosage is the same as that for the sulfonamide without phenazopyridine (see the appropriate evaluation). Treatment with the fixed-ratio combination products should not exceed two days. The sulfonamide should be given alone after this period.

Azo Gantanol (Roche), ***Generic.*** Each tablet contains sulfamethoxazole 500 mg and phenazopyridine hydrochloride 100 mg.

Azo Gantrisin (Roche), ***Generic.*** Each tablet contains sulfisoxazole 500 mg and phenazopyridine hydrochloride 50 mg.

Because proof of efficacy is lacking, the following product is not recommended:

Urobiotic-250 (Roerig). Each capsule contains sulfamethizole 250 mg, oxytetracycline hydrochloride equivalent to oxytetracycline 250 mg, and phenazopyridine hydrochloride 50 mg.

ERYTHROMYCIN ETHYLSUCCINATE AND SULFISOXAZOLE ACETYL

[Eryzole, Pediazole]

This fixed-ratio combination is used to treat acute otitis media and also may be effective in acute bacterial sinusitis. The most likely causative organisms of these infections are *Streptococcus pneumoniae* and *Haemophilus influenzae. Moraxella (Branhamella) catarrhalis* also is an important pathogen in some geographic locations. Amoxicillin (or ampicillin) traditionally has been preferred, but the increasing emergence of resistant (β lactamase-producing) strains of *H. influenzae* (or *M. catarrhalis*) is becoming a major problem in some areas. Erythromycin plus sulfisoxazole is an alternative therapy for patients in whom amoxicillin-resistant *H. influenzae* (or *M. catarrhalis*) is a possibility or for those who cannot tolerate penicillins. For additional discussion, see index entry Otitis Media, Treatment.

There is no unique antibacterial advantage when erythromycin and sulfisoxazole are combined in a fixed-ratio preparation; administration of the two agents separately should be equally effective. However, the fixed-ratio combination is more convenient to administer, a possible advantage in young children with acute otitis media.

The actions, pharmacokinetics, and adverse effects associated with erythromycin ethylsuccinate/sulfisoxazole acetyl are the same as those expected from equivalent doses of the individual agents (see the evaluation on Sulfisoxazole in this chapter and on Erythromycin in the chapter on Macrolides and Lincosamides).

DOSAGE AND PREPARATIONS.

Oral: *Children over 2 months* may be given the drug every six hours for ten days according to the following schedule suggested by the manufacturer: *Less than 8 kg*, dosage is adjusted according to body weight (erythromycin component, 50 mg/kg/day; sulfisoxazole component, 150 mg/kg/day to a maximum of 6 g/day); *8 kg*, 2.5 ml; *16 kg*, 5 ml; *24 kg*, 7.5 ml; and *more than 45 kg*, 10 ml. These doses are administered every six hours.

Eryzole (Alra), ***Pediazole*** (Ross), ***Generic.*** Granules for reconstitution in 100, 150, 200, and 250 (***Pediazole*** only) ml containers. Reconstituted suspension contains erythromycin ethylsuccinate equivalent to 200 mg erythromycin activity and sulfisoxazole acetyl equivalent to 600 mg sulfisoxazole/5 ml.

DIHYDROFOLATE REDUCTASE INHIBITORS

Trimethoprim, a 2,4-diaminopyrimidine, is the prototype of a group of nonsulfonamide drugs that inhibit dihydrofolate reductases of bacterial (also protozoal) cells, thus preventing the formation of tetrahydrofolic acid. Mammalian dihydrofolate reductases are much less inhibited by these compounds. This ability to selectively inhibit an enzyme that is essential to the growth of certain bacteria results in antibacterial activity with limited toxicity to the host. Furthermore, the combination of trimethoprim with a sulfonamide (eg, sulfamethoxazole) results in a synergistic antibacterial effect due to the sequential blockade of two steps in the same biosynthetic pathway (see Figure 2 in the Introduction and the evaluation on Trimethoprim/Sulfamethoxazole).

TRIMETHOPRIM

[Proloprim, Trimpex]

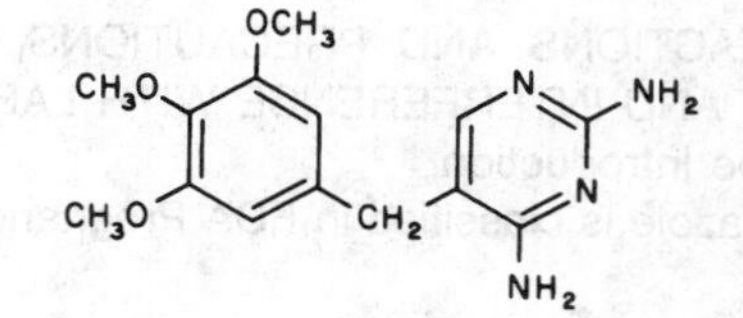

MECHANISM OF ACTION. Trimethoprim competitively inhibits the conversion of dihydrofolic acid to tetrahydrofolic acid by blocking the action of bacterial dihydrofolate reductase (see Figure 2 in the Introduction). Trimethoprim is about 50,000 times more active against bacterial dihydrofolate reductase than against the human enzyme. Lack of tetrahydrofolic acid prevents the one-carbon transfer reactions necessary for the synthesis of certain amino acids (eg, glycine, methionine), purines, and thymidine and, ultimately, DNA, RNA, and protein. Since thymidine biosynthesis by thymidylate synthetase requires stoichiometric amounts of tetrahydrofolic acid, this is believed to be the critical reaction that is prevented by trimethoprim. Trimethoprim may be bacteriostatic or bactericidal depending on the growth conditions. Because pus contains thymine and thymidine, the action of trimethoprim may be inhibited in necrotic wounds containing pus and other cellular debris.

ANTIMICROBIAL SPECTRUM. Trimethoprim is active in vitro against many gram-positive cocci, including *Staphylococcus aureus*, *S. saprophyticus*, *Streptococcus pyogenes*, *S. pneumoniae,* and viridans streptococci. Activity against *Enterococcus faecalis* is variable. Some gram-positive bacilli, such as *Corynebacterium diphtheriae* and *Listeria monocytogenes*, also are susceptible. *Clostridium perfringens* and most anaerobes are resistant, however.

The gram-negative cocci, *Neisseria meningitidis* and *N. gonorrhoeae*, show a variable response, but many strains are resistant.

The majority of clinically important aerobic gram-negative bacilli, including *Escherichia coli*, *Klebsiella*, *Enterobacter*, *Proteus mirabilis*, *Salmonella*, *Shigella*, and *Haemophilus influenzae*, are susceptible. *Pseudomonas aeruginosa, Bacteroides,* and other anaerobes are resistant, however.

Nocardia asteroides is variably susceptible. Trimethoprim acts synergistically with sulfamethoxazole against *Pneumo-*

cystis carinii, an organism of uncertain taxonomic status (probably protozoan or fungus).

Treponema pallidum, Mycoplasma species, and *Mycobacterium tuberculosis* are resistant. Trimethoprim is not effective against fungi or viruses.

RESISTANCE. Resistance to trimethoprim can occur by several mechanisms, which may be plasmid or chromosome mediated. Chromosomal resistance mechanisms include: qualitative alteration in bacterial dihydrofolate reductase resulting in decreased affinity for trimethoprim; overproduction of the bacterial dihydrofolate reductase enzyme; decreased bacterial cell wall permeability to the drug; and thymine- or thymidine-dependent bacterial mutants that are intrinsically resistant to trimethoprim because they lack thymidylate synthetase and, thus, depend on exogenous thymine or thymidine for growth (Burchall et al, 1982; Goldstein et al, 1986; Huovinen, 1987). These mechanisms usually confer on the bacteria a low-level resistance to trimethoprim (Goldstein et al, 1986).

Clinically, the most important type of acquired resistance to trimethoprim results from the production of novel trimethoprim-resistant dihydrofolate reductases (eg, type I DHFR, type II DHFR). These additional dihydrofolate reductase enzymes are encoded on transferable plasmids or transposons and confer on the bacteria a high-level resistance to trimethoprim (Burchall et al, 1982; Mayer et al, 1985; Murray et al, 1985; Goldstein et al, 1986; Huovinen, 1987). At least nine different trimethoprim-resistant plasmid-encoded bacterial dihydrofolate reductase enzymes or their genes have been described in Enterobacteriaceae, other gram-negative bacteria, and staphylococci (Huovinen, 1987; Zinner and Mayer, 1990).

Emergence of resistance to trimethoprim (alone or as a component of trimethoprim/sulfamethoxazole) varies among countries, cities within countries, and individual hospitals. Results from sequential surveys generally suggest that trimethoprim resistance, particularly high-level plasmid-mediated resistance, has been gradually increasing in developed countries, such as Finland (Huovinen et al, 1985; Huovinen, 1987; Heikkilä et al, 1990 A), Great Britain (Towner, 1982; Brumfitt et al, 1983; Hamilton-Miller and Purves, 1986; Towner and Slack, 1986), and the United States (Mayer et al, 1985; Murray et al, 1985). Most of these surveys indicate that 3% to 20% of *E. coli* strains are now resistant to this drug in these developed countries. In contrast, resistance to trimethoprim (or trimethoprim/sulfamethoxazole) is widespread in many developing countries (Murray et al, 1985) and in certain cities (Goldstein et al, 1986), hospitals (Acar and Goldstein, 1982; Huovinen et al, 1986; Heikkilä et al, 1990 B), and day care centers (Reves et al, 1987, 1990).

Considerable controversy has revolved around whether trimethoprim alone is more likely to cause the development of resistant bacterial strains than the combination of trimethoprim and sulfamethoxazole. The combination was originally marketed in preference to trimethoprim alone because of the drugs' synergistic action and because it was believed that the exclusive use of the combination would prevent the emergence of organisms resistant to either agent. Although considerable clinical work has been conducted to test the latter premise, the controversy has not been completely resolved. Clearly, trimethoprim resistance has spread in developing countries where the drug combination has been used primarily (Murray et al, 1985). Furthermore, in Finland, where trimethoprim alone has been used to treat outpatient urinary tract infections for nearly 20 years, although resistance among *E. coli* strains to this drug has increased, the proportion of trimethoprim-resistant, but sulfonamide-susceptible *E. coli* isolates has not increased (Heikkilä et al, 1990 A). In contrast, an increase in trimethoprim-resistant but sulfonamide-sensitive clinical isolates of Enterobacteriaceae in Nottingham (United Kingdom) has been reported (Towner, 1982; Towner and Slack, 1986). To date, significant resistance has not developed to either the combination or to trimethoprim alone in the United States (Murray et al, 1985; Reves et al, 1987, 1990). In summary, there is no strong evidence that there has been a more rapid increase in resistance to trimethoprim as the result of its use alone. However, continued surveillance of resistance patterns combined with appropriate use of both trimethoprim alone and the trimethoprim/sulfamethoxazole combination are necessary (see also the evaluation on Trimethoprim/Sulfamethoxazole).

USES. Trimethoprim alone is labeled only for the initial treatment of acute, uncomplicated urinary tract infections (eg, cystitis) caused by susceptible organisms, particularly *E. coli*, *P. mirabilis*, *K. pneumoniae*, *Enterobacter* species, and *S. saprophyticus*. Urinary concentrations of the drug greatly exceed those required to inhibit sensitive pathogens, and trimethoprim appears to be as effective as trimethoprim/sulfamethoxazole for initial episodes of acute, uncomplicated urinary tract infections. Trimethoprim has been associated with fewer side effects than the combination, presumably because of the absence of the sulfa component (see Brogden et al, 1982; Johnson and Stamm, 1987). Trimethoprim has been used as an alternative to trimethoprim/sulfamethoxazole for short-course therapy (eg, three days) as well as conventional therapy (7 to 14 days) of acute, uncomplicated lower urinary tract infections (see Johnson and Stamm, 1987; see also index entry Urinary Tract Infections).

A single daily dose of trimethoprim also is effective for the prophylaxis of recurrent urinary tract infections in women. Presently, however, trimethoprim/sulfamethoxazole is preferred for this indication (see this evaluation and index entry Urinary Tract Infections).

Trimethoprim, a relatively lipophilic compound, is one of the few antibacterial agents that adequately penetrates into the uninflamed prostate gland. Therefore, it is useful in the treatment of chronic bacterial prostatitis, an infection that is difficult to cure. Presently, trimethoprim/sulfamethoxazole or a fluoroquinolone (ciprofloxacin [Cipro], ofloxacin [Floxin]) is the regimen of choice for this infection. Some infectious disease experts believe that trimethoprim alone should be preferred to the combination for chronic prostatitis because sulfamethoxazole fails to achieve therapeutic concentrations in the uninflamed prostate (Friesen et al, 1981; Reeves, 1982). See also the evaluation on Trimethoprim/Sulfamethoxazole and index entry Prostatitis.

Trimethoprim appears to be an effective alternative to trimethoprim/sulfamethoxazole in certain patients (eg, sulfonamide-allergic) for both the treatment and prophylaxis of travelers' diarrhea (DuPont et al, 1982, 1983). The fluoroquinolones (ciprofloxacin, ofloxacin, norfloxacin) also are very effective for these indications (see index entry Diarrhea, Travelers').

Trimethoprim should not be used alone for treatment of *Pneumocystis carinii* pneumonia. However, the combination of trimethoprim/sulfamethoxazole is preferred for both treatment and prophylaxis of this infection. Trimethoprim plus dapsone also has been effective for mild or moderate *P. carinii* pneumonia (Medina et al, 1990). Presently, this regimen is a second-line therapy, however (see index entry Pneumocystis Pneumonia).

ADVERSE REACTIONS AND PRECAUTIONS. Trimethoprim generally is well tolerated. The overall frequency of side effects with this drug alone has been less than for trimethoprim/sulfamethoxazole when these regimens have been compared in the treatment of urinary tract infections (see Brogden et al, 1982).

The most common adverse effects are pruritus and skin rash. Maculopapular and morbilliform rashes have been reported most often, but exfoliative dermatitis and toxic epidermal necrolysis also have been observed rarely. Gastrointestinal reactions are common and include epigastric distress, nausea, vomiting, and glossitis. Hematologic reactions, including thrombocytopenia, leukopenia, neutropenia, megaloblastic anemia, and methemoglobinemia, are rare and occur most often when large doses and/or prolonged therapy are used or when the drug is administered to patients with folate deficiencies. Fever and elevated levels of serum transaminases, bilirubin, blood urea nitrogen, and serum creatinine have been noted. A case of cholestatic jaundice has been reported (Tanner, 1986). Symptoms of aseptic meningitis have been associated with the use of trimethoprim alone (Carlson and Wiholm, 1987).

Trimethoprim should be used with caution in patients with possible folate deficiency (eg, alcoholics, malnourished or debilitated patients, pregnant women, patients receiving phenytoin, patients with malabsorption syndromes). Folinic acid can be administered concomitantly to prevent the antifolate effects of trimethoprim without decreasing its antibacterial efficacy.

Caution is recommended in patients with impaired renal or hepatic function. Dosage reductions are necessary when creatinine clearance is between 15 and 30 ml/minute. The use of trimethoprim in patients with a creatinine clearance below 15 ml/min is not recommended.

Since trimethoprim is a folate antagonist, it might be expected to cause teratogenic effects. Fetal malformations have occurred in rats given large doses (40 times the human dose) but have not yet been reported clinically. Nevertheless, because of the lack of published data on use of the drug in pregnant women and because folate levels are probably marginal during pregnancy, trimethoprim is generally contraindicated in pregnant women or should be used only when the potential benefit justifies the potential risk to the fetus (FDA Pregnancy Category C). Caution should be exercised when trimethoprim is administered to nursing mothers since it is excreted in human milk and may interfere with folate metabolism in the nursing infant. Infants younger than 2 months should not be given the drug since its safety has not been established in this age group.

DRUG INTERACTIONS. Trimethoprim can inhibit the hepatic metabolism of phenytoin and delay its elimination (increased half-life; reduced metabolic clearance). When these drugs are administered concurrently, the plasma phenytoin concentration should be monitored and the patient observed for symptoms of phenytoin toxicity (eg, nystagmus, ataxia). The phenytoin dosage should be adjusted, if necessary, accordingly (see Tatro, 1991).

Trimethoprim has been reported to increase the plasma concentration of procainamide and its active N-acetyl metabolite by decreasing their renal clearance (Kosoglou et al, 1988; Vlasses et al, 1989). Although these studies were done in healthy male volunteers, it is recommended that clinical and antiarrhythmic plasma level monitoring be done for patients (especially the elderly) receiving trimethoprim and maintenance doses of procainamide (see Tatro, 1991).

A bidirectional drug interaction was observed between dapsone and trimethoprim, resulting in higher plasma concentrations of each in the presence of the other, in patients with the acquired immunodeficiency syndrome (AIDS) being treated for *P. carinii* pneumonia (Lee et al, 1989).

PHARMACOKINETICS. Trimethoprim is absorbed rapidly and completely from the gastrointestinal tract. Peak serum concentrations are attained one to four hours after oral administration. Mean peak serum levels of approximately 1 mcg/ml can be attained after an initial dose of 100 mg.

Approximately 44% of circulating trimethoprim is bound to plasma protein. The drug is widely distributed in the body and the volume of distribution is 1.8 ± 0.2 L/kg (Benet and Williams, 1990). This compound is relatively lipophilic and diffuses well into tissues and body fluids (Brumfitt and Hamilton-Miller, 1980; Friesen et al, 1981; Brogden et al, 1982). Concentrations equal to or greater than serum levels occur in prostate tissue and fluid, saliva, sputum, lung tissue, bronchial and vaginal secretions, and synovial fluid. Therapeutic concentrations also can be achieved in middle ear fluid, bile, seminal fluid, bone tissue, and aqueous humor. In patients with uninflamed meninges, cerebrospinal fluid concentrations are approximately 20% to 40% of serum concentrations. Trimethoprim readily crosses the placenta.

The kidneys are the main organs of excretion through glomerular filtration and tubular secretion. The half-life in adult patients with normal renal function is 9 to 11 hours; in children, shorter elimination half-lives (1 to 3 years, 3.7 hours; 8 to 10 years, 5.4 hours) have been reported (Hoppu, 1987). The half-life of trimethoprim is prolonged in those with severe renal impairment. After oral administration, 50% to 60% of a dose is recovered in the urine within 24 hours; about 80% is unchanged drug and the remainder is inactive oxidized or hydroxylated metabolites. Urinary concentrations of trimethoprim are considerably higher than serum levels. After a single oral dose of 100 mg, urine concentrations ranged from 30 to

160 mcg/ml during the first four hours and declined to between 18 and 91 mcg/ml from 8 to 24 hours.

DOSAGE AND PREPARATIONS.

Oral: For acute, uncomplicated urinary tract infections, *adults and children over 12 years*, 100 mg every 12 hours or 200 mg every 24 hours, each for ten days. The use of trimethoprim in patients with creatinine clearance of less than 15 ml/min is not recommended. When creatinine clearance is between 15 and 30 ml/min, a dose of 50 mg every 12 hours should be employed.

For prophylaxis of recurrent urinary tract infections in women, *adults*, 50 to 100 mg once daily at bedtime; 50 to 100 mg every other day was considered adequate by some infectious disease experts. The duration of prophylaxis generally is six months.

For chronic prostatitis (eg, in sulfonamide-allergic patients), *adults*, 200 mg twice daily for 12 weeks.

For the treatment of travelers' diarrhea, *adults*, 200 mg twice daily for five days (DuPont et al, 1982). For the prophylaxis of travelers' diarrhea, *adults*, 200 mg once daily beginning on day of travel and continuing two days after return home (DuPont et al, 1983; Satterwhite and DuPont, 1983).

Proloprim (Burroughs Wellcome), ***Generic.*** Tablets 100 and 200 mg.

Trimpex (Roche). Tablets 100 mg.

Mixture

TRIMETHOPRIM/SULFAMETHOXAZOLE

[Bactrim, Cotrim, Septra]

MECHANISM OF ACTION. Trimethoprim/sulfamethoxazole (also called co-trimoxazole) inhibits sequential steps in the synthesis of tetrahydrofolic acid, an essential metabolic cofactor in the bacterial synthesis of purines, thymidine, glycine, and methionine. Sulfonamides, including sulfamethoxazole, are structural analogues of PABA and block the synthesis of dihydropteroic acid, the immediate precursor of dihydrofolic acid, from PABA and pteridine. Trimethoprim subsequently acts to inhibit the reduction of dihydrofolic acid to the metabolically active tetrahydrofolic acid by the enzyme, dihydrofolate reductase (see Figure 2 in the Introduction). The most important consequence of this sequential enzymatic inhibition appears to be the interruption of thymidine synthesis.

Combining the two antimetabolites has the following theoretical advantages. Antibacterial synergism is observed in vitro, ie, most bacteria are considerably more susceptible to the combination than to either of the agents used alone. Whereas the individual drugs are primarily bacteriostatic at therapeutic concentrations, the combination is usually bactericidal. The concomitant use of the two drugs also may reduce the rate of emergence of resistant bacterial strains.

Since mammalian cells do not produce folic acid, the sulfamethoxazole-induced inhibition of folic acid synthesis does not take place in humans. Also, the affinity of trimethoprim for bacterial dihydrofolate reductase is about 50,000 times greater than for the human enzyme. Thus, a high therapeutic/toxic ratio is obtained with trimethoprim/sulfamethoxazole.

ANTIMICROBIAL SPECTRUM. Trimethoprim/sulfamethoxazole is active in vitro against a variety of gram-negative and gram-positive bacteria. Among aerobic gram-negative enteric bacteria, *Escherichia coli, Proteus mirabilis, Salmonella* (including *S. typhi*), *Shigella,* and *Citrobacter* are very susceptible. Indole-positive *Proteus, Morganella morganii, Serratia marcescens, Klebsiella pneumoniae, Enterobacter,* and *Providencia stuartii* are moderately susceptible.

Other gram-negative bacilli that are very susceptible to trimethoprim/sulfamethoxazole include *Haemophilus influenzae, Vibrio cholerae,* and *Yersinia pestis. Acinetobacter, Bordetella pertussis, Brucella, Gardnerella (Haemophilus) vaginalis, H. ducreyi, Pseudomonas pseudomallei, P. cepacia, Flavobacterium meningosepticum, Yersinia enterocolitica, Aeromonas hydrophila, Legionella pneumophila,* and *L. micdadei* also are susceptible. *Bacteroides* and *Fusobacterium,* gram-negative anaerobic bacteria, are usually resistant. *Pseudomonas aeruginosa* is resistant.

Most strains of *Neisseria meningitidis* and *N. gonorrhoeae*, gram-negative cocci, are susceptible. *Moraxella (Branhamella) catarrhalis* also are susceptible (Kallings, 1986; Nicotra et al, 1986).

Most gram-positive bacteria are susceptible to trimethoprim/sulfamethoxazole in vitro, but there are only limited clinical data regarding treatment of systemic infections caused by these organisms. Among gram-positive cocci, *Staphylococcus aureus* (including many methicillin-resistant strains), *S. epidermidis, Streptococcus pneumoniae, S. pyogenes*, and viridans streptococci frequently are susceptible in vitro. Trimethoprim/sulfamethoxazole usually is only bacteriostatic against staphylococci, however. The activity in vitro against *Enterococcus faecalis* is variable, and trimethoprim/sulfamethoxazole should not be relied on clinically for enterococcal urinary tract infections. *Corynebacterium diphtheriae* and *Listeria monocytogenes,* gram-positive bacilli, are susceptible in vitro.

Nocardia and *Chlamydia trachomatis* are susceptible. Trimethoprim/sulfamethoxazole has been effective in the treatment of *Pneumocystis carinii* pneumonia (see below). Certain atypical mycobacteria (eg, *Mycobacterium marinum*) are susceptible. *Mycoplasma* species and *Treponema pallidum* are resistant.

The maximum synergistic interaction between trimethoprim and sulfamethoxazole is observed when the microorganism is susceptible to both drugs. However, synergistic activity also has been observed when organisms are sulfamethoxazole-resistant and trimethoprim-susceptible or moderately trimethoprim-resistant. Intrinsic susceptibility to trimethoprim is a major factor in determining the efficacy of the combination for most organisms. An exception is *N. gonorrhoeae*, which is more susceptible to the sulfonamide.

RESISTANCE. The frequency of development of bacterial resistance to trimethoprim/sulfamethoxazole is considered to be lower than it is to either of the agents alone. Resistance to trimethoprim has received the most attention. Clinically, the most important mechanism is due to the production of novel dihydrofolate reductases that are highly resistant to trimethoprim. These enzymes differ from native dihydrofolate reductase in molecular weight, subunit structure, and kinetic properties. This type of resistance is mediated by transferable plasmids or transposons. Other mechanisms of resistance, usually chromosome mediated, include increased levels of dihydrofolate reductase and production of an altered dihydrofolate reductase with a decreased binding affinity for trimethoprim. Decreased permeability of the bacterial cell to trimethoprim has been reported rarely (eg, for *Pseudomonas aeruginosa*). For a more detailed discussion, see the evaluation on Trimethoprim. For mechanisms of resistance to sulfonamides, see the Introduction.

USES. Trimethoprim/sulfamethoxazole is a preferred or alternative antimicrobial regimen for a number of infectious diseases as outlined below. For additional discussion, see index entries on these infections.

Urinary Tract Infections: This combination is recommended for the treatment of upper or lower urinary tract infections due to susceptible strains of *Escherichia coli, Klebsiella, Enterobacter, Proteus mirabilis, P. vulgaris,* and *Morganella morganii.* Intravenous administration may be necessary for severe infections (eg, acute pyelonephritis).

Many infectious disease experts consider oral trimethoprim/sulfamethoxazole to be the preferred therapy for acute uncomplicated urinary tract infections in outpatients (see Johnson and Stamm, 1987; Sobel and Kaye, 1990; Johnson et al, 1991; *Med Lett Drugs Ther*, 1992 B). In addition to conventional (multiple-dose) treatment (7 to 14 days), this combination has been shown to be particularly useful in short-course therapy for three days, or alternatively as a single dose, for initial attacks of acute cystitis in nonpregnant women with no renal parenchymal involvement and who are available for follow-up. The recommended dosage for adults is trimethoprim 160 mg/sulfamethoxazole 800 mg (ie, one double-strength tablet) twice daily for three days (or alternatively, trimethoprim 320 mg/sulfamethoxazole 1.6 g [ie, two double-strength tablets] as a single dose).

Trimethoprim (40 mg)/sulfamethoxazole (200 mg), ie, one-half regular-strength tablet, at bedtime three times per week on Sunday, Wednesday, and Friday (some experts prefer daily administration) is preferred for the long-term (eg, six months or longer) prophylaxis of recurrent urinary tract infections in selected women.

Trimethoprim/sulfamethoxazole or a fluoroquinolone (ciprofloxacin, ofloxacin) is the therapy of choice for acute and chronic bacterial prostatitis. Chronic bacterial prostatitis requires a prolonged course of therapy (eg, adults, trimethoprim 160 mg/sulfamethoxazole 800 mg [ie, one double-strength tablet] twice daily for 12 weeks). Trimethoprim alone is another alternative for chronic prostatitis.

Respiratory Tract Infections: Trimethoprim/sulfamethoxazole is useful for the treatment of acute otitis media and acute sinusitis caused by susceptible strains of *Streptococcus pneumoniae, Haemophilus influenzae,* and *Moraxella (Branhamella) catarrhalis* when there are advantages over amoxicillin, the usual drug of choice (eg, in penicillin-allergic patients, presence of amoxicillin-resistant *H. influenzae* or *M. catarrhalis* strain). This combination also has been used as an alternative to sulfisoxazole or ampicillin for long-term (eg, six months) prophylaxis of recurrent otitis media in selected children.

Trimethoprim/sulfamethoxazole is recommended for acute exacerbations of chronic bronchitis caused by susceptible strains of *S. pneumoniae* and *H. influenzae* when there are advantages over single agents (eg, amoxicillin, tetracycline). Based on currently available data, however, the effectiveness of antimicrobial drug therapy for this indication is uncertain.

Although not the therapy of choice, trimethoprim/sulfamethoxazole can be effective in pneumonias caused by susceptible strains of *H. influenzae* or other gram-negative bacteria. Intravenous administration should be used in seriously ill patients.

Trimethoprim/sulfamethoxazole is an alternative to erythromycin for the elimination of *B. pertussis* carriage in patients with pertussis.

Trimethoprim/sulfamethoxazole is *not* recommended for pharyngitis due to *Streptococcus pyogenes* because failures have been reported.

Gastrointestinal Infections: Trimethoprim/sulfamethoxazole or a fluoroquinolone (ciprofloxacin, ofloxacin) is a preferred regimen for shigellosis caused by susceptible strains of *Shigella flexneri* and *S. sonnei*. Antibacterial agents shorten the duration of illness and decrease the relapse rate in this disease.

Antibacterial agents usually are not useful for simple gastroenteritis caused by *Salmonella*. However, they are indicated for typhoid fever (*S. typhi*) or for systemic infections (eg, bacteremia) caused by other species of *Salmonella*. Presently, trimethoprim/sulfamethoxazole is an alternative for these infections. Third generation cephalosporins (eg, cefotaxime [Claforan], ceftriaxone [Rocephin]), ampicillin, chloramphenicol, and the fluoroquinolones (ciprofloxacin, ofloxacin) are other drugs used to treat salmonelloses. Trimethoprim/sulfamethoxazole also may be effective in eliminating chronic *Salmonella* carriage.

Travelers' diarrhea is most frequently caused by enterotoxigenic strains of *Escherichia coli* (about 50% of cases); *Shigella* and other enteric pathogens are less common causes of this disease. Trimethoprim/sulfamethoxazole has been shown to be effective in the treatment of travelers' diarrhea (DuPont et al, 1982) and is a recommended regimen for more severe cases (National Institutes of Health Consensus Development Conference, 1985). Adding the antimotility agent, loperamide [Imodium], to this combination has been reported to hasten relief of diarrhea and enteric symptoms (Ericsson et al, 1990, 1992). The fluoroquinolones (ciprofloxacin, ofloxacin) also are effective for travelers' diarrhea and are preferred by many experts (see index entry Diarrhea, Travelers').

Trimethoprim/sulfamethoxazole also is effective for the prophylaxis of travelers' diarrhea (DuPont et al, 1983). Prophylaxis generally is not recommended, however, because of the potential for adverse drug reactions and the emergence of resistant bacterial strains (National Institutes of Health Consensus Development Conference, 1985).

Trimethoprim/sulfamethoxazole is a preferred regimen for infections caused by *Yersinia enterocolitica* and *Aeromonas hydrophila*; this combination is an alternative to tetracycline in cholera. Trimethoprim/sulfamethoxazole is recommended in isosporiasis (*Isospora belli*).

Sexually Transmitted Diseases: Although many strains of *Neisseria gonorrhoeae* are susceptible to trimethoprim/sulfamethoxazole, single-dose regimens of other drugs (eg, ceftriaxone [Rocephin], a fluoroquinolone) usually are preferred for uncomplicated gonococcal infections. Larger oral doses of trimethoprim/sulfamethoxazole (ie, a single daily dose of nine regular strength [80 mg/400 mg] tablets for five days) have been effective in pharyngeal gonococcal infections caused by penicillinase-producing *N. gonorrhoeae* (PPNG) strains and may be used when ceftriaxone, the preferred drug, cannot be tolerated (eg, due to hypersensitivity) (see *MMWR*, 1989; Moran and Zenilman, 1990; and index entry Sexually Transmitted Diseases).

Trimethoprim/sulfamethoxazole is an alternative to ceftriaxone or erythromycin (preferred regimens) for chancroid in geographic areas where *H. ducreyi* strains are susceptible. Although chlamydial infections and granuloma inguinale may respond to this combination, tetracyclines are preferred. This preparation is not active in syphilis or *Ureaplasma urealyticum* infections (eg, urethritis).

Other Infections: Trimethoprim/sulfamethoxazole is a therapy of choice for *Pseudomonas cepacia* and *Xanthomonas maltophilia* infections. This combination also is effective for nocardiosis, and some experts prefer it to single-entity sulfonamides (eg, sulfadiazine, sulfisoxazole). Trimethoprim/sulfamethoxazole, in combination with ceftazidime or with tetracycline and chloramphenicol, has been useful for melioidosis. Trimethoprim/sulfamethoxazole is an alternative regimen for brucellosis (a tetracycline with either streptomycin or rifampin is preferred); *Legionella* infections (erythromycin with or without rifampin is preferred); and infections caused by *Mycobacterium marinum* (minocycline is preferred).

Trimethoprim/sulfamethoxazole may be useful in serious infections, including meningitis, osteomyelitis, bacteremia, and endocarditis, caused by susceptible gram-negative bacteria when other antibacterial agents are ineffective or not tolerated. Of particular note, gram-negative bacillary meningitis caused by organisms only moderately susceptible to third generation cephalosporins (eg, *Enterobacter cloacae, Serratia marcescens*) or resistant to these antibiotics (*Acinetobacter, Pseudomonas cepacia*) may be candidates for trimethoprim/sulfamethoxazole therapy if the organisms are susceptible (Levitz and Quintiliani, 1984). This combination may be an effective alternative to ampicillin (or penicillin G) with or without an aminoglycoside for the treatment of meningitis and bacteremia caused by *Listeria monocytogenes* (Levitz and Quintiliani, 1984; Spitzer et al, 1986). Trimethoprim/sulfamethoxazole may be useful for the treatment of infective endocarditis caused by *Coxiella burnetii* (Street and Durack, 1988).

In a double-blind, randomized, prospective study, intravenous trimethoprim/sulfamethoxazole (320 mg/1.6 g twice daily) was shown to be less effective than vancomycin in the treatment of intravenous drug users with serious *Staphylococcus aureus* infections, including bacteremias, endocarditis, septic arthritis, and osteomyelitis. However, all treatment failures with trimethoprim/sulfamethoxazole occurred in patients with methicillin-sensitive *S. aureus*. No treatment failures were recorded in patients with methicillin-resistant *S. aureus* infections (Markowitz et al, 1992). The investigators concluded that this combination may be a useful alternative to vancomycin in selected cases of methicillin-resistant *S. aureus* infection caused by susceptible isolates. However, some consultants have expressed concern about the use of trimethoprim/sulfamethoxazole in deep-seated staphylococcal infections (eg, endocarditis) because this combination may only be bacteriostatic against this organism.

Trimethoprim/sulfamethoxazole prophylaxis has been beneficial in the management of chronic granulomatous disease (Weening et al, 1983; Margolis et al, 1990). Trimethoprim/sulfamethoxazole also has been used to treat a few patients with Wegener's granulomatosis (DeRemee, et al, 1985; West et al, 1987), but its efficacy in this disease has not been observed by others (Hoffman et al, 1992).

Pneumocystis carinii Pneumonia: This opportunistic protozoal (or fungal) infection frequently occurs in immunocompromised patients. High-dose oral or intravenous trimethoprim/sulfamethoxazole is considered to be the therapy of choice for this disease in children and adults with cancer or organ transplants because it is at least as effective but less toxic than the available alternative, pentamidine isethionate [Pentam 300] (Hughes et al, 1978; Winston et al, 1980; Sattler and Remington, 1981; Hughes, 1982, 1987; Young, 1982; Siegel et al, 1984). This combination also is effective in the prevention of *P. carinii* pneumonia (Hughes et al, 1977, 1987), and prophylaxis is indicated in selected patients (eg, children with acute lymphocytic leukemia who are at high risk for this infection).

P. carinii pneumonia also is one of the most common opportunistic infections in patients with the acquired immunodeficiency syndrome (AIDS). Oral or intravenous trimethoprim/sulfamethoxazole (alternative, pentamidine isethionate intravenously) has been shown to be effective in AIDS-associated *P. carinii* pneumonia, although it generally requires a longer course of therapy than is necessary in other immunocompromised patients with the disease (Hughes, 1987; Sattler et al, 1988; Davey and Masur, 1990; Glatt and Chirgwin, 1990; *Med Lett Drugs Ther*, 1991). Furthermore, its use has been associated with a high incidence of adverse reactions (see the section on Adverse Reactions and Precautions; see also Jaffe et al, 1983; Mitsuyasu et al, 1983; Gordin et al, 1984; Kovacs et al, 1984; Wharton et al, 1986; Hughes, 1987; Sattler et al, 1988; Davey and Masur, 1990; Glatt and Chirgwin, 1990). The toxicity associated with trimethoprim/sulfamethoxazole may be diminished, and therapy successfully completed, when the dosage is modified by pharmacokinetic monitoring to maintain serum trimethoprim concentrations of 5 to 8 mcg/ml (Sattler et al, 1988). If an adverse reaction requires discontinuation of trimethoprim/sulfamethoxazole, the course of treatment may be successfully completed with pentamidine isethionate (Davey and Masur, 1990; Glatt and

Chirgwin, 1990). In contrast, AIDS patients who have failed to respond to trimethoprim/sulfamethoxazole after five to seven days of therapy also are unlikely to respond to pentamidine (Small et al, 1985; Sattler et al, 1988; Davey and Masur, 1990; Glatt and Chirgwin, 1990). Possible alternative regimens for *P. carinii* pneumonia in AIDS patients include atovaquone [Mepron], dapsone plus trimethoprim (for mild to moderate disease), clindamycin plus primaquine, and trimetrexate (with leucovorin to prevent bone marrow suppression) (see Davey and Masur, 1990; Glatt and Chirgwin, 1990; Falloon et al, 1991; *Med Lett Drugs Ther*, 1991). Adjunctive corticosteroid therapy is indicated for moderate to severe *P. carinii* pneumonia with hypoxia (room air $PO_2 \leq 70$ mm Hg or Aa gradient ≥ 35 mm Hg) (see *Med Lett Drugs Ther*, 1991). For additional discussion, see index entry Pneumocystis Pneumonia.

Prevention of *P. carinii* pneumonia, either primary or secondary, is a preferred alternative to treating HIV-infected patients for successive episodes of this disease. In a randomized controlled trial in adults receiving zidovudine [Retrovir] (100 mg every four hours) and who had recovered from an initial episode of *P. carinii* pneumonia (AIDS Clinical Trials Group trial 021), oral trimethoprim (160 mg)/sulfamethoxazole (800 mg) once daily was significantly more effective than aerosolized pentamidine for the prophylaxis of *P. carinii* pneumonia. Severe adverse effects occurred in approximately 30% of patients receiving trimethoprim/sulfamethoxazole (see *MMWR*, 1992). Based on the results of this clinical trial, the U.S. Public Health Service Task Force on Antipneumocystis Prophylaxis for Patients with Human Immunodeficiency Virus Infection currently recommends this once-daily trimethoprim (160 mg)/sulfamethoxazole (800 mg) regimen for lifetime prophylaxis against *P. carinii* pneumonia, unless drug intolerance or contraindications exist, for any HIV-infected adult or adolescent ($\geq$13 years of age) who has recovered from a documented episode of *P. carinii* pneumonia (secondary prophylaxis) and for HIV-infected adults or adolescents who have never had an episode of *P. carinii* pneumonia (primary prophylaxis) if their CD4+ T-lymphocyte cell count is <200 cells/microliter or who present with constitutional symptoms such as thrush or unexplained fever >100° F for $\geq$2 weeks, regardless of CD4+ T-lymphocyte cell count (*MMWR*, 1992).

Trimethoprim/sulfamethoxazole also is the drug of choice for prophylaxis against *P. carinii* pneumonia in infants and children. The Working Group on PCP Prophylaxis in Children recommends initiation of primary prophylaxis for children $\geq$1 month of age who are HIV-infected, HIV-seropositive or, if <12 months old, born to an HIV-infected mother, and who have the following age-adjusted CD4+ T-lymphocyte cell count indicator levels:

<1,500 cells/microliter for children 1 to 11 months;
<750 cells/microliter for children 12 to 23 months;
<500 cells/microliter for children 24 months to 5 years;
<200 cells/microliter for children 6 years or older.

A CD4+ T-lymphocyte percentage of <20% of total lymphocytes, regardless of absolute count, or a history of a prior episode of *P. carinii* pneumonia also are indications for the initiation of prophylaxis. The recommended dosage of trimethoprim/sulfamethoxazole in children is trimethoprim 150 mg/M^2/day with sulfamethoxazole 750 mg/M^2/day given orally in divided doses twice daily, three times per week, on consecutive days (eg, Monday, Tuesday, Wednesday) (*MMWR*, 1991).

Prophylaxis in Neutropenic Patients: Trimethoprim/sulfamethoxazole has been reported to be effective in reducing the incidence of gram-negative rod bacteremia in neutropenic patients, usually those with acute leukemias, in a number of clinical studies (Gurwith et al, 1979; Dekker et al, 1981; Kauffman et al, 1983; Wade et al, 1983; Riben et al, 1983; Estey et al, 1984; Kovatch et al, 1985). Some studies have failed to show a benefit from prophylaxis, however (Gaya et al, 1980; Henry et al, 1984; Kramer et al, 1984). Also, infections with trimethoprim/sulfamethoxazole-resistant organisms and prolongation of neutropenia in patients treated with this antimicrobial combination have been reported (Dekker et al, 1981; Wade et al, 1983; Woods et al, 1984; Kovatch et al, 1985). The role of trimethoprim/sulfamethoxazole in the prophylaxis of gram-negative bacillary infection in neutropenic cancer patients remains controversial.

Prevention of Infections in Transplantation: Prophylaxis with trimethoprim/sulfamethoxazole has been shown to reduce the incidence of bacterial infections in renal transplant patients (Fox et al, 1990); side effects were minimal and drug interactions with cyclosporine [Sandimmune] were not observed (Maki et al, 1992). Prophylaxis with this regimen currently is used in many transplant (eg, renal, heart, bone marrow) programs (Sinnott and Rubin, 1990).

ADVERSE REACTIONS AND PRECAUTIONS. Trimethoprim/sulfamethoxazole usually is well tolerated by adults (Lawson and Paice, 1982; Wormser et al, 1982) and children (Gutman, 1984); however, severe, including fatal, adverse reactions have been reported rarely (*FDA Drug Bull*, 1984). Any adverse effect reported with the use of sulfonamides or trimethoprim may occur following administration of the combination (see the Introduction and the evaluation on Trimethoprim).

Skin rashes are among the most common adverse effects caused by trimethoprim/sulfamethoxazole and are most often due to hypersensitivity to the sulfonamide component. These are usually mild, diffuse, maculopapular rashes that are reversible upon discontinuation of the drug. Serious skin reactions, including toxic epidermal necrolysis, erythema multiforme, exfoliative dermatitis, and the Stevens-Johnson syndrome, have occurred rarely.

Sulfonamides have caused leukopenia, thrombocytopenia, eosinophilia, agranulocytosis, bone marrow aplasia, and hemolytic anemia (both related to hypersensitivity and to G6PD deficiency). Some of these are hypersensitivity reactions. Because blood dyscrasias have been reported, blood tests should be performed at regular intervals during prolonged therapy. Although such tests detect the milder leukopenias, the sudden appearance of sore throat, fever, pallor, purpura, or jaundice may be an indication of a serious blood disorder, and blood counts should be obtained.

Increased incidences of hematologic abnormalities, most commonly a transient and reversible neutropenia, in children receiving oral or intravenous trimethoprim/sulfamethoxazole have been reported by some investigators (Ardati et al, 1979; Asmar et al, 1981; see also Worsmer et al, 1982). However, it is unclear whether many of these observed hematologic abnormalities were actual adverse reactions caused by trimethoprim/sulfamethoxazole or were due to some other cause, such as an underlying viral illness (see Gutman, 1984; Feldman et al, 1985).

In addition to hypersensitivity reactions involving the skin and blood, trimethoprim/sulfamethoxazole has been associated with chills, drug fever, allergic vasculitis, a lupus erythematosus-like syndrome, and anaphylaxis. The sulfonamide component probably is the causative drug. Patients who are allergic to either component of the combination should not be given trimethoprim/sulfamethoxazole.

Trimethoprim has caused megaloblastosis due to its folate-depleting effect. This is uncommon and usually occurs in patients prone to folate deficiency including alcoholics, malnourished or debilitated patients, pregnant women, patients receiving phenytoin, and patients with malabsorption syndromes. The administration of folinic acid reverses or prevents the adverse effect without affecting antimicrobial effectiveness.

Trimethoprim/sulfamethoxazole has caused mild reversible increases in serum creatinine levels. Interstitial nephritis is an uncommon, reversible adverse effect more frequently seen in patients with renal disease. Crystalluria can occur; therefore, patients taking this medication should maintain an adequate fluid intake. The dosage should be reduced in patients with impaired renal function. Liver damage (eg, inflammation, cholestatic jaundice) develops rarely, but may progress to fulminant hepatic failure if the drug is not discontinued. Drug-associated acute pancreatitis has been reported in a renal transplant patient (Antonow, 1986). Also, a case of combined fulminant liver failure and acute hemorrhagic pancreatitis, resulting in death, has been reported (Alberti-Flor et al, 1989).

Upper gastrointestinal irritation, manifested by anorexia, nausea, and vomiting, is common. Glossitis and stomatitis also have occurred. Diarrhea is relatively uncommon; pseudomembranous colitis has been reported rarely. Trimethoprim/sulfamethoxazole causes minimal change in the composition of the anaerobic fecal flora.

Headache, depression, hallucinations, and neuritis have occurred and are probably caused by the sulfonamide. Ataxia (Liu et al, 1986) and acute psychosis (Mermel et al, 1986) have been reported in isolated patients receiving large intravenous doses. Rarely, trimethoprim/sulfamethoxazole has been reported to cause aseptic meningitis (Kremer et al, 1983; Derbes, 1984; Streiffer et al, 1986; Joffe et al, 1989).

Isolated cases of adult respiratory distress syndrome (Cass, 1987) and QT-interval prolongation and torsades de pointes (Lopez et al, 1987) have been reported following oral administration of trimethoprim/sulfamethoxazole.

Sulfonamides are similar chemically to some goitrogens and oral hypoglycemic agents. Goiters and hypoglycemia have occurred rarely.

This combination should not be used during pregnancy unless the potential benefits outweigh the risks (FDA Pregnancy Category C). Because of the risk of kernicterus, it should not be given to pregnant women at term, nursing mothers, or infants less than 2 months. Use of trimethoprim/sulfamethoxazole should be restricted in all patients considered to have marginal or reduced levels of folates, such as pregnant women, alcoholics, or malnourished individuals.

Pain and irritation at the site of administration have been reported infrequently following intravenous administration.

Patients with HIV disease have a higher incidence of adverse reactions to trimethoprim/sulfamethoxazole than other patient populations. In some studies, as many as 80% of AIDS patients exhibited adverse reactions to this combination (Jaffe et al, 1983; Mitsuyasu et al, 1983; Gordin et al, 1984; Kovacs et al, 1984; Wharton et al, 1986; Fischl et al, 1988; Sattler et al, 1988). These adverse reactions have included nausea and vomiting, fever, cutaneous reactions (erythroderma, morbilliform rash, toxic epidermal necrolysis, Stevens-Johnson syndrome), peripheral cytopenias (neutropenia, thrombocytopenia, anemia), hepatitis, and azotemia. Many of these are believed to be hypersensitivity reactions because they recur with drug rechallenge; in a few cases, re-exposure has resulted in life-threatening hypotension (Kelly et al, 1992). However, some of the serious toxic reactions associated with trimethoprim/sulfamethoxazole, such as myelosuppression, appear to be dose-related (Sattler et al, 1988). Concomitant zidovudine may exacerbate the myelosuppression.

Discontinuation of trimethoprim/sulfamethoxazole therapy frequently is necessary in AIDS patients who experience serious adverse reactions. However, Sattler et al (1988) did not observe severe myelosuppression and were able to successfully complete trimethoprim/sulfamethoxazole therapy in AIDS patients by monitoring and maintaining serum trimethoprim concentrations of 5 to 8 mcg/ml. Acetaminophen, diphenhydramine, and lorazepam (or prochlorperazine) may alleviate the symptoms of fever, pruritus, and nausea, respectively.

Another option, oral trimethoprim/sulfamethoxazole desensitization, has been performed successfully for purposes of both intravenous therapy for active *P. carinii* pneumonia and for oral prophylaxis (see Bayard et al, 1992).

DRUG INTERACTIONS. Trimethoprim/sulfamethoxazole may potentiate the anticoagulant effect of warfarin and result in bleeding complications. Prothrombin time should be monitored. Trimethoprim/sulfamethoxazole can displace certain drugs from plasma protein binding sites. In particular, the combination has been shown to potentiate the bone marrow depressant effect of methotrexate. The hypoglycemic effect of oral antidiabetic drugs may be increased due to both displacement from plasma protein binding sites and inhibition of hepatic metabolism. The half-life of phenytoin also is prolonged by concomitant trimethoprim/sulfamethoxazole administration. Sulfamethoxazole can be displaced from plasma protein binding sites by certain acidic drugs including phenylbutazone, dicumarol, and salicylic acid. Thrombocytopenia has occurred more frequently in elderly patients when sulfonamides and thiazide diuretics were administered concomitantly. Hyponatremia has been reported with concomitant trimethoprim and diuretic administration (Eastell and Edmonds, 1984).

It has been suggested that trimethoprim/sulfamethoxazole may produce additive nephrotoxicity with cyclosporine or reduce plasma cyclosporine concentrations (see Tatro, 1991). However, a prospective, randomized, double-blind study of trimethoprim/sulfamethoxazole for prophylaxis of infection in renal transplant patients showed no effect of this antimicrobial on cyclosporine plasma concentrations and only a modest (15%) and reversible elevation in serum creatinine concentrations with concomitant administration. The elevation was caused by inhibition of tubular excretion of creatinine by trimethoprim in the presence of cyclosporine (Maki et al, 1992).

PHARMACOKINETICS. Although the pharmacokinetics of trimethoprim and sulfamethoxazole are not identical, they are sufficiently similar that the administration of the fixed-ratio combination is rational in this regard.

Both trimethoprim and sulfamethoxazole are well absorbed from the upper intestinal tract. When administered in the standard 1:5 ratio tablet containing 80 mg of trimethoprim and 400 mg of sulfamethoxazole, peak plasma concentrations (of free drugs) of approximately 1 mcg/ml trimethoprim and 20 mcg/ml sulfamethoxazole are achieved in one to four hours. In vitro, the 1:20 ratio appears to provide optimum synergy against a number of bacterial species. When the drug combination is administered every 12 hours, a steady-state is achieved in two to three days at concentrations approximately 50% higher than those achieved with a single dose.

Trimethoprim/sulfamethoxazole also can be administered intravenously for more severe infections. Following repeated intravenous administration of 160 mg trimethoprim and 800 mg sulfamethoxazole every eight hours, the steady-state peak and trough plasma concentrations were 8.8 and 5.6 mcg/ml for trimethoprim and 106 and 71 mcg/ml for sulfamethoxazole, respectively.

Approximately 44% of trimethoprim and 70% of sulfamethoxazole are bound to plasma proteins. The volume of distribution of trimethoprim (1.8 L/kg) is considerably greater than that of sulfamethoxazole (0.21 L/kg). Because of the lipophilic properties of trimethoprim, it reaches considerably higher concentrations in various tissues and fluids when compared to sulfamethoxazole. These include prostatic fluid and tissue, vaginal secretions, middle ear fluid, cerebrospinal fluid, sputum, pleural effusions, lung tissue, bile, and aqueous humor. Because of differences in distribution between the two drugs, the 1:20 plasma ratio between trimethoprim and sulfamethoxazole is not obtained in these other body tissues and fluids. However, synergism occurs at other ratios. Trimethoprim/sulfamethoxazole crosses the placenta and is excreted in breast milk.

Both trimethoprim and sulfamethoxazole are eliminated primarily by the kidneys; both glomerular filtration and tubular secretion are involved. Approximately 50% to 60% of a dose of trimethoprim is recovered in the urine within 24 hours, 80% of which appears as unchanged drug; the remainder is excreted as inactive metabolites. In contrast, only about 20% to 30% of sulfamethoxazole is excreted into urine as active drug; acetylated and glucuronide-conjugated metabolites make up the rest. Although the urinary concentrations of both bioactive trimethoprim and sulfamethoxazole are greater than the serum levels, the ratio of trimethoprim to sulfamethoxazole in the typically acidic urine of most patients is about 1:1. In an alkaline urine, the trimethoprim:sulfamethoxazole ratio will decrease.

The half-lives of trimethoprim and sulfamethoxazole are about 9 to 11 hours and 10 to 12 hours, respectively, in adults with normal renal function. The trimethoprim half-life is shorter in children (see the evaluation). In those with renal failure, trimethoprim/sulfamethoxazole can accumulate if the dosage is not reduced. Therapeutic levels of trimethoprim (but not sulfamethoxazole) usually can be achieved in the urine of patients with severe renal insufficiency. Trimethoprim and nonacetylated sulfamethoxazole can be removed by hemodialysis, although metabolites of sulfamethoxazole can accumulate and cause crystalluria.

DOSAGE AND PREPARATIONS.

Oral: The following dosages are for patients with normal renal function: *Adults,* for urinary tract infections, one double-strength (DS) tablet, two regular strength tablets, or four teaspoonsful (20 ml) of suspension every 12 hours for 10 to 14 days. For shigellosis, the same dosage is administered for five days. For acute exacerbations of chronic bronchitis, the same dosage is administered for 14 days. For the treatment of travelers' diarrhea, the same dosage is administered for three to five days (DuPont et al, 1982; National Institutes of Health Consensus Development Conference, 1985). For prophylaxis of travelers' diarrhea, one DS tablet or two regular strength tablets once daily beginning on day of travel and continuing two days after return home (DuPont et al, 1983; Satterwhite and DuPont, 1983). See the Uses section for dosages in short-course (three-day or single-dose) treatment of initial attacks of acute cystitis in women; prophylaxis of recurrent urinary tract infections in women; chronic prostatitis; and pharyngeal gonococcal infections caused by PPNG.

Children, for urinary tract infections or acute otitis media, 8 mg/kg of trimethoprim and 40 mg/kg of sulfamethoxazole daily in two divided doses every 12 hours for 10 days. The same dosage can be given for five days to treat shigellosis. The following table may be used as a guideline in *children 2 months or older:*

Weight		Dose (every 12 hours)	
lb	**kg**	**teaspoonsful**	**tablets***
22	10	1 (5 ml)	½
44	20	2 (10 ml)	1
66	30	3 (15 ml)	1½
88	40	4 (20 ml)	2 (or 1 *DS* tablet)

** regular strength*

The oral preparation is contraindicated in *infants under 2 months.*

For severe infections, the daily amount may be increased by one-half and given in three divided doses.

The dosage for treatment of *Pneumocystis carinii* pneumonia is 20 mg/kg of trimethoprim and 100 mg/kg of sulfamethoxazole daily in equally divided doses every six hours for 14 days. A longer course of therapy, usually 21 days, is required in AIDS patients (Davey and Masur, 1990; *Med Lett Drugs Ther*, 1991). Furthermore, monitoring of serum trimethoprim concentrations to maintain levels of 5 to 8 mcg/ml may decrease the incidence of serious adverse reactions in AIDS patients and allow successful completion of therapy (Sattler et al, 1988). The following table can be used as a guideline in *children*:

Weight		Dose (every 6 hours)	
lb	**kg**	**teaspoonsful**	**tablets***
18	8	1 (5 ml)	½
35	16	2 (10 ml)	1
53	24	3 (15 ml)	1½
70	32	4 (20 ml)	2 (or 1 *DS* tablet)

* *regular strength*

For prophylaxis of *P. carinii* infection in high-risk immunocompromised (not HIV-infected) patients, 5 mg/kg of trimethoprim and 25 mg/kg of sulfamethoxazole daily (Hughes, 1982; Wormser et al, 1982). Alternatively, trimethoprim (150 mg/M^2) and sulfamethoxazole (750 mg/M^2) in two divided doses on three consecutive days of the week (Monday, Tuesday, Wednesday) was shown to be as effective as a daily regimen in children with acute lymphocytic leukemia, and the three-day regimen resulted in fewer fungal infections and was less expensive (Hughes et al, 1987). The maximum daily dose used was 320 mg trimethoprim and 1.6 g sulfamethoxazole.

For primary and secondary prophylaxis of *P. carinii* pneumonia in HIV-infected adults and children, see the Uses section for dosages. See also *MMWR*, 1991, 1992.

For patients with impaired renal function, it is recommended that the usual dose be given if creatinine clearance is >30 ml/min; that the dose be reduced to one-half the usual amount if creatinine clearance is between 15 and 30 ml/min; and that the combination not be used if creatinine clearance is <15 ml/min. All patients should maintain an adequate urine volume to prevent crystalluria.

Bactrim (Roche), ***Cotrim*** (Lemmon), ***Septra*** (Burroughs Wellcome), ***Generic.*** Each 5 ml of suspension contains sulfamethoxazole 200 mg and trimethoprim 40 mg; each tablet contains sulfamethoxazole 400 mg and trimethoprim 80 mg; each double-strength tablet contains sulfamethoxazole 800 mg and trimethoprim 160 mg (***Bactrim-DS***, ***Cotrim-DS***, ***Septra-DS***).

Intravenous: *Adults and children over 2 months with normal renal function*, for severe urinary tract infections and shigellosis. 8 to 10 mg/kg daily (based on the trimethoprim component) in two to four equally divided doses at intervals of 6, 8, or 12 hours for up to 14 days for severe urinary tract infections or five days for shigellosis.

For *P. carinii* pneumonia, 15 to 20 mg/kg daily (based on the trimethoprim component) in three or four equally divided doses at six- or eight-hour intervals for up to 14 days. A longer course of therapy, usually 21 days, is required in AIDS patients (Davey and Masur, 1990; *Med Lett Drugs Ther*, 1991). Furthermore, monitoring of serum trimethoprim concentrations to maintain levels of 5 to 8 mcg/ml may decrease the incidence of serious adverse reactions in AIDS patients and allow successful completion of therapy (Sattler et al, 1988).

The intravenous preparation is contraindicated in *infants under 2 months.*

For patients with impaired renal function, it is recommended that the usual dose be given if creatinine clearance is >30 ml/min; that the dose be reduced to one-half the usual amount if creatinine clearance is between 15 and 30 ml/min; and that the combination not be used if creatinine clearance is <15 ml/min. All patients should maintain an adequate urine volume to prevent crystalluria.

Bactrim I.V. (Roche), ***Generic.*** Solution (sterile) containing trimethoprim 16 mg/ml and sulfamethoxazole 80 mg/ml in 5, 10, and 30 and 50 ml (***Bactrim I.V.*** only) containers.

Septra I.V. (Burroughs Wellcome). Solution (sterile) containing trimethoprim 16 mg/ml and sulfamethoxazole 80 mg/ml in 5, 10, 20, and 50 ml containers.

Cited References

Human drugs; combination drug containing sulfamethoxazole and phenazopyridine hydrochloride and related combination drugs; drug efficacy study implementation; conditions for approval and marketing phenazopyridine-containing drug products; labeling requirements. *Federal Register* 48:34516-34519, 1983.

Serious adverse reactions with sulfonamides. *FDA Drug Bull* 14:5-6, 1984.

Drugs for AIDS and associated infections. *Med Lett Drugs Ther* 33:95-102, 1991.

Drugs for parasitic infections. *Med Lett Drugs Ther* 34:17-26, 1992 A.

Choice of antibacterial drugs. *Med Lett Drugs Ther* 34:49-56, 1992 B

1989 Sexually transmitted diseases treatment guidelines. *MMWR* (suppl 8):1-43, 1989.

Guidelines for prophylaxis against *Pneumocystis carinii* pneumonia for children infected with human immunodeficiency virus. *MMWR* 40(No. RR-2):1-13, 1991.

Recommendations for prophylaxis against *Pneumocystis carinii* pneumonia for adults and adolescents infected with human immunodeficiency virus. *MMWR* 41 (No. RR-4):1-11, 1992.

Acar JF, Goldstein FW: Genetic aspects and epidemiologic implications of resistance to trimethoprim. *Rev Infect Dis* 4:270-275, 1982.

Alberti-Flor JJ, et al: Fulminant liver failure and pancreatitis associated with the use of sulfamethoxazole/trimethoprim. *Am J Gastroenterol* 84:1577-1579, 1989.

Antonow DR: Acute pancreatitis associated with trimethoprim/sulfamethoxazole. *Ann Intern Med* 104:363-365, 1986.

Araujo OE, Flowers FP: Stevens-Johnson syndrome. *J Emerg Med* 2:129-135, 1984.

Ardati KO, et al: Intravenous trimethoprim/sulfamethoxazole in treatment of serious infections in children. *J Pediatr* 95:801-806, 1979.

Asmar BI, et al: Hematologic abnormalities after oral trimethoprim/sulfamethoxazole therapy in children. *Am J Dis Child* 135:1100-1103, 1981.

Bayard PJ, et al: Drug hypersensitivity reactions and human immunodeficiency virus disease. *J Acquir Immune Defic Syndr* 5:1237-1257, 1992.

Benet LZ, Williams RL: Design and optimization of dosage regimens: Pharmacokinetic data, in Gilman AG, et al (eds): *The Pharmacological Basis of Therapeutics*, ed 8. New York, Pergamon Press, 1990, 1713.

Bernard PAM, et al: Randomized, controlled trial comparing long-term sulfonamide therapy to ventilation tubes for otitis media with effusion. *Pediatrics* 88:215-222, 1991.

Brogden RN, et al: Trimethoprim: Review of its antibacterial activity, pharmacokinetics and therapeutic use in urinary tract infections. *Drugs* 23:405-430, 1982.

Brumfitt W, Hamilton-Miller JMT: Trimethoprim. *Br J Hosp Med* 23:283-288, 1980.

Brumfitt W, et al: Evidence for slowing in trimethoprim resistance during 1981: Comparison with earlier years. *J Antimicrob Chemother* 11:503-509, 1983.

Burchall JJ, et al: Molecular mechanisms of resistance to trimethoprim. *Rev Infect Dis* 4:246-254, 1982.

Carlson J, Wiholm BE: Trimethoprim associated aseptic meningitis. *Scand J Infect Dis* 19:687-691, 1987.

Cass RM: Adult respiratory distress syndrome and trimethoprim/sulfamethoxazole, letter. *Ann Intern Med* 106:331, 1987.

Davey RT, Masur H: Recent advances in the diagnosis, treatment, and prevention of *Pneumocystis carinii* pneumonia. *Antimicrob Agents Chemother* 34:499-504, 1990.

Dekker AW, et al: Prevention of infection by trimethoprim-sulfamethoxazole plus amphotericin B in patients with acute nonlymphocytic leukemia. *Ann Intern Med* 95:555-559, 1981.

Derbes SJ: Trimethoprim-induced aseptic meningitis. *JAMA* 252:2865-2866, 1984.

DeRemee RA, et al: Wegener's granulomatosis: Observations on treatment with antimicrobial agents. *Mayo Clin Proc* 60:27-32, 1985.

DuPont HL, et al: Treatment of travelers' diarrhea with trimethoprim-sulfamethoxazole and with trimethoprim alone. *N Engl J Med* 307:841-844, 1982.

DuPont HL, et al: Prevention of travelers' diarrhea with trimethoprim-sulfamethoxazole and trimethoprim alone. *Gastroenterology* 84:75-80, 1983.

Eastell R, Edmonds CJ: Hyponatremia associated with trimethoprim and a diuretic. *BMJ* 289:1658-1659, 1984.

Ericsson CD, et al: Treatment of traveler's diarrhea with sulfamethoxazole and trimethoprim and loperamide. *JAMA* 263:257-261, 1990.

Ericsson CD, et al: Optimal dosing of trimethoprim-sulfamethoxazole when used with loperamide to treat traveler's diarrhea. *Antimicrob Agents Chemother* 36:2821-2824, 1992.

Estey E, et al: Infection prophylaxis in acute leukemia: Comparative effectiveness of sulfamethoxazole and trimethoprim, ketoconazole, and combination of the two. *Arch Intern Med* 144:1562-1568, 1984.

Falloon J, et al: A preliminary evaluation of 566C80 for the treatment of pneumocystis pneumonia in patients with the acquired immunodeficiency syndrome. *N Engl J Med* 325:1534-1538, 1991.

Feldman S, et al: Similar hematologic changes in children receiving trimethoprim/sulfamethoxazole or amoxicillin for otitis media. *J Pediatr* 106:995-1000, 1985.

Fischl MA, et al: Safety and efficacy of sulfamethoxazole and trimethoprim chemoprophylaxis for *Pneumocystis carinii* pneumonia in AIDS. *JAMA* 259:1185-1189, 1988.

Friesen WT, et al: Trimethoprim: Clinical use and pharmacokinetics. *DICP* 15:325-330, 1981.

Fox BC, et al: A prospective, randomized, double-blind study of trimethoprim-sulfamethoxazole for prophylaxis of infection in renal transplantation: Clinical efficacy, absorption of trimethoprim-sulfamethoxazole, effects on the microflora, and the cost-benefit of prophylaxis. *Am J Med* 89:255-274, 1990.

Gaya H, et al: Double-blind placebo controlled trial of prophylactic trimethoprim and sulfamethoxazole (TMP-SMX) for prevention of infection in granulocytopenic patients, abstract 331. *20th Interscience Conference on Antimicrobial Agents and Chemotherapy*. New Orleans, Sept 22-24, 1980.

Glatt AE, Chirgwin K: *Pneumocystis carinii* pneumonia in human immunodeficiency virus-infected patients. *Arch Intern Med* 150:271-279, 1990.

Goldstein FW, et al: Changing pattern of trimethoprim resistance in Paris, with review of worldwide experience. *Rev Infect Dis* 8:725-737, 1986.

Gordin FM, et al: Adverse reactions to trimethoprim-sulfamethoxazole in patients with acquired immunodeficiency syndrome. *Ann Intern Med* 100:495-499, 1984.

Gurwith MJ, et al: Prospective controlled investigation of prophylactic trimethoprim/sulfamethoxazole in hospitalized granulocytopenic patients. *Am J Med* 66:248-256, 1979.

Gutman LT: Use of trimethoprim-sulfamethoxazole in children: Review of adverse reactions and indications. *Pediatr Infect Dis* 3:349-357, 1984.

Hamilton-Miller JMT, Purves D: Trimethoprim resistance and trimethoprim usage in and around the Royal Free Hospital in 1985, letter. *J Antimicrob Chemother* 18:643-644, 1986.

Heikkilä E, et al: Emergence and mechanisms of trimethoprim resistance in *Escherichia coli* isolated from outpatients in Finland. *J Antimicrob Chemother* 25:275-283, 1990 A.

Heikkilä E, et al: Trimethoprim resistance in *Escherichia coli* isolates from a geriatric unit. *Antimicrob Agents Chemother* 34:2013-2015, 1990 B.

Henry SA, et al: Oral trimethoprim/sulfamethoxazole in attempt to prevent infection after induction chemotherapy for acute leukemia. *Am J Med* 77:663-666, 1984.

Hoffman GS, et al: Wegener granulomatosis: An analysis of 158 patients. *Ann Intern Med* 116:488-498, 1992.

Hoppu K: Age differences in trimethoprim pharmacokinetics: Need for revised dosing in children? *Clin Pharmacol Ther* 41:336-343, 1987.

Hughes WT: Trimethoprim-sulfamethoxazole therapy for *Pneumocystis carinii* pneumonitis in children. *Rev Infect Dis* 4:602-607, 1982.

Hughes WT: *Pneumocystis carinii* pneumonitis, editorial. *N Engl J Med* 317:1021-1023, 1987.

Hughes WT, et al: Successful chemoprophylaxis for *Pneumocystis carinii* pneumonitis. *N Engl J Med* 297:1419-1426, 1977.

Hughes WT, et al: Comparison of pentamidine isethionate and trimethoprim-sulfamethoxazole in treatment of *Pneumocystis carinii* pneumonia. *J Pediatr* 92:285-291, 1978.

Hughes WT, et al: Successful intermittent chemoprophylaxis for *Pneumocystis carinii* pneumonitis. *N Engl J Med* 316:1627-1632, 1987.

Huovinen P: Trimethoprim resistance. *Antimicrob Agents Chemother* 31:1451-1456, 1987.

Huovinen P, et al: Trimethoprim resistance of *Escherichia coli* in outpatients in Finland after ten years use of plain trimethoprim. *J Antimicrob Chemother* 16:435-441, 1985.

Huovinen P, et al: Emergence of trimethoprim resistance in relation to drug consumption in a Finnish hospital from 1971 through 1984. *Antimicrob Agents Chemother* 29:73-76, 1986.

Jaffe HS, et al: Complications of co-trimoxazole in treatment of AIDS-associated *Pneumocystis carinii* pneumonia in homosexual men. *Lancet* 2:1109-1111, 1983.

Joffe A, et al: Trimethoprim/sulfamethoxazole-associated aseptic meningitis: Case reports and review of the literature. *Am J Med* 87:332-338, 1989.

Johnson JR, Stamm WE: Diagnosis and treatment of acute urinary tract infections. *Infect Dis Clin North Am* 1:773-791, 1987.

Johnson JR, et al: Therapy for women hospitalized with acute pyelonephritis: A randomized trial of ampicillin versus trimethoprim-sulfamethoxazole for 14 days. *J Infect Dis* 163:325-330, 1991.

Kallings I: Sensitivity of *Branhamella catarrhalis* to oral antibiotics. *Drugs* 31 (suppl 3):17-22, 1986.

Kauffman CA, et al: Trimethoprim/sulfamethoxazole prophylaxis in neutropenic patients: Reduction of infections and effect on bacterial and fungal flora. *Am J Med* 74:599-607, 1983.

Kelly JW, et al: Severe unusual reaction to trimethoprim/sulfamethoxazole in patients infected with human immunodeficiency virus. *Clin Infect Dis* 14:1034-1039, 1992.

Kosoglou T, et al: Trimethoprim alters disposition of procainamide and N-acetylprocainamide. *Clin Pharmacol Ther* 44:467-477, 1988.

Kovacs JA, et al: *Pneumocystis carinii* pneumonia: Comparison between patients with acquired immunodeficiency syndrome and patients with other immunodeficiencies. *Ann Intern Med* 100:663-671, 1984.

Kovatch AL, et al: Oral trimethoprim/sulfamethoxazole for prevention of bacterial infection during induction phase of cancer chemotherapy in children. *Pediatrics* 76:754-760, 1985.

Kramer BS, et al: Prophylaxis of fever and infection in adult cancer patients: Placebo-controlled trial of oral trimethoprim-sulfamethoxazole plus erythromycin. *Cancer* 53:329-335, 1984.

Kremer I, et al: Aseptic meningitis as adverse effect of co-trimoxazole, letter. *N Engl J Med* 308:1481, 1983.

Lawson DH, Paice BJ: Adverse reactions to trimethoprim-sulfamethoxazole. *Rev Infect Dis* 4:429-433, 1982.

Lee BL, et al: Dapsone, trimethoprim, and sulfamethoxazole plasma levels during treatment of *Pneumocystis* pneumonia in patients with acquired immunodeficiency syndrome (AIDS): Evidence of drug interactions. *Ann Intern Med* 110:606-611, 1989.

Levitz RE, Quintiliani R: Trimethoprim-sulfamethoxazole for bacterial meningitis. *Ann Intern Med* 100:881-890, 1984.

Liu LX, et al: Intravenous trimethoprim/sulfamethoxazole and ataxia, letter. *Ann Intern Med* 104:448, 1986.

Lopez JA, et al: QT prolongation and torsades de pointes after administration of trimethoprim/sulfamethoxazole. *Am J Cardiol* 59:376-377, 1987.

Maki DG, et al: Prospective, randomized, double-blind study of trimethoprim/sulfamethoxazole for prophylaxis of infection in renal transplantation: Side effects of trimethoprim/sulfamethoxazole, interaction with cyclosporine. *J Lab Clin Med* 119:11-24, 1992.

Mandell GL, Sande MA: Antimicrobial agents: Sulfonamides, trimethoprim-sulfamethoxazole, quinolones, and agents for urinary tract infections, in Gilman AG, et al (eds): *The Pharmacological Basis of Therapeutics,* ed 8. New York, Pergamon Press, 1990, 1047-1064.

Margolis DM, et al: Trimethoprim-sulfamethoxazole prophylaxis in the management of chronic granulomatous disease. *J Infect Dis* 162:723-726, 1990.

Markowitz N, et al: Trimethoprim-sulfamethoxazole compared with vancomycin for the treatment of *Staphylococcus aureus* infection. *Ann Intern Med* 117:390-398, 1992.

Mayer KH, et al: Trimethoprim resistance in multiple genera of Enterobacteriaceae at a U.S. hospital: Spread of type II dihydrofolate reductase gene by single plasmid. *J Infect Dis* 151:783-789, 1985.

Medina I, et al: Oral therapy for *Pneumocystis carinii* pneumonia in the acquired immunodeficiency syndrome. *N Engl J Med* 323:776-782, 1990.

Mermel LA, et al: Acute psychosis in patient receiving trimethoprim/sulfamethoxazole intravenously. *J Clin Psychiatry* 47:269-270, 1986.

Mitsuyasu R, et al: Cutaneous reaction to trimethoprim-sulfamethoxazole in patients with AIDS and Kaposi's sarcoma, letter. *N Engl J Med* 308:1535-1536, 1983.

Moran JS, Zenilman JM: Therapy for gonococcal infections: Options in 1989. *Rev Infect Dis* 12(suppl 6):S633-S644, 1990.

Murray BE, et al: Increasing resistance to trimethoprim/sulfamethoxazole among isolates of *Escherichia coli* in developing countries. *J Infect Dis* 152:1107-1113, 1985.

National Institutes of Health Consensus Development Conference: Travelers' diarrhea. *JAMA* 253:2700-2704, 1985.

Nicotra B, et al: *Branhamella catarrhalis* as lower respiratory tract pathogen in patients with chronic lung disease. *Arch Intern Med* 146:890-893, 1986.

Pratt WB, Fekety R: *The Antimicrobial Drugs*. New York, Oxford University Press, 1986, 229-251.

Reeves D: Sulfonamides and trimethoprim. *Lancet* 2:370-373, 1982.

Reves RR, et al: Children with trimethoprim- and ampicillin-resistant fecal *Escherichia coli* in day care centers, *J Infect Dis* 156:758-762, 1987.

Reves RR, et al: Risk factors for fecal colonization with trimethoprim-resistant and multiresistant *Escherichia coli* among children in day-care centers in Houston, Texas. *Antimicrob Agents Chemother* 34:1429-1434, 1990.

Riben PD, et al: Reduction in mortality from gram-negative sepsis in neutropenic patients receiving trimethoprim/sulfamethoxazole therapy. *Cancer* 51:1587-1592, 1983.

Satterwhite TK, DuPont HL: Infectious diarrhea in office practice. *Med Clin North Am* 67:203-220, 1983.

Sattler FR, Remington JS: Intravenous trimethoprim-sulfamethoxazole therapy for *Pneumocystis carinii* pneumonia. *Am J Med* 70:1215-1221, 1981.

Sattler FR, et al: Trimethoprim/sulfamethoxazole compared with pentamidine for treatment of *Pneumocystis carinii* pneumonia in acquired immunodeficiency syndrome: Prospective, noncrossover study. *Ann Intern Med* 109:280-287, 1988.

Shear NH, et al: Differences in metabolism of sulfonamides predisposing to idiosyncratic toxicity. *Ann Intern Med* 105:179-184, 1986.

Siegel SE, et al: Treatment of *Pneumocystis carinii* pneumonitis: Comparative trial of sulfamethoxazole-trimethoprim versus pentamidine in pediatric patients with cancer; Report from the Childrens Cancer Study Group. *Am J Dis Child* 138:1051-1054, 1984.

Sinnott JV, Rubin RH: Infections in transplantation, in Reese RE, Betts RF (eds): *Practical Approach to Infectious Diseases,* ed 3. Boston, Little Brown, 1990, 619-642.

Small CB, et al: Treatment of *Pneumocystis carinii* pneumonia in acquired immunodeficiency syndrome. *Arch Intern Med* 145:837-840, 1985.

Sobel JD, Kaye D: Urinary tract infections, in Mandell GL, et al (eds): *Principles and Practice of Infectious Diseases,* ed 3. New York, Churchill Livingstone, 1990, 582-611.

Spitzer PG, et al: Treatment of *Listeria monocytogenes* infection with trimethoprim/sulfamethoxazole: Case report and review of literature. *Rev Infect Dis* 8:427-430, 1986.

Street AC, Durack DT: Experience with trimethoprim/sulfamethoxazole in treatment of infective endocarditis. *Rev Infect Dis* 10:915-921, 1988.

Streiffer RH, et al: Aseptic meningitis and trimethoprim/sulfamethoxazole, letter. *J Fam Pract* 23:314, 1986.

Tanner AR: Hepatic cholestasis induced by trimethoprim. *BMJ* 293:1072-1073, 1986.

Tatro DS(ed): *Drug Interaction Facts.* St Louis, JB Lippincott, 1991, 240, 241, 403, 596b.

Then R, Angehrn P: Sulfonamide-induced "thymineless death" in *Escherichia coli. J Gen Microbiol* 76:255-263, 1973 A.

Then R, Angehrn P: Nature of bactericidal action of sulfonamides and trimethoprim, alone and in combination. *J Infect Dis* 128(suppl):S498-S501, 1973 B.

Towner KJ: Resistance to trimethoprim among urinary tract isolates in United Kingdom. *Rev Infect Dis* 4:456-460, 1982.

Towner KJ, Slack RCB: Effect of changing selection pressures on trimethoprim resistance in *Enterobacteriaceae. Eur J Clin Microbiol* 5:502-506, 1986.

Vlasses PH, et al: Trimethoprim inhibition of the renal clearance of procainamide and N-acetylprocainamide. *Arch Intern Med* 149:1350-1353, 1989.

Wade JC, et al: Selective antimicrobial modulations as prophylaxis against infection during granulocytopenia: Trimethoprim-sulfamethoxazole versus nalidixic acid. *J Infect Dis* 147:624-634, 1983.

Weening RS, et al: Continuous therapy with sulfamethoxazole-trimethoprim in patients with chronic granulomatous disease. *J Pediatr* 103:127-130, 1983.

West BC, et al: Wegener granulomatosis and trimethoprim/sulfamethoxazole: Complete remission after twenty-year course. *Ann Intern Med* 106:840-842, 1987.

Wharton JM, et al: Trimethoprim/sulfamethoxazole or pentamidine for *Pneumocystis carinii* pneumonia in acquired immunodeficiency syndrome: Prospective randomized trial. *Ann Intern Med* 105:37-44, 1986.

Winston DJ, et al: Trimethoprim-sulfamethoxazole for treatment of *Pneumocystis carinii* pneumonia. *Ann Intern Med* 92:762-769, 1980.

Woods WG, et al: Myelosuppression associated with co-trimoxazole as prophylactic antibiotic in maintenance phase of childhood acute lymphocytic leukemia. *J Pediatr* 105:639-644, 1984.

Wormser GP, et al: Co-trimoxazole (trimethoprim-sulfamethoxazole): Updated review of its antibacterial activity and clinical efficacy. *Drugs* 24:459-518, 1982.

Young LS: Trimethoprim-sulfamethoxazole in treatment of adults with pneumonia due to *Pneumocystis carinii. Rev Infect Dis* 4:608-613, 1982.

Zinner SH, Mayer KH: Sulfonamides and trimethoprim, in Mandell GL, et al (eds): *Principles and Practice of Infectious Diseases*, ed 3. New York, Churchill Livingstone, 1990, 325-334.

Other Selected References

Trimethoprim. *Med Lett Drugs Ther* 22:69-70, 1980.

Update and advances in intravenous therapy with trimethoprim/sulfamethoxazole. *Rev Infect Dis* 9 (suppl 2):S153-S229, 1987 (8 papers).

Cockerill FR III, Edson RS: Trimethoprim-sulfamethoxazole. *Mayo Clin Proc* 66:1260-1269, 1991.

Finland M, et al (eds): Trimethoprim-sulfamethoxazole revisited. *Rev Infect Dis* 4:185-618, 1980 (56 papers).

Foltzer MA, Reese RE: Trimethoprim/sulfamethoxazole and other sulfonamides. *Med Clin North Am* 71:1177-1194, 1987.

Gleckman R, et al: Intravenous sulfamethoxazole-trimethoprim: Pharmacokinetics, therapeutic indications, and adverse reactions. *Pharmacotherapy* 1:206-211, 1981.

Hughes WT: Trimethoprim/sulfamethoxazole. *Pediatr Clin North Am* 30:27-30, 1983.

Hughes WT: Sulfonamides and trimethoprim, in Peterson PK, Verhoef J (eds): *The Antimicrobial Agents Annual/3*. New York, Elsevier, 1988, 229-237.

Reese RE, Betts RF: Antibiotic use: Sulfonamides and trimethoprim-sulfamethoxazole; trimethoprim, in Reese RE, Betts RF (eds): *Practical Approach to Infectious Diseases*, ed 3. Boston, Little Brown, 1990, 954-964.

Rubin RH, Swartz MN: Trimethoprim-sulfamethoxazole. *N Engl J Med* 303:426-432, 1980.

Smith LG, Sensakovic J: Trimethoprim-sulfamethoxazole. *Med Clin North Am* 66:143-156, 1982.

Fluoroquinolone Antimicrobial Drugs 70

The fluoroquinolone antimicrobial drugs are synthetic 6-fluoro-7-piperazino-4-quinolone derivatives that are considerably more potent and have broader spectra of activity against bacterial pathogens than their precursors, nalidixic acid [NegGram] and cinoxacin [Cinobac]. Although the latter two drugs are available in the United States, they have been replaced by the fluoroquinolones and are not considered further in this chapter. Five fluoroquinolones are available in the United States: ciprofloxacin [Cipro], enoxacin [Penetrex], lomefloxacin [Maxaquin], norfloxacin [Noroxin], and ofloxacin [Floxin]. All can be administered orally, and two (ciprofloxacin, ofloxacin) are available in parenteral formulations. The chemical structures of these fluoroquinolones are shown in the Figure.

MECHANISM OF ACTION. The fluoroquinolones inhibit bacterial DNA gyrase (topoisomerase II) and are usually rapidly bactericidal for susceptible bacteria, but the exact mechanism of cell killing is not entirely understood (Hooper and Wolfson, 1991 A).

ANTIMICROBIAL SPECTRUM. The fluoroquinolones have similar antimicrobial spectra that include most aerobic gram-negative and some gram-positive bacteria. Ciprofloxacin generally is the most active fluoroquinolone in vitro, especially against susceptible gram-negative bacteria (eg, *Pseudomonas* species). It is less active against gram-positive organisms. Specific differences in potency among the fluoroquinolones exist for some organisms; however, the clinical significance of these differences depends on factors such as the pharmacokinetic properties and relative toxicities of the various agents (see the other sections of this Introduction and the evaluations; see also Andriole, 1990; Fitton, 1992; Hooper and Wolfson, 1991 A; Neu, 1991 A, 1991 B; Walker and Wright, 1991).

The fluoroquinolones are highly active against most Enterobacteriaceae, including *Escherichia coli, Klebsiella, Enterobacter, Proteus mirabilis, P. vulgaris, Morganella morganii, Providencia, Citrobacter,* and *Serratia.* Most isolates worldwide are inhibited in vitro by concentrations ranging from 0.002 to 2 mcg/ml. Many organisms that are resistant to aminoglycosides and cephalosporins are susceptible to the fluoroquinolones.

These agents are active against *Pseudomonas aeruginosa,* including strains that are resistant to other antibacterial agents (Venezio et al, 1986). Ciprofloxacin is the most potent fluoroquinolone in vitro against *P. aeruginosa*; in most studies, 90% of isolates were reported to be inhibited by 1 mcg/ml or less (Hooper and Wolfson, 1991 A; Neu, 1991 A, 1991 B). *P. maltophilia* and *P. cepacia* appear to be less susceptible to the fluoroquinolones; ciprofloxacin is the most active derivative against these organisms. Most strains of *Acinetobacter,* another nonfermentative, aerobic, gram-negative bacillus, are susceptible to 1 mcg/ml or less of ciprofloxacin or ofloxacin. Norfloxacin, enoxacin, and lomefloxacin are less active.

The fluoroquinolones are highly active against most gram-negative bacterial pathogens of the gastrointestinal tract, including enterotoxigenic *E. coli, Shigella, Salmonella, Yersinia enterocolitica, Aeromonas* species, and *Vibrio* species. *Campylobacter jejuni* is somewhat less susceptible (Wolfson and Hooper, 1989 A).

CHEMICAL STRUCTURES OF FLUOROQUINOLONES

Norfloxacin

Ciprofloxacin

Enoxacin

Ofloxacin

Lomefloxacin

The gram-negative coccobacilli, *Haemophilus influenzae* and *H. ducreyi*, and the gram-negative cocci, *Neisseria meningitidis, N. gonorrhoeae,* and *Moraxella (Branhamella) catarrhalis,* are highly susceptible to the fluoroquinolones. The β-lactamase-producing strains of these organisms also are susceptible.

The fluoroquinolones are active against some gram-positive bacteria, although inhibitory concentrations generally are higher than for gram-negative bacteria. All of the fluoroquinolones are active against staphylococci (*S. aureus, S. epidermidis*), including methicillin-resistant strains. Ciprofloxacin and ofloxacin are the most active; 90% of isolates were inhibited by 1 mcg/ml or less in most studies (Neu, 1991 A). However, in some centers, there has been a substantial increase in the percentage of isolates of methicillin-resistant *S. aureus* that are resistant to ciprofloxacin and other fluoroquinolones (Blumberg et al, 1991). All of these agents inhibit *S. saprophyticus,* a common urinary pathogen, at concentrations achieved in urine. Streptococci, including *S. pyogenes* (group A), *S. agalactiae* (group B), *S. pneumoniae,* and viridans streptococci, are usually highly susceptible. *Enterococcus faecalis* (enterococci) are only moderately susceptible to ciprofloxacin and ofloxacin. Norfloxacin, enoxacin, and lomefloxacin are less active, although concentrations achieved in urine are usually adequate for urinary tract infections caused by *E. faecalis*.

The fluoroquinolones are active in vitro against *Legionella pneumophila,* the causative organism of legionnaires' disease. Ciprofloxacin and ofloxacin are active against *Mycobacterium tuberculosis* and certain atypical mycobacteria (eg, *M. fortuitum*) (Wallace et al,1990). Although other mycobacteria (eg, *M. avium-intracellulare, M. chelonae*) are moderately to highly susceptible to ciprofloxacin, they frequently are resistant to ofloxacin (Fenlon and Cynamon, 1986; Wallace et al, 1990). Ciprofloxacin, enoxacin, lomefloxacin, and ofloxacin have activity in vitro against *Chlamydia trachomatis* and mycoplasmas (eg, *M. pneumoniae*) (Andriole, 1990; Hooper and Wolfson, 1991 A).

In general, anaerobic bacteria have shown limited susceptibility to the fluoroquinolones, although ciprofloxacin and ofloxacin are active against some species (Andriole, 1990; Neu, 1991 A, 1991 B; Hooper and Wolfson, 1991 A). The anaerobic gram-positive bacillus, *Clostridium difficile*, is resistant.

The activities of the fluoroquinolones are unaffected by the presence of serum but are decreased in acidic urine. Factors, such as the concentration of multivalent cations (Wolfson and Hooper, 1989 A), in addition to pH, appear to be involved. Although the clinical significance of this phenomenon is not completely clear, concentrations of drugs achieved in urine appear to be more than sufficient for most urinary pathogens. Inoculum size or type of medium has little effect on the in vitro activities of the fluoroquinolones against most organisms. A significant postantibiotic suppressive effect (PAE) has been demonstrated against Enterobacteriaceae, *P. aeruginosa,* and staphylococci but not enterococci (Neu, 1991 A).

RESISTANCE. Resistance to the fluoroquinolones is caused by chromosomal mutations. Plasmid-mediated, transferable resistance has not been reported. The mechanisms of resistance involve alterations in DNA gyrase (Hooper and Wolfson, 1991 A) or changes in outer membrane proteins that affect bacterial membrane permeability (Bryan and Bedard, 1991; Hooper et al, 1989). Enzymatic inactivation of these drugs has not been demonstrated. All quinolone derivatives exhibit cross resistance with one another in vitro (Sanders et al, 1984; Hooper and Wolfson, 1991 B; Barry and Fuchs, 1991). The development of cross resistance between fluoroquinolones and other classes of antimicrobial agents (eg, β lactams, imipenem) is less common but has been reported (Sanders et al, 1984; Aubert et al, 1992).

It is not known whether acquired resistance to the fluoroquinolones will become a major problem clinically, as it is for nalidixic acid. These agents do not appear to readily select for spontaneous, single-step mutations that cause high-level resistance. Although gradual, stepwise decreases in susceptibility to the fluoroquinolones have been produced in vitro by serial exposure of gram-negative bacilli to subinhibitory concentrations of these agents, the increases in minimal inhibitory concentrations (MICs) usually were not sufficient to be of clinical significance in urinary tract infections. Whether resistance would be clinically important in systemic infections is less clear. A number of resistant bacterial strains, primarily *S. pneumoniae, P. aeruginosa,* and *Staphylococcus aureus,* but also *Serratia marcescens, Enterococcus faecalis, Campylobacter jejuni, C. coli,* and *E. coli,* have been isolated from patients during therapy (eg, for cystic fibrosis, osteomyelitis) (Aguiar et al, 1992; Jonsson et al, 1990; Harnett et al, 1991; Nakanishi et al, 1991; Rautelin et al, 1991; Trucksis et al, 1991).

USES. Because of their pharmacokinetic properties (eg, superior oral bioavailability, tissue distribution, and penetration), broad spectrum, and bactericidal potency against most aerobic gram-negative and many aerobic gram-positive bacteria, the fluoroquinolones have significant potential in the therapy of infections at a wide variety of anatomical sites. Treatment guidelines for indications in which these drugs are preferred (rare) or alternative therapy appear in the section, Anti-Infective Therapy. See the chapters in that section and/or index entries on specific indications for additional information. The following discussion summarizes the current role of the fluoroquinolones in pharmacotherapy by site of infection (for reviews, see *Med Lett Drugs Ther,* 1991 A, 1991 B; 1992; Sanders, 1992 A, 1992 B; Todd and Faulds, 1991; Walker and Wright, 1991; Wadworth and Goa, 1991; Neu, 1991 A, 1991 B; Hooper and Wolfson, 1991 B; Outman, 1990; Andriole, 1990; Jaber et al, 1989; Wolfson and Hooper, 1989 A).

Bacteremia and Sepsis: On the basis of their excellent oral bioavailability and distribution, rapid bactericidal activity against most gram-negative (including *P. aeruginosa*) and some gram-positive aerobic bacteria, and the low incidence of adverse reactions associated with their use, the fluoroquinolones have significant potential both for prophylaxis and use in empiric regimens for treatment of febrile episodes in neutropenic patients (Hughes et al, 1990; Maiche, 1991).

In a randomized double-blind trial, norfloxacin was superior to placebo in preventing gram-negative infections in granulocytopenic adults with acute leukemia. Resistance to norfloxacin did not occur, the drug had no significant effect on the frequency of gram-positive or fungal infections, and overall there was no difference in the duration of survival (Karp et al, 1987). Results of a placebo-controlled, randomized trial in neutropenic oncology patients undergoing bone marrow transplantation showed that oral ofloxacin delayed the onset of fever and prevented clinically or bacteriologically documented infections except colonization by fungi (Lew et al, 1991). However, because of the small number of subjects in this study, the results cannot be generalized. In another randomized trial, ciprofloxacin (plus amphotericin B) was significantly more effective than trimethoprim/sulfamethoxazole [Bactrim, Cotrim, Septra] plus colistin [Coly-Mycin] in preventing both gram-negative bacillary infections and colonization with resistant gram-negative bacilli in neutropenic adults with acute leukemia, and it was better tolerated (Dekker et al, 1987).

In other randomized trials, ofloxacin has been compared with trimethoprim/sulfamethoxazole for prophylaxis of bacterial infections in neutropenic patients with acute leukemia and other hematologic malignancies (Liang et al, 1990; Kern and Kurrle, 1991). Ofloxacin was superior in reducing the incidence of gram-negative bacillary infection and the duration of fever, was well tolerated, and did not appear to select for fluoroquinolone-resistant strains or predispose patients to gram-positive bacterial infections. However, as reported in studies with ciprofloxacin and norfloxacin, the majority of ofloxacin recipients were colonized with quinolone-resistant coagulase-negative staphylococci and viridans group streptococci. In general, the fluoroquinolones seem to be effective for prophylaxis of febrile episodes and bacterial infection in neutropenic adults; however, because widespread prophylactic use of these drugs might select for resistance among bacterial isolates, thus reducing their effectiveness as therapeutic agents, no recommendation can yet be made on this indication (Hughes et al, 1990).

The emergence of gram-positive bacteria (eg, staphylococci, streptococci) as major nosocomial pathogens in neutropenic patients warrants caution when fluoroquinolones are considered for use as monotherapy in the treatment of these patients because these agents are less active against such organisms. There also is risk of selecting for resistant strains. This observation is supported by data indicating that intravenous ciprofloxacin 200 to 300 mg twice daily was significantly less effective than piperacillin [Pipracil] plus amikacin [Amikin] as empiric therapy in febrile, neutropenic cancer patients (Meunier et al, 1991). The unsatisfactory success rate of ciprofloxacin in this study probably resulted in part from insufficient dosing and was attributed to a poor outcome among patients with single organism gram-positive coccal bacteremia. In contrast, those with gram-negative infections responded equally well to both regimens, although the small number of subjects makes it difficult to generalize the findings. These results contrast with those of a study in which oral ofloxacin was as effective as standard empiric parenteral therapy (eg, amikacin plus carbenicillin [Geocillin], cloxacillin [Cloxapen, Tegopen], piperacillin) in neutropenic febrile patients, especially those whose neutropenia was of short duration (Malik et al, 1992).

Additional studies indicate that the therapeutic range of the fluoroquinolones may be extended when they are used with other antibacterial drugs, thereby enhancing their efficacy in febrile granulocytopenic patients. Ciprofloxacin has been given with vancomycin [Vancocin, Vancoled] (Smith et al, 1988), netilmicin [Netromycin] (Chan et al, 1989), penicillin G (Kelsey et al, 1990), and azlocillin [Azlin] (Hyatt et al, 1991), and ofloxacin has been given with cefotaxime [Claforan] (Maiche and Teerenhovi, 1991). In these studies, combination therapy was comparable or superior to the single-drug regimen and was generally better tolerated. Although the available data suggest that fluoroquinolones are an excellent option for empiric antibacterial therapy in febrile neutropenic adults, as with their prophylactic use, additional comparative studies are required before these drugs can be recommended as primary therapy for this indication (Hughes et al, 1990).

Bone and Joint Infections: Oral fluoroquinolones have been effective in the treatment of osteomyelitis (eg, contiguous infection, vascular insufficiency, postoperative infection) caused by various Enterobacteriaceae, *P. aeruginosa*, and *S. aureus* (Gentry, 1991; Wolfson and Hooper, 1989 A). In a randomized, comparative trial, oral ciprofloxacin was as safe and effective as parenteral antibiotics (eg, ceftazidime [Fortaz, Tazicef, Tazidime], nafcillin [Nafcil, Nallpen, Unipen] plus an aminoglycoside) in chronic osteomyelitis caused by susceptible organisms (Gentry and Rodriquez, 1990). Oral ofloxacin was similarly effective in a randomized trial when compared with parenteral cefazolin [Ancef, Kefzol] or ceftazidime in biopsy-confirmed nonprosthetic chronic osteomyelitis caused by susceptible organisms (Gentry and Rodriguez-Gomez, 1991). However, because of the small number of patients in these studies, differences between the treatment regimens are difficult to detect. Overall, for cases that are microbiologically proven and thoroughly debrided, oral therapy with fluoroquinolones should be as effective as parenteral treatment, except in patients with underlying conditions such as diabetes mellitus or severe peripheral vascular insufficiency; the latter may require an initial course of parenteral therapy. These results are encouraging because the use of oral fluoroquinolones in outpatients may significantly reduce the expense, discomfort, and inconvenience associated with long-term therapy of this infection. However, the emergence of ciprofloxacin-resistant strains of staphylococci could diminish the utility of this drug for this indication.

Gastrointestinal Tract/Intra-Abdominal Infections: The fluoroquinolones are potentially very useful for the treatment of infectious diarrhea because they are active against all important aerobic gram-negative bacillary enteropathogens but have little activity against the normal anaerobic fecal flora, and plasmid-mediated transfer of resistance does not occur (see Antimicrobial Spectrum and Resistance; see also Neu 1991 A ; DuPont, 1991; Hooper and Wolfson, 1991 A; Wolfson and Hooper, 1989 A). Ciprofloxacin, enoxacin (Calderón et al, 1991), lomefloxacin (Wadworth and Goa, 1991), norfloxacin, and ofloxacin (DuPont et al, 1992) shorten the clinical course and eradicate various gram-negative bacillary enteropathogens (eg, *Shigella*) from patients with acute infectious diarrhea.

In a randomized, double-blind trial, ciprofloxacin was comparable to oral ampicillin in resolving diarrhea and systemic symptoms caused by ampicillin-sensitive isolates of *Shigella* species and was markedly superior to ampicillin in patients infected with isolates that were resistant in vitro to the β-lactam antibiotic (Bennish et al, 1990). Results of a small randomized trial in adults with acute invasive diarrhea suggested that norfloxacin was equivalent to nalidixic acid in patients who were infected with strains of *Shigella* that are sensitive to nalidixic acid, and it may be superior in patients with isolates that are resistant in vitro to nalidixic acid (Bhattacharya et al, 1991). However, the small number of patients in this study precludes generalizations about the relative efficacy of these agents in shigellosis.

In a placebo-controlled, randomized, double-blind trial, ciprofloxacin was comparable to trimethoprim/sulfamethoxazole, and both were significantly more effective than placebo in the treatment of mild-to-moderate and moderate-to-severe travelers' diarrhea in adults. Both regimens were efficacious in treating diarrhea caused by enterotoxigenic *E. coli*, invasive enteropathogens (usually *Shigella*), and unknown enteropathogens (Ericsson et al, 1987).

Thus, based on the available data, ciprofloxacin, norfloxacin, and ofloxacin appear to be equivalent or superior to other drugs (eg, trimethoprim/sulfamethoxazole, trimethoprim alone, ampicillin) for empiric treatment of acute infectious diarrhea (including travelers' diarrhea) caused by the majority of enteric pathogens, including isolates resistant to multiple agents (see the section on Antimicrobial Spectrum above). Because of the pharmacokinetics, bactericidal efficacy, and relative lack of adverse effects of the fluoroquinolones, many infectious disease experts consider them drugs of choice for this indication in adults. Loperamide [Imodium] may be used concomitantly if desired, although current evidence indicates that combined therapy with loperamide and ciprofloxacin is not superior to use of the fluoroquinolone alone (Petruccelli et al, 1992; Taylor et al, 1991), and this is probably also true of combined therapy using loperamide with other fluoroquinolones. Two potential limitations of fluoroquinolone therapy have been found, however. Empiric treatment of acute gastroenteritis may result in drug resistance among *Campylobacter* and *Salmonella* species and may prolong the carriage of *Salmonella* in the stool (Wiström et al, 1992).

In a prospective, randomized double-blind trial involving U.S. students in Mexico, norfloxacin was superior to placebo in preventing travelers' diarrhea, and norfloxacin-resistant aerobic gram-negative bacilli did not emerge (Johnson et al, 1986). Currently, however, the use of antimicrobial agents for the prophylaxis of travelers' diarrhea is discouraged (National Institutes of Health Consensus Development Conference, 1985; see also index entry Diarrhea, Travelers').

Because the fluoroquinolones have excellent activity in vitro against typhoidal and nontyphoidal species of *Salmonella*, including isolates that are resistant to chloramphenicol [Chloromycetin], ampicillin, and trimethoprim/sulfamethoxazole, and have excellent penetration into bile, gallbladder, liver, and phagocytes, these drugs have been extensively investigated for activity in *Salmonella* infections (Asperilla et al, 1990; Trujillo et al, 1991). The fluoroquinolones, including norfloxacin, ciprofloxacin, and ofloxacin, are effective in the treatment of typhoid fever when given for 7 to 10 days (Velmonte and Montalban, 1988; Ramirez et al, 1985; Wang et al, 1989) and probably are the drugs of choice for this disease in areas where *S. typhi* are resistant to chloramphenicol (Limson and Littaua, 1989; Akhtar et al, 1989).

The fluoroquinolones currently are considered the treatment of choice for *S. typhi* carriers. This observation is based on results of two studies demonstrating the value of norfloxacin and ciprofloxacin in the management of *S. typhi* carriers in Peru and Chile. In the first study, norfloxacin (400 mg twice daily for 28 days) eradicated intestinal carriage of typhoid organisms in 18 of 23 patients (78%) (Gotuzzo et al, 1988). In the second, ciprofloxacin (750 mg twice daily for 28 days) terminated carriage in 11 of 12 carriers (92%) (Ferreccio et al, 1988). The fluoroquinolones appear to eliminate intestinal carriage of typhoid organisms in patients with and without gallbladder disease (Gotuzzo et al, 1988).

In general, the fluoroquinolones alleviate and shorten the duration of clinical signs and symptoms in acute uncomplicated nontyphoid *Salmonella* enterocolitis and may terminate the fecal excretion of organisms, although the latter effect may depend on the dosage and duration of treatment and follow-up (Neill et al, 1991). Fluoroquinolones eradicate biliary and intestinal carriage of *Salmonella* species more effectively than trimethoprim/sulfamethoxazole, ampicillin, and amoxicillin (based on historical comparisons) and are effective and well tolerated for bacteremia and invasive salmonelloses in both immunocompetent and immunocompromised (eg, those with AIDS) patients, although only small numbers of patients were studied (see Trujillo et al, 1991). Prophylaxis for an indefinite duration to prevent relapse in AIDS patients has been advocated. Additional controlled trials are required to define the optimal therapeutic regimens for these drugs.

Current evidence suggests that fluoroquinolones (primarily ciprofloxacin) may be effective in the treatment of various gram-negative intra-abdominal infections, including biliary sepsis (Westphal et al, 1991), peritonitis associated with chronic ambulatory peritoneal dialysis (Dryden et al, 1991), and in combination with metronidazole for intra-abdominal sepsis primarily associated with operative procedures (Yoshioka et al, 1991). In the latter randomized study, ciprofloxacin plus metronidazole was well tolerated and equivalent in effectiveness to amoxicillin plus clavulanic acid [Augmentin]. Despite the apparent usefulness of the fluoroquinolones, their advantages in the management of intra-abdominal infections are primarily due to their pharmacokinetic properties; rational use of these drugs for these indications must take into account the possibility of the presence of anaerobic pathogens and enterococci, and further therapy with additional appropriate (eg, anti-anaerobic) drugs must be considered (Smith, 1991).

Respiratory Tract Infections: Generally, clinical responses have been good when ciprofloxacin, enoxacin, or ofloxacin was used to treat lower respiratory tract infections, including acute exacerbations of chronic bronchitis (or chronic lung disease) and acute pneumonias (Gentry et al, 1992; Sanders et al, 1991; Thys et al, 1991; Wolfson and Hooper, 1989 A). Single daily doses of lomefloxacin were equivalent to a twice-daily regimen of this drug in patients with acute exacerbations of chronic bronchitis caused by gram-negative organisms (Kemper and Kohler, 1992). In comparative trials in patients with similar exacerbations of chronic bronchitis caused by gram-negative bacilli, lomefloxacin once daily was more effective than amoxicillin (Grassi et al, 1992) and clinically equivalent but bacteriologically superior to cefaclor [Ceclor] (Gotfried and Ellison, 1992).

Infections caused by aerobic gram-negative bacteria, such as *H. influenzae, M. catarrhalis,* and various Enterobacteriaceae (eg, *Klebsiella pneumoniae*), usually are very susceptible to all of the available fluoroquinolones. However, there is concern about the empiric use of these agents in community-acquired pneumonia in adults, because *S. pneumoniae,* the most commonly involved organism, is less susceptible to the fluoroquinolones than to the penicillins and other established drugs and has persisted in the sputum of some patients who were treated with fluoroquinolones. Hence, these agents are not recommended for empiric use in community-acquired pneumonias. Furthermore, except for patients who are allergic (eg, with IgE-mediated hypersensitivity) to β-lactam agents or those who have received multiple courses of antibiotics and may be colonized with resistant gram-negative bacteria, the fluoroquinolones should be considered alternative therapy to established, less expensive drugs of choice (eg, aminopenicillins, penicillin G, erythromycin) for most respiratory tract infections. In the special case of nosocomial gram-negative bacillary pneumonia in hospitalized patients, combination (ideally, synergistic) therapy (which may include a fluoroquinolone) is frequently recommended because of the significant morbidity and mortality associated with improper or ineffective treatment of this type of infection. For additional information, see index entry Respiratory Tract Infections.

Oral ciprofloxacin has produced clinical improvement when used alone in cystic fibrosis patients with acute pulmonary exacerbations of their disease caused by infection with *P. aeruginosa* (LeBel, 1991; Wolfson and Hooper, 1989 A), and it appears to be as effective as intravenous combination therapy with an antipseudomonal penicillin plus an aminoglycoside. However, although short-term reductions in sputum colony counts of *P. aeruginosa* were observed, ciprofloxacin failed to produce long-term *P. aeruginosa* eradication, and ciprofloxacin-resistant strains of this organism emerged during therapy. This is consistent with results obtained with other antipseudomonal antimicrobial agents. Thus, ciprofloxacin appears to be promising as an alternative for short-term oral therapy in patients with cystic fibrosis who are infected with *P. aeruginosa*.

Data are inadequate to evaluate the efficacy of the other fluoroquinolones in the therapy of recurrent bacterial exacerbations in cystic fibrosis patients. Furthermore, prolonged use of oral fluoroquinolones in outpatients with cystic fibrosis appears to be inappropriate because emergence of highly resistant strains of *P. aeruginosa* is likely.

Fluoroquinolones do not prevent pneumonia due to *Pneumocystis carinii.*

Sexually Transmitted Diseases: Single-dose (in some studies, two-dose) oral regimens of ciprofloxacin, enoxacin, lomefloxacin, norfloxacin, and ofloxacin are highly effective in the treatment of uncomplicated urethral and endocervical gonorrhea caused by susceptible strains, including infections caused by penicillinase-producing strains (PPNG) (Wadworth and Goa, 1991; Hooper and Wolfson, 1989). Based on results achieved in limited numbers of patients in these trials, the fluoroquinolones also appear to be effective in rectal and pharyngeal gonococcal infections, but additional studies are needed. Similarly, although complicated or disseminated gonococcal and chlamydial infections (eg, salpingitis, septic arthritis) have responded to oral fluoroquinolones (Wendel et al, 1991; Hooper and Wolfson, 1989), their role in these infections is not established (see index entry Sexually Transmitted Diseases for treatment guidelines for these indications).

None of these agents, given in single doses, is useful in nongonococcal urethritis (NGU) or in mucopurulent cervicitis due to *Chlamydia trachomatis* (Ronald and Peeling, 1991; Hooper and Wolfson, 1989). Studies with 7- to 10-day courses of ofloxacin (Hooton et al, 1992; Corrado, 1991 A; Boslego et al, 1988) or ciprofloxacin (Oriel, 1986) suggest that these fluoroquinolones are, respectively, comparable to or less effective than doxycycline in *C. trachomatis* genital infections. A 10-day course of norfloxacin was ineffective against chlamydial infections (Bowie et al, 1986). Although preliminary data indicate that 7- to 14-day courses of oral lomefloxacin eradicate *C. trachomatis* in patients with NGU (Wadworth and Goa, 1991), additional studies are required to establish the role of this drug in these infections. In male patients with NGU caused by *U. urealyticum,* norfloxacin was only moderately effective (63%) in eradicating the organism from the urethra; in a comparative study in patients with NGU caused by the same organism, ciprofloxacin was similar in activity to norfloxacin and slightly superior to doxycycline. Additional comparative studies are required to establish the role of the oral fluoroquinolones in the therapy of NGU caused by *U. urealyticum*.

Preliminary studies indicate that both ciprofloxacin and enoxacin are comparable to trimethoprim/sulfamethoxazole against chancroid (*H. ducreyi*), a common cause of genital ulcers in developing countries (Bodhidatta et al, 1988; Hooper and Wolfson, 1991 B).

Skin and Soft Tissue Infections: Oral fluoroquinolones have been effective in serious skin and soft tissue infections (eg, wound infections, cellulitis, scrotal abscesses, lower extremity ulcers) caused by various Enterobacteriaceae, *P. aeruginosa*, and *S. aureus* (Gentry, 1992; Wolfson and Hooper, 1989 A). In randomized, comparative trials, oral ciprofloxacin or ofloxacin was comparable to parenteral third-generation cephalosporins (eg, cefotaxime, ceftazidime) in serious skin and soft tissue infections (Gentry, 1992). These results are encouraging because use of oral fluoroquinolones may permit outpatient treatment of soft tissue infections that currently require long-term intravenous therapy in a hospital. Use of these drugs in a sequential intravenous/oral regimen may significantly reduce the costs associated with prolonged inpatient therapy of serious skin or soft tissue infections (see Gentry, 1992). It should be noted, however, that resistant organisms, especially *P. aeruginosa* and *S. aureus,* have emerged during therapy of these infections with ciprofloxacin. Studies on use of enoxacin in serious skin and soft tissue infections are limited (see Henwood and Monk, 1988).

Although the currently available fluoroquinolones may provide effective therapy for common skin pyodermas caused by *Streptococcus pyogenes* or methicillin-susceptible *S. aureus,* none of them should replace conventional antibiotics (eg, oral penicillins, erythromycin, cephalosporins) for these indications.

Urinary Tract Infections: All of the fluoroquinolones appear to be effective when given orally for urinary tract infections, particularly those caused by *P. aeruginosa* and other multiple drug-resistant aerobic gram-negative bacilli. (For reviews, see Neu, 1992; Andriole, 1991; Corrado, 1991 B; Wolfson and Hooper, 1989 B.) They are excellent agents for nosocomial urinary tract infections, pyelonephritis (upper tract diseases), and complicated urinary tract infections. The fluoroquinolones have the advantages of not altering the anaerobic intestinal flora (see below), and they do not select plasmid-resistant strains. Thus far, the emergence of fluoroquinolone-resistant bacterial strains has been uncommon during treatment of urinary tract infections with these agents. However, except for complicated infections caused by *P. aeruginosa* or other resistant gram-negative bacteria, the fluoroquinolones should be considered alternatives to established agents for most urinary tract infections in adults who tolerate and respond to those drugs (Hooper and Wolfson, 1991 A). See also index entry Urinary Tract Infections.

The fluoroquinolones penetrate prostatic tissue, prostatic fluid, and seminal fluid in concentrations approaching or exceeding those in serum. Ciprofloxacin, enoxacin, and lomefloxacin penetrate prostatic tissue to a similar extent, followed in descending order by norfloxacin and ofloxacin. Results of clinical studies suggest that ciprofloxacin, enoxacin, lomefloxacin, norfloxacin, and ofloxacin may be effective in treating acute and chronic bacterial prostatitis. Response rates that are comparable or superior to those obtained with nonquinolone drugs (eg, trimethoprim/sulfamethoxazole, carbenicillin indanyl, tetracyclines) have been reported, especially in patients with infections caused by *E. coli* and other nonpseudomonal gram-negative bacilli. In contrast, prostatitis caused by gram-positive cocci, especially *E. faecalis,* or by *P. aeruginosa* may be less responsive to fluoroquinolones (Andriole, 1991; Naber, 1991). Thus, although some clinicians prefer fluoroquinolones for primary use in some cases of bacterial prostatitis (eg, acute infections due to *E. coli* or other highly susceptible gram-negative bacilli), additional clinical studies are required to establish these agents as clearly superior to other drugs for infections caused by other bacteria.

Miscellaneous Infections: Oral ciprofloxacin is an effective, convenient, and nontoxic agent for the treatment of malignant external otitis caused by *P. aeruginosa* (Barza, 1991). In the largest study to date, most patients responded to six weeks of oral ciprofloxacin 1.5 g/day following adequate debridement of infected tissues (Lang et al, 1990). However, because relief of signs and symptoms may require considerably more time than eradication of the infecting pathogen(s) from the external ear canal, the dosage and duration of therapy must be individualized.

Other potential uses of ciprofloxacin (and probably other fluoroquinolones) for which there are limited clinical data include treatment of upper respiratory tract colonization with methicillin-resistant *S. aureus* (Mulligan et al, 1987), *Neisseria meningitidis* (Dworzack et al, 1988; Gaunt and Lambert, 1988), or *H. influenzae* type b; serious infections caused by methicillin-resistant staphylococci when vancomycin cannot be used (Piercy et al, 1989); and respiratory tract infections caused by *Legionella* species or *Mycobacterium tuberculosis.* Ciprofloxacin has been used in combination with other agents (eg, rifampin [Rifadin, Rimactane], ethambutol [Myambutol], and clofazimine [Lamprene]; clarithromycin [Biaxin] and amikacin) in the treatment of *M. avium-intracellulare* bacteremia in patients with AIDS (Kemper et al, 1992; De Lalla et al, 1992); however, what effect, if any, the fluoroquinolone has in these regimens has not been determined. Additional data are required to establish the role of these drugs in the treatment of mycobacterial infections.

DRUG SELECTION. For many of the infections discussed above, other antimicrobial drugs are equally effective and, in most cases, less expensive than the fluoroquinolones. Furthermore, clinical experience and other accumulated information on the older drugs (eg, penicillins, trimethoprim/sulfamethoxazole, early generation cephalosporins, macrolides) are far more extensive than they are for the fluoroquinolones. Ciprofloxacin is the best known and most widely used fluoroquinolone among those currently available in the United States. However, this drug has been used inappropriately (Frieden and Mangi, 1990), and such misuse has resulted in selection of resistant isolates and subsequent loss of therapeutic efficacy. To forestall the loss of these drugs as therapeutic options if their misuse continues, the following list provides six indications for which a fluoroquinolone is *preferred* over other agents (Hooper and Wolfson, 1991 A): (1) complicated urinary tract infections, particularly those caused by *P. aeruginosa* or resistant gram-negative pathogens, for which few other oral agents are effective; (2) suspected bacterial gastroenteritis in patients sufficiently ill for empiric therapy to be considered; (3) eradication of chronic fecal carriage of *S. typhi*; (4) mild bacterial exacerbations associated with *P. aeruginosa* in the sputum of patients with cystic fibrosis; (5) invasive external otitis caused by *P. aeruginosa* (in conjunction with adequate surgical debridement); and (6) chronic gram-negative bacillary osteomyelitis (in conjunction with adequate surgical debridement), with therapy perhaps initiated with parenteral formulations, followed by oral therapy for four or more weeks.

The fluoroquinolones also may be rationally considered (1) for infections caused by susceptible pathogens when the drug(s) of choice is more toxic or less efficacious; (2) for patients who cannot tolerate older, conventional drugs because of severe allergy or other adverse reactions; (3) for infections that are caused by multiple bacteria and that would require multiple drug therapy; (4) to allow use of an oral agent rather than a parenteral one (eg, an aminoglycoside) in infections that are resistant to other oral drugs; and (5) as an oral drug to complete a course of parenteral therapy in outpatients (see above; see also Walker and Wright, 1991).

ADVERSE REACTIONS AND PRECAUTIONS. Based on current clinical studies, the fluoroquinolones are well tolerated and adverse reactions seldom are severe enough to require discontinuation of therapy (for reviews, see Jaber et al, 1989; Wolfson and Hooper, 1989 A; Andriole, 1990; Norrby, 1991; Hooper and Wolfson, 1991 B; Todd and Faulds, 1991; Wadworth and Goa, 1991).

Adverse reactions most frequently affect the gastrointestinal tract and the central nervous system. Nausea, headache, and dizziness occur most commonly. Adverse effects on the gastrointestinal tract include abdominal pain, dyspepsia, flatulence, vomiting, diarrhea, and stomatitis. Pseudomembranous colitis has been reported rarely. Adverse reactions affecting the central nervous system include malaise, drowsiness, weakness, insomnia, restlessness, and agitation. Rarely, depression, hallucinations, visual disturbances, psychosis, and convulsive seizures have been reported. These drugs should be used with caution in patients with cerebral arteriosclerosis or epilepsy.

Although hypersensitivity reactions, usually skin rash, are uncommon, anaphylaxis has occurred after the first dose of ciprofloxacin. Swelling of joints, tendinitis, facial edema, interstitial nephritis, vasculitis, and photosensitivity reactions have been reported.

Vaginitis caused by overgrowth of *Candida* has developed.

Laboratory abnormalities also occur infrequently and are minor and reversible. These include eosinophilia, leukopenia, and elevations in hepatic transaminases (ALT, AST), blood urea nitrogen, and serum creatinine levels.

Crystalluria has been reported when large doses of norfloxacin and ciprofloxacin were given to normal volunteers, but this has not been observed with the lower doses used clinically. Alkalizing the urine with sodium bicarbonate increased the incidence of crystalluria with ciprofloxacin.

The fluoroquinolones currently are contraindicated in children because of potential adverse effects on developing bone and cartilage. However, recent studies have indicated efficacy and lack of arthropathy in pediatric patients who received fluoroquinolones for prophylaxis of bacterial infections and other indications (Douidar and Snodgrass, 1989; Schaad, 1991; Schaad and Wedgwood, 1992). Additional data are required to confirm these findings before recommendations can be made for the use of these drugs in children under 18 years.

These agents are not recommended for use in pregnant or nursing women.

DRUG INTERACTIONS: Some fluoroquinolones increase plasma theophylline concentrations, presumably by interfering with its hepatic metabolism. This may result in symptoms of theophylline toxicity, including nausea, vomiting, central nervous system stimulation (eg, nervousness, insomnia), cardiovascular instability, and convulsions. Elevated theophylline concentrations and symptoms of toxicity have been most frequently seen with enoxacin and, to a much lesser extent, with ciprofloxacin (Radandt et al, 1992). The effect of lomefloxacin (Nix et al, 1989; Wijnands et al, 1990), norfloxacin, and ofloxacin on serum theophylline concentrations appears to be minimal (Radandt et al, 1992). Nevertheless, it is advisable to use fluoroquinolones, particularly enoxacin, with caution in all patients receiving theophylline. Furthermore, because interpatient variability in metabolic disposition may be significant, plasma theophylline concentrations should be monitored in patients who also are receiving a fluoroquinolone (see Radandt et al, 1992).

Ciprofloxacin and enoxacin reduce the clearance of caffeine (see Radandt et al, 1992); this interaction has not been observed with lomefloxacin (Healy et al, 1991), norfloxacin, or ofloxacin. Enoxacin decreased the clearance of the pharmacologically less active (R)-warfarin, but had no effect on (S)-warfarin or on prothrombin time. Concurrent administration of ciprofloxacin with cyclosporine has been associated with elevated serum creatinine concentrations in two patients (Avent et al, 1988; Elston and Taylor, 1988). Because these observations have not been confirmed by others and the available data are limited, physicians should be aware of the possibility of reduced drug clearance resulting in adverse effects whenever the fluoroquinolones are administered with drugs that depend on hepatic metabolism for their elimination (Radandt et al, 1992).

The divalent and trivalent cations (eg, aluminum, magnesium, calcium) in antacid products and the antiulcer agent, sucralfate, appear to significantly reduce the gastrointestinal absorption of fluoroquinolones (Radandt et al, 1992; Shimada et al, 1992). This inhibition of absorption probably results from the chelation of the antimicrobial agent with the cation, forming an insoluble complex; it does not appear to be due to alteration of the gastric pH by the antacid. Because serum concentrations of the fluoroquinolones may be reduced, simultaneous use of cation-containing antacids or sucralfate should be avoided.

Nitrofurantoin may antagonize the antibacterial effect of the fluoroquinolones in the urinary tract, and concurrent use is not recommended.

PHARMACOKINETICS. Some pharmacokinetic values for the fluoroquinolones in healthy volunteers are shown in the Table.

Absorption. The fluoroquinolones are rapidly, but variably, absorbed following oral administration. In general, these drugs exhibit linear pharmacokinetics (see Wolfson and Hooper, 1989 A; Andriole, 1990; Hooper and Wolfson, 1991 B). Oral bioavailability approximates 40% to 50% for norfloxacin; 60% to 70% for ciprofloxacin; and 90% to 100% for enoxacin, lomefloxacin, and ofloxacin. The time to peak serum concentration (T_{max}) usually ranges from one to two hours for all of these agents. However, for any given dose, the peak serum concentrations (C_{max}) and areas under the serum concentration-time curves (AUC) differ; highest values are obtained with ofloxacin, followed by lomefloxacin, enoxacin, ciprofloxacin, and norfloxacin (see the Table). These differences are due, in part, to differences in gastrointestinal absorption. The presence of food appears to delay the absorption of the fluoroquinolones so that serum peaks appear later than under fasting conditions; however, there is only a slight effect on the total amount absorbed.

Ciprofloxacin and ofloxacin also are available in parenteral formulations for intravenous infusion. The distribution and elimination of these preparations are linear and similar to those of the oral compounds. In general, a peak serum concentration of approximately 1 mcg/ml is achieved for each 100 mg of ciprofloxacin or ofloxacin infused intravenously.

SELECTED PHARMACOKINETIC VALUES FOR FLUOROQUINOLONES[1,2]

Fluoroquinolone [Trade Name]	Maximal Serum Concentration (mcg/ml)	Time to Maximal Serum Concentration (hrs)	Terminal Serum Half-Life (hrs)	Volume of Distribution (liters)	Renal Excretion (%)[3]
Ciprofloxacin [Cipro]	1.5[4]	1.1	3.3	348	29
Enoxacin [Penetrex]	2.3	1.6	4.9	175	44
Lomefloxacin [Maxaquin]	3.7	2.0	7.8	127	66
Norfloxacin [Noroxin]	1.5	1.5	3.3	225	27
Ofloxacin [Floxin]	4.0	1.4	5.0	102	73

[1]*Adapted from Wolfson and Hooper, 1989 A; Andriole, 1990; Hooper and Wolfson, 1991 B.*

[2]*Values obtained following a single 400-mg oral dose in healthy volunteers.*

[3]*Cumulative percentage of dose excreted in 24 hrs for ciprofloxacin, lomefloxacin, norfloxacin, ofloxacin, 72 hrs for enoxacin.*

[4]*Extrapolated value.*

Distribution. Plasma protein binding of the fluoroquinolones is relatively low (9% for lomefloxacin; 14% to 25% for ciprofloxacin, norfloxacin, and ofloxacin; 18% to 54% for enoxacin) (Wolfson and Hooper, 1989 A). All of the fluoroquinolones appear to distribute widely in body fluids and tissues. The large apparent volumes of distribution suggest that these drugs are concentrated in certain tissues, regardless of the route of administration.

Fluoroquinolones adequately penetrate into blister fluid, bile, saliva, sputum, peritoneal fluid, macrophages, polymorphonuclear neutrophils, lung, liver, kidney, gallbladder, skeletal muscle, uterus, cervix, vagina, and bone (see Wolfson and Hooper, 1989 A; Andriole, 1990; Hooper and Wolfson, 1991 B; Neu, 1991 A). In the urine, all of the fluoroquinolones reach concentrations that exceed the minimum inhibitory concentrations (MICs) of most urinary tract pathogens for at least 12 hours. Gastrointestinal secretion of these drugs also results in high intestinal concentrations. Concentrations equal to or greater than those in serum have been measured in prostatic tissue and fluids for each of these agents (Andriole, 1991; Naber, 1991).

In patients with inflamed meninges, ciprofloxacin and ofloxacin may reach concentrations in the cerebrospinal fluid (CSF) that exceed the MIC90 for most gram-negative pathogens that cause bacterial meningitis, including *P. aeruginosa, Salmonella* species, and other Enterobacteriaceae. However, concentrations of these drugs achieved in the CSF are not adequate to treat meningitis caused by staphylococci, *S. pneumoniae,* group B streptococci, and *Listeria monocytogenes* (Modai, 1991). Data on the other fluoroquinolones are extremely limited. None of these drugs is recommended for the treatment of bacterial meningitis.

Metabolism and Excretion. The metabolism and excretion of the fluoroquinolones are not completely understood. Both renal and nonrenal (hepatic and gastrointestinal) routes are involved in the elimination of norfloxacin, ciprofloxacin, lomefloxacin, and enoxacin; ofloxacin is almost entirely removed by the kidneys (see Table).

All of the fluoroquinolones are excreted renally, and unchanged drugs and their metabolites are recovered in the urine (see Table). The mechanisms include both glomerular filtration and active tubular secretion (renal clearance exceeds creatinine clearance for all of these agents). The bile appears to be a minor route of elimination, although high concentrations of ciprofloxacin, norfloxacin, and ofloxacin may accumulate there. High concentrations of ciprofloxacin, enoxacin, norfloxacin, and ofloxacin are found in feces; this appears to be due to incomplete absorption and gastrointestinal secretion.

The half-lives of the fluoroquinolones vary; lomefloxacin, ofloxacin, and enoxacin have longer half-lives than ciprofloxacin and norfloxacin in adults with normal renal function (see Table). The half-lives of the fluoroquinolones increase in patients with renal impairment, but again there are differences. In anuric patients (creatinine clearance less than 10 ml/min), the half-lives of norfloxacin, enoxacin, and ciprofloxacin only increase to approximately eight or nine hours. For these drugs, dosage reductions are necessary only in those with more severe renal impairment (eg, creatinine clearance less than 30 ml/min for norfloxacin and less than 50 ml/min for ciprofloxacin). In contrast, the half-life of ofloxacin is approximately 40 hours in anuric patients and that of lomefloxacin may reach 48 hours. Greater dosage reductions are necessary in all patients with renal impairment who receive either of these agents. Hemodialysis has only a modest effect on removal of fluoroquinolones, and dosage supplementations are probably unnecessary.

The pharmacokinetics of oral ciprofloxacin have been investigated in adults with cystic fibrosis; values were similar to those in normal volunteers (Goldfarb et al, 1986; Smith et al, 1986; Davis et al, 1987). However, in one study a shorter mean elimination half-life, due to smaller apparent volumes of distribution, was reported for cystic fibrosis patients (LeBel et al, 1986).

Drug Evaluations

CIPROFLOXACIN
[Cipro I.V.]

CIPROFLOXACIN HYDROCHLORIDE
[Cipro]

Ciprofloxacin is the most potent fluoroquinolone in vitro against most bacterial pathogens (eg, Enterobacteriaceae, *Pseudomonas aeruginosa,* gram-positive cocci, *Mycobacterium tuberculosis, Chlamydia trachomatis*).

USES. Ciprofloxacin is effective in complicated urinary tract infections, bacterial prostatitis, uncomplicated gonorrhea (including PPNG infections), bacterial gastroenteritis, and in the prevention of aerobic gram-negative bacillary infections in adult neutropenic patients. In addition, ciprofloxacin provides effective oral therapy for serious systemic infections caused by aerobic gram-negative bacilli, including *P. aeruginosa* and organisms that are resistant to other antimicrobial agents (eg, third generation cephalosporins, aminoglycosides) in immunocompetent and neutropenic patients. It is effective for lower respiratory tract infections (when *Streptococcus pneumoniae* or staphylococci are known or suspected not to be involved), including short-term treatment of acute pulmonary exacerbations of cystic fibrosis, as well as for joint infections, osteomyelitis, skin and soft tissue infections, and malignant external otitis caused by *P. aeruginosa.* Other potential uses of ciprofloxacin include typhoid fever and infections caused by quinolone-susceptible methicillin-resistant staphylococci, *Legionella* species, and *M. tuberculosis.* However, current data are limited and additional clinical studies are required to properly assess the role of ciprofloxacin in those infections. The possibility of using an oral antimicrobial drug instead of intravenous therapy (or to complete a course of intravenous therapy) for serious gram-negative bacillary infections (eg, osteomyelitis) is appealing. However, ciprofloxacin-resistant bacterial strains, particularly *Staphylococcus aureus* and *P. aeruginosa*, have emerged during therapy with the drug. An intravenous formulation of ciprofloxacin is available and may be useful in a sequential parenteral/oral regimen for most infections.

PRECAUTIONS. This drug is not recommended for empiric treatment of community-acquired pneumonia that may be caused by *S. pneumoniae* or for pneumonia when a diagnostic Gram stain indicates the presence of gram-positive cocci. The drug should not be used in pregnant or nursing women or prepubertal children. It is classified in FDA Pregnancy Category C.

See the Introduction for a complete discussion of the actions, antimicrobial spectrum, uses, pharmacokinetics, adverse reactions and precautions, and drug interactions of ciprofloxacin.

DOSAGE AND PREPARATIONS.

CIPROFLOXACIN:

Intravenous: *Adults,* for mild to moderate urinary tract infections, 200 mg every 12 hours; for severe or complicated urinary tract infections or mild to moderate lower respiratory tract, skin and skin structure, or bone and joint infections, 400 mg every 12 hours. As with oral ciprofloxacin, the duration of treatment depends on the severity of the infection; in general, the drug should be continued for at least two days after the signs and symptoms of infection have disappeared. The usual duration of therapy is 7 to 14 days but may be six weeks or longer for some infections (eg, bone and joint, prostatitis). The preparation is infused over a period of 60 minutes.

Adults with creatinine clearance 30 ml/min or greater, usual dose; creatinine clearance 5 to 29 ml/min, 200 to 400 mg every 18 to 24 hours. For patients with changing renal function or those with renal insufficiency or hepatic impairment, see oral dosage.

Cipro I.V. (Miles). Solution containing 200 or 400 mg in 20 and 40 ml of water, respectively, for dilution, in single-use containers or in 5% dextrose for direct infusion in 100 or 200 ml flexible containers.

CIPROFLOXACIN HYDROCHLORIDE:

Oral: *Adults,* for mild to moderate urinary tract infections, 250 mg every 12 hours. For severe or complicated urinary tract infection; bacterial prostatitis; mild to moderate respiratory tract, bone and joint, and skin and skin structure infections; and infectious diarrhea, 500 mg every 12 hours. This dosage is also given to patients with typhoid fever (Ramirez et al, 1985). For severe or complicated respiratory tract, bone and joint, and skin and skin structure infections, 750 mg every 12 hours. Determination of dosage for the individual patient depends on the nature and severity of infection, susceptibility of causative organism, integrity of patient's host-defense mechanisms, and status of renal function (see below). The usual duration of therapy is 7 to 14 days, but more prolonged therapy may be required for severe or complicated infections. Bone and joint infections may require treatment for four to six weeks or longer. Infectious diarrhea may be treated for five to seven days. Three days of therapy may be adequate for acute cystitis in women.

Adults with creatinine clearance >50 ml/min, see usual dosages (above); creatinine clearances of 30 to 50 ml/min, 250 to 500 mg every 12 hours; creatinine clearances of 5 to 29 ml/min, 250 to 500 mg every 18 hours; and for patients on hemodialysis or peritoneal dialysis, 250 to 500 mg every 24 hours (after dialysis). In patients with severe infections and severe renal impairment, a unit dose of 750 mg may be administered at the intervals noted above. However, patients should be monitored carefully and the serum concentration should be measured periodically. Peak concentrations (one to two hours after dosing) above 5 mcg/ml should be avoided. For patients with changing renal function or those with renal impairment and hepatic insufficiency, measurement of serum concentrations may provide additional guidance for adjusting dosage.

For uncomplicated urethral, endocervical, rectal, and pharyngeal gonorrhea (including PPNG infections), 500 mg as a single dose (*MMWR,* 1989).

For chancroid, 500 mg every 12 hours for three days.

For prevention of gram-negative bacillary infection in neutropenic adults with acute leukemia, 500 mg every 12 hours (Dekker et al, 1987).

Oral ciprofloxacin can be taken with or without meals. The preferred time of dosing is two hours after a meal with a glass of water. Patients should be well hydrated. Concurrent use of antacids or sucralfate should be avoided.

Cipro (Miles). Tablets 250, 500, and 750 mg.

ENOXACIN

[Penetrex]

This fluoroquinolone is very similar to norfloxacin with regard to antimicrobial spectrum and potency in vitro, but orally administered enoxacin is better absorbed and has a longer half-life.

USES. There are few published clinical studies on enoxacin. This drug appears to be effective for complicated urinary tract infections. Single doses have been beneficial in uncomplicated urethral and endocervical gonorrhea.

Further clinical trials with enoxacin are necessary to determine its spectrum of indications, dosage range, and relative usefulness compared with the other fluoroquinolones. At present, enoxacin does not appear to have any significant advantage over the other fluoroquinolones and is not recommended for general use.

PRECAUTIONS. Enoxacin is not recommended for infections of the respiratory tract. Nausea and central nervous system side effects (eg, agitation, dizziness, hallucinations, epileptiform attacks), presumably due to an interaction with concomitant use of theophylline, have been reported when enoxacin 400 to 600 mg twice daily was administered with this xanthine.

Enoxacin should not be used in pregnant or nursing women or prepubertal children. It is classified in FDA Pregnancy Category C.

See the Introduction for a complete discussion of the actions, antimicrobial spectrum, uses, pharmacokinetics, adverse reactions and precautions, and drug interactions of enoxacin.

DOSAGE AND PREPARATIONS.

Oral: *Adults,* for mild to moderate acute urinary tract infections, 200 mg every 12 hours for seven days. For complicated or severe urinary tract infections, 400 mg every 12 hours for 14 days. For uncomplicated gonococcal urethritis or cervicitis, 400 mg in a single dose for one day. The manufacturer recommends reducing the dose by 50% in patients with creatinine clearances below 30 ml/min. Concurrent use of antacids or sucralfate should be avoided.

Penetrex (Rhone-Poulenc Rorer). Tablets 200 and 400 mg.

LOMEFLOXACIN HYDROCHLORIDE
[Maxaquin]

The in vitro bactericidal spectrum and potency of lomefloxacin are equivalent to those of the other available fluoroquinolones, with the exception of ofloxacin and ciprofloxacin.

USES. In acute exacerbations of chronic bronchitis of mixed etiology that does not involve *Streptococcus pneumoniae* and in uncomplicated and complicated infections of the upper and lower urinary tract, lomefloxacin 400 mg once daily appears to be comparable to standard therapy (eg, amoxicillin, trimethoprim/sulfamethoxazole). Although data are limited, this drug appears to be effective in the treatment of acute and chronic bacterial prostatitis, infectious diarrhea, bone and joint infections, infections of the skin and skin structures, and sexually transmitted diseases (eg, chancroid due to *Haemophilus ducreyi*).

The primary advantage of lomefloxacin over the other fluoroquinolones is its longer half-life, which allows once-daily administration for all indications studied thus far. In contrast to enoxacin (and, to a lesser extent, ciprofloxacin), lomefloxacin does not significantly alter theophylline clearance and serum concentrations in patients receiving both drugs concomitantly; therefore, it is not necessary to adjust the dosage of theophylline in these patients.

Comparative studies of lomefloxacin and other fluoroquinolones have not been conducted and thus rigorous assessment of potential therapeutic differences within this class of drugs is not yet possible. Furthermore, until data demonstrating the superiority of lomefloxacin over other drugs are available, it should be regarded as an alternative to well-established nonquinolone drugs for most infections (see the section Drug Selection in the Introduction).

PRECAUTIONS. Lomefloxacin is not recommended for empiric use in patients with community-acquired pneumonia in which gram-positive cocci are confirmed or suspected.

This drug should not be used in pregnant or nursing women or prepubertal children. It is classified in FDA Pregnancy Category C.

See the Introduction to this chapter for a complete discussion of the actions, antimicrobial spectrum, uses, pharmacokinetics, adverse reactions and precautions, and drug interactions of lomefloxacin.

DOSAGE AND PREPARATIONS. Lomefloxacin may be taken with or without meals. Concurrent use of antacids or sucralfate should be avoided.

Oral: *Adults,* for mild to moderate acute exacerbation of chronic bronchitis or cystitis, 400 mg once daily for 10 days; for complicated urinary tract infections, 400 mg once daily for 14 days; for prophylaxis for transurethral surgical procedures, 400 mg two to six hours prior to surgery.

Adults with renal impairment (creatinine clearance 10 to 40 ml/min), an initial loading dose of 400 mg followed by maintenance doses of 200 mg once daily for the duration of treatment; hemodialysis patients should receive the same regimen as those with impaired renal function. Serial determination of lomefloxacin serum concentrations is recommended to guide dosage adjustments.

Maxaquin (Searle). Tablets 400 mg.

NORFLOXACIN
[Noroxin]

USES. This orally administered antibacterial agent is indicated primarily for uncomplicated and complicated urinary tract infections caused by susceptible bacteria. In particular, it is useful for complicated urinary tract infections caused by multiple antibiotic-resistant Enterobacteriaceae, *Pseudomonas aeruginosa,* and enterococci. Potential uses of norfloxacin include bacterial prostatitis, uncomplicated gonorrhea (including PPNG infections), bacterial gastroenteritis, and prevention of aerobic gram-negative bacillary infections in adult neutropenic patients. However, norfloxacin is not recommended for systemic infections (eg, respiratory tract infections, osteomyelitis), primarily because its pharmacokinetic properties are inferior to those of the other fluoroquinolones.

PRECAUTIONS. This drug should not be used in pregnant or nursing women or prepubertal children. It is classified in FDA Pregnancy Category C.

See the Introduction for a complete discussion of the actions, antimicrobial spectrum, uses, pharmacokinetics, adverse reactions and precautions, and drug interactions of norfloxacin.

DOSAGE AND PREPARATIONS. Norfloxacin is taken one hour before or two hours after meals with a glass of water. Patients should be well hydrated. Concurrent use of antacids or sucralfate should be avoided.

Oral: *Adults,* for uncomplicated urinary tract infections, 400 mg twice daily for 7 to 10 days; for complicated urinary tract infections, 400 mg twice daily for 10 to 21 days (maximum, 800 mg/day). *Adults with renal impairment,* 400 mg once daily when creatinine clearance is $\leq$30 ml/min/1.73 M^2. When creatinine clearance is $>$30 ml/min/1.73 M^2, dosage modification is unnecessary.

For acute bacterial prostatitis, 400 mg twice daily for at least 10 days (Andriole, 1991); four to six weeks of therapy is usually required for chronic prostatitis.

For uncomplicated urethral or endocervical gonorrhea, 800 mg as a single dose (*MMWR,* 1989).

For bacterial gastroenteritis, 400 mg twice daily for three to five days (DuPont et al, 1987). For prevention of gram-negative bacillary infections in neutropenic adults with acute leukemia, 400 mg twice daily (Karp et al, 1987).

Noroxin (Merck Sharp & Dohme). Tablets 400 mg.

OFLOXACIN

[Floxin, Floxin I.V.]

USES. The antimicrobial spectrum of this fluoroquinolone is similar to that of ciprofloxacin. In vitro, the two drugs have comparable potency against staphylococci and streptococci, but ciprofloxacin is more potent against most gram-negative bacteria (eg, Enterobacteriaceae, *Pseudomonas aeruginosa*). In contrast, orally administered ofloxacin has better pharmacokinetic properties, including greater bioavailability and a longer half-life.

Ofloxacin is effective in uncomplicated and complicated urinary tract infections, uncomplicated gonorrhea (including PPNG infections), chlamydial urethritis and cervicitis, and lower respiratory tract infections caused by gram-negative pathogens. Other possible indications include infectious diarrhea (including travelers' diarrhea), typhoid fever, bone and joint and skin and skin structure infections, bacterial prostatitis (acute and chronic), tuberculosis, atypical mycobacterial infections, and prophylactic and empiric use alone or in combination regimens for neutropenic patients. Clinical trials comparing ofloxacin with ciprofloxacin are necessary to determine whether one drug offers significant advantages over the other for various infections.

PRECAUTIONS. This drug is not recommended for empiric treatment of community-acquired pneumonia that may be caused by *Streptococcus pneumoniae* or for pneumonia when a diagnostic Gram stain indicates the presence of gram-positive cocci.

Ofloxacin should not be used in pregnant or nursing women or prepubertal children. It is classified in FDA Pregnancy Category C.

See the Introduction for a complete discussion of the actions, antimicrobial spectrum, uses, pharmacokinetics, adverse reactions and precautions, and drug interactions of ofloxacin.

DOSAGE AND PREPARATIONS. Because the bioavailability of the intravenous and oral formulations of ofloxacin are equivalent, dosage recommendations are the same.

Oral, Intravenous: *Adults,* for uncomplicated urinary tract infections, 200 mg every 12 hours for three to seven days; for complicated urinary tract infections, 200 mg every 12 hours for 10 days; for mild to moderate infections of the lower respiratory tract (eg, acute exacerbations of chronic bronchitis or pneumonia not due to gram-positive cocci) and skin and skin structures, 400 mg every 12 hours for 10 days; for bacterial prostatitis, 300 mg every 12 hours for six weeks; for cervicitis or urethritis due to *Chlamydia trachomatis* and *Neisseria gonorrhoeae,* 300 mg every 12 hours for seven days; for uncomplicated gonorrhea, 400 mg in a single dose for one day.

For *adults with renal impairment,* increasing the dosage interval to 24 hours when creatinine clearance is between 10 and 50 ml/min and halving the normal dose and increasing the dosage interval to 24 hours when creatinine clearance is less than 10 ml/min are recommended.

Floxin (Ortho). Tablets 200, 300, and 400 mg.

Floxin I.V. (Ortho). Solution (concentrate) in single-use vials containing 400 mg in 10 or 20 ml of water for dilution prior to use (see package insert for compatible diluents) and 200 or 400 mg in 50 or 100 ml flexible containers or bottles with 5% dextrose solution (both for direct infusion).

Cited References

The choice of antibacterial drugs. *Med Lett Drugs Ther* 34:49-56, 1992.

Intravenous ciprofloxacin. *Med Lett Drugs Ther* 33:75-76, 1991 A.

Ofloxacin. *Med Lett Drugs Ther* 33:71-73, 1991 B.

1989 Sexually transmitted diseases treatment guidelines. *MMWR* 38(suppl 8):1-43, 1989.

Aguiar JM, et al: The emergence of highly fluoroquinolone-resistant *Escherichia coli* in community-acquired urinary tract infections. *J Antimicrob Chemother* 29:349-350, 1992.

Akhtar MA, et al: Efficacy of ofloxacin in typhoid fever, particularly in drug-resistant cases. *Rev Infect Dis* 11(suppl 5):1193, 1989.

Andriole VT: Quinolones, in Mandell GL, et al (eds): *Principles and Practice of Infectious Diseases,* ed 3. New York, Churchill Livingstone, 1990, 334-345.

Andriole VT: Use of quinolones in treatment of prostatitis and lower urinary tract infections. *Eur J Clin Microbiol Infect Dis* 10:342-350, 1991.

Asperilla MO, et al: Quinolone antibiotics in the treatment of Salmonella infections. *Rev Infect Dis* 12:873-889, 1990.

Aubert G, et al: Emergence of quinolone-imipenem cross-resistance in *Pseudomonas aeruginosa* after fluoroquinolone therapy. *J Antimicrob Chemother* 29:307-312, 1992.

Avent CK, et al: Synergistic nephrotoxicity due to ciprofloxacin and cyclosporine. *Am J Med* 85:452-453, 1988.

Barry AL, Fuchs PC: Cross-resistance and cross-susceptibility between fluoroquinolone agents. *Eur J Clin Microbiol Infect Dis* 10:1013-1018, 1991.

Barza M: Use of quinolones for treatment of ear and eye infections. *Eur J Clin Microbiol Infect Dis* 10:296-303, 1991.

Bennish ML, et al: Therapy for shigellosis: II. Randomized, double-blind comparison of ciprofloxacin and ampicillin. *J Infect Dis* 162:711-716, 1990.

Bhattacharya SK, et al: Randomized clinical trial of norfloxacin for shigellosis. *Am J Trop Med Hyg* 45:683-687, 1991.

Blumberg HM, et al: Rapid development of ciprofloxacin resistance in methicillin-susceptible and -resistant *Staphylococcus aureus. J Infect Dis* 163:1279-1285, 1991.

Bodhidatta L, et al: Evaluation of 500- and 1,000-mg doses of ciprofloxacin for treatment of chancroid. *Antimicrob Agents Chemother* 32:723-725, 1988.

Boslego JW, et al: Prospective randomized trial of ofloxacin vs doxycycline in treatment of uncomplicated male urethritis. *Sex Transm Dis* 15:186-191, 1988.

Bowie WR, et al: Failure of norfloxacin to eradicate *Chlamydia trachomatis* in nongonococcal urethritis. *Antimicrob Agents Chemother* 30:594-597, 1986.

Bryan LE, Bedard J: Impermeability to quinolones in gram-positive and gram-negative bacteria. *Eur J Clin Microbiol Infect Dis* 10:232-239, 1991.

Calderón E, et al: Treatment of acute diarrhea in adults. *Curr Ther Res* 49:792-800, 1991.

Chan CC, et al: Randomized trial comparing ciprofloxacin plus netilmicin versus piperacillin plus netilmicin for empiric treatment of fever in neutropenic patients. *Antimicrob Agents Chemother* 33:87-91, 1989.

Corrado ML: The clinical experience with ofloxacin in the treatment of sexually transmitted diseases. *Am J Obstet Gynecol* 164:1396-1400, 1991 A.

Corrado ML: Worldwide clinical experience with ofloxacin in urologic cases. *Suppl Urol* 37:28-32, 1991 B.

Davis RL, et al: Pharmacokinetics of ciprofloxacin in cystic fibrosis. *Antimicrob Agents Chemother* 31:915-919, 1987.

Dekker AW, et al: Infection prophylaxis in acute leukemia: A comparison of ciprofloxacin with trimethoprim/sulfamethoxazole and colistin. *Ann Intern Med* 106:7-12, 1987.

De Lalla F, et al: Clarithromycin-ciprofloxacin-amikacin for therapy of *Mycobacterium avium-Mycobacterium intracellulare* bacteremia in patients with AIDS. *Antimicrob Agents Chemother* 36:1567-1569, 1992.

Douidar SM, Snodgrass WR: Potential role of fluoroquinolones in pediatric infections. *Rev Infect Dis* 11:878-889, 1989.

Dryden MS, et al: Low dose intraperitoneal ciprofloxacin for the treatment of peritonitis in patients receiving continuous ambulatory peritoneal dialysis (CAPD). *J Antimicrob Chemother* 28:131-139, 1991.

DuPont HL: Use of quinolones in the treatment of gastrointestinal infections. *Eur J Clin Microbiol Infect Dis* 10:325-329, 1991.

DuPont HL, et al: Use of norfloxacin in treatment of acute diarrheal disease. *Am J Med* 82 (suppl 6B):79-83, 1987.

DuPont HL, et al: Five versus three days of ofloxacin therapy for traveler's diarrhea: A placebo-controlled study. *Antimicrob Agents Chemother* 36:87-91, 1992.

Dworzack DL, et al: Evaluation of single-dose ciprofloxacin in eradication of *Neisseria meningitidis* from nasopharyngeal carriers. *Antimicrob Agents Chemother* 32:1740-1741, 1988.

Elston RA, Taylor J: Possible interaction of ciprofloxacin with cyclosporin A. *J Antimicrob Chemother* 21:679-680, 1988.

Ericsson CD, et al: Ciprofloxacin or trimethoprim/sulfamethoxazole as initial therapy for travelers' diarrhea: Placebo-controlled, randomized trial. *Ann Intern Med* 106:216-220, 1987.

Fenlon CH, Cynamon MH: Comparative in vitro activities of ciprofloxacin and other 4-quinolones against *Mycobacterium tuberculosis* and *Mycobacterium intracellulare*. *Antimicrob Agents Chemother* 29:386-388, 1986.

Ferreccio C, et al: Efficacy of ciprofloxacin in the treatment of chronic typhoid carriers. *J Infect Dis* 157:1235-1239, 1988.

Fitton A: The quinolones: An overview of their pharmacology. *Clin Pharmacokinet* 22 (suppl 1):1-11, 1992.

Frieden TR, Mangi RJ: Inappropriate use of oral ciprofloxacin. *JAMA* 264:1438-1440, 1990.

Gaunt PN, Lambert BE: Single dose ciprofloxacin for eradication of pharyngeal carriage of *Neisseria meningitidis*. *J Antimicrob Chemother* 21:489-496, 1988.

Gentry LO: Oral antimicrobial therapy for osteomyelitis, editorial. *Ann Intern Med* 114:986-987, 1991.

Gentry LO: Therapy with newer oral β-lactam and quinolone agents for infections of the skin and skin structures: A review. *Clin Infect Dis* 14:285-297, 1992.

Gentry LO, Rodriguez GG: Oral ciprofloxacin compared with parenteral antibiotics in the treatment of osteomyelitis. *Antimicrob Agents Chemother* 34:40-43, 1990.

Gentry LO, Rodriguez-Gomez G: Ofloxacin versus parenteral therapy for chronic osteomyelitis. *Antimicrob Agents Chemother* 35:538-541, 1991.

Gentry LO, et al: Parenteral followed by oral ofloxacin for nosocomial pneumonia and community-acquired pneumonia requiring hospitalization. *Am Rev Respir Dis* 145:31-35, 1992.

Goldfarb J, et al: Single-dose pharmacokinetics of oral ciprofloxacin in patients with cystic fibrosis. *J Clin Pharmacol* 26:222-226, 1986.

Gotfried MH, Ellison WT: Safety and efficacy of lomefloxacin versus cefaclor in the treatment of acute exacerbations of chronic bronchitis. *Am J Med* 92 (suppl 4A):4A-108S-4A-113S, 1992.

Gotuzzo E, et al: Use of norfloxacin to treat chronic typhoid carriers. *J Infect Dis* 157:1221-1225, 1988.

Grassi C, et al: Lomefloxacin versus amoxicillin in the treatment of acute exacerbations of chronic bronchitis: An Italian multicenter study. *Am J Med* 92 (suppl 4A):4A-103S-4A-107S, 1992.

Harnett N, et al: Emergence of quinolone resistance among clinical isolates of methicillin-resistant *Staphylococcus aureus* in Ontario, Canada. *Antimicrob Agents Chemother* 35:1911-1913, 1991.

Healy DP, et al: Lack of interaction between lomefloxacin and caffeine in normal volunteers. *Antimicrob Agents Chemother* 35:660-664, 1991.

Henwood JM, Monk JP: Enoxacin: Review of its antibacterial activity, pharmacokinetic properties and therapeutic use. *Drugs* 36:32-66, 1988.

Hooper DC, Wolfson JS: Treatment of genitourinary tract infections with fluoroquinolones: Clinical efficacy in genital infections and adverse effects. *Antimicrob Agents Chemother* 33:1662-1667, 1989.

Hooper DC, Wolfson JS: Fluoroquinolone antimicrobial agents. *N Engl J Med* 324:384-394, 1991 A.

Hooper DC, Wolfson JS: Mode of action of the new quinolones: New data. *Eur J Clin Microbiol Infect Dis* 10:223-231, 1991 B.

Hooper DC, et al: Mechanisms of quinolone resistance in *Escherichia coli*: Characterization of *nfxB* and *cfxB*, two mutant resistance loci decreasing norfloxacin accumulation. *Antimicrob Agents Chemother* 33:283-290, 1989.

Hooton TM, et al: Ofloxacin versus doxycycline for treatment of cervical infection with *Chlamydia trachomatis*. *Antimicrob Agents Chemother* 36:1144-1146, 1992.

Hughes WT, et al: Guidelines for the use of antimicrobial agents in neutropenic patients with unexplained fever. *J Infect Dis* 161:381-396, 1990.

Hyatt DS, et al: A randomized trial of ciprofloxacin plus azlocillin versus netilmicin plus azlocillin for the empirical treatment of fever in neutropenic patients. *J Antimicrob Chemother* 28:324-325, 1991.

Jaber LA, et al: Enoxacin: A new fluoroquinolone. *Clin Pharm* 8:97-107, 1989.

Johnson PC, et al: Lack of emergence of resistant fecal flora during successful prophylaxis of travelers' diarrhea with norfloxacin. *Antimicrob Agents Chemother* 30:671-674, 1986.

Jonsson M, et al: First clinical isolate of highly fluoroquinolone-resistant *Escherichia coli* in Scandinavia. *Eur J Clin Microbiol Infect Dis* 9:851-853, 1990.

Karp JE, et al: Oral norfloxacin for prevention of gram-negative bacterial infections in patients with acute leukemia and granulocytopenia: A randomized, double-blind, placebo-controlled trial. *Ann Intern Med* 106:1-7, 1987.

Kelsey SM, et al: A comparative study of intravenous ciprofloxacin and benzylpenicillin versus netilmicin and piperacillin for the empirical treatment of fever in neutropenic patients. *J Antimicrob Chemother* 25:149-157, 1990.

Kemper P, Kohler D: A double-blind study of two dosage regimens of lomefloxacin in bacteriologically proven exacerbations of chronic bronchitis of gram-negative etiology. *Am J Med* 92 (suppl 4A): 4A-98S-4A-102S, 1992.

Kemper CA, et al: Treatment of *Mycobacterium avium* complex bacteremia in AIDS with a four-drug oral regimen: Rifampin, ethambutol, clofazimine, and ciprofloxacin. *Ann Intern Med* 116:466-472, 1992.

Kern W, Kurrle E: Ofloxacin versus trimethoprim-sulfamethoxazole for prevention of infection in patients with acute leukemia and granulocytopenia. *Infection* 19:73-80, 1991.

Lang R, et al: Successful treatment of malignant external otitis with oral ciprofloxacin: Report of experience with 23 patients. *J Infect Dis* 161:537-540, 1990.

LeBel M: Fluoroquinolones in the treatment of cystic fibrosis: A critical appraisal. *Eur J Clin Microbiol Infect Dis* 10:316-324, 1991.

LeBel M, et al: Pharmacokinetics and pharmacodynamics of ciprofloxacin in cystic fibrosis patients. *Antimicrob Agents Chemother* 30:260-266, 1986.

Lew MA, et al: Prophylaxis of bacterial infections with ciprofloxacin in patients undergoing bone marrow transplantation. *Transplantation* 51:630-636, 1991.

Liang RHS, et al: Ofloxacin versus co-trimoxazole for prevention of infection in neutropenic patients following cytotoxic chemotherapy. *Antimicrob Agents Chemother* 34:215-218, 1990.

Limson BM, Littaua RT: Comparative study of ciprofloxacin versus cotrimoxazole in the treatment of salmonella enteric fever. *Infection* 17:105-106, 1989.

Maiche AG: Use of quinolones in the immunocompromised host. *Eur J Clin Microbiol Infect Dis* 10:361-367, 1991.

Maiche AG, Teerenhovi L: Empiric treatment of serious infections in patients with cancer: Randomised comparison of two combinations. *Infection* 19 (suppl 6):S326-S329, 1991.

Malik IA, et al: Randomised comparison of oral ofloxacin alone with combination of parenteral antibiotics in neutropenic febrile patients. *Lancet* 339:1092-1096, 1992.

Meunier F, et al: Prospective randomized evaluation of ciprofloxacin versus piperacillin plus amikacin for empiric antibiotic therapy of febrile granulocytopenic cancer patients with lymphomas and solid tumors. *Antimicrob Agents Chemother* 35:873-878, 1991.

Modai J: Potential role of fluoroquinolones in the treatment of bacterial meningitis. *Eur J Clin Microbiol Infect Dis* 10:291-295, 1991.

Mulligan ME, et al: Ciprofloxacin for eradication of methicillin-resistant *Staphylococcus aureus* colonization. *Am J Med* 82 (suppl 4A):215-219, 1987.

Naber KG: The role of quinolones in the treatment of chronic bacterial prostatitis. *Infection* 19 (suppl 3):S170-S177, 1991.

Nakanishi N, et al: Mechanisms of clinical resistance to fluoroquinolones in *Enterococcus faecalis. Antimicrob Agents Chemother* 35:1053-1059, 1991.

National Institutes of Health Consensus Development Conference: Travelers' diarrhea. *JAMA* 253:2700-2704, 1985.

Neill MA, et al: Failure of ciprofloxacin to eradicate convalescent fecal excretion after acute salmonellosis: Experience during an outbreak in health care workers. *Ann Intern Med* 114:195-199, 1991.

Neu HC: The place of quinolones in bacterial infections. *Adv Intern Med* 36:1-32, 1991 A.

Neu HC: Microbiologic aspects of fluoroquinolones. *Am J Ophthalmol* 112:15S-24S, 1991 B.

Neu HC: Urinary tract infections. *Am J Med* 92 (suppl 4A):4A-63S-4A-70S, 1992.

Nix DE, et al: Effect of lomefloxacin on theophylline pharmacokinetics. *Antimicrob Agents Chemother* 33:1006-1008, 1989.

Norrby SR: Side-effects of quinolones: Comparisons between quinolones and other antibiotics. *Eur J Clin Microbiol Infect Dis* 10:378-383, 1991.

Oriel JD: Ciprofloxacin in treatment of gonorrhea and non-gonococcal urethritis. *J Antimicrob Chemother* 18 (suppl D):129-132, 1986.

Outman WR: Enoxacin: A new fluoroquinolone antibiotic. *Hosp Formul* 25:32-40, 1990.

Petruccelli BP, et al: Treatment of traveler's diarrhea with ciprofloxacin and loperamide. *J Infect Dis* 165:557-560, 1992.

Piercy EA, et al: Ciprofloxacin for methicillin-resistant *Staphylococcus aureus* infections. *Antimicrob Agents Chemother* 33:128-130, 1989.

Radandt JM, et al: Interactions of fluoroquinolones with other drugs: Mechanisms, variability, clinical significance, and management. *Clin Infect Dis* 14:272-284, 1992.

Ramirez CA, et al: Open, prospective study of clinical efficacy of ciprofloxacin. *Antimicrob Agents Chemother* 28:128-132, 1985.

Rautelin H, et al: Emergence of fluoroquinolone resistance in *Campylobacter jejuni* and *Campylobacter coli* in subjects from Finland. *Antimicrob Agents Chemother* 35:2065-2069, 1991.

Ronald AR, Peeling RW: Chlamydial infections and the quinolones. *Eur J Clin Microbiol Infect Dis* 10:351-354, 1991.

Sanders CC: Review of preclinical studies with ofloxacin. *Clin Infect Dis* 14:526-538, 1992 A.

Sanders WE Jr: Oral ofloxacin: A critical review of the new drug application. *Clin Infect Dis* 14:539-554, 1992 B.

Sanders CC, et al: Selection of multiple antibiotic resistance by quinolones, β-lactams, and aminoglycosides with special reference to cross-resistance between unrelated drug classes. *Antimicrob Agents Chemother* 26:797-801, 1984.

Sanders WE Jr, et al: Oral ofloxacin for the treatment of acute bacterial pneumonia: Use of nontraditional protocol to compare experimental therapy with 'usual care' in a multicenter clinical trial. *Am J Med* 91:261-266, 1991.

Schaad UB: Use of quinolones in pediatrics. *Eur J Clin Microbiol Infect Dis* 10:355-360, 1991.

Schaad UB, Wedgwood J: Lack of quinolone-induced arthropathy in children. *J Antimicrob Chemother* 30:414-416, 1992.

Shimada J, et al: Effect of antacid on absorption of the quinolone lomefloxacin. *Antimicrob Agents Chemother* 36:1219-1224, 1992.

Smith JA: Treatment of intra-abdominal infections with quinolones. *Eur J Clin Microbiol Infect Dis* 10:330-333, 1991.

Smith MJ, et al: Pharmacokinetics and sputum penetration of ciprofloxacin in patients with cystic fibrosis. *Antimicrob Agents Chemother* 30:614-616, 1986.

Smith GM, et al: A clinical, microbiological and pharmacokinetic study of ciprofloxacin plus vancomycin as initial therapy of febrile episodes in neutropenic patients. *J Antimicrob Chemother* 21:647-655, 1988.

Taylor DN, et al: Treatment of travelers' diarrhea: Ciprofloxacin plus loperamide compared with ciprofloxacin alone: A placebo-controlled, randomized trial. *Ann Intern Med* 114:731-734, 1991.

Thys JP, et al: Role of quinolones in the treatment of bronchopulmonary infections, particularly pneumococcal and community-acquired pneumonia. *Eur J Clin Microbiol Infect Dis* 10:304-315, 1991.

Todd PA, Faulds D: Ofloxacin: A reappraisal of its antimicrobial activity, pharmacology and therapeutic use. *Drugs* 42:825-876, 1991.

Trucksis M, et al: Emerging resistance to fluoroquinolones in staphylococci: An alert, editorial. *Ann Intern Med* 114:424-426, 1991.

Trujillo IZ, et al: Fluoroquinolones in the treatment of typhoid fever and the carrier state. *Eur J Clin Microbiol Infect Dis* 10:334-341, 1991.

Velmonte MA, Montalban CS: Norfloxacin in the treatment of infections caused by *Salmonella typhi. Scand J Infect Dis* 56 (suppl): 46-48, 1988.

Venezio FR, et al: Activity of ciprofloxacin against multiply resistant strains of *Pseudomonas aeruginosa, Staphylococcus epidermidis,* and group JK corynebacteria. *Antimicrob Agents Chemother* 30:940-941, 1986.

Wadworth AN, Goa KL: Lomefloxacin: A review of its antibacterial activity, pharmacokinetic properties and therapeutic use. *Drugs* 42:1018-1060, 1991.

Walker RC, Wright AJ: The fluoroquinolones. *Mayo Clin Proc* 66:1249-1259, 1991.

Wallace RJ Jr, et al: Activities of ciprofloxacin and ofloxacin against rapidly growing mycobacteria with demonstration of acquired resistance following single-drug therapy. *Antimicrob Agents Chemother* 34:65-70, 1990.

Wang F, et al: Treatment of typhoid fever with ofloxacin. *J Antimicrob Chemother* 23:786-788, 1989.

Wendel GD Jr, et al: A randomized trial of ofloxacin versus cefoxitin and doxycycline in the outpatient treatment of acute salpingitis. *Am J Obstet Gynecol* 164:1390-1396, 1991.

Westphal JF, et al: Management of biliary tract infections: Potential role of the quinolones. *J Antimicrob Chemother* 28:486-490, 1991.

Wijnands GJA, et al: The effect of multiple-dose oral lomefloxacin on theophylline metabolism in man. *Chest* 98:1440-1444, 1990.

Wiström J, et al: Empiric treatment of acute diarrheal disease with norfloxacin: A randomized, placebo-controlled study. *Ann Intern Med* 117:202-208, 1992.

Wolfson JS, Hooper DC: Fluoroquinolone antimicrobial agents. *Clin Microbiol Rev* 2:378-424, 1989 A.

Wolfson JS, Hooper DC: Treatment of genitourinary tract infections with fluoroquinolones: Activity in vitro, pharmacokinetics, and clinical efficacy in urinary tract infections and prostatitis. *Antimicrob Agents Chemother* 33:1655-1661, 1989 B.

Yoshioka K, et al: A randomized prospective controlled study of ciprofloxacin with metronidazole versus amoxicillin/clavulanic acid with metronidazole in the treatment of intra-abdominal infection. *Infection* 19:25-29, 1991.

Miscellaneous Antibacterial Drugs

71

VANCOMYCIN HYDROCHLORIDE

TEICOPLANIN (Investigational drug)

RIFAMPIN

METRONIDAZOLE

SPECTINOMYCIN HYDROCHLORIDE

POLYMYXINS

BACITRACIN

URINARY TRACT ANTIMICROBIAL AGENTS

VANCOMYCIN HYDROCHLORIDE

[Vancocin, Vancoled]

Vancomycin is a glycopeptide antibiotic derived from *Amycolatopsis orientalis* (formerly *Streptomyces orientalis*). This drug was introduced in the late 1950s because of its efficacy against penicillin-resistant staphylococci, but it was largely replaced by the less toxic antistaphylococcal penicillins and cephalosporins in the 1960s. A resurgence in the use of vancomycin has occurred in recent years, primarily because of the increase in methicillin-resistant staphylococcal infections and because of the recognition of *Clostridium difficile* as the major cause of antibiotic-associated pseudomembranous colitis.

MECHANISM OF ACTION. Vancomycin inhibits the biosynthesis of peptidoglycan polymers during the second stage of bacterial cell wall formation. This is its primary site of action, and it is distinct from that of the β-lactam antibiotics (Pratt and Fekety, 1986 A; Nagarajan, 1991; see also index entry Penicillins). Vancomycin also injures protoplasts by altering their cytoplasmic membranes and inhibits ribonucleic acid (RNA) synthesis. The drug usually is bactericidal for multiplying organisms.

ANTIMICROBIAL SPECTRUM. Vancomycin is active only against gram-positive bacteria. It is one of the most potent antibiotics against *Staphylococcus aureus* and *S. epidermidis*, including methicillin- and cephalothin-resistant strains. The minimal inhibitory concentration (MIC) for most strains is ≤ 5 mcg/ml. Although the minimal bactericidal concentration (MBC) usually is similar to the MIC, some strains of staphylococci may be tolerant to the bactericidal effect of vancomycin. These strains appear to be deficient in autolysins that are necessary to kill the bacterial cell.

Streptococcus pyogenes and *S. pneumoniae* (including penicillin G-resistant strains) are highly susceptible to vancomycin. It usually inhibits the growth of viridans streptococci, *S. bovis, S. agalactiae* (group B), and enterococci (eg, *E. faecalis*) at concentrations attainable in vivo. However, vancomycin may not be bactericidal against some strains of these species, particularly the enterococci. Antibacterial synergism against enterococci is usually obtained when vancomycin is combined with an aminoglycoside, particularly gentamicin or streptomycin. Anaerobic or microaerophilic streptococci are usually susceptible.

Gram-positive bacilli that are susceptible to vancomycin include clostridia (including *C. difficile*), corynebacteria (including the penicillin-resistant group JK diphtheroids), *Bacillus anthracis, Listeria monocytogenes, Actinomyces* species, and lactobacilli. *Flavobacterium meningosepticum* is susceptible in vitro at concentrations between 16 and 25 mcg/ml, but other gram-negative bacilli, mycobacteria, *Bacteroides*, and fungi are completely resistant.

For additional discussion, see Fekety, 1990 A; Wilhelm, 1991; Phillips and Golledge, 1992.

RESISTANCE. Resistance to vancomycin was not a serious clinical problem during the first 30 years of its use. However, since about 1986, vancomycin-resistant gram-positive bacteria have been isolated from patients who were treated with this drug (for reviews, see Johnson et al, 1990; Woodford et al, 1991). Resistance to vancomycin or other glycopeptides (eg, teicoplanin) has been observed in six genera of gram-positive bacteria: *Enterococcus, Erysipelothrix, Lactobacillus, Leuconostoc, Pediococcus*, and *Staphylococcus.* Among all but the enterococci and staphylococci, resistance is an intrinsic and constitutively expressed property. However, this is not considered a serious clinical problem because, although the infections caused by these bacteria can be severe, their incidence is relatively low and the bacteria are often susceptible to other antibiotics, including clindamycin, erythromycin, gentamicin, and penicillins. In contrast, resistance to glycopeptides among enterococci (and perhaps some coagulase-negative staphylococci) is emerging as a potentially significant clinical problem (for review, see Courvalin, 1990). This property arises through selective pressure and is expressed in two different forms based on MIC. High-level (MIC for vancomycin 64 mcg/ml or greater) resistance is coded by plasmid-borne genes that are transferable in vitro to other gram-positive bacteria by conjugation. Low-level (MIC for vancomycin 16 to 32 mcg/ml) resistance does not appear to be transferable and is probably chromosomally encoded. High-level resistance may be induced by vancomycin or teicoplanin; low-level resistance is induced only by vancomycin. Enterococcal isolates that exhibit high-level resistance to vancomycin (eg, strains of *E. faecalis, E. faecium*, and *E. avium*) also are cross-resistant to teicoplanin (MIC 16 mcg/ml or greater) and frequently to a number of other drugs, including penicillins and aminoglycosides. Strains with low-level resistance (eg, *E. faecalis, E. faecium, E. gallinarum*) remain susceptible to teicoplanin (see Courvalin, 1990). Although glycopeptide resistance in enterococci is relatively uncommon at the present time, susceptibility testing of clinical isolates using revised standards is recommended, especially in settings where glycopeptide usage may be high (eg, renal units with large numbers of ambulatory patients receiving continuous peritoneal dialysis) (Woodford et al, 1991).

Because glycopeptide antimicrobial drugs are chemically unrelated to other antimicrobial agents and act at a unique site, cross-resistance does not occur between glycopeptides and nonglycopeptides.

USES. The use of intravenous vancomycin should be restricted to serious infections caused by susceptible gram-positive bacteria when other antibiotics are ineffective or not tolerated. Vancomycin is recommended for serious methicillin-sensitive staphylococcal infections only in patients who cannot receive (eg, due to immediate-type hypersensitivity) or have not responded to penicillins and cephalosporins. However, physicians must be cautious in their interpretation or determination of penicillin hypersensitivity in all patients with severe gram-positive infections that may be more responsive to a penicillinase-resistant penicillin (eg, nafcillin) than to vancomycin (see index entry Hypersensitivity, Drug-induced, for additional information on penicillin hypersensitivity).

Vancomycin is the drug of choice for serious infections caused by methicillin-resistant *S. aureus* (MRSA) and coagulase-negative staphylococci, including methicillin-resistant *S. epidermidis* (MRSE). These infections include septicemia, endocarditis, osteomyelitis, pneumonia, lung abscesses, soft tissue infections, wound infections, and meningitis. Lumbar intrathecal or intraventricular administration may be required to treat meningitis. The clinical response to vancomycin may be slow when this drug is used alone to treat patients with acute native valve endocarditis and bacteremia due to *S. aureus*, including MRSA (Levine et al, 1991) and methicillin-susceptible isolates (Small and Chambers, 1990). Because of this, the addition of other drugs (eg, rifampin, gentamicin) to a vancomycin regimen initially may be considered (Karchmer, 1991).

MRSE (and other coagulase-negative staphylococci) has become an important cause of infections associated with indwelling devices, including prosthetic heart valves, prosthetic hips, cerebrospinal fluid shunts, and intravenous (eg, Hickman) catheters. Vancomycin is the drug of choice for treatment of these infections. For prosthetic valve endocarditis caused by MRSE, intravenous vancomycin in combination with rifampin and gentamicin for two weeks, followed by vancomycin plus rifampin for an additional four weeks, has been recommended (Karchmer, 1985; Bisno et al, 1989). Surgical intervention frequently is required.

The combination of vancomycin with gentamicin or streptomycin (for susceptible strains) is the regimen of choice for enterococcal endocarditis in penicillin-allergic patients. Although vancomycin can be used to treat endocarditis caused by viridans streptococci in penicillin-allergic patients, first generation cephalosporins (eg, cefazolin, cephalothin, cephapirin) usually are preferred unless there also is cephalosporin hypersensitivity.

Intravenous vancomycin is useful for prophylaxis of infective endocarditis in high-risk patients who are allergic to penicillin and are undergoing dental or certain other surgical procedures. (See index entry Endocarditis, Chemoprophylaxis.)

Vancomycin is an alternative to first-generation cephalosporins or antistaphylococcal penicillins for prophylaxis during certain surgical procedures (eg, cardiac valve replacement, total hip replacement) in patients allergic to penicillins and cephalosporins. (See index entry Cardiac Surgery.)

Vancomycin is the drug of choice for the uncommon pneumococcal infections that are resistant to penicillin G. For example, meningitis caused by penicillin-resistant *S. pneumoniae* has been successfully treated with intravenous vancomycin (Viladrich et al, 1991). However, because of the narrow therapeutic margin of vancomycin and the substantial variability in cerebrospinal fluid (CSF) concentrations obtained with intravenous administration, its routine use in this manner for this infection is not recommended. Adjunctive intrathecal injection may be considered for this indication. Regardless of the route of administration, vancomycin should be reserved for those patients who exhibit immediate-type (eg, IgE-mediated) anaphylactic reactions to β-lactam drugs and for those with infections caused by multiply resistant isolates that have previously not responded to other therapy (eg, chloramphenicol, penicillins, third-generation cephalosporins). Vancomycin also may be effective for serious infections (eg, prosthetic valve endocarditis) caused by the penicillin-resistant JK strains of corynebacteria and *Flavobacterium meningosepticum* meningitis that is resistant to other antimicrobial agents.

When administered intravenously or intraperitoneally, this drug is useful in the management of peritonitis associated with continuous ambulatory peritoneal dialysis (CAPD). Gram-positive bacteria, particularly staphylococci, are the most common causative organisms of these infections.

Oral vancomycin is a drug of choice for the treatment of confirmed antibiotic-associated pseudomembranous colitis (AAPMC) caused by *Clostridium difficile*, especially in seriously ill patients. In asymptomatic patients, vancomycin may temporarily eliminate fecal excretion of *C. difficile,* but such treatment may result in a higher rate of *C. difficile* carriage (Johnson et al, 1992). Thus, use of vancomycin for this indication in asymptomatic patients is not recommended. Oral metronidazole may be equally effective in patients with confirmed AAPMC, and it is not as expensive as vancomycin.

There is considerable controversy regarding the role of vancomycin in empiric antibacterial regimens for adults or children who become febrile and develop infections as a sequela of neutropenia caused by cytotoxic chemotherapy for cancer (see Hughes et al, 1990; Pizzo et al, 1991). During the past decade, the spectrum of bacteria infecting these patients has changed from predominantly gram-negative bacilli to primarily gram-positive isolates, especially *S. aureus* (including MRSA), coagulase-negative staphylococci (*S. epidermidis*, including MRSE), alpha-hemolytic streptococci, and *Corynebacterium* species. Because of this evolution, which is presumed to have occurred for a number of reasons related to advances in cancer chemotherapy, the necessity for vancomycin in management of these infections is not disputed. Rather, the timing of its administration is a matter of debate: some investigators believe that routine inclusion of vancomycin in the initial regimen is appropriate, while others contend that this drug can be added later if gram-positive bacteria are isolated in culture or if the patient does not respond to the initial antibiotic(s) (see Hughes et al, 1990). The results of several recent prospective, randomized trials do not support the routine inclusion of vancomycin in an empiric therapeutic regimen consisting primarily of ceftazidime (European Organization for Research and Treatment of Cancer [EORTC] International Antimicrobial Therapy Cooperative Group, 1991; Viscoli et al, 1991; Ramphal et al, 1992). However, empiric use of vancomycin has been recommended in centers that experience a high frequency of infections with MRSA, in patients who have evidence of infection at the exit or tunnel sites of central venous catheters and other indwelling lines, or in those with nonpatent vascular lines (Hughes et al, 1990; Pizzo et al, 1991; see also index entry Bacteremia, Treatment). Although both approaches to therapy have merit, the clinician also should consider the clinical status of the patient, the local prevalence and patterns of bacterial resistance to β-lactam drugs, the results of clinical bacterial susceptibility assays (if available), and the possible added expense if toxicity is associated with administration of vancomycin.

For additional discussion, see *Med Lett Drugs Ther,* 1986; Levine, 1987; Fekety, 1990 A.

ADVERSE REACTIONS AND PRECAUTIONS. In general, the purified preparations of vancomycin now available are well tolerated when properly administered. Frequent reports of certain adverse reactions (eg, fever, chills) with early preparations of the drug appear to have been caused by impurities. In addition, there is now a better awareness of the hazards of rapid intravenous administration.

The most common adverse reaction to vancomycin, the so-called "red neck" or "red man" syndrome (RMS), has recently been termed glycopeptide-induced anaphylactoid reaction (GIAR) (Polk, 1991). This nonimmunologic, dose-dependent response may occur in adults or children and is characterized by one or more of the following signs or symptoms: an erythematous macular rash involving the face, neck, upper torso, back and arms; flushing; pruritus; pain and muscle spasms in the chest; tachycardia; or hypotension (Levy et al, 1990; Sahai et al, 1990; Wallace et al, 1991). Profound hypotension and, rarely, cardiac arrest have been reported after inadvertent bolus injection (Glicklich and Figura, 1984; Mayhew and Deutsch, 1985). Although slow intravenous infusion of vancomycin over 60 minutes in a large volume of fluid reduces the incidence of these symptoms and is the recommended method of administration, RMS has been reported in patients and normal volunteers receiving 60-minute infusions of vancomycin, particularly when a 1-g dose was administered (Wallace et al, 1991; Healy et al, 1990). The frequency and severity of RMS may be further reduced by extending the infusion time to two hours (Healy et al, 1990). In most instances, the signs and symptoms of RMS resolve promptly on discontinuation of the infusion and may begin to disappear during the infusion. Thus, although some manifestations of RMS may be severe and require the institution of supportive measures, it is not generally considered to be a significant deterrent to the use of vancomycin in most patients for whom this drug may be indicated (Polk, 1991).

Despite extensive study, the exact mechanism of RMS remains unknown. Its occurrence has been associated with elevations in plasma histamine concentrations in healthy adult subjects (Healy et al, 1990). This correlation is further supported by data showing that pretreatment with the histamine H_1 blocking drugs, hydroxyzine (Sahai et al, 1989) or diphenhydramine (Wallace et al, 1991), is highly effective in preventing RMS in healthy volunteers and hospitalized patients with various infections who subsequently received a standard 1-g dose of vancomycin during a 60-minute infusion. However, because the available studies only indicate an association between elevations of plasma histamine concentrations and the occurrence of RMS secondary to vancomycin administration, additional clinical data are necessary to determine its exact mechanism.

It appears that the frequency of infusion-related anaphylactoid reactions increases with concomitant administration of anesthetic agents (Odio et al, 1984; Slight et al, 1985; Southorn et al, 1986). The manufacturer suggests that these events may be reduced by administering vancomycin as a 60-minute infusion prior to induction of anesthesia.

Ototoxicity has been considered a serious adverse effect of vancomycin since 1958. This conclusion was largely derived from reports describing a connection between various manifestations of ototoxicity and the administration of vancomycin in only 28 patients (for reviews, see Bailie and Neal, 1988;

Brummett and Fox, 1989). Because of inexactitude with regard to the dosage of vancomycin used, its serum concentrations, the definition of hearing loss and its measurement, the extent of post-treatment follow-up, and the concomitant use of other potentially ototoxic drugs (eg, aminoglycosides, erythromycin) in some subjects, it is not possible to correlate the use of this drug and the occurrence of ototoxicity precisely. Nevertheless, on the basis of the sum of these data, it is reasonable to conclude that, in certain patients (eg, those with impaired renal function, the aged, those also receiving other potentially ototoxic drugs [especially aminoglycosides], those with pre-existing hearing loss), a standard regimen of vancomycin could produce some loss of hearing acuity, which may proceed from tinnitus and loss of high frequency (>4 kHz) acuity to threshold increases in the conversational frequency range. To reduce this risk, it is recommended that serum concentrations of vancomycin be carefully monitored and adjusted to maintain them within the recommended peak and trough ranges (see section on Dosage below) and that concomitant use of other drugs in patients receiving this glycopeptide be evaluated critically.

Dose-dependent nephrotoxicity was relatively common with earlier preparations of vancomycin, but now occurs infrequently and is reversible when currently available preparations are administered appropriately (see Bailie and Neal, 1988). In one retrospective study, the concomitant administration of vancomycin and an aminoglycoside resulted in significantly elevated serum creatinine concentrations in 35% of patients (Farber and Moellering, 1983), but contradictory data also have been reported (Cimino et al, 1987).

Fever, chills, and chemical thrombophlebitis are less common with the purified preparations currently available. However, phlebitis at the site of infusion still occurs, particularly when vancomycin is administered through peripheral venous catheters (see Sorrell and Collignon, 1985). This may be avoided by changing the site of infusion frequently or by infusing the drug through central venous catheters.

Other adverse effects include skin rash in 3% to 5% of patients, reversible neutropenia, transient thrombocytopenia, and eosinophilia. Nausea and an unpleasant taste have been reported after oral administration. Stevens-Johnson syndrome and vasculitis associated with use of vancomycin have been reported rarely.

Renal function should be monitored frequently in patients receiving intravenous vancomycin. Caution should be exercised in patients over 60 years, neonates (due to incompletely developed renal function), patients with pre-existing renal or otic disease, and when certain other drugs (eg, aminoglycosides) are administered concurrently. Measurement of vancomycin serum concentrations is recommended for those at high risk. Serial audiograms are recommended for certain high-risk patients, including those with renal failure or on prolonged therapy. The safety of vancomycin during pregnancy is not established (FDA Pregnancy Category C).

For additional discussion, see Fekety, 1990 A; Sorrell and Collignon, 1985; *Med Lett Drugs Ther,* 1986; Levine, 1987.

DRUG INTERACTIONS. Other ototoxic or nephrotoxic drugs should be given cautiously when vancomycin is administered because of the potential for additive effects (see above; Pauly et al, 1990).

Vancomycin has been reported to be incompatible in intravenous solution with many drugs, including heparin, chloramphenicol, methicillin, adrenal corticosteroids, aminophylline, barbiturates, chlorothiazide, phenytoin, sodium bicarbonate, sulfisoxazole diolamine, and warfarin (Cheung and DiPiro, 1986; see also Trissel, 1986).

Cholestyramine and oral vancomycin should not be given concurrently to treat pseudomembranous colitis because the anion exchange resin binds and inactivates the antibiotic.

PHARMACOKINETICS. Vancomycin is poorly absorbed from the gastrointestinal tract after oral administration, although clinically significant serum concentrations have been reported in patients with pseudomembranous colitis and severely impaired renal function (Thompson et al, 1983; Dudley et al, 1984; Spitzer and Eliopoulos, 1984; Matzke et al, 1987). High concentrations of vancomycin are attained in stool following oral but not intravenous administration. Intramuscular injection causes severe pain and is not recommended. Vancomycin must be given intravenously to treat systemic infections.

Peak serum concentrations of 20 to 50 mcg/ml and trough levels of 5 to 10 mcg/ml are observed following slow intravenous infusion of 1 g. Approximately 55% of circulating vancomycin is bound to plasma proteins. The steady-state volume of distribution in adult and pediatric subjects may range from 0.39 to 0.92 L/kg and 0.45 to 0.97 L/kg, respectively. Therapeutic concentrations of drug are attained in pleural, ascitic, pericardial, and synovial fluids. However, low levels are found in bile. Vancomycin does not penetrate the uninflamed meninges, but therapeutic levels may be attained in cerebrospinal fluid in the presence of meningitis. Supplemental lumbar intrathecal or intraventricular administration may be necessary in patients who respond poorly to intravenous treatment. Information on concentrations in human tissues is very limited. Therapeutic concentrations of vancomycin have been observed in peritoneal dialysis fluid after intravenous administration in patients undergoing continuous ambulatory peritoneal dialysis (Blevins et al, 1984).

Vancomycin is eliminated by the kidneys, primarily by glomerular filtration; 80% to 90% of a dose appears in the urine of healthy subjects as unchanged drug within 24 hours. The usual elimination half-life in adults with normal renal function ranges from three to nine hours (mean, six hours). In one study (Cutler et al, 1984), longer elimination half-lives were reported for men older than 60 years compared with men between 20 and 26 years (mean half-lives, 12.1 and 7.2 hours, respectively). Elimination half-lives are 5.9 to 9.8 hours in newborns, 4.1 hours in older infants, and 2.2 to 3 hours in children; indomethacin may decrease the clearance of vancomycin in neonates. In anuric patients, the half-life may be prolonged to eight or nine days. Dosage reductions are necessary in patients with renal insufficiency. Although it has been reported that elimination is prolonged in patients with impaired hepatic function (Brown et al, 1983), nonrenal elimination is minor (less than 5%) and dosage reductions are unnecessary.

Elimination of vancomycin is not significantly affected by hemodialysis or peritoneal dialysis, although total body clearance of drug may be significant in some patients on prolonged peritoneal dialysis. Vancomycin clearance may be increased during hemofiltration, continuous arteriovenous hemodialysis, and hemodialysis using high flux dialysis membranes. Hemoperfusion with charcoal and Amberlite resin XAD-4 has been reported to remove vancomycin rapidly (Ahmad et al, 1982).

For additional discussion, see Moellering, 1984; Cheung and DiPiro, 1986; Matzke et al, 1986.

MONITORING OF SERUM VANCOMYCIN CONCENTRATIONS. Because of significant interpatient variability in vancomycin pharmacokinetics (eg, volume of distribution; rate of elimination) and the potential for ototoxicity and nephrotoxicity, serum concentrations should be monitored when feasible, especially in high-risk patients (the elderly, the morbidly obese, neonates, those with renal impairment, individuals given other ototoxic and/or nephrotoxic agents concurrently). Peak concentrations should be determined in serum samples obtained one hour after infusion. At steady state (24 to 36 hours following initiation of therapy), peak concentrations of 30 to 40 mcg/ml and trough concentrations of 5 to 10 mcg/ml generally are recommended for most patients; however, data supporting this recommendation are inconsistent. A correlation between higher transient peak serum concentrations of vancomycin (eg, 80 mcg/ml or greater) and the occurrence of toxicity has not been confirmed (Matzke et al, 1984). Thus, it has been suggested that clinicians may seek to achieve peak concentrations up to 80 mcg/ml in low-risk patients (see Cheung and DiPiro, 1986). In practice, this may be difficult to control because vancomycin pharmacokinetics are complex. Furthermore, the optimal time for drawing serum samples for determination of peak concentrations has not been defined. Use of samples obtained one hour after drug administration appears to be acceptable and is recommended by some authorities.

Monitoring trough concentrations alone may be adequate to avoid toxicity in most patients. Because there is no evidence that fewer toxic reactions occur in patients when trough concentrations are maintained below 10 mcg/ml, it may be reasonable to maintain these in a range of 10 to 15 mcg/ml, depending on the risk factors of the individual patient and the susceptibility (if known) of the clinical bacterial isolate. The regimen may then be modified by adjusting the dose interval or the dose based on the measured trough concentrations rather than by attempting to achieve a specific peak (see Cheung and DiPiro, 1986). Trough concentrations should be determined in serum samples taken immediately prior to administering the next dose. When these conditions are met, the desired percentage of increase or decrease can be accomplished using an equivalent proportional change in the dose. Whichever method is used, it is essential that the dose, infusion time, and sampling times be controlled precisely to obtain accurate and reproducible results. Various assay methods (eg, bioassay, high-pressure liquid chromatography, fluorescence polarization immunoassay [FPIA]) are available to measure serum vancomycin concentrations. However, FPIA may falsely indicate elevated serum concentrations in patients with renal insufficiency. Therefore, a confirmatory assay using another methodology should be performed when FPIA indicates that vancomycin levels are higher than expected.

For a detailed discussion of therapeutic monitoring of vancomycin, see the reviews by Cheung and DiPiro, 1986, and Matzke, 1986; see also Healy et al, 1987.

DOSAGE AND PREPARATIONS. Refrigerated reconstituted solutions are stable for 96 hours (intravenous) or two weeks (oral).

Intravenous: At the time of use, 500-mg and 1-g vials are initially reconstituted with 10 ml and 20 ml, respectively, of sterile water for injection. Reconstituted vials containing 500 mg and 1 g then should be diluted with at least 100 and 200 ml, respectively, of 0.9% sodium chloride injection, 5% dextrose injection, or other compatible intravenous fluid (see manufacturer's literature) and administered slowly by intermittent infusion over a period of at least 60 minutes to reduce the risk of thrombophlebitis and hypotension. Continuous infusion should be used only when intermittent infusion is not feasible.

In *adults of average size with normal renal function*, the usual dosage is 1 g (15 mg/kg) every 12 hours (preferred) or 500 mg (6.5 to 8 mg/kg) every six hours. Monitoring of serum concentrations is recommended in the elderly. In severely ill patients, such as those with meningitis, 1 g may be given every eight hours for two to three days until the infection is under control. Intrathecal administration also may be necessary in central nervous system infections (see below). Morbidly obese patients may require higher doses, which should be based on total body weight, creatinine clearance, and the measurement of serum concentrations. In *children and infants older than 1 month with normal renal function*, the usual dosage is 40 mg/kg daily given in four divided doses. Larger doses (eg, 60 mg/kg daily in four divided doses) may be required in patients with central nervous system infections; intrathecal administration also may be necessary (see below). In *infants 8 days to 1 month with normal renal function*, the manufacturer suggests an initial dose of 15 mg/kg followed by 10 mg/kg every eight hours. In *infants 0 to 7 days with normal renal function*, the manufacturer suggests an initial dose of 15 mg/kg followed by 10 mg/kg every 12 hours. Because of interpatient variability in pharmacokinetics (Schaad et al, 1980; Alpert et al, 1984; Naqvi et al, 1986), monitoring of serum vancomycin concentrations is recommended in neonates.

Patients with impaired renal function must receive reduced dosages. Monitoring of peak and trough vancomycin serum concentrations to achieve peak concentrations of 30 to 40 mcg/ml and trough concentrations between 5 and 10 mcg/ml is recommended (see above).

Other methods also are available for administration of vancomycin to patients with impaired renal function. In one method, following a loading dose of 15 mg/kg in adults, the daily maintenance dose in milligrams is 150 plus 15 times the creatinine clearance (Ccr) in milliliters per minute (see index entry Drug Response Variation for calculation of Ccr). This produces a vancomycin steady-state serum concentration of 20 mcg/ml (Nielsen et al, 1975). Another method is to give 1 g to adults every 36 hours when the serum creatinine concentration is between 1.5 and 5 mg/dL and 1 g every 10 to 14 days when the serum creatinine concentration is greater than 5 mg/dL (see Fekety, 1990 A). Still another approach is to use a published nomogram that is designed to yield vancomycin steady-state serum concentrations of 15 mcg/ml (Moellering et al, 1981; see also the manufacturer's literature). Nomograms also have been published by Matzke et al (1984) and Lake and Peterson (1985). However, each of these methods provides only an estimation of the optimal dose in patients with impaired renal function. If administration of the drug is to be continued beyond two to three days, the serum concentrations should be measured to adjust the dosage in the individual patient (see Zokufa et al, 1989).

Because hemodialysis usually removes little or no vancomycin, 1 g (15 mg/kg) every 7 to 10 days usually provides adequate serum concentrations in functionally anephric adults, but monitoring of serum concentrations is recommended. Adults on continuous ambulatory peritoneal dialysis can be given the drug intravenously (loading dose, 23 mg/kg; maintenance dose, 17 mg/kg every seven days [Blevins et al, 1984]) or intraperitoneally (loading dose, 30 mg/kg; maintenance dose, 7 mg/kg once daily or 1.5 mg/kg every six hours [Bunke et al, 1983]). Monitoring of serum concentrations is recommended.

See index entry Endocarditis, Chemoprophylaxis, for dosage in chemoprophylaxis of infective endocarditis. See index entries Cardiac Surgery, Orthopedic Surgery, for dosages in perioperative prophylaxis of cardiovascular and orthopedic surgical procedures.

Generic. Powder equivalent to 500 mg or 1 g of base.

Vancocin (Lilly), ***Vancoled*** (Lederle). Powder equivalent to 500 mg, 1, 5 (***Vancoled*** only), or 10 (***Vancocin*** only) g of base.

Intrathecal: Experience with lumbar intrathecal and intraventricular therapy with vancomycin in refractory bacterial meningitis is limited. These routes of administration should be considered if cerebrospinal fluid cultures remain positive after 24 to 48 hours of intravenous therapy alone. Suggested dosages (Gump, 1981) for lumbar intrathecal administration are *adults,* 20 mg/day and *neonates and children,* 5 to 20 mg/day. If intraventricular instillation is employed, the initial dose should not exceed 5 mg because of the relatively small volume of distribution within the cerebrospinal fluid. Cerebrospinal fluid vancomycin concentrations should be monitored to make certain that levels are adequate but not excessive. See the product labeling for instructions on preparing vancomycin solutions for intrathecal use.

Oral: *Adults*, an aqueous solution or capsule(s) containing 125 to 500 mg may be given every six hours. The lower dose is effective for most cases of confirmed pseudomembranous colitis caused by *C. difficile* (Fekety et al, 1989; see also index entry Colitis, Pseudomembranous, Treatment). *Children,* 50 mg/kg daily in divided doses every six hours (maximum, 2 g/day).

Vancocin (Lilly). Powder equivalent to 1 or 10 g of base; capsules 125 and 250 mg.

TEICOPLANIN (Investigational drug)
[Targocid]

Teicoplanin (originally called teichomycin A_2) is a tetracyclic glycopeptide antimicrobial complex that is produced by the actinomycete, *Actinoplanes teichomyceticus,* and is structurally similar to vancomycin. It consists of 6 components designated as teicoplanin-A_2 (1 through 5) and teicoplanin-A_3. The five components of the former complex account for approximately 90% to 95% of the drug mixture.

MECHANISM OF ACTION. The mechanism of action of teicoplanin is similar to that of vancomycin (for reviews, see Campoli-Richards et al, 1990; Nagarajan, 1991; Phillips and Golledge, 1992). It binds to the terminal acyl-D-alanyl-D-alanine moiety of peptidoglycan, thus inhibiting polymerization of the major structural component of the nascent bacterial cell wall. The bactericidal effect is presumed to result from the action of released autolytic enzymes (eg, autolysins) similar to that observed with β-lactam antibiotics. However, because of their differing sites of action, cross-resistance does not occur between these drug classes. Because of its mechanism, teicoplanin, like vancomycin and the β lactams, is active only against dividing cells. Further, it is a large, polar molecule. As such, it cannot penetrate the external lipid bilayer that surrounds gram-negative organisms and thus is generally not active against this group of bacteria.

ANTIMICROBIAL SPECTRUM. The in vitro antimicrobial spectrum of teicoplanin is qualitatively equivalent to that of vancomycin (see the above evaluation on Vancomycin Hydrochloride; see also Campoli-Richards et al, 1990; Phillips and Colledge, 1992). Thus, it is highly active against almost all aerobic and anaerobic gram-positive bacteria; MIC values are 4 mcg/ml or lower against the majority of susceptible species. However, compared with vancomycin, teicoplanin is several times more potent against streptococci and enterococci, generally equipotent against staphylococci (including methicillin-resistant *Staphylococcus aureus*), and frequently is less active against coagulase-negative staphylococci (eg, *S. epidermidis, S. haemolyticus*) (Goldstein et al, 1990). Against most susceptible gram-positive anaerobes, MIC values are generally below 1 mcg/ml and are usually equivalent to twofold lower than those observed with vancomycin. Although teicoplanin is bactericidal against most susceptible bacteria at clinically attainable concentrations, it may be bacteriostatic against some isolates of coagulase-negative, penicillin-tolerant staphylococci, enterococci, and *L. monocytogenes* (see Campoli-Richards et al, 1990).

RESISTANCE. Resistance to teicoplanin has been observed among staphylococcal and enterococcal isolates in Europe and the United States (Dutka-Malen et al, 1990; Chomarat et al, 1991). For a detailed discussion of glycopeptide resistance and additional references, see the evaluation on Vancomycin Hydrochloride.

USES. The indications for teicoplanin are similar to those for vancomycin. These include serious gram-positive bacterial infections that are caused by penicillin- and cephalosporin-resistant strains (eg, methicillin-resistant *S. aureus* and *S.*

epidermidis; JK corynebacteria) or that are present in penicillin-allergic patients (eg, enterococcal endocarditis; osteomyelitis); prophylaxis of endocarditis in high-risk patients allergic to penicillin; as a component of empiric regimens in febrile, neutropenic patients; and, administered orally, antibiotic-associated pseudomembranous colitis caused by *C. difficile*.

The results of early clinical trials of teicoplanin therapy for gram-positive infections were inconsistent and sometimes conflicting (for reviews, see Pryka et al, 1988; Calain and Waldvogel, 1990; Campoli-Richards et al, 1990; Phillips and Golledge, 1992). In large, open, noncomparative multicenter trials in patients with suspected or proven skin and soft tissue, bone or joint, pulmonary, urinary tract, intra-abdominal, and endocardial infections and bacterial septicemia, this drug was effective (defined as cure or improvement) in 67% to 96% of those who received daily dosages of 200 to 400 mg (depending on the severity of the infection) following a 400-mg loading dose. Most patients received teicoplanin alone, but 28% also were given aminoglycosides, β lactams, or rifampin. However, with the exception of endocarditis, clinical outcomes in these studies did not correlate with the dose of teicoplanin. These generally favorable results contrasted with those obtained by other investigators, who found that a similar 200-mg daily maintenance regimen of teicoplanin produced unsatisfactory outcomes in patients with severe, deep-seated infections caused by gram-positive bacteria, primarily staphylococci (Glupczynski et al, 1986; Calain et al, 1987; Galanakis et al, 1988). In these studies, only approximately 45% of patients with bacteremia, endocarditis, or osteomyelitis responded to teicoplanin. Despite the fact that serum concentrations of the drug reached and frequently exceeded by manyfold the MIC of the infecting isolate in most patients, wide variation in the data makes it difficult to infer a precise dose-response relationship.

Because of these results, it was hypothesized that higher doses of teicoplanin would be necessary for effective treatment of severe gram-positive infections. This idea is supported by a recent re-evaluation of data from early European open trials of teicoplanin therapy in patients with endocarditis and *S. aureus* bacteremia, which indicates that this drug apparently was effective when the daily maintenance dosage was at least 6 mg/kg rather than the typical 3 mg/kg dose used in most of the early, unsuccessful trials (Davey and Williams, 1991 A). The results of subsequent trials suggest that daily maintenance doses of 7 to 15 mg/kg (yielding peak serum concentrations >30 mcg/ml) are required for successful treatment of serious gram-positive infections, especially bacteremia and endocarditis involving staphylococci and enterococci (Leport et al, 1989; Martino et al, 1989; Greenberg, 1990; Gilbert et al, 1991; Schmit, 1992; Venditti et al, 1992).

Teicoplanin was reported to be a safe, effective alternative to vancomycin for gram-positive infections associated with Hickman catheters in neutropenic patients with hematologic malignancies (Smith et al, 1989). Because 85% of the patients in this study also received gentamicin and piperacillin, however, it is difficult to determine the efficacy of the glycopeptide alone. A subsequent report indicated that teicoplanin alone (3 to 6 mg/kg daily) was equivalent to vancomycin in producing clinical and bacteriologic cures of severe gram-positive bacteremia and skin and soft tissue bacterial infections (predominantly due to *S. epidermidis* and *S. aureus*) in immunocompromised oncology patients (Van der Auwera et al, 1991). In additional studies, it was concluded that teicoplanin appeared to be effective and well tolerated for the empiric treatment of gram-positive infections when combined with tobramycin and piperacillin (Kureishi et al, 1991), amikacin and piperacillin (Martino et al, 1992), and ciprofloxacin (Kelsey et al, 1992). However, in another study, the empiric use of teicoplanin with ceftazidime did not markedly improve the final outcome in febrile, granulocytopenic patients when compared with the cephalosporin alone (Nováková et al, 1991). Further, patients who received the combination initially were more prone to develop subsequent infective complications and have adverse reactions to the two drugs. The authors of this study concluded that the inclusion of teicoplanin in the initial empiric regimen for febrile, neutropenic patients is unnecessary in the absence of signs and symptoms of gram-positive infections. This is consistent with the guidelines given for the use of vancomycin in this clinical situation (see the evaluation of Vancomycin Hydrochloride; see also index entry Bacteremia, Treatment). It is recommended that clinicians apply these criteria in deciding when to use teicoplanin in empiric regimens for febrile, neutropenic patients.

The preceding discussion provides strong evidence that teicoplanin may be an effective alternative to vancomycin for the treatment and prophylaxis of serious gram-positive bacterial infections at a variety of sites. However, at the present time, specific indications and the optimal dosage range for teicoplanin have not been established. Moreover, it is not clear whether toxic reactions to this drug given at daily doses of 10 mg/kg or more are less prevalent than those associated with use of the newer, affinity-purified preparations of vancomycin. Therefore, additional well-controlled trials comparing teicoplanin at higher doses with vancomycin are required to define the role of this drug in the treatment and prophylaxis of infectious diseases.

ADVERSE REACTIONS AND PRECAUTIONS. Teicoplanin is well tolerated when given intravenously or intramuscularly at daily doses up to 10 mg/kg; the overall incidence of drug-related adverse events is approximately 10%. Those that occur most commonly include nonspecific constitutional symptoms (eg, fatigue, headache, diarrhea); injection site intolerance (pain, redness, phlebitis); cutaneous reactions (maculopapular rash, pruritus, urticaria); reversible hematologic abnormalities (eosinophilia, neutropenia, thrombocytopenia); and asymptomatic elevations of liver transaminase levels (for reviews, see Campoli-Richards et al, 1990; Davey and Williams, 1991 B). In general, these adverse effects are not serious and should not deter use of this drug when it is needed. However, recent data indicate that the risk of adverse events (eg, drug fever, rash, perhaps ototoxicity) (see below), may be dose-related, with a higher incidence in patients who receive daily amounts greater than 10 mg/kg (Greenberg, 1990; Venditti et al, 1992).

Ototoxicity is extremely rare in patients given teicoplanin at doses of <10 mg/kg and, because of a lack of controlled data on this subject, there is uncertainty whether it can be related to treatment with this drug per se (see Davey and Williams, 1991 B). Similarly, although nephrotoxicity manifested primarily as reversible increases in plasma creatinine concentrations has been reported in a small number of patients who received teicoplanin at <10 mg/kg, it occurred primarily in those who also received an aminoglycoside (Kureishi et al, 1991), which makes it difficult to assess the effect of this drug alone on renal function. In contrast, in one comparative trial, teicoplanin alone at a dose of 6 mg/kg had no effect on serum creatinine concentrations, which were elevated in a small proportion of those who received vancomycin (Van der Auwera et al, 1991). Additional controlled data are required to determine the true risk of ototoxicity and nephrotoxicity in patients who receive teicoplanin therapy.

In contrast to vancomycin, teicoplanin does not cause the release of histamine in patients or healthy volunteers and only rarely causes red man syndrome (RMS) (for review, see Polk, 1991). This has been shown in studies using teicoplanin at doses of 3 to 6 mg/kg (Smith et al, 1989), 15 mg/kg (Sahai et al, 1990), and 30 mg/kg (Rybak et al, 1992). Thus, on the basis of these data and reports from other clinical trials (see Campoli-Richards et al, 1990), it can be inferred that RMS is not a significant problem associated with the use of teicoplanin.

Because anaphylactoid cross-reactivity with vancomycin does not appear to be common, patients who cannot tolerate the latter drug may usually be safely treated with teicoplanin. In contrast, those who respond to vancomycin with true IgE-mediated hypersensitivity, which is rare, may not tolerate teicoplanin (McElrath et al, 1986; Lewis et al, 1992). However, this observation is controversial (Schlemmer et al, 1988); and additional comparative clinical trials are required to resolve this disparity.

DRUG INTERACTIONS. Like vancomycin, teicoplanin is bound and inactivated by cholestyramine (Pantosti et al, 1985).

PHARMACOKINETICS. Teicoplanin is not absorbed from the gastrointestinal tract after oral administration. Unlike vancomycin, it can be administered intramuscularly deep into a large muscle mass. Intramuscular injection of 3 mg/kg produced a peak plasma concentration of 7 mcg/ml at two hours; bioavailability by this route was 90% (Verbist et al, 1984).

About 90% of circulating teicoplanin is protein bound, principally by albumin. Its volume of distribution at steady state ranges from 0.56 to 1.1 L/kg (see Rowland, 1990). Teicoplanin is widely distributed and reaches therapeutic concentrations in the following body fluids and tissues after a single 400-mg (6 mg/kg) bolus dose: blister fluid, gallbladder wall, bile, tonsils, cartilage, mucosa, liver, pancreas, and bone; lower concentrations are attained in fat, skin, and cerebrospinal fluid (see Campoli-Richards et al, 1990).

In early studies, the pharmacokinetics of intravenously administered teicoplanin were determined using plasma sampling periods of three to four days (for a review, see Rowland, 1990). In more recent investigations, plasma and urine samples have been collected for periods of 14 to 72 days after intravenous infusion (Carver et al, 1989; Lam et al, 1990; Outman et al, 1990; Rybak et al, 1991; Del Favero et al, 1991; Smithers et al, 1992; Thompson et al, 1992). Because of the increased length of the sampling period, the terminal elimination half-life of teicoplanin has now been found to be approximately 150 hours, with a range of 83 to 176 hours, based on a three-compartment pharmacokinetic model.

With single- or multiple-dose administration to normal volunteers, the other pharmacokinetic parameters of teicoplanin are essentially linear over a dosage range of 3 to 30 mg/kg. In contrast, total and renal clearances in bacteremic intravenous drug abusers receiving intravenous teicoplanin for bacterial endocarditis are significantly greater and more variable than in healthy subjects (Rybak et al, 1991). Consequently, serum concentrations of teicoplanin may vary widely in such patients, thus necessitating individualization of the dosage regimen to ensure that adequate treatment is provided.

Mean peak serum concentrations of approximately 30 mcg/ml are obtained immediately after a 30-minute infusion of 3 mg/kg (Lam et al, 1990). Average peak concentrations of 194, 197, and 253 mcg/ml have been reported immediately after a 30-minute infusion of 15, 20, or 25 mg/kg, respectively; 24 hours after these doses, mean plasma concentrations were 10.5, 13.6, and 19.8 mcg/ml, respectively (Del Favero et al, 1991).

Teicoplanin is cleared from the plasma almost entirely by glomerular filtration; 95% to 100% of a dose can be recovered unchanged in the urine of subjects with normal renal function (Carver et al, 1989; Smithers et al, 1992). In patients with impaired renal function, the drug accumulates in the serum, its half-life is prolonged, and a smaller amount is recovered in the urine (Lam et al, 1990). Therefore, dosage reductions are necessary in these patients. A nomogram to accomplish this is available (Lam et al, 1990). Teicoplanin is not removed by hemodialysis or peritoneal dialysis (Bonati et al, 1987).

DOSAGE AND PREPARATIONS.

Intravenous, Intramuscular: In *adults with normal renal function,* four intravenous loading doses of 6 mg/kg at 12-hour intervals (Outman et al, 1990) followed by single daily doses of 6 to 7 mg/kg have been suggested for serious infections caused by gram-positive bacteria (Bibler et al, 1987; Smith et al, 1989). Some investigators recommend monitoring the serum teicoplanin concentrations with adjustment of daily doses to maintain steady-state trough concentrations of approximately 10 mcg/ml. Higher dosages (eg, 12 to 15 mg/kg twice daily) are necessary for some deep tissue infections, such as endocarditis and osteomyelitis (see Greenberg, 1990; Gilbert et al, 1991). In *children under 12 years with normal renal function*, the usual adult loading dose (see above) is recommended, followed by daily doses of 6 to 10 mg/kg depending on the severity of the infection (Campoli-Richards et al, 1990). In granulocytopenic pediatric patients, doses of up to 12 mg/kg daily are recommended. Because efficacy and toxicity data are limited, the use of teicoplanin in *children under 3 years* is not recommended.

Dosing regimens for patients with impaired renal function have not been established (Lam et al, 1990). It has been recommended that, after the normal loading doses, the dosage interval be doubled (or the dose halved and given at 24-hour intervals) for individuals with mild-to-moderate renal impairment (creatinine clearance, 40 to 60 ml/min); for individuals with severe renal impairment (creatinine clearance, <40 ml/min), the maintenance regimen is one-third the usual daily dose, or the dosage interval is tripled (eg, the usual dose every third day) (Rowland, 1990).

Targocid (Marion Merrell Dow).

RIFAMPIN

[Rifadin, Rimactane, Rifadin I.V.]

For chemical formula, see index entry Rifampin, In Tuberculosis, Atypical Mycobacterial Infections.

MECHANISM OF ACTION AND ANTIMICROBIAL SPECTRUM. Rifampin binds to the β subunit of bacterial DNA-dependent RNA polymerase and blocks initiation of RNA synthesis in susceptible bacteria. The drug is bactericidal.

Rifampin is highly potent against *Staphylococcus aureus* and *S. epidermidis*, including methicillin-resistant strains. The minimal inhibitory concentration (MIC) for most strains is less than 0.015 mcg/ml (Thornsberry et al, 1983). However, some strains of methicillin-resistant *S. epidermidis* (MRSE) also are resistant to rifampin.

Most streptococci, including *S. pyogenes* (group A), *S. pneumoniae, S. agalactiae* (group B), and viridans streptococci, are susceptible. The drug is somewhat less active against enterococci (*E. faecalis*).

Other susceptible bacteria include *Listeria monocytogenes, Clostridium difficile,* most other anaerobes (including the *Bacteroides fragilis* group), *Neisseria gonorrhoeae, N. meningitidis, Haemophilus influenzae,* and *Legionella pneumophila*. In vitro, rifampin is considerably more potent than erythromycin against *L. pneumophila*. *Chlamydia trachomatis* and *C. psittaci* are also susceptible. Rifampin is active against *Mycobacterium tuberculosis* and certain atypical mycobacteria (eg, *M. avium, M. kansasii, M. marinum, M. leprae*). Most aerobic, gram-negative bacilli (eg, *Escherichia coli, Klebsiella, Proteus, Pseudomonas*) are resistant.

RESISTANCE. High-level resistance to rifampin develops rapidly due to mutations that alter the β subunit of RNA polymerase. Cross-resistance with other antimicrobial agents generally does not occur. Because of the rapid emergence of resistance, *rifampin should not be used alone to treat established infections*. However, in some patients, resistant strains have emerged even with combination drug therapy (Simon et al, 1983; Karchmer et al, 1984).

USES. Rifampin is a first-line drug in the treatment of tuberculosis. For a discussion of its role in this and other mycobacterial infections, see index entry Rifampin, In Tuberculosis, Atypical Mycobacterial Infections.

Rifampin eliminates nasopharyngeal carriage of *Neisseria meningitidis* and currently is the preferred drug for chemoprophylaxis of close contacts of patients with meningococcal meningitis. Similarly, this drug also eliminates oropharyngeal carriage of *H. influenzae* type b and is recommended by the American Academy of Pediatrics to prevent secondary *H. influenzae* type b disease in all household contacts, regardless of their age or immunization status, in those households with at least one contact younger than 48 months (American Academy of Pediatrics, 1991; see also index entry Haemophilus Influenzae Type b Infections, Chemoprophylaxis). However, rifampin generally is not indicated for the treatment of meningitis caused by either of these pathogens. Short-term prophylaxis of meningitis is the only indication for rifampin monotherapy.

Rifampin, always in combination with one or more other antibiotics, also may be used in a variety of staphylococcal infections for which treatment with more conventional drugs has been less than satisfactory (see Farr and Mandell, 1990; Kapusnik et al, 1984; Kapusnik and Sande, 1986). Selection of an appropriate antistaphylococcal drug to combine with rifampin has been somewhat controversial. Although some rifampin-containing combinations exhibit antagonistic or indifferent effects in vitro, such a result may not be predictive of efficacy in vivo (see Van der Auwera et al, 1983; Kapusnik et al, 1984).

Intravenous vancomycin plus oral rifampin for six weeks, with the addition of gentamicin for the initial two weeks, is the currently preferred regimen to treat prosthetic valve endocarditis caused by MSRE, although surgical intervention also is frequently required to cure this disease (Karchmer, 1985; Bisno et al, 1989; see also index entry Endocarditis, Treatment). The addition of gentamicin significantly decreased the emergence of rifampin-resistant strains of *S. epidermidis* during therapy compared with the two-drug combination (Karchmer et al, 1984).

The combined use of rifampin plus a penicillinase-resistant penicillin (eg, nafcillin) or vancomycin may be useful in *S. aureus* endocarditis complicated by metastatic abscesses or in patients who do not respond to single-agent therapy. However, clinical data are minimal.

Based on limited clinical data, the combination of rifampin and nafcillin or vancomycin may improve response rates in chronic staphylococcal osteomyelitis (Gentry, 1990). The use of rifampin with a penicillinase-resistant penicillin or vancomycin may be appropriate in the treatment of other serious staphylococcal infections that fail to respond to single-agent therapy, although such combinations must be considered investigational.

Rifampin can eradicate nasal carriage of staphylococci (Wheat et al, 1983; McAnally et al, 1984), and the combination of rifampin and an oral antistaphylococcal penicillin (to prevent emergence of resistance to rifampin) may be useful in some patients with recurrent furunculosis. Rifampin plus trimethoprim/sulfamethoxazole (or vancomycin) eradicated or reduced nasal carriage of methicillin-resistant *S. aureus* (MRSA) during nosocomial outbreaks (Ward et al, 1981; Locksley et al, 1982; Ellison et al, 1984). The results of a recent small, uncontrolled trial suggest that a regimen consisting of oral rifampin plus minocycline and intranasal mupirocin ointment was highly effective and comparable to rifampin plus trimethoprim/sulfamethoxazole or other antimicrobials in eradicating nasal carriage of MRSA among patients in a spinal cord injury unit (Darouiche et al, 1991). Although these data require confirmation in controlled trials, they support a role for rifampin in controlling the nosocomial outbreak and spread of MRSA (see Rahal, 1986).

The use of rifampin with erythromycin generally is indicated in the treatment of *L. pneumophila* infections that fail to respond to erythromycin alone. Some experts recommend combination therapy for all severe infections caused by this pathogen.

Rifampin can kill susceptible intracellular bacteria. It has eradicated staphylococci present in neutrophils of patients with chronic granulomatous disease and may be useful in this disease. Its role in diseases such as brucellosis is unclear. However, in one comparative trial for the treatment of brucellosis (Ariza et al, 1985), the relapse rate following 30 days of rifampin plus doxycycline (38.8%) was significantly greater than with tetracycline plus streptomycin (7.1%), and a longer treatment duration was recommended.

ADVERSE REACTIONS AND PRECAUTIONS. Rifampin has caused very few adverse reactions when used for short-term prophylaxis of meningitis. Red discoloration of the urine or other secretions is common, and permanent staining of soft contact lenses has been reported.

See index entry Rifampin, In Tuberculosis, Atypical Mycobacterial Infections, for adverse reactions and precautions associated with prolonged daily and/or intermittent therapy.

Rifampin is classified in FDA Pregnancy Category C.

DRUG INTERACTIONS. See index entry Rifampin, Drug Interactions.

PHARMACOKINETICS. Rifampin is well absorbed from the gastrointestinal tract after oral administration. Elimination is primarily via the biliary route following desacetylation (to an active metabolite) in the liver. Rifampin is highly lipid soluble and exhibits excellent penetration into most tissues and body fluid compartments, including cerebrospinal fluid, abscesses, and leukocytes. See index entry Rifampin, In Tuberculosis, Atypical Mycobacterial Infections, for a detailed discussion of pharmacokinetics.

DOSAGE AND PREPARATIONS. An extemporaneous oral suspension may be prepared for adults and children who have difficulty swallowing capsules; see the package insert for instructions.

Oral: *Adults*, 600 mg daily as a single dose or divided into two doses; in life-threatening infections (eg, prosthetic valve endocarditis), a maximum daily dose of 1.2 g may be given. *Children*, 10 to 20 mg/kg daily.

For prophylaxis of meningococcal disease, *adults*, 600 mg twice daily for two days; *children 1 month to 12 years*, 10 mg/kg twice daily for two days; *newborns less than 1 month*, 5 mg/kg twice daily for two days.

For prophylaxis of *H. influenzae* type b disease, *adults and children*, 20 mg/kg once daily (maximum, 600 mg daily) for four days. For young infants, dosage has not been established. Some experts administer 10 mg/kg once daily for four days to *infants less than 1 month*.

Rifadin (Marion Merrell Dow). Capsules 150 and 300 mg.
Rimactane (CIBA). Capsules 300 mg.

Intravenous: *Adults*, dosage is the same as for the oral preparation and should be reserved for patients who cannot take this drug orally.

Rifadin I.V. (Marion Merrell Dow). Powder (lyophilized) 600 mg.

METRONIDAZOLE

[Flagyl, Flagyl I.V. RTU, Metric 21, Metro I.V., Protostat]

METRONIDAZOLE HYDROCHLORIDE

[Flagyl I.V.]

For chemical formula, see index entry Metronidazole, In Protozoal Infections.

MECHANISM OF ACTION AND ANTIMICROBIAL SPECTRUM. The selective bactericidal action of metronidazole is due to the preferential reduction of the 5′-nitro group of the parent drug by anaerobic organisms, presumably by a ferredoxin-like system. An anaerobic environment is required for reduction to proceed. The short-lived active intermediate products formed subsequently interact with bacterial DNA and perhaps other macromolecules. Although the exact mechanism of action is unknown, double strand scissions in DNA probably are produced. Metronidazole is not activated by, and therefore fails to inhibit, most aerobic and facultative organisms.

Unlike other drugs, metronidazole is consistently bactericidal to susceptible anaerobic bacteria. Clinically important susceptible anaerobic bacteria include *Bacteroides, Prevotella, Porphyromonas, Fusobacterium, Clostridium* (including *C. difficile*), *Veillonella*, *Peptococcus,* and *Peptostreptococcus.* Of particular importance is the essentially uniform susceptibility of the commonly encountered *Bacteroides fragilis* group, anaerobic gram-negative bacilli that often are resistant to other antibacterial agents (see Tally et al, 1985). Only one-fourth of the strains of *Actinomyces* and *Arachnia,* the causative agents of actinomycosis, are susceptible. Most strains of other nonsporulating, gram-positive, anaerobic rods that seldom cause infection are resistant to metronidazole. Except for *Gardnerella* (*Haemophilus*) *vaginalis* and *Campylobacter fetus,* facultative anaerobes, microaerophilic bacteria, and obligate aerobes usually are not susceptible to metronidazole (see Finegold and Mathisen, 1990).

RESISTANCE. Acquired resistance to metronidazole is rare. Since it is not related chemically to other available drugs used in anaerobic bacterial infections, cross resistance does not occur.

USES. A wide variety of anaerobic bacterial infections respond to metronidazole. These include brain abscess, intra-abdominal infections (eg, peritonitis secondary to bowel perforation, abscess, liver abscess), gynecologic pelvic infections (eg, endometritis, endomyometritis, tubo-ovarian abscess), soft tissue infections (eg, necrotizing fasciitis, infected decubitus ulcers), bacteremias, osteomyelitis, septic arthritis, and endocarditis. However, many foci that are infected with anaerobic bacteria also are infected by aerobic pathogens that are not susceptible to metronidazole. These mixed infections (eg, aspiration pneumonia, lung abscess, empyema) must be treated with metronidazole and other drugs (eg, an aminoglycoside) to eradicate the aerobic bacteria.

Metronidazole is the drug of first choice in the rare case of endocarditis caused by penicillin-resistant *Bacteroides* species, most commonly *B. fragilis*. Although chloramphenicol may still be preferred by some infectious disease experts for anaerobic infections of the central nervous system (eg, subdural empyema, brain abscess), metronidazole is very effective because of its excellent penetration into the central nervous system and its consistent bactericidal activity. It appears to be as effective as clindamycin (or other drugs active against *B. fragilis*) in intra-abdominal, pelvic, skin, and soft tissue infections and is considered a good choice for infections caused by organisms, particularly *B. fragilis*, that are resistant to other drugs.

In addition to antimicrobial drug therapy, surgical debridement of necrotic tissue and drainage of abscesses are important for the successful treatment of anaerobic infections.

For a more detailed discussion on the management of anaerobic infections, see Bartlett, 1990; see also index entries Antimicrobial Drugs; Sexually Transmitted Diseases, Treatment.

The efficacy of metronidazole in surgical prophylactic regimens, particularly in patients undergoing colon or gynecologic surgery, has been established by well-controlled clinical trials. Although the drug is widely used for this purpose in Europe, there is less experience with metronidazole for surgical prophylaxis in the United States (Kaiser, 1986; see also index entry Antimicrobial Drugs, Chemoprophylaxis for Surgical Patients). In this country, it is labeled for prophylaxis in elective colorectal surgery.

Oral metronidazole is the preferred drug to treat bacterial vaginosis (formerly called nonspecific vaginitis), a syndrome now believed to be caused by the interaction of several species of vaginal bacteria, including anaerobes (see *MMWR*, 1989, and index entry Vaginosis, Bacterial). The results of a recent meta-analysis suggest that a single 2-g dose is as effective as a five- or seven-day course of this drug (Lugo-Miro et al, 1992). The potential clinical advantages of the one-day regimen include increased compliance, reduced incidence of adverse effects, and lower cost.

Oral metronidazole is very effective in the treatment of antibiotic-associated colitis (AAPMC) caused by *Clostridium difficile* (Teasley et al, 1983), and is equivalent to oral vancomycin for this indication. Many infectious disease experts recommend metronidazole as first-line therapy for mildly to moderately ill patients with AAPMC because it is considerably less expensive than vancomycin (see index entry Colitis, Pseudomembranous). Metronidazole also may be effective when used intravenously to treat AAPMC in patients who cannot take oral therapy. Oral metronidazole is ineffective in eradicating fecal excretion of *C. difficile* in asymptomatic patients and is not recommended in the latter patients (Johnson et al, 1992).

Metronidazole is considered a crucial component of the triple therapy regimen (metronidazole, a bismuth salt [eg, bismuth subsalicylate, Pepto Bismol], and either amoxicillin or tetracycline) that is currently recommended for the treatment of *Helicobacter pylori* gastric infection (see Blaser, 1992). This regimen is successful in 80% of patients who are infected with a metronidazole-sensitive strain of *H. pylori*. However, if the isolate is resistant to metronidazole, eradication rates fall to <20%. This resistance has been associated with previous exposure to metronidazole, in some cases as long as 18 years prior to the subsequent use. Because of the problem of metronidazole resistance, it is currently recommended that the susceptibility of an *H. pylori* isolate to this drug be determined prior to instituting this regimen.

For other uses, see index entry Metronidazole.

ADVERSE REACTIONS AND PRECAUTIONS. Metronidazole is generally well tolerated. The most common adverse effects are minor gastrointestinal disturbances (eg, nausea, epigastric distress, anorexia). Vomiting and diarrhea are less common. Isolated cases of pseudomembranous colitis caused by *C. difficile* have been reported. Other untoward effects include dryness of the mouth, bitter metallic taste, maculopapular rash, urticaria, urethral and vaginal burning, darkening of the urine, headache, dizziness, confusion, fever, and thrombophlebitis after intravenous infusion.

The most serious adverse effects involve the central nervous system and include convulsions and peripheral neuropathy, which is characterized mainly by numbness or paresthesia of an extremity. These effects are rare unless large doses or prolonged therapy is employed (eg, in Crohn's disease). If neurologic symptoms are observed, the drug must be discontinued immediately. Metronidazole should be used cautiously in individuals with a history of seizures or other central nervous system disorders.

Reversible neutropenia occurs in less than 1% of patients receiving metronidazole. Total and differential leukocyte counts are recommended before and after therapy.

Isolated cases of metronidazole-induced pancreatitis (Corey et al, 1991) and gynecomastia (Fagan et al, 1985) have been reported.

Because metronidazole is metabolized slowly in patients with impaired hepatic function, the drug may accumulate in plasma. Therefore, the dosage should be reduced in these patients, particularly if renal function also is impaired. Metronidazole should be used with caution in patients with clinically evident jaundice.

Metabolites of metronidazole excreted in the urine in humans have been shown to be mutagenic in in vitro bacterial systems, but there is no evidence of mutagenicity in mammalian cells. The drug is carcinogenic in mice and possibly in rats, but not in hamsters, when large doses are administered for very prolonged periods. In at least one study, treated rats survived longer than controls; this may have contributed to the increased incidence of tumors. Although there is no evidence that the incidence of cancer is increased in humans exposed to metronidazole, the available data are sufficient only to exclude a high risk of cancer because of the long latent period associated with chemical carcinogenesis.

Metronidazole crosses the placenta and is excreted in breast milk. Although the drug has not been shown to be teratogenic in animals or humans, benefits and risks should be weighed carefully before it is given to pregnant women or nursing mothers. Generally, it is not recommended during pregnancy, particularly during the first trimester. It is classified in FDA Pregnancy Category B.

Metronidazole has been reported to lower serum cholesterol and triglyceride levels (Davis et al, 1983). The mechanism and clinical significance of this effect are unknown.

DRUG INTERACTIONS AND INTERFERENCE WITH LABORATORY TESTS. Metronidazole inhibits the metabolism of warfarin and other coumarins, which potentiates their anticoagulant effect. Therefore, concomitant use should be avoided or the dosage of the anticoagulant should be reduced to maintain the desired prothrombin time.

Metronidazole appears to reduce the clearance and thus possibly increase the toxicity of fluorouracil.

Metronidazole has caused an intolerance to alcohol similar to that produced by disulfiram. Although not all patients exhibit a reaction, individuals receiving metronidazole should be advised not to drink alcohol because abdominal cramps, nausea, vomiting, headaches, and flushing may occur. This drug should never be administered concomitantly with disulfiram; acute psychotic reactions have been reported.

Cimetidine prolongs the plasma clearance of metronidazole, presumably by inhibiting metabolic enzymes (Gugler and Jensen, 1983); toxic concentrations of metronidazole may be produced. Drugs that induce microsomal liver enzymes (eg, phenobarbital) may accelerate the elimination of metronidazole, resulting in reduced plasma concentrations.

Metronidazole may interfere with certain types of determinations of serum chemistry values, such as aspartate aminotransferase (AST), alanine aminotransferase (ALT), lactate dehydrogenase (LDH), triglycerides, and hexokinase glucose. Values of zero may be observed. All of the assays in which interference has been reported involve enzymatic coupling of the assay to oxidation-reduction of nicotine adenine dinucleotide. Interference is due to the similarity in absorbance peaks of NADH (340 nm) and metronidazole (322 nm) at pH 7.0.

PHARMACOKINETICS. Metronidazole is well absorbed following oral administration. Peak plasma concentrations occur one to two hours after administration and are proportional to the dose (eg, oral administration of 250, 500, and 2,000 mg produced peak plasma levels of 6, 12, and 40 mcg/ml, respectively). Absorption is not significantly affected by food, although the time to peak plasma concentrations is increased. Metronidazole is variably absorbed when administered rectally (suppository).

Intravenous infusion is recommended initially for serious anaerobic bacterial infections. Plasma concentrations also are proportional to dose with this method of administration. Using a standard intravenous dosage regimen (15 mg/kg loading dose, followed by 7.5 mg/kg every six hours), peak and trough steady-state plasma concentrations average 25 and 18 mcg/ml, respectively.

Plasma concentrations of metronidazole are similar during the elimination phase after equivalent intravenous and oral doses.

Less than 20% of circulating metronidazole is bound to plasma proteins. The drug is widely distributed throughout all body tissues, and the volume of distribution is 0.8 L/kg.

Bactericidal concentrations are achieved in vaginal secretions, seminal fluid, saliva, empyema fluid, hepatic abscesses, pelvic tissues (eg, myometrium), bone, and bile. Metronidazole penetrates well into the central nervous system, including cerebrospinal fluid and brain abscesses. It crosses the placenta and is excreted in breast milk.

Metronidazole is metabolized primarily in the liver. The major metabolites are 1-(2-hydroxyethyl)-2-hydroxymethyl-5-nitroimidazole, which has approximately 30% of the bioactivity of the parent drug; 2-methyl-5-nitroimidazole-1-yl-acetic acid; and glucuronide conjugates.

Metronidazole and its metabolites are eliminated primarily in the urine (60% to 80% of the dose); 6% to 15% is excreted in the feces. Less than 20% of a dose is excreted as unchanged drug.

The normal half-life of metronidazole is approximately eight hours. In patients with impaired hepatic function, the plasma clearance of metronidazole is decreased, and dosage adjustment is likely to be necessary. Although the half-life of parent metronidazole is not increased in patients with renal failure (in the absence of hepatic disease), dosage adjustment may be considered in some patients with renal insufficiency because of the retention of biologically active metabolites (eg, 1-[2-hydroxyethyl]-2-hydroxymethyl-5-nitroimidazole). However, it is not known whether the metabolites are neurotoxic, because most instances of severe neurotoxicity have occurred in association with excessive doses of drug or hepatic dysfunction. Metronidazole and its metabolites are rapidly removed from serum by hemodialysis.

DOSAGE AND PREPARATIONS. The intravenous route is recommended initially in the treatment of most serious anaerobic bacterial infections. Oral therapy may be substituted when conditions warrant.

Intravenous: Metronidazole hydrochloride [Flagyl I.V.] or metronidazole intravenous solution [Flagyl I.V. RTU, Metro I.V.] must be administered slowly, either as a continuous or intermittent infusion. Metronidazole hydrochloride cannot be administered by direct intravenous injection (intravenous bolus) because of its low pH (0.5 to 2.0) after reconstitution. The reconstituted drug should be diluted further with intravenous fluid to a concentration not exceeding 8 mg/ml, neutralized to pH 6.0 to 7.0 with sodium bicarbonate, and administered by intravenous infusion. Metronidazole intravenous solution [Flagyl I.V. RTU, Metro I.V.] is a ready-to-use isotonic solution that does not require dilution or buffering before infusion.

Adults, for anaerobic infections, a loading dose of 15 mg/kg is infused over one hour, followed by maintenance doses of 7.5 mg/kg infused over a one-hour period every six to eight hours (maximum, 4 g/24-hour period). Accumulation may occur if treatment is prolonged, and the dosage may have to be reduced, particularly in patients with hepatic insufficiency. The usual duration of therapy is 7 to 21 days but may be longer for some infections (eg, joints, bone, endocardium).

METRONIDAZOLE:
Flagyl I.V. RTU (Schiapparelli Searle), ***Metro I.V.*** (McGaw), ***Generic.*** Solution (sterile) 5 mg/ml in 100 ml containers.
METRONIDAZOLE HYDROCHLORIDE:
Flagyl I.V. (Schiapparelli Searle). Powder (sterile, lyophilized) equivalent to 500 mg of base.

Oral: *Adults,* for anaerobic infections, 7.5 mg/kg every six hours.

For bacterial vaginosis, *adults,* a single 2-g dose or 500 mg twice daily for seven days.

For pseudomembranous colitis caused by *C. difficile, adults,* 500 mg three times daily for 7 to 15 days; alternative dosage, 250 mg four times daily for 10 days.

METRONIDAZOLE:
Generic, Flagyl (Searle), ***Protostat*** (Ortho). Tablets 250 and 500 mg.
Metric 21 (Fielding). Tablets 250 mg.

SPECTINOMYCIN HYDROCHLORIDE
[Trobicin]

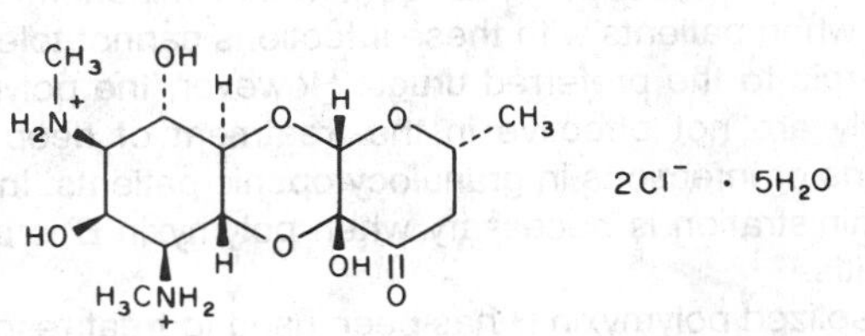

$2Cl^- \cdot 5H_2O$

Spectinomycin is an aminocyclitol antibiotic produced by a strain of *Streptomyces spectabilis.* It differs structurally and biologically from the aminoglycosides.

MECHANISM OF ACTION AND ANTIMICROBIAL SPECTRUM. Spectinomycin interacts with the bacterial 30S ribosomal subunit to inhibit protein synthesis, but the mechanism is unknown. It does not cause misreading of polyribonucleotides as do the aminoglycosides. It is usually bacteriostatic but appears to be bactericidal for some pathogens, including *Neisseria gonorrhoeae.*

Spectinomycin is active against most strains of *N. gonorrhoeae*, including penicillinase-producing strains (PPNG), chromosomal-mediated resistant *N. gonorrhoeae* (CMRNG), and high-level tetracycline-resistant *N. gonorrhoeae* (TRNG). Although a number of other gram-positive and gram-negative bacteria are susceptible, the presence of naturally resistant strains and the rapid emergence of acquired resistance to this antibiotic have limited its usefulness in treating gonococcal infections. *Chlamydia trachomatis* and *Treponema pallidum*, other common pathogens of sexually transmitted diseases, are resistant to spectinomycin. Some strains of *Ureaplasma urealyticum* are susceptible.

RESISTANCE. Spectinomycin-resistant strains of gonococci can be selected in vitro. Resistance can be relative or absolute, and both plasmid-mediated enzyme inactivation and chromosomal mutations that alter the 30S ribosome have been observed.

Spectinomycin-resistant clinical isolates have been reported, including a few strains that also produced penicillinase (Ashford et al, 1981; *MMWR*, 1983; Pon et al, 1986). The occurrence of spectinomycin-resistant *N. gonorrhoeae* usually has been uncommon and sporadic. However, a high prevalence of such strains with associated treatment failures (8.2%) was observed in U.S. military personnel stationed in the Republic of Korea, an area where spectinomycin had become the primary treatment for gonococcal infections (Boslego et al, 1987). Thus far, clinically resistant strains, including those from the Republic of Korea, appear to be the result of chromosomal mutations.

USES. Spectinomycin is used primarily to treat uncomplicated anogenital gonorrhea (urethritis and proctitis in men, cervicitis and proctitis in women) caused by susceptible strains of *N. gonorrhoeae*. Because this agent is effective against PPNG, CMRNG, and TRNG strains, the Centers for Disease Control and Prevention recommends spectinomycin, intramuscularly, as primary alternative therapy to ceftriaxone, the current drug of choice, for patients who cannot tolerate this cephalosporin (eg, due to hypersensitivity) (*MMWR*, 1989; see also index entry Gonococcal Infections).

Spectinomycin should not be used to treat pharyngeal gonococcal infections, since it does not eradicate the infection in more than 50% of patients. If the ceftriaxone regimen cannot be used, ciprofloxacin is the preferred alternative. Spectinomycin is not effective in syphilis or nongonococcal urethritis caused by *C. trachomatis.* Because of the high frequency of coexisting chlamydial and gonococcal infections, the CDC recommends that spectinomycin be followed by a seven-day course of doxycycline or tetracycline (alternative, erythromycin) to treat coexisting chlamydial infection (*MMWR,* 1989).

In the CDC guidelines for disseminated gonococcal infections, intramuscular spectinomycin is recommended as an alternative to ceftriaxone for patients who are allergic to cephalosporins (*MMWR,* 1989).

ADVERSE REACTIONS AND PRECAUTIONS. Adverse effects occur infrequently and include pain at the site of injection, nausea, vomiting, abdominal cramps, chills, fever, dizziness, insomnia, pruritus, urticaria, and oliguria. A few cases of systemic anaphylaxis or anaphylactoid reactions have been reported (Bender et al, 1983). Unlike the aminoglycosides, spectinomycin does not appear to cause cochlear or vestibular toxicity. In single- and multiple-dose studies in normal volunteers, a reduction in urine output was noted. However, in extensive renal function studies, no consistent changes indicative of renal toxicity were demonstrated.

Results of laboratory tests may be abnormal following multiple doses; decreased hemoglobin, hematocrit, and creatinine clearance and elevated alkaline phosphatase, blood urea nitrogen (BUN), and serum glutamic pyruvic transaminase (ALT) levels have been reported.

Although the safety of spectinomycin during pregnancy has not been established, this drug does not appear to be teratogenic. Therefore, it is recommended by the CDC (*MMWR,* 1989) for use in pregnant women who are allergic to other antigonococcal drugs (eg, ceftriaxone) or who do not respond to other treatment. Spectinomycin has been used successfully to treat gonorrhea in prepubertal children. The safety of spectinomycin in infants and children has not been established. However, the diluent provided by the manufacturer of Trobicin contains benzyl alcohol, which has been associated with a fatal gasping syndrome in infants.

Because spectinomycin does not eliminate incubating syphilis, serologic tests for syphilis should be performed at the time of treatment with spectinomycin and again in two to three months.

PHARMACOKINETICS. Spectinomycin is rapidly and completely absorbed following intramuscular injection. Mean peak serum concentrations of 100 mcg/ml are achieved one hour after administration of a single 2-g dose; at eight hours, mean serum concentrations are 15 mcg/ml. A single 4-g dose produces peak serum concentrations averaging 160 mcg/ml at two hours; at eight hours, mean serum concentrations are 31 mcg/ml. The drug is weakly bound to plasma proteins. It is concentrated in the urine where levels of 1,000 to 2,000 mcg/ml can be attained. Penetration into saliva is poor, which accounts for its poor efficacy in pharyngeal gonorrhea. The elimination half-life in individuals with normal renal function is approximately two hours (range, 1.2 to 2.8 hours); it is increased in patients with renal impairment. Approximately 80% of the dose is excreted in the urine as unchanged drug and in a biologically active form.

DOSAGE AND PREPARATIONS.

Intramuscular: For uncomplicated gonorrhea, *adults,* 2 g as a single dose; this dose also is indicated for retreatment after other antibiotic therapy has failed. For patients living in areas where antibiotic resistance is known to be prevalent, 4 g is preferred and should be divided between two gluteal sites. The safety of spectinomycin in *infants and children* has not been established; 40 mg/kg, administered as a single dose, has been used in *children weighing less than 45 kg* (*MMWR,* 1989).

For disseminated gonococcal infection, *adults,* 2 g twice a day for seven days (three days may be adequate) (see index entry Gonococcal Infections).

Trobicin (Upjohn). Powder (sterile, for solution) 2 and 4 g with 3.2 and 6.2 ml of diluent, respectively (contains 400 mg/ml when reconstituted).

POLYMYXINS

The polymyxins are a group of related polypeptides elaborated by strains of *Bacillus polymyxa.* Only polymyxin B [Aerosporin] and E (colistin [Coly-Mycin S]) have a sufficient margin of safety to be useful therapeutically. Colistimethate sodium [Coly-Mycin M], a sulfomethyl derivative of colistin, is the parenteral form of polymyxin E.

MECHANISM OF ACTION AND ANTIMICROBIAL SPECTRUM. The polymyxins are cationic surface-active compounds at physiologic pH. They exert their bactericidal effect by interacting with phospholipid components in the cytoplasmic membranes of susceptible bacteria and, therefore, disrupt the osmotic integrity of the cell membrane. However, their biochemical mechanism is unclear.

Polymyxins are almost exclusively active against aerobic gram-negative bacilli. In particular, they exhibit excellent activity against *Pseudomonas aeruginosa*. Other organisms that are usually susceptible include *Escherichia coli*, *Klebsiella pneumoniae*, *Enterobacter*, *Salmonella*, *Shigella*, *Haemophilus*, *Bordetella*, *Pasteurella*, and *Vibrio*. *Proteus*, *Providencia*, *Neisseria*, and *Serratia marcescens* are resistant. Polymyxins are not active against gram-positive bacteria, most obligate anaerobes, or fungi (for review, see Hoeprich, 1970).

RESISTANCE. Acquired bacterial resistance develops rarely, and the overall efficacy of the polymyxins has remained fairly constant. Resistant bacteria usually have cell walls that prevent access of the drug to the cytoplasmic membrane. Complete cross-resistance occurs between polymyxin B and colistin, but not with other classes of antibiotics.

USES. Indications for parenteral polymyxin B or colistimethate sodium are extremely limited; they are not drugs of choice for any infection. Their primary use is in serious, life-threatening infections (eg, bacteremia) caused by strains of *P. aeruginosa* (or other aerobic gram-negative bacilli) that are resistant to other drugs (eg, aminoglycosides, antipseudomonal β-lactams, including aztreonam and imipenem/cilastatin), or when patients with these infections cannot tolerate or are allergic to the preferred drugs. However, the polymyxins generally are not effective in the treatment of deep tissue infections or infections in granulocytopenic patients. Intrathecal administration is necessary when polymyxin B is used in meningitis.

Aerosolized polymyxin B has been used to treat respiratory infections due to *Pseudomonas* in patients with cystic fibrosis or bronchiectasis and to prevent *Pseudomonas* infections in respiratory intensive care units. Its effectiveness is limited, however, because pneumonias due to resistant organisms frequently develop.

Polymyxin B, in combination with neomycin, has been used as a bladder irrigant to prevent urinary tract infections in patients with indwelling catheters.

Oral colistin sulfate has been used in infants and children to treat diarrhea caused by enteropathogenic *E. coli.*

Polymyxin B is most commonly used topically for infections of the eye, ear, and skin, frequently as a component of an antibiotic mixture (see index entry Polymyxin B, As Antibacterial Agent). Colistin sulfate also has been used topically for certain infections of the ear.

ADVERSE REACTIONS AND PRECAUTIONS. Parenteral polymyxins can cause serious nephrotoxicity and neurotoxicity, which have significantly limited the usefulness of these antibiotics for systemic use.

Dose-dependent nephrotoxicity is a common and serious adverse effect. This is usually manifested by elevated blood urea nitrogen (BUN) and serum creatinine concentrations. Mild nephrotoxicity is usually reversible after the drug is discontinued, but some patients develop renal failure and acute tubular necrosis. This is more likely to occur with large doses or prolonged therapy and appears to be due to cumulative binding of polymyxins to renal tubular epithelium. Patients with pre-existing renal disease or receiving other nephrotoxic drugs (eg, aminoglycosides) are at increased risk. Renal function should be monitored frequently when polymyxins are given. Polymyxins should be administered cautiously to patients with impaired renal function and dosage adjustments are necessary.

Neurotoxicity also is a common and serious adverse effect of the polymyxins. Transient neurologic disturbances, including dizziness, vertigo, ataxia, slurred speech, blurred vision, drowsiness, confusion, circumoral paresthesias, and numbness of the extremities, have been observed following parenteral administration. These adverse reactions are dose related and disappear soon after the drugs have been discontinued. However, larger doses can cause neuromuscular blockade and respiratory arrest. Neuromuscular blockade is not reversed by neostigmine but may respond to calcium gluconate. Neurotoxicity is most likely to occur in patients with impaired renal function or pre-existing neuromuscular disease (eg, myasthenia gravis). See also Drug Interactions.

Respiratory arrest has been reported following administration of polymyxins as irrigants into serous cavities (eg, peritoneum) or as aerosols.

Allergic reactions are rare, but urticaria and shock due to histamine release have occurred with too rapid intravenous infusion.

Polymyxin B causes pain at the site of intramuscular injection and this route of administration is not recommended. When intramuscular injection of polymyxin B is necessary, the inclusion of a local anesthetic may decrease the pain.

DRUG INTERACTIONS. The concomitant use of polymyxins with other nephrotoxic drugs (eg, aminoglycosides) should be avoided, if possible, because nephrotoxicity may be additive.

Drugs that may impair neuromuscular transmission also should not be given with polymyxins, if possible, because respiratory arrest may occur. Such drugs include the neuromuscular blocking agents (eg, tubocurarine), aminoglycosides, anesthetics with prominent muscle relaxant properties (eg, enflurane), and parenteral quinidine, quinine, or magnesium.

PHARMACOKINETICS. Polymyxins are not absorbed from the gastrointestinal tract following oral administration except in neonates. Polymyxin B is usually given intravenously, but intrathecal administration is required to treat meningitis. Intravenous infusion of polymyxin B (2.5 mg/kg) yields peak serum concentrations of about 5 mcg/ml. The intramuscular route is not recommended.

Colistimethate sodium can be administered intravenously or intramuscularly, and it is preferred to polymyxin B when intramuscular administration is desired. Following intramuscular injection of 150 mg, peak serum levels of 5 to 6 mcg/ml are achieved after about two hours. Colistimethate sodium is partially metabolized in the body to the more active colistin.

Colistin sulfate is used orally for a local antibacterial effect.

Polymyxins do not pass readily into cerebrospinal fluid or other body compartments (eg, pleural, synovial, brain tissue), but they cross the placenta. High concentrations are achieved in urine. Plasma protein binding may be as high as 75%. Effectiveness is reduced in the presence of pus or other organic material.

Polymyxins are excreted renally, primarily by glomerular filtration. In patients with normal renal function, the plasma half-lives of polymyxin B and colistimethate sodium are 6 to 7 hours and 2 to 4.5 hours, respectively.

DOSAGE AND PREPARATIONS.

POLYMYXIN B SULFATE:

Intravenous: *Adults and children with normal renal function,* 1.5 to 2.5 mg (15,000 to 25,000 units)/kg daily. The total daily dose generally should not exceed 2.5 mg (25,000 units)/kg, although *infants* usually tolerate up to 4 mg (40,000 units)/kg daily if needed. Dextrose injection 5% may be used as a vehicle, and one-half of the daily dose should be given by continuous intravenous drip every 12 hours. To avoid widespread neuromuscular blockade, this drug should not be injected rapidly as a single bolus.

Intramuscular: This route is not recommended because marked pain occurs at the site of injection.

Intrathecal: For *P. aeruginosa* meningitis, *adults and children over 2 years with normal renal function,* 5 mg (50,000 units) once daily for three to four days, followed by 5 mg (50,000 units) once every other day; *children under 2 years with normal renal function,* 2 mg (20,000 units) once daily for three to four days, or 2.5 mg (25,000 units) once every other day. These amounts are given for at least two weeks after cultures of the cerebrospinal fluid become negative and the sugar content has returned to normal.

In *patients with impaired renal function,* the parenteral dosage of polymyxin B should be reduced in proportion to the degree of renal impairment as determined by measurement of creatinine clearance or blood creatinine levels. The following guidelines may be used (Hoeprich, 1970; Fekety, 1990 B):

Creatinine Clearance (Ccr)	Daily Dosage
Normal or ≥80% of normal	2.5-3 mg/kg
80% to ≥30% of normal	First day: 2.5 mg/kg Daily thereafter: 1-1.5 mg/kg
< 30% of normal	First day: 2.5 mg/kg Every 2-3 days thereafter: 1-1.5 mg/kg
Anuric	First day: 2.5 mg/kg Every 5-7 days thereafter: 1 mg/kg

Aerosporin (Burroughs Wellcome), ***Generic***. Powder (sterile) 500,000 units equivalent to 50 mg of polymyxin B sulfate.

COLISTIMETHATE SODIUM:

Intramuscular, Intravenous: The intravenous dose should be administered slowly by intravenous drip. *Adults and children with normal renal function,* 2.5 to 5 mg/kg daily in divided doses every 8 or 12 hours (maximum, 300 mg daily). *Adults with impaired renal function,* following an initial dose of 2.5 to 5 mg/kg, the dosage should be modified according to the following schedule (see the manufacturer's literature for further information):

	RENAL IMPAIRMENT		
	Mild	Moderate	Marked
Serum Creatinine (mg/dL)	1.3-1.5	1.6-2.5	2.6-4
Daily Dose (mg/kg)	2.5-3.8	2.5	1.5
Dosage Interval (hours)	12	12-24	36

Coly-Mycin M (Parke-Davis). Powder (sterile, lyophilized) equivalent to 150 mg base.

COLISTIN SULFATE:

Oral: *Infants and children,* 5 to 15 mg/kg daily in three divided doses.

Coly-Mycin S (Parke-Davis). Powder for oral suspension equivalent to 300 mg of base, providing the equivalent of 25 mg of base/5 ml when suspended in 37 ml of distilled water.

BACITRACIN

Bacitracin is a mixture of polypeptide antibiotics produced by a strain of *Bacillus subtilis* (Tracey).

MECHANISM OF ACTION AND ANTIMICROBIAL SPECTRUM. Bacitracin inhibits the formation of the linear peptidoglycan chains that are major components of the bacterial cell wall. It is bactericidal.

Most gram-positive bacteria, including staphylococci, streptococci, and *Clostridium difficile*, are susceptible to bacitracin. Although this agent is active against *Neisseria* and *Haemophilus influenzae*, most gram-negative bacteria are resistant.

RESISTANCE. Acquired bacterial resistance to bacitracin is rare.

USES. Indications for systemic (intramuscular) bacitracin are extremely limited due to its nephrotoxicity and the availability of more effective drugs. It may be used as a drug of last resort in infants with serious staphylococcal pneumonia with empyema that is resistant to all other antibiotics.

Bacitracin is only negligibly absorbed from the gastrointestinal tract and has been used orally to resolve the symptoms of pseudomembranous colitis caused by *C. difficile*. See also index entry on this disorder.

Bacitracin is most commonly used topically for infections of the eye and skin caused by susceptible gram-positive bacteria (eg, staphylococci, streptococci). It frequently is combined with other antibiotics (eg, neomycin, polymyxin B) to increase the antibacterial spectrum. For additional discussion, see index entry Bacitracin.

ADVERSE REACTIONS AND PRECAUTIONS. *Bacitracin is highly nephrotoxic and systemic administration should be avoided, if possible.* Nephrotoxic reactions include albuminuria, cylindruria, and azotemia. Glomerular and tubular necrosis have occurred after systemic use. Renal function should be monitored if bacitracin must be used systemically, and the drug should be discontinued at the first sign of nephrotoxicity.

Other adverse reactions include nausea, vomiting, and skin rash; allergic contact dermatitis and postirrigation anaphylaxis have been reported.

Intramuscular injection of bacitracin is quite painful.

PHARMACOKINETICS. Bacitracin is not absorbed from the gastrointestinal tract following oral administration. If systemic administration is necessary, the drug is injected intramuscularly. Absorption is rapid and complete after intramuscular injection; peak blood concentrations are reached in one to two hours.

Distribution is relatively widespread after parenteral administration. However, only traces are found in the cerebrospinal fluid unless the meninges are inflamed.

Bactericidal plasma concentrations may be present for four to six hours after a single intramuscular dose. The drug is eliminated slowly by glomerular filtration; the quantity recovered in the urine varies from 10% to 40% in the first 24 hours.

DOSAGE AND PREPARATIONS. Injections should be given in the upper outer quadrant of the buttocks, alternating right and left and avoiding multiple injections in the same region.

Intramuscular: When parenteral administration is essential, the following amounts may be given: *Infants weighing less than 2.5 kg,* 900 units/kg daily in two or three divided doses. *Infants over 2.5 kg,* 1,000 units/kg daily in two or three divided doses.

Generic. Powder (for injection) 50,000 and 5,000,000 units.

URINARY TRACT ANTIMICROBIAL AGENTS

Methenamine and nitrofurantoin are used only to treat or prevent urinary tract infections. These agents are active against common urinary tract pathogens and, because they are concentrated only in the urine, have been classified as urinary tract antimicrobial agents.

METHENAMINE

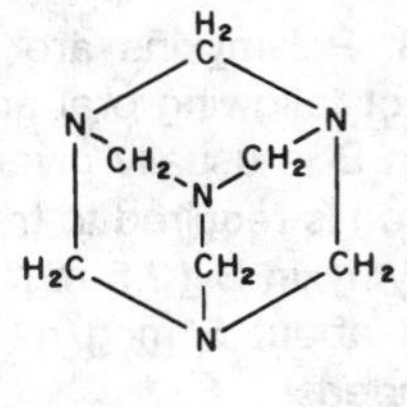

METHENAMINE HIPPURATE
[Hiprex, Urex]

METHENAMINE MANDELATE
[Mandelamine]

MECHANISM OF ACTION AND ANTIMICROBIAL SPECTRUM. Methenamine itself does not exert an antibacterial effect. In an acid medium (pH $\leq$5.5), this tertiary amine is hydrolyzed to ammonia and formaldehyde, the active degradation product. Formaldehyde kills bacteria by denaturing proteins. For additional discussion, see Mayrer and Andriole, 1982; Andriole, 1990.

Virtually all bacteria and fungi are susceptible to formaldehyde (at approximately 20 mcg/ml). However, certain urease-positive bacteria (eg, *Proteus*) can convert urea to ammonium hydroxide, which can prevent the conversion of methenamine to formaldehyde.

RESISTANCE. Resistance to formaldehyde does not develop; thus, methenamine-resistant organisms are unknown.

USES. Methenamine is used for prophylaxis of recurrent urinary tract infections, but other drugs (eg, trimethoprim/sulfamethoxazole, trimethoprim alone, nitrofurantoin) generally are preferred. However, when residual urine is present (eg, prostatism, neurogenic bladder), methenamine is an excellent drug for long-term prophylaxis because there is sufficient time to generate formaldehyde in bladder urine and no formaldehyde-resistant organisms are known.

Methenamine is not recommended for treatment of acute urinary tract infections.

For additional discussion on the treatment and prophylaxis of urinary tract infections, see index entry on this subject.

ADVERSE REACTIONS AND PRECAUTIONS. Methenamine and its salts are relatively safe and usually well tolerated. Gastrointestinal irritation and nausea have occurred, presumably caused by the generation of formaldehyde, an irritant, in the acid milieu of the stomach; the use of enteric-coated tablets may decrease these effects. Similarly, bladder irritation, characterized by dysuria, frequency, and hematuria, has been reported. Large doses can cause acute inflammation of the urinary tract, which necessitates discontinuation of therapy and administration of an alkalizing salt (eg, sodium bicarbonate). Skin rashes have occurred.

Because ammonia is generated during methenamine hydrolysis, this drug should not be administered to patients with hepatic insufficiency.

Methenamine base is not contraindicated in the presence of renal insufficiency, and azotemic patients readily convert urinary methenamine to formaldehyde. However, the salts of methenamine (eg, hippurate, mandelate preparations) are contraindicated in dehydrated patients and in those with severe renal disease. When the urinary output is decreased severely, methenamine salts may precipitate and cause crystalluria. Methenamine salts also should be avoided in patients with gout, since urate crystals may be precipitated in the urine.

The pH of the urine should be monitored to assure that an acidic medium is present for the hydrolysis of methenamine to formaldehyde. Patients should be instructed to avoid ingesting substances that could increase urinary pH (eg, citrus fruits, milk and milk products, antacids containing sodium carbonate or bicarbonate). Likewise, the ingestion of copious amounts of fluid may be counterproductive because the increased diuresis may increase urinary pH and dilute urinary formaldehyde concentrations to subinhibitory levels. Protein-rich diets with liberal amounts of cranberries, plums, prunes, and, possibly, the ingestion of acidifying agents (eg, ascorbic acid, ammonium chloride) are often recommended to maintain an acid urine. However, the value of these acidifying agents in the usual amounts ingested is questionable. The contributions of mandelic acid and hippuric acid to the antibacterial effect of methenamine, when administered in the commercially available acid salt forms, are probably negligible.

Methenamine is classified in FDA Pregnancy Category C.

For additional discussion, see Mayrer and Andriole, 1982; Andriole, 1990.

DRUG INTERACTIONS AND INTERFERENCE WITH LABORATORY TESTS. Drugs that increase urinary pH (eg, acetazolamide, sodium bicarbonate) prevent the hydrolysis of methenamine to formaldehyde. Methenamine should not be given to patients receiving these drugs.

The concomitant administration of sulfamethizole or sulfathiazole with methenamine has resulted in crystalluria. Methenamine should not be used with sulfonamides.

Formaldehyde interferes with (1) fluorometric procedures for determination of urinary catecholamines and vanillylmandelic acid (VMA) yielding falsely elevated values; (2) acid hydrolysis methods for determination of urinary estriol yielding falsely low values; (3) the Porter-Silber method for determination of 17-hydroxycorticosteroids yielding falsely elevated values; and (4) nitrosonaphthol methods for determination of 5-hydroxy indoleacetic acid (5-HIAA) yielding falsely low values.

PHARMACOKINETICS. Methenamine and its salts are absorbed rapidly from the gastrointestinal tract following oral administration. Between 10% and 30% of a dose may be hydrolyzed in the acid of the stomach. Enteric-coated preparations decrease formaldehyde generation in the stomach.

Methenamine is distributed throughout total body water, including red blood cells; cerebrospinal, synovial, and pericardial fluids; and aqueous and vitreous humors. However, the drug has no antibacterial activity in these fluids because formaldehyde is not generated at physiologic pH.

Over 90% of methenamine is excreted in the urine within 24 hours; up to 20% of this is hydrolyzed to free formaldehyde. The transit time through the kidney is too brief for adequate formaldehyde generation; thus, activity is limited to the bladder. At pH 5.0 to 5.5, about two hours are required to generate bactericidal levels of formaldehyde, which can be maintained for up to six hours or until the patient voids. The intake of copious amounts of fluids with methenamine may increase diuresis and urine pH and dilute the formaldehyde concentration to subinhibitory levels (see Mayrer and Andriole, 1982).

DOSAGE AND PREPARATIONS.

METHENAMINE, METHENAMINE MANDELATE:

Oral: *Adults,* 1 g four times daily after each meal and at bedtime. Pediatric dosages recommended by the manufacturers of methenamine mandelate are: *children 6 to 12 years,* 500 mg four times daily; *children under 6 years,* 18.3 mg/kg four times daily. Alternatively, *children,* 50 to 75 mg/kg daily in divided doses every six hours (The Medical Letter, 1992).

METHENAMINE:

Generic. Granules 500 and 2,500 g.

METHENAMINE MANDELATE:

Generic. Suspension (Forte) 500 mg/5 ml; tablets (plain, enteric coated) 500 mg and 1 g.

Mandelamine (Parke-Davis). Suspension 250 mg/5 ml; tablets (plain) 500 mg and 1 g.

METHENAMINE HIPPURATE:

Oral: *Adults and children over 12 years,* 1 g twice daily. *Children 6 to 12 years,* 500 mg to 1 g twice daily (manufacturers' recommendation) or, alternatively, 25 to 50 mg/kg daily in divided doses every 12 hours (The Medical Letter, 1992).

Hiprex (Marion Merrell Dow), ***Urex*** (3M Pharmaceuticals). Tablets 1 g. (NOTE: Hiprex tablets contain tartrazine.)

NITROFURANTOIN

[Furadantin (microcrystalline), Macrodantin (macrocrystalline)]

MECHANISM OF ACTION AND ANTIMICROBIAL SPECTRUM. The mechanism of action of this synthetic nitrofuran compound is unclear. There is evidence that nitrofurantoin inhibits a variety of enzyme systems in bacteria, including those of the tricarboxylic acid cycle. It also has been suggested that reduction of nitrofurantoin in bacterial cells produces short-lived, highly reactive intermediates that can cause DNA damage and cell death (see Pratt and Fekety, 1986 B).

Nitrofurantoin is active against common urinary tract pathogens. Bacteria with a minimum inhibitory concentration (MIC) of $\leq$32 mcg/ml are considered susceptible.

Most strains of *Escherichia coli* are susceptible. About two-thirds of the strains of other coliforms, but only one-third of *Klebsiella-Enterobacter* strains, are susceptible. Most *Proteus* and *Serratia* species are moderately to completely resistant. *Pseudomonas aeruginosa* and other *Pseudomonas* species are resistant.

Staphylococcus aureus, S. saprophyticus, and *Enterococcus faecalis* (enterococci) also are susceptible to nitrofurantoin.

Although in vitro susceptibility of *Salmonella*, *Shigella*, *Neisseria*, *Streptococcus pyogenes*, *S. pneumoniae*, *Corynebacterium*, and many anaerobes has been demonstrated, nitrofurantoin is of little importance clinically for infections caused by these organisms.

For additional discussion, see Mayrer and Andriole, 1982; Andriole, 1990.

RESISTANCE. Susceptible bacteria do not readily develop resistance to nitrofurantoin during therapy. However, plasmid-mediated, transferable resistance has been demonstrated (Breeze and Obaseiki-Ebor, 1983).

USES. Nitrofurantoin is one of a number of alternative antibacterial agents (eg, trimethoprim/sulfamethoxazole, sulfisoxazole, ampicillin, amoxicillin, fluoroquinolones) recommended for the treatment of uncomplicated lower urinary tract infections (eg, cystitis) caused by susceptible bacteria.

Nitrofurantoin also is one of the recommended drugs (trimethoprim/sulfamethoxazole and trimethoprim alone are others) for the prophylaxis of recurrent lower urinary tract infections. An advantage of this drug is that resistant bacterial strains rarely emerge during long-term use. However, serious adverse reactions rarely have been associated with prolonged administration of nitrofurantoin (see below).

Although nitrofurantoin may be active in upper urinary tract infections, other agents usually are preferred. Nitrofurantoin is not useful for infections outside the urinary tract.

For additional discussion on the treatment and prophylaxis of urinary tract infections, see index entry on this subject.

ADVERSE REACTIONS AND PRECAUTIONS. The overall incidence of adverse effects is relatively high (10% or more). Gastrointestinal irritation is most common. Symptoms include anorexia, nausea, and vomiting; diarrhea and abdominal pain occur less frequently. Gastrointestinal intolerance is less frequent with the macrocrystalline preparation. Administration of the drug with food or milk may control these side effects. Superinfection is rare.

Acute, subacute, and chronic pulmonary reactions have occurred. Acute pneumonitis was reported frequently in one Swedish study (Holmberg et al, 1980), but the incidence of this adverse reaction in other countries appears to be quite low (see D'Arcy, 1985). Acute pneumonitis is manifested by sudden onset of fever, chills, cough, chest pain, dyspnea, pulmonary infiltration with consolidation or pleural effusion on x-ray, and eosinophilia. The elderly are more likely to be affected. The acute reaction usually occurs during the first week of therapy, is reversible on discontinuation of treatment, and may respond to a corticosteroid. It is believed to be a hypersensitivity reaction because it quickly recurs with drug rechallenge. Symptoms of subacute pneumonitis are more insidious; fever and eosinophilia are less common, and symptoms resolve more slowly.

Chronic pulmonary reactions are rare and usually occur in patients receiving prolonged therapy (eg, more than six months). Common findings are malaise, dyspnea on exertion, cough, and altered pulmonary function. Diffuse interstitial pneumonitis and/or fibrosis are common. The severity and reversibility of the chronic pulmonary reaction usually correlate with the duration of therapy after symptoms first appear. Permanent impairment of pulmonary function may occur, and fatalities have been reported. It is unclear whether this chronic reaction also is allergic in origin or is a toxic effect that is due to the production of active species of oxygen (eg, superoxide anion), which damage tissue (Martin, 1983; see also Pratt and Fekety, 1986 B; Andriole, 1990).

If any of these pulmonary reactions occur, nitrofurantoin should be discontinued and appropriate treatment should be instituted. Patients on long-term therapy should be monitored.

Other types of hypersensitivity reactions occur less frequently but may be severe. Rash and urticaria are most common, but chills and fever are sometimes seen. Hepatotoxicity, manifested as hepatitis (including chronic active hepatitis) and cholestatic jaundice, develops rarely. Chronic active hepatitis primarily occurs in women receiving prolonged therapy; fatalities have been reported (Black et al, 1980; Sharp et al,

1980; Tolman, 1980; Young et al, 1985). Arthralgia, angioedema, a lupus erythematosus-like syndrome, and anaphylaxis also have been reported.

Headache, drowsiness, dizziness, nystagmus that is readily reversible, and peripheral polyneuropathy have been reported. The peripheral neuritis, an ascending sensorimotor neuropathy, may be progressive and is one of the most serious adverse effects of nitrofurantoin. It is more common in patients with renal failure or in elderly patients receiving prolonged therapy (see Andriole, 1990). Anemia, diabetes, electrolyte imbalance, vitamin B deficiency, and debilitating disease are other predisposing conditions for this adverse reaction.

Leukopenia, granulocytopenia, eosinophilia, and megaloblastic anemia have been reported. Acute hemolytic anemia may occur in individuals with glucose-6-phosphate dehydrogenase (G6PD) deficiency (eg, 10% of blacks have this defect). A similar reaction may occur in infants with premature red cell enzyme systems (glutathione instability). Therefore, nitrofurantoin should not be administered to patients with G6PD deficiency, to infants less than 1 month of age, or to pregnant women at term because of the possibility of hemolytic anemia.

Large doses of nitrofurantoin depress spermatogenesis through a direct action on seminiferous tubules. Usual therapeutic doses do not appear to have this effect.

Nitrofurantoin may cause brown discoloration of urine.

DRUG INTERACTIONS. A fall in serum phenytoin concentration with recurrence of seizures was observed in a single patient following nitrofurantoin administration (Heipertz and Pilz, 1978); however, this finding has not been confirmed. Magnesium trisilicate, a component of some antacids, has been shown to adsorb nitrofurantoin and may decrease its gastrointestinal absorption, but the clinical significance is unknown. In vitro, nitrofurantoin antagonized the antimicrobial action of nalidixic and oxolinic acids; these urinary tract antimicrobial agents probably should not be given concomitantly. For additional discussion of drug interactions, see D'Arcy, 1985.

PHARMACOKINETICS. Nitrofurantoin is administered orally, and it is rapidly and completely absorbed from the gastrointestinal tract. Both a microcrystalline and a macrocrystalline form are available. The larger macrocrystals dissolve more slowly in the small intestine, and this form is more slowly absorbed than the microcrystalline formulation. This appears to result in a lower incidence of gastrointestinal intolerance, although the therapeutic efficacies of the two formulations are the same.

The presence of food in the intestine decreases the rate of absorption but appears to increase bioavailability. The duration of therapeutic urinary concentrations is prolonged by about two hours when the drug is administered with food.

Serum concentrations of nitrofurantoin are low (<2 mcg/ml) when usual doses are given, and the drug does not accumulate in the serum of patients with normal renal function. Therapeutic concentrations are not achieved in most body tissues. Although nitrofurantoin crosses the blood-brain barrier and the placenta, it does so to a very small extent. About 60% of a dose is reversibly bound to plasma proteins.

The serum half-life is approximately 20 minutes in patients with normal renal function. About two-thirds of a dose is rapidly metabolized in all body tissues, especially the liver. The remaining one-third is rapidly excreted into the urine by glomerular filtration and tubular secretion in a therapeutically active, unchanged form; an average dose of nitrofurantoin yields a urine concentration of approximately 200 (range, 50 to 250) mcg/ml in patients with normal renal function. In acid urine, nitrofurantoin, a weak acid, is partially reabsorbed in the unionized form, resulting in lower urinary concentrations. However, the urine should not be alkalized to increase drug levels because antibacterial activity is significantly diminished at the higher pH (see Andriole, 1990).

Recovery of nitrofurantoin from urine is linearly related to creatinine clearance. If creatinine clearance is less than 40 ml/min, urinary concentrations of nitrofurantoin are inadequate and blood levels of the drug are elevated, which increases the danger of toxicity. Therefore, nitrofurantoin should not be administered to patients with significantly diminished renal function.

For additional discussion, see Mayrer and Andriole, 1982; Andriole, 1990.

DOSAGE AND PREPARATIONS.

Oral: The manufacturers recommend administration of nitrofurantoin with food to enhance drug absorption and improve gastrointestinal tolerance. *Adults,* 50 to 100 mg three or four times daily. Most uncomplicated urinary tract infections caused by susceptible bacteria in patients with normal renal function are adequately treated with 50 mg three times daily. *Children,* 5 to 7 mg/kg every 24 hours in four divided doses.

For prophylaxis of frequently recurring urinary tract infections in *adults*, 50 to 100 mg at bedtime may be adequate; in *children*, doses as low as 1 mg/kg daily, given in a single or in two divided doses, may be adequate.

NITROFURANTOIN:

Generic (microcrystalline). Capsules, tablets 50 and 100 mg.

Furadantin (microcrystalline) (Procter & Gamble). Suspension 25 mg/5 ml; tablets 50 and 100 mg.

Macrodantin (macrocrystalline) (Procter & Gamble). Capsules 25, 50, and 100 mg.

PHENAZOPYRIDINE HYDROCHLORIDE

[Pyridium]

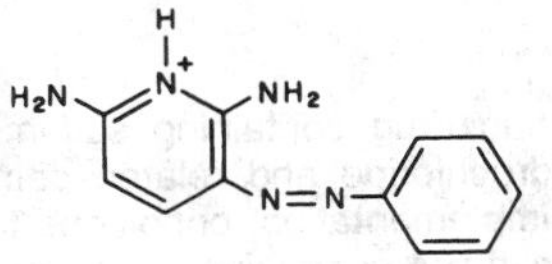

ACTIONS AND USES. Phenazopyridine is *not* a urinary tract antiseptic. However, it is excreted in the urine where it has an analgesic effect on the urinary tract mucosa. Thus, it is used to relieve pain, burning, urgency, and frequency of urination associated with irritation of the lower urinary tract. These symptoms can result from infection (eg, cystitis), trauma, surgery, catheterization, and endoscopy. Because this drug provides only symptomatic relief, prompt appropriate treatment of the cause of the pain must be instituted. Phenazopyridine should be discontinued when symptoms are controlled. It should not be continued beyond the first 48 hours in urinary tract infections because no evidence exists that the combined administration of phenazopyridine and an antibacterial agent provides greater benefit than the latter alone after two days (*Federal Register,* 1983).

Many fixed-ratio combinations containing antibacterial agents and phenazopyridine are available, but separate drug administration is preferred.

ADVERSE REACTIONS AND PRECAUTIONS. The principal adverse reactions are gastrointestinal disturbances and headache, which occur occasionally. A yellowish tinge to the skin or sclerae may indicate accumulation due to impaired renal excretion; therapy should be discontinued. A few cases of hemolytic anemia, transient acute renal failure, and hepatic toxicity have been reported, usually at overdose levels. Overdosage or prolonged use in patients with diminished renal function may produce methemoglobinemia. The use of phenazopyridine is contraindicated in patients with renal insufficiency or severe hepatitis. The drug is an azo dye and colors the urine red or orange; clothing is likely to be stained, and the stain is difficult to remove from fabric.

Long-term administration of phenazopyridine has induced neoplasia in rats and mice. Although no association between phenazopyridine and cancer in humans has been reported, adequate epidemiologic studies have not been conducted (*Federal Register*, 1983).

Phenazopyridine is classified in FDA Pregnancy Category B.

INTERFERENCE WITH LABORATORY TESTS. Because of its properties as an azo dye, phenazopyridine may interfere with urinalysis based on spectrometry or color reactions.

PHARMACOKINETICS. Following oral administration, approximately 90% of the dose is eliminated in the urine within 24 hours, about 40% as unchanged drug and 50% as aniline and its metabolites, mainly p-aminophenol and N-acetyl-p-aminophenol (acetaminophen).

DOSAGE AND PREPARATIONS.

Oral: *Adults,* 200 mg three times daily after meals; *children 6 to 12 years,* 100 mg three times daily after meals.

Pyridium (Parke-Davis), ***Generic.*** Tablets 100 and 200 mg.

Cited References

Human drugs; combination drug containing sulfamethoxazole and phenazopyridine hydrochloride and related combination drugs; drug efficacy study implementation; conditions for approval and marketing phenazopyridine-containing drug products; labelling requirement. *Federal Register* 48:34516-34519, 1983.

New preparations of vancomycin. *Med Lett Drugs Ther* 28:121-122, 1986.

Spectinomycin-resistant penicillinase-producing *Neisseria gonorrhoeae. MMWR* 32:51-52, 1983.

1989 Sexually transmitted diseases treatment guidelines. *MMWR* 38(suppl 8):1-43, 1989.

Report of the Committee on Infectious Diseases: *American Academy of Pediatrics Redbook*, ed 22. Elk Grove Village, Ill, American Academy of Pediatrics, 1991, 220-229.

Ahmad R, et al: Vancomycin: Reappraisal. *BMJ* 284:1953-1954, 1982.

Alpert G, et al: Vancomycin dosage in pediatrics reconsidered. *Am J Dis Child* 138:20-22, 1984.

Andriole VT: Urinary tract agents: Nitrofurantoin and methenamine, in Mandell GL, et al (eds): *Principles and Practice of Infectious Diseases,* ed 3. New York, Churchill Livingstone, 1990, 345-349.

Ariza J, et al: A comparative trial of rifampin-doxycycline versus tetracycline-streptomycin in therapy of human brucellosis. *Antimicrob Agents Chemother* 28:548-551, 1985.

Ashford WA, et al: Spectinomycin-resistant penicillinase-producing *Neisseria gonorrhoeae. Lancet* 2:1035-1037, 1981.

Bailie GR, Neal D: Vancomycin ototoxicity and nephrotoxicity: A review. *Med Toxicol* 3:376-386, 1988.

Bartlett JG: Anaerobic bacteria: General concepts, in Mandell GL, et al (eds): *Principles and Practice of Infectious Diseases*, ed 3. New York, Churchill Livingstone, 1990, 1828-1842.

Bender BS, et al: Systemic anaphylaxis caused by parenteral spectinomycin. *South Med J* 76:1456-1457, 1983.

Bibler MA, et al: Clinical evaluation of efficacy, pharmacokinetics, and safety of teicoplanin for serious gram-positive infections. *Antimicrob Agents Chemother* 31:207-212, 1987.

Bisno AL, et al: Antimicrobial treatment of infective endocarditis due to viridans streptococci, enterococci, and staphylococci. *JAMA* 261:1471-1477, 1989.

Black M, et al: Nitrofurantoin-induced chronic active hepatitis. *Ann Intern Med* 92:62-64, 1980.

Blaser MJ: *Helicobacter pylori:* Its role in disease. *Clin Infect Dis* 15:386-393, 1992.

Blevins RD, et al: Pharmacokinetics of vancomycin in patients undergoing continuous ambulatory peritoneal dialysis. *Antimicrob Agents Chemother* 25:603-606, 1984.

Bonati M, et al: Teicoplanin pharmacokinetics in patients with chronic renal failure. *Clin Pharmacokinet* 12:292-301, 1987.

Boslego JW, et al: Effect of spectinomycin use on prevalence of spectinomycin-resistant and of penicillinase-producing *Neisseria gonorrhoeae. N Engl J Med* 317:272-278, 1987.

Breeze AS, Obaseiki-Ebor EE: Transferable nitrofuran resistance conferred by R-plasmids in clinical isolates of *E. coli. J Antimicrob Chemother* 12:459-467, 1983.

Brown N, et al: Effects of hepatic function on vancomycin clinical pharmacology. *Antimicrob Agents Chemother* 23:603-609, 1983.

Brummett RE, Fox KE: Vancomycin- and erythromycin-induced hearing loss in humans. *Antimicrob Agents Chemother* 33:791-796, 1989.

Bunke CM, et al: Vancomycin kinetics during continuous ambulatory peritoneal dialysis. *Clin Pharmacol Ther* 34:631-637, 1983.

Calain P, Waldvogel F: Clinical efficacy of teicoplanin. *Eur J Clin Microbiol Infect Dis* 9:127-129, 1990.

Calain P, et al: Early termination of prospective, randomized trial comparing teicoplanin and flucloxacillin for treating severe staphylococcal infections. *J Infect Dis* 155:187-191, 1987.

Campoli-Richards DM, et al: Teicoplanin: A review of its antibacterial activity, pharmacokinetic properties and therapeutic potential. *Drugs* 40:449-486, 1990.

Carver PL, et al: Pharmacokinetics of single- and multiple-dose teicoplanin in healthy volunteers. *Antimicrob Agents Chemother* 33:82-86, 1989.

Cheung RPF, DiPiro JT: Vancomycin: An update. *Pharmacotherapy* 6:153-169, 1986.

Chomarat M, et al: Coagulase-negative staphylococci emerging during teicoplanin therapy and problems in the determination of their sensitivity. *J Antimicrob Chemother* 27:475-480, 1991.

Cimino MA, et al: Relationship of serum antibiotic concentrations to nephrotoxicity in cancer patients receiving concurrent aminoglycoside and vancomycin therapy. *Am J Med* 83:1091-1097, 1987.

Corey WA, et al: Metronidazole-induced acute pancreatitis. *Rev Infect Dis* 13:1213-1215, 1991.

Courvalin P: Resistance of enterococci to glycopeptides. *Antimicrob Agents Chemother* 34:2291-2296, 1990.

Cutler NR, et al: Vancomycin disposition: The importance of age. *Clin Pharmacol Ther* 36:803-810, 1984.

D'Arcy PF: Nitrofurantoin. *Drug Intell Clin Pharm* 19:540-547, 1985.

Darouiche R, et al: Eradication of colonization by methicillin-resistant *Staphylococcus aureus* by using oral minocycline-rifampin and topical mupirocin. *Antimicrob Agents Chemother* 35:1612-1615, 1991.

Davey PG, Williams AH: Teicoplanin monotherapy of serious infections caused by gram-positive bacteria: A re-evaluation of patients with endocarditis or *Staphylococcus aureus* bacteraemia from a European open trial. *J Antimicrob Chemother* 27 (suppl B):43-50, 1991 A.

Davey PG, Williams AH: A review of the safety profile of teicoplanin. *J Antimicrob Chemother* 27 (suppl B):69-73, 1991 B.

Davis JL, et al: Metronidazole lowers serum lipids. *Ann Intern Med* 99:43-44, 1983.

Del Favero A, et al: Pharmacokinetics and tolerability of teicoplanin in healthy volunteers after single increasing doses. *Antimicrob Agents Chemother* 35:2551-2557, 1991.

Dudley MN, et al: Absorption of vancomycin. *Ann Intern Med* 101:144, 1984.

Dutka-Malen S, et al: Phenotypic and genotypic heterogeneity of glycopeptide resistance determinants in gram-positive. *Antimicrob Agents Chemother* 34:1875-1879, 1990.

Ellison RT, et al: Oral rifampin and trimethoprim/sulfamethoxazole therapy in asymptomatic carriers of methicillin-resistant *Staphylococcus aureus* infections. *West J Med* 140:735-740, 1984.

European Organization for Research and Treatment of Cancer (EORTC) International Antimicrobial Therapy Cooperative Group and the National Cancer Institute of Canada—Clinical Trials Group: Vancomycin added to empirical combination antibiotic therapy for fever in granulocytopenic cancer patients. *J Infect Dis* 163:951-958, 1991.

Fagan TC, et al: Metronidazole-induced gynecomastia. *JAMA* 254:3217, 1985.

Farber BF, Moellering RC Jr: Retrospective study of toxicity of preparations of vancomycin from 1974 to 1981. *Antimicrob Agents Chemother* 23:138-141, 1983.

Farr B, Mandell GL: Rifamycins, in Mandell GL, et al (eds): *Principles and Practice of Infectious Diseases,* ed 3. New York, Churchill Livingstone, 1990, 295-303.

Fekety R: Vancomycin and teicoplanin, in Mandell GL, et al (eds): *Principles and Practice of Infectious Diseases*, ed 3. New York, Churchill Livingstone, 1990 A, 317-323.

Fekety R: Polymyxins, in Mandell GL, et al (eds): *Principles and Practice of Infectious Diseases*, ed 3. New York, Churchill Livingstone, 1990 B, 323-325.

Fekety R, et al: Treatment of antibiotic-associated *Clostridium difficile* colitis with oral vancomycin: A comparison of two dosage regimens. *Am J Med* 86:15-19, 1989.

Finegold SM, Mathisen GE: Metronidazole, in Mandell GL, et al (eds): *Principles and Practice of Infectious Diseases,* ed 3. New York, Churchill Livingstone, 1990, 303-308.

Galanakis N, et al: Poor efficacy of teicoplanin in treatment of deep-seated staphylococcal infections. *Eur J Clin Microbiol Infect Dis* 7:130-134, (April) 1988.

Gentry LO: Antibiotic therapy for osteomyelitis. *Infect Dis Clin North Am* 4:485-499, 1990.

Gilbert DN, et al: Failure of treatment with teicoplanin at 6 milligrams/kilogram/day in patients with *Staphylococcus aureus* intravascular infection. *Antimicrob Agents Chemother* 35:79-87, 1991.

Glicklich D, Figura I: Vancomycin and cardiac arrest. *Ann Intern Med* 101:880-881, 1984.

Glupczynski Y, et al: Clinical evaluation of teicoplanin for therapy of severe infections caused by gram-positive bacteria. *Antimicrob Agents Chemother* 29:52-57, 1986.

Goldstein FW, et al: Percentages and distributions of teicoplanin- and vancomycin-resistant strains among coagulase-negative staphylococci. *Antimicrob Agents Chemother* 34:899-900, 1990.

Greenberg RN: Treatment of bone, joint, and vascular-access-associated gram-positive bacterial infections with teicoplanin. *Antimicrob Agents Chemother* 34:2392-2397, 1990.

Gugler R, Jensen JC: Interaction between cimetidine and metronidazole, letter. *N Engl J Med* 309:1518-1519, 1983.

Gump DW: Vancomycin for treatment of bacterial meningitis. *Rev Infect Dis* 3 (suppl):S289-S292, 1981.

Healy DP, et al: Comparison of steady-state pharmacokinetics of two dosage regimens of vancomycin in normal volunteers. *Antimicrob Agents Chemother* 31:393-397, 1987.

Healy DP, et al: Vancomycin-induced histamine release and 'red man syndrome': Comparison of 1- and 2-hour infusions. *Antimicrob Agents Chemother* 34:550-554, 1990.

Heipertz R, Pilz H: Interaction of nitrofurantoin with diphenylhydantoin. *J Neurol* 218:297-301, 1978.

Hoeprich PD: The polymyxins. *Med Clin North Am* 54:1257-1265, 1970.

Holmberg L, et al: Adverse reactions to nitrofurantoin: An analysis of 921 reports. *Am J Med* 69:733-738, 1980.

Hughes WT, et al: Guidelines for the use of antimicrobial agents in neutropenic patients with unexplained fever. *J Infect Dis* 161:381-396, 1990.

Johnson AP, et al: Resistance to vancomycin and teicoplanin: An emerging clinical problem. *Clin Microbiol Rev* 3:280-291, 1990.

Johnson S, et al: Treatment of asymptomatic *Clostridium difficile* carriers (fecal excretors) with vancomycin or metronidazole: A randomized, placebo-controlled trial. *Ann Intern Med* 117:297-302, 1992.

Kaiser AB: Antimicrobial prophylaxis in surgery. *N Engl J Med* 315:1129-1138, 1986.

Kapusnik JE, Sande MA: Rifampin, in Peterson PK, Verhoef J (eds): *The Antimicrobial Agents Annual/1.* New York, Elsevier, 1986, 179-187.

Kapusnik JE, et al: Use of rifampin in staphylococcal infections: A review. *J Antimicrob Chemother* 13 (suppl C):61-66, 1984.

Karchmer AW: Staphylococcal endocarditis: Laboratory and clinical basis for antibiotic therapy. *Am J Med* 78 (suppl 6B):116-127, 1985.

Karchmer AW: *Staphylococcus aureus* and vancomycin: The sequel. *Ann Intern Med* 115:739-741, 1991.

Karchmer AW, et al: Methicillin-resistant *Staphylococcus epidermidis* (SE) prosthetic valve (PV) endocarditis (E). Therapeutic trial, abstract 476. *24th Interscience Conference on Antimicrobial Agents and Chemotherapy*. Washington, DC, Oct 8-10, 1984.

Kelsey SM, et al: Teicoplanin plus ciprofloxacin versus gentamicin plus piperacillin in the treatment of febrile neutropenic patients. *Eur J Clin Microbiol Infect Dis* 11:509-514, 1992.

Kureishi A, et al: Double-blind comparison of teicoplanin versus vancomycin in febrile neutropenic patients receiving concomitant tobramycin and piperacillin: Effect on cyclosporin A-associated nephrotoxicity. *Antimicrob Agents Chemother* 35:2246-2252, 1991.

Lake KD, Peterson CD: Simplified dosing method for initiating vancomycin therapy. *Pharmacotherapy* 5:340-344, 1985.

Lam YWF, et al: The pharmacokinetics of teicoplanin in varying degrees of renal function. *Clin Pharmacol Ther* 47:655-661, 1990.

Leport C, et al: Evaluation of teicoplanin for treatment of endocarditis caused by gram-positive cocci in 20 patients. *Antimicrob Agents Chemother* 33:871-876, 1989.

Levine JF: Vancomycin: A review. *Med Clin North Am* 71:1135-1145, 1987.

Levine DP, et al: Slow response to vancomycin or vancomycin plus rifampin in methicillin-resistant *Staphylococcus aureus* endocarditis. *Ann Intern Med* 115:674-680, 1991.

Levy M, et al: Vancomycin-induced red man syndrome. *Pediatrics* 86:572-580, 1990.

Lewis EW, et al: Teicoplanin administration in patients with vancomycin hypersensitivity, in: *Program and Abstracts of the 32nd Interscience Conference on Antimicrobial Agents and Chemotherapy.* Anaheim, Calif: American Society for Microbiology, 1992.

Locksley RM, et al: Multiply antibiotic-resistant *Staphylococcus aureus*: Introduction, transmission, and evolution of nosocomial infection. *Ann Intern Med* 97:317-324, 1982.

Lugo-Miro VI, et al: Comparison of different metronidazole therapeutic regimens for bacterial vaginosis: A meta-analysis. *JAMA* 268:92-95, 1992.

Martin WJ: Nitrofurantoin: Evidence for oxidant injury of lung parenchymal cells. *Am Rev Respir Dis* 127:482-486, 1983.

Martino P, et al: Teicoplanin in the treatment of gram-positive-bacterial endocarditis. *Antimicrob Agents Chemother* 33:1329-1334, 1989.

Martino P, et al: Piperacillin plus amikacin vs. piperacillin plus amikacin plus teicoplanin for empirical treatment of febrile episodes in neutropenic patients receiving quinolone prophylaxis. *Clin Infect Dis* 15:290-294, 1992.

Matzke GR: Vancomycin, in Evans WE, et al (eds): *Applied Pharmacokinetics: Principles of Therapeutic Drug Monitoring*, ed 2. Spokane, Wash, Applied Therapeutics, 1986, 399-436.

Matzke GR, et al: Pharmacokinetics of vancomycin in patients with various degrees of renal function. *Antimicrob Agents Chemother* 25:433-437, 1984.

Matzke GR, et al: Clinical pharmacokinetics of vancomycin. *Clin Pharmacokinet* 11:257-282, 1986.

Matzke GR, et al: Systemic absorption of oral vancomycin in patients with renal insufficiency and antibiotic-associated colitis. *Am J Kidney Dis* 9:422-425, 1987.

Mayhew JF, Deutsch S: Cardiac arrest following administration of vancomycin. *Can Anaesth Soc J* 32:65-66, 1985.

Mayrer AR, Andriole VT: Urinary tract antiseptics. *Med Clin North Am* 66:199-208, 1982.

McAnally TP, et al: Effect of rifampin and bacitracin on nasal carriers of *Staphylococcus aureus*. *Antimicrob Agents Chemother* 25:422-426, 1984.

McElrath MJ, et al: Allergic cross-reactivity of teicoplanin and vancomycin. *Lancet* 1:47, 1986.

The Medical Letter: *Handbook of Antimicrobial Therapy*. New Rochelle, NY, The Medical Letter, Inc, 1992, 124-139.

Moellering RC Jr: Pharmacokinetics of vancomycin. *J Antimicrob Chemother* 14(suppl D):43-52, 1984.

Moellering RC Jr, et al: Vancomycin therapy in patients with impaired renal function: A nomogram for dosage. *Ann Intern Med* 94:343-346, 1981.

Nagarajan R: Antibacterial activities and modes of action of vancomycin and related glycopeptides. *Antimicrob Agents Chemother* 35:605-609, 1991.

Naqvi SH, et al: Vancomycin pharmacokinetics in small, seriously ill infants. *Am J Dis Child* 140:107-110, 1986.

Nielsen HE, et al: Renal excretion of vancomycin in kidney disease. *Acta Med Scand* 197:261-264, 1975.

Nováková I, et al: Ceftazidime as monotherapy or combined with teicoplanin for initial empiric treatment of presumed bacteremia in febrile granulocytopenic patients. *Antimicrob Agents Chemother* 35:672-678, 1991.

Odio C, et al: Adverse reactions to vancomycin used as prophylaxis for CSF shunt procedures. *Am J Dis Child* 138:17-19, 1984.

Outman WR, et al: Teicoplanin pharmacokinetics in healthy volunteers after administration of intravenous loading and maintenance doses. *Antimicrob Agents Chemother* 34:2114-2117, 1990.

Pantosti A, et al: Comparison of in vitro activities of teicoplanin and vancomycin against *Clostridium difficile* and their interactions with cholestyramine. *Antimicrob Agents Chemother* 28:847-848, 1985.

Pauly DJ, et al; Risk of nephrotoxicity with combination vancomycin-aminoglycoside antibiotic therapy. *Pharmacotherapy* 10:378-382, 1990.

Phillips G, Golledge CL: Vancomycin and teicoplanin: Something old, something new. *Med J Aust* 156:53-57, 1992.

Pizzo PA, et al: The child with cancer and infection: 1. Empiric therapy for fever and neutropenia, and preventive strategies. *J Pediatr* 119:679-694, 1991.

Polk RE: Anaphylactoid reactions to glycopeptide antibiotics. *J Antimicrob Chemother* 27(suppl B):17-29, 1991.

Pon E, et al: Unusual case of penicillinase-producing *Neisseria gonorrhoeae* resistant to spectinomycin in California. *Sex Transm Dis* 13:47-49, 1986.

Pratt WB, Fekety R: *The Antimicrobial Drugs*. New York, Oxford University Press, 1986 A, 85-112.

Pratt WB, Fekety R: *The Antimicrobial Drugs*. New York, Oxford University Press, 1986 B, 262-276.

Pryka RD, et al: Teicoplanin: An investigational glycopeptide antibiotic. *Clin Pharm* 7:647-658, 1988.

Rahal JJ: Treatment of methicillin-resistant staphylococcal infections, in Peterson PK, Verhoef J (eds): *The Antimicrobial Agents Annual/1*. New York, Elsevier, 1986, 489-514.

Ramphal R, et al: Vancomycin is not an essential component of the initial empiric treatment regimen for febrile neutropenic patients receiving ceftazidime: A randomized prospective study. *Antimicrob Agents Chemother* 36:1062-1067, 1992.

Rowland M: Clinical pharmacokinetics of teicoplanin. *Clin Pharmacokinet* 18:184-209, 1990.

Rybak MJ, et al: Teicoplanin pharmacokinetics in intravenous drug abusers being treated for bacterial endocarditis. *Antimicrob Agents Chemother* 35:696-700, 1991.

Rybak MJ, et al: Absence of 'red man syndrome' in patients being treated with vancomycin or high-dose teicoplanin. *Antimicrob Agents Chemother* 36:1204-1207, 1992.

Sahai J, et al: Influence of antihistamine pretreatment on vancomycin-induced red man syndrome. *J Infect Dis* 160:876-881, 1989.

Sahai J, et al: Comparison of vancomycin- and teicoplanin-induced histamine release and 'red man syndrome'. *Antimicrob Agents Chemother* 34:765-769, 1990.

Schaad UB, et al: Clinical pharmacology and efficacy of vancomycin in pediatric patients. *J Pediatr* 96:119-126, 1980.

Schlemmer B, et al: Teicoplanin for patients allergic to vancomycin, letter. *N Engl J Med* 318:1127-1128, 1988.

Schmit JL: Efficacy of teicoplanin for enterococcal infections: 63 cases and review. *Clin Infect Dis* 15:302-306, 1992.

Sharp JR, et al: Chronic active hepatitis and severe hepatic necrosis associated with nitrofurantoin. *Ann Intern Med* 92:14-19, 1980.

Simon GL, et al: Emergence of rifampin-resistant strains of *Staphylococcus aureus* during combination therapy with vancomycin and rifampin: Report of two cases. *Rev Infect Dis* *J*(suppl 3):S507-S508, 1983.

Slight PH, et al: Trial of vancomycin for prophylaxis of infections after neurosurgical shunts, letter. *N Engl J Med* 312:921, 1985.

Small PM, Chambers HF: Vancomycin for *Staphylococcus aureus* endocarditis in intravenous drug users. *Antimicrob Agents Chemother* 34:1227-1231, 1990.

Smith SR, et al: Randomized prospective study comparing vancomycin with teicoplanin in the treatment of infections associated with Hickman catheters. *Antimicrob Agents Chemother* 33:1193-1197, 1989.

Smithers JA, et al: Pharmacokinetics of teicoplanin upon multiple-dose intravenous administration of 3, 12, and 30 milligrams per kilogram of body weight to healthy male volunteers. *Antimicrob Agents Chemother* 36:115-120, 1992.

Sorrell TC, Collignon PJ: Prospective study of adverse reactions associated with vancomycin therapy. *J Antimicrob Chemother* 16:235-241, 1985.

Southorn PA, et al: Adverse effects of vancomycin administered in perioperative period. *Mayo Clin Proc* 61:721-724, 1986.

Spitzer PG, Eliopoulos GM: Systemic absorption of enteral vancomycin in a patient with pseudomembranous colitis. *Ann Intern Med* 100:533-534, 1984.

Tally FP, et al: Nationwide study of susceptibility of *Bacteroides fragilis* group in United States. *Antimicrob Agents Chemother* 28:675-677, 1985.

Teasley DG, et al: A prospective randomized trial of metronidazole versus vancomycin for *Clostridium difficile*-associated diarrhoea and colitis. *Lancet* 2:1043-1046, 1983.

Thompson CM, et al: Absorption of oral vancomycin: Possible associated toxicity. *Int J Pediatr Nephrol* 4:1-4, 1983.

Thompson GA, et al: Pharmacokinetics of teicoplanin upon multiple dose intravenous administration to normal healthy male volunteers. *Biopharm Drug Dispos* 13:213-220, 1992.

Thornsberry C, et al: Rifampin: Spectrum of antibacterial activity. *Rev Infect Dis* 5(suppl 3):S412-S417, 1983.

Tolman KG: Nitrofurantoin and chronic active hepatitis, editorial. *Ann Intern Med* 92:119-120, 1980.

Trissel LA: *Handbook on Injectable Drugs*, ed 4. Bethesda, Md, American Society of Hospital Pharmacists, 1986, 582-584.

Van der Auwera P, et al: Clinical study of combination therapy with oxacillin and rifampin for staphylococcal infections. *Rev Infect Dis* 5(suppl 3):S515-S522, 1983.

Van der Auwera P, et al: Randomized study of vancomycin versus teicoplanin for the treatment of gram-positive bacterial infections in immunocompromised hosts. *Antimicrob Agents Chemother* 35:451-457, 1991.

Venditti M, et al: 4-week treatment of streptococcal native valve endocarditis with high-dose teicoplanin. *Antimicrob Agents Chemother* 36:723-726, 1992.

Verbist L, et al: In vitro activity and human pharmacokinetics of teicoplanin. *Antimicrob Agents Chemother* 26:881-886, 1984.

Viladrich PF, et al: Evaluation of vancomycin for therapy of adult pneumococcal meningitis. *Antimicrob Agents Chemother* 35:2467-2472, 1991.

Viscoli C, et al: Ceftazidime plus amikacin versus ceftazidime plus vancomycin as empiric therapy in febrile neutropenic children with cancer. *Rev Infect Dis* 13:397-404, 1991.

Wallace MR, et al: Red man syndrome: Incidence, etiology, and prophylaxis. *J Infect Dis* 164:1180-1185, 1991.

Ward TT, et al: Observations relating to inter-hospital outbreak of methicillin-resistant *Staphylococcus aureus*: The role of antimicrobial therapy in infection control. *Infect Control* 2:453-459, 1981.

Wheat LJ, et al: Long-term studies of effect of rifampin on nasal carriage of coagulase-positive staphylococci. *Rev Infect Dis* 5(suppl 3):S459-S462, 1983.

Wilhelm MP: Vancomycin. *Mayo Clin Proc* 66:1165-1170, 1991.

Woodford N, et al: Detection of glycopeptide resistance in clinical isolates of gram-positive bacteria. *J Antimicrob Chemother* 28:483-490, 1991.

Young TL, et al: Chronic active hepatitis induced by nitrofurantoin. *Cleve Clin Q* 52:253-256, 1985.

Zokufa HZ, et al: Simulation of vancomycin peak and trough concentrations using five dosing methods in 37 patients. *Pharmacotherapy* 9:10-16, 1989.

Drugs Used Topically in Eye and Ear Infections

72

EYE INFECTIONS

Bacteria are implicated as causative pathogens in a large proportion of eye infections; in order of frequency, viruses, fungi, and amebae also cause these infections (Pavan-Langston, 1983). Vision-threatening corneal infections caused by *Acanthamoeba* species are uncommon and are usually associated with improper contact lens care (ie, use of homemade saline solutions that do not contain preservatives).

Primary care physicians can manage most superficial infections of the eyelids and conjunctiva. More severe infections (those that threaten vision, those that respond poorly to therapy, or those that involve the cornea, orbit, or intraocular structures) require immediate management by an ophthalmologist.

The differential diagnosis of the inflamed eye ("red eye") is challenging (Donshik, 1986; Elkington and Khaw, 1988; Stratton, 1988; Cykiert, 1989). Superficial ocular infections must be distinguished from allergic reactions (classically associated with clear discharge, itching, presence of eosinophils in the tear film) and reactions caused by contact chemical irritants. The differential diagnosis of an acute "red eye" due to iritis, acute glaucoma, or external ocular infections, including keratitis, is especially important in the preservation of vision. Slit-lamp examination, use of fluorescein and rose bengal dyes, Giemsa and Gram stains, and cultures from conjunctival swabs and corneal scrapings may be indicated to assist in the diagnosis of infections.

LID AND OCULAR INFECTIONS

Drug therapy for these infections is based on the site of involvement, the susceptibility of the ocular tissues, the offending organism, and the severity of infection. Discussion in this section is limited to infections of the lids, conjunctiva, and cornea. Some of these infections may require additional systemic antibiotic therapy. Involvement of other ocular structures (eg, retinitis, endophthalmitis, periorbital and orbital cellulitis) will almost always require intraocular or systemic therapy.

Blepharitis

CHRONIC BACTERIAL BLEPHARITIS. In most instances, this infectious condition affects the margins of the eyelids; it is caused by *Staphylococcus aureus* or *S. epidermidis* and is referred to as staphylococcal blepharitis. Chronically erythematous lid margins, broken or misdirected eyelashes, crusting of the eyelashes, presence of fibrinous scales surrounding individual cilia, and lid ulcerations are common. Conjunctivitis also may occur. In addition, plugging of the meibomian gland ducts that open along the posterior margin of the lids may lead to an acute focal infection or a chronic granulomatous reaction (chalazion) and meibomian gland dysfunction. A sty (external hordeolum) is an abscess of the sebaceous glands (glands of Zeiss and Moll) associated with eyelash follicles; an internal hordeolum is an abscess of a meibomian gland.

Therapy for staphylococcal blepharitis consists of daily lid scrubs and topical application of antibiotics (eg, bacitracin, gentamicin, tobramycin, erythromycin). Treatment for at least one month is recommended to minimize recurrences. Physicians should be aware that an over-the-counter ophthalmic ointment preparation, yellow mercuric oxide 1%, has long been used by the public for the treatment of blepharitis (Kastl et al, 1987).

Most hordeola resolve spontaneously or respond to topical therapy. The management of an acute internal hordeolum or chalazion includes application of hot compresses with or without use of topical antibiotics for three to four weeks (Smythe et al, 1990). Patients with underlying sebaceous gland inflammation (usually rosacea) may require systemic preparations of doxycycline or tetracycline. In nonresponsive patients, outpatient surgery may be necessary to drain an acute abscess or remove a persistent granuloma. After local anesthesia with lidocaine and epinephrine (if not contraindicated), incision and drainage using a conjunctival approach is performed with use of a chalazion clamp. An antibiotic or steroid ointment is then applied; an eyepatch may be worn for 12 hours thereafter. For chronic chalazia, corticosteroids may be injected intralesionally.

CHRONIC SEBORRHEIC BLEPHARITIS. This condition is commonly associated with a seborrheic scalp condition. Older adults are most commonly affected, and the disease may persist for years. In addition to the chronically erythematous lid margins and scaling, meibomian gland activity is usually excessive and this gives the scales and tear film an oily appearance. Manifestations of seborrhea may be present in other regions (postauricular and anterior chest areas). Eyelid hygiene similar to that described for staphylococcal blepharitis is desirable; shampoos containing antiseborrheic agents are recommended for the scalp but are not used on the lids and lashes. Baby shampoo diluted 1:2 or 1:5 with water or a commercial ophthalmic cleansing solution may be used on the lids and lashes and then rinsed off with water. One drop of an artificial tears preparation applied to each eye two to four times daily also may reduce debris and oil in the tear film. (See also index entry Seborrhea.)

A mixed form, staphylococcal and seborrheic blepharoconjunctivitis, which almost always involves the conjunctiva and possibly the cornea, also may occur. The therapy described for both types of blepharitis will be required to eliminate the organisms.

Conjunctivitis

ACUTE BACTERIAL CONJUNCTIVITIS. This relatively common infection is caused by a variety of organisms that produce an erythematous conjunctiva, purulent or mucopurulent conjunctival discharge, eyelid edema, a foreign body sensation, and sticking shut of the lids on awakening. The causative organism depends on the age group of the patient (Gigliotti et al, 1984; Fisher, 1987; Limberg, 1991): In adults, *Staphylococcus aureus* is a frequent and *S. epidermidis* an occasional cause of both acute and chronic bacterial conjunctivitis worldwide. Conjunctivitis caused by *Haemophilus influenzae* and *Streptococcus pneumoniae* is most common in children and often is self-limited. When infection with *S. pneumoniae* is associated with subconjunctival petechial hemorrhages, antibiotics may be applied to shorten the duration of the infection and enhance eradication of the causative organism. Conjunctivitis caused by *Chlamydia* occurs predominantly in neonates and sexually active young adults.

Neisseria gonorrhoeae and *N. meningitidis* (rare) produce a characteristic fulminant or hyperpurulent discharge (hyperacute bacterial conjunctivitis) that drips out of the eye; other manifestations include aching pain, tenderness, chemosis, and marked lymphadenopathy at the involved site.

Pseudomembrane formation is an uncommon sign in acute bacterial conjunctivitis but may be seen in association with conjunctivitis caused by streptococci or adenoviruses.

Drug Selection: Because of the extremely high antibiotic concentrations achieved at the ocular surface, most cases of bacterial conjunctivitis will respond to topical antibiotics even when in vitro tests indicate antibiotic resistance. Sodium sulfacetamide is widely used to treat mild and moderate infections. Single-entity topical anti-infectives (eg, bacitracin, chlortetracycline, erythromycin, gentamicin, sulfisoxazole, tobramycin) administered four times daily also are effective in most patients with acute bacterial conjunctivitis caused by susceptible organisms. Bacitracin, chlortetracycline, and erythromycin are available commercially only in ointment formulations. Alternatively, combinations such as trimethoprim-polymyxin B (eyedrops), bacitracin-polymyxin B (ointment), or gramicidin-neomycin-polymyxin B (eyedrops) can be prescribed. Because chloramphenicol rarely is associated with bone marrow aplasia, it is usually reserved for conjunctivitis that does not respond to conventional therapy in the United States; however, it is a drug of choice in much of Europe. The more recently introduced antibiotics, ciprofloxacin and norfloxacin, also are effective, especially in patients with severe bacterial conjunctivitis.

Acute gonococcal or chlamydial conjunctivitis will require systemic therapy because the causative organisms affect other organ systems (see index entry Gonococcal Infections and the following section on Acute Chlamydial Conjunctivitis).

More frequent administration of topical solutions or suspensions generally is recommended for severe conjunctivitis. Drops are instilled every two hours initially; the interval can be extended to every four hours during waking hours as the infection is controlled. Ointments are useful as nighttime medication or for treatment of younger children whose tearing induced by instillation of eyedrops may rapidly wash away a solution. Generally, adults prefer eyedrops to ointments except at bedtime because the latter blur vision.

Most patients with bacterial conjunctivitis respond to topical antibacterial therapy within one week. Referral is indicated for any patient with infectious conjunctivitis that persists without improvement for longer than one week, is worsening or spreading to the cornea, reduces vision, or produces severe pain.

ACUTE CHLAMYDIAL CONJUNCTIVITIS (INCLUSION CONJUNCTIVITIS). The causative agent of this infection is the intracellular bacterium, *Chlamydia trachomatis.* The disease is most common in sexually active adults, particularly those who have acquired a new sexual partner in recent months. Diagnosis may be delayed in adults because genital symptoms of a chlamydial infection are commonly not present at the time of eye involvement. The follicular conjunctivitis and less common superficial keratitis caused by acute chlamydial conjunctivitis may be difficult to distinguish from that seen with adenoviral-induced epidemic keratoconjunctivitis, except that a vascular pannus may be present superiorly and chlamydial infection is not self-limiting. Since chlamydial conjunctivitis often lasts for months if untreated, this infection should be suspected in any viral-like conjunctivitis that persists for more than three weeks or any follicular conjunctivitis that does not respond to topical antibiotics. Diagnosis is confirmed by identification of chlamydial antigen by immunofluorescence (IF) tests utilizing direct fluorescent antibody or enzyme-linked immunosorbent assay [ELISA] or by culture of conjunctival scrapings.

The preferred regimen for chlamydial conjunctivitis is oral tetracycline 250 mg four times daily or doxycycline 100 mg twice daily for one week. Oral erythromycin should be substituted for the tetracycline preparation in children under 8 years. The newer systemic antibiotics, ofloxacin, clarithromycin, and azithromycin, are active against *Chlamydia* and are alternative choices. Sexual partners also should be treated.

The diagnosis, clinical course, and treatment of this disease in both adults and neonates has been reviewed (Stenberg and Mårdh, 1990).

ACUTE CHLAMYDIAL CONJUNCTIVITIS IN THE NEONATE (INCLUSION BLENNORRHEA OF THE NEWBORN). At present, *C. trachomatis* is the most common cause of neonatal conjunctivitis. It is acquired by the newborn during passage through the infected cervix. Bilateral eye involvement is most common. A papillary palpebral rather than a bulbar conjunctivitis is typical; in addition, a purulent discharge develops 5 to 14 days after delivery.

Prophylaxis with topical silver nitrate, erythromycin, or tetracycline does not eliminate nasopharyngeal colonization with *C. trachomatis* and does not protect against neonatal chlamydial pneumonia (Hammerschlag et al, 1980; Rettig et al, 1981; *MMWR,* 1989). Because topical prophylaxis is ineffective, either antenatal diagnosis of chlamydia infection in the mother or prompt culture of the suspected organism followed by systemic treatment with erythromycin is encouraged to minimize chronic chlamydial infection (Chandler, 1989; Hammerschlag et al, 1989).

The Centers for Disease Control guidelines for treating culture-proven pediatric chlamydial conjunctivitis recommend erythromycin syrup 50 mg/kg/day divided into four doses for at least two weeks; topical therapy is not required. For resistant cases (about 20% of the infants), a second course is recommended. Parents of infected neonates also should be treated with oral tetracycline or erythromycin 500 mg four times daily for two to four weeks; if compliance is a problem, doxycycline 100 mg twice daily for at least seven days or a single 1-g dose of azithromycin is an alternative therapy.

PREVENTION OF GONOCOCCAL CONJUNCTIVITIS IN THE NEONATE (OPHTHALMIA NEONATORUM). Topical application of silver nitrate (Credé's prophylaxis) is legally required in many states for the prevention of gonococcal ophthalmia neonatorum. One drop of a 1% solution (preferably packaged in wax ampuls) is instilled in the conjunctival sac of each eye immediately after delivery. It should not be rinsed from the eyes. Silver nitrate prophylaxis has greatly reduced the incidence of gonococcal conjunctivitis in the newborn, but it may cause local irritation. Improved prenatal screening and treatment of maternal gonococcal infection also is an important strategy to minimize neonatal gonococcal conjunctivitis (Chandler, 1989; Hammerschlag et al, 1989).

Either erythromycin or tetracycline ophthalmic ointment is considered by the Centers for Disease Control and others as an acceptable alternative to silver nitrate in the prophylaxis of gonococcal ophthalmia neonatorum (Chandler, 1989; Hammerschlag et al, 1989; *MMWR,* 1989); some states permit any one of these three agents to be used for prophylaxis. Although tetracycline appears to be as effective as silver nitrate for prophylaxis if it is applied properly within 30 minutes after birth (Laga et al, 1988), some authorities speculate that the visual blurring caused by the ointment may interfere with mother-infant bonding (Chandler, 1989). Topical application of these agents is not useful in established gonococcal infections of the conjunctiva in neonates, but the smaller inoculum of organisms received during birth is presumably eliminated.

ACUTE VIRAL CONJUNCTIVITIS. Adenoviruses characteristically produce one of three clinical forms of this disorder. All forms of adenovirus-induced conjunctivitis are manifested by a follicular conjunctivitis of the tarsal surface of the palpebral conjunctiva. The follicles are avascular and translucent; this is presumed to be a gross manifestation of lymphoid aggregates. Moderate conjunctival redness, discomfort, and tearing often occur in one eye and usually extend to the second eye later. The course of the disease is self-limited and seldom exceeds two weeks.

In the first form of acute viral conjunctivitis (ie, pharyngoconjunctivitis), fever occurs, especially in children, and the conjunctivitis is associated with an upper respiratory infection and anterior cervical lymphadenopathy. The second form is indistinguishable from the pharyngoconjunctival form except that the conjunctivitis and upper respiratory signs and symptoms tend to be milder. This nonspecific follicular conjunctivitis is the most commonly observed adenoviral infection and is termed "pink eye." Characteristically, a preauricular lymph node is palpable. Treatment is symptomatic unless a conjunctival pseudomembrane forms. In such instances, referral to an ophthalmologist may be indicated for possible topical corticosteroid therapy. None of the antiviral agents discussed under viral keratitis is effective against these adenoviruses.

The third form of adenoviral-induced conjunctivitis, epidemic keratoconjunctivitis (EKC), frequently is produced by adenovirus 8 or 19 but many other subtypes also may be causative. The disorder typically occurs in older children and adults. The adenoviruses are highly contagious, but the course is usually self-limited with a duration of two to four weeks. Signs range from a mildly red eye to pronounced keratoconjunctivitis. Most commonly, onset is rapid in one eye; manifestations include discomfort, tearing, foreign body sensation, photophobia, and blurring of vision. A follicular conjunctivitis is typical. Tender preauricular lymphadenopathy and pseudomembranes are occasionally associated with the diffuse superficial keratitis that is commonly present. Slit-lamp examination reveals slightly elevated focal epithelial lesions. In about 10 to 14 days, subepithelial opacities form under some of the epithelial lesions in approximately 50% of patients. Although the epithelial lesions fade away gradually within two weeks, the subepithelial opacities may persist for months to several years without producing symptoms of irritation, although they occasionally cause blurred vision. Subepithelial opacities are the distinctive feature of EKC.

Treatment of EKC is symptomatic. Use of artificial tear preparations may be helpful. Topical antibiotics are commonly prescribed to prevent secondary bacterial infection or when the disease cannot be distinguished from bacterial conjunctivitis. The routine application of topical corticosteroids is discouraged even though these preparations will clear the opacities, because steroids may prolong the duration of the disease. Their use is reserved for patients with significant discomfort and impairment of vision.

Keratitis

Corneal ulcers are a medical emergency. They may be caused by bacteria, viruses, fungi, or protozoa. Predisposing risk factors include abrasion from contact lenses, especially extended-wear soft lenses; other ocular trauma (including foreign bodies); eyelid and conjunctival infections; intraocular surgery; use of topical ophthalmic corticosteroids; corneal disorders; immunosuppression (including diabetes); hygienic or nutritional deficiencies; ocular surface disorders (eg, pemphigoid, Stevens-Johnson syndrome); and keratoconjunctivitis sicca, the "dry eye" often associated with many systemic diseases (eg, Sjogren's syndrome, systemic lupus erythematosus, lymphomas) (Musch et al, 1983). Moderate to severe pain is a prominent symptom of all corneal ulcers unless corneal sensation is impaired (eg, herpes zoster or herpes simplex infection). Recurrent herpetic infections may be less painful due to nerve destruction during the primary infection.

The four major classes of infecting organisms are discussed separately because the signs, symptoms, course, and prognosis of the keratitis and anti-infective drug treatment differ considerably. Depending on the severity of the keratitis and the presence of iridocyclitis, mydriatic-cycloplegic drugs may be used to decrease the pain of ciliary muscle spasm and to prevent posterior adhesions of the iris to the lens (see index entries Miotics; Mydriatics; Cycloplegics). Local anesthetics are contraindicated because they worsen keratitis by diminishing the protective mechanism of ocular sensation and are toxic to the corneal epithelium when used repeatedly.

BACTERIAL KERATITIS. The signs and symptoms of bacterial corneal ulcers include pain, foreign body sensation, photophobia, distinct epithelial ulceration covered with mucopurulent exudate, focal stromal infiltration and ulceration, and possibly iridocyclitis or hypopyon.

The most common causative pathogens in bacterial keratitis in adults vary among countries but include *Staphylococcus aureus, S. epidermidis, Pseudomonas aeruginosa, Streptococcus pneumoniae, Klebsiella pneumoniae*, and other Enterobacteriaceae *(Escherichia coli, Proteus, Citrobacter, Enterobacter,* and *Serratia)* (Limberg, 1991). *P. aeruginosa* is the pathogen most frequently isolated from corneal ulcers of patients wearing soft contact lenses.

An accurate diagnosis is desirable in the management of suppurative bacterial keratitis but is often difficult to attain. Initially, corneal scrapings should be examined and the causative organism identified by culture. Examination of the scrapings by Gram stain is less satisfactory for diagnosis but has served as the basis for initial therapy. Only 53% to 73% of organisms will be identified even with culture (Maske et al, 1986); therefore, the initial decision to use an antimicrobial agent and choice of the agent frequently must be made without the benefit of microbiologic data.

Drug Selection: With the exception of ciprofloxacin [Ciloxan] 0.3% and norfloxacin [Chibroxin] 0.3%, commercially available strengths of antibiotic eyedrops are considered inadequate for initial treatment of bacterial keratitis (Stern, 1988; Steinert, 1991). Consequently, for other antibacterial agents, solutions or suspensions containing fortified concentrations are preferred to standard concentrations and are prepared from sterile products intended for parenteral use (see Tables 1 and 3 in the section on Ophthalmic Anti-Infective Preparations).

Two antibiotics (eyedrop formulations) that are active against gram-positive and gram-negative organisms are chosen for initial empiric therapy. An initial loading dose (one drop every minute for five minutes) will increase antibiotic concentrations in the cornea rapidly (Glasser et al, 1985). In one recommended regimen, one drop of the first drug is applied every minute for five minutes, followed by a five-minute interval to avoid washout before the second drug (if required) is applied in the same manner. Application of the second drug is followed by a 45- to 55-minute interval, after which the sequence is repeated around the clock for 48 hours.

If the ulcer does not heal, further treatment is based on the antibiotic sensitivity of the organism. Empiric therapy with gentamicin or tobramycin drops plus a topical cephalosporin is useful, especially if a gram-negative infection is suspected. However, the risk of toxicity is greater with fortified concentrations of an aminoglycoside than with standard concentrations (Davison et al, 1991). Symptoms of toxicity may be difficult to distinguish from those produced by the keratitis; a toxicologic finding of great concern is conjunctival necrosis (approximate incidence, $<0.1\%$), which heals within five days to two weeks after the aminoglycoside is withdrawn. In vitro studies evaluating antimicrobial activity suggest that fluoroquinolones may be preferred to the aminoglycosides; these drugs also may be less toxic to the corneal epithelium (Cutarelli et al, 1991).

Indications for hospitalization include a large ulcer near the visual axis, an ulcer that is progressing despite aggressive therapy, unreliable setting for instillation of drops, potential noncompliance, a patient with only one eye, and corneal infections in children.

Because of their poor penetration into the cornea, systemic administration of antibiotics generally is not indicated except for gonococcal and chlamydial infections at any age, scleral extension of the infection, or impending perforation of the cornea. Adjunctive subconjunctival injection is controversial because it has not been definitively established that this route provides additional benefit and the injection is often painful. Nevertheless, subconjunctival injections may be useful when compliance is questionable or in infants and young children who cry, because topical medication is diluted by tears and the drops are squeezed out of the eye. Once the infection is under control, commercial strength topical antibiotics can be administered less frequently.

Guidelines have been proposed for the use of corticosteroids in patients with bacterial keratitis (Stern and Buttross, 1991): (1) Corticosteroids should not be used until the causative organism has been identified, the effectiveness of the antibiotic has been confirmed, and the patient has responded favorably to antibiotic therapy. (2) If the eye continues to improve without their use, corticosteroids should be withheld. (3) If inflammation persists, corticosteroids may be added to the regimen after several days of antibiotic therapy when the eye is totally or nearly sterilized. (4) In all cases, concomitant use of appropriate antibiotics should be continued. (5) Because of potential activation of collagenolytic enzymes and/or suppression of collagen resynthesis, corticosteroids should not be used when perforation is a threat because of corneal thinning.

Corticosteroids are used in the treatment of any form of infectious keratitis before therapeutic penetrating keratoplasty. In this instance, it is assumed that the surgical procedure will eliminate the infectious organisms, and pretreatment with topical corticosteroids for up to 24 hours before surgery may lessen postsurgical inflammation and improve the likelihood of a successful corneal graft.

VIRAL KERATITIS. DNA viruses that affect the eye include herpes simplex virus (HSV), varicella-zoster virus, cytomegalovirus, Epstein-Barr virus, adenovirus, and papillomavirus.

A primary viral infection may be caused by HSV in patients without prior exposure. It is most common in children between 8 months and 5 years. The infection is subclinical in approximately 90% of patients, but a nonspecific keratoconjunctivitis or blepharitis may occur. Primary viral keratitis is even less common, but it is more likely to occur in patients with atopic disease. Recurrent symptomatic HSV infections are common in adults. A recurrence rate of 40% for ocular infection during a five-year period is similar to that observed for orolabial infection from HSV, type 1, but this rate is only about one-half that observed for genital infection with HSV, type 2 (Cobo, 1988). An estimated 300,000 to 500,000 cases of HSV eye infections occur yearly in the United States. In most affected patients, only one eye is involved.

Symptomatic primary ocular HSV infection is characterized by follicular conjunctivitis (except in infants and young children) and vesicular lesions of the eyelids that may be accompanied by punctate keratitis. Recurrent infection is generally manifested by epithelial keratitis, usually in the form of dendritic ulceration or, less commonly, as geographic ulcers. Stromal keratitis and uveitis develop in 10% to 20% of patients; most forms are believed to be caused by immune mechanisms.

Drug Selection: Although a considerable number of antiviral drugs are being developed and evaluated clinically for systemic administration (see index entry Antiviral Agents), available antiviral agents used topically in the eye are limited to the treatment of HSV, types 1 and 2. Acyclovir [Zovirax] is administered orally for the treatment of acute herpes zoster ophthalmicus, and it is being evaluated topically in the treatment of acute and recurrent resistant HSV ocular infections.

Actions. The three antiviral agents commercially available in the United States for topical ophthalmic use are idoxuridine (IDU) [Herplex] (ointment and eyedrops), vidarabine [Vira-A] (ointment), and trifluridine [Viroptic] (eyedrops). Acyclovir is available as an ophthalmic ointment 3% only from the manufacturer (Burroughs Wellcome) on a compassionate-use basis (Richards et al, 1983; Lass, 1987).

All of these agents disrupt viral synthesis of DNA. Acyclovir is activated by being phosphorylated by virus-specific thymidine-kinase; other antiviral drugs are phosphorylated nonspecifically. Their degree of activation in normal cells determines their toxicity.

Uses. These agents are efficacious topically in HSV epithelial infections of the conjunctiva and cornea and in uncomplicated dendritic keratitis. Trifluridine eyedrops are preferred to idoxuridine eyedrops, however, because the latter compound has more limited solubility, greater systemic toxicity, and more rapid metabolism, and treatment failures approach 25%. These agents have been used with some success to treat vaccinia infections of the eye. No cross sensitivity or cross resistance appears to exist among these drugs, and patients who are allergic or resistant to one may benefit from treatment with another.

Epithelial disease has been treated successfully by mechanical debridement, but a topical antiviral agent with or without debridement is utilized currently. The management of ocular HSV epithelial keratitis has been reviewed (Liesegang, 1988). The principles of medical therapy emphasized include the following: (1) The status of the epithelium should be assessed with rose bengal rather than fluorescein dye to optimize diagnosis and monitoring. (2) Corticosteroids should be avoided in active epithelial disease and trophic ulcers, because they enhance infection and create larger ulcers that are less responsive to antiviral therapy and may result in loss of vision (see below for guidelines for corticosteroid use). (3) Antiviral therapy should be deferred for a short observation period if equivocal replicating virus is present or other causal mechanisms are suspected (eg, indolent ulceration, trophic ulceration, drug toxicity). (4) If active viral epithelial disease has not responded after seven days of treatment, a different antiviral agent should be selected. (5) If the epithelium has not healed in 21 days, the diagnosis should be reconsidered. See Table 1 for preparations and Table 4 for dosage of antiviral agents used to treat ocular HSV epithelial keratitis.

Acyclovir is effective orally and topically in many cases of herpetic stromal keratitis and uveitis. None of the other antiviral drugs penetrate sufficiently to affect HSV infections in these ocular structures and thus they are ineffective. Corticosteroids have the potential to enhance viral replication within the corneal stroma and to promote recurrence of an epithelial keratitis; therefore, the use of topical corticosteroids in HSV stromal keratitis is controversial. Most ophthalmologists prescribe them to suppress the excessive inflammation, but a minority believe this inflammation is necessary to terminate the infection and that corticosteroids prolong the course of the disease. When ophthalmologists do prescribe corticosteroids, certain principles are recognized (Liesegang, 1988): (1) Their use should be avoided in mild stromal keratitis. (2) Topical corticosteroid therapy should not be initiated prior to administration of prophylactic antiviral treatment. (3) The least amount of corticosteroid needed to suppress inflammation should be used. (4) The dose should be reduced gradually to avoid a rebound stromal response.

Adverse Reactions and Precautions. Idoxuridine, vidarabine, and trifluridine may cause local irritation (toxic and/or allergic), photophobia, follicular conjunctivitis, lid margin thickening and keratinization, protrusion of the meibomian glands, ptosis, edema of the eyelids and cornea, punctal occlusion, and superficial punctate keratopathy. The risk of corneal toxicity is increased by long-term treatment or administration to patients with dry-eye syndromes; sequelae may include permanent punctal occlusion, conjunctival cicatrization, and corneal scarring. Antiviral drugs also inhibit stromal and epithelial wound healing.

In clinical trials, the adverse reactions observed with topical ophthalmic preparations of acyclovir have been essentially limited to reversible superficial punctate keratitis and conjunctivitis, but only short-term use in limited numbers of patients has been employed (Høvding, 1989). Systemic acyclovir also is generally well tolerated. For a more detailed discussion of adverse reactions, see index entry Acyclovir.

FUNGAL KERATITIS. Fungal corneal ulcers occur most commonly in warm climates after injury or surgery (usually filamentous fungi), or when host resistance is decreased (usually yeast-type fungi). The increased incidence of oculomycosis observed in recent years has been attributed to the widespread use of corticosteroids and, possibly, broad spectrum antibiotics but may be related to improved isolation techniques.

More than 100 varieties of fungi have been identified as ocular pathogens. The fungi most frequently cultured from mycotic corneal ulcers are *Aspergillus* (usually *A. fumigatus*), *Fusarium solani, Candida albicans, Cephalosporium,* and *Curvularia.*

The signs and symptoms of fungal infection of the eye are only minimally diagnostic; they are more similar to bacterial than viral infections or allergic inflammation.

Drug Selection: Fungal corneal ulcers often respond slowly or poorly to topical antifungal therapy. Because of the poor penetration of some agents, any extension of the infection into the anterior chamber or vitreous of the eye will require subconjunctival, intraocular, and/or systemic administration of antifungal agents (Cobo, 1987; Pflugfelder et al, 1988). Some patients will require an excisional keratoplasty to resolve the infection.

The only commercially available topical ophthalmic antifungal drug is natamycin, a polyene that is related to amphotericin B. Its spectrum of action is somewhat more limited and, when applied topically, it usually is less toxic than amphotericin B. Natamycin is especially effective against superficial keratomycoses caused by *Fusarium* and *Cephalosporium* species.

A compounded dilute solution of amphotericin B prepared from the parenteral product is frequently used topically when natamycin is ineffective or clinical judgment on sensitivity studies suggests that amphotericin B is the drug of choice (0.05% to 0.15% concentrations are preferred to the 0.5% to 1.5% concentrations formerly recommended, because local toxicity and eye pain caused by the deoxycholate used to solubilize the drug are reduced and efficacy is usually adequate). Amphotericin B has significant activity against *Candida*, *Coccidioides*, *Cryptococcus*, *Histoplasma*, *Blastomyces*, and *Sporotrichum*, as well as the filamentous fungi, *Fusarium* and *Cephalosporium* species, which are the most common causes of fungal keratitis.

Miconazole, an imidazole, also is used topically in the eye; a 1% solution must be compounded from the parenteral product. Penetration is somewhat better than with the polyenes, and this drug is principally used for *Candida* and *Aspergillus* infections (Foster, 1981). Miconazole has not been compared with amphotericin B in large controlled studies; the latter remains the standard. A once popular extemporaneously prepared topical solution of the polyene antifungal drug, nystatin, is now seldom employed. Occasionally, flucytosine is used both topically and systemically in *Candida* keratitis. Development of resistance is a problem, and topical solutions must be compounded from the parenteral product. Flucytosine is usually used with topical amphotericin B, because the two drugs act synergistically against *Candida*.

See Table 1 for preparations and Table 5 for dosage of antifungal agents.

Results of one prospective controlled study suggest that silver sulfadiazine 1% ophthalmic ointment (investigational formulation) was at least as safe and effective as miconazole 1% ophthalmic ointment (investigational formulation) in 43 patients with documented positive corneal fungal ulcers, and it was effective in a few patients who did not respond to miconazole (Mohan et al, 1988). In another study on 31 patients with culture-documented fungal infection, the cure rate with topical silver sulfadiazine was 77.8% (Vajpayee et al, 1990); those who did not respond to topical silver sulfadiazine also did not respond to topical miconazole. Two other antifungal agents, itraconazole and fluconazole, are undergoing evaluation to determine their usefulness in the treatment of ocular fungal infections.

Most serious fungal infections of the eye will require systemic therapy (see index entry Mycoses, Subcutaneous, Systemic).

AMEBIC KERATITIS. Three protozoan genera cause serious ocular infections. *Toxoplasma gondii* and *Microsporidia* species, both obligate intracellular protozoans, produce a chorioretinitis (see index entry Toxoplasmosis) and a keratoconjunctivitis (Didier et al, 1991), respectively, particularly in immunocompromised patients. *Acanthamoeba,* a nonflagellated free-living ameba that is ubiquitous in the environment and has both a trophozoite and dormant cyst form, causes severe keratitis.

The most serious complication associated with use of contact lenses is microbial keratitis, particularly that caused by *Pseudomonas* and other gram-negative organisms. *Acanthamoeba* species cause a rare but especially devastating keratitis that has resulted in enucleation in 10% to 15% of patients. Early recognition and initiation of therapy are essential for successful eradication of the organism. The infection was first associated with contact lens wear in 1973, and approximately 150 cases were documented by the end of 1988; the incidence has expanded considerably in the last few years, probably because of improved diagnosis (Stehr-Green et al, 1989). The infection occurs rarely in individuals who do not wear contact lenses.

Acanthamoeba keratitis is associated most often with improper care of all types of soft and hard contact lenses but is more common with daily-wear soft contact lenses (Cohen et al, 1987; Wiens and Jackson, 1988). Other risk factors include swimming with contact lens in place, preparation of preservative-free homemade saline or tap water solutions for lens care, chemical rather than heat sterilization, contact lens trauma, and use of contaminated lens-care solutions, particularly those containing gram-negative organisms (*Acanthamoeba* grow best in a culture overlaid with *E. coli* because the bacteria serve as a food source).

A number of strains of *Acanthamoeba* can produce keratitis; however, they vary in pathogenicity. The diagnosis should be suspected in any patient who wears contact lenses and has herpes simplex virus-like keratitis that produces severe pain out of proportion to the apparent degree of corneal involvement. Most commonly, pseudodendrites, fine epithelial opacities, radial neuritis, and microcysts associated with edema are observed early in the infection. Progression of the disease is characterized by persistent or recurrent epithelial defects, microcysts developing into bullae, stromal edema, and corneal ring infiltrates. The presence of a 360° ring infiltrate or abscess is an important but, unfortunately, late diagnostic sign. Descemetoceles and frank corneal perforation are late manifestations of inadequately treated or resistant infection.

Initially, scrapings of corneal lesions touched to slides, air-dried, and stained with one of the available microbiologic stains or formalin-fixed and stained with calcofluor white often provide a diagnosis; however, definitive diagnosis is based on culture and isolation of the organism or microscopic identification of corneal biopsy tissue.

Drug Selection: A cycloplegic is commonly instilled initially; epithelial debridement is performed on occasion. The amebicidal drugs of choice are two stilbamidine derivatives, dibrompropamidine ointment 0.15% and propamidine isethionate [Brolene] solution 0.1%. The most effective dosage schedules have not been established. One schedule utilizes propamidine isethionate solution plus the combination product, neomycin, polymyxin B, and gramicidin, given alternately every 15 to 30 minutes around the clock for the first three days and then every hour during the day and every two hours at night for one week (Moore, 1988; Moore and McCulley, 1989). If tolerated, topical applications then are reduced in frequency to four times a day and continued for one year. Administration is then discontinued, and the patient is observed for recurrences. The combination product is effective against trophozoites but not cysts.

Topical miconazole 1% (prepared from the parenteral product) had been used as an alternative therapy in patients who did not respond, but topical clotrimazole 1% is now preferred by some clinicians as an alternative or is used with the stilbamidine drugs and the neomycin combination (Driebe et al, 1988).

Another regimen that has been evaluated consists of topical instillation of propamidine isethionate 0.1% every hour, a mixture of neomycin-polymyxin B-gramicidin plus miconazole 1% every two hours, and dibrompropamidine isethionate ointment 0.15% applied at bedtime (Berger et al, 1990). The course of treatment necessary to resolve the infection ranged from 4 to 17 months in six of seven patients in either early or late stages of infection. Earlier penetrating keratoplasty may be required to relieve intractable pain or actual or threatened corneal perforation. In this study, penetrating keratoplasty was required to eradicate a persistent (although improved) active keratitis in the seventh patient. Although topical corticosteroids were used in five of the seven patients, their effectiveness and possible negative effects remain controversial.

Prevention and early recognition of symptoms are paramount. Patients who wear contact lenses must be educated in their proper care; this includes heat sterilization and the use of commercial saline solutions. Soaking the lens in hydrogen peroxide for at least two hours is also acceptable for sterilization. Other helpful guidelines for lens care to prevent this serious infection are available (Moore et al, 1987).

Viral Retinitis

Cytomegalovirus causes viral retinitis in approximately 10% of patients with AIDS. Parenterally administered ganciclovir is the drug of choice to treat the disease providing the macula has not been destroyed (see index entry Ganciclovir). About 20% of patients cannot tolerate ganciclovir or develop resistance to this agent after prolonged treatment. Parenteral administration of foscarnet also is effective, and this drug may be considered an alternative to ganciclovir (see index entry, Foscarnet). Intravitreal administration of ganciclovir also appears to be effective if intravenous administration causes unacceptable toxicity (Goldschmidt and Dong, 1991).

Bacterial Endophthalmitis

Bacterial endophthalmitis is an uncommon but devastating complication that most frequently occurs after ocular surgery but may develop following penetrating eye trauma or as a metastasis from a distant primary infection. It involves the uveal tract, vitreous body, and retina and produces eye pain, loss of vision, conjunctival and ciliary injection, chemosis, lid swelling, corneal edema, hypopyon, and decreased or absent red reflex on ophthalmoscopic examination. The major causative bacteria are *Staphylococcus aureus, S. epidermidis, Streptococcus, Pseudomonas,* and *Proteus. Bacillus cereus* is an increasingly recognized and important bacterial pathogen in penetrating eye trauma.

Prompt and aggressive management with subconjunctival, intravitreal, and systemic antibacterial agents plus subconjunctival injection and oral administration of corticosteroids is needed to minimize loss of vision (Forster et al, 1980). Sampling of aqueous and vitreous compartments for culture is imperative. A combination of intravitreal vancomycin and amikacin is recommended for infections caused by *B. cereus*. The cephalosporins are ineffective against this organism (Kervick et al, 1990). Topical antibacterial agents alone are of little value in initial treatment because the infection is in the uvea, vitreous, and retina.

OPHTHALMIC ANTI-INFECTIVE PREPARATIONS

Routes of Administration

OCULAR. Ointments and topical suspensions or solutions often are adequate for the treatment of superficial infections of the lids and conjunctiva. With the exception of ciprofloxacin 0.3% and norfloxacin 0.3%, commercial strengths of topical antibiotics generally are inadequate for the initial treatment of bacterial keratitis. Therefore, frequent application of fortified antibiotic solutions are recommended for such infections; these strengths are not commercially available and thus must be formulated from parenteral solutions.

Although it is controversial, periocular injection of certain drugs occasionally is employed adjunctively along with topical fortified solutions in order to deliver additional amounts of antibiotics to the cornea and anterior chamber. Direct diffusion to the anterior structures of the eye occurs after subconjunctival administration; however, some of the antibiotic leaks from the site of deposition back through the injection site and is absorbed from the conjunctival tear film. Intravitreal injections, which deliver antibiotics to the posterior structures of the eye (ie, vitreous, retina), are used when systemic therapy is inadequate. Periocular or intravitreal injections for infections involving the vitreous and retina may have to be repeated every 12 to 24 hours at different sites, depending on the infection and its severity.

SYSTEMIC. Systemic antibiotics are used, sometimes in conjunction with topical therapy, to treat some forms of severe bacterial conjunctivitis, particularly those associated with systemic effects (eg, gonococcal and chlamydial conjunctivitis at any age, *Pseudomonas* and *Haemophilus* conjunctivitis in infants). Systemic therapy for bacterial keratitis does not enhance outcome; therefore, it is not necessary for most patients who are being treated with an appropriate regimen of a topical fortified antibiotic formulation. When actual corneal perforation occurs or extension of the infection into the limbus or sclera is suspected, systemic therapy is advisable to prevent endophthalmitis. Systemic administration also is recommended for retinitis due to cytomegalovirus or *Toxoplasma gondii* and in infections of the soft tissues of the lids, ocular adnexa, and orbit.

Topical Formulations and Pharmacokinetics

Available topical ophthalmic formulations of antibacterial, antiviral, and antifungal drugs include solutions, suspensions, and ointments. In general, aqueous solutions are more stable than ointments; however, drugs in lipid-soluble ointments are absorbed better than drugs in water-soluble solutions or ointments; absorption is least with the latter. The permeability and bioavailability of suspensions tend to be variable. The advantages of ointments include a longer tissue contact time, lessened dilution by tears, and reduced nasolacrimal drainage. Their disadvantages include the ointment film's interference with vision and with the bioavailability of some concurrently used topical agents; the necessity for the active component to pass into and dissolve in the tear film, which delays onset of action; and the tendency of hydrophilic components to crystallize. Moreover, fortified ointment preparations are not yet available because of problems with solubility and stability.

An eye dropper delivers 20 to 70 microliters/drop of solution or suspension. The fluid volume that the tear film can contain is about 30 microliters; however, when adjusted for blinking, this amount may be as little as 10 microliters. Thus, applying more than one drop at a time appears to be of little value. Lacrimal drainage is rapid (about 15% of the applied volume/minute). Only about 2% of the active drug remains in the eye 30 minutes after topical administration (Gardner, 1987).

Whether or not a loading dose regimen is used for a particular infection, subsequent doses generally are applied hourly around the clock for several days during the early treatment of severe bacterial keratitis. The number of applications can be decreased gradually as control of the infection is achieved; hourly administration of fortified solutions may be necessary for a few days.

The many factors that affect the pharmacokinetics of topical ophthalmic formulations have been reviewed (Gardner, 1987).

Topical Anti-Infective Drugs

Antibacterial, antiviral, antifungal, and antiprotozoal drugs are used topically to treat lid and ocular infections. Bacitracin, gramicidin, neomycin, and polymyxin B are poorly absorbed and rarely administered systemically. They are available commercially for topical use as single-entity preparations or in mixtures. Although sulfacetamide sodium is better absorbed, it likewise is rarely used systemically. Commercial ophthalmic preparations containing chloramphenicol, chlortetracycline, ciprofloxacin, gentamicin, norfloxacin, sulfisoxazole, tetracycline, and tobramycin also are available.

Single-entity topical antibacterial preparations are listed in Tables 1 and 3 and mixtures in Table 2. Antiviral and antifungal preparations appear in Tables 4 and 5, respectively.

TABLE 1. TOPICAL OPHTHALMIC ANTI-INFECTIVE PREPARATIONS (SINGLE-ENTITY)

Preparation	Preservatives	Container Size
ANTIBACTERIAL AGENTS		
Bacitracin		
Ophthalmic Ointment		
AK-Tracin (Akorn), Generic 500 units/g	Preservative-free	3.5 g
Chloramphenicol		
Ophthalmic Ointment 1%		
AK-Chlor (Akorn)	Preservative-free	3.5 g
Chloromycetin (Parke-Davis)	Preservative-free	3.5 g
Chloroptic (Allergan)	Chlorobutanol 0.5%	3.5 g
Ocu-Chlor (Ocumed)	Preservative-free	3.5 g
Ophthalmic Solution 0.5%		
AK-Chlor (Akorn)	Chlorobutanol 0.5%	7.5 and 15 ml
Chloromycetin (Parke-Davis)	Preservative-free	15 ml
Chloroptic (Allergan)	Chlorobutanol 0.5%	2.5 and 7.5 ml
I-Chlor (Akorn)	Chlorobutanol 0.5%	7.5 and 15 ml
Ocu-Chlor (Ocumed)	Preservative-free	7.5 and 15 ml
Chlortetracycline		
Ophthalmic Ointment 1%		
Aureomycin (Lederle)	Preservative-free	3.5 g
Ciprofloxacin		
Ophthalmic Solution 0.3%		
Ciloxan (Alcon)	Benzalkonium chloride, EDTA	2.5, 5, and 10 ml
Erythromycin		
Ophthalmic Ointment 0.5%		
AK-Mycin (Akorn)	Preservative-free	3.5 g
Erythromycin (Bausch & Lomb)	Preservative-free	3.5 g
Ilotycin (Dista)	Preservative-free	1 and 3.5 g
Gentamicin		
Ophthalmic Ointment 0.3%		
Garamycin (Schering)	Methylparaben, propylparaben	3.5 g
Genoptic S.O.P. (Allergan)	Methylparaben, propylparaben	3.5 g
Gentacidin (Iolab)	Preservative-free	3.5 g
Gentak (Akorn)	Methylparaben, propylparaben	3.5 g
Gentrasul (Bausch & Lomb)	Methylparaben, propylparaben	3.5 g
Ocu-Mycin (Ocumed)	Methylparaben, propylparaben	3.5 g
Ophthalmic Solution 0.3%		
Garamycin (Schering)	Benzalkonium chloride	5 ml
Genoptic (Allergan)	Benzalkonium chloride, EDTA	1 and 5 ml
Gentacidin (Iolab)	Benzalkonium chloride	5 ml
Gentak (Akorn)	Benzalkonium chloride	5 and 15 ml
Gentrasul (Bausch & Lomb)	Benzalkonium chloride	5 and 15 ml
I-Gent (Akorn)	Benzalkonium chloride	5 ml
Ocu-Mycin (Ocumed)	Benzalkonium chloride	5 and 15 ml
Norfloxacin		
Ophthalmic Solution 0.3%		
Chibroxin (Merck Sharp & Dohme)	Benzalkonium chloride, EDTA	5 ml

(table continued on next page)

TABLE 1 (Continued)

Preparation	Preservatives	Container Size
ANTIBACTERIAL AGENTS (continued)		
Silver Nitrate		
Ophthalmic Solution 1%		
Generic	—	Single-dose ampuls
Sulfacetamide Sodium		
Ophthalmic Ointment 10%		
AK-Sulf (Akorn)	Methylparaben, propylparaben	3.5 g
Bleph-10 S.O.P. (Allergan)	Phenylmercuric acetate 0.0008%	3.5 g
Cetamide (Alcon)	Methylparaben, propylparaben	3.5 g
Ocu-Sul-10 (Ocumed)	Methylparaben, propylparaben	3.5 g
Sodium Sulamyd (Schering)	Methylparaben, propylparaben, benzalkonium chloride	3.5 g
Ophthalmic Solution		
AK-Sulf (10%, 15%, 30%) (Akorn)	Methylparaben, propylparaben	2, 5, and 15 ml
Bleph-10 (10%) (Allergan)	EDTA, benzalkonium chloride	2.5, 5, and 15 ml
Isopto Cetamide (15%) (Alcon)	Methylparaben, propylparaben	5 and 15 ml
Ocu-Sul (10%, 15%, 30%) (Ocumed)	Methylparaben, propylparaben	15 ml
Sodium Sulamyd (10%, 30%) (Schering)	Methylparaben, propylparaben	10%—5 and 15 ml 30%—15 ml
Sulf-10 (10%) (Iolab)	Thimerosal 0.01%	15 ml
Sulten-10 (10%) (Bausch & Lomb)	EDTA, methylparaben, propylparaben	15 ml
Sulfisoxazole Diolamine		
Ophthalmic Solution 4%		
Gantrisin (Roche)	Phenylmercuric nitrate 1:100,000	15 ml
Tetracycline Hydrochloride		
Ophthalmic Ointment 1%		
Achromycin (Lederle)	Preservative-free	3.7 g
Ophthalmic Suspension 1%		
Achromycin (Lederle)	Preservative-free	4 ml
Tobramycin		
Ophthalmic Ointment 0.3%		
Tobrex (Alcon)	Chlorobutanol 0.5%	3.5 g
Ophthalmic Solution 0.3%		
Tobrex (Alcon)	Benzalkonium chloride 0.01%	5 ml
ANTIFUNGAL AGENT		
Natamycin		
Ophthalmic Suspension 5%		
Natacyn (Alcon)	Benzalkonium chloride 0.02%	15 ml
ANTIVIRAL AGENTS		
Idoxuridine		
Ophthalmic Solution 0.1%		
Herplex (Allergan)	Benzalkonium chloride, EDTA	15 ml
Trifluridine		
Ophthalmic Solution 1%		
Viroptic (Burroughs Wellcome)	Thimerosal 0.001%	7.5 ml
Vidarabine		
Ophthalmic Ointment 3%		
Vira-A (Parke-Davis)	Preservative-free	3.5 g

TABLE 2.
ANTIBACTERIAL MIXTURES FOR TOPICAL OPHTHALMIC THERAPY

Drugs	Preparations	Preservatives	Container Size
Ophthalmic Ointments			
Bacitracin Zinc 500 units and Polymyxin B Sulfate 10,000 units/g	AK-Poly-Bac (Akorn)	preservative-free	3.7 g
	Ocumycin (Bausch & Lomb)	preservative-free	3.7 g
	Polysporin Ophthalmic (Burroughs Wellcome)	preservative-free	3.7 g
Bacitracin Zinc 400 units, Neomycin Sulfate (equivalent to 3.5 mg base), and Polymyxin B Sulfate 10,000 units/g	AK-Spore (Akorn)	preservative-free	3.5 g
	Neosporin (Burroughs Wellcome)	preservative-free	3.5 g
	Neotricin (Bausch & Lomb)	preservative-free	3.5 g
	Ocu-Spor-B (Ocumed)	preservative-free	3.5 g
	Ocutricin (Bausch & Lomb)	preservative-free	3.5 g
Ophthalmic Solutions			
Gramicidin 0.025 mg, Neomycin Sulfate (equivalent to 1.75 mg base), and Polymyxin B Sulfate 10,000 units/ml	AK-Spore (Akorn)	thimerosal 0.001%	2 and 10 ml
	Neosporin (Burroughs Wellcome)	thimerosal 0.001%	10 ml
	Neotricin (Bausch & Lomb)	thimerosal 0.001%	2 and 10 ml
	Ocu-Spor-G (Ocumed)	thimerosal 0.001%	10 ml
	Ocutricin (Bausch & Lomb)	thimerosal 0.001%	2 and 10 ml
Polymyxin B Sulfate 10,000 units and Trimethoprim Sulfate 1 mg/ml	Polytrim (Allergan)	benzalkonium chloride 0.004%	10 ml

In addition to these commercial preparations, eyedrops may be formulated for treatment of bacterial keratitis by diluting parenteral antibiotics with sterile water for injection or artificial tears and adjusting for isotonicity (see Table 3). The solubility and stability of antibiotics prepared in this manner may vary. Because these solutions are not stable, they should be prepared just prior to dispensing. Most of these solutions remain stable for three to four days, except for the aminoglycosides, which may remain stable for up to 30 days (Glasser and Hyndiuk, 1987).

A number of products contain a fixed-dose combination of a corticosteroid and an antibacterial agent, and these are prescribed by some ophthalmologists to treat conditions in which both may be required. These mixtures should *not* be used to treat keratitis of unknown origin because they may worsen viral or fungal infections (Stern and Buttross, 1991; O'Day, 1991).

INDICATIONS FOR ANTIBACTERIAL DRUGS. The antibacterial spectrum of *bacitracin* is similar to that of penicillin G except that it is more effective against staphylococci. This drug is preferred to penicillin for topical treatment of superficial staphylococcal and streptococcal infections because few strains of organisms are resistant, allergic reactions occur less frequently, and future sensitization to penicillin is avoided.

Gramicidin is similar in activity to bacitracin, but it is available only in combination products.

Neomycin is bactericidal and is active against many gram-positive and gram-negative organisms, including *Proteus*. Sensitivity or toxicity develops more readily than with other topical antibiotics, particularly when neomycin is used for longer than five or six days. In sensitized individuals, the development of allergic conjunctivitis may worsen signs and symptoms, causing the unwary physician to intensify therapy instead of discontinuing the drug.

Polymyxin B and *colistin* are bactericidal against most gram-negative organisms, including *Pseudomonas aeruginosa, Escherichia coli, Klebsiella pneumoniae*, and *Enterobacter aerogenes*. They are not effective against *Proteus* or gram-positive organisms. The minimal effective concentration of polymyxin B is 10,000 units/ml (*Federal Register*, 1980). Organisms resistant to polymyxin B often are resistant to colistin.

Combinations containing bacitracin, gramicidin, neomycin, polymyxin B, and trimethoprim are widely used in ocular therapy because of their broad spectrum of activity. See also Table 2.

Sulfacetamide sodium is effective against some gram-positive and gram-negative organisms. It is bacteriostatic, not bactericidal, and many organisms are resistant. This drug is commonly used to treat chronic blepharitis and mild to moderate acute bacterial conjunctivitis (eg, that caused by *Haemophilus aegyptius, Streptococcus pneumoniae*, and many strains of *Staphylococcus aureus*) (Lohr et al, 1988).

Gentamicin and *tobramycin* are aminoglycosides that are active against a wide variety of gram-negative and gram-positive organisms. These agents are particularly useful because of their significant activity against *Pseudomonas, Proteus, Klebsiella, E. coli*, and *Staphylococcus*. Streptococci are relatively resistant. Since occasional strains of *Pseudomonas* are

TABLE 3.
FORTIFIED ANTIBACTERIAL DRUG FORMULATIONS FOR KERATITIS

Drug	Commercially Available Solution or Suspension[1]	Commercially Available Ointment[1]	Compounded Fortified Solutions or Suspensions for Keratitis
Amikacin	—	—	50 mg/ml[2]
Ampicillin	—		50 mg/ml[2]
Bacitracin	—	500 units/g	10,000 units/ml[2] 9,600 units/ml[3]
Carbenicillin	—		4 mg/ml[2] 6.2 mg/ml[2]
Cefamandole	—		50 mg/ml[2]
Cefazolin	—		50 mg/ml[2] 33 mg/ml[3]
Cephalothin	—		65 mg/ml[3]
Chloramphenicol	0.5%	1%	—
Chlortetracycline	—	1%	—
Ciprofloxacin	0.3%	—	0.3%[4]
Erythromycin	—	0.5%	10 mg/ml[3]
Gentamicin	0.3%	0.3%	20 mg/ml[2] 14 mg/ml[3]
Methicillin	—		50 mg/ml[2]
Moxalactam	—		50 mg/ml[2]
Neomycin	—		33 mg/ml[3]
Norfloxacin	0.3%		0.3%[4]
Oxacillin	—	—	66 mg/ml[3]
Penicillin G	—	—	100,000 units/ml[2]
Polymyxin B	—	—	50,000 units/ml[2] 25,000 units/ml[3]
Sulfacetamide	10%, 15%, 30%	10%	—
Sulfisoxazole	4%	—	—
Tetracycline	1%	1%	—
Ticarcillin	—	—	6.3 mg/ml[3]
Tobramycin	0.3%	0.3%	20 mg/ml[2] 14 mg/ml[3]
Vancomycin	—		50 mg/ml[2,3]

[1] *See Table 1 for preparations.*
[2] *See Glasser and Hyndiuk, 1987, for preparation.*
[3] *See Baum, 1987, for preparation.*
[4] *Commercial strength adequate for keratitis.*

resistant, polymyxin B and antipseudomonal penicillins or cephalosporins may be considered as additional therapy for pseudomonal keratitis.

Chloramphenicol is used topically to treat acute conjunctivitis caused by *Haemophilus* and *Moraxella*. Topical application rarely causes sensitization. Because blood dyscrasias have been reported during or several months after continuous or intermittent use of chloramphenicol eyedrops or ointment (Fraunfelder and Meyer, 1985), it is preferable to use less toxic agents whenever possible (Glasser and Hyndiuk, 1987). This opinion is not shared by all physicians, however. Chloramphenicol is the most popular topical antibiotic prescribed for acute conjunctivitis by general practitioners in Britain (McDonnell, 1988).

Erythromycin, available topically only as an ointment, is well tolerated and is effective against many gram-positive organisms, including *Streptococcus pneumoniae* and *S. pyogenes*. Staphylococci occasionally are resistant to this antibiotic initially, and many strains become resistant during long-term therapy. Erythromycin is effective in the treatment of neonatal chlamydial conjunctivitis. (See the discussion on Acute Chlamydial Conjunctivitis in the Neonate.)

The *tetracyclines* are bacteriostatic and are active against a wide range of gram-positive and gram-negative organisms that affect the eye, including *Chlamydia*. Because of their high lipid solubility, the tetracyclines (especially minocycline) penetrate well into ocular tissues after systemic administration. However, systemic forms are contraindicated in pregnant women and children under 8 years. Ophthalmic ointment preparations are most commonly used in the treatment of mild bacterial conjunctivitis and in the treatment of chlamydial and gonorrheal infections in neonates.

Two fluoroquinolone antibiotics, *ciprofloxacin* [Ciloxan] and *norfloxacin* [Chibroxin], are available as topical ophthalmic solutions for the treatment of bacterial conjunctivitis and keratitis. Their pharmacology and antibacterial spectrum are presented elsewhere (see index entry Fluoroquinolones). In general, this class of antibiotics is active against a wide spec-

TABLE 4.
ANTIVIRAL AGENTS FOR TOPICAL OPHTHALMIC THERAPY[1]

Drug	Concentration	Dosage
Idoxuridine	0.1% solution	One drop every hour during the day and every 2 hours at night until definite improvement occurs as demonstrated by lack of staining with fluorescein; dosage is then reduced to 1 drop every 2 hours during the day and every 4 hours at night. Treatment should be continued for 3-5 days after healing appears to be complete but not for more than 14-21 days.
Trifluridine	1% solution	Initially, 1 drop every 2 hours while awake (maximum, 9 drops daily). When healing begins, treatment should be continued for 7 days at a dosage of 1 drop 5 times daily. Therapy generally should not be continued for more than 14-21 days.
Vidarabine	3% ointment	One-half inch applied 5 times daily at 3-hour intervals. When healing appears to be complete, treatment should be continued for 7 days at a reduced dosage (eg, twice daily). Therapy generally should not be continued for more than 14-21 days.
Acyclovir[2]	3% ointment	One-half inch applied 5 times daily at 3- to 4-hour intervals and continued for at least 3 days after complete healing. Therapy generally should not be continued for more than 14-21 days.

[1]*See Table 1 for preparations.*

[2]*Only available on a compassionate-use basis. The dermal ointment 5% should not be used in place of the ophthalmic ointment 3% formulation.*

trum of gram-positive and gram-negative organisms, including penicillin-resistant strains of *Neisseria gonorrhoeae* and methicillin-resistant staphylococci. Ciprofloxacin was effective in more than 90% of patients with bacterial keratitis (Leibowitz, 1991 A, 1991 B; *Med Lett Drugs Ther*, 1991). Adverse effects of both agents are limited to mild burning and stinging, conjunctival hyperemia, and chemosis.

Vancomycin is bactericidal and is especially effective against gram-positive cocci and bacilli. It is an alternative drug if the penicillins, cephalosporins, or fluoroquinolones cause allergic reactions, are ineffective, or are poorly tolerated. In eye infections, vancomycin's primary use is limited to topical application (must be prepared from parenteral product and topical concentrations should not exceed 50 mg/ml). Subconjunctival injection may cause conjunctival necrosis and sloughing. Vancomycin is administered with an aminoglycoside by intravitreal injection for endophthalmitis (concentrations for intraocular injection should not exceed 1 mg/0.1 ml).

TABLE 5.
ANTIFUNGAL AGENTS FOR TOPICAL OPHTHALMIC THERAPY

Drug	Concentration	Dosage
Amphotericin B	0.025%-0.15% suspension[1]	One drop every 30 minutes and then every hour until the infection is under control. If effective, lower concentrations are associated with less toxicity. Higher concentrations have been associated with severe local irritation.
Miconazole	1% solution[1]	Initially, one drop every hour day and night for 4-10 days, followed by one drop every hour during the day for 2-4 weeks, then one drop six times daily for 3-7 weeks.
Natamycin[2]	5% suspension[3]	For fungal keratitis, initially one drop every hour during the day and every 2 hours at night. After 3-4 days, the frequency of instillation may be reduced to 6-8 times daily. Therapy should be continued for 14-21 days.

[1] *Compounding necessary.*

[2] *See Table 1 for preparations.*

[3] *Available in this concentration as ophthalmic product.*

See Tables 1 and 3 for available single-entity antibacterial preparations.

ADVERSE REACTIONS AND PRECAUTIONS. The adverse reactions of topical antibiotics are related to the antibiotic itself or to the weakly active bacteriostatic preservatives used in the formulation (Glasser and Hyndiuk, 1987). Epithelial toxicity (ie, punctate epithelial keratitis, delayed epithelial healing) and hypersensitivity reactions are the principal manifestations of antibiotic or preservative toxicity. Fortified solutions or suspensions are likely to be more toxic (Davison et al, 1991). Neomycin appears to be the most allergenic. Other aminoglycosides also may produce an allergic reaction or pseudomembranous conjunctivitis in addition to epithelial toxicity. In vitro studies evaluating corneal epithelial toxicity suggest that fluoroquinolones may be less toxic than fortified solutions of aminoglycosides (Cutarelli et al, 1991).

Although the antibiotic components in these fortified solutions or suspensions are more prone to cause toxicity than the preservative components because of dilution, preservatives always must be considered as a cause of adverse events associated with topical ophthalmic drug use. Chlorobutanol and chlorhexidine may be toxic to the corneal epithelium and endothelium, respectively. Benzalkonium is contraindicated for intraocular use because it is especially toxic to the corneal endothelium. Its toxicity is characterized by loss of superficial epithelial cells and delayed healing caused by impaired epithelial adhesion. Hypersensitivity reactions occur infrequently. Thimerosal has been associated with hypersensitivity reactions that cause keratoconjunctivitis with coarse punctate epithelial keratopathy, calcific band keratopathy, and stromal infiltrates.

When systemic toxicity is a concern, such as during pregnancy or lactation, systemic absorption can be decreased by occlusion of the nasolacrimal duct for three to five minutes after topical application and removal of excess tears or medication with absorbent material prior to release of pressure.

There is little evidence to suggest that topical ophthalmic medications of any type are teratogenic in humans (Samples and Meyer, 1988).

The *National Registry of Drug-induced Ocular Side Effects* contains the relevant world medical literature, the Food and Drug Administration's reports on adverse ocular effects, and data from 24 countries concerning topically or ocularly administered drugs that have been reported to cause adverse ocular or systemic effects in humans (Fraunfelder, 1990). Most of the clinical cases were recorded since the Registry began in 1974, but the compilation of world literature includes the earliest reports on each drug. This database is available as a service of the American Academy of Ophthalmology; information may be obtained from the Oregon Health Sciences University, 503/494-5686.

EAR DISORDERS

External Otitis

External otitis is an inflammatory condition involving the lining of the external auditory canal and pinnae. Common causative factors are trauma from attempts at cleaning or other manipulation by the patient, environmental factors (eg, high temperature and humidity), accumulation of cerumen, and frequent exposure to water (swimmer's ear) (Strauss and Dierker, 1987). The normal pH of the ear canal is slightly acidic (4.0-5.0); breakdown of this acid mantle with subsequent elevation of the pH into the alkaline range allows pathogenic organisms to overwhelm the normal flora and cause infection. The vast majority of cases of acute external otitis are caused by gram-negative bacteria or fungi. The most common infecting gram-negative bacteria are *Pseudomonas aeruginosa* and species of *Proteus*. *Candida* and *Aspergillus* are the most common causes of otomycosis and account for about 10% of all cases of external otitis. Herpes zoster occasionally produces a viral eruption. Infections may be localized (furuncle) or diffuse, deep or superficial, and may involve any part of the external ear.

The signs and symptoms of external otitis vary according to etiologic agent, chronicity, extension, and specific location and include pruritus, pain, tenderness, erythema, edema, hearing loss, ulceration, granulation tissue, and odoriferous discharge. A feeling of fullness and some reversible hearing loss may result when the ear canals fill with debris and pus. Tinnitus may be present if the ear drum is directly or indirectly involved.

In addition to use of antibacterial and antifungal preparations, the management of external otitis requires removal of purulent secretions, cerumen, foreign bodies, polyps, and granulation tissue.

The local anesthetic, benzocaine 20% in glycerin 1% [Americaine Otic Solution], may relieve the pain that usually accompanies acute external otitis when the tympanic membrane is intact. However, since its absorption from the skin or tympanic membrane generally is poor and depends partially on the preparation, effectiveness is unpredictable. Benzocaine also may cause hypersensitivity reactions and macerate the keratin layer of skin, obscuring important clinical signs and making diagnosis and monitoring of progress difficult. Most important, pain control is secondary to treatment of the underlying infection; pain usually diminishes rapidly following specific therapy.

Topical preparations containing antipyrine alone or with benzocaine are not recommended for external otitis; systemic analgesics (eg, aspirin, acetaminophen, codeine) are preferred to relieve pain.

DRUG SELECTION. Antibacterial and antifungal agents are used empirically to treat external ear infections.

Antibacterial Agents: Several single-entity topical antibacterial preparations appear to be effective for bacterial infections of the external ear.

Acetic acid solutions (2% to 5%) have antibacterial and antifungal activity, particularly against *Pseudomonas aeruginosa, Candida,* and *Aspergillus.* The antimicrobial action of acetic acid reduces inflammation and edema and thus relieves signs and symptoms of external otitis. It is also recommended in the prophylaxis of swimmer's ear (Marcy, 1985). Some authorities prefer the acetic acid 2% and isopropyl alcohol 70% solution [VōSol Otic] because the alcohol provides an additional drying effect. This mixture is especially effective in preventing external otitis in high-risk groups (eg, competitive swimmers, surfers, scuba divers). It is commonly used after each day's aquatic activities have been concluded.

Acetic acid solution is well tolerated, nonsensitizing, and does not produce resistant organisms. It does, however, have an unpleasant vinegar-like odor and can be very painful when applied to the middle ear through a tympanostomy tube or a perforation. If irritation or symptoms of sensitivity to the vehicle occur, the medication should be discontinued.

When the ear canal is swollen, weeping, and inflamed, a solution containing *aluminum acetate* is useful; it has anti-inflammatory, antipruritic, astringent, and limited antibacterial properties and is nonsensitizing.

The aminoglycoside antibiotic, *neomycin*, is effective against *Escherichia, Enterobacter aerogenes,* and most species of *Klebsiella, Salmonella, Shigella,* and *Proteus;* many strains of *Staphylococcus aureus* also are sensitive. It has only weak activity against many strains of *Pseudomonas,* which is the most common bacterial isolate in external otitis. Therefore, topical preparations containing neomycin also contain polymyxin B or colistin (polymyxin E), which have antipseudomonal activity. These preparations are often considered drugs of choice for empiric therapy of acute external otitis (Fairbanks, 1980; Cody et al, 1981), as well as in the treatment of external otitis caused by susceptible organisms.

Neomycin is a topical sensitizer, and cutaneous hypersensitivity reactions may result from its use in the ear. If irritation or sensitivity develops, the drug should be discontinued. The physician must always be alert for these reactions, since they frequently mimic the disease being treated. Such reactions usually can be recognized because the inflammatory process spreads to the tragus, antitragus, and lobule of the ear and the infection worsens rather than improves with continued treatment. Cross-sensitization can occur between neomycin and other aminoglycosides and may prevent the subsequent use of these antibacterial agents.

Another aminoglycoside, *gentamicin*, also may be used in the ear (ophthalmic drop dosage form) when patients do not respond to less toxic therapy.

Aminoglycosides are ototoxic when given systemically, and ototoxicity has been demonstrated in laboratory animals after *topical* application of gentamicin and neomycin to the round window membrane and middle ear. Despite the ototoxic and neurotoxic properties of polymyxin, colistin, and the aminoglycosides, hearing loss due to topical use of these antibiotics, even in the presence of tympanic perforation or tympanostomy tubes, has not been clearly established (Marcy, 1985). Nevertheless, in 1987 the FDA directed all manufacturers of aminoglycosides to revise their labeling to include the statement: "Perforated tympanic membrane is considered a contraindication to the use of any medication in the external ear." In general, these medications are only required for severe complicated infections of the external ear. For further information on antibacterial activity and adverse reactions, see index entry Aminoglycosides.

Polymyxin B and *colistin* are effective against *Pseudomonas aeruginosa, Escherichia,* and some other gram-negative organisms that commonly infect the ear. They lack ototoxic properties and therefore are particularly useful in patients with perforated ear drums or tubes. However, they are not active against other organisms that often cause external otitis, such as *Proteus*, or gram-positive bacteria. A polymyxin is commonly included in otic mixtures that are indicated for external otitis caused by susceptible organisms. Adverse reactions are uncommon, but treatment should be discontinued if irritation or sensitivity occurs.

Chloramphenicol generally is reserved for patients refractory to less toxic therapy. It has a broad spectrum of activity against many organisms; strains of *Staphylococcus aureus, Escherichia coli,* and *Proteus* species are susceptible. It is useful topically to treat resistant superficial infections of the external auditory canal caused by these organisms. Signs of local irritation have been reported in patients sensitive to this preparation. If these occur, chloramphenicol should be discontinued. It should be kept in mind that blood dyscrasias have been associated with systemic use of this drug and have been reported after prolonged therapy with a topical ophthalmic preparation. For further information on antibacterial activity and adverse reactions, see index entry Chloramphenicol.

See Tables 6 and 7 for dosage and preparations.

Infections may be inadequately treated with topical otologic formulations due to the limited number of antibiotics available and the potential adverse effect of an acidic pH on antibacterial activity. Furthermore, discomfort associated with acidic preparations, particularly when the tympanic membrane is perforated, can be severe. Thus, the use of topical ophthalmic antibiotic formulations may be considered in selected patients with external otitis who did not benefit from therapy with otologic preparations (Hoffman and Goldofsky, 1991).

Preparations that contain a corticosteroid in addition to an antibacterial agent may be useful when external otitis is complicated by severe inflammation or allergic dermatitis. However, there is no evidence that the corticosteroid enhances the efficacy of the antibiotic. Topical otic preparations that contain a corticosteroid often contain more than one antibacterial agent. The proposed rationale for these mixtures is that they have a wide antibacterial spectrum that includes both gram-positive and gram-negative organisms. Such fixed-ratio mixtures for topical use have reasonable therapeutic value but may cause the adverse reactions associated with each ingredient. Formulations containing a corticosteroid are contraindicated in patients with herpes simplex, vaccinia, and varicella. See Table 7 for preparations. For further information on actions and adverse reactions of topical adrenal corticosteroids, see index entry Adrenal Corticosteroids, Adverse Reactions, Topical. Topical ophthalmic corticosteroid formulations provide a higher concentration of the active agent than otologic formulations and can be used if the latter preparations are inadequate.

Systemic antibiotics are rarely needed to treat external otitis. Their use should be limited to those occasions when there is a positive identification of the pathogen and resolution with topical medication seems delayed.

Patients who do not respond to the usual treatment, especially the elderly or those with diabetes, should be observed

TABLE 6.
ANTIBACTERIAL AND ANTIFUNGAL AGENTS FOR TOPICAL OTIC THERAPY

Preparation	Concentration	Other Ingredients	Dosage	Container Size
ANTIBACTERIAL AGENTS				
Acetic Acid				
VōSol Otic Solution (Wallace), Generic	2%	Propylene glycol diacetate 3%, isopropyl alcohol 70%	*Adults and children,* four to six drops are instilled every two or three hours.	15 and 30 ml
Otic Domeboro Solution (Miles)	2%	Aluminum acetate (modified Burow's solution)	*Adults and children,* initially, when possible a cotton wick is saturated, inserted into the ear canal, and kept moist for 24 hours; the wick is then removed and five drops are instilled directly into the ear canal three or four times daily.	60 ml
Chloramphenicol	0.5%	Propylene glycol	*Adults and children,* two or three drops are instilled three times daily.	15 ml
Chloromycetin Otic (Parke-Davis)				
Gentamicin Sulfate	0.3%	Benzalkonium (solution)	*Adults and children,* one or two drops instilled every four hours. This preparation should not be used in patients with perforated tympanic membranes or tympanostomy tubes.	5 ml
Garamycin Ophthalmic Solution (Schering)				
m-Cresyl Acetate	25%	Propylene glycol, isopropanol 25%, chlorobutanol 1%, benzyl alcohol 1%, castor oil 5%, acetic acid 0.5%	*Adults and children,* three to five drops three or four times daily. A drug-impregnated ear wick can also be used.	15 ml
Cresylate Solution (Recsei)				
ANTIFUNGAL AGENTS				
Acetic Acid				
VōSol Otic Solution (Wallace), Generic	2%	See above	See above	15 and 30 ml
Amphotericin B	3%	Propylene glycol	*Adults and children,* three to four drops applied to lesions two to four times daily. Duration of therapy depends on patient response.	30 ml
Fungizone Lotion (Squibb)				
Clotrimazole	1%	Polyethylene glycol	*Adults and children,* three or four drops instilled three times daily with weekly or biweekly cleaning of the ear canal.	10 and 30 ml
Lotrimin Solution (Schering)				
Mycelex Solution (Miles)				
m-Cresyl Acetate	25%	See above	See above	15 ml
Cresylate Solution (Recsei)				

TABLE 7. ANTI-INFECTIVE/ANTI-INFLAMMATORY MIXTURES FOR TOPICAL OTIC THERAPY*

Preparation	Anti-infective Agent(s)	Corticosteroid	Other Ingredients	Container Size
Coly-Mycin S Otic with Neomycin and Hydrocortisone Suspension (Parke-Davis)	Colistin sulfate (equivalent to 3 mg base), neomycin sulfate (equivalent to 3.3 mg base/ml), acetic acid	Hydrocortisone acetate 1%	Thonzonium bromide 0.05%, thimerosal 0.002%, polysorbate 80	5 and 10 ml
Cortisporin Otic Solution (Burroughs Wellcome)	Neomycin sulfate (equivalent to 3.5 mg base), polymyxin B sulfate 10,000 units/ml	Hydrocortisone 1%	Cupric sulfate, glycerin, propylene glycol, potassium metabisulfite 0.1%	10 ml
Cortisporin Otic Suspension (Burroughs Wellcome)	Neomycin sulfate (equivalent to 3.5 mg base), polymyxin B sulfate 10,000 units/ml	Hydrocortisone 1%	Cetyl alcohol, propylene glycol, polysorbate 80, thimerosal 0.01%	10 ml
Otic Tridesilon Solution (Miles)	Acetic acid 2%	Desonide 0.05%	Propylene glycol	10 ml
Otobiotic Solution (Schering)	Polymyxin B sulfate 10,000 units/ml	Hydrocortisone 0.5%	Propylene glycol	15 ml
Otocort Solution (Lemmon)	Neomycin sulfate (equivalent to 3.5 mg base), polymyxin B sulfate 10,000 units/ml	Hydrocortisone 1%	Propylene glycol, glycerin, potassium metabisulfite	10 ml
Otocort Suspension (Lemmon)	Neomycin sulfate (equivalent to 3.5 mg base), polymyxin B sulfate 10,000 units/ml	Hydrocortisone 1%	Cetyl alcohol, propylene glycol, polysorbate 80, thimerosal 0.01%	10 ml
Pedi-Otic Suspension (Burroughs Wellcome)	Neomycin sulfate (equivalent to 3.5 mg base), polymyxin B sulfate 10,000 units/ml	Hydrocortisone 1%	Cetyl alcohol, propylene glycol, thimerosal 0.001%	7.5 ml
Pyocidin-Otic Solution (Forest)	Polymyxin B sulfate 10,000 units/ml	Hydrocortisone 0.5%	Propylene glycol	10 ml
VōSol HC Otic Solution (Wallace)	Acetic acid 2%	Hydrocortisone 1%	Propylene glycol diacetate, benzethonium chloride 0.02%	10 ml

* *Dosage: Solutions and Suspensions, Adults, four drops; children, three drops. The preparation is instilled three or four times daily or may be applied on a wick and inserted into the ear canal. The wick should be kept moist and changed every 24 hours.*

more closely, because they may develop malignant or necrotizing external otitis caused by *Pseudomonas aeruginosa* (Scherbenske et al, 1988). This begins in the soft tissues of the external auditory canal, progresses to involve the cartilage and perichondrium of the canal, and eventually leads to osteitis of the temporal bone and base of the skull. If the patient is not given systemic antipseudomonal antibiotics, complications such as facial nerve palsy, multiple cranial nerve palsies, osteomyelitis, and intracranial infection may result (Meyers et al, 1987). Surgical debridement of infected cartilage and bone is often required in addition to systemic antibiotic and hyperbaric oxygen therapy. (Also see index entry Otitis External, Malignant.)

Antifungal Agents: Most fungi, particularly those infecting superficial layers of skin, require a warm, moist, dark area and dead tissue for growth. Mycotic infections also may follow the use of certain antibiotics (eg, aminoglycosides) or prolonged topical application of corticosteroids.

Otomycoses are characterized by the cotton-like appearance of the surface in different colors, pruritus, and desquamation. The white, black, brown, or bluish color identifies the different families of fungi. The precise nature of the fungus may be determined by culture on appropriate media or appearance on a potassium hydroxide-treated slide. *Candida* and *Aspergillus* most often cause otomycosis.

Most important in the management of fungal infections is meticulous, gentle cleansing of the skin of the ear canal; keratolytic agents also may be helpful. After cleansing, an antifungal preparation is instilled or applied to the skin of the ear canal. Treatment should continue for one or two weeks after disappearance of all clinical symptoms and evidence of the disease, because fungal infections often recur. When there is a mixed infection of fungus and bacteria, a preparation containing both antifungal and antibacterial agents is useful.

Amphotericin B [Fungizone] is one of the most effective topical antifungal agents; it is active against a variety of fungi, particularly *Candida. Clotrimazole* [Lotrimin, Mycelex] drops are very effective in the local treatment of refractory fungal external otitis. Other antifungal agents present in some preparations include *acetic acid, cresyl acetate,* and *parachlorometaxylenol. Propylene glycol* is dehydrating to fungi, and this ingredient enhances the effectiveness of antifungal agents. In addition, the low pH of some otic preparations provides an unsuitable medium for growth of many fungi.

See Table 6 for dosage and preparations.

Impacted Cerumen

Cerumen (ear wax) is produced by the apocrine and sebaceous glands in the outer one-third of the external ear canal. Because it is hydrophobic and probably bacteriostatic and fungistatic, the wax provides a protective coating for the external auditory canal. The type of wax produced is genetically determined; individuals in western countries produce moist cerumen, while those in eastern countries produce dry cerumen. Normally, the canal is self-cleaning, but the physiologic mechanism for removing cerumen occasionally becomes inefficient and excessive amounts accumulate. The most frequent causes of breakdown of this mechanism are an individual's misguided attempts to remove wax, narrow tortuous ear canals, or excessive hair growth in the ear. Occlusion of the ear canal by a large mass of cerumen can produce significant conductive hearing loss and predispose to the development of external otitis.

Patients who have chronic difficulty with hard, but not impacted, cerumen should instill light mineral oil (baby oil) or glycerin into the ear canal occasionally to soften the cerumen and promote normal removal.

Professional cleaning may be needed occasionally to remove wax and epithelial debris. This can be performed painlessly and efficiently. Some otologists advise their patients to fill the canal with mineral oil, which is inexpensive and nonallergenic, and plug the ear at night with cotton, which is removed in the morning. This oil treatment is initiated three nights before the office visit for professional cleaning and may be repeated nightly one to three times. In addition to softening the debris, oil separates the dead skin from the living surface, permitting almost the entire mass to be removed gently with a number 5 or 7 French suction tube. Thus, rapid removal of wax and debris with a minimum of discomfort and instrumentation is possible. A nonprescription solution of carbamide peroxide in glycerin [Debrox Drops] (Marion Merrell Dow) also may aid in the removal of excessive or hardened cerumen. It is available in 15 and 30 ml containers. Glycerin softens the wax, and the effervescent oxygen released from peroxide loosens tissue debris. Use of an ear bulb syringe to irrigate the canal gently with water at body temperature or normal saline also may facilitate removal of the cerumen. After treatment, the ear canal should be dried chemically with a solution containing isopropyl alcohol 70% and acetic acid 2% [VōSol Otic]).

If external otitis is present in addition to impacted cerumen, it should be treated as discussed above. The instillation of an antibiotic-steroid preparation to reduce inflammation also may aid in softening the wax.

If impacted cerumen causes little or no inflammation, removal under direct visualization with a ring curette, wire loop, or another suitable instrument is preferable to irrigation. Extreme care should be taken not to traumatize the canal, since this portion of the ear is very sensitive to instrumentation. If the wax cannot be removed mechanically, a wax-softening or, rarely, a cerumenolytic agent may be used, followed by irrigation. One such preparation is a solution of triethanolamine polypeptide oleate-condensate in propylene glycol [Cerumenex] (Purdue Frederick). This solution can cause severe contact dermatitis.

Cited References

Ophthalmic ciprofloxacin. *Med Lett Drugs Ther* 33:52-53, 1991.

Oligosaccharide, peptide, and certain other antibiotic drugs. *Federal Register* 45:57735-57737, 1980.

Prevention of ophthalmia neonatorum. *MMWR* 38:27, (Sept 1) 1989.

Baum J: Appendix 1: Preparation of antibiotics for topical use, in Lamberts DW Potter DE (eds): *Clinical Ophthalmic Pharmacology.* Boston, Little Brown, 1987, 519-522.

Berger ST, et al: Successful medical management of *Acanthamoeba* keratitis. *Am J Ophthalmol* 110:395-403, 1990.

Chandler JW: Controversies in ocular prophylaxis of newborns, editorial. *Arch Ophthalmol* 107:814-815, 1989.

Cobo LM: Antifungals, in Lamberts DW, Potter DE (eds): *Clinical Ophthalmic Pharmacology.* Boston, Little Brown, 1987, 97-106.

Cobo LM: Ocular herpes simplex infections, editorial. *Mayo Clin Proc* 63:1154-1156, 1988.

Cody DTR, et al: *Diseases of the Ear, Nose, and Throat: A Guide to Diagnosis and Management.* Chicago, Year Book Medical Publishers, 1981.

Cohen EJ, et al: Medical and surgical treatment of *Acanthamoeba* keratitis. *Am J Ophthalmol* 103:615-625, 1987.

Cutarelli PE, et al: Topical fluoroquinolones: Antimicrobial activity and *in vitro* corneal epithelial toxicity. *Curr Eye Res* 10:557-563, 1991.

Cykiert RC: Reading and righting a red eye. *Emerg Med* 100-111, (Jan 15) 1989.

Davison CR, et al: Conjunctival necrosis after administration of topical fortified aminoglycosides. *Am J Ophthalmol* 111:690-693, 1991.

Didier ES, et al: Isolation and characterization of a new human microsporidian, *Encephalitozoon hellem* (n. sp.), from three AIDS patients with keratoconjunctivitis. *J Infect Dis* 163:617-621, 1991.

Donshik P: Evaluating the red eye. *Infect Med* 3:269-272, 282-286, 1986.

Driebe WT Jr, et al: *Acanthamoeba* keratitis: Potential role for topical clotrimazole in combination chemotherapy. *Arch Ophthalmol* 106:1196-1201, 1988.

Elkington AR, Khaw PT: The red eye. *BMJ* 296:1720-1724, 1988.

Fairbanks DNF: Otic topical agents. *Otolaryngol Head Neck Surg* 88:327-331, 1980.

Fisher MC: Conjunctivitis in children. *Pediatr Clin North Am* 34:1447-1456, 1987.

Forster RK, et al: Management of infectious endophthalmitis. *Ophthalmology* 87:313-318, 1980.

Foster CS: Miconazole therapy for keratomycosis. *Am J Ophthalmol* 91:622-629, 1981.

Fraunfelder FT: National Registry of Drug-induced Ocular Side Effects. *Am J Ophthalmol* 110:426, 1990.

Fraunfelder FT, Meyer SM: Side effects of drugs, in Reinecke RD (ed): *Ophthalmology Annual*. Norwalk, Conn, Appleton-Century-Crofts, 1985, vol 1, 179-191.

Gardner SK: Ocular drug penetration and pharmacokinetic principles, in Lamberts DW, Potter DE (eds): *Clinical Ophthalmic Pharmacology*. Boston, Little Brown, 1987, 1-52.

Gigliotti F, et al: Efficacy of topical antibiotic therapy in acute conjunctivitis in children. *J Pediatr* 104:623-626, 1984.

Glasser DB, Hyndiuk RA: Antibiotics, in Lamberts DW, Potter DE (eds): *Clinical Ophthalmic Pharmacology*. Boston, Little Brown, 1987, 53-95.

Glasser DB, et al: Loading doses and extended dosing intervals in topical gentamicin therapy. *Am J Ophthalmol* 99:329-333, 1985.

Goldschmidt RH, Dong BJ: Current report—HIV: Treatment of AIDS and HIV-related conditions. *J Am Board Fam Pract* 4:178-191, (May-June) 1991.

Hammerschlag MR, et al: Erythromycin ointment for ocular prophylaxis of neonatal chlamydial infection. *JAMA* 244:2291-2293, 1980.

Hammerschlag MR, et al: Efficacy of neonatal ocular prophylaxis for the prevention of chlamydial and gonococcal conjunctivitis. *N Engl J Med* 320:769-772, 1989.

Hoffman RA, Goldofsky E: Topical ophthalmologics in otology. *Ear Nose Throat J* 70:201-205, 1991.

Høvding G: Comparison between acyclovir and trifluorothymidine ophthalmic ointment in the treatment of epithelial dendritic keratitis: A double blind, randomized parallel group trial. *Acta Ophthalmol* 67:51-54, 1989.

Kastl PR, et al: Placebo-controlled, double-blind evaluation of the efficacy and safety of yellow mercuric oxide in suppression of eyelid infections. *Ann Ophthalmol* 19:376-379, 1987.

Kervick GN, et al: Antibiotic therapy for *Bacillus* species infections. *Am J Ophthalmol* 110:683-687, 1990.

Laga M, et al: Prophylaxis of gonococcal and chlamydial ophthalmia neonatorum: Comparison of silver nitrate and tetracycline. *N Engl J Med* 318:653-657, 1988.

Lass JH: Antivirals, in Lamberts DW, Potter DE (eds): *Clinical Ophthalmic Pharmacology*. Boston, Little Brown, 1987, 107-155.

Leibowitz HM: Antibacterial effectiveness of ciprofloxacin 0.3% ophthalmic solution in the treatment of bacterial conjunctivitis. *Am J Ophthalmol* 112 (suppl):29S-33S, 1991 A.

Leibowitz HM: Clinical evaluation of ciprofloxacin 0.3% ophthalmic solution for treatment of bacterial keratitis. *Am J Ophthalmol* 112:34S-47S, 1991 B.

Liesegang TJ: Ocular herpes simplex infection: Pathogenesis and current therapy. *Mayo Clin Proc* 63:1092-1105, 1988.

Limberg MB: A review of bacterial keratitis and bacterial conjunctivitis. *Am J Ophthalmol* 112 (suppl):2S-9S, 1991.

Lohr JA, et al: Comparison of three topical antimicrobials for acute bacterial conjunctivitis. *Pediatr Infect Dis J* 7:626-629, 1988.

Marcy SM: Infections of the external ear. *Pediatr Infect Dis* 4:192-201, 1985.

Maske R, et al: Management of bacterial corneal ulcers. *Br J Ophthalmol* 70:199-201, 1986.

McDonnell PJ: How do general practitioners manage eye disease in the community? *Br J Ophthalmol* 72:733-736, 1988.

Meyers BR, et al: Malignant external otitis: Comparison of monotherapy vs combination therapy. *Arch Otolaryngol Head Neck Surg* 113:974-978, 1987.

Mohan M, et al: Topical silver sulphadiazine—new drug for ocular keratomycosis. *Br J Ophthalmol* 72:192-195, 1988.

Moore MB: *Acanthamoeba* keratitis, editorial. *Arch Ophthalmol* 106:1181-1183, 1988.

Moore MB, McCulley JP: Acanthamoeba keratitis associated with contact lenses: Six consecutive cases of successful management. *Br J Ophthalmol* 73:271-275, 1989.

Moore MB, et al: *Acanthamoeba* keratitis: A growing problem in soft and hard contact lens wearers. *Ophthalmology* 94:1654-1661, 1987.

Musch DC, et al: Demographic and predisposing factors in corneal ulceration. *Arch Ophthalmol* 101:1545-1548, 1983.

O'Day DM: Corticosteroids: An unresolved debate, editorial. *Ophthalmology* 98:845-846, 1991.

Pavan-Langston D: Diagnosis and therapy of common eye infections: Bacterial, viral, fungal. *Compr Ther* 9:33-42, (May) 1983.

Pflugfelder SC, et al: Exogenous fungal endophthalmitis. *Ophthalmology* 95:19-30, 1988.

Rettig PJ, et al: Postnatal prophylaxis of chlamydial conjunctivitis, letter. *JAMA* 246:2321-2322, 1981.

Richards DM, et al: Acyclovir: Review of its pharmacodynamic properties and therapeutic efficacy. *Drugs* 26:378-438, 1983.

Samples JR, Meyer SM: Use of ophthalmic medications in pregnant and nursing women. *Am J Ophthalmol* 106:616-623, 1988.

Scherbenske JM, et al: Acute pseudomonas infection of the external ear (malignant external otitis). *J Dermatol Surg Oncol* 14:165-169, 1988.

Smythe D, et al: The management of chalazion: A survey of Ontario ophthalmologists. *Can J Ophthalmol* 25:252-255, 1990.

Stehr-Green JK, et al: Epidemiology of *Acanthamoeba* keratitis in the United States. *Am J Ophthalmol* 107:331-336, 1989.

Steinert RF: Current therapy for bacterial keratitis and bacterial conjunctivitis. *Am J Ophthalmol* 112:10S-14S, 1991.

Stenberg K, Mårdh P-A: Chlamydial conjunctivitis in neonates and adults: History, clinical findings and follow-up. *Acta Ophthalmol* 68:651-657, 1990.

Stern GA: Update on the medical management of corneal and external eye diseases, corneal transplantation, and keratorefractive surgery. *Ophthalmology* 95:842-854, 1988.

Stern GA, Buttross M: Use of corticosteroids in combination with antimicrobial drugs in the treatment of infectious corneal disease. *Ophthalmology* 98:847-853, 1991.

Stratton CW: Common infections of the eye. *Infect Dis Newslett* 7:33-36, (May) 1988.

Strauss MB, Dierker RL: Otitis externa associated with aquatic activities (swimmer's ear). *Clin Dermatol* 5:103-111, 1987.

Vajpayee RB, et al: Ocular atopy and mycotic keratitis. *Ann Ophthalmol* 22:369-372, 1990.

Wiens JJ, Jackson WB: *Acanthamoeba* keratitis: Update. *Can J Ophthalmol* 23:107-110, 1988.

Drugs Used for Superficial Infections of the Skin and Mucous Membranes

73

BACTERIAL INFECTIONS

Pyodermas

Rosacea

Burn Infections

FUNGAL INFECTIONS

Dermatophytosis

Tinea Versicolor

Candidiasis

Cutaneous Candidiasis

Candidiasis Affecting Mucous Membranes

Oropharyngeal Candidiasis

Vaginal Candidiasis

VIRAL INFECTIONS

Warts

BACTERIAL INFECTIONS

Pyodermas

Skin infections (pyodermas) caused by bacteria are classified as primary or as secondary when they occur in conjunction with skin disorders, such as insect, animal, or human bites; burns; breaks in the skin; defects in leukocyte function; excessive skin hydration; presence of foreign bodies; other dermatoses; and fungal or viral infections. The most common serious secondary pyodermas are observed in patients with second- or third-degree burns, skin ulcers, eczematous dermatitis, or intertrigo and in diabetic, debilitated, or immunocompromised patients.

PATHOGENESIS. Group A beta-hemolytic *Streptococcus* (*S. pyogenes*) and coagulase-positive *Staphylococcus aureus* are the most common causative organisms (Blumer et al, 1987; Hirschmann, 1988; Feingold et al, 1989; Scott, 1989; Aly, 1990). Coagulase-negative *Staphylococcus epidermidis* and *S. hominis* are isolated from about 10% of all pyodermas and about one-half of these are a pure culture. Gram-negative pathogens, both aerobic and anaerobic, are much less common etiologic agents, but they may cause some secondary pyodermas (eg, infected burns, infected dermal stasis ulcers in the elderly). Erythrasma is caused by the gram-positive organism, *Corynebacterium minutissimum*.

The most common primary pyodermas include impetigo, ecthyma, erysipelas, folliculitis, furunculosis, carbuncles, and cellulitis. Evidence continues to accumulate that the predominant organism of the common or crusted form of nonbullous impetigo is *Staphylococcus aureus* (Britton et al, 1990; Demidovich et al, 1990; Grossman and Rasmussen, 1991; Barnett and Frieden, 1992). Other clinicians support the historical concept that streptococci are the predominant causative organisms but only early in the disease course. Staphylococci predominate in cultures of older lesions, which suggests secondary colonization of skin sites already traumatized by infection (Aly, 1990). The bullous form of superficial impetigo is caused by the local action of *S. aureus*-elaborated epidermolytic toxins A and B (exfoliatin), which produce dyshesion of keratinocytes along the cell layers of the epidermis (Resnick, 1992).

Ecthyma (a deeper, ulcerative form of impetigo) and erysipelas (a superficial form of cellulitis) are caused by Group A β-hemolytic streptococci. Folliculitis, furunculosis, and carbuncles are caused by staphylococci. Cellulitis may be produced by either gram-positive or gram-negative bacteria. Scarlatiniform rashes associated with phage group I *S. aureus* infection have been reported. These bacteria produce an epidermolytic toxin that is distinct from that of phage group II strains (eg, staphylococcal scalded skin syndrome) but has some common features. Hidradenitis suppurativa is a chronic suppurative disease of the apocrine glands that begins with obstruction of the ducts. Staphylococci, streptococci, and gram-negative rods have been identified as causative.

DRUG SELECTION. The general management and topical antibiotic therapy for uncomplicated bacterial pyodermas are presented in this section. For information on pyodermas associated with burns, see the discussion on burn therapy in this chapter. Systemic therapy for skin infections is discussed elsewhere; see index entry Pyodermas, Antimicrobial Treatment.

Warm moist compresses or soaks and antimicrobial soaps for wound cleansing, debridement, and promotion of drainage are useful adjuncts to drug therapy in pyodermas.

Older conventional topical antibiotics are primarily used for the prevention of infection in superficial wounds and, along with local cleansing, may be sufficient for the treatment of uncomplicated superficial pyodermas, especially when the patient or family members are able to perform gentle debridement of the thick crusts prior to application of the antibiotic.

Topical rather than systemic antibiotic therapy more often leads to the emergence of resistance by encouraging the persistence, transfer, and selection of plasmids between strains of organisms; therefore, it has been recommended that parenteral antibiotics that are used for serious systemic infections not be used topically (Noble, 1990). The topical antibiotics that are seldom given systemically are widely used in uncomplicated pyodermas, although comparative data on efficacy are limited. The antibiotics not available for systemic administration include neomycin [Myciguent] and mupirocin [Bactroban]; bacitracin and polymyxin B are rarely used systemically. Tetracycline [Achromycin] is used both topically and systemically.

Neomycin has the broadest spectrum of activity and is effective against both gram-positive and gram-negative organisms. Streptococci and other gram-positive organisms are especially susceptible to bacitracin. Many gram-negative organisms, except *Proteus* and *Serratia*, are susceptible to polymyxin B.

Topical antibiotics that are effective against gram-positive organisms are usually satisfactory for erythrasma.

Because culturing of skin infections often reveals the presence of multiple organisms, mixtures of topical antibiotics frequently are used to improve the spectrum of antibacterial activity.

Coagulase-negative staphylococci are the most common causative organisms in skin infections associated with the use of prosthetic materials in immunocompromised patients. Results of a study that compared a single application of a number of antiseptics (povidone-iodine 10%, aqueous iodine 2%, tincture of iodine 2%, ethanol 70%, chlorhexidine-ethanol 0.5%), mupirocin ointment, and an antibiotic ointment (neomycin, bacitracin, and polymyxin) showed that only the latter eradicated these organisms from all layers of the skin and prevented repopulation over a 12- to 24-hour period (Hendley and Ashe, 1991).

Mupirocin, which is unrelated chemically to other available topical antibiotics (Dobson, 1990), is effective in primary and secondary skin infections (Rumsfield et al, 1986; Ward and Campoli-Richards, 1986; Leyden, 1987; Parenti et al, 1987; *Med Lett Drugs Ther*, 1988). It is the only topical agent that has been effective in uncomplicated impetigo due to staphylococci (especially methicillin-resistant) or streptococci. Results of a few controlled studies indicate that topical mupirocin is as safe and effective as oral erythromycin (Mertz el al, 1989; McLinn, 1990). Systemic preparations of mupirocin probably will not be marketed because this antibiotic is metabolized too rapidly.

Gentamicin cream or ointment [Garamycin] has a more limited spectrum of activity and is available only on prescription. It is useful occasionally for *Pseudomonas* infections unresponsive to poorly absorbed topical antibiotics (eg, limited infection in burns or venous stasis ulcers).

Clioquinol (iodochlorhydroxyquin) [Vioform] is not an antibiotic, and it has only limited antibacterial and antifungal activity. Single-entity nonprescription preparations are available in cream and ointment forms; a systemic preparation is not marketed. Clioquinol also is used occasionally in combination with a corticosteroid [Hysone, Vioform-Hydrocortisone] in localized bacterial infections and dermatophytoses associated with certain inflammatory skin conditions. In view of its limited efficacy, extensive absorption, and potential toxicity, the benefit-risk ratio of topical clioquinol is unfavorable, especially in children (see the evaluation in the section on Fungal Infections).

Furuncles, carbuncles, or abscesses with surrounding cellulitis caused by staphylococci usually require a systemic antibiotic. Systemic administration also is usually preferred for extensive streptococcal skin infections (eg, ecthyma, erysipelas) (Odom, 1989). When used adjunctively with systemic antibiotics, topical agents can help to reduce contagion. However, a study conducted in mice to evaluate prophylactic antibacterial therapy following surgery concluded that the additive effect of combined topical and systemic antibiotic therapy is useful only when contamination is severe or extensive (Scher and Peoples, 1991). Surgical incision and drainage are necessary for purulent furuncles and carbuncles that have abscessed.

Special formulations of erythromycin [A/T/S, EryDerm, Erugel, Erymax, Erycette, Staticin], tetracycline [Topicycline, T-Stat], meclocycline sulfosalicylate [Meclan], and clindamycin [Cleocin T] are used mainly in acne vulgaris to suppress *Propionibacterium acnes*, thereby reducing the inflammatory response to chemotactic factors derived from fatty acids produced by *P. acnes*. These preparations are not used for pyodermas (see index entry Acne Vulgaris).

Drug Evaluations

BACITRACIN
[Baciguent]

ACTIONS AND USES. This polypeptide antibiotic is rarely used systemically. Topical preparations contain bacitracin alone or the zinc salt in combination with other poorly absorbed antibiotics and/or corticosteroids.

Bacitracin is bactericidal against gram-positive organisms, including the most common skin pathogens, staphylococci and streptococci. It is inactive against most gram-negative organisms, including *Pseudomonas.* Acquired bacterial resistance is rare.

Topical bacitracin is beneficial in limited uncomplicated primary pyodermas (eg, superficial folliculitis) and limited secondary pyodermas not caused by gram-negative organisms. It is used with systemic antibiotics in more extensive gram-positive pyodermas to control infection, promote healing, and reduce contagion locally.

ADVERSE REACTIONS AND PRECAUTIONS. When given systemically, hypersensitivity reactions, usually manifested as allergic dermatitis (urticaria) or conjunctivitis, may be severe. These reactions are rare when bacitracin is applied topically, but anaphylaxis has been reported.

Bacitracin sensitization may be increasing in frequency. This finding may be more apparent than real because patch tests for bacitracin sensitivity designated in the past as negative at 48 hours often do not become positive until 96 hours (current recommendation) (Katz and Fisher, 1987).

Bacitracin is not absorbed significantly from the skin; therefore, it may be used during pregnancy and lactation.

DOSAGE AND PREPARATIONS.

Topical: *Adults and children*, the ointment is applied to lesions one to three times daily.

Generic. Ointment 500 units/g in 15 and 30 g containers (nonprescription).

Baciguent (Roberts). Ointment 500 units/g in 15 and 30 g containers (nonprescription).

MUPIROCIN
[Bactroban]

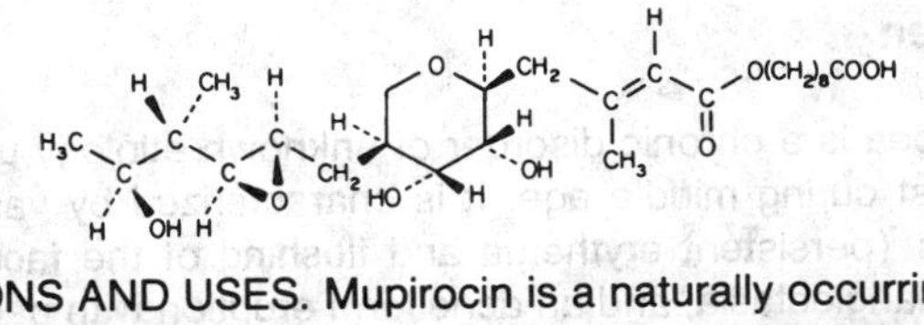

ACTIONS AND USES. Mupirocin is a naturally occurring antibiotic whose mechanism of action differs from that of other poorly absorbed topical antibiotics. Mupirocin inhibits protein and RNA synthesis in *S. aureus* by suppressing the activity of bacterial isoleucyl-t-RNA synthetase, but it has little affinity for the comparable mammalian synthetase. Activity is pH-dependent; acidity enhances effectiveness. It is not likely that this topical antibiotic will be marketed for systemic use because it is metabolized too rapidly.

Most staphylococci (including *S. epidermidis* and methicillin-resistant staphylococci) and streptococci (except for *S. faecalis*) are sensitive to mupirocin. A few gram-negative organisms are susceptible (eg, *Escherichia coli, Haemophilus influenzae, Neisseria meningitidis, N. gonorrhoeae*). Mupirocin has little activity against *Chlamydia*, fungi, and organisms constituting normal skin flora. The drug is bactericidal at concentrations attained when it is applied locally as a 2% ointment with polyethylene glycol as the vehicle; the vehicle also has some antibacterial activity.

Mupirocin is used topically for the treatment of impetigo due to *Staphylococcus aureus* and *Streptococcus pyogenes.* It is effective in primary as well as many types of secondary skin infections when compared to placebo (Rumsfield et al, 1986; Pappa, 1987; Ward and Campoli-Richards, 1986; Leyden, 1987; Parenti et al, 1987). Results of clinical studies suggest that the effectiveness of topical mupirocin in primary and secondary skin infections may in some circumstances be equal to that of a number of orally administered antibiotics, including erythromycin, dicloxacillin, cloxacillin, and amoxicillin, or a combination of topically applied poorly absorbed antibiotics *(Med Lett Drugs Ther,* 1988; Parenti et al, 1987; Arredondo, 1987; Goldfarb et al, 1988; Mertz et al, 1989; Britton et al, 1990; McLinn, 1990). However, when the infection is extensive, cellulitis is present, or systemic effects of infection occur, systemic antibiotic therapy is recommended.

Because mupirocin has a novel chemical structure, it is anticipated that little cross resistance will occur between it and other poorly absorbed topical and systemic antibiotics used to treat skin infections, and studies appear to support this assumption. Unfortunately, development of resistance to mupirocin itself by *S. aureus* has been noted with prolonged administration (months) (Rahman et al, 1989; Cookson, 1990).

A preparation of mupirocin in soft paraffin is being evaluated in clinical trials for eradication of nasal carriage of *S. aureus* (Aly and Bayles, 1991).

ADVERSE REACTIONS AND PRECAUTIONS. Mupirocin is well tolerated; only a few individuals have had to discontinue the drug because of local adverse reactions. Burning, stinging, contact dermatitis, pruritus, xerosis, and erythema have been observed in no more than 2% of patients in most studies. No systemic signs or symptoms or alterations of laboratory values have been attributed to the drug. Photosensitivity and contact sensitization have not been reported. In view of mupirocin's lack of systemic absorption, drug interactions are not anticipated.

Because of the potential hazard of nephrotoxicity due to the polyethylene glycol content of the vehicle, care should be exercised if this product is used in premature neonates or to treat extensive burns, trophic ulceration, and other extensive conditions in which absorption of large quantities of polyethylene glycol is possible.

Treatment should be discontinued if a reaction suggesting sensitivity or chemical irritation occurs.

PREGNANCY AND LACTATION. Reproduction studies in rats and rabbits using systemic doses up to 100 times those employed topically in humans have revealed no evidence of impaired fertility or harm to the fetus. No well-controlled studies in pregnant women are available. Mupirocin is classified in FDA pregnancy Category B.

PHARMACOKINETICS. Following topical application to human forearm skin with occlusion for 24 hours, detectable amounts of mupirocin were not found in blood, urine, or feces. When administered systemically, mupirocin (pseudomonic acid A) is 95% bound to serum protein and is rapidly converted to monic acid, an inactive metabolite (Leyden, 1987).

DOSAGE AND PREPARATIONS.

Topical: A small amount of ointment is applied to the affected area three times daily. The area may be covered with a gauze dressing if desired. Patients who do not respond within three to five days should be re-evaluated.

Bactroban (SmithKline Beecham). Ointment 2% in 1, 15, and 30 g containers.

NEOMYCIN SULFATE
[Myciguent]

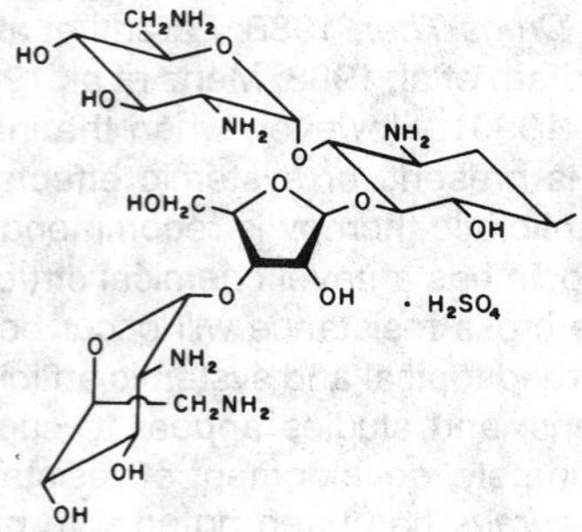

USES. This broad spectrum aminoglycoside antibacterial agent is too toxic for parenteral use and is poorly absorbed orally. Therefore, neomycin is used only topically on the skin alone or in combination with other poorly absorbed antibiotics and/or corticosteroids.

Neomycin may be beneficial when used alone in limited uncomplicated primary pyodermas (eg, superficial folliculitis) and limited secondary pyodermas (eg, infected dermal ulcers, intertrigo), but hypersensitivity is a concern (see below). Infections caused by staphylococci are most responsive. Systemic antibiotics are preferred by most physicians for more extensive pyodermas.

ADVERSE REACTIONS AND PRECAUTIONS. In one investigational study, hypersensitivity to topical neomycin 20% (a 3.5 mg/g concentration of neomycin sulfate as the base is available commercially) occurred in 3.7% to 60% of individuals with contact dermatitis or chronically damaged skin (eg, stasis dermatitis). However, the incidence was only about 1% after application to undamaged skin if treatment was limited to seven days. Cross sensitivity with other aminoglycoside antibiotics may occur and limit their use. Patch tests utilizing 20% neomycin in petrolatum should be read at 48 and 96 hours.

Neomycin is not absorbed significantly from the skin; therefore, it may be used during pregnancy and lactation.

DOSAGE AND PREPARATIONS.

Topical: An appropriate preparation is applied one to three times daily.

Generic. Ointment 5 mg/g in 15 and 30 g containers (nonprescription).

Myciguent (Roberts). Cream 5 mg (equivalent to 3.5 mg of base)/g in 15 g containers; ointment 5 mg (equivalent to 3.5 mg of base)/g in 15 and 30 g containers (nonprescription).

POLYMYXIN B SULFATE

USES. This cationic surface-active polypeptide antibiotic is rarely used systemically. Polymyxin B is not available as a single-entity preparation for topical application because its spectrum of action is limited to gram-negative organisms, including *Pseudomonas*, that are less commonly involved in pyodermas. It is combined with other poorly absorbed antibiotics and/or corticosteroids to treat limited uncomplicated primary pyodermas (eg, superficial folliculitis) and secondary pyodermas; such preparations also may be used with systemic antibiotics in more extensive pyodermas to control infection, promote healing, and reduce contagion locally. Bacterial resistance to polymyxin B develops slowly.

ADVERSE REACTIONS AND PRECAUTIONS. Although uncommon, hypersensitivity is the most frequent adverse reaction to topical polymyxin B. Patch tests should be read at 48 and 96 hours. Polymyxin is not absorbed significantly from the skin; therefore, it may be used during pregnancy and lactation.

PREPARATIONS. Single-entity preparations are not available. See following listing for mixtures (all forms nonprescription).

BACITRACIN AND POLYMYXIN B:
Generic. Ointment.
Polysporin (Burroughs Wellcome). Powder, aerosol, and ointment.

BACITRACIN, POLYMYXIN B, AND NEOMYCIN:
Mycitracin Ointment (Upjohn), ***Neosporin Ointment*** (Burroughs Wellcome), ***N-B-P.*** (Forest), ***Generic***. Ointment.

NEOMYCIN AND POLYMYXIN B:
Neosporin Cream (Burroughs Wellcome).

OXYTETRACYCLINE AND POLYMYXIN B:
Terramycin with Polymyxin B Powder (Leeming).

Rosacea

Rosacea is a chronic disorder of unknown etiology usually seen first during middle age. It is characterized by vascular changes (persistent erythema and flushing of the face and neck; telangiectasia; and an acneiform eruption with papules, pustules, cysts, and sebaceous gland hyperplasia, especially on the nose [rhinophyma]) (Arndt, 1989). Unlike acne vulgaris, sebum excretion does not correlate with sebaceous gland hyperplasia.

Except for the telangiectasia, at least 50% of the signs and symptoms of rosacea respond to systemic antibiotics, especially tetracycline; erythromycin, ampicillin, and metronidazole also are effective. A topical preparation of metronidazole

[MetroGel] is available. Limited data suggest that it may have slightly less efficacy than oral tetracycline; however, the frequency and speed of relapse upon discontinuation of therapy may be lower with topical metronidazole (Hirschmann, 1988). Because of metronidazole's effectiveness, it is assumed that anaerobic bacteria may have a contributory or causative role in the pathogenesis of rosacea.

Drug Evaluation

METRONIDAZOLE
[MetroGel]

For chemical formula, see index entry Metronidazole, In Protozoal Infections.

ACTIONS AND USES. Metronidazole is widely used systematically (see index entry Metronidazole). The topical form was developed originally as an orphan drug for the treatment of rosacea. Its mechanism of action in rosacea is unknown, but an anti-inflammatory or antibacterial action against anaerobic bacteria is proposed. Inflammatory erythema, papules, pustules, cysts, and sebaceous gland hyperplasia associated with rosacea may respond to metronidazole; however, the telangiectasia is not affected.

ADVERSE REACTIONS AND PRECAUTIONS. Since serum concentrations of metronidazole are minimal with topical application, the side effects and drug interactions associated with systemically administered metronidazole should be minimized with this preparation, and they have not been reported.

Transient redness, mild dryness, burning, and skin irritation have been observed (incidence, less than 2%). Contact with the eyes should be avoided, because tearing has been reported. The drug is contraindicated in individuals with a history of hypersensitivity to metronidazole or parabens, which are present in the formulation.

Data on the use of topical metronidazole in pregnant or lactating patients are limited. The topical form of metronidazole is classified in FDA Pregnancy Category B.

DOSAGE AND PREPARATIONS.
Topical: *Adults,* a thin film of the gel is applied twice daily to affected areas after washing. If effective, a response should be observed within three weeks.

MetroGel (Curatek). Gel 0.75% in 30 g containers.

Burn Infections

Burns are classified on the basis of severity (ie, superficial partial thickness, deep partial thickness, full thickness); extent (percentage of body surface area); etiology (ie, thermal, electrical, chemical); and area of involvement (eg, perineal, facial). The infected burn wound represents a unique therapeutic problem (Boswick, 1987). Since blood supply to the injured skin is usually compromised, topical administration is necessary to distribute the antimicrobial compound at the involved site.

The principal gram-positive bacteria isolated from infected burn wounds are staphylococci (predominant) and beta-hemolytic streptococci. The most common gram-negative organisms are *Pseudomonas aeruginosa* and *Escherichia coli*; *Klebsiella, Enterobacter, Proteus, Providencia*, and *Serratia* also may be causative organisms. Fungi, especially *Candida albicans*, are present in 10% to 15% of infected burns (Grube et al, 1988).

MANAGEMENT. Nondrug procedures are helpful in the general management of burns (Jacoby, 1984; Luterman et al, 1986; Peate, 1992; Robson et al, 1992). These include prompt washing with clean, cool water; avoidance of bacterial contamination; debridement under strict aseptic conditions; avoidance of alcohol-based, scented, deodorant soaps to minimize irritation and sensitization; fluid and electrolyte replacement; and metabolic and nutritional management (Molnar and Burke, 1984) when indicated. When necessary, medications for pain and tetanus prophylaxis are indicated. Oxygen may be necessary to support respiratory function. Additional special considerations are important for selected pediatric (Coren, 1987; Stuart et al, 1987) and geriatric patients (Hammond and Ward, 1991).

Use of prophylactic topical antibacterial therapy is controversial. Some clinicians do not recommend topical antibacterial preparations in burns smaller than 20% of total body surface area when sepsis is not a threat. Most clinicians feel that topical antibacterials are indicated for prophylaxis to maintain low bacterial tissue counts pending debridement and wound closure, especially when burns increase the risk of infection, as in (1) burns of the hands, feet, or perineum; (2) burns in poor-risk patients (eg, the elderly, children, diabetics, alcoholics, patients with congestive heart failure, those receiving corticosteroid therapy); (3) burns complicated by fractures or soft tissue injury; (4) electrical burns; (5) inhalation burns; (6) partial-thickness burns of more than 15% (adults) or 10% (children) or full-thickness burns over more than 2% to 3% of the body surface area. Many physicians recommend topical antibacterial agents for heavily colonized but not obviously infected burns, and most physicians recommend them for infected burns. If bacteremia is present or anticipated, systemic antibiotic therapy may be necessary (see index entry Burns). The use of Biobrane, a semisynthetic dressing material, may be a useful alternative (Gerding et al, 1990) in more superficial, noncontaminated wounds that do not have complex anatomic contours (eg, genitalia). Early wound closure may be associated with lower rates of infection and mortality (Wolfe et al, 1983; Demling, 1985).

DRUG SELECTION FOR TOPICAL APPLICATION. Topical preparations of silver sulfadiazine [SSD, SSD AF, Silvadene], mafenide [Sulfamylon], povidone-iodine [ACU-dyne, Betadine, Efodine, Pharmadine, Polydine], nitrofurazone [Furacin], silver nitrate, and gentamicin [Garamycin] are available for the prevention and treatment of infected burns (MacMillan, 1980; Luterman et al, 1986). Silver sulfadiazine is widely used for severe extensive burns. It does not penetrate the eschar as well as mafenide, but it does not produce the often severe pain on application or the occasional acid-base disturbances that are characteristic of the latter drug. Although nitrofurazone is bactericidal for many gram-positive organisms (especially staphylococci) present in surface infections, strains of *Pseudomonas* and other gram-negative organisms often are not sufficiently susceptible. Povidone-iodine may cause mild pain on application and it does not penetrate eschar as well as mafenide.

Gentamicin is recommended only when the causative organism is *Pseudomonas* or other sensitive gram-negative species resistant to silver sulfadiazine and mafenide, because resistance to gram-negative organisms develops rapidly in the burn wound and significant systemic absorption may produce nephrotoxicity and/or ototoxicity. Although silver nitrate solution is economical and effective, the frequent applications required to minimize drying, pain on application, staining, and occasional hyponatremia and hyperchloremic acidosis have limited its use.

Nystatin is often combined with topical antibacterials to prevent *Candida* infections in burn patients.

For systemic therapy for infected burns, see index entry Burns, Infection.

Drug Evaluations

SILVER SULFADIAZINE

[SSD, SSD AF, Silvadene]

Ag^+ H_2N–C_6H_4–SO_2N^-–(pyrimidinyl)

ACTIONS AND USES. This topical sulfonamide is the drug of choice to treat infected burn wounds and grafts and to prevent burn wound infections in selected patients at high risk (Peate, 1992). Its use in the management of soft tissue wound infections is promising (Smoot and Kucan, 1987). Silver sulfadiazine is effective against a wide variety of gram-positive and gram-negative organisms, as well as *Candida*. Some strains of *Klebsiella, Enterobacter*, staphylococci, and *Pseudomonas* are resistant. The bactericidal action of silver sulfadiazine does not appear to be entirely attributable to the sulfonamide content; silver also has bacteriostatic properties (Fox, 1983).

ADVERSE REACTIONS AND PRECAUTIONS. Silver sulfadiazine does not cause electrolyte disturbances, even after prolonged contact with the burned area. Application is usually painless, unlike that of mafenide, although a burning sensation, rash, and pruritus have been reported in approximately 2.5%, 0.2%, and 0.1% of patients, respectively. Leukopenia in the peripheral circulation is transient and does not usually require discontinuation of silver sulfadiazine.

Significant quantities of sulfadiazine can be absorbed following prolonged treatment of extensive burns. Accordingly, all adverse reactions attributable to systemic sulfonamides may occur (see index entry Sulfonamides). Monitoring of serum levels during prolonged treatment is not necessary except, possibly, in patients with extensive burn wounds or impaired renal or hepatic function. Individuals with a deficiency of glucose 6-phosphate dehydrogenase may develop hemolysis on exposure to silver sulfadiazine.

Silver sulfadiazine is classified in FDA Pregnancy Category B. This agent should not be used near term, on premature infants, or on newborns during the first two months of life to avoid kernicterus.

Cross sensitivity between silver sulfadiazine and other sulfonamides is possible. Thus, silver sulfadiazine should be used cautiously in patients who have a history of sulfonamide sensitivity.

DOSAGE AND PREPARATIONS.

Topical: Topical therapy should begin as soon as possible. Following cleansing and debridement of the wound, the cream is applied with a sterile gloved hand to a thickness of 1 to 3 mm; all interstices and crevices of the irregular burn surface should be covered. Because of the drug's low solubility, the antimicrobial action persists for many hours; thus, once-daily application is usually adequate, although some patients may require twice-daily application. Silver sulfadiazine should be applied more frequently to burned areas from which the cream might be removed by movement of the patient. Therapy is continued until satisfactory healing has occurred or the burn site is ready for grafting.

Although dressings are unnecessary, a layer of fine mesh gauze covered with a roller bandage will help ensure contact of the drug with the wound and is more comfortable than no dressing to most patients.

Silver sulfadiazine softens eschar but, by decreasing local bacterial action, it decreases its autolysis. Therefore, hydrotherapy and debridement should be performed daily for removal of eschar, especially in patients with full-thickness burns.

SSD, SSD AF (Boots). Cream (water-miscible) 10 mg/g with cetyl alcohol in 25, 50, 85, 400, and 1,000 g containers (***SSD***) and without cetyl alcohol in 50, 400, and 1,000 g containers (***SSD AF***).

Silvadene (Marion Merrell Dow). Cream (water-miscible) 10 mg/g in 20, 50, 85, 400, and 1,000 g containers.

MAFENIDE ACETATE

[Sulfamylon]

$H_3\overset{+}{N}CH_2$–C_6H_4–SO_2NH_2 CH_3COO^-

ACTIONS AND USES. Mafenide is not a true sulfonamide chemically but has essentially the same antibacterial spectrum as silver sulfadiazine and is particularly effective against susceptible strains of *Pseudomonas aeruginosa*. Its action, unlike that of most sulfonamides, is not inhibited by pus and body fluids. Mafenide is highly soluble and diffuses into and through eschar. It may be the drug of choice if thick eschar is present (eg, electrical burns). Because of the pain produced on application and its potential for adverse reactions, some authorities do not recommend mafenide as a first-line drug for acute burns. It is used principally as a less preferred alternative to silver sulfadiazine to prevent infection in selected high-risk patients with heavily colonized burns or in wounds with resistant organisms, especially *Pseudomonas* infections.

ADVERSE REACTIONS AND PRECAUTIONS. Unlike silver sulfadiazine, mafenide causes pain that can be severe at the site of application. Allergic skin reactions and acid-base disturbances (metabolic acidosis with tachypnea and hyperventilation) also may develop. The acid-base disturbances result from the inhibition of carbonic anhydrase by mafenide and its principal metabolite. Its use in elderly patients who have burns on more than 40% of the body surface area may overwhelm inadequate respiratory reserves necessary to compensate for the metabolic acidosis.

This drug is classified in FDA Pregnancy Category C.

DOSAGE AND PREPARATIONS.

Topical: Following cleansing and debridement of the wound, the cream is applied with a sterile gloved hand to a thickness of 1 mm two or three times daily. It should be applied more frequently to burned areas from which the cream might be removed by movement of the patient. Therapy is continued until satisfactory healing has occurred or until the burn site is ready for grafting. Dressings can be applied over the cream, although this is unnecessary. Because the drug's antibacterial activity delays separation of eschar, daily hydrotherapy and mechanical debridement are advisable, especially in patients with full-thickness burns.

Sulfamylon (Hickam). Cream (water-miscible) equivalent to 85 mg of base/g in 56.7, 113.4, and 411 g containers.

NITROFURAZONE

[Furacin]

NO_2–(furan)–CH = NNHCONH$_2$

Nitrofurazone, a synthetic nitrofuran, is bactericidal for many gram-positive organisms. However, because strains of *Pseudomonas* are often not susceptible, use of this drug is restricted to the treatment of limited infected burns. Silver sulfadiazine is preferred.

Nitrofurazone may be effective in the treatment of resistant staphylococcal burn infections. It should be used with caution in patients with renal impairment.

ADVERSE REACTIONS. Allergic contact dermatitis has been reported (the overall rate is about 1.1%); hypersensitivity is more common on damaged skin. Under normal conditions of topical use, significant amounts of nitrofurazone are not absorbed into the systemic circulation. Nitrofurazone is classified in FDA Pregnancy Category C.

DOSAGE AND PREPARATIONS.

Topical: Once-daily application is usually adequate. Therapy is continued until satisfactory healing has occurred.

Generic. Ointment (soluble dressing) 0.2% in 30 and 454 g containers; solution 0.2% in 400 and 3,840 ml containers.

Furacin (Roberts). Cream (water-miscible) 0.2% in 28 g containers; ointment (soluble dressing) 0.2% in 28, 56, and 454 g containers; solution 0.2% in 473 ml containers.

POVIDONE-IODINE

[ACU-dyne, Betadine, Efodine, Pharmadine, Polydine]

[–CHCH$_2$–(N-pyrrolidone)–]$_n$ · xI

ACTIONS AND USES. Povidone-iodine, an iodophor, is a complex of iodine and the nonsurfactant polymer, polyvinylpyrrolidone. The iodophor complex releases free iodine gradually and in low concentration and it has a broad antimicrobial spectrum in vitro.

Povidone-iodine is used to prevent and treat burn wound infections. However, its use is limited because of pain on application and failure to control infections caused by gram-negative organisms. Silver sulfadiazine or mafenide is generally preferred for most burn infections, especially moderately extensive partial- and full-thickness burns. Povidone-iodine does not penetrate eschar as well as mafenide.

ADVERSE REACTIONS AND PRECAUTIONS. Mild pain may occur on application to burns. Povidone-iodine is less irritating and less toxic than aqueous and alcoholic solutions of elemental iodine. Although the frequency of hypersensitivity reactions varies, sensitization appears to be uncommon (Lachapelle, 1984).

Under normal conditions of use in burns of less than 15% to 20% of body surface area, povidone-iodine is not significantly absorbed into the systemic circulation. Systemic absorption of iodine may occur if the burned area is extensive (Zellner and Bugyi, 1985). The blood iodine concentration peaks in two to three days, and the value returns to normal about one week after discontinuation of povidone-iodine. No clinically significant adverse reactions related to blood iodine concentrations have been noted.

DOSAGE AND PREPARATIONS.

Topical: See manufacturers' recommendations.

(All forms nonprescription)

Generic. Ointment in 1, 1.2, 1.5, 30, 100, and 500 g containers; solution in 15, 30, 60, 120, 240, 480, 960, and 3,840 ml containers.

ACU-dyne (Acme United). Ointment in 1.2, 2.7, and 454 g containers.

Betadine (Purdue-Frederick). Aerosol spray in 90 ml containers; aerosol foam (Helafoam solution) in 270 g containers; cream in 15 g containers; ointment in 0.94, 3.8, 30, and 454 g containers; solution in 15, 30, 120, 240, 480, 948, and 3,840 ml containers; concentrate (for whirlpool) in 3,840 ml containers.

Efodine (Fougera). Ointment in 0.94, 30, and 454 g containers.

Pharmadine (Sherwood). Ointment in 1, 1.5, 2, and 30 g containers; solution in 15, 120, 240, 480, 948, and 3,840 ml containers; solution (for whirlpool) in 3,840 ml containers.

Polydine (Century). Ointment in 30, 120, and 454 g containers; solution in 30, 120, 240, 480, and 3,840 ml containers.

FUNGAL INFECTIONS

This section discusses the therapy used for superficial dermatophytic and candidal infections and tinea versicolor. Drugs used for subcutaneous and systemic mycoses and chronic mucocutaneous candidiasis are discussed elsewhere; see index entry Mycoses, Subcutaneous, Systemic.

Important factors in the choice of an antifungal agent for these infections include whether the mycosis is a dermatophytic or candidal infection (some therapeutic agents are specific for these organisms), its location and severity, the probability of patient compliance, and cost (Odom, 1987). The common use of nonprescription antifungal products prior to consultation of a physician also is an important consideration in the treatment of these mycoses. When self-therapy has not been satisfactory, the physician initially should confirm the patient's diagnosis and, if correct, should determine that the nonprescription medication (often as potent as some prescription preparations) has been used properly before another antifungal agent is substituted. Because of the importance of these considerations, the prescription status of the antifungal agents and the type and location of the infection are noted where appropriate in the following discussion, as well as in Tables 1 and 2 and the evaluations.

Dermatophytosis

Dermatophytic infections, the most common superficial mycoses, involve the skin, hair, and nails and are caused by species of *Epidermophyton, Trichophyton*, and *Microsporum*. When these fungal infections affect the skin, they are usually treated with topical agents. Resistant fungi or involvement of the hair or nails usually requires the prolonged (months) oral administration of griseofulvin, ketoconazole [Nizoral], or fluconazole [Diflucan]; the investigational antifungal agents, itraconazole [Sporanox] and terbinafine [Lamisil], also have been used.

DRUG SELECTION: Mild to Moderate Tinea Infections: Clotrimazole and miconazole, broad spectrum antifungal imidazoles, are effective in these infections when applied for 14 to 28 days, depending on the extent and site of involvement. These drugs are available in both prescription and nonprescription formulations (see Table 1 and the evaluations). Tioconazole [Vagistat], another broad spectrum imidazole, appears to be equally effective (East, 1983; Clissold and Heel, 1986; Fromtling, 1988). It has been approved for over-the-counter use in dermatophytic skin infections but is only marketed for the treatment of vaginal candidiasis in the United States.

Other nonprescription drugs for the treatment of mild, cutaneous tinea infections of the trunk, groin, or soles include tolnaftate [Aftate, Tinactin] and compound undecylenic acid [Desenex]. Controlled clinical trials support the effectiveness of tolnaftate in athlete's foot, jock itch, and ringworm and compound undecylenic acid in athlete's foot.

Haloprogin [Halotex] has limited effectiveness against tinea compared with the azoles.

Any antifungal effect of salicylic acid observed clinically is attributed to its keratolytic effect. This agent may be sufficient for mild cases of tinea pedis and also may be useful to make infections in deeper layers accessible to more potent antifungal agents. An older remedy, salicylic acid 3% and benzoic acid 6% in ointment (Whitfield's ointment) or cream form, is useful in the management of chronic moccasin-type tinea pedis (Logan et al, 1987).

Triacetin [Fungacetin] cream, a nonprescription product, is used topically in limited cutaneous fungal infections. Its antifungal action may be partly due to alteration of pH and the keratolytic action of acetic acid, which is released slowly from triacetin by esterases in fungi, skin, and serum.

Carbol-fuchsin solution (Castellani's Paint) is still used on occasion to treat chronic intertrigo of the toes but causes stinging and staining. More effective and acceptable agents are available.

In addition to its limited antibacterial activity, clioquinol (iodochlorhydroxyquin) [Vioform] has some antifungal activity; however, there is concern about excessive topical absorption, especially in infants and small children (see the evaluation).

Moderately Severe Tinea Infections: These infections usually respond to topical clotrimazole [Lotrimin, Mycelex], econazole [Spectazole], ketoconazole [Nizoral Cream], miconazole [Monistat-Derm], oxiconazole [Oxistat], or sulconazole [Exelderm]. All of these imidazoles are about equally effective in eradicating the infection when used under comparable conditions of patient selection and compliance, although some differences in response time may be noted (Benfield and Clissold, 1988; Fromtling, 1988).

In controlled studies, the spectrum of activity and efficacy of ciclopirox olamine [Loprox], a hydroxypyridone, in tinea infections are comparable to those of the imidazoles. In tinea pedis and versicolor, ciclopirox olamine produced a more rapid and complete clinical response than clotrimazole in some studies (Kligman et al, 1985; Cullen et al, 1985).

Another nonimidazole antifungal agent, naftifine [Naftin], is one of a number of novel synthetic allylamines and is applied topically. The closely related and more potent allylamine, terbinafine, is being evaluated in advanced clinical trials and is used both orally and topically. Both agents are effective against some fungal species resistant to the imidazoles (Ryder, 1987; Monk and Brogden, 1991; Balfour and Faulds, 1992). The fungicidal action of the allylamines is due to their much greater allosteric inhibition of the fungal enzyme, squalene epoxidase, compared with the mammalian form of the enzyme (Rippon, 1986). The allylamines are especially effective against many dermatophytic organisms that cause tinea infections. The indications for naftifine include the treatment of tinea pedis, cruris, and corporis. Since there is minimal interaction with cytochrome P450, orally active antifungal allylamines do not interfere with the synthesis of steroidal hormones and prostaglandins.

Severe Tinea Infections: Infections of the palms, soles, and fingernails usually respond to oral griseofulvin or oral ketoconazole. Depending on the site and extent of infection, treatment may be required for months. Griseofulvin is the drug of choice for tinea barbae and tinea capitis when the causative organism is *Trichophyton tonsurans*, *Microsporum audouinii*, or *M. canis* (Laude et al, 1982; Krowchuk et al, 1983; Gan et al, 1987). Biweekly selenium sulfide shampoos may shorten the period of contagion (Gan et al, 1987). A systemic corticosteroid has been recommended if kerions are present; however, one controlled study showed that adjunctive use of intralesional corticosteroids did not improve outcome over that achieved with griseofulvin alone (Ginsburg et al, 1987). At least one month but often three to six months of therapy is required for clinical cure. Oral ketoconazole is an alternative to griseofulvin. Some dermatologists reserve this drug for treatment of severe dermatophytic infections when griseofulvin is ineffective in higher doses (2 g/day) or is contraindicated (Odom, 1987; Faergemann and Maibach, 1987; Tanz et al, 1988) because of its potential for drug interactions and for producing hepatitis. Because these oral drugs are absorbed systemically, they are not recommended for trivial tinea infections that usually are relieved by topical therapy alone.

A number of antifungal bis-triazoles are being evaluated clinically. One, terconazole [Terazol], is marketed for topical treatment of vulvovaginal candidiasis. Two others, itraconazole and fluconazole, are given orally; itraconazole is investigational but has been studied extensively for dermatophytic infection; data on oral fluconazole are limited and, in the United States, this drug has been principally used in the treatment of systemic mycoses (see index entry Fluconazole, Uses, Subcutaneous, Systemic Mycoses) and mucosal candidiasis.

These agents have greater selectivity for fungal than mammalian enzymes, a lesser effect on mammalian steroid biosynthesis, and a higher affinity for the skin than ketoconazole (Cauwenbergh et al, 1988; Cauwenbergh and Degreef, 1990). These findings probably explain why itraconazole has been safer and more effective in the treatment of dermatophytic infections than ketoconazole. Oral itraconazole (given for three to six months) ameliorates signs and symptoms in patients with indolent chronic *T. rubrum* infections known to be resistant to griseofulvin and oral ketoconazole. The drug is well tolerated (Hanifin and Tofte, 1988) (see the evaluation).

Tinea Versicolor

Tinea versicolor (pityriasis) is caused by the hyphal form, *Malassezia furfur*, of the pathogenic lipophilic yeast, *Pityrosporum orbiculare*, which is present on normal skin. A number of nonprescription drugs are used in tinea versicolor. They include the antidandruff agents, zinc pyrithione shampoo [Danex, DHS-Zinc, Head and Shoulders, Zincon, ZNP Bar] (applied for five minutes daily for 14 days) and selenium sulfide suspension [Exsel, Selsun] (applied for 15 to 30 minutes daily for 7 to 14 days). Sodium thiosulfate 25% with salicylic acid 1% [Tinver] also is effective when applied to affected areas twice a day for several weeks. Topical prescription drugs that eradicate tinea versicolor when used for an adequate length of time include ciclopirox olamine, haloprogin, clotrimazole, econazole, ketoconazole cream and ketoconazole antidandruff shampoo (investigational use), miconazole, and sulconazole.

A single dose of oral ketoconazole 400 mg usually is effective in eliminating tinea versicolor; it may be necessary to use the drug prophylactically in immunocompromised patients (Borelli et al, 1991; Goodless et al, 1991). Griseofulvin is ineffective in tinea versicolor.

Candidiasis

CUTANEOUS CANDIDIASIS. *Candida albicans* most often causes this infection, but *C. tropicalis* and *C. glabrata* also can be implicated. Cutaneous candidiasis is confined to dry skin and nails or moist skin in intertriginous areas; involvement may be limited or extensive. Candidiasis around the mouth, anus, and vulva almost always affects the contiguous mucous membranes (see the following discussion on candidiasis affecting the mucous membranes for treatment of these areas as well as for infections involving mucous membranes exclusively).

Drug Selection: Cutaneous candidiasis responds to topical preparations of the polyene antibiotics, amphotericin B [Fungizone] and nystatin [Mycostatin, Nilstat]; haloprogin [Halotex]; ciclopirox olamine [Loprox]; and the imidazoles (clotrimazole [Lotrimin, Mycelex], econazole [Spectazole], miconazole [Micatin, Monistat-Derm, Zeasorb-AF], oxiconazole [Oxistat], and sulconazole [Exelderm] (investigational use). Once-daily application of ketoconazole cream 2% [Nizoral] is effective and may improve compliance in some patients (Greer and Jolly, 1988). Recurrences were not observed at a two-week follow-up. Only limited data are available on the use of the newer antifungal allylamines, naftifine and terbinafine, for the treatment of cutaneous candidiasis. However, both drugs appear to be quite effective in this condition and are well tolerated (Monk and Brogden, 1991; Balfour and Faulds, 1992).

Candidiasis limited to the skin does not respond to topical undecylenic acid, topical tolnaftate, or oral griseofulvin. Clioquinol has only limited antifungal activity, and excessive topical absorption has raised concerns (see the evaluation).

CANDIDIASIS AFFECTING MUCOUS MEMBRANES. *Candida albicans* and, less often, *C. tropicalis* and *C. glabrata* also affect moist skin and adjacent mucous membranes (eg, orocutaneous at the corners of the mouth [perleche], perianal, vulvovaginal) or mucous membranes exclusively (eg, oropharyngeal [thrush; moniliasis], esophageal).

The following patients are predisposed to candidiasis of intertriginous areas and mucous membranes: those with certain forms of cancer, acquired or congenital immunodeficiency syndrome, poor nutrition, severe burns, diabetes mellitus, hepatic and/or renal failure; those known to abuse narcotics; those undergoing dialysis; and those receiving adrenal corticosteroids, antineoplastic drugs, cyclosporine, or broad spectrum antibacterial agents. Pregnancy predisposes to candidal vulvovaginitis.

Chronic cutaneous candidiasis associated with chronic mucocutaneous candidiasis is uncommon and most often devel-

TABLE 1.
THERAPY FOR DERMATOPHYTIC AND CUTANEOUS CANDIDAL INFECTIONS

Drug	Route of Administration	Preparations	Site of Dermatophytic (Tinea) Infection: Body Perineum Foot Hand	Site of Dermatophytic (Tinea) Infection: Scalp Nails Beard	Tinea Versicolor	Cutaneous Candidal Infection
Ciclopirox olamine			+		+	+
Loprox	Topical	Cream, lotion				
Clioquinol			+			+
Vioform*	Topical	Cream, ointment				
Griseofulvin[1]			+[2]	+[3]		
Generic	Oral	Capsules				
Fulvicin U/F, P/G	Oral	Tablets				
Grisactin	Oral	Capsules, tablets				
Grisactin Ultra	Oral	Tablets				
Grifulvin V	Oral	Suspension, tablets				
Gris-PEG	Oral	Tablets				
Haloprogin			+		+	+
Halotex	Topical	Cream, solution				
Pyrithione zinc					+	
Danex,* DHS-Zinc,* Head and Shoulders,* Zincon* ZNP Bar*	Topical	Shampoo				
Selenium sulfide					+	
Generic*, Exsel, Selsun*	Topical	Shampoo				
Tolnaftate			+			
Aftate*	Topical	Aerosol powder, gel, powder, liquid aerosol, liquid spray				
Tinactin*	Topical	Aerosol powder, cream, liquid aerosol, powder, solution				
Compound Undecylenic Acid			+			
Generic*	Topical	Ointment				
Desenex*	Topical	Aerosol powder, cream, ointment, powder, foam, soap				
ALLYLAMINES						
Naftifine			+			+
Naftin	Topical	Cream, gel				
Terbinafine[4]						
Lamisil	Topical	Cream	+			
	Oral			+		+

(table continued on next page)

TABLE 1 (Continued)

Drug	Route of Administration	Preparations	Site of Dermatophytic (Tinea) Infection: Body Perineum Foot Hand	Site of Dermatophytic (Tinea) Infection: Scalp Nails Beard	Tinea Versicolor	Cutaneous Candidal Infection
AZOLES						
Imidazoles						
Clotrimazole			+		+	+
Lotrimin, Lotrimin-AF*	Topical	Cream, solution, lotion				
Mycelex, Mycelex OTC*	Topical	Cream, solution				
Econazole			+		+	+
Spectazole	Topical	Cream				
Ketoconazole						
Nizoral	Oral	Tablets	+	+	+	+
	Topical	Cream, shampoo	+		+	+
Miconazole nitrate			+			+
Generic	Topical	Cream				
Micatin*	Topical	Cream, powder, aerosol powder, liquid aerosol				
Monistat-Derm	Topical	Cream				
Zeasorb-AF*	Topical	Powder				
Oxiconazole nitrate			+		+	
Oxistat	Topical	Cream				
Sulconazole nitrate			+		+	
Exelderm	Topical	Cream, solution				
Bis-triazoles						
Fluconazole[5]			+	+	+	+
Diflucan	Oral					
Itraconazole[4]			+	+	+	+
Sporanox	Oral					
POLYENE ANTIBIOTICS						
Amphotericin B						+
Fungizone	Topical	Cream, lotion, ointment				
Nystatin						+
Generic	Topical	Cream				
Mycostatin	Topical	Cream, ointment, powder				
Nilstat	Topical	Cream, ointment, powder				

* *Nonprescription.*
[1] *The preparations of griseofulvin listed are not interchangeable; dosage recommendations are based on differences in absorption based principally on particle size and formulation.*
[2] *Griseofulvin is not recommended for trivial dermatophytic infections that usually respond to topical therapy alone.*
[3] *Oral griseofulvin is the drug of choice for infection that does not respond to topical therapy.*
[4] *Investigational drug.*
[5] *Limited published data.*

ops in immunocompromised or debilitated patients. The skin, scalp, nails, and mucous membranes are extensively involved, and a systemic antifungal agent is usually required. Oral ketoconazole should be used for severe infections, for which it is the drug of choice. Topical antifungal therapy may be required in addition. Intravenous amphotericin B is effective for chronic mucocutaneous candidiasis; however, the relapse rate is very high when the drug is stopped, and prolonged administration can cause serious adverse reactions (see also index entry Mycoses, Subcutaneous, Systemic).

Oropharyngeal Candidiasis (Thrush): When present temporarily (eg, myelosuppression during chemotherapy, short-term steroid therapy, use of orally administered broad spectrum antibiotics), oropharyngeal candidiasis usually responds to local lozenge (troche) therapy with clotrimazole [Mycelex] or oral suspensions or lozenges (pastilles) of nystatin [Mycostatin, Nilstat]. Extemporaneously compounded solutions of amphotericin B are effective in candidiasis that does not respond to conventional therapy (Brandell et al, 1988). Oropharyngeal and esophageal candidiasis that develops during prolonged immunosuppression usually is treated more effectively with systemically administered antifungal agents (see index entry, Mycoses, Subcutaneous, Systemic).

Vaginal Candidiasis: Seventy-five percent of women will experience an episode of vulvovaginal candidiasis during their lifetime, and 13 million cases occur annually in the United States (Horowitz, 1991). Most cases of vulvovaginal candidiasis are caused by *Candida albicans*; *C. tropicalis* and *C. glabrata* are responsible for a large percentage of the remaining cases. Bacterial vaginosis, trichomoniasis, vulvar vestibulitis, and other noninfectious causes of symptoms (eg, pudendal neuralgia) should be excluded before the diagnosis is made.

Drug Selection: Many equally effective antifungal agents and a variety of formulations (eg, creams, suppositories in the form of tablets or gelatin capsules, pessaries) are available to treat this infection. Patient compliance often depends on formulation acceptability. Other significant factors in drug selection include the severity and duration of the illness, history of chronic or recurrent vaginal candidiasis, history of local hypersensitivity reaction or irritation after use of a topical anticandidal agent, and pregnancy status.

Vaginal candidiasis responds to topical preparations of nystatin [Mycostatin, Nilstat, O-V Statin], butoconazole [Femstat], clotrimazole [Gyne-Lotrimin, Mycelex-G], miconazole [Monistat 3, Monistat 7], terconazole [Terazol 3, Terazol 7], and tioconazole [Vagistat-1]. The duration of therapy depends on the formulation and dosage employed. Miconazole 200 mg/day for three days [Monistat 3] or 100 mg/day for seven days [Monistat 7]; clotrimazole 500 mg as a single dose, 200 mg/day for three days, or 100 mg/day for seven days (Hughes and Kriedman, 1984; Fleury et al, 1985); and tioconazole 300 mg as a single dose are effective. The single-dose treatment with clotrimazole and tioconazole appears to be as effective as the three-day regimens with miconazole, terconazole, or butoconazole for mild to moderate infections. Nystatin may be slightly less effective than the imidazoles, and a longer treatment period (14 days) is required for clinical cure.

Sufficient clinical experience has accumulated with selected imidazoles to establish their overall safety; thus, clotrimazole and miconazole are now available in cream and suppository form [Gyne-Lotrimin, Monistat 7] as nonprescription drugs for infections that recur. These preparations should not be used initially without confirmation of the diagnosis by a physician. Although symptoms often disappear rapidly, the patient should continue treatment for seven days with these nonprescription products. If symptoms are not controlled within three days, she should contact her physician for confirmation of the diagnosis and further advice.

Surveys in a number of countries reveal that as many as 45% to 90% of women prefer oral to topical therapy for this infection (Kovacs et al, 1990; Merkus, 1990; Sobel, 1990; Van Heusden et al, 1991). Oral ketoconazole is used to treat acute vaginal candidiasis. The recommended dose is 200 mg twice daily for five days or until the infection has cleared. However, some concern exists about the potential for serious adverse reactions and drug interactions with systemic therapy with this agent. Single 150-mg daily doses of the orally effective bis-triazole antifungal agents, itraconazole and fluconazole, have been effective. These triazoles have much less effect on mammalian cytochrome P450 enzymes; therefore, the potential for drug interactions and more serious adverse reactions may be less than with some imidazole antifungal agents.

Vulvovaginal candidiasis is common during pregnancy, and neonatal oral candidiasis and dermatitis may occur when vulvovaginal candidiasis is present at the time of delivery. Intravaginal nystatin, the imidazoles, and the triazole, terconazole, are safe during the second and third trimester of pregnancy. The Centers for Disease Control currently advises that the six- or seven-day topical antifungal regimens of the imidazoles and terconazole may be preferred. Only nystatin is recommended during the first trimester. This limitation has received some support from results of a small study that suggest, but do not establish, that the imidazoles may be associated with an increase in the risk of spontaneous abortions when they are used during the first trimester (Rosa et al, 1987); this association has not been observed with nystatin.

It can be quite difficult to determine the etiology and management of chronic or recurrent vulvovaginal candidiasis. The diagnosis should be confirmed and all reversible causes (eg, uncontrolled diabetes) eliminated. If the condition is still uncorrected (idiopathic), therapy should be initiated with either oral or topical antifungal agents and continued until the candidiasis is in remission (ie, asymptomatic and culture-negative). A maintenance or prophylactic regimen should then be given in sufficient dosage and frequency to keep the patient in remission. If immunosuppression continues or cannot be minimized sufficiently, long-term topical and/or oral prophylactic antifungal therapy is essential in therapeutic management, although the effects may be only palliative. Low-dose oral ketoconazole administered daily or clotrimazole 500 mg administered weekly is suitable and may be required for long periods, since relapse is common after withdrawal of the drug (Sobel, 1986, 1990, 1992 A, 1992 B; Sobel et al, 1989). The

TABLE 2
THERAPY FOR OROPHARYNGEAL AND VAGINAL CANDIDAL INFECTIONS

Drug	Route of Administration	Preparations	Site of Candidal Infection	
			Oropharynx	Vagina
AZOLES				
Imidazoles				
Butoconazole				+
Femstat	Intravaginal	Cream		
Clotrimazole				
Mycelex Troche	Oral	Troches (lozenge)	+	
Gyne-Lotrimin[1]	Intravaginal	Cream, tablets		+
Mycelex G, Mycelex Twin Pack	Intravaginal	Cream, tablets		+
Ketoconazole			+	+
Nizoral	Oral	Tablets		
Miconazole nitrate				+
Monistat 7[1]	Intravaginal	Cream, suppositories		
Monistat 3; Monistat Dual Pack	Intravaginal	Suppositories; cream/ suppositories		
Tioconazole				+
Vagistat-1	Topical	Cream		
Bis-triazoles				
Fluconazole				
Diflucan	Oral	Tablets	+	+
Itraconazole[2]				
Sporanox	Oral		+	+
Terconazole				+
Terazol 3	Intravaginal	Suppositories		
Terazol 7	Intravaginal	Cream		
POLYENE ANTIBIOTIC				
Nystatin				
Generic	Oral (nonabsorbed)	Tablets, oral suspension	+	
	Intravaginal	Tablets		+
Mycostatin	Oral (nonabsorbed)	Tablets, pastilles (lozenges), oral suspension	+	
	Intravaginal	Tablets		+
Nilstat	Oral (nonabsorbed)	Tablets, oral suspension	+	
	Intravaginal	Tablets		+
O-V Statin	Oral (nonabsorbed)	Tablets	+	
	Intravaginal	Tablets		+

[1] *Nonprescription.*
[2] *Investigational drug.*

decision to use ketoconazole prophylactically must be weighed against the slight (1:10,000) but serious risk of hepatotoxicity that can occur with such a regimen. The orally administered triazoles, itraconazole and fluconazole, may prove to be as effective as oral ketoconazole and may cause less or no hepatotoxicity (Sobel, 1992 A, 1992 B). Boric acid 600 mg in gelatin capsules twice daily intravaginally for two weeks (Sobel, 1992 A, 1992 B) is an alternative.

The benefit of treating male sexual partners is controversial, but if candidal balanitis is present, it should be treated with a topical preparation of clotrimazole or miconazole.

A gastrointestinal tract reservoir in vaginal candidiasis has been proposed; however, no conclusive evidence exists that orally administered nystatin or the azoles diminish the rate of occurrence.

Drug Evaluations

CICLOPIROX OLAMINE
[Loprox]

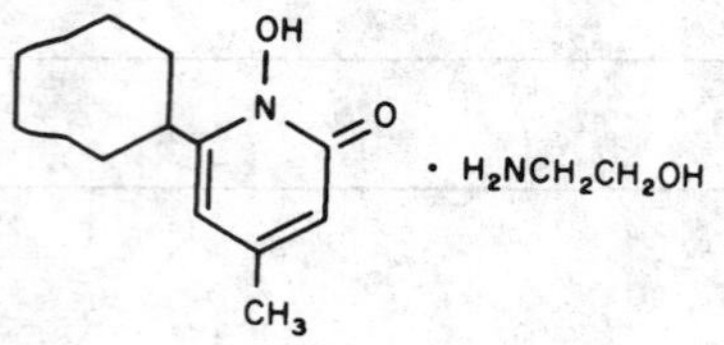

ACTIONS AND USES. This antifungal agent, a hydroxypyridone, is chemically unrelated to the broad spectrum imidazoles (Jue et al, 1985). Its action is attributed to inhibition of uptake of precursors of macromolecular synthesis from the medium (Sakurai et al, 1978).

Ciclopirox appears to be as effective as clotrimazole in the treatment of dermatophytic and cutaneous candidal infections, as well as tinea versicolor. Its optimal role in tinea capitis, tinea barbae, and moderately severe tinea infections of the palms, soles, or nails remains to be determined.

ADVERSE REACTIONS AND PRECAUTIONS. Side effects are reported to be infrequent and minor (eg, pruritus, burning). The drug appears to be nonsensitizing. Systemic toxicity has not been reported following topical application.

Safety and effectiveness in children under 10 years have not been established.

PREGNANCY AND LACTATION. Reproduction studies in mice, rats, rabbits, and monkeys utilizing various routes of administration and doses ten or more times the topical human dose have had no effect on fertility or the fetus. However, no adequate or well-controlled studies have been performed in pregnant women. This drug is classified in FDA Pregnancy Category B.

It is not known whether ciclopirox is excreted in human milk, but, because many drugs are, caution should be exercised when ciclopirox is administered to nursing women.

PHARMACOKINETICS. Tagged studies of ciclopirox in polyethylene glycol 400 showed that an average of 1.3% of the dose was absorbed when this formulation was applied to 750 cm^2 on the back, followed by six hours of occlusion. Of the amount absorbed, the biologic half-life was 1.7 hours and excretion occurred via the kidney.

DOSAGE AND PREPARATIONS.

Topical: The preparation is applied to the affected area twice daily. The use of occlusive wrappings or dressings is not recommended. Although improvement may be noted in one week, clinical cure usually requires a minimum of two to four weeks, depending on the site and extent of involvement.

Loprox (Hoechst-Roussel). Cream 1% in 15, 30, and 90 g containers; lotion 1% in 30 ml containers.

CLIOQUINOL (Iodochlorhydroxyquin)
[Vioform]

ACTIONS AND USES. Clioquinol, an 8-hydroxyquinolone, is related to the amebicide, iodoquinol. Like the latter, it has limited antibacterial and antifungal activity when applied topically. The oral preparation was withdrawn from the United States market because it has an appreciable potential for producing subacute myelo-optic neuropathy (SMON).

Clioquinol is available as a single-entity nonprescription agent and in mixtures with hydrocortisone for topical application in the treatment of limited fungal infections of the skin, such as tinea pedis (athlete's foot), and limited primary and secondary bacterial pyodermas (eg, superficial folliculitis, uncomplicated impetigo, infected dermal ulcers, infectious eczematoid dermatitis, intertrigo). It is not used topically on the mucous membranes.

Based on a review of the combination product containing clioquinol and hydrocortisone conducted by the National Academy of Science-National Research Council, the FDA has listed this mixture as only "possibly effective" for all of its indications.

Studies on the topical absorption of clioquinol have raised serious concerns about the risk/benefit ratio of this agent (Ezzedeen et al, 1984). In one study, absorption was rapid and extensive following use on intact adult human skin for 12 hours. The drug was detectable in the blood at two hours and reached a stable blood concentration by four hours; an average of 40% ± 6.5% of the dose was absorbed (Stohs et al, 1984).

ADVERSE REACTIONS AND PRECAUTIONS. Irritation and hypersensitivity reactions occur only rarely, but patients who are hypersensitive to iodine should not receive this medication.

The drug should not be used in children under 2 years.

The hydroxy group of clioquinol interacts with the ferric chloride test for phenylketonuria to yield a false-positive result if the compound is present on the diaper or in the urine. Clioquinol stains hair and fabrics.

DOSAGE AND PREPARATIONS.

Topical: An appropriate preparation is applied to the affected area two or three times a day.

Generic. Cream 3% in 30 and 454 g containers (nonprescription).

Vioform (CIBA). Cream, ointment 3% in 30 g containers (nonprescription).

Available Mixtures.

CLIOQUINOL AND HYDROCORTISONE:

Generic. Cream and ointment containing hydrocortisone 0.5% or 1% and clioquinol 3%.

Hysone (Hauck). Cream containing hydrocortisone 1% and clioquinol 3% in 20 g containers.

Vioform-Hydrocortisone (CIBA). Cream containing hydrocortisone 0.5% and clioquinol 3% in 15 and 30 g containers or hydrocortisone 1% and clioquinol 3% in 5 and 20 g containers; lotion containing hydrocortisone 1% and clioquinol 3% in 15 ml containers; ointment containing hydrocortisone 0.5% and clioquinol 3% in 30 g containers or hydrocortisone 1% and clioquinol 3% in 20 g containers.

Similar Mixture.

IODOQUINOL AND HYDROCORTISONE:

Vytone (Dermik). Cream containing hydrocortisone 1% and iodoquinol 1% in 30 g containers.

GRISEOFULVIN

[*Microcrystalline:* Fulvicin-U/F, Grifulvin V, Grisactin; *Ultramicrocrystalline:* Fulvicin P/G, Grisactin Ultra, Gris-PEG]

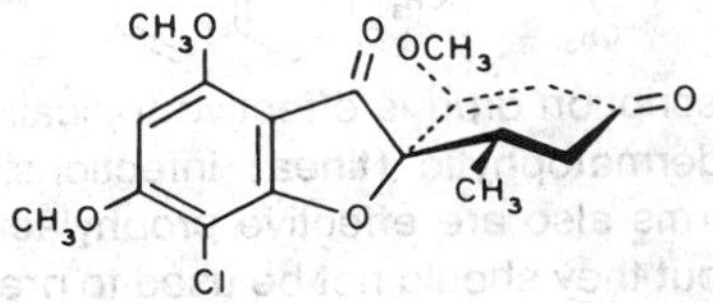

ACTIONS. Griseofulvin is derived from a species of *Penicillium*. Its fungicidal effect is limited to actively growing organisms, since one of the major cellular effects of griseofulvin is to inhibit fungal mitosis by binding to intracellular microtubular protein.

USES. Griseofulvin is effective orally for dermatophytic (tinea) infections but is not useful in tinea versicolor. It is not recommended routinely for trivial fungal infections that usually respond to a topical agent alone and is ineffective for candidal infections.

Griseofulvin is the drug of choice for tinea barbae and tinea capitis caused by *Trichophyton tonsurans*, *Microsporum audouinii*, or *M. canis* (Laude et al, 1982; Krowchuk et al, 1983). It is especially useful when extensive or multiple sites of infection are present. A systemic corticosteroid has been recommended if kerions are present; however, in one controlled study, adjunctive intralesional corticosteroids did not improve outcome over that achieved with griseofulvin alone (Ginsburg et al, 1987). At least two months of therapy usually is required for clinical cure. Biweekly shampoos containing selenium sulfide, a sporicidal agent active against the causative organism of tinea capitis, are effective adjunctively in combination with oral griseofulvin (Gan et al, 1987).

Dermatophytic infections of the palms usually require two to three months of treatment; the fingernails usually respond within six months, although nine months may be necessary. If the response is based on lack of recurrence of the infection, only about 15% of toenail infections respond. Treatment with griseofulvin must be continued until infected keratinous structures have been eradicated as determined by clinical and laboratory examinations. In stubborn infections, concomitant treatment with topical antifungal and/or keratolytic agents in areas of hyperkeratosis may be helpful. Some forms of onychomycosis are almost completely resistant to therapy.

Oral ketoconazole is recommended for severe infections of the scalp, beard, and nails when griseofulvin is contraindicated or the organism is resistant (see index entry Mycoses, Subcutaneous, Systemic).

ADVERSE REACTIONS, PRECAUTIONS, AND INTERACTIONS. The most common minor reaction is headache, which usually disappears in a few days, even with continued therapy. Other reactions include dysgeusia, dryness of the mouth, gastrointestinal disturbances (nausea, vomiting, diarrhea), arthralgia, peripheral neuritis, vertigo, and fever. Griseofulvin occasionally causes syncope, blurred vision, insomnia, and rash. Rarely, it may cause serum sickness, angioedema, confusion, lapses of memory, and impaired judgment that may affect the performance of routine tasks. This compound also may produce estrogen-like effects in children.

Serious reactions associated with the use of griseofulvin occur infrequently. Leukopenia is observed occasionally and granulocytopenia may develop after use of large doses and/or prolonged therapy. It may be advisable to perform blood counts occasionally during therapy.

Griseofulvin rarely causes hepatotoxicity, and it is contraindicated in patients with acute intermittent porphyria or a history of that condition, hepatocellular failure, and hypersensitivity to the drug.

Urticaria and fixed drug eruption have been reported rarely. Exacerbation of systemic lupus erythematosus may occur.

The safe use of griseofulvin during pregnancy has not been established. Therefore, potential benefits must be weighed against the possible hazards if this agent is considered for use in women of childbearing age.

Griseofulvin may decrease the activity of coumarin-type anticoagulants (eg, warfarin), cyclosporine, and estrogen-containing oral contraceptives, and dosage adjustments may be required. Since these interactions probably result from induction of cytochrome P450 enzymes, other drugs that are metabolized by this system of oxidation also may require dosage adjustment. Conversely, barbiturates and primidone depress griseofulvin activity by decreasing its systemic absorption and/or enhancing metabolism, and an increase in dosage of the latter may be required.

PHARMACOKINETICS. Griseofulvin is only administered orally. During long-term administration, the drug is deposited in the skin, hair, and nails and is actively secreted from eccrine sweat glands. Griseofulvin appears to move in and out of the stratum corneum rapidly, and lesions begin to heal within a few days after treatment is initiated. The stratum corneum is cleared of drug two to three days after therapy is discontinued.

Griseofulvin is extensively metabolized by the liver. The half-life ranges from 24 to 36 hours; therefore, once-daily administration is usually adequate. However, administration every six hours is recommended to maintain effective serum concentrations and lessen side effects when large doses are required initially to control severe infections. Plasma levels can be detected for four days after therapy has ceased.

DOSAGE AND PREPARATIONS. Griseofulvin was marketed originally in a macrocrystalline form that required the use of large doses to achieve and maintain effective blood levels. A microcrystalline form has now replaced the macrocrystalline preparations, and the same blood levels can be achieved with smaller doses. An ultramicrocrystalline form produces the same blood levels as the microcrystalline form at a further one-third reduction in dosage (Straughn et al, 1980). However, there is no convincing evidence that further reducing the particle size confers any significant advantage. Therefore, there appears to be no practical therapeutic difference between the microcrystalline and ultramicrocrystalline forms. The dosage required to assure comparable blood levels of the ultramicrocrystalline form of griseofulvin are cited below.

MICROCRYSTALLINE FORM:

Oral: *Adults,* for less serious infections, 500 mg daily in single or divided doses with meals; 750 mg to 1 g daily in divided doses has been recommended for severe infections. *Children,* approximately 15 mg/kg daily in single or divided doses with meals. Divided dosage regimens usually are indicated only if the patient cannot tolerate a single daily dose or large initial doses are required.

Fulvicin-U/F (Schering). Tablets 250 and 500 mg.
Grifulvin V (Ortho). Suspension (pediatric) 125 mg/5 ml; tablets 250 and 500 mg.
Grisactin (Wyeth-Ayerst). Capsules 250 mg; tablets 500 mg.

ULTRAMICROCRYSTALLINE FORM:

Oral: *Adults,* 330 mg daily in single or divided doses with meals is satisfactory in most patients with tinea corporis, tinea cruris, and tinea capitis. For fungal infections that are more difficult to eradicate, such as tinea pedis and tinea unguium, 660 mg in divided doses is recommended. Approximately 10 mg/kg/day is effective for most *children.* On this basis, the following dosages are suggested for administration in single or divided amounts: *Children weighing 16 to 23 kg,* 125 to 165 mg daily; *23 to 34 kg,* 165 to 250 mg daily; *over 34 kg,* 250 to 330 mg daily; *2 years or younger,* dosage has not been established. Clinical experience with griseofulvin in children with tinea capitis indicates that a single daily dose is effective.

Clinical relapse will occur if the medication is discontinued before the infecting organism is eradicated.

Fulvicin P/G (Schering). Tablets 125, 165, 250, and 330 mg.
Grisactin Ultra (Wyeth-Ayerst). Tablets 125, 250, and 330 mg.
Gris-PEG (ALLERGAN Herbert). Tablets 125 and 250 mg.

HALOPROGIN

[Halotex]

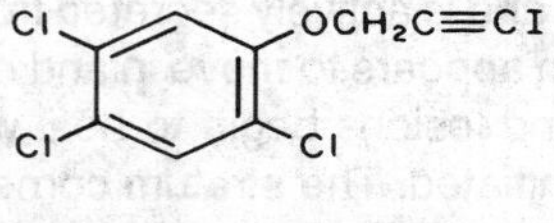

USES. Haloprogin is a synthetic topical antifungal agent used to treat dermatophytic (tinea) infections and tinea versicolor. The cure and relapse rates with haloprogin are similar to those with tolnaftate; however, unlike tolnaftate, haloprogin is effective in cutaneous candidal infections as well; the latter use is investigational.

ADVERSE REACTIONS AND PRECAUTIONS. Adverse reactions include local irritation, burning sensation, and vesicle formation. If sensitization is noted, the drug should be discontinued and not used again. Contact with the eyes should be avoided.

Haloprogin is classified in FDA Pregnancy Category B.

DOSAGE AND PREPARATIONS.

Topical: The preparation is applied liberally to the affected area twice daily for two to four weeks. Interdigital lesions may require up to four weeks of therapy. If there is no improvement after four weeks, haloprogin should be discontinued and the diagnosis reconfirmed.

Halotex (Westwood-Squibb). Cream 1% in 15 and 30 g containers; solution 1% in 10 and 30 ml containers.

TOLNAFTATE

[Aftate, Tinactin]

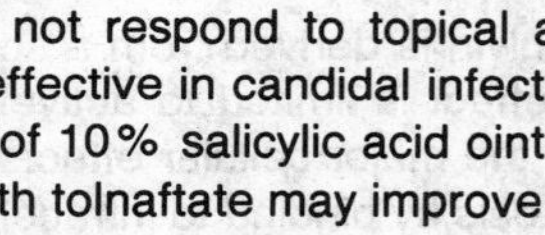

This nonprescription drug is effective topically in the treatment of mild dermatophytic (tinea) infections. The powder and aerosol forms also are effective prophylactically against athlete's foot, but they should not be used to prevent jock itch and ringworm. Fungal infections of the scalp, nails, soles, and palms usually do not respond to topical antifungal agents. Tolnaftate is not effective in candidal infections.

Alternating use of 10% salicylic acid ointment (as needed for keratolysis) with tolnaftate may improve the effectiveness of the latter in hyperkeratotic lesions. Topical haloprogin, clotrimazole, or miconazole is recommended for lesions refractory to tolnaftate.

Tolnaftate is well tolerated. Sensitization is rare, and irritation occurs infrequently.

DOSAGE AND PREPARATIONS.

Topical: One or two drops of solution or a small amount of cream or powder is rubbed into lesions twice daily for two to three weeks; treatment for four to six weeks may be required. The powder or powder aerosol may be used following the original treatment period to help maintain remission in patients susceptible to tinea.

Aftate (Schering-Plough). Gel 1% in 15 g containers; powder 1% in 45 and 67.5 g containers; powder (aerosol) 1% in 150 g containers; liquid (aerosol) 1% in 120 ml containers; liquid (pump spray) 1% in 45 ml containers (all forms nonprescription).
Tinactin (Schering-Plough). Cream 1% in 15 and 30 g containers; liquid (aerosol) 1% in 120 ml containers; powder 1% in 45 and 90 g containers; powder (aerosol) 1% in 100 g containers; solution 1% in 10 ml containers (all forms nonprescription).

COMPOUND UNDECYLENIC ACID

This nonprescription mixture of undecylenic acid and zinc undecylenate is effective topically in mild dermatophytic (tinea) infections, but it is not effective in tinea versicolor or candidal infections (Landau, 1983).

The most extensive use of compound undecylenic acid has been for tinea pedis (athlete's foot). Its effectiveness in this condition is reported to compare favorably with that of tolnaftate.

Compound undecylenic acid is well tolerated, but it should be discontinued if irritation develops. Under normal conditions of topical use, clinically significant quantities of this mixture are not absorbed from the skin.

DOSAGE AND PREPARATIONS.

Topical: The ointment or powder is applied once or twice daily to the involved area. A common practice is to apply powder or aerosol in the morning and an ointment or aerosol at night.

Generic. Ointment containing undecylenic acid 5% and zinc undecylenate 20% (nonprescription).

Available Trademark.

Desenex Cream, Ointment, Powder, Aerosol Powder, Solution, Foam, Soap (Fisons) (all forms nonprescription).

Allylamines

NAFTIFINE HYDROCHLORIDE

[Naftin]

ACTIONS AND USES. Naftifine is the first antifungal agent of the new antifungal class of synthetic allylamines to be approved for the topical treatment of tinea corporis and tinea cruris (Ryder, 1987; Monk and Brogden, 1991). Although results of clinical investigations support a broader spectrum of antifungal action against many organisms that cause dermatophytic and candidal infections, data on tinea pedis and cutaneous candidiasis are limited. In initial limited controlled studies, naftifine was significantly more effective than econazole in various dermatomycoses and than clotrimazole in tinea pedis.

Naftifine may have an advantage over conventional topical antifungal agents, especially in noncompliant patients, because once-daily application appears to be adequate in some controlled trials; the manufacturer's recommendation currently is for twice-daily application (gel) and once-daily application (cream). More data are needed to determine whether naftifine's anti-inflammatory action will be an additional advantage in inflammatory dermatomycoses.

The fungicidal action of this agent is based on its allosteric inhibition of the fungal enzyme, squalene epoxidase, which is associated with an accumulation of toxic quantities of squalene and a decrease in the concentrations of ergosterol. The comparable mammalian enzyme is much less affected.

ADVERSE REACTIONS AND PRECAUTIONS. Results of controlled clinical trials indicate that both allylamines are well tolerated (Plotkin et al, 1990; Smith et al, 1990). The typical adverse reactions of naftifine cream are similar to those of the imidazoles, ie, burning and stinging (6%), dryness (3%), erythema (2%), pruritus 2%, and local irritation (2%). Adverse reactions associated with naftifine gel during clinical trials were burning/stinging (5%), pruritus (1%), and erythema, rash, or skin tenderness (0.5%). Allergic contact eczema has been reported with administration of naftifine; however, as with the imidazoles, the reaction is rare.

PREGNANCY AND LACTATION. Reproduction studies in rats and rabbits using oral doses 150 times or more than the topical human dose revealed no significant evidence of impaired fertility or harm to the fetus. Naftifine is classified in FDA Pregnancy Category B.

Since it is not known whether naftifine is excreted in breast milk and since it is known that up to 6% of a topical dose can be absorbed systemically, consideration should be given to discontinuing nursing temporarily while using naftifine cream or gel and for several days after the last application.

PHARMACOKINETICS. Following a single topical application of naftifine 1% to the skin of healthy subjects, approximately 6% of the dose of the cream and 4.2% of the gel were absorbed. Naftifine and/or its metabolites are excreted in the urine and feces; the half-life is about two to three days.

DOSAGE AND PREPARATIONS.

Topical: A sufficient quantity of gel is gently massaged into the affected area and surrounding skin twice daily (morning and evening); the cream is applied once daily. Treatment is continued for one to two weeks after symptoms have subsided in order to assure healing and reduce the possibility of recurrence. Four weeks of treatment are usually adequate.

Naftin (Herbert). Cream 1% in 15 and 30 g containers; gel 1% in 20, 40, and 60 g containers.

TERBINAFINE (Investigational Drug)

[Lamisil]

ACTIONS AND USES. Terbinafine is the first antifungal agent of the class of synthetic allylamines that is effective both topically and orally. Like naftifine, its fungicidal action is based on allosteric inhibition of the fungal enzyme, squalene epoxidase, which is associated with accumulation of toxic quantities of squalene and a decrease in the concentration of ergosterol, which is required for cell membrane integrity. This agent's principal fungicidal action against dermatophytes is due to its inhibition of squalene epoxidase; however, the deficiency of ergosterol may be more responsible for its effect on Candida (Birnbaum, 1990).

Terbinafine is especially effective in tinea infections (tinea corporis, tinea cruris) (Cole and Stricklin, 1989; Greer and Jolly, 1990; Millikan, 1990). Both the oral and topical forms are superior to griseofulvin in relieving signs and symptoms of moccasin-type tinea pedis and eradicating the causative organism (Savin and Zaias, 1990; Smith et al, 1990). In an uncontrolled open study, oral terbinafine was effective in 24 patients with onychomycosis, 7 of whom had not responded to griseofulvin (Goodfield et al, 1989); no recurrences were noted in a 12-month follow-up period. Terbinafine also has been effective topically in cutaneous candidal infections (Balfour and Faulds, 1992).

ADVERSE REACTIONS AND PRECAUTIONS. Dyspepsia was the only adverse effect noted and was more common in patients with a prior history of the disorder. Routine function tests of the kidney, liver, and hematopoietic system were normal.

PHARMACOKINETICS. Terbinafine is highly lipophilic and is well absorbed orally; peak plasma concentrations are achieved within two hours. The drug is distributed from the blood via diffusion through the dermis and epidermis and is transported via the sebum to sites of cutaneous fungal infections. After six months of dosing, the concentration in the hair, skin, and nails of primates was tenfold greater than peak plasma concentrations. Three inactive metabolites are formed (Birnbaum, 1990). Less than 5% of the total cytochrome P450 capacity of the liver is involved in this metabolism compared with 60% for ketoconazole.

DOSAGE AND PREPARATIONS.

Topical: In investigational studies, a 1% cream has been applied twice daily for two weeks (tinea corporis) or four weeks (tinea pedis).

Oral: For tinea pedis and onychomycosis, 125 mg twice daily for three months (fingernails) or six months (toenails).

Lamisil (Sandoz).

Imidazoles

BUTOCONAZOLE NITRATE

[Femstat]

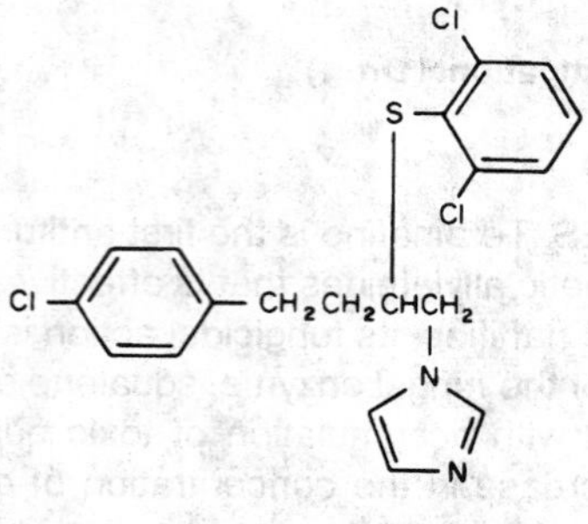

ACTIONS AND USES. Like other imidazoles, butoconazole is fungistatic and depends on the immune response of the host to effect a clinical cure (Bradbeer et al, 1985; Kaufman, 1986). This agent is known to inhibit ergosterol biosynthesis in the cytoplasmic membrane of fungi; however, this mechanism of action probably is not primary or exclusive (Fromtling, 1988). Although its spectrum of action is broad and is similar to that of the related imidazole, ketoconazole, only a topical intravaginal preparation has been studied extensively and approved by the FDA for the local treatment of vulvovaginal infections caused by Candida.

Compared with other available imidazoles used for the treatment of vaginal candidiasis and at comparable doses based on length of treatment, topical butoconazole is at least equivalent to clotrimazole and miconazole in the limited studies available (*Med Lett Drugs Ther,* 1986; Fromtling, 1988; Tatum and Eggleston, 1988). No significant differences among these imidazoles were determined with regard to the incidence and severity of local adverse reactions; however, some patients preferred butoconazole because of minimal leakage from the vagina. Strains of *C. albicans* known to be resistant to other imidazoles clinically also appear to be resistant to butoconazole in vitro.

ADVERSE REACTIONS AND PRECAUTIONS. Butoconazole is well tolerated. In controlled clinical trials, the principal adverse reactions reported following vaginal administration were vulvovaginal burning and itching (2.3%), vulvar itching (0.9%), and discharge, swelling, and soreness (0.2%). Therapy was discontinued in 1.6% of patients because of adverse reactions. No systemic effects have been observed; hepatic dysfunction has not been reported. Patients should be instructed to complete the full course of therapy even if prompt symptomatic relief or menstruation occurs.

PREGNANCY AND LACTATION. This drug is classified in FDA Pregnancy Category C based on the observation that rats who received three to seven times the human dose of butoconazole intravaginally during the period of organogenesis had an increase in resorption rate and a decrease in litter size. However, no teratogenic effects were noted. Since there are no adequate and well-controlled studies in pregnant women during the first trimester, the manufacturer recommends that the drug's use be limited to the second and third trimesters. It is not known whether butoconazole is excreted in human milk; however, metabolic products representing about 5% of the dose are present equally in urine and feces following intravaginal administration and absorption.

PHARMACOKINETICS. An average of 5.5% of a dose is absorbed slowly from the vagina, and plasma levels of the drug and its metabolites were detected between two to eight hours after administration. Maximum plasma concentrations of butoconazole and metabolites were achieved 24 hours after application (range, 19 to 44 ng/ml) and were undetectable after 96 to 120 hours. The elimination half-life of radiolabeled butoconazole was 21 to 24 hours. The drug probably is metabolized in the liver, and the metabolic derivatives are eliminated equally in the urine and feces.

DOSAGE AND PREPARATIONS.

Intravaginal: In nonpregnant patients, one applicatorful of cream is applied at bedtime for three days. Treatment can be extended for an additional three days if necessary. In pregnant patients in the second and third trimesters, the duration of treatment is six days.

Femstat (Syntex). Cream (vaginal) 2% in 28 g container with three disposable dose applicators or three prefilled single-dose applicators (***Femstat Prefill***).

CLOTRIMAZOLE

[Lotrimin, Gyne-Lotrimin, Mycelex, Mycelex-G]

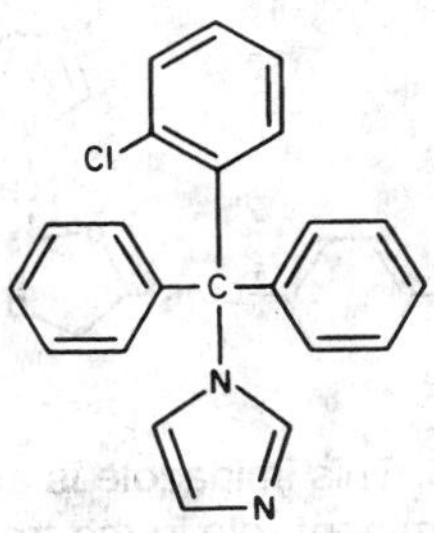

ACTIONS AND USES. The imidazole, clotrimazole, is closely related chemically to miconazole (Sawyer et al, 1975). It affects the permeability of fungi by interfering with the biosynthesis of ergosterol, which causes disorganization of the plasma membrane (Beggs et al, 1981). Systemic preparations are not available.

Clotrimazole is useful when applied topically in dermatophytic (tinea) infections and tinea versicolor, cutaneous candidiasis, and candidal infections of the mucous membranes and mucocutaneous junctions (eg, orocutaneous [perleche]; oropharyngeal [thrush]; perianal, intertriginous, and vulvovaginal areas). Clinical cure of dermatophytic and candidal infections of the skin, mucous membranes, and mucocutaneous junctions usually requires two weeks to one month, depending on the site and extent of involvement. The time required for clinical cure of vaginal candidiasis depends on the size of the dose, the dosage schedule, and the severity of infection.

Studies support the prophylactic use of the lozenge (troche) form in selected patients (eg, those receiving cytotoxic and immunosuppressant drugs) (Owens et al, 1984; Shectman et al, 1984; Cuttner et al, 1986). This dosage form also may be adequate for mild to moderate involvement of the esophagus; however, systemic therapy with amphotericin B (with or without flucytosine), oral ketoconazole, or fluconazole may be necessary in patients with more severe infections (Mathieson and Dutta, 1983; Kodsi and Goldberg, 1983).

In order to improve compliance and minimize relapses and recurrent infections, treatment of vulvovaginal candidiasis has been modified to reduce exposure time by utilizing the highest dose possible commensurate with acceptable side effects. Treatment periods have been reduced from seven to three to one day (single dose) and doses increased from 100 to 200 to 500 mg, respectively. All regimens appear to be equally effective in mild to moderate infections, but a conventional one-week regimen of therapy is preferred for more severe episodes. Some physicians prefer to use the lower daily doses for three or seven days in pregnant women and only during the second and third trimesters to limit peak blood concentrations. A nonprescription preparation is available for a seven-day course of treatment for recurrent, uncomplicated cases of vaginal candidiasis.

ADVERSE REACTIONS AND PRECAUTIONS. Adverse effects after topical use of clotrimazole include erythema; stinging, blistering, and peeling of the skin; edema; pruritus; and urticaria. Preparations of clotrimazole should be used with caution around the eyes.

Adverse reactions after use of the troche form include nausea and vomiting (incidence, about 5%). Reversible elevation of AST to abnormal levels has occurred in 15% of patients receiving troches. The manufacturer recommends periodic assessment of hepatic function, particularly in patients with pre-existing hepatic impairment. The safety and effectiveness of clotrimazole troches in children less than 3 years have not been established; therefore, use of this dosage form in these patients is not recommended.

Following vaginal application, mild vaginal burning, erythema, and irritation have occurred.

PREGNANCY AND LACTATION. Clotrimazole is embryotoxic in rats and mice when given in amounts 100 times the adult human dose (in mg/kg), possibly secondary to maternal toxicity. The drug was not teratogenic in mice, rabbits, and rats when given in amounts up to 200 times the human dose. There are no adequate, well-controlled reproductive studies in pregnant women.

Pregnancy is not a contraindication to the topical cutaneous application of clotrimazole or to its use intravaginally during the second and third trimesters. Its use during the first trimester is not recommended because of its embryotoxic action in animals and a study suggesting the drug may be associated with spontaneous abortions (Rosa et al, 1987). Cutaneous and intravaginal preparations are classified in FDA Pregnancy Category B and the oral troche in FDA Pregnancy Category C.

Clotrimazole is poorly and erratically absorbed, and it would not be expected to be present in sufficient amounts in breast milk to cause a problem.

DOSAGE AND PREPARATIONS.

Topical: A sufficient amount of cream, solution, or lotion to cover the affected and surrounding areas is applied twice daily (morning and evening).

Lotrimin (Schering), ***Mycelex*** (Miles). Cream 1% in 15, 30, 45 (***Lotrimin*** only), and 90 g containers; solution 1% in 10 and 30 ml containers; and lotion 1% (***Lotrimin*** only) in 30 ml containers.

Available Mixture.

Lotrisone (Schering). Cream containing clotrimazole 1% and betamethasone dipropionate 0.05% in 15 and 45 g containers.

Intravaginal: One tablet (100 mg) is inserted into the vagina nightly for seven days or one applicatorful of cream is inserted into the vagina nightly for 7 to 14 days.

For nonpregnant patients with mild to moderate infections, an alternative, equally effective regimen is two tablets (200 mg) inserted into the vagina nightly for three days; studies also support the efficacy of a single 500-mg vaginal tablet (Hughes and Kriedman, 1984; Fleury et al, 1985) or 5 g of a 10% cream (investigational) (Sposetti et al, 1987). A seven-day regimen may be preferable for severe infections.

Gyne-Lotrimin (Schering-Plough). Cream (vaginal) 1% in 45 g containers with applicator (nonprescription); tablets (vaginal) 100 mg (nonprescription).

Mycelex-G (Miles). Cream (vaginal) 1% in 45 and 90 g containers with applicator; tablets (vaginal) 100 and 500 mg with applicator and 500 mg with cream 1% in 7 g containers (Twin Pack).

Oral: One troche five times a day for 14 consecutive days; the troche must be dissolved slowly in the mouth.

Mycelex (Miles). Troche 10 mg.

ECONAZOLE NITRATE

[Spectazole]

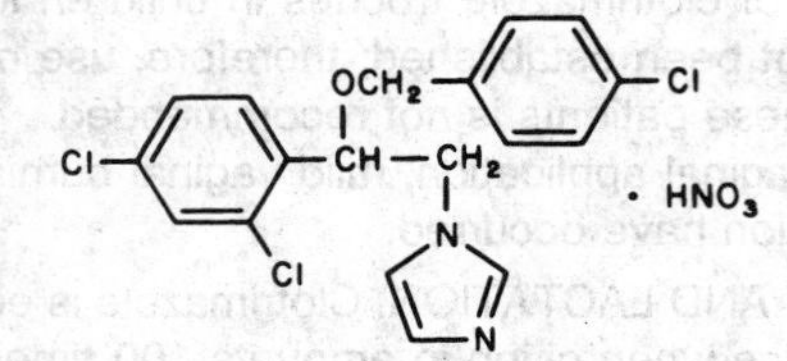

ACTIONS AND USES. This imidazole affects the permeability of fungi by interfering with the biosynthesis of ergosterol, which causes disorganization of the plasma cell membrane (Beggs et al, 1981).

Econazole is available for topical application in the treatment of dermatophytic skin infections, as well as tinea versicolor and cutaneous candidiasis (Fromtling, 1988). Comparative studies with other topical imidazoles suggest that it is equally effective in these infections.

ADVERSE REACTIONS AND PRECAUTIONS. Side effects in controlled studies are reported to be infrequent (3.3%) and minor (eg, pruritus, burning and stinging, erythema). The incidence of sensitization is very low. Overdose of econazole has not been reported. No systemic toxicity has occurred following topical administration because of limited absorption.

PREGNANCY AND LACTATION. Econazole was not teratogenic when administered orally to mice, rabbits, or rats. Fetotoxic or embryotoxic effects were observed in mice, rabbits, and/or rats receiving oral doses 80 or 40 times the human dermal dose. Econazole should be used during the first trimester only when administration is considered essential (FDA Pregnancy Category C).

It is not known whether econazole is excreted in human milk. Oral administration to lactating rats resulted in excretion of econazole and/or metabolites in milk and these substances were found in nursing pups. Therefore, caution should be exercised when econazole is administered to nursing women.

PHARMACOKINETICS. Econazole is not used systemically, and clinically insignificant amounts (less than 1%) are absorbed after topical application to the skin.

DOSAGE AND PREPARATIONS.

Topical: The preparation is applied to affected areas once daily in patients with tinea pedis, tinea cruris, tinea corporis, tinea versicolor and twice daily in those with cutaneous candidiasis. Candidal infections and tinea cruris and corporis should be treated for two weeks and tinea pedis for one month to reduce the possibility of recurrence.

Spectazole (Ortho). Cream 1% in 15, 30, and 85 g containers.

KETOCONAZOLE

[Nizoral]

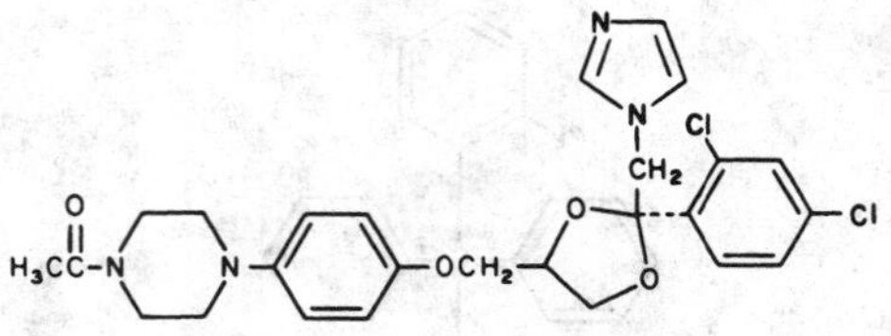

ACTIONS AND USES. This imidazole is adequately absorbed orally and plays a prominent role in the treatment of a number of systemic mycoses. It is at least as effective as other imidazoles in the treatment of dermatophytic infections and is the drug of choice for chronic mucocutaneous candidiasis. (See index entry Ketoconazole for a more complete discussion of the oral form.) Because of the potential for adverse reactions following systemic administration, oral ketoconazole should be reserved for extensive lesions or superficial infections that do not respond to conventional topical drugs.

A topical cream preparation of ketoconazole is available for use in superficial fungal infections of the skin, including tinea cruris and corporis, tinea versicolor, cutaneous candidiasis, and seborrheic dermatitis (Shear, 1987). The shampoo preparation, which is used for dandruff, is being investigated for tinea versicolor.

One mechanism of action of ketoconazole is to interfere with fungal ergosterol biosynthesis. Preliminary data from animal studies suggest that topical ketoconazole cream may have an anti-inflammatory action (Van Cutsem et al, 1991). Infrequently, resistant strains of *Trichophyton tonsurans* and *T. rubrum* have been noted.

ADVERSE REACTIONS AND PRECAUTIONS. No systemic effects after topical application have been reported; systemic absorption has not been observed following use of topical ketoconazole 2%. This agent is well tolerated, and side effects are limited to irritation, pruritus, and stinging. All of these reactions occasionally can be severe, but usually occur in no more than 5% of patients; in comparison, in clinical studies the placebo reaction was about 2%. Phototoxicity and photosensitivity have not been reported.

See index entry Ketoconazole for potential reactions after oral administration.

PREGNANCY AND LACTATION. Ketoconazole is teratogenic in the rat when given orally in a dose ten times that recommended in humans; however, when applied to human skin, significant systemic absorption has not been demonstrated in concentrations above the detectable concentration in blood. This drug is classified in FDA Pregnancy Category C.

DOSAGE AND PREPARATIONS.

Topical: The cream should be applied once daily to affected areas. The recommended duration for treatment of fungal infections of the skin is generally two weeks, even if symptomatic relief occurs more promptly, in order to minimize recurrence.

Nizoral (Janssen). Cream 2% in 15, 30, and 60 g containers; shampoo 2% in 120 g container.

Oral: See index entry Ketoconazole, Uses, Subcutaneous, Systemic Mycoses.

MICONAZOLE NITRATE

[Micatin, Monistat-Derm, Monistat 3, Monistat 7, Zeasorb-AF]

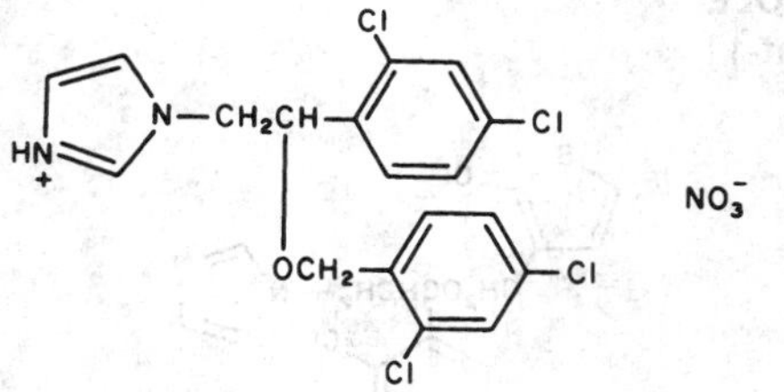

ACTIONS AND USES. Miconazole is a synthetic imidazole with broad in vitro antifungal activity. This drug affects fungal permeability by interfering with the biosynthesis of ergosterol to cause disorganization of the plasma membrane (Beggs et al, 1981).

Miconazole is effective topically in dermatophytic infections of the intertriginous and glabrous skin and in tinea versicolor. However, griseofulvin is preferred in moderate to severe dermatophytoses of the scalp, beard, palms, and fingernails. Miconazole also is useful in cutaneous and vaginal candidal infections. A nonprescription preparation is available for treatment of recurrent, uncomplicated cases of vaginal candidiasis.

ADVERSE REACTIONS AND PRECAUTIONS. Side effects after topical application consist of irritation, burning, or maceration. If these reactions appear to be caused by hypersensitivity or if undue discomfort occurs, the drug should be discontinued. Miconazole should be used cautiously around the eyes.

After vulvovaginal application of 100 mg/day for seven days, burning, pruritus, or irritation occurred in 6% to 7% of patients in controlled studies but required discontinuation in only 0.9%. Doses of 200 mg/day for three days caused burning, pruritus, or irritation in 2% of patients in controlled studies; urticaria and skin rash occurred in less than 0.5%. Only 0.3% of patients discontinued therapy.

PREGNANCY AND LACTATION. Small amounts of miconazole are absorbed from the vagina; however, no adverse effects or complications attributable to the drug have been reported in infants of women treated for vulvovaginal candidiasis during pregnancy.

Use of miconazole should be limited to the second and third trimesters of pregnancy. A recent study suggests that a slightly increased risk of spontaneous abortion may be associated with the use of miconazole during the first trimester (Rosa et al, 1987).

DOSAGE AND PREPARATIONS.

Topical: A sufficient amount of cream to cover the affected area is applied once daily. Two weeks of therapy are usually sufficient, but four weeks are recommended for infections of the soles. If no improvement is seen after one month of therapy, the diagnosis should be reconfirmed.

Generic. Cream 2% in 15 and 30 g containers (nonprescription).

Micatin (Ortho). Cream 2% in 15 and 30 g containers; powder (aerosol) 2% in 90 g containers; powder 2% in 45 g containers; liquid (aerosol) 2% in 105 ml containers (nonprescription).

Monistat-Derm (Ortho). Cream 2% in 15, 30, and 85 g containers.

Zeasorb-AF (Stiefel). Powder 2% in 70 g containers (nonprescription).

Intravaginal: One applicatorful of cream is inserted high in the vagina or one 100-mg suppository is inserted nightly for seven days; alternatively, to increase compliance, one 200-mg suppository may be inserted nightly for three days. In resistant cases, the course of therapy may be repeated after the diagnosis has been reconfirmed.

Monistat 3 (Ortho). Suppositories 200 mg with applicator; cream 2% in 15 g container with three 200-mg suppositories (Dual Pack).

Monistat 7 (Ortho). Cream 2% in 45 g containers with applicator; suppositories 100 mg with applicator (both forms nonprescription).

OXICONAZOLE NITRATE

[Oxistat]

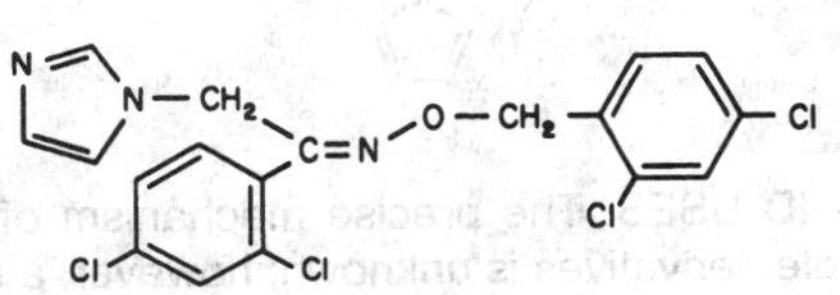

ACTIONS AND USES. The fungistatic activity of this synthetic imidazole presumably results in part from the inhibition of ergosterol synthesis that is required for fungal membrane integrity. Oxiconazole has a broad spectrum of microbiological activity; however, it is marketed only for topical application in the treatment of dermatophytic skin infections (Ellis et al, 1989). Although this imidazole is effective against selected strains of *Candida* and *Malassezia furfur*, clinical data on its use in cutaneous candidiasis and tinea versicolor are limited. Results of two- to four-week studies comparing oxiconazole with miconazole and econazole in other tinea infections suggest that oxiconazole is equally effective and safe, and relapse rates are similar with administration once daily.

ADVERSE REACTIONS AND PRECAUTIONS. Oxiconazole was well tolerated in clinical studies. About 4% of patients had adverse reactions, which included pruritus (1.6%), burning (1.4%), irritation (0.4%), erythema (0.2%), and maceration and fissuring (0.1%). About 0.3% of the drug is absorbed systemically, but this finding is based on urinary excretion alone, not fecal excretion. Contact sensitization has been reported with oxiconazole, but appreciable clinical experience with other topical imidazoles indicates that contact sensitization among the imidazole antifungals is rare (Jelen and Tennstedt, 1989).

The cream formulation is for use on the skin; it should not be applied intravaginally or in the eye.

PREGNANCY AND LACTATION. Reproduction studies using oxiconazole orally in rabbits, rats, and mice have revealed no evidence of harm to the fetus. Nevertheless, adequate and well-controlled studies in pregnant women have not been conducted. Therefore, oxiconazole should be used during pregnancy only if clearly needed (FDA Pregnancy Category B). Studies indicate that any amount absorbed after topical application would be excreted in human milk; therefore caution is advised when the drug is given to nursing women.

DOSAGE AND PREPARATIONS.

Topical: In patients with tinea pedis, tinea corporis, and tinea cruris, a sufficient amount of the preparation should be applied to cover affected areas once daily in the evening. Tinea corporis and tinea cruris should be treated for two weeks and tinea pedis for one month to reduce the possibility of recurrence.

Oxistat (Glaxo). Cream 1% in 15, 30, and 60 g containers.

SULCONAZOLE NITRATE

[Exelderm]

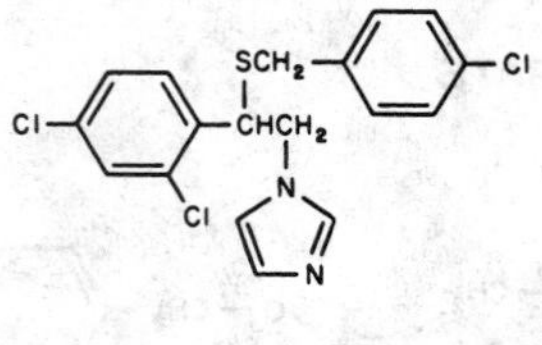

ACTIONS AND USES. The precise mechanism of action of most imidazole derivatives is unknown; however, a fungistatic action on the cell membrane with loss of selective permeability is most likely. Although sulconazole has a relatively broad antifungal spectrum, it is available only for topical application in the treatment of dermatophytic skin infections and tinea versicolor. In comparative clinical trials with clotrimazole, econazole, and miconazole for dermatophytic infections of the body, groin, or feet, the efficacy of sulconazole was similar to that of the other antifungal imidazoles (Benfield and Clissold, 1988). Relapse rates were also comparable.

ADVERSE REACTIONS AND PRECAUTIONS. Sulconazole is well tolerated; the dropout rate in clinical trials because of adverse reactions was negligible. Less than 3% of patients complained of erythema, irritation, and pruritus. Allergic contact dermatitis, phototoxicity, or photoallergy has not been observed. About 12% of a dose is absorbed from the forearm of healthy male volunteers (Franz and Lehman, 1988); however, no systemic adverse effects have been reported.

Because sulconazole produced embryotoxic, not teratogenic, effects in rats when given large (hundredfold) doses of sulconazole orally, the drug is classified in FDA Pregnancy Category C. It should be used during pregnancy only if clearly needed. It is not known whether sulconazole is excreted in human milk. Its safety and efficacy in children have not been established.

DOSAGE AND PREPARATIONS.

Topical: The cream or solution is applied to affected areas once or twice daily in patients with tinea cruris, tinea corporis, and tinea versicolor; application twice daily is recommended for tinea pedis. Although relief and clinical improvement are usually observed within a few days to one week, treatment should continue for three weeks (four weeks recommended for tinea pedis) to minimize the risk of relapse.

Exelderm (Westwood-Squibb). Cream 1% in 15, 30, and 60 g containers; solution 1% in 30 ml containers.

TIOCONAZOLE

[Vagistat-1]

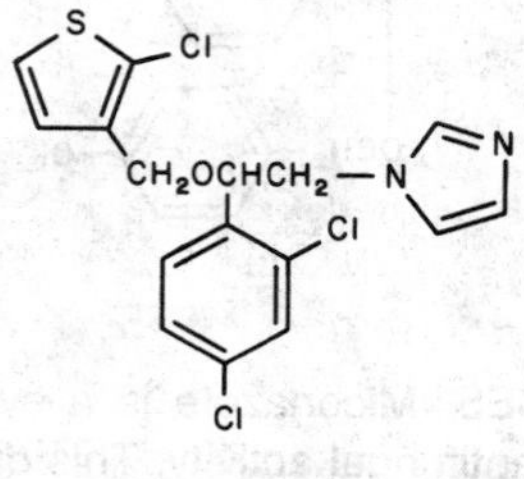

ACTIONS AND USES. Like other imidazoles, tioconazole inhibits ergosterol biosynthesis in the cytoplasmic membrane of fungi. This imidazole is approved for topical treatment of dermatophytic skin infections and vulvovaginal candidiasis, but it is marketed only for the latter indication in the United States. Its broad-spectrum antifungal activity against dermatophytes is similar to that of miconazole (East, 1983; Clissold and Heel, 1986; Fromtling, 1988). Studies comparing this agent with other imidazoles and triazoles in the treatment of vaginal candidiasis are limited.

ADVERSE REACTIONS AND PRECAUTIONS. Burning and pruritus were the most common side effects observed in clinical trials (incidence, about 5%). Local irritation, vaginal pain, vulvar edema, dysuria, and reduced vaginal secretions occurred infrequently (incidence, <1%).

Based on the results of animal studies, tioconazole is classified in FDA Pregnancy Category C; therefore, it should be used during pregnancy only if the potential benefit justifies the potential risk to the fetus.

DOSAGE AND PREPARATIONS.

Topical: The manufacturer's recommended dose is a single applicatorful of ointment (300 mg) inserted into the vagina just prior to bedtime.

Vagistat-1 (Mead Johnson). Ointment 6.5% in 4.6 g prefilled vaginal applicator.

Bis-triazoles

FLUCONAZOLE

[Diflucan]

For chemical formula, see index entry Fluconazole, Uses, Subcutaneous, Systemic Mycoses.

ACTIONS AND USES. This bis-triazole fungistatic agent is available for oral and parenteral administration. Fluconazole inhibits lanosterol 14-demethylase, one of the superfamily of cytochrome P450 enzymes. It has a greater specificity for fungal cytochrome P450 enzyme systems than for mammalian species, and this difference is probably responsible for the low toxicity of this drug compared with the orally administered imidazole, ketoconazole (Back and Tjia, 1991). Fluconazole is used for cryptococcal meningitis and systemic deep infections due to *Candida*, including oropharyngeal and esophageal candidiasis.

Evidence from clinical trials also supports the effectiveness of fluconazole in vulvovaginal candidiasis (Multicentre Study Group, 1988). Controlled comparative studies were conducted in Europe in approximately 2,000 patients with acute vulvovaginal candidiasis who were randomly assigned to receive one of four regimens: a single oral dose of fluconazole 150 mg, ketoconazole 200 mg orally twice daily for five days (Kutzer et al, 1988), clotrimazole 200 mg intravaginally daily for three days (*Br J Obstet Gynecol*, 1989), or a single intravaginal application of econazole 150 mg (Osser et al, 1991). Clinical and mycologic cure and failure rates in the short (two weeks) and long (four to six weeks) term were essentially the same in all treatment arms. All regimens were generally well tolerated. Another comparative study using clotrimazole 200 mg/day intravaginally or fluconazole 50 mg/day orally, each given for three consecutive days, yielded similar results (Stein et al, 1991). The higher potency, longer half-life, and persistence of fluconazole in vaginal secretions probably account for the effectiveness observed with single-dose oral therapy. It is likely that fluconazole also will be evaluated as an alternative to oral ketoconazole in the prophylaxis of recurrent vaginal candidiasis (Sobel, 1992 A, 1992 B).

Pregnant women have been excluded from studies of fluconazole in vaginal candidiasis to date; therefore, no clinical data are available on these patients.

Although there is some evidence to suggest that fluconazole is effective in selected dermatophytoses, data are too limited to determine the role of this agent in these conditions.

ADVERSE REACTIONS AND PRECAUTIONS. The overall incidence of side effects in the single-dose 150 mg- or three-dose 50 mg-regimens has varied from 6% to 10.9%. The most common untoward effects involve the gastrointestinal system (eg, nausea [most common], diarrhea, dyspepsia, abdominal pain, vomiting). Headache and rash also have been reported. See index entry, Fluconazole, Uses, Subcutaneous, Systemic Mycoses for potential adverse effects on the liver.

DRUG INTERACTIONS AND PHARMACOKINETICS. See index entry Fluconazole, Uses, Subcutaneous, Systemic Mycoses.

DOSAGE AND PREPARATIONS.

Oral: In clinical trials to date, the most common dosage schedule used for the treatment of acute vulvovaginal candidiasis has been 150 mg as a single dose.

Diflucan (Pfizer). Tablets 50, 100, and 200 mg.

ITRACONAZOLE (Investigational drug)

[Sporanox]

For chemical formula, see index entry Itraconazole, Uses.

ACTIONS AND USES. Itraconazole, a bis-triazole antifungal agent, has been used primarily for oral treatment of subcutaneous and systemic fungal diseases (see above index entry). It also is effective orally in the treatment of superficial mycoses, including dermatophytosis and oropharyngeal and vaginal candidiasis (Cauwenbergh and Degreef, 1990; Van Heusden et al, 1991). Results of controlled and uncontrolled studies have demonstrated that itraconazole is more effective than placebo when given orally in the treatment of tinea versicolor (Delescluse, 1990); tinea corporis, cruris, pedis, and manuum (Hay et al, 1990; Legendre and Esola-Macre, 1990; Saul and Bonifaz, 1990); tinea unguium (Hay et al, 1990); and oropharyngeal (Blatchford, 1990) and vaginal (Merkus, 1990) candidiasis.

Itraconazole inhibits lanosterol 14-demethylase, one of the superfamily of cytochrome P450 enzymes. Itraconazole has a greater specificity for fungal cytochrome P450 enzyme systems than for mammalian species, and this difference is probably responsible for the relatively low toxicity of this orally administered bis-triazole compared with the orally administered imidazole, ketoconazole (Back and Tjia, 1991).

ADVERSE REACTIONS AND PRECAUTIONS. Itraconazole is well tolerated following oral administration even for periods of up to nine months. Headache, dizziness, and gastrointestinal discomfort (abdominal pain, nausea, dyspepsia, diarrhea, vomiting) occurred in 6% of patients; however, no correlation was observed between gastrointestinal side effects and daily dose levels of 50, 100, and 200 mg or the time of administration. Some patients with gastrointestinal discomfort improved with continued administration of the drug. Occasionally, rashes were noted; these disappeared on cessation of itraconazole therapy. No change in results of tests for hematologic, hepatic, or renal function were observed.

Itraconazole is teratogenic in rats at doses higher than those effective clinically. It should not be used during pregnancy or in women of childbearing age if contraception cannot be assured.

DRUG INTERACTIONS AND PHARMACOKINETICS. See index entry Itraconazole, Uses, Subcutaneous, Systemic Mycoses.

DOSAGE AND PREPARATIONS.

Oral: In clinical trials, the following dosage schedules have been utilized for superficial mycoses. However, these schedules may need to be modified if symptoms and signs of infection persist; in chronic or disseminated mycoses; in tinea modified by corticosteroid therapy; or in the presence of an additional pathogen(s) (eg, *Candida*), especially in immunocompromised patients. For tinea versicolor, 200 mg daily for 5 to 7 days; tinea corporis and tinea cruris, 100 mg daily for 15 days; tinea manuum and tinea pedis, 100 mg daily for 30 to 45 days (however, more chronic *T. rubrum* infections of toe webs, palms, soles, and nails may require six to nine months of therapy); oropharyngeal candidiasis, 200 mg daily for 14 to 30 days; vaginal candidiasis, 200 mg daily for two days.

Sporanox (Janssen).

TERCONAZOLE

[Terazol 3, Terazol 7]

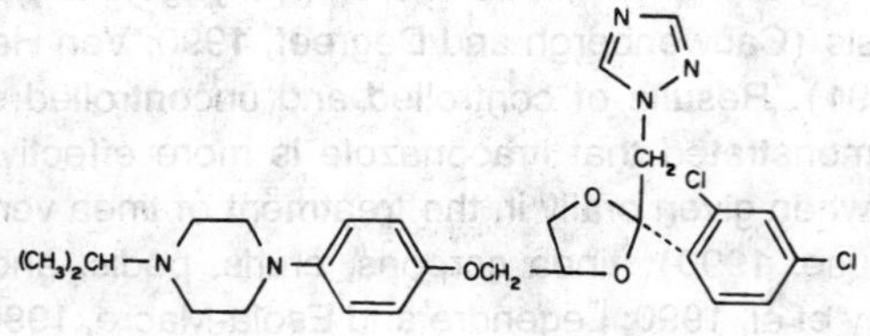

ACTIONS AND USES. This fungistatic agent of the azole class is a bis-triazole derivative; therefore, it is more similar to fluconazole and itraconazole than to the imidazole antifungal agents (Rippon, 1986). Although terconazole is active against dermatophytes, it is marketed only for topical application in the treatment of vulvovaginal candidiasis. It is quite effective against many species of *Candida*. Its precise mechanism of action is unknown; however, like the other azole antifungal agents, the drug inhibits cytochrome P450 lanosterol 14-demethylase in susceptible fungi to cause a decrease in the amount of ergosterol needed by the organism for membrane development and maintenance of selective permeability.

Terconazole has cured at least 80% of patients with vulvovaginal candidiasis whether the three-day or seven-day regimen was used. It is as effective as clotrimazole and miconazole in both pregnant and nonpregnant patients (Wiesmeier, 1989). The relapse rate three to four weeks following treatment is reported to be 3% to 17%, but the rates are much higher in patients with chronic severe vulvovaginal candidiasis (Schmitt et al, 1990).

Terconazole is not recommended for use during the first trimester. The CDC recommends that the seven-day regimen be used during the second and third trimester.

Organism resistance is not significant clinically.

ADVERSE REACTIONS AND PRECAUTIONS. Terconazole is generally well tolerated. Local vulvovaginal burning, irritation, and pruritus occur in no more and usually in less than 5% of patients. Headache (26% versus 17% with placebo) and body pain (2.1% versus none with placebo) also have been observed. A one- to two-day "flu-like" syndrome consisting of transient headache, fever, chills, and hypotension has been reported. The syndrome is dose dependent and is similar to that observed infrequently with ketoconazole. Discontinuation of therapy because of adverse reactions is reported to be less than 2%.

The base present in the suppository formulation may interact with certain rubber or latex products, such as those used in vaginal contraceptive diaphragms; therefore, concurrent use is not recommended.

No teratogenicity has been reported for terconazole. A decrease in litter size, fetal weight, and number of viable young and a delay in fetal ossification in rats given terconazole orally were observed. These embryotoxic effects occurred at doses that result in a mean peak plasma concentration fortyfold greater than that attained in adult humans following intravaginal administration. Terconazole is classified in FDA Pregnancy Category C. It is not known whether this agent is excreted in breast milk. Safety and efficacy in children have not been established.

PHARMACOKINETICS. Following intravaginal administration of terconazole in humans, absorption ranged from 5% to 8% in three hysterectomized subjects and 12% to 16% in two nonhysterectomized subjects with tubal ligations. Terconazole is extensively metabolized; the blood elimination half-life is 6.9 hours (4.0 to 11.3).

DOSAGE AND PREPARATIONS.

Topical: One applicatorful of cream (20 mg) of Terazol 7 or 40 mg of Terazol 3 inserted into the vagina once daily at bedtime for three consecutive days (Terazol 3) or seven consecutive days (Terazol 7), or one suppository (80 mg) inserted into the vagina once daily at bedtime for three consecutive days.

Terazol 3 (Ortho). Cream 0.8% in 20 g containers; suppositories 80 mg in packages of three.

Terazol 7 (Ortho). Cream 0.4% in 45 g containers.

Polyene Antibiotics

AMPHOTERICIN B

[Fungizone]

For chemical formula, see index entry Amphotericin B, Uses, Systemic Mycoses.

Although intravenous amphotericin B has a broad spectrum of activity in systemic mycoses, its topical application is limited to the treatment of cutaneous and some acute mucocutaneous candidal infections (eg, diaper rash, otomycosis, perleche, intertrigo); no vaginal preparation is available. Amphotericin B is not effective in dermatophytic (tinea) infections.

Topical amphotericin B is not well absorbed and no systemic effects have been observed. Local irritation (pruritus, burning, erythema) occurs occasionally, most often after application on intertriginous areas.

DOSAGE AND PREPARATIONS.

Topical: Formulations are applied two to four times daily for an appropriate length of time, depending on the degree of involvement, its location, and the patient's response (see manufacturer's literature).

Fungizone (Apothecon). Cream and ointment 3% in 20 g containers; lotion 3% in 30 ml containers.

NYSTATIN

[Mycostatin, Nilstat, O-V Statin]

ACTIONS AND USES. Nystatin is an antifungal polyene antibiotic derived from *Streptomyces noursei*. This drug has no effect on the normal flora of the intestine and is not absorbed from the gastrointestinal tract. Its use usually is limited to infections of the skin and mucous membranes of the mouth, esophagus, and vagina caused by all species of *Candida*. Nystatin is administered vaginally, topically to the skin, and orally as tablets to be swallowed for their effect on *Candida* in the gastrointestinal tract or orally as lozenges or suspensions for their effect on oropharyngeal-esophageal candidiasis; it is too toxic for parenteral use.

Vaginal candidiasis responds well to topical nystatin, but the tablet form appears to be somewhat less effective than miconazole cream and usually requires at least 14 days of treatment to effect a cure and minimize recurrences. Nystatin is safe for use during the first trimester of pregnancy.

ADVERSE REACTIONS. Adverse reactions occur infrequently and are mild and transitory. Nausea, vomiting, and diarrhea may develop after oral administration. Irritation occurs rarely after topical application. The Stevens-Johnson syndrome has been associated with use of nystatin in two patients (Kiev and Hale, 1991; Gantz, 1991). Resistance to nystatin has not been reported clinically.

No adverse effects or complications have been attributed to nystatin in infants born to women treated with nystatin vaginal tablets during pregnancy. Vaginal preparations are classified in FDA Pregnancy Category A and the powder for oral suspension and troches in FDA Pregnancy Category C.

DOSAGE AND PREPARATIONS.

Oral: *Adults* (tablets), 500,000 to 1,000,000 units three times daily. *Adults and children* (suspension), 400,000 to 600,000 units four times daily (one-half of dose in each side of mouth), retained in the mouth for a time before swallowing; *infants,* 200,000 units four times daily; *premature and low-birth-weight infants,* 100,000 units four times daily. Treatment should be continued for at least 48 hours after disappearance of symptoms. *Adults and children* (lozenge), 200,000 to 400,000 units allowed to dissolve slowly in the mouth four or five times a day, continued for at least 48 hours after disappearance of symptoms.

Mycostatin (Apothecon), ***Nilstat*** (Lederle), ***Generic.*** Drops (oral suspension) 100,000 units/ml; tablets (oral) 500,000 units.

Mycostatin (Bristol-Myers). Lozenge (pastille) 200,000 units.

Vaginal: 100,000 to 200,000 units daily for two weeks.

Generic. Tablets (vaginal) 100,000 units.

Mycostatin (Mead Johnson), ***Nilstat*** (Lederle). Tablets (vaginal) 100,000 units with applicator.

O-V Statin (Apothecon). Oral/vaginal therapy pack containing 42 tablets (oral) 500,000 units and 14 tablets (vaginal) 100,000 units.

Topical: The ointment or cream is applied to lesions twice daily (the ointment should not be used in hairy intertriginous areas). The powder is preferred for moist lesions and is applied two or three times daily; however, caking may occur and result in local irritation.

Generic. Cream and ointment 100,000 units/g in 15 and 30 g containers.

Mycostatin (Westwood-Squibb). Cream and ointment 100,000 units/g in 15 and 30 g containers; powder 100,000 units/g in 15 g containers.

Nilstat (Lederle). Cream 100,000 units/g in 15 and 240 g containers; ointment 100,000 units/g in 15 g containers.

VIRAL INFECTIONS

Certain DNA and RNA viruses primarily affect the skin (Berman and Berman, 1988; Highet, 1988). DNA viruses commonly associated with skin disease include herpesviruses, poxviruses (eg, molluscum contagiosum), and papovaviruses (eg, human papillomavirus). Human papillomavirus (HPV) causes a number of verrucous diseases (warts), including condyloma acuminatum, and is strongly associated with a number of genital, laryngeal, and esophageal cancers. RNA viruses are exemplified by picornaviruses (enteroviruses) that include Coxsackie A and B viruses, which are responsible for hand, foot, and mouth disease; viral exanthemas and enanthemas (vesicular stomatitis); and togavirus (arborvirus) and paramyxovirus, which cause rubella and rubeola, respectively.

Warts

The discussion on topical antiviral drug therapy in this section is limited to the treatment of molluscum contagiosum, nongenital cutaneous warts, and genital warts (eg, condyloma acuminatum). The latter also are referred to by the trivial names, venereal or moist warts. Vaccines to prevent rubella and rubeola are discussed elsewhere; see index entry Vaccines. For the treatment of herpes infections, see index entry Antiviral Agents.

Based on DNA homology, more than 70 distinct genotypes of HPV have been identified and associated with the various forms of warts (Berman and Berman, 1988; Howley and Schlegel, 1988; Cripe, 1990). One classification system is based on anatomical location (eg, facial, oral, palmar, plantar, paronychial, periungual, laryngeal, esophageal, anogenital). Another classification system is based on clinical morphology (eg, keratotic [verruca vulgaris], flat, papular, filiform [digitate], hyperplastic [condyloma acuminatum], mosaic, myrmecia [anthill], confluent) (Rees, 1984).

Common warts (verruca vulgaris) on the skin are generally caused by HPV types 1-4, 7, 10, and 28. Genital, oral, and laryngeal condylomas are commonly caused by HPV types 6 and 11, both of which have a low risk for producing malignancy; however, condylomas associated with HPV types 16, 18, 31, 33 and others are associated with lesions that have a high potential for malignant carcinoma of the vulva, cervix, penis, esophagus, and anus. Condylomas are considered to be sexually transmitted; therefore, affected individuals should be screened for associated sexually transmitted diseases and partners should be systematically evaluated. Papanicolaou smears for women with external genital warts and/or partners of men with genital warts also are recommended.

The typical exophytic warty growth of a condyloma draws attention away from the fact that nearby normal-appearing tissue also is commonly affected (subclinical HPV infection). Colposcopy and androscopy utilizing 5% acetic acid may identify such areas of subclinical infection in the cervix and glans penis; it is probable that these areas account for the high rates of "recurrence" among patients with condylomas. The latent nature of HPV infection also is a major factor in recurrence.

THERAPY. The therapy selected depends on the type and size of wart, number of lesions, risk of scarring, immunocompetence and age of the patient, and anatomic location (Eron, 1988). Reviews discussing options and techniques for the treatment of nongenital (Goldfarb et al, 1991) and genital warts (Trofatter, 1991; Greene, 1992) are available.

Nongenital Warts: Common cutaneous warts disappear spontaneously in about 50% of patients after one year; the same odds apply again in the following year. The spontaneous resolution of warts is presumed to depend on the release of antigen systemically during the keratolytic process, which results in antibody formation and/or cell-mediated immunity (Rees, 1984). Intervention is indicated when warts are painful, subject to trauma or secondary infection, or cosmetically objectionable. Therapy that produces little or no scarring is preferred (Bunney, 1986; Gellis, 1987; Bolton, 1991).

Application of topical keratolytic agents, with periodic paring of lesions, is employed for most common cutaneous warts. Keratolytic agents should be applied carefully and treatment repeated to minimize destruction of normal tissue.

Salicylic acid 5% to 17% with or without lactic acid is effective, especially in collodion solution, because application is easily confined to the wart; salicylic acid is well tolerated by most individuals. A cure rate for cutaneous warts approximating 70% to 80% has been obtained with daily applications; therefore, it is the drug of choice. A salicylic acid 40% plaster also is available but is primarily used to remove palmar and plantar warts. Bichloroacetic acid (Kahlenberg solution) and trichloroacetic acid are effective caustic agents in concentrations of 30% to 50%, but salicylic acid is less destructive to surrounding skin and is usually preferred. Bichloroacetic and trichloroacetic acid are best reserved for deep plantar warts.

The cure rate with cryotherapy of common cutaneous warts is similar to that with salicylic acid and lactic acid. Carbon dioxide snow (dry ice) molded into stick form, liquid nitrogen, or Freon-12 (dichlorodifluoromethane) can be used. Liquid nitrogen has been used most frequently, but the higher freezing temperature of Freon-12 may cause fewer complications. The recommended interval between treatments is two weeks and no more than three weeks; three treatments are sufficient for most patients.

Electrodesiccation with curettage is acceptable. Good cosmetic results have been obtained with carbon dioxide laser treatment, and it is being used much more frequently in the treatment of cutaneous warts (Goldfarb et al, 1991; Trofatter, 1991). Laser treatment should be performed only by qualified physicians who are knowledgeable about safety guidelines. Local anesthesia is required for both electrodesiccation and laser treatment.

Cantharidin [Cantharone, Verr-Canth] is useful for almost all nongenital warts, including periungual common warts and molluscum contagiosum, a benign, self-limited cutaneous poxvirus disease that may not require treatment (Gellis, 1987).

Bleomycin sulfate is effective when administered by the intralesional route for recalcitrant nongenital warts. Since injection of bleomycin is usually painful, a bleomycin-lidocaine mixture can be used to minimize discomfort (Manz and Pelachyk, 1991). No systemic effects have been observed; however, local complications occasionally occur (eg, a persisting Raynaud's phenomenon following injection of warts on the finger; scarring; nail dystrophy when used for periungual warts).

Genital Warts: Cryotherapy is useful for the treatment of distal urethral and anogenital condyloma acuminatum. Laser treatment is being used frequently as well, especially during pregnancy if avoidance of chemotherapy is desirable (Goldfarb et al, 1991; Trofatter, 1991). As for nongenital warts, laser treatment should be performed only by qualified physicians who are knowledgeable about safety guidelines.

Podophyllin resin [Pod-Ben-25, Podoben] is an extract that is chemically nonhomogeneous, which may account for its variable effectiveness. This preparation has been commonly used to treat condyloma acuminatum; the CDC currently recommends it as an alternative to podofilox. Podophyllin is more effective for multiple or cauliflower-like lesions than for lesions in nonmoist areas (eg, penile shaft, proximal thighs).

Podofilox [Condylox] is a distinct chemical entity that offers the advantage of self-application by the patient. It appears to be equally effective on moist and keratinized lesions (Beutner et al, 1989).

Vaginal condylomas that are numerous and widespread usually respond well to topical trichloroacetic acid, and this agent can be used in pregnant patients. Most ectocervical lesions also can be treated with trichloroacetic acid. Lesions in the transformation (endocervical) region are probably best treated with cryotherapy or laser ablation.

Because of variable efficacy and toxicity, intralesional use of alpha interferons (interferon alfa-2b and interferon alfa-n3) for condyloma acuminatum should be reserved for patients who do not respond satisfactorily to conventional agents or procedures; who have chronic disease (longer than 18 months); or who have an unusual condition, such as Buschke-Löwenstein giant condyloma. Extensive anogenital condylomas in children acquired as the result of sexual abuse probably warrant systemic rather than intralesional therapy to minimize additional physical and psychological trauma (Trofatter, 1991). The use of interferons as adjunctive therapy with other therapeutic modalities (eg, laser ablation, cryotherapy) is currently being evaluated; however, guidelines for patient selection must be developed.

Interferon beta has been investigated on a limited basis; it is given intramuscularly for genital warts and appears to be more effective than placebo (Trofatter, 1991).

Drug Evaluations

CANTHARIDIN

[Cantharone, Verr-Canth]

Cantharidin produces intraepidermal vesiculation by disrupting oxidative phosphorylation. It resolves various types of warts caused by the human papilloma virus, especially the periungual variety and the flat wart-like lesions (smooth, waxy, umbilicated papules) of molluscum contagiosum caused by the poxvirus. This agent is not used for genital warts. An occlusive bandage is applied after use of cantharidin and is removed in 24 hours. The blister that forms will break, crust, and fall off in about ten days.

Burning and stinging may be noted after blister formation. A severe inflammatory response may occur in patients with molluscum contagiosum. Cantharidin is quite toxic if taken orally; it should not be prescribed for home use.

Cantharone (Seres). Liquid containing cantharidin 0.7% in a vehicle containing ether 35%, acetone, ethocel, and flexible collodion in 7.5 ml containers.

Verr-Canth (Palisades). Liquid containing cantharidin 0.7% in an adherent film-forming base containing ethylcellulose, cellosolve, castor oil, penederm, and acetone in 7.5 ml containers.

INTERFERON ALFA-2b
[Intron A]

INTERFERON ALFA-n3
[Alferon N]

TYPES AND SOURCES. The interferons are a family of naturally occurring glycoproteins with molecular weights of approximately 15,000 to 21,000 daltons. The three types of interferon that are recognized include alpha (leukocyte interferon), beta (fibroblast interferon), and gamma (immune interferon) (Baron et al, 1991).

Alpha interferons are produced by two different techniques. In the first, a human leukocyte cell line is stimulated by an avian (Sendai) virus to produce a combination of at least 16 subtypes of interferon that are then purified by chromatography to yield a "natural" interferon, interferon alfa-n1. This product is marketed only in Canada (as Wellferon). Interferon alfa-n3 [Alferon N] is a mixture of 14 alpha interferon subtypes that are obtained from pooled human leukocytes stimulated by Sendai virus. In the second technique, recombinant molecular technology is used to insert human DNA coding for interferon into *Escherichia coli* to produce a single alpha interferon subtype that is also purified by chromatography. Two alpha subtypes are manufactured: If lysine or arginine is present in position 23, the product is interferon alfa-2a [Roferon A] or interferon alfa-2b [Intron A], respectively (Galvani et al, 1988).

ACTIONS AND USES. The use of alpha interferons for warts has been limited essentially to the treatment of those genotypes of HPV that cause genital HPV infection (condyloma acuminatum) and laryngeal infection (laryngeal papillomatosis). The most established direct antiviral action of alpha interferons is cellular stimulation of 2′, 5′ oligoadenylate synthetase; this in turn breaks down viral RNA through an endonuclease, thus inhibiting viral replication. Other antiproliferative and immunomodulatory mechanisms probably are involved in the antiviral action of alpha interferons (Baron et al, 1991). See also index entry Interferons, Actions.

When indicated (see discussion on Therapy in this section), intralesional injection of interferon alfa-2b and interferon alfa-n3 is employed for the treatment of genital warts. Limited comparative studies support the effectiveness of intralesional injection of alpha interferons over placebo. In a comparative controlled trial, about twice as many anogenital warts injected with interferon alfa-2b, interferon alfa-n1, or interferon beta regressed compared with placebo injections. Improvement in uninjected lesions occurred in approximately 50% of these patients (Reichman et al, 1990). Similar results have been observed in patients treated with interferon alfa-n3 (Friedman-Kien et al, 1988). No significant clinical differences in efficacy and safety among the interferons has been confirmed (Trofatter, 1991; Greene, 1992).

Topical application of alpha interferons appears to be no more effective than placebo (Keay et al, 1988). The systemic administration (subcutaneous) of interferon alfa-2b has been used investigationally in immunocompromised patients with warts (eg, allograft recipients), in patients with resistant or recurrent lesions, and in sexually abused children.

Considerable evidence (eg, spontaneous remissions, enhanced HPV infection in the immunocompromised patient) supports the view that an intact host immune response augments the response to interferon therapy. It is likely that relapse rates (25% to 40%) are related to undetected but involved skin or mucous membrane (subclinical wart) infection associated with overt lesions. Androscopy or colposcopy using acetic acid to identify areas of subclinical wart infection has been recommended for both males (glans penis) and females to minimize relapses (Berman and Berman, 1988). It has not been established that interferon therapy has eliminated the viral genome from all cells even in the presence of a clinical cure or remission lasting for years.

ADVERSE REACTIONS AND PRECAUTIONS. Systemic side effects are common even with intralesional administration (Eron et al, 1986; Friedman-Kien et al, 1988; Welander et al, 1990). The most common symptoms include a "flu-like" syndrome associated with fever, chills, fatigue, headache, and myalgias, and mild to moderate leukopenia and occasionally thrombocytopenia. Some tolerance develops to the systemic side effects, and analgesics are useful to minimize their severity; acetaminophen (adults, 650 mg) or ibuprofen (adults, 600 to 800 mg) is recommended. Local reactions tend to be mild and are well tolerated. In most studies, the percentage of patients discontinuing interferon therapy did not exceed 5%.

Drug interactions should be anticipated when one of the alpha interferons is used with other agents that cause central nervous system depression, leukopenia, or thrombocytopenia. Patients who are sensitive to mouse immunoglobulin may be sensitive to interferon alfa-2a and alfa-n3; however, antibodies to alfa-n3 were not detected in one clinical trial (Friedman-Kien et al, 1988). Interferon alfa-n3 also contains egg protein and neomycin.

Prior to intralesional injection, baseline urinalysis; complete blood count; and blood chemistry profile including serum creatinine, blood urea nitrogen, uric acid, electrolyte concentrations, and liver function tests are recommended (Trofatter, 1991). These tests probably should be repeated at least every other week after initiation of therapy.

Interferon alfa-2b is classified in FDA Pregnancy Category C. Avoidance of breast feeding should be considered when alpha interferons are being administered.

PHARMACOKINETICS. Although side effects associated with alpha interferons occur less frequently and are less severe with intralesional than with systemic administration (subcutaneous, intramuscular), some systemic absorption occurs even with intralesional administration. The portion of an alpha interferon that is absorbed systemically following intralesional injection is completely cleared by glomerular filtration, and it undergoes rapid degradation during tubular reabsorption. Prolonged half-lives may be observed in patients with impaired renal function. For more complete information, see index entry Interferons.

DOSAGE AND PREPARATIONS.

A 30-gauge needle is recommended for intradermal injection at the base of the lesions.

INTERFERON ALFA-2b:

Intralesional: Only the 10-million IU/ml preparation should be used for intralesional injection for condyloma because dilution of other sizes (ie, 3, 5, and 25 million IU/ml) would produce a hypertonic solution.

The following dosage is recommended by the manufacturer: *Adults,* 1 million IU per wart (up to five warts) three times a week on alternate days for three weeks. If the response is not satisfactory 12 to 16 weeks after the initial treatment course, a second course may be given. Patients with 6 to 10 warts may be given a second (sequential) course of treatment at the same dose to treat up to five additional warts per course. For patients with more than 10 warts, additional courses may be given as needed with up to five additional warts per course. Alternatively, the following doses are based on lesion size and are administered two or three times weekly (Trofatter, 1991).

Lesion Area	Dose (MIU)*
≤16 mm^2	0.25
17-36 mm^2	0.5
37-64 mm^2	0.75
65-100 mm^2	1.0

** Million International Units*

Dosages for larger lesions can be calculated by combining the amounts for smaller lesions and then dividing the injection among several areas at the base of the lesion. If the patient has fewer than 10 warts, larger doses (eg, 0.5 to 1 million IU) per lesion can be administered, but the total dose should not exceed 6 million IU/day. Generally, treatment courses of four weeks alternating with four weeks of observation are practical and efficacious.

Intron A (Schering). Solution 10 million IU/ml in 1 ml containers. Reconstitute with diluent (bacteriostatic water).

INTERFERON ALFA-n3:

Intralesional: *Adults,* 250,000 IU injected at the base of the wart two times weekly for up to eight weeks. For large warts, this amount may be injected at several points around the periphery of the lesion. No more than 2.5 million IU are recommended by the manufacturer per usual treatment session. *Children,* dosage has not been established.

Alferon N (Purdue Frederick). Solution 5 million IU/ml in 1 ml containers.

PODOPHYLLIN RESIN

[Pod-Ben-25, Podoben]

Podophyllin resin is an extract of *Podophyllum peltatum* (May apple) or *P. emodi* and is used principally to treat external anogenital warts (condyloma acuminatum). Podophyllin contains a number of unidentified ingredients, and its activity may vary widely depending on the source of the material.

ADVERSE REACTIONS AND PRECAUTIONS. Podophyllin resin should be applied sparingly on extensive lesions because it can be absorbed and produce psychotoxic confusional states, severe peripheral neuropathy, adynamic ileus, renal damage, leukopenia, and thrombocytopenia; fatalities have been reported (Cassidy et al, 1982; Conard et al, 1990). Because podophyllin is embryotoxic and teratogenic, its use during pregnancy is contraindicated (Karol et al, 1980). *Podophyllin should not be given to the patient for self-administration.*

DOSAGE AND PREPARATIONS.

Topical: Podophyllin resin is applied by the clinician at weekly intervals. The patient should be instructed to wash the resin off after a few hours to minimize local reactions.

Pod-Ben-25 (Palisades), ***Generic.*** Liquid containing podophyllin resin 25% in compound benzoin tincture in 0.5 and 30 ml containers.

Podoben Liquid (American). Liquid containing podophyllin 25% in compound benzoin tincture 10% and isopropyl alcohol 72% in 5 ml containers.

Available Mixtures:

Cantharone Plus (Seres). Liquid containing podophyllin resin 2%, cantharidin 1%, and salicylic acid 30% in octylphenylpolyethylene glycol 0.5%, cellosolve, ethocel, collodion, castor oil, and acetone in 7.5 ml containers.

Verrex (Palisades). Liquid containing podophyllin resin 10% and salicylic acid 30% in an adherent film-forming vehicle in 7.5 ml containers.

Verrusol (Palisades). Liquid containing podophyllin resin 5%, cantharidin 1%, and salicylic acid 30% in an adherent film-forming vehicle in 7.5 ml containers.

PODOFILOX

[Condylox]

Podofilox (formerly podophyllotoxin), a distinct chemical entity, is the principal active ingredient of podophyllin resin (von Krogh, 1983, 1987; Beutner, 1987). Podofilox inhibits microtubule function by combining with free dimers of tubulin, the main structural component of microtubules (Norberg and Back, 1987). Unlike podophyllin resin, the 0.5% podofilox solution is pharmaceutically standardized and has a shelf-life of two years. Application in the treatment of external anogenital warts (condyloma acuminatum) is safer than with podophyllin resin, and podofilox can be self-administered (Beutner et al, 1989; Baker et al, 1990). In a controlled study on 70 patients, podofilox was self-applied twice daily for three days, followed by a four-day drug-free period. The treated warts disappeared in 79% of patients, and 60% remained free of warts at six weeks (Greenberg et al, 1991).

ADVERSE REACTIONS AND PRECAUTIONS. Mild to moderate pain, burning, pruritus, and erosion were reported in over

50% of patients after application of podofilox. Inflammation, vesiculation, edema, malodor, and skin sloughing were observed in less than 20%; however, all local reactions were transient and reversible. No systemic toxicity was observed. Podofilox is embryotoxic but not teratogenic (FDA Pregnancy Category C).

DOSAGE AND PREPARATIONS.

Topical: *Adults,* podofilox is applied every 12 hours (morning and evening) for three consecutive days followed by a four-day drug-free period. This cycle can be repeated up to four continuous weeks, depending on the response of the patient.

Condylox (Oclassen). Solution 0.5% in lactate-buffered alcohol in 3.5 ml containers.

SALICYLIC ACID

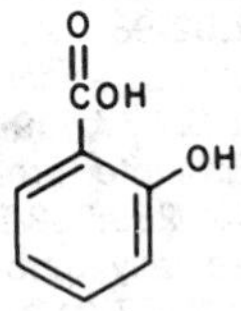

USES. Salicylic acid 3% to 6% in an ointment base is a keratolytic agent that is useful for thinning or removing calluses. Concentrations of 5% to 17% in collodion are effective and well tolerated by most patients for the removal of common warts. Combinations of salicylic acid 10% to 20% and lactic acid 10% to 20% in flexible collodion also have been used (Bunney, 1986). Controlled studies are required to determine if lactic acid enhances the effect of salicylic acid. A concentration of 40% has been applied as a plaster, principally for removal of palmar and plantar warts; efficacy is variable. This acid is not effective in a zinc oxide paste (eg, Lassar's Plain Zinc Paste) because it forms zinc salicylate, which is pharmacologically inactive.

ADVERSE REACTIONS AND PRECAUTIONS. Salicylic acid is absorbed readily and is excreted slowly in the urine. Thus, it should not be applied over large areas, in high concentrations, or for prolonged periods. Caution must be exercised when a 40% plaster is used, particularly on the extremities; in diabetics; or in patients with peripheral vascular disease, since acute inflammation and ulceration may occur after excessive use.

Ointments containing salicylic acid are odorless and do not stain the skin.

Salicylic acid is classified in FDA Pregnancy Category C.

DOSAGE AND PREPARATIONS. The collodion solution is applied to warts. After drying, an adhesive moleskin is applied to the affected area and is left on for one to three days. The softened necrotic tissue is pared with a scalpel blade or scissors. Applications and parings are repeated as necessary. Plantar warts generally require longer exposures and more frequent debridement.

SALICYLIC ACID, U.S.P.:

Generic. Powder.

Occlusal (GenDerm). Solution containing salicylic acid 17% in a polyacrylic vehicle in 15 ml containers.

Occlusal-HP (GenDerm). Solution containing salicylic acid 26% in a polyacrylic vehicle in 10 ml containers.

SALICYLIC ACID COLLODION, U.S.P.:

Duofilm (Schering-Plough). Solution containing salicylic acid 17%, alcohol 15.8%, and ether 42.6% in a collodion vehicle in 15 ml containers (nonprescription).

Freezone (Whitehall). Solution containing salicylic acid 13.6%, alcohol 20.5%, and ether 64.8% in a collodion vehicle in 9.3 ml containers (nonprescription).

Wart-Off (Pfizer). Solution containing salicylic acid 17% and alcohol 26.35% in a flexible collodion vehicle in 15 ml containers (nonprescription).

SALICYLIC ACID GEL, U.S.P.:

Duoplant (Schering-Plough). Gel containing salicylic acid 17% in an ethyl lactate, hydroxypropylcellulose, polybutene, and collodion vehicle in 15 g containers.

Hydrisalic (Pedinol). Gel containing salicylic acid 6% in a propylene glycol, ethyl alcohol, and hydroxypropylcellulose vehicle in 28.4 g containers.

Keralyt (Westwood-Squibb). Gel containing salicylic acid 6% in a propylene glycol, alcohol 19.4%, and hydroxypropylcellulose vehicle in 28.4 g containers.

SALICYLIC ACID PLASTER, U.S.P.:

Numerous commercial products containing salicylic acid 40% available for wart and callus treatment. Selected concentrations (usually 5% to 17%) also can be compounded by a pharmacist.

LACTIC AND SALICYLIC ACIDS:

Lactisol (Palisades). Flexible collodion containing salicylic acid 16.7% and lactic acid 16.7% in 15 ml containers and salicylic acid 20% and lactic acid 20% in 15 ml containers (***Lactisol-Forte***).

Salactic Film (Pedinol), ***Viranol*** (American Dermal). Flexible collodion containing salicylic acid 16.7% and lactic acid 16.7% in 10 ml (***Viranol*** only) and 15 ml (***Salactic Film*** only) containers.

BENZOIC AND SALICYLIC ACIDS OINTMENT:

Mixture available generically under the name Whitfield's Ointment in 30, 45, and 454 g containers.

Cited References

Butoconazole for vulvovaginal candidiasis. *Med Lett Drugs Ther* 28:68, 1986.

A comparison of single-dose oral fluconazole with 3-day intravaginal clotrimazole in the treatment of vaginal candidiasis: Report of an international multicentre trial. *Br J Obstet Gynecol* 26:226-232, 1989.

Mupirocin: New topical antibiotic. *Med Lett Drugs Ther* 30:55-56, 1988.

Aly R: The pathogenic staphylococci. *Semin Dermatol* 9:292-299, (Dec) 1990.

Aly R, Bayles C: The effect of mupirocin ointment on the nasal carriage of *S. aureus. Clin Res* 39, No. 1, 1991.

Arndt KA: *Manual of Dermatologic Therapeutics with Essentials of Diagnosis,* ed 4. Boston, Little Brown, 1989.

Arredondo JL: Efficacy and tolerance of topical mupirocin compared with oral dicloxacillin in the treatment of primary skin infections *Curr Ther Res* 41:121-127, 1987.

Back DJ, Tjia JF: Comparative effects of the antimycotic drugs ketoconazole, fluconazole, itraconazole and terbinafine on the metabolism of cyclosporin by human liver microsomes. *Br J Clin Pharmacol* 32:624-626, 1991.

Baker DA, et al: Topical podofilox for the treatment of condylomata acuminata in women. *Obstet Gynecol* 76:656-659, 1990.

Balfour JA, Faulds D: Terbinafine: A review of its pharmacodynamic and pharmacokinetic properties, and therapeutic potential in superficial mycoses. *Drugs* 43:259-284, 1992.

Barnett BO, Frieden IJ: Streptococcal skin diseases in children. *Semin Dermatol* 11:3-10, (March) 1992.

Baron S, et al: The interferons: Mechanisms of action and clinical applications. *JAMA* 266:1375-1383, 1991.

Beggs WH, et al: Action of imidazole-containing antifungal drugs. *Life Sci* 28:111-118, 1981.

Benfield P, Clissold SP: Sulconazole: Review of its antimicrobial activity and therapeutic use in superficial dermatomycoses. *Drugs* 35:143-153, 1988.

Berman A, Berman JE: New concepts in viral wart infection. *Compr Ther* 14:19-24, 1988.

Beutner KR: Podophyllotoxin in treatment of genital human papillomavirus infection: Review. *Semin Dermatol* 6:10-18, 1987.

Beutner KR, et al: Patient-applied podofilox for treatment of genital warts. *Lancet* 1:831-833, 1989.

Birnbaum JE: Pharmacology of the allylamines. *Suppl J Am Acad Dermatol* 23:782-785, 1990.

Blatchford NR: Treatment of oral candidosis with itraconazole: A review. *J Am Acad Dermatol* 23:565-567, 1990.

Blumer JL, et al: Changing therapy for skin and soft tissue infections in children: Have we come full circle? *Pediatr Infect Dis J* 6:117-122, 1987.

Bolton RA: Nongenital warts: Classification and treatment options. *Am Fam Physician* 43:2049-2056, 1991.

Borelli D, et al: Tinea versicolor: Epidemiologic, clinical, and therapeutic aspects. *J Am Acad Dermatol* 25:300-305, 1991.

Boswick JA Jr (ed): *The Art and Science of Burn Care.* Rockville, Md, Aspen Publishers, 1987.

Bradbeer CS, et al: Butoconazole and miconazole in treating vaginal candidiasis. *Genitourinary Med* 61:270-272, 1985.

Brandell R, et al: Treatment of oral candidiasis with amphotericin B solution. *Clin Pharm* 7:70-72, 1988.

Britton JW, et al: Comparison of mupirocin and erythromycin in the treatment of impetigo. *J Pediatr* 117:827-829, 1990.

Bunney MH: Viral warts: New look at an old problem. *BMJ* 293:1045-1047, 1986.

Cassidy DE, et al: Podophyllum toxicity: Report of fatal case and review of literature. *J Toxicol Clin Toxicol* 19:35-44, 1982.

Cauwenbergh G, Degreef H (eds): Clinical use of itraconazole in fungal infections. *Suppl J Am Acad Dermatol* 23 (No. 3, part 2):549-614, 1990.

Cauwenbergh G, et al: Pharmacokinetic profile of orally administered itraconazole in human skin. *J Am Acad Dermatol* 18:263-268, 1988.

Clissold SP, Heel RC: Tioconazole: Review of its antimicrobial activity and therapeutic use in superficial mycoses. *Drugs* 31:29-51, 1986.

Cole GW, Stricklin G: A comparison of a new oral antifungal, terbinafine, with griseofulvin as therapy for tinea corporis. *Arch Dermatol* 125:1537-1539, 1989.

Conard PF, et al: Delayed recognition of podophyllum toxicity in a patient receiving epidural morphine. *Anesth Analg* 71:191-193, 1990.

Cookson BD: Mupirocin resistance in staphylococci. *J Antimicrob Chemother* 25:497-501, 1990.

Coren CV: Burn injuries in children. *Pediatr Ann* 16:328-339, 1987.

Cripe TP: Human papillomaviruses: Pediatric perspectives on a family of multifaceted tumorigenic pathogens. *Pediatr Infect Dis J* 9:836-844, 1990.

Cullen SI, et al: Treatment of tinea versicolor with new antifungal agent, ciclopirox olamine cream 1%. *Clin Therapeut* 7:574-583, 1985.

Cuttner J, et al: Clotrimazole treatment for prevention of oral candidiasis in patients with acute leukemia undergoing chemotherapy. *Am J Med* 81:771-774, 1986.

Delescluse J: Itraconazole in tinea versicolor: A review. *J Am Acad Dermatol* 23:551-554, 1990.

Demidovich CW, et al: Current etiology and comparison of penicillin, erythromycin, and cephalexin therapies. *Am J Dis Child* 144:1313-1315, 1990.

Demling RH: Burns. *N Engl J Med* 313:1389-1398, 1985.

Dobson RL: Antimicrobial therapy for cutaneous infections. *Suppl J Am Acad Dermatol* 22:871-873, 1990.

East MO (ed): Tioconazole: Review of clinical studies in dermatology. *Dermatologica* 166 (suppl 1):1-33, (June) 1983.

Ellis CN, et al: Placebo-controlled evaluation of once-daily versus twice-daily oxiconazole nitrate (1%) cream in treatment of tinea pedis. *Curr Ther Res* 46:269-276, 1989.

Eron LJ: Update: Prevention and therapy of genital warts. *Compr Ther* 14:7-11, (Nov) 1988.

Eron LJ, et al: Interferon therapy for condylomata acuminata. *N Engl J Med* 315:1059-1064, 1986.

Ezzedeen FW, et al: Percutaneous absorption and disposition of iodochlorhydroxyquin in dogs. *J Pharmaceut Sci* 73:1369-1372, 1984.

Faergemann J, Maibach H: Griseofulvin and ketoconazole: Review with special emphasis on dermatology. *Semin Dermatol* 6:31-42, 1987.

Feingold DS, et al: Bacterial infections of the skin. *J Am Acad Dermatol* 20:469-475, 1989.

Fleury F, et al: Therapeutic results obtained in vaginal mycoses after single dose treatment with 500 mg clotrimazole vaginal tablets. *Am J Obstet Gynecol* 152 (part 2):968-970, 1985.

Fox CL Jr: Topical therapy and development of silver sulfadiazine. *Surg Gynecol Obstet* 157:82-88, 1983.

Franz TJ, Lehman P: Percutaneous absorption of sulconazole nitrate in humans. *J Pharmaceut Sci* 77:489-491, 1988.

Friedman-Kien AE, et al: Natural interferon alfa for treatment of condylomata acuminata. *JAMA* 259:533-538, 1988.

Fromtling RA: Overview of medically important antifungal azole derivatives. *Clin Microbiol Rev* 1:187-217, 1988.

Galvani D, et al: Interferon for treatment: The dust settles. *BMJ* 296:1554-1556, 1988.

Gan VN, et al: Epidemiology and treatment of tinea capitis: Ketoconazole vs. griseofulvin. *Pediatr Infect Dis J* 6:46-49, 1987.

Gantz BZ: Stevens Johnson syndrome associated with nystatin treatment. *Arch Dermatol* 127:741-742, 1991.

Gellis SE: Warts and molluscum contagiosum in children. *Pediatr Ann* 16:69-76, 1987.

Gerding RL, et al: Outpatient management of partial-thickness burns: Biobrane versus 1% silver sulfadiazine. *Ann Emerg Med* 19:121-124, (Feb) 1990.

Ginsburg CM, et al: Randomized controlled trial of intralesional corticosteroid and griseofulvin vs griseofulvin alone for treatment of kerion. *Pediatr Infect Dis J* 6:1084-1087, 1987.

Goldfarb J, et al: Randomized clinical trial of topical mupirocin versus oral erythromycin for impetigo. *Antimicrob Agents Chemother* 32:1780-1783, 1988.

Goldfarb MT, et al: Office therapy for human papillomavirus infection in nongenital sites. *Dermatol Clin* 9:287-296, 1991.

Goodfield MJD, et al: Treatment of dermatophyte infection of the finger- and toe-nails with terbinafine (SF 86-327, Lamisil), an orally active fungicidal agent. *Br J Dermatol* 121:753-757, 1989.

Goodless DR, et al: Ketoconazole in the treatment of pityriasis versicolor: International review of clinical trials. *DICP* 25:395-398, 1991.

Greenberg MD, et al: A double-blind, randomized trial of 0.5% podofilox and placebo for the treatment of genital warts in women. *Obstet Gynecol* 77:735-739, 1991.

Greene I: Therapy for genital warts. *Dermatol Clin* 10:253-267, 1992.

Greer D, Jolly HW: Topical ketoconazole treatment of cutaneous candidiasis. *J Am Acad Dermatol* 18:748-750, 1988.

Greer DL, Jolly HW Jr: Treatment of tinea cruris with topical terbinafine. *Suppl J Am Acad Dermatol* 23:800-804, 1990.

Grossman KL, Rasmussen JE: Recent advances in pediatric infectious disease and their impact on dermatology. *J Am Acad Dermatol* 24:379-389, 1991.

Grube BJ, et al: Candida: Decreasing problem for the burned patient? *Arch Surg* 123:194-196, 1988.

Hammond J, Ward CG: Burns in octogenarians. *South Med J* 84:1316-1319, 1991.

Hanifin JM, Tofte SJ: Itraconazole therapy for recalcitrant dermatophyte infections. *J Am Acad Dermatol* 18:1077-1080, 1988.

Hay RJ, et al: Itraconazole in the management of chronic dermatophytosis. *J Am Acad Dermatol* 23:561-564, 1990.

Hendley JO, Ashe KM: Effect of topical antimicrobial treatment on aerobic bacteria in the stratum corneum of human skin. *Antimicrob Agent Chemother* 35:627-631, 1991.

Highet AS: Viral warts. *Semin Dermatol* 7:53-57, 1988.

Hirschmann JV: Topical antibiotics in dermatology. *Arch Dermatol* 124:1691-1700, 1988.

Horowitz BJ: Mycotic vulvovaginitis: A broad overview. *Am J Obstet Gynecol* 165:1188-1192, 1991.

Howley PM, Schlegel R: Human papillomaviruses. *Am J Med* 85(suppl 2A):155-158, 1988.

Hughes D, Kriedman T: Treatment of vulvovaginal candidiasis with 500-mg vaginal tablet of clotrimazole. *Clin Ther* 6:662-668, 1984.

Jacoby F: Care of massive burn wound. *Crit Care Q* 44-53, (Dec) 1984.

Jelen G, Tennstedt D: Contact dermatitis from topical imidazole antifungals: 15 new cases. *Contact Dermatitis* 21:6-11, 1989.

Jue SG, et al: Ciclopirox olamine 1% cream: Preliminary review of its antimicrobial activity and therapeutic use. *Drugs* 29:330-341, 1985.

Karol MD, et al: Podophyllum: Suspected teratogenicity from topical application. *Clin Toxicol* 16:283-286, 1980.

Katz BE, Fisher AA: Bacitracin: Unique topical antibiotic sensitizer. *J Am Acad Dermatol* 17:1016-1024, 1987.

Kaufman RH (ed): Vulvovaginal candidiasis: Symposium. *J Reprod Med* 31(suppl):639-669, 1986.

Keay S, et al: Topical interferon for treating condyloma acuminata in women. *J Infect Dis* 158:934-939, 1988.

Kiev J, Hale J: Stevens-Johnson syndrome and nystatin. *Complications Surg* 10:30-33, (Nov) 1991.

Kligman AM, et al: Evaluation of ciclopirox olamine cream for the treatment of tinea pedis: Multicenter double-blind comparative studies. *Clin Ther* 7:409-417, 1985.

Kodsi BE, Goldberg PK: Therapeutic strategy for esophageal candidiasis. *Drug Ther* 13:199-213, (April) 1983.

Kovacs GT, et al: A prospective study to assess the efficacy of ketoconazole in the treatment of recurrent vaginal candidiasis. *Med J Aust* 153:328-330, (Sept) 1990.

Krowchuk DP, et al: Current status of identification and management of tinea capitis. *Pediatrics* 72:625-631, 1983.

Kutzer E, et al: A comparison of fluconazole and ketoconazole in the oral treatment of vaginal candidiasis; report of a double-blind multicentre trial. *Eur J Obstet Gynecol Reprod Biol* 29:305-313, 1988.

Lachapelle JM: Occupational allergic contact dermatitis to povidone-iodine. *Contact Dermatitis* 11:189-190, 1984.

Landau JW: Commentary: Undecylenic acid and fungous infections. *Arch Dermatol* 119:351-353, 1983.

Laude TA, et al: Tinea capitis in Brooklyn. *Am J Dis Child* 136:1047-1050, 1982.

Legendre R, Esola-Macre J: Itraconazole in the treatment of tinea capitis. *J Am Acad Dermatol* 23:559-560, 1990.

Leyden JJ: Mupirocin: New topical antibiotic. *Semin Dermatol* 6:48-54, 1987.

Logan RA, et al: Antifungal efficacy of combination of benzoic and salicylic acids in novel aqueous vanishing cream formulation, letter. *J Am Acad Dermatol* 16:136-138, 1987.

Luterman A, et al: Infections in burn patients. *Am J Med* 81(suppl 1A):45-52, 1986.

MacMillan BG: Infections following burn injury. *Surg Clin North Am* 60:186-196, 1980.

Manz LA, Pelachyk JM: Bleomycin-lidocaine mixture reduces pain of intralesional injection in the treatment of recalcitrant verrucae. *J Am Acad Dermatol* 25:524-526, 1991.

Mathieson R, Dutta SK: Candida esophagitis. *Dig Dis Sci* 28:365-370, 1983.

McLinn S: A bacteriologically controlled, randomized study comparing the efficacy of 2% mupirocin ointment (Bactroban) with oral erythromycin in the treatment of patients with impetigo. *Suppl J Am Acad Dermatol* 22:883-885, 1990.

Merkus JMWM: Treatment of vaginal candidiasis: Orally or vaginally? *J Am Acad Dermatol* 23:568-572, 1990.

Mertz PM, et al: Topical mupirocin treatment of impetigo is equal to oral erythromycin therapy. *Arch Dermatol* 125:1069-1073, 1989.

Millikan LE: Efficacy and tolerability of topical terbinafine in the treatment of tinea cruris. *Suppl J Am Acad Dermatol* 23:795-799, 1990.

Molnar JA, Burke JF: Metabolic and nutritional management: Avoiding pitfalls. *Drug Ther (Hosp)* 9:45-54, (Oct) 1984.

Monk JP, Brogden RN: Naftifine: A review of its antimicrobial activity and therapeutic use in superficial dermatomycoses. *Drugs* 42:659-672, 1991.

Multicentre Study Group: Treatment of vaginal candidiasis with a single oral dose of fluconazole. *Eur J Clin Microbiol Infect Dis* 7:364-367, 1988.

Noble WC: Topical and systemic antibiotics: Is there a rationale? *Semin Dermatol* 9:250-254, (Dec) 1990.

Norberg BO, Back O: Biological activity of high-grade podophyllotoxin in neutrophil leukocyte assay *Curr Ther Res* 41:173-178, 1987.

Odom R: Practical review of antifungals. *Mod Med* 55:59-64, 1987.

Odom R: Effective drug therapy in streptococcal skin infections. *Mod Med* 57:130-139, 1989.

Osser S, et al: Treatment of candidal vaginitis: A prospective randomized investigator-blind multicenter study comparing topically applied econazole with oral fluconazole. *Acta Obstet Gynecol Scand* 70:73-78, 1991.

Owens NJ, et al: Prophylaxis of oral candidiasis with clotrimazole troches. *Arch Intern Med* 144:290-293, 1984.

Pappa KA: Comment: Topical mupirocin, letter. *Drug Intell Clin Pharm* 21:466, 1987.

Parenti MA, et al: Mupirocin: Topical antibiotic with unique structure and mechanism of action. *Clin Pharm* 6:761-770, 1987.

Peate WF: Outpatient management of burns. *Am Fam Physician* 45:1321-1332, 1992.

Plotkin EL, et al: Naftifine cream 1% versus clotrimazole cream 1% in the treatment of tinea pedis. *J Am Podiatr Med Assoc* 80:314-318, 1990.

Rahman M, et al: Transmissible mupirocin resistance in *Staphylococcus aureus. Epidemiol Infect* 102:261-270, 1989.

Rees RB: Treatment of warts. *Semin Dermatol* 3:130-135, 1984.

Reichman RC, et al: Treatment of condyloma acuminatum with three different interferon-α preparations administered parenterally: A double-blind, placebo-controlled trial. *J Infect Dis* 162:1270-1276, 1990.

Resnick SD: Staphylococcal toxin-mediated syndromes in childhood. *Semin Dermatol* 11:11-18, (March) 1992.

Rippon JW: New era in antimycotic agents, editorial. *Arch Dermatol* 122:399-402, 1986.

Robson MC, et al: Acute management of the burned patient. *Plast Reconstr Surg* 85:1155-1168, 1992.

Rosa FW, et al: Pregnancy outcomes after first-trimester vaginitis drug therapy. *Obstet Gynecol* 69:751-755, 1987.

Rumsfield J, et al: Topical mupirocin in the treatment of bacterial skin infections. *Drug Intell Clin Pharm* 20:943-948, 1986.

Ryder NS: Mechanism of action of allylamine antimycotics, in Fromtling RA (Chairman): *Recent Trends in the Discovery, Development and Evaluation of Antifungal Agents: Proceedings of an International Telesymposium.* Barcelona, J.R. Prous Science Publishers, 1987.

Sakurai K, et al: Mode of action of 6-cyclohexyl-1-hydroxy-4-methyl-2(1H)-pyridone ethanolamine salt (Hoe 296). *Chemotherapy* 24:68-76, 1978.

Saul A, Bonifaz A: Itraconazole in common dermatophyte infections of the skin: Fixed treatment schedules. *J Am Acad Dermatol* 23:554-558, 1990.

Savin RC, Zaias N: Treatment of chronic moccasin-type tinea pedis with terbinafine: A double-blind, placebo-controlled trial. *Suppl J Am Acad Dermatol* 23:804-807, 1990.

Sawyer PR, et al: Clotrimazole: Review of its antifungal activity and therapeutic efficacy. *Drugs* 9:424-447, 1975.

Scher KS, Peoples JB: Combined use of topical and systemic antibiotics. *Am J Surg* 161:422-425, 1991.

Schmitt C, et al: Comparison of 0.8% and 1.6% terconazole cream in severe vulvovaginal candidiasis. *Obstet Gynecol* 76:414-416, 1990.

Scott MA: Bacterial skin infections. *Prim Care* 16:591-602, (Sept) 1989.

Shear NH: Ketoconazole in superficial fungal infections. *Semin Dermatol* 6:58-61, 1987.

Shectman LB, et al: Clotrimazole treatment of oral candidiasis in patients with neoplastic disease. *Am J Med* 76:91-94, 1984.

Smith EB, et al: A clinical trial of topical terbinafine (a new allylamine antifungal) in the treatment of tinea pedis. *Suppl J Am Acad Dermatol* 23:790-794, 1990.

Smoot EC III, Kucan JO: Management of soft tissue wound infections with topical antibacterials. *Res Staff Physician* 33:27-35, 1987.

Sobel JD: Recurrent vulvovaginal candidiasis: Prospective study of the efficacy of maintenance ketoconazole therapy. *N Engl J Med* 315:1455-1458, 1986.

Sobel JD: Individualizing treatment of vaginal candidiasis. *J Am Acad Dermatol* 23:572-576, 1990.

Sobel JD: Vulvovaginitis. *Dermatol Clin* 10:339-359, 1992 A.

Sobel JD: Pathogenesis and treatment of recurrent vulvovaginal candidiasis. *Clin Infect Dis* 14 (suppl 1):S148-S153, 1992 B.

Sobel JD, et al: Clotrimazole treatment of recurrent and chronic candida vulvovaginitis. *Obstet Gynecol* 73:330-334, 1989.

Sposetti R, et al: Comparison between two local clotrimazole formulations for single administration in vaginal candidiasis: Controlled clinical trial. *Clin Trials J* 24:147-155, 1987.

Stein GE, et al: Comparative study of fluconazole and clotrimazole in the treatment of vulvovaginal candidiasis. *DICP* 25:582-585, 1991.

Stohs SJ, et al: Percutaneous absorption of iodochlorhydroxyquin in humans. *J Invest Dermatol* 82:195-198, 1984.

Straughn AB, et al: Bioavailability of microsize and ultramicrosize griseofulvin products in man. *J Pharmacokinet Biopharm* 8:347-362, 1980.

Stuart JD, et al: Pediatric burn. *Am Fam Physician* 36:139-146, (Oct) 1987.

Tanz RR, et al: Treating tinea capitis: Should ketoconazole replace griseofulvin? *J Pediatr* 112:987-991, 1988.

Tatum DM, Eggleston M: Butoconazole nitrate. *Infect Control Hosp Epidemiol* 9:122-124, 1988.

Trofatter KF Jr: Interferon treatment of anogenital human papillomavirus: Related diseases. *Dermatol Clin* 9:343-352, 1991.

Van Cutsem J, et al: The antiinflammatory effects of ketoconazole: A comparative study with hydrocortisone acetate in a model using living and killed *Staphylococcus aureus* on the skin of guinea-pigs. *J Am Acad Dermatol* 25:257-261, 1991.

Van Heusden AM, et al: Single-dose oral fluconazole versus single-dose topical miconazole for the treatment of acute vulvovaginal candidosis. *Acta Obstet Gynecol Scand* 69:557-559, 1991.

von Krogh G: Condylomata acuminata 1983. *Semin Dermatol* 2:109-129, 1983.

von Krogh G: Topical self-treatment of penile warts with 0.5% podophyllotoxin in ethanol for four or five days. *Sex Transm Dis* 14:135-140, 1987.

Ward A, Campoli-Richards DM: Mupirocin: Review of its antibacterial activity, pharmacokinetic properties and therapeutic use. *Drugs* 32:425-444, 1986.

Welander CE, et al: Intralesional interferon alfa-2b for the treatment of genital warts. *Am J Obstet Gynecol* 162:348-354, 1990.

Wiesmeier E: Terconazole: Summary of clinical studies. *Curr Ther Res* 46:342-351, 1989.

Wolfe RA, et al: Mortality differences and speed of wound closure among specialized burn care facilities. *JAMA* 250:763-766, 1983.

Zellner PR, Bugyi S: Povidone-iodine in treatment of burn patients. *J Hosp Infect* Suppl A:139-146, (Mar 6) 1985.

Drugs Used Topically for Infestations

74

Organisms from the phylum, Arthropoda, that parasitize man belong to one of two main classes (ie, Arachnida, Insecta). The principal parasite of Arachnida that infests man is known by the trivial name itch mite and causes scabies. The principal parasites of the class Insecta that infest man and cause pediculosis are *Pediculus humanus* var *capitis* (head lice), *Pediculus humanus* var *corporis* (body lice), and *Pthirus pubis* (pubic lice, crabs).

SCABIES

Scabies occurs when the gravid female itch mite, *Sarcoptes scabiei* var hominis, invades the skin. Adult female mites are approximately 0.4 x 0.3 mm and attack warm, moist areas (folds) of the skin. The newly fertilized female takes about one hour to bury herself in the horny layer of the skin and then proceeds to make a tortuous burrow at the rate of 2 to 3 mm/day for a distance of about 15 mm. She lays one or two eggs daily for the last 14 days of her entire life span (about one month). The eggs hatch in about three to four days; the larvae migrate to the skin surface where they mature in 10 to 17 days. The total number of mites on an infested human averages 11 or 12 in adults and 20 in children.

TRANSMISSION. Skin-to-skin contact, usually prolonged, is necessary to transmit scabies. However, prolonged nonsexual contact accounts for most transmission, especially between children and adults and between patients and medical staff. Children sleeping with infested parents can acquire the disease. In crusted (Norwegian) scabies, mite populations are prodigious (thousands), and the shedding of epidermal scales in fomites containing numerous mites causes rapid spread of the disease, even to individuals who are exposed briefly to infested skin or only to fomites.

Scabies epidemics are alleged to occur in 25- to 30-year cycles, which are hypothesized to result from a form of "immunity" that develops during infestation. However, this immunity is not absolute and lasts only for several months after infestation (Orkin and Maibach, 1985). Further, a reassessment of all of the evidence does not support the occurrence of cycles (Burkhart, 1983).

SIGNS AND SYMPTOMS. Pruritus occurs after scabies is fully developed and usually is accompanied by papular dermatitis. During severe infestations, induration, crusting, and even nodules may occur. Irritation and pruritus are caused by sensitization to the organism and/or its excretions. Scratching can lead to excoriation and secondary infection.

Burrows may not be visible or may not appear in the classic form. When burrows are apparent, they appear as wavy lines several millimeters long, usually surrounded by mild inflammation and erythema. In adults, burrows are observed most frequently on the sides and webs of fingers, the ulnar border of the hand, the volar aspects of the wrists, the points of the elbows, the axillary folds, the margins of the feet, the areolae of the nipples and intertriginous folds of the breasts in women, and the genitalia in men. In infants, small children, and bedridden individuals, scabietic eruptions are common on the head, neck, and buttocks, and the symptoms of secondary infection are more likely to obscure the characteristic lesion than in adults. In the tropics and many areas of the United States in summer months, burrows are uncommon or absent. Erythematous papules, 1 to 2 mm, may be the only sign.

Crusted (Norwegian) scabies is characterized by a crusting and hyperkeratotic psoriasiform dermatitis on the hands and feet associated with dystrophic nails. Inflammation and pruritus are much less common. This rare form of scabies is highly contagious and is observed most often in elderly or mentally retarded patients in institutions who are unable to care for themselves and in physically or immunologically debilitated individuals (eg, patients with AIDS). Crusted scabies differs so markedly from classic scabies that it often is not diagnosed until attending personnel begin to develop scabies.

See Orkin and Maibach, 1985, for a detailed discussion of scabies.

DIAGNOSIS. Classic scabies often is diagnosed easily in adults, but diagnosis can be difficult in infants, children, and the elderly. The pathognomonic lesion is the burrow produced by the gravid female. Secondary lesions include vesicles, pustules, excoriations, and crusts. Identification of the mite from direct skin scrapings or cutaneous biopsy ensures a definitive diagnosis, which is not always attainable, especially if the physician is inexperienced in searching for the parasite.

Since scabietic lesions can mimic any pruritic skin disease, differential diagnosis must exclude such common conditions as atopic dermatitis, impetigo, ecthyma, seborrheic dermatitis, eczematous dermatitis, dermatitis herpetiformis, psoriasis, papular urticaria, pediculosis, chickenpox, and prickly heat (miliaria).

MANAGEMENT. The first goal of treatment is to identify the source of the infestation and avoid or remove it. Treatment of an infested individual also should include the simultaneous administration of a scabicide to the sexual partner(s) of the patient and all household members or those in close contact in nursing homes. Such therapy may prevent the "ping-pong" passing of the disease from one individual to another.

Disinfestation of Fomites: Away from the human body, the scabies mite survives in a moist environment usually for only two or three days. Fomites may play a significant role in the transmission of scabies (Burkhart, 1983). If disinfestation of fomites is necessary, intimate clothing and bedding used within the previous 48 hours may be machine washed and dried. No other measures are necessary, except for crusted scabies.

Secondary Bacterial Infection: This is the most common complication of scabietic infestations. Although there may be only a dozen mites, hundreds of inflammatory papules may be present. Scratching, particularly in individuals with poor personal hygiene, can lead to dermatoses that range from pustules to furunculosis. If secondary infection with beta-hemolytic *Streptococcus* occurs, acute glomerulonephritis may develop. Appropriate topical antibacterial preparations may be effective in mild secondary infections, but systemic antibiotics occasionally are required for moderate to severe pyodermas.

Drug Application: Medication is curative only when correctly utilized. Claims by a patient that he has undergone scabicidal therapy at an earlier date should not lead a physician to a misdiagnosis. Often an individual may undertake self-medication, which ameliorates symptoms without curing the infestation. Moreover, during self-medication, the patient may apply the drug erratically or only on areas that exhibit definite pruritus, thereby allowing some infested areas to escape treatment.

Pruritus may persist for several days after treatment because of residual eggs and feces, which prompts patients to apply preparations more frequently and for longer periods than prescribed. Physicians should, therefore, give careful instructions on the use of scabicides and prescribe only the amount needed for a given course of therapy with *no refills*. If a preparation is used too often or for too long a period, it may cause dermatitis that is mistaken for persistence of the infestation which, in turn, is aggravated by further application of the drug. The patient should be instructed not to use topical preparations other than those prescribed.

Drug Selection: Lindane (gamma benzene hexachloride) [Kwell, Scabene], permethrin 5% [Elimite], and crotamiton [Eurax] are the principal drugs available in the United States for treating scabies. There are no definitive data to determine the degree to which these drugs are ovicidal in vivo; therefore, it is important that the patient be observed for at least one month. This is sufficiently long for all original lesions to heal and for any eggs that are still viable after treatment to hatch and reach maturity (Taplin et al, 1986).

All exposed family members should be treated. The scabicide should be applied to all skin surfaces, including nail edges, from the top of the head to the soles of the feet in infants, children, and elderly adults. It usually is not necessary to treat the head of younger adults. A single 8- to 14-hour exposure is often successful. A second application may be necessary after two to four weeks in symptomatic patients (those with persistent pruritus, dermatitis) or after one week in those with signs of continued infestation (live lice, eggs).

A 5% concentration of permethrin was more effective for treating scabies than lindane in a controlled clinical trial in which resistance to lindane may have been a confounding factor. This concentration, left on the skin for 12 to 18 hours, was well tolerated (Taplin et al, 1986; Taplin and Meinking, 1987, 1990).

When used properly (ie, good physician education of the patient and patient compliance), lindane has a satisfactory record of safety (Rasmussen, 1981). However, some clinicians remain concerned about occasional reports of neurotoxicity associated with this agent, especially in children, when an excessive amount of the lotion is applied (Schultz et al, 1990). Furthermore, clusters of resistance to lindane have occurred (Purvis and Tyring, 1991), especially in immigrant children or in travelers who have returned recently from Central and South America or Asia. These patients usually respond to one application of permethrin 5% if the preparation is applied correctly.

Cure rates for crotamiton tend to be lower with the same number of applications than for lindane and permethrin 5%

(Taplin et al, 1990); therefore, the latter two agents are preferred.

Sulfur ointment is reported to be effective, but it is messy, has a bad odor, and stains clothing.

Benzyl benzoate is effective in scabies but can produce primary irritation, especially in warm humid climates. It is rarely used in the United States. Monosulfiram [Tetmosol] is used in England as a substitute for benzyl benzoate, particularly in children, since benzyl benzoate often stings when applied to the skin. Monosulfiram is diluted with two to three parts of water before application. Adults using this drug must be warned to avoid alcohol immediately before and during therapy since monosulfiram is related to disulfiram [Antabuse].

An emulsion concentrate (NBIN) containing chlorophenothane 6%, benzyl benzoate 68%, benzocaine 12%, and polysorbate 80 14% is recommended by the World Health Organization as a relatively inexpensive scabicide that can be compounded from materials readily obtainable even in developing countries. The preparation requires a 1:15 dilution with water before application. Thiabendazole, given orally or applied topically as a 10% solution (Hernández-Pérez, 1976), also is used in other countries.

PEDICULOSIS

Pediculosis in man is caused by three types of lice: *Pthirus pubis* (crab louse), which primarily infests the pubic skin and hair; *Pediculus humanus* var *corporis* (body louse), which inhabits clothing and infests the trunk and limbs only to feed; and *Pediculus humanus* var *capitis* (head louse), which affects the scalp.

Differences in the habits of crab, body, and head lice produce three distinct public health problems. The distinction is most evident in countries with high standards of hygiene, where regular laundering of clothing has almost eliminated body louse infestations. In the United States today, people harboring body lice are mostly vagrants or those living in substandard housing with poor facilities for maintaining cleanliness; the most serious cases often involve elderly, infirm, or mentally retarded individuals.

Louse infestations per se generally are not injurious to health. *P. capitis* has never been established as a primary vector for any disease. Body lice can transmit the Rickettsia that cause typhus, relapsing fever, and, rarely, trench fever. Louse-borne diseases now occur only in a few parts of the world, since they can spread only where there is a high proportion of infested individuals.

INCIDENCE. The frequency of head and crab louse infestations is increasing, but there is no evidence that body louse infestations are on the rise. Regular bathing and shampooing do not ensure freedom from crab or head lice. However, poor personal hygiene by those already infested may increase the possibility of secondary bacterial infection.

Head louse infestations are prominent in some industrial areas and are not restricted to any race or socioeconomic group. However, blacks are rarely infested with head lice; the reason for this decreased prevalence has not been totally explained, but it may be because the oval cross-section structure of hair in blacks is difficult for head lice to grasp. Children are affected more often than adults, and girls or young women are infested more commonly than boys or young men. Long hair and complex hairdos are of contributory importance only when they impede early detection of an infestation or make combing to eliminate the nits difficult or when amounts of pediculicide are insufficient to saturate long hair.

The population affected by crab lice cannot be defined clearly, but they are likely to be sexually active or belong to a family with a promiscuous member.

TRANSMISSION. Crab lice are transferred from one individual to another by sexual contact, and occasionally by infested towels or clothing. Children can acquire the disease from infested adults through close personal contact, such as sleeping with an infested parent.

Body lice are transmitted by contact with infested clothing or bedding, since the louse lives in garment seams and visits the body only to feed. Thus, the body louse can be removed from the host by removing infested clothing. The continued existence of the louse depends on the continuous wearing of infested clothing for a major portion of each day.

Head lice move from the head of one host to that of another, and direct person-to-person spread is believed to be the predominant mode of transmission. Exchange of combs, headwear, or other wearing apparel also may play a role.

SIGNS AND SYMPTOMS. Pruritus with scratching, excoriation, and, sometimes, secondary bacterial infection are associated with louse infestations. Symptoms are caused by an allergic reaction to saliva deposited on the skin by the parasite. Lightly infested individuals are often asymptomatic.

DIAGNOSIS. Pediculosis pubis and capitis may be diagnosed by identifying the adult louse or, more commonly, eggs (nits) attached to the hair shaft initially close to the hair-skin junction. Pediculosis pubis usually involves the pubic and perianal regions but can spread to the trunk, legs, and axillae and rarely involves the margins of the eyebrows and eyelashes (mainly in children), scalp, and mustache. Pediculosis capitis generally is found on the scalp; the occipital and postauricular regions are most commonly involved. In rare instances, the beard and other exceptionally hairy areas may harbor head lice.

Pediculosis corporis can be confirmed by the presence of lice or nits in the seams of clothing, usually where clothing comes in contact with the axillae and perineum, or at the beltline and collar. Except in heavily infested individuals, parasites may be almost absent from the body.

MANAGEMENT. Pediculosis capitis, pubis, and corporis are managed by disinfestation of fomites and proper application of agents that kill the lice and nits.

Disinfestation of Fomites: General decontamination procedures have been described for all three kinds of lice. Heat is lethal to lice and their eggs; therefore, personal articles can be disinfested by machine washing in hot water and/or drying using the hot cycle of the dryer. Eggs are killed after five minutes at 51.5° C (135° F) or 30 minutes at 49.5° C (117° F), and adult lice succumb to slightly lower temperatures.

Combs and brushes can be disinfested by soaking for one hour in saponated cresol solution 2% or the equivalent (eg, Lysol, Pine-Sol) or heating in water to about 60° C for five to ten minutes. Clothing or bedding that cannot be washed may be dry cleaned or placed in a plastic bag and sealed for two weeks (head lice and crab lice). Head lice die in about 24 hours without a blood meal, crab lice separated from the host die in less than 36 hours, and body lice may survive for four to ten days away from the host. Eggs remaining in warm, humid environments may hatch up to 30 days after removal from the host. Shaving or cutting the hair is not necessary.

Cleaning of houses, wards, or other rooms inhabited by infested individuals should be limited to thorough vacuuming. Fumigation of living areas generally is not necessary, but may be a useful alternative procedure to decontaminate the clothing of individuals with body louse infestation. If fumigation is necessary, clothing or bedding can be placed in an air-tight metal container or plastic bag and exposed to ethyl formate 2 ml/L (60 ml/ft^3) for one hour. Longer exposure times (five hours or more) achieve the same results with lower concentrations of ethyl formate (0.5 ml/L, 15 ml/ft^3). In either case, the cost is low. Clothing temporarily retains a slight odor of ethyl formate upon removal from the fumigating container. Small quantities of ethyl formate can be handled safely. An aerosol preparation containing pyrethrins sprayed on clothing and other inanimate objects is effective and much easier to use than most fumigation procedures. The aerosol spray should not be used directly on humans or animals.

Drug Selection: The treatment for head and crab lice is somewhat similar because these insects live directly on the patient. Although the procedures differ, the contact insecticides used are similar.

Lindane shampoo, permethrin 1% [Nix], and preparations containing pyrethrins synergized with piperonyl butoxide [A-200 Pediculicide Shampoo Concentrate Pyrinate, R & C Shampoo, RID] are equally effective when used as directed for the treatment of head and pubic lice (Rasmussen, 1983; Brandenburg et al, 1986; Bowerman et al, 1987; Fusia et al, 1987; Taplin and Meinking, 1987, 1990). Lindane is a prescription product; preparations of permethrin 1% used for head and pubic lice are nonprescription products. The recommended exposure is four minutes for lindane shampoo and ten minutes for permethrin and the pyrethrins. There is little probability of significant absorption for permethrin or the pyrethrins; however, lindane may be difficult to wash off completely, and there is some concern about absorption when it is used in excessive amounts.

Permethrin 1% is highly ovicidal (70% to 80%) in clinical studies and is detectable on the hair for at least ten days following a single application; these findings probably are responsible for the observation that a single treatment is sufficient to eliminate head lice infestation in most patients (DiNapoli et al, 1988). Cure rates reported after a single application range from 97% to 99% in uncomplicated cases.

The same outcome should not necessarily be expected in the treatment of pubic lice in all population groups. Although both lindane shampoo and permethrin 1% were equally effective and well tolerated in a partially controlled study, each agent was associated with a failure rate of about 40% among predominantly male homosexual patients, many of whom were unresponsive to previous therapy (Kalter et al, 1987). A single retreatment with pyrethrins seven days following initial therapy for pubic lice is recommended by the manufacturers. For lindane, retreatment is recommended after two to four weeks in symptomatic patients and after at least one week in those with signs of continued infestation (nits, live lice).

Malathion aqueous emulsion 0.5% [Prioderm], one of the least toxic organophosphorus insecticides, has been used widely in Europe to treat head and pubic lice but was commercially unsuccessful and was withdrawn from the United States market in 1985. It has been reintroduced in the United States as a lotion in 78% alcohol [Ovide] *(Med Lett,* 1989). The ovicidal activity of malathion exceeds that of the pyrethrins and lindane (Meinking et al, 1986). It is highly effective against both head and pubic lice. A 15-minute exposure time is sufficient to kill both lice and eggs (Meinking et al, 1986). Allowing malathion to remain on the hair for 8 to 12 hours produces a residual pediculicidal effect that may persist for several weeks. However, many patients find the odor objectionable, and the lotion is flammable.

Petrolatum ophthalmic ointment is used to treat crab louse (*P. pubis*) infestation of the eyelashes. The ointment is applied thickly twice daily for eight days. An ophthalmic ointment containing physostigmine 0.25% also has been applied, but undesirable effects on vision, pupillary size, and accommodation have limited its usefulness.

Chlorophenothane (DDT) was one of the first synthetic insecticides used against lice. However, body lice have become resistant in many countries, and head lice are resistant in some areas outside the United States. DDT is not ovicidal and furnishes no residual protection. Anxiety about environmental contamination with DDT has restricted its use, and it is no longer available in the United States.

Powder preparations of DDT are often useful in managing head lice during epidemics or in developing countries where houses are poorly heated and hot running water is not available. The latter conditions make wetting the hair unacceptable to patients, especially in the winter. Powders also are more convenient than lotions or shampoos in controlling head lice in jails and prisons where the daily admission and discharge rate is high. Under these circumstances, it is easier to shake on a powder than it is to ensure that a recalcitrant or inebriated person will apply a lotion or shampoo properly. Powders also control body lice when a change of clothes or laundry facilities are not readily available.

As with scabicides, patients tend to use pediculicides more frequently than necessary. To avoid toxicity and/or irritant dermatitis, pediculicides should not be applied more than twice, and seven to ten days should elapse between treatments.

Drug Evaluations

BENZYL BENZOATE

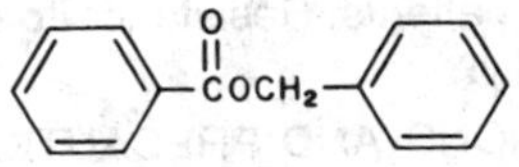

This agent has been widely used to treat scabies in developing countries, especially in veterinary medicine.

Benzyl benzoate is relatively nontoxic but may irritate the skin and eyes. Increased pruritus and irritation (manifested by burning and stinging, particularly of the genitalia and scalp) are common and may be severe in hot humid climates. Contact with the eyes and urethral meatus should be avoided. There is no evidence that this drug is absorbed through the skin in amounts sufficient to cause systemic toxicity. Even when ingested, benzyl benzoate is converted to hippuric acid and systemic toxic symptoms have not been described in humans. In animals, this agent has been reported to cause progressive incoordination, central nervous system excitation, convulsions, and death.

DOSAGE AND PREPARATIONS. The commercially available 50% benzyl benzoate preparation should be diluted before topical application.

Topical: After thorough cleansing of the skin with soap and water for ten minutes, the diluted preparation containing approximately 25% of the drug is applied to the entire body below the neck; after this application has dried, the medication may be reapplied and the residue washed off 24 hours later. Benzyl benzoate may be applied nightly or every other night for a total of three applications.

Generic. Emulsion 50% in pint and gallon containers (nonprescription).

CROTAMITON
[Eurax]

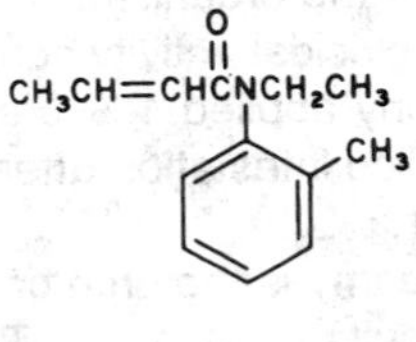

Crotamiton is effective in scabies, but cure rates tend to be lower for the same number of applications than with lindane and permethrin. It is claimed to have antipruritic activity independent of its scabietic effects, but this has been questioned (Smith et al, 1985).

Crotamiton rarely causes allergic contact dermatitis but occasionally produces irritant contact dermatitis and may be particularly irritating to denuded skin.

This drug is classified in FDA Pregnancy Category C.

DOSAGE AND PREPARATIONS.

Topical: The preparation is massaged into the skin of the whole body, working from the chin down. When the head and face are involved (eg, infants), these areas also should be treated. Particular attention should be given to the body folds, hands, feet (including the soles), and intertriginous areas. Contact with the eyes, mouth, and urethral meatus should be avoided. Two or more applications at 24-hour intervals eradicate most scabietic infestations. A cleansing bath should be taken 48 hours following the last application. In resistant cases, treatment may be repeated one week later or an alternative drug used.

Eurax (Westwood-Squibb). Cream 10% in 60 g containers; lotion 10% in 60 and 454 ml containers.

LINDANE (Gamma Benzene Hexachloride)
[Kwell, Scabene]

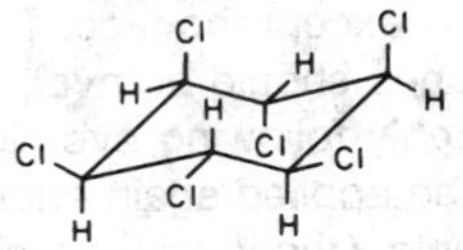

USES. Lindane is one of the drugs of choice for the treatment of scabies. The shampoo is highly effective for killing adult head and pubic lice, and it may have some ovicidal activity. In the last decade, clusters of patients have become resistant to lindane in some countries (eg, Central and South America, Asia); therefore, some immigrants or travelers may not respond to this agent (Purvis and Tyring, 1991).

ADVERSE REACTIONS AND PRECAUTIONS. The potential for serious toxicity is considerable if the preparation is misused; therefore, it is important that the patient or family be given adequate instructions in use of lindane (Rasmussen, 1981, 1983).

As usually formulated, lindane is irritating to the eyes and mucosa. Allergic contact dermatitis has not been documented, but irritant contact dermatitis has occurred when the drug was applied in excessive amounts, too frequently, or for extended periods. If irritation becomes evident, the drug should be washed off and not used again.

Lindane is absorbed through intact skin and is toxic if absorbed in excessive amounts; hydrated skin may increase absorption. Since occasional cases of neurotoxicity have been observed when an excessive amount of the lotion was applied (Schultz et al, 1990), some authorities have expressed concern about the absorption of lindane cream or lotion after the recommended 8- to 12-hour exposure time for scabies, especially in children. When used as an insecticide (in concentrations greater than the prescription strength of 1%), lindane has been implicated in 13 cases of aplastic anemia and 5 cases of other blood dyscrasias. One case of aplastic anemia has been reported when lindane was used as a scabicide in a 1% concentration (Rauch et al, 1990). This agent is excreted slowly in the urine (half-life, approximately 20 hours) when absorbed.

If accidental ingestion occurs, prompt gastric lavage eliminates much of the preparation. Oil-type laxatives should be avoided since they enhance absorption. Systemic toxicity is usually manifested as central nervous system stimulation progressing to convulsions; intravenous diazepam or barbiturates counteract this effect. Intravenous calcium gluconate also may be beneficial. Epinephrine should be avoided.

Lindane has been used in pregnant women for head and pubic lice; however, definitive data on safety for the fetus are not available (FDA Pregnancy Category B).

DOSAGE AND PREPARATIONS. The lotion and cream are used only for scabies; the shampoo is recommended for head and pubic lice. Careful adherence to recommended dosage is advised.

Topical: For scabies, a warm bath prior to application is helpful if crusted lesions are present; however, the skin should be dry and cool before the medication is applied to minimize skin absorption. *Adults (excluding pregnant or lactating women) and children*, no more than 30 g of lotion or cream is applied to all parts of the body except the face. The eyes, eyelashes, and mucous membranes should be avoided. The medication is washed off thoroughly following overnight exposure (8 to 12 hours). It should be applied again after two to four weeks in symptomatic patients (those with persistent pruritus, dermatitis) or after one week in those with signs of continued infestation (live lice, eggs). When used in *infants,* the manufacturers' recommended dose should not be exceeded.

For head lice, *adults and children*, up to 30 ml of shampoo is massaged into the hair for four minutes. The hair is then thoroughly rinsed with warm water and towel dried. Treatment is repeated in one week in symptomatic patients or those with signs of continued infestation (live lice, eggs).

For pubic lice, *adults and children,* the shampoo is applied to the affected and adjacent hairy areas, particularly the pubic mons and perianal region, and is removed after four minutes; in hairy individuals, the thighs, trunk, and axillary regions also should be shampooed. When the hair is dry, any remaining nits or nit shells should be removed with a fine-toothed comb and tweezers. Retreatment in seven days is indicated if signs of continued infestation (live lice, eggs) are present or after two to four weeks in patients with persistent pruritus or dermatitis. Lindane should not be used for *P. pubis* infestations of the eyelashes (see the discussion on Drug Selection in the section on Pediculosis).

Generic. Lotion and shampoo 1% in 60, 480, and 3,840 ml containers.

Kwell (Reed & Carnrick). Cream 1% in 60 g containers; lotion 1% in 60 and 480 ml containers; shampoo 1% in 60 and 480 ml containers.

Scabene (Stiefel). Lotion and shampoo 1% in 60 and 480 ml containers.

MALATHION

[Ovide]

ACTIONS AND USES. The mechanism of action of this organophosphate insecticide and acaricide is inhibition of cholinesterase. Malathion is almost exclusively used as a pediculicide rather than as a scabicide.

The ovicidal activity of malathion exceeds that of crotamiton, the pyrethrins, and lindane. A 15-minute exposure time is sufficient to kill both lice and eggs (Meinking et al, 1986). Allowing malathion to remain on the hair for 8 to 12 hours produces a residual pediculicidal effect that may persist for several weeks. Many patients find the odor of malathion and the oily terpene excipients it contains objectionable. These excipients appear to enhance the ovicidal activity of malathion (Burgess, 1991). Retreatment after one week may be necessary in some patients. Resistance to malathion has developed occasionally.

ADVERSE REACTIONS AND PRECAUTIONS. Malathion is one of the least toxic organophosphates. Scalp irritation has been reported occasionally; allergic contact dermatitis is rare. Although all of the signs and symptoms of systemic organophosphate absorption are potentially a concern, they have not been reported when this preparation was applied appropriately. Because of the alcohol content of this product, exposure of hair to open flames and hair dryers must be avoided.

Malathion is classified in FDA Pregnancy Category B. Breast feeding probably should be avoided during treatment, although no data are available to validate this precaution.

PHARMACOKINETICS. Data on the degree of systemic absorption of malathion after use of the 0.5% lotion are not available; however, no reports of clinically significant systemic signs and symptoms of organophosphate inhibition of cholinesterase following the recommended topical therapeutic dosage regimen have appeared in the literature.

DOSAGE AND PREPARATIONS.

Topical: Small amounts of the lotion are sprinkled on dry hair until the hair is thoroughly wet. After 8 to 12 hours, the hair is washed and rinsed and nits are removed with a fine-toothed comb. Application may be repeated in one week if necessary.

Ovide (GenDerm). Lotion 0.5% in 60 ml containers.

PERMETHRIN

[Elimite, Nix]

ACTIONS AND USES. Permethrin, a pyrethroid, is active against lice, ticks, fleas, mites, and other arthropods. It acts on the nerve cell membrane to disrupt the sodium channel current by which polarization of the membrane is regulated, resulting in paralysis of the organism.

Because of its high ovicidal activity against lice and persistence on hair, a properly applied 1% cream rinse eliminates most head and pubic lice infestation after a single application (DiNapoli et al, 1988).

Permethrin 5% (cream) is the drug of choice for the treatment of scabies (Schultz et al, 1990; Taplin and Meinking, 1990; *Med Lett Drugs Ther*, 1992).

ADVERSE REACTIONS AND PRECAUTIONS. In general, the preparations are well tolerated, and systemic signs or symptoms have not been a problem. Mild, limited pruritus occurs in about 6% of patients after use of the 1% cream rinse. Transient burning, stinging, tingling, numbness, or scalp discomfort occurs in approximately 3.4% of patients, and 2.1% experience mild transient erythema, edema, or rash of the scalp.

In clinical trials of the 5% cream for scabies, generally mild, transient burning and stinging followed application in 10% of patients and was correlated with the severity of infestation. Erythema, numbness, tingling, and rash were reported in ≤2% of those treated.

Treatment with permethrin 5% may temporarily exacerbate the pruritus, edema, and erythema that often accompany scabies. Patients should be advised that itching, mild burning, and/or stinging may occur after application of the cream. In clinical trials, pruritus occurred in 7% of patients and ceased after two to four weeks in approximately 75% of these patients. If irritation persists, the physician should be consulted. Permethrin cream may be mildly irritating to the eyes; if contact occurs, the eyes should be flushed with water immediately.

The potential for contact dermatitis and photosensitization is very low. The safety and effectiveness of permethrin in children less than 2 months have not been established. Patients who cannot tolerate pyrethrins and other synthetic pyrethroids may not tolerate permethrin.

PREGNANCY AND LACTATION. In reproductive studies in mice, rats, and rabbits, oral doses of 200 to 400 mg/kg had no effect on the fetus. This drug is classified in FDA Pregnancy Category B. Although it is not known whether permethrin is excreted in human milk, less than 2% of the dose applied topically is absorbed. Some evidence of tumorigenicity has been observed in animal studies. Therefore, discontinuing nursing should be considered.

PHARMACOKINETICS. Permethrin is rapidly metabolized by ester hydrolysis to inactive metabolites that are excreted in the urine. It persists on hair for at least ten days.

DOSAGE AND PREPARATIONS.

Topical: For scabies, *adults and children*, the 5% cream is thoroughly massaged into the skin from the head to the soles of the feet; 30 g usually is sufficient for an average adult. Infants and elderly patients should be treated on the scalp, temples, and forehead as well. The cream should be removed by washing (shower or bath) after 8 to 14 hours. A second application may be necessary after two to four weeks in symptomatic patients (those with persistent pruritus, dermatitis) or after one week in those with continued signs of infestation (live lice, eggs).

For head lice, after the hair has been shampooed, rinsed, and towel dried, a sufficient volume of the 1% cream rinse is applied to saturate the scalp, hair, the area behind the ears, and the nape of the neck. The preparation should remain on the hair and skin for ten minutes before being rinsed off with water. A single application is usually sufficient to eliminate head lice infestations; retreatment is not required in most patients who follow instructions properly. Because the cream rinse formulation leaves the hair easier to comb, combing to remove nits is also facilitated.

For pubic lice, the 1% cream rinse is applied to the hair and surrounding skin and is rinsed off with water after ten minutes. A single retreatment seven days following initial therapy is recommended.

Elimite (Allergan Herbert). Cream 5% in 60 g containers.

Nix (Burroughs Wellcome). Cream rinse 1% in 60 ml containers (nonprescription).

PYRETHRINS AND PIPERONYL BUTOXIDE

[A-200 Pediculicide Shampoo Concentrate Pyrinate, R & C Shampoo, RID]

Pyrethrins synergized with piperonyl butoxide are available without prescription in liquid form in concentrations ranging from 0.17% to 0.3%. These contact insecticides are alternative preparations of choice for the treatment of head and pubic lice (Taplin and Meinking, 1990).

A partially controlled study utilizing pyrethrins (outcome evaluator blinded) demonstrated that a shampoo is much more effective than a lotion, probably because the detergent action of the shampoo augments the ability of the active agent to penetrate nits (Cordero and Zaias, 1987).

Topical absorption from intact skin is poor. Toxicology studies in animals indicate that pyrethrins are among the safest insecticides available.

Impurities in extracts of pyrethrins may cause allergic dermatitis, especially in individuals sensitive to ragweed. Pharmaceutical formulations generally do not cross react in patch tests on humans sensitized to ragweed pollen, but caution is advised.

Because commercial formulations are irritating to the eyes and mucous membranes, they should not be used to treat *P. pubis* infestations of the eyelashes (see the discussion on Drug Selection in the section on Pediculosis).

DOSAGE AND PREPARATIONS.

Topical: Liquid preparations are applied to the hair, scalp, or other infested area until the hair is thoroughly wet. After ten minutes, the insecticide is removed by shampooing and rinsing with warm water. Remaining nits or nit shells should be removed with a fine-toothed comb and tweezers. Treatment should be repeated in one week.

A-200 Pediculicide Shampoo Concentrate Pyrinate (SmithKline Beecham). Liquid containing pyrethrins 0.3%, piperonyl butoxide 3%, and petroleum distillates in 60 and 120 ml containers (nonprescription).

R & C Shampoo (Reed & Carnrick). Shampoo containing pyrethrins 0.3%, piperonyl butoxide 3%, and petroleum distillate 1.2% in 60 and 120 ml containers (nonprescription).

RID (Pfizer). Liquid containing pyrethrins 0.3%, piperonyl butoxide 3%, and petroleum distillate 1.2% in 60 and 120 ml containers (nonprescription).

SULFUR

This compound is applied topically as a 6% (range, 5% to 10%) ointment of precipitated sulfur in petrolatum or in Cetaphil lotion (which is less messy) to treat scabies. Only a few authorities consider sulfur to be a preferred scabicide for infants, young children, and pregnant women.

Sulfur ointment has staining properties and an unpleasant odor; rarely, it causes irritation and dermatitis. Systemic adverse effects from topically applied sulfur are uncommon (Lin et al, 1988).

DOSAGE AND PREPARATIONS.

Topical: Following a cleansing scrub using tepid water and soap, the skin is dried and sulfur ointment is applied nightly for three nights. The patient may bathe each night prior to application of the drug or once 24 hours after the last application.

No pharmaceutical dosage form is available; compounding is necessary for prescription. The usual formulation is a 6% ointment of precipitated sulfur in petrolatum.

Cited References

Drugs for parasitic infections. *Med Lett Drugs Ther* 34:17-26, (March 6) 1992.

Malathion for head lice. *Med Lett* 31:110-111, 1989.

Bowerman JG, et al: Comparative study of permethrin 1% creme rinse and lindane shampoo for the treatment of head lice. *Pediatr Infect Dis J* 6:252-255, 1987.

Brandenburg K, et al: 1% permethrin cream rinse vs 1% lindane shampoo in treating pediculosis capitis. *Am J Dis Child* 140:894-896, 1986.

Burgess I: Malathion lotions for head lice: A less reliable treatment than commonly believed. *Pharm J* 630-632, (Nov) 1991.

Burkhart CG: Scabies: Epidemiologic reassessment. *Ann Intern Med* 98:498-503, 1983.

Cordero C, Zaias N: Clinical evaluation of pediculicidal and ovicidal efficacy of two pyrethrin-piperonyl-butoxide formulations. *Clin Ther* 9:461-465, 1987.

DiNapoli JB, et al: Eradication of head lice with a single treatment. *Am J Public Health* 78:978-980, 1988.

Fusia JF, et al: Nationwide comparative trial of pyrethrins and lindane for pediculosis in children: Experience in northeastern United States. *Curr Ther Res* 41:881-890, 1987.

Hernández-Pérez E: Topically applied thiabendazole in treatment of scabies. *Arch Dermatol* 112:1400-1401, 1976.

Kalter DC, et al: Treatment of pediculosis pubis: Clinical comparison of efficacy and tolerance of 1% lindane shampoo vs 1% permethrin creme rinse. *Arch Dermatol* 123:1315-1319, 1987.

Lin AN, et al: Sulfur revisited. *J Am Acad Dermatol* 18:553-558, 1988.

Meinking TL, et al: Comparative efficacy of treatments of pediculosis capitis infestations. *Arch Dermatol* 122:267-271, 1986.

Orkin M, Maibach HI (eds): *Cutaneous Infestations and Insect Bites.* New York, Marcel Dekker, 1985.

Purvis RS, Tyring SK: An outbreak of lindane-resistant scabies treated successfully with permethrin 5% cream. *J Am Acad Dermatol* 25:1015-1016, 1991.

Rasmussen JE: Problem of lindane. *J Am Acad Dermatol* 5:507-516, 1981.

Rasmussen JE: Advances in treatment of head and public lice. *Drug Ther* 13:185-192, (Nov) 1983.

Rauch AE, et al: Lindane (Kwell)-induced aplastic anemia. *Arch Intern Med* 150:2393-2395, 1990.

Schultz MW, et al: Comparative study of 5% permethrin cream and 1% lindane lotion for the treatment of scabies. *Arch Dermatol* 126:167-170, 1990.

Smith EB, et al: Crotamiton lotion in pruritus. *Int Dermatol* 23:684-685, 1985.

Taplin D, Meinking TL: Pyrethrins and pyrethroids for treatment of scabies and pediculosis. *Semin Dermatol* 6:125-135, 1987.

Taplin D, Meinking TL: Pyrethrins and pyrethroids in dermatology. *Arch Dermatol* 126:213-221, 1990.

Taplin D, et al: Permethrin 5% dermal cream: New treatment for scabies. *J Am Acad Dermatol* 15:995-1001, 1986.

Taplin D, et al: Comparison of crotamiton 10% cream (Eurax) and permethrin 5% cream (Elimite) for the treatment of scabies in children. *Pediatr Dermatol* 7:67-73, (March) 1990.

Antiseptics and Disinfectants 75

Antiseptics

These antimicrobial agents are applied topically to living tissues (usually intact skin, mucous membranes, or wounds) to destroy microorganisms or inhibit their reproduction or metabolic activities. Antiseptics are included in some formulations employed by health care personnel as surgical hand scrubs, as handwashes to reduce the risk of cross contamination, and for preoperative skin preparation. Deodorant soaps contain antimicrobials to reduce skin bacteria for a deodorant effect.

Skin cleansers and protectants for the laity may contain antiseptics to minimize the potential for infection associated with minor cuts, abrasions, burns, or insect bites. However, such use is of limited value. These agents should be considered, at best, only adjuncts to adequate removal of dirt and organic matter by sudsing, emulsification, irrigation, and debridement techniques (Larson, 1985, 1988) and use of protective dressings that assure adequate drainage.

For health care personnel, the use of antiseptics is more effective than nonmedicated control vehicles in reducing the number of microorganisms (Bartzokas et al, 1987); however, controversy exists as to which antiseptics are most effective and safe (Sebben, 1983; Rutala and Cole, 1984; Larson, 1988; Laufman, 1989). Although it is known that effectiveness is dependent on formulation, concentration, and quantity (Larson et al, 1987), large-scale, comparative trials among rather than between products are needed to resolve the selection process (Bjerke, 1987).

The antiseptics most widely employed by health care personnel include ethyl and isopropyl alcohols; cationic surface-active agents (eg, benzalkonium); the biguanide, chlorhexidine; iodine compounds (ie, iodine solution, iodine tincture, povidone-iodine); triclocarban, a substituted carbanilide; and the phenolic compounds, triclosan, parachlorometaxylenol, and hexachlorophene. These antiseptics, except for hexachlorophene, are incorporated into over-the-counter (OTC) products. Also available are chlorine compounds (eg, sodium hypochlorite, oxychlorosene); hydrogen peroxide; the organic mercurial compound, thimerosal; and other phenolic compounds (eg, phenol, hexylresorcinol).

Silver nitrate is used prophylactically for ophthalmia neonatorum. Triclosan and triclocarban are used principally as components of antimicrobial soaps for deodorant purposes.

Disinfectants

These substances are used on inanimate objects to destroy microorganisms and prevent infection. Some disinfectants are used as antiseptics if they can be diluted sufficiently to avoid injuring living tissues while retaining antimicrobial activity. The principal disinfectants available are the aldehydes, formaldehyde and glutaral; hypochlorites; and the phenolic compound, cresol, and selected quaternary ammonium compounds.

Sterilization is the elimination of all viable microbes, including vegetative bacteria, spores, fungi, and viruses. Ethylene oxide, glutaraldehyde, peroxyacetic acid, hydrogen peroxide, and sodium hypochlorite can act as chemical sterilizing agents for objects that cannot be heated or sterilized by other physical methods (eg, radiation).

ETHYL ALCOHOL

ISOPROPYL ALCOHOL

Alcohols are applied to reduce local microbial flora prior to penetration with needles or other sharp instruments and as a preoperative wash. Their antiseptic action can be enhanced by prior mechanical cleansing of the skin with water and a detergent and gentle rubbing with sterile gauze during application.

Ethyl alcohol is widely used for skin antisepsis, especially when an immediate reduction in colony-forming units is desired; little if any substantive or cumulative effect is observed with repeated use. The bactericidal effects of ethyl alcohol result from rapid coagulation of protein. The 70% aqueous solution is more effective in reducing the surface tension of bacterial cells than absolute alcohol; the latter precipitates protoplasm at the periphery of the cell and thus tends to retard penetration of the agent. Isopropyl alcohol has slightly greater bactericidal activity than ethyl alcohol due to its greater reduction of surface tension. It rapidly kills vegetative forms of most bacteria when used as a 60% to 70% aqueous solution. In one study, both ethyl alcohol and isopropyl alcohol were more effective than chlorhexidine and povidone-iodine in producing antisepsis on the hands in the presence of blood (Larson and Bobo, 1992).

Ethyl and isopropyl alcohol are used as cleansers, lubricants, and rubefacients for bedridden patients. Rubbing alcohol contains about 70% (by volume) isopropyl alcohol. Alcohol is applied to cool the skin but it may irritate inflamed or denuded tissue, especially after repeated use. Application of an emollient after an alcohol rub alleviates the dry feeling.

Ethyl and isopropyl alcohol are potent virucidal agents (Klein and Deforest, 1983). Neither has reliable fungicidal or sporicidal activity in any concentration and they are not useful for sterilization of instruments.

Alcohols should not be used to disinfect wounds because they irritate tissues, resulting in painful burning and stinging, and they precipitate protein to form a coagulated mass in which bacteria may grow.

ETHYL ALCOHOL:
Alcohol, U.S.P., Diluted Alcohol, U.S.P.
ISOPROPYL ALCOHOL:
Isopropyl Alcohol, N.F. (nonprescription), Rubbing Alcohol, N.F. (nonprescription).

FORMALDEHYDE

GLUTARAL

Formaldehyde is a potent, volatile, wide-spectrum germicide that has been used as a vapor and as a solution in water (formalin). The vapor is irritating when inhaled or applied to the skin in the concentrations required for antisepsis. Therefore, formaldehyde is used principally as a disinfectant in concentrations of 2% to 8%.

Glutaral (glutaraldehyde) is a potent dialdehyde with a wide range of antimicrobial activity; it is sporicidal and possesses tuberculocidal activity. A 2% aqueous solution buffered with sodium carbonate 0.3% to a pH of 7.5 to 8.5 disinfects and sterilizes surgical and endoscopic instruments and plastic and rubber apparatus used for respiratory therapy and anesthesia. Glutaral loses activity within two weeks after preparation because it tends to polymerize in alkaline solution, which is the optimum pH for germicidal activity. Several alkaline solutions that are stabilized with surfactants [Cidex-7, Cidex Plus, Vespore] have longer use lives (four to six weeks). This disinfectant may cross-react with formaldehyde.

FORMALDEHYDE SOLUTION, U.S.P.:
Solution containing 37% by weight of formaldehyde with methanol added to prevent polymerization.
GLUTARAL:
Calgocide (Calgon Vestal), ***Cidex Solution, Cidex-7*** (J & J Medical), ***Vespore*** (Calgon Vestal). Solution 2% (nonprescription).
Cidex Plus (J & J Medical). Solution 3.2% (nonprescription).

TRICLOCARBAN

This carbanilide is used as an antimicrobial in bar soap; it has antibacterial and antifungal actions. The FDA has approved triclocarban 1.5% as safe and effective for daily topical use.

Coast (Procter & Gamble), ***Dial*** (Armour-Dial), ***Jergens Clear Complexion Bar*** (Jergens), ***Safeguard*** (Procter & Gamble), ***Zest*** (Procter & Gamble) (all nonprescription).

ETHYLENE OXIDE

Ethylene oxide is readily diffusible, noncorrosive, and has antimicrobial activity against all organisms at room temperature. This gaseous alkylating agent is widely used as an alternative to heat sterilization of drugs and medical devices. It reacts with chloride and water to produce two active germicides, 2-chloroethanol and ethylene glycol. Special sterilizing chambers are required because the gas must remain in contact with the objects for several hours. *Adequate airing* of sterilized materials is important to minimize skin irritation in nonsensitized individuals who come into contact with such materials. The presence of ethylene oxide in dialysis tubing has been suggested as a possible cause of allergic reactions in some patients (Patterson et al, 1986). Ethylene oxide also is a pulmonary irritant when inhaled. It is too toxic to be applied topically as an antiseptic.

Ethylene oxide and 2-chloroethanol (but not ethylene glycol, an alkylating agent) are mutagenic and carcinogenic in some animals, and some concern exists about the current Occupational Safety and Health Administration's exposure limit for workers of 1 ppm over an eight-hour period.

HYDROGEN PEROXIDE

When hydrogen peroxide comes into contact with catalase, an enzyme found in blood and most tissues, it rapidly decomposes into oxygen and water. This occurs in wounds and on mucous membranes. The liberated oxygen has little bactericidal effect except, possibly, on anaerobes, but it does loosen masses of infected detritus in wounds. Hydrogen peroxide has little effect on intact skin because the oxygen is released so slowly.

When diluted with one or more parts of water, hydrogen peroxide is sometimes employed as a mouthwash, but its use to treat stomatitis and gingivitis may irritate the tongue and buccal mucosa. The 3% solution or a solution diluted to 1.5% often is instilled in the external ear tc aid in removal of cerumen. The use of solutions stronger than 3% in open or recent wounds is discouraged, because this concentration may be toxic to fibroblasts. Hydrogen peroxide should never be instilled in closed body cavities or abscesses from which the gas has no free egress. Hemiplegia has followed its use to irrigate the pleural cavity; presumably this is caused by the passage of the gas into the vascular system, resulting in cerebral embolism.

Generic. Solution 3% (nonprescription).

CHLORHEXIDINE GLUCONATE

[Hibiclens, Hibistat, Peridex Oral Rinse]

Chlorhexidine is a chlorophenyl biguanide with a relatively broad spectrum of antimicrobial activity (Aly and Maibach, 1983; Goldblum et al, 1983; Sebben, 1983). At pH 5.0 to 8.0, it is most effective against gram-positive (10 mcg/ml) and gram-negative (50 mcg/ml) bacteria. The development of resistance is not a significant problem. Bacterial spores are prevented from germinating but are not killed except at elevated temperatures. High concentrations of serum proteins reduce the bacteriostatic and bactericidal effects of chlorhexidine. Its effectiveness is slightly reduced by blood and other organic matter (Sheikh, 1986). Although high levels of surfactants also may reduce the bacteriostatic and bactericidal effects of chlorhexidine, this problem may be minimized by careful formulation. Since chlorhexidine is cationic, formulations that contain anionic-based chemicals may neutralize its effect.

Chlorhexidine has a slower onset of action than the alcohols; however, it has considerable skin persistence or substantivity (residual adherence) and is the agent of choice when continued chemical antimicrobial activity on the skin is desirable (Larson and Laughon, 1987). Chlorhexidine has low potential for producing contact sensitivity and photosensitivity with long-term clinical use, and it is not absorbed through intact skin, even after many daily hand washings.

Low concentrations of chlorhexidine are widely used as a preservative in eye formulations and contact lens solution. Products containing chlorhexidine gluconate 4% in a sudsing base formulation (eg, Hibiclens) are used as antiseptic superficial wound and general skin cleansers, for preoperative preparation of the skin, as surgical scrubs, and as handwashes for health care personnel. Hibistat is a germicidal hand rinse; the clear, colorless liquid contains 0.5% weight/weight chlorhexidine gluconate in 70% isopropyl alcohol with emollients.

Peridex is used to prevent oral infections in immunocompromised patients (Ferretti, et al, 1987) and is safe and effective for the treatment of gingivitis and periodontal disease (Grossman et al, 1986). It is available only on prescription and contains chlorhexidine 0.12% in a mouthrinse formulation.

ADVERSE REACTIONS AND PRECAUTIONS. Corneal exposure to high concentrations of chlorhexidine for durations of 5 to 15 minutes (preoperative skin preparation using chlorhexidine gluconate 4%) has resulted in serious keratitis and progressive diminution of vision experimentally and clinically (Hamed et al, 1987; Phinney et al, 1988). Therefore, it is imperative that contact of the 4% solution with the eyes be avoided when health care personnel apply skin antiseptic preparations on the face or head.

Six patients have developed anaphylaxis following exposure to chlorhexidine (Okano et al, 1989). An analysis of the cases suggests that anaphylaxis is most likely to occur following application of concentrations ≥0.5% to open wounds or mucous membranes.

Hibiclens Skin Cleanser, Hibistat Hand Rinse (Stuart) (nonprescription); ***Peridex Oral Rinse*** (Procter & Gamble).

MERCURIAL COMPOUNDS

Although organic mercurial compounds generally are less irritating and less toxic than inorganic compounds, some are more readily absorbed than inorganic compounds and can cause serious central nervous system toxicity. Organic mercurial compounds have only weak bacteriostatic activity and are less effective than ethyl alcohol. Serum and tissue proteins reduce antimicrobial activity, and skin sensitization is common. Consequently, the antiseptic and disinfectant uses of mercurial compounds are limited, and only thimerosal is available.

A tentative final monograph published by the FDA in 1991 proposes to ban mercury-containing antiseptics, and the Agency has reclassified thimerosal as Category II (ineffective). This action of the FDA is in concert with an earlier OTC Review Panel's recommendation. Thus, products containing thimerosal, such as Mercurochrome, Merosal, or Merthiolate, would either have to be reformulated or be removed from the market when the final rule goes into effect.

CATIONIC SURFACTANTS

Soaps are anionic and organic quaternary ammonium compounds are cationic surface-active agents. Both classes of detergents emulsify sebaceous material, which is then removed with dirt and microbes. The mild desquamating effect of the quaternary ammonium compounds aids in cleansing. Their antimicrobial properties are limited and solutions are prone to contamination; thus, their usefulness as antiseptics is often less than desired (Sebben, 1983). Nevertheless, these compounds are widely used as industrial and home detergents, emulsifiers, and sanitizers. Their antimicrobial action is ascribed to alteration of microbial membrane permeability.

The quaternary ammonium compounds are adsorbed and inactivated by cotton fabrics, cellulose sponges, certain plastics (particularly polyvinyl chloride), or other porous materials. For this reason, these agents should not be used for cold sterilization of catheters, flexible endoscopes, or other instruments.

BENZALKONIUM CHLORIDE
[Ionax, Zephiran]

Benzalkonium chloride is the prototype of the organic quaternary ammonium compounds. It is active against gram-positive and gram-negative bacteria, some fungi (including yeasts), and certain protozoa (eg, *Trichomonas vaginalis*). Strains of *Pseudomonas aeruginosa* are more resistant and require longer exposure. Aqueous solutions are ineffective against *Mycobacterium tuberculosis, Clostridium,* and other spore-forming bacteria and viruses.

Benzalkonium chloride is applied to minor lacerations, wounds, and abrasions to limit infection. Organic material, soap, and other anionic substances inactivate this agent. The following concentrations are recommended: For use on intact skin, minor wounds, and abrasions, 1:750 (tincture or aqueous solutions); for use on mucous membranes and broken or diseased skin, 1:2,000 to 1:5,000 (aqueous solution).

Concentrated solutions can produce corrosive skin lesions with deep necrosis and scarring. Properly diluted solutions are not ordinarily irritating or sensitizing; however, if they are used under occlusive dressings, casts, or packs, irritation may occur. Caution is advisable when irrigating body cavities with benzalkonium chloride, for systemic absorption may cause muscle weakness.

Benzalkonium chloride also is used as a disinfectant for surgical instruments, catheters, and other devices in a concentration of 1:750. An anti-rust agent should be added to retard corrosion of metallic instruments. Solutions should be checked periodically for contamination by resistant bacteria and spores and replenished frequently to maintain effective bactericidal concentrations.

(All forms nonprescription)
Generic. Solution, concentrate.
Ionax (Owen). Foam aerosol, scrub paste.
Zephiran (Sanofi Winthrop). Solution (aqueous), concentrate, tincture, tincture spray.

METHYLBENZETHONIUM CHLORIDE
[Diaparene]

This cationic surfactant is effective against gram-positive and gram-negative organisms. It is commonly used as a rinse for diapers and for bed linen and underclothes of incontinent adults to prevent irritant contact dermatitis; articles should be free of soap to avoid inactivation of the antiseptic. Methylbenzethonium also is applied topically as a dusting powder around the genitalia, rectum, and thighs and in intertriginous areas to prevent and treat perianal dermatitis, miliaria rubra, and intertrigo. It seldom produces irritation.

Diaparene (Lehn & Fink). Powder, perianal cream, ointment (all forms nonprescription).

CHLORINE COMPOUNDS

CHLORINE

SODIUM HYPOCHLORITE SOLUTION

OXYCHLOROSENE
[Clorpactin XCB, Clorpactin WCS-90]

Chlorine is a potent germicidal agent used to disinfect inanimate objects, water supplies, and swimming pools. It is not recommended for disinfecting medical instruments because of its corrosive properties. The germicidal action is primarily due to the hypochlorous acid that forms in aqueous solution; elemental chlorine also plays a role. Organic matter and an alkaline pH decrease the germicidal effect.

Sodium hypochlorite solution is used to disinfect utensils. The undiluted solution contains approximately 5% sodium hypochlorite and is too irritating for use as an antiseptic except in root canal therapy. Sodium hypochlorite solution diluted (modified Dakin's solution) contains 0.5% sodium hypochlorite adjusted to a neutral pH with sodium bicarbonate. It once was widely used to treat suppurating wounds, but its solvent action delays clotting.

Sodium hypochlorite may cause irritant contact dermatitis.

The germicidal chlorophor, oxychlorosene, is a mixture of hypochlorous acid and alkylbenzene sulfonates. The sulfonates appear to enhance the germicidal activity of hypochlorous acid by causing its slow release. The sodium salt is used as a topical antiseptic for preoperative preparation of the skin and for wound irrigation in a concentration of 0.2% to 0.4%. Concentrations of 0.1% to 0.2% are useful for urologic and ophthalmologic irrigations or applications.

SODIUM HYPOCHLORITE SOLUTION, N.F.:
Available generically and as household bleach (nonprescription).
DILUTED SODIUM HYPOCHLORITE SOLUTION, N.F.
OXYCHLOROSENE:
Clorpactin XCB (Guardian). Powder 5 g (for solution) (nonprescription).
OXYCHLOROSENE SODIUM:
Clorpactin WCS-90 (Guardian). Powder 2 g (for solution) (nonprescription).

IODINE COMPOUNDS

Elemental iodine is a powerful antimicrobial agent; adequate concentrations and duration of exposure can destroy most known bacteria, fungi, viruses, protozoa, and yeasts. Bacterial resistance to iodine is unknown. Elemental iodine is poorly soluble in water or alcohol, and a saturated solution of about 0.03% (300 ppm) is formed in both. Soluble iodine is referred to as free iodine. Additional iodine can be made soluble only by conversion to triiodide ion with an iodide salt, such as the inclusion of sodium iodide in U.S.P. iodine solution and U.S.P. iodine tincture. This reaction is reversible when the concentration of elemental iodine falls below the saturation level. The potentially reversible inorganic triiodide ion plus free iodine are together referred to as "available iodine," whereas free and complexed elemental iodine (I_2) in organic iodophors (eg, povidone-iodine) are together referred to as "available iodine." However, only free iodine appears to possess significant antimicrobial activity (Favero, 1982).

Free iodine is an avid collector of electrons to form iodide ion. Iodine captures electrons from many organic molecules, such as glucose, starches, glycols, lipids, amino acids, and proteins, which is the basis for its rapid antimicrobial action. Once iodine is converted to iodide ion, antimicrobial activity is lost. Iodine cannot penetrate tissue without undergoing rapid conversion to inactive iodide ion, ie, it is active only on tissue surfaces. Nevertheless, iodophors remain active in the presence of blood, pus, serum, mucosal secretions, other tissue fluids, and soap.

Iodine can be used to disinfect water when other methods are not available; three drops of tincture of iodine added to one quart of water kills bacteria and amebae within 15 minutes.

Hypersensitivity reactions may occur after application of any of these compounds. Iodine solutions occasionally are taken with suicidal intent. The caustic action of elemental iodine affects the gastrointestinal mucosa. Suspensions of starch or protein or solutions of sodium thiosulfate may be ingested as antidotes.

IODINE SOLUTION, U.S.P.

IODINE TINCTURE

Iodine solution U.S.P. contains approximately 2% iodine and 2.4% sodium iodide in water (2% available iodine and 0.03% free iodine). It is preferred for superficial lacerations to prevent microbial infections, since it is effective and nonirritating. (Iodine Solution should not be confused with Strong Iodine Solution, U.S.P. [Lugol's solution], which is used to treat thyroid disease.) Irrigation of the wound with saline and application of iodine solution around the wound is preferable to applying it directly to the wound, because iodine is toxic to fibroblasts and epithelial cells and may retard healing.

Iodine tincture is a 2% solution of elemental iodine with 2.4% sodium iodide in water and 44% to 50% alcohol (2% available iodine and 0.03% free iodine). It is preferred to the older 7% iodine tincture, which caused severe burns, and to iodine solution for the decontamination of intact skin prior to intravenous injection or obtaining blood for microbial culture studies. The concentration of alcohol in iodine tincture is irritating to wounds.

IODINE SOLUTION, U.S.P.
IODINE TINCTURE, U.S.P.

Iodophors

Iodophors are complexes of iodine and organic compounds that gradually release low concentrations of free iodine from a reservoir of available iodine. In addition to their medical use as antiseptics, iodophors are extensively employed as general disinfectants for household, industrial, farming, and veterinary purposes. Medical use is limited to the nonsurfactant aqueous and alcohol-soluble povidone-iodine (polyvinylpyrrolidine-iodine complex).

POVIDONE-IODINE

For chemical formula, see index entry Povidone-Iodine, In Burns.

The iodine complexed with povidone has no antimicrobial activity until it is released as free iodine in solution. It has the same broad antimicrobial spectrum as iodine solution and iodine tincture (the standard undiluted 10% aqueous povidone-iodine solutions are formulated to contain 1% available iodine but only 0.0002% [2 ppm] free iodine).

Although diluting the standard 10% aqueous povidone-iodine solution with water 1:10 increases the liberation of elemental iodine four- to fivefold (Berkelman et al, 1982), fewer organisms are eliminated. Moreover, dilute solutions are less stable, deteriorate rapidly on standing, and are more susceptible to inactivation by organic materials. Therefore, full strength povidone-iodine preparations (7.5% to 10%) should be used to ensure optimal antisepsis. Antiseptic activity ceases when povidone-iodine in dressings or on the skin becomes dry.

Povidone-iodine preparations are used as handwashes for health care personnel; as surgical scrubs; to prepare skin prior to surgery, injection, or aspiration; to treat minor cuts and abrasions; to treat burns (see the section on Chemotherapeutic Agents for Burns); and as a disinfectant for urinary catheters and peritoneal dialysis equipment. Povidone-iodine may be used locally as a vaginal disinfectant in the treatment of trichomoniasis. Its topical vaginal application elevates serum iodine concentrations; therefore, this drug should not be used repeatedly during pregnancy to avoid goiter and hypothyroidism in the fetus and newborn infant (see also index entry Povidone-Iodine, In Trichomoniasis).

Clinically significant systemic absorption of iodine after topical application of povidone-iodine is usually related to its use in burns that cover more than 20% to 25% of body surface area (Zamora, 1986) (see the Section on Chemotherapeutic Agents for Burns). However, possible metabolic complications arising from systemic iodine absorption has been reported in an elderly patient following topical application of povidone-iodine to decubitus ulcers (Dela Cruz et al, 1987).

Povidone-iodine is less irritating and less toxic than aqueous and alcoholic solutions of elemental iodine (Rodeheaver et al, 1982); however, irritation occurs occasionally, especially with use of solutions containing detergents. Local hypersensitivity reactions are uncommon, but individuals with a history of iodine sensitization should not use this agent.

(All forms nonprescription)
Generic. Ointment, liquid, solution, surgical scrub, vaginal douche.
Aerosol Spray:
Betadine (Purdue Frederick).
Mouthwash and Gargle:
Betadine (Purdue Frederick).
Cream:
Betadine (Purdue Frederick).

Ointment:
ACU-dyne (Acme United), ***Betadine*** (Purdue Frederick), ***Efodine*** (Fougera), ***Pharmadine*** (Sherwood), ***Polydine*** (Century).

Skin Cleanser:
ACU-dyne (Acme United), ***Betadine Liquid, Foam*** (Purdue Frederick), ***Pharmadine*** (Sherwood).

Solution:
ACU-dyne (Acme United), ***Betadine*** (Purdue Frederick), ***Pharmadine*** (Sherwood), ***Polydine*** (Century).

Surgical Scrub:
Betadine (Purdue Frederick), ***Mallisol*** (Hauck), ***Pharmadine*** (Sherwood).

PHENOLIC COMPOUNDS

PHENOL

SAPONIFIED CRESOL SOLUTION

HEXYLRESORCINOL

PARACHLOROMETAXYLENOL

PARABENS

Phenol and substituted phenols vary greatly in their antiseptic and disinfectant efficacy and safety. Phenol is bacteriostatic in concentrations of 1:500 to 1:800 and bactericidal and fungicidal in concentrations of 1:50 to 1:100. It is not effective against spores. Phenol is seldom used as an antiseptic or disinfectant. Because it possesses local anesthetic activity and has an antipruritic effect at concentrations of 0.5% to 1.5%, its primary use is as a component of topical antipruritic formulations.

Under certain conditions, phenol damages skin, which increases the rate of penetration; therefore, it should be applied only on small areas of skin, and occlusive dressings, bandages, or diapers should not be used. Phenol is not recommended for use in pregnant women, in infants under 6 months, or for diaper rash. Phenolic disinfectants have produced epidemics of neonatal hyperbilirubinemia when used to clean bassinets and mattresses in poorly ventilated nurseries. Fatalities have been documented in infants. Phenol has been implicated as a tumor promoter in rodent models in concentrations above 5%. Tumorigenicity has not been reported in humans.

Cresol is a mixture of the three methyl isomers of phenol saponified in linseed oil. It is as toxic as phenol but three times more potent as a bactericide. Because of its irritating effect on the skin, use of cresol is limited to disinfection. However, neither phenol nor cresol should be used to disinfect rubber, plastic, or fabrics that may adsorb the agent, because burns may result when these come into contact with the skin.

Hexylresorcinol is a more effective and less toxic bactericide than phenol. It is used in antiseptic mouthwashes and as a skin wound cleanser, but it may be irritating.

Parachlorometaxylenol (PCMX) 0.5% to 2% also is a more effective bactericide than phenol. It is a component of handwashes used by health care personnel and of OTC mixtures used for acne, seborrhea, and otic infections. Published data on efficacy, safety, and cost of PCMX have been reviewed (Larson and Talbot, 1986). The FDA has requested additional data on absorption, distribution, metabolism, and excretion of this agent before granting category I (safe and efficacious) status.

The short alkyl esters of *p*-hydroxybenzoic acid are known as the *parabens*. Although they are seldom used as antiseptics, methylparaben and its homologues are included in many topical and some parenteral preparations as preservatives. The parabens may sensitize the skin, but the incidence is low.

PHENOL, U.S.P.

SAPONIFIED CRESOL SOLUTION:
Lysol.

HEXYLRESORCINOL, N.F.

PARACHLOROMETAXYLENOL, U.S.P.:
Medicated Lotion Soap (Moore H.L.) 0.5%.

HEXACHLOROPHENE
[pHisoHex, Septisol]

This chlorinated bisphenol compound has strong bacteriostatic activity and is most effective against gram-positive bacteria, including staphylococci. It has little activity against most gram-negative bacteria or spores. Hexachlorophene is used for handwashing by hospital personnel, as a surgical hand scrub, and for preoperative preparation of the skin.

Although single washings of the skin are no more effective than soap in reducing the number of bacteria, regularly repeated scrubs steadily decrease bacterial flora. Cleansing with alcohol or washing with soap removes the antibacterial residue.

ADVERSE REACTIONS AND PRECAUTIONS. Hexachlorophene may produce irritation, but hypersensitivity reactions are rare. Preparations may cause a burning sensation on the skin and in the eyes, and suds containing this agent should be rinsed promptly from the eyes with water.

Hexachlorophene is absorbed through intact skin and mucosal surfaces. Since amounts sufficient to produce neurotoxic effects may be absorbed, it should not be applied in compresses, and special precautions should be taken to avoid extensive application to broken, denuded, or burned skin. Systemic absorption causes symptoms characteristic of cerebral irritability and seizures. Hexachlorophene should not be used routinely for prophylactic total body bathing, especially for infants. When it is applied to clean small areas of pyoderma in infants, the residue should be rinsed off thoroughly. The drug is available only on prescription.

Hexachlorophene is classified in FDA Pregnancy Category C.

pHisoHex (Sanofi Winthrop). Emulsion 3% in 150, 480, and 3,785 ml containers.

Septisol (Calgon Vestal). Foam 0.23% with alcohol 46% in 180 and 600 ml containers.

TRICLOSAN

This 5-chloro-2-(2,4-dichlorophenoxy) phenol is an antimicrobial ingredient of bar soaps limited to concentrations no greater than 1%. It is also present in antiseptic, wound cleanser, and wound protectant products. The FDA is expected to reclassify triclosan as safe and effective for hand washes, surgical hand scrubs for health care personnel, and for preoperative skin preparation. Products containing triclosan should not be used in infants under 6 months because the cumulative effects of cutaneous absorption have not been determined.

Antimicrobial soaps such as ***Lifebuoy, Liquid Safeguard, Phase III***; also with triclocarban as ***Irish Spring*** (all nonprescription).

SILVER COMPOUNDS

Silver nitrate and silver sulfadiazine [Silvadene] are the only silver compounds widely used. Colloidal silver preparations (eg, mild silver protein [Argyrol S.S. 10%]) are less corrosive, but their disinfecting properties do not equal those of the silver salts because less of the active free silver ion is available; therefore, they are not recommended for such use.

Silver sulfadiazine is used in burn therapy and in the treatment of chronic pressure ulcers (Kucan et al, 1981). See index entry Silver Sulfadiazine, In Burns.

SILVER NITRATE

This silver salt is strongly bactericidal when applied topically in relatively low concentrations; most microorganisms are destroyed rapidly by a 1:1,000 solution, and a 1:10,000 solution is bacteriostatic.

In many states, instillation of two drops of 1% solution into the conjunctival sac of newborn infants is required by law to prevent ophthalmia neonatorum. (See index entry Silver Nitrate, In Neonatal Conjunctivitis.)

Since silver nitrate is an effective germicide and astringent, a 0.1% to 0.5% solution is used on wet dressings, but it may stain tissue black due to reduction of silver deposits upon exposure to sunlight. Occasionally, 0.01% to 0.03% solutions are applied to irrigate the urethra and bladder.

Aqueous solutions of 0.5% silver nitrate are sometimes applied as dressings on second- and third-degree burns to prevent infections caused by *Pseudomonas aeruginosa*, *Proteus*, or other gram-negative and gram-positive organisms. The most important adverse effect with such use is depletion of sodium and chloride caused by precipitation of insoluble silver chloride; this is particularly likely if silver nitrate is applied to extensive areas over prolonged periods. Small amounts of silver nitrate may be absorbed through the skin after prolonged use, resulting in argyria, a permanent bluish-black discoloration of the skin (only one case of argyria has been reported in association with burn therapy). Pain lasting for one-half to one hour after application of dressings is common with concentrations exceeding 0.5% and occasionally with lower concentrations. Drying of the dressings may result in higher concentrations of silver nitrate, which will produce chemical cauterization of the wound.

A solid preparation in a pencil-form applicator (toughened silver nitrate) or a cotton pledget dipped in 10% silver nitrate solution is used to cauterize wounds, fissures, aphthae, and granulomatous tissue.

Generic. Solution (ophthalmic) 1%; ointment; toughened stick applicators.

Cited References

Aly R, Maibach HI: Comparative evaluation of chlorhexidine gluconate (Hibiclens) and povidone-iodine (E-Z Scrub) sponge/brushes for presurgical hand scrubbing. *Curr Ther Res* 34:740-745, 1983.

Bartzokas CA, et al: Evaluation of skin disinfecting activity and cumulative effect of chlorhexidine and triclosan handwash preparations on hands artificially contaminated with *Serratia marcescens*. *Infect Control* 8:163-167, 1987.

Berkelman RL, et al: Increased bactericidal activity of dilute preparations of povidone-iodine solutions. *J Clin Microbiol* 15:635-639, 1982.

Bjerke NB: Handwashing agents. *Infect Control* 8:384-385, 1987.

Dela Cruz F, et al: Iodine absorption after topical administration. *West J Med* 146:43-45, 1987.

Favero MS: Iodine: Champagne in tin cup. *Infect Control* 3:30-32, 1982.

Ferretti GA, et al: Chlorhexidine for prophylaxis against oral infections and associated complications in patients receiving bone marrow transplants. *J Am Dent Assoc* 114:461-467, 1987.

Goldblum SE, et al: Comparison of 4% chlorhexidine gluconate in detergent base (Hibiclens) and povidone-iodine (Betadine) for skin preparation of hemodialysis patients and personnel. *Am J Kidney Dis* 11:548-552, 1983.

Grossman E, et al: Six-month study of the effects of a chlorhexidine mouthrinse on gingivitis in adults. *J Periodont Res* (suppl) 33-43, 1986.

Hamed LM, et al: Hibiclens keratitis. *Am J Ophthalmol* 104:50-56, 1987.

Klein M, Deforest A: Principles of viral inactivation, in Block SS (ed): *Disinfection, Sterilization, and Preservation,* ed 3. Philadelphia, Lea & Febiger, 1983, 422-434.

Kucan JO, et al: Comparison of silver sulfadiazine, povidone-iodine, and physiological saline in treatment of chronic pressure ulcers. *J Am Geriatr Soc* 29:232-235, 1981.

Larson E: Handwashing and skin: Physiologic and bacteriologic aspects. *Infect Control* 6:14-23, 1985.

Larson E: Guideline for use of topical antimicrobial agents. *Am J Infect Control* 16:253-266, 1988.

Larson E, Bobo L: Effective hand degermination in the presence of blood. *J Emerg Med* 10:7-11, 1992.

Larson EL, Laughon BE: Comparison of four antiseptic products containing chlorhexidine gluconate. *Antimicrob Agents Chemother* 31:1572-1574, 1987.

Larson EL, Talbot GH: Approach for selection of health care personnel handwashing agents. *Infect Control* 7:419-424, 1986.

Larson EL, et al: Quantity of soap as variable in handwashing. *Infect Control* 8:371-375, 1987.

Laufman H: Current use of skin and wound cleansers and antiseptics. *Am J Surg* 157:359-365, 1989.

Okano M, et al: Anaphylactic symptoms due to chlorhexidine. *Arch Dermatol* 125:50-52, 1989.

Patterson R, et al: Ethylene oxide (ETO) as possible cause of allergic reaction during peritoneal dialysis and immunologic detection of ETO from dialysis tubing. *Am J Kidney Dis* 8:64-66, 1986.

Phinney RB, et al: Corneal edema related to accidental Hibiclens exposure. *Am J Ophthalmol* 106:210-215, 1988.

Rodeheaver G, et al: Bactericidal activity and toxicity of iodine-containing solutions in wounds. *Arch Surg* 117:181-186, 1982.

Rutala WA, Cole EC: Antiseptics and disinfectants: Safe and effective? Editorial. *Infect Control* 5:215-218, 1984.

Sebben JE: Surgical antiseptics. *J Am Acad Dermatol* 9:759-765, 1983.

Sheikh W: Comparative antibacterial efficacy of Hibiclens and Betadine in the presence of pus derived from human wounds. *Curr Ther Res* 40:1096-1102, 1986.

Zamora JL: Chemical and microbiologic characteristics and toxicity of povidone-iodine solutions. *Am J Surg* 151:400-406, 1986.

Antimycobacterial Drugs 76

TUBERCULOSIS

Tuberculosis is caused by *Mycobacterium tuberculosis*, a bacillus that can remain dormant in the human host for years. This disease appears to have been with mankind since prehistoric time, for paleopathologic evidence of spinal tuberculosis in neolithic and pre-Columbian skeletons has been reported. Tuberculosis appears to have become a major public health problem during the industrial revolution when poor living and working conditions favored its spread. Today it is one of the most widespread infections; 1.7 billion persons (one-third of the world's population) harbor the tubercle bacillus. Each year there are 8 million new cases; of these, 3.6 million are infectious pulmonary tuberculosis (ie, sputum smear-positive), an equal number are smear-negative pulmonary tuberculosis, and 800,000 are extrapulmonary tuberculosis. The fatality rate for untreated tuberculosis is over 50%, and it has been estimated that worldwide nearly three million persons die each year from the disease. Statistics from the developing world suggest that one-quarter of avoidable adult deaths (age 15 to 59 years) are due to tuberculosis. Today tuberculosis is the most common cause of death from a single infectious agent in the world.

In recent years two problems with tuberculosis have developed: the epidemic of human immunodeficiency virus (HIV) infection and the transmission of multiple-drug resistant (MDR) strains of tuberculosis. HIV infection is the most important risk factor identified for reactivation of latent tuberculosis and progression to active disease, and it has exacerbated the epidemiologic problem of tuberculosis throughout the world. In Africa, nearly 50% of HIV-seropositive individuals also are infected with the tubercle bacillus and, of these, it is estimated that 5% to 8% will develop clinical tuberculosis each year. Worldwide, tuberculosis is one of the most common opportunistic infections affecting AIDS patients.

The Centers for Disease Control and Prevention (CDC) has estimated that from 1985 through 1992 over 51,700 excess cases of tuberculosis accumulated in the United States. The largest increase (54.5%) occurred among those 25 to 44 years. The increase in cases in this age group very likely was due to the occurrence of tuberculosis in persons with HIV infection, but epidemiologic data linking these two diseases were difficult to obtain because of confidentiality laws. Evidence suggesting such linkage was reported (Barnes et al, 1991; Bloch et al, 1989; *MMWR*, 1986, 1989). In the United States, approximately 4% of AIDS patients have had tuberculosis. HIV seroprevalence surveys of tuberculosis patients in several cities have shown HIV-seropositive rates ranging from 1.4% to 46.3% (Centers for Disease Control, 1990).

Currently, approximately 10 million persons in the United States are asymptomatically infected with tubercle bacilli. More than 90% of the cases reported annually to the CDC are estimated to develop in these infected asymptomatic individuals and less than 10% in individuals with recently acquired infection. Since 1990 approximately 25,000 new cases of tuberculosis and 2,000 deaths have been reported annually. In addition to persons infected with HIV, the following groups have been identified by the CDC as potentially at high risk of tuberculous infection and symptomatic disease: the homeless, recent immigrants, Hispanics, blacks, Native Americans, Asians/Pacific Islanders, intravenous drug users, and residents of correctional institutions and nursing homes. About two-thirds of tuberculosis cases occur among racial and ethnic minorities. More than 80% of cases of tuberculosis in children under 15 years occur in minorities; the significant increase in tuberculosis in this age group in recent years suggests increased transmission of tuberculous infection in this country.

The association between tuberculosis and AIDS is quite striking among intravenous drug users. In a prospective study of 520 intravenous drug users, 20% of HIV-seronegative and 23% of HIV-seropositive persons had a positive tuberculin skin test before entry into the study. The incidence of tuberculosis was 7.9%/year among those who were initially HIV-seropositive; in contrast, no cases were observed in HIV-seronegative individuals (Selwyn et al, 1989). Tuberculosis spreads very rapidly among HIV-infected persons housed in the same facility. In an outbreak that occurred between December 1990 and April 1991, tuberculosis was diagnosed in 12 residents of a housing facility for HIV-infected patients. Time from diagnosis of the first case to the last was only 106 days; in one patient, disease developed within four weeks of exposure (*MMWR*, 1991 A; Daley et al, 1992).

Outbreaks of multiple drug-resistant tuberculosis (MDR-TB) were reported before the beginning of the AIDS epidemic, but these appear to have been isolated phenomena (Steiner et al, 1970; *MMWR*, 1977). During the 1980s, reports of outbreaks of MDR-TB not associated with HIV infection occurred in immunocompetent persons. These outbreaks were not confined to any specific geographic area and in two cases involved interstate transmission (*MMWR,* 1985, 1983, 1987, 1990 A). The first documentation of the nosocomial transmission of MDR-TB among HIV-infected patients was reported in 1990. In this outbreak, transmission of tubercle bacilli resistant to at least isoniazid and rifampin among HIV-infected patients as well as in health care workers occurred in an urban hospital in Florida (*MMWR*, 1990 B, 1991 B). During 1990 and 1991, outbreaks of MDR-TB in three hospitals in New York city were reported by the CDC (*MMWR*, 1991 B); approximately 90% of the MDR-TB cases occurred in HIV-infected persons in whom mortality rates up to 90% were reported with a median of 4 to 16 weeks from diagnosis to death. Characteristics of the outbreaks in New York and Florida were very similar and included late diagnosis of tuberculosis and recognition of drug resistance, ineffective patient isolation, and the nosocomial transmission to patients and health care workers.

Thus, physicians today are not only faced with an upsurge in tuberculosis, but also with the additional complications of the HIV epidemic, the occurrence of MDR-TB for which a truly efficacious therapeutic regimen is difficult to devise, and the maintenance of adequate infection control procedures in treatment facilities.

In the United States, it is mandatory in all states for physicians to report newly diagnosed tuberculosis cases as well as patients who prematurely discontinue therapy. Detailed records of therapy must be kept, including changes in regimen, all bacteriologic reports, and the results of drug susceptibility tests.

Transmission and Pathogenesis

Tuberculosis is typically transmitted by inhalation of aerosols of sputum in droplet nuclei containing the tubercle bacilli. Rarely, infection may occur from inhalation of aerosols formed during the processing of tissue specimens or secretions. Aerosolized droplets are formed when persons with pulmonary tuberculosis speak, sneeze, cough, or sing. Patients with cavitary disease are particularly likely to be infectious. The droplet nuclei are so small (<5 microns) that normal room air currents can keep them airborne for long periods. Persons at highest risk of acquiring infection from actively infected, untreated patients are the close contacts (household members and close friends or fellow workers who regularly breathe the potentially infectious air). Over the past decade, transmission rates have been relatively stable with about 29% of close contacts and 15% of other contacts estimated to be infected.

Following inhalation, a droplet nucleus is deposited in a respiratory bronchiole beyond the mucociliary system where the bacilli multiply with little initial host resistance. Subsequently, the organisms are slowly engulfed by alveolar macrophages but remain viable and continue replication within the macrophages unless the macrophage is activated by prior exposure to the tubercle bacillus. The infected, nonactivated macrophage may actually aid in the spread of the organisms to regional lymph nodes, sometimes producing ipsilateral hilar and mediastinal lymphadenopathy. The organisms in the infected lymph node then are disseminated via the blood stream to more distant sites, such as the upper lung, kidneys, bones, and brain, where the environment favors their growth. Many replication cycles can occur before specific immunity develops to limit replication. Specific cell-mediated immunity develops in 2 to 10 weeks; this interval corresponds with the development of a positive tuberculin skin test. In most persons, the immunity is usually adequate to restrict further multiplication of the bacilli; the host remains asymptomatic and the lesions heal.

Extrapulmonary tuberculosis usually results from the hematogenous spread of the organisms and is a common form of the disease in the United States. Its incidence increased by 20% from 1984 to 1989; this may have been due to the HIV epidemic. Tuberculosis lymphadenitis (scrofula) is the most common and tuberculosis pleurisy the second most common extrapulmonary forms of disease in this country. Pleural effusion may occur any time after the initial infection. It is caused by the release of tuberculoprotein from the infected lung into the pleural space, which in turn produces an inflammatory response and clear, protein-rich fluid accumulates. Miliary tuberculosis may occur as part of the early infection or it may develop later during the course of the disease; any age group can be affected. Miliary tuberculosis develops when a necrotic focus erodes a blood vessel permitting a number of bacilli to enter the vascular system in a brief period of time; as a result, many organs may be seeded. Among pregnant women, lymphohematogenous transmission or endometritis can spread the tubercle bacilli to the fetus or to the newborn at the time of delivery. Hematogenous spread also may occur through the placenta via the umbilical vein.

Infected individuals who do not have active disease are not infectious to others. About 10% of infected persons will develop active tuberculosis at some time in their lives, approximately 5% within the first two years. In the absence of treatment, the fatality rate from active disease is about 50% in five years. Infected persons who also are immunocompromised (eg, those with HIV infection) are at considerably greater risk of developing active disease and experiencing accelerated disease progression and may have a much higher fatality rate.

ENDOGENOUS REACTIVATION. Although the acquisition of cell-mediated immunity leads to the resolution of the primary infection in most persons, they remain at risk of disease reactivation for life. Reactivation tuberculosis can occur at any site seeded with bacilli at the time of the primary infection, but it is most common in the upper lobes of the lungs, perhaps due to the relatively high oxygen tension there. Endogenous reactivation probably accounts for up to 90% of tuberculosis cases in the United States.

Necrosis is a conspicuous feature of reactivation tuberculosis and is due to tissue destruction following the allergic inflammatory reaction to tuberculin. The lesion is localized because cellular immunity limits bacterial multiplication and dissemination. However, the disease may spread to adjacent tissue. Erosion of an infected bronchus may lead to bronchogenic spread or, if a blood vessel is affected, to hematogenous spread of the bacilli. Macrophages and lymphocytes do not function or survive in necrotic areas and, therefore, the benefits of acquired cellular immunity are lost at these sites.

REINFECTION TUBERCULOSIS. This occurs when individuals who have been infected previously have delayed hypersensitivity to tuberculin and are infected again, presumably with a new strain. Clinically, it is indistinguishable from reactivation tuberculosis. Except in elderly persons who may be infected again after losing the immunity they once had (Stead et al, 1985, 1987), reinfection tuberculosis is rare in the United States; however, it is relatively common in developing countries where disease prevalence is high. Using the restriction fragment length polymorphism technique, investigators have demonstrated reinfection with MDR-TB in patients with AIDS (Small et al, 1993).

TUBERCULOSIS AND HIV INFECTION. The immunosuppression that follows infection with HIV is a very important risk factor for the development of mycobacterial disease. The *M. avium* complex (MAC) is the mycobacterial species most frequently isolated from AIDS patients, but of greater public health concern is the increasing frequency with which disease caused by *M. tuberculosis* is being recognized in these patients, especially in groups in which the organism is prevalent, eg, intravenous drug abusers, Haitians. However, tuberculosis related to HIV infection also has been reported in homosexual and bisexual men, sexual contacts of bisexual men, and in one person with transfusion-associated AIDS. Concern has been expressed that further transmission of HIV among populations with a high prevalence of tuberculous infection may result in dramatic increases in the disease unless recommended control measures are successful.

The relative contribution of HIV-related tuberculosis to the overall incidence of this disease reported nationally is not known, but infection with HIV has had substantial impact in some areas. Tuberculosis is usually diagnosed preceding or coincident with the diagnosis of AIDS. If tuberculosis occurs before another opportunistic infection develops, 75% to 100% of the patients will have pulmonary disease. Between 25% and 75% of the patients also will have extrapulmonary disease. Lymphatic and disseminated tuberculosis are common among HIV-infected patients; apical pulmonary disease is less common.

Because of the overlap of risk groups, the index of suspicion for tuberculosis should be high in HIV-infected persons and, similarly, the suspicion of HIV infection should be high for those who are diagnosed with tuberculosis. HIV antibody status should be determined for all persons diagnosed with tuberculosis. A Mantoux skin test with 5 units of PPD should be performed on all HIV-infected patients; a reaction of 5 mm or more induration is considered indicative of tuberculous infection. All HIV-infected patients who have respiratory or constitutional symptoms also should be given chest radiographs. Mycobacterial stains and cultures should be performed on all diagnostic specimens to aid in the establishment of a diagnosis of tuberculosis. A positive acid-fast smear should be presumed to be *M. tuberculosis*, and therapy should be started while awaiting culture results.

All patients with pulmonary tuberculosis, including those who are HIV-infected, are potentially infectious. Contact tracing is very important in tuberculosis control programs, and all cases must be reported to the local health department so that standard procedures for contact investigation can be followed. Close contacts should be given a tuberculin skin test and, if there is an independent risk of HIV infection, HIV antibody testing and counseling should be offered.

It has been recommended that chemotherapy for tuberculosis be initiated whenever acid-fast bacilli are observed in a respiratory tract specimen of an HIV-infected person or in a person at increased risk for HIV infection whose antibody status is not known and who declines to be tested. Although it is impossible to distinguish tuberculosis from MAC disease other than by culture, it is important to consider treatment of such patients with a regimen effective against the tubercle bacillus because of the public health implications of tuberculosis. Therapy should be given for a minimum of nine months and should continue for at least six months following documented culture conversion as demonstrated by three negative cultures (*MMWR*, 1989). Chemoprophylaxis with isoniazid is recommended for HIV seropositive individuals who have a significant reaction to 5 units of PPD (*MMWR*, 1989). The recommended duration is 12 months, but some experts favor lifelong isoniazid chemoprophylaxis because of the inevitable deterioration of immune function in HIV-infected persons (*MMWR*, 1989).

BCG vaccine is not recommended for immunocompromised adults, including those with HIV infection. However, the World Health Organization recommends that asymptomatic HIV-infected children in populations in whom the risk of tuberculosis is high should receive the vaccine at birth or as soon as possible thereafter (*MMWR*, 1988). However, this recommendation has been questioned (Reichman, 1989).

Diagnosis

Classically, diagnosis of active tuberculosis is made on the basis of a positive tuberculin skin test, positive acid-fast bacilli (AFB) smear or culture, and a compatible chest radiograph. The traditional method of demonstrating infection with *M. tuberculosis* has been the tuberculin skin test. Although current tests are considerably less than 100% sensitive and specific, no better diagnostic test has yet been devised. The standard test is performed with 5 tuberculin units of PPD contained in a 0.1 mcg/0.1 ml dose of a PPD preparation (PPD-S). The test is read at 48 or 72 hours after injection, and the basis of interpretation is the presence or absence of induration. Although not precise, in general the larger the reaction, the greater the probability that it represents infection with the tubercle bacillus.

Because delayed hypersensitivity may wane in some elderly patients who were exposed to tuberculosis in the past, a negative initial skin test reaction may be misleading. To avoid this, a two-step PPD test can be performed with the second dose given one week after the first in these individuals and others in whom a false-negative reaction is suspected. If the reaction to the second test is positive, presumably this is due to the "booster phenomenon" and not because the patient was exposed to tuberculosis in the intervening week between tests. Although the booster phenomenon can occur at any age, it increases with age and is encountered most frequently among persons over 55 years. Repeated testing of uninfected persons does not sensitize them to tuberculin.

BCG vaccination and HIV infection can complicate the interpretation of a tuberculin skin test. There is no reliable method of distinguishing a positive PPD reaction caused by BCG vaccination from that caused by a natural mycobacterial infection. It has been suggested, however, that large reactions in BCG-vaccinated individuals may indicate infection with *M. tuberculosis*, especially among persons from countries with a high prevalence of the disease (American Thoracic Society, 1990 A).

Anergy to tuberculin, which confounds interpretation of the skin test and could lead to misdiagnosis, is often encountered in HIV-infected patients. The usefulness of the two-step testing procedure described above in these individuals is unknown. Thus, negative tests must be interpreted with caution in HIV-infected patients. Guidelines for anergy testing and management of anergic persons at risk of tuberculosis have been published (*MMWR*, 1991 C).

For recommendations for persons in whom skin testing is indicated, see Table 1, and for classification of positive skin test reactions, see Table 2.

TABLE 1.
PERSONS IN WHOM TUBERCULIN TESTING IS INDICATED*

1. Persons with signs (eg, radiographic abnormality) and/or symptoms (eg, cough, hemoptysis, weight loss) suggestive of current tuberculosis disease
2. Recent contacts with known tuberculosis cases or persons suspected of having tuberculosis
3. Persons with abnormal chest roentgenograms compatible with past tuberculosis
4. Persons with medical conditions that increase the risk of tuberculosis (eg, silicosis, gastrectomy, diabetes, immunosuppressive therapy, lymphomas)
5. Persons with HIV infection
6. Groups at high risk of recent infection with *M. tuberculosis*, such as immigrants from Asia, Africa, Latin America, and Oceania; some inner-city and homeless populations; personnel and long-term residents in some hospitals, nursing homes, mental institutions, and prisons

** Adapted from the American Thoracic Society, 1990 A.*

TABLE 2.
GENERAL CLASSIFICATION OF POSITIVE INTRACUTANEOUS MANTOUX REACTIONS*

Size of Reaction Considered Positive (mm Induration)	Risk Category
≥5 mm	HIV+ patients. Persons with risk factors for HIV infection whose serostatus is unknown; with recent close contact with infectious TB cases; or with chest radiographs consistent with previous but healed TB.
≥10 mm	Persons not meeting above criteria but who have other risk factors including (1) foreign-born from high prevalence countries (Asia, Africa, Latin America); (2) intravenous drug users; (3) medically underserved populations, including ethnic minorities; (4) residents of long-term care facilities (eg, correctional institutions, nursing homes, mental institutions); (5) persons with medical conditions reported to increase risk of TB; (6) other high-risk populations as identified by local public health authorities.
≥15 mm	All other persons not listed above.

** Adapted from the American Thoracic Society, 1990 A.*

Drug Selection

The objectives of antituberculous chemotherapy are to eliminate tubercle bacilli rapidly and to prevent relapse. Ideally, therapy for pulmonary tuberculosis would render the sputum negative by both smear and culture and would keep the sputum consistently negative thereafter. The goal is to make the patient noninfectious as rapidly as possible and to maintain the noninfectious state permanently. There is general agreement that an effective therapeutic regimen should produce a failure-relapse rate of less than 5%.

There are two main principles of therapy for tuberculosis: (1) Therapy must consist of two or more drugs to which the tubercle organisms are susceptible. (2) Treatment must continue long enough (at least three to six months after the sputum becomes negative) to sterilize the lesions and prevent relapse.

Tubercle bacilli are killed by antituberculous drugs only during replication. *Mycobacterium tuberculosis* is an obligate aerobe and the frequency of multiplication, as well as the level of metabolic activity, varies with the concentration of oxygen. In addition, the bacilli are affected by the pH of their environment. Three replicating populations of tubercle bacilli are hypothesized to exist in the host: (1) those in cavitary lesions; (2) those in closed caseous lesions; and (3) those within macrophages.

In cavities, the oxygen tension is fairly high, the medium is neutral or slightly alkaline, and multiplication is active. In closed caseous lesions, the oxygen tension is low, the medium is neutral, and replication is slow and intermittent. The intracellular milieu of macrophages is acidic and multiplication is relatively slow. There is evidence that the efficacy of antituberculous drugs differs among these various bacterial populations (see Table 3). In addition, the host may harbor bacilli that are not replicating, have a low level of metabolic activity, and are not affected by antituberculous drugs.

Because there are basically three different populations of bacilli (rapidly dividing, slowly dividing, and intermittently dividing) and antituberculous drugs differ in their ability to kill these populations, during the past decade chemotherapy has been based on the hypothesis that at least two bactericidal drugs are needed to prevent the emergence of resistant tubercle bacilli. This is the basis for the currently recommended six-month regimen for drug-susceptible tuberculosis consisting of the bactericidal drugs isoniazid, rifampin, and pyrazinamide for two months, followed by four months of isoniazid and rifampin. With current regimens, patients usually cease to be infectious within two to four weeks after the initiation of chemotherapy, assuming that the patient is compliant with therapy and the organisms are susceptible to the drugs being employed. Because this is not always the case, it is important to monitor patients to document conversion of sputum cultures to negative and other signs of response to therapy.

In the United States, ethambutol and streptomycin are alternative first-line drugs recommended for the initial treatment of tuberculosis in adults and children. Second-line drugs include capreomycin, kanamycin, ethionamide, aminosalicylic acid, and cycloserine. The latter drugs are less effective, more toxic, or less acceptable to patients, and they usually are reserved for use when organisms exhibit multiple resistance or when one or more of the first-line drugs cannot be tolerated.

Isoniazid and rifampin are the most potent antituberculous drugs available; they are thought to be bactericidal for extracellular (including cavitary) bacteria, intracellular (macrophages) bacteria, and bacteria in closed caseous lesions; rifampin and pyrazinamide appear to be more active than isoniazid against slowly or intermittently replicating bacilli in macrophages and closed caseous lesions.

Isoniazid distributes well into body tissues and fluids, including cerebrospinal fluid, which explains its efficacy in treating extrapulmonary disease. It is generally well tolerated and is inexpensive. Hepatic and peripheral nervous system disturbances are the most common adverse reactions seen with isoniazid therapy. Increasing age and alcoholism are associated with an increased risk of hepatitis. Hepatotoxicity is age-related and is rarely present in those under age 20; once hepatitis becomes established, the mortality rate is 7% (see

TABLE 3.
ACTION OF DRUGS DEPENDING ON THE METABOLIC ACTIVITY OF TUBERCLE BACILLI

	Metabolic Activity of Tubercle Bacilli		
		Slowly multiplying	
Drug	Actively multiplying (usually extracellular)	At acid pH (intracellular)	At neutral pH (extracellular)
Streptomycin	+ + +	0	0
Isoniazid	+ +	+	±
Rifampin	+ +	+	+
Pyrazinamide	+ or ±	+ +	0
Ethambutol	±	±	0

NOTE: Metabolic activity is expressed on a scale of 0 to + + + as follows: 0 = no activity; ± = bacteriostatic activity; and +, + +, and + + + = bactericidal activity of increasing intensity.

From Dutt AK, Stead WW: Present chemotherapy for tuberculosis. J Infect Dis *146:698-704, 1982. Reprinted with permission.*

Table 4). *However, if therapy is terminated at the first signs of hepatotoxicity, many cases of hepatitis resolve without sequelae.* Peripheral neuropathy is most often seen in patients taking isoniazid who are diabetic, alcoholic, malnourished, pregnant, or have seizures. In these patients, concurrent administration of pyridoxine 6 to 50 mg daily is recommended; 10 to 25 mg daily is the most commonly used dose. Another concern with isoniazid is the development of increasing resistance to the drug throughout the world. Resistance may be present in 7% to 10% of individuals who have previously taken isoniazid; this should be taken into account when the drug is prescribed for such patients.

TABLE 4.
HEPATITIS RATES OF PATIENTS TAKING ISONIAZID BY AGE GROUP*

	Age (years)				
	<20	20-34	35-49	50-64	>65
Approximate Case Rate	0	3	12	23	8

** Based on 1,000 individuals.*

Rifampin has broad antimicrobial activity but is best known for its potent activity in tuberculosis and leprosy. It is well distributed throughout the body, including the central nervous system. Use of the drug in treatment regimens has increased the response of seriously ill patients and significantly shortened the duration of therapy. The most frequently seen adverse effect is gastrointestinal upset. Other adverse effects include hepatotoxicity and skin eruptions. Rifampin is a powerful inducer of liver microsomal enzymes and will accelerate the clearance of drugs that are metabolized at that site. Therefore, the requirement for methadone for those in drug abuse maintenance programs may increase, oral contraceptives may not prevent pregnancy, and the requirement for corticosteroids for patients on maintenance therapy may increase.

Pyrazinamide, although not very active in vitro, is believed to be quite active against intracellular bacilli in the acidic environment of the macrophages. These are the bacilli that are likely to cause relapses. Worldwide, pyrazinamide has become the most important drug after isoniazid and rifampin and is used in combination with them. The most important therapeutic contribution of pyrazinamide is its ability to increase the sterilizing power of tuberculosis regimens as indicated by the prevention of relapses after initially successful treatment. Furthermore, it can be administered orally. Clinical studies have shown that pyrazinamide is most useful during the initial phase of therapy. It is an important component of short-course therapy and also is used for retreatment in patients with isoniazid-resistant bacilli.

Streptomycin is believed to be bactericidal only for the large, rapidly multiplying, extracellular population of tubercle bacilli in cavitary lesions. This drug must be administered parenterally, has significant ototoxicity, and is nephrotoxic. In the United States, streptomycin currently is used for the treatment of infections with resistant organisms, in certain multidrug short-course regimens, and in situations in which an injectable agent or one not metabolized by the liver is indicated. When streptomycin is used as a single agent, resistance develops rapidly.

Ethambutol [Myambutol] is considered to be bacteriostatic at the usual dose of 15 mg/kg/day but bactericidal at a dose of 25 mg/kg/day. Its greatest value in multidrug regimens is its ability to prevent or delay the emergence of organisms resistant to the other drugs in the regimen. The most common adverse effect is optic neuritis; this effect is dose-related and occurs infrequently at the dose commonly used in the United States (15 mg/kg) after the first two months of therapy.

Drug Resistance: An important consideration in drug selection is the likelihood that drug-resistant organisms are present. The incidence of resistant strains varies with different population groups. In certain developing countries, tuberculosis is common and the incidence of resistance to isoniazid and streptomycin is high, especially in patients who contracted disease in the Far East, Africa, or Central and South America.

Recent outbreaks involving the transmission of MDR-TB in the United States have raised concern. Transmission has been reported in families, household contacts, correctional institutions, and in shelters for the homeless; community outbreaks have been reported in several states. During 1991, a collaborative study on drug resistance conducted by the CDC and the NYC Department of Health involved 465 patients—238 previously treated patients (PTP) and 227 patients not previously treated (NTP). In the PTP group, 44% were resistant to at least one drug; 36% were resistant to isoniazid, 34% were resistant to rifampin, and 30% were resistant to isoniazid and rifampin. Among NTP, 23% were resistant to at least one drug; 15% were resistant to isoniazid, 9% were resistant to rifampin, and 7% were resistant to both isoniazid and rifampin. In a follow-up national survey conducted by the CDC, susceptibility testing was performed on 2,720 cases. Of these, 389 cases were resistant to one or more drugs, 163 cases were resistant to two or more drugs, and 90 cases were resistant to both isoniazid and rifampin. In a survey conducted at the Kings County Hospital in Brooklyn, NY, which serves a population in which homelessness and substance abuse are prevalent, the overall resistance rate to one or more drugs was 30.9%, with primary resistance 22.6% and secondary resistance 49.2%. Of the resistant isolates, 56.6% were multiply resistant. Isoniazid resistance was noted in 90.7% and rifampin resistance in 50% of the resistant isolates. Prior treatment with antituberculous drugs was highly predictive of drug resistance (Chawla et al, 1992).

There is consensus that the single most important factor associated with drug resistance is prior drug treatment, especially erratic or ineffective drug therapy. In general, persons with secondary resistance harbor organisms that are resistant to a greater number of drugs. The factors that influence the probability of drug resistance are summarized in Table 5. As a strategy to avoid inadequate therapy in patients at increased risk for drug resistance, the gathering of historical and epidemiologic data is a logical first step.

TABLE 5.
FACTORS THAT INFLUENCE THE CHANCE FOR DRUG RESISTANCE

INCREASED CHANCE

1. Previous treatment for tuberculosis:
   - (a) Greatest risk if treatment fails or disease relapses while patient is still on drugs.
   - (b) Significant risk if treatment was inadequate (weak drug regimens and/or inappropriate duration).
   - (c) Treatment received while living in a high tuberculosis incidence area (closely related to [b]).
2. Birth and/or recent residence in a high tuberculosis incidence area.
   - (a) Particularly Asia, South and Central America, and Africa.
   - (b) Certain localized areas within developed countries (skid row, barrios, etc.)
   - (c) The younger the age, the greater the risk.
3. Recent exposure to a known case of drug-resistant disease.

DECREASED CHANCE

1. No previous treatment for tuberculosis.
2. Birth and/or residence in a low tuberculosis incidence area—the longer, the less likely.
3. Recent exposure to a known case of drug-susceptible disease.

Adapted from Davidson, 1987.

Mutants naturally resistant to two drugs are rare (frequency about 10^{-11} organisms) and, to avoid their growth, it is imperative that dual *bactericidal* drug therapy be used initially in patients with active tuberculosis and be continued long enough to eliminate populations that multiply infrequently.

Progress is being made in understanding the molecular mechanism by which the tubercle bacillus develops resistance to isoniazid, rifampin, and streptomycin. Researchers reported that they identified a single *M. tuberculosis* gene, *katG*, that restored sensitivity to isoniazid in a resistant mutant of *M. smegmatis* and conferred isoniazid susceptibility in some strains of *E. coli*, an organism that is intrinsically resistant to the drug. The *katG* gene encodes for both catalase and peroxidase. Deletion of this gene was associated with isoniazid resistance in two patient isolates of *M. tuberculosis*. The investigators suggested that the enzyme encoded by the gene may chemically convert the drug to a biologically active form, that the active metabolite might be useful in therapy, and that search for the target(s) of the activated drug could be a strategy for development of new drugs (Zhang et al, 1992).

Rifampin is considered to act by binding to the β subunit of RNA polymerase in a locus formed by the appropriate complexing of the different RNA polymerase subunits. Development of resistance to rifampin in tubercle bacilli follows a single-step high-level resistance pattern. Mutants arise spontaneously at a rate of one mutation per 10^7 to 10^8 organisms. Resistance has been attributed to changes in the RNA polymerase following substitution of key amino acids in the enzyme. In *E. coli*, resistance to rifampin has been shown to be associated with specific nucleic acid substitutions in the gene encoding for RNA polymerase subunit β (*rpoβ*). In a recent study, workers cloned the *rpoβ* subunit of *M. tuberculosis* and determined that resistance was due to mutations involving eight conserved amino acids in a region containing 23 amino acids encoded by the subunit. Mutations at serine$_{531}$ and histidine$_{526}$ were most common; they accounted for 80% of detected mutations. Thus, substitution of a limited number of highly conserved amino acids encoded by the *rpoβ* gene was determined to be the primary molecular mechanism responsible for the single-step high-level resistance to rifampin in tubercle bacilli. These workers also established a polymerase chain reaction single-strand conformation polymorphism (PCR-SSCP) technique that could identify all rifampin-resistant strains in which mutations had been demonstrated (Telenti et al, 1993). The PCR-SSCP technique yields results within 48 to 72 hours compared to the three to eight weeks required for susceptibility testing by standard techniques.

In the case of *M. leprae*, rifampin resistance that emerged in nine patients with lepromatous leprosy stemmed from mutation in the *rpoβ* gene. In all but one, missense mutations were found to affect a serine residue, ser$_{425}$; in the remaining mutant, a small insertion was found close to this site (Honore and Cole, 1993).

A ribosomal gene mutation in streptomycin-resistant *M. tuberculosis* isolates also has been identified. An A-G mutation at position 866 in the 16S rRNA gene of streptomycin-resistant clinical isolates was identified through a PCR technique (the amplification refractory mutation system) and appeared to be the primary mechanisms of resistance (Douglass and Steyn, 1993).

The foregoing findings hold promise for the development of rapid screening procedures that involve the polymerase chain reaction to identify rifampin-resistant *M. tuberculosis* and *M. leprae* strains and thus should considerably shorten the interval needed to make an informed decision regarding effective regimens for treatment of the diseases caused by these organisms.

The choice of antituberculous agents depends primarily on whether the organism can be presumed to be susceptible to the first-line drugs. If there is any possibility of previous treatment with an antituberculous drug or if infection with drug-resistant organisms is suspected, special consideration must be given to selection of the initial chemotherapeutic agents. If drugs were given previously, it has been recommended that at least two drugs that the patient has not received previously be used until results of sensitivity studies are available. Because it is difficult at times to obtain accurate information on previous treatment, some clinicians advise that the four-drug regimen currently recommended by the ACET be employed initially in these patients (see the section on Treatment of Drug-Resistant Tuberculosis). There is evidence that in patients who relapse (rather than fail to benefit from therapy) after apparently successful treatment with regimens containing isoniazid and rifampin, usually the strains involved in the relapse remain susceptible to these drugs if initially they were fully susceptible. In these cases, the appropriate retreatment regimen may well be the original regimen, which can be reinitiated until the results of susceptibility studies are available.

In addition to the use of multiple drugs, adequate doses must be administered for sufficient periods to effect a cure. Supervised drug administration or reliable patient compliance is essential for successful therapy. With optimal treatment of drug-susceptible cases, the rate of cure approaches 100%.

A number of effective and safe multiple-drug regimens have been utilized to individualize treatment of active disease. Expanded knowledge of pharmacokinetics and pharmacodynamics and the availability of bactericidal drugs have altered approaches to drug selection and treatment, especially with respect to dosage schedules and duration of therapy. Authorities agree that the best chance to bring about rapid and complete recovery is when the diagnosis is first made, when the organisms are multiplying rapidly, and before chronic, often irreversible, changes occur.

A single drug should never be added to an initial regimen that may be failing. In this situation (which occurs rarely if optimal treatment is prescribed initially), at least two effective agents not previously administered should be added. It may be best to substitute an entirely new regimen of two or more drugs on the basis of dependable bacterial susceptibility studies. Such specialized studies are readily available through many state health departments or large independent laboratories.

The less commonly used second-line antituberculous drugs (capreomycin, kanamycin, ethionamide, and cycloserine) are generally considered to be bactericidal. These drugs are reserved for use when organisms exhibit multiple resistance to the first-line drugs or when the latter are not tolerated or are contraindicated. They are more commonly employed in the retreatment of tuberculosis. Use of aminosalicylic acid is undesirable because of the gastrointestinal distress it produces, especially in adults, but it may play an important role in the treatment of MDR-TB and has been used safely in adults. This drug is well tolerated in children under 2 years and may be an alternative to ethambutol in these patients, who cannot be monitored satisfactorily for retrobulbar neuritis. However, ethionamide usually is advised as a substitute for ethambutol in children.

PREVENTIVE THERAPY. Preventive therapy of tuberculosis has three goals: (1) to prevent latent (asymptomatic) infection from progressing to clinical disease, (2) to prevent recurrence of past disease, and (3) to prevent initial infection. The first goal is the primary one for which preventive therapy is usually recommended. It is prescribed to prevent active disease in an individual who is infected but does not have overt disease (significant reaction to the Mantoux skin test but no evidence of active disease; therefore, subclinical infection is presumed). Prophylactic therapy reduces the bacterial population in the radiographically invisible lesions to prevent the development of disease. For the third goal, therapy is given in an attempt to prevent the establishment of infection, and the recipient is protected only so long as drug therapy is continued.

In the United States, isoniazid is highly effective and is the drug of choice for chemoprophylaxis; it is the only drug approved by the FDA for this purpose. It is bactericidal, safe (when used as recommended), easily administered, and inexpensive. In controlled trials conducted by the U.S. Public Health Service, isoniazid preventive therapy reduced the incidence of disease by 54% to 88% (Comstock and Woolpert, 1984). In a European clinical trial, isoniazid given for 12 months was 75% effective in all persons assigned to the regimen and 93% effective in those who were compliant (International Union Against Tuberculosis, 1982). Isoniazid preventive therapy was 98% efficacious in children and recently infected nursing home patients who were compliant with therapy (Hsu, 1984; Stead, 1987).

Without chemoprophylaxis, approximately 5% of immunocompetent patients recently infected with tubercle bacilli will develop clinically detectable disease within the first two years and an additional 5% sometime during their lifetime. In HIV-infected individuals with a positive tuberculin skin test, the risk may be as high as 8% per year. There also is a public health reason for prophylaxis with isoniazid: Infected, asymptomatic persons become part of a reservoir of infection and have a lifelong risk of development of disease. Approximately 22% of the contacts of diagnosed tuberculosis patients have been estimated to be infected when examined and, in 1% of these, the infection will have progressed to clinical disease (Farer et al, 1988).

Everyone with a significant tuberculin skin test reaction is at some risk of developing the disease and, therefore, presumably could benefit from preventive therapy with isoniazid. However, not all are at equal risk, and patients can be grouped into categories with different probabilities of developing tuberculous disease. Recommended priorities for isoniazid preventive therapy take into account the risk of developing tuberculosis compared with the risk of developing hepatotoxicity during the preventive treatment period (American Thoracic Society/Centers for Disease Control, 1986; *MMWR*, 1990 C). The categories of persons for whom isoniazid chemoprophylaxis is recommended are listed in Table 6. The risk for young children and adolescents who are household contacts of active tuberculosis cases may be twice that for adults. Some contacts may have insignificant tuberculin skin test reactions, but should still be considered for preventive therapy; for example, children who are contacts of bacteriologically confirmed patients are at high risk of developing disease.

The CDC has identified as priority candidates for preventive therapy persons belonging to any of the following risk groups (*MMWR*, 1990 C): (1) Those with HIV infection as well as those with risk factors for HIV infection whose HIV infection status is unknown but is suspect; (2) close contacts of persons with newly diagnosed infectious tuberculosis as well as tuberculin-negative children and adolescents who have been close contacts of infectious patients within the previous three months (until a repeat skin test is done 12 weeks after contact with the infectious source); (3) recent skin test converters ($\geq$10 mm increase within a two-year period for those $<$35 years old; $\geq$15 mm increase for those $\geq$35 years old); (4) persons with abnormal chest radiographs demonstrating fibrotic lesions representing old, healed tuberculosis; (5) HIV-seronegative intravenous drug users; and (6) persons with medical conditions that have been reported to increase the risk of tuberculosis.

In addition to the above, persons <35 years old in the following high incidence groups are considered candidates for preventive therapy if their skin test reaction is ≥10 mm: Foreign-born persons from high-prevalence countries; medically underserved low-income populations (high-risk racial or ethnic minorities); and residents of facilities for long-term care (eg, correctional institutions, nursing homes, mental institutions).

Public health officials may identify other high-risk populations in specific communities. Staff in facilities where an infectious person would pose a risk to large numbers of susceptible persons also may be considered for preventive therapy if their skin test reaction is ≥10 mm induration.

For regimens for preventive therapy, see Table 7. The physician should make efforts to ensure patient compliance.

Because there is an increased risk of isoniazid hepatotoxicity in patients >35 years, transaminase levels should be obtained both before and during the course of therapy. Discontinuation of isoniazid should be considered if any test result exceeds the upper limit of normal by a factor of 3 to 5. Patients should be fully informed and monitored monthly by appropriately trained personnel. Isoniazid preventive therapy should not be undertaken if monthly monitoring is not possible. Because clinical data suggest that women, especially black and Hispanic women, may be at greater risk of serious or fatal adverse effects caused by isoniazid, they should be monitored more closely (Kopanoff et al, 1978; Franks et al, 1989; Moulding et al, 1989; Snider and Caras, 1992).

Rifampin alone has been recommended as an alternative to isoniazid when the infecting strain is isoniazid-resistant but susceptible to rifampin (American Thoracic Society/Centers for Disease Control, 1986; Table 7). Many, if not all, of the *M.*

TABLE 6.
CRITERIA FOR DETERMINING NEED FOR PREVENTIVE THERAPY FOR PERSONS WITH POSITIVE TUBERCULIN REACTIONS, BY CATEGORY AND AGE GROUP*

Category	Age Group (yrs) <35	≥35
With risk factor	Treat at all ages if reaction to 5TU purified protein derivative (PPD) ≥10 mm (or ≥5 mm and patient is recent contact, HIV-infected, *or* has radiographic evidence of old TB)	
No risk factor High-incidence group	Treat if PPD ≥10 mm	Do not treat
No risk factor Low-incidence group	Treat if PPD ≥15 mm†	Do not treat

* *From* MMWR, *1990 C.*

† *Lower or higher cut points may be used for identifying positive reactions, depending upon the relative prevalence of* M. tuberculosis *infection and nonspecific cross-reactivity in the population.*

TABLE 7.
PREVENTIVE THERAPY FOR TUBERCULOSIS

Risk Group	Regimen	Comments
1. Immunocompetent, contact with isoniazid-sensitive strain likely	*Adults,* isoniazid (orally, 4 to 5 mg/kg or 300 mg daily). *Children,* isoniazid (orally, 10 to 14 mg/kg daily to a maximum of 300 mg/day). Continue treatment for at least six months; persons with an abnormal radiograph (stable parenchymal lesions) should receive 12 months of therapy. Isoniazid also can be given twice weekly at a dosage of 15 mg/kg (maximum, 900 mg) when therapy must be directly monitored and resources for daily therapy are inadequate.	Pyridoxine (orally, 15 to 50 mg daily) should be given to persons in whom neuropathy is commonly associated with isoniazid administration (diabetes, uremia, alcoholism, malnutrition). Pyridoxine also is recommended for persons receiving isoniazid who are pregnant or have a seizure disorder. Pyridoxine is rarely necessary in younger children.
2. Immunocompetent, high probability of contact with isoniazid-resistant strain (eg, immigrants from Asia) and those particularly susceptible to tuberculosis (eg, immunocompromised)	*Adults,* rifampin orally, 10 to 20 mg/kg or 600 mg daily; *children,* rifampin, 10 to 20 mg/kg, maximum 600 mg daily. Continue regimen for 12 months.	Some clinicians add another drug to which the organisms are thought to be susceptible (eg, ethambutol) in standard therapeutic doses for 6 to 12 months.
3. HIV-infected, positive tuberculin skin test (≥ 5 mm induration)	*Adults and children,* isoniazid orally as for (1) for a minimum of 12 months.	Some clinicians advocate isoniazid preventive therapy beyond 12 months; others favor lifelong therapy.

tuberculosis isolates from MDR-TB outbreaks have been resistant to both isoniazid and rifampin; some have been resistant to other drugs also. When the infecting strain is resistant to both drugs, treatment options are problematic. No clinical data exist on regimens for preventive therapy that do not include isoniazid or rifampin. Preventive therapy with more than one drug has been recommended, since efficacy of monotherapy with alternative drugs has not been shown (*MMWR*, 1992).

The clinician should be aware of a number of considerations when selecting a drug regimen for a person exposed to MDR-TB (see Figure). Drug susceptibility testing of an *M. tuberculosis* isolate from the presumed source case is important. Alternative drugs should be chosen only after susceptibility to these drugs has been demonstrated. Those suggested for preventive therapy of MDR-TB (*MMWR*, 1992) include (1) a combination of pyrazinamide (25 to 30 mg/kg/day) and ethambutol (15 to 25 mg/kg/day); (2) pyrazinamide plus a fluoroquinolone with in vitro activity against *M. tuberculosis*. Both ofloxacin and ciprofloxacin have been reported to have similar in vitro potency against mycobacteria. Suggested doses are ofloxacin 400 mg twice daily and ciprofloxacin 750 mg twice daily. Short-term administration of the fluoroquinolones is well tolerated, but therapy for six months or longer has not been adequately studied; and (3) aminoglycosides (streptomycin, kanamycin, amikacin) or the polypeptide antibiotic, capreomycin, should be considered for inclusion in a preventive treatment regimen. These drugs are partially bactericidal but require injection, thus creating logistical problems.

Patients on alternative regimens should receive periodic medical and radiographic evaluation for the first two years after tuberculous infection (eg, every three months for HIV-positive and every six months for HIV-negative patients). The suggested duration is six months for HIV-negative and 12 months for HIV-positive patients (*MMWR*, 1992). Physicians who are unfamiliar with management of MDR-TB patients should seek expert consultation. (See Figure.)

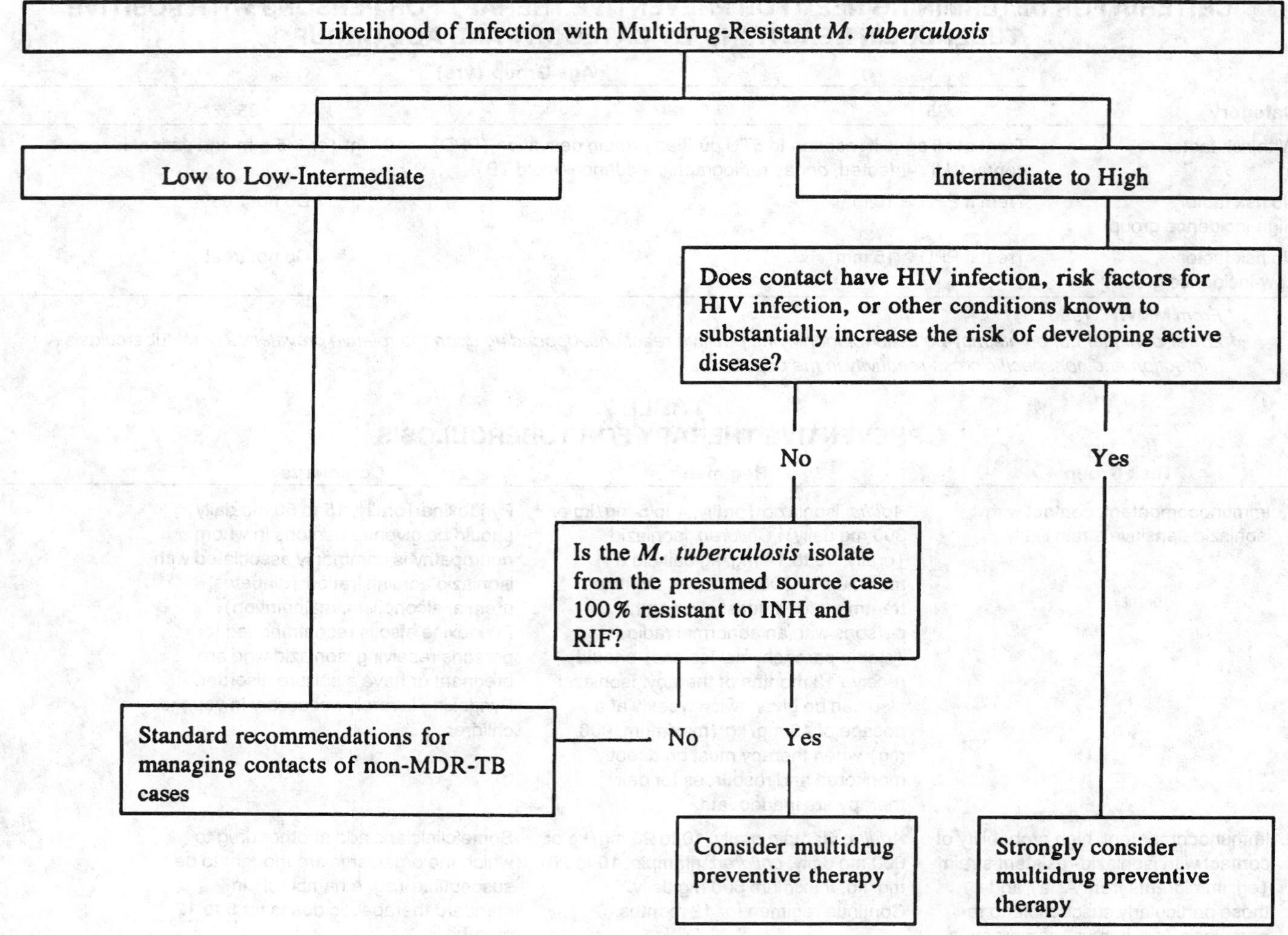

Approach to selecting drug regimens for preventive therapy candidates by likelihood of infection with multidrug-resistant M. tuberculosis *and by likelihood that persons will develop active tuberculosis. From* MMWR, *1992.*

Recommendations for isoniazid prophylaxis during pregnancy have been somewhat controversial. In both rats and rabbits, isoniazid has an embryocidal effect; however, there is no evidence that the drug has teratogenic effects or causes an increase in the incidence of congenital defects in humans (Snider et al, 1980; Coleman and Slutkin, 1984). Therefore, since preventive therapy is elective, it has been recommended that administration of isoniazid generally should be deferred until after delivery. Pregnant women likely to have been infected recently and all HIV seropositive women are an exception; in these women, prophylactic isoniazid therapy should begin when infection is documented but after the first trimester (American Thoracic Society/Centers For Disease Control, 1986).

ACTIVE DISEASE TREATMENT. At one time, standard therapy consisted of 18 months or more of administration of two drugs such as isoniazid, streptomycin, or ethambutol, which produced excellent results. However, limitations of this prolonged regimen include increased cost, difficulties with compliance, and possible toxicity. Therefore, there was a major effort in the 1980s to shorten the overall length of therapy. The availability of the bactericidal drug, rifampin, was of considerable aid in achieving this goal. A nine-month course of chemotherapy with isoniazid and rifampin has been effective in adults and children with pulmonary and extrapulmonary tuberculosis, provided that the organisms are susceptible to both drugs. The drugs may be administered daily for the duration of therapy or, if directly observed therapy is used, twice weekly after one month of daily treatment (Dutt et al, 1979, 1984, 1986). Although the nine-month course of isoniazid-rifampin therapy was quite successful, results of one study demonstrated that a six-month course employing these two drugs alone was inadequate for smear-positive patients (Snider et al, 1984 A). A more recent study, however, demonstrated that six months of therapy with isoniazid and rifampin was adequate for pulmonary tuberculosis when the tubercle bacilli were less numerous (ie, smear-negative, culture-positive); an overall success rate of 99% was achieved. However, the authors recommended that this regimen not be used when drug resistance is suspected or in patients with HIV infection (Dutt et al, 1992).

The current consensus is that the minimal acceptable duration of therapy for sputum-positive patients receiving isoniazid, rifampin, and pyrazinamide is six months; relapse rates with therapy of shorter duration are unacceptably high. With regimens shorter than nine months, isoniazid, rifampin, and pyrazinamide for the initial two months of intensive therapy appear necessary. Because of its overall effectiveness and low cost, isoniazid is always administered for the duration of therapy unless adverse effects or resistance develops. Rifampin also must be given for the duration of therapy. Pyrazinamide enhances the efficacy of short-term therapy during the intensive phase (usually two months) but does not noticeably improve the efficacy of regimens containing isoniazid and rifampin beyond this initial period. The same may be said of streptomycin. Substituting streptomycin or ethambutol for pyrazinamide appears to decrease the effectiveness of a regimen and results in the need to continue treatment for a longer period (American Thoracic Society/Centers for Disease Control, 1986). After an initial phase of intensive daily treatment, intermittent administration of drugs in appropriately adjusted doses appears to produce results equivalent to those with daily administration.

A six-month regimen for drug-susceptible tuberculosis consisting of isoniazid, rifampin, and pyrazinamide daily for two months, followed by isoniazid and rifampin daily for four months, is effective for pulmonary tuberculosis and, because the duration is shorter, it is preferred by many clinicians provided compliance is carefully monitored. If isoniazid resistance is suspected, ethambutol or streptomycin should be included in the initial phase (American Thoracic Society/Centers for Disease Control, 1986). Following the two-month intensive phase, combined chemotherapy can be administered two times weekly with little or no loss of effect if the mean daily dose of each agent is increased (except for rifampin, the daily dose of which is not increased when given two or more times weekly). In a study comparing the effectiveness, toxicity, and acceptability of the six-month regimen with those of the nine-month regimen, patients on the former regimen converted sputums more rapidly than patients on the latter regimen, had similar adverse drug reaction rates, had lower noncompliance rates, and had similar relapse rates 96 weeks after completing therapy. A significantly higher proportion of patients given the six-month regimen successfully completed therapy (Combs et al, 1990).

Intermittent outpatient chemotherapy is most useful in areas with a high incidence of tuberculosis and limited facilities for treatment, as in developing countries. In the United States, intermittent administration is very useful in recalcitrant patients, alcoholics, and others in whom compliance must be supervised closely. It is essential that directly observed therapy be employed whenever intermittent administration is used.

A primarily biweekly 62-dose, six-month regimen for pulmonary and extrapulmonary tuberculosis has been described that is efficacious and is especially useful for patients in whom directly observed therapy is indicated. Isoniazid, rifampin, pyrazinamide, and streptomycin are administered daily for two weeks and then are given in higher doses twice weekly for six weeks. This is followed by isoniazid and rifampin twice weekly for 18 weeks. The time at which sputum samples became culture-negative in patients with pulmonary tuberculosis ranged from 1 to 19 weeks (median, 4.6 weeks); 100% were culture-negative after 20 weeks. The regimen was at least 87% ± 5.5% effective (Cohn et al, 1990).

Although a six-month course of combination therapy is adequate for otherwise healthy patients with drug-susceptible tuberculosis, it may not be adequate for those in certain high-risk groups. In a controlled clinical comparison of six and eight months of therapy for the treatment of patients with silicotuberculosis in Hong Kong, isoniazid, rifampin, pyrazinamide, and streptomycin were given three times weekly for either six or eight months. Those with a history of previous antituberculous therapy also received ethambutol for the first three months. During the three years of assessment, bacteriologic relapse occurred in 22% of the patients in the six-month regimen compared with 7% in the eight-month regimen (Hong

Kong Chest Service/Tuberculosis Research Centre, Madras/ British Medical Research Council, 1991).

Treatment of Drug-Resistant Tuberculosis: For patients with pulmonary tuberculosis caused by bacilli resistant to isoniazid and rifampin, even the best available treatment often is not successful. In a retrospective study, the clinical courses were determined for 171 patients with pulmonary disease due to tubercle bacilli resistant to at least isoniazid and rifampin. Regimens for these patients were selected individually and preferably included three drugs that had not been previously administered and to which the strain was fully susceptible. These patients had previously received a median of six drugs and shed organisms that were resistant to a median of six drugs. Of 134 patients with sufficient follow-up data, only 65% responded to chemotherapy (negative sputum cultures for at least three consecutive months). Twelve of the patients who responded subsequently relapsed. The overall response rate was 56% over a mean period of 51 months. Of the 171 patients, 63 died and 37 of these deaths were attributable to tuberculosis (Goble et al, 1993).

Because of the increasing prevalence of drug-resistant tuberculosis in the United States, recent recommendations from the Advisory Council for the Elimination of Tuberculosis (ACET) have emphasized three points for the initial therapy of tuberculosis: (1) initial four-drug regimens should be used for treatment, (2) initial directly observed therapy (DOT) should be considered for all persons with tuberculosis, and (3) in vitro drug susceptibility testing of initial *M. tuberculosis* isolates from all patients should be performed and the results reported to the health department (*MMWR*, 1993). Drug susceptibility testing also should be performed on any additional isolates from patients whose culture does not convert to negative within three months of therapy initiation or if therapy is unsuccessful.

A four-drug regimen (isoniazid, rifampin, pyrazinamide, and streptomycin or ethambutol) is recommended for the initial treatment of tuberculosis (see Tables 8 and 9) for the following reasons: When adherence to the regimen is assured, the four-drug regimen is highly effective, even in patients with isoniazid-resistant bacilli. Data collected by the CDC suggest that 98% of patients would receive at least two drugs to which the organisms are susceptible; sputum conversion is faster with a four-drug regimen than with a three-drug regimen of isoniazid, rifampin, and pyrazinamide; DOT is easier to administer with the four-drug regimen because compliance is enhanced with an intermittent regimen; and a patient who defaults on a four-drug regimen is more likely to be cured and not relapse than a patient treated with a three-drug regimen.

The initial phase of treatment should include the above drugs during the first two months. When drug susceptibility results are available, the regimen should be appropriately altered. Unless the likelihood of isoniazid or rifampin resistance is very low, it is recommended that the foregoing four-drug regimen be given to all patients. Analysis of the local rates of drug resistance will provide the best basis for decisions in situations in which a four-drug regimen might not be necessary. Community rates of drug resistance below 4% may be an indication that an initial regimen with fewer than four drugs

TABLE 8.
REGIMEN OPTIONS FOR THE INITIAL TREATMENT OF TUBERCULOSIS IN CHILDREN AND ADULTS WITHOUT HIV INFECTION*

Option 1	Option 2	Option 3
Administer daily isoniazid, rifampin, and pyrazinamide for 8 weeks followed by 16 weeks of isoniazid and rifampin daily or 2-3 times/week.† In areas where the isoniazid resistance rate is not documented to be <4%, ethambutol or streptomycin should be added to the initial regimen until susceptibility to isoniazid and rifampin is demonstrated. Continue treatment for at least 6 months and 3 months beyond culture conversion. Consult a tuberculosis medical expert if the patient is symptomatic or smear- or culture-positive after 3 months.	Administer daily isoniazid, rifampin, pyrazinamide, and streptomycin or ethambutol for 2 weeks followed by 2 times/week† administration of the same drugs for 6 weeks (by DOT‡) and, subsequently, with 2 times/week administration of isoniazid and rifampin for 16 weeks (by DOT). Consult a tuberculosis medical expert if the patient is symptomatic or smear- or culture-positive after 3 months.	Treat by DOT, 3 times/week† with isoniazid, rifampin, pyrazinamide, and ethambutol or streptomycin for 6 months.§ Consult a tuberculosis medical expert if the patient is symptomatic or smear- or culture-positive after 3 months.

* *Adapted from* MMWR, *1993.*

† *All regimens administered 2 times/week or 3 times/week should be monitored by DOT for the duration of therapy.*

‡ *DOT—Directly observed therapy.*

§ *The strongest evidence from clinical trials is the effectiveness of all four drugs administered for the full 6 months. There is weaker evidence that streptomycin can be discontinued after 4 months if the isolate is susceptible to all drugs. The evidence for stopping pyrazinamide before the end of 6 months is equivocal for the 3 times/week regimen, and there is no evidence on the effectiveness of this regimen with ethambutol for less than the full 6 months.*

TABLE 9. DOSAGE RECOMMENDATIONS FOR THE INITIAL TREATMENT OF TUBERCULOSIS IN CHILDREN* AND ADULTS†

	Dosage					
	Daily		2 times/week		3 times/week	
Drugs	Children	Adults	Children	Adults	Children	Adults
Isoniazid	10-20 mg/kg Max. 300 mg	5 mg/kg Max. 300 mg	20-40 mg/kg Max. 900 mg	15 mg/kg Max. 900 mg	20-40 mg/kg Max. 900 mg	15 mg/kg Max. 900 mg
Rifampin	10-20 mg/kg Max. 600 mg	10 mg/kg Max. 600 mg	10-20 mg/kg Max. 600 mg	10 mg/kg Max. 600 mg	10-20 mg/kg Max. 600 mg	10 mg/kg Max. 600 mg
Pyrazinamide	15-30 mg/kg Max. 2 g	15-30 mg/kg Max. 2 g	50-70 mg/kg Max. 4 g	50-70 mg/kg Max. 4 g	50-70 mg/kg Max. 3 g	50-70 mg/kg Max. 3 g
Ethambutol‡	15-25 mg/kg Max. 2.5 g	15-25 mg/kg Max. 2.5 g	50 mg/kg	50 mg/kg	25-30 mg/kg	25-30 mg/kg
Streptomycin	20-30 mg/kg Max. 1 g	15 mg/kg Max. 1 g	25-30 mg/kg Max. 1.5 g	25-30 mg/kg Max. 1.5 g	25-30 mg/kg Max. 1 g	25-30 mg/kg Max. 1 g

** Children ≤ 12 years of age.*

† From MMWR, *1993.*

‡ Ethambutol is generally not recommended for children whose visual acuity cannot be monitored (<6 years of age). However, ethambutol should be considered for all children with organisms resistant to other drugs when susceptibility to ethambutol has been demonstrated or is likely.

is acceptable. In certain situations (eg, in institutions experiencing MDR-TB outbreaks), five- and six-drug regimens may be required as initial therapy. If so, these regimens should include four drugs as previously described, plus one or two other drugs; it is also recommended that the regimen include at least three drugs to which the MDR-TB strain is believed to be susceptible to maximize the probability that the patient receives a minimum of two effective drugs. Regimens should be individualized on the basis of the results of drug susceptibility tests.

Regimens that are adequate for the treatment of pulmonary tuberculosis in adults and children also will usually be effective in extrapulmonary disease. However, some experts lengthen the duration of therapy for patients with disseminated disease, miliary disease, disease involving the bones or joints, or tuberculous lymphadenitis. Occasionally, the use of adjunctive therapies, such as surgery and corticosteroids, may be required.

Although pediatric tuberculosis may be treated with one of the aforementioned regimens, ethambutol usually is not employed in children whose visual acuity cannot be monitored; streptomycin is an alternative. However, when the child is infected with organisms resistant to other drugs and susceptibility to ethambutol has been demonstrated, this drug should be considered for inclusion in the treatment regimen. Because tuberculosis in an infant is likely to disseminate, prompt and vigorous treatment should be initiated as soon as tuberculosis is suspected.

It is essential that effective regimens be used in pregnant women who have active disease. The preceding recommendations must be altered in the pregnant patient, however. Because streptomycin interferes with in utero development of the ear and may cause congenital deafness, it should not be used. Routine use of pyrazinamide also is not recommended because teratogenicity data are inadequate. Therefore, the preferred regimen in pregnant women is isoniazid, rifampin, and ethambutol. In addition, a minimum of nine months of therapy should be given. When resistance to other drugs and susceptibility to pyrazinamide are likely, the use of pyrazinamide should be considered and the risks and benefits of the drug carefully evaluated.

Patients with resistant bacilli should be treated in consultation with physicians familiar with such therapy; consultation often is available through state and local health departments.

Because of the increased incidence of resistant organisms, there is heightened interest in new drugs for the treatment of tuberculosis, such as the fluoroquinolones. The in vitro activity of ciprofloxacin and ofloxacin against mycobacteria is independent of resistance to other antimycobacterial agents. These drugs readily penetrate macrophages, which is important for the treatment of intracellular pathogens such as the tubercle bacilli (Young, et al, 1987; Van Caekenberghe, 1990). Lomefloxacin also has good in vitro activity against *M. tuberculosis* and has the advantage of possessing a relatively long elimination half-life (seven to eight hours); it has therefore been proposed as a potential supplementary drug for the treatment of tuberculosis (Kavi et al, 1989; Piersimoni et al, 1992). The investigational fluoroquinolone, sparfloxacin, was reported to have a broad spectrum of action against mycobacteria and its in vitro efficacy against *M. tuberculosis* was better than that of ofloxacin and ciprofloxacin (Rastogi et al, 1991).

Clinical trials on the fluoroquinolones have been initiated. In one prospective trial, the efficacy of ofloxacin, rifampin, and isoniazid was compared with the regimen of ethambutol, rifampin, and isoniazid for the primary treatment of pulmonary tuberculosis in 124 patients. All of the drugs were given orally daily for nine months. After three months, culture conversion rates were 98% in the ofloxacin group and 94% in the ethambutol group; all patients in both groups were culture-negative by six months. No relapse in either group was observed during a two-year follow-up period after cessation of therapy (Kohno et al, 1992).

Recently, treatment strategies of patients with tuberculosis with various patterns of drug resistance have been published (Iseman, 1993). The author emphasized that their efficacy depends on the careful performance of laboratory studies to confirm the resistance pattern of a new isolate and that a careful history of previous drug administration is very important.

Chemotherapy for Tuberculosis in HIV-Infected Persons: HIV infection seriously compromises the immune system and significantly increases the risk of tuberculosis. Selection of an effective regimen for the treatment of tuberculosis in HIV-infected patients is further complicated by the potential for infection with drug-resistant organisms and rapid disease progression and death. Data on the course and outcome of tuberculosis in HIV-infected patients is limited. Some early studies indicated that the initial therapeutic response was not impaired, but no long-term results were reported. In one retrospective study on 132 patients listed in both the AIDS and tuberculosis case registries in San Francisco from 1981 through 1988, patients were treated with either six- or nine-month conventional regimens consisting of isoniazid, rifampin, ethambutol, and pyrazinamide. The intended duration of treatment for patients whose regimen included pyrazinamide was six months and for those who did not receive pyrazinamide, nine months. In compliant patients, conventional therapy resulted in rapid sterilization of sputum, radiographic improvement, and low rates of relapse (Small et al, 1991).

Although data were not sufficient to determine the optimal treatment of tuberculosis in HIV-infected patients, the ACET previously recommended treatment for at least nine months and for at least six months beyond the time that sputum cultures become negative. The regimen consisted of isoniazid, rifampin, and pyrazinamide for two months followed by isoniazid and rifampin for an additional seven months; ethambutol was added to the regimen for patients with central nervous system involvement or disseminated tuberculosis or when resistance to isoniazid was suspected (*MMWR*, 1989).

More recently, ACET has considered intermittent therapy two or three times weekly to be as effective for treatment of tuberculosis in HIV-infected patients as in those without HIV infection (Table 8) (*MMWR*, 1993). Because of concern about drug resistance and the risk of rapid disease progression when immunocompromised patients receive inadequate therapy, ACET also recommended that use of ethambutol or streptomycin be continued for the entire course if drug susceptibility tests are not available.

Persons with HIV infection or those at increased risk whose infection status is unknown and who decline testing should be given chemotherapy whenever acid-fast bacilli are seen in a specimen from the respiratory tract. Although it is impossible to distinguish the tubercle bacilli from *M. avium* except from culture, it is nonetheless imperative to initiate therapy against *M. tuberculosis* because of the public health implications of the latter; persons with both HIV infection and tuberculosis generally respond well to antituberculous therapy, but the incidence of adverse effects to antituberculous drugs is higher in these patients (Chaisson et al, 1987; Small et al, 1991).

Adrenal Corticosteroids: These drugs had been reported to have a mixed effect in tuberculosis and, until recently, there was no consensus on their role in treating this disease.

Steroids exert significant immunosuppressive and anti-inflammatory effects resulting in impairment of antibody production and cell-mediated immunity, and they affect many cells of the immune system. The effects on immune system cells are most evident when doses exceed 0.3 mg/kg/day of prednisone or its equivalent. When doses exceed 1 mg/kg/day, there is a marked increase in susceptibility to a wide variety of infections. Thus, the risk/benefit ratio for steroids in the therapy of infections must be weighed carefully.

Processes that are influenced by steroids include the intrinsic activation of mediator cascades, such as the complement system, the kallikrein-bradykinin system, and the coagulation cascade, as well as the recruitment of inflammatory cells and their activation to generate and excrete mediators, such as interleukins and cytokines. Inflammatory pathways can be activated by intact bacteria as well as by their breakdown products (eg, those released by bactericidal antibiotics). This inflammatory response, which may be detrimental to the host, may be lessened by steroid treatment. In tuberculosis, the inflammatory response is thought to be due principally to tuberculoprotein.

In 1992, the Antimicrobial Agents Committee of the Infectious Diseases Society of America issued guidelines for the use of systemic glucocorticoids in the management of infections, including tuberculosis (McGowan et al, 1992). The working group classified the strength of each recommendation for or against the use of steroid therapy and the quality of the evidence available to support a given recommendation. With regard to tuberculosis, the group found that there was good evidence to support a recommendation for use of corticosteroids in pericarditis to limit fibrotic sequelae and prevent constriction and moderate evidence to support a recommendation for their use in meningitis. They found poor evidence for steroid use in debilitated patients or in those with severe constitutional symptoms such as severe hypoxia, pleurisy, or peritonitis.

In a randomized, placebo-controlled, double-blind trial with a two-year follow-up, patients with active tuberculosis and constrictive pericarditis receiving a six-month, four-drug antituberculous regimen plus prednisolone had significantly more rapid improvement than those who did not receive the steroid. Only 4% of those in the prednisolone group versus 11% of those in the placebo group died as a result of pericarditis; this suggests that the steroid may have prevented death in a small percentage of patients. Furthermore, 21% of the prednisolone-treated group versus 30% of those receiving a placebo required pericardiectomy, suggesting that the drug also decreased the need for this procedure (Strang et al, 1987). Suggested treatment regimens begin with prednisone 40 to 80 mg daily, with the dose gradually decreased over several weeks as effusion subsides.

In tuberculous meningitis, steroids have been reported to improve the clinical condition acutely (Kendig, 1989; *Lancet*, 1986). In one open, prospective, randomized trial, mortality and morbidity were reduced to a greater extent in patients treated with dexamethasone and antituberculous drugs than in those treated with the latter alone (Girgis et al, 1991). In a controlled double-blind study, dexamethasone therapy added to isoniazid and streptomycin decreased cerebrospinal fluid pressure earlier than in patients treated with isoniazid and streptomycin alone (O'Toole et al, 1969). Steroid therapy has been recommended for patients with elevated intracranial pressure, focal neurologic abnormalities, altered consciousness, or impending cerebrospinal outflow obstruction (Molavi et al, 1985). Recommended doses for adults begin at 60 mg of dexamethasone daily (children, 1 to 3 mg/kg/day) and are gradually reduced after one or two weeks using clinical symptoms as a guide to the rapidity with which the doses should be tapered over four to six weeks (Girgis et al, 1991; Molavi et al, 1985).

When considering the use of these agents in tuberculous patients, the physician is reminded that rifampin increases the metabolism of steroids; therefore, the dose of a corticosteroid must be increased accordingly when rifampin is used.

For preparations, see index entry Adrenal Corticosteroids, Uses, Immune Disorders.

EVALUATION OF TREATMENT. The response to therapy in patients with a positive pretreatment sputum test is best evaluated by monthly sputum examinations until conversion is documented. More than 90% of these patients should have converted to negative within three months when contemporary regimens containing both isoniazid and rifampin are used. Those who have not must be carefully re-evaluated. Drug susceptibility tests should be performed and direct observation of drug administration to assure patient compliance should be considered. In the absence of demonstrated resistance, the same regimen should be continued with emphasis on compliance. If resistance is encountered, the regimen should be modified to include at least two drugs to which the organism is susceptible. Evaluations of sputum are then conducted monthly until conversion is observed. Patients completing the six- and nine-month regimens previously described who have had a prompt response do not need routine follow-up. Follow-up evaluations for patients who had resistant organisms must be individualized.

In patients with an initial negative sputum, chest radiographs and clinical evaluation are the best indicators of therapeutic response. If the radiograph does not reveal improvement after three months of chemotherapy, the abnormality may be the result of previous tuberculosis or some other process. However, if there is a positive tuberculin reaction, therapy with isoniazid alone for one year or with the addition of rifampin for six months should be given. The necessity for repeat evaluations in patients with extrapulmonary disease is determined by the site of involvement.

Adverse Reactions

Although most antituberculous agents are well tolerated, all have some potential toxicity. The most serious error made by physicians is failure to recognize true toxicity promptly. A more common error is failure to distinguish between drug reactions and adverse events produced by the plethora of signs and symptoms of the disease that are not related to chemotherapy. The physician who diagnoses drug toxicity erroneously may delete one drug after another from the regimen, sometimes making inappropriate substitutions. Loss of drug susceptibility and therapeutic failure may be the end result.

Physicians must be familiar with the major adverse effects of the drugs included in any regimen employed and routinely monitor the patient. Baseline measurements of liver enzymes, bilirubin, serum creatinine, or blood urea nitrogen and a complete blood and platelet count should be performed on all adult patients. If pyrazinamide is to be given, baseline levels of serum uric acid also should be determined. Visual acuity and color vision should be determined for patients who will receive ethambutol, and audiometry is recommended for those receiving streptomycin. These baseline tests are necessary in order to detect any abnormality that may occur during therapy. Baseline tests for children are usually unnecessary except for those who are to receive ethambutol.

Hypersensitivity reactions occur most often between the third and eighth week of treatment. If a drug or group of drugs is tolerated well for at least four months, a full course of chemotherapy usually can be completed. The most common early signs and symptoms of hypersensitivity are skin rashes; fever, which increases over a period of several days; and tachycardia. At this time, results of laboratory studies are usually within normal limits, but eosinophilia and other abnormalities are observed rarely. If the offending drug is discontinued promptly, the patient soon recovers. If not, the reaction becomes progressively worse and is often accompanied by cutaneous reactions, including exfoliative dermatitis; hepatitis, renal abnormalities; and, occasionally, acute blood dyscrasias. Severe reactions can be fatal.

Patients who develop hypersensitivity to one antituberculous drug may be at greater than usual risk of reacting to others. When such reactions occur, all chemotherapy should be discontinued unless the disease is life-threatening (in which case, drugs least likely to produce these reactions are continued, possibly in conjunction with corticosteroids if indicated). When the reaction has subsided, treatment should be resumed with one drug at a time, beginning with a test dose, then adding other drugs as rapidly as they can be tolerated until the patient is again receiving adequate chemotherapy. With the number of effective agents available to treat drug-susceptible disease, it is not advisable to risk continuing treatment with a drug that has caused a serious reaction (eg, hepatitis).

Some of the adverse reactions reported in the literature have been noted infrequently, sometimes only once and without verification. Also, in combined chemotherapy, toxicity ascribed to one drug may actually have been caused by another or by a drug-drug interaction. In the evaluations that follow, emphasis is placed on those adverse reactions that are well documented and occur more than rarely; however, significant rare reactions also are cited.

Precautions

Many toxic effects of the antimycobacterial agents, particularly those related to dosage, can be avoided by taking into account the patient's age, weight, and general health. Renal status is especially important, since impaired function may lead to proportionately high serum concentrations with increased danger of toxicity.

Relatively small doses may be sufficient to produce therapeutic serum concentrations in elderly or unusually small adults. Some antimycobacterial agents are prescribed routinely on the basis of body weight, and consideration should be given to this factor when prescribing all drugs, especially those administered to children.

Although most agents are metabolized in the liver, evidence of hepatic dysfunction is seldom a deterrent in selecting a regimen. When a history of alcoholism, infectious hepatitis, jaundice, or other hepatic disease is present, it is advisable to obtain a complete profile of liver function before beginning treatment. In fact, in any new case in which the patient has not been under regular medical supervision, it is wise to obtain baseline studies of the renal, hepatic, and hematopoietic systems.

Since most treatment is now given on an outpatient basis, the patient should receive information on the potential toxicity of the drugs in the regimen. Patients also must be monitored at regular intervals throughout treatment. Laboratory studies should be performed promptly if indicated by symptoms suggestive of hepatitis.

Drug Evaluations

AMINOSALICYLIC ACID

AMINOSALICYLATE SODIUM

ACTIONS AND USES. Aminosalicylic acid (PAS) is bacteriostatic for *M. tuberculosis* in therapeutic doses, although its exact mechanism of action is unknown. Because it is an analogue of aminobenzoic acid (PABA), it is thought to suppress growth and reproduction of tubercle bacilli by competitively inhibiting formation of folic acid.

PAS is indicated for the treatment of active pulmonary and extrapulmonary tuberculosis when the infecting organisms are known or strongly suspected to be susceptible to this drug and resistant to the first-line drugs; the sodium salt is used most commonly. PAS is much less effective than other antituberculous drugs. When used alone, its antimycobacterial effect is scarcely discernible and bacterial resistance may develop rapidly. Therefore, it should be used only with other agents, with the combination based on drug susceptibility patterns of the infecting strain. When included in a regimen with isoniazid and rifampin, it may delay the development of resistance to these drugs. In the past, PAS was used almost exclusively as a substitute for ethambutol in regimens for children under 2 years. (These patients cannot be tested for ocular toxicity when ethambutol is administered.) Renewed interest in this drug is due to the appearance of multiple-drug resistant tuberculosis and the paucity of effective drugs for its treatment.

ADVERSE REACTIONS AND PRECAUTIONS. The most common adverse effect is gastrointestinal irritation. Hypersensitivity reactions may occur, usually between the second and seventh week of drug administration. Loeffler's syndrome and perifocal infiltration of the lung may develop. Liver dysfunction, including hepatitis, may be caused by a direct effect of PAS or a hypersensitivity reaction. The drug suppresses the formation of prothrombin, but this is rarely clinically significant unless underlying liver disease is present. Thyroid dysfunction is a rare direct biological effect of PAS. A goiter may result from high-dose therapy, and irreversible anatomic degeneration has occurred in those with underlying thyroid disease. Other adverse effects observed infrequently include crystalluria, hemolytic anemia, and an infectious mononucleosis-like syndrome.

Patient acceptance and tolerance of PAS are poor in adults; children are less affected. Therapy must be discontinued in approximately 20% of patients (15% because of intolerable gastrointestinal [GI] disturbances, particularly nausea, vomiting, and diarrhea, and 4% because of hypersensitivity reactions that occasionally are very serious or even fatal). Most of the GI adverse effects are increased when the drug is taken in a fasting state; ingestion of PAS after meals or with 10 to 15 ml of aluminum hydroxide will reduce the irritative effects. Reduction of the dose ameliorates the problem in some patients. In others, it may be necessary to discontinue therapy for up to 14 days to allow a respite from GI distress. Therapy should be resumed at low doses (2 g/day) and gradually increased to the full daily dose as tolerated. Patient compliance may be poor.

Patients should be monitored closely, especially those with renal insufficiency. Because PAS preparations contain sodium, fluid retention may occur in patients with vascular and cardiac insufficiency, and dosage reduction, administration of diuretics, or discontinuation of the drug may be necessary if intractable fluid retention occurs.

The risk/benefit ratio should be considered before administration of the drug to patients with congestive heart failure or gastric ulcer.

DRUG INTERACTIONS. The bacteriostatic action of PAS may be antagonized by aminobenzoates because they may be absorbed by bacteria preferentially over PAS; concurrent use is not recommended. The effects of coumarin or indandione anticoagulants may be increased when used with PAS because of decreased hepatic synthesis of procoagulant factors; dosage adjustments may be necessary during and after PAS therapy. Renal tubular secretion of PAS may be decreased if probenecid or sulfinpyrazone are used concurrently. The dose of PAS may have to be reduced during and after concurrent therapy with sulfinpyrazone to avoid increased and prolonged serum concentrations and/or adverse effects. Patients should be monitored. (Concomitant use of probenecid is not recommended.)

PAS may impair the absorption of rifampin resulting in decreased serum concentrations of the latter. The two drugs should be administered at least six hours apart. PAS also may impair the absorption of vitamin B_{12} from the GI tract, and the requirements for the vitamin may be increased in patients receiving PAS.

A cumulative effect of GI irritation will occur if the drug is administered with aspirin or aspirin-like drugs. PAS should not be given to patients with a history of previous allergic reactions to aminosalicylates, other salicylates, or sulfonamides.

PHARMACOKINETICS. PAS is readily absorbed from the GI tract. After oral ingestion of 4 g, a peak serum level of 750 mcg/ml is reached in one to two hours; the volume of distribution is 0.23 L/kg. Blood levels are negligible within four to five hours after a single usual dose. Appreciable concentrations are found in all organ tissues, and high concentrations occur in pleural fluid and caseous tissue; however, low concentrations appear in the cerebrospinal fluid. PAS exhibits low protein binding (15%), and it undergoes hepatic metabolism with greater than 50% acetylated to inactive metabolites.

PAS is rapidly excreted in the urine by glomerular filtration. Over 80% of a dose is excreted in urine in the first 10 hours; 14% to 33% is excreted unchanged in the urine. The half-life is 45 to 60 minutes in patients with normal renal function; it is up to 23 hours in those with impaired renal function.

PAS is excreted in breast milk; however, adverse effects in nursing infants have not been documented.

DOSAGE AND PREPARATIONS.

AMINOSALICYLATE SODIUM:

The following doses are expressed in terms of the base.

Oral: *Adults,* in combination with other antimycobacterial drugs, 3 to 4 g every eight hours or 5 to 6 g every 12 hours after meals (maximum, 20 g daily). *Children,* in combination with other antimycobacterial drugs, 50 to 75 mg/kg every six hours or 66.7 to 100 mg/kg every eight hours after meals (maximum, 12 g daily).

Generic. Granules in 4-g packets. Available from the Division of Tuberculosis Elimination, Centers for Disease Control and Prevention, Atlanta, Georgia 30333.

CAPREOMYCIN SULFATE
[Capastat Sulfate]

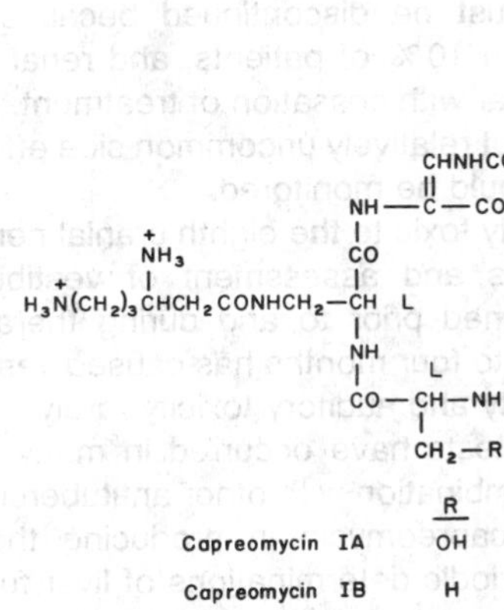

	R	
Capreomycin IA	OH	$C_{25}H_{44}N_{14}O_8$
Capreomycin IB	H	$C_{25}H_{44}N_{14}O_7$

ACTIONS AND USES. Capreomycin is a polypeptide antibiotic isolated from a species of *Streptomyces.* It is a complex of four microbiologically active components that have been only partially characterized. This drug is indicated in pulmonary infections caused by susceptible strains when the primary agents (isoniazid, streptomycin, ethambutol, pyrazinamide, and rifampin) cannot be used because of toxicity or the presence of resistant bacilli. Resistance may develop rapidly when capreomycin is administered alone; therefore, it only should be given with other antituberculous drugs. This agent usually is reserved for retreatment regimens when parenteral therapy is indicated; it is given by deep intramuscular injection.

Capreomycin has a marked suppressive effect against *Mycobacterium tuberculosis* and *M. bovis* in vitro and in vivo. Most strains of *M. kansasii* also are susceptible, but other nontuberculous mycobacteria often are resistant. No cross resistance has been observed between capreomycin and isoniazid, aminosalicylic acid, cycloserine, streptomycin, ethionamide, or ethambutol. Cross resistance occurs to varying degrees between capreomycin and kanamycin or neomycin.

Compared with kanamycin (an antibiotic derived from another species of *Streptomyces*), capreomycin is less toxic and has a somewhat greater bacteriostatic effect. Capreomycin approaches streptomycin in therapeutic efficacy and, since there is no cross resistance between the two, it is useful in patients with streptomycin-resistant strains of tubercle bacilli. Nevertheless, because of potential nephrotoxicity, capreomycin cannot be substituted routinely for streptomycin.

When capreomycin is used with other effective agents that are administered orally every day, its prolonged daily use is rarely necessary. After two to four months, it can be given two or three times a week to reduce the risk of permanent renal damage without appreciably affecting efficacy.

ADVERSE REACTIONS, PRECAUTIONS, AND INTERACTIONS. Extensive experimental and clinical studies have demonstrated that renal damage is the most consistent and significant toxic effect of capreomycin. This is manifested by elevated urea nitrogen levels, decreased creatinine clearance, albuminuria, and cylindruria. Fatal toxic nephritis has been reported in a patient with portal cirrhosis who was given both capreomycin and aminosalicylic acid for one month. However, capreomycin must be discontinued because of nephrotoxicity in fewer than 10% of patients, and renal abnormalities usually disappear with cessation of treatment. Hypokalemia is a significant but relatively uncommon side effect; blood potassium levels should be monitored.

Capreomycin is potentially toxic to the eighth cranial nerve. Audiometric measurements and assessment of vestibular function should be performed prior to and during therapy. However, daily use for two to four months has caused vestibular toxicity only infrequently and auditory toxicity rarely.

Abnormal liver function tests have occurred in many patients taking the drug in combination with other antituberculosis agents. The role of capreomycin in producing these changes is unclear, but periodic determinations of liver function are recommended.

Because of its potential toxicity for the kidneys and eighth cranial nerve, capreomycin is rarely prescribed for patients with renal disease and should not be administered with other nephrotoxic or ototoxic agents (eg, amikacin, colistin, gentamicin). It is advisable to obtain pertinent baseline laboratory data before beginning treatment with capreomycin. There is no evidence that previous damage to the eighth nerve precludes treatment with capreomycin, but impaired renal function must be considered, particularly with respect to dosage and frequency of administration.

Caution should be employed when neuromuscular blocking agents are used concurrently with capreomycin. Neuromuscular blockade may be enhanced with resulting skeletal muscular weakness and respiratory depression or paralysis. A partial neuromuscular block has been demonstrated after large intravenous doses of capreomycin. This adverse effect was enhanced by ether anesthesia and antagonized by neostigmine.

Eosinophilia often occurs during treatment and occasionally has been marked. Leukocytosis and leukopenia also have been observed; rare cases of thrombocytopenia have been reported. Definite hypersensitivity reactions, manifested by fever and rash, apparently are uncommon and are not severe.

In teratogenic studies, a questionable rib abnormality was reported in rats only. Capreomycin crosses the placenta. Data in humans are insufficient to evaluate this drug's safety during pregnancy or lactation (FDA Pregnancy Category C). Its safety in infants and children has not been established.

PHARMACOKINETICS. The oral bioavailability of capreomycin is negligible. Peak serum concentrations after intramuscular administration are achieved rapidly (one to two hours), and the half-life is three to six hours. Capreomycin accumulates in the serum of patients with impaired renal function. Only an insignificant amount is metabolized, and the drug is eliminated unchanged in the urine. The drug does not enter the cerebrospinal fluid; however, high concentrations are achieved in the urine.

DOSAGE AND PREPARATIONS. Capreomycin should be dissolved in 2 ml of sodium chloride injection or sterile water for injection; two to three minutes should be allowed for complete dissolution.

Intramuscular (deep): *Adults,* 15 mg/kg (approximately 1 g) daily for two to four months, followed by 1 g two or three times weekly for 6 to 12 months or longer, if necessary. Most patients tolerate 1 g daily for two to four months and occasionally for as long as six months. A dose of 20 mg/kg/day should not be exceeded. Information is inadequate to establish a dosage for *children.*

Capastat Sulfate (Lilly). Powder (sterile) 1 g (equivalent to base) in 10 ml containers.

CYCLOSERINE

[Seromycin]

ACTIONS AND USES. Cycloserine is an analogue of D-alanine and interferes with an early step in cell wall synthesis in susceptible bacteria. It competitively inhibits the enzymes L-alanine racemase, which forms D-alanine from L-alanine, and D-alanine-D-alanine synthetase, which incorporates D-alanine into the pentapeptide necessary for peptidoglycan formation and bacterial cell wall synthesis.

Although cycloserine is derived from a species of *Streptomyces*, it is chemically unrelated to and therefore exhibits no cross resistance with the aminoglycosides or capreomycin. This broad spectrum antibiotic also has been synthesized. It may be either bactericidal or bacteriostatic, depending on serum concentrations. *M. tuberculosis* as well as both gram-positive and gram-negative bacteria are susceptible. Cycloserine is administered orally and, when tolerated, has proven to be an effective antimycobacterial agent. This secondary drug is indicated for the treatment of active pulmonary and extrapulmonary tuberculosis caused by susceptible strains and is used only when treatment with the primary antituberculous drugs (isoniazid, ethambutol, rifampin, pyrazinamide, streptomycin) has proved inadequate. Cycloserine should be administered with other effective agents.

ADVERSE REACTIONS AND PRECAUTIONS. The limiting factor in the use of cycloserine is its central nervous system toxicity, including both neurologic and psychic disturbances. Neurologic reactions vary from muscular twitching to seizures. The value of pyridoxine in preventing CNS toxicity produced by cycloserine has not been proved. Concurrent administration of ethionamide or isoniazid may potentiate neurotoxic effects, and dosage adjustments may be necessary.

Psychic disturbances range from nervousness to frank psychotic episodes. These effects occasionally are related to excessive serum concentrations, especially if the total daily dose exceeds 500 mg, but more often they cannot be predicted or prevented. Psychotic episodes occur in nearly 10% of patients treated with cycloserine and require prompt cessation of treatment. These reactions are nearly always reversible within two weeks. Large doses of chlorpromazine may hasten recovery. Until the patient's condition returns to normal, he or she should be watched closely and security measures taken if necessary. Suicide has occurred occasionally during a drug-induced psychotic reaction.

Cycloserine is contraindicated in those with seizure disorders, depression, severe anxiety or psychosis, or renal insufficiency; with excessive concurrent use of alcoholic beverages; and in patients who are hypersensitive.

Blood levels should be determined weekly in patients with reduced renal function.

Data in humans are insufficient to evaluate the safety of cycloserine during pregnancy or lactation (FDA Pregnancy Category C). The decision on whether to discontinue nursing or the drug should take into account the importance of cycloserine for the mother and the potential for serious adverse effects in nursing infants. Safety and dosage have not been established for children.

DRUG INTERACTIONS. If possible, isoniazid or ethionamide should not be given with cycloserine because of potential additive central nervous system toxicity. Requirements for pyridoxine may be increased in patients taking cycloserine.

PHARMACOKINETICS. Cycloserine is readily absorbed from the gastrointestinal tract with peak blood levels occurring in four to eight hours. Blood levels of 25 to 30 mcg/ml can generally be maintained with the usual dosage of 250 mg twice daily. The drug is widely distributed throughout body fluids and tissues, including cerebrospinal fluid. Concentrations in the cerebrospinal fluid, pleural fluid, fetal blood, and breast milk approach those found in serum. One-third of an administered dose is metabolized to an unidentified substance, and the remainder is eliminated unchanged in the urine. Because cycloserine is highly concentrated in the urine, large doses are not required in urinary tract tuberculosis. Maximum excretion occurs two to six hours after administration, and 50% of the drug is eliminated in 12 hours.

DOSAGE AND PREPARATIONS.

Oral: *Adults,* initially, 250 mg twice daily at 12-hour intervals for the first two weeks. The dose may be increased by 250 mg every few days (if tolerated) until therapeutic serum levels are obtained. The usual dosage is 500 mg to a maximum of 1 g daily in divided doses. It may be possible to administer a smaller total dose once daily without loss of therapeutic effect when cycloserine is used with other agents that are also prescribed once daily. Blood levels should be monitored during therapy. Best results occur with peak serum concentrations of 25 to 30 mcg/ml. Serum levels in excess of 30 mcg/ml have been associated with toxicity and should be avoided. Blood used to determine serum drug concentrations should be drawn before the patient's first dose of the day.

Seromycin (Lilly). Capsules 250 mg.

ETHAMBUTOL HYDROCHLORIDE

[Myambutol]

$$CH_3CH_2 - \overset{CH_2OH}{\underset{H}{C}} - \overset{+}{N}H_2CH_2CH_2\overset{+}{N}H_2 - \overset{H}{\underset{CH_2OH}{C}} - CH_2CH_3 \quad 2Cl^-$$

SPECTRUM AND ACTIONS. *Mycobacterium tuberculosis, M. bovis,* and most strains of *M. kansasii* are highly susceptible to ethambutol, and some nonphotochromogens (mycobacterial group III organisms) are susceptible to this drug in vitro; the mechanism of action is not completely understood. Ethambutol inhibits the synthesis of cell metabolites, which inhibits cell metabolism and results in cell death; its effects appear to be mediated through interference with RNA synthesis. Ethambutol has a bactericidal action against *M. tuberculosis,* which is dependent on the replication activity of the organism, the drug concentration, and the period of exposure (Gangadharam et al, 1990). No cross resistance between ethambutol and other antituberculous drugs has been demonstrated.

USES. This synthetic antimycobacterial compound is used in short-course chemotherapy to preclude monotherapy when resistance to isoniazid or rifampin is suspected (see the Introduction). In retreatment and cases of primary resistance, ethambutol is of great value when combined with other effective antimycobacterial agents.

ADVERSE REACTIONS AND PRECAUTIONS. The most significant adverse effect produced by ethambutol is dose-related ocular toxicity; with initial doses of 25 mg/kg daily for two months followed by 15 mg/kg daily, the incidence is 0.8%. The visual changes generally are reversible over a period of weeks or months but, rarely, recovery is delayed for one year or more or the effects are irreversible. Eye involvement usually is bilateral and consistent with retrobulbar neuritis (decreased visual acuity, loss of color discrimination, constriction of visual fields, and central and peripheral scotomata). Currently recommended doses produce ocular toxicity only rarely in patients with normal renal function; the drug should be used cautiously in those with impaired renal function, and the dose should be reduced as determined by drug serum levels.

Regular ophthalmologic examinations are not necessary during treatment with the lower dose (15 mg/kg), but the patient should be instructed to report any visual changes promptly and should be questioned about vision during each regularly scheduled visit. Symptoms often precede objective evidence of toxicity. If a patient complains of blurring or fading of vision, a complete ophthalmologic examination should be performed at once. Ethambutol should be discontinued immediately if symptoms persist or visual acuity decreases significantly. It is prudent that visual acuity and color vision be determined periodically in all patients throughout the treatment period.

If the patient has cataracts or other ocular abnormalities that make changes in vision difficult to detect or evaluate, a complete ophthalmologic examination is mandatory to establish a baseline before beginning treatment with ethambutol. However, pretreatment examinations are not indicated routinely in patients with normal vision or simple errors of refraction corrected by glasses.

The incidence of hypersensitivity to ethambutol is very low (about 0.1%) and reactions tend to be mild. Serum uric acid levels may be elevated, and precipitation of acute gout has been reported. Peripheral neuritis has developed rarely.

Patients treated with ethambutol have included many pregnant women, most of whom were already receiving chemotherapy before conception. The drug is excreted in breast milk in concentrations approximating those in maternal serum; however, no adverse effects in nursing infants have been documented.

No toxic effects have been observed in children receiving therapeutic doses of ethambutol. In severe disease, particularly disseminated tuberculosis caused by highly resistant strains of bacilli, young children have received ethambutol for up to five years without evidence of toxicity. However, many clinicians do not recommend this drug for use in children under 2 years, for they cannot be monitored for visual acuity.

PHARMACOKINETICS. Ethambutol is absorbed rapidly from the gastrointestinal tract (time to peak effect, two to four hours; bioavailability, 77% ± 8%). Except for the cerebrospinal fluid, it is widely distributed to most tissues and fluids. Volume of distribution is 1.6 ± 2 L/kg. Protein binding is 20% to 30%. Ethambutol is excreted mainly by the kidneys; up to 80% is excreted in the urine in 24 hours, 50% as unchanged drug and 15% as inactive metabolites. About 20% is excreted unchanged in the feces. Clearance is 8.6 ± 0.8 ml/min/kg, and the elimination half-life is 3.1 ± 0.4 hours. Ethambutol does not penetrate intact meninges but 10% to 15% may be detected in the cerebrospinal fluid of patients with tuberculous meningitis.

DOSAGE AND PREPARATIONS. The dose of ethambutol must be determined on the basis of body weight. The amount must be calculated carefully and adjusted if there are appreciable changes in the patient's weight. However, in the interest of compliance, doses should be rounded off to the nearest whole tablet. In patients with renal failure in whom ethambutol must be used, the dose must be reduced, with adjustments determined by the serum concentration.

Oral: *Adults and children,* daily regimen, 15 to 25 mg/kg (maximum, 2.5 g) given in one dose. For alternative regimens, see Table 9.

Myambutol (Lederle). Tablets 100 and 400 mg.

ETHIONAMIDE

[Trecator-SC]

N
CH_2CH_3
CNH_2
S

ACTIONS AND USES. This drug is the thioamide of isonicotinic acid and is related chemically to isoniazid. Ethionamide is about one-tenth as active as isoniazid. Like the latter drug, it is widely distributed in the body, including the cerebrospinal fluid. It is effective against human and bovine strains of mycobacteria and against *M. kansasii*. The mechanism of action is not known, but the drug appears to inhibit peptide synthesis. Depending on its concentration and the susceptibility of the organism, its action may be either bacteriostatic or bactericidal.

Ethionamide is indicated in any form of active tuberculosis following therapeutic failure after adequate treatment with the primary drugs. It should be given only with other effective antituberculous drugs. Its usefulness in tuberculosis is limited because many patients cannot tolerate therapeutic doses. In approximately one-third of patients, ethionamide must be discontinued or the dose reduced. Most patients tolerate one-half to two-thirds of the usual total daily dose, but the therapeutic efficacy of these amounts is uncertain, particularly since ethionamide is used in retreatment regimens, often in combination with drugs having marginal antimycobacterial activity. Ethionamide also is used in the treatment of leprosy and atypical mycobacterial infections.

ADVERSE REACTIONS AND PRECAUTIONS. Ethionamide almost invariably causes gastrointestinal disturbances, most frequently anorexia, nausea, and vomiting. These effects are thought to be caused by its central nervous system actions rather than direct gastric irritation. Their severity may limit the total dosage to 250 mg twice daily in up to 50% of patients.

Ethionamide is potentially toxic to the liver. Abnormal results of liver function studies are noted in 9% of patients, and jaundice occurs in 1% to 3%. However, recovery is usually rapid when the drug is discontinued. Determinations of serum transaminase should be conducted prior to and every two to four weeks during therapy.

Hypersensitivity reactions are infrequent. Like isoniazid, ethionamide may cause peripheral neuritis, particularly in susceptible patients, by acting as a pyridoxine antagonist or increasing the renal excretion of pyridoxine; thus, dosage requirements for pyridoxine may be increased. Mental depression and hypothyroidism have occasionally been attributed to treatment with this agent. Seizures and, rarely, gynecomastia, impotence, and purpura have been reported. Seizures associated with cycloserine therapy may be aggravated by the concomitant use of ethionamide.

Teratogenic effects were produced in animals given doses higher than those used clinically. Ethionamide crosses the placenta, and its use is not recommended during pregnancy. Data in humans are insufficient to evaluate the safety of ethionamide during lactation.

PHARMACOKINETICS. Ethionamide is well absorbed orally (time to peak effect is about three hours) and is widely distributed (including cerebrospinal fluid). Bioavailability is 100%, and the volume of distribution is approximately 2.8 L/kg. The drug is metabolized to sulfoxide (active) and to inactive metabolites. The half-life is approximately three hours and the time to peak serum concentration is 1.8 hours. Ethionamide is excreted by the kidneys; 1% is excreted unchanged, 5% as active metabolite, and the remainder as inactive metabolites.

DOSAGE AND PREPARATIONS.

Oral: *Adults,* 0.5 to 1 g daily in one to three doses after meals. Variations in dose and timing of administration may be tried. Some patients tolerate the drug best when a single dose is given at bedtime, whereas others prefer a single dose after the evening meal. When the total amount can be tolerated in one dose, serum concentrations are higher and a therapeutic effect is more likely than when small doses are administered two or three times a day. *Children*, 4 to 5 mg/kg every eight hours (maximum daily dose, 750 mg).

Trecator-SC (Wyeth-Ayerst). Tablets 250 mg.

ISONIAZID (INH)

[INH, Nydrazid]

N

$CNHNH_2$
‖
O

ACTIONS AND USES. Isoniazid (isonicotinic acid hydrazide, INH) is indicated for all forms of tuberculosis. It is bactericidal for both extracellular and intracellular bacteria, primarily those that are actively dividing. Its exact mechanism of action is unknown, but isoniazid may act by interfering with cell wall mycolic acid biosynthesis. This synthetic compound probably remains the best single antimycobacterial agent with respect to efficacy, toxicity, cost, ease of administration, and patient acceptance. It is administered alone for prophylaxis and is commonly used in combination regimens for chemotherapy of disease. See the sections on Preventive Therapy and Active Disease Treatment in the Introduction.

ADVERSE REACTIONS AND PRECAUTIONS. The two most common adverse effects are peripheral neuropathy and hepatitis. The metabolism of isoniazid is characterized by increased excretion of pyridoxine, which may result in peripheral neuritis, particularly when large doses are prescribed and in malnourished patients. The incidence in adults has been reported to be about 10% when 8 to 10 mg/kg of isoniazid is given. Peripheral neuritis occasionally produces bizarre symptoms and, therefore, may not be recognized promptly. In adults, it may be treated with pyridoxine 50 to 100 mg orally; in severe cases, parenteral administration may be more effective. Since peripheral neuritis is not always completely reversible, some clinicians routinely administer pyridoxine 10 to 25 mg (range, 6 to 50 mg) daily to patients receiving usual doses of isoniazid, especially those with diabetes mellitus, alcoholism, or malnutrition. Those receiving larger doses of isoniazid or individuals with pre-existing symptoms of peripheral neuritis should receive 100 to 300 mg of pyridoxine daily.

Convulsions have occurred in less than 1% of patients treated with isoniazid, and this drug has been administered without difficulty to many individuals being treated for convulsive disorders. Since the action of phenytoin may be potentiated by isoniazid, particularly in slow isoniazid acetylators, the blood level of phenytoin should be monitored when the two drugs are given simultaneously and the dose of the anticonvulsant reduced if indicated.

Reversible psychotic episodes may be precipitated in a small percentage of patients treated with very large doses of isoniazid. Arthralgia or arthritis has been noted infrequently. Gastrointestinal, hematologic, metabolic, and endocrine reactions have been reported.

Optic neuropathy has been reported rarely, but a causal relationship has not been established. This is true of many other abnormalities listed in the labeling of isoniazid preparations. It is probable that some of the reactions reported, including vasculitis with antinuclear antibodies, may be manifestations of a hypersensitivity reaction simulating systemic lupus erythematosus.

The most serious adverse effect of isoniazid is hepatitis. The incidence of this reaction increases with age; it is uncommon in individuals less than 35 years (see Table 4). The daily consumption of alcohol increases the risk of isoniazid-related hepatitis during therapy.

Patients should be monitored periodically for signs or symptoms of hepatitis or other significant adverse reactions. They should be informed of the prodromal symptoms of hepatitis (fatigue, weakness, malaise, anorexia, nausea, vomiting) and told to report any that occur immediately. Discontinuation of the drug at this point will help to prevent progression of hepatitis. Established hepatitis has a mortality rate of 7%. It is well known that serum transaminase levels are elevated during the first few months of treatment in at least 10% of patients, and more specific evidence of liver dysfunction sometimes is noted. All values usually return to normal and are not an indication for discontinuing treatment without clinical evidence of hepatitis. However, some clinicians routinely monitor serum transaminase levels and discontinue isoniazid therapy when the transaminase levels exceed three to five times normal.

Isoniazid is contraindicated in patients who develop severe hypersensitivity or drug-induced hepatitis.

In reproductive studies on mammals, no isoniazid-related congenital anomalies were observed (FDA Pregnancy Category C). The concentration of isoniazid in breast milk is about 20% of serum levels, but no adverse effects in nursing infants have been reported.

PHARMACOKINETICS. Isoniazid is rapidly absorbed following oral administration; however, a significant first-pass effect may occur. Bioavailability is generally reported to be about 90%, and time to peak serum concentration is one to two hours. This drug is widely distributed to all tissues and fluids, including the cerebrospinal fluid; it crosses the placenta and is excreted in breast milk. The volume of distribution is 0.57 to 0.76 L/kg. Protein binding is clinically insignificant ($<10\%$). Approximately 75% to 95% of the drug is excreted in the urine, primarily as inactive metabolites.

Isoniazid is almost completely metabolized by enzymatic acetylation and dehydrazination. Because of genetic heterogeneity, about one-half of the population in the United States acetylates isoniazid rapidly (mean half-life, 1.1 $\pm$ 0.2 hours; clearance, 7 ml/min/kg) and the other half slowly (mean half-life, 3 $\pm$ 0.8 hours; clearance, 2.5 ml/min/kg). Isoniazid is acetylated by N-acetyl transferase to N-acetylisoniazid and subsequently is metabolized to isonicotinic acid and monoacetylhydrazine. The latter compound is associated with hepatotoxicity when it is N-hydroxylated by the cytochrome P450 mixed oxidase system to form a reactive intermediate metabolite. Slow acetylators have a lower level of N-acetyl transferase. The rate of acetylation does not significantly affect the efficacy of isoniazid, but slow acetylation may lead to higher blood levels of the drug and thus to an increase in toxic reactions.

Pyridoxine deficiency is probably due to competition by isoniazid for the enzyme, apotryptophanase.

DRUG INTERACTIONS. Isoniazid is thought to affect cytochrome P450, and drugs that affect or are affected by this enzyme system may in turn affect isoniazid activity or be affected by the drug. Isoniazid inhibits the metabolism of phenytoin resulting in increased plasma levels, especially in slow acetylators. There is some evidence that inducers of cytochrome P450 (eg, carbamazepine, rifampin, phenobarbital, primidone, alcohol) increase the formation of hepatotoxic metabolites and the subsequent risk of hepatitis and/or hepatic necrosis. Use of ketoconazole and miconazole also may increase the potential for hepatotoxicity. Concurrent use of acetaminophen may increase the potential for hepatotoxicity and nephrotoxicity. Concurrent use of prednisolone and possibly other adrenal corticosteroids may increase hepatic metabolism and/or excretion resulting in decreased plasma concentrations and effectiveness, especially in patients who are fast acetylators; dosage adjustments may be necessary. Concomitant use of anticoagulants (ie, coumarin and indandione derivatives) with isoniazid may result in enhanced anticoagulant effect due to the inhibition of the enzymatic metabolism of anticoagulants. Isoniazid may decrease the hepatic metabolism of benzodiazepines (eg, diazepam, chlordiazepoxide, flurazepam, prazepam) that are metabolized by phase I reactions (N-methylation and hydroxylation). Isoniazid also may impair the oxidation of triazolam to increase plasma benzodiazepine concentrations. First-pass metabolism and elimination of midazolam in the liver may be decreased by isoniazid due to inhibition at the cytochrome P450 binding sites to result in increased steady-state plasma concentrations of midazolam. Theophylline plasma concentrations may be increased if isoniazid is used concurrently.

Additive central nervous system effects (dizziness, drowsiness) occur when cycloserine or ethionamide are used with isoniazid.

Aluminum-containing antacids decrease the absorption of isoniazid and lower serum concentrations of orally administered isoniazid. Patients should be advised to allow at least one hour after an oral dose of isoniazid before taking these antacids.

Isoniazid is closely related to monoamine oxidase inhibitors. Ingestion of certain fish (eg, tuna, skipjack, Sardinella) or cheese (eg, Parmesan) may induce a typical tyramine syndrome of palpitations, severe general flushing, conjunctival injection, headache, dyspnea, tightness of the chest, tachypnea, and sweating. The reaction is thought to be due to the inhibition of plasma monoamine oxidase and diamine oxidase by isoniazid, thus interfering with the metabolism of tyramine and histamine found in fish and cheese.

DOSAGE AND PREPARATIONS.
Oral, Intramuscular: *Adults*, for chemoprophylaxis, 5 mg/kg daily (up to 300 mg daily) is given orally in a single dose. For chemotherapy, 5 mg/kg/day is given with other antimycobacterial agents (maximum, 300 mg daily). For alternative regimens, see Table 9.

Infants and children, for active tuberculosis, 10 to 20 mg/kg daily, depending on the severity of the infection, in one or more doses; for preventive therapy, 10 to 15 mg/kg daily (maximum, 300 mg daily). For alternative regimens, see Table 9.

Generic. Tablets 100 and 300 mg.
INH (CIBA). Tablets 300 mg.
Nydrazid (Apothecon). Solution (for injection) 100 mg/ml in 10 ml containers.
The combination preparations listed below may be more convenient to use than multiple single-entity preparations and have been reported to enhance compliance in some patients.
Rifamate (Marion Merrell Dow). Capsules containing isoniazid 150 mg and rifampin 300 mg.
Rimactane/INH (CIBA). Tablets containing isoniazid 300 mg and rifampin 300 mg.

PYRAZINAMIDE (PZA)

ACTIONS AND USES. Pyrazinamide, an amide derivative of pyrazine-2-carboxylic acid, is not water soluble and exhibits antimycobacterial activity in vitro only in an acid medium. *M. tuberculosis* strains susceptible to pyrazinamide produce the enzyme, pyrazinamidase; the enzyme is absent in resistant strains. Pyrazinamide itself is not active, but must be transformed by pyrazinamidase to the active compound, pyrazinoic acid, which itself has antituberculosis activity in vitro. The currently used in vitro pyrazinamide susceptibility test is a pyrazinamidase assay, and susceptibility of tubercle bacilli strains correlates with activity of this enzyme (McClatchy et al, 1981; Trividi, 1987). Such correlation, however, does not apply to *M. avium* complex (MAC), which suggests that pyrazinamide is not appropriate for therapy of MAC disease (Heifets et al, 1986). The in vivo activity of pyrazinamide was believed to arise from the acidic environment of the macrophage phagolysosomes where tubercle bacilli produce the amidase that converts pyrazinamide to pyrazinoic acid. Inhibition of tubercle bacilli by pyrazinamide in cultured human macrophages has been reported to be as active as that observed clinically (Crowle et al, 1986). However, a more recent study has questioned the hypothesis of the intracellular action of pyrazinamide (Rastogi et al, 1988).

Despite its pronounced clinical activity, pyrazinamide was much less bactericidal in broth cultures against drug-susceptible *M. tuberculosis* strains than other antituberculous drugs. The investigators suggest that the clinical efficacy of pyrazinamide may be due to its bacteriostatic effects combined with unfavorable acidic conditions within the macrophages (Heifets et al, 1990).

Pyrazinamide is indicated for the initial treatment of active tuberculosis in adults and children and should be used only in combination with other antituberculous agents. It also is indicated after treatment failure with other primary drugs in any form of active tuberculosis.

Pyrazinamide was once considered a second-line agent and was used in the United States primarily for retreatment and only when the disease was a greater threat than the drug's potential toxicity. However, the addition of pyrazinamide to treatment regimens has allowed the conventional nine-month regimen of isoniazid and rifampin to be shortened to six months with good results, increased patient compliance, and reduction of cost.

ADVERSE REACTIONS AND PRECAUTIONS. Pyrazinamide can cause hepatotoxicity, which apparently is dose-related. Early studies indicated that a dose of 3 g daily was effective when given with isoniazid in the initial treatment of tuberculosis, but the incidence of hepatotoxicity with this regimen was approximately 14% and one death occurred from acute yellow atrophy of the liver. These reports led to abandonment of pyrazinamide as a first-line drug for the treatment of tuberculosis. Doses used then were higher (40 to 70 mg/kg) than those employed in combination regimens today (15 to 30 mg/kg), and there has not been a significant increase in hepatotoxicity when pyrazinamide was used in the latter dosage range in regimens containing isoniazid and rifampin. Liver damage produced by pyrazinamide is rarely serious, especially when the drug is discontinued after two months. Pretreatment laboratory studies should include a complete liver function profile.

The most frequently observed adverse effect is nongouty polyarthralgia (incidence, approximately 40%). Pyrazinamide inhibits renal excretion of urates and almost routinely causes hyperuricemia, which is usually asymptomatic; serum uric acid levels of 12 to 14 mg/dL are not uncommon. Baseline serum uric acid levels should be determined. Pyrazinamide should be discontinued if hyperuricemia accompanied by acute gouty arthritis develops. A complete blood count, urinalysis, and serum profile screening should be performed monthly.

Other adverse effects reported include mild arthralgia and myalgia (frequent) and fever, hypersensitivity, acne, photosensitivity, porphyria, dysuria, thrombocytopenia, sideroblastic anemia, and interstitial nephritis (infrequent). Nausea, vomiting, and anorexia also have been reported.

Pyrazinamide is contraindicated in patients with severe hepatic damage, acute gout, or those with a hypersensitivity to the drug.

Data in humans are insufficient to evaluate the safety of pyrazinamide during pregnancy (FDA Pregnancy Category C) or lactation; however, adverse effects in nursing infants have not been documented.

PHARMACOKINETICS. Pyrazinamide is well absorbed orally (time to peak effect is about two hours) and is widely distributed, including the cerebrospinal fluid. The volume of distribution is 0.57 to 0.74 L/kg. Protein binding is low. Plasma pyrazinoic acid levels exceed those of the parent compound and peak four to eight hours after an oral dose. The half-life of pyrazinamide is 9 to 10 hours. Excretion is primarily via the kidney; 3% of the administered dose is excreted unchanged in the urine and 36% is excreted as pyrazinoic acid. The major metabolic pathway of pyrazinamide is conversion to pyrazinoic acid followed by subsequent conversion to hydroxypyrazinoic acid, a reaction catalyzed by xanthine oxidase. The elimination half-life is 10 to 16 hours.

DOSAGE AND PREPARATIONS.

Oral: *Adults and children,* 15 to 30 mg/kg daily in one or more doses (maximum, 2 g daily). For alternative regimens, see Table 9.

Pyrazinamide (Lederle). Tablets 500 mg.

RIFAMPIN

[Rifadin, Rimactane]

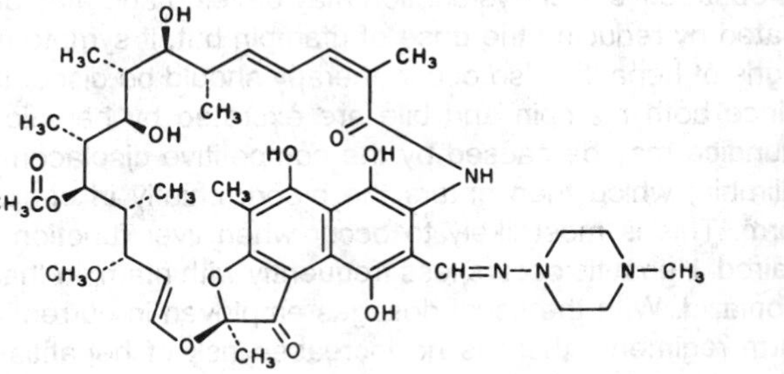

SPECTRUM, ACTIONS, AND USES. Rifampin is a semisynthetic derivative of rifamycin B. This antibiotic represents the greatest contribution to the chemotherapy of tuberculosis since the introduction of isoniazid. In vitro and in vivo, rifampin has a marked bactericidal effect against extracellular and intracellular *Mycobacterium tuberculosis*, *M. bovis*, and nearly all strains of *M. kansasii*. Some strains of scotochromogens (mycobacterial group II) and a few strains of nonphotochromogens (mycobacterial group III) are inhibited by low concentrations of the drug. The in vitro bactericidal activity of rifampin was reported to be substantially lower against *M. avium* than *M. tuberculosis* (Heifets et al, 1990). This drug is indicated in the initial treatment and retreatment of tuberculosis in combination with other antituberculous drugs.

Rifampin is most active during cell multiplication, but it also appears to have some effect on resting cells. It inhibits bacterial RNA synthesis by binding to the B-subunit of DNA-dependent RNA polymerase, thus inhibiting the attachment of the enzyme to DNA and resulting in a block of RNA transcription and elongation. Rifampin does not inhibit the counterpart mammalian enzyme. Cross resistance has only been shown with other rifamycins. Mycobacterial resistance can develop rapidly when the drug is used as monotherapy and can be reduced markedly by combination therapy with isoniazid, ethambutol, streptomycin, or other effective antimycobacterial agents administered in therapeutic doses; thus, rifampin is always administered with one or more of these drugs in active treatment or retreatment regimens.

Rifampin alone is used for preventive therapy as an alternative to isoniazid in patients who cannot tolerate the latter drug or who have a high probability of contact with an isoniazid-resistant strain (Table 7). It is used for the treatment of asymptomatic carriers of *N. meningitidis* to eliminate the organism from the nasopharynx but is not indicated for the treatment of meningococcal infection. Rifampin also is effective in the treatment of leprosy (see the section on Leprosy).

ADVERSE REACTIONS AND PRECAUTIONS. The most commonly observed adverse effect is gastrointestinal disturbance. However, most patients tolerate and accept rifampin well. Abdominal distress, aching in muscles and joints, and cramping in the legs occur occasionally, especially during the first few weeks of treatment. During this period, asymptomatic jaundice is noted rarely but usually subsides without interruption of therapy. The subsidence may be caused by the increased biliary excretion of rifampin due to enzyme induction that occurs during the first few weeks of use, which reduces the half-life by about 40%. Jaundice with laboratory evidence of obstructive liver dysfunction may develop and may be alleviated by reducing the dose of rifampin but, if symptoms and signs of hepatitis also occur, therapy should be discontinued. Since both rifampin and bile are excreted by hepatic cells, jaundice may be caused by the competitive displacement of bilirubin, which then enters the blood, chiefly in conjugated form. This is most likely to occur when liver function is impaired. Hepatitis occurs less frequently with rifampin than with isoniazid. With the usual dosages employed in current short-term regimens, there is no increased risk of hepatitis when rifampin and isoniazid are given together.

When rifampin is administered to patients with impaired liver function, they should be kept under close medical supervision; serum enzyme levels should be monitored in alcoholics and those with pre-existing liver disease for at least the first two or three months of treatment.

Hypersensitivity reactions have been reported. Pruritus with or without rash has been noted in less than 3% of patients. Rifampin and its metabolites impart a reddish orange color to urine, feces, saliva, sweat, and tears; there may be discoloration of soft contact lenses in patients taking this drug. Patients should be informed of these problems to prevent anxiety.

Thrombocytopenia, transient leukopenia, and hemolytic anemia have been reported occasionally. Elevations in BUN and serum uric acid have occurred. Interstitial nephritis has developed rarely.

Intermittent treatment with rifampin and other agents has been employed for years without significant toxicity. However, a serious reaction, assumed to be immunologic in nature, has occurred in about 1% of patients who received large doses (900 mg to 1.2 g) intermittently or in whom treatment was resumed after a lapse of days or weeks. The mechanism is unknown, but rifampin-dependent antibodies have been demonstrated in the serum of some patients. The reaction is characterized by a severe "flu-like" syndrome with dyspnea, sometimes accompanied by wheezing; purpura associated with thrombocytopenia; leukopenia; and, occasionally, a state similar to true anaphylaxis. Rarely, hemolysis, hemoglobinuria, hematuria, and renal insufficiency also occurred. Treatment with rifampin had to be discontinued in only 3% of the patients, and most were able to tolerate the drug when the dose was reduced or when daily treatment was substituted for intermittent therapy.

Teratogenic effects have not been reported in humans, even after inadvertent administration during the first trimester of pregnancy. However, rifampin crosses the placenta, and it has caused postnatal hemorrhage in the mother and infant when administered during the last few weeks of pregnancy; vitamin K may be indicated (FDA Pregnancy Category C). The drug is excreted in milk; however, adverse effects in nursing infants have not been documented.

DRUG INTERACTIONS. Rifampin is a potent inducer of hepatic cytochrome P450 enzymes and has produced clinically important interactions with anticoagulants, oral contraceptives, methadone and other opioids, nonopioid analgesics, sulfonylureas, barbiturates, glucocorticoids, quinidine, digoxin, digitoxin, theophylline, cyclosporine, chloramphenicol, beta blockers, verapamil, diltiazem, nifedipine, haloperidol, ciprofloxacin, diazepam, clofibrate, progestins, disopyramide, mexiletine, and phenytoin and other anticonvulsants. Therefore, adjustments in dosages of these agents may be indicated.

Rifampin may increase the likelihood of isoniazid-induced hepatotoxicity in slow isoniazid acetylators. Dapsone concentrations may be reduced, but it is generally considered unnecessary to adjust the dosage recommended for concurrent therapy with rifampin for leprosy. The bentonite excipients in some aminosalicylic acid preparations may interfere with the oral absorption of rifampin; therefore, the drugs should be taken eight hours apart.

Patients should be advised to use an alternative contraceptive method while taking rifampin if they had been taking an oral contraceptive.

Blood levels of rifampin are increased by probenecid. Halothane given concurrently with rifampin increases the hepatotoxicity of both drugs. When given with rifampin, ketoconazole diminishes the serum concentrations of both drugs; dosage adjustment may be required. Daily use of alcohol may result in an increase in the incidence of rifampin-induced hepatotoxicity and increase the metabolism of rifampin; dosage adjustments may be necessary. Concurrent use with clofazamine has resulted in reduced absorption of rifampin with a delay in time to peak concentration and increased half-life. Use of antiarrhythmic drugs (eg, tocainide, propaphenone) with rifampin may enhance the metabolism of these drugs and result in significantly lower serum concentrations of the former; serum concentrations of these drugs should be monitored and dosage adjustments made if necessary.

The plasma concentration of fluconazole may be lowered when this drug is used with rifampin, and the dose may need to be increased. Concurrent use of rifampin with other hepatotoxic medications may increase the potential for hepatotoxicity. Use of trimethoprim with rifampin may significantly increase the elimination of trimethoprim and shorten its elimination half-life.

PHARMACOKINETICS. Although the oral bioavailability of rifampin is reported to be 90% to 95%, repeated administration causes enzyme induction that increases the clearance of plasma rifampin and increases biliary excretion of the major metabolite, 2,5-*o*-desacetyl-rifamycin. Food interferes with the rate and extent of absorption. Rifampin diffuses freely into body tissues and fluids, including cerebrospinal fluid. About 80% of the drug is protein-bound. The drug also crosses the placenta. Currently recommended doses produce peak serum levels in 1.5 to 4 hours; levels above the minimal inhibitory concentration persist for at least six hours. The volume of distribution is 1.6 ± 0.2 L/kg.

Rifampin is metabolized by the liver and is excreted in the bile; approximately 60% to 65% of the dose appears in the feces. As much as 33% of a dose is eliminated in the urine as parent drug (50%) and active metabolites; therefore, therapeutic concentrations appear in the urine. Rifampin also is excreted in breast milk.

The half-life of the parent molecule is 1.5 to 5 hours, and the major metabolite is active. Initially, the mean half-life is 2.3 to 5.1 hours but decreases after repeated administration over a two-week period to approximately two hours because of enzyme induction.

DOSAGE AND PREPARATIONS. Both oral and intravenous formulations are available. The latter is indicated when the drug cannot be taken by mouth.

Oral: *Adults,* 10 mg/kg daily or biweekly (maximum, 600 mg/day); *children,* 10 to 20 mg/kg daily or biweekly (maximum, 600 mg/day). The drug should be given in a single dose one hour before a meal (usually breakfast) or two hours afterward (see also Table 9).

Rifadin (Marion Merrell Dow). Capsules 150 and 300 mg.

NOTE: Instructions on the preparation of an extemporaneous oral suspension for use in pediatric and adult patients in whom swallowing is difficult or when lower doses are needed are available from the manufacturer.

Rimactane (CIBA). Capsules 300 mg.

The combination preparations listed below may be more convenient to use than multiple single-entity preparations and have been reported to enhance compliance in some patients.

Rifamate (Marion Merrell Dow). Capsules containing isoniazid 150 mg and rifampin 300 mg.

Rimactane/INH (CIBA). Tablets containing isoniazid 300 mg and rifampin 300 mg.

Intravenous: *Adults,* 600 mg in a single daily dose. *Children,* 10 to 20 mg/kg (maximum, 600 mg/day).

Rifadin I.V. (Marion Merrell Dow). Powder 600 mg.

STREPTOMYCIN SULFATE

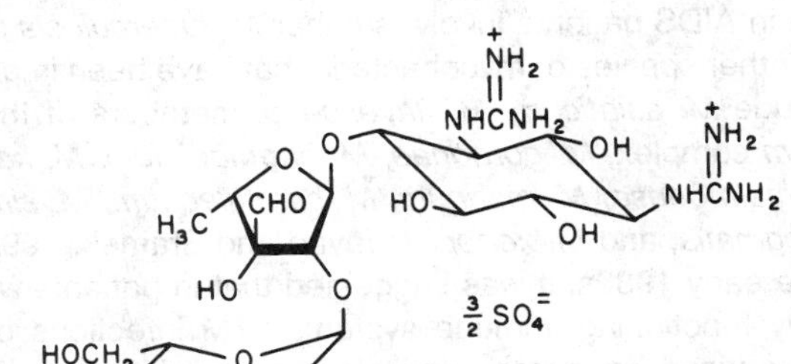

ACTIONS AND USES. Streptomycin was the first chemotherapeutic agent of undeniable efficacy in the treatment of tuberculosis. It must be administered intramuscularly, which limits its usefulness in long-term therapy. Streptomycin is the most effective and least toxic of the parenterally administered antibiotics derived from *Streptomyces*. It is bactericidal, principally for extracellular (including cavitary) tubercle bacilli, probably through a direct action on the bacterial ribosome to inhibit protein synthesis. An alkaline environment enhances the drug's bactericidal activity.

Streptomycin is of greatest value in the early weeks or months of therapy. Possibly because it is administered parenterally and high serum concentrations are produced rapidly, this drug appears to enhance the effect of agents administered orally, even such effective agents as ethambutol and isoniazid. The combination of intramuscular streptomycin and isoniazid has an immediate, marked, suppressive effect on susceptible organisms and often has been lifesaving in critical situations.

Studies have indicated that a four-drug regimen, selected to provide maximal bactericidal activity, consisting of streptomycin, rifampin, isoniazid, and pyrazinamide for two months followed by four months of isoniazid and rifampin produced results comparable to any other drug regimen given for any duration in drug-susceptible infections (Algerian Working Group/British Medical Research Council, 1984; Snider et al, 1984 B, 1986). More recently, a six-month, 62-dose regimen employing isoniazid, rifampin, pyrazinamide, and streptomycin was reported to be at least 87% ±5.5% effective (Cohn et al, 1990).

Parenteral administration of streptomycin also is valuable when oral medication with other drugs is contraindicated or when gastrointestinal absorption is impaired. When used alone, resistance develops rapidly. Streptomycin also is useful in intermittent therapy, and it is one of the few agents that is effective against nonphotochromogens (mycobacterial group III organisms) in vitro.

ADVERSE REACTIONS, PRECAUTIONS, AND DRUG INTERACTIONS. When administered correctly, streptomycin is rarely toxic and most individuals tolerate this agent well. Occasionally, transient headache or malaise occurs soon after injection. Clinically unimportant facial paresthesia, particularly around the mouth, is noted in approximately 15% of patients and may be accompanied by a tingling sensation in the hands.

Ototoxicity is the most serious adverse reaction of streptomycin. It may frequently affect the vestibular branch of the auditory nerve to produce nausea, vomiting, and vertigo. The incidence of ototoxicity is directly related to dose and duration of treatment. Old age and renal impairment are predisposing conditions. Loss of hearing may occur and, when extensive, is usually permanent. The neurotoxicity of streptomycin can result in respiratory paralysis from neuromuscular blockade, especially following anesthesia and use of muscle relaxants.

Nephrotoxicity occurs only occasionally with streptomycin but may be increased in patients with pre-existing renal insufficiency or when other nephrotoxic drugs (eg, cephalosporins, polymyxin) are used simultaneously. Therefore, concurrent or sequential use of other neurotoxic and/or nephrotoxic drugs should be avoided.

Since both ototoxicity and nephrotoxicity are more common in persons over 65 years, streptomycin should be avoided in this age group, if possible. For all patients, baseline and periodic audiograms and caloric test of vestibular function are recommended. Ototoxicity and nephrotoxicity are related both to cumulative dose and peak serum concentrations. A total dose of 120 g should not be exceeded unless other therapeutic options are not available.

Hypersensitivity reactions occur occasionally during the early weeks of treatment but are less common than with aminosalicylic acid and usually are less serious than with aminosalicylic acid or isoniazid. A few reports of anaphylactic and hematopoietic reactions, including eosinophilia, agranulocytosis, and aplastic anemia, have been reported.

Teratogenicity has been documented in laboratory animals. This drug should not be administered during the first trimester of pregnancy or in total doses exceeding 20 g during the last half of pregnancy to minimize the possibility of congenital deafness. Streptomycin is classified in FDA Pregnancy Category D.

Minimal amounts of streptomycin appear in breast milk when therapeutic serum levels are achieved in the mother.

PHARMACOKINETICS. Oral bioavailability of streptomycin is less than 1%. The drug is rapidly (time to peak effect 60 minutes) and well absorbed after intramuscular injection and its effect diminishes to approximately 50% after five to six hours. High concentrations are found in all organs except the brain; significant amounts are found in tuberculous cavities and in pleural fluid. There is inadequate penetration into cells, including the tubercle bacillus, and into cerebrospinal fluid, even when the meninges are inflamed. Volume of distribution is 0.25 L/kg. Metabolism is negligible, and the drug is almost entirely eliminated by glomerular filtration. The rate of clearance approximates two-thirds of the simultaneous creatinine clearance. The elimination half-life is about five hours; however, tissue-bound streptomycin may be released slowly over many days. Streptomycin crosses the placenta; small amounts are excreted in milk, saliva, and sweat.

DOSAGE AND PREPARATIONS.
(Doses and strengths expressed in terms of the base)

Intramuscular: *Adults,* 15 mg/kg daily (maximum, 1 g). *Children,* 20 to 30 mg/kg daily (maximum, 1 g). For alternative regimens for adults and children, see Table 9. A total dose of 120 g should not be exceeded.

Generic. Solution 1 g (400 mg/ml) in 2.5 ml containers. Distributed free to physicians by Pfizer Pharmaceuticals.

NONTUBERCULOUS (ATYPICAL) MYCOBACTERIAL INFECTIONS

Mycobacteria other than *M. tuberculosis* may cause disease in humans. On culture, these bacteria form colonies that are not typical of *M. tuberculosis*, hence the term "atypical mycobacteria" has been employed. Currently, the terms nontuberculous mycobacteria (NTM) and mycobacteria other than tuberculosis (MOTT) are more commonly used. Runyon (1965) classified NTM into four large groups on the basis of pigment production or rapid growth in culture. After publication of a preliminary report of Runyon's classification system, a number of patients in the southeastern United States were reported to have disease attributable to NTM. These patients were epidemiologically distinct from the usual tuberculosis patients in that they were older, more frequently were white, often had an underlying chronic lung disease, and responded poorly to existing antituberculous drugs. An epidemiologic study conducted from 1981 to 1983 to determine the incidence of NTM disease in the United States found that the prevalence rates were highest for *M. avium* complex (MAC) followed by *M. kansasii* and *M. fortuitum-M. chelonae* (O'Brien et al, 1987 A). In some parts of the United States, NTM disease may be as common as tuberculosis. Mycobacteria in the environment appear to be the source of infection in humans.

Nontuberculous mycobacteria vary in their susceptibility to drugs; some are completely susceptible and others are markedly resistant. Some strains of *M. kansasii* may be as susceptible to chemotherapy as *M. tuberculosis*, whereas others are resistant.

Routine testing for susceptibility to antituberculous drugs using the single low drug concentrations designed for routine tuberculosis testing has no clinical value for four species of the NTM: *M. marinum, M. avium* complex, *M. fortuitum,* and *M. chelonae*. However, it has been recommended that susceptibility testing using the standard antituberculous methodology be performed in the following circumstances: (1) All initial isolates of *M. kansasii* in which prior drug therapy cannot be excluded or when a history of prior drug therapy is not available; (2) cases of *M. kansasii* disease in which sputum fails to convert after four months of regimens containing rifampin or when relapses have occurred; (3) recovery of an infrequently isolated species of NTM that appears to be clinically significant, but for which drug therapy and susceptibility patterns are uncertain; (4) smear-positive samples in a clinical setting suspicious for tuberculosis; and (5) cases of *M. marinum* infection in which there has been no response to regimens containing rifampin or relapses have occurred (American Thoracic Society, 1990 B).

Shortly after the recognition of AIDS as a clinical entity, physicians observed that the profound suppression of cell-mediated immunity allowed disseminated mycobacteriosis to occur in these patients. Approximately 90% of the mycobacteriosis in AIDS patients involves either *M. tuberculosis* or *M. avium*; other species of mycobacteria that have been implicated include *M. asiaticum, M. flavescens*, members of the *M. fortuitum* complex, *M. gordonae, M. haemophilum, M. kansasii, M. malmoense, M. marinum, M. scrofulaceum, M. simiae, M. smegmatis*, and *M. xenopi* (Wayne and Sramek, 1992).

In the early 1980s, it was suggested that in patients with a normally functioning immune system, NTM infections could be categorized as either relatively easy or difficult to treat (Bailey, 1983). Included in the former group are the following slow growing mycobacteria (ie, requiring >7 days for visible growth to appear from dilute inoculum): *M. kansasii, M. marinum, M. szulgai*, and *M. xenopi. M. kansasii* may be considered as the prototype for the "easy-to-treat" group and has been used as the model for therapy of these mycobacteria.

THERAPEUTICALLY SUSCEPTIBLE NTM. *M. kansasii* (the "yellow bacillus") is the most important pathogen of Runyon's Group I (photochromogens, slow grower) and is often associated with pulmonary disease. It is usually susceptible in vitro to commonly used antituberculous drugs and disease caused by the organism is almost as easily treated as uncomplicated tuberculosis. Previously untreated strains of *M. kansasii* are susceptible to rifampin, isoniazid, ethambutol, ethionamide, and streptomycin at serum concentrations readily achievable with usual therapeutic doses. The organism also is susceptible in vitro to erythromycin, sulfamethoxazole, amikacin, and rifabutin, but there is little information on the clinical usefulness of these drugs. Isolates usually are resistant to achievable levels of aminosalicylic acid, capreomycin, and pyrazinamide. Acquired resistance to rifampin, ethambutol, and isoniazid has occurred in isolates from treatment-failure cases.

There have been no randomized controlled clinical trials comparing one drug regimen with another or with no drug treatment. However, several retrospective and prospective studies have provided a good basis for drug therapy recommendations. Currently, the American Thoracic Society recommends that pulmonary and extrapulmonary disease caused by *M. kansasii* be treated with isoniazid 300 mg, rifampin 600 mg, and ethambutol 15 mg/kg daily for 18 months. For patients who cannot tolerate isoniazid, administration of rifampin and ethambutol with or without streptomycin for the first three months is thought to be a reasonable alternative; however, the effectiveness of this regimen has not been established by clinical trials. Pyrazinamide is not acceptable as an alternative or third drug because all strains of *M. kansasii* are resistant to this drug. Short-course or intermittent drug treatment has not been sufficiently studied to permit a recommendation (American Thoracic Society, 1990 B).

In general, the regimen employed for patients with drug-resistant organisms should consist of those agents to which in vitro susceptibility has been demonstrated. In patients in whom organisms have become resistant to rifampin as a result of previous therapy, a regimen consisting of isoniazid (900 mg/day), pyridoxine (50 mg/day), high-dose ethambutol (25 mg/kg/day), and sulfamethoxazole (1 g/day) or trimethoprim/sulfamethoxazole (160 to 800 mg two or three times/day) has been studied. The regimen also included streptomycin or amikacin given daily or five times per week for two to three months, followed by intermittent streptomycin or amikacin for at least six months. Preliminary results indicated sputum conversion in seven of eight patients after a mean of 10 weeks (Ahn et al, 1987).

Infection with *M. kansasii* also can appear as a late complication of HIV infection when CD4 cell counts are <200/microliter and usually is associated with pulmonary disease. It has not been established whether drugs should be prescribed differently or for a longer period in patients with AIDS. The regimen of isoniazid, rifampin, and ethambutol was reported to be effective in patients with *M. kansasii* and HIV infection. Clinical resolution of pulmonary disease, sputum conversion, and prevention of deaths attributed to *M. kansasii* pneumonia has been achieved (Levine and Chaisson, 1991).

Disseminated *M. kansasii* disease has occurred in AIDS patients and is the second most common disseminated NTM disease in this population; most cases have been fatal. The regimen of isoniazid, rifampin, and ethambutol used for pulmonary disease did not appear to be effective in HIV-infected patients with disseminated disease (Carpenter and Parks, 1991).

M. marinum, another NTM considered easy to treat, typically causes cutaneous disease after trauma in an aquatic setting; the syndrome is referred to as "swimming pool granuloma." Isolates have been reported to be susceptible to rifampin and ethambutol; of intermediate susceptibility to streptomycin; and resistant to isoniazid and pyrazinamide. Isolates frequently also are susceptible to sulfonamides or trimethoprim/sulfamethoxazole and susceptible or of intermediate sensitivity to doxycycline and minocycline. A number of regimens have been employed; those reported to be effective include minocycline or doxycycline 100 mg twice daily; trimethoprim/sulfamethoxazole 160 to 800 mg twice daily; or rifampin 600 mg/day plus ethambutol 15 mg/kg/day. Each regimen is administered for a minimum of three months (Black and Eykyn, 1986; American Thoracic Society, 1990 B). Surgical debridement also may be important.

THERAPEUTICALLY RESISTANT NTM. The "difficult-to-treat" NTMs are members of the *M. fortuitum* complex and *M. avium* complex (MAC). The former includes the species *M. fortuitum* and *M. chelonae,* each of which is further subdivided into subspecies and biovars. The complex is composed of strains that produce visible growth from diluted inoculum in <7 days and the aryl sulfatase test is positive (Wayne and Sramek, 1992).

Both of these rapidly growing NTMs cause a wide spectrum of clinical disease, the most common being cutaneous infection following open trauma or puncture wounds. Other infections with which they have been associated include sternal osteomyelitis, wound infections, corneal ulceration, meningitis, pericarditis, disseminated disease, pulmonary infections, intestinal mycobacteriosis, dialysis-related infections, prosthetic valve endocarditis, and infection of prosthetic breast implants.

M. fortuitum *Complex:* Some strains of the *M. fortuitum* complex are highly resistant to antituberculous drugs. Antibacterial drugs to which these organisms have been reported to be susceptible include fluoroquinolones, sulfonamides, cefoxitin, doxycycline, erythromycin, clarithromycin, amikacin, and imipenem/cilastatin. No controlled clinical trials on therapy for diseases caused by this group of organisms have been reported. In several studies, patients with cutaneous disease who were treated on the basis of in vitro susceptibilities had a good response. Proper susceptibility testing of all clinically significant isolates is essential for proper patient management. However, susceptibility testing methods used for these organisms differ from the single low drug concentration method routinely employed with *M. tuberculosis*.

For serious cutaneous disease caused by all subgroups of *M. fortuitum* except *M. chelonae* subspecies *chelonae*, the American Thoracic Society has recommended as initial therapy a regimen consisting of intravenous amikacin (400 mg twice daily) plus intravenous cefoxitin (12 g/day) administered for two to four weeks until clinical improvement is evident. If the organisms are susceptible to oral agents, one or more of the following drugs (doxycycline 100 mg twice daily, sulfamethoxazole 1 g three times/day, or ciprofloxacin 500 mg twice daily) can be substituted. A minimum of three months and, for bone infections, six months of therapy is needed to provide a high likelihood of cure (American Thoracic Society, 1990 B). Surgery is indicated when there is extensive disease or abscess formation or when drug therapy is difficult. Removal of foreign bodies (eg, breast implants, catheters) may be essential.

Monotherapy with clarithromycin also has been reported to be safe and effective for cutaneous disease, especially disseminated disease, due to *M. chelonae*. Fourteen patients (10 with disseminated disease) were enrolled in an open, noncomparative trial in which 500 mg of clarithromycin was given orally twice daily for six months. Underlying diseases included rheumatoid arthritis, other autoimmune disorders, and organ transplantation. All patients were receiving either corticosteroids (93%) or cyclophosphamide (7%). These patients were reported to have an excellent response with only mild adverse effects. Therapy was discontinued in 9 of 11 patients who received therapy for at least six months with no evidence of relapse. The authors concluded that clarithromycin may be the drug of choice for cutaneous (disseminated) disease due to *M. chelonae*, but cautioned that long-term clinical follow-up of more patients was needed (Wallace et al, 1993).

Pulmonary disease caused by the rapidly growing mycobacteria is uncommon, and most such infections are caused by *M. chelonae* subspecies *abscessus*. The most useful agents for these infections are amikacin, cefoxitin, and imipenem/cilastatin. For patients infected with *M. fortuitum* or an erythromycin-sensitive strain of *M. chelonae*, oral therapy should be attempted using a two- or three-drug regimen consisting of ciprofloxacin, doxycycline, erythromycin, or sulfonamides. There are anecdotal reports of successful treatment of pulmonary infections with trimethoprim/sulfamethoxazole or cefoxitin plus ciprofloxacin (Pacht, 1990; Singh and Yu, 1992).

M. avium *Complex (MAC):* This group of slow-growing nonchromogenic mycobacteria was previously thought to consist only of *M. avium* and *M. intracellulare*, but it has been suggested that the group also should include *M. paratuberculosis* and a possible new species, *M. lepraemurium*, the "wood pigeon" bacillus (Wayne and Sramek, 1992). For many years the distinction between *M. avium* and *M. intracellulare* was blurred and no phenotypic properties provided definitive resolution. However, recent reports on primary, secondary, and tertiary semantide have confirmed that the two groups are distinct species and has led to the redistribution of agglutinating serovars between the two species. On the evolutionary scale, they are quite different from *M. scrofulaceum* and from other species of mycobacteria. Other recent studies of mycobacterial semantides have suggested that *M. lepraemurium* and *M. paratuberculosis* should be reduced to subspecies of *M. avium* (Wayne and Sramek, 1992).

Before the AIDS epidemic, MAC infection was uncommon and occurred primarily as a slowly progressive pneumonitis in elderly patients with chronic pulmonary disorders. Rarely, disseminated MAC infection was found in immunocompromised patients. With the onset of the AIDS epidemic, the incidence of MAC infection, principally disseminated disease, has increased dramatically, and it is now one of the most common infections in AIDS patients. It occurs in 4.2% of HIV-infected patients at the time of AIDS diagnosis and in up to 50% of AIDS patients at the time of autopsy. The incidence of the infection increases linearly by approximately 20% per year each year after a patient's first AIDS-defining opportunistic event, and the incidence of MAC bacteremia increases exponentially as the CD4 count approaches zero. Disseminated MAC disease is rarely observed in AIDS patients with CD4 counts $>100/mm^3$; the mean number of cells in patients with this infection is <60 cells/mm^3. The gastrointestinal tract probably is the most frequent source of MAC infection in HIV-infected patients; however, in one study, the presence of MAC in respiratory specimens had substantial predictive value for subsequent disseminated infection (Jacobson et al, 1991).

Using species-specific nucleic acid probes, investigators have reported that 98% of a series of 45 AIDS patients with disease caused by species of MAC harbored only *M. avium*, whereas 40% of a series of patients without AIDS yielded *M. intracellulare* on culture. Isolation of *M. avium* from patients without AIDS was considered to be more likely to represent colonization than infection (Guthertz et al, 1989). The major *M. avium* serovars associated with AIDS patients in the United States are 1, 4, and 8, with serovar 8 dominant in southern California and serovar 4 dominant in northern California and the eastern United States.

Prophylaxis. Both *M. avium* and *M. intracellulare* are ubiquitous in the environment, being found in water, dust, soil, and food. The immunocompromised state of AIDS patients is an important predisposing factor in acquiring and developing disseminated MAC disease. Therefore, prophylactic measures to prevent this disease in these patients is a worthy goal. Chemoprophylaxis with rifabutin [Mycobutin] is now available for HIV-positive patients with CD4 counts $<100/mm^3$. Two randomized, double-blind, multicenter trials of daily prophylactic treatment with either rifabutin (300 mg daily) or placebo were reported recently (Nightingale et al, 1993). In the first trial, MAC bacteremia developed in 51 of 298 patients (17%) receiving placebo and in 24 of 292 patients (8%) receiving rifabutin. In the second trial, bacteremia developed in 51 of 282 patients in the placebo group (18%) and in 24 of 274 patients in the rifabutin group (9%). Several symptoms were significantly reduced in patients receiving rifabutin; although survival was not significantly prolonged, there was a trend in that direction. A U.S. Public Health Service Task Force has recommended lifelong prophylaxis with rifabutin (300 mg/day) for HIV-infected patients with CD4 counts <100 per mm^3 unless multiple drug therapy for MAC becomes necessary because of the development of MAC disease (Masur and the Public Health Service Task Force on Prophylaxis and Therapy for *Mycobacterium avium* Complex, 1993). A controlled study on clarithromycin and a randomized double-blind study (AIDS Clinical Trials Group, protocol 196) comparing rifabutin, clarithromycin, and the combination of the two for the prevention of disseminated MAC are being conducted.

Treatment. In immunocompetent individuals, MAC most commonly affects the lungs in those with pre-existing pulmonary disorders. Many strains of MAC are 10 to 100 times less sensitive than *M. tuberculosis* to antituberculous drugs.

Early experience with chemotherapy for *pulmonary disease* caused by MAC was disappointing. In 1990, the American Thoracic Society recommended a four-drug regimen consisting of isoniazid, rifampin, ethambutol, and streptomycin for initial therapy in patients with pulmonary disease for whom treatment is indicated (American Thoracic Society, 1990 B). Since then other regimens have been tried. A regimen consisting of clarithromycin (500 mg twice daily), ethambutol (15 mg/kg/day), and rifampin (600 mg/day) with treatment continued for six months after sputum conversion now is preferred by many clinicians for the treatment of this disease.

Disseminated disease caused by MAC is rare in immunocompetent individuals but is the most common form in AIDS patients. The response to therapy and long-term prognosis of patients with AIDS have generally been poor because disseminated disease occurs as a late opportunistic infection in these severely immunosuppressed patients. In early studies, evidence that chemotherapy improved microbiologic indicators or survival was not convincing. Thus, some physicians questioned whether MAC shortened survival time and whether treatment resulted in any clinical improvement. Subsequent studies have shown that survival is significantly shorter in those with disseminated MAC infection (median, 4 months) than in those without the disease (median, 11 months) and that treated patients survive longer than untreated patients (mean 9.5 months versus 5.6 months, respectively) (Horsburgh et al, 1991; Jacobson et al, 1991).

In recent years, the development of new treatment regimens and extension of treatment duration has yielded encouraging results. Two macrolide antibiotics, azithromycin and clarithromycin, appear to possess favorable ratios of toxic to therapeutic effects and are active against MAC in vitro and in animal models. Although minimum inhibitory concentrations against MAC are in excess of achievable serum concentrations, at high concentrations azithromycin accumulates in phagocytes where mycobacteria persist and multiply; in addition, it has a long half-life and excellent tissue distribution. Experimentally infected mice have been treated successfully with this antibiotic. For these reasons, an uncontrolled Phase I trial of azithromycin monotherapy was conducted in 24 evaluable male homosexuals with AIDS and disseminated MAC disease (Young et al, 1991). Patients were given azithromycin 500 mg/day orally for 10 (3 patients), 20 (5 patients), or 30 days (16 patients). Blood cultures showed a mean reduction in bacteremia from 118 colony-forming units (CFU)/ml to 43 CFU/ml in the 3 patients treated for 10 days and from 2028 CFU/ml to 136 CFU/ml in the 21 patients treated for 20 or 30 days. In most patients, fever and night sweats were reduced and performance status improved modestly, but fatigue, weight loss, and appetite were unchanged. The principal adverse effects were loose stools or diarrhea (Young et al, 1991).

Clarithromycin also has good in vitro and in vivo activity against MAC and high levels are attained intracellularly and in tissue. An AIDS Clinical Trial Group study (ACTG 157) evaluated the efficacy and safety of this drug for treating disseminated MAC disease. A total of 108 patients were randomized to receive clarithromycin 500 mg, 1 g, or 2 g twice daily. The antibiotic was highly active as monotherapy for suppressing disseminated MAC bacteremia over a period of 12 weeks. Median decreases in bacteremia were 2.6 to 2.8 logs of CFU in the blood over three months. Patients receiving clarithromycin 2 g twice daily became culture-negative significantly faster than those receiving either of the other two doses. Median times to sterilization of cultures were 55 days (500 mg group), 43 days (1 g group), and 27 days (2 g group). At the highest dose, however, there was substantial drug intolerance. In a quality-of-life survey in 68 of the 108 participants, overall health improved significantly and severity of symptoms decreased. Resistance to the drug developed in 47% of patients within 12 weeks; the earliest resistance occurred within eight weeks (mean time to resistance, 104 days). No relationship between dosage level and time to resistance was demonstrated. Resistance was associated with a re-emergence of MAC symptoms, and it was suggested that a combination regimen with other drugs active against MAC would be necessary to prevent the emergence of resistance (Chaisson et al, 1992).

Studies conducted in Europe using clarithromycin with other antibiotics have been reported. In one randomized, double-blind, placebo-controlled trial using a modified crossover design, 15 males with late AIDS were divided into two groups. During the first phase of the study (six weeks), eight patients in Group I received clarithromycin 1 g orally twice daily and seven patients in Group II received placebo. At the end of the six-week period, patients were crossed over to Phase 2 (also six weeks). Group I patients were given placebo plus a combination of rifampin (10 mg/kg/day), isoniazid (5 mg/kg/day), ethambutol (20 mg/kg/day), and clofazamine (100 mg daily), and patients in Group II were given clarithromycin (1 g twice daily) plus the same four-drug regimen described above. (Because of two early deaths, the activity of clarithromycin could be evaluated in only five patients in Group II.) All eight patients in Group I had marked declines in blood MAC CFU; in six patients, CFU decreased to zero. When seven patients in this group were switched to placebo plus the four-drug regimen in the second phase of the study, the CFU rose in four patients and remained undetectable in three. The five evaluable patients in Group II had progressive CFU increases; when three were switched to clarithromycin plus the four-drug regimen in Phase 2, the CFU declined (Dautzenberg et al, 1991).

A multicenter open trial was conducted by the above investigators to further assess the clinical efficacy of clarithromycin against disseminated MAC in 77 patients with late-stage AIDS. The patients were divided into two groups: Group I (n=21) received low-dose clarithromycin (500 mg or 1 g daily) and those in Group II (n=56) received high-dose clarithromycin (1.5 or 2 g daily); all but five patients received other antimycobacterial agents concomitantly. MAC was eliminated from the blood in 11 of 16 (63%) evaluable patients in Group I and in 45 of 46 (98%) patients in Group II. Acquired resistance to clarithromycin occurred after two to seven months of treatment and was associated with relapse. The overall relapse rate after initial negative blood cultures was

25%. The mean delay before relapse was 127±68.1 days (Dautzenberg et al, 1993).

A pilot study evaluated the combination of clarithromycin, ciprofloxacin, and amikacin in 12 AIDS patients with persistent MAC bacteremia. The regimen consisted of amikacin (7.5 mg/kg intravenously twice daily for three weeks), clarithromycin (1 g orally twice daily), and ciprofloxacin (500 mg orally three times daily); the latter two drugs were continued indefinitely (range, 10 to 44 weeks). Eight patients had previously received other antimycobacterial drugs for periods ranging from 2 to 32 weeks (mean, 11.8 weeks); however, by the start of the experimental protocol, all patients had discontinued the use of other antimycobacterial agents for at least two weeks. Mycobacteremia cleared in all patients and symptoms resolved after two to eight weeks. Four patients died, but all had negative blood cultures until the time of death. Disseminated MAC disease was not considered the primary cause of death in these patients (de Lalla et al, 1992).

In a randomized double-blind study, nine bacteremic patients with AIDS and disseminated MAC infection received clarithromycin (n=4) 1 g twice daily or placebo (n=5) in addition to a basic regimen that included daily doses of isoniazid (300 mg), ethambutol (25 mg/kg; maximum dose, 1.6 g), and clofazamine (300 mg). The study had three phases: a six-week intensive-treatment phase was randomized and placebo-controlled, while both maintenance phases were conducted in an open format without placebo. During maintenance therapy, clarithromycin was given with rifabutin for 24 weeks, after which clarithromycin was given alone lifelong. All four patients receiving clarithromycin in the initial phase showed blood culture conversion and clinical response. Of the five patients not given clarithromycin in the initial phase, two showed blood culture conversion of bacteremia and clinical response, while two others died without having demonstrated a response. The fifth patient deteriorated until clarithromycin was substituted, after which there was blood culture conversion and rapid clinical improvement. One patient had a relapse during the maintenance phase when monotherapy with clarithromycin was employed; the relapse was associated with acquired resistance to the drug (Ruf et al, 1992).

After a review of the studies to date, the Public Health Service Task Force on Prophylaxis and Therapy for MAC made the following recommendations (Masur and the Public Health Service Task Force on Prophylaxis and Therapy for *Mycobacterium avium* Complex, 1993): (1) Treatment regimens used outside a clinical trial should include at least two agents. (2) Every regimen should include either azithromycin or clarithromycin. Many experts prefer ethambutol as a second drug. Potential third-line drugs include clofazamine, rifabutin, rifampin, ciprofloxacin, and, in some situations, amikacin. Isoniazid and pyrazinamide are not effective for the therapy of MAC. (3) Therapy should continue for the lifetime of the patient if clinical and microbiologic improvement is observed. It is not recommended that in vitro drug susceptibilities be relied on as a guide in the selection of the initial treatment regimen.

Drug Evaluations

CLARITHROMYCIN

[Biaxin]

For chemical formula, see index entry Macrolides, Chemical Structures.

USES. Clarithromycin recently has been approved for the treatment of disseminated mycobacterial infections due to *Mycobacterium avium* and *M. intracellulare.* The drug has been recommended by the U.S. Public Health Service Task Force on Prophylaxis and Therapy for MAC as a primary agent for the treatment of disseminated infection due to *M. avium* complex. It should be used in combination with other antimycobacterial drugs that have shown activity against MAC, including ethambutol, clofazamine, and rifampin (see the preceeding section). It has been recommended that clarithromycin therapy be continued for life if clinical and mycobacterial improvement are observed (Masur and the Public Health Service Task Force on Prophylaxis and Therapy for *Mycobacterium avium* Complex, 1993).

ADVERSE REACTIONS. Adverse events with an incidence ≥5% seen in clinical trials in AIDS and other immunocompromised patients with MAC disease treated with a dose of 500 mg twice daily were nausea (9% to 28%), taste perversion (0.4% to 18.9%), and vomiting (3.9% to 24.5%); abdominal pain, diarrhea, flatulence, headache, and rash were reported less frequently. For further information on clarithromycin, see index entry Clarithromycin, As Antibiotic.

DOSAGE AND PREPARATIONS.

Oral: *Adults*, for disseminated disease due to MAC, 500 mg twice daily; *children*, 7.5 mg/kg twice daily (maximum, 500 mg twice daily).

Biaxin (Abbott). Tablets (film-coated) 250 and 500 mg.

RIFABUTIN

[Mycobutin]

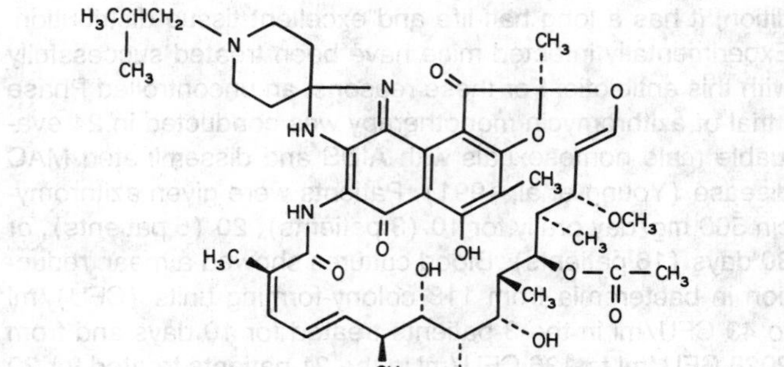

ACTIONS. Rifabutin is a semisynthetic ansamycin antibiotic that is derived from rifamycin S. Like rifampin, rifabutin is believed to exert its primary bacteriostatic effect by inhibiting DNA-dependent RNA polymerase activity in susceptible cells but not in mammalian cells. It is active against a wide variety of gram-positive and gram-negative bacteria in vitro (O'Brien et al, 1987 B); the drug also is active in vitro against a variety of mycobacteria, including both *Mycobacterium tuberculosis* and atypical species (Heifets and Iseman, 1985). It is not known whether this activity is dependent on inhibition of DNA-dependent RNA polymerase. Rifabutin was reported to be more active than rifampin against *M. avium* complex (MAC) (Woodley and Kilburn, 1982).

USES. Rifabutin is indicated to prevent disseminated MAC disease in patients in the advanced stages of AIDS; the overall clinical benefit is modest. This drug was evaluated for prevention of MAC bacteremia in two placebo-controlled, double-blind multicenter trials involving 1,146 patients with CDC-defined AIDS and CD4 counts $<200/mm^3$. The incidence of MAC bacteremia was 8% to 9% in patients taking rifabutin 300 mg daily and 17% to 18% in placebo recipients. Although rifabutin prophylaxis reduced the incidence, signs, and symptoms of MAC bacteremia in patients with advanced AIDS, it did not have a significant effect on survival (Nightingale et al, 1993). Rifabutin, in combination with other drugs, also has been used with some success to treat established MAC infection in AIDS patients (Agins et al, 1989); the optimal dosage has not been established. Rifabutin currently is being investigated for treatment of tuberculosis.

ADVERSE REACTIONS AND PRECAUTIONS. In general, rifabutin is well tolerated at doses of 300 mg/day. Primary reasons for discontinuation of therapy in clinical trials were rash (4%), gastrointestinal intolerance (3%), and neutropenia (2%). Other reactions with an incidence of at least 1% in excess of placebo responses were impairment of taste (2%) and abdominal pain, eructation, nausea and vomiting, myalgia, and fever (1%). Rifabutin appears to be a probable cause of the following adverse events that occurred in less than 1% of treated patients: flu-like syndrome, hepatitis, hemolysis, arthralgia, myositis, and chest pressure or pain with dyspnea.

Neutropenia was reported in a significantly larger number of patients treated with rifabutin (25/566 or 4.4%) than with placebo (20/580 or 3.4%). Because thrombocytopenia also may occur in patients receiving rifabutin, periodic hematologic screening may be advisable.

Use of rifabutin may color the skin and bodily secretions or excretions orange-brown; soft contact lenses may be permanently stained.

Rifabutin should not be used as a single agent for prophylaxis against MAC disease in patients with active tuberculosis. Patients who develop symptoms consistent with active tuberculosis while receiving rifabutin should be evaluated immediately so that an effective antituberculous regimen may be initiated in those with active disease.

Rifabutin is classified in FDA Pregnancy Category B.

DRUG INTERACTIONS. Because rifabutin is structurally similar to rifampin and, like the latter, also induces hepatic isoforms of P450, both drugs may have some effect on the disposition of other agents also affected by this enzyme. Although rifabutin appears to be two to three times less potent in this respect than rifampin, dosage adjustment may be necessary when affected agents are administered with rifabutin. (See index entry, Rifampin, Drug Interactions.)

Concurrent administration of rifabutin decreased the steady-state concentration of zidovudine by 48% during Phase I clinical trials; this interaction was not apparent in patients who received both drugs in Phase III trials. The kinetics of didanosine and fluconazole appear to be unaffected.

PHARMACOKINETICS. Rifabutin is fairly well absorbed after oral administration; however, data obtained in a limited number of HIV-positive patients indicate that bioavailability is only approximately 20%. Administration with a high-fat meal decreases the rate but not the extent of absorption after oral administration. Peak plasma concentrations (mean, 375 ng/ml) are achieved within two to four hours following a single oral dose of 300 mg.

Because it is highly lipophilic, rifabutin is widely distributed and concentrated intracellularly; plasma protein binding is approximately 85%. Elimination occurs largely by hepatic metabolism. The two major metabolites are 25-O-deacetyl and 31-hydroxy derivatives. The activity of the former is equal to that of the parent drug and is responsible for up to 10% of the antimicrobial effect associated with administration of rifabutin.

The mean terminal elimination half-life of rifabutin is 45 hours. During long-term therapy, steady-state concentrations may decrease by 38%, presumably due to induction of intestinal and/or hepatic metabolism. Steady-state kinetics of rifabutin in HIV-positive patients with minimal symptoms are similar to those in healthy volunteers and are only slightly modified (but more variable) in patients over age 70 and in those with hepatic dysfunction. Renal excretion of unchanged drug is a minor route of elimination; however, impaired renal function may decrease the extravascular distribution of rifabutin and therefore result in faster elimination and a lower plasma concentration.

DOSAGE AND PREPARATIONS.
Oral: *Adults,* 300 mg once daily; a dosage of 150 mg twice daily may be used in patients who experience symptoms of gastrointestinal intolerance. Rifabutin can be taken with food. *Children and adolescents,* a wide dosage range has been used in a small number of pediatric and adolescent patients (range, 2.8 to 25 mg/kg/day). The current suggested dose is 5 mg/kg. Studies are ongoing to determine the optimum dose for MAC prophylaxis in pediatric patients.

Mycobutin (Adria). Capsules 150 mg.

LEPROSY

Epidemiology: It has been estimated that 3 million people worldwide have leprosy (Hansen's disease); the estimated annual incidence is approximately 800,000 new cases. About 62% of the cases are in Asia and 34% in Africa; the majority occur in India and Africa; India alone has about 1.2 million registered cases. In some sections of developing countries prevalence may be as high as 40/1,000 population.

There are approximately 6,000 cases of leprosy in the United States, and 200 to 250 new cases are reported each year. New York, California, Hawaii, Florida, Louisiana, and Texas have the largest number. In Los Angeles, the number rose dramatically between 1968 and 1985 and was attributed to immigration rather than to secondary infection (Modlin and Rea, 1987). Endemic foci exist in Texas, Louisiana, and Hawaii. The increased incidence of leprosy in this country appears to be attributable entirely to immigrants, particularly those from Mexico, the Philippines, and Southeast Asia. In the United States, 33% of patients are Hispanic. Forty percent of all cases occur in individuals 20 to 40 years.

Although the leprosy bacillus, *Mycobacterium leprae,* was first identified by Hansen in 1874, the bacteria still cannot be cultivated on artificial media. It is cultivable in animals, however; the mouse (via footpad inoculation), the nine-banded armadillo, and both the sooty mangabey and rhesus monkey are susceptible to laboratory infection. Natural infection of wild armadillos has been described; there have been anecdotal reports of human leprosy following contact with these animals, but the relationship is unclear. Most cases of human leprosy occur in areas where armadillos do not exist (eg, India).

Provided that the disease is under therapeutic control, leprosy is no longer a reason to deny an immigrant entry into the United States. Therefore, although the possibility is still remote, the likelihood of a physician encountering a patient with leprosy is greater today than ever before because of the ease of intercontinental travel and the steady influx of immigrants from endemic areas.

As noted, mycobacterial infections, including tuberculosis, have been associated with HIV infection. It appears that high-grade pathogens, such as *M. tuberculosis,* may develop earlier in AIDS patients than low-grade pathogens, such as *M. avium,* which become apparent when immune deficiency is more advanced. There have been a few reports of an association between HIV infection and leprosy, a disease that is associated with a defect in cell-mediated immunity (Lamfers et al, 1987; Turk and Rees, 1988; Meeran, 1989). In a study conducted in Zambia, 6 of 18 newly diagnosed patients with leprosy were HIV seropositive; in comparison, 27 of 54 suspected tuberculosis patients were seropositive. The prevalence of HIV infection was significantly higher among patients with leprosy than among blood donors or surgical patients (Meeran, 1989). Further epidemiologic studies must be conducted to confirm this reported association and to assess whether it indicates a change in the epidemiologic characteristics of leprosy. However, it is interesting to note that infection with the simian immunodeficiency virus (SIV) has been reported to increase the susceptibility of rhesus monkeys to leprosy, an event possibly related to loss of T-helper cell function (Gormus et al, 1989).

There is little reason to fear that leprosy will spread throughout the United States because patient infectivity declines markedly with chemotherapy. In recent years, no spread attributable to imported cases has been reported.

Although other possibilities exist, the most widely held view is that leprosy is spread by bacilli from the upper respiratory tract of infected persons that enter through the respiratory tract of susceptible individuals. As many as 200 individuals may become infected for every overt case that develops and is detected; however, only 5% may develop active disease and 80% of those that do will have paucibacillary infection. The chief source of infection is the untreated or inadequately treated patient with multibacillary disease. The infectivity rate does not appear to be high, and it is believed that the incubation period varies from three to ten years. The clinical attack rate in close family contacts of multibacillary cases is 5% to 10%. Hospitalization is usually unnecessary and, since therapy rapidly renders the patient noninfectious, isolation is not required.

The World Health Organization has proclaimed the goal of eliminating leprosy as a public health problem by the year 2000 (elimination is defined as a prevalence of one case/10,000 population or less).

Types: There are two major polar types of leprosy: tuberculoid and lepromatous. Intermediate between the two is the borderline or dimorphous type. Indeterminate leprosy is an early form manifested by a hypopigmented macule; it has a variable course. In about 75% of patients, the lesion heals spontaneously; other patients remain indeterminate for a prolonged period. Without treatment, the condition may progress to tuberculoid, borderline, or lepromatous leprosy. Tuberculoid leprosy characteristically consists of one to a few well-circumscribed skin lesions with profound anesthesia; there also may be an enlarged nerve nearby. Lepromatous leprosy consists of widespread, usually symmetrical, distribution of skin lesions and is characterized by anergy. Skin lesions consist of massive numbers of macrophages that contain large numbers of bacilli. Worldwide, tuberculoid leprosy is the most common form; however, in the United States, 67% of cases reported in 1981 were of the borderline-lepromatous type.

The different forms of leprosy are thought to be due to differences in cell-mediated immunity to *M. leprae*. The relative degree of host resistance to *M. leprae* is greatest in tuberculoid and most indeterminate forms; in the lepromatous type, resistance is severely compromised.

The different clinical forms of leprosy have been classified into five different groups (Ridley and Jopling, 1966) by subdividing the borderline type into three subgroups: borderline-tuberculoid (BT), borderline-lepromatous (BL), and mid-borderline (BB) between the two. The characteristics of these forms are shown in Table 10.

Paucibacillary leprosy includes the indeterminate, tuberculoid (TT), and borderline-tuberculoid (BT) groups; multibacillary leprosy includes the lepromatous (LL), borderline-lepromatous (BL), and mid-borderline (BB) groups. This classification is very useful for prognosis and for determining therapy and duration of treatment.

Clinical Aspects: Skin lesions, skin anesthesia, and enlarged nerves are three cardinal signs of infection with *M. leprae.* These features are related to bacterial proliferation, host immunologic responses to leprotic antigens, and peripheral neuritis due to the preceding two processes. In the skin, hypopigmented and hypoanesthetic patches appear as macules, plaques, or nodules. Skin biopsy reveals a granuloma consisting of macrophages and lymphocytes. Tuberculoid granulomas are well organized and consist of a central core of mature macrophages and a surrounding mantle of lymphocytes, whereas lepromatous granulocytes are disorganized and principally consist of immature macrophages (histio-

**TABLE 10.
A CLINICAL CLASSIFICATION OF HANSEN'S DISEASE BASED ON THE RIDLEY-JOPLING CLASSIFICATION**

	Type of HD			
Observation or Test	**TT**	**BT**	**BB-BL**	**LL**
Number of skin lesions	Single usually	Single or few	Several or many	Very many
Size of lesions	Variable	Variable	Variable	Small
Surface of lesions	Very dry, sometimes scaly	Dry	Shiny	Shiny
Hair growth in lesions	Absent	Moderately diminished	Slightly diminished	Not affected
Sensation in lesions (not face)	Completely lost	Moderate-marked loss	Slight-moderate loss	No loss
AFB in smears	Nil	Nil or scanty	Several or many	Very many
AFB in nasal scrapings or in nose-blows	Nil	Nil	Nil (scanty rarely)	Very many
Lepromin test	Strongly positive (+ + +)	Weakly positive (+ or + +)	Negative	Negative

From Jopling WH: Clinical classification of Hansen's disease. The Star, *Carville, Louisiana, May-June 1983. Reprinted with permission.*
AFB = acid-fast bacilli; TT = tuberculoid; BT = borderline-tuberculoid; BB-BL = mid-borderline and borderline-lepromatous; LL = lepromatous

cytes) and a sprinkling of lymphocytes. Numerous acid-fast bacilli are found in lepromatous lesions, but few are present in tuberculoid lesions. In advanced cases, the former may contain as many as 10^{10} bacilli per gram of tissue. The large number of bacilli in macrophages in lepromatous lesions results in a foamy appearance; large fatty droplets of aggregated organisms in these cells are called "globi."

Leprosy always involves the peripheral nerves; tuberculoid patients characteristically have anesthetic lesions, while lepromatous patients typically have an acrodistal symmetric anesthesia. Damage to nerves occurs as a result of episodic, immunologically mediated inflammation directed against leprotic antigens and to bacterial growth, most likely in Schwann cells and neighboring macrophages. This results in a loss of sensation and motor control, wasting, and acute deformities. Deformities also are associated with the loss of protective sensation and resulting traumatization of extremities, open wounds, and secondary infection. Acute neuritis always requires the administration of corticosteroids (eg, prednisolone). Rarely, neurosurgical procedures such as neurolysis may be needed for relief of pain and improvement in nerve function caused by constriction of swollen nerves. Corrective surgery may be of value in reducing deformity and reconstituting limb function.

The course of infection appears to be directly related to the host's innate cell-mediated immune (CMI) response to the leprosy bacillus. When the host's CMI response is poor, multibacillary (lepromatous) disease develops; when the CMI response is adequate, bacillary replication is inhibited and a localized lesion develops that has a tendency to heal without treatment (indeterminate tuberculoid leprosy). In multibacillary disease, anterior uveitis is a common complication and requires mydriatic and corticosteroid drops; when untreated, blindness occurs.

CMI response may have a genetic basis. Intradermal skin tests with lepromin, a heat-killed suspension of *M. leprae* prepared from infected armadillo tissue, is uniformly negative in lepromatous patients and remains so even after years of chemotherapy. The lepromin test has no diagnostic value, but it may be of prognostic significance. The exact defect in the CMI response is not known but may exist at the lymphocyte or macrophage level. In lepromatous leprosy, specific T-helper cells may be absent or fail to function (clonal deletion hypothesis). *M. leprae*-specific T-suppressor cell activity has been hypothesized to inhibit the activity of T-helper cells. In leprosy, macrophages have been shown to inhibit T-cell responses and to be defective in antigen presentation and in the production of interleukin 1. The failure of the macrophage to kill the leprosy bacillus is key to understanding the mechanisms of host resistance.

Antibodies to leprotic antigens directly correlate with bacillary load and inversely with CMI response. The highest titers are found in lepromatous patients; tuberculoid patients have the lowest. Thus, these antibodies do not appear to be protective; however, they could play a role in the pathogenesis of erythema nodosum leprosum reactions.

Leprosy Reactions: Reactions occur during the treatment of leprosy in up to 50% of patients. Two types are seen: Type 1 (reversal) reactions in the borderline and tuberculoid forms and Type 2 (erythema nodosum leprosum [ENL]) reactions in the lepromatous and, occasionally, borderline forms.

Type 1 reactions commonly occur during the first six months of treatment. Neuritis is the predominant symptom and may become severe and lead to sensorimotor loss. Skin lesions may become erythematous, edematous, and occasionally ulcerate. There may be edema of the face, hands, or feet. This type of reaction is generally considered to be a phenomenon of delayed hypersensitivity associated with an increase in the cell-mediated immune response to *M. leprae*.

Type 2 reactions are associated most commonly with lepromatous leprosy. They usually occur later in the course of treatment than type 1 reactions. Crops of erythematous nodules may appear anywhere on the skin, often accompanied by fever and malaise. Neuritis, orchitis, iridocyclitis, arthritis, proteinuria, and lymphadenopathy also may occur. In severe reactions, lesions may become vesicular or bullous and break down. Muscle paralysis is less common and severe than in type 1 reactions. Type 2 reactions are thought to be caused by changes in the CMI response to *M. leprae* and are mediated through increased production of tumor necrosis factor (TNF) and interleukin 2 (IL-2).

Patients with mild leprosy reactions may require no treatment or can be treated with analgesic doses of aspirin or other nonsteroidal anti-inflammatory agents, such as ibuprofen.

Severe leprosy reactions of either type respond to corticosteroids; prednisone 60 mg daily is usually sufficient for initial control (larger doses may be necessary in patients receiving rifampin), and the dose often can be reduced gradually to an alternate-day schedule if prolonged therapy is required. Corticosteroids should be used whenever neuritis occurs or a skin ulceration appears.

Thalidomide is the treatment of choice for type 2 reactions and is available only for this investigational use in the United States. It is of no value in type 1 reactions. After an initial dose of up to 400 mg daily (adults), the amount often can be decreased over two weeks to a maintenance level of 100 mg daily. Periodic attempts should be made to discontinue the drug; the course can be repeated if symptoms recur. Except under unusual circumstances, thalidomide is contraindicated in women of child-bearing age who might conceive during therapy. When it is used in these patients, effective birth control must be guaranteed, preferably through the use of implantable contraceptives.

Clofazimine given daily may slowly control leprosy reactions of either type but is not useful in the acute management of serious reactions. The manufacturer recommends a dosage of 100 to 200 mg daily for up to three months; the dose should be tapered to 100 mg daily as soon as possible after the reactive episode is controlled.

In general, chemotherapy should be continued despite the appearance of a leprosy reaction because discontinuing or reducing the dose of dapsone or any other medication will not immediately ameliorate the reactive episode. Withdrawal of therapy may have been responsible, at least in part, for the appearance of sulfone-resistant strains of *M. leprae*.

The treatment of leprosy or leprosy reactions is difficult and complex and should be undertaken only by specialists or in consultation with them. Assistance is available at all times from the experts at the National Hansen's Disease Center (NHDC).

See the evaluations for adverse reactions and precautions.

Household Contacts: A household contact has been defined as "anyone who has lived with the patient for at least one month since the onset of his symptoms." It has been established that 20% to 45% of leprosy cases may be traced to household contacts. Family members are said be eight times more likely to develop lepromatous leprosy and four times more likely to develop tuberculoid leprosy (Hendrick and Wilkin, 1982). It is recommended that all family members be screened once yearly for at least five years.

Drug Selection

Generally, leprosy is best managed by specialists who, in the United States, are usually associated with the NHDC or with various outpatient clinics associated with the NHDC located in states where the disease is most prevalent. Indeed, the resources of these facilities are usually required to establish a diagnosis.

Biopsies will be examined, at no cost, at the NHDC. The biopsy should be taken entirely from within the lesion and preserved in neutral formalin. Once the diagnosis is established, the attending physician must report the case to the state health department whether he decides to treat the patient himself or refers the patient to NHDC facilities.

Current recommendations for the treatment of leprosy may be obtained from the NHDC at Carville, Louisiana ([800] 642-2477). This institution and its clinics provide free care to any leprosy patient irrespective of nationality or citizenship. Outpatient leprosy clinics are located in Los Angeles, San Francisco, San Diego, Seattle, Boston, Staten Island, Miami, San Antonio, and Chicago.

Regimens: Chemotherapy is the mainstay in the treatment of leprosy. The broad objectives of chemotherapy are (1) to render the patient noninfectious; (2) to prevent further bacterial multiplication; and (3) to avoid or treat reactions.

Treatment of leprosy with sulfones was introduced in 1943. For many years, monotherapy with dapsone was the treatment of choice; in the early years, small initial doses were given and the amount was increased gradually to maintenance levels. In subsequent years, full dosage levels were used throughout treatment. However, the widespread use of dapsone as monotherapy has resulted in the emergence of resistant *M. leprae*. Primary and secondary resistance to dapsone has been increasing since it was first reported in 1964. In some countries, primary resistance has been reported to be as high as 40%. In the United States, the problem of primary resistance is not as great as that of secondary resistance. At the NHDC, secondary resistance has been as high as 10%.

An additional problem in leprosy chemotherapy is the presence of "persisters." These viable, fully drug-susceptible *M. leprae* are able to survive for many years in the patient, despite the presence of bactericidal concentrations of an antileprosy drug. They are dormant bacilli that escape the action of antileprosy drugs and may cause relapses after the cessation of chemotherapy. No single drug eliminates these persisting organisms.

The persistence of *M. leprae* and the development of primary and secondary resistance to dapsone have led to recommendations that multiple-drug therapy be used for the treatment of leprosy. It is hoped that combination drug regimens will prevent the development of resistant strains of *M. leprae* where they do not already exist and/or shorten the treatment period.

The NHDC currently advises the regimens described in Tables 11 and 12.

TABLE 11.
NHDC[1] STANDARD REGIMENS FOR CHEMOTHERAPY OF LEPROSY

PAUCIBACILLARY FORMS (I, TT, BT)[2]

Sulfone-sensitive strains

Dapsone: 100 mg daily for six months; *for I and TT forms,* drug is continued for three years after negative skin tests; *for BT form*, drug is continued for five years after negative skin tests

Rifampin: 600 mg daily for six months (I, TT, and BT)

Sulfone-resistant strains

Clofazimine: 50 to 100 mg daily is given in place of dapsone in the above regimen

MULTIBACILLARY FORMS (BB, BL, LL)[3]

Sulfone-sensitive strains

Dapsone: 100 mg daily for three years; *for BB,* drug is continued for 10 years beyond negative skin tests; *for BL and LL*, drug is continued indefinitely

Rifampin: 600 mg daily for three years

Sulfone-resistant strains

Clofazimine:[4] *For BB, BL, and LL*, 50 to 100 mg daily indefinitely

Rifampin: *For BB, BL, and LL*, 600 mg daily for three years

[1] *National Hansen's Disease Center*
[2] *I = indeterminate; TT = tuberculoid; BT = borderline-tuberculoid*
[3] *BB = mid-borderline; BL = borderline-lepromatous; LL = lepromatous*
[4] *Ethionamide 250 mg daily and rifampin 600 mg daily given indefinitely may be substituted for clofazimine for those who refuse it because of the pigmentation produced.*

TABLE 12.
NHDC[1] INVESTIGATIONAL REGIMENS FOR CHEMOTHERAPY OF LEPROSY

PAUCIBACILLARY FORMS (I, TT, BT)[2]

Dapsone: 100 mg (1 to 2 mg/kg) daily

Rifampin: 600 mg daily or once monthly

Treatment is continued for 12 months and then is discontinued.

MULTIBACILLARY FORMS (BB, BL, LL)[3]

Dapsone: 100 mg (1 to 2 mg/kg) daily

Rifampin: 600 mg daily or once monthly for patients weighing >35 kg; 450 mg daily or once monthly for those weighing <35 kg.

Clofazamine: 300 mg once monthly plus 50 mg daily

Treatment is continued for two years and then is discontinued.

[1] *National Hansen's Disease Center*
[2] *I = indeterminate; TT = tuberculoid; BT = borderline-tuberculoid*
[3] *BB = mid-borderline; BL = borderline-lepromatous; LL = lepromatous*

In reviewing the existing world situation, particularly that in underdeveloped countries where cost and compliance are significant factors, the World Health Organization Study Group on Chemotherapy for Leprosy (World Health Organization, 1982) felt that the widespread prevalence of dapsone resistance precluded the recommendation of dapsone plus *one* additional drug for multibacillary leprosy, since this was likely to give rise to multiple drug resistance. It therefore recommended that two additional drugs be combined with dapsone, one of which is rifampin because of its great potency. The Study Group also felt that multidrug regimens should allow a shortened course of therapy, noting that long-term treatment (up to lifelong) is not feasible in most developing countries. The multibacillary regimen (Table 13) was designed for the treatment of all patients with multibacillary leprosy, including those who are newly diagnosed and previously untreated, as well as those previously treated with dapsone monotherapy regardless of therapeutic outcome.

The World Health Organization Study Group (World Health Organization, 1982) also has recommended only four drugs for combined chemotherapy: dapsone, rifampin, clofazimine, and ethionamide. (When available, protionamide may replace the latter, although it has no particular advantage.) Dapsone is inexpensive and nontoxic in recommended dosages and is weakly bactericidal against *M. leprae* in humans. Although expensive, rifampin is rapidly bactericidal for *M. leprae*; toxic effects have not occurred after monthly administration, although adverse effects may be encountered when this drug is given at shorter intervals. Clofazimine also is expensive and its major adverse effect is skin pigmentation. It is weakly bactericidal against the leprosy bacillus. Ethionamide has less bactericidal activity than rifampin; it is an alternative to clofazimine when the latter is unacceptable.

The WHO Study Group recommended short-course chemotherapy with rifampin and dapsone for all patients with paucibacillary leprosy (see Table 13). The recommendations take into account the practical constraints under which field programs have to operate, the cost, and the fact that precise classification of patients might not be possible. Therefore, the patients were divided into two groups: paucibacillary and multibacillary. It was presumed that sulfone resistance is common and, therefore, that any regimen should be effective against both sensitive and resistant strains. A low percentage of relapses is considered acceptable. In order to assure patient compliance, regimens should be fully supervisable.

The Study Group reasoned that, since the bacterial load in paucibacillary leprosy is much lower than that in the multibacillary type, the probability of encountering drug-resistant mutants is insignificant. Also, bacterial persisters are likely to be contained by cell-mediated immunity, which is adequate in these patients. Therefore, short-course chemotherapy is feasible, especially with the bactericidal drug, rifampin. Patients are not expected to harbor rifampin-resistant *M. leprae* bacilli. The regimen should not be interrupted if reversal reactions occur.

TABLE 13.
WHO RECOMMENDED STANDARD REGIMENS FOR CHEMOTHERAPY OF LEPROSY[1]

PAUCIBACILLARY FORMS[2] (I, TT, BT)[3]

Rifampin: 600 mg once monthly for six months. Supervised.

Dapsone: 100 mg (1 to 2 mg/kg) daily for six months. Self-administered.

Follow-up should be continued for a minimum of four years.

MULTIBACILLARY FORMS[2] (LL, BL, BB)[4]

Rifampin: 600 mg once monthly for patients >35 kg; 450 mg once monthly for those <35 kg. Supervised.

Dapsone: 100 mg/day (1 to 2 mg/kg). Self-administered.

Clofazimine:[5] 300 mg once monthly, supervised, and 50 mg daily, self-administered.

Treatment Period: Minimum two years (preferably to smear negativity).

[1] *World Health Organization, 1982.*
[2] *These regimens still have to be evaluated in a significantly large number of patients over a long-term period.*
[3] *I = indeterminate; TT = tuberculoid; BT = borderline-tuberculoid*
[4] *LL = lepromatous; BL = borderline-lepromatous; BB = mid-borderline*
[5] *When clofazimine is unacceptable, it may be replaced by ethionamide 250 to 375 mg (5 to 10 mg/kg) daily, self-administered.*

The WHO regimens have become the standard treatment for leprosy throughout most of the world. Data from WHO indicate that the relapse rate in patients treated with these regimens is very low (approximately 1% overall with up to nine years of followup).

Investigational Therapy: Antimicrobial resistance has resulted in the use of multidrug therapy as a standard practice for the treatment of leprosy. Currently recommended regimens employ rifampin, clofazamine, and dapsone. However, because clofazamine and dapsone are only weakly active against *M. leprae*, new bactericidal agents with different mechanisms of action have been sought. Two classes of drugs that seem to hold promise are the tetracycline, minocycline, and the fluoroquinolones, pefloxacin and ofloxacin [Floxin]. These drugs are bactericidal for *M. leprae*, but significantly less than rifampin. Tetracyclines interfere with protein synthesis by blocking the attachment of aminoacyl transfer RNA to the messenger RNA-ribosome complex, while fluoroquinolones inhibit the enzyme DNA gyrase that controls supercoiling of DNA in bacteria. Results of clinical trials conducted with these agents have been encouraging.

In one recent study, eight patients (five with lepromatous leprosy, three with borderline lepromatous leprosy) who had been previously untreated (six patients) or whose leprosy had relapsed (two patients) were given minocycline (100 mg/day) for three months. After one week of treatment, improvement in either skin erythema or induration was observed in six patients and improvement in both manifestations was observed in two patients. After three months, skin lesions had noticeably improved in all patients and six patients had complete resolution of erythema and induration. *M. leprae* organisms were isolated from skin biopsies and inoculated into the footpads of mice; no patient was found to harbor any viable organisms at either two or three months after starting treatment (Gelber et al, 1992).

A six-month trial of pefloxacin was conducted in previously untreated lepromatous patients in Africa. Among the 10 patients selected, seven were classified as polar lepromatous and three as borderline lepromatous; all had active skin lesions with a high bacterial index. Pefloxacin was given as monotherapy (400 mg twice daily) for six months. After this period, all patients were placed on the WHO regimen for multibacillary leprosy for a minimum of two years. Definite clinical improvement was seen in all patients as early as two months after the initiation of therapy with pefloxacin, and there was a relatively rapid bactericidal effect as determined by serial mouse footpad inoculations; approximately 99% of the bacilli were killed during the first two months of treatment. Pefloxacin was well tolerated throughout the six-month trial (N'Deli et al, 1990).

A subsequent study compared pefloxacin and ofloxacin, both given orally, in the treatment of lepromatous leprosy. Among 21 previously untreated patients selected for the study, 19 were classified as lepromatous and 2 as borderline lepromatous. The patients were randomly assigned to two groups: 11 to receive pefloxacin and 10 ofloxacin. All patients received 800 mg of either pefloxacin or ofloxacin on day 1 and stopped treatment from day 2 to 7. On day 7, monotherapy was resumed with daily administration of either pefloxacin 800 mg or ofloxacin 400 mg until day 56. Thereafter, the WHO regimen for multibacillary leprosy was given in addition to either pefloxacin or ofloxacin until day 180. A definite improvement in clinical manifestations was observed in all patients in both groups on day 28 (after 22 doses), and the killing rate of *M. leprae* ranged from 99% to 99.999% for both groups. The clinical response continued during the period of combined therapy, and marked improvement was seen in all patients six months after initiation of the trial. By day 56 of monotherapy, no viable organisms could be isolated from skin biopsies by the mouse footpad technique. Both fluoroquinolones were well tolerated (Grosset el al, 1990).

These results prompted the WHO to organize a large-scale, multicenter field trial to compare the efficacy, safety, and acceptability of combined regimens containing ofloxacin with the regimens currently recommended by WHO in patients with both multibacillary and paucibacillary leprosy. Of particular interest is the combination of ofloxacin and rifampin because of its potential to shorten the duration of treatment to one month. A double-blind, randomized, controlled, seven-nation trial involving 4,000 patients is now underway. Results are expected by 1996 or 1997.

Drug Evaluations

CLOFAZIMINE
[Lamprene]

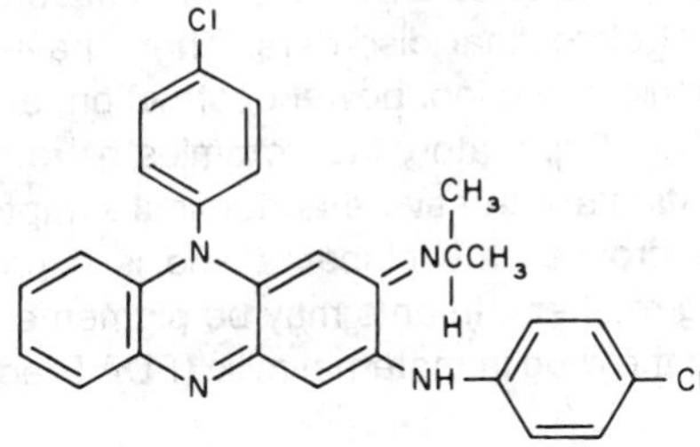

ACTIONS AND USES. This fat-soluble aminophenazine dye has been used for the treatment of leprosy since the early 1960s but was approved for this use in the United States only in the late 1980s. It has been used investigationally in combination with other antimycobacterial drugs to treat *Mycobacterium avium* infections in AIDS patients. Clofazimine has a bactericidal effect similar to that of dapsone and rifampin and is the treatment of choice (given with rifampin) when sulfone-resistant *M. leprae* are present. Clofazimine also has a marked anti-inflammatory effect and is given to control the leprosy reaction, erythema nodosum leprosum.

The mechanism of its antibacterial action is uncertain. It preferentially binds to mycobacterial DNA and interferes with growth. Clofazimine is slowly bactericidal for *M. leprae;* a delay of 50 days is required before bactericidal activity can be demonstrated in biopsy tissue from leprosy patients. The drug is active against *M. avium* isolates in vitro with an MIC varying from 1 to 5 mcg/ml. Clofazimine does not show cross resistance with either dapsone or rifampin. Resistance to clofazimine has been reported only rarely. The mechanism of action of this drug in controlling erythema nodosum leprosum reaction is unknown.

ADVERSE REACTIONS AND PRECAUTIONS. Clofazimine, a red-colored compound that is deposited in the tissues, may discolor the skin and conjunctivae in 75% to 100% of patients. The skin first develops a reddish hue that may progress to mahogany brown, while the leprosy lesions become even more pigmented and appear mauve, slate gray, or black. The degree of pigmentation varies from patient to patient; generally, the larger the dose and the more advanced the disease, the more pronounced the pigmentation. The conjunctivae become varying shades of red-brown. In addition, a red tint may appear in the urine, sputum, and sweat. All of these effects clear slowly after therapy is discontinued. Skin discoloration may cause depression in patients.

Diminished sweating and tear production due to an anticholinergic effect may be noted, and photosensitivity reactions have been reported.

Gastrointestinal disturbances are the most serious adverse effects of clofazimine and develop in about 50% of patients. Nausea, vomiting, and diarrhea are uncommon if the dose is 100 mg or less daily. Larger doses sometimes produce abdominal pain and, because of extensive deposition of the drug in the wall of the small bowel, which may become edematous, symptoms suggesting bowel obstruction occasionally develop. Clofazimine should be used with caution in patients who have gastrointestinal disorders. There have been rare reports of splenic infarction, bowel obstruction, and gastrointestinal bleeding. Exploratory laparotomies have been needed in some patients with severe abdominal symptoms.

Clofazimine crosses the placenta and is excreted in the milk of nursing mothers. Infants may be pigmented at birth or after ingesting the drug in maternal milk (FDA Pregnancy Category C).

PHARMACOKINETICS. The absorption of clofazimine is quite variable, ranging from 45% to 62% after oral administration. The drug has a long half-life; after repeated administration, it is about 70 days. Clofazimine is widely, but unevenly, distributed throughout the body. It is highly lipophilic. High concentrations are found in the reticuloendothelial system, subcutaneous fat, and distal small bowel. It is excreted slowly, largely unmetabolized; less than 1% appears in the urine.

DOSAGE AND PREPARATIONS.

Oral: *Adults,* 50 to 100 mg daily. The WHO Study Group (World Health Organization, 1982) has recommended 300 mg once monthly, supervised, and 50 mg daily, self-administered, for treatment of multibacillary leprosy. Control of leprosy reactions may require 100 mg three times daily, but the dose must be reduced at once if symptoms of gastrointestinal toxicity develop.

Lamprene (Geigy). Capsules 50 and 100 mg.

DAPSONE

H_2N–⟨benzene ring⟩–SO_2–⟨benzene ring⟩–NH_2

ACTIONS. Dapsone is an analogue of p-aminobenzoic acid and inhibits the synthesis of folic acid. It is principally bacteriostatic, although in the mouse footpad test it appears to have some bactericidal properties also.

USES. This sulfone continues to be a drug of choice for all patients infected with sulfone-sensitive *Mycobacterium leprae*. Dapsone is inexpensive and nontoxic in the usual dosage range. A dose of 100 mg/day produces peak serum levels that exceed the MIC by a factor of approximately 500 and has some bactericidal activity against the leprosy bacillus. Maximum dosage should be used from the initiation of therapy and continued during leprosy reactions.

Dapsone has been administered alone for the treatment of all forms of leprosy and has been suggested for prophylaxis of household contacts of borderline and lepromatous patients. However, the increasing incidence of sulfone-resistant organisms has precipitated a re-evaluation of dapsone monotherapy, and it is now recommended that other antileprosy drugs (most commonly rifampin and clofazimine) be given with dapsone.

Dapsone has been used investigationally for both prophylaxis and treatment of *Pneumocystis carinii* pneumonia in AIDS patients (Mills et al, 1988).

ADVERSE REACTIONS AND PRECAUTIONS. Adverse reactions are usually mild and occur infrequently with the doses used to treat leprosy. Nausea, vomiting, headache, dizziness, and tachycardia are uncommon, and methemoglobinemia, leukopenia, and agranulocytosis are rare with therapeutic doses. Peripheral neuropathy has been reported as a rare complication of dapsone therapy in nonleprosy patients.

The major adverse effects of dapsone are dose-dependent hemolytic anemias. Many patients receiving 100 mg/day experience an increased rate of erythrocyte destruction; however, this is severe only in occasional patients with glucose-6-phosphate dehydrogenase (G6PD) deficiency.

Deaths from agranulocytosis, aplastic anemia, and other blood dyscrasias have been associated with dapsone. The manufacturer recommends that complete blood counts should be performed frequently: weekly for the first month, monthly for six months, and semimonthly thereafter in conjunction with baseline and periodic liver function tests.

A hypersensitivity reaction, termed the "sulfone syndrome," also occurs rarely. It begins one to four weeks after administration (Tomecki and Catalano, 1981) and is characterized by fever, malaise, exfoliative dermatitis, jaundice with hepatic necrosis, lymphadenopathy, methemoglobinemia, and anemia. The condition improves if dapsone is withdrawn and corticosteroid therapy is given.

Dapsone is carcinogenic in laboratory rodents. However, no teratogenic effect has been reported to date in humans, although neonatal mortality may be higher than normal; careful observation of the neonate is recommended (Farb et al,

1982). This drug is classified in FDA Pregnancy Category C. Dapsone is excreted in breast milk in large quantities. Mild reversible hemolytic anemia transmitted through breast milk has been reported in one infant (Sanders et al, 1982).

PHARMACOKINETICS. Dapsone is rapidly (time to peak effect is four to eight hours) and almost completely absorbed after oral administration. The drug is 50% bound to plasma protein. The plasma elimination half-life ranges from 10 to 50 hours with a mean of 28 hours. About 70% to 80% of a dose is excreted as N-glucuronide or N-sulfamate conjugates. Dapsone is acetylated in the liver, and enterohepatic circulation accounts for appreciable tissue levels three weeks after therapy is terminated. Rifampin lowers dapsone levels seven- to tenfold by increasing plasma clearance.

DOSAGE AND PREPARATIONS.

***Oral:** Adults and children,* 100 mg (1 to 2 mg/kg) daily. Dapsone is usually given with other antileprosy drugs, most commonly rifampin and clofazimine. It is advisable to screen the patient for G6PD deficiency prior to initiation of therapy. If deficiency is found, the drug should be given more cautiously, starting with a dosage of 25 mg twice weekly. If the patient cannot tolerate the drug and severe hemolysis occurs, clofazimine should be used instead.

Generic. Tablets 25 and 100 mg.

ETHIONAMIDE (Investigational indication)

[Trecator-SC]

The use of this drug for the treatment of leprosy is investigational in the United States. Ethionamide has been shown to be bactericidal for *Mycobacterium leprae* in mice; in humans, its bactericidal effect is intermediate between that of dapsone and rifampin. It is used as an alternative to clofazimine in the triple-drug regimen (dapsone, rifampin, clofazimine) recommended by the WHO Study Group (World Health Organization, 1982) when the latter is not acceptable. Ethionamide also has been used in combination regimens for the treatment of both sulfone-sensitive and sulfone-resistant leprosy.

The major adverse effect of ethionamide in leprosy patients is hepatotoxicity, especially when this drug is given with rifampin.

DOSAGE AND PREPARATIONS.

***Oral:** Adults,* for multibacillary leprosy, 250 to 375 mg daily in combination with other antileprosy drugs (dapsone, rifampin) for at least two years.

Trecator-SC (Wyeth-Ayerst). Tablets 250 mg.

RIFAMPIN (Investigational indication)

[Rifadin, Rimactane]

USES. Rifampin is effective in the treatment of leprosy, but this use is investigational in the United States. It is much more rapidly bactericidal for *Mycobacterium leprae* than the other currently used drugs.

Reports indicate that oral doses of 300 to 600 mg daily (adults) render bacilli noninfective for the mouse footpad and, therefore, presumably noninfectious for contacts more rapidly than dapsone or clofazimine (several days versus two to three months). However, in humans, the longer term response, as measured by clearance of skin lesions and reduction in the number of bacilli in skin smears, is no better.

Some patients have taken rifampin alone for as long as 10 years without problems. On the other hand, resistant strains of *M. leprae* have appeared in three to four years in patients given rifampin monotherapy. Thus, it is now recommended that rifampin be used only in combination drug regimens. Usually these utilize rifampin plus dapsone (plus clofazimine in some patients) for infections with sulfone-sensitive *M. leprae* and rifampin plus either clofazimine or ethionamide for infections with sulfone-resistant *M. leprae*.

ADVERSE REACTIONS AND PRECAUTIONS. The adverse effects of rifampin in the treatment of leprosy are the same as those observed when the drug is used to treat tuberculosis (see the evaluation in the section on Tuberculosis). The induction of P450 enzymes by rifampin may require that larger doses of corticosteroids be given to control leprosy reactions if rifampin is being given daily. Also, methods of contraception other than oral contraceptives are required with a daily rifampin regimen in women of childbearing age who request such protection.

DOSAGE AND PREPARATIONS.

***Oral:** Adults,* the usual dose is 600 mg daily. The WHO Study Group has recommended 600 mg once monthly under supervision in a regimen consisting of rifampin, dapsone, and clofazimine (World Health Organization, 1982).

Rifadin (Marion Merrell Dow). Capsules 150 and 300 mg.

Rimactane (CIBA). Capsules 300 mg.

Cited References

Management of non-respiratory tuberculosis. *Lancet* 1:1423-1424, 1986.

Drug-resistant tuberculosis—Mississippi. *MMWR* 26:417-423, 1977.

Interstate outbreak of drug-resistant tuberculosis involving children—California, Montana, Nevada, Utah. *MMWR* 32:5516-5518, 1983.

Drug-resistant tuberculosis among the homeless—Boston. *MMWR* 34:429-431, 1985.

Tuberculosis and acquired immunodeficiency syndrome—Florida. *MMWR* 35:587-590, 1986.

Multi-drug-resistant tuberculosis—North Carolina. *MMWR* 35:785-787, 1987.

Use of BCG vaccines in control of tuberculosis: Joint statement by the ACIP and the Advisory Committee for the Elimination of Tuberculosis. *MMWR* 37:663-675, 1988.

Tuberculosis and human immunodeficiency virus infection: Recommendations of the Advisory Committee for the Elimination of Tuberculosis (ACET). *MMWR* 38:236-238, 243-250, 1989.

Outbreak of multidrug-resistant tuberculosis—Texas, California, and Pennsylvania. *MMWR* 39:369-372, 1990 A.

Nosocomial transmission of multidrug-resistant tuberculosis to health-care workers and HIV-infected patients in an urban hospital—Florida. *MMWR* 39:718-722, 1990 B.

The use of preventive therapy for tuberculous infection in the United States: Recommendations of the Advisory Committee for Elimination of Tuberculosis. *MMWR* 39(No. RR-8):9-12, 1990 C.

Tuberculosis outbreak among persons in a residential facility for HIV-infected persons—San Francisco. *MMWR* 40:649-652, 1991 A.

Nosocomial transmission of multidrug-resistant tuberculosis among HIV-infected persons—Florida and New York, 1988-1991. *MMWR* 40:585-591, 1991 B.

Purified protein derivative (PPD)-tuberculin anergy and HIV infection: Guidelines for anergy testing and management of anergic persons at risk of tuberculosis. *MMWR* 40(No. RR-5):27-33, 1991 C.

Management of persons exposed to multidrug-resistant tuberculosis. *MMWR* 41(No. RR-11):61-71, 1992.

Initial therapy for tuberculosis in the era of multidrug resistance: Recommendations of the Advisory Council for the Elimination of Tuberculosis. *MMWR* 42(No. RR-7):1-8, 1993.

Agins BD, et al: Effect of combined therapy with ansamycin, clofazimine, ethambutol, and isoniazid for *Mycobacterium avium* infection in patients with AIDS. *J. Infect Dis* 159:784-787, 1989.

Ahn CH, et al: Sulfonamide-containing regimens for disease caused by rifampin-resistant *Mycobacterium kansasii. Am Rev Respir Dis* 135:10-16, 1987.

Algerian Working Group/British Medical Research Council Cooperative Study: Controlled clinical trial comparing 6-month and 12-month regimen in treatment of pulmonary tuberculosis in the Algerian Sahara. *Am Rev Respir Dis* 129:921-928, 1984.

American Thoracic Society: Diagnostic standards and classification of tuberculosis. *Am Rev Respir Dis* 142:725-735, 1990 A.

American Thoracic Society: Diagnosis and treatment of disease caused by nontuberculous mycobacteria. *Am Rev Respir Dis* 142:940-953, 1990 B.

American Thoracic Society/Centers for Disease Control: Treatment of tuberculosis and tuberculous infection in adults and children. *Am Rev Respir Dis* 134:355-363, 1986.

Bailey WC: Treatment of atypical mycobacterial disease. *Chest* 84:625-628, 1983.

Barnes PF, et al: Tuberculosis in patients with human immunodeficiency virus infection. *N Engl J Med* 234:1644-1650, 1991.

Black MM, Eykyn S: The successful treatment of tropical fish tank granuloma *(Mycobacterium marinum* infections). *Arch Intern Med* 146:902-904, 1986.

Bloch AB, et al: The epidemiology of tuberculosis in the United States. *Semin Respir Infect* 4:157-170, 1989.

Borcherding SM, et al: Update on rifampin drug interactions II. *Arch Intern Med* 152:711-716, 1992.

Carpenter JL, Parks JM: *Mycobacterium kansasii* infections in patients positive for human immunodeficiency virus. *Rev Infect Dis* 13:789-796, 1991.

Centers for Disease Control: *National HIV Seroprevalence Surveys: Summary of Results: Data From Serosurveillance Activities Through 1989*. Washington, DC, US Dept of Health and Human Services, publication HIV/CID/9-90/006, 1990.

Chaisson RE, et al: Tuberculosis in patients with the acquired immunodeficiency syndrome: Clinical features, response to therapy, and survival. *Am Rev Respir Dis* 36:570-574, 1987.

Chaisson RE, et al: Clarithromycin therapy for disseminated *Mycobacterium avium* complex (MAC) in AIDS, abstract 891. Interscience Conference on Antimicrobial Agents and Chemotherapy (ICACC), Washington, DC, American Society for Microbiology, 1992.

Chawla PK, et al: Drug-resistant tuberculosis in an urban population including patients at risk for human immunodeficiency virus infection. *Am Rev Respir Dis* 146:280-284, 1992.

Cohn DL, et al: A 62-dose, 6-month therapy for pulmonary and extrapulmonary tuberculosis: A twice-weekly, directly observed, and cost-effective regimen. *Ann Intern Med* 112:407-415, 1990.

Coleman DL, Slutkin G: Chemoprophylaxis against tuberculosis. *West J Med* 140:106-110, 1984.

Combs DL, et al: USPHS tuberculosis short-course chemotherapy trial 21: Effectiveness, toxicity, and acceptability: The report of final results. *Ann Intern Med* 112:397-406, 1990.

Comstock GW, Woolpert SF: Preventive therapy, in Kubica GP, Wayne LG (eds): *The Mycobacteria: A Sourcebook*. New York, Marcel Dekker, 1984, 1071-1082.

Crowle AJ, et al: Inhibition by pyrazinamide of tubercle bacilli within cultured human macrophages. *Am Rev Respir Dis* 134:1052-1055, 1986.

Daley CL, et al: An outbreak of tuberculosis with accelerated progression among persons infected with the human immunodeficiency virus. *N Engl J Med* 326:231-235, 1992.

Dautzenberg B, et al: Activity of clarithromycin against *Mycobacterium avium* infection in patients with the acquired immune deficiency syndrome: A controlled clinical trial. *Am Rev Respir Dis* 144:564-569, 1991.

Dautzenberg B, et al: Clarithromycin and other antimicrobial agents in the treatment of disseminated *Mycobacterium avium* infections in patients with acquired immunodeficiency syndrome. *Arch Intern Med* 153:368-372, 1993.

Davidson PT: Drug resistance and the selection of therapy for tuberculosis. *Am Rev Respir Dis* 136:255-257, 1987.

de Lalla F, et al: Clarithromycin-ciprofloxacin-amikacin for therapy of *Mycobacterium avium-Mycobacterium intracellulare* bacteremia in patients with AIDS. *Antimicrob Agents Chemother* 36:1567-1569, 1992.

Douglass J, Steyn LM: A ribosomal gene mutation in streptomycin-resistant *Mycobacterium tuberculosis* isolates, correspondence. *J Infect Dis* 167:1505-1506, 1993.

Dutt AK, et al: Short course chemotherapy for tuberculosis with largely twice-weekly INH-RIF: Results up to 30 months. *Chest* 5:441-447, 1979.

Dutt AK, et al: Short-course chemotherapy for tuberculosis with mainly twice-weekly isoniazid and rifampin: Community physicians' experience with mainly outpatients. *Am J Med* 77:233-242, 1984.

Dutt AK, et al: Short-course chemotherapy for extrapulmonary tuberculosis: Nine years' experience. *Ann Intern Med* 104:7-12, 1986.

Dutt AK, et al: Tuberculous pleural effusion: 6-month therapy with isoniazid and rifampin. *Am Rev Respir Dis* 145:1429-1432, 1992.

Farb H, et al: Clofazimine in pregnancy complicated by leprosy. *Obstet Gynecol* 59:122-123, 1982.

Farer LS, et al: Tuberculosis: Current recommendations for cure and control. *Postgrad Med* 84:58-73, 1988.

Franks AL, et al: Isoniazid hepatitis among pregnant and postpartum Hispanic patients. *Public Health Rep* 104:151-155, 1989.

Gangadharam PRJ, et al: The effects of exposure time, drug concentration, and temperature on the activity of ethambutol versus *Mycobacterium tuberculosis. Am Rev Respir Dis* 141:1478-1482, 1990.

Gelber RH, et al: A clinical trial of minocycline in lepromatous leprosy. *BMJ* 304:91-92, 1992.

Girgis NI, et al: Dexamethasone adjunctive treatment for tuberculous meningitis. *Pediatr Infect Dis J* 10:179-183, 1991.

Goble M, et al: Treatment of 171 patients with pulmonary tuberculosis resistant to isoniazid and rifampin. *N Engl J Med* 328:527-532, 1993.

Gormus BJ, et al: Interactions between simian immunodeficiency virus and *Mycobacterium leprae* in experimentally inoculated rhesus monkeys. *J Infect Dis* 160:405-413, 1989.

Grosset JH, et al: Clinical trial of pefloxacin and ofloxacin in the treatment of lepromatous leprosy. *Int J Leprosy* 58:281-295, 1990.

Guthertz LS, et al: *Mycobacterium avium* and *Mycobacterium intracellulare* infections in patients with and without AIDS. *J Infect Dis* 160:1037-1041, 1989.

Heifets LB, Iseman MD: Determination of *in vitro* susceptibility of mycobacteria to ansamycin. *Am Rev Respir Dis* 132:710-711, 1985.

Heifets LB, et al: Pyrazinamide is not active in vitro against Mycobacterium avium complex. *Am Rev Respir Dis* 134:1287-1288, 1986.

Heifets LB, et al: Bactericidal activity *in vitro* of various rifamycins against *Mycobacterium avium* and *Mycobacterium tuberculosis. Am Rev Respir Dis* 141:626-630, 1990.

Hendrick SS, Wilkin JK: Leprosy. *Am Fam Physician* 26:161-166, 1982.

Hong Kong Chest Service/Tuberculosis Research Centre, Madras/British Medical Research Council: A controlled clinical comparison of 6 and 8 months of antituberculosis chemotherapy in the treatment of patients wih silicotuberculosis in Hong Kong. *Am Rev Respir Dis* 143:262-267, 1991.

Honore N, Cole ST: Molecular basis of rifampin resistance in *Mycobacterium leprae. Antimicrob Agents Chemother* 37:414-418, 1993.

Horsburgh CR Jr, et al: Survival of patients with acquired immune deficiency syndrome and disseminated *Mycobacterium avium* complex infection with and without antimycobacterial chemotherapy. *Am Rev Respir Dis* 144:557-559, 1991.

Hsu KH: Thirty years after isoniazid: Its impact on tuberculosis in children and adolescents. *JAMA* 251:1283-1285, 1984.

International Union Against Tuberculosis: Committee on Prophylaxis: Efficacy of various durations of isoniazid preventive therapy for tuberculosis: Five years of follow-up in the IUAT trial. *Bull WHO* 60:555-564, 1982.

Iseman MD: Treatment of multidrug-resistant tuberculosis. *N Engl J Med* 329:784-791, 1993.

Jacobson MA, et al: Natural history of disseminated *Mycobacterium avium* complex infection in AIDS. *J Infect Dis* 164:994-998, 1991.

Kavi J, et al: Tissue penetration and pharmacokinetics of lomefloxacin following multiple doses. *Eur J Clin Microbiol Infect Dis* 8:168-170, 1989.

Kendig EL Jr: Steroids for meningitis: Tuberculous and bacterial. *Pediatr Infect Dis J* 8:541-542, 1989.

Kohno S, et al: Prospective comparative study of ofloxacin or ethambutol for the treatment of pulmonary tuberculosis. *Chest* 102:1815-1818, 1992.

Kopanoff DE, et al: Isoniazid related hepatitis. *Am Rev Respir Dis* 117:991-1001, 1978.

Lamfers EJP, et al: Leprosy in the acquired immunodeficiency syndrome, letter. *Ann Intern Med* 107:111-112, 1987.

Levine B, Chaisson RE: *Mycobacterium kansasii*: A cause of treatable pulmonary disease associated with advanced human immunodeficiency virus (HIV) infection. *Ann Intern Med* 114:861-868, 1991.

Masur H, Public Health Service Task Force on Prophylaxis and Therapy for *Mycobacterium avium* Complex: Recommendations on prophylaxis and therapy for disseminated *Mycobacterium avium* complex disease in patients infected with the human immunodeficiency virus. *N Engl J Med* 329:898-904, 1993.

McClatchy JK, et al: Use of pyrazinamidase activity in Mycobacterium tuberculosis as a rapid method for determination of pyrazinamide susceptibility. *Antimicrob Agents Chemother* 20:556-557, 1981.

McGowan JE Jr, et al: Guidelines for the use of systemic glucocorticosteroids in the management of selected infections. *J Infect Dis* 165:1-13, 1992.

Meeran K: Prevalence of HIV infection among patients with leprosy and tuberculosis in rural Zambia. *BMJ* 298:364-365, 1989.

Mills J, et al: Dapsone treatment of *Pneumocystis carinii* pneumonia in the acquired immunodeficiency syndrome. *Antimicrob Agents Chemother* 32:1057-1060, 1988.

Modlin RL, Rea TH: Leprosy: New insight into an ancient disease. *J Am Acad Dermatol* 17:1-13, 1987.

Molavi A, et al: Tuberculous meningitis. *Med Clin North Am* 69:315-331, 1985.

Moulding TS, et al: Twenty isoniazid-associated deaths in one state. *Am Rev Respir Dis* 140:700-705, 1989.

N'Deli L, et al: Effectiveness of pefloxacin in the treatment of lepromatous leprosy. *Int J Leprosy* 58:12-18, 1990.

Nightingale SD, et al: Two controlled trials of rifabutin prophylaxis against *Mycobacterium avium* complex infection in AIDS. *N Engl J Med* 329:828-833, 1993.

O'Brien RJ, et al: Epidemiology of nontuberculous mycobacterial diseases in the United States: Results from a national survey. *Am Rev Respir Dis* 135:1007-1014, 1987 A.

O'Brien RJ, et al: Rifabutin (ansamycin LM 427): A new rifamycin-S derivative for the treatment of mycobacterial diseases. *Rev Infect Dis* 9:519-530, 1987 B.

O'Toole RD, et al: Dexamethasone in tuberculous meningitis: Relationship of cerebrospinal fluid effects to therapeutic efficacy. *Ann Intern Med* 70:39-48, 1969.

Pacht ER: *Mycobacterium fortuitum* lung abscess: Resolution with prolonged trimethoprim/sulfamethoxazole therapy. *Am Rev Respir Dis* 141:1599-1601, 1990.

Piersimoni C, et al: *In vitro* activity of the new quinolone lomefloxacin against *Mycobacterium tuberculosis. Am Rev Respir Dis* 146:1445-1447, 1992.

Rastogi N, et al: Pyrazinamide is not effective against intracellularly growing Mycobacterium tuberculosis, letter. *Antimicrob Agents Chemother* 32:287, 1988.

Rastogi N, et al: *In vitro* activity of the new fluorinated quinolone sparfloxacin (AT-4140) against *Mycobacterium tuberculosis* compared with activities of ofloxacin and ciprofloxacin. *Antimicrob Agents Chemother* 35:1933-1936, 1991.

Reichman LB: Why hasn't BCG proved dangerous in HIV-infected patients? *JAMA* 261:3246, 1989.

Ridley DS, Jopling WH: Classification of leprosy according to immunity: Five-group system. *Int J Lepr* 34:255-273, 1966.

Ruf B, et al: Effectiveness of the macrolide clarithromycin in the treatment of *Mycobacterium avium* complex infection in HIV-infected patients. *Infection* 20:267-272, 1992.

Runyon EH: Pathogenic mycobacteria. *Bibl Tuberc Med Thorac* 21:235-237, 1965.

Sanders SW, et al: Hemolytic anemia induced by dapsone transmitted through breast milk. *Ann Intern Med* 96:465-466, 1982.

Selwyn PA, et al: A prospective study of the risk of tuberculosis among intravenous drug users with human immunodeficiency virus infection. *N Engl J Med* 320:545-550, 1989.

Singh N, Yu VL: Successful treatment of pulmonary infection due to *Mycobacterium chelonae*: Case report and review. *Clin Infect Dis* 14:156-161, 1992.

Small PM, et al: Treatment of tuberculosis in patients with advanced human immunodeficiency virus infection. *N Engl J Med* 324:289-294, 1991.

Small PM, et al: Exogenous reinfection with multidrug-resistant *Mycobacterium tuberculosis* in patients with advanced HIV infection. *N Engl J Med* 328:1137-1144, 1993.

Snider DE Jr, Caras GJ: Isoniazid-associated hepatitis deaths: A review of available information. *Am Rev Respir Dis* 145:494-497, 1992.

Snider DE Jr, et al: Treatment of tuberculosis during pregnancy. *Am Rev Respir Dis* 122:65-79, 1980.

Snider DE Jr, et al: Six-months isoniazid-rifampin therapy for pulmonary tuberculosis: Report of United States Public Health Service cooperative trial. *Am Rev Respir Dis* 129:573-579, 1984 A.

Snider DE, et al: Supervised six-months' treatment of newly diagnosed pulmonary tuberculosis using isoniazid, rifampin, and pyrazinamide with and without streptomycin. *Am Rev Respir Dis* 130:1091-1094, 1984 B.

Snider DE, et al: Short course tuberculosis chemotherapy studies conducted in Poland during the past decade. *Eur J Respir Dis* 68:12-18, 1986.

Stead WW: Significance of the tuberculin skin test in elderly persons. *Ann Intern Med* 107:837-842, 1987.

Stead WW, et al: Tuberculosis as an endemic and nosocomial infection among the elderly in nursing homes. *N Engl J Med* 312:1483-1487, 1985.

Stead WW, et al: Benefit-risk considerations in preventive treatment for tuberculosis in elderly persons. *Ann Intern Med* 107:843-845, 1987.

Steiner M, et al: Primary drug-resistant tuberculosis: Report of an outbreak. *N Engl J Med* 283:1353-1358, 1970.

Strang JIG, et al: Controlled trial of prednisolone as adjuvant in treatment of tuberculosis constrictive pericarditis in Transkei. *Lancet* 2:1418-1422, 1987.

Telenti A, et al: Detection of rifampicin-resistance mutations in *Mycobacterium tuberculosis. Lancet* 341:647-650, 1993.

Tomecki KJ, Catalano CJ: Dapsone hypersensitivity: Sulfone syndrome revisited. *Arch Dermatol* 117:38-39, 1981.

Trividi S: Pyrazinamidase activity of Mycobacterium tuberculosis: Test of sensitivity to pyrazinamide. *Tubercle* 68:221-224, 1987.

Turk JL, Rees RJW: AIDS and leprosy. *Lepr Rev* 59:193-194, 1988.

Van Caekenberghe D: Comparative in-vitro activities of ten fluoroquinolones and fusidic acid against *Mycobacterium* spp. *J Antimicrob Chemother* 26:381-386, 1990.

Wallace RJ Jr, et al: Clinical trial of clarithromycin for cutaneous (disseminated) infection due to *Mycobacterium chelonae. Ann Intern Med* 119:482-486, 1993.

Wayne LG, Sramek HA: Agents of newly recognized or infrequently encountered mycobacterial diseases. *Clin Microbiol Rev* 5:1-25, 1992.

Woodley CL, Kilburn JO: In vitro susceptibility of *Mycobacterium avium* complex and *Mycobacterium tuberculosis* strains to a spiropiperidyl rifamycin. *Am Rev Respir Dis* 126:586-587, 1982.

World Health Organization: *Chemotherapy of Leprosy for Control Programmes.* WHO Technical Report Series No. 675, Publication No. ISBN 92 4 120675 6, Geneva, Switzerland, 1982.

Young LS, et al: Activity of ciprofloxacin and other fluorinated quinolones against mycobacteria. *Am J Med* 82 (suppl 4A):23-26, 1987.

Young LS, et al: Azithromycin for treatment of *Mycobacterium avium-intracellulare* complex infection in patients with AIDS. *Lancet* 338:1107-1109, 1991.

Zhang Y, et al: The catalase-peroxidase gene and isoniazid resistance of *Mycobacterium tuberculosis*, letter. *Nature* 358:591-593, 1992.

Drugs Used for Systemic Mycoses

77

For therapeutic purposes, fungal infections (mycoses) may be classified as superficial, subcutaneous, and systemic. This chapter describes the antifungal agents used for subcutaneous mycoses (relatively localized to regions other than the skin or mucous membranes), systemic (disseminated) mycoses, and chronic mucocutaneous candidiasis. For discussion of agents used for superficial mycoses, see index entry Mycoses, Superficial.

Organisms that cause aspergillosis, blastomycosis, coccidioidomycosis, cryptococcosis, histoplasmosis, mucormycosis (zygomycosis), and paracoccidioidomycosis usually enter the body by inhalation. The infection is generally limited to the lung (eg, blastomycosis, coccidioidomycosis, histoplasmosis) or other airway passages (eg, mucormycosis of the nose and sinuses). The fungus may spread hematogenously, usually to specific organs (eg, cutaneous blastomycosis, cryptococcal meningitis) or, in the case of mucormycosis, by direct extension to the orbits and/or brain. Disseminated candidiasis is thought to originate at a mucocutaneous or gastrointestinal tract site rather than in the lung. It also may originate from an infected intravascular catheter. Organisms causing chromoblastomycosis, mycetoma, phaeohyphomycosis, and sporotrichosis commonly enter the body through the skin and spread only to contiguous tissues; therefore, they are often referred to as subcutaneous mycoses. Organisms causing phaeohyphomycosis and sporotrichosis also may be acquired by inhalation. Sporotrichosis often disseminates by way of lymphatic channels but only rarely hematogenously. Chronic mucocutaneous candidiasis is uncommon except in immunocompromised hosts. The skin, scalp, nails, and mucous membranes are usually involved.

Blastomycosis, chromoblastomycosis, coccidioidomycosis, histoplasmosis, mycetoma, paracoccidioidomycosis, and sporotrichosis may develop in immunocompetent individuals. The organisms that cause aspergillosis, candidiasis, cryptococcosis, fusariosis, mucormycosis, and pseudallescheriasis often are termed *opportunistic* pathogens. They occur predominantly in immunocompromised (eg, leukemic, neutropenic) or debilitated patients (eg, those with severe burns, patients who have had major surgery) (Lucente, 1988; Musial et al, 1988). The incidence of opportunistic fungal infections is high in patients with acquired immunodeficiency syndrome (AIDS); up to 90% can be expected to develop at least one fungal infection. Candidiasis is the most common and, with esophageal invasion, is considered a hallmark of AIDS in adults (incidence, up to 50%). Cryptococcal meningitis develops in about 6% to 10% of AIDS patients (Dismukes et al, 1987; Dismukes, 1988). In some geographic areas, disseminated histoplasmosis (Wheat et al, 1985; Graybill, 1988 A) and coccidioidomycosis (Ampel et al, 1989; Galgiani and Ampel, 1990) are observed with increasing frequency in AIDS patients. In recognition of these findings, the Centers For Disease Control (CDC) includes esophageal and mucocutaneous candidiasis and the disseminated forms of coccidioidomycosis, cryptococcosis, and histoplasmosis among its indicator criteria for the diagnosis of AIDS.

Aspergillosis, blastomycosis, candidiasis, coccidioidomycosis, cryptococcosis, histoplasmosis, and sporotrichosis occur in the United States. However, blastomycosis, coccidioidomycosis, and histoplasmosis are endemic in nature and may occur in those who visit or travel through an endemic area as well as in residents. Thus, a complete travel history is essential for an accurate diagnosis of fungal disease. See Table 1 for information on causative organisms, synonyms, and geographic distribution.

TABLE 1.
MEDICALLY IMPORTANT SUBCUTANEOUS AND SYSTEMIC MYCOSES

Infection [Alternative Names]	Organism	Geographic and Demographic Distribution
Aspergillosis	*Aspergillus* species (especially *A. fumigatus* and *A. flavus*)	Worldwide. Neutropenic patients are most susceptible.
Blastomycosis [North American Blastomycosis]	*Blastomyces dermatitidis*	North America (endemic in southeastern and north central United States); occasionally in Africa.
Candidiasis [Moniliasis; Thrush; Candidosis]	*Candida albicans* *C. kruzei* *C. parapsilosis* *C. tropicalis* *C. lusitaniae*	Worldwide. Immunocompromised patients are most susceptible. Invasive disease occurs in neutropenic patients. Mucosal disease occurs in patients with defective CMI.*
Chromoblastomycosis [Chromomycosis]	*Fonsecaea (Hormodendrum) pedrosoi* *F. (H.) compactum* *F. (H.) dermatitidis* *Phialophora verrucosa* *Cladosporium carrioni*	Subcutaneous fungal infection found worldwide. Most common in subtropical countries. Men age 30 to 50 years working in agricultural areas are most commonly infected.
Coccidioidomycosis [San Joaquin Fever; Valley Fever]	*Coccidioides immitis*	Endemic in California (San Joaquin Valley) and other dry regions of southwestern United States (Arizona, New Mexico, Texas, Nevada, and southern Utah), northern Mexico, Central and South America (especially northern Argentina and Paraguay). Severe disease most prevalent in men age 25 to 55 years.
Cryptococcosis [Torulosis]	*Cryptococcus neoformans*	Worldwide. Most commonly affects men age 40 to 60 years. Immunocompromised patients are most susceptible.
Histoplasmosis	*Histoplasma capsulatum*	Principally North America in the central United States, particularly the Mississippi Valley. An African variant of the organism also exists. The young, elderly, and hosts with defective CMI* are most susceptible to disseminated infection.
Mucormycosis	*Rhizopus, Mucor, Rhizomucor, Cunninghamella*, and *Absidia* genera are examples from the Order Mucorales and Class Zygomycetes	Worldwide. Malnourished, neutropenic, diabetic patients are most susceptible. Hemodialysis and deferoxamine therapy are additional risk factors.
Paracoccidioidomycosis [South American Blastomycosis]	*Paracoccidioides brasiliensis*	South and Central America (most common in Brazil), especially in male agricultural workers age 20 to 50 years.
Pseudallescheriasis	*Pseudallescheria boydii*	Worldwide. Recognized as the major etiologic agent of mycetoma in North America. Immunocompromised and debilitated patients are most susceptible.
Sporotrichosis	*Sporothrix schenckii*	Subcutaneous fungal infection found worldwide. Most common in Central and South America. Agricultural workers, especially horticulturists, are most often affected.

**CMI = cell-mediated immunity*

DRUG SELECTION

Treatment: Systemic mycoses are often difficult to diagnose. Since most antifungal agents are not active against bacteria and it is not always possible to differentiate between bacterial, fungal, and mixed infections solely on the basis of signs and symptoms, the causative organism should be identified before initiating treatment. Serologic tests are helpful in the diagnosis and management of coccidioidomycosis, cryptococcosis, histoplasmosis, and paracoccidioidomycosis. Histologic or cultural proof usually is required for diagnosis of a subcutaneous mycosis (Penn et al, 1983). Correct diagnosis is especially important because some antifungal drugs have a considerable potential for adverse reactions.

Amphotericin B [Fungizone] and flucytosine (5-fluorocytosine) [Ancobon], which are sometimes given together, have traditionally been used for subcutaneous and systemic mycoses. A newer group of antifungal drugs, those containing azole rings, are further divided into imidazoles and triazoles. The imidazoles, ketoconazole [Nizoral] and miconazole [Monistat], also have been administered to treat subcutaneous and systemic mycoses. However, with the possible exception of pseudallescheriasis caused by *P. boydii*, miconazole is not commonly used for these infections. The triazoles include fluconazole [Diflucan] and the investigational agents, itraconazole [Sporanox] and saperconazole (Fromtling, 1988; Graybill, 1989).

Amphotericin B has been the drug of choice for the treatment of most life-threatening, disseminated forms of aspergillosis, blastomycosis, candidiasis, chromoblastomycosis, coccidioidomycosis, cryptococcosis, histoplasmosis, mucormycosis, and sporotrichosis and, until recently, was the only effective drug available for these conditions (Graybill, 1988 B). The discovery that flucytosine acts synergistically with amphotericin B against many experimental fungal infections (see Medoff, 1987 for review) led to studies assessing this drug combination in patients with disseminated, life-threatening cryptococcosis (Bennett et al, 1979; Dismukes et al, 1984; 1987) and disseminated candidiasis (Smego et al, 1984). The combination of amphotericin B and flucytosine was at least as effective in cryptococcal meningitis as larger doses of amphotericin B given alone. However, controversy exists about the routine use of the combination in non-AIDS patients. Furthermore, although it is generally agreed that combination therapy with amphotericin B and flucytosine is effective in AIDS patients with meningeal cryptococcosis, the latter drug must be used with extreme caution because these patients cannot tolerate the myelosuppressive effects that frequently occur when serum concentrations of flucytosine exceed 100 mcg/ml (Stamm et al, 1987; Chuck and Sande, 1989; Clark et al, 1990). In addition, it is not clear that the inclusion of flucytosine in the regimen with amphotericin B increases treatment efficacy and improves the clinical outcome in AIDS patients. Thus, amphotericin B alone in large doses is preferred; flucytosine should be administered to these patients only with extreme caution and careful monitoring.

Flucytosine is sometimes used alone for treatment of chromoblastomycosis, but it is not used alone in other fungal infections because resistant organisms may be selected out rapidly. Only smaller lesions of chromoblastomycosis respond to this drug when it is administered as initial therapy; larger lesions should be resected and amphotericin B (with or without flucytosine) should then be administered.

Based on extensive clinical experience, many authorities consider ketoconazole the drug of choice for treatment of chronic mucocutaneous candidiasis and paracoccidioidomycosis. It also is effective in the treatment of some patients with nonlife-threatening extrameningeal blastomycosis, coccidioidomycosis, and histoplasmosis. It is marginally effective in chromoblastomycosis and has shown variable effectiveness in sporotrichosis. However, because of the high incidence of undesirable side effects during long-term administration, newer azoles (eg, fluconazole, itraconazole) may supplant ketoconazole as preferred therapy for several indications.

Miconazole has rarely been used as an alternative to amphotericin B in coccidioidomycosis since ketoconazole became available. Some authorities consider miconazole the drug of choice for pseudallescheriasis caused by *P. boydii* (Lutwick et al, 1979).

Fluconazole is the first of the new, orally active triazole derivatives to be approved for use against fungal infections in the United States. Recent data indicate that its efficacy in active cryptococcal meningitis in AIDS patients is similar to that of amphotericin B, although the latter may sterilize cerebrospinal fluid (CSF) faster than fluconazole (Stratton, 1990). To prevent the recurrence of cryptococcal meningitis in AIDS patients following eradication of active disease with amphotericin B, oral fluconazole is clearly superior to placebo (Bozzette et al, 1991) or intravenous maintenance therapy with amphotericin B, especially in those who generally cannot tolerate the debilitating side effects associated with long-term amphotericin B therapy. However, additional comparative studies are required to determine the optimal dosage and duration of treatment for active and maintenance therapy of cryptococcal meningitis. Fluconazole may be regarded as the drug of choice for therapy and prophylaxis of oropharyngeal/esophageal candidiasis and has excellent efficacy for chronic mucocutaneous candidiasis. However, the clinical data do not support its use as preferred therapy in acute hematogenously disseminated, invasive candidal infections. Fluconazole also has shown some efficacy in blastomycosis, coccidioidomycosis, and histoplasmosis, but because available clinical data are limited, it can only be considered alternative therapy in these infections (Grant and Clissold, 1990).

The pharmacokinetics and antifungal spectrum of itraconazole, an investigational orally active triazole, are similar to those of ketoconazole (Grant and Clissold, 1989). In noncomparative clinical trials, itraconazole has had good to excellent efficacy in aspergillosis, blastomycosis, oropharyngeal candidiasis, chromoblastomycosis, coccidioidomycosis, cryptococcosis, histoplasmosis, paracoccidioidomycosis, and sporotrichosis. Other data indicate that itraconazole is promising for prophylaxis of opportunistic fungal infections in patients at risk (eg, those receiving immunosuppressants, neutropenic patients, patients with AIDS). This drug may be considered primary therapy for chromoblastomycosis caused by *F. pedrosoi* and *C. carrioni*, nonlife-threatening forms of histoplasmosis, cutaneous-lymphatic manifestations of paracoccidioidomycosis and sporotrichosis, and possibly nonlife-threatening blastomycosis and phaeohyphomycoses.

Immunocompromised patients with subcutaneous or systemic mycoses are more resistant to therapy than immunocompetent individuals with the same mycoses (Bodey, 1984; Hawkins and Armstrong, 1985; Wheat et al, 1985). See Table 2 for suggested therapy for subcutaneous and systemic mycoses. For further information on these mycoses and their differential diagnosis and treatment, see the texts by Mandell et al, 1990; Hoeprich, 1983 A, as well as reviews of drug treatment (Terrell and Hermans, 1987; Bodey, 1988; Benson and Nahata, 1988; Fromtling, 1988; Graybill, 1988 B; Walsh and Pizzo, 1988; *Med Lett Drugs Ther,* 1990).

TABLE 2.
ANTIFUNGAL THERAPY FOR SUBCUTANEOUS AND SYSTEMIC MYCOSES

Infection	Recommended Therapy	Alternative Treatment	Comments
ASPERGILLOSIS			
Disseminated or Pulmonary (invasive)	Amphotericin B (intravenous)	Itraconazole* (oral)	Immunosuppressed patients have required up to 1 mg/kg/day of amphotericin B.
Pulmonary (noninvasive)			Therapy usually is not required.
BLASTOMYCOSIS			
Disseminated or Pulmonary (chronic)	Amphotericin B (intravenous)	Itraconazole* (oral) Ketoconazole (oral)	Azoles are often preferred in patients with nonlife-threatening extrameningeal disease.
Pulmonary (acute, self-limited)			Therapy often is not required.
CANDIDIASIS			
Disseminated or Invasive	Amphotericin B (intravenous) with or without flucytosine (oral)	Fluconazole (oral) Itraconazole* (oral)	In non-AIDS patients, the combination of flucytosine 150 mg/kg/day with reduced doses of amphotericin B (0.3 mg/kg/day) may minimize the adverse reactions caused by the larger dose of amphotericin B required when used alone. Flucytosine should be used with extreme caution in AIDS patients, who require amphotericin B 0.6-1 mg/kg/day.
Chronic Mucocutaneous	Ketoconazole (oral)	Amphotericin B (intravenous) Fluconazole* (oral) Itraconazole* (oral)	Ketoconazole is effective and is safer than amphotericin B; however, either drug must be given for prolonged periods to avoid relapses, and this is especially difficult with amphotericin B because it is toxic. Fluconazole and itraconazole are much less toxic oral alternatives to either ketoconazole or amphotericin B. A topical candicidal agent may be useful as an adjunct.
Oropharyngeal/Esophageal (immunocompromised patients)	Fluconazole (oral)	Itraconazole* (oral) Ketoconazole (oral) Amphotericin B (intravenous)	
CHROMOBLASTOMYCOSIS			
Subcutaneous	Itraconazole* (oral)	Flucytosine (oral) with or without amphotericin B (intravenous) Ketoconazole (oral)	Only small lesions respond to drugs alone; larger lesions are resected, and flucytosine (with or without amphotericin B) is given after resection. Intralesional injection of amphotericin B is reported to be effective in some patients.

(continued on next page)

TABLE 2 (continued)

Infection	Recommended Therapy	Alternative Treatment	Comments
COCCIDIOIDOMYCOSIS			
Meningeal	Amphotericin B (intrathecal plus intravenous)	Fluconazole* (oral or intravenous)	
Chronic (progressive) or Disseminated (nonmeningeal)	Amphotericin B (intravenous)	Itraconazole* (oral) Ketoconazole (oral) Fluconazole* (oral)	Ketoconazole usually is not employed in patients with rapidly progressing coccidioidomycosis, but is often used as initial therapy in more indolent progressive pulmonary, skeletal, or soft tissue infections. Itraconazole is as effective as ketoconazole, but much less toxic.
Pulmonary (acute, self-limited)			Therapy usually is not required.
CRYPTOCOCCOSIS			
Disseminated or Meningeal	Amphotericin B (intravenous) with or without flucytosine (oral)	Fluconazole (oral or intravenous) Itraconazole* (oral)	In non-AIDS patients, reduced doses of amphotericin B (0.3 mg/kg/day) plus flucytosine (150 mg/kg/day) may be less toxic than amphotericin B given alone in higher doses. Patients with AIDS should receive higher doses of amphotericin B (0.6-1 mg/kg/day), with or without flucytosine (100-150 mg/kg/day). Oral fluconazole 200 mg daily is given for maintenance therapy following completion of amphotericin B induction regimen; determination of its role in therapy of active disease awaits further clinical data.
Localized (nonmeningeal)	Amphotericin B (intravenous) with or without flucytosine (oral)	Ketoconazole* (oral) Fluconazole* (oral) Itraconazole* (oral)	Although ketoconazole is effective in some patients with less severe infections of the lung, bone, and skin, it has not consistently prevented cryptococcal meningitis.
HISTOPLASMOSIS			
Disseminated or Chronic Cavitary	Amphotericin B (intravenous)	Itraconazole* (oral) Ketoconazole (oral) Fluconazole* (oral)	Itraconazole is the drug of choice in less severe, nonlife-threatening disease.
Pulmonary (acute, self-limited)			Nonprogressive pulmonary infection usually does not require therapy.
MUCORMYCOSIS			
Rhinocerebral Pulmonary Gastrointestinal or Disseminated	Amphotericin B (intravenous)		Amphotericin B should be used promptly and the dose increased to 1-1.5 mg/kg/day as soon as possible. Surgical debridement is usually required. Azoles have no role in therapy.
PARACOCCIDIOIDOMYCOSIS			
Cutaneous-lymphatic and/or Visceral-lymphatic	Itraconazole* (oral)	Ketoconazole (oral) Amphotericin B (intravenous)	Amphotericin B is preferred in severe, life-threatening infections or when ketoconazole is ineffective.

(continued on next page)

TABLE 2 (continued)

Infection	Recommended Therapy	Alternative Treatment	Comments
PSEUDALLESCHERIASIS			
Disseminated or Pulmonary	Miconazole (intravenous)	Ketoconazole* (oral)	*P. boydii* may be intrinsically resistant to amphotericin B.
SPOROTRICHOSIS			
Disseminated or Extracutaneous	Amphotericin B (intravenous)	Itraconazole* (oral) Ketoconazole* (oral)	
Cutaneous-lymphatic	Potassium Iodide (oral) or Itraconazole* (oral)	Ketoconazole* (oral)	Limited data suggest that ketoconazole is effective in some patients. Local heat may be beneficial adjunctively.

* *Investigational use*

Empiric Antifungal Therapy: Empiric antifungal therapy is now routinely considered for febrile, neutropenic patients in whom broad spectrum antibacterial treatment does not cause defervescence (Sugar, 1990). In these patients, infectious complications are responsible for the majority of deaths not related to the underlying condition. Although bacterial infections are frequent causes of morbidity and mortality in neutropenic patients, fungal infections are increasingly common causes of death in this group (incidence, 60% in one study) (Pizzo et al, 1982). The risk of fungal infections is substantial for a number of reasons in patients who are seriously ill with underlying disease (eg, cancer, diabetes); they may be receiving immunosuppressants following organ transplantation, adrenal corticosteroid therapy, long-term antibacterial therapy, or parenteral nutrition; they may have an indwelling vascular catheter; or they may be debilitated due to major surgery or extensive burns or trauma. The common element in these patients is a major impairment of the normal phagocyte response to fungal infection, usually as a consequence of profoundly depressed neutrophil counts (< 500 per mm^3) for prolonged periods (ie, more than one week).

Opportunistic fungal pathogens are frequent infectious agents in neutropenic patients (Musial et al, 1988; Anaissie et al, 1989 A; Denning and Stevens, 1990; Milliken and Powles, 1990). Species of *Candida* and *Aspergillus* predominate, often in combination. Other pathogens include those causing mucormycosis, *Torulopsis glabrata, Cryptococcus neoformans,* as well as less common fungi such as *Alternaria, Fusarium, Geotrichum, Kluveromyces, Penicillium, Saccharomyces, Scopulariopsis, Trichophyton*, and *Trichosporon.*

The large number of opportunistic fungal pathogens underscores the necessity for using broad-spectrum empiric antifungal treatment in febrile, neutropenic patients. Intravenous amphotericin B has been reported to reduce the occurrence of invasive fungal infections (Pizzo et al, 1982; Walsh and Pizzo, 1988; EORTC International Antimicrobial Cooperative Group, 1989). In another study, intravenous miconazole produced similar results in patients with prolonged neutropenia (Wingard et al, 1987); however, miconazole is not used routinely because of the frequency of adverse reactions.

Recently it has been suggested that amphotericin B may be overused in empiric therapy for fungal infections (Gross et al, 1987; Wingard et al, 1987). The variability in outcome of clinical trials assessing the empiric efficacy of the drug may be a consequence of differences in patient populations due to inconsistent patient selection criteria and the variable regimens employed. (See Sugar, 1990, for a review of patient selection criteria and guidelines for amphotericin B therapy and management of toxicity.)

In general, febrile (temperature >38°C), neutropenic (<500 polymorphonuclear leukocytes per mm^3) patients who have not responded to a four- to seven-day course of broad spectrum antibacterial therapy should be considered candidates for empiric antifungal therapy with amphotericin B. If the specific fungal pathogen has not been identified, amphotericin B 0.5 to 0.6 mg/kg/day should be administered until defervescence occurs and the neutrophil count increases. The patient should be closely observed during the treatment period to ensure adequate management of any complications of therapy. When the fungal organism has been identified, specific therapy should be instituted.

Prophylactic Antifungal Therapy: Invasive fungal infections are a significant cause of morbidity and mortality in immunocompromised patients whether they are neutropenic due to iatrogenic causes or have AIDS. Since diagnosis and adequate therapy of these infections can be extremely difficult in the immunocompromised host, prophylaxis is an attractive alternative for their control (Meunier, 1987; Meunier and Klastersky, 1988; Bodey et al, 1990).

As noted above, the most frequently encountered opportunistic fungal pathogens are species of *Candida* and *Aspergillus*. Basic strategy for preventing fungal infections in immunocompromised patients can be divided into general measures designed to prevent acquisition of causative organisms and chemoprophylaxis with oral antifungal drugs. The general measures include maintenance of personal hygiene, hand-washing, adherence to a restricted diet consisting of cooked foods, and avoidance as much as possible of invasive procedures, such as placement of venous or indwelling urinary catheters. Orally administered agents used for chemoprophylaxis include nonabsorbable polyenes (nystatin, [Mycostatin, Nilstat] amphotericin B), imidazoles (miconazole, ketoconazole), and triazoles (fluconazole, itraconazole), most commonly to prevent various forms of candidiasis and aspergillosis. Prevention of the development of the invasive pulmonary form of aspergillosis may be accomplished by isolation of patients in rooms equipped with high-efficiency particulate air (HEPA) filters and the prophylactic use of nebulized amphotericin B (Meunier, 1987; Conneally et al, 1990).

Although results of studies on chemoprophylaxis for invasive fungal infections have been disappointing in general, recent data indicate that fluconazole is highly effective in preventing oropharyngeal candidiasis in patients with various metastatic malignancies (Samonis et al, 1990). However, it appears that reliable regimens for chemoprophylaxis of invasive fungal infections have not been clearly established and that prophylactic therapy may have to be designed for specific diseases in specific host environments.

Drug Evaluations

AMPHOTERICIN B

[Fungizone]

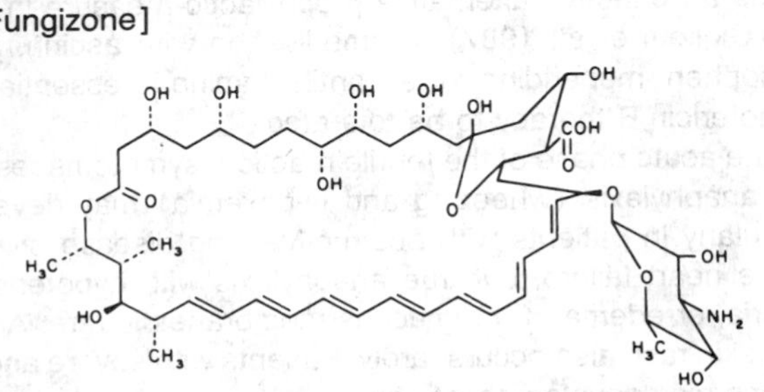

ACTIONS. Amphotericin B is a polyene antibiotic produced by *Streptomyces nodosus*. Low concentrations inhibit the growth of fungi, protozoa, and algae. Amphotericin B is principally fungistatic; concentrations near the upper limits of tolerance in man are fungicidal to some strains. Although amphotericin B binds to sterols in fungal and mammalian membranes, it binds more avidly to ergosterol in fungal membranes than to cholesterol in mammalian membranes. Binding to ergosterol in fungal cell membranes alters membrane selective permeability.

USES. Amphotericin B (frequently given with flucytosine) is considered a primary therapeutic option for non-AIDS patients with disseminated cryptococcosis (Bennett et al, 1979; Dismukes et al, 1984). The combination also may be used to treat disseminated candidiasis (Smego et al, 1984), although many authorities prefer amphotericin B alone for this indication (*Med Lett Drugs Ther*, 1990). In the original study comparing the combination of amphotericin B plus flucytosine with amphotericin B alone in cryptococcal meningitis (Bennett et al, 1979), the dose of amphotericin B was 0.4 mg/kg/day, an amount now considered too low to be effective; this may have led to the conclusion that the combination drug regimen was more effective in this disease. Results of a subsequent controlled study utilizing a low dose of amphotericin B with a maximal dose of flucytosine suggested that four weeks of treatment might be adequate for some non-AIDS patients with cryptococcal meningitis who do not have neurologic complications or other underlying diseases, are not receiving immunosuppressive therapy, have a pretreatment CSF white cell count $>20/mm^3$, have a pretreatment serum cryptococcal antigen titer $<1:32$, and, after four weeks of therapy, have a negative CSF india ink preparation and CSF culture and serum, as well as CSF cryptococcal antigen titers $<1:8$. Patients with cryptococcal meningitis who do not meet these criteria should receive at least six weeks of therapy (Dismukes et al, 1987).

Flucytosine must be used with extreme caution in AIDS patients, since serious hematologic abnormalities occur frequently when the serum concentration exceeds 100 mcg/ml (Stamm et al, 1987). In these patients, a high dose regimen (up to 1 mg/kg/day) of amphotericin B alone may be given for 8 to 12 weeks, followed by maintenance therapy with oral fluconazole (*Med Lett Drugs Ther*, 1990).

Amphotericin B is an alternative to oral azoles in nonlife-threatening blastomycosis, histoplasmosis, and paracoccidioidomycosis but is the drug of choice in patients with life-threatening infections or when azoles are ineffective (National Institute of Allergy and Infectious Diseases Mycoses Study Group, 1985; Grant and Clissold, 1989, 1990). It is the drug of choice for mucormycosis and other diseases caused by organisms from the class Zygomycetes (Benbow and Stoddart, 1986), although these infections, as well as invasive aspergillosis and coccidioidomycosis, may not respond well to drug therapy. Amphotericin B is indicated in disseminated and extracutaneous sporotrichosis, but itraconazole or potassium iodide is preferred for the cutaneous-lymphatic form. The subcutaneous mycoses, mycetoma (Mahgoub, 1985) and chromoblastomycosis, appear to be least affected by amphotericin B. Intralesional injection has been reported to be effective in some patients with chromoblastomycosis.

Intravenous amphotericin B has been used empirically to prevent fungal superinfection and control clinically undetected fungal invasion in febrile granulocytopenic patients who have been receiving broad-spectrum antibacterial therapy (Pizzo et al, 1982; EORTC International Antimicrobial Cooperative Group, 1989). This potentially toxic therapy is advocated in these patients because of the difficulty of diagnosing fungal infections, which may be rapidly progressive and are frequently fatal (Meunier, 1987; Anaissie et al, 1989 A). However, determination of appropriate indications for empiric therapy has been difficult due to differences in patient populations and drug regimens. At present, the consensus is that the patient who remains febrile and profoundly neutropenic (<500 neutrophils/mm^3) for one week despite receiving adequate doses of broad-spectrum antibacterial agents is a candidate for empiric amphotericin B therapy. However, each case must be considered individually and every effort should be made (lesion biopsy, chest and sinus roentgenograms, cultures, serologic tests for fungal antibody and antigens, computed tomography of abdomen and chest) to identify a fungal pathogen infection prior to initiating empiric therapy. Patient selection criteria and treatment algorithms for empiric use of amphotericin B have been outlined (Hughes et al, 1990; Sugar, 1990).

Liposome-encapsulated amphotericin B (ampholiposomes) is a promising new therapy for disseminated fungal infections (Lopez-Berestein, 1987; Wiebe and DeGregorio, 1988; Meunier, 1989). Antifungal efficacy in vivo is enhanced and toxicity is reduced due to altered tissue distribution of the drug, the ability to administer a larger amount without toxicity, and possibly other factors. Results of limited clinical studies using investigational formulations of liposomes containing amphotericin B in patients refractory to traditional antifungal medications (including standard amphotericin B preparations) are encouraging (Lopez-Berestein, 1987; Lopez-Berestein et al, 1989; Wiebe and DeGregorio, 1988). Although this novel carrier system was ineffective in about one-third of such patients, at least one-third responded partially and one-third were cured. Side effects and serious adverse reactions were reduced in most patients. In another limited nonrandomized study, higher blood levels, improved efficacy, and diminished toxicity were reported in patients with fungal infections and solid or hematologic malignancies who received an investigational formulation of liposomes containing amphotericin B (Sculier et al, 1988).

It is apparent that technology must yet be developed for the large-scale production of uniform liposome products, especially since preliminary data indicate that specific alteration of the lipid composition may provide a means for tissue-specific drug delivery (Brajtburg et al, 1990 A). Controlled clinical studies are underway to determine the definitive role of this technology versus traditional amphotericin B therapy for candidiasis, coccidioidomycosis, and cryptococcosis. Preliminary data indicate that the liposome-encapsulated preparation can be given at substantially higher dosages than previously used.

RESISTANCE. The isolation of fungi resistant to amphotericin B has been reported rarely since this drug's introduction over 30 years ago. However, it is difficult to ascertain precisely the incidence of fungal resistance to this agent, since susceptibility studies may not be performed routinely and inconsistencies in test methodology have hindered interlaboratory comparison of data (Pfaller et al, 1990). Fungal resistance to amphotericin B frequently has been ascribed to quantitative or qualitative alterations in cell membrane lipid composition (Brajtburg et al, 1990 B). Resistant pathogens include rare spontaneous mutants of *C. albicans* and *P. boydii*, which have increased or reduced membrane ergosterol content. Acquired resistance has been observed in other isolates of *C. albicans*, *C. tropicalis*, *C. parapsilosis*, and *C. lusitaniae*. Clinical data indicate that the emergence of amphotericin B-resistant yeast in immunocompromised patients receiving the drug for long periods is correlated with poor, usually fatal, outcome (Powderly et al, 1988). In general, however, organisms responsible for the major mycoses have remained sensitive to amphotericin B.

ADVERSE REACTIONS AND PRECAUTIONS. Intravenous amphotericin B produces formidable toxic effects and should be used only when the potential benefits outweigh the risks. In general, amphotericin B-induced toxic reactions can be categorized as frequent or infrequent (Cleary et al, 1988) and further subdivided into frequent infusion-related reactions, frequent dose-related reactions, infrequent idiosyncratic reactions, and infrequent dose-related reactions. Frequent infusion-related adverse reactions include fever, chills, headache, nausea, vomiting, and phlebitis; frequent dose-related reactions include renal dysfunction, hypokalemia, and anemia. Infrequent idiosyncratic reactions include anaphylaxis, thrombocytopenia, acute liver dysfunction, flushing, vertigo, pain, and tonic-clonic seizures; and infrequent dose-related effects include ventricular fibrillation and cardiac arrest. Renal dysfunction is regarded as the use-limiting reaction but usually is reversible upon discontinuation of the drug.

An acute febrile reaction is the most prominent untoward reaction early in therapy. A shaking chill is often the initial symptom of the typical febrile reaction, which begins precipitously about two hours after an infusion is started. Fever is maximal about one hour after onset and subsides within the next two hours. Intravenous infusion of hydrocortisone sodium succinate 25 to 50 mg prior to or during the infusion may decrease the intensity of known reactions in patients not already receiving corticosteroids. Hydrocortisone should not be given routinely, however, because its immunosuppressant action may worsen the course of the mycosis. Ibuprofen 10 mg/kg was an effective alternative prophylactic measure in one trial (Gigliotti et al, 1987). Premedication with aspirin, acetaminophen, meperidine, or an antihistamine is essential for amphotericin B therapy to be tolerated.

In the acute phase of the febrile reaction, symptoms resembling anaphylaxis (wheezing and hypoxemia) may develop, particularly in patients with obstructive lung disease or congestive heart failure, but true anaphylaxis with hypotension, urticaria, or edema of the mucous membranes is rare. An allergic skin rash also occurs rarely. Patients with severe angina pectoris may develop chest pain.

Transient, dose-dependent azotemia is observed as a later reaction in almost all patients. There is minimal permanent renal damage in those without prior renal dysfunction, but impairment may become permanent in patients with pre-existing renal disease or in those receiving a total dose of more than 3 g. In patients without prior renal disease, the usual daily dose of 0.4 to 0.6 mg/kg eventually produces a serum creatinine level of 1.7 to 3.5 mg/dL and a blood urea nitrogen level of 25 to 50 mg/dL. Renal function should be monitored frequently if the serum creatinine level rises rapidly to 2 mg/dL or more, and serum electrolytes should be monitored at least twice weekly. Renal tubular acidosis or hypokalemia may require treatment. Avoidance of dehydration and supplemental sodium loading (100 to 150 mEq/day) have been reported to decrease nephrotoxicity and allow administration of a full dose of amphotericin B (Branch, 1988). Controlled studies are still required to confirm these findings and provide guidelines for sodium supplementation to minimize nephrotoxicity. More severe azotemia (creatinine level >3 mg/dL) may require reduction of dosage, alternate-day therapy, sodium supplementation, improved hydration, and avoidance or elimination of diuretics (eg, furosemide) or nephrotoxic drugs (eg, cyclosporine, aminoglycosides). Hemodialysis or peritoneal dialysis may be necessary if the fungal infection is life-threatening and no alternative therapy exists.

Amphotericin B often causes hypokalemia. When this drug is given with other drugs that commonly produce hypokalemia (eg, corticosteroids, potassium-depleting diuretics) or whose toxicity is enhanced by hypokalemia (eg, digoxin), serum potassium concentrations should be monitored frequently. Hypomagnesemia also has been reported (Barton et al, 1984).

The hematocrit often falls during therapy to a stable level between 20% and 30%. Transfusion ordinarily should be avoided. A slight decrease in leukocyte count and, rarely, thrombocytopenia may occur. Nausea, vomiting, anorexia, and weight loss are common.

Heparin 1,000 units (10 mg) is often added to the drug suspension in an attempt to decrease phlebitis when peripheral veins are used for the infusion. As intravenous therapy continues, patients may experience less phlebitis and anorexia if a double dose of amphotericin B on alternate days is substituted gradually.

Intrathecal injection of amphotericin B may cause nausea and vomiting; urinary retention; pain in the back, legs, or abdomen; headache; radiculitis; paresis (usually transient); paresthesias; and vertigo.

In pregnant women or those of childbearing age, therapy with amphotericin B should be limited to those with life-threatening infections. At least six pregnant patients have been treated successfully without obvious teratogenic effects. Parenteral amphotericin B is classified in FDA Pregnancy Category B.

PHARMACOKINETICS. Amphotericin B is not adequately absorbed when given orally. It is injected intravenously for systemic fungal infections and sometimes intrathecally (into the CSF of the lumbar spine, cisterna magna, or cerebral ventricle) for coccidioidal and cryptococcal meningitis.

Amphotericin B is highly protein bound (90% to 95%), predominantly to β-lipoproteins. The large volume of distribution (4.0 ± 0.4 L/kg) probably reflects binding to cell membranes. The drug accumulates in highest concentrations in the liver and spleen, with lesser amounts in the kidneys, lung, and heart (Collette et al, 1989); it penetrates extravascular compartments poorly. An initial plasma half-life of about 24 hours is followed by a slower terminal elimination half-life of about 15 days (Daneshmend and Warnock, 1983). After therapy is discontinued, amphotericin B can be detected in the serum for seven to eight weeks because it is released slowly from tissue depots. Metabolic pathways are unknown. Peak serum concentrations following conventional intravenous doses are 0.5 to 2 mcg/ml but rapidly decrease to reach a plateau of 0.2 to 0.5 mcg/ml. The concentration in the urine is similar to that in serum. The serum concentration is not elevated in patients with impaired or absent renal function. Neither hemodialysis nor peritoneal dialysis removes a significant amount of drug.

DOSAGE AND PREPARATIONS. Detailed instructions for storage, preparation, and administration should be followed closely, because this drug is unstable under certain conditions (eg, exposure to heat, prolonged exposure to sunlight, pH below 4.2). The powder should be refrigerated, and preparations for infusion should be used within 24 hours. The preparation is a colloidal suspension; thus, any in-line membrane filter used during the infusion should have a mean pore diameter of at least 1.0 micron. Suspensions are prepared by adding 10 ml of water for injection to 50 mg of amphotericin B and shaking the vial until the contents are clear. The desired dose is then added to 5% dextrose injection. The pH of the suspension should be 4.2 or above. The dose should not be added to infusions that contain bacteriostatic agents (eg, benzyl alcohol), potassium chloride, sodium chloride, or other electrolytes because they may cause the drug to precipitate. Cloudy solutions may produce low serum levels and should be discarded.

Intravenous (infusion): Daily dosage must be individualized on the basis of the severity of the disease and tolerance of the patient. The total daily dose of amphotericin B is administered as an infusion that usually is given over two to four hours. However, data indicate that a 45-minute infusion is well tolerated and is not associated with a higher incidence of adverse reactions (Cleary et al, 1988). A small, randomized, double-blind trial comparing one- and four-hour infusion rates showed that both were equally well tolerated, although controllable side effects appeared more rapidly in those patients receiving the one-hour infusion (Oldfield et al, 1990). However, this study did not address the safety of one-hour infusions, especially the cardiovascular effects. Thus, infusion of amphotericin B over shorter periods than usual should be performed cautiously, with consideration given to the potential for life-threatening cardiac complications such as asystole and ventricular fibrillation (Craven and Gremillion, 1985; DeMonaco and McGovern, 1983).

An initial test dose in *adults and children* usually should not exceed 0.25 mg/kg. Often only 1 mg is administered over two to four hours initially to test for an acute reaction, although some investigators may use a shorter period for this infusion. The dose may be increased by 5 to 10 mg daily to 0.4 to 0.6 mg/kg/day. In critically ill patients and those with AIDS, many experts recommend 0.6 to 1 mg/kg/day immediately following the test dose. Some clinicians prefer to give 1 mg/kg/day initially for several days to severely ill, immunocompromised patients; however, continued administration of this dose usually causes formidable problems in management. An alternate-day regimen is satisfactory for most chronic mycoses and reduces the frequency of phlebitis and acute reactions.

A total dose of 30 mg/kg (1 to 3 g) for a course of therapy usually can be administered over a period of six to ten weeks, depending on the illness. Several months may be necessary to achieve a cure. Shorter treatment periods may be inadequate and lead to relapse. Whenever administration is interrupted for longer than seven days, therapy should be resumed gradually according to the above schedule.

When given with flucytosine for disseminated candidiasis or cryptococcosis in non-AIDS patients with normal renal function, the initial regimen is amphotericin B 0.3 mg/kg/day plus flucytosine 37.5 mg/kg at six-hour intervals. Alternatively, because of its long half-life, flucytosine 75 mg/kg may be given at 12-hour intervals. If renal function remains stable, some clinicians increase the dose of amphotericin B to 0.4 or 0.6 mg/kg/day as needed. Patients with AIDS may receive amphotericin B 0.6 to 1 mg/kg/day plus flucytosine 100 to 150 mg/kg/day. However, they must be closely monitored for the occurrence of hematologic toxicity, in which case flucytosine must then be given at a lower dose or withdrawn. Usually six weeks of therapy are required, depending on the mycosis. Some clinicians decrease the daily maintenance dose of flucytosine to 25 mg/kg at six-hour intervals depending on the tolerance and response of the patient.

For *low-birth-weight, high-risk neonates* with systemic candidal infections, institution of therapy immediately after clinical diagnosis has been recommended; the initial dose is 0.5 mg/kg/day every 24 hours (cumulative dose, 20 to 30 mg/kg) (Baley et al, 1990). The benefit of the addition of flucytosine in neonatal therapy is controversial at present (Baley et al, 1990; Butler et al, 1990).

Intrathecal: The suspension for lumbar intrathecal injection may be diluted in 10% dextrose. The patient is placed in a 30° Trendelenburg position for 30 to 45 minutes immediately after the injection to allow downward flow of the hyperbaric solution. Hydrocortisone sodium succinate 10 to 15 mg may be added to the solution to decrease chemical arachnoiditis, although the extra volume necessitates use of enough dextrose to maintain a hyperbaric final concentration. For injections in the lateral cerebral ventricle employing a subcutaneous reservoir, the solution is diluted in 5% dextrose with or without hydrocortisone sodium succinate 10 to 15 mg.

The initial dose is approximately 0.05 mg; subsequent doses are increased by 0.1 mg three times a week until a maintenance dose of 0.5 mg two or three times weekly is achieved.

Fungizone (Squibb), ***Generic*** (Lyphomed). Powder (lyophilized, sterile) 50 mg.

FLUCYTOSINE
[Ancobon]

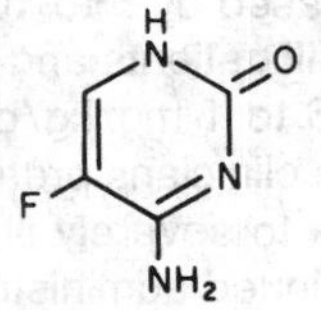

ACTIONS AND USES. Flucytosine, a synthetic agent, is administered orally to treat subcutaneous chromoblastomycosis. Smaller lesions respond to flucytosine alone but larger lesions must be resected before this drug is used. Amphotericin B may be given concomitantly when the response to flucytosine alone is inadequate or the disease is extensive.

Flucytosine has been used alone extensively to treat *Candida* urinary tract infections; it is usually efficacious if no urinary catheter, stents, or stones are present.

Flucytosine is used with amphotericin B to treat subcutaneous or systemic infections caused by *Candida* or *Cryptococcus neoformans*, because resistance may develop rapidly when flucytosine is given alone; 5% to 15% of pretreatment isolates of *Candida* are resistant to this antimetabolite. Some geographic variation in drug response may be due to differential species distribution. Combined use of these agents also permits reduction in the dose of amphotericin B (for discussion and dosage, see evaluation on Amphotericin B).

Flucytosine is metabolized to fluorouracil and fluorodeoxyuridine monophosphate. Fluorouracil is incorporated into fungal RNA and inhibits protein synthesis; it is the probable metabolic moiety responsible for bone marrow depression. Fluorodeoxyuridine monophosphate inhibits DNA synthesis.

ADVERSE REACTIONS AND PRECAUTIONS. The most common serious adverse reactions are leukopenia and thrombocytopenia, either of which can be fatal. These reactions are dose related, are more likely to develop when amphotericin B is used concurrently or the serum concentration of flucytosine exceeds 100 mcg/ml, and are usually reversible on discontinuing the drug (Stamm et al, 1987). Flucytosine also may cause rash, nausea, vomiting, and diarrhea. Diarrhea can become protracted if therapy is continued. Perforation of the bowel as a result of colonic ulcers has been reported (Kerkering, 1982).

If it must be used, flucytosine must be administered cautiously to patients with AIDS and bone marrow depression (eg, that caused by certain hematologic diseases, radiation, or drugs). An allergic skin reaction occurs occasionally.

Flucytosine does not cause renal toxicity. However, because it is excreted primarily by the kidneys, the dosage should be adjusted to prevent accumulation of active drug in patients with impaired renal function. Serum concentrations should be monitored frequently in those with severe or rapidly developing azotemia. Special caution is advised when flucytosine is administered with amphotericin B, because the latter's potential for inducing renal impairment may interfere with the elimination of flucytosine (Stamm et al, 1987). The serum creatinine concentration should be monitored twice weekly; if indicated, the creatinine clearance may be useful to adjust the dose when this combination is used.

Elevation of hepatic alanine and aspartate aminotransferases and alkaline phosphatase is noted occasionally. Three cases of patchy hepatic cell necrosis have been reported (Kerkering, 1982); fatal hepatitis also has occurred.

The safety of flucytosine during pregnancy has not been established (FDA Pregnancy Category C). Therefore, the drug should be given to pregnant patients only when serious or life-threatening systemic fungal infections exist, and contraceptive measures should be considered in women of childbearing age.

PHARMACOKINETICS. More than 80% of a dose of flucytosine is absorbed from the gastrointestinal tract, and peak serum levels of 70 to 80 mcg/ml are achieved within one to two hours after a dose of 37.5 mg/kg in patients with normal renal function (Daneshmend and Warnock, 1983; Bennett et al, 1979). The drug is widely distributed in body water; protein binding is negligible. The volume of distribution approximates total body water. Levels in the cerebrospinal fluid and central nervous system are about 80% of those in the serum. About 63% to 84% of a dose is eliminated principally unchanged in the urine; concentrations are 200 to 500 mcg/ml. Clearance is approximately 75% of creatinine clearance. The serum half-life is three to six hours.

DOSAGE AND PREPARATIONS.

Oral: *Adults and children with normal renal function,* usually 37.5 mg/kg at six-hour intervals. For dosages employed in combination regimens with amphotericin B, see that evaluation.

Serum concentrations of flucytosine should be monitored and the dosage adjusted accordingly, especially in AIDS patients. The serum concentration should be determined two hours after an oral dose once a week, and the dose should be adjusted to maintain the desired peak concentration of 50 to 100 mcg/ml. The following guidelines are recommended for patients with renal impairment (Stamm et al, 1987). Creatinine clearance of 26 to 50 ml/min, the dosing interval is doubled or the dose is halved; creatinine clearance of 13 to 25 ml/min, the interval is quadrupled or the dose is reduced fourfold. Patients undergoing hemodialysis should receive 37.5 mg/kg after each hemodialysis session, and those on continuous peritoneal dialysis should receive a single daily dose of 37.5 mg/kg.

Ancobon (Roche). Capsules 250 and 500 mg. An intravenous preparation is available from the manufacturer on a compassionate-use basis.

AZOLE ANTIFUNGAL AGENTS

Imidazole

KETOCONAZOLE

[Nizoral]

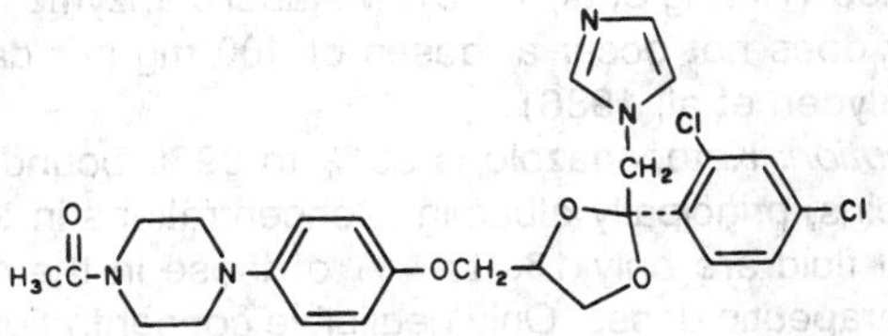

ACTIONS. Ketoconazole is an antifungal imidazole (Smith and Henry, 1984; Van Tyle, 1984; Graybill, 1988 C; Saag and Dismukes, 1988). Like other imidazoles (clotrimazole, econazole, and miconazole), ketoconazole inhibits the cytochrome P-450 enzyme system that catalyzes the 14-demethylation of lanosterol, the precursor of ergosterol, and thus it interferes with ergosterol synthesis. This effect alters the permeability of the fungal cell membrane. High concentrations are required to inhibit the biosynthesis of cholesterol in mammals. Since yeast forms of *Candida albicans* are more susceptible to phagocytosis by leukocytes than are pseudohyphae, an additional action of the drug in *Candida* infections may be inhibition of the transformation of yeast to hyphal forms. Ketoconazole is fungistatic at lower concentrations and fungicidal at higher concentrations.

USES. ***Candidiasis:*** Ketoconazole is the drug of choice for chronic mucocutaneous candidiasis, but it must be given for prolonged periods to avoid relapse (Graybill et al, 1980; Petersen et al, 1980; Jorizzo, 1982). It also is effective in oropharyngeal and esophageal candidiasis. Patients with disseminated or invasive disease often respond poorly; amphotericin B alone or with flucytosine is the therapy of choice.

Blastomycosis and Histoplasmosis: Ketoconazole is usually effective in patients with blastomycosis and histoplasmosis (National Institute of Allergy and Infectious Diseases Mycoses Study Group, 1985); therefore, it is an alternative to amphotericin B except in patients with severe immunosuppression, AIDS, or meningitis.

Coccidioidomycosis: Ketoconazole is effective in nonmeningeal coccidioidomycosis. However, when the disease is severe, amphotericin B is preferred in spite of the greater frequency and severity of adverse reactions. Ketoconazole 1.2 g/day has been used for meningitis, but fluconazole is effective and much less toxic than ketoconazole in high doses (Tucker et al, 1990 A).

Cryptococcosis (investigational): Ketoconazole has been used in only a small number of patients with nonmeningeal and possibly self-limiting forms of cryptococcosis; therefore, its efficacy cannot be assessed. Because ketoconazole does not penetrate the central nervous system or cerebrospinal fluid, it is not recommended for cryptococcal meningitis.

Chromoblastomycosis: Ketoconazole occasionally may cause slight improvement, but it is usually ineffective in this mycosis. Oral itraconazole is the therapy of choice.

Paracoccidioidomycosis: Ketoconazole is useful in mild to moderate disease; amphotericin B is preferred in severe, life-threatening disease.

Sporotrichosis (investigational): Ketoconazole is only marginally effective in cutaneous-lymphatic sporotrichosis; itraconazole (or saturated potassium iodide solution) is the drug of choice. Amphotericin B remains the drug of choice for disseminated sporotrichosis. However, a recent report shows that ketoconazole can be effective in the treatment of systemic sporotrichosis when given for prolonged periods in relatively large doses (400 to 800 mg daily) (Calhoun et al, 1991).

Miscellaneous: Ketoconazole is reported to be effective in stable patients with pulmonary pseudallescheriasis (Galgiani et al, 1984); however, miconazole is preferred when deep visceral pseudallescheriasis is present (Walsh and Pizzo, 1988). Patients with aspergillosis and mucormycosis do not respond to ketoconazole; amphotericin B is the drug of choice.

RESISTANCE. Resistance has been encountered only rarely in normally susceptible species. However, susceptible species of *Candida* may be replaced by *Torulopsis glabrata*, a normally nonpathogenic fungus that is usually resistant to ketoconazole and may be lethal in neutropenic patients who are treated with this drug (Graybill, 1988 B). Efficacy cannot be predicted on the basis of in vitro susceptibility tests.

ADVERSE REACTIONS AND PRECAUTIONS. Gastrointestinal toxicity (nausea and vomiting) is dose related and occurs in about 50% of patients receiving more than 800 mg daily

(Sugar et al, 1987). Headache, pruritus, dysfunctional uterine bleeding, dizziness, abdominal pain, constipation, diarrhea, somnolence, and nervousness have been reported less frequently (<1%), especially when lower doses (400 mg daily) are used (National Institute of Allergy and Infectious Diseases Mycoses Study Group, 1985).

The drug elevates hepatic alanine and aspartate aminotransferase levels temporarily in 2% to 5% of patients, but they remain asymptomatic. Abrupt onset of hepatic dysfunction with symptoms that resemble viral hepatitis occurs in about 1 in 15,000 patients, especially middle-aged women, and appears to be idiosyncratic. Fatalities have been reported in a few individuals who developed hepatic necrosis (Smith and Henry, 1984; Lake-Bakaar et al, 1987). Patients should be informed of the symptoms of hepatitis and told to return for consultation and blood testing if the condition is suspected.

Gynecomastia, infertility, decreased libido, or oligospermia occur in some males. The effect is dose dependent and is most likely to develop when doses exceed 600 mg/day. Ketoconazole suppresses the activity of cytochrome P-450 (Sonino, 1987). Since testosterone synthesis is dependent on that enzyme system, gonadal testosterone and adrenal androgen synthesis are inhibited. The decrease in serum testosterone results in a reflex increase in the serum concentrations of LH and FSH (Glass, 1986). Doses of 600 to 800 mg/day transiently inhibit adrenal steroidogenesis by blocking the 11-hydroxylation step of synthesis. Hypoadrenalism has been observed and occasionally may be prolonged (Best et al, 1987; Tucker et al, 1985; Sonino, 1987) or result in adrenal crisis (Khosla et al, 1989).

Ketoconazole inhibits the deposition of methylprednisolone, prednisone, and prednisolone by inhibiting 6β-hydroxylase, thereby prolonging the adrenal suppressive effect of these corticosteroids (Glynn et al, 1986; Zürcher et al, 1989). It also inhibits the synthesis of endogenous cortisol.

Ketoconazole also inhibits cholesterol synthesis by blocking the conversion of lanosterol to cholesterol (Kraemer and Pont, 1986). A decrease in total cholesterol of 20% to 30% is related to a change in the LDL cholesterol concentration. Serum lanosterol concentrations increase, but the effects of prolonged elevations are unknown.

Hypothyroidism may be a rare, genetically determined side effect of ketoconazole (Kitching, 1986).

Doses of 80 mg/kg/day have caused syndactyly and oligodactyly in the offspring of rats. Data are insufficient to evaluate this drug's safety in pregnant women; therefore, ketoconazole should not be used during pregnancy unless the potential benefit justifies the risk to the fetus (FDA Pregnancy Category C). The drug is present in breast milk.

DRUG INTERACTIONS. Ketoconazole is reported to increase cyclosporine blood concentrations and the serum creatinine concentration resulting in nephrotoxicity. This interaction probably occurs at the level of cytochrome P-450 drug metabolizing enzymes (Brown et al, 1985).

Ketoconazole has increased the prothrombin time in a few patients receiving coumarin derivatives (Smith, 1984). Cimetidine and probably ranitidine markedly decrease ketoconazole blood concentrations. Ketoconazole may reduce the clearance of chlordiazepoxide, theophylline, and cyclosporine.

When isoniazid or rifampin is administered with ketoconazole, therapeutic blood concentrations of the latter may not be obtainable (Engelhard et al, 1984). Therefore, alternative antifungal therapy or increased dosage of ketoconazole is recommended in patients taking these drugs (Doble et al, 1988). Conversely, ketoconazole may depress the blood concentration of rifampin. Phenytoin and ketoconazole are alleged to have a similar reciprocal effect.

PHARMACOKINETICS. *Absorption:* Approximately one to two hours after a single 200-mg dose, the serum concentration ranges from 1.6 to 6.9 mcg/ml and can be maintained with a single daily dose. Relative bioavailability of the tablet formulation is about 80% (Huang et al, 1986).

Controversy exists as to whether higher serum levels are achieved if the drug is given without food (Lelawongs et al, 1988). The absence of gastric hydrochloric acid will lead to poor absorption of ketoconazole. Thus, especially in the elderly and in patients with AIDS, who frequently have achlorhydria, serum levels of ketoconazole may not attain expected levels. Since bioavailability depends on gastric acidity, glutamic acid capsules may provide an effective, convenient method of enhancing ketoconazole's absorption in patients with reduced gastric acidity (Lelawongs et al, 1988). Anticholinergic agents and H_2 blocking agents (eg, cimetidine, ranitidine) should be avoided. Antacids may not interfere with absorption if they are given no less than two hours after ketoconazole.

Metabolism: Extensive hepatic degradation by microsomal enzymes occurs, and little active drug is excreted in the bile. Only 2% to 4% of a dose is eliminated unchanged in the urine. Dose-dependent kinetics were observed in humans with doses of 200, 400, and 800 mg; the cause remains to be determined (Huang et al, 1986). Metabolic enzyme induction probably does not occur at doses of 400 mg per day in humans (Blyden et al, 1986).

Distribution: Ketoconazole is 95% to 99% bound to plasma proteins, principally albumin. Concentrations in the cerebrospinal fluid are only 1% to 4% of those in the serum at usual therapeutic doses. Only negligible concentrations occur in the peritoneal fluid of patients undergoing peritoneal dialysis.

Elimination: An initial half-life of one to four hours is probably more meaningful than the beta terminal half-life of 6 to 10 hours in view of the low serum concentrations associated with the longer half-life (Daneshmend and Warnock et al, 1988).

DOSAGE AND PREPARATIONS. The most effective dose and duration of therapy must be determined in each individual.

Oral: *Adults,* for subcutaneous or systemic infection, the usual initial dose is 400 mg daily. The amount may be increased to 600 to 800 mg daily, given in divided doses if necessary. The minimum duration of therapy is six months, and treatment for one year is not uncommon. The high incidence of relapse or failure in some subcutaneous mycoses, such as coccidioidomycosis, has led to use of larger doses (up to 1.6 g) and longer courses of treatment (Dismukes et al, 1983; Hoeprich,

1983 B; Goodpasture et al, 1985), but large doses are poorly tolerated (Sugar et al, 1987). Continuous maintenance therapy is required for chronic mucocutaneous candidiasis.

Children over 2 years, 3.3 mg/kg once daily; for subcutaneous infections, at least 6.6 mg/kg once daily for a minimum of six months.

Nizoral (Janssen). Tablets 200 mg.

Triazoles

FLUCONAZOLE
[Diflucan]

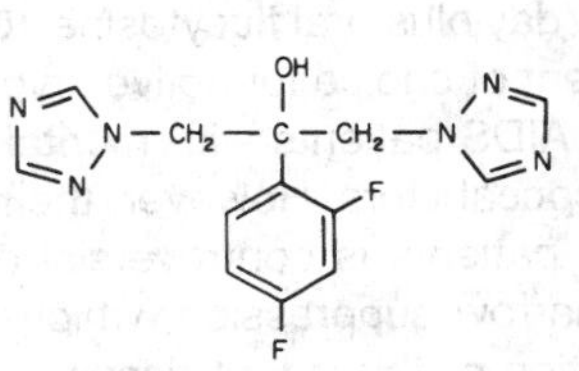

ACTIONS. This triazole compound is primarily fungistatic and apparently acts by inhibiting ergosterol biosynthesis. The demethylation of 14α-methylsterol to produce ergosterol (a component of fungal cell membranes) is catalyzed by enzymes of the cytochrome P-450 family. Fluconazole binds to fungal cytochrome P-450 with high affinity, but it binds only weakly to the counterpart mammalian enzyme. It is believed that this difference in binding accounts for the reduced toxicity of fluconazole compared with the imidazoles such as ketoconazole (Shaw et al, 1987).

In vitro, the minimum inhibitory concentrations of fluconazole for a variety of fungal species vary considerably, and data generally are unreliable in predicting efficacy in vivo. In animal models, fluconazole is active in blastomycosis, candidiasis, coccidioidomycosis, cryptococcosis, dermatophytosis, histoplasmosis, and paracoccidioidomycosis. However, activity against a number of infections (eg, aspergillosis) is seen only at very high drug concentrations that are not attained with therapeutic doses (Grant and Clissold, 1990).

USES. ***Candidiasis:*** In a noncomparative, randomized, double-blind, placebo-controlled study, the prophylactic efficacy of oral fluconazole 50 mg/day for four weeks was tested in 112 evaluable cancer patients at risk of developing oropharyngeal candidal infection (Samonis et al, 1990). In patients given fluconazole, candidiasis developed in 2% of 58 patients; in contrast, 28% of 54 patients given placebo developed the infection. Adverse reactions possibly due to fluconazole therapy occurred in only four patients, and consisted of nausea and vomiting in one patient and transient abnormalities in liver function tests in three patients; cessation of drug therapy was required in all. These and other data (Hay, 1990 A, 1990 B) indicate that fluconazole is effective chemoprophylaxis for subgroups who are at highest risk of infection, including patients in whom *Candida* species are colonized, in those receiving adrenal corticosteroids, and in those who are neutropenic or otherwise immunocompromised (Roilides et al, 1990; Vuddhakul et al, 1990).

In an open noncomparative study of cancer patients with oropharyngeal candidiasis, a therapeutic response rate of 90% was attained in 31 evaluable patients who received oral fluconazole 50 mg/day (Meunier et al, 1987). In a subsequent randomized, double-blind study, oral fluconazole 100 mg/day and ketoconazole 400 mg/day were compared for treatment of oropharyngeal candidal infection in cancer patients (Meunier et al, 1990). Cure was observed in 15 of 19 (78.9%) and in 14 of 18 (77.8%) patients given fluconazole and ketoconazole, respectively. Pathogenic fungi were eradicated in 10 patients in each group. The number of relapses and occurrence of adverse reactions were similar in both groups. However, in patients who relapsed (recurrence of signs and symptoms), the interval between cessation of treatment and relapse was markedly shorter for those who received ketoconazole (no relapses occurred >15 days following cessation) compared with those who received fluconazole (no relapses occurred <30 days after treatment was stopped).

Another randomized, double-blind trial compared fluconazole 50 mg/day and ketoconazole 200 mg/day in the treatment of oropharyngeal candidiasis in patients with AIDS and AIDS-related complex (DeWit et al, 1989). Cure was observed in 100% (17/17) of patients given fluconazole versus 75% (12/16) of patients who were treated with ketoconazole ($p = 0.044$). Mycologic cultures were negative in 87% (13/15) of patients given fluconazole and in 69% (9/13) of those receiving ketoconazole after a mean duration of therapy of 27 and 22 days, respectively.

Adverse reactions caused by fluconazole or ketoconazole were not a serious problem in the patients in these studies. However, because of other factors associated with ketoconazole therapy (eg, unreliable gastrointestinal absorption, inhibition of corticosteroid and testosterone biosynthesis, generally unfavorable pharmacokinetics compared with fluconazole [Cleary et al, 1990]), fluconazole is regarded as the drug of choice for treatment and prophylaxis of oropharyngeal/esophageal candidiasis in both immunocompromised and immunocompetent patients.

Cryptococcosis: Two early open, noncomparative, nonrandomized investigational studies on fluconazole (50 to 400 mg/day) concentrated on immunocompromised patients with cryptococcal meningitis. Results reported in those studies were encouraging and indicated that fluconazole was efficacious in active infection as well as in the long-term suppression of disease after active infection was eradicated with amphotericin B (Stern et al, 1988; Sugar and Saunders, 1988). In another noncomparative study, a 400-mg loading dose of oral fluconazole followed by 200 mg once daily was effective in 74% of 58 patients with active cryptococcal disease who had not tolerated, had not responded to, or had relapses with other drugs, including amphotericin B, ketoconazole, itraconazole, and flucytosine (Robinson et al, 1990). Fluconazole was well tolerated in this group of patients.

In a recent open-label, multicenter study, AIDS patients with active cryptococcal meningitis received fluconazole orally as initial therapy (Sugar et al, 1990). After a 400-mg loading dose, 35 patients received fluconazole 150 to 200 mg/day or 400 mg/day for 45 to 60 days. After 60 days of treatment, 26 of 29 evaluable patients (90%) were asymptomatic or improved regardless of dosage. However, mycologic evaluations clearly indicated that the larger dose was more effective than the smaller dose in eradicating the infectious agent from the CSF. Fluconazole was well tolerated, and no patients were forced to discontinue therapy because of adverse reactions.

In view of the promising data regarding the role of fluconazole in the treatment of cryptococcal meningitis, two prospective, randomized clinical trials were initiated by the Mycoses Study Group and the AIDS Clinical Trials Units of the National Institute of Allergy and Infectious Diseases. One study compared fluconazole 200 mg daily with low-dose amphotericin B (≥0.3 mg/kg/day), with or without flucytosine, primarily in AIDS patients with active cryptococcal meningitis. The other study evaluated fluconazole 200 mg daily versus amphotericin B 1 mg/kg/week as suppressive maintenance therapy for cryptococcal meningitis in AIDS patients whose cultures were negative following primary therapy with ≥15 mg/kg amphotericin B. Results reported in the former study indicated that clinical response in the patients who adhered to the protocol was similar, with 34% responding to fluconazole and 40% to amphotericin B (see Galgiani, 1990). Overall mortality was 23% within each treatment group. However, CSF cryptococcal cultures converted to negative at a significantly slower rate in patients who received fluconazole compared with those given amphotericin B. Moreover, patients treated with fluconazole died at a rate three times higher during the first week of therapy compared with those given amphotericin B. In contrast to the results of the Mycoses Study Group trial, the results of a small comparative, randomized clinical trial suggested that the mycologic and clinical efficacy of oral fluconazole 400 mg/day was inferior to that of amphotericin B plus flucytosine in the treatment of active cryptococcal meningitis in patients with AIDS (Larsen et al, 1990). However, those results must be interpreted cautiously, due to the small sample size (20 patients total) and uncharacteristically high response to amphotericin B plus flucytosine (100% versus approximately 60% historically).

The results of the Mycoses Study Group trial comparing maintenance therapy with fluconazole versus amphotericin B were unequivocal in showing the superiority of the triazole for this indication. Disease relapse occurred in 8% of patients receiving fluconazole and in approximately 33% of those receiving amphotericin B ($p<0.01$). Significantly, fluconazole was much better tolerated than amphotericin B. Since maintenance therapy for cryptococcal meningitis in AIDS patients must continue indefinitely, the relative absence of significant toxicity caused by fluconazole should result in a higher compliance rate in patients given this drug than in those who receive amphotericin B. When compared with placebo, fluconazole also is highly efficacious for maintenance therapy in cryptococcal infection (meningeal and urinary tract) in AIDS patients following clinical resolution of disease with amphotericin B alone or with flucytosine (Bozzette et al, 1991). In this study, oral fluconazole 100 or 200 mg daily reduced the cumulative risk of meningeal recurrence from 25% to 0% and the risk of recurrence at any site from 100% to 5% after one year when compared with placebo treatment. Significantly, the results achieved suggest that the detection and eradication of persistent, occult urinary tract cryptococcal infection are critical in reducing the risk of meningeal disease recurrence. Fluconazole was well tolerated by patients in this study. However, for suppression of cryptococcal meningitis, the drug is frequently given in doses larger than 100 or 200 mg daily, which usually produce proportionally more severe adverse reactions (Grant and Clissold, 1990). Nevertheless, this drug is the best treatment available for this indication, and its therapeutic benefit outweighs the potential for deleterious reactions that may accompany its use.

Clinical data presently available indicate that amphotericin B 0.5 to 1 mg/kg/day plus oral flucytosine 100 to 150 mg/kg/day is the treatment of choice for active cryptococcal meningitis in critically ill AIDS patients with mental obtundation and high CSF cryptococcal titers. However, the routine use of flucytosine in AIDS patients is controversial due to the occurrence of bone marrow suppression, which frequently forces early discontinuation of this agent despite close medical observation. For patients who are less critically ill, fluconazole alone may be considered as alternative therapy for active cryptococcal meningitis. Regardless of the induction therapy used, however, oral fluconazole is clearly the drug of choice for indefinite maintenance therapy following eradication of active cryptococcal infection.

Recent data suggest that fluconazole also is effective and well tolerated in non-AIDS patients with cryptococcal meningitis (Sugar et al, 1990) and may be efficacious in treating soft-tissue cryptococcal infections (Shuttleworth et al, 1989). However, data on the use of fluconazole in non-AIDS patients with cryptococcal infections are limited, and further trials are required to establish its efficacy in these patients.

Coccidioidomycosis: In a recent open study, oral fluconazole was administered for treatment of meningitis caused by *Coccidioides immitis* in patients whose disease progressed because of failure of or intolerance to conventional therapy, in those in whom avoidance of the toxic side effects of amphotericin B was desirable because of limited life expectancy, and in those who relapsed following successful conventional treatment (Tucker et al, 1990 A). Some patients in this study received intrathecal amphotericin B (eight patients) or miconazole (one patient) concurrently; none received other systemic therapy. After receiving daily doses of 50 to 400 mg of fluconazole for a mean duration of 10 months, 10 of 15 evaluable patients (67%) had responded, 1 (7%) had partially responded, and 4 (27%) were unresponsive. Of eight evaluable patients who received fluconazole as sole therapy, five (63%) responded fully or partially. Two patients discontinued fluconazole after initially responding to therapy, and both subsequently relapsed. No patient experienced severe toxic effects with daily doses of 400 mg. Other data indicate that fluconazole is promising as therapy for extraneural coccidioidal infection (Catanzaro and Fierer, 1988). Despite the encouraging early results, however, additional comparative trials are necessary to establish the therapeutic role of fluconazole in coccidioidal infections.

Miscellaneous Systemic Fungal Infections: Fluconazole has been reported to be effective for chronic disseminated candidiasis (hepatosplenic) in leukemia patients who received prior treatment with amphotericin B (Anaissie et al, 1989 B). It also has been effective in the treatment of small numbers of patients who have serious systemic and invasive fungal infections of the urinary tract, peritoneum, and lungs (Hay and Clayton, 1988; Van't Wout et al, 1988; Cohen, 1989; Dave et al, 1989; Warnock, 1989; Grant and Clissold, 1990). It is being evaluated in patients with blastomycosis, histoplasmosis, and paracoccidioidomycosis. However, at present, data are too limited to determine the role of fluconazole in treating these mycoses.

ADVERSE REACTIONS AND PRECAUTIONS. In general, fluconazole is well tolerated. The most common side effects associated with its use are nausea, vomiting, bloating, and abdominal discomfort. Elevated hepatic alanine and aspartate aminotransferase levels have been reported in less than 5% of patients and were reversible upon discontinuation of the drug. Stevens-Johnson reaction has been noted in at least seven patients who were treated with fluconazole. However, this effect cannot be attributed to fluconazole, since the patients were also taking other drugs associated with the condition (Grant and Clissold, 1990). Rashes occur occasionally, and reversible thrombocytopenia has been reported rarely. Fluconazole has no significant effect on plasma levels of testosterone or on the response to adrenocorticotrophic hormone in healthy volunteers receiving usual therapeutic dosages (eg, 100, 200, or 400 mg/day) for 14 days (Lazar and Wilner, 1990).

Since fluconazole is excreted in unchanged form, primarily by glomerular filtration, renal dysfunction will result in an increase in serum levels of the drug. Thus, it is essential to monitor renal function (eg, creatinine clearance) in patients receiving this agent and to adjust the dosage accordingly (see Dosage and Preparations below).

Because pregnant women generally are excluded from investigational studies, no clinical data are available on these patients. Fluconazole should be administered to pregnant women only when the benefits outweigh the potential risks (FDA Pregnancy Category C).

DRUG INTERACTIONS. Fluconazole interacts with members of the cytochrome P-450 family of drug-metabolizing enzymes. Therefore, it is likely to affect the metabolic disposition of other drugs. Results of investigational studies to date indicate that potentially deleterious pharmacokinetic interactions may occur when fluconazole is given to patients who are also receiving cyclosporine, glipizide, glyburide, tolbutamide, rifampin, warfarin, or phenytoin, particularly when the dosage of the triazole is ≥200 mg/day. Prothrombin time has increased in patients given warfarin plus fluconazole when compared with those given warfarin alone. Concomitant treatment with fluconazole and phenytoin, cyclosporine, glyburide, glipizide, or other sulfonylureas can result in elevated serum levels of the latter drugs. Blood glucose levels should be monitored in patients who are receiving oral hypoglycemic agents and fluconazole. Conversely, coadministration of rifampin and fluconazole can reduce fluconazole serum levels and half-life through enhancement of hepatic metabolism of the latter drug (Grant and Clissold, 1990; Lazar and Wilner, 1990; Howitt and Oziemski, 1989; Sugar et al, 1989; Collignon et al, 1989).

PHARMACOKINETICS. Fluconazole is reliably and well absorbed (>90% bioavailability) when given orally in the fed or fasting state and independent of gastric acidity. A plasma concentration peak of approximately 2 mcg/ml can be expected in healthy persons one to two hours after a single 100-mg dose. Peak plasma concentrations and AUC values are linearly proportional to dose. Fluconazole is approximately 12% protein bound and is widely distributed as free drug to all types of tissues. In humans, the apparent volume of distribution approaches that of total body water (0.8 L/kg). The concentration of fluconazole in CSF approximates 70% to 90% of that in plasma, depending on the dose (Brammer et al, 1990; Shiba et al, 1990). Fluconazole is metabolically stable. About 91% of a dose is eliminated in the urine (80% unchanged, 11% metabolites). The plasma elimination half-life is approximately 30 hours. Therefore, once-daily dosing is adequate. Five to seven days of therapy at usual dosage are required to achieve a steady state plasma concentration, which approximates 2.5 times that achieved after a single dose (Brammer et al, 1990). However, some experts indicate that a loading dose of 400 mg twice daily for two days will result in a steady state blood level by the second day. Pharmacokinetic data on fluconazole in children are unavailable at the present time.

DOSAGE AND PREPARATIONS.

Intravenous, Oral: Since the oral bioavailability of fluconazole is >90%, oral and intravenous dosages are equivalent (Brammer et al, 1990). In general, selection of the dosage is based on the infectious organism, the site of infection, and patient response. The duration of therapy is determined by the disappearance of clinical signs of infection or negative culture results. Since fluconazole is fungistatic rather than fungicidal when given in usual therapeutic doses, the duration of therapy must be sufficient to avoid recurrence of infection. In the patient who is severely immunocompromised (eg, by AIDS) or has cryptococcal meningitis, long-term maintenance therapy is usually required.

For active cryptococcal meningitis, *adults,* an oral loading dose of 400 mg is administered, followed by 200 mg daily for at least 10 to 12 weeks after the CSF culture becomes negative. However, some clinicians prefer to use 400 mg (or more) daily when response to therapy is not evident (Sugar et al, 1990). For chronic suppressive therapy of cryptococcal meningitis in immunocompromised patients, at least 200 mg/day is given orally. The efficacy of larger doses for both active and suppressive therapy is being studied.

For oropharyngeal or esophageal candidiasis, a loading dose of 200 mg is followed by 100 mg/day. Although improvement is usually evident within several days to one week, treatment of oropharyngeal candidiasis should continue for at least two weeks, and esophageal infection may require three to five weeks of therapy. Immunocompromised patients usually require long-term maintenance therapy to avoid relapse.

For systemic, subcutaneous, or invasive candidal infections, a 400-mg loading dose is followed by 200 to 400 mg daily for at least one month and administration is continued for two weeks following clinical resolution of infection. However, some authorities caution that the efficacy of fluconazole in these infections is not well established.

Patients with impaired renal function should receive the recommended dose at the following intervals based on creatinine clearance: >40 ml/min, once every 24 hours; 21 to 40 ml/min, once every 48 hours; 10 to 20 ml/min, once every 72 hours; dialysis patients, once following each dialysis session (Brammer et al, 1990).

Children, specific recommendations are not available. However, a recent study of fluconazole efficacy in patients with life-threatening fungal infections included some children as young as 5 to 7 years. Fluconazole was administered at a dosage of approximately 3 mg/kg/day to those patients who weighed <50 kg (Robinson et al, 1990).

Diflucan (Roerig). Solution (sterile, for intravenous infusion) 2 mg/ml in 100 and 200 ml containers; tablets 50, 100, and 200 mg. The manufacturer of fluconazole will provide the drug free of charge to uninsured AIDS patients. Physicians who wish to apply for oral fluconazole for these patients should contact the Diflucan Reimbursement Information Program at 800/869-9979, Monday through Friday, from 9:00 AM to 5:00 PM EST.

ITRACONAZOLE (Investigational drug)

[Sporanox]

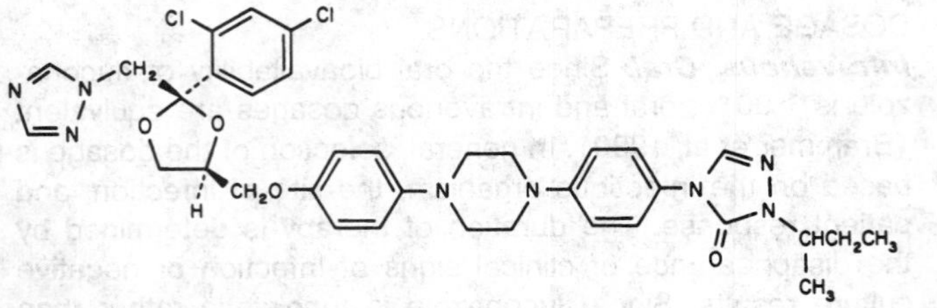

ACTIONS. Like fluconazole, itraconazole inhibits the fungal cytochrome P-450 enzyme system that causes the 14-demethylation of lanosterol, the precursor of ergosterol. Thus, it interferes with ergosterol synthesis and cell membrane integrity. Also like fluconazole, itraconazole has a greater specificity for fungal cytochrome P-450 enzyme systems than for mammalian species. This difference may account for the relatively low toxicity of triazoles when compared with imidazoles in clinical trials. In addition, itraconazole interferes with chitin synthesis in both yeast budding and hyphal growth of fungi.

USES. Itraconazole is effective orally in a number of subcutaneous and systemic mycotic infections.

Aspergillosis: In an open, noncomparative study of 34 Italian patients with various forms of aspergillosis, 20 patients were considered cured and four markedly improved following treatment with oral itraconazole 100 to 400 mg daily (Viviani et al, 1990). In a subgroup of patients with invasive pulmonary aspergillosis, 15 of 18 (83.3%) were cured. The response in those with other forms of aspergillosis was less pronounced: two of three patients with chronic necrotizing pulmonary disease were cured; one of five with the pulmonary form associated with cystic fibrosis was cured; none of four with aspergilloma were cured; and one patient with allergic bronchopulmonary disease was not cured. Similar results were described in another open, noncomparative study (Dupont, 1990). In 21 patients with invasive aspergillosis, 15 were cured when given oral itraconazole 200 or 400 mg daily: itraconazole alone (six patients), following amphotericin B plus flucytosine (five patients), or with amphotericin B plus flucytosine for a short period (four patients). Two of 14 patients with aspergilloma were cured, eight improved, and two showed no change following oral itraconazole 200 or 400 mg daily. Of 14 patients with chronic necrotizing pulmonary aspergillosis, seven were healed clinically, biologically, and mycologically; six showed marked clinical, radiologic, and biologic improvement; and one stabilized with no improvement.

A third open, nonrandomized study evaluated the efficacy of oral itraconazole 100 to 400 mg daily in various forms of aspergillosis (Denning et al, 1990). Fifteen of 21 patients were assessable and 12 had a favorable outcome: four of five with invasive pulmonary aspergillosis, two of two with skeletal disease, one of two with pleural disease, and one of one each with other forms of aspergillosis. In all of the studies described, the vast majority of patients with aspergillosis were immunocompromised, and predisposing factors included organ transplantation, various leukemias and lymphomas, and AIDS (one patient). With the exception of hypokalemia in one patient (Viviani et al, 1990), itraconazole was well tolerated even in patients who received the drug for periods exceeding one year.

The efficacy of itraconazole in most cases of invasive aspergillosis appears to be similar to that of amphotericin B, with or without flucytosine, especially in pulmonary invasive aspergillosis and bone and joint disease (Denning and Stevens, 1990). In contrast, its efficacy in other forms of aspergillosis (cerebral, sinusitis, aspergilloma) is not established, and amphotericin B is the preferred therapy in these diseases. With the possible exception of flucytosine, itraconazole is the only orally administered drug that is efficacious in the treatment of documented invasive aspergillosis. However, its therapeutic role (primary, maintenance, salvage) is not yet clear because of lack of experience with its use in the most lethal forms of invasive aspergillosis and limited follow-up data to assess relapse versus cure rates.

Candidiasis: Oral itraconazole has been evaluated in a number of different patient populations with oropharyngeal and esophageal candidiasis (Blatchford, 1990). In a double-blind, placebo-controlled study of oral candidiasis in immunosuppressed patients, itraconazole 100 or 200 mg was given daily for two weeks. Clinical cure was observed in 5 of 17 patients given placebo, 10 of 12 given itraconazole 100 mg daily, and 13 of 18 given itraconazole 200 mg daily. Mycologic cures occurred in 20%, 54%, and 56% of the patients, respectively. Oral itraconazole 200 mg daily was compared to clotrimazole troches 10 mg five times daily in a 14-day, double-blind study of oral candidiasis. At the end of treatment, 14 of 14 patients in the itraconazole group and 13 of 14 patients in the clotrimazole group were clinically and mycologically cured. This study also showed that oral candidiasis responded faster and relapses occurred at a slower rate in patients given itraconazole than in those given clotrimazole.

In a small, open study of patients with chronic mucocutaneous candidiasis, eight of eight patients given itraconazole 100 mg daily for 3 to 12 weeks responded to therapy. After a mean follow-up period of ten weeks, two patients had relapses. Finally, in a double-blind, randomized trial, itraconazole 200 mg daily was compared with ketoconazole 200 mg twice daily for treatment of oropharyngeal and esophageal candidiasis in patients with AIDS or AIDS-related complex. At the end of 28 days of therapy, 39 of 40 patients given itraconazole had complete cure of oropharyngeal candidiasis compared with 38 of 38 who received ketoconazole. Twenty-two of these patients had esophageal involvement, of whom 11 of 12 responded to itraconazole and 10 of 10 responded to ketoconazole, as confirmed by endoscopic examination. Relapse rates three months after completion of therapy were 82% in itraconazole-treated patients and 80% in those given ketoconazole. In all studies, itraconazole was well tolerated; only eight patients reported adverse effects. The reactions were primarily gastrointestinal and included diarrhea, nausea, and abdominal discomfort. Two cases of rash were also reported.

The data indicate that itraconazole may be an alternative to fluconazole or ketoconazole in the treatment of oropharyngeal and esophageal candidiasis in susceptible patients. However, comparative trials are necessary to determine the relative efficacies of the azoles in this disease and in chronic mucocutaneous candidiasis.

Chromoblastomycosis: This subcutaneous mycosis is characterized by progressive, disfiguring granulomatous lesions of the skin and subcutaneous tissues and has been refractory to treatment. Treatment has included surgical resection and local heat (small lesions only); intralesional injection of amphotericin B; and flucytosine alone or with ketoconazole, thiabendazole, or amphotericin B. Results have been variable. However, response to itraconazole has been excellent in chromoblastomycosis. In a small series of patients with chromoblastomycosis caused by *C. carrionii* (nine patients) and *F. pedrosoi* (five patients) oral itraconazole 100 to 400 mg was given daily for four to eight months (Borelli, 1987). Cure was obtained in eight of nine cases due to *C. carrionii* and in two of five cases due to *F. pedrosoi*. In the latter patients, one cure was achieved using local heat plus itraconazole; in the other patient, flucytosine was given concurrently. None of the patients reported any adverse reaction due to itraconazole, including those who received 400 mg per day. Transient hypokalemia and an increase in serum alkaline phosphatase were observed in one patient and resolved after treatment was stopped.

In another study of chromoblastomycosis due to *F. pedrosoi*, ten patients received itraconazole 100 to 200 mg daily (Restrepo et al, 1988). Symptomatic improvement was not apparent until after six months of therapy; minor to major improvement was attained in nine patients after 12 to 24 months of treatment. Six of the patients were mycologically negative, but fungal eradication could be confirmed in only three. In two additional studies on four patients with chromoblastomycosis due to *F. pedrosoi* who were treated with oral itraconazole (Ganer et al, 1987; Lavalle et al, 1987), marked improvement or clinical cure was achieved with itraconazole 100 to 200 mg daily for 7 to 12 months. Drug toxicity was limited; hypokalemia was noted in one man who received 200 mg (Ganer et al, 1987).

Although clinical experience with itraconazole is limited in the therapy of chromoblastomycosis, the data available show that this drug is the best available for disease caused by *C. carrionii* and, in combination with heat or flucytosine, appears efficacious for disease caused by *F. pedrosoi*.

Coccidioidomycosis: In a recent open study, administration of itraconazole 100 to 400 mg daily for periods up to 39 months was evaluated for treatment of nonmeningeal coccidioidomycosis in non-AIDS patients (Graybill et al, 1990). At completion of therapy, clinical remission was achieved in 6 patients with osteoarticular disease, 12 patients with chronic pulmonary disease, and 7 patients with soft tissue disease out of 44 evaluable patients (57% remission rate). Sixteen patients (43%) did not achieve remission and three (7%) discontinued therapy because of toxicity. Significantly, of the 25 patients who achieved remission, only four had relapsed 4 to 21 months after completing therapy. In this study, the most common adverse reactions to itraconazole were nausea and vomiting, which caused discontinuation of therapy in only one patient. One patient discontinued therapy because of leukopenia and one discontinued therapy because of the development of nephrotic syndrome.

In another open study of nonmeningeal coccidioidomycosis, itraconazole was given to 72 patients in 75 courses at dosages of 50 to 400 mg daily (Tucker et al, 1990 B). Of 58 assessable courses, 42 (72%) patients responded and 16 (28%) were considered nonresponders. Among the former, 17 responded within three months, 16 within three to six months, and 9 between six and nine months. Mild gastrointestinal intolerance was the most frequently noted side effect. Hypertriglyceridemia was observed in 11% of patients, but the cause was unclear because serum was not obtained from all fasting patients. Overall, itraconazole was well tolerated; toxicity caused discontinuation of therapy in two patients and dosage reduction in two others. Among 38 assessable patients who had received prior antifungal therapy (amphotericin B, ketoconazole, or both), 16 (42%) did not benefit from itraconazole treatment in contrast to 0 of 18 who had not received previous therapy (Tucker et al, 1990 B). Of 26 patients who completed a course of therapy, five (19%) relapsed within a year. This relapse rate is similar to that observed by other investigators (Graybill et al, 1990).

In an open, nonrandomized trial of itraconazole therapy (300 to 400 mg/day) for chronic coccidioidal meningitis, the drug was given to ten patients with culture or serologic evidence of disease previously refractory to therapy with other agents, including intrathecal amphotericin B (ten patients), ketoconazole (seven patients), miconazole (two patients); or fluconazole (one patient) (Tucker et al, 1990 C). Of five patients who received itraconazole as sole therapy, four responded clinically and mycologically with decline of CSF antibody titer to *C. immitis*. Three patients who received concurrent intrathecal amphotericin B and itraconazole also responded clinically, so that amphotericin B could be discontinued. Thus, of eight evaluable patients, seven (88%) responded to itraconazole. Toxicity was minimal; mild nausea without vomiting occurred in one patient and was tolerated without dosage reduction. Because this study has not been concluded, data on relapse are not available.

These data indicate that itraconazole is highly efficacious as sole therapy for disseminated, nonmeningeal coccidioidomycosis and is highly promising for the meningeal form of the disease. The remission rates of 57% and 72% in disseminated disease overlap the 50% to 75% range of remission estimated for amphotericin B (Drutz, 1983), which has been the mainstay of therapy for the past 20 years when given by a variety of parenteral routes. Antifungal azoles, including miconazole, ketoconazole, and fluconazole, have been used in coccidioidomycosis with variable success. However, miconazole is seldom administered because it must be given intravenously several times daily, is very toxic, and does not routinely produce cures (Stevens, 1983). Ketoconazole has been tested for efficacy in a large number of trials, and response rates range from 30% to 88%, depending on the scoring system used to determine therapeutic outcome and the disease site (Knoper and Galgiani, 1988). Fluconazole alone or in combination with intrathecal amphotericin B or miconazole induced a 67% response rate in 15 patients treated for coccidioidal meningitis; toxicity was minimal (Tucker et al, 1990 A).

Although ketoconazole may be considered a reasonable alternative to amphotericin B for treatment of coccidioidomycosis, doses of 400 mg daily cause significant toxicity and more severe, therapy-limiting effects occur at doses of 800 mg daily; furthermore, a high percentage of patients experience relapse (Galgiani et al, 1988). In contrast, itraconazole is relatively nontoxic at doses of 400 mg daily, which are sufficient to cure disseminated coccidioidomycosis at rates equivalent to or higher than are achieved with ketoconazole, and fewer relapses are observed. Thus, itraconazole may be considered the first alternative to amphotericin B for treatment of nonmeningeal coccidioidomycosis. However, further comparative studies are necessary to assess the relative efficacies of itraconazole, fluconazole, and amphotericin B in life-threatening meningeal disease.

Cryptococcosis: The efficacy of oral itraconazole for active or maintenance therapy of cryptococcosis, including meningitis in AIDS patients, has recently been evaluated in several open studies. Of 28 evaluable patients with cryptococcal meningitis who were given itraconazole 200 mg twice daily, 18 (64%) responded completely, 6 (21%) had partial responses, and 4 (14%) did not respond. Of 24 assessable AIDS patients with meningitis who received itraconazole alone, 16 responded (67%), 5 (21%) partially responded, and 3 (13%) did not respond (Denning et al, 1989; 1990). Cryptococcemia, pulmonary disease, osteomyelitis, and soft tissue disease all responded to treatment. However, meningitis recrudesced during therapy in 42% of responding patients. Partial responses or failures correlated with failure of previous therapy, severe disease, low serum concentrations of itraconazole, or resistance of cultured organisms to the drug. Possible drug-induced side effects included nausea, vomiting, elevated triglyceride levels (four patients), elevated liver enzymes (three patients), hypokalemia and lethargy (two patients each), and drug rash (one patient).

In another study of AIDS patients with active cryptococcal meningitis, 9 of 12 responded to itraconazole alone (200 to 400 mg daily) and 8 of 10 responded to itraconazole (200 to 400 mg daily) plus flucytosine (150 to 200 mg/kg/day) (Viviani et al, 1990). Symptoms resolved within 7 to 30 days with itraconazole alone and within 7 to 20 days with combination therapy; clinical outcome generally paralleled declines in serum cryptococcal antigen titers and negative CSF cultures. A second group of patients received maintenance therapy with itraconazole 200 mg daily following eradication of active infection with itraconazole alone (nine patients), itraconazole with flucytosine (eight patients), or other antifungal drugs (14 patients). Relapse during maintenance therapy was observed in four patients within 12 months; 14 (45%) did not relapse (serum antigen declined in 12) and 13 (42%) were completely cured, as evidenced by nondetectable serum antigen titers. Hypokalemia in one patient was related to administration of itraconazole and necessitated substitution of another antifungal agent. Tolerance to the drug regimen was otherwise acceptable.

These data and others (Grant and Clissold, 1989) indicate that itraconazole is an attractive alternative to weekly administration of amphotericin B for maintenance therapy in cryptococcal meningitis, particularly in AIDS patients. However, large, comparative trials of itraconazole and fluconazole are required to assess their relative efficacies in this role; the latter is currently considered the treatment of choice. Additional data also are required to assess the relative efficacy of itraconazole in active cryptococcosis.

Histoplasmosis: The efficacy of oral itraconazole in chronic, disseminated manifestations of histoplasmosis has been studied in a small, open trial and in individual patients. In 17 patients with chronic pulmonary or disseminated histoplasmosis, itraconazole 100 mg was given daily until clinical cure was established, followed by 50 mg daily until six months of therapy was completed (Negroni et al, 1987). Clinical cure or striking improvement was achieved in 16 patients (94%). One patient relapsed after therapy was completed, but a second six-month course of itraconazole was successful. The drug was well tolerated; a transient and asymptomatic increase in hepatic enzyme levels occurred in two patients. Significantly, the disease was cured using itraconazole in doses four to eight times lower than those necessary for cure with oral ketoconazole. One patient with disseminated mucocutaneous lesions, which recurred following resolution with amphotericin B and ketoconazole, was cured after receiving oral itraconazole 50 mg daily for 6.5 months (Dupont and Drouhet, 1987). Clinical and biochemical tolerance were excellent, and no relapses occurred after nine months of follow-up. Two patients received itraconazole therapy for recurrent histoplasmosis following prior ketoconazole treatment (Ganer et al, 1987). One patient with oral disease was cured after receiving itraconazole 100 mg daily for 14 months; another with biopsy-proven adrenal involvement received itraconazole 200 mg daily for nine months, at which time computerized tomographic scan showed resolution of the lesion.

Cumulative data in an overview of experience with itraconazole indicate an 81% success rate in 42 patients treated with 100 to 200 mg daily for 2 to 12 months (Cauwenbergh and De Doncker, 1987). This suggests that oral itraconazole therapy is equivalent to standard intravenous amphotericin B (57% to 100% success rate) in non-AIDS patients with various forms of histoplasmosis, although the relative efficacies of the two drugs have not been determined directly. Similarly, the data indicate that itraconazole is equivalent to ketoconazole in immunocompetent patients (National Institute of Allergy and Infectious Diseases Mycoses Study Group, 1985). However, controlled clinical trials have not critically evaluated the relative efficacies of ketoconazole and itraconazole in non-AIDS disseminated histoplasmosis. Nevertheless, itraconazole can be considered the first alternative to amphotericin B in life-threatening histoplasmosis, and, based on efficacy and relative lack of toxicity, is superior to ketoconazole in nonlife-threatening forms of the disease. In AIDS patients with disseminated histoplasmosis, itraconazole may be given as maintenance therapy, after aggressive induction therapy with high-dose amphotericin B (McKinsey et al, 1989; Larsen, 1990). Ketoconazole is not effective for this indication in AIDS patients (National Institute of Allergy and Infectious Diseases Mycoses Study Group, 1985).

Paracoccidioidomycosis: Itraconazole has been evaluated in 51 patients with various forms of paracoccidioidomycosis that was diagnostically confirmed by direct visualization of *P. brasiliensis* in all but one case (Borelli, 1987; Negroni et al, 1987; Restrepo et al, 1987). The majority of patients had disseminated disease with multiple lesions in the larynx, lungs, lymph nodes, oral cavity, and skin. Itraconazole 50 or 100 mg was given daily for 6 to 12 months. In ten patients (Borelli, 1987), amelioration of symptoms was noted within days after starting therapy at 50 mg daily. Cicatrization of visible, ulcerated lesions occurred during the first two weeks; pulmonary lesions responded at later, variable times. Patients regained weight that had been lost due to their infection. No adverse drug-related effects were reported.

In another study of 25 patients with disseminated paracoccidioidomycosis, 19 achieved clinical cure and 6 showed striking improvement after three to six months of therapy with itraconazole 50 mg daily (Negroni et al, 1987). Two patients subsequently relapsed and were successfully treated with a second course of the drug. Adverse reactions were reported to be insignificant. In another study, itraconazole 100 mg daily for six months resolved clinical symptoms, improved chest roentgenographic findings, and eliminated *P. brasiliensis* from clinical culture samples in 13 patients who completed therapy (Restrepo et al, 1987). No adverse reactions were reported by the patients, and no toxic effects on bone marrow or liver function were observed. Relapse was not observed among seven patients who were followed for six months after therapy, which suggests that itraconazole cured the infection.

At this time, available data indicate that itraconazole is highly effective in paracoccidioidomycosis, with efficacy equivalent to that of ketoconazole. However, itraconazole may be given in much smaller dosage than ketoconazole, thus possibly reducing the required length of therapy (Restrepo et al, 1987; Negroni et al, 1987). In addition, itraconazole appears to be more active than ketoconazole in ameliorating pulmonary lesions (Restrepo et al, 1987). The relative efficacies of ketoconazole and itraconazole in this disease have not been established by comparative clinical trials. Nevertheless, the available data indicate that itraconazole may be superior to ketoconazole in nonlife-threatening forms of paracoccidioidomycosis, especially when relative toxicity and required duration of therapy as well as efficacy are considered in choosing treatment. Intravenous amphotericin B is the drug of choice for life-threatening infections in patients who require hospitalization and parenteral therapy (Sugar, 1988).

Sporotrichosis: Itraconazole 100 mg daily was used to treat 17 patients with cutaneous and lymphangitic manifestations of sporotrichosis (Restrepo et al, 1986). Cure was reported in all patients after six months of therapy; lesions disappeared and mycologic eradication was documented by negative cultures. Clinical responses and mycologic clearance were observed as early as three months after institution of treatment; mean duration of therapy was 130 days. No significant adverse reactions were reported; two patients experienced transient elevation of hepatic aminotransferase levels, which resolved after a month. Follow-up for an average of 115 days detected no evidence of relapse, which indicates that cure was complete. The efficacy and low toxicity of itraconazole 100 to 200 mg daily also have been demonstrated in additional studies (Borelli, 1987; Lavalle et al, 1987; Graybill, 1989; Viviani et al, 1990) and in a summary of clinical experience in sporotrichosis (Cauwenbergh and De Doncker, 1987).

Potassium iodide has long been considered the drug of choice for cutaneous and lymphangitic sporotrichosis. However, dose titration often is necessary to control the many unpleasant side effects that occur during iodide therapy and that frequently cause patients to discontinue treatment. Ketoconazole therapy is not recommended in cutaneous and lymphangitic sporotrichosis, and the efficacy of fluconazole has not been critically evaluated (Winn, 1988). Thus, current data indicate that itraconazole is the preferred therapy in cutaneous and lymphangitic sporotrichosis. However, when cost is a major consideration in choice of therapy, as in many developing countries, potassium iodide may be preferred in cutaneous and lymphangitic forms of sporotrichosis. Disseminated life-threatening manifestations of this infection must be treated with intravenous amphotericin B (Winn, 1988).

Blastomycosis: Clinical data on use of itraconazole in blastomycosis are limited. In a small number of patients, doses of 100 to 400 mg daily have yielded response rates approximating 90%, including patients who did not respond to previous therapy with other drugs, including ketoconazole, or relapsed following treatment (Dismukes et al, 1986; Cauwenbergh and De Doncker, 1987; Bradsher, 1987, 1988; Saag et al, 1988). These data were obtained primarily in patients with nonmeningeal, nonlife-threatening disease. Tolerance was excellent at the doses employed. The presently available data indicate that itraconazole may be superior to ketoconazole in nondisseminated disease, especially when all aspects of therapy (efficacy, toxicity, compliance) are considered in choosing a drug. However, direct comparative trials are required to establish relative efficacies of these agents. Intravenous amphotericin B is the drug of choice in life-threatening blastomycosis (Bradsher, 1988).

Phaeohyphomycosis: A recent study showed that itraconazole 50 to 600 mg daily for one to 48 months was effective in 19 patients with phaeohyphomycosis caused by fungi of seven different genera (Sharkey et al, 1990). Clinical outcome was assessable in 17 patients with disease of the skin (9), soft tissue (9), sinuses (8), bone (5), joints (2), and lungs (2). Fourteen patients had not benefitted from previous therapy, including amphotericin B, ketoconazole, or miconazole or a combination of amphotericin B and an azole. Clinical improvement or remission was achieved in nine patients; two had disease stabilization, six did not respond, and one relapsed after successful therapy. Drug reactions were mild and infrequent; only one patient discontinued treatment and one patient developed hypokalemia that required potassium supplementation. Excellent responses in phaehyphomycosis have been reported by other investigators (Graybill, 1989). Although itraconazole appears to be highly effective in these infections, additional data are required to fully establish its role.

RESISTANCE. Itraconazole is active in vitro against a wide variety of fungi. Its spectrum of activity is similar to that of ketoconazole and includes dimorphic fungi, yeasts, dermatophytes, and agents of chromoblastomycosis and aspergillosis. With the exception of species of *Madurella*, the majority of mycetoma fungi are resistant in vitro to itraconazole at all but the highest concentrations tested, as are zygomycetes, most species of *Fusarium,* and actinomycetales (Grant and Clissold, 1989). Itraconazole resistance has been documented in isolates of *Candida* from patients who were treated with ketoconazole for a prolonged period. Although itraconazole is more potent than ketoconazole in vitro, results of assays vary considerably, depending on culture medium, inoculum size, incubation conditions, and other factors. Thus, in vitro assay results may not reflect in vivo efficacy.

ADVERSE REACTIONS AND PRECAUTIONS. Adverse effects have been infrequent (2.8%) and minor in initial studies and include headache, heartburn, and nausea. Too few patients have been studied to determine if the idiosyncratic hepatitis induced by ketoconazole (1:15,000 patients) also is produced by itraconazole; however, reversible alterations of liver function values have been documented in less than 5% of patients. Isolated cases of hypokalemia have been reported in patients receiving 400 and 600 mg daily for four to five months (Grant and Clissold, 1989).

Itraconazole does not appear to inhibit cytochrome P-450 enzymes in mice. Thus, it is expected that testosterone and cortisol biosynthesis will not be affected by this drug (Damanhouri et al, 1988); clinical reports to date confirm these suppositions. However, since these findings are based on early investigational studies with low doses of itraconazole, they may need to be revised as larger doses are used to achieve maximal antifungal efficacy.

Itraconazole is teratogenic in rats in doses higher than those effective clinically. Its use during pregnancy or in women of childbearing age is not recommended.

DRUG INTERACTIONS. In a number of in vivo models, itraconazole apparently does not induce cytochrome P-450 drug metabolizing enzymes, nor does it appear to inhibit drug metabolism. However, rifampin, phenobarbital, and phenytoin have been reported to reduce itraconazole serum levels in several patients who received one of these agents concurrently with the latter drug (Grant and Clissold, 1989; Blomley et al, 1990). Conversely, itraconazole was shown to increase cyclosporine serum concentrations to levels that were toxic to the kidneys in transplant patients (Kramer et al, 1990).

PHARMACOKINETICS. Itraconazole is poorly soluble in aqueous solution and thus is administered orally. Peak plasma concentrations occur within 1.5 to 4 hours of administration and are maximal when the drug is ingested with food. Steady-state plasma levels are achieved after two weeks, with the peak concentration approximating 0.6 mcg/ml after doses of 100 mg daily. The drug is widely distributed in the body and accumulates in certain tissues or organs at concentrations up to tenfold that attained in plasma. Itraconazole penetration of CSF is negligible. This drug is 95% protein bound in serum, primarily to albumin. It is eliminated primarily in the urine and bile after extensive hepatic metabolism. Biotransformation thus is a saturable process, which may explain the dose and duration dependence of the elimination half-life. In healthy volunteers, the terminal half-life is 20 hours after a 100-mg oral dose and increases to approximately 30 hours following two to four weeks of treatment with 100 mg daily. Neither renal nor hepatic impairment appears to mandate dosage adjustment, but additional data are required to clarify their relationship to the disposition of itraconazole (Grant and Clissold, 1989).

DOSAGE AND PREPARATIONS. The dose and duration of therapy depend on the pathogenic fungus and its site(s) of involvement.

Oral: *Adults,* for systemic fungal infections, investigational studies generally employ doses of 100 to 400 mg daily for 3 to 12 months or longer, as determined by the clinical or mycologic response.

Sporanox (Janssen).

Cited References

Drugs for treatment of fungal infections. *Med Lett Drugs Ther* 32:58-60, 1990.

Ampel NM, et al: Coccidioidomycosis: Clinical update. *Rev Infect Dis* 11:897-911, 1989.

Anaissie E, et al: New spectrum of fungal infections in patients with cancer. *Rev Infect Dis* 11:369-378, 1989 A.

Anaissie E, et al: Fluconazole: A new, safe and effective oral agent for hepatosplenic candidiasis in patients with leukemia and prior amphotericin B therapy, abstract. Program and Abstracts of the 31st Annual Meeting of the American Society of Hematology. Atlanta, Ga, Dec 1-5, 1989 B, 890.

Baley JE, et al: Pharmacokinetics, outcome of treatment, and toxic effects of amphotericin B and 5-fluorocytosine in neonates. *J Pediatr* 116:791-797, 1990.

Barton CH, et al: Renal magnesium wasting associated with amphotericin B therapy. *Am J Med* 77:471-474, 1984.

Benbow EW, Stoddart RW: Systemic zygomycosis. *Postgrad Med J* 62:985-996, 1986.

Bennett JE, et al: Comparison of amphotericin B alone and combined with flucytosine in treatment of cryptococcal meningitis. *N Engl J Med* 301:126-131, 1979.

Benson JM, Nahata MC: Clinical use of systemic antifungal agents. *Clin Pharm* 7:424-438, 1988.

Best TR, et al: Persistent adrenal insufficiency secondary to low-dose ketoconazole therapy. *Am J Med* 82:676-680, 1987.

Blatchford NR: Treatment of oral candidosis with itraconazole: A review. *J Am Acad Dermatol* 23:565-567, 1990.

Blomley M, et al: Itraconazole and anti-tuberculosis drugs. *Lancet* 336:1255, 1990.

Blyden GT, et al: Ketoconazole does not impair antipyrine clearance in humans. *Int J Clin Pharmacol Ther Toxicol* 24:225-226, 1986.

Bodey GP: Candidiasis in cancer patients. *Am J Med* 77(4D):13-19, 1984.

Bodey GP: Topical and systemic antifungal agents. *Med Clin North Am* 72:637-658, 1988.

Bodey GP, et al: Prophylaxis of candidiasis in cancer patients. *Semin Oncol* 17:24-28, 1990.

Borelli D: A clinical trial of itraconazole in the treatment of deep mycoses and leishmaniasis. *Rev Infect Dis* 9(suppl 1):S57-S63, 1987.

Bozzette SA, et al: A placebo-controlled trial of maintenance therapy with fluconazole after treatment of cryptococcal meningitis in the acquired immunodeficiency syndrome. *N Engl J Med* 324:580-584, 1991.

Bradsher RW: Itraconazole therapy of blastomycosis: Cure after failure of ketoconazole, abstract. Program and Abstracts of the 27th Interscience Conference on Antimicrobial Agents and Chemotherapy. New York, Oct 4-7, 1984, 332.

Bradsher RW: Blastomycosis. *Infect Dis Clin North Am* 2:877-898, 1988.

Brajtburg J, et al: Amphotericin B: Delivery systems. *Antimicrob Agents Chemother* 34:381-384, 1990 A.

Brajtburg J, et al: Amphotericin B: Current understanding of mechanisms of action. *Antimicrob Agents Chemother* 34:183-188, 1990 B.

Brammer KW, et al: Pharmacokinetics and tissue penetration of fluconazole in humans. *Rev Infect Dis* 12(suppl 3):S318-S326, 1990.

Branch RA: Prevention of amphotericin B-induced renal impairment: Review on the use of sodium supplementation. *Arch Intern Med* 148:2389-2394, 1988.

Brown MW, et al: Effect of ketoconazole on hepatic oxidative drug metabolism. *Clin Pharmacol Ther* 37:290-297, 1985.

Butler KM, et al: Amphotericin B as a single agent in the treatment of systemic candidiasis in neonates. *Pediatr Infect Dis J* 9:51-56, 1990.

Calhoun DL, et al: Treatment of systemic sporotrichosis with ketoconazole. *Rev Infect Dis* 13:47-51, 1991.

Catanzaro A, Fierer J: Fluconazole treatment of coccidioidomycosis. *Am Rev Respir Dis* 137:218, 1988.

Cauwenbergh G, De Doncker P: The clinical use of itraconazole in superficial and deep mycoses, in Fromtling RA (ed): *Recent Trends in the Discovery, Development and Evaluation of Antifungal Agents.* Barcelona, Spain, JR Prous Scientific Publishers, 1987, 273-284.

Chuck SL, Sande MA: Infections with *Cryptococcus neoformans* in the acquired immunodeficiency syndrome. *N Engl J Med* 321:794-799, 1989.

Clark RA, et al: Spectrum of *Cryptococcus neoformans* infection in 68 patients infected with human immunodeficiency virus. *Rev Infect Dis* 12:768-777, 1990.

Cleary JD, et al: Effect of infusion rate on amphotericin B-associated febrile reactions. *Drug Intell Clin Pharm* 22:769-772, 1988.

Cleary JD, et al: Imidazoles and triazoles in antifungal therapy. *DICP* 24:148-152, 1990.

Cohen J: Treatment of systemic yeast infection with fluconazole. *J Antimicrob Chemother* 23:294-295, 1989.

Collette N, et al: Tissue concentrations and bioactivity of amphotericin B in cancer patients treated with amphotericin B-deoxycholate. *Antimicrob Agents Chemother* 33:362-368, 1989.

Collignon P, et al: Interaction of fluconazole with cyclosporin, letter. *Lancet* 1:1262, 1989.

Conneally E, et al: Nebulized amphotericin B as prophylaxis against invasive aspergillosis in granulocytopenic patients. *Bone Marrow Transplant* 5:403-406, 1990.

Craven PC, Gremillion DH: Risk factors of ventricular fibrillation during rapid amphotericin B infusion. *Antimicrob Agents Chemother* 27:868-871, 1985.

Damanhouri Z, et al: In-vivo effects of itraconazole on hepatic mixed-function oxidase. *J Antimicrob Chemother* 21:187-194, 1988.

Daneshmend TK, Warnock DW: Clinical pharmacokinetics of systemic antifungal drugs. *Clin Pharmacokinet* 8:17-42, 1983.

Daneshmend TK, Warnock DW: Clinical pharmacokinetics of ketoconazole. *Clin Pharmacokinet* 14:13-34, 1988.

Dave J, et al: Fluconazole in renal candidosis, letter. *Lancet* 1:163-164, 1989.

DeMonaco JH, McGovern B: Transient asystole associated with amphotericin B infusion. *Drug Intell Clin Pharm* 17:547-548, 1983.

Denning DW, Stevens DA: Antifungal and surgical treatment of invasive aspergillosis: Review of 2,121 published cases. *Rev Infect Dis* 12:1147-1201, 1990.

Denning DW, et al: Itraconazole therapy for cryptococcal meningitis and cryptococcosis. *Arch Intern Med* 149:2301-2308, 1989.

Denning DW, et al: Itraconazole in opportunistic mycoses: Cryptococcosis and aspergillosis. *J Am Acad Dermatol* 23:602-607, 1990.

DeWit S, el al: Comparison of fluconazole and ketoconazole for oropharyngeal candidiasis in AIDS. *Lancet* 1:746-748, 1989.

Dismukes WE: Cryptococcal meningitis in patients with AIDS. *J Infect Dis* 157:624-628, 1988.

Dismukes WE, et al: Treatment of systemic mycoses with ketoconazole: Emphasis on toxicity and clinical response in 52 patients. *Ann Intern Med* 98:13-20, 1983.

Dismukes WE, et al: Comparison of two different treatment regimens of flucytosine and amphotericin B in cryptococcal meningitis, abstract. Program and Abstracts of the 24th Interscience Conference on Antimicrobial Agents and Chemotherapy. Washington, DC, Oct 8-10, 1984, 286.

Dismukes W, et al: Itraconazole therapy for blastomycosis and histoplasmosis, abstract. Program and Abstracts of the 26th Interscience Conference on Antimicrobial Agents and Chemotherapy. New Orleans, La, Sept 28-Oct 1, 1986, 242.

Dismukes WE, et al: Treatment of cryptococcal meningitis with combination amphotericin B and flucytosine for four as compared with six weeks. *N Engl J Med* 317:334-341, 1987.

Doble N, et al: Pharmacokinetic study of the interaction between rifampicin and ketoconazole. *J Antimicrob Chemother* 21:633-635, 1988.

Drutz DJ: Amphotericin B in the treatment of coccidioidomycosis. *Drugs* 26:337-346, 1983.

Dupont B: Itraconazole therapy in aspergillosis: Study in 49 patients. *J Am Acad Dermatol* 23:607-614, 1990.

Dupont B, Drouhet E: Early experience with itraconazole in vitro and in patients: Pharmacokinetic studies and clinical results. *Rev Infect Dis* 9(suppl 1):S71-S76, 1987.

Engelhard D, et al: Interaction of ketoconazole with rifampin and isoniazid. *N Engl J Med* 311:1681-1683, 1984.

EORTC (European Organization for Research and Treatment of Cancer) International Antimicrobial Cooperative Group: Empiric antifungal therapy in febrile granulocytopenic patients. *Am J Med* 86:668-672, 1989.

Fromtling RA: Overview of medically important antifungal azole derivatives. *Clin Microbiol Rev* 1:187-217, 1988.

Galgiani JN: Fluconazole, a new antifungal agent, editorial. *Ann Intern Med* 113:177-179, 1990.

Galgiani JN, Ampel NM: Coccidioidomycosis in human immunodeficiency virus-infected patients. *J Infect Dis* 162:1165-1169, 1990.

Galgiani JN, et al: *Pseudallescheria boydii* infections treated with ketoconazole. *Chest* 86:219-224, 1984.

Galgiani JN, et al: Ketoconazole therapy of progressive coccidioidomycosis: Comparison of 400- and 800-mg doses and observations at higher doses. *Am J Med* 84:603-610, 1988.

Ganer A, et al: Initial experience in therapy for progressive mycoses with itraconazole, the first clinically studied triazole. *Rev Infect Dis* 9 (suppl 1):S77-S86, 1987.

Gigliotti F, et al: Induction of prostaglandin synthesis as the mechanism responsible for the chills and fever produced by infusing amphotericin B. *J Infect Dis* 156:784-789, 1987.

Glass AR: Ketoconazole-induced stimulation of gonadotropin output in men: Basis for potential test of gonadotropin reserve. *J Clin Endocrinol Metab* 63:1121-1125, 1986.

Glynn AM, et al: Effects of ketoconazole on methylprednisolone pharmacokinetics and cortisol secretion. *Clin Pharmacol Ther* 39:654-659, 1986.

Goodpasture HC, et al: Treatment of central nervous system fungal infection with ketoconazole. *Arch Intern Med* 145:879-880, 1985.

Grant SM, Clissold SP: Itraconazole: A review of its pharmacodynamic and pharmacokinetic properties, and therapeutic use in superficial and systemic mycoses. *Drugs* 37:310-344, 1989.

Grant SM, Clissold SP: Fluconazole: A review of its pharmacodynamic and pharmacokinetic properties, and therapeutic potential in superficial and systemic mycoses. *Drugs* 39:877-916, 1990.

Graybill JR: Histoplasmosis and AIDS. *J Infect Dis* 158:623-626, 1988 A.

Graybill JR: Therapeutic agents. *Infect Dis Clin North Am* 2:805-825, 1988 B.

Graybill JR: Antifungal agents of the 1980's. *Antimicrob Newslett* 5:45-52, (July) 1988 C.

Graybill JR: New antifungal agents. *Eur J Clin Microbiol Infect Dis* 8:402-412, 1989

Graybill JR, et al: Ketoconazole treatment of chronic mucocutaneous candidiasis. *Arch Dermatol* 116:1137-1141, 1980.

Graybill JR, et al: Itraconazole treatment of coccidioidomycosis. *Am J Med* 89:282-290, 1990.

Gross MH, et al: Retrospective review of amphotericin B use in a tertiary-care medical center. *Am J Hosp Pharm* 44:1353-1357, 1987.

Hawkins CC, Armstrong D: Opportunistic organisms in the immunocompromised. *Consultant* 25:93-127, (May) 1985.

Hay RJ: Overview of studies of fluconazole in oropharyngeal candidiasis. *Rev Infect Dis* 12 (suppl 3):S334-S337, 1990 A.

Hay RJ: Fluconazole, editorial. *J Infect* 21:1-6, 1990 B.

Hay RJ, Clayton YM: Fluconazole in the management of patients with chronic mucocutaneous candidosis. *Br J Dermatol* 119:683-684, 1988.

Hoeprich PD (ed): *Infectious Diseases: A Modern Treatise of Infectious Processes*, ed 3. Philadelphia, JB Lippincott, 1983 A.

Hoeprich PD: Ketoconazole in systemic mycoses, editorial. *Ann Intern Med* 98:105, 1983 B.

Howitt KM, Oziemski MA: Phenytoin toxicity induced by fluconazole. *Med J Aust* 151:603-604, 1989.

Huang Y-C, et al: Pharmacokinetics and dose proportionality of ketoconazole in normal volunteers. *Antimicrob Agents Chemother* 30:206-210, 1986.

Hughes WT, et al: Guidelines for the use of antimicrobial agents in neutropenic patients with unexplained fever. *J Infect Dis* 161:381-396, 1990.

Jorizzo JL: Chronic mucocutaneous candidosis: Update, editorial. *Arch Dermatol* 118:963-965, 1982.

Kerkering TM: Present status of flucytosine therapy. *Drug Ther* 12:75-79, 1982.

Khosla S, et al: Adrenal crisis in the setting of high-dose ketoconazole therapy. *Arch Intern Med* 149:802-804, 1989.

Kitching NH: Hypothyroidism after treatment with ketoconazole. *Br Med J* 293:993-994, 1986.

Knoper SR, Galgiani JN: Coccidioidomycosis. *Infect Dis Clin North Am* 2:861-874, 1988.

Kraemer FB, Pont A: Inhibition of cholesterol synthesis by ketoconazole. *Am J Med* 80:616-622, 1986.

Kramer MR, et al: Cyclosporine and itraconazole interaction in heart and lung transplant recipients. *Ann Intern Med* 113:327-329, 1990.

Lake-Bakaar G, et al: Hepatic reactions associated with ketoconazole in the United Kingdom. *Br Med J* 294:419-422, 1987.

Larsen RA: Azoles and AIDS. *J Infect Dis* 162:727-730, 1990.

Larsen RA, et al: Fluconazole compared with amphotericin B plus flucytosine for cryptococcal meningitis in AIDS: A randomized trial. *Ann Intern Med* 113:183-187, 1990.

Lavalle P, et al: Itraconazole for deep mycoses: Preliminary experience in Mexico. *Rev Infect Dis* 9 (suppl 1):S64-S70, 1987.

Lazar JD, Wilner KD: Drug interactions with fluconazole. *Rev Infect Dis* 12 (suppl 3):S327-S333, 1990.

Lelawongs P, et al: Effect of food and gastric acidity on absorption of orally administered ketoconazole. *Clin Pharm* 7:228-235, 1988.

Lopez-Berestein G: Liposomes as carriers of antimicrobial agents. *Antimicrob Agents Chemother* 31:675-678, 1987.

Lopez-Berestein G, et al: Treatment of systematic fungal infections with liposomal amphotericin B. *Arch Intern Med* 149:2533-2536, 1989.

Lucente FE (ed): Mycoses of the head and neck. *Ear Nose Throat J* 67:794-855, 1988.

Lutwick LI, et al: Deep infections due to *Petriellidium boydii* treated with miconazole. *JAMA* 241:272-273, 1979.

Mahgoub ES: Mycetoma. *Semin Dermatol* 4:230-239, 1985.

Mandell GL, et al (eds): Mycoses, in: *Principles and Practice of Infectious Diseases*, ed 3. New York, Churchill Livingstone, 1990, 1942-2034.

McKinsey DS, et al: Long-term amphotericin B therapy for disseminated histoplasmosis in patients with the acquired immunodeficiency syndrome (AIDS). *Ann Intern Med* 111:655-659, 1989.

Medoff G: Controversial areas in antifungal chemotherapy: Short-course and combination therapy with amphotericin B. *Rev Infect Dis* 9:403-407, 1987.

Meunier F: Prevention of mycoses in immunocompromised patients. *Rev Infect Dis* 9:408-416, 1987.

Meunier F: New methods for delivery of antifungal agents. *Rev Infect Dis* 11 (suppl 7):S1605-S1612, 1989.

Meunier F, Klastersky J: Recent developments in prophylaxis and therapy of invasive fungal infections in granulocytopenic cancer patients. *Eur J Cancer Clin Oncol* 24:539-544, 1988.

Meunier F, et al: Fluconazole therapy of oropharyngeal candidiasis in cancer patients, in Fromtling RA (ed): *Recent Trends in the Discovery, Development and Evaluation of Antifungal Agents.* Barcelona, Spain, JR Prous Scientific Publishers, 1987, 169-174.

Meunier F, et al: Therapy for oropharyngeal candidiasis in the immunocompromised host: A randomized double-blind study of fluconazole vs. ketoconazole. *Rev Infect Dis* 12 (suppl 3):S364-S368, 1990.

Milliken ST, Powles RL: Antifungal prophylaxis in bone marrow transplantation. *Rev Infect Dis* 12 (suppl 3):S374-S379, 1990.

Musial CE, et al: Fungal infections of the immunocompromised host: Clinical and laboratory aspects. *Clin Microbiol Rev* 1:349-364, 1988.

National Institute of Allergy and Infectious Diseases Mycoses Study Group: Treatment of blastomycosis and histoplasmosis with ketoconazole: Results of prospective randomized clinical trial. *Ann Intern Med* 103:861-872, 1985.

Negroni R, et al: Oral treatment of paracoccidioidomycosis and histoplasmosis with itraconazole in humans. *Rev Infect Dis* 9 (suppl 1): S47-S50, 1987.

Oldfield EC, et al: Randomized, double-blind trial of 1- versus 4-hour amphotericin B infusion durations. *Antimicrob Agents Chemother* 34:1402-1406, 1990.

Penn RL, et al: Invasive fungal infections: Use of serologic tests in diagnosis and management. *Arch Intern Med* 143:1215-1220, 1983.

Petersen EA, et al: Treatment of chronic mucocutaneous candidiasis with ketoconazole. *Ann Intern Med* 93:791-795, 1980.

Pfaller MA, et al: Collaborative investigation of variables in susceptibility testing of yeasts. *Antimicrob Agents Chemother* 34:1648-1654, 1990.

Pizzo PA, et al: Empiric antibiotic and antifungal therapy for cancer patients with prolonged fever and granulocytopenia. *Am J Med* 72:101-110, 1982.

Powderly WG, et al: Amphotericin B-resistant yeast infection in severely immunocompromised patients. *Am J Med* 84:826-832, 1988.

Restrepo A, et al: Itraconazole therapy in lymphangitic and cutaneous sporotrichosis. *Arch Dermatol* 122:413-417, 1986.

Restrepo A, et al: Itraconazole in the treatment of paracoccidioidomycosis: A preliminary report. *Rev Infect Dis* 9(suppl 1): S51-S56, 1987

Restrepo A, et al: Treatment of chromoblastomycosis with itraconazole. *Ann NY Acad Sci* 544:504-516, 1988.

Robinson PA, et al: Fluconazole for life-threatening fungal infections in patients who cannot be treated with conventional antifungal agents. *Rev Infect Dis* 12(suppl 3):S349-S363, 1990.

Roilides E, et al: Effects of antifungal agents on the function of human neutrophils in vitro. *Antimicrob Agents Chemother* 34:196-201, 1990.

Saag MS, Dismukes WE: Azole antifungal agents: Emphasis on new triazoles. *Antimicrob Agents Chemother* 32:1-8, 1988.

Saag M, et al: Itraconazole (I) therapy (Rx) for blastomycosis (B), histoplasmosis (H), and sporotrichosis (S), abstract. Program and Abstracts of the 28th Interscience Conference on Antimicrobial Agents and Chemotherapy. Los Angeles, Oct 23-26, 1988, 210.

Samonis G, et al: Prophylaxis of oropharyngeal candidiasis with fluconazole. *Rev Infect Dis* 12(suppl 3):S369-S373, 1990.

Sculier JP, et al: Pilot study of amphotericin B entrapped in sonicated liposomes in cancer patients with fungal infections. *Eur J Cancer Clin Oncol* 24:527-538, 1988.

Sharkey, et al: Itraconazole treatment of phaeohyphomycosis. *J Am Acad Dermatol* 23:577-586, 1990.

Shaw JTB, et al: Cytochrome P-450 mediated sterol synthesis and metabolism: Differences in sensitivity to fluconazole and other azoles, in Fromtling RA (ed): *Recent Trends in the Discovery, Development and Evaluation of Antifungal Agents.* Barcelona, Spain, JR Prous Scientific Publishers, 1987, 125-139.

Shiba K, et al: Safety and pharmacokinetics of single oral and intravenous doses of fluconazole in healthy subjects. *Clin Ther* 12:206-215, 1990.

Shuttleworth D, et al: Cutaneous cryptococcosis: Treatment with oral fluconazole. *Br J Dermatol* 20:683-687, 1989.

Smego RA Jr, et al: Combined therapy with amphotericin B and 5-fluorocytosine for *Candida meningitis*. *Rev Infect Dis* 6:791-801, 1984.

Smith AG: Potentiation of oral anticoagulants by ketoconazole. *Br Med J* 288:188-189, 1984.

Smith EB, Henry JC: Ketoconazole: Orally effective antifungal agent: Mechanism of action, pharmacology, clinical efficacy and adverse effects. *Pharmacotherapy* 4:199-204, 1984.

Sonino N: Use of ketoconazole as inhibitor of steroid production. *N Engl J Med* 317:812-818, 1987.

Stamm AM, et al: Toxicity of amphotericin B plus flucytosine in 194 patients with cryptococcal meningitis. *Am J Med* 83:236-242, 1987.

Stern JJ, et al: Oral fluconazole therapy for patients with acquired immunodeficiency syndrome and cryptococcosis: Experience with 22 patients. *Am J Med* 85:477-480, 1988.

Stevens DA: Miconazole in treatment of coccidioidomycosis. *Drugs* 26:347-354, 1983.

Stratton CW: Antifungal agents: The old and the new. *Infect Dis Newslett* 9:41-45, 1990.

Sugar AM: Paracoccidioidomycosis. *Infect Dis Clin North Am* 2:913-924, 1988.

Sugar AM: Empiric treatment of fungal infections in the neutropenic host: Review of the literature and guidelines for use. *Arch Intern Med* 150:2258-2264, 1990.

Sugar AM, Saunders C: Oral fluconazole as suppressive therapy of disseminated cryptococcosis in patients with acquired immunodeficiency syndrome. *Am J Med* 85:481-489, 1988.

Sugar AM, et al: Pharmacology and toxicity of high-dose ketoconazole. *Antimicrob Agents Chemother* 31:1874-1878, 1987.

Sugar AM, et al: Interaction of fluconazole and cyclosporine, letter. *Ann Intern Med* 110:844, 1989.

Sugar AM, et al: Overview: Treatment of cryptococcal meningitis. *Rev Infect Dis* 12(suppl 3):S338-S348, 1990.

Terrell CL, Hermans PE: Antifungal agents used for deep-seated mycotic infections. *Mayo Clin Proc* 62:1116-1128, 1987.

Tucker WS Jr, et al: Reversible adrenal insufficiency induced by ketoconazole. *JAMA* 253:2413-2414, 1985.

Tucker RM, et al: Treatment of coccidioidal meningitis with fluconazole. *Rev Infect Dis* 12(suppl 3):S380-S389, 1990 A.

Tucker RM, et al: Itraconazole therapy for nonmeningeal coccidioidomycosis: Clinical and laboratory observations. *J Am Acad Dermatol* 23:593-601, 1990 B.

Tucker RM, et al: Itraconazole therapy for chronic coccidioidal meningitis. *Ann Intern Med* 112:108-112, 1990 C.

Van't Wout JW, et al: A prospective study of the efficacy of fluconazole (UK-49,858) against deep-seated fungal infections. *J Antimicrob Chemother* 21:665-672, 1988.

Van Tyle JH: Ketoconazole: Mechanism of action, spectrum of activity, pharmacokinetics, drug interactions, adverse reactions and therapeutic use. *Pharmacotherapy* 4:343-373, 1984.

Viviani MA, et al: European experience with itraconazole in systemic mycoses. *J Am Acad Dermatol* 23:587-593, 1990.

Vuddhakul V, et al: Suppression of neutrophil and lymphoproliferative responses *in vitro* by itraconazole but not fluconazole. *Int J Immunopharmacol* 12:639-645, 1990.

Walsh TJ, Pizzo A: Treatment of systemic fungal infections: Recent progress and current problems. *Eur J Clin Microbiol Infect Dis* 7:460-475, 1988.

Warnock DW: Itraconazole and fluconazole: New drugs for deep fungal infection. *J Antimicrob Chemother* 24:275-277, 1989.

Wheat LJ, et al: Histoplasmosis in acquired immune deficiency syndrome. *Am J Med* 78:203-210, 1985.

Wiebe VJ, DeGregorio MW: Liposome-encapsulated amphotericin B: Promising new treatment for disseminated fungal infections. *Rev Infect Dis* 10:1097-1101, 1988.

Wingard JR, et al: Prevention of fungal sepsis in patients with prolonged neutropenia: Randomized, double-blind, placebo-controlled trial of intravenous miconazole. *Am J Med* 83:1103-1110, 1987.

Winn RE: Sporotrichosis. *Infect Dis Clin North Am* 2:899-911, 1988.

Zürcher RM, et al: Impact of ketoconazole on the metabolism of prednisolone. *Clin Pharmacol Ther* 45:366-372, 1989.

Antiprotozoal Drugs 78

All four classes of protozoa include pathogenic organisms. The *Sarcodina* (eg, *Entamoeba histolytica*) cause amebic disease. The *Mastigophora* (flagellates) produce dientamebiasis, giardiasis (lambliasis), leishmaniasis, trichomoniasis, and trypanosomiasis. The *Ciliophora* (ciliates) include at least one organism, *Balantidium coli*, that produces disease (balantidiasis). The *Apicocomplexa* (formerly termed *Sporozoa*) cause coccidiosis (isosporiasis and cryptosporidiosis), malaria, and toxoplasmosis. *Pneumocystis carinii* pneumonia (PCP) is caused by an organism of uncertain taxonomic status, and it has been suggested that it may be more closely related to fungi than to protozoa (Edman et al, 1988).

Drug therapy for protozoal infections has improved markedly during the last three decades. Nevertheless, the indications and use of these drugs may differ considerably between developed and developing countries, especially for diseases that are endemic to specific areas. The management of patients with most parasitic infections is quite satisfactory in the United States but presents more difficulties in developing countries. Chemotherapy may be a significant economic burden for countries with limited resources, and programs of mass chemoprophylaxis have had only limited success. More effective measures include control of the nonhuman vector (when one exists), elimination of the reservoir of infection, and improvement of sanitation and living conditions. Unfortunately, the people at risk are spread over large, sometimes inaccessible, areas and often cannot comply with instructions given by a physician or health worker. Moreover, they are frequently infected with several organisms, which makes diagnosis, therapy, and follow-up complex. Even when individual cures are achieved, the patient returns to an environment where reinfection is almost a certainty.

Drugs noted in this chapter as being available from the Centers for Disease Control (CDC) may be obtained by contacting the Drug & Immunobiologics Service, CDC, 1600 Clifton Road, Bldg 1, Room 1259, Atlanta, GA 30333. During regular business hours (8 AM to 4:30 PM EST, Monday through Friday), the telephone number is 404/639-3670; the emergency number is 404/639-2888 (nights, weekends, or holidays). In Canada, help in obtaining exotic drugs is available from the Bureau of Human Prescription Drugs, Ottawa (day 613/993-3105; after hours 613/992-0123).

AMEBIASIS

Entamoeba histolytica is present in the gastrointestinal tract of 10% of the world's population. In the United States, the prevalence rate among homosexuals is 25% to 32%, although invasive disease does not appear to have increased proportionately. Amebiasis is a leading parasitic cause of death in the world (Walsh, 1986).

Amebiasis is transmitted when mature cysts are ingested (Guerrant, 1986; Ravdin, 1987) or, rarely, introduced by colonic irrigation. Pregnant, malnourished, or immunocompromised individuals are at greater risk of developing severe disease. Each cyst develops into eight trophozoites, usually in the ileocecal region of the intestine. A colony is established in the cecum and later extends throughout the colon.

Trophozoites penetrate the mucosa and cause ulceration of the intestinal wall that may simulate idiopathic ulcerative colitis. Bloody mucoid diarrhea, abdominal pain, weight loss, bloating, tenesmus, and cramps are common in those with invasive disease. Leukocytosis, mild anemia, and an elevated sedimentation rate occur frequently. A test for occult blood in the stool is usually positive. Leukocytes may not be present in the feces. Most individuals remain asymptomatic while transmitting amebae by passing mature cysts in formed stools. *E. histolytica* occasionally invades the liver, and this is manifested by abscess formation and elevation of alkaline phosphatase. Rarely, amebic abscesses occur in other locations (eg, the pleural space, pericardium, brain).

Definitive diagnosis is based on finding the organism in fresh or preserved stool specimens or in colonic tissue biopsies obtained by endoscopy. The indirect hemagglutinin test is highly specific and is most commonly used, especially in those with liver involvement or severe colonic disease (Healy, 1986). Serologic tests can aid in screening; in the presence of fever, leukocytosis, or hepatic dysfunction, a positive serologic test is sufficient to make a presumptive diagnosis and initiate treatment. However, results may remain positive for years following invasive disease.

Strains of *E. histolytica* vary in virulence. Tissue invasion by *E. histolytica* is facilitated by secreted proteolytic enzymes, cytotoxins, contact-dependent cytolysis, and phagocytosis (Ravdin, 1986). Immunity apparently does not develop to asymptomatic intestinal colonization; however, there is some evidence that cell-mediated immunity develops after cure of invasive amebiasis (Salata and Ravdin, 1986).

CLASSIFICATION OF AMEBICIDES. Some drugs act on amebae only within the lumen of the bowel (luminal amebicide), whereas others affect the parasite in the intestinal wall or other organs (tissue amebicide).

Diloxanide [Furamide] and iodoquinol (diiodohydroxyquin) [Yodoxin] act in the intestinal lumen. These agents and the nonabsorbable aminoglycoside antibiotic, paromomycin [Humatin], are termed oral luminal or contact amebicides. Most authorities consider paromomycin a less effective luminal amebicide than iodoquinol.

Metronidazole [Flagyl, Protostat] has a relatively low toxic potential and is effective against tissue amebae. Although it also exerts an effect in the colonic lumen, its actions are most pronounced in tissue because most of the compound is absorbed during passage through the small intestine. For this reason, iodoquinol or paromomycin is usually given after administration of metronidazole to eradicate organisms in the intestine and avoid relapse. Other nitroimidazoles (flunidazole, tinidazole) that are related to metronidazole but have appreciably longer half-lives are being investigated for use in amebiasis (Rossignol et al, 1984).

Emetine; its analogue, dehydroemetine [Mebadin] (which is as effective as emetine and probably less toxic); and chloroquine [Aralen] also are tissue amebicides. The emetines are given parenterally and affect amebae in the intestinal wall and liver. As with metronidazole, iodoquinol or paromomycin is often administered after the emetines. Chloroquine is given orally and acts principally in the liver. It is appreciably less effective than the emetines but also is less toxic. It is not indicated for intestinal infection. Chloroquine alone probably is inadequate for amebic abscess but can be given with iodoquinol and the emetines.

DRUG SELECTION. The choice of amebicide(s) depends principally on the severity of disease and site of involvement (luminal or extraintestinal); other factors influencing drug selection are pregnancy (eg, avoidance of metronidazole during the first trimester if possible), drug allergy, intolerance, and relative toxicity.

Within endemic areas, asymptomatic carriers generally are not treated. Elsewhere, the asymptomatic cyst carrier is treated with a luminal amebicide. The drug of choice is iodoquinol; paromomycin and diloxanide are suitable alternatives. Some authorities prefer diloxanide, but it is available only from the CDC. Because metronidazole is less effective as a luminal amebicide than as a tissue amebicide, this agent is not generally recommended to treat asymptomatic amebiasis. The recommended dose of iodoquinol and duration of therapy should not be exceeded because of the possibility of causing optic neuritis.

In symptomatic, invasive intestinal amebiasis, *E. histolytica* are present in the intestinal lumen, on the mucosal surface of the bowel, and in the walls of the intestine. Metronidazole is the drug of choice in combination with iodoquinol or paromomycin.

Emetine or dehydroemetine (preferred) with iodoquinol is an alternative regimen to metronidazole with iodoquinol for severe disease. Paromomycin plus iodoquinol may be useful when metronidazole or the emetines are not effective, not tolerated, or contraindicated. Because of the potential cardiotoxicity of the emetines, patients receiving these drugs should be monitored by electrocardiography and remain sedentary during therapy.

Tissue abscesses can be treated with metronidazole. A luminal amebicide (usually iodoquinol) also is indicated to eliminate the primary source of infection and prevent relapses. Chloroquine is occasionally used with this regimen, especially in infants with hepatic abscesses. Alternative therapy consists of emetine or dehydroemetine and iodoquinol with or without chloroquine. Drainage of liver abscesses should be avoided because of the high morbidity and mortality associated with amebic peritonitis. However, occasionally liver abscesses

TABLE 1.
RECOMMENDED THERAPY FOR AMEBIASIS*

Type of Infection	Therapy of Choice	Alternative Therapy
Asymptomatic (cyst carrier state)	Iodoquinol[1]	Paromomycin[3] or Diloxanide furoate[2]
Mild to moderate intestinal disease	Metronidazole[4] followed by Iodoquinol[1]	Metronidazole[4] followed by Paromomycin[3]
Severe intestinal disease	Metronidazole[4] followed by Iodoquinol[1]	Dehydroemetine[5] or Emetine[6] followed by Iodoquinol[1]
Tissue abscess (usually hepatic)	Metronidazole[4] followed by Iodoquinol[1]	Dehydroemetine[5] or Emetine[6] plus Iodoquinol[1] with or without Chloroquine phosphate[7]

**Except for emetine and dehydroemetine, all drugs are given orally.*

[1]Adults, 650 mg three times daily for 20 days. Children, 30 to 40 mg/kg/day in two or three doses for 20 days (maximum, 2 g/day). Do not exceed dose or duration.

[2]Adults, 500 mg three times daily for 10 days. Children, 20 mg/kg/day in three doses for 10 days.

[3]Adults and children, 25 to 35 mg/kg/day in three doses for 7 to 10 days.

[4]Adults, 750 mg three times daily for 10 days. Children, 35 to 50 mg/kg/day in three doses for 10 days.

[5]Adults, 1 to 1.5 mg/kg/day (maximum, 90 mg/day) for five days. Children, no more than 1 to 1.5 mg/kg/day in two doses for five days.

[6]Adults, 1 mg/kg/day (maximum, 60 mg/day) for five days. Children, no more than 0.5 mg/kg twice daily for five days. Monitor during therapy by electrocardiography.

[7]Adults, 1 g (600 mg base) daily for two days, then 500 mg (300 mg base) daily for two to three weeks. Children, 10 mg (base)/kg/day for 21 days (maximum, 300 mg (base)/day).

may require drainage depending on the size and response to therapy; closed aspiration is preferred when there is uncertainty regarding the diagnosis, a palpable mass (especially when the left lobe impinges on the diaphragm with potential pericardial involvement), persistent local tenderness, or markedly raised hemidiaphragm (Basile et al, 1983; Thompson et al, 1985). Ultrasound or CT is useful to locate the abscesses. Liver abscesses sometimes rupture, contaminating the lungs, pleura, pericardium, or peritoneum. These complications are treated by drainage and administration of the same regimen used for hepatic amebiasis.

Complications of intestinal amebiasis include ameboma (a tumor-like mass of granulomatous tissue in the intestinal wall), stricture, perforation, intussusception, and toxic megacolon. These conditions are treated with metronidazole alone or with emetine or dehydroemetine and a luminal amebicide. Intussusception must be reduced surgically during therapy. Peritonitis is a serious complication. Ulcerative postdysenteric colitis usually responds to maintenance of an adequate fluid and electrolyte balance, blood transfusion, and a high-calorie diet.

Dosage recommendations appear in the individual drug evaluations and in Table 1. For a detailed discussion of adverse reactions, precautions, and contraindications, see the evaluations.

BALANTIDIASIS

Balantidiasis is caused by the ciliate protozoan, *Balantidium coli*, which infects the terminal ileum and cecum of the large intestine. Pigs may be reservoirs of infection, and people who handle these animals may become infected from ingestion of the cyst form. However, the parasite also is transmitted between humans. The incidence of human balantidiasis is low, and many individuals are asymptomatic, although diarrhea and abdominal pain may occur. In severe infections, a dysenteric syndrome similar to that observed in amebiasis develops.

Balantidiasis is treated with tetracycline. Iodoquinol and metronidazole are being investigated for use in this infection.

COCCIDIOSIS

CRYPTOSPORIDIOSIS. *Cryptosporidium*, an intracellular coccidian parasite, commonly produces mild, self-limited nonbloody, noninflammatory diarrhea of two to four weeks' duration and a mild "flu-like" state in immunocompetent persons (Angus, 1983; Wolfson et al, 1985; Soave and Armstrong, 1986); an asymptomatic carrier phase also occurs. In severely malnourished or immunocompromised individuals, especially those with acquired immunodeficiency syndrome (AIDS), enteritis or enterocolitis with severe chronic diarrhea characterized by watery (cholera-like) or frothy nonbloody stools develops. Nausea, vomiting, weakness, low-grade fever, anorexia, and severe abdominal cramps also are present. However, symptoms initially may be mild in many AIDS patients. Esophageal, gastric, biliary, or bronchial involvement is noted in a small percentage of patients with severe infection. Definitive diagnosis is based on identification of oocysts in stool specimens.

Cryptosporidium develops within a single host (monoxenous life cycle) and is highly infectious. The organism produces a similar infection in many animals but is not highly species-specific. The disease may be spread through contact with pets, farm animals, and certain wild animals. Like giardiasis, *Cryptosporidium* has caused diarrhea in day-care centers (*MMWR*, 1984; Taylor et al, 1985) and has been identified as the cause of waterborne outbreaks of disease (Hayes et al, 1989). Clearance of the parasite from the stool often lags two to three weeks behind resolution of the clinical illness.

Supportive measures are usually adequate for treating immunocompetent patients. Moderate to severe diarrhea can develop in immunocompromised patients and is very resistant to therapy. Cryptosporidia have become a prominent gastrointestinal pathogen in AIDS patients. Most anti-infective agents are ineffective in treating this disease. In a small, randomized, placebo-controlled trial, oral spiramycin [Rovamycine], a macrolide antibiotic similar to erythromycin, shortened the duration of diarrhea and promoted the excretion of oocysts in the stools of immunocompetent infants (Sáez-Llorens et al, 1989). However, in another controlled trial this drug was ineffective in relieving diarrhea produced by *Cryptosporidium* in infants (Wittenberg et al, 1989). Its use for treatment of cryptosporidiosis does not have strong support among infectious disease authorities, and it is not generally administered for this purpose.

Nonopioid antidiarrheal agents have had little effect in relieving the severe diarrhea associated with cryptosporidiosis in AIDS patients, and they may even worsen the condition. Opioid antidiarrheal agents have been anecdotally reported to be effective. Their use is not contraindicated in patients with a limited life span, because they improve the quality of life in many of these individuals (Connolly et al, 1988).

Total parenteral nutrition (TPN) may be indicated to reduce stool volume in some patients. Two case reports describe the long-term effectiveness of the investigational use of octreotide [Sandostatin], a long-acting somatostatin analogue, for this secretory type of diarrhea (Katz et al, 1988; Cook et al, 1988). It is given by intravenous infusion (10 to 75 mcg/hr) or subcutaneously (100 to 300 mcg three times daily) and has markedly reduced stool frequency and volume. The rationale for this use is based on octreotide's effectiveness in the severe secretory diarrheas associated with carcinoid syndrome, vasoactive intestinal polypeptide (VIP)-secreting tumors, and ileostomies. Mild gastrointestinal disturbances (abdominal cramping and bloating) were well tolerated. However, most infectious disease experts believe the data on octreotide are not adequate to support its use in this illness.

ISOSPORIASIS. This coccidiosis is caused by *Isospora belli*, a human intracellular parasite that is harbored in the gut after transmission by contact with contaminated human excreta. The infection usually resolves in two to four weeks without treatment. A subacute febrile syndrome, headache, anorexia, and gastrointestinal symptoms (nonbloody diarrhea, abdominal tenderness and distension) are characteristic. Chronic diarrhea in patients with adult T-cell leukemia may be caused by isosporiasis (Greenberg et al, 1988). In immunocompromised individuals, severe cholera-like diarrhea accompanied by malabsorption and weight loss of 10% or more may occur. This disorder is not common in patients with AIDS in this country (incidence <0.2%); however, Haitian patients with AIDS are at high risk (incidence 15%). The reason for the difference has not been identified.

Oral trimethoprim 160 mg and sulfamethoxazole 800 mg [Bactrim-DS, Septra-DS] given four times daily for 10 days and then twice daily for three weeks appeared to be quite effective in an open study (DeHovitz et al, 1986). Since the diarrhea was controlled within two days after treatment began and the recurrence rate was 47%, the investigators suggest that an initial course of one to two weeks should be followed by prophylactic daily doses for an indefinite period. The combination of pyrimethamine and sulfadiazine also appears to be effective. Weekly prophylactic doses of pyrimethamine/sulfadoxine [Fansidar] also have been suggested, but the benefit should be weighed against the potential toxicity of this drug combination.

DIENTAMEBIASIS

Dientamebiasis is caused by the flagellate parasite, *Dientamoeba fragilis* (Millet et al, 1983). No cyst form of this organism exists, and the trophozoite is highly labile and easily overlooked unless stools are examined immediately or preserved for later examination. Dientamebiasis is often associated with enterobiasis; most investigators believe that the trophozoite is transmitted within the pinworm egg.

The role of *D. fragilis* as a pathogen remains unsettled (Oxner et al, 1987). Those authorities who believe that it causes chronic, mild lower intestinal symptoms, including persistent diarrhea, recommend treatment with either iodoquinol or tetracycline. No controlled treatment trials have been reported. Recommended regimens include iodoquinol 40 mg/kg (maximum, 2 g) in divided doses three times daily for 20 days or tetracycline 500 mg four times daily for 20 days (Panosian, 1988).

GIARDIASIS

The terms, giardiasis and lambliasis, refer to colonization and/or infection of the gastrointestinal tract by *Giardia intestinalis* (*G. lamblia*). The infection can be transmitted by sexual practices involving fecal exposure, but person-to-person contact and ingestion of the organism that is present on fecal-contaminated surfaces or in water or food is most common. Man is the principal host and main source of infection.

G. intestinalis is the most common flagellate in the human gastrointestinal tract worldwide. It is often found in individuals returning to the United States following foreign travel; young children are especially susceptible to infection. Giardiasis has occurred in endemic form in the United States (prevalence rate, 2% to 10% in high-risk cohorts [eg, children in day-care centers, indigent and institutionalized populations] and 6% to 18% in homosexuals); 20% to 80% of infected persons may be asymptomatic. Day-care centers are considered a reservoir for infection (Child Day Care Infectious Disease Study Group, 1985).

The motile trophozoite of *G. intestinalis* attaches to the mucosa of the small intestine. No enterotoxins have been identified; however, damage to intestinal epithelial cells and their brush border has been observed in morphologic studies.

Biochemical differences have been noted among strain isolates of *Giardia*. It has now been established conclusively that strain variation in the pathogenicity of *Giardia* infections in humans also exists (Nash et al, 1987). Epidemiologic studies suggest that cellular and humoral immune responses provide protection from illness and help eliminate the parasite. The majority of patients exhibit increased serum IgM, IgG, IgA, and intestinal fluid IgA antibody responses to the parasite. Trophozoites occasionally are present in the bile ducts and gallbladder. Cysts, the usual infective stage, are passed in formed stools; trophozoites are passed by some, but not all, individuals with frank diarrhea.

Infections that coexist with giardiasis and that are normally sensitive to antibiotics may not respond to treatment because oral absorption of the drugs may be impaired by *Giardia* (Craft et al, 1987). In a rat model of giardiasis, absorption of amoxicillin, ampicillin, cefaclor, cephalexin, erythromycin, and penicillin was significantly impaired, but absorption of chloramphenicol and sulfamethoxazole was not affected.

DIAGNOSIS. Symptoms of giardiasis commonly include foul diarrhea (with or without episodes of constipation), abdominal distention, foul flatulence, bloating, foul belching, heartburn, nocturnal borborygmi, vomiting, colicky pain related to food ingestion, lactose intolerance, and profound malaise. Symptoms lasting longer than two weeks help differentiate giardiasis from other causes of acute gastroenteritis. Weight loss is common in giardiasis with chronic diarrhea, and its occurrence can be helpful in differentiating this condition from the irritable bowel syndrome. Because vitamin A is poorly absorbed and steatorrhea may be present, the infection may resemble celiac syndrome or kwashiorkor. The pain associated with giardiasis may mimic that of appendicitis, cholelithiasis, ulcer, or hiatal hernia.

For positive diagnosis, trophozoites or cysts must be identified in fresh or preserved stool specimens, in aspirates obtained by duodenal intubation, with use of the "string test" (Entero-test, Hedeco, Palo Alto, CA), or by biopsy of small intestine mucosa. A fluorescent antibody test and a test for *Giardia* antigen in stools are commercially available.

Chronic giardiasis may be more common than previously believed (Chester et al, 1985). Increased frequency of constipation and upper gastrointestinal disturbances that persist for a mean duration of 3.3 years distinguish chronic from acute giardiasis (symptoms less than six months) and may be an indication for duodenal aspiration or biopsy.

MANAGEMENT/DRUG SELECTION. Environmental sanitation is essential to limit the spread of giardiasis (eg, personal hygiene, examination of household contacts). Guidelines are available for the prevention and management of outbreaks in day-care centers (Child Day Care Infectious Disease Study Group, 1985).

Metronidazole has become the drug of choice in giardiasis because it has good activity and usually is well tolerated in both children and adults. The tablets can be formulated into a suspension (Holtan, 1988). Other related nitroimidazoles (tinidazole, ornidazole, secnidazole) have appreciably longer half-lives and also are being investigated for use in giardiasis (Rossignol et al, 1984). Of these, tinidazole has been used most commonly; a single dose of 1.5 or 2 g has been as effective as two doses of metronidazole (Jokipii and Jokipii, 1982), and a single 2-g dose of tinidazole was more effective than a single 2.4-g dose of metronidazole (Speelman, 1985).

Quinacrine [Atabrine] can be given to severely affected adults who can tolerate it; however, severe nausea and vomiting, skin disorders, psychosis, or other toxic effects often preclude its use. Combined therapy with quinacrine and metronidazole should be considered in individuals who do not respond to repeated courses of single-drug therapy (Taylor et al, 1987).

Furazolidone [Furoxone] also is an effective antigiardial agent. Cure rates of 75% to 85% with few relapses have been reported, but the drug has not been as widely used as quinacrine in the United States. Furazolidone is available as a suspension, and it is usually well tolerated by children, for whom it is an alternative drug of choice. At least seven and preferably ten days of therapy with this drug are recommended (Murphy and Nelson, 1983).

LEISHMANIASIS

This disease remains largely *tropical* and *subtropical* in distribution because it is transmitted by blood-sucking insect vectors indigenous to these areas. The reticuloendothelial cells are invaded by the amastigote form of *Leishmania*, which is transmitted to man by sandflies of the genus *Phlebotomus* (Old World) or *Lutzomyia* (New World) from a reservoir of organisms borne in rodents or other small animals.

The onset of visceral leishmaniasis, which is caused by *L. donovani*, is usually gradual, and symptoms can range from severe to mild and self-limiting. They include fever, weight loss, hepatosplenomegaly with mild hepatocellular dysfunction, hypoalbuminemia, hypergammaglobulinemia, pancytopenia, hemorrhage, and lymphadenopathy. In some untreated patients who are asymptomatic or have mild symptoms, the infection does not progress; however, established infection is usually fatal if left untreated. After cure or recovery from visceral infection, the organism can remain dormant in the immunocompetent host for many years; disease can recur when the host's immunologic system is severely suppressed for any reason. Malnutrition is a definite risk factor for the development of visceral leishmaniasis (Cerf et al, 1987). Progressive, fatal visceral leishmaniasis (kala-azar) can occur in many patients without obvious immunosuppression.

In South America, mucocutaneous leishmaniasis (espundia) is principally caused by *L. braziliensis*. Treatment of this infection is recommended because marked disfiguration usually occurs due to progressive ulceration of mucous membranes in the mouth, palate, pharynx, and nose.

Cutaneous leishmaniasis begins as a nodule that develops at the site of the insect bite, may crust or ulcerate, and is very slow to heal. This form is caused by *L. tropica* or *L. major* (Old World leishmaniasis) and *L. braziliensis*, *L. mexicana*, or *L. peruviana* (New World leishmaniasis). Recent evidence suggests that an endemic focus of disease caused by *L. mexicana* is present in south central Texas (Furner, 1990).

DRUG SELECTION. Since the mucocutaneous and visceral forms of leishmaniasis rarely are self-limited, treatment is indicated. Parenteral administration of the pentavalent antimonial compounds, sodium stibogluconate [Pentostam] (available in the United States only from the Centers for Disease Control) and meglumine antimoniate [Glucantime] (not available in the United States), are recommended as initial therapy for 28 to 30 days (Berman, 1988). Because of side effects, it may be necessary to shorten the course of therapy (but to no less than 20 days). Physicians who use these agents are urged to consult the CDC to obtain treatment information (see the evaluation for the address and telephone number).

In primary visceral leishmaniasis, lack of response to sodium stibogluconate ranges from 2% to 8% in most areas; the failure rate is higher in Kenya (Pearson and De Queiroz Sousa, 1990). These patients may benefit from additional courses of therapy. Severe mucocutaneous leishmaniasis is even more resistant to standard antimonial therapy (Franke et al, 1990). The diamidine, pentamidine [Pentam 300], and amphotericin B [Fungizone] may be suitable alternatives if the antimonial agents are not effective or cannot be tolerated (World Health Organization, 1984; Mishra et al, 1991).

Liposomal formulations of the antimonials and amphotericin B show much promise in experimental animal models of infection. Liposomal formulations of antimonials have the potential to greatly increase efficacy over the currently available preparations (Coune, 1988; Hunter et al, 1988). With liposomal formulations of amphotericin B, toxicity is lower than with conventional formulations (Berman et al, 1986; Davidson et al, 1991).

In limited open studies, allopurinol [Lopurin, Zyloprim] has been somewhat effective in mucocutaneous and visceral leishmaniasis (Berman, 1988; Croft, 1988; Dellamonica et al, 1989); however, it is excreted rapidly. Synthesis of longer-acting derivatives (eg, allopurinol riboside), combination with stibogluconate, and administration with probenecid are being explored to exploit the obvious advantages of oral effectiveness and low toxicity that are characteristic of allopurinol. Allopurinol riboside has been shown to halt the progression of leishmaniasis (Saenz et al, 1989).

The standard treatment for mucocutaneous and visceral leishmaniasis also has been used for cutaneous leishmaniasis, although until recently it was not known whether therapy for this milder, frequently self-limiting form of the disease resulted in a significantly faster cure rate than would occur with no treatment (Berman, 1988). Results of a recent randomized trial showed that both oral ketoconazole [Nizoral] (600 mg daily for 28 days) and pentavalent antimonials (20 mg/kg/day for 20 days) accelerated healing of cutaneous ulcers caused by *L. braziliensis panamensis* (Saenz et al, 1990). Cure rates were 76% and 68%, respectively, in patients treated with either drug, compared with 0% in those given placebo. Systemic treatment of cutaneous leishmaniasis is indicated when lesions are slow to heal or are caused by organisms with a propensity to metastasize and produce mucocutaneous disease. If a considerable number of disfiguring scars in cosmetically important areas are anticipated, intralesional therapy may be indicated (Sharquie et al, 1988). The duration of treatment for cutaneous leishmaniasis is shorter than for the mucocutaneous and visceral forms (usually 20 days). If stibogluconate is not well tolerated at the conventional dose, some patients will respond to 15 mg Sb/kg/daily. Local ultrasound-induced hyperthermia is an alternative (Aram and Leibovici, 1987).

MALARIA

Malaria is a worldwide, common cause of morbidity and mortality. Diminution in spraying programs and the emergence of insecticide-resistant strains of mosquitoes and drug-resistant strains of *Plasmodium falciparum* in many areas have resulted in resurgence of this disease. Malaria caused by *P. falciparum* produces the highest mortality among all types of this disease that affect man.

In the United States, malaria can result from exposure to infected mosquitoes abroad, transmittal by immigrants, induction by accidental blood inoculation among drug addicts or by transfusion of infected blood, or rarely by mosquitoes (*MMWR*, 1991 A).

PARASITE LIFE CYCLE AND CLINICAL COURSE. The four species of *Plasmodium* that cause malaria in man are *P. falciparum*, *P. vivax*, *P. ovale*, and *P. malariae*. The human phase of the life cycle begins when an infected female anopheline mosquito bites the host and injects sporozoites from her salivary glands. The sporozoites enter the circulation and rapidly reach the liver where they invade cells, develop into primary tissue schizonts (the primary exoerythrocytic forms), and mature into tissue merozoites. This asexual multiplication is termed pre-erythrocytic schizogony. The asymptomatic (prepatent) period lasts 8 to 21 days, depending on the species. At the end of the prepatent period, the merozoites of all species enter the blood stream, invade red cells, develop into trophozoites (blood schizonts), and begin the erythrocytic cycle of schizogony. The erythrocytic cycle ends when the infected red cells rupture, releasing parasites (that reinvade other red cells), pigments, and other products. The clinical attack of malaria (ie, chills, fever, profuse sweating) occurs at this time.

In individuals infected with *P. vivax* and *P. ovale*, dormant hepatic forms (hypnozoites) are subsequently activated to initiate schizogony that causes clinical relapse months to years after a primary infection (Krotoski, 1985). This does not occur with *P. falciparum* and *P. malariae*.

After several cycles, some erythrocytic parasites develop into gametocytes, the sexual forms of the organism. When the infected person is then bitten by a female anopheline mosquito, gametocytes enter the mosquito. In the intestinal tract of the mosquito, a fertilized form is produced (ie, a zygote) that develops into an oocyst, which eventually produces sporozoites. The latter migrate to the salivary glands of the insect vector, from where they are inoculated into a human host during the taking of a blood meal. Thus, the cycle from human host to vector is completed and the disease is perpetuated.

Definitive diagnosis of malaria is made by the presence of parasites on thick or thin peripheral blood films. The classical cycles of malarial paroxysms take place when the maturation phase of erythrocytic parasites becomes synchronized, although this may not be observed until after several attacks have occurred. In falciparum malaria, cyclic fever may not occur.

Untreated or inadequately treated patients who survive initial attacks of malaria become partially immune, especially those with *P. falciparum* infection. These individuals may experience recrudescences and can transmit malaria by blood transfusion. Immunity wanes over a period of a few years, and frequent re-exposure is required for it to be maintained. Treatment should not be withheld to stimulate the immune response, even if the patient returns to the endemic area. Immunity may be suppressed as a consequence of severe illness, pregnancy, treatment with immunosuppressive drugs, or major surgery.

The natural duration of infection with *P. vivax*, *P. ovale*, and *P. falciparum* in untreated patients who do not die from the disease is one to four years, and survivors are essentially cured after these intervals. Infections due to *P. malariae* persist lifelong in the absence of antimalarial therapy.

CLASSIFICATION OF ANTIMALARIAL AGENTS. Antimalarial agents are classified on the basis of their action against plasmodia at different stages in their life cycle in the human. Drugs that eliminate the erythrocytic asexual forms of the parasite are known as blood schizonticides and are used to cure the asexual attack form of malaria. None of the blood schizonticides eliminate exoerythrocytic forms of the parasite. However, these drugs completely cure (*radical cure*) *P. falciparum* and *P. malariae* infections because, unlike *P. ovale* and *P. vivax*, the former two organisms do not have parasitic forms that persist in the liver for years and cause relapses. A tissue schizonticide is necessary to produce a radical cure for *P. ovale* and *P. vivax* infections; however, it is usually administered following therapy with a blood schizonticide.

Blood schizonticides available in the United States include chloroquine [Aralen], hydroxychloroquine [Plaquenil], pyrimethamine [Daraprim], sulfadiazine, pyrimethamine/sulfadoxine [Fansidar], quinine sulfate (oral), quinidine gluconate (intravenous), tetracycline, mefloquine [Lariam], and clindamycin [Cleocin]. Some blood schizonticides are not available in the United States; they are used only for chemoprophylaxis and include proguanil [Paludrine] and pyrimethamine/dapsone [Maloprim].

Primaquine is the only agent used as a tissue schizonticide.

TREATMENT. Patients with mild to moderate malaria require supportive therapy and chemotherapy. Bedrest, antipyretics (aspirin or related analgesics) and/or sponging with tepid water, and maintenance of adequate fluid and salt balance may be required during acute attacks. Hypovolemia and hyponatremia are often associated with moderate to severe acute malaria and require fluid and electrolyte replacement.

Infection caused by *P. falciparum* in a nonimmune individual can be cured if appropriate antimalarial therapy is initiated before overwhelming parasitemia develops. Complications of falciparum malaria include hemolytic anemia, encephalopathy with confusion or coma ("cerebral malaria"), hemoglobinuria with renal failure (blackwater fever), noncardiac pulmonary edema, or hypoglycemia (White et al, 1983) associated with marked hyperinsulinemia (especially during pregnancy and severe disease). Prompt ancillary measures to treat these complications may be useful (Peters and Hall, 1985); packed red cells, antipyretics, assisted ventilation, exchange transfusions, plasma volume expanders or low-molecular-weight dextran, or dialysis also may be necessary. Antiepileptic drugs may be required for seizures due to cerebral malaria. A single intramuscular injection of phenobarbital 3.5 mg/kg is inexpensive and effective in preventing seizures (White et al, 1988 B). In a controlled trial, high-dose dexamethasone was of no value in cerebral malaria (Hoffman et al, 1988).

Drug Selection: The clinical use (Warhurst, 1987; Herwaldt et al, 1988; Krogstad et al, 1988 A; Krogstad and Herwaldt, 1988) and mechanism of action (Warhurst, 1986; Schlesinger et al, 1988) of antimalarial drugs have been reviewed. Drug selection for treatment of confirmed malaria (Table 2) depends on the prevalence of drug resistance in the area visited (ie, chloroquine-resistant or pyrimethamine/sulfadoxine [Fansidar]-resistant falciparum malaria), the probability of persisting exoerythrocytic forms (ie, *P. vivax*, *P. ovale*), whether the patient is pregnant, and the existence of drug allergy or intolerance.

Four levels of chloroquine resistance manifested by *P. falciparum* have been described (Weniger et al, 1982; Wernsdorfer, 1984): R0 or S (no resistance—clearance of the organism from the blood usually within three but no longer than seven days without recrudescence); RI (mild resistance—clearance as described for R0, but with recrudescence not produced by reinfection within 28 days); RII (moderate resistance—parasitemia decreased within seven days but complete clearance not achieved); and RIII (complete resistance—chloroquine has no effect on the parasitemia). For drug selection, RI, RII, and RIII are considered resistant to chloroquine.

Cure of an acute attack of malaria caused by *P. vivax*, *P. ovale*, *P. malariae*, or chloroquine-sensitive strains of *P. falciparum* is readily accomplished with a three-day course of chloroquine phosphate. If oral administration is not feasible, chloroquine hydrochloride may be administered intravenously until an oral preparation can be used. Alternatively, oral quinine sulfate can be given or, in severe attacks, quinidine gluconate can be administered by slow intravenous infusion if parenteral chloroquine hydrochloride is unavailable. No additional treatment is usually required in patients infected with chloroquine-sensitive *P. falciparum* and *P. malariae* but, to prevent relapses and to achieve radical cure of *P. vivax* and *P. ovale* infections, a two-week course of primaquine must be given after consideration of the fact that primaquine causes

TABLE 2.
TREATMENT OF CONFIRMED MALARIA: DRUG THERAPY IN THE UNITED STATES[1,2]

Preferred Therapy[3]	Alternative Therapy
Chloroquine-Sensitive Strains of *Plasmodium falciparum, P. malariae, P. ovale,* and *P. vivax*	
Chloroquine phosphate (oral) or Hydroxychloroquine phosphate (oral) or Chloroquine hydrochloride (parenteral)[4]	Quinine sulfate (oral) Pyrimethamine/sulfadoxine [Fansidar] (oral) Mefloquine (oral)
Chloroquine-Resistant Strains of *Plasmodium falciparum*	
Quinine sulfate (oral) or Quinidine gluconate (parenteral)[5] or Quinine or quinidine plus an oral or parenteral tetracycline or Quinine or quinidine plus an oral or parenteral antifolate: Pyrimethamine and sulfadiazine (or sulfisoxazole) or Pyrimethamine/sulfadoxine [Fansidar]	Mefloquine (oral) Clindamycin[6] (oral or parenteral) (alone or with quinine)

[1]*Following any regimen of therapy for* P. vivax *and* P. ovale, *a course of primaquine should be given to eradicate exoerythrocytic forms. A G6PD level must be obtained before primaquine is prescribed.*

[2]*Selection of a regimen from within categories is dependent principally on the severity of illness. Oral therapy is adequate for mild to moderate uncomplicated infection, but parenteral therapy is required initially for severe or complicated infection (eg, vomiting, coma, or >5% parasitemia). Oral therapy should be substituted for parenteral therapy as soon as possible. For suggested doses, see individual evaluations.*

[3]*When quinine or quinidine is used alone, seven to ten days of therapy is generally recommended; only three days of therapy is recommended for quinine or quinidine when oral tetracycline or an antifolate is also administered.*

[4]*Chloroquine hydrochloride may be difficult to obtain in the United States. Quinidine gluconate should be substituted as needed for this drug.*

[5]*Quinine dihydrochloride is no longer available from the CDC.*

[6]*Investigational indication.*

hemolysis in G6PD-deficient individuals. Geographic variants of *P. vivax* may be less sensitive to primaquine; however, larger dosages frequently are effective (see the evaluation on Primaquine). Clinicians also should be aware of possible infections with chloroquine-resistant strains of *P. vivax* among travelers returning to North America from Indonesia and Oceania (Schwartz et al, 1991). See Table 2.

Malaria caused by *P. falciparum* from an area in which multiple drug resistance is known to occur should be assumed to be resistant to chloroquine and treated as such. Treatment should be initiated with oral quinine sulfate, if possible. In severe life-threatening attacks, when parenteral administration is necessary, the administration of quinidine gluconate by slow intravenous infusion is the treatment of choice (Miller et al, 1989; *MMWR*, 1991 B). Quinine dihydrochloride is no longer available from the CDC. When oral medication can be tolerated, sulfadiazine and pyrimethamine or the combination of pyrimethamine/sulfadoxine [Fansidar] can be given with quinine sulfate. Alternatively, tetracycline plus quinine or quinidine may be substituted for the sulfonamide/pyrimethamine combination (Reacher et al, 1981). These regimens are also effective against chloroquine-sensitive strains, but chloroquine alone is preferable. See Table 2.

Mefloquine [Lariam], a 4-quinoline methanol derivative of quinine and a long-acting blood schizonticide, is used for both chemoprophylaxis and treatment of malaria. It is indicated for the treatment of mild to moderate acute malaria caused by mefloquine-sensitive strains of *P. falciparum* (both chloroquine-sensitive and chloroquine-resistant strains) or by *P. vivax.* Data are insufficient to determine its efficacy in malaria caused by *P. ovale* and *P. malariae.* The principal use of mefloquine is malaria chemoprophylaxis in travelers to areas where chloroquine-resistant and/or pyrimethamine/sulfadoxine-resistant strains of *P. falciparum* are most likely to be present (see below). It also may be used for oral therapy in patients with malaria acquired in such areas (Harinasuta et al, 1985).

Clindamycin is known to have antiplasmodial activity (Kremsner, 1990). It has eliminated parasitemia slowly in patients with uncomplicated malaria acquired in an endemic malarial area in Africa where chloroquine- or pyrimethamine/sulfadoxine-resistant *P. falciparum* infection is common; these patients received an oral dose of 5 mg/kg twice a day for five days (Wakeel et al, 1985). It has been used successfully with quinine in patients with complications of severe malaria. A definitive role has not been established for clindamycin alone

TABLE 3.
RECOMMENDED ANTIMALARIAL PROPHYLACTIC REGIMENS BY GEOGRAPHIC AREA[1, 2]

Regimen A— Routine weekly prophylaxis with chloroquine alone, beginning 1 to 2 weeks prior to travel and continuing for 4 weeks after leaving the malarious area.

Regimen B— Routine weekly prophylaxis with mefloquine [Lariam][3] beginning 1 week prior to travel and continuing for 4 weeks after leaving the malarious area.

Recommended Regimen	Geographic Area of Exposure
B	AFGHANISTAN
None	ALBANIA
None	ALGERIA Very limited risk in Sahara region.
None	ANDORRA
B	ANGOLA
None	ANTIGUA AND BARBUDA
A	ARGENTINA Rural areas near Bolivian border; Salta and Jujuy Provinces.
None	AUSTRALIA
None	AUSTRIA
None	AZORES (PORTUGAL)
None	BAHAMAS
None	BAHRAIN
B	BANGLADESH All areas, except no risk in city of Dhaka. Chloroquine resistance widespread in areas along northern and eastern borders.
None	BARBADOS
None	BELGIUM
A	BELIZE (formerly BRITISH HONDURAS) Rural areas, except no risk in central coastal district of Belize.
B	BENIN (formerly DAHOMEY)
None	BERMUDA (U.K.)
B	BHUTAN Rural areas in districts bordering India.
B	BOLIVIA Rural areas only, except no risk in highland areas; Oruro Dept. and Prov. of Ingavi, Los Andes, Omasuyos, and Pacajes (La Paz Dept.) and southern and central Potosi Department.
B	BOTSWANA Northern part of country (North of 21 ° S)
B	BRAZIL Acre and Rondonia States, Territory of Amapá and Roraima; part of rural areas of Amazonas, Goiás, Maranhao, Mato Grosso, and Pará States. Travelers who will only visit the coastal States from the horn to the Uruguay border are not at risk and need no prophylaxis.
None	BRUNEI DARUSSALAM
None	BULGARIA
B	BURKINA FASO (formerly UPPER VOLTA)
	BURMA (see MYANMAR)
B	BURUNDI
B	CAMEROON
None	CANADA
None	CAPE VERDE
None	CAYMAN ISLANDS (U.K.)
B	CENTRAL AFRICAN REPUBLIC

1 *Adapted from annual monograph on* Health Information for International Travel 1990 *(Centers for Disease Control, 1990).*

2 *Particularly between dusk and dawn, the use of protective clothing, insect repellants, insecticide sprays, mosquito net and/or screens is recommended. See evaluations for dosage regimens, precautions, and adverse drug reactions.*

3 *See text and Table 4 for alternatives depending on the traveler's age, drug sensitivity, length of exposure, and pregnancy status.*

(table continued on next page)

TABLE 3 (continued)

Recommended Regimen	Geographic Area of Exposure
B	CHAD
None	CHILE
A/B	CHINA Rural areas only, except no risk in northern provinces bordering Mongolia and in the western provinces of Heilungkiang, Kirin, Ningsia Hui Tibet, and Tsinghai. North of 33 ° N latitude transmission occurs July to November; between 33 ° and 25 ° N latitude transmission occurs May to December; south of 25 ° N latitude transmission occurs year-round. Travelers visiting cities and popular rural sites on usual tourist routes are generally not at risk, and chemoprophylaxis is not recommended. Travelers on special scientific, educational, or recreational visits should determine whether their itineraries include evening or nighttime exposure in areas of risk or in areas of chloroquine resistance. Travelers to most areas of risk within China should follow Regimen A; travelers to areas of chloroquine resistance should follow Regimen B.
None	CHRISTMAS ISLAND (AUSTRALIA)
B	COLOMBIA Rural areas only, except no risk in Bogota and vicinity. Risk in rural areas of Uraba (Antioquia Dept.); Bajo Cauca-Nechi (Cauca and Antioquia Dept.); Magdalena Medio, Caqueta (Caqueta Intendencia); Sarare (Arauca Intendencia); Catatumbo (Norte de Santander Dept.). Pacifico Central and Sur, Putumayo (Putumayo Intendencia); Ariari (Meta Dept.); Alto Vaupes (Vaupes Comisaria); Amazonas and Guainia (Comisarias).
B	COMOROS
B	CONGO
None	COOK ISLANDS (NEW ZEALAND)
A	COSTA RICA Limited risk in rural areas except the central highlands; Cartago and San Jose Provinces.
B	COTE D'IVOIRE (formerly IVORY COAST)
None	CUBA
None	CYPRUS
None	CZECHOSLOVAKIA
None	DENMARK
A	DJIBOUTI
None	DOMINICA
A	DOMINICAN REPUBLIC All rural areas except tourist resorts. Highest risk in provinces bordering Haiti.
B	ECUADOR All areas in the provinces along the eastern border and the Pacific coast; Esmeraldas, El Oro, Guayas (including Guayaquil), Los Rios, Manabi, Morona-Santiago, Napo, Pastaza, Pichincha, and Zamora-Chinchipe provinces. Travelers who will only visit Quito and vicinity, the central highland tourist areas, or the Galapagos Islands are not at risk and need no prophylaxis.
A	EGYPT Rural areas of Nile Delta, El Faiyum area, the oases, and part of southern (upper) Egypt.
A	EL SALVADOR Rural areas only.
B	EQUATORIAL GUINEA
B	ETHIOPIA All areas, except no risk in Addis Ababa and above 2,000 meters.
None	FALKLAND ISLANDS (U.K.)
None	FAROE ISLANDS (DENMARK)
None	FIJI
None	FINLAND
None	FRANCE
B	FRENCH GUIANA
None	FRENCH POLYNESIA (TAHITI)
B	GABON
B	GAMBIA
None	GERMANY
B	GHANA
None	GIBRALTAR (U.K.)
None	GREECE

(table continued on next page)

TABLE 3 (continued)

Recommended Regimen	Geographic Area of Exposure
None	GREENLAND (DENMARK)
None	GRENADA
None	GUADELOUPE (FRANCE)
None	GUAM (U.S.)
A	GUATEMALA Rural areas only, except no risk in central highlands.
B	GUINEA
B	GUINEA-BISSAU
B	GUYANA Rural areas in the southern interior and northwest coast; Rupununi and North West Regions.
A	HAITI
A	HONDURAS
None	HONG KONG (U.K.)
None	HUNGARY
None	ICELAND
B	INDIA
B	INDONESIA In general, rural areas only, except high risk in all areas of Irian Jaya (western half of island of New Guinea). No risk in resort areas of Bali. Malaria transmission in Indonesia (except for Irian Jaya) is largely confined to rural areas not visited by most travelers; most travel to rural areas of Indonesia is during daytime hours when there is minimal risk of exposure. Chemoprophylaxis is recommended only for those travelers who will have outdoor exposure during evening and nighttime hours in rural areas.
B	IRAN (ISLAMIC REPUBLIC OF) Rural areas only in the provinces of Sistan-Baluchestan and Hormozgan, the southern parts of Fars, Kohgiluyeh-Boyar, Lorestan, and Chahar Mahal-Bakhtiari, and the northern section of Khuzestan.
A	IRAQ All areas in northern region: Duhok, Erbil, Kirkuk, Ninawa, Sulaimaniya Provinces.
None	IRELAND
None	ISRAEL
None	ITALY
None	JAMAICA
None	JAPAN
None	JORDAN
B	KAMPUCHEA, DEMOCRATIC (formerly CAMBODIA)
B	KENYA All areas (including game parks), except no risk in Nairobi and areas above 2,500 meters.
None	KIRIBATI (FORMERLY GILBERT ISLANDS)
None	KOREA, DEMOCRATIC PEOPLE'S REPUBLIC OF (NORTH)
None	KOREA, REPUBLIC OF (SOUTH)
None	KUWAIT
B	LAO PEOPLE'S DEMOCRATIC REPUBLIC All areas, except no risk in city of Vientiane.
None	LEBANON
None	LESOTHO
B	LIBERIA
None	LIBYAN ARAB JAMAHIRIYA Very limited risk in two small foci in southwest of country.
None	LIECHTENSTEIN
None	LUXEMBOURG
None	MACAO (PORTUGAL)
B	MADAGASCAR All areas, highest risk in coastal areas.
None	MADEIRA (PORTUGAL)

(table continued on next page)

TABLE 3 (continued)

Recommended Regimen	Geographic Area of Exposure
B	MALAWI
B	MALAYSIA Peninsular Malaysia and Sarawak (NW Borneo) malaria is limited to the rural hinterland; urban and coastal areas are malaria free. Sabah (NE Borneo) has malaria throughout. Malaria transmission in Malaysia (except Sabah) is largely confined to rural areas not visited by most travelers; most travel to rural areas is during daytime hours when there is minimal risk of exposure. Chemoprophylaxis is recommended only for those travelers who will have outdoor exposure during evening and nighttime hours in rural areas.
None	MALDIVES Rural areas only, except no risk in Male Island, Kaafu Atoll, and resort areas.
B	MALI
None	MALTA
None	MARTINIQUE (FRANCE)
B	MAURITANIA All areas except no risk in northern region: Dakhlet-Nouadhibou, Inchiri, Adrar, and Tiris-Zemour.
A	MAURITIUS Rural areas only, except no risk on Rodriguez Island.
A	MEXICO Rural areas, except no risk in the Distrito Federal and the states directly north and northeast of the capital (Guanajuato, Hidalgo, Mexico, Queretaro, Tiaxcala) and the U.S. border states of Baja California Norte, Sonora, and Coahuila. Although chemoprophylaxis is not recommended for travel to the major resort areas on the Pacific and Gulf Coasts, all travelers should be advised to use insect repellants and other personal protection measures.
None	MONACO
None	MONGOLIA
None	MONTSERRAT (U.K.)
None	MOROCCO Very limited risk in rural areas of coastal provinces.
B	MOZAMBIQUE
B	MYANMAR (formerly BURMA) Rural areas only. Malaria transmission is largely confined to rural areas not visited by most travelers; most travel is during daytime hours when there is minimal risk of exposure.
B	NAMIBIA All areas of Ovamboland and Caprivi Strip.
None	NAURU
B	NEPAL Rural areas in Terai Dist. and Hill Districts below 1,200 meters; no risk in Katmandu.
None	NETHERLANDS
None	NETHERLANDS ANTILLES
None	NEW CALEDONIA (FRANCE)
None	NEW ZEALAND
A	NICARAGUA Rural areas only; however, risk exists in outskirts of Chinandega, Leon, Granada, Managua, Nandaime, and Tipitapa.
B	NIGER
B	NIGERIA
None	NIUE (NEW ZEALAND)
None	NORTHERN MARIANA ISLANDS (U.S.)
None	NORWAY
A	OMAN
None	PACIFIC ISLANDS, TRUST TERRITORY OF THE U.S.A.
B	PAKISTAN
A/B	PANAMA Rural areas of the eastern provinces (Darien and San Blas) and the northwestern provinces (Boca Del Toro and Veraguas). There is no risk in the Canal Zone or in Panama City and vicinity. Travelers to rural areas west of the Canal Zone should follow Regimen A; travelers to areas east of the Canal Zone (including the San Blas Islands) should follow Regimen B.
B	PAPUA NEW GUINEA
A	PARAGUAY Rural areas bordering Brazil.

(table continued on next page)

TABLE 3 (continued)

Recommended Regimen	Geographic Area of Exposure
A/B	PERU Rural areas. Travelers who will visit only Lima and vicinity, coastal area south of Lima, or the highland tourist areas (Cuzco, Machu Picchu, Lake Titicaca) are not at risk and need no prophylaxis. Risk exists in rural areas of Departments of Amazonas, Cajamarca (except Hualgayoc Province), La Libertad (except Otuzco, Santiago de Chuco Provinces), Lambayeque, Loreto, Piura (except Talara Province), San Martin and Tumbes; Provinces of Santa (Ancash Dept.); parts of La Convension (Cuzco Dept.), Tayacaja (Huancavelica Dept.), Satipo (Junin Dept.). Travelers to most areas of risk within Peru should follow Regimen A; travelers to the northern provinces bordering Brazil who will have rural exposure during evening and nighttime hours should follow Regimen B.
B	PHILIPPINES Rural areas only, except there is no risk in Provinces of Bohol, Catanduanes, Cebu, and Leyte. Malaria transmission in the Philippines is largely confined to rural areas not visited by most travelers; most travel to rural areas in the Philippines is during daytime hours when there is minimal risk of exposure. Chemoprophylaxis is recommended only for those travelers who will have outdoor exposure during evening and nighttime hours in rural areas. Travelers at risk should use Regimen A, unless they will be at risk in areas of chloroquine resistance, in which case they should follow Regimen B.
None	PITCAIRN (U.K.)
None	POLAND
None	PORTUGAL
None	PUERTO RICO (U.S.)
None	QATAR
None	REUNION (FRANCE)
None	ROMANIA
B	RWANDA
None	SAINT CHRISTOPHER (SAINT KITTS) AND NEVIS (U.K.)
None	SAINT HELENA (U.K.)
None	SAINT LUCIA
None	SAINT PIERRE AND MIQUELON (FRANCE)
None	SAINT VINCENT AND THE GRENADINES
None	SAMOA (formerly WESTERN SAMOA)
None	SAMOA, AMERICAN (U.S.)
None	SAN MARINO
A	SAO TOME AND PRINCIPE
A	SAUDI ARABIA All areas in the western provinces except no risk in the high altitude areas of Asir Province (Yemen border) and the urban areas of Jeddah, Mecca, Medina, and Taif.
B	SENEGAL
None	SEYCHELLES
B	SIERRA LEONE
None	SINGAPORE
B	SOLOMON ISLANDS
B	SOMALIA
B	SOUTH AFRICA Rural areas (including game parks) in the north, east, and western low altitude areas of Transvaal and in the Natal coastal areas north of 28° S.
None	SPAIN
B	SRI LANKA (formerly CEYLON) All areas except Colombo. Risk exists in districts of Amparai, Anuradhapura, Badulla (part), Batticaloa, Hambantota, Jaffna, Kandy, Kegalle, Kurungala, Mannar, Matale, Matara, Moneragala, Polonnaruwa, Puttalam, Ratnapura, Trincomalee, and Vavuniya.
B	SUDAN
B	SURINAME Rural areas only, except no risk in Paramaribo District and coastal areas north of 5° N.
B	SWAZILAND All lowland areas.
None	SWEDEN
None	SWITZERLAND
A	SYRIAN ARAB REPUBLIC Rural areas only, except no risk in the southern and western Districts of Deir-es-zor and Sweida.

(table continued on next page)

TABLE 3 (continued)

Recommended Regimen	Geographic Area of Exposure
None	TAIWAN
B	TANZANIA, UNITED REPUBLIC OF
B	THAILAND Rural areas only. Malaria transmission in Thailand is largely confined to forested rural areas principally along the borders of Kampuchea (Cambodia) and Myanmar (Burma) not visited by most travelers; most travel to rural areas of Thailand is during daytime hours when there is minimal risk of exposure.
B	TOGO
None	TONGA
None	TRINIDAD AND TOBAGO
None	TUNISIA
A	TURKEY Southeast Anatolia from coastal city of Mersin to the Iraqi border (Cukorova/Amikova areas).
None	TUVALU
B	UGANDA
None	UNION OF SOVIET SOCIALIST REPUBLICS
A	UNITED ARAB EMIRATES Northern Emirates, except no risk in cities of Dubai, Sharjah, Ajman, Umm al Qaiwan, and Emirate of Abu Dhabi.
None	UNITED KINGDOM (including CHANNEL ISLANDS and the ISLE OF MAN)
None	UNITED STATES OF AMERICA
None	URUGUAY
B	VANUATU (formerly NEW HEBRIDES) All areas, except no risk on Fortuna Island.
B	VENEZUELA Rural areas of all border states and territories and the southeastern states of Barinas, Merida, and Portuguesa.
B	VIETNAM Rural areas only, except no risk in the Red and Mekong deltas.
None	VIRGIN ISLANDS, BRITISH
None	VIRGIN ISLANDS, U.S.
None	WAKE ISLAND (U.S.)
A	YEMEN All areas, except no risk in two northwestern provinces, Sada and Hajja.
A	YEMEN, DEMOCRATIC All areas, except no risk in city of Aden or airport perimeter.
None	YUGOSLAVIA
B	ZAIRE
B	ZAMBIA
B	ZIMBABWE (formerly RHODESIA) All areas, except no risk in city of Harare.

in the treatment of malaria; concern exists about its slow onset of action and the potential for development of pseudomembranous colitis in patients who receive this drug.

Halofantrine [Halfan], an investigational phenanthrene methanol derivative similar to mefloquine, also is effective against chloroquine-resistant *P. falciparum* and has been well tolerated in early studies (Watkins et al, 1988; Wirima et al, 1988).

Another investigational substance, artemisinin (qinghaosu), is a novel sesquiterpene peroxide that acts rapidly as a blood schizonticide; it is effective in the treatment of chloroquine-resistant strains of *P. falciparum* (Klayman, 1985), but the recrudescence rate is high. The synthesis and development of better oral and injectable derivatives are being studied (Luo and Shen, 1987).

Chloroquine-sensitive and chloroquine-resistant parasites take up chloroquine at the same rate; however, chloroquine efflux occurs 40 to 50 times more rapidly in resistant strains than in sensitive strains. This drug efflux is inhibited in vitro by high concentrations of calcium channel blockers (eg, verapamil, diltiazem), vinblastine, daunorubicin (Krogstad et al, 1988 B; Ward, 1988), and desipramine (Bitonti et al, 1988). Therapeutic strategies based on these observations are being pursued to determine if nontoxic concentrations of similar inhibitors can reduce chloroquine resistance.

For more complete information, see the evaluations.

CHEMOPROPHYLAXIS. The morbidity and mortality of malaria can be significantly reduced by the judicious use of chemoprophylactic drugs (Keystone, 1990). The CDC publishes guidelines for drug selection (*MMWR*, 1990 A, 1990 B, 1991 C) and annually updates geographic information indicating the prevalence and drug sensitivity of malarial organisms (USPHS Centers for Disease Control monograph, *Health Information for International Travel,* publication number 90-8280, available from the Superintendent of Documents, US Government Printing Office, Washington, DC 20402, 202/783-3238). Some of this information is summarized in Table 3. Information also is available from the CDC malaria information hotline, 404/332-4555.

Mefloquine has supplanted chloroquine as the drug of choice for malaria chemoprophylaxis in areas where chloroquine-resistant *P. falciparum* malaria is endemic. Recommendations for its use recently have been updated (*MMWR*, 1991 C). Those travelers who cannot use mefloquine or elect to use chloroquine in locations where resistance to the latter drug is known to occur (see Table 3) should be given a single dose (three tablets) of pyrimethamine/sulfadoxine [Fansidar] to be used for self-treatment of a febrile illness when medical care is unavailable within 24 hours (presumptive malarial treatment). However, since the combination of pyrimethamine/sulfadoxine can cause serious toxic reactions (see the evaluation) (Miller et al, 1986; Pearson and Hewlett, 1987), presumptive treatment with these agents should be considered temporary and, following medical evaluation, weekly chloroquine prophylaxis should be resumed. Further, Fansidar and similar combinations are no longer useful in preventing or treating *P. falciparum* malaria in Thailand and other parts of Southeast Asia because of the prevalence of multiple drug resistance in these areas (Nosten et al, 1991).

Doxycycline [Vibramycin] has been reported to be more effective than chloroquine for prophylaxis of malaria (Pang et al, 1987). However, it is not recommended for routine use in individuals traveling to areas where chloroquine-sensitive organisms are prevalent. In these areas, chloroquine is the drug of choice (see Table 4).

TABLE 4.
DRUG SELECTION FOR CHEMOPROPHYLAXIS OF MALARIA[1,2]

	Dosage	
Preferred Drugs	**Adults**	**Children**
TRAVEL TO GEOGRAPHIC AREAS WHERE PRINCIPAL MALARIAL ORGANISMS ARE:		
Chloroquine-sensitive *Plasmodium falciparum, P. malariae, P. ovale, P. vivax*		
Chloroquine phosphate	300 mg of base per week beginning one week prior to entering the area of risk and continuing for four weeks after leaving malarious area	5 mg of base/kg/week (maximum, 300 mg) using the same dosage schedule as for adults
Chloroquine-resistant *Plasmodium falciparum*		
Mefloquine hydrochloride[3]	250 mg of base (1 tablet) weekly beginning one week prior to entering the area of risk and continuing for four weeks after leaving malarious area	15-19 kg, ¼ tablet/wk[4] 20-30 kg, ½ tablet/wk 31-45 kg, ¾ tablet/wk >45 kg, 1 tablet/wk
Doxycycline hydrochloride	100 mg/day beginning one to two days prior to entering the area of risk and continuing for four weeks after leaving malarious area	Do not use in children under 8 years; over 8 years, 2 mg/kg/day (maximum, 100 mg)
Chloroquine phosphate[5]	300 mg of base per week beginning one week prior to entering the area of risk and continuing for four weeks after leaving malarious area	5 mg of base/kg/week (maximum, 300 mg) using the same dosage schedule as for adults

[1]MMWR, *1990 A, 1990 B, 1991 C.*
[2]*The use of protective clothing, insect repellants, insecticide sprays, and mosquito net and/or screens is recommended, particularly between dusk and dawn.*
[3]*Mefloquine hydrochloride is not recommended for use by travelers with known hypersensitivity to this agent; children <15 kg (30 lbs); pregnant women; travelers using beta blockers; travelers involved in tasks requiring fine coordination and spatial discrimination, such as airline pilots; and travelers with histories of epilepsy or psychiatric disorders.*
[4]*Children should be given the drugs according to adult dosage schedule.*
[5]*Travelers who elect to use chloroquine should be given a treatment dose of Fansidar (adults: 3 tablets, each containing 75 mg pyrimethamine and 1.5 g sulfadoxine; children: 5-10 kg, ½ tablet; 11-20 kg, 1 tablet; 21-31 kg, 1½ tablets; 31-45 kg, 2 tablets; >45 kg, 3 tablets) for use* only *when a febrile illness arises and medical care is unavailable within 24 hours; weekly chloroquine prophylaxis should be continued after presumptive treatment with Fansidar.*

In addition to the presence of chloroquine-resistant *P. falciparum*, selection of appropriate agents for chemoprophylaxis also depends on drug hypersensitivity, age, and whether a woman is pregnant. Fansidar is not recommended for use in infants under 2 months, and doxycycline is not recommended for use in pregnant women or children under 8 years.

Proguanil and the combination product, pyrimethamine/dapsone [Maloprim], are alternative chemoprophylactic agents that can be obtained outside the United States. Amodiaquine is no longer recommended because its use is associated with an unacceptably high incidence of agranulocytosis and hepatitis (*MMWR*, 1986).

Proguanil is a short-acting precursor of an active blood schizonticide that inhibits dihydrofolate reductase. It has had considerable use and is one of the safer antimalarial drugs. In 1984, the World Health Organization recommended proguanil (200 mg daily) for chemoprophylaxis of malaria. Because *P. falciparum* and *P. vivax* develop resistance rapidly to its active metabolite, cycloguanil, proguanil generally is used with chloroquine if possible. Proguanil is not recommended for use in New Guinea or Thailand because *P. falciparum* is highly resistant to it in these countries. In a randomized open study conducted in Africa, in which proguanil plus chloroquine was compared with chloroquine plus pyrimethamine/sulfadoxine, the former regimen was as effective as the latter and side effects were reduced by about 40% (Fogh et al, 1988). Results of recent open trials in Cameroon also suggest that the combination of chloroquine and proguanil may be effective in the prophylaxis of chloroquine-resistant *P. falciparum* malaria; side effects occurred frequently but were minor (Gozal et al, 1991 A, 1991 B). However, in the absence of controlled trials, the efficacy of these regimens remains uncertain.

The combination product, pyrimethamine/dapsone, is used by some physicians in other countries in preference to Fansidar. However, it should be employed cautiously in individuals with a history of hypersensitivity to sulfonamides; neutropenia also has been observed with dapsone.

The development of a vaccine to prevent malaria still progresses, but much more work will be needed before an effective vaccine becomes available (Certa, 1991; Good, 1991; Siddiqui, 1991).

Compliance: *Travelers should be informed that no prophylactic regimen is absolutely effective and instructed to consult a physician if any symptoms appear, especially during the first two months following their return.* If symptoms of malaria are noted, blood tests should be performed immediately to screen for plasmodia, especially potentially drug-resistant *P. falciparum*.

Surveys of American (Lobel et al, 1987 A, 1987 B) and British (Phillips-Howard et al, 1986; Williams and Lewis, 1987) travelers returning from countries with endemic malaria revealed that only 42.4% and 48%, respectively, were in complete compliance with the chemoprophylaxis program. A Canadian survey (Keystone et al, 1984) also revealed that less than 50% of physicians interviewed could give accurate information about drug regimens for chemoprophylaxis of malaria. The results of these surveys emphasize the need for practitioners to be well informed and to give clear written directions to the traveler. The latter should include information on drug usage, dosage, early "flu-like" signs and symptoms, susceptibility of the pregnant patient, emphasis on follow-up therapy after return to minimize relapse of *P. vivax* and *P. ovale* malaria, and the importance of insect repellants (eg, those containing DEET), protective clothing, well-screened sleeping locations, and avoidance of rural areas when possible.

Adverse Reactions and Precautions. See the individual drug evaluations.

PNEUMOCYSTIS CARINII PNEUMONIA

Pneumocystis pneumonia (PCP) is caused by *Pneumocystis carinii*, an organism of uncertain taxonomic status (Edman et al, 1988). Although this organism colonizes more than 75% of healthy U.S. children (Hughes, 1991), it usually does not cause illness in adults or children unless their immune responses are impaired by disease, drugs, or protein-calorie malnutrition (Peters and Prakash, 1987). (However, a small cluster of cases recently has been described in adults with no identifiable risk factors [Jacobs et al, 1991].) The incidence of PCP is remarkably high in individuals with AIDS in North America and Europe. PCP is a major cause of morbidity and mortality in patients with AIDS. It is the diagnostic indicator for approximately 60% of cases and will occur in 75% to 85% of all patients with AIDS; in addition, the expected incidence of PCP in children with acute lymphatic leukemia is about 20% (Hughes, 1991). Evidence supports the concept that *P. carinii* organisms are detectable in AIDS patients only when clinical pneumonia is present, regardless of its severity; treatment is required when organisms are identified (Ognibene et al, 1988).

Clinical signs and symptoms of PCP are usually nonspecific; they include frequent nonproductive cough, dyspnea and/or tachypnea, chest discomfort, pallor, fever, and cyanosis. Rales are infrequent. Definitive diagnosis is made by identification of the organism (pleomorphic trophozoite or cyst) in induced liquefied sputum (Zaman et al, 1988), bronchoalveolar lavage fluid, or lung biopsy material. Quantitative estimation of T-helper (CD4+) cells (<200/microliter indicates severe immunosuppression), chest radiograph, gallium lung scan (especially when the chest radiograph cannot differentiate between new and residual lesions), blood gases, and pulmonary function studies may be helpful in the diagnosis (Hopewell, 1988). No reliable serologic tests for PCP are available.

A diffuse alveolitis usually is present in patients with this disease. The alveoli are infiltrated with organisms and alveolar macrophages. When it is untreated, the pneumonia is fatal in more than 90% of patients. Death may be sudden with few, if any, premonitory signs. Because of advances in the diagnosis and treatment of PCP, survival in patients with mild to moderate disease is ≥90%; however, mortality ranges from 20% to 40% in individuals with severe disease manifested by significant impairment of pulmonary oxygen exchange.

TREATMENT. In the last decade, trimethoprim/sulfamethoxazole replaced pentamidine as the therapy of choice for PCP because it was equally effective and was believed to be less toxic than the latter agent (Davey and Masur, 1990). However, since at least 30% and as many as 50% to 80% of patients with AIDS and PCP cannot tolerate or are hypersensitive to trimethoprim/sulfamethoxazole (Gordin et al, 1984; Sattler et al, 1988; Wormser et al, 1991), the need for pentamidine therapy is still quite substantial. The reverse is true if pentamidine is selected as initial therapy. These agents should be substituted cautiously, because the signs and symptoms of PCP in patients receiving either preparation frequently worsen during the first several days of treatment before showing improvement. Adverse reactions to trimethoprim/sulfamethoxazole or parenteral pentamidine are much more common and severe in patients with AIDS than in those without this disease (Glatt and Chirgwin, 1990). Since there is no evidence that coadministration of pentamidine and trimethoprim/sulfamethoxazole is more effective than the use of either preparation alone, and since adverse effects (neutropenia, thrombocytopenia, and renal and hepatic dysfunction) occur more frequently and are more pronounced if the two preparations are given together, such treatment is not recommended.

For more detailed information, see index entries Trimethoprim/Sulfamethoxazole; Pentamidine.

Data recently accumulated from case reports and uncontrolled and randomized trials suggest that aerosolized pentamidine may be as effective as standard regimens in treating mild cases of PCP (see reviews by Monk and Benfield, 1990; Wong and Hardy, 1990; Wispelwey and Pearson, 1991). The advantages of inhalation therapy with aerosolized pentamidine compared with systemic pentamidine or trimethoprim/sulfamethoxazole include the delivery of drug to pulmonary sites at greater concentrations but significantly lower (sometimes undetectable) plasma levels, low systemic toxicity, and increased patient compliance. However, relapse and recrudescence of disease, as well as an increase in the incidence of pneumothorax and dissemination of pneumocystis infection to extrapulmonary sites, have been reported in patients receiving aerosolized pentamidine (Telzak et al, 1990). In addition, more severe disease does not respond well to pentamidine inhalation therapy (Conte et al, 1990; Soo Hoo et al, 1990), and this mode of drug delivery is extremely expensive. Thus, the relative role of this treatment modality in PCP is not well defined, and it is recommended for use only in patients with relatively mild disease manifestations.

Results of limited open studies suggested that the combination of trimethoprim and dapsone is as effective and well tolerated as trimethoprim/sulfamethoxazole in AIDS patients with mild to moderate PCP (Leoung et al, 1986; Mills et al, 1988). A subsequent randomized, double-blind, placebo-controlled trial in a limited number of subjects confirmed these findings in AIDS patients with mild to moderate first episodes of PCP (Medina et al, 1990). With the exception of anemia and methemoglobinemia, serious adverse reactions were less common and therapy was better tolerated in patients given trimethoprim and dapsone. Substitution of intravenous pentamidine was necessary because of severe toxic effects in 57% of patients receiving trimethoprim/sulfamethoxazole and in 30% of those receiving dapsone and trimethoprim ($p < 0.025$). However, it is recognized that trimethoprim/sulfamethoxazole is toxic in a high proportion of AIDS patients when given at the dosage used in the study cited above (20 mg/kg of the trimethoprim component daily); a lower dose may be equally effective and less toxic in those patients (Sattler et al, 1988). Although other data suggest that patients who are hypersensitive to sulfamethoxazole may not cross-react when given dapsone, dapsone alone is less effective than when it is given with trimethoprim. Thus, although the data now available are promising, trimethoprim/dapsone cannot be recommended as first-line therapy until further data accumulate on the relative efficacy, prevalence and severity of adverse reactions, and cross-sensitivity of this combination.

The investigational agent, trimetrexate glucuronate, has been approved for Treatment Investigational New Drug status by the FDA for use in AIDS patients with confirmed PCP who cannot tolerate or do not respond to approved therapies (*Med Lett Drugs Ther*, 1989). Trimetrexate is a much more potent inhibitor of *P. carinii* dihydrofolate reductase than trimethoprim. Initial uncontrolled studies suggested that trimetrexate, which must be given with leucovorin, is as effective in treating PCP as either trimethoprim/sulfamethoxazole or pentamidine, whether used alone or combined with sulfadiazine (Allegra et al, 1987; Zar, 1991). However, an unacceptably high rate of early relapse has occurred in patients who received this drug. Furthermore, a large, controlled trial of trimetrexate and trimethoprim/sulfamethoxazole in patients with moderate to severe PCP was recently halted prematurely by an independent data and safety monitoring board because the survival rate among those receiving trimetrexate was lower than that in patients receiving the standard drug combination two months after completion of therapy. Additional concerns about appropriate dose ratios of trimetrexate and leucovorin have been discussed in a dosage evaluation study in patients with PCP (Sattler et al, 1990). Thus, the therapeutic role of trimetrexate in these patients is unclear at present, and its routine use cannot be recommended.

Eflornithine [Ornidyl], a specific irreversible inhibitor of polyamine biosynthesis, has been used with some success (primarily as salvage therapy) in the treatment of PCP in AIDS patients who could not tolerate or did not respond to trimethoprim/sulfamethoxazole or pentamidine treatment (Schechter et al, 1987; Sjoerdsma, 1987; Sahai and Berry, 1989; Zar, 1991). However, the available data are from uncontrolled studies, and it is premature to recommend the use of eflornithine except in those in whom conventional therapy has failed.

Other agents have shown promise in the treatment of PCP in AIDS patients. The investigational hydroxynaphthoquinone, BW566C80, which was originally developed as an antimalarial drug, was effective in animals (Hughes et al, 1990) and in the treatment of mild to moderate PCP in Phase I and II studies. In uncontrolled trials, clindamycin plus oral or intravenous primaquine has been used successfully for treatment of mild to moderate episodes as well as for salvage therapy (Black et al, 1991; Ruf et al, 1991; Toma et al, 1989; Toma, 1991). Both BW566C80 and the clindamycin/primaquine regimen are now being compared with trimethoprim/sulfamethoxazole for mild to moderate PCP in ongoing multicenter trials.

Adjunctive Corticosteroid Therapy: The adjunctive use of corticosteroids in AIDS patients being treated for PCP has received considerable attention and is now recommended for specific patients as delineated in a consensus statement from The National Institutes of Health—University of California Expert Panel for Corticosteroids as Adjunctive Therapy for Pneumocystis Pneumonia (1990). This statement is based on results from five randomized clinical trials (Bozzette et al, 1990; Gagnon et al, 1990; Montaner et al, 1990; Clement et al, 1989; The National Institutes of Health—University of California Expert Panel for Corticosteroids as Adjunctive Therapy for Pneumocystis Pneumonia, 1990). The results of recent case reports and uncontrolled retrospective series in AIDS patients also suggest that corticosteroids are beneficial when given adjunctively during salvage or primary therapy for PCP (Kovacs and Masur, 1990). Together, the accumulated data clearly indicate that adjunctive corticosteroid therapy can reduce the likelihood of deterioration of oxygenation, respiratory failure, and death in AIDS patients receiving antimicrobial therapy for moderate to severe PCP (Bozzette, 1990).

Patients who are selected to receive corticosteroids should be adults or adolescents (>13 years old) with proved or suspected HIV infection and PCP and moderate to severe pulmonary dysfunction, based on an arterial oxygen pressure <70 mm Hg or an arterial-alveolar difference >35 mm Hg obtained while the patient is breathing room air. Corticosteroid treatment should be initiated within 72 hours of beginning specific therapy for PCP. Delay of steroid administration beyond 72 hours will probably not be beneficial; however, this has not been established definitively, since none of the studies reviewed in the consensus statement specified initiation of corticosteroid administration beyond this time frame. The following regimen using oral prednisone is recommended: days 1 through 5, 40 mg twice daily; days 6 through 10, 40 mg daily; day 11 through the end of primary treatment, 20 mg daily. If parenteral administration is necessary, methylprednisolone can be given intravenously at 75% of the above doses.

Although no study has assessed the benefit of adjunctive corticosteroid therapy in PCP in immunocompromised patients without AIDS or in HIV-infected pregnant women, it appears reasonable to consider such treatment in these two groups, according to the entry criteria described above.

CHEMOPROPHYLAXIS. Despite recent advances in prophylaxis and treatment (Glatt et al, 1988; Buckley et al, 1990), recurrence of this infection in AIDS patients continues to be a significant problem. Without the institution of specific prophylaxis, relapse of PCP can be expected in 50% of zidovudine-treated patients within six months (Montaner et al, 1991), with a mortality in excess of 20% in severe cases (Fischl et al, 1990). Thus, chemoprophylaxis of PCP should be considered for both adults (*MMWR*, 1989) and children (*MMWR*, 1991 D) who are known to be infected with HIV or are immunosuppressed and susceptible for other reasons.

A CD4+ T-lymphocyte cell count of <200/mm^3 or a CD4+ count of <20% of total lymphocytes constitutes the indications for the institution of primary prophylaxis (ie, indicating no prior PCP episodes) in adults (*MMWR*, 1989). Other factors that indicate substantial risk for the development of PCP include oral candidiasis and persistent fever (>100°F) in patients with AIDS (Phair et al, 1990).

According to guidelines published by the Working Group on PCP Prophylaxis in Children (*MMWR*, 1991 D), the recommended threshold CD4+ T-lymphocyte cell count (per mm^3) for institution of prophylaxis in children varies with age: <1,500 for children 1 to 11 months; <750 for children 12 to 23 months; <500 for children 24 months through 5 years; <200 for children 6 years and older. However, as in adults, a CD4+ T-lymphocyte percentage <20% also should be regarded as an indication for prophylaxis. Prophylaxis should be instituted in all adults and children who have experienced a prior episode of PCP (ie, secondary prophylaxis).

Aerosolized pentamidine has been widely used for chemoprophylaxis of PCP in AIDS patients, and adverse reactions have been minimal when compared with those observed with systemic administration of this drug (Davey and Masur, 1990; Leoung et al, 1990; Hirschel et al, 1991; Montaner et al, 1991; Murphy et al, 1991). Aerosol delivery of drug yields bronchoalveolar fluid concentrations that may be five or six times higher than those attained by intravenous administration of the same dose. However, limited absorption of pentamidine from the lungs produces mean peak plasma concentrations that are approximately 5% of those that occur following systemic administration, and the half-life in bronchoalveolar fluid ranges from one to four months (Conte and Golden, 1988). The success of this treatment depends on the total amount of drug delivered to the lungs and the distribution within the lungs. These factors are directly related to the efficiency of aerosolization and the particle size produced in the aerosol (Monk and Benfield, 1990). A primary prophylactic regimen of aerosolized pentamidine 300 mg once monthly using the Respirgard II Nebulizer (Marquest, Englewood, CO), with administration of a bronchodilator as needed to alleviate severe coughing or bronchospasm during treatment, appears to be most effective (Leoung et al, 1990). This regimen has been approved by the FDA and is recommended by the United States Public Health Service Task Force on Pneumocystis Prophylaxis for use in patients who fulfill the criteria listed above for oral prophylaxis; it also is recommended as an alternative to trimethoprim/sulfamethoxazole in children >5 years (Working Group on PCP Prophylaxis in Children, *MMWR*, 1991 D).

Although aerosolized pentamidine is efficacious in chemoprophylaxis of PCP, recent reports indicate that signs and symptoms of disease recurrence may be atypical in patients who receive this treatment (Edelstein and McCabe, 1990; Jules-Elysee et al, 1990). These include unusual roentgenographic findings (upper lobe predominant infiltrates, cystic changes, pleural effusion), pneumothorax (Sepkowitz et al, 1991), and false-negative bronchoalveolar lavage and induced-sputum organism yields. As a result, diagnosis of recurrent PCP may be more difficult than usual. Other problems that may occur with administration of aerosolized pentamidine are disease breakthrough with dissemination of PCP infection to extrapulmonary sites and pulmonary reactions (bronchospasm, cough) (Telzak et al, 1990).

Based on results of controlled prophylaxis studies in individuals with leukemia (Hughes et al, 1987) and AIDS (Fischl et al, 1988), trimethoprim/sulfamethoxazole is effective for prophylaxis when given orally (trimethoprim 160 mg and sulfamethoxazole 800 mg) twice daily with leucovorin calcium (folinic acid) 5 mg once daily. This regimen also was effective when administered on an intermittent schedule (eg, three consecutive days per week), and the incidence of fungal infections, fever, or other adverse reactions was lower (Hughes et al, 1987). In a subsequent retrospective analysis, the same dose of trimethoprim/sulfamethoxazole three times weekly on alternate days, without leucovorin, was shown to prevent the development of PCP during a mean follow-up period of 18 months in patients with AIDS or AIDS-related complex who were at high risk of developing the infection (Ruskin and LaRiviere, 1991). In this study, the overall adverse reaction rate of 28% represents a significant improvement over the 50% rate observed by other investigators (Fischl et al, 1988). Trimethoprim/sulfamethoxazole 150 mg/M^2/day and 750 mg/M^2/day, respectively, in two divided doses given orally three times weekly on consecutive days (eg, Monday-Tuesday-Wednesday) is the recommended regimen for children 1 month or older (Working Group on PCP Prophylaxis in Children, *MMWR*, 1991 D). However, alternative regimens for this combination have been suggested for use when these dosages are not well tolerated.

TOXOPLASMOSIS

Toxoplasmosis is caused by the obligate intracellular parasite, *Toxoplasma gondii.* This protozoan is distributed worldwide and infects a wide variety of creatures ranging from poikilotherms to man. Felines are definitive hosts, harboring the enteric sexual cycle (oocysts are shed in the feces) and extraintestinal asexual forms. Other animals, including man, are intermediate hosts in which only the asexual forms develop (ie, tachyzoites or proliferative forms; bradyzoites or encysted forms). Many animals and man may harbor and pass the parasite without clear evidence of disease. The infection can be contracted by ingesting oocysts from cat feces that contaminate soil, food, and hands; by ingestion of tissue cysts in inadequately cooked or raw meat; or by congenital transmission from mother to fetus. The infection also may be transmitted by blood, blood products, bone marrow, organs used for transplantation, and exposure in the research laboratory.

TOXOPLASMOSIS IN IMMUNOCOMPETENT PATIENTS. Acquired infection usually is subclinical and remains latent for years with the live organisms dormant in tissue cysts. The most common signs and symptoms are lymphadenopathy, fatigue, and fever. A mild to moderate mononucleosis-like syndrome (prolonged low-grade fever, malaise, and enlarged lymph nodes) associated with a persistently negative heterophil antibody test suggests either toxoplasmosis or cytomegalovirus infection as the most likely diagnosis. The most serious consequence of disease is encephalitis, including chorioretinitis. Toxoplasmosis may mimic other diseases, including atypical pneumonia, and may cause myocarditis progressing to heart failure.

The most reliable diagnostic test for the determination of recent infection in immunocompetent patients is the double-sandwich IgM capture enzyme-linked immunosorbent assay. The IgM-IFA (immunofluorescent antibody) test is more helpful than a single-determination IgG-IFA test in recent infection because of the high prevalence of positive IgG titers in the general population. CT and MRI scans (for central nervous system disease) also are useful for diagnosis and for monitoring therapy.

TOXOPLASMOSIS IN IMMUNOCOMPROMISED PATIENTS. Toxoplasmosis in the immunocompromised patient has a predilection for the central nervous system (Navia et al, 1986; Holliman, 1988; Haverkos, 1987), and infections in patients with AIDS may be severe. Most cases of cerebral toxoplasmosis are believed to result principally from reactivation of latent infection in patients who are seropositive for toxoplasma antibodies (Zangerle et al, 1991). However, toxoplasmosis also is observed commonly in heart transplant patients who received the organ from a seropositive donor. Acute or subacute deterioration in mental status, reduced level of consciousness, focal neurologic signs, fever, and persistent headache are common signs and symptoms. The absence of specific IgM antibody and/or no elevation in IgG titer to *T. gondii* is commonly noted in patients with AIDS and does not exclude toxoplasmosis in the immunocompromised host.

The need for brain biopsy to diagnose CNS toxoplasmosis in AIDS patients is controversial. The CDC and commonly accepted clinical practice suggest that empiric therapy with pyrimethamine and a sulfonamide be employed if a patient is known to be infected with HIV and has clinical signs and symptoms, radiographic evidence consistent with the diagnosis, and any positive titer for IgG toxoplasma antibody. If the patient improves clinically, no biopsy is necessary. However, the sensitivity and specificity of these clinical criteria are not clear. Several other disorders may mimic CNS toxoplasmosis, particularly CNS lymphoma. In addition, serologic evidence of toxoplasma infection is common in our society, and many patients treated with pyrimethamine and a sulfonamide also are treated with steroids and other antimicrobial agents, which may confound the results of the therapeutic challenge by production of "false" improvement in signs and symptoms of lymphoma or other conditions.

MATERNAL AND FETAL TOXOPLASMOSIS. Women who have had toxoplasmosis before pregnancy develop immunity and their fetuses are not at risk for congenital toxoplasmosis.

Acute maternal toxoplasmosis occurs in 2 to 8/1,000 pregnancies; in about one-third, the infection is transmitted to the fetus (Carter and Frank, 1986). Thus, about one in 1,000 live newborns have congenital toxoplasmosis. The fetus is at highest risk of infection during the third trimester, but manifestations are most pronounced when infection occurs during the first trimester. Clinical manifestations are present at birth in only 10% to 20% of exposed fetuses, and only 10% of those affected develop severe signs and symptoms. One-half of these infants will die at or shortly after birth. The eyes, brain, and other organs may be damaged severely; the characteristic syndrome consists of hydrocephalus, hepatosplenomegaly with jaundice, mental retardation, and bilateral retinochoroiditis, occasionally with microcephaly and cerebral calcification. Many (8% to 23%) affected children who were asymptomatic at birth develop chorioretinitis. Approximately 20% experience visual impairment, and their intelligence also may be adversely affected.

A large study has examined the distribution of toxoplasma antibody titers in 22,845 pregnant women (predominantly from northeastern and northwestern states) in relation to the clinical findings for both mothers and children over a seven-year period (Sever et al, 1988). Toxoplasma antibody was present in 38.7% of the pregnant women; 2.3% of the total number of patients had seroconversions, significant increases in antibody during pregnancy, or were in the highest titer ranges. Among those in the latter group, the most common associated clinical findings in their children at 7 years of age were visual impairment, bilateral deafness, microcephaly, and low IQ.

DRUG SELECTION. An acute uncomplicated case of toxoplasmosis in the nonpregnant patient with intact immunity requires treatment only if there is chorioretinitis or organ involvement, particularly of the liver or brain. In these patients, the treatment of choice is sulfadiazine or trisulfapyrimidines with pyrimethamine. Leucovorin calcium (folinic acid) should be given with pyrimethamine (a folic acid antagonist); however, the former should not be given if acute leukemia is associated with toxoplasmosis, because leucovorin may worsen the leukemia (see the evaluation).

In AIDS patients, toxoplasmosis is a life-threatening opportunistic infection (Holliman, 1988; Luft and Remington, 1988). Although the drugs of choice remain the same, a more aggressive regimen of treatment is recommended (Leport et al, 1988). Following an oral loading dose of pyrimethamine 100 to 200 mg daily in two divided doses for one to two days, large daily doses of pyrimethamine (50 to 100 mg) and sulfadiazine (2 to 6 g) are given for six to ten weeks or until CNS signs and symptoms abate or are significantly resolved. Since current clinical evidence indicates that the cyst form of the parasite is not sensitive to this therapy, relapses usually occur in 80% or more of patients. Low doses of pyrimethamine (25 to 50 mg daily) and sulfadiazine (1 to 4 g daily) plus leucovorin (5 to 10 mg daily depending on the white blood cell count) are recommended for lifelong maintenance therapy.

When it is necessary to discontinue sulfadiazine because of adverse effects, including Stevens-Johnson syndrome, severe rash, drug fever, or bone marrow suppression, clindamycin (1.2 to 4.8 g daily) plus pyrimethamine has been effective as alternative therapy (Dannemann et al, 1991; Katlama, 1991; Ruf and Pohle, 1991). Pyrimethamine also has been used alone; however, substantially higher plasma concentrations are required for successful therapy of CNS disease than when it is used in combination with a sulfonamide. If possible, monitoring serum pyrimethamine concentrations may be helpful to minimize toxicity in view of the considerable variation that exists among individuals and that cannot be reliably predicted from the daily dose (Weiss et al, 1988).

The macrolide antibiotic, spiramycin, has had considerable use in Europe for the treatment of toxoplasmosis, especially during pregnancy (see below). Although its effectiveness in immunocompetent patients has been reported in a few studies, the results have been disappointing in AIDS patients (Cook, 1987; Luft and Remington, 1988; Chang and Pechère, 1988; Holliman, 1988). Doses range from 500 to 750 mg four times daily or 1 g three times daily. Newer macrolides (eg, azithromycin, clarithromycin) may hold greater promise for the treatment of toxoplasmosis, possibly by eradicating the cyst form of the parasite (Huskinson-Mark et al, 1991) if adequate cerebrospinal fluid or neural tissue penetration can be attained.

The intracellular accumulation of methotrexate, an inhibitor of *T. gondii* dihydrofolate reductase, requires an active transport system that is lacking in *T. gondii*. Trimetrexate, a novel lipid-soluble investigational analogue of methotrexate, requires no such transport system. It is similar to the available, clinically useful antifolates, pyrimethamine and trimethoprim. Trimetrexate alone or with sulfadiazine prolonged survival in a mouse model of toxoplasmosis (Kovacs et al, 1987). In limited, uncontrolled studies in AIDS patients who had not benefitted from standard therapy, clinical and radiologic improvement was observed initially but was not sustained.

BW566C80, an investigational hydroxynaphthoquinone, has been used successfully as salvage therapy in a limited number of AIDS patients who failed to respond to or could not tolerate conventional treatment.

Systemic corticosteroids are used adjunctively for chorioretinitis and occasionally for cerebral toxoplasmosis to reduce cerebral edema. They must be administered with antiprotozoal agents and preferably in brief courses with rapid tapering of the dose.

TOXOPLASMOSIS AND PREGNANCY. A recent prospective study of 746 documented cases of maternal toxoplasma infection described a treatment regimen that decreases the incidence of congenital toxoplasmosis (Daffos et al, 1988). Diagnosis was based on the identification of acute infection in the mother, followed by culture of fetal blood and amniotic fluid, serologic testing of fetal blood for toxoplasma-specific IgM and nonspecific measures of infection, and ultrasound examination of the fetal brain. In all of these cases of maternal infection, spiramycin 1 g three times daily was given as soon as the diagnosis was made in the mother and was continued throughout pregnancy. Infection was transmitted to the fetus in only 42 of 746 pregnancies, a rate approximately 70% less than would have been predicted based on previous reports; this suggests that spiramycin is efficacious in preventing transplacental transmission of infection from mother to fetus. In 15 pregnancies with infected fetuses that were diagnosed antenatally and not terminated, the mother received pyrimethamine, a sulfonamide (preferably sulfadiazine), and leucovorin in addition to spiramycin. Although initial outcomes are encouraging, it is too early to determine the prognosis of these infants.

TRICHOMONIASIS

Vaginal infections caused by *Trichomonas vaginalis* are common and occur most frequently during the reproductive years when estrogen levels are high. Infections often recur, which indicates that trichomonads may persist in extravaginal foci. However, *T. vaginalis* has been found in the urine rather than the vaginal mucus and may be present in the male urethra and the periurethral glands and ducts (McCue, 1989), which suggests that reinfection from a sexual partner is a more likely cause of recurrence.

Trichomonal vaginitis, urethritis, and prostatovesiculitis are classified as sexually transmitted diseases. Although, in theory, infections may be acquired from contaminated items (eg, toilet articles, toilet seats), no well-documented cases of nonvenereal transmission have been reported.

DIAGNOSIS. Diagnosis is established by direct microscopic examination of a preparation containing fresh exudate from the vagina, semen, or prostatic fluid obtained by massage or examination of urinary sediment. Trichomonal flagella usually are identified easily in fresh preparations, but special stains are required to identify them in fixed smears. When symptoms suggest trichomoniasis (eg, wet, pruritic, inflamed vagina; "strawberry" cervix; a thin, yellow, slightly alkaline, frothy, malodorous discharge) but parasites cannot be identified, empiric therapy is indicated. Culture of *T. vaginalis* is the most sensitive technique to establish the diagnosis; however, culture systems are not widely available. Generally, males are asymptomatic when infected and are treated empirically when the female sexual partner is found to be infected (Saultz and Toffler, 1989). When signs and symptoms disappear and results of microscopic examination of appropriate samples are negative, initial infection is presumed to be controlled; however, cultures are necessary to confirm cures in patients of either sex. Intercourse should be avoided until a cure is confirmed or a course of adequate therapy has been completed.

DRUG SELECTION. Metronidazole [Flagyl, Protostat] is the drug of choice. Other nitroimidazoles (tinidazole, ornidazole, secnidazole) have been tested in other countries (Rossignol et al, 1984).

The locally acting anti-infective preparation, povidone-iodine [Betadine], may be useful. Restoration of the normal vaginal pH by periodic vinegar douching may eliminate mild infections. It has been claimed that the vaginal instillation of lactobacilli is beneficial in vaginitis of any etiology by reducing the vaginal pH. However, lactobacilli do not restore vaginal flora to normal nor eradicate specific pathogens and, therefore, have limited value.

A number of combination products are available for local application in the treatment of trichomoniasis. There is little objective evidence of their efficacy, and none of these mixtures is as effective as metronidazole. Some preparations are recommended not only for trichomoniasis but also for other vaginal infections characterized as bacterial, candidal, mixed, or "nonspecific."

The estrogen present in some mixtures may not be appropriate for some women. The quinoline derivatives in some mixtures may be useful, but aminacrine is of doubtful value. Some preparations contain alleged debriding agents (eg, allantoin) but these have little value. Detergents and surfactants may exert some cleansing effect and improve the action of other ingredients, but this synergism has not been proved. For these reasons, the following mixtures are not recommended for trichomoniasis: ***AAS*** (Rugby), ***Aci Jel*** (Ortho), ***AVC*** (Marion Merrell Dow), ***Vagisec*** (Schmid), ***Vagisec Plus*** (Schmid).

Adverse Reactions and Precautions: See the individual drug evaluations.

TRYPANOSOMIASIS

AFRICAN TRYPANOSOMIASIS. Sleeping sickness is caused by the bite of a tsetse fly infected by *Trypanosoma*. Two clinical types of African sleeping sickness are caused by two subtypes of *Trypanosoma brucei*: West African or Gambian (*T. gambiense*) transmitted by riverine tsetse flies, and East African or Rhodesian (*T. rhodesiense*) transmitted by savannah tsetse flies. Both subtypes produce similar symptoms, but the onset and progression of disease are more rapid with *T. rhodesiense* infection. The chancre that is produced at the site of the bite is an important clinical sign. In the earlier stages of disease, the organism localizes in the lymphatic system and causes intermittent attacks of fever, lymphadenopathy, hepatosplenomegaly, dyspnea, and tachycardia (hemolymphatic stage). When the organisms reach the central nervous system, the chronic, so-called sleeping sickness state begins, characterized by headache, disturbances in coordination, mental dullness, and apathy. As the disease progresses, the patient sleeps constantly, becomes emaciated, and, if untreated, will die.

Although Gambian trypanosomiasis is responsive to both pentamidine and suramin, the hemolymphatic stage of this disease is traditionally treated with pentamidine because this agent is somewhat less toxic than suramin. Conversely, the hemolymphatic stage of Rhodesian trypanosomiasis is treated with suramin because some strains are resistant to pentamidine. This therapy should only be used for patients in whom a spinal tap has been done to rule out CSF involvement. The trivalent arsenical compound, melarsoprol [Arsobal], is the conventional drug of choice to eliminate organisms of either geographic subtype in the central nervous system.

Eflornithine [2-(difluoromethyl)-D,L-ornithine] is an inhibitor of ornithine decarboxylase, the rate-limiting enzyme involved in cellular polyamine biosynthesis (McCann et al, 1987). It has been effective in all stages of West African (Gambian) trypanosomiasis (Doua et al, 1987; Pepin et al, 1987; Schechter et al, 1987; Sjoerdsma, 1987; Taelman et al, 1987; Petru et al, 1988) and is safer than melarsoprol. In the absence of unexpected toxicity and as more clinical experience is gained with eflornithine, it may become the drug of choice for Gambian trypanosomiasis. Limited animal studies suggest that a more lipid-soluble derivative of eflornithine, alpha-monofluoro-methyldehydroornithine methyl ester, may be even more effective in a shorter regimen and at lower doses (Bacchi et al, 1987).

The availability of eflornithine for treatment of the late encephalitic stages of Gambian trypanosomiasis is especially noteworthy, since a vaccine that would be effective against trypanosomiasis is not likely to become available soon. The surface of the trypanosome is covered by the variable surface glycoprotein (VSG). Trypanosomes evade their host's immune defenses through a process called antigenic variation, ie, by regularly changing the VSG in their surface coat (Donelson, 1987).

SOUTH AMERICAN TRYPANOSOMIASIS. South American trypanosomiasis (Chagas' disease) is transmitted to man by reduviid bugs infected with *T. cruzi*. Urine and feces deposited by the insects while they are feeding are rubbed into the bite area or eye by the host while scratching the site. These parasites have been found in reservoir hosts as far north as the state of Maryland. *T. cruzi* is distinct from the organisms that cause African trypanosomiasis.

Chagas' disease is often asymptomatic but, when present, symptoms vary from region to region. Signs of acute Chagas' disease are local swelling (chagoma) with severe inflammation at the site of the bite, rash, fever, and edema of the eyelids and face. In some acute infections, acute myocarditis and/or meningoencephalitis develop.

Chronic Chagas' disease may be asymptomatic or, in certain geographic locations, may produce organomegaly, particularly megaesophagus and megacolon. *T. cruzi* damages the nerve cells in the parasympathetic nervous system of the gastrointestinal tract in a manner not entirely understood and also has affinity for cardiac parenchymal cells. Complications affecting the central nervous system, such as meningoencephalitis, are occasionally fatal, especially in young children. The most common manifestation is cardiomyopathy that occurs many years after the initial infection. Chronic cardiopathy is the usual cause of death in long-standing Chagas' disease.

Acute or chronic Chagas' disease is difficult to treat, and no drug is suitable for general therapy of this infection. Primaquine may be effective against extracellular trypanosomes (trypomastigotes) in the blood but is ineffective against intracellular forms (amastigotes); it is not used clinically. Nifurtimox [Lampit, Bayer 2502] also acts against extracellular parasites, but gastrointestinal reactions and peripheral neuritis limit its usefulness. It is beneficial only for therapy of acute disease and is the only drug available for this indication in the United States. Benznidazole, an analogue of metronidazole, is effective but toxic effects (hypersensitive skin reactions, dose-dependent polyneuropathy) are common. A better understanding of the mechanisms of action of nifurtimox and benznidazole is expected to lead to compounds that are less toxic and/or more effective.

Itraconazole [Sporanox] is a promising member of the azole class of antifungal agents. In mice infected with *T. cruzi*, itraconazole rapidly produced a parasitologic cure as determined by negative hemocultures and serology and absence of parasites in the tissues. Effective doses are well tolerated by patients with systemic mycoses (McCabe et al, 1986).

For a review of the chemotherapy of Chagas' disease, see Marr and Docampo, 1986.

Drug Evaluations

CHLOROQUINE HYDROCHLORIDE
[Aralen]

CHLOROQUINE PHOSPHATE
[Aralen Phosphate]

H
Cl N+
CH_2CH_3
$HNCH(CH_2)_3\overset{+}{N}H$ $2H_2PO_4^-$
CH_3 CH_2CH_3

USES. Chloroquine, a 4-aminoquinoline, is a blood schizonticide and is the drug of choice for prophylaxis and treatment of acute attacks of malaria caused by *Plasmodium vivax*, *P. ovale*, *P. malariae*, and susceptible strains of *P. falciparum*. It also is a component of the combination, Aralen Phosphate with Primaquine Phosphate. The combination has no advantage over the individual drugs used in sequence. (See the evaluation.)

Chloroquine occasionally is combined with emetine or dehydroemetine and iodoquinol for the treatment of hepatic amebiasis. It is less effective than other drugs when used alone.

ADVERSE REACTIONS AND PRECAUTIONS. Most adverse effects of antimalarial doses of chloroquine are relatively mild, since the amounts used for clinical prophylaxis are small and the larger doses employed to treat acute attacks are given only for short periods. Adverse effects are dose related and include gastrointestinal discomfort with nausea and diarrhea, pruritus, rash, headache, and central nervous system stimulation. Most gastrointestinal reactions can be minimized by administering the drug with meals. There is no evidence that administration once weekly for treatment of malaria is associated with development of retinal damage.

Ingestion of more than 5 g of chloroquine may be fatal. Early mechanical ventilation with the administration of diazepam and ephinephrine appears to markedly reduce mortality (Riou et al, 1988).

Adverse reactions and precautions associated with the use of chloroquine in patients with amebiasis resemble those occurring with its use in malaria patients, except that daily administration for a longer period may increase the frequency of gastrointestinal disturbances. When chloroquine is given in large daily doses for prolonged periods as an anti-inflammatory agent, severe visual and cardiac reactions may occur (see index entry Hydroxychloroquine, In Arthritis, for a discussion of toxicity after long-term use).

Rapid intravenous injection causes dizziness, nausea, visual disturbances, and a transient fall in blood pressure. Overdosage can cause circulatory failure, convulsions, respiratory and cardiac arrest, and death. Patients with epilepsy may be very sensitive to seizures induced by chloroquine.

In controlled studies, cimetidine (but not ranitidine) decreased the clearance and metabolism of chloroquine and increased the elimination half-life, all by about 50% (Ette et al, 1987).

Chloroquine is safe when used during pregnancy in the low doses employed for malaria chemoprophylaxis. Less than 5% of the maternal dose is found in breast milk.

The efficacy of the human diploid cell vaccine for rabies may be reduced when it is given by the intradermal route concurrently with chloroquine (or mefloquine). When these antimalarial agents must be given during rabies immunization, the vaccine should be injected intramuscularly (Centers for Disease Control, 1990).

PHARMACOKINETICS. The pharmacokinetics of chloroquine have been reviewed (Walker et al, 1987). Absorption is essentially complete and rapid. Taking chloroquine with food may augment its bioavailability. The volume of distribution is greater than 100 L/kg. Approximately 50% of circulating drug is bound to plasma proteins. The initial plasma half-life is 6 to 12 days, but the drug is retained in certain tissues (eg, lungs, kidney, liver, eyes), has a high affinity for tissue melanin, and is detectable in the urine months and even years after therapy is discontinued. About 30% of a dose is metabolized to monodesethylchloroquine and bisdesethylchloroquine (major metabolite).

Renal clearance is approximately 55% of the total systemic clearance (1.8 ml/min/kg). Chloroquine and its major metabolite account for 70% of the total urinary output. The renal excretion of unchanged chloroquine is increased in acidic urine. Patients with severely depressed renal function (glomerular filtration rate <10 ml/minute) who require prolonged therapy should receive a reduced dose (50 to 100 mg daily).

When chloroquine is given by intravenous injection over 10 to 12 minutes, transiently high plasma concentrations may result from relatively slow distribution into a very large apparent volume (>100 L/kg). Significant hypotension, tachycardia, and prolongation of the QRS interval may occur at this rate of injection; therefore, intravenous infusion over four hours is recommended to minimize toxicity. When intravenous equipment is not readily available, intramuscular injection in divided doses (assuming the patient is not in shock), adjusted for weight, may accomplish the same purpose (Phillips et al, 1986 C).

DOSAGE AND PREPARATIONS. Chloroquine can be administered orally, intramuscularly, or intravenously. The phosphate salt is given only orally; the hydrochloride salt is given parenterally to patients with severe nausea or vomiting, when drug absorption may be impaired, or when the infection is particularly severe. Special caution is necessary when using the parenteral form in children. Oral administration should be substituted as soon as practicable.

CHLOROQUINE PHOSPHATE:

Oral: For treatment of amebiasis, *adults,* 600 mg of base (1 g salt) daily for two days, followed by 300 mg of base (500 mg salt) daily for two to three weeks. *Children,* 10 mg of base/kg (maximum, 300 mg of base) daily for three weeks.

For treatment of a clinical attack of malaria, adults, 600 mg of base (1 g salt), followed by 300 mg of base (500 mg salt) in six hours and daily for the next two days. *Children,* 10 mg of base/kg initially (maximum, 600 mg base), followed by 5 mg of base/kg in six hours and daily for the next two days. Chloroquine resistance should be considered if an adequate response is not noted in two or three days.

For prophylaxis of malaria, *adults,* 300 mg of base (500 mg salt); *children,* 5 mg of base/kg. The dose is given once weekly on the same day of the week beginning one to two weeks before the individual enters the malarious area, during, and for four weeks after leaving the area. Primaquine should be added to the regimen immediately after the individual has left an area endemic for *P. vivax* or *P. ovale*, particularly if exposure has been heavy and prolonged and if the individual is not G6PD deficient (see that evaluation).

Generic. Tablets 250 and 500 mg (equivalent to 150 and 300 mg of base).

Aralen Phosphate (Winthrop). Tablets 500 mg (equivalent to 300 mg of base).

CHLOROQUINE HYDROCHLORIDE:

Intramuscular, subcutaneous: For treatment of a clinical attack of malaria, *adults,* 2.5 mg of base/kg every four hours or 3.5 mg of base/kg every six hours, repeated, if necessary (maximum, 25 mg/kg/day). The usual dose is 200 to 250 mg base every six hours for three days. An oral preparation should be substituted as soon as possible. Intramuscular or subcutaneous administration should be used in *infants and children* only when absolutely necessary because of the potential for local irritation and even necrosis. The suggested dose is 3.5 mg base/kg every six hours (White et al, 1988 A). Oral chloroquine should be substituted as soon as the condition of the child improves sufficiently.

Intravenous: For treatment of a clinical attack of malaria, *adults*, 10 mg of base/kg preferably infused over four hours, while monitoring cardiovascular status to detect hypotension or arrhythmias; 5 mg of base/kg is then given every 12 hours, preferably infused over two hours (maximum, 25 mg/kg/day), until the patient is alert. *Children*, initially 1.25 mg of base/kg/hr is infused continuously for eight hours, immediately followed by 0.62 mg of base/kg for 24 hours (White et al, 1988 A). Close monitoring of blood glucose, blood pressure, heart rate, and the electrocardiogram is advisable. If parenteral administration is impossible, chloroquine suspension or syrup should be given in conventional oral doses through a nasogastric tube, because the drug is well absorbed from this site even in comatose children.

Aralen (Winthrop). Solution (injection) 50 mg (equivalent to 40 mg of base)/ml in 5 ml containers.

DEHYDROEMETINE (Investigational drug)
[Mebadin]

EMETINE HYDROCHLORIDE

ACTIONS AND USES. These salts of an ipecac alkaloid have a direct amebicidal effect against trophozoites of *Entamoeba histolytica* in tissues but are not active against cysts. Extraintestinal (tissue) forms of *E. histolytica* also are affected. These agents are used with iodoquinol for severe intestinal amebiasis and extraintestinal amebiasis (usually hepatic abscess); chloroquine phosphate occasionally is added to this regimen. However, metronidazole plus iodoquinol is the preferred regimen for all forms of symptomatic amebiasis. Emetine should not be used unless the nitroimidazoles are ineffective or contraindicated.

Emetines inhibit polypeptide chain elongation, thereby blocking protein synthesis in eukaryotic but not prokaryotic cells. Therefore, protein synthesis is inhibited in parasitic and mammalian cells but not in bacteria.

ADVERSE REACTIONS AND PRECAUTIONS. Adverse reactions are common, especially when the emetines are used for a prolonged period. The incidence of toxicity is similar with both drugs, although dehydroemetine is slightly less cardiotoxic than emetine. The drugs accumulate in the body, and untoward effects are more frequent with repeated courses.

Cardiovascular reactions are the most serious and include precordial pain, dyspnea, tachycardia, hypotension, gallop rhythm, cardiac dilatation, congestive failure, and death. Electrocardiographic changes are those of conduction delay and can be of long duration (average, six weeks); alterations include widening of the QRS complex, prolongation of the P-R and Q-T intervals, alteration of the S-T segment, and flattening or inversion of the T wave. If these changes are observed, the drug should be discontinued immediately. Injury to the myocardium and other organs may occur.

Nausea, vomiting, and diarrhea are sometimes seen, even when the drugs are administered parenterally, and may make it difficult to assess the response to therapy in amebic dysentery. Headache, skeletal muscle weakness, stiffness, pain and muscle weakness at the site of injection, as well as eczematous, urticarial, or purpuric lesions also have been observed.

Patients receiving the emetines should be hospitalized and remain in bed during treatment. An electrocardiogram should be performed before therapy is initiated and repeated daily; the heart rate and blood pressure also should be monitored. The emetines should not be used during pregnancy, in patients with heart or kidney disease, or in children unless other therapy is ineffective. These drugs must be used with caution in debilitated or elderly patients. If a ten-day course of therapy is not successful, six weeks to two months should elapse before a second course is started to prevent cumulative toxicity.

PHARMACOKINETICS. The emetines are concentrated in the liver, kidney, spleen, and lung, which may contribute to their efficacy in hepatic amebiasis. It is assumed that the kidney is the major route of excretion in man, but documentation for this is not adequate.

DOSAGE AND PREPARATIONS. The emetines usually are administered by subcutaneous or deep intramuscular injection. They are not given intravenously because severe toxic reactions may occur.

EMETINE HYDROCHLORIDE:

Intramuscular (deep), Subcutaneous: *Adults,* 1 mg/kg daily (maximum, 60 mg daily) in one dose (two divided doses may be given if the patient cannot tolerate one dose) for up to five days; symptoms often improve after three days. The dose should be reduced by one-half in *underweight, elderly, or debilitated patients. Children,* no more than 1 mg/kg (maximum, 60 mg) daily in two doses for not more than five days. Multiple injection sites should be used to avoid abscesses.

Generic. Solution 65 mg/ml in 1 ml containers.

DEHYDROEMETINE:

Intramuscular (deep), Subcutaneous: *Adults,* 1 to 1.5 mg/kg (maximum, 90 mg) daily in one dose for up to five days; *children,* 1 to 1.5 mg/kg (maximum, 90 mg) daily in two divided doses for up to five days.

Mebadin. Drug available from the Drug & Immunobiologics Service, Centers for Disease Control, Atlanta, GA 30333.

DILOXANIDE FUROATE (Investigational drug)
[Furamide]

USES. This amebicide is an alternative to iodoquinol in asymptomatic cyst carriers but is available only through the

Centers for Disease Control. Diloxanide is less effective in symptomatic patients with intestinal amebiasis who are passing trophozoites or in those with acute amebic dysentery; the combination of metronidazole and iodoquinol is preferred. Diloxanide is of no value in extraintestinal amebiasis. Its mechanism of action is unknown.

ADVERSE REACTIONS AND PRECAUTIONS. Diloxanide is relatively safe, and discontinuation of therapy because of adverse reactions is only rarely necessary. Excessive flatulence is the most common side effect. Infrequently reported adverse reactions include esophagitis, nausea, vomiting, diarrhea, abdominal cramps, vague tingling sensations, pruritus, urticaria, and albuminuria. Abnormal results of hematologic and blood chemistry tests have not been noted.

Since the safety of diloxanide during pregnancy has not been determined, this drug should not be given to pregnant women. Also, it should not be administered to children under 2 years.

PHARMACOKINETICS. Diloxanide is rapidly and significantly absorbed from the gastrointestinal tract after oral administration. The ester is largely hydrolyzed in the intestine, and only diloxanide appears in the systemic circulation. Time to peak effect is approximately one hour. The elimination half-life is approximately six hours, and the major portion of diloxanide appears in the urine as the glucuronide.

DOSAGE AND PREPARATIONS.

Oral: *Adults,* 500 mg three times daily for ten days. *Children 2 years or older,* 20 mg/kg daily in three divided doses for ten days. Treatment may be repeated if the initial course is unsuccessful.

Furamide. In the United States, this preparation is available from the Drug & Immunobiologics Service, Centers for Disease Control, Atlanta, GA 30333.

EFLORNITHINE HYDROCHLORIDE

[Ornidyl]

ACTIONS AND USES. The polyamines, putrescine, spermidine, and spermine, are polycations of low molecular weight that play an essential role in the growth, differentiation, and replication of animal cells by functioning in nucleic acid and protein synthesis. Eflornithine [2-(difluoromethyl)-D,L-ornithine] is a potent irreversible inhibitor of ornithine decarboxylase, the rate-limiting enzyme of the polyamine biosynthesis pathway (McCann et al, 1987).

Trypanosomal ornithine decarboxylase is sensitive to the action of eflornithine. Intracellular concentrations of putrescine and spermidine are significantly reduced in trypanosomes exposed to this agent. Studies in animals suggest that the action of eflornithine is cytostatic rather than cytolytic; therefore, a host antibody response is probably necessary to eliminate the trypanosomes. Organisms are cleared from the blood within four days after initiating therapy.

Animal studies showed that when eflornithine was combined with suramin, its effectiveness against *Trypanosoma brucei* was 100%. In open studies in patients with severe trypanosomiasis affecting the central nervous system, eflornithine alone was effective (Doua et al, 1987; Schechter et al, 1987; Sjoerdsma, 1987; Taelman et al, 1987; Petru et al, 1988). Side effects of eflornithine are minimal compared with those produced by melarsoprol, the only other drug available for the treatment of late-stage meningoencephalitis associated with West African (Gambian) trypanosomiasis.

Eflornithine also is being evaluated for use in cryptosporidiosis, leishmaniasis, and malaria, but data are too fragmentary to determine its role in any of these diseases. This drug also has been effective in *Pneumocystis carinii* pneumonia (PCP) (Sahai and Berry, 1989). Data from a series of case reports indicate that eflornithine was effective in about 35% of patients with PCP who were unresponsive to or could not tolerate other therapy. However, patients received this agent during various stages of disease and were treated for different periods of time. Until results of controlled clinical trials become available, eflornithine can only be recommended as salvage therapy for PCP.

ADVERSE REACTIONS AND PRECAUTIONS. Eflornithine has been well tolerated in the human studies conducted to date, whether given orally or intravenously (Schechter et al, 1987; Sjoerdsma, 1987). Nausea and vomiting, loose stools, anemia, thrombocytopenia and leukopenia, and hearing loss have been reported (Sahai and Berry, 1989). All side effects were spontaneously reversible.

Eflornithine is classified in FDA Pregnancy Category C.

PHARMACOKINETICS. Eflornithine is well absorbed after oral administration but is approved only for intravenous use. After administration of 100 mg/kg intravenously, approximately 80% of the dose is excreted unchanged in the urine within 24 hours and the terminal plasma half-life is approximately three hours. Since clearance of eflornithine through the kidney approximates that of creatinine, dosage adjustment is necessary in patients with impaired renal function. This drug does not bind appreciably to plasma proteins and penetrates cerebrospinal fluid well (CSF:blood ratios of 0.13 to 0.51). At steady-state, peak serum concentrations in patients receiving 100 mg/kg ranged from 196.6 to 317.9 mcg/ml; the volume of distribution is 0.43 L/kg.

DOSAGE AND PREPARATIONS. Prior to use, the hypertonic drug solution must be diluted with sterile water for injection, USP, to a concentration of 40 mg/ml (5 g eflornithine in 125 ml total volume). The diluted drug must be stored at 4° C (39° F) and used within 24 hours to minimize the risk of microbial proliferation.

Intravenous, Oral: For Gambian trypanosomiasis, *adults,* 100 mg/kg is infused every six hours for 14 days (minimum infusion period, 45 minutes).

For PCP (investigational use), *adults,* 100 mg/kg infused every six hours for 14 days (minimum infusion period, 45 minutes), followed by 75 mg/kg orally every six hours for four to six weeks (Sahai and Berry, 1989). The total daily dose should not exceed 30 g. (Oral eflornithine may be obtained from the Marion Merrell Dow Research Institute, 2110 E. Galbraith Rd, Cincinnati, OH 45212, after internal review board approval and informed consent by the patient or guardian.)

Ornidyl (Marion Merrell Dow). Solution 200 mg/ml in 100 ml containers (as the monohydrate). This preparation should be stored at *room temperature*, preferably below 30° C (86° F), and protected from freezing and light.

FURAZOLIDONE

[Furoxone]

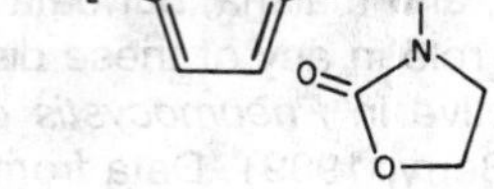

ACTIONS AND USES. Furazolidone's mechanism of antigiardial action is unclear, but this drug is known to interfere with several bacterial enzyme systems. Resistance to this agent is minimal.

This nitrofuran is effective in the treatment of giardiasis. Although cure rates in excess of 90% and few relapses have been reported, furazolidone has not been widely used for giardiasis in the United States because metronidazole or quinacrine is preferred. However, the liquid formulation of furazolidone may be preferred in children.

Furazolidone has been used investigationally in the treatment of persistent isosporiasis.

ADVERSE REACTIONS AND PRECAUTIONS. Furazolidone usually is well tolerated, but nausea and vomiting occur occasionally and vesicular morbilliform pruritic rash has been reported. It may cause acute hemolysis in individuals with G6PD deficiency. Traces of the drug and its metabolites may tint the urine brown.

Furazolidone produces a disulfiram-type reaction in some patients if taken with alcohol. Its administration markedly inhibits the activity of monoamine oxidase, and a hypertensive reaction may occur if the drug is given with adrenergic agents, tricyclic compounds, or foods containing significant amounts of tyramine (eg, cheeses, red wines).

DOSAGE AND PREPARATIONS.

Oral: *Adults,* 100 mg four times daily for seven to ten days. *Children,* 6 mg/kg daily divided into four doses for seven to ten days. Alternatively, up to 8 mg/kg/24 hours divided into three equal doses is taken at mealtime for at least seven and preferably ten days (Murphy and Nelson, 1983). The drug should not be given to *infants under 1 month.*

Furoxone (Roberts). Liquid 50 mg/15 ml; tablets 100 mg.

HYDROXYCHLOROQUINE SULFATE

[Plaquenil Sulfate]

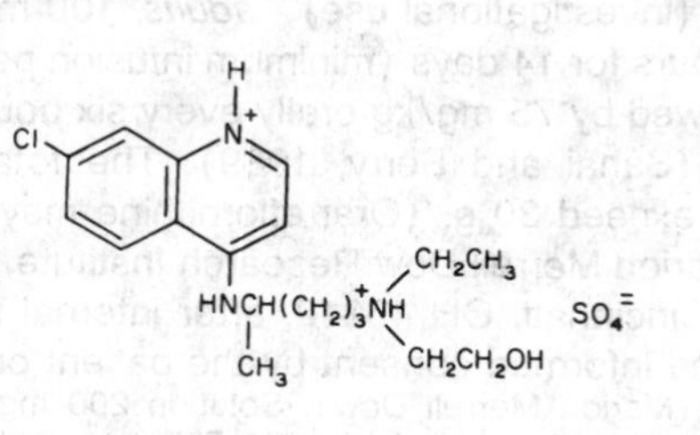

Hydroxychloroquine, a 4-aminoquinoline, can be used orally for both prophylaxis and clinical cure of malaria caused by *Plasmodium vivax*, *P. malariae*, *P. ovale*, and susceptible strains of *P. falciparum*. However, although hydroxychloroquine is as effective and safe as chloroquine, it has no therapeutic advantage over this drug and is seldom used for this indication. Traditionally, hydroxychloroquine is more commonly used than chloroquine as an anti-inflammatory agent for arthritis, lupus erythematosus, and other connective tissue disorders. For further information on adverse reactions, precautions, and pharmacokinetics, see index entry Hydroxychloroquine, In Arthritis.

Adverse reactions caused by hydroxychloroquine are the same as those for chloroquine (see that evaluation).

DOSAGE AND PREPARATIONS.

Oral: For treatment of malaria, *adults,* 620 mg of base (800 mg salt) initially, followed by 310 mg of base (400 mg salt) in six hours and daily for the next two days. *Children,* 10 mg of base/kg initially, followed by 5 mg of base/kg in six hours and daily for the next two days.

For prophylaxis of malaria, *adults,* 310 mg of base (400 mg salt); *children,* 5 mg of base/kg (maximum, 310 mg of base [400 mg salt]/week). The dose is given once weekly on the same day of the week beginning one to two weeks before the individual enters the malarious area, during, and for eight weeks after leaving the area.

Plaquenil Sulfate (Winthrop). Tablets 200 mg (equivalent to 155 mg of base).

IODOQUINOL (Diiodohydroxyquin)

[Diquinol, Yodoxin]

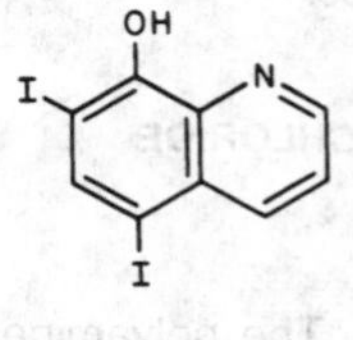

USES. This organic iodine compound acts against amebae in the intestinal lumen and is the drug of choice for the treatment of asymptomatic intestinal amebiasis (cyst carrier state). Diloxanide is preferred by some authorities, but it is available only from the Centers for Disease Control. Iodoquinol alone is not effective in symptomatic or extraintestinal amebiasis, but it is given to eliminate luminal organisms after a course of metronidazole (preferred regimen).

Iodoquinol is reported to be effective in some patients with *Dientamoeba fragilis* and *Balantidium coli* infections.

ADVERSE REACTIONS AND PRECAUTIONS. Occasional adverse reactions include nausea, abdominal cramps, pruritus ani, rash, acne, and slight enlargement of the thyroid gland.

Iodoquinol has caused subacute myelo-optic neuropathy (SMON) when doses larger than those recommended for amebiasis were given for three weeks. SMON is characterized by muscle pain and weakness, usually below the T-12 vertebra; painful dysesthesias, especially of the limbs, often associated with significant alteration of gait; and, in some instances, optic atrophy and blindness. Although these symptoms may regress following discontinuation of the drug, they are not always completely reversible. Children appear to be most susceptible. Iodoquinol has not produced SMON as often as clioquinol, which is no longer available for systemic use in the United States.

The safety of iodoquinol during pregnancy or lactation has not been established.

Iodoquinol is contraindicated in patients hypersensitive to iodine and interferes with the results of some thyroid function tests; therefore, it is relatively contraindicated in patients with thyroid disorders.

DOSAGE AND PREPARATIONS.

Oral: For amebiasis, dientamebiasis (investigational use), and balantidiasis (investigational use), *adults,* 650 mg three times daily after meals; *children,* 30 to 40 mg/kg daily in three doses (maximum, 2 g daily). The duration of therapy should not exceed 20 days. If required, the course may be repeated after a two- or three-week interval.

Generic. Tablets 650 mg; powder 25, 100, and 1,000 g.

Diquinol (Consolidated Midland). Tablets 650 mg.

Yodoxin (Glenwood). Tablets 210 and 650 mg; powder 25 g.

MEFLOQUINE HYDROCHLORIDE

[Lariam]

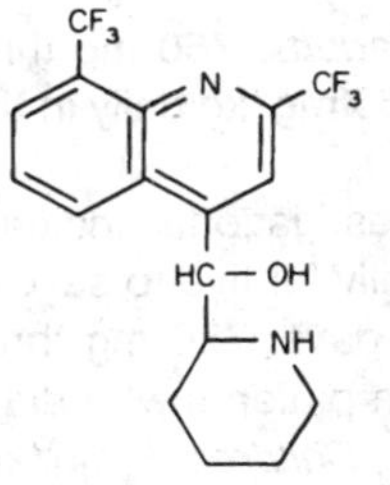

ACTIONS AND USES. Mefloquine, a 4-quinoline methanol derivative of quinine, is employed for both chemoprophylaxis and treatment of malaria. It has no clinical activity against exoerythrocytic forms of *P. vivax,* but kills the asexual erythrocytic forms of *P. falciparum* and *P. vivax* (blood schizonticide) (Harinasuta et al, 1985).

Mefloquine is indicated for the treatment of mild to moderate acute malaria caused by mefloquine-susceptible strains of *P. falciparum* or *P. vivax.* Administration of primaquine is necessary to eliminate exoerythrocytic (hepatic phase) *P. vivax* parasites and avoid relapses. Insufficient data are available to support the clinical efficacy of mefloquine in malaria caused by *P. malariae* or *P. ovale.* Its primary use is chemoprophylaxis of malaria in travelers to areas where there is risk of chloroquine-resistant *P. falciparum* infection or where *P. falciparum* infection is resistant to both chloroquine and pyrimethamine/sulfadoxine [Fansidar], as well as in the treatment of malaria acquired in such areas (*MMWR,* 1990 A, 1990 B, 1991 C).

ADVERSE REACTIONS AND PRECAUTIONS. Mefloquine is well tolerated in doses used for chemoprophylaxis or treatment of malaria. The most common side effects are nausea, vomiting, myalgia, abdominal pain, anorexia, diarrhea, dizziness, tinnitus, headache, and rashes. Side effects occurring in less than 1% of patients include bradycardia, emotional disturbances, pruritus, asthenia, severe vertigo, and loss of resting-phase hair (telogen effluvium). Seizures and psychosis also have been reported. Occasionally, alterations of hematologic profiles and chemistry (eg, decreased hematocrit, transient elevation of transaminases, leukopenia, thrombocytopenia) have occurred.

If mefloquine is to be administered for a prolonged period, periodic liver function tests have been advocated by some clinicians. However, these evaluations are not recommended by the CDC. Although the retinal abnormalities seen in humans with long-term chloroquine use have not been observed with mefloquine, long-term feeding of doses of 12.5 mg/kg/day and higher to rats produced ocular lesions (retinal degeneration, retinal edema, and lenticular opacity). Periodic ophthalmic examinations have been suggested by some investigators, but they are not recommended by the CDC.

Rarely, asymptomatic bradycardia and prolonged QT interval have been associated with administration of mefloquine; avoiding concurrent use of beta blockers, calcium channel blockers, or other drugs that may prolong or alter cardiac conduction is advisable.

Mefloquine generally should not be given with quinine or quinidine. If these drugs are to be used in the initial treatment of severe malaria, administration of mefloquine should be delayed at least 12 hours after the last dose of either of these drugs.

Patients taking mefloquine while also taking valproic acid had loss of seizure control and lower than expected blood levels of valproic acid. Therefore, in patients receiving both drugs, the blood level of valproic acid should be monitored and the dosage adjusted appropriately.

PREGNANCY. Mefloquine has been teratogenic in rats and mice at doses of 100 mg/kg/day. In rabbits, a dose of 160 mg/kg/day was embryotoxic and teratogenic, and a dose of 80 mg/kg/day was teratogenic but not embryotoxic. There are no adequate and well-controlled studies in pregnant women. Mefloquine should be used during pregnancy only if the potential benefit justifies the potential risk to the fetus. This agent is classified in FDA Pregnancy Category C.

PHARMACOKINETICS. Mefloquine is well absorbed from the gastrointestinal tract. Peak plasma concentrations occur within 2 to 12 hours. The drug is highly protein bound in the plasma (approximately 98%). The erythrocyte/plasma concentration ratio is 2. In a few studies in healthy individuals, the mean elimination half-life was about three weeks. Large differences in pharmacokinetic parameters between ethnic groups (Swiss and Thai) have been observed (Looareesuwan et al, 1987); however, all of the Thai patients had malaria. The drug is metabolized in the liver, and the principal route of excretion is in the bile, partially as a glucuronide; enterohepatic cycling occurs. The total clearance of mefloquine, which is essentially hepatic, is 30 ml/min.

DOSAGE AND PREPARATIONS. Mefloquine is available only in an oral formulation. If possible, this drug should not be taken on an empty stomach, and it should be given with at least 8 ounces (240 ml) of water in adults.

Oral: For prophylaxis of malaria, *adults,* 250 mg of base weekly, beginning one week prior to entering the area of risk and continuing for four weeks after leaving the area (*MMWR,* 1991 C). *Children (>30 lb),* 4 mg/kg (maximum, 250 mg) weekly, beginning one week prior to entering the area of risk and continuing for four weeks after leaving the area (*MMWR,* 1990 A, 1991 C).

For treatment of malaria, *adults,* 1.25 g of base given as a single oral dose; *children,* 25 mg/kg in a single dose.

Lariam (Roche). Tablets 274 mg (equivalent to 250 mg base).

MELARSOPROL (MEL-B) (Investigational drug)
[Arsobal]

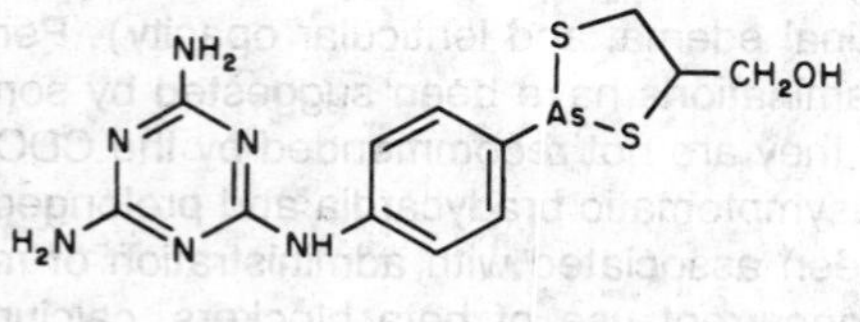

USES. This trivalent arsenical compound traditionally has been the drug of choice for meningoencephalitis associated with the late stages of Gambian or Rhodesian trypanosomiasis. Because of its greater margin of safety and effectiveness in clinical trials to date, eflornithine probably will replace melarsoprol as the drug of choice, especially in the Gambian form of trypanosomiasis. Melarsoprol is somewhat effective in the earlier stages but, because of its potential to cause encephalopathy, is not used until later in the course of disease.

ADVERSE REACTIONS AND PRECAUTIONS. Melarsoprol is very toxic and many adverse effects are those of arsenic poisoning. Potentially fatal reactive encephalopathy develops in 3% to 5% of patients. Other reactions include abdominal pain, vomiting, hypotension, albuminuria, peripheral neuropathy, arthralgia, angioedema, and rashes. A Herxheimer-like reaction may follow the first dose of melarsoprol. Patients receiving this drug should be hospitalized and monitored closely.

The drug is given intravenously but is irritating to tissues and care must be taken to avoid extravasation.

Arsobal. Information on dosage and precautions is available from the Drug & Immunobiologics Service, Centers for Disease Control, Atlanta, GA 30333.

METRONIDAZOLE
[Flagyl, Protostat]

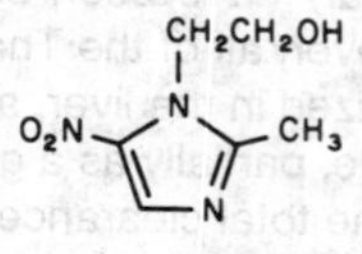

USES. This synthetic nitroimidazole compound is amebicidal for *Entamoeba histolytica* at both intestinal (luminal) and extraintestinal (tissue) sites, and currently it is the preferred drug for amebiasis except in asymptomatic cyst carriers. Because most of an oral dose is absorbed, another luminal amebicide (generally iodoquinol) must be given to eradicate organisms in the intestine and avoid relapse. See also the section on Amebiasis in the Introduction to this chapter.

Metronidazole is effective in the treatment of giardiasis and has largely replaced quinacrine in this role. It has been shown to be synergistic with quinacrine against *Giardia,* and this combination has been useful in the management of patients with diffuse hypogammaglobulinemia in whom giardiasis has been very difficult to eradicate.

Metronidazole is the drug of choice in the treatment of *Trichomonas vaginalis* infection in men and women. This drug is active in semen, urine, and extravaginal (eg, prostate, seminal vesicles, epididymis), as well as vaginal, foci. It is active against *Gardnerella vaginalis* vaginitis but is inactive against *Candida* species that cause vaginitis.

Metronidazole also is the drug of choice for many serious anaerobic bacterial infections and is an alternative to tetracycline in the treatment of balantidiasis. For further information on uses, adverse reactions and precautions, pharmacokinetics, and use in pregnancy and lactation, see index entry Metronidazole.

DOSAGE AND PREPARATIONS. When necessary, metronidazole tablets can be formulated into a suspension (Holtan, 1988).

Oral: For amebiasis, *adults,* 750 mg three times daily for ten days. *Children,* 35 to 50 mg/kg daily in three divided doses for ten days.

For giardiasis (investigational indication), *adults*, 250 to 500 mg three times daily for five to seven days or 2 g daily in a single dose for three days; 750 mg three times daily for ten days has been used in patients who did not respond to lower doses (Holtan, 1988). *Children*, 5 mg/kg three times daily for five to seven days. To simplify the dosage schedule and improve compliance, an alternative schedule, based on the patient's weight, is recommended by some authorities: *25 to 40 kg*, 50 mg/kg in a single daily dose for three days; *< 25 kg,* 35 mg/kg in a single daily dose for three days.

For balantidiasis (investigational indication), *adults*, 750 mg three times daily for five to ten days; *children*, 35 to 50 mg/kg/day divided into three doses for five to ten days.

For trichomoniasis, treatment is the same for men and women. The dosage should be individualized to ensure compliance and minimize reinfection. One-day treatment, 2 g as a single dose (preferred if tolerated by the patient) or in two equally divided doses; seven-day treatment, 250 mg three times daily for seven consecutive days. *Children (prepubertal)*, 15 mg/kg daily divided into three doses for seven to ten days. (Child abuse should be considered and evaluated.) *Infants 1 month or older,* 10 to 30 mg/kg daily for five to eight days.

Flagyl (Searle), ***Protostat*** (Ortho), ***Generic.*** Tablets 250 and 500 mg.

Additional Trademarks.
Metric 21 (Fielding), ***Metryl*** (Lemmon).

NIFURTIMOX (Investigational drug)
[Lampit]

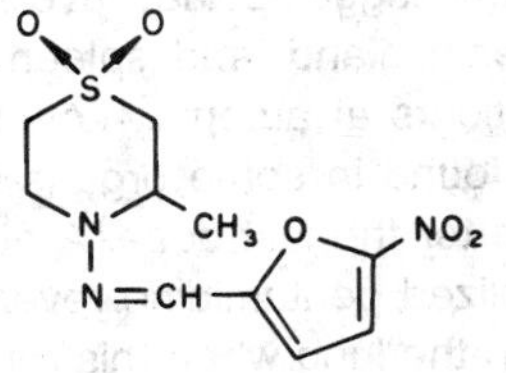

ACTIONS AND USES. This nitrofuran derivative is potentially curative in the acute stage of South American trypanosomiasis (Chagas' disease), because, in tolerated therapeutic doses, it inhibits the extracellular but not the intracellular forms of *Trypanosoma cruzi* and reduces parasitemia. However, nifurtimox must be taken for months, and gastric upset makes compliance difficult. Nifurtimox is more effective against Argentinean and Chilean strains of the parasite than against Brazilian strains.

The cytotoxic action of nifurtimox on *T. cruzi* is mediated by the generation of oxygen reduction products (Marr and Docampo, 1986). The same effect probably causes toxicity in the host.

ADVERSE REACTIONS. Adverse reactions are more common in adults (incidence, 40% to 70%) than in children. They usually consist of anorexia, nausea, vomiting, abdominal pain, excitement, vertigo, headache, myalgia, insomnia, and skin rashes. Peripheral neuritis and psychoses also may be seen.

PHARMACOKINETICS. After oral administration, nifurtimox is extensively metabolized; the metabolites are excreted primarily by the kidney.

Lampit. Information on dosage and preparations is available from the Drug & Immunobiologics Service, Centers for Disease Control, Atlanta, GA 30333.

PAROMOMYCIN SULFATE
[Humatin]

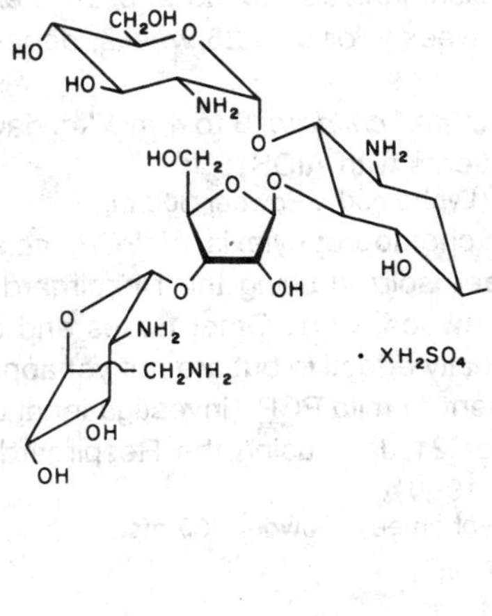

Paromomycin is a luminal amebicide. This aminoglycoside generally is administered as an alternative to metronidazole in the treatment of mild to moderate intestinal amebiasis caused by *Entamoeba histolytica*. Paromomycin also is an alternative to iodoquinol in the asymptomatic carrier state. Occasionally, it is used to treat giardiasis during pregnancy.

For use of paromomycin in intestinal tapeworm infections, see index entry Paromomycin, As Anthelmintic.

ADVERSE REACTIONS AND PRECAUTIONS. Frequently reported adverse reactions include nausea, increased gastrointestinal motility, abdominal pain, and diarrhea. Rash, headache, vertigo, and vomiting occur occasionally. Patients should be observed for signs of superinfection.

Paromomycin is poorly absorbed from the intact gastrointestinal tract, and most of a single dose is eliminated in the feces. Nevertheless, to avoid excessive absorption (which may cause ototoxicity and nephrotoxicity), the drug should be used with caution in patients with renal failure, intestinal inflammation, or ulcerations.

DOSAGE AND PREPARATIONS.
Oral: *Adults and children,* 25 to 35 mg/kg daily in three divided doses with meals for seven to ten days. The course may be repeated after a two-week interval.

Humatin (Parke-Davis). Capsules equivalent to 250 mg of base.

PENTAMIDINE ISETHIONATE
[NebuPent, Pentam 300]

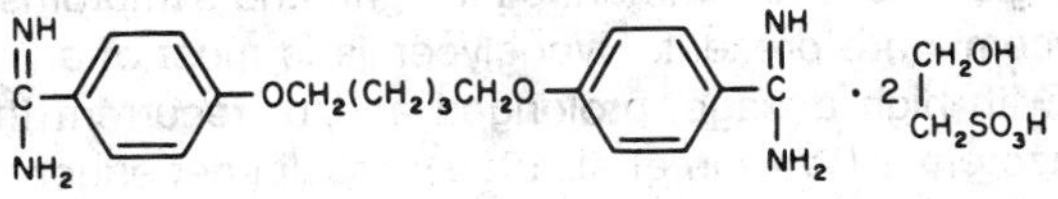

ACTIONS AND USES. This diamidine eliminates the organisms that cause trypanosomiasis, leishmaniasis, and *Pneumocystis carinii* pneumonia (PCP) (Sands et al, 1985; Monk and Benfield, 1990). Its mechanism of action may involve one or more of the following: inhibition of oxidative phosphorylation, nucleic acid and protein synthesis, glucose metabolism, or dihydrofolate reductase activity.

Pentamidine is effective in the treatment of early Gambian sleeping sickness caused by *Trypanosoma gambiense* when the central nervous system is not affected, although the response rate may not be as high as that attained with suramin. It is an alternative drug for early-stage Rhodesian sleeping sickness when suramin is contraindicated, but some *T. rhodesiense* infections do not respond. Some experts caution against the prophylactic use of pentamidine for this disease, because the drug may suppress the hemolymphatic stage and central nervous system involvement may be the first manifestation of disease. Melarsoprol currently is the preferred agent for either form of African trypanosomiasis when the central nervous system is involved. Recent success with eflornithine (see the evaluation) may alter the roles of pentamidine, suramin, and melarsoprol in the treatment of hemolymphatic (*T. gambiense*) and CNS (*T. gambiense* and *T. rhodesiense*) African trypanosomiasis. Pentamidine is ineffective in South American trypanosomiasis (Chagas' disease).

This drug is an alternative in cutaneous and visceral leishmaniasis if the preferred antimonial agents are ineffective or not tolerated.

Intravenous pentamidine is an effective alternative to trimethoprim/sulfamethoxazole in pneumonia caused by *Pneumocystis carinii*. Pentamidine in aerosol form can be used alone for the treatment of those with mild to moderate disease or to complete a course of conventional treatment of serious infection. The aerosolized drug also is effective when used alone in the chemoprophylaxis of *P. carinii* infection in patients with HIV infection or other profound immunosuppression (see the discussion on *Pneumocystis carinii* Pneumonia in the Introduction).

ADVERSE REACTIONS AND PRECAUTIONS. Pentamidine may cause pain at the site of intramuscular injection, followed by tissue necrosis and abscess formation. Other adverse reactions include nausea, vomiting, hypotension, tachycardia, and arrhythmias. Severe hypotension has been reported even after the administration of a single dose of pentamidine, whether given by the intravenous or intramuscular route; this can be minimized or eliminated by giving the drug intravenously over a period of at least one hour.

Pentamidine-induced severe hypoglycemia has been associated with pancreatic beta islet cell necrosis and inappropriately high plasma concentrations of insulin; monitoring of blood glucose is recommended if signs and symptoms of hypoglycemia are present. Hypoglycemia is most often associated with high dosage, prolonged and/or recurrent therapy, and azotemia (Waskin et al, 1988). Insulin-dependent diabetes mellitus may result.

Many patients develop renal and hepatic dysfunction and leukopenia that is usually reversible when the drug is discontinued. Thrombocytopenia, confusion, hallucinations, anemia, rash, pancreatitis, fever, hypocalcemia, and Stevens-Johnson syndrome also have occurred. In general, adverse drug reactions are more common in patients with AIDS than in other immunocompromised patients.

Although aerosolized pentamidine is effective in the chemoprophylaxis of PCP, recent reports indicate that signs and symptoms of recurrence of the disease may be atypical in patients who receive this treatment (Edelstein and McCabe, 1990; Jules-Elysee et al, 1990). These include unusual roentgenographic findings (upper lobe predominant infiltrates, cystic changes, pleural effusion), pneumothorax, and false-negative bronchoalveolar lavage and induced-sputum organism yields. As a result, diagnosis of recurrent PCP may be more difficult than usual. Other problems that may occur with the use of aerosolized pentamidine include disease breakthrough with dissemination of PCP infection to extrapulmonary sites (Telzak et al, 1990) and pulmonary reactions (bronchospasm, cough).

Animal reproduction studies have not been conducted. Pentamidine should be used during pregnancy only if diagnosis is definitive and the agent is clearly needed (FDA Pregnancy Category C).

PHARMACOKINETICS. Since pentamidine is poorly absorbed from the gastrointestinal tract, it must be administered parenterally. The volume of distribution is about 3 L/kg. A bioassay procedure suggests that levels are highest in the liver, kidney, adrenal gland, and spleen but are low in the lungs of AIDS patients at autopsy. Low but detectable concentrations were found in some organs but not the lung as late as one year after the last dose. A number of studies on the use of aerosolized pentamidine reveal that the drug can be concentrated in the lung when this route of administration is used, and this reduces systemic toxicity (see the Introduction). Mean peak plasma concentrations achieved after intramuscular and intravenous administration are 209 ng/ml and 612 ng/ml, respectively.

Elimination of pentamidine from the plasma is rapid, with mean half-lives after intramuscular and intravenous administration of 6.4 and 9.4 hours, respectively. However, the drug accumulates in selected tissues and clearance from these sites is slow. Pentamidine appears in the urine for six to eight weeks after cessation of systemic therapy. The major path of excretion is via the kidney (about 80%), and the dose should be adjusted in patients with renal dysfunction (Conte et al, 1987). If the glomerular filtration rate (GFR) is 10 to 35 ml/min, the dosage interval should be 24 to 36 hours. If the GFR is less than 10 ml/min, the dosage interval should be 48 hours.

DOSAGE AND PREPARATIONS.

Intravenous (preferred), Intramuscular: Fatalities due to arrhythmias and severe hypotension have occurred, even after the administration of a single dose of pentamidine, whether given intravenously or intramuscularly. Therefore, the dose should be infused over at least 60 to 120 minutes to avoid hypotension and the blood pressure should be monitored until it is stable. Dividing the dose may minimize the local reaction when the drug is administered by deep intramuscular injection.

For the hemolymphatic stage of Gambian or Rhodesian trypanosomiasis, *adults and children*, 4 mg/kg/day for 10 days.

For visceral leishmaniasis, *adults and children*, 4 mg/kg/day three times weekly for 5 to 25 weeks, depending on the response.

For PCP, *adults and children*, 3 to 4 mg/kg/day for 14 days (21 days for patients with AIDS).

Pentam 300 (Lyphomed). Powder 300 mg.

Inhalation: For chemoprophylaxis of PCP, *adults,* 300 mg once a month aerosolized using the Respirgard II Nebulizer (Marquest, Englewood, CO). Other doses and delivery systems may be equally effective but are not yet approved by the FDA. For treatment of mild PCP (investigational use), *adults*, 8 mg/kg daily for 21 days using the Respirgard II nebulizer (Soo Hoo et al, 1990).

NebuPent (Lyphomed). Powder 300 mg.

POVIDONE-IODINE
[Betadine]

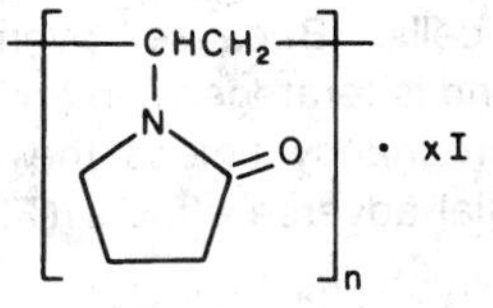

Clinical evidence indicates that this water-soluble complex of polyvinylpyrrolidone and iodine may be beneficial in vaginal infections caused by *Trichomonas vaginalis* when extravaginal sources of reinfection are not present. Metronidazole is preferred for this indication.

ADVERSE REACTIONS AND PRECAUTIONS. Although povidone-iodine does not produce the degree of local irritation associated with use of tincture of iodine, adverse reactions may occur in patients allergic to iodine.

Topical vaginal application of povidone-iodine elevates serum concentrations of iodine. Euthyroid women showed no evidence of thyroid dysfunction (Safran and Braverman, 1982); however, this drug should not be used repeatedly as a vaginal disinfectant during pregnancy to avoid goiter and hypothyroidism in the fetus and newborn (Vorherr et al, 1980).

DOSAGE AND PREPARATIONS.

Topical (vaginal): Initially the cervix and vulvovaginal areas are swabbed with a povidone-iodine solution in the physician's office. Thereafter, one applicatorful of the gel is inserted nightly, followed by use of the douche preparation the next morning. Daily applications of gel and douche should be continued for at least two weeks. Infections may resolve in 10 to 15 days, or therapy may be required for two or three menstrual cycles.

Generic. Douche; gel; solution (nonprescription).

Betadine (Purdue Frederick). Douche 10% in 15, 30, 120, and 240 ml containers; gel 10% in 18 g containers; solution 10% in 15, 30, and 240 ml containers (all forms nonprescription).

PRIMAQUINE PHOSPHATE

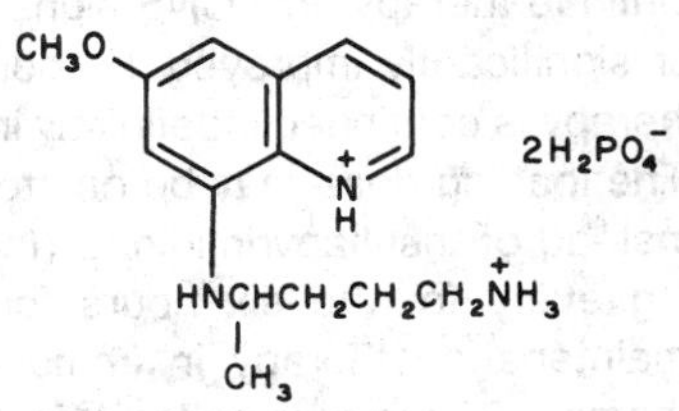

USES. Primaquine is the most effective and least toxic of the available 8-aminoquinolines. It is used almost exclusively as a tissue schizonticide to provide radical cure of malaria caused by the exoerythrocytic hepatic (hypnozoite) forms of *Plasmodium vivax* or *P. ovale*. Because it may cause hemolysis in certain patients (see below), most experts advise that post-travel prophylactic use of primaquine be employed only when exposure to *P. vivax* and *P. ovale* was prolonged.

Resistance to primaquine occurs in about one-third of patients infected with the Chesson strain of *P. vivax* in southeastern Asia and Oceania. Approximately 10% of Asian strains of *P. vivax* also are resistant to this agent. If relapses occur in patients infected with these strains, retreatment with 1.5 to 2 times the standard dose is indicated.

Although primaquine is effective against the erythrocytic forms of plasmodia, it is not used for prophylaxis because of its slow onset of action and short half-life.

Primaquine controls parasitemia in South American trypanosomiasis (Chagas' disease), but is ineffective against intracellular parasites (nifurtimox is preferred).

Primaquine has been used in combination with clindamycin for therapy of PCP in AIDS patients (see the section on *Pneumocystis carinii* Pneumonia).

ADVERSE REACTIONS AND PRECAUTIONS. The most serious adverse effect is intravascular hemolysis manifested as acute hemolytic anemia in patients with glucose-6-phosphate dehydrogenase (G6PD) deficiency. Rarely, primaquine also may induce hemolysis in individuals with other defects of the erythrocytic pentose phosphate pathway of glucose metabolism and certain hemoglobinopathies. In healthy individuals with G6PD deficiency, the severity of hemolysis varies directly with the dose of primaquine and degree of enzyme deficiency. There are many molecular variations and degrees of G6PD deficiency found among all races. In individuals with the African variant, the hemolytic anemia induced by a standard course of primaquine therapy is relatively mild, self-limited, and often asymptomatic. In those with the Mediterranean variant, clinically evident hemolysis with the usual dosage schedule is likely. Thus, in patients whose ethnic origin indicates the possibility of G6PD deficiency (those from the Mediterranean area, blacks, and Asians), screening for this deficiency prior to primaquine administration is necessary. Monitoring of the hemogram, including reticulocyte counts and bilirubin, is recommended, especially during the first and second weeks of therapy. The urine should be examined as well.

Primaquine also may cause abdominal discomfort, nausea, headache, interference with visual accommodation, and pruritus. Methemoglobinemia is common but rarely necessitates interruption of therapy. Leukopenia and agranulocytosis occur rarely. Primaquine may exacerbate psoriasis.

Although it has not been established conclusively that primaquine causes teratogenic effects in humans, use of this agent probably should be postponed until after delivery. This drug may cause hemolysis in G6PD-deficient fetuses.

PHARMACOKINETICS. Limited studies suggest that primaquine is rapidly and completely absorbed, extensively distributed (apparent volume of distribution is 243 ± 70 L), and converted principally to carboxyprimaquine. The drug is not subject to extensive first-pass metabolism. Clearance is 24 ± 7.4 L/hour (Mihaly et al, 1985). Less than 5% of the administered dose is found in the urine (White, 1985).

DOSAGE AND PREPARATIONS. All doses are expressed in terms of the base.

Oral: For treatment of malaria (radical cure) due to *P. vivax* and *P. ovale* or to prevent relapses in travelers after their return from malarious areas when exposure to *P. vivax* and *P. ovale* was prolonged, *adults,* 15 mg, and *children,* 0.3 mg/kg. This dose is given daily for 14 days, preferably *consecutively* with chloroquine or other therapy, which is given on the first three days of an acute attack.

The following regimens are equally effective and reduce the risk of hemolysis; however, use of chloroquine for treatment of relapses or prophylaxis (6 to 12 months) may be preferable. For those with the African variant of G6PD deficiency, 45 mg of primaquine once weekly for eight weeks; for those with the Caucasian or Oriental variant, 30 mg once weekly for 15 weeks.

No pediatric formulation of primaquine is available, and it is necessary to break the tablet into the approximate dose portion for children.

Generic (Winthrop). Tablets 26.3 mg (equivalent to 15 mg of base). Primaquine phosphate is no longer available from the CDC Drug Service and should be obtained from the manufacturer.

PYRIMETHAMINE
[Daraprim]

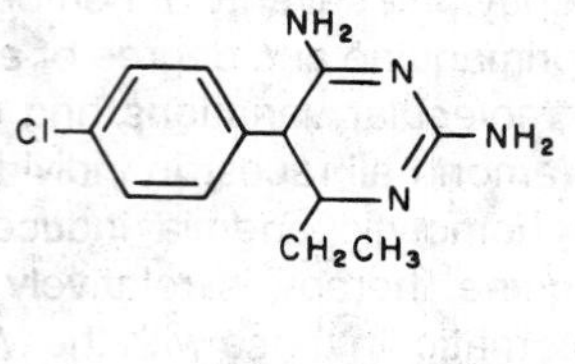

ACTIONS AND USES. This potent dihydrofolate reductase inhibitor has been used for the prophylaxis and treatment of malaria caused by susceptible species of *Plasmodium*, including chloroquine-resistant *P. falciparum*. However, because parasites readily develop resistance to this drug when it is given alone and the combined activity of folic acid antagonists and sulfonamides is many times greater than that of either type of drug alone, pyrimethamine is rarely administered alone for therapy or prophylaxis of malaria (see Keystone, 1990). It is given principally in combination with sulfadiazine. A product combining sulfadoxine with pyrimethamine [Fansidar] also is available. It is used for single-dose, one time presumptive treatment of chloroquine-resistant strains of *P. falciparum* malaria (see the evaluation on Pyrimethamine/Sulfadoxine and the Introduction to this chapter).

The combination of pyrimethamine, a sulfonamide, and quinine is a regimen of choice in the treatment of an acute attack of malaria due to a chloroquine-resistant organism where Fansidar resistance is not known to occur. For dosage, see the evaluation on Quinine Sulfate.

Pyrimethamine with sulfadiazine or trisulfapyrimidines is the treatment of choice for toxoplasmosis. The combination of pyrimethamine and sulfadiazine is used investigationally to treat persistent isosporiasis and has been used for prophylaxis of PCP.

ADVERSE REACTIONS AND PRECAUTIONS. The hazards from small, suppressive, antimalarial doses of pyrimethamine are minimal. Eosinophilic pneumonitis has been reported. However, prolonged administration of this drug may produce toxicity. Toxic symptoms mainly reflect interference with folic acid metabolism. The effects, therefore, are most evident in rapidly dividing cells. Because pyrimethamine has an antifolate action and is teratogenic in animals, it is not recommended during pregnancy unless the risk of malaria outweighs the potential adverse effects (FDA Pregnancy Category C).

If hematologic abnormalities appear, pyrimethamine administration should be stopped and leucovorin calcium (folinic acid) should be given intramuscularly or intravenously (3 to 9 mg) or orally (10 mg) each day until the blood cell count returns to acceptable levels. Alternatively, concomitant administration of 3 to 9 mg daily of leucovorin calcium with pyrimethamine usually prevents anemia, thrombocytopenia, and leukopenia without affecting the antiprotozoal action of pyrimethamine. Leucovorin is often beneficial during treatment of AIDS patients with folic acid antagonists because they frequently have baseline neutropenia caused by their underlying condition.

PHARMACOKINETICS. Pyrimethamine is well absorbed; peak plasma concentrations are achieved within two to six hours. Plasma protein binding is 87%. The drug is eliminated slowly by the kidney (half-life, approximately four days).

DOSAGE AND PREPARATIONS.

Oral: For prophylaxis of malaria, the following doses are given once weekly on the same day of the week: *Adults and children over 10 years,* 25 mg; *children 2 years and under,* 6.25 to 12.5 mg; *3 to 10 years,* 12.5 to 25 mg. Since adequate blood levels are obtained within a few hours after ingestion, administration need not be started until the day before entering an endemic area and should be continued for four weeks after return or six to ten weeks after exposure.

For toxoplasmosis, *adults*, initially, a loading dose of 100 to 150 mg in two equal doses daily for three days, followed by 25 to 50 mg/day for three to four weeks plus trisulfapyrimidines 2 to 6 g daily in four to six divided doses for three to four weeks. For treatment of CNS toxoplasmosis in patients with AIDS, some clinicians have used pyrimethamine 50 to 100 mg/day and continue therapy until CNS signs and symptoms are resolved or significantly improved (Leport et al, 1988). Maintenance therapy is continued indefinitely in AIDS patients (see below). The loading dose may be omitted. Sulfadiazine may be used instead of trisulfapyrimidines (initially, 2 to 6 g, followed by 1 g every four to six hours for three to four weeks). For maintenance therapy in immunocompromised *adults*, pyrimethamine 25 mg plus sulfadiazine 2 g is given in four divided doses daily for three to five days per week indefinitely. In AIDS patients, leucovorin calcium (folinic acid) 10 mg/day is added. *Children*, 2 mg/kg/day (maximum, 25 mg/day) for three days, then 1 mg/kg/day (maximum, 25 mg/day) for four weeks. This should be given with 100 to 200 mg/kg/day of trisulfapyrimidines in four to six divided doses for three to four weeks. *Infants*, 2 mg/kg/day for three days, then 1 mg/kg/day every two to three days for four weeks.

Daraprim (Burroughs Wellcome). Tablets 25 mg.

QUINACRINE HYDROCHLORIDE

[Atabrine Hydrochloride]

$2Cl^- \cdot 2H_2O$

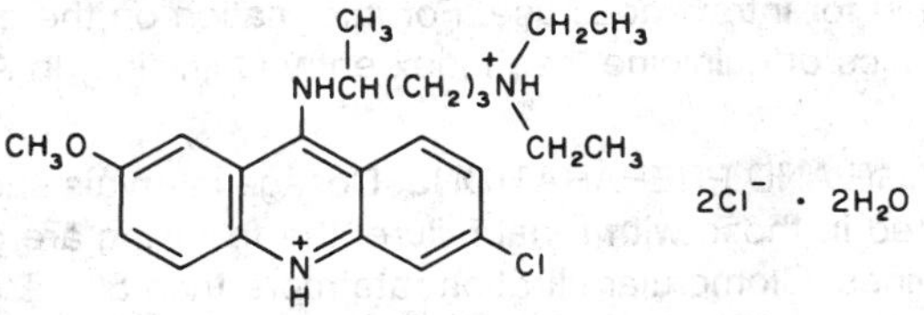

ACTIONS AND USES. Even though metronidazole remains an investigational agent for the treatment of giardiasis, it and other nitroimidazole compounds have replaced quinacrine as the therapy of choice, because these drugs are more effective and are less toxic in children, who do not tolerate quinacrine well. Thus, in giardiasis, quinacrine now is an alternative for patients who should not receive or cannot tolerate metronidazole.

Quinacrine is obsolete in the treatment of malaria. It is no longer marketed in Canada.

ADVERSE REACTIONS AND PRECAUTIONS. Nausea and vomiting are the most common adverse effects of quinacrine. Its prolonged administration stains the skin yellow and produces a deep yellow urine, which can be confused with symptoms of hepatitis. Toxic psychosis has been reported in 1.5% to 2% of adults taking this drug. Transient dizziness also may occur. Aplastic anemia, exfoliative dermatitis, atypical lichen planus, and acute hepatic necrosis occur rarely.

Quinacrine should be used cautiously in patients over 60 years and in those with a history of psychosis. This drug should not be used in patients with psoriasis, because it may exacerbate this condition. Treatment of pregnant women should be postponed until after delivery because giardiasis generally is not life-threatening and quinacrine poses a hazard to the fetus. However, since malnutrition and weight loss caused by severe giardial infection also may be detrimental to the fetus, the individual clinical situation must be evaluated to determine if the relative risks are equivalent.

PHARMACOKINETICS. Quinacrine is well absorbed from the intestinal tract. It is widely distributed in tissues where it accumulates and is liberated slowly. Quinacrine is excreted in the urine; significant amounts can be detected in the urine two months after therapy is discontinued.

DOSAGE AND PREPARATIONS.

Oral: For giardiasis, *adults*, 100 mg three times daily after meals for five days. *Children* (not commonly used), 2 mg/kg three times daily after meals for five days (maximum, 300 mg/day).

Atabrine Hydrochloride (Winthrop). Tablets 100 mg.

QUININE SULFATE

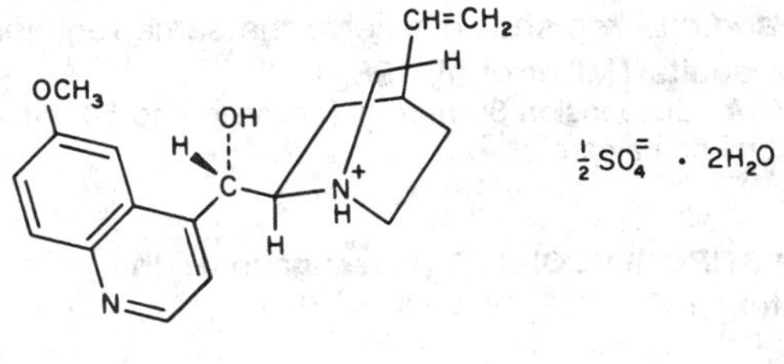

$\frac{1}{2}SO_4^= \cdot 2H_2O$

QUINIDINE GLUCONATE

USES. Quinine with or without pyrimethamine and a sulfonamide (eg, sulfadoxine, sulfadiazine) or tetracycline are the regimens of choice to treat uncomplicated infections with chloroquine-resistant strains of *Plasmodium falciparum* (see also Table 2). Quinine alone has been effective for treatment of *P. falciparum* malaria in Africa but not in Southeast Asia. The preferred regimen for severe infections is intravenous quinidine gluconate, which has supplanted quinine dihydrochloride for this indication (*MMWR*, 1991 B; Phillips et al, 1985; Philpott and Keystone, 1987; Miller et al, 1989); the FDA and the manufacturer have amended the labeling of this drug to include therapy for life-threatening *P. falciparum* malaria among its indications. Unless they are not tolerated or are contraindicated, the safer and more rapid-acting 4-aminoquinolines should be used instead of quinine in the treatment of malaria caused by other species or chloroquine-sensitive *P. falciparum*. Quinine is not used for prophylaxis of malaria because of its short half-life, toxicity, and lack of patient compliance.

Quinine can be administered orally (quinine sulfate) or intravenously (quinidine gluconate). The intravenous route is preferred in patients with severe attacks of malaria when absorption of quinine sulfate cannot be assured. The parenteral preparation of quinine (dihydrochloride salt) is no longer available from the Centers for Disease Control (*MMWR*, 1991 B).

Quinine has been used in the treatment of myotonia congenita, as an antipyretic-analgesic, and as a local anesthetic or sclerosing agent. More effective drugs are available for these uses. It is also used for the prevention of nocturnal leg cramps (see index entry Quinine).

ADVERSE REACTIONS AND PRECAUTIONS. The adverse reactions associated with quinine also occur with the other cinchona alkaloids, although there may be quantitative differences in the various responses. The usual antimalarial dose of quinine sulfate (and other cinchona alkaloids) may cause mild to moderate cinchonism (tinnitus, headache, altered auditory acuity, blurred vision, nausea, diarrhea), but symptoms seldom necessitate cessation of treatment. Severe symptoms develop only rarely (except with overdosage), most often when plasma levels of the drug exceed 10 mg/dL. Asthma may be precipitated in susceptible individuals. Urticaria is the most frequent allergic reaction, and pruritus may develop with or without rash. Signs of hematologic toxicity include acute hemolysis, hypoprothrombinemia, thrombocytopenic purpura, and agranulocytosis. The precise role played by quinine in precipitating blackwater fever is unknown.

In volunteers or patients receiving quinine or quinidine for the treatment for falciparum malaria, significant hyperinsulinemia associated with hypoglycemia has been observed (Phillips et al, 1986 B). This occurrence may be life-threatening, especially in patients with severe malaria, in pregnant women, or in children, but it can be minimized or eliminated by infusing the drug over a period of at least three to four hours (Taylor et al, 1988). However, since hypoglycemia can be a manifestation of severe malaria, it is difficult to discern the basis of this phenomenon and ascribe it to quinine treatment per se.

Blindness or other visual disturbances occurred within 4 to 14 hours after an overdose in 6 of 48 patients; the effect is reversible in most patients, but long-term visual impairment can result (Bateman and Dyson, 1986).

Intravenous administration of quinidine gluconate may produce hypotension and acute circulatory failure. A number of potentially fatal cardiac effects (widening of the QRS complex and Q-T_C interval, SA block or arrest, high-grade AV block, ventricular tachyarrhythmias, asystole) also may occur as the concentration of quinidine in plasma rises above 2 mcg/ml. Thus, when this drug is given intravenously, the ECG should be monitored and appropriate supportive measures for management of severe manifestations of cardiac toxicity should be readily available. The CDC has recommended that patients receiving this drug be treated in intensive-care facilities (*MMWR*, 1991 B). Very dilute solutions should be infused slowly, and oral administration of quinine sulfate should be substituted as soon as possible. Other adverse reactions associated with quinine sulfate also may occur with quinidine gluconate.

Cinchona alkaloids should be given with caution to patients who have preexisting atrial fibrillation or rapid ventricular rate and to those who experience idiosyncratic reactions of cutaneous angioedema or visual or auditory symptoms. These drugs are contraindicated in patients with optic neuritis and tinnitus. For other adverse reactions and precautions, see index entry Quinidine, In Arrhythmias.

Quinine sulfate is classified in FDA Pregnancy Category X. However, since the oxytocic effect of this drug is observed only when larger than recommended doses are given, pregnant patients with presumed chloroquine-resistant malaria should not be denied treatment with quinine. In a recent study in eight pregnant patients, none developed painful uterine contractions or went into labor during the intravenous infusion of quinine over at least four hours (Phillips et al, 1986 A). Drug-induced hypoglycemia is more threatening than induction of labor (Looareesuwan, 1985).

PHARMACOKINETICS.

QUININE SULFATE:

Quinine is readily absorbed whether given intramuscularly or orally. Over 80% of an oral dose is absorbed primarily in the proximal small intestine. Peak plasma concentrations are reached one to three hours after an oral dose; the half-life is approximately 11 hours. Concentrations in plasma between 8 and 15 mcg/ml are clinically effective, generally nontoxic, and usually achieved with therapeutic doses of the drug. Quinine is widely distributed in the body and has an apparent volume of distribution of about 2 L/kg; approximately 90% is bound to plasma proteins. The concentration of the drug in the cerebrospinal fluid is about 2% to 5% of that in the plasma. The compound freely crosses the placenta and reaches fetal tissues. Quinine is extensively metabolized in the liver; about 10% of urinary excretion products is unaltered drug. Metabolites are excreted in the urine, and this drug does not accumulate in the body with continued administration. Excretion is more rapid in acidic than in alkaline urine.

QUINIDINE GLUCONATE:

Although this drug may be administered orally, it is recommended for intravenous use. For information on the pharmacokinetics of quinidine, see index entry Quinidine, In Arrhythmias.

DOSAGE AND PREPARATIONS. Dosage intervals should be adjusted in those with renal failure; the following are general guidelines: Glomerular filtration rate more than 50 ml/minute, 8-hour interval; 10 to 50 ml/minute, 8- to 12-hour interval; less than 10 ml/minute, 24-hour interval.

QUININE SULFATE:

Oral: For treatment of chloroquine-sensitive malaria when chloroquine is contraindicated or not tolerated, *adults,* 650 mg of salt (or 10 mg/kg) every eight hours for three days. *Children,* 25 mg/kg/day in divided doses every eight hours for three days. *P. falciparum* infections acquired in Southeast Asia, particularly Thailand, should be treated for seven days.

For treatment of chloroquine-resistant *P. falciparum* malaria in *adults*, the above dose is given. To prevent recrudescences, pyrimethamine 25 mg twice daily is added for the first three days and sulfadiazine 500 mg four times daily for five days, or the fixed-dose combination of pyrimethamine and sulfadoxine [Fansidar] (three tablets as a single dose) can be added to the regimen. Alternatively, quinine may be given for three days and tetracycline (investigational use) administered in a dose of 1 g daily in divided amounts every six hours for seven days. Infections acquired in Thailand should be treated with quinine for seven days and tetracycline given as noted above. In *children under 8 years or pregnant women,* clindamycin (investigational use) can be used in place of tetracycline: *Adults,* 900 mg three times daily for three days; *children,* 20 to 40 mg/kg/daily in three doses for three days. For *children*, quinine 25 mg/kg/day is given in divided doses every eight hours for three days, pyrimethamine 0.5 to 1 mg/kg/day is given in divided doses every 12 hours for three days (with supplemental leucovorin calcium), and sulfadiazine 120 to 150 mg/kg/day (maximum, 2 g/day) is given in divided doses every six hours for five days, or the fixed-dose combination of pyrimethamine and sulfadoxine [Fansidar] should be added to the regimen (see the evaluation).

Generic. Capsules 200, 300, 325, and 1,260 mg; tablets 260 and 300 mg.

QUINIDINE GLUCONATE:

Intravenous: For treatment of severe malaria, *adults,* a loading dose of 10 mg of salt/kg (equivalent to 6.2 mg quinidine base) is infused over one to two hours while monitoring for hypotension and widening of the QRS interval; if either occurs, the rate should be decreased or the infusion discontinued. A constant infusion of 0.02 mg of salt/kg/min is given after the loading dose (Miller et al, 1989; *MMWR*, 1991 A). *Infants and children* should receive the same regimen that is used for adults (Miller et al, 1989).

Generic. Suspension 80 mg/ml (equivalent to 50 mg/ml base) in 10 ml containers.

SODIUM STIBOGLUCONATE (Investigational drug)

[Pentostam]

MEGLUMINE ANTIMONIATE (Investigational drug)
[Glucantime]

ACTIONS AND USES. The pentavalent antimonial, sodium stibogluconate, is a drug of choice in treating all forms of leishmaniasis. The antimonial compounds may inhibit *Leishmania* bioenergetics, but their exact mode of action has not been fully established. Meglumine antimoniate [Glucantime] is not available in the United States.

ADVERSE REACTIONS AND PRECAUTIONS. Sodium stibogluconate is better tolerated than trivalent antimonials. Common side effects are cardiotoxicity, usually manifested as T-wave depression on ECG and hepatotoxicity manifested as two- to fivefold elevation of hepatocellular enzyme levels. Prolongation of the QT_C interval beyond 0.5 seconds and concave ST segments are rare but require termination of treatment. Impairment of kidney function is rare. Milder reactions include nausea, vomiting, rash, headache, syncope, dyspnea, facial edema, and abdominal pain. Pain in joints and muscles occurs frequently toward the end of a therapeutic course.

Pentavalent antimonials are generally contraindicated in patients with cardiac, hepatic, or renal disease; pneumonia; tuberculosis; pregnant women; or infants under 18 months. However, because of lack of suitable alternative therapy for leishmaniasis, antimonials may be used in these circumstances with frequent monitoring for toxicity.

PHARMACOKINETICS. Pentavalent antimonial compounds are not absorbed when given orally. Up to 90% of the dose is excreted in the urine following injection; the half-life is approximately two hours.

DOSAGE AND PREPARATIONS.

Intramuscular, Intravenous: Previously recommended dosages of these antimonials have been shown to be inadequate in a number of patients (Ballou et al, 1987). Because higher doses are more efficacious and equally safe, in 1991 the CDC revised the World Health Organization guidelines. (For dosing information, contact the CDC at the telephone number given below.) For cutaneous leishmaniasis, *adults and children*, 66 mg of sodium stibogluconate equivalent to 20 mg antimony (Sb)/kg/day is given for 20 days. For mucocutaneous or visceral leishmaniasis, 20 mg Sb/kg/day is given for 28 days. Lower daily doses may be considered on an individual basis if the physician determines that 20 mg/kg/day of sodium stibogluconate could be excessive. An expert in the Parasitic Diseases Branch of the CDC should be consulted.

Intralesional: For cutaneous leishmaniasis, intralesional administration of sodium stibogluconate may be equally efficacious and is associated with fewer serious side effects than parenteral administration. Reviews of this technique are available (Kellum, 1986; Sharquie et al, 1988).

Pentostam. Sodium antimony gluconate (sodium stibogluconate) is available from the Drug & Immunobiologics Service, Centers for Disease Control, Atlanta, GA 30333 (404/639-3670; 404/488-4050). Solution (sterile, aqueous) for parenteral administration containing 330 mg equivalent to 100 mg of antimony/ml in 100 ml containers. For intravenous administration, the appropriate volume is diluted in 50 ml of D5W and infused over approximately 10 minutes.

SURAMIN (Investigational drug)

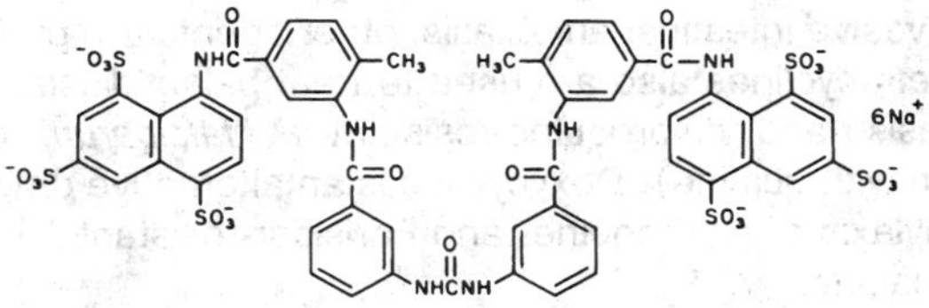

ACTIONS AND USES. Suramin is trypanosomicidal and is the drug of choice for the treatment of early (hemolymphatic) Rhodesian sleeping sickness when the central nervous system is not involved. It is an alternative drug in early Gambian sleeping sickness (pentamidine is preferred). When the parasite is entrenched within the central nervous system, melarsoprol or eflornithine is the drug of choice for Gambian trypanosomiasis. Suramin appears to be selectively absorbed into trypanosomes, perhaps by pinocytosis, where it binds with enzymes, often in a reversible fashion. The exact mechanism of action has not been determined.

Suramin also is used to destroy adult worms in onchocerciasis (see index entry Suramin, As Anthelmintic).

ADVERSE REACTIONS AND PRECAUTIONS. Suramin should be administered only in a hospital under close medical supervision. Adverse effects on the central nervous system are common and include paresthesias, hyperesthesia of the palms and soles, peripheral neuropathy, and photophobia. Loss of consciousness and seizures occur in approximately 0.3% of patients. Pruritus and urticaria may develop quickly, even with therapeutic doses, and other types of rashes, including exfoliative dermatitis, may develop later. Suramin is nephrotoxic and causes proteinuria, hematuria, and cylindruria. Rarely, blood dyscrasias and hemolytic anemia have been reported. Occasionally, a shock-like reaction characterized by nausea, vomiting, hypotension, and unconsciousness occurs immediately after injection.

PHARMACOKINETICS. Suramin is not well absorbed orally. It is tightly bound to proteins and persists in the circulation for months. This drug is released slowly from plasma proteins and excreted by the kidney.

DOSAGE AND PREPARATIONS.

Intravenous: For trypanosomiasis, a 100- to 200-mg test dose should be administered before the first full therapeutic injection is given. If a severe reaction does not occur, therapy can be initiated. *Adults,* following the test dose, 10 to 15 mg/kg is given on days 1, 3, 7, 14, and 21. *Children,* 20 mg/kg given on the same days as for adults. A fresh solution must be prepared before each injection.

Suramin is available from the Drug & Immunobiologics Service, Centers for Disease Control, Atlanta, GA 30333.

TETRACYCLINES

These broad spectrum antibiotics are partially active against amebae in the intestinal lumen and wall. They may be indirectly amebicidal in that they modify the intestinal flora necessary for amebic viability. Tetracycline and oxytetracycline are the most effective members of this group. Although they have been used with other drugs to treat mild to moderate invasive intestinal amebiasis, other agents are preferred. The tetracyclines also are used to treat balantidiasis, dientamebiasis, and chloroquine-resistant *P. falciparum* malaria (given with quinine). Doxycycline is an alternative drug in the prophylaxis of chloroquine- and Fansidar-resistant *P. falciparum* malaria.

For adverse reactions, precautions, and other uses, see index entry Tetracyclines.

DOSAGE AND PREPARATIONS.

OXYTETRACYCLINE, TETRACYCLINE:

Oral: *Adults,* for dientamebiasis (investigational use), 500 mg four times daily for ten days. For treatment of chloroquine-resistant *P. falciparum* malaria (investigational use), 1 g daily in divided doses every six hours for seven days.

DOXYCYCLINE:

Oral: For prophylaxis of chloroquine-resistant *P. falciparum* malaria (investigational use), *adults*, 100 mg/day during the exposure period and for four weeks afterward; *children over 8 years*, 2 mg/kg/day, up to 100 mg/day.

For preparations, see index entry Tetracyclines.

TRIMETREXATE GLUCURONATE (Investigational drug)

ACTIONS AND USES. Trimetrexate is a potent inhibitor of dihydrofolate reductase; it is 1,500 times more potent than trimethoprim as an inhibitor of this enzyme in *Pneumocystis carinii*. It is more lipophilic than methotrexate and this is assumed to account for its better penetration into *P. carinii*. The drug can produce considerable myelosuppression due to its antifolate action; however, administration with leucovorin allows differential rescue of host tissues without reversal of the antiprotozoal effect.

Trimetrexate has received FDA Treatment Investigational New Drug status for the therapy of *P. carinii* pneumonia (PCP) (*Med Lett Drugs Ther*, 1989). Until more adequate data on safety are available, the agency recommends that the drug be used in those patients (1) who have failed to respond to at least five days of treatment with each of the recommended approved drugs (ie, trimethoprim/sulfamethoxazole and pentamidine) or (2) who have failed to respond to at least five days of treatment with one of the approved drugs and have developed a serious adverse reaction to the other. The FDA's recommendation is based in part on an open study in which response and survival rates with trimetrexate were improved in patients who did not respond to trimethoprim/sulfamethoxazole or who had a history of hypersensitivity to sulfonamides; trimetrexate also was effective when combined with sulfadiazine (Allegra et al, 1987; Hughes, 1987). At least 66% of patients in each of the three groups receiving trimetrexate had satisfactory response and survival rates. These preliminary data compared favorably with similar results in patients receiving either trimethoprim/sulfamethoxazole or pentamidine. However, a subsequent large, controlled trial of trimetrexate and trimethoprim/sulfamethoxazole in patients with moderate to severe PCP was halted prematurely by an independent data and safety monitoring board because the survival rate among those receiving trimetrexate was lower two months after completion of therapy. Thus, although additional studies of trimetrexate in therapy of PCP are in progress, its role is unclear at present and it cannot be recommended except as salvage therapy.

ADVERSE REACTIONS AND PRECAUTIONS. Trimetrexate was well tolerated in early studies (Allegra et al, 1987; Eisenhauer et al, 1988). Fluctuating leukopenia and thrombocytopenia, anemia, and transient increases in serum concentrations of aspartate and alanine aminotransferases are observed commonly. Bone marrow suppression generally responds promptly to lowering the dose by 50% or increasing the dose of leucovorin twofold. Initial three- to fivefold increases in serum concentrations of aminotransferases gradually are reversed when therapy is continued. Mucositis (stomatitis), increases in alkaline phosphatase, and skin rashes occur occasionally; diarrhea, arthralgia, fever, bleeding, anorexia, nausea, and vomiting are reported even less frequently. Patients with hypoproteinemia and/or liver disease would be expected to be more sensitive to the drug, and dosage adjustment should be considered.

PHARMACOKINETICS. Trimetrexate has a mean oral bioavailability of 44% (range, 19% to 67%); therefore, it is administered intravenously (Rogers et al, 1988). The drug is extensively protein bound (95%). Unlike methotrexate, which is excreted mainly unchanged in the urine, trimetrexate is extensively metabolized by the liver (Bertino et al, 1988). At least two metabolites are active and two are conjugated with glucuronic acid. The hepatic degradation may account for the low and variable oral absorption. The terminal elimination half-life is 15 to 20 hours (approximately 12 hours in AIDS patients with PCP).

DOSAGE AND PREPARATIONS. The 50-mg lyophilized preparation is reconstituted in 1.9 ml of sterile water, then diluted in 150 ml of 5% dextrose in water and infused intravenously over 30 minutes.

Intravenous: For PCP in AIDS patients, *adults,* 30 to 45 mg/M^2 daily is given for 21 days (Sattler et al, 1990). Leucovorin 20 to 40 mg/M^2 is administered either as an intravenous bolus or orally every six hours for 23 days.

Trimetrexate Glucuronate (US Bioscience). Lyophilized powder 25 mg. Information about availability of trimetrexate under the Treatment IND may be obtained by calling 800/537-9978.

Mixtures

CHLOROQUINE/PRIMAQUINE PHOSPHATES

[Aralen Phosphate with Primaquine Phosphate]

This combination of chloroquine and primaquine is suitable and safe for the prophylaxis of malaria when used for at least four weeks after the individual has left a malarious area. It has been especially useful in the long-term prophylaxis of vivax malaria in military personnel but has never achieved widespread acceptance for civilian use.

The same adverse effects and precautions apply to the combination as for either drug used alone. See the evaluations for details.

DOSAGE AND PREPARATIONS.

Oral: For prophylaxis of malaria, *adults and children over 45 kg,* one tablet weekly on the same day of each week, starting two weeks before entering the malarious area, during, and for six weeks after leaving. For younger children, a suspension of the tablets is made in chocolate syrup or fruit juice so that each 5 ml contains 40 mg of chloroquine base and 6 mg of primaquine base. The following amounts are then given once weekly on the same day of each week: *Children 5 to 7 kg,* 2.5 ml; *8 to 11 kg,* 5 ml; *12 to 15 kg,* 7.5 ml; *16 to 20 kg,* 10 ml; *21 to 24 kg,* 12.5 ml; and *25 to 45 kg,* one-half tablet. These doses should not be exceeded.

Aralen Phosphate with Primaquine Phosphate (Winthrop). Tablets containing chloroquine phosphate 500 mg (equivalent to 300 mg of base) and primaquine phosphate 79 mg (equivalent to 45 mg of base).

PYRIMETHAMINE/SULFADOXINE

[Fansidar]

ACTIONS AND USES. This combination contains pyrimethamine and sulfadoxine in a fixed ratio of 1:20, respectively. It is indicated for the treatment of malaria caused by susceptible strains of plasmodia. This regimen is effective against many strains of chloroquine-resistant *P. falciparum*, but resistance to Fansidar occurs in widespread areas of Southeast Asia, East Africa, and the Amazon Basin in Brazil. Because of increasing resistance and this mixture's toxicity, it no longer is used routinely for prophylaxis of this form of malaria. Mefloquine is now recommended for this purpose. Pyrimethamine/sulfadoxine is now recommended only for presumptive treatment of travelers in remote areas who suspect infection but do not have ready access to medical attention (ie, within 24 hours). Most strains of *P. vivax* do not respond to this combination.

This mixture acts by sequential blockade of two consecutive steps in the formation of folinic acid from para-aminobenzoic acid (PABA) by the parasite. Sulfadoxine prevents the parasite from utilizing PABA to synthesize folic acid; pyrimethamine, a dihydrofolate reductase inhibitor, inhibits the enzyme, dihydrofolate reductase, thereby preventing formation of tetrahydrofolic acid (folinic acid).

ADVERSE REACTIONS. The adverse effects of the mixture are those characteristic of the sulfonamides (see index entry Sulfonamides) and pyrimethamine (see the evaluation).

The combination should be avoided in patients who are sensitive to or cannot tolerate the sulfonamides, because erythema multiforme, Stevens-Johnson syndrome, and toxic epidermal necrolysis have been reported. The incidence of these reactions during prophylactic use by American travelers ranges from 1:5,000 to 1:8,000, and fatal reactions occur in 1:11,000 to 1:25,000 users (Miller et al, 1986). Recommendations for American travelers have been revised because of these findings. Other serious reactions include serum sickness, exfoliative dermatitis, urticaria, and hepatitis.

Because the most severe cutaneous reactions have been associated only with multiple doses of Fansidar, individuals with renal insufficiency or liver damage may be particularly susceptible. Further, accumulation of the drugs and their metabolites increases not only the potential risk for direct toxicity but also allergic reactions. Prophylactic (repeated) use of Fansidar is contraindicated in patients with severe renal insufficiency, marked liver parenchymal damage, or blood dyscrasias.

Overdosage may result in acute intoxication manifested by anorexia, nausea, vomiting, and central nervous system stimulation, including convulsions. Megaloblastic anemia, leukopenia, thrombocytopenia, glossitis, and crystalluria also may develop.

Pyrimethamine/sulfadoxine is classified in FDA Pregnancy Category C.

PHARMACOKINETICS. Both drugs are absorbed orally and achieve peak plasma concentrations at about the same time (eg, 2.5 to 6 hours for sulfadoxine, 1.5 to 8 hours for pyrimethamine). Elimination half-life is about 100 to 230 hours for sulfadoxine and 50 to 150 hours for pyrimethamine; these drugs are excreted primarily by the kidney.

DOSAGE AND PREPARATIONS. This combination is no longer recommended for routine prophylaxis of malaria or for sole treatment of documented chloroquine-resistant *P. falciparum* malaria. For the latter condition, the combination should be administered following an initial course of quinine or quinidine gluconate.

Oral: For self-treatment of an acute attack of chloroquine-resistant *P. falciparum* malaria, a single dose should be given according to the following schedule: *Adults,* three tablets; *children 9 to 14 years*, two tablets; *4 to 8 years*, one tablet; *1 to 3 years*, one-half tablet; *less than 1 year*, one-quarter tablet.

Fansidar (Roche). Tablets containing sulfadoxine 500 mg and pyrimethamine 25 mg.

TRIMETHOPRIM/SULFAMETHOXAZOLE

See the evaluation in the chapter, Sulfonamides and Trimethoprim.

Cited References

Cryptosporidiosis among children attending day-care centers: Georgia, Pennsylvania, Michigan, California, New Mexico. *MMWR* 33:599-601, 1984.

Agranulocytosis associated with use of amodiaquine for malarial prophylaxis. *MMWR* 35:165-166, 1986.

Guidelines for prophylaxis against *Pneumocystis carinii* pneumonia for persons infected with human immunodeficiency virus. *MMWR* 38(S-5):1-9, 1989.

Recommendations for the prevention of malaria among travelers. *MMWR* 39(No. RR-3):1-10, 1990 A.

Revised dosing regimen for malaria prophylaxis with mefloquine. *MMWR* 39:630, 1990 B.

Mosquito-transmitted malaria—California and Florida, 1990. *MMWR* 40:106-108, 1991 A.

Treatment of severe *Plasmodium falciparum* malaria with quinidine gluconate: Discontinuation of parenteral quinine from CDC drug service. *MMWR* 40:240, 1991 B.

Change of dosing regimen for malaria prophylaxis with mefloquine. *MMWR* 40 (No. 4):72-73, 1991 C.

Guidelines for prophylaxis against *Pneumocystis carinii* pneumonia for children infected with human immunodeficiency virus. *MMWR* 40 (No. RR-2):1-13, 1991 D.

The Leishmaniases. Geneva, World Health Organization, Technical Report Series 701, 1984.

Trimetrexate for *Pneumocystis carinii* pneumonia. *Med Lett Drugs Ther* 31:5-6, 1989.

Allegra CJ, et al: Trimetrexate for the treatment of *Pneumocystis carinii* pneumonia in patients with the acquired immunodeficiency syndrome. *N Engl J Med* 317:978-985, 1987.

Angus KW: Cryptosporidiosis in man, domestic animals and birds: Review. *J R Soc Med* 76:62-70, 1983.

Aram H, Leibovici V: Ultrasound-induced hyperthermia in the treatment of cutaneous leishmaniasis. *Cutis* 40:350-353, 1987.

Bacchi CJ, et al: Effects of ornithine decarboxylase inhibitors DL-alpha-difluoromethylornithine and alphamonofluoromethyldehydroornithine methyl ester alone and in combination with suramin against *Trypanosoma brucei brucei* central nervous system models. *Am J Trop Med Hyg* 36:46-52, 1987.

Ballou WR, et al: Safety and efficacy of high-dose sodium stibogluconate therapy of American cutaneous leishmaniasis. *Lancet* 2:13-16, 1987.

Basile JA, et al: Amebic liver abscess: The surgeon's role in management. *Am J Surg* 146:67-71, 1983.

Bateman DN, Dyson EH: Quinine toxicity. *Adverse Drug React Acute Poisoning Rev* 4:215-233, 1986.

Berman JD: Chemotherapy for leishmaniasis: Biochemical mechanisms, clinical efficacy, and future strategies. *Rev Infect Dis* 10:560-586, 1988.

Berman JD, et al: Antileishmanial activity of liposome-encapsulated amphotericin B in hamsters and monkeys. *Antimicrob Agents Chemother* 30:847-851, 1986.

Bertino JR, et al: Clinical pharmacology and metabolism of trimetrexate. *Semin Oncol* 15 (suppl 2):8-9, 1988.

Bitonti AJ, et al: Reversal of chloroquine resistance in malaria parasite *Plasmodium falciparum* by desipramine. *Science* 242:1301-1303, 1988.

Black JR, et al: Clindamycin and primaquine as primary treatment for mild and moderately severe *Pneumocystis carinii* pneumonia in patients with AIDS. *Eur J Clin Microbiol Infect Dis* 10:204-207, 1991.

Bozzette SA: The use of corticosteroids in *Pneumocystis carinii* pneumonia. *J Infect Dis* 162:1365-1369, 1990.

Bozzette SA, et al: A controlled trial of early adjunctive treatment with corticosteroids for *Pneumocystis carinii* pneumonia in the acquired immunodeficiency syndrome. *N Engl J Med* 323:1451-1457, 1990.

Buckley RM, et al: Opportunistic infections in the acquired immunodeficiency syndrome. *Semin Oncol* 17:335-349, 1990.

Carter AO, Frank JW: Congenital toxoplasmosis: Epidemiologic features and control. *Can Med Assoc J* 135:618-623, 1986.

Centers for Disease Control: *Health Information for International Travel 1990*. Washington, DC, Superintendent of Documents, US Government Printing Office, 1990.

Cerf BJ, et al: Malnutrition as a risk factor for severe visceral leishmaniasis. *J Infect Dis* 156:1030-1033, 1987.

Certa U: Malaria vaccine. *Experientia* 47:157-163, 1991.

Chang HR, Pechère JCF: Activity of spiramycin against *Toxoplasma gondii* in vitro, in experimental infections and in human infection. *J Antimicrob Chemother* 22 (suppl B):87-92, 1988.

Chester AC, et al: Giardiasis as a chronic disease. *Dig Dis Sci* 30:215-218, 1985.

Child Day Care Infectious Disease Study Group: Considerations of infectious diseases in day care centers. *Pediatr Infect Dis* 4:124-136, 1985.

Clement M, et al: Corticosteroids as adjunctive therapy in severe *Pneumocystis carinii* pneumonia: A prospective placebo-controlled trial. *Am Rev Respir Dis* 139 (suppl A):abstract 250, 1989.

Connolly GM, et al: Cryptosporidial diarrhea in AIDS and its treatment. *Gut* 29:593-597, 1988.

Conte JE Jr, Golden JA: Concentrations of aerosolized pentamidine in bronchoalveolar lavage, systemic absorption, and excretion. *Antimicrob Agents Chemother* 32:1490-1493, 1988.

Conte JE Jr, et al: Pentamidine pharmacokinetics in patients with AIDS with impaired renal function. *J Infect Dis* 156:885-890, 1987.

Conte JE Jr, et al: Intravenous or inhaled pentamidine for treating *Pneumocystis carinii* pneumonia in AIDS: A randomized trial. *Ann Intern Med* 113:203-209, 1990.

Cook GC: Opportunistic parasitic infections associated with the acquired immune deficiency syndrome (AIDS): Parasitology, clinical presentation, diagnosis and management. *Q J Med* 65:967-983, 1987.

Cook DJ, et al: Somatostatin treatment for cryptosporidial diarrhea in a patient with the acquired immunodeficiency syndrome (AIDS). *Ann Intern Med* 108:708-709, 1988.

Coune A: Liposomes as drug delivery system in the treatment of infectious diseases: Potential applications and clinical experience. *Infection* 16:141-147, 1988.

Craft JC, et al: Malabsorption of oral antibiotics in humans and rats with giardiasis. *Pediatr Infect Dis* 6:832-836, 1987.

Croft SL: Recent developments in the chemotherapy of leishmaniasis. *Trends Pharmacol Sci* 9:376-381, 1988.

Daffos F, et al: Prenatal management of 746 pregnancies at risk for congenital toxoplasmosis. *N Engl J Med* 318:271-275, 1988.

Dannemann BR, et al: Treatment of acute toxoplasmosis with intravenous clindamycin. *Eur J Clin Microbiol Infect Dis* 10:193-195, 1991.

Davey RT Jr, Masur H: Recent advances in the diagnosis, treatment, and prevention of *Pneumocystis carinii* pneumonia. *Antimicrob Agents Chemother* 34:499-504, 1990.

Davidson RN, et al: Liposomal amphotericin B in drug-resistant visceral leishmaniasis. *Lancet* 337:1061-1062, 1991.

DeHovitz JA, et al: Clinical manifestations and therapy of *Isospora belli* infection in patients with the acquired immunodeficiency syndrome. *N Engl J Med* 315:87-90, 1986.

Dellamonica P, et al: Allopurinol for treatment of visceral leishmaniasis in patients with AIDS. *J Infect Dis* 160:904-905, 1989.

Donelson JE: Evading host defenses: The African trypanosome. *Infect Med* 4:323-329, 1987.

Doua F, et al: Treatment of human late-stage gambiense trypanosomiasis with alpha-difluoromethylornithine (eflornithine): Efficacy and tolerance in 14 cases in Cote d'Ivoire. *Am J Trop Med Hyg* 37:525-533, 1987.

Edelstein H, McCabe RE: Atypical presentations of *Pneumocystis carinii* pneumonia in patients receiving inhaled pentamidine prophylaxis. *Chest* 98:1366-1369, 1990.

Edman JC, et al: Ribosomal RNA sequence show *Pneumocystis carinii* to be a member of the fungi, letter. *Nature* 334:519-522, 1988.

Eisenhauer EA, et al: Trimetrexate: Predictors of severe or life-threatening toxic effects. *J Natl Cancer Inst* 80:1318-1322, 1988.

Ette EI, et al: Effect of ranitidine on chloroquine disposition. *Drug Intell Clin Pharm* 21:732-734, 1987.

Fischl MA, et al: Safety and efficacy of sulfamethoxazole and trimethoprim chemoprophylaxis for *Pneumocystis carinii* pneumonia in AIDS. *JAMA* 259:1185-1189, 1988.

Fischl MA, et al: A randomized controlled trial of a reduced daily dose of zidovudine in patients with the acquired immunodeficiency syndrome. *N Engl J Med* 323:1009-1014, 1990.

Fogh S, et al: Malaria chemoprophylaxis in travellers to East Africa: A comparative prospective study of chloroquine plus proguanil with chloroquine plus sulfadoxine-pyrimethamine. *Br Med J* 296:820-822, 1988.

Franke ED, et al: Efficacy and toxicity of sodium stibogluconate for mucosal leishmaniasis. *Ann Intern Med* 113:934-940, 1990.

Furner BB: Cutaneous leishmaniasis in Texas: Report of a case and review of the literature. *J Am Acad Dermatol* 23:368-371, 1990.

Gagnon S, et al: Corticosteroids as adjunctive therapy for severe *Pneumocystis carinii* pneumonia in the acquired immunodeficiency syndrome: A double-blind, placebo-controlled trial. *N Engl J Med* 323:1444-1450, 1990.

Glatt AE, Chirgwin K: *Pneumocystis carinii* pneumonia in human immunodeficiency virus-infected patients. *Arch Intern Med* 150:271-279, 1990.

Glatt AE, et al: Treatment of infections associated with human immunodeficiency virus. *N Engl J Med* 318:1439-1448, 1988.

Good MF: Towards the development of the ideal malaria vaccine: A decade of progress in a difficult field. *Med J Aust* 154:284-289, 1991.

Gordin FM, et al: Adverse reactions to trimethoprim-sulfamethoxazole in patients with the acquired immunodeficiency syndrome. *Ann Intern Med* 100:495-499, 1984.

Gozal D, et al: Prolonged malaria prophylaxis with chloroquine and proguanil (chloroguanide) in a nonimmune resident population of an endemic area with a high prevalence of chloroquine resistance. *Antimicrob Agents Chemother* 35:373-376, 1991 A.

Gozal D, et al: Long-term chloroquine-proguanil malaria prophylaxis in a nonimmune pediatric population. *J Pediatr* 118:142-145, 1991 B.

Greenberg SJ, et al: *Isospora belli* enteric infection in patients with human T-cell leukemia virus type I-associated adult T-cell leukemia. *Am J Med* 85:435-438, 1988.

Guerrant RL: The global problem of amebiasis: Current status, research needs, and opportunities for progress. *Rev Infect Dis* 8:218-226, 1986.

Harinasuta T, et al: Trials of mefloquine in vivax and of mefloquine plus 'Fansidar' in falciparum malaria. *Lancet* 1:885-888, 1985.

Haverkos HW (coordinator): Assessment of therapy for toxoplasma encephalitis: The TE study group. *Am J Med* 82:907-914, 1987.

Hayes EB, et al: Large community outbreak of cryptosporidiosis due to contamination of a filtered public water supply. *N Engl J Med* 320:1372-1376, 1989.

Healy GR: Immunologic tools in the diagnosis of amebiasis: Epidemiology in the United States. *Rev Infect Dis* 8:239-246, 1986.

Herwaldt BL, et al: Antimalarial agents: Specific chemoprophylaxis regimens. *Antimicrob Agents Chemother* 32:953-956, 1988.

Hirschel B, et al: A controlled study of inhaled pentamidine for primary prevention of *Pneumocystis carinii* pneumonia. *N Engl J Med* 324:1079-1083, 1991.

Hoffman SL, et al: High-dose dexamethasone in quinine-treated patients with cerebral malaria: A double-blind, placebo-controlled trial. *J Infect Dis* 158:325-331, 1988.

Holliman RE: Toxoplasmosis and the acquired immune deficiency syndrome. *J Infect* 16:121-128, 1988.

Holtan NR: Giardiasis: A crimp in the life-style of campers, travelers, and others. *Postgrad Med* 83:54-60, (April) 1988.

Hopewell PC: *Pneumocystis carinii* pneumonia: Diagnosis. *J Infect Dis* 157:1115-1119, 1988.

Hughes WT: *Pneumocystis carinii* pneumonitis, editorial. *N Engl J Med* 317:1021-1023, 1987.

Hughes WT: *Pneumocystis carinii* pneumonia: New approaches to diagnosis, treatment and prevention. *Pediatr Infect Dis J* 10:391-399, 1991.

Hughes WT, et al: Successful intermittent chemoprophylaxis for *Pneumocystis carinii* pneumonitis. *N Engl J Med* 316:1627-1632, 1987.

Hughes WT, et al: Efficacy of a hydroxynaphthoquinone, 566C80, in experimental *Pneumocystis carinii* pneumonitis. *Antimicrob Agents Chemother* 34:225-228, 1990.

Hunter CA, et al: Vesicular systems (niosomes and liposomes) for delivery of sodium stibogluconate in experimental murine visceral leishmaniasis. *J Pharm Pharmacol* 40:161-165, 1988.

Huskinson-Mark J, et al: Evaluation of the effect of drugs on the cyst form of *Toxoplasma gondii*. *J Infect Dis* 164:170-177, 1991.

Jacobs JL, et al: A cluster of *Pneumocystis carinii* pneumonia in adults without predisposing illnesses. *N Engl J Med* 324:246-250, 1991.

Jokipii L, Jokipii AMM: Treatment of giardiasis: Comparative evaluation of ornidazole and tinidazole as single oral dose. *Gastroenterology* 83:399-404, 1982.

Jules-Elysee KM, et al: Aerosolized pentamidine: Effect on diagnosis and presentation of *Pneumocystis carinii* pneumonia. *Ann Intern Med* 112:750-757, 1990.

Katlama C: Evaluation of the efficacy and safety of clindamycin plus pyrimethamine for induction and maintenance therapy of toxoplasmic encephalitis in AIDS. *Eur J Clin Microbiol Infect Dis* 10:189-191, 1991.

Katz MD, et al: Treatment of severe cryptosporidium-related diarrhea with octreotide in a patient with AIDS. *Drug Intell Clin Pharm* 22:134-136, 1988.

Kellum RE: Treatment of cutaneous leishmaniasis with an intralesional antimonial drug (Pentostam). *J Am Acad Dermatol* 15:620-622, 1986.

Keystone JS: Prevention of malaria. *Drugs* 39:337-354, 1990.

Keystone JS, et al: Counselling travellers about malaria chemoprophylaxis. *Can Med Assoc J* 131:715-716, 1984.

Klayman DL: Qinghaosu (artemisinin): An antimalarial drug from China. *Science* 228:1049-1055, 1985.

Kovacs JA, Masur H: Are corticosteroids beneficial as adjunctive therapy for pneumocystis pneumonia in AIDS? Editorial. *Ann Intern Med* 113:1-3, 1990.

Kovacs JA, et al: Potent effect of trimetrexate, a lipid-soluble antifolate, on *Toxoplasma gondii*. *J Infect Dis* 155:1027-1040, 1987.

Kremsner PG: Clindamycin in malaria treatment. *J Antimicrob Chemother* 25:9-14, 1990.

Krogstad DJ, Herwaldt BL: Chemoprophylaxis and treatment of malaria. *N Engl J Med* 319:1538-1540, 1988.

Krogstad DJ, et al: Antimalarial agents: Specific treatment regimens. *Antimicrob Agents Chemother* 32:957-961, 1988 A.

Krogstad DJ, et al: Antimalarial agents: Mechanism of chloroquine resistance. *Antimicrob Agents Chemother* 32:799-801, 1988 B.

Krotoski WA: Discovery of the hypnozoite and a new theory of malarial relapse. *Trans R Soc Trop Med Hyg* 79:1-11, 1985.

Leoung GS, et al: Dapsone-trimethoprim for *Pneumocystis carinii* pneumonia in the acquired immunodeficiency syndrome. *Ann Intern Med* 105:45-48, 1986.

Leoung GS, et al: Aerosolized pentamidine for prophylaxis against *Pneumocystis carinii* pneumonia: The San Francisco Community Prophylaxis Trial. *N Engl J Med* 323:769-775, 1990.

Leport C, et al: Treatment of central nervous system toxoplasmosis with pyrimethamine/sulfadiazine combination in 35 patients with the acquired immunodeficiency syndrome: Efficacy of long-term continuous therapy. *Am J Med* 84:94-100, 1988.

Lobel HO, et al: Use of prophylaxis for malaria by American travelers to Africa and Haiti. *JAMA* 257:2626-2627, 1987 A.

Lobel HO, et al: Efficacy of malaria prophylaxis in American and Swiss travelers to Kenya. *J Infect Dis* 155:1205-1209, 1987 B.

Looareesuwan S, et al: Quinine and severe falciparum malaria in late pregnancy. *Lancet* 2:4-7, 1985.

Looareesuwan S, et al: Studies of mefloquine bioavailability and kinetics using a stable isotope technique: A comparison of Thai patients with falciparum malaria and healthy Caucasian volunteers. *Br J Clin Pharmacol* 24:37-42, 1987.

Luft BJ, Remington JS: Toxoplasmic encephalitis. *J Infect Dis* 157:1-6, 1988.

Luo X-D, Shen C-C: The chemistry, pharmacology, and clinical applications of qinghaosu (artemisinin) and its derivatives. *Med Res Rev* 7:29-52, 1987.

Marr JJ, Docampo R: Chemotherapy for Chagas' disease: A perspective of current therapy and considerations for future research. *Rev Infect Dis* 8:884-903, 1986.

McCabe RE, et al: In vitro and in vivo effects of itraconazole against *Trypanosoma cruzi*. *Am J Trop Med Hyg* 35:280-284, 1986.

McCann PP, et al (eds): *Inhibition of Polyamine Metabolism: Biological Significance and Basis for New Therapies*. San Diego, Academic Press, 1987.

McCue JD: Evaluation and management of vaginitis: An update for primary care practitioners. *Arch Intern Med* 149:565-568, 1989.

Medina I, et al: Oral therapy for *Pneumocystis carinii* pneumonia in the acquired immunodeficiency syndrome. *N Engl J Med* 323:776-782, 1990.

Mihaly GW, et al: Pharmacokinetics of primaquine in man: I. Studies of the absolute bioavailability and effects of dose size. *Br J Clin Pharmacol* 19:745-750, 1985.

Miller KD, et al: Severe cutaneous reactions among American travelers using pyrimethamine-sulfadoxine (Fansidar) for malaria prophylaxis. *Am J Trop Med Hyg* 35:451-458, 1986.

Miller KD, et al: Treatment of severe malaria in the United States with a continuous infusion of quinidine gluconate and exchange transfusion. *N Engl J Med* 321:65-70, 1989.

Millet V, et al: *Dientamoeba fragilis*, a protozoan parasite in adult members of a semicommunal group. *Dig Dis Sci* 28:335-339, 1983.

Mills J, et al: Dapsone treatment of *Pneumocystis carinii* pneumonia in the acquired immunodeficiency syndrome. *Antimicrob Agents Chemother* 32:1057-1060, 1988.

Mishra M, et al: Amphotericin B for second-line treatment of Indian kala-azar. *Lancet* 337:926, 1991.

Monk JP, Benfield P: Inhaled pentamidine: An overview of its pharmacological properties and a review of its therapeutic use in *Pneumocystis carinii* pneumonia. *Drugs* 39:741-756, 1990.

Montaner JSG, et al: Corticosteroids prevent early deterioration in patients with moderately severe *Pneumocystis carinii* pneumonia and the acquired immunodeficiency syndrome (AIDS). *Ann Intern Med* 113:14-20, 1990.

Montaner JSG, et al: Aerosol pentamidine for secondary prophylaxis of AIDS-related *Pneumocystis carinii* pneumonia: A randomized, placebo-controlled study. *Ann Intern Med* 114:948-953, 1991.

Murphy TV, Nelson JD: Five versus ten days' therapy with furazolidone for giardiasis. *Am J Dis Child* 137:267-270, 1983.

Murphy RL, et al: Aerosol pentamidine prophylaxis following *Pneumocystis carinii* pneumonia in AIDS patients: Results of a blinded dose-comparison study using an ultrasonic nebulizer. *Am J Med* 90:418-426, 1991.

Nash TE, et al: Experimental human infections with *Giardia lamblia. J Infect Dis* 156:974-984, 1987.

The National Institutes of Health—University of California Expert Panel for Corticosteroids as Adjunctive Therapy for Pneumocystis Pneumonia: Consensus statement on the use of corticosteroids as adjunctive therapy for pneumocystis pneumonia in the acquired immunodeficiency syndrome. *N Engl J Med* 323:1500-1504, 1990.

Navia BA, et al: Cerebral toxoplasmosis complicating the acquired immune deficiency syndrome: Clinical and neuropathological findings in 27 patients. *Ann Neurol* 19:224-238, 1986.

Nosten F, et al: Mefloquine-resistant falciparum malaria on the Thai-Burmese border. *Lancet* 337:1140-1143, 1991.

Ognibene FP, et al: Nonspecific interstitial pneumonitis without evidence of *Pneumocystis carinii* in asymptomatic patients infected with human immunodeficiency virus (HIV). *Ann Intern Med* 109:874-879, 1988.

Oxner RBG, et al: Dientamoeba fragilis: A bowel pathogen? *N Z Med J* 100:64-65, 1987.

Pang LW, et al: Doxycycline prophylaxis for falciparum malaria. *Lancet* 1:1161-1164, 1987.

Panosian CB: Parasitic diarrhea. *Infect Dis Clin North Am* 2:685-703, 1988.

Pearson RD, De Queiroz Sousa A: Leishmania species: Visceral (kala-azar), cutaneous, and mucosal leishmaniasis, in Mandell GL, et al (eds): *Principles and Practice of Infectious Diseases*, ed 3. New York, Churchill Livingstone, 1990, 2066-2077.

Pearson RD, Hewlett EL: Use of pyrimethamine-sulfadoxine (Fansidar) in prophylaxis against chloroquine-resistant *Plasmodium falciparum* and *Pneumocystis carinii. Ann Intern Med* 106:714-718, 1987.

Pepin J, et al: Difluoromethylornithine for arseno-resistant *Trypanosoma brucei gambiense* sleeping sickness. *Lancet* 2:1431-1433, 1987.

Peters W, Hall AP: The treatment of severe falciparum malaria. *Br Med J* 291:1146-1147, 1985.

Peters SG, Prakash JBS: Pneumocystis carinii pneumonia: Review of 53 cases. *Am J Med* 82:73-78, 1987.

Petru AM, et al: African sleeping sickness in the United States: Successful treatment with eflornithine. *Am J Dis Child* 142:224-228, 1988.

Phair J, et al: The risk of *Pneumocystis carinii* pneumonia among men infected with human immunodeficiency virus type I. *N Engl J Med* 322:161-165, 1990.

Phillips RE, et al: Intravenous quinidine for the treatment of severe falciparum malaria: Clinical and pharmacokinetic studies. *N Engl J Med* 312:1273-1278, 1985.

Phillips RE, et al: Quinine pharmacokinetics and toxicity in pregnant and lactating women with falciparum malaria. *Br J Clin Pharmacol* 21:677-683, 1986 A.

Phillips RE, et al: Hypoglycaemia and antimalarial drugs: Quinidine and release of insulin. *Br Med J* 292:1319-1321, 1986 B.

Phillips RE, et al: Divided dose intramuscular regimen and single dose subcutaneous regimen for chloroquine: Plasma concentrations and toxicity in patients with malaria. *Br Med J* 293:13-15, 1986 C.

Phillips-Howard PA, et al: Malaria prophylaxis: Survey of the response of British travellers to prophylactic advice. *Br Med J* 293:932-934, 1986.

Philpott J, Keystone JS: Severe falciparum malaria. *Can Med Assoc J* 137:135-136, 1987.

Ravdin JI: Pathogenesis of disease caused by *Entamoeba histolytica*: Studies of adherence, secreted toxins, and contact-dependent cytolysis. *Rev Infect Dis* 8:247-260, 1986.

Ravdin JI: Diagnosis and management of *Entamoeba histolytica* infection. *Infect Med* 4:155-165, 1987.

Reacher M, et al: Drug therapy for *Plasmodium falciparum* malaria resistant to pyrimethamine-sulfadoxine (Fansidar): A study of alternate regimens in Eastern Thailand, 1980. *Lancet* 2:1066-1069, 1981.

Riou B, et al: Treatment of severe chloroquine poisoning. *N Engl J Med* 318:1-6, 1988.

Rogers P, et al: Bioavailability of oral trimetrexate in patients with acquired immunodeficiency syndrome. *Antimicrob Agents Chemother* 32:324-326, 1988.

Rossignol J-F, et al: Nitroimidazoles in the treatment of trichomoniasis, giardiasis, and amebiasis. *Int J Clin Pharmacol Ther Toxicol* 22:63-72, 1984.

Ruf B, Pohle HD: Role of clindamycin in the treatment of acute toxoplasmosis of the central nervous system. *Eur J Clin Microbiol Infect Dis* 10:183-186, 1991.

Ruf B, et al: Efficacy of clindamycin/primaquine versus trimethoprim/sulfamethoxazole in primary treatment of *Pneumocystis carinii* pneumonia. *Eur J Clin Microbiol Infect Dis* 10:207-210, 1991.

Ruskin J, LaRiviere M: Low-dose co-trimoxazole for prevention of *Pneumocystis carinii* pneumonia in human immunodeficiency virus disease. *Lancet* 337:468-471, 1991.

Saenz RE, et al: Treatment of American cutaneous leishmaniasis with orally administered allopurinol riboside. *J Infect Dis* 160:153-157, 1989.

Saenz RE, et al: Efficacy of ketoconazole against *Leishmania braziliensis panamensis* cutaneous leishmaniasis. *Am J Med* 89:147-155, 1990.

Sáez-llorens X, et al: Spiramycin vs. placebo for treatment of acute diarrhea caused by *Cryptosporidium. Pediatr Infect Dis J* 8:136-140, 1989.

Safran M, Braverman LE: Effect of chronic douching with polyvinylpyrrolidone-iodine on iodine absorption and thyroid function. *Obstet Gynecol* 60:35-40, 1982.

Sahai J, Berry AJ: Eflornithine for the treatment of *Pneumocystis carinii* pneumonia in patients with the acquired immunodeficiency syndrome: A preliminary review. *Pharmacotherapy* 9:29-33, 1989.

Salata RA, Ravdin JI: Review of human immune mechanisms directed against *Entamoeba histolytica. Rev Infect Dis* 8:261-272, 1986.

Sands M, et al: Pentamidine: A review. *Rev Infect Dis* 7:625-634, 1985.

Sattler FR, et al: Trimethoprim-sulfamethoxazole compared with pentamidine for treatment of *pneumocystis carinii* pneumonia in the acquired immunodeficiency syndrome: A prospective, noncrossover study. *Ann Intern Med* 109:280-287, 1988.

Sattler FR, et al: Trimetrexate-leucovorin dosage evaluation study for treatment of *Pneumocystis carinii* pneumonia. *J Infect Dis* 161:91-96, 1990.

Saultz JW, Toffler WL: Trichomonas infections in men. *Am Fam Physician* 39:177-180, (Feb) 1989.

Schechter PJ, et al: Clinical aspects of inhibition of ornithine decarboxylase with emphasis on therapeutic trials of eflornithine (DFMO) in cancer and protozoan diseases, in McCann PP, et al (eds): *Inhibition of Polyamine Metabolism: Biological Significance and Basis for New Therapies.* San Diego, Academic Press, 1987, 345-364.

Schlesinger PH, et al: Antimalarial agents: Mechanisms of action. *Antimicrob Agents Chemother* 32:793-798, 1988.

Schwartz IK, et al: Chloroquine-resistant *Plasmodium vivax* from Indonesia. *N Engl J Med* 324:927, 1991.

Sepkowitz KA, et al: Pneumothorax in AIDS. *Ann Intern Med* 114:455-459, 1991.

Sever JL, et al: Toxoplasmosis: Maternal and pediatric findings in 23,000 pregnancies. *Pediatrics* 82:181-192, 1988.

Sharquie KE, et al: Intralesional therapy of cutaneous leishmaniasis with sodium stibogluconate antimony. *Br J Dermatol* 119:53-57, 1988.

Siddiqui WA: Where are we in the quest for vaccines for malaria? *Drugs* 41:1-10, 1991.

Sjoerdsma A: New class of chemotherapeutic agents: Inhibitors of polyamine biosynthesis, in Rand MJ, Raper C (eds): *Excerpta Medica International Congress Series 750.* Amsterdam, Elsevier Science Publishers, 1987, 643-652.

Soave R, Armstrong D: *Cryptosporidium* and cryptosporidiosis. *Rev Infect Dis* 8:1012-1023, 1986.

Soo Hoo GW, et al: Inhaled or intravenous pentamidine therapy for *Pneumocystis carinii* pneumonia in AIDS: A randomized trial. *Ann Intern Med* 113:195-202, 1990.

Speelman P: Single-dose tinidazole for treatment of giardiasis. *Antimicrob Agents Chemother* 27:227-229, 1985.

Taelman H, et al: Difluoromethylornithine, an effective new treatment of Gambian trypanosomiasis: Results in five patients. *Am J Med* 82:607-614, 1987.

Taylor JP, et al: Cryptosporidiosis outbreak in a day-care center. *Am J Dis Child* 139:1023-1025, 1985.

Taylor GD, et al: Combined metronidazole and quinacrine hydrochloride therapy for chronic giardiasis. *Can Med Assoc J* 136:1179-1180, 1987.

Taylor TE, et al: Blood glucose levels in Malawian children before and during the administration of intravenous quinine for severe falciparum malaria. *N Engl J Med* 319:1040-1047, 1988.

Telzak EE, et al: Extrapulmonary *Pneumocystis carinii* infections. *Rev Infect Dis* 12:380-386, 1990.

Thompson JE Jr, et al: Amebic liver abscess: A therapeutic approach. *Rev Infect Dis* 7:171-179, 1985.

Toma E: Clindamycin/primaquine for treatment of *Pneumocystis carinii* pneumonia in AIDS. *Eur J Clin Microbiol Infect Dis* 10:210-213, 1991.

Toma E, et al: Clindamycin with primaquine for *Pneumocystis carinii* pneumonia. *Lancet* 1:1046-1048, 1989.

Vorherr H, et al: Vaginal absorption of povidone-iodine. *JAMA* 244:2628-2629, 1980.

Wakeel ESE, et al: Clindamycin for the treatment of falciparum malaria in Sudan. *Am J Trop Med Hyg* 34:1065-1068, 1985.

Walker O, et al: The disposition of chloroquine in healthy Nigerians after single intravenous and oral doses. *Br J Clin Pharmacol* 23:295-301, 1987.

Walsh JA: Problems in recognition and diagnosis of amebiasis: Estimation of the global magnitude of morbidity and mortality. *Rev Infect Dis* 8:228-238, 1986.

Ward SA: Mechanisms of chloroquine resistance in malarial chemotherapy. *Trends Pharmacol Sci* 9:241-246, 1988.

Warhurst DC: Antimalarial drugs: Mode of action and resistance. *J Antimicrob Chemother* 18 (suppl B):51-59, 1986.

Warhurst DC: Antimalarial drugs: An update. *Drugs* 33:50-65, 1987.

Waskin H, et al: Risk factors for hypoglycemia associated with pentamidine therapy for *Pneumocystis* pneumonia. *JAMA* 260:345-347, 1988.

Watkins WM, et al: Efficacy of multiple-dose halofantrine in treatment of chloroquine-resistant falciparum malaria in children in Kenya. *Lancet* 2:247-250, 1988.

Weiss LM, et al: Pyrimethamine concentrations in serum and cerebrospinal fluid during treatment of acute toxoplasma encephalitis in patients with AIDS. *J Infect Dis* 157:580-583, 1988.

Weniger BG, et al: High-level chloroquine resistance of *Plasmodium falciparum* malaria acquired in Kenya. *N Engl J Med* 307:1560-1562, 1982.

Wernsdorfer WH: Drug resistant malaria. *Endeavour* 8:166-171, 1984.

White NJ: Clinical pharmacokinetics of antimalarial drugs. *Clin Pharmacokinet* 10:187-215, 1985.

White NJ, et al: Severe hypoglycemia and hyperinsulinemia in falciparum malaria. *N Engl J Med* 309:61-66, 1983.

White NJ, et al: Chloroquine treatment of severe malaria in children: Pharmacokinetics, toxicity, and new dosage recommendations. *N Engl J Med* 319:1493-1500, 1988 A.

White NJ, et al: Single dose phenobarbitone prevents convulsions in cerebral malaria. *Lancet* 2:64-66, 1988 B.

Williams A, Lewis DJM: Malaria prophylaxis: Postal questionnaire survey of general practitioners in south east Wales. *Br Med J* 295:1449-1452, 1987.

Wirima J, et al: Clinical trials with halofantrine hydrochloride in Malawi. *Lancet* 2:250-252, 1988.

Wispelwey B, Pearson RD: Pentamidine: A review. *Infect Control Hosp Epidemiol* 12:375-382, 1991.

Wittenberg DF, et al: Spiramycin is not effective in treating cryptosporidium diarrhea in infants: Results of a double-blind randomized trial. *J Infect Dis* 159:131-132, 1989.

Wolfson JS, et al: Cryptosporidiosis in immunocompetent patients. *N Engl J Med* 312:1278-1282, 1985.

Wong RJ, Hardy WD: Focus on aerosolized pentamidine: An agent for prophylaxis of *Pneumocystis carinii* pneumonia. *Hosp Formul* 25:1061-1075, 1990.

Wormser GP, et al: Low-dose intermittent trimethoprim-sulfamethoxazole for prevention of *Pneumocystis carinii* pneumonia in patients with human immunodeficiency virus infection. *Arch Intern Med* 151:688-692, 1991.

Zaman MK, et al: Rapid noninvasive diagnosis of *Pneumocystis carinii* from induced liquefied sputum. *Ann Intern Med* 109:7-10, 1988.

Zangerle R, et al: High risk of developing toxoplasmic encephalitis in AIDS patients seropositive to *Toxoplasma gondii. Med Microbiol Immunol* 180:59-66, 1991.

Zar FA: Formulary aspects of therapy and prevention of *Pneumocystis carinii* pneumonia. *Hosp Formul* 26:36-46, 1991.

New Evaluation

ATOVAQUONE
[Mepron]

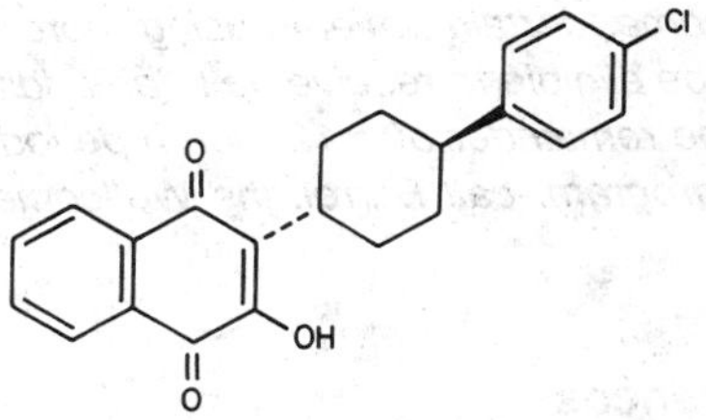

ACTIONS AND USES. This hydroxy 1,4-naphthoquinone, which was originally identified in a screening test for antimalarial activity, is classified as an antiprotozoal drug that appears to interfere with the mitochondrial electron transport chain by acting as an analogue of ubiquinone (Araujo et al, 1992). Atovaquone blocks dihydro-orotate dehydrogenase, a key enzyme of the pyrimidine biosynthesis pathway, to inhibit pyrimidine production. Because it acts by a mechanism other than folate antagonism, atovaquone represents a new class of drugs for the treatment of *Pneumocystis carinii* pneumonia (PCP).

Atovaquone is indicated for patients with mild to moderate PCP, which is defined by an alveolar-arterial oxygen diffusion gradient (A-a) $DO_2 \leq 45$ mm Hg and/or a $PO_2 \geq 60$ mm Hg (on room air) and/or clinical signs and symptoms consistent with mild to moderate PCP. Because a higher mortality rate was associated with atovaquone than with trimethoprim/sulfamethoxazole in the principal controlled trial, atovaquone is indicated for use only in patients who cannot tolerate trimethoprim/sulfamethoxazole therapy. Similarly, atovaquone is an alternative to parenteral pentamidine, which also is reserved for patients with mild to moderate PCP who cannot tolerate trimethoprim/sulfamethoxazole. The published early clinical trials using atovaquone have been reviewed and the drug compared with other alternatives (Hughes, 1992).

Atovaquone was previously available under a Treatment IND protocol for mild to moderate PCP and under an open-label protocol for severe PCP. The controlled clinical trial discussed below was the principal source of data for full approval of the drug by the FDA.

In a randomized, double-blind, multicenter clinical study of 322 patients, success rates with atovaquone and trimethoprim/sulfamethoxazole were comparable (62% and 64%, respectively); however, lack of response was more common in those treated with atovaquone (18%) than with trimethoprim/sulfamethoxazole (6%) and mortality rates were higher with atovaquone (8%) than with trimethoprim/sulfamethoxazole (0.6%). Therapeutic failures were attributed to intolerable adverse reactions in 20% of patients receiving trimethoprim/sulfamethoxazole but in only 7% of those treated with atovaquone. The following dosages were given orally three times daily for 21 days: atovaquone 750 mg; trimethoprim 320 mg/sulfamethoxazole 1.6 g (Hughes et al, in press).

When atovaquone was compared with intravenous infusion of pentamidine in an unblinded, randomized clinical trial in 109 patients being treated for primary PCP, success rates were 57% in those treated with atovaquone and 40% in those receiving pentamidine. Lack of response was more common in those treated with atovaquone (29%) than with pentamidine (17%); mortality rates were comparable. Therapeutic failures were attributed to intolerable adverse reactions in 36% of patients receiving pentamidine but in only 3.6% of those treated with atovaquone. The dosage schedule was atovaquone 750 mg orally three times daily for 21 days or pentamidine 3 to 4 mg/kg administered as a single intravenous infusion daily for 21 days.

Oral trimethoprim/sulfamethoxazole is the drug of choice for prophylaxis of PCP and aerosolized pentamidine is an alternative in high-risk patients. Atovaquone has not been systematically evaluated for use as a long-term suppressive agent to prevent the development of PCP. Studies to evaluate this possible use of atovaquone will be conducted when a more bioavailable formulation is available.

Limited studies suggest that atovaquone also may be effective in the treatment of ocular and cerebral toxoplasmosis in patients with AIDS (Araujo et al, 1992; Kovacs and The NIAID-Clinical Center Intramural AIDS Program, 1992; Lopez et al, 1992).

ADVERSE REACTIONS AND PRECAUTIONS. Adverse drug reaction data were obtained from clinical trial participants, all of whom had advanced AIDS. The most frequently (≥10%) reported adverse reactions in descending order of frequency were rash, nausea, diarrhea, headache, vomiting, fever, and insomnia. The rash is usually mild and often resolves with continued treatment. No life-threatening or fatal reactions were reported in clinical trials prior to drug approval. Although 2% of patients in the controlled trial developed transient mild elevations of liver enzymes and atovaquone was discontinued, trimethoprim/sulfamethoxazole was discontinued in 7% of patients for the same reason. Weekly monitoring of hematologic, renal, and hepatic function is desirable until more data are available (Hughes, 1992).

No drug interactions were documented during clinical trials. Atovaquone is more than 99% bound to plasma proteins; therefore, the potential for displacement by other highly plasma protein-bound drugs exists. However, no significant adverse interaction occurs between atovaquone and phenytoin.

Preliminary studies by the manufacturer suggest that caution should be used in patients receiving drugs that may impede the absorption of atovaquone (eg, metoclopramide, rifampin).

No adequate and well-controlled trials in pregnant women have been performed. Although teratogenic effects have not been observed in animals given atovaquone, maternal toxicity was reported at the highest doses used in pregnant rabbits. No mutagenic effects were observed during routine in vitro testing. Atovaquone is classified in FDA Pregnancy Category C. In rats, atovaquone concentrations in the milk were 30% of the concentration in the maternal plasma; no data in humans are available.

PHARMACOKINETICS. Atovaquone is highly lipophilic, and bioavailability is quite low and variable; however, bioavailability can be increased threefold when the drug is taken with meals. Fat significantly enhances atovaquone absorption. Even with meals, steady-state plasma concentrations in patients with AIDS (13.9 mcg/ml in adults taking 750 mg three times daily with food and 14 mcg/ml in children taking 40 mg/kg daily with food) are only one-third to one-half of those achieved in healthy individuals. Increasing the dose above the currently recommended total of 2.25 g daily for adults does not appreciably increase absorption. The peak concentration in plasma occurs in one to eight hours; however, a second peak occurs in 24 to 96 hours, which suggests that there is considerable enterohepatic cycling of the drug.

More than 94% of the dose can be recovered from the feces as unchanged drug. The mean half-life of atovaquone is 2.2 days in patients with AIDS and 2.9 days in healthy subjects.

DOSAGE AND PREPARATIONS.

Oral: For mild to moderate PCP, *adults*, 750 mg taken with food three times daily for 21 days. *Children,* Phase I studies suggest that 40 mg/kg/day administered with food is necessary to achieve steady-state plasma concentrations comparable to those attained with the total daily dose used in adults. Tablets may be crushed and mixed with water or cut in half to achieve the appropriate dose. Alternatively, a suspension can be prepared using a commercially available syrup.

Mepron (Burroughs Wellcome). Tablets 250 mg.

Note: In a program established by the manufacturer, Burroughs Wellcome, certain patients using more than 411 g of Mepron may be eligible to receive up to an additional 684 g at no cost for the remainder of a 12-month period. For information on this program, call Burroughs Wellcome at 800/722-9294.

Cited References

Araujo FG, et al: In vitro and in vivo activities of the hydroxynaphthoquinone 566C80 against the cyst of *Toxoplasma gondii. Antimicrob Agents Chemother* 36:326-330, 1992.

Hughes WT: A new drug (566C80) for the treatment of *Pneumocystis carinii* pneumonia. *Ann Intern Med* 116:953-954, 1992.

Hughes WT, et al: Comparison of atovaquone (566C80) with trimethoprim/sulfamethoxazole for the treatment of *Pneumocystis carinii* pneumonia in patients with the acquired immunodeficiency syndrome (AIDS). *N Engl J Med* In press.

Kovacs JA, The NIAID-Clinical Center Intramural AIDS Program: Efficacy of atovaquone in treatment of toxoplasmosis in patients with AIDS. *Lancet* 340:637-638, 1992.

Lopez JS, et al: Orally administered 566C80 for treatment of ocular toxoplasmosis in a patient with the acquired immunodeficiency syndrome, letter. *Am J Ophthalmol* 13:331-333, (March) 1992.

Anthelmintics

79

Parasitic worm infections are a major cause of disease and disability in many areas of the world. Helminthiases often occur in humans living in squalid conditions, but poor sanitation is not an absolute prerequisite to infection.

With few exceptions (eg, *Strongyloides stercoralis, Hymenolepis nana, Capillaria philippinensis*), adult helminths do not multiply directly in the human host. Individuals who harbor many helminths but are not re-exposed lose worms over time; therefore, anthelmintics are not essential to cure some parasitic infestations, especially if the intensity of infection or the burden of worms is light (eg, whipworm, hookworm). However, in countries with a relatively high standard of living where individualized therapy is available, patients should be treated for most diagnosed helminthic infections unless specific contraindications for therapy exist. Individualized treatment is often impractical in developing countries because of the prohibitive costs of medication, limited medical facilities and access to health care, and the great potential for reinfection in endemic areas. It is apparent, therefore, that control of helminthiases involves more than application of chemotherapeutic measures. Equally important adjunctive techniques may include removal of patients from the infected environment or cleansing the environment of the parasite or transmission vector. Similarly, knowledge of when to treat and what signs or symptoms precede complications is of considerable value to the physician.

Disease Classification: The helminths that commonly infect man belong to two phyla: (1) the Nemathelminthes, which includes the class, Nematoda (roundworms), and (2) the Platyhelminthes (flatworms), which encompasses the classes, Cestoda (tapeworms) and Trematoda (flukes). For disease classification and suggested drug therapy, see Table 1.

Therapy: Anthelmintic drugs act locally on worms in the gastrointestinal tract or systemically on those that have migrated into various body tissues. Most common intestinal parasites can be eliminated easily and safely with an appropriate luminal anthelmintic agent. Tissue infections (eg, muscle, liver, lung) may be more difficult to treat, are often of longer duration (subchronic to chronic), and occasionally require

TABLE 1.
CLASSIFICATION OF THE MAJOR HELMINTHS AND DRUGS USED TO TREAT HELMINTHIASIS

Disease Name (s)	Parasite	Geographical Distribution	Usual Source and Route of Infection
CESTODES (Tapeworms)			
Intestinal Infections			
Diphyllobothriasis	*Diphyllobothrium latum* Fish Tapeworm	Cosmopolitan (more common in temperate areas)	Freshwater Crustacea to fish to man
Dipylidiasis	*Dipylidium caninum* Dog Tapeworm	Cosmopolitan	Dog or cat fleas to mouth
Hymenolepiasis	*Hymenolepis nana* Dwarf Tapeworm	Cosmopolitan	Human feces to soil to food. Fecal contamination
Taeniasis	*Taenia saginata* Beef Tapeworm	Cosmopolitan (mainly Middle East, Kenya, Ethiopia, South America, Mexico, Russia)	Beef as food
Taeniasis	*Taenia solium* Pork Tapeworm	Cosmopolitan (common in Mexico, Central and South America), India, China, South Africa	Pork as food
Tissue Infections			
Cysticercosis (Neurocysticercosis)	*Cysticercus cellulosae* Cysticercoid stage of *Taenia solium*	Cosmopolitan (common in Mexico, Central and South America, India, China)	*T. solium* eggs in fecal-contaminated food or soil, carrier self-contamination, or reverse peristalsis
Echinococcosis			
Alveolar Hydatid Disease	*Echinococcus multilocularis*	Cosmopolitan (domestic cycle involving dogs and domestic herbivores; sylvatic cycle involving foxes and rodents [primarily in Northern hemisphere])	Canine fecal contamination
Cystic Hydatid Disease	*Echinococcus granulosus*	Cosmopolitan (primarily involving domestic dogs and herbivores; northern sylvatic cycle also exists)	Canine fecal contamination
NEMATODES (Roundworms)			
Intestinal Infections			
Ascariasis	*Ascaris lumbricoides* Roundworm	Cosmopolitan (more common in tropics)	Human feces to soil to food
Enterobiasis	*Enterobius vermicularis* Pinworm, Seatworm	Cosmopolitan (less common in tropics)	Anal contact Fecal or soil contamination to food
Strongyloidiasis (Cochin-China Diarrhea)	*Strongyloides stercoralis* Threadworm	Tropics and subtropics (more common in tropics)	Human feces to soil to skin
Trichuriasis	*Trichuris trichiura* Whipworm	Cosmopolitan (more common in tropics)	Human feces to soil to food
Uncinariasis (Ancylostomiasis, Miner's Anemia)	*Ancylostoma duodenale* Old World, European, or Common Hookworm	Tropics and subtropics (Europe, North Africa, Middle and Far East, South America)	Human feces to soil to skin or food
Uncinariasis (Necatoriasis)	*Necator americanus* New World or American Hookworm	Tropics and subtropics (Americas, Italy, tropical Africa, Asia)	Human feces to soil to skin

Vector or Intermediate Host	Stage(s) in Man	Site(s) of Involvement	Drug(s) of Choice	Alternative Drugs
Freshwater Crustacea to fish to man	Adults	Ileum	Niclosamide or Praziquantel	None
Dog or Cat flea	Adults	Small Intestine	Niclosamide or Praziquantel	None
None	Larvae and Adults	Small Intestine	Praziquantel	Niclosamide
Cattle	Adults	Small Intestine	Niclosamide or Praziquantel	Albendazole[1]
Swine	Adults	Small Intestine	Niclosamide or Praziquantel	Albendazole[1]
Swine	Larvae	Any tissue, especially skeletal muscle, central nervous system, and eye	Albendazole[1]	Praziquantel
Wild rodents (lemmings, mice, shrews, voles) Humans (abnormal host)	Larvae	Liver, with contiguous structural invasion and metastasis to distant sites (brain, lung, mediastinum)	Surgery plus adjunctive use of Albendazole[1] or Mebendazole	Albendazole[1] or Mebendazole for inoperable cases
Herbivores (camels, goats, horses, pigs, sheep, yaks) Humans	Larvae	Primarily liver, lung; other sites including muscle, bone, kidney, spleen, brain; noninvasive encapsulated cysts	Surgery plus adjunctive Albendazole[1] or Mebendazole	Albendazole[1] or Mebendazole for inoperable cases
None	Larvae and Adults	Small Intestine	Pyrantel pamoate or Mebendazole	Albendazole[1] Piperazine citrate
None	Larvae and Adults	Cecum, Ascending Colon, Ileum	Pyrantel pamoate or Mebendazole	Albendazole[1] Piperazine citrate
None	Larvae and Adults	Small Intestine, Lung	Thiabendazole[2]	Albendazole[1] Mebendazole Ivermectin
None	Larvae and Adults	Cecum, Upper Colon, Rectum, Appendix	Mebendazole[2]	Albendazole[1]
None	Larvae and Adults	Small Intestine	Pyrantel pamoate or Mebendazole	Albendazole[1]
None	Larvae and Adults	Small Intestine	Pyrantel pamoate or Mebendazole	Albendazole[1]

(table continued on next page)

TABLE 1 (continued)

Disease Name (s)	Parasite	Geographical Distribution	Usual Source and Route of Infection
NEMATODES (continued)			
Tissue Infections			
Cutaneous Larva Migrans (Creeping Eruption)	*Ancylostoma braziliense*	Tropics and subtropics (Asia, Africa, Americas, Pacific)	Cat and dog feces to soil to skin
Dracunculiasis (Dracontiasis, Dirofilariasis, Guinea Worm Infection)	*Dracunculus medinensis* Guinea Worm	Subsaharan Africa, India, Pakistan	Ingesting infected water fleas
Filariasis			
Brugiasis	*Brugia* (species unknown)	North American (Eastern United States)	Insect bite
Brugiasis (Lymphatic, Malayan, or Brug's Filariasis)	*Brugia malayi, B. timori*	Southeast Asia (Malaya, Borneo, India, Ceylon, tropical China)	Insect bite
Loiasis (Eyeworm Disease of Africa, Calabar Swelling Disease)	*Loa loa*	West and Central Africa (Rain Forest)	Insect bite
Lymphatic Filariasis (Bancroftian or Wuchereriasis)	*Wuchereria bancrofti*	Asia, Africa, Pacific, South America	Insect bite
Mansonellosis (Dipetalonemiasis)	*Mansonella perstans*	West and Central Africa, South America	Insect bite
Onchocerciasis (River Blindness)	*Onchocerca volvulus*	Africa, Yemen, Central and South America	Insect bite
Ozzardi Filariasis	*Mansonella ozzardi*	South America, West Indies	Insect bite
Pulmonary Dirofilariasis	*Dirofilaria immitis*	Cosmopolitan	Insect bite
Toxocariasis (Visceral Larva Migrans)	*Toxocara canis, T. cati*	Cosmopolitan (common in North America and Europe)	Cat and dog feces to soil to skin
Trichinosis (Trichinelliasis)	*Trichinella spiralis* Pork Roundworm	Cosmopolitan (more common in Northern Hemisphere than in tropics)	Meat as food (usually pork)

Vector or Intermediate Host	Stage(s) in Man	Site(s) of Involvement	Drug(s) of Choice	Alternative Drugs
Cats, Dogs	Larvae only (in epidermis)	Skin	Thiabendazole (oral and topical)	Albendazole[1] (oral)
Cyclops water flea	Larvae and Adults	Loose Connective Tissue and Skin	Anthelmintic therapy not indicated.[3] Topical antibiotics and tetanus toxoid may be useful.	
Unknown	Adults (macrofilariae)	Lymph Nodes	Drug therapy not indicated: surgery when necessary	None
Mansonoides mosquito	Larvae (microfilariae in blood) and Adults (macrofilariae)	Lymphatics, Blood	Diethylcarbamazine citrate	None
Chrysops fly	Larvae (microfilariae in blood) and Adults (macrofilariae)	Lymphatics, Blood, Subcutaneous Tissue, Skin	Diethylcarbamazine citrate	Mebendazole
Culex, Aedes, and *Anopheles* mosquitoes	Larvae (microfilariae in blood) and Adults (macrofilariae)	Lymphatics, Blood	Diethylcarbamazine citrate	Ivermectin[1]
Culicoides midge	Larvae (microfilariae in blood) and Adults (macrofilariae)	Lymphatics, Blood, Serous Cavities	Diethylcarbamazine citrate	Mebendazole
Simulium (Black fly)	Larvae (microfilariae) migrate and Adults (macrofilariae) in skin	Lymphatics, Blood, Skin, Subcutaneous Tissue, Eye	Ivermectin[1]	Diethylcarbamazine citrate followed by Suramin[1]
Culicoides and *Simulium*	Larvae (microfilariae in blood) and Adults (macrofilariae)	Lymphatics, Blood, Visceral Adipose Tissue	Ivermectin[1]	None
Mosquito	Adults only	Lung	Drug therapy not indicated; surgery when necessary	
Dogs, Cats	Larvae only	Liver, Lungs; occasionally Kidney, Brain, Eye	Mebendazole or Thiabendazole plus Corticosteroids[4] if symptoms are severe, especially if there is ocular involvement	Albendazole[1] Diethylcarbamazine citrate
Swine (mainly)	Larvae and Adults	Small Intestine	Thiabendazole plus Corticosteroids[4]	Mebendazole[5] Pyrantel pamoate (kills only adult worms) Albendazole[1]

(table continued on next page)

TABLE 1 (continued)

Disease Name(s)	Parasite	Geographical Distribution	Usual Source and Route of Infection
TREMATODES (FLUKES)			
Clonorchiasis	*Clonorchis sinensis* Chinese Liver Fluke	Far East, mainly Japan, Korea, China, Vietnam	Human and animal feces to water to snail to soil to fish as food
Fascioliasis	*Fasciola hepatica* Sheep Liver Fluke	Cosmopolitan (more common in Europe, Cuba, and Chile)	Sheep feces to water to snail to wild watercress and other pasture food plants
Fasciolopsiasis	*Fasciolopsis buski* Giant Intestinal Fluke	China, India, Indonesia, Thailand, Malaya, Taiwan	Swine feces to soil to snail to water plants (eg, water chestnuts)
Opisthorchiasis	*Opisthorchis viverrini* Liver Fluke	Far East, mainly Japan, Korea, China, Vietnam	Human and animal feces to water to snail to soil to fish as food
Paragonimiasis	*Paragonimus westermani* Lung Fluke	Far East, Central and South America	Human sputum and feces to soil to snail to freshwater crabs used as food
Schistosomiasis (African)	*Schistosoma intercalatum* African Blood Fluke	Africa	Skin penetration from contaminated water
Schistosomiasis (Chinese or Oriental)	*Schistosoma japonicum*, *S. mekongi* Oriental Blood Fluke	Japan, China, Philippines, Celebes	Skin penetration from contaminated water
Schistosomiasis (Intestinal)	*Schistosoma mansoni* Blood Fluke	Africa, West Indies, South America, Middle East	Skin penetration from contaminated water
Schistosomiasis (Urinary)	*Schistosoma haematobium* Blood Fluke	Iraq, Africa, Near East, Madagascar	Skin penetration from contaminated water

[1] *Investigational drug in the United States*

[2] *Follow-up therapy with pyrantel pamoate may be indicated if multiple infection with* Ascaris *roundworms and pinworms also present.*

[3] *Although nitroimidazoles (eg, metronidazole, niridazole) are used in this disease, their beneficial effect appears to be unrelated to any antiparasitic action; they probably minimize the high risk of secondary skin infection and inflammation that accompany the primary lesion.*

additional supportive procedures, including surgery, for cure. The efficacy of therapy may be difficult to evaluate in complex infections, such as schistosomiasis. Criteria for satisfactory progress include relief of signs and symptoms; absence of the parasite in blood, stool, or tissue; reduction of the fecal egg count; correction of biochemical or hematologic abnormalities; and resolution of lesions shown by various imaging techniques (eg, CT or MRI scans in cerebral cysticercosis; CT, ultrasonography, and roentgenography in echinococcosis).

Because of the relative specificity of some anthelmintic drugs, accurate diagnosis is necessary for optimal therapy of many infections. However, this may be less essential with broader spectrum agents, such as albendazole [Zentel] (not approved in the United States), mebendazole [Vermox], pyrantel pamoate [Antiminth], or praziquantel [Biltricide]. Parasites occasionally can be identified by gross examination of the stool, but more often an appropriate specimen (stool, blood, urine, sputum, aspirate, or biopsy) must be submitted to a parasitology laboratory for definitive diagnosis.

When the initial course of therapy with the drug of choice has not effected a cure and alternative therapy is more hazardous, retreatment with the first drug should be undertaken before another anthelmintic agent is prescribed. In mixed infections, which are very common and often unrecognized, the effect of therapy on each of the species present must be considered.

For sources of anthelmintic drugs, see Table 2. Drugs that are noted as being available from the CDC may be obtained

Vector or Intermediate Host	Stage(s) in Man	Site(s) of Involvement	Drug(s) of Choice	Alternative Drugs
Snail, Fish (other definitive hosts are cats, dogs, rats)	Larvae and Adults	Biliary Tract	Praziquantel	None
Snail (sheep and cattle are definitive hosts)	Larvae and Adults	Biliary Tract	Praziquantel	Bithionol[1]
Snail, Freshwater plants	Adults	Small Intestine	Praziquantel	Niclosamide
Snail, Fish (other definitive hosts are cats, dogs, rats)	Larvae and Adults	Biliary Tract	Praziquantel	None
Snail, Freshwater crabs	Larvae and Adults	Lung; occasionally Central Nervous and Gastrointestinal Systems	Praziquantel	Bithionol[1]
Freshwater snail	Larvae (penetrate the skin) and Adults	Veins of Small and Large Intestine, Other Tissues	Praziquantel	None
Freshwater snail	Larvae (penetrate the skin) and Adults	Veins of Small and Large Intestine, Other Tissues	Praziquantel	None
Freshwater snail	Larvae (penetrate the skin) and Adults	Veins of Small and Large Intestine, Other Tissues	Praziquantel	Oxaminiquine
Freshwater snail	Larvae (penetrate the skin) and Adults	Veins of Urinary Bladder, Other Tissues	Praziquantel	Metrifonate[1]

[4] *Thiabendazole is nematocidal in conventional doses during early larval migration; corticosteroids reduce the marked inflammation that usually occurs during the migration.*

[5] *Mebendazole, used in a larger dose and for a longer duration than for intestinal worms, kills encysted larvae (Levin, 1983).*

by contacting the Drug and Immunobiologics Center, Centers for Disease Control, 1600 Clifton Road, Bldg 1, Room 1259, Atlanta, GA 30333. During regular business hours (8 AM to 4:30 PM), the telephone number is (404) 329-3670; the emergency number is (404) 329-2888.

CESTODE INFECTIONS

Intestinal Cestode Infections

DIPHYLLOBOTHRIASIS (FISH TAPEWORM INFECTION). Diphyllobothrium infections are acquired by eating undercooked or raw fish containing a plerocercoid, which is the form infective to man. Once the adult worm develops, eggs are excreted in the feces. If deposited in water, a ciliated embryo hatches and may be eaten by a freshwater flea, which, in turn, is eaten by various freshwater fish.

Most infected individuals harbor a single tapeworm and may remain asymptomatic for years. Infections with multiple tapeworms only occasionally cause minor complaints of abdominal discomfort, malaise, or weight loss. *D. latum* utilizes vitamin B_{12} and folic acid in unusually large quantities and may cause megaloblastic anemia, but this manifestation is uncommon. Therefore, infection, particularly with the larger species, often first becomes apparent when a segment (proglottid) is passed in the stool.

TABLE 2.
ANTHELMINTIC DRUGS

Generic Name	Source: U.S.	Source: Foreign	Principal Use (s)
DRUGS OF CHOICE AND PRIMARY ALTERNATIVE DRUGS			
Albendazole[1]	Zentel [SmithKline Beecham]	United Kingdom, France (Zentel [SmithKline Beecham])	Ascariasis Cutaneous Larva Migrans Cysticercosis Echinococcosis Enterobiasis Strongyloidiasis Taeniasis Toxocariasis Trichinosis Trichuriasis Uncinariasis
Bithionol[1]	CDC (Bitin, Lorothidol)	Japan (Bitin)	Fascioliasis Paragonimiasis
Diethylcarbamazine citrate	Hetrazan[2] [Lederle]	Canada, United Kingdom (Banocide), Australia, West Germany (Hetrazan [Lederle]), France (Notezine)	Brugiasis Loiasis Mansonellosis Onchocerciasis Toxocariasis Wuchereriasis
Ivermectin[1]	CDC (Mectizan)	France (Mectizan [Merck Sharp & Dohme])	Onchocerciasis Ozzardi Filariasis Strongyloidiasis Wuchereriasis
Mebendazole	Vermox [Janssen]	Canada, United Kingdom, Australia, South Africa, West Germany (Vermox [Janssen])	Ascariasis Dipetalonemiasis Echinococcosis Enterobiasis Loiasis Strongyloidiasis Toxocariasis Trichinosis Trichuriasis Uncinariasis
Niclosamide	Niclocide [Miles]	Canada, United Kingdom, Argentina, Australia, South Africa, West Germany (Yomesan [Bayer]), France (Tredemine)	Cestodiasis
Oxamniquine	Vansil [Pfizer]	South Africa (Vansil [Pfizer]), Brazil (Mansil [Pfizer])	Schistosomiasis *(S. mansoni)*
Piperazine citrate	Vermizine [Vortech]	Switzerland (Helmizin, Wurmsirup [Siegfried]), France (Piperol Forte), Japan (Pipenin)	Ascariasis Enterobiasis

[1] *Investigational drug in the U.S.*

[2] *Hetrazan is available without charge from the manufacturer. Contact Professional Medical Services, Lederle Laboratories, Middletown Road, Pearl River, NY 10965 (914) 735-5000.*

(table continued on next page)

TABLE 2 (continued)

Generic Name	Source: U.S.	Source: Foreign	Principal Use(s)
DRUGS OF CHOICE AND PRIMARY ALTERNATIVE DRUGS (continued)			
Praziquantel	Biltricide [Miles]	West Germany (Biltricide [Bayer])	Clonorchiasis Cysticercosis Diphyllobothriasis Dipylidiasis Fascioliasis Fasciolopsiasis Hymenolepiasis Opisthorchiasis Paragonimiasis Schistosomiasis (all types) Taeniasis
Pyrantel pamoate	Antiminth [Pfizer]	Canada, South Africa, Argentina, France (Combantrin [Pfizer]), West Germany (Helmex [Pfizer])	Ascariasis Enterobiasis Trichinosis Uncinariasis
Suramin[1]	CDC (Fourneau 309, Bayer 205, Belganyl, Naphuride, Naganol)	West Germany (Germanin [Bayer]), United Kingdom (Antrypol [ICI]), France (Moranyl [Specia])	Onchocerciasis
Thiabendazole	Mintezol [Merck Sharp & Dohme]	Canada, United Kingdom, Australia, South Africa (Mintezol [Merck Sharp & Dohme]), Argentina (Foldan)	Cutaneous Larva Migrans Strongyloidiasis Toxocariasis Trichinosis
SECONDARY ALTERNATIVE DRUGS[3]			
Antimony potassium tartrate	—	United Kingdom	Schistosomiasis *(S. haematobium, S. mansoni, S. japonicum)*
Bephenium hydroxynaphthoate	—	United Kingdom, South Africa, West Germany (Alcopar [Burroughs Wellcome])	Ascariasis Uncinariasis
Hycanthone mesylate	—	United Kingdom, South Africa (Etrenol [Winthrop])	Schistosomiasis *(S. haematobium, S. mansoni)*
Levamisole	Ergamisol [Janssen]	United Kingdom (Ketrax [ICI]), Argentina (Meglum, Stimamizol), South Africa (Ergamisol)	Ascariasis
Metrifonate	—	West Germany (Bilarcil [Bayer])	Schistosomiasis *(S. haematobium)*
Niridazole	—	United Kingdom, South Africa (Ambilhar [CIBA])	Dracontiasis Schistosomiasis *(S. japonicum)*
Paromomycin	Humatin [Parke-Davis]	Argentina (Gabbromicina [Montedison]), West Germany (Gabbromycin [Farmitalia])	Cestodiasis
Pyrvinium pamoate	—	Canada, Australia (Vanquin [Parke-Davis]), Argentina (Tru [Elea])	Enterobiasis

(table continued on next page)

TABLE 2 (continued)

Generic Name	Source: U.S.	Source: Foreign	Principal Use(s)
SECONDARY ALTERNATIVE DRUGS (continued)			
Stibocaptate	—	United Kingdom (Astiban [Roche])	Schistosomiasis *(S. haematobium, S. japonicum, S. mansoni)*
Tetrachloroethylene[4]	Nema Worm Capsules [Parke-Davis][4]	United Kingdom (Perklone [ICI])	Fasciolopsiasis

[3] *These anthelmintics generally are less effective, have a limited spectrum of action, and/or possess a greater potential for serious adverse reactions. They are not generally available for human use in the United States. Since availability and cost are important in the selection of drugs, they may be used in developing countries in certain endemic regions.*

[4] *Veterinary product*

DIPYLIDIASIS (DOG TAPEWORM INFECTION). *Dipylidium caninum* has an obligate intermediate host, the flea. More rarely, a louse or other arthropod may be the intermediate host. Larval fleas feed on eggs in proglottids passed by infected dogs or cats. The infection occurs primarily in children, who ingest fleas infected with the larval form (cysticercoid) of the organism. The adult worm develops in the small intestine in three to four weeks.

Patients often are asymptomatic but may complain of anorexia, abdominal pain, anal pruritus, weight loss, and irritability. Gravid segments (proglottids in short chains) may be observed in stool or on the perineum. These segments often are confused with pinworms (Hamrick et al, 1983).

HYMENOLEPIASIS (DWARF TAPEWORM INFECTION). This disease is acquired by fecal contamination of the hands or food or from contact with contaminated soil. Man can serve as the definitive or intermediate host for *Hymenolepis nana*. Eggs are immediately infective and, after hatching, the embryos enter the cells of intestinal villi where they develop into cercocysts (an intermediate stage), from which the adult tapeworm hatches.

H. nana is the most common tapeworm affecting man in the United States. Infections involving large numbers of worms (up to 1,000) have been reported, particularly in mental hospitals or schools for young children where fecal-oral exposure is difficult to control. Anorexia, diarrhea, abdominal pain, headache, dizziness, and occasional seizures have been reported but are not well documented.

TAENIASIS (BEEF AND PORK TAPEWORM INFECTION). These tapeworm infections occur worldwide and result from ingestion of raw or undercooked meat containing live cysticerci; man is the only definitive host. The adult worm fastens itself to the intestinal wall by means of suckers and hooks on the scolex (head) and develops a long strobilum (body) composed of segmental proglottids. Eggs pass out of the bowel, either free or in gravid segments, and, following ingestion by the appropriate intermediate host, hatch to form the larval stage. These larvae penetrate the intestinal mucosa, migrate to the muscles, and develop into encysted forms, thereby completing the cycle. Intermediate hosts for *Taenia saginata* are cattle, llamas, buffalo, and related species. *T. saginata* rarely produces severe symptoms; reports of abdominal discomfort, pruritus ani, weight loss, and excessive hunger are not well documented. The usual intermediate hosts for *T. solium* are domestic swine. Although the adult form of *T. solium* rarely causes signs and symptoms, the development of cysticercosis is a danger that should be prevented (see below).

Therapy: Tapeworm infections should be treated when diagnosed. A single oral dose of niclosamide [Niclocide] is effective in the therapy of beef, pork, fish, and dog tapeworm infections. Praziquantel also is effective in all intestinal tapeworm infections (King and Mahmoud, 1989) and is the drug of choice for the dwarf tapeworm infection because a single dose kills both the cercocyst and adult worm; in comparison, five days of niclosamide treatment are required to produce this effect. Unlike niclosamide, praziquantel is absorbed systemically and appears to be safe (Pearson and Guerrant, 1983; Weniger and Schantz, 1984). Albendazole is an acceptable alternative to niclosamide or praziquantel for tapeworm infections caused by both species of *Taenia* (Jagota, 1986). Other secondary drugs are less effective (eg, paromomycin) or are potentially more toxic (eg, aspidium extract).

Tissue Cestode Infections

CYSTICERCOSIS. This disease is prevalent in areas where humans and domestic swine coexist in close proximity under unhygienic living conditions. Man may be both the definitive and intermediate host of *Taenia solium* and *T. saginata*; however, cysticercosis due to *T. saginata* is extremely rare in humans. Cysticercosis caused by *T. solium* can be acquired by ingestion of parasite eggs present in contaminated food or soil or through direct contact with a tapeworm carrier. Autoinfection can occur, but the mechanisms for this route are unclear. The ingested eggs hatch in the small intestine, releasing larvae that penetrate into the blood stream. The larvae most commonly infect the brain, subcutaneous tissues, skeletal muscles, and eye and form cysts to cause cysticercosis.

In light infections, only mild fever and slight muscular pain may be present during migration of the oncospheres. Encysted cysticerci in the muscles and subcutaneous tissues generally are well tolerated. Although severe symptoms may occur in patients with ocular, cardiac, and muscular involvement, symptoms are most common with nervous system cysticercosis (neurocysticercosis). The clinical manifestations of neurocysticercosis are pleomorphic and depend on the sites of involvement in the nervous system (Earnest et al, 1987; Del Brutto and Sotelo, 1988; Crimmins et al, 1990). *Parenchymal* brain involvement is usually manifested by seizures, focal neurologic deficits, and occasionally by intellectual deterioration; *subarachnoid* and *intraventricular* sites of involvement are commonly associated with nonlocalizing neurologic signs of meningitis or hydrocephalus and increased intracranial pressure caused by inflammatory occlusion of subarachnoid spinal fluid pathways or ventricular obstruction due to ependymitis or ventricular cysts. The clinical signs and symptoms of *spinal* neurocysticercosis usually are similar to those of chronic aseptic meningitis, but cysts also may compress the spinal cord causing paraplegia. Diagnosis of neurocysticercosis relies heavily on the integration of data obtained from CT and MRI scans and antibody detection in serum and cerebrospinal fluid (CSF).

Therapy: Patients with calcified cysts or granulomata and no inflammatory changes in the CSF probably should not receive anticysticercal drugs. They need only symptomatic treatment (eg, antiepileptic drugs) to control any clinical signs. Patients with multiple viable cysts are usually considered candidates for anticysticercal therapy.

Praziquantel and albendazole are effective for the treatment of neurocysticercosis when viable cysts are present in brain parenchymal tissue (Cruz et al, 1991). However, albendazole is preferred for this indication, because it is more effective than praziquantel and can be given in shorter courses (Sotelo et al, 1990). If patients do not respond well to albendazole, praziquantel may be substituted to eliminate any remaining lesions. Praziquantel also may be used as initial therapy if albendazole is not available. Albendazole should be used when cysts are present in the ventricles (Vasconcelos et al, 1987) because the concentration of praziquantel in the CSF is only 10% to 20% of that in serum.

Although either albendazole or praziquantel may appear to elicit or exacerbate neurologic signs or symptoms (eg, headache, nausea, seizures), these manifestations are considered to be a result of the strong inflammatory reaction produced by the host in response to antigen liberated by damage and destruction of viable cysts; they may be ameliorated by the use of analgesics, antiemetics, and antiepileptic drugs. Concomitant administration of corticosteroids for the first several days of treatment with albendazole or praziquantel may relieve headache, especially in patients who have elevated intracranial pressure due to large lesions (Cruz et al, 1991).

The use of the anticysticercal drugs is less clear in patients with calcified, nonviable parenchymal brain cysts with prominent edema and inflammation on CT and a long history of seizures. The acute inflammatory encephalitic phase reflects the host's immune reaction against the lesions. Widespread lesions are occasionally associated with diffuse brain swelling and may cause cysticercotic encephalitis, especially in children. When the swelling is severe, patients with these signs and symptoms should receive corticosteroids and diuretics. Those with less severe inflammation may require only corticosteroids, especially if intracranial pressure is elevated. Many of these lesions will disappear spontaneously, especially in children, in whom a solitary inflamed parenchymal lesion is common (Mitchell and Crawford, 1988). Follow-up monitoring with CT is advisable to determine the need for anticysticercal drugs in adults. Anticysticercal therapy is recommended only if lesions persist for more than three months (Del Brutto and Sotelo, 1988). Ventricular shunting and anticysticercal therapy may be required for patients with hydrocephalus, and surgical removal of intraventricular cysts has been advocated (Madrazo et al, 1983).

ECHINOCOCCOSIS. The term "echinococcosis" encompasses two distinct diseases that are caused by the larval form of different species of tissue cestodes: cystic hydatid disease (CHD, hydatidosis) and alveolar hydatid disease (AHD). The epidemiology, manifestations, prognosis, and treatment of these echinococcoses are quite different. Neither resolves spontaneously, and AHD is 100% fatal if it is not treated.

CHD, which is caused by *Echinococcus granulosus,* is prevalent in Central and South America, but most cases occur in Argentina, Brazil, Chile, Peru, and Uruguay. Asian, European, and Middle Eastern countries with high endemic prevalence of this infection include China, Cyprus, Iraq, Lebanon, Sardinia, Turkey, USSR, Bulgaria, and Yugoslavia; in Africa, it is endemic in parts of Ethiopia, Kenya, Libya, and Sudan. CHD is rare in the contiguous United States but does occur in limited geographic areas, including parts of Utah, the central valley of California, and areas of Arizona and New Mexico. A northern sylvatic strain of *E. granulosus* infects Aleuts, Eskimos, and other Native Americans in Alaska and Canada.

The life cycle of *E. granulosus* involves two hosts and is dependent on the food chain and great fecundity of the cestode for continuation. Members of the family Canidae, including domestic dogs, wolves, and foxes, are the definitive hosts for *E. granulosus*. Typically, they become infected by consuming cyst-containing tissues or organs of herbivores, such as camels, cows, goats, horses, pigs, sheep, and yaks. The herbivorous intermediate hosts acquire the organism by ingesting vegetation that has been contaminated with canid fecal material containing viable cestode eggs. Humans become infected by ingesting eggs of the cestode, which may be present in their immediate environment or in food supplies due to contamination with excrement from infected canines. In certain geographic areas where the disease is hyperendemic (eg, parts of Kenya), cultural, occupational, and religious practices facilitate its transmission to humans from domestic dogs.

Clinical signs of CHD depend on the location and number of cysts present in a particular organ or tissue and are generally considered to be a consequence of functional deficiency resulting from the mass effect of the growing lesion. However, because of the slow rate of growth and small size (usually less than 10 cm in diameter) of the cysts, a majority of cases of CHD remain undetected until discovered by ultrasound, CT, or roentgenographic analysis or at autopsy.

Single cysts are found in 80% of affected patients; the liver and lung are the most commonly affected organs. Cysts also have been observed in muscle, bone, kidney, spleen, and brain. Chronic signs of hepatic CHD include hepatomegaly and obstructive jaundice with gastric distress. A hepatic cyst may become infected with bacteria and present as an abscess. Pulmonary involvement may be indicated by coughing, dyspnea, fever, and hemoptysis. Lesions in the central nervous system may increase intracranial pressure and cause epilepsy, blindness, and paralysis. Allergic manifestations, which include asthma, dyspnea, edema, pruritus, and urticaria, may be caused by cyst leakage. Cyst rupture with sudden release of the contents rarely may induce acute, fatal anaphylaxis; cyst rupture in the abdominal cavity may cause peritonitis and secondary CHD in the form of disseminated or locally recurrent disease.

The inclusion of CHD in a differential diagnosis is warranted by the occurrence of a space-filling, well-defined (sometimes calcified), nonmalignant cystic lesion in a patient with appropriate symptoms and a history of travel or residence in an endemic area. Serologic tests may help confirm the diagnosis.

The cestode, *E. multilocularis*, which causes AHD, was first detected in the United States in 1964, and its range now includes a number of north central states and adjacent provinces of Canada. It is endemic in Alaska, and the vast majority of North American cases of AHD occur among Eskimos (for review, see Wilson and Rausch, 1980). Outside of North America, AHD is endemic to regions of central Europe, Siberia, the northern islands of Japan, and western China.

E. multilocularis can be maintained and propagated through either of two life cycles. In the sylvatic life cycle, foxes serve as the definitive host and wild rodents (eg, voles, lemmings, shrews, mice) are intermediate hosts. A domestic cycle in which dogs and cats serve as the definitive hosts, with rodents as intermediate hosts, also can maintain the parasite. The domestic cycle is considered to be the primary means of disease transmission in Eskimo villages, where large numbers of sled dogs are kept in close proximity to humans. Like CHD, AHD occurs in individuals who ingest viable cestode eggs present in canid fecal material that contaminates their immediate environment or food supplies. However, humans are poor and unusual intermediate hosts for this cestode, a factor that influences lesion development and the course of the disease compared to CHD (see below).

Although the primary lesion of AHD always occurs in the liver, it differs from CHD in that it has the characteristics of a malignant neoplastic growth, including the ability to invade contiguous vital abdominal structures (eg, inferior vena cava, portal vein, common bile duct) and metastasize to distant sites (eg, brain, lungs, mediastinum). Symptoms and signs of disease may include a palpable liver, right upper quadrant pain, an abdominal mass in the liver, jaundice, and shortness of breath. Since the multilocular cysts grow slowly in humans, 20 to 30 years may elapse before symptoms of disease become evident, and AHD may be incurable upon discovery. The disease is usually diagnosed in patients 50 years of age or older who have a history of residence in an endemic area.

Radiographic analysis of the liver reveals diffuse, space-filling lesions, some of which may be calcified (Rausch et al, 1987). Serologic assays can help confirm the diagnosis in patients with the appropriate clinical, surgical (eg, laparoscopic biopsy), and historical indicators of disease (for a review, see Wilson and Rausch, 1980).

The treatment of echinococcosis depends on the causative organism and the number and location of cysts. Surgical resection of lesions remains the treatment of choice for uncomplicated CHD but is not indicated in patients with multiple localized hydatid cysts or cysts located in bone or brain or in those who are very ill or debilitated. Surgery also has been the traditional approach to management of patients with AHD. However, since the multilocular AHD lesion is pleomorphic, infiltrates in all directions, and cannot be separated from the surrounding tissue or organ, surgical cure is frequently uncertain. Furthermore, recurrence of either disease at rates ranging from 11% to 30% within five years of resection of a primary cyst and substantially increased morbidity and mortality in patients undergoing subsequent procedures pose considerable problems in the management of the echinococcoses by surgery alone.

Therapy: In patients with inoperable echinococcosis caused by either cestode or in those who are poor surgical candidates, benzimidazole carbamate derivatives can be used as primary therapy. Mebendazole has been variably effective in such patients (Davis et al, 1986, 1989) and has been used as an adjunct to surgery to shrink cysts preoperatively or to prevent secondary disease caused by intraoperative spillage of cyst contents (Kune et al, 1983). The inconsistent results observed with use of this drug as primary treatment of the echinococcoses are probably related to the dose, duration of therapy, patient age, size and location of cysts, duration of follow-up, and difficulty of monitoring the response to therapy. In particular, mebendazole is not well absorbed when given orally and thus therapeutic serum levels are not attained in many patients. The drug also appears to have a parasitostatic rather than parasiticidal effect on *E. multilocularis* (Ammann et al, 1990), which suggests that maintenance therapy is necessary in AHD to preclude disease relapse. Long-term follow-up is essential in the management of all patients with AHD or CHD.

In a recent study, large doses of mebendazole (100 to 200 mg/kg daily versus a normal daily dosage of 10 to 15 mg/kg) given over a short period of time were reported to be effective and relatively nontoxic in the treatment of children with CHD (Messaritakis et al, 1991). In this study, a mean plasma concentration of 116 ng/ml was attained, which exceeds the therapeutic threshold (100 ng/ml) for this drug. These promising results must be sustained throughout a longer follow-up period and additional confirmatory data are required before the therapeutic role of this high-dose regimen can be established in CHD patients. More studies also are required to determine an effective dosage and duration for primary therapy in patients with echinococcosis of either type so that mebendazole's ultimate role in the management of these diseases can be established.

Although albendazole has the same mechanism of action as mebendazole, it is more consistently absorbed systemically. In addition, albendazole sulfoxide, the principal protoscolicidal metabolite of albendazole, attains cyst-to-serum concentration ratios that exceed those of mebendazole (Morris et al, 1987). The results of a number of trials have shown that albendazole is effective in the treatment of AHD and CHD (for review, see Horton, 1989; see also Davis et al, 1986, 1989; Golematis et al, 1989; De Rosa and Teggi, 1990). In a comparative study in patients with unresectable CHD, albendazole was generally more effective than mebendazole and produced similar adverse reactions (Davis et al, 1989). Data directly comparing the efficacy of albendazole with that of mebendazole in patients with AHD are not available. However, because it has a more predictable and reliable pharmacokinetic profile and, when compared to mebendazole, similar efficacy in patients with CHD, albendazole is regarded as the drug of choice for use as primary therapy in patients with AHD and CHD. To reduce the risk of dissemination or local recurrence of disease, albendazole, or alternatively, mebendazole, should be considered for all patients with echinococcosis who undergo surgical resection as primary treatment.

NEMATODE INFECTIONS

Intestinal Nematode Infections

ASCARIASIS (ROUNDWORM INFECTION). Infection with the roundworm, *Ascaris lumbricoides*, is the most common helminthiasis in the world. It has been estimated that more than one billion people are infected with this nematode. Roundworms are cosmopolitan in distribution, with greatest prevalence in tropical regions. In the United States, an estimated 4 million persons are infected, mainly in the rural southeast. Although the infection may occur in people of any age, it is most prevalent in children of preschool or grade school age. It is usually transmitted from hand to mouth by ingestion of embryonated eggs that are present on contaminated foodstuffs (eg, raw vegetables) or in soil.

Adult worms inhabit the lumen of the small intestine and have a life span of one to two years. Fecund female worms may produce up to 20,000 eggs daily, which are passed in feces. Under favorable environmental conditions, infective embryos develop from the eggs in five to ten days. Embryos that are ingested by humans hatch and release larvae in the small intestine. The larvae penetrate the intestinal walls and migrate via the venous and lymphatic vessels to the lungs. Within the lungs, the larvae penetrate the alveoli, ascend through the bronchi and trachea to the epiglottis, are swallowed, and return to the duodenum. There the larvae develop into mature adult worms. Approximately two months are required for the development of gravid female worms.

Most individuals who are infected with roundworms are asymptomatic. Acute signs and symptoms of infection, which occur during the period of larval migration, may include fever, cough, and pulmonary infiltration. A clinical diagnosis usually cannot be made on the basis of these symptoms, although pneumonitis associated with eosinophilia and generalized allergic manifestations (Loeffler's syndrome) may be suggestive of ascariasis. Detection of eggs in a stool sample is required for definitive diagnosis. Abdominal distress, epigastric pain, anorexia, nausea, and vomiting are likely to be associated with intestinal obstruction due to masses of worms; this complication is commonly seen in children with heavy infections. Complete obstruction of the appendix or intestinal lumen may occur, and asphyxia or aspiration pneumonia may result from vomiting. Serious complications also may arise following migration of adult worms into the pancreatic and biliary ducts (most frequently the common duct), gallbladder, and liver (Khuroo et al, 1990). In addition, roundworms may be found in atypical sites, including umbilical and hernial fistulas, fallopian tubes, and the urinary bladder.

Therapy: Because of the possibility of serious complications, ascariasis should always be treated. Pyrantel pamoate and mebendazole are drugs of choice. Piperazine citrate [Vermizine] and albendazole are alternatives. Levamisole [Ergamisol], diethylcarbamazine, and bephenium hydroxynaphthoate also are effective but are used principally in other parts of the world. (See index entry Levamisole, As Immunostimulant). When treating mixed infections that include ascariasis, agents that are ineffective against ascarids should be avoided initially, because the worms may be stimulated to migrate, possibly exacerbating the symptoms of infection.

ENTEROBIASIS (PINWORM INFECTION). Enterobiasis is caused by the pinworm *Enterobius vermicularis*. It is prevalent throughout the world but occurs more often in temperate than tropical regions. Pinworm infections are the most common of the helminthiases in the United States, with the estimated number of cases exceeding 40 million. Although this infection is primarily considered a childhood ailment, adults also are susceptible. Enterobiasis is not associated with any socioeconomic class. It is transmitted by the oral ingestion of infective eggs and is commonly spread among susceptible groups (institutionalized individuals and in areas of high population density) and members of the same family by direct contact with contaminated hands, bedding, nightclothes, toys, and house dust.

The life cycle of pinworms is similar to that of whipworms (see below). The larvae hatch from mature eggs in the duodenum, molt twice, and develop into mature adults in five to eight weeks. The adults migrate to the cecum and adjacent gut, where they have a life span of 11 to 35 days. Gravid adult females migrate at night to the perianal and perineal regions and deposit eggs on the skin. Embryos develop from the eggs and become infective within six hours, and they may remain viable for up to 20 days after being deposited. The adherence of eggs to transparent adhesive tape that has been pressed against the perianal region early in the morning is indicative of pinworm infection; a single examination in this manner may detect 50% of infections, three examinations detect 90%, and five examinations detect 99%. If eggs are found in one family member, other members should be tested for their presence.

Most patients with enterobiasis are asymptomatic. Pruritus ani and vulvae may occur. There may be eosinophilia of up to 12%, but it is seldom a significant diagnostic sign. Rare serious complications caused by ectopic deposition of eggs and subsequent inflammation and fibrosis include intra-abdominal inflammation, appendicitis, peritoneal granulomas, and allergic urticaria. Migration of worms may cause vaginitis and, rarely, endometritis or salpingitis. Enterobiasis is often associated with dientamebiasis.

Because of the relative ubiquity of *Enterobius vermicularis*, it is important that good personal hygiene, including nail cleaning and careful hand washing following defecation or urination, be instituted with drug therapy to prevent reinfection.

Therapy: Mebendazole and pyrantel pamoate are drugs of choice in pinworm infection. Albendazole, piperazine citrate, and pyrvinium pamoate are alternatives. All members of a family should be treated with an appropriate drug at least once. Since developing larvae and eggs may not be killed with a single dose, retreatment with a second dose in two or three weeks has been recommended.

STRONGYLOIDIASIS (THREADWORM INFECTION). Infection with the nematode, *Strongyloides stercoralis*, is endemic in tropical and subtropical regions, including areas of the southeastern United States, primarily Louisiana, Kentucky, and Tennessee (Berk et al, 1987). Its prevalence in developing tropical countries (85%) is much higher than that observed in the United States (0.4% to 4%). Risk factors include foreign residence; the use of antacids, histamine receptor antagonists, or immunosuppressive agents (eg, corticosteroids) to prevent allograft rejection; and the presence of underlying diseases or conditions that cause immunosuppression (DeVault et al, 1990; Kramer et al, 1990; Zygmunt, 1990). The prevalence of strongyloidiasis is above normal in institutionalized populations (eg, mentally retarded children), among whom it is transmitted primarily by the fecal-oral route.

The worm can exist in soil in the parasitic or free-living form. Infection of humans occurs when invasive filariform larvae penetrate the skin, enter the cutaneous blood vessels, are carried to the pulmonary veins, and penetrate the alveoli. After molting twice in the alveoli, the immature adults ascend the tracheobronchial tree to the posterior pharynx and are swallowed. They develop into mature adults in the small intestine. Adult female worms burrow into the mucosa of the duodenum and jejunum and, after approximately 28 days, begin to produce eggs that hatch into rhabditiform larvae. The latter are passed in the feces and, under favorable soil conditions, molt and differentiate into free-living adult males or females or metamorphose into infectious third-stage larvae, which can survive for about two weeks. These larvae are sensitive to dryness, excessive moisture, or temperatures below 8° C. The free-living adults may produce invasive filariform larvae, which can infect humans and continue the cycle.

In contrast to most other helminths, *S. stercoralis* can multiply within the human host, which can lead to two derangements of the normal life cycle: autoinfection and hyperinfection, which frequently coexist. Cyclic autoinfection results when rhabditiform larvae prematurely develop into invasive filariform larvae, which penetrate the intestinal mucosa (internal autoinfection) or perianal mucosa (external autoinfection), migrate through the systemic circulation, invade the lungs, ascend the tracheobronchial tree to be swallowed and thus re-enter the intestine. This process may result in chronic infection and a massive worm burden. In chronic disseminated disease, a serpiginous creeping urticarial eruption caused by the intradermal migration of filariform larvae is characteristic of some strains (von Kuster and Genta, 1988). The disseminated form of strongyloidiasis has been observed in patients with various cancers (lymphomas, leukemias), leprosy, or AIDS and in transplant recipients receiving immunosuppressant drugs to prevent organ rejection, and it can be fatal if untreated (Davidson et al, 1984; DeVault et al, 1990). However, disseminated strongyloidiasis has not emerged in epidemic proportions among AIDS patients as was initially feared, and it was removed from the CDC list of AIDS indicator diseases in 1987 (Genta, 1989).

Hyperinfection is marked by an increase in total worm burden without subsequent spread of the larvae outside the normal migratory pattern. It is rare in an immunocompetent host.

Definitive diagnosis of strongyloidiasis is established by the detection of larvae in the feces or duodenal contents. Stool concentration techniques (eg, zinc sulfate method) should be used to examine stool samples. Samples of duodenal contents can be obtained by use of the string test (Enterotest, Health Development Company, Palo Alto, CA). Detection of filarial antibodies in individuals at high risk of infection may be accomplished by the use of an enzyme-linked immunoassay (ELISA) procedure (Genta et al, 1987).

Despite the potential severity of strongyloidiasis in certain hosts (see above), the infection usually is asymptomatic in those who do not have the aforementioned risk factors for severe disease. Mild infection occasionally is associated with abdominal bloating and/or pain, intermittent diarrhea, and eosinophilia. A petechial and purpuric rash, especially over the thighs and buttocks, and intense pruritus may occur for a few days after infiltration of the parasite, followed by mild chest pains and cough. Symptoms of moderate infection include diarrhea, malabsorption duodenitis (resembling peptic ulcer), and eosinophilia. Transient pneumonitis also has been observed. The manifestations of severe infection, hyperinfection syndrome, or disseminated strongyloidiasis include vomiting, acute abdominal pain, voluminous foul-smelling stools, malabsorption syndrome, dehydration, electrolyte imbalance, and secondary bacteremia. Edema and adynamic ileus may develop, and the mortality rate is high in certain patients (eg, an immunocompromised host) (Davidson et al, 1984; Cook, 1987).

Therapy: Thiabendazole [Mintezol] usually controls the infection. In immunocompromised patients, repeated courses may be necessary to maintain suppression of the infection. In serious infections that do not respond to thiabendazole or in patients who cannot tolerate this drug, albendazole or mebendazole may be effective alternatives. Ivermectin also has been effective (Naquira et al, 1989), but, it should be reserved for use in patients who cannot tolerate or do not respond to thiabendazole or the benzimidazole carbamates.

TRICHURIASIS (WHIPWORM INFECTION) Infection with *Trichuris trichiura* occurs worldwide, most commonly in warm, moist climates, and it often is found in immigrants and travelers returning from areas where the worm is endemic. It has been estimated that approximately one billion people harbor the parasite that causes trichuriasis, including several million in the United States, predominantly in rural areas of the southeast. Infection results from ingestion of embryonated eggs, usually via contaminated hands, food, or drinking water. Larvae hatch in the upper small intestine and penetrate the mucosa, where they develop for an additional three to ten days. Immature worms usually inhabit the superficial mucosa of the cecum but also may be found in the upper colon, rectum, or appendix. Within one to three months of hatching, female worms begin to produce 5,000 to 20,000 eggs per day. Adult worms have a mean expected life span of one year but may survive for ten years or longer. Since the adults do not multiply in the definitive human host, an existing infection can become heavier only by the ingestion of additional embryonated eggs.

Trichuriasis seldom produces discernible symptoms in hosts with small worm burdens. Eosinophilia, which is usually insignificant (up to 15%), is not usually useful diagnostically. Individuals with heavy infections may develop diarrhea or dysentery, and children may suffer from growth retardation. When the worm burden is extremely large, rectal prolapse may occur, especially in children, and expose a mucosa covered with small, white worms. Blood may be lost at the rate of 0.005 ml of blood/worm/day from the inflamed intestinal mucosa. Although this amount of blood loss is not usually clinically significant, heavily infected, malnourished persons with inadequate iron intake may become anemic.

Since the level of egg output is so high, fecal examination by the simple smear technique without use of concentration methods is usually sufficient for diagnosis of infection.

Therapy: Patients with large worm burdens must be treated. Mebendazole is the drug of choice for treatment of trichuriasis; the cure rate is 60% to 85% and the reduction in egg excretion is 90% to 99%. Albendazole is an alternative and produces similar cure rates when given as a single dose or in a three-day course.

UNCINARIASIS (HOOKWORM INFECTION). The two major hookworm diseases that affect man, *ancylostomiasis* and *necatoriasis,* occur in the tropics and subtropics. Both are common in Africa, Asia, and South America and to a lesser extent in northern Australia, Japan, and Portugal. *Necator* species also are found in the southern United States and West Indies and *Ancylostoma* species exist in Italy and the North African littoral. Hookworm infection is most common in rural areas where there is abundant rainfall and shade, low standards of sanitation, and the inhabitants often go barefoot.

Infection of humans occurs when third-stage larvae penetrate the skin or are swallowed (frequent with *A. duodenale*). Larvae migrate by way of the lymphatics, venules, and the venous bloodstream via the heart to the lungs where they penetrate the alveoli, ascend the bronchi and trachea, and are swallowed. When larvae reach the small intestine, they attach themselves by means of a buccal capsule to the luminal walls where they suck blood. As tissue erodes and is digested, the worms move to new sites. Blood may be lost through shallow ulcerations that are created at the site of worm attachment. Blood also passes from the anus of the worm. Segmented eggs are passed in the feces. If eggs are deposited on soil, the first-stage larvae hatch in 24 hours, feed on organic material or bacteria, and molt twice to form the third-stage, nonfeeding, filariform larvae. These larvae can survive for about four weeks in shaded, moist, sandy soil.

A process of arrested development has been described for *Ancylostoma* organisms in India. Larvae that invade the body during the latter part of the monsoon season may remain dormant until the following year when they develop into adults. Thus, an infection may be manifested many months after an individual has left the endemic area.

Nausea, vomiting, and abdominal pain may occur in patients with acute infections. Chronic blood loss is characteristic of hookworm infections, and individuals with marginal iron intake or inadequate iron stores (eg, malnourished children, some menstruating women) are especially prone to anemia. Patients with satisfactory iron intake may develop anemia if loss of red blood cells cannot be compensated by the normal erythropoietic mechanisms. Thus, symptoms and signs of progressive iron deficiency anemia may occur, and this condition must be corrected at the same time that anthelmintic therapy is begun. Additional symptoms of infection include abdominal fullness, epigastric pain, and cough due to pneumonitis that occurs when large numbers of worms are migrating through the lungs. Local erythema and pruritus ("ground itch") may develop at the site of skin penetration.

The incidence of hookworm infection has decreased markedly in the United States (except for some areas in the South), but, when present, is almost universally caused by *Necator americanus*. Some cases of hookworm are imported, and the species usually is unknown at the time of treatment. Individuals with light worm burdens are asymptomatic and may not require treatment unless they are anemic.

Therapy: Pyrantel pamoate and mebendazole are the drugs of choice for treating heavy infections. Albendazole is an excellent alternative for hookworm infections caused by *A. duodenale* (Maisonneuve et al, 1984) and *N. americanus* (Nahmias et al, 1989). Bephenium hydroxynaphthoate and tetrachloroethylene also are effective, but they are used principally in other parts of the world.

Tissue Nematode Infections

CUTANEOUS LARVA MIGRANS (CREEPING ERUPTION). This skin infection most often is caused by *Ancylostoma braziliense*, a species of hookworm common in cats and dogs, but also may be caused by *Uncinaria stenocephala* or *A. caninum*. It occurs on the southeastern and gulf coasts of the United States and in many tropical and subtropical areas, including tropical South America, Africa, and the Malay peninsula.

Individuals often become infected when filariform larvae present in cat or dog feces penetrate the skin of the feet, legs, and hands. Because man is an aberrant rather than a definitive host, the larvae migrate around in the skin at the rate of 1 to 2 cm daily for several months but usually do not penetrate beyond the dermis where they enter vascular or lymphatic channels. Rarely, some larvae reach the bowel or lungs and cause isolated eosinophilia and/or patchy pulmonary infiltration and bronchospasm (Loeffler's syndrome). An allergic reaction to the worm causes intense pruritus ("ground itch") that leads to scratching, excoriation of the skin, and secondary infection. The appearance of the lesion left by the entrance of the larvae and the occurrence of an erythematous, serpiginous, intracutaneous tract or burrow usually are diagnostic.

Therapy: Oral or topical thiabendazole eradicates this parasite. However, since oral administration may cause significant side effects, topical therapy is preferred. Recent data suggest that albendazole, a derivative of thiabendazole, is effective orally in the treatment of this disease and produces few reactions (Jones et al, 1990). In countries where infection is common, ethyl chloride spray is used with topical formulations containing bacitracin, polymyxin B, and neomycin (eg, Mycitracin, Neosporin) to control associated bacterial skin infections.

DRACUNCULIASIS (DRACONTIASIS, GUINEA WORM INFECTION). This disease is acquired by an estimated 10 million persons yearly in tropical regions, particularly Africa, the Middle East, and parts of India and Pakistan, by the ingestion of water that contains water fleas harboring infective larvae of the guinea worm, *Dracunculus medinensis* (Imtiaz et al, 1990; *MMWR*, 1990, 1991 A). Following their release from the infected copepods in the host stomach, infective larvae pass into the small intestine, penetrate the mucosa, and migrate to the retroperitoneum where they mature and mate. The male worm dies after copulation. The gravid adult female migrates to the subcutaneous tissues, primarily of the foot or leg, and after approximately one year the anterior end emerges through an ulceration of the overlying skin and discharges a whitish material that contains first-stage larvae.

Immediately prior to the emergence of the worm, patients often develop a generalized reaction manifested by urticaria, nausea, vomiting, diarrhea, and dyspnea. Intense, painful inflammatory reactions, and often secondary bacterial infections including tetanus, may occur if the disease is untreated or treated improperly. In addition to secondary bacterial infections of the cutaneous lesions, other complications include acute abscesses, cellulitis, arthritis, synovitis, epididymo-orchitis, fibrous ankylosis of joints, and contractures of tendons. As many as 40% of patients may become totally incapacitated by this disease and its complications for up to six weeks.

After the worms emerge through the skin surface, they may be extracted with a forceps; usually, an emerging worm is gradually wound around a small stick at a few centimeters per day until free. However, if worms are encapsulated in subcutaneous tissues and do not emerge, it is difficult to detect their presence. A recently developed serologic ELISA eventually may be valuable for diagnosis of prepatent dracunculiasis (Fagbemi and Hillyer, 1990), and the early detection has great potential to help reduce the associated morbidity of this disease.

Therapy: Although the benzimidazole, niridazole, and the nitroimidazole, metronidazole [Flagyl, Metryl], are used in the treatment of this disease, their beneficial action appears to be unrelated to any antiparasitic effect. Instead, their main role may be minimization of secondary skin infections and inflammation (*Lancet*, 1983). Large, potentially toxic doses of thiabendazole may ameliorate inflammation and facilitate worm removal. Mebendazole has been reported to kill the worm directly when given at doses likely to be toxic (*Med Lett Drugs Ther*, 1990).

FILARIASIS. Filariases are transmitted to humans via the bites of insects. They are largely restricted to tropical and subtropical regions because the arthropods that serve as vectors or reservoirs of infection are found principally in these areas. The life cycles of the various filarial parasites are similar (for review, see Nanduri and Kazura, 1989). Infective larvae carried by the insect vector enter the human host through a breach produced in the skin when the insect vector takes a blood meal, molt to later-stage larvae, and develop into sexually mature adults in the lymphatic system or subcutaneous tissues (see Table 1). For the major filariases, the prepatent period extends from the time of infection until the point at which microfilariae can be detected in the blood of the host and ranges from four months to one year.

When microfilariae present in the human blood stream or subepidermis are ingested by the appropriate insect vector, they migrate to the arthropod gut, penetrate its wall, and eventually reach the thoracic musculature or fatty tissues. In these environments, the microfilariae metamorphose, molt, and finally mature into infective larvae. The latter migrate to the proboscis of the vector, from where they enter a new host during the taking of a blood meal. Within the insect vector, the developmental period for infective larvae is 10 to 14 days for agents that produce lymphatic filariases and five to eight days for those that produce onchocerciasis (see below). Adult worms may live for 7 to 10 years in the human host, although 40-year life spans have been reported. For therapeutic purposes, microfilariae generally represent the pathogenic stage of onchocerciasis, and adult worms cause chronic illness in the lymphatic and cutaneous filariases.

Although the diseases caused by these tissue-invasive nematodes are prevalent in endemic areas, travelers returning to the United States from these areas rarely harbor parasites (*Loa loa* may be an exception). However, North American species of *Brugia* (eg, *B. beaveri*, *B. lepori*) are found in racoons, rabbits, and woodchucks. Nine patients on the East Coast of the United States, not all of whom had traveled abroad, were reported to be infected with acquired autochthonous brugian filariasis (Baird et al, 1986).

Loiasis, Mansonellosis, Ozzardi Filariasis: Microfilariae of *Loa loa*, *Mansonella perstans*, and *M. ozzardi* may be found in the blood of individuals who have lived in an endemic area for a significant period of time. Loiasis is the most important of the three infections clinically. Localized painful swelling of the extremities becomes evident 3 to 12 months following infection and often subsides in several days. Swelling around the eyes of infected persons usually signifies the presence of adult worms in the subcutaneous tissues of this area. Neurologic manifestations of infection are rare, but may be associated with heavy infestations or produced by therapy. Eosinophilia may be noted, especially following the institution of therapy.

Patients with mansonellosis usually are asymptomatic, but fever, headache, lymphadenitis, erythematous rashes, arthritis, hepatomegaly with abdominal pain, and hypereosinophilia may occur.

Therapy: Diethylcarbamazine is the drug of choice to treat infection with *Loa loa*. Its actions appear to be both microfilaricidal and macrofilaricidal. Moreover, in a controlled study in Peace Corps volunteers, a dose of 300 mg weekly for two years was well tolerated and highly effective in the prophylaxis of loiasis (Nutman et al, 1988). Mebendazole also is effective in reducing microfilaremia and eosinophilia in patients with loiasis (Van Hoegaerden et al, 1987).

Although diethylcarbamazine has limited effectiveness against *M. perstans*, it is regarded as the drug of choice for this indication because no more effective drug is currently available. However, mebendazole has been somewhat successful in treating this infection (Van Hoegaerden et al, 1987) and is an alternative to diethylcarbamazine. Ivermectin has produced a satisfactory response in the treatment of *M. ozzardi* filariasis (Nutman et al, 1987), an infection for which reliable therapy has not been established. Diethylcarbamazine is not useful for this indication.

Lymphatic Filariasis (Brugiasis, Wuchereriasis): Brugiasis (caused by *Brugia malayi* and *B. timori*) and wuchereriasis (caused by *Wuchereria bancrofti*) are serious diseases that have been estimated to afflict some 90 million people worldwide (WHO Expert Committee on Filariasis, 1984). Approximately 67% of these persons reside in China, India, and Indonesia. The greatest numbers of infections with *W. bancrofti* are found in tropical and subtropical Africa, Asia, and the South Pacific; endemic foci also exist in Caribbean nations, such as Haiti, and coastal areas of Brazil. Brugiasis due to *B. malayi* is limited to southern China, Malaysia, a few areas of India, and the Philippines. Infections with *B. timori* are found exclusively on the Indonesian islands of Flores and Timor.

Persons with light infections, even those living in endemic areas, may be asymptomatic despite the presence of microfilaremia. Heavier infections may produce a syndrome known as "filarial fevers" or paroxysmal inflammatory filariasis (Weller and Arnow, 1983). Chronic obstruction of the afferent lymphatic channels of the legs and scrotum occurs as a consequence of endothelial proliferation; fibrin deposition; and production of a granulomatous inflammatory infiltrate consisting of eosinophils, lymphocytes, and macrophages, all induced by the presence of molting and dead adult worms. Obstruction of lymph flow results in edema and the debilitating and disfiguring sequelae of elephantiasis and hydrocele.

The syndrome of tropical pulmonary eosinophilia may develop and is characterized by nocturnal paroxysmal cough, hypereosinophilia (3,000 to 50,000 cells/mm^3), elevated sedimentation rate, radiologic evidence of diffuse miliary lesions or increased bronchovascular markings, high titers of filarial and IgE antibodies, and impaired (restrictive-type) pulmonary function. Hepatosplenomegaly and lymphadenopathy have been observed. Chronic pulmonary fibrosis may result if the disease is untreated.

Inflammatory filariasis is characterized by chills and fever lasting two to ten days and is associated with headache, nausea, vomiting, diaphoresis, constipation, urticarial rash, lymphadenitis, and lymphangitis that develops in a retrograde manner. These episodes occur in paroxysmal fashion and may recur over a period of many years.

Therapy: Diethylcarbamazine rapidly clears microfilariae of *W. bancrofti*, *B. malayi*, and *B. timori* from the blood of infected persons, and it has been the drug of choice for treatment of these infections for more than 40 years (Ottesen, 1985). However, when this drug is given in microfilaricidal doses, the beneficial effect is transient, probably because not all of the adult worms harbored in the lymphatics are killed or sterilized. Although this problem theoretically may be overcome by optimizing the dosage regimens of this drug for different populations, the usefulness of diethylcarbamazine in mass treatment programs to eradicate these diseases in endemic areas is limited by the requirement for multiple microfilaricidal doses or prolonged administration of large macrofilaricidal doses. Thus, recent data indicating that a single oral dose of ivermectin is comparable to the standard multiple doses of diethylcarbamazine in eliminating microfilariae of these lymphatic-dwelling species from the blood of infected persons (Kumaraswami et al, 1988; Ottesen et al, 1990; Richards et al, 1991) provide hope that transmission of the lymphatic filariases may one day be controlled as simply and effectively as onchocerciasis (see below). However, there is no evidence for macrofilaricidal activity of ivermectin in lymphatic filariases that is comparable to that of diethylcarbamazine.

Onchocerciasis (River Blindness): This potentially devastating disease is caused by the filarial tissue nematode, *Onchocerca volvulus*, for which man is the definitive host. Details of its life cycle and development in humans have been summarized succinctly in a recent review (Nelson, 1991). Onchocerciasis is endemic to regions of West and Central Africa and Central and South America. Since these regions are not generally frequented by tourists and prolonged exposure to the vector (black flies of the genus *Simulium*) that transmits the parasite is required for infection, this disease is rare among travelers returning to the United States from tropical areas. However, immigrants from endemic areas or long-term residents may be infected and symptomatic on entry to this country.

The disease manifests itself as pruritus and skin irritation (onchocercal dermatitis) about one year after the infection is acquired, and these are the major causes of morbidity among infected persons (Pacqué et al, 1991 A). Skin nodules containing macrofilariae (adult worms) and ocular pathology (corneal opacities) caused by microfilariae are evident in persons with heavy infections. In addition, microfilariae can migrate to many other tissues and cause severe signs and symptoms. Serious chronic inflammatory responses may be provoked by degeneration of microfilariae in the skin and eyes; this frequently causes blindness (hence the colloquial name, "river blindness"), primarily in heavily infested individuals who have lived in an endemic region for years. Active infiltration of injured microfilariae into tissues of the eye (eg, the cornea) is postulated to be the cause of blindness (Dadzie et al, 1987).

Therapy: Ivermectin is the drug of choice for therapy of onchocerciasis and is given orally (for reviews, see Taylor and Greene, 1989; Ette et al, 1990). A single yearly dose of ivermectin 150 mcg/kg has significantly reduced the microfilarial load and disease transmission among study populations in endemic areas and is safe, practical, and well accepted for administration on a community-wide basis (Taylor et al, 1990; Pacqué et al, 1990, 1991 A, 1991 B). The administration of 150 mcg/kg biannually also appears to be very effective in suppressing microfilarial levels, is well tolerated, and is a practical regimen for use in mass treatment programs (Greene et al, 1991). Ivermectin has supplanted diethylcarbamazine in this role primarily because, in contrast to that agent, ivermectin does not cause mobilization and degradation of microfilariae within the eye (Dadzie et al, 1987; Taylor et al, 1989), does not require administration in multiple doses over a period of a week or two, and produces little or no Mazzoti reaction.

There is no evidence that ivermectin has macrofilaricidal activity when given as a single dose of 150 mcg/kg. However, one recent report showed that treatment of Guatemalan patients with 12 monthly doses of ivermectin 150 mcg/kg killed 22% of nodular adult female and 12% of adult male worms; it had no effect on the remaining worms (Duke et al, 1990). If confirmed, this result has significant therapeutic implications, since adult worms live for years and, following single-dose treatment, resume the production of microfilariae within 12 months. However, a monthly regimen is impractical for use in a mass treatment program because patient compliance may be difficult to ensure.

Until the advent of ivermectin, the administration of diethylcarbamazine followed by suramin was the most widely used regimen for treatment of onchocerciasis (Edwards, 1984). Diethylcarbamazine is effective only against microfilariae of *O. volvulus*, while suramin is primarily macrofilaricidal. Intermittent administration of diethylcarbamazine controls the signs and symptoms of disease (eg, when reinfection is prevalent and suramin is not readily available, practical, or warranted because of toxicity). Diethylcarbamazine is well tolerated and relatively safe when given orally, but patients with severe onchocerciasis frequently experience allergic skin reactions (eg, Mazzoti reaction) and ocular complications caused by the drug-induced redistribution and disintegration of microfilariae. The concomitant use of corticosteroids minimizes the allergic phenomena and increases tolerance to the drug. Stepwise escalation of the dosage of diethylcarbamazine also appears to minimize the severity of these reactions.

Suramin, which is primarily a macrofilaricide for *O. volvulus*, also has some microfilaricidal activity, but its use alone may induce a severe allergic reaction affecting the eye. In addition, it is relatively more toxic (substantial nephrotoxicity) than diethylcarbamazine citrate and must be given intravenously.

PULMONARY DIROFILARIASIS (DOG HEARTWORM INFECTION). The dog heartworm, *Dirofilaria immitis*, is the causative agent of a pulmonary form of dirofilariasis in humans. The dog is the definitive host and humans are secondary hosts of this parasite. It is transmitted by a mosquito vector, and, in dogs, adult worms usually inhabit the right ventricle of the heart and the pulmonary arteries; microfilariae are present in the blood. In humans, the disease is characterized by benign lung nodules (Ciferri, 1982). About 50% of patients experience chest discomfort, malaise, cough, fever, and occasionally hemoptysis; microfilariae are not found in the circulation. Radiographic examination usually is required for diagnosis in asymptomatic individuals. Serologic methods are available to assist in diagnosis of patients with symptoms and pulmonary lesions suggestive of this disease (Glickman et al, 1986), but they are not widely used because this condition is seldom considered in differential diagnosis. Microfilaricides are used to control the disease in dogs. In humans, surgery is the only definitive therapy.

TOXOCARIASIS (VISCERAL LARVA MIGRANS). Toxocariasis in humans results from the invasion of visceral organs by larval forms of roundworms that normally infect dogs (*Toxocara canis*) or cats (*T. cati*). Since humans are not the definitive host for these nematode species, development beyond the larval stage is halted. Humans become infected by ingesting embryonated eggs, which are shed with cat or dog feces and thus may contaminate soil or raw vegetables in areas where these animals have been present. After hatching in the small intestine, larvae migrate via the blood stream or peritoneal serosa to the lungs or liver. The larvae are very thin and sometimes pass through the sinusoids to the kidney, brain, or eyes (ocular toxocariasis). In the United States, risk factors for infection include dog ownership, pica, low socioeconomic status, and residence in the Southeast (Ellis et al, 1986). Seropositivity for *Toxocara canis* antibodies is widely variable in the United States; it ranges from about 3% to 54%, depending on the population and region. In general, toxocariasis is a disease of children and occurs most commonly in those under 6 years. Because they are frequented by cats, sandboxes in public playgrounds are a common source of infection in young children.

Persons infected with small numbers of larvae may be asymptomatic or complain of recurrent abdominal pain. Cough, fever, wheezing, and other generalized symptoms are common among infected persons seeking medical attention. Moderate to severe infection is manifested by persistent eosinophilia, leukocytosis, hepatomegaly, and pneumonitis, particularly in children. The diagnosis in a young child is usually suggested by the presence of eosinophilia accompanied by leukocytosis and hepatomegaly and signs and symptoms of other organ involvement. It is confirmed by the histologic detection of larvae in affected tissues or by serologic methods (ELISA).

Therapy: Toxocariasis is usually self-limiting, and most patients recover without specific therapy. When the infection is severe, mebendazole or thiabendazole, plus a corticosteroid to minimize inflammatory reactions due to injury to the parasite (especially in ocular disease), may be effective. Diethylcarbamazine or albendazole are alternatives and are used with corticosteroids if necessary.

TRICHINOSIS (TRICHINELLIASIS, PORK ROUNDWORM INFECTION). Trichinosis is caused by infection with *Trichinella spiralis*. Although this infection occurs worldwide, areas of high incidence include eastern Europe, especially Poland and Yugoslavia, and parts of western Europe. Cases also have been reported in the Arctic, South America, Asia, and East Africa. The incidence of infection in the United States has decreased markedly in the past few years. However, recurrent outbreaks of trichinosis in this country have occurred among recent immigrants from Southeast Asia (*MMWR*, 1991 B), indicating that persons who consume raw pork are at risk. Infection is uncommon in Great Britain. Trichinosis in swine does not occur in Australia.

The most common reservoir of this infection for man is the domestic pig, but other carnivores may host *Trichinella spiralis*, including the wild boar, bear, fox, wildcat, weasel, martin, lynx, badger, and rat. Human infection typically is acquired when undercooked pork or pork products or other infected meat (bear, wild boar, walrus) containing encysted larvae is ingested. The cyst wall is digested in the stomach, and first-stage larvae invade the mucosa of the duodenum where they molt four times. Fertilized females appear in the intestinal lumen in less than two days and begin to produce first-stage larvae that are deposited in the ileal mucosa. Adult females live for only a few weeks. The larvae penetrate the mucosa and are carried to skeletal muscle by the blood stream and lymphatics and become encysted in a muscle cell in about 17 days. Thus, three weeks are required before encysted larvae appear in a press preparation or digested specimen of a muscle biopsy or the ELISA serologic test becomes strongly positive. Some encysted larvae live for years, while others die and are calcified within a few months.

Initially, trichinosis may cause diarrhea lasting one to three weeks, followed by fatigue, myalgia, periorbital edema, sore throat, fever, and eosinophilia (25% to 50%) lasting one to two weeks. The great majority of affected individuals recover following the use of aspirin and supportive therapy, but cysts remain in the muscles. A small percentage of patients develop life-threatening complications, such as congestive heart failure, meningitis, neuritis, or a Guillain-Barré-type syndrome.

Therapy: Trichinosis is usually self-limited, and most people recover within several months. If treatment is necessary, it can be directed at two distinct phases based on the biology of the parasite and the duration and intensity of infection: In the first phase, adult worms are killed within the intestine, thereby reducing the worm burden and preventing the production of invasive larvae. In the second phase, extraintestinal migrating and encysted larval forms are killed, thus relieving symptoms and preventing the development of systemic complications.

Adult worms can be killed in the intestine by benzimidazoles, such as thiabendazole, albendazole, or mebendazole, or by pyrantel pamoate. Thiabendazole has some effect on migrating larvae but does not eliminate encapsulated forms. Mebendazole has been administered in large doses for prolonged periods to kill encysted larvae (Levin, 1983). Conventional doses of albendazole also may eliminate residual larvae, as indicated by a reduction in antibody titers during prolonged follow-up of patients (Fourestié et al, 1988). Ketoconazole [Nizoral], a related imidazole, was as effective as mebendazole in a mouse model of trichinosis (Hess et al, 1986). The use of corticosteroids is essential during the larval migratory stage to reduce the inflammatory response and alleviate symptoms.

TREMATODE INFECTIONS

CLONORCHIASIS AND OPISTHORCHIASIS (CHINESE OR ORIENTAL LIVER FLUKE INFECTION). Infection with these organisms (*Clonorchis sinensis* and *Opisthorchis viverrini*, respectively) rarely occurs in travelers to the Far East but is common in Southeast Asian and Chinese immigrants in the United States (see Table 1). The disease is acquired by eating undercooked, raw, dried, or pickled freshwater fish that contains infective metacercariae of these trematodes. The excysted larvae ascend the biliary tree from the duodenum and mature in the bile ducts. The disease is usually asymptomatic, but ascending cholangitis, biliary stones, and cholangiocarcinoma may complicate the infection. Malaise, epigastric pain, tender hepatomegaly, and eosinophilia may develop. The parasite may live for 40 years in man.

Therapy: Praziquantel is effective and appears to be safe in the treatment of clonorchiasis and opisthorchiasis (Pearson and Guerrant, 1983; Weniger and Schantz, 1984; O'Keefe and Edgett, 1986; Mahmoud, 1987; Yangco et al, 1987). Biliary obstruction may require surgery.

FASCIOLIASIS (SHEEP LIVER FLUKE INFECTION). The sheep liver fluke, *Fasciola hepatica*, is the only fluke that is indigenous to the continental United States. Humans usually acquire fascioliasis by ingesting watercress and other aquatic plants that are contaminated by encysted metacercarial forms of this organism; a snail is required as an intermediate host (see Table 1).

Symptoms of this infection appear within one to three months after the disease is acquired; their severity depends on the worm burden. The usual pattern is loss of appetite, slight fever, lassitude, and a dull ache in the hepatic area. The liver may be tender and enlarged. Urticaria also may be present and there may be a considerable eosinophilia.

Therapy: Oral bithionol is effective and is considered the drug of choice by some authorities (*Med Lett Drugs Ther*, 1990), but it has potentially serious toxicity and is not readily available in the United States (it can be obtained only from the CDC). Praziquantel appears to be somewhat effective in treating this infection, although experience with its use is limited (Pearson and Guerrant, 1983; Weniger and Schantz, 1984; Mahmoud, 1987). Treatment failures, especially in children, have been reported. Limited data indicate that triclabendazole [Fasinex], a veterinary fasciolicide, may be useful in treating fascioliasis (Loutan et al, 1989), and it is being investigated by the WHO for this indication. Albendazole also may have some value in this condition. Although no drug is consistently reliable in treating fascioliasis, a rational approach is to initiate therapy with praziquantel, and if it is not effective, substitute bithionol. Other agents should be used only if the first two choices do not improve or cure the disease.

FASCIOLOPSIASIS (GIANT INTESTINAL FLUKE INFECTION). The giant intestinal fluke, *Fasciolopsis buski*, occurs primarily in Southeast Asia and is normally found in pigs. Parasite eggs are passed in the feces of the host, and a snail acts as an intermediate vector. Humans acquire the infection by eating raw vegetables (eg, water chestnuts) grown in contaminated water (see Table 1).

Most humans with these infections are asymptomatic. Heavy infections may produce abdominal symptoms that can mimic those of peptic ulcer. Alternating diarrhea and constipation may be noted. Edema of the face and trunk sometimes occurs, especially in children. In the most severe cases, intestinal stasis, ulceration, and complete bowel obstruction requiring surgical intervention have been reported.

Therapy: Fasciolopsiasis is more responsive to therapy than some related infections. An early study demonstrated a 100% cure rate with praziquantel (Bunnag et al, 1983), which is the drug of choice. Niclosamide and tetrachloroethylene are alternatives, but the latter drug is available only as a veterinary product in the United States and has significant toxicity. Piperazine citrate is least effective.

PARAGONIMIASIS (LUNG FLUKE INFECTION). *Paragonimus westermani*, which occurs in the Far East and Central and South America, is the most common etiologic agent of this disease in man (see Table 1). *P. kellicotti* appears to be limited to the Americas, but this species, and others (eg, *P. skrjabini*, *P. heterotremus*, *P. africanus*) that are found in Africa and China and other Far Eastern countries, only infrequently infect man. Pulmonary symptoms, often with hemoptysis, are the primary manifestations of disease but gastrointestinal and central nervous system symptoms also may develop.

Therapy: Currently available data suggest that praziquantel is the drug of choice; it is safer than the alternative drug, bithionol (Pearson and Guerrant, 1983; Pachucki et al, 1984; Weniger and Schantz, 1984; Mahmoud, 1987). Bithionol is not effective when the parasite is localized in the brain or spinal cord.

SCHISTOSOMIASIS (BLOOD FLUKE INFECTION). Freshwater snails are the intermediate hosts for these flukes, which differ primarily in their geographic distribution and the specific sites at which they produce chronic infection (Table 1). Humans acquire the disease when infective cercariae present in contaminated water penetrate the skin. Transmission of the disease does not occur in the United States because the appropriate snails are not indigenous to this country. Swimmers' itch is sometimes seen in the United States. This irritation is caused by an animal schistosome that penetrates the skin but does not fully develop before it dies.

Acute Schistosomiasis: Dermatitis, which results from cercarial penetration of the skin, develops two to eight days after an individual is infected (Nash et al, 1982; King, 1991). Acute schistosomiasis (Katayama fever) may resemble serum sickness and follows deposition of eggs by adult worms. Fever accompanied by cough, lymphadenopathy, anorexia, weight loss, malaise, angioedema, myalgia, urticaria, hepatosplenomegaly, and eosinophilia may develop in two to eight weeks. Leukocytosis and elevated levels of alkaline phosphatase, IgG, IgE (Hagan et al, 1991), and especially IgM are characteristic signs of infection. Serologic testing is very helpful in diagnosing this disease. Definitive diagnosis is based on identification of eggs in the feces five to six weeks after exposure. Stool sedimentation may be necessary because the eggs are so few in number. Signs and symptoms of infection abate over three to four months without treatment even though the adult worms and eggs persist; generally only supportive therapy is required. Praziquantel is effective in treating patients with severe acute schistosomiasis; however, an inflammatory reaction that is produced by the destructive effects of the drug may be severe enough to require administration of corticosteroids (Monson, 1987).

Chronic Schistosomiasis: The vasculature of the intestinal tract, biliary system, and, less commonly, the lungs may be sites of involvement in chronic schistosomiasis.

Chronic schistosomiasis produced by *Schistosoma mansoni, S. japonicum,* and *S. mekongi* affects the liver and is characterized by the gradual development of asymptomatic hepatosplenomegaly (DeCock, 1986). Hepatic fibrosis (Symmers' clay pipestem fibrosis of the liver) and granulomata are typical pathologic findings. Variceal bleeding may be a late finding and is caused by portal hypertension. Splenomegaly results from portal hypertension or reticuloendothelial hyperplasia. Chronic salmonellosis and chronic schistosomiasis can coexist. The bacteria may be harbored by the parasite, and antischistosomal therapy may be required before antibiotics can be effective. Spinal cord involvement (eg, transverse myelitis) is rare and appears to be caused by deposition of eggs in spinal cord vessels. *S. japonicum* invades the brain in 2% to 4% of patients.

The urinary tract is most commonly involved in infection caused by *S. haematobium*. Painless hematuria, dysuria, and white cells in the urine are characteristic symptoms of this disease. Definitive diagnosis is based on identification of eggs in the urine. An association between bladder cancer and endemic schistosomiasis has been demonstrated, but the exact role of the schistosome is unknown (Hicks, 1983).

Therapy: Chronic schistosomiasis usually responds to chemotherapy. Praziquantel is the drug of choice for treatment of all forms of the disease (Nash et al, 1982; Pearson and Guerrant, 1983; Weniger and Schantz, 1984; King and Mahmoud, 1989). Oxamniquine [Vansil] is an alternative in *S. mansoni* infections, and metrifonate [Bilarcil] can be used in *S. haematobium* infection. In developing countries where *S. haematobium* is endemic and cost is a major consideration in selecting a drug for mass treatment programs, metrifonate appears to be the agent of choice (King et al, 1990). Antimony potassium tartrate and niridazole are more toxic than other available drugs and only somewhat effective in the treatment of *S. japonicum, S. mekongi,* and *S. intercalatum* infections. In addition, since there is considerable concern about niridazole's potential carcinogenicity, the use of these agents to eliminate these organisms generally is not recommended in the United States. Although the end-stage hepatic fibrosis that occurs in chronic schistosomiasis cannot be reversed by drug therapy, the prevalence of Symmers' periportal fibrosis was reported to be two to three times lower in patients who received chemotherapy for their infections than in those who were not so treated (Homeida et al, 1988).

Drug Evaluations

ALBENDAZOLE (Investigational drug)
[Zentel]

ACTIONS. Albendazole is one of the most potent broad spectrum benzimidazole carbamate anthelmintics. It is effective against adult and larval forms of many nematodes and cestodes and acts by interfering with their uptake of glucose, which leads to depletion of glycogen and adenosine triphosphate stores. Tubulin binding that disrupts the aggregation of microtubules and diminishes intracellular transport may be the mechanism of action.

USES. When given in single or multiple doses, albendazole is a very effective alternative to mebendazole or pyrantel pamoate for the treatment of intestinal nematode infections, including ascariasis, enterobiasis, trichuriasis, and uncinariasis, and can be considered an alternative to thiabendazole for the treatment of strongyloidiasis (see the Introduction). A number of tissue nematode infections respond to albendazole and, because it is less toxic, this also is an alternative to thiabendazole for the treatment of cutaneous larva migrans (Jones et al, 1990), toxocariasis, and trichinosis. Although the usefulness of this drug in the treatment of taeniasis caused by beef or pork tapeworms is variable, it is a reasonable alternative to niclosamide or praziquantel for these indications.

Because albendazole is more effective than praziquantel and may be given in a shorter course, it is the drug of choice for cerebral cysticercosis caused by larvae of *T. solium*, although praziquantel may be preferred by some clinicians. However, praziquantel is not indicated for patients who have intraventricular cysticercal lesions; these should be treated with albendazole. In patients with echinococcosis caused by *E. granulosus* or *E. multilocularis*, albendazole is preferred to mebendazole for primary therapy of unresectable lesions and as an adjunct to prevent dissemination or relapse of disease in patients who undergo surgical resection for removal of cysts (see the Introduction).

ADVERSE REACTIONS AND PRECAUTIONS. When given orally in doses of 5 to 8 mg/kg daily for one to three days to patients with intestinal helminthiases, albendazole has been well tolerated. Constipation, abdominal pain, diarrhea, nausea, and dizziness were reported infrequently. Reversible alopecia has been reported rarely in patients given large doses (eg, > 800 mg/day) for prolonged periods. However, placebo effect or disease-induced adverse reactions were not assessed in these initial studies.

When administered orally in doses of 9 to 15 mg/kg (eg, 600 to 800 mg) daily for 28 days to patients with hepatic, alveolar, or cystic hydatidosis, significant reversible hepatotoxicity was manifested by gradually increasing concentrations of AST and ALT (Wilson et al, 1987; Steiger et al, 1990); these effects were not reported when comparable doses were administered to patients with neurocysticercosis (Escobedo et al, 1987; Cruz et al, 1991). It is not known whether elevated enzyme levels are caused by the gradual accumulation of a hepatotoxic metabolite of albendazole (eg, albendazole sulfoxide) or are peculiar to the type of cestodal tissue infection being treated. It is important to monitor hepatic function closely in patients given prolonged therapy.

Other reversible adverse reactions in patients who receive albendazole for the treatment of neurocysticercosis, but not echinococcosis, include severe headache, intracranial hypertension, meningeal signs, diplopia, hypertension, and seizures. These adverse reactions are not due to direct effects of albendazole, but are a result of a host inflammatory reaction to antigen release that follows death of or damage to the parasite.

PHARMACOKINETICS. The absorption of oral albendazole is low, and the unchanged drug is essentially undetectable in plasma. However, when it is given orally, the portion that is absorbed is rapidly converted to the active metabolite, albendazole sulfoxide. Supratherapeutic concentrations of the latter are evident in plasma four hours after oral administration of the parent drug (Wilson et al, 1987). Significant quantities of albendazole sulfoxide appear in lung and liver tissues and in cyst fluid of patients receiving albendazole for the treatment of echinococcosis (Saimot et al, 1983). Stable plasma concentrations of the metabolite are reached after two to four days of treatment. The elimination half-life of albendazole sulfoxide is reported to be three to four hours (Morris et al, 1985). Albendazole sulfoxide is the primary metabolite found in urine; urinary excretion represents the primary mechanism of clearance.

With long-term treatment, albendazole significantly inhibits aminopyrine-N-demethylation and induces its own metabolism (Steiger et al, 1990). These findings suggest that albendazole may interact with other drugs that are metabolized by microsomal enzymes and provides a rationale for administering this drug cyclically rather than continuously.

Pharmacokinetic data on pregnant patients are unavailable.

DOSAGE AND PREPARATIONS.
Oral: *Adults and children >2 years*, for ascariasis, enterobiasis, strongyloidiasis, trichuriasis, and uncinariasis, 400 mg as a single dose; for cutaneous larva migrans, some cases of strongyloidiasis, and for taeniasis, 400 mg daily for three days; for toxocariasis, 600 mg daily in divided doses for five days (Stürchler et al, 1989); for trichinosis, 800 mg daily in divided doses for six days (Kocięcka et al, 1989).

For primary therapy of inoperable alveolar or cystic echinococcosis, three 28-day cycles of 400 mg twice daily with 14-day drug-free intervals between each cycle (Horton, 1989). Patients with hepatic or pulmonary lesions should receive only three cycles initially to demonstrate a response; those with bone or brain lesions will usually require more courses. For patients undergoing surgical resection of echinococcal lesions, presurgical prophylaxis may be given for up to six weeks; postsurgical prophylaxis may include up to three cycles (Horton, 1989). Cyclic therapy has been beneficial in echinococcosis caused by *E. granulosus*, but it may be only parasitostatic in disease caused by *E. multilocularis* (Davis et al, 1986, 1989). For neurocysticercosis, 15 mg/kg daily is given for eight days (Sotelo et al, 1990); treatment may continue for up to 30 days if necessary (Sotelo et al, 1988; Cruz et al, 1991). Corticosteroids are administered during albendazole therapy for neurocysticercosis (Cruz et al, 1991). Periodic monitoring of hepatic function is recommended in patients receiving therapy for echinococcosis or neurocysticercosis.

Children <2 years, for intestinal nematode infections, 200 mg as a single dose (Pamba et al, 1987). Pediatric doses for other indications have not been established.

Zentel (SmithKline Beecham).

DIETHYLCARBAMAZINE CITRATE

[Hetrazan]

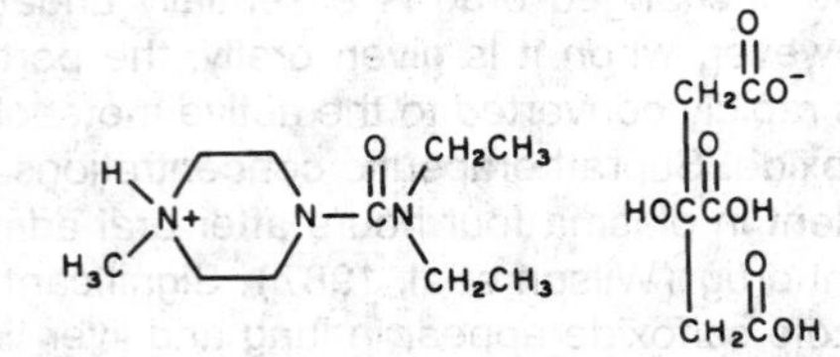

ACTIONS AND USES. Diethylcarbamazine citrate destroys the microfilariae of *Wuchereria bancrofti, Brugia malayi, B. timori, Loa loa, Onchocerca volvulus*, and, to a lesser extent, those of *Mansonella perstans* (Ottesen, 1985). It is the drug of choice for all of these filariases, with the exception of onchocerciasis (see below). Large doses of this drug given for prolonged periods kill or sterilize adult females of these species (except *Onchocerca*) and, therefore, usually are curative. Diethylcarbamazine and its metabolites are not active against microfilariae in vitro. The in vivo microfilaricidal action of diethylcarbamazine is produced by enhanced adhesion of granulocytes to microfilariae through antibody dependent and independent mechanisms (King et al, 1983). The adults of *O. volvulus* must be removed surgically or treated with suramin sodium; otherwise, microfilariae generally reappear a few months after treatment with diethylcarbamazine.

The microfilaricide, ivermectin, is preferred to diethylcarbamazine for onchocerciasis because it can be given in single doses, produces fewer allergic ocular complications, acts more slowly, and does not induce migration of microfilariae to ocular sites (see the evaluation on Ivermectin).

Diethylcarbamazine has been used in the treatment of toxocariasis. It is effective against *Ascaris lumbricoides* but is less useful in patients with strongyloidiasis, paragonimiasis, and dracunculiasis (see Ottesen, 1985). Since more effective drugs are available, diethylcarbamazine generally is not used for therapy of the latter infections.

ADVERSE REACTIONS. Adverse reactions attributable to diethylcarbamazine are usually mild and consist of headache, dizziness, weakness, nausea, and vomiting.

Allergic reactions caused by substances released when microfilariae are damaged or destroyed are usually less deleterious in patients with lymphatic filariases than in those with severe onchocerciasis and loiasis. Effects include pedal edema that may be severe, intense pruritus, dermatitis, fever, colic, arthritis, and lymphadenitis. In patients with lymphatic filariases especially, testicular and spermatic cord pain may be substantial if the dosage is escalated too rapidly. Ocular complications include punctate keratitis, uveitis, retinal pigment atrophy, chorioretinitis, and optic atrophy. Tachycardia sometimes occurs. Allergic encephalopathy (reaction to dead microfilariae) may develop in patients treated for loiasis, especially when large numbers of microfilariae are present. These reactions usually subside within three to seven days, and doses larger than those that initiated the adverse effects may be administered without further problems.

PHARMACOKINETICS. Diethylcarbamazine is absorbed rapidly from the gastrointestinal tract, and its volume of distribution is well in excess of total body water. Peak blood concentrations are reached in approximately four hours. The plasma half-life is approximately 10 to 12 hours. Plasma protein binding is negligible. Diethylcarbamazine is rapidly and extensively metabolized. Renal excretion of unchanged compound (approximately 52% of a dose) and metabolites is complete 48 hours after a single dose and can be reduced by alkalization of the urine. Diethylcarbamazine does not appear in breast milk (Edwards and Breckenridge, 1988).

DOSAGE AND PREPARATIONS. A gradual increase in dosage and/or the concomitant administration of corticosteroids is advisable to minimize allergic effects, particularly when there is ocular involvement in patients with onchocerciasis. If reactions are severe, the dose of diethylcarbamazine should be reduced or treatment interrupted. In general, the dosage used for treatment of filarial infections is determined empirically and has varied considerably. Suggested dosage regimens may be altered to reflect local conditions.

Oral: *Adults*, for infections caused by *Loa loa*, *W. bancrofti*, *B. malayi*, *B. timori*, and *M. perstans:* day 1, 50 mg; day 2, 50 mg three times; day 3, 100 mg three times; day 4 through day 21, 2 mg/kg three times a day. *Children:* day 1, 25 to 50 mg; day 2, 25 to 50 mg three times; day 3, 50 to 100 mg three times; day 4 through day 21, 2 mg/kg three times a day *(Med Lett Drugs Ther*, 1990).

Because severe ocular reactions are likely when treating heavy *O. volvulus* infections, the dosage schedule for either systemic or ocular onchocerciasis is: *Adults*, initially, 25 mg daily for three days, then 50 mg/day for five days, 100 mg/day for three days, and maintenance doses of 150 mg/day for two to three weeks. *Infants and small children*, 0.5 mg/kg three times daily (maximum, 25 mg daily) for three days, 1 mg/kg three times daily (maximum, 50 mg daily) for three or four days; 1.5 mg/kg three times daily (maximum, 100 mg daily) for three or four days, and maintenance doses of 2 mg/

kg three times daily (maximum, 150 mg daily) for two to three weeks. An alternative maintenance dose for adults and children is 3 mg/kg three times daily for three weeks.

See the evaluation on Suramin Sodium for follow-up treatment of onchocerciasis. Some experts believe that heavy *Loa loa* infections should be treated in the same manner as *O. volvulus* infections because of the potential for severe reactions.

Hetrazan (Lederle). Tablets 50 mg (available without charge; see Table 2).

IVERMECTIN (Investigational drug)
[Mectizan]

ACTIONS. Ivermectin, a semisynthetic macrocyclic lactone drug that is produced by an actinomycete, *Streptomyces avermitilis* (Campbell et al, 1983), has nematocidal and ectoparasiticidal actions. It produces flaccid paralysis in nematodes and ectoparasites (insects, ticks, and mites) through inhibition of the neurotransmitter, gamma aminobutyric acid (GABA). It has been postulated that this drug is ineffective against cestodes and trematodes because these parasites do not possess a GABAergic-mediated neuromuscular mechanism for muscle contraction (Campbell et al, 1983).

USES. Ivermectin is the drug of choice in the treatment of onchocerciasis, particularly when there is ocular involvement (for reviews, see Taylor and Greene, 1989; Ette et al, 1990). This orally administered microfilaricide is safe, practical, and well accepted for use in mass treatment eradication programs in onchocerciasis endemic areas (Pacqué et al, 1990, 1991 B; Taylor et al, 1990). Unlike diethylcarbamazine, ivermectin does not penetrate the eye in significant concentrations; therefore, the ocular reaction to dying and damaged microfilariae that is associated with functional visual deficit, ocular changes, and blindness are minimized in heavily infected persons who receive this drug (Dadzie et al, 1987; Taylor et al, 1989). A single oral dose of ivermectin is as effective in reducing the microfilarial load as the standard seven- to ten-day course of diethylcarbamazine. The concentration of microfilariae in the skin of infected persons given an annual dose is sufficiently reduced within one to two years following treatment to interrupt the transmission of *O. volvulus* by the black fly vector (Taylor et al, 1990). However, administration of a single dose once yearly does not appear to be efficacious for treatment of heavily infected persons with severe ocular disease (Rothova et al, 1990). Although an annual dose of 150 mcg/kg does not kill adult worms, data from a recent report showed that the same dose given monthly over a one-year period killed a small proportion of adult male and female worms that were harbored within nodules (Duke et al, 1990).

Although data are limited, ivermectin appears to be as effective as diethylcarbamazine against microfilariae of other filarial parasites, such as *Wuchereria bancrofti* (Kumaraswami et al, 1988; Ottesen et al, 1990; Richards et al, 1991) and *Mansonella ozzardi* (Nutman et al, 1987); its advantages over the latter drug include lower toxicity (both inherent and induced allergic manifestations) and convenience of administration. These factors also enhance patient compliance.

Ivermectin also appears to be effective against strongyloidiasis (Naquira et al, 1989). However, because data are limited, ivermectin should be considered an alternative in patients who cannot tolerate or do not respond to thiabendazole or other benzimidazoles (eg, albendazole, mebendazole).

ADVERSE REACTIONS AND PRECAUTIONS. Single oral doses of 100 to 200 mcg/kg are well tolerated. Fever, glandular tenderness, pruritus, muscle aching, and headaches have been reported. However, the frequency and severity of these symptoms are no greater than these observed in patients given diethylcarbamazine, and they can be controlled by the use of analgesics. The classical acute febrile polyarthritis caused by diethylcarbamazine has not been observed in patients treated with ivermectin. Orthostatic hypotension has been reported but has not required therapeutic intervention.

In rabbits and rats, ivermectin 1.5 mg/kg is neither teratogenic nor fetotoxic; however, the drug produced cleft palate and unexplained maternal mortality in mice when given in doses higher than those used therapeutically in humans. Ivermectin has been found in breast milk of rats. No data are available on the safety of this drug in children under 5 years, in pregnant and lactating women, and in patients with liver disease (for review, see Ette et al, 1990). Pregnant women generally have been excluded from studies of ivermectin in the therapy of filariases. The use of this drug in pregnant women or children under age 5 is not recommended.

PHARMACOKINETICS. Pharmacokinetic data in humans are limited (see Ette et al, 1990). Orally administered ivermectin is well absorbed. Peak plasma concentrations are reached two to four hours after its administration. The drug is widely distributed and is found unchanged in tissues (liver, kidney, fat). The half-life is about 28 hours. The major hepatic metabolite is a hydroxylated derivative; minor hydroxylated derivatives as well as monosaccharide conjugates have been documented in animal studies (Chiu et al, 1986).

DOSAGE AND PREPARATIONS.
Oral: *Adults*, for onchocerciasis, doses as large as 200 mcg/kg have been used, but 150 mcg/kg in a single dose annually appears to be equally effective for reducing microfilarial loads and causes fewer side effects (White et al, 1987). This dose also may be effective in reducing the morbidity of severe onchodermatitis (Pacqué et al, 1991 A). In patients with severe ocular involvement, a single annual dose of 150 mcg/kg may not be sufficient to halt progression of ocular disease (Rothova et al, 1990). Although some data are available to indicate that repeated doses of 150 mcg/kg are well tolerated (Duke et al, 1990), no systematic studies have been performed to assess the efficacy and safety of multiple doses of ivermectin in these patients. Current data suggest that filarial parasitic diseases caused by *W. bancrofti* and *M. ozzardi* are at least as responsive to ivermectin as onchocerciasis. Thus, a single annual dose of ivermectin 20 to 200 mcg/kg may be effective in treating these filariases, and few side effects are associated with the lower doses (Nutman et al, 1987; Kumaraswami et al, 1988; Ottesen et al, 1990; Richards et al, 1991). Therapy may be tailored to reflect local conditions and sensitivities of organisms and patients.

Mectizan (Merck Sharp & Dohme). This drug has been approved by the French Directorate of Pharmacy and Drugs for the treatment of onchocerciasis. Merck Sharp & Dohme distributes it without charge in developing countries where the disease is endemic. The manufacturer and the World Health Organization (Onchocerciasis Control Program) have collaborated in a study in some 140,000 individuals in 12 countries. In the United States, Merck Sharp & Dohme cooperates with the Centers for Disease Control in allowing this organization to distribute the drug free of charge to physicians who register as clinical investigators by completing FDA form FD-1573 (Investigational New Drug) and who have patients with an appropriate indication.

MEBENDAZOLE
[Vermox]

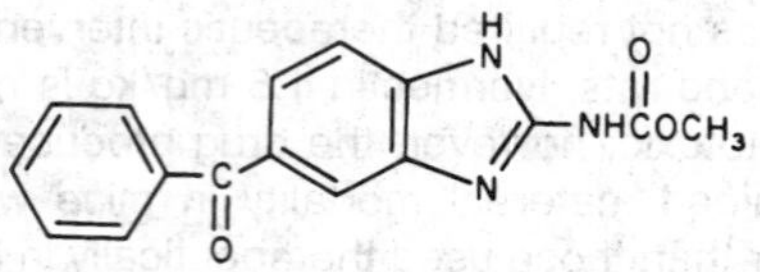

ACTIONS AND USES. Mebendazole is a broad spectrum anthelmintic that inhibits microtubule assembly and irreversibly blocks the uptake of glucose, thereby depleting the parasites' glycogen stores. It is the drug of choice in trichuriasis (whipworm infection). Multiple doses have produced cure rates ranging from 65% to 85% (particularly in children). Retreatment may be necessary in massive whipworm infections (more than 40,000 eggs/g of feces); the drug may decrease the fecal egg count by 70% to 99% even in refractory infections.

Mebendazole also is a drug of choice for treating enterobiasis (pinworm infection); single doses have produced cure rates of 90% to 100%. Cure rates exceeding 85% are attained after multiple doses are given to treat hookworm infections. However, those caused by *N. americanus* may be more responsive to albendazole than to mebendazole if a single-dose regimen is used (Holzer and Frey, 1987).

Mebendazole is very effective in ascariasis, but caution is necessary because worms may be stimulated to migrate to the mouth of heavily infected patients. Pyrantel pamoate is equally effective against ascariasis and also can be considered a drug of choice for this indication.

Because of its broad spectrum of anthelmintic activity, mebendazole may be particularly useful in mixed intestinal nematode infections. In addition, it is given in large doses as alternative therapy for trichinosis (thiabendazole preferred) and is a drug of choice for toxocariasis (thiabendazole alternative drug of choice).

Inoperable cystic hydatid disease caused by *E. granulosus* has been treated successfully with mebendazole, but albendazole is preferred. Mebendazole has not been reliably efficacious in alveolar hydatidosis caused by *E. multilocularis*, and albendazole also is preferred for this disease (see the Introduction and evaluation on Albendazole).

ADVERSE REACTIONS AND PRECAUTIONS. Occasional adverse effects include transient abdominal pain, diarrhea, fever, pruritus, and skin rash.

Reversible neutropenia may occur, especially when larger than usual doses are given to treat echinococcosis (Davis et al, 1986) or trichinosis (Levin et al, 1983).

Teratogenic effects have occurred in rats but not in dogs, sheep, or horses. This anthelmintic is classified in FDA Pregnancy Category C. There is no evidence that mebendazole is secreted in breast milk.

DRUG INTERACTIONS. Mebendazole is reported to increase the secretion of insulin, which potentiates the action of exogenously administered insulin and oral hypoglycemic drugs (Caprio et al, 1984). Carbamazepine and phenytoin decrease the plasma concentration of mebendazole when the latter is used in large doses for the treatment of hydatidosis. Conversely, cimetidine increases the serum concentration of mebendazole by inhibiting its metabolism; therefore, cimetidine has been used to enhance and prolong the effectiveness of mebendazole in the treatment of hydatid cysts (Bekhti and Pirotte, 1987).

PHARMACOKINETICS. Because mebendazole has very low aqueous solubility, it is poorly and variably (< 5% to 10%) absorbed. Oral bioavailability is only 2% to 3% because of very high first-pass elimination (Dawson et al, 1985), but is enhanced by the concomitant ingestion of lipid-containing foods. Following a single oral dose of 10 mg/kg, peak plasma concentrations ranged from 17.5 to 500 ng/ml in 1.5 to 7.5 hours. The mean peak concentration after an initial dose (69.5 ng/ml) increased to 137.4 ng/ml following prolonged therapy (Braithwaite et al, 1982).

The elimination half-life of mebendazole has ranged from 2.8 to 9 hours; however, based on studies in which the drug was given intravenously, these values may be more related to variations in absorption than elimination half-life. The elimination half-life is prolonged in patients with impaired hepatic function. Small amounts of unchanged mebendazole and its major metabolites are eliminated in the urine. Three polar metabolites that undergo extensive enterohepatic recycling have been identified. Mebendazole is highly (95%) bound to plasma protein. Concentrations in tissue and hydatid cyst material from two patients ranged from 59.5 to 206.6 ng/g (Braithwaite et al, 1982).

DOSAGE AND PREPARATIONS.
Oral: *Adults and children,* for uncinariasis, ascariasis, and trichuriasis infections, 100 mg morning and evening for three consecutive days; enterobiasis is usually cured by a single 100-mg dose. If cure is not achieved with initial therapy or if re-exposure is likely, a second course may be given two weeks later (*Med Lett Drugs Ther,* 1990). The manufacturer recommends retreatment three weeks after the initial dose.

For trichinosis, *adults*, 200 to 400 mg three times daily for three days, then 400 to 500 mg three times daily for ten days.

For inoperable echinococcosis caused by *E. granulosus* or *E. multilocularis*, 40 to 50 mg/kg/day in four divided doses for three to eight months to shrink cysts; the same dose can be given for three weeks postoperatively if there is spillage of cyst contents during surgery. The white blood cell count should be monitored frequently, especially during the first few weeks of therapy (Levin et al, 1983). A gradual increase in dosage may be indicated to determine individual tolerance.

Some physicians recommend up to 200 mg/kg/day in four divided doses to achieve a blood concentration of 80 ng/ml, which appears to correlate well with drug efficacy.

Mebendazole has not been extensively investigated in *children under 2 years,* and the relative benefit:risk ratio must be considered when it is used in these patients.

Vermox (Janssen). Tablets (chewable) 100 mg.

METRIFONATE (Investigational drug)

[Bilarcil]

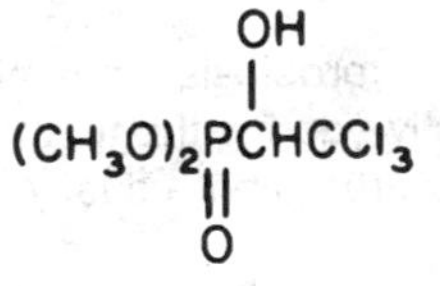

$$(CH_3O)_2P(=O)CH(OH)CCl_3$$

ACTIONS AND USES. Metrifonate, an organophosphorus cholinesterase inhibitor, acts by paralyzing worm musculature. It is slowly metabolized to dichlorvos in man.

Metrifonate is an alternative to praziquantel, the drug of choice, in the treatment of *Schistosoma haematobium* infection. The cure rate with metrifonate in this condition is 70% to 85%.

ADVERSE REACTIONS AND PRECAUTIONS. When it is given in therapeutic doses, metrifonate is usually well tolerated. Side effects usually are mild and transient and include abdominal discomfort, diarrhea, vomiting, weakness, headache, dizziness, and vertigo. These effects probably are unrelated to effects on plasma cholinesterase levels, which are depressed to approximately 5% of pretreatment values within six hours after the drug is administered and return to normal within four to six weeks. Therefore, metrifonate should be avoided when cholinesterase levels are already depressed (eg, in patients with genetic variants, severe liver disease, those living in areas where there is extensive use of organophosphorus insecticides). Furthermore, cholinesterase-inhibiting muscle relaxants should be avoided during surgery in any patient taking metrifonate unless ventilation is assisted.

Organ damage developed in animals after prolonged use of large doses of this drug. Toxicity from overdose is related to metrifonate's anticholinesterase action (see index entry Poisoning.)

DOSAGE AND PREPARATIONS.

Oral: 5 to 15 mg/kg every two weeks for three doses.

Bilarcil (Bayer). Not available in the United States. See Table 2 for foreign sources.

NICLOSAMIDE

[Niclocide]

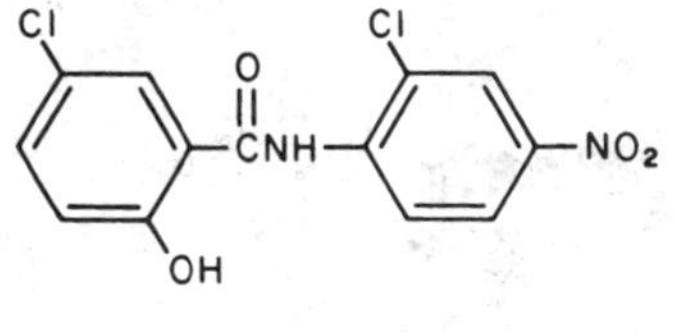

(Structure: 5-chloro-salicyl-CNH- linked to 2-chloro-4-nitrophenyl; labels: Cl, O, CNH, Cl, NO_2, OH)

ACTIONS AND USES. Inhibition of oxidative phosphorylation in the mitochondria of cestodes is the proposed mechanism of action of this anthelmintic. Niclosamide or praziquantel is a drug of choice for intestinal tapeworm infections produced by *Taenia saginata*, *T. solium*, *Diphyllobothrium latum*, and *Dipylidium caninum*. Niclosamide is an alternative to praziquantel for dwarf tapeworm (*H. nana*) infections (the latter drug is preferred because a single-dose regimen is effective).

Niclosamide can be given orally, and its use does not require hospitalization. Concomitant use of a laxative is not necessary except possibly in *T. solium* infections. Niclosamide destroys *T. solium* segments during therapy, releasing viable eggs that theoretically could cause cysticercosis. Therefore, some clinicians suggest that the laxative be administered one to two hours after the anthelmintic to avoid reinfection. However, no documented cases of cysticercosis have occurred with this route.

ADVERSE REACTIONS AND PRECAUTIONS. Absorption of niclosamide from the gastrointestinal tract is minimal and no serious adverse reactions have been reported. Up to 10% of patients may experience malaise, mild abdominal pain, and nausea on the day the drug is administered. Since tapeworm infections generally are not life-threatening, treatment of pregnant women should be postponed until after delivery (FDA Pregnancy Category B).

DOSAGE AND PREPARATIONS. For intestinal tapeworm infections except *H. nana* (eg, diphyllobothriasis, dipylidiasis, taeniasis), the patient should omit breakfast but may eat two hours after the last dose. *The tablets should be chewed thoroughly and swallowed with a little water.*

Oral: *Adults,* 2 g (four tablets) as a single dose. *Children weighing more than 34 kg (75 lb),* 1.5 g (three tablets) as a single dose; *11 to 34 kg (25 to 75 lb),* 1 g (two tablets) as a single dose (*Med Lett Drugs Ther*, 1990).

For *H. nana* infections in *adults,* 2 g (four tablets) on day 1, followed by 1 g (two tablets) daily for six days. *Children weighing more than 34 kg (75 lb),* 1.5 g (three tablets) on day 1, then 1 g (two tablets) daily for six days; *11 to 34 kg (25 to 75 lb),* 1 g (two tablets) on day 1, then 0.5 g (one tablet) for six days (*Med Lett Drugs Ther*, 1990).

Niclocide (Miles). Tablets (chewable) 500 mg.

OXAMNIQUINE

[Vansil]

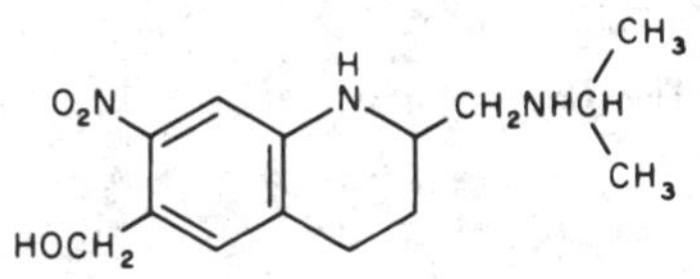

(Structure: tetrahydroquinoline with O_2N, $HOCH_2$, N–H, $CH_2NHCH(CH_3)_2$)

ACTIONS AND USES. The mechanism of action of oxamniquine, a tetrahydroquinoline derivative, is not established. However, it causes muscular paralysis that impairs the adult worm's suckers. This induces a shift of the worms in the liver; males remain in the liver and die, and females return to the mesenteric veins but are incapable of releasing eggs.

Oxamniquine has schistosomicidal activity and is an alternative to praziquantel in the treatment of individuals with *Schistosoma mansoni* infections and for mass treatment and control programs. Although praziquantel is preferred, millions of patients have responded to oxamniquine (Sleigh et al, 1986). This drug can be given intramuscularly as well as orally (the oral route is preferred), and the course of treatment is relatively short. In South America, especially Brazil, a 100% cure rate has been reported following single doses. In Africa, the drug must be administered for several days to produce a 90% to 100% cure rate. Resistance to oxamniquine has been documented in Brazil and Kenya (Yeang et al, 1987).

ADVERSE REACTIONS AND PRECAUTIONS. The most common side effects are dizziness and somnolence. Nausea, vomiting, fever, eosinophilia, transient pulmonary infiltration, liver function test abnormalities, electroencephalographic changes, hallucinations, and seizures also have been reported. Oxamniquine should not be given to patients with epilepsy, decompensated congestive heart failure, or renal failure. Orange discoloration of the urine may occur.

Although there is no evidence showing that oxamniquine is teratogenic or carcinogenic, these effects have been reported with related compounds. Thus, this drug should not be given to pregnant women (FDA Pregnancy Category C).

PHARMACOKINETICS. Oxamniquine is well absorbed after oral administration, and time to peak plasma concentration is about three hours. The presence of food in the gastrointestinal tract may retard absorption and reduce plasma concentrations of the drug. Most of an administered dose is extensively metabolized to inactive compounds in the liver, principally by a first-pass mechanism, and approximately 70% of a dose is excreted in the urine. The elimination half-life of parent drug is 1 to 2.5 hours.

DOSAGE AND PREPARATIONS. Intrinsic differences in organism susceptibility in various endemic areas must be taken into consideration when determining dosage.

Oral: *Adults (western hemisphere),* 15 mg/kg as a single dose given after a meal or late in the day to minimize side effects; *(East Africa),* 15 mg/kg twice daily for one day; (*Egypt and South Africa*), 15 mg/kg twice daily for two days. *Children (western hemisphere),* 20 mg/kg in two equally divided doses two to eight hours apart; *(Africa)* 15 mg/kg twice daily for two days.

Intramuscular: *(South America only),* 7.5 mg/kg as a single dose given after a meal or late in the day.

Vansil (Pfizer). Capsules 250 mg.

PIPERAZINE CITRATE

[Vermizine]

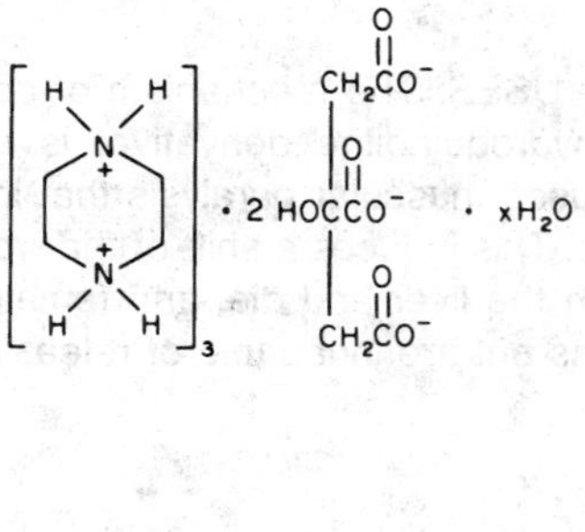

ACTIONS AND USES. Piperazine citrate causes reversible muscle paralysis in intestinal nematodes, presumably by causing hyperpolarization of nerve endings. It is an alternative drug for the treatment of ascariasis and enterobiasis. Pyrantel pamoate or mebendazole is preferred to piperazine citrate for therapy of both infections. A single dose of piperazine citrate cures approximately 70% of individuals with ascariasis. Two doses given on successive days increase the cure rate to between 90% and 100%. Roundworms are passed, paralyzed and alive, one to three days after treatment. Although a laxative is not needed, it may help to expel the worms from the gut.

In patients with enterobiasis, the majority of worms are passed alive and active during the first four days of therapy. A seven-day course of treatment usually is needed for optimal effects.

ADVERSE REACTIONS AND PRECAUTIONS. Therapeutic doses do not usually cause adverse effects, but nausea, vomiting, diarrhea, and allergic reactions may develop. With larger doses, as in inadvertent overdosage or when the drug accumulates in the presence of renal insufficiency, muscular incoordination or weakness, vertigo, dysphasia, confusion, and myoclonic contractions have been reported. These effects usually disappear when the drug is discontinued. Piperazine citrate may induce or exacerbate epileptic seizures in predisposed patients. For these reasons, it is contraindicated in patients with renal or hepatic insufficiency or epilepsy.

No harmful effects on the fetus have been reported after use of piperazine citrate in pregnant women.

PHARMACOKINETICS. Information on the pharmacokinetics of this drug is limited. Piperazine citrate is rapidly absorbed from the small intestine. A substantial proportion of a dose is eliminated unchanged in the urine within 24 hours (Edwards and Breckenridge, 1988).

DOSAGE AND PREPARATIONS. (Doses and strengths expressed in terms of the hexahydrate salt that is formed in solution from the citrate salt.)

Oral: For ascariasis, *adults and children*, 75 mg/kg (maximum, 3.5 g) once daily for two consecutive days. For enterobiasis, *adults and children,* 65 mg/kg (maximum, 2.5 g) once daily for seven consecutive days. The course should be repeated after a one-week interval. Fasting before treatment is not necessary.

Generic. Syrup 500 mg/5 ml; tablets 250 mg.

Vermizine (Vortech). Syrup 500 mg/5 ml.

PRAZIQUANTEL

[Biltricide]

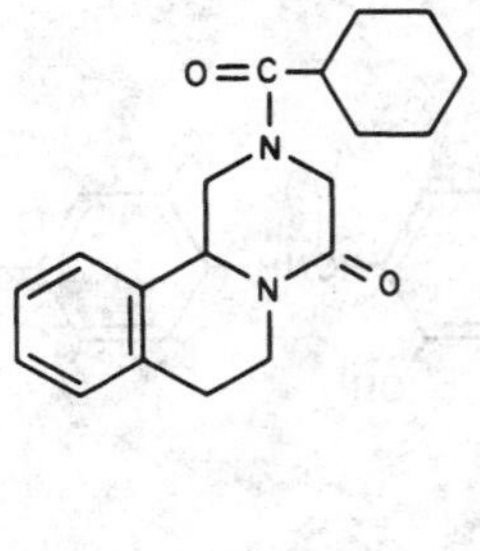

ACTIONS. Praziquantel, a pyrazinoisoquinoline, has a broad spectrum of activity against trematodes (flukes) and cestodes (tapeworms) (for review, see King and Mahmoud, 1989). It causes efflux of intracellular calcium resulting in tetanic paralysis and subsequent dislodgement of worms from their various sites of attachment. Bleb formation on the worm integument is followed by extensive vacuolization and rupture, which appears to facilitate phagocytic attachment and lysis of the parasite.

USES. ***Schistosomiasis (Blood Flukes):*** Praziquantel is the drug of choice for treating all pathogenic *Schistosoma* infections in man, ie, those caused by *S. mansoni, S. haematobium, S. japonicum, S. mekongi,* and *S. intercalatum* (Nash et al, 1982; Pearson and Guerrant, 1983; Weniger and Schantz, 1984; King and Mahmoud, 1989). Alternative chemotherapy for *S. mansoni* (oxamniquine) and *S. haematobium* (metrifonate) infections are available if other factors militate against the use of praziquantel.

Praziquantel is equally effective in both acute and chronic schistosomiasis. End-stage hepatic fibrosis is not reversed by drug treatment; however, the pathogenic process usually can be halted and fecal egg counts markedly reduced or eliminated. Standard single-day therapy is safe and very effective in cerebral schistosomiasis (Watt et al, 1986).

Clonorchiasis, Opisthorchiasis, Fascioliasis, Paragonimiasis, Fasciolopsiasis: A single oral dose of praziquantel is considered the treatment of choice in infections caused by *Clonorchis* and *Opisthorchis* species (Chinese or Oriental liver flukes) (O'Keefe and Edgett, 1986; Yangco et al, 1987). A second course of therapy occasionally is necessary to effect a cure. It has been suggested that praziquantel replace bithionol as the drug of choice in the treatment of paragonimiasis (Pachucki et al, 1984). Limited data show that praziquantel is probably more effective than tetrachloroethylene in treating fasciolopsiasis (Bunnag et al, 1983), and it has been effective in fascioliasis (Schiappacasse et al, 1985).

Diphyllobothriasis, Dipylidiasis, Hymenolepiasis, Taeniasis: Praziquantel is as effective as niclosamide and appears to be quite safe in treating intestinal infections caused by *Taenia saginata, T. solium*, *Diphyllobothrium latum*, and *Dipylidium caninum*. Doses as low as 2.5 mg/kg are effective against taeniasis and may be safer and more economical for community-based mass treatment programs (Pawlowski, 1990). In dwarf tapeworm infection, a single dose of praziquantel seems to be as effective as a seven-day regimen of niclosamide. Thus, praziquantel is the drug of choice in treating patients with hymenolepiasis.

Cysticercosis: Praziquantel is effective in the treatment of cysticercosis caused by *Taenia solium* when it is given daily for two weeks (Del Brutto and Sotelo, 1988; Sotelo et al, 1990; Cruz et al, 1991). Albendazole is preferred for therapy of parenchymal cysticercosis because it has equivalent activity and can be given in a shorter course than praziquantel (Sotelo et al, 1990). Adjunctive therapy with antiepileptic drugs, corticosteroids, and/or surgery may be required. Praziquantel is only partially effective or ineffective in patients with a malignant form of the disease (cysticercotic encephalitis). When cysts are located in the ventricular fluid, surgery or albendazole is a more definitive treatment (Vasconcelos et al, 1987).

ADVERSE REACTIONS AND PRECAUTIONS. The following adverse reactions have been associated with the use of large doses of praziquantel. Dizziness, headache, malaise, abdominal pain, and nausea are relatively common but generally mild and transient. Lassitude, diarrhea, urticaria, pruritus, fever, sweating, pruritic rash, and mild to moderate increases in AST and ALT levels occur less frequently, but also are usually transient and reversible. Vomiting also may occur.

Praziquantel is related chemically to sedative and antianxiety agents. Because drowsiness develops relatively frequently, the patient should be advised to use caution while driving or performing activities that require mental alertness until one day after the last dose is taken.

A syndrome consisting of headache, hyperthermia, seizures, intracranial hypertension, and/or arachnoiditis develops in many patients given praziquantel for neurocysticercosis, especially in those with multiple brain cysts. This syndrome is presumed to result from an inflammatory response to dead and dying organisms in cerebrospinal fluid and central nervous system tissue. The symptoms may be prevented by prior and/or concurrent corticosteroid therapy. Since destruction of parasites within the eye may cause irreparable lesions, the use of praziquantel in the treatment of ocular cysticercosis is contraindicated.

No serious drug interactions have been reported.

Experience with acute praziquantel overdosage in humans is limited. The oral LD_{50} in animals ranges from 1 to 2.8 g/kg.

The safety of praziquantel in children under 4 years has not been established.

PREGNANCY AND LACTATION. Reproduction studies performed in rats and rabbits using up to 40 times the human dose revealed no evidence of impaired fertility or harm to the fetus. The abortion rate in rats increased when three times the single human therapeutic dose was given. There are no well-controlled studies in pregnant women. This drug should be used during pregnancy only if clearly needed (FDA Pregnancy Category B).

Praziquantel appears unchanged in human breast milk in concentrations about one-fourth those in maternal serum. Women should not nurse on the day praziquantel is given and for 72 hours thereafter.

PHARMACOKINETICS. About 80% of an oral dose is absorbed; however, extensive first-pass hepatic hydroxylation occurs and probably accounts for considerable interindividual variation in pharmacokinetics (Ofori-Adjei et al, 1988). A single 50-mg oral dose in healthy adults results in peak serum concentrations of 1 mcg/ml of unchanged drug in one to two hours. The anthelmintic activity of metabolites is less than that of the parent drug. Distribution in the tissues is not well documented, but the concentration in cerebrospinal fluid is 10% to 20% of that in the serum (free and bound).

Hepatic metabolites of praziquantel are excreted (80%) in the urine. The unchanged drug has a serum half-life of 0.8 to 1.5 hours. This may be extended in some individuals. Metabolites have a half-life of four to five hours. A higher plasma concentration that is associated with a higher incidence of side effects occurs in those with hepatic disease (Watt et al, 1988).

DOSAGE AND PREPARATIONS. Since praziquantel has a bitter taste, the tablets should not be chewed before swallowing to avoid gagging and emesis.

Oral: For *Schistosoma intercalatum, S. japonicum,* and *S. mekongi* infections, *adults and children over 4 years,* 60 mg/kg in three equal doses separated by not less than four or more than six hours. For *S. haematobium* and *S. mansoni* infections, *adults and children over 4 years,* 40 mg/kg in two doses separated by not less than four or more than six hours.

For clonorchiasis, fascioliasis, fasciolopsiasis, opisthorchiasis, and paragonimiasis, *adults and children over 4 years*, 75 mg/kg daily given in three equal doses separated by not less than four or more than six hours. The drug is given for one day in clonorchiasis, fascioliasis, fasciolopsiasis, and opisthorchiasis and for one to three days in paragonimiasis; the course may be repeated for clonorchiasis, fascioliasis, or opisthorchiasis if required.

For taeniasis, diphyllobothriasis, and dipylidiasis, *adults and children over 4 years*, 10 to 20 mg/kg in a single dose.

For hymenolepiasis, *adults and children over 4 years*, 25 mg/kg in a single dose.

For cysticercosis, *adults and children over 4 years*, 50 mg/kg/day in three equal doses every four to six hours for 14 days. Concomitant corticosteroid treatment (eg, dexamethasone 6 to 16 mg daily, prednisone 30 to 40 mg daily) is recommended in selected patients with cerebral involvement and elevated intracranial pressure. Therapy may be repeated in three to six months if necessary.

Biltricide (Miles). Tablets 600 mg.

PYRANTEL PAMOATE

[Antiminth]

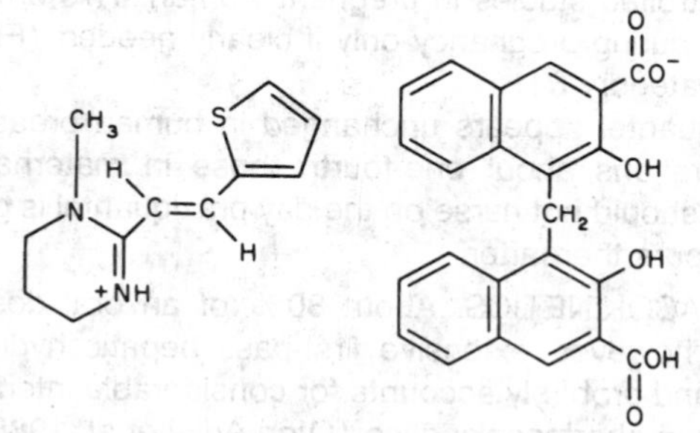

ACTIONS AND USES. Pyrantel pamoate acts as a depolarizing neuromuscular blocking agent that paralyzes the worms, which are then expelled from the body, usually without requiring the adjunctive use of a laxative. It is a drug of choice for therapy of ascariasis and enterobiasis; cure rates are 90% to 100% following a single dose. Most authorities consider pyrantel pamoate to be a drug of choice for uncinariasis (hookworm infections). Cure rates ranging from 48% to 93% for infections caused by *Necator americanus* and 92% to 93% for those due to *Ancylostoma duodenale* have been reported with conventional doses. This drug is not used in therapy of trichuriasis (whipworm) and strongyloidiasis (threadworm). Pyrantel pamoate kills only the adult form of *Trichinella spiralis*; it has no effect on encysted larvae.

ADVERSE REACTIONS AND PRECAUTIONS. Systemic adverse reactions to pyrantel pamoate include anorexia, nausea, headache, dizziness, drowsiness, and rash. Other untoward effects that probably result from local activity in the gut are abdominal pain, vomiting, and diarrhea. Transient elevation of the AST level may occur; therefore, pyrantel pamoate should be used with caution in patients with pre-existing liver dysfunction.

There has been little experience with the drug in children under 2 years, and its safety during pregnancy has not been determined.

PHARMACOKINETICS. Pyrantel pamoate is poorly and incompletely absorbed from the gastrointestinal tract; most of an oral dose is excreted unchanged in the feces and about 7% is excreted unchanged in the urine. Significant amounts have not been detected in breast milk.

DOSAGE AND PREPARATIONS. (Dosage expressed in terms of the base)

Oral: *Adults and children,* for ascariasis and enterobiasis, a single dose of 11 mg/kg (maximum, 1 g); for enterobiasis, the dose is repeated after two weeks. For uncinariasis, the above dose is given for three consecutive days. Fasting before treatment is not necessary. For the intestinal stage of trichinosis, 10 mg/kg daily for four days.

Antiminth (Pfizer). Oral suspension 250 mg/5 ml (equivalent to base).

SURAMIN SODIUM (Investigational drug)

[Fourneau 309]

For chemical formula, see index entry Suramin, In Trypanosomiasis.

USES. Suramin sodium, a complex derivative of urea, is used parenterally in the treatment of African trypanosomiasis (see index entry Trypanosomiasis). It also has been used with diethylcarbamazine citrate to kill the adult forms of *Onchocerca volvulus.* Multiple doses of suramin sodium kill adult female *O. volvulus* within two to four months, but males remain alive longer. Microfilariae disappear over a period of several months. The mechanism of action of suramin sodium is unknown. Ivermectin is the drug of choice for onchocerciasis.

ADVERSE REACTIONS AND PRECAUTIONS. The need for multiple doses and the potentially dangerous adverse reactions limit the usefulness of suramin sodium; close medical supervision during treatment is essential.

Suramin sodium may cause nausea, vomiting, colic, urticaria, severe local irritation or extravasation, and, in very sensitive persons, shock, syncope, acute circulatory failure, and seizures. Because suramin sodium has some microfilaricidal activity, allergic reactions to proteins released by degenerating microfilariae (eg, pruritus, rash, fever, edema, burning and hyperesthesia of the soles, photophobia, iritis, lacrimation) occur but generally are less intense than those that develop in patients treated with diethylcarbamazine. It is advisable to reduce the microfilarial load by treatment with ivermectin prior to initiating therapy with suramin. This drug may cause albuminuria, casts, hematuria, and, rarely, agranulocytosis or hemolytic anemia, exfoliative dermatitis, chronic diarrhea, nephritis, and renal failure. It is contraindicated in patients with severe renal or ocular disease.

PHARMACOKINETICS. Since suramin sodium is not absorbed from the gastrointestinal tract, it must be administered parenterally. It is extensively and tightly bound to plasma protein; low plasma concentrations persist for as long as three months after terminating administration. Suramin is taken up by Kupffer's cells of the liver and epithelial cells of the proximal convoluted tubule of the kidney.

DOSAGE AND PREPARATIONS.
Intravenous: A 10% solution in water for injection is used. For onchocerciasis, *adults,* 100 mg initially to test tolerance, then 1 g weekly for five weeks. The total dose should not exceed 5.5 g, since larger doses may cause renal toxicity. *Children,* 100 mg initially to test tolerance, then 10 to 15 mg/kg weekly for five weeks. Severe local irritation results from extravasation. Suramin may be administered intramuscularly, but only if the intravenous route is contraindicated or not feasible.

Fourneau 309. Available from the Drug Service, Centers for Disease Control only for the treatment of African trypanosomiasis (see the Introduction for address and telephone numbers).

THIABENDAZOLE
[Mintezol]

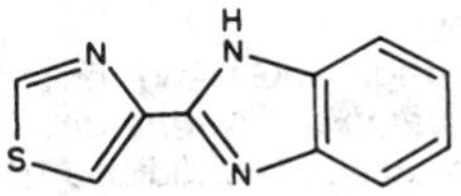

ACTIONS AND USES. It has been suggested that thiabendazole acts by inhibiting the helminth-specific enzyme, fumarate reductase. However, recent evidence suggests that, like other benzimidazoles (eg, albendazole, mebendazole), it inhibits microtubule assembly.

Thiabendazole is a broad spectrum drug that is ovicidal and larvicidal, and it is the drug of choice for the treatment of *Strongyloides stercoralis* (threadworm) infection. It may be lifesaving in patients with disseminated strongyloidiasis (hyperinfection syndrome), which occurs primarily in those who are immunocompromised for any reason. It also is the drug of choice for oral and topical therapy of cutaneous larva migrans caused by *Ancylostoma braziliense* and is an alternative drug for oral therapy in toxocariasis due to *Toxocara canis* and *T. cati*. However, a recent report suggests that oral albendazole, a less toxic benzimidazole carbamate, is effective for cutaneous larva migrans (Jones et al, 1990) and thus may be preferred.

Thiabendazole is the drug of choice in patients with trichinosis. It reduces the number of developing and migrating larvae of *Trichinella spiralis*; activity also has been demonstrated against adult female *T. spiralis* in the intestine. Thiabendazole is ineffective against encysted larvae.

Although this drug is effective in treating other nematode infections (ie, ascariasis, enterobiasis, trichuriasis, uncinariasis), safer and more effective drugs are available. Thiabendazole should be used for these infections only if the preferred drugs are unavailable or contraindicated.

ADVERSE REACTIONS AND PRECAUTIONS. Common untoward effects of thiabendazole are dizziness, drowsiness, giddiness, anorexia, nausea, and vomiting. Diarrhea, fever, epigastric distress, flushing, chills, angioedema, pruritus, lethargy, rash, and headache occur less frequently. Additional adverse reactions include tinnitus, conjunctival injection, blurred vision, hypotension, syncope, anaphylaxis, numbness, seizures, transient leukopenia, lymphadenopathy, enuresis, hyperglycemia, cholestasis probably due to a hypersensitivity-mediated idiosyncratic reaction, xanthopsia, crystalluria, and hematuria. A few cases of erythema multiforme and Stevens-Johnson syndrome have been reported.

Thiabendazole should be used cautiously in patients with impaired liver or kidney function. It may interfere with the metabolism of xanthine derivatives and increase the blood concentration of theophylline (Schneider et al, 1990).

The safety of this drug during pregnancy and lactation has not been established (FDA Pregnancy Category C).

PHARMACOKINETICS. Thiabendazole is well absorbed after oral administration; time to peak plasma concentration is about one hour. Much of the drug is metabolized to 5-hydroxythiabendazole, which is then conjugated to form a glucuronide or sulfate. The inactive metabolites are excreted in the urine within 24 hours.

DOSAGE AND PREPARATIONS.
Oral: *Adults and children,* for strongyloidiasis, 25 mg/kg twice daily (maximum, 3 g/day) for two successive days. In some studies, a significant number of patients required more than two days of therapy to achieve negative stool samples; follow-up stool samples should be obtained. Therapy should be continued for at least five days in patients with disseminated infections (hyperinfection syndrome). Immunocompromised patients may require more prolonged therapy.

For patients with cutaneous larva migrans, topical therapy alone is preferred except when lesions are widespread. (A topical formulation is not available; however, the tablets may be crushed and compounded in a 15% water-soluble base or petroleum jelly and applied three times daily for five days. Alternatively, if available, the oral suspension can be applied directly on a 5- to 7.5-cm area over the end of the larval burrow or tunnel in the skin three times daily for five days.) If oral therapy is required, 25 mg/kg is given twice daily (maximum, 3 g/day) for two to five successive days. (This dose may have to be reduced because of toxicity.) If active lesions are still present two days after completion of therapy, a second course is recommended. Concomitant topical therapy also is recommended.

For toxocariasis, 25 mg/kg is given twice daily (maximum, 3 g/day) for five successive days. For trichinosis, 25 mg/kg is given twice daily for five successive days. When the drug is used to treat trichinosis or toxocariasis involving the eye, concomitant administration of corticosteroids may be needed to minimize the severe inflammatory reaction to the dying larvae.

For ascariasis, enterobiasis, trichuriasis, and uncinariasis, 25 mg/kg is given twice daily (maximum, 3 g/day) for two successive days.

Mintezol (Merck Sharp & Dohme). Suspension (oral) 500 mg/5 ml; tablets (chewable) 500 mg.

Cited References

After smallpox, guineaworm? editorial. *Lancet* 1:161-162, 1983.

Drugs for parasitic infections. *Med Lett Drugs Ther* 32:23-32, 1990.

Update: Dracunculiasis Eradication—Worldwide, 1989. *MMWR* 38:882-885, 1990.

Update: Dracunculiasis Eradication—Ghana and Nigeria, 1990. *MMWR* 40:245-247, 1991 A.

Trichinella spiralis infection—United States, 1990. *MMWR* 40:57-60, 1991 B.

Ammann RW, et al: Recurrence rate after discontinuation of long-term mebendazole therapy in alveolar echinococcosis (preliminary results). *Am J Trop Med Hyg* 43:506-515, 1990.

Baird JK, et al: North American brugian filariasis: Report of nine infections of humans. *Am J Trop Med Hyg* 35:1205-1209, 1986.

Bekhti A, Pirotte J: Cimetidine increases serum mebendazole concentrations: Implications for treatment of hepatic hydatid cysts. *Br J Clin Pharm* 24:390-392, 1987.

Berk SL, et al: Clinical and epidemiologic features of strongyloidiasis: Prospective study in rural Tennessee. *Arch Intern Med* 147:1257-1261, 1987.

Braithwaite PA, et al: Clinical pharmacokinetics of high dose mebendazole in patients treated for cystic hydatid disease. *Eur J Clin Pharmacol* 22:161-169, 1982.

Bunnag D, et al: Field trial on treatment of fasciolopsiasis with praziquantel. *Southeast Asian J Trop Med Public Health* 14:216-219, 1983.

Campbell WC, et al: Ivermectin: A potent new antiparasitic agent. *Science* 221:823-828, 1983.

Caprio S, et al: Improvement of metabolic control in diabetic patients during mebendazole administration: Preliminary studies. *Diabetologia* 27:52-55, 1984.

Chiu S-HL, et al: Metabolic disposition of ivermectin in tissues of cattle, sheep, and rats. *Drug Metab Disp* 14:590-600, 1986.

Ciferri F: Human pulmonary dirofilariasis in the United States: Critical review. *Am J Trop Med Hyg* 31:302-308, 1982.

Cook GC: *Strongyloides stercoralis* hyperinfection syndrome: How often is it missed? *Q J Med* 64:625-629, 1987.

Crimmins D, et al: Neurocysticercosis: An under-recognized cause of neurological problems. *Med J Aust* 152:434-438, 1990.

Cruz M, et al: Albendazole versus praziquantel in the treatment of cerebral cysticercosis: Clinical evaluation. *Trans R Soc Trop Med Hyg* 85:244-247, 1991.

Dadzie KY, et al: Ocular findings in a double-blind study of ivermectin versus diethylcarbamazine versus placebo in the treatment of onchocerciasis. *Br J Ophthalmol* 71:78-85, 1987.

Davidson RA, et al: Risk factors for strongyloidiasis: Case-control study. *Arch Intern Med* 144:321-324, 1984.

Davis A, et al: Multicentre clinical trials of benzimidazolecarbamates in human echinococcosis. *Bull WORLD Health Organ* 64:383-388, 1986.

Davis A, et al: Multicentre clinical trials of benzimidazole-carbamates in human cystic echinococcosis (phase 2). *Bull WORLD Health Organ* 67:503-508, 1989.

Dawson M, et al: Pharmacokinetics and bioavailability of tracer dose of [^{3}H]-mebendazole in man. *Br J Clin Pharmacol* 19:79-86, 1985.

DeCock KM: Hepatosplenic schistosomiasis: Clinical review. *Gut* 27:734-745, 1986.

Del Brutto OH, Sotelo J: Neurocysticercosis: An update. *Rev Infect Dis* 10:1075-1087, 1988.

De Rosa F, Teggi A: Treatment of *Echinococcus granulosus* hydatid disease with albendazole. *Ann Trop Med Parasitol* 84:467-472, 1990.

DeVault GA Jr, et al: Opportunistic infections with *Strongyloides stercoralis* in renal transplantation. *Rev Infect Dis* 12:653-671, 1990.

Duke BOL, et al: Effects of multiple monthly doses of ivermectin on adult *Onchocerca volvulus*. *Am J Trop Med Hyg* 43:657-664, 1990.

Earnest MP, et al: Neurocysticercosis in the United States: 35 cases and a review. *Rev Infect Dis* 9:961-979, 1987.

Edwards G: Recent advances in chemotherapy of onchocerciasis. *TIPS* 192-195, (May) 1984.

Edwards G, Breckenridge AM: Clinical pharmacokinetics of anthelmintic drugs. *Clin Pharmacokinet* 15:67-93, 1988.

Ellis GS Jr, et al: *Toxocara canis* infestation: Clinical and epidemiological associations with seropositivity in kindergarten children. *Ophthalmology* 93:1032-1037, 1986.

Escobedo F, et al: Albendazole therapy for neurocysticercosis. *Arch Intern Med* 147:738-741, 1987.

Ette EI, et al: Ivermectin: A long-acting microfilaricidal agent. *DICP* 24:426-433, 1990.

Fagbemi BO, Hillyer GV: Immunodiagnosis of dracunculiasis by Falcon assay screening test-enzyme-linked immunosorbent assay (FAST-ELISA) and by enzyme-linked immunoelectrotransfer blot (EITB) technique. *Am J Trop Med Hyg* 43:665-668, 1990.

Fourestié V, et al: Randomized trial of albendazole versus tiabendazole plus flubendazole during an outbreak of human trichinellosis. *Parasitol Res* 75:36-41, 1988.

Genta RM: Global prevalence of strongyloidiasis: Critical review with epidemiologic insights into the prevention of disseminated disease. *Rev Infect Dis* 11:755-767, 1989.

Genta RM, et al: Strongyloidiasis in US veterans of the Vietnam and other wars. *JAMA* 258:49-52, 1987.

Glickman LT, et al: Serologic diagnosis of zoonotic pulmonary dirofilariasis. *Am J Med* 80:161-164, 1986.

Golematis B, et al: Albendazole in the conservative management of multiple hydatid disease. *Mt Sinai J Med* 56:53-55, 1989.

Greene BM, et al: A comparison of 6-, 12-, and 24-monthly dosing with ivermectin for treatment of onchocerciasis. *J Infect Dis* 163:376-380, 1991.

Hagan P, et al: Human IgE, IgG4 and resistance to reinfection with *Schistosoma haematobium*. *Nature* 349:243-245, 1991.

Hamrick HJ, et al: Two cases of dipylidiasis (dog tapeworm infection) in children: Update on old problem. *Pediatrics* 72:114-117, 1983.

Hess JA, et al: Comparative efficacy of ketoconazole and mebendazole in experimental trichinosis. *Antimicrob Agents Chemother* 30:953-954, 1986.

Hicks RM: Canopic worm: Role of bilharziasis in aetiology of human bladder cancer. *J R Soc Med* 76:16-22, 1983.

Holzer BR, Frey FJ: Differential efficacy of mebendazole and albendazole against *Necator americanus* but not for *Trichuris trichiura* infestations. *Eur J Clin Pharmacol* 32:635-637, 1987.

Homeida MA, et al: Effect of antischistosomal chemotherapy on prevalence of Symmers' periportal fibrosis in Sudanese villages. *Lancet* 2:437-440, 1988.

Horton RJ: Chemotherapy of *Echinococcus* infection in man with albendazole. *Trans R Soc Trop Med Hyg* 83:97-102, 1989.

Imtiaz R, et al: Permanent disability from dracunculiasis. *Lancet* 336:630, 1990.

Jagota SC: Albendazole, a broad-spectrum anthelmintic, in the treatment of intestinal nematode and cestode infection: A multicenter study in 480 patients. *Clin Therapeut* 8:226-231, 1986.

Jones SK, et al: Oral albendazole for the treatment of cutaneous larva migrans. *Br J Dermatol* 122:99-101, 1990.

Khuroo MS, et al: Hepatobiliary and pancreatic ascariasis in India. *Lancet* 335:1503-1506, 1990.

King CH: Acute and chronic schistosomiasis. *Hosp Pract* 26:117-130, 1991.

King CH, Mahmoud AAF: Drugs five years later: Praziquantel. *Ann Intern Med* 110:290-296, 1989.

King CH, et al: Diethylcarbamazine citrate, antifilarial drug, stimulates human granulocyte adherence. *Antimicrob Agents Chemother* 24:453-456, 1983.

King CH, et al: Chemotherapy-based control of schistosomiasis haematobia: II, Metrifonate vs. praziquantel in control of infection-associated morbidity. *Am J Trop Med Hyg* 42:587-595, 1990.

Kocięcka W, et al: Clinical evaluation of albendazole in the therapy of human trichinellosis. *Wiad Parazytol* 35:457-465, 1989.

Kramer MR, et al: Disseminated strongyloidiasis in AIDS and non-AIDS immunocompromised hosts: Diagnosis by sputum and bronchoalveolar lavage. *South Med J* 83:1226-1229, 1990.

Kumaraswami V, et al: Ivermectin for the treatment of *Wuchereria bancrofti* filariasis. *JAMA* 259-3150-3153, 1988.

Kune GA, et al: Hydatid disease in Australia: Prevention, clinical presentation, and treatment. *Med J Aust* 2:385-388, 1983.

Levin ML: Treatment of trichinosis with mebendazole. *Am J Trop Med Hyg* 32:980-983, 1983.

Levin MH, et al: Severe, reversible neutropenia during high-dose mebendazole therapy for echinococcosis. *JAMA* 249:2929-2931, 1983.

Loutan L, et al: Single treatment of invasive fascioliasis with triclabendazole. *Lancet* 2:383, 1989.

Madrazo I, et al: Intraventricular cysticercosis. *Neurosurgery* 12:148-152, 1983.

Mahmoud AAF: Praziquantel for the treatment of helminthic infections. *Adv Intern Med* 32:193-206, 1987.

Maisonneuve H, et al: A pediatric suspension of albendazole in the treatment of ascariasis, ancylostomiasis and trichuriasis (167 patients). *Curr Ther Res* 36:404-408, 1984.

Messaritakis J, et al: High mebendazole doses in pulmonary and hepatic hydatid disease. *Arch Dis Child* 66:532-533, 1991.

Mitchell WG, Crawford TO: Intraparenchymal cerebral cysticercosis in children: Diagnosis and treatment. *Pediatrics* 82:76-82, 1988.

Monson MH: Praziquantel in acute schistosomiasis. *Trans R Soc Trop Med Hyg* 81:777, 1987.

Morris DL, et al: Albendazole: Objective evidence of response in human hydatid disease. *JAMA* 253:2053-2057, 1985.

Morris DL, et al: Penetration of albendazole sulphoxide into hydatid cysts. *Gut* 28:75-80, 1987.

Nahmias J, et al: Evaluation of albendazole, pyrantel, bephenium, pyrantel-praziquantel and pyrantel-bephenium for single-dose mass treatment of necatoriasis. *Ann Trop Med Parasitol* 83:625-629, 1989.

Nanduri J, Kazura JW: Clinical and laboratory aspects of filariasis. *Clin Microbiol Rev* 2:39-50, 1989.

Naquira C, et al: Ivermectin for human strongyloidiasis and other intestinal helminths. *Am J Trop Med Hyg* 40:304-309, 1989.

Nash TE, et al: Schistosome infections in humans: Perspectives and recent findings. *Ann Intern Med* 97:740-754, 1982.

Nelson GS: Human onchocerciasis: Notes on the history, the parasite and the life cycle. *Ann Trop Med Parasitol* 85:83-95, 1991.

Nutman TB, et al: Ivermectin in the successful treatment of a patient with *Mansonella ozzardi* infection. *J Infect Dis* 156:662-665, 1987.

Nutman TB, et al: Diethylcarbamazine prophylaxis for human loiasis: Results of a double-blind study. *N Engl J Med* 319:752-756, 1988.

Ofori-Adjei D, et al: Oral praziquantel kinetics in normal and *Schistosoma haematobium*-infected subjects. *Ther Drug Monitor* 10:45-49, 1988.

O'Keefe P, Edgett H: Efficacy and safety of praziquantel in treatment of *Clonorchis sinensis/Opisthorchis viverrini:* Results of double-blind, placebo-controlled trial in Southeast Asian refugees. *Curr Ther Res* 40:411-417, 1986.

Ottesen EA: Efficacy of diethylcarbamazine in eradicating infection with lymphatic-dwelling filariae in humans. *Rev Infect Dis* 7:341-356, 1985.

Ottesen EA, et al: A controlled trial of ivermectin and diethylcarbamazine in lymphatic filariasis. *N Engl J Med* 322:1113-1117, 1990.

Pachucki CT, et al: American paragonimiasis treated with praziquantel. *N Engl J Med* 311:582-583, 1984.

Pacqué M, et al: Safety of and compliance with community-based ivermectin therapy. *Lancet* 335:1377-1380, 1990.

Pacqué M, et al: Improvement in severe onchocercal skin disease after a single dose of ivermectin. *Am J Med* 90:590-594, 1991 A.

Pacqué M, et al: Community-based treatment of onchocerciasis with ivermectin: Safety, efficacy, and acceptability of yearly treatment. *J Infect Dis* 163:381-385, 1991 B.

Pamba HO, et al: Albendazole (Zentel) in the treatment of helminthiasis in children below two years of age: A preliminary report. *East Afr Med J* 448-452, (July) 1987.

Pawlowski ZS: Efficacy of low doses of praziquantel in taeniasis. *Acta Trop* 48:83-88, 1990.

Pearson RD, Guerrant RL: Praziquantel: Major advance in anthelmintic therapy. *Ann Intern Med* 99:195-198, 1983.

Rausch RL, et al: Spontaneous death of *Echinococcus multilocularis*: Cases diagnosed serologically (by EM_2 ELISA) and clinical significance. *Am J Trop Med Hyg* 36:576-585, 1987.

Richards FO Jr, et al: Comparison of high dose ivermectin and diethylcarbamazine for activity against bancroftian filariasis in Haiti. *Am J Trop Med Hyg* 44:3-10, 1991.

Rothova A, et al: Ocular involvement in patients with onchocerciasis after repeated treatment with ivermectin. *Am J Ophthalmol* 110:6-16, 1990.

Saimot AG, et al: Albendazole as potential treatment for human hydatidosis. *Lancet* 2:652-656, 1983.

Schiappacasse RH, et al: Successful treatment of severe infection with *Fasciola hepatica* with praziquantel. *J Infect Dis* 152:1339-1340, 1985.

Schneider D, et al: Theophylline and antiparasitic drug interactions: A case report and study of the influence of thiabendazole and mebendazole on theophylline pharmacokinetics in adults. *Chest* 97:84-87, 1990.

Sleigh AC, et al: Manson's schistosomiasis in Brazil: 11-year evaluation of successful disease control with oxamniquine. *Lancet* 1:635-637, 1986.

Sotelo J, et al: Short course of albendazole therapy for neurocysticercosis. *Arch Neurol* 45:1130-1133, 1988.

Sotelo J, et al: Comparison of therapeutic regimen of anticysticercal drugs for parenchymal brain cysticercosis. *J Neurol* 237:69-72, 1990.

Steiger U, et al: Albendazole treatment of echinococcosis in humans: Effects on microsomal metabolism and drug tolerance. *Clin Pharmacol Ther* 47:347-353, 1990.

Stürchler D, et al: Thiabendazole *vs.* albendazole in treatment of toxocariasis: A clinical trial. *Ann Trop Med Parasitol* 83:473-478, 1989.

Taylor HR, Greene BM: The status of ivermectin in the treatment of human onchocerciasis. *Am J Trop Med Hyg* 41:460-466, 1989.

Taylor HR, et al: Ivermectin treatment of patients with severe ocular onchocerciasis. *Am J Trop Med Hyg* 40:494-500, 1989.

Taylor HR, et al: Impact of mass treatment of onchocerciasis with ivermectin on the transmission of infection. *Science* 250:116-118, 1990.

Van Hoegaerden M, et al: The use of mebendazole in the treatment of filariases due to *Loa loa* and *Mansonella perstans. Ann Trop Med Parasitol* 81:275-282, 1987.

Vasconcelos D, et al: Selective indications for use of praziquantel in treatment of brain cysticercosis. *J Neurol Neurosurg Psychiatry* 50:383-388, 1987.

von Kuster LC, Genta RM: Cutaneous manifestations of strongyloidiasis. *Arch Dermatol* 124:1826-1830, 1988.

Watt G, et al: Praziquantel in treatment of cerebral schistosomiasis. *Lancet* 2:529-532, 1986.

Watt G, et al: Praziquantel pharmacokinetics and side effects in *Schistosoma japonicum*-infected patients with liver disease. *J Infect Dis* 157:530-535, 1988.

Weller PF, Arnow PM: Paroxysmal inflammatory filariasis: Filarial fevers, editorial. *Arch Intern Med* 143:1523-1524, 1983.

Weniger BG, Schantz PM: Praziquantel and refugee health. *JAMA* 251:2391-2392, 1984.

White AT, et al: Controlled trial and dose-finding study of ivermectin for treatment of onchocerciasis. *J Infect Dis* 156:463-470, 1987.

WHO Expert Committee on Filariasis: *Lymphatic Filariasis.* Geneva, World Health Organization, Technical Report Series 702, 1984.

Wilson JF, Rausch RL: Alveolar hydatid disease: A review of clinical features of 33 indigenous cases of *Echinococcus multilocularis* infection in Alaskan Eskimos. *Am J Trop Med Hyg* 29:1340-1355, 1980.

Wilson JF, et al: Albendazole therapy in alveolar hydatid disease: A report of favorable results in two patients after short-term therapy. *Am J Trop Med Hyg* 37:162-168, 1987.

Yangco BG, et al: Clinical study evaluating efficacy of praziquantel in clonorchiasis. *Antimicrob Agents Chemother* 31:135-138, 1987.

Yeang FSW, et al: Oxamniquine resistance in *Schistosoma mansoni*. *Ann Trop Med Parasitol* 81:337-339, 1987.

Zygmunt DJ: *Strongyloides stercoralis*. *Infect Control Hosp Epidemiol* 11:495-497, 1990.

Antiviral Drugs

80

Compared with the remarkable progress made in the treatment of bacterial diseases in the past four decades, notable advances in the chemotherapy of viral diseases, while apparent, have been less remarkable. Only a few antiviral agents of proved clinical value are available for a limited number of indications. Although they are much simpler organisms than bacteria, viruses are obligate intracellular parasites that utilize many biochemical pathways of the infected host cell. Through recent advances in molecular virology, it has been possible to identify enzymes unique for the replicating viruses. The exploitation of these observations for the development of virus-specific inhibitors has received more attention recently. With nonselective inhibitors of viral replication, it is difficult to achieve clinically useful antiviral activity without also affecting some aspect of normal host cell metabolism and thus potentially causing toxic effects in noninfected host cells. It is anticipated that host-cell toxicity can be minimized with the development of selective inhibitors of viral replication; therefore, the therapeutic index (ratio of efficacy to toxicity) can be enhanced.

Failure to demonstrate the activity of potentially useful antiviral compounds often reflects the natural history of the disease. Namely, by the time explicit symptoms appear, several cycles of virus multiplication usually have occurred and viral replication is waning. This is particularly true in acute infections of short duration, such as the common cold and influenza, in which rapid multiplication of the virus occurs prior to the development of clinical illness. With the appearance of illness, the host usually is succeeding in the control of viral replication. Obviously, immunocompromised individuals fail to control viral replication as promptly as the normal host. Agents that inhibit viral replication may be ineffective unless they are given very early during the stage of progeny virion multiplication. Therefore, antiviral agents should be given as early as possible during the course of infection or even prophylactically (eg, influenza).

A specific diagnosis is essential prior to the initiation of antiviral therapy. Historically, the lack of rapid diagnostic tests allowed only those diseases with overt cutaneous manifestations (eg, shingles, herpes simplex labialis) to be targets for antiviral therapy. Fortunately, the development of useful reagents for diagnostic purposes has changed this observation to some extent. The availability of both monoclonal and polyclonal antibodies to many respiratory pathogens has expedited the initiation of treatment of respiratory syncytial virus infection, among others. However, further improvements are mandatory if therapeutic advances are to be achieved.

The first drugs tested as antivirals, idoxuridine [Herplex, Stoxil] and cytarabine [Cytosar-U], had limited clinical usefulness because of low therapeutic indices. These drugs do not act selectively on the events of viral replication, but they inhibit defined host cell functions. As a consequence, they have been considered "first-generation" antiviral drugs. Toxicity, specifically bone marrow suppression, prevented the parenteral administration of either of these compounds, and only idoxuridine is considered useful today; it is a second or third choice agent for the topical treatment of herpes simplex keratoconjunctivitis. In two studies, topical idoxuridine was reported to be beneficial in the treatment of herpes labialis. In a double-blind trial conducted on 86 patients with herpes labialis or nasalis, idoxuridine in a glycyrrhizinic acid gel reduced time to crust formation and relieved pain (Segal et al, 1987). In 301 evaluable patients with recurrent herpes labialis, early application of topical idoxuridine 15% in 80% dimethylsulfoxide reduced the duration of pain and accelerated the mean healing time to loss of hard crust (Spruance et al, 1990 A). Vidarabine [Vira-A], a third "first generation" antiviral drug, is acceptable for parenteral therapy in certain life-threatening diseases. Since it has a higher therapeutic index than idoxuridine, vidarabine also is used for topical therapy in herpes simplex infections of the eye.

As understanding of viral replication has increased regarding the essential enzymes, as well as structural and nonstructural proteins and their assembly, processing events that are unique to viruses have been identified. Examples include: (1) host cell-surface receptors to which viruses attach and that probably mediate absorption, and (2) viral-encoded enzymes (eg, herpesvirus-induced thymidine kinases, human immunodeficiency virus-induced reverse transcriptase). Exploitation of such functions in retrospect has led to the development of such antiviral drugs as amantadine [Symmetrel], acyclovir [Zovirax], ribavirin [Virazole], and zidovudine [Retrovir], all of which are available for clinical use. With increased understanding of the molecular biology of virus multiplication, additional virus-specific functions should be discovered that will serve as targets for attack by future highly effective antiviral drugs.

CLASSIFICATION AND BIOLOGY OF VIRUSES

Viruses are composed of a nucleic acid core surrounded by a protein-containing outer coat. The viral genome contains either ribonucleic acid (RNA) or deoxyribonucleic acid (DNA), but never both. The number of nucleic strands (either one or two) and the type of nucleic acid provide the basis for classification of viruses. Viruses can be subdivided further by characteristics such as morphology, whether the virus shell has an envelope, whether viral multiplication occurs in the nucleus or cytoplasm of the infected cell, and serologic type.

Selected viruses that infect humans and the typical diseases that they cause are as follows (classification is initially by virus family) (Melnick, 1980):

RNA Viruses:
Picornaviridae—polioviruses (poliomyelitis), coxsackieviruses and echoviruses (aseptic meningitis), and rhinoviruses (common cold).
Reoviridae—rotaviruses (diarrhea).
Togaviridae—various mosquito-borne encephalitis viruses (encephalitis), yellow fever virus (yellow fever), and rubella virus (rubella).
Orthomyxoviridae—influenza viruses (influenza).
Paramyxoviridae—parainfluenza viruses (croup, pneumonia, bronchitis), mumps virus (mumps), measles virus (measles), and respiratory syncytial virus (bronchiolitis, pneumonia).
Rhabdoviridae—rabies virus (rabies).
Coronaviridae—coronaviruses (respiratory illnesses).
Bunyaviridae—California encephalitis viruses (encephalitis).
Retroviridae—human T-cell lymphotropic viruses (leukemia/lymphoma; HTLV-I, HTLV-II), human immunodeficiency virus types 1 and 2 (HIV-1, HIV-2) (acquired immunodeficiency syndrome).

DNA Viruses:
Papovaviridae—papilloma viruses (warts, progressive multifocal leukoencephalopathy).
Adenoviridae—adenoviruses (acute respiratory diseases, keratitis).
Herpesviridae—herpes simplex types 1 and 2 ("cold" sores, keratitis, genital infections, encephalitis), varicella-zoster (chickenpox, shingles), cytomegalovirus (cytomegalic inclusion disease, chorioretinitis, pneumonitis), Epstein-Barr virus (infectious mononucleosis, association with Burkitt's lymphoma), and human herpesvirus type 6 and 7 (unknown disease association).
Chordopoxviridae—variola virus (smallpox).

Although the precise mechanisms of infection are often different and quite specific for individual viruses, the general cellular infective process proceeds along the following scheme: Initially, viruses adsorb onto the surface of a host cell by electrostatic interaction. It is likely that most viruses attach to virus-specific receptors, accounting for cell and tissue tropism; this has been demonstrated for influenza virus, poliovirus, and HIV. Viruses then penetrate the host cell membrane by pinocytosis, and their nucleic acid is released after an uncoating process. Following uncoating, the replication, transcription, and translation of the viral genome occur either in the cytoplasm or nucleus, depending on the virus. These events result in the production of sufficient quantities of viral nucleic acid and protein to form a new generation of virions (ie, complete infectious virus particles). In the classic cytolytic infection, the replicative mechanisms of the host cell are turned off and the host cell dies. Once the viral components have been manufactured, they are assembled and released as mature virions to begin the cycle again. The processes involved are numerous and complex and utilize not only cellular enzyme systems, but also viral enzymes produced for specialized functions.

Certain viruses (eg, adenoviruses, papovaviruses, retroviruses, herpesviruses) are capable of transforming cells into a malignant state at least in vitro. All or part of the viral genome is integrated into the host cell genome, thus creating a new cell type that, under certain conditions, may express features of a malignant cell. (For further information, see Klein, 1980; Dulbecco and Ginsberg, 1980.)

Although some viral infections are chronic (eg, hepatitis B and non-A/non-B, warts, molluscum contagiosum), the overwhelming majority of those seen clinically are acute. They may remain localized (eg, common cold, influenza) or disseminate via the blood stream to other parts of the body (eg, chickenpox, smallpox). It should be remembered that, for the most part, viral infection is frequently asymptomatic, and symptoms may appear only after an incubation period when a secondary target organ becomes involved. Acute viral infections usually terminate when a sufficient immune response develops to the infecting virus; for some viruses, this immunity may persist for the entire lifetime of the host. However, recurrences or reinfections of certain viral infections are common, because (1) the virus persists within the host in a latent state (eg, herpesviruses, HIV), (2) multiple viral serotypes exist that do not exhibit significant cross-immunity (eg, rhinoviruses), or (3) antigenic shift occurs (eg, influenza viruses).

NONDRUG TREATMENT OF VIRAL INFECTIONS

Supportive Care

Since chemotherapeutic approaches are still limited, symptomatic and supportive treatment (eg, bed rest, analgesics, antipyretics) is the only means of management for many viral diseases, particularly acute respiratory infections.

One nonspecific approach to management of herpes zoster and acute mononucleosis infections has included the use of corticosteroids. This form of therapy is designed to decrease the frequency of postherpetic neuralgia as well as alleviate the pain associated with acute neuritis. Opinions weigh both in favor of and against their use (Eaglstein et al, 1970; Esmann et al, 1987), but at the present time steroid therapy does not seem indicated.

Immunization

Active Immunization: Active immunization employing either live attenuated or killed viral vaccines to stimulate the normal host defense mechanisms remains the most effective means of controlling many viral diseases. Vaccination prevents measles, rubella, mumps, poliomyelitis, yellow fever, smallpox, and hepatitis B. In addition, it has proved effective for prevention of such exotic viral infections as Japanese encephalitis and Venezuelan equine encephalitis among others. Despite the problems of antigenic shifts, vaccination against influenza often provides short-term protection and is recommended annually for high-risk individuals (eg, patients with underlying chronic cardiovascular and pulmonary diseases, the elderly). Unfortunately, vaccines have not been developed for all viruses, and this would appear to be impractical in some cases. For example, the rhinoviruses have 100 known antigenically distinct serotypes.

Passive Immunization: Passive immunization with human immune globulin or equine antiserum is another nondrug approach to combat viral infections. For example, hyperimmune globulins are very useful in the prophylaxis of varicella, rabies, and hepatitis B. Use of these hyperimmune products will continue even with the availability of vaccines.

For detailed discussion of active and passive immunization, see index entry Immunization.

Interferons

Vaccines and available antiviral drugs possess narrow spectrums of activity. Consequently, their uses are limited to selected viral infections. Clinically effective, broad spectrum antiviral agents are generally unavailable.

One of the attractive features of the antiviral substances, interferons, is their broad spectrum. Naturally occurring interferons refer to a family of glycoproteins produced by animal (including human) cells infected with viruses or stimulated by various other natural and synthetic substances. The current nomenclature for the three principal types of interferons appears in Table 1.

The advances in molecular biology during the past decade have led to the recognition that there are several interferon (IFN) subtypes. More than 20 IFN-α genes have been postulated, but not all have been clearly identified with a product. Nevertheless, at least 14 distinct subtypes of IFN-α have been cloned using recombinant DNA techniques. Up to five IFN-β mRNAs have been identified, but only two gene products, IFN-β_1 and IFN-β_2, have been established. IFN-β_1 represents over 90% of the interferon produced by fibroblasts. Thus far, only one type of IFN-γ has been described. This interferon bears little homology to the IFN-α or IFN-β species but shares many of their biological functions. In humans, the main cluster of IFN-producing genes is on chromosome 9 (IFN-α and IFN-β_1). Chromosomes 2 and 5 have been associated with the production of IFN-β_2, while chromosome 12 is associated with IFN-γ production.

Actions: Binding of interferon to the intact cell membrane is the first step in establishing an antiviral effect. IFN binds to specific cell surface receptors; IFN-γ appears to have a different receptor from either IFN-α or -β, which may explain the synergistic antiviral and antitumor effects sometimes observed when IFN-γ is given with either of the other two IFN species.

A prevalent view of interferon action (Preble and Friedman, 1983) is that, following binding, there is synthesis of new cellular RNAs and proteins, which mediate the antiviral effect. Chromosome 21 is required to develop the antiviral state in humans no matter which species of IFN is employed. At least three of the newly synthesized proteins in IFN-treated cells appear to be associated with the development of the antiviral state: (1) a 2′-5′ oligoadenylate (2-5A) synthetase, (2) a protein kinase, and (3) an endonuclease. The antiviral state is not fully expressed until these primed cells are infected with virus.

Double-stranded RNA, which is produced during the replication of many viruses, activates 2-5A synthetase and protein kinase. The activated 2-5A synthetase catalyzes the polymerization of ATP into 2′-5′ oligonucleotides that in turn activate endogenous cellular endoribonuclease, which degrades viral RNA. The activated protein kinase phosphoryl-

TABLE 1.
HUMAN INTERFERON NOMENCLATURE

New Nomenclature	Old Nomenclature
IFN-α	Le (leukocyte), type I, pH 2 stable, foreign cell-induced, classical
IFN-β	F (fibroblast), Fi, type I, pH 2 stable
IFN-γ	IIF (immune), type II, T, pH 2 labile, antigen-induced, mitogen-induced

Adapted from Stiehm et al, 1982.

ates the alpha subunit of eukaryotic initiation factor 2 resulting in inhibition of viral protein synthesis. The combined effects of protein kinase and endonuclease in IFN-treated cells are thought to result in inhibition of virus protein synthesis and, hence, virus replication. However, it is not yet known how these enzymes discriminate between host and virus protein synthesis.

Although the foregoing postulate on IFN's mechanism of action explains its inhibition of virus replication, interferon does not appear to act by inhibiting virus-specific RNA or protein synthesis in all virus systems. For example, interferon appears to inhibit the final maturation of retroviruses in infected cells so that they are not released into the medium but instead accumulate on the cell surface. If interferon is removed, virus release proceeds normally. Other enzymes and proteins have been described in IFN-treated cells. For a detailed review of the actions of interferons, see Becker, 1984.

In addition to their antiviral effect, interferons have a number of other biological properties, both useful and potentially deleterious, including inhibition of cell proliferation and enhancement of the cytotoxic activities of lymphocytes, the expression of cell surface antigens, and the phagocytic and tumoricidal activities of macrophages. These properties may play an important role in the in vivo antiviral and antitumor effects of the interferons.

Sources: Although interferons exhibit broad spectrum antiviral activity, they are relatively species-specific, usually having maximal activity only in cells from the same or closely related species. Previously, the amount of human interferons available for clinical trials was limited and preparations were impure. To circumvent the early limited supply of exogenous human interferon, compounds that stimulate the endogenous production of interferon by host cells were investigated. Interferon inducers include certain microorganisms (eg, viruses, *Rickettsia*, *Mycoplasma*, coliform bacteria), microbial extracts, certain dyes (eg, methylene blue, acridine orange), tilorone, and synthetic polymers; however, none of these agents have been shown to be safe or effective in man. Currently, all three species of IFN are produced by recombinant DNA technology.

Clinical Trials: A number of clinical investigations with exogenous human interferons are ongoing. Most of the early studies utilized semipurified interferon (HuIFN-α) from buffy-coat leukocytes stimulated with Sendai virus. These leukocytes were obtained from outdated blood bank stores. A few studies employed fibroblast interferon from poly rI:rC-induced human fibroblasts grown in culture.

The general consensus has been that these preparations have some antiviral effects in a number of infections, although this role remains to be defined. For example, leukocyte IFN administered prophylactically as a nasal spray reduced the incidence and severity of colds caused by rhinoviruses (Greenberg et al, 1982; Scott et al, 1982) and suppressed varicella in immunocompromised children with cancer (Arvin et al, 1982 A). When given prophylactically, leukocyte IFN significantly reduced the incidence of cytomegalovirus reactivation as well as associated syndromes and opportunistic infections in renal transplant patients (Hirsch et al, 1983). However, in infants with congenital rubella, treatment decreased pharyngeal virus excretion only temporarily (Arvin et al, 1982 B). Treatment of women with primary genital herpes simplex virus infection resulted in a statistically significant accelerated rate of healing but not relief of pain (Pazin et al, 1987). Leukocyte IFN used either alone (Garcia et al, 1987) or in combination with synthetic antiviral agents was effective in chronic hepatitis B infection (Smith et al, 1982; Garcia et al, 1987), herpetic keratitis (Colin et al, 1983), and progressive cutaneous herpes simplex infection (Shalev et al, 1984). However, in each instance in which IFN demonstrated clinical benefit, fever, malaise, and, in a few patients, neutropenia were encountered. Tachyphylaxis was observed with continued administration.

As with leukocyte interferon from buffy coats, recombinant leukocyte interferon (rHuIFN-α_2) given prophylactically in the form of nasal spray or drops prevented infection and reduced the severity and frequency of illness and virus shedding in experimentally challenged subjects (Samo et al, 1983; Hayden and Gwaltney, 1983) and in patients naturally infected with rhinoviruses (Herzog et al, 1983; Farr et al, 1984). In two other studies, rHuIFN-α_2 self-administered for seven days by healthy individuals exposed to another family member with cold-like symptoms reduced the symptoms of respiratory illness in recipients by 39% to 41%. This beneficial effect was confined to rhinovirus infections. When rhinoviral colds alone were considered, the IFN prevented colds in 78% to 79% of patients or shortened the course of the colds with 76% fewer symptom days (Douglas et al, 1986; Hayden et al, 1986). In addition, intranasal rHuIFN-α_2 was effective in reducing the incidence of colds, the severity of symptoms, and viral multiplication in experimental respiratory coronavirus infection (Higgins et al, 1983). Although clinical benefit was demonstrated in these studies, administration of rHuIFN-α_2 for two to three weeks or longer led to hemorrhagic mucosa of the nasal passages.

Recent studies suggest that IFN has a role in the treatment of hepatitis. In a small study, the administration of rHuIFN-α_2 to patients with chronic hepatitis B temporarily suppressed Dane particle-associated polymerase activity (Smith et al, 1983). In a larger study performed at the National Institutes of Health, suppression of hepatitis B DNA polymerase was demonstrated in 10 of 31 (32%) patients who received IFN for four months compared with 1 of 14 (7%) placebo recipients (Hoofnagle et al, 1988). Although these results were not statistically different, probably because of small numbers, they have prompted additional multicenter United States and European trials (Perrillo, 1989; Lok et al, 1989). An important observation during these initial studies was the potential value of prednisone for "immune priming" (Perrillo et al, 1988). In these studies, significant benefit (loss of hepatitis B DNA polymerase) was observed in 50% (nine of the treated patients) ($p=0.035$ as compared to controls). Further studies also have suggested the beneficial effect of rHuIFN-α_2 in the treatment of non-A, non-B (type C) hepatitis (Hoofnagle et al, 1986; Davis et al, 1989; Di Bisceglie et al, 1989). Results of both studies have prompted a large controlled trial to define the clinical usefulness of this compound in these diseases. In addition, the treatment of delta hepatitis with IFN is being investigated (Rizzetto et al, 1986; Rosina et al, 1987, 1989).

Several large controlled trials have demonstrated the clinical benefit of rHuIFN-α_2 for condylomata accuminata. Both the intralesional (Eron et al, 1986; Reichman et al, 1988) and parenteral (Reichman et al, 1988) administration of this IFN have resulted in a complete response rate of approximately 60% in the IFN recipients compared with almost 20% in the placebo recipients. These regimens involved the administration of IFN three times a week for three to six weeks. A relapse rate of approximately 20% was noted in both groups, and toxicity was not a limiting factor. Studies utilizing the intralesional or parenteral administration of either rHuIFN-α or rHuIFN-β have been performed on only limited numbers of patients, and larger controlled studies are required. There have been no well-controlled trials to demonstrate the antiviral efficacy of HuIFN-γ, although one pharmacokinetic study in cancer patients has been published (Gutterman et al, 1984). Future controlled studies probably will employ combinations of forms of IFN.

It should be noted that when rHuIFN-α_2 was administered to bone marrow transplant patients with serious cytomegalovirus or adenovirus infection, no favorable effect was observed (Meyers et al, 1983). Treatment of recurrent genital herpes simplex infections also has been of no therapeutic value (Gnann et al, 1984). Similarly, the administration of IFN in combination with synthetic antiviral drugs has not yet been shown to be of clinical value. As discussed elsewhere, rHuIFN-α has antitumor activity (see index entry Interferon Alfa-2a, -2b, In Cancer).

Adverse Reactions: Not only are the clinical antiviral activities of cell culture and recombinant interferon preparations similar, if not identical, but so are their adverse effects. Fever has occurred in most patients receiving interferons intramuscularly or intravenously. Headache and myalgia also are common. Malaise and fatigue have been observed and become more pronounced with additional doses. Interferons produced reversible dose-related leukopenia and thrombocytopenia. Nausea and vomiting, erythema and pain at the site of intramuscular injection, and transient alopecia also have been observed.

In clinical studies employing rHuIFN-α_2 intranasally, nasal irritation with discharge of blood-tinged mucus, superficial erosions of the nasal mucosa, and transient leukopenia were reported (Hayden and Gwaltney, 1983; Samo et al, 1983; Farr et al, 1984; Douglas et al, 1986; Hayden et al, 1986).

In pharmacokinetic studies in humans who were given rHuIFN-α_2 intravenously, intramuscularly, and subcutaneously, the severity of adverse effects was related to the route of administration (Willis et al, 1984). However, it has been suggested that neutralizing antibodies will develop to the rHuIFNs with repeated administration. This is potentially of greater concern, and the occurrence of this phenomenon will require careful monitoring in the planned prospective studies to determine efficacy.

DRUG THERAPY FOR VIRAL INFECTIONS

Classification and Uses

PYRIMIDINE AND PURINE ANTIMETABOLITES. Many compounds considered to be potential antiviral drugs are antimetabolites that inhibit nucleic acid synthesis. The clinical usefulness of these pyrimidine and purine derivatives is related directly to their ability to selectively block viral, as opposed to host, nucleic acid synthesis. Particular emphasis has been placed on the development of such drugs to treat herpesvirus and human immunodeficiency virus infections.

Cytarabine: Cytarabine [Cytosar-U], a cytidine analogue used to treat acute myelogenous leukemia, was originally developed as an antiviral drug. This agent inhibits herpesvirus DNA synthesis but has a greater inhibitory effect on dividing host cells, causing severe bone marrow and gastrointestinal toxicity. Therefore, cytarabine is not used clinically as an antiviral drug.

Idoxuridine and Trifluridine: Idoxuridine [Herplex, Stoxil] and trifluridine [Viroptic] are analogues of thymidine. When administered systemically, these substituted nucleosides are phosphorylated by both viral and cellular thymidine kinases to the active triphosphorylated derivatives, which inhibit viral and cellular DNA synthesis. The result is both antiviral activity and sufficient host cytotoxicity to prevent their systemic use for viral infections. The poor therapeutic index of idoxuridine therapy for herpes simplex encephalitis is illustrated by the significant toxicity (bone marrow suppression) encountered following parenteral administration (Boston Interhospital Antiviral Study Group and the NIAID Cooperative Antiviral Clinical Study Group, 1975). The toxicity is not significant, however, when idoxuridine and trifluridine are applied topically to the eye to treat herpes simplex keratitis. Most authorities consider trifluridine superior to idoxuridine (see index entry Eye Infection, Keratitis). In England and other countries, the topical application of idoxuridine dissolved in dimethyl sulfoxide (DMSO) has been reported to be effective in cutaneous herpes simplex and herpes zoster lesions. Results of two clinical studies conducted in the United States indicated that topical idoxuridine in a glycyrrhizinic acid gel or 80% dimethyl sulfoxide solution was effective in reducing pain and accelerating healing time (Segal et al, 1987; Spruance et al, 1990 A). However, in a randomized, double-blind, controlled trial, 30% idoxuridine in DMSO had no effect on the clinical manifestations of initial or recurrent genital herpesvirus infections (Silvestri et al, 1982). No idoxuridine-DMSO formulations are marketed in the United States.

Vidarabine: Vidarabine [Vira-A] is a purine nucleoside analogue with selective activity against herpesviruses. It is phosphorylated by host kinases to the active 5′-triphosphate (ara-ATP). This triphosphate competitively inhibits DNA-dependent DNA polymerases of DNA viruses approximately 40 times more than those of host cells. In addition, vidarabine is incorporated into terminal positions of both cellular and herpesvirus DNA, thus inhibiting completion of DNA chains. Therefore, viral DNA synthesis is blocked at lower doses of drug than is host cell DNA synthesis, resulting in a relatively selective antiviral effect. However, large doses of vidarabine are cytotoxic to dividing host cells because antiviral selectivity is not absolute.

When administered intravenously, vidarabine is effective in biopsy-proven herpes simplex encephalitis (Whitley et al, 1977, 1981), neonatal herpes simplex infection (Whitley et al, 1980, 1986 B), and herpes zoster (Whitley et al, 1976, 1982 D) and varicella (Whitley et al, 1982 A) infections in immunocompromised patients. This drug also is used topically to treat herpes simplex keratitis (see index entry Vidarabine, In Ophthalmic Infection). It has limited effect in mucocutaneous herpesvirus infections in immunocompromised hosts (Whitley et al, 1984). In chronic hepatitis B infection, vidarabine decreased Dane particle-associated polymerase activity temporarily but pretreatment levels were observed following cessation of therapy (Pollard et al, 1978; Bassendine et al, 1981; Hoofnagle et al, 1984). In two separate trials, cytomegalovirus (CMV) infections in bone marrow (Kraemer et al, 1978) or renal transplant (Marker et al, 1980) patients did not respond to vidarabine. However, in one small study of progressive CMV retinitis, 20 mg/kg/day of vidarabine seemed to alter the course of the disease, although significant adverse effects were observed (Pollard et al, 1980). The drug is not useful in genital herpesvirus or smallpox infections. From a practical standpoint, it has for the most part been replaced by acyclovir for the treatment of herpes simplex and varicella-zoster virus infections.

A major disadvantage of vidarabine is its poor solubility, which necessitates the use of large volumes of intravenous fluid and prolonged infusion times (see the evaluation). Vidarabine is rapidly deaminated by adenosine deaminase to hypoxanthine arabinoside, which has much weaker antiviral activity. This observation led to the search for derivatives resistant to deamination by this enzyme. Cyclaradine, a carbocyclic analogue, is as potent as vidarabine in vitro and is resistant to deamination by adenosine deaminase (Vince and Daluge, 1977). However, although cyclaradine is a promising compound (Vince et al, 1983), clinical trials have not yet been initiated.

Acyclovir and Derivatives: Acyclovir [Zovirax], a nucleoside analogue of guanosine, is probably the best example of a drug with selective antiviral activity. In infected cells, herpesvirus thymidine kinase converts acyclovir to acyclovir monophosphate, a nucleotide analogue. In uninfected host cells (eg, Vero, HeLa), this phosphorylation is limited; depending on the virus strain/host cell system employed, the rate is 30 to 120 times faster in extracts prepared from infected cells than in those from uninfected host cells. (Notably, uninfected cells apparently contain a kinase enzyme that differs from the viral thymidine kinase and that phosphorylates acyclovir to a limited extent.) Following conversion to the monophosphate derivative, the compound is further converted to the diphosphate by cellular guanylate kinase and finally to the triphosphate (acyclo-GTP) by a number of cellular enzymes. The latter is the active form of the drug. Once formed, acyclo-GTP may remain in the cell for a prolonged period.

The initial reaction in the phosphorylation sequence is critical, for the specificity of the viral enzyme is quite different from that of thymidine kinase from the uninfected cell. The herpesvirus thymidine kinase binds 200 times more strongly to acyclovir and phosphorylates it 3 million times faster than does host cell thymidine kinase.

Acyclo-GTP is a potent and selective inhibitor of viral DNA polymerase; it inhibits cellular alpha-DNA polymerase to a much lesser degree, and cellular beta-DNA polymerase is insensitive to the compound. Acyclo-GTP can be incorporated into growing chains of DNA by viral and, to a much lesser extent, cellular DNA polymerase. When this incorporation occurs, DNA chain growth is terminated, apparently because acyclovir does not have a 3′-hydroxyl group on which chain elongation can continue, and the acyclo-GMP-terminated template binds and inactivates the viral DNA polymerase.

Acyclovir is available in intravenous, topical, and oral forms. Intravenous acyclovir has been effective in immunocompromised patients with mucocutaneous herpes (Mitchell et al, 1981; Chou et al, 1981; Wade et al, 1982 A; Meyers et al, 1982) and for the treatment and prophylaxis of herpes simplex (Spector et al, 1982; Saral et al, 1981, 1983) and herpes zoster infections (Selby et al, 1979; Spector et al, 1982; Balfour et al, 1983; Serota et al, 1982; Meyers et al, 1984; Shepp et al, 1986; Jura et al, 1989). In one study, acyclovir was more effective than vidarabine for the treatment of localized zoster infection following bone marrow transplantation (Shepp et al, 1986). In a randomized double-blind trial, prophylaxis with intravenous acyclovir (5 mg/kg, three times daily) and oral acyclovir (800 mg, four times daily) initiated the day prior to bone marrow transplantation and continued for six months significantly reduced the incidence of both herpes simplex and varicella-zoster infections when compared with placebo. Although reactivation of infections followed quickly after discontinuation of therapy, the patients had re-established bone marrow function and immunity and recurrences of infection were much less severe. Prophylactic therapy did not reduce the incidence of cytomegalovirus infections (Selby et al, 1989). In immunocompetent patients, intravenous acyclovir has been effective in primary genital herpes (Mindel et al, 1982; Corey et al, 1983) and herpes zoster infections (Peterslund et al, 1981, 1984; Bean et al, 1982; Esmann et al, 1982).

A collaborative study that compared intravenous acyclovir and vidarabine in the treatment of herpes simplex encephalitis concluded that acyclovir was the treatment of choice. Mortality in the vidarabine and acyclovir groups was, respectively, 43% versus 13% at one month, 54% versus 19% at six months, and 54% versus 28% overall. In patients less than 30 years old, the mortality rate was 6% for those treated with acyclovir and 45% for those treated with vidarabine. Six months after therapy, 14% of those in the vidarabine group and 38% of those in the acyclovir group were functionally normal (Whitley et al, 1986 A).

A number of clinical studies on oral acyclovir have been conducted. In immunocompromised patients, oral acyclovir suppressed symptomatic attacks of mucocutaneous and other herpes simplex virus infections (Straus et al, 1982, 1984 A), prevented herpes simplex virus reactivation after transplantation (Wade et al, 1984), and was credited with eliminating the dissemination of varicella-zoster virus in children (Prober et al, 1982; Novelli et al, 1984). Short-term prophylaxis prevented the development of recurrent herpes labialis in skiers (Spruance, 1988). A randomized, placebo-controlled, double-blind trial of acyclovir for the prevention of cytomegalovirus disease in recipients of cadaveric renal allografts was conducted in 118 patients. The results of this study indicated that oral administration of acyclovir beginning before and continuing for 12 weeks after transplantation reduced the rate of cytomegalovirus infection and disease but did not affect the survival rate of either grafts or patients. The greatest prophylactic benefit was observed in seronegative patients who had received a kidney from a seropositive donor. The incidence of cytomegalovirus infection in patients who received placebo was 61%; in comparison, the incidence was 36% in patients who received acyclovir. Among acyclovir-treated patients, virus recovery rates from blood and urine were significantly reduced (Balfour et al, 1989).

In immunocompetent patients, oral acyclovir was effective in primary herpes genitalis (Nilsen et al, 1982; Bryson et al, 1983; Mertz et al, 1984). Continuous oral treatment reduced the incidence of recurrences and significantly increased the mean time to the first recurrent herpes outbreak in patients with frequent episodes of genital herpes (Straus et al, 1984 B; Douglas et al, 1984; Mindel et al, 1984, 1988; Mertz et al, 1988 A and B; Mattison et al, 1988; Straus et al, 1988; Baker et al, 1989). Long-term oral acyclovir treatment (exceeding one year) was reported to have a significant effect in preventing the signs and symptoms of recurrent genital herpes or reduce their frequency or severity but did not eliminate virus shedding; treatment reduced the rate of symptomatic but not of asymptomatic shedding (Straus et al, 1989). Thus, virus transmission is possible during such therapy, even in the absence of signs and symptoms. The efficacy of oral acyclovir for genital herpes simplex infections was suggested in earlier studies as well (Thin et al, 1985; Ruhnek-Forsbeck et al, 1985). In one double-blind, randomized trial of oral acyclovir in 174 immunocompetent adults with herpes labialis, drug therapy reduced pain and healing time but did not prevent new lesion development (Spruance et al, 1990 B).

Oral and intravenous acyclovir were reported to be equally effective in reducing pain and accelerating the rate of healing in herpes zoster (Peterslund et al, 1984; Huff et al, 1988; Morton et al, 1989). A randomized, placebo-controlled, double-blind trial of oral acyclovir conducted on 105 otherwise healthy children age 5 to 16 years found that patients treated with acyclovir within 24 hours of developing varicella exanthem had defervescence sooner, had accelerated cutaneous lesion healing, and had fewer skin lesions. The drug did not appear to significantly influence the rate of varicella complications; however, the incidence of such complications was low for all patients. No adverse drug effects were reported (Balfour et al, 1990). The intravenous formulation is now approved for the treatment of varicella-zoster infections in immunocompromised adults and children, and the oral formulation is approved for the treatment of varicella-zoster infections in immunocompetent patients.

Topical acyclovir has been efficacious in the treatment of mucocutaneous herpesvirus infections in immunocompromised patients (Spruance et al, 1982; Whitley et al, 1982 B) but not in many immunocompetent patients (Spruance et al, 1982, 1984). In the latter, topical administration has been useful for the management of primary, but not recurrent, genital herpes infections (Corey et al, 1982 A and B; Luby et al, 1984). However, because the oral route is more effective than topical application, oral acyclovir is the treatment of choice. Many studies support the efficacy of topical acyclovir in the treatment of herpes simplex keratitis; approval of an ophthalmic formulation is under consideration by the Food and Drug Administration.

The acyclic nucleoside, ganciclovir (DHPG; 9-[1,3-dihydroxy-2-propoxymethyl] guanine), is an analogue of acyclovir with considerably more activity against CMV. In vitro, it inhibited the replication of HSV-1 and -2, CMV, and Epstein-Barr virus (EBV). In mice, it was more active than acyclovir against herpesvirus encephalitis and genitalis. In vitro studies have shown that replication of human herpesvirus type 6 is strongly inhibited by ganciclovir; acyclovir was much less active, with only the highest concentration showing an antiviral effect (Russler et al, 1989).

The activity of ganciclovir in herpesvirus-infected cells depends on phosphorylation by a virus-induced cellular kinase (not, however, the enzyme thymidine kinase). Like acyclovir, ganciclovir monophosphate is further converted to the di- and triphosphate by additional cellular kinases. In cells infected by HSV-1 or -2, the triphosphate (DHPGTP) competitively inhibits the incorporation of GTP into virus DNA; DHPGTP is incorporated at internal and terminal sites of viral DNA, thus inhibiting DNA synthesis. The mode of action of ganciclovir against CMV is believed to be due to the competitive inhibition of viral DNA polymerase and direct incorporation of the triphosphate into viral DNA, resulting in termination of DNA chain elongation. Cellular DNA polymerase is inhibited at higher concentrations. In vitro, ganciclovir-TP levels produced by CMV-infected cells are more than tenfold higher than those in uninfected cells. These elevated levels persist and may even increase in infected cells long after the drug is discontinued.

Ganciclovir is of clinical interest because of its great potency and broad spectrum of activity against herpesviruses, particularly CMV. However, its potential toxicity dampens enthusiasm for widespread use. In contrast to nucleoside analogues with a similar structure, such as acyclovir, ganciclovir has a terminal 3′ hydroxy group on the ribose ring and, as a consequence, is incorporated into both the host cell and viral DNA. This structural characteristic of the drug is relevant in defining the therapeutic index. Its structure alone would indicate the potential for suppression of rapidly proliferating cell lines, particularly of the gastrointestinal tract and bone marrow. In fact, such toxicity, including gonadal toxicity, has been documented in animals. Available information indicates that gonadal toxicity occurs at any dose tested, regardless of how low that dose might be.

Ganciclovir has been approved for use in CMV retinitis in immunocompromised patients.

In studies of AIDS patients with chorioretinitis, the virus is cleared from the blood, sputum, and throat in more than 80% of patients after 10 to 14 days of therapy with doses of 7.5 to 15 mg/kg/day. After short courses, visual acuity improves in more than 50% of patients with chorioretinitis; the disease stabilizes in an additional 35% of patients. Visual acuity can be stabilized for up to four months in approximately 50% of patients on maintenance regimens. Representative reports summarizing these experiences include Bach et al, 1985; The Collaborative DHPG Treatment Study Group, 1986; Felsenstein et al, 1985; Laskin et al, 1987 A, 1987 B. Maintenance regimens consisting of two to five doses of 2.5 mg/kg weekly did not prevent relapses, either because of clinical reactivation or the development of leukopenia requiring cessation of therapy (Masur et al, 1986).

In a company-sponsored trial, patients with CMV retinitis and AIDS were treated with ganciclovir under open-label guidelines. The most common dose employed was 5 mg/kg twice daily given intravenously over a one-hour period for 14 to 21 days. Of 254 treated patients, 141 (56%) were judged to have improved and 67 (26%) to have stabilized. In 61 untreated patients, only 2 (3%) showed stabilization and 59 (97%) experienced progressive disease (Syntex, unpublished data, CL 4197). In another study employing similar doses, 22 of 34 (65%) treated patients had a complete response and 5 of 34 (15%) had a partial response (Jabs et al, 1989).

Reactivation of retinal infection commonly occurs when ganciclovir treatment is stopped. Therefore, most patients have received maintenance therapy of 5 to 6 mg/kg/day given as a single intravenous infusion five to seven days per week for a total dose of 30 to 35 mg/kg/week. Results of randomized trials indicate that maintenance therapy delays but does not prevent reactivation of infection. In one small study, following a ten-day induction course of ganciclovir (2.5 mg/kg every eight hours), AIDS patients with CMV retinitis received either immediate or deferred maintenance therapy. The results indicated that long-term therapy with the drug retarded the progression of CMV retinitis, and the investigators recommended that maintenance dosing begin immediately following induction therapy and suggested an optimum dose of 6 to 7.5 mg/kg/day, which should be adjusted to maintain an absolute neutrophil count above 800 cells/microliter (Jacobson et al, 1990). This dose is higher than that suggested by the manufacturer.

Treatment-associated myelosuppression prohibits maintenance therapy in a number of AIDS patients with CMV retinitis; in many, zidovudine therapy must be discontinued. Therefore, the usefulness of intravitreal ganciclovir has been investigated as an alternative to the intravenous route. Repeated intravitreal injections of ganciclovir in ten patients resolved necrotizing retinitis in all patients after induction therapy (six injections over two to three weeks); vision was stabilized or improved in all but one eye. Local effects were minimal. The investigators concluded that intravitreal ganciclovir is a safe and effective alternative in patients who cannot tolerate the drug systemically (Cantrill et al, 1989).

Therapy appears to be less useful for CMV pneumonia, but it is not without some benefit. In one study on ten bone marrow transplant recipients with biopsy-proven CMV pneumonia treated with ganciclovir, viruria and viremia ceased after four days of treatment in all patients with initially positive urine or blood cultures. Also, CMV was eliminated from respiratory secretions after a median of eight days; however, only one patient survived the pneumonia (Shepp et al, 1985). More recent studies tend to favor ganciclovir therapy for this disease, but results are limited by the number of patients in the studies as well as by the number of suitable controls (Frank and Friedman, 1988; Emanuel et al, 1988; Reed et al, 1988). Results of animal experiments suggest that the combination of ganciclovir and anti-CMV antiserum is more effective for the treatment of CMV disease than either agent alone. Because of the severity of CMV pneumonia and the poor results obtained with other regimens, the potential of this combined regimen has been investigated. Results of several small studies suggest that this regimen significantly alters the outcome of patients with CMV pneumonia (Emanuel el al, 1988; Reed et al, 1988; Schmidt et al, 1988; D'Alessandro et al, 1989). However, the addition of CMV immune globulin did not appear to add markedly to the efficacy of ganciclovir in AIDS-associated CMV retinitis (Jacobson et al, 1990).

Zidovudine: Zidovudine (3′-azido-2′, 3′ dideoxythymidine; azidothymidine; AZT) [Retrovir] is a thymidine analogue that inhibits HIV replication in vitro. It is converted to the mono-, di,- and triphosphate by the same cellular enzymes that catalyze the phosphorylation of thymidine and thymidine nucleosides. Zidovudine triphosphate is then terminally incorporated into the growing DNA chains via the viral reverse transcriptase. As with acyclovir triphosphate, zidovudine triphosphate is an obligate chain terminator. It also is a highly efficient substrate of thymidine kinase and produces zidovudine monophosphate, which accumulates in cells as the major metabolite (Furman et al, 1986; Mitsuya et al, 1985).

In Phase I studies, zidovudine was administered both intravenously and orally and was well tolerated over a six-week period. There was evidence suggestive of clinical improvement (Yarchoan et al, 1986). In these small pilot studies, it was determined that demonstrable levels of zidovudine appeared in the cerebrospinal fluid (CSF/plasma ratio, 20% to 50%) and that it could at least transiently reverse HIV-induced dementia.

A subsequent placebo-controlled study of 282 patients with AIDS demonstrated the efficacy of zidovudine therapy. Therapy consisted of zidovudine 250 mg or placebo administered orally every four hours for 24 weeks; however, an independent Data Safety and Monitoring Board terminated the trial because of evidence of efficacy of zidovudine. At the time of termination, 19 placebo and one zidovudine recipient had died ($p=0.001$). In addition, 45 placebo and 24 zidovudine recipients developed opportunistic infections ($p=0.001$). The decrease in the frequency of opportunistic infections was paralleled by weight gain and enhancement of the baseline Karnofsky performance score ($p=0.001$). Variations in CD4 counts were observed. Overall, CD4 counts in the zidovudine-treated patients increased; however, the CD4 counts of AIDS patients decreased after 12 weeks of therapy but remained stable in those with AIDS-related complex (Fischl et al,

1987). In spite of evidence of a beneficial drug effect, serious adverse reactions, particularly bone marrow suppression, were observed and appeared to correlate with severity of underlying HIV disease. Anemia with hemoglobin concentrations below 7.5 g/dL developed in 24% of zidovudine recipients and in 4% of placebo recipients ($p=0.001$). In the initial study conducted in patients with advanced HIV disease, a total of 21% and 4% of zidovudine and placebo recipients, respectively, required multiple red blood cell transfusions ($p=0.001$). Absolute granulocytopenia ($\leq$500 cells/mm^3) developed in 16% and in 2% of the two treatment groups, respectively (Richman et al, 1987). The appearance of myalgia, nausea, and insomnia occurred more frequently in the zidovudine recipients.

Additional studies have demonstrated the usefulness of zidovudine in patients with asymptomatic HIV infection and those with early symptomatic disease (Volberding et al, 1990; Fischl et al, 1990) (see also the evaluation). However, the drug had no effect on the extent of Kaposi's sarcoma in AIDS patients (Lane et al, 1989).

Although serious hematologic effects may occur, including neutropenia, leukopenia, and anemia (usually macrocytic), the marrow-suppressive effects are dependent on both dose and the patient's underlying marrow reserve. Low doses of zidovudine (500 to 600 mg/day) have generally been better tolerated, particularly in patients with less advanced disease.

Capsule, syrup, and intravenous formulations of zidovudine are available for use in adults and children. For children with HIV disease, 180 mg/M^2 every six hours (720 mg/M^2/day) is equivalent to 200 mg every four hours in adults. The efficacy of lower doses in children is being studied.

Ribavirin: Ribavirin [Virazole] exhibits a broad antiviral spectrum that includes both RNA and DNA viruses. The mechanisms of its antiviral effect are poorly understood and probably are not the same for all viruses; however, its ability to alter nucleotide pools and the packaging of mRNA appears to be important. This process is not totally virus specific, but there is a certain selectivity in that infected cells produce more mRNA than noninfected cells. A major action is the inhibition by ribavirin-5′-monophosphate of inosine monophosphate dehydrogenase, an enzyme essential for DNA synthesis. This inhibition may have direct effects on the intracellular level of GMP; other nucleotide levels may be altered, but the mechanisms are presently unknown. Also, the 5′-triphosphate of ribavirin inhibits the formation of the 5′-guanylation capping on the mRNA of vaccinia and Venezuelan equine encephalitis viruses. In addition, the triphosphate is a potent inhibitor of viral mRNA (guanine-7-) methyltransferase of vaccinia virus. The capacity of viral mRNA to support protein synthesis is markedly reduced by ribavirin. Of note, high concentrations of ribavirin also inhibit cellular protein synthesis. It has been suggested that ribavirin may inhibit influenza A RNA-dependent RNA polymerase.

Results of clinical trials employing oral ribavirin suggest that this form is marginally effective in the prophylaxis of influenza A and B infections and, possibly, in the treatment of influenza A. Aerosolized ribavirin has been more effective in controlling influenza infections. In an early study on influenza A infections (Knight et al, 1981), fever and illness disappeared more rapidly and virus shedding was reduced in treated patients compared to controls; in a later study, the duration of fever was shorter and recovery was more rapid with use of ribavirin aerosol (Wilson et al, 1984). More rapid defervescence, resolution of clinical illness, and reduction of viral shedding in nasal secretions also were observed in patients with influenza B infections treated with aerosolized ribavirin (McClung et al, 1983).

Ribavirin therapy is indicated in respiratory syncytial virus (RSV) infections. Use of aerosolized ribavirin in adults and children with RSV infections reduced the severity of illness and virus shedding (Hall et al, 1983 A and B). In a double-blind, placebo-controlled trial, this form was evaluated in RSV lower respiratory tract disease in 26 infants, including those with underlying cardiopulmonary disease. Treated infants improved significantly faster as measured by illness severity score, arterial blood gas values, and amount of virus shed from nasal washes. In addition, a generally good outcome was observed in 27 nonrandomized severely ill infants with congenital heart disease who were treated with ribavirin aerosol. Notably, about one-third of infants with congenital heart disease may die from RSV infection. No adverse effects were observed in any of the infants studied, and no ribavirin-resistant RSV strains were isolated despite prolonged treatment in some infants (Hall et al, 1985). Aerosol therapy with ribavirin appears to have the advantage of producing very high pulmonary drug levels with little systemic absorption. In patients receiving eight or more hours of continuous therapy, the mean peak level in tracheal secretions may be 100 times greater than the minimum inhibitory concentration preventing the RSV replication in vitro (Connor et al, 1984). Furthermore, repeated courses eliminated simultaneous infection with both parainfluenza and RSV in an infant with severe combined immunodeficiency syndrome (McIntosh et al, 1984). However because of the small number of patients evaluated in controlled trials, the use of ribavirin for the treatment of RSV infections is not without controversy (Wald et al, 1988).

Ribavirin has been reported to be effective by other routes in several other viral infections, including measles, genital herpes infections, herpes zoster, and acute hepatitis types A and B (Fernandez, 1980; Uylangco et al, 1981; Bierman et al, 1981; Minkoff et al, 1980). When given intravenously or orally, it has been reported to reduce mortality significantly in patients with Lassa fever (McCormick et al, 1986). Of perhaps greater interest for Eastern countries, ribavirin was recently demonstrated to be useful for epidemic hemorrhagic fever (Huggins et al, 1988).

At high concentrations, ribavirin inhibits the replication of HIV. However, clinical trials sponsored by the National Institutes of Health have not provided evidence of its efficacy.

Bromovinyldeoxyuridine and Fluoroiodoaracytosine: The investigational agent, bromovinyldeoxyuridine (BVDU), is a potent inhibitor of herpes simplex virus type 1 (HSV-1) and varicella-zoster virus (VZV). In vitro, it is somewhat more potent than acyclovir against HSV-1 and approximately 1,000 times more potent against VZV; however, it is about 50 times less potent than acyclovir against HSV-2. It is also effective against several herpesviruses infecting animals.

Like acyclovir, the selectivity of BVDU is based on the phosphorylation of the parent compound by herpesvirus thymidine kinase, which restricts its action to virus-infected cells. When added to cells infected with HSV-1 and HSV-2, virus-encoded thymidine kinase rapidly converts the parent compound to the 5′-monophosphate form. In cells infected with HSV-1, but not HSV-2, the monophosphate is rapidly phosphorylated to the 5′-diphosphates and 5′-triphosphates. The triphosphate inhibits viral DNA polymerase much more than cellular DNA polymerases. In addition, the triphosphate is incorporated into viral DNA, which also may contribute to its antiviral activity. The difference in sensitivity of HSV-1 and HSV-2 to BVDU is thought to be due to the induction of a dTMP kinase by HSV-1 but not HSV-2. This kinase catalyzes the phosphorylation of BVDU monophosphate to the diphosphate. The triphosphate of BVDU inhibits HSV-1 and HSV-2 DNA polymerases equally; thus, the differential susceptibility of the two viruses is at the level of the dTMP kinase rather than of the DNA polymerase.

In preliminary, uncontrolled clinical trials, topical BVDU appeared to be effective in treating herpetic keratitis (Maudgal et al, 1981 A), and the oral form appeared to be beneficial in mucocutaneous herpes simplex and zoster infections in immunocompromised patients (de Clercq et al, 1980; Wildiers and de Clercq, 1984), VZV infections in leukemic children (Benoit et al, 1985), and ophthalmic zoster infections in the elderly (Maudgal et al, 1981 B). No adverse effects were reported in any of these studies. However, two potential problems have been identified in the drug's development. First, when BVDU is administered parenterally to man, the principal plasma metabolite is bromovinyl uracil and not BVDU. The former metabolite has very little antiviral activity. Second, preclinical toxicologic studies identified a higher frequency of tumor generation after long-term exposure in treated as compared to control animals. This latter problem has not been further clarified. Thus, controlled trials must be limited to high-risk patients or the elderly until potential toxicologic problems have been solved.

Fluoroiodoaracytosine (FIAC) is another potent selective inhibitor of herpesviruses. Related compounds include fluoromethylarauracil (FMAU) and fluoroethylarauracil (FEAU), the principal metabolite of FIAC. Like acyclovir and BVDU, its activity depends on phosphorylation by herpesvirus thymidine kinase. FIAC is phosphorylated 1,200 to 9,000 times better by the virus enzyme than by enzymes of normal host cells. The parent compound is converted rapidly to the triphosphate in infected cells, is selectively utilized by virus DNA polymerase, and is incorporated into viral DNA, resulting in the formation of very short chains. In vitro, FIAC has greater antiviral activity than acyclovir against HSV-1; it also is active against HSV-2, VZV, and CMV. Although it is highly active against the latter, its mechanism of action against this virus is not well understood. CMV does not produce its own thymidine kinase, but does increase the production of the cellular enzyme. In vitro, the therapeutic index of the drug has been calculated to be about 500 against CMV.

An uncontrolled clinical trial with FIAC suggested that this agent was effective in the treatment of VZV infections in immunocompromised patients (Young et al, 1983). The related compounds initially were considered too toxic for further evaluation after Phase I studies but currently are being re-evaluated.

AMANTADINE AND DERIVATIVES. Amantadine [Symmetrel] is a highly selective antiviral drug that inhibits the growth of known subtypes of influenza A viruses (H1 N1, H2 N2, and H3 N2). Because it has no clinical activity against influenza B viruses, this drug is used prophylactically and therapeutically only in infections caused by influenza type A virus (see the evaluation). It also is widely used in Parkinson's disease (see index entry Amantadine, In Parkinsonism).

Amantadine's mechanism of action in inhibiting influenza and in Parkinson's disease is similar, ie, it serves as an ion channel blocker. In Parkinson's disease, the nicotinic-acetylcholine receptor (an ion channel) is blocked; in influenza, the drug blocks acidification of the virus core via the M2 protein ion channel. Amantadine also inhibits virus assembly indirectly by affecting the conformation of the hemagglutinin during virus assembly. The latter mechanism predominates in avian myxovirus strains, and the former mechanism predominates in human influenza virus strains. Amantadine blocks the acidification process that occurs during adsorption and penetration of the virus into cells via endosomes. Indirect conformational change in the hemagglutinin, followed by acidification of the virus core, is thought to be necessary to allow the dissociation to matrix protein and release of RNA into the cytoplasm of infected cells (Belshe et al, 1989 B).

There is general agreement that at 200 mg/day the efficacy of amantadine when used prophylactically in influenza A infections averages 70% to 80% (range, 0% to 100%), approximately the same as with influenza vaccines. At a lower dose (100 mg/day) the drug has been reported to protect against influenza A strains in children and in the elderly (Payler et al, 1984; Betts et al, 1987; Arden et al, 1988). When given therapeutically, amantadine will accelerate defervescence and resolution of acute disease symptoms.

Rimantadine, an investigational analogue of amantadine, has a spectrum and mechanism of action identical to those of the parent drug (Belshe et al, 1988). In laboratory studies, rimantadine is two to four times more active than amantadine against influenza A (Belshe et al, 1989 B), but appreciable differences in clinical efficacy have not been demonstrated.

Several early clinical studies conducted in the United States demonstrated the prophylactic and therapeutic efficacy of rimantadine (200 mg/day) in influenza A infections (Dolin et al, 1982; Quarles et al, 1981; Van Voris et al, 1981). Results of studies in children and the elderly indicate that a dose of 100 mg/day also is effective prophylactically against influenza A outbreaks (Clover et al, 1986; Betts et al, 1987; Crawford et al, 1988). Rimantadine has no effect on influenza B infections at concentrations achieved clinically.

Most investigators agree that rimantadine causes fewer adverse effects than amantadine after use of identical dosages; higher plasma drug levels are obtained with amantadine, which could account for the higher incidence of adverse effects with this drug. In the elderly, however, plasma levels of amantadine were nearly three times higher than those in younger adults, possibly due to decreased renal function in older individuals; therefore, a reduction of dosage of amantadine may be necessary to reduce the incidence of adverse effects (Patriarca et al, 1984).

MISCELLANEOUS INVESTIGATIONAL DRUGS. Many compounds are being evaluated for selective antiviral activity. The following have shown some potential for clinical use.

Isoprinosine, a combination of inosine and dimepranol acedoben, is being used in Europe to treat a number of viral diseases, including herpesvirus, rhinovirus, and influenza A infections and viral hepatitis, but results of clinical studies are equivocal (Chang and Heel, 1981). Isoprinosine has been investigated in the United States for use in influenza, rhinovirus, herpes simplex, and herpes zoster infections with variable results. It was reported to be effective in the long-term treatment of subacute sclerosing panencephalitis, but this finding is controversial (Dyken et al, 1982; Durant et al, 1982; Haddah and Risk, 1980). At the present time, in the absence of data from properly conducted large-scale studies, it cannot be determined whether the drug has any value in the treatment of viral infections in humans.

The mechanism of action is not known. It was postulated early that Isoprinosine modifies ribosomes so that binding of virus mRNA occurs, but translation of the message is inhibited. Claims also have been made that Isoprinosine is an immunomodulator, since the drug potentiates in vitro lymphocyte responses to mitogens. Principally because of its purported immunomodulatory activities, Isoprinosine has been studied for its effect in AIDS patients (Table 2). The results of a recent randomized, double-blind, placebo-controlled trial on 866 HIV-infected patients without manifestations of AIDS lead the investigators to conclude that treatment with this drug delays the progression to AIDS (Pedersen et al, 1990). However, a number of concerns about this study were expressed by the Food and Drug Administration's Division of Antiviral Products, which concluded that more clinical investigation is needed before the drug's value can be properly assessed (Kweder et al, 1990). It has been suggested that Isoprinosine has a dual antiviral effect in that it supports lymphocyte functions by promoting cellular RNA synthesis and translational ability but suppresses viral RNA synthesis (Ohnishi et al, 1982). In humans, the drug is rapidly metabolized; the half-life is 50 minutes after oral administration and 3 minutes after intravenous injection.

Enviroxime is a benzimidazole derivative that is being evaluated for use against rhinoviruses, the primary causative organisms of the common cold. In vitro, it inhibits the replication of a wide range of rhinoviruses and also has antiviral effects against coxsackieviruses, echoviruses, and polioviruses. The proposed mechanism of action is interference with macromolecular synthesis in infected cells through inhibition of a viral RNA polymerase. In vitro studies have shown that enviroxime added to cell cultures a few hours after virus inoculation still significantly inhibits replication, thus suggesting a primary action during a late phase of replication. Some efficacy was observed against experimentally induced rhinovirus type 9 infection after combined oral and intranasal administration (Phillpotts et al, 1981), but other studies failed to demonstrate significant effects on artificially induced rhinovirus infections when the drug was administered only intranasally (Hayden and Gwaltney, 1982; Levandowski et al, 1982; Phillpotts et al, 1983).

Oral enviroxime is not well tolerated; adverse effects include nausea, vomiting, diarrhea, abdominal pain, and headache. However, the drug is well tolerated when given intranasally. Further studies are needed before the potential clinical usefulness of this compound can be determined.

Foscarnet sodium (trisodium phosphonoformate, PFA), a pyrophosphate analogue of phosphonoacetic acid (PAA), has potent in vitro and in vivo activity against herpesvirus. Background data are available on initial studies of this drug as an inhibitor of herpesvirus replication. In laboratory animals, PAA produced liver degeneration, gingivitis, and severe dermal toxicity, and it accumulated in bone. Thus, it was considered too toxic for human use. PFA is considerably less toxic and no dermal effects have been observed.

Both PAA and PFA inhibit the DNA polymerases of all human herpesviruses through similar mechanisms of action. These drugs are thought to act by blocking the pyrophosphate binding site, thus inhibiting the formation of the 3′-5′-phosphodiester bond between primer and substrate and preventing chain elongation. In addition to inhibiting herpesvirus DNA polymerase, PFA recently has attracted attention as an inhibitor of HIV replication. It also inhibits influenza A RNA-dependent RNA polymerase. Notably, PFA inhibits the reverse transcriptases of several other animal and human retroviruses. The cellular DNA polymerase α is approximately 80 times more resistant to this action than herpesvirus DNA polymerases. The antiviral spectrum of PFA in vitro includes herpes simplex virus types 1 and 2, VZV, CMV, EBV, African swine fever, HIV as noted, and various animal retroviruses (avian myeloblastosis, visna, and murine leukemia virus).

There have been few clinical trials with PFA. In one preliminary study in patients with recurrent herpes labialis, topical application of a 3% cream significantly shortened the vesicular period and decreased the development of new vesicles (Wallin et al, 1980). However, it was of no value in the treatment of genital herpes (Sacks et al, 1987). PFA also is undergoing clinical trials in patients with AIDS. A drawback to its use is that, like PAA, it is deposited in bone; however, in mice, 50% of bound PFA is released within three weeks. Results of preliminary studies in patients with AIDS suggest the possibility of nephrotoxicity at dosages required to inhibit viral replication. Additional clinical trials are necessary to evaluate the therapeutic potential of PFA more extensively.

Newer Antiviral Agents Used to Treat AIDS: The development of drugs to inhibit HIV replication is proliferating rapidly. The compounds listed in Table 2 are being studied.

Two compounds not discussed previously, *dideoxycytosine* and *dideoxyinosine,* appear promising and are currently being evaluated in Phase II and III trials. The mechanism of action of these drugs is very similar to that of zidovudine. Initial trials of dideoxycytidine showed that it had an antiviral effect, but peripheral neuropathy was the dose-limiting adverse effect. The potential usefulness of these compounds must be demonstrated in the expanded studies.

TABLE 2.
SOME HIV ANTIVIRAL AGENTS IN CLINICAL TRIALS FOR AIDS

Agent	Mechanism of Action	Manufacturer or Sponsor
Acemannan [Carrisyn]	Binds to viral thymidine; immunomodulator	Carrington Laboratories
AL-721	Alteration of viral envelope or host cell membrane	Ethigen Corp.
Amphotericin B methyl ester	Irreversible binding to sterols	Waksman Institute
Ampligen (mismatched RNA)	Interferon inducer	HEM Research, Inc. E.I. Dupont de Nemours
Castanospermine	Inhibits glycosylation	GD Searle
Soluble CD_4 (rST_4)	Inhibits viral attachment	Biogen Genentech Smith Kline & French
Dextran sulfate (UA 001)	Inhibits viral adsorption	Ueno Fine Chemicals
Dideoxycytidine (ddC)	Reverse transcriptase inhibitor; DNA chain termination	Hoffmann-LaRoche, NCI
Dideoxyinosine (ddI)	Reverse transcriptase inhibitor; DNA chain termination	Bristol Myers, NCI
Didihydro-dideoxythymidine (D4T)	Inhibits viral DNA chain elongation	Bristol Myers
Foscarnet sodium (PFA, trisodium phosphonoformate)	Reverse transcriptase inhibitor	Astra Pharmaceuticals
Fusidic acid	Unknown; possibly protease inhibitor	Leo Lovens
HPA-23	Reverse transcriptase inhibitor	Rhone-Poulenc
Interferons (alpha, beta, gamma)	Antiviral; antiproliferative; immunomodulators	Burroughs Wellcome Genentech Hoffmann-LaRoche Schering Plough Triton Bioscience
Isoprinosine	Antiviral action unknown; immunomodulator	Newport Pharmaceuticals International
Penicillamine	Metal chelating agent; cross-links disulfide groups; inactivates viral proteins	Carter Wallace Degussa Pharmaceutical
Peptide T (octapentide sequence)	Inhibits viral binding to receptor	Peninsula Laboratories
Ribavirin [Virazole]	Probably interference with viral mRNA synthesis	Viratek/ICN Pharmaceuticals
Rifabutin (ansamycin)	Reverse transcriptase inhibitor	Adria Laboratories
Zidovudine (azidothymidine, AZT) [Retrovir]	Reverse transcriptase inhibitor; DNA chain termination	Burroughs Wellcome

Resistance

As with other microorganisms, virus mutants may arise that have decreased sensitivity to certain antiviral drugs. Resistance must be evaluated in two contexts: in vitro laboratory studies and problems related to clinical use.

For herpesviruses, two encoded enzymes, thymidine kinase (TK) and DNA polymerase, are intimately involved in the action of antiherpesvirus drugs in current use or being investigated (acyclovir, vidarabine, BVDU, FIAC, PFA). As might be expected, loss or reduction of thymidine kinase activity or subtle alterations in viral thymidine kinase or DNA polymerase markedly reduces the sensitivity of herpesviruses to these drugs. For example, five types of mutants have been isolated by passage of virus in cell cultures maintained in the presence of acyclovir: (1) mutants with absent or low production of TK, (2) mutants producing altered TK, (3) mutants with altered DNA polymerase, (4) mutants deficient in TK and with altered DNA polymerase, and (5) mutants with altered TK and DNA polymerase.

Acquired resistance in mutants isolated from cell cultures, animals, and man has been reported for idoxuridine, vidarabine, cytarabine, trifluorothymidine, acyclovir, ganciclovir, zidovudine, BVDU, FIAC, PAA, and PFA. From a laboratory perspective, TK-defective mutants are inherently resistant to all drugs whose action is mediated through this enzyme; thus, TK-mutants have been described that are cross resistant to idoxuridine, cytarabine, acyclovir, and BVDU (Field et al, 1981). It is rather facile to isolate a TK-resistant mutant in cell culture; a single passage of virus in cells cultured in the presence of any of the TK-mediated drugs is sufficient to isolate TK-resistant viruses.

Resistance through alterations in herpesvirus DNA polymerase may lead to cross resistance, but this point is not well defined. For example, it was reported early that mutants resistant to PAA were always resistant to the analogue, PFA. Although mutants resistant to PAA have been reported to be resistant to acyclovir, this has not been well established. The physical map limits of sequences within the HSV-1 DNA polymerase locus that contain mutations conferring resistance to BVDU have been defined. The region of resistance mutation for vidarabine is closely linked to that for PAA and acyclovir and overlaps with that for BVDU; however, the latter can be transferred separately (Crumpacker et al, 1982 A and B). Thus, cross resistance to the herpesvirus drugs, PAA, PFA, acyclovir, and vidarabine, due to an altered DNA polymerase can be expected, at least in vitro. The resistance of herpesvirus DNA polymerase to BVDU appears to be independent of its resistance to PAA, acyclovir, and vidarabine.

Fortunately, resistant herpesvirus mutants do not emerge frequently in humans or animals undergoing chemotherapy, even though they arise readily in drug-treated cell cultures. Attempts to isolate resistant viruses from experimentally infected animals treated with acyclovir have been generally unsuccessful. It is thought that conditions exist in vivo that limit the development of resistance. By far the most frequently isolated resistant mutants from infected cell cultures or patients are those that are defective in TK production. These TK- mutants appear to be present in clinical isolates both before and after therapy with acyclovir. TK-deficient mutants are less virulent than the wild strains and considerably less capable of establishing latency in experimental animals. A clinical isolate of an HSV mutant with resistance due to an altered TK has been reported. Such resistance appears to be increasingly problematic in AIDS patients. Acyclovir resistance with VZV also has been reported in AIDS patients. Clinical isolates of resistant mutants with an altered DNA polymerase have not yet been reported. As might be anticipated, resistant strains of herpesviruses have been encountered more frequently in immunocompromised patients receiving acyclovir; all such isolates have been TK-deficient mutants. The greater extent of virus multiplication in these patients may be a factor in the selection of resistant strains. Administration of acyclovir by continuous infusion has been suggested as an alternative to traditional intermittent therapy for infections due to acyclovir-resistant mutants (Fletcher et al, 1989).

CMV strains resistant to ganciclovir have been isolated from the blood of three hospitalized patients who had received prolonged therapy with the drug and had CMV disease refractory to ganciclovir therapy. However, the sequence of events, as determined by genetic analysis, was distinctly different in each case. One patient was infected with a resistant virus, another was infected with a susceptible virus that became resistant, and the third was infected first by a susceptible strain and subsequently by a genetically distinct resistant one (Erice et al, 1989).

Herpesviruses also exhibit a different type of resistance that poses a major problem. Latent herpesviruses persist for prolonged periods in certain areas of the body (eg, neural cells of ganglia for herpes simplex and varicella-zoster viruses). This latent infection is punctuated by episodes of active viral replication and disease recurrence. Unfortunately, the currently available antiherpesvirus drugs must be given during active viral multiplication to be effective. None are active against latent virus and, therefore, active infections can be expected once treatment is stopped.

Strains of influenza A resistant to amantadine have emerged following a single passage in cell cultures containing the compound. Resistance of influenza A virus to amantadine or rimantadine is easily developed in the laboratory by serial passage of the virus in cultures containing low concentrations of either drug, and such isolates are cross resistant (Oxford et al, 1980). Resistant mutants of influenza A also have been isolated from infected mice treated with amantadine. Mutants with increased resistance to the drug were observed after a single passage; after six passages, most of the isolated strains were completely resistant to amantadine and rimantadine (Oxford et al, 1970). Amantadine- and rimantadine-resistant influenza strains have been isolated from patients in whom neither compound was used prophylactically (Heider et al, 1981). Rimantadine-resistant mutants have been recovered from children receiving treatment and from family members receiving postexposure prophylaxis (Hall et al, 1987; Belshe et al, 1988; Hayden et al, 1989). In one study, there was apparent transmission of drug-resistant strains (Hayden et al, 1989). In a ten-year study of amantadine and rimantadine resistance in one community, naturally occurring resistant strains were not detected in untreated patients; however, rimantadine-resistant strains were recovered from members of one family undergoing therapy or prophylaxis with the drug (Belshe et al, 1989 A).

Resistance to either drug has been associated with point mutations in the RNA sequence coding for the M2 polypeptide, a 97 amino acid protein coded by a second mRNA transcribed from the same viral gene that codes for the matrix protein. This mutation results in a single amino acid change in the membrane opening portion (Belshe et al, 1988; Hay et al, 1979, 1986).

Isolates of HIV-1 with increased resistance to zidovudine in vitro have been obtained from patients receiving long-term therapy with the drug. Isolates from several patients showed a 100-fold increase in resistance; these isolates also were insensitive to 3′-azido-2′,3′-dideoxyuridine (AZdU) but remained sensitive to dideoxycytidine (ddC), 2′,3′-dideoxy-2′,3′ didehydrothymidine (D4T), and foscarnet (trisodium phosphonoformate). However, the clinical significance of this finding is unknown (Larder et al, 1989).

Drug Evaluations

ACYCLOVIR SODIUM (Parenteral)
[Zovirax]

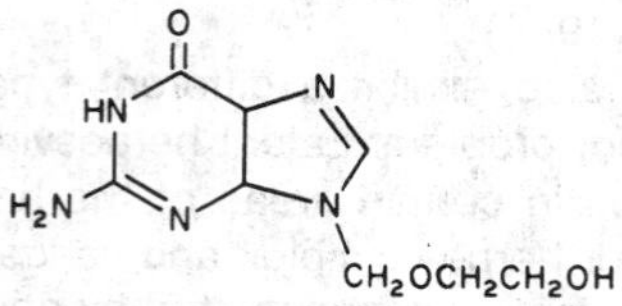

ACTIONS. The antiviral spectrum of acyclovir is limited to herpesviruses. In vitro, the order of decreasing susceptibility to its antiviral activity is HSV-1, HSV-2, varicella-zoster virus (VZV), Epstein-Barr virus (EBV), and cytomegalovirus (CMV). Acyclovir is 160 times more potent than vidarabine against herpes simplex type 1 in tissue culture experiments. The specific activation of acyclovir by herpesvirus thymidine kinase and the subsequent preferential inhibition of viral DNA polymerase by acyclo-GTP provide the drug with a high degree of selective activity (see the Introduction). A 3,000-fold greater concentration of acyclovir is required to inhibit the growth of host cells than to inhibit viral replication.

The mechanism of action of acyclovir against CMV and EBV appears to be somewhat different than against herpes simplex or varicella-zoster viruses. Unlike the latter viruses, neither CMV nor EBV code for their own thymidine kinase. In cells infected by these viruses, acyclovir is poorly phosphorylated; however, once phosphorylated to the triphosphate, both CMV and EBV DNA polymerase are quite sensitive to the drug.

USES. A number of double-blind, placebo-controlled studies support the efficacy of acyclovir both systemically and topically in various herpesvirus infections (see also the following evaluations on oral and topical acyclovir).

Acyclovir is indicated for the treatment of initial and recurrent mucosal and cutaneous herpes simplex (HSV-1 and HSV-2) and varicella-zoster (shingles) infections in immunocompromised patients. It is also indicated for the treatment of severe initial episodes of herpes genitalis in immunocompetent patients and for herpes simplex encephalitis in patients over age 6 months. In immunocompromised patients with mucocutaneous herpes simplex infections, the median times to cessation of new lesion formation, lesion crusting, lesion healing, cessation of pain, and termination of viral shedding were shorter in patients in the acyclovir group than in those in the placebo group (Mitchell et al, 1981; Chou et al, 1981; Wade et al, 1982 B; Meyers et al, 1982).

Acyclovir also appears to be effective in other herpes simplex infections in immunocompromised patients. When intravenous acyclovir was given to herpes simplex virus-seropositive recipients of bone marrow transplants for 18 days beginning three days before transplantation, no patient developed lesions during the course of therapy (Saral et al, 1981). One-half of the treated patients developed mild herpes simplex infections after cessation of therapy, however, indicating that acyclovir cannot eradicate latent infection. Similarly, acyclovir prevented reactivation of HSV infections when given prophylactically to leukemic patients receiving timed sequential chemotherapy (Saral et al, 1983), but infection recurred in many patients after cessation of acyclovir when cancer chemotherapy was resumed.

The efficacy of acyclovir against herpes zoster infections in immunocompromised patients has been demonstrated in several clinical trials (Selby et al, 1979; Spector et al, 1982; Serota et al, 1982; Balfour et al, 1983; Meyers et al, 1984). In one trial, 40 marrow transplant patients were treated with acyclovir for VZV infections (Meyers et al, 1984) and a rapid antiviral effect was noted; the median times to cessation of virus positivity, new lesion formation, and total pustulation were shorter than those reported for vidarabine. In a prospective randomized trial, acyclovir and vidarabine given intravenously were compared in 22 severely compromised patients who presented within 72 hours of onset of VZV infection. Cutaneous dissemination of infection did not occur in any of the 10 evaluable patients treated with acyclovir; in comparison, 5 of the evaluable 10 recipients of vidarabine developed localized dermatomal disease. Acyclovir also was superior to vidarabine in shortening the period of virus shedding, new lesion formation, the median interval until the first decrease in pain, the pustulation and crusting of all lesions, and the complete healing of lesions and in reducing the incidence of fever. The investigators concluded that acyclovir was the drug of choice for the treatment of VZV infection in immunocompromised patients (Shepp et al, 1986).

Studies also have suggested that acyclovir is effective in immunocompetent patients with herpes zoster (Peterslund et al, 1981, 1984; Bean et al, 1982; Esmann et al, 1982; Huff et al, 1988; Morton et al, 1989). Reduction in pain and erythema, prevention of new lesion formation, and decrease in healing time were reported.

As noted above, acyclovir for biopsy-proven herpes simplex virus encephalitis is superior to vidarabine as demonstrated by increased survival and a greater likelihood of return to normal function. Acyclovir is still being evaluated for neonatal herpes simplex virus infections.

In patients with normal immune systems, acyclovir has been effective in primary genital herpesvirus infections. When compared to placebo controls, patients receiving acyclovir showed more rapid healing, earlier cessation of pain and pruritus, and earlier termination of viral shedding (Corey et al, 1983; Mindel et al, 1982; Peacock et al, 1988).

Results of clinical studies employing acyclovir to treat CMV disease in immunocompromised patients are equivocal. In one study, organ transplant patients with CMV disease were given acyclovir 500 mg/M^2 three times daily intravenously for seven days (Balfour et al, 1982). These patients experienced more rapid defervescence and clinical improvement than placebo controls. In a second study, however, marrow transplant patients with CMV pneumonia were given doses ranging from 400 to 1,200 mg/M^2 without favorable effect (Wade et al, 1982 B). In a more recent study, an indirect clinical benefit was suggested (eg, a decrease in fever and time to onset of CMV excretion) in these high-risk patients; a larger controlled study appears to be necessary (Meyers et al, 1988).

ADVERSE REACTIONS AND PRECAUTIONS. In general, intravenous acyclovir has not produced serious adverse effects. Elevations in blood urea nitrogen and creatinine concentrations have been reported and were more common when the drug was administered as an intravenous bolus. The elevations returned to normal after cessation of therapy and, in some cases, despite continued therapy. Increasing the infusion time, decreasing the dose, or increasing water intake reversed the effect. The proposed mechanism for this nephrotoxic action is crystallization of acyclovir in renal tubules, which was observed previously in animal studies. Therefore, it is recommended that acyclovir be administered by infusion over one hour. Caution should be exercised in dehydrated patients or in those with impaired renal function.

Phlebitis at the injection site and delirium in two patients also have been reported. This drug is classified in FDA Pregnancy Category C.

PHARMACOKINETICS. Following intravenous administration, acyclovir exhibits dose-independent pharmacokinetics in the range of 0.5 to 15 mg/kg. In adults, when 5 mg/kg was given in one-hour infusions every eight hours, mean steady-state peak and trough concentrations of 9.8 mcg/ml and 0.7 mcg/ml, respectively, were achieved.

Acyclovir is widely distributed in tissues and body fluids. Concentrations attained in the cerebrospinal fluid are approximately 50% of those in the plasma. Plasma protein binding is low (9% to 33%). The drug is excreted by glomerular filtration and tubular secretion, primarily in unchanged form. The half-life is about 2.5 hours in adults and children with normal renal function.

DOSAGE AND PREPARATIONS.

Intravenous: Acyclovir should be administered by intravenous infusion. Rapid or bolus intravenous, intramuscular, or subcutaneous injection must be avoided. Therapy should be initiated as early as possible following onset of symptoms. Dosage adjustments are necessary in patients with renal impairment (see the manufacturer's recommendations).

For mucosal and cutaneous herpes simplex (HSV-1 and HSV-2) infections in immunocompromised patients, *adults,* 5 mg/kg infused at a constant rate over a one-hour period every eight hours (15 mg/kg/day) for seven days; *children under 12 years,* 250 mg/M^2 infused at a constant rate over a one-hour period every eight hours (750 mg/M^2/day) for seven days.

For severe initial episodes of herpes genitalis in immunocompetent patients, the same dosages as above are administered for five days.

For herpes zoster infections in immunocompromised patients, *adults and children over 12 years,* 10 mg/kg over a one-hour period every eight hours for seven days. For immunocompetent *adults* (investigational indication), 5 mg/kg over a one-hour period every eight hours for seven days. In *children under 12 years,* equivalent plasma concentrations are attained by infusing 500 mg/M^2 at a constant rate over a one-hour period every eight hours for seven days. Obese patients should receive 10 mg/kg. The maximum dose is 500 mg/M^2 every eight hours.

For herpes simplex encephalitis, *adults,* 10 mg/kg infused at a constant rate over a one-hour period every eight hours for ten days. For *children 6 months to 12 years,* more accurate dosing is achieved by infusing 500 mg/M^2 for the same period.

Zovirax (Burroughs Wellcome). Powder (sterile) equivalent to 500 mg base in 10 ml containers, or 1 g base in 20 ml containers.

ACYCLOVIR (Oral)
[Zovirax]

USES. Oral acyclovir is indicated for the treatment of initial episodes of genital herpes virus infections and management of recurrences in certain patients. It is also indicated for acute treatment of herpes zoster infection.

Treatment of primary genital herpes infection with oral acyclovir 200 mg given five times daily for five to ten days significantly reduced viral shedding, time to crusting, duration of local pain, and severity of symptoms (Nilsen et al, 1982; Bryson et al, 1983; Mertz et al, 1984); however, recurrence rates did not appear to be influenced.

Oral acyclovir also has been beneficial in the treatment of recurrent genital herpes infections. In a multicenter trial involving 250 patients with recurrent genital herpes, oral acyclovir 200 mg given five times daily for five days reduced virus shedding and shortened the time to healing of lesions by approximately 24 to 48 hours. The effects were more pronounced when therapy was initiated early in the course of recurrences. However, therapy did not appear to affect the latent state, for there was no difference in times to the next recurrence between drug and placebo groups (Reichman et al, 1984).

In a randomized, double-blind trial, acyclovir 200 mg four times daily for 12 weeks reduced the mean monthly recurrence rate and median time to first recurrence (Mindel et al, 1984). In other studies in which acyclovir was administered in two, three, or five daily doses over a four-month period, significantly fewer recurrences were reported in treated patients compared to placebo-controlled groups (Straus et al, 1984 B; Douglas et al, 1984). In one study, the time to first recurrence was similar in both drug- and placebo-controlled groups (Straus et al, 1984 B). In other studies, the median time to first recurrence was significantly shorter in the treated groups (Douglas et al, 1984; Mindel et al, 1984). However, more recent studies clearly have established the value of oral therapy (Mertz et al, 1988 A and B; Mattison et al, 1988; Straus et al, 1988).

Long-term (12 months) therapy does not appear to have any lasting effect on the natural history of the disease; recurrences return to pretreatment frequencies following cessation of therapy (Douglas et al, 1984). Longer therapy has been reported to be of value (Straus et al, 1988; Mertz et al, 1988 A). In addition, lesions in treated patients contained resistant virus, although in later recurrences the virus appeared to be drug-sensitive (Straus et al, 1984 B). Thus, studies to date suggest that oral acyclovir is useful for maintenance therapy rather than for cure of genital herpes, but no recommendations can be made regarding episodic versus continuous therapy until further studies are completed.

In a number of clinical trials, oral acyclovir had significant efficacy against other herpesvirus infections in both immunocompromised and immunocompetent patients. Symptomatic attacks of mucocutaneous herpes simplex infections were suppressed in immunocompromised patients during the course (up to 65 days) of drug administration (Straus et al, 1982). In recurrent infections in immunodeficient patients, 200 mg five times daily for five days reduced virus shedding, alleviated signs and symptoms, and increased time to recurrence (Straus et al, 1984 A). In the clinical trials, however, recurrences always followed cessation of therapy. In the latter study, however, expected recurrences were suppressed by the administration of 200 mg twice daily.

In a prospective, randomized, double-blind, placebo-controlled trial, oral acyclovir was reported to be safe and effective in preventing herpesvirus reactivation after marrow transplantation when 400 mg was given five times daily from one week before to four weeks after transplantation (Wade et al, 1984). It is also being employed for suppression of mucocutaneous recurrences following renal transplantation.

In an uncontrolled study, dissemination of VZV in immunocompromised children was prevented by oral acyclovir 400 mg five times daily for ten days (Novelli et al, 1984). In a double-blind, randomized trial in elderly patients with acute zoster infections, oral acyclovir 400 mg five times daily for five days was as effective as intravenous acyclovir in shortening the duration of pain and accelerating the healing rate (Peterslund et al, 1984). In a double-blind, placebo-controlled trial conducted in immunocompetent patients over 50 years old with herpes zoster, the only statistically significant difference demonstrated by a similar regimen of oral acyclovir was a decrease in the number of days of new lesion formation within the affected dermatome after day zero (McKendrick et al, 1984). However, results of two subsequent double-blind, placebo-controlled trials showed that oral acyclovir shortened the time to lesion scabbing, healing, and complete cessation of pain; reduced the duration of new lesion formation; and reduced the prevalence of zoster-associated neurologic symptoms (Huff et al, 1988; Morton et al, 1989).

ADVERSE REACTIONS. Acyclovir is well tolerated when given orally. The most frequently reported reactions during short-term administration are nausea and/or vomiting (incidence 2.7%) and headache (0.6%); the most common reactions during long-term administration are headache (1.9%), diarrhea (2.4%), nausea and/or vomiting (4.8%), and rash (1.7%). Acyclovir has not affected results of laboratory tests, except for one report of increased mean corpuscular volume of erythrocytes and mean corpuscular hemoglobin concentrations (Straus et al, 1984 A) and another report of elevated bilirubin levels (Douglas et al, 1984). These data, however, have not been confirmed in larger clinical trials (Mertz et al, 1988 A and B).

Large doses of acyclovir decreased spermatogenesis in some animals and, in some acute studies, were reported to produce mutagenic effects. It was not possible to confirm the spermatogenic effects in humans (Douglas et al, 1988). Because chromosome breaks may occur at high drug concentrations, acyclovir should not be used during pregnancy unless the potential benefits outweigh the risks to the fetus (FDA Pregnancy Category C). No adequate controlled studies have been done in pregnant women. The drug has been found in breast milk following oral administration; concentrations are 0.6 to 4.1 times higher than corresponding plasma levels.

PHARMACOKINETICS. Acyclovir is slowly and variably absorbed; peak levels are achieved in one to four hours. Bioavailability is 15% to 30%. Depending on the dose employed, peak plasma levels range from 0.3 to 2 mcg/ml. The half-life of oral acyclovir is 3.3 hours. After administration of 200 mg orally, levels of 0.19 mcg/ml and 0.8 mcg/ml, respectively, were attained in saliva and vaginal secretions. Ten to fifteen percent of the administered dose is excreted unchanged in the urine, and 15% to 25% is excreted unchanged in stools. A single-dose bioavailability study showed that acyclovir capsules 200 mg are bioequivalent to acyclovir 200 mg in aqueous solution.

DOSAGE AND PREPARATIONS.

Oral: *Adults,* for initial episodes of genital herpes, 200 mg every four hours five times daily for ten days (one 200-mg capsule or one teaspoonful of suspension). For chronic suppressive therapy for recurrent disease, 400 mg two times daily for up to 12 months, followed by re-evaluation. Alternative regimens have included doses ranging from 200 mg three times daily to 200 mg five times daily. For intermittent therapy for recurrent disease, 200 mg every four hours five times daily for five days. Therapy should begin at the earliest sign of recurrence, ie, at the onset of prodrome. For treatment of immunocompetent patients with herpes zoster, 800 mg every four hours five times daily for seven to ten days. In patients with renal impairment (creatinine clearance ≤10 ml/min/1.73 M^2), 200 mg should be given every 12 hours; creatinine clearance between 10 and 25 ml/min/1.73 M^2, 200 mg (one teaspoonful of the suspension) should be given every eight hours.

Zovirax (Burroughs Wellcome). Capsules 200 mg; suspension 200 mg/5 ml.

ACYCLOVIR (Topical)

[Zovirax Ointment]

USES. A topical ointment containing acyclovir 5% in polyethylene glycol is used for the management of initial genital herpes infections. A double-blind, placebo-controlled study showed that the application of acyclovir ointment to lesions four or six times a day promoted healing, relieved pain and pruritus, and decreased the duration of viral shedding in patients with initial infections (Corey et al, 1982 A and B). In contrast, no benefit was noted in patients with recurrent herpes genitalis, although some decrease in the duration of viral shedding was observed (Luby et al, 1984). Oral acyclovir is the treatment of choice for genital herpes infections, because it prevents the development of new lesions and shortens the duration of dysuria whereas topical application does not. Acyclovir does not eradicate latent herpesvirus and, therefore, does not prevent recurrences of active disease (see also the Introduction). The use of topical acyclovir in genital herpes is limited to active initial infections, although experts recommend oral therapy.

Topical acyclovir also has been used for limited, nonlife-threatening, mucocutaneous herpes simplex infections, mainly herpes labialis, in immunocompromised patients. The duration of viral shedding was reduced and the duration of pain was decreased slightly (Whitley et al, 1982 B). No evidence of clinical benefit has been observed in immunocompetent patients with herpes labialis, although some decrease in the duration of viral shedding has been noted (Spruance et al, 1982, 1984).

A number of clinical trials have established the effectiveness of an ophthalmic ointment containing acyclovir 3% in the treatment of herpes simplex keratitis. However, this use is currently investigational.

ADVERSE REACTIONS AND PRECAUTIONS. The most common adverse effect is mild pain, including transient burning and stinging, at the site of application. Pruritus, rash, and vulvitis also have been reported. These adverse effects probably are caused by the application of ointment to tender lesions, since placebo-treated patients also experienced these undesirable effects.

The topical form of acyclovir is classified in FDA Pregnancy Category C.

DOSAGE AND PREPARATIONS.

Topical: Sufficient ointment to cover all lesions should be applied every three hours six times a day for seven days. The dose/application depends on the total lesion area but should approximate a one-half inch ribbon of ointment/4 in^2 of surface area. A finger cot or rubber glove should be used to prevent autoinoculation of other body sites and transmission of infection to other persons. Therapy should be initiated as early as possible following onset of signs and symptoms.

Zovirax (Burroughs Wellcome). Ointment 5% (50 mg/g) in a polyethylene glycol base in 3 and 15 g containers.

AMANTADINE HYDROCHLORIDE

[Symmetrel]

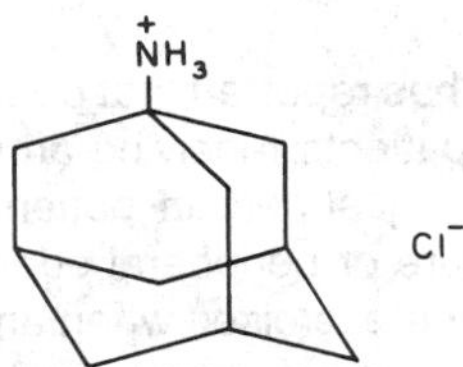

ACTIONS AND USES. Amantadine has a narrow antiviral spectrum. All influenza A subtypes and some C strains are inhibited in vitro; influenza B strains are rarely sensitive. Strains of influenza A differ in sensitivity; in vitro inhibitory concentrations vary from 0.2 to 30 mcg/ml, depending on the assay system employed. Sendai and rubella viruses also are sensitive to amantadine in vitro. Early studies suggested that amantadine acted by inhibiting viral penetration and/or uncoating, but more recent studies indicate that its inhibitory effect may involve interaction with the virion M (matrix) protein (see the Introduction).

Amantadine is useful in the prophylaxis and treatment of influenza A infections (National Institutes of Health Consensus Development Conference, 1980). Approximately 70% of recipients exposed to influenza A viruses are protected. Although early immunization is preferred, amantadine is recommended when vaccine is unavailable or contraindicated, particularly in children and adults at high risk because of underlying diseases, elderly patients in semiclosed institutional environments, and individuals with vital community functions (eg, policemen, firemen, hospital personnel). Since amantadine does not interfere with the immune response to influenza A vaccine, it can be administered concomitantly to provide interim protection or to augment the prophylactic effect in a previously vaccinated individual.

Amantadine also is effective in the treatment of active influenza A infection when administered within 48 hours after the onset of symptoms. This drug is of no clinical value in infections caused by influenza B or other myxoviruses.

ADVERSE REACTIONS AND PRECAUTIONS. Amantadine is well tolerated by most patients during short- and long-term use. Central nervous system side effects are most common and include difficulty in thinking, confusion, lightheadedness, hallucinations, anxiety, and insomnia. These symptoms are mild, usually occur shortly after therapy is started, are reversible on discontinuation of the drug, and often cease even when administration is continued. Activities requiring mental alertness (eg, driving) should be avoided until it is reasonable to assume that these symptoms will not occur. More severe adverse effects, such as mental depression and psychosis, are usually associated with doses exceeding 200 mg daily. Less common untoward effects include anorexia, nausea, vomiting, and orthostatic hypotension. Rarely, leukopenia and neutropenia are observed; other hematologic disorders have not been reported.

Livedo reticularis occasionally associated with ankle edema has occurred with use of amantadine in Parkinson's disease, particularly in women given the drug for a month or longer (see index entry Amantadine, In Parkinsonism). This reaction has not been observed with the smaller doses used for influenza.

The manufacturer has reported that congestive heart failure developed in a few patients receiving amantadine. The dose may require careful adjustment in patients with pre-existing congestive heart failure or peripheral edema.

Caution also must be exercised when amantadine is administered to patients with impaired renal function, liver disease, epilepsy, and psychosis or severe psychoneurosis not controlled by psychotropic agents.

In certain laboratory animals, large doses have been embryotoxic and teratogenic. Thus, amantadine should be used in pregnant women only after the risks to the fetus are weighed against the benefit to the patient (FDA Pregnancy Category C). Amantadine is excreted in milk and thus should not be given to nursing mothers.

DRUG INTERACTIONS. The peripheral and central adverse effects of anticholinergic drugs are increased by the concomitant use of amantadine. Acute psychotic reactions identical to those caused by atropine poisoning have occurred with combined therapy. Psychotic reactions also have developed occasionally in patients receiving amantadine and levodopa. If signs of central toxicity develop, the dose of anticholinergic drug or levodopa should be reduced while the patient is receiving amantadine.

PHARMACOKINETICS. Amantadine is absorbed rapidly and completely after oral administration; peak serum levels of approximately 0.3 mcg/ml are achieved two to four hours after administration of 2.5 mg/kg. The half-life in the serum averages 20 hours (range, 9 to 37 hours). When the usual adult dose of 100 mg is given every 12 hours, maximal tissue concentrations are reached in approximately 48 hours. Amantadine is not metabolized in humans, and about 90% of an administered dose is excreted unchanged in the urine. The drug crosses the blood-brain barrier, and a cerebrospinal fluid concentration approximating 60% of that in the plasma may be attained.

The clearance of amantadine is significantly reduced in adults with renal insufficiency. The elimination half-life increases up to threefold when creatinine clearance is less than 40 ml/min/1.73 M^2 and averages eight days in patients receiving prolonged maintenance hemodialysis. Therefore, the dose should be decreased or therapy discontinued in these patients. In patients 65 years and older, renal clearance is reduced and plasma levels are increased. In elderly patients taking 100 mg daily, plasma levels have approximated those in younger patients taking 200 mg daily.

DOSAGE AND PREPARATIONS.

Oral: For prophylaxis of influenza A infections, *adults under age 65 and children older than 9 years,* 100 mg twice daily; *adults over 65 years*, 100 mg daily; *children 1 to 9 years,* 4.4 to 8.8 mg/kg daily in two or three equal doses (maximum, 150 mg daily).

Prophylactic administration should be started in anticipation of contact or as soon as possible after exposure to influenza A viruses. Amantadine should be given for at least ten days following a known exposure or throughout the risk period, which in most communities is four to six weeks. Dosage can be continued for up to 90 days in cases of possible repeated and unknown exposures. When used with inactivated influenza A vaccine (to provide interim protection until adequate antibody titers develop), amantadine is continued for two to three weeks after administration of vaccine.

For treatment of established influenza A, the same dosage used for prophylaxis should be administered within 48 hours after onset of illness and continued for four to five days.

Symmetrel (DuPont), ***Generic.*** Capsules 100 mg; syrup 50 mg/5 ml.

GANCICLOVIR SODIUM

[Cytovene]

Ganciclovir (DHPG, BW-759U), a synthetic acyclic nucleoside analogue of 2′-deoxyguanosine, is a potent inhibitor of herpesviruses, including cytomegalovirus (CMV).

ACTIONS. The principal action of ganciclovir against CMV is the inhibition of viral DNA synthesis by ganciclovir-5′-triphosphate (ganciclovir-TP), which is caused by a quantitatively selective inhibition of viral DNA polymerase. Inhibition of cellular DNA polymerase alpha is weaker. Ganciclovir is metabolized to the triphosphate by the action of three cellular enzymes: a deoxyguanosine kinase produced in CMV-infected cells, guanylate kinase, and phosphoglycerate kinase. Other nucleotide-metabolizing enzymes may be involved. The antiviral activity of the triphosphate is due to the inhibition of viral DNA synthesis because of competitive inhibition with deoxyguanosine triphosphate for binding to viral DNA polymerase and to direct incorporation into viral DNA resulting in the termination of chain elongation.

USES. Ganciclovir is indicated for the treatment of CMV retinitis in immunocompromised patients, including those with AIDS. Diagnosis should be made by indirect ophthalmoscopy. Differential diagnosis includes candidiasis, toxoplasmosis, and cotton wool spots, any of which may produce a similar retinal appearance. Diagnosis may be supported by culture of CMV, but a negative culture does not rule out CMV retinitis.

The safety and efficacy of ganciclovir have not been established for congenital or neonatal CMV disease, for treatment of other CMV infections (eg, pneumonitis, colitis), or for use in immunocompetent patients. The drug is administered only by intravenous infusion.

Also see the Introduction.

ADVERSE REACTIONS. During clinical trials, ganciclovir was withdrawn or therapy was interrupted in 32% of patients because of adverse effects. The most frequent adverse reactions involved the hematopoietic system. Granulocytopenia occurred in 40% and thrombocytopenia in 20% of the patients. Withdrawal of the drug has resulted in increased neutrophil or platelet counts in most patients; however, some individuals experienced irreversible neutropenia or sepsis during neutropenic episodes. Approximately 40% of AIDS patients with CMV retinitis may be unable to tolerate ganciclovir because of marrow toxicity. Other than leukopenia and thrombocytopenia, the most frequent adverse events reported by the manufacturer are anemia, fever, rash, and abnormal liver function values, which developed in approximately 2% of the patients. However, in one study of 314 immunocompromised patients, additional adverse effects included those affecting the central nervous system (18%); nausea, fever, and rash (6%); and vomiting, diarrhea, anemia, and pain at the infusion site (4%) (Buhles et al, 1988).

PRECAUTIONS. Ganciclovir should be used with caution in patients with preexisting cytopenias or a history of cytopenic reactions to other drugs. Granulocytopenia usually occurs during the first or second week of therapy, but may occur at any time. Ganciclovir should not be administered if the absolute neutrophil count is less than 500 cells/mm^3 or the platelet count is less than 25,000/mm^3. Cell counts usually start to recover within three to seven days following drug withdrawal.

Administration of ganciclovir to laboratory animals has caused inhibition of spermatogenesis and subsequent infertility. Therefore, it is probable that at the recommended doses the drug causes temporary or permanent inhibition of spermatogenesis and also may suppress fertility in females. In laboratory studies, this drug has been shown to be both mutagenic and carcinogenic. Therefore, pregnancy should be avoided during treatment and for at least 90 days following treatment (FDA Pregnancy Category C). It is not known if ganciclovir is excreted in human milk, but since many drugs are and the drug is both mutagenic and carcinogenic, nursing should be discontinued during ganciclovir treatment and not resumed until 72 hours after the last dose. Use of the drug in children should be undertaken only with extreme caution because of the probability of long-term carcinogenicity and reproductive toxicity and only if the potential benefits clearly outweigh the risks.

The patient should be adequately hydrated, for ganciclovir is excreted by the kidney and adequate renal function is necessary for normal drug clearance. Dosage adjustments are required if renal function is impaired (see Dosage and Preparations). Elderly patients frequently have reduced glomerular filtration; therefore, it is particularly important that renal function be assessed in these patients.

Since acyclovir and ganciclovir are chemically similar, patients hypersensitive to one also may be allergic to the other.

Because of the frequency with which granulocytopenia and thrombocytopenia occur in patients receiving ganciclovir, it is recommended that neutrophil and platelet counts be performed every two days during twice-daily administration and at least weekly thereafter. Neutrophil counts should be determined daily in patients whose counts are less than 1,000 cells/mm^3 at the initiation of treatment or in those in whom ganciclovir or other nucleoside analogues previously have caused leukopenia.

Viral resistance has been reported for CMV isolates obtained from ganciclovir-treated patients. Some patients may be infected with CMV strains resistant to the drug. Therefore, the possibility of viral resistance should be considered in those who respond poorly or in whom viral excretion persists during therapy.

DRUG INTERACTIONS. Since both ganciclovir and zidovudine cause granulocytopenia, these drugs should not be given concomitantly. Concurrent use with zidovudine also may cause additive or synergistic myelosuppression. Drugs that inhibit renal tubular secretion, such as probenicid, may reduce renal clearance of ganciclovir. Generalized seizures have been reported in patients who received ganciclovir and imipenem/cilastin. Drugs that inhibit replication of rapidly dividing cells, such as bone marrow, may have an additive toxic effect when given with ganciclovir.

PHARMACOKINETICS. Ganciclovir is poorly absorbed following oral administration; bioavailability is only 3% to 4.6%. When given intravenously to patients with normal renal function, the plasma half-life is 2.9 ± 1.3 hours and systemic clearance is 3.64 ± 1.86 ml/kg/min. In patients with impaired renal function, plasma half-life was 4.6 to 10.7 hours and systemic clearance varied from 30 to 128 ml/1.73 M^2/min. Ganciclovir is widely distributed; concentrations in the lungs and liver are 99% and 92% of corresponding blood levels, respectively. High concentrations also appear in the kidneys. Binding of ganciclovir to plasma proteins is low (1% to 2%). Limited evidence suggests that the drug crosses the blood-brain barrier. The intraocular concentration of ganciclovir following intravenous administration has been reported for two patients: In one given 6 mg/kg, subretinal and aqueous humor concentrations were 3.6 and 2.4 micromolar, respectively, and the corresponding plasma concentration was 6 micromolar. In a second patient given 5 mg/kg by intravenous infusion, subretinal fluid concentration was 7.16 micromolar and the plasma level was 8.16 micromolar. Little ganciclovir is metabolized, and renal excretion of unchanged drug by glomerular filtration is the major route of elimination. In patients with normal renal function, more than 90% of the administered dose is recovered in the urine.

DOSAGE AND PREPARATIONS. Since ganciclovir solutions reconstituted from powder have a high pH, they should be infused only into veins with adequate blood flow to permit rapid dilution and distribution.

Intravenous: *For adults with normal renal function, induction treatment,* 5 mg/kg given at a constant rate over one hour every 12 hours for 14 to 21 days; *maintenance treatment,* 5 mg/kg over one hour once daily for seven days each week; alternatively, 6 mg/kg once daily may be given for five days each week. Patients in whom retinitis progresses while receiving maintenance therapy may be re-treated with the twice-daily regimen. For *patients with impaired renal function,* see the following table.

Creatinine Clearance* (ml/1.73 M^2/min)	Dose (mg/kg)	Dosing Interval (hours)
>80	5.0	12
50-79	2.5	12
25-49	2.5	24
<25	1.25	24

**Creatinine clearance can be related to serum creatinine by the following formulas:*

Creatinine clearance for males =

$$\frac{(140 - \text{age [yrs]})\ (\text{body wt [kg]}) \times 1.73\ M^2}{(72)\ (\text{serum creatinine [mg/dl]})}$$

Creatinine clearance for females = 0.85 × male value

A pediatric dose has not been established.

Cytovene (Syntex). Powder (sterile) 500 mg in 10 ml containers.

RIBAVIRIN

[Virazole]

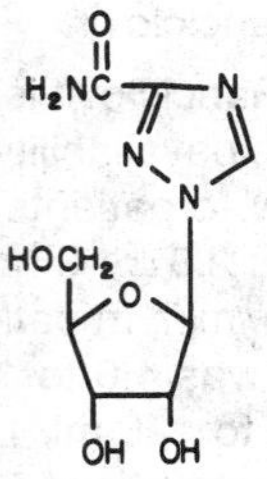

ACTIONS AND USES. Ribavirin (1-β-D-ribofuranosyl-1,3,4-triazole-3-carboxamide) has antiviral inhibitory activity in vitro against respiratory syncytial virus (RSV), influenza virus, and herpes simplex virus. It also is active against RSV in experimentally infected cotton rats. In cell cultures, the inhibitory activity of ribavirin for RSV is selective. The mechanism of action is unknown. Reversal of the in vitro antiviral activity by guanosine or xanthosine suggests that ribavirin may act as an analogue of these cellular metabolites.

Several clinical isolates of RSV were evaluated for ribavirin susceptibility by plaque reduction in tissue culture. Plaques were reduced 85% to 98% by 16 mcg/ml; however, the degree of reduction varies with the test system. The clinical significance of these data is unknown.

Ribavirin in aerosol form is indicated solely for the treatment of carefully selected hospitalized infants and young children with severe lower respiratory tract infections due to RSV. In two placebo-controlled trials in hospitalized infants this drug had a therapeutic effect, as judged by a reduction in the severity of clinical manifestations of RSV lower respiratory tract infection by treatment day three. In one of these studies, virus titers in respiratory secretions were also significantly reduced.

The vast majority of infants and children with RSV infection have no lower respiratory tract disease or have disease that is mild and self-limited and does not require hospitalization or antiviral treatment. Moreover, many children with mild lower respiratory tract involvement will require shorter hospitalization than would be required for a full course of ribavirin (three to seven days) and should not be treated with the drug. Thus, the decision to use ribavirin aerosol should be based on the severity of the RSV infection, and treatment should be continued only when there is documentation of RSV infection.

The presence of an underlying condition such as prematurity or cardiopulmonary disease may increase the severity of the infection and its risk to the patient. High-risk infants and young children with these underlying conditions may benefit from ribavirin therapy, although efficacy has been evaluated in only a small number of such patients. Use of ribavirin must be accompanied by and does not replace standard supportive respiratory and fluid management for infants and children with severe respiratory tract infection.

ADVERSE REACTIONS AND PRECAUTIONS. Approximately 200 patients have been treated with ribavirin aerosol in controlled or uncontrolled clinical studies. Pulmonary function significantly deteriorated during ribavirin therapy in six of six adults with chronic obstructive lung disease and in four of six adults with asthma. Dyspnea and chest soreness also were reported in the latter group. Minor abnormalities in pulmonary function also were seen in healthy adult volunteers.

Several serious adverse effects occurred in severely ill infants with life-threatening underlying disease, many of whom required assisted ventilation. Pulmonary reactions include worsening of respiratory status, bacterial pneumonia, pneumothorax, apnea, and ventilator dependence. Cardiovascular reactions include cardiac arrest, hypotension, and digitalis toxicity. The causative role of ribavirin in these reactions has not been determined.

Seven deaths occurred during or shortly after treatment with ribavirin, but no death was attributed to this antiviral agent by the investigators. Some patients requiring assisted ventilation have experienced serious difficulties, which may jeopardize adequate ventilation and gas exchange. Precipitation of drug within the ventilatory apparatus, including the endotracheal tube, has resulted in increased positive expiratory pressure and increased positive inspiratory pressure. Accumulation of fluid in tubing ("rain out") also has been noted. Although anemia has not been reported with use of the aerosol, it occurs frequently with oral and intravenous ribavirin, and most infants treated with the aerosol have not been evaluated one to two weeks after treatment, which is when anemia is likely to occur. Reticulocytosis, rash, and conjunctivitis have been associated with the use of ribavirin aerosol.

Patients with lower respiratory tract infection due to RSV require close monitoring and attention to respiratory and fluid status.

The use of ribavirin aerosol is not indicated in nursing mothers because RSV infection is self-limited in this population. Ribavirin is toxic to lactating animals and their offspring. It is not known whether the drug is excreted in human milk.

Ribavirin is contraindicated in women or girls who are or may become pregnant during exposure to the drug, for it may cause fetal harm and RSV infection is self-limited in this population (FDA Pregnancy Category X). Ribavirin can accumulate in erythrocytes and is not completely cleared from human blood even four weeks after administration. Although there are no pertinent human data, ribavirin has been found to be teratogenic and/or embryolethal in nearly all species in which it has been tested. Teratogenicity was evident after a single oral dose of 2.5 mg/kg in the hamster and after daily oral doses of 10 mg/kg in the rat. Malformations of skull, palate, eye, jaw, skeleton, and gastrointestinal tract were noted in animal studies. Survival of fetuses and offspring was reduced. The drug causes embryolethality in the rabbit at daily oral dose levels as low as 1 mg/kg.

Ribavirin induces cell transformation in an in vitro mammalian system (Balb/C 3T3 cell line). However, in vivo carcinogenicity studies are incomplete. Results thus far, although inconclusive, suggest that chronic feeding of ribavirin to rats at dose levels of 16 to 60 mg/kg can induce benign mammary, pancreatic, pituitary, and adrenal tumors. Ribavirin is mutagenic to mammalian (15178Y) cells in culture. Results of microbial mutagenicity assays and a dominant lethal assay (mouse) were negative. Ribavirin causes testicular lesions (tubular atrophy) in adult rats at oral dose levels as low as 16 mg/kg/day (lower doses not tested), but fertility of ribavirin-treated animals (male or female) has not been adequately investigated.

Ribavirin administered by aerosol produced cardiac lesions in mice and rats after doses of 30 and 36 mg/kg, respectively, for four weeks and after oral administration of 120 mg/kg in monkeys and 154 to 200 mg/kg in rats for one to six months. In developing ferrets, ribavirin aerosol administered in doses of 60 mg/kg for 10 or 30 days resulted in inflammatory and possibly emphysematous changes in the lungs. Proliferative changes were observed with doses of 131 mg/kg for 30 days. The significance of these findings for humans is unknown.

DRUG INTERACTIONS. Interactions with administration of ribavirin and other drugs such as digoxin, bronchodilators, other antiviral agents, antibiotics, or antimetabolites have not been evaluated.

PHARMACOKINETICS. Assay for ribavirin in human materials is performed by a radioimmunoassay that detects ribavirin and at least one metabolite. When administered by aerosol, ribavirin is absorbed systemically. Four pediatric patients who inhaled the aerosol by face mask for 2.5 hours each day for three days had plasma concentrations ranging from 0.44 to 1.55 micrometers (mean, 0.76 micrometer). The plasma half-life was reported to be 9.5 hours. Three pediatric patients who inhaled the aerosol by face mask or mist tent for 20 hours each day for five days had plasma concentrations ranging from 1.5 to 14.3 micrometers (mean, 6.8 micrometers). It is probable that the concentration of ribavirin in respiratory tract secretions is much higher than that in plasma in view of the route of administration.

The bioavailability of ribavirin is unknown and may depend on the mode of delivery. After inhalation, peak plasma concentrations are less than the concentration that reduced RSV plaque formation in tissue culture by 85% to 98%, and respiratory tract secretions are likely to contain ribavirin in concentrations many times higher than those required to reduce plaque formation. However, RSV is an intracellular virus, and serum concentrations may reflect intracellular concentrations in the respiratory tract better than respiratory secretion concentrations.

In man, rats, and rhesus monkeys, accumulation of ribavirin and/or metabolites in the red blood cells has been noted; the amount plateaus in red cells in man in about four days and gradually declines. The apparent half-life is 40 days. The extent of accumulation of ribavirin following inhalation therapy is not well defined.

DOSAGE AND PREPARATIONS. Ribavirin is administered by the Viratek Small Particle Aerosol Generator (SPAG), Model SPAG-2. It should not be used with any other aerosol generating device or with other aerosolized medications and should not be given to patients requiring simultaneous assisted ventilation. Administration by face mask or oxygen tent may be necessary if a hood cannot be employed. However, the volume of distribution and condensation area are larger in a tent and the efficacy of this method of drug delivery has been evaluated in only a small number of patients.

Inhalation: A total of 6 g of lyophilized drug in a 100 ml-vial for aerosol administration only is used. By sterile technique, the drug is diluted in the 100-ml vial with sterile water for injection or inhalation. The medication is transferred to the clean, sterilized 500-ml wide-mouth Erlenmeyer flask (SPAG-2 Reservoir) and further diluted to a final volume of 300 ml with sterile water for injection or inhalation (no preservatives added). The final concentration should be 20 mg/ml. The average aerosol concentration in the drug reservoir of the SPAG unit for a 12-hour period is 190 mcg/L (0.19 mg/L) of air. Treatment is continued 12 to 18 hours per day for at least three and no more than seven days.

Virazole (ICN). Aerosol powder (sterile, lyophilized) 6 g in 100-ml glass vials. Vials containing the powder should be stored in a dry place at 15 to 25° C (59 to 78° F). Reconstituted solutions may be stored, under sterile conditions, at room temperature (20 to 30° C, 68 to 86° F) for 24 hours. Solutions that have been placed in the SPAG-2 unit should be discarded at least every 24 hours.

VIDARABINE

[Vira-A]

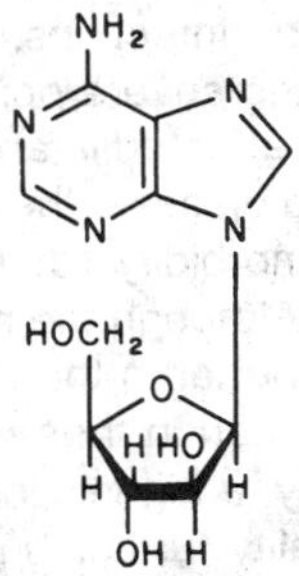

ACTIONS AND USES. Vidarabine is converted to ara-ATP, the active metabolite, which preferentially inhibits viral DNA polymerase (see the Introduction). In vitro, the drug is active against herpes simplex types 1 and 2, varicella-zoster, cytomegalovirus (CMV), and vaccinia viruses. CMV and vaccinia virus are most resistant. Vidarabine is inactive against adenoviruses. Among the RNA viruses, only rhabdoviruses (vesicular stomatitis and rabies viruses) and retroviruses (Rous sarcoma, Gross murine leukemia, and Rauscher murine leukemia viruses) are susceptible.

When administered by intravenous infusion, vidarabine is useful in the treatment of herpes simplex encephalitis. In a multicenter, double-blind, placebo-controlled study (Whitley et al, 1977), vidarabine 15 mg/kg/day for ten days decreased overall mortality from 70% to 28% and reduced debilitating neurologic sequelae in individuals who exhibited only lethargy when therapy was begun. Although vidarabine reduced mortality in semicomatose and comatose patients, it did not alter morbidity or prevent serious neurologic sequelae in these patients. The results of this trial were confirmed in a later study (Whitley et al, 1981).

Early and accurate diagnosis of herpes simplex encephalitis is essential to achieve maximum benefits. This disease should be suspected whenever there is a history of febrile encephalopathy, disordered mental state, reduced consciousness, and focal cerebral signs. Examination of the cerebrospinal fluid, electroencephalography, and a brain scan using computerized axial tomography may be helpful, but a brain biopsy is essential to confirm the diagnosis (see Whitley et al, 1982 C). Specimens are negative in over one-half of patients suspected of having this disease. Treating such patients with vidarabine not only subjects them to the adverse effects of the drug but, more importantly, may deprive them of effective therapy for other diseases.

Intravenous acyclovir is more effective than vidarabine for the treatment of herpes simplex encephalitis and is the drug of choice for this infection (Whitley et al, 1986 A). Thus, it has been suggested that vidarabine be restricted to patients who have not responded to acyclovir, those with acyclovir-resistant strains, or individuals who relapse after acyclovir therapy.

Intravenous vidarabine has been effective for other severe herpesvirus infections in double-blind, placebo-controlled clinical trials. In neonatal herpes simplex infections, vidarabine decreased both mortality and morbidity (Whitley et al, 1980, 1983). Once again, however, efficacy was related inversely to the severity of the disease. In neonates who experienced only localized skin, eye, or oral infections, vidarabine 15 mg/kg/day for ten days prevented severe ocular and neurologic sequelae. In more severely affected infants with central nervous system and disseminated disease, the drug reduced mortality from 74% to 38% and morbidity (at 1 year of age) in survivors from 89% to 71%. Although the number of patients was small, the outcome was better in those with localized central nervous system disease than in those with disseminated disease. In a follow-up study, a higher dosage (30 mg/kg/day) failed to decrease mortality further but did prevent progression of the disease in a greater number of children than with the 15 mg/kg/day dosage. Thus, with a larger dose, vidarabine appears to slow the process of neurologic impairment but cannot reverse existing damage.

Vidarabine also is indicated to treat localized herpes zoster and chickenpox infections in immunocompromised adults and children, respectively. Results in patients with herpes zoster who received vidarabine within 72 hours after onset of symptoms were compared to those achieved in untreated controls; the former experienced faster rates of healing (ie, earlier cessation of new vesicle formation, shorter times to total pustulation and scabbing), decreased cutaneous dissemination and visceral complications, and reduced duration of postherpetic neuralgia (Whitley et al, 1976; Whitley et al, 1982 D). Efficacy was similar in immunocompromised children with chickenpox (Whitley et al, 1982 A). However, a more recent clinical trial compared intravenous vidarabine with acyclovir for the treatment of localized zoster infections in bone marrow transplant patients and concluded that acyclovir was more effective in these patients (Shepp et al, 1986).

Intravenous vidarabine has not been effective in cytomegalovirus or smallpox infections.

A topical ophthalmic preparation of vidarabine [Vira-A] is effective in herpes simplex keratitis (see index entry Vidarabine, In Ophthalmic Infection). However, vidarabine is not useful in herpes simplex labialis or genitalis. It is of limited value for the treatment of mucocutaneous HSV infection in immunocompromised patients in whom it may be a second choice to acyclovir.

ADVERSE REACTIONS AND PRECAUTIONS. When therapeutic doses are given intravenously, vidarabine causes minimal or no adverse effects in most patients. The most common side effects (incidence, 10% to 15%) are gastrointestinal disturbances (eg, anorexia, nausea, vomiting, diarrhea), which are usually mild. Central nervous system disturbances noted occasionally include tremors, dizziness, confusion, hallucinations, ataxia, and psychoses. Doses of 20 mg/kg/day or more cause more pronounced central nervous system effects; cytotoxic effects, leukopenia, and thrombocytopenia also become apparent.

Patients with impaired renal function (eg, renal transplant patients) excrete arabinosyl hypoxanthine (ara-Hx), the major metabolite of vidarabine, slowly, and dosage reduction may be required to avoid accumulation and severe adverse reactions. Liver function and hematologic tests are recommended because elevated AST and bilirubin levels and/or decreased hemoglobin, hematocrit, and white blood cell counts occasionally have been associated with vidarabine therapy.

Supportive care may be required in patients who are susceptible to fluid overload or cerebral edema, which is a common consequence of herpes simplex encephalitis. Measures to combat increased intracranial pressure should be utilized; elevation of the head, administration of mannitol and/or glycerin, and hyperventilation to maintain a decreased arterial PCO_2 level are recommended.

Vidarabine is teratogenic in laboratory animals. Therefore, its use in pregnant women should be avoided if possible (FDA Pregnancy Category C).

DRUG INTERACTIONS. Increased neurotoxicity has been reported in patients receiving allopurinol with vidarabine. This is probably due to increased blood levels of ara-Hx resulting from inhibition of xanthine oxidase by allopurinol. A reduction in vidarabine dosage should be considered when these two drugs are given together.

PHARMACOKINETICS. Because of its poor aqueous solubility, vidarabine must be administered in large volumes of fluid by continuous intravenous infusion over a 12- to 24-hour period. It is rapidly deaminated to arabinosylhypoxanthine (ara-Hx), which has much weaker antiviral activity. Peak plasma levels of ara-Hx and vidarabine range from 3 to 6 mcg/ml and 0.2 to 0.4 mcg/ml, respectively, after slow infusion of 10 mg/kg of vidarabine. These levels reflect the slow rate of infusion and lack of accumulation. The plasma half-life of ara-Hx is approximately four hours, and excretion is primarily via the kidneys. Approximately 60% of a daily dose is recovered in urine as ara-Hx; only 1% to 3% is parent drug. Ara-Hx levels in cerebrospinal fluid are about one-third of those in plasma.

DOSAGE AND PREPARATIONS.

Intravenous: The solubility of vidarabine in intravenous solutions is limited; a maximum of 450 mg can be dissolved in 1 L of fluid. The drug should be administered by slow, continuous infusion over a 12- to 24-hour period. Rapid or bolus injection must be avoided.

Adults and children, for herpes simplex encephalitis, 15 mg/kg daily for ten days. For herpes simplex infection in *neonates*, 15 mg/kg/day for ten days. For varicella-zoster in immunocompromised patients, 10 mg/kg/day for five days.

Vira-A (Parke-Davis). Suspension (sterile) 200 mg monohydrate (equivalent to 187.4 mg of base)/ml in 5 ml containers.

ZIDOVUDINE (AZT)
[Retrovir]

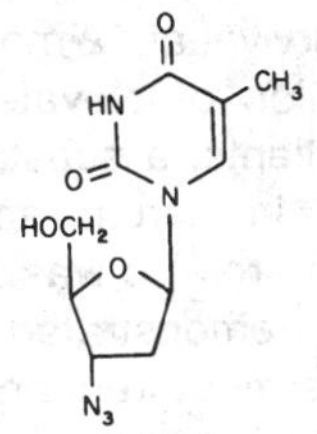

Zidovudine is an antiretroviral agent with clinical activity against HIV-1. The capsule and syrup formulations are bioequivalent.

ACTIONS. In vitro, zidovudine inhibits the replication of all retroviruses against which it has been tested, including HIV. This drug is a thymidine analogue in which the 3′-hydroxy (-OH) group is replaced by an azido (-N_3) group. Cellular thymidine kinase converts zidovudine into zidovudine monophosphate. This monophosphate is further phosphorylated to the diphosphate and triphosphate derivatives by cellular thymidylate kinase and by other cellular enzymes. Zidovudine triphosphate interferes with the HIV viral RNA-dependent DNA polymerase (reverse transcriptase); thus, it inhibits viral replication. The triphosphate derivative of zidovudine can be incorporated into the enlarging DNA chain but acts as a DNA chain terminator. Chain termination occurs with much higher concentrations of AZT-triphosphate (concentrations 100-fold higher than those required to inhibit reverse transcriptase) when cellular α-DNA polymerase is the enzyme employed.

AZT-triphosphate has been reported to act as an efficient inhibitor of cellular DNA polymerase gamma but at concentrations tenfold higher than those required to inhibit the reverse transcriptase of HIV-1. Cellular DNA polymerase alpha-primase and DNA polymerase beta were not inhibited (König et al, 1989). Of the eukaryotic DNA polymerases, DNA polymerase gamma is the most sensitive to inhibition by dideoxynucleotides. This enzyme is responsible for the replication of the mitochondrial genome and is needed to maintain a sufficient level of mitochondria in growing cells. It has been speculated that some of the adverse effects seen in AIDS patients treated with zidovudine may be due in part to the inhibition of this vital enzyme (König et al, 1989).

Although the in vitro sensitivity results vary according to the test assay and the cell line employed, zidovudine blocked 90% of detectable HIV replication in vitro at concentrations of ≤0.13 mcg/ml (ID_{90}) and 0.013 mcg/ml (ID_{50}), as measured by determining HIV replication in H9 cells. At the former drug concentrations, p24 gag protein expression was also undetectable. Cells chronically infected with HIV are generally not amenable to zidovudine therapy. Partial inhibition of virus replication in these cells (presumed to carry integrated HIV DNA) required concentrations approximately 100 times higher than those necessary to block HIV replication in acutely infected cells.

The major metabolite of zidovudine, 3′-azido-3′-deoxy-5′-O-B-D-glucopyranuronosylthymidine (GAZT), does not inhibit HIV replication in vitro nor does it antagonize the antiviral effect of zidovudine.

Development of resistance during treatment has been reported, but the frequency of resistant isolates in the general population is unknown. From the small number of patients studied, it could not be determined whether development of a less sensitive phenotype resulted in clinical resistance (Larder et al, 1989). More extensive studies are needed to determine the clinical significance of these observations.

USES. Zidovudine is indicated for the treatment of HIV-infected adult patients who have evidence of impaired immunity (CD_4 cell count ≤500/mm^3) before therapy is started. This use is based on the results of three randomized, double-blind, placebo-controlled trials of oral zidovudine in HIV-infected patients with CD_4 counts ≤500/mm^3. Separate studies evaluated zidovudine therapy in asymptomatic HIV-infected patients, in patients with early symptomatic HIV disease, and in patients with advanced symptomatic HIV disease (AIDS or advanced ARC). Zidovudine also is indicated for HIV-infected children over age 3 months who have HIV-related symptoms or who are asymptomatic but have abnormal laboratory values indicating significant HIV-related immunosuppression. This use is based on two open-label studies involving 124 children age 3.5 months to 12 years with HIV-associated disease (AIDS or advanced ARC).

Asymptomatic HIV Infection in Adults: Entry into this trial, conducted at 32 collaborating medical centers, was dependent on the absence of signs and symptoms consistent with HIV disease. In this study, 1,338 asymptomatic patients with T4 lymphocyte counts <500/mm^3 received either zidovudine 100 or 300 mg or placebo, each given five times daily. Participants were monitored for the development of the signs and symptoms of HIV disease and tolerance to the regimens employed. The study was terminated early because a statistically significant difference in progression to AIDS or advanced ARC was observed between the group receiving 500 mg/day and the placebo group. Of the patients enrolled in the study, 38 of 428 receiving placebo, 17 of 453 receiving zidovudine 500 mg/day, and 19 of 457 receiving zidovudine 1.5 g/day developed symptoms of advanced HIV disease after a mean of 55 weeks of treatment. Changes in immunologic and virologic parameters (T4 lymphocyte count and serum p24 antigen level) paralleled the observed clinical benefits (Volberding et al, 1990). Although early treatment delayed progression of disease, it is not yet known whether it prolongs survival.

Early Symptomatic HIV Disease in Adults: In this trial, conducted at 29 medical centers, 713 patients were studied;

these patients had early manifestations of HIV disease (baseline T4 lymphocyte count of 200 to 800/mm^3 and symptoms such as oral candidiasis, oral hairy leukoplakia, or intermittent diarrhea). This trial was terminated early because there was a statistically significant difference in the rate of development of advanced symptomatic HIV disease between the treated and placebo groups. Of the 352 patients receiving placebo, 36 progressed to advanced symptomatic disease (21 to AIDS), but only 13 of 361 zidovudine recipients progressed to advanced symptomatic disease (5 to AIDS) (Fischl et al, 1990).

Advanced Symptomatic HIV Disease in Adults: A randomized, double-blind, multicenter, placebo-controlled trial evaluated 281 patients with AIDS or advanced ARC for an average of 4.5 months. Of the total, 160 patients had AIDS (85 received zidovudine and 75 placebo) and 121 ARC (59 received zidovudine and 62 placebo) (Fischl et al, 1987; Richman et al, 1987). The majority of patients (221 or 79% overall) had less than 200 CD_4 cells/mm^3 at entry. A dose of 250 mg was given every four hours; this dosage was reduced or the drug discontinued if serious bone marrow toxicity developed. Based on the premature determination of a reduction in mortality, the trial was terminated by a Data Safety and Monitoring Board. There were 19 deaths in the placebo group and 1 in the zidovudine group ($p < 0.001$). All deaths were apparently due to opportunistic infections or other complications of HIV infection. The initial duration of treatment ranged from 12 to 16 weeks, with a mean and median duration of 17 and 18 weeks, respectively. Zidovudine also significantly reduced the risk of acquiring an AIDS-defining opportunistic infection after six weeks of treatment ($p < 0.001$).

At the conclusion of the placebo-controlled trial, 80% of zidovudine and placebo recipients volunteered to enroll in an uncontrolled extension protocol in which all patients received 200 mg of the drug every four hours. These patients have been followed for variable periods of time. Benefits of therapy were observed during this extended period, although opportunistic infections continued to occur and more patients died. Survival for all patients was 96.5% at six months, 84.7% at one year, 68.3% at 18 months, and 41.2% at two years. Untreated AIDS patients diagnosed in San Francisco in 1985 who had survived 60 days after PCP had a one-year survival rate of 34.7% and a two-year survival rate of 4.2% from the time of diagnosis of PCP. In a more recent study of AIDS patients diagnosed in the same city in 1986 and 1987, median survival for patients receiving zidovudine was 21.6 months compared with 14.9 months for those who did not receive this drug.

Results of a dose comparison study in adults with AIDS indicated that an induction dose of zidovudine 200 mg orally every four hours (1.2 g/day) for one month followed by long-term administration of 100 mg every four hours (600 mg/day) produced survival rates and frequency of opportunistic infections comparable to those seen in patients given larger doses. The incidence of hematologic toxicity also was decreased with this regimen; its effectiveness in improving neurologic dysfunction associated with HIV infection is unknown.

Pediatric Symptomatic HIV Disease: Two open-label studies evaluated the efficacy, safety, and pharmacokinetics of zidovudine in 124 children with advanced HIV disease. In the majority of these children, HIV was acquired perinatally from the mother. In the Phase I study, three intravenous regimens were given for four to eight weeks and, subsequently, oral zidovudine (180 mg/M^2) every six hours was substituted. These children have been followed for a mean of 465 days. In the Phase II study, oral zidovudine 180 mg/M^2 was given every six hours.

Clinical, immunologic, and virologic improvement was observed in some of the children. These included reductions in hepatosplenomegaly and increases in weight percentiles in previously growth-retarded children. The probability of being free of opportunistic infections for up to 12 months was 0.76, and the probability of survival at 12 months was 0.87. A tendency toward normalization of elevated IgG concentrations was noted. In some patients, a substantial reduction in p24 antigen concentrations in serum and cerebrospinal fluid (CSF) was observed. There also was a reduction in the number of patients with HIV demonstrated in CSF cultures.

The adverse reactions most frequently reported were anemia and neutropenia, which occurred in 46% of the children. Because of the development of hematologic abnormalities, dose modification was required in 36% of the patients and 30% received transfusions for anemia. Zidovudine therapy was discontinued in a few patients because of neutropenia.

ADVERSE REACTIONS AND PRECAUTIONS. The frequency and severity of adverse reactions associated with zidovudine are greater in patients with more advanced disease at the time of initiation of therapy and in those receiving larger doses. In all of the clinical trials, anemia and granulocytopenia were the most significant reactions observed, especially in the original trial involving patients with advanced symptomatic HIV disease. In that trial, bone marrow suppression was a significant complication, specifically granulocytopenia (<750 cells/mm^3, 47% of zidovudine and 10% of placebo recipients) and anemia (25% hemoglobin reduction, 45% of zidovudine and 14% of placebo recipients). The occurrence of these hematologic reactions correlated inversely to the number of CD_4 lymphocytes, hemoglobin, and granulocytes at study entry and directly with the dose and duration of therapy (Richman et al, 1987). The manufacturer's findings on the frequency of granulocytopenia and anemia in the three trial groups are summarized in the following tables.

Other adverse effects that occurred in 5% or more of patients at significantly greater rates in those who received zidovudine include severe headache, insomnia, nausea, vomiting, and myalgia. Nausea and headache often subside after a few weeks of therapy, but in some patients they may be severe enough to warrant discontinuation of therapy. A few patients who received zidovudine for a number of months developed myositis with muscular wasting and elevations of creatinine kinase, which may be due to zidovudine's ability to inhibit mitochondrial DNA polymerase. Rare but potentially fatal adverse reactions include seizures, a Wernicke-like encephalopathy, and Stevens-Johnson syndrome (Creagh-Kirk et al, 1988). Some patients receiving large doses, particularly blacks, develop a bluish pigmentation of the fingernails.

ADULT ASYMPTOMATIC HIV INFECTION Study (n = 1338)

	Granulocytopenia (<750/mm³)			Anemia (Hgb <8 g/dl)		
	Zidovudine		Placebo	Zidovudine		Placebo
Dose	1.5 g*	500 mg	---	1.5 g*	500 mg	---
CD4 ≤500	6.4% (n = 457)	1.8% (n=453)	1.6% (n=428)	6.4% (n=457)	1.1% (n=453)	0.2% (n=428)

ADULT EARLY SYMPTOMATIC HIV DISEASE Study (n = 713)

	Granulocytopenia (<750/mm³)		Anemia (Hgb <8 g/dl)	
	Zidovudine	Placebo	Zidovudine	Placebo
Dose	1.2 g	---	1.2 g	---
CD4 >200	4% (n = 361)	1% (n=352)	4% (n=361)	0% (n=352)

ADULT ADVANCED SYMPTOMATIC HIV DISEASE Study (n = 281)

	Granulocytopenia (<750/mm³)		Anemia (Hgb <7.5 g/dl)	
	Zidovudine	Placebo	Zidovudine	Placebo
Dose	1.5 g*	---	1.5 g*	---
CD4 >200	10% (n = 30)	3% (n=30)	3% (n=30)	0% (n=30)
CD4 <200	47% (n = 114)	10% (n=107)	29% (n=114)	5% (n=107)

** Three times the currently recommended dose in asymptomatic patients.*

ADVANCED PEDIATRIC HIV DISEASE (n = 124)

	Granulocytopenia (<750/mm³)		Anemia (Hgb <7.5 g/dL)	
	N	%	N	%
Dose of Zidovudine (see text)	48	39	28†	23

† Twenty-two children received one or more transfusions due to a decline in hemoglobin to <7.5 g/dL; an additional 15 children received transfusions for hemoglobin levels >7.5 g/dL. Fifty-nine percent of the patients who received transfusions had a prestudy history of anemia or transfusion requirement.

Zidovudine should be used with extreme caution in patients who have a granulocyte count <1,000/mm³ or a hemoglobin level <9.5 g/dL. Since significant anemia most commonly occurred after four to six weeks of therapy and required dose adjustment or discontinuation of therapy, frequent blood counts (at least every two weeks) are recommended. If anemia or granulocytopenia develops, dosage adjustments may be necessary (see Dosage and Preparations).

In an in vitro mammalian cell transformation assay, zidovudine was positive at concentrations of 0.5 mcg/ml and higher. No evidence of mutagenicity was observed in the Ames test. In a mutagenicity assay conducted in L5178Y/TK+/− mouse lymphoma cells, zidovudine was weakly mutagenic in the absence of metabolic activation only at the highest concentrations tested (4,000 and 5,000 mcg/ml). In long-term carcinogenicity studies conducted in rodents, vaginal neoplasms devloped in mice given the highest does and a vaginal squamous cell papilloma developed in one who received a median dose. No vaginal tumors were found in those who received the lowest dose. Non-metastasizing vaginal squamous cell carcinomas occurred in rats given the highest dose. No vaginal tumors occurred at lower doses.

No effect on male or female fertility has been observed in rats receiving oral doses of up to 450 mg/kg/day, and studies in rats and rabbits receiving zidovudine orally have revealed no evidence of teratogenicity. Zidovudine is classified in FDA Pregnancy Category C.

There is insufficient evidence to recommend a dosing regimen for infants under 3 months. Zidovudine clearance may be reduced in children under 1 month. It is not known whether zidovudine is excreted in human milk, but since many drugs are and since the potential for serious adverse reactions is high in nursing infants, mothers should be advised to discontinue nursing if they are taking this drug. Zidovudine should be given to pregnant women only if clearly needed.

DRUG INTERACTIONS. The administration of zidovudine with other drugs metabolized by glucuronidation (eg, acetaminophen, aspirin, indomethacin) should be avoided because the toxicity of either drug may be potentiated. Probenecid may inhibit glucuronidation and/or reduce renal excretion of zidovudine. Drugs that are nephrotoxic, cytotoxic, or that interfere with RBC/WBC number or function (eg, dapsone, pentamidine, amphotericin B, flucytosine, vincristine, vinblastine, doxorubicin, interferon) may increase the risk of toxicity. Some nucleoside analogues may affect RBC/WBC number or function and hence may increase the hematologic toxicity of zidovudine. Concurrent use with ganciclovir may cause additive or synergistic myelosuppression (see the evaluation on Ganciclovir). Drugs such as trimethoprim/sulfamethoxazole, pyrimethamine, and acyclovir may be necessary for the management or prevention of opportunistic infections. In the controlled trial in patients with advanced HIV disease, increased toxicity was not observed when exposure to these drugs was limited.

Phenytoin levels have been reported to be altered in some patients given zidovudine, which suggests that phenytoin levels should be carefully monitored in such patients because many AIDS patients have central nervous system disorders that may predispose to seizure activity.

In vitro studies have demonstrated that ribavirin has an antagonistic effect on the inhibition of HIV-1 by zidovudine. This antagonistic effect is apparently due to the inhibition of phosphorylation of zidovudine by ribavirin. Although the clinical significance of this is unknown, the results suggest these agents should not be administered simultaneously (Vogt et al, 1987).

PHARMACOKINETICS. ***Adults:*** The pharmacokinetics of zidovudine have been evaluated in a Phase I dose-escalation study. Zidovudine was infused intermittently in doses of 1 to 2.5 mg/kg/day for 14 to 28 days followed by one of several oral dosing regimens (Yarchoan et al, 1986). Following intravenous administration, dose-independent kinetics were observed in the range of 1 to 5 mg/kg with a mean zidovudine half-life of 1.1 hours (range, 0.48 to 2.86 hours). Total body clearance averaged 1,900 ml/70 kg/min, and the apparent volume of distribution was 1.6 L/kg. Renal clearance is estimated to be 400 ml/70 kg/min, which indicates glomerular filtration and active tubular secretion by the kidneys. Plasma protein binding is 34% to 38%, which suggests that drug interactions involving binding site displacement are not anticipated.

Zidovudine is well absorbed from the gastrointestinal tract after oral administration (bioavailability, average 65%; range 52% to 75%); peak serum concentrations occur within 0.5 to 1.5 hours. The kinetics were dose-independent within the range of 2 mg/kg every eight hours to 10 mg/kg every four hours. The mean half-life was approximately one hour (range, 0.78 to 1.93 hours) following oral administration. Steady-state serum concentrations following prolonged oral administration of 250 mg every four hours were 0.16 mcg/ml predose (range, 0 to 84 mcg/ml) and 0.62 mcg/ml 1.5 hours postdose (range, 0.05 to 1.46 mcg/ml). Of note is the fact that zidovudine can be detected in the cerebrospinal fluid after oral administration.

Zidovudine is rapidly metabolized to 3′-azido-3′-deoxy-5′-O-B-D-glucopyranuronosylthymidine (GAZT), which has an apparent elimination half-life of one hour (range, 0.61 to 1.73 hours). Following oral administration, 14% of the dose excreted in the urine was identified as zidovudine and 74% as GATZ; the total amount averaged 90% (range, 63% to 95%).

Zidovudine is eliminated primarily by renal excretion following glucuronidation in the liver. The pharmacokinetics of zidovudine have been evaluated in some patients with impaired renal function following a single 200-mg dose. In anuric patients, the half-life was 1.4 hours compared with one hour in control subjects with normal renal function. In anuric patients, the half-life of GATZ was 8 hours vs 0.9 hours for controls, and the plasma concentration-time curve (AUC) was 17 times higher than that for control subjects. Hemodialysis has a negligible effect on removal of the parent compound, but elimination of GATZ is enhanced.

In a multiple-dose bioavailability study conducted in HIV-infected adults receiving 100 or 200 mg every four hours, zidovudine syrup was bioequivalent to the capsules with respect to the AUC. The rate of absorption of zidovudine from the syrup, however, was greater than that from the capsules.

Children: The pharmacokinetics of zidovudine have been studied in children age 6 months to 12 years following intravenous doses (80 to 160 mg/M^2) given every six hours and after oral doses (90 to 240 mg/M^2) of the intravenous solution given every six hours. Zidovudine plasma concentrations fell exponentially after discontinuation of the infusion, which is consistent with two-compartment pharmacokinetics. The mean terminal half-life and total body clearance with all doses were 1.5 hours and 30.9 ml/min/kg, respectively. The mean oral availability was 65% and was independent of dose. The mean CSF/plasma ratio after intermittent intravenous and oral administration varied from 0.68 to 0.85 in Phase I and Phase II studies, respectively. During continuous intravenous infusion, the mean steady state CSF/plasma ratio was 0.26. As in adults, the major route of elimination was by metabolism to GAZT. Following intravenous administration, approximately 29% of the dose is excreted unchanged in the urine and about 45% as GAZT. Thus, overall the pharmacokinetics of zidovudine in children over 3 months is similar to that in adults.

DOSAGE AND PREPARATIONS.

Oral: *Adults with symptomatic HIV infection,* initially, 200 mg (two 100-mg capsules or four teaspoonsful [20 ml] of syrup) administered every four hours (1.2 g total daily dose). After one month, the dose may be reduced to 100 mg every four hours (600 mg total daily dose). *For adults with asymptomatic HIV infection,* 100 mg administered every four hours while awake (500 mg/day). *Children 3 months to 12 years*, 180 mg/M^2 every six hours (720 mg/M^2/day) (maximum, 200 mg every six hours).

Careful monitoring of hematologic indices every two weeks is recommended to detect serious anemia or granulocytopenia. In patients with hematologic toxicity, reduction in the hemoglobin level may occur as early as two to four weeks after treatment is begun; granulocytopenia usually occurs after six to eight weeks.

If significant anemia (hemoglobin level <7.5 g/dL or reduction of $>25\%$ below baseline) and/or significant granulocytopenia (granulocyte count $<750/mm^3$ or reduction of $>50\%$ below baseline) occur, the manufacturer recommends that therapy be interrupted until some evidence of marrow recovery is observed. Dose modification does not necessarily eliminate the need for transfusion if there is significant anemia. When anemia or granulocytopenia is less severe, a reduction in daily dose may be adequate. If marrow recovery occurs after dose modification, gradual increases in dosage may be appropriate depending on hematologic indices and patient tolerance.

Retrovir (Burroughs Wellcome). Capsules 100 mg; syrup 50 mg/5 ml.

Intravenous: 1 to 2 mg/kg is infused over one hour at a constant rate every four hours around the clock (six times daily). Rapid infusion and bolus injection should be avoided. The intravenous route should only be used until oral therapy can be substituted. The intravenous dose equivalent to oral administration of 100 mg every four hours is approximately 1 mg/kg every four hours.

Retrovir (Burroughs Wellcome). Solution (sterile) 10 mg/ml in 20 ml containers.

Cited References

Arden NH, et al: The roles of vaccination and amantadine prophylaxis in controlling an outbreak of influenza A (H3N2) in a nursing home. *Arch Intern Med* 148:865-868, 1988.

Arvin AM, et al: Human leukocyte interferon for treatment of varicella in children with cancer. *N Engl J Med* 306:761-765, 1982 A.

Arvin AM, et al: Alpha interferon administration to infants with congenital rubella. *Antimicrob Agents Chemother* 21:259-261, 1982 B.

Bach MC, et al: 9-(1,3 dihydroxy-2-propoxymethyl) guanine for cytomegalovirus infections in patients with acquired immunodeficiency syndrome. *Ann Intern Med* 103:381-384, 1985.

Baker DA, et al: One-year suppression of frequent recurrences of genital herpes with oral acyclovir. *Obstet Gynecol* 73:84-87, 1989.

Balfour HH Jr, et al: Acyclovir in immunocompromised patients with cytomegalovirus disease: Controlled trial at one institution. *Am J Med* 73(1A):241-248, 1982.

Balfour HH Jr, et al: Acyclovir halts progression of herpes zoster in immunocompromised patients. *N Engl J Med* 308:1448-1453, 1983.

Balfour HH Jr, et al: A randomized, placebo-controlled trial of oral acyclovir for the prevention of cytomegalovirus disease in recipients of renal allografts. *N Engl J Med* 320:1381-1387, 1989.

Balfour HH Jr, et al: Acyclovir treatment of varicella in otherwise healthy children. *J Pediatr* 116:633-639, 1990.

Bassendine MF, et al: Adenine arabinoside therapy in HBsAG-positive chronic liver disease: Controlled study. *Gastroenterology* 80:1016-1022, 1981.

Bean B, et al: Acyclovir therapy for acute herpes zoster. *Lancet* 2:118-121, 1982.

Becker Y (ed): *Antiviral Drugs and Interferon: The Molecular Basis of Their Activity.* Boston, Martinus Nijhoff, 1984.

Belshe RB, et al: Genetic basis of resistance to rimantadine emerging during treatment of influenza virus infection. *J Virol* 62:1508-1512, 1988.

Belshe RB, et al: Resistance of influenza A virus to amantadine and rimantadine: Results of one decade of surveillance. *J Infect Dis* 159:430-435, 1989 A.

Belshe RB, et al: Drug resistance and mechanisms of action on influenza A viruses. *J Respir Dis* 10(suppl):S52-S61, 1989 B.

Benoit Y, et al: Oral BVDU treatment of varicella and zoster in children with cancer. *Eur J Pediatr* 143:198-202, 1985.

Betts RF, et al: Antiviral agents to prevent or treat influenza in the elderly. *J Respir Dis* 8(suppl 11A):S56-S59, 1987.

Bierman SM, et al: Clinical efficacy of ribavirin in treatment of genital herpes simplex virus infection. *Chemotherapy* 27:139-145, 1981.

Boston Interhospital Virus Study Group and the NIAID-Sponsored Cooperative Antiviral Clinical Study Group: Failure of high dose 5-iodo-2′-deoxyuridine in therapy of herpes simplex virus encephalitis: Evidence of unacceptable toxicity. *N Engl J Med* 292:599-603, 1975.

Bryson YJ, et al: Treatment of first episodes of genital herpes simplex virus infection with oral acyclovir. *N Engl J Med* 308:916-921, 1983.

Buhles WC, et al: Ganciclovir treatment of life- or sight-threatening cytomegalovirus infection: Experience in 314 immunocompromised patients. *Rev Infect Dis* 10(suppl 3):495-506, 1988.

Cantrill HL, et al: Treatment of cytomegalovirus retinitis with intravitreal ganciclovir: Long term results. *Ophthalmology* 96:367-374, 1989.

Chang T-W, Heel RC: Ribavirin and inosiplex: Review of their present status in viral diseases. *Drugs* 22:111-128, 1981.

Chou S, et al: Controlled clinical trial of intravenous acyclovir in heart-transplant patients with mucocutaneous herpes simplex infections. *Lancet* 1:1392-1394, 1981.

Clover RD, et al: Effectiveness of rimantadine prophylaxis of children within families. *Am J Dis Child* 140:706-709, 1986.

Colin J, et al: Combination therapy for dendritic keratitis with human leukocyte interferon and acyclovir. *Am J Ophthalmol* 95:346-348, 1983.

Collaborative DHPG Treatment Study Group: Treatment of serious cytomegalovirus infections with 9-(1,3-dihydroxy-2-propoxymethyl) guanine in patients with AIDS and other immunodeficiencies. *N Engl J Med* 314:801-805, 1986.

Connor JD, et al: Ribavirin pharmacokinetics in children and adults during therapeutic trials, in Smith RA, et al (eds): *Clinical Applications of Ribavirin.* Orlando, Fla, Academic Press, 1984, 107-123.

Corey L, et al: Trial of topical acyclovir in genital herpes simplex virus infections. *N Engl J Med* 306:1313-1319, 1982 A.

Corey L, et al: Double-blind controlled trial of topical acyclovir in genital herpes simplex infection. *Am J Med* 73(1A):326-334, 1982 B.

Corey L, et al: Intravenous acyclovir for treatment of primary genital herpes. *Ann Intern Med* 98:914-921, 1983.

Crawford SA, et al: Rimantadine prophylaxis in children: A follow-up study. *Pediatr Infect Dis* 7:379-383, 1988.

Creagh-Kirk T, et al: Survival experience among patients with AIDS receiving zidovudine. *JAMA* 260:3009-3015, 1988.

Crumpacker CS, et al: Resistance of herpes simplex virus to adenine arabinoside and E-5-(2-bromovinyl)-2′-deoxyuridine: Physical analysis. *J Infect Dis* 146:167-172, 1982 A.

Crumpacker CS, et al: Resistance to antiviral drugs of herpes simplex virus isolated from patient treated with acyclovir. *N Engl J Med* 306:343-346, 1982 B.

D'Alessandro AM, et al: Successful treatment of severe cytomegalovirus infections with ganciclovir and CMV hyperimmune globulin in liver transplant recipients. *Transplant Proc* 21:3560-3561, 1989.

Davis GL, et al: Treatment of chronic hepatitis C with recombinant interferon alfa. *N Engl J Med* 321:1501-1506, 1989.

de Clercq E, et al: Oral (E)-5-(2-bromovinyl)-2′-deoxyuridine in severe herpes zoster. *Br Med J* 281:1178, 1980.

Di Bisceglie AM, et al: Recombinant interferon alfa therapy for chronic hepatitis C. *N Engl J Med* 321:1506-1510, 1989.

Dolin R, et al: Controlled trial of amantadine and rimantadine in prophylaxis of influenza A infections. *N Engl J Med* 307:580-584, 1982.

Douglas JM, et al: Double-blind study of oral acyclovir for suppression of recurrences of genital herpes simplex virus infection. *N Engl J Med* 310:1551-1556, 1984.

Douglas RM, et al: Prophylactic efficacy of intranasal alpha$_2$-interferon against rhinovirus infections in family setting. *N Engl J Med* 314:65-70, 1986.

Douglas JM, et al: Double-blind, placebo-controlled trial of effect of chronically administered oral acyclovir on sperm production in men with frequently recurrent genital herpes. *J Infect Dis* 157:588-593, 1988.

Dulbecco R, Ginsberg HS: *Virology.* Hagerstown, Md, Harper & Row, 1980.

Durant RH, et al: Influence of inosiplex treatment on neurological disability of patients with subacute sclerosing panencephalitis. *J Pediatr* 101:288-293, 1982.

Dyken PR, et al: Long-term follow-up of subacute sclerosing panencephalitis patients treated with inosiplex. *Ann Neurol* 11:359-364, 1982.

Eaglstein WH, et al: Effects of early corticosteroid therapy on skin eruption and pain of herpes zoster. *JAMA* 211:1681-1683, 1970.

Emanuel D, et al: Cytomegalovirus pneumonia after bone marrow transplantation successfully treated with the combination of ganciclovir and high-dose intravenous immune globulin. *Ann Intern Med* 109:777-782, 1988.

Erice A, et al: Progressive disease due to ganciclovir-resistant cytomegalovirus in immunocompromised patients. *N Engl J Med* 320:289-293, 1989.

Eron LJ, et al: Interferon therapy for condyloma acuminata. *N Engl J Med* 315:1059-1064, 1986.

Esmann V, et al: Therapy of acute herpes zoster with acyclovir in non-immunocompromised host. *Am J Med* 73 (1A):320-325, 1982.

Esmann V, et al: Prednisolone does not prevent post-herpetic neuralgia. *Lancet* 2:126-129, 1987.

Farr BM, et al: Intranasal interferon-∞2 for prevention of natural rhinovirus colds. *Antimicrob Agents Chemother* 26:31-34, 1984.

Felsenstein D, et al: Treatment of cytomegalovirus retinitis with 9-[2-hydroxy-1-(hydroxymethyl) ethoxymethyl] guanine. *Ann Intern Med* 103:377-380, 1985.

Fernandez H: Ribavirin: Summary of clinical trials—Herpes genitalis and measles, in Smith RA, Kirkpatrick W (eds): *Ribavirin: A Broad Spectrum Antiviral Agent*. New York, Academic Press, 1980, 215-230.

Field H, et al: Sensitivity of acyclovir-resistant mutants of herpes simplex virus to other antiviral drugs. *J Infect Dis* 143:281-285, 1981.

Fischl MA, et al: Efficacy of 3′-azido-3′-deoxythymidine (azidothymidine) in treatment of patients with AIDS and AIDS-related complex: Double-blind placebo-controlled trial. *N Engl J Med* 317:185-191, 1987.

Fischl MA, et al: The safety and efficacy of zidovudine (AZT) in the treatment of subjects with mildly symptomatic human immunodeficiency virus type 1 (HIV) infection: A double-blind, placebo-controlled trial. *Ann Intern Med* 112:727-737, 1990.

Fletcher CV, et al: Continuous infusion of high-dose acyclovir for serious herpesvirus infections. *Antimicrob Agents Chemother* 33:1375-1378, 1989.

Frank I, Friedman HM: Progress in the treatment of cytomegalovirus pneumonia, editorial. *Ann Intern Med* 109:769-771, 1988.

Furman PA, et al: Phosphorylation of 3′-azido-3′-deoxythymidine and selective interaction of the 5′-triphosphate with human immunodeficiency virus reverse transcriptase. *Proc Natl Acad Sci USA* 83:8333-8337, 1986.

Garcia G, et al: Adenine arabinoside monophosphate in combination with human leukocyte interferon in treatment of chronic hepatitis B: Randomized, double-blind placebo controlled trial. *Ann Intern Med* 107:278-285, 1987.

Gnann JW, et al: Controlled trial of parenteral interferon alpha$_2$ in treatment of recurrent genital herpes, abstract 1024. Washington, DC, Interscience Conference on Antimicrobial Agents and Chemotherapy, 1984.

Greenberg SB, et al: Prophylactic effect of low doses of human leukocyte interferon against infection with rhinovirus. *J Infect Dis* 145:542-546, 1982.

Gutterman JU, et al: Pharmacokinetic study of partially pure γ-interferon in cancer patients. *Cancer Res* 44:4164-4170, 1984.

Haddah FS, Risk WS: Isoprinosine treatment in 18 patients with subacute sclerosing panencephalitis: Controlled study. *Ann Neurol* 7:185-188, 1980.

Hall CB, et al: Aerosolized ribavirin Treatment of infants with respiratory syncytial viral infection: Randomized double-blind study. *N Engl J Med* 308:1443-1447, 1983 A.

Hall CB, et al: Ribavirin treatment of experimental respiratory syncytial viral infection: Controlled double-blind study in young adults. *JAMA* 249:2666-2670, 1983 B.

Hall CB, et al: Ribavirin treatment of respiratory syncytial virus infection in infants with underlying cardiopulmonary disease. *JAMA* 254:3047-3051, 1985.

Hall CB, et al: Children with influenza A infection: Treatment with rimantadine. *Pediatrics* 80:275-282, 1987.

Hay AJ, et al: Matrix protein gene determines amantadine-sensitivity of influenza viruses. *J Gen Virol* 42:189-191, 1979.

Hay AJ, et al: Molecular basis of resistance of influenza A viruses to amantadine. *J Antimicrob Chemother* 18 (suppl B): 19-29, 1986.

Hayden FG, Gwaltney JM Jr: Prophylactic activity of intranasal enviroxime against experimentally induced rhinovirus type 39 infection. *Antimicrob Agents Chemother* 21:892-897, 1982.

Hayden FG, Gwaltney JM Jr: Intranasal interferon ∞2 for prevention of rhinovirus infection and illness. *J Infect Dis* 148:543-550, 1983.

Hayden FG, et al: Prevention of natural colds by contact prophylaxis with intranasal alpha$_2$-interferon. *N Engl J Med* 314:71-75, 1986.

Hayden FG, et al: Emergence and apparent transmission of rimantadine-resistant influenza A virus in families. *N Engl J Med* 321:1696-1702, 1989.

Heider H, et al: Occurrence of amantadine- and rimantadine-resistant influenza A virus strains during 1980 epidemic. *Acta Virol* 25:395-400, 1981.

Herzog C, et al: Intranasal interferon for contact prophylaxis against common cold in families, letter. *Lancet* 2:962, 1983.

Higgins PG, et al: Intranasal interferon as protection against experimental respiratory coronavirus infection in volunteers. *Antimicrob Agents Chemother* 24:713-715, 1983.

Hirsch MS, et al: Effects of interferon-alpha on cytomegalovirus reactivation syndromes in renal-transplant recipients. *N Engl J Med* 308:1489-1493, 1983.

Hoofnagle JH, et al: Randomized controlled trial of adenine arabinoside monophosphate for chronic type B hepatitis. *Gastroenterology* 86:150-157, 1984.

Hoofnagle JH, et al: Treatment of chronic non-A, non-B hepatitis with recombinant human alpha interferon. *N Engl J Med* 315:1575-1578, 1986.

Hoofnagle JH, et al: Randomized, controlled trial of recombinant human alpha interferon in patients with chronic hepatitis B. *Gastroenterology* 95:1318-1325, 1988.

Huff JC, et al: Therapy of herpes zoster with oral acyclovir. *Am J Med* 85 (2A):85-89, 1988.

Huggins JW, et al: Effective therapy of epidemic hemorrhagic fever patients with ribarivin: Decreasing mortality and reversible anemia, abstract 4. Williamsburg, Va, International Society for Antiviral Research, 1988.

Jabs DA, et al: Cytomegalovirus retinitis and acquired immunodeficiency syndrome. *Arch Ophthalmol* 107:75-80, 1989.

Jacobson MA, et al: Failure of adjunctive cytomegalovirus intravenous immune globulin to improve efficacy of ganciclovir in patients with acquired immunodeficiency syndrome and cytomegalovirus retinitis: A Phase 1 study. *Antimicrob Agents Chemother* 34:176-178, 1990.

Jura E, et al: Varicella-zoster virus infections in children infected with human immunodeficiency virus. *Pediatr Infect Dis J* 8:586-560, 1989.

Klein G (ed): *Viral Oncology*. New York, Raven Press, 1980.

König H, et al: Azidothymidine triphosphate is an inhibitor of both human immunodeficiency virus type 1 reverse transcriptase and DNA polymerase gamma. *Antimicrob Agents Chemother* 33:2109-2114, 1989.

Knight V, et al: Ribavirin aerosol in influenza A infections, abstract 876. Chicago, 21st Interscience Conference on Antimicrobial Agents and Chemotherapy, (Nov 4-6) 1981.

Kraemer KG, et al: Prophylactic adenine arabinoside following marrow transplantation. *Transplant Proc* 10:237-240, 1978.

Kweder SL, et al: Inosine pranobex: Is a single positive trail enough? *N Engl J Med* 322:1807-1809, 1990.

Lane HC, et al: Zidovudine in patients with human immunodeficiency virus (HIV) infection and Kaposi sarcoma: A Phase II randomized, placebo-controlled trial. *Ann Intern Med* 111:41-50, 1989.

Larder BA, et al: HIV with reduced sensitivity to zidovudine (AZT) isolated during prolonged therapy. *Science* 243:1731-1734, 1989.

Laskin OL, et al: Use of ganciclovir to treat serious cytomegalovirus infections in patients with AIDS. *J Infect Dis* 155:323-327, 1987 A.

Laskin OL, et al: Ganciclovir for treatment and suppression of serious infections caused by cytomegalovirus. *Am J Med* 83:201-207, 1987 B.

Levandowski RA, et al: Topical enviroxime against rhinovirus infection. *Antimicrob Agents Chemother* 22:1004-1007, 1982.

Lok ASF, et al: Treatment of chronic hepatitis B with interferon: Experience with Asian patients. *Semin Liver Dis* 9:249-253, 1989.

Luby JP, et al: Collaborative study of patient-initiated treatment of recurrent genital herpes with topical acyclovir or placebo. *J Infect Dis* 150:1-6, 1984.

Marker SC, et al: Trial of vidarabine for cytomegalovirus infection in renal transplant patients. *Arch Intern Med* 140:1441-1444, 1980.

Masur H, et al: Effect of 9-(1, 3-dihydroxy-2-propoxymethyl) guanine on serious cytomegalovirus disease in eight immunosuppressed homosexual men. *Ann Intern Med* 104:41-44, 1986.

Mattison HR, et al: Double-blind, placebo-controlled trial comparing long-term suppressive with short-term oral acyclovir for management of recurrent genital herpes. *Am J Med* 85(suppl 2A):20-25, 1988.

Maudgal PC, et al: Efficacy of (E)-5-(2-bromovinyl)-2′-deoxyuridine in topical treatment of herpes simplex keratitis. *Graefes Arch Clin Exp Ophthalmol* 216:261-268, 1981 A.

Maudgal PC, et al: Preliminary results of oral BVDU treatment of herpes zoster ophthalmicus. *Bull Soc Belge Ophtalmol* 193:49-56, 1981 B.

McClung HW, et al: Ribavirin aerosol treatment of influenza B virus infection. *JAMA* 249:2671-2674, 1983.

McCormick JB, et al: Lassa fever: Effective therapy with ribavirin. *N Engl J Med* 314:20-26, 1986.

McIntosh K, et al: Treatment of respiratory viral infection in immunodeficient infant with ribavirin aerosol. *Am J Dis Child* 138:305-308, 1984.

McKendrick MW, et al: Oral acyclovir in herpes zoster. *J Antimicrob Chemother* 14:661-665, 1984.

Melnick JL: Taxonomy of viruses, 1980. *Prog Med Virol* 26:214-232, 1980.

Mertz GJ, et al: Double-blind placebo-controlled trial of oral acyclovir in first-episode genital herpes simplex virus infection. *JAMA* 252:1147-1151, 1984.

Mertz GJ, et al: Long-term acyclovir suppression of frequently recurring genital herpes simplex virus infection: Multicenter double-blind trial. *JAMA* 260:201-206, 1988 A.

Mertz GJ, et al: Prolonged continuous versus intermittent oral acyclovir in normal adults with frequently recurring genital herpes simplex virus infection. *Am J Med* 85(suppl 2A):14-19, 1988 B.

Meyers JD, et al: Multicenter collaborative trial of intravenous acyclovir for treatment of mucocutaneous herpes simplex virus infection in immunocompromised host. *Am J Med* 73(1A):229-235, 1982.

Meyers JD, et al: Recombinant leukocyte A interferon for treatment of serious viral infections after marrow transplant: Phase I study. *J Infect Dis* 148:551-556, 1983.

Meyers JD, et al: Acyclovir treatment of varicella-zoster virus infection in compromised host. *Transplantation* 37:571-574, 1984.

Meyers JD, et al: Acyclovir for prevention of cytomegalovirus infection and disease after allogenic marrow transplantation. *N Engl J Med* 318:70-75, 1988.

Mindel A, et al: Intravenous acyclovir treatment for primary genital herpes. *Lancet* 1:697-700, 1982.

Mindel A, et al: Prophylactic oral acyclovir in recurrent genital herpes. *Lancet* 2:57-59, 1984.

Mindel A, et al: Dosage and safety of long-term suppressive acyclovir therapy for recurrent genital herpes. *Lancet* 1:926-928, 1988.

Minkoff DI, et al: Clinical use of ribavirin and treatment of herpes zoster in otherwise normal adults, in Smith RA, Kirkpatrick W (eds): *Ribavirin: A Broad Spectrum Antiviral Agent*. New York, Academic Press, 1980, 185-199.

Mitchell CD, et al: Acyclovir therapy for mucocutaneous herpes simplex infections in immunocompromised patients. *Lancet* 1:1389-1392, 1981.

Mitsuya H, et al: 3′-azido-3′-deoxythymidine (BW A509U): Antiviral agent that inhibits the infectivity and cytopathic effect of human T-lymphotropic virus type III/lymphadenopathy-associated virus in vitro. *Proc Natl Acad Sci USA* 82:7096-7100, 1985.

Morton P, et al: Oral acyclovir in the treatment of herpes zoster in general practice. *NZ Med J* 102:93-95, 1989.

National Institutes of Health Consensus Development Conference: Amantadine: Does it have role in prevention and treatment of influenza? *Ann Intern Med* 92:256-258, 1980.

Nilsen AE, et al: Efficacy of oral acyclovir in treatment of initial and recurrent genital herpes. *Lancet* 2:571-573, 1982.

Novelli VM, et al: Acyclovir administered perorally in immunocompromised children with varicella-zoster infections. *J Infect Dis* 149:478, 1984.

Ohnishi H, et al: Mechanism of host defense suppression induced by viral infection: Mode of action of inosiplex as antiviral agent. *Infect Immun* 38:243-250, 1982.

Oxford JS, et al: In vivo selection of influenza A2 strain resistant to amantadine. *Nature* 226:82-83, 1970.

Oxford JS, et al: Antiviral activity of amantadine: A review of laboratory and clinical data. *Pharmacol Ther* 11:181-262, 1980.

Patriarca PA, et al: Safety of prolonged administration of rimantadine hydrochloride in prophylaxis of influenza A virus infections in nursing homes. *Antimicrob Agents Chemother* 26:101-103, 1984.

Payler DK, et al: Influenza A prophylaxis with amantadine in a boarding school. *Lancet* 1:502-504, 1984.

Pazin GJ, et al: Leukocyte interferon for treating first episodes of genital herpes in women. *J Infect Dis* 156:891-898, 1987.

Peacock JE Jr, et al: Intravenous acyclovir therapy of first episodes of genital herpes: Multicenter double-blind, placebo-controlled trial. *Am J Med* 85:301-306, 1988.

Pedersen C, et al: The efficacy of inosine pranobex in preventing the acquired immunodeficiency syndrome in patients with human immunodeficiency virus infection. *N Engl J Med* 322:1757-1763, 1990.

Perrillo RP: Treatment of chronic hepatitis B with interferon: Experience in Western countries. *Semin Liver Dis* 9:240-248, 1989.

Perrillo RP, et al: Prednisone withdrawal followed by recombinant alpha interferon in treatment of chronic type B hepatitis: Randomized, controlled trial. *Ann Intern Med* 109:95-100, 1988.

Peterslund NA, et al: Acyclovir in herpes zoster. *Lancet* 2:827-830, 1981.

Peterslund NA, et al: Oral and intravenous acyclovir are equally effective in herpes zoster. *J Antimicrob Chemother* 14:185-189, 1984.

Phillpotts RJ, et al: Activity of enviroxime against rhinovirus infection in man. *Lancet* 1:1342-1344, 1981.

Phillpotts RJ, et al: Therapeutic activity of enviroxime against rhinovirus infection in volunteers. *Antimicrob Agents Chemother* 23:671-675, 1983.

Pollard RB, et al: Effect of vidarabine on chronic hepatitis B virus infection. *JAMA* 239:1648-1650, 1978.

Pollard RB, et al: Cytomegalovirus retinitis in immunosuppressed hosts: I. Natural history and effects of treatment with adenine arabinoside. *Ann Intern Med* 93:655-664, 1980.

Preble OT, Friedman RM: Interferon-induced alterations in cells: Relevance to viral and nonviral diseases. *Lab Invest* 49:4-18, 1983.

Prober CG, et al: Acyclovir therapy of chickenpox in immunosuppressed children: A collaborative study. *J Pediatr* 101:622-625, 1982.

Quarles JM, et al: Comparison of amantadine and rimantadine for prevention of type A (Russian) influenza. *Antiviral Res* 1:149-155, 1981.

Reed EC, et al: Treatment of cytomegalovirus pneumonia with ganciclovir and intravenous cytomegalovirus immunoglobulin in patients with bone marrow transplants. *Ann Intern Med* 109:783-788, 1988.

Reichman RC, et al: Treatment of recurrent genital herpes simplex infections with oral acyclovir: Controlled trial. *JAMA* 251:2103-2107, 1984.

Reichman RC, et al: Treatment of condyloma acuminatum with three different interferons administered intralesionally: Multicentered, placebo-controlled trial. *Ann Intern Med* 108:675-679, 1988.

Richman DD, et al: Toxicity of azidothymidine (AZT) in treatment of patients with AIDS and AIDS-related complex: Double-blind, placebo-controlled trial. *N Engl J Med* 317:192-197, 1987.

Rizzetto M, et al: Treatment of chronic delta hepatitis with α-2 recombinant interferon. *J Hepatol* 3 (suppl 2):S229-S233, 1986.

Rosina F, et al: Alpha 2 recombinant interferon in treatment of chronic delta hepatitis. *Prog Clin Biol Res* 234:299-303, 1987.

Rosina F, et al: Treatment of chronic type D (delta) hepatitis with alpha interferon. *Semin Liver Dis* 9:264-266, 1989.

Ruhnek-Forsbeck M, et al: Treatment of recurrent genital herpes simplex infections with oral acyclovir. *J Antimicrob Chemother* 16:621-628, 1985.

Russler SK, et al: Susceptibility of human herpesvirus 6 to acyclovir and ganciclovir. *Lancet* 2:382, 1989.

Sacks SL, et al: Clinical course of recurrent genital herpes and treatment with foscarnet cream: Results of a Canadian multicenter trial. *J Infect Dis* 155:178-186, 1987.

Samo TC, et al: Efficacy and tolerance of intranasally applied recombinant leukocyte A interferon in normal volunteers. *J Infect Dis* 148:535-542, 1983.

Saral R, et al: Acyclovir prophylaxis of herpes simplex virus infections: Randomized, double-blind controlled trial in bone marrow transplant recipients. *N Engl J Med* 305:63-67, 1981.

Saral R, et al: Acyclovir prophylaxis against herpes simplex virus infection in patients with leukemia: Randomized, double-blind, placebo-controlled study. *Ann Intern Med* 99:773-776, 1983.

Schmidt GM, et al: Ganciclovir/immunoglobulin combination therapy for the treatment of human cytomegalovirus-associated interstitial pneumonia in bone marrow allograft recipients. *Transplantation* 46:905-907, 1988.

Scott GM, et al: Purified interferon as protection against rhinovirus infection. *Br Med J* 284:1822-1825, 1982.

Segal R, et al: Glycyrrhizin gel as a vehicle for idoxuridine, I: Clinical investigations. *J Clin Pharm Ther* 12:165-171, 1987.

Selby PJ, et al: Parenteral acyclovir therapy for herpesvirus infections in man. *Lancet* 2:1267-1270, 1979.

Selby PJ, et al: The prophylactic role of intravenous and long-term oral acyclovir after allogeneic bone marrow transplantation. *Br J Cancer* 59:434-438, 1989.

Serota FT, et al: Acyclovir treatment of herpes zoster infections: Use in children undergoing bone marrow transplantation. *JAMA* 247:2132-2135, 1982.

Shalev Y, et al: Progressive cutaneous herpes simplex infection in acute myeloblastic leukemia: Successful treatment with interferon and cytarabine. *Arch Dermatol* 120:922-926, 1984.

Shepp DH, et al: Activity of 9-[2-hydroxy-1-(hydroxymethyl) ethoxymethyl] guanine in treatment of cytomegalovirus pneumonia. *Ann Intern Med* 103:368-373, 1985.

Shepp DH, et al: Treatment of varicella-zoster virus infection in severely immunocompromised patients: Randomized comparison of acyclovir and vidarabine. *N Engl J Med* 314:208-212, 1986.

Silvestri DL, et al: Ineffectiveness of topical idoxuridine in dimethyl sulfoxide for therapy for genital herpes. *JAMA* 248:953-959, 1982.

Smith CI, et al: Vidarabine monophosphate and human leukocyte interferon in chronic hepatitis B infection. *JAMA* 247:2261-2265, 1982.

Smith CI, et al: Acute Dane particle suppression with recombinant leukocyte A interferon in chronic hepatitis B virus infection. *J Infect Dis* 148:907-913, 1983.

Spector SA, et al: Treatment of herpes virus infections in immunocompromised patients with acyclovir by continuous intravenous infusion. *Am J Med* 73 (1A):229-235, 1982.

Spruance SL, et al: Treatment of herpes simplex labialis with topical acyclovir in polyethylene glycol. *J Infect Dis* 146:85-90, 1982.

Spruance SL, et al: Early, patient-initiated treatment of herpes labialis with topical 10% acyclovir. *Antimicrob Agents Chemother* 25:553-555, 1984.

Spruance SL: Cutaneous herpes simplex virus lesions induced by ultraviolet radiation: Review of model systems and prophylactic therapy with oral acyclovir. *Am J Med* 85 (suppl 2A):43-48, 1988.

Spruance SL, et al: Early application of topical 15% idoxuridine in dimethylsulfoxide shortens the course of herpes simplex labialis: A multicenter placebo-controlled trial. *J Infect Dis* 161:191-197, 1990 A.

Spruance SL, et al: Treatment of recurrent herpes simplex labialis with oral acyclovir. *J Infect Dis* 161:185-190, 1990 B.

Stiehm ER, et al: Interferon: Immunobiology and clinical significance. *Ann Intern Med* 96:80-93, 1982.

Straus SE, et al: Acyclovir for chronic mucocutaneous herpes simplex virus infection in immunosuppressed patients. *Ann Intern Med* 96:270-277, 1982.

Straus SE, et al: Oral acyclovir to suppress recurring herpes simplex virus infections in immunodeficient patients. *Ann Intern Med* 100:522-524, 1984 A.

Straus SE, et al: Suppression of frequently recurring genital herpes: Placebo-controlled double-blind trial of oral acyclovir. *N Engl J Med* 310:1545-1550, 1984 B.

Straus SE, et al: Acyclovir suppression of frequently recurring genital herpes: Efficacy and diminishing need during successive years of treatment. *JAMA* 260:2227-2230, 1988.

Straus SE, et al: Effect of oral acyclovir treatment on symptomatic and asymptomatic virus shedding in recurrent genital herpes. *Sex Transm Dis* 16:107-113, 1989.

Thin RN, et al: Recurrent genital herpes suppressed by oral acyclovir: Multicentre double blind trial. *J Antimicrob Chemother* 16:219-226, 1985.

Uylangco CV, et al: Double-blind placebo-controlled evaluation of ribavirin in treatment of acute measles. *Clin Ther* 3:389-396, 1981.

Van Voris LP, et al: Successful treatment of naturally occurring influenza A/USSR/77 147NI. *JAMA* 245:1128-1131, 1981.

Vince R, Daluge S: Carbocyclic arabinosyladenine: Adenosine deaminase resistant antiviral agent. *J Med Chem* 20:612-613, 1977.

Vince R, et al: Carbocyclic arabinofuranosyladenine (Cyclaradine): Efficacy against genital herpes in guinea pigs. *Science* 221:1405-1406, 1983.

Vogt MW, et al: Ribavirin antagonizes effect of azidothymidine on HIV replication. *Science* 235:1376-1379, 1987.

Volberding PA, et al: Zidovudine in asymptomatic human immunodeficiency virus infection: A controlled trial in persons with fewer than 500 CD4-positive cells per cubic millimeter. *N Engl J Med* 322:941-949, 1990.

Wade JC, et al: Intravenous acyclovir to treat mucocutaneous herpes simplex virus infection after marrow transplantation: Double-blind trial. *Ann Intern Med* 96:265-269, 1982 A.

Wade JC, et al: Treatment of cytomegalovirus pneumonia with high-dose acyclovir. *Am J Med* 73 (1A):249-256, 1982 B.

Wade JC, et al: Oral acyclovir for prevention of herpes simplex virus reactivation after marrow transplantation. *Ann Intern Med* 100:823-828, 1984.

Wald ER, et al: *In re* ribavirin: Case of premature adjudication? *J Pediatr* 112:154-158, 1988.

Wallin J, et al: Treatment of recurrent herpes labialis with trisodium phosphonoformate, in Nelson JD, Grassi C (eds): *Current Chemotherapy and Infectious Disease*. Washington, DC, American Society for Microbiology, 1980, 1361-1362.

Whitley RJ, et al: Adenine arabinoside therapy of herpes zoster in immunosuppressed: NIAID Collaborative Antiviral Study. *N Engl J Med* 294:1193-1199, 1976.

Whitley RJ, et al: Adenine arabinoside therapy of biopsy-proved herpes simplex encephalitis: NIAID Collaborative Antiviral Study. *N Engl J Med* 297:289-294, 1977.

Whitley RJ, et al: Vidarabine therapy of neonatal herpes simplex infection. *Pediatrics* 66:495-501, 1980.

Whitley RJ, et al: Herpes simplex encephalitis: Vidarabine therapy and diagnostic problems. *N Engl J Med* 304:313-318, 1981.

Whitley R, et al: Vidarabine therapy of varicella in immunosuppressed patients. *J Pediatr* 101:125-131, 1982 A.

Whitley RJ, et al: Mucocutaneous herpes simplex virus infections in immunocompromised patients: Model for evaluation of topical antiviral agents. *Am J Med* 73 (1A):236-240, 1982 B.

Whitley RJ, et al: Herpes simplex encephalitis: Clinical assessment. *JAMA* 247:317-320, 1982 C.

Whitley RJ, et al: Early vidarabine therapy to control complications of herpes zoster in immunosuppressed patients. *N Engl J Med* 307:971-975, 1982 D.

Whitley RJ, et al: Neonatal herpes simplex virus infection: Follow-up evaluation of vidarabine therapy. *Pediatrics* 72:778-785, 1983.

Whitley RJ, et al: Vidarabine therapy for mucocutaneous herpes simplex virus infections in immunocompromised host. *J Infect Dis* 149:1-8, 1984.

Whitley RJ, et al: Vidarabine versus acyclovir therapy in herpes simplex encephalitis. *N Engl J Med* 314:144-149, 1986 A.

Whitley RJ, et al: Vidarabine versus acyclovir therapy of neonatal herpes simplex virus infection, abstract 987. Washington, DC, Society for Pediatric Research, 1986 B.

Wildiers J, de Clercq E: Oral (E)-5-(2-bromovinyl)-2′-deoxyuridine treatment of severe herpes zoster in cancer patients. *Eur J Cancer Clin Oncol* 20:471-476, 1984.

Willis RJ, et al: Interferon kinetics and adverse reactions after intravenous, intramuscular, and subcutaneous injection. *Clin Pharmacol Ther* 35:722-727, 1984.

Wilson SZ, et al: Treatment of influenza A(H1N1) virus infection with ribavirin aerosol. *Antimicrob Agents Chemother* 26:200-203, 1984.

Yarchoan R, et al: Administration of 3′-azido-3′-deoxythymidine, an inhibitor of HTLV-III/LAV replication, to patients with AIDS or AIDS-related complex. *Lancet* 1:575-580, 1986.

Young CW, et al: Phase I evaluation of 2′-fluoro-5-iodo-1-β-D-arabinofuranosylcytosine in immunosuppressed patients with herpesvirus infection. *Cancer Res* 43:5006-5009, 1983.

Other Selected References

Belshe RB (ed): *Textbook of Human Virology*. Littleton, Mass, PSG Publishing Company, 1984.

Galasso G, et al (eds): *Antiviral Agents and Therapy of Human Viral Infections*. New York, Raven Press, 1985.

Stuart-Harris CH, Oxford J (eds): *Problems of Antiviral Therapy*. New York, Academic Press, 1983.

New Evaluations

DIDANOSINE (ddI)
[Videx]

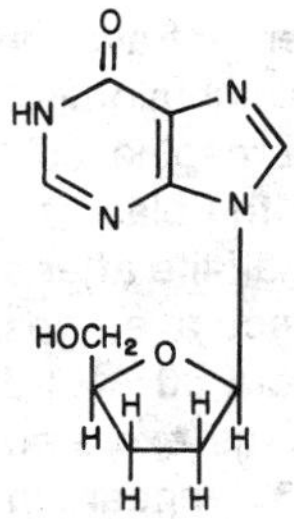

ACTIONS AND USES. Didanosine, 2′,3′-dideoxyinosine (ddI), is a nucleoside analogue of deoxyadenosine and an inhibitor of the replication of the human immunodeficiency virus (HIV). After entry into the cell it is converted by cellular enzymes to dideoxyadenosine triphosphate (ddATP), the active metabolite. In vitro, the intracellular half-life of ddATP varies from 12 to >24 hours. Since ddATP lacks the free 3′-hydroxyl group to which 5′-monophosphate nucleosides subsequently attach, the incorporation of this compound into the growing viral DNA chain leads to chain termination and, hence, cessation of viral replication. In addition, ddATP inhibits HIV reverse transcriptase by competing with the natural nucleoside triphosphate, dATP, for binding to the active site of the enzyme.

In vitro, didanosine is active against HIV-1 in a variety of infected T-cell and monocyte/macrophage cell cultures and is active against HIV-2 in human cell cultures. The drug also inhibits the replication of human hepatitis B virus in cell cultures; the clinical significance of this finding is not known.

Didanosine is indicated for the treatment of adults and pediatric patients (>6 months) with advanced HIV infection who either cannot tolerate zidovudine or have experienced significant clinical or immunologic deterioration during zidovudine therapy. Unless it is contraindicated, zidovudine should be considered as initial therapy for the treatment of advanced HIV infection since it has been shown to prolong survival and to decrease the incidence of opportunistic infections.

ADVERSE REACTIONS. In phase I studies in which adults received doses ≤12.5 mg/kg/day (approximately 1.75 times the recommended dose), the major adverse effects were pancreatitis (9%) and peripheral neuropathy (34%). In other studies, adverse effects reported were headache (36%), diarrhea (34%), peripheral neuropathy (42%), asthenia (25%), insomnia (25%), nausea/vomiting (25%), rash/pruritus (24%), abdominal pain (21%), central nervous system depression (19%), constipation (16%), stomatitis (14%), myalgia (13%), arthritis (11%), taste loss/perversion (10%), pain (10%), dry mouth (9%), alopecia (8%), and dizziness (7%). These reactions were reported less frequently in the didanosine Expanded Access program in which the median duration of treatment was shorter than in the combined adult phase I studies (5 versus 8.5 months). The most common adverse event reported in the Expanded Access patients was diarrhea (incidence, 18%).

Serious laboratory abnormalities reported in adult phase I patients included leukopenia, granulocytopenia, and thrombocytopenia; abnormal elevations of ALT, AST, alkaline phosphatase, bilirubin, uric acid, and amylase also were observed. The incidence of these effects was higher in patients who had abnormal baseline values.

In pediatric phase I trials, pancreatitis occurred in 3% of patients treated at entry with doses <300 mg/M²/day and in 13% of those receiving larger doses. Other adverse reactions reported in 25% or more of the children (n=60) given <300 mg/M²/day included malaise, anorexia, asthenia, chills/fever, pain, liver abnormalities, abdominal pain, diarrhea, nausea/vomiting, nervousness, headache, asthma, cough, dyspnea, rhinitis, and rash/pruritus. Since no comparative controlled data for HIV-infected, untreated children was reported in these studies, the adverse events should be regarded as *potential* hazards of didanosine treatment.

Serious laboratory abnormalities that occurred in some pediatric patients who received doses ≤300 mg/M²/day (n=60) were leukopenia (3%), granulocytopenia (24%), thrombocytopenia (2%), and anemia (4%). Bilirubin was elevated in 2% of the patients. As with adults, the incidence was higher in those who had abnormal baseline values.

PRECAUTIONS. Patients should be informed that the major toxicities of didanosine are pancreatitis and peripheral neuropathy, and they should be advised to report any symptoms related to pancreatitis (abdominal pain, nausea, vomiting) or peripheral neuropathy (tingling, burning, numbness or pain in the hands or feet). Dosage modification and/or discontinuation of the drug may be required. Alcohol consumption may increase the risk for the development of pancreatitis.

Opportunistic infections and other complications of HIV infection may continue to develop in patients receiving didanosine. Therefore, these individuals should be closely supervised by a physician experienced in the treatment of HIV-infected patients.

Didanosine tablets should be used with caution in patients with phenylketonuria, for the tablets contain 33.7 mg of phenylalanine in the 150-mg size and 22.5 mg in all other sizes.

Because didanosine is rapidly degraded at acidic pH, all oral formulations contain buffering agents to increase the pH of the stomach. Each dose for adults and children >1 year must consist of two tablets to achieve adequate acid-neutralizing capacity; a one-tablet dose is sufficient in infants <1 year.

In phase I studies in adults, didanosine buffered powder for oral solution was associated with diarrhea in 34% of the patients. If diarrhea develops in a patient receiving this product, substitution of buffered tablets should be considered.

Physicians who treat patients on sodium-restricted diets should be aware that each buffered tablet contains 264.5 mg of sodium and each single-dose packet of buffered powder for oral solution contains 1.38 g of sodium.

Patients with impaired renal function (serum creatinine >1.5 mg/dL or creatinine clearance ≤60 ml/min) may be at increased risk of toxicity, and a reduction in dose should be considered. The magnesium hydroxide content of each tablet is 15.7 mEq, which may be excessive for patients with significant renal impairment. A dose reduction also may be necessary for patients with hepatic impairment, although this has not been evaluated.

At high doses, didanosine has been associated with asymptomatic hyperuricemia; discontinuation of treatment may be necessary if efforts to reduce uric acid levels fail.

PREGNANCY AND LACTATION. In animal reproduction studies, rats and rabbits received doses 12 to 14.2 times higher than the human dose and there was no evidence of impaired fertility or fetal harm. However, at doses 12 times higher than the human dose, anorexia was observed in female rats and their offspring. There are no adequate controlled studies in pregnant women, and the drug should be used during pregnancy only if it is clearly indicated (FDA Pregnancy Category B).

It is not known whether didanosine is excreted in human milk. Since many drugs are and there is potential for serious adverse effects in nursing infants, mothers should be advised to discontinue nursing when taking the drug.

OVERDOSAGE. There is no known antidote for didanosine overdosage, and it is not known whether the drug is removed by peritoneal dialysis or hemodialysis. Experience in clinical studies in which the initial dose was 10 times that currently recommended suggests that chronic overdosage would produce pancreatitis, peripheral neuropathy, diarrhea, hyperuricemia, and hepatic dysfunction.

DRUG INTERACTIONS. Drugs whose absorption can be affected by stomach acidity (eg, ketoconazole, dapsone) should be administered at least two hours prior to didanosine. Administration with drugs that also cause pancreatitis and peripheral neuropathy may increase the risk of these toxicities. Didanosine products contain magnesium and/or aluminum and should not be administered with any form of tetracycline. Plasma concentrations of some quinolone antibiotics are decreased when they are given with antacids containing magnesium or aluminum. Thus, quinolone antibiotics should not be administered within two hours of a dose of didanosine.

PHARMACOKINETICS. *Adults.* Although the tablet preparation of didanosine is 20% to 25% more bioavailable than the solution, both formulations have produced similar plasma concentrations (C_{max}, 1.6 mcg/ml). The mean area under the plasma concentration versus time curve (AUC) is 3±0.8 mcg/hr/ml for the buffered solution and 2.6±0.7 mcg/hr/ml for the tablet. Although there is significant variability among patients, the C_{max} and AUC values are proportional to dose over the range of amounts given clinically. At doses ≤7 mg/kg, the bioavailability is 33% (±14%) after a single dose and 37% (±14%) after a four-week dosing period.

Pharmacokinetic parameters at steady state are not significantly different from values obtained after an initial oral or intravenous dose. After intravenous administration, the steady state volume of distribution is 54 L. The concentration of didanosine in the cerebrospinal fluid one hour after infusion averages 21% of that in the plasma.

The usual elimination half-life after oral administration is 1.6 hours. Total body clearance averages 800 ml/min, and renal clearance represents about 50% of this. After a single intravenous dose, about 55% is excreted in the urine; after oral administration, about 20% appears in the urine.

There have been no studies in humans to evaluate the metabolism of didanosine. Extensive metabolism has been observed in dogs after a single intravenous or oral dose. The major metabolite identified in urine, allantoin, accounted for 61% of an oral dose. Other urinary metabolites identified were hypoxanthine, xanthine, and uric acid. Presumably the metabolism of didanosine in humans occurs by the same pathways involved in the elimination of endogenous purines.

Human plasma protein binding in vitro is less than 5%; this suggests that drug interactions at the binding site are not likely.

Children. As in adults, C_{max} and AUC values increase in proportion to dose. The absolute bioavailability in one clinical study varied from 32%±12% to 42%±18% after the first oral dose and at steady state, respectively. In a second study, the oral absorption of didanosine also varied significantly; the average absolute bioavailability was 19%±17%. After the administration of oral doses of 80, 120, and 180 mg/M^2 in one study, the usual steady-state AUC was 1.4±0.4, 1.6±0.9, and 2.3±0.9 mcg/hr/ml, respectively. The corresponding steady-state C_{max} values were 0.8±0.4, 1.4±0.7, and 1.7±0.9 mcg/ml, respectively.

After intravenous administration, the volume of distribution was 35.6 l/M^2 and the cerebrospinal fluid levels corresponded to 12% to 85% of the plasma concentration. Total body clearance was 532 ml/min/M^2.

After oral administration, the elimination half-life averaged 0.8 hours. Mean renal clearance was 190 to 319 ml/min/M^2 after the first oral dose and 231 to 265 ml/min/M^2 at steady state. Urinary recovery was 17% at steady state. There was no evidence of the accumulation of adenosine after administration of oral doses for an average of 26 days.

DOSAGE AND PREPARATIONS. All formulations should be administered on an empty stomach; ingestion with food reduces absorption by as much as 50%. A 12-hour dosing schedule should be employed.

Oral: *Adults*, the initial dose depends on weight (see the following table:

ADULT DOSING

Patient Weight	Tablets (Buffered)*	Powder (Buffered)
≥75 kg	300 mg twice daily	375 mg twice daily
50-74 kg	200 mg twice daily	250 mg twice daily
35-49 kg	125 mg twice daily	167 mg twice daily

**Two tablets should be taken at each dose to provide adequate buffering to prevent gastric acid degradation of the drug.*

Children, the recommended dose in children depends on body surface area (see the following table):

PEDIATRIC DOSING (based on average recommended dose of pediatric powder 200 mg/M²/day)

Body Surface Area (M²)	Tablets (Buffered)*	Pediatric Powder (Buffered) (Vol/10 mg/ml admixture)
1.1-1.4	100 mg twice daily	125 mg (12.5 ml) twice daily
0.8-1	75 mg twice daily	94 mg (9.5 ml) twice daily
0.5-0.7	50 mg twice daily	62 mg (6 ml) twice daily
≤0.4	25 mg twice daily	31 mg (3 ml) twice daily

**To prevent gastric acid degradation,* children older than one year *should receive a two-tablet dose;* children less than one year *should receive a one-tablet dose.*

Videx (Bristol-Myers Squibb). Tablets (chewable, buffered, water dispersible) 25, 50, 100, and 150 mg; powder (buffered, for oral solution) 100, 167, 250, and 375 mg in single-dose packets; powder (pediatric, for oral solution) 2 and 4 g.

FOSCARNET SODIUM

[Foscavir]

$$(NaO)_2\overset{\overset{O}{\|}}{P}COONa$$

Foscarnet (trisodium phosphonoformate), a pyrophosphate analogue of phosphonoacetic acid (PAA), has potent in vitro and in vivo activity against herpesviruses. Because PAA produced liver degeneration, gingivitis, and severe dermal toxicity and accumulated in bone in laboratory animals, it was considered too toxic for human use. Foscarnet is considerably less toxic and, therefore, was selected for clinical development.

ACTIONS. In vitro, foscarnet inhibits the replication of all known herpesviruses, including cytomegalovirus (CMV); herpes simplex virus (HSV) types 1 and 2; human herpesvirus 6; and Epstein-Barr and varicella-zoster viruses. Recently, this drug also has been shown to inhibit HIV replication; it inhibits the reverse transcriptase activity of HIV, other human retroviruses, and several animal retroviruses (avian myeloblastosis, visna, and murine leukemia virus). It also inhibits influenza A RNA-dependent RNA polymerase and has been reported to have activity against hepatitis B virus. Foscarnet is active against acyclovir- and ganciclovir-resistant herpesviruses, including CMV.

Foscarnet inhibits the DNA polymerases of all human herpesviruses and retrovirus reverse transcriptases by blocking the pyrophosphate binding site, thus inhibiting the formation of the 3′-5′-phosphodiester bond between primer and substrate and preventing chain elongation. The drug does not require activation (phosphorylation) by thymidine kinase or any other kinase, which explains its activity against resistant herpesvirus mutants that are deficient in thymidine kinase. It also has been reported to be active against HSV DNA polymerase mutants resistant to acyclovir. However, HSV mutants resistant to both acyclovir and foscarnet have been isolated from AIDS patients previously treated with both drugs.

CMV mutants resistant to foscarnet have emerged both in vitro and in vivo. The latent state of any human herpesvirus is not known to be sensitive to the drug, and reactivation of CMV occurs after foscarnet therapy is terminated.

USES. Foscarnet is indicated for the treatment of CMV retinitis in patients with AIDS. The diagnosis of CMV retinitis should be established by indirect ophthalmoscopy by an ophthalmologist familiar with the retinal symptoms. Although a CMV culture may support the diagnosis, a negative culture does not rule it out.

Many of the clinical studies on the use of foscarnet for the treatment of CMV retinitis have been open-label trials involving comparison with untreated historical controls or patients treated with ganciclovir. In most studies, therapy was begun with an induction dose of 60 mg/kg/every eight hours for the first two to three weeks, followed by once-daily administration of 60 to 120 mg/kg. In one early trial, 31 AIDS patients with CMV retinitis received foscarnet as a continuous infusion for up to three weeks of induction therapy. The retinitis improved in 93.5% of the patients and completely resolved in 62%. However, all patients who did not receive maintenance therapy relapsed within three weeks of cessation of foscarnet therapy. In six patients given maintenance therapy, the rate of relapse was 50% within the first five weeks. Use of foscarnet with zidovudine prolonged the duration of remission to 12 weeks (LeHoang et al, 1989).

In a later study in patients with CMV retinitis, intermittent intravenous administration appeared to be effective and relatively nontoxic. Ten patients with AIDS and newly diagnosed CMV retinitis were given 60 mg/kg as a two-hour infusion every eight hours for 14 days. At the end of the induction period, the retinitis stabilized or improved in 9 of the patients; 8 who had CMV in urine or blood upon entry into the study had negative urine and blood cultures. In 6 of 7 patients given maintenance therapy (60 mg/kg as a single daily infusion five days/week), retinal lesions increased in size after 2 to 32 weeks (Jacobson et al, 1989).

In a randomized, controlled trial of foscarnet in the treatment of CMV retinitis, 24 previously untreated AIDS patients at low risk for loss of visual acuity were randomly assigned to receive either no treatment (delayed treatment, control group) or immediate induction therapy with foscarnet (60 mg/kg three times per day for three weeks), followed by a maintenance regimen (90 mg/kg once daily). The mean time to progression of retinitis was 3.2 weeks in the control group (n=11) compared with 13.3 weeks in the treatment group (n=13). Nine patients in the latter group had positive blood cultures for CMV at entry and all showed clearing of the virus from blood by the end of the induction period versus 1 of 6 patients in the control group. There was no reduction in HIV p24 antigen levels in the control group compared with a 50% reduction in the treated group (Palestine et al, 1991).

Foscarnet therapy also appears to be effective in ganciclovir-resistant CMV retinitis in AIDS patients. In one trial, 170 AIDS patients with CMV retinitis who either could not tolerate or became resistant to ganciclovir received foscarnet induction therapy (60 mg/kg intravenously every eight hours for 14 days) and were then randomized to receive 60, 90, or 120 mg/kg/day for maintenance. The median times to progression of retinitis in the three groups were 9, 9, and 15 weeks, respectively. The length of remission correlated with increased doses of the drug without any obvious increase in toxicity (Jacobson et al, 1991 A).

Foscarnet and zidovudine have a synergistic effect against HIV in vitro and may have an additive effect against the virus in AIDS patients (Eriksson and Schinazi, 1989; Jacobson et al, 1991 B). In a multicenter, randomized, nonblinded clinical trial designed to compare foscarnet with ganciclovir in AIDS patients with CMV retinitis, no significant difference in the rate of progression of retinitis was observed in the two treatment groups. The median time to disease progression was 59 days in the foscarnet group versus 56 days in the ganciclovir group, and there was no significant difference in visual acuity scores. However, the mortality rate was 79% higher among the patients given ganciclovir and the investigators felt that this could not be associated with any identifiable subgroup of patients. The median survival time for those in the ganciclovir group was 8.5 months, while in the foscarnet group it was 12.6 months (Studies of Ocular Complications of AIDS Research Group and the AIDS Clinical Trials Group, 1992). These results are viewed by some authorities as preliminary and controversial for the following reasons: (1) the foscarnet recipients were able to tolerate substantially more zidovudine than were the ganciclovir recipients; (2) among those who received neither zidovudine nor other antiretroviral therapy, there was little difference in mortality between foscarnet and ganciclovir recipients; (3) significantly greater numbers of foscarnet-treated patients had to be switched to ganciclovir because of adverse effects than the reverse (Hirsch, 1992). In addition, the longer survival of the foscarnet recipients was noted in only one group; ganciclovir recipients with decreased creatinine clearance survived longer.

Although the number of patients involved in trials on the use of foscarnet in the treatment of resistant herpesvirus and varicella-zoster infections has been small, the results have been encouraging. For example, in a randomized trial that compared foscarnet with vidarabine in 14 AIDS patients with mucocutaneous herpetic lesions unresponsive to acyclovir, the lesions in all eight patients receiving foscarnet healed completely within 10 to 24 days. The time to complete healing, to 50% reduction in the size of the lesions, and to the end of viral shedding, as well as the pain score, were significantly reduced in the patients given foscarnet. However, after foscarnet was discontinued, the infection recurred in every patient within a median of 42.5 days (Safrin et al, 1991 A).

In an uncontrolled cohort study of foscarnet therapy in five AIDS patients with varicella-zoster virus (VZV) infection resistant to acyclovir, therapy for 14 to 25 days (median, 21 days) resulted in complete healing with cessation of viral shedding in three patients and nearly complete healing in one patient in whom serial cultures were not performed. Relapse of VZV infection at the original lesion site occurred in two patients 7 to 14 days after discontinuing foscarnet treatment; isolates from both patients were sensitive to acyclovir in vitro. VZV isolates resistant to foscarnet were obtained in one patient who experienced complete healing (Safrin et al, 1991 B). Although foscarnet is a potentially effective antiviral agent for patients with acyclovir-resistant herpesvirus infections, the optimal dosage and duration of therapy require further study.

The efficacy or safety of foscarnet in the treatment of other CMV infections (eg, pneumonitis, gastroenteritis, colitis, esophagitis, congenital or neonatal disease) or its use in nonimmunocompromised patients has not been established.

ADVERSE REACTIONS AND PRECAUTIONS. The most frequent adverse reactions reported in clinical trials were fever (65%), nausea (47%), diarrhea (30%), abnormal renal function (27%), vomiting (26%), headache (26%), and seizures (10%). Anemia (33%) and granulocytopenia (17%) have been observed in patients receiving foscarnet. Anemia usually has been corrected with transfusions. Discontinuation of foscarnet has been required in only 1% of patients developing anemia or neutropenia. Hypomagnesemia, hypophosphatemia, hyperphosphatemia, hypocalcemia, hypokalemia, polydipsia, polyuria, and nephrogenic diabetes insipidus also have developed. Hypertension has been reported, but probably was due to fluid overload. The most serious reactions were death (14%), abnormal renal function (14%), bone marrow suppression (10%), severe anemia (9%), and seizures (7%). The complications of renal impairment, electrolyte abnormalities, and seizures may have contributed to patient deaths.

Nephrotoxicity manifested by increased serum creatinine concentrations ≥2.0 mg/dL) in patients with previously normal renal function usually is reversible. Since renal impairment may occur at any time during therapy with foscarnet, renal function should be monitored closely and the dose adjusted if decreased or altered renal function is observed. The severity and incidence of nephrotoxicity are less with intermittent than with continuous intravenous administration. Maintenance of adequate hydration can decrease the extent of renal damage caused by foscarnet.

A transient, dose-related decrease in ionized serum calcium concentration is associated with foscarnet therapy; it may be due to chelation of divalent metal cations, such as calcium. Physicians should be prepared to treat patients who complain of symptoms associated with low ionized calcium (perioral tingling, numbness in the extremities, paresthesias), as well as more severe manifestations, such as tetany and seizures. Since the rate of infusion may affect the decrease in ionized calcium, slowing the rate may prevent or lessen symptoms. The risk of cardiac disturbances and seizures may be increased with changes in levels of calcium and other electrolytes. The drug should be used cautiously in patients who have altered calcium or other electrolyte levels prior to therapy, in those with neurologic or cardiac abnormalities, and in those receiving other drugs known to influence electrolytes and minerals. If factors predisposing a patient to seizures are present, electrolyte levels must be monitored carefully.

Asymptomatic hyperphosphatemia may be common due to the effect of foscarnet on renal elimination of phosphate or to the replacement of phosphate in the bone matrix by foscarnet.

Foscarnet has been reported to cause painful ulceration of the oral mucosa and penis. The latter appears to be due to high concentrations of unchanged drug in the subpreputial space.

Foscarnet solutions should be infused only into veins with an adequate blood flow to permit rapid dilution and distribution and to avoid local irritation. The rate of infusion must not exceed 1 mg/kg/min and should be controlled by use of an infusion pump.

There are no adequate well-controlled studies in pregnant women; foscarnet should be used during pregnancy only if clearly indicated (FDA Pregnancy Category C). Although it is not known whether foscarnet is secreted in human milk, many drugs are and caution should be exercised if the drug is administered to a nursing woman.

The safety and efficacy of this drug in children have not been evaluated. It should be administered to children only if the potential benefits outweigh the risks. There have been no studies on the safety and efficacy of foscarnet in patients over 65 years.

OVERDOSAGE. Overdosage has been reported in 10 patients, and all experienced seizures, impairment of renal function, paresthesias, and electrolyte disturbances. All but one patient recovered completely. That patient died after experiencing a grand mal seizure after receiving a total daily dose of 12.5 g for three days rather than the intended 10.9 g; the cause of death was listed as respiratory/cardiac arrest. The other nine patients received an average of four times their recommended doses.

There is no specific antidote for foscarnet overdose. Hemodialysis and hydration may reduce drug plasma levels; however, this has not been evaluated clinically.

DRUG INTERACTIONS. Drugs that inhibit renal tubular secretion may impair the elimination of foscarnet. Its use with potentially nephrotoxic drugs, such as aminoglycosides, amphotericin B, and intravenous pentamidine, should be avoided. Particular caution should be exercised when foscarnet is given with other drugs known to affect serum calcium levels.

Four patients who received foscarnet and intravenous pentamidine developed hypocalcemia; one patient died. No interaction between aerosolized pentamidine and foscarnet has been reported.

In one clinical study, concomitant use of foscarnet and zidovudine appeared to have an additive effect and cause anemia, but there was no evidence of increased myelosuppression. In a more recent study, the concurrent use of these two drugs appeared to have an additive neutropenic effect (Palestine et al, 1991).

PHARMACOKINETICS. Only 12% to 22% of an orally administered dose is absorbed, and serum concentrations are too low to inhibit either CMV or HIV. From 14% to 17% of the drug is bound to plasma protein at plasma-drug concentrations of 1 to 1,000 μM. Intermittent administration of foscarnet as a two-hour intravenous infusion (60 mg/kg every eight hours) has produced peak and trough serum drug concentrations on the 14th day of sampling of approximately 520 and 100 μM, respectively. Mean plasma clearance ranged from 130 to 178 ml/min when the drug was given by intermittent infusion. When determined on days 1 or 3 of therapy, the plasma half-life of foscarnet is about three hours. The terminal half-life is 18 to 42 hours.

In animal studies, approximately 40% of an intravenous dose is deposited in the bone of young animals and 7% appears in the bone of adults. Foscarnet accumulates in the bone in humans, but the extent is unknown. The mean volume of distribution of foscarnet at steady state is 0.3 to 0.6 L/kg. Although the drug distributes rapidly into the cerebrospinal fluid, there is variable penetration; this may be caused by disease-related defects in the blood-brain barrier. The main route of excretion is the kidney. There are no known metabolites, and the renal clearance is about 80% of the plasma clearance.

DOSAGE AND PREPARATIONS.

Intravenous: *Induction therapy for adults with normal renal function,* 60 mg/kg given at a constant rate over a minimum of one hour every eight hours for two to three weeks depending on clinical response. Adequate hydration is recommended to establish diuresis both prior to and during treatment. *Maintenance therapy for adults with normal renal function,* 90 to 120 mg/kg/day given as an infusion over two hours; because higher plasma concentrations may be associated with increased toxicity, most patients should be given the 90 mg/kg/day regimen initially. *All doses must be individualized on the basis of the patient's renal function* (see following table). If creatinine clearance falls below the limits of the dosing nomograms (0.4 ml/min/kg), foscarnet should be discontinued until renal function improves.

Foscarnet Dosing Guide for Induction

CrCl (ml/min/kg)	Dose every 8 hours (equivalent to 60 mg/kg)
≥1.6	60
1.5	57
1.4	53
1.3	49
1.2	46
1.1	42
1.0	39
0.9	35
0.8	32
0.7	28
0.6	25
0.5	21
0.4	18

Foscarnet Dosing Guide for Maintenance

CrCl (ml/min/kg)	Dose every 24 hours (equivalent to 90 mg/kg)	Dose every 24 hours (equivalent to 120 mg/kg)
≥1.4	90	120
1.2-1.4	78	104
1.0-1.2	75	100
0.8-1.0	71	94
0.6-0.8	63	84
0.4-0.6	57	76

To use the foregoing dosing guide, actual 24-hour creatinine clearance (ml/min) must be divided by body weight (kg) or *the estimated creatinine clearance in ml/min/kg can be calculated from serum creatinine (mg/dL) using the following formula* (modified Cockcroft and Gault equation):

$$\text{For Males: } \frac{140 - \text{age}}{\text{Serum creatinine} \times 72} \text{ (x 0.85 for females)}$$

Foscavir (Astra). Solution (for intravenous infusion) 24 mg/ml in 250 and 500 ml containers.

Cited References

Eriksson BFH, Schinazi RF: Combinations of 3′-azido-3′-deoxythymidine (zidovudine) and phosphonoformate (foscarnet) against human immunodeficiency virus type 1 and cytomegalovirus replication in vitro. *Antimicrob Agents Chemother* 33:663-669, 1989.

Hirsch MS: The treatment of cytomegalovirus in AIDS: More than meets the eye. *N Engl J Med* 326:264-266, 1992.

Jacobson MA, et al: Foscarnet treatment of cytomegalovirus retinitis in patients with the acquired immunodeficiency syndrome. *Antimicrob Agents Chemother* 33:736-741, 1989.

Jacobson MA, et al: Phase 2 dose-ranging study of foscarnet (PFA) salvage therapy for CMV retinitis in patients intolerant of or resistant to ganciclovir. Presented at the 31st Interscience Conference on Antimicrobial Agents and Chemotherapy, Chicago, 1991 A, abstract 296.

Jacobson MA, et al: In vivo additive antiretroviral effect of combined zidovudine and foscarnet therapy for human immunodeficiency virus infection (ACTG Protocol 053). *J Infect Dis* 163:1219-1222, 1991 B.

LeHoang P, et al: Foscarnet in the treatment of cytomegalovirus retinitis in acquired immune deficiency syndrome. *Ophthalmology* 96:865-873, 1989.

Palestine AG, et al: A randomized, controlled trial of foscarnet in the treatment of cytomegalovirus retinitis in patients with AIDS. *Ann Intern Med* 115:665-673, 1991.

Safrin S, et al: A controlled trial comparing foscarnet with vidarabine for acyclovir-resistant mucocutaneous herpes simplex in the acquired immunodeficiency syndrome. *N Engl J Med* 325:551-555, 1991 A.

Safrin S, et al: Foscarnet therapy in five patients with AIDS and acyclovir-resistant varicella-zoster virus infection. *Ann Intern Med* 115:19-21, 1991 B.

Studies of Ocular Complications of AIDS Research Group, in Collaboration with the AIDS Clinical Trials Group: Mortality in patients with the acquired immunodeficiency syndrome treated with either foscarnet or ganciclovir for cytomegalovirus retinitis. *N Engl J Med* 326:213-220, 1992.

New Evaluation 80

INTERFERON ALFA-2b
[Intron A]

Interferon alfa-2b (IFNα-2b) is a recombinant molecule that is obtained from the fermentation products of an *Escherichia coli* strain bearing a genetically engineered plasmid containing an IFNα-2b gene from human leukocytes. The specific activity of recombinant IFNα-2b is about 2×10^8 international units (IU) per milligram of protein. This agent can be administered intramuscularly, subcutaneously, or intralesionally.

ACTIONS. Interferons (IFNs) exert their cellular effects by binding to specific receptors on cell membranes. Human IFN receptors have been demonstrated on human lymphoblastoid cells and appear to be highly asymmetric membrane proteins. These receptors show selectivity for human, but not murine IFNs, thus suggesting species specificity. Results of studies on other IFNs have shown varying degrees of species specificity.

Once bound to cell membrane receptors, IFNs initiate a complex series of events that includes induction of certain enzymes (see the introduction to this chapter). The responses that result include inhibition of virus replication, suppression of cell growth, and immunomodulating activities such as enhanced cytocidal activity of lymphocytes for target cells and increased phagocytic activity of macrophages (see also index entry interferons, Actions). Any or all of these activities may contribute to the therapeutic effects of IFNs in vivo.

USES. Interferon α-2b is indicated for the treatment of selected cases of condyloma acuminatum involving external surfaces of the genital and perianal areas. However, other therapies often are preferred (see index entry Condyloma Acuminatum). Interferon α-2b also is used for chronic non-A, non-B (type C) hepatitis in patients 18 years or older with compensated liver disease who have a history of blood or blood product exposure and/or are antibody-positive for hepatitis C virus (HCV). For other uses of this agent, see index entry interferon Alfa-2b.

Condyloma Acuminatum: Genital warts are sexually transmitted and commonly occur on the anus, penis, perineum, urethra, vulva, vagina, and cervix. Their incidence is increasing in the United States; about three million new and recurrent cases occur each year. Human papilloma virus (HPV) is the etiologic agent and may be present, occasionally with dysplastic changes, in areas where there are no detectable warts. HPV types 6 and 11 are most prevalent in genital warts, while types 16, 18, 31, and other higher types have been associated with genital malignancies, especially carcinoma of the cervix. Spontaneous resolution may occur during the first year of infection, but the rate of recurrence is high with all methods of treatment for genital warts. Use of a condom is recommended during treatment and follow-up; sexual partners with clinically apparent HPV infection also should be treated.

Results of a randomized, double-blind, placebo-controlled, multicenter trial of natural (leukocyte) INF-α demonstrated that this agent is effective intralesionally in the treatment of condyloma acuminatum. Eighty-six patients received IFN-α and 72 were given placebo. Warts were completely eliminated in 62% of the patients treated with IFN-α and in 21% of the placebo-treated patients; however, relapse occurred in 25% of the patients successfully treated with INF-α (Friedman-Kien et al, 1988).

The efficacy and toxicity of intralesionally administered recombinant (α-2b), lymphoblastoid, and human fibroblast (beta) interferons in the treatment of patients with condyloma acuminatum refractory to conventional therapy were assessed in a randomized, placebo-controlled, double-blind, multicenter trial. Forty-seven percent of the warts injected with IFNα-2b resolved completely compared with 22% of placebo-treated warts. No differences in response rates were reported among the groups receiving interferon. About one-third of successfully treated warts recurred within four months. Intralesional administration appeared to be nontoxic and was well tolerated (Reichman et al, 1988).

A three-week course of intralesional IFNα-2b (1.5 million IU/lesion/week) has been employed investigationally in combination with podophyllin for the treatment of anogenital warts. Patients receiving the combination had a significantly greater decrease in wart site volume from baseline compared with monotherapy recipients (63% versus 29% at week 11). In addition, there was complete clearance of treated warts in 67% of recipients of the combination therapy versus 42% of those who received monotherapy. Approximately 65% of the patients in each group experienced recurrences, and the median time to recurrence was not significantly longer for patients receiving the combination (40 versus 31 days). Clearance rates were higher in women, in patients with warts of less than 12 months' duration, and in those who were HIV seronegative (Douglas et al, 1990). Additional trials are needed before a final assessment of combination therapy can be made.

Chronic Hepatitis Non-A, Non-B (Type C): Recent studies indicate that IFNα-2b has clinically significant effects on this disease. In a preliminary study, ten patients with chronic non-A, non-B hepatitis were treated with IFNα-2b in varying doses (0.5 to 5 million IU) daily, on alternate days, or three times weekly for up to 12 months. In eight of ten patients, elevated serum alanine aminotransferase (ALT) concentrations decreased rapidly during therapy and eventually fell into the normal range. The improvement in ALT levels was sustained during prolonged therapy and was further sustained in six of the ten patients after therapy was discontinued (Hoofnagle et al, 1986).

More recent studies have confirmed and extended the results of this preliminary report. In a multicenter, randomized, controlled trial, 166 patients with chronic hepatitis C received 1 or 3 million IU of IFNα-2b three times weekly for 24 weeks or received no treatment. The probability of normalization or near normalization of serum ALT concentrations after six months was 46% in patients treated with the higher dose (85% of whom had complete normalization), 28% in those treated with the lower dose, and only 8% in untreated patients. Hepatic histology improved in patients who received the higher dose, as reflected by regression of lobular and periportal inflammation. However, relapse after the cessation of therapy occurred within six months in 51% of the patients treated with the higher dose and in 44% of those treated with the lower dose (Davis et al, 1989).

A randomized, double-blind, placebo-controlled trial studied the effects IFNα-2b in patients with well-documented chronic non-A, non-B hepatitis. IFNα-2b (2 million IU) was administered subcutaneously three times weekly to 21 patients for six months; 20 patients were given placebo. Mean serum ALT concentrations and histologic features of the liver improved significantly in the IFN-treated patients but not in those given placebo. However, after termination of treatment, serum ALT concentrations often returned to pretreatment levels, and 6 to 12 months later only 10% of the responding patients still had normal ALT levels (Di Bisceglie et al, 1989).

ADVERSE REACTIONS AND PRECAUTIONS. Adverse reactions are dose dependent. The most frequently reported reactions are "flu-like" symptoms that occur within the first two weeks of treatment. These include fever (incidence, up to 56%), headache (up to 47%), myalgia (up to 44%), and chills (45%). Less common adverse effects include fatigue (approximately 25%), depression, confusion, nausea, diarrhea, and alopecia. Pruritus, transient reversible cardiomyopathy, sweating, and irritability also have been observed. The induction of autoimmune thyroid disease has been noted in some patients. Abnormal laboratory test values that have been reported include reduced hemoglobin concentrations and leukocyte, granulocyte, and platelet counts.

Moderate to severe adverse reactions may require modification of dosage or termination of therapy. IFNα-2b should be used cautiously in patients with a history of severe cardiovascular or pulmonary disease, diabetes mellitus prone to ketoacidosis, coagulation disorders, or severe myelosuppression. Patients with a history of psychiatric disorders should not be treated with IFNs, and therapy should be discontinued in any patient who develops severe depression during treatment. IFNs should not be used in persons with a pre-existing thyroid abnormality if thyroid function cannot be maintained in the normal range by medication; therapy should be discontinued in those who develop thyroid abnormalities that are unresponsive to medication.

Prior to use of IFNα-2b for the treatment of chronic non-A, non-B (type C) hepatitis, a liver biopsy should be performed to confirm the diagnosis and document the severity of hepatic inflammation; patients also should be tested for the presence of anti-HCV antibodies. IFNα-2b therapy currently is not recommended for individuals with decompensated liver disease or for immunocompromised transplant recipients. Those with autoimmune hepatitis or a history of autoimmune disease should not receive this agent. Complete blood count and platelet baseline levels should be established before therapy begins, and these measurements should be repeated one and two weeks after therapy is initiated and monthly thereafter in order to monitor potential toxicity. To assess response to treatment, ALT concentrations should be evaluated after 2, 16, and 24 weeks of therapy.

The safety and efficacy of IFNα-2b have not been assessed in patients under 18 years. IFNα-2b has affected the menstrual cycle and decreased serum estradiol and progesterone levels in human females; studies in nonhuman primates have shown menstrual cycle abnormalities. At high doses, IFNα-2b has abortifacient effects in rhesus monkeys; it should be used during pregnancy only if the potential benefit outweighs the potential risk to the fetus (FDA Pregnancy Category C).

Serum neutralizing antibodies have been detected in 0.3% to 15% of treated patients, but their clinical significance is unknown.

DRUG INTERACTIONS. There may be a synergistic adverse interaction between interferon and zidovudine. Patients who have received both drugs have experienced a higher incidence of neutropenia than when zidovudine is given alone. Interferon inhibits the activity of hepatic cytochrome p 450 function and, therefore, may cause other drug interactions.

PHARMACOKINETICS. Studies have been conducted in healthy male volunteers who received single doses of 5 million IU/M^2 of IFNα-2b given intramuscularly, subcutaneously, and as a 30-minute intravenous infusion. Mean serum concentrations following intramuscular and subcutaneous injections were comparable; the maximum concentration (18 to 116 IU/ml) occurred 3 to 12 hours after administration and fell below the detectable limit (10 IU/ml) by 16 hours. Elimination half-lives with these routes were two to three hours.

With intravenous infusion, serum concentrations peaked (135 to 273 IU/ml) by the end of the infusion and were not detectable four hours later. The elimination half-life was approximately two hours. IFNα-2b was not detectable in the urine.

DOSAGE AND PREPARATIONS. The 10 million IU-preparation is used for condyloma accuminatum and the 3-million IU preparation for chronic non-A, non-B hepatitis.

Intralesional: For condyloma acuminatum in *adults over 18 years,* 1 million IU injected into each lesion three times weekly on alternate days for three weeks. The injection should be directed at the center of the base of the wart and at an angle nearly parallel to that of the skin. As many as five lesions can be treated at one time. The maximum response occurs four to eight weeks after initial treatment; however, the optimum dose and duration of therapy have not been established. A second course may be given to patients who do not respond or respond poorly after 12 to 16 weeks. Patients with 6 to 10 warts also may receive a second course of treatment and those with more than 10 warts may receive additional courses.

Subcutaneous, intramuscular: For chronic non-A, non-B (type C) hepatitis, *adults over 18 years,* 3 million IU three times weekly. The optimum dose and duration of therapy have not been established. The manufacturer recommends six months of treatment. Consideration may be given to discontinuing therapy in patients whose ALT levels do not decrease after 16 weeks of therapy.

Intron A (Schering). Powder 3 and 10 million IU in 1 ml containers. Reconstitute with diluent (bacteriostatic water). Preparations should be stored between 2° and 8° C both before and after reconstitution.

Cited References

Davis GL, et al: Treatment of chronic hepatitis C with recombinant interferon alfa: A multicenter randomized, controlled trial. *N Engl J Med* 321:1501-1506, 1989.

Di Bisceglie AM, et al: Recombinant interferon alfa therapy for chronic hepatitis C: A randomized, double-blind, placebo-controlled trial. *N Engl J Med* 321:1506-1510, 1989.

Douglas JM Jr, et al: A randomized trial of combination therapy with intralesional interferon α_{2b} and podophyllin versus podophyllin alone for the therapy of anogenital warts. *J Infect Dis* 162:52-59, 1990.

Friedman-Kien AE, et al: Natural interferon alfa for treatment of condylomata acuminata. *JAMA* 259:533-538, 1988.

Hoofnagle JH, et al: Treatment of chronic non-A, non-B hepatitis with recombinant human alpha interferon: A preliminary report. *N Engl J Med* 315:1575-1578, 1986.

Reichman RC, et al: Treatment of condyloma acuminatum with three different interferons administered intralesionally: A double-blind, placebo-controlled trial. *Ann Intern Med* 108:675-679, 1988.

THIS EVALUATION WAS PREPARED AFTER COMPLETION OF THIS CHAPTER

New Evaluation 80

RIMANTADINE HYDROCHLORIDE
[Flumadine]

CH_3
$CHNH_2$
H_2C CH_2 • HCl
CH_2

ACTIONS. Rimantadine, the α-methyl derivative of amantadine, has a spectrum of antiviral activity and mechanism of action similar to those of the parent drug. In vitro, it appears to be a more potent inhibitor of influenza A viruses than amantadine; however, both drugs are apparently equally effective clinically. Rimantadine inhibits the in vitro replication of influenza A isolates from all three human subtypes (H1N1, H2N2, and H3N2). It has no significant activity against influenza B or other respiratory viruses at pharmacologic concentrations and does not appear to interfere with the immunogenicity of inactivated influenza vaccines. Treated patients can develop drug-resistant strains that may be transmitted and cause typical influenza disease.

Rimantadine and amantadine appear to exert their inhibitory effect at two points in the viral replicative cycle through their activity as ion channel blockers. Susceptibility to these drugs is determined principally by the viral M2 protein, which is present on the surface of infected cells as well as in the virion. This protein forms ion channels through which H+ protons pass across the membranes of intracellular endocytic and exocytic vesicles. Early in the cycle, during virus uncoating, the protons are transferred from the endocytic vesicle to the virion, causing a fall in pH that is necessary to release replication-competent viral RNA into the cell cytoplasm. Later in the cycle, during virus assembly, the protons are transferred out of the exocytic vesicle, thus maintaining the pH above the level at which the viral hemagglutinin would lose its structural integrity and fail to be incorporated into the viral envelope. Thus, both rimantadine and amantadine block the M2-mediated transfer of protons and thereby inhibit viral uncoating, viral assembly, or both depending on the virus strain (also see the Introduction to this chapter). These observations are supported by results of studies on resistant viruses.

Complete cross-resistance between amantadine and rimantadine has been reported frequently, and the genetic basis for resistance is identical for the two drugs, ie, a single amino acid change in one of five amino acid residues in the transmembrane portion of the M2 protein results in high-level resistance to both drugs.

USES. Rimantadine is indicated for the prophylaxis and treatment of influenza type A in adults and for the prophylaxis of these infections in children over 1 year; prophylactic studies have not been performed in children less than 1 year. The drug's efficacy in the treatment of symptomatic influenza in children has been inconsistent; viral shedding, which may include resistant variants, may be prolonged in treated children.

Rimantadine was safe and effective in preventing the signs and symptoms of infection caused by influenza A viruses in controlled studies in children over 1 year, adults, and elderly patients. When administered prior to and throughout an epidemic period, both rimantadine and amantadine were 70% to 90% effective in preventing illness due to influenza type A. However, immunization with influenza vaccine prior to the influenza season is preferred for prophylaxis unless the vaccine is contraindicated. Rimantadine does not prevent the development of an immune response to influenza and, therefore, individuals taking the drug may have some immune protection against a subsequent exposure to the same virus strain. Since rimantadine does not interfere with the antibody response to influenza vaccine, it may be given with the vaccine to provide interim protection until a protective level of antibodies is reached or to augment the prophylactic effect in a previously vaccinated individual.

Treatment with rimantadine should be considered for adults who develop an influenza-like disease during a known or suspected outbreak of influenza A in a community. Its administration within 48 hours of the onset of signs and symptoms has reduced the duration of fever and other symptoms. This drug's efficacy in the prevention of complications or in the treatment of severe influenza (eg, pneumonia) is uncertain.

ADVERSE REACTIONS. The most frequently reported adverse events with rimantadine at the recommended dose (200 mg/day) involve the central nervous and gastrointestinal systems; these include insomnia, dizziness, headache, nervousness, and fatigue (incidence, 1% to 2.1%) and nausea, vomiting, anorexia, dry mouth, and abdominal pain (1.4% to 2.8%). Their incidence increases significantly when doses exceed 200 mg/day. Less frequently reported adverse events (0.3% to 1%) at recommended doses include diarrhea, dyspepsia, impairment of concentration, ataxia, somnolence, agitation, depression, rash, tinnitus, and dyspnea. Adverse events reported rarely (<0.3%) include gait abnormality, euphoria, hyperkinesia, tremor, hallucinations, confusion, convulsions, bronchospasm, cough, pallor, palpitation, hypertension, cerebrovascular disorder, cardiac failure, pedal edema, heart block, tachycardia, syncope, nonpuerperal lactation, taste loss or change, and parosmia. Adverse reactions resolve rapidly after the drug is discontinued.

Results of clinical studies comparing rimantadine and amantadine show that the frequencies of central and peripheral nervous system adverse reactions are significantly lower with rimantadine.

In clinical trials, the incidence of adverse reactions after conventional doses was higher in the elderly than in younger adults and children. In controlled studies on prophylactic use, the incidence of adverse reactions at the recommended dose in persons over 65 years compared with controls was, for central and peripheral nervous systems, 12.5% versus 8.7%, and for the gastrointestinal system, 17% versus 11.3%. Consequently, many authorities recommend that a reduced dose (100 mg/day) be used in elderly patients.

PRECAUTIONS. Rimantadine is contraindicated in patients with a known hypersensitivity to drugs of the adamantane class.

As with amantadine, in clinical trials, seizure-like activity was observed in a small number of patients with a history of seizures who were not receiving antiepileptic therapy. Thus, rimantadine should be used with caution in patients with a prior history of seizures and discontinued if seizures develop.

Patients with renal or severe hepatic insufficiency should be treated cautiously because of the potential for the accumulation of rimantadine and its metabolites in plasma (see the section on Pharmacokinetics).

Strains of influenza virus that are resistant to rimantadine can emerge during treatment and can be transmitted to susceptible persons and cause typical influenza disease. Results of several studies have demonstrated that 10% to 30% of patients with initially sensitive virus may shed resistant virus after treatment with rimantadine. Although the response to rimantadine is slower in patients who subsequently shed resistant virus, no data on humans are available regarding the effectiveness of the drug in those who are initially infected with resistant virus. However, both amantadine and rimantadine have been found to be ineffective in experimental animals infected with resistant strains.

PREGNANCY AND LACTATION. Rimantadine is classified in FDA Pregnancy Category C. This drug crosses the placenta in mice, and a dose 11 times higher than the recommended human dose was embryotoxic (increased fetal resorption) in rats. No embryotoxic effects were observed in rabbits given a dose five times the recommended human dose. Maternal toxicity was observed in pregnant rats who received doses exceeding the recommended human dose by 1.7 to 6.8 times peri- and postnatally; at the highest dose, there was an increase in pup mortality during the first two to four days postpartum. Decreased fertility of the F_1 generation was observed at the two highest doses.

Because of the adverse reactions observed in offspring of rats given rimantadine during the nursing period, it is recommended that the drug not be given to nursing mothers. In rats, rimantadine concentrated in breast milk in a dose-related manner; two to three hours after administration, the levels in milk were about twice those observed in serum.

OVERDOSAGE. There is no known specific antidote for rimantadine overdosage; supportive therapy should be administered as indicated. Overdoses of the parent drug, amantadine, have caused agitation, hallucinations, arrhythmias, and death; the intravenous administration of physostigmine, 1 to 2 mg in adults and 0.5 mg in children, repeated as needed (maximum, 2 mg/hour), was reported anecdotally to be beneficial in patients with CNS effects due to amantadine overdoses.

DRUG INTERACTIONS. When a single 100-mg dose of rimantadine was given to normal healthy adults one hour after the initiation of cimetidine therapy (300 mg four times daily), total rimantadine clearance was reduced by 18%.

Concomitant administration of acetaminophen or aspirin (650 mg four times daily) has been reported to reduce the peak plasma concentration and the area under the curve (AUC) of rimantadine by approximately 10%.

PHARMACOKINETICS. The tablet and syrup formulations of rimantadine are equally and well absorbed after oral administration. In clinical studies, the mean peak plasma concentration after a single 100-mg dose was 74 ± 22 ng/ml (range, 45 to 138 ng/ml) and the time to peak concentration was 6 ± 1 hours in 20- to 44-year-old adults. In this group, the single-dose elimination half-life was 25.4 ± 6.3 hours (range, 13 to 65 hours). In a group of healthy adults aged 71 to 79 years, the single-dose elimination half-life was 32 ± 16 hours (range, 20 to 65 hours).

After the administration of rimantadine 100 mg twice daily for 10 days to healthy adults 18 to 70 years, the AUC values were about 30% higher than predicted from single-dose studies. At steady state, plasma trough levels ranged from 118 to 468 ng/ml. In a comparative study on three groups of healthy older adults (50 to 60, 61 to 70, and 71 to 79 years), subjects in the oldest group had average AUC values, peak plasma concentrations, and elimination half-life values at steady state that were 20% to 30% higher than in the other two groups. In nursing home patients (68 to 102 years), steady-state concentrations were two- to fourfold higher than those observed in healthy younger adults taking comparable doses (ie, 200 mg/day).

The pharmacokinetics of rimantadine in children is not well defined. However, in one study on 10 children 4 to 8 years who were given a single dose of rimantadine syrup (6.6 mg/kg), plasma concentrations ranged from 446 to 988 ng/ml at 5 to 6 hours and from 170 to 424 ng/ml at 24 hours. In some of these children, the drug was detectable in the plasma 72 hours after the last dose.

Rimantadine is extensively metabolized in the liver following oral administration, and less than 25% of the dose is excreted unchanged in the urine. Three hydroxylated metabolites of the drug appear in the plasma. These, an additional conjugated metabolite, and parent drug account for approximately 75% of a single 200-mg dose excreted in the urine over 72 hours.

The pharmacokinetics of rimantadine were not appreciably changed in patients with chronic liver disease, the majority of whom had stabilized cirrhosis, compared with healthy subjects who were sex, age, and weight matched. However, after administration of a single 200-mg dose to patients with severe hepatic dysfunction, the AUC was reported to be threefold larger, the elimination half-life about twofold longer, and the apparent clearance approximately 50% lower compared with historic data from healthy subjects.

Following the administration of a single 200-mg dose of rimantadine to eight patients with a creatinine clearance (CL_{cr}) of 31 to 50 ml/min and six patients with a CL_{cr} of 11 to 30 ml/min, the apparent clearance was 37% and 16% lower, respectively, and plasma metabolite concentrations were higher compared with matched healthy subjects (CL_{cr}, >50 ml/min). In a study on eight hemodialysis patients (CL_{cr}, 0 to 10 ml/min) who received a single 200-mg dose of rimantadine, there was a 1.6-fold increase in the elimination half-life and a 40% decrease in apparent clearance compared with age-matched healthy controls.

In vitro, the human plasma protein binding of rimantadine is approximately 40% greater than typical plasma concentrations. Albumin is the major binding protein. No pharmacokinetic data exist that establish a correlation between plasma concentration of rimantadine and its antiviral effect.

DOSAGE AND PREPARATIONS.

Oral: *Adults*, for prophylaxis and treatment, 100 mg twice daily or 200 mg once daily. For patients with severe hepatic dysfunction or renal failure (CL_{cr}, ≤10 ml/min) and elderly nursing home patients, 100 mg/day. For treatment, therapy preferably should be initiated within 48 hours after the onset of signs and symptoms of influenza infection and should continue for approximately five days.

For prophylaxis in *children 1 to 10 years*, 5 mg/kg (maximum, 150 mg) once daily; *over 10 years*, the adult dose is used.

Flumadine (Forest). Tablets 100 mg; syrup 50 mg/5 ml.

New Evaluation 80

ZALCITABINE (ddC)
[Hivid]

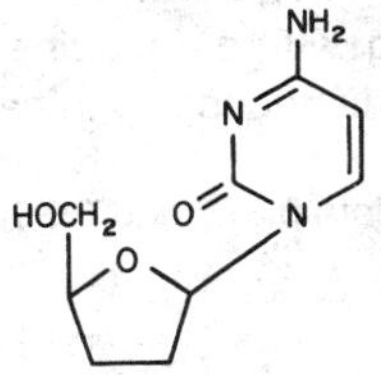

ACTIONS. Zalcitabine (2′,3′-dideoxycytidine) is a synthetic analogue of the naturally occurring nucleoside, 2′-deoxycytidine. Within cells, zalcitabine is converted by cellular enzymes into dideoxycytidine 5′-triphosphate (ddCTP), which serves as an alternative substrate for the reverse transcriptase of human immunodeficiency virus (HIV), thereby halting viral DNA synthesis and resulting in cessation of viral replication (Mitsuya and Broder, 1986). ddCTP also inhibits mitochondrial DNA polymerase, a polymerase involved in DNA repair, and, to a lesser degree, cellular DNA polymerase. The half-life of ddCTP in established cell lines and in human peripheral blood mononuclear cells in culture ranges from 2.6 to 10 hours.

USES. Zalcitabine is used with zidovudine to treat adults with advanced AIDS (CD4 cell count ≤300 cells/mm^3) who have symptoms of significant clinical and immunologic deterioration (Lipsky, 1993).

In a Phase I study, administration of zalcitabine 0.03 to 0.09 mg/kg every four hours produced transient immunologic improvement in 20 patients with AIDS or AIDS-related complex (ARC) (Yarchoan et al, 1988). Circulating serum p24 antigen levels were reduced. However, patients often developed a severe, painful peripheral neuropathy. In addition, a syndrome of maculovesicular cutaneous eruptions, aphthous ulcers, fever, and malaise developed in many patients after four to six weeks of therapy, but the symptoms often subsided with continued treatment. In one study on 15 patients, toxicity was reduced at a dosage of 0.005 mg/kg every four hours (Merigan et al, 1989). Although an antiviral effect was still observable at the lower dosage, p24 antigen levels were suppressed less frequently and onset of therapeutic action was slower. Patients with ARC appeared to be more responsive to the p24 antigen suppressive action of zalcitabine and appeared to experience greater enhancement of CD4 cell counts than those with AIDS. In a pilot study on 15 children with AIDS, low doses of zalcitabine produced similar antiviral effects, as indicated by increased appetite, weight, and CD4 cell counts and decreased p24 antigen levels (Pizzo et al, 1990).

In patients with advanced AIDS, long-term administration of zidovudine did not prevent a decline in CD4 lymphocytes or retard disease progression, probably because of incomplete inhibition of HIV replication and emergence of viral isolates with reduced in vitro susceptibility to the drug. Studies were carried out on these zidovudine-resistant patients to test the feasibility of combination or alternating regimens of zidovudine and zalcitabine (Yarchoan et al, 1988; Bozzette and Richman, 1990; Meng et al, 1992). Results of a Phase I/II trial on 56 patients that compared five different zalcitabine/zidovudine combinations and one regimen using zidovudine alone showed that zalcitabine 0.005 mg/kg plus zidovudine 50 mg significantly increased CD4 cell counts more than monotherapy with zidovudine 50 mg (Meng et al, 1992). Combined therapy also produced weight gain and improvement in p24 antigenemia. The regimen of zalcitabine 0.01 mg/kg and zidovudine 200 mg produced the best responses and is being used in Phase II/III trials.

ADVERSE REACTIONS AND PRECAUTIONS. A major adverse reaction to zalcitabine is peripheral neuropathy. Other serious toxicities include pancreatitis, esophageal ulcers, cardiomyopathy, congestive heart failure, and anaphylactoid reactions.

In Phase II/III trials, peripheral neuropathy occurred in 17% to 31% of patients who received monotherapy with zalcitabine compared with 0% to 12% of patients treated with zidovudine alone. The frequency of occurrence of neuropathy in patients treated with both drugs has not been determined. Zalcitabine-related peripheral neuropathy is a sensorimotor disorder that is characterized initially by numbness and burning dysesthesia involving the distal extremities. These symptoms may be followed by sharp shooting pains or severe continuous burning pain. The neuropathy may progress to severe pain that requires opioid analgesics and is potentially irreversible if zalcitabine is not withdrawn without delay. With prompt discontinuation of the drug, the neuropathy usually is slowly reversible although it may worsen in the first few weeks of drug abstinence. Thus, it is imperative that zalcitabine be withdrawn immediately when numbness, tingling, burning, or pain in the extremities develops or any related symptoms occur.

Pancreatitis or asymptomatic elevated serum amylase concentrations has been observed in <1% of those receiving zalcitabine monotherapy. Fatalities have occurred in patients with fulminant pancreatitis. Zalcitabine should be given cautiously to individuals with known risk factors for or a history of pancreatitis, and treatment with zalcitabine and zidovudine should be stopped immediately if nausea, vomiting, abdominal pain, or other symptoms suggesting the onset of pancreatitis develop. If the diagnosis of pancreatitis is confirmed, zalcitabine should be discontinued permanently.

Information on the safety of combined use of zalcitabine and zidovudine is limited. The toxicity of zalcitabine in children younger than 13 years and in asymptomatic HIV-infected individuals has not been established.

Patients receiving zalcitabine or any other antiretroviral therapy may continue to develop opportunistic infections and other complications of HIV infection and should be closely observed by physicians experienced in HIV-associated diseases; this precaution is especially important in those with impaired renal and/or hepatic function.

Zalcitabine is teratogenic in mice and rats. There are no adequate, well-controlled studies on use of this drug in pregnant women; therefore, it should not be administered during pregnancy unless the potential benefit outweighs the possible risk to the fetus. This drug is classified in FDA Pregnancy Category C.

It is not known whether zalcitabine is excreted in human milk. In the United States, it is currently recommended that HIV-infected women not breastfeed their infants whether or not they are using antiretroviral agents.

PHARMACOKINETICS. Following oral administration to HIV-infected adults, the mean absolute bioavailability of zalcitabine was >80%. When this drug was administered with food, the absorption rate was reduced, resulting in decreases of 39% and 14% in the mean maximum plasma concentration and total amount absorbed, respectively.

Following intravenous administration, the steady-state volume of distribution averaged 0.53 L/kg. At 2 to 3.5 hours, measurable concentrations of the drug appeared in cerebral fluids; the cerebral/plasma concentration ratio ranged from 9% to 37%, indicating that zalcitabine penetrated the blood-brain barrier.

Zalcitabine is phosphorylated intracellularly to ddCTP. Renal excretion appears to be the main route of elimination, accounting for 70% of an orally administered dose. The mean elimination half-life is two hours. Total body clearance averages 285 ml/min. Zalcitabine probably is eliminated more slowly in patients with impaired renal function. Less than 10% of the drug appears in the feces.

The pharmacokinetic parameters in children are similar to those reported in adults receiving doses of 0.03 to 0.5 mg/kg (Pizzo et al, 1990).

DOSAGE AND PREPARATIONS.

Oral: *Adults,* 0.75 mg with zidovudine 200 mg every eight hours. Dose reduction is necessary in patients who weigh less than 30 kg.

Hivid (Roche). Tablets 0.375 and 0.75 mg.

Cited References

Bozzette SA, Richman DD: Salvage therapy for zidovudine-intolerant HIV-infected patients with alternating and intermittent regimens of zidovudine and dideoxycytidine. *Am J Med* 88(suppl 5B):5B-24S-5B-26S, 1990.

Lipsky JJ: Zalcitabine and didanosine. *Lancet* 341:30-32, 1993.

Meng T-C, et al: Combination therapy with zidovudine and dideoxycytidine in patients with advanced human immunodeficiency virus infection: A Phase I/II study. *Ann Intern Med* 116:13-20, 1992.

Merigan TC, et al: Circulating p24 antigen levels and responses to dideoxycytidine in human immunodeficiency virus (HIV) infections: A Phase I and II study. *Ann Intern Med* 110:189-194, 1989.

Mitsuya H, Broder S: Inhibition of the in vitro infectivity and cytopathic effect of human T-lymphotrophic virus type III/lymphadenopathy-associated virus (HTLV-III/LAV) by 2′,3′-dideoxynucleosides. *Proc Natl Acad Sci USA* 83:911-915, 1986.

Pizzo PA, et al: Dideoxycytidine alone and in an alternating schedule with zidovudine in children with symptomatic human immunodeficiency virus infection. *J Pediatr* 117:799-808, 1990.

Yarchoan R, et al: Phase I studies of 2′,3′-dideoxycytidine in severe human immunodeficiency virus infection as a single agent and alternating with zidovudine (AZT). *Lancet* 1:76-81, 1988.

Antiarthritic Drugs

ARTHRITIS

Most arthritic diseases are characterized by some degree of inflammation and tissue damage at joints. Arthritis occurs in diffuse connective tissue diseases (eg, rheumatoid and juvenile arthritis, polymyositis/dermatomyositis, systemic lupus erythematosus, systemic sclerosis, vasculitides, Sjögren's syndrome, polymyalgia rheumatica) and may be associated with spondylitis (eg, ankylosing spondylitis, Reiter's syndrome, psoriatic arthritis, inflammatory bowel disease, the seronegative spondylarthropathies), degenerative joint disease (osteoarthritis), and infection (eg, bacterial or viral arthritis). Joint inflammation may be secondary to metabolic and endocrine diseases, bone and cartilage disorders, neuropathic disorders, and, rarely, neoplasm. Drug therapy of selected arthritic conditions (rheumatoid arthritis, juvenile arthritis, seronegative arthropathies, osteoarthritis, crystal-induced joint disease) is discussed in this chapter. For information on the treatment of dermatomyositis, polymyositis, and rheumatic fever, see index entries on these disorders.

Although the following discussion is limited to drug therapy, it should be recognized that mechanical problems seldom respond to drugs alone and that other measures must be employed (ie, physical therapy, exercise, surgery, adaptive devices). Furthermore, the impact of the disease on all aspects of the patient's life may require assessment by a social worker, occupational therapist, physical therapist, vocational rehabilitation specialist, and sometimes behavioral health services. Educating patients to understand the disease and its management, including realistic expectations from drug therapy, is important in achieving therapeutic success.

Rheumatoid Arthritis

This chronic inflammatory autoimmune disease occurs in about 1% of the adult population and is two and one-half times more common in women than in men. The incidence peaks in the fourth and fifth decades, but rheumatoid arthritis (RA) can appear from childhood to old age. In women, it often begins after menopause. The incidence of disease for both sexes may equalize after age 60.

PATHOGENESIS. RA is characterized by persistent inflammation of the synovium in multiple diarthrodial joints, local destruction of bone and cartilage, and a variety of systemic manifestations. Despite intensive research over the past few decades, the specific cause of RA remains unknown. However, recent advances in immunology and molecular biology have contributed to a better understanding of its pathogenetic mechanisms and have encouraged the development of investigational treatments.

Various infectious agents have been suggested to have a primary causative role. The possibility that a virus (eg, parvovirus, Epstein Barr) or proteins from other infectious agents are involved continues to receive considerable attention (Harris, 1990).

Identical twins have an increased concordance for disease, and first-degree relatives of patients with seropositive RA also are at increased risk. Individuals with RA are more likely to express one of a number of HLA-DR molecules (DR4 [Dw4, Dw14, Dw15] and DR1) that are similar in the third hypervariable region of the beta chain, a portion of the molecule that plays a major role in presentation of peptide antigens to T-lymphocytes.

Many observations support the view that local activation of T-cells is the primary factor in persistent rheumatoid inflammation. The synovial tissue mononuclear cell infiltrate is composed of perivascular aggregates of macrophages surrounded by CD4+ "memory" helper T-cells; the number of CD8+ suppressor T-cells is decreased in patients with RA. Although few synovial T-cells are in mitosis, surface markers indicate that they are activated. Immunosuppressive drugs (eg, cyclosporine [Sandimmune], cytotoxic agents) and investigational forms of immunotherapy that target T-cells or the interleukin 2 receptor (IL-2R) are variably effective in reducing disease activity. In addition, the onset of AIDS in which CD4+ cells are markedly reduced usually leads to remission of RA.

In early stages of the disease, histopathologic findings include endothelial cell injury and obliteration of small blood vessels by inflammatory cells or thrombi, vascular congestion, and edema. Under the influence of a variety of effector molecules produced by stimulated synovial and endothelial cells, neutrophils, mononuclear cells, and lymphocytes bind to postcapillary venules and migrate through the vascular endothelium to the inflammatory site. The use of monoclonal antibodies directed against cell surface structures (anti-CD4, anti-CD7, intercellular adhesion molecule [I-CAM]) that facilitate this process is being investigated.

Subsequently, over a period of several weeks, the number of cells lining the synovial tissue increases in association with synovial membrane angiogenesis and intense mononuclear cell infiltration. Nodular aggregates that contain numerous lymphoblasts and plasma cells often can be observed in the rheumatoid synovium. These and other polyclonally activated B-cells secrete immunoglobulins, including autoantibody rheumatoid factors (RFs), which can be identified in about 80% of affected individuals using standard tests for IgM RF. RFs are the product of a distinct subset of B-cells that express the CD5 marker (Burastero et al, 1988) and are composed of all Ig isotypes (not just IgM), indicating participation by T-cells in antibody maturation.

The inflammatory process in synovial fluid involves a variety of mediators (eg, complement cleavage products, leukotrienes and prostaglandins, histamine, serotonin, proteases, platelet-activating factor). Synovial fluid contains a much greater number of neutrophils than synovial tissue. Exposure of neutrophils to immune complexes, RF, and cytokines in the synovial fluid results in release of granule contents, toxic oxygen metabolites, and proinflammatory products of the arachidonic acid cascade. Some of the inflammatory products produced by this reaction probably contribute to the cartilage and bone destruction seen in RA; other substances are chemoattractants for blood-borne inflammatory cells and thus may help perpetuate intra-articular inflammation.

Locally produced cytokines probably are important mediators of acute and chronic inflammation, connective tissue destruction, and some of the extra-articular manifestations (fever, constitutional symptoms, hepatic production of acute phase reactants). In general, macrophage/monocyte-derived products such as IL-1, IL-6, IL-9, platelet-derived growth factor (PDGF), granulocyte-macrophage colony stimulating factor (GM-CSF), and tumor necrosis factor alpha (TNFα) are elevated in the rheumatoid synovium, whereas T-cell-derived cytokines such as IL-2, IL-3, IL-4, TNFβ, and interferon gamma (IFNγ) are rarely detectable.

In progressive disease, granulation tissue or pannus develops within the joint. Pannus is a highly vascularized connective tissue containing a variety of cell types, including lymphocytes, macrophages, histiocytes, fibroblast-like cells, and mast cells, that encroaches on articular cartilage, tendon sheaths, and subchondral bone. A host of factors secreted by the inflammatory tissue (eg, angiogenin, TNFα, fibroblast growth factor, TGFβ, PDGF, GM-CSF) contribute to the pronounced neovascularization. Cytokines, particularly IL-1, stimulate the synthesis and release of neutral proteinases (eg, collagenase, stromelysin) from rheumatoid synovial cells and chondrocytes. These enzymes are capable of destroying matrix proteins within articular cartilage and bone. Activation of complement by locally generated immune complexes may accelerate the development of bone and cartilage damage and contribute to the extra-articular manifestations of RA.

DIAGNOSIS. The diagnosis of RA is based on clinical observations. Early manifestations may include fatigue, weight loss, anorexia, and general malaise. The major manifestations, which develop later, are diffuse and prolonged morning stiffness; pain on motion; warmth, tenderness and/or swelling of multiple joints, usually symmetrical; subcutaneous nodules; and roentgenographic changes. The hands are involved in more than 90% of patients. Extra-articular manifestations, such as anemia, vasculitis, scleritis, pleurisy, pericarditis, and peripheral neuropathy, also may develop.

Diagnostic criteria were revised most recently in 1987 by the American College of Rheumatology (Arnett et al, 1988). These criteria are as follows: (1) morning stiffness in and around joints lasting at least one hour before maximal improvement; (2) soft tissue swelling of three or more joint areas; (3) swelling of the proximal interphalangeal, metacarpophalangeal, or wrist joints; (4) symmetric arthritis; (5) presence of rheumatoid nodules; (6) presence of RF; and (7) radiographic erosions and/or periarticular osteopenia in hand and/or wrist joints. RA is defined by the presence of four or more criteria; criteria 1 through 4 must have been present for at least six weeks.

Serologic testing for RF helps confirm the diagnosis, since at least 80% of affected patients are seropositive; however, RF, usually in low titers, is expressed in many other disease states. Some patients with RA produce autoantibodies against nuclear proteins, collagen, proteoglycans, and various other cellular components. Erythrocyte sedimentation rates, C-reactive protein levels, circulating immune complexes, and platelet counts often are elevated in RA and the hemoglobin concentration often is low with normal red blood cell indices; all are common indicators of disease activity.

THERAPY. The primary aims in the treatment of RA are to reduce joint pain and inflammation, maintain joint mobility and range of motion, and prevent deformity. A potential goal is to retard disease progression. Traditionally, the early stages of RA have been managed conservatively with a "pyramid" approach based on rest, patient education, appropriate exercise and physical therapy, and the use of anti-inflammatory agents (eg, aspirin, salicylates, other NSAIDs) as "first-line" therapy. Although these drugs relieve pain and inflammation rapidly, their benefit is primarily symptomatic and they usually do not arrest the course of the disease. With this strategy, "second-line" agents are reserved for disease progression. In contrast to anti-inflammatory agents, these drugs have a slow onset of action. Most also can be more toxic, but they have the potential to retard disease progression or induce remission; thus, they also have been referred to as slow-acting antirheumatic drugs (SAARDs) or disease-modifying antirheumatic drugs (DMARDs). Drugs in this category are the injectable gold compounds, aurothioglucose [Solganal] and gold sodium thiomalate [Myochrysine], and the oral gold compound, auranofin [Ridaura]; penicillamine [Cuprimine, Depen]; the antimalarial, hydroxychloroquine [Plaquenil]; sulfasalazine [Azulfidine]; the antimetabolite, methotrexate [Rheumatrex]; and the immunosuppressive drugs, azathioprine [Imuran], cyclophosphamide [Cytoxan], and cyclosporine. Methotrexate may exert beneficial effects within two to four weeks; however, several weeks to months of therapy with other second-line agents often are required before clinical benefit becomes apparent. Because of this slow onset of action, NSAID therapy often remains a component of the therapeutic regimen.

Although their use is controversial, low-dose corticosteroid therapy has been given as a bridge between first- and second-line therapies or to reduce pain and inflammation in patients in whom salicylates and other NSAIDs are contraindicated or not tolerated. In many patients, corticosteroids are used in combination regimens. They often are given orally, but many RA patients benefit from intra-articular injection of corticosteroids into a particularly troublesome joint.

The conservative pyramid approach was based on the assumption that RA is a heterogeneous, nonfatal disease that primarily affects function and is characterized by remission and exacerbation. Indeed, patients with RA often experience substantial improvement during the first several months of treatment with anti-inflammatory agents, and results of numerous controlled trials have demonstrated the beneficial effects of second-line agents on measures of disease activity and use of some drugs also have been associated with a decrease in the rate of cartilage erosion. However, such trials usually lasted one year or less and therefore provide little information on long-term outcome. In addition, although many patients respond to a second-line agent, therapy often must be discontinued within one to two years due to adverse effects or decreased response to a particular drug. Thus, it is now recognized that in most patients with moderate to severe RA, the disease is progressive and causes long-term morbidity and increased mortality. Observational studies suggest that pyramid treatment strategies have not measurably improved long-term disability outcome (Pincus et al, 1984; Scott et al, 1987; Kushner, 1989). Furthermore, in patients who develop erosive rheumatoid disease, the first two years of persistent synovitis (ie, the time of gradually moving through the treatment pyramid) may be the critical period during which a disproportionate amount of the joint damage occurs.

These observations have prompted many rheumatologists to consider the use of more aggressive strategies, including immunotherapy, in an attempt to control inflammation before erosive lesions develop. Protocols have been proposed that invert the pyramid by using second-line agents early (Wilske and Healey, 1989; Fries, 1990; Bensen et al, 1990; McCarty, 1990; Wilke and Clough, 1991). The interval between diagnosis and initiation of second-line therapies has shortened (ie, weeks or less) in the hope of providing more effective long-term modification of disease activity. However, it is not known whether treatment with second-line agents that is started within one or two months of disease onset (before erosions occur) prevents or slows disease progression.

Based on experience in oncology, some rheumatologists advocate combined use of second-line agents in the hope that the therapeutic response may be enhanced, toxicity decreased, and refractoriness avoided. Results of a number of open, uncontrolled, or retrospective trials suggest that combination therapy in RA is highly effective and warrants evaluation by controlled studies (for review see Schwarzer et al, 1990; Jaffe, 1990; Boehrs and Ramsden, 1991; Wilke and Clough, 1991). In randomized controlled studies, the combination of parenteral gold with penicillamine or hydroxychloroquine or the combination of penicillamine with sulfasalazine was reported to be more effective than either drug used alone (Bitter, 1984; Taggart et al, 1987; Scott et al, 1989). However, the combination of penicillamine and an antimalarial agent is less effective than either drug alone (Bunch et al, 1984; Gibson et al, 1987). In one study, the combination of methotrexate and azathioprine was somewhat more effective than methotrexate alone, but the difference was not statistically significant (Willkens et al, 1992). The lack of understanding of the mechanism of action of the second-line drugs precludes precise determination of the best drug combination or sequence of administration other than that dictated by shared toxicities. Thus, drug selection is still empiric and based on clinical experience. Randomized treatment studies of patients with early disease are required.

NSAIDs: Acetylated or nonacetylated salicylates are the preferred anti-inflammatory drugs for initial therapy. They are least expensive and no other NSAID has been proven to be more effective. Doses larger than those required for analgesia must be given to reduce inflammation. Although the latter action is most important in arthritis, the analgesic effect of salicylates may enhance their therapeutic value. The lowest dosage that controls symptoms should be prescribed and should be taken regularly for as long as symptoms persist. Dosage must be individualized because of differences in body weight and variations in the pharmacokinetics of salicylates among individuals. Serum salicylate concentrations usually are not employed to establish the dose, but the most satisfactory anti-inflammatory concentration is 15 to 30 mg/dL. Pain and stiffness are alleviated to some degree in more than 90% of patients; objective improvement also can be documented. However, additional drug therapy will be required in more than one-half of these patients.

Based on cost considerations, aspirin is the initial drug of choice. However, this agent can be toxic to the gastrointestinal tract. Some rheumatologists are concerned that the risk of gastric hemorrhage or perforation and the complexities of aspirin's pharmacokinetics make this drug less desirable for the long-term treatment of RA, especially since newer NSAIDs are more convenient and may have fewer adverse effects.

When prolonged use of large doses of regular aspirin cannot be tolerated because of gastric irritation, nonacetylated alternatives (eg, salsalate, choline salicylate) or aspirin in enteric-coated, matrix-release, or rectal suppository formulations may be tried. All preparations produce similar salicylate concentrations in the plasma. The enteric-coated preparations cause fewer gastric lesions than uncoated or buffered aspirin, and other salicylates (choline magnesium trisalicylate, magnesium salicylate, salsalate) may cause fewer gastrointestinal side effects than aspirin. Choline magnesium trisalicylate and salsalate may interfere less with prothrombin time and renal function. These drugs and possibly enteric-coated aspirin preparations offer the additional advantage of administration twice daily.

One of the other NSAIDS (see Table) may be tried in patients who cannot tolerate or do not respond to salicylates. Preference for one drug over another varies among patients and physicians. Like aspirin, these agents have anti-inflammatory, analgesic, and antipyretic actions; however, compounds vary in their specific properties. They appear to be about as effective as aspirin in RA, but equieffective doses may produce fewer gastrointestinal reactions and less gastrointestinal bleeding. Although controversial, there may be differences in the overall risk of peptic ulcer complications among these agents (Savage et al, 1993) (see discussion on Adverse Reactions). Nevertheless, all should be used with extreme caution in patients with a history of peptic ulcer or upper gastrointestinal bleeding. Less common but potentially serious adverse reactions (eg, hepatotoxicity, fluid retention and edema, hypersensitivity reactions) should be kept in mind when these drugs are considered for long-term therapy. Serum creatinine levels can increase. More serious renal toxicity, including nephrotic syndrome, acute oliguric renal failure, and interstitial nephritis, has been reported.

CHEMICAL CLASSIFICATION OF NSAIDS

Salicylic acids	
Acetylated	Aspirin
Nonacetylated	Diflunisal [Dolobid]
	Choline salicylate [Arthropan]
	Magnesium salicylate [Magan, Mobidin]
	Choline-Magnesium Trisalicylate [Trilisate]
	Sodium salicylate
	Salsalate [Disalcid]
Propionic acids	Fenoprofen [Nalfon]
	Flurbiprofen [Ansaid]
	Ibuprofen [Motrin, Rufen]
	Ketoprofen [Orudis]
	Naproxen [Anaprox, Naprosyn]
	Oxaprozin [Daypro]
Acetic acids	Diclofenac [Voltaren]
	Etodolac [Lodine]
	Indomethacin [Indocin]
	Sulindac [Clinoril]
	Tolmetin [Tolectin]
Enolic acids	
Oxicam	Piroxicam [Feldene]
Pyrazole	Phenylbutazone
Fenamic acids	Meclofenamate [Meclomen]
Nonacidic compound	Nabumetone [Relafen]

Different drugs and dosages can be tried to determine the optimum regimen for each individual. It should be kept in mind that adequate doses must be given for sufficient periods (two to four weeks) to evaluate efficacy before substitution of a different drug is considered. If the first NSAID fails, one or two more should be tried in succession. The concurrent use of aspirin and other NSAIDs may produce drug interactions that decrease the anti-inflammatory response and increase gastric toxicity and therefore is contraindicated.

Indomethacin [Indocin], an older NSAID, is effective in moderate to severe RA, including acute exacerbations of chronic disease, but it is often of more value in osteoarthritis of the hip, ankylosing spondylitis, and acute gouty arthritis. Small doses are given initially and the amount increased gradually to the level of tolerance (see the evaluation).

Opioid Analgesics: The management of chronic pain syndromes that can accompany RA may require adjunctive doses of analgesic medication. Opioid analgesics may relieve severe articular pain, but drugs with high abuse potential should be prescribed only rarely and for short periods of time. However, those with low abuse potential (eg, propoxyphene [Darvon]) may be useful.

Second-Line Drugs: If the symptoms of active RA do not improve adequately after a sufficient trial (four to six weeks) with NSAIDs, a second-line drug should be added to the regimen. Anti-inflammatory drugs should be continued adjunctively.

Because *hydroxychloroquine* partially suppresses disease in 40% to 60% of patients with RA and those with earlier and milder disease are likely to have the best response (Weinblatt and Maier, 1991), this antimalarial may be indicated even in patients with mild disease (Davis et al, 1991). The potential for visual impairment is low but has limited the use of this agent; however, hydroxychloroquine is probably one of the safest second-line drugs. Total dose appears to be the most important factor in development of retinal toxicity, and small doses can be given for long periods without toxic effects. Ocular reactions occur only rarely when doses <6.5 mg/kg/day are prescribed and usually are reversible if detected in the early stages by periodic ophthalmologic monitoring. Preferably, the dosage should be determined on the basis of lean body weight, particularly in children (Mackenzie, 1983). Administration two or three times a week may be as effective as daily therapy (Maksymowych and Russell, 1987). Hydroxychloroquine must be given for at least three to six months before maximal beneficial effects are noted. If response is inadequate after a trial of at least six months, another second-line agent should be substituted or added to the regimen. If the therapeutic goals are achieved and toxicity is absent, hydroxychloroquine may be continued indefinitely.

The parenteral *gold compounds*, aurothioglucose and gold sodium thiomalate, may be the first gold preparations employed because there has been more experience with their use. A therapeutic response occurs within six months in approximately 40% to 60% of patients receiving weekly 50-mg injections. Meta-analysis of four randomized trials found that the mean response to gold injections was a 30% reduction in the number of inflamed joints and erythrocyte sedimentation rate and a 14% increase in grip strength; adverse events occurred in approximately 40% of patients, but only 11% discontinued therapy because of toxicity (Clark et al, 1989). The frequency of side effects of the oral drug, auranofin, appears to be comparable to those of injectable gold, but there are fewer serious adverse reactions. Auranofin rarely causes blood dyscrasias or proteinuria, but diarrhea can be a limiting side effect (Chaffman et al, 1984). Parenteral gold is more effective and some patients respond only to that form. In either case, patients should be informed of the potential adverse effects of gold therapy and the fact that beneficial effects are usually delayed. If significant improvement is observed and the agent is tolerated, therapy should be continued for several years and, possibly, indefinitely.

Results of controlled studies have established the effectiveness of *penicillamine* as an alternative to gold (Hochberg, 1986); however, its use has declined in recent years as methotrexate has been recognized as more effective and less toxic. With current dosage regimens for penicillamine (eg, 250 mg/day for several weeks, increasing to a total daily dose of 750 mg at bedtime), the prevalence of adverse reactions appears to be lower than in early trials using larger doses; however, more than 50% of patients do not tolerate the drug. Patients must be monitored carefully.

Sulfasalazine was formulated in the late 1930s to be a disease-modifying drug for RA. After the publication of unfavorable results in a comparative trial with gold in 1948, interest in sulfasalazine declined except for its use in inflammatory bowel disease. In 1978, its action in RA was reinvestigated and it was shown to be effective (McConkey et al, 1978). Subsequently, a number of investigators confirmed sulfasalazine's value as a disease-modifying drug in the long-term management of RA (Bax and Amos, 1985; Pinals et al, 1986). In addition to clinical improvement, radiographic evidence suggests that there may be slower deterioration of the joint (Pullar et al, 1987) and a beneficial effect on nonarticular manifestations, such as subcutaneous nodules (Englert et al, 1987).

The usefulness of sulfasalazine can be determined within two to three months after initiation of therapy. The principal side effects are nausea and vomiting, abdominal pain, and dizziness. Gastrointestinal side effects can be minimized by employing enteric-coated preparations in small doses (500 mg/day) with a gradual increase to 2 g daily (Farr et al, 1986). The next most prominent reactions affect the skin; a pruritic maculopapular generalized eruption is most common (Amos et al, 1986). The most serious adverse effect is reversible neutropenia that is not dose related; it may be more common in patients with JRA. Onset is precipitous, and this reaction usually occurs during the first two or three months of therapy (Capell et al, 1986).

Methotrexate or *azathioprine*, or some combination of second-line agents, should be considered in patients with systemic manifestations of RA, evidence of erosive disease, very high erythrocyte sedimentation rate, nodules, or high RF titers.

In the United States, methotrexate has evolved from its position as a drug of last resort in patients with RA to one that is favored first by many rheumatologists. Long-term observational studies suggest that this drug is well tolerated and retains efficacy in a significant number of patients. Methotrexate often has a more rapid onset of therapeutic effect than other disease-modifying agents. Weekly administration of 2.5 mg every 12 hours for three doses or 7.5 to 15 mg orally as a single dose is effective. The risk/benefit ratio of low-dose therapy for RA requires further study, especially the long-term risks of cirrhosis, but this is substantially reduced by low-dose pulse therapy (see the evaluation).

Small doses of azathioprine (1.5 mg/kg/day) given for up to three years were effective in some cases of severe RA not responsive to other therapy. The low-dosage regimen reduced the risk of serious adverse reactions, including oncogenesis (Van Wanghe and Dequeker, 1982); however, the risk/benefit ratio of azathioprine is not as favorable as that of methotrexate.

In small clinical trials, methotrexate and azathioprine (Hamdy et al, 1987) or gold sodium thiomalate (Morassut et al, 1989; Rau et al, 1991 A) were equally effective in RA. In larger, double-blind comparative studies, methotrexate was more effective and better tolerated than oral gold or azathioprine (Weinblatt, 1989 A; Jeurissen et al, 1991).

Use of the cytotoxic agent, *cyclophosphamide,* in RA has been studied extensively. Although controlled trials have shown that cyclophosphamide may be very beneficial in selected patients, because of its potential serious toxicity, this drug should be reserved for patients with severe disease refractory to other disease-modifying therapy. Cyclophosphamide appears to be more toxic than azathioprine or methotrexate. Bone marrow suppression, increased incidence of infections, mucous membrane lesions, hemorrhagic cystitis, bladder cancer, and an overall increased incidence of neoplastic disease have occurred (Kovarsky, 1983).

Corticosteroids: Systemic corticosteroids usually improve functional capacity, relieve pain and stiffness, and control inflammation, although joint destruction may continue. However, their usefulness is limited because of numerous adverse effects. Therefore, systemic use of these drugs often is reserved for patients with moderately severe, rapidly progressing RA that responds poorly to other antirheumatic agents; for those threatened with severe disability or unemployability; and for those with significant extra-articular involvement. These agents also may be used temporarily during initiation of second-line therapy, but the difficulty of withdrawing the steroid must be considered. Prednisone and prednisolone are most commonly used systemically. The minimum dosage that improves symptoms and signs should be prescribed; when these drugs are used as "bridge therapy," the initial dose should be low and increased to 7.5 mg of prednisone or equivalent daily if necessary for extra-articular manifestations. Complete relief is not sought; therefore, amelioration of disability may be the major indication for these agents unless extra-articular signs are present. Larger doses may be required in the presence of vasculitis.

When only one or two joints are affected or present a major problem, synovitis often can be relieved for long periods by injecting long-acting corticosteroids intra-articularly. The dose and frequency of injections must be individualized; the smallest amount should be administered as infrequently as possible to provide relief. It is suggested that injection into a single joint should not be repeated more than three or four times yearly. For other uses of corticosteroids in rheumatic disease, see index entry Prednisone.

Cyclosporine: There have been several short-term controlled trials of cyclosporine in the treatment of severe, advanced, or intractable RA (for review see Dijkmans et al, 1992). Results of early trials confirmed the beneficial effects of this agent at daily doses of 5 mg/kg in patients with severe RA; however, significant gastrointestinal and renal toxicity occurred. RA patients may be more susceptible to cyclosporine-induced renal damage, especially those treated concurrently with NSAIDs or other nephrotoxic agents (eg, gold, penicillamine). Results of another controlled study suggest that lower initial doses (ie, 2.5 mg/kg/day increased to 3.8 mg/kg/day) may provide the best balance between efficacy and toxicity (Tugwell et al, 1990).

IMMUNOTHERAPY. Immunotherapy will probably play an important role in the management of RA in the future. Results of a number of open, uncontrolled studies that used monoclonal antibodies directed against pan T-cell antigens (CD5, CDw52 [CAMPATH]), T-helper cell antigen (CD4), and T-cell activation antigens (anti-CD25) have verified that single doses of monoclonal antibodies are capable of inducing short-term clinical improvement in patients with RA.

Antibodies that target all mature T-cells include anti-CD5 and anti-CDw52 (CAMPATH-1H). The CD5 antigen also is present on B-cell subsets, which are believed to be important in the pathogenesis of RA. In a Phase II study, 41 of 79 patients treated with CD5+ (a murine CD5 antibody linked to ricin A toxin) improved significantly within one month after start of treatment (Strand et al, 1991). In an open trial of humanized monoclonal antibody CAMPATH-1H in eight patients (Watts and Isaacs, 1992), significant clinical benefit was observed in seven and was sustained for eight months in one. Although this form of treatment reduces immunogenicity compared with use of murine antibodies, anti-idiotype responses still may occur with repeated therapy. Five murine and one chimeric CD4 mAB have been used for the treatment of RA in open trials (for review, see Watts and Isaacs, 1992). Although short-term beneficial effects were reported, antibody immunogenicity that may restrict repetition of administration also was apparent in many patients. A rat antibody directed against the interleukin 2 receptor (anti-CD25; CAMPATH-6) also is being studied. Another investigational approach involves the use of a genetically engineered fusion protein consisting of diphtheria toxin and IL-2; clinical trials are being conducted with such an agent (DAB_{389}IL-2). Studies also are underway examining the effects of anti-TNFα and an antibody (BIRR 1) that binds specifically to intercellular adhesion molecule (ICAM-1).

Juvenile Arthritis

SYMPTOMS. By definition, onset of this form of arthritis occurs prior to age 16; it is the most common connective tissue disease affecting children. The type is determined by manifestations that appear during the first six months of disease and varies with respect to age at onset, sex, number and distribution of joints affected, results of serologic tests, extra-articular manifestations, and prognosis. Juvenile patients with chronic arthritis may be either seropositive (juvenile rheumatoid arthritis) or seronegative. Seronegative juvenile arthritis has three main onset types: (1) systemic (acute febrile or Still's disease), (2) pauciarticular (four or fewer joints affected), and (3) polyarticular (five or more joints affected). Pauciarticular is most common. For appropriate therapy, juvenile arthritis must be differentiated (usually by exclusion) from several other diseases with similar manifestations commonly seen in children (eg, rheumatic fever, juvenile ankylosing spondylitis, septic arthritis, trauma, malignancy, Lyme disease).

During the first ten years of disease, chronic iridocyclitis develops in about 25% of patients who have the pauciarticular type and a positive test for antinuclear antibody (ANA); young girls are most commonly affected. Since iridocyclitis is frequently asymptomatic at onset and may be detected only by slit-lamp examination, children with the pauciarticular form should have an ophthalmologic evaluation at least every six months so that therapy can be instituted when necessary. Corticosteroids (topical or systemic) and the nightly instillation of mydriatics prevent further complications and loss of vision. Concomitant administration of NSAIDs may permit reduction of corticosteroid dosage (Olson et al, 1988). Careful monitoring is required because of the risk of glaucoma, cataract, or band keratopathy.

The prognosis is good for most children with juvenile rheumatoid arthritis (JRA). Overall, more than 75% have remissions without joint damage. However, severe destructive arthritis occurs in more than 50% of patients with polyarticular disease who have a positive test for RF. Polyarticular disease usually begins in late childhood and resembles severe adult-onset RA. Severe arthritis develops in only about 10% to 15% of children in the seronegative group and in about 20% of those in the systemic (acute febrile) group. The arthritis is only rarely severe in those with the pauciarticular type; however, more severe polyarticular disease develops in later years in some of these children, usually boys. The incidence of HLA-B27 is high (75%) and serologic tests for ANA and RF are negative. These patients are likely to develop ankylosing spondylitis or sacroiliitis with increasing duration of disease.

THERAPY. Drug therapy for juvenile arthritis is only one part of total management, which includes a home program of supportive measures performed by parents and regular follow-up care by the physician. Treatment is most effective when initiated early. Aspirin often is preferred initially, regardless of the onset subtype, although concern about its association with Reye's syndrome (see index entry Analgesics, Nonopioid) has restricted its use somewhat. Beneficial effects may not appear for one to two weeks, and significant changes may not be observed for several months. Aspirin should be administered for at least six months after articular signs and symptoms have subsided. The drug then may be discontinued gradually but should be reinstituted if symptoms recur.

Since tinnitus, the usual sign of aspirin toxicity, may be difficult to determine in young children, serum salicylate concentrations should be monitored to establish optimal dosage. Concentrations of 20 to 30 mg/dL are generally safe and effective, and many children experience maximum benefit at lower levels.

Hepatotoxicity may be dose-related and occurs more frequently when serum salicylate levels exceed 25 mg/dL (Calabro, 1985). Hepatic function tests should be performed before aspirin therapy is initiated and when the salicylate serum concentration is determined approximately 10 days later. Minor elevations of AST and ALT are common and require monitoring but not discontinuation of the salicylate. Lethargy and episodic hyperpnea are early signs of aspirin toxicity; if these occur, the drug should be discontinued until the signs abate, and administration should be resumed at a slightly lower dose. Gastrointestinal disturbances are uncommon in children but, if they occur, other preparations (eg, enteric-coated aspirin, choline salicylate) can be tried.

Ibuprofen (30 to 40 mg/kg daily in three divided doses) (Giannini et al, 1990 A) or naproxen (10 to 15 mg/kg daily in two divided doses) is preferred to aspirin for initial therapy in Great Britain and by some clinicians in the United States (Stiehm, 1988). In the United States, only naproxen and tolmetin are labeled for this indication, but daily doses of fenoprofen (900 mg to 1.8 g/M^2), ibuprofen, ketoprofen (100 to 200 mg/M^2), sodium meclofenamate (3 to 7.5 mg/kg), piroxicam (0.33 mg/kg), and diclofenac (2 to 3 mg/kg) have been used as well (Williams et al, 1986; Leak et al, 1988; Fink, 1990). Because of the potentially serious adverse reactions of indomethacin and phenylbutazone, these drugs should be avoided in children under 14 years.

If polyarticular disease progresses and no improvement is noted after three to six months of NSAID therapy, a second-line drug generally should be added to the regimen (Duffy et al, 1989; Rosenberg, 1989; Fink, 1990). Except for methotrexate, there have been few placebo-controlled trials of these agents in the treatment of JRA. Results of retrospective and open comparative studies suggest that other second-line drugs are about equally effective, but ease of use and adverse effects differ (Grondin et al, 1988).

Results of uncontrolled studies suggest that parenteral gold therapy is of considerable value in many children, although its efficacy may not be apparent for several months. Toxic effects are similar to those in adults; patients should be observed closely and appropriate laboratory tests should be performed prior to each injection (see the evaluations on Gold Compounds). Similarly, results of uncontrolled studies of oral gold in children with JRA suggest that efficacy and the frequency of side effects are similar to those reported in adults (Brewer at al, 1983). However, in a double-blind, randomized controlled trial, addition of the oral gold compound, auranofin [Ridaura], to NSAID therapy did not significantly improve the response over that achieved with NSAIDs alone (Giannini et al, 1990 B). In a long-term follow-up of this study, auranofin was well tolerated but adequate long-term control was observed in only a small percentage of patients (Giannini et al, 1991).

Hydroxychloroquine also is used in children, and some clinicians prefer to employ it before gold compounds. As in adults, the dosage must be calculated carefully based on lean body weight. The effectiveness of hydroxychloroquine in JRA has been questioned (Rynes, 1989); trials have supported (Kvien et al, 1985) and not supported (Brewer et al, 1986) its value. This drug should be discontinued if beneficial effects are not observed within six to nine months (van Kerckhove et al, 1988). Side effects in children are similar to those in adults, with ocular toxicity the chief hazard (Schaller, 1985).

Penicillamine was approximately as effective as gold in a few open studies (Ansell and Hall, 1981). In one controlled study, penicillamine was more effective than placebo and its use permitted a reduction in the dose of corticosteroid (Prieur et al, 1985). However, results of another study indicated that when an NSAID also was administered, penicillamine was no better than placebo (Brewer et al, 1986). Thus, because of potential toxicity, penicillamine should be used only under carefully controlled conditions and should be discontinued if no benefit is obtained in four months (van Kerckhove et al, 1988).

Several uncontrolled trials have indicated that methotrexate was effective in JRA patients who did not benefit from other therapy (Truckenbrodt and Häfner, 1986; Wallace et al, 1989; Speckmaier et al, 1989). Results of a randomized, six-month double-blind controlled trial confirmed the short-term efficacy of methotrexate 10 mg/M^2/week in children with resistant JRA (Giannini et al, 1992), and the drug appears to be well tolerated (Graham et al, 1992). However, questions remain about the long-term efficacy and safety of low-dose methotrexate in these patients (Halle and Prieur, 1991; White and Ansell, 1992). Azathioprine has not been particularly effective in such children.

In a preliminary open study of 18 patients with systemic JRA, pulse therapy with methylprednisolone and cyclophosphamide in addition to oral methotrexate significantly suppressed systemic and articular manifestations in 100% (Shaikov et al, 1992).

Oral corticosteroids should not be administered routinely because of their potential adverse reactions, including growth retardation, and the problems associated with withdrawal. They should be reserved for seriously ill children with polyarticular disease who do not respond to aspirin and other anti-inflammatory drugs (eg, naproxen, tolmetin) or for those with myocarditis, and the duration of therapy should not exceed a few months consecutively (Baum, 1983). Alternate-day therapy may be useful for some patients. Intra-articular injection also may be useful, but no more than three or four injections should be made into the same joint each year. Topical corticosteroids are essential in the treatment of chronic iridocyclitis; rarely, local injection or systemic administration is needed when topical application does not control inflammation.

Osteoarthritis

SYMPTOMS. Osteoarthritis is characterized by joint pain, tenderness, limitation of movement, occasional effusion, and variable degrees of local inflammation. It is not considered a systemic disease and may be confined to a single joint. Weight-bearing joints (knee and hip) are most commonly affected; the spine is involved less frequently. In the fingers, involvement generally is limited to the distal interphalangeal joints (Heberden's nodes) and less commonly the proximal interphalangeal joints (Bouchard's nodes). The carpometacarpal joint in the thumb often is affected.

The exact pathogenesis is unknown. Certain kindreds with premature polyarticular osteoarthritis possess a discrete abnormality in the collagen 2A gene (Palotie et al, 1989; Knowlton et al, 1990), but it is not known whether defects in cartilage structure or function are primary risk factors for other patients. The disorder may be secondary to other diseases that cause joint deformity or to repeated joint trauma, but in many patients no such association is present. The incidence of osteoarthritis increases with age, but the disease is not caused solely by aging of articular tissues.

Loss of cartilage occurs in areas of increased load along with alteration of the tensile, compressive, and shear properties and hydraulic permeability of the cartilage. Cartilage degradation is accompanied by variable degrees of inflammation and repair. Biochemical changes also are noted in proteoglycans, collagen, and other matrix molecules. In later stages, severe cartilage loss is accompanied by sclerosis and focal osteonecrosis of the subchondral bone. Various cytokines (eg, IL-1, IL-6, TNFα) have been implicated in promoting matrix degradation (Morales and Hascall, 1989).

Symptoms are referable to the joint involved; the most common is pain that becomes worse with use of the joint. Pain at night is common; stiffness in the morning and after sitting ("gelling") also occurs often but, unlike RA, lasts less than 30 minutes. Diagnosis is based on symptoms, analysis of joint fluid to exclude a WBC $>$2,000/mm^3, and radiographic findings.

THERAPY. Measures to reduce strain on weight-bearing joints, physical therapy (passive range of motion exercises; application of heat or cold to reduce pain), appropriate exercise to preserve muscle strength, rest, weight loss, joint protection (cane, crutches, walker, orthotic shoes), and drug therapy are all important in the management of osteoarthritis.

Results of large, double-blind placebo-controlled study of acetaminophen (4 g daily) versus ibuprofen at either analgesic (1.2 g/day) or anti-inflammatory (2.4 g/day) doses did not demonstrate any increased benefit from the NSAID (Bradley et al, 1991); thus, some practitioners recommend that if analgesia is required, acetaminophen should be used at maximum dosage before an NSAID is substituted (Jones and Doherty, 1992). Other analgesics (eg, propoxyphene, codeine) are sometimes used in combination with acetaminophen or anti-inflammatory drugs, but drugs with abuse potential should be avoided if possible. In patients in whom inflammation contributes significantly to symptoms, NSAIDs are more effective than simple analgesics because of their combined activity. Other NSAIDs may be better tolerated than aspirin, especially by older patients (see the evaluations). If pain is not relieved by one of these agents, indomethacin may be used; it has been particularly effective in osteoarthritis involving the hip, hands, knees, and shoulders.

Systemic corticosteroids generally are not indicated in this condition and may cause serious adverse effects. Intra-articular injection of long-acting preparations may relieve symptoms in a contracted joint, permitting institution of physical therapy to restore function. Surgical procedures utilizing total joint replacement are preferred when the joint deteriorates to instability or, in patients with severe, persistent pain, when there is loss of function.

Seronegative Spondylarthropathies

The spondylarthropathies include the prototype disorder, ankylosing spondylitis, as well as Reiter's syndrome and other reactive arthritides, adult-onset Still's disease, enteropathic sacroiliitis (ie, Crohn's disease, ulcerative colitis), psoriatic arthritis, and the rare disorders, acute anterior uveitis, Behcet's syndrome, and Whipple's disease. There is considerable evidence of clinical overlap among the various seronegative spondylarthropathies. These disorders are characterized by a high frequency of spinal inflammation (spondylitis and/or sacroiliitis), inflammatory lesions at ligamentous and joint capsular attachments to bone (ie, enthesopathy), and peripheral synovitis. Compared with RA, the associated synovitis has a relatively good prognosis and, except for psoriatic arthritis, joint inflammation typically is oligoarticular and the lower limb is predominantly affected.

The distribution of ankylosing spondylitis in the general population follows that of the HLA-B27 gene. More than 95% of Caucasian patients with ankylosing spondylitis are HLA-B27 positive. A similar but less strong correlation (80%) has been observed for Reiter's syndrome. The degree of association between HLA-B27 and other seronegative arthropathies is related to the population involved, but it is generally higher when sacroiliitis coexists. Much attention has been directed to a possible link between infection and synovitis. Various hypotheses (eg, pathogenic peptide, molecular mimicry, altered self) have been proposed to explain the mechanism of the HLA-B27-spondylarthropathy association (see Schwartz, 1990; Maclean, 1992). A possible role for *Klebsiella pneumoniae* in the pathogenesis of ankylosing spondylitis has been proposed, and various bacteria (eg, *Chlamydia trachomatis, Ureaplasma urealyticum, Yersinia enterocolitica, Salmonella* and *Shigella* species) have been implicated in the development of Reiter's syndrome and other reactive arthritides. In addition to the part played by acute infective enterocolitis, it has been suggested that the gastrointestinal tract may be involved based on the association between chronic inflammatory bowel disease, alterations in bowel permeability, and development of arthritis.

ANKYLOSING SPONDYLITIS. Symptoms: This form of seronegative arthritis differs in many respects from RA. It is characterized by involvement of the sacroiliac joints, the spinal apophyseal joints, and the paravertebral soft tissues. The hips and shoulders also may be affected in about 30% of patients. The history often includes insidious onset of back discomfort and early morning stiffness that persists for more than three months and is associated with decreased spinal mobility. This disorder also may affect other body systems; acute anterior uveitis occurs in about 25% of patients and bilateral pulmonary fibrosis in the upper lung fields may mimic tuberculosis. A mild normocytic normochromic anemia may be present.

The prevalence of ankylosing spondylitis in Caucasians is probably similar to that of RA, but the disease occurs much less frequently in blacks. Disease onset is observed most often during the second or third decade of life and is about three times more common in men. Symptoms tend to progress and the disease becomes chronic.

The erythrocyte sedimentation rate (ESR) is elevated in many patients but may be normal despite severe disease; tests for RF and ANA are negative. Diagnosis is confirmed by roentgenographic examination.

Therapy: Early recognition and initiation of appropriate therapy are important for successful treatment of ankylosing spondylitis. Although progression of the disease may not be modified by any available therapy, relief of pain and inflammation and maintenance of function usually are possible. Spontaneous remissions and exacerbations occur, and the prognosis generally is good.

The mainstay of treatment is a daily exercise regimen to maintain spinal mobility and muscle strength. NSAIDs aid in these goals by minimizing pain and stiffness.

Although aspirin may be effective for mild attacks, it usually does not relieve severe pain. Indomethacin has been considered the drug of choice, but some of the other NSAIDs (eg, diclofenac, naproxen, piroxicam, sulindac) also are effective and may be better tolerated. In individual patients, preferences are often strong for one NSAID over another. Many patients report that only a few days to a week are needed to identify the drug that they consider superior. Such patient self-selection will provide better compliance and presumably a better clinical outcome (Wasner et al, 1981). Phenylbutazone may provide symptomatic relief but, because of its potential to produce severe blood dyscrasias, it should be used only after other drugs have failed (see the evaluation). The anti-inflammatory drugs should be withdrawn slowly and only after active disease has been suppressed for several months.

A meta-analysis of five randomized controlled trials comparing the short-term use of sulfasalazine (2 to 3 g/day) with placebo determined that treatment with this drug reduced morning stiffness, pain, and the ESR and improved the patient's sense of well being (Ferraz et al, 1990). Thus, the addition of sulfasalazine may benefit those who do not experience adequate relief from NSAIDs alone. Long-term studies are necessary to determine whether the course of the disease is affected.

Systemic corticosteroids are rarely useful unless iridocyclitis or vasculitis occurs, and should be avoided, if possible. Topical corticosteroids and mydriatics usually are useful for anterior uveitis. Steroids may be injected intra-articularly if one or two peripheral joints are severely affected and interfere with the exercise program. Neither penicillamine nor gold compounds are effective in ankylosing spondylitis or the spondylitis in other HLA-B27-associated arthropathies.

PSORIATIC ARTHRITIS. Symptoms: This seronegative spondylarthropathy occurs in about 5% of patients with psoriasis. Onset is insidious and the characteristic asymmetric enthesopathy commonly involves only a few joints. With polyarticular involvement, which is the most common form of established disease, small- to medium-sized joints are affected, and the pattern can be either symmetrical or asymmetrical (Gladman, 1992). Sacroiliitis and spondylitis develop in about 20% of patients with psoriatic arthritis. The risk of back involvement is higher in individuals with HLA-B27 antigen. Psoriasis also has been associated with HLA-B13 and Bw17; Bw38, HLA DR4, and DR7 have been associated with peripheral joint disease.

Therapy: The psoriatic and arthritic components are treated separately (see index entry Psoriasis). Prognosis for psoriatic arthritis generally is good because this disease is not severe or disabling in most patients (Vasey et al, 1982). However, those with polyarticular disease may develop progressive, destructive arthritis and some develop arthritis mutilans, a severe resorptive arthropathy. Remissions and exacerbations of peripheral arthritis probably only coincidently parallel those of the skin disease.

In general, treatment of arthritic symptoms is similar to that for RA (Goupille et al, 1992). The anti-inflammatory drugs provide adequate management in 80% to 90% of patients. Aspirin is not as effective as in RA, but it may be helpful in mild cases. Indomethacin controls pain and increases the range of spinal motion. Another NSAID may be substituted when there is no response or the patient cannot tolerate indomethacin.

Methotrexate or azathioprine suppresses the dermal lesions as well as the arthritis but should be reserved for use in patients who do not respond adequately to other medication.

Parenteral (Dorwart et al, 1978; Richter et al, 1980) and oral (Carette et al, 1989) gold compounds are beneficial in some patients. In one double-blind comparative trial, parenteral gold was more effective than auranofin (Palit et al, 1990).

Results of two open studies suggest that sulfasalazine 2 g/day may be effective for patients with psoriatic arthritis not controlled by NSAIDs, particularly in those with polyarticular disease and spondylitis (Farr et al, 1988 A; Newman et al, 1991). Results of small open studies also suggest that cyclosporine has beneficial effects on both the arthritis and the skin lesions (Goupille et al, 1992). Larger, double-blind studies are required to determine the relative safety and efficacy of cyclosporine for the arthritic component.

Some clinicians avoid the use of hydroxychloroquine in psoriasis because of the belief that it may exacerbate dermal lesions and because of the remote possibility that it may induce a life-threatening exfoliative dermatitis (Kuflik, 1980). However, in one prospective study on 100 patients, hydroxychloroquine was well tolerated and only rarely caused cutaneous adverse effects (Kammer et al, 1979).

Although systemic corticosteroids may improve both the skin and joint disease, the dosage required usually is so large that adverse reactions result and withdrawal of steroids may exacerbate the psoriasis; thus, except for intra-articular administration, they have virtually no role in the treatment of this condition.

REITER'S SYNDROME. Symptoms: This seronegative spondyloarthropathy occurs primarily in young adult males. The etiology is unknown, but two epidemiologic forms are recognized: the epidemic form that follows dysentery and the more common (in the United States) endemic or venereal form. Enteric (eg, *Yersinia, Shigella, Salmonella* species) and genitourinary (eg, *Chlamydia trachomatis, Mycoplasma* species) organisms are among the many bacteria associated with Reiter's syndrome. The genitourinary, ocular, skeletal, and mucocutaneous systems may be affected. *Chlamydia trachomatis* has emerged as the primary pathogen associated with the disease in young men, but the triad of nongonococcal urethritis, conjunctivitis, and arthritis frequently is not present in these patients.

The term "reactive arthritis" may be applied when the arthritogenic organism (eg, *Borrelia burgdorferi, Campylobacter jejuni, Neisseria gonorrhoeae, Streptococcus*) is known, whether or not the complete triad of Reiter's syndrome is present. Attention currently is focused on the possibility that microorganisms or antigenic determinants from them gain access to the joint and play a central role in the initiation of synovitis; live organisms, antigenic fragments, and nucleic acid sequences have been found occasionally.

Rheumatologic features include arthralgias, tendonitis, plantar fasciitis, spondylitis and other enthesopathies, as well as arthritis. Initial episodes of Reiter's syndrome may be self-limiting within six months, but the syndrome can recur, become chronic, and produce disability. The HLA-B27 antigen is present in about 80% of patients with Reiter's syndrome, and its identification may aid in determination of the prognosis; its presence suggests chronic disease.

Therapy: There is no specific treatment for Reiter's syndrome. Accompanying urethritis or cervicitis is treated with antibiotics; however, there is little evidence that this therapy will affect the severity or duration of the arthritis. Anti-inflammatory drugs suppress pain, but the musculoskeletal symptoms are less responsive. Indomethacin should be considered in the selection of an initial agent. Another NSAID may be tried as an alternative. Aspirin does not appear to be as effective as other NSAIDs. Phenylbutazone is effective, but the potential for serious adverse reactions must be considered.

Patients with severe recurrent uveitis may require corticosteroid eye drops or subconjunctival preparations. Systemic corticosteroids should be avoided because they are usually less effective, although intra-articular injection of a long-acting steroid preparation is useful when inflammation of one or two joints persists. Sulfasalazine has been reported to be effective in Reiter's syndrome. Cytotoxic therapy may be indicated in patients with chronic severe disease. Oral methotrexate 7.5 to 10 mg weekly (Lally and Ho, 1985) and azathioprine 1 to 2.5 mg/kg/day (Calin, 1986) are beneficial in some patients resistant to other therapy (Gerber, 1984). Gold, penicillamine, and hydroxychloroquine are ineffective.

NONSTEROIDAL ANTI-INFLAMMATORY AGENTS

Currently available NSAIDs vary chemically (see Table). As a group, the NSAIDs have anti-inflammatory, analgesic, antipyretic, and platelet-inhibitory actions (for review see Brooks and Day, 1991). They are used primarily in the treatment of chronic arthritic conditions and certain soft tissue disorders associated with pain and inflammation. These drugs are effective in RA, JRA, ankylosing spondylitis, Reiter's syndrome, psoriatic arthritis, osteoarthritis, and acute gouty arthritis. Some of these drugs also are used to relieve pain (see index entry Analgesics) and headache (see index entry Headache), to treat proteinuria and dysmenorrhea, and to prevent thrombosis.

MECHANISM OF ACTION. NSAIDs block the synthesis of prostaglandins by inhibiting cyclo-oxygenase, which converts arachidonic acid to cyclic endoperoxides, precursors of prostaglandins. Inhibition of prostaglandin synthesis accounts for their analgesic, antipyretic, and platelet-inhibitory actions; other mechanisms may contribute to their anti-inflammatory effects. Compared with aspirin, salicylate is a weak inhibitor of cyclo-oxygenase activity yet retains its anti-inflammatory efficacy. Doses required for peak analgesic and anti-inflammatory effects differ for most of these agents, particularly aspirin. At anti-inflammatory doses, NSAIDs inhibit various neutrophil functions and membrane-bound enzymes, perhaps by interfering with G protein-mediated signal transduction (Abramson and Weissmann, 1989). Certain NSAIDs also may inhibit lipoxygenase enzymes or phospholipase C or may modulate T-cell function.

PHARMACOKINETICS. All NSAIDs are absorbed rapidly after oral administration, but, when taken with food, the rate and sometimes the extent of absorption are decreased (see the evaluations). The onset of analgesic effects generally occurs within one hour, and time to peak serum concentration ranges from 0.5 to 5 hours (Porter, 1984). The antirheumatic action may not be apparent for one to two weeks and time to peak effect varies from one to four weeks.

Plasma concentrations of aspirin and naproxen have been shown to correlate with therapeutic efficacy; this relationship is not established for other NSAIDs. Plasma salicylate concentrations of 20 to 30 mg/dL tend to correlate with anti-inflammatory activity.

These drugs are highly bound to plasma proteins, especially albumin, and have small volumes of distribution. These features increase the possibility of drug interactions with concomitant administration of anticoagulants or oral hypoglycemic agents, which also are extensively bound to plasma proteins. In the usual therapeutic dosage range, plasma protein binding is saturable for salicylates and some other NSAIDs (naproxen, phenylbutazone, ibuprofen); thus, increases in dosage may yield disproportionate increases in the free plasma concentration.

The liver is the major site for metabolism of the NSAIDs, which for the most part are characterized by low, nonflow-dependent hepatic clearance and negligible first-pass metabolism. The major pathway for excretion is the kidney, but significant amounts of most of these drugs are excreted in the feces. Indomethacin and sulindac undergo significant enterohepatic circulation. The clearance of ketoprofen, fenoprofen, and naproxen is decreased in patients with renal failure or with concomitant administration of probenecid.

Plasma elimination half-lives vary greatly; the longest is that of piroxicam (37 to 86 hours) (Lipman, 1982; Porter, 1984). The frequency of administration necessary to achieve anti-inflammatory activity can affect compliance. Studies have demonstrated that compliance is poor (40% to 57.5%) in arthritic patients treated with multiple doses. Some of the newer NSAIDs and prolonged-release forms of the older drugs require less frequent administration. Piroxicam, oxaprozin, and nabumetone require administration only once daily, choline magnesium trisalicylate can be given once or twice daily, and salsalate [Disalcid], diclofenac, naproxen, and sulindac can be given twice daily. Diflunisal also may be administered twice daily, although it is more useful in painful conditions other than arthritis. The prolonged-release preparation of indomethacin sustains therapeutic drug concentrations up to 12 hours. Aspirin can sometimes be given two or three times daily, especially the prolonged-release preparations.

ADVERSE REACTIONS. NSAIDs have been associated with a broad spectrum of adverse reactions. Prolonged administration of large doses of these drugs, as in rheumatic disease, enhances the probability and potential severity of reactions. Indeed, NSAIDs account for approximately one-third of all adverse reactions reported to the Food and Drug Administration.

The most frequent or severe adverse reactions are gastrointestinal, dermatologic, renal, hepatic, hematologic, and immunologic in nature. Although such reactions have been associated with all NSAIDs, there are differences that often provide the basis for drug selection.

Gastrointestinal Reactions: These are the most common side effects caused by aspirin and other NSAIDs and are widely recognized as a serious problem. Prostaglandin-sparing agents, such as the nonacetylated salicylates (Roth, 1988) and the newer NSAID, nabumetone, appear to be associated with fewer peptic ulcers; however, similar claims have been made for several other NSAIDs. To date, there is no convincing evidence that any one NSAID produces fewer ulcers than another in clinical practice (Soll et al, 1991). In one case-control study, treatment with piroxicam was associated with a greater risk of perforation and hemorrhage of peptic ulcer than some other NSAIDs (eg, diclofenac, ketoprofen, sulindac) (Savage et al, 1993). Further controlled studies are required to confirm this finding. NSAIDs appear to both exacerbate existing peptic diathesis and cause new ulcers (Soll, 1992); however, there is poor correlation between gastrointestinal symptoms (eg, dyspepsia, abdominal pain) and the presence of ulcers or erosions.

The point prevalence of "ulcers" identified with surveillance endoscopy is 10% to 25%; however, only 1% to 4% of patients taking NSAIDs continuously for one year will develop clinically significant peptic ulcer disease. Results of a recent meta-analysis and nested case-control study indicate that the relative risk for its development is three to eight times higher among current users of NSAIDs (Griffin et al, 1991; Gabriel et al, 1991). Risk was increased during the first three months of therapy, in patients over 60 years, and in those receiving higher dosage or using corticosteroids concomitantly; additional risk factors suggested from other studies include smoking, alcohol use, and stress. Older age may constitute a special risk factor, not only because of the age-related loss of renal function, but because ulcers tend to be painless initially in the elderly; most fatal gastrointestinal events occur in this age group (Carson et al, 1987; Paulus, 1988; Griffin et al, 1988).

Although the absolute risk of gastrointestinal complications attributable to NSAIDs use is small, when the number of patients exposed annually is considered, NSAID use may account for over 70,000 hospitalizations and 7,600 deaths in patients with (probable) RA and osteoarthritis (Fries et al, 1989). FDA estimates of annual mortality that is NSAID-induced are even higher (Paulus, 1985).

The FDA now requires that the labeling on all NSAIDs indicate that "bleeding, ulcers, and perforations can occur at any time, with or without symptoms, in patients treated chronically." The labeling also must suggest that physicians inform the patient of these possible risks, including a potential fatal outcome, and be aware of alternative therapy.

The concomitant administration of antacids, sucralfate, [Carafate], or H_2 receptor blocking agents (eg, cimetidine [Tagamet], ranitidine [Zantac]) does not prevent aspirin- or other NSAID-induced ulcers (Soll et al, 1991). The prostaglandin analogue, misoprostol [Cytotec] may offer some protection for patients at risk for gastropathy (Graham et al, 1988, Roth et al, 1989), but periodic evaluation is still essential. Estimation of the benefit obtained from prophylaxis with misoprostol was based on the prevention of endoscopic lesions of uncertain clinical significance, not on the perforation or hemorrhage; efficacy has not been adequately tested in patients with a history of gastrointestinal disease (Soll et al, 1991). Nevertheless, prophylaxis with misoprostol may be indicated in high-risk, NSAID-dependent patients (eg, age over 60 years, history of ulcer disease, large NSAID dose, concomitant corticosteroid or anticoagulant use, those who are poor surgical risks or otherwise in poor health) (Soll et al, 1991; Gabriel, 1991). For additional information on the prophylaxis and treatment of NSAID-induced ulcers, see index entry Ulcer, Drug-induced.

Therapy with NSAIDs also increases the risk of esophageal strictures and may alter intestinal or bowel permeability.

Problems involving the lower gastrointestinal tract, particularly severe diarrhea and/or bleeding, are reported occasionally. Such patients should be evaluated for de novo or occult inflammatory bowel disease (Kaufmann and Taubin, 1987; Hochberg, 1989).

Central Nervous System Reactions: These have been observed with all NSAIDs and include dizziness, lightheadedness, drowsiness, headache, and confusion. Indomethacin causes headache in more than 10% of patients. Behavioral disturbances, such as depersonalization and depression, also have been reported occasionally with this drug. Aseptic meningitis has been reported rarely with ibuprofen, sulindac, and tolmetin, primarily in patients with systemic lupus erythematosus.

Dermatologic Reactions: Cutaneous effects occur with the use of NSAIDs; cited frequencies vary. These reactions are common with tolmetin, sulindac, naproxen, meclofenamate sodium, and piroxicam. Urticaria, exanthema, photosensitivity, and pruritus are reported most often. Toxic epidermal necrolysis and erythema multiforme have occurred. Rarely, rash may presage an anaphylactic reaction, which has been noted in a very small percentage of patients taking aspirin and even less often in those taking other NSAIDs.

Renal Reactions: The effects of NSAIDs on renal function probably are mediated by inhibition of renal prostaglandin synthesis. Prostaglandins participate in the autoregulation of renal blood flow and glomerular filtration and also inhibit the tubular transport of ions and water. In normal individuals, inhibition of prostaglandin synthesis does not significantly affect renal function; however, caution is warranted in patients at risk of compromised renal function, in whom prostaglandins are important in maintaining renal blood flow.

Renal reactions induced by NSAIDs include reversible decline of the glomerular filtration rate, edema, acute or chronic renal insufficiency or failure, nephrotic syndrome with interstitial nephritis, papillary necrosis, and hyperkalemia. All NSAIDs can impair renal function in patients at risk. Those with (1) renal impairment (eg, due to age, hypertension, atherosclerosis, or other chronic renal disease), (2) congestive heart failure or ascites, and (3) volume depletion (eg, sodium depletion, diuretic therapy, hypoalbuminemia) are more likely to experience drug-induced renal insufficiency.

Nephrotic syndrome (with acute interstitial nephritis) and acute tubular necrosis are rare; they have been reported most often with fenoprofen and probably represent an idiosyncratic reaction. Indomethacin and phenylbutazone have produced significant edema, especially in the lower extremities.

Hepatic Reactions: Hepatic dysfunction caused by aspirin and other NSAIDs occurs occasionally. Drug-related abnormalities in liver function tests (elevated levels of ALT, AST, and total bilirubin) have been produced most frequently by aspirin, especially in female patients with JRA, systemic lupus erythematosus, or other connective tissue disorders. The liver damage usually has been mild, reversible, and dose dependent. However, there is a slight risk of serious, acute liver injury associated with use of NSAIDs (Rodríguez et al, 1992). Predisposing factors include advanced age, impaired renal function, large doses, prolonged therapy, and coexistent viral illness.

A number of NSAIDs have been tested in animals for their effect on aminolevulinic acid synthase activity (McColl et al, 1987). The following drugs did not increase ALA synthase activity and are presumed to be well tolerated by patients with hepatic porphyria: aspirin, ibuprofen, indomethacin, ketoprofen, naproxen, and phenylbutazone.

Hematologic Reactions: Serious hematologic reactions are rare. All of these agents except the nonacetylated salicylates inhibit platelet aggregation, but only aspirin's effect is irreversible. Although very small, the risk of agranulocytosis and aplastic anemia is believed to be greatest with phenylbutazone. Aplastic anemia, agranulocytosis, and related blood dyscrasias have been reported rarely with other NSAIDs. Due to the low rate of occurrence (<1/100,000), it is not established whether treatment with other NSAIDs also increases the risk of blood dyscrasias.

Idiosyncratic Reactions: Aspirin and NSAIDs evoke two types of idiosyncratic reactions: bronchospasm with rhinoconjunctivitis and urticaria, angioedema, or both together. Such reactions are termed "aspirin intolerance" to differentiate them from immune-mediated phenomena. A history of adult-onset asthma, chronic rhinitis, nasal polyps, or chronic urticaria/angioedema predisposes to these reactions (see index entry Aspirin, Intolerance). Generally, cross sensitivity to other NSAIDs and the yellow food dye, tartrazine, occurs, and the administration of all NSAIDs and aspirin-containing medications is contraindicated in these patients. The nonacetylated salicylates can be given, with appropriate precautions, to these individuals (Roth, 1988).

Anaphylactoid reactions also have been reported after ingestion of aspirin or other NSAIDs (Manning et al, 1992).

These reactions usually occur within minutes of ingesting the drug and are characterized by hypotension, laryngeal edema, generalized pruritus, tachypnea, and lapses in consciousness; specific IgEs have not been demonstrated but, in contrast to those with intolerance to aspirin, there is a lack of cross reactivity between individual NSAIDs and aspirin and the need for prior sensitizing exposure.

Miscellaneous Side Effects: Tinnitus, hearing loss, blurred vision, taste dysfunction, tachycardia, and palpitations have been reported with the NSAIDs. See the evaluations on the individual drugs for more specific information.

PRECAUTIONS. Ingestion of medication with food or after meals can reduce gastrointestinal discomfort. When the patient has a history of or an active peptic ulcer, the benefits of an NSAID must be weighed carefully against the risks. All patients should be informed about the signs and symptoms of serious gastrointestinal toxicity and the steps to take if these occur.

Patients with atherosclerosis, hepatic cirrhosis (especially if ascites is present), or renal insufficiency and those receiving diuretic therapy concurrently require close monitoring. Additionally, the elderly usually have reduced renal function and should be monitored. In patients at risk, the BUN and creatinine levels should be determined at the initiation of therapy and the tests should be repeated at regular intervals during prolonged therapy. Proteinuria, hematuria, and cells and casts in the urine are important early signals of compromised renal function. Consideration should be given to reducing the dose in patients at risk.

Precautions should be taken to avoid hepatotoxicity. The ALT level appears to be the most sensitive indicator of liver function. Patients with signs or symptoms suggesting liver impairment should be evaluated further. If abnormal test results persist or worsen or if signs and symptoms of liver disease develop, the drug should be discontinued.

Because the NSAIDs impair platelet aggregation and prolong bleeding time, they should be used cautiously in patients with bleeding disorders. The presence of a bleeding disorder is a relative contraindication to the use of aspirin. Furthermore, aspirin should be discontinued seven to ten days prior to surgery. Most nonsteroidal drugs need not be stopped until 24 to 48 hours before surgery, but those with a long half-life (eg, piroxicam, oxaprozin, nabumetone) may need to be discontinued earlier. Serious consideration should be given to the potential for severe hematologic reactions.

If tinnitus or hearing loss occurs, the dose of the NSAID should be reduced.

Overdose of NSAIDs, other than the salicylates and phenylbutazone, rarely presents a serious problem (Court and Volans, 1984; Meredith and Vale, 1986). For specific information, see the evaluations on the individual drugs.

USE DURING PREGNANCY AND LACTATION. Although many women experience remission of RA during pregnancy, it may be necessary to continue medication for this and other arthritic conditions. The actions of these drugs on the fetus and neonate have been reviewed extensively (Byron, 1987). Large prospective studies indicate that salicylates do not produce fetal malformations, result in reduced birth weight, or increase perinatal mortality. Less data in humans are available for the other NSAIDs. There is no evidence of teratogenicity in animal studies for ibuprofen, flurbiprofen, naproxen, sulindac, diflunisal, diclofenac, or piroxicam.

Administration of aspirin and other salicylates or any of the other NSAIDs during the last six months of pregnancy may prolong gestation and labor. Aspirin is associated with greater blood loss at delivery and antepartum and postpartum hemorrhage. Its use within a few days of delivery has been associated with intracranial hemorrhage in the premature neonate. Exposure to the anti-inflammatory agents has caused persistent pulmonary hypertension in the newborn, with or without premature closure of the ductus arteriosus.

Although side effects with use of these drugs during breast feeding are uncommon, metabolic acidosis in infants has been reported with salicylates.

DRUG INTERACTIONS. Concomitant administration of NSAIDs and anticoagulants can produce significant adverse effects. The actions of anticoagulants may be enhanced by their displacement from plasma protein binding sites, increased prothrombin times, or inhibition of metabolism. It has been suggested that certain NSAIDs can be used with anticoagulants if appropriate precautions are taken, including measurement of prothrombin time daily for the first five days of combined therapy (Rodnan et al, 1983). However, all NSAIDs can damage the gastrointestinal mucosa and inhibit platelet aggregation, both of which increase the risk of gastrointestinal bleeding in patients receiving anticoagulants. Thus, all NSAIDs should be avoided in these patients when possible.

The hypoglycemic effect of the sulfonylureas may be enhanced by administration with salicylates or phenylbutazone. Displacement from plasma protein binding sites and inhibition of renal tubular secretion are the postulated mechanisms with salicylates; displacement from binding sites and inhibition of degradative metabolism may account for the interaction with phenylbutazone. Moderate to large doses of these drugs should be given cautiously to patients receiving oral hypoglycemic agents. Phenylbutazone also may inhibit the metabolism of phenytoin. Salicylates may inhibit the metabolism of valproate.

Antacids may alter the absorption and sometimes the disposition of a NSAID. Aspirin prolongs the half-life of penicillin G and inhibits the uricosuric effect of sulfinpyrazone [Anturane]. Indomethacin, and to a lesser extent other NSAIDs, inhibits the diuretic effect of furosemide and may decrease the antihypertensive activity of beta-blocking agents and ACE inhibitors. Patients receiving diuretics or other antihypertensive drugs should be monitored for clinical signs of fluid retention and have their blood pressure checked often if NSAIDs are used concomitantly.

The coadministration of diclofenac or ketoprofen with large doses of methotrexate has been reported to prolong and increase serum methotrexate concentrations (Thyss et al, 1986). In three of four patients observed with such increased concentrations, severe methotrexate toxicity resulted in death. These interactions with methotrexate also occur with salicylates and a number of other NSAIDs (Furst, 1988). The most serious responses developed with antineoplastic doses; thus, NSAIDs are contraindicated when large doses of methotrexate are being taken. There is little data to suggest that the concomitant use of NSAIDs with antirheumatic doses of methotrexate (ie, up to 15 mg per week) results in a meaningful increase in toxicity.

NSAIDs and lithium share a common excretory pathway in the proximal tubule, thereby diminishing lithium clearance; their concomitant administration, especially that of diclofenac, has resulted in lithium toxicity. Probenecid may reduce the metabolism and renal clearance of NSAIDs.

The potential for NSAIDs to cause renal dysfunction must be considered in patients receiving drugs that are eliminated primarily by the kidney and have a low therapeutic index (eg, digoxin, aminoglycosides). The risk of renal toxicity may be increased in patients also receiving diuretics or other drugs that are nephrotoxic (eg, cyclosporine). The combination of triamterene and indomethacin is contraindicated.

Administration of two NSAIDs together confers no additional benefit over the use of an individual agent.

Drug Evaluations

SALICYLATES

USES. The salicylates have a long history of efficacy in relieving pain and stiffness and improving routine task performance in patients with arthropathies. Of the salicylates, aspirin is the drug of choice in active RA, juvenile arthritis, and osteoarthritis. It is less effective in ankylosing spondylitis, Reiter's syndrome, and psoriatic arthritis.

Aspirin is used primarily for its anti-inflammatory effect in RA and must be administered in maximally tolerated doses; smaller doses, primarily for relief of pain, may be adequate in osteoarthritis.

Salsalate is the "pure" salicylate. Its double salicylate moiety uncouples only in the alkaline medium of the bowel. Thus, it bypasses an upper gastrointestinal tract susceptible to its irritating properties and is the only prodrug of the salicylate series (Roth, 1985). In a multicenter study comparing salsalate with aspirin in RA, the drugs were equally effective but salsalate was associated with fewer gastrointestinal disturbances and had the theoretical advantages of not affecting platelet function and of having less effect on prostaglandin-dependent renal function (Multicenter Salsalate/Aspirin Comparison Study Group, 1989).

ADVERSE REACTIONS AND PRECAUTIONS. Gastrointestinal disturbances are the most common adverse reactions. See discussion and FDA-mandated warning for gastrointestinal disturbances under Adverse Reactions in the section on Nonsteroidal Anti-Inflammatory Agents.

Reversible tinnitus, a feeling of fullness in the ear, and hearing loss are the most common initial signs of toxicity (salicylism) in adults and may help determine the maximal tolerated daily dose. However, they are not a reliable indication of toxicity in children or some elderly patients, who may not develop tinnitus even with large doses, or in patients with preexisting hearing impairment. The initial signs of overdosage in children and occasionally in adults include hyperventilation or episodic hyperpnea and lethargy. When initiating therapy, the dosage for children and elderly patients should be increased gradually and cautiously, and these patients should be observed closely for early signs of ototoxicity.

A very small percentage of patients are intolerant of aspirin and may develop an asthmatic-type reaction, which can be life-threatening (see index entry Aspirin, Intolerance). Patients sensitive to aspirin also are variably sensitive to other NSAIDs that inhibit prostaglandin synthesis; however, asthmatic-type reactions have not been associated with usual doses of nonacetylated salicylates.

Large doses of salicylates prolong prothrombin time, but this effect is clinically insignificant. Since aspirin (but not sodium salicylate or other nonacetylated salicylates) inhibits platelet aggregation irreversibly and prolongs bleeding time, it should be avoided in patients receiving heparin or coumarin anticoagulants and in those with bleeding disorders (eg, hemophilia).

Reversible, usually mild, hepatotoxicity has been associated with the large doses of aspirin given to children with juvenile arthritis and to adults with RA or systemic lupus erythematosus. The effect is dependent on salicylate blood concentrations (levels exceeding 25 mg/dL are likely to cause hepatic injury after one to four weeks of treatment), the disease state (eg, rheumatic or collagen disease), and pre-existing liver disease. Most patients remain asymptomatic; therefore, AST, ALT, alkaline phosphatase, and bilirubin should be measured periodically in patients with these conditions. Aspirin should not be used in those with severe liver disease.

Large doses of aspirin taken over extended periods rarely are associated with serious nephropathy; renal damage is more common in those with lupus erythematosus, who may have decreased creatinine clearance with elevated serum creatinine and blood urea nitrogen, or in those with active renal disease. Renal papillary necrosis has been reported in a few individuals.

Patients on a sodium-restricted diet should not be given sodium salicylate. Individuals with renal insufficiency may develop hypermagnesemia after use of magnesium salicylate.

DRUG INTERACTIONS. Since the renal clearance of salicylates is increased by corticosteroids, toxicity may occur when corticosteroids are discontinued in patients receiving large doses of salicylates concomitantly. The use of aspirin with another NSAID may reduce the anti-inflammatory action and increase gastrointestinal side effects.

A number of other drug interactions occur when salicylates are used concomitantly but do not affect their application in arthritis therapy. However, the following precautions should be observed. The uricosuric action of probenecid and sulfinpyrazone may be diminished by low doses of salicylates; however, high plasma concentrations of salicylates exert a uricosuric effect. The effectiveness of furosemide is reduced; the cardiac status of patients receiving furosemide for the management of congestive heart failure may worsen. The hypoglycemic action of some of the oral sulfonylureas is enhanced. Salicylates increase the toxicity of large doses (ie, cancer chemotherapy) of methotrexate by increasing its plasma concentration. Increased toxicity has not been demonstrated when low doses of methotrexate (<0.2 mg/kg/week) are used with salicylates in the treatment of RA.

CHRONIC INTOXICATION. Chronic aspirin overdosage is the result of accumulation of drug because of its nonlinear saturable elimination kinetics at higher doses. "Chronic salicylism" usually is detected when the patient complains of tinnitus, a sensation of fullness in the ears, and muffled hearing. These effects may be abolished within 24 hours by reducing the dose. Otic symptoms may not occur in patients with pre-existing hearing loss, in infants, in young children, or in the elderly. It is advisable to determine if tinnitus already is present before beginning a course of salicylate therapy.

In general, other symptoms of severe chronic overdosage are similar to those of acute overdosage, but hyperventilation, dehydration (particularly in children), acidosis, and CNS manifestations (agitation, hyperactivity, slurred speech, tremor, hallucinations, seizures, and coma) are encountered more frequently; nausea, vomiting, lethargy, and disorientation (particularly in elderly patients) occur with equal frequency but less often. At equivalent serum concentrations of salicylate in children, chronic salicylism produces greater morbidity than acute ingestion. For comprehensive reviews of acute and chronic salicylate intoxication, see Temple, 1981; Gaudreault et al, 1982; Lovejoy, 1987; and McGuigan, 1987.

For additional information on adverse reactions and interactions, see index entry Salicylates.

PHARMACOKINETICS. The pharmacokinetics of salicylates are complex. The half-life increases with dosage so that an increase in dose may produce a disproportionate increase in plasma drug levels. There is considerable individual variation in metabolism. See index entry Salicylates.

DOSAGE AND PREPARATIONS. The dose should be individualized and adjusted to the amount that produces an adequate anti-inflammatory effect. Blood salicylate concentration and therapeutic effect do not correlate well with dose. A plasma concentration greater than 15 mg/dL is usually required for efficacy; levels above 30 mg/dL are frequently toxic and should be avoided. If there is any uncertainty about the adequacy of dosage, toxicity, or patient compliance, salicylate concentrations should be determined. Because elevated doses of salicylate are associated with a prolonged half-life, 7 to 10 days are required after initiation or change in dosage to reach steady-state concentration.

Oral, Rectal: *Adults,* for RA, initially 2.4 to 3 g of aspirin or the equivalent salicylate daily in three or four divided doses. The total daily dose can be increased at the rate of one to two 300-mg tablets every one to two weeks until the desired therapeutic effect is attained or signs of toxicity appear. For osteoarthritis, doses usually can be reduced. For juvenile arthritis of pauciarticular or polyarticular onset, *children weighing 25 kg or less,* up to 100 mg/kg daily; *children weighing more than 25 kg,* 2.4 to 3.6 g daily. Larger doses may be required in those with the systemic (acute febrile) onset type. Since these doses may be toxic, it is advisable to start with two-thirds of the anticipated optimal dose and increase this amount gradually to attain plasma concentrations of 20 to 30 mg/dL.

Administration during meals and with a small meal at bedtime reduces gastrointestinal symptoms. Alternatively, a larger fraction of the daily dose may be given at bedtime or enteric-coated preparations may be used.

ASPIRIN:

NOTE: Because most manufacturers express dosage sizes of aspirin in grains rather than milligrams, the grain sizes with approximate milligram equivalents are given.

Generic. Tablets 5, 7 1/2, and 10 gr (325, 500, and 650 mg); tablets (buffered) 5 gr (325 mg); tablets (enteric-coated) 5, 7.5, 10, and 15 gr (325, 500, 650, and 975 mg); suppositories 1, 2, 3, 5, 10, and 20 gr (60, 120, 200, 300, and 600 mg and 1.2 g) (all forms nonprescription).

Arthritis Pain Formula (Whitehall). Tablets 500 mg with magnesium and aluminum hydroxide (nonprescription).

Ascriptin (Rhone-Poulenc Rorer). Tablets 325 mg with magnesium and aluminum hydroxide 100 mg or 150 mg (***Ascriptin A/D***) and 500 mg with magnesium and aluminum hydroxide and calcium carbonate 160 mg (***Ascriptin ES***) (nonprescription).

Bayer-8 Hour (Sterling). Tablets (prolonged-release) 650 mg (nonprescription).

Bufferin (Bristol-Myers). Tablets 324 mg with magnesium carbonate 97.2 mg and aluminum glycinate 48.6 mg (nonprescription).

Cama (Sandoz). Tablets 500 mg with magnesium oxide 150 mg and aluminum hydroxide 150 mg (nonprescription).

Easprin (Parke-Davis). Tablets (enteric-coated) 975 mg.

Ecotrin (SmithKline Beecham Consumer). Tablets (enteric-coated) 325 and 500 mg (nonprescription).

ZORprin (Boots). Tablets (prolonged-release) 800 mg.

SODIUM SALICYLATE:

Generic. Tablets (plain, enteric-coated) 325 and 650 mg (nonprescription).

CHOLINE SALICYLATE:

Arthropan (Purdue Frederick). Each 5 ml of liquid is equivalent in salicylate content to 870 mg of aspirin (nonprescription).

CHOLINE MAGNESIUM TRISALICYLATE:

Generic. Tablets 500, 750, and 1,000 mg.

Trilisate (Purdue Frederick), ***Tricosal*** (Duramed). Each tablet contains choline salicylate 293, 440, or 587 mg (***Trilisate*** only) and magnesium salicylate 362, 544, or 725 mg to provide 500, 750, or 1,000 mg (***Trilisate*** only) of salicylate; each 5 ml of liquid contains choline salicylate 293 mg and magnesium salicylate 362 mg to provide 500 mg of salicylate.

MAGNESIUM SALICYLATE:

Magan (Savage). Tablets 545 mg.

Mobidin (Ascher). Tablets 600 mg.

SALSALATE (Salicylsalicylic Acid):

Disalcid (3M Pharmaceuticals). Capsules 500 mg; tablets 500 and 750 mg.

Mono-Gesic (Central), ***Generic.*** Tablets 750 mg.

Salflex (Carnrick), ***Generic.*** Tablets 500 and 750 mg.

DIFLUNISAL

[Dolobid]

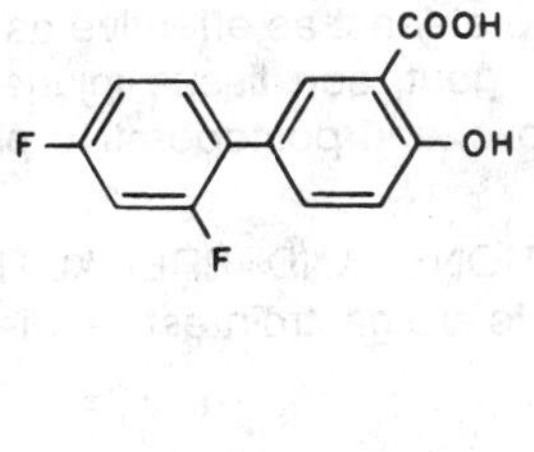

COOH

F — — OH

F

ACTIONS AND USES. Diflunisal is a fluoridated salicylic acid derivative. Like aspirin, it has analgesic, anti-inflammatory, and antipyretic activities and inhibits prostaglandin synthesis. This peripherally acting, nonopioid analgesic has a long duration of action. Diflunisal is effective in the symptomatic treatment of osteoarthritis and RA.

For other uses, see index entry Diflunisal, As Analgesic.

ADVERSE REACTIONS. Diflunisal is generally well tolerated. Gastrointestinal disturbances are the most common adverse reactions. See discussion and FDA-mandated warning for gastrointestinal disturbances under Adverse Reactions in the section on Nonsteroidal Anti-Inflammatory Agents. Acute renal failure and Stevens-Johnson syndrome have been reported. Cross sensitivity may occur in patients sensitive to aspirin.

Other adverse reactions are similar to those of the NSAIDs in general (see the Introduction on this section). For further information on adverse reactions, poisoning, and drug interactions, see index entry Diflunisal, As Analgesic.

Diflunisal is classified in FDA Pregnancy Category C.

PHARMACOKINETICS. Diflunisal is rapidly absorbed after oral administration; peak plasma concentrations occur one to three hours after ingestion (Verbeeck et al, 1983; Davies, 1983). Diflunisal exhibits dose-dependent kinetics; the elimination half-life ranges from 5 to 20 hours. Ingestion every 12 hours produces steady-state plasma levels within three to nine days. For further information, see index entry Diflunisal, As Analgesic.

DOSAGE AND PREPARATIONS.

Oral: *Adults*, for osteoarthritis and RA, 500 mg to 1 g daily in two divided doses. Dosage may be increased or decreased according to the patient's response. Maintenance doses should not exceed 1.5 g daily.

Dolobid (Merck). Tablets 250 and 500 mg.

DICLOFENAC SODIUM

[Voltaren]

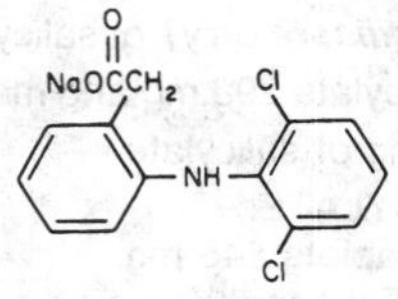

ACTIONS AND USES. This phenylacetic acid reduces production of prostaglandins, thromboxane, and leukotrienes and inhibits the release of arachidonic acid, the precursor of the prostaglandins.

Diclofenac is indicated for the treatment of RA, osteoarthritis, and the seronegative spondylarthropathies. Like other NSAIDs, it possesses analgesic, anti-inflammatory, and antipyretic activity. Results of investigational studies suggest that diclofenac would be at least as effective as other NSAIDs for the following: JRA, gout, soft tissue injuries, dysmenorrhea, renal and biliary colic, and postoperative pain (eg, following dental surgery).

ADVERSE REACTIONS AND PRECAUTIONS. The most common side effects are gastrointestinal disturbances, particularly abdominal pain, indigestion, nausea, and either diarrhea or constipation. See discussion and FDA-mandated warning for gastrointestinal disturbances under Adverse Reactions in the section on Nonsteroidal Anti-Inflammatory Agents.

The next most common adverse effects are headache, dizziness, and fluid retention. Because of the latter, care should be exercised in administering the drug to patients with heart failure or hypertension.

Elevations in one or more hepatic function tests, particularly ALT, may occur. In clinical trials, elevations of AST greater than three times the upper limit of normal occurred in 2% of diclofenac-treated patients. In one open trial, this degree of elevated ALT and/or AST appeared in about 4% of the patients, and elevations greater than eight times the upper limit of normal were observed in 1%. Rarely, the drug may precipitate overt hepatic failure. These results suggest a greater need for transaminase monitoring with diclofenac than with other NSAIDs. Since this adverse response is most likely to occur during the first two months of therapy, the manufacturer recommends that the first transaminase determination be made no later than eight weeks after initiation of therapy. Patients should be advised to notify their physician if they experience signs and symptoms that might indicate hepatotoxicity (nausea, fatigue, lethargy, pruritus, jaundice, right upper quadrant tenderness, or "flu-like" symptoms). Interestingly, diclofenac-associated transaminase elevations were found most frequently in patients with osteoarthritis. Since the drug can precipitate an acute exacerbation of hepatic porphyria, it should be avoided in patients with this genetic condition.

As with other NSAIDs, administration of diclofenac has been associated with dermatologic, renal, hematologic, idiosyncratic, and other miscellaneous reactions. For further information, see Adverse Reactions and Precautions in the section on Nonsteroidal Anti-Inflammatory Agents.

Diclofenac is classified in FDA Pregnancy Category B. In daily doses below 100 mg, diclofenac does not appear in the milk of nursing mothers, but it may be present at higher doses (Todd and Sorkin, 1988). It is recommended that nursing mothers requiring large amounts of NSAIDs not be given diclofenac.

OVERDOSAGE. The manufacturer of diclofenac has recorded 27 cases of overdose; all of these patients recovered. The highest overdose was 2.5 g in a 20-year-old man who developed transient renal failure, with recovery in two days following three dialysis sessions. The next highest dose was 2.35 g ingested by a 17-year-old woman who experienced vomiting and drowsiness.

DRUG INTERACTIONS. Most drug interactions involving diclofenac also occur with other NSAIDs (see the discussion under Drug Interactions in the section on Nonsteroidal Anti-Inflammatory Agents).

Diclofenac may alter the response to insulin or oral hypoglycemic agents, unpredictably enhancing or diminishing their activity. It is recommended that such patients have their blood glucose monitored more frequently until the effect, if any, is determined.

Aspirin has diminished the plasma concentration of diclofenac; their combined use is not recommended.

PHARMACOKINETICS. Diclofenac is well absorbed from the gastrointestinal tract, but about 40% to 50% of a dose is lost due to first-pass metabolism by the liver. Peak plasma concentrations occur in 10 to 30 minutes with an uncoated preparation (not commercially available) and, in fasting patients, in two to three hours with an enteric-coated preparation. More than 99.5% is bound to serum proteins, mostly albumin. The apparent volume of distribution is 0.12 to 0.55 L/kg.

Approximately 90% of a single dose of diclofenac is metabolized and excreted within 96 hours. The principal metabolite is 4′-hydroxydiclofenac, which possesses weak anti-inflammatory activity. The other metabolites are inactive. Only about 5% to 10% of conjugated but otherwise unchanged diclofenac is excreted by the kidney and less than 5% is excreted in the bile. Age, rheumatic disorders, or hepatic impairment does not appear to affect diclofenac pharmacokinetics. Dosage adjustment is not required in the presence of diminished renal function. Clearance is approximately 15.8 to 21 L/hr (Willis et al, 1979; manufacturer's literature, 1988). The elimination half-life is two to three hours.

DOSAGE AND PREPARATIONS.

Oral: *Adults,* for osteoarthritis, 50 mg two or three times daily or 75 mg twice daily; for RA, 50 mg three or four times daily or 75 mg twice daily. For ankylosing spondylitis, the manufacturer recommends 25 mg four times daily with an additional 25 mg at bedtime if necessary; alternatively, the same dosage schedule as that for osteoarthritis may be used. *Children,* dosage has not been established.

Voltaren (Geigy). Tablets (enteric-coated) 25, 50, and 75 mg.

ETODOLAC

[Lodine]

ACTIONS AND USES. Like other NSAIDs, etodolac inhibits prostaglandin synthesis at the cyclo-oxygenase level. The marketed preparation is a racemic mixture of R- and S-etodolac. As with other NSAIDs, the S-form is biologically active but the R-form is not. Both enantiomers are stable, and there is no R-to-S conversion in vivo.

This NSAID is indicated for acute and long-term use in the management of osteoarthritis and also is used as a general purpose analgesic. Although it is not indicated for the treatment of RA, etodolac appeared to be as effective as other NSAIDs in the treatment of this disease in several clinical trials (Jacob et al, 1986; Waltham-Weeks, 1987; Balfour and Buckley, 1991).

In early studies, etodolac was reported to be as effective as aspirin for the treatment of osteoarthritis and was better tolerated (Sanda et al, 1983; Andelman et al, 1983). The results of double-blind, randomized clinical trials in patients with osteoarthritis of the knee indicated that etodolac 600 mg/day was equivalent to piroxicam 20 mg/day or diclofenac 150 mg/day in relieving symptoms (Platt, 1989). In another double-blind study on similar patients, etodolac 300 mg twice daily was more effective than indomethacin 50 mg three times daily (Karbowski, 1991).

ADVERSE REACTIONS AND PRECAUTIONS. The most frequently reported adverse effects are abdominal pain and dyspepsia. It is not known whether etodolac is less likely to cause serious gastrointestinal bleeding than other NSAIDs used to treat osteoarthritis. There is a serious risk of gastrointestinal ulceration, bleeding, and perforation with NSAID therapy that can occur at any time with or without premonitory symptoms in patients receiving long-term therapy. See discussion and FDA-mandated warning for gastrointestinal disturbances under Adverse Reactions in the section on Nonsteroidal Anti-Inflammatory Agents.

Borderline elevations in the results of one or more liver tests may occur in up to 15% of patients; meaningful elevations of ALT or AST have been reported in only 1% of patients. Patients receiving etodolac may have a false-positive urine test for bilirubin due to the presence of phenolic metabolites of the drug.

As with other NSAIDs, administration of etodolac has been associated with dermatologic, renal, hematologic, central nervous system, idiosyncratic, and other miscellaneous reactions. For further information, see Adverse Reactions and Precautions in the section on Nonsteroidal Anti-Inflammatory Agents.

No adequate studies with etodolac have been performed in pregnant women. NSAIDs affect parturition and the fetal cardiovascular system (closure of the ductus arteriosus). Consequently, etodolac should be used during pregnancy only if the expected benefits justify the potential risk to the fetus (FDA Pregnancy Category C). Its effects on labor and delivery are not known. It also is not known whether etodolac is secreted in human milk. The safety and efficacy of the drug in children have not been established.

OVERDOSAGE. Symptoms following acute NSAID overdose are generally limited to lethargy, drowsiness, nausea, vomiting, and epigastric pain; these are usually reversible with supportive care. There are no specific antidotes for etodolac overdosage; patients should be managed with symptomatic and supportive care.

DRUG INTERACTIONS. When administered with aspirin, the protein binding of etodolac is reduced, although the clearance of the free drug is not altered.

All NSAIDs can damage the gastrointestinal mucosa and inhibit platelet aggregation, both of which increase the risk of gastrointestinal bleeding in patients receiving anticoagulants. Administration of warfarin with etodolac results in reduced protein binding of the anticoagulant, but there is no change in the clearance of free warfarin or in its pharmacodynamic effects on prothrombin time; thus, no dosage adjustment of either drug should be required, but regular monitoring of the prothrombin time after initiation of etodolac therapy should be and warfarin should be avoided if possible.

Interactions between etodolac and drugs eliminated by renal excretion are similar to those reported for other NSAIDs, and administration of etodolac has the same potential for other drug interactions as other NSAIDs. For further information, see the discussion under Drug Interactions in the section on Nonsteroidal Anti-Inflammatory Agents.

PHARMACOKINETICS. Etodolac is well absorbed and does not undergo significant first-pass metabolism. After oral administration, bioavailability is about 80%. Peak concentrations are proportional to the dose for both total and free drug when amounts up to 400 mg are given every 12 hours; with a 600-mg dose, the peak is approximately 20% higher than anticipated on the basis of lower doses. The plasma levels achieved after recommended doses vary considerably among subjects. Food intake reduces the peak concentration by about 50% and increases the time to peak concentration by 1.4 to 3.8 hours. Antacids decrease the peak concentration by about 20% but have no effect on the time to peak concentration.

Etodolac is >99% bound to plasma proteins. The drug is extensively metabolized in the liver. About 72% of a dose is recovered in the urine, principally as metabolites, and about 16% is excreted in the feces. The terminal elimination half-life is 7.3 ± 4 hours.

DOSAGE AND PREPARATIONS.

Oral: For osteoarthritis, *adults,* initially, 800 mg to 1.2 g/day given in divided doses. For maintenance, the dose ranges from 600 mg to 1.2 g/day given in divided amounts. For acute pain, *adults,* 200 to 400 mg every six to eight hours as needed. (For specific details on individualization of dosage, see the manufacturer's literature.) The total daily dose should not exceed 1.2 g (20 mg/kg for patients weighing ≤60 kg).

Lodine (Wyeth-Ayerst). Capsules 200 and 300 mg.

FENOPROFEN CALCIUM

[Nalfon]

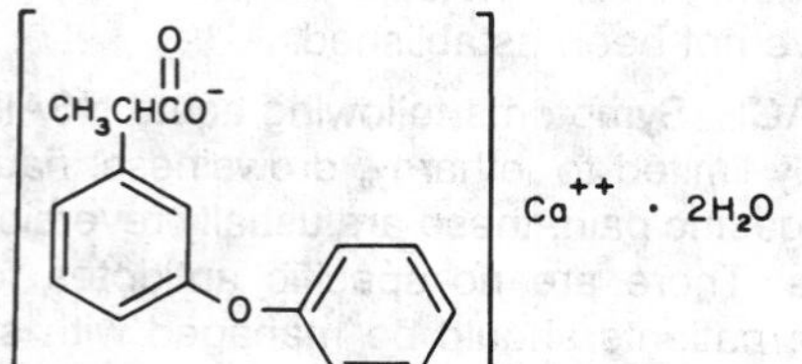

CH_3CHCO^- (O) ... $]_2$ $Ca^{++} \cdot 2H_2O$

ACTIONS AND USES. Fenoprofen is chemically and pharmacologically similar to ibuprofen. It is effective as initial therapy or as an alternative to aspirin in RA and osteoarthritis. Results of comparative studies in patients with RA indicated that fenoprofen 2.4 g/day was approximately equivalent to aspirin 3.9 g/day. In osteoarthritis, the benefit of fenoprofen 1.2 to 1.8 g/day was similar to that obtained with aspirin 2 to 3 g. Fenoprofen relieved symptoms in a few patients with ankylosing spondylitis, but additional studies are needed to establish its comparative efficacy in this condition. Fenoprofen may prove useful as alternative therapy in psoriatic or gouty arthritis and Reiter's syndrome.

ADVERSE REACTIONS AND PRECAUTIONS. The most common adverse reactions are gastrointestinal disturbances (eg, dyspepsia, constipation, nausea, vomiting). See discussion and FDA-mandated warning for gastrointestinal disturbances under Adverse Reactions in the section on Nonsteroidal Anti-Inflammatory Agents.

Fenoprofen has produced nephrotic syndrome with interstitial nephritis. Because the reaction is idiosyncratic, it is not possible to predict patients at risk. The syndrome can occur days or months following institution of therapy. There is evidence that it is the result of disordered T-lymphocyte function (Stachura et al, 1983).

As with other NSAIDs, administration of fenoprofen has been associated with other renal, dermatologic, hepatic, hematologic, neurologic, idiosyncratic, and miscellaneous reactions. For further information, see Adverse Reactions and Precautions and Use During Pregnancy and Lactation in the section on Nonsteroidal Anti-Inflammatory Agents.

OVERDOSE. Overdosage (0.3 to 3 g in children, 2 to 15 g in adults) with fenoprofen is rare and symptoms usually are mild. Manifestations include hypotension, tachycardia, and difficulty in breathing. Two cases of severe toxicity have been reported. Gastric lavage, activated charcoal, and a cathartic produced a favorable response in one patient. In the other, hypothermia, coma, and respiratory depression culminated in fatal cardiac arrest (Court and Volans, 1984).

DRUG INTERACTIONS. Aspirin enhances the metabolic clearance of fenoprofen, thus reducing plasma concentrations of the drug. See the discussion under Drug Interactions in the section on Nonsteroidal Anti-Inflammatory Agents for other potential drug interactions involving fenoprofen.

PHARMACOKINETICS. Fenoprofen is rapidly absorbed after oral administration, and peak plasma levels occur within 90 minutes. Absorption and availability are not affected by the concomitant administration of antacids containing aluminum and magnesium. Fenoprofen is highly bound (more than 99%) to plasma protein; thus, at therapeutic concentrations, significant amounts do not appear in breast milk, amniotic fluid, cord blood, or saliva. Vd is 0.08 to 0.1 L/kg. The drug is almost completely metabolized, primarily to glucuronide conjugates; small amounts of a hydroxylated metabolite (4-hydroxyprofen) are formed. The elimination half-life is two to three hours. Metabolites are excreted by the kidney; small amounts of unchanged drug are recovered in the feces.

DOSAGE AND PREPARATIONS.

Oral: *Adults,* for RA or osteoarthritis, 300 to 600 mg three or four times daily. Total daily dosage should not exceed 3.2 g. After a satisfactory response is obtained, the dose is adjusted to the patient's needs. If gastrointestinal reactions occur, fenoprofen may be given with meals. *Children,* dosage has not been established.

Nalfon (Dista), ***Generic.*** Capsules 200 and 300 mg; tablets 600 mg (strengths expressed in terms of the base).

FLURBIPROFEN

[Ansaid]

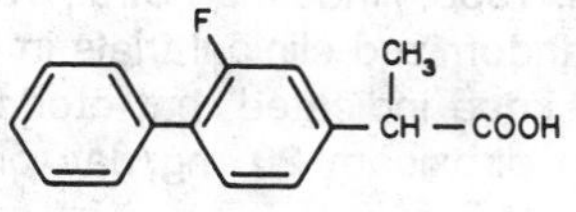

F CH_3 CH — COOH

ACTIONS AND USES. This phenylpropionic acid derivative is related chemically to ibuprofen, fenoprofen, and ketoprofen and is effective as initial therapy or as an alternative to salicylates or other NSAIDs for the symptomatic management of RA and osteoarthritis. In addition to its anti-inflammatory activity, flurbiprofen possesses antipyretic and analgesic properties but is labeled only for RA and osteoarthritis.

In controlled studies, flurbiprofen 100 mg twice a day was equivalent to naproxen 250 mg twice a day in RA (Brown et al, 1986 A) and 50 mg twice a day was equivalent to sulindac 150 mg twice a day in osteoarthritis (Brown et al, 1986 B).

ADVERSE REACTIONS AND PRECAUTIONS. The most common complaints are indigestion, nausea, diarrhea, and abdominal pain. See discussion and FDA-mandated warning for gastrointestinal disturbances under Adverse Reactions in the section on Nonsteroidal Anti-Inflammatory Agents.

As with other NSAIDs, administration of flurbiprofen has been associated with renal, hepatic, dermatologic, hematologic, neurologic, idiosyncratic, and miscellaneous reactions. Renal papillary necrosis induced by flurbiprofen has been reported (Nafria et al, 1991). Relatively common miscellaneous adverse effects include headache, blurred vision, signs and symptoms suggesting urinary tract infection, and dermatitis. Borderline elevations of hepatic transaminase concentrations may occur in up to 15% of patients; these may progress, remain unchanged, or disappear with continued medication. For further information, see Adverse Reactions and Precautions in the section on Nonsteroidal Anti-Inflammatory Agents.

This drug is classified in FDA Pregnancy Category B. Since it is excreted in breast milk, flurbiprofen is not recommended for use in nursing mothers.

OVERDOSE. The manufacturer's literature (1988) indicates that overdosage has been reported in 13 children and 12 adults. Nine of the 13 children were below age 6. Drowsiness occurred after ingestion of 150 to 800 mg in three of the children; mydriasis occurred in one, and a 2-year-old became semiconscious and had miosis, diminished muscle tone, and elevated hepatic transaminases. The remaining children, who ingested 200 mg to 2.5 g, remained asymptomatic.

Dizziness, drowsiness, headache, nausea, epigastric pain, coma, and respiratory depression have occurred after ingestion of 3 to 6 g in adults. Many of the adult case reports also involved the ingestion of alcohol or other drugs.

DRUG INTERACTIONS. Concurrent administration of aspirin and flurbiprofen reduces the serum concentration of the latter by 50%; thus, combination therapy is not recommended. Pretreatment with cimetidine slightly decreases the systemic clearance of flurbiprofen. See the discussion under Drug Interactions in the section on Nonsteroidal Anti-Inflammatory Agents for other potential drug interactions involving flurbiprofen.

PHARMACOKINETICS. Flurbiprofen is well absorbed following oral administration; a peak serum concentration is attained in about 1.5 hours. The drug is 99% bound to plasma proteins. It undergoes metabolic oxidation in the liver to form at least three different intermediates hydroxylated on the unsubstituted phenyl ring. These, along with unchanged flurbiprofen, then are eliminated by the kidney, mostly as sulfate and glucuronide conjugates (Kaiser et al, 1986). The elimination half-life is 5.7 hours and does not differ appreciably with age. The pharmacokinetics of flurbiprofen in patients with hepatic disease have not been assessed.

DOSAGE AND PREPARATIONS.

Oral: *Adults,* for RA and osteoarthritis, 200 to 300 mg daily in two to four divided doses. Individual doses should not exceed 100 mg, and a total daily dose above 300 mg is not recommended.

Ansaid (Upjohn). Tablets 50 and 100 mg.

IBUPROFEN

[Children's Advil Suspension, Motrin, PediaProfen, Rufen]

$$CH_3CHCH_2(CH_3)\text{—}C_6H_4\text{—}CH(CH_3)COOH$$

ACTIONS AND USES. Ibuprofen is a phenylpropionic acid derivative with analgesic, anti-inflammatory, and antipyretic actions. Like aspirin and other NSAIDs, it inhibits prostaglandin synthesis. Ibuprofen is effective for the symptomatic treatment of RA and osteoarthritis and has been reported to be useful in ankylosing spondylitis and gouty and psoriatic arthritis. It also may be useful as an alternative agent in Reiter's syndrome.

In RA, ibuprofen is as effective as aspirin, piroxicam, indomethacin, and tolmetin. It may be administered with maintenance doses of gold salts for additional symptomatic relief and also may be given with corticosteroids.

In osteoarthritis, therapeutic doses of ibuprofen are as effective as aspirin, aspirin and acetaminophen, sulindac, and indomethacin.

ADVERSE REACTIONS AND PRECAUTIONS. The overall incidence of adverse reactions is low, and ibuprofen appears to be one of the better-tolerated NSAIDs. The most common reactions are nausea and vomiting; diarrhea, constipation, heartburn, and epigastric pain occur less frequently. See discussion and FDA-mandated warning for gastrointestinal disturbances under Adverse Reactions in the section on Nonsteroidal Anti-Inflammatory Agents.

Central nervous system reactions reported occasionally include dizziness, lightheadedness, and headache. Aseptic meningitis has been reported rarely, primarily in patients with underlying connective tissue disorders. Maculopapular, erythematous, or urticarial rashes and generalized pruritus also have occurred.

Toxic amblyopia, characterized by reduced visual acuity and difficulty in color discrimination, has been observed in a few patients. Although a definite cause-and-effect relationship was not established, the symptoms disappeared after ibuprofen was discontinued. Ophthalmologic examination of numerous patients did not reveal similar visual disturbances. Nevertheless, patients receiving ibuprofen should have a complete ophthalmologic examination if they experience any visual disturbances.

As with other NSAIDs, administration of ibuprofen has been associated with hepatic, renal, idiosyncratic, and miscellaneous reactions. Meaningful (three times the upper limit of normal) elevations of serum transaminases occurred in less than 1% of patients in controlled clinical trials. Hyperuricemia has occurred sporadically. For further information, see Adverse Reactions and Precautions in the section on Nonsteroidal Anti-Inflammatory Agents.

There is no evidence that ibuprofen has any teratogenic effect in rabbits and rats. However, since this agent was found in the fetal circulation of animals after administration to the mothers during late pregnancy, it appears to cross the placenta. Ibuprofen was not detectable in the breast milk of human mothers taking 2 g daily (Townsend et al, 1984). Nevertheless, administration of ibuprofen is not recommended during pregnancy or lactation.

OVERDOSE. More than 100 cases of overdosage have been reported; the estimated intake varied from 1.2 g in children to 16 g in an adult. Symptoms included dizziness, nystagmus, apnea, unconsciousness, and hypotension. The latter may be alleviated by administration of fluid. Most patients recovered with no apparent sequelae. No deaths from overdosage have been reported when ibuprofen was the sole drug ingested in a single dose. No specific antidote is known; standard supportive treatment should be instituted. The stomach should be emptied by induced vomiting or lavage, activated charcoal instilled, and urine output maintained.

DRUG INTERACTIONS. Measurements of clotting function were not affected when doses up to 2.4 g/day of ibuprofen were given to patients receiving warfarin sodium, but larger amounts may displace warfarin from protein binding sites. Ibuprofen may be one of the least hazardous NSAIDs for concurrent use with anticoagulants (Hansten, 1983).

The concomitant administration of single doses of ibuprofen and aspirin had no effect on the availability or elimination of either drug; however, multiple doses of these drugs decreased blood levels of ibuprofen. See the discussion under Drug Interactions in the section on Nonsteroidal Anti-Inflammatory Agents for other potential drug interactions involving ibuprofen.

PHARMACOKINETICS. See index entry Ibuprofen, As Analgesic-Antipyretic.

DOSAGE AND PREPARATIONS.

Oral: *Adults,* for RA and osteoarthritis, including flare-ups of chronic disease, 1.2 to 3.2 g daily in divided doses. Because of variability in response, the optimal dose for each patient must be individualized. Daily dosage should not exceed 3.2 g. The dosage for osteoarthritis may be smaller than that for RA. *Children*, for juvenile arthritis, 30 to 40 mg/kg/day divided into three or four doses.

Children's Advil Suspension (Wyeth-Ayerst), ***PediaProfen*** (McNeil Consumer). Suspension 100 mg/5 ml.

Motrin (Upjohn), ***Generic.*** Tablets 300, 400, 600, and 800 mg.

Rufen (Boots). Tablets 400, 600, and 800 mg.

INDOMETHACIN
[Indocin]

CH_3O — CH_2COOH — CH_3 — N — C=O — Cl

ACTIONS AND USES. Indomethacin is a NSAID of the indole group with analgesic, anti-inflammatory, and antipyretic effects. Like aspirin and other NSAIDs, indomethacin inhibits prostaglandin synthesis; other actions (eg, interference with migration of leukocytes, inhibition of phosphodiesterase) may contribute to its anti-inflammatory effect.

Because of its potential to cause severe adverse effects, this agent is not recommended as a simple analgesic or antipyretic. Indomethacin is the drug of choice in the treatment of ankylosing spondylitis and should be considered for initial use in Reiter's syndrome. It also is useful as an anti-inflammatory agent in moderate to severe RA and osteoarthritis, particularly of the hands, hips, knees, and shoulders. It may be effective as an alternative agent in the treatment of psoriatic arthritis. The prolonged-release formulation is comparable to the other formulations in efficacy and patient tolerance, and it offers the advantage of once- or twice-daily dosing. Indomethacin is used to treat attacks of acute gouty arthritis, but the prolonged-release preparation should not be used for this indication. (See the evaluation in the section on Gout and Hyperuricemia.) Indomethacin also is effective in bursitis, tendinitis, and traumatic synovitis.

ADVERSE REACTIONS. Gastrointestinal disturbances (nausea, vomiting, abdominal distress, indigestion, epigastric burning, constipation, diarrhea) have been observed in 3% to 9% of patients and may be lessened by giving the drug with food. The frequency of gastrointestinal and other side effects is similar with comparable doses of the regular and prolonged-release preparations (Rhymer et al, 1982). See discussion and FDA-mandated warning for gastrointestinal disturbances under Adverse Reactions in the section on Nonsteroidal Anti-Inflammatory Agents.

Central nervous system effects (headaches, vertigo, dizziness, somnolence, depression, and fatigue) are common. Headaches occur in more than 10% of patients and are usually severe in the morning; if they persist, treatment should be discontinued. Convulsions, peripheral neuropathy, lightheadedness, syncope, confusion, coma, and behavioral disturbances, such as depersonalization, also have been reported occasionally.

Ocular complications (corneal deposits and retinal disturbances) have been observed after prolonged use of indomethacin. A thorough ophthalmologic examination is required if blurred vision develops. Tinnitus occurs commonly, but deafness is infrequent.

As with other NSAIDs, renal, hepatic, hematologic, and dermatologic reactions may occur in association with the use of indomethacin. For further information, see Adverse Reactions and Precautions in the section on Nonsteroidal Anti-Inflammatory Agents.

PRECAUTIONS AND CONTRAINDICATIONS. Indomethacin is contraindicated in pregnant women, nursing mothers, and children 14 years and under, since safe conditions for use in these individuals have not been established. The drug also is contraindicated in patients with active gastrointestinal lesions or a history of recurrent gastrointestinal lesions. Indomethacin should be used with caution in the elderly and in those with epilepsy, parkinsonism, or emotional or psychiatric problems, since it may aggravate these conditions.

OVERDOSE. Overdose (75 to 175 mg in children, 175 mg to 1.5 g in adults) is manifested by drowsiness, gastric irritation, nausea, headache, feelings of dissociation, and tinnitus. Sixty-one percent of patients remained asymptomatic after taking up to 2.5 g (Court and Volans, 1984). The elimination half-life is not prolonged with overdose.

DRUG INTERACTIONS. The plasma concentration of indomethacin may be increased by the concomitant administration of probenecid; thus, lower doses of indomethacin may be used in patients receiving both drugs. The combination of triamterene and indomethacin impaired renal function in healthy subjects (Favre et al, 1982). See the discussion under Drug Interactions in the section on Nonsteroidal Anti-Inflammatory Agents for other potential drug interactions involving indomethacin.

PHARMACOKINETICS. Indomethacin is rapidly and almost completely absorbed after oral administration. About 90% of a dose is bound to plasma proteins. Indomethacin is metabolized in the liver by demethylation, deacetylation, and glucuronide conjugation; the metabolites and unchanged drug are excreted in the bile and urine. About 60% of the dose is recovered in the urine and 33% in the feces.

Absorption is slower when the drug is taken with meals, but the extent of absorption is not affected. The half-life of indomethacin is 5 to 10 hours (Helleberg, 1981), but there is marked inter- and intraindividual variation (Verbeeck et al, 1983). This variation is due to extensive enterohepatic recycling through excretion of the glucuronide metabolite in the bile followed by reabsorption of indomethacin after hydrolysis (Yeh, 1982).

Bioavailability studies on the prolonged-release preparation (containing 75 mg of the drug, of which 25 mg is released immediately) showed that there is a statistically significant reduction (55%) in peak plasma concentration and significantly less variation in plasma concentrations.

DOSAGE AND PREPARATIONS.

Oral: For ankylosing spondylitis, osteoarthritis, and RA, *adults,* initially, 25 mg two or three times daily. If well tolerated, the daily dose may be increased by 25 or 50 mg at weekly intervals until a maximum of 150 to 200 mg daily is reached. The 200-mg maximal dose should be reserved for patients of large stature. Some patients may respond in four to six days while others require up to one month of therapy. In acute exacerbations, it may be necessary to increase the daily dose by 25 or 50 mg. After the acute phase is controlled, the daily dose should be reduced until the smallest effective amount is given or the drug can be discontinued.

For painful shoulder (bursitis, tendinitis), 25 mg three or four times daily, usually for 7 to 14 days. After the signs and symptoms of inflammation have been controlled for several days, the drug should be discontinued.

The prolonged-release preparation can be taken once daily to sustain plasma concentrations comparable to those obtained with 25 mg three times daily. In addition, one prolonged-release capsule taken in the morning and one in the evening were as effective as the conventional 50-mg capsule taken three times daily.

Indocin (Merck), ***Generic.*** Capsules 25 and 50 mg; capsules (prolonged-release) 75 mg (***Indocin SR***); suspension 25 mg/5 ml.

Rectal: *Adults,* 50 mg up to four times daily; *children,* 1.5 to 2 mg/kg daily administered in divided doses up to a maximum of 4 mg/kg/day or 150 to 200 mg/day, whichever is less.

Indocin (Merck). Suppositories 50 mg.

KETOPROFEN

[Orudis]

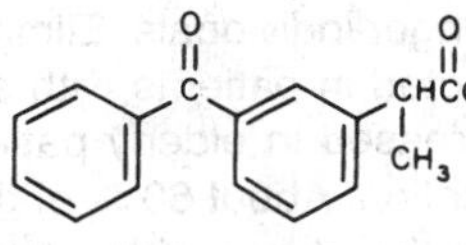

ACTIONS AND USES. Ketoprofen is a propionic acid derivative with analgesic, anti-inflammatory, and antipyretic actions. It is effective for the treatment of RA, ankylosing spondylitis, acute gout, and osteoarthritis. As with other NSAIDs, the therapeutic effects of ketoprofen are thought to be mediated, at least in part, by inhibition of prostaglandin synthesis.

ADVERSE REACTIONS AND PRECAUTIONS. The most common adverse reactions are dyspepsia, nausea, vomiting, abdominal pain, headache, dizziness, tinnitus, visual disturbance, rash, and impairment of renal function. See discussion and FDA-mandated warning for gastrointestinal disturbances under Adverse Reactions in the section on Nonsteroidal Anti-Inflammatory Agents.

As with other NSAIDs, hepatic, hematologic, dermatologic, idiosyncratic, and other miscellaneous reactions have occurred in association with the use of ketoprofen. For further information, see Adverse Reactions and Precautions in the section on Nonsteroidal Anti-Inflammatory Agents.

Studies in rats and rabbits have not demonstrated teratogenic effects. However, since studies in animals do not always predict the occurrence of teratogenicity in humans, ketoprofen should be used only when the risk justifies the benefit. This drug is classified in FDA Pregnancy Category B. Data on the concentration of ketoprofen in human breast milk are not available, but this drug is not recommended for use in nursing mothers.

OVERDOSE. Only mild symptoms have been observed in the 20 patients who received an overdose of ketoprofen. Vomiting and drowsiness were most prominent in four of these patients. One individual ingested 5 g without sequelae. Supportive measures should be instituted. The stomach should be emptied by induced vomiting or lavage followed by instillation of activated charcoal. Since the drug undergoes significant enterohepatic circulation, serial doses of activated charcoal may be indicated.

DRUG INTERACTIONS. The concomitant administration of ketoprofen and aspirin decreased the protein binding and increased the clearance of ketoprofen from plasma. Although the clinical significance of this interaction has not been established, these two drugs should not be used together. See the discussion under Drug Interactions in the section on Nonsteroidal Anti-Inflammatory Agents for other potential drug interactions involving ketoprofen.

PHARMACOKINETICS. Ketoprofen is rapidly absorbed following oral administration; peak plasma concentrations occur in 0.5 to 2 hours. When ketoprofen is taken immediately after meals, its absorption is delayed but the total amount absorbed is not affected. The drug is highly bound (99%) to plasma protein. Following absorption, the parent compound and hydroxylated metabolites and their respective glucuronides appear in plasma.

The mean elimination half-life is five hours in the elderly and three hours in younger individuals. Elimination of ketoprofen is relatively unaffected in patients with alcoholic cirrhosis but is moderately decreased in elderly patients and in those with impaired renal function. About 60% of the dose is excreted in urine primarily as the glucuronide metabolite.

DOSAGE AND PREPARATIONS.

Oral: *Adults,* for RA and osteoarthritis, initially, 75 mg three times daily or 50 mg four times daily. Minor side effects may be relieved by using a lower dose, which may produce an adequate therapeutic effect. If the drug is well tolerated, the dose may be increased to a maximum of 300 mg daily.

Elderly patients and those with impaired renal function, the dose should be reduced by one-half with further adjustments guided by response (Williams and Upton, 1988).

Orudis (Wyeth-Ayerst). Capsules 25, 50, and 75 mg.

MECLOFENAMATE SODIUM MONOHYDRATE

[Meclomen]

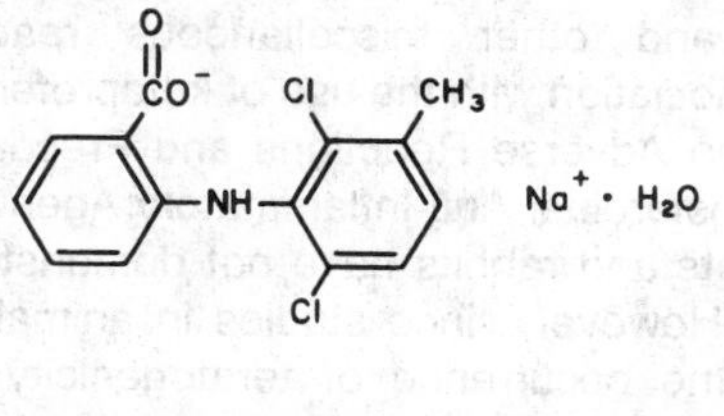

ACTIONS AND USES. This halogenated anthranilic acid derivative is related chemically to mefenamic acid. Both compounds have analgesic, anti-inflammatory, and antipyretic activities, but meclofenamate had a more potent anti-inflammatory effect in animal studies. Like aspirin and other NSAIDs, meclofenamate inhibits prostaglandin synthesis; it also competes for binding at prostaglandin receptor sites. These actions probably significantly influence its clinical effects. In several controlled studies, meclofenamate was effective in the symptomatic treatment of RA and osteoarthritis.

ADVERSE REACTIONS AND PRECAUTIONS. Gastrointestinal reactions were reported most frequently. Diarrhea occurred in 10% to 33% of patients and was severe enough to require discontinuation of treatment in about 4%. This adverse reaction is most likely to occur early in therapy and usually is reversible when the dose is reduced. Nausea with or without vomiting occurred in about 10% and abdominal pain in about 7% of patients. Less common gastrointestinal reactions include pyrosis and flatulence. Symptoms usually can be controlled by reducing the dose or temporarily discontinuing therapy. See discussion and FDA-mandated warning for gastrointestinal disturbances under Adverse Reactions in the section on Nonsteroidal Anti-Inflammatory Agents.

The incidence of central nervous system reactions, such as headache and dizziness, was less than with indomethacin. The incidence of rashes of various types was about the same as with aspirin (4%).

The hematocrit, hemoglobin, and erythrocyte count decreased in about 10% of patients, but discontinuation of the drug was rarely required. Low white cell counts were observed rarely. The relationship between these changes and administration of the drug is not understood. If anemia is suspected in patients receiving long-term therapy, hemoglobin and hematocrit values should be determined. In contrast to aspirin, meclofenamate did not prolong bleeding time or reduce collagen-induced platelet aggregation after repeated administration.

Increased serum alkaline phosphatase, transaminases, creatinine, and blood urea nitrogen levels occurred occasionally but usually returned to normal even when administration of the drug was continued.

Meclofenamate should not be used during pregnancy because there is no experience with its use in pregnant women. Some fetotoxicity, but no major teratogenicity, was observed in animals.

OVERDOSE. Overdose may produce central nervous system stimulation marked by agitation and generalized seizures. Renal toxicity, manifested by oliguria, anuria, or azotemia, may follow. Management includes induced emesis or lavage and instillation of activated charcoal into the stomach. Intravenous diazepam (adults, 5 to 10 mg; children, 0.1 to 0.3 mg/kg), if necessary, can be given to manage prolonged or repetitive seizures.

DRUG INTERACTIONS. When meclofenamate was administered to patients already receiving warfarin sodium, the dose of warfarin had to be reduced. Prothrombin time should be monitored during simultaneous use, which should be avoided if possible.

The concomitant administration of aspirin and meclofenamate decreased the plasma level of the latter drug, but the plasma salicylate concentration was not affected. Meclofenamate did not affect the uricosuric action of sulfinpyrazone when the two drugs were given together. See the discussion under Drug Interactions in the section on Nonsteroidal Anti-

Inflammatory Agents for other potential drug interactions involving meclofenamate.

PHARMACOKINETICS. Following a single oral dose, peak plasma concentrations occur in one-half to one hour. When taken with food, absorption is delayed, but the total amount absorbed is not altered. The absorption of meclofenamate was not affected by the concurrent administration of a magnesium-aluminum hydroxide antacid. Meclofenamate is highly bound (99%) to plasma proteins. The plasma half-life following a single dose is two hours; the half-life after multiple doses for four days is 3.3 hours. The drug does not accumulate in the body. It is metabolized to a hydroxymethyl derivative (25%), which also has anti-inflammatory activity, and a carboxy derivative (6%); both metabolites are excreted as glucuronide conjugates. A small amount of drug is excreted unchanged. Approximately two-thirds of the dose is excreted in the urine and one-third in the feces.

DOSAGE AND PREPARATIONS. Dosage should be individualized on the basis of the patient's needs and response. A low dose should be given initially and increased as necessary.

Oral: *Adults,* for RA and osteoarthritis, 200 to 400 mg daily in three or four equal doses. The drug may be taken with meals or milk. After a satisfactory response is obtained, the dosage should be adjusted as necessary. If a severe adverse reaction occurs, meclofenamate should be discontinued. *Children,* dosage has not been established.

Generic. Capsules and tablets 50 and 100 mg.

Meclomen (Parke-Davis). Capsules 50 and 100 mg of meclofenamic acid in the form of meclofenamate sodium monohydrate.

NABUMETONE

[Relafen]

$CH_2CH_2COCH_3$

CH_3O

ACTIONS AND USES. This NSAID is indicated for acute and chronic treatment of the signs and symptoms of osteoarthritis and RA. Its mode of action is not known but, as with other NSAIDs, is probably related to inhibition of prostaglandin synthesis at the cyclo-oxygenase level. The parent compound is a prodrug that undergoes hepatic biotransformation to the active compound, 6 methoxy-2-naphthylacetic acid (6 MNA), which is a potent inhibitor of prostaglandin synthesis.

In double-blind controlled trials involving more than 1,000 patients with osteoarthritis, nabumetone 1 g/day for six weeks to six months was comparable in efficacy to naproxen 500 mg/day or aspirin 3.6 g/day. In randomized, double-blind controlled trials involving 770 patients with RA, these same doses of nabumetone, naproxen, and aspirin administered for three weeks to six months also were comparable in efficacy. Nabumetone also has been used in combination regimens with gold compounds, penicillamine, and corticosteroids.

Clinical studies conducted in healthy males showed no difference in fecal blood loss after three to four weeks of administration of nabumetone 1 or 2 g/day when compared with placebo-treated or untreated subjects. In contrast, the administration of aspirin 3.6 g/day increased fecal blood loss compared with nabumetone-treated, placebo-treated, or untreated subjects.

In studies conducted in 488 patients who had baseline and post-treatment endoscopy, fewer patients who received nabumetone 1 to 2 g/day had detectable lesions than those who received naproxen 250 or 500 mg twice daily, piroxicam 10 to 20 mg/day, indomethacin 100 to 150 mg/day, or ibuprofen 2.4 g/day. Results comparable to those observed with nabumetone were reported with a regimen consisting of ibuprofen 2.4 g/day plus misoprostol 800 mcg/day.

In one-week, repeat-dose studies, nabumetone 1 g/day had little to no effect on collagen-induced platelet aggregation or bleeding time. In contrast, naproxen 500 mg/day inhibited the former and significantly increased the latter.

ADVERSE REACTIONS AND PRECAUTIONS. The adverse effects most frequently reported are diarrhea (14%), dyspepsia (13%), and abdominal pain (12%). Serious gastrointestinal toxicity (eg, ulceration, bleeding, perforation) can occur at any time with or without warning signs or symptoms in patients treated with NSAIDs for prolonged periods. In controlled clinical trials with nabumetone, the cumulative incidence of peptic ulcers was 0.3% at three to six months, 0.5% at one year, and 0.8% at two years. Physicians must weigh the potential benefits of therapy with nabumetone against possible hazards, especially when large doses are being considered, and should monitor the patient's progress carefully. See discussion and FDA-mandated warning for gastrointestinal disturbances under Adverse Reactions in the section on Nonsteroidal Anti-Inflammatory Agents.

Nabumetone may increase photosensitivity.

As with other NSAIDs, renal, hepatic, hematologic, dermatologic, neurologic, idiosyncratic, and other miscellaneous reactions have occurred in association with use of nabumetone. For further information, see Adverse Reactions and Precautions in the section on Nonsteroidal Anti-Inflammatory Agents.

No adequate controlled studies have been performed in pregnant women. Use of nabumetone during the third trimester of pregnancy is not recommended, and this drug should be used during the first and second trimester only if clearly needed (FDA Pregnancy Category C). The effects of nabumetone on labor and delivery are unknown. It also is not known whether nabumetone or its metabolites are secreted in human milk; however, its major metabolite, 6 MNA, is secreted in the milk of lactating rats.

The safety and efficacy of nabumetone in children have not been established. No differences in efficacy or safety have been observed between elderly and younger patients.

OVERDOSAGE. If overdosage occurs, it is recommended that the stomach be emptied and general supportive measures be instituted as necessary; there are no specific antidotes.

DRUG INTERACTIONS. Laboratory studies have shown that 6 MNA may displace other protein-bound drugs from their binding sites. Antacids have no effect on the bioavailability of 6 MNA.

See the discussion under Drug Interactions in the section on Nonsteroidal Anti-Inflammatory Agents for other potential drug interactions involving nabumetone.

PHARMACOKINETICS. Nabumetone is well absorbed from the gastrointestinal tract. Administration with food or milk increases the rate of absorption and subsequent appearance of 6 MNA in the plasma. However, it does not affect the conversion of the parent compound to 6 MNA, although peak plasma concentrations are increased by about 33%. Approximately 35% of a 1-g oral dose is converted to 6 MNA and 50% to unidentified metabolites that are subsequently excreted in the urine. Over 99% of 6 MNA is bound to plasma proteins. The free fraction (range, 0.2% to 0.8%) is dependent on the total concentration of this metabolite and is proportional to dose when 1 to 2 g is given. 6 MNA undergoes biotransformation in the liver; the inactive metabolites produced are eliminated as both free metabolites and as conjugates. After oral administration of 1- or 2-g doses to steady state, the mean plasma elimination half-life of 6 MNA is about 24 hours. The elimination half-life is increased in patients with severe renal dysfunction (creatinine clearance <30 ml/min/1.73 M^2).

DOSAGE AND PREPARATIONS.

Oral: For osteoarthritis and RA, *adults*, initially, 1 g/day as a single dose with or without food; however, dyspeptic symptoms may be alleviated by taking the drug with food. Some patients may require 1.5 to 2 g daily; doses exceeding 2 g/day have not been studied. There is considerable interpatient variation in response to nabumetone. The lowest effective amount should be used for long-term treatment. Patients weighing <50 kg are less likely to require doses >1 g/day. (For details on individualization of dosage, see the manufacturer's literature.)

Relafen (SmithKline Beecham). Tablets 500 and 750 mg.

NAPROXEN

[Naprosyn]

CH_3
CHCOOH
O
CH_3O

NAPROXEN SODIUM

[Anaprox]

ACTIONS AND USES. Naproxen is chemically related to the phenylpropionic acid group of drugs. It has analgesic, anti-inflammatory, and antipyretic actions and, like other NSAIDs, inhibits prostaglandin synthesis. This drug is effective in the symptomatic treatment of RA, JRA, ankylosing spondylitis, osteoarthritis, and acute gouty arthritis. It also may be useful as an alternative agent in the treatment of psoriatic arthritis and Reiter's syndrome.

Results of comparative studies in patients with RA demonstrated that naproxen 500 mg daily was as effective as aspirin 3.6 to 4.8 g and that naproxen was equally or more effective than ibuprofen, fenoprofen, or indomethacin in this disorder. The drug's steroid-sparing effect was demonstrated in a limited number of individuals who were also receiving a corticosteroid for RA. When naproxen was given to patients receiving gold therapy, it enhanced the therapeutic effect. Naproxen was as effective as aspirin, indomethacin, or sulindac in patients with osteoarthritis.

ADVERSE REACTIONS AND PRECAUTIONS. Naproxen is one of the better tolerated NSAIDs. The most common adverse reactions are gastrointestinal disturbances. See discussion and FDA-mandated warning for gastrointestinal disturbances under Adverse Reactions in the section on Nonsteroidal Anti-Inflammatory Agents.

Like aspirin, naproxen inhibits platelet aggregation and prolongs bleeding time; however, this effect is reversible on discontinuation of naproxen.

Central nervous system effects reported occasionally are headache, drowsiness, and dizziness or vertigo. Other adverse reactions occurring occasionally include pruritus, rash, urticaria, sweating, tinnitus, edema, and visual and hearing disturbances. As with other prostaglandin inhibitors, glomerulonephritis (rare), interstitial nephritis, and nephrotic syndrome have been reported with naproxen. Since the drug is eliminated largely by the kidney, it should be used with caution in patients with impaired renal function. Both pulmonary infiltration with eosinophils and pulmonary edema have been reported. These complications should be considered when pulmonary involvement is a component of the underlying disease (Reeve et al, 1987).

Naproxen readily crosses the placenta following oral administration to pregnant women and is excreted in the milk of lactating women. Thus, this drug should not be used during pregnancy or lactation. Naproxen is classified in FDA Pregnancy Category B.

OVERDOSE. Overdose usually causes only mild to moderate symptoms (eg, nausea, hypoprothrombinemia). There is a single report of a seizure in a patient who ingested 35 g.

DRUG INTERACTIONS. Naproxen is highly bound to plasma protein (99%) and may displace other albumin-bound drugs from their binding sites. Therefore, patients receiving such drugs (eg, oral anticoagulants, sulfonylureas, hydantoins) should be observed for interactions. The concomitant administration of probenecid increases the plasma concentration and half-life of naproxen. The rate of absorption is decreased slightly by magnesium and aluminum hydroxide and is increased by sodium bicarbonate. See the discussion under Drug Interactions in the section on Nonsteroidal Anti-Inflammatory Agents for other potential drug interactions involving naproxen.

PHARMACOKINETICS. Naproxen and naproxen sodium are rapidly absorbed after oral administration; the peak plasma concentration of the naproxen anion occurs within two to four hours after administration of naproxen and within one to two hours after administration of naproxen sodium. Absorption is not significantly delayed by the presence of food. Naproxen is highly bound (99%) to plasma proteins at plasma concentrations between 23 and 40 mcg/ml. The drug is metabolized by demethylation and subsequent glucuronide conjugation. The elimination half-life is 12 to 15 hours and excretion occurs largely in the urine.

DOSAGE AND PREPARATIONS.

Oral: *Adults,* the daily dosage for RA, osteoarthritis, and ankylosing spondylitis is 500 mg to 1 g of naproxen or 550 mg to 1.1 g of naproxen sodium divided into two doses (morning and evening). Doses do not have to be of equal size; 750 mg to 1 g daily of naproxen usually is required for treatment of RA and ankylosing spondylitis. The dose may be increased or decreased during long-term use, depending on the patient's response. If necessary, those who tolerate lower doses well may be given 1.5 g/day of naproxen or 1.65 g/day of naproxen sodium for limited periods. *Children,* for JRA, a total daily dose of 10 mg/kg (base equivalent) is given in two divided doses.

NAPROXEN:

Naprosyn (Syntex). Tablets 250, 375, and 500 mg; suspension 125 mg/5 ml in 480 ml containers.

NAPROXEN SODIUM:

Anaprox (Syntex). Tablets 275 mg (equivalent to 250 mg base) and 550 mg (***Anaprox DS***) (equivalent to 500 mg base).

OXAPROZIN

[Daypro]

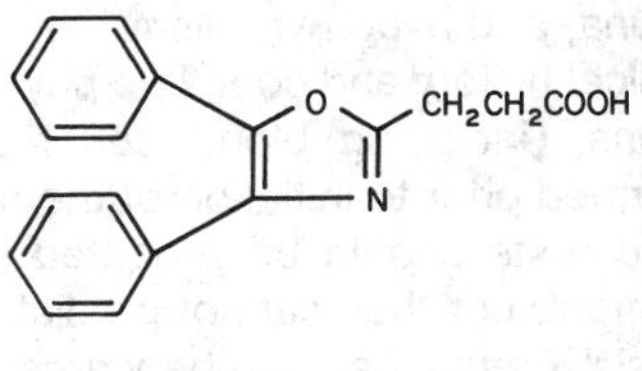

ACTIONS AND USES. Oxaprozin is a propionic acid derivative with analgesic, anti-inflammatory, and antipyretic actions. Analgesic effects are apparent after a single 1.2 g dose, but repeated doses are required to produce reliable anti-inflammatory effects. Like other NSAIDs, oxaprozin inhibits prostaglandin synthesis and this is presumed to be related to its therapeutic effects.

In most controlled trials on patients with RA, oxaprozin 1.2 g/day was as effective as aspirin 2.6 to 3.9 g/day or naproxen 500 mg/day (Schorn, 1981; *Semin Arthritis Rheum*, 1986; Miller, 1992). Like many other NSAIDs, oxaprozin may be better tolerated than aspirin and also may be effective in patients who do not respond adequately to that drug (Vreede et al, 1986). Oxaprozin also appears to be comparable to aspirin, piroxicam, and naproxen in the treatment of osteoarthritis (Ginsberg and Famaey, 1984; Kolodny et al, 1986; Powell et al, 1986). Results of controlled studies indicate that doses of 1.2 g may be effective in the treatment of ankylosing spondylitis (Caldwell et al, 1986), tendinitis and bursitis (Bono et al, 1986), and postoperative oral surgery pain (Winter and Post, 1983). Results of open trials suggest that oxaprozin also may be useful in the treatment of acute gout (Mease and Willkens, 1986), Behcet's disease (Takeuchi et al, 1984), and JRA (10 to 20 mg/kg/day) (Bass et al, 1985).

ADVERSE REACTIONS AND PRECAUTIONS. The most common adverse reactions reported in clinical trials were gastrointestinal disturbances (ie, nausea, dyspepsia, constipation) and rash. Adverse effects that were reported in more than 1% of patients were other gastrointestinal disturbances (ie, abdominal pain, anorexia, flatulence, vomiting), central nervous system dysfunction (ie, depression, somnolence, confusion, sleep disturbance), urogenital dysfunction (ie, dysuria, frequency), and tinnitus. Other adverse effects associated with use of oxaprozin and the precautions to be observed are similar to those noted with most other NSAIDs (see the Introduction to the section on Nonsteroidal Anti-Inflammatory Agents).

DRUG INTERACTIONS. Total body clearance of oxaprozin is reduced approximately 20% by concomitant administration of cimetidine or ranitidine. Oxaprozin may decrease the antihypertensive effects of beta-adrenergic blocking agents. Although the anticoagulant effect of warfarin is not affected by the concomitant administration of oxaprozin 1.2 g/day, all NSAIDs can damage the gastrointestinal mucosa and inhibit platelet aggregation, both of which increase the risk of gastrointestinal bleeding in patients receiving anticoagulants. For information on other potential drug interactions, see the Introduction to the section on Nonsteroidal Anti-Inflammatory Agents.

PHARMACOKINETICS. Oxaprozin is well absorbed after oral administration; bioavailability is approximately 95%, and peak plasma concentrations are achieved within three to five hours. Food decreases the rate but not extent of absorption of oxaprozin. Antacids do not affect absorption.

Like most other NSAIDs, oxaprozin is highly protein bound (99.9%) and has a relatively small volume of distribution, which reflects its limited extravascular distribution. Therapeutic doses saturate plasma protein binding sites; accordingly, use of larger doses (within the clinical range) results in a less than proportional increase in the plasma concentration of unbound drug because, as the free fraction increases, total systemic clearance also increases.

Oxaprozin is eliminated primarily by hepatic oxidation and conjugation with glucuronic acid. A portion of conjugated metabolite is secreted into the bile and eliminated in the feces, but enterohepatic recycling of oxaprozin is insignificant. Phenolic hydroxylation yields a small number and amount of active metabolites, but these do not contribute significantly to the overall pharmacologic activity. The renal clearance of oxaprozin is low. Because hepatic clearance of oxaprozin also is relatively low, this drug has a long elimination half-life (approximately 50 hours). Limited data suggest that clearance and half-life are not significantly altered in patients with cirrhosis (Lasseter et al, 1985).

According to the manufacturer's literature, age, gender, and well-compensated cardiac failure do not affect the plasma protein binding or pharmacokinetics of oxaprozin. In one study, oxaprozin clearance was slightly decreased in healthy elderly men but not in women (Greenblatt et al, 1985). Renal dysfunction appears to alter oxaprozin binding, resulting in a reduction in intrinsic clearance and Vd. Other reports indicate that the unbound fraction of oxaprozin is increased in patients with renal dysfunction and in those undergoing hemodialysis (Chiang et al, 1982; Jusko and Chiang, 1982).

DOSAGE AND PREPARATIONS.

Oral: *Adults*, the usual initial dose is 1.2 g/day for RA and 600 mg/day for osteoarthritis; divided doses may be used in patients who cannot tolerate once-daily dosing. If indicated, a loading dose of 1.2 to 1.8 g (not to exceed 26 mg/kg) can be administered. Daily maintenance doses larger than 1.2 g should be reserved for patients who have not experienced gastrointestinal, renal, hepatic, or dermatologic adverse events and who have not responded adequately to lower doses. In addition, criteria for patients receiving larger doses should include severe disease, weight >50 kg, normal renal and hepatic function, and low risk of peptic ulcer. The maximum recommended total daily dosage is 1.8 g in divided doses.

Daypro (Searle). Tablets 600 mg.

PHENYLBUTAZONE

$CH_3CH_2CH_2CH_2$

ACTIONS AND USES. Phenylbutazone has anti-inflammatory, antipyretic, and analgesic activities. It is especially effective in the treatment of ankylosing spondylitis. It also is useful in RA and Reiter's syndrome. Although phenylbutazone is effective in gouty arthritis, risk/benefit considerations indicate that this drug should not be employed for this disease.

Use of this drug poses a significant risk of agranulocytosis and aplastic anemia that counterbalances the benefits of its potent anti-inflammatory activity. As a general rule, phenylbutazone should be prescribed only after other NSAIDs have failed and when the severity of symptoms warrants the risk of a blood disorder.

ADVERSE REACTIONS AND PRECAUTIONS. Furst and Paulus (1987) have reviewed a number of epidemiologic reports of adverse reactions from controlled studies, spontaneous reporting to the manufacturer, and published case studies involving phenylbutazone in a number of clinical applications, including analgesia. Unfortunately, dose size or duration was not recorded in a number of these reports. Patients with RA were more susceptible to phenylbutazone-induced renal damage than the general population. Likewise, the incidence of aplastic anemia was significantly higher in patients with osteoarthritis, and 48% of severe skin reactions occurred in those with nonspecific rheumatologic conditions. The incidence of certain side effects was influenced by the sex of the patient. About 80% of the dermal reactions and 78% of the cases of salivary enlargement occurred in women, while the proportion of severe gastrointestinal reactions was higher in men. Almost one-half of the adverse events occurred within the first three months of therapy, 28% in the first week. All cases of salivary gland enlargement or inflammation and cardiovascular side effects occurred within three months; 64% of the instances of gastrointestinal bleeding occurred within three weeks. Thyroid and renal toxicity usually did not develop until after more than three months of treatment. Dermal reactions were unaffected by age. However, the incidence of gastrointestinal side effects, agranulocytosis, aplastic anemia, and thrombocytopenia was increased in older patients.

The most serious adverse reactions associated with phenylbutazone are blood dyscrasias (leukopenia, agranulocytosis, and aplastic anemia), which occur infrequently. The fatality rate from such effects has been estimated to be 2.2/100,000 patients (Hart and Huskisson, 1984). Agranulocytosis may occur shortly after initiation of therapy, but aplastic anemia usually appears after prolonged treatment. Hematologic toxicity may develop abruptly or gradually and may become apparent days or weeks after cessation of therapy. In patients older than 60 years, especially women, phenylbutazone should be restricted to short-term use (one week maximum) if possible.

Rashes, water retention and edema, and gastrointestinal disturbances ranging from mild irritation to ulceration occur and can be serious (eg, toxic epidermal necrolysis, gastrointestinal hemorrhage). See discussion and FDA-mandated warning for gastrointestinal disturbances under Adverse Reactions in the section on Nonsteroidal Anti-Inflammatory Agents. Other adverse reactions include jaundice, hepatitis, purpura, hematuria, and hypothyroidism.

A careful medical history and complete physical and laboratory examinations (including blood count and urinalysis) should be performed prior to initiation of therapy with phenylbutazone. These tests should be repeated regularly during prolonged treatment, but they cannot predict the occurrence of blood dyscrasia. Patients should be warned not to exceed the recommended dose and to discontinue the drug and report to the physician when fever, sore throat, oral lesions, dyspepsia, epigastric pain, unusual bleeding or bruising, black or tarry stools, symptoms of anemia, rashes, significant weight gain, or edema occurs. If long-term treatment is needed, the lowest effective dose should be used and patients should be informed of the risks.

Phenylbutazone is contraindicated in children under 14 years and in elderly patients. It also is contraindicated in individuals with gastrointestinal lesions or a history of recurrent lesions; in those with renal, hepatic, or cardiovascular disease; and in patients with a history of blood dyscrasias. Phenylbutazone also is contraindicated in patients with pancreatitis, parotitis, stomatitis, temporal arteritis, and polymyalgia rheumatica. This drug should be used with extreme caution, if at all, in patients with borderline or overt congestive heart failure because it may produce severe fluid retention.

This drug is classified in FDA Pregnancy Category C.

OVERDOSE. Mild poisoning with phenylbutazone has been associated with nausea, abdominal pain, and drowsiness. The urine may be pink due to a metabolite, rubazonic acid. In more severe cases, hyperpyrexia, respiratory alkalosis and metabolic acidosis, hypotension, coma, convulsions, and acute renal failure may occur (Meredith and Vale, 1986). Hypoprothrombinemia, thrombocytopenia, and leukopenia may follow. In all cases of overdose, gastric lavage and activated charcoal should be administered immediately.

DRUG INTERACTIONS. Since phenylbutazone may prolong the prothrombin time in patients receiving coumarin anticoagulants concomitantly, combined use should be avoided. Phenylbutazone may increase the hypoglycemic effect of insulin and the oral hypoglycemic agents. It also reduces iodine uptake by the thyroid. See the discussion under Drug Interactions in the section on Nonsteroidal Anti-Inflammatory Agents for other potential drug interactions involving phenylbutazone.

PHARMACOKINETICS. Phenylbutazone is rapidly and completely absorbed following oral administration. Peak plasma concentrations occur within 2.5 ± 1.4 hours, and the drug is highly bound to plasma protein. The major metabolite of phenylbutazone is the active form, oxyphenbutazone, which undergoes glucuronidation and is excreted mainly in the urine. The elimination half-life of phenylbutazone is 84 ± 23 hours, and there is significant inter- and intraindividual variation.

DOSAGE AND PREPARATIONS.

Oral: *Adults,* for RA, ankylosing spondylitis, and acute attacks of degenerative joint disease, 300 to 600 mg daily in three or four equally divided doses. A one-week trial period is considered adequate to determine response; if a favorable response does not occur, the drug should be discontinued. If symptoms can be controlled with a maintenance dose of 100 to 200 mg daily, the drug may be given for longer periods under careful and close supervision. The maximum maintenance dose is 300 to 400 mg daily. In patients 60 years and older, phenylbutazone should be avoided if possible.

Generic. Capsules and tablets 100 mg.

PIROXICAM

[Feldene]

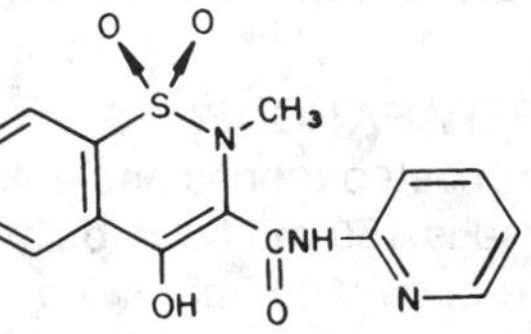

ACTIONS. Piroxicam differs chemically from other NSAIDs but has similar anti-inflammatory, analgesic, and antipyretic activities. Like other NSAIDs, piroxicam inhibits prostaglandin synthesis by blocking cyclo-oxygenase; it has no effect on lipoxygenase. The drug also inhibits chemotaxis, release of lysosomal enzymes, and neutrophil aggregation. Piroxicam has been reported to have a greater effect than other NSAIDs in inhibiting the production of RF. It increases the percentage of suppressor T-cells in peripheral blood and their in vitro response to phytohemagglutinin stimulation (Goodwin et al, 1983). The significance of these effects on its anti-inflammatory and antiarthritic actions is not clear.

USES. In controlled clinical studies, this agent was effective in the symptomatic treatment of RA and osteoarthritis. It also appears to be useful in ankylosing spondylitis and acute gouty arthritis, but additional studies are needed to establish comparative effectiveness and dosages in these conditions. Piroxicam can be administered once daily.

ADVERSE REACTIONS AND PRECAUTIONS. Gastrointestinal reactions occurred in about 20% of patients. Epigastric distress and nausea were noted most frequently; abdominal discomfort, constipation, diarrhea, and flatulence also were reported. The incidence of gastric irritation and ulcer increases with doses greater than 20 mg daily. See discussion and FDA-mandated warning for gastrointestinal disturbances under Adverse Reactions in the section on Nonsteroidal Anti-Inflammatory Agents.

Since hemoglobin and hematocrit levels were decreased in some patients, these should be determined periodically. Like aspirin, piroxicam inhibits platelet aggregation and prolongs bleeding time. Aplastic anemia has been associated with piroxicam therapy.

Peripheral edema has occurred in about 2% of patients receiving piroxicam. Congestive heart failure (five cases) and myocardial infarction also have been reported (Fowler and Arnold, 1983). Thus, piroxicam should be used very cautiously in patients with impaired cardiac function, hypertension, or other conditions predisposing to fluid retention. Elevation of BUN levels (reversible), interstitial nephritis, acute renal failure, and hyperkalemia have occurred. Because piroxicam and its metabolites are excreted primarily by the kidney, this drug should be used cautiously in those with impaired renal function.

Severe dermatologic reactions (eg, exfoliative dermatitis, fatal pemphigus vulgaris) have been reported rarely. Erythema multiforme has been observed occasionally and there have been a number of reports of photosensitivity (McKerrow and Greig, 1986; Gerber, 1987).

Cross sensitivity with aspirin and other prostaglandin inhibitors may occur; therefore, piroxicam is contraindicated in patients with a history of nasal polyps and angioedema or bronchospasm induced by aspirin or other anti-inflammatory drugs.

OVERDOSE. In adults, doses of 300 to 400 mg usually produce no symptoms of poisoning; doses of 500 mg to 1.8 g have produced hyperventilation, hyperreflexia, and convulsions. Doses of 100 mg in 2-year-old children have resulted in severe electrolyte disturbances, edema, and, in one instance, marrow aplasia (Meredith and Vale, 1986).

DRUG INTERACTIONS. Aspirin and piroxicam should not be used concomitantly. Piroxicam is highly bound to plasma proteins and may displace other albumin-bound drugs from binding sites. An interaction with warfarin has been reported. Patients receiving oral antidiabetic agents or phenytoin should be monitored carefully. See the discussion under Drug Interactions in the section on Nonsteroidal Anti-Inflammatory Agents for other potential drug interactions involving piroxicam.

PHARMACOKINETICS. Following oral administration, piroxicam is rapidly absorbed; peak plasma levels occur in three to five hours. With repeated daily doses of 20 mg, steady-state plasma levels of 3 to 5 mcg/ml are attained in 7 to 12 days. Plasma levels of piroxicam are not affected by the administration of antacids.

Concentration of the drug in synovial fluid is about 40% of that in plasma but the significance of this is not known. The apparent volume of distribution ranges from 0.12 to 0.14 L/kg, and the mean half-life is about 50 hours (range, 30 to 86 hours). The drug is extensively bound (99%) to plasma proteins. Piroxicam is metabolized predominantly by hydroxylation and subsequent conjugation with glucuronic acid. The metabolites are excreted primarily in the urine; a small amount is excreted in the feces, and about 2% to 5% of the drug is excreted unchanged. Piroxicam clearance is unaffected or increased (due to decreased protein binding leading to more rapid hepatic metabolism) in patients with renal impairment.

DOSAGE AND PREPARATIONS.

Oral: *Adults*, for RA and osteoarthritis, 20 mg daily as a single dose or in divided doses; the incidence of gastrointestinal reactions is likely to increase with doses in excess of 20 mg/day (maximum recommended by the manufacturer). Assessment of the drug's efficacy should be delayed for about two weeks to allow time for attainment of steady-state plasma levels. *Children,* dosage has not been established.

Feldene (Pfizer), ***Generic***. Capsules 10 and 20 mg.

SULINDAC
[Clinoril]

ACTIONS AND USES. Sulindac is a substituted indene analogue of indomethacin and has similar analgesic and antipyretic properties but less anti-inflammatory activity. It is as effective as aspirin in RA and osteoarthritis and appears to be comparable to phenylbutazone in ankylosing spondylitis. Sulindac may be useful as an alternative agent in the treatment of psoriatic or gouty arthritis or Reiter's syndrome.

ADVERSE REACTIONS AND PRECAUTIONS. The most common reactions are abdominal pain, dyspepsia, nausea, constipation, and diarrhea. See discussion and FDA-mandated warning for gastrointestinal disturbances under Adverse Reactions in the section on Nonsteroidal Anti-Inflammatory Agents.

Central nervous system effects include dizziness, drowsiness, and headache; the incidence of these is about the same as with aspirin and ibuprofen but less than with indomethacin. Other common adverse reactions are rash, pruritus, edema, and tinnitus.

Other serious reactions associated with sulindac include Stevens-Johnson syndrome, which may progress to toxic epidermal necrolysis, and pancreatitis. As with other NSAIDs, renal, hepatic, hematologic, idiosyncratic, and other miscellaneous reactions have occurred in association with the use of sulindac. For further information, see Adverse Reactions and Precautions in the section on Nonsteroidal Anti-Inflammatory Agents.

Pregnant and nursing women should avoid the use of sulindac.

OVERDOSE. Few cases of overdose with sulindac have been reported and symptoms have not been severe.

DRUG INTERACTIONS. Although sulindac and its sulfide metabolite are highly bound to plasma protein, no clinically significant interaction with oral anticoagulants or oral hypoglycemic agents has been reported in normal patients. Plasma levels of the active sulfide were depressed by the concomitant administration of aspirin but not acetaminophen or propoxyphene. See the discussion under Drug Interactions in the section on Nonsteroidal Anti-Inflammatory Agents for other potential drug interactions involving sulindac.

PHARMACOKINETICS. About 90% of a dose is absorbed rapidly following oral administration, and the drug's disposition is complex. The parent drug (sulfoxide) is inactive but is reduced reversibly to the sulfide (active metabolite) and oxidized irreversibly to the sulfone (inactive metabolite). Sulindac, sulfone, and their conjugates are excreted primarily in the urine; less than 1% of a dose appears in the urine as the sulfide metabolite. The sulfide, which is responsible for the biological activities of the parent drug, is eliminated slowly from plasma (half-life, about 16 hours). Sulindac and its metabolites are excreted in the bile to varying degrees; thus, they may be reabsorbed unchanged, biotransformed, or excreted.

DOSAGE AND PREPARATIONS.

Oral: For *adults* with osteoarthritis and ankylosing spondylitis, the usual initial dose is 150 mg twice daily with food. Patients with RA usually require 200 mg twice daily. The dosage should be adjusted on the basis of the patient's response. A single dose of 300 mg at breakfast is a satisfactory alternative dosage schedule. Doses over 400 mg/day are not recommended. *Children*, dosage has not been established.

Clinoril (Merck), ***Generic***. Tablets 150 and 200 mg.

TOLMETIN SODIUM
[Tolectin]

$$\cdot\ 2H_2O$$

ACTIONS AND USES. Like other NSAIDs, tolmetin inhibits prostaglandin synthetase in vitro and may alter lymphocyte function. In patients with RA, tolmetin has been as effective as aspirin, indomethacin, ibuprofen, and phenylbutazone. This agent also is comparable to aspirin in JRA. Its effectiveness in osteoarthritis is similar to that of aspirin, ibuprofen, and indomethacin. In a limited number of studies, tolmetin was comparable to indomethacin in ankylosing spondylitis. In addition, it has been reported to reduce pain in nonarticular and traumatic painful conditions. Tolmetin may be useful as an alternative agent in the treatment of psoriatic arthritis and Reiter's syndrome. It is not effective for the treatment of gout.

ADVERSE REACTIONS AND PRECAUTIONS. A postmarketing study of 8,000 outpatients receiving tolmetin showed that no serious adverse reactions (allergic, hematopoietic, dermal, or central nervous system disturbances) occurred within 90 days (Jick et al, 1989). The most frequently reported adverse reactions are gastrointestinal disturbances. See discussion and FDA-mandated warning for gastrointestinal disturbances under Adverse Reactions in the section on Nonsteroidal Anti-Inflammatory Agents.

Central nervous system reactions include headache, dizziness, lightheadedness, nervousness, and drowsiness. These effects occurred less frequently than with indomethacin.

Since tolmetin causes pseudoproteinuria in tests involving acid precipitation, other methods for detecting proteinuria should be used in patients receiving this drug.

Tolmetin is a chemical analogue of the analgesic, zomepirac, which was withdrawn from the market because it was associated with a substantial number of cases of anaphylaxis, some of which were fatal. The incidence of anaphylaxis with tolmetin also has been higher than with other NSAIDs. As with other NSAIDs, renal, dermatologic, hepatic, hematologic, idiosyncratic, and other miscellaneous reactions have occurred in association with the use of tolmetin. For further information, see Adverse Reactions and Precautions in the section on Nonsteroidal Anti-Inflammatory Agents.

This drug is classified in FDA Pregnancy Category C.

OVERDOSE. No serious side effects have occurred in patients reported to have taken an overdose of tolmetin.

DRUG INTERACTIONS. Tolmetin does not affect the anticoagulant activity of warfarin or the hypoglycemic effect of insulin or sulfonylureas. See the discussion under Drug Interactions in the section on Nonsteroidal Anti-Inflammatory Agents for potential drug interactions involving tolmetin.

PHARMACOKINETICS. Tolmetin is rapidly and completely absorbed after oral administration; peak plasma concentrations occur in 30 to 60 minutes. Absorption is not significantly affected by the short- or long-term administration of an antacid mixture of magnesium and aluminum hydroxides. The drug is highly bound (99%) to plasma protein. It undergoes biotransformation by oxidation of its aromatic methyl group, and 70% of the dose is recovered in the urine as this oxidized metabolite (Verbeeck et al, 1983). The elimination half-life is one to three hours.

DOSAGE AND PREPARATIONS.

Oral: *Adults,* for RA, initially, 400 mg three times daily. After a therapeutic response is achieved, the dose is adjusted to the patient's needs; 600 mg to 1.8 g daily is optimal for most patients. For osteoarthritis, 600 mg to 1.6 g daily usually is adequate. *Children over 2 years,* 20 mg/kg daily in divided doses initially; for maintenance, 15 to 30 mg/kg daily.

Tolectin (McNeil), ***Generic***. Capsules 400 mg (***Tolectin DS***); tablets 200 and 600 mg ***(Tolectin 600)*** (strengths expressed in terms of the base).

SECOND-LINE DRUGS

The second-line drugs employed for RA are dissimilar chemically and vary widely in their proposed mechanism of action and toxicity. The terms that have been used to refer to these drugs include disease-modifying antirheumatic drug (ie, DMARD), slow-acting antirheumatic drug (ie, SAARD), and second-line antirheumatic drug. None of these terms are entirely satisfactory. In long-term observational studies, it has been questioned whether these drugs are truly disease-modifying. However, whether the disappointing long-term outcome of patients with moderate to severe RA has resulted from the traditional practice of withholding these agents until later in the course of the disease or is primarily a reflection of their inadequate long-term efficacy is controversial.

Traditionally, second-line drugs are separated from anti-inflammatory agents (eg, salicylates and other NSAIDs, corticosteroids) in part because the latter "first-line" agents provide rapid symptomatic relief. However, methotrexate and sulfasalazine do not require several months for onset of action (hence, they are not SAARDs) and, in many patients, discontinuation of these and other second-line agents results in a rapid return of symptoms, suggesting that at least part of their acton is "anti-inflammatory." Although second-line implies that these agents are not used initially or are less effective than first-line agents, many rheumatologists now employ these agents in the early stages of RA, and they often provide at least short-term improvement in measures of disease activity in patients who have not responded to first-line therapy. For information on current patterns of use and for comparative comments, see discussion on RA in the Introduction.

In doses of 15 to 20 mg/day of prednisone or equivalents, corticosteroids may be disease modifying (Empire Rheumatism Council, 1955); however, long-term toxicity with these amounts makes such use undesirable.

Drug Evaluations

HYDROXYCHLOROQUINE SULFATE

[Plaquenil Sulfate]

For chemical formula, see index entry Hydroxychloroquine, In Malaria.

ACTIONS AND USES. The 4-aminoquinoline compound, hydroxychloroquine, is used to treat RA, usually as second-line therapy. This drug also is employed in JRA, lupus erythematosus, and other inflammatory connective tissue diseases. When it is administered in appropriate doses, its toxicity is minimal. Beneficial effects obtained are variable; approximately 70% of patients with RA experience moderate relief of symptoms but relatively few achieve adequate long-term control. Thus, hydroxychloroquine generally is used in patients with early disease refractory to NSAIDs alone. Since clinical improvement is slow, a 6- to 12-month trial is necessary to obtain maximal benefits. The recommended dosage must not be exceeded.

Because of its good patient acceptance and relative safety compared with other second-line agents, this agent also has been added to other second-line agents in combination regimens. (The combination of hydroxychloroquine and penicillamine is not recommended.)

ADVERSE REACTIONS AND PRECAUTIONS. Ocular toxicity is the only very serious complication noted; most other side effects are reversible, although dermal pigmentation may be permanent. Serious retinal changes occur very infrequently with hydroxychloroquine; however, progressive impairment of vision and eventual blindness, even after the drug is discontinued, may develop. The retinopathy starts in the area of the macula and appears to affect pigmentation; increased granularity and edema of the retina are the earliest findings. Retinopathy appears to be dose related; the risk is greater with larger doses, even when given for short periods, than with small doses administered over a prolonged period. Daily doses less than 6.5 mg/kg appear to be relatively safe.

In patients under age 60, an ophthalmologic examination (eg, visual acuity, visual fields [testing with a 5 mm red test object is particularly sensitive], retinal and corneal biomicroscopy) should be performed after six months to one year of hydroxychloroquine therapy or after a cumulative dose of 100 g (there are no reported cases of ocular toxicity at a lower dose) and at 6- to 12-month intervals thereafter. In patients over age 60, a baseline eye examination should be conducted to determine if senile macular degeneration or drusen are present. Senile macular degeneration resembles the retinopathy produced by this drug and is a contraindication to its use, since the patient cannot be monitored adequately (Runge, 1989). It has been suggested that eye examinations be performed semiannually in patients over age 60. The use of an Amsler grid once a month by the patient at home with instructions as to what changes require prompt notification of the physician has been recommended as a sensitive, inexpensive monitoring procedure (Easterbrook, 1988; Runge, 1989) but may cause undue anxiety.

Hydroxychloroquine should be discontinued at the first sign of pigmentary change in the ocular fundus or if visual field examination demonstrates a 5° constriction compared with the initial baseline or a developing paracentral scotoma (Rynes, 1989). Since this drug is deposited in the uveal tissue of the fetus, institution of hydroxychloroquine therapy is contraindicated during pregnancy (Parke, 1988).

Other adverse reactions include mild headache, gastrointestinal disturbances (diarrhea, nausea, abdominal cramps), rash, and neuropsychiatric effects (eg, emotional changes). Acute intermittent porphyria and neuromyopathy also may occur. The skin lesions of psoriasis may be aggravated and exfoliative dermatitis has been reported rarely; therefore, hydroxychloroquine should be used in patients with psoriatic arthritis only after they have been informed of the possible consequences. Patients with G6PD deficiency should be observed closely for development of hemolytic anemia. Discontinuation of therapy because of side effects is necessary in approximately 3% to 7% of patients. Routine hematologic and urinary examinations are not required.

OVERDOSE. After acute overdosage, hypotension, myocardial depression, impaired cardiac conduction, and, less frequently, convulsions may be noted within 30 minutes and death may occur. Treatment is largely supportive; no specific antagonists are known (Ellenhorn and Barceloux, 1988). Children are especially sensitive to hydroxychloroquine; therefore, the drug must be kept out of their reach.

PHARMACOKINETICS. Hydroxychloroquine is readily absorbed from the gastrointestinal tract. The plasma half-life during prolonged therapy is six to seven days. The drug is deposited in tissues (eg, lungs, kidney, eyes), and 50% is excreted in one week. Because 3% to 5% of the drug in tissue is more firmly bound, complete excretion may take months or even years after therapy is discontinued.

DOSAGE AND PREPARATIONS.

Oral: *Adults,* 200 mg once or twice daily with meals. Dosage should be calculated on the basis of ideal body weight and should not exceed 6.4 mg/kg/day. For maintenance, if a good response is obtained (usually in 4 to 12 weeks), the daily dosage should be reduced by 50% and continued at that level. *Children,* 6.4 mg/kg/day. Dosage should be based on lean body weight and should not exceed 200 mg/M^2/day.

Plaquenil Sulfate (Sanofi Winthrop). Tablets 200 mg (equivalent to 155 mg of base).

METHOTREXATE

[Rheumatrex]

For chemical formula, see index entry Methotrexate, Uses, Cancer.

ACTIONS AND USES. Results of short-term, placebo-controlled (Weinblatt et al, 1985; Anderson et al, 1985) and comparative trials (Hamdy et al, 1987; Morassut et al, 1989; Jeurissen et al, 1991; Rau et al, 1991 B) have established that methotrexate is effective in patients with active RA. Its mechanism of action in this disease is unknown. Most studies of immune function in RA patients treated with methotrexate reveal only marginal effects on humoral or cellular immune responses; however, improvement in measures of disease activity are noted. Inhibition of cytokines (eg, IL-1) (Chang et al, 1992) and synovial enzymes (eg, metalloproteinases, serine proteases) may be contributory.

Methotrexate has a more rapid onset of action (two to six weeks) than other second-line agents. A plateau in clinical response may occur after approximately six months of therapy, but results of long-term prospective trials indicate that efficacy is sustained in the majority of patients (Kremer and Phelps, 1992; Weinblatt et al, 1992). Treatment generally must be continued to maintain efficacy.

In the past, use of methotrexate generally was reserved for patients with severe RA refractory to salicylates or other NSAIDs, often after a trial with other second-line agents, such as hydroxychloroquine, gold, or penicillamine. However, because of its perceived effectiveness and tolerability, many rheumatologists advocate that methotrexate therapy be instituted earlier in the course of the disease, prior to or in combination with traditional therapies such as gold.

In long-term studies, disease progression confirmed by radiography generally has been observed, but some patients experience stabilization of disease (Kremer, 1989; Rau et al, 1991 B; Weinblatt et al, 1992).

Methotrexate also is used in the treatment of psoriatic arthritis. Results of a recent controlled study suggest that it may be useful in the treatment of JRA (Giannini et al, 1992), but further trials are necessary to document its safety and efficacy in this disease.

ADVERSE REACTIONS AND PRECAUTIONS. Although the dosage of methotrexate employed in arthritic patients is considerably below that used in cancer chemotherapy, a potential for serious, life-threatening toxicity exists. Since a great deal of experience has accumulated with the drug in the treatment of psoriasis, guidelines developed for the safe use of methotrexate in the management of that condition (Roenigk et al, 1988) plus observations with its use in a number of arthritic patients (Weinblatt, 1989 B; Fehlauer et al 1989; McKendry and Cyr, 1989; Kremer, 1992) can be utilized.

Low-dose, pulse (once-a-week), oral administration of methotrexate is associated with few serious side effects. Nausea and vomiting, anorexia, diarrhea, mucosal ulcers, and stomatitis are most common. Headache, malaise, fatigue, and lightheadedness also occur frequently on the day following drug administration.

Long-term effects on hepatic function in patients with RA receiving methotrexate appear to be significantly more benign than in those with psoriasis (Brick et al, 1989). Nevertheless, the potential for serious liver disease in these patients exists (Phillips et al, 1992). Transient elevations of the transaminase or alkaline phosphatase levels are common and are not predictive of hepatic disease; however, a long-term prospective study of sequential liver biopsies in patients receiving methotrexate showed that the number of monthly AST levels that were in the abnormal range was the best predictor of liver biopsy outcome (Kremer et al, 1989). Baseline biopsies may be indicated in those with a previous history of hepatic disease or with other risk factors (eg, alcohol abuse). Repeated biopsies on the basis of cumulative dose (eg, after 1.5 g) are not recommended. Instead, frequent elevations of AST or a decline in serum albumin have been suggested as indicators for biopsy (Kremer, 1992).

There appears to be no correlation between sex, seriousness or duration of arthritis, or the use of other drugs *(except alcohol)* and the development of hepatotoxicity. In addition to alcohol use, morbid obesity, pulmonary fibrosis, glucose intolerance, and insulin-dependent diabetes are significant risk factors for methotrexate-associated hepatotoxicity (Shergy et al, 1988). Results of a recent case control study suggest that serious liver disease in patients with RA is an age- and dose-related but uncommon complication of low-dose methotrexate therapy (Walker et al, in press). It is recommended that methotrexate therapy not be instituted in patients with significant pre-existing liver dysfunction or active or recent hepatitis. It should be administered with caution in obese patients or those with diabetes (Furst and Kremer, 1988).

Nephrotoxicity is rarely a problem with low-dose pulse therapy. It results from precipitation of methotrexate in the renal tubule. Because this is promoted in an acid urine, a diet providing a more alkaline urine is protective, but there are no data that indicate that alkalization of urine is necessary with the lower doses used in arthritis. The half-life of methotrexate is influenced by the creatinine clearance. Renal function, which may include creatinine clearance, should be determined in all patients prior to instituting therapy whether or not there is a history of renal disease. There is a greater incidence of adverse drug reactions in patients with higher initial serum creatinine and blood urea nitrogen concentrations (Fehlauer et al, 1989). Methotrexate should be used with great caution when creatinine clearance is below 50 ml/min.

Interstitial pneumonitis is a well-recognized but infrequent complication of methotrexate therapy. It appears to be a hypersensitivity reaction and is not dose related. It is characterized by dyspnea, cough, fever, acute changes in pulmonary function, and the appearance of infiltrates on radiographic examination. Most cases have been reported in men, and elderly patients with RA seem predisposed to develop pneumonitis, even with low doses (Green et al, 1988). The patient may recover spontaneously with discontinuation of therapy. Some patients, however, will require high-dose corticosteroid therapy, and fatalities have been reported. Pre-existing pulmonary abnormalities should be considered relative contraindications to methotrexate use.

Reversible myelosuppression, usually manifested as leukopenia, is induced by methotrexate. Thrombocytopenic anemia and pancytopenia also may occur. Leucovorin (folinic acid) should be administered as soon as possible to minimize any hematologic abnormality if methotrexate overdose occurs inadvertently. Opportunistic infections, including herpes zoster and *Pneumocystis carinii* pneumonia have been reported during therapy. Reversible alopecia has occurred in a small number of patients.

Altered menstrual function has been reported rarely in women with RA who have received methotrexate. Transient oligospermia may occur in men. Pregnancy should be avoided if either partner is receiving methotrexate and for a minimum of three months after therapy for male patients and for at least one ovulatory cycle after therapy for female patients (FDA Pregnancy Category X).

DRUG INTERACTIONS. Renal elimination may be delayed by the concurrent administration of salicylates and other NSAIDs, particularly in patients with diminished renal function (Ahern et al, 1988); this usually is not significant with the low doses of methotrexate employed for arthritis but is an indication for additional caution. Concomitant administration of trimethoprim or trimethoprim/sulfamethoxazole with methotrexate may increase bone marrow suppression, probably as an additive antifolate effect. Use of methotrexate with probenecid or phenylbutazone is not recommended.

DOSAGE AND PREPARATIONS. There is no compelling therapeutic advantage for the use of intramuscular rather than oral methotrexate. However, the intramuscular route may be preferable in the noncompliant patient or if doses >15 mg/week are necessary. Reduced dosage has been suggested in elderly patients. In the treatment of arthritis, there is no advantage to the use of the traditional weekly regimen of three doses at 12-hour intervals that was designed for maximal benefit in psoriasis (Furst and Kremer, 1988).

Oral: For rheumatoid and psoriatic arthritis, *adults,* 7.5 mg/week as a single dose. This can be increased to 15 mg/week after six weeks, if necessary.

Rheumatrex (Lederle), ***Generic.*** Tablets 2.5 mg.

Intramuscular: *Adults,* initially 5 mg/week increased by 5 mg/week to a total of 20 mg/week, if necessary.

(Strengths expressed in terms of base)

Folex PFS (Adria). Solution (preservative-free) 25 mg/ml in 2, 4, 8, and 10 ml containers.

Methotrexate (Lederle). Powder (lyophilized, preservative-free) in 20 and 50 mg and 1 g containers; solution (injection) 25 mg/ml in 2 and 10 ml containers (alcohol 0.9%) and in 2, 4, 8, and 10 ml containers (preservative-free) (***Methotrexate LPF***).

PENICILLAMINE

[Cuprimine, Depen]

For chemical formula see index entry Penicillamine, Uses, Metal Poisoning.

ACTIONS AND USES. Comparative studies indicate that penicillamine, a chelating drug, may be as effective as parenteral gold compounds or azathioprine in RA. It also is beneficial in many patients with seropositive or seronegative juvenile polyarticular arthritis (Ansell and Hall, 1981) and has been recommended as therapy for diffuse scleroderma. This drug is not useful in ankylosing spondylitis, psoriatic arthritis, or other HLA-B27 associated diseases.

The mechanism of action is not known, but penicillamine has immunosuppressive activity and appears to affect immune complex levels, possibly by exerting an effect on T-cells. Many of this drug's clinical effects are similar to those of the gold compounds.

Because it may cause serious adverse reactions, penicillamine should be reserved for patients with severe, active disease that has not responded adequately to more conservative drug therapy. Physicians who prescribe this drug should be familiar with its action, and patients should be supervised closely.

ADVERSE REACTIONS AND PRECAUTIONS. The incidence of adverse reactions is high (CSSRD Group, 1987). Some effects are related to the rate of dosage increase and may be prevented by titrating the dose carefully. The risk of adverse reactions may be greater in patients with a limited sulfoxidation capacity (Emery et al, 1984).

The most common adverse reactions are pruritus, rash, anorexia, epigastric pain, nausea, vomiting, or occasional diarrhea and an alteration in taste that may be transient. Serious reactions involving the hematologic system (thrombocytopenia, leukopenia, agranulocytosis, aplastic anemia) and renal system (proteinuria, hypoalbuminemia, nephrotic syndrome) have been observed. Proteinuria and/or hematuria may develop during therapy and may be warning signs of membranous glomerulopathy, which can progress to a nephrotic syndrome. Close observation of these patients is essential. In some patients, proteinuria disappears with continued therapy; in others, penicillamine must be discontinued. When proteinuria or hematuria develops, the physician must ascertain whether it is drug-induced or is unrelated to penicillamine therapy.

Blood tests should be performed periodically, and complete blood cell counts, including platelets, must be obtained at two-week intervals during the first six months of treatment and monthly thereafter. A white cell count below 3,000 or a platelet count below 100,000 requires that penicillamine be discontinued while the patient is evaluated. The risk of developing hematologic toxicity appears to be greater in patients over 65 years. Blood urea nitrogen and creatinine levels should be monitored occasionally. If urinary protein excretion is greater than 1 g/24 hours, the drug should be discontinued or the dose reduced. Reduction of dosage corrects proteinuria in some patients after several months. Penicillamine must be discontinued if significant hypoalbuminemia, nephrotic syndrome, hematuria, drug fever, or other symptoms of toxicity develop.

Other serious reactions reported occasionally are lupus-like disease, pemphigus, Goodpasture's syndrome, myasthenia gravis, and dermatomyositis or polymyositis. If any of these autoimmune syndromes appear, penicillamine must be discontinued and the patient should not receive the drug again.

PHARMACOKINETICS. Penicillamine is rapidly absorbed from the intestine after oral administration; the peak plasma concentration usually occurs in about two hours. Metabolism is complex; five forms appear in plasma and the percentage of each urinary metabolite varies somewhat with the disease being treated. Plasma elimination half-life is 60.7 ± 8.2 minutes. Urinary excretion is 21.2% ± 2.3% within 24 hours; 50% of an oral dose is excreted in the feces, but the metabolites have not been identified (Perrett, 1981; Wiesner et al, 1981).

DOSAGE AND PREPARATIONS. The dose must be individualized on the basis of clinical response and adverse reactions. There is no apparent correlation between serum levels of penicillamine and clinical course or many of the side effects (Muijsers et al, 1984). Because of the long latent period of the clinical response, changes in dosage should not be made at intervals of less than two to three months. Gold compounds, antimalarial agents, cytotoxic drugs, and phenylbutazone should not be administered concomitantly. Penicillamine should be given on an empty stomach (about one hour before meals) to ensure maximum absorption. Iron supplements should be avoided since they interfere with the uptake of penicillamine.

Oral: *Adults,* initially, 125 mg/day as a single dose; the amount may be increased by increments of 125 mg/day at one- to three-month intervals to 500 mg/day and then at three-month intervals to a maximum of 750 mg/day. *Children,* initially 5 mg/kg/day; the dosage may be increased to 10 to

15 mg/kg/day after two months if no effect is seen with the lower amounts (Baum, 1983). Administration should be discontinued if response is inadequate within four months after the maximum dose is reached (van Kerckhove et al, 1988).

Cuprimine (Merck). Capsules 125 and 250 mg.
Depen (Wallace). Tablets 250 mg.

SULFASALAZINE
[Azulfidine]

For chemical formula, see index entry Sulfasalazine, In Inflammatory Bowel Disease.

ACTIONS AND USES. Results of placebo-controlled (Pinals, et al, 1986) and comparative trials (Pullar et al, 1983; Williams et al, 1988 A) have established sulfasalazine as a useful second-line agent in the treatment of RA. Results of a limited number of short-term comparative studies and one meta-analysis (Felson et al, 1990) suggest that sulfasalazine is as effective as hydroxychloroquine or penicillamine but is less likely to produce serious toxic effects than the latter; open (Bax and Amos, 1985) and controlled (Pullar et al, 1983; Williams et al, 1988 A) comparisons with injectable gold compounds yielded conflicting results, but most clinicians feel that sulfasalazine is somewhat less effective than parenteral gold. Sulfasalazine has been combined with other second-line agents (eg, hydroxychloroquine, parenteral gold) in the treatment of RA (Taggart et al, 1987; Farr et al, 1988 B). In short-term studies, these combinations appeared to be more effective than monotherapy but caused greater toxicity.

Sulfasalazine also may be effective in the treatment of ankylosing spondylitis and psoriatic arthritis. Limited open studies suggest that the drug also may be beneficial as a second-line agent for JRA.

ADVERSE REACTIONS AND PRECAUTIONS. Considerable experience has accumulated in the long-term use of this drug for chronic inflammatory bowel disease (see index entry Sulfasalazine, In Inflammatory Bowel Disease). The spectrum of side effects in patients with RA is similar to that observed in patients with bowel disease, but reactions appear to occur more frequently (Farr et al, 1986; Amos et al, 1986). The principal adverse reactions requiring discontinuation of therapy are nausea, vomiting, abdominal pain, and dizziness. Mucocutaneous reactions also are common, particularly a pruritic maculopapular generalized eruption and, less commonly, photosensitivity. Patients exhibiting the latter should be advised to avoid exposure to sunlight and other UV sources. Urticarial lesions, oral ulcers, and a lupus-like reaction occur rarely. Patients with elevated hepatic enzyme concentrations should discontinue use of this agent.

The most serious reaction is nondose-related, reversible neutropenia (Capell et al, 1986). It has been recommended that the blood be examined at two-week intervals during the first 12 weeks of therapy and at six-week intervals thereafter for the first year.

Sulfasalazine should not be used in patients with hepatic porphyria, glucose-6-phosphate dehydrogenase deficiency, or a history of hypersensitivity to salicylates or sulfonamides. Care should be exercised in patients with hepatic or renal dysfunction. Because kernicterus is a theoretical possibility, the drug should not be used during pregnancy (FDA Pregnancy Category B) or breast feeding. (See index entry Sulfasalazine, In Inflammatory Bowel Disease, for additional precautions.)

DOSAGE AND PREPARATIONS.
Oral: *Adults,* for RA, it is recommended that an enteric-coated preparation be used and that therapy be initiated with doses of 500 mg/day and gradually increased to 2 g/day or occasionally 3 g/day. A favorable response may permit reduction in the maintenance dose to between 1 and 2 g daily. Because of a genetic esterase deficiency, a few patients may eliminate the enteric-coated preparation unchanged.

Azulfidine EN-tabs (Kabi Pharmacia), ***Generic.*** Tablets (enteric-coated) 500 mg. For additional preparations, see index entry Sulfasalazine, In Inflammatory Bowel Disease.

Gold Compounds

AUROTHIOGLUCOSE
[Solganal]

CH_2OH, O, HO, HO, OH, SAu

GOLD SODIUM THIOMALATE
[Myochrysine]

$CH_2CO^-Na^+$ / $AuSCHCO^-Na^+$ · H_2O

ACTIONS AND USES. Active adult and juvenile RA are the principal indications for these agents, but beneficial effects also have been obtained in some patients with psoriatic arthritis. Although the exact mechanism of action is not known, there is evidence that gold alters the function of monocytes at the site of inflammation; decreased titers of RF and immunoglobulins often are observed (Tsokos, 1987).

Gold compounds frequently are used in the treatment of RA that progresses despite adherence to a conservative program of salicylates or other NSAIDs, rest, and physical therapy. Therapy should be initiated before irreversible changes have occurred in the involved joints. In some short-term studies, use of parenteral gold has reduced bone erosions. The injectable gold compounds appear to be equally effective, but there is some evidence that aurothioglucose is less toxic (Lawrence, 1976), although the injections are more painful.

ADVERSE REACTIONS AND PRECAUTIONS. The usefulness of chrysotherapy is limited by toxicity, especially dermatologic, hematologic, and renal reactions. Approximately 20%

of patients must discontinue the drug because of intolerance (Gray and Gottlieb, 1986).

Toxic effects may be observed after the first injection, during the course of therapy, or several months after chrysotherapy has been discontinued; these effects have been reviewed in detail (Gray and Gottlieb, 1986; Cohen, 1988). The incidence and severity of adverse reactions appear to depend on dosage; severe effects are most common after a cumulative dose of 400 to 800 mg has been administered. Since these reactions are unpredictable, patients should be questioned about symptoms of toxicity (eg, rash, purple blotches, pruritus, stomatitis, metallic taste) prior to each injection. A complete blood count, including platelet count, should be performed before the first injection to serve as a baseline value and should be repeated on a regular schedule throughout the period of treatment. Hematologic reactions (eg, eosinophilia, leukopenia, thrombocytopenia, agranulocytosis, hypoplastic or aplastic anemia) are rare; some fatalities have occurred. Gold therapy should be discontinued if the white blood cell count falls below 3,500.

Dermatitis (ranging from macular, papular, or urticarial rashes to exfoliative dermatitis) and lesions of the mucous membranes (stomatitis and, more rarely, proctitis and vaginitis) occur in about 20% of patients; the mucocutaneous effects may occur at any time but are usually seen during the first six months of therapy. Pruritus or eosinophilia may signify the early development of a skin reaction. When a pruritic skin lesion of uncertain etiology appears, gold therapy should be discontinued temporarily. Dermatologic side effects may be aggravated by sunlight.

Hepatitis, cholestatic jaundice, severe enterocolitis, interstitial lung disease, peripheral neuritis, and encephalopathy have developed rarely.

Anaphylactoid or "nitritoid-type" reactions (eg, flushing, syncope, dizziness, sweating), as well as nausea, vomiting, and weakness may occur with gold sodium thiomalate, but they are probably caused by the vehicle rather than the gold. Substituting aurothioglucose usually alleviates these symptoms.

Some patients experience a transient flare-up of disease within 24 hours after the injection; however, it is thought that most of these patients eventually respond well to gold therapy. In a few individuals, this reaction is so severe that prednisone must be given for a few days to control it.

Renal damage manifested as proteinuria (less commonly, microscopic hematuria) accounts for approximately 12% of all adverse reactions. Proteinuria may develop at any time. Before initiating gold therapy, renal function should be assessed; any patient with pretreatment proteinuria is not a candidate for this therapy. Urine protein estimates should be made before each injection, and the serum creatinine and urea concentrations should be determined every three months. Proteinuria (1 g/24 hours or more) generally mandates cessation of gold therapy, which is all that may be necessary for resolution in more than 70% of patients. The remaining affected patients develop a nephrotic syndrome. This can be treated by dietary measures and diuretics, even when the proteinuria is severe. Corticosteroid therapy is ineffective and may be harmful (Hall, 1988).

Gold compounds should be used with extreme caution in patients with impaired renal or hepatic function, blood disorders, rash, marked hypertension, or systemic lupus erythematosus. They are contraindicated in patients with severe debilitation or previous signs of gold and, possibly, penicillamine toxicity. Diabetes mellitus or heart failure should be under control before initiating gold therapy. These agents are seldom needed during pregnancy but, if their use is contemplated, the benefit/risk ratio should be considered (FDA Pregnancy Category C). Gold is excreted in the milk of nursing mothers. Because of the potential for adverse reactions in nursing infants, either nursing or the gold therapy should be discontinued.

PHARMACOKINETICS. Gold is stored in the body tissues, particularly the reticuloendothelial system. It is excreted over a period of six months or more. Following administration, the serum half-life is about six days. About 70% is excreted by the kidney and the remainder in the feces.

DOSAGE AND PREPARATIONS.

Intramuscular (gluteal): *Adults,* initially, single weekly injections of 10 mg the first week, 25 mg the second week, and 25 or 50 mg the third week and each week thereafter until a total dose of 800 mg to 1 g has been administered. If there is no response after 1 to 1.5 g has been given, the patient may be considered unresponsive and the drug discontinued. If the patient has improved and no toxic effects have developed, dosage may be reduced. If the clinical course remains stable, 25 to 50 mg may be given every two to three weeks and then at monthly intervals.

Comparative studies have demonstrated that 10 or 25 mg is as effective as the usual 50-mg dose and that the response is not related to serum level of gold (Sharp et al, 1977). A remission after one year of maintenance therapy had been considered an indication for complete withdrawal of the drug, but many rheumatologists now feel that gold therapy probably should be continued indefinitely on a reduced dosage schedule. If relapse occurs when the interval between doses is increased or the drug is discontinued, the former schedule should be reinstituted.

For JRA, recommendations vary; the initial intramuscular dose of aurothioglucose or gold sodium thiomalate usually is 0.2 mg/kg, with the amount increased after one week by 0.5 mg/kg. If no adverse reactions (rash, oral ulcers, leukopenia, or proteinuria) occur, 1 mg/kg may be given in the third week (Nelson, 1982). This amount usually is administered weekly for about 20 weeks and then at increasing intervals, leading to a once-monthly maintenance dose for as long as therapy is beneficial and there are no signs of toxicity. Single doses for children and all but the largest adolescents should not exceed 50 mg.

AUROTHIOGLUCOSE:

Solganal (Schering). Suspension (sterile) 50 mg/ml in sesame oil with aluminum monostearate 2% and propylparaben 1 mg/ml in 10 ml containers.

GOLD SODIUM THIOMALATE:

Generic. Solution 50 mg/ml in 1 ml containers.

Myochrysine (Merck). Solution (sterile, aqueous) 25 mg/ml with benzyl alcohol 0.5% in 1 ml containers and 50 mg/ml with benzyl alcohol 0.5% in 1 and 10 ml containers.

AURANOFIN

[Ridaura]

$(C_2H_5)_3P \rightarrow Au{-}S$, H_3CCO, $OCCH_3$, $OCCH_3$, CH_2OCCH_3

ACTIONS AND USES. Auranofin differs chemically and in some pharmacologic actions from the older gold compounds (Walz et al, 1982 A). Unlike the latter preparations, which must be given parenterally, auranofin is effective when administered orally for RA. Like the other gold compounds, auranofin can modify the disease process. Thus, it is a useful alternative to parenteral gold compounds in patients with milder RA.

Auranofin decreases morning stiffness and the number of painful and swollen joints and increases grip strength. In addition, a decrease in weakness, fatigue, and progressive weight loss was reported by some patients. A reduction in erythrocyte sedimentation rate and RF paralleled the clinical response to auranofin. In comparative studies, auranofin was less toxic than parenteral gold preparations (Gray and Gottlieb, 1986). Although it is less effective, auranofin appears to be capable of sustaining the response induced by parenteral gold (Williams et al, 1988 B).

Like other gold compounds, auranofin has an immunomodulator action, although some effects differ from those of gold sodium thiomalate. The mechanism of these actions and their exact relationship to the therapeutic effects of auranofin in RA are not known (Walz et al, 1982 B).

ADVERSE REACTIONS AND PRECAUTIONS. The most frequent adverse reactions to auranofin are gastrointestinal disturbances (changes in bowel habits, loose stools, diarrhea, flatulence). Diarrhea was reported in about 50% of patients. Other gastrointestinal reactions include abdominal pain, nausea, dyspepsia, and anorexia. These reactions generally occur within the first three months of therapy and usually are transient. If they persist, reduction of the dosage may relieve symptoms. A mild enterocolitis is more common with oral than parenteral gold. Skin reactions (eg, pruritus, nonpruritic rash) are mild and occur in about 30% of patients; stomatitis occurs in 10%. Alopecia and conjunctivitis have been reported in 2% and 10% of patients, respectively.

Proteinuria was reported in about 4% of patients but required discontinuation of therapy in only 0.7%. The same precautions should be observed as with parenteral gold preparations (see that evaluation). Proteinuria should be evaluated every two to four weeks. Abnormal results of liver function tests occurred in 0.4% of patients in U.S. studies. Anemia, leukopenia, eosinophilia, and thrombocytopenia developed infrequently and were reversible on discontinuation of the drug. Aplastic anemia and pure red cell aplasia have been reported very rarely.

Auranofin is contraindicated in patients with a history of gold-induced anaphylactic reactions, necrotizing enterocolitis, pulmonary fibrosis, exfoliative dermatitis, bone marrow aplasia, or other severe hematologic disorders.

This drug is classified in FDA Pregnancy Category C.

PHARMACOKINETICS. Following oral administration of a single dose (6 mg), peak plasma levels occurred in 1.5 to 2.5 hours; approximately 25% of the dose was absorbed. With repeated daily doses, little day-to-day variation occurred in blood gold levels once steady state was achieved. The mean levels after three and six months of therapy (6 mg/day) were approximately the same: 0.62 ± 0.19 mcg/ml and 0.68 ± 0.45 mcg/ml, respectively. Blood gold levels following auranofin administration were about one-third of those reported with parenteral gold compounds, although the serum half-life of the latter was shorter. The gold from auranofin appeared to be more rapidly and completely excreted.

A major portion of the blood gold content was found to be associated with the cellular elements. After six months of administration (3 mg twice daily), the mean plasma terminal half-life was 17 to 25.5 days and the mean total body terminal half-life was 80.8 days. About 85% of the recoverable gold is excreted in the feces and 15% in the urine. Approximately 100% of a single dose of Au^{195}-labeled auranofin was excreted over six months. (See reviews by Gottlieb, 1982; Blocka et al, 1986.)

DOSAGE AND PREPARATIONS.

Oral: The optimal therapeutic dose appears to be 6 mg/day given in one or two doses. Smaller doses can be used if this amount is not tolerated. Blood gold levels are dose-related, but there appears to be no correlation between blood levels and therapeutic efficacy. Larger dosages (9 mg/day) caused a higher incidence of gastrointestinal adverse reactions but have been tolerated by some patients.

Ridaura (SmithKline Beecham). Capsules 3 mg.

Immunosuppressive Agents

ADRENAL CORTICOSTEROIDS

Of the systemic corticosteroids, prednisone and prednisolone are most commonly used in rheumatic disorders and are equally effective when given orally. The use of low-dose systemic corticosteroid therapy (ie, no more than 7.5 mg prednisone equivalent daily) in the management of RA has increased in recent years. Corticosteroids are sometimes substituted for NSAIDs in the elderly and in patients with gastrointestinal or other intolerance to NSAIDs. They frequently are used to maintain patients who have not benefitted from initial therapy with salicylates or NSAIDs until the therapeutic effects of a second-line agent become apparent. Short-term use of low-dose prednisone often benefits patients with RA and produces few side effects (Harris et al, 1983). Increasingly, corticosteroids are used by some clinicians in combination regimens for early RA. As the disease progresses, these agents often remain a component of the therapeutic regimen (Paulus, 1991).

Despite their clinical acceptance, long-term efficacy and safety in RA are not well documented (Caldwell and Furst, 1991). Alterations in glucose metabolism, cutaneous atrophy, cataracts, and glaucoma may occur; osteoporosis, steroid-induced myopathy, and dysfunction of the hypothalamic-pituitary adrenal axis develop in some patients. Thus, although systemic corticosteroids are effective for short-term therapy, such use often evolves into long-term therapy, because efforts to discontinue steroids commonly are complicated by disease flare-up. Long-term studies are needed to confirm that such use is appropriate (Paulus, 1991).

For equivalency and adverse reactions, see index entry Adrenal Corticosteroids.

Intra-articular injection of a long-acting corticosteroid (eg, prednisolone tebutate [Hydeltra-T.B.A.], betamethasone sodium phosphate and acetate [Celestone Soluspan], dexamethasone acetate [Decadron-LA] triamcinolone acetonide [Kenalog], triamcinolone hexacetonide [Aristospan], methylprednisolone acetate [depMedalone, Depo-Medrol]) temporarily relieves pain when only a few joints are markedly affected. Effects last several weeks to months, depending on the preparation used, but it is suggested that injections not be repeated more than three or four times yearly. Several rheumatologists have reported that triamcinolone preparations are the most potent and have the longest duration of action (Gray et al, 1981).

DOSAGE AND PREPARATIONS.

PREDNISONE, PREDNISOLONE:

Oral: *Adults,* for RA, the daily dose should not exceed 7.5 mg of prednisone or the equivalent or 5 mg or the equivalent in postmenopausal women (Roth, 1984). The amount should be adjusted at three- to seven-day intervals, depending on response, to the maintenance level. Discontinuation of therapy should be gradual (ie, dosage reductions of 1 mg/month).

For *children,* small doses (as little as 2 to 3 mg/day) sometimes improve juvenile polyarticular arthritis with severe inflammation that is unresponsive to other medications (Baum, 1983). If possible, 1-mg tablets should be given as a single dose in the morning. Alternate-day therapy is preferred and can be utilized if symptoms are controlled satisfactorily during the day on which no medication is given.

For preparations, see index entries Prednisolone; Prednisone.

AZATHIOPRINE

[Imuran]

For chemical formula, see index entry Azathioprine, Uses, Immune Disorders.

ACTIONS AND USES. Azathioprine, an imidazolyl derivative of mercaptopurine, is rapidly metabolized to the latter, which also is active and accounts for most of the effects of this compound. The exact mechanism of the immunosuppressant and anti-inflammatory actions of azathioprine in RA is not known.

Results of short-term, randomized, placebo-controlled (Urowitz et al, 1973) and comparative trials (Paulus et al, 1984; Hamdy et al, 1987) have established that azathioprine (1 to 2.5 mg/kg/day) is effective in patients with active RA. Therapeutic response usually is evident in 6 to 12 weeks, but 12 to 24 weeks is considered the appropriate time frame for an adequate trial. Because of potential toxic effects, use of azathioprine generally has been limited to severe, active progressive disease that has not responded to conventional management, including other drug therapy. Anti-inflammatory antirheumatic drugs (eg, NSAIDs, prednisone) generally are continued when azathioprine is given, although the required dose of prednisone often can be decreased.

Azathioprine is approximately as effective as gold or penicillamine. Comparisons with methotrexate have produced varied results. Two short-term randomized trials with one- (Arnold et al, 1990) or two-year (Hamdy et al, 1987) follow-up indicated that azathioprine and methotrexate were similar in efficacy. In contrast, results of a double-blind randomized trial showed methotrexate to be superior (Jeurissen et al, 1991). The effects of combined use of azathioprine with other second-line agents has not been adequately studied in controlled trials. Results of one controlled trial suggest that the combination of azathioprine and methotrexate does not offer significant additional benefit over use of methotrexate alone (Willkens et al, 1992).

ADVERSE REACTIONS AND PRECAUTIONS. The incidence of adverse reactions is less when azathioprine is given for RA than when it is used as an immunosuppressant in renal homotransplantation. As with other second-line agents, the risk of side effects increases with the length of exposure to azathioprine. In a multicenter prospective study in patients with RA, the most common adverse effects attributed to azathioprine were gastrointestinal distress (ie, nausea, vomiting, diarrhea, abdominal pain), mucosal ulcers, rash, and leukopenia (Singh et al, 1991). The gastrointestinal disturbances usually are mild and occur soon after treatment is begun. Hematologic reactions (anemia) occur most frequently. These are dose-related and usually are mild, but leukopenia is occasionally severe. Severe bone marrow depression occurs infrequently. Therefore, complete blood counts, including platelets, should be performed periodically during therapy (eg, weekly during the first month, twice monthly during the second and third months, and monthly thereafter). If there is a rapid fall, a persistent low leukocyte count, or other evidence of bone marrow depression, the dose should be reduced or the drug discontinued.

Hepatotoxicity is uncommon (incidence, <1%), but it may be severe; the effects generally are reversible after discontinuation of the drug.

Although serious infections are a potential hazard of immunosuppressant therapy, the incidence of infections has not increased in patients receiving azathioprine for RA.

An increase in lymphoma, reticulum cell sarcoma, and other neoplasms has been noted in renal transplant patients receiving azathioprine. Although the risk of malignancies is less in patients with RA, acute myelogenous leukemia, non-Hodgkin's lymphoma, and solid tumors have been reported. However, patients with moderate to severe RA may be at increased risk of malignancy, particularly lymphoproliferative disorders (Matteson et al, 1991). Data to date indicate that the increased risk of lymphoma (and probably other cancers) associated with azathioprine therapy in these patients is probably low compared with their innate risk (Silman et al, 1988; Hickey et al, 1992).

Azathioprine is teratogenic in animals and, since it crosses the placenta in humans, the drug should not be used during pregnancy.

If azathioprine is given with allopurinol, the dose should be reduced to about one-third or one-fourth the usual amount because the inhibition of xanthine oxidase by allopurinol reduces the conversion of mercaptopurine to its major inactive metabolite, 6-thiouric acid. Since this metabolite is excreted in the urine, the dose of azathioprine also should be reduced in patients with renal dysfunction.

For other adverse reactions and precautions, see index entry Azathioprine, Uses, Immune Disorders.

DOSAGE AND PREPARATIONS.

Oral: *Adults*, initially, about 1 mg/kg (50 to 100 mg) as a single dose or in two divided doses daily. This may be increased after six to eight weeks by 0.5 mg/kg/day at four-week intervals to a maximum of 2.5 mg/kg/day. A therapeutic response may not be observed for six to eight weeks; thus, at least 12 weeks should be allowed to determine whether the patient is refractory to treatment. If the response is satisfactory and there are no toxic effects, the drug may be continued for long-term therapy, but the smallest effective maintenance dose should be used and the patient should be monitored carefully.

Imuran (Burroughs Wellcome). Tablets 50 mg.

GOUT AND HYPERURICEMIA

Gout is characterized biochemically by hyperuricemia and clinically by episodes of severe, acute arthritis. The untreated disease may develop through four stages: (1) asymptomatic hyperuricemia, which infrequently progresses to acute gout; (2) acute gouty arthritis, which is usually monoarticular but may be polyarticular; (3) asymptomatic intercritical (interval) period; and (4) chronic tophaceous gout with chronic arthritis (30% to 40% of patients with gout develop tophi). If the disease is diagnosed early and appropriate therapy is employed promptly, gout usually can be arrested and complications (eg, destructive joint lesions, urolithiasis) can be prevented.

Interstitial nephritis may occur in some patients with gout. More commonly, the nephropathy is secondary to vascular disease, hypertension, lead intoxication, or is an independent renal disease. Nephrolithiasis can result from hyperuricosuria. Therapy with uric acid-lowering drugs will not reverse the progressive renal insufficiency, which is independent of the hyperuricemia (Beck, 1986).

The hyperuricemia that underlies the clinical manifestations of acute gouty arthritis commonly is classified as primary or secondary. Primary hyperuricemia may result from overproduction of uric acid, decreased renal excretion of uric acid, or both. The precise mechanism of uric acid overproduction is undefined in most cases. Obesity, excessive weight gain in young adulthood, and hypertension are risk factors for development of gout in white males (Roubenhoff et al, 1991). In some patients, a deficiency of hypoxanthine-guanine-phosphoribosyl transferase or increased activity of phosphoribosyl-pyrophosphate synthetase may lead to elevated levels of 5-phosphoribosyl-1-pyrophosphate, which promotes the synthesis of uric acid (Rodnan et al, 1983).

Impaired renal clearance of uric acid is much more common than overproduction. In many patients with gout, the renal capacity to excrete uric acid is defective. This capacity depends on the integrity of a four-component model of filtration, reabsorption, secretion, and postsecretory reabsorption. Decreased tubular secretion or enhanced tubular reabsorption are the most likely mechanisms in primary hyperuricemia.

Secondary hyperuricemia develops during the course of another disease or is the consequence of some external precipitating event (eg, drug therapy). Like primary hyperuricemia, the underlying causes of secondary hyperuricemia are the overproduction and/or decreased renal excretion of uric acid. For example, in patients with myeloproliferative disorders, increased bone marrow activity results in increased production and turnover of both cells and nucleic acids, which lead to elevated blood concentrations of uric acid. Renal elimination of uric acid may be compromised by diuretic therapy or chronic ingestion of alcohol, which also may lead to elevated blood concentrations.

Symptoms of acute gout usually develop at serum uric acid concentrations above 7 mg/dL in males or postmenopausal females as measured by the uricase method. These concentrations characteristically promote deposition of monosodium urate crystals in synovial tissue or fluid, which eventually causes an acute inflammatory attack. Although the precise mechanism is not known, events responsible for an attack include leukocytic phagocytosis of crystals, activation of the kallikrein and complement systems, disruption of lysosomes within the leukocytes, and subsequent disruption of whole cells with release of lysosomal enzymes into the synovial fluid (Kelley and Palella, 1987).

Gout is uncommon in women, who represent only about 5.2% of the cases. Diuretic therapy, renal insufficiency, and postmenopausal status are significant associations. Otherwise, the spectrum of the disease, including mean serum urate concentration, is similar to gout in men (Krane, 1986; Lally et al, 1986).

Many disorders are associated with hyperuricemia, and the symptoms of acute gout may resemble those of several other types of arthritis. Demonstration of monosodium urate crystals in synovial fluid leukocytes or tophi is diagnostic of gout. In addition, the combination of hyperuricemia, monoarticular arthritis that resolves with an intercritical period, and a prompt response to colchicine usually differentiates gout from similar conditions.

Drug Therapy

The principal objectives of the treatment of gout are: (1) to terminate the inflammatory process of an acute attack, and (2) to reduce hyperuricemia in order to prevent formation of urate deposits and recurrent attacks and to promote the resolution of tophi in tophaceous gout. There is some disagreement on the necessity of reducing hyperuricemia in all patients with gout. In high-risk patients with secondary hyperuricemia, particularly those with neoplasm-related hyperuricemia who are receiving antineoplastic agents, reduction of hyperuricemia may be necessary to avoid obstructive uropathy.

NSAIDs are most commonly used to treat attacks of acute gouty arthritis. Colchicine rarely is indicated. Drugs employed to reduce hyperuricemia are probenecid [Benemid] and sulfinpyrazone [Anturane], which increase the renal excretion of uric acid, and allopurinol [Lopurin, Zyloprim], which decreases the formation of uric acid. These agents should not be used to treat acute attacks because they are ineffective and may exacerbate or precipitate an acute attack.

Acute Gouty Arthritis: Drug selection depends on the physician's or patient's experience with a certain drug. Medication is most effective when given early during an acute attack, and patients should be advised to take the drug at the first signs of an impending acute attack.

NSAIDs (eg, indomethacin [Indocin], naproxen [Anaprox, Naprosyn]) are the preferred agents for the treatment of acute gouty arthritis and subsequent attacks. Because of its adverse reactions, including blood dyscrasias, phenylbutazone should be reserved for patients with a history of severe treatment-resistant attacks that have responded favorably to the drug in the past and should be used only after therapeutic measures, including other NSAIDs, have been unsatisfactory. Phenylbutazone should be taken for no longer than seven days.

Intramuscular or intravenous administration of corticotropin (ACTH) or oral or intra-articular injection of a corticosteroid rarely is necessary except in very severe acute attacks or in patients who do not respond to or cannot tolerate other anti-inflammatory agents. Colchicine should be given with and after discontinuation of corticotropin or steroids to prevent rebound attacks.

Intercritical (Interval) Period: Proper management of patients with gout during the intercritical (asymptomatic) period includes drug therapy, attention to diet for control of body weight and excess intake of purines, and avoidance of precipitating factors, including alcohol. Many patients do well during the intercritical phase without drug therapy. This discussion is limited to a consideration of appropriate drug therapy.

Small daily doses of colchicine (0.5 to 1.5 mg) can be used to prevent recurrent acute attacks. Some clinicians do not initiate prophylactic therapy unless two or three attacks occur within a one-year period. If symptoms of an impending acute attack occur during prophylactic therapy, the dose of colchicine should be increased. An attack usually can be aborted with a few tablets. As an alternative to colchicine, a small dose of indomethacin (25 mg twice daily) or another NSAID may be used for prophylaxis.

After the inflammation of an acute attack has subsided, the administration of drugs that decrease serum uric acid (allopurinol, probenecid, sulfinpyrazone) should be considered to avoid the other physiologic manifestations of gout. Opinions vary regarding the time in the treatment program when antihyperuricemic therapy, if indicated, should be started. Most clinicians prefer to withhold these drugs after only one or two attacks if hyperuricemia is mild and renal function is normal; others believe that hyperuricemia severe enough to produce one acute attack should be treated. Serum urate levels should not be reduced suddenly, because the rapid mobilization of urate from body pools may precipitate an acute attack.

Since uricosuric agents and allopurinol may precipitate an attack of acute gouty arthritis during initial treatment, small doses should be used initially and the amount increased gradually.

The choice between allopurinol or a uricosuric is based on the production and, thus, excretion of uric acid. Patients consuming a normal diet who have normal renal function (creatinine clearance greater than 80 ml/min is ideal, but never less than 50 ml/min) and in whom the 24-hour urinary uric acid excretion on a regular diet is less than 800 mg should be treated with a uricosuric. However, uricosuric agents are not used ordinarily in patients over 60 years. When uric acid excretion is persistently above 800 mg, overproduction of uric acid can be presumed and the patient should be treated with allopurinol. Allopurinol also is preferred in those with renal insufficiency, nephrolithiasis, or large tophi. The objective of treatment in these patients is to maintain normal serum and urinary uric acid levels.

Regardless of which drug is used to treat hyperuricemia, the serum urate concentration should be measured regularly to determine the efficacy of treatment. To help avoid urate renal calculi during uricosuric therapy, a large flow of less acid urine (pH 6.0 to 6.5) should be maintained by increasing fluid intake. Renal function should be assessed periodically during this therapy.

Tophaceous Gout: The objective of treatment in tophaceous gout is to decrease the serum uric acid concentration to about 5 mg/dL, or at least to less than 7 mg/dL in males and 6 mg/dL in females, thereby allowing tophi to be reduced in size without precipitating crystals in the kidneys or joints. Because allopurinol reduces the load of uric acid excreted by the kidney and because the amount of uric acid that is mobilized from tophi is extremely high, this drug is preferred. In the rare patient with adequate renal function who is not controlled by a single medication, allopurinol may be used with probenecid. Such combination therapy does not necessitate changing the dose of either drug and usually lowers serum urate concentration (Kelley and Palella, 1987). Effectiveness of therapy can be assessed by observing the frequency of acute gouty attacks as well as the reduction in tophi and prevention of joint deformity. Periodic radiographic assessments may be necessary to confirm the response to therapy (McCarthy et al, 1991).

Secondary Hyperuricemia: Secondary hyperuricemia may result from excessive production and/or decreased renal excretion of uric acid. Overproduction occurs in various myeloproliferative disorders, such as polycythemia vera, myeloid metaplasia, leukemia, or lymphoma, as well as during the treatment of these diseases with drugs that cause a breakdown of cellular nucleic acid. Patients with these diseases should be given allopurinol prior to treatment with cytotoxic drugs (see the evaluation on Allopurinol for precautions). Decreased renal excretion of uric acid occurs in conditions such as lead nephropathy, glycogen storage disease, and sickle cell disease; the endogenous production of uric acid also is increased in the latter two conditions.

Several drugs, including salicylates in low doses, pyrazinamide, niacin, ethambutol [Myambutol], cyclosporine, and alcohol, may increase the serum uric acid level. Hyperuricemia often is induced by diuretics that are widely used to treat hypertension, but the routine use of drugs to reduce serum uric acid in these patients is unnecessary. Antihypertensive therapy should be the primary treatment in patients with both gout and hypertension, since studies suggest that renal disease is a more common complication of uncontrolled hypertension than uncontrolled hyperuricemia. Some clinicians believe that hyperuricemia should be treated with a uricosuric agent if the serum urate level exceeds 10 mg/dL in females and 13 mg/dL in males (Simkin, 1979) and that colchicine should be given concomitantly during the early months of therapy to prevent attacks of acute gout.

Asymptomatic Hyperuricemia: The risk of developing gouty arthritis is proportional to the degree of hyperuricemia. Mild hyperuricemia with no clinical manifestations of gout should not be treated. Treatment should be instituted if symptoms of gout develop; if there is a family history of gout, nephrolithiasis, or renal failure; or if there is marked overproduction of uric acid as indicated by the daily urinary excretion of more than 1.1 g (Kelley and Palella, 1987).

Pseudogout: Pseudogout is a term used to describe deposition of calcium pyrophosphate in the joint, often associated with chondrocalcinosis. Clinically, it resembles acute gouty arthritis and is characterized by acute inflammation and pain in one or more joints that lasts several days or more. It is thought to result from an inflammatory response to calcium pyrophosphate crystals in the synovial fluid similar to that seen in patients with acute gout caused by accumulation of urate crystals. The magnitude of this inflammatory response is generally less than that seen in acute gouty arthritis.

The NSAIDs are effective in relieving inflammation and pain. When large joints are affected acutely, thorough aspiration alone or with concomitant injection of corticosteroids may be beneficial. Colchicine can be useful for acute attacks when administered intravenously in usual therapeutic doses; however, caution is required because of its potential toxicity. Oral administration generally is less effective for acute attacks of pseudogout (Rodnan et al, 1983) but is useful for prophylaxis.

Drug Evaluations

DRUGS USED IN ACUTE GOUTY ARTHRITIS

COLCHICINE

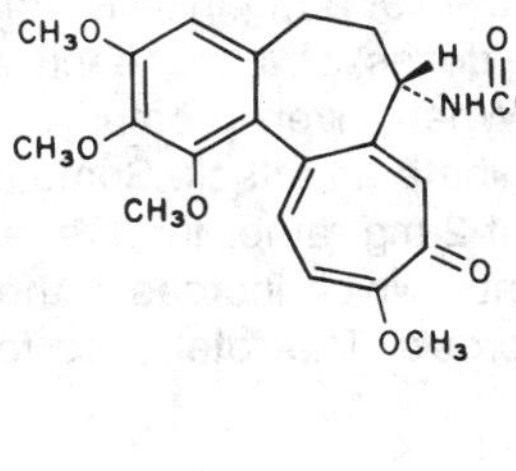

CH_3O H O $NHCCH_3$ CH_3O CH_3O O OCH_3

ACTIONS AND USES. Colchicine inhibits microtubular formation and migration of neutrophils to inflamed areas. It also may inhibit the generation and release of inflammatory mediators formed by phagocytes in response to exposure to urate crystals. This drug usually is reserved for patients who cannot tolerate or do not respond satisfactorily to NSAIDs. Therapy should begin at the first sign of an attack and continue until symptoms subside, gastrointestinal distress develops, or the maximal dose is given.

This drug may be administered orally or intravenously. The oral route is not used as frequently as in the past because of gastrointestinal disturbances and the availability of other drugs. When colchicine is given intravenously, care must be taken to prevent extravasation, which causes sloughing of skin and subcutaneous tissues. Some rheumatologists prefer this route because it produces a more rapid response and the incidence of gastrointestinal disturbances is lower. Relief of pain and inflammation usually occurs within 24 to 48 hours after oral therapy and 6 to 12 hours after intravenous injection, but several days may elapse before swelling subsides completely. It may be difficult to obtain prompt relief with nontoxic doses if there is delay in treatment or inconsistency in the dosage schedule.

Use of small doses of oral colchicine during the intercritical period may prevent acute attacks or diminish their severity and facilitate treatment. This drug also is given to prevent attacks of acute gouty arthritis that may be precipitated during the initial months of treatment with uricosurics or allopurinol, but this combined therapy should be individualized. Colchicine should be given until all visible or radiographically demonstrated tophi are dissolved. In the absence of tophi, it is advisable to continue therapy for one year. The dosage should be adjusted to provide maximal freedom from acute attacks without adverse reactions. Patients receiving colchicine prophylaxis sometimes respond to small additional therapeutic doses, thus terminating an acute attack without unpleasant reactions.

Intravenous colchicine may be used to control acute attacks of pseudogout (Tabatabai and Cummings, 1980; Spilberg et al, 1980).

In one small placebo-controlled, double-blind, crossover study, administration of colchicine 0.5 mg three times daily for 16 weeks was beneficial in patients with psoriatic arthritis (Seideman et al, 1987).

When taken prophylactically, colchicine may prevent the episodic attacks of painful serositis characteristic of familial Mediterranean fever and may improve the symptoms of amyloidosis (Zemer et al, 1986). Alternatively, short courses of colchicine taken at the earliest onset of symptoms may abort attacks in some patients.

Colchicine has been reported to be effective in dermatitis herpetiformis (Silvers et al, 1980), the cutaneous and ocular manifestations of Behçet's disease (Miyachi et al, 1981), acute febrile neutrophilic dermatosis (Suehisa et al, 1983), erythema nodosum leprosum (Sarojini and Mshana, 1983), idiopathic thrombocytopenic purpura resistant to standard treatment (Strother et al, 1984), and primary biliary cirrhosis

(Kaplan et al, 1986). It also has been employed in sarcoid, scleroderma, and Still's disease in adults.

ADVERSE REACTIONS AND PRECAUTIONS. Colchicine causes gastrointestinal reactions about 8 to 12 hours after oral administration in approximately 80% of patients, especially when maximal doses are used. These include nausea and vomiting or abdominal pain, as well as the limiting therapeutic endpoint of diarrhea. The warning provided by gastrointestinal intolerance tends to protect the patient from toxic doses. As soon as symptoms of intolerance occur, administration should be discontinued, irrespective of the status of joint symptoms. Oral colchicine often causes diarrhea before relieving gout in elderly patients. Drugs to control vomiting and diarrhea may be given.

Gastrointestinal distress rarely develops after slow intravenous administration of therapeutic amounts, but extravasation produces inflammation and necrosis of the skin and soft tissues. Severe toxicity and death from arrhythmias can occur due to too rapid administration. Intravenous administration is contraindicated in patients with leukopenia, extrahepatic biliary obstruction, creatinine clearance rate less than 10 ml/min, or combined renal and hepatic disease. The dosage (oral or intravenous) should be reduced in the presence of renal or hepatic disease and in elderly patients with apparently normal renal function (Wallace and Singer, 1988). Colchicine should be avoided, if possible, in patients with active peptic ulcer. Intravenous and oral administration should not be employed concurrently.

Diminished renal function, causing increasing plasma concentrations of colchicine, is most often responsible for side effects associated with long-term therapy. Other reactions include rashes, alopecia, thrombocytopenia, and occasionally neutropenia. These patients also may exhibit reversible myopathy (proximal muscle weakness) and irreversible neuropathy (diminished deep tendon reflexes and abnormal sensory and motor electromyography). Elevated serum creatine kinase activity is a sensitive measure of this condition, with the enzyme activity paralleling the severity (Kuncl et al, 1987).

Colchicine is classified in FDA Pregnancy Category D.

OVERDOSAGE AND POISONING. Severe reactions have been reported and generally have been associated with therapeutic or suicidal overdosage (Stapczynski et al, 1981). The fatal oral dose of colchicine in adults is approximately 20 mg. A second stage of intoxication, usually heralded by fever, appears about 24 to 72 hours after the overdose. A number of organs are affected. Signs and symptoms include respiratory distress with diffuse interstitial and alveolar edema; ileus; elevated hepatic transaminases and amylase; bone marrow hypoplasia with peripheral granulocytopenia and thrombocytopenia; prolonged coagulation time or disseminated intravascular coagulation; fluid, electrolyte, and renal disorders, including frank hematuria and proteinuria, hypocalcemia, hypokalemia, and hypophosphatemia; and metabolic acidosis. Acute circulatory failure occurring within 72 hours after ingestion is the cause of nearly all fatalities. Its etiology is not clear, but it may represent direct myocardial injury. Although hypovolemia secondary to intestinal loss of water and to intravascular fluid shift is present in almost all patients, its correction may not improve the cardiac index.

Management of the intoxication is symptomatic: repeated doses of activated charcoal orally, treatment of hypovolemia with central venous pressure monitoring, combating hypothermia, administration of phytonadione (vitamin K_1) or fresh frozen plasma for coagulation deficiencies and platelets or red blood cells if indicated, parenteral nutrition, correction of electrolyte imbalance, and administration of intravenous benzodiazepines if convulsions occur. Patients who survive serious colchicine intoxication usually demonstrate a rebound leukocytosis during recovery of bone marrow function in about one week. Reversible alopecia is common, usually beginning about 7 to 12 days after the incident.

PHARMACOKINETICS. Following oral administration of 2 mg, a mean peak plasma level of 2.2 ng/ml is reached after two hours; however, absorption is variable. Following intravenous injection of a 1-mg bolus in normal subjects, the mean elimination half-life is 65 ± 15 minutes and total clearance is 601 ± 155 ml/min. The apparent volume of distribution is 2 L/kg. Colchicine levels decline biexponentially, fitting a two-compartment open-body model. Protein binding is minimal. The drug is concentrated in peripheral leukocytes and may persist there for ten days. The metabolism of colchicine is not known. Colchicine undergoes significant biliary and intestinal secretion following absorption and is excreted primarily in the feces. About 5% to 20% of a single dose is eliminated by the kidney.

DOSAGE AND PREPARATIONS.

Oral: For acute attacks, *adults,* 0.5 or 0.6 mg (one tablet) is administered hourly; alternatively, 1 or 1.2 mg (two tablets) may be given initially, followed by 0.5 or 0.6 mg every two hours until articular symptoms subside or gastrointestinal distress occurs. A maximum dose of 6 mg in 24 hours may be administered to an otherwise healthy patient, but most patients cannot tolerate this amount. For prophylaxis, the dosage depends on the sensitivity of the patient to gastrointestinal reactions. Usually 0.5 to 1 mg daily is given (Yü, 1982); 0.5 mg should be given every two hours for several days if symptoms of an impending attack occur.

Generic. Tablets 0.5 and 0.6 mg.

Intravenous: To minimize sclerosis of the vein and the risk of arrhythmias, the contents of the 2-ml vial should be diluted to 20 ml with sterile normal sodium chloride injection and administered slowly over no less than five minutes. Solutions containing a bacteriostatic agent or 5% dextrose should not be used; any solution containing a precipitate should be discarded. Caution should be exercised and the risk/benefit ratio should be considered for each patient; attention should be given to the guidelines developed to reduce drug-related morbidity (Roberts et al, 1987; Wallace and Singer, 1988).

For acute attacks, *adults,* 2 mg initially, followed by one or rarely two additional doses of 1 mg each at 6- to 12-hour intervals if needed. When given promptly, one or two slow infusions usually terminate an attack. Some clinicians recommend a single dose of 2 mg rather than repeated administration of smaller amounts, which increases the risk of extravasation and tissue necrosis. The total dose for one course of treatment should never exceed 4 mg. Colchicine should not be administered by any route for seven days after patients receive a full intravenous course. In the elderly, a maximum dose for one course of treatment is 2 mg with an interval of at least three weeks between courses. In patients with impaired renal or hepatic function, the total dose for one course of therapy should be decreased. If creatinine clearance is <50 ml/min, the total dose should not exceed 2 mg; intravenous colchicine is contraindicated if creatinine clearance is less than 10 ml/min.

Generic. Solution 0.5 mg/ml in 2 ml containers.

Anti-Inflammatory Drugs

ADRENAL CORTICOSTEROIDS

CORTICOTROPIN (ACTH)

[Acthar]

Although needed only infrequently, corticotropin or systemic corticosteroids may be effective in unusually severe acute attacks when other agents are contraindicated or patients do not respond to other anti-inflammatory drugs. These agents should not be administered for more than a few days and should not be given to treat chronic gout.

A single intramuscular dose of 40 units of corticotropin is not associated with side effects and can be utilized in those who cannot tolerate indomethacin. About 20% of patients will experience a rebound attack after single-dose therapy (Preston and Axelrod, 1987) if other prophylactic therapy is not provided. To prevent rebound attacks, colchicine 0.5 or 0.6 mg two or three times daily should be given with and for seven days after discontinuation of corticotropin or steroids. If the acute attack is limited to a single joint, a corticosteroid injected intra-articularly usually relieves pain.

For adverse reactions and precautions, see index entries Adrenal Corticosteroids; Corticotropin, In Adrenal Dysfunction.

DOSAGE AND PREPARATIONS.

CORTICOTROPIN:

Intramuscular: *Adults,* 40 to 80 units every six to eight hours for two or three days; the dose then is reduced gradually until the medication can be withdrawn completely. Also see the use of single-dose therapy in the preceding discussion.

Available generically and as ***ACTH***. Gel (repository) 40 and 80 units/ml in 5 ml containers; powder 40 and 80 units.

Acthar (Rhone-Poulenc Rorer). Gel (repository) 40 and 80 units/ml in 1 and 5 ml containers (***H.P. Acthar Gel***); powder (sterile, lyophilized) 25 and 40 units.

ADRENAL CORTICOSTEROIDS:

The doses vary greatly depending on the individual preparation, but oral doses of 20 to 30 mg daily of prednisone and intra-articular injection of 8 to 40 mg of prednisolone tebutate or 2 to 20 mg of triamcinolone hexacetonide, depending on the size of joint, are suggested (Simkin, 1979; Talbott, 1980; Holmes, 1981).

For preparations, see index entry Adrenal Corticosteroids.

INDOMETHACIN

[Indocin]

For chemical formula, see evaluation in section on Arthritis.

USES. Indomethacin's anti-inflammatory properties are useful in the short-term treatment of attacks of acute gouty arthritis, and it or one of the other NSAIDs is the drug of choice when the diagnosis is well established. Efficacy is comparable to that of colchicine. Indomethacin also may be beneficial in acute pseudogout.

ADVERSE REACTIONS AND PRECAUTIONS. The adverse reactions produced by indomethacin, some of which may be serious, generally are dose and time dependent. Gastrointestinal effects (nausea, vomiting, dyspepsia, diarrhea, abdominal pain, constipation) or central nervous system effects (headache, a mild confusional state, vertigo, somnolence, depression, and fatigue) are most common.

Indomethacin should not be given to patients with an active ulcer, a history of recurrent gastrointestinal lesions, nasal polyps associated with angioedema, a history of bronchospastic reaction to aspirin or other NSAIDs, or renal insufficiency. This drug should be used cautiously in the elderly, since the incidence of adverse reactions appears to be higher in these patients.

When indomethacin is administered with probenecid, the tubular secretion of indomethacin is inhibited and the plasma concentration is increased; thus, a smaller dose of indomethacin may be satisfactory. Indomethacin also may interact with aspirin, lithium, and furosemide.

DOSAGE AND PREPARATIONS. Oral indomethacin should be taken with food, immediately after meals, or with antacids to reduce gastrointestinal irritation. The prolonged-release preparation should not be used for acute gout.

Oral: For attacks of acute gout, *adults,* initially, 50 mg, followed by 25 mg three or four times daily until symptoms subside. Pain usually is relieved within two to four hours, tenderness and heat in 24 to 36 hours, and swelling gradually disappears, usually in three to five days. The dose is then reduced rapidly to cessation of therapy. Alternatively, some clinicians prefer a fixed-dose, nine-day schedule of 50 mg three times daily for the first three days followed by 50 mg twice daily for three days and 50 mg once daily for the final three days. The drug may be withdrawn at any time if the attack is terminated before the full nine days.

Indocin (Merck), ***Generic.*** Capsules 25 and 50 mg; suspension 25 mg/5 ml

Rectal: *Adults,* 25 to 50 mg two to four times daily. *Children,* dosage has not been established.

Indocin (Merck). Suppositories 50 mg.

FENOPROFEN CALCIUM

IBUPROFEN

NAPROXEN, NAPROXEN SODIUM

SULINDAC

For chemical formulas, see evaluations in the section on Arthritis.

These NSAIDs were developed primarily to treat RA but, because of their anti-inflammatory and analgesic actions, are also useful in acute gout. Although only sulindac and naproxen are labeled for use in gout, results of clinical studies have demonstrated that the others also are effective. There is insufficient evidence to indicate that any of these drugs is superior to the others as the initial agent in an acute attack. However, any of them may be tried as substitutes for colchicine, especially if the diagnosis has been confirmed.

These NSAIDs also are alternatives to colchicine for prophylaxis prior to and during initial therapy with allopurinol or uricosurics. They may be effective as nonspecific therapy in acute pseudogout.

For a discussion of adverse reactions, precautions, and interactions, see the evaluations on these drugs in the section on Arthritis.

DOSAGE AND PREPARATIONS.

FENOPROFEN CALCIUM:

Oral: For acute attacks, dosage has not been established. In investigational studies, 800 mg was given every six hours for three to eight days, depending on response.

IBUPROFEN:

Oral: For acute attacks, dosage has not been established. In investigational studies, 800 mg was given every eight hours initially; the amount was reduced to 400 mg every six hours for 24 to 72 hours after symptoms subsided.

NAPROXEN, NAPROXEN SODIUM:

Oral: For acute attacks, initially, naproxen 750 mg or naproxen sodium 875 mg, followed by naproxen 250 mg or naproxen sodium 275 mg every eight hours until the attack subsides.

SULINDAC:

Oral: For acute attacks, *adults,* 200 mg twice a day. The dose can be reduced after a satisfactory response has occurred; seven days of therapy are usually sufficient.

For preparations, see the evaluations in the section on Arthritis.

DRUGS USED FOR TOPHACEOUS GOUT AND OTHER HYPERURICEMIAS

ALLOPURINOL

[Lopurin, Zyloprim]

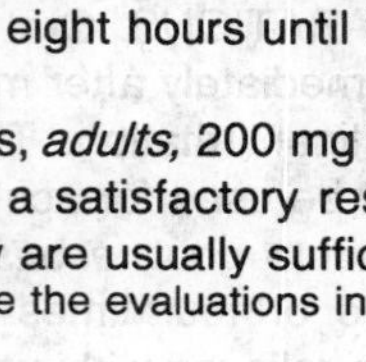

ACTIONS. Allopurinol decreases the production of uric acid by inhibiting xanthine oxidase, which converts hypoxanthine to xanthine and xanthine to uric acid; plasma and urine concentrations of uric acid are thus reduced. Allopurinol also inhibits de novo purine synthesis through a feedback mechanism. This action requires the presence of hypoxanthine-guanine phosphoribosyltransferase. Children with Lesch-Nyhan syndrome, who lack this enzyme, and the few adults with a partial deficiency do not benefit from this effect.

Allopurinol is itself metabolized by xanthine oxidase to oxipurinol, which also inhibits xanthine oxidase. Oxipurinol has a considerably longer plasma half-life than allopurinol, thus accounting for the latter's long duration of action, which permits administration of allopurinol once daily. Unlike uricosuric agents, allopurinol decreases the renal excretion of uric acid and its action is not antagonized by salicylates.

USES. Allopurinol is the preferred drug in the treatment of chronic tophaceous gout; it reduces serum urate levels, usually within a few days to two weeks. Prolonged treatment inhibits the formation of tophi and mobilizes stored urates, which causes a gradual regression in the size of tophi already formed. Allopurinol is especially useful in patients with chronic gout complicated by renal insufficiency or uric acid renal calculi, although careful titration of dose is important.

This drug also is used to treat hyperuricemia associated with excessive production of uric acid (urinary uric acid excretion more than 800 mg/24 hours). This often occurs in patients with polycythemia vera, myeloid metaplasia, leukemia, or lymphoma, as well as during the treatment of these conditions with cytotoxic agents that break down cellular nucleic acids, which leads to acute uric acid nephropathy. Patients with these disorders should receive allopurinol prior to cytotoxic drug therapy. In patients with the Lesch-Nyhan syndrome, allopurinol controls blood uric acid levels and prevents nephropathy, tophi, and arthritis but has no effect on the neurologic and behavioral manifestations.

Like the uricosurics, allopurinol may increase the frequency of attacks of acute gouty arthritis during the early stages of treatment; therefore, colchicine or an NSAID should be given prophylactically during the initial months of therapy (see the evaluation on Colchicine), and patients should receive appropriate treatment if acute attacks occur. Attacks usually diminish in number and severity after several months of treatment with allopurinol.

ADVERSE REACTIONS AND PRECAUTIONS. Allopurinol is well tolerated by most patients, and most adverse reactions can be attributed to excessive dosage (McInnes et al, 1981). However, a toxic syndrome associated with hypersensitivity has been reported (Hande et al, 1984). Manifestations include a diffuse, erythematous, desquamating rash; pruritus; gastrointestinal distress; diarrhea; fever; hepatic dysfunction; eosinophilia; and renal dysfunction. Of the 78 reported cases of severe allopurinol toxic syndrome, 16 have resulted in death. Most patients who developed this syndrome took 200 to 400 mg daily for two to four weeks and had renal insufficiency. The causative factor may be allopurinol's active metabolite, oxipurinol, since its long half-life is prolonged further in patients with impaired renal function. In a study of six cases (Hande et al, 1984), the serum oxipurinol half-life was related inversely to renal creatinine clearance.

Of the 78 cases reported, 52 patients were being treated for asymptomatic hyperuricemia. Thus, the incidence of toxicity could be reduced by avoiding use of this drug in patients with asymptomatic hyperuricemia and by avoiding or reducing the dose in those with renal insufficiency. If a rash and/or fever develop, allopurinol should be discontinued. Some patients recover spontaneously after drug withdrawal, while others require steroids or hemodialysis. If the use of allopurinol is imperative in a patient who has exhibited a hypersensitivity reaction to the drug, an oral desensitization regimen may be attempted (Webster and Panush, 1985; Fam et al, 1992).

The long-term administration of allopurinol has been associated with cataracts in a few patients (Fraunfelder et al, 1982; Lerman et al, 1982, 1984); however, a causal relationship has not been established. It is recommended that patients receiving allopurinol be advised to undergo periodic ophthalmologic examinations and, if lens opacity is present, the drug should be discontinued.

Reactions that occur occasionally include nausea, vomiting, diarrhea, abdominal discomfort, drowsiness, headache, and a metallic taste. Rare reactions for which a causal relationship has not been established include peripheral neuritis, precipitation of peptic ulcer or increase in ulcer symptoms, tachycardia, pancreatitis, pyelonephritis, increased blood urea nitrogen levels, anemia, retinopathy, and macular degeneration. One death associated with bone marrow depression has been reported.

Hepatic effects ranging from altered liver function (increased serum levels of alkaline phosphatase and transaminases) to hepatitis, which may be part of a generalized hypersensitivity reaction, have been reported frequently. Granulomatous hepatitis has been reported rarely. If anorexia, weight loss, or pruritus develops in patients taking allopurinol, liver function should be evaluated. This drug is relatively contraindicated in patients with liver disease and bone marrow suppression.

Xanthine renal calculus formation occurs rarely, even in patients with Lesch-Nyhan syndrome.

Studies in animals have shown that allopurinol has no teratogenic effects. However, there is no information on the effects of xanthine oxidase inhibition on the human fetus, and the potential benefits should be weighed against the possible risk to the fetus before allopurinol is used in pregnant women or women of childbearing age (FDA Pregnancy Category C).

DRUG INTERACTIONS. Because allopurinol inhibits the oxidation of mercaptopurine, the dose of the latter must be reduced to one-third or one-fourth of the usual amount when both drugs are given concomitantly. Since mercaptopurine is a metabolite of azathioprine, similar precautions should be observed when using the latter drug. Allopurinol also appears to increase the toxicity of other cytotoxic agents (eg, cyclophosphamide). Anemia, nausea, pain, pruritus, and tremors have developed in patients receiving allopurinol and vidarabine. Thus, caution is advised when these two drugs are administered concomitantly (Friedman and Grasela, 1981).

The incidence of rash after administration of ampicillin is unusually high in patients receiving allopurinol concomitantly. Allopurinol should be discontinued promptly when rash occurs, since this reaction may become serious if treatment is continued.

Allopurinol inhibits hepatic drug metabolizing enzymes; thus, drugs metabolized by these enzymes (eg, coumarin derivatives) should be given in lower doses.

PHARMACOKINETICS. Following a single oral dose of 300 mg, about 80% of the dose is absorbed. Peak serum concentrations of 1.4 ± 0.23 ng/ml are reached in one to two hours; oxipurinol, the major metabolite, reaches a peak concentration of 5.2 ± 0.65 ng/ml in 5.2 to 6.5 hours. The half-life of allopurinol is 1.3 ± 0.1 hours and that of oxipurinol is 21.2 ± 0.4 hours (Chang et al, 1981). Most of the oxipurinol is excreted unchanged by the kidney.

DOSAGE AND PREPARATIONS. Allopurinol is better tolerated if taken after meals.

Oral: *Adults,* dosage must be individualized to establish the minimal effective dose that maintains the serum urate level below 7 mg/dL (males) or 6 mg/dL (females). Initially, 100 mg/day, increased by 100 mg at intervals of one month or longer until the serum uric acid level is normal or near normal. An effective range for most patients with normal renal function is 200 to 500 mg daily. The maintenance dosage should be reduced in patients with renal insufficiency: creatinine clearance 10 to 20 ml/min, maximum daily dosage, 200 mg; <10 ml/min, maximum daily dosage, 100 mg. In patients with severe renal impairment (creatinine clearance <3 ml/min), the interval between doses also may need to be lengthened.

For secondary hyperuricemias, the optimal dose is the smallest amount necessary to maintain serum uric acid levels within the normal range. *Adults,* 100 to 200 mg daily is the minimum effective dose (maximum, 800 mg); *children 6 to 10 years with malignancies,* 300 mg daily; *under 6 years,* 150 mg daily.

Lopurin (Boots), ***Zyloprim*** (Burroughs Wellcome), ***Generic.*** Tablets 100 and 300 mg.

Rectal: Extemporaneous rectal suppositories have been prepared from tablets for use in patients unable to take oral medications; however, absorption of the drug in suppository form was poor and erratic. Although clinical efficacy, as determined by the decrease in serum uric acid level, has been reported, additional studies are needed to confirm these results. Therefore, this route does not appear to be an effective alternative to oral administration (Chang et al, 1981).

PROBENECID

[Benemid]

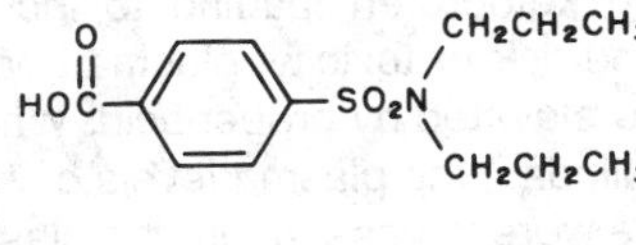

$HO\overset{O}{\overset{\|}{C}}-C_6H_4-SO_2N(CH_2CH_2CH_3)_2$

ACTIONS AND USES. This effective uricosuric agent is used to prevent or reduce the joint changes and tophi that occur in chronic gout; it is chosen primarily for patients with normal renal function whose 24-hour urinary uric acid excretion is less than 800 mg. Its uricosuric effect is attributed to inhibition of the tubular reabsorption of filtered urate. Probenecid usually has no significant uricosuric activity when the glomerular filtration rate is less than 30 ml/min and thus may not be effective in patients with chronic renal insufficiency. It has been used in patients with renal impairment, but an increase in dosage may be required. Probenecid is not usually used in those over 60 years. This drug is not indicated in acute attacks of gouty arthritis.

Since acute attacks of gout may occur during the initial months of therapy, colchicine should be given concomitantly during this period. (See the evaluation on Colchicine.)

ADVERSE REACTIONS AND PRECAUTIONS. Probenecid is well tolerated by most patients. Gastrointestinal reactions (anorexia, nausea, vomiting), headache, hypersensitivity reactions (including anaphylaxis, dermatitis, pruritus, and fever), urinary frequency, anemia, dizziness, and flushing have occurred. Hemolytic anemia, which may be related to G6PD deficiency; aplastic anemia; nephrotic syndrome; and hepatic necrosis have been reported rarely.

During the first few weeks of therapy, a large volume (2 to 3 L/day) of alkaline urine should be maintained to minimize urate precipitation. This is especially important for patients living in hot, dry climates. Probenecid is contraindicated in those with a history of renal calculi, especially uric acid stones, because it may aggravate or precipitate this condition. The drug also should not be used in patients whose glomerular filtration rate is less than 50% of normal.

DRUG INTERACTIONS. Salicylates and some of the NSAIDs (but not ibuprofen or indomethacin) diminish the effect of probenecid and should not be used concomitantly. The patient must be warned about this interaction, since it is estimated to be the cause of about 25% of treatment failures. The very small doses of aspirin (80 mg/day) used as prophylaxis in myocardial infarction apparently may be employed without affecting the uricosuric action of probenecid. Probenecid inhibits the renal transport of aminosalicylic acid, chlorpropamide, dapsone, dyphylline, sulfinpyrazone, sulfonamides (mostly as inactive conjugates), and zidovudine. The drug has been reported to increase plasma levels of rifampin and methotrexate and to markedly increase the anticoagulant activity of heparin. The dosage of these agents should be modified when they are administered with probenecid.

Since probenecid increases the renal excretion of oxipurinol, inhibition of xanthine oxidase is reduced when probenecid is given with allopurinol. However, in tophaceous gout, it can be given with allopurinol for more rapid dissolution of tophi. Probenecid inhibits the renal and hepatic clearance of indomethacin and ketoprofen leading to increased plasma concentrations and risk of toxicity; plasma concentrations of ketorolac also are elevated by probenecid. When probenecid was given with sulindac, the plasma levels of sulindac and its sulfone metabolite were increased, but the plasma sulfide levels were only slightly affected. Probenecid slows the clearance of naproxen by inhibiting hepatic metabolism; thus, concomitant use results in higher plasma concentrations of naproxen (Runkel et al, 1978).

Probenecid reduces the renal clearance of some antibiotics (eg, most penicillins, cephalosporins, fluoroquinolones, captopril, furosemide). These interactions probably are not clinically significant except for penicillins, with which probenecid is sometimes employed to enhance the therapeutic effect.

PHARMACOKINETICS. Probenecid is readily absorbed following oral administration. Peak plasma concentrations are observed three to four hours after a 0.5-g dose. The elimination half-life is dose dependent: 4.2 hours after the 0.5-g dose and 6 to 12 hours with larger doses. Probenecid is metabolized by side chain oxidation and glucuronidation. It is excreted in urine principally as acylglucuronides and oxidized metabolites. Only a small amount is excreted unchanged in urine (Selen et al, 1982).

DOSAGE AND PREPARATIONS.

Oral: Dosage should be individualized to obtain the desired serum urate level. *Adults,* 250 mg daily for one week or more depending on response; the amount is then increased slowly at one- to two-week intervals to the minimum dose necessary to maintain normal serum urate levels. Usually 1 g/day is sufficient, but some patients may require 1.5 g/day or more. Amounts in excess of 250 mg are given in divided doses twice daily (every 12 hours) or three times daily (every 8 hours).

Benemid (Merck), ***Generic.*** Tablets 500 mg.

SULFINPYRAZONE

[Anturane]

ACTIONS AND USES. Sulfinpyrazone is a congener of phenylbutazone, but it lacks the latter's anti-inflammatory, analgesic, and sodium-retaining properties. This effective uricosuric agent is used to treat tophaceous gout and hyperuricemia during the intercritical period. It is more potent than probenecid on a weight basis and is chosen primarily for patients with normal renal function whose 24-hour urinary uric acid excretion is less than 800 mg. It is of no value in relieving acute attacks of gouty arthritis and is not usually used in those over 60 years.

Because acute attacks of gout may increase in frequency or severity during the initial months of therapy with sulfinpyrazone, colchicine or a NSAID should be given concomitantly during this period. (See the evaluation on Colchicine.)

Since it inhibits thromboxane synthesis, sulfinpyrazone inhibits platelet function and has been used as an antithrombotic agent (see index entry Sulfinpyrazone, Uses).

ADVERSE REACTIONS AND PRECAUTIONS. The most frequently reported adverse reactions are abdominal pain and nausea. Since reactivation or exacerbation of peptic ulcer also has been reported, sulfinpyrazone should be used cautiously in patients with a history of ulcer and is contraindicated in those with active peptic ulcer. Rash is uncommon; anemia, leukopenia, agranulocytosis, and thrombocytopenia have occurred rarely.

An adequate fluid intake and alkalization of the urine should be maintained to minimize the renal deposition of urate during the first few weeks of therapy until the serum urate level is within the normal range. It is especially important to maintain an adequate urine flow in patients living in hot, dry climates. The drug should be used with caution in patients with impaired renal function or a history of renal calculi, especially uric acid stones, because of the possibility of aggravating or precipitating the condition. Renal calculi are somewhat more common after initiation of therapy with this drug than with probenecid. Sulfinpyrazone should not be used when the glomerular filtration rate is less than 50% of normal. Patients with significant renal impairment should have periodic evaluations of their renal function. Sulfinpyrazone is contraindicated in patients with a history of blood dyscrasias.

DRUG INTERACTIONS. Sulfinpyrazone reduces the renal tubular excretion of salicylic acid while salicylates and some of the other NSAIDs diminish the effect of sulfinpyrazone; thus, these agents should not be used concomitantly. The patient should be warned of this interaction because it is a frequent cause of treatment failure.

Like phenylbutazone, sulfinpyrazone may potentiate the actions of insulin and oral hypoglycemic agents; therefore, it should be used with caution in patients receiving these drugs. The antiprothrombin activity of oral anticoagulants may be enhanced. Because of its chemical relationship to phenylbutazone and the similarity of some adverse effects, sulfinpyrazone should be used cautiously, if at all, in patients known to be sensitive to phenylbutazone; however, serious reactions are less common than with phenylbutazone. Sulfinpyrazone has no effect on sodium reabsorption.

PHARMACOKINETICS. Sulfinpyrazone is rapidly and completely absorbed following oral administration. Peak blood levels occur in about one hour and the half-life is one to three hours. This drug is highly bound to plasma protein. About 20% to 45% of a dose is excreted unchanged in urine; the remainder is metabolized to the parahydroxyl analogue, which also has uricosuric activity.

DOSAGE AND PREPARATIONS.

Oral: *Adults,* 100 to 200 mg two times daily given with meals or milk. The dose is increased gradually over a one-week period until the dosage required to control blood urate levels is reached, usually 200 to 400 mg (maximum, 800 mg). The dose then may be reduced to the minimal effective amount.

Generic. Capsules 200 mg; tablets 100 and 200 mg.

Anturane (CIBA). Capsules 200 mg; tablets 100 mg.

Mixture

PROBENECID AND COLCHICINE

[ColBENEMID]

This mixture of probenecid and colchicine is designed to facilitate maintenance therapy in patients with chronic gout, but its usefulness is limited because the amount of each ingredient cannot be individualized. If the usual dosage of probenecid were used, this mixture would provide a greater amount of colchicine than needed by many patients and less than that needed by some.

For adverse reactions and precautions, see the evaluations on Colchicine and Probenecid.

DOSAGE AND PREPARATIONS. The dosage is based on the patient's requirement for the individual ingredients, provided that these have been established individually and are consistent with the ratio present in this preparation. (See the evaluations on Probenecid and Colchicine.)

ColBENEMID (Merck), ***Generic.*** Each tablet contains probenecid 500 mg and colchicine 0.5 mg.

Cited References

Oxaprozin: A new nonsteroidal antiinflammatory drug. *Semin Arthritis Rheum* 15(suppl 2):1-107, 1986.

Abramson SB, Weissmann G: The mechanisms of action of nonsteroidal antiinflammatory drugs. *Arthritis Rheum* 32:1-9, 1989.

Ahern M, et al: Methotrexate kinetics in rheumatoid arthritis: Is there an interaction with nonsteroidal anti-inflammatory drugs? *J Rheumatol* 15:1356-1360, 1988.

Amos RS, et al: Sulphasalazine for rheumatoid arthritis: Toxicity in 774 patients monitored for one to 11 years. *BMJ* 293:420-423, 1986.

Andelman SY, et al: Etodolac, aspirin, and placebo in patients with degenerative joint disease: A twelve-week study. *Clin Ther* 5:651-661, 1983.

Anderson PA, et al: Weekly pulse methotrexate in rheumatoid arthritis: Clinical and immunologic effects in a randomized double blind study. *Ann Intern Med* 103:489-496, 1985.

Ansell BM, Hall MA: Penicillamine in chronic arthritis of childhood. *J Rheumatol* 8(suppl 7):112-115, 1981.

Arnett FC, et al: The American Rheumatism Association 1987 revised criteria for the classification of rheumatoid arthritis. *Arthritis Rheum* 31:315-324, 1988.

Arnold MH, et al: Comparative controlled trial of low-dose weekly methotrexate versus azathioprine in rheumatoid arthritis: 3-year prospective study. *Br J Rheumatol* 29:120-125, 1990.

Balfour JA, Buckley MM-T: Etodolac: A reappraisal of its pharmacology and therapeutic use in rheumatic diseases and pain states. *Drugs* 42:274-299, 1991.

Bass JC, et al: A once-daily antiinflammatory drug, oxaprozin, in the treatment of juvenile rheumatoid arthritis. *J Rheumatol* 2:384-386, 1985.

Baum J: Pharmacologic treatment of juvenile arthritis. *Compr Ther* 9:8-13, (Sept) 1983.

Bax D, Amos R: Sulphasalazine: A safe, effective agent for prolonged control of rheumatoid arthritis: A comparison with sodium aurothiomalate. *Ann Rheum Dis* 44:194-198, 1985.

Beck LH: Requiem for gouty nephropathy. *Kidney Int* 30:280-287, 1986.

Bensen WG, et al: Remodelling the pyramid: The therapeutic target of rheumatoid arthritis, editorial. *J Rheumatol* 17:987-989, 1990.

Bitter T: Combined disease modifying chemotherapy for intractable rheumatoid arthritis. *Clin Rheum Dis* 10:413-428, 1984.

Blocka KLN, et al: Clinical pharmacokinetics of oral and injectable gold compounds. *Clin Pharmacokinet* 11:133-143, 1986.

Boehrs M, Ramsden M: Longacting drug combinations in rheumatoid arthritis: A formal overview. *J Rheumatol* 18:316-324, 1991.

Bono RF, et al: Oxaprozin in the treatment of patients with tendinitis and bursitis: Comparison with phenylbutazone and placebo. *Semin Arthritis Rheum* 15(suppl 2):90-94, 1986.

Bradley JD, et al: Comparison of an antiinflammatory dose of ibuprofen, an analgesic dose of ibuprofen, and acetaminophen in the treatment of patients with osteoarthritis of the knee. *N Engl J Med* 325:87-91, 1991.

Brewer EJ Jr, et al: Early experiences with auranofin in juvenile rheumatoid arthritis. *Am J Med* 75(suppl 6A):152-156, 1983.

Brewer EJ, et al: Penicillamine and hydroxychloroquine in the treatment of severe juvenile rheumatoid arthritis: Results of the USA-

USSR double-blind placebo-controlled trial. *N Engl J Med* 314:1269-1276, 1986.

Brick JE, et al: Prospective analysis of liver biopsies before and after methotrexate therapy in rheumatoid patients. *Semin Arthritis Rheum* 19:31-44, (Aug) 1989.

Brooks PM, Day RO: Nonsteroidal antiinflammatory drugs: Differences and similarities. *N Engl J Med* 324:1716-1725, 1991.

Brown BL, et al: Flurbiprofen versus naproxen in the treatment of rheumatoid arthritis. *Am J Med* 80 (suppl 3A):105-109, 1986 A.

Brown BL, et al: Double-blind comparison of flurbiprofen and sulindac for the treatment of osteoarthritis. *Am J Med* 80:112-117, 1986 B.

Bunch TW, et al: Controlled trial of hydroxychloroquine singly and in combination in the treatment of rheumatoid arthritis. *Arthritis Rheum* 27:267-276, 1984.

Burastero SE, et al: Monoreactive high affinity and polyreactive low affinity rheumatoid factors are produced by CD5+ B-cells from patients with rheumatoid arthritis. *J Exp Med* 168:1979, 1988.

Byron MA: Treatment of rheumatic diseases. *BMJ* 294:236-238, 1987.

Calabro JJ: Juvenile rheumatoid arthritis, in Roth SH (ed): *Rheumatic Therapeutics.* New York, McGraw-Hill, 1985, 19-40.

Caldwell JR, Furst DE: The efficacy and safety of low-dose corticosteroids for rheumatoid arthritis. *Semin Arthritis Rheum* 21:1-11, (Aug) 1991.

Caldwell JR, et al: Treatment of ankylosing spondylitis with oxaprozin: A comparison with indomethacin. *Semin Arthritis Rheum* 15 (suppl 2):95-100, 1986.

Calin A: Placebo controlled, crossover study of azathioprine in Reiter's syndrome. *Ann Rheum Dis* 45:653-655, 1986.

Capell HA, et al: Comparison of white blood cell dyscrasias during sulphasalazine therapy of rheumatoid arthritis and inflammatory bowel disease. *Drugs* 32 (suppl 1):44-48, 1986.

Carette S, et al: A double-blind placebo controlled study of auranofin in patients with psoriatic arthritis. *Arthritis Rheum* 32:158-165, 1989.

Carson JL, et al: Association of nonsteroidal anti-inflammatory drugs with upper gastrointestinal tract bleeding. *Arch Intern Med* 147:85-88, 1987.

Chaffman M, et al: Auranofin: Preliminary review of its pharmacological properties and therapeutic use in rheumatoid arthritis. *Drugs* 27:378-424, 1984.

Chang S-L, et al: Bioavailability of allopurinol oral and rectal dosage forms. *Am J Hosp Pharm* 38:365-368, 1981.

Chang DM, et al: The effects of methotrexate on interleukin-1 in patients with rheumatoid arthritis. *J Rheumatol* 19:1678-1682, 1992.

Chiang ST, et al: Oxaprozin disposition in renal disease. *Clin Pharmacol Ther* 31:509-515, 1982.

Clark P, et al: Meta-analysis of injectable gold in rheumatoid arthritis. *J Rheumatol* 16:442-447, 1989.

Cohen MAH: Adverse reactions to gold compounds. *Adverse Drug React Acute Poisoning Rev* 4:163-178, 1988.

Court H, Volans GN: Poisoning after overdose with non-steroidal anti-inflammatory drugs. *Adverse Drug React Acute Poisoning Rev* 3:1-21, 1984.

CSSRD (Cooperative Systematic Studies of Rheumatic Disease) Group: Toxicity of long term low dose D-penicillamine therapy in rheumatoid arthritis. *J Rheumatol* 14:67-73, 1987.

Davies RO: Review of animal and clinical pharmacology of diflunisal. *Pharmacotherapy* 3 (suppl 1):9S-22S, 1983.

Davis MJ, et al: Should disease modifying agents be used in mild rheumatoid arthritis? *Br J Rheumatol* 30:451-454, 1991.

Dijkmans BAC, et al: Cyclosporine in rheumatoid arthritis. *Semin Arthritis Rheum* 22:30-36, (Aug) 1992.

Dorwart BB, et al: Cryotherapy in psoriatic arthritis. *Arthritis Rheum* 21:513-515, 1978.

Duffy CM, et al: Drug therapy for juvenile arthritis. *Compr Ther* 15:48-59, (Oct) 1989.

Easterbrook M: Ocular effects and safety of antimalarial agents. *Am J Med* 85 (suppl 4A):23-29, 1988.

Ellenhorn MJ, Barceloux DG: *Medical Toxicology: Diagnosis and Treatment of Human Poisoning.* New York, Elsevier, 1988, 341-347.

Emery P, et al: D-penicillamine induced toxicity in rheumatoid arthritis: Role of sulphoxidation status and HLA-DR3. *J Rheumatol* 11:626-632, 1984.

Empire Rheumatism Council: Multi-centre controlled trial comparing cortisone acetate and acetyl salicylic acid in the long-term treatment of rheumatoid arthritis. *Ann Rheum Dis* 14:353-367, 1955.

Englert HJ, et al: Sulphasalazine and regression of rheumatoid nodules. *Ann Rheum Dis* 46:244-245, 1987.

Fam AG, et al: Desensitization to allopurinol in patients with gout and cutaneous reactions. *Am J Med* 93:299-302, (Sept) 1992.

Farr M, et al: Side effect profile of 200 patients with inflammatory arthritides treated with sulfasalazine. *Drugs* 32 (suppl 1):49-53, 1986.

Farr R, et al: Treatment of psoriatic arthritis with sulphasalazine: A one year open study. *Clin Rheumatol* 7:372-377, 1988 A.

Farr R, et al: Sulfasalazine in rheumatoid arthritis: Combination therapy with D-penicillamine or sodium aurothiomalate. *Clin Rheumatol* 7:242-248, 1988 B.

Favre L, et al: Reversible acute renal failure from combined triamterene and indomethacin: Study in healthy subjects. *Ann Intern Med* 96:317-320, 1982.

Fehlauer CS, et al: Methotrexate therapy in rheumatoid arthritis: 2-year retrospective followup study. *J Rheumatol* 16:307-312, 1989.

Felson DT, et al: The comparative efficacy and toxicity of second-line drugs in rheumatoid arthritis: Results of two metaanalyses. *Arthritis Rheum* 33:1449-1461, 1990.

Ferraz MB, et al: Meta-analysis of sulfasalazine in ankylosing spondylitis. *J Rheumatol* 17:1482-1486, 1990.

Fink CM: Medical treatment of juvenile arthritis. *Clin Orthop Rel Res* 259:60-69, (Oct) 1990.

Fowler RW, Arnold KG: Non-steroidal analgesic and anti-inflammatory agents, letter. *BMJ* 287:835, 1983.

Fraunfelder FT, et al: Cataracts associated with allopurinol therapy. *Am J Ophthalmol* 94:137-140, 1982.

Friedman HM, Grasela T: Adenine arabinoside and allopurinol: Possible adverse drug interaction, letter. *N Engl J Med* 304:423, 1981.

Fries JF: Reevaluating the therapeutic approach to rheumatoid arthritis: The 'sawtooth' strategy. *J Rheumatol* 17 (suppl 22):12-15, 1990.

Fries JF, et al: Toward an epidemiology of gastropathy associated with nonsteroidal anti-inflammatory drug use. *Gastroenterology* 96:647-655, 1989.

Furst DE: Clinically important interactions of nonsteroidal antiinflammatory drugs with other medications. *J Rheumatol* 15:58-62, 1988.

Furst DE, Kremer JM: Methotrexate in rheumatoid arthritis. *Arthritis Rheum* 31:305-314, 1988.

Furst DE, Paulus HE: Phenylbutazone, in Paulus HE, et al (eds): *Drugs for Rheumatic Disease.* New York, Churchill Livingstone, 1987, 265-284.

Gabriel SE: Is misoprostol prophylaxis indicated for NSAID induced adverse gastrointestinal events? An epidemiologic opinion, comment. *J Rheumatol* 18:958-960, 1991.

Gabriel SE, et al: Risk for serious gastrointestinal complications related to use of nonsteroidal anti-inflammatory drugs: A meta-analysis. *Ann Intern Med* 115:787-796, 1991.

Gaudreault P, et al: Relative severity of acute versus chronic salicylate poisoning in children: Clinical comparison. *Pediatrics* 70:566-569, 1982.

Gerber RC: Diagnosis and management of Reiter's syndrome. *Compr Ther* 10:51-57, (Aug) 1984.

Gerber D: Adverse reactions of piroxicam. *DICP* 9:707-710, 1987.

Giannini EH, et al: Ibuprofen suspension in the treatment of juvenile rheumatoid arthritis. *J Pediatr* 117: 645-652, 1990 A.

Giannini EH, et al: Auranofin in the treatment of juvenile rheumatoid arthritis: Results of the USA-USSR double-blind, placebo-controlled trial. *Arthritis Rheum* 33:466-476, 1990 B.

Giannini EH, et al: Auranofin therapy for juvenile rheumatoid arthritis: Results of the five-year open label extension trial. *J Rheumatol* 18:1240-1242, 1991.

Giannini EH, et al: Methotrexate in resistant juvenile rheumatoid arthritis: Results of the U.S.A.-U.S.S.R. double-blind, placebo-controlled trial. *N Engl J Med* 326:1043-1049, 1992.

Gibson T, et al: Combined D-penicillamine and chloroquine treatment of rheumatoid arthritis: A comparative study. *Br J Rheumatol* 26:279-284, 1987.

Ginsberg F, Famaey JP: A double-blind, parallel trial of oxaprozin versus naproxen in the treatment of osteoarthritis. *Curr Med Res Opin* 10:689-695, 1984.

Gladman DD: Psoriatic arthritis: Recent advances in pathogenesis and treatment. *Rheum Dis Clin North Am* 1:247-255, 1992.

Goodwin JS, et al: Administration of nonsteroidal anti-inflammatory agents in patients with rheumatoid arthritis: Effects on indexes of cellular immune status and serum rheumatoid factor levels. *JAMA* 250:2485-2488, 1983.

Gottlieb NL: Comparative pharmacokinetics of parenteral and oral gold compounds. *J Rheumatol* 9 (suppl 8):99-109, 1982.

Goupille P, et al: Treatment of psoriatic arthropathy. *Semin Arthritis Rheum* 21:355-367, (June) 1992.

Graham DY, et al: Prevention of NSAID-induced gastric ulcer with misoprostol: Multicentre, double-blind, placebo-controlled trial. *Lancet* 2:1277-1280, 1988.

Graham LD, et al: Morbidity associated with long-term methotrexate therapy in juvenile rheumatoid arthritis. *J Pediatr* 120:468-473, 1992.

Gray RG, Gottlieb NL: Toxicity from injectable and oral gold compounds, in Blau SP (ed): *Emergencies in Rheumatoid Arthritis.* Mount Kisco, NY, Futura, 1986, 375-405.

Gray RG, et al: Local corticosteroid injection treatment in rheumatic disorders. *Semin Arthritis Rheum* 10:231-254, 1981.

Green L, et al: Severe reversible interstitial pneumonitis induced by low dose methotrexate: Report of a case and review of the literature. *J Rheumatol* 15:110-112, 1988.

Greenblatt DJ, et al: Oxaprozin pharmacokinetics in the elderly. *Br J Clin Pharmacol* 19:373-378, 1985.

Griffin MR, et al: Nonsteroidal anti-inflammatory drug use and death from peptic ulcer in elderly persons. *Ann Intern Med* 109:359-363, 1988.

Griffin MR, et al: Nonsteroidal anti-inflammatory drug use and increased risk for peptic ulcer disease in elderly persons. *Ann Intern Med* 114:257-263, 1991.

Grondin C, et al: Slow-acting antirheumatic drugs in chronic arthritis of childhood. *Semin Arthritis Rheum* 18:38-47, 1988.

Hall CL: Gold nephropathy. *Nephron* 50:265-272, 1988.

Halle F, Prieur AM: Evaluation of methotrexate in the treatment of juvenile chronic arthritis according to subtype. *Clin Exp Rheumatol* 9:297-302, 1991.

Hamdy H, et al: Low-dose methotrexate compared with azothioprine in the treatment of rheumatoid arthritis: Twenty-four-week controlled clinical trial. *Arthritis Rheum* 30:361-368, 1987.

Hande KR, et al: Severe allopurinol toxicity: Description and guidelines for prevention in patients with renal insufficiency. *Am J Med* 76:47-56, 1984.

Hansten PD: Nonsteroidal anti-inflammatory drugs and oral anticoagulants. *Drug Interact Newslett* 3:49-53, (Nov) 1983.

Harris ED Jr: Rheumatoid arthritis: Pathophysiology and implications for therapy. *N Engl J Med* 322:1277-1289, 1990.

Harris ED, et al: Low dose prednisone therapy in rheumatoid arthritis: A double-blind study. *J Rheumatol* 10:713-721, 1983.

Hart FD, Huskisson EC: Non-steroidal anti-inflammatory drugs: Current status and rational therapeutic use. *Drugs* 27:232-255, 1984.

Helleberg L: Clinical pharmacokinetics of indomethacin. *Clin Pharmacokinet* 6:245-258, 1981.

Hickey AR, et al: Monitoring cancer incidence in the rheumatoid arthritis azathioprine registry, abstract D49, in: *American College of Rheumatology Arthritis Health Professionals Association, 56th Annual Meeting, Atlanta, Ga, October 11-15.* 1992, 5222.

Hochberg MC: Auranofin or D-penicillamine in treatment of rheumatoid arthritis. *Ann Intern Med* 105:528-535, 1986.

Hochberg MC: Diarrhea associated with nonsteroidal anti-inflammatory drugs. *JAMA* 261:3081, 1989.

Holmes EW Jr: Rational approach to gout. *Drug Ther* 11:117-124, (Feb) 1981.

Jacob G, et al: Minimum effective dose of etodolac for the treatment of rheumatoid arthritis. *J Clin Pharmacol* 26:195-202, 1986.

Jaffe IA: Combination therapy of rheumatoid arthritis: Rationale and overview. *J Rheumatol* 17 (suppl 25):24-27, 1990.

Jeurissen M, et al: Methotrexate versus azathioprine in the treatment of rheumatoid arthritis: A forty-eight week randomized, double-blind trial. *Arthritis Rheum* 34:961-972, 1991.

Jick H, et al: Follow-up study of tolmetin users. *Pharmacotherapy* 9:91-94, 1989.

Jones AC, Doherty M: The treatment of osteoarthritis. *Br J Clin Pharmacol* 33:357-363, 1992.

Jusko WJ, Chiang ST: Distribution volume related to body weight and protein binding. *J Pharm Sci* 71:649-670, 1982.

Kaiser DG, et al: Pharmacokinetics of flurbiprofen. *Am J Med* 80 (suppl 3A):10-15, 1986.

Kammer GM, et al: Psoriatic arthritis: A clinical, immunologic and HLA study of 100 patients. *Semin Arthritis Rheum* 9:75-97, 1979.

Kaplan MM, et al: Prospective trial of colchicine for primary biliary cirrhosis. *N Engl J Med* 315:1448-1454, 1986.

Karbowski A: Double-blind, parallel comparison of etodolac and indomethacin in patients with osteoarthritis of the knee. *Curr Med Res Opin* 12:309-317, 1991.

Kaufmann HJ, Taubin HL: Nonsteroidal anti-inflammatory drugs activate quiescent inflammatory bowel disease. *Ann Intern Med* 107:513-516, 1987.

Kelley WM, Palella TD: Gout and other disorders of purine metabolism, in Braunwald E, et al (eds): *Harrison's Principles of Internal Medicine,* ed 11. New York, McGraw-Hill, 1987, 1623-1632.

Knowlton RG, et al: Genetic linkage of a polymorphism in the type II procollagen gene (C0L2A1) to primary osteoarthritis associated with mild chondrodysplasia. *N Engl J Med* 322:526-530, 1990

Kolodny AL, et al: The efficacy and safety of single daily doses of oxaprozin in the treatment of osteoarthritis: A comparison with aspirin. *Semin Arthritis Rheum* 15 (suppl 2):72-79, 1986.

Kovarsky J: Clinical pharmacology and toxicology of cyclophosphamide: Emphasis on use in rheumatic disease. *Semin Arthritis Rheum* 12:359-372, 1983.

Krane SM: Crystal-induced joint disease. *Sci Am Med* Sect. 15, Part 9 (May) 1986.

Kremer JM: Methotrexate 1989—the evolving story, editorial. *J Rheumatol* 16:261-263, 1989.

Kremer JM: Liver biopsies in patients with rheumatoid arthritis receiving methotrexate: Where are we going? Editorial. *J Rheumatol* 19:189-191, 1992.

Kremer JM, Phelps CT: Long-term prospective study of the use of methotrexate in the treatment of rheumatoid arthritis: Update after a mean of 90 months. *Arthritis Rheum* 35:138-145, 1992.

Kremer JM, et al: Liver histology in rheumatoid arthritis patients receiving long-term methotrexate therapy: A prospective study with baseline and sequential biopsy samples. *Arthritis Rheum* 32:121-127, 1989.

Kuflik EG: Effect of antimalarial drugs on psoriasis. *Cutis* 26:153-155, 1980.

Kuncl RW, et al: Colchicine myopathy and neuropathy. *N Engl J Med* 316:1562-1568, 1987.

Kushner I: Does aggressive therapy of rheumatoid arthritis affect outcome? Editorial. *J Rheumatol* 16:1-4, 1989.

Kvien TK, et al: Slow acting antirheumatic drugs in patients with juvenile rheumatoid arthritis: Evaluated in a randomized, parallel 50-week clinical trial. *J Rheumatol* 12:533-539, 1985.

Lally EV, Ho G Jr: Review of methotrexate therapy in Reiter syndrome. *Semin Arthritis Rheum* 15:139-145, 1985.

Lally EV, et al: Clinical spectrum of gouty arthritis in women. *Arch Intern Med* 146:2221-2225, 1986.

Lasseter KC, et al: Pharmacokinetics of oxaprozin in patients with hepatic impairment. *Clin Res* 33:284A, 1985.

Lawrence JS: Comparative toxicity of gold preparations in treatment of rheumatoid arthritis. *Ann Rheum Dis* 35:171-173, 1976.

Leak AM, et al: A crossover study of naproxen, diclofenac and tolmetin in juvenile chronic arthritis. *Clin Exp Rheumatol* 6:157-160, 1988.

Lerman S, et al: Allopurinol therapy and cataractogenesis in humans. *Am J Ophthalmol* 94:141-146, 1982.

Lerman S, et al: Further studies on allopurinol therapy and human cataractogenesis. *Am J Ophthalmol* 97:205-209, 1984.

Lipman AG: Anti-inflammatories: Overview of subtle differences. *Mod Med* 50:227-228, (Sept) 1982.

Lovejoy FH Jr: Aspirin (salicylate) poisoning, in Rudolph AM, Hoffman JIE (eds): *Pediatrics,* ed 18. Norwalk, Conn, Appleton & Lange, 1987, 720-722.

Mackenzie AH: Dose refinements in long-term therapy of rheumatoid arthritis with antimalarials. *Am J Med* 75 (suppl 1A):40-45, 1983.

Maclean L: HLA-B27 subtypes: Implications for the spondyloarthropathies. *Ann Rheum Dis* 51:929-931, 1992.

Maksymowych W, Russell AS: Antimalarials in rheumatology: Efficacy and safety. *Semin Arthritis Rheum* 16:206-221, 1987.

Manning ME, et al: Reactions to aspirin and other nonsteroidal anti-inflammatory drugs. *Immunol Allergy Clin North Am* 12:611-631, 1992.

Matteson EL, et al: Occurrence of neoplasia in patients with rheumatoid arthritis in a DMARD registry. *J Rheumatol* 18:809-814, 1991.

McCarthy GM, et al: Influence of antihyperuricemic therapy on the clinical and radiographic progression of gout. *Arthritis Rheum* 34:1489-1494, 1991.

McCarty DJ: Suppress rheumatoid inflammation early and leave the pyramid to the Egyptians, editorial. *J Rheumatol* 17:1115-1118, 1990.

McColl KEL, et al: Studies in laboratory animals to assess the safety of anti-inflammatory agents in acute porphyria. *Ann Rheum Dis* 46:540-542, 1987.

McConkey B, et al: Salazopyrin in rheumatoid arthritis. *Agents Actions* 8:438-441, 1978.

McGuigan MA: Two-year review of salicylate deaths in Ontario. *Arch Intern Med* 147:510-512, 1987.

McInnes GT, et al: Acute adverse reactions attributed to allopurinol in hospitalised patients. *Ann Rheum Dis* 40:245-249, 1981.

McKendry RJR, Cyr M: Toxicity of methotrexate compared with azathioprine in the treatment of rheumatoid arthritis: Case control study of 131 patients. *Arch Intern Med* 149:685-689, 1989.

McKerrow KJ, Greig DE: Piroxicam-induced photosensitive dermatitis. *J Am Acad Dermatol* 15:1237-1241, 1986.

Mease PJ, Willkens RF: Treatment of acute gout with oxaprozin. *Semin Arthritis Rheum* 15 (suppl 2):86-89, 1986.

Meredith TJ, Vale JA: Non-narcotic analgesics: Problems of overdosage. *Drugs* 32 (suppl 4):177-205, 1986.

Miller LG: Oxaprozin: A once-daily nonsteroidal anti-inflammatory drug. *Clin Pharm* 11:591-603, 1992.

Miyachi Y, et al: Colchicine in treatment of cutaneous manifestations of Behçet's disease. *Br J Dermatol* 104:67-69, 1981.

Morales TI, Hascall VC: Factors involved in the regulation of proteoglycan metabolism in articular cartilage. *Arthritis Rheum* 32:1197-1201, 1989.

Morassut P, et al: Gold sodium thiomalate compared to low dose methotrexate in the treatment of rheumatoid arthritis: Randomized, double blind 26-week trial. *J Rheumatol* 16:302-306, 1989.

Muijsers AO, et al: D-penicillamine in patients with rheumatoid arthritis: Serum levels, pharmacokinetic aspects, and correlation with clinical course and side effects. *Arthritis Rheum* 27:1362-1369, 1984.

Multicenter Salsalate/Aspirin Comparison Study Group: Does the acetyl group of aspirin contribute to the anti-inflammatory efficacy of salicylic acid in the treatment of rheumatoid arthritis? *J Rheumatol* 16:321-327, 1989.

Nafria EC, et al: Renal papillary necrosis to flurbiprofen. *DICP* 25:870, 1991.

Nelson AM: Juvenile rheumatoid arthritis: Drug therapy plan and look at prognosis. *Mod Med* 50:187-196, (Nov) 1982.

Newman ED, et al: Sulfasalazine therapy in psoriatic arthritis: Clinical and immunologic response. *J Rheumatol* 18:1379-1382, 1991.

Olson NY, et al: Nonsteroidal anti-inflammatory drug therapy in chronic childhood iridocyclitis. *Am J Dis Child* 142:1289-1292, 1988.

Palit J, et al: A multicentre double-blind comparison of auranofin, intramuscular gold thiomalate and placebo in patients with psoriatic arthritis. *Br J Rheumatol* 29:280-283, 1990.

Palotie A, et al: Predisposition to familial osteoarthritis linked to type II collagen gene. *Lancet* 1:924-927, 1989.

Parke A: Antimalarial drugs and pregnancy. *Am J Med* 85 (suppl 4A):30-33, 1988.

Paulus HE: FDA Arthritis Advisory Committee meeting: Post-marketing surveillance of non-steroidal anti-inflammatory drugs. *Arthritis Rheum* 28:1168-1169, 1985.

Paulus HE: FDA Arthritis Advisory Committee meeting: Serious gastrointestinal toxicity of nonsteroidal anti-inflammatory drugs; drug-containing renal and biliary stones; diclofenac and carprofen approved. *Arthritis Rheum* 31:1450-1451, 1988.

Paulus HE: Current medicinal approaches to the treatment of rheumatoid arthritis. *Clin Orthop Rel Res* 265:96-115, 1991.

Paulus HE, et al: Azathioprine versus D-penicillamine in rheumatoid arthritis patients who have been treated unsuccessfully with gold. *Arthritis Rheum* 27:721, 1984.

Perrett D: Metabolism and pharmacology of D-penicillamine in man. *J Rheumatol* 8 (suppl 7):41-50, 1981.

Phillips CA, et al: Clinical liver disease in patients with rheumatoid arthritis taking methotrexate. *J Rheumatol* 19:229-233, 1992.

Pinals RS, et al: Sulfasalazine in rheumatoid arthritis: A double-blind, placebo-controlled trial. *Arthritis Rheum* 29:1427-1434, 1986.

Pincus T, et al: Severe functional decline, work disability, and increased mortality in seventy-five rheumatoid arthritis patients studied over nine years. *Arthritis Rheum* 27:864-871, 1984.

Platt PN: Recent experience with etodolac in the treatment of osteoarthritis of the knee. *Clin Rheumatol* 8 (1 suppl):54-62, 1989.

Porter RS: Factors determining efficacy of NSAIDs. *Drug Intell Clin Pharm* 18:42-51, 1984.

Powell WR, et al: Once-daily oxaprozin and piroxicam compared in osteoarthritis. *Semin Arthritis Rheum* 15 (suppl 2):80-85, 1986.

Preston SA, Axelrod DA: Comparison of parenteral ACTH vs oral indomethacin in treatment of acute gout, abstract. *Arthritis Rheum* 30 (suppl 1):S38, 1987.

Prieur AM, et al: Evaluation of D-penicillamine in juvenile chronic arthritis. *Arthritis Rheum* 28:376-382, 1985.

Pullar T, et al: Sulphasalazine in rheumatoid arthritis: A double blind comparison of sulphasalazine with placebo and sodium aurothiomalate. *BMJ* 287:1102-1104, 1983.

Pullar T, et al: Effect of sulphasalazine on radiological progression of rheumatoid arthritis. *Ann Rheum Dis* 46:398-402, 1987.

Rau R, et al: A double blind randomized parallel trial of intramuscular methotrexate and gold sodium thiolmalate in early erosive rheumatoid arthritis. *J Rheumatol* 18:328-333, 1991 A.

Rau R, et al: Retardation of radiologic progression in rheumatoid arthritis with methotrexate therapy: A controlled study. *Arthritis Rheum* 34:1236-1244, 1991 B.

Reeve PA, et al: Pulmonary oedema, jaundice and renal impairment with naproxen, letter. *Br J Rheumatol* 26:70-71, 1987.

Rhymer AR, et al: Double-blind trial comparing indomethacin sustained release capsules (Indocid-R) with indomethacin capsules in patients with rheumatoid arthritis. *Rheumatol Rehabil* 21:101-106, 1982.

Richter MB, et al: Gold in psoriatic arthropathy. *Ann Rheum Dis* 39:279-280, 1980.

Roberts WN, et al: Colchicine in acute gout: Reassessment of risks and benefits. *JAMA* 257:1920-1922, 1987.

Rodnan GP, et al (eds): Gout, in: *Primer on the Rheumatic Diseases,* ed 8. Atlanta, Ga, Arthritis Foundation, 1983, 120-128.

Rodríguez LAG, et al: The role of non-steroidal anti-inflammatory drugs in acute liver injury. *BMJ* 305:865-868, 1992.

Roenigk HH Jr, et al: Methotrexate in psoriasis: Revised guidelines. *J Am Acad Dermatol* 19:145-156, 1988.

Rosenberg AM: Advanced drug therapy for juvenile rheumatoid arthritis. *J Pediatr* 114:171-178, 1989.

Roth SH: Arthritis and rheumatism: Old questions, new answers. *Compr Ther* 10:58-64, (Aug) 1984.

Roth SH: Salicylates, in Roth SH (ed): *Rheumatic Therapeutics.* New York, McGraw-Hill, 1985, 309-323.

Roth SH: NSAID and gastropathy: A rheumatologist's review. *J Rheumatol* 15:912-919, 1988.

Roth S, et al: Misoprostol heals gastroduodenal injury in patients with rheumatoid arthritis receiving aspirin. *Arch Intern Med* 149:775-779, 1989.

Roubenoff R, et al: Incidence and risk factors for gout in white men. *JAMA* 266:3004-3007, 1991.

Runge LA: Antimalarials, in McCarty DJ (ed): *Arthritis and Allied Conditions: A Textbook of Rheumatology,* ed 11. Philadelphia, Lea & Febiger, 1989, 556-562.

Runkel R, et al: Naproxen-probenecid interaction. *Clin Pharmacol Ther* 24:706-713, 1978.

Rynes RI: Antimalarial drugs, in Kelley WN, et al (eds): *Textbook of Rheumatology,* ed 3. Philadelphia, WB Saunders, 1989, 792-803.

Sanda M, et al: Three-month multicenter study of etodolac (Ultradol) in patients with osteoarthritis of the hip. *Curr Ther Res* 33:782-792, 1983.

Sarojini PA, Mshana RN: Use of colchicine in management of erythema nodosum leprosum (ENL), letter. *Lepr Rev* 54:151-156, 1983.

Savage RL, et al: Variation in the risk of peptic ulcer complications with nonsteroidal antiinflammatory drug therapy. *Arthritis Rheum* 36:84-90, 1993.

Schaller JG: Treatment of juvenile rheumatoid arthritis, in McCarty DJ (ed): *Arthritis and Allied Conditions: Textbook of Rheumatology,* ed 10. Philadelphia, Lea & Febiger, 1985, 811-818.

Schorn D: A comparison between oxaprozin and naproxen in rheumatoid arthritis. *S Afr Med J* 14:768, 1981.

Schwartz BD: Infectious agents, immunity, and rheumatic diseases. *Arthritis Rheum* 33:457-465, 1990.

Schwarzer AC, et al: The cycling of combination antirheumatic drug therapy in rheumatoid arthritis. *Br J Rheumatol* 29:445-450, 1990.

Scott DL, et al: Longterm outcome of treating rheumatoid arthritis: Results after 20 years. *Lancet* 1:1108-1111, 1987.

Scott DL, et al: Combination therapy with gold and hydroxychloroquine in rheumatoid arthritis: A prospective, randomized, placebo-controlled study. *Br J Rheumatol* 28:128-133, 1989.

Seideman P, et al: Psoriatic arthritis treated with oral colchicine. *J Rheumatol* 14:777-779, 1987.

Selen A, et al: Pharmacokinetics of probenecid following oral doses in human volunteers. *J Pharmaceut Sci* 71:1238-1242, 1982.

Shaikov AV, et al: Repetitive use of pulse therapy with methylprednisolone and cyclophosphamide in addition to oral methotrexate in children with systemic juvenile rheumatoid arthritis: Preliminary results of a longterm study. *J Rheumatol* 19:612-616, 1992.

Sharp JT, et al: Comparison of two dosage schedules of gold salts in treatment of rheumatoid arthritis. *Arthritis Rheum* 20:1179-1187, 1977.

Shergy WJ, et al: Methotrexate-associated hepatotoxicity: Retrospective analysis of 210 patients with rheumatoid arthritis. *Am J Med* 85:771-774, 1988.

Silman AJ, et al: Lymphoproliferative cancer and other malignancy in patients with rheumatoid arthritis treated with azathioprine: A 20 year follow up study. *J Rheum Dis* 47:988-992, 1988.

Silvers DN, et al: Treatment of dermatitis herpetiformis with colchicine. *Arch Dermatol* 116:1373-1374, 1980.

Simkin PA: Management of gout. *Ann Intern Med* 90:812-816, 1979.

Singh G, et al: Toxicity profiles of disease modifying antirheumatic drugs in rheumatoid arthritis. *J Rheumatol* 18:188-194, 1991.

Soll AH: Nonsteroidal anti-inflammatory drugs and ulcers, editorial. *West Med J* 157:465-468, 1992.

Soll AH, et al (moderator): Nonsteroidal anti-inflammatory drugs and peptic ulcer disease. *Ann Intern Med* 114:307-319, 1991.

Speckmaier M, et al: Low dose methotrexate in systemic onset juvenile chronic arthritis. *Clin Exp Rheum* 7:647-650, 1989.

Spilberg I, et al: Colchicine and pseudogout. *Arthritis Rheum* 23:1062-1063, 1980.

Stachura I, et al: T and B lymphocyte subsets in fenoprofen nephropathy. *Am J Med* 75:9-16, 1983.

Stapczynski JS, et al: Colchicine overdose: Report of two cases and review of the literature. *Ann Emerg Med* 10:364-369, 1981.

Stiehm ER: Nonsteroidal anti-inflammatory drugs in pediatric patients, editorial. *Am J Dis Child* 142:1281, 1988.

Strand V, et al; Treatment of rheumatoid arthritis with an anti-CD5 immunoconjugate: Final results of Phase II studies. *Arthritis Rheum* 34:S91, 1991.

Strother SV, et al: Colchicine therapy for refractory idiopathic thrombocytopenic purpura. *Arch Intern Med* 144:2198-2200, 1984.

Suehisa S, et al: Colchicine in treatment of acute febrile neutrophilic dermatosis (Sweet's syndrome). *Br J Dermatol* 108:99-101, 1983.

Tabatabai MR, Cummings NA: Intravenous colchicine in treatment of acute pseudogout. *Arthritis Rheum* 23:370-374, 1980.

Taggart AJ, et al: Sulphasalazine alone or in combination with D-penicillamine in rheumatoid arthritis. *Br J Rheumatol* 26:32-36, 1987.

Takeuchi A, et al: Efficacy of oxaprozin in the treatment of articular symptoms of Behcet's disease. *Clin Rheumatol* 3:397-399, 1984.

Talbott JH: Gouty arthritis: Disease for all ages. *Geriatrics* 35:69-78, (May) 1980.

Temple AR: Acute and chronic effects of aspirin toxicity and their treatment. *Arch Intern Med* 141:364-369, 1981.

Thyss A, et al: Clinical and pharmacokinetic evidence of life-threatening interaction between methotrexate and ketoprofen. *Lancet* 1:256-258, 1986.

Todd PA, Sorkin EM: Diclofenac sodium: Reappraisal of its pharmacodynamic and pharmacokinetic properties, and therapeutic efficacy. *Drugs* 35:244-285, 1988.

Townsend RJ, et al: Excretion of ibuprofen into breast milk. *Am J Obstet Gynecol* 149:184-186, 1984.

Truckenbrodt H, Häfner R: Methotrexate therapy in juvenile rheumatoid arthritis: Retrospective study. *Arthritis Rheum* 29:801-807, 1986.

Tsokos GC: Immunomodulatory treatment in patients with rheumatic diseases: Mechanisms of action. *Semin Arthritis Rheum* 17:24-38, (Aug) 1987.

Tugwell P, et al: Low-dose cyclosporin versus placebo in patients with rheumatoid arthritis. *Lancet* 335:1051-1055, 1990.

Urowitz MB, et al: Azathioprine in rheumatoid arthritis: A double-blind, cross-over study. *Arthritis Rheum* 16:411, 1973.

van Kerckhove C, et al: Temporal patterns of response to D-penicillamine, hydroxychloroquine, and placebo in juvenile rheumatoid arthritis patients. *Arthritis Rheum* 31:1252-1258, 1988.

Van Wanghe P, Dequeker J: Compliance and long-term effect of azathioprine in 65 rheumatoid arthritis cases. *Ann Rheum Dis* 41(suppl):40-43, 1982.

Vasey FB, et al: Clinical aspects of psoriatic arthritis. *Compr Ther* 8:34-39, (April) 1982.

Verbeeck RK, et al: Clinical pharmacokinetics of non-steroidal anti-inflammatory drugs. *Clin Pharmacokinet* 8:297-331, 1983.

Vreede PD, et al: Use of oxaprozin in the treatment of aspirin failures in rheumatoid arthritis. *Semin Arthritis Rheum* 15(suppl 2):66-71, 1986.

Walker AM, et al: Determinants of serious liver disease among patients receiving low-dose methotrexate for rheumatoid arthritis. *Arthritis Rheum* In press.

Wallace SL, Singer JZ: Review: Systemic toxicity associated with the intravenous administration of colchicine: Guidelines for use. *J Rheumatol* 15:495-499, 1988.

Wallace CA, et al: Toxicity and serum levels of methotrexate in children with juvenile rheumatoid arthritis. *Arthritis Rheum* 32:677-681, 1989.

Waltham-Weeks CD: Etodolac versus naproxen in rheumatoid arthritis: A double-blind crossover study. *Curr Med Res Opin* 10:540-547, 1987.

Walz DT, et al: Comparative pharmacology and biological effects of different gold compounds. *J Rheumatol* 9(suppl 8):54-60, 1982 A.

Walz DT, et al: Mechanisms of action of auranofin: Effects on human immune response. *J Rheumatol* 9(suppl 8):32-36, 1982 B.

Wasner C, et al: Nonsteroidal anti-inflammatory agents in rheumatoid arthritis and ankylosing spondylitis. *JAMA* 246:2168-2172, 1981.

Watts RA, Isaacs JD: Immunotherapy of rheumatoid arthritis. *Ann Rheum Dis* 51:577-579, 1992.

Webster E, Panush RS: Allopurinol hypersensitivity in a patient with severe, chronic, tophaceous gout. *Arthritis Rheum* 28:707-709, 1985.

Weinblatt ME: Oral methotrexate (MTX) versus gold therapy (auranofin) in active rheumatoid arthritis: 36-week multicentre trial, abstract 16. *Arthritis Rheum* 32 (suppl):S43, 1989 A.

Weinblatt ME: Methotrexate, in Kelley WN, et al (eds): *Textbook of Rheumatology,* ed 3. Philadelphia, WB Saunders, 1989 B, 833-844.

Weinblatt ME, Maier AL: Disease-modifying agents and experimental treatments of rheumatoid arthritis. *Clin Orthop Rel Res* 265:103-115, (April) 1991.

Weinblatt ME, et al: Efficacy of low-dose methotrexate in rheumatoid arthritis. *N Engl J Med* 312:818-822, 1985.

Weinblatt ME, et al: Long-term prospective study of methotrexate in the treatment of rheumatoid arthritis: 84-month update. *Arthritis Rheum* 35:129-137, 1992.

White PH, Ansell BM: Methotrexate for juvenile rheumatoid arthritis, editorial. *N Engl J Med* 326:1077-1078, 1992.

Wiesner RH, et al: Pharmacokinetics of D-penicillamine in man. *J Rheumatol* 8 (suppl 7):51-55, 1981.

Wilke WS, Clough JD: Therapy for rheumatoid arthritis: Combinations of disease-modifying drugs and new paradigms of treatment. *Semin Arthritis Rheum* 21:21-34, (Oct) 1991.

Williams RL, Upton RA: Clinical pharmacology of ketoprofen. *J Clin Pharmacol* 28:S13-S22, 1988.

Williams PL, et al: Multicentre study of piroxicam versus naproxen in juvenile arthritis with special reference to problem areas in clinical trials of nonsteroidal anti-inflammatory drugs in childhood. *Br J Rheumatol* 25:67-71, 1986.

Williams H, et al: A controlled trial comparing sulphasalazine, gold sodium thiomalate and placebo in rheumatoid arthritis. *Arthritis Rheum* 31:702-713, 1988 A.

Williams HJ, et al: One-year experience in patients treated with auranofin following completion of a parallel, controlled trial comparing auranofin, gold sodium thiomalate, and placebo. *Arthritis Rheum* 31:9-14, 1988 B.

Willis JV, et al: Pharmacokinetics of diclofenac sodium following intravenous and oral administration. *Eur J Clin Pharmacol* 16:405-410, 1979.

Willkens RF, et al: Comparison of azathioprine, methotrexate, and the combination of both in the treatment of rheumatoid arthritis: A controlled clinical trial. *Arthritis Rheum* 35:849-856, 1992.

Wilske KR, Healey LA: Remodeling the pyramid: A concept whose time has come, editorial. *J Rheumatol* 16:565-567, 1989.

Winter L, Post A: Double-blind comparison of single oral doses of oxaprozin, aspirin, and placebo for relief of postoperative oral surgery pain. *J Int Med Res* 11:308-314, 1983.

Yeh KC: Indomethacin and indomethacin sustained release: Comparison of their pharmacokinetic profiles. *Semin Arthritis Rheum* 12 (suppl 1):136-141, 1982.

Yü TF: Efficacy of colchicine prophylaxis in articular gout: Reappraisal after 20 years. *Semin Arthritis Rheum* 12:256-264, 1982.

Zemer D, et al: Colchicine in prevention and treatment of the amyloidosis of familial Mediterranean fever. *N Engl J Med* 314:1001-1005, 1986.

Histamine and Antihistamines 82

HISTAMINE

Histamine is a low-molecular-weight amine that is stored in tissue mast cells and circulating basophils throughout the body. Its release is precipitated by antigen-IgE antibody reactions or exposure to various substances, including drugs, chemicals, dyes, foods, alkaloids, venoms, and physical stimuli such as cold dry air.

Histamine interacts with specific H_1, H_2, and H_3 receptors in various target tissues. Stimulation of H_1 receptors causes smooth muscle contraction and increases vascular permeability and mucus secretion; some of these effects may be mediated by increased levels of intracellular cyclic guanosine monophosphate (cGMP). In the central nervous system, histamine probably serves as a neurotransmitter.

Stimulation of both H_1 and H_2 receptors contributes to vascular dilation and flushing. In bronchial smooth muscle, H_1 and H_2 receptors mediate opposing responses to histamine. Stimulation of H_2 receptors causes acid secretion within the gastric mucosa due to an increase in the concentration of cyclic adenosine monophosphate (cAMP) and a decrease in the levels of cGMP. H_2 antihistamines block these actions. See index entry Histamine-2 Receptor Antagonists for discussion of these drugs.

H_3 receptors appear to regulate the feedback control of histamine synthesis and release in nonmast cell sites. Stimulation of H_3 receptors inhibits cholinergic and noncholinergic excitatory nerves in the airways (Hill, 1990). Blockade of these receptors limits the bronchoconstriction induced by histamine challenge.

Important clinical effects of histamine that are mediated primarily by H_1 receptors include (1) vasodilation of small blood vessels and increased capillary permeability, which occur when large amounts of histamine enter the circulation rapidly and may be severe enough to cause vascular shock; (2) pruritus (eg, that associated with allergic rhinitis or urticaria); (3) bronchospasm (both naturally occurring and that resulting from inhalation challenge with histamine solutions); and (4) mediation of the wheal and flare component of the triple response in skin; histamine often is used as a positive control during skin testing for allergic conditions.

ANTIHISTAMINES

The antihistamines discussed in this chapter are H_1 receptor blocking agents and are among the most widely used drugs. Like histamine, H_1 antagonists contain a substituted ethylamine moiety, but, unlike histamine, most H_1 antagonists have other groupings in place of the primary amino structure and single aromatic ring. Traditional (first-generation) antihistamines are often classified according to these other groupings as amino alkyl ethers (diphenhydramine, clemastine), ethylenediamines (pyrilamine, tripelennamine), alkylamines (brompheniramine, chlorpheniramine, dexchlorpheniramine, triprolidine), and phenothiazines (methdilazine, promethazine, trimeprazine). Several agents have widely varying added groupings. Cyproheptadine and its derivative, azatadine, contain a tricyclic nucleus with an attached piperidine side ring.

The following newer drugs are regarded as second-generation antihistamines. Although structurally related to cyproheptadine and azatadine, loratadine has different pharmacologic properties. Cetirizine is a metabolite of hydroxyzine, a piperazine. Astemizole and terfenadine do not have any of the traditional structural groupings. Levocabastine, a cyclohexylpiperidine derivative, also is structurally unrelated to other antihistamines. (See Tables 1 and 2.)

TABLE 1.
ACTIONS OF GROUPS OF ANTIHISTAMINES[1]

Class	Antihistaminic Activity	Sedative Effects	Anticholinergic Activity	Antiemetic Effects	Gastrointestinal Side Effects	Duration of Action
FIRST-GENERATION ANTIHISTAMINES						
AMINO ALKYL ETHERS (Ethanolamines)	+ to + +[2]	+ to + + +	+ + +	+ + to + + +	+	4 to 6 hours
ETHYLENEDIAMINES	+ to + +	+ to + +	0 to +	0	+ + +	4 to 6 hours
ALKYLAMINES (Propylamines)	+ + to + + +	+ to + +	+ +	0	+	4 to 25 hours
PHENOTHIAZINES	+ to + + +	+ + +	+ + +	+ + + +	0	4 to 24 hours
SECOND-GENERATION ANTIHISTAMINES	+ + to + + +	0 to +	0 to +	0	0	12 to 24 hours

[1]Adapted from Ziment, 1978.
[2]0 to + + + + = scale of activity; 0 represents an effect similar to that of placebo.

Actions and Physiologic Effects

Antihistamines probably act by competing reversibly for histamine receptor sites on target organ cells, thus preventing the actions of histamine. In addition to H_1 receptor blockade, many H_1 antagonists prevent the release of inflammatory mediators in allergen challenge tests; however, clinical benefits resulting from inhibition of mediator release have not been demonstrated. Cetirizine has antiallergic early- and late-phase inhibitory actions in the skin, but late-phase effects produced by this drug have not been observed in the upper respiratory tract (Campoli-Richards et al, 1990; Simons, 1992).

In addition to $histamine_1$ receptor blockade, first-generation antihistamines produce variable degrees of sedation, which patients may not be aware of. These drugs also may have anticholinergic, antiemetic, and local anesthetic actions and gastrointestinal side effects. Drugs that lack these effects (second-generation antihistamines) are now available (astemizole, levocabastine, loratadine, terfenadine) or are being investigated (acrivastine, azelastine, cetirizine, ebastine). Structural modifications limit the ability of second-generation agents to cross the blood-brain barrier in appreciable amounts; as a result, in recommended doses they do not impair coordination or have other effects on the central nervous system (CNS) in most patients. In controlled clinical trials using recommended doses, the incidence and extent of sedation and other CNS adverse effects did not differ significantly from those of placebo (Mann et al, 1989; Sutherland, 1989). (See Tables 1 and 2.)

Antihistamines help suppress the vasodilation, increased capillary permeability, tissue edema, and pruritus that occur in urticaria and angioedema and that are induced by skin tests. Usual doses do not inhibit bronchospasm in patients with asthma; however, these drugs do inhibit histamine-mediated bronchoconstriction in histamine or allergen inhalation challenge tests.

Although many symptoms of allergic disease can be prevented or ameliorated by antihistamines, relief often is incomplete, probably because other mediator substances not affected by antihistamines are released with histamine. Some first-generation antihistamines also relieve symptoms mediated by the cholinergic system. In addition, dose-related adverse effects may make it difficult to achieve concentrations at receptor sites large enough to compete with histamine.

The potency and adverse effects of the H_1 receptor blocking agents vary. One first-generation antihistamine is sometimes substituted for another because of ineffectiveness or presumed tolerance, and the substituted drug is chosen from a different chemical group; however, the substitution usually is unsuccessful. In some patients, administration of a single dose of a long-acting first-generation antihistamine in the evening may relieve symptoms without producing noticeable sedation or other adverse effects in patients whose symptoms are prominent in the morning (Drouin, 1985; Goetz et al, 1991). Second-generation antihistamines are the drugs of choice for patients who are sensitive to or cannot tolerate the CNS effects of the first-generation antihistamines.

Some agents (eg, the investigational drugs, azelastine and ketotifen) have considerable H_1 blocking activity and are often classified as antihistamines, but their antiallergic late-phase actions may predominate. Thus, these agents cannot be classified only as antihistamines. (See index entries Azelastine, Ketotifen, Uses, Asthma.)

Oral administration of all the antihistamines (with the exception of levocabastine) usually is recommended.

Uses

Upper Respiratory Disorders: First-generation antihistamines prevent and relieve mild symptoms of allergic rhinitis (sneezing, rhinorrhea, and pruritus of the nose, eyes, and throat) of recent onset, but they are less effective when not taken regularly or when nasal congestion is pronounced or prolonged. Seasonal allergic rhinitis (hay fever) is more responsive than the nonseasonal chronic form. Antihistamines are less likely to be helpful in vasomotor rhinitis, and their

TABLE 2.
ANTIHISTAMINES

Drug/Chemical Structure	Usual Dosage	Preparations	Comment
FIRST-GENERATION ANTIHISTAMINES			
AMINO ALKYL ETHERS			
Diphenhydramine Hydrochloride	*Oral: Adults,* 25-50 mg 3 or 4 times daily. *Children under 12 years,* 5 mg/kg in 4 divided doses over a 24-hour period. *Intravenous (preferred), Intramuscular (deep): Adults,* 10-50 mg (maximum, 400 mg daily). *Children,* 5 mg/kg daily in 4 divided doses (maximum, 300 mg daily). *Topical:* Cream or solution applied as indicated to affected area.	*Generic.* Capsules, elixir, syrup, tablets, solution (for injection) *Benadryl* (Parke-Davis). Capsules 25 (nonprescription) and 50 mg; elixir 12.5 mg/5 ml (alcohol 5.6%) (nonprescription); solution (for injection) 10 mg/ml in 10 and 30 ml containers and 50 mg/ml in 1 and 10 ml containers; spray (topical) 1% and 2% in 60 ml containers (nonprescription); cream 1% and 2% in 15 and 30 g containers (nonprescription)	Most widely used antihistamine for parenteral administration in treatment of anaphylactic and other allergic reactions. May be given with epinephrine but is not a substitute for it. Incidence of drowsiness high. Diphenhydramine and other antihistamines applied topically may cause sensitization (contact dermatitis). Drug should not be given to premature and newborn infants. Drug should not be used with ototoxic antibiotics, as the ototoxicity may be masked.
Clemastine Fumarate	*Oral: Adults,* 1.34-2.68 mg 2 or 3 times daily (maximum, 8.04 mg daily). *Children 6 to 12 years,* for allergic rhinitis, 0.5 mg twice daily (maximum, 3 mg/day); for urticaria, 1 mg twice daily (maximum, 3 mg/day).	*Tavist* (Sandoz), *Generic.* Syrup 0.5 mg/5 ml (alcohol 5.5%); tablets 1.34 (*Tavist-1*) (nonprescription) and 2.68 mg	Drowsiness is most frequent side effect, but incidence of central sedative effects is generally low. Anticholinergic effect very weak.
ETHYLENEDIAMINES			
Tripelennamine Hydrochloride	*Oral: Adults,* 25-50 mg every 4 to 6 hours (tablets) or 100 mg 2 or 3 times daily (prolonged-release form). *Children,* 5 mg/kg/24 hours in 4 to 6 divided doses (tablets) or, for *children over 5 years,* 50 mg 2 or 3 times daily (prolonged-release form). *Topical:* Cream applied as needed.	*Generic.* Tablets, cream *PBZ* (Geigy). Tablets 25 and 50 mg *PBZ-SR* (Geigy). Tablets (prolonged-release) 100 mg	Topical application may cause sensitization (contact dermatitis), and this route of administration is not recommended.
Pyrilamine Maleate	*Oral: Adults,* 75-100 mg daily in 3 or 4 divided doses. *Children,* information is inadequate to establish dose.	*Generic.* Powder	Incidence of drowsiness low.

(table continued on next page)

TABLE 2 (Continued)

Drug/Chemical Structure	Usual Dosage	Preparations	Comment
ALKYLAMINES			
Chlorpheniramine Maleate	*Oral: Adults,* 4 mg every 4 to 6 hours (maximum, 24 mg/day) (tablets, syrup) or 8 mg 1 to 3 times daily or 12 mg 1 or 2 times daily (prolonged-release form). *Children under 12 years,* 0.35 mg/kg daily divided into 4 doses; *7 years and older,* 8 mg every 12 hours (prolonged-release form). *Intramuscular, Intravenous, Subcutaneous: Adults,* 5 to 40 mg (intravenous injection should be made over period of 1 minute). *Subcutaneous: Children under 12 years,* 0.35 mg/kg daily divided into 4 doses.	*Generic.* Capsules and tablets (plain, prolonged-release); solution (for injection); syrup *Chlor-Trimeton* (Schering-Plough). Syrup 2 mg/5 ml (alcohol 7%) (nonprescription); tablets 4 mg (nonprescription); tablets (prolonged-release) 8 mg (nonprescription) and 12 mg; solution (for injection) 10 mg/ml in 1 ml containers *Teldrin* (SmithKline Beecham). Capsules (prolonged-release) 12 mg (nonprescription)	Drowsiness most common reaction, but overall incidence low. Common ingredient in cold remedies.
Brompheniramine Maleate	*Oral: Adults,* 4 mg every 4 to 6 hours (maximum, 24 mg daily) (tablets, elixir) or 8 to 12 mg 2 or 3 times daily (prolonged-release form). *Children 6 to 12 years,* 2 mg every 4 to 6 hours (maximum, 12 mg daily) (tablets, elixir) or 8 to 12 mg every 12 hours (prolonged-release form); *2 to 6 years,* 1 mg every 4 to 6 hours (maximum, 6 mg daily) (elixir). *Intramuscular, Intravenous, Subcutaneous: Adults,* 10 mg (range, 5 to 20 mg) every 3 to 12 hours (maximum, 40 mg daily). *Children under 12 years,* 0.5 mg/kg daily divided into 3 or 4 doses.	*Generic.* Elixir, tablets (nonprescription), solution (for injection) *Chlor-Phed* (Roberts). Solution (for injection) 10 mg/ml in 10 ml containers *Dimetane* (Robins). Elixir 2 mg/5 ml (alcohol 3%); tablets 4 mg; tablets (prolonged-release) 8 and 12 mg (all forms nonprescription)	Most common reaction is drowsiness, but overall incidence low.
Dexchlorpheniramine Maleate	*Oral: Adults,* 2 mg every 4 to 6 hours (maximum, 12 mg/day) (tablets, syrup) or 4 or 6 mg 2 times daily; for resistant cases, 8 mg 2 times daily or 6 mg 3 times daily (prolonged-release form). *Children under 12 years,* 0.15 mg/kg daily divided into 4 doses.	*Generic.* Syrup, tablets (plain, prolonged-release) *Polaramine* (Schering). Syrup 2 mg/5 ml (alcohol 6%); tablets 2 mg; tablets (prolonged-release) 4 and 6 mg	Incidence of reactions low; most common reaction is drowsiness.

(table continued on next page)

TABLE 2 (Continued)

Drug/Chemical Structure	Usual Dosage	Preparations	Comment
Triprolidine Hydrochloride 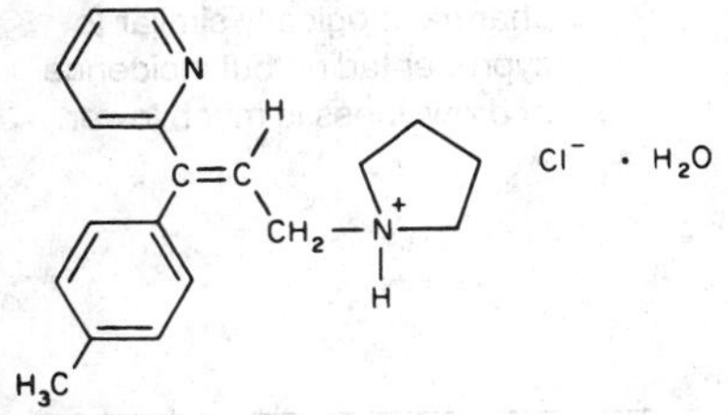	*Oral:* The following amounts are given every 6 hours (maximum, 4 doses a day). (tablets) *Adults,* 2.5 mg. (syrup) *Children 6 to 12 years,* 1.25 mg; *4 to 6 years*, 0.9 mg; *2 to 4 years*, 0.6 mg; *1 to 2 years*, 0.3 mg.	*Generic.* Syrup, tablets	Incidence of reactions low; most common reaction is drowsiness.
PHENOTHIAZINES Methdilazine Methdilazine Hydrochloride 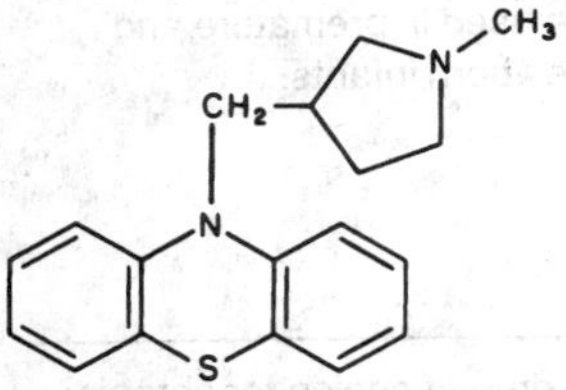	*Oral: Adults,* 16 to 32 mg daily divided into 2 to 4 doses. *Children over 3 years,* 4 mg 2 to 4 times daily.	*Tacaryl* (Westwood-Squibb). Tablets (chewable) 3.6 mg (equivalent to 4 mg of hydrochloride) *Tacaryl [hydrochloride]* (Westwood-Squibb). Syrup 4 mg/5 ml (alcohol 5.7%); tablets 8 mg	Used primarily as antipruritic. Drowsiness less prominent than with other phenothiazines used as antihistamines. Most serious adverse reactions of other phenothiazines not reported with methdilazine.
Promethazine Hydrochloride 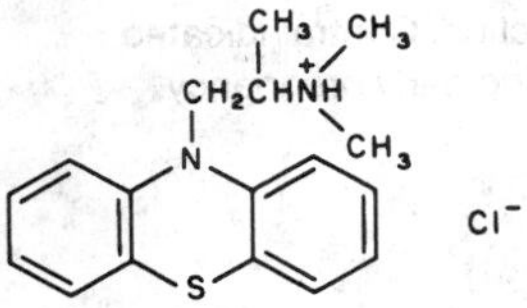	*Oral: Adults,* 25 mg at bedtime or 12.5 mg 4 times daily. *Children,* 25 mg at bedtime or 6.25 to 12.5 mg 3 times daily. *Rectal, Intramuscular, Intravenous: Adults,* 25 mg repeated in 2 hours if necessary. *Intramuscular: Children under 12 years,* no more than one-half adult dose.	*Generic.* Tablets, solution (for injection), syrup, suppositories *Phenergan* (Wyeth-Ayerst). Syrup 6.25 and (fortis) 25 mg/5 ml; tablets 12.5, 25, and 50 mg; suppositories 12.5, 25, and 50 mg; solution (for injection) 25 and 50 mg/ml in 1 ml containers	Pronounced sedative effect limits use in many ambulatory patients. Most precautions applicable to phenothiazines should be observed (see index entry Phenothiazines). Photosensitization is contraindication to further use.
Trimeprazine Tartrate 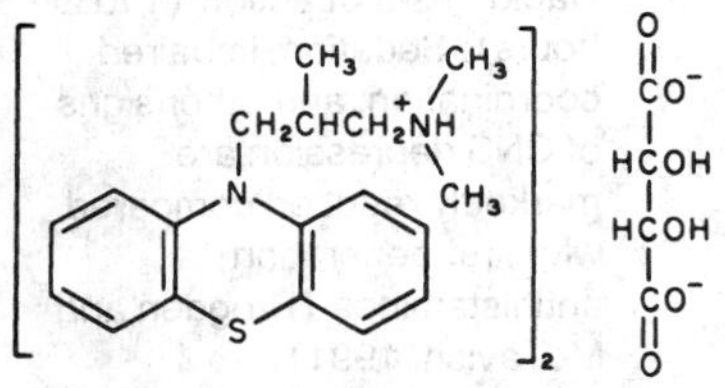	*Oral: Adults,* 10 mg daily divided into 4 doses (tablets, syrup) or 2 doses 12 hours apart (prolonged-release form). *Children 6 months to 3 years,* 1.25 mg at bedtime or 3 times daily if required (syrup); *3 to 12 years,* 2.5 mg at bedtime or 3 times daily if required (tablets, syrup).	*Generic.* Syrup *Temaril* (Allergan Herbert). Capsules (prolonged-release) 5 mg; syrup 2.5 mg/5 ml (alcohol 5.7%); tablets 2.5 mg	Used primarily as antipruritic. Drowsiness most common reaction. All precautions applicable to phenothiazines should be observed (see index entry Phenothiazines).

(table continued on next page)

TABLE 2 (Continued)

Drug/Chemical Structure	Usual Dosage	Preparations	Comment
MISCELLANEOUS Azatadine Maleate	*Oral: Adults,* 1 to 2 mg twice daily. *Children,* dosage has not been established.	*Optimine* (Schering). Tablets 1 mg	Chemically and pharmacologically similar to cyproheptadine but incidence of drowsiness is much lower.
Cyproheptadine Hydrochloride	*Oral: Adults,* 4 to 20 mg daily in divided doses. Dosage must be individualized and should not exceed 0.5 mg/kg daily. *Children 2 to 6 years,* 2 mg 2 or 3 times daily (maximum, 12 mg daily); *7 to 14 years,* 4 mg 2 or 3 times daily (maximum, 16 mg daily).	*Generic.* Syrup, tablets *Periactin* (Merck). Syrup 2 mg/5 ml (alcohol 5%); tablets 4 mg	Used to relieve pruritus. Reported to be especially useful in cold urticaria. Drowsiness most common reaction. Increases appetite and weight. Drug should not be used in premature and newborn infants.
Hydroxyzine Hydrochloride Hydroxyzine Pamoate	*Oral: Adults,* initially, 25 mg 3 times daily, increased if necessary to 100 mg 4 times daily. *Children under 6 years,* 50 mg daily divided into 3 or 4 doses; *over 6 years,* 50 to 100 mg daily divided into 3 or 4 doses.	*Generic.* Syrup, tablets (hydrochloride); capsules (pamoate) *Atarax [hydrochloride]* (Roerig). Syrup 10 mg/5 ml (alcohol 0.5%); tablets 10, 25, 50, and 100 mg *Vistaril [pamoate]* (Pfizer). Capsules 25, 50, and 100 mg; suspension (oral) equivalent to 25 mg hydrochloride/5 ml	A drug of choice for chronic urticaria and many dermatologic allergies. Drowsiness most common reaction. Contraindicated during early pregnancy.
SECOND-GENERATION ANTIHISTAMINES Acrivastine (Investigational) 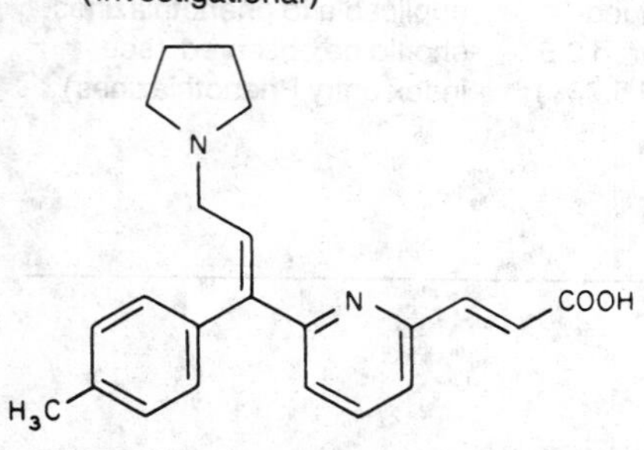	*Oral: Adults and children over 12 years,* 8 mg 3 or 4 times daily.	*Prolert* (Burroughs Wellcome).	Rapid onset of action (1 to 2 hours). Sedation, impaired coordination, and other signs of CNS depression are markedly reduced compared with first-generation antihistamines (Brogden and McTavish, 1991).

(table continued on next page)

TABLE 2 (Continued)

Drug/Chemical Structure	Usual Dosage	Preparations	Comment
Astemizole F–C₆H₄–CH₂ (benzimidazole)–NH–(piperidine)N–CH₂CH₂–C₆H₄–OCH₃	*Oral: Adults and children over 12 years,* a maximum of 10 mg once daily taken on an empty stomach. *Children 6 to 12 years,* data are insufficient to recommend a dosage; however, one-half the adult dose has been used.	*Hismanal* (Janssen). Tablets 10 mg	Slow onset of action (1 to 6 days); thus, most useful for prophylaxis. This and other second-generation antihistamines may be as effective as hydroxyzine for chronic urticaria and many dermatologic allergies. Sedation, impaired coordination, and other signs of CNS depression do not occur. Efficacy is not enhanced by giving larger doses. Rare, potentially lethal arrhythmias have occurred with overdose or may develop when recommended doses are used with ketoconazole, itraconazole, erythromycin, clarithromycin, troleandomycin, or other agents that inhibit hepatic drug metabolism or prolong the QT interval; concomitant use with these drugs or in patients with severe hepatic dysfunction is contraindicated. Weight gain has been observed with prolonged use (more than two weeks). Astemizole should be discontinued six weeks prior to skin testing.
Cetirizine Hydrochloride (Investigational) Cl–C₆H₄–CH(C₆H₅)–N(piperazine)N–$CH_2CH_2OCH_2COOH$ · 2HCl	*Oral: Adults and children over 12 years,* 5 to 20 mg once daily.	*Reactine* (Pfizer).	Rapid onset of action (1 hour). The incidence of sedation, impaired coordination, and other signs of CNS depression is markedly reduced compared with first-generation antihistamines but may be greater than with terfenadine (Backhouse et al, 1990). It is unclear whether overdosage or drug interactions cause arrhythmias; more data are needed. The unmetabolized drug is excreted primarily by the kidneys.
Levocabastine Hydrochloride NC, H, H, CH_3, CO_2H, N, F · HCl	*Topical: Adults,* 2 sprays of nasal preparation (investigational) in each nostril 2 to 4 times daily; 1 drop of ophthalmic preparation in each eye 4 times daily (Dechant and Goa, 1991).	*Livostin* (Iolab). Suspension (sterile, ophthalmic) 0.05% with benzalkonium chloride 0.01%, disodium edetate, hydroxypropyl methylcellulose, and purified water in 5 ml containers	Rapid onset of action (5 minutes). First antihistamine developed as a single agent for nasal and ophthalmic application. Well tolerated. Topical preparations appear to be nonsedating.

(table continued on next page)

TABLE 2 (Continued)

Drug/Chemical Structure	Usual Dosage	Preparations	Comment
Loratadine 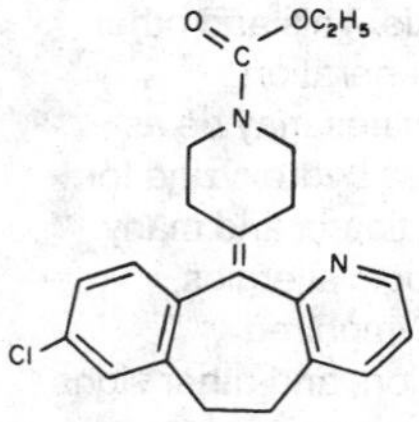	*Oral: Adults and children over 12 years,* 10 mg once daily.	*Claritin* (Schering). Tablets 10 mg	Rapid onset of action (1 to 2 hours). Similar in actions and efficacy to terfenadine. Sedation and other signs of CNS depression are not observed with usual doses. It is unclear whether overdosage or drug interactions cause arrhythmias; more data are needed.
Terfenadine 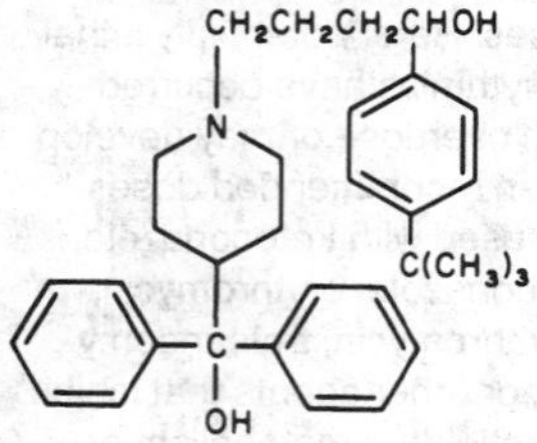	*Oral: Adults and children 12 years or over,* 60 mg twice daily. Administration of 120 mg once daily may be effective for some patients (Henauer et al, 1987; Yamate et al, 1988; McTavish et al, 1990; Ratner et al, 1992). A daily dose of 120 mg should not be exceeded. *Children 6 to 12 years,* 30 to 60 mg twice daily adjusted according to weight; *3 to 5 years,* 15 mg twice daily.	*Seldane* (Marion Merrell Dow). Tablets 60 mg	Rapid onset of action (1 to 3 hours). This and other second-generation antihistamines may be as effective as hydroxyzine for chronic urticaria and many dermatologic allergies. Sedation, impaired coordination, and other signs of CNS depression do not commonly occur. Efficacy is not enhanced by giving larger doses. Rare, potentially lethal arrhythmias have occurred with overdose or when recommended doses are used with ketoconazole, itraconazole, erythromycin, clarithromycin, troleandomycin, or other agents that inhibit hepatic drug metabolism or prolong the QT interval; concomitant use with these drugs or in patients with severe hepatic or cardiovascular dysfunction is contraindicated.

value in infectious rhinitis is very limited. The symptomatic relief sometimes experienced by patients with vasomotor or infectious rhinitis can be attributed to the drying effect on nasal mucosa caused by the anticholinergic action of some first-generation antihistamines.

The second-generation antihistamines appear to be as effective as the first-generation antihistamines in allergic disorders (Richards et al, 1984; Sorkin and Heel, 1985; Aaronson, 1991; Simons and Simons, 1991; Ryhal and Fletcher, 1991; Kaliner, 1992). In patients with seasonal allergic rhinitis, terfenadine and loratadine have a more rapid onset of action (one to three hours) than astemizole (one to six days) and thus may be more useful when rapid relief is required (Girard et al, 1985; Sussman and Kobric, 1985; Gutkowski et al, 1988; Clissold et al, 1989; Simons, 1988; Quercia and Broisman, 1993). The investigational drugs, cetirizine and acrivastine, are similar in efficacy and actions to terfenadine; cetirizine has a longer duration of action than acrivastine (Berman et al, 1988; Grossman et al, 1988; Broide et al, 1988; Campoli-Richards et al, 1990; Brogden and McTavish, 1991).

Because of their anti-inflammatory actions, intranasal preparations of corticosteroids (eg, beclomethasone dipropionate) generally are more effective than antihistamines in patients with acute or chronic allergic rhinitis, particularly for severe symptoms (Simons and Simons, 1991; Welch, 1991). The combination of terfenadine (or another antihistamine) and a topical corticosteroid may provide significantly better control of nasal and ocular symptoms than terfenadine alone (Backhouse et al, 1986).

A renewed interest in the use of topical antihistamine nasal preparations was prompted by the results of clinical studies on the second-generation antihistamine, levocabastine, and the investigational antiallergy agent, azelastine. Short-term use of both of these drugs provided protection against antigen-provoked allergic rhinitis and allergic rhinoconjunctivitis

(Simons and Simons, 1991). Levocabastine is a highly specific H_1 receptor antagonist. It is the first antihistamine developed for use alone in a nasal spray preparation (investigational). In clinical trials, intranasal levocabastine administered four times daily significantly relieved symptoms in patients with allergic rhinitis (Palma-Carlos et al, 1991; Schata et al, 1991; Schuermans et al, 1993). An eye-drop preparation is now available and is effective for allergic conjunctivitis (Dechant and Goa, 1991); in a limited number of studies, topical application in low doses did not appear to be sensitizing. Additional studies are required to verify its lack of sensitization. Like other second-generation agents, topical levocabastine appears to be well tolerated and produces little sedation (Dechant and Goa, 1991; Rombaut et al, 1991). However, the oral preparation of this drug (investigational) is sedating.

The efficacy of antihistamines in the common cold and other upper respiratory infections has been reviewed (West et al, 1975). More current evidence indicates that neither first- nor second-generation antihistamines prevent colds or significantly shorten the duration of infection, although mild symptomatic relief has been reported in some patients (Bluestone, 1988; Welliver, 1990). Despite this lack of evidence of substantial effectiveness, antihistamines are common ingredients of cold remedies (Hendeles, 1993) (see index entry Cold Remedies).

Lower Respiratory Disorders: Although H_1 antagonists may have a slight bronchodilating effect, at best these antihistamines offer only mild protection against bronchospasm. They generally are not useful for the treatment of acute, moderate, or severe asthma. In patients with both seasonal allergic rhinitis and asthma, the first-generation antihistamines can be used to treat symptoms of the former, since it is no longer believed that the anticholinergic drying actions aggravate asthma.

Dermatologic Conditions: Acute urticaria and atopic dermatitis, particularly the pruritic component, often are alleviated by oral H_1 antagonists. It has generally been believed that the pruritus associated with atopic or contact dermatitis may be relieved by first-generation antihistamines as a result of their CNS depressant actions. In patients with severe pruritus, the dual effects of sedation and histamine receptor blockade can be particularly helpful, especially if these drugs are used at bedtime. Although the second-generation antihistamines appear to be less effective in pruritic dermatoses other than urticaria, the fact that these drugs do provide some degree of relief suggests that H_1 receptor antagonism also may be involved in these disorders (Doherty et al, 1989).

In one study on patients with acute urticaria, it was reported that H_2 antagonists (eg, cimetidine) were effective when used with H_1 antagonists (Moscati and Moore, 1990); it is possible that an increase in the serum concentration of H_1 antagonists induced by the H_2 antagonists may be the mechanism for the antiurticarial action of the latter drugs (Simons et al, in press).

Recurrent episodes of urticaria lasting longer than six weeks are defined as chronic idiopathic urticaria; often no cause can be found and treatment is difficult (Soter, 1990). Results of studies comparing different drugs have varied. Hydroxyzine has been a drug of choice for treatment of this condition but the tricyclic antidepressant, doxepin, and the second-generation antihistamines, astemizole, loratadine, and terfenadine, appear to be equally effective (Bernstein and Bernstein, 1986; Sussman and Jancelewicz, 1991; Drouin, 1985; Grant et al, 1988; Boggs et al, 1989; Clissold et al, 1989; Belaich et al, 1990). The investigational drug cetirizine significantly reduced the occurrence of wheals, erythema, and pruritus compared with placebo in patients with chronic idiopathic urticaria (Juhlin and Arendt, 1988; Kietzmann et al, 1990; Maddin et al, 1991). Results of some studies indicate that astemizole or cetirizine may be more effective than terfenadine (Monroe, 1988; Kietzmann et al, 1990). The relatively long half-lives of hydroxyzine, astemizole, and terfenadine permit administration once or twice daily, which enhances compliance.

The combination of an H_1 and H_2 antagonist also may be beneficial in some patients with chronic urticaria refractory to H_1 blockers alone (Choy and Middleton, 1991). An H_2 blocker is not recommended for patients with chronic urticaria who respond adequately to an H_1 blocker, and, as with their use in acute urticaria, H_2 blockers should not be given alone (Beauchamp and Millares, 1985). A one-month trial will probably identify patients who respond to the combination.

Antihistamines prevent physical urticaria such as that produced by cold or exercise (Wanderer et al, 1986). Compared with placebo, cetirizine had a significant effect in preventing pressure-induced dermographism and cold-induced urticaria (Juhlin et al, 1987). The combination of H_1 and H_2 antagonists also may be beneficial in this form of urticaria (Irwin et al, 1985; Duc et al, 1986; Theoharides, 1989).

See Table 3 for treatment guidelines for chronic urticaria, physical urticaria, and atopic dermatitis.

Hypersensitivity Reactions: Antihistamines aid in the treatment of urticaria and pruritus associated with allergic reactions (eg, penicillin or other drug sensitivity; food allergies; wasp, yellow jacket, and hornet stings; acute reactions to drugs and allergen injections). However, these drugs are ineffective in combating severe symptoms of hypersensitivity resulting in anaphylaxis (eg, hypotension, upper respiratory obstruction due to laryngeal edema). Epinephrine is the only recommended immediate treatment for anaphylaxis and other allergic emergencies (see index entry Shock, Anaphylactic), but antihistamines can be used as adjuncts to control secondary effects on skin and mucosa.

Antihistamines may help prevent allergic reactions to contrast media. Diphenhydramine has been employed most commonly, usually in conjunction with corticosteroids; when indicated, both are given parenterally prior to the intravenous administration of contrast media. The addition of ephedrine may further reduce such reactions (Greenberger and Patterson, 1991; Marshall and Lieberman, 1991).

Antihistamines are sometimes used topically to treat allergic conjunctivitis, allergic dermatitis, pruritus caused by insect stings, and similar conditions. However, with the possible exception of levocabastine or azelastine, local application of antihistamines for long periods may cause sensitization. Accordingly, oral administration is preferred.

TABLE 3.
GUIDELINES FOR USE OF ANTIHISTAMINES IN TREATMENT OF IDIOPATHIC CHRONIC URTICARIA, PHYSICAL URTICARIA, AND ATOPIC DERMATITIS

Idiopathic Chronic Urticaria

1. Prescribe an H_1-blocker with little or no sedative effect (eg, terfenadine 120 mg/day in 1 or 2 doses, astemizole or loratadine 10 mg/day in 1 dose taken in the morning).
2. If treatment fails or is inadequate, prescribe another H_1-blocker from a different group or an H_1-blocker *plus* an H_2-blocker.
3. If step 2 fails, consider use of another type of treatment.

Physical Urticaria

1. Persuade the patient to avoid the causative factor.
2. If this is impossible, prescribe an H_1-blocker. *Special situations:* cold urticaria, prescribe cyproheptadine; cholinergic urticaria, prescribe hydroxyzine.

Atopic Dermatitis

1. Topical corticosteroids are the drugs of choice.
2. First-generation antihistamines with marked sedative properties (eg, hydroxyzine, diphenhydramine, promethazine, cyproheptadine) appear to be more effective for relief of pruritus than the second-generation, relatively nonsedating antihistamines.

Adapted from Advenier and Queille-Roussel, 1989.

Transfusion Reactions: Antihistamines may ameliorate histamine-induced flushing, urticaria, and pruritus associated with mild transfusion reactions not caused by incompatibility or pyrogens, but these agents do not prevent such reactions. Antihistamines should not be given routinely to patients receiving blood or blood products but may be administered prophylactically to those with a history of transfusion reactions. They should never be added to blood being transfused.

Miscellaneous Uses: The sedative effect of the first-generation antihistamines, particularly hydroxyzine and promethazine, is the basis for their use for preoperative medication (see index entry Adjuncts to Anesthesia).

The first-generation antihistamines are the principal components of most over-the-counter sleep aids. The amount of antihistamine permitted in each dose generally is limited, and tolerance to the sedative effect may develop. (See also index entry Insomnia.)

The piperazine antihistamines (buclizine [Bucladin-S], cyclizine [Marezine], and meclizine [Antivert, Bonine]) and the amino alkyl ether, dimenhydrinate [Dramamine], are used principally for motion sickness and dizziness. Some antihistamines are used in Parkinson's disease and in the treatment of acute dystonia. (See index entries on these disorders.)

For information on specific antihistamines, see Table 2.

Cost

As shown in Table 4, second-generation agents are considerably more expensive than first-generation antihistamines with the exception of clemastine and azatadine (*Intern Med Alert*, 1992); this may be a factor in drug selection for some patients.

TABLE 4.
APPROXIMATE RETAIL COST OF ANTIHISTAMINES*

	Number of Tablets	Cost of Daily Dose
First-Generation Antihistamines		
Chlorpheniramine	4	$0.15
Diphenhydramine	4	$0.25
Brompheniramine	4	$0.43
Promethazine	4	$0.37
Triprolidine	4	$0.19
Hydroxyzine	3	$0.42
Cyproheptadine	3	$0.29
Azatadine	2	$2.44
Clemastine	3	$2.01
Second-Generation Antihistamines		
Terfenadine	2	$1.78
Astemizole	1	$1.66
Loratadine	1	$1.70

* *Adapted from* Intern Med Alert, *1992.*

Adverse Reactions and Drug Interactions

First-Generation Antihistamines: Therapeutic doses of these H_1 antagonists cause adverse effects that rarely are serious and often disappear after a few days of continued usage. However, there is marked variation in tolerance among individuals.

The most common adverse effects are drowsiness and sedation. Daytime drowsiness may be a problem, especially while driving or operating machinery. Some patients believe that they are alert, but performance and reaction times may be significantly impaired (Gengo and Manning, 1990; Meltzer, 1990). Some patients become tolerant of the drowsiness or sedative effect within a few days or weeks. Administration of the antihistamines with relatively long serum half-lives (eg, chlorpheniramine, brompheniramine, hydroxyzine) as a single dose at bedtime may prevent or decrease daytime sedation in adults (Drouin, 1985; Goetz et al, 1991; Simons et al, 1990). Patients should be warned that simultaneous ingestion of alcohol or other CNS depressants increases somnolence. Other untoward effects include dizziness, lassitude, incoordination, fatigue, tinnitus, and diplopia. Paradoxically, euphoria, nervousness, irritability, insomnia, tremors, and increased tendency toward convulsions also may occur, especially in children and the elderly.

Arrhythmias rarely have been reported with overdose of some first-generation antihistamines.

Gastrointestinal symptoms, such as loss of appetite, nausea, vomiting, abdominal discomfort, constipation, or diarrhea, are the next most common side effects.

Many first-generation antihistamines have anticholinergic actions that are manifested as dryness of the mouth, throat, and nasal airway; glaucoma; tightness of the chest; palpitations; headache; and prostatism (urinary retention) or dysuria. Monoamine oxidase inhibitors prolong and intensify the anticholinergic drying effects of antihistamines.

Allergic dermatitis is more common after topical application. Leukopenia and agranulocytosis occur rarely.

Second-Generation Antihistamines: In therapeutic doses, sedation and other CNS adverse effects do not occur in most patients taking second-generation antihistamines. In addition, these drugs usually do not potentiate the sedative actions of CNS depressants (eg, alcohol, benzodiazepines) or impair psychomotor performance. However, in an occasional patient, drowsiness, sedation, and other manifestations of CNS impairment occur when doses exceed the recommended amount (Simons and Simons, 1991; Backhouse et al, 1990; Gendron and Kirkwood, 1990; Woodward, 1990; Falliers et al, 1991; Renton et al, 1991; Hugonot et al, 1986).

The incidence of anticholinergic effects is negligible with second-generation antihistamines. The use of astemizole for longer than two weeks may increase appetite and cause weight gain (Wilson and Hillas, 1982).

Transient arrhythmias occur rarely in both adults and children. A potentially lethal complication observed in patients treated with astemizole or terfenadine is the development of a prolonged QT interval, most commonly with overdosage. The disturbances in cardiac rhythm include an atypical ventricular tachycardia, torsades de pointes (TdP), and ventricular fibrillation (*Med Lett Drugs Ther*, 1992; *FDC Reports*, 1992; Simons et al, 1988 A; Hoppu et al, 1991; Simons and Simons, 1991; Tobin et al, 1991; Janssen, 1992; MacConnell and Stanners, 1991). As of May 1993, fewer than 300 cases of serious arrhythmias in patients treated with astemizole or terfenadine have been reported worldwide.

Use of recommended doses of astemizole or terfenadine in patients receiving drugs that inhibit hepatic metabolism (eg, imidazole antifungals such as ketoconazole, itraconazole; macrolides such as troleandomycin, erythromycin, clarithromycin) also may prolong the QT interval and precipitate TdP (Davies et al, 1989; Eller and Okerholm, 1991; Cantilena et al, 1991; Mathews et al, 1991; Monahan et al, 1990; *FDC Reports*, 1992). Therefore, concomitant use of terfenadine or astemizole in patients treated with such drugs is contraindicated. Furthermore, patients with severe hepatic dysfunction (eg, hepatitis, alcoholic cirrhosis), those receiving other drugs that prolong the QT interval, and those susceptible to a prolonged QT interval (eg, those with hypokalemia or congenital QT syndrome) also should not receive terfenadine or astemizole (Marion Merrell Dow, 1992; Janssen, 1992; Morganroth et al, 1993). Cardiac disturbances associated with terfenadine and astemizole also may occur with first-generation antihistamines (Morganroth et al, 1993).

The arrhythmogenic action of terfenadine appears to result from inhibition of the potassium channel, which slows repolarization; the active metabolite, terfenadine carboxylate, has no effect on potassium currents in vitro and does not appear to have arrhythmogenic effects (Woosley et al, 1993).

TdP frequently terminates spontaneously. Effective regimens to suppress the arrhythmia in patients treated with either terfenadine or astemizole include discontinuation of the drug and institution of supportive measures, infusion of intravenous magnesium sulfate, and temporary rapid atrial or ventricular pacing (Vukmir, 1991; Ben-David and Zipes, 1993). If pacing is not available, an alternative is the temporary cautious use of intravenous isoproterenol, which also decreases the QT interval. Magnesium corrects abnormal repolarization by a different mechanism; rather than the QT interval, sites of its action appear to be in the Na^+, K^+-ATPase system and potassium flux in the myocardial cell membrane (Vukmir, 1991). Magnesium is much safer than isoproterenol. Lidocaine, a Class 1B antiarrhythmic, also decreases the QT interval and can be tried if necessary, but it has variable effectiveness. Quinidine and other Class 1A drugs cause TdP, and their use is contraindicated.

Current data indicate that loratadine, cetirizine, and acrivastine, alone or in combination with other agents, do not prolong the QT interval (Affrime et al, 1993; Sale et al, 1993; Frosolono et al, 1993). However, additional data are needed to determine the potential of these or other newer antihistamines to cause cardiac disturbances.

There has been concern that loratadine produced tumors in animals and that cetirizine may have carcinogenic potential in doses higher than those used in investigational studies in animals. However, an FDA advisory committee has determined that it is unlikely that either drug produces tumors in humans (*FDC Reports*, 1991).

Acute Overdosage

Although the first-generation antihistamines have a relatively large margin of safety, their widespread use makes acute poisoning common, especially in children. Drowsiness, dizziness, and ataxia are the most common symptoms of acute overdosage, and anticholinergic effects (flushing, dilated pupils, and hyperthermia) often occur within two hours following ingestion. Paradoxical CNS stimulant effects predominate in children, and hallucinations, toxic psychosis, and/or delirium tremens may be observed. Eventually, convulsions, which may be resistant to therapy, may ensue (Iserson and Hackney, 1983). CNS stimulation is observed less frequently in adults after acute overdosage, but seizures can occur, especially in the elderly. In adults, a latent period may be followed by respiratory depression, cardiovascular depression, and death.

Treatment of acute overdosage is symptomatic and generally supportive. Induction of emesis (in a conscious patient within one hour after ingestion) or gastric lavage (when emesis is inadvisable) is followed by administration of activated charcoal and cathartics to prevent further absorption. After overdose of first-generation agents, physostigmine is often recommended for treatment of symptoms caused by anticholinergic activity. However, the cholinergic action of physostigmine can be dangerous, and this drug should be avoided except in young children with delirium or hyperthermia that does not respond to external cooling.

After astemizole or terfenadine overdose, cardiac function should be monitored. For specific treatment of arrhythmias that may occur with overdosage, see the discussion under Adverse Reactions.

Precautions

Recent evidence suggests that in some patients, H_1 receptor antagonists taken within one week before allergy skin testing may affect the extent of the reaction. Astemizole should be withdrawn six weeks prior to testing (Wyse, 1987). Compliance can be verified by documenting suppression of the histamine-mediated wheal and flare reaction. Antihistamines should not be given prophylactically to patients receiving allergen injections because they may mask mild symptoms, and severe anaphylactic reactions may occur if dosage of the allergen is increased.

There are no clear guidelines for safe use of antihistamines in pregnant women.

Tolerance: Although there is some evidence that prolonged administration of some first-generation antihistamines may produce subsensitivity (Bantz et al, 1987), other data suggest that subsensitivity of an H_1 receptor blocker does not occur as a result of autoinduction of enzyme systems, more rapid clearance of the drug, or lower concentrations of the drug in serum or tissue (Simons and Simons, 1987, 1991). Long-term administration of second-generation antihistamines has not been associated with the development of subsensitivity (Simons et al, 1988 B; Kemp, 1989; Bousquet et al, 1990; Simons and Simons, 1991).

Pharmacokinetics

The clinical pharmacokinetics of antihistamines have been reviewed (Paton and Webster, 1985; Simons et al, 1987).

First-Generation Antihistamines: The first-generation antihistamines, brompheniramine, chlorpheniramine, promethazine, diphenhydramine, and hydroxyzine, have been studied extensively. These drugs are metabolized by the liver and thus may accumulate in patients with severe hepatic disease. The elimination half-lives of these agents are: diphenhydramine, about eight hours; hydroxyzine, about 20 hours; promethazine, 10 to 14 hours; chlorpheniramine, 14 to 25 hours; and brompheniramine, about 25 hours. Total body clearances in adults range from 5 to 12 ml/kg/min, and apparent volumes of distribution are large (>4 L/kg).

Following oral administration of most first-generation agents, effects begin within 15 to 30 minutes and persist for 4 to 24 hours. Alkylamines, piperazines, and phenothiazines may have a considerably longer duration of action (see Table 1). In single-dose studies, the serum half-lives of chlorpheniramine, brompheniramine, and hydroxyzine exceeded 20 hours in adults; therefore, administration of these drugs once or twice daily may be feasible if the results with single doses can be extrapolated to prolonged administration (Drouin, 1985; Goetz et al, 1991). The serum half-lives of these drugs are shorter in children, and administration two or three times daily may be required. Intramuscular or intravenous injection produces a more prompt action, but rapid intravenous administration may cause hypotension. The duration of action of an antihistamine cannot be predicted by its half-life and must be determined by assessment of clinical effects and duration of wheal suppression (Aaronson, 1991).

Second-Generation Antihistamines: Extensive pharmacokinetic data are available for terfenadine (Sorkin and Heel, 1985), loratadine (Hilbert et al, 1987), cetirizine (Wood et al, 1987; Simons et al, 1987; Simons and Simons, 1991), acrivastine (Brogden and McTavish, 1991), levocabastine (Dechant and Goa, 1991), and astemizole (Richards et al, 1984). The chemical structures and high levels of serum protein binding of these drugs prevent their passage across the blood-brain barrier. This inability to enter the CNS is the primary reason for their lack of CNS adverse reactions with usual doses. The affinity of second-generation agents for histamine receptors in the central and peripheral nervous systems is similar.

Terfenadine and loratadine are well absorbed, and peak serum concentrations occur one to two hours after an oral dose. Both drugs are extensively and rapidly metabolized and well distributed to the tissues. Two major metabolites of terfenadine have been identified; one, a carboxylic acid metabolite, has significant antihistaminic activity and is being studied as a therapeutic agent (*FDC Reports*, 1993). Loratadine also has an active major metabolite. Both drugs are highly bound to plasma proteins, which contributes to difficulty in crossing the blood-brain barrier. About 60% of a dose of terfenadine or loratadine is eliminated in the feces; most of the remainder is recovered in the urine. The single-dose elimination half-life of the carboxylic acid metabolite of terfenadine in healthy adults is about 17 hours (Simons and Simons, 1991). In adults given a single dose, loratadine has a relatively long elimination half-life (8 to 20 hours), and a single daily dose provides an adequate serum concentration (Hilbert et al, 1987).

Acrivastine is well absorbed after oral administration; peak serum concentrations occur in two to three hours. About 16% of an oral dose is metabolized; most of the remainder is excreted unchanged by the kidneys (Brogden and McTavish, 1991). Hepatic metabolism of levocabastine is minimal; 75%

to 90% of the drug is excreted unchanged in the urine and feces (Dechant and Goa, 1991).

Cetirizine is the major metabolite of hydroxyzine. Following oral administration to healthy adults, peak serum concentrations occur in one hour. The drug is excreted in the urine essentially unchanged. Its mean elimination half-life is 7.4 hours (Wood et al, 1987).

After oral administration of astemizole, peak serum levels occur in one to four hours. Initially, it was believed that the absorption of astemizole from the gastrointestinal tract was decreased in the presence of food, but this is no longer accepted (Simons and Simons, 1991). Astemizole undergoes extensive first-pass metabolism in the liver to several active and inactive metabolites; it is well distributed in the tissues and is slowly displaced from receptor sites. In human volunteers, the drug was 96% bound to plasma proteins. Astemizole and its metabolites are excreted slowly following a single oral dose; 54% to 73% of the dose is recovered in the feces within 14 days. The apparent elimination half-life of unchanged drug and metabolites is about 9.5 days.

Mixtures

Many fixed-ratio mixtures containing a first-generation antihistamine with other agents, most commonly adrenergic nasal decongestants and analgesics, are marketed for the symptomatic treatment of allergies and upper respiratory infections. The combination of more than one ingredient in an individual dosage form can be recommended for convenience only. It is unlikely that all of the drugs in the mixture are provided in the exact dose needed. For a listing of commonly prescribed mixtures containing antihistamines, see index entry Cold Remedies.

Fixed-dose preparations containing a second-generation antihistamine and a long-acting nasal decongestant (eg, pseudoephedrine) are being evaluated (Simons and Simons, 1991). One such preparation containing terfenadine and pseudoephedrine [Seldane-D] is now available. The incidence of CNS stimulation (including insomnia) appears to be higher with this type of preparation than when the second-generation agent is used alone.

Cited References

First- and second-generation antihistamines in allergies. *Intern Med Alert* 26-28, (March 15) 1992.

Hismanal 'Dear Doctor' letter and revised labeling on heart risks. Titusville, NJ, Janssen, (Oct) 1992.

Janssen's *Hismanal* (astemizole) labeling adopts drug interaction warnings; new contraindications against erythromycin, ketoconazole and itraconazole use. *FDC Reports* 3-4, (Nov 2) 1992.

Marion Merrell Dow developing noncardiotoxic *Seldane* metabolite. *FDC Reports* 11-12, (March 29) 1993.

Safety of terfenadine and astemizole. *Med Lett Drugs Ther* 34:9-10, (Feb) 1992.

Schering-Plough's Claritin and Pfizer's Reactine human carcinogenicity "not likely"—Advisory Cmte.; OTC doxylamine should carry cancer warning. *FDC Reports* 7-9, (June 24) 1991.

Seldane 'Dear Doctor' letter and revised labeling on heart risks. Cincinnati, Marion Merrell Dow, 1992.

Aaronson DW: Comparative efficacy of H_1 antihistamines. *Ann Allergy* 67:541-547, 1991.

Advenier C, Queille-Roussel C: Rational use of antihistamines in allergic dermatological conditions. *Drugs* 38:634-644, 1989.

Affrime MB, et al: Three month evaluation of electrocardiographic effects of loratadine in humans, abstract. *J Allergy Clin Immunol* 91:259, 1993.

Backhouse CI, et al: Treatment of seasonal allergic rhinitis with flunisolide and terfenadine. *J Int Med Res* 14:35-41, 1986.

Backhouse CI, et al: Multicentre, double-blind comparison of terfenadine and cetirizine in patients with seasonal allergic rhinitis. *Br J Clin Pract* 44:88-91, 1990.

Bantz EW, et al: Chronic chlorpheniramine therapy: Subsensitivity, drug metabolism, and compliance. *Ann Allergy* 59:341-346, 1987.

Beauchamp C, Millares M: H_2 antagonists in hives and urticaria. *Drug Intell Clin Pharm* 19:662-663, 1985.

Belaich S, et al: Comparative effects of loratadine and terfenadine in the treatment of chronic idiopathic urticaria. *Ann Allergy* 64:191-194, 1990.

Ben-David J, Zipes DP: Torsades de pointes and proarrhythmia. *Lancet* 341:1578-1582, 1993.

Berman B, et al: Cetirizine therapy of perennial allergic rhinitis, abstract. *J Allergy Clin Immunol* 81:177, 1988.

Bernstein IL, Bernstein DI: Efficacy and safety of astemizole, long-acting and nonsedating H_1 antagonist for treatment of chronic idiopathic urticaria. *J Allergy Clin Immunol* 77:37-42, 1986.

Bluestone CD (moderator): Symposium: Questioning the efficacy and safety of antihistamines in the treatment of upper respiratory infection. *Pediatr Infect Dis J* 7:215-242, 1988.

Boggs PB, et al: Double-blind, placebo-controlled study of terfenadine and hydroxyzine in patients with chronic idiopathic urticaria. *Ann Allergy* 63:616-620, 1989.

Bousquet J, et al: Lack of subsensitivity to loratadine during long-term dosing during 12 weeks. *J Allergy Clin Immunol* 86:248, 1990.

Brogden RN, McTavish D: Acrivastine: A review of its pharmacological properties and therapeutic efficacy in allergic rhinitis, urticaria and related disorders. *Drugs* 41:927-940, 1991.

Broide DH, et al: Evaluation of cetirizine in the treatment of patients with seasonal allergic rhinitis, abstract. *J Allergy Clin Immunol* 81:176, 1988.

Campoli-Richards DM, et al: Cetirizine: A review of its pharmacological properties and clinical potential in allergic rhinitis, pollen-induced asthma, and chronic urticaria. *Drugs* 40:762-781, 1990.

Cantilena LR Jr, et al: Torsades de pointes occurring in association with terfenadine use, letter. *JAMA* 266:2375-2376, 1991.

Choy M, Middleton RK: Cimetidine in idiopathic urticaria. *DICP* 25:609-612, 1991.

Clissold SP, et al: Loratadine: A preliminary review of its pharmacodynamic properties and therapeutic efficacy. *Drugs* 37:42-57, 1989.

Davies AJ, et al: Cardiotoxic effect with convulsions in terfenadine overdose. *BMJ* 298:325, 1989.

Dechant KL, Goa KL: Levocabastine: A review of its pharmacological properties and therapeutic potential as a topical antihistamine in allergic rhinitis and conjunctivitis. *Drugs* 41:202-224, 1991.

Doherty V, et al: Treatment of itching in atopic eczema with antihistamines with a low sedative profile. *BMJ* 298:96, 1989.

Drouin MA: H_1 antihistamines: Perspective on use of conventional and new agents. *Ann Allergy* 55:747-752, 1985.

Duc J, et al: Successful treatment of idiopathic cold urticaria with association of H_1 and H_2 antagonists. *Ann Allergy* 56:355-357, 1986.

Eller MG, Okerholm RA: Pharmacokinetic interaction between terfenadine and ketoconazole. *Clin Pharmacol Ther* 49:130, 1991.

Falliers CJ, et al: Double-blind comparison of cetirizine and placebo in the treatment of seasonal rhinitis. *Ann Allergy* 66:257-262, 1991.

Frosolono MF, et al: Chronic administration of acrivastine does not affect cardiac repolarization, abstract. *Ann Allergy* 70:48, 1993.

Gendron CN, Kirkwood CF: Loratadine: A nonsedating antihistamine. *Drug Ther* 79-81, (May) 1990.

Gengo FM, Manning C: A review of the effects of antihistamines on mental processes related to automobile driving. *J Allergy Clin Immunol* 186:1034-1039, 1990.

Girard JP, et al: Double-blind comparison of astemizole, terfenadine and placebo in hay fever with special regard to onset of action. *J Int Med Res* 13:102-108, 1985.

Goetz DW, et al: Objective antihistamine side effects are mitigated by evening dosing of hydroxyzine. *Ann Allergy* 67:448-454, 1991.

Grant JA, et al: Double-blind comparison of terfenadine, chlorpheniramine, and placebo in the treatment of chronic idiopathic urticaria. *J Allergy Clin Immunol* 81:574-579, 1988.

Greenberger PA, Patterson R: The prevention of immediate generalized reactions to radiocontrast media in high-risk patients. *J Allergy Clin Immunol* 87:867-872, 1991.

Grossman J, et al: Cetirizine vs terfenadine in the treatment of seasonal allergic rhinitis, abstract. *Int Congress Allerg Clin Immunol* 9:370, 1988.

Gutkowski A, et al: Comparison of the efficacy and safety of loratadine, terfenadine and placebo in the treatment of seasonal allergic rhinitis. *J Allergy Clin Immunol* 81:902-907, 1988.

Henauer S, et al: Multi-centre double-blind comparison of terfenadine once daily versus twice daily in patients with hay fever. *J Int Med Res* 15:212-223, 1987.

Hendeles L: Efficacy and safety of antihistamines and expectorants in nonprescription cough and cold preparations. *Pharmacotherapy* 13(2):154-158, 1993.

Hilbert J, et al: Pharmacokinetics and dose proportionality of loratadine. *J Clin Pharmacol* 27:694-698, 1987.

Hill SJ: Distribution, properties, and functional characteristics of three classes of histamine receptor. *Pharmacol Rev* 42:45-83, 1990.

Hoppu K, et al: Accidental astemizole overdose in young children. *Lancet* 338:538-540, 1991.

Hugonot L, et al: A double-blind comparison of terfenadine and mequitazine in the symptomatic treatment of acute pollinosis. *J Int Med Res* 14:124-130, 1986.

Irwin RB, et al: Mediator release in local heat urticaria: Protection with combined H_1 and H_2 antagonists. *J Allergy Clin Immunol* 76:35-39, 1985.

Iserson KV, Hackney KU: Antihistamines, in Haddad LM, Winchester JF (eds): *Clinical Management of Poisoning and Drug Overdosage*. Philadelphia, WB Saunders, 1983, 503-509.

Juhlin L, Arendt C: Treatment of chronic urticaria with cetirizine dihydrochloride, a non-sedating antihistamine. *Br J Dermatol* 119:67-72, 1988.

Juhlin L, et al: Inhibiting effect of cetirizine on histamine-induced and 48/80-induced wheals and flares, experimental dermographism, and cold-induced urticaria. *J Allergy Clin Immunol* 80:599-602, 1987.

Kaliner MA: Nonsedating antihistamines: Pharmacology, clinical efficacy and adverse effects. *Am Fam Physician* 45:1337-1342, 1992.

Kemp JP: Tolerance to antihistamines: Is it a problem? *Ann Allergy* 63:621-623, 1989.

Kietzmann H, et al: Comparison of cetirizine and terfenadine in the treatment of chronic idiopathic urticaria. *Ann Allergy* 65:498-500, 1990.

MacConnell TJ, Stanners AJ: Torsades de pointes complicating treatment with terfenadine. *BMJ* 302:1469, 1991.

Maddin S, et al: Treatment of chronic idiopathic urticaria: Cetirizine vs. terfenadine and placebo. *Can J Dermatol* 3:147-152, (July/Aug) 1991.

Mann KV, et al: Nonsedating histamine H_1-receptor antagonists. *Clin Pharm* 8:331-344, 1989.

Marshall GD Jr, Lieberman PL: Comparison of three pretreatment protocols to prevent anaphylactoid reactions to radiocontrast media. *Ann Allergy* 67:70-74, 1991.

Mathews DR, et al: Torsades de pointes occurring in association with terfenadine use. *JAMA* 266:2375-2376, 1991.

McTavish D, et al: Terfenadine: An updated review of its pharmacological properties and therapeutic efficacy. *Drugs* 39:552-574, 1990.

Meltzer EO: Performance effects of antihistamines. *J Allergy Clin Immunol* 86:613-619, 1990.

Monahan BP, et al: Torsades de pointes occurring in association with terfenadine use. *JAMA* 264:2788-2790, 1990.

Monroe EW: Chronic urticaria: Review of nonsedating H_1 antihistamines in treatment. *J Am Acad Dermatol* 19:842-849, 1988.

Morganroth J, et al: Variability of the QT_c interval: Impact on defining drug effect and low-frequency cardiac event. *Am J Cardiol* 72:26B-31B, 1993.

Moscati RM, Moore GP: Comparison of cimetidine and diphenhydramine in the treatment of acute urticaria. *Ann Emerg Med* 19:12-15, 1990.

Palma-Carlos AG, et al: Double-blind comparison of levocabastine nasal spray with sodium cromoglycate nasal spray in the treatment of seasonal allergic rhinitis. *Ann Allergy* 67:394-398, 1991.

Paton DM, Webster DR: Clinical pharmacokinetics of H_1-receptor antagonists (antihistamines). *Clin Pharmacokinet* 10:477-497, 1985.

Quercia RA, Broisman L: Focus on loratadine: A new second-generation nonsedating H_1-receptor antagonist. *Hosp Formul* 28:137-153, (Feb) 1993.

Ratner PH, et al: A placebo controlled double-blind randomized parallel study comparing the safety and efficacy of terfenadine 60 mg BID and terfenadine 120 mg (2x60 mg) QD in the treatment of patients with seasonal allergic rhinitis, abstract. *Ann Allergy* 68:110, 1992.

Renton R, et al: Multicenter, crossover study of the efficacy and tolerability of terfenadine, 120 mg, versus cetirizine, 10 mg, in perennial allergic rhinitis. *Ann Allergy* 67:416-420, 1991.

Richards DM, et al: Astemizole: Review of its pharmacodynamic properties and therapeutic efficacy. *Drugs* 28:38-61, 1984.

Rombaut N, et al: Effects of topical administration of levocabastine on psychomotor and cognitive function. *Ann Allergy* 67:75-79, 1991.

Ryhal BT, Fletcher MP: The second-generation antihistamines: What makes them different? *Postgrad Med* 89:87-99, (May) 1991.

Sale ME, et al: Lack of electrocardiographic effects of cetirizine in healthy humans, abstract. *J Allergy Clin Immunol* 91:258, 1993.

Schata M, et al: Levocabastine nasal spray better than sodium cromoglycate and placebo in the topical treatment of seasonal allergic rhinitis. *J Allergy Clin Immunol* 87:873-878, 1991.

Schuermans V, et al: Meta-analysis of the global evaluation of levocabastine nasal spray versus placebo. *Drug Info J* 27:575-584, 1993.

Simons FER: Loratadine, a non-sedating H_1-receptor antagonist (antihistamine). *Ann Allergy* 63:266-268, 1988.

Simons FER: The antiallergic effects of antihistamines (H_1-receptor antagonists). *J Allergy Clin Immunol* 90:705-715, 1992.

Simons KJ, Simons FER: The effect of chronic administration of hydroxyzine on hydroxyzine pharmacokinetics in dogs. *J Allergy Clin Immunol* 79:928-932, 1987.

Simons FER, Simons KJ: Second-generation H_1-receptor antagonists. *Ann Allergy* 66:5-16, 1991.

Simons FE, et al: Comparative pharmacokinetics of H_1-receptor antagonists. *Ann Allergy* 63:20-24, 1987.

Simons FER, et al: Astemizole overdose: Torsade de pointes: Case report. *Lancet* 2:624, 1988 A.

Simons FER, et al: Lack of subsensitivity to terfenadine during long-term terfenadine treatment. *J Allergy Clin Immunol* 82:1068-1075, 1988 B.

Simons KJ, et al: Pharmacokinetics and pharmacodynamics of terfenadine and chlorpheniramine in the elderly. *J Allergy Clin Immunol* 85:540-547, 1990.

Simons FER, et al: The effect of the H_2-antagonist cimetidine (C) on the pharmacokinetics (PK) and pharmacodynamics (PD) of the H_1-antagonist hydroxyzine (H) in patients with chronic urticaria. In press.

Sorkin EM, Heel RC: Terfenadine: Review of its pharmacodynamic properties and therapeutic efficacy. *Drugs* 29:34-56, 1985.

Soter NA: Urticaria: Current therapy. *J Allergy Clin Immunol* 86:1009-1014, 1990.

Sussman G, Jancelewicz Z: Controlled trial of H_1 antagonists in the treatment of chronic idiopathic urticaria. *Ann Allergy* 67:433-439, 1991.

Sussman GL, Kobric M: Treatment of seasonal allergic rhinitis with astemizole, non-sedating antihistamine: Results of open, multicenter clinical trial. *Todays' Ther Trends* 2:11-19, 1985.

Sutherland DC: Antihistamine agents: New options or just more drugs? *Med J Aust* 151:158-162, 1989.

Theoharides TC: Histamine$_2$ (H_2)-receptor antagonists in the treatment of urticaria. *Drugs* 37:345-355, 1989.

Tobin JR, et al: Astemizole-induced cardiac conduction disturbances in a child. *JAMA* 266:2737-2740, 1991.

Vukmir RB: Torsades de pointes: A review. *Am J Emerg Med* 9:250-255, 1991.

Wanderer AA, et al: Clinical characteristics of cold-induced systemic reactions in acquired cold urticaria syndromes: Recommendations for prevention of this complication and proposal for diagnostic classification of cold urticaria. *J Allergy Clin Immunol* 78:417-423, 1986.

Welch MJ: New-generation antihistamines. *West J Med* 154:455, 1991.

Welliver RC: The role of antihistamines in upper respiratory tract infections. *J Allergy Clin Immunol* 86:633-637, 1990.

West S, et al: Review of antihistamines and common cold. *Pediatrics* 56:100-107, 1975.

Wilson JD, Hillas JL: Astemizole: New long-acting antihistamine in treatment of seasonal allergic rhinitis. *Clin Allergy* 12:131-140, 1982.

Wood SG, et al: Metabolism and pharmacokinetics of ^{14}C-cetirizine in humans. *Ann Allergy* 59:31-34, 1987.

Woodward JK: Pharmacology of antihistamines. *J Allergy Clin Immunol* 86:606-612, 1990.

Woosley RL, et al: Mechanism of the cardiotoxic actions of terfenadine. *JAMA* 269:1532-1536, 1993.

Wyse D: Efficacy of skin test suppression by astemizole, abstract. *J Allergy Clin Immunol* 79:205, 1987.

Yamate M, et al: Comparison of terfenadine in two dosage regimens in the treatment of seasonal allergic rhinitis. *J Allergy Clin Immunol* 81:228, 1988.

Ziment I: *Respiratory Pharmacology and Therapeutics.* Philadelphia, WB Saunders, 1978.

Immunomodulating Agents 83

Immunomodulators adjust the immune response to a desired level of activity through the processes of immunosuppression (eg, corticosteroids, cytotoxic drugs, T-cell specific inhibitors, antiserums), induction of tolerance (desensitization, unresponsiveness), or immunopotentiation (eg, immune globulin replacement therapy).

Exposure to foreign antigen elicits a complex response in which the immune system plays a major role. The sequence of events comprising the immune response can be divided into five stages: (1) uptake and processing of antigen; (2) transfer of information (antigen presentation) and triggering of effector cells of the immune system; (3) proliferation, differentiation, and maturation of involved lymphocytes; (4) synthesis and release of mediator substances (cytokines) and antibodies; and (5) responses to mediators, antibodies, and effector cells.

It is theoretically possible to regulate the immune response at each of these levels, but many drugs are cytotoxic compounds that were originally tested for use in cancer chemotherapy and act by interfering with production of involved lymphocytes (stage 3).

IMMUNOSUPPRESSION. The immune response can be suppressed by producing tolerance to a specific antigen. Immunologic tolerance (unresponsiveness) is defined as failure of the immune system to respond to a specific antigen after prior exposure to that antigen and is thought to be due to either elimination of responding lymphocyte clones or inhibition of the immune system by regulatory mechanisms. It is possible to produce tolerance to both cell-mediated and humoral immune responses. The nature of the antigen, the amount, and the route of administration influence the degree of tolerance. In general, the greater the immunocompetence of the organism, the more difficult it is to induce tolerance. Nevertheless, irradiation or administration of antilymphocyte globulin followed by exposure to antigen may produce tolerance to specific antigens.

Specific IgE antibody can be suppressed in the allergic patient by repeated administration of specific antigen; the technique produces a "tolerance" to this antigen, which has been referred to as allergen immunotherapy. It is not known to what extent this "tolerance" is due to suppression of IgE formation or, more likely, to induction of IgG molecules that compete with IgE for the allergen. Desensitization to insect venom, for example, is an important immunotherapeutic measure for sensitive individuals who may respond to bee stings with anaphylaxis.

Injection of antibodies produced elsewhere and passively transferred can inhibit or suppress specific antibody production by a negative feedback mechanism or by masking the antigen with the exogenous antiserum. Thus, if anti-Rh_o antibody is given to an Rh-negative mother at the time of delivery of her Rh-positive child, sensitization and anti-Rh_o antibody production can be avoided.

Immunosuppressive agents inhibit immune responses. Their action is usually nonspecific, but some agents have a degree of specificity. For example, antilymphocyte serum suppresses T-lymphocyte activity more than B-lymphocyte activity, and cyclosporine [Sandimmune] also primarily affects T-lymphocyte function by inhibiting the production of lymphokines. The monoclonal antibody, muromonab-CD3 [Orthoclone OKT3], reacts with and blocks the function of a 20,000-dalton molecule (CD3) associated with the T-cell receptor for specific antigen recognition that is essential for signal transduction. In this manner, it blocks the generation and function of T-effector cells that participate in graft rejection (see the evaluation). Some nonspecific suppressants, such as methotrexate [Folex], are cell cycle specific; others, like cyclophosphamide [Cytoxan, Neosar], are not specific for any phase of the cell cycle. The cellular responses to these agents vary widely. The immunosuppressive action of all nonspecific drugs is obtained only at doses close to toxic levels. (For detailed information about immunosuppressants in cancer chemotherapy, see index entry Cancer, Treatment, Immunologic.)

Corticosteroid therapy is the mainstay in the treatment of many immune diseases. Corticosteroids and cyclosporine have a wider margin of safety than the cytotoxic drugs. Combination therapy with a corticosteroid and the immunosuppressant, cyclosporine, with or without azathioprine [Imuran], is used to suppress allograft rejection.

The cytotoxic drugs, cyclophosphamide, chlorambucil [Leukeran], and methotrexate, are effective antineoplastic agents, especially when used in a large-dose, pulsed regimen: The larger doses enhance neoplastic cytotoxicity, and pulsed therapy permits recovery of the immune response. Conversely, smaller doses of these drugs are effective in conventional regimens to maintain immunosuppression with minimal toxicity. In view of their considerable potential toxicity, antineoplastic drugs usually are reserved for autoimmune, immune complex, or granulomatous diseases and vasculitides that do not respond adequately to corticosteroid therapy.

Two factors that determine a cytotoxic drug's ability to reduce a population of immunoreactive cells are the cell cycle specificity of the agent and the proliferative status of the target cell. The former refers to the phase of the mitotic cycle in which the drug exerts its effect; the latter refers to the proportion of target cells in the various phases of the mitotic cycle. Cytotoxic agents can be classified as: (1) *Phase-specific drugs*, which are toxic only during a specific phase of the mitotic cycle. Examples include azathioprine, cytarabine [Cytosar-U, Tarabine PFS], mercaptopurine [Purinethol], and methotrexate, all of which are primarily S phase (stage of DNA synthesis) inhibitors. (2) *Cycle-specific drugs* (eg, cyclophosphamide), which affect both intermitotic and cycling cells, although there is preferential toxicity for proliferating cells. (3) *Cycle-nonspecific drugs* (eg, mechlorethamine [Mustargen]), which are toxic to both intermitotic and proliferating cells.

Prior to antigen challenge, lymphocytes are predominantly in the intermitotic phase; after contact with antigen, they actively proliferate. Cycle-nonspecific drugs are most inhibitory when given just prior to antigen challenge. Phase-specific drugs are only active when cells are replicating (after antigen challenge). Cycle-specific drugs are effective before and after antigen challenge. (See Table 1.)

SUPPRESSION OF ALLOGRAFT REJECTION. The most common rejection response to a histoincompatible kidney, marrow, liver, or heart graft is the development of cytotoxic and lymphokine-producing T-lymphocytes. Monocytes and B-lymphocytes also play a role; the latter are especially prominent during accelerated vascular rejection. Corticosteroids are indispensable to attenuate rejection episodes. Lymphocyte immune globulin [Atgam] seems to be useful in allotransplantation because it markedly suppresses T-lymphocyte mediated immune responses.

TABLE 1.
SUMMARY OF USES OF CYTOTOXIC IMMUNOSUPPRESSIVE DRUGS

DISORDERS IN WHICH CYTOTOXIC DRUGS ARE PROBABLY CLINICALLY BENEFICIAL:
Rheumatoid arthritis
Systemic lupus erythematosus
Lipoid nephrosis
Nephrotic syndrome
Psoriasis
Polydermatomyositis
Wegener's granulomatosis
Chronic active hepatitis
Inflammatory bowel disease
Autoimmune hemolytic anemia
Immune thrombocytopenia
Circulating anticoagulants
Systemic necrotizing vasculitis
Goodpasture's syndrome

Cyclosporine: The immunosuppressive agent, cyclosporine, has proved very useful in suppressing allograft rejection. This potent drug prolonged the survival of allografts and even xenografts in laboratory animals. Heart, lung, kidney, pancreas, liver, skin, muscle, nerve cells, bone marrow, small intestine, cornea, islets of Langerhans, ovaries, and fallopian tubes have been transplanted successfully in cyclosporine-treated animals. In humans, cyclosporine has greatly improved the success of transplantation and is the drug of choice for maintenance of heart, liver, and cadaveric kidney allografts. In kidney transplants from perfectly matched, living, related donors, some clinicians have been satisfied with graft and patient survival in those receiving azathioprine and steroids.

Cyclosporine suppresses T-lymphocyte functions without producing myelosuppression. For optimal suppression of T-cell function, cyclosporine must be present in the early phase of the immune response; maximum suppression occurs during the first 24 hours of antigen stimulation. The critical period is during induction of the immune response against the allograft, since T-cells already primed by antigen are resistant to cyclosporine. Maintenance of adequate immunosuppression with cyclosporine also remains a critical determinant of long-term transplant survival. (For reviews, see Kahan, 1989, and Borel, 1989.)

For a discussion of the mechanism of action and the serious adverse effects that limit use of cyclosporine, see the evaluation.

FK-506: The macrolide antibiotic, FK-506, is among the most promising of the new immunosuppressive drugs under investigation for the treatment of autoimmune disorders. It is produced by the bacterium, *Streptomyces tsukubaensis*, and was discovered during routine screening of fermentation broths for inhibitory effects on murine mixed lymphocyte reaction (MLR), an in vitro correlate for allograft rejection. FK-506 suppresses alloantigen or T-cell mitogen-induced lymphocyte proliferation at concentrations 100-fold lower than effective concentrations of cyclosporine. Like cyclosporine, it selectively inhibits CD4+ T-lymphocyte activation and cytokine production (see the evaluation on Cyclosporine) but it binds to a different immunophylin (immunosuppressant binding protein), referred to as FKBP (Macleod and Thomson, 1991; Schreiber, 1991; Thomson and Starzl, 1992). FK-506 also inhibits the generation of cytotoxic and suppressor T cells in human MLR, but does not affect antigen recognition or antigen processing and presentation by human monocytes at concentrations that suppress T-cell proliferation. It does not affect natural killer cell activity or antibody-dependent cytotoxicity. Like cyclosporine, FK-506 inhibits pro-inflammatory mediator release from human basophils (Thomson and Starzl, 1992).

FK-506 significantly prolongs survival of various organ and skin grafts in rodents, dogs, rabbits, and primates. It has reversed cardiac and renal rejection in rats and dogs and, in humans, has reversed acute or early chronic liver rejection, a property that distinguishes it from cyclosporine. In rodents, xenograft survival has been prolonged by FK-506, and this drug also has been beneficial in models of insulin-dependent diabetes mellitus, rheumatoid arthritis, posterior uveitis, allergic encephalomyelitis, and glomerulonephritis.

Severe but reversible thymic medullary atrophy following administration of FK-506 has occurred in rodents; this also is seen with cyclosporine. Minor renal impairment and hyperglycemia also have been observed in this species. Anorexia, vascular lesions, hepatocellular swelling, renal proximal tubular cell vacuolation, and pancreatic cell degeneration have been observed in dogs. However, as with cyclosporine, these animal toxicology studies may be an inadequate and misleading guide to the risk/benefit ratio of this drug in clinical practice (Macleod and Thomson, 1991).

The first report on FK-506's ability to reverse rejection in patients with liver allografts who were unresponsive to therapy with conventional immunosuppressive drugs was published in 1989 (Starzl et al, 1989). It has since been used as primary immunosuppressive therapy in adult recipients of liver transplants, 92% of whom were alive 6 to 12 months after surgery. Compared with cyclosporine-treated historical controls, patient survival was greatly improved, there were fewer episodes of rejection, and steroid requirements were reduced in FK-506 recipients (Macleod and Thomson, 1991). The drug is now considered equal or superior to cyclosporine in primary liver transplantation. Results with FK-506 as rescue therapy in liver transplants have been encouraging; up to 50% of the grafts that were failing with cyclosporine therapy were rescued. Use of FK-506 in these patients has allowed reduced usage of steroids compared with administration of cyclosporine.

Experience with FK-506 in kidney and heart transplantation is more limited, but results to date indicate that it can reverse rejection of these organs; however, further data are needed to determine whether FK-506 is as effective as cyclosporine. FK-506 also is being investigated in autoimmune diseases; in animal models of autoimmune disease, it has shown activity in uveitis, arthritis, insulin-dependent diabetes, spontaneous autoimmune lupus erythematosus, experimental autoimmune glomerulonephritis, autoimmune thyroiditis, and allergic encephalomyelitis (Thomson and Starzl, 1992).

The pharmacokinetics of FK-506 are problematic. After oral administration, drug absorption is highly variable (range, 6% to 57%; mean 25%). Unlike cyclosporine, absorption is not dependent on the availability of bile in the gut. Peak plasma levels are reached one to four hours after an oral dose. The drug is highly bound to erythrocytes with a mean blood:plasma trough concentration ratio of 10:1. The half-life ranges from 3.5 to 40.5 hours (mean, 8.7 hours). The drug is chiefly metabolized by the liver by N-demethylation and hydroxylation and is excreted in bile, urine, and feces within 48 hours. In patients with hepatic dysfunction, half-life is increased and clearance is reduced. Trough plasma concentrations of FK-506 are increased by coadministration of erythromycin, fluconazole [Diflucan], and clotrimazole [Lotrimin] (Thomson and Starzl, 1992).

Major adverse reactions include impairment of renal function (main dose-limiting toxicity), alterations in glucose metabolism, and neurotoxicity. The overall incidence of post-transplant lymphoproliferative disorder at one center was 1.6%. These effects are similar to those occurring with cyclosporine administration; however, the incidence of hypertension is lower than with cyclosporine, and gum hyperplasia and hirsutism have not been observed (Thomson and Starzl, 1992).

A comprehensive survey on the mechanism of action, pharmacology, clinical efficacy, and safety of FK-506 has been published (Starzl et al, 1991).

Muromonab-CD3: The first monoclonal antibody to be approved by the Food and Drug Administration for therapeutic use was muromonab-CD3, which is indicated for the treatment of acute allograft rejection in renal transplant patients. This murine antibody is a product of a hybridoma produced by the somatic cell hybridization technique of Köhler and Milstein (1975). It is a purified IgG_2 immunoglobulin that is directed to the CD3 molecule of the T-cell antigen receptor complex located on the surface membranes of T-cells, and it acts by blocking the function of all T-cells that play a major role in acute renal rejection. Following intravenous administration, muromonab-CD3 produces a rapid and concomitant decrease in CD3-, CD4-, and CD8-expressing T-cells within minutes. Studies have suggested that 74% to 94% of acute renal rejection episodes that have not responded to steroid therapy can be reversed by this agent. Investigational studies indicate that anti-CD3 therapy also may be useful in preventing or treating rejection of cardiac, liver, and pancreatic transplants (Luke, 1988). The drug is not myelosuppressive but it is a murine immunoglobulin and does induce the production of both isotypic and antiidiotypic antibodies; the latter inhibit its binding to T-cells, thereby reducing or abrogating its therapeutic activity (Chatenoud et al, 1986), which suggested that its use might be limited to a single course in a patient. In practice, however, this has applied only to individuals with high titers of those antibodies (<33% of treated patients). Several testing systems to detect antimurine antibodies are available and may be employed to guide therapeutic decisions.

IMMUNOLOGIC AUGMENTATION. It is possible to reconstitute a deficient immune system by transplanting bone marrow and thymus tissue, but these techniques are not in widespread clinical use. Immune globulin also augments the immune response. Transfer factor, a dialyzable extract of immune lymphocytes, has been investigated as a method of transferring cell-mediated immunity in humans.

Some agents amplify the production of antibodies. These adjuvants are administered with antigen to increase the immune response to that antigen. Aluminum phosphate is an example of a specific immunostimulant of this type; when added to tetanus toxoid, this mineral salt markedly enhances the ability of the toxoid to stimulate antibody production. Other methods employed experimentally in animals to enhance antibody production include (1) use of antigen with water-in-oil emulsions containing killed mycobacteria (complete Freund's adjuvant) or without mycobacteria (incomplete Freund's adjuvant), and (2) use of synthetic polynucleotides and bacterial endotoxins.

The exact mechanisms of action of these techniques are obscure, but some facts are apparent. Mineral salts provoke granulomas at the site of injection, which stimulates macrophage activity and slows antigen absorption. Freund's adjuvant markedly slows antigen absorption and increases dispersal while stimulating T-cell activity; the mycobacteria contained in complete Freund's adjuvant strongly stimulate macrophages and T-cells. Endotoxins stimulate DNA synthesis and differentiation in B-lymphocytes. Cellular actions of the adjuvants are being investigated.

Interferons: The interferons (IFNs) are immunomodulatory agents that have both anticancer and antiviral activity. Although they were discovered in 1957, it was not until the early 1980s, through recombinant DNA technology, that IFNs became available in sufficient quantities for widespread clinical evaluation.

Initially, it was thought that only a single type of interferon existed. The material was characterized as a broad spectrum, antiviral, species-specific glycoprotein produced by all nucleated animal cells, which acted by inducing a refractory state to virus infection. It is now known that there are three major classes of interferons (alpha, beta, and gamma) with broad biological activities. These include inhibition of DNA synthesis, cell multiplication, antibody synthesis, delayed hypersensitivity, and tumor growth. On the other hand, interferons enhance the activity of cytolytic T-cells and natural killer (NK) cells, the expression of HLA antigens and β_2-microglobulin on lymphocytes, HLA and tumor-associated antigens on cancer cells, and tumoricidal and phagocytic activity of macrophages. All three types of interferon enhance the expression of HLA class I antigens, but interferon-γ appears to be the most potent inducer. Expression of class II HLA molecules is associated only with interferon-γ. All three classes enhance the production of IL-1.

Recombinant IFN-α2 has been approved by the FDA for use in hairy cell leukemia, AIDS-related Kaposi's sarcoma, condyloma acuminatum, and chronic non-A, non-B (type C) hepatitis. In certain other malignancies, complete and/or partial objective responses have been observed in patients with advanced disease treated with the drug (Table 2). The activity of IFN-α against cancer cells is probably due to direct antiproliferative effects at all stages of the cell cycle, inhibition of oncogene expression, induction of differentiation in cancer cells, and immunologic enhancement of macrophage activity and lymphocyte cytotoxicity (see index entry Interferons, Uses).

TABLE 2.
CLINICAL ACTIVITY OF ALPHA INTERFERON AGAINST VARIOUS MALIGNANCIES AND VIRAL DISEASES

Malignancies	
	Hairy cell leukemia
	Non-Hodgkin's lymphoma
	Mycosis fungoides (cutaneous T-cell lymphoma)
	Kaposi's sarcoma (AIDS-associated)
	Multiple myeloma
	Malignant melanoma
	Renal cell cancer
	Basal cell carcinoma
	Bladder cancer (superficial tumors)*
	Carcinoid syndrome
	Ovarian cancer*
	Chronic myelogenous leukemia
Viral diseases	
	Juvenile laryngeal papillomatosis
	Condylomata acuminata
	Prophylaxis of upper respiratory infection
	Coronavirus colds
	Genital herpes
	Chronic non-A, non-B hepatitis
	Hepatitis B
	Acute fulminant hepatitis
	Varicella in cancer patients

**Activity has been seen primarily with local or regional administration.*

Both recombinant and natural (leukocyte) IFN-α have been used investigationally with various degrees of success for the treatment of certain viral diseases (Table 2). The antiviral activities of the IFNs following binding to cell receptors are mediated by synthesis of new cellular RNAs and proteins that are responsible for the development of the antiviral state (see index entry Antiviral Agents). Enzyme-linked immunosorbent assays (ELISA) have detected serum antibodies in 3% to 27% of all patients given IFN-α, but neutralizing activity has been demonstrated only rarely. No clinical sequelae attributable to these antibodies have been documented, although theoretically they could abrogate therapeutic effects.

IFN-α was the first interferon produced in sufficient quantities for clinical trials, and testing of IFN-β and IFN-γ has been less extensive. As a group, IFNs differ in both in vitro and in vivo activities. Both IFN-β and IFN-γ have been reported to be superior to IFN-α in inhibiting the growth of certain tumor cell lines in vitro. IFN-α and IFN-β have different tissue specificities: IFN-α may have preferential effects on hematopoietic cells and IFN-β may have greater effects on nonhematopoietic cells (Krown, 1986). Clinical studies with recombinant IFN-β have been conducted in patients with melanoma and multiple sclerosis, but thus far success has been limited or results are inconclusive. Effective inhibition of DNA polymerase activity was noted in five patients with chronic hepatitis B infection (Sarna et al, 1986; Eisenberg et al, 1986).

IFN-γ currently is indicated to reduce the frequency and severity of serious infections associated with chronic granulomatous disease (see the evaluation in this chapter). It has other interesting clinical activities. In one study, recombinant IFN-γ was effective in chronic rheumatoid arthritis and was well tolerated: 58 of 80 patients receiving either natural or recombinant drug improved clinically; 40 were classified as very improved and 18 as improved (Obert and Hofschneider, 1985). However, intramuscular administration of recombinant IFN-γ produced only minimal improvement in a few patients with psoriasis (Morhenn et al, 1987). In contrast, recombinant IFN-α has exacerbated this disease (Quesada and Gutterman, 1986).

For further information on the use of IFNs in cancer, multiple sclerosis, or as antiviral agents, see index entry Interferons, Uses.

Interleukin 2: Interleukin 2 (IL-2) is a lymphokine produced principally by activated helper T-lymphocytes in response to antigen or mitogen stimulation. It is a growth factor required for the proliferation of T-lymphocytes, and it stimulates proliferation of B-lymphocytes and activates and supports the growth of cytotoxic effector cells, including CD8 T-lymphocytes, NK cells, and lymphokine-activated killer (LAK) cells. In certain T-cells, IL-2 also may enhance the production of other T-cell lymphokines, including granulocyte-macrophage colony stimulating factor (GM-CSF), B-cell growth and differentiation factors, and interferon (γ). Impaired IL-2 production has been observed in systemic lupus erythematosus, primary immunodeficiency diseases, AIDS, and advanced metastatic malignancies. Activation of NK cells has been reported to be due to the induction of IFN-γ, which mediates the enhanced killing (Kawase et al, 1983; Weigent et al, 1983; Ortaldo et al, 1984; Itoh et al, 1985). However, other investigators have suggested that INF-γ is not the mediator of the IL-2 effect. LAK cells are important in tumor-cell killing and respond to IL-2 not only with proliferation and increased cytotoxicity to malignant cells, but also with some enhancement of the ability to lyse other modified cells (eg, lectin-activated lymphoblasts). Thus, LAK cells differ from cytotoxic T-lymphocytes and NK cells by the broader range of cells they are capable of lysing. Most LAK cells generated from blood or spleen are IL-2-activated NK cells rather than a distinct or unique cell type.

In 1985, an adoptive immunotherapy method was described for the production of human LAK cells from peripheral blood lymphocytes incubated with IL-2 (Rosenberg, 1985). Therapeutic regimens employing this technique had clinical activity in patients with metastatic melanoma and renal cell carcinoma. For further information, see the evaluation on Aldesleukin and index entry Interleukin-2, In Cancer.

Hematopoietic Growth Factors: Use of these factors augments the immune response. These substances, sometimes referred to as hematologic growth hormones, are glycoproteins that stimulate the proliferation and differentiation of hematopoietic progenitor cells in the bone marrow. Some of these cytokines have been cloned and purified to homogeneity, including erythropoietin, interleukin-3 (IL-3), granulocyte-macrophage colony stimulating factor (GM-CSF, sargramostim [Leukine, Prokine], molgramostim [Leucomax]), granulocyte colony stimulating factor (G-CSF, filgrastim [Neupogen]), and macrophage colony stimulating factor (M-CSF).

Erythropoietin is principally produced in the kidneys of adults and in the liver of the fetus; it is necessary for normal production of erythrocytes and is specific for their generation only. Erythropoietin is not known to be an immunomodulating agent; however, because it is a hematologic growth hormone, it is discussed here briefly. The usefulness of recombinant human erythropoietin (epoetin alfa [Epogen]) has been clearly demonstrated in the treatment of the anemia associated with chronic renal failure and zidovudine [Retrovir] therapy in HIV-infected patients. In investigational studies, epoetin had activity in the treatment of anemia associated with multiple myeloma and other advanced cancers (Ludwig et al, 1990; Abels et al, 1991). In addition, this agent was reported to significantly increase the ability of patients to donate autologous blood prior to elective surgery (Goodnough et al, 1989). See also index entries Erythropoietin, Epoetin Alfa.

The other four hematologic growth hormones are lymphokines that stimulate leukocyte production and activity. These are often referred to as colony stimulating factors (CSF) because of their ability to stimulate colony formation when bone marrow cells are cultured in vitro. *IL-3* is produced by T-lymphocytes and is a multicolony stimulating factor. It is thought to act at an early stage of stem cell differentiation and acts on all cells stimulated by G-CSF and GM-CSF, as well as on precursors of T-lymphocytes and mast cells. It can support the growth of multi-lineage colonies (erythrocytes, granulocytes, monocytes, megakaryocytes at various stages of differentiation) that are derived from a single stem cell. IL-3 is being investigated in the treatment of AIDS and for promotion of recovery from and prevention of infections in patients with burns or after cancer chemotherapy or bone marrow transplantation.

GM-CSF is also a multi-CSF, but it exerts its major effect later in the maturation sequence by supporting the growth and differentiation of cells committed to becoming granulocytes and monocytes. It also stimulates the activity of erythroid and megakaryocyte progenitors. GM-CSF stimulates the functional activities of polymorphonuclear leukocytes and macrophages, including their phagocytic and antitumor cytotoxic activities. For further discussion, see index entries GM-CSF and Sargramostim.

G-CSF promotes the growth of a smaller number of leukocytes than GM-CSF. It appears to stimulate the growth of granulocytes specifically and also may induce differentiation and maturation of the immature leukocytes that are characteristic of leukemia. Thus, it is of interest for the treatment of leukemia patients. For further information, see index entries G-CSF and Filgrastim.

M-CSF causes macrophages to proliferate and may induce them to produce GM-CSF. Because M-CSF boosts the production of macrophages, there is interest in it, for these cells not only attack bacteria- and virus-infected cells but also cancer cells. (For further discussion, see index entry M-CSF.)

A number of other natural and synthetic immunomodulators are being investigated for their ability to enhance the immune response in various immunodeficiency disorders, including AIDS and malignancies. These are discussed in the section on Investigational Agents.

IMMUNOLOGIC REPLACEMENT. There is currently no synthetic drug to treat immunodeficiency diseases, but various forms of immunotherapy are available and some may even have a curative effect on the underlying disease. Marrow transplant has been beneficial in marrow failure and other immunodeficiencies. Thymic hormones have been administered in an attempt to stimulate the immune system in very young and very old patients. The usefulness of bone marrow or thymus transplantation is limited by the availability of appropriate donors. Nevertheless, they do offer a therapeutic avenue of approach.

When there is a deficiency in the immune system, replacement with immune globulin (gamma globulin) sometimes has been helpful. Immune globulin is derived from human plasma and contains most of the antibodies found in whole blood. The preparation consists primarily of IgG with lesser amounts of IgM. Since IgA, found mostly in mucosal surfaces, is not present in significant amounts in these preparations, immune globulin cannot be used for IgA deficiency. It is administered most commonly for replacement therapy in agammaglobulinemia and for the prevention of measles and hepatitis A. Recommended uses of immune globulin for the treatment of immunodeficiency conditions appear in Table 3. Specific immune globulin is preferred for prophylaxis after exposure to known infectious agents (see index entry Immune Globulin).

PLASMAPHERESIS. Plasmapheresis has been used to manage immunopathologic diseases, such as myasthenia gravis; some types of hepatitis; and rheumatic, autoimmune, and immune complex disorders. The efficacy of this technique has been demonstrated in a limited number of conditions, including myasthenia gravis, Goodpasture's syndrome, and thrombotic thrombocytopenic purpura; its usefulness in systemic lupus erythematosus is controversial.

In plasmapheresis, dialysis equipment can remove 6 to 8 L of plasma in two to four hours and exchange this with reconstituted plasma, albumin, or purified plasma protein fraction. Theoretically, plasmapheresis will remove specific autoantibodies; nonspecific inflammatory mediators, such as complement or fibrinogen; and immune complexes. However, the technique is costly, there are no prospective controlled studies, and the side effects are not completely known. Thus, plasmapheresis is principally considered an investigational technique, although it is of demonstrated value for hyperviscosity syndrome associated with Waldenström's macroglobulinemia or myeloma. (See also index entry Plasmapheresis.)

TABLE 3. TREATMENT OF IMMUNODEFICIENCY WITH IMMUNE GLOBULIN (GAMMA GLOBULIN)

B-CELL DISORDERS (intramuscular or intravenous preparations may be used)

- Acquired hypogammaglobulinemia
- Secondary hypogammaglobulinemia when associated with infection
- X-linked hypogammaglobulinemia
- DO NOT use in selective IgA deficiency.

T-CELL DISORDERS (intramuscular or intravenous preparations may be used)

- Use only when an antibody response has been demonstrated to be absent (intravenous preparation may be given).
- Wiskott-Aldrich syndrome (intramuscular preparation is not recommended)

PHAGOCYTIC DISORDERS

- Not recommended

COMPLEMENT DISORDERS

- Not recommended

OTHER

- Children with AIDS

Adapted from Ammann, 1984.

ADVERSE REACTIONS AND PRECAUTIONS

Reactions peculiar to each drug are discussed in the evaluations, but certain general statements can be made. Suppression of bone marrow by cytotoxic agents inhibits the function of phagocytes, neutrophils, and, to a lesser degree, lymphocytes and monocytes. Suppression of these final effector cells increases the risk of overwhelming infection. The more subtle forms of a drug's ability to inhibit immunoinflammatory responses emerge clinically as infection with unusual pathogens, such as *Pneumocystis carinii, Listeria monocytogenes,* cytomegalovirus, or *Toxoplasma gondii.* Resistance to the more common but serious gram-negative bacteremia or *Streptococcus pneumoniae* infection also is reduced.

Although the risk of infection in a compromised host is well appreciated, the risk of neoplasia in patients undergoing immunomodulator therapy is less clear but of great importance. The incidence of neoplasia, particularly skin cancer and lymphoma, is higher in transplant patients. This may represent a complex situation involving multiple immunosuppressive agents, fundamental drug-induced alterations in normal cytokine patterns, and the stimulatory presence of a foreign graft. For example, evidence suggests that infections with certain viruses, such as Epstein-Barr virus, may cause lymphoproliferative disorders, and this process may be enhanced by immunosuppression and altered levels of cytokines such as IL-4, IL-6, and IL-10. Data exist concerning the emergence of tumors in patients treated with low-dose, immunosuppressive, cytotoxic therapy. Reports of lymphoproliferative disease, including lymphomas, predominate, but solid tumors in young patients also have been described. The confounding variable is that often the diseases being treated cause abnormal immune responses and, on that basis alone, are associated with a high risk of neoplasia.

Alkylating agents produce oligospermia and sometimes permanent azoospermia. To assure future fertility, males should be informed that cryogenic storage of spermatozoa prior to the initiation of therapy is available.

Use of naturally occurring immunomodulators (interleukins, interferons, colony stimulating factors) is not without adverse effects. Serious reactions, including death, have been associated with interleukin-2 therapy. However, compared with the cytotoxic drugs, adverse reactions produced by these natural substances are usually mild and readily reversible. The dose-limiting adverse effects of alpha interferons are influenza-like symptoms; although bone marrow suppression can occur, it is usually mild in most patients. Interferon toxicity is rapidly reversible (usually within two to three days) upon drug withdrawal; in comparison, three to four weeks are required for recovery from the marrow suppression produced by many cytotoxic drugs. In addition, the latter have the potential for cumulative toxicity, which has not been observed with the interferons. In clinical trials conducted thus far, the colony stimulating factors, like the interferons, have produced only mild adverse effects.

The use of any immunomodulator entails both theoretical and actual risks to the patient. The risk/benefit ratio should be determined, and informed consent should be obtained.

Drug Evaluations

ANTI-INFLAMMATORY AGENTS

Glucocorticoids

The anti-inflammatory and immunomodulating effects of glucocorticoids become apparent only when pharmacologic doses are administered. Patients receiving systemic corticosteroids for nonendocrine disorders are at risk of developing adverse effects, such as cushingoid features, increased susceptibility to infection, and suppression of the hypothalamic-pituitary-adrenal (HPA) axis. Therefore, the expected benefits must be weighed against the possible adverse effects before initiating therapy. Guidelines for the judicious use of corticosteroids include the following:

(1) The presence of a steroid-responsive condition must be ascertained initially.

(2) Corticosteroid therapy should be initiated only after less toxic therapy has been ineffective.

(3) Dosage should be based on the severity of the disease; the smallest amount that controls a specific symptom or sign should be used. The purpose of therapy is to achieve an acceptable degree of palliation; complete remission is usually not an appropriate therapeutic goal.

(4) Dosage, frequency of administration, duration of therapy, and corticosteroid preparations influence the therapeutic response and the frequency of adverse reactions. Systemic administration of a single large dose (ie, 1 to 2 mg/kg of prednisone or equivalent) is virtually without ill effects and may decrease morbidity; this justifies the use of such therapy in life-threatening emergencies when the diagnosis is only tentative. Generally, the severity of adverse reactions increases with the duration of therapy and size of the dose and is directly related to the degree of immunosuppressive anti-inflammatory effect.

(5) When possible, the corticosteroid should be administered locally to concentrate therapeutic effects on the diseased tissue and minimize adverse effects.

(6) To avoid adrenal crisis before HPA axis responsiveness returns after prolonged therapy, pharmacologic doses of corticosteroids must be reduced gradually over weeks to months except in unusual circumstances. In some cases, adrenal responsiveness to corticotropin (ACTH) should be tested (see index entry Cosyntropin).

(7) When possible, once the underlying disease is in remission, alternate-day therapy should be used to minimize adverse effects.

ACTIONS. At the molecular level, glucocorticoids act by passively entering a target cell and rapidly binding to intracellular cytoplasmic steroid receptors. After the steroid-receptor complexes undergo conformational changes termed "activation," they cross the nuclear membrane and bind to DNA directly at sites known as glucocorticoid response elements (GRE). GRE-binding controls transcription of specific genes by either promoting or inhibiting the production of specific mRNAs. Consequently, there are changes in the rates of synthesis of protein translated from these hormone-regulated mRNAs, which, in turn, mediate the response to glucocorticoids.

Glucocorticoids act at multiple sites. They do not block the interaction of antibodies with sensitized lymphocytes or the release of histamine or kinins that is initiated by this process. Rather, they block the multiple tissue responses to these stimuli. Glucocorticoids prevent the initiation of the cascade of reactions leading to the production of certain prostaglandins and leukotrienes by inducing the production and release of a protein (macrocortin, lipomodulin) that inhibits phospholipase A_2, an enzyme that releases free arachidonic acid from membrane phospholipids. At high tissue concentrations, they may stabilize lysosomal enzymes, thus preventing the spillage of hydrolytic enzymes. Glucocorticoids increase the number of beta-agonist receptors on cell membranes. They help to maintain capillary integrity and interfere with the movement of immune complexes across basement membranes. Glucocorticoids maintain vascular tone, possibly by potentiating the action of vasoconstrictors.

Glucocorticoids have broad effects on both immune and inflammatory processes. Human lymphocytes are relatively resistant to lysis by corticosteroids, and effects are not based on the cytotoxicity of these agents. Upon immune activation, however, human lymphocytes become more sensitive and lysis of antigen-activated lymphocytes may occur when glucocorticoids are used for treatment of graft rejection. There is evidence that proliferating lymphocytes are sensitive to steroids but become resistant after reaching the effector stage. Except at extremely high doses, the cytotoxic process is not inhibited by corticosteroids unless they are added during the early sensitization phase of cytotoxic cells.

Normal human lymphocytes, monocytes, neutrophils, and eosinophils contain specific glucocorticoid receptors. Although heterogeneity of receptors has been reported for different lymphocyte populations, a functional significance for this variability has not been established except in preliminary studies; the results of these studies suggest that production of lymphokines, such as interleukin-2 (IL-2) and macrophage mitogenic factor, may be receptor-mediated.

Glucocorticoids may alter lymphocyte traffic and induce peripheral blood lymphopenia. Lymphocytopenia is more pronounced for T-cells; it does not appear to result from selective depression of T-subsets (Schuyler et al, 1984) but rather from redirection of normal lymphocyte traffic. B-cells are less affected. B-cells have been reported to metabolize cortisol more rapidly than T-cells, which suggests a mechanism for their relative resistance (Klein et al, 1980). Lymphocytes tend to sequester within lymph nodes and bone marrow, but total body lymphocyte mass is probably not decreased.

Although other circulating leukocytes decrease in number or remain relatively unchanged, the number and proportion of neutrophils increase temporarily. This increase has been attributed to release of mature neutrophils from the bone marrow coupled with decreased egress from the blood. The latter may account for failure of neutrophils and leukocytes to accumulate at inflamed sites.

Production of IL-1 by monocytes and IL-2 by lymphocytes is suppressed by glucocorticoids. There is also evidence that corticosteroids render IL-2-producing T-cells unresponsive to IL-1. Because IL-1 also is responsible for the production of fever, glucocorticoid-mediated inhibition of IL-1 explains the potent antipyretic activity of glucocorticoids. The production or actions of other lymphokines, such as tumor necrosis factor (α), granulocyte-macrophage colony stimulating factor, and platelet activating factor, are inhibited by glucocorticoids.

The bactericidal activity of monocytes is reduced substantially in patients receiving glucocorticoids; delayed-type hypersensitivity responses measured by skin tests also are reduced. T-lymphocyte responses to mitogens and antigens are suppressed by these agents. Suppressor cells that spontaneously appear in vivo also are inhibited by glucocorticoids, although studies have indicated that suppressor cells are resistant in vitro. Serum levels of IgG, IgA, and, to a lesser degree, IgM are suppressed by glucocorticoids; maximal suppression occurs two to four weeks after administration. Serum IgE levels appear to be minimally affected, but late-phase components of immediate hypersensitivity are altered. Thus, some B-cell responses are affected but it is not known whether the effect is direct or mediated through some other component of the immune system.

Glucocorticoids do not inhibit the release of histamine or protect against histamine shock.

USES. A wide variety of immunologically mediated diseases have been treated with corticosteroids: connective tissue diseases (eg, systemic lupus erythematosus, rheumatoid arthritis), asthma, vasculitides, granulomatous diseases, autoimmune hemolytic anemia, inflammatory bowel disease, and organ transplant rejection. Chronic disease may require the prolonged use of suppressive doses, and careful consideration must be given to the selection of a therapeutic regimen. Choice will depend on the severity of the disorder, the anticipated dose and duration of therapy, presence of factors predisposing to complications, and alternative modes of therapy to reduce glucocorticoid requirements. In most patients, a shorter acting drug, eg, prednisone, is preferred since it can be used in a manner that closely resembles the diurnal cortisol cycle.

Allergic Disorders: Systemically administered glucocorticoids promptly relieve symptoms in many allergic states, including bronchial asthma; nonseasonal allergic rhinitis; seasonal allergic rhinitis (hay fever, pollinosis); reactions to drugs, serum, and transfusions; and allergic dermatoses. In the past, they have been reserved for control of acute, severe episodes and not as a substitute for other medication (eg, beta-adrenergic agonists for asthma, antihistamines for hay fever) or avoidance of allergens. However, the use of inhalant steroids is increasingly being advocated as first-line therapy for mild to moderate asthma. For anaphylactic reactions, steroids should be employed as adjuncts to epinephrine and cardiorespiratory support. Topical preparations have been used for maintenance therapy when a glucocorticoid effect is desired without the risks associated with systemic administration. (See also index entries Bronchial Disorders; Shock; Dermatologic Disorders, Treatment.)

Cerebral Edema: Glucocorticoids are most effective when edema is of the vasogenic type, such as that caused by brain tumors, especially metastases and glioblastomas; they are somewhat less effective in edema caused by astrocytomas and meningiomas. Edema resulting from brain abscesses responds to glucocorticoid therapy; that produced by closed head injury is least responsive. There is doubt about the benefit of glucocorticoids in ischemic brain edema; these agents appear to have a deleterious effect in patients with malaria (Warrell et al, 1982).

The role of glucocorticoids in the treatment of severe head injury remains controversial. In animal studies, functional recovery improved in dogs and cats receiving massive doses (ie, methylprednisolone 15 to 30 mg/kg, dexamethasone 3 to 6 mg/kg) within one hour of induced spinal cord injury (Braughler and Hall, 1985); smaller doses or delayed therapy was ineffective. However, in clinical studies, glucocorticoids lack beneficial activity and are detrimental in some instances. For example, in one study, patients receiving "large" doses of methylprednisolone (a bolus of 1 g intravenously, repeated daily for ten days) fared worse than patients receiving "standard" doses (a bolus of 100 mg intravenously, repeated daily for ten days) (Bracken et al, 1984). Further studies are needed to determine the role of glucocorticoids in head trauma.

These steroids have been used for brain edema associated with stroke, but opinion is divided on their efficacy. They also are sometimes used with mannitol to treat brain edema associated with Reye's syndrome.

Bacterial Meningitis: An estimated 15,000 infants and children develop bacterial meningitis each year, and, despite advances in antimicrobial therapy, up to 10% of the cases are fatal. As many as 30% of the survivors have long-term sequelae, most commonly hearing loss, which occurs in 5% to 20% of patients. Cytokines, such as tumor necrosis factor (α) and interleukin-1 (β), appear to have a seminal role in the initial events that lead to meningeal inflammation. This results in increased cerebral pressure, reduction in cerebral blood flow, and cerebral ischemia. Microbial products, in part released by lysis of microbial cells in response to antibiotics, play a critical role in triggering these cytokine cascades. In studies in animals, endotoxin provoked much of the inflammatory response leading to increases in tumor necrosis factor, lactate, and interleukin-1 in the cerebrospinal fluid (CSF).

Many of the components of the inflammatory response are down-regulated by adrenal corticosteroids given in pharmacologic doses, and their administration decreases the hydrostatic pressure of the CSF. Anti-inflammatory mechanisms of steroids in meningitis include reduction in brain edema and decreased lactate, tumor necrosis factor α, interleukin-1, and prostaglandin E_2 concentrations in the CSF. Although early studies did not substantiate a clear benefit, results of more recent studies in pediatric patients have confirmed the beneficial effects of corticosteroids when used as adjuncts to antimicrobial therapy in the treatment of acute, nontuberculous bacterial meningitis (American Academy of Pediatrics, Committee on Infectious Diseases, 1990; Odio et al, 1991). For treatment guidelines, see index entry Meningitis, Treatment.

Collagen Disorders: Generally, steroids are most beneficial when large doses (1 to 2 mg/kg of prednisone or the equivalent) are given during acute exacerbations; the effectiveness of long-term maintenance therapy varies. Some manifestations of *systemic lupus erythematosus* may be controlled by glucocorticoids. Topical preparations are used if dermatologic symptoms predominate, and systemic therapy is appropriate when nephritis, central nervous system disturbances, and hematologic complications, such as hemolytic anemia or thrombocytopenia, are present. Symptoms and serologic values (eg, serum complement, anti-DNA antibodies) may aid in determining the minimum dosage that improves survival rates (Urman and Rothfield, 1977).

Short-term use of large doses (1 to 2 mg/kg of prednisone or the equivalent) may be required for remission, particularly when the central nervous system is involved. High-dose pulse therapy (methylprednisolone 500 mg to 1 g intravenously [alternative, 1 g/day for three days]) also has been used to treat severe acute lupus nephritis or central nervous system syndromes. Clinical studies are in progress to determine if long-term intermittent pulse therapy is beneficial. Fewer exacerbations were reported to occur if the daily dose is reduced 10% per week after the patient's condition stabilizes (Yount et al, 1975). If serum complement levels rise during therapy and then decrease as the dose is reduced, the amount should be increased and the rate of reduction slowed.

The combination of an immunosuppressive agent, such as azathioprine or cyclophosphamide, with a glucocorticoid appears to be more beneficial than either type of agent alone in slowing the progression of renal failure in some patients with lupus nephritis (Carette et al, 1983). Azathioprine or cyclophosphamide also can be added to allow reduction in the steroid dose in some patients who are resistant to withdrawal of glucocorticoids.

Polymyositis and *dermatomyositis* are idiopathic inflammatory myopathies thought to result from an autoimmune response triggered by an environmental factor in a genetically susceptible host. The primary indication for treatment is muscle weakness severe enough to cause disability. Corticosteroids are the initial agents used to treat these myopathies, and they produce at least partial improvement in approximately 75% to 90% of patients. Other immunosuppressive agents have been used in severe acute disease and when patients do not respond adequately or cannot tolerate corticosteroid therapy. For treatment guidelines, see index entries on these disorders.

Polyarteritis nodosa (systemic necrotizing vasculitis) is usually not treated with steroids alone. Patients who have multiple organ involvement are treated with a combination of a steroid and a cytotoxic drug, such as cyclophosphamide. (Fauci et al, 1978, 1979; Leib et al, 1979). Patients with limited disease (eg, local skin manifestations without organ involvement) may respond to steroid therapy alone. Steroid therapy is initiated with prednisone 40 to 60 mg daily; the dose is then reduced to the lowest effective amount for maintenance. Hypertension must be controlled but is not a contraindication to steroid therapy. Residual hypertension is common.

Polymyalgia rheumatica usually occurs in individuals over 60 years and is improved by glucocorticoid therapy to suppress symptoms and maintain the erythrocyte sedimentation rate below 30 mm/hour (Behn et al, 1983). In one regimen, small doses (eg, prednisone 10 to 20 mg daily) are used initially with the amount reduced by 1 mg/month in patients taking 10 mg daily or less. The incidence of *temporal arteritis* (giant cell arteritis) is high in patients with polymyalgia rheumatica, and they generally require larger doses to control the disease (initial dose, prednisone 60 mg daily). Because of the high risk of temporal arteritis, some practitioners favor treating all patients who have polymyalgia rheumatica with high-dose steroid therapy.

Patients with less severe forms of *mixed connective tissue disease* (MCTD) may respond well to glucocorticoids; most symptoms can be controlled with alternate-day therapy and steroids often can be discontinued eventually. Those with more severe manifestations may require the addition of cytotoxic drugs. Differential diagnosis of MCTD and systemic scleroderma is essential, however, because glucocorticoids do not improve the vascular lesions or fibrosis produced by the latter.

Hematologic Disorders: Idiopathic and acquired *autoimmune hemolytic anemia* may respond to glucocorticoids, which are sometimes the sole therapeutic agents employed. Glucocorticoids do not reduce hemolysis in transfusion reactions, although they may lessen drug-induced hemolysis. In *erythroblastopenia* (pure erythrocyte aplasia, congenital hypoplastic anemia, Blackfan-Diamond syndrome), small maintenance doses given on alternate days may eliminate dependence on transfusion and may be the treatment of choice.

Rarely, glucocorticoids produce remissions of variable length in *aplastic anemia*. They may be useful when a suitable donor for bone marrow transplantation is not available and in patients with less severe disease. Following immunosuppression and pending the availability of a suitable donor, androgens and anabolic steroids also may be utilized.

Although their effectiveness has not been proved in controlled trials, glucocorticoids are recommended as initial therapy for *idiopathic thrombocytopenic purpura* (ITP). ITP is considered an autoimmune disease, and antibodies (most commonly IgG) adhere to platelets in up to 90% of patients. Glucocorticoids are thought to act by inhibiting the phagocytosis of antibody-associated platelets, thus increasing platelet life span. Doses of 1 to 1.5 mg/kg of prednisone or the equivalent produce remission in 40% to 60% of patients (Rote and Lau, 1985; Burns and Saleem, 1983). Danazol [Danocrine] has been reported to induce remissions in patients with ITP and to reduce the need for glucocorticoids (Ahn et al, 1983; Weinblatt et al, 1988; Nalli et al, 1988; Mueller-Eckhardt, 1988). It is unclear whether glucocorticoids reduce the risk of life-threatening intracranial hemorrhage. Long-term steroid therapy has no role in the treatment of ITP.

The treatment of ITP during pregnancy usually is conservative. Many pregnant women with moderate disease do not require treatment, but those with severe ITP do. Most clinicians prescribe the lowest dose of glucocorticoid that increases the platelet count and returns the bleeding time to normal (Kelton, 1983). Infants of mothers with ITP are at risk for thrombocytopenia. Use of steroids during pregnancy may protect the fetus, but generalizations cannot be made concerning their effectiveness in controlling the fetal platelet count. If the neonatal platelet count falls below 50,000 to 75,000 platelets/mm^3, prednisone 1 to 2 mg/kg/day, exchange transfusions, and immune globulin should be considered (Rote and Lau, 1985). Intravenous immune globulin has been established as a treatment for ITP in adults and children. This drug is classified in FDA Pregnancy Category C. (See index entry Immune Globulin.)

Hepatic Diseases: The effectiveness and safety of glucocorticoids in the treatment of liver disease depend on the form involved and the condition of the patient. These agents are used in the initial therapy of *subacute hepatic necrosis* (prednisolone 60 to 100 mg/day) and autoimmune *chronic active hepatitis* (prednisone 20 to 60 mg/day). Traditionally, medication is withdrawn gradually when there are signs of maximal improvement; if relapse occurs, more prolonged therapy is required. However, recent data indicate that not all patients with chronic active hepatitis who initially responded to steroids will respond to these drugs again if relapse occurs. Therefore, some experts suggest life-long maintenance steroid therapy (ie, prednisone 5 to 15 mg/day) for selected patients with chronic active hepatitis. Concomitant administration of azathioprine sometimes allows reduction of the glucocorticoid dose. See index entry Hepatitis, Chronic.

Patients with hepatitis B surface antigens who have chronic active hepatitis should *not* receive glucocorticoid therapy, because remission is delayed, complications occur more frequently, and the mortality rate is higher.

In *alcoholic hepatitis*, survival rates are enhanced when glucocorticoids are given to seriously ill patients with encephalopathy who do not have active gastrointestinal bleeding. These agents may be used in *sarcoidosis* when acute inflammatory changes coexist with functional abnormalities as demonstrated by liver biopsy. Glucocorticoids also may be effective in other types of hepatic granulomata except those due to infections or neoplasms.

Glucocorticoids may be beneficial in drug-induced hepatic disorders, but controlled studies are lacking. Whether these agents are effective in biliary cirrhosis or infectious mononucleosis has not been demonstrated adequately. They are *not* indicated for the treatment of acute viral hepatitis or inactive postnecrotic cirrhosis. It has been noted that the effect of corticosteroids is enhanced in patients with cirrhosis.

Renal Disease: In patients less than 16 years, the most common subtype of idiopathic *nephrotic syndrome* is minimal change nephrosis, which generally responds to glucocorticoids. The initial dosage is prednisone 1 to 1.5 mg/kg/day or the equivalent. Both daily and alternate-day administration have been utilized; 80% to 90% of children respond within four to eight weeks, although a three-month course is usual. Two-thirds of those who respond never experience relapse or do so no more than once yearly; courses of glucocorticoids may be repeated in the latter. The remaining responsive patients relapse two to four times yearly and may require more prolonged therapy, preferably on an alternate-day schedule. The addition of an alkylating agent (cyclophosphamide or chlorambucil) to the regimen may maintain remission in children with frequent relapses; these drugs also may be used in steroid-resistant patients. Alkylating agents should be administered only when necessary because of their side effects (Martinez-Maldonado and Garcia, 1981).

Adults with nephrotic syndrome may respond to daily or alternate-day prednisone therapy, depending on the subtype present; in decreasing order of responsiveness these are: minimal change nephrosis, membranous nephropathy, diffuse proliferative nephritis, and focal sclerosis (Bolton et al, 1977).

The following regimens, alternated monthly for six months, were reported to relieve proteinuria and preserve renal function in adults with idiopathic membranous nephropathy: intravenous methylprednisolone 1 g daily for 3 days, followed by either oral methylprednisolone 0.4 mg/kg/day or prednisone 0.5 mg/kg/day for 27 days, then oral chlorambucil 0.2 mg/kg/day for 30 days (Ponticelli et al, 1984).

Respiratory Disorders: Glucocorticoids have palliative effects in *pulmonary sarcoidosis* but apparently have little influence on the development of pulmonary fibrosis or the eventual outcome of the disease. They generally are reserved for patients in whom functioning of a vital extrapulmonary organ is impaired and those with stage 2 or 3 pulmonary sarcoidosis. Patients with a differential count of pretreatment bronchoalveolar lavage (BAL) specimens containing greater than 35% lymphocytes are more likely to respond favorably than patients with BAL lymphocytes less than 35% (Hollinger et al, 1985). Therapy is initiated with prednisone 30 to 40 mg (or 40 to 60 mg on alternate days) for six to eight weeks; the dose then is reduced to the lowest effective amount.

Respiratory distress syndrome (RDS) is a significant cause of death in premature neonates. Antenatal administration of glucocorticoids reduces the incidence, severity, and mortality rate. Glucocorticoids have been of significant benefit in infants of 26 to 34 weeks' gestation when delivery occurred at least 24 hours after initiating treatment. In pregnancies of this length, the mother may be treated if the lecithin/sphingomyelin ratio is less than 2 or if amniotic fluid analysis is unavailable. No definite effect has been noted during pregnancies with longer gestation periods. In children monitored for four years after prophylactic steroid treatment for RDS, no significant alterations in growth or development were observed. The possibility that a long latent period or a rare adverse effect may be identified eventually cannot be ignored, however, and monitoring of these children must continue before this form of therapy can be accepted unequivocally. The availability of surfactant preparations has markedly improved the management of RDS. In both prophylactic and treatment ("rescue") trials, the severity of RDS has been significantly diminished and the number of deaths decreased (see index entry Respiratory Distress Syndrome). Antenatal administration of corticosteroids to the mother may have synergistic beneficial effects in infants receiving surfactant.

In pregnancies complicated by severe pre-eclampsia, the number of fetal deaths increased after glucocorticoid therapy, and neonatal hypoglycemia was observed. Apgar scores and onset of lactation were unaffected. Although the neonatal cortisol level was suppressed for several days, adrenal insufficiency was not reported. In some studies, the incidence of maternal infection increased, particularly when there was premature rupture of membranes. Prophylactic administration of glucocorticoids for RDS is not indicated in women with severe pre-eclampsia or when immediate delivery is required for maternal or neonatal survival (ie, maternal infection, fetal distress, abruptio placentae, placenta previa).

Recent studies suggest that the administration of corticosteroids as adjunctive therapy for *Pneumocystis carinii* pneumonia (PCP) in AIDS patients is beneficial. For treatment guidelines, see index entry Pneumocystis Pneumonia.

Caution should be exercised before prescribing these drugs for certain populations of HIV-infected patients. It is not clear that they are beneficial for those in whom conventional treatments for PCP have failed and respiratory failure has developed. No benefit associated with steroid treatment was observed in a prospective trial in which 41 patients received intravenous methylprednisolone 60 mg or placebo every six hours when the PaO_2 declined to <51 mm Hg. In the majority of these patients, corticosteroids were given as salvage therapy more than 72 hours after specific therapy for PCP was initiated (Clement et al, 1989).

Considerable caution should be exercised when prescribing corticosteroids for HIV-infected patients who are at increased risk for tuberculosis. These patients may be anergic and/or infected with multidrug-resistant organisms (Centers for Disease Control, 1991 A, 1991 B), and the immunosuppressive effect of corticosteroids could be catastrophic. A definitive diagnosis of PCP should be attempted; if this is not possible, preventive therapy with isoniazid should be considered for persons at increased risk for tuberculosis (eg, evidence of past exposure to tuberculosis; certain ethnic groups; intravenous drug users).

Finally, corticosteroids may cause acute exacerbations of pulmonary and cutaneous Kaposi's sarcoma (Sattler, 1991). A significant proportion of AIDS patients with pulmonary Kaposi's sarcoma have interstitial infiltrates similar to PCP, and the diagnosis of the former must be established by bronchoscopy. Therefore, corticosteroids should be prescribed cautiously in patients with cutaneous Kaposi's sarcoma, and withholding their use in patients with typical radiographic features or evidence of pulmonary Kaposi's sarcoma should be considered.

DRUG SELECTION. Localized therapy is generally preferred because it minimizes adverse effects. It should be noted, however, that local or topical administration of highly potent agents (eg, clobetasol propionate, betamethasone dipropionate) can have systemic effects (see the section on Adverse Reactions). When systemic administration is required, the oral route is preferred for ease in regulation of dose and the variety of regimens.

Prednisone is the usual preparation of choice for oral administration, because it has the longest history of use and is reliable, readily available, and inexpensive. Prednisone is metabolized to the active metabolite, prednisolone, by the liver. This conversion was thought to be impeded in patients with acute liver disease, and it was suggested that prednisolone may be preferred in this situation. However, further studies show that the conversion of prednisone to prednisolone is not impaired significantly in these patients (Uribe et al, 1982). Thus, there appears to be little real advantage in using one preparation over another in patients with liver disease or hypoalbuminemia from other causes (Pickup, 1979).

Prednisone has slight but significant mineralocorticoid activity. In patients with hypertension, congestive heart failure, or other conditions in which salt retention is a problem, a preparation with even less mineralocorticoid activity may be chosen (see Table 4). This is particularly important when unusually large doses must be prescribed.

Cortisone and hydrocortisone have the most potent mineralocorticoid activity among the available glucocorticoids. Systemic administration should be limited to short-term use because prolonged administration of pharmacologic doses may result in sodium and water retention, hypertension, and hypo-

TABLE 4. RELATIVE POTENCIES OF GLUCOCORTICOIDS

	Glucocorticoid Potency	Equivalent Dose (mg)	Mineralocorticoid Potency
SHORT-ACTING			
Hydrocortisone	1	20.0	2+
Cortisone	0.8	25.0	2+
INTERMEDIATE-ACTING			
Meprednisone	4-5	4.0	0
Methylprednisolone	5	4.0	0
Prednisolone	4	5.0	1+
Prednisone	4	5.0	1+
Triamcinolone	5	4.0	0
LONG-ACTING			
Betamethasone	20-30	0.60	0
Dexamethasone	20-30	0.75	0
Paramethasone	10	2.0	0

kalemia; sodium restriction and potassium supplementation may be necessary.

Dexamethasone has minimal mineralocorticoid activity and is commonly chosen to treat vasogenic cerebral edema. Mild diuresis with sodium loss may occur in patients who had been receiving other glucocorticoids.

Triamcinolone often produces a mild diuresis with sodium loss during the first days of treatment whether or not the patient is frankly edematous; conversely, edema may occur in patients with a decreased glomerular filtration rate. Certain adverse reactions are unique to triamcinolone; myopathy is encountered more frequently, and this agent tends to cause anorexia (with resultant weight loss) rather than stimulation of appetite, and sedation and depression rather than euphoria.

ALTERNATE-DAY THERAPY. Glucocorticoid therapy may be initiated with a single daily dose or multiple daily doses. After symptoms are controlled by daily therapy, most chronic diseases respond to alternate-day administration of intermediate-acting glucocorticoids (prednisone, prednisolone, methylprednisolone). The advantages are less suppression of the HPA axis, convenience that may enhance compliance, and a lower incidence of adverse effects. For example, when pharmacologic doses of glucocorticoids are given daily to children, the rate of growth is decreased; however, normal growth patterns are maintained with alternate-day therapy. Alternate-day therapy produces less inhibition of intestinal calcium absorption and results in less bone loss.

There are many methods of transferring patients from daily to alternate-day therapy. One approach is to reduce the daily dose to prednisone 40 to 50 mg (or the equivalent amount of an intermediate-acting agent) (Kehrl and Fauci, 1983). Then, the daily dose on the day designated as "on" is doubled to 80 to 100 mg. The dose on the "off" day is decreased gradually by 5 to 10 mg. Tapering is continued until the dose on the "off" day is 20 mg, at which point the dose is reduced by 2.5 mg until the patient receives no steroid on the "off" day. If remission is maintained, the dose on the "on" day is reduced to the least amount that controls symptoms. If a relapse occurs, the dose on the "on" day is increased sufficiently to reinduce remission.

The most common reasons for failure of transfer from daily to alternate-day therapy are too rapid conversion and inadequate dose on the "on" day. Although not all patients can be adequately controlled, the benefits of alternate-day therapy justify trial in most patients receiving prolonged glucocorticoid therapy.

With the alternate-day regimen, the steroid is administered every other morning between 7 and 8 AM. This simulates the natural circadian rhythm of glucocorticoid secretion (early morning peak, evening nadir) and produces less suppression of the HPA axis. Ideally, the level of *exogenous* hormone is high on the morning of treatment and that of *endogenous* hormone is normal on the morning that medication is withheld, for the HPA axis is not suppressed on that day.

Alternate-day therapy is reported to be particularly effective in asthma, systemic lupus erythematosus, uveitis, and nephrotic syndrome. Alternate-day therapy may not be adequate in severe conditions, such as renal transplantation or certain hematologic and malignant disorders. Some patients, especially those with rheumatoid arthritis and adults with ulcerative colitis, may become symptomatic or experience an exacerbation on the day that the glucocorticoid is withheld. If symptoms persist despite an increase in dose, a single morning dose is preferred to a more suppressive daily divided-dose schedule.

ADVERSE REACTIONS. Corticosteroids have many potential adverse effects that are often extensions of their pharmacologic actions. The incidence of adverse reactions correlates with the dose, frequency and route of administration, duration of therapy, age and condition of the patient, and underlying disease. The risks versus benefits for each patient should be considered before treatment is initiated.

Gastrointestinal Reactions: Glucocorticoids decrease the protection provided by the gastric mucus barrier, interfere with tissue repair, and, in some patients, increase gastric acid and pepsinogen production. There has been some question on whether steroids per se are responsible for the peptic ulcers encountered during therapy. It has been suggested that corticosteroids cause peptic ulcer only in patients receiving NSAIDs concomitantly (Guslandi and Tittobello, 1992). However, glucocorticoid therapy may mask the symptoms of peptic ulcer so that perforation or hemorrhage occurs without antecedent pain; therefore, periodic examination of the stools for occult blood is suggested.

Clinical data have shown that corticosteroids caused peptic ulcers in only 1 in 100 patients (0.8/100 controls had ulcers, 1.8/100 treated patients had ulcers—an increase of 1 patient per 100). Therefore, antiulcer drugs should not be prescribed routinely for patients receiving corticosteroids. Instead, therapy to prevent ulcers should be used only when other medications that increase the risk of peptic ulcer disease (eg, nonsteroidal anti-inflammatory drugs) are taken concomitantly or if the patient has a confirmed history of ulcer. If an ulcer occurs, the corticosteroid should be discontinued slowly if possible, and antiulcer therapy should be prescribed (Spiro, 1983). For treatment of ulcers, see index entry Peptic Ulcer.

Steroids should be used cautiously in patients with nonspecific ulcerative colitis if there is a probability of impending perforation, abscess, or other pyogenic infection or in the presence of diverticulitis, fresh intestinal anastomoses, active or latent peptic ulcer, renal insufficiency, hypertension, osteoporosis, or myasthenia gravis.

Edema: Since glucocorticoids with little or no mineralocorticoid activity are now available, electrolyte imbalance is observed less frequently. Edema is best treated by restricting dietary sodium at the inception of therapy. If edema occurs, sodium intake should be reduced sharply; if it persists, the patient should receive a glucocorticoid with less mineralocorticoid activity. However, caution is required if average or large doses of any corticosteroid are given for prolonged periods to patients with cardiovascular or renal disease because even slight fluid retention may be dangerous.

Hypokalemia: Severe hypokalemia may cause asthenia, paralysis, or arrhythmias that may proceed to cardiac arrest. The incidence of hypokalemia is related to the mineralocorticoid activity of a specific glucocorticoid and can be avoided in most patients by restricting dietary sodium, consuming foods rich in potassium (eg, spinach, raisins, orange juice, cantaloupe, bananas), supplementing the diet with oral potassium, and using a steroid with minimal mineralocorticoid activity. Concurrent use of potassium-wasting diuretics (eg, thiazides) may exacerbate potassium loss. See also index entry Hypokalemia.

Hypophosphatemia: Rarely, the administration of steroids can result in extremely low levels of phosphate, which may cause severe muscle weakness, cardiac dysfunction, and hemolysis. Serum phosphate levels should be monitored in patients receiving long-term, high-dose therapy and in children and the elderly. Ingestion of milk or equivalent dairy products is suggested, but potassium or sodium phosphate preparations will be required in those more severely affected.

Osteoporosis: This common but inadequately recognized adverse effect is associated with long-term use of glucocorticoids. All corticosteroids increase calcium excretion and should be administered with caution to patients with osteoporosis. The morphologic findings are bone loss in areas with a high content of trabecular bone, such as the ribs and vertebrae, and enlargement of the marrow cavity. Fractures are most common in these bones. Glucocorticoids appear to decrease bone formation directly through suppression of osteoblastic formation. They also act indirectly by inhibiting calcium absorption from the gastrointestinal tract and reabsorption from the renal tubules; hypocalcemia results and increases the plasma parathyroid hormone concentration, which ultimately increases bone resorption (Baylink, 1983). Rising parathyroid hormone levels also may increase renal phosphate wasting and contribute to the development of hypophosphatemia.

The amount of bone loss is related to the dose and duration of steroid therapy. Doses as low as prednisone 5 mg daily (or equivalent) or 25 mg every other day result in demonstrable bone loss within one year in a significant number of patients.

Patients should be monitored with bone densitometry if available, and those at risk for osteoporosis should receive vitamin D 50,000 IU twice weekly or calcifediol 40 to 60 mcg daily and elemental calcium 1.5 g daily for prophylaxis. For treatment of this disorder, see index entry Osteoporosis.

Osteonecrosis: Corticosteroid-induced osteonecrosis most commonly affects the femoral head but also may involve the head of the humerus, femoral condyles, tibial plateau, talus, and capitulum. A number of mechanisms have been suggested, including fat embolism, hypercoagulability, increased intraosseous pressure, and swelling of fat cells, but none has been proven. The first symptoms (joint pain and stiffness) are often noted 12 to 24 months after first exposure. Techniques recommended for early diagnosis are bone marrow pressure recordings and intraosseous venography (Nixon, 1984).

Osteonecrosis of bone is most commonly associated with prolonged corticosteroid therapy but also has occurred following brief high-dose treatment (McCluskey and Gutteridge, 1982; Sambrook et al, 1984; Taylor, 1984). Data suggest that large doses contribute to osteonecrosis in predisposed patients (Zizic et al, 1985).

It has been suggested that the increased medullary fat deposition induced by steroids also may be influenced by diet. Because weight gain and development of cushingoid facial features can be reduced if patients follow a low-fat, high-protein diet and because of alterations in glucose metabolism, lipid levels, and nitrogen balance (see below), it is reasonable to recommend a low-fat diet for all patients receiving long-term steroid therapy.

Negative Nitrogen Balance: Negative nitrogen balance results from the excessive breakdown of protein by glucocorticoids; this may be modified somewhat by administration of anabolic agents and a high-protein diet. However, there is no evidence that anabolic agents protect tissues from atrophy and osteoporosis.

Carbohydrate and Lipid Metabolism: Glucocorticoids elevate plasma glucose concentrations 10% to 20% by increasing gluconeogenesis and decreasing cellular sensitivity to insulin. They aggravate diabetes, but ketosis generally is not a problem and diabetes can be controlled by modifying the diet or adjusting the dose of hypoglycemic agents. Glucocorticoids also can make latent diabetes chemically apparent. However, patients with normal pancreatic insulin production and response are not affected. Serum triglyceride concentrations frequently are elevated. These alterations in lipid metabolism are of concern in transplant patients receiving long-term steroid therapy because they are associated with an increased incidence of cardiovascular disease in these individuals.

Central Nervous System Effects: Large doses of glucocorticoids cause behavioral and personality changes, usually manifested by euphoria. Other signs include insomnia, increased appetite, nervousness, irritability, and hyperkinesia. Psychotic episodes, including manic-depressive and paranoid states and acute toxic psychoses, have been reported occasionally. Symptoms may occur within days to two weeks after initiating therapy or may develop in a subsequent course of therapy. They may disappear partly or completely on dosage reduction. Treatment of steroid-induced psychosis with haloperidol [Haldol] (1 to 10 mg two or three times daily) appears to be effective and is well tolerated.

Patients sometimes become psychologically dependent on corticosteroids. Glucocorticoid abuse also occurs when the drug is taken for an inappropriate indication. Pre-existing psychiatric illness does not appear to increase the risk of mental problems during steroid therapy; however, this history may influence the character of the emotional manifestation. In some instances, it may be impossible to determine whether psychiatric symptoms are caused by steroid therapy or the underlying condition (eg, systemic lupus erythematosus) (Ling et al, 1981).

Growth Suppression: Because growth is suppressed in children receiving long-term, daily, divided-dose glucocorticoid therapy, use of such regimens in children should be restricted to the most urgent indications. Alternate-day therapy with a short-acting agent usually avoids or minimizes growth suppression. When daily administration is required, a short-acting steroid taken as a single dose at 7 to 8 AM minimizes growth suppression and is preferred over multiple daily doses. Growth and development of infants and children receiving prolonged corticosteroid therapy should be monitored carefully.

Myopathy: Pharmacologic doses of corticosteroids cause protein catabolism and can lead to myopathy and loss of muscle mass. This disorder develops slowly, and the weakness primarily involves the proximal musculature of the upper and lower extremities. Myopathy responds to a reduction in dosage, and recovery occurs slowly over a period of months. This disorder is most often associated with use of 9α-fluorinated steroids, such as triamcinolone; it rarely occurs in patients receiving less than 30 mg daily of prednisone or the equivalent. It has been suggested that myopathy may be reversed by physical exercise.

Ocular Effects: Systemic administration and ocular application of glucocorticoids occasionally elevate intraocular pressure by decreasing outflow facility (open-angle glaucoma). The tendency to develop these symptoms is inherited in a recessive autosomal pattern and occurs most frequently in patients with primary open-angle glaucoma and their relatives, especially homozygous individuals. An exaggerated intraocular pressure response also is common among diabetics and myopes. Glucocorticoid therapy may be continued if topical ophthalmic preparations control the ocular hypertension.

Prolonged use of corticosteroids may enhance the development of secondary ocular infections due to fungi or viruses. These drugs should be used cautiously in patients with ocular herpes simplex infections because of possible corneal perforation. Exophthalmos has been reported with use of steroids.

Posterior subcapsular cataracts (PSCC) are common in patients receiving prolonged systemic or topical glucocorticoid therapy. There is disagreement on whether PSCC is associated with dose, duration of therapy, or the patient's age. Some experts think that patients receiving prednisone 10 mg daily (or the equivalent) or less or those treated for less than six months to one year are unlikely to develop PSCC. In contrast, others believe that the most important factor in PSCC may be individual susceptibility rather than extent of exposure. Children (especially those treated for rheumatoid arthritis) are affected more often than adults.

Miscellaneous Reactions: Secondary adrenocortical failure (pituitary unresponsiveness), particularly in times of stress (eg, trauma, surgery, illness), as well as the development of the cushingoid state, petechiae, and ecchymoses, have been reported. Other reactions include facial erythema; increased sweating; impaired wound healing; urticaria and other allergic, anaphylactic, or hypersensitivity reactions; acne; hirsutism; menstrual disorders; facial rounding; thin and shiny skin; supraclavicular fat pads; weight gain due to increased appetite; headache; pseudotumor cerebri; hypertension; impotence; flushing; vertigo; chronic pancreatitis; intestinal perforation; hepatomegaly; and acceleration of atherosclerosis.

PRECAUTIONS. Pharmacologic doses of glucocorticoids may suppress the signs and symptoms of disease that are required for diagnosis through their anti-inflammatory and anti-immunologic actions. The presence of systemic fungal infections and known hypersensitivity to components in the steroid formulation are contraindications to glucocorticoid therapy. Perforation of a peptic ulcer may occur with minimal discomfort. Septicemia may progress without fever.

The degradation of glucocorticoids is increased markedly in patients with hyperthyroidism. Pharmacologic doses have been given empirically to some patients with thyrotoxic crises (thyroid storm) because the compensatory increase in adrenal secretion may be inadequate in this condition. Steady-state glucocorticoid plasma concentrations may be increased in patients with hypothyroidism or hepatic damage.

Infection and Other Stress: Resistance to infection is decreased during prolonged treatment with pharmacologic doses of glucocorticoids because the same mechanisms that prevent the destruction of tissue by inflammation also may increase vulnerability to infectious agents and mask some signs of infection. The patient is predisposed to all types of infection (bacterial, viral, fungal, parasitic), and susceptibility is often increased by the underlying disease (eg, systemic lupus erythematosus, leukemia). Fewer infections may occur when the dosage interval is increased (as in alternate-day therapy) so that immunologic defenses remain intact.

Reactivation of latent tuberculosis in patients receiving glucocorticoids is well documented. If these drugs are indicated in such patients, close observation is necessary because the disease may be reactivated. These patients should receive chemoprophylactic therapy during prolonged corticosteroid therapy. Since skin sensitivity to tuberculin usually is lost during treatment with moderate to large daily doses of glucocorticoids (about 20 mg of prednisone or the equivalent daily), tuberculin skin testing is recommended for all patients before initiating long-term, daily, high-dose therapy. (Patients on alternate-day therapy may not be affected.) Those with positive skin tests may be candidates for appropriate chemotherapy. In addition, because of the immunosuppressive regimens to be employed, potential organ transplant recipients with a history of significant exposure to tuberculosis are candidates for chemoprophylaxis with antituberculosis drugs.

In active tuberculosis, use of glucocorticoids should be restricted to individuals with fulminating or disseminated disease in whom the steroid is given with an appropriate antituberculosis regimen. There are insufficient data to recommend isoniazid chemoprophylaxis for patients treated with low doses of glucocorticoids (less than 10 mg of prednisone daily) (see index entry Tuberculosis).

Large doses of steroids also diminish or inhibit the positive reaction to antigens that elicit a delayed hypersensitivity reaction (purified protein derivative [PPD], histoplasmin, mumps virus) and suppress the reaction to patch tests for cutaneous contact allergy (nickel, chrome, phenylenediamine).

Drug-induced secondary adrenocortical insufficiency may be minimized by a gradual reduction of the dosage. This type of relative insufficiency may persist for months after discontinuation of therapy; therefore, therapy should be reinstituted in any situation of stress occurring during that period. Since mineralocorticoid secretion may be impaired, salt and/or a mineralocorticoid should be administered concurrently.

Individuals with normal adrenal function secrete larger amounts of corticosteroids during the early phase of most conditions of stress, including infectious illnesses. Those dependent on exogenous steroids (whether for replacement or nonendocrine indications) require larger doses during stress since they are unable to secrete adequate additional amounts of endogenous hormone. When infection occurs in patients treated for a prolonged period with pharmacologic doses of glucocorticoids, a dilemma occurs: Administering the larger doses needed for the nonspecific, stress-related functions of glucocorticoids may further compromise resistance to infection. For mild illness, if the maintenance dose is low, the usual solution is to double the normal dose. In patients already receiving doses exceeding the amount produced endogenously under maximum stress (approximately 60 mg or more of prednisone or the equivalent daily), probably no additional steroid is necessary for mild illness. All patients should be treated concomitantly with an appropriate antimicrobial agent.

Normal adults may secrete 250 to 300 mg of cortisol daily in response to major stress (eg, trauma, surgery). When patients taking pharmacologic doses of glucocorticoids undergo such stress, the suppressed pituitary secretes insufficient ACTH and the adrenal glands may be unable to secrete the extra hormone required. Additional exogenous corticosteroid is given in the dosage and for the duration appropriate for the severity of the stress. For example, for major surgery, hydrocortisone 100 mg intravenously every six hours is given on the day of surgery, after which the dose is reduced by 20% to 30% daily for three days. For minor surgery, a similar regimen is administered for one day. For procedures such as colonoscopy or dental extractions, hydrocortisone 100 mg may be given with preoperative medications, followed by 20 mg orally that evening (Collins and Byyny, 1980).

Hypothalamic-Pituitary-Adrenal Axis Suppression: Administration of exogenous glucocorticoids will result in some degree of suppression (through negative feedback of glucocorticoid) of the hypothalamic-pituitary-adrenal (HPA) axis. The suppression generally is proportional to the size of the dose, relative glucocorticoid activity, biological half-life, and, most importantly, duration of therapy. Prolonged therapy produces adrenal atrophy and inhibits pituitary function (which requires more time for recovery). If patients have been receiving pharmacologic doses for more than one month, it may be assumed that they are unable to secrete normal amounts of hormone or to respond to stress by increasing secretion. However, there is wide individual variation in the dose and duration of treatment required to produce HPA suppression. Significant adrenal suppression may occur within one week after large doses of a glucocorticoid are given. In general, however, less than 5 mg of prednisone daily or the equivalent causes little suppression. Divided doses (three or four daily) are more suppressive than single daily doses, and doses administered just before or at bedtime are more suppressive than those given earlier in the day.

The same precautions exercised by patients receiving adrenal replacement therapy, such as carrying a steroid identification card and bracelet and keeping emergency supplies of medication, also apply to those receiving large doses of these hormones for nonendocrine conditions. (See also index entry Adrenocortical Insufficiency, Treatment.)

Pregnancy and Lactation: The placenta has extensive 11-beta-ol-dehydrogenase activity, an enzyme that metabolizes glucocorticoids to their inactive 11-ketosteroid counterparts. In studies using perfused human placenta, cortisol, prednisolone, prednisone, and dexamethasone all were extensively metabolized before crossing the placenta and entering the fetus. Thus, there appears to be no significant advantage of one preparation over the others in raising fetal circulatory concentrations of glucocorticoids (Levitz et al, 1978).

Prenatal administration of glucocorticoids to animal fetuses retarded somatic growth and compromised central nervous system development. The dose and duration of administration exceeded those used in humans. When betamethasone 12 mg is administered to women prenatally, fetal blood levels of glucocorticoid are similar to those observed during stress. The steroid is cleared from the fetal circulation within three days.

When very large pharmacologic doses must be used for prolonged periods during pregnancy, fetal adrenal hypoplasia may occur. The state of neonatal adrenal function must be assessed and replacement therapy provided if necessary. When steroids are discontinued, normal adrenal function is recovered eventually. Infants born to mothers who have received substantial doses during pregnancy should be carefully observed for signs of hypoadrenalism.

These drugs are classified in FDA Pregnancy Category C.

Corticosteroids are found in the breast milk of lactating women receiving systemic therapy. However, it is probably safe for a lactating mother to nurse her infant if she is taking small doses.

Drug Interactions: See Table 5.

TABLE 5. CLINICALLY IMPORTANT ADVERSE INTERACTIONS OF CORTICOSTEROIDS

Agent	Interactions
Dosage of corticosteroids should be decreased:	
Antibiotics (eg, erythromycin, troleandomycin)	Reduce methylprednisolone clearance in asthmatic patients resulting in therapeutic enhancement or cushingoid side effects
Cyclosporine	Reduces the plasma clearance of prednisolone in renal transplant patients
Estrogen	Increases levels of corticosteroid-binding globulin, resulting in increased bound (inactive) fraction; also decreases metabolism
Isoniazid	Inhibits the metabolism of corticosteroids
Ketoconazole	Inhibits the metabolism of corticosteroids and reduces methylprednisolone elimination
Dosage of corticosteroids should be increased:	
Aminoglutethimide, carbamazepine, phenobarbital, phenytoin, rifampin	Increase metabolism of corticosteroids by the induction of hepatic metabolizing enzymes
Cholestyramine	Decreases gastrointestinal absorption of corticosteroids
Dosage of cited drug should be adjusted:	
Antianxiety and antipsychotic agents	Recurrence or poor control of central nervous system symptoms due to inherent corticosteroid effects
Anticholinesterases (eg, neostigmine, pyridostigmine)	Concurrent use with corticosteroid may precipitate myasthenic crises
Anticoagulants	Corticosteroids decrease effectiveness of anticoagulant by either increasing or decreasing clotting
Antihypertensive agents	Partial loss of hypertensive control when administered with corticosteroids due to the steroid's mineralocorticoid effect
Cyclosporine	Large doses of IV methylprednisolone increase plasma cyclosporine concentrations in renal transplant patients
Hypoglycemic drugs	Corticosteroids have a hyperglycemic effect
Live or killed virus vaccine	Corticosteroids may induce immunosuppression that reduces ability to respond to a killed vaccine and or enhances susceptibility to live virus vaccine; this could result in disseminated disease
Pancuronium	Neuromuscular blockade partially reversed by corticosteroids
Salicylates	Corticosteroids increase clearance of salicylates
Sympathomimetic agents	Corticosteroids increase responses to these agents resulting in increased efficacy and potential toxicity

Effects on Laboratory Tests: Corticosteroids may increase the blood level of glucose, sometimes resulting in diabetes mellitus and glycosuria. This reflects not only elevated blood glucose but a lowered renal threshold for glucose. Potent glucocorticoids (eg, dexamethasone) decrease urinary levels of 17-ketosteroids and 17-hydroxysteroids due to the negative feedback effect on secretion of endogenous hormones.

WITHDRAWAL FROM THERAPY. Several patterns of response to steroid withdrawal have been described (Dixon and Christy, 1980). These include HPA suppression with or without symptoms, exacerbation of the disease being treated, and physical or psychological dependence with otherwise normal function.

The length of time and the rate of dosage reduction necessary for withdrawal from pharmacologic steroid therapy depend on the degree of HPA suppression (related to dose and duration of therapy) and the response of the underlying disease. A variety of schedules have been suggested (Byyny, 1976; Fass, 1979; Collins and Byyny, 1980; Chamberlain and Meyer, 1981). The lowest possible dose of corticosteroid should be used to control the condition being treated, and, when reduction in dosage is possible, the reduction should be gradual.

Glucocorticoids given in large doses for one to three days probably suppress HPA function only temporarily and they can be withdrawn suddenly or gradually over one week. After one month or more of treatment, dosage reduction usually begins by administering a single dose in the morning to minimize adrenal suppression. The dose may be reduced by up to 5 mg of prednisone or the equivalent every three to seven days until 5 mg/day is given. At this time, hydrocortisone 20 mg daily is substituted and the dose is reduced by 2.5 mg at weekly intervals to reach a daily dose of 10 mg (see Table 6). Alternatively, the dose may be reduced by 25% weekly until 10 mg/day of prednisone or the equivalent is given. This amount is administered on alternate days and finally discontinued. The maximum rate of dosage reduction is limited by the patient's response; too rapid withdrawal may exacerbate symptoms of the underlying disease or lead to withdrawal symptoms.

TABLE 6.
PROTOCOL FOR GLUCOCORTICOID WITHDRAWAL[1]

Step	Interval	Observation	Result	Glucocorticoid and Dose
I	Variable	Underlying disease present	Worsening of underlying disease	Variable; gradually decrease dose to hydrocortisone 20 mg/day or equivalent
			Symptoms and signs of steroid withdrawal	Increase dose if disease worsens; continue if disease is quiescent; increase dose for stress
II	4 weeks	8 AM plasma cortisol	Plasma cortisol: When <10 mcg/100 ml	Begin hydrocortisone 20 mg/day; decrease by 2.5 mg/day once/week to 10 mg each morning and continue this dosage; increase dose for stress
			When >10 mcg/100 ml	Stop hydrocortisone; supplemental dose for stress
III	4 weeks—Indefinite	8 AM 250 mcg IM cosyntropin[2] test	When plasma cortisol increased by <6 mcg/100 ml or maximum <20 mcg/100 ml (or both)	Supplemental dose for stress
IV	4 weeks—Indefinite	8 AM 250 mcg IM cosyntropin[2] test	When plasma cortisol increased by >6 mcg/100 ml or maximum >20 mcg/100 ml	Stop supplementation for stress
V	Indefinite	Routine	——	As indicated

[1]*See text for discussion.*
[2]*Synthetic (1 to 24 amino acids) corticotropin (ACTH)*
Adapted from Byyny, 1976.

Short- or intermediate-acting agents (eg, hydrocortisone, prednisone) should be employed, since long-acting agents (eg, betamethasone, dexamethasone) offer no therapeutic advantage but cause more prolonged adrenal and HPA axis suppression. The adrenal gland begins to regain the ability to respond to corticotropin stimulation at daily doses of 5 to 7.5 mg of prednisone or the equivalent.

The entire process of recovery of HPA axis function occurs in stages and may be rapid or may require one year or more for completion. Children tend to recover function more quickly than adults (Chamberlain and Meyer, 1981). During the first phase of recovery, plasma ACTH levels normalize, followed by secretion of normal basal levels of cortisol. This is usually achieved within several months and indicates recovery of adrenal responsiveness to corticotropin and resumption of the cortisol feedback mechanism. This stage of recovery is indicated by a morning (before taking the morning dose of corticosteroid, or on the morning of no medication when using alternate-day therapy) plasma cortisol level greater than 10 mcg/dL. In the second phase, normal corticotropin and cortisol secretory responses to stressful stimuli return. This can be demonstrated in patients with normal morning cortisol levels by a normal response to an ACTH stimulation test (see Table 6). A few patients with normal responses to ACTH stimulation tests have had an abnormal serum cortisol response to insulin tolerance tests, which may indicate acute adrenal insufficiency (Borst et al, 1982). Because extended suppression is possible, those who received systemic glucocorticoid therapy during the previous year should be given appropriate doses of steroids during stress unless recovery of the HPA axis has been confirmed by appropriate tests.

Corticotropin injections should not be used to accelerate recovery from adrenal atrophy because further HPA suppression occurs even though adrenal secretion is stimulated.

In addition to HPA suppression, withdrawal of glucocorticoid therapy may be accompanied by malaise, fever, myalgia, arthralgia, fatigue, and restlessness. This syndrome may be mistaken for an exacerbation of the underlying disease, particularly in patients with rheumatoid arthritis. Gradual reduction of the dose and treatment with nonsteroidal anti-inflammatory drugs minimizes these problems.

Some patients become psychologically dependent on glucocorticoids (Flavin et al, 1983), particularly those given repeated courses of therapy for recurring symptoms (eg, those with asthma or certain dermatologic conditions). Dependence also may occur when the underlying disease is inactive. Since euphoria and rapid relief occur when glucocorticoid therapy is initiated, it may be difficult to convince the patient to accept repeated attempts to withdraw medication with its attendant discomforts.

ADRENAL CORTICOSTEROIDS

Numerous synthetic corticosteroids have been developed by modifying the chemical structure of hydrocortisone (cortisol, Compound F) (see the Figure). The analogues thus produced may differ from the parent compound in half-life, potency, and sodium-retaining activity. Prednisone and prednisolone were produced by introducing a double bond between carbon atoms 1 and 2 (Δ-1 analogues) of cortisone and hydrocortisone, respectively; this increased glucocorticoid activity while decreasing mineralocorticoid effects. Other synthetic preparations have either glucocorticoid (dexamethasone, betamethasone) or mineralocorticoid (desoxycorticosterone) activity almost exclusively; most have been synthesized primarily for their glucocorticoid effects and are widely used in nonendocrine diseases. See also preceding discussion on Glucocorticoids.

GLUCOCORTICOID STRUCTURES

CH_2OH, C=O, CH_3, ---OH, CH_3, 1, 2, 6, 9, 11, 16, O

	$C_1—C_2$	C_6	C_9	C_{11}	C_{16}
Short-acting					
Cortisone	single bond	—H	—H	=O	—H
Hydrocortisone	single bond	—H	—H	◄OH	—H
Intermediate-acting					
Fludroprednisolone	double bond	---F	—H	◄OH	—H
Methylprednisolone	double bond	---CH_3	—H	◄OH	—H
Prednisolone	double bond	—H	—H	◄OH	—H
Prednisone	double bond	—H	—H	=O	—H
Triamcinolone	double bond	—H	---F	◄OH	---OH
Long-acting					
Betamethasone	double bond	—H	---F	◄OH	---CH_3
Dexamethasone	double bond	—H	---F	◄OH	---CH_3
Paramethasone	double bond	---F	—H	◄OH	---CH_3

When considering the therapeutic efficacy of the corticosteroids, it is important to remember that separation of glucocorticoid and mineralocorticoid activity is incomplete. Some agents that are considered to be primarily glucocorticoids (eg, hydrocortisone, cortisone, prednisone, prednisolone) possess variable mineralocorticoid activity as well and, therefore, cause sodium retention and potassium depletion when used in pharmacologic amounts.

The plasma half-lives of the synthetic glucocorticoids are variable and often are considerably longer than that of hydrocortisone. The tissue half-lives determine biological effectiveness. Although they generally correlate with plasma half-lives, the relationship is not linear: tissue half-lives always exceed plasma half-lives. The relative potency is a measure of anti-inflammatory and HPA suppressive activities. However, the degree and duration of HPA suppression caused by the long-acting glucocorticoids, betamethasone and dexamethasone, are greater than would be predicted on the basis of their plasma half-lives and relative potencies. Table 7 lists the properties of glucocorticoids currently marketed in the United States.

DOSAGE AND PREPARATIONS. Glucocorticoids may be administered by a number of routes, depending on the nature of the disease and the condition of the patient. The intravenous route is preferred in emergencies, and the intramuscular route may be employed temporarily when oral medication cannot be taken, but the oral route is used for systemic administration whenever possible. Depot preparations may be injected intra-articularly (eg, in rheumatoid arthritis), extra-articularly (eg, in bursitis, tenosynovitis, localized noninfectious tissue inflammatory disorders), and intralesionally (eg, keloids, psoriasis). Intrasynovial injection of a corticosteroid may produce systemic as well as local effects. Local injection of a steroid into a previously inflamed joint should be avoided, and these drugs should not be injected into unstable joints. Rectal preparations are employed in inflammatory bowel disorders, topical preparations are used for dermatologic or ocular disorders, and inhalant preparations are used for respiratory disorders (see index entries on these disorders).

Oral, Parenteral: Prednisone 1 to 2 mg/kg (or the equivalent) provides tissue and serum concentrations with lymphoid, neutrophil, and monocyte effects. Doses higher than 2 mg/kg probably do not increase the therapeutic effect but do increase drug-related morbidity.

A common regimen employs a single morning dose of prednisone. The lowest dose should be given in the least toxic interval that is sufficient to control the disease. However, for active diseases, a dose sufficient to produce remission should be employed (eg, 1 mg/kg/day of prednisone in up to three divided doses). The dose is then adjusted until the lowest effective amount is determined; the patient then can be converted to alternate-day therapy until the drug can be discontinued.

For specific routes employed, see Table 7.

BETAMETHASONE:

Celestone (Schering). Syrup 0.6 mg/5 ml (alcohol <1%); tablets 0.6 mg.

BETAMETHASONE SODIUM PHOSPHATE:

Celestone Phosphate (Schering), ***Generic.*** Solution 3 mg/ml in 5 ml containers.

BETAMETHASONE ACETATE AND BETAMETHASONE SODIUM PHOSPHATE:

Celestone Soluspan (Schering). Each ml of suspension contains betamethasone acetate 3 mg and betamethasone sodium phosphate 3 mg in 5 ml containers.

CORTISONE ACETATE:

Generic. Suspension 25 mg/ml in 10 and 20 ml containers and 50 mg/ml in 10 ml containers; tablets 5, 10, and 25 mg.

Cortone Acetate (Merck Sharp & Dohme). Suspension 50 mg/ml in 10 ml containers; tablets 25 mg.

DEXAMETHASONE:

Generic. Elixir 0.5 mg/5 ml (alcohol 5%); solution (oral) 0.5 mg/5 ml (alcohol-free) and 0.5 mg/0.5 ml (alcohol 30%); tablets 0.25, 0.5, 0.75, 1, 1.5, 2, 4, and 6 mg.

TABLE 7.
GLUCOCORTICOID PROPERTIES AND ROUTES OF ADMINISTRATION

Drug	Effect[1]			Half-life (hours)	
	Onset	Peak (hours)	Duration[2]	Plasma	Biological
SHORT-ACTING					
Cortisone				0.5	8-12
Acetate					
Oral	Rapid	2	1.25-1.5 days		
IM	Slow	20-48			
Hydrocortisone				1.5-2	8-12
Oral		1	1.25-1.5 days		
IM[3]		4-8			
Rectal (retention enema)	3-5 days				
Acetate					
IA, IS, IB, IL, ST		24-48	3-28 days		
Rectal (foam)	5-7 days				
Cypionate					
Oral	Slower than tablet	1-2			
Sodium Phosphate					
IV	Rapid				
IM	Rapid	1			
Sodium Succinate					
IV	Rapid				
IM	Rapid	1	Variable		
INTERMEDIATE-ACTING					
Methylprednisolone				>3.5	18-36
Oral		1-2	1.25-1.5 days		
Acetate					
IM	Slow (6-48 hours)	4-8 days	7-28 days		
IA, IL, ST	Very slow	7 days	7-35 days		
Sodium Succinate					
IV	Rapid				
IM	Rapid				
Prednisolone				2.1-3.5	18-36
Oral		1-2	1.25-1.5 days		
Acetate					
IM	Slow				
Acetate/Sodium Phosphate					
IM			Up to 28 days		
IB, IS, IA, ST			3-28 days		
Sodium Phosphate					
IV	Rapid	1			
IM	Rapid	1			
IA, IL, ST			3-21 days		
Tebutate					
IA, IL, ST	Slow (1-2 days)		7-21 days		

(Continued on next page)

TABLE 7 (continued)

Drug	Effect[1] Onset	Peak (hours)	Duration[2]	Half-life (hours) Plasma	Biological
INTERMEDIATE-ACTING (continued)					
Prednisone				3.4-3.8	18-36
Oral		1-2	1.25-1.5 days		
Triamcinolone				2->5	18-36
Oral		1-2	2.25 days		
Acetonide					
IM	Slow (24-48 hours)		7-42 days		
IB, IA, IS, IL, ST			7-42 days		
Diacetate					
Oral		1-2			
IM	Slow		4-28 days		
IL			7-14 days		
IA, IS, ST			7-56 days		
Hexacetonide					
IA, IL			21-28 days		
LONG-ACTING					
Betamethasone				3-5	36-54
Oral		1-2	3.25 days		
Sodium Phosphate					
IV	Rapid				
IM	Rapid				
Acetate/Sodium Phosphate					
IM	1-3 hours		7 days		
IA, IS			7-14 days		
IL, ST			7 days		
Dexamethasone				3-4.5	36-54
Oral		1-2	2.75 days		
Acetate					
IM		8	6 days		
IA, ST, IL			7-21 days		
Sodium Phosphate					
IV	Rapid				
IM	Rapid				
IA, IS, IL, ST			3-21 days		
Paramethasone				3-4.5	36-54
Acetate					
Oral		1-2	2 days		

Adapted from USP Dispensing Information. Rockville, Md, The United States Pharmacopeial Convention, Inc, vol I, 1992.

Abbreviations: IA = intra-articular IB = intrabursal IL = intralesional IM = intramuscular IS = intrasynovial IV = intravenous SC = subcutaneous ST = soft tissue

[1]Actual onset, peak, and duration of action depend on route and site of administration, solubility of dosage form, dose administered, and condition being treated.

[2]Duration of action is based on biological half-life.

[3]Parenteral dosage form not commercially available in the United States.

Decadron (Merck Sharp & Dohme). Elixir 0.5 mg/5 ml (alcohol 5%); tablets 0.25, 0.5, 0.75, 1.5, 4, and 6 mg.
Dexone (Solvay). Tablets 0.5, 0.75, 1.5, and 4 mg.
Hexadrol (Organon). Elixir 0.5 mg/5 ml (alcohol 5%); tablets 4 mg.

DEXAMETHASONE ACETATE:
Generic. Suspension 8 mg/ml in 5 ml containers.
Dalalone D.P. (Forest). Suspension (repository) 16 mg/ml in 1 and 5 ml containers (not for intralesional use).
Dalalone L.A. (Forest), ***Decaject-L.A.*** (Mayrand), ***Dexone-LA*** (Keene). Suspension (repository) 8 mg/ml in 5 ml containers.
Decadron-LA (Merck Sharp & Dohme). Suspension (repository) 8 mg/ml in 1 and 5 ml containers.

DEXAMETHASONE SODIUM PHOSPHATE:
Generic. Solution 4 mg/ml in 1, 5, 10, and 30 ml containers, 10 mg/ml in 1 and 10 ml containers, and 24 mg/ml in 5 ml containers (for intravenous use only).
Decaject (Mayrand). Solution 4 mg/ml in 5 and 10 ml containers.
Dalalone (Forest). Solution 4 mg/ml in 5 ml containers.
Decadron Phosphate (Merck Sharp & Dohme). Solution 4 mg/ml in 1, 2.5, 5, and 25 ml containers and 24 mg/ml in 5 and 10 ml containers (for intravenous use only).
Hexadrol Phosphate (Organon). Solution 4 mg/ml in 1 and 5 ml containers, 10 mg/ml in 1 and 10 ml containers (intravenous or intramuscular use only).

Available Mixture:
Decadron Phosphate with Xylocaine (Merck Sharp & Dohme). Each milliliter of solution contains dexamethasone sodium phosphate 4 mg and lidocaine hydrochloride 10 mg in 5 ml containers.

HYDROCORTISONE:
Cortef (Upjohn). Tablets 5, 10, and 20 mg.
Hydrocortone (Merck Sharp & Dohme), ***Generic.*** Tablets 10 and 20 mg.

HYDROCORTISONE ACETATE:
Generic. Suspension 25 and 50 mg/ml in 10 ml containers.
Hydrocortone Acetate (Merck Sharp & Dohme). Suspension 25 and 50 mg/ml in 5 ml containers.

HYDROCORTISONE CYPIONATE:
Cortef (Upjohn). Suspension (oral) 10 mg/5 ml.

HYDROCORTISONE SODIUM PHOSPHATE:
Hydrocortone Phosphate (Merck Sharp & Dohme), ***Generic.*** Solution 50 mg/ml in 2 and 10 ml containers.

HYDROCORTISONE SODIUM SUCCINATE:
A-hydroCort (Abbott), ***Solu-Cortef*** (Upjohn), ***Generic.*** Powder 100, 250, and 500 mg and 1 g.

METHYLPREDNISOLONE:
Generic. Tablets 4, 16, 24, and 32 mg.
Medrol (Upjohn). Tablets 2, 4, 8, 16, 24, and 32 mg.

METHYLPREDNISOLONE ACETATE:
Generic. Suspension 20 mg/ml in 5 and 10 ml containers, 40 mg/ml in 1, 5, and 10 ml containers, and 80 mg/ml in 1 and 5 ml containers.
depMedalone (Forest). Suspension 40 and 80 mg/ml in 5 ml containers.
Depo-Medrol (Upjohn). Suspension 20 mg/ml in 5 ml containers, 40 mg/ml in 5 and 10 ml containers, and 80 mg/ml in 5 ml containers.
Duralone (Hauck). Suspension 40 mg/ml in 10 ml containers and 80 mg/ml in 5 ml containers.

METHYLPREDNISOLONE SODIUM SUCCINATE:
Solu-Medrol (Upjohn), ***Generic.*** Powder 40, 125, and 500 mg and 1 and 2 g (***Solu-Medrol*** only).

PARAMETHASONE ACETATE:
Haldrone (Lilly). Tablets 2 mg.

PREDNISOLONE:
Generic. Tablets 5 mg.
Prelone (Muro). Syrup 15 mg/5 ml (alcohol 5%).

PREDNISOLONE ACETATE:
Generic. Suspension 25 and 50 mg/ml in 10 and 30 ml containers.
Predalone (Forest). Suspension 50 mg/ml in 10 ml containers.

PREDNISOLONE ACETATE AND PREDNISOLONE SODIUM PHOSPHATE:
Generic. Each ml of suspension contains prednisolone acetate 80 mg and prednisolone sodium phosphate 20 mg in 10 ml containers.

PREDNISOLONE SODIUM PHOSPHATE:
Generic. Solution 20 mg/ml in 10 ml containers.
Hydeltrasol (Merck Sharp & Dohme). Solution 20 mg/ml in 2 and 5 ml containers.

PREDNISOLONE TEBUTATE:
Generic. Suspension 20 mg/ml in 10 ml containers.
Hydeltra-T.B.A. (Merck Sharp & Dohme). Suspension 20 mg/ml in 1 and 5 ml containers.

PREDNISONE:
Deltasone (Upjohn). Tablets 2.5, 5, 10, 20, and 50 mg.
Liquid-Pred (Muro), ***Generic.*** Solution (oral) 5 mg/5 ml (alcohol 5%); solution (oral concentrate) 5 mg/ml (alcohol 30%); tablets 1, 2.5, 5, 10, 20, 25, and 50 mg.
Meticorten (Schering). Tablets 1 mg.
Orasone (Solvay). Tablets 1, 5, 10, 20, and 50 mg.
Prednicen-M (Central). Tablets 5 mg.
Sterapred (Mayrand). Tablets 10 mg.

TRIAMCINOLONE:
Generic. Tablets 4 mg.
Aristocort (Fujisawa). Tablets 1, 2, 4, and 8 mg.
Kenacort (Apothecon). Tablets 4 and 8 mg.

TRIAMCINOLONE ACETONIDE:
Generic. Suspension 40 mg/ml in 1 and 5 ml containers.
Kenalog (Westwood-Squibb). Suspension 10 mg/ml in 5 ml containers and 40 mg/ml in 1, 5, and 10 ml containers.

TRIAMCINOLONE DIACETATE:
Generic. Suspension 40 mg/ml in 5 and 10 ml containers.
Aristocort Diacetate (Fujisawa). Suspension 25 mg/ml in 5 ml containers (intralesional) and 40 mg/ml in 1 and 5 ml containers ***(Forte)***.
Kenacort Diacetate (Apothecon). Syrup 4 mg/5 ml.

TRIAMCINOLONE HEXACETONIDE:
Aristospan (Fujisawa). Suspension 5 mg/ml in 5 ml containers (intralesional) and 20 mg/ml in 1 and 5 ml containers (intra-articular).

CYTOTOXIC DRUGS

Immunosuppression can be achieved by agents that kill immunologically competent cells. These agents, like those used for cancer chemotherapy, are not selectively toxic for lymphocytes but are capable of killing any cell that can replicate. The activity of cytotoxic drugs may depend on the phase of the mitotic cycle in which the drug exerts its effect (see the Introduction). Cytotoxic drugs inhibit both B-cell and T-cell responses, but they do not inhibit all immune responses equally. The primary immune response is more readily inhibited than a secondary one; drugs that are effective in an unsensitized situation may have little or no effect in a sensitized system.

Cytotoxic drugs are often used to treat autoimmune disorders. Their generalized cytotoxicity is a hazard, particularly to rapidly dividing cells of the bone marrow.

The undesired effects of cytotoxic immunosuppressive drugs include bone marrow suppression with neutropenia, thrombocytopenia, and anemia; gastrointestinal disturbances; sterility; infections resulting from generalized suppression of immune responses; and increased risk of malignancies, especially lymphoma.

AZATHIOPRINE
[Imuran]

AZATHIOPRINE SODIUM
[Imuran]

ACTIONS. Azathioprine is a derivative of mercaptopurine, to which it is converted rapidly after administration, and has similar biological activity. Mercaptopurine is an S-phase specific compound that acts by competitive enzyme inhibition to inhibit purine biosynthesis and thus decreases the rate of cell replication (see index entry Mercaptopurine, As Antineoplastic Agent). Azathioprine and mercaptopurine have similar in vivo immunosuppressive activity, but the former is less toxic at immunosuppressive doses and therefore has a higher therapeutic index. Azathioprine inhibits delayed hypersensitivity and causes variable alterations in antibody production. It suppresses T-cell more than B-cell activity and has limited anti-inflammatory properties. Clinically, the number of mononuclear and granulocytic cells available for migration to an area of inflammation is decreased. Azathioprine also inhibits the proliferation of promyelocytes within bone marrow, thus decreasing the number of circulating monocytes available to become macrophages in the peripheral blood.

Azathioprine exerts its maximum immunosuppressive effect when given immediately after immunologic challenge (induction phase). When given prior to antigen challenge (preinduction phase), it may augment antibody response in specific immunoglobulin classes. Azathioprine is not effective when given in the effector phase (proliferation and maturation phases). Therefore, the compound has no effect on established graft rejections or secondary responses.

USES. Azathioprine is indicated as an adjunct for the prevention of graft rejection in renal transplantation and for the management of severe, active rheumatoid arthritis unresponsive to conventional treatment.

The introduction of cyclosporine for immunosuppression in transplants has not eliminated the use of azathioprine for this purpose. Combination regimens that include azathioprine have permitted lower doses of cyclosporine, thus reducing the risk of cyclosporine-induced nephrotoxicity (Simmons et al, 1986; First et al, 1986). In addition, the adverse effects of long-term steroid therapy have been reported to be avoided by the substitution of azathioprine for the steroid in cyclosporine-treated renal transplant patients (Kupin et al, 1988).

Azathioprine is indicated for rheumatoid arthritis only in adults who meet established criteria for classic or definite rheumatoid arthritis as specified by the American Rheumatism Association (McEwen, 1972). For further information on its use in this condition, see index entry Azathioprine, Uses, Arthritis.

Azathioprine has been administered in systemic lupus erythematosus and other collagen, vascular, and systemic inflammatory states. A combined corticosteroid-azathioprine regimen was reported to be safe and effective and has resulted in long-term remissions in patients with pemphigus vulgaris (Aberer et al, 1987). In a preliminary, unblinded study, early administration of a regimen of azathioprine and prednisone improved metabolic control in some patients with insulin-dependent diabetes mellitus of recent onset (Silverstein et al, 1988). This drug also has been used in patients with polymyositis or dermatomyositis, myasthenia gravis, multiple sclerosis, inflammatory bowel disease, and biliary cirrhosis. For further information, see index entry Azathioprine, Uses.

ADVERSE REACTIONS AND PRECAUTIONS. The frequency and severity of adverse effects depend on the dose and duration of administration and on any underlying disease or concomitant therapy. Toxic effects on the gastrointestinal tract and hematologic systems are most common. In addition, the risk of secondary infection and neoplasia is increased. The incidence of hematologic toxicity, neoplasia, and infection is significantly higher in renal transplantation than in rheumatoid arthritis (eg, infection rate is 50 to 60 times higher in renal transplant patients). The high incidence of toxicity following renal transplantation may be due to the accumulation of metabolites normally eliminated by the kidney. The concomitant use of steroids and induction therapies employing antilymphocyte globulins also may be factors.

Although bone marrow depression, the most serious adverse reaction, is uncommon with conventional doses of azathioprine, it occurs more frequently with larger doses. Hematologic toxicity is usually limited to mild leukopenia and thrombocytopenia and, less frequently, to megaloblastic anemia, pure red blood cell aplasia, and reticulocytopenia. Typically, myelosuppression is delayed, and hematologic disorders appear 7 to 14 days after initiation of therapy. A few cases of acute idiosyncratic aplastic anemia have occurred shortly after initiation of therapy or suddenly during a previously stable course.

Since severe leukopenia and/or thrombocytopenia may develop in patients receiving azathioprine, complete blood and platelet counts should be performed at regular intervals. Prompt reduction in dosage or withdrawal of the drug may be necessary if there is evidence of serious bone marrow depression. Azathioprine is slow-acting and effects may persist after this drug is discontinued.

Nausea, vomiting, and gastrointestinal discomfort are common during the first few months of azathioprine therapy and usually respond to dosage adjustment. Symptoms of gastrointestinal toxicity most often develop within the first few weeks of therapy and are reversible on discontinuation of the drug. However, a gastrointestinal hypersensitivity reaction characterized by severe nausea and vomiting also has been described. These symptoms may be accompanied by diarrhea, rash, fever, malaise, myalgia, liver enzyme elevation, and, occasionally, hypotension. This reaction can recur within hours after rechallenge with a single dose of azathioprine (Assini et al, 1986; Cox et al, 1988).

Enzyme changes characteristic of hepatocellular necrosis and cholestasis may occur relatively early (one or two weeks) but also extremely late (years) during treatment and usually require discontinuing azathioprine. Most often, hepatotoxicity develops within the first six months of transplantation, but it is usually reversible after azathioprine is discontinued. If administration must be continued, close observation is essential, since deaths from hepatic decompensation have occurred. Periodic measurement of serum transaminases, alkaline phosphatase, and bilirubin is indicated to detect hepatotoxicity promptly. Azathioprine should be permanently withdrawn if hepatic veno-occlusive disease is suspected. Patients with chronic liver disease may not tolerate full doses and should be observed closely until they are stable. Acute liver dysfunction often requires significant reduction in dose.

Pancreatitis and hypersensitivity-type interstitial pneumonitis have been reported occasionally. Uncommon adverse effects are skin rash, alopecia, fever, arthralgia, steatorrhea, and negative nitrogen balance.

Azathioprine is carcinogenic in animals and is associated with increased risk of neoplasia, mainly lymphoproliferative disease, in transplant patients. There may be a prohibitive risk of neoplasia in patients with rheumatoid arthritis who have been treated with alkylating agents.

Azathioprine is mutagenic and teratogenic in laboratory animals, and transplacental transmission of drug and metabolites has been reported in humans. Therefore, risk versus benefit should be assessed carefully before administering this drug to pregnant patients and, whenever possible, its use should be avoided (FDA Pregnancy Category D). Precautions should be taken to avoid conception for at least 12 weeks following discontinuation of azathioprine. Azathioprine is not recommended for treating arthritis in pregnant women.

DRUG INTERACTIONS. Because allopurinol inhibits xanthine oxidase, the enzyme required for 6-mercaptopurine metabolism, the dose of azathioprine should be reduced to one-third or one-fourth the usual maintenance amount in patients taking this drug concomitantly. The use of angiotensin-converting enzyme inhibitors in patients receiving azathioprine has been reported to cause severe leukopenia (Kirchertz et al, 1981). Drugs known to induce (phenytoin, phenobarbital, rifampin) or inhibit (ketoconazole, erythromycin) hepatic microsomal enzymes may alter the clearance of azathioprine.

PHARMACOKINETICS. Oral azathioprine is efficiently absorbed. After oral administration of 35-S-azathioprine, maximum serum radioactivity occurs at one to two hours and the half-life is five hours (decay rate for all 35-S-containing metabolites).

Azathioprine is cleaved in vivo to mercaptopurine, which is then catabolized to various oxidized and methylated derivatives, including 6-thiouric acid, the major metabolite. The latter is formed after oxidation of mercaptopurine by xanthine oxidase in the liver. About 10% of azathioprine is cleaved between the sulfur and purine ring to form 1-methyl-4-nitro-5-thioimidazole. Proportions of metabolites differ in individual patients, which may account for variability in drug effects.

Azathioprine is mainly eliminated by metabolic degradation. Small amounts of unchanged drug and mercaptopurine are eliminated by the kidney. Following oral administration, no azathioprine or mercaptopurine is detectable in the urine after eight hours.

Mercaptopurine derived from the metabolism of azathioprine is widely distributed in body tissues, but only a small percentage enters the cerebrospinal fluid. About 30% of both azathioprine and mercaptopurine is bound to serum protein. Usual doses of azathioprine produce low blood levels (less than 1 mcg/ml) of both the foregoing compounds and both quickly leave the circulation. Neither the magnitude nor the duration of the clinical response can be predicted from the blood levels, since these correlate with thiopurine nucleotide levels in tissues rather than in blood. The effects of azathioprine may persist long after clearance is complete.

DOSAGE AND PREPARATIONS. Azathioprine is a potent immunosuppressive agent and should only be used under the direction of a physician familiar with the risks associated with this type of therapy. The patient should be evaluated carefully and monitored adequately during treatment.

Oral, Intravenous: For allotransplantation, initially, 3 to 5 mg/kg/day as a single dose beginning on the day of transplant. For maintenance, 1 to 3 mg/kg/day. Intravenous administration is used in patients who are unable to tolerate oral medication; the oral form is substituted as soon as possible.

AZATHIOPRINE:
Imuran (Burroughs Wellcome). Tablets 50 mg.

AZATHIOPRINE SODIUM:
Imuran (Burroughs Wellcome), ***Generic.*** Powder (lyophilized, sterile) equivalent to azathioprine 100 mg.

CHLORAMBUCIL

[Leukeran]

For chemical formula, see index entry Chlorambucil, As Antineoplastic Agent.

This bifunctional alkylating agent has not been used extensively for immunosuppression in the United States. Behcet's syndrome, systemic lupus erythematosus, and Wegener's granulomatosis have been reported to respond to low doses of chlorambucil.

Chlorambucil is a slow-acting nitrogen mustard that is cell cycle nonspecific but has a marked lympholytic effect. The induction time for an immunologic effect is longer than for cyclophosphamide, but serious hematologic depression appears to occur less frequently and urinary excretion is not impaired. Chlorambucil is a very potent alkylator and is carcinogenic in humans. It can produce infertility and is probably mutagenic and teratogenic in humans (FDA Pregnancy Category D). Bone marrow suppression is the most common adverse effect. Chlorambucil should not be used as an immunosuppressive agent except in life-threatening disease.

See index entry Chlorambucil, As Antineoplastic Agent, for a more detailed discussion.

DOSAGE AND PREPARATIONS.

Oral: 0.05 to 0.1 mg/kg daily.

Leukeran (Burroughs Wellcome). Tablets 2 mg.

CYCLOPHOSPHAMIDE

[Cytoxan, Neosar]

For chemical formula, see index entry Cyclophosphamide, Uses, Cancer.

ACTIONS AND USES. Cyclophosphamide is an alkylating agent of the cyclic mustard group. It is a prodrug that requires metabolic activation by liver enzymes before it can alkylate cellular substances. It has greater effect on B- than T-cell lymphocytes. A possible mechanism of immunosuppression is direct cytotoxicity on immunocompetent lymphocytes, especially those that have undergone antigenic differentiation and division or an abrogation of suppressor cell function by blockage at the CD4, 2H4+ cell level (Ehrke et al, 1987). Cyclophosphamide inhibits an established immune response, which usually is present in patients considered to be candidates for immunomodulatory therapy.

Cyclophosphamide can be given orally and intravenously. It does not cause severe tissue necrosis after inadvertent subcutaneous injection. Oral administration for 7 to 14 days is required before a clinically detectable immunomodulatory effect occurs.

Since cyclophosphamide can suppress the immune response of both T- and B-lymphocytes, many investigators have used this drug in patients with various nonmalignant inflammatory diseases (eg, rheumatoid arthritis, systemic lupus erythematosus, Wegner's granulomatosis, multiple sclerosis). However, use of this agent has been severely limited because of the numerous adverse effects observed, including alopecia, bone marrow suppression, hemorrhagic cystitis, gonadal failure, and malignancy. In a long-term, case-control, follow-up study, the rate of development of malignancy was reported to be significantly greater in treated patients than in control patients six years following initiation of therapy, and this increased rate persisted even at 13 years (Baker et al, 1987). Large cumulative doses were associated with the greatest risk of secondary malignancies.

Although prednisone traditionally has been the initial drug of choice for most patients with severe systemic lupus erythematosus, it is not effective in some patients with severe renal or central nervous system involvement and may predispose patients to serious complications; thus, alternative therapy has been sought. Evidence suggests that cytotoxic agents, such as cyclophosphamide, may be more effective than prednisone alone in some individuals. In one preliminary, uncontrolled study in nine individuals, monthly intravenous administration of cyclophosphamide substantially ameliorated severe symptoms and produced discrete changes in T-lymphocyte markers and function (McCune et al, 1988).

Investigators also have reported that cyclophosphamide may be beneficial for multiple sclerosis. For further information, see index entry Multiple Sclerosis, Drug Therapy.

Because of its low cost and ready availability, cyclophosphamide has been investigated as an alternative to azathioprine in renal allotransplantation. This alternative has special relevance for developing countries. In a retrospective study of 29 recipients of living-related donor renal transplants, cyclophosphamide replaced azathioprine in a regimen that included prednisolone. It was concluded that cyclophosphamide was a safe and effective alternative to azathioprine (Yadav et al, 1988).

ADVERSE REACTIONS AND PRECAUTIONS. Cyclophosphamide produces the same adverse effects as other cytotoxic agents, including reversible alopecia, nausea, and vomiting. Life-threatening reactions include bone marrow suppression, acute hemorrhagic cystitis, bladder telangiectasia, and abnormal urinary cytology. Adverse reactions involving the bladder can be minimized by increasing the fluid intake and emptying the bladder prior to sleep or by the concomitant use of mesna [Mesnex] (Luce et al, 1988). Long-term use is associated with bladder fibrosis and carcinoma. Impaired urinary excretion has been reported only with large doses. Cyclophosphamide should be discontinued if hematuria occurs. Massive urinary bleeding may require supravesicular diversion. Acute myopericarditis, which can be fatal, may occur following large doses of cyclophosphamide given prior to bone marrow transplantation.

When cyclophosphamide therapy is contemplated in young patients, the probability of drug-induced infertility must be considered. Ovulation is inhibited and permanently impaired in 30% to 50% of women after continuous low-dose therapy; aspermia is common after three to six months of therapy. The teratogenic potential of cyclophosphamide appears to be low, but contraception should be encouraged during treatment (FDA Pregnancy Category D).

For other indications, adverse reactions, and dosages, see index entry Cyclophosphamide, Uses.

Generic. Powder 100, 200, and 500 mg and 1 g.

Cytoxan (Bristol-Myers). Powder 100, 200, and 500 mg and 1 and 2 g; tablets 25 and 50 mg.

Neosar (Adria). Powder 100, 200, and 500 mg and 1 and 2 g.

METHOTREXATE

[Rheumatrex]

METHOTREXATE SODIUM

[Folex PFS]

For chemical formula, see index entry Methotrexate, Uses, Cancer.

ACTIONS AND USES. Methotrexate is a phase-specific compound that acts by inhibiting folate metabolism. It has a marked affinity for dihydrofolate reductase, thus inhibiting the conversion of dihydrofolic acid to tetrahydrofolic acid. The latter and other reduced folates participate in a number of biochemical reactions that result in the synthesis of DNA, RNA, and various protein molecules. Reduced folates are needed for the metabolic transfer of one-carbon units in various biochemical reactions. As a consequence of methotrexate's action, the biosynthesis of inosinic acid, the precursor of purines needed for DNA and RNA synthesis, and thymidylic acid, the nucleotide specific to DNA, are inhibited. These effects inhibit cellular replication. The reaction is cell-cycle specific and occurs during the proliferative phase of mitosis. The drug's mechanism of action in rheumatoid arthritis is unknown but may be more anti-inflammatory than immunosuppressive (Segal et al, 1990).

Methotrexate is indicated for the treatment of certain neoplastic diseases; for the symptomatic control of severe, recalcitrant, disabling psoriasis not responsive to other forms of therapy; and for the management of selected adults with severe, active, classical rheumatoid arthritis. The drug also has been used in patients with polymyositis or dermatomyositis. Methotrexate has been added to the regimens of patients with inflammatory muscle disease when no clinical response occurred after three to six months of therapy with prednisone 1 mg/kg. Methotrexate also has been used investigationally for juvenile rheumatoid arthritis and has been recommended for early consideration for patients who are not responding adequately to usual antiarthritic therapy (Truckenbrodt and Häfner, 1986; Rose et al, 1990).

This folic acid analogue also has been administered for immunosuppression in organ transplant recipients. Clinical transplant groups have used a 17-dose, 102-day methotrexate regimen for graft-versus-host disease (GVHD) in bone marrow recipients. A four-dose regimen (10 mg/M^2/day on post-transplant days 1, 3, 6, and 11 only) was reported to be as effective as the 102-day regimen in preventing both acute and chronic GVHD (Smith et al, 1985). In one study, methotrexate was reported to be effective as an adjunct in the treatment of persistent low-grade cardiac allograft rejection and produced minimal morbidity (Olsen et al, 1990).

See index entry Methotrexate, for a more detailed discussion of other uses and dosages for this drug.

ADVERSE REACTIONS AND PRECAUTIONS. The most common adverse effects are ulcerative stomatitis, leukopenia, nausea, and abdominal distress. Other side effects include marked myelosuppression with anemia, leukopenia, and thrombocytopenia. Pulmonary fibrosis also has developed.

Methotrexate may be hepatotoxic, especially when large doses or prolonged therapy is employed. Since early signs of hepatotoxicity may be absent, hepatic function tests should be performed both prior to and during therapy. Concomitant use of other hepatotoxic drugs (including alcohol) should be avoided. An intermittent dosage schedule appears to be less toxic than a continuous one.

Methotrexate has been reported to act as an abortifacient and has caused congenital abnormalities. Therefore, it is not recommended for women of childbearing potential (FDA Pregnancy Category D).

METHOTREXATE:
Rheumatrex (Lederle). Tablets 2.5 mg.

METHOTREXATE SODIUM:
(Strengths expressed in terms of the base)
Folex PFS (Adria). Solution (for injection) 25 mg/ml in 2, 4, 8, and 10 ml containers (preservative-free).
Methotrexate (Lederle). Powder (cryodesiccated) 20 and 50 mg and 1 g containers (preservative-free); solution (for injection) 25 mg/ml in 2 and 10 ml containers (with preservative) and 25 mg/ml in 2, 4, 8, and 10 ml containers (preservative-free) (***Methotrexate LPF***).

T-LYMPHOCYTE SUPPRESSANTS

CYCLOSPORINE (Cyclosporin A)
[Sandimmune]

Ala — D — Ala — MeLeu — MeLeu — MeVal — N — C — CO — Abu — MeGly — MeLeu — Val — MeLeu
1 2 3 4 5 6 7 8 9 10 11

ACTIONS. Cyclosporine is a metabolite produced by the fungus, *Tolypocladium inflatum gams.* The compound is a cyclic polypeptide consisting of 11 amino acids. This drug inhibits cell-mediated reactions such as allograft rejection, delayed hypersensitivity, allergic encephalomyelitis, adjuvant arthritis, and graft-versus-host disease (GVHD) in animals, but it does not produce bone marrow suppression in animals or humans. Cyclosporine suppresses primary and, to a lesser degree, secondary antibody responses to T-cell dependent antigens; it also strongly inhibits antibody responses to some T-independent antigens (eg, trinitrophenylated-Ficoll) but not others (eg, dextran, lipopolysaccharide). It is not clear whether its effect on B-cell responses is separate or different from that on T-cells, for the response may be a consequence of impaired T-cell function that is required for B-cell growth and differentiation. This agent depletes medullary thymocytes and splenic T-lymphocytes. Its effectiveness is due to specific and reversible inhibition of T-lymphocytes in the G_0 or G_1 phase of the cell cycle; it does not inhibit mature, proliferative T-cells. The T-helper cell is the main target, but the T-suppressor cell may be inhibited to a degree.

The exact molecular mechanism of action is unclear; the drug appears to act on several aspects of the immune response of T-cells. Cyclosporine has been reported to inhibit the production of interleukin (IL)-2 and -3 and interferon-γ as a result of blockage in the transcription of lymphokine genes. Inhibition of IL-2 appears to be of paramount importance for its immunosuppressive effect. It is not clear whether the expression of IL-2 receptors is also inhibited. Cyclosporine does not affect expression of the T-cell antigen receptor or the proliferative responses of T-helper or cytotoxic T-cells induced by IL-2 (Herold et al, 1986).

Binding of cyclosporine to calmodulin, a protein with a central regulatory role in Ca^{2+}-mediated cellular processes, was thought to be responsible for its immunosuppressive effect (Colombani et al, 1985). However, subsequent studies did not support this hypothesis (LeGrue et al, 1986; Hait et al, 1986), and other studies suggested that cyclosporine exerts many of its effects by the specific inhibition of T-cell receptor (TCR)-mediated activation events (Shevach, 1985; Jenkins et al, 1988).

More recently, considerable insight has been gained into the molecular action of cyclosporine. Following the binding of TCR to a major histocompatibility complex (MHC)-associated antigen, stimulation of the T-cell results in activation of a TCR signal transmission pathway. The signal is transduced through the cytoplasm and activates specific nuclear transcription factors, such as the nuclear factor of activated T-cells (NF-AT). These nuclear factors regulate the transcription of T-cell activation genes, such as the gene for IL-2. NF-AT is formed when a signal from the TCR induces a pre-existing cytoplasmic subunit to translocate to the nucleus and combine with a newly synthesized subunit of NF-AT. Cyclosporine binds to cyclophilin, a cytoplasmic protein with cis-trans prolyl isomerase activity, and recent evidence suggests that the immunosuppressive effects of the drug are mediated by the cyclosporine-cyclophilin complex. The complex binds to calcineurin, a cytoplasmic protein with serine phosphatase activity. Binding inhibits the phosphatase activity of the enzyme and the translocation of the cytoplasmic component of NF-AT from the cytosol to the nucleus, thus preventing transcription of IL-2 mRNA (Flanagan et al, 1991; Liu et al, 1991; Schreiber, 1991; Thomson, in press).

Cyclosporine may have multiple sites of action. In vitro studies indicate that it inhibits release of preformed histamine from human basophils and de novo synthesis of inflammatory mediators (Cirillo et al, 1990). This suggests that in addition to its effects on lymphokine gene expression, cyclosporine also can interfere with the release of mediators from human inflammatory cells.

Although cyclosporine prevents GVHD in animals, irradiated species who received syngeneic bone marrow transplants and subsequently were treated with this agent developed autoimmunity on drug withdrawal (Hess et al, 1985). This same phenomenon has been observed in humans (Hood et al, 1987). Administration of cyclosporine to newborn mice has produced organ-specific autoimmune disease (Sakaguchi and Sakaguchi, 1989). Removal of the thymus in animals prior to the administration of the drug prevented the induction of autoimmunity; this suggests that this organ is necessary for the development of autoimmunity. A reduction in MHC class II molecule expression in the thymic medulla or effects on the development of suppressor cells that regulate autoreactive T-cell clones have been postulated to explain the phenomenon (Cheney and Sprent, 1985; Sakaguchi and Sakaguchi, 1988). Cyclosporine inhibits the development of TCR-$\alpha\beta^+$ thymocytes without discernibly affecting TCR-$\gamma\delta^+$ thymocytes or interfering with deletion of cells bearing self-reactive TCRs in the population of single positive thymocytes that do develop; this suggests a direct mechanism for cyclosporine-induced autoimmunity (Jenkins et al, 1988).

Cyclosporine is extensively metabolized, and some of these metabolites may have immunosuppressive properties (Rosano et al, 1986).

USES. This potent immunosuppressant is indicated to prevent organ rejection in kidney, liver, and heart allogeneic transplants. The manufacturer's package insert states that it should always be used with adrenal corticosteroids. However, some transplant centers, particularly in Europe, reserve use of corticosteroids for treatment of acute rejection.

Cyclosporine also may be used to prevent chronic rejection in patients previously treated with other immunosuppressants. It is the drug of choice for maintenance of kidney, liver, heart, pancreas, and lung allografts. One-year kidney transplant survival has increased from approximately 50% (for conventional therapy) to more than 75%, hospitalization time has decreased, and patient survival has increased to 95% to 98% beyond one year. Survival of liver transplants has improved from about 30% to more than 75% after one year. One-year survival rates for heart transplants have increased to more than 75%.

Investigationally, cyclosporine has been used to treat established GVHD in bone marrow transplant patients and to prevent bone marrow transplant rejection. When used alone, it has had no advantage over conventional immunosuppressive measures in segmental pancreatic allograft recipients. However, a significant reduction in the incidence of GVHD occurred in marrow transplant patients who received both methotrexate and cyclosporine compared with those who received cyclosporine alone (33% and 54%, respectively). In addition, the actuarial survival rates for the two groups at 1.5 years were 80% and 55%, respectively (Storb et al, 1986). A more recent report updated the results of this randomized prospective trial with follow-up of 3 to 4.5 years after transplantation. The incidence of chronic GVHD was nearly identical in the two groups (26% and 24%). The disease-free three-year survival rate was slightly better in the methotrexate/cyclosporine group (65% versus 54%), but this was observed only in patients with chronic myelocytic leukemia (73% versus 54%); no improvement was seen in those with acute nonlymphoblastic leukemia (Storb et al, 1989).

Cyclosporine is being investigated for a number of autoimmune diseases, including diabetes mellitus, multiple sclerosis, myasthenia gravis, ocular inflammation (eg, uveitis, Behcet's disease), psoriasis, rheumatoid arthritis, nephrotic syndrome, and ulcerative colitis. Other autoimmune diseases in which cyclosporine has been investigated include Grave's ophthalmopathy, biliary cirrhosis, pulmonary sarcoidosis, Wegner's granulomatosis, systemic lupus erythematosus, amyotrophic lateral sclerosis, aplastic anemia, dermatomyositis, polymyositis, Crohn's disease, pure red cell aplasia, pemphigus, glomerular diseases, and alopecia areata.

Cyclosporine also has been effective in the treatment of schistosomiasis; malaria; filariasis; and *Coccidioides immitis, Giardia, Leishmania,* and *Cryptococcus* infections in experimental animals (Bout et al, 1986; Belosevic et al, 1986; Solbach et al, 1986; Mody et al, 1988).

See also index entry Cyclosporine, Uses.

ADVERSE REACTIONS. The most frequent adverse reactions are renal dysfunction, hypertension, hirsutism, and neurotoxicity; other effects include thromboembolism, hepatotoxicity, diabetogenesis, and gingival hyperplasia. Some patients who develop hypertension may require antihypertensive therapy.

Nephrotoxicity (incidence 25% to 38%) is the most frequent and important toxic effect of cyclosporine. Renal dysfunction can occur immediately after transplant, especially if cyclosporine is administered intravenously; this effect may be enhanced by cadaveric renal allograft ischemia. In renal transplant patients, a major difficulty is differentiating drug-induced nephrotoxicity from acute rejection episodes; the diagnosis is generally one of exclusion. This adverse reaction has been defined as an increase in serum creatinine levels of more than 25% over several days that is reversed by decreasing the dose of cyclosporine. In patients with acute renal allograft rejection, there is a sudden increase in serum creatinine associated with fever, graft tenderness, and decreased urine output and renal blood flow, and cellular infiltrate is observable on biopsy (Ptachcinski et al, 1985 A). The mechanism by which cyclosporine exerts its nephrotoxic effects is unknown, but intrarenal vasoconstriction appears to be an important component. Histologic studies reveal glomerular thromboses, severe tubular damage, and giant mitochondria; fine needle biopsies reveal deposits of the drug.

Neurotoxic effects associated with cyclosporine include hallucinations (Noll and Kulkarni, 1984), limb paresthesias (incidence, 50%); fine distal upper extremity tremor (incidence, 20%), and seizures (Shah et al, 1984; Powell-Jackson et al, 1984; Beaman et al, 1985). The latter tend to occur within the first month of treatment. Some seizures appear to be due to profound hypomagnesemia and renal magnesium wasting (Thompson et al, 1984; June et al, 1985). Adequate magnesium replacement has resolved seizures and prevented recurrences (Thompson et al, 1984).

Hepatotoxicity (incidence 4% to 7%) also occurs in patients given cyclosporine. This is accompanied by an increase in both direct and total bilirubin concentrations; serum transaminases and alkaline phosphatase are increased in approximately 50% of patients with hyperbilirubinemia. A reduction in cyclosporine dosage rapidly reverses the hepatotoxic effects.

In a retrospective study on 90 recipients of cadaveric kidney allografts who were treated with cyclosporine, 17 thromboembolic complications occurred in 13 patients. Increased concentrations of factor VIII:C, fibrinogen, antithrombin III, and protein C were found in treated patients, and adenosine-5′-diphosphate-induced platelet aggregation was enhanced (Vanrenterghen et al, 1985). However, in a subsequent report, no increase in deep vein thrombosis could be associated with use of cyclosporine (Bergentz et al, 1985). Cyclosporine-related thrombosis is mainly a feature of renal allografts; the association with thrombosis elsewhere is doubtful. Some investigators believe that thromboembolic complications are not a common problem in patients receiving cyclosporine; however, such complications have been common in renal transplant patients treated with azathioprine and prednisolone (Zazgornik et al, 1985).

Lymphoproliferative disease has developed in patients receiving cyclosporine. These neoplasms do not appear to be specific to cyclosporine therapy but probably are due to immunosuppression per se. Infections have been observed in transplant recipients receiving cyclosporine, but compared with patients receiving conventional immunosuppressive therapy, the incidence generally has been lower (Hofflin et al, 1987).

Rarely, patients have developed a hypersensitivity reaction to intravenous cyclosporine, but no reactions have occurred with subsequent oral administration using the soft-gelatin capsule formulation. Hypersensitivity reactions after use of the oral solution have been reported rarely.

PRECAUTIONS. Therapeutic levels may be difficult to achieve in patients with malabsorption. Oral absorption is erratic, and blood levels should be monitored. Subsequent dosage adjustments may be required to avoid toxicity due to overdose or organ rejection due to low drug levels.

Renal and liver function tests should be performed regularly during cyclosporine therapy. Blood urea nitrogen (BUN) levels may be elevated; this may be related to concomitant administration of steroids. In renal transplant patients, this does not necessarily indicate rejection and each patient must be evaluated individually before any dosage adjustment is made. Persistently high levels of BUN and creatinine that do not respond to adjustment in dosage may suggest that other immunosuppressive therapy should be considered. However, in addition to dose adjustment, other procedures, such as biopsy, renal flow scan, or ultrasound, are indicated prior to substituting other immunosuppressive therapy.

If there are signs of chronic unremitting rejection, it is preferable to remove the transplanted kidney rather than to increase dosage to a high level in an attempt to inhibit the rejection. Cyclosporine has not been proven effective in reversing established graft rejection. However, large doses may be indicated in some patients because of the highly variable pharmacokinetics of this agent.

Monitoring of blood or plasma concentrations of cyclosporine has been recommended as a means of limiting toxicity while ensuring sufficient immunosuppression. Critical issues in cyclosporine monitoring have been reviewed and three major consensus statements regarding assay, specimen, frequency of testing, and therapeutic range have been published (*Clin Chem*, 1987; *Transplant Proc*, 1990; Shaw et al, 1990).

Large oral doses of cyclosporine are embryotoxic and fetotoxic in rats and rabbits. This drug should be used during pregnancy only if the potential benefit justifies the potential risk to the fetus (FDA Pregnancy Category C). Successful pregnancies in patients receiving cyclosporine have been reported. Cyclosporine is excreted in human milk; therefore, nursing should be avoided.

DRUG INTERACTIONS. Synergistic effects may occur when cyclosporine is used with other nephrotoxic drugs. Interactions with the following drugs are well substantiated: gentamicin, tobramycin, vancomycin, amphotericin B, ketoconazole, melphalan, cimetidine, ranitidine, diclofenac, trimethoprim with sulfamethoxazole, and apazone (azapropazon). Combined use with ciprofloxacin also has been reported to cause nephrotoxicity.

Drugs that affect the mixed-function oxidase system can alter the metabolism of cyclosporine. The drug is extensively metabolized by the liver, and circulating levels may be altered by drugs that affect hepatic microsomal enzymes, especially the cytochrome P450 system. Substances that inhibit these enzymes decrease hepatic metabolism and therefore increase cyclosporine levels, whereas substances that induce cytochrome P450 activity increase hepatic metabolism and thus decrease drug levels. Cyclosporine blood levels must be monitored and dosage adjustment made as needed when such drugs are used concomitantly.

Drugs that are reported to increase cyclosporine levels include diltiazem, nicardipine, verapamil, ketoconazole, fluconazole, itraconazole, danazol, bromocriptine, metoclopramide, erythromycin, and methylprednisolone. Oral contraceptives and anabolic steroids also have been reported to increase blood levels. Drugs that decrease cyclosporine levels include rifampin, phenytoin, phenobarbital, and carbamazepine.

Reduced clearance of prednisolone, digoxin, and lovastatin has been observed when these drugs were administered with cyclosporine. Several cases of reversible myopathy with rhabdomyolysis have been reported during combined therapy with lovastatin and cyclosporine. The apparent volume of distribution of digoxin has decreased after cyclosporine administration; severe digitalis toxicity occurred in several patients within a few days after cyclosporine administration. Cyclosporine should not be used with potassium-sparing diuretics because hyperkalemia can occur. Vaccination may be less effective in patients given cyclosporine; the use of live virus vaccines should be avoided in these individuals. Gingival hyperplasia has occurred frequently when cyclosporine was administered with nifedipine. Convulsions have been induced when large doses of methylprednisolone were given with cyclosporine. (See the manufacturer's literature for further information on drug interactions.)

PHARMACOKINETICS. Absorption of cyclosporine from the gastrointestinal tract is incomplete and variable. Although kinetics are highly variable, the manufacturer's literature indicates that peak blood and plasma concentrations (C_{max}) occur in approximately 3.5 hours; C_{max} is about 1 ng/ml/mg of dose for plasma and 1.4 to 2.7 ng/ml/mg of dose for blood (for low to high doses). Compared with intravenous infusion, the absolute bioavailability of the oral solution is about 30%. Administration of cyclosporine with food has been reported to increase peak and trough blood concentrations, as well as the area under the blood concentration versus time curve (mean increase, 60%) (Ptachcinski et al, 1985 B). Malabsorption of oral cyclosporine is a common problem after orthotopic liver transplantation.

The volume of distribution of cyclosporine ranges from less than 1 to 13 L/kg. Most of the drug is distributed outside the blood volume. Distribution is concentration-dependent in blood; 33% to 47% is in plasma, 4% to 9% in leukocytes, 5% to 12% in granulocytes, and 41% to 58% in erythrocytes. Uptake by leukocytes and erythrocytes becomes saturated at high concentrations. Approximately 90% of a dose is bound to plasma proteins, primarily lipoproteins.

Cyclosporine is extensively metabolized but there is no major metabolic pathway. Only 0.1% of a dose is excreted as unchanged drug in the urine; 15 metabolites have been characterized in human urine. The cytochrome P450 liver enzyme systems are responsible for metabolism. The rate of cyclosporine clearance is low to intermediate and is highly variable. The rate appears to be higher in the late evening and morning; thus, trough levels should be determined at the same time each day.

Disposition of the drug from blood is biphasic with a terminal half-life ranging from 10 to 27 hours. Cyclosporine is eliminated primarily in the bile, and only 6% of a dose is excreted in the urine.

DOSAGE AND PREPARATIONS.

Intravenous, Oral: The dose should be determined carefully for each patient. The absorption of cyclosporine is erratic; therefore, blood concentrations should be monitored frequently and the dosage adjusted accordingly. Cyclosporine is routinely administered with adrenal corticosteroids; its use with other immunosuppressive agents is investigational.

Different transplant centers have employed different protocols. Some centers do not administer cyclosporine to renal transplant patients until after postoperative diuresis. For further information, see the manufacturer's package insert.

Sandimmune (Sandoz). Capsules (soft gelatin) 25 and 100 mg (alcohol 12.7%); solution (intravenous) 50 mg/ml in 5 ml containers (alcohol 32.9%); solution (oral) 100 mg/ml (alcohol 12.5%).

MUROMONAB-CD3 (Murine Monoclonal Antibody, Anti-CD3, Human T-Cell Inhibitor)

[Orthoclone OKT3]

Muromonab-CD3 is a monoclonal antibody to the T3 (CD3) antigen of human T-lymphocytes (Kung et al, 1979; Van Wauwe et al, 1980). The T_3 molecule is associated with the antigen recognition site of T-cells and is essential for signal transduction (Chang et al, 1981). The monoclonal antibody is purified IgG_{2a} and contains two heavy chains of about 50,000 daltons and two light chains of approximately 25,000 daltons.

ACTIONS. Muromonab-CD3 reverses acute allograft rejection in renal transplant patients by blocking the function and generation of cytotoxic T-lymphocytes responsible for renal inflammation and destruction during acute renal rejection. The antibody combines with and blocks the function of a 20,000-dalton molecule (CD3) located in the cytoplasmic membrane of T-cells associated with the antigen recognition structure and essential for signal transduction. Circulating T-lymphocytes bearing the CD3 antigen, including CD4 and CD8 expressing cells, are removed from the circulation within minutes following intravenous administration of muromonab-CD3. Complement is not involved in this reaction, and removal probably results from phagocytic activity of the reticuloendothelial system that follows opsonization by the monoclonal antibody. After one week of daily administration, there is a gradual return of lymphocytes expressing the CD4 and CD8 antigens but a continued absence of cells expressing the CD3 antigen; this suggests a modulation and blockage of the Ti/CD3 TCR. Evidence indicates that muromonab-CD3 exerts its in vivo immunosuppressive effects in part by antigenic modulation of the T3/Ti cell receptor complex. Modulated cells reversibly lose the expression of the CD3 TCR complex and have been shown to be functionally immunoincompetent. Antigenic modulation is maintained as long as significant levels of anti-CD3 levels are present. In the absence of this antibody, T-cells re-express the CD3-Ti receptor complex. This induced antigenic modulation takes place within the allograft and thus appears to represent a major mechanism contributing to the clinical efficacy of muromonab-CD3 (Caillat-Zucman et al, 1990).

Two other mechanisms for the immunosuppressive effect of muromonab-CD3 have been proposed: (1) mediation of cytolysis by inter-T cell bridging, and (2) apoptosis (programmed cell death). In the former, there is evidence that anti-CD3 antibodies (which are divalent) cross-link CD3 antigen on two different cells and induce TCR-dependent, antibody-bridged, cell-mediated cytolysis between T-cells; thus, this is a mechanism whereby T-cells lyse other T-cells in the presence of anti-CD3 monoclonal antibodies (Wong et al, 1990). Apoptosis is characterized by the cleavage of DNA into small fragments. This fragmentation is initiated by exogenous signals that activate calcium-dependent endonucleases and drive the cells to an internal "suicide." Data have been published demonstrating that monoclonal antibody directed against the TCR/CD3 complex, including muromonab-CD3, induces apoptosis in preactivated human TCR-α/β as well as γ/δ-positive T-cells. Apoptosis, then, may be an important mechanism affecting the removal of activated T-cells by this monoclonal antibody (Janssen et al, 1992). These two mechanisms may help to explain further the sustained action and efficacy of muromonab-CD3.

Increased numbers of CD3 cells have been observed in patients during the second week of therapy with muromonab-CD3, possibly as a consequence of the development of host antibodies to the monoclonal antibody resulting in reduced immunosuppressive activity. The incidence of such antibodies is 21% for IgM, 86% for IgG, and 29% for IgE. The mean time of appearance of these antibodies is about 20 days. Between days 2 and 7, circulating CD4 and CD8 cell numbers increase.

Leukocytes have been observed in cerebrospinal and peritoneal fluid following administration of muromonab-CD3; the mechanism for this effect is unknown.

USES. In an early study, established renal allograft rejection episodes in eight patients were reversed within two to seven days by muromonab-CD3 antibody despite continued reduction of the steroid dosages employed (Cosimi et al, 1981). Similar success occurred in a second study that also involved a small number of patients. In the latter study, production of human antimurine antibodies was observed, which suggested that administration of muromonab-CD3 may be limited to a single short course in each patient (Burton et al, 1982). In a prospective, randomized, multicenter trial involving 123 patients experiencing acute rejection of cadaveric renal transplants, muromonab-CD3 reversed 94% of the rejections compared to 75% with conventional steroid treatment. The superior reversal rate with muromonab-CD3 was reflected by an improved one-year graft survival of 62% for the muromonab-CD3-treated group versus 45% for the steroid-treated group (Ortho Multicenter Transplant Study Group, 1985). At two-year follow up, the rates were 56% and 42%, respectively. Patient survival at one and two years did not differ significantly between the two groups.

In additional open clinical trials, the reversal rate for acute renal allograft rejection was 92% with muromonab-CD3 therapy. This antibody preparation also reversed rejections in 65% of patients in whom steroids and lymphocyte immune globulin were contraindicated or not used.

Although host antibodies to the injected monoclonal antibody have been observed, they have not severely limited the efficacy of muromonab-CD3 following retreatment or caused serious adverse reactions. Between 40% and 80% of transplant patients initially treated with muromonab-CD3 develop host antibodies to the idiotypic region, and host antimurine antibody has developed in as many as 28% of the patients. The antimurine antibody has been of special concern since it could prevent the use of other murine monoclonals. However, successful retreatment of allograft rejection has been reported in patients who had either no or only low-titer antiidiotypic or antimurine antibodies, although re-exposure to the monoclonal antibody further stimulated antimonoclonal antibody production and broadened the specificity of the antibodies produced (Mayes et al, 1988; Norman et al, 1988; First et al, 1989). It has been recommended that retreatment with muromonab-CD3 not be considered unless the antibody status of the patient is known and that alternative antirejection therapy be used in patients with a high-titer antimurine response. A larger dose of the monoclonal antibody also has been necessary for the successful retreatment of patients with low-titer antimurine antibody (First et al, 1989).

Investigationally, muromonab-CD3 is being used to treat rejection of other organ transplants (eg, liver, pancreas, heart) (D'Alessandro et al, 1990; Stratta et al, 1991). A multi-institutional randomized trial comparing muromonab-CD3 with steroids concluded that the former was superior in reversing liver allograft rejection and greatly reduced the need for retransplantation (Cosimi et al, 1987). Retreatment also was reported to reverse rejection of liver transplants (Millis et al, 1989). Similarly, muromonab-CD3 has been reported to be safe and effective in reversing cardiac allograft rejection refractory to conventional therapy with high-dose steroids and antithymocyte globulin (Gilbert et al, 1987; Klein et al, 1988).

ADVERSE REACTIONS AND PRECAUTIONS. Determinations of adverse reactions have been obtained primarily from patients who were simultaneously receiving low-dose immunosuppressive therapy, principally azathioprine and corticosteroids. A high incidence of adverse effects (pyrexia, chills, and dyspnea) has been observed following the first dose of this monoclonal antibody. The most serious first-dose reaction is severe pulmonary edema; because this has been observed in approximately 2% of patients, it is recommended that muromonab-CD3 not be given to hypervolemic patients and that all patients be closely supervised after administration of the first dose. First-dose reactions may be minimized by using the regimens in Table 8.

In addition to the pyrexia and chills experienced as part of the first-dose reaction, a number of other adverse reactions occur primarily within the first three days of therapy. These include chest pain (14%), dyspnea (21%), wheezing

TABLE 8.
PREVENTION AND TREATMENT OF MUROMONAB-CD3 FIRST-DOSE EFFECTS

Adverse Reaction	Prevention or Palliation	Supportive Treatment
Severe pulmonary edema	Clear chest x-ray within 24 hours preinjection	Prompt intubation and oxygenation; 24 hours close observation
	Weight restriction to ≤3% gain over 7 days preinjection	
Fever, chills	10 mg/kg methylprednisolone sodium succinate preinjection	Cooling blanket
	Fever reduction below 37.8 °C (100° F) preinjection	Acetaminophen as required
Respiratory effects	100 mg hydrocortisone sodium succinate 30 minutes postinjection	Additional 100 mg hydrocortisone sodium succinate as required

(13%), nausea (19%), vomiting (19%), diarrhea (14%), tremor (13%), headache (11%), and tachycardia (10%). Hypotension, abnormal chest sounds, pruritus, and hypoventilation also have been reported. The incidence of infections was modestly increased in renal transplant patients receiving muromonab-CD3 compared with those receiving conventional therapy, and the infections were more likely to be serious (Oh et al, 1988).

The dosages of other immunosuppressive agents used with muromonab-CD3 should be reduced to minimal levels.

Muromonab-CD3 should not be given to patients who are hypersensitive to this or any product of murine origin. Patients who have fluid overload confirmed by chest x-ray or whose weight has increased by >3% in the previous week also should not receive this agent. Antibodies (IgM, IgG, and IgE) to this preparation have been observed during and following its use. One report of anaphylaxis and two possible cases of serum sickness have been associated with these antibodies.

Therapy should be conducted in facilities equipped and staffed with adequate laboratory and supportive medical resources. The product should not be administered to patients whose temperature exceeds 100° F; antipyretics may be used to reduce the temperature.

This product contains polysorbate 80 and must not be used for the in vitro treatment of bone marrow.

The safety and efficacy of muromonab-CD3 in children have not been established, but patients as young as 2 years have received the drug with no unusual effects (for review, see Ryckman et al, 1991).

Muromonab-CD3 monoclonal antibody should be given to pregnant women only if clearly needed (FDA Pregnancy Category C).

An aseptic meningitis syndrome was identified in a postmarketing survey. Reported symptoms were fever (89%), headache (44%), neck stiffness (14%), and photophobia (10%); a combination of these symptoms occurred in 5% of patients.

PHARMACOKINETICS. Following treatment with 5 mg/day for 14 days, mean serum trough levels increased during the first three days and then averaged 0.9 mcg/ml on days 3 to 14. The levels attained during therapy block T-cell effector functions in vitro.

DOSAGE AND PREPARATIONS.
Intravenous: *Adults*, for the treatment of acute renal allograft rejection, 5 mg/day by intravenous push for 10 to 14 days using a low protein-binding (0.2 or 0.22 micron) filter. The dosage of conventional immunosuppressive therapy given concomitantly should be decreased to minimal levels during the administration of muromonab-CD3. The manufacturer should be consulted for information on measures to decrease the incidence of first-dose reactions. See also Table 8.

Orthoclone OKT3 (Ortho Biotech). Solution (sterile, buffered) 1 mg/ml in 5 ml containers.

AGENTS FOR IMMUNOENHANCEMENT

ALDESLEUKIN (Interleukin 2)
[Proleukin]

Interleukin 2 (IL-2), a lymphokine produced by activated helper T-lymphocytes, induces the proliferation of T-cells and promotes the differentiation of lymphocytes into cytotoxic cells. IL-2 also induces the production of interferon-γ and activates natural killer (NK) cells and other lymphokine-activated killer (LAK) cells.

IL-2 has been cloned in bacteria through recombinant DNA technology, thus allowing the production of large amounts. No functional difference was observed between native and recombinant IL-2 in supporting the growth of IL-2-dependent cell lines, enhancing the generation of cytolytic cells in vitro, or generating LAK cells from lymphocyte preparations (Rosenberg et al, 1984). Studies with natural and recombinant materials suggest that IL-2 can sustain proliferation but not differentiation of B-cells, that activated B-lymphocytes carry functional IL-2 receptors at their surface, and that IL-2 appears to increase the production of IL-1 (Jacques and Soulillou, 1985).

In vitro studies on animal and human cells have shown that T-cell responses are potentiated and restored by IL-2. Sufficient quantities of IL-2 are now available, and a number of clinical studies are currently being conducted.

Lymphocytes from patients with AIDS produce significantly less IL-2 than cells from healthy controls and have a greatly decreased proliferative response to mitogen induction. Addition of IL-2 to lymphocyte cultures from AIDS patients partially or fully restored this response in approximately 50% of treated cultures. Clinical trials of IL-2 in combination with antiviral drugs are currently in progress in AIDS patients. Adoptive immunotherapy employing LAK cells and repeated injections of recombinant IL-2 (aldesleukin) was reported to be highly effective in reducing the numbers and size of established pulmonary sarcoma metastases in mice (Mulé et al, 1984).

IL-2 (aldesleukin) is indicated for the treatment of renal cell carcinoma. Malignant melanoma and colorectal carcinoma also have been reported to be sensitive to IL-2/LAK therapy (Rosenberg et al, 1987; Oliver, 1988). For further information, see index entry Interleukin 2, In Cancer.

Proleukin (Cetus).

BCG VACCINE

BCG vaccine is an attenuated strain of *Mycobacterium bovis*. It has been used in the past to induce immunity against tuberculosis but results were variable. This agent also has been administered as a nonspecific stimulator of the immune system in patients with cancer. Success in the treatment of tumors with BCG is most likely when the neoplasm is small and localized, the patient has a normally functioning immune system, there is close contact between BCG and tumor cells, and a sufficient number of viable organisms is administered. (See index entry BCG, In Cancer.)

In many subjects, BCG appears to act principally by nonspecifically stimulating the reticuloendothelial system. It is not known whether this is a primary effect or secondary to T-cell activation and lymphokine production. This agent activates natural killer cells and enhances the production of hematopoietic stem cells. BCG has been reported to cross-react with melanoma, leukemia, and hepatoma cells, which could explain reports of specific effects on these types of tumors. Macrophages affected by BCG become more active killer cells and more efficiently clear antigen and immune complexes and recruit other cells involved in the destruction of cancer cells.

The precise mechanism of action of BCG in the treatment of carcinoma in situ of the urinary bladder is unknown. It promotes a local inflammatory response with histiocytic and leukocytic infiltration in the urinary bladder, and this effect is associated with elimination or reduction of the cancerous cells. An HLA-restricted T-cell response may be involved in the treatment of superficial bladder cancer with intravesicular BCG, for it was found to induce HLA class II antigen expression on tumor cells (Prescott et al, 1989). In addition, a direct correlation between the amount of interleukin-2 released into the urine following BCG therapy and the treatment response has been reported (Ratliff et al, 1986; Fleischmann et al, 1987, 1989).

Under certain circumstances, BCG may enhance tumor growth, apparently due to formation of immune complexes (BCG/anti-BCG) that block the cytotoxic action of lymphocytes and stimulation of antigen-specific T-suppressor cells. However, this has not been clearly demonstrated in the treatment of cancer of the urinary bladder.

See also index entry BCG Vaccine.

INTERFERON GAMMA-1b

[Actimmune]

Interferon gamma-1b is a single-chain polypeptide containing 140 amino acids. This recombinant interferon is produced by fermentation of genetically engineered *Escherichia coli* containing the relevant DNA and is purified by conventional column chromatography.

ACTIONS. The interferons (IFNs) consist of three families of protein molecules (alpha, beta, and gamma) whose production can be induced in most eukaryotic cells in response to a variety of stimuli, including viruses. All the IFNs have antiviral activity, but there are important differences between the three classes. For example, there are at least 17 human IFN-α genes, but only one IFN-β gene and one IFN-γ gene.

Several characteristics distinguish IFN-γ from IFN-α and IFN-β. IFN-γ is produced by sensitized T-lymphocytes and natural killer (NK) cells, whereas IFN-α is produced by several types of leukocytes and IFN-β is produced by fibroblasts, epithelial cells, and macrophages. IFN-γ has potent phagocyte-activating effects that have not been reported for the other interferons. It is the principal macrophage-activating factor, and it enhances the production of reactive oxygen intermediates and the killing of bacterial and protozoan pathogens both in vitro and in vivo. In addition to the enhancement of the oxidative burst in macrophages, IFN-γ enhances antibody-dependent cellular cytotoxicity and NK cell activity. In addition, it affects the expression of both the Fc receptor and the major histocompatibility antigens.

There is a growing consensus that IFN-γ should be characterized as a lymphokine of the interleukin (IL) type and that all of the interleukins form part of a complex lymphokine regulatory network. For example, IFN-γ activates macrophages by inducing the production of tumor necrosis factor (TNF). TNF can have an antiviral effect through the induction of IFNβ, and this antiviral activity may be enhanced by IFN-γ. IFN-γ also can enhance the cytolytic activity of TNF. Enhancement of NK cell activity by IL-2 is correlated with the induction of IFN-γ, which itself may be directly cytolytic. IL-1 can induce IL-2, which in turn induces IFN-γ or IFN-β. Finally, IFN-γ and IL-4 may act reciprocally to suppress IgE levels in humans.

The principal action of IFN-γ in chronic granulomatous disease (CGD) appears to be most directly related to elevation of superoxide levels in macrophages, which results in improved killing of ingested bacterial cells. Although phagocytes of CGD patients ingest microorganisms normally, killing is deficient due to the failure of a membrane-associated enzyme complex, nicotinamide-adenine dinucleotide phosphate (NADPH), to produce superoxide and related oxygen metabolites. NADPH is involved in the production of the superoxide necessary to generate bactericidal agents such as hydrogen peroxide, hypochlorous acid, and chloramine.

USES. Interferon gamma-1b is indicated to reduce the frequency and severity of serious infections associated with CGD.

CGD is a rare (incidence, 1 case/million persons), inherited disease that results in pediatric immunodeficiency and, when untreated, can be life-threatening. About two-thirds of the patients inherit the disease according to an X-linked pattern, while the remainder follow an autosomal recessive pattern. Most patients experience chronic and recurring infections; granulomas formed as a result of these chronic infections can lead to obstruction of the gastrointestinal and genitourinary tracts.

Preclinical studies demonstrated that the addition of IFN-gamma-1b to in vitro cultures of granulocytes and monocytes from patients with various genetic types of CGD partially corrected the defect in superoxide production. In an early clinical trial on four patients with the X-linked form of the disease, IFN-gamma-1b 0.1 mg/M^2 was administered subcutaneously on two consecutive days. This treatment produced a five- to tenfold increase in superoxide production by the patients' granulocytes and monocytes, and the increased function was sustained for more than two weeks. Granulocyte bactericidal activity rose proportionally, there was an increase in the cellular contents of phagocyte cytochrome b (a critical component of the superoxide-producing oxidase) and in the immunoreactive cytochrome b heavy chain (the product of the gene defective in X-linked CGD), and levels of cytochrome b rose from zero to 10% to 50% of normal values (Ezekowitz et al, 1988).

More recently, in a randomized, double-blind, placebo-controlled study on 128 patients (median age, 15 years) with CGD, IFN-gamma-1b 50 mcg/M^2 or placebo was administered subcutaneously three times weekly for up to one year. Most of the patients also received prophylactic antibiotics. With respect to time to serious infection, the primary endpoint of the investigation, a mean of 77% of patients in the IFN-gamma-1b-treated group were free of serious infection 12 months after randomization compared with 30% in the placebo group. Further, 14/63 patients in the IFN-gamma-1b group versus 30/65 patients in the placebo group had serious infections; there was also a reduction in the total number of serious infections in the IFN-gamma-1b group (20 versus 56). Treatment with IFN-gamma-1b was beneficial regardless of patient age, gender, the use of prophylactic antibiotics, or whether the disease was of the X-linked or autosomal recessive type. However, the investigators could not detect any significant changes in superoxide production by the patients' phagocytes. IFN-gamma-1b was well tolerated, and no serious toxicity was reported. These results strongly suggested that IFN-gamma-1b, in conjunction with prophylactic antibiotics, be considered the recommended treatment for patients with CGD (The International Chronic Granulomatous Disease Cooperative Study Group, 1991). However, similar results were not obtained in a European study on a smaller number of patients (58) who appear to have had milder disease, which suggests that in this subgroup, aggressive antibiotic prophylaxis should be considered as the initial treatment of choice and that IFN-gamma-1b be reserved for adjuvant therapy at the time of serious infection (Mouy et al, 1991; Ezekowitz, 1991).

IFN-gamma-1b has been used investigationally for the treatment of dermatologic diseases such as atopic dermatitis, genital warts, and keloids (Mahrle and Schulze, 1990; Gross, 1991). Rationale for its use in prevention or treatment of AIDS-related opportunistic infections has been published (Murray, 1990).

ADVERSE REACTIONS AND PRECAUTIONS. Since intravenous or intramuscular administration of IFN-gamma-1b was associated with increased adverse effects, it now is given only subcutaneously. The most common adverse events are "flu-like" or constitutional symptoms that may decrease in severity as treatment continues. These symptoms may be minimized by administration at bedtime; acetaminophen may be employed to prevent or partially alleviate fever and headache. The following adverse effects were more common than with placebo in CGD patients given IFN-gamma-1b 50 mcg/M^2 three times weekly: fever (52%), headache (33%), erythema or tenderness at the injection site (14%), and chills (14%). Rash, vomiting, nausea, and myalgia occurred less frequently.

IFN-gamma-1b should be used cautiously in patients with pre-existing cardiac disease; doses of 250 mcg/M^2/day or larger may exacerbate these conditions. Patients with seizure disorders and/or compromised central nervous system (CNS) function also should be treated with caution. CNS reactions, particularly in patients receiving doses >250 mcg/M^2/day, include increased mental impairment, gait disturbance, and dizziness. Most of these effects are mild and reversible with dose reduction or discontinuation of therapy. Reversible neutropenia and elevation of hepatic enzymes can be dose limiting at amounts >250 mcg/M^2/day. The drug should be used cautiously in patients with myelosuppression. The long-term effects of IFN-gamma-1b therapy on growth, development, or other parameters are not known.

Hematologic tests, blood chemistries, and urinalysis are recommended for all patients prior to the initiation of IFN-gamma-1b therapy and at three-month intervals thereafter.

PREGNANCY AND LACTATION. IFN-gamma-1b should be used during pregnancy only if the potential benefit justifies the risk to the fetus (FDA Pregnancy Category C). The incidence of abortions was increased in primates when IFN-gamma-1b was given in doses approximately 100 times higher than the human dose. However, no teratogenic activity could be demonstrated in pregnant primates treated with intravenous doses 2 to 100 times higher than the human dose.

It is not known whether IFN-gamma-1b is excreted in human milk. Because of the potential for serious adverse reactions in infants, nursing should be discontinued or the drug withdrawn.

DRUG INTERACTIONS. Although interactions between IFN-gamma-1b and other drugs have not been fully evaluated, caution is advised when administering this drug with other potentially myelosuppressive agents. Studies in rodents using species-specific IFN-γ demonstrated a decrease in hepatic microsomal cytochrome P450 concentrations. Potentially, this could lead to depression of the hepatic metabolism of some drugs that use this degradative pathway.

PHARMACOKINETICS. Following the injection of a single dose (100 mcg/M^2), IFN-gamma-1b is rapidly cleared after intravenous administration (1.4 L/min) and slowly absorbed after intramuscular or subcutaneous administration. The mean elimination half-life after intravenous administration is 38 minutes and 2.9 and 5.9 hours after intramuscular or subcutaneous administration, respectively. The apparent fraction of dose absorbed after intramuscular or subcutaneous injection is greater than 89%. Peak plasma concentrations occur about four hours after intramuscular administration and seven hours after subcutaneous administration. IFN-gamma-1b has not been detected in the urine of healthy human volunteers after the administration of 100 mcg/M^2 by the intravenous, intramuscular, or subcutaneous routes.

DOSAGE AND PREPARATIONS.

Subcutaneous: For CGD, 50 mcg/M^2 (1.5 million units/M^2) for patients with a body surface area >0.5 M^2 and 1.5 mcg/kg/dose for patients with a body surface area ≤ 0.5 M^2. Larger doses are not recommended. The drug should be injected three times weekly; the optimum sites are the right and left deltoid and anterior thigh.

Intramuscular, Intravenous: In other diseases, IFN-gamma-1b has been administered by intravenous infusion or intramuscular injection at generally higher doses (>100 mcg/M^2/day) than are used currently in CGD.

Actimmune (Genentech). Solution (injection) containing 100 mcg (3 million units) in 0.5 ml vials (preservative free). The vial is suitable for a single dose only; the unused portion should be discarded.

LEVAMISOLE

[Ergamisol]

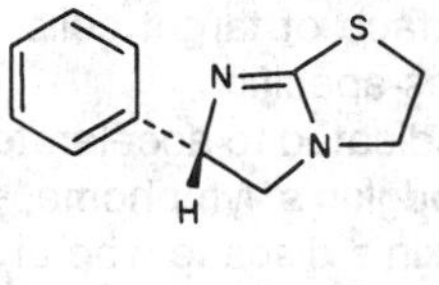

Levamisole, the levo-isomer of tetramisole and an established anthelmintic drug, was first reported to be an immunostimulant in 1972. Since then, it has been investigated in a large variety of disease states.

ACTIONS. The mechanism of action of levamisole is not completely understood. Depending on the dose and time of administration, it either augments or depresses immune responses; it usually acts as an immunopotentiator. Immunopotentiation generally requires the simultaneous administration of a primary stimulus, such as antigen. Levamisole has been referred to as an "immunonormalizing" agent since a normal immune system is not stimulated. T-cell function is enhanced more than B-cell function. Delayed hypersensitivity reactions have been restored or increased in the elderly and in patients with malignant and nonmalignant diseases.

The drug appears to act directly on lymphocytes, macrophages, and granulocytes to modify their proliferation, mobility, and secretion. The maturation and proliferation of T-cells are enhanced, but NK or K cells do not appear to be affected. Some investigators consider the principal action of levamisole to be facilitation of monocyte chemotaxis; the drug has been reported to enhance monocyte phagocytosis. It also increases neutrophil mobility, adherence, and chemotaxis. Defective Fc receptor activity of neutrophils has been restored (Patrone et al, 1985; Luzi et al, 1983). Levamisole has other pharmacologic properties including inhibition of alkaline phosphatase and cholinergic activity.

The mechanism of action of levamisole in combination with fluorouracil as a treatment regimen for stage III (Duke's stage C) colon cancer is unknown.

USES. Levamisole is indicated as adjuvant treatment in combination with fluorouracil after surgical resection in patients with stage III (Duke's stage C) colon cancer. It is not useful for the treatment of advanced or metastatic disease (see index entry Levamisole, In Cancer).

Levamisole also has been used to maintain steroid-free remission in children with steroid-responsive but dependent nephrotic syndrome. Alternative therapies are needed for children with this disease because alkylating drugs often do not maintain remission, and chronic steroid treatment may be complicated by drug toxicity. Children receiving alternate-day prednisolone therapy for corticosteroid-responsive but dependent nephrotic syndrome were randomly assigned to receive levamisole (2.5 mg/kg on alternate days) or placebo for a maximum of 112 days. The prednisolone dosage was gradually reduced and the drug was discontinued after 56 days. Forty-five percent of the patients in the levamisole group versus 13% in the placebo group remained in remission at 112 days despite the lack of steroid treatment; no significant adverse effects were reported (British Association for Paediatric Nephrology, 1991).

See also index entry Levamisole.

Ergamisol (Janssen).

PEGADEMASE BOVINE

[Adagen]

ACTIONS. Severe combined immunodeficiency disease (SCID) is a rare, inherited, and frequently fatal disease that is associated with a deficiency of the enzyme, adenosine deaminase (ADA). In the absence of this enzyme, the purine substrates, adenosine and 2′-deoxyadenosine, and their metabolites accumulate in lymphocytes causing metabolic disturbances that are toxic to the cells. Pegademase corrects this deficiency and, hence, the metabolic abnormalities. This drug is of no benefit to patients with immunodeficiency due to other causes. Pegademase is a conjugate of numerous strands of monomethoxypolyethylene glycol covalently attached to ADA. The ADA enzyme used in the manufacture of the product is derived from bovine intestine.

Improvement in immune function and decreased frequency of opportunistic infections occurs only after the metabolic abnormalities are corrected. The time between correction of the metabolic abnormalities and improvement in immune function ranges from a few weeks to six months.

USES. Pegademase is indicated for enzyme replacement therapy for ADA deficiency in patients with SCID who are not suitable candidates for or who have not benefitted from bone marrow transplantation. It is recommended for use in newborns as well as other children at the time of diagnosis. It is not intended as a replacement for HLA-identical bone marrow transplantation therapy. It also is not intended as a replacement for other therapies (eg, antibiotic, nutrition, oxygen, immune globulin) as indicated for intercurrent illnesses.

ADVERSE REACTIONS AND PRECAUTIONS. Clinical experience with pegademase is limited. Adverse reactions that have been observed include headache and pain at the injection site.

Pegademase should be used only by physicians knowledgeable in the treatment of immunodeficiency diseases. Because this agent is administered by intramuscular injection, it should be used with caution in patients with thrombocytopenia and not used at all if the condition is severe.

The optimal dosage and schedule of administration should be established for each individual patient based on monitoring of plasma ADA activity levels, biochemical markers of ADA deficiency, and parameters of immune function. Plasma ADA activity and erythrocyte dATP (deoxyadenosine nucleotide) levels should be determined prior to the initiation of therapy and monitored during therapy according to the manufacturer's instructions.

Antibody to pegademase may develop in some patients and may cause more rapid clearance of the drug. This should be suspected if preinjection levels of plasma ADA fall to 10 μmol/hr/ml or less and persist. If no other cause for such a decline can be determined, a specific assay for antibody to pegademase should be performed. If antibody is the cause of the fall, adjustment of the dose and other measures should be taken to induce tolerance and restore adequate ADA activity.

PREGNANCY AND LACTATION. This drug is classified in FDA Pregnancy Category C. Animal reproduction studies have not been conducted with this product, and it should be used in pregnant women only if clearly needed.

It is not known whether pegademase is excreted in human milk, but caution should be exercised if the drug is administered to nursing women.

DRUG INTERACTIONS. There have been no reported drug interactions with pegademase. However, vidarabine is a substrate for ADA and 2[1]-deoxycoformycin is a potent inhibitor of ADA. The activities of these drugs and pegademase could be altered if they are used in combination.

PHARMACOKINETICS. The pharmacokinetics of pegademase have been studied in 6-week-old to 12-year-old children with SCID associated with ADA deficiency. After intramuscular injection, peak plasma levels of ADA were reached two to three days after administration. The plasma elimination half-life was variable, ranging from three to >six days. Following weekly injections, the average trough level of plasma ADA activity was 20 to 35 μmol/hr/ml.

DOSAGE AND PREPARATIONS. Because potency of each lot of the product cannot be assured, any indication of a decrease in potency should be reported to the manufacturer immediately.

Intramuscular: The manufacturer recommends that the dosage be individualized. The recommended initial schedule is 30 units/kg twice weekly. Dosage in severely ill patients should be based on ideal body weight (ie, 50th percentile for a normal child of the same age). When the patient is stable and shows evidence of improving immune function, the frequency of injections is reduced to 30 units/kg once weekly. Maintenance dosage should be aimed at achieving (1) plasma ADA activity in the range of 20 to 35 μmol/hr/ml, and (2) decline in red blood cell dATP to 0.005 to 0.015 μmol/ml or less of packed erythrocytes or 1% or less of the total erythrocyte adenine nucleotide (ATP + dATP) content as determined in a preinjection sample.

Adagen (Enzon). Solution (injection) 250 units/ml in single-use 1.5 ml containers. The product should be kept refrigerated but not frozen.

SARGRAMOSTIM (GM-CSF)
[Leukine, Prokine]

ACTIONS AND USES. Sargramostim is a human granulocyte-macrophage colony stimulating factor (GM-CSF). This hematopoietic growth factor supports the growth and differentiation of stem cells into granulocytes and macrophages. It also is capable of activating mature granulocytes and macrophages and can promote the proliferation of megakaryocytes and erythroid progenitors, although other factors are required to induce the complete maturation of these two lineages. The chemotactic, antifungal, and antiparasitic activity of granulocytes and monocytes are enhanced by this agent. In vitro exposure of monocytes to the drug increases their cytotoxicity for certain neoplastic cells, and similar exposure of polymorphonuclear neutrophils activates their inhibition of tumor cell growth. Activity of GM-CSF is mediated through its binding to specific receptors on the surface of target cells. The biologic activity of GM-CSF is species-specific.

Sargramostim is indicated to accelerate myeloid recovery in patients with nonHodgkin's lymphoma, acute lymphoblastic leukemia, and Hodgkin's disease who are undergoing autologous bone marrow transplantation (see index entry Sargramostim, Uses).

FILGRASTIM (G-CSF)
[Neupogen]

ACTIONS AND USES. Filgrastim is a human granulocyte colony stimulating factor (G-CSF) produced in *Escherichia coli* by recombinant DNA technology. Natural human G-CSF is a glycoprotein produced by monocytes, fibroblasts, and endothelial cells and regulates the production of neutrophils within the bone marrow. It has a minimal effect on the production of other hematopoietic cell types. Because filgrastim is produced in *E. coli*, it is nonglycosylated and thus differs from the natural substance.

G-CSF is a lineage-specific colony stimulating factor with selectivity for the neutrophil lineage, but it is not species-specific. It primarily affects the proliferation and differentiation of neutrophil progenitor cells and certain functional activities of mature neutrophils including enhanced phagocytosis, priming of cellular metabolism, antibody-dependent cell killing, and increased expression of functions associated with certain cell surface antigens. G-CSF has been reported to enhance the phagocytic and bactericidal activity of normal and defective human neutrophils. Bacterial phagocytosis and bactericidal activity of neutrophils from both normal individuals and patients infected with HIV-1 were significantly enhanced in vitro by preincubation with G-CSF; however, neither phagocytosis nor fungicidal activity of normal neutrophils against *Candida albicans* blastoconidia was increased (Roilides et al, 1991).

Filgrastim is indicated to decrease the incidence of infection, as manifested by febrile neutropenia, in patients with nonmyeloid malignancies who are receiving myelosuppressive drugs associated with a significant incidence of severe neutropenia and fever. It has accelerated recovery of neutrophil cell counts following a number of different chemotherapeutic regimens. In these studies, benefits of therapy included reduction of febrile neutropenia, decreased number and duration of hospitalizations, and decreased antibiotic usage. However, no difference in survival or disease progression was observed.

Also see Introduction and index entry Filgrastim.

AGENT FOR REPLACEMENT THERAPY

IMMUNE GLOBULIN

Immune globulin (gamma globulin, immune serum globulin) is derived from human plasma and contains most of the antibodies found in whole blood. Only plasma units that are nonreactive for HBsAg and HIV antibodies are employed. The preparation consists primarily of IgG with lesser amounts of IgM. Since IgA, which is found mostly on mucosal surfaces, is not present in significant amounts in the preparation, immune globulin cannot be used for IgA deficiency.

Immune globulin is used most commonly for replacement therapy in congenital and acquired hypogammaglobulinemia and for the prevention of measles and hepatitis A. It also is used prophylactically when hepatitis B and varicella-zoster immune globulin are not available. Both intramuscular and intravenous formulations have been employed to treat B- and T-cell disorders (see Table 3). An advantage of the intravenous preparation is that large amounts of immune globulin can be administered. The intramuscular preparation has been used principally for prophylaxis.

An intravenous formulation of immune globulin (IGIV) is used to treat patients with idiopathic thrombocytopenic purpura and B-cell chronic lymphocytic leukemia. IGIV also has been used investigationally to treat various autoimmune diseases, such as neutropenia, hemolytic anemia, antibody-mediated pure red cell aplasia, neonatal autoimmune thrombocytopenia, and chronic polymyositis (Pollack et al, 1988; Lakos and Timar, 1987; Leickly and Buckley, 1987; McGuire et al, 1987; Ballin et al, 1988; Roifman et al, 1987). The mode of action of IGIV in these immunologic disorders is not well understood.

Results of several studies indicate that IGIV is useful in the treatment and prevention of acute infections in HIV-infected pediatric patients, and many pediatricians routinely use this product prophylactically in this patient group (Grossman, 1988; Ochs, 1987; Ohno et al, 1988; Steele et al, 1988; Yap and Williams, 1988 A, 1988 B).

Of considerable interest is IGIV's success in reducing coronary artery abnormalities in infants with Kawasaki disease (Newburger et al, 1986; Rowley and Shulman, 1988). Results of surveys conducted in the United States and Canada in 1987 demonstrated widespread acceptance of this treatment modality, and it has been recommended that all infants diagnosed with Kawasaki disease within 10 days of onset of fever receive large doses of IGIV as soon as possible (Rowley and Shulman, 1988). Although it is widely accepted that IGIV (400 mg/kg daily for four days) should be administered to any infant under 12 months of age with Kawasaki disease, its efficacy in patients over 12 months is controversial (Nishihara et al, 1988).

Frequently recurring upper respiratory infection in children should not be treated with immune globulin unless an immunodeficiency has been demonstrated. When interpreting blood levels in children, close attention must be paid to age-adjusted standards.

See also Table 3; for further discussion see index entry Immune Globulin.

AGENT FOR ERYTHROBLASTOSIS FETALIS

Rh_o(D) IMMUNE GLOBULIN
[Gamulin Rh, HypRho-D, RhoGAM]

Rh_o(D) IMMUNE GLOBULIN (Microdose)
[HypRho-D Mini Dose, MICRhoGAM, Mini-Gamulin Rh]

Rh_o(D) immune globulin (RhIG) is a sterile, concentrated solution of immune globulin. It is prepared by cold alcohol fractionation of human plasma obtained from donors immunized to produce high levels of Rh_o(D) antibodies. Only plasma units nonreactive in tests for HBsAg and HIV antibodies are used.

ACTIONS AND USES. RhIG is indicated to prevent Rh hemolytic disease of the newborn (erythroblastosis fetalis). It is administered to the Rh_o(D)-negative, D^u-negative mother within 72 hours after the birth of an Rh_o(D)-positive or D^u-positive infant when the following criteria are met: (1) The mother is Rh_o(D)- and D^u-negative and is not already sensitized to the Rh_o(D) factor. (2) The infant is Rh_o(D)-positive or D^u-positive and has a negative direct Coombs' test due to anti-Rh_o(D). (A positive direct Coombs' test may be caused by antibodies other than anti-Rh_o(D); although therapy with RhIG is not contraindicated, the cause should be investigated.) If the fetal Rh status cannot be determined, it should be presumed to be Rh-positive.

RhIG is indicated for all unimmunized Rh_o(D)-negative, D^u-negative women after abortion or ectopic pregnancy (unless the fetus or the father is shown to be Rh-negative), following amniocentesis or other abdominal trauma that allows fetal cells to enter the maternal circulation, and following transfusion with Rh_o(D)-positive or D^u-positive red blood cells or blood components prepared from blood containing such cells in an Rh_o(D)-negative or D^u-negative premenopausal female.

The routine use of RhIG during the 28th week of gestation in all Rh-negative women was favored by a large number of medical centers surveyed by the Committee on Obstetrics, Maternal and Fetal Medicine of the American College of Obstetricians and Gynecologists (Nichols, 1984).

RhIG acts by suppressing the specific immune response of Rh-negative individuals to Rh-positive red blood cells. Exposure to these red blood cells may result from pregnancy, abortion, delivery, amniocentesis, or transfusion. Prevention of sensitization to the Rh_o(D) factor in pregnant Rh_o(D)-negative women prevents hemolytic disease of the newborn. Injection of RhIG suppresses the antibody response and the formation of anti-Rh_o(D). Although the mechanism of action is unclear, it has been proposed that binding of passive antibody to circulating antigen prevents stimulation of antigen-sensitive cells and subsequent production of anti-Rh_o(D).

Primary immunization occurs most often during labor and delivery in about 15% of the women at risk. Rh_o immunoprophylaxis fails to prevent sensitization in 10% to 15% of these women. Reasons for these therapeutic failures may include previous undetected or overlooked Rh-positive pregnancies or transfusions or the administration of an inadequate dose of RhIG. The most frequent cause of apparent failure of postpartum prophylaxis is probably Rh immunization early during pregnancy.

The administration of RhIG within 72 hours of delivery of a full-term infant reduces the incidence of Rh isoimmunization as a result of pregnancy from 12% to 13% to 1% to 2%. The incidence of isoimmunization can be reduced further to less than 0.1% by administering the product in two doses, one at 28 weeks gestation and another following delivery. Protection against isoimmunization is decreased when the Rh antibody is administered more than 72 hours following delivery.

ADVERSE REACTIONS AND PRECAUTIONS. Adverse reactions are infrequent, mild, and generally confined to the site of injection. Slight elevations of temperature have been reported following injection. Other adverse effects are the same as those encountered with similar human immune globulin preparations (see index entry Immune Globulins).

RhIG is contraindicated in Rh-positive patients and in Rh-negative patients who have already developed Rh antibodies. It must not be administered intravenously or given to the neonate. A broad spectrum compatibility test capable of detecting "incomplete" antibodies should be performed to determine if the patient already has been sensitized to the Rh_o(D) factor.

This agent is classified in FDA Pregnancy Category C.

DOSAGE AND PREPARATIONS. RhIG should be stored at 2° to 8° C but not frozen.

STANDARD PREPARATION:

Intramuscular: Postpartum, prophylaxis, miscarriage, abortion, ectopic pregnancy, *adults*, the entire contents of one vial is administered. This is sufficient to suppress the immunizing potential of 15 ml of red blood cells or approximately 30 ml of whole blood. RhIG should be administered within 72 hours of the fetomaternal hemorrhage.

Transfusion accident, one vial will suppress the immune response to 15 ml of Rh-positive red blood cells. To calculate the volume of red blood cells in whole blood transfusions, the total volume of blood transfused is multiplied by the hematocrit of the donor; alternatively, the volume may be approximated by multiplying the total volume by 0.45.

Generic. Unit-dose containers.

Gamulin Rh (Armour), ***HypRho-D*** (Miles-Cutter), ***RhoGAM*** (Ortho). Packages containing a single dose.

MICRODOSE PREPARATION:

Intramuscular: This preparation contains approximately one-sixth the Rh_o(D) antibody present in the standard preparation and is indicated only for Rh_o(D)-negative women undergoing abortion or miscarriage up to 12 weeks' gestation, unless the father is Rh negative. *Adults,* one vial is usually sufficient and should be administered within 72 hours of the termination of pregnancy.

Generic. Unit-dose containers.

HypRho-D Mini Dose (Miles-Cutter), ***MICRhoGAM*** (Ortho), ***Mini-Gamulin Rh*** (Armour). Single (microdose) containers.

IMMUNOSUPPRESSIVE ANTISERUM

LYMPHOCYTE IMMUNE GLOBULIN (Antithymocyte Globulin [Equine])

[Atgam]

ACTIONS. Lymphocyte immune globulin is obtained from serum Ig of horses immunized with lymphocytes from human thymus tissue. This preparation is a selective immunosuppressant that reduces the number of circulating, thymus-dependent lymphocytes (T-cells) that are partly responsible for graft rejection; it has little effect on B-cells and is not associated with severe lymphopenia. Immunosuppressive activity may vary from patient to patient due to imprecise laboratory methods of measuring potency. Since it is usually administered with other immunosuppressants, such as corticosteroids and antimetabolites, the patient's response to the equine globulin is minimal and the incidence of hypersensitivity reactions is reduced.

USES. Lymphocyte immune globulin has been used primarily to minimize allograft rejection in renal transplant patients. Administration at the time of rejection enhances resolution of acute episodes. It now usually is administered as an adjunct to other immunosuppressive therapy to delay the onset of the first rejection episode. Efficacy and safety have not been demonstrated in renal transplant patients who are not receiving other immunosuppressive therapy concomitantly.

Lymphocyte immune globulin also is indicated for the treatment of moderate to severe aplastic anemia in patients who are unsuitable for bone marrow transplantation; it may induce partial to complete hematologic remission when given with a regimen of supportive care. Lymphocyte immune globulin has not been demonstrated to be useful in patients who are suitable candidates for bone marrow transplantation or in patients with aplastic anemia secondary to neoplastic disease, storage disease, myelofibrosis, or Fanconi's syndrome or in those exposed to myelotoxic agents or radiation. This preparation has been used investigationally in patients with T-cell malignancies or GVHD. To date, safety and efficacy have not been established in circumstances other than renal transplantation and aplastic anemia.

ADVERSE REACTIONS AND PRECAUTIONS. Common adverse effects (incidence 10% to 50%) include chills, fever, vertigo, leukopenia, thrombocytopenia, systemic infections, and dermatologic reactions (rash, pruritus, urticaria, wheal and flare). Other reactions (incidence 1% to 5%) include arthralgia, chest or back pain, headache, nausea and/or vomiting, diarrhea, peripheral thrombophlebitis, stomatitis, dyspnea, hypotension, night sweats, and pain at the infusion site. Rarely (incidence less than 5%), anaphylaxis, serum sickness, tachycardia, laryngospasm, pulmonary edema, herpes simplex virus reactivation, local and systemic infections, or myalgias may occur.

In studies in patients with aplastic anemia and other hematologic abnormalities, liver (AST, ALT, alkaline phosphatase) and renal (serum creatinine) function tests have been abnormal. In some trials, clinical and laboratory findings of serum sickness were seen in most patients.

Since lymphocyte immune globulin is of equine origin, the usual precautions should be observed (see index entry Immune Globulins). Caution should be exercised when giving repeated doses of this preparation, and patients should be observed for signs of allergy. It is recommended that only physicians experienced in immunosuppressive therapy use this product and that patients be treated in facilities equipped and staffed with adequate laboratory and supportive medical resources. A skin test for sensitivity to equine serum is recommended prior to the first infusion. A systemic reaction, such as generalized rash, tachycardia, dyspnea, hypotension, or anaphylaxis, precludes further administration. Some previously masked reactions to the antiserum (hypersensitivity) may appear if doses of other immunosuppressants given concomitantly are reduced. Patients should be monitored carefully for leukopenia and thrombocytopenia, especially when the antiserum is used with other immunosuppressive agents. Treatment should be discontinued if symptoms of anaphylaxis develop or if severe, unremitting thrombocytopenia or leukopenia occurs. This antiserum is *contraindicated* in patients who previously experienced a severe systemic reaction to lymphocyte immune globulin or any equine immunoglobulin preparation.

Administration during pregnancy is not recommended (FDA Pregnancy Category C). The antiserum has not been tested in pregnant or lactating women.

The patient should be observed carefully for signs of concurrent infection and treated promptly if infection develops. Results of several studies suggest that the incidence of cytomegalovirus infection is increased in patients who receive this product.

DOSAGE AND PREPARATIONS. The dosage varies from patient to patient. The maximum tolerated dose has not been determined. The following dosages are examples of immunosuppressive regimens that have been employed. Lymphocyte immune globulin is used with other immunosuppressive agents. The manufacturer's instructions for pretesting and infusion procedures should be followed carefully. Dilution of the product in dextrose or acidic solutions is not recommended. A dose should not be infused in less than four hours. A systemic reaction such as generalized rash, tachycardia, dyspnea, hypotension, or anaphylaxis precludes any additional administration. The package insert should be consulted for information on the management of potential adverse reactions.

Intravenous: Renal allograft recipients, *adults*, 10 to 30 mg/kg daily; *children*, 5 to 25 mg/kg (experience with children is limited).

To delay rejection, *adults*, 15 mg/kg daily for 14 days, then every other day for 14 days for a total of 21 doses in 28 days. The first dose should be administered 24 hours before or after transplant.

For treatment of rejection, *adults*, the first dose can be delayed until diagnosis of the first rejection episode. The recommended dose is 10 to 15 mg/kg daily for 14 days. Additional alternate-day therapy up to a total of 21 doses may be given.

Aplastic anemia, *adults*, 10 to 20 mg/kg daily for 8 to 14 days. Additional alternate-day therapy up to a total of 21 doses may be administered. Since thrombocytopenia has been associated with this product, patients with aplastic anemia may need prophylactic platelet transfusions.

Atgam (Upjohn). Each milliliter of solution contains equine gamma globulin 50 mg stabilized in 0.3 molar glycine to a pH of about 6.8 in 5 ml containers (preservative, thimerosal 0.01%). This product should be stored at 2° to 8° C but not frozen.

VENOM ALLERGENS FOR IMMUNOTHERAPY

The sting of the bee, wasp, hornet, or yellow-jacket poses a serious hazard for sensitive individuals who may respond to a second exposure with anaphylaxis. Anaphylactic shock caused by insect sting is no less hazardous than that caused by other allergens. There is much clinical experience to indicate that immunotherapeutic injections of protein extracts from *Hymenoptera* can produce a refractory state. However, for treatment of acute anaphylaxis, epinephrine is the drug of choice (see index entry Epinephrine, In Anaphylactic Shock). Hymenoptera venoms have not been fully characterized, but they contain a complex mixture of allergenic proteins, antigens, peptides, and a number of vasoactive substances.

For many years, hyposensitization therapy against the sting of *Hymenoptera* employed a whole body extract. However, results of investigations indicated that whole body extracts were ineffective or less effective than extracts from pure venom or venom sacs only, and whole body extracts were withdrawn from the market by order of the Food and Drug Administration.

The diagnosis of insect hypersensitivity depends on history, physical examination when possible, and determination of IgE antibody against *Hymenoptera* protein through skin or radioallergosorbent (RAST) testing. Skin testing was more sensitive than RAST in one study (Small et al, 1983). Any adult with a history of a systemic allergic reaction (cutaneous, respiratory, or cardiovascular) who has a positive skin or RAST test is a candidate for venom immunotherapy (Lichtenstein et al, 1979). Venom immunotherapy is 97% effective in reducing the danger of anaphylaxis from stings in adults who had previous systemic reactions (Hunt et al, 1978). Without therapy, approximately 60% of such adults will experience systemic reactions if stung again; in contrast, the reaction rate is less than 2% among those immunized with venom (Valentine et al, 1990).

Children with severe systemic reactions (not limited to the skin) also should be considered for immunotherapy. Those whose reactions are confined to the skin have a more favorable prognosis without immunotherapy than do adults. In a study of 242 such children 2 to 16 years old, immunotherapy resulted in significantly fewer systemic reactions after a subsequent sting; however, since only 9.2% of stings in untreated children led to a systemic reaction and there was no progression to a more severe reaction, the investigators concluded that venom immunotherapy was not indicated or cost effective in children in this age group (Valentine et al, 1990). Patients who experienced severe local reactions with a positive skin or RAST test should be considered for immunotherapy only if the reactions are incapacitating or there is clear progression of symptoms following repeated stings.

Neither the degree of reactivity to skin testing nor the level of response to RAST testing correlates with the degree of sensitivity to insect sting. There is a very narrow range between the diagnostic and irritant concentrations of the skin test antigens. Some individuals, particularly children, lose their sensitivity after several years without exposure. However, immunotherapy stimulates the production not only of protective IgG-blocking antibodies but also of IgE antibodies, which may tend to maintain the sensitivity. In most cases, IgE levels rise initially and then decrease. In some patients, protection does not appear to be related to IgG antibodies, which raises the possibility that other mechanisms may be involved during immunotherapy, such as stimulation of antigen-specific T-suppressor cells.

The degree of protection achieved with venom extract is not clear. No endpoint has been established; the prevailing view appears to be that a minimum of three years' therapy is necessary.

ADVERSE REACTIONS AND PRECAUTIONS. Because severe systemic reactions may occur, *Hymenoptera* venom preparations should be given only by a physician experienced in administering allergens and/or after allergy consultation. In highly sensitive individuals, even the small dose used for skin tests may precipitate an anaphylactic reaction.

An anaphylactic reaction is always possible with use of any immunotherapeutic agent. For that reason, a tourniquet, epinephrine, and agents to treat shock and bronchospasm should be available. In addition, patients should remain in the office under close observation for one hour after an injection (see index entry Shock, Anaphylactic).

Systemic reactions have been noted in about 16% of adults receiving immunotherapy. These may occur while increasing the dosage or after a maintenance dose. Symptoms include any of the following: pruritus, urticaria, sneezing, nasal discharge, hoarseness, coughing, wheezing, tachycardia, gastrointestinal discomfort and nausea, neck or chest pain, sweating, or lacrimation. Systemic reactions commonly occur shortly after injection; however, a serum sickness-like reaction manifested by fever, malaise, joint pain, and myalgia can appear up to 48 hours following injection. Local and systemic reactions are less common in children.

Because of the risks, the patient should be fully informed and should be instructed in emergency self-injection procedures with subcutaneous epinephrine. Emergency insect sting treatment kits containing prepackaged doses of epinephrine and antihistamines and instructions for use are available commercially [Ana-Kit, EpiPen]. These kits should be prescribed for patients at risk from insect sting anaphylaxis and should be readily available at all times of possible exposure. Patients should be instructed by the physician regarding the proper use of the kits.

Because antihistamines may interfere with skin test responses, they should not be taken for at least 72 hours prior to skin testing.

The risk of treatment failure is increased if the venom-specific IgG antibody response is less than 3.5 mcg/ml.

Safety during pregnancy has not been established (FDA Pregnancy Category C). The benefit/risk ratio must be evaluated carefully because of the risk of serious systemic reactions.

ADMINISTRATION. The regimens for immunotherapy vary according to the recommendation of the manufacturer. Recommended dosage schedules may have to be adjusted for highly sensitive patients. Current guidelines recommend venom immunotherapy at four-week intervals for an indefinite period; however, studies have suggested that this interval may be extended safely to at least six weeks (Goldberg and Reisman, 1988). A prick test followed by an intradermal test is recommended for diagnostic skin testing. The subcutaneous route is preferred for immunotherapy injections. It is important to include a negative control with diluent and a positive control with histamine to interpret the significance of the wheal and erythema reaction if it occurs. The product information sheet should be consulted for recommended diluent, dilutions, and interpretation of the skin test response.

VENOM EXTRACT KITS:

Albay (Hollister-Stier). Diagnostic kits, maintenance kits, and bulk vials are available. Each vacuum-sealed bulk vial contains venom protein 550 mcg. When reconstituted with 5.5 ml of the appropriate diluent (50% glycerin, normal saline, or Hollister-Stier albumin-saline diluent), each vial contains 100 mcg/ml of venom protein (honey bee, yellow jacket, yellow hornet, white-faced hornet, wasp, and mixed vespid). The manufacturer's recommendation for reconstitution should be followed closely.

Pharmalgen (Alk Laboratories). The diagnostic kit contains one vial each of 100 mcg of honey bee, yellow jacket, yellow hornet, white-faced hornet, and wasp venoms. Treatment kits containing 6 x 100 mcg are available for all venoms included in the diagnostic kit, as well as for mixed vespids (6 x 300 mcg). Multiple dose vials containing 1,000 mcg are available for honey bee, yellow jacket, yellow hornet, white-faced hornet, and wasp, and one containing 3,000 mcg is available for mixed vespids. All products are supplied freeze dried; the appropriate diluent is available separately. When refrigerated, all freeze-dried preparations are stable for at least 30 months. Solutions containing 100 mcg/ml are stable for one year. Lower concentrations are stable for shorter periods.

EPINEPHRINE KITS:

Ana-Kit (Miles). Kit containing epinephrine injection 1:1,000 (1 mg/ml) in a 1-ml sterile syringe designed to deliver two 0.3-ml doses plus four 2-mg chewable tablets of chlorpheniramine maleate. Kit also contains two sterile alcohol pads and one tourniquet.

EpiPen (Center). Kit containing epinephrine injection 1:1,000 (1 mg/ml) or 1:2,000 (0.5 mg/ml [pediatric]) (***EpiPen Jr.***) in 2 ml containers (Auto-Injector syringes) designed to deliver a 0.3-mg or 0.15-mg (***EpiPen Jr.***) dose.

INVESTIGATIONAL AGENTS

MURAMYL DIPEPTIDE

Because BCG immunotherapy occasionally causes severe adverse effects, attempts have been made to use subfractions of the bacterium in the hope of reducing these complications. Muramyl dipeptide (MDP) is the smallest active component of the mycobacterial cell wall and retains the immunoadjuvant activity of BCG. This water-soluble fragment is administered orally. A large number of MDP analogues have been prepared, and the parent compound and derivatives have been studied extensively as adjuvants for immunization.

In animals, MDP induces tumoricidal and bactericidal activities of macrophages and increases the secretion of monokines. When incorporated into oil with antigen, it augments the development of both cellular and humoral immunity. In vitro studies have shown that T-cell function and B-cell proliferation are enhanced.

Data on the activity of MDP in humans are limited. In vitro, MDP encapsulated in liposomes enhanced the tumoricidal activity of human monocytes; a significantly smaller amount was required if MDP was incorporated into liposomes (Sone et al, 1984). Liposomes containing a derivative, muramyl tripeptide, have been reported to protect mice from fatal herpes simplex type 2 infection (Koff et al, 1985). When administered intraperitoneally, MDP inhibited the ascitic growth of four of five thymoma cell lines in mice (Phillips et al, 1983).

THYMIC HORMONES

The epithelium of the thymus gland synthesizes many hormone-like factors that appear to play a major role in the regulation and differentiation of T-lymphocytes. Several active factors have been isolated from the thymus, including thymosin fraction 5 (TF-5), thymosin α-1, thymopentin (TP), thymic humoral factor (THF), serum thymic factor (facteur thymique serique, FTS), and thymostimulin (TS). These thymic hormones are involved in the maturation of T-cell precursors and promote the differentiation and proliferation of mature T-cells. Blood levels are highest in childhood, decline during the third or fourth decade, and are low in the elderly. Levels are undetectable in patients with complete DiGeorge syndrome who lack the thymus. Because of the low levels in the elderly, thymic hormones previously have been evaluated in this group to enhance immune responsiveness.

Thymosin fraction 5 is an extract of calf thymus and contains over 20 peptides with molecular weights ranging from 2 to 15,000 daltons. The activity of TF-5 varies from lot to lot and the extract may contain toxic contaminants. Although TF-5 is generally nonreactogenic in humans, hypersensitivity reactions to bovine antigens have been reported.

TF-5 induces the expression of antigens associated with maturation on precursor T-cells, stimulates terminal deoxynucleotidyl transferase (TdT, a DNA-polymerase present only in prothymocytes and hence a marker for immature cells), and enhances the production of IL-2. TF-5 also augments the functions of both T-helper (Th) and T-suppressor (Ts) cells and accordingly either increases or decreases cytotoxic T-cell activity. It does not appear to affect NK cell activity. In experimental models, TF-5 has some antitumor effects, but no significant reproducible effect has been demonstrated in human studies. Because of the variable responses that have been obtained, research has focused primarily on the isolation, purification, and characterization of the individual polypeptides in TF-5.

Thymosin alpha-1 (T-α_1) is a polypeptide found in TF-5; its gene has been cloned and it also has been synthesized. This peptide contains 28 amino acids and has a molecular weight of 3,100 daltons. T-α_1 enhances several T-cell functions in vitro, including the synthesis of migration inhibitory factor, the proliferative response to T-cell mitogens (but not alloantigens), Th cell activity, antibody synthesis in secondary responses to T-dependent antigens, and the number of high affinity IL-2 receptors expressed by human peripheral blood lymphocytes, and it promotes the production of alpha and gamma interferon as well as IL-2. It also induces the expression of T-cell surface antigens and TdT at considerably lower doses than TF-5. While T-α_1 appears to augment the development of cytotoxic T-cells, it does not appear to activate NK cells. The maturation of T-precursor cells in vivo is induced by T-α_1 at significantly lower doses than TF-5. In animal models, it has demonstrated some efficacy in preventing experimental and spontaneous metastases.

The administration of T-α_1 to woodchucks infected with the woodchuck hepatitis virus was reported to decrease virus levels several hundredfold without any obvious toxic effects; however, when treatment was discontinued, the virus levels rebounded in several of the animals (Korba et al, 1990). More recently, the safety and efficacy of TF-5 and T-α_1 was investigated in a prospective, placebo-controlled trial in 12 patients with chronic hepatitis B. Seven patients received TF-5 and T-α_1 and five patients received placebo twice weekly for six months. By the end of the study, serum aminotransferase levels had improved significantly in the thymosin-treated patients but not in the placebo group; 86% of those receiving thymosin versus 20% of those receiving placebo cleared HBV DNA from the serum, and therapy was associated with significant improvement in lymphocyte CD3 and CD4 counts. No significant adverse effects were observed in patients given the thymosin preparations (Mutchnick et al, 1991).

Thymopentin is a pure polypeptide (molecular weight, 5,260) obtained from human thymus extract. Thymopentin pentapeptide (TP-5) has been synthesized and found to have the same biologic activity as the whole native molecule. TP-5 appears to be related to the active site on the native molecule. In vivo, it has a half-life of 30 minutes. In vitro, TP-5 has increased the NK cell activity of mouse bone marrow, and its administration to healthy elderly individuals has been associated with a significant enhancement of human NK cell activity (Hu et al, 1990). The mechanism responsible for the immunopotentiating activity of TP-5 is unknown, but recent data indicate that the administration of the drug to immunocompromised elderly subjects enhances the production of IL-2.

In small clinical trials, TP-5 has been reported to induce clinical and immunologic improvement in such diseases as DiGeorge's syndrome, rheumatoid arthritis, insulin-dependent diabetes mellitus, and progressive systemic sclerosis.

Thymic humoral factor (THF) is isolated from calf thymus by dialysis and may be similar to thymosin fraction 5. It increases the production of T-lymphocytes in animals and humans and leads to T-cell differentiation and maturation.

Serum thymic factor (FTS), a nonapeptide produced by the thymus, has been synthesized. It modulates NK cell activity in mice; it increases activity, but decreases the abnormally high level of NK activity in thymectomized mice. In vivo studies on human cells have shown that low concentrations increased and high concentrations decreased NK activity.

Thymostimulin (TS) is another extract of calf thymus that enhances T-cell proliferation and differentiation. In vitro studies have indicated that TS increases lymphoproliferative responses and NK cell activity. In vivo, TS appears to have a strong, multifaceted effect on the immune system, including the activity of T-suppressor cells. In clinical pilot studies, it has been reported to boost age-related immunodepression, to decrease the number and severity of recurrences of herpes simplex labialis in immunodeficient patients, and to increase remission rates in insulin-dependent diabetes mellitus.

The use of thymic hormones to treat human disease requires further clinical studies. The extent to which a thymic deficiency may contribute to the pathogenesis of any disease is important in defining the probable efficacy of these agents. Studies employing purified materials derived from recombinant DNA technology or from chemical synthesis should not only identify the specific active factors, but eliminate the lot-to-lot variation in thymic extracts that has made the determination of appropriate dosage a significant problem.

Cited References

Consensus document: Hawk's Cay meeting on therapeutic drug monitoring of cyclosporine. *Transplant Proc* 22:1357-1361, 1990.

Critical issues in cyclosporine monitoring: Report of the Task Force on Cyclosporine Monitoring. *Clin Chem* 33:1269-1288, 1987.

Abels RI, et al: Recombinant human erythropoietin (r-HuEPO) for the treatment of the anemia of cancer in Murphy MJ Jr (ed): *Blood Cell Growth Factors: Their Present and Future Use in Hematology and Oncology.* Dayton, Ohio, AlphaMed Press, 1991, 121-141.

Aberer W, et al: Azathioprine in the treatment of pemphigus vulgaris: Long-term follow-up. *J Am Acad Dermatol* 16:527-533, 1987.

Ahn YS et al: Danazol for treatment of idiopathic thrombocytopenic purpura. *N Engl J Med* 308:1396-1399, 1983.

American Academy of Pediatrics, Committee on Infectious Diseases: Dexamethasone therapy for bacterial meningitis in infants and children. *Pediatrics* 86:130-133, 1990.

Ammann AJ: Immunodeficiency diseases, in Stites DP, et al (eds): *Basic & Clinical Immunology,* ed 5. Los Altos, Calif, Lange Medical Publications, 1984, 384-422.

Assini JF, et al: Adverse reactions to azathioprine mimicking gastroenteritis. *J Rheumatol* 13:1117-1118, 1986.

Baker GL, et al: Malignancy following treatment of rheumatoid arthritis with cyclophosphamide: Long-term case-control follow-up study. *Am J Med* 83:1-9, 1987.

Ballin A, et al: High-dose intravenous gammaglobulin therapy for neonatal autoimmune thrombocytopenia. *J Pediatr* 112:789-792, 1988.

Baylink DJ: Glucocorticoid-induced osteoporosis, editorial. *N Engl J Med* 309:306-308, 1983.

Beaman M, et al: Convulsions associated with cyclosporin A in renal transplant recipients. *BMJ* 290:139-140, 1985.

Behn AR, et al: Polymyalgia rheumatica and corticosteroids: How much for how long? *Ann Rheum Dis* 42:374-378, 1983.

Belosevic M, et al: Effects of cyclosporin A on the course of infection with Giardia muris in mice. *Am J Trop Med Hyg* 35:496-500, 1986.

Bergentz SE, et al: Venous thrombosis and cyclosporin. *Lancet* 2:101-102, 1985.

Bolton WK, et al: Therapy of idiopathic nephrotic syndrome with alternate day steroids. *Am J Med* 62:60-70, 1977.

Borel JF: Pharmacology of cyclosporine (Sandimmune): IV. Pharmacological properties in vivo. *Pharmacol Rev* 41:260-351, 1989.

Borst GC, et al: Discordant cortisol response to exogenous ACTH and insulin-induced hypoglycemia in patients with pituitary disease. *N Engl J Med* 306:1462-1464, 1982.

Bout D, et al: Antischistosomal effect of cyclosporin A: Cure and prevention of mouse and rat schistosomiasis mansoni. *Infect Immun* 52:823-827, 1986.

Bracken MB, et al: Efficacy of methylprednisolone in acute spinal cord injury. *JAMA* 251:45-52, 1984.

Braughler JM, Hall ED: Current application of "high-dose" steroid therapy for CNS injury: Pharmacological perspective. *J Neurosurg* 62:806-810, 1985.

British Association for Paediatric Nephrology: Levamisole for corticosteroid-dependent nephrotic syndrome in childhood. *Lancet* 337:1555-1557, 1991.

Burns TR, Saleem A: Idiopathic thrombocytopenic purpura. *Am J Med* 75:1001-1007, 1983.

Burton RC, et al: Monoclonal antibodies to human T cell subsets: Use for immunologic monitoring and immunosuppression in renal transplantation. *J Clin Immunol* 2(suppl):142S-147S, (July) 1982.

Byyny RL: Withdrawal from glucocorticoid therapy. *N Engl J Med* 295:30-32, 1976.

Caillat-Zucman S, et al: The OKT3 immunosuppressive effect: In situ antigenic modulation of human graft-infiltrating T cells. *Transplantation* 49:156-160, 1990.

Carette S, et al: Controlled studies of oral immunosuppressive drugs in lupus nephritis. *Ann Intern Med* 99:1-8, 1983.

Centers for Disease Control: Purified protein derivative (PPD)-tuberculin anergy and HIV infection: Guidelines for anergy testing and management of anergic persons at risk of tuberculosis. *MMWR* 40(no. RR-5):27-33, 1991 A.

Centers for Disease Control: Nosocomial transmission of multidrug-resistant tuberculosis among HIV-infected persons—Florida and New York, 1988-1991. *MMWR* 40(no. 34):585-591, 1991 B.

Chamberlain P, Meyer WJ III: Management of pituitary-adrenal suppression secondary to corticosteroid therapy. *Pediatrics* 67:245-251, 1981.

Chang TW, et al: Does OKT3 monoclonal antibody react with an antigen-recognition structure on human T cells? *Proc Natl Acad Sci USA* 78:1805-1808, 1981.

Chatenoud L, et al: Restitution of the human in vivo immune response against the mouse monoclonal OKT3. *J Immunol* 137:830-838, 1986.

Cheney RT, Sprent J: Capacity of cyclosporine to induce auto-graft-versus-host disease and impair intrathymic T cell differentiation. *Transplant Proc* 17:528-530, 1985.

Cirillo R, et al: Cyclosporin A rapidly inhibits mediator release from human basophils presumably by interacting with cyclophilin. *J Immunol* 144:3891-3897, 1990.

Clement M, et al: Corticosteroids as adjunctive therapy in severe *Pneumocystis carinii* pneumonia: A prospective placebo-controlled trial, abstract. *Am Rev Respir Dis* 139 (suppl):A250, 1989.

Collins TR, Byyny RL: Clinical use of glucocorticoids. *Compr Ther* 6:63-72, (Nov) 1980.

Colombani PM, et al: Cyclosporin A binding to calmodulin: A possible site of action on T lymphocytes. *Science* 228:337-339, 1985.

Cosimi AB, et al: Treatment of acute renal allograft rejection with OKT3 monoclonal antibody. *Transplantation* 32:535-539, 1981.

Cosimi AB, et al: Randomized clinical trial comparing OKT3 and steroids for treatment of hepatic allograft rejection. *Transplantation* 43:91-95, 1987.

Cox J, et al: Devastating diarrhoea caused by azathioprine: Management difficulty in inflammatory bowel disease. *Gut* 29:686-688, 1988.

D'Alessandro AM, et al: Use of OKT3 in kidney, pancreas, and liver transplantation. *Transplant Proc* 22:1748-1749, 1990.

Dixon RB, Christy NP: On various forms of corticosteroid withdrawal syndrome. *Am J Med* 68:224-230, 1980.

Ehrke MJ, et al: Effects of anticancer drugs on the immune system in humans. *Semin Oncol* 16:230-253, 1987.

Eisenberg M, et al: Preliminary trial of recombinant fibroblast interferon in chronic hepatitis B virus infection. *Antimicrob Agents Chemother* 29:122-126, 1986.

Ezekowitz RAB: Interferon gamma for chronic granulomatous disease, letter. *N Engl J Med* 325:1516-1517, 1991.

Ezekowitz RAB, et al: Partial correction of the phagocyte defect in patients with X-linked chronic granulomatous disease by subcutaneous interferon gamma. *N Engl J Med* 319:146-151, 1988.

Fass B: Glucocorticoid therapy for nonendocrine disorders: Withdrawal and "coverage." *Pediatr Clin North Am* 26:251-256, 1979.

Fauci AS, et al: Cyclophosphamide-induced remissions in advanced polyarteritis nodosa. *Am J Med* 84:890-894, 1978.

Fauci AS, et al: Cyclophosphamide therapy of severe systemic necrotizing vasculitis. *N Engl J Med* 301:235-238, 1979.

First MR, et al: Use of low doses of cyclosporine, azathioprine, and prednisone in renal transplantation. *Transplant Proc* 18 (suppl 1):132-135, 1986.

First MR, et al: Successful retreatment of allograft rejection with OKT3. *Transplantation* 47:88-91, 1989.

Flanagan WM, et al: Nuclear association of a T-cell transcription factor blocked by FK-506 and cyclosporin A, letter. *Nature* 352:803-807, 1991.

Flavin DK, et al: Corticosteroid abuse: Unusual manifestation of drug dependence. *Mayo Clin Proc* 58:764-766, 1983.

Fleischmann J, et al: Clinical response to intravesical BCG correlated with urine acidity and consistent interleukin-2 (IL-2) production. *J Urol* 137:145A, 1987.

Fleischmann JD, et al: Urinary interleukins in patients receiving intravesical bacillus Calmette-Guerin therapy for superficial bladder cancer. *Cancer* 64:1447-1454, 1989.

Gilbert EM, et al: Treatment of refractory cardiac allograft rejection with OKT3 monoclonal antibody. *Am J Med* 82:202-206, 1987.

Goldberg A, Reisman RE: Prolonged interval maintenance venom immunotherapy. *Ann Allergy* 61:177-179, (Sept) 1988.

Goodnough LT, et al: Increased preoperative collections of autologous blood with recombinant human erythropoietin therapy. *N Engl J Med* 321:1163-1168, 1989.

Gross G: Recombinant interferon gamma in condylomata acuminata, letter. *JAMA* 266:2706, 1991.

Grossman M: Children with AIDS. *Infect Dis Clin North Am* 2:533-541, 1988.

Guslandi M, Tittobello A: Steroid ulcers: A myth revisited. Steroids cause peptic ulcers only when given together with non-steroidal anti-inflammatory drugs. *BMJ* 304:655-656, 1992.

Hait WN, et al: Calmodulin, cyclophilin, and cyclosporin A. *Science* 233:987-988, 1986.

Herold KC, et al: Immunosuppressive effects of cyclosporin A on cloned T cells. *J Immunol* 136:1315-1321, 1986.

Hess AD, et al: Development of graft-vs-host disease-like syndrome in cyclosporine-treated rats after syngeneic bone marrow transplantation: I. Development of cytotoxic T lymphocytes with apparent polyclonal anti-Ia specificity, including autoreactivity. *J Exp Med* 161:718-730, 1985.

Hofflin JM, et al: Infectious complications in heart transplant recipients receiving cyclosporine and corticosteroids. *Ann Intern Med* 106:209-216, 1987.

Hollinger WM, et al: Prediction of therapeutic response in steroid-treated pulmonary sarcoidosis: Evaluation of clinical parameters, bronchoalveolar lavage, gallium-67 lung scanning, and serum angiotensin-converting enzyme levels. *Am Rev Respir Dis* 132:65-69, 1985.

Hood AF, et al: Acute graft-vs-host disease: Development following autologous and syngeneic bone marrow transplantation. *Arch Dermatol* 123:745-750, 1987.

Hu C, et al: *In vivo* enhancement of NK-cell activity by thymopentin. *Int J Immunopharmacol* 12:193-197, 1990.

Hunt KJ, et al: A controlled trial of immunotherapy in insect hypersensitivity. *N Engl J Med* 299:157-161, 1978.

The International Chronic Granulomatous Disease Cooperative Study Group: A controlled trial of interferon gamma to prevent infection in chronic granulomatous disease. *N Engl J Med* 324:509-516, 1991.

Itoh K, et al: Generation of activated killer (AK) cells by recombinant interleukin 2 (rIL 2) in collaboration with interferon-γ (IFN-γ). *J Immunol* 134:3124-3129, 1985.

Jacques Y, Soulillou J-P: Third French workshop on interleukin-2: Joint report. *Lymphokine Res* 4:159-167, 1985.

Janssen O, et al: Immunosuppression by OKT3—Induction of programmed cell death (apoptosis) as a possible mechanism of action. *Transplantation* 53:233-234, 1992.

Jenkins MK, et al: Effects of cyclosporine A on T cell development and clonal deletion. *Science* 241:1655-1658, 1988.

June CH, et al: Profound hypomagnesemia and renal magnesium wasting associated with use of cyclosporine for marrow transplantation. *Transplantation* 39:620-624, 1985.

Kahan BD: Cyclosporine. *N Engl J Med* 321:1725-1738, 1989.

Kawase I, et al: Interleukin 2 induces γ-interferon production: Participation of macrophages and NK-like cells. *J Immunol* 131:288-292, 1983.

Kehrl JH, Fauci AS: Clinical use of glucocorticoids. *Ann Allergy* 50:2-8, 1983.

Kelton JG: Management of pregnant patient with idiopathic thrombocytopenic purpura. *Ann Intern Med* 99:796-800, 1983.

Kirchertz EJ, et al: Successful low dose captopril rechallenge following drug-induced leucopenia. *Lancet* 1:1362-1363, 1981.

Klein A, et al: Difference between human B and T lymphocytes regarding their capacity to metabolize cortisol. *J Steroid Biochem* 13:517-520, 1980.

Klein JB, et al: Use of OKT3 monoclonal antibody in the treatment of acute cardiac allograft rejection. *Transplantation* 45:727-729, 1988.

Koff WC, et al: Protection of mice against fatal herpes simplex type 2 infection by liposomes containing muramyl tripeptide. *Science* 228:495-497, 1985.

Köhler G, Milstein C: Continuous cultures of fused cells secreting antibody of predefined specificity. *Nature* 256:495-497, 1975.

Korba BE, et al: Treatment of chronic woodchuck hepatitis virus infection with thymosin alpha-1, abstract. *Hepatology* 12:880, 1990.

Krown SE: Interferons: Not just alpha. *Cancer Treat Rep* 70:1353-1355, 1986.

Kung PC, et al: Monoclonal antibodies defining distinctive human T cell surface antigens. *Science* 206:347-349, 1979.

Kupin W, et al: Complete replacement of methylprednisolone by azathioprine in cyclosporine-treated primary cadaveric renal transplant recipients. *Transplantation* 45:53-55, 1988.

Lakos A, Timar L: Treatment of idiopathic chronic neutropenia with high-dose intravenous immunoglobulin, letter. *Am J Dis Child* 141:12-13, 1987.

LeGrue SJ, et al: Does the binding of cyclosporine to calmodulin result in immunosuppression? *Science* 234:68-71, 1986.

Leib ES, et al: Immunosuppressive and corticosteroid therapy of polyarteritis nodosa. *Am J Med* 67:941-947, 1979.

Leickly FE, Buckley RH: Successful treatment of autoimmune hemolytic anemia in common variable immunodeficiency with high-dose intravenous gamma globulin. *Am J Med* 82:159-162, 1987.

Levitz M, et al: Transfer and metabolism of corticosteroids in perfused human placenta. *Am J Obstet Gynecol* 132:363-366, 1978.

Lichtenstein LM, et al: Insect allergy: State of the art. *J Allergy Clin Immunol* 64:5-12, 1979.

Ling MHM, et al: Side effects of corticosteroid therapy: Psychiatric aspects. *Arch Gen Psychiatry* 38:471-477, 1981.

Liu J, et al: Calcineurin is a common target of cyclophilin-cyclosporin A and FKBP-FK506 complexes. *Cell* 66:807-815, 1991.

Luce JK, et al: Efficacy of mesna in preventing further cyclophosphamide-induced hemorrhagic cystitis. *Med Pediatr Oncol* 16:372-374, 1988.

Ludwig H, et al: Erythropoietin treatment of anemia associated with multiple myeloma. *N Engl J Med* 322:1693-1699, 1990.

Luke RG: Summary: Non renal uses. *Am J Kidney Dis* 11:153, 1988.

Luzi G, et al: Levamisole therapy: Clinical and immunological evaluation in herpetic keratitis. *Int J Immunopharm* 5:197-199, 1983.

Macleod AM, Thomson AW: FK 506: An immunosuppressant for the 1990s? *Lancet* 337:25-27, 1991.

Mahrle G, Schulze H-J: Recombinant interferon-gamma (rIFN-gamma) in dermatology. *J Invest Dermatol* 95:132S-137S, 1990.

Martinez-Maldonado M, Garcia A: Practical approach to nephrotic syndrome. *Drug Ther* 11:79-91, (March) 1981.

Mayes JT, et al: Reexposure of OKT3 in renal allograft recipients. *Transplantation* 45:349-353, 1988.

McCluskey J, Gutteridge DH: Avascular necrosis of bone after high doses of dexamethasone during neurosurgery. *BMJ* 284:333-334, 1982.

McCune WJ, et al: Clinical and immunologic effects of monthly administration of intravenous cyclophosphamide in severe systemic lupus erythematosus. *N Engl J Med* 318:1423-1431, 1988.

McEwen C: Diagnosis and differential diagnosis of rheumatoid arthritis, in: *Arthritis and Allied Conditions,* Philadelphia, Lea & Febiger, 1972, 403-418.

McGuire WA, et al: Treatment of antibody-mediated pure red-cell aplasia with high-dose intravenous gamma globulin. *N Engl J Med* 317:1004-1008, 1987.

Millis JM, et al: Randomized prospective trial of OKT3 for early prophylaxis of rejection after liver transplantation. *Transplantation* 47:82-88, 1989.

Mody CH, et al: Cyclosporin A inhibits the growth of Cryptococcus neoformans in a murine model. *Infect Immun* 56:7-12, 1988.

Morhenn VB, et al: Use of recombinant interferon gamma administered intramuscularly for the treatment of psoriasis. *Arch Dermatol* 123:1633-1637, 1987.

Mouy R, et al: Interferon gamma for chronic granulomatous disease, letter. *N Engl J Med* 325:1516, 1991.

Mueller-Eckhardt C: Autoimmune thrombocytopenic purpura: Diagnostic and therapeutic actualities. *Curr Stud Hematol Blood Transfus* 55:69-80, 1988.

Mulé JJ, et al: Adoptive immunotherapy of established pulmonary metastases with LAK cells and recombinant interleukin-2. *Science* 225:1487-1489, 1984.

Murray HW: Interferon-γ therapy in AIDS for mononuclear phagocyte activation. *Biotherapy* 2:149-159, 1990.

Mutchnick MG, et al: Thymosin treatment of chronic hepatitis B: A placebo-controlled pilot trial. *Hepatology* 14:409-415, 1991.

Nalli G, et al: Danazol therapy for idiopathic thrombocytopenic purpura (ITP). *Haematologica (Pavia)* 73:55-57, 1988.

Newburger JW, et al: Treatment of Kawasaki syndrome with intravenous gamma globulin. *N Engl J Med* 315:341-347, 1986.

Nichols EE: Routine antepartum Rh immune globulin administration. *JAMA* 252:2763, 1984.

Nishihara S, et al: Intravenous gammaglobulin and reduction of coronary artery abnormalities in children with Kawasaki disease, letter. *Lancet* 2:973, 1988.

Nixon JE: Early diagnosis and treatment of steroid induced avascular necrosis of bone. *BMJ* 288:741-744, 1984.

Noll RB, Kulkarni R: Complex visual hallucinations and cyclosporine. *Arch Neurol* 41:329-330, 1984.

Norman DJ, et al: Effectiveness of a second course of OKT3 monoclonal anti-T cell antibody for treatment of renal allograft rejection. *Transplantation* 46:523-529, 1988.

Obert H-J, Hofschneider PH: Interferon bei chronischer polyarthritis. *Dtsch Med Wockenscht* 110:1766-1769, 1985.

Ochs HD: Intravenous immunoglobulin in treatment and prevention of acute infections in pediatric acquired immunodeficiency patients. *Pediatr Infect Dis J* 6:509-511, 1987.

Odio CM, et al: The beneficial effects of early dexamethasone administration in infants and children with bacterial meningitis. *N Engl J Med* 324:1525-1531, 1991.

Oh C-S, et al: Increased infections associated with the use of OKT3 for treatment of steroid-resistant rejection in renal transplantation. *Transplantation* 45:68-73, 1988.

Ohno T, et al: Effect of immunoglobulin preparation on course of AIDS-related complex (ARC). *Tohuku J Exp Med* 156:415-416, 1988.

Oliver RTD: Clinical potential of interleukin-2. *Br J Cancer* 58:405-409, 1988.

Olsen SL, et al: Methotrexate as an adjunct in the treatment of persistent mild cardiac allograft rejection. *Transplantation* 50:773-775, 1990.

Ortaldo JR, et al: Effects of natural and recombinant IL 2 on regulation of IFN γ production and natural killer activity: Lack of involvement of TAC antigen for these immunoregulatory effects. *J Immunol* 133:779-783, 1984.

Ortho Multicenter Transplant Study Group: Randomized clinical trial of OKT3 monoclonal antibody for acute rejection of cadaveric renal transplants. *N Engl J Med* 313:337-342, 1985.

Patrone F, et al: Restoration of defective EA_G-rosetting capacity of cancer patient neutrophils by levamisole. *Cancer* 55:1668-1672, 1985.

Phillips NC, et al: Modulation of murine lymphoma growth by MDP, MDP(D-D) and cyclophosphamide: 1. Inhibition of growth in vivo. *Int J Immunopharm* 5:219-227, 1983.

Pickup ME: Clinical pharmacokinetics of prednisone and prednisolone. *Clin Pharmacokinet* 4:111-128, 1979.

Pollack S, et al: High-dose intravenous gamma globulin for autoimmune neutropenia, letter. *N Engl J Med* 307:253, 1988.

Ponticelli C, et al: Controlled trial of methylprednisolone and chlorambucil in idiopathic membranous nephropathy. *N Engl J Med* 310:946-950, 1984.

Powell-Jackson PR, et al: Adult respiratory distress syndrome and convulsions associated with administration of cyclosporine in liver transplant recipients. *Transplantation* 38:341-343, 1984.

Prescott S, et al: HLA DR expression by high grade superficial bladder cancer treated with BCG. *Br J Urol* 63:264-269, 1989.

Ptachcinski RJ, et al: Cyclosporine. *Drug Intell Clin Pharm* 19:90-100, 1985 A.

Ptachcinski RJ, et al: Effect of food on cyclosporine absorption. *Transplantation* 40:174-176, 1985 B.

Quesada JR, Gutterman JU: Psoriasis and alpha-interferon. *Lancet* 1:1466-1468, 1986.

Ratliff TL, et al: Interleukin-2 production during intravesical bacille Calmette-Guerin therapy for bladder cancer. *Clin Immunol Immunopathol* 40:375-379, 1986.

Roifman CM, et al: Reversal of chronic polymyositis following intravenous immune serum globulin therapy. *JAMA* 258:513-515, 1987.

Roilides E, et al: Granulocyte colony-stimulating factor enhances the phagocytic and bactericidal activity of normal and defective human neutrophils. *J Infect Dis* 163:579-583, 1991.

Rosano TG, et al: Immunosuppressive metabolites of cyclosporine in the blood of renal allograft recipients. *Transplantation* 42:262-267, 1986.

Rose CD, et al: Safety and efficacy of methotrexate therapy for juvenile rheumatoid arthritis. *J Pediatr* 117:653-659, 1990.

Rosenberg SA: Lymphokine activated killer cells: New approach to the immunotherapy of cancer. *J Natl Cancer Inst* 75:595-603, 1985.

Rosenberg SA, et al: Biological activity of recombinant human interleukin-2 produced in *Escherichia coli*. *Science* 223:1412-1415, 1984.

Rosenberg SA, et al: Progress report on the treatment of 157 patients with advanced cancer using lymphokine-activated killer cell and interleukin-2 or high-dose interleukin-2 alone. *N Engl J Med* 316:889-897, 1987.

Rote NS, Lau RJ: Immunologic thrombocytopenic purpura. *Clin Obstet Gynecol* 28:84-100, 1985.

Rowley AH, Shulman ST: What is the status of intravenous gammaglobulin for Kawasaki syndrome in the United States and Canada. *Pediatr Infect Dis J* 7:463-466, 1988.

Ryckman FC, et al: Use of monoclonal antibody immunosuppressive therapy in pediatric renal and liver transplantation. *Clin Transplant* 5:186-190, 1991.

Sakaguchi S, Sakaguchi N: Thymus and autoimmunity: Transplantation of the thymus from cyclosporin A-treated mice causes organ-specific autoimmune disease in athymic nude mice. *J Exp Med* 167:1479-1485, 1988.

Sakaguchi S, Sakaguchi N: Organ-specific autoimmune disease inducted in mice by elimination of T cell subsets. *J Immunol* 142:471-480, 1989.

Sambrook PN, et al: Osteonecrosis after high dosage, short term corticosteroid therapy. *J Rheumatol* 11:514-516, 1984.

Sarna G, et al: Phase I study of recombinant β ser 17 interferon in the treatment of cancer. *Cancer Treat Rep* 70:1365-1372, 1986.

Sattler FR: Who should receive corticosteroids as adjunctive treatment for *Pneumocystis carinii* pneumonia, editorial. *Chest* 99:1058-1060, 1991.

Schreiber SL: Chemistry and biology of the immunophilins and their immunosuppressive ligands. *Science* 251:283-287, (Jan) 1991.

Schuyler RM, et al: Prednisone and T-cell subpopulations. *Arch Intern Med* 144:973-975, 1984.

Segal R, et al: Methotrexate: Mechanism of action in rheumatoid arthritis. *Arthritis Rheum* 20:190-199, 1990.

Shah D, et al: Generalised epileptic fits in renal transplant recipients given cyclosporin A. *BMJ* 289:1347-1348, 1984.

Shaw LM, et al: Canadian consensus meeting on cyclosporine monitoring: Report of the consensus panel. *Clin Chem* 36:1842-1846, 1990.

Shevach EM: Effects of cyclosporin A on the immune system. *Annu Rev Immunol* 3:397-423, 1985.

Silverstein J, et al: Immunosuppression with azathioprine and prednisone in recent-onset insulin-dependent diabetes mellitus. *N Engl J Med* 319:599-604, 1988.

Simmons RL, et al: New immunosuppressive drug combination for mismatched related and cadaveric renal transplantation. *Transplant Proc* 18 (suppl 1):76-81, 1986.

Small P, et al: Venom immunotherapy: Critical evaluation of in vitro techniques. *Ann Allergy* 50:256-259, 1983.

Smith BR, et al: Efficacy of short course (four doses) of methotrexate following bone marrow transplantation for prevention of graft-versus-host disease. *Transplantation* 39:326-329, 1985.

Solbach W, et al: Suppressive effect of cyclosporin A on the development of Leishmania tropica-induced lesions in genetically susceptible BALB/c mice. *J Immunol* 137:702-707, 1986.

Sone S, et al: Potentiating effect of muramyl dipeptide and its lipophilic analog encapsulated in liposomes on tumour cell killing by human monocytes. *J Immunol* 132:2105-2110, 1984.

Spiro HM: Is the steroid ulcer a myth? Editorial. *N Engl J Med* 309:45-47, 1983.

Starzl TE, et al: FK-506 for liver, kidney, and pancreas transplantation. *Lancet* 2:1000-1004, 1989.

Starzl TE, et al (eds): Proceedings of the First International Congress on FK 506. *Transplant Proc* 23:2709-2750, 1991.

Steele RW, et al: Intravenous immunoglobulin: New clinical applications. *Ann Allergy* 60:89-94, 1988.

Storb R, et al: Methotrexate and cyclosporine compared with cyclosporine alone for prophylaxis of acute graft versus host disease after marrow transplantation for leukemia. *N Engl J Med* 314:729-735, 1986.

Storb R, et al: Methotrexate and cyclosporine versus cyclosporine alone for prophylaxis of graft-versus-host disease in patients given HLA-identical marrow grafts for leukemia: Long-term follow-up of a controlled trial. *Blood* 73:1729-1734, 1989.

Stratta R, et al: Experience with OKT3 after orthotopic liver transplantation. *Transplant Proc* 23:1970, 1991.

Taylor LJ: Multifocal avascular necrosis after short-term high-dose steroid therapy: Report of three cases. *J Bone Joint Surg* 66-B:431-433, 1984.

Thomson AW: Immunological effects of cyclosporin A, in Bach J-F (ed): *T Cell-Directed Immunosuppression.* Oxford, Blackwell Scientific Publications, in press.

Thomson AW, Starzl TE: FK 506 and autoimmune disease: Perspective and prospects. *Autoimmunity* 12:303-313, 1992.

Thompson CB, et al: Association between cyclosporin neurotoxicity and hypomagnesaemia. *Lancet* 2:1116-1120, 1984.

Truckenbrodt H, Häfner R: Methotrexate therapy in juvenile rheumatoid arthritis: A retrospective study. *Arthritis Rheum* 29:801-807, 1986.

Uribe M, et al: Comparative serum prednisone and prednisolone concentrations following administration to patients with chronic active liver disease. *Clin Pharmacokinet* 7:452-459, 1982.

Urman JD, Rothfield NF: Corticosteroid treatment in systemic lupus erythematosus: Survival studies. *JAMA* 238:2272-2276, 1977.

Valentine MD, et al: The value of immunotherapy with venom in children with allergy to insect stings. *N Engl J Med* 323:1601-1603, 1990.

Vanrenterghen Y, et al: Thromboembolic complications and haemostatic changes in cyclosporin-treated cadaveric kidney allograft recipients. *Lancet* 1:999-1002, 1985.

Van Wauwe JP, et al: OKT3: Monoclonal antihuman T lymphocyte antibody with potent mitogenic properties. *J Immunol* 124:2708-2713, 1980.

Warrell DA, et al: Dexamethasone proves deleterious in cerebral malaria: Double-blind trial in 100 comatose patients. *N Engl J Med* 306:313-319, 1982.

Weigent DA, et al: Interleukin 2 enhances natural killer cell activity through induction of gamma interferon. *Infect Immun* 41:992-997, 1983.

Weinblatt ME, et al: Danazol for children with immune thrombocytopenic purpura. *Am J Dis Child* 142:1317-1319, 1988.

Wong JT, et al: The mechanism of anti-CD3 monoclonal antibodies: Mediation of cytolysis by inter-T cell bridging. *Transplantation* 50:683-689, 1990.

Yadav RVS, et al: Cyclophosphamide in renal transplantation. *Transplantation* 45:421-424, 1988.

Yap PL, Williams PE: Immunoglobulin preparations for HIV-infected patients. *Vox Sang* 55:65-74, 1988 A.

Yap PL, Williams PE: Treatment of HIV-infected patients with intravenous immunoglobulin. *J Hosp Infect* (Suppl D):35-46, (Aug) 1988 B.

Yount WJ, et al: Corticosteroid therapy of collagen vascular disorders, in Azarnoff DL (ed): *Steroid Therapy.* Philadelphia, WB Saunders, 1975, 269-286.

Zazgornik J, et al: Venous thrombosis and cyclosporin, letter. *Lancet* 2:102, 1985.

Zizic TM, et al: Corticosteroid therapy associated with ischemic necrosis of bone in systemic lupus erythematosus. *Am J Med* 79:596-609, 1985.

Agents for Active and Passive Immunity: General Recommendations

84

Immunization is an inclusive term denoting the process of inducing immunity or providing it artificially through administration of a vaccine, toxoid, or preformed antibody. Active immunization is induced by natural infection or by a vaccine or toxoid that causes the recipient to produce specific antibodies and antitoxins. The immunologic mechanism responsible for protection is unknown for some vaccines (eg, bacillus Calmette-Guerin [BCG]) but may be due in part to cell-mediated immunity. In the case of BCG, empiric observations of protection following vaccine administration have served as a guide. In passive immunization, temporary immunity is provided through administration of preformed antibodies produced in another individual by natural infection or active immunization. Three types of agents are employed for passive immunization: pooled human immune globulin, specific immune globulin, and antiserums produced in animals.

The ultimate goal of many immunization programs is the eradication of communicable diseases through the use of vaccines and antiserums. For example, an effective worldwide immunization program with smallpox vaccine has eradicated the natural disease, and international efforts to eradicate poliomyelitis are now underway. Immunization also may have the immediate goal of preventing specific diseases in selected individuals and groups.

Attainment of a high proportion of immune individuals in a community is the most effective means of preventing communicable disease. Universal immunization is an important part of good health care and should be pursued actively through routine and intensive programs to ensure that all children and other susceptible persons are immunized. In the United States, universal immunization of children with diphtheria/tetanus/pertussis (DTP), poliovirus, *Haemophilus influenzae* type b (Hib), measles/mumps/rubella (MMR), and hepatitis B vaccines has been recommended.

The Advisory Committee on Immunization Practices (ACIP) of the United States Public Health Service regularly updates information on vaccines and antiserums and periodically revises recommendations for their use; it also provides general immunization recommendations (*MMWR*, 1994). ACIP advisories and recommendations are published in the widely circulated *Morbidity and Mortality Weekly Report* (*MMWR*), and the pertinent articles routinely appear in *The Journal of the American Medical Association*. Physicians should consult these publications for updated information on vaccines and antiserums. The American Academy of Pediatrics and the American College of Physicians also publish recommendations for the use of vaccines. The physician also should consult the manufacturer's package insert.

VACCINES

Vaccines are suspensions of living or killed microorganisms (bacteria, viruses), components, or products thereof employed to induce active immunity. Some vaccines consist of highly defined antigens (eg, the polysaccharide antigens of *Haemophilus influenzae* type b or pneumococci, the hepatitis B surface antigen) while others contain crude antigens or are incompletely defined (eg, pertussis vaccine, BCG, live attenuated virus vaccines). Certain vaccines (DTP, MMR, poliovirus, hepatitis B, and Hib) are used routinely for pediatric immunization, while others (eg, rabies, influenza, meningococcal, pneumococcal, BCG, plague, anthrax, typhoid, cholera, yellow fever) are indicated primarily for those at special risk. Most vaccines are intended for use in normal, healthy individuals, although they may be safe and effective in persons with some underlying diseases or conditions.

Vaccines are used prophylactically, usually before exposure to infectious disease, but some are effective in individuals previously exposed to a specific disease. For example, pre-exposure rabies immunization is given only to selected individuals at high risk (eg, veterinarians, animal handlers); however, rabies vaccine also is administered routinely after potential contact with the virus, as through an animal bite. Measles vaccine given within 72 hours after exposure may prevent disease. This is thought to be due to the shorter incubation period for vaccine measles (seven days) compared with natural or wild type measles (11 days).

VIRAL VACCINES. These are composed of live attenuated viruses (eg, measles, mumps, rubella vaccines; oral poliovirus vaccine [OPV]), inactivated nonliving whole viruses (eg, influenza, rabies, inactivated poliovirus vaccine [IPV]), or antigenic components of the virus particle (eg, influenza "split-virus" vaccine, hepatitis B vaccine). They may contain a single agent (eg, measles, hepatitis B) or a combination (eg, MMR).

In normal recipients, vaccines containing live, attenuated microorganisms produce a mild or subclinical infection that results in active immunity. Replication of the virus in the recipient is essential to the induction of immunity. Most vaccines containing live, attenuated viruses require only a single dose to provide long-term protection. However, three doses of live OPV and two doses of MMR vaccine are currently recommended to ensure seroconversion. A high level of seroconversion is thought to be associated with long-term protection. In addition to systemic protection, OPV also appears to stimulate local immunity by inducing IgA at the portal of entry and in the intestine.

Inactivated vaccines must contain a sufficient antigenic mass in the injected bolus to induce the desired immune response, since the organisms in these preparations cannot replicate in the host. Repeated administration is usually necessary to induce long lasting immunity. The primary immunization schedule usually consists of two or three doses, with booster doses to maintain immunity.

BACTERIAL VACCINES. These are prepared from whole bacteria (eg, pertussis vaccine), from purified products of whole cell vaccine (eg, acellular pertussis vaccine), from purified capsular polysaccharides of certain bacteria (eg, pneumococcal vaccine, meningococcal vaccine), or from purified polysaccharides conjugated to protein carriers to improve immunogenicity (eg, Hib vaccine). Except for BCG and oral typhoid vaccine Ty21a, bacterial vaccines are composed of nonliving agents. The live, attenuated bacterial vaccines act in a manner analogous to that described for live virus vaccines.

Bacterial vaccines stimulate the production of various antibodies; those that play a protective role are directed against antigens on the surface of a bacterial cell or its exotoxin. Coating of these bacterial surface antigens with antibodies renders the organisms more susceptible to phagocytosis (opsonins) or to lysis by complement (lytic antibodies) or may cause aggregation or interfere with the function of a critical bacterial surface structure.

Inactivated bacterial vaccines are usually given in two to four doses. However, polysaccharide vaccines provide long-term protection after a single dose, except in children less than two years.

TOXOIDS. Toxoids are modified bacterial exotoxins that have been rendered nontoxic by chemical treatment. They retain the ability to stimulate the production of antibodies that combine with toxin. The two agents used clinically are tetanus and diphtheria toxoids. They are available in combination with each other (pediatric: DT; adult: Td) and with whole cell or acellular pertussis vaccines (DTP, DTaP). Although tetanus toxoid is available as a single agent, the combined preparations are preferred.

COMPONENTS OF VACCINES AND TOXOIDS. Physicians should be familiar with the major constituents of vaccines and toxoids, since they may cause adverse effects (eg, hypersensitivity reactions).

Immunizing Antigen(s): In some preparations (eg, recombinant hepatitis B vaccine, tetanus toxoid), this is a single, well-defined material, while in others (eg, pertussis vaccine, live virus vaccines), the material is crude and less well defined.

Suspending Fluid: This may be simple (sterile water or saline) or complex (eg, tissue culture fluid). Small amounts of proteins and other material derived from the biological system or medium of preparation (eg, egg protein, serum protein, cell culture antigens) may be included.

Preservatives, Stabilizers, Antibiotics: Mercurials, glycine, lactose, dextrose, and certain antibiotics are present to prevent bacterial growth or stabilize the antigen. These materials occasionally cause hypersensitivity reactions in some individuals.

Adjuvants: Certain vaccines contain an aluminum compound to intensify the immune response and to aid in retention of the antigen at the depot site, which prolongs the stimulant effect. Adjuvants are employed in vaccines containing inactivated microorganisms or their products (eg, toxoids, hepatitis B). Vaccines containing adjuvants should not be injected subcutaneously or intracutaneously, since local irritation, inflammation, granuloma, or necrosis may follow. They should be injected deep into muscle masses.

ANTISERUMS AND IMMUNE GLOBULINS

These substances are used both prophylactically and therapeutically to provide temporary immunity against infectious agents, microbial exotoxins, and snake and insect venoms. Antiserums provide protection by the passive transfer of antibodies produced in another individual either by natural infection (eg, hepatitis B immune globulin) or by active immunization with a known immunogen (eg, rabies antiserum, human or equine). The protection may be specific, as with diphtheria antitoxin, or useful for prophylaxis against two or more conditions, as with immune globulin (IG, gamma globulin).

Antiserums are commonly used when (1) no vaccine is available and use of antibody prevents or modifies the disease (eg, hepatitis A); (2) protection is needed immediately, and there is insufficient time to stimulate the patient's own antibodies through active immunization (eg, hepatitis B, rabies prophylaxis, certain exposures to measles); (3) a disease caused by a specific microbial toxin (eg, botulism) is best managed by administration of antibody; (4) clinical disease is present and an antibody is known to neutralize the effect of the unfixed toxin (eg, diphtheria, tetanus, snake or spider envenomation); or (5) the patient has diminished or absent capacity to produce antibodies (eg, immunosuppression caused by cancer chemotherapy or radiation treatment, immunodeficiency disease).

Antiserums for clinical use are of human or equine origin. Serious hypersensitivity reactions (serum sickness, anaphylaxis) occur much more often with equine antiserums. In addition, antibodies from heterologous species, such as those in equine antiserums, disappear from the blood rapidly; often none remain after seven to ten days. In contrast, the half-life of human antiserums is approximately four weeks.

IG is a sterile serum protein solution (15% to 18%) containing antibodies from human blood. It is derived from pooled human serum by cold ethanol fractionation and consists primarily of immunoglobulin G (95% IgG); small amounts of other immunoglobulins (IgM, IgA) and other serum proteins also are present. IG contains antibodies in proportion to those in the population from which it was derived, and large numbers of donors are employed to ensure that adequate amounts of desired antibodies (eg, measles, hepatitis A) are included. IG is primarily indicated to maintain immunity in immunodeficient patients and for passive immunization against measles and hepatitis A. It is intended for intramuscular use only.

Specific IG preparations are obtained from plasma donors preselected for high titers of the desired antibody (eg, cytomegalovirus, hepatitis B, varicella-zoster, rabies, vaccinia, tetanus). Some preparations are obtained from individuals hyperimmunized with a specific vaccine (eg, vaccinia, tetanus, rabies), while others are obtained from pooled plasma drawn from subjects with naturally high antibody titers to a specific antigen (eg, varicella-zoster, hepatitis B). In all other respects, specific IG preparations conform to the description of IG.

IG for intravenous administration is specially treated and delivered in vehicles that minimize aggregate formation. It contains a lower concentration of immunoglobulin (generally, 5%) than the IG preparation for intramuscular use and is indicated for replacement therapy in primary antibody deficiency disorders and for the treatment of Kawasaki disease, immune thrombocytopenic purpura, and hypogammaglobulinemia in chronic lymphocytic leukemia. IG preparations intended for intramuscular use must *never* be given intravenously; similarly, intravenous preparations are inappropriate for intramuscular or subcutaneous use.

Antitoxins are antibodies directed against a toxin (eg, microbial exotoxin, snake or spider venom) that combine specifically with it to neutralize toxicity. Antitoxins for human use are principally of equine origin (antivenins; diphtheria, botulism, and tetanus antitoxins), but tetanus antitoxin of human origin (tetanus immune globulin) is more commonly used.

Antivenins are antitoxins directed against the venom of a snake (eg, North American coral snake) or insect (black widow spider). All antivenins for human use are of equine origin and are given only after envenomation has occurred.

Antiserums and IG preparations contain antibodies that combine with antigenic sites on the infectious organism or toxin, resulting in anti-invasive, neutralizing, or antitoxic activity. Passive immunization with these materials results in protection of short duration (one to three months). Protective antiviral (neutralizing) antibodies inhibit adsorption, penetration, and normal uncoating of the virus. Since antibodies do not penetrate the intact cell, they act only on extracellular viruses. Antitoxins combine avidly with specific toxins. Once combined with antibody, the toxin's action is inhibited and it is said to be neutralized; however, antitoxin cannot affect toxin already fixed to cells or reverse its prior effect.

ADVERSE REACTIONS

VACCINES. Adverse reactions have been reported for all vaccines. These are usually local and transient but may be systemic and immediate or delayed. Local inflammatory reactions at the site of injection are most common. Systemic reactions (eg, fever, rash, hypersensitivity) occur infrequently and most subside within 48 hours; they usually can be managed with symptomatic treatment only. The following types of adverse reactions have been encountered with vaccines.

Mild Local Reactions: These effects are the most common and occur after use of most vaccines. A local inflammatory reaction (eg, erythema, tenderness) develops at the site of injection. Induration is seen less often.

Severe Local Reactions: These are most commonly encountered with certain live vaccines, such as smallpox and BCG, which produce a lesion at the injection site that leaves a scar. With BCG vaccine, severe ulceration and keloidal scars may result.

Mild Systemic Reactions: Following vaccination, transient fever, malaise, or mild headache may occur, but these reactions usually subside within 48 hours and require symptomatic treatment only.

Severe, Nonallergic Systemic Reactions: These reactions are rare and may be characterized by a severe febrile response, severe headache, febrile convulsions, or paralysis. Examples include the high fevers and febrile convulsions that develop occasionally in children after pertussis vaccination; reactions to vaccination or booster doses of typhoid, cholera, or plague vaccine; and the rare instances of paralytic poliomyelitis that develop after administration of live oral poliovirus vaccine. Infrequently, events such as afebrile seizures and encephalopathy or encephalitis are reported after vaccination. Whether these events are caused by vaccination or are coincidental is often difficult to determine. See the evaluations in the chapter, Agents for Immunization, for information on these and other adverse events.

TABLE 1.
TREATMENT OF ANAPHYLACTIC SHOCK

Route	Epinephrine Dosage	
	Adults	Children
Initial (repeated every 20 to 30 minutes as necessary, up to 3 doses):		
Subcutaneous (preferred), Intramuscular (epinephrine 1:1,000)	0.3-0.5 ml	0.01 ml/kg (maximum, 0.3 ml)
Severe shock or inadequate response to intramuscular or subcutaneous administration:		
Intravenous (epinephrine 1:10,000)*	3 to 5 ml at 5 to 10 min intervals	0.1 ml/kg every 5 to 10 min, as needed

** Solution diluted 1:10,000 by adding 1 ml of 1:1,000 solution to syringe containing 9 ml of physiologic saline injection. A ready-made 1:10,000 solution is available from several manufacturers. Administer slowly over a period of 4 to 5 minutes.*

Hypersensitivity Reactions: These reactions occur very rarely. Allergic reactions are thought to be due to the following vaccine constituents: (1) Trace amounts of egg protein in influenza, measles, mumps, and yellow fever vaccines. (2) Antibiotic(s) in the vaccines; for example, MMR vaccine contains a small amount of neomycin, and some individuals who are allergic to neomycin may experience a delayed-type local reaction (erythematous, pruritic papule) 48 to 72 hours after injection of the vaccine. (3) Some component of the infectious agent itself or one of its products. Rarely, urticarial reactions have been observed in individuals receiving tetanus or diphtheria toxoid, and these are thought to be hypersensitivity reactions to the immunogens themselves.

ANTISERUMS AND IMMUNE GLOBULINS. Adverse reactions to antiserums are much more common than to vaccines or IG preparations. Serious hypersensitivity reactions occur with much greater frequency with use of antiserums of equine origin than to those of human origin. Three types of sensitivity reactions occur: (1) Anaphylactic reactions develop seconds to minutes after injection and consist of urticaria, dyspnea, cyanosis, and shock. (See following discussion.) (2) Serum sickness consisting of rash, urticaria, arthritis, adenopathy, and fever occurs hours or days after injection. It is more common and has a more rapid onset in persons who received prior serum injections or large doses and may be managed with salicylates, antihistamines, or corticosteroids. (3) Acute febrile reactions are usually mild and may be treated with antipyretics. Rarely, they may result in death due to hyperpyrexia.

Serious reactions to IG preparations are uncommon, although anaphylaxis and systemic collapse have been reported. These reactions may be caused by previous sensitization to foreign antigens in the IG preparation. They occur most frequently in IgA-deficient individuals (incidence, 1:300 to 1:800 in the general population) who experience an immune response to the small amount of normal IgA contained in IG. The most common reaction is discomfort on administration, which often can be alleviated by using several sites for injection (intramuscular) or slowing the rate of administration (intravenous). Organic mercurials (eg, thimerosal) are used as preservatives in these products and may accumulate in patients given some IG preparations over a prolonged period. However, only one instance of proven mercury sensitivity has been reported.

ANAPHYLACTIC SHOCK. Anaphylaxis is an acute systemic manifestation of immediate hypersensitivity and is often life-threatening. IgE-dependent release of preformed mediators (eg, histamine) from mast cells and basophils and secondary synthesis of other vasoactive compounds (eg, prostaglandins, leukotrienes, platelet-activating factor) are responsible for the many complex and varied reactions. Histamine and various membrane-derived lipid mediators alter venule permeability, and the cysteinyl leukotrienes (eg, LTD_4) constrict both vascular and nonvascular smooth muscle.

The onset of anaphylactic shock is frequently marked by generalized pruritus, flushing, and urticaria and/or angioedema. Laryngeal edema, hypotension, bronchospasm, and arrhythmias may follow and are the most common life-threatening complications. Generalized reactions are rare and occur primarily when vaccines containing egg protein are used; systemic reactions to equine antiserum are more common.

The aim of initial therapy is to prevent or reverse complications and includes administration of epinephrine, cardiac monitoring, establishing intravenous access, and immediate attention to the upper airway. The latter is imperative, for most fatal reactions involve obstruction at this site. Hypoxia should be treated by establishing a patent airway and administering oxygen. Endotracheal intubation may be necessary; emergency tracheostomy is indicated in the presence of laryngeal edema sufficient to impede passage of an endotracheal tube.

The usual treatment for vascular shock (eg, maintaining body temperature, elevating the lower extremities) also may be needed. For severe cardiovascular collapse, it may be necessary to administer epinephrine directly into the heart and to initiate cardiopulmonary resuscitation. Intravenous fluids should be administered, and intravenous infusion of norepinephrine [Levophed] may be required to support blood pressure (for adults, 2 to 8 ml of solution added to 500 ml of

TABLE 2.
VACCINE INJURY TABLE[1]

Vaccine/Toxoid	Event	Interval from Vaccination
DTP, Pertussis, DTP/Polio Combined	A. Anaphylaxis or anaphylactic shock	24 hours
	B. Encephalopathy (or encephalitis) *	7 days
	C. Shock-collapse or hypotonic-hyporesponsive collapse*	7 days
	D. Residual seizure disorder*	(See Aids to Interpretation*)
	E. Any acute complication or sequela (including death) of above events	No limit
	F. Events in vaccinees described in manufacturer's package insert as contraindications to additional doses of vaccine† (such as convulsions)	(See package insert)
Measles, Mumps, and Rubella; DT, Td, Tetanus Toxoid	A. Anaphylaxis or anaphylactic shock	24 hours
	B. Encephalopathy (or encephalitis) *	15 days for measles, mumps, and rubella vaccines; 7 days for DT, Td, and Tetanus toxoids
	C. Residual seizure disorder*	(See Aids to Interpretation*)
	D. Any acute complication or sequela (including death) of above events	No limit
	E. Events in vaccinees described in manufacturer's package insert as contraindications to additional doses of vaccine†	(See package insert)
Oral Poliovirus Vaccine	A. Paralytic poliomyelitis	
	—in a non-immunodeficient recipient	30 days
	—in an immunodeficient recipient	6 months
	—in a vaccine-associated community case	No limit
	B. Any acute complication or sequela (including death) of above events	No limit
	C. Events in vaccinees described in manufacturer's package insert as contraindications to additional doses of vaccine†	(See package insert)
Inactivated Poliovirus Vaccine	A. Anaphylaxis or anaphylactic shock	24 hours
	B. Any acute complication or sequela (including death) of above event	No limit
	C. Events in vaccinees described in manufacturer's package insert as contraindications to additional doses of vaccine†	(See package insert)

*** Aids to Interpretation:**

Shock-collapse or hypotonic-hyporesponsive collapse may be evidenced by signs or symptoms such as decrease in or loss of muscle tone, paralysis (partial or complete), hemiplegia, hemiparesis, loss of color or turning pale white or blue, unresponsiveness to environmental stimuli, depression of or loss of consciousness, prolonged sleeping with difficulty arousing, or cardiovascular or respiratory arrest.

Residual seizure disorder may be considered to have occurred if no other seizure or convulsion unaccompanied by fever or accompanied by a fever of less than 102° F occurred before the first seizure or convulsion after the administration of the vaccine involved,

AND, if in the case of measles-, mumps-, or rubella-containing vaccines, the first seizure or convulsion occurred within 15 days after vaccination

OR in the case of any other vaccine, the first seizure or convulsion occurred within three days after vaccination,

AND, if two or more seizures or convulsions unaccompanied by fever or accompanied by a fever of less than 102°F occurred within one year after vaccination.

The terms seizure and convulsion include grand mal, petit mal, absence, myoclonic, tonic-clonic, and focal motor seizures and signs.

Encephalopathy means any significant acquired abnormality of, injury to, or impairment of function of the brain. Among the frequent manifestations of encephalopathy are focal and diffuse neurologic signs, increased intracranial pressure, or changes lasting at least 6 hours in level of consciousness, with or without convulsions. The neurologic signs and symptoms of encephalopathy may be temporary with complete recovery, or they may result in various degrees of permanent impairment. Signs and symptoms such as high-pitched and unusual screaming, persistent inconsolable crying, and bulging fontanel are compatible with an encephalopathy, but in and of themselves are not conclusive evidence of encephalopathy. Encephalopathy usually can be documented by slow wave activity on an electroencephalogram.

†The health care provider must refer to the CONTRAINDICATION section of the manufacturer's package insert for each vaccine.

1 From MMWR, *1988.*

5% dextrose injection is given at a rate adjusted to maintain satisfactory blood pressure).

Epinephrine 1:1,000 is the primary drug used in anaphylaxis because of its combined alpha- and beta-adrenergic agonist properties. The alpha component increases peripheral resistance and decreases urticaria. The beta component increases cyclic adenosine monophosphate (cAMP) levels to inhibit further release of mediators, relax bronchial smooth muscle, and increase cardiac rate and contractility. The dosages in Table 1 should be given at the earliest sign of anaphylaxis.

Antihistamines (eg, diphenhydramine) are usually considered part of the standard treatment of anaphylactic reactions but play no role in immediate treatment because they do not reverse effects already produced by histamine. Antihistamines act by competitively inhibiting histamine at receptor sites but have no effect on SRS-A (slow reacting substance of anaphylaxis) and, thus, bronchospasm is not reversed. However, these agents do reverse such cutaneous manifestations as pruritus and thus may be used adjunctively. Diphenhydramine can be given orally after reversal of reactions by epinephrine, but it should be given parenterally for life-threatening episodes.

Patients who develop severe wheezing without vascular shock should be treated initially with epinephrine, which may be followed by use of theophylline or a sympathomimetic bronchodilator (see index entry Bronchodilators).

Since corticosteroids neither prevent nor reverse anaphylactic symptoms, they are not useful in emergencies but are often given to shorten the course of the reaction. Those who advocate their use in refractory cases (when hypotension or bronchospasm is present) believe that corticosteroids may decrease the duration or severity of symptoms in prolonged reactions. Steroids may prevent the effects of (1) some mediators (prostaglandins, leukotrienes) that are not preformed but are released after antigen stimulation and may have extended effects, and (2) circulating antigen that may persist and cause a recurrence of symptoms. However, results of clinical studies do not conclusively support the use of steroids in anaphylaxis or determine an agent of choice.

Hypotensive patients who do not respond to repeated doses of epinephrine, intravenous fluids, and antihistamines may be treated with pressor agents. Although the agent of choice is controversial, some investigators prefer dopamine. Acidosis may result from hypoxia and decreased cardiac output; treatment with sodium bicarbonate has been recommended. For a more detailed discussion on anaphylaxis and its treatment, see Sheffer and Pennoyer, 1984; Reuben, 1986; Lichtenstein, 1988; Yunginger, 1992 A, 1992 B; Fisher, 1992; Bochner and Lichtenstein, 1991.

ADVERSE REACTION REPORTING AND STANDARDS FOR IMMUNIZATION PRACTICE

NATIONAL CHILDHOOD VACCINE INJURY ACT (NCVIA). The National Childhood Vaccine Injury Act of 1986 (Title XXIII of the Public Health Service Act) requires reporting to the Department of Health and Human Services selected adverse events that occur following administration of DTP or its components, MMR or its components, OPV, or IPV (see Table 2). Details of the NCVIA requirements have been published by the U.S. Public Health Service (*MMWR*, 1988). In addition, other significant reactions following receipt of these *and all other vaccines* should be reported to the Vaccine Adverse Event Reporting System (VAERS) using the pre-addressed and postage-paid VAERS reporting form, which is available by calling 800/822-7967. A copy appears at the end of this chapter for the reader's reference. The adverse events that must be reported are listed in Table 2. Written notification of report receipt by VAERS will be sent to those who send in a form. For certain serious adverse events, the health provider or vaccine administrator will be contacted by VAERS for a follow-up of the patient's condition at 60 days and at one year.

National Vaccine Injury Compensation Program: The National Vaccine Injury Compensation Program, under which compensation can be paid on behalf of a person who was injured or died as a result of being given one of the covered vaccines, was established by the NCVIA of 1986 and became effective in October 1988. It is intended as an alternative to civil litigation under the traditional tort system in that negligence need not be proven. The legislation establishing the program also established a vaccine injury table (see Table 2) that lists the specific vaccines covered by the program as well as the conditions for which compensation may be paid. Persons may be compensated for an injury listed in Table 2 or one that can be demonstrated to result from administration of one of the listed vaccines. Injuries resulting from the administration of vaccines that are not listed in Table 2 are not eligible for compensation through the program. For additional information, contact the National Vaccine Injury Compensation Program, Health Resources and Services Administration, Parklawn Building, Room 8-05, 5600 Fishers Lane, Rockville, MD, 20857 (301/443-6593 or 800/338-2382). Individuals who wish to file a claim for vaccine injury should contact U.S. Claims Court, 717 Madison Place, NW, Washington, DC, 20005 (202/633-7257).

Required Vaccine Information: The NCVIA requires that informational materials be developed for each vaccine covered by the Act. Vaccine informational pamphlets have been prepared by the U.S. Public Health Service and should be used by all public and private vaccine providers. Copies are available from state health authorities responsible for immunization. Alternatively, private providers may develop their own materials, but these must contain the specific elements required by the Act. The CDC has developed Important Information Statements for vaccines not covered by the NCVIA; these must be used in public health clinics and other settings where federally purchased vaccines are administered. Copies are available from state health authorities responsible for immunization.

Immunization Records: Providers who administer one or more of the vaccines covered by the NCVIA are required to ensure that the recipients' permanent medical records state the date the vaccine was administered; the vaccine manufacturer; the vaccine lot number; and the name, address, and title of the person administering the vaccine. (The ACIP rec-

TABLE 3.
STANDARDS FOR PEDIATRIC IMMUNIZATION PRACTICES*

1. Immunization services are readily available.
2. There are no barriers or unnecessary prerequisites to the receipt of vaccines.
3. Immunization services are available free or for a minimal fee.
4. Providers utilize all clinical encounters to screen and, when indicated, immunize children.
5. Providers educate parents and guardians about immunization in general terms.
6. Providers question parents or guardians about contraindications and, before immunizing a child, inform them in specific terms about the risks and benefits of the immunizations their child is to receive.
7. Providers follow only true contraindications.
8. Providers administer simultaneously all vaccine doses for which a child is eligible at the time of each visit.
9. Providers use accurate and complete recording procedures.
10. Providers coschedule immunization appointments in conjunction with appointments for other child health services.
11. Providers report adverse events following immunization promptly, accurately, and completely.
12. Providers operate a tracking system.
13. Providers adhere to appropriate procedures for vaccine management.
14. Providers conduct semiannual audits to assess immunization coverage levels and to review immunization records in the patient populations they serve.
15. Providers maintain up-to-date, easily retrievable medical protocols at all locations where vaccines are administered.
16. Providers operate with patient-oriented and community-based approaches.
17. Vaccines are administered by properly trained individuals.
18. Providers receive ongoing education and training on current immunization recommendations.

* *Ad Hoc Working Group for the Development of Standards of Pediatric Immunization Practices, 1993.*

ommends that the foregoing information be kept for all vaccines.) In addition, it is recommended that parents establish a permanent immunization record card for each newborn infant and that it be maintained continuously.

Frequently, persons without adequate documentation of immunizations are encountered by vaccine providers. Immunizations should not be postponed if records cannot be found; such persons should be considered susceptible and an appropriate immunization schedule should be initiated.

STANDARDS FOR IMMUNIZATION PRACTICES. Standards for both pediatric and adult immunization programs have been published (Ad Hoc Working Group for the Development of Standards for Pediatric Immunization Practices, 1993; *MMWR*, 1990 A). The pediatric standards were developed by the CDC in collaboration with a 35-member working group representing 22 public and private agencies involved in clinical care and prevention health services. They reflect the consensus of the National Vaccine Advisory Committee and the Ad Hoc Working Group on the most appropriate immunization practices in an immunization service for both the public and private sectors (Table 3). These standards, which have been endorsed by a variety of medical and public health organizations, including the American Medical Association, are goals that all providers should strive to attain; they include elimination of unnecessary prerequisites to the receipt of vaccines and missed opportunities so that all eligible children are appropriately vaccinated. (See also Table 4.)

TABLE 4.
GUIDE TO CONTRAINDICATIONS AND PRECAUTIONS TO IMMUNIZATIONS*

True Contraindications and Precautions	Not True (Vaccines May Be Given)
General for All Vaccines (DTP/DTaP, OPV, IPV, MMR, Hib, Hepatitis B)†	
Anaphylactic reaction to a vaccine contraindicates further doses of that vaccine. Anaphylactic reaction to a vaccine constituent contraindicates the use of vaccines containing that substance. Moderate or severe illnesses with or without a fever	Mild to moderate local reaction (soreness, redness, swelling) following a dose of an injectable antigen Mild acute illness with or without low-grade fever Current antimicrobial therapy Convalescent phase of illnesses Prematurity (same dosage and indications as for normal, full-term infants) Recent exposure to an infectious disease History of penicillin or other nonspecific allergies or fact that relatives have such allergies
DTP/DTaP	
Encephalopathy within 7 days of administration of dose of DTP Precaution: Fever of ≥40.5° C (105° F) within 48 hours after vaccination with a dose of DTP‡ Precaution: Collapse or shocklike state (hypotonic-hyporesponsive episode) within 48 hours of receiving a prior dose of DTP‡ Precaution: Seizures within 3 days of receiving a prior dose of DTP‡ (see footnote § regarding management of children with a personal history of seizures at any time) Precaution: Persistent, inconsolable crying lasting ≥3 hours, within 48 hours of receiving a dose of DTP‡	Temperature of <40.5° C (105° F) following a previous dose of DTP Family history of convulsions§ Family history of an adverse event following DTP administration Family history of sudden infant death syndrome
OPV‖	
Infection with HIV or a household contact with HIV Known altered immunodeficiency (hematologic and solid tumors; congenital immunodeficiency; and long-term immunosuppressive therapy) Immunodeficient household contact Precaution: Pregnancy‡	Breast-feeding Current antimicrobial therapy Diarrhea
IPV	
Anaphylactic reaction to neomycin or streptomycin Precaution: Pregnancy‡	None identified
MMR‖	
Anaphylactic reactions to egg ingestion and to neomycin¶ Pregnancy Known altered immunodeficiency (hematologic and solid tumors, congenital immunodeficiency, and long-term immunosuppressive therapy) Precaution: Recent (within 3 months) immunoglobulin administration‡	Tuberculosis or positive for purified protein derivative (PPD) of tuberculin Simultaneous tuberculosis skin testing# Breast-feeding Pregnancy of mother of recipient Immunodeficient family member or household contact Infection with HIV Nonanaphylactic reactions to eggs or neomycin

(table continued on next page)

TABLE 4. (continued)

True Contraindications and Precautions	Not True (Vaccines May Be Given)
Hib	
None identified	History of Hib disease
Hepatitis B	
Anaphylactic reaction to common baker's yeast	Pregnancy

Ad Hoc Working Group for the Development of Standards for Pediatric Immunization Practices, 1993. This information is based on the recommendations of the Advisory Committee on Immunization Practices (ACIP) and those of the Committee on Infectious Diseases (Red Book Committee) of the American Academy of Pediatrics (AAP). Sometimes these recommendations vary from those contained in the manufacturers' package inserts. For more detailed information, providers should consult the published recommendations of the ACIP, the AAP, the American Academy of Family Physicians, and the manufacturers' package inserts.

†*DTP indicates diphtheria and tetanus toxoids and pertussis vaccine; DTaP, diphtheria, tetanus, and acellular pertussis vaccine; OPV, oral poliovirus vaccine; IPV, inactivated poliomyelitis vaccine; MMR, measles, mumps, and rubella vaccine; Hib,* Haemophilus influenzae *b vaccine; and HIV, human immunodeficiency virus.*

‡*Although not a contraindication, this should be carefully reviewed. The benefits and risks of administering a specific vaccine to an individual under the circumstances should be considered. If the risks are believed to outweigh the benefits, the immunization should be withheld; if the benefits are believed to outweigh the risks (for example, during an outbreak or foreign travel), the immunization should be given. Whether and when to administer DTP to children with proven or suspected underlying neurologic disorders should be decided on an individual basis. It is prudent on theoretical grounds to avoid vaccinating pregnant women. However, if immediate protection against poliomyelitis is needed, OPV, not IPV, is recommended.*

§*Acetaminophen given prior to administering DTP and thereafter every 4 hours for 24 hours should be considered for children with a personal or family history of convulsions in siblings or parents.*

‖*There is a theoretical risk that the administration of multiple live virus vaccines (OPV and MMR) within 30 days of one another if not given on the same day will result in a suboptimal immune response. There are no data to substantiate this.*

¶*Persons with a history of anaphylactic reactions following egg ingestion should be vaccinated only with extreme caution. Protocols have been developed for vaccinating such persons and should be consulted (Herman et al, 1983; and Greenberg and Birx, 1988).*

#*Measles vaccination may temporarily suppress tuberculin reactivity. If testing cannot be done the day of MMR vaccination, the test should be postponed for 4 to 6 weeks.*

The National Coalition for Adult Immunization (NCAI) has developed standards for adult immunization that outline basic strategies; if these strategies are fully implemented, they could markedly improve delivery of vaccines to adults and help achieve national health objectives by the year 2000 (Table 5). Adults who were not infected or immunized during childhood may be at increased risk for vaccine-preventable diseases because of advanced age, occupation, lifestyle, or development of certain chronic diseases. All adults should have completed a primary series of tetanus and diphtheria toxoids and subsequently receive a booster dose every 10 years. All adults 65 years and older and those with medical conditions that place them at risk for pneumococcal disease or serious complications of influenza should receive the pneumococcal polysaccharide vaccine and annual immunization with influenza vaccine. Immunization programs for adults also should provide MMR vaccine to anyone who is believed to be susceptible to measles, mumps, or rubella. All young adults should have documentation of receiving at least one dose of measles vaccine on or after their first birthday or other evidence of immunity. Persons born after 1956 who are attending post-high school educational institutions or who are newly employed in situations that place them at high risk of measles transmission should have documentation of having received two doses of MMR on or after their first birthday or have other evidence of immunity. Widespread use of hepatitis B vaccine in adults and adolescents is encouraged for those who may be at risk.

PRECAUTIONS

The physician should be aware of the following general recommendations and precautions when administering a vaccine, immune globulin, or serum of animal origin.

STORAGE AND HANDLING OF IMMUNOBIOLOGICS. Immunobiologics (vaccines, toxoids, antibody-containing preparations) must be stored and handled properly to maintain their immunologic activity. Each manufacturer includes in its package insert important information on storage and handling, and these recommendations should be followed closely to assure the potency of the product at the time of administration. Immediately on receipt, vaccines should be checked to assure that the "cold chain" has been maintained during shipping, and they should be stored at the recommended temperatures. Some vaccines (eg, OPV, yellow fever vaccine) are very sensitive to heat, while others (diphtheria and tetanus toxoids with pertussis vaccine [DTP]; diphtheria and tetanus

TABLE 5.
NATIONAL COALITION FOR ADULT IMMUNIZATION (NCAI)*
STANDARDS FOR ADULT IMMUNIZATION PRACTICE, 1990†

The NCAI

1. Encourages the promotion of appropriate vaccine use through information campaigns for health care practitioners and trainees, employers, and the public about the benefits of immunizations; and
2. Encourages physicians and other health care personnel (in practice and in training) to protect themselves and prevent transmission to patients by assuring that they themselves are completely immunized; and
3. Recommends that all health providers routinely determine the immunization status of their adult patients, offer vaccines to those for whom they are indicated, and maintain complete immunization records; and
4. Recommends that all health care providers identify high-risk patients in need of influenza vaccine and develop a system to recall them for annual immunization each autumn; and
5. Recommends that all health care providers and institutions identify high-risk adult patients in hospitals and other treatment centers and assure that appropriate vaccination is considered either prior to discharge or as part of discharge planning; and
6. Recommends that all licensing/accrediting agencies support the development by health care institutions of comprehensive immunization programs for staff, trainees, volunteer workers, inpatients, and outpatients; and
7. Encourages states to establish pre-enrollment immunization requirements for colleges and other institutions of higher education; and
8. Recommends that institutions that train health care professionals, deliver health care, or provide laboratory or other medical support services require appropriate immunizations for persons at risk of contracting or transmitting vaccine-preventable illnesses; and
9. Encourages health care benefit programs, third-party payers, and governmental health care programs to provide coverage for adult immunization services; and
10. Encourages the adoption of a standard personal and institutional immunization record as a means of verifying the immunization status of patients and staff.

** Full text of these standards and additional information about the NCAI is available from NCAI, 4733 Bethesda Avenue, Suite 750, Bethesda, MD 20814; (301) 656-0003.*

†MMWR, *1990 A.*

toxoids with acellular pertussis vaccine [DTaP]; diphtheria and tetanus toxoids [DT, Td]; enhanced-potency inactivated poliovirus vaccine [eIPV]; *Haemophilus influenzae* type b conjugate vaccine [Hib]; hepatitis B vaccine; influenza vaccine; pneumococcal vaccine) are quite sensitive to freezing temperatures. If there is any doubt about the appropriate handling of the agent, the manufacturer should be contacted.

VACCINES. Intervals between doses of vaccines that are longer than recommended do not reduce final antibody titers; however, doses administered at less than the recommended minimum intervals should not be considered part of a primary series.

In general, an inactivated vaccine can be administered before, after, or with a different inactivated or live vaccine if given at separate sites. Simultaneous administration of most live and inactivated vaccines at separate sites has not resulted in impaired antibody responses or increased the rate or severity of adverse reactions. The simultaneous administration of vaccines recommended in childhood immunization programs increases the probability that a child will be fully immunized at the appropriate age and is particularly important if it is thought that the child may not return for subsequent vaccinations. Therefore, infants and children who are at the recommended age to receive DTP (or DTaP), MMR, OPV (or IPV), Hib, and hepatitis B vaccine and in whom no specific contraindication exists at the time of the office visit may be given these vaccines simultaneously (*MMWR*, 1994).

The simultaneous administration of other vaccines also is possible. A satisfactory antibody response without an increase in the incidence or severity of adverse reactions in adults has been reported with the simultaneous administration of pneumococcal polysaccharide and whole-virus influenza vaccine (DeStefano et al, 1982), hepatitis B and yellow fever vaccines (Yvonnet et al, 1986), and measles and yellow fever vaccines (*MMWR*, 1990 B). However, the antibody response to yellow fever and cholera vaccines is decreased when these vaccines are administered together or within a short time of each other; thus, these vaccinations should be given at least three weeks apart. In addition, if inactivated vaccines commonly associated with local or systemic reactions (eg, cholera, parenteral typhoid, plague) are given at the same time, adverse reactions may be accentuated. It is preferable to administer such vaccines on separate occasions.

TABLE 6.
GUIDELINES FOR SPACING THE ADMINISTRATION OF LIVE AND KILLED ANTIGENS*

Antigen Combination	Recommended Minimum Interval Between Doses
≥ 2 Killed antigens	None. May be administered simultaneously or at any interval between doses.†
Killed and live antigens	None. May be administered simultaneously or at any interval between doses.‡
≥ 2 Live antigens	4-week minimum interval if not administered simultaneously.§ However, OPV can be administered at any time before, with, or after MMR, if indicated.

* MMWR, *1994.*

† *If possible, vaccines associated with local or systemic side effects (eg, cholera, parenteral typhoid, and plague vaccines) should be administered on separate occasions to avoid accentuated reactions.*

‡ *Cholera vaccine with yellow fever vaccine is the exception. If time permits, these antigens should not be administered simultaneously, and at least 3 weeks should elapse between administration of yellow fever vaccine and cholera vaccine. If the vaccines must be administered simultaneously or within 3 weeks of each other, the antibody response may not be optimal.*

§ *If oral live typhoid vaccine is indicated (eg, for international travel undertaken on short notice), it can be administered before, simultaneously with, or after OPV.*

There is a theoretical possibility that the immune response to one live virus vaccine may be impaired if it is administered within 30 days of another live virus vaccine. Thus, it has been recommended that live virus vaccines *administered on different days* should be given at least 30 days apart (*MMWR*, 1994). An exception to this is that OPV and MMR vaccines can be administered at any time before, with, or after each other. See Table 6 for guidelines for spacing the administration of live and killed vaccines.

Some vaccines contain preservatives (eg, thimerosal) or trace amounts of antibiotics (eg, neomycin) to which some patients may be hypersensitive. However, no currently recommended vaccine contains penicillin or a derivative. The most common animal protein allergen encountered in vaccines is egg protein, which is found in vaccines prepared in chicken eggs or cell cultures (influenza, measles, mumps, and yellow fever vaccines). Persons who can safely eat eggs or egg products can be given these vaccines; in general, those with a history of anaphylaxis to eggs should not receive these products. However, protocols have been described for testing and vaccinating persons who have had anaphylactic reactions to egg ingestion with measles, mumps and MMR vaccines (*American Academy of Pediatrics Redbook*, 1991; Lavi et al, 1990; Greenberg and Birx, 1988; Herman et al, 1983). A regimen for administering influenza vaccine to children with severe asthma and hypersensitivity to eggs also has been reported (Murphy and Strunk, 1985).

Immunosuppressed patients, such as those with AIDS, leukemia, lymphoma, or generalized malignancy, generally should not receive live virus vaccines because virus replication may be enhanced in these individuals. An exception is live, attenuated MMR vaccine for children with HIV infection. All asymptomatic HIV-infected children should receive this vaccine, and it also should be considered for those with symptoms because of the severity of measles in these children and the apparent low risk of vaccine-related adverse events (*MMWR*, 1994).

Live vaccine should not be administered to patients undergoing immunosuppressive therapy until three months after all such therapy has been discontinued. Inactivated vaccines can be administered to all immunocompromised patients. Because immunodeficient patients may not have an adequate response to vaccination, it is advisable, if possible, to determine antibody levels to assess the efficacy of immunization and to guide future management. OPV should not be given to any immunocompromised patient or to a member of a household in which there is a family history of immunodeficiency until the immune competence of the recipient and other family members is known. Vaccine virus excreted by the recipient may be communicated to an immunodeficient person and complications may result.

Live virus vaccines (eg, MMR) may interfere with the tuberculin skin test response; therefore, testing should be done on the same day or four to six weeks after vaccine administration.

Immunization of persons with neurologic disorders may present special problems with certain vaccines (eg, pertussis vaccine). Recommendations for each vaccine should be consulted. Individuals with moderate to severe illnesses, whether febrile or not, should not be immunized until they have recovered from the acute phase of the illness.

In general, live virus vaccines are not recommended for pregnant women or those likely to become pregnant within three months of vaccination. However, both OPV and yellow fever vaccine can be administered to pregnant women who are at substantial risk of imminent exposure to natural infection. Although OPV is preferred, IPV may be considered if the complete vaccination series can be administered before the anticipated exposure. Pregnant women who must travel to areas where the risk for yellow fever is high should receive yellow fever vaccine since the slight risk from vaccination is far outweighed by the risk of yellow fever infection (*MMWR*, 1994). Pregnancy is a contraindication to administration of rubella, measles, and mumps vaccines. There is no convinc-

TABLE 7.
GUIDELINES FOR SPACING THE ADMINISTRATION OF IG PREPARATIONS* AND VACCINES†

Simultaneous Administration		Nonsimultaneous Administration		
		Immunobiologic Administered		
Immunobiologic Combination	Recommended Minimum Interval Between Doses	First	Second	Recommended Minimum Interval Between Doses
IG and killed antigen	None. May be given simultaneously at different sites or at any time between doses.	IG	Killed antigen	None
		Killed antigen	IG	None
IG and live antigen	Should generally not be administered simultaneously.‡ If simultaneous administration of measles-mumps-rubella [MMR], measles-rubella, and monovalent measles vaccine is unavoidable, administer at different sites and revaccinate or test for seroconversion after the recommended interval (Table 8).	IG	Live antigen	Dose related‡,§
		Live antigen	IG	2 weeks

* *Blood products containing large amounts of IG (such as serum IG, specific IGs [eg, TIG, HBIG], intravenous IG [IGIV], whole blood, packed red blood cells, plasma, and platelet products).*

† MMWR, *1994.*

‡ *Oral poliovirus, yellow fever, and oral typhoid (Ty21a) vaccines are exceptions to these recommendations. These vaccines may be administered at any time before, after, or simultaneously with an IG-containing product without substantially decreasing the antibody response (Kaplan et al, 1984).*

§ *The duration of interference of IG preparations with the immune response to the measles component of the MMR, measles-rubella, and monovalent measles vaccine is dose-related (Table 8).*

ing evidence of risk to the fetus from immunizing pregnant women with inactivated viral or bacterial vaccines.

IMMUNE GLOBULINS. IG preparations should be given only for diseases in which their efficacy has been established.

Since IG preparations may contain trace amounts of IgA, patients selectively deficient for IgA may develop antibody to it and subsequently react to IG preparations, serum, plasma, or whole blood. Normal individuals may develop antibodies to genetic types of IgG that differ from their own.

Aggregates of IgG may form on standing and rarely may cause systemic reactions (eg, anaphylaxis) after administration of IG preparations.

Isoimmunization is a possibility in immunocompetent individuals given IG .

Intramuscular or intravenous IG, as well as specific immune globulins and certain blood products (whole blood, packed red blood cells, plasma) can diminish the immune response to MMR or its individual component vaccines. Thus, these vaccines should not be administered before the recommended interval when an IG preparation or blood product has been given (see Tables 7 and 8). Vaccine virus replication and stimulation of immunity usually occurs one to two weeks after vaccination. If the interval between vaccine and IG administration is <14 days, the vaccination should be repeated after the recommended interval (Tables 7 and 8) unless serologic testing indicates an adequate immune response. Recent evidence suggests that large doses of IG can inhibit the immune response to measles vaccine for more than three months; IG also can inhibit the response to rubella vaccine. However, the postpartum vaccination of rubella-susceptible women with rubella or MMR vaccine should not be delayed because of the administration of anti-Rho(D) IG or any other blood product during the last trimester of pregnancy or at delivery.

MMR or its component vaccines can be administered simultaneously with an IG preparation if necessary because of imminent exposure to disease; however, immunity may be compromised. MMR or a component vaccine should be given at a site remote from that used for the IG inoculation. It is recommended that vaccination be repeated after the recommended interval (Tables 7 and 8) unless serologic testing demonstrates that an adequate immune response was obtained.

Inactivated vaccines and toxoids are less likely to interfere with IG preparations and, therefore, they may be given with, before, or after an IG preparation provided different sites are used for administration.

ANIMAL SERUMS. Because of their potential for causing serious hypersensitivity reactions, animal serums should be used only when other forms of therapy or prophylaxis (eg, IG) are not available. IG preparations have replaced most animal serums. Before administration of any animal serum, a careful inquiry should be made into the prospective recipient's history of hypersensitivity, and appropriate tests for hypersensitivity (intracutaneous skin or eye test) should be performed. (See following discussion.)

No serum should be injected or any test for hypersensitivity performed unless there is a syringe containing 0.5 ml of aqueous epinephrine 1:1,000 (maximum initial dose) within immediate reach.

TESTS FOR HYPERSENSITIVITY. Antigens in vaccines and antiserums may cause hypersensitivity reactions. Certain constituents of vaccines (eg, egg protein, antibiotics) may cause

TABLE 8.
SUGGESTED INTERVALS BETWEEN ADMINISTRATION OF IG PREPARATIONS FOR VARIOUS INDICATIONS AND VACCINES CONTAINING LIVE MEASLES VIRUS*

Indication	Dose (including mg IgG/kg)	Suggested interval before measles vaccination (months)
Tetanus (TIG)	250 units (10 mg IgG/kg) IM	3
Hepatitis A (IG)		
Contact prophylaxis	0.02 ml/kg (3.3 mg IgG/kg) IM	3
International travel	0.06 ml/kg (10 mg IgG/kg) IM	3
Hepatitis B prophylaxis (HBIG)	0.06 ml/kg (10 mg IgG/kg) IM	3
Rabies prophylaxis (HRIG)	20 IU/kg (22 mg IgG/kg) IM	4
Varicella prophylaxis (VZIG)	125 units/10 kg (20-40 mg IgG/kg) IM (maximum 625 units)	5
Measles prophylaxis (IG)		
Normal contact	0.25 ml/kg (40 mg IgG/kg) IM	5
Immunocompromised contact	0.50 ml/kg (80 mg IgG/kg) IM	6
Blood transfusion		
Red blood cells (RBCs), washed	10 ml/kg (negligible IgG/kg) IV	0
RBCs, adenine-saline added	10 ml/kg (10 mg IgG/kg) IV	3
Packed RBCs (Hct 65%)†	10 ml/kg (60 mg IgG/kg) IV	6
Whole blood (Hct 35-50%)†	10 ml/kg (80-100 mg IgG/kg) IV	6
Plasma/platelet products	10 ml/kg (160 mg IgG/kg) IV	7
Replacement of humoral immune deficiencies	300-400 mg/kg IV§ (as IGIV)	8
Treatment of:		
ITP¶	400 mg/kg IV (as IGIV)	8
ITP¶	1,000 mg/kg IV (as IGIV)	10
Kawasaki disease	2 g/kg IV (as IGIV)	11

* *This table is not intended for determining the correct indications and dosage for the use of immune globulin preparations. Unvaccinated persons may not be fully protected against measles during the entire suggested interval and additional doses of immune globulin and/or measles vaccine may be indicated following measles exposure. The concentration of measles antibody in a particular immune globulin preparation can vary by lot. The rate of antibody clearance following receipt of an immune globulin preparation can also vary. The recommended intervals are extrapolated from an estimated half-life of 30 days for passively acquired antibody and an observed interference with the immune response to measles vaccine for 5 months following a dose of 80 mg IgG/kg (Siber et al, 1993)* (MMWR, *1994).*

† *Assumes a serum IgG concentration of 16 mg/ml.*

§ *Measles vaccination is recommended for children with HIV infection but is contraindicated in patients with congenital disorders of the immune system.*

¶ *Immune (formally, idiopathic) thrombocytopenic purpura.*

allergic reactions, and individuals known to have severe reactions (eg, anaphylaxis) to a vaccine component should not receive that vaccine.

An intracutaneous skin test preceded by an eye (conjunctival) test must be performed before injection of any animal serum, regardless of whether or not the patient has ever received the serum species. For any of the following sensitivity tests, the concomitant use of antihistamines may invalidate the testing procedure. Epinephrine should always be available during testing, desensitization, or administration.

Conjunctival Test: One drop of a 1:10 dilution of the test serum in isotonic sodium chloride solution is instilled into one conjunctival sac. One drop of isotonic sodium chloride solution is instilled into the other to serve as a control. A positive test is manifested by lacrimation and conjunctival injection in 10 to 30 minutes.

Intradermal Test: This test is performed only if the conjunctival test is negative. INDIVIDUALS WITH NO KNOWN ALLERGIES, 0.1 ml of a 1:100 dilution of the serum in saline is injected. As a control, the saline diluent only is injected at a distant site. A positive reaction consists of wheal formation in 10 to 30 minutes. INDIVIDUALS WITH A HISTORY OF ALLERGY, the test dose is reduced to 0.05 ml of a 1:1,000 dilution.

The physician is cautioned that intradermal skin tests have resulted in fatalities but eye tests have not. *Skin tests should never be performed unless a syringe containing 0.5 ml of aqueous epinephrine 1:1,000 (maximum initial dose) is within immediate reach.*

A negative eye or skin test is *not* an absolute guarantee that sensitivity is absent, but only indicates that sensitivity is probably lacking.

Desensitization for Serum Reactions: If a test for hypersensitivity is positive or if there is a history of allergy in a patient whose need for animal serum is imperative, it is still possible to proceed with passive immunization. In such instances, the following desensitization procedure may increase the patient's tolerance to the foreign protein. However, it is dangerous to assume that true desensitization occurs.

The following doses are injected every 15 minutes if they can be tolerated without local or systemic reaction: (1) 0.05 ml of 1:20 dilution subcutaneously, (2) 0.1 ml of 1:10 dilution subcutaneously, (3) 0.3 ml of 1:10 dilution subcutaneously, (4) 0.1 ml of undiluted serum subcutaneously, (5) 0.2 ml of undiluted serum intramuscularly, (6) 0.5 ml of undiluted serum intramuscularly, and (7) the remaining therapeutic dose intramuscularly. It is recommended that a written record be maintained of pulse, blood pressure, and respiration taken before each succeeding injection.

ROUTE, SITE, AND TECHNIQUE OF IMMUNIZATION

Each immunobiologic agent has a recommended route of administration based on prior clinical trials and experience. To avoid untoward local or systemic effects and to ensure optimal efficacy, the practitioner should not deviate from the recommended route.

Injectable immunobiologics should be given in an area with minimal opportunity for local, neural, vascular, or tissue injury. Usually, *subcutaneous injections* are administered into the thigh of infants and the deltoid area of older children and adults. *Intradermal injections* are generally given on the volar surface of the forearm, except for human diploid cell rabies vaccine, which is given in the deltoid area to avoid severe reactions. At the present time, the preferred sites for *intramuscular injection* are the anterolateral aspect of the upper thigh for children under 3 years and the deltoid muscle of the upper arm for older children and adults. However, for children older than 1 year, the site may be determined individually based on the volume of material to be injected and the size of the muscle mass. Vaccines that contain adjuvants must be injected deep into the muscle mass; subcutaneous or intradermal administration may cause local irritation.

Under most circumstances, the upper, outer aspect of the buttocks should not be used for routine immunizations. In those rare instances when this site must be used (eg, for administration of large volumes of IG), the upper outer mass of the gluteus maximus away from the central region of the buttocks should be selected to avoid injury to the sciatic nerve.

A separate sterile disposable syringe and needle should be used for each vaccine injected to minimize contamination. If different vaccines are given at the same time, each injection should be at a different site.

As noted in the previous section on Precautions, most widely used vaccines are both safe and effective when given simultaneously. This is practical in certain circumstances: imminent exposure to several infectious diseases, preparation for foreign travel or uncertainty of patient return, and integration with other health care activities (eg, well-infant visits). However, vaccines commonly associated with adverse reactions (eg, cholera, parenteral typhoid, plague) preferably should be given on separate occasions when feasible.

Cited References

National Childhood Vaccine Injury Act: Requirements for permanent vaccination records and for reporting of selected events after vaccination. *MMWR* 37:197-200, 1988.

Public health burden of vaccine-preventable diseases among adults: Standards for adult immunization practice. *MMWR* 39(No. 41): 725-729, 1990 A.

Yellow fever vaccine: Recommendations of the Immunization Practices Advisory Committee (ACIP). *MMWR* 39(No. RR-6):1-6, 1990 B.

General recommendations on immunization: Recommendations of the Advisory Committee on Immunization Practices (ACIP). *MMWR* 43(No. RR-1):1-38, 1994.

Ad Hoc Working Group for the Development of Standards for Pediatric Immunization Practices: Standards for pediatric immunization practices. *JAMA* 269:1817-1822, 1993.

Report of the Committee on Infectious Diseases: *American Academy of Pediatrics Redbook*, ed 22. Elk Grove Village, Ill, American Academy of Pediatrics, 1991.

Bochner BS, Lichtenstein LM: Anaphylaxis. *N Engl J Med* 324:1785-1790, 1991.

DeStefano F, et al: Simultaneous administration of influenza and pneumococcal vaccines. *JAMA* 247:2551-2554, 1982.

Fisher M: Treating anaphylaxis with sympathomimetic drugs: In severe anaphylaxis adrenaline by any route is better than none. *BMJ* 305:1107-1108, 1992.

Greenberg MA, Birx DL: Safe administration of mumps-measles-rubella vaccine in egg-allergic children. *J Pediatr* 13:504-506, 1988.

Herman JJ, et al: Allergic reactions to measles (rubeola) vaccine in patients hypersensitive to egg protein. *J Pediatr* 102:196-199, 1983.

Kaplan JE, et al: The effect of immune globulin on the response to trivalent oral poliovirus and yellow fever vaccinations. *Bull WHO* 62:585-590, 1984.

Lavi S, et al: Administration of measles, mumps, and rubella virus vaccine (live) to egg-allergic children. *JAMA* 263:269-271, 1990.

Lichtenstein LM: Anaphylaxis, in Wyngaarden JB, Smith LH (eds): *Cecil Textbook of Medicine,* ed 18. Philadelphia, WB Saunders, 1988, 1956-1958.

Murphy KR, Strunk RC: Safe administration of influenza vaccine in asthmatic children hypersensitive to egg proteins. *J Pediatr* 106:931-933, 1985.

Reuben DB: Office management of anaphylaxis. *Am Fam Physician* 34:179-183, 1986.

Sheffer AL, Pennoyer DS: Management of adverse drug reactions. *J Allergy Clin Immunol* 74:580-588, 1984.

Siber GR, et al: Interference of immune globulin with measles and rubella immunization. *J Pediatr* 122:204-211, 1993.

Yunginger JW: Anaphylaxis: *Ann Allergy* 69:87-96, (Aug) 1992 A.

Yunginger JW: Anaphylaxis: *Curr Probl Pediatr* 130-146, (March) 1992 B.

Yvonnet B, et al: Simultaneous administration of hepatitis B and yellow fever vaccinations. *Bull WHO* 19:307-311, 1986.

Other Selected References

Venomous bites and stings. *J Toxicol Clin Toxicol* 21:417-560, 1983-1984.

Advisory Committee on Immunization Practices (ACIP): *Adult Immunization.* Atlanta, Centers for Disease Control, 1990.

American College of Physicians Task Force on Adult Immunization and Infectious Disease Society of America: *Guide for Adult Immunization,* ed 3. Philadelphia, American College of Physicians, 1994.

Lerner RA, et al (eds): *Vaccines 85: Molecular and Chemical Basis of Resistance to Parasitic, Bacterial, and Viral Diseases.* New York, Cold Spring Harbor Laboratory, 1985.

Plotkin SA, Mortimer EA Jr (eds): *Vaccines,* ed 2. Philadelphia, WB Saunders, 1994.

VACCINE ADVERSE EVENT REPORTING SYSTEM

VAERS

24 Hour Toll-free information line 1-800-822-7967

Patient identity kept confidential

For CDC/FDA Use Only

VAERS Number ______

Date Received ______

Patient Name:

Last First M.I.

Address

City State Zip

Telephone no. (____)______

Vaccine administered by (Name):

Responsible Physician ______

Facility Name/Address

City State Zip

Telephone no. (____)______

Form completed by (Name):

Relation to Patient ☐ Vaccine Provider ☐ Patient/Parent ☐ Manufacturer ☐ Other

Address *(if different from patient or provider)*

City State Zip

Telephone no. (____)______

1. State
2. County where administered
3. Date of birth __/__/__ (mm dd yy)
4. Patient age
5. Sex ☐ M ☐ F
6. Date form completed __/__/__ (mm dd yy)
7. Describe adverse event(s) (symptoms, signs, time course) and treatment, if any
8. Check all appropriate:
   - ☐ Patient died (date __/__/__ mm dd yy)
   - ☐ Life threatening illness
   - ☐ Required emergency room/doctor visit
   - ☐ Required hospitalization (____days)
   - ☐ Resulted in prolongation of hospitalization
   - ☐ Resulted in permanent disability
   - ☐ None of the above
9. Patient recovered ☐ YES ☐ NO ☐ UNKNOWN
10. Date of vaccination __/__/__ (mm dd yy) Time ______ AM PM
11. Adverse event onset __/__/__ (mm dd yy) Time ______ AM PM
12. Relevant diagnostic tests/laboratory data
13. Enter all vaccines given on date listed in no. 10

	Vaccine (type)	Manufacturer	Lot number	Route/Site	No. Previous doses
a.					
b.					
c.					
d.					

14. Any other vaccinations within 4 weeks of date listed in no. 10

	Vaccine (type)	Manufacturer	Lot number	Route/Site	No. Previous doses	Date given
a.						
b.						

15. Vaccinated at:
    - ☐ Private doctor's office/hospital
    - ☐ Military clinic/hospital
    - ☐ Public health clinic/hospital
    - ☐ Other/unknown
16. Vaccine purchased with:
    - ☐ Private funds
    - ☐ Military funds
    - ☐ Public funds
    - ☐ Other /unknown
17. Other medications
18. Illness at time of vaccination (specify)
19. Pre-existing physician-diagnosed allergies, birth defects, medical conditions (specify)
20. Have you reported this adverse event previously? ☐ No ☐ To health department ☐ To doctor ☐ To manufacturer
21. Adverse event following prior vaccination (check all applicable, specify)

	Adverse Event	Onset Age	Type Vaccine	Dose no. in series
☐ In patient				
☐ In brother or sister				

Only for children 5 and under

22. Birth weight ____ lb. ____ oz.

23. No. of brothers and sisters

Only for reports submitted by manufacturer/immunization project

24. Mfr. / imm. proj. report no.

25. Date received by mfr. / imm. proj.

26. 15 day report? ☐ Yes ☐ No

27. Report type ☐ Initial ☐ Follow-Up

Health care providers and manufacturers are required by law (42 USC 300aa-25) to report reactions to vaccines listed in the Vaccine Injury Table. Reports for reactions to other vaccines are voluntary except when required as a condition of immunization grant awards.

Form VAERS -1

"Fold in thirds, tape & mail - DO NOT STAPLE FORM"

NO POSTAGE
NECESSARY
IF MAILED
IN THE
UNITED STATES
OR APO/FPO

BUSINESS REPLY MAIL
FIRST CLASS MAIL PERMIT NO. 1895 ROCKVILLE, MD

POSTAGE WILL BE PAID BY ADDRESSEE

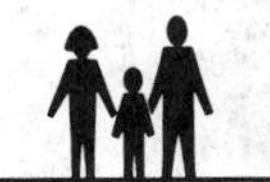

VAERS
c/o ERC BioServices Corporation
A Division of Ogden Biomedical Services Group
1055 First Street, Suite 130
Rockville MD 20850-9788

DIRECTIONS FOR COMPLETING FORM

(Additional pages may be attached if more space is needed.)

GENERAL

- Use a separate form for each patient. Complete the form to the best of your abilities. Items 3, 4, 7, 8, 10, 11, and 13 are considered essential and should be completed whenever possible. Parents/Guardians may need to consult the facility where the vaccine was administered for some of the information (such as manufacturer, lot number or laboratory data.)
- Refer to the Vaccine Injury Table (VIT) for events mandated for reporting by law. Reporting for other serious events felt to be related but not on the VIT is encouraged.
- Health care providers other than the vaccine administrator (VA) treating a patient for a suspected adverse event should notify the VA and provide the information about the adverse event to allow the VA to complete the form to meet the VA's legal responsibility.
- These data will be used to increase understanding of adverse events following vaccination and will become part of CDC Privacy Act System 09-20-0136, "Epidemiologic Studies and Surveillance of Disease Problems". Information identifying the person who received the vaccine or that person's legal representative will not be made available to the public, but may be available to the vaccinee or legal representative.

SPECIFIC INSTRUCTIONS

Form Completed By: To be used by parents/guardians, vaccine manufacturers/distributors, vaccine administrators, and/or the person completing the form on behalf of the patient or the health professional who administered the vaccine.

Item 7: Describe the suspected adverse event. Such things as temperature, local and general signs and symptoms, time course, duration of symptoms diagnosis, treatment and recovery should be noted.

Item 9: Check "YES" if the patient's health condition is the same as it was prior to the vaccine, "NO" if the patient has not returned to the pre-vaccination state of health, or "UNKNOWN" if the patient's condition is not known.

Item 10: and 11: Give dates and times as specifically as you can remember. If you do not know the exact time, please indicate "AM" or "PM" when possible if this information is known. If more than one adverse event, give the onset date and time for the most serious event.

Item 12: Include "negative" or "normal" results of any relevant tests performed as well as abnormal findings.

Item 13: List ONLY those vaccines given on the day listed in Item 10.

Item 14: List ANY OTHER vaccines the patient received within four weeks of the date listed in Item 10.

Item 16: This section refers to how the person who gave the vaccine purchased it, not to the patient's insurance.

Item 17: List any prescription or non-prescription medications the patient was taking when the vaccine(s) was given.

Item 18: List any short term illnesses the patient had on the date the vaccine(s) was given (i.e., cold, flu, ear infection).

Item 19: List any pre-existing physician-diagnosed allergies, birth defects, medical conditions (including developmental and/or neurologic disorders) the patient has.

Item 21: List any suspected adverse events the patient, or the patient's brothers or sisters, may have had to previous vaccinations. If more than one brother or sister, or if the patient has reacted to more than one prior vaccine, use additional pages to explain completely. For the onset age of a patient, provide the age in months if less than two years old.

Item 26: This space is for manufacturers' use only.

Summer 1994

Recommended Immunizations and Schedules

IMMUNIZATION SCHEDULES

Schedules for routine primary active immunization of children against diphtheria, tetanus, pertussis (whooping cough), poliomyelitis, measles, rubella, mumps, hepatitis B virus (HBV), and *Haemophilus influenzae* type b have been developed by the U.S. Public Health Services Advisory Committee on Immunization Practices (ACIP) and the Committee on Infectious Diseases of the American Academy of Pediatrics (see Tables 1, 2, and 3). These recommendations are based on the following factors: Vaccines that every normal infant and child should receive, optimal and practical ages for effective immunization, efficacy and tolerance of combinations of vaccines, current epidemiology of the diseases, possibility of integrating vaccinations with other health care activities (well-child visits), and other practical aspects of administration.

Schedules for the routine immunization of adults against influenza and pneumococcal disease and for tetanus-diphtheria booster doses are provided by the ACIP and the American College of Physicians.

IMMUNIZATION RECORDS. Every physician should maintain a permanent record of the immunization history of each patient so that information can be updated regularly and those in need of immunization can be identified easily and recalled.

In addition to good medical practice, the National Childhood Vaccine Injury Act (NCVIA) requires that all health providers who administer vaccines against diphtheria, tetanus, pertussis, poliomyelitis (live or inactivated), measles, mumps, and/or rubella maintain permanent and readily available records of each dose administered including date given, manufacturer and lot number, and the individual who administered the vaccine. In addition, the law requires that vaccine informational materials be distributed to the guardians of all minors who are to receive a vaccine.

All providers should take all necessary precautions in the administration of any vaccine, not only to provide optimum medical care but also to protect themselves against unwarranted litigation. Specifically, in addition to honoring the requirements of the NCVIA, all providers of vaccines should adhere to the following guidelines:

1. The responsible provider should be knowledgeable about the nature, the expected benefits and risks, and the indications and contraindications for each vaccine administered.

2. The anticipated benefits and risks of the vaccine should be communicated in understandable language to the patient or the child's guardian. Obtaining a signed information form is helpful, if only as evidence that a provider was aware of the need to inform the recipient, but by itself is inadequate in the absence of a verbal explanation.

3. A brief statement that such a discussion was conducted should be recorded in the record.

4. When the patient returns for a subsequent vaccine dose, such as with DTP, careful inquiry should be made about any untoward events that occurred following the prior dose, and any reactions should be recorded in the patient's record. As a corollary, any adverse events about which the provider is notified in the interim, such as by telephone a day or two following a dose of DTP, should be recorded and, if indicated, carefully investigated. Adverse events should be reported to the Vaccine Adverse Events Reporting System (see the chapter on Agents for Active and Passive Immunity: General Recommendations).

Permanent, comprehensive immunization records also should be maintained by the parent. In addition, immunization records (containing at least immunization dates and vaccine administered) should be kept by institutions, such as schools and day care centers. Since persons frequently relocate, it is

TABLE 1.
RECOMMENDED SCHEDULE FOR ROUTINE ACTIVE VACCINATION OF INFANTS AND CHILDREN*

Vaccine	At birth (before hospital discharge)	1-2 months	2 months†	4 months	6 months	6-18 months	12-15 months	15 months	4-6 years (before school entry)
Diphtheria-tetanus-pertussis§			DTP	DTP	DTP			DTaP/DTP¶	DTaP/DTP
Polio, live oral			OPV	OPV	OPV**				OPV
Measles-mumps-rubella							MMR		MMR††
Haemophilus influenzae type b conjugate									
HbOC/PRP-T§,§§			Hib	Hib	Hib		Hib¶¶		
PRP-OMP§§			Hib	Hib			Hib¶¶		
Hepatitis B***									
Option 1	HepB	HepB†††				HepB†††			
Option 2		HepB†††		HepB†††		HepB†††			

**From:* MMWR, *1994. See Table 2 for the recommended immunization schedule for infants and children up to their seventh birthday who do not begin the vaccination series at the recommended times or who are > 1 month behind in the immunization schedule.*

†Can be administered as early as 6 weeks of age.

§Two DTP and Hib combination vaccines are available (DTP/HbOC [TETRAMUNE] and PRP-T [ActHIB, OmniHIB]; the latter can be reconstituted with DTP vaccine produced by Connaught).

¶This dose of DTP can be administered as early as 12 months of age provided that the interval since the previous dose of DTP is at least 6 months. Diphtheria and tetanus toxoids and acellular pertussis vaccine (DTaP) is currently recommended only for use as the fourth and/or fifth doses of the DTP series among children aged 15 months through 6 years (before the seventh birthday). Some experts prefer to administer these vaccines at 18 months of age.

***The American Academy of Pediatrics (AAP) recommends this dose of vaccine at 6 to 18 months of age.*

††The AAP recommends that two doses of MMR be administered by 12 years of age with the second dose being administered preferentially at entry to middle school or junior high school.

§§HbOC: [HibTITER] (Lederle-Praxis). PRP-T: [ActHIB, OmniHIB] (Pasteur Merieux). PRP-OMP: [PedvaxHIB] (Merck). A DTP/Hib combination vaccine can be used in place of HbOC/PRP-T.

¶¶After the primary infant Hib conjugate vaccine series is completed, any of the licensed Hib conjugate vaccines may be used as a booster dose at age 12 to 15 months.

****For use in infants born to HBsAg-negative mothers. The first dose should be administered during the newborn period, preferably before hospital discharge, but no later than age 2 months. Premature infants of HBsAg-negative mothers should receive the first dose of the HepB series at the time of hospital discharge or when the other routine childhood vaccines are initiated. (All infants born to HBsAg-positive mothers should receive immunoprophylaxis for hepatitis B as soon as possible after birth.)*

†††HepB can be administered simultaneously at the same visit with DTP (or DTaP), OPV, Hib, and/or MMR.

recommended that personal immunization records be maintained by all individuals.

PEDIATRIC IMMUNIZATIONS. The recommendations in Tables 1, 2, and 3 are influenced by: (1) the risks of the disease and its complications for specific age groups; (2) the risk of vaccine reactions; (3) the ability of an age group to respond to a vaccine; and (4) the possible presence of maternal antibody, which could interfere with the expected immune response.

Current recommendations for routine pediatric immunizations before school entry specify that nine different virus antigens be given at five to seven different periods starting as early as birth (Table 1). Two of the products are combination vaccines that are familiar to all physicians: DTP (diphtheria and tetanus toxoids with pertussis vaccine) and MMR (measles, mumps, and rubella vaccine). Recently, two combination DTP-Hib vaccines have been introduced: TETRAMUNE (Lederle-Praxis), which consists of a licensed DTP vaccine [TRI-IMMUNOL] plus a Haemophilus b conjugate vaccine [HibTITER] and a PRP-T [Act HIB, OmniHIB]/DTP vaccine that is prepared by reconstituting the lyophilized Hib vaccine with Connaught's DTP vaccine in the same syringe.

HBV: Universal immunization of all infants with hepatitis B vaccine (HepB) was recommended by the Immunization Practices Advisory Committee (ACIP) in 1991 (*MMWR*, 1991 A). The first dose is administered during the neonatal period, preferably before hospital discharge, but no later than 2 months of age. Either one of two schedules has been recommended for infants born to HBsAg (hepatitis B surface antigen)-negative mothers (Table 1). The currently licensed

TABLE 2.
RECOMMENDED ACCELERATED IMMUNIZATION SCHEDULE FOR INFANTS AND CHILDREN <7 YEARS OF AGE WHO START THE SERIES LATE* OR WHO ARE >1 MONTH BEHIND IN THE IMMUNIZATION SCHEDULE† (IE, CHILDREN FOR WHOM COMPLIANCE WITH SCHEDULED RETURN VISITS CANNOT BE ASSURED)§

Timing	Vaccine (s)	Comments
First visit (≥ 4 mos of age)	DTP¶, OPV, Hib¶,**, HepB, MMR (should be given as soon as child is age 12-15 mos)	All vaccines should be administered simultaneously at the appropriate visit.
Second visit (1 month after first visit)	DTP¶, Hib¶**, HepB	
Third visit (1 month after second visit)	DTP¶, OPV, Hib¶,**	
Fourth visit (6 weeks after third visit)	OPV	
Fifth visit (≥6 mos after third visit)	DTaP¶ or DTP, Hib¶,**, HepB	
Additional visits		
(Age 4-6 yrs)	DTaP¶ or DTP, OPV, MMR	Preferably at or before school entry.
(Age 14-16 yrs)	Td	Repeat every 10 yrs throughout life.

* *If initiated in the first year of life, administer DTP doses 1, 2, and 3 and OPV doses 1, 2, and 3 according to this schedule; administer MMR when the child reaches 12 to 15 months of age.*

† *See individual ACIP recommendations for detailed information on specific vaccines.*

§ *From:* MMWR, *1994. DTP indicates diphtheria-tetanus-pertussis; DTaP, diphtheria-tetanus-acellular pertussis; Hib,* Haemophilus influenzae *type b conjugate; HepB, hepatitis B; MMR, measles-mumps-rubella; OPV, poliovirus vaccine, live oral, trivalent; and Td, tetanus and diphtheria toxoids (for use in persons ≥ 7 years of age).*

¶ *Two DTP and Hib combination vaccines are available (DTP/HbOC [TETRAMUNE] and PRP-T [ActHIB, OmniHIB] can be reconstituted with DTP vaccine produced by Connaught). DTaP preparations are currently recommended only for use as the fourth and/or fifth doses of the DTP series among children age 15 months through 6 years (before the seventh birthday). DTP and DTaP should not be used on or after the seventh birthday.*

** *The recommended schedule varies by vaccine manufacturer. For information specific to the vaccine being used, consult the package insert and ACIP recommendations. Children beginning the Hib vaccine series at age 2 to 6 months should receive a primary series of three doses of HbOC [HibTITER] (Lederle-Praxis), PRP-T [ActHIB, OmniHIB] (Pasteur Merieux; SmithKline Beecham; Connaught), or a licensed DTP-Hib combination vaccine; or two doses of PRP-OMP [PedvaxHIB] (Merck). An additional booster dose of any licensed Hib conjugate vaccine should be administered at 12 to 15 months of age and at least 2 months after the previous dose. Children beginning the Hib vaccine series at 7 to 11 months of age should receive a primary series of two doses of an HbOC, PRP-T, or PRP-OMP-containing vaccine. An additional booster dose of any licensed Hib conjugate vaccine should be administered at 12 to 18 months of age and at least 2 months after the previous dose. Children beginning the Hib vaccine series at ages 12 to 14 months should receive a primary series of one dose of an HbOC, PRP-T, or PRP-OMP-containing vaccine. An additional booster dose of any licensed Hib conjugate vaccine should be administered 2 months after the previous dose. Children beginning the Hib vaccine series at ages 15 to 59 months should receive one dose of any licensed Hib vaccine. Hib vaccine should not be administered after the fifth birthday except for special circumstances as noted in the specific ACIP recommendations for the use of Hib vaccine.*

vaccines produce high rates of seroconversion (>95%) and induce adequate levels of anti-HBs whether given to infants (1) at birth, 2 months, and 6 months or (2) at 2 months, 4 months, and 6 months.

The immunization schedule for HepB most often used for adults and children over 7 years consists of three intramuscular injections, the second and third given one and six months, respectively, after the first (Table 4). An alternative schedule consisting of four doses given at 0, 1, 2, and 12 months has been approved for one vaccine [Engerix-B] and may induce immunity more rapidly; however, there are no data to suggest that this regimen provides greater protection than the standard three-dose schedule. If the four-dose regimen is employed, the last dose (at 12 months) is necessary to ensure the highest final antibody level.

If the vaccination series is interrupted after the first dose of HepB, the second dose should be administered as soon as possible, and the third dose separated by at least two months and given after the age of four months. If only the third dose is delayed, it may be given whenever convenient. The recom-

TABLE 3.
RECOMMENDED IMMUNIZATION SCHEDULE FOR PERSONS ≥ 7 YEARS OF AGE NOT VACCINATED AT THE RECOMMENDED TIME IN EARLY INFANCY*

Timing	Vaccine (s)	Comments
First visit	Td†, OPV§, MMR¶, and Hep B**	Primary poliovirus vaccination is not routinely recommended for persons ≥ 18 years of age.
Second visit (6-8 weeks after first visit)	Td, OPV, MMR¶,††, Hep B**	
Third visit (6 months after second visit)	Td, OPV, Hep B**	
Additional visits	Td	Repeat every 10 years throughout life.

* *From:* MMWR, *1994. See individual ACIP recommendations for details. HepB indicates hepatitis B vaccine, recombinant; MMR, measles-mumps-rubella; OPV, poliovirus vaccine, live oral, trivalent; Td, tetanus and diphtheria toxoids (for use among persons ≥ 7 years of age).*

† *The DTP and DTaP doses administered to children < 7 years of age who remain incompletely vaccinated at age ≥ 7 years should be counted as prior exposure to tetanus and diphtheria toxoids (eg, a child who previously received two doses of DTP needs only one dose of Td to complete a primary series for tetanus and diphtheria).*

§ *When polio vaccine is administered to previously unvaccinated persons ≥ 18 years of age, inactivated poliovirus vaccine (IPV) is preferred. For the immunization schedule for IPV, see specific ACIP statement on the use of polio vaccine.*

¶ *Persons born before 1957 can generally be considered immune to measles and mumps and need not be vaccinated. Rubella (or MMR) vaccine can be administered to persons of any age, particularly to nonpregnant women of childbearing age.*

** *Selected high-risk groups for whom vaccination is recommended include persons with occupational risk, such as health care and public safety workers who have occupational exposure to blood, clients and staff of institutions for the developmentally disabled, hemodialysis patients, recipients of certain blood products (eg, clotting factor concentrates), household contacts and sex partners of hepatitis B virus carriers, injecting drug users, sexually active homosexual and bisexual men, certain sexually active heterosexual men and women, inmates of long-term correctional facilities, certain international travelers, and families of HBsAg-positive adoptees from countries where HBV infection is endemic. Because risk factors are often not identified directly among adolescents, universal HepB vaccination of teenagers should be implemented in communities where injecting drug use, pregnancy among teenagers, and/or sexually transmitted diseases are common.*

†† *The ACIP recommends a second dose of measles-containing vaccine (preferably MMR to assure immunity to mumps and rubella) for certain groups. Children with no documentation of live measles vaccination after the first birthday should receive two doses of live measles-containing vaccine not less than 1 month apart. In addition, the following persons born in 1957 or later should have documentation of measles immunity (ie, two doses of measles-containing vaccine [at least one of which is MMR], physician-diagnosed measles, or laboratory evidence of measles immunity): (a) those entering post-high school educational settings; (b) those beginning employment in health care settings who will have direct patient contact; and (c) travelers to areas with endemic measles.*

mended dose varies by product, the recipient's age, and, in the case of infants, by the mother's HBsAg status (see the chapter on Agents for Immunization). Larger amounts or an increased number of doses are necessary to induce protective antibody levels in a high percentage of hemodialysis patients and also may be necessary for other immunocompromised individuals (see the chapter on Agents for Immunization).

Hepatitis delta virus (HDV) is a defective virus that can replicate only in the presence of HBV; thus, prevention of HBV infection through immunization also prevents HDV infection in susceptible persons.

DTP: Since the late 1940s, immunization of infants and children by simultaneous vaccination against diphtheria, tetanus, and pertussis (DTP vaccine) has been a routine practice in the United States. Currently recommended schedules are presented in Tables 1 and 2. Children who receive all four of the primary vaccination doses before their fourth birthday should receive a fifth booster dose of DTP before entering elementary school. This booster dose is not necessary if the fourth dose was given on or after the fourth birthday. Two combination DTP-Hib vaccines have been licensed for use in infants and may be administered whenever these vaccines are scheduled to be given at the same visit.

Two combination products containing an acellular pertussis vaccine (DTaP) are now available: ACEL-IMUNE (Lederle Laboratories) and TRIPEDIA (Connaught Laboratories). These vaccines are licensed only for use as the fourth and fifth doses of the DTP series in children age 15 months to 6 years. They are not recommended for children who have received fewer than three doses of whole-cell DTP vaccine, regardless of age; questions remain as to whether sole use of acellular pertussis vaccines confers protection when administered early in infancy and whether protection so induced at any age is equivalent to that of whole-cell pertussis vaccine preparations. The ACIP has recommended the use of DTaP for the fourth and fifth doses because it substantially reduces local reactions, fever, and other common systemic events that often follow administration of whole-cell DTP. In addition, when used for the fourth and fifth doses, the immunogenicity of the antigens included in the acellular vaccines is comparable to that of whole-cell DTP. DTP or DTaP can be used interchangeably for the fourth and fifth doses of the routine series of vaccination against these diseases (*MMWR*, 1991 B, 1992 A, 1992 B).

Pertussis vaccination is not recommended for adults or children after their seventh birthday because the severity of pertussis decreases with age and adverse reactions caused by the vaccine may be increased. For this group, a series of three intramuscular injections of tetanus and diphtheria toxoid vaccine for adult use (Td) should be given. The Td vaccine, which contains a reduced dose of diphtheria toxoid, is employed rather than the DT vaccine in children >7 years because adverse effects from the higher dose of diphtheria toxoid contained in the latter are more common in this group than in younger children.

For children <7 years in whom pertussis vaccine is contraindicated, DT should be used instead of DTP. Previously unvaccinated infants who receive their first DT dose when <1 year should receive a total of four doses of DT as the primary series, the first three doses at four- to eight-week intervals and the fourth dose 6 to 12 months later. If additional doses of pertussis vaccine are contraindicated after a DTP series is begun in the first year of life, DT should be substituted for each of the remaining scheduled DTP doses.

Children ≥1 year who are unvaccinated and for whom pertussis vaccine is contraindicated should receive two doses of DT four to eight weeks apart, followed by a third dose 6 to 12 months later to complete the primary series. Children who received one or two doses of DT or DTP after their first birthday and for whom further pertussis vaccine is contraindicated should receive a total of three doses of a preparation containing diphtheria and tetanus toxoids appropriate for their age, with the third dose given 6 to 12 months after the second dose. Children completing a primary series of DT before their fourth birthday should receive a fifth dose before entering elementary school; this dose is not needed if the fourth dose was given after the fourth birthday. A monovalent pertussis vaccine (Michigan Department of Health) can be used to complete vaccination against pertussis for children <7 years who have received fewer than the recommended number of doses of pertussis vaccine but have received the recommended number of doses of diphtheria and tetanus toxoids for their age.

Infants and children with certain underlying neurologic conditions present a special problem for the administration of DTP vaccine because they appear to be at increased risk of developing manifestations of the underlying neurologic disorder within two to three days after vaccination. However, protection against diphtheria, tetanus, and pertussis is at least as important for these children as for other children and may be even more important. On the basis of these considerations, the ACIP has recommended the following approaches (*MMWR*, 1991 B):

A. *Infants and children with previous convulsions:* It is prudent to delay DTP vaccination until the child's status has been fully assessed, a treatment regimen established, and the condition stabilized.

B. *Unvaccinated infants who are suspected of having underlying neurologic disorder:* Until further observation and study have clarified the child's neurologic status and the effect of treatment, it is prudent to delay initiation of vaccination with DTP or DT, but not other vaccines.

C. *Children who have not received a complete vaccine series and who have a neurologic event occurring between doses:* If the seizure or other disorder occurs before the first birthday and before completion of the first three doses of the primary series of DTP, further doses of DTP or DT should be deferred until the infant's status has been clarified. The decision to complete the series with DTP or DT should be made before the first birthday and the nature of the problem and the benefits and possible risks of the vaccine should be considered. If the seizure or other disorder occurs after the first birthday, the neurologic status should be evaluated to ensure that the disorder is stable before another dose of DTP is administered.

D. *Infants and children with stable neurologic conditions:* These children may be vaccinated. The occurrence of a single seizure temporally unassociated with DTP does not contraindicate DTP vaccination, especially if the seizure can be satisfactorily explained. Parents of children with a history of convulsions should be informed of the increased risk of postvaccination seizures. Acetaminophen (15 mg/kg at the time of vaccination and every four hours for the next 24 hours) should be given to these children to reduce the possibility of postvaccination fever.

E. *Children with resolved or corrected neurologic disorders:* DTP vaccination is recommended for infants with certain neurologic problems that have been corrected or have subsided without sequelae. A family history of convulsions or other central nervous system disorders is not a contraindication to pertussis vaccination. It is, however, recommended that acetaminophen 15 mg/kg be given at the time of vaccination and every four hours for the next 24 hours to reduce the possibility of postvaccination fever.

Hib: Use of Haemophilus b conjugate vaccine (Hib) for the routine immunization of infants and children ≥2 months has been recommended by the ACIP since 1991 (*MMWR*, 1991 C). Currently, four types of Hib vaccines are licensed for use in children ≥15 months: PRP-D [Prohibit], HbOC [HIBTITER], PRP-OMP [PedvaxHIB], and PRP-T [ActHIB, OmniHib]. The latter three vaccines also are licensed for use in children ≥2 months. Specific characteristics of the four conjugated vaccines vary, including the type of protein carrier, the size of the polysaccharide, and the chemical linkage between the polysaccharide antigen and carrier. After the primary series of three injections, antibody levels decline following administration of any of the conjugate vaccines to infants; therefore, the ACIP recommends a booster dose at 12 to 15 months (*MMWR*, 1991 C). Ideally, the same conjugate vaccine should be used throughout the entire vaccination series; however, if different vaccines are used, a total of three doses for the primary series in infants is adequate. A booster dose with any of the four conjugate vaccines is likely to provide a good response in children ≥12 months. Unvaccinated children 15 to 59 months may be given any one of the Hib vaccines licensed for this age group. A detailed immunization schedule for each of the four Hib vaccines is presented in Table 2.

Two combination vaccines are now available to provide protection against diphtheria, tetanus, pertussis, and *Haemophilus influenzae* type b (Hib), [TETRAMUNE] (Lederle-Praxis) and a PRP-T [ActHIB, OmniHIB] combination. The former vaccine is made by a combination of DTP vaccine [TRI-IMMUNOL] and HbOC [HIBTITER], while the latter is prepared by the user by reconstituting the lyophilized PRP-T vaccine with the Connaught DTP vaccine. Immunogenicity studies indicate that antibody responses to Hib PRP, diphtheria, and tetanus toxins were comparable to separate, concurrent administration of DTP and HbOC vaccines when these vaccines were administered to infants at 2, 4, 6, or 15 to 18 months of age. Either of the combination vaccines may be used for the routine vaccination of infants to prevent diphtheria, tetanus, pertussis, and Hib disease beginning at 2 months of age (but not earlier than 6 weeks). If one of these vaccines is used, unvaccinated infants 2 to 6 months of age should receive three doses given at least two months apart, followed by an additional dose at 12 to 15 months after at least a six-month interval following the third dose or as soon as possible thereafter. They also may be used for the first and second doses of the vaccine series for infants who received both Hib and DTP vaccines late. In these infants, additional doses of DTP (without Hib) may be necessary to assure that all four recommended doses of DTP are administered.

Infants age 7 to 11 months who have not been immunized with DTP or Hib vaccines may receive two doses of combination vaccine given at least two months apart. (They also may receive the single antigen Hib and DTP separately.) This should be followed by a dose of DTP four to eight weeks after the second dose of the combination vaccine. An additional dose of DTP and Hib vaccines should then be administered, the former given at least six months after the third dose of DTP and the latter at 12 to 18 months of age with an interval of at least two months after the last Hib dose.

A combination vaccine may be used to complete an infant immunization series begun with any Hib and any DTP vaccine if both vaccines are due to be administered simultaneously. Conversely, any DTP vaccine may be used to complete a series initiated with a combination vaccine.

ADULT IMMUNIZATIONS. Immunization programs have primarily targeted children in order to achieve long-term universal immunity; thus, vaccination is a routine part of pediatric practice. However, a substantial portion of adolescents and adults who escaped natural infection or were not immunized with vaccines recommended during childhood remain susceptible to one or more common communicable diseases. In addition, certain vaccines are recommended for routine use in adults. It has been recommended that health care providers for adults and older adolescents provide vaccinations as a routine part of their practice. Adults in certain groups (eg, age, occupational, environmental, life-style), those with special health problems, and travelers to certain countries as well as foreign students and immigrants in this country also may be susceptible to these diseases and should be vaccinated. See Table 4 for ACIP recommendations for immunizations for these individuals.

Age Groups: The ACIP recommends that all adults age 18 to 24 years complete a primary series of Td vaccine if this was not given during childhood. In addition, they should be immune to measles, mumps, and rubella (*MMWR*, 1991 D). Those attending post-high school educational institutions or who are newly employed in situations that put them at high risk of measles transmission should have documentation of having received two doses of MMR on or after their first birthday or other evidence of immunity (ie, documentation of physician-diagnosed disease, laboratory evidence of immunity). Because the risk of acquiring measles outside the United States is greater than the risk incurred in the United States, travelers should be immune to measles before leaving the country. Consideration should be given to providing a dose of measles vaccine to persons born during or after 1957 who travel abroad, who have not previously received two doses of measles vaccine, and who do not have other evidence of measles immunity. During outbreaks of measles, mumps, or rubella, all exposed persons should have evidence of immunity or be given a dose of MMR vaccine.

All adults age 25 to 64 years also should complete a primary series of Td if not received previously. All adults born after 1956 should receive one dose of measles vaccine (preferably as MMR) unless they have documentation of the receipt of measles vaccine on or after their first birthday or other evidence of immunity as stated above. This is especially important for certain adults (eg, college students, persons working in health care facilities, international travelers) born after 1956; these individuals are at increased risk of measles and should have evidence of having received two doses of measles vaccine or other evidence of immunity. In addition, mumps vaccine should be given to adults who are considered susceptible. Rubella vaccine is recommended for adults, especially women of childbearing age, unless there is proof of prior immunization or laboratory evidence of immunity.

Adults $\geq$65 years old should have completed a primary series of diphtheria and tetanus toxoids; if not, a primary series of three doses of Td should be initiated. Annual influenza vaccination is recommended for all adults in this age group. Pneumococcal polysaccharide vaccine given as a single initial dose also is recommended; a booster dose administered six or more years after the first dose should be strongly considered for those at highest risk of either a fatal pneumococcal disease (eg, asplenic patients) or a rapid decline in antibody levels (eg, transplant recipients, those with chronic renal failure, those with nephrotic syndrome).

For all adults and adolescents who have completed a primary series of immunization, a booster dose of Td should be given every 10 years.

Routine poliovirus vaccination of adults residing in the United States is not recommended. Most adults are already immune, and the risk of exposure is very low. However, adults at increased risk of exposure include (1) travelers to areas where poliomyelitis is prevalent, (2) members of population

TABLE 4.
IMMUNOBIOLOGICS RECOMMENDED FOR SPECIAL OCCUPATIONS, LIFE-STYLES, ENVIRONMENTAL CIRCUMSTANCES, TRAVEL, FOREIGN STUDENTS, IMMIGRANTS, AND REFUGEES, UNITED STATES*

Indication	Immunobiologic
OCCUPATION	
Hospital, laboratory, and other health care personnel	Hepatitis B Influenza Measles Rubella Mumps Polio
Public safety personnel	Hepatitis B Influenza
Staff of institutions for the developmentally disabled	Hepatitis B Influenza
Veterinarians and animal handlers	Rabies Plague
Selected field workers (those who come into contact with possibly infected animals)	Rabies Plague
Selected occupations (those who work with imported animal hides, furs, wool, animal hair, and bristles)	Anthrax
LIFE-STYLES	
Homosexual males	Hepatitis B
Injecting drug users	Hepatitis B
Heterosexual persons with multiple sexual partners or recently acquired sexually transmitted disease	Hepatitis B
ENVIRONMENTAL SITUATION	
Inmates of long-term correctional facilities	Influenza Pneumococcal polysaccharide Hepatitis B
Residents of institutions for the developmentally disabled	Hepatitis B
Household contacts of HBV carriers	Hepatitis B
Homeless persons	Tetanus/diphtheria§ Measles Mumps Rubella Influenza
TRAVEL†	Measles Mumps Rubella Polio Influenza Hepatitis B Japanese encephalitis Rabies Meningococcal polysaccharide Tetanus/diphtheria§ Yellow fever Typhoid Cholera Plague¶ Immune globulin**

(table continued on next page)

TABLE 4 (continued)

Indication	Immunobiologic
FOREIGN STUDENTS, IMMIGRANTS, AND REFUGEES	Measles Rubella Diphtheria Tetanus Mumps Polio Hepatitis B

* *Adapted from* MMWR, *1991 D.*

† *Vaccines needed for travelers will vary depending on individual itineraries; travelers should refer to* Health Information for International Travelers *for more detailed information.*

§ *If not received within 10 years.*

¶ *In or during travel to areas with enzootic or epidemic plague in which exposure to rodents cannot be prevented.*

** *For Hepatitis A prophylaxis.*

groups with disease caused by poliovirus, (3) certain laboratory personnel working with virulent polioviruses, (4) health care workers in frequent contact with poliomyelitis patients (eg, those working in developing countries), and (5) unimmunized or inadequately immunized parents or other adults residing in the same household as children to be given OPV. (Susceptible adult contacts are at slight risk of paralytic disease resulting from fecal excretion of revertant viruses.) Adults who are household contacts of children to be given OPV may wish to follow the most appropriate schedule as outlined below before the vaccine is administered to the child.

For adults at increased risk of exposure to wild poliovirus, the following recommendations are based on the immune status of the individual:

A. *Unvaccinated or uncertain immune status*: Primary vaccination with enhanced-potency inactivated poliovirus vaccine (eIPV). If time does not permit administration of at least three doses, the following schedules are recommended: (1) Less than eight weeks, but more than four: Two doses of eIPV at least four weeks apart. (2) Less than four weeks: A single dose of OPV or eIPV. In both instances, the remaining doses of vaccine should be given later at the recommended interval if the person remains at increased risk.

B. *Incompletely immunized*: Adults who have received less than a full course of either OPV or eIPV should be given the remaining doses of either vaccine regardless of the interval since the last dose.

C. *Completion of a primary course of either poliovirus vaccine*: Those who have completed a primary course of OPV may be given another dose of the same vaccine. Those who have completed a primary course of eIPV may be given a dose of either the oral or inactivated vaccine.

The nonimmunized or inadequately immunized parent whose child is scheduled for OPV represents a special problem because of the remote risk of acquiring paralytic poliomyelitis from contact with the child. Because this risk is so remote, the recommended and usual practice in the United States is to administer OPV to the child regardless of the immunization history of the parents. An alternative approach for the unimmunized parent is to delay immunization of the child until the parent has received two doses of eIPV. This requires a delay of several months in administering OPV to the infant and should be undertaken only if there is complete confidence that the infant will receive the full course of vaccine. For the partially immunized parent, the primary series can be completed.

Occupations: Adults in certain occupations may be at increased risk of exposure to certain vaccine-preventable diseases and may need selected vaccines in addition to those routinely recommended for their age group. (ACIP recommendations for immunizations for special occupations, lifestyles, environmental circumstances, and for travelers, foreign students, immigrants, and refugees are presented in Table 4 [*MMWR*, 1991 D]).

MMR and annual influenza vaccinations are recommended for physicians, nurses, and other personnel in hospital, chronic care, and outpatient care settings who have contact with high-risk patients in all age groups. Such immunizations protect the individual vaccinee and reduce the possibility of nosocomial transmission of these diseases to patients, especially those at high risk (eg, rubella in pregnant women).

HBV infection is a major occupational hazard for health care and public safety workers and they should be vaccinated with HepB vaccine; the risk of acquiring the infection depends on the frequency of exposure to blood and blood products. Among health care workers with frequent exposure to blood, the prevalence of serologic evidence of HBV infection ranges from 15% to 30%; in comparison, prevalence in the general population is 5%.

Although not routinely recommended for persons over 18 years, poliovirus vaccine should be given to hospital personnel who do not have satisfactory evidence of completing a full series of polio immunizations and who have close contact with patients who may be excreting virulent poliovirus and laboratory personnel who may handle specimens containing virulent poliovirus. If they are not already immune, these persons should complete a primary series of poliovirus vaccine. eIPV is preferred for adults because they have a slightly increased risk of vaccine-associated paralysis after receiving OPV and because vaccine polioviruses may be excreted by OPV recipients for 30 days or more, thus increasing the risk of acquiring vaccine-associated paralytic poliomyelitis among susceptible immunocompromised OPV recipients and/or their close contacts.

In health care and research settings, plague, anthrax, and rabies vaccines are indicated only for laboratory personnel working with, isolating, or testing these infectious agents. Smallpox vaccine is indicated only for those laboratory workers involved with orthopox viruses or in clinical trials of vaccinia-recombinant vaccines.

Veterinarians, animal handlers, and selected field workers are at risk of rabies exposure because of occupational contact with domestic and wild animals and, consequently, should receive pre-exposure rabies immunization. Plague vaccine should be considered in the western United States for veterinarians and their assistants because they may be exposed to bubonic and pneumonic infection in the animals they treat, particularly domestic cats. Plague and pre-exposure rabies vaccines also are indicated for field personnel who may be exposed to potentially plague- or rabies-infected animals.

Anthrax vaccine is indicated for workers who come in contact with imported animal hides, furs, bonemeal, wool, animal hair (especially goat), and bristles.

Special Groups: HepB vaccine is recommended for homosexual males, injecting drug users, and heterosexual persons with multiple sexual partners or recently acquired sexually transmitted disease. From 35% to 80% of homosexually active males have serologic evidence of HBV infection. Therefore, HepB vaccine should be administered to susceptible homosexual males as soon as possible after they begin homosexual activity because 10% to 20% can be expected to acquire the infection each year. Evidence of HBV infection also has been found in 60% to 80% of injecting drug users, and 10% to 20% can be expected to acquire the infection each year after becoming drug abusers.

Laboratory evidence of HBV infection has been found in 10% to 80% of male prisoners. Thus, HepB vaccination should be considered for inmates of long-term correctional facilities because of the likelihood of homosexual behavior and of injecting drug use. Annual influenza vaccination and immunization with the pneumococcal polysaccharide vaccine also are advised for prisoners ≥65 years and those with high-risk medical conditions.

From 35% to 80% of residents of institutions for the developmentally disabled have serologic evidence of HBV infection; therefore, newly admitted individuals should be vaccinated as soon as possible and current residents should be screened for evidence of immunity and vaccinated if susceptible. Finally, household contacts of HBV carriers are at high risk of infection and should be tested for evidence of immunity; all susceptible contacts should be vaccinated.

Homeless persons are susceptible to a number of vaccine-preventable diseases and, therefore, their vaccination status should be assessed whenever possible. Appropriate vaccines include Td, MMR, and influenza.

In many countries, pediatric immunization with DTP, MMR, and poliovirus vaccines is not routine; hence, persons entering the United States as students, immigrants, or refugees may be susceptible to one or more of these diseases. Unless such persons can document receipt of these vaccines at appropriate ages and intervals or provide laboratory evidence of immunity, they should receive the recommended vaccines for their age group. Vaccines that should be considered include MMR, Td, and HepB.

Special Health Problems: Adults with special health problems may need to be vaccinated, but because of an underlying health condition, some vaccines may be contraindicated while others may be indicated. To minimize concern about possible teratogenicity, it is prudent to delay the administration of any vaccine to pregnant women until the second or third trimester. Live virus vaccines should not be given to pregnant women or to those likely to become pregnant within three months. Pregnant women not previously vaccinated should receive two properly spaced doses of Td; those who have previously received one or two doses should complete their primary series during pregnancy. The ACIP recommends that rubella vaccine be given in the postpartum period to women not known to be immune, preferably before discharge from the hospital. Influenza and pneumococcal polysaccharide vaccine should be given to those at increased risk. Influenza vaccine may be safely administered to pregnant women, but it is advisable to administer pneumococcal polysaccharide vaccine before pregnancy.

Persons receiving hemodialysis are at high risk of infection with HBV. An estimated 15% of these individuals have serologic evidence of infection, and routine serologic screening is currently recommended. Larger and increased numbers of doses are generally recommended for these patients because of lower vaccine immunogenicity. Therefore, three doses of HepB vaccine should be given as soon as possible and revaccination with one or more doses should be considered for persons who do not respond serologically to vaccination.

Patients with clotting disorders who receive factor VII or IX concentrates also are at increased risk of HBV infection and should be vaccinated appropriately before receiving any blood products. Prevaccination serologic screening for HBV markers is recommended for those who have already received infusions of these products.

Immunocompromised individuals present a special problem for immunizations. Recently, the ACIP published recommendations on the use of vaccines and immune globulins for persons with altered immunocompetence (*MMWR*, 1993 A); these are based primarily on the degree to which a patient is immunocompromised and the nature of the immunosuppression. In general, killed or inactivated vaccines do not constitute a danger to immunocompromised persons and may be administered as recommended for immunocompetent persons. Vaccines given to immunocompromised individuals should be assumed to be less effective than in healthy persons. Because virus replication may be enhanced in severely immunocompromised patients receiving live vaccines, in general, such vaccines should not be given. An important exception to this rule is MMR vaccination, which is recommended for all children and adults when otherwise indicated, regardless of their HIV status.

Live vaccines usually can be given to those receiving steroids if therapy is short term (<2 weeks) or low to moderate doses are given. The immunosuppressive effects of steroid treatment vary, but many clinicians consider a dose equivalent to either 2 mg/kg or a total of 20 mg/day of prednisone sufficiently immunosuppressive to cause concern about the safety of live virus vaccine administration. At least three months should elapse after discontinuation of steroid therapy before administration of a live virus vaccine to patients who have received large doses of systemic steroids for two or more weeks.

The ACIP has divided persons with immunocompromising conditions into three groups: (1) those who are severely immunocompromised, but not as a result of HIV infection; (2) those with HIV infection; and (3) those with conditions that cause limited immune deficits (eg, asplenia, renal failure, diabetes). Recommendations on routine immunization of immunocompromised children and adults appear in Tables 5 and 6; recommendations on nonroutine immunization of immunocompromised persons appear in Table 7.

OPV should not be administered to any household contact of a severely immunocompromised patient because of the danger of transmitting vaccine virus to the patient and subsequent reversion to the wild type. MMR vaccine is not contraindicated for the close contacts of immunocompromised persons because vaccine virus transmission and reversion has not been demonstrated with this vaccine. Persons with leukemia in remission who have not received chemotherapy for at least three months may be given live virus vaccines. Ideally, vaccination should precede the initiation of chemotherapy or immunosuppression by two or more weeks. For certain immunocompromised patients, passive immunoprophylaxis with immune globulin may be indicated instead of or in addition to vaccination.

HIV-infected patients usually should not receive live vaccines. However, limited studies with MMR vaccine in both asymptomatic and symptomatic HIV-infected patients did not demonstrate serious or unusual adverse events. Therefore, MMR vaccination is recommended for all HIV-infected children and adults in the same schedules as for uninfected persons. Pneumococcal vaccine is indicated for all HIV-infected persons >2 years. Annual influenza vaccination also is indicated for HIV-infected persons. When needed, eIPV is the preferred poliovirus vaccine for HIV-infected patients. HIV-infected children <2 years should receive Hib vaccine according to the routine schedule. Use of Hib vaccine also should be considered in HIV-infected adults, for the disease may be severe in these patients.

Certain conditions (eg, renal failure, diabetes, alcoholic cirrhosis, asplenia) may increase the risk for some diseases. Selected vaccines, especially bacterial polysaccharide vaccines, are recommended for these patients; larger or more frequent doses may be required to maintain adequate immunity (see Table 6). Generally, persons in this category are not considered seriously immunosuppressed for the purposes of vaccination and should receive routine vaccinations with both live and inactivated vaccines according to the usual schedules.

IMMUNIZATIONS FOR TRAVELERS

The risk of acquiring a vaccine-preventable disease during international travel depends on the areas visited and the extent of possible exposure. Requirements and recommendations for specific immunizations and health practices for travel to various countries change yearly. The best source of up-to-date information is *Health Information for International Travel,*

TABLE 5.
SUMMARY OF ACIP RECOMMENDATIONS ON IMMUNIZATION OF IMMUNOCOMPROMISED INFANTS AND CHILDREN*

Vaccine	Routine (not immunocompromised)	HIV infection/ AIDS	Severely immunocompromised (non-HIV related)†	Asplenia	Renal Failure	Diabetes
ROUTINE INFANT IMMUNIZATIONS						
DTP (DT/T/Td)§	Recommended	Recommended	Recommended	Recommended	Recommended	Recommended
OPV	Recommended	**Contraindicated**	**Contraindicated**	Recommended	Recommended	Recommended
eIPV	Use if indicated	Recommended	Recommended	Use if indicated	Use if indicated	Use if indicated
MMR (MR/M/R)	Recommended	Recommended/ considered¶	**Contraindicated**	Recommended	Recommended	Recommended
Hib	Recommended	Recommended	Recommended	Recommended	Recommended	Recommended
HepB**	Recommended	Recommended	Recommended	Recommended	Recommended	Recommended
OTHER CHILDHOOD IMMUNIZATIONS						
Pneumococcal††	Use if indicated	Recommended	Recommended	Recommended	Recommended	Recommended
Influenza§§	Use if indicated	Recommended	Recommended	Recommended	Recommended	Recommended

* *From* MMWR, *1993 A.*
† *Severe immunosuppression can be the result of congenital immunodeficiency, HIV infection, leukemia, lymphoma, aplastic anemia, generalized malignancy, or therapy with alkylating agents, antimetabolites, radiation, or large amounts of corticosteroids.*
§ *Including DTaP boosters.*
¶ *See discussion of MMR.*
** *HepB vaccine is now recommended for all infants.*
†† *Recommended for persons ≥2 years of age.*
§§ *Not recommended for infants <6 months of age.*

TABLE 6.
SUMMARY OF ACIP RECOMMENDATIONS ON IMMUNIZATION OF IMMUNOCOMPROMISED ADULTS*

Vaccine	Routine (not immuno-compromised)	HIV infection/ AIDS	Severely immuno-compromised (non-HIV related)**	Post-solid organ transplant or chronic immuno-suppressive therapy	Asplenia	Renal failure	Diabetes	Alcoholism and alcoholic cirrhosis
Td	Recommended	Recommended	Recommended	Recommended	Recommended	Recommended	Recommended	Recommended
MMR (MR/M/R)	Use if indicated	Recommended/ considered†	Contraindicated	Contraindicated	Use if indicated	Use if indicated	Use if indicated	Use if indicated
HepB	Use if indicated	Use if indicated	Use if indicated	Use if indicated	Use if indicated	Recommended	Use if indicated	Use if indicated
Hib	Not recommended	Considered	Recommended	Recommended	Recommended	Use if indicated	Use if indicated	Use if indicated
Pneumococcal	Recommended if ≥65 years	Recommended	Recommended	Recommended	Recommended	Recommended	Recommended	Recommended
Meningococcal	Use if indicated	Use if indicated	Use if indicated	Use if indicated	Recommended	Use if indicated	Use if indicated	Use if indicated
Influenza	Recommended if ≥65 years	Recommended	Recommended	Recommended	Recommended	Recommended	Recommended	Recommended

*From MMWR, *1993 A.*

†*Severe immunosuppression can be the result of congenital immunodeficiency, HIV infection, leukemia, lymphoma, generalized malignancy, or therapy with alkylating agents, antimetabolites, radiation, or large amounts of corticosteroids.*

§*See discussion of MMR.*

¶*Patients with renal failure on dialysis should have their anti-Hbs response tested after vaccination, and those found not to respond should be revaccinated.*

***See discussion of HIV in the section on Special Health Problems.*

TABLE 7.
SUMMARY OF ACIP RECOMMENDATIONS ON NONROUTINE IMMUNIZATION OF IMMUNOCOMPROMISED PERSONS*

Vaccine	Not immunocom-promised	HIV infection/AIDS	Severely immunocompromised (non-HIV related)†	Post-solid organ transplant or chronic immuno-suppressive therapy	Asplenia, renal failure, diabetes, alcoholism, and alcoholic cirrhosis
LIVE VACCINES					
BCG	Use if indicated	Contraindicated	Contraindicated	Contraindicated	Use if indicated
OPV	Use if indicated	Contraindicated	Contraindicated	Contraindicated	Use if indicated
Vaccinia	Use if indicated	Contraindicated	Contraindicated	Contraindicated	Use if indicated
Typhoid, Ty21a	Use if indicated	Contraindicated	Contraindicated	Contraindicated	Use if indicated
Yellow fever§	Use if indicated	Contraindicated	Contraindicated	Contraindicated	Use if indicated
KILLED OR INACTIVATED VACCINES					
eIPV	Use if indicated	Use if indicated	Use if indicated	Use if indicated	Use if indicated
Cholera	Use if indicated	Use if indicated	Use if indicated	Use if indicated	Use if indicated
Plague	Use if indicated	Use if indicated	Use if indicated	Use if indicated	Use if indicated
Typhoid, inactivated	Use if indicated	Use if indicated	Use if indicated	Use if indicated	Use if indicated
Rabies	Use if indicated	Use if indicated	Use if indicated	Use if indicated	Use if indicated
Anthrax	Use if indicated	Use if indicated	Use if indicated	Use if indicated	Use if indicated

*From MMWR, *1993 A.*

† *Severe immunosuppression can be the result of congenital immunodeficiency, HIV infection, leukemia, lymphoma, aplastic anemia, generalized malignancy, or therapy with alkylating agents, antimetabolites, radiation, or large amounts of corticosteroids.*

§ *Yellow fever vaccine should be considered for patients when exposure to yellow fever cannot be avoided.*

which is published annually by the Centers for Disease Control and Prevention and can be obtained from the Superintendent of Documents, U.S. Government Printing Office, Washington, DC 20402. The CDC also maintains an international traveler's hotline that provides information on vaccine requirements and recommendations by geographic area (404/332-4559). Additionally, the CDC informs all state and many city and county health departments twice monthly about changing risks and requirements for international travelers.

Infants <6 months are usually exempt from requirements for certain vaccines, but they should receive the usual pediatric immunizations at the recommended intervals.

Immunizations that should be considered for travelers to foreign countries are listed in Table 4. In the following discussion, immunizations are divided into three groups: (1) Prerequisite for entry into a country or area, (2) commonly recommended, and (3) occasionally recommended.

Immunizations Required for Entry

Yellow Fever: At present, this disease occurs only in Africa and South America. Vaccination is required in some African countries for entering travelers; other countries require vaccination only for those entering from areas considered to harbor the infection. The vaccine is usually recommended for all persons >9 months who travel in areas where the disease exists. Vaccination should be considered for pregnant women and infants >4 months if travel to a high-risk area is anticipated and cannot be postponed. Infants <4 months should never be given yellow fever vaccine because of the risk of developing encephalitis due to the vaccine virus. Since protection is effective for at least 10 years, booster doses should be given at 10-year intervals. The vaccine must be administered at an approved Yellow Fever Vaccination Center (consult state or local health departments).

Studies indicate that antibody titers to both yellow fever and cholera are reduced if the vaccines are given simultaneously or within three weeks of each other.

Cholera: Cholera is a continuing health risk in Africa, Asia, and Latin America. The outbreak of epidemic cholera in Central and South America during the early 1990s focused attention on the continuing need for surveillance of this problem. In 1992, 339,561 cases and 2,321 cholera-related deaths were reported for 21 countries in the Western Hemisphere, with a total of 731,312 cases and 6,323 deaths reported since the beginning of the epidemic in January 1991 (*MMWR*, 1993 B). The traveler's best protection against the disease is avoidance of food and water that might be contaminated.

Cholera vaccines have limited effectiveness; field trials demonstrate that the currently available vaccine is only 50% effective in preventing clinical illness for a three- to six-month period and does not prevent transmission of the infection. Booster doses may be given every six months but enhance protection only temporarily. Thus, the World Health Organization no longer recommends cholera vaccination for travel to or from cholera-infected areas. However, some countries affected or threatened by the disease may require evidence of vaccination as a condition of entry. A single dose meets international requirements and is valid for six months.

Immunizations Commonly Recommended

Typhoid Fever: Immunization is recommended for travelers to areas where typhoid fever and poor sanitation exist. The killed vaccine is about 70% effective but often causes local reaction of one to two days' duration at the injection site, fever, malaise, and headache. Protection may last up to three years; booster doses are recommended every three years.

A live oral typhoid vaccine (Ty21a) is available in the United States. It is essentially nonreactogenic and appears to be at least as effective as the killed vaccine (Levine et al, 1987). The manufacturer of Ty21a recommends revaccination with the entire four-dose series every five years. An early field trial of an injectable acellular vaccine containing the capsular polysaccharide (Vi antigen) of *Salmonella typhi* showed negligible reactivity and comparable efficacy (Acharya et al, 1987). Subsequent trials demonstrated that a single injection of the purified polysaccharide vaccine is highly immunogenic and provides protection against blood culture-confirmed typhoid fever in about 74% of vaccinees. FDA approval is pending.

Hepatitis A: This disease occurs worldwide and is spread by the fecal-oral route. Immune globulin (IG) is recommended for travelers who will visit areas with primitive sanitation where exposure to potentially contaminated food and water is anticipated. A single intramuscular dose provides protection for up to three months. IG should be given within a few days of departure. All active immunizations should be completed (at least two weeks prior to the administration of IG). Inactivated vaccines to prevent hepatitis A have been reported to be highly effective when given as a two- or three-dose series. One vaccine has been licensed for use in some countries in Europe. An application for license in the United States is pending at the FDA.

Poliomyelitis: Vaccination is recommended for nonimmune or inadequately immunized travelers to areas where poliomyelitis is prevalent and sanitation is poor. Depending on immune status and history, either the eIPV or OPV may be employed. Unvaccinated adults preferably should complete a primary series of at least three doses of eIPV given one month apart before traveling to a country where poliomyelitis is endemic. If travel plans do not allow for these intervals, a single dose of either OPV or eIPV should be administered. For adults who were incompletely immunized with OPV or IPV, the remaining doses required for completion of the primary series should be administered regardless of the time since the last dose or type of vaccine previously received. Travelers who previously completed a primary series of OPV should receive a single supplementary dose of OPV; those who previously received a primary series of IPV should receive a single supplementary dose of either OPV or eIPV.

Tetanus: Tetanus immunization is recommended for everyone at home or traveling abroad. A booster injection combined with diphtheria toxoid (Td) should be given every 10 years to those who have completed the primary series.

Immunizations Occasionally Recommended

Diphtheria: The bacteria causing diphtheria are distributed throughout the world. In spite of immunization programs, many adults are susceptible. Travelers at high risk of infection are those in contact with children in poorer areas in underdeveloped nations. Since 1990, a large outbreak of diphtheria has been occurring in the countries of the former Soviet Union, especially Russia and Ukraine. A tetanus/diphtheria toxoid (Td) booster injection is recommended every 10 years for those who have completed the primary series.

Rabies: Vaccination with rabies vaccine is recommended only for travelers anticipating contact with animals or prolonged residence (one month or more) in areas where exposure to rabies is a constant threat.

Plague: Immunization is generally recommended only for travelers who expect to have contact with rodents, rabbits, or fleas in areas where plague is endemic (eg, Southeast Asia, Africa, South America). The risk of exposure is highest in rural or semirural areas.

Hepatitis B: Although not ordinarily recommended for travelers, HepB vaccine should be considered for certain individuals traveling to areas where the disease is prevalent (Southeast Asia, sub-Saharan Africa, the Amazon basin of South America, most of the Middle East, and countries of the former Soviet Union) and who plan to reside there for six months or more. Health care personnel whose work requires handling of body fluids and individuals expecting to have sexual contact with persons at risk are candidates for the vaccine. In order to complete the full immunization series, vaccination ideally should begin six months in advance of the anticipated travel date.

Measles: Many adolescents and young adults are susceptible to measles, and measles in adults is often more serious than in children. Foreign travel, including to Europe, may place these individuals at increased risk of exposure. All persons traveling abroad should be immune to measles in order to reduce the importation of the disease into the United States. More than 650 measles cases reported from 1985 to 1992 occurred among U.S. citizens returning from international travel. It is suggested that anyone born after 1956 who has not previously received two doses of measles vaccine receive one dose of live vaccine unless there is evidence of measles immunity (eg, physician-diagnosed measles, demonstrable serum antibody). If the traveler also is likely to be susceptible to mumps or rubella, MMR is the vaccine of choice. It is especially important that women of childbearing age be immune to rubella before leaving the United States.

Meningococcal Disease: Immunization is not usually recommended for adults, but travelers to countries where meningococcal disease is endemic (eg, sub-Saharan Africa from Mauritania to Ethiopia) are candidates for the vaccine. Outbreaks of group A meningococcal disease occurred in India, Nepal, and Saudi Arabia in 1987. Because the worldwide epidemiology of the disease varies from year to year, physicians should consult local or state health departments or the CDC for timely information.

Influenza: Persons at increased risk of complications from influenza who are planning travel to the tropics at any time or to the southern hemisphere during April through September should review their influenza vaccination history. If these persons were not vaccinated during the previous fall or winter, they should consider immunization before travel. Persons at high risk who were given the previous season's vaccine in preparation for travel should be revaccinated in the fall or winter with the currently recommended vaccine; such persons may, therefore, receive two doses of influenza vaccine within one year.

Japanese Encephalitis: Japanese encephalitis (JE), a mosquito-borne arboviral infection, is the leading cause of viral encephalitis in Asia. Sporadic and epidemic cases of JE are reported annually in China, Korea, Japan, Southeast Asia, the Indian subcontinent, and parts of Oceania; overt encephalitis develops in 1 to 20 per 1,000 cases. Encephalitis usually is severe, resulting in death in 25% of the cases and residual neuropsychiatric sequelae in 30%. JE infection acquired during the first or second trimester of pregnancy causes intrauterine infection and spontaneous abortion.

JE virus is transmitted in an enzootic cycle among mosquitoes and vertebrate-amplifying hosts, chiefly domestic pigs and wading birds. Culex mosquitoes are the principal vectors, and viral infection rates are up to 3% in these insects. This species is prolific in rural areas where the larvae breed in ground pools and rice fields, and infections in humans occur principally in this setting. In endemic areas, the annual incidence is 1 to 10 per 10,000.

The risk of acquiring JE among most travelers to Asia is very low. However, the risk for an individual is highly variable and depends on the season, locations and duration of travel, and the activities of the individual. The estimated risk for JE for travelers to an endemic area (incidence rate 1/5,000) for a one-month period during the transmission season is 1/5,000 or 1/20,000 per week (*MMWR*, 1993 C).

A vaccine for JE, derived from infected mouse brain, was licensed in 1992 to meet the needs of the U.S. military and of U.S. residents traveling to Asia. Its efficacy has been estimated to be from 80% to 91%. The JE vaccine is *not* recommended for all travelers to Asia; it should be offered to individuals spending one month or longer in endemic areas during the transmission season, especially if travel will include rural areas.

Cited References

Hepatitis B virus: A comprehensive strategy for eliminating transmission in the United States through universal childhood vaccination: Recommendations of the Immunization Practices Advisory Committee (ACIP). *MMWR* 40(No. RR-13):1-25, 1991 A.

Diphtheria, tetanus, and pertussis: Recommendations for vaccine use and other preventive measures: Recommendations of the Immunization Practices Advisory Committee (ACIP). *MMWR* 40(No. RR-10):1-28, 1991 B.

Haemophilus b conjugate vaccines for prevention of *Haemophilus influenzae* type b disease among infants and children two months of age and older: Recommendations of the Immunization Practices Advisory Committee (ACIP). *MMWR* 40(No. RR-1):1-7, 1991 C.

Update on adult immunization: Recommendations of the Immunization Practices Advisory Committee (ACIP). *MMWR* 40 (No. RR-12):1-94, 1991 D.

Pertussis vaccination: Acellular pertussis vaccine for reinforcing and booster use—supplementary ACIP statement: Recommendations of the Immunization Practices Advisory Committee (ACIP). *MMWR* 41(No. RR-1):1-10, 1992 A.

Pertussis vaccination: Acellular pertussis vaccine for the fourth and fifth doses of the DTP series: Update to supplementary ACIP statement: Recommendations of the Advisory Committee on Im-

munization Practices (ACIP). *MMWR* 41(No. RR-15):1-5, 1992 B.
Use of vaccines and immune globulins in persons with altered immunocompetence: Recommendations of the Advisory Committee on Immunization Practices (ACIP). *MMWR* 42(No. RR-4):1-18, 1993 A.
Update: Cholera—Western Hemisphere, 1992. *MMWR* 42:89-91, 1993 B.
Inactivated Japanese encephalitis virus vaccine: Recommendations of the Advisory Committee on Immunization Practices (ACIP). *MMWR* 42(No. RR-1):1-15, 1993 C.
General Recommendations on Immunization: Recommendations of the Advisory Committee on Immunization Practices (ACIP). *MMWR* 43(No. RR-1):1-38, 1994.
Acharya IL, et al: Prevention of typhoid fever in Nepal with the Vi capsular polysaccharide of *Salmonella typhi:* Preliminary report. *N Engl J Med* 317:1101-1104, 1987.
Levine MM, et al: Large-scale field trial of Ty21a live oral typhoid vaccine in enteric-coated capsule formulation. *Lancet* 1:1049-1052, 1987.

Agents for Immunization 86

Many effective vaccines continue to be produced by established, classic methods. These include whole organism vaccines such as pertussis, influenza, killed typhoid, and inactivated poliovirus vaccine as well as naturally occurring strains that induce immunity in the host without causing clinical disease (eg, live poliovirus; measles, mumps, rubella; BCG vaccines). Influenza split-virus, hepatitis B, and Haemophilus influenzae type b vaccines are subcellular components of pathogens that also are used to induce immunity. Still other vaccines are chemically modified exotoxins that have been inactivated without destroying their immunogenic potential (eg, tetanus and diphtheria toxoids).

Recent advances in immunology and biotechnology provide new approaches to vaccine development. The recently approved live oral typhoid vaccine (Ty21a) is one product of this new surge in vaccine development. Another promising agent is live attenuated varicella vaccine. The ability of molecular biologists to use recombinant DNA technology to replicate important epitopes of pathogens has allowed the creation of new vaccines by inserting genomic material into suitable vectors (eg, yeast cells) to yield safe and effective vaccines (eg, recombinant hepatitis B vaccines).

Classically produced and genetically engineered vaccines, as well as agents for passive immunity, are evaluated in this chapter.

ROUTINE IMMUNIZING AGENTS

Diphtheria

Diphtheria is primarily a disease of childhood, but it may occur in all age groups. Since the advent of immunization on a large scale, diphtheria is no longer a problem in the United States. However, the disease remains a threat due to its ubiquity in other countries and waning immunity in U.S. populations, probably because of lack of continuing exposure and inconsistent immunization of adults. The disease is caused by invasion of the skin or upper respiratory tract by *Corynebacterium diphtheriae,* which produces toxins that cause systemic manifestations, including peripheral neuropathy and myocarditis.

Active immunization is achieved with the use of diphtheria toxoid, a preparation of formaldehyde-inactivated toxins of *C. diphtheriae*. It is usually given in combination with tetanus toxoid and pertussis vaccine (DTP) for primary immunization of infants and young children. In addition, diphtheria toxoid is available in combination with tetanus toxoid without pertussis vaccine in a pediatric preparation (DT) or an adult preparation (Td).

Despite mass vaccination against diphtheria, a substantial portion of the population may have levels of antibody that are not protective. A major outbreak of diphtheria occurred in Sweden (where universal immunization is practiced) during 1984 to 1986, and the death/case ratio was quite high (Rappuoli et al, 1988). Such reports underscore the importance of reimmunization schedules for adults. It has been recommended that diphtheria toxoid be given to all adults at age 15 and every 10 years thereafter; in addition, adults should receive a tetanus-diphtheria toxoid booster prior to traveling abroad (Karzon and Edwards, 1988).

Diphtheria antitoxin is used with appropriate antibiotic therapy to treat clinical diphtheria. The most important aspect of treatment is to give the appropriate dose of antitoxin at the earliest possible moment. The dose depends on the severity and duration of the disease and is substantially increased if the diphtheritic membrane is extensive or the illness is prolonged (see the evaluation).

DIPHTHERIA AND TETANUS TOXOIDS AND PERTUSSIS VACCINE ADSORBED (DTP)

This combination of diphtheria and tetanus toxoids with pertussis vaccine is the recommended preparation for routine primary immunization and recall (booster) injections in children under 7 years.

The combined triple antigens are not recommended for use on or after the seventh birthday because: (1) both the incidence and severity of disease decrease with age and the vaccine may cause undesirable adverse reactions, and (2) the diphtheria component is present in a high dose that is not recommended for individuals over 7 years. Tetanus and diphtheria toxoids, adult type (Td), is used for primary immunization of older patients (7 years or more); diphtheria and tetanus toxoids, pediatric type (DT), may be used in younger children when pertussis vaccine is contraindicated.

ADVERSE REACTIONS AND PRECAUTIONS. Reactions attributed to DTP may be considered in three categories. The most frequent untoward effects of DTP are local reactions, including redness and swelling at the site of injection, rarely with the induction of a sterile abscess. Mild, transient systemic reactions (eg, fever, irritability, anorexia, drowsiness, vomiting) often occur (Cody et al, 1981). Fever of 39° C or more may develop in about 6% of recipients and of 40.5° C or more in 0.3%. Because these reactions are seen less frequently with DT, the major contributor appears to be the pertussis component of DTP.

The second category of reactions is more worrisome and includes inconsolable crying that may persist for more than three hours (about 1%), an unusual hypotonic-hyporesponsive state that may also persist for hours, and a short-lived febrile convulsion. Both the hypotonic-hyporesponsive episodes and febrile convulsions have been observed following about 1 in 1,750 doses (95% confidence intervals 1:925 to 1:3,850). These reactions have not been associated with permanent sequelae.

The third and most important category of untoward events temporally related to DTP is acute, severe encephalopathy, sometimes with permanent brain damage, that appears within three days after receipt of the vaccine. In an early comprehensive study of children with such episodes, it was suggested that most, if not all, represent simple coincidence or the precipitation of inevitable manifestations of an underlying central nervous system disorder by the known systemic effects of DTP. Results of this study indicated that, if it occurs at all, DTP rarely may produce encephalopathy with permanent brain damage once per 330,000 doses with very wide confidence intervals (Miller et al, 1981; Ross and Miller, 1986).

Findings of the foregoing study have been challenged in other studies. In one prospective study of 538 children observed from age 2 to 20 months, no convulsion, hypotonic-hyporesponsive episode, encephalopathy, or temperature over 40.5° C occurred; age was reported to affect the type and rate of adverse events more than the number of vaccine doses (Long et al, 1990). Additional studies have not provided evidence to support a causal relationship between DTP vaccination and either serious acute neurologic illness or permanent neurologic injury. These include: (1) the North West Thames Study in England, conducted from 1975 to 1981, in which 17,000 children, each of whom received three doses of DTP, were compared with 18,000 children, each of whom received three doses of DT vaccine (Pollock et al, 1983); (2) a study conducted from 1974 to 1983 in which children in the Group Health Cooperative of Puget Sound received a total of 106,000 doses of DTP vaccine (Walker et al, 1988); and (3) a study conducted from 1974 to 1984 in which 38,171 Tennessee Medicaid children received 107,154 doses of DTP vaccine (Griffin et al, 1990). Results of a large study in Denmark of approximately 150,000 children, among whom there were 554 cases of epilepsy, failed to demonstrate any relationship between the age at onset of epilepsy and the age at administration of DTP vaccine (Shields et al, 1988). While each of these studies was not of sufficient size to provide a definitive answer to the question of the possible causation of neurologic injury by DTP vaccine, results of the foregoing studies taken together are in contrast to the findings of the British studies cited above. Further, a recent pilot study of neurologic illness in children conducted from 1987 to 1988 in Washington and Oregon did not provide evidence of a statistically significant increased risk of serious acute neurologic illness within 7, 14, or 28 days of DTP immunization. However, as a pilot effort, the ability of this study to detect significant increases in individual neurologic conditions was limited. Review of data from the National Childhood Encephalopathy Study indicates that pertussis vaccine has not been proven to have a role in causing brain damage (Griffith, 1989).

Other studies have indicated that DTP is not causally related to the sudden infant death syndrome (SIDS) or infantile spasms.

The vaccine is contraindicated in patients with acute febrile disease. DTP vaccination should be delayed in those undergoing immunosuppressive therapy if cessation of therapy is anticipated in the immediate future to enhance the likelihood of an adequate immune response to the vaccine.

Contraindications to continuing the series of injections include the occurrence of the following adverse events after DTP or monovalent pertussis vaccination: (1) an immediate anaphylactic reaction; (2) temperature of 105° F or higher within 48 hours; (3) collapse or shock-like state within 48 hours; (4) encephalopathy occurring within seven days, including severe alterations in consciousness with generalized or focal neurologic signs that persist for more than 12 hours. Immunization may be continued with DT in such children.

The decision to give subsequent doses of a vaccine containing the pertussis component should be carefully considered if any of the following events occurs in temporal relationship to receipt of DTP: (1) persistent, inconsolable crying lasting three hours or more or an unusual, high pitched cry occurring within 48 hours; and (2) convulsion(s) with or without fever occurring within three days. Although these events were considered absolute contraindications in previous recommendations, there may be circumstances, such as a high incidence of pertussis, that outweigh the possible risks involved, particularly in view of the fact that these adverse effects are unlikely to produce permanent sequelae (Immunization Practices Advisory Committee, 1991 A).

Because data suggest that infants and young children with a history of convulsions are more likely to develop seizures after pertussis immunization, it has been recommended that immunization with any vaccine containing pertussis be deferred in these patients until it can be determined that there is no evolving neurologic disorder; a family history of seizures is not a contraindication (Immunization Practices Advisory Committee, 1985 B, 1987 A) (see also the chapter on Immunization Practices). However, when DTP is to be given to an infant or a child with a family or personal history of febrile seizures, consideration should be given to the use of an antipyretic drug for the ensuing 48 to 72 hours (Immunization Practices Advisory Committee, 1987 A). Infants and children with suspected or proven underlying neurologic disorders represent special problems that have been reviewed in detail (Immunization Practices Advisory Committee, 1985 B).

DOSAGE.
Intramuscular: *Children 2 months to the seventh birthday,* initially, 0.5 ml, followed by two more doses at four- to eight-week intervals. A fourth dose is given at 15 to 18 months of age (Immunization Practices Advisory Committee, 1986 A), and a booster dose is given when the child is 4 to 6 years old. This booster dose is not necessary if the fourth dose in the primary series was given on or after the fourth birthday. DTP should not be used after the seventh birthday.

Each 0.5 ml of DTP contains approximately 4 protective units of pertussis antigen. Eighty to 90% of exposed immunized individuals will be protected from pertussis.

(See the manufacturer's recommendations for further information.)

Manufacturers: Connaught, Lederle (***Tri-Immunol***).

DIPHTHERIA AND TETANUS TOXOIDS ADSORBED (PEDIATRIC) (DT)

Diphtheria and tetanus toxoids pediatric (DT) may be used for primary immunization and recall injections in children up to 7 years of age when pertussis vaccine is contraindicated. It should not be used in older individuals. Primary immunization with DT ensures protection in more than 95% of recipients. Following primary immunization, booster doses given for tetanus-prone wounds ensure protective levels of antitoxin within five to seven days.

ADVERSE REACTIONS AND PRECAUTIONS. As with other routine immunization procedures, administration of combined diphtheria and tetanus toxoids should be deferred in the presence of moderate or severe febrile illness. A history of a neurologic or severe hypersensitivity reaction following a previous dose is a contraindication to further use. Erythema, induration, and tenderness at the injection site develop in some patients. Systemic reactions, such as fever, drowsiness, fretfulness, vomiting, anorexia, and persistent crying, are sometimes observed. Neurologic complications following tetanus toxoid administration have been reported rarely.

DOSAGE.
Intramuscular: *Children less than 12 months,* three 0.5-ml injections administered at different sites at four- to eight-week intervals, followed by a fourth dose 6 to 12 months later. *Children over 12 months,* two doses four to eight weeks apart, followed by a third dose 6 to 12 months later (Immunization Practices Advisory Committee, 1985 B). A booster dose is given when the child is 4 to 6 years old, but it is not necessary if the fourth dose in the primary series was given on or after the fourth birthday.

Manufacturers: Connaught, Lederle, Sclavo, Wyeth-Ayerst.

TETANUS AND DIPHTHERIA TOXOIDS ADSORBED FOR ADULT USE (Td)

Tetanus and diphtheria toxoids adsorbed for adult use (Td) is used for primary immunization or recall (booster) injections in adults and children 7 years and older. This preparation contains the same amount of tetanus toxoid as DTP but only one-sixth to one-twelfth of the diphtheria toxoid contained in pediatric preparations. It is preferred to tetanus toxoid alone in wound management (see Table 1).

Serum antibody responses are similar to those seen with the pediatric vaccine (DT). High levels of immunity to diphtheria are attained in recipients after primary immunization. These levels can be maintained by booster immunization with Td at ten-year intervals.

ADVERSE REACTIONS. Reactions to Td are usually mild. They include erythema, induration, and tenderness at the site of injection; fever and malaise also may occur. Booster injections rarely may produce severe reactions to either component. These are most likely to occur in persons who have received large numbers of booster doses and usually reflect pre-existing high antibody titers. Neurologic complications following tetanus toxoid administration have been reported rarely.

DOSAGE.
Intramuscular: *Adults and children 7 years and older,* two injections of 0.5 ml with an interval of four to eight weeks between injections. A reinforcing dose to complete basic immunization is given 6 to 12 months later and every ten years thereafter.

Manufacturers: Connaught, Lederle, Sclavo, Wyeth-Ayerst.

DIPHTHERIA TOXOID ADSORBED (Pediatric). This product is no longer marketed in the United States.

DIPHTHERIA ANTITOXIN

This antitoxin is a sterile solution of enzyme-treated antibodies obtained from the serum of horses immunized with diphtheria toxoid alone or in conjunction with diphtheria toxin. It is used to treat active cases of diphtheria, and a few experts believe it should be considered for prophylaxis in exposed, nonimmunized, susceptible individuals who are not under close surveillance. For active cases, antitoxin should be administered on the basis of a clinical diagnosis of diphtheria without waiting for bacteriologic confirmation. Appropriate antimicrobial therapy (eg, penicillin, erythromycin) helps eliminate bacteria from the infected sites but is of no value against the toxin. Antibiotics are *not* a substitute for antitoxin. Appropriate material for culture should be obtained before antibiotics are given. Active immunization with diphtheria toxoid, using a different site, should be initiated at the same time that diphtheria antitoxin is given, because recovery from the disease does not necessarily confer immunity.

ADVERSE REACTIONS AND PRECAUTIONS. Serum sickness (urticaria, fever, pruritus, malaise, arthralgia) may occur in 7 to 14 days. The incidence of serum sickness caused by the currently available enzyme-treated serum is about 5%. The extent and severity of reactions depend on the amount of horse serum administered, the hypersensitivity of the patient, and the history of previous serum injections. Life-threatening anaphylaxis may occur in persons who have been previously sensitized to equine serum. Before injecting diphtheria antitoxin, it is essential to determine whether the patient has received a previous injection of animal serum or has a history of asthma or allergy. A skin or conjunctival test for sensitivity should be performed in all patients (see the chapter, Agents for Active and Passive Immunity: General Recommendations).

DOSAGE. The entire dose required should be given at one time if possible. Enough antitoxin must be administered to neutralize all the circulating toxin and any that may continue to be produced; usually one-half is given intravenously and one-half intramuscularly.

Intramuscular: *Adults and children*, all contacts of patients with diphtheria who are not appropriately immunized should receive diphtheria toxoid promptly for prophylaxis and be under surveillance for seven days. A few experts continue to suggest that those who cannot be monitored also should be given diphtheria antitoxin as follows:

If sensitivity tests are negative or desensitization has been completed, 2,000 to 10,000 units of antitoxin is given, depending on the length of time since exposure and extent of exposure.

For treatment, dosage of antitoxin depends on the site, severity, and duration of infection. Suggested ranges for *adults and children* are: pharyngeal or laryngeal disease of 48 hours' duration, 20,000 to 40,000 units; nasopharyngeal lesions, 40,000 to 60,000 units; extensive disease of three or more days' duration, 80,000 to 120,000 units.

Intravenous (slow infusion): *Adults and children*, for treatment only, same as intramuscular dose.

Manufacturer: Connaught.

Tetanus

Tetanus is not communicable; it results from the introduction of *Clostridium tetani,* a spore-forming anaerobic bacillus, into an area of injury. Under certain local tissue conditions (eg, low oxygen tension), the spore is converted to the vegetative form, which produces an exotoxin, tetanospasmin, which acts on the nervous system. Although tetanus is rare in the United States, the mortality rate may be 30% or greater. Fortunately, the disease is completely preventable by adequate immunization. Most cases occur in adults who have not received the primary immunization series or the necessary boosters to maintain adequate immunity. All military personnel beginning with World War II and nearly everyone born since the late 1940s has received the primary series. For these reasons, women born prior to 1947 are at special risk.

Since there is no natural immunity to tetanus, prophylaxis must be achieved by immunization: actively with tetanus toxoid, passively with tetanus immune globulin, or both. To provide adequate protection, it is important (1) that all children receive the recommended primary immunizations, (2) that booster injections be given every ten years, (3) that a history of immunizations be obtained from adult patients and primary immunization or booster injections be given as necessary, and (4) that an injured patient receive appropriate treatment of wounds and tetanus prophylaxis when indicated.

Primary immunization schedules appear in Tables 1, 2, and 3 in the previous chapter, Immunization Practices. Schedules for the use of prophylactic agents in wound management appear in Table 1 in this chapter.

Prophylaxis: Since complete primary immunization with tetanus toxoid protects for ten years or more, boosters are required only every ten years in those who have completed the primary series. For tetanus prophylaxis following a wound, it is necessary to determine whether a patient completed primary immunization and, if not, how many doses were given. If a wound is "tetanus prone" and the person has not completed a primary series, tetanus immune globulin should be administered simultaneously with tetanus toxoid. Primary immunization should be completed in patients who received fewer than the recommended doses, including those given as part of wound management. Because the response to tetanus toxoid in fully immunized persons is excellent, even if no booster dose has been received within ten years, a single booster as part of routine preventive care may be expected to restore protection no matter how many years have elapsed since the last dose.

The preparation of choice for tetanus immunization in persons 7 years and older is Td (tetanus and diphtheria toxoids adsorbed, for adult use). Many adults are susceptible to diphtheria and simultaneous administration of diphtheria toxoid will enhance protection against this disease.

For children less than 7 years, the products employed are diphtheria and tetanus toxoids and pertussis vaccine adsorbed (DTP) or diphtheria and tetanus toxoids adsorbed (for pediatric use) (DT) if pertussis vaccine is contraindicated.

Clinical Tetanus: Treatment of tetanus includes injection of tetanus immune globulin (human). (Equine antitoxin caused hypersensitivity reactions and is no longer available.) Other measures include appropriate wound management with debridement if necessary; administration of antibiotics (penicillin or tetracycline), sedatives, and muscle relaxants; and other supportive therapy (eg, quiet environment, adequate nutrition).

TABLE 1.
GUIDE TO TETANUS PROPHYLAXIS IN ROUTINE WOUND MANAGEMENT[1]

History of adsorbed tetanus toxoid (doses)	Clean, minor wounds		All other wounds[2]	
	Td[3]	TIG	Td[3]	TIG
Unknown or < 3	Yes	No	Yes	Yes
≥ 3[4]	No[5]	No	No[6]	No

[1] *Adapted from Immunization Practices Advisory Committee, 1985 B.*

[2] *Such as, but not limited to, wounds contaminated with dirt, feces, soil, and saliva; puncture wounds; avulsions; and wounds from missiles, crushing, burns, and frostbite.*

[3] *For children under 7 years, DTP (DT if pertussis vaccine is contraindicated) is preferred to tetanus toxoid alone. For persons 7 years old and older, Td is preferred to tetanus toxoid alone.*

[4] *If only three doses of fluid toxoid have been received, a fourth dose of toxoid, preferably adsorbed toxoid, should be given.*

[5] *Yes, if more than 10 years since last dose.*

[6] *Yes, if more than 5 years since last dose. (More frequent boosters are not needed and can accentuate side effects.)*

TETANUS TOXOID

TETANUS TOXOID ADSORBED

Tetanus toxoid is a sterile preparation of inactivated toxin of *Clostridium tetani.* It is available in fluid or adsorbed form; *the latter is preferred* because it usually induces higher antitoxin titers and a longer duration of protection.

An immunizing course of tetanus toxoid is highly effective, produces few adverse reactions, and provides long-lasting protection against tetanus. This agent usually is given with diphtheria toxoid and pertussis vaccine (DTP) for primary immunization of infants and children under 7 years of age. For primary immunization of adults and children 7 years and older, Td (tetanus and diphtheria toxoids adsorbed for adult use) is preferred to tetanus toxoid alone to maintain protection against diphtheria. For children under 7 years in whom the pertussis component is contraindicated, DT is recommended. (See these evaluations.)

DT or Td is recommended for wound management in incompletely immunized individuals with tetanus-prone injuries because of the "priming" effect of prior doses of tetanus toxoid and the need to maintain diphtheria immunity. Additional considerations in treatment are the condition of the wound and whether to use tetanus toxoid alone for active immunization or to use tetanus immune globulin in addition for passive immunization. (See Table 1.)

At least three injections of tetanus toxoid are needed to induce sufficient levels of neutralizing antibody. Immunity lasts up to ten years in 95% of vaccinees, and a blood level equal to or greater than 0.01 IU tetanus antitoxin will be maintained.

ADVERSE REACTIONS AND PRECAUTIONS. Adverse reactions occur infrequently and include erythema, induration, and tenderness at the site of injection; fever, malaise, and neurologic complications are rare. The incidence of adverse reactions may be higher in persons over 25 years of age. High antibody levels following too frequent booster doses of tetanus toxoid have been associated with hypersensitivity reactions. (See also the evaluations on the combinations of tetanus toxoid with diphtheria toxoid and pertussis vaccine.)

DOSAGE.
Intramuscular: The adsorbed form is preferred to the fluid preparation. Tetanus toxoid adsorbed, for *adults and children* not previously immunized, three injections of 0.5 ml; the second injection is given four to six weeks after the first and the third injection is given six months to one year after the second. A booster dose is given every ten years.

Manufacturers: Connaught, Lederle, Sclavo, Wyeth-Ayerst.

TETANUS IMMUNE GLOBULIN (TIG)

Tetanus immune globulin is a sterile solution of globulins obtained from the plasma of adults hyperimmunized with tetanus toxoid. It is indicated in the prophylaxis and treatment of persons with wounds potentially contaminated by *Clostridium tetani.*

Passive immunization is indicated for individuals with tetanus-prone wounds who have never completed a primary series with tetanus toxoid or whose immune status is uncertain and cannot be established conclusively.

TIG induces longer lasting protective levels of circulating antitoxin with considerably lower doses than the previously available equine antitoxin. It has a half-life of approximately four weeks, and appreciable serum levels are maintained for up to 14 weeks. Antibiotic therapy supplements, but does not replace, TIG prophylaxis for management of wounds. Active immunization with tetanus toxoid should be initiated concomitantly using a different injection site and different syringe.

ADVERSE REACTIONS. Because tetanus immune globulin is of human origin, it is relatively free from the risk of hypersensitivity reactions. As with other gamma globulin preparations, pain and erythema may occur at the site of injection.

DOSAGE. Tetanus immune globulin should be given intramuscularly only.
Intramuscular: For prophylaxis, *adults and children*, 250 to 500 units by deep intramuscular injection. (Tetanus toxoid adsorbed may be given concurrently in a separate syringe and at a different site.) If threat of tetanus infection persists (eg, in patients with severe burns or other open wounds of long duration), the dose may be repeated at four-week intervals.

For treatment, the optimum dose has not been established but the following amounts are recommended: *Adults*, 3,000 to 6,000 units; *children*, a single dose of 500 to 3,000 units. Part of the dose may be placed in the wound area (American Academy of Pediatrics, 1988).

Available Trademark.
Hyper-Tet (Cutter/Miles).

Pertussis

Pertussis is a highly communicable disease caused by the bacterium, *Bordetella pertussis.* About 70% of reported clinical cases occur during the first five years of life, and most deaths occur in infants less than 1 year. The disease is becoming more common in those older than 15 years, probably as a result of both waning immunity and improved reporting, but fatalities are rare in older patients. Vaccination early in life is strongly recommended, preferably as part of the routine primary immunization program (see Tables 1, 2, and 3 in the previous chapter, Immunization Practices). Although the immune mechanisms of infection and vaccination are not yet completely understood, the widespread use of pertussis vaccine during the past 40 years has markedly reduced morbidity and mortality from the disease.

PERTUSSIS VACCINE ADSORBED

Pertussis vaccine adsorbed is a preparation of whole killed bacteria. It is a sterile suspension of killed *Bordetella pertussis* in saline solution containing aluminum phosphate and thimerosal. Recent research has resulted in identification and isolation of components of the organism that undoubtedly are important for induction of clinical immunity, and field trials of less toxic acellular vaccines containing one or more of these components are in progress (Hinman and Onorato, 1987).

Pertussis vaccine adsorbed is used in rare circumstances when immunization with the monovalent vaccine is preferred. It also has been used to a limited extent as a booster during outbreaks of pertussis. Pertussis vaccine appears to be more effective in protecting against clinical pertussis than against subclinical infection with *Bordetella pertussis*. Short-lived protection may be mediated through secretory IgA in respiratory epithelium.

This vaccine is usually administered with diphtheria and tetanus toxoids as DTP (see that evaluation). Since the incidence and mortality of pertussis decrease with age, pertussis immunization is only rarely recommended for those over 7 years.

ADVERSE REACTIONS AND PRECAUTIONS. Convulsions (primarily febrile) following use of DTP occur in infants but have not been associated with permanent sequelae. Accordingly, although a convulsion following a dose of DTP previously had been considered a contraindication to further doses, there are circumstances under which subsequent doses may be indicated, including the local epidemiology of pertussis disease. Rare, severe encephalopathic reactions also have been described. If pertussis vaccine does induce such reactions, the incidence is exceedingly rare and is clearly lower than that of similar effects produced by the disease.

Common adverse reactions include induration, local tenderness, fever, and malaise. Formation of sterile abscesses is rare. (See also the evaluations on DTP vaccine and other individual components.)

DOSAGE.
Intramuscular: *Children 2 months to 6 years,* three injections of 0.5 ml each given four to eight weeks apart and a fourth dose at 15 to 18 months of age. A booster dose of 0.5 ml should be given at 4 to 6 years of age. Recall injections after intimate exposure may be given to children up to 7 years. *Adults*, 0.25-ml booster has been given to medical personnel exposed during pertussis epidemics.

Monovalent pertussis vaccine may be obtained from the Biologic Products Division, Michigan Department of Health, PO Box 30035, Lansing, MI 48909 ([517]-335-8050).

Measles

Prior to the development of an effective vaccine, measles was a common childhood disease and was associated with pneumonia, acute encephalitis, subacute sclerosing panencephalitis, and death. Measles is often complicated by middle ear infection or bronchopneumonia. Encephalitis occurs in about 1/1,000 reported cases, and survivors frequently have permanent brain damage and mental retardation. The disease is fatal in 1/1,000 reported cases, usually as a result of respiratory or neurologic complications. Since the use of live attenuated measles virus vaccine, morbidity and mortality have decreased markedly. Before the first measles vaccine was available, more than 400,000 cases were reported annually in the United States. Since vaccine licensure in 1963, vaccination programs resulted in a 99% reduction in the number of reported cases. However, where immunization efforts have lapsed, there has been a resurgence of cases. After reaching an all-time low of 1,497 cases in 1983, the number of cases increased to more than 18,000 in 1989.

At present, programs are under way to eliminate measles from the United States. However, in recent years two major types of outbreaks have occurred in this country among unvaccinated preschool-age children and among vaccinated school-age children. In the latter, outbreaks have occurred in schools with vaccination levels exceeding 98%. In addition, a large number of cases have occurred in students and personnel on college campuses, even though many of these persons had been vaccinated. Setbacks in the national goal of measles elimination have been due to failure to implement recommended vaccination strategies and vaccine failure. Vaccine failure may be either primary (ie, an inadequate response to immunization) or secondary (ie, due to waning immunity). Although the measles vaccine currently available is considered to be at least 95% effective for children vaccinated at age 15 months, efficacy may be lower for those vaccinated between 12 and 14 months. Secondary vaccine failure appears to affect only a small percentage of individuals who are immunized. To help achieve the goal of elimination of measles nationwide, a routine two-dose measles vaccination schedule is now recommended (Immunization Practices Advisory Committee, 1989 A).

Measles vaccination may be accomplished with the individual measles virus vaccine or with a combination product con-

TABLE 2. RECOMMENDATIONS FOR MEASLES VACCINATION[1]

Routine Childhood Schedule, United States Most areas	Two doses[2,3] first dose at 15 months second dose at 4-6 years (entry to kindergarten or first grade)[4]
High-risk areas[5]	Two doses[2,3] first dose at 12 months second dose at 4-6 years (entry to kindergarten or first grade)[4]
Colleges and other educational institutions post-high school	Documentation of receipt of two doses of measles vaccine after the first birthday[3] or other evidence of measles immunity[6]
Medical personnel beginning employment	Documentation of receipt of two doses of measles vaccine after the first birthday[3] or other evidence of measles immunity[6]

[1]From Immunization Practices Advisory Committee, 1989 A.
[2]Both doses should preferably be given as combined measles, mumps, rubella vaccine (MMR).
[3]No less than 1 month apart. If no documentation of any dose of vaccine, vaccine should be given at the time of school entry or employment and no less than 1 month later.
[4]Some areas may elect to administer the second dose at an older age or to multiple age groups. The American Academy of Pediatrics (1989) recommends administration of the second dose of MMR at entry to middle school.
[5]A county with more than five cases among preschool-aged children during each of the last 5 years, a county with a recent outbreak among unvaccinated preschool-aged children, or a county with a large inner-city urban population. These recommendations may be applied to an entire county or to identified risk areas within a county.
[6]Prior physician-diagnosed measles disease, laboratory evidence of measles immunity, or birth before 1957.

TABLE 3. RECOMMENDATIONS FOR MEASLES OUTBREAK CONTROL[1]

Outbreaks in preschool-aged children	Lower age for vaccination to as low as 6 months of age in outbreak area if cases are occurring in children <1 year of age[2,3]
Outbreaks in institutions: day-care centers, K-12th grades, colleges, and other institutions	Revaccination of all students and their siblings and of school personnel born in or after 1957 who do not have documentation of immunity to measles[4]
Outbreaks in medical facilities	Revaccination of all medical workers born in or after 1957 who have direct patient contact and who do not have proof of immunity to measles.[4] Vaccination may also be considered for workers born before 1957 Susceptible personnel who have been exposed should be relieved from direct patient contact from the 5th to the 21st day after exposure (regardless of whether they received measles vaccine or IG) or—if they become ill—for 7 days after they develop rash

[1]From Immunization Practices Advisory Committee, 1989 A.
[2]Mass revaccination of entire populations is not necessary. Revaccination should be limited to populations at risk, such as students attending institutions where cases occur.
[3]Children initially vaccinated before the first birthday should be revaccinated at 15 months of age. A second dose should be administered at the time of school entry or according to local policy.
[4]Documentation of physician-diagnosed measles disease, serologic evidence of immunity to measles, or documentation of receipt of two doses of measles vaccine on or after the first birthday.

taining measles with rubella or measles with mumps and rubella. The last is more commonly employed for routine immunization programs because it requires only a single injection and provides protection against all three diseases.

MEASLES VIRUS VACCINE LIVE

This vaccine is a bacteriologically sterile preparation containing a highly attenuated strain of measles (rubeola) virus grown in chick embryo cell cultures. The Moraten strain is currently used in the United States. A noncommunicable, mild measles virus infection develops in susceptible individuals and results in the production of protective antibodies. The vaccine is highly immunogenic, and seroconversion rates of 90% to 95% are expected. Little or no virus is excreted, and secondary spread to contacts does not occur.

Vaccine-induced antibody levels may decline over time, but studies to date suggest that protection is usually permanent. The chief factors responsible for primary vaccine failure are thermal inactivation of the live virus or neutralization by preexisting antibodies that may inhibit viral replication and the subsequent development of host immunity. The simultaneous administration of immune globulin to reduce adverse reactions is not recommended, since this may interfere with the immunogenicity of the vaccine.

Immunization with live measles vaccine, preferably combined with mumps and rubella vaccines (MMR), is recommended for all children at or after 15 months of age when transplacental passive immunity has dissipated (Immunization Practices Advisory Committee, 1989 A). (See Table 2.) During outbreaks or in communities where measles is endemic, a two-dose strategy is recommended for infants: monovalent measles vaccine is recommended for infants as young as 6 months and should be repeated in combination with mumps and rubella vaccines (MMR) at 15 months and again at school entry (Immunization Practices Advisory Committee, 1989 A). The vaccine is also recommended for all persons who received inactivated measles vaccine or vaccine of unknown type between 1963 and 1967. Most adults born prior to 1957 are considered to be immune to measles. Measles outbreaks have reappeared in recent years and, consequently, both the ACIP and the American Academy of Pediatrics currently recommend that all children receive a second dose of measles vaccine, preferably given as MMR, at kindergarten, first grade, or middle school entry (American Academy of Pediatrics, 1989; Immunization Practices Advisory Committee, 1989 A). (See Table 3.)

HIV-infected persons, including children, who are in need of measles immunization should receive the MMR vaccine. This vaccine also should be considered for all HIV-infected children who are symptomatic, since measles in these children can be severe. Vaccination of either asymptomatic or symptomatic HIV-infected children has not been associated with severe or unusual adverse events, but antibody responses have been unpredictable.

Although the vast majority of individuals who have received live attenuated measles vaccine remain clinically immune and the current outbreaks are small compared with those in the pre-vaccine era, it is clear that the anticipated control of measles has not been achieved with a single-dose regimen. There are many possible reasons for this, and they are not precisely defined. Nevertheless, a routine second dose of measles vaccine as MMR represents the most logical approach. However, the optimum schedule for the initial and second dose remains unsettled and may depend on local circumstances such as regional measles epidemiology. Physicians should be aware that these recommendations continue to evolve, and they should be alert to updated information from the U.S. Public Health Service, state health departments, the American Medical Association, the American Academy of Pediatrics, and other authorities.

ADVERSE REACTIONS AND PRECAUTIONS. Approximately 5% to 15% of vaccinees develop fever ≥103° F and about 5% develop mild rash. Both occur about 5 to 12 days after administration of the vaccine and generally last approximately one to two days. Febrile convulsions also occur occasionally. Because children with a family or personal history of seizures are at slightly increased risk of a febrile seizure, it may be desirable to administer a nonaspirin-containing antipyretic drug prophylactically beginning five days after inoculation and continuing for six days. Other central nervous system effects observed rarely include encephalitis and encephalopathy, but the risk of these reactions is less than with natural measles and may represent coincidence. Although subacute sclerosing panencephalitis has been reported rarely in children who received the vaccine, this late complication of the disease has nearly disappeared with widespread use of the vaccine.

Anaphylactic reactions rarely have been reported after administration of measles vaccine, which is prepared in chick embryo cell culture, to persons with a prior history of severe anaphylactic reactions following ingestion of egg proteins. A procedure for desensitization of children with positive skin tests to both egg albumin and vaccine has been described (Herman et al, 1983; Greenberg et al, 1988).

Exposure to measles is not a contraindication to vaccination. If the vaccine is given within 72 hours after exposure, protection may be provided. Immune globulin may be used to modify measles in a susceptible person (see that evaluation) but should not be administered concurrently with the vaccine.

The vaccine should not be given to pregnant females, and pregnancy should be avoided for three months following vaccination.

DOSAGE.

Subcutaneous: *Children 15 months or older,* a single dose of 0.5 ml of reconstituted vaccine is injected, preferably into the outer aspect of the upper arm. It is essential that only the diluent supplied with the vaccine be used for reconstitution. (See also Tables 2 and 3.)

Available Trademark.
Attenuvax (Merck Sharp & Dohme).

Mumps

Historically, mumps occurred primarily in children 5 to 9 years of age; more recently, the peak incidence appears to have shifted to adolescents and young adults. It is a relatively benign, self-limited disease. The principal clinical manifestation, parotitis, may be unpleasant or debilitating, although many infections are asymptomatic. Orchitis occurs in up to 20% of postpubertal males, but sterility is rare. Meningoencephalitis occurs occasionally, but permanent sequelae are also uncommon. Nerve deafness, usually unilateral, may result from infection but is a rare complication. Since the introduction of live mumps virus vaccine in 1967, the incidence of clinical mumps and morbidity due to complications have declined markedly.

MUMPS VIRUS VACCINE LIVE

Live mumps virus vaccine is a suspension of the attenuated Jeryl Lynn strain of virus grown in chick embryo culture. It produces a subclinical, noncommunicable infection. The vaccine produces seroconversion in over 97% of susceptible vaccinees and is 95% efficacious in preventing disease. Estimates of vaccine efficacy during outbreaks have ranged from 75% to 95%. Levels of circulating antibodies are significantly lower than following natural infection, but are adequate to provide protection for many years, probably for life. Primary vaccine failures may be due to virus inactivation during storage or to pre-existing neutralizing antibody.

Immunization is recommended for all children ≥12 months of age (Immunization Practices Advisory Committee, 1989 D). Mumps vaccine may be given alone or in combination with rubella or with live measles and rubella virus vaccines (MMR); the triple combination is commonly used in routine immunization programs and is the preparation of choice. (Mumps and measles combined vaccine is not marketed in the United States.) If administered as MMR, it should be given at 15 months of age. A second dose of MMR is recommended at entry into elementary or middle school for measles control. Immunization is not recommended for children under 12 months since persisting maternal antibodies may interfere with seroconversion. The vaccine is of particular value in susceptible individuals approaching puberty, adolescents, and adults. Persons born before 1957 are generally considered to be immune. It is not necessary, however, to test for susceptibility before vaccination. It has been recommended that all HIV-infected children receive mumps vaccine as MMR at age 15 months.

Mumps vaccine may not provide protection when given after exposure to the disease; however, if exposure did not result in infection, the vaccine will protect against subsequent infection. Immune globulin does not provide postexposure prophylaxis and is not recommended.

ADVERSE REACTIONS AND PRECAUTIONS. Mumps vaccine produces very few adverse reactions. Low-grade fever or tenderness at the site of injection has been reported. Parotitis has occurred occasionally. Allergic reactions are uncommon and usually are mild and brief. As with measles vaccine, mumps vaccine should be administered with extreme caution to persons who have had anaphylactic reactions to egg products. There is no evidence of increased risk in persons with allergies to eggs that are not anaphylactic in nature or in persons with allergies to chickens or feathers. In addition, persons who have experienced anaphylactic reactions to neomycin should not receive mumps vaccine. Manifestations of central nervous system involvement are very rare. There is no evidence that mumps vaccine produces diabetes.

The vaccine should not be used during pregnancy, in patients with hypogammaglobulinemia or dysgammaglobulinemia, in those receiving immunosuppressive therapy (eg, corticosteroids, irradiation, antineoplastic agents), in those with severe febrile illness, or in those with leukemia, lymphomas, or malignant neoplasms. However, HIV infection is not a contraindication. It should be given at least two weeks before and deferred until three months after administration of immune globulin, whole blood, or any antibody-containing products.

DOSAGE.
Subcutaneous: *Adults and children 12 months or older,* the total volume (0.5 ml) of reconstituted vaccine is administered. The reconstituted vaccine should be stored at 2° to 8° C in the dark; it should be discarded if not used within eight hours. Only the diluent supplied should be used for reconstitution.

Available Trademark.
Mumpsvax (Merck Sharp & Dohme).

Rubella

The primary objective of immunization against rubella is to prevent infection in pregnant women because fetal infection may cause serious congenital abnormalities. Rubella in children generally is benign and self-limited, but this age group may be a source of infection for pregnant women.

Following the introduction of live attenuated rubella virus vaccines, the number of cases of rubella and congenital rubella syndrome decreased by over 98%; also, the anticipated periodic epidemics of rubella have not occurred.

Immunization recommendations include: (1) All persons ≥12 months of age should receive rubella vaccine, preferably in combination with measles and mumps vaccines, as part of their routine immunization program. When administered as MMR, it usually should be given at 15 months. A second dose of MMR is recommended at entry to elementary or middle school to provide protection to those who did not respond to their initial measles immunization. (2) School records should be audited annually to permit identification and vaccination of children before puberty. (3) All females of childbearing age should receive rubella vaccine unless they were previously vaccinated or serologic testing reveals that they are immune. Females in this age group should be asked if they are pregnant and excluded from immunization with rubella if they are. The theoretical risks should be explained to these individuals and they should understand that pregnancy must be avoided for three months after immunization. (4) Susceptible mothers should be vaccinated in the immediate postpartum period before discharge from the hospital. (5) All children, adolescents, and adults (especially women) who are considered to be susceptible should be vaccinated if there are no contraindications (Immunization Practices Advisory Committee, 1984 B).

RUBELLA VIRUS VACCINE LIVE

Live rubella virus vaccine is a suspension of attenuated rubella virus derived from the Wistar Institute RA 27/3 strain grown in human diploid cell (WI-38) culture. The vaccine produces a mild infection in susceptible persons, which results in the production of protective antibodies. Excretion of small amounts of live virus from the nose or throat occurs in most vaccinees 7 to 28 days after vaccination. Nevertheless, contact spread is not known to occur. Thus, there is no hazard for susceptible pregnant females exposed to vaccinated children.

Antibody response induced by this vaccine resembles natural rubella more closely than that produced by the earlier vaccines. Rubella antibody levels are detectable in over 95% of patients within four to six weeks following vaccination and persist for as long as 16 years, suggesting active immunity of long duration. Antibody levels may decline over time. Reinfection following exposure to wild rubella virus, as evidenced by increased antibody levels, is rare. Over 90% of vaccinees are protected against both clinical rubella and viremia for at least 15 years and probably for life.

ADVERSE REACTIONS AND PRECAUTIONS. Data indicate that only susceptible vaccinees experience adverse reactions; these occur more frequently in postpubertal women than in men. Adverse reactions include low-grade fever; rash, induration, erythema, and tenderness at the site of injection; and regional adenopathy. Transient arthritis, arthralgia, and polyneuritis may occur within two months after immunization. Up to 3% of children have experienced arthralgia, but arthritis has been rare in these patients. In contrast, approximately 25% of susceptible postpubertal women experience arthralgias and about 10% report arthritis following vaccination. Very rarely, subsequent chronic arthritis has been reported in susceptible women, but the relationship to rubella vaccine is not entirely clear. Encephalitis also has been reported very rarely, but a causal association has not been demonstrated.

Rubella virus vaccine is contraindicated in pregnant women (FDA Pregnancy Category C). However, if a pregnant woman is inadvertently given the vaccine, experience to date indicates that the risk of vaccine-associated malformations is nonexistent or negligible (Centers for Disease Control, 1989). Because of the importance of rubella immunity for females of childbearing age, women known to be susceptible should be vaccinated during the immediate postpartum period.

For theoretical reasons, vaccination should be avoided in patients with leukemia, lymphomas, generalized malignancy, or immunodeficiencies and in those receiving immunosuppressive therapy (corticosteroids, antineoplastic drugs, or irradiation). Mild illnesses, even with slight fever, such as a cold, are not contraindications. Individuals who have had anaphylactic reactions to neomycin should not receive rubella vaccine. However, HIV infection is not a contraindication.

Rubella vaccine should be given at least two weeks before or deferred until approximately three months after the individual has received immune globulin, whole blood, or other antibody-containing products.

DOSAGE.

Subcutaneous: *Adults and children 12 months or older*, 0.5 ml of the reconstituted vaccine should be injected into the outer aspect of the upper arm. It should not be given intravenously or intranasally.

The vaccine should be refrigerated at 2° C to 8° C and protected from light. It must remain refrigerated after reconstitution and should be discarded if not used within eight hours. Only the diluent supplied should be used to reconstitute the vaccine.

Available Trademark.
Meruvax II (Merck Sharp & Dohme).

MEASLES, MUMPS, AND RUBELLA VIRUS VACCINE LIVE (MMR)

Live measles, mumps, and rubella virus vaccine is a suspension of the same attenuated viruses present in the monovalent vaccines. It is indicated for simultaneous routine immunization of children 15 months of age or older and may be used in adolescents and adults who have not been vaccinated against or experienced any or all of the natural infections. Clinical studies have shown that the vaccine produces antibody levels comparable to those obtained with the use of each monovalent vaccine given at properly spaced intervals. Persistence of immunity is similar to that observed with the live, attenuated monovalent vaccines.

There is no evidence that prior immunity to any one of the three constituents, whether from natural infection or immunization, is associated with enhanced risk of reactions to MMR. Adverse reactions and precautions generally are the same as those associated with the monovalent vaccines (see the evaluations). The vaccine is usually well tolerated, but malaise, mild fever, and regional lymphadenopathy occur occasionally.

Because the measles and mumps components are prepared in chick embryo culture, MMR should not be given to a person with a history of anaphylaxis following ingestion of egg products.

DOSAGE.

Subcutaneous: *Children 15 months of age or older,* the total volume of reconstituted vaccine (0.5 ml) is injected into the outer aspect of the upper arm. The AAP and ACIP have recommended that a second dose be given to all children at school entry or after entry into middle or junior high school.

Available Trademark.
M-M-R II (Merck Sharp & Dohme).

MEASLES AND RUBELLA VIRUS VACCINE LIVE

Live measles and rubella virus vaccine is a suspension of the same attenuated viruses present in equivalent monovalent vaccines. Available evidence indicates that it produces a serologic response equivalent to that induced by the individual measles and rubella vaccines. It is used for simultaneous immunization against measles and rubella in children from 15 months of age to puberty and in adults when simultaneous immunization against mumps is unnecessary or is contraindicated.

Adverse reactions and precautions are the same as those associated with the monovalent vaccines (see the evaluations).

DOSAGE.

Subcutaneous: *Adults and children 15 months of age or older,* 0.5 ml of the reconstituted vaccine is injected into the outer aspect of the upper arm.

Available Trademark.
M-R-VAX II (Merck Sharp & Dohme).

RUBELLA AND MUMPS VIRUS VACCINE LIVE

Live rubella and mumps virus vaccine is a suspension of the same attenuated viruses present in equivalent monovalent vaccines. The vaccine is used for the simultaneous routine immunization of children ≥12 months of age who have been appropriately vaccinated against measles or experienced the natural disease but who have no history of immunizing exposure to rubella and mumps viruses. The vaccine produces antibody levels comparable to those stimulated by the monovalent vaccines given separately; the degree of protection against natural disease is also comparable.

Contraindications, precautions, and adverse reactions are the same as those associated with the monovalent vaccines (see the evaluations).

DOSAGE.

Subcutaneous: *Children 12 months of age to puberty,* the total volume of reconstituted vaccine (0.5 ml) is injected into the outer aspect of the upper arm. The reconstituted vaccine should be stored at 2° to 8° C and discarded if not used within eight hours.

Available Trademark.
Biavax II (Merck Sharp & Dohme).

Poliomyelitis

The virtual elimination of poliomyelitis from the United States by the use of vaccines is one of the most important medical achievements in recent years. Although the risk of poliomyelitis in the United States is very small, epidemics are to be expected if the immunity of the population is not maintained by immunizing all children beginning in the first year of life. Subclinical infection with wild strains is no longer a significant natural means of establishing or maintaining immunity and thus universal vaccination of infants and children is increasingly important.

Oral poliovirus vaccine (OPV) and an enhanced-potency inactivated poliovirus vaccine (IPV) are available in the United States. The oral vaccine is the agent of choice for routine immunization of children. For nonimmunized adults at risk, primary immunization with IPV is recommended. If protection is needed in less than four weeks, a dose of OPV or IPV is recommended. If the person remains at increased risk, a three-dose primary series should be completed.

POLIOVIRUS VACCINE INACTIVATED (IPV)

Inactivated poliovirus vaccine (IPV) consisting of all three types of poliovirus, produced in monkey kidney cells and rendered noninfectious by formalin treatment, became available in the United States in 1955 and was widely used until the early 1960s when it was replaced by live, attenuated poliovirus vaccine (OPV). During these years IPV reduced the incidence of paralytic poliomyelitis considerably. Epidemiologic studies show that IPV also diminished the spread of wild poliovirus in vaccinated communities. However, some IPV-vaccinated individuals have developed abortive infections with both wild and attenuated vaccine viruses and have excreted these strains in their feces. IPV is used in some areas of Canada as well as in several European countries, including Sweden, where it has been used exclusively and has essentially eradicated poliomyelitis.

In 1988, enhanced-potency IPV replaced the previously licensed conventional preparation. This newer IPV, prepared in human diploid cells, requires fewer doses to achieve protective levels of serum antibody in 99% or more of recipients, as determined by studies in European and U.S. children. Although the duration of protection and the need for booster doses have not been determined conclusively, serologic evidence indicates that protection persists for at least five years (Immunization Practices Advisory Committee, 1987 B). Because IPV is noninfectious, it is safe for use in immunodeficient patients and their household contacts, but the immune response may be inadequate in the immunodeficient. Nevertheless, the vaccine may be administered to the latter patients in an attempt to provide some degree of protection.

The vaccine may be given to susceptible adults at risk of exposure by reason of travel. Physicians may administer a primary series of vaccinations or, when constrained by time, at least two doses one month apart. If less than one month remains before travel is to take place, a single dose of either IPV or OPV is recommended.

No serious adverse effects have been reported. IPV is classified in FDA Pregnancy Category C.

DOSAGE.

PRIMARY IMMUNIZATION:

Subcutaneous: *Infants,* when IPV is indicated, immunization should be started at the initial visit (6 to 12 weeks of age). Two doses of 0.5 ml each are administered into the subcutaneous tissue near the insertion of the deltoid muscle at intervals of four to eight weeks; a third 0.5-ml dose is given 6 to 12 months after the second dose, and it may be given at the same time as DTP and MMR at 15 to 18 months of age if feasible (see Table 1 in the previous chapter, Immunization Practices). *Older children and adults at increased risk of exposure who are unvaccinated* are given the same regimen. *Adults with incomplete primary immunization* may complete the series regardless of the interval since the last dose.

REINFORCING (BOOSTER) IMMUNIZATION:

Children who have received three primary immunization doses should be given a booster dose of 0.5 ml prior to entering school, unless the third dose was given after the fourth birthday. The need for subsequent booster doses has not yet been determined. *Adults over 18 years* at increased risk of exposure who have completed primary immunization may be given a 0.5-ml booster dose.

Manufacturer: Connaught.

POLIOVIRUS VACCINE LIVE ORAL TRIVALENT (OPV)

This vaccine contains attenuated poliovirus types I, II, and III and stimulates production of mucosal antibodies in the digestive tract as well as circulating antibodies. Oral poliovirus vaccine is the agent of choice for the routine prevention of paralytic poliomyelitis. It is easily administered and long-lasting immunity is achieved (Immunization Practices Advisory Committee, 1982, 1987 B, and 1989 C).

In susceptible individuals, the type-specific, serum-neutralizing antibody titer begins to increase about one week after ingestion and reaches a peak about three weeks later. A three-dose primary series produces an immune response to each of the three virus types in more than 95% of recipients.

OPV is recommended routinely for all infants and children who do not have immunodeficiency diseases or altered immune states and do not live with persons having these disorders.

Initial vaccination is not recommended routinely prior to 6 weeks of age because of persistence of maternal antibodies. However, in certain tropical areas where poliomyelitis is endemic, it may be advisable to start immunization when the infant is discharged from the hospital. This dose is not considered part of the primary series.

Routine immunization of adults living in the continental United States is unnecessary because most are immune, exposure to wild virus is unlikely, and there may be a slightly greater risk of vaccine-associated paralysis in adults than in children. However, any nonimmunized adult who might be exposed to poliovirus by traveling to epidemic or endemic areas should receive OPV or IPV (see the chapter on Immunization Practices). If there is not sufficient time for at least two doses of IPV, one dose of either vaccine is preferred.

ADVERSE REACTIONS AND PRECAUTIONS. OPV rarely has been associated with paralytic disease. Most authorities believe that a causal relationship exists between the development of paralytic poliomyelitis in certain recipients and their close contacts (contact within 75 days after administration) and the reversion to greater neurovirulence of vaccine progeny. However, the risk of vaccine-associated paralysis is extremely small for recipients and their close contacts (1 in approximately 2.6 million doses), especially when weighed against the benefits. Over two-thirds of vaccine-related paralytic diseases in recipients and contacts occurs following the first dose.

Tonsillectomy, adenoidectomy, and pregnancy are not contraindications to the use of vaccine when immunization is required, as during an epidemic. The vaccine should not be administered if the patient has marked diarrhea. Immunization with OPV is contraindicated when the immune state of the recipient may be altered, as in those with HIV infection, dysgammaglobulinemia, lymphoma, leukemia, or generalized malignancies, as well as in patients receiving therapeutic regimens that may impair cellular immunity (eg, corticosteroids, antineoplastic agents, immunosuppressive agents, irradiation). OPV should not be given to a member of a household in which there is a history of immunodeficiency until the immune status of the recipient and other children in the family is determined to be normal. It also is prudent to recommend that vaccine recipients avoid close household-type contact with all immunosuppressed persons for at least one month.

OPV is classified in FDA Pregnancy Category C.

DOSAGE. This vaccine is never administered by injection.

Oral: For primary immunization, three doses are administered. *Infants,* the primary series of three doses is usually administered at 2, 4, and 15 to 18 months of age (American Academy of Pediatrics, 1988). Some authorities prefer to administer an extra dose at age 6 months to those who live in or travel to endemic areas.

Children and adolescents, two doses administered not less than six and preferably eight weeks apart; the third dose is given 12 months later. Children who have completed primary immunization should be given a single additional dose of vaccine prior to entering elementary school unless the third dose was administered after the fourth birthday. *Children and adults who have completed primary immunization and are at increased risk* by virtue of contact, travel, or occupation may be given a single additional dose.

Available Trademark.

Orimune (Lederle).

Haemophilus influenzae Type b Infections

Haemophilus influenzae type b (Hib) is a principal cause of serious systemic bacterial disease in children and is the most common cause of bacterial meningitis in the United States. Approximately 12,000 cases of Hib meningitis occur yearly, primarily in children under 5 years. The mortality rate ranges from 5% to 10% and neurologic sequelae develop in 25% to 35% of survivors. Other diseases caused by Hib include epiglottitis, pneumonia, septic arthritis, cellulitis, osteomyelitis, pericarditis, and sepsis. Although *H. influenzae* is a major cause of otitis media, only 5% to 10% of cases are produced by type b strains; the majority of cases are caused by nonencapsulated (nontypeable) strains.

In the United States, the cumulative risk of systemic Hib disease during the first five years of life is estimated to be 1 in 200. Rates are highest between age 6 and 12 months, but 30% to 35% of systemic Hib disease occurs in children over 18 months and approximately 25% occurs in children over 24 months. Groups at increased risk are Native Americans, blacks, persons in lower socioeconomic classes, and patients with asplenia, sickle cell disease, Hodgkin's disease, or antibody immunodeficiency syndromes. In addition, children who attend day care centers may have a substantially increased risk of Hib disease (Redmond and Pichichero, 1984).

HAEMOPHILUS b POLYSACCHARIDE VACCINES

Haemophilus b polysaccharide vaccine is derived from the purified polysaccharide capsule of *Haemophilus influenzae* type b (Hib); it is a linear copolymer of ribose-ribitol-phosphate (PRP). Two types of haemophilus b vaccines have been available in the past: (1) *polysaccharide* vaccines consisting only of the capsular polysaccharide, and (2) *conjugate* vaccines (HbCV) consisting of the purified capsular polysaccharide covalently bound to diphtheria toxoid (PRP-D), diphtheria CRM_{197} protein (PRP-HbOC), or to an outer membrane protein complex of the B 11 strain of *Neisseria meningitidis* serogroup B (PRP-OMP). The latter type has replaced the former.

Polysaccharides are T-independent antigens and do not require direct T-lymphocyte participation to induce antibody production; instead, they directly stimulate B-lymphocytes to do so. Further, the antibody response to these antigens shows poor immunologic memory. By conjugating Hib capsular polysaccharide to a protein antigen, the new conjugated antigen acts as a T-dependent antigen, which results in enhanced antibody response and immunologic memory. In addition, the conjugated antigen is more immunogenic in infants who usually do not respond well to polysaccharide antigens. This allows the conjugate vaccine to be given to infants at a younger age (2 to 15 months) than the polysaccharide-only vaccine (24 months). See Tables 4, 5, and 6.

TABLE 4. IMMUNOGENICITY STUDIES OF CONJUGATE AND POLYSACCHARIDE VACCINES[1]

Vaccine	Age (Months)	No. of Subjects	Post-Vaccination Anti-PRP GMT[2] (mcg/ml)	Subjects Responding with >1.0 mcg/ml (%)
PRP-D[3]	18-21	173	2.85	75
	22-26	37	2.96	73
Polysaccharide	18-20	51	0.100	24
	24-27	84	0.520	43
PRP-OMP[4]	15-17	71	3.29	80
	18-23	64	7.16	97
	24-71	61	10.29	93
Polysaccharide	18-23	13	0.39	15
	24-71	47	0.87	36
PRP-HbOC[5]	15-17	236	10.82	97.9
	18-23	141	12.29	97.2
Polysaccharide	22-26	42	2.07	61.9

[1]*Because of interlaboratory variability in antibody assays for the capsular polysaccharide (PRP), definitive comparisons between vaccines cannot be based on these data.*
[2]*Geometric mean titer 4 to 8 weeks after vaccination.*
[3]*Haemophilus b Conjugate Vaccine (Diphtheria Toxoid Conjugate). Source: Connaught Laboratories, Inc., unpublished data.*
[4]*Haemophilus b Conjugate Vaccine (Meningococcal Protein Conjugate). Source: Merck Sharp & Dohme, unpublished data.*
[5]*Haemophilus b Conjugate Vaccine (Diphtheria CRM_{197} Protein Conjugate). Source: Praxis Biologics, unpublished data.*

TABLE 5. HAEMOPHILUS B CONJUGATE VACCINES: DIFFERENCES IN IMMUNOGENICITY BY AGE OF CHILD AT VACCINATION[1]

Vaccine	Children 15-17 mos.			Children 18-23 mos.		
	No.	% >1 mcg/ml[2]	GMT[3]	No.	% >1 mcg/ml[2]	GMT[3]
PRP-D[4]	43	53[5]	1.2	180	73[5]	3.1
PRP-HbOC[6]	236	98[7]	10.8	141	97[7]	12.3
PRP-OMP[8]	71	80[5]	3.3	84	97[5]	7.2

[1]*From Immunization Practices Advisory Committee, 1990 A. Because of interlaboratory variability in assays for antibody to the capsular polysaccharide of* Haemophilus influenzae *type b (PRP), definitive comparisons between vaccines cannot be made based on these data.*
[2]*Percentage of children with >1 mcg/ml PRP antibody 4-8 weeks after vaccination.*
[3]*Geometric mean titer of PRP antibody (mcg/ml).*
[4]*Haemophilus b Conjugate Vaccine (Diphtheria Toxoid Conjugate). Source: Connaught Laboratories, Inc., unpublished data.*
[5]*$p < 0.05$ (15-17 months vs. 18-23 months). PRP-D data for "children 18-23 mos." column are from children 18-24 months at vaccination.*
[6]*Haemophilus b Conjugate Vaccine (Diphtheria CRM_{197} Protein Conjugate). Source: Praxis Biologics, unpublished data.*
[7]*Not significant (15-17 months vs. 18-23 months).*
[8]*Haemophilus b Conjugate Vaccine (Meningococcal Protein Conjugate). Source: Merck Sharp & Dohme, unpublished data.*

TABLE 6. HAEMOPHILUS B CONJUGATE VACCINE (DIPHTHERIA CRM_{197} PROTEIN CONJUGATE): IMMUNOGENICITY IN INFANTS RECEIVING FIRST DOSE AT 1-2 MONTHS[1]

Infant Age at Initial Vaccination	Mo After Initial Vaccination	Vaccination Schedule[2]	No. of Subjects	Geometric Mean (SD) Anti-HbPs, mcg/mL	% of Subjects With ≥ 1 mcg/mL
1-2 mos	0	+	187	0.20 (0.07-0.57)	11.8
	2	+	187	0.30 (0.10-0.88)	15.0
	4	+	185	5.11 (1.04-25.21)	83.8
	5	−	163	16.84 (5.57-50.92)	98.2
	10	−	88	7.41 (2.32-23.66)	94.3
	24 mo of age	−	65	3.20 (0.78-13.19)	80.0

[1]*Adapted from Madore et al, 1990.*
[2]*Vaccine administered at two-month intervals.*

In vitro, antibodies to the Hib polysaccharide antigen mediate complement-dependent bacteriolysis and opsonization; in vivo, they protect animals from experimental infection. Studies in Finland indicated that the unconjugated vaccine reduced the rate of bacteremic Hib disease by 90% in children age 18 months to 5 years; the vaccine was not effective in younger children (Peltola et al, 1984). In 1985 the unconjugated vaccine was recommended for routine use in the United States in children 24 months to 6 years of age. However, results of postmarketing studies in the United States were disparate; variable efficacy was observed in a series of post-licensure studies. One study showed no efficacy and four showed efficacies ranging from 41% to 88% (Ward et al, 1988). Thus, it was concluded that the vaccine was not as efficacious as indicated by the original trials in Finland.

Any of the three conjugated Hib vaccines that are available in the United States is preferred to the unconjugated preparation because antibody titers following immunization have been shown to be considerably higher in studies involving Finnish and U.S. children (Immunization Practices Advisory Committee, 1988 A). In Finland, protection against clinical disease in infants was demonstrated with the vaccine conjugated with diphtheria toxoid. In studies conducted at various locations in the United States, 73% or more of children 18 months or older who were given a single dose of conjugate vaccine subsequently had an antibody level ≥1 mcg/ml, which is indicative of long-term protection (see Tables 4, 5, and 6).

Of the three HbCV vaccines currently licensed in the United States for administration to children ≥15 months of age, one, diphtheria CRM_{197} protein conjugate (PRP-HbOC), was approved in late 1990 for routine immunization of infants beginning at 2 months of age (Table 6). Other HbCV vaccines may be so licensed in the future; efficacy trials are being conducted. The Immunization Practices Advisory Committee recently issued the following recommendations for the HbCV vaccines (Immunization Practices Advisory Committee, 1991 B): (1) All infants should receive the conjugated vaccine, PRP-HbOC, at 2, 4, and 6 months of age; (2) unvaccinated infants 7 to 11 months of age should receive two doses of PRP-HbOC two months apart; (3) unvaccinated children 12 to 14 months of age should receive a single dose of PRP-HbOC vaccine; (4) a booster dose of any of the three currently licensed HbCV vaccines should be given to all children at 15 months of age at an interval not less than two months after the previous dose; (5) unvaccinated children 15 to 60 months old should receive a single dose of any of the licensed HbCV vaccines and do not require a booster. Children who had invasive haemophilus b disease when less than 2 years of age should receive the vaccine because they may have failed to develop adequate immunity. Similar recommendations have been made by the American Academy of Pediatrics (1990).

Concomitant administration of conjugate vaccines with diphtheria and tetanus toxoids, DTP, MMR, or OPV given at different sites has not impaired the immune response to the individual antigens or affected the type, frequency, and severity of adverse effects compared with those seen when the individual vaccines are given alone.

Although the vaccine may be given to protect against future exposure, it is not a substitute for rifampin prophylaxis in unimmunized contacts of those with Hib disease.

This vaccine is classified in FDA Pregnancy Category C.

ADVERSE REACTIONS AND PRECAUTIONS. The preparations appear to cause few reactions. Fever (101° F) and erythema and induration at the injection site occur in 1% to 2% of recipients. The vaccine is contraindicated if there is hypersensitivity to any of its components, including the protein component of the conjugate (eg, diphtheria toxoid). The expected immune response may not be achieved in patients who are immunocompromised. Vaccination should be delayed in the presence of any febrile illness or active infection. Hib disease may occur during the week following vaccination prior to the onset of the protective effects of the vaccine. Even though there may be some immune response to the diphtheria toxoid component of the conjugate, this preparation should not be considered a substitute for routine diphtheria immunization. Similarly, immunization with the meningococcal conjugate should not be considered to confer protection against meningococcal disease.

INTERACTIONS. Sensitive tests (eg, latex agglutination kits) may detect PRP derived from the vaccine in the urine of some vaccinees for up to seven days following vaccination with conjugate vaccine.

DOSAGE AND PREPARATIONS.
Intramuscular: *Children 2 months to 5 years,* 0.5 ml of reconstituted vaccine. See preceding text for schedule.

Licensed for use at 2 months:

HibTITER (Lederle). 10 mcg capsular oligosaccharide and 25 mcg diphtheria CRM_{197} protein per dose.

Licensed for use at 15 months:

PedvaxHIB (Merck Sharp & Dohme). 15 mcg capsular polysaccharide and 250 mcg *N. meningitidis* OMP per dose.

ProHIBIT (Connaught). 25 mcg capsular polysaccharide and 18 mcg conjugated diphtheria toxoid protein per dose.

Viral Hepatitis

Several clinically similar diseases are included under this term, but each is etiologically and epidemiologically distinct: hepatitis A ("infectious" hepatitis); hepatitis B ("serum" hepatitis); non-A, non-B hepatitis (NANB), which includes two epidemiologically distinct types, parenterally and enterically transmitted NANB hepatitis; and delta hepatitis.

Hepatitis A is caused by an RNA-containing virus and is classified as a picornavirus. It is transmitted primarily by the fecal-oral route and produces an illness characterized by fever, malaise, abdominal discomfort, dark urine, and jaundice. Transmission by blood transfusion has been reported, but this is uncommon. The incubation period is 15 to 50 days; the case fatality rate is approximately 0.6%. In the United States, this infection is common in older children and adults. In 1988, 50% of the cases of hepatitis reported in this country were due to hepatitis A.

Hepatitis B infection is caused by hepatitis B virus (HBV), a DNA-containing virus that is classified as a hepadnavirus. Several well-characterized antigen-antibody systems are associated with infection. The incubation period is long (45 to 160 days). Signs and symptoms include anorexia, malaise, nausea, vomiting, abdominal pain, and jaundice. Skin rashes, arthralgias, and arthritis also can occur as extrahepatic manifestations of the disease. Like human immunodeficiency virus (HIV), HBV is transmitted by sexual contact, by infected blood products, from infected mother to infant, and by close contact with infected body fluids. It is not usually transmitted by the fecal-oral route. The case fatality rate is about 1.4%. A variable proportion of infected individuals become chronically infected with HBV; this is central to the epidemiology of the transmission of the virus.

HBV infection is highly prevalent in certain groups in the United States. The lifetime risk varies from about 5% for the general population to nearly 100% for those in the highest risk groups (see Table 7). About 300,000 persons are infected with HBV each year in the United States and 25% subsequently develop jaundice. Between 6% and 10% of infected young adults become carriers and 25% of these develop chronic active hepatitis. (A carrier has been defined as a person who is HBsAg-positive on at least two occasions six months apart or who is HBsAg-positive and IgM anti-HBc negative on a single specimen.) There are 500,000 to 1 million carriers in the United States, and the number is thought to be more than 200 million worldwide. The carrier state may lead to chronic liver disease, including massive hepatic necrosis, chronic active hepatitis, cirrhosis, and hepatocellular carcinoma. The disease is highly endemic in China, Southeast Asia, sub-Saharan Africa, most Pacific islands, and the Amazon basin.

Among those who become HBV carriers, about 25% develop chronic persistent or chronic active hepatitis or chronic active hepatitis with cirrhosis. The five-year survival rates have been estimated to be 97% for patients with chronic persistent hepatitis, 86% for those with chronic active hepatitis, and 55% for individuals with chronic active hepatitis with cirrhosis (Weissberg et al, 1984).

TABLE 7. EXPECTED HEPATITIS B VIRUS (HBV) PREVALENCE IN VARIOUS POPULATION GROUPS

Population Group: Spectrum of Risk	Prevalence of Serologic Markers of HBV Infection: HBsAg* (%)	Any markers (%)
Immigrants/refugees from areas of high HBV endemicity	13	70-85
Alaskan natives/Pacific islanders	5-15	40-70
Clients in institutions for the developmentally disabled	10-20	35-80
Users of illicit parenteral drugs	7	60-80
Homosexually active men	6	35-80
Household contacts of HBV carriers	3-6	30-60
Patients in hemodialysis units	3-10	20-80
Health-care workers—frequent blood contact	1-2	15-30
Prisoners (male)	1-8	10-80
Staff of institutions for the mentally retarded	1	10-25
Heterosexuals with multiple partners	0.5	5-20
Health-care workers—no or infrequent blood contact	0.3	3-10
General Population		
Blacks	0.9	14
Whites	0.2	3

* *HB surface antigen*

Adapted from Immunization Practices Advisory Committee, 1990 B.

Several viruses are responsible for NANB hepatitis. *Parenterally transmitted NANB* hepatitis is the most common form of transfusion-related hepatitis and may be caused by at least two viruses. The genome of one (proposed as hepatitis C) has been partially cloned, which has led to development of an antibody assay to identify infected individuals (Choo et al, 1989; Kuo et al, 1989). Although parenterally transmitted NANB hepatitis traditionally has been considered a transfusion-associated disease, most reported cases have not been associated with transfusions. Other groups at risk include dialysis patients, parenteral drug abusers, and health care workers who have frequent contact with blood. It is unclear whether sexual or perinatal transmission of this type of hepatitis occurs.

Epidemics of *enterically transmitted NANB* (ET-NANB) hepatitis, spread by the fecal-oral route, have been described in Asia, Africa, and Mexico; young to middle-aged adults are most often affected, and mortality is high among pregnant women. The virus of ET-NANB hepatitis is serologically distinct from other known hepatitis viruses. It has been postulated that a single virus is responsible for the majority of cases of ET-NANB hepatitis, and it may be a member of the calcivirus family. Recent studies of a cDNA clone from virus-infected monkeys suggest that the infectious agent of ET-NANB hepatitis has a plus-stranded RNA genome with a size of 7.6 Kb that is polyadenylated. The name hepatitis E virus (HEV) has been proposed for this agent (Reyes et al, 1990).

Delta hepatitis virus (also called hepatitis D virus [HDV]) contains a single strand of RNA and an internal protein antigen (delta antigen [HDAg]), and its 35-nm viral particle is coated with an HBV surface antigen (HBsAg) as the surface protein. HDV is a defective virus and is dependent on HBV for replication. Therefore, prevention of HBV infection in a susceptible individual prevents HDV infection in that individual. The manner of transmission of HDV is similar to that of HBV. Infection with HDV is associated with episodes of acute hepatitis as well as chronic active hepatitis; fulminant hepatitis also may result.

Each of the foregoing types of viral hepatitis, except hepatitis A and ET-NANB, often is associated with a chronic carrier state. In 1988, 28,500 cases of hepatitis A; 23,200 cases of hepatitis B; 2,620 cases of NANB hepatitis; and 2,470 cases of unspecified hepatitis type were reported in the United States.

PREVENTIVE MEASURES. Sanitation and other hygienic measures are of major importance in the prevention of all varieties of hepatitis. Passive immunoprophylaxis employing intramuscular immune globulin (IG) may be effective in preventing hepatitis A and hepatitis B. Although there are no definitive studies, the administration of IG 0.06 ml/kg as soon as possible after exposure may be a reasonable course of action for persons with percutaneous exposure to blood from a patient with parenterally transmitted NANB hepatitis (Immunization Practices Advisory Committee, 1990 B). There is no evidence that IG will prevent infection with enterically transmitted NANB hepatitis. Only IG prepared for intramuscular administration should be employed for prophylaxis. Hepatitis B may also be prevented by active immunization; no vaccine is available for any of the other viruses causing hepatitis. Because of the dependence of delta hepatitis on concomitant hepatitis B infection, prevention of hepatitis B should prevent delta hepatitis.

Hepatitis A: Immune globulin is effective for prophylaxis against hepatitis A, especially when given within a few days of exposure, although it may have some effect up to two weeks after exposure. Prophylactic value is greatest when this agent is given early in the incubation period and declines thereafter. It is recommended for travelers to high-risk areas. For those who will reside in such areas less than three months, a single dose of 0.02 ml/kg is sufficient. Persons who will reside in developing countries for long periods should receive IG (0.06 ml/kg) every five months. IG produced in developing countries may not meet U.S. standards. IG also has been recommended for postexposure prophylaxis (one intramuscular dose of 0.02 ml/kg) for household and sexual contacts of infected persons and for outbreaks in day-care centers, schools, institutions for custodial care, and hospitals; specific recommendations depend on the nature of the exposure (Immunization Practices Advisory Committee, 1990 B). It is not indicated in patients with clinical manifestations of the disease or in those exposed more than two weeks previously. (See the section on Immune Globulins.)

Hepatitis B: There is no treatment for chronic hepatitis. However, hepatitis B can be prevented through vaccination and administration of hepatitis B immune globulin (HBIG). In the United States, the present strategy for preventing HBV is to immunize those persons at high risk of infection. Universal HBsAg screening of pregnant women has been recommended to prevent perinatal transmission of HBV. The universal vaccination of infants and adolescents is under consideration as another strategy to control transmission of this disease.

Postexposure prophylaxis with HBV vaccine to prevent infection with HBV should be employed in the following situations: perinatal exposure of a neonate born to a mother known to be positive for hepatitis B surface antigen (HBsAg), accidental exposure (percutaneous or permucosal) to HBsAg-positive blood, sexual exposure to an HBsAg-positive person, and household exposure of an infant under 12 months to a primary care giver who has acute hepatitis B (Immunization Practices Advisory Committee, 1990 B).

Neonatal Exposure. The principal objective of postexposure prophylaxis in neonates is to prevent the establishment of an HBV carrier state. Approximately 80% to 90% of infants born to HBsAg- and HBeAg-positive mothers become infected with HBV, and about 90% of infected infants become chronic HBV carriers. Approximately 25% of these carriers eventually die of cirrhosis or primary hepatocellular carcinoma. If the mother is HBsAg-positive but HBeAg-negative or if anti-HBe is present, transmission of HBV to the infant occurs in less than 25% and 12% of cases, respectively. In such cases, transmission rarely leads to chronic infection, but severe acute disease, including fatal fulminating hepatitis in the neonate, has been observed. Studies have demonstrated that a combination of HBV vaccine and HBIG prevents chronic HBV infection in approximately 90% of infants born to HBsAg-positive mothers.

TABLE 8.
RECOMMENDATIONS FOR HEPATITIS B PROPHYLAXIS FOLLOWING PERCUTANEOUS OR PERMUCOSAL EXPOSURE[1]

	Treatment When Source Is Found to be:		
Exposed Person	**HBsAg-Positive**	**HBsAg-Negative**	**Source Not Tested or Unknown**
Unvaccinated	HBIG × 1[2] and initiate HBV vaccine[3]	Initiate HBV vaccine[3]	Initiate HBV vaccine[3]
Previously vaccinated Known responder	Test exposed for anti-HBs 1. If adequate,[4] no treatment 2. If inadequate, HBV vaccine booster dose	No treatment	No treatment
Known nonresponder	HBIG × 2 or HBIG × 1 plus 1 dose HBV vaccine	No treatment	If known high-risk source, *may treat as if source were HBsAg-positive*
Response unknown	Test exposed for anti-HBs 1. If inadequate,[4] HBIG × 1 plus HBV vaccine booster dose 2. If adequate, no treatment	No treatment	Test exposed for anti-HBs 1. If inadequate[4], HBV vaccine booster dose 2. If adequate, no treatment

[1]*From Immunization Practices Advisory Committee, 1990 B.*
[2]*HBIG dose 0.06 ml/kg IM.*
[3]*HBV vaccine dose—see text. First dose within 1 week; second and third doses, 1 and 6 months later.*
[4]*Adequate anti-HBs is ≥ 10 SRU by RIA or positive by EIA.*

In 1988, the Immunization Practices Advisory Committee recommended that for each pregnancy all women be routinely tested for HBsAg during an early prenatal visit. HBIG 0.5 ml and HBV vaccine 0.5 ml should be given intramuscularly to all babies born to HBsAg-seropositive mothers. Women who present for delivery without prenatal care or medical records documenting HBsAg screening results should have the test performed as soon as possible after admission; delay in the administration of HBIG to infants of seropositive mothers will decrease the efficacy of treatment. If the mother is identified as HBsAg-seropositive a month or more after delivery, the infant should be tested for HBsAg and, if negative, should receive both HBIG and HBV vaccine. It has been estimated that screening of the approximately 3.5 million pregnant women in the United States per year would identify 16,500 as HBsAg-positive and permit early treatment that would prevent 3,500 infants from becoming HBV carriers (Immunization Practices Advisory Committee, 1988 B, 1990 B).

Household members and sexual partners of women identified as HBsAg-positive through prenatal screening should be tested to determine susceptibility and, if susceptible, should receive HBV vaccine (Immunization Practices Advisory Committee, 1990 B).

Implementation of the foregoing recommendations requires that initial administration of HBIG and HBV vaccine be given to newborns of HBsAg-positive mothers *in the hospital* as soon as possible after birth (HBIG within 12 hours; HBV vaccine in first week). Subsequent doses of HBV vaccine should be given at 1 and 6 months of age. In certain populations in whom HBV infection is highly endemic and transmission occurs principally in childhood, such as in Alaskan natives and Pacific islanders, universal immunization of newborn infants with HBV vaccine is recommended to prevent transmission during both the perinatal period and childhood (Immunization Practices Advisory Committee, 1988 B, 1990 B). In these populations, prenatal screening is impractical and control of HBV infection is best achieved by universal vaccination.

Other pediatric vaccinations should not be postponed because of immunization with HBV vaccine. Similarly, administration of HBIG soon after birth should not interfere with the DTP and poliovirus vaccines usually administered at 2 months of age.

Sexual Exposure. For susceptible persons who have had sexual contact with an HBsAg-positive partner and those who continue to have such contact with a person who has acute disease but soon becomes HBsAg-negative, a single intramuscular dose of HBIG (0.06 ml/kg) given within 14 days of last sexual contact is recommended. The first dose of HBV vaccine should also be given either simultaneously or within seven days of exposure. When HBV vaccine is not given initially, a second dose of HBIG should be given for heterosexual exposures if the index patient remains HBsAg-positive three months after detection, and the HBV vaccine series should be started. Regular sexual partners of known HBV carriers or index patients who remain HBsAg-positive for three months should receive HBV vaccine. The vaccine is recommended for all susceptible homosexual men.

Percutaneous Exposure. Factors that must be considered before instituting prophylaxis following percutaneous or permucosal exposure to blood known or suspected of being HBsAg-positive are (1) the vaccination status of the exposed person, (2) the source of the blood, and (3) the HBsAg status of the source. Table 8 summarizes the recommendations for HBV prophylaxis after percutaneous or mucous membrane exposure.

TABLE 9. RECOMMENDED DOSES AND SCHEDULES OF CURRENTLY LICENSED HB VACCINES[1]

Group	Vaccine Dose					
	Heptavax-B[2,3]		Recombivax HB[2]		Engerix-B[2,4]	
	(mcg)	(ml)	(mcg)	(ml)	(mcg)	(ml)
Infants of HBV-carrier mothers	10	(0.5)	5	(0.5)	10	(0.5)
Other infants and children <11 years	10	(0.5)	2.5	(0.25)	10	(0.5)
Children and adolescents 11-19 years	20	(1.0)	5	(0.5)	20	(1.0)
Adults >19 years	20	(1.0)	10	(1.0)	20	(1.0)
Dialysis patients and other immunocompromised persons	40	(2.0)[5]	40	(1.0)[6]	40	(2.0)[5,7]

[1]*From Immunization Practices Advisory Committee, 1990 B.*
[2]*Usual schedule: three doses at 0, 1, 6 months.*
[3]*Available only for hemodialysis and other immunocompromised patients and for persons with known allergy to yeast.*
[4]*Alternative schedule: four doses at 0, 1, 2, 12 months.*
[5]*Two 1.0-ml doses given at different sites.*
[6]*Special formulation for dialysis patients.*
[7]*Four-dose schedule recommended at 0, 1, 2, 6 months.*

For all exposed persons who have never received HBV vaccine, immunization should be initiated within a week regardless of the HBsAg status of the source. Additionally, if the source is positive, a single dose of HBIG should be given as soon as possible after exposure. If the source is known to be HBsAg-negative or is untested, HBIG is not recommended.

If the exposed individual has been previously vaccinated and is known to have responded, the source need not be tested for HBsAg and no treatment is indicated. If the exposed individual was vaccinated but failed to respond, the source should be tested for HBsAg and, if positive, the exposed individual should be given a dose of HBIG promptly (within seven days) and a second dose one month later. Treatment is unnecessary if the source is HBsAg-negative or of unknown status. If the response of the exposed individual to HBV immunization is unknown, no treatment is needed if the source is HBsAg-negative or cannot be tested. If the source is positive, an exposed person who was immunized but whose response is unknown should be tested for anti-HBs. If immune, no treatment is required. If antibody levels are inadequate, a single dose of HBIG and a booster dose of HBV vaccine should be given promptly.

Household Contacts. Prophylaxis of infants under age 12 months with HBIG 0.5 ml and HBV vaccine is indicated if the mother or primary care giver has acute HBV infection. Prophylaxis for other household contacts is not indicated unless they have been exposed to the blood of the index patient. If the index patient becomes a carrier, all household contacts should be given HBV vaccine (Immunization Practices Advisory Committee, 1990 B).

HEPATITIS B VACCINE INACTIVATED (HBV Vaccine)

Three preparations of hepatitis B vaccine are available. One, licensed in 1981, is a noninfectious formalin-inactivated preparation derived from the surface antigen (HBsAg) of hepatitis B virus. HBsAg is harvested and purified from HBsAg-positive blood donated by carriers of hepatitis B virus. Each ml of HBV vaccine contains 20 mcg of HBsAg protein and is formulated in an alum adjuvant. Initially, it is purified by ultracentrifugation. This is then followed by a three-step inactivation process, which inactivates HBV and representative viruses from all known groups, including retroviruses. With nearly 5 million doses distributed, there is no evidence that acquired immunodeficiency syndrome (AIDS) can be transmitted by this product. This plasma-derived vaccine is no longer being produced in this country, and its use is now limited to hemodialysis and immunocompromised patients and persons with an allergy to yeast.

Two additional genetically engineered hepatitis B vaccines are available in the United States (Immunization Practices Advisory Committee, 1990 B). In both, the antigen is produced in *Saccharomyces cerevisiae* (baker's yeast) by inserting a plasmid containing the gene for HBsAg. After incubation, HBsAg is separated from the yeast, filter-sterilized, inactivated with formalin, and adsorbed onto aluminum hydroxide. Yeast components constitute *less than* 5% of the final product. The safety and efficacy (as measured by antibody studies) of these newer preparations are comparable to the older preparation except that the recombinant vaccines appear to be less efficacious in immunocompromised and hemodialysis patients. Therefore, except for these individuals, recommendations for use are similar. A vaccine with greater potency has been prepared for use in immunocompromised and hemodialysis patients [Recombivax HB], and additional recombinant vaccines are expected to be licensed in the near future.

These HBV vaccines contain 10 to 40 mcg HBsAg protein/ml and are adsorbed with aluminum hydroxide. The usual primary vaccination schedule is three intramuscular doses of the vaccine given at 0, 1, and 6 months. Adults and children over 10 years are given the full dose, and children under 10 years are given a half dose. An alternative four-dose schedule has been approved for one vaccine [Engerix-B], which may be administered at 0, 1, 2, and 12 months. Higher doses or an increased number of doses are required to induce protective levels of antibody in hemodialysis and other immunocom-

TABLE 10.
PERSONS FOR WHOM HEPATITIS VACCINE IS INDICATED OR SHOULD BE STRONGLY CONSIDERED

Pre-exposure

PERSONS FOR WHOM VACCINE IS RECOMMENDED:
- Health-care workers having blood or needle-stick exposures
- Clients and staff of institutions for the developmentally disabled
- Hemodialysis patients
- Homosexually active men
- Users of illicit injectable drugs
- Recipients of certain blood products
- Household members and sexual contacts of HBV carriers
- Populations with high endemicity of HBV infection
- Heterosexually active persons with multiple sexual partners

PERSONS FOR WHOM VACCINE SHOULD BE CONSIDERED:
- Long-term inmates of correctional facilities
- International travelers to HBV endemic areas

Postexposure

PERSONS FOR WHOM VACCINE IS RECOMMENDED:
- Infants born to HBV-positive mothers
- Health-care workers having percutaneous or permucosal exposures to infected human blood
- Sexual exposure to an infected person
- Household contacts exposed to the blood of an infected person

Adapted from Immunization Practices Advisory Committee, 1990 B. See text.

promised patients. If the primary series is interrupted after the first dose, the second and third dose should be given separated by a three- to five-month interval. Optimal protection is not conferred until after the third dose (Immunization Practices Advisory Committee, 1990 B). See Table 9 for complete information on age-specific dosages of available vaccines.

HBV vaccine is indicated for immunization against infection caused by all known B virus subtypes. Vaccination is recommended for all persons who are at increased risk of infection, such as populations with a high incidence of disease (eg, Alaskan Eskimos, Indochinese and Haitian refugees), health care personnel, hematology and hemodialysis patients and staff, patients and staff of institutions for the mentally retarded, blood bank and fractionation workers, recipients of blood clotting factor concentrates, homosexual males, household and sexual contacts of HBV carriers, prostitutes, heterosexually active persons with multiple sexual partners, illicit drug users, prisoners, and international travelers who will be in highly endemic areas for more than six months (see Tables 7 and 10). Vaccination is also recommended for maternally exposed newborn infants in combination with hepatitis B immune globulin (HBIG).

The three-dose regimen stimulates production of detectable antibodies in 85% to 96% of vaccinees, and clinical protection lasts at least seven years in adults. Establishment of the need for booster doses, if any, awaits the results of ongoing surveillance of immunized persons. However, in hemodialysis patients, immunogenicity and efficacy are much lower than in normal adults and the duration of protection in these patients is unknown. The immunologic response of infants and children to a course of three doses has been excellent. A suboptimal response may follow injection into the buttock, because injections into this site may inadvertently be deposited in fat where the vaccine is less well mobilized.

Adverse effects to either type of vaccine are mainly local, mild, and transitory. Slight tenderness at the injection site is most common (10% of adults and 4% of children). Pregnancy is not a contraindication to use of the vaccine, which is classified in FDA Pregnancy Category C.

DOSAGE.

Intramuscular: Because the antigenic contents of licensed hepatitis B vaccines differ and because the volume injected is not always the same for different products, Table 9 should be consulted prior to administration. The manufacturer's package insert also should be consulted because dosage and schedule recommendations may change as more information becomes available.

Available Trademarks.
Engerix B (Smith Kline & French), ***Heptavax-B*** (Merck Sharp & Dohme), ***Recombivax HB*** (Merck Sharp & Dohme).

HEPATITIS B IMMUNE GLOBULIN (HBIG)

This sterile solution of immune globulin is prepared from the pooled plasma of donors with high titers of antibody to hepatitis B surface antigen (anti-HBs). Only plasma free of HBsAg and HIV antibody is used to prepare immune globulins.

HBIG is indicated for postexposure prophylaxis following parenteral exposure (eg, accidental "needle-stick," direct mucous membrane contact [accidental splash]), or oral ingestion (pipetting accident) of HBsAg-positive materials, such as blood, plasma, or serum. It is also indicated for infants born to HBsAg-positive mothers (especially those who also are HBeAg-positive), since these infants are at risk of acquiring hepatitis B infection. Susceptible persons who are sexual contacts of HBsAg-positive individuals also are candidates for the antiserum. This product is of no value in the treatment of fulminant acute or chronic active hepatitis B. (See section on Hepatitis B and Immunization Practices Advisory Committee, 1990 B.)

Adverse reactions include local pain and tenderness at the injection site, urticaria, and angioedema.

HBIG is classified in FDA Pregnancy Category C.

DOSAGE.

Intramuscular: For *adults and children*, 0.06 ml/kg or 5 ml to adults, administered as soon as possible (within seven days) after exposure. If HBV vaccination is initiated, no additional doses are needed. If HBV vaccination is not initiated, HBIG should be readministered 28 to 30 days later to those with a single percutaneous exposure and 90 days later to those with continuing sexual exposure to an HBsAG-positive partner.

For *newborn infants,* the usual dose is 0.5 ml given as soon after birth as possible and no later than 12 hours, and active immunization with hepatitis B vaccine should be initiated.

HBIG should not be given intravenously.

Available Trademarks.
H-BIG (Abbott), ***Hep-B-Gammagee*** (Merck Sharp & Dohme), ***HyperHep*** (Cutter/Miles).

TABLE 11. INFLUENZA VACCINE* DOSAGE BY PATIENT AGE

Age Group	Product†	Dosage	No. Doses	Route§
6-35 mos.	Split virus only	0.25 ml	1 or 2¶	IM
3-8 yrs.	Split virus only	0.50 ml	1 or 2¶	IM
9-12 yrs.	Split virus only	0.50 ml	1	IM
>12 yrs.	Whole or split virus	0.50 ml	1	IM

** Contains 15 mcg each of A/Taiwan/1/86-like (H1N1), A/Shanghai/16/89 (H3N2), and B/Yamagata/16/88-like hemagglutinin antigens in each 0.5 ml. Manufacturers include: Connaught Laboratories, Inc. (distributed by E.R. Squibb & Sons, Inc.) (Fluzone whole or split); Evans Medical Ltd.-Lederle Laboratories (distributed by Lederle Laboratories) (Flu-Imune purified surface antigen vaccine); Parke-Davis (Fluogen split); and Wyeth-Ayerst Laboratories (Influenza Virus Vaccine, Trivalent split). For further product information call Connaught, 800/822-2463; Lederle, 800/533-3753; Parke-Davis, 800/223-0432; Wyeth-Ayerst, 800/950-5099.*

† Because of the lower potential for causing febrile reactions, only split-virus vaccines should be used in children. They may be labeled as "split," "subvirion," or "purified-surface-antigen" vaccine. Immunogenicity and side effects of split- and whole-virus vaccines are similar in adults when vaccines are used at the recommended dosage.

§ The recommended site of vaccination is the deltoid muscle for adults and older children. The preferred site for infants and young children is the anterolateral aspect of the thigh.

¶ Two doses are recommended for children <9 years of age who are receiving influenza vaccine for the first time.

Source: Centers for Disease Control, 1990.

Influenza

INFLUENZA VIRUS VACCINE

This trivalent vaccine is prepared from types A and B influenza viruses grown in embryonated chicken eggs. It is available as an inactivated whole virus, subvirion, or purified surface antigen product. All current influenza vaccines contain the same two type A and one type B strains that are considered likely to be spread in the United States in the upcoming winter. For safety reasons, only the subvirion or purified surface antigen preparation should be used in children less than 13 years; any type may be used in adults. Infants less than 6 months should not receive any influenza vaccine. Most children over 9 years and young adults develop high postvaccination antibody titers within four weeks after a single dose. Two doses are required in children 6 months to 8 years old. Booster doses should not be given except in this age group. The elderly and patients with certain chronic diseases may develop lower titers and remain susceptible to upper respiratory tract infections due to influenza virus. However, in many of these individuals the vaccine is effective in preventing lower respiratory tract involvement and other influenza complications, thus reducing the risk of hospitalization and death. In one study conducted on residents of nursing homes, influenza immunization was reported to attenuate infection; unvaccinated persons were more likely to develop pneumonia, be hospitalized, and/or die of influenza-like illness (Patriarca et al, 1985).

The vaccine is recommended for anyone 6 months or older who is at increased risk for complications due to influenza illness. Such groups include all persons 65 years or older; residents of nursing homes; adults and children with chronic disorders of the pulmonary or cardiovascular systems; adults and children with chronic metabolic diseases, renal dysfunction, hemoglobinopathies, or impaired immune response; and children and adolescents who are receiving long-term aspirin therapy and are at risk of developing Reye's syndrome. The vaccine also has been recommended for those who can transmit influenza virus to individuals at high risk (eg, physicians, nurses, nursing home employees, home care providers, household members). In addition, the vaccine may be given to anyone who desires immunization. Vaccination is a prudent precaution in persons infected with HIV, for influenza may result in more serious illness and complications. However, these individuals may have a relatively low antibody response to the vaccine, and a booster dose does not improve their immune response. Travelers to foreign countries during times of influenza outbreaks may wish to consider influenza vaccination before leaving the United States.

The vaccine is known to induce production of antibodies to the H (hemagglutinin) antigen of each of the virus strains contained in the vaccine. Efficacy is about 80%. Although efficacy is lower when new antigenic variants appear, in most years this is not a major problem.

ADVERSE REACTIONS AND PRECAUTIONS. Currently available vaccines are partially purified and well tolerated. Split virus vaccines appear to cause fewer adverse effects than whole virus vaccines in children. The most frequent adverse effect is soreness at the injection site. Fever, malaise, myalgia, and other systemic symptoms are more common in children than in adults. Reactions may appear within 6 to 12 hours and disappear within one to two days. Allergic reactions are rare because current vaccines contain very small quantities of egg protein.

The vaccine may be given with other vaccines, though at a different site. It also may be given to pregnant women, but it is prudent to wait until the second or third trimester unless this would leave a pregnant woman with a high-risk medical condition unprotected when influenza is beginning to cause widespread outbreaks (FDA Pregnancy Category C).

DOSAGE.

Intramuscular: See Table 11 and the manufacturers' literature. Recommendations for vaccine composition and administration are widely publicized each year.

Available Trademarks.

Fluogen (Parke-Davis), ***Fluzone*** (Connaught), ***Influenza Virus Vaccine Trivalent, Subvirion type*** (Wyeth-Ayerst), ***Flu-Imune*** (Lederle).

Pneumococcal Pneumonia

PNEUMOCOCCAL POLYSACCHARIDE VACCINE

The incidence of serious pneumococcal disease remains high. Pneumococcal pneumonia occurs in all age groups; the incidence gradually increases in adults over 40 years and increases twofold in those over 60 years. Despite antibiotic therapy, death occurs in approximately 20% of patients with bacteremic pneumococcal pneumonia and 30% of patients with meningitis. Mortality is highest in patients with certain underlying medical conditions and in older persons; in high-risk patients, mortality may be as high as 40% for those with bacteremic disease and 55% for those with meningitis. Prophylaxis with pneumococcal vaccines may reduce mortality and morbidity (Immunization Practices Advisory Committee, 1989 B).

The current formulation of polyvalent vaccine contains purified capsular polysaccharides from 23 of the most common pneumococcal types frequently associated with disease in adults and children (see manufacturers' package insert). These cause about 87% of the cases of bacteremic pneumococcal disease in the United States, including nearly 100% of cases in children. Each 0.5-ml dose of vaccine contains 25 mcg of the purified capsular material from each type dissolved in isotonic saline solution with 0.25% phenol [Pneumovax] or 0.01% thimerosal [Pnu-Imune] as preservative.

Persons in the following special groups should be immunized with pneumococcal polysaccharide vaccine: (1) Immunocompetent children over 2 years and adults who are at increased risk of pneumococcal disease or its complications because of chronic illnesses (eg, cardiovascular disease, pulmonary disease, diabetes mellitus, alcoholism, cirrhosis, cerebrospinal fluid leaks) or adults 65 years and older. (2) Immunocompromised children over 2 years and adults at increased risk of pneumococcal disease or its complications (eg, splenic dysfunction or anatomic asplenia, Hodgkin's disease, lymphoma, multiple myeloma, chronic renal failure, nephrotic syndrome, conditions such as organ transplantation associated with immunosuppression). (3) Children over 2 years and adults with asymptomatic or symptomatic HIV infection. (4) Persons living in special environments or social settings with an identified risk of pneumococcal disease or its complications (eg, certain Native American populations).

Recurrent pneumococcal otitis media or sinusitis in children is not an indication for vaccination. The vaccine should be given at least two weeks before elective splenectomy. The interval between vaccine administration and subsequent initiation of immunosuppressive therapy should be as long as possible. Influenza vaccine may be given simultaneously with pneumococcal vaccine if different injection sites and different syringes are used.

The duration of protection provided by pneumococcal vaccine is unknown. Antibody levels are detectable five years after immunization but fall to prevaccination levels within 10 years. Revaccination with the 23-valent vaccine is recommended for persons at high risk of fatal pneumococcal infection (eg, asplenia) who previously received the 14-valent vaccine or who received the 23-valent vaccine ≥ six years earlier. Revaccination also is indicated for those in whom the decline in pneumococcal antibody levels is rapid (eg, patients with nephrotic syndrome or renal failure; transplant recipients).

Only a few studies have utilized pneumococcal vaccine in children. One study employed octavalent vaccine in patients 2 to 25 years old with sickle cell disease or asplenia; the occurrence of bacteremic pneumococcal disease was reduced significantly (Ammann et al, 1977). Children less than 2 years of age have an unsatisfactory antibody response.

Using distribution of serotypes of invasive isolates from unvaccinated and vaccinated groups as a basis of comparison, the overall efficacy of a 14-valent pneumococcal vaccine was estimated to be 64% and did not appear to differ significantly with age; in persons over 65 years with or without underlying illness, efficacy was reported to be 61% (Bolan et al, 1986).

In a case-control study of 90 patients with systemic evidence of pneumococcal infection and matched controls, vaccine efficacy was 0% for severely immunocompromised patients, 70% for patients 55 years or older, and 77% for patients at moderately increased risk of pneumococcal infections (Shapiro and Clemens, 1984). In another case-control study of 122 patients with systemic pneumococcal infection, vaccine efficacy was 70% in immunocompetent patients (Sims et al, 1988). One study has shown that vaccination against pneumococcal pneumonia is cost-effective and that benefits would be enhanced if the vaccine were more widely used (Sisk and Riegelman, 1986). In a position paper, the Health and Public Policy Committee of the American College of Physicians (1986) concluded that pneumococcal vaccine was underutilized in patients who clearly could be expected to benefit from it. However, two studies conducted in military veterans failed to demonstrate efficacy (Simberkoff et al, 1986; Forrester et al, 1987). Enrollment of an inadequate number of subjects in one study and incomplete ascertainment of vaccination status in the other may have contributed to this divergence from other studies.

ADVERSE REACTIONS AND PRECAUTIONS. Serious adverse effects to pneumococcal vaccines are rare. The most common reactions are local erythema and tenderness at the injection site, which usually subside within one to two days; local induration is noted less frequently. Fever may occur. Anaphylactic reactions have been reported rarely. The vaccine is contraindicated in those with febrile respiratory illness or active infection, children under 2 years, and during pregnancy (FDA Pregnancy Category C).

DOSAGE.

Subcutaneous, Intramuscular: A single 0.5-ml dose. Intravenous inoculation should be avoided.

Available Trademarks.
Pneumovax 23 (Merck Sharp & Dohme), ***Pnu-Imune 23*** (Lederle).

Rabies

Pre-exposure Immunization: Pre-exposure immunization is advised for persons at high risk of exposure to rabies virus

TABLE 12.
CRITERIA FOR PRE-EXPOSURE RABIES IMMUNIZATION

Risk Category	Nature of Risk	Typical Populations	Pre-exposure Regimen
Continuous	Virus present continuously, often in high concentrations. Aerosol, mucous membrane, bite, or nonbite exposure possible. Specific exposures may go unrecognized.	Rabies research lab workers[1] Rabies biologics production workers	Primary pre-exposure immunization course[2] Serology every 6 months Booster immunization when antibody titer falls below acceptable level
Frequent	Exposure usually episodic, with source recognized, but may also be unrecognized. Aerosol, mucous membrane, bite, or nonbite exposure.	Rabies diagnostic lab workers[1], spelunkers, veterinarians, and animal control and wildlife workers in rabies epizootic areas Certain travelers to foreign rabies epizootic areas	Primary pre-exposure immunization course Booster immunization or serology every 2 years[3]
Infrequent (greater than population-at-large)	Exposure nearly always episodic with source recognized. Mucous membrane, bite, or nonbite exposure.	Veterinarians and animal control and wildlife workers in areas of low rabies endemicity Veterinary students	Primary pre-exposure immunization course Booster immunization or serology
Rare (population-at-large)	Exposure always episodic with source recognized. Mucous membrane or bite exposure.	U.S. population-at-large, including individuals in rabies epizootic areas	No pre-exposure immunization

[1] Judgment of relative risk and extra monitoring of immunization status of laboratory workers is the responsibility of the laboratory supervisor.

[2] Pre-exposure immunization consists of three doses of HDCV or RVA 1 ml IM (ie, deltoid area) one each on days 0, 7, and 28. Administration of routine booster doses of vaccine depends on exposure risk category as noted above. Pre-exposure immunization of immunosuppressed persons is not recommended.

[3] Pre-exposure booster immunization recommended consists of one dose of HDCV 1 ml/dose IM (deltoid area). Boost if titer falls below 1:5. RVA is a suitable alternative to HDCV.

Adapted from Immunization Practices Advisory Committee, 1984 C.

(eg, veterinarians, animal handlers, certain laboratory workers, persons spending one month or more in countries where rabies is a constant threat, spelunkers) and others whose vocation or avocation brings them into contact with potentially rabid domestic or wild animal species (Table 12). Pre-exposure prophylaxis is given to (1) protect against inapparent exposure to rabies, (2) protect persons when postexposure therapy might be delayed, and (3) simplify postexposure therapy by eliminating the need for immune globulin and decreasing the number of required doses of vaccine. It should be noted that pre-exposure immunization does not eliminate the need for postexposure prophylaxis following exposure; it only reduces the extent of the needed regimen.

For pre-exposure immunization regimens, see Table 12.

Postexposure Prophylaxis: Clinical rabies is rare in humans in the United States, but many persons receive prophylactic treatment because of possible exposure. Although dog and cat bites are the principal reasons for treatment, rabies in domestic animals has decreased considerably since the widespread use of veterinary vaccines. However, rabies in wildlife has become more widespread in recent years and wild animals now constitute the most important source of infection for both humans and domestic animals. In the United States, only Hawaii remains free of rabies.

Appropriate management depends on assessment of the risk of infection and proper employment of prophylactic therapy. Carnivorous animals (especially skunks, foxes, coyotes, raccoons, and bobcats) and bats are more likely to be infective than other animals. Bites of rabbits, squirrels, chipmunks, gerbils, hamsters, rats, and mice rarely, if ever, call for rabies prophylaxis. Properly immunized domestic animals are not likely to develop rabies. In doubtful or unusual cases, the local health authority should be consulted. Even in areas where rabies is enzootic, if adequate data indicate that infection is not present in the particular species, the local authority may recommend that no specific rabies immunoprophylaxis be given.

The management of patients exposed to possibly rabid animals should follow the guidelines given in Table 13. It is more likely that an animal is rabid if the attack is unprovoked. (Bites following attempts to handle or feed an apparently healthy animal should generally be regarded as provoked.) Nonbite exposure to rabies virus, such as a scratch or other contamination of an open wound or mucus membrane with potentially infectious material (eg, saliva) from a rabid animal or an infectious aerosol (eg, in bat caves), also is possible. Thus, each case must be evaluated individually. Dogs and cats should be restrained and observed for ten days after the bite.

TABLE 13.
RABIES POSTEXPOSURE PROPHYLAXIS GUIDE

Animal Species	Condition of Animal at Time of Attack	Treatment of Exposed Person[1]
DOMESTIC		
Dog and cat	Healthy and available for 10 days of observation	In the United States, none, unless animal develops rabies[2]
	Rabid or suspected rabid	RIG[3] and HDCV or RVA
	Unknown (escaped)	Consult public health officials. If treatment is indicated, give RIG[3] and HDCV
WILD		
Skunk, bat, fox, coyote, raccoon, bobcat, and other carnivores	Regard as rabid unless proven negative by laboratory tests[4]	RIG[3] and HDCV or RVA
OTHER		
Livestock, rodents, and lagomorphs (rabbits and hares)	Consider individually. Local and state public health officials should be consulted about the need for rabies prophylaxis. Bites of squirrels, hamsters, guinea pigs, gerbils, chipmunks, rats, mice, other rodents, rabbits, and hares almost never call for antirabies prophylaxis.	

The above recommendations are only a guide. In applying them, take into account the animal species involved, the circumstances of the bite or other exposure, the vaccination status of the animal, and presence of rabies in the region. Local or state public health officials should be consulted if questions arise about the need for rabies prophylaxis.

[1] All bites and wounds should immediately be thoroughly cleansed with soap and water. If antirabies treatment is indicated, both rabies immune globulin (RIG) and human diploid cell rabies vaccine (HDCV) or RVA should be given as soon as possible, regardless of the interval after exposure. Local reactions to vaccines are common and do not contraindicate continuing treatment. Discontinue vaccine if fluorescent antibody tests of the animal are negative.

[2] During the usual holding period of 10 days, begin treatment with RIG and HDCV or RVA at first sign of rabies in a dog or cat that has bitten someone. The symptomatic animal should be killed immediately and tested.

[3] If RIG is not available, use antirabies serum, equine (ARS). Do not use more than the recommended dosage.

[4] The animal should be killed and tested as soon as possible. Holding for observation is not recommended.

Adapted from Immunization Practices Advisory Committee, 1984 C.

If no clinical signs of rabies develop during this period, it can be considered that no exposure to rabies occurred. However, if the animal is killed or dies, the head should be sent to the local health authorities for confirmatory diagnosis.

As part of the postexposure prophylactic treatment, all bite wounds, as well as scratches and skin abrasions exposed to licks of animals, should be immediately and thoroughly flushed with copious amounts of soap and water. If available, 20% tincture of green soap should be used; subsequent use of 70% alcohol may increase the efficacy of local treatment. If debridement is necessary, the wound area may be infiltrated with a local anesthetic. If possible, bite wounds should not be sutured immediately. Antibiotic therapy and appropriate tetanus prophylaxis should be initiated if indicated.

Postexposure prophylaxis should be initiated as soon as possible after exposure. Two types of immunoprophylactic agents employed in the United States are: (1) human diploid cell rabies vaccine (HDCV) and rabies vaccine adsorbed (RVA), which are used to induce active immunity but require seven to ten days for a measurable antibody response, and (2) human rabies immune globulin (RIG), which is used to provide rapid protection for a short time (half-life, about 21 days). Human rabies immune globulin is prepared from the plasma of donors hyperimmunized with rabies vaccine. Adverse effects are rare with RIG.

Postexposure antirabies immunization for both bite and nonbite exposures usually includes administration of both rabies immune globulin (RIG) and vaccine (see Table 13). The first dose of vaccine should be given as soon as possible after exposure of a previously immunized person, with additional doses given on days 3, 7, 14, and 28. RIG is administered only at the beginning of prophylaxis to provide passive immunity until the patient starts to produce his own antibodies. If possible, up to one-half the dose of RIG should be used to infiltrate the wound. If RIG administration is delayed for some reason, it may be given up to the eighth day after the first dose of vaccine; it is not indicated after this time as it can be presumed that an antibody response to the vaccine has occurred. RIG never should be given at the same site as the rabies vaccine.

A person who previously has been fully immunized with HDCV or RVA vaccine or, if immunized previously with a rabies vaccine other than these, had a documented adequate rabies antibody titer, should receive only two doses of the vaccine (three days apart). If the immune status of a previously vaccinated person who did not receive the recommended HDCV regimen is not known, the full primary postexposure regimen (RIG plus five doses of HDCV or RVA) should be initiated. However, if antibody is present in a serum sample collected prior to vaccine administration, treatment may be discontinued after two doses of HDCV or RVA.

HUMAN DIPLOID CELL RABIES VACCINE (HDCV)

This inactivated virus vaccine is prepared from fixed rabies virus grown in human diploid cell cultures.

Pre-exposure prophylaxis provides the basis for a rapid anamnestic response to booster doses of the vaccine. The antibody response requires 7 to 14 days to develop, but persists for more than a year; multiple doses are required to reach 100%. Booster doses at two-year intervals are sometimes necessary to maintain adequate antibody titers. In persons working with live rabies virus or involved in vaccine production, rabies antibody titers should be measured every six months and boosters given as needed to maintain adequate antibody levels.

In 1986 the FDA licensed a human diploid cell rabies vaccine for intradermal use [Imovax Rabies ID] produced by the Merieux Institute and packaged in a single-dose syringe (Immunization Practices Advisory Committee, 1986 B) for pre-exposure immunization. *The intradermal preparation must not be used for postexposure prophylaxis.*

ADVERSE REACTIONS AND PRECAUTIONS. Reactions are principally mild local (incidence 25% to 75%) or systemic (incidence 20%) effects. The vaccine is considerably less reactogenic than the earlier vaccines.

An immune complex-like reaction sometimes occurs 2 to 21 days after HDCV boosters; symptoms include generalized urticaria, arthralgia, arthritis, angioedema, nausea, vomiting, fever, and malaise. It occurs in up to 6% of persons receiving booster doses but is much less frequent in those given primary immunization. In none of the reported cases has the reaction been life-threatening. These reactions have been attributed to the presence in the vaccine of human serum albumin rendered allergenic by the β-propiolactone used to inactivate the virus. The reaction appears to be less common with RVA. Persons who experience these reactions should not receive further doses of HDCV unless they are likely to have been exposed and have inadequate rabies antibody titers.

Once treatment with rabies vaccine has been initiated, it should not be interrupted because of local or mild systemic reactions. These usually can be managed with anti-inflammatory and antipyretic agents. Serious systemic anaphylactic or neuroparalytic reactions are extremely rare and must be evaluated carefully; assistance may be sought from state health departments or the vaccine manufacturer and should be reported to these bodies.

Pregnancy is not a contraindication to postexposure prophylaxis and, if there is substantial risk, pre-exposure prophylaxis may be indicated. HDCV is classified in FDA Pregnancy Category C.

DRUG INTERACTIONS. In a randomized, controlled clinical trial, chloroquine 300 mg per week significantly reduced the mean antibody response to immunization with intradermal HDCV rabies vaccine (Pappaioanou et al, 1986). Corticosteroids, antineoplastic drugs, and immunosuppressive agents may interfere with the development of active immunity. Unless these agents are essential, they should be discontinued during postexposure vaccine therapy. Serum antibody levels should be measured in these patients and rabies immune globulin should be given.

DOSAGE.

Intramuscular: *Adults and children*, for pre-exposure immunoprophylaxis, 1 ml is injected into the deltoid area on days 0, 7, and 28. Individuals at risk should have a serum antibody test two years later to determine if revaccination is necessary. If antibody levels are inadequate, for booster immunization in *adults* and *children*, a single 1-ml dose may be given in the deltoid area and the level measured again in two to three weeks.

Available Trademark.
Imovax Rabies (Merieux).

Intradermal: The schedule for the intradermal preparation is identical except that each dose consists of 0.1 ml.

For postexposure immunization, see Table 14.

Available Trademark.
Imovax Rabies ID (Merieux).

RABIES VACCINE, ADSORBED (RVA)

A rabies vaccine adsorbed onto an aluminum salt was licensed in 1988 for both pre-exposure and postexposure prophylaxis (Centers for Disease Control, 1988). It is produced and distributed by the Michigan Department of Public Health

TABLE 14.
POSTEXPOSURE RABIES IMMUNIZATION PROCEDURES*

Persons not previously immunized:	RIG, 20 IU/kg body weight, one-half infiltrated at bite site (if possible), remainder IM; 5 doses of HDCV or RVA, 1 ml IM (ie, deltoid area), one each on days 0, 3, 7, 14 and 28
Persons previously immunized†:	Two doses of HDCV or RVA, 1 ml IM (ie, deltoid area), one each on days 0 and 3. RIG should not be administered.

The intradermal preparation of rabies vaccine must not be used for postexposure prophylaxis.

** All postexposure treatment should begin with immediate thorough cleansing of all wounds with soap and water.*

† Pre-exposure immunization with HDCV, prior postexposure prophylaxis with HDCV, or persons previously immunized with any other type of rabies vaccine and a documented history of positive antibody response to the prior vaccination.

Adapted from Immunization Practices Advisory Committee, 1984 C, and Centers for Disease Control, 1988.

and is now available for out-of-state distribution. The vaccine consists of the Kissling strain of rabies virus produced from a diploid cell line derived from fetal rhesus monkey lung. It is inactivated with β-propiolactone and concentrated by adsorption onto aluminum phosphate, which also serves as an adjuvant. Acceptable levels of neutralizing antibody have been found in more than 99% of vaccinated individuals. The recommended vaccination intervals are identical to those of HDCV.

ADVERSE REACTIONS AND PRECAUTIONS. Adverse reactions after primary vaccination are similar to those after use of HDCV. However, systemic allergic reactions have been observed in less than 1% of persons who received a booster dose of RVA (Centers for Disease Control, 1988). See also the evaluation on HDCV.

DOSAGE. See the evaluation on HDCV.

Rabies Vaccine, Adsorbed (Michigan Department of Public Health).

RABIES IMMUNE GLOBULIN (RIG)

RIG is a sterile solution of antirabies immunoglobulin prepared by cold ethanol fractionation of plasma from donors hyperimmunized with the rabies vaccine. The globulin solution is stabilized with glycine and contains thimerosal as a preservative. The product is standardized to contain an average of 150 IU/ml.

RIG is indicated for all persons with known or suspected exposure to rabies virus and is given in conjunction with rabies vaccine. However, individuals who were previously immunized with rabies vaccine and had a documented positive antibody response should be given only two doses of the vaccine. Repeated doses of RIG should not be administered once rabies vaccine has been injected, for this could prevent full development of active immunity. (See the section on Rabies and Tables 13 and 14.)

RIG is classified in FDA Pregnancy Category C.

DOSAGE.

Intramuscular: 20 IU/kg; one-half of the material should be infiltrated around the wound if feasible. RIG is used as soon as possible after a suspected exposure to rabies and always in conjunction with rabies vaccine. (See Tables 13 and 14.)

Available Trademarks.

Hyperab (Cutter), ***Imogam*** (Merieux).

VACCINES USED UNDER SPECIAL CIRCUMSTANCES

BCG VACCINE

BCG vaccine is a standardized preparation of a living BCG (Bacillus Calmette-Guerin) strain used for active immunization against tuberculosis. BCG is an attenuated strain of bovine tubercle bacillus (*Mycobacterium bovis*). All BCG vaccines are derived from the original strain, but genetic mutations have occurred leading to differences in immunogenicity and efficacy. Data on these vaccines have been obtained primarily from other countries and do not necessarily pertain to the vaccines available in the United States. Efficacy of current vaccines has not been clearly established. Vaccines currently available in the United States have been evaluated only for their ability to induce hypersensitivity.

Only one strain of BCG vaccine (Tice) is currently licensed in the United States for the prevention of tuberculosis. The Tice strain is available from Bionetics Research, Inc., Chicago, and Antigen Supply House, Northridge, California, and is given percutaneously. There are no available data concerning the clinical efficacy of this vaccine strain.

BCG vaccine is not recommended for routine immunization in the United States, for the general population is at low risk of acquiring tuberculosis. In addition, the disease usually can be successfully controlled by case detection, chemotherapy, and preventive therapy. BCG vaccine is recommended only for children with negative tuberculin skin tests (1) who cannot receive isoniazid or rifampin preventive therapy but are repeatedly exposed to persons with infectious tuberculosis, (2) who are exposed to infectious patients with tubercle bacilli resistant to isoniazid and rifampin, or (3) who are members of groups with annual infection rates of more than 1% among whom the usual measures of case detection, chemotherapy, and preventive therapy have failed or cannot be applied effectively. BCG is no longer recommended for adults, including health-care workers, who may be at high risk for acquiring the disease (Immunization Practices Advisory Committee, 1988 C).

In normal tuberculin-negative recipients, proper intradermal injection of vaccine results in localized skin infection. A lesion appears within seven to ten days, reaches a maximum diameter of about 8 mm after five weeks, then gradually regresses to form a scar in approximately three months. Postvaccination tuberculin skin tests do not reliably predict the degree of protection afforded by BCG vaccination.

BCG vaccine also has been used as an adjuvant to enhance antibody formation and to treat certain types of localized cancer (see index entry BCG Vaccine, In Cancer).

ADVERSE REACTIONS AND PRECAUTIONS. The frequency and severity of adverse reactions vary with the BCG substrain employed. Adverse effects occur in 1% to 10% of recipients. Lymphadenitis (incidence, less than 1%), local ulceration that may become severe and persistent, ulcers resulting from autoinoculation, granulomas, and transient urticaria of the limbs and trunk may occur. Keloidal scars develop in some individuals. Osteomyelitis occurs more frequently in neonates than in adults (adults, 1/1,000,000 vaccinees; neonates, 5/100,000 vaccinees). Isolated cases of disseminated BCG infection and death have been reported (1 to 10/10,000,000 vaccinees), principally in children with an impaired immune response.

BCG vaccine is *contraindicated* in individuals with an impaired immune response due to congenital immunodeficiency, HIV infection, leukemia, lymphoma, or generalized malignancy. It should not be given to pregnant women or patients with extensive skin infections (FDA Pregnancy Category C). It is also contraindicated in patients receiving immunosuppressive agents, including corticosteroids or radiation. The effectiveness of BCG in patients taking isoniazid, rifampin, streptomycin, or other drugs that inhibit the growth of the organism is not known.

BCG vaccine has not been reported to cause disseminated infection in individuals, including children, with asymptomatic HIV infection. The World Health Organization has recommended that asymptomatic children who are members of populations at high risk of both tuberculosis and HIV infection should receive the vaccine at birth or as soon as possible thereafter. However, the vaccine should not be given to children with symptomatic HIV infection or members of populations at increased risk of HIV infection but with a low risk of tuberculosis (World Health Organization, 1987).

DOSAGE. BCG vaccine should be protected from light and refrigerated during long-term storage (<10° C).

Percutaneous: *Children with negative tuberculin skin tests* who are at risk from continued exposure to active disease may be given the freshly reconstituted vaccine. See the manufacturer's instructions for further information on dosage and administration.

Manufacturer: Organon.

CHOLERA VACCINE

This combined bacterial vaccine consists of the Ogawa and Inaba strains of *Vibrio cholerae,* inactivated by phenol and suspended in a saline solution containing 0.5% phenol as a preservative. Many public health officials feel that killed whole cell cholera vaccines are minimally effective and do not prevent disease transmission. Clinical immunity develops in only about 50% of recipients and lasts a short time. The low level of immunity begins to recede in three to six months. Consequently, a booster dose should be administered every six months as long as there is risk of exposure. Use of the vaccine in community immunization programs is of limited value in controlling a cholera outbreak, for it does not prevent transmission of infection. The most important control measures are optimum food and water hygiene.

The U.S. Public Health Service does not require cholera vaccination for entry into the United States from infected areas, and the World Health Organization no longer recommends routine vaccination for travel to or from infected areas. Nevertheless, some countries in Asia, the Middle East, and Africa still require evidence of cholera vaccination for entry. The vaccine is not recommended for infants under 6 months of age.

Persons given yellow fever and cholera vaccines simultaneously or one to three weeks apart have had diminished antibody responses to both vaccines, but the clinical importance of this data is unknown. However, whenever possible, these two vaccines should be given at least three weeks apart (Immunization Practices Advisory Committee, 1988 D).

Malaise, fever, and induration and erythema at the site of injection may occur. Serious reactions are extremely rare.

Cholera vaccine is classified in FDA Pregnancy Category C.

DOSAGE.

Intramuscular, Subcutaneous: Primary immunization consists of two doses given one week to one month apart; booster doses of identical size are advised at six-month intervals so long as there is risk of exposure. The amounts given in each dose are: *adults and children over 10 years,* 0.5 ml; *children 5 to 10 years,* 0.3 ml; *6 months through 4 years,* 0.2 ml.

A single dose (primary or booster) by either of the foregoing routes within six months of travel will satisfy international health regulations where immunization is required.

Intradermal: *Adults and children 5 years or older,* 0.2 ml for both primary immunization or booster doses.

Manufacturers: Lederle, Moore, Wyeth-Ayerst.

MENINGOCOCCAL POLYSACCHARIDE VACCINES

Meningococcal disease is both endemic and epidemic. It is largely endemic in the United States, although small localized outbreaks occur occasionally in closed populations of infants, children, and military recruits, and there is a high incidence of secondary cases among household contacts. Despite antimicrobial therapy, the case-fatality rate can be as high as 10% for meningococcal meningitis and 20% for meningococcemia.

Endemic meningococcal disease is most common in the pediatric age group, especially infants 6 to 12 months of age. The causative organism, *Neisseria meningitidis,* has at least seven serogroups based on differing capsular polysaccharides. Groups B, C, and W-135 cause 85% to 95% of meningococcal infections in the United States. The vaccine containing Groups A, C, Y, and W-135 polysaccharide antigen is immunogenic. However, serogroup B polysaccharide antigen does not readily induce antibody production. Group B strains are responsible for 50% to 55% of all *N. meningitidis* cases in the United States. Although serogroup A is responsible for only a few cases in the United States, it is the most frequent cause of epidemics in other countries. Areas experiencing epidemic diseases may be determined by contacting travelers' clinics or the CDC quarantine facility. Certain chronic conditions (asplenia, complement deficiency) appear to predispose to severe meningococcal infections. Military recruits were once considered to be at very high risk for meningococcal disease, particularly group C, but routine use of an A/C/Y/W-135 vaccine has greatly reduced the incidence of the disease.

Routine immunization with meningococcal polysaccharide vaccines is not recommended, but it should be considered for individuals with terminal complement component deficiencies, those with anatomic or functional asplenia, travelers to countries where meningococcal disease is epidemic, and military recruits. Individuals receiving cancer chemotherapy respond poorly to meningococcal vaccine; in patients requiring splenectomy for Hodgkin's disease, immunization should be completed before surgery, if possible.

The vaccine available for civilian and military use in the United States is quadrivalent and contains serogroups A, C, Y, and W-135 (Immunization Practices Advisory Committee, 1985 A). It contains 50 mcg of each of the purified capsular polysaccharides. Clinical studies have demonstrated the immunogenicity and efficacy of the A and C components in military personnel in the United States and other countries. However, children less than 2 years old respond poorly to the C, Y, and W-135 components; infants 3 months and older do respond to the A component when the vaccine is given in two doses at a 3-month interval. The Y and W-135 components have been shown to be immunogenic in adults and children over 2 years of age. It is thought that the clinical protection induced by the quadrivalent vaccine persists for at least three years, although antibody titers to the A and C components diminish markedly during this time, especially in young children.

ADVERSE REACTIONS AND PRECAUTIONS. Adverse reactions are more common in children and include erythema, induration, malaise, low-grade fever, and axillary adenopathy.

Meningococcal vaccine has been given to pregnant women in Brazil, and no adverse effects were reported in their infants. However, on theoretical grounds, it should be avoided during pregnancy except when the risk of exposure is high (FDA Pregnancy Category C).

DOSAGE.

A/C/Y/W-135 QUADRIVALENT VACCINE:

Subcutaneous: *Adults and children over 2 years,* 0.5 ml as a single injection. Booster injections may be indicated for children first vaccinated when less than 4 years of age who remain at high risk.

Available Trademark.
Menomune A/C/Y/W-135 (Connaught).

PLAGUE VACCINE

Plague vaccine is prepared from *Yersinia pestis* grown on media containing beef, protein, soy, and casein, killed with formaldehyde, and preserved with 0.5% phenol. Plague vaccine is recommended for laboratory personnel engaged in aerosol experimentation and those persons whose occupation or circumstances make avoidance of fleas and rodents difficult when they are traveling or working in rural or urban areas where plague is known to be active in wild rodents or has been reported in humans and/or commensal rats.

It is generally believed that immunization greatly increases the chance of recovery from bubonic plague, but there are no data that have proven the vaccine's efficacy. The extent to which the vaccine protects against the pneumonic form is unknown. Plague vaccine should not be relied upon as a principal preventive measure. Control of rodents and their ectoparasites is most effective.

ADVERSE REACTIONS. Adverse reactions include local erythema and induration, malaise, mild lymphadenopathy, hyperpyrexia, and, occasionally, headache. Booster injections increase the incidence and severity of adverse reactions. Sensitivity reactions (urticaria, asthma) are rare. The vaccine should be avoided in persons sensitive to constituents of the medium.

DOSAGE.

Intramuscular: *Adults and children over 10 years,* for primary vaccination, one 1-ml dose, followed in four weeks by a second dose of 0.2 ml. A third injection of 0.2 ml three to six months after the first injection completes the primary series. If essential, an accelerated schedule of three doses of 0.5 ml each at weekly intervals may be given; however, the efficacy of this schedule has not been determined. Booster injections of 0.1 to 0.2 ml every six months are recommended for individuals who remain at risk. After three such doses, boosters at one- to two-year intervals should provide the needed protection. *Children under 10 years* receive the same series at the same intervals, but at a reduced dosage as follows: *Infants 1 year or less,* first dose 0.2 ml, second and third doses 0.04 ml, booster dose 0.02 to 0.04 ml; *1 to 4 years,* first dose 0.4 ml, second and third doses 0.08 ml, booster dose 0.04 to 0.08 ml; *5 to 10 years,* first dose 0.6 ml, second and third doses 0.12 ml, booster dose 0.06 to 0.12 ml.

Manufacturer: Cutter.

SMALLPOX VACCINE

In 1980, the World Health Organization declared the world free of smallpox in the natural state, which attested to the highly effective worldwide smallpox immunization programs. All countries in the world have officially discontinued routine smallpox vaccination. International Certificates of Vaccination are not required for travelers. In the United States, routine vaccination was abandoned in 1971 and vaccination for hospital personnel was abandoned in 1976. It is still used in some military personnel. General distribution of the vaccine to the civilian population was discontinued in May 1983 to end its misuse in diseases such as warts and herpes. The only currently recommended nonmilitary use of the vaccine is for laboratory personnel who work with the virus or a closely related orthopox virus and those involved in vaccine production.

Vaccinia immune globulin is available through the Centers for Disease Control to treat the clinical complications of smallpox vaccination in civilians.

SOURCE. At present, smallpox vaccine is no longer available in the United States for use in the general public. However, the Department of Defense has a policy of immunizing some personnel on active duty. At the present time, the Centers for Disease Control is the only source of smallpox vaccine for civilians. Requests for the vaccine to be used in the laboratory workers noted above should be sent to: Drug, Immunobiologic and Vaccine Service, Center for Infectious Diseases, Mailstop D09, Centers for Disease Control, Atlanta, GA 30333 (404) 639-3356.

VACCINIA IMMUNE GLOBULIN

Vaccinia immune globulin (VIG) is a solution of immunoglobulins prepared from the serum of persons recently immunized with vaccinia virus. VIG is used to treat the clinical complications (eczema vaccinatum, vaccinia necrosum, ocular vaccinia, generalized vaccinia) of smallpox vaccination. VIG is of no benefit in patients with postvaccinal encephalitis. This immune globulin should be administered as soon as possible after the onset of symptoms. Doses may be large and should be given over 24 to 36 hours. More detailed information may be obtained from the Centers for Disease Control, Division of Immunization (404) 639-1870.

DOSAGE.

Intramuscular: For prevention or modification of vaccinia infection, *adults and children*, 0.3 ml/kg should be given as soon as possible after exposure. Doses over 10 ml should be injected at two or more sites.

For treatment of postvaccinal complications, *adults and children*, 0.6 ml/kg administered as soon as possible after symptoms appear. Doses over 10 ml should be injected at two or more sites. The dose may be repeated, depending on severity of symptoms and response to treatment.

Vaccinia immune globulin is only available through Drug Immunobiologics and Vaccine Service, Center for Infectious Diseases, Centers for Disease Control. Requests from physicians for VIG should be made to (404) 639-3356 Monday through Friday, 8 am to 4:30 pm Eastern time or (404) 639-2888 at all other times.

Vaccines for Typhoid Fever

Typhoid fever remains a major problem worldwide; approximately 12.5 million cases are reported annually. In the United States, the incidence declined steadily between 1900 and 1960 and has remained low since then. Between 1975 and 1984, an average of 464 cases were reported annually. During that period, more than 50% of the cases occurred in patients older than 20 years and 62% were in travelers to other countries. In contrast, from 1967 to 1976, 33% of the cases occurred in individuals who had traveled abroad. Travelers to Chile, Peru, India, and Pakistan appear to have the greatest risk of infection.

Of those cases acquired in the United States, 23% have been associated with typhoid carriers, 24% with food outbreaks, 23% with the ingestion of contaminated food or water, 6% with household contact with an infected person, and 4% with laboratory exposure to *Salmonella typhi*. The majority of typhoid patients respond favorably to antibiotic therapy, but this does not eradicate the carrier state. The emergence of chloramphenicol- or ampicillin-resistant strains has complicated therapy.

Two vaccines are currently available for use by civilians in the United States: a parenteral phenol and heat-inactivated vaccine and a live attenuated oral vaccine, Ty21a. The former has protected 50% to 77% of recipients in various field trials. In several field trials, the efficacy of an acetone-inactivated vaccine (available only to the military) has ranged from 70% to 93%, but it is considerably more reactogenic than the phenol and heat-inactivated vaccine. In recent studies employing both types of whole cell killed vaccine, 67% of recipients were protected after challenge with a moderate dose of typhoid bacilli, but the vaccines had little efficacy after a high-dose challenge. In controlled trials in Chile, three doses of the Ty21a live oral vaccine also protected 67% of recipients against clinical infection for at least four years.

Selective immunization with typhoid vaccine is indicated for (1) travelers to areas where typhoid fever is endemic, (2) persons with intimate exposure to a documented typhoid carrier, and (3) laboratory workers who have frequent contact with *S. typhi*. Typhoid vaccine does not appear to be useful in controlling common-source outbreaks and is not indicated in areas that have experienced a natural disaster (eg, a flood) or for persons attending summer camps.

TYPHOID VACCINE

Typhoid vaccine is a sterile saline suspension of phenol and heat-killed typhoid bacilli (*S. typhi*) of a strain (Ty-2) selected for high antigenicity. The vaccine contains 0.5% phenol as a preservative. The current inactivated vaccine is approximately 70% effective against infectious doses commonly found in contaminated water and milk, but it may not protect against large doses, such as those present in heavily contaminated foods.

The administration of the vaccine is followed by the production of agglutinins and bactericidal antibodies, which eliminate bacteria from the blood. However, intracellular bacteria inaccessible to these antibodies may multiply and produce endotoxins that have injurious effects even in the presence of circulating antibodies. The fecal carriage load of typhoid bacilli is not reduced by circulating antibodies.

Immunity wanes with time, and booster doses should be given every three years to those who are continuously at risk. Although a natural infection increases resistance, second attacks of typhoid have occurred.

ADVERSE REACTIONS AND PRECAUTIONS. Adverse reactions to typhoid vaccine are frequent and include local erythema, tenderness at the site of injection, malaise, myalgia, headache, and fever. Reactions usually begin within 24 hours after administration and persist for one or two days. Administration of the vaccine should be delayed in the presence of acute respiratory illness or other active infections and is contraindicated in those who have previously experienced an allergic reaction to the vaccine. The vaccine should be used with caution in patients with a severe febrile illness or a history of febrile convulsions following vaccine administration (especially children). Safety of the vaccine during pregnancy has not been established, and its use should be individualized to reflect actual need.

DOSAGE.

Subcutaneous: *Adults and children over 10 years,* two 0.5-ml doses four or more weeks apart or, if insufficient time exists, three 0.5-ml doses at weekly intervals, but this schedule may be less effective. *Children 6 months to 10 years,* two 0.25-ml doses four or more weeks apart or three doses at weekly intervals. If there is continued or repeated exposure, a booster dose should be given at least every three years; *adults and children over 10 years* should receive 0.5 ml and *children under 10 years,* 0.25 ml.

Manufacturer: Wyeth-Ayerst.

TYPHOID VACCINE LIVE ORAL Ty21a

The protection provided by parenterally administered killed typhoid vaccines is inadequate against large numbers of organisms, and adverse reactions are common. In addition, the relative importance of humoral immunity to typhoid has been questioned, and it has been suggested that local defense mechanisms at the intestinal mucosa are the dominant immune determinants.

Oral vaccines have stimulated local immunity in other diseases and, in general, have been nonreactogenic. A live oral typhoid vaccine consisting of a mutant strain (Ty21a) of *S. typhi* is now available. This mutant lacks the enzyme, uridine diphosphate (UDP)-galactose-4-epimerase, and contains greatly reduced levels of two other enzymes involved in galactose metabolism (Germanier and Fürer, 1975). Consequently, immunogenic lipopolysaccharides that act as antigens are synthesized in amounts inadequate to maintain cell wall integrity. More important, galactose-1-phosphate and UDP-galactose accumulate. These events result in bacterial lysis. Thus, the oral vaccine is quite antigenic, but the organism has limited viability in man due to its autodestructive nature. The Ty21a mutant is stable, and reversion to the wild type has not been observed in laboratory or field trials.

In the first clinical trial of the Ty21a vaccine, it was 87% effective in protecting vaccinees challenged with virulent typhoid bacilli five to nine weeks after immunization (Gilman et al, 1977). Excretion of *S. typhi* Ty21a was not observed after the third day, there was no evidence of reversion to the wild type, and significantly fewer virulent *S. typhi* bacilli (emanating from the challenge dose) were excreted in the feces.

A series of double-blind field trials in children have demonstrated the effectiveness of Ty21a vaccine. The first was performed in Alexandria, Egypt, with a study population of 32,388 children aged 6 to 7 years. Three doses, which were given in suspension form, were administered after ingestion of bicarbonate; these resulted in a 95% decrease in the incidence of typhoid fever over a three-year period (Wahden et al, 1982). In a subsequent trial in school-aged children in Santiago, Chile, the vaccine in enteric-coated capsules had an efficacy of 21% with a single dose and 54% with a two-dose schedule after a 33-month surveillance program (Levine et al, 1986). In another field trial utilizing a three-dose schedule (enteric-coated capsules administered on alternate days) in school-aged children, the incidence of typhoid fever decreased 67% (Levine et al, 1987). The relative efficacy of two, three, or four doses of enteric-coated capsules administered to children on alternate days indicated that efficacy was highest for the four-dose regimen and persisted for five years (Ferreccio et al, 1989).

USES. Typhoid vaccine live oral Ty21a is indicated for the immunization of adults and children over 6 years against disease caused by *S. typhi*. However, not all vaccine recipients will be fully protected against typhoid fever, and the vaccine does not protect against other *Salmonella* species or other bacteria causing enteric disease.

ADVERSE REACTIONS. Adverse effects are infrequent, transient, and resolve spontaneously. Reported reactions include nausea, abdominal cramps, vomiting, and skin rash or urticaria in the trunk and/or extremities.

PRECAUTIONS. Since the vaccine is not 100% effective, travelers to endemic areas should take all necessary precautions to avoid contact with or ingestion of potentially contaminated food or water. The vaccine should not be administered to persons who are immunodeficient or who are undergoing immunosuppressive therapy, and it should not be taken during an acute febrile or gastrointestinal illness. The vaccine should not be administered to patients receiving antibiotics or sulfonamides because these may interfere with multiplication of the vaccine strain and the subsequent development of immunity. It should not be administered to any person with a known hypersensitivity to any of the vaccine components.

Pregnant women should receive the vaccine only if it is clearly indicated (FDA Pregnancy Category C). Its safety and efficacy have not been established in children under 6 years and, therefore, the vaccine is not recommended for this age group.

DOSAGE AND ADMINISTRATION.

Oral: *Children over 6 years and adults,* one capsule ingested with a cold or lukewarm drink one hour before a meal on days 1, 3, 5, and 7. *Booster dose*, one capsule taken on alternate days for four doses every five years when exposure to *S. typhi* continues.

Available Trademark.

Virotif Berna (Swiss Serum and Vaccine Institute, Berne, Switzerland. Distributed by Berna Products, Inc., Coral Gables, FL 33134.)

Yellow Fever

YELLOW FEVER VACCINE

This live, attenuated virus vaccine is prepared from the 17D strain grown in chicken embryos. When the vaccine is administered subcutaneously, infection develops, followed by low-grade viremia in three to nine days. Virus multiplication is believed to occur chiefly in lymphoreticular cells. Immunity develops by the seventh day and lasts for ten years or more. Revaccination is required after ten years by countries that require a vaccination certificate.

Yellow fever vaccine must meet standards established by the World Health Organization and must be administered at approved centers located in most cities in the United States; information on specific locations can be obtained from state, city, or county public health officers.

Vaccination is recommended for persons 9 months of age or older traveling to or living in rural or semirural areas of countries where yellow fever is endemic (currently parts of Africa and South America) and in areas of the yellow fever belt, even though recent cases may not have been reported. Travel to large urban areas currently does not pose a risk, although specific countries may require vaccination (Immunization Practices Advisory Committee, 1990 C). Pregnant women and infants over 4 months should be considered for immunization if travel in epidemic areas is absolutely necessary and exposure to mosquitoes cannot be avoided. The vaccine is contraindicated in infants under 4 months because of risk of vaccine-related encephalitis. Vaccination is also recommended for laboratory personnel who might be exposed to the virulent yellow fever virus.

A certificate of vaccination against yellow fever is required by certain countries for all entering travelers or for travelers who have visited any country thought to harbor endemic disease. Since requirements and disease epidemiologic patterns may change, all travelers should seek current information from state health departments or from the division of Vector-Borne Viral Diseases, CDC, Fort Collins, Colorado (303/221-6400).

Available evidence suggests that yellow fever vaccine may be administered concomitantly with other live virus vaccines without impairment of antibody response or increase in adverse effects. If not given concurrently, four weeks should elapse between administration of live virus vaccines. Simultaneous administration of cholera and yellow fever vaccines reduces the antibody levels to both vaccines. When possible, these agents should be given at a minimal interval of three weeks. If not possible, it is recommended that they be given simultaneously. Immune serum globulin and chloroquine given concurrently with yellow fever vaccine do not adversely affect the immune response.

ADVERSE REACTIONS AND PRECAUTIONS. Adverse reactions are generally mild and consist of headache, myalgia, or low-grade fever in 2% to 5% of vaccinees. The vaccine is contraindicated in individuals with a history of any signs or symptoms of an anaphylactic reaction after eating eggs; those with febrile illnesses, dysgammaglobulinemia, or AIDS; or those receiving immunosuppressive therapy. There is a theoretical risk of encephalitis from the vaccine virus infection in AIDS and other immunosuppressed patients. Such patients should not be given the vaccine. After counseling, asymptomatic HIV-infected persons who must travel to endemic areas should be offered the choice of vaccination. It is prudent to avoid vaccinating pregnant women (FDA Pregnancy Category C). If the sole reason for vaccinating a pregnant woman or an individual with known allergy is to satisfy international travel requirements, efforts should be made to obtain a letter of waiver clearly stating the contraindication to the vaccine.

DOSAGE.

Subcutaneous: *Adults and children over 6 months,* 0.5 ml of reconstituted vaccine. International regulations do not require revaccination more frequently than every ten years.

Available Trademark.
YF-Vax (Connaught).

OTHER IMMUNE GLOBULINS

IMMUNE GLOBULIN (IG)

Immune globulin (formerly immune serum globulin) is a sterile solution of immunoglobulin, primarily IgG, containing 16.5% ± 1.5% protein that is prepared by cold ethanol precipitation of pooled human plasma. Only plasma units nonreactive for hepatitis B surface antigen (HBsAg) and antibodies to HIV are employed. IG contains glycerin and the preservative, thimerosal. There is no risk of HIV infection.

IG preparations consist of a pool of antibodies that neutralize or otherwise modify the activity of the agents (eg, measles virus) to which their specificities are directed and, hence, protect the host. These protective antibodies to common infectious agents reflect those of the donor population from which the IG preparations are made. Thus, different lots of IG vary in specific antibody titer. IG should be distinguished from special immune globulin preparations, such as HBIG or VZIG, that are derived from the plasma of persons hyperimmunized against a specific infectious agent.

IG contains all four immunoglobulin subclasses and all of the known IgG genetic groups. Although 95% of the preparation is IgG, traces of IgA, IgM, and other serum proteins are present.

USES. ***Hepatitis:*** Immune globulin contains antibodies to both the hepatitis A virus and the hepatitis B surface antigen (anti-HBs). Studies have shown that IG is protective if given before exposure or during the incubation period of hepatitis A. It is not indicated in patients with clinical manifestations of the disease or in those exposed more than two weeks previously. It is recommended for travelers to countries where there is a significant risk of infection with hepatitis A and is given prior to departure. It is also recommended for postexposure prophylaxis against hepatitis A, for household and sexual contacts of infected patients, and for individuals at risk during outbreaks in day care centers, schools, institutions for custodial care, and hospitals. When there is a common source of exposure, such as an infected food handler, IG prophylaxis may be considered if it can be administered within two weeks of exposure.

IG has no role in postexposure prophylaxis of hepatitis B.

IG also has been suggested for prophylaxis after percutaneous exposure to blood from patients with non-A, non-B (NANB) hepatitis.

Measles: IG is indicated to prevent or modify measles (rubeola) in susceptible persons exposed less than six days previously, especially household contacts of measles patients (particularly infants under 1 year and pregnant women) for whom the risk of complications is high. Susceptible children whose immune systems are compromised, such as those with generalized malignancy, immunodeficiency disease, or those receiving immunosuppressive therapy who are exposed to measles, should receive IG immediately. Children with symptomatic infection with HIV who are exposed to measles should receive IG regardless of prior vaccination status.

Immunoglobulin Deficiency: IG is used prophylactically in patients with immunoglobulin (IgG) deficiency to prevent serious infection. It may not prevent infections in the respiratory or gastrointestinal tract or other secretory tissues. Prophylactic use, especially against encapsulated bacteria, is effective in Bruton-type, sex-linked, congenital agammaglobulinemia; agammaglobulinemia with thymoma; and acquired agammaglobulinemia.

Rubella: Some studies have indicated that the use of IG in exposed, susceptible women may lessen the likelihood of infection and fetal damage. However, the routine use of IG for prophylaxis during early pregnancy is of dubious value and can be justified only when the exposed woman will not accept therapeutic abortion if she develops rubella.

ADVERSE REACTIONS AND PRECAUTIONS. Adverse reactions consist of local pain, tenderness at the injection site, urticaria (occasional), and angioedema. Because of the possibility of systemic reactions, epinephrine should be readily available to treat acute allergic symptoms immediately.

Because IG contains IgA and because patients with isolated IgA deficiency may develop antibodies to any IgA-containing preparation, they may, on future exposure to products containing IgA, develop an anaphylactic reaction. IG aggregates in vitro; therefore, intravenous use is contraindicated, for it may cause severe, even fatal, reactions.

Immune globulin is classified in FDA Pregnancy Category C.

DOSAGE.

Intramuscular: For hepatitis A postexposure prophylaxis (household or close personal contacts of infected individuals), *adults and children*, 0.02 ml/kg as soon as possible after exposure. The use of IG two weeks after exposure or after onset of symptoms is not indicated.

For travel in areas where hepatitis A is common (pre-exposure prophylaxis), *adults and children*, 0.02 ml/kg for less than two-month length of stay; 0.06 ml/kg repeated every five months for longer visits. For postexposure prophylaxis, 0.02 ml/kg (Immunization Practices Advisory Committee, in press, 1991).

For prevention of measles in exposed susceptible *adults and children*, 0.25 ml/kg (maximum, 15 ml) administered less than six days following exposure. No more than 5 ml should be injected at any one site. *Immunocompromised susceptible individuals and symptomatic HIV-infected persons*, 0.5 ml/kg.

For prophylaxis in *adults and children* with immunoglobulin deficiency, initially, 1.32 ml/kg, followed by 0.66 ml/kg every three to four weeks. Frequency of administration should be determined by clinical response (absent or infrequent infections).

Available Trademark.
Gammar IM (Armour).

IMMUNE GLOBULIN INTRAVENOUS (IGIV)

Intravenous immune globulin is a sterile solution of plasma proteins containing IgG antibodies from pooled human plasma. Only plasma units nonreactive for hepatitis B surface antigen and antibodies to HIV are used. It is prepared for intravenous use either by treatment with pepsin at acid pH [Sandoglobulin I.V.], by diafiltration and ultrafiltration [Gamimune N], by chromatography [Gammagard], or cold ethanol at normal pH (Gammar IV). The preparation contains no less than 90% immunoglobulin consisting of all the IgG subclasses and trace amounts of IgA and IgM. IGIV is used in place of intramuscular immune globulin preparations when an immediate increase or higher levels of circulating immunoglobulin are required or when intramuscular injections are contraindicated.

USES. IGIV is indicated to treat congenital and acquired immunodeficiency disease, such as agammaglobulinemia, hypogammaglobulinemia, and combined immunodeficiency. Its use in these conditions and in a variety of other disorders has been reviewed (Stiehm et al, 1987). It is used by many physicians as a prophylactic measure against sepsis in HIV-infected neonates, but this use is investigational.

Experimental studies in animals and trials in humans suggest that IGIV may be of use in the management of severe bacterial sepsis with both gram-negative and gram-positive organisms. It has been indicated for chronic lymphocytic leukemia patients with recurrent bacterial infections and/or hypogammaglobulinemia (Cooperative Group for the Study of Immunoglobulin in Chronic Lymphocytic Leukemia, 1988). However, because an adverse outcome has been observed in a few instances, therapy for such uses remains investigational and is not currently recommended. Trials designed to assess the prophylactic value of IGIV in high-risk premature and other newborn infants have yielded promising, but unconfirmed results. Similarly, preliminary studies of its use in the treatment of certain neonatal viral infections indicate the need for further evaluation. Immunoglobulins containing high titers of antibody against cytomegalovirus (CMV) have been shown to reduce by 50% or more the incidence of severe CMV infections when they were given prophylactically to patients with bone marrow or kidney transplants; however, they appear to be of no value once infection is established.

IGIV also is indicated in idiopathic thrombocytopenic purpura, particularly for the acute form and especially in children. For reasons that are not clear, treatment with IGIV effectively reduces the incidence of coronary artery disease that occurs in Kawasaki disease. It also appears to be of at least transient benefit in myasthenia gravis. It has been evaluated in several other autoimmune disorders; clarification of its effects must await further study. It should be emphasized that treatment of any disorder with IGIV requires supervision by a physician experienced with its use.

Approximately three days after intravenous administration, IGIV is evenly distributed in the intra- and extravascular compartments. It has an intravascular half-life of about three weeks. As with physiologic IgG, IGIV may cross the placenta but only during the final weeks of pregnancy. It should be used during pregnancy only if clearly indicated.

ADVERSE REACTIONS AND PRECAUTIONS. IGIV is *contraindicated* in patients known to have experienced an anaphylactic reaction or severe systemic response to IG and in individuals with selective IgA deficiencies or class-specific anti-IgA. A precipitous fall in blood pressure and signs and symptoms of anaphylaxis have been observed in some patients. These events appear to be related to infusion rate, which should be carefully controlled and monitored.

IGIV should be given only intravenously (the intramuscular route has not been evaluated) through a separate line and *not* mixed with other fluids or medications. Inflammatory reactions due to antigen overload occur in less than 1% of patients with normal immune functions. If the initial infusion rate exceeds 1 ml/minute, adverse reactions (eg, flushing, chills, wheezing, malaise, dizziness) develop in approximately 10%

of patients. Rarely, anaphylactic reactions occur in patients previously sensitized to antigens in the preparation.

IGIV is classified in FDA Pregnancy Category C.

DOSAGE.

GAMIMUNE N:

Intravenous: For prophylaxis in immunodeficiency syndromes, *adults and children*, 100 to 200 mg/kg (2 to 4 ml/kg) at a rate of 0.01 to 0.02 ml/kg/min for 30 minutes. If there is no discomfort, the rate may be increased up to 0.08 ml/kg/min. If side effects occur, the rate should be reduced or the infusion interrupted until symptoms subside. The infusion may then be resumed at a rate that is tolerated by the patient.

Immune globulin may be administered once a month. If the clinical response is inadequate or the level of IgG achieved in the circulation is insufficient, the dose may be increased to 400 mg/kg (8 ml/kg) or the infusion may be given more than once a month.

For treatment of idiopathic thrombocytopenic purpura, 400 mg/kg daily for five days. If the platelet count decreases to clinically hazardous levels, a maintenance dose of 400 mg/kg administered as a single dose every several weeks may be of benefit.

GAMMAGARD:

Intravenous: For prophylaxis in immunodeficiency syndromes, *adults and children,* initially, 200 to 400 mg/kg. At least 100 mg/kg is given monthly thereafter. The frequency and amount of immunoglobulin therapy may vary from patient to patient. The minimum serum concentration of IgG necessary for protection has not been established.

For treatment of idiopathic thrombocytopenic purpura, *adults and children,* 1 g/kg. The need for additional doses should be determined by clinical response and platelet count. If required, up to three doses may be given on alternate days.

For patients with hypogammaglobulinemia and/or recurrent bacterial infections due to B-cell chronic lymphocytic leukemia, a dose of 400 mg/kg every three to four weeks is recommended.

GAMMAR IV:

Intravenous: The usual dose is directed toward restoration of the immune-deficient patient's circulating IgG level to near normal levels; 100 to 200 mg/kg every three to four weeks is recommended. An initial loading dose of at least 200 mg/kg at more frequent intervals, proceeding to 100 to 200 mg/kg at three-week intervals once a therapeutic plasma level has been established, can be used. However, treatment must be individualized due to variation in the catabolic rate of IgG among patients.

SANDOGLOBULIN I.V.:

Intravenous: For prophylaxis in immunodeficiency syndromes, *adults and children*, 200 mg/kg once monthly. If the clinical response or the level of serum IgG is insufficient, the dose may be increased to 300 mg/kg or the infusion may be repeated more frequently. The initial infusion must be given as a 3% solution at a rate of 0.5 to 1 ml/min. After 15 to 30 minutes, the infusion rate may be increased to 1.5 to 2.5 ml/min. If, after the first dose, large doses must be administered repeatedly, a 6% solution may be given at an initial infusion rate of 1 to 1.5 ml/min. Systems for self-administration of IGIV by patients at home have been developed (Stiehm et al, 1987). For induction treatment of idiopathic thrombocytopenic purpura, 400 mg/kg on two to five consecutive days. If after induction therapy the platelet count falls to less than 30,000/microliter and/or the patient manifests clinically significant bleeding, 0.4 g/kg may be given as a single infusion. If an adequate response does not result, the dose can be increased to 0.8 to 1 g/kg given as a single infusion (Fehr et al, 1982; Bussel et al, 1983).

Available Trademarks.

Gamimune N (Cutter), ***Gammagard*** (Hyland), ***Gammar IV*** (Armour), ***Sandoglobulin I.V.*** (Sandoz).

VARICELLA-ZOSTER IMMUNE GLOBULIN (HUMAN) (VZIG)

VZIG is a sterile 16% to 18% solution of the globulin fraction of human plasma of which not less than 99% is IgG; trace amounts of IgA and IgM also are present. VZIG is derived from plasma having high titers of varicella-zoster antibodies. Only plasma units nonreactive for hepatitis B surface antigen and antibodies to HIV are employed. The plasma pools are fractionated by cold ethanol precipitation of the proteins, and the final product contains 100 to 180 mg/ml of protein.

VZIG is not the same as zoster immune globulin (ZIG), although the terms have been used synonymously. The two preparations are derived from different donor populations: ZIG was derived from the serum of convalescent zoster patients, whereas VZIG is derived from the plasma of healthy adults. VZIG has replaced ZIG commercially.

VZIG is intended for passive immunization of selected, susceptible individuals (eg, immunocompromised children, AIDS patients) at high risk of varicella-associated complications following significant exposure to the virus (see Table 15). Effectiveness is maximal when treatment is initiated as soon as possible after exposure; VZIG has not been evaluated for efficacy beyond 96 hours after initial exposure.

There is no evidence that VZIG modifies established varicella-zoster infections. Its principal use in pregnancy is to prevent complications of varicella in susceptible women rather than to prevent intrauterine infection.

The decision to administer VZIG should be evaluated on an individual basis; most adults are probably immune. Postexposure administration of VZIG may ameliorate but not prevent illness, in which case varicella may still be contagious. The incubation period for varicella infection in immunocompromised patients may be prolonged an additional 14 to 18 days, and healthy individuals who receive VZIG should be considered contagious for 10 to 28 days following exposure or until all lesions have healed.

VZIG should never be administered intravenously.

DOSAGE.

Intramuscular: *Adults*, 125 units/10 kg (see following table). Each 125 units (2.5 ml) must be injected into a different site. [Data do not exist from which a calculation of the most appropriate dose for adults can be made. The Immunization Practices Advisory Committee (1984 A) states that a dose of

TABLE 15.
INDICATIONS AND GUIDELINES FOR USE OF VARICELLA-ZOSTER IMMUNE GLOBULIN (VZIG) FOR PROPHYLAXIS OF CHICKENPOX (VARICELLA)

I. Exposure criteria for which VZIG is indicated (patients must meet both criteria)
   1. One of the following types of exposure to chickenpox or zoster patient(s):
      a. Continuous household contact
      b. Playmate contact (>1 hour play indoors)
      c. Hospital contact (in same 2- to 4-bed room or adjacent beds in a large ward or prolonged face-to-face contact with an infectious staff member or patient)
      d. Newborn contact (newborn of mother who had onset of chickenpox ≤ 5 days before delivery or within 48 hours after delivery, regardless of prior administration of VZIG to the mother)
   2. Exposure occurred ≤96 hours prior to contemplated administration of VZIG

II. Persons for whom VZIG is indicated (all four criteria should be met)
   1. Susceptible to varicella-zoster infection
   2. Significant exposure (see I above)
   3. Age <15 years; administration to immunocompromised adolescents and adults and other older patients on an *individual* basis
   4. One of the following underlying illnesses or conditions:
      a. Leukemia or lymphoma
      b. Congenital or acquired immunodeficiency
      c. Immunosuppressive treatment
      d. Newborn of mother who had onset of chickenpox < 5 days before delivery or within 48 hours after delivery
      e. Premature infants (≥28 weeks' gestation born to a mother with a negative history of chickenpox)
      f. Premature infant (<28 weeks' gestation or birthweight ≤ 1 kg) regardless of maternal history
      g. Symptomatic HIV infection (AIDS)

Adapted from Immunization Practices Advisory Committee, 1984 A.

625 units is probably sufficient for healthy adults, but larger doses may be necessary in immunocompromised patients.]

Body Weight (kg)	Units	Vials	Injection Sites
0–10	125	1	1
10.1 to 20	250	2	2
20.1 to 30	375	3	3
30.1 to 40	500	4	4
Over 40	625	5	5

It has been recommended that postexposure prophylaxis with VZIG be repeated at three-week intervals in persons with continued or repeated exposure to varicella until such risk is no longer present unless there is laboratory evidence of adequate immunity at the time of re-exposure (Immunization Practices Advisory Committee, 1984 A).

VZIG is produced by the Massachusetts Public Health Biologic Laboratories, which distributes the preparation in that state. It is distributed elsewhere by the American Red Cross Blood Services-Northeast Region through regional blood centers. The Centers for Disease Control (404/639-1870) maintains a listing of telephone numbers of these distribution centers and continues to provide consultation regarding the indications for VZIG.

EQUINE ANTISERUMS

BOTULISM ANTITOXIN TRIVALENT

Botulism antitoxin is a refined, concentrated preparation of globulins obtained from horses immunized with botulinus toxins types A, B, and E and modified by enzymatic digestion. It may be administered by intramuscular or intravenous injection.

Botulism antitoxin neutralizes circulating (or unbound) toxin produced by *Clostridium botulinum* in persons who have ingested contaminated foods or acquired toxin through other means ("wound" botulism). It is not employed for the treatment of botulism in infants because efficacy in this age group has not been demonstrated.

The incubation period of botulism is usually 12 to 48 hours after ingestion of contaminated food. The outcome of the illness depends largely on the quality of supportive care, particularly mechanical ventilation. Antitoxin is an adjunct to these measures. Experimental data on the amount of circulating antitoxin needed to neutralize circulating toxin in humans are imprecise. Because of the serious nature of the disease, it is important to administer antitoxin as soon as possible to symptomatic patients in an effort to prevent progression of symptoms. Antitoxin will not reverse manifestations of the disease that have already appeared.

Because the amount or type of botulinus toxin ingested is not usually known, the entire contents of two vials of trivalent antitoxin should be given intravenously. The half-life of antitoxin is five to seven days; therefore, the administration of part of this dose intramuscularly to provide a reservoir is not recommended. Assays of circulating antitoxin in humans after administration of this preparation, as well as studies in mice, indicate that two vials are ample for almost all cases of botulism.

In addition to antitoxin and optimum respiratory management, initial therapy should include elimination of toxin by such means as induced vomiting, intubation, gastric lavage, rapid purgation, and high enemas. Signs and symptoms may progress for some hours after initiation of treatment and should not be considered as an indication for additional antitoxin.

ADVERSE REACTIONS AND PRECAUTIONS. Adverse effects are those associated with any equine globulin preparation, especially hypersensitivity reactions. The antitoxin should never be administered without conducting appropriate sensitivity tests. Patients who appear to be sensitive to equine serum should be desensitized first and the antitoxin then should be administered over several hours until the total dose has been given. See index entries Antiserums; Immune Globulins.

DOSAGE AND PREPARATIONS.

Intravenous, Intramuscular: For symptomatic botulism, *adults*, after sensitivity testing, two vials intravenously. For prophylaxis after ingestion of food contaminated with the toxin, one-fifth to one vial, intramuscularly. If symptoms appear, full therapeutic dosage should be administered. In addition, induction of vomiting and purging of the gastrointestinal tract may decrease absorption of toxin.

Botulism Antitoxin Trivalent is supplied in vials of 7 to 10 ml containing the following amounts of antitoxin: Type A, 7,500 IU; Type B, 6,600 IU; Type E, 8,500 IU. To procure antitoxin, the state epidemiologist should be contacted. If the state epidemiologist is unavailable, it may be obtained through the Centers for Disease Control, Atlanta, GA, 30333 (404/639-3670; off-duty hours 404/639-2888).

ANTIVENINS

Snakebites

It has been estimated that about 8,000 people are bitten by snakes annually but only 12 to 15 of these bites are fatal. Pit vipers or crotalids (rattlesnakes, cottonmouths [water moccasins], and copperheads) are responsible for most of the bites in the United States. Rattlesnake bites are the most serious, followed by those of the cottonmouth and copperhead. Copperhead envenomation usually does not cause major systemic injury. Envenomation does not necessarily occur after snakebite; about one of five pit viper bites is "dry," ie, not associated with injection of venom. Furthermore, the amount of venom injected with each bite varies.

Polyvalent crotalidae antivenin and North American coral snake antivenin neutralize the venoms of certain poisonous snakes indigenous to the United States. Venoms of snakes found outside the United States usually require other antivenins. The Oklahoma Poison Information Center (405/271-5454), in cooperation with the Oklahoma City Zoo, maintains an Antivenin Index (Rappolt et al, 1978) and can provide information on the availability of snake antivenins; it also maintains a snakebite consultation service for physicians. The physician also is encouraged to consult the literature (eg, Russell, 1983) and manufacturers of antivenin preparations for recommended methods of management of venomous snakebite and precautions regarding the use of antivenin.

Antivenins are prepared by injecting horses with venoms to induce the production of antibodies. Their administration carries the risk inherent in the injection of foreign protein; thus, it is important to observe the criteria for use of these agents carefully.

Since there is some risk of sensitization or reaction to antivenin, careful evaluation of the patient's condition should precede the decision to begin treatment. Signs and symptoms of envenomation include fang marks, swelling, and edema that develop within 20 minutes and pain, which is not always severe. Systemic signs and symptoms include weakness, syncope, paresthesia, and hypotension; blurred vision and ecchymoses are less common. Treatment with antivenin should be initiated as soon as the diagnosis is established.

The antivenins are diluted in normal saline and usually administered intravenously. Small amounts may be given intramuscularly, but these agents should never be injected into the fingers or toes. Adequate dosage is critical and prompt administration is essential. Children may require larger doses than adults.

In addition to antivenins, management of envenomation should include appropriate antitetanus therapy and adequate supportive management.

ANTIVENIN (CROTALIDAE) POLYVALENT

Antivenin (Crotalidae) polyvalent is an antiserum prepared from refined and concentrated serum globulins obtained from horses immunized against the venoms of the pit vipers, *Crotalus adamanteus* (eastern diamond rattlesnake), *C. atrox* (western diamond rattlesnake), *C. durissus terrificus* (tropical rattlesnake, Cascabel), and *Bothrops atrox* (fer-de-lance).

This antivenin is indicated only to treat envenomation due to bites of the specified crotalids (pit vipers): rattlesnakes (*Crotalus, Sistrurus*); copperhead and cottonmouth moccasins (*Agkistrodon*), including *A. halys* of Korea and Japan; fer-de-lance and other species of *Bothrops*; tropical rattler (*Crotalus durissus* and similar species); Cantil (*A. bilineatus*); and bushmaster (*Lachesis mutus*) of Central and South America. It is ineffective against coral snake venom.

The severity of envenomation should be estimated as soon as possible and before antivenin is administered. The amount of the first dose is based on this estimate (none, minimal, moderate, or severe). (See Dosage and Preparations.)

The antivenin is most effective when given within four hours of the bite, less effective after eight hours, and of questionable value after 12 hours. Nevertheless, in severe poisonings, antivenin therapy should be given even 24 hours after the snakebite.

ADVERSE REACTIONS AND PRECAUTIONS. The principal adverse effect is hypersensitivity to the equine serum proteins in the preparation. Since severe envenomation can be fatal, this risk must be weighed carefully against the risk of withholding antivenin. Testing for sensitivity to equine serum must be carried out prior to injection (see index entry Hypersensitivity, Tests). A procedure has been described for use in severely envenomated patients with positive sensitivity tests (see Wingert and Wainschel, 1975).

DOSAGE AND PREPARATIONS. Lyophilized preparations are active for at least five years; they are readily soluble in water for injection and should be reconstituted immediately prior to administration. For intravenous use, a 1:1 or 1:10 dilution is made of antivenin reconstituted in sodium chloride or 5% dextrose injection. The initial 5 to 10 ml should be infused over a three- to five-minute period. If no signs of a systemic reaction appear, intravenous infusion may be continued at the maximum rate. The intravenous route usually is preferred and is mandatory in the case of shock. Maximum blood levels of antivenin are not reached until eight or more hours after intramuscular administration.

Intravenous: *Adults and children*, initial dosage is based on the extent of envenomation; envenomation by large snakes in children or small adults requires larger doses. The amount administered to a child is not based on weight. For minimum envenomation, 20 to 40 ml; moderate envenomation, 50 to 90 ml; severe envenomation, 100 to 150 ml or more. The need for additional antivenin must be based on the clinical response to the initial dose and continuing assessment of the patient's condition. If warranted, an additional 10 to 50 ml may be administered.

See the manufacturer's literature for more detailed dosage information.

Antivenin (Crotalidae) Polyvalent (Equine Origin) (Wyeth-Ayerst). Lyophilized preparation with 10 ml of bacteriostatic water for reconstitution and injection; 1 ml of normal horse serum as sensitivity testing material is also provided.

NORTH AMERICAN CORAL SNAKE ANTIVENIN

This is a refined, concentrated, and lyophilized preparation of serum globulins obtained from the fractionated blood of horses immunized with the venom of the eastern coral snake (*Micrurus fulvius fulvius*). This antivenin neutralizes venom of *M. f. tenere* (Texas coral snake) but *not* that of *Micruroides euryxanthus* (Arizona or Sonoran coral snake). Each 10-ml vial contains sufficient material to neutralize approximately 250 mouse LD_{50} or about 2 mg of *M. f. fulvius* venom.

Although they rarely bite people, are small with short fangs, and often do not inject much venom, coral snakes can be dangerous. Death from respiratory paralysis may occur within four hours, but in some persons symptoms may not occur for many hours. Coral snake venom is chiefly paralytic (neurotoxic) in action and, customarily, only minimal to moderate tissue reaction and pain occur at the site of the bite. The adult LD_{100} has been estimated to be 4 to 5 mg of the dried venom. Under laboratory conditions, bites of the coral snake (*M.f. fulvius*) have yielded 1 to 28 mg of venom, depending on the size of the snake. Some patients require ten or more vials to neutralize the venom dose injected by the snake.

The intravenous route is preferred and antivenin should be given as soon as possible and before signs and symptoms occur. If signs and symptoms are already present when the patient is first seen, antivenin should be given promptly. The rate of infusion is determined by the severity of signs and symptoms and tolerance to the antivenin.

With vigorous treatment and careful observation, patients with complete respiratory paralysis have recovered, indicating that this effect is reversible. The use of morphine or other opioids that depress respiration is *contraindicated*. Sedatives should be used with extreme caution.

DOSAGE AND PREPARATIONS. Appropriate history and testing should be conducted prior to administration, since this antivenin is prepared from horse serum. In the event of sensitivity (if the history is positive and either the skin or conjunctival test is strongly positive), administration is contraindicated in all but acute emergencies. See index entry Hypersensitivity, Tests.

Intravenous: *Adults and children*, an intravenous drip of 250 to 500 ml of sodium chloride injection is begun, and the contents of three to five vials of antivenin (30 to 50 ml) are administered directly into the intravenous tubing or added to the reservoir bottle. In either case, the first 1 to 2 ml should be injected over a three- to five-minute period with careful observation of the patient for anaphylactic reaction. If no evidence of sensitivity appears, the infusion may be continued at an appropriate rate until the equivalent of 30 to 50 ml of undiluted antivenin in 250 to 500 ml of sodium chloride injection has been given (30 minutes in previously healthy adults). Additional antivenin may be given if required.

Antivenin (Micrurus fulvius) (Wyeth-Ayerst). Lyophilized preparation with 10 ml bacteriostatic water for reconstitution and injection.

Arthropod Bites

Biting or stinging insects possess venoms that contain deleterious substances. Unlike snakebite, the volume of toxin injected by insects and most spiders and scorpions usually is too small to cause serious problems except in hypersensitive individuals. In these individuals, insect stings cause anaphylactic shock, and prophylactic hyposensitization is essential for management.

Spider bites and scorpion stings cause injury by envenomation and are, therefore, the only arthropod-caused injuries currently amenable to treatment with antivenin. The only spider antivenin readily available is black widow spider antivenin.

The venom of the Arizona bark scorpion contains several potent components that act at the neuromuscular junction and also may affect the sympathetic nervous system. Symptoms include marked restlessness, especially in children; hypertonicity; pharyngeal spasms; drooling; fecal and urinary incontinence; hyperthermia; and sometimes paralysis. Beta-adrenergic blocking agents have been suggested for tachycardia and hypertension. Many patients are unable to locate the site of the sting, since most scorpion venoms produce minimal local reaction. An antivenin against the Arizona bark scorpion produced from goat serum is available in Arizona only. For the most part, treatment is symptomatic and most stings do not require medical care.

Like scorpion venom, the lethal fraction of black widow spider venom is a protein that causes destabilization of cell membranes and degranulation of nerve terminals resulting in the release of neurotransmitters. Central and peripheral nervous system excitement, autonomic activity, muscle spasm, vasoconstriction, and hypertension result from envenomation.

BLACK WIDOW SPIDER ANTIVENIN

Black widow spider antivenin is prepared from the serum of horses immunized against the venom of the black widow spider (*Lactrodectus mactans*). Each vial contains not less than 6,000 antivenin units (1 unit of antivenin will neutralize one murine lethal dose of venom).

The earliest possible use of antivenin is recommended for greatest effectiveness. If possible, the patient should be hospitalized. Supportive therapy may include warm baths, intravenous methocarbamol or 10% calcium gluconate solution to control myalgia, and diazepam to lessen extreme restlessness. Morphine may be required for pain, but since the spider venom is a neurotoxin and may cause respiratory paralysis, caution should be employed when considering the use of morphine or a barbiturate. Corticosteroids also have been used with varying results. No apparent benefit is gained by local treatment (eg, tourniquets, incision, suction).

The antivenin is indicated *only* for the treatment of envenomation due to the bite of the black widow spider. In individuals between age 16 and 60, antivenin use may be deferred and treatment with muscle relaxants considered.

A test for hypersensitivity to horse serum must be performed prior to use of this preparation (see index entry Hypersensitivity, Tests).

Black widow spider antivenin is classified in FDA Pregnancy Category C.

DOSAGE AND PREPARATIONS.

Intramuscular (anterolateral thigh): *Adults and children*, the entire contents of one container (2.5 ml restored serum) is administered. One dose usually relieves symptoms in one to three hours; a second dose may be needed.

Intravenous: This is the preferred route in severe cases, in children under 12 years, or in those in shock. The contents of the container is diluted in 10 to 50 ml of saline and administered over a 15-minute period.

Antivenin (Lactrodectus mactans) (Equine Origin) (Merck Sharp & Dohme). Powder (for suspension) containing not less than 6,000 Antivenin Units with 2.5 ml of sterile water for injection and 1 ml of normal horse serum for sensitivity testing.

VACCINES UNDER INVESTIGATION

ROTAVIRUS VACCINE LIVE ORAL ATTENUATED. In the United States, it is estimated that nearly three million children less than 5 years old experience rotavirus diarrhea each year. Of these, more than one million will have severe diarrhea, 24,000 will require hospitalization, and 150 will die (Institute of Medicine, 1985 A). Among the approximately 400 million children less than 5 years in the developing world, it is believed that about 130 million incur rotavirus diarrhea annually; in more than 18 million, the disease is at least moderately severe, and nearly 900,000 will die (Institute of Medicine, 1985 B). Although the more widespread use of oral rehydration may reduce mortality by 50%, it is obvious that an effective vaccine would be of major benefit. Field trials of at least two live attenuated vaccines employing related bovine and monkey-derived viruses have yielded promising though somewhat variable results (Institute of Medicine, 1985 B; Hanlon et al, 1987; Flores et al, 1987; Senturia et al, 1987; Biryahwaho, 1987).

VARICELLA-ZOSTER VACCINE LIVE ATTENUATED. Although a number of live varicella vaccines have been developed, the attenuated vaccine derived from the Oka strain has been most widely tested and is considered the leading candidate for licensure. The Oka strain was originally isolated in 1974 in Japan from a child with varicella. It was attenuated by passage at 34° C on human embryo fibroblasts, followed by passages at 37° C in cell cultures of guinea pig embryo cells and human diploid (WI-38) cells. Studies performed in Japan on normal and immunocompromised children and children with leukemia in remission or with solid tumors demonstrated that the vaccine was well tolerated, immunogenic, and protective against natural varicella infection.

A double-blind, placebo-controlled trial of attenuated Oka vaccine was conducted on 956 children 1 to 14 years old with no history of varicella. The vaccine was well tolerated and produced few adverse reactions in the 468 children who received it, and there was no clinical evidence of viral spread. Seroconversion was observed in 94% of vaccinated children. During a nine-month surveillance period, no vaccinated child developed varicella, whereas 39 cases occurred in placebo recipients; thus, within the limits of the study, the vaccine appeared to be 100% effective (Weibel et al, 1984). Another study in healthy children showed 96% protection upon exposure (Johnson et al, 1988). Vaccine efficacy rates of 94% to 98% have been reported in uncontrolled studies in Japan, Europe, and the United States after observation periods up to ten years (Arbeter et al, 1986). The duration of immunity following VZV immunization in healthy children was determined in a three-year study of 140 OKA/Merck vaccine recipients. Although there was a significant overall decrease in antibody titer over time, persistence of antibody for two years was observed, and the few reinfections that did occur were greatly attenuated (Johnson et al, 1989). Immunization with VZV vaccine also has induced VZV-specific memory cytotoxic T-lymphocyte responses comparable to those observed in naturally immune subjects; these responses persisted long after the primary VZV infection (Diaz et al, 1989).

The vaccine was well tolerated after administration to several thousand healthy children. Adverse reactions, which occur in 4% to 10% of vaccinees, consist of rashes, mild temperature elevations, and local reactions at the injection site. In a placebo-controlled trial in which healthy children (mean age, 16 months) were given MMR vaccine in conjunction with VZV, antibodies to all four viruses appeared in amounts comparable to those found when each of the vaccines was given alone; no significant difference was observed in the rate or extent of adverse reactions (Englund et al, 1989). Asymptomatic seroconversion after exposure to healthy vaccinees has been reported (Weibel et al, 1984). Vaccinated immunocompromised children also have been found to transmit the vaccine virus to healthy siblings, although at a low rate.

The safety and efficacy of Oka vaccine has also been investigated in children with leukemia in remission. In a study involving 191 children (mean age 6 years), there was serologic evidence of immunogenicity after one dose in about 80% of recipients and after two doses in more than 90%. The major adverse effect was a mild rash, which occurred in 36% of recipients after the first dose and in 14% after the second dose. Those with rash were more likely to transmit vaccine virus to others. The vaccine was considered to be about 80% effective in preventing clinical varicella and 100% effective in preventing severe varicella in these leukemic children (Gershon et al, 1984). A more recent study in 437 children with leukemia in remission found that seroconversion occurred in 88% after the first dose and in 98% after two doses. Some of the vaccinated patients who initially became seropositive subsequently became seronegative. The incidence of seronegativity increased with the length of time since immunization and reached 30% after five years. Varicella occurred in 8% of seropositive patients after household exposure to a family member with varicella, and in 29% of vaccinated patients who were seronegative at the time of exposure. These attack rates are considerably lower than the 80% to 90% reported for susceptible children with household exposures. Breakthrough varicella in seronegative patients was mild, with an average of 128 vesicles compared with the 250 to 500 vesicles commonly seen in otherwise healthy children with varicella. Thus, there is evidence of residual immunity in vaccinated but seronegative patients (Gershon et al, 1989). This may be a function of cell-mediated immunity, which has been reported to be long-lasting (Diaz et al, 1989).

A major uncertainty regarding the licensing of varicella vaccine in the United States is the extent to which zoster will occur later in life due to reactivation of the vaccine virus.

Zoster has occurred rarely in recipients of live varicella vaccine; only two cases were found in 4,000 or more recipients of the attenuated Oka vaccine in Japan. In the United States, one case of vaccine-induced zoster occurred in a child with acute lymphocytic leukemia almost two years after administration of the vaccine (Williams et al, 1985). More recently, two cases of zoster have occurred in healthy children vaccinated with the OKA/Merck strain approximately four years after initial immunization. Lesions were atypical, progressed from papules to crusted lesions more rapidly, and were few in number; the children were otherwise asymptomatic (Plotkin et al, 1989). A multi-institutional study in children with underlying acute lymphoblastic leukemia vaccinated with live attenuated VZV vaccine concluded that the incidence of zoster following immunization was no greater than that following natural varicella infection (Lawrence et al, 1988). Both the vaccine virus and strains isolated from vaccinated patients with malignancies who developed either varicella or zoster are as susceptible to acyclovir as wild type viruses (Shiraki et al, 1984).

Cited References

American Academy of Pediatrics: *Report of the Committee on Infectious Diseases*, ed 21. Elk Grove Village, Ill, American Academy of Pediatrics, 1988.

American Academy of Pediatrics: Policy statement. Measles: Reassessment of current immunization policy. *AAP News* 5(7):6-7, 1989.

American Academy of Pediatrics: Policy statement. Haemophilus influenzae type b conjugate vaccines: Immunization of children 2 to 15 months of age. *AAP News* 6(11):19, 23, 1990.

Ammann AJ, et al: Polyvalent pneumococcal-polysaccharide immunization of patients with sickle-cell anemia and patients with splenectomy. *N Engl J Med* 297:897-900, 1977.

Arbeter AM, et al: Varicella studies in healthy children and adults. *Pediatrics* 78(suppl):748-756, 1986.

Biryahwaho B: Trial of an attenuated bovine rotavirus vaccine (RIT 4237). *Lancet* 2:344, 1987.

Bolan G, et al: Pneumococcal vaccine efficacy in selected populations in the United States. *Ann Intern Med* 104:1-6, 1986.

Bussel JB, et al: Intravenous use of gammaglobulin in the treatment of chronic immune thrombocytopenic purpura as a means to defer splenectomy. *J Pediatr* 103:651-654, 1983.

Centers for Disease Control: Rabies vaccine, adsorbed: New rabies vaccine for use in humans. *MMWR* 37:217-218, 223, 1988.

Centers for Disease Control: Rubella vaccination during pregnancy—United States, 1971-1988. *MMWR* 38:289-293, 1989.

Centers for Disease Control: Clarification. *MMWR* 39:469, 1990.

Choo Q-L, et al: Isolation of a cDNA clone derived from a blood-borne non-A, non-B hepatitis genome. *Science* 244:359-362, 1989.

Cody CL, et al: Nature and rates of adverse reactions associated with DTP and DT immunizations in infants and children. *Pediatrics* 68:650-676, 1981.

Cooperative Group for the Study of Immunoglobulin in Chronic Lymphocytic Leukemia: Intravenous immunoglobulin for the prevention of infection in chronic lymphocytic leukemia: Randomized controlled clinical trial. *N Engl J Med* 319:902-907, 1988.

Diaz PS, et al: T lymphocyte cytotoxicity with natural varicella-zoster virus infection and after immunization with live attenuated varicella vaccine. *J Immunol* 142:636-641, 1989.

Englund JA, et al: Placebo-controlled trial of varicella vaccine given with or after measles-mumps-rubella vaccine. *J Pediatr* 114:37-44, 1989.

Fehr J, et al: Transient reversal of thrombocytopenia in idiopathic thrombocytopenic purpura by high dose intravenous gamma globulin. *N Engl J Med* 306:1254-1258, 1982.

Ferreccio C, et al: Comparative efficacy of two, three, or four doses Ty21a live oral vaccine in enteric-coated capsules: A field trial in an endemic area. *J Infect Dis* 159:766-769, 1989.

Flores J, et al: Protection against severe rotavirus diarrhea by Rhesus rotavirus vaccine in Venezuelan infants. *Lancet* 1:882-884, 1987.

Forrester HL, et al: Inefficacy of pneumococcal vaccine in high-risk populations. *Am J Med* 83:425-430, 1987.

Germanier R, Fürer E: Isolation and characterisation of Gal E mutant Ty21a of *Salmonella typhi*: A candidate strain for a live, oral typhoid vaccine. *J Infect Dis* 131:553-558, 1975.

Gershon AA, et al: Live attenuated varicella vaccine: Efficacy for children with leukemia in remission. *JAMA* 252:355-362, 1984.

Gershon AA, et al: Persistence of immunity to varicella in children with leukemia immunized with live attenuated varicella vaccine. *N Engl J Med* 320:892-897, 1989.

Gilman RH, et al: Evaluation of UPD-glucose-4-epimeraseless mutant of *Salmonella typhi* as live oral vaccine. *J Infect Dis* 136:717-723, 1977.

Greenberg MA, et al: Safe administration of mumps-measles-rubella vaccine in egg-allergic children. *J Pediatr* 113:504-506, 1988.

Griffin MR, et al: Risk of seizures and encephalopathy after immunization with the diphtheria-tetanus-pertussis vaccine. *JAMA* 263:1641-1645, 1990.

Griffith AH: Permanent brain damage and pertussis vaccination: Is the end of the saga in sight? *Vaccine* 7:199-210, 1989.

Hanlon P, et al: Trial of an attenuated bovine rotavirus vaccine (RIT 4237) in Gambian infants. *Lancet* 1:1342-1345, 1987.

Health and Public Policy Committee, American College of Physicians: Pneumococcal vaccine. *Ann Intern Med* 104:118-120, 1986.

Herman JJ, et al: Allergic reactions to measles (rubeola) vaccine in patients hypersensitive to egg protein. *J Pediatr* 102:196-198, 1983.

Hinman AR, Onorato IM: Acellular pertussis vaccines. *Pediatr Infect Dis J* 6:341-343, 1987.

Immunization Practices Advisory Committee (ACIP): Poliomyelitis prevention. *MMWR* 31:22-26, 31-34, 1982.

Immunization Practices Advisory Committee (ACIP): Varicella-zoster immune globulin for prevention of chickenpox. *MMWR* 33:84-100, 1984 A.

Immunization Practices Advisory Committee (ACIP): Rubella prevention. *MMWR* 33:301-310, 315-318, 1984 B.

Immunization Practices Advisory Committee (ACIP): Rabies prevention—United States, 1984. *MMWR* 33:393-402, 408, 1984 C.

Immunization Practices Advisory Committee (ACIP): Meningococcal vaccines. *MMWR* 34:255-259, 1985 A.

Immunization Practices Advisory Committee (ACIP): Diphtheria, tetanus, and pertussis: Guidelines for vaccine prophylaxis and other preventive measures. *MMWR* 34:405-426, 1985 B.

Immunization Practices Advisory Committee (ACIP): New recommended schedule for active immunization of normal infants and children. *MMWR* 35:577-579, 1986 A.

Immunization Practices Advisory Committee (ACIP): Rabies prevention: Supplementary statement on the preexposure use of human diploid rabies vaccine by the intradermal route. *MMWR* 35:767-768, 1986 B.

Immunization Practices Advisory Committee (ACIP): Pertussis immunization: Family history of convulsions and use of antipyretics—supplementary ACIP statement. *MMWR* 36:281-282, 1987 A.

Immunization Practices Advisory Committee (ACIP): Poliomyelitis prevention: Enhanced-potency inactivated poliomyelitis vaccine—supplementary statement. *MMWR* 36:795-897, 1987 B.

Immunization Practices Advisory Committee (ACIP): Update: Prevention of *Haemophilus influenzae* type b disease. *MMWR* 37:13-16, 1988 A.

Immunization Practices Advisory Committee (ACIP): Prevention of perinatal transmission of hepatitis B virus: Prenatal screening of all pregnant women for hepatitis B surface antigen. *MMWR* 37:341-351, 1988 B.

Immunization Practices Advisory Committee (ACIP): Use of BCG vaccines in the control of tuberculosis: A joint statement by the ACIP and the advisory committee for elimination of tuberculosis. *MMWR* 37:663-675, 1988 C.

Immunization Practices Advisory Committee (ACIP): Cholera vaccine. *MMWR* 37:617-624, 1988 D.

Immunization Practices Advisory Committee (ACIP): Measles prevention: Recommendations of the Immunization Practices Advisory Committee (ACIP). *MMWR* 38 (suppl S-9):1-18, 1989 A.

Immunization Practices Advisory Committee (ACIP): Pneumococcal polysaccharide vaccine. *MMWR* 38:64-68, 73-76, 1989 B.

Immunization Practices Advisory Committee (ACIP): General recommendations on immunization. *MMWR* 38:205-214, 219-227, 1989 C.

Immunization Practices Advisory Committee (ACIP): Mumps prevention. *MMWR* 38:388-392, 397-400, 1989 D.

Immunization Practices Advisory Committee (ACIP): Supplementary statement: Change in administration schedule for haemophilus b conjugate vaccines. *MMWR* 39:232-233, 1990 A.

Immunization Practices Advisory Committee (ACIP): Protection against viral hepatitis: Recommendations of the Immunization Practices Advisory Committee (ACIP). *MMWR* 39 (No. RR-2):1-26, 1990 B.

Immunization Practices Advisory Committee (ACIP): Yellow fever vaccine: Recommendations of the Immunization Practices Advisory Committee (ACIP). *MMWR* 39 (No. RR-6):1-6, 1990 C.

Immunization Practices Advisory Committee (ACIP): Diphtheria, tetanus, and pertussis: Guidelines for vaccine use and other preventive measures. *MMWR* (in press) 1991 A.

Immunization Practices Advisory Committee (ACIP): Haemophilus b conjugate vaccine for prevention of *Haemophilus influenzae* type b disease in infants 2 months of age and older. *MMWR* (in press) 1991 B.

Institute of Medicine: *New Vaccine Development. Establishing Priorities. Vol I. Diseases of Importance in the United States.* Washington, DC, National Academy Press, 1985 A, 410-423.

Institute of Medicine: *New Vaccine Development. Establishing Priorities. Vol II. Diseases of Importance in Developing Countries.* Washington, DC, National Academy Press, 1985 B, 308-318.

Johnson CE, et al: Live attenuated varicella vaccine in 12 to 24 month-old children. *Pediatrics* 81:512-518, 1988.

Johnson C, et al: Humoral immunity and clinical reinfections following varicella vaccine in healthy children. *Pediatrics* 84:418-421, 1989.

Karzon DT, Edwards KM: Diphtheria outbreaks in immunized populations, editorial. *N Engl J Med* 318:41-43, 1988.

Kuo G, et al: An assay for circulating antibodies to a major etiologic virus of human non-A, non-B hepatitis. *Science* 244:362-364, 1989.

Lawrence R, et al: The risk of zoster after varicella vaccination in children with leukemia. *N Engl J Med* 318:543-548, 1988.

Levine MM, et al: The efficacy of attenuated *S. typhi* oral vaccine strain Ty21a evaluated in controlled field trials, in Holmgren J, et al (eds): *Development of Vaccines and Drugs Against Diarrhea.* Lund, Sweden, Studentlitteratur, 1986, 90-101.

Levine MM, et al: Large-scale field trial of Ty21a live oral typhoid vaccine in enteric-coated capsule formulation. *Lancet* 1:1049-1052, 1987.

Long SS, et al: Longitudinal study of adverse reactions following diphtheria-tetanus-pertussis vaccine in infancy. *Pediatrics* 85:294-302, 1990.

Madore DC, et al: Safety and immunologic response to *Haemophilus influenzae* type b oligosaccharide-CRM_{197} conjugate vaccine in 1- to 6-month-old infants. *Pediatrics* 85:331-337, 1990.

Miller DL, et al: Pertussis immunization and serious acute neurological illness in children. *Br Med J* 282:1595-1599, 1981.

Pappaioanou M, et al: Antibody response to preexposure human diploid-cell rabies vaccine given concurrently with chloroquine. *N Engl J Med* 314:280-284, 1986.

Patriarca PA, et al: Efficacy of influenza vaccine in nursing homes: Reduction in illness and complications during influenzae A (H3N2) epidemic. *JAMA* 253:1136-1139, 1985.

Peltola H, et al: Prevention of *Haemophilus influenzae* type b bacteremic infections with the capsular polysaccharide vaccine. *N Engl J Med* 310:1561-1566, 1984.

Plotkin SA, et al: Zoster in normal children after varicella vaccine. *J Infect Dis* 159:1000-1001, 1989.

Pollock TM, et al: A seven year study of disorders attributed to vaccination in the North West Thames region. *Lancet* 1:753-757, 1983.

Rappolt RT, et al: Medical toxicologist's notebook: Snakebite treatment and international antivenin index. *Clin Toxicol* 13:409-438, 1978.

Rappuoli R, et al: Molecular epidemiology of the 1984-1986 outbreak of diphtheria in Sweden. *N Engl J Med* 318:12-14, 1988.

Redmond SR, Pichichero ME: *Haemophilus influenzae* type b disease: Epidemiologic study with special reference to day-care centers. *JAMA* 252:2581-2584, 1984.

Reyes GR, et al: Isolation of a cDNA from the virus responsible for enterically transmitted non-A, non-B hepatitis. *Science* 247:1335-1339, 1990.

Ross E, Miller D: Risk and pertussis vaccine, letter. *Arch Dis Child* 61:98-99, 1986.

Russell FE: *Snake Venom Poisoning.* Great Neck, NY, Scholium International, 1983.

Senturia, et al: Live attenuated rotavirus vaccines. *Lancet* 2:1091-1092, 1987.

Shapiro ED, Clemens JD: Controlled evaluation of protective efficacy of pneumococcal vaccine for patients at high risk of serious pneumococcal infections. *Ann Intern Med* 101:325-330, 1984.

Shields WD, et al: Relationship of pertussis immunization to the onset of neurologic disorders: A retrospective epidemiologic study. *Pediatrics* 113:801-805, 1988.

Shiraki K, et al: Susceptibility to acyclovir of Oka-strain varicella vaccine and vaccine-derived viruses isolated from immunocompromised patients, letter. *J Infect Dis* 150:306-307, 1984.

Simberkoff MS, et al: Efficacy of pneumococcal vaccine in high-risk patients: Results of a Veterans Administration Cooperative Study. *N Engl J Med* 315:1318-1327, 1986.

Sims RV, et al: The clinical effectiveness of pneumococcal vaccine in the elderly. *Ann Intern Med* 108:653-657, 1988.

Sisk JE, Riegelman RK: Cost effectiveness of vaccination against pneumococcal pneumonia: Update. *Ann Intern Med* 104:79-86, 1986.

Stiehm ER, et al: Intravenous immunoglobulins as therapeutic agents. *Ann Intern Med* 107:367-382, 1987.

Wahden MH, et al: A controlled field trial of live *Salmonella typhi* strain Ty21a oral vaccine against typhoid: Three-year results. *J Infect Dis* 145:292-296, 1982.

Walker AM, et al: Neurologic events following diphtheria-tetanus-pertussis immunization. *Pediatrics* 81:345-349, 1988.

Ward JI, et al: *Haemophilus influenzae* type b vaccines: Lessons for the future. *Pediatrics* 81:886-893, 1988.

Weibel RE, et al: Live attenuated varicella virus vaccine: Efficacy trial in healthy children. *N Engl J Med* 310:1409-1415, 1984.

Weissberg JI, et al: Survival in chronic hepatitis B: Analysis of 379 patients. *Ann Intern Med* 101:613-616, 1984.

Williams DL, et al: Herpes zoster following varicella vaccine in child with acute lymphocytic leukemia. *J Pediatr* 106:259-261, 1985.

Wingert WA, Wainschel J: Diagnosis and management of envenomation by poisonous snakes. *South Med J* 68:1015-1026, 1975.

World Health Organization: Special programme on AIDS and expanded programme on immunization—joint statement: Consultation on human immunodeficiency virus (HIV) and routine childhood immunization. *Wkly Epidemiol Rec* 62:297-299, 1987.

Other Selected References

Venomous bites and stings. *J Toxicol Clin Toxicol* 21:417-560, 1983-1984.

American College of Physicians Task Force on Adult Immunization and Infectious Disease Society of America: *Guide for Adult Immunization*, ed 2. Philadelphia, American College of Physicians, 1990.

Immunization Practices Advisory Committee (ACIP): *Adult Immunization*. Atlanta, Centers for Disease Control, 1985.

Lerner RA, et al (eds): *Vaccines 85: Molecular and Chemical Basis of Resistance to Parasitic, Bacterial, and Viral Diseases*. New York, Cold Spring Harbor Laboratory, 1985.

Plotkin SA, Mortimer EA Jr (eds): *Vaccines*. Philadelphia, WB Saunders, 1988.

New Evaluation

CYTOMEGALOVIRUS IMMUNE GLOBULIN INTRAVENOUS (HUMAN)
[CytoGam]

Cytomegalovirus (CMV) infection is a significant hazard for recipients of bone marrow, liver, or cardiac allografts and is the major viral pathogen encountered in renal transplant recipients. In immunosuppressed patients, CMV can cause retinitis, gastrointestinal ulcerations, leukopenia, hepatitis, and life-threatening pneumonitis. In renal transplant patients, CMV infection also has been associated with fungal or parasitic superinfections and loss of the graft. Attempts at active immunization with CMV vaccine generally have been disappointing. Passive immunization with CMV immune globulin provides an alternative approach.

In 1979, a method was devised to extract CMV immune globulin from selected normal donor blood and to concentrate specific antibody by about 20-fold (Zaia et al, 1979). Subsequently, a preparation suitable for intravenous administration was found to be safe and to raise CMV serum antibody titers significantly (Snydman et al, 1984). The current product, CMV immune globulin intravenous (CMV-IGIV), is a sterile lyophilized powder of IgG stabilized with sucrose 5% and human albumin 1%. It contains no preservative. The purified IgG is derived from pooled adult human plasma selected for high antibody titers for CMV. The pooled plasma is fractionated by ethanol precipitation of the proteins according to Cohn methods 6 and 9, modified to yield a product suitable for intravenous administration. Each milliliter of the reconstituted product contains 50 ± 10 mg of immunoglobulin, principally IgG, and trace amounts of IgA and IgM.

ACTIONS AND USES. In seronegative individuals who may be exposed to CMV, CMV-IGIV raises the relevant antibodies to levels sufficient to attenuate or reduce the incidence of serious CMV disease associated with renal transplantation. It is indicated for recipients who are seronegative for CMV and who receive a kidney from a CMV seropositive donor. Approximately 60% of untreated, seronegative recipients of kidneys from seropositive donors would be expected to develop CMV disease; clinical studies have shown that when such recipients are given CMV-IGIV, there is a 50% reduction in the expected incidence of primary CMV disease.

The effectiveness of CMV-IGIV prophylaxis in renal transplant recipients has been demonstrated in two clinical trials. In the first, a randomized clinical trial, the overall incidence of virologically confirmed CMV-associated disease was reduced from 60% in the controls to 21% in recipients of CMV-IGIV and of serious CMV disease from 46% to 13% (Snydman et al, 1987). This included reduction in the frequency of leukopenia, hepatitis, CMV pneumonia, and thrombocytopenia. Fungal and parasitic infections did not develop in the immunoglobulin recipients but occurred in 20% of the controls. In a subsequent nonrandomized prospective trial, the incidence of virologically confirmed CMV-associated syndrome in renal transplant patients was 36% in the CMV-IGIV recipients. The results in seronegative recipients were the same as in the preceding trial with regard to CMV-associated pneumonia, hepatitis, and concomitant fungal and parasitic superinfection (Snydman et al, 1988).

The efficacy of CMV-IGIV in liver, bone marrow, or cardiac allograft recipients or in preventing reactivation of latent infection in CMV-seropositive renal transplant patients has not been established.

ADVERSE REACTIONS. Flushing, chills, muscle cramps, back pain, fever, nausea, vomiting, and wheezing were observed most frequently during clinical trials. The incidence was <5% for all infusions, and these minor reactions most often were related to infusion rates. Angioedema and anaphylactic shock are possibilities, although neither has been observed in clinical trials.

PRECAUTIONS. CMV-IGIV should not be given to individuals with a history of a prior severe reaction associated with the administration of a human immunoglobulin preparation. Individuals with selective IgA deficiency have the potential ability to develop antibodies to IgA and, therefore, could have anaphylactic reactions to subsequent administration of blood products containing IgA. The patient's vital signs should be monitored continuously throughout the infusion. If hypotension or anaphylaxis occurs, the infusion should be discontinued immediately and epinephrine and diphenhydramine administered. The infusion schedule should be adhered to closely.

Animal reproduction studies have not been conducted with CMV-IGIV. Also, it is not known whether this product can harm the fetus if it is administered to a pregnant woman or can affect reproductive function. CMV-IGIV should be given to pregnant women only if clearly indicated (FDA Pregnancy Category C).

DRUG INTERACTIONS. Antibodies present in this and other immunoglobulin preparations may interfere with the immune response to live virus vaccines and, therefore, vaccination with live virus vaccines should be deferred until three months after the administration of CMV-IGIV. Revaccination may be necessary if the vaccine was administered shortly after this product was given. Admixtures of CMV-IGIV with other drugs have not been evaluated; thus, it is recommended that CMV-IGIV be administered separately.

DOSAGE AND PREPARATIONS. The infusion should begin within six hours after reconstitution of the lyophilized powder and completed within 12 hours. CMV-IGIV should be administered through an intravenous line (preferably a separate intravenous line) using a constant infusion pump (ie, IVAC pump or equivalent). Predilution is not recommended.

Intravenous: *Adults,* the maximum recommended dosage per infusion is 150 mg/kg administered according to the following schedule:

Within 72 hours of transplant:	150 mg/kg
2 weeks post-transplant:	100 mg/kg
4 weeks post-transplant:	100 mg/kg
6 weeks post-transplant:	100 mg/kg
8 weeks post-transplant:	100 mg/kg
12 weeks post-transplant:	50 mg/kg
16 weeks post-transplant:	50 mg/kg

The initial dose is given at a rate of 15 mg/kg/hr. If no untoward reactions occur within 30 minutes, the infusion rate may be increased to 30 mg/kg/hr. If no untoward reactions occur within a subsequent 30 minutes, the infusion rate may be increased to 60 mg/kg/hr. For subsequent doses, CMV-IGIV may be administered at a rate of 15 mg/kg/hr for 15 minutes. If no untoward reactions occur, the rate may be increased to 30 mg/kg/hr for 15 minutes and then to a final maximum rate of 60 mg/kg/hr. For both initial and subsequent doses, *the rate of administration should not exceed 75 ml/hr.*

CytoGam (Massachusetts Public Health Biologic Laboratories [manufacturer], Connaught Laboratories, Inc [distributor]). Powder (lyophilized) containing 2.5 g ± 250 mg in single-dose vials for reconstitution with 50 ml sterile water for injection, U.S.P.

Cited References

Snydman DR, et al: A pilot trial of a novel cytomegalovirus immune globulin in renal transplant recipients. *Transplantation* 38:553-557, 1984.

Snydman DR, et al: Use of cytomegalovirus immune globulin to prevent cytomegalovirus disease in renal transplant recipients. *N Engl J Med* 317:1049-1054, 1987.

Snydman DR, et al: A further analysis of primary cytomegalovirus disease prevention in renal transplant recipients with a cytomegalovirus immune globulin: Interim comparison of a randomized and an open-label trial. *Transplant Proc* 20(suppl 8):24-30, (Dec) 1988.

Zaia JA, et al: Cytomegalovirus immune globulin: Production from selected normal donor blood. *Transplantation* 27:66-67, 1979.

Principles of Cancer Chemotherapy

87

In the past half century, since the reduction of death rates due to infectious diseases, cancer has emerged as one of the leading causes of death in industrial societies. In the United States, cancer ranks second to heart disease in overall mortality and is the leading cause of death in women age 35 to 74 years and in nonaccidental deaths of children age 1 to 14 years (Silverberg et al, 1990). Research during the past decade has significantly increased understanding of the molecular, genetic, and cellular factors that contribute to the development of cancer. Of particular note is the convergence of formerly disparate lines of investigation that suggests similarities in the mechanisms of neoplastic transformation by carcinogenic chemicals and tumor-causing viruses (Bishop, 1987). Novel therapeutic approaches resulting from this new knowledge are being investigated and, in a few instances, have progressed to clinical trials. Although many forms of cancer can be cured with the therapeutic modalities available at this time, achievements for many others (mostly solid tumors) are limited to modest increases in lifespan or palliation of symptoms. In the next decade, increased understanding of the molecular and cellular biology of cancer should result in more effective therapy and improved cure rates.

All cancers are malignant tumors characterized by an unlimited growth potential that is not under normal regulatory controls and an ability to expand locally by invasion of surrounding tissues and systemically by metastasis to distant sites. There is disagreement at present on whether the primary defects in malignant cells are in the mechanisms regulating cell proliferation or in those responsible for terminal differentiation. It seems likely that both are important but that malignancies may vary in the relative contributions of unrestrained growth or arrested differentiation to the underlying process of neoplastic transformation. Although this issue is not resolved, induction of tumor cell differentiation is an active area of investigation for new antineoplastic drug development (Pierce and Speers, 1988), and several agents that possess this ability are now in clinical trials.

Studies on the molecular and cellular biology of cancer have identified a large number of normal cellular genes (termed proto-oncogenes or c-*onc* genes) whose expression at quantitatively increased levels, in inappropriate tissues, or in an untimely fashion can lead to neoplastic transformation (Bishop, 1987; Weinberg, 1989; Park and Vande Woude, 1989). Altered expression can result from chemically induced mutations in DNA sequences that regulate transcription of these genes (Weinstein, 1988) or from chromosomal rearrangements that either remove normal regulatory sequences or introduce aberrant regulatory elements near the gene in question (Croce, 1986; Rowley, 1989, 1990). In addition, amplification of a c-*onc* gene, which can multiply its copy number manyfold, can lead to its overexpression and possibly to neoplasia (Seemayer and Cavenee, 1989). Alternatively, viral transduction can juxtapose c-*onc* genes with viral regulatory elements to generate a transforming viral oncogene (v-*onc*) (Bishop, 1987; Weinberg, 1989; Howley, 1989).

Cancer also can result from mutations induced by chemicals (Weinstein, 1988; Pitot, 1989) or by ionizing radiation (Fry, 1989) in the coding sequences of some c-*onc* genes that alter the function of their protein gene products. Similarly, viral transduction of gene fragments, which retain sequences coding for the catalytic portions of the corresponding c-*onc* proteins but have lost those segments involved in regulating the proteins' activity, also can lead to the production of v-*onc* genes (Bishop, 1987; Weinberg, 1989; Howley, 1989). In addition, inactivation of genes whose products have a negative effect on rates of cell proliferation (often termed tumor suppressor genes or anti-oncogenes) can contribute to oncogenesis (Sager, 1989; Skuse and Rowley, 1989). The multistep nature of carcinogenesis, which includes initiation, promotion, and progression of tumor growth, suggests that sequential genetic alterations resulting in two or more activated oncogenes (or activated oncogenes and inactivated suppressor genes) are required for development of a malignancy (Weinstein, 1988; Weinberg, 1989).

The intracellular functions of many of the oncogene-encoded proteins can be divided into four broad categories (Druker et al, 1989; Park and Vande Woude, 1989; Roberts and Sporn, 1989). A number of oncogenes code either for growth factors (eg, *sis*, which codes for a subunit of platelet-derived growth factor) or for transmembrane receptors for growth factors (eg, *erb*B, which codes for the epidermal growth factor receptor). There also is one known oncogene that codes for a cytoplasmic hormone receptor (*erb*A, the thyroid hormone receptor). A large number of oncogene proteins are involved in transducing signals originating with ligand binding at membrane receptors in the interior of the cell; their presence ultimately results in altered expression of specific regulated genes within the nucleus. This group includes enzymatic activities associated with various transmembrane proteins (eg, the protein tyrosine kinases of the *src* family of oncogenes); membrane-associated guanine nucleotide binding proteins, which regulate the activities of other signal-transducing enzymes (eg, the *ras* oncogenes); and cytoplasmic enzymes involved in signal transduction (eg, the serine/threonine protein kinases such as those encoded by the *mos* oncogene). The final group includes a number of nuclear proteins that are thought to act as regulators of transcription for specific classes of genes involved in regulating either proliferation or differentiation (eg, the *myc* and *fos* oncogenes). As research into the basic molecular and cellular biology of cancer progresses, therapeutic agents that attack each of these altered steps of the signal transduction pathways in a tumor-specific fashion should become available (Roberts and Sporn, 1989).

Depending on the organ system and cell type involved, each form of cancer has a unique natural history, pattern of spread, and response to therapy. Therefore, the physician treating cancer is faced with not one but a multiplicity of diseases with a broad range of prognoses and potential treatments. When additional factors, such as extent of disease (eg, size of primary tumor, status of lymph nodes, presence or absence of metastasis) and patient characteristics, are considered for each case, it becomes apparent that the treatment of cancer is challenging even to the experienced oncologist.

The most important decision in developing a treatment plan for the patient with cancer is to determine whether the goal is cure or palliation (eg, increased survival time, alleviation of symptoms, maintenance of close to normal function). When cure is considered possible, therapy must be appropriate and aggressive. The underlying principle of curative cancer therapy is the removal or eradication of the last neoplastic cell, since it appears that a single clonogenic malignant cell is capable of multiplying and eventually killing the host by the volume of its progeny (Skipper et al, 1964). Palliative therapy should provide benefits to the patient that outweigh the risks of treatment, and it ranges from aggressive chemotherapy to no treatment at all.

Three major therapeutic modalities are currently employed in cancer treatment: surgery, radiation therapy (including hyperthermia), and chemotherapy (including hormones). Surgery and/or radiation usually are the initial treatment modalities for most solid cancers, particularly when cure is anticipated. However, surgical extirpation or irradiation of malignant tissue only eliminates localized and regional disease. Of the 930,000 patients with cancer diagnosed in 1986 (the most recent year for which follow-up data are available), 598,000 (64%) had what appeared to be localized or operable cancer and were initially treated by surgery and/or local irradiation. Of these, 373,000 (62%) are likely to remain tumor-free five years after treatment (DeVita, 1989). The remaining 225,000 patients, whose tumors did or will recur after localized therapy, undoubtedly harbored undetectable disseminated tumor (micrometastases) at the time of diagnosis. They, together with the 332,000 patients with inoperable tumors or with metastases detected at the time of diagnosis (or 60% of all new cases), cannot be cured by localized therapy alone and are candidates for systemic chemotherapy.

Anticancer drugs can be effective in systemic neoplastic disease. Increased understanding of the pharmacology and mechanisms of action of a number of antineoplastic agents has led to the rational application of these drugs, most often in combination chemotherapy. Chemotherapy has been the primary treatment modality for most patients with hematologic malignancies (eg, leukemia, lymphomas) for some time. By the early 1970s, combination chemotherapy had improved five-year survival rates to approximately 50% or more for newly diagnosed patients with disseminated Hodgkin's disease, childhood acute lymphocytic leukemia, and Burkitt's lymphoma. By the end of that decade, five-year survival rates also approached or exceeded 50% for some forms of disseminated non-Hodgkin's lymphoma (Frei, 1985; Silverberg et al, 1990).

Curative regimens for treatment of some hematologic malignancies were developed rather early in the history of cancer chemotherapy. In contrast, during much of that period chemotherapy for solid neoplasms was limited to those tumors unresponsive to surgery and radiation therapy. Although antineoplastic drugs are still widely used for palliation of certain disseminated cancers, for more than a decade greater emphasis has been placed on optimal chemotherapy to produce a cure. Germ cell tumors were found to be particularly sensitive to antineoplastic drugs, and approximately 70% of disseminated testicular cancers were curable by combination chemotherapy following orchiectomy (Einhorn, 1981; for more recent reviews see Loehrer et al, 1988; Williams et al, 1989). Chemotherapy combined with surgery and/or irradiation, termed combined modality therapy, has increased survival rates for a number of solid tumors. Although the greatest success has been achieved with relatively uncommon solid tumors in children (eg, Wilms' tumor, Ewing's sarcoma, embryonal rhabdomyosarcoma), survival also has been prolonged in many other cancers (eg, osteogenic sarcoma, breast cancer, colorectal carcinoma, uterine cancer, prostatic adenocarcinoma, bladder cancer) (Silverberg et al, 1990).

This chapter is divided into three sections: determinants of response to cancer chemotherapy; drug selection, with a brief overview of current chemotherapy for a number of cancers, including combination and adjuvant chemotherapy; and shared toxicities associated with the use of antineoplastic agents. Evaluations of individual antineoplastic drugs, including investigational agents, are presented in the following four chapters.

DETERMINANTS OF RESPONSE TO CANCER CHEMOTHERAPY

The goal of cancer chemotherapy is to achieve selective toxicity against malignant tumor cells and to spare normal host cells. Selective toxicity of the degree associated with bacterial chemotherapy has not been possible in chemotherapy of cancers, however, because the differences between normal and malignant cells are much more subtle. With few exceptions, antineoplastic agents suppress proliferating cells, and toxicity to dividing normal cells (eg, bone marrow, gastrointestinal and germinal epithelia, hair follicles, lymphoid organs) is a routine consequence of cancer chemotherapy. Thus, successful treatment depends on killing malignant tumor cells with doses that allow recovery of normal proliferating cells. Although many successes in cancer chemotherapy have been the result of empiricism, rationales for drug treatment based on tumor determinants, particularly cell kinetics, and pharmacologic and host factors have clearly evolved. For more detailed discussions, see Pratt and Ruddon, 1979; Carter et al, 1981; Lane, 1985; Riggs, 1986 A and B; DeVita, 1989; Chabner and Myers, 1989; Tannock, 1989; Haskell, 1990 A; Chabner, 1990; Collins, 1990.

Tumor Determinants

Growth Fraction, Gompertzian Growth Curves: Rapidly growing cancers (eg, certain leukemias and lymphomas, choriocarcinoma, testicular cancer) are more susceptible to killing by antineoplastic agents than slower growing cancers (eg, non-small cell lung, colon, breast). A major determinant of the time required for a malignant tumor to double its volume, ie, the mass doubling time, is its growth fraction, which is defined as the percentage of viable cells in active cell division. For most solid tumors, the growth fraction declines as the tumor grows larger. Actively dividing tumor cells usually are most sensitive to cytotoxic anticancer drugs. Certain normal tissues (eg, bone marrow, gastrointestinal mucosa, hair follicles) with high growth fractions also are susceptible to these drugs. Thus, the difference in growth fractions between tumor and normal cell populations may be an important factor in determining the outcome of chemotherapy. When active drugs are given in the proper schedule, tumors with a high growth fraction can be treated successfully with acceptable toxicity to normal tissues. This usually is not the case for tumors with low growth fractions, however.

Based on experimental tumor models, the growth curves of most cancers follow a Gompertzian function, ie, growth at every instant is exponential but with a growth constant that simultaneously is exponentially slowing. Thus, the doubling time increases as the tumor volume increases. This is probably due to depletion of nutrients resulting in both increased cell loss and, more important, decreased growth fraction. Because it is estimated that a tumor must be 1 cm in diameter and contain approximately 1×10^8 to 1×10^9 cells to be diagnosed clinically, many human cancers, particularly solid tumors, are approaching the plateau phase of the Gompertzian growth curve when they are diagnosed. Thus, the effectiveness of chemotherapy is further diminished by the smaller growth fractions associated with the relatively large tumors present at initial diagnosis.

The model implies that smaller tumors are more sensitive to chemotherapy and has provided a rationale for the treatment approaches now employed clinically. One approach is to remove large tumor volumes by surgery or irradiation (debulking) in the hope that the remaining cells will be stimulated into active division and, therefore, be susceptible to chemotherapy. This has been termed recruitment. Another approach (adjuvant chemotherapy) is to treat certain high-risk patients who have apparently local or regional disease with chemotherapy shortly after removing the primary tumor by surgery or irradiation (Salmon, 1987). Because it is common for metastases to develop eventually after surgery or irradiation alone, adjuvant chemotherapy is initiated when metastases are too small to be detected (micrometastases) and presumed to have large growth fractions.

Tumor Burden, Fractional Cell-kill Hypothesis: In addition to a decreased growth fraction, a large tumor burden imposes additional problems for effective chemotherapy: therapeutic concentrations of drug may not be able to penetrate large tumors, metastases are more likely to have occurred, greater heterogeneity within the tumor cell population increases the potential for drug resistance, and there are more tumor cells that must be killed. The last point deserves particular attention. In animal tumor models, it has been shown that antineoplastic drugs kill tumor cells by first-order kinetics, ie, a given dose of drug kills a constant fraction, rather than a constant number, of tumor cells. In other words, the same dose that can reduce the tumor burden from 1×10^{12} to 1×10^9 cells would be required to lower the number from 1×10^9 to 1×10^6 cells. Furthermore, one remaining viable tumor cell has the ability to repopulate and eventually kill the host.

The clinical implication of these cytokinetic data is that successful chemotherapy is most likely when the tumor burden is low. Also, since the dose-response curves for most antineoplastic drugs are quite steep, the use of maximally tolerated doses with optimal scheduling is critical to obtain the highest log kill of tumor cells compatible with recovery of normal proliferating cells. Even when other reasons for treatment failure are disregarded, cure of cancer by chemotherapy cannot be accomplished if tumor cells repopulate more quickly than normal cells.

Presently, quantitative cytokinetic data on human cancers are considerably less accurate than those on experimental tumors. Estimation of total tumor burden, particularly for solid tumors, can be subject to considerable error. This is also true for estimates of cell kill (eg, by measuring numbers of remaining leukemia cells or the decrease in size of a solid tumor) and rate of tumor cell repopulation (eg, by determining time to recurrence). Heterogeneity within tumor cell populations increases the imprecision. Furthermore, although the steep dose-response relationships observed for most anticancer drugs in experimental systems, which are the basis for the use of high-dose intermittent treatment scheduling, appear to hold true for human cancers, some exceptions have been observed. Thus, it is difficult to determine optimal dose, interval, and duration of treatment clinically. Although past knowledge should be utilized, certain assumptions and empiric decisions are often necessary.

Antineoplastic Agents and the Cell Cycle: To understand why only certain cells in a tumor are susceptible to some drugs and how different drugs act, the phases of the cell cycle must be considered. All actively dividing cells pass through certain phases from one mitosis to the next. The first part of the interphase after completion of cell division is the G_1 phase, during which DNA synthesis has not yet begun but RNA and protein synthesis continue normally. In late G_1, there is a burst of RNA synthesis and the S phase begins, during which cellular DNA is replicated. After completion of the S phase, a cell enters the G_2 period. During this phase, the cell is tetraploid (ie, it contains twice the DNA content) and continues to synthesize RNA and protein. In mitosis (M phase), RNA and protein synthesis diminish abruptly while genetic material is condensed into chromosomes and then segregated into daughter cells. After completion of mitosis, a cell may re-enter the G_1 phase and continue to proliferate, or the cell may enter a resting state, usually termed the G_0 phase. Some resting cells lose their ability to proliferate and are irreversibly out of cycle; others retain the potential to produce an unlimited line of descendants and are the so-called clonogenic or stem cells. The sensitivity of actively dividing cells to cytotoxic antineoplastic agents and the importance of a large growth fraction to the success of chemotherapy have been discussed. Resting clonogenic cells also are very important because they are most likely to survive chemotherapy and are necessary for the recovery of proliferating normal tissues; however, they also can repopulate the tumor, resulting in disease recurrence. Thus, the persistence of resting clonogenic tumor cells is a likely cause of chemotherapeutic failures.

A number of antineoplastic drugs are effective primarily during a specific part of the cell cycle and are classified as cell cycle phase specific drugs. For example, cytarabine and hydroxyurea are S phase specific, ie, they exert their cytotoxic effects only on dividing cells in the S phase of the cell cycle. Other drugs, such as methotrexate and mercaptopurine, are also S phase specific, but their effects are self-limiting because they have other inhibitory actions that slow the entry of cells into the S phase. The mitotic spindle inhibitors, vincristine and vinblastine, are M phase specific drugs. Phase specific anticancer drugs are only effective against actively dividing cells; therefore, cytotoxic concentrations of these drugs must be maintained long enough to expose a sufficient fraction of the tumor cells during their passage through the sensitive phase. Some phase specific drugs (fluorouracil, cytarabine, and occasionally vinblastine) are administered by continuous infusion rather than as a bolus because of their cell cycle specificity.

The remaining antineoplastic drugs usually are considered to be cell cycle phase nonspecific and include alkylating agents, most antitumor antibiotics, platinum complexes, and procarbazine. Distinctions are more relative than absolute, however, and many phase nonspecific agents are somewhat more effective against proliferating cells or those in a specific phase of the cell cycle. For example, if alkylated DNA of a resting clonogenic tumor cell is repaired prior to entry of the cell into the DNA replicative cycle, that cell will be unaffected by the alkylating agent. Thus, quiescent tumor cells are relatively resistant to the cytocidal effects of most alkylating agents (with the exception of the chloroethylnitrosoureas).

In animal tumor models, effective chemotherapeutic regimens have been developed on the basis of known cell cycle specificities of various antineoplastic agents. For example, when mice bearing L1210 leukemia cells were given vinblastine followed 16 hours later by cytarabine, therapeutic effectiveness was enhanced markedly (Vadlamudi and Goldin, 1971). Enhanced activity was not observed when the drugs were given at the same time. The explanation for these observations was that vinblastine transiently arrested cells in the M phase resulting in a synchronized cell population. About 16 hours later, essentially all of the cells entered the S phase and were sensitive to the effects of cytarabine. Thus, sequencing and timing of this two-drug combination were critical to its enhanced effectiveness. Clinical application of this approach requires a tumor with a large growth fraction. In addition, concomitant synchronization of normal proliferating cells (eg, bone marrow) should be avoided to obtain a selective antitumor effect. In practice, it is unclear whether combination regimens that utilize schedules designed to achieve and exploit partial in vivo tumor cell synchronization can be administered in a tumor-selective manner. It also is unclear whether such regimens have contributed significantly to longer survival time.

Tumor Cell Heterogeneity, Phenotypic Instability: It is now well established that human tumors do not consist of a collection of identical cells but instead are composed of various subpopulations that differ from each other in a number of important characteristics (Heppner and Miller, 1989). Neoplastic cells within individual tumors are both genetically (clonally) and structurally or organizationally (secularly) heterogeneous. Secular heterogeneity results from microenvironmental variations within the tumor (eg, concentration gradients of nutrients, growth factors, oxygen, cellular waste products). Some of these variations are, at least partially, due to irregular vascularization within solid tumors. Secular heterogeneity affects rates of cell proliferation, intracellular drug concentrations, cell cycle phase distributions, growth fractions, and other parameters in different regions within a solid tumor. These variations, in turn, may alter the antitumor drug sensitivity of cells located in different microenvironments.

Sensitivity to antineoplastic agents within tumors also may differ because of clonal heterogeneity. Variations in expression of antitumor drug targets, drug activating or inactivating enzymes, growth factors and their receptors, and surface antigens are among the more obvious examples of phenotypic differences within a tumor that can contribute to heterogeneity in drug sensitivity between cells. Other cell-to-cell differences that may affect clinical outcome include karyotypes, morphologies, and metastatic potentials. Furthermore, interaction between the various subpopulations within a tumor may affect the responses of individual cells to chemotherapeutic drugs.

Undoubtedly, the inherent genetic and phenotypic instability (clonal evolution) of tumors (Nowell, 1989), which results in progressive changes in their biologic behavior, also contributes to tumor heterogeneity and differential drug sensitivity. The observation that many malignant tumors are aneuploid and that aneuploidy may be a reliable prognostic indicator for some tumors (Merkel and McGuire, 1990) may be related to clonal evolution and phenotypic instability in human cancer. Tumor evolution may, in turn, contribute to the increase in metastatic potential during tumor progression (Killion and Fidler, 1989). It also is possible that mutations induced by DNA-damaging antitumor drugs in cells that survive initial treatment can further exacerbate clonal evolution and tumor cell heterogeneity. Together, the various sources and mechanisms of tumor cell heterogeneity provide a sound rationale for combination chemotherapy to minimize the survival of drug-resistant cells within tumors.

Resistance: The presence of drug-resistant tumor cells is an important factor in the success or failure of cancer chemotherapy. A mathematical model has been developed (Goldie and Coldman, 1979) for drug resistance in tumor cell populations, in which the likelihood of finding a single cell with resistance to a specific drug is related to both population size and frequency of mutation. Given the number of cells present within most tumors at the time of diagnosis, it seems likely that a resistant subpopulation will be present for each individual chemotherapeutic drug. Antineoplastic agents exert a positive selective pressure on tumor cell populations; replication of drug-resistant clones can result in drug-resistant tumors and therapeutic failures. In addition to such acquired resistance, some tumors may be intrinsically resistant to certain antineoplastic drugs.

Some identified mechanisms of resistance are decreased cellular uptake or enhanced efflux (many drugs), increased (methotrexate) or decreased (etoposide) levels of target enzyme, altered affinity for target enzyme (methotrexate), decreased activation of drug (mercaptopurine and fluorouracil), increased inactivation of drug (cytarabine), increased DNA repair (alkylating agents), and increased utilization of salvage pathways for purine and pyrimidine biosynthesis (antimetabolites).

Tumor cells may develop multiple drug resistance (Moscow and Cowan, 1988). Exposure to a single drug may result in selection of cells that are cross-resistant to a number of structurally unrelated compounds with different mechanisms of action. It appears that in one form of multiple drug resistance the surviving cells have impaired ability to accumulate and retain drug. A high-molecular-weight "P-glycoprotein" is present in elevated levels in the plasma membrane of the resistant cells and functions as a drug efflux pump (Deuchars and Ling, 1989; van der Bliek and Borst, 1989). A related protein is a carrier for histidine and other small molecules in bacteria. This type of multiple drug resistance may be an example of mechanisms that have evolved to protect organisms against naturally occurring toxins. Reversal of efflux-mediated drug resistance has been reported using calcium channel blocking agents (Dalton et al, 1989) and calmodulin inhibitors. The basis for this reversal involves competitive inhibition of P-glycoprotein pump activity.

Two other mechanisms that contribute to multiple drug resistance have been identified (Moscow and Cowan, 1988). In the first, increased concentrations of glutathione may lead to enhanced formation of inactive glutathione-drug conjugates for some alkylating agents, platinum compounds, and certain antibiotics (Arrick and Nathan, 1984; Kramer et al, 1988). In the second, reduced levels of the enzyme DNA topoisomerase II lead to decreased DNA damage on treatment with one of the many drugs (eg, anthracyclines, epipodophyllotoxins) that inhibit the enzyme (Ross et al, 1988; Liu, 1989).

To minimize the effects of drug resistance, combinations of drugs having different mechanisms of action that are individually effective against the specific tumor are employed and therapy is initiated when the tumor burden is small (see the section on Combination Chemotherapy).

Pharmacologic Determinants

The effectiveness of an antineoplastic agent is related directly to its pharmacologic disposition in the patient. For cytotoxic antineoplastic agents, tumoricidal concentrations must reach the tumor cells and remain there for a sufficient time to kill these cells. Agents such as interferon and other biological response modifiers may act by noncytotoxic mechanisms, and their effects on tumor cells may persist after concentrations fall below minimally active levels.

As with other drug classes, basic principles of pharmacology apply to anticancer drugs. The attainment of therapeutic concentrations inside the tumor cell depends on absorption (eg, for oral preparations), plasma protein binding, distribution to various organs, rates of excretion (eg, renal, biliary) and metabolic transformation, and a drug's ability to penetrate into the (solid) tumor and cross individual tumor cell membranes. The following examples illustrate the importance of these factors.

Cyclophosphamide is a prodrug that must be metabolized by the hepatic mixed-function oxidase system before active drug can be generated. Mechlorethamine, dactinomycin, daunorubicin, and doxorubicin are very reactive chemically and must be administered intravenously to obtain a systemic effect and avoid local tissue necrosis. Cytarabine has an extremely short serum half-life (eg, 12 minutes for the initial phase) due to rapid inactivation by cytidine deaminase, particularly in the liver. Thus, this drug often is administered by continuous intravenous infusion to maintain effective concentrations. Continuous infusion of a variety of chemotherapeutic agents is now relatively common in the treatment of certain tumors; a review is available (Lokich, 1990).

Nitrosoureas and procarbazine are among the few antineoplastic drugs that cross the blood-brain barrier in sufficient concentrations to be useful in brain tumors. High-dose methotrexate and cytarabine also may reach potentially cytotoxic concentrations in the central nervous system. When most other antineoplastic agents are used systemically, the central nervous system may provide a pharmacologic sanctuary for tumor cells, which can lead to relapse. For this reason, in addition to systemic therapy, intrathecal methotrexate and/or cytosine arabinoside and central nervous system radiation therapy are given prophylactically to prevent relapses in the central nervous system in children with acute lymphocytic leukemia. However, invasive tumors may disrupt the blood-brain barrier allowing for greater drug delivery.

Low blood flow to parts of large (ischemic) tumors often prevents adequate drug penetration to all tumor cells in the mass. For tumors confined to the pleural or peritoneal cavities, intracavitary chemotherapy may allow high local concentrations of drug with acceptable systemic levels (Markman, 1985; Markman et al, 1989). Other approaches to regional administration of antitumor drugs include intravesical delivery for bladder cancer; intra-arterial infusion for liver metastases (hepatic artery), brain tumors (carotid artery), and other cancers; and intraportal vein delivery for liver metastases. Some of these approaches to treatment (eg, hepatic artery or portal vein delivery) have not yet been conclusively shown to improve survival compared with systemic chemotherapy and thus should only be used in controlled clinical trials (O'Connell, 1990).

Finally, a sufficient concentration of most drugs must cross the individual tumor cell membrane to reach the site of action inside the cell. If the permeability barrier is too formidable, the drug will not be effective. Large doses of methotrexate are necessary to attain effective concentrations in cultured osteogenic sarcoma cells, in part because of poor transport across the sarcoma cell membrane. Usually, such amounts would be prohibitively toxic to normal cells (eg, bone marrow). However, the subsequent administration of leucovorin, which enters normal and malignant cells via the carrier-mediated transport mechanism that is more active in normal cells than in sarcoma cells, bypasses the inhibition of dihydrofolate reductase by methotrexate in normal cells and "rescues" them from the cytotoxic antimetabolite. Thus, differences in membrane transport have been exploited to therapeutic advantage, although the clinical efficacy of this approach remains controversial (see index entry Methotrexate, Uses, Cancer).

The attainment of selectively tumoricidal or growth inhibitory concentrations of an antineoplastic drug requires consideration of additional complicating factors. As discussed earlier, not all tumor cells are susceptible to a specific anticancer drug at any given time (eg, only S phase cells are sensitive to cytarabine), and a certain percentage of dividing normal cells are likely to be killed. Furthermore, both tumor and normal cell growth kinetics will be perturbed by drug administration and subsequent drug sensitivities may be altered. Thus, dosage schedules must be optimized to yield a maximum tumor cell kill with minimum lethality to normal cells.

Host Determinants

A number of host factors also influence the response to cancer chemotherapy. Among the most important is the overall performance status (eg, Karnofsky scale) of the patient. Generally, individuals who are asymptomatic and ambulatory and who show no evidence of disease (eg, performance score of 100) are likely to have the best response to chemotherapy. As disease symptoms increase and the ability to function normally decreases, the prognosis for successful therapy diminishes. Patients who are disabled and require special care and assistance (eg, performance score of 40 or less) are less likely to improve significantly with chemotherapy. Thus, for most cancers, patients who are diagnosed early have a greater chance for prolonged survival and possible cure.

The patient's immune status, particularly cell-mediated immunity, is another important correlate of response to chemotherapy; among patients with some types of tumors, immunocompetent individuals appear to respond more favorably than immunocompromised patients. Determination of immune status is complicated because the neoplastic disease produces immunologic defects, and most antineoplastic drugs are immunosuppressive due to their antiproliferative effect on blood cell-forming tissues. Generally, maintenance of immunocompetence has been accomplished most often by using intensive, intermittent, chemotherapy regimens in which time is allowed for recovery of these normal tissues.

Patients who have not received prior radiation or chemotherapy almost invariably experience a better response than previously treated patients. Prior treatments that reduce bone marrow reserves usually decrease tolerance of myelosuppression caused by antineoplastic agents. The immune status also is more likely to be compromised. Furthermore, prior chemotherapy may result in selection of multiple-drug resistant cells. As a result, the first attempt at therapy should be with maximally tolerated doses and optimal scheduling, particularly when cure is anticipated. Supportive measures, including transfusions (see index entry Transfusion Therapy), autologous or allogeneic bone marrow transplantation, administration of recombinant human hematopoietic colony-stimulating factors to decrease the severity and duration of neutropenia (see index entry Growth Factors, Hematopoietic), antimicrobial chemotherapy, total parenteral nutrition, therapy for the hypercalcemia of malignancy (see index entry Hypercalcemia, Treatment), and administration of allopurinol to prevent uric acid-induced renal disease, may increase the likelihood of success.

Other patient characteristics that influence the response to chemotherapy include age, sex, race, organ function, and the presence of other diseases. For example, the functional status of organs that are involved in drug elimination or are particularly susceptible to drug toxicity must be considered. The dosage of methotrexate and vincristine may have to be reduced in patients with impaired renal or hepatic function, respectively, because these drugs are eliminated primarily by the kidneys or liver. Similarly, doxorubicin, bleomycin, and cisplatin are examples of drugs that must be administered with caution or avoided in patients with pre-existing cardiac, pulmonary, or renal disease, respectively, because of their direct toxic effects on these organs.

DRUG SELECTION

A large number of antineoplastic agents are currently available for use in various cancers. The individual drugs are listed in Table 1 according to class, and important properties of each drug are summarized. Some antineoplastic drugs (eg, cyclophosphamide, methotrexate, vincristine, doxorubicin) have broad spectrums of activity and are used in the treatment of many hematologic and solid cancers. In contrast, the use of other drugs is limited due to their narrow spectrum of activity (eg, mitotane for adrenocortical tissue, streptozocin for beta cells of the islets of Langerhans) or undesirable toxicologic (eg, plicamycin) or pharmacologic (eg, mechlorethamine) properties.

A primary determinant of antineoplastic drug selection clinically is the sensitivity of a particular cancer to the various drugs. General knowledge of tumor sensitivities primarily has been obtained empirically in clinical trials. Although a reasonably reliable prediction can be made, individual tumors may not respond, resulting in chemotherapeutic failure. Analogous to susceptibility testing for bacteria, specific in vitro chemosensitivity testing for an individual patient's tumor has been investigated for some time (Von Hoff, 1990), and both clonogenic and nonclonogenic assays have been adapted for this purpose. Only two prospective trials have compared patient responses when treatment was based on the results of in vitro predictive assays with those in patients treated empirically with standard drug regimens (Von Hoff et al, 1990; Gazdar et al, 1990). Patient selection for the two treatment strategies was random only in the first trial (Von Hoff et al, 1990). Neither trial focused on previously untreated patients whose initial therapy was chosen either empirically or on the basis of results of in vitro testing.

For second-line therapy in patients with advanced metastatic malignancies, the rate of objective responses (partial remissions) was significantly higher in those for whom drug choice was based on in vitro test results than in those treated empirically (Von Hoff et al, 1990). However, the improved response rate did not result in increased survival time for patients given drugs to which their tumors responded when cultured. Nevertheless, analysis of a large number of retrospective studies correlating the results of in vitro assays with patient responses to chemotherapy suggests that predictive drug sensitivity assays to choose initial therapy may increase the response rates and may ultimately lead to improved survival time for patients with some cancers (Von Hoff, 1990). A prospective trial to test this hypothesis is in progress. At present, however, the usefulness of routine drug sensitivity testing in cancer patients has not been established.

In contrast to the status of chemosensitivity assays, predictions of patient responses to therapy based on measurement of drug receptors in biopsy specimens are more established in the management of endocrine-responsive tumors. The first assay that provided clinically useful predictive information was the measurement of estrogen receptor (ER) levels in breast tumor specimens (Jordan et al, 1988).

Patients with ER-negative tumors (about one-third of all breast cancers in postmenopausal women) are not likely to respond to hormonal therapy and such patients are usually treated with cytotoxic chemotherapy. Patients with ER-positive tumors often receive hormonal therapy, although the presence of estrogen receptors accurately predicts response in only about 50% of these cases. More recent studies suggest that concomitant measurement of tumor progesterone receptors may improve predictive capability, since the presence of both indicates that the ER is functional in the breast tumor cells.

Certain cancers, particularly those with a high growth fraction, are quite sensitive to chemotherapy. These include acute leukemias, lymphomas, many pediatric solid tumors, germ cell tumors, and small cell lung, ovarian, and breast carcinomas. Patients, even those with a poorer performance status, who have these types of cancers usually should be treated because of the possibility of a complete response leading to prolonged survival and, in some cases, cure. Consistent with the principles outlined in the preceding section, the first attempt at therapy should aim for maximal effectiveness, even if it is likely to be the most toxic. Drugs should be used in the largest possible doses to ensure an optimal tumor cell kill and should be administered by the routes and in the schedules designed to provide optimal selective toxicity to the tumors.

Many solid cancers, including renal, pancreatic, colorectal, and non-small cell lung carcinomas and melanomas, remain relatively refractory to chemotherapy. For patients with these types of cancers, other factors (eg, performance status, age, extent of disease, expected drug-induced toxicity) must be considered before initiating chemotherapy. If chemotherapy is elected, participation in a therapeutic research protocol is the best approach.

Some of the currently preferred regimens for various cancers are listed in Table 2, which provides an overview of the role of chemotherapy in the treatment of different neoplastic diseases and gives the reader some knowledge of the drugs and drug combinations being used most often. For many of the diseases listed, chemotherapy is neither the first nor the only therapeutic measure used. Comprehensive texts such as those listed under Other Selected References should be consulted for detailed information on global treatment strategies for individual tumor types. Also, for many cancers (eg, non-Hodgkin's lymphomas) the number and variety of combination regimens currently are too large to allow for their com-

TABLE 1.
SPECIFIC AGENTS USED IN CANCER CHEMOTHERAPY[1]

Drug	Cell Cycle Specificity	Route (s) of Administration	Elimination
DNA DAMAGING AGENTS			
Nitrogen Mustards			
Chlorambucil [Leukeran]	Phase nonspecific	Oral	Hepatic metabolism
Cyclophosphamide (CTX) [Cytoxan, Neosar]	Phase nonspecific	Intravenous, oral	Hepatic metabolism
Ifosfamide [Ifex]	Phase nonspecific	Intravenous	Hepatic metabolism
Mechlorethamine Hydrochloride (HN_2, Nitrogen Mustard) [Mustargen]	Phase nonspecific	Intravenous, intracavitary, topical	Chemical decomposition (hydrolysis)
Melphalan (L-PAM, Phenylalanine Mustard) [Alkeran]	Phase nonspecific	Oral, intravenous	Hepatic metabolism
Aziridine Derivative			
Thiotepa	Phase nonspecific	Intravenous, intracavitary, intravesical, intrathecal	Hepatic metabolism
Alkyl Sulfonate			
Busulfan [Myleran]	Phase nonspecific	Oral	Hepatic metabolism and chemical decomposition
Methyl Hydrazine Derivative			
Procarbazine Hydrochloride [Matulane]	Phase nonspecific	Oral	Hepatic metabolism

Major Toxicity[2]		
Acute	**Delayed**	**Indications**
Mild nausea and vomiting; seizures	*Bone marrow depression* (leukopenia, thrombocytopenia, anemia); carcinogenesis (secondary malignancies); immunosuppression; hepatic toxicity; sterility; pulmonary infiltrates and fibrosis (rare)	Chronic lymphocytic leukemia; Hodgkin's and non-Hodgkin's lymphomas
Nausea and vomiting; hemorrhagic cardiomyopathy when used in large doses to ablate the bone marrow before transplantation	*Bone marrow depression* (primarily leukopenia; thrombocytopenia is less severe); alopecia; hemorrhagic cystitis; carcinogenesis (secondary malignancies); sterility; immunosuppression; teratogenesis; inappropriate ADH secretion; pulmonary infiltrates and fibrosis	Acute and chronic leukemias; in large doses, marrow ablation in preparation for bone marrow transplants; Hodgkin's, non-Hodgkin's, and Burkitt's lymphomas; multiple myeloma; choriocarcinoma; testicular cancer; breast, lung, ovarian, endometrial, and cervical carcinomas; Ewing's and soft tissue sarcomas; rhabdomyosarcoma; neuroblastoma
Nausea and vomiting; central nervous system effects including temporary confusion, mutism, and extrapyramidal symptoms; nephrotoxicity; metabolic acidosis	*Bone marrow depression;* hemorrhagic cystitis (risk is reduced by simultaneous administration of mesna); alopecia; inappropriate ADH secretion; neurotoxicity; teratogenesis; sterility; rickets in children	Lung, breast, ovarian, and testicular carcinomas; embryonal rhabdomyosarcoma; Ewing's, soft tissue, and osteogenic sarcomas; Hodgkin's and non-Hodgkin's lymphomas; acute leukemias
Nausea and vomiting; local reactions and phlebitis due to vesicant action	*Bone marrow depression* (leukopenia, thrombocytopenia); alopecia; diarrhea; oral ulcers; sterility; carcinogenesis (secondary malignancies); venous hyperpigmentation; immunosuppression	Hodgkin's, non-Hodgkin's, mycosis fungoides, and cutaneous T-cell lymphomas
Mild nausea and vomiting; hypersensitivity reactions; renal damage when used in large doses to ablate the bone marrow before transplantation	*Bone marrow depression* (leukopenia, thrombocytopenia, anemia); pulmonary infiltrates and fibrosis; carcinogenesis (secondary malignancies); sterility; immunosuppression	Multiple myeloma; breast and ovarian carcinomas; in large doses, marrow ablation in preparation for bone marrow transplants
Mild nausea and vomiting; local pain	*Bone marrow depression* (leukopenia, thrombocytopenia, anemia); menstrual dysfunction; interference with spermatogenesis; sterility	Hodgkin's disease; breast and ovarian carcinomas; bladder (intravesically); carcinomatous meningitis; in large doses, marrow ablation in preparation for bone marrow transplants
Mild nausea and vomiting; diarrhea (rare); seizures when used in large doses to ablate the bone marrow before transplantation	*Bone marrow depression* (leukopenia, thrombocytopenia, anemia); pulmonary fibrosis; hyperpigmentation of skin; alopecia; gynecomastia; ovarian failure; azoospermia; cataracts; Addisonian syndrome; sterility	Chronic myelogenous leukemia; in large doses, marrow ablation in preparation for bone marrow transplants
Nausea and vomiting; CNS depression; disulfiram-like effect with alcohol; hypertensive reactions and other interactions with sympathomimetic agents and tricyclic antidepressants resulting from monoamine oxidase inhibition	*Bone marrow depression* (leukopenia, thrombocytopenia, anemia; myelosuppression may be delayed); stomatitis; neurologic toxicity (CNS depression, peripheral neuropathy, myalgia, arthralgia); dermatitis; pneumonitis; sterility; carcinogenesis (secondary malignancies); teratogenesis; immunosuppression	Hodgkin's and non-Hodgkin's lymphomas; brain tumors; small cell lung carcinoma

(table continued on next page)

TABLE 1 (continued)

Drug	Cell Cycle Specificity	Route(s) of Administration	Elimination
Nitrosoureas			
Carmustine (BCNU) [BiCNU]	Phase nonspecific	Intravenous	Chemical decomposition and hepatic metabolism
Lomustine (CCNU) [CeeNU]	Phase nonspecific	Oral	Chemical decomposition and hepatic metabolism
Streptozocin (Streptozotocin) [Zanosar]	Phase nonspecific	Intravenous	Renal
Platinum Complexes			
Cisplatin (Cis-platinum, CDDP) [Platinol]	Phase nonspecific	Intravenous	Renal
Carboplatin (CBDCA) [Paraplatin]	Phase nonspecific	Intravenous	Chemical reaction and renal excretion
Triazenes			
Dacarbazine (DIC, DTIC) [DTIC-Dome]	Phase nonspecific	Intravenous	Metabolic
Altretamine (Hexamethylmelamine) [Hexalen]	Phase nonspecific	Oral	Hepatic metabolism and renal excretion
Sulfhydryl Uroprotective Agent			
Mesna [Mesnex]		Intravenous	Renal
ANTIMETABOLITES			
Folic Acid Analogues			
Methotrexate, Methotrexate Sodium (MTX, Amethopterin) [Folex, Mexate]	S phase specific but self-limiting	Intravenous, intramuscular, oral, intrathecal	Primarily renal; some hepatic

Major Toxicity[2]		
Acute	**Delayed**	**Indications**
Nausea and vomiting; local phlebitis	*Delayed leukopenia and thrombocytopenia* (may be prolonged, myelosuppression is cumulative); pulmonary fibrosis (may be irreversible); delayed renal damage; hepatic toxicity; sterility; hemolytic-uremic syndrome	Brain tumors; Hodgkin's and non-Hodgkin's lymphomas; multiple myeloma; advanced gastric and colorectal carcinomas refractory to other therapies; melanoma
Nausea and vomiting	*Delayed (4 to 6 weeks) leukopenia and thrombocytopenia* (may be prolonged, myelosuppression is cumulative); renal and hepatic toxicity; neurologic reactions; pulmonary fibrosis; sterility	Brain tumors; Hodgkin's and non-Hodgkin's lymphomas; advanced lung and colorectal carcinomas refractory to other drugs; melanoma
Nausea and vomiting; local pain; chills and fever	*Renal toxicity* (common); bone marrow depression (uncommon and usually mild); hepatotoxicity; hyperglycemia; hypoglycemia; diarrhea; eosinophilia; sterility	Islet cell carcinoma; malignant carcinoid; pancreatic carcinoma; Hodgkin's disease
Nausea and vomiting (often severe and prolonged); fever; hypersensitivity reactions including anaphylaxis	*Nephrotoxicity including renal failure;* ototoxicity including hearing loss; bone marrow depression (leukopenia, thrombocytopenia, anemia); peripheral neuropathy; hypomagnesemia and hypocalcemia; hypokalemia; hemolytic anemia; Raynaud's syndrome; sterility; hemolytic-uremic syndrome	Testicular cancer; ovarian, bladder, cervical, head and neck, small cell and non-small cell lung, uterine, gastric, breast, and esophageal carcinomas; osteogenic sarcoma; non-Hodgkin's lymphomas; brain tumors
Mild nausea and vomiting	*Myelosuppression* (thrombocytopenia); peripheral neuropathy (uncommon); hearing deficits; hemolytic anemia	Primary and recurrent ovarian cancer; small cell and non-small cell lung cancer; head and neck and testicular carcinomas
Nausea and vomiting; local pain; diarrhea; anaphylaxis (rare)	*Bone marrow depression* (leukopenia, thrombocytopenia); "flu-like" syndrome; alopecia; renal impairment; hepatic necrosis; photosensitivity; paresthesia; facial flushing; rash; hepatic vein thrombosis (Budd-Chiari syndrome)	Hodgkin's disease; melanoma; soft tissue sarcomas; neuroblastoma; islet cell carcinoma; malignant carcinoid syndrome
Nausea and vomiting; anorexia; diarrhea	Neurotoxicity (peripheral neuropathy, weakness, paresthesias, mood alterations); mild myelosuppression (leukopenia, thrombocytopenia)	Second line therapy for palliation of persistent or recurrent ovarian cancer
Nausea and vomiting; diarrhea	None	Prophylaxis of ifosfamide- or cyclophosphamide-induced hemorrhagic cystitis
Mild nausea and vomiting; diarrhea; acute hypersensitivity reactions; fever; renal toxicity with large doses	*Bone marrow depression* (leukopenia, anemia, thrombocytopenia); oral and gastrointestinal ulceration; renal tubular necrosis; hepatic fibrosis; pneumonitis; osteoporosis	Choriocarcinoma; acute lymphocytic and myeloid leukemias; Hodgkin's and non-Hodgkin's lymphomas; osteogenic sarcoma; rhabdomyosarcoma; head and neck, breast, lung, cervical, ovarian, and bladder carcinomas; medulloblastoma; meningeal leukemia

(table continued on next page)

TABLE 1 (continued)

Drug	Cell Cycle Specificity	Route(s) of Administration	Elimination
Leucovorin Calcium (Folinic acid) [Wellcovorin]	Phase nonspecific	Oral, intramuscular, intravenous	Metabolic and renal
Pyrimidine Analogues			
Cytarabine (Ara C, Cytosine Arabinoside) [Cytosar-U, Tarabine PFS]	S phase specific	Intravenous, subcutaneous, intrathecal	Metabolic; renal after large doses
Floxuridine [FUDR]	Phase nonspecific but acts on proliferating cells (cycle specific)	Intrahepatic artery; intravenous	Metabolic
Fluorouracil (5-FU) [Adrucil]	Phase nonspecific but acts on proliferating cells (cycle specific)	Intravenous; intrahepatic artery	Metabolic
Purine Analogues			
Cladribine (2-chlorodeoxyadenosine; 2-CldA) [Leustatin]	Cycle nonspecific	Intravenous	Some renal; remainder not known
Fludarabine Phosphate (2-Fl-AMP) [Fludara]	S phase specific	Intravenous	Metabolic followed by renal clearance of metabolite(s)
Mercaptopurine (6-MP) [Purinethol]	S phase specific but self-limiting	Oral, intravenous	Metabolic
Pentostatin (2-deoxycoformycin) [Nipent]	Phase nonspecific	Intravenous	Primarily renal; some metabolic

Major Toxicity[2]		
Acute	**Delayed**	**Indications**
Allergic reactions (rash, hives, pruritus, wheezing) (uncommon)	None	Rescue after high-dose methotrexate therapy for osteogenic or Ewing's sarcoma, non-Hodgkin's lymphomas and gestational trophoblastic, breast, or head and neck tumors; for biochemical modulation of tumor responses to fluorouracil therapy for advanced colon, head and neck, squamous cell, gastric, and breast carcinomas; protection of bone marrow after intrathecal methotrexate
Nausea and vomiting; fever; anaphylaxis (hypersensitivity) (rare); diarrhea	*Bone marrow depression* (leukopenia, thrombocytopenia, anemia, megaloblastosis); stomatitis; hepatic dysfunction; conjunctivitis; pulmonary edema, encephalopathy, pancreatitis, and cerebellar toxicity with high doses	Acute lymphocytic and myeloid leukemias; non-Hodgkin's lymphomas; meningeal leukemia
Nausea and vomiting; diarrhea	*Bone marrow depression* (leukopenia, thrombocytopenia, anemia); *oral and gastrointestinal ulceration;* alopecia; hyperpigmentation; dermatitis; cerebellar ataxia; hepatotoxicity; sclerosing cholangitis	Liver metastases of gastrointestinal tumors; hepatocellular carcinoma; gastrointestinal carcinoma
Nausea and vomiting; diarrhea; hypersensitivity reaction (rare)	*Bone marrow depression* (leukopenia, thrombocytopenia, anemia); *oral and gastrointestinal ulceration;* cholestasis and rarely hepatic necrosis; alopecia; hyperpigmentation; dermatitis; cerebellar ataxia; "hand-foot" syndrome (palmar-plantar erythrodysesthesia); conjunctivitis; arrhythmias; coronary artery spasm with angina or myocardial infarction (rare); gastrointestinal toxicity may be exacerbated when used with biochemical modulators (eg, leucovorin)	Breast, colorectal, anal, gastric, pancreatic, esophageal, hepatocellular, ovarian, endometrial, cervical, prostate, bladder, and head and neck carcinomas; liver metastases of gastrointestinal tumors
Occasional chills, fatigue, or headache; nausea with larger doses	*Bone marrow depression* (neutropenia, thrombocytopenia); fever; neurologic toxicity and renal damage with larger doses	Hairy cell leukemia; refractory chronic lymphocytic leukemia; refractory low-grade non-Hodgkin's or cutaneous T-cell lymphomas
Nausea and vomiting (mild); fever, chills, fatigue, pain, diarrhea, weakness, rash (all rare)	*Bone marrow depression* (neutropenia, anemia, thrombocytopenia); immunosuppression; stomatitis; central nervous system toxicity and renal damage with higher doses	Chronic lymphocytic leukemia (refractory to standard therapy); refractory low-grade non-Hodgkin's lymphomas
Nausea, vomiting, and diarrhea (can be dose-limiting with bolus injection)	*Bone marrow depression* (particularly leukopenia; also thrombocytopenia, anemia); hepatotoxicity; allopurinol may increase half-life	Acute lymphocytic and myeloid leukemias; chronic myelogenous leukemia
Nausea and vomiting (mild); fever, fatigue, rash, pain, diarrhea, headache, chills (all rare)	*Bone marrow depression* (leukopenia, anemia, thrombocytopenia); immunosuppression; nephrotoxicity, central nervous system depression, hepatic and/or renal dysfunction, anorexia, respiratory failure, arthralgia, myalgia, photophobia, conjunctivitis (all rare at usual doses, more frequent at larger doses)	Hairy cell leukemia

(table continued on next page)

TABLE 1 (continued)

Drug	Cell Cycle Specificity	Route(s) of Administration	Elimination
Thioguanine (6-TG)	S phase specific	Oral, intravenous	Metabolic
Ribonucleotide Reductase Inhibitor			
Hydroxyurea [Hydrea]	S phase specific	Oral	Primarily renal
NATURAL PRODUCTS AND THEIR ANALOGUES			
Antibiotics and Synthetic Derivatives			
Bleomycin Sulfate [Blenoxane]	Phase nonspecific	Intravenous, intramuscular, subcutaneous, intracavitary	Primarily renal; some metabolic
Dactinomycin (Actinomycin D) [Cosmegen]	Cycle nonspecific	Intravenous, isolation-perfusion	Biliary and renal
Daunorubicin Hydrochloride [Cerubidine]	Cycle nonspecific but S phase most sensitive	Intravenous	Metabolic and biliary; some renal
Doxorubicin Hydrochloride [Adriamycin]	Cycle nonspecific but S phase most sensitive	Intravenous	Metabolic and biliary
Idarubicin Hydrochloride [Idamycin]	Cycle nonspecific but S phase probably most sensitive	Intravenous	Metabolism followed by biliary and renal excretion
Mitomycin [Mutamycin]	Cycle nonspecific but late G_1 and early S phases most sensitive	Intravenous	Metabolic

Major Toxicity[2]		
Acute	**Delayed**	**Indications**
Occasional nausea and vomiting	*Bone marrow depression* (leukopenia, thrombocytopenia, anemia); cholestasis; stomatitis	Acute myeloid, chronic myelogenous, and acute lymphocytic leukemias
Mild nausea and vomiting	*Bone marrow depression* (leukopenia, thrombocytopenia, anemia, megaloblastosis); stomatitis; alopecia; hyperpigmentation; neurologic disturbances (rare)	Chronic myelogenous leukemia; cervical carcinoma; polycythemia vera; essential thrombocythemia
Mild nausea and vomiting (uncommon); fever; anaphylaxis and other hypersensitivity reactions	*Pneumonitis and pulmonary fibrosis;* rash and hyperpigmentation; stomatitis; alopecia; Raynaud's phenomenon; synergistic enhancement of oxygen-induced pulmonary damage in patients treated with cumulative doses ≥360 mg	Hodgkin's and non-Hodgkin's lymphomas; testicular cancer; squamous cell carcinomas (eg, head and neck, cervix, esophagus)
Nausea and vomiting; diarrhea; local irritation and phlebitis; anaphylactoid reaction	*Bone marrow depression* (leukopenia, thrombocytopenia, anemia); *oral and gastrointestinal mucositis;* alopecia; folliculitis; dermatitis in previously irradiated areas	Choriocarcinoma; Wilms' tumor; Ewing's, osteogenic, and soft tissue sarcomas; rhabdomyosarcoma; testicular cancer
Nausea and vomiting, diarrhea; red urine (drug metabolite; not hematuria); transient EKG changes; severe local tissue damage and necrosis on extravasation	*Bone marrow depression* (leukopenia, thrombocytopenia, anemia); cardiac toxicity including irreversible congestive heart failure (total cumulative dose should not exceed 750 mg/M^2); alopecia; stomatitis; fever and chills; dermatitis on previously irradiated areas	Acute myeloid and lymphocytic leukemias; neuroblastoma
Nausea and vomiting; diarrhea; red urine (drug metabolite; not hematuria); transient EKG changes; severe local tissue damage and necrosis on extravasation; ventricular arrhythmia	*Bone marrow depression* (leukopenia, thrombocytopenia, anemia); cardiac toxicity including irreversible congestive heart failure (total cumulative dose should not exceed 550 mg/M^2); alopecia; stomatitis; fever and chills; pigmentation in extremities; dermatitis in previously irradiated areas	Acute myeloid and lymphocytic leukemias; Hodgkin's and non-Hodgkin's lymphomas; multiple myeloma; breast, lung, gastric, pancreatic, hepatocellular, bladder, prostatic, ovarian, endometrial, cervical, and thyroid carcinomas; osteogenic, Ewing's, and soft tissue sarcomas; rhabdomyosarcoma; Wilms' tumor; neuroblastoma
Nausea and vomiting; diarrhea and abdominal cramps; transient EKG changes; severe local tissue damage and necrosis on extravasation; ventricular arrhythmia; headache; red urine (not hematuria)	*Bone marrow depression* (leukopenia more frequent than thrombocytopenia); cardiac toxicity including irreversible congestive heart failure (maximal cumulative dose not yet established); alopecia; mucositis and stomatitis; transient changes in tests of renal and hepatic function; pulmonary toxicity; dermatologic toxicity; impaired mental status; fever	Acute myeloid leukemia in adults
Nausea and vomiting; local irritant	*Bone marrow depression* (cumulative leukopenia, thrombocytopenia; also anemia); alopecia; stomatitis; renal toxicity; pulmonary toxicity; hemolytic-uremic syndrome; worsens anthracycline-induced cardiomyopathy	Gastric, colorectal, anal, pancreatic, esophageal, lung, breast, cervical, and bladder carcinomas

(table continued on next page)

TABLE 1 (continued)

Drug	Cell Cycle Specificity	Route(s) of Administration	Elimination
Mitoxantrone Hydrochloride [Novantrone]	Cycle nonspecific but late G_1 and G_2 phases most sensitive	Intravenous	Biliary and renal
Plicamycin (Mithramycin) [Mithracin]	Cycle nonspecific; S phase probably most sensitive	Intravenous	Metabolic
Plant Alkaloids and Derivatives			
Vinblastine Sulfate (VLB) [Velban, Velsar]	M phase specific	Intravenous	Metabolic and biliary
Vincristine Sulfate (VCR) [Oncovin, Vincasar]	M phase specific	Intravenous	Metabolic and biliary
Etoposide (VP-16, VP-16-213) [VePesid]	Appears to act primarily in G_2 phase; possibly in late S or M phases as well	Intravenous, oral	Liver and renal (uncertain)
Paclitaxel [Taxol]	M phase specific	Intravenous	Not known
Teniposide (VM-26) [Vumon]	Late S or early G_2 phases	Intravenous	Metabolic and renal
Enzyme			
Asparaginase [Elspar]	Postmitotic G_1 phase specific	Intravenous, intramuscular	Metabolic

Major Toxicity[2]		
Acute	**Delayed**	**Indications**
Blue-green coloration of urine and sclera; nausea, vomiting, and diarrhea; stomatitis	*Bone marrow depression* (leukopenia and thrombocytopenia); cardiotoxicity; alopecia; hepatotoxicity; renal failure	Acute myeloid leukemias; breast cancer; non-Hodgkin's lymphomas
Nausea and vomiting; diarrhea; fever	*Bone marrow depression* (thrombocytopenia most marked; also, leukopenia and anemia); coagulation defects resulting in *hemorrhagic diathesis* (can occur in the absence of thrombocytopenia); hepatotoxicity; hypocalcemia; CNS toxicity; skin rashes and fever; renal toxicity	Hypercalcemia of malignancy; embryonal cell carcinoma of the testes (no longer recommended for this indication since other less toxic, more effective regimens are available)
Nausea and vomiting; local reaction and phlebitis with extravasation	*Bone marrow depression* (primarily leukopenia); mucositis; alopecia; neurologic toxicity as for vincristine but much less common; muscle pain; paralytic ileus; jaw pain	Hodgkin's and non-Hodgkin's lymphomas; testicular cancer; choriocarcinoma; breast carcinoma; mycosis fungoides; Kaposi's sarcoma (AIDS-related); Langerhans cell histiocytosis (histiocytosis X or Letterer-Siwe disease); non-small cell lung cancer
Local irritant	*Neurologic toxicity* including peripheral neuropathy (eg, areflexia, muscular weakness, peripheral neuritis), paralytic ileus, cranial nerve palsies; alopecia; inappropriate ADH secretion (rare); negligible bone marrow depression	Acute and chronic lymphocytic leukemias; Hodgkin's and non-Hodgkin's lymphomas; small cell lung and breast carcinomas; Ewing's, Kaposi's (AIDS-related), and soft tissue sarcomas; rhabdomyosarcoma; Wilms' tumor; neuroblastoma
Mild nausea and vomiting; hypotension with rapid infusion; diarrhea; fever; metabolic acidosis (large doses)	*Bone marrow depression* (primarily leukopenia; also thrombocytopenia, anemia); alopecia; peripheral neuropathy; hepatic damage at high concentrations; stomatitis (after large doses)	Testicular cancer; lung carcinoma (particularly small cell); choriocarcinoma; acute myeloid leukemia; non-Hodgkin's lymphomas; embryonal rhabdomyosarcoma; Ewing's and Kaposi's (AIDS-related) sarcomas; in large doses, marrow ablation in preparation for bone marrow transplants for relapsed or refractory Hodgkin's disease
Hypersensitivity reactions (hypotension, bronchospasm, urticaria, diaphoresis, abdominal and extremity pain, pruritus, and erythema); nausea and vomiting (rare)	*Neutropenia*; peripheral neurotoxicity (numbness and paresthesias); cardiotoxicity (asymptomatic bradycardia); alopecia; transient myalgias or arthralgias; mucositis	Advanced ovarian cancer unresponsive to first-line or subsequent therapy; advanced breast cancer
Hypersensitivity reactions (chills, fever, urticaria, tachycardia, bronchospasm, dyspnea, hypertension or hypotension, facial flushing); diarrhea; nausea and vomiting	*Bone marrow depression* (leukopenia, neutropenia, thrombocytopenia, anemia); mucositis; alopecia; peripheral neuropathy	Acute lymphoblastic leukemia in children (induction of remission in patients refractory to standard regimens)
Nausea and vomiting; fever; chills; hypersensitivity reactions including anaphylaxis; headache; hyperglycemia leading to coma	Cerebral dysfunction (eg, disorientation, coma, seizures); acute hemorrhagic pancreatitis; coagulation defects; hepatic dysfunction; thrombosis; renal damage; decreased protein synthesis	Acute lymphocytic leukemia

(table continued on next page)

TABLE 1 (continued)

Drug	Classification	Route(s) of Administration	Elimination
HORMONALLY DIRECTED AGENTS[3]			
Prednisone [Deltasone] Prednisolone	Adrenal corticosteroid	Oral	Metabolic
Dexamethasone [Decadron, Dexone, Hexadrol] Methylprednisolone [Medrol, Solu-Medrol, Depo-Medrol]	Adrenal corticosteroid	Oral, intramuscular, intravenous	Metabolic
Diethylstilbestrol (DES) Chlorotrianisene Conjugated estrogens Esterified estrogens Estrone	Estrogen	Oral	Metabolic
Ethinyl Estradiol [Estinyl]	Estrogen	Oral	Metabolic
Estramustine Phosphate Sodium [Emcyt]	Estradiol mustard	Oral	Metabolic
Tamoxifen Citrate [Nolvadex]	Antiestrogen	Oral	Metabolic
Fluoxymesterone [Halotestin] Methyltestosterone	Androgen	Oral	Metabolic
Testolactone [Teslac]	Androgen	Oral	Metabolic
Testosterone Propionate	Androgen	Intramuscular	Metabolic
Flutamide [Eulexin]	Antiandrogen	Oral	Metabolic and renal

Major Toxicity[2]		
Acute	**Delayed**	**Indications**
Gastric irritation	Hyperadrenocorticism; adverse reactions expected with corticosteroids, including sodium retention (edema, hypertension), glucose intolerance, accumulation of fat on face and trunk, osteoporosis, psychoses and euphoria, insomnia, loss of skin collagen, increased susceptibility to infection, weight gain, growth retardation in children, gastric ulceration, hypokalemia, muscle wasting, bruising, immunosuppression	Acute and chronic lymphocytic leukemias; Hodgkin's and non-Hodgkin's lymphomas; multiple myeloma; breast carcinoma
Perineal irritation after rapid intravenous infusion	Same as prednisone, prednisolone	Primary and metastatic brain tumors (to reduce cerebral edema); Hodgkin's and non-Hodgkin's lymphomas
Occasional nausea	Fluid retention; hypercalcemia; feminization; uterine bleeding; increased frequency of vascular accidents (especially with large doses); bladder atony; vaginal carcinoma in offspring of pregnant women given drug; thromboembolism; nipple hyperpigmentation and tenderness; gynecomastia in males	Advanced prostatic and breast carcinomas
None	Fluid retention; hypercalcemia; feminization; uterine bleeding; increased frequency of vascular accidents (especially at high doses); thromboembolism	Advanced prostatic and breast carcinomas
Nausea and vomiting; diarrhea	Fluid retention, gynecomastia; abnormal liver function tests; pulmonary infiltrates and fibrosis	Advanced prostatic and breast carcinomas
Mild nausea and vomiting; hot flashes; transient increased bone or tumor pain	Vaginal bleeding; skin rashes; transient leukopenia and thrombocytopenia; hypercalcemia; pruritus vulvae; weight gain; headache; retinopathy and corneal opacities with high-dose, long-term use	Breast carcinoma, melanoma
None	Fluid retention; masculinization including hirsutism and painful clitoral hypertrophy; cholestatic jaundice; hypercalcemia	Breast carcinoma
None	Fluid retention; masculinization (usually minimal); hypercalcemia	Breast carcinoma
None	Fluid retention; masculinization; hypercalcemia	Breast carcinoma
Occasional diarrhea, nausea, and vomiting; transient elevations in serum levels of hepatic enzymes	Gynecomastia; may cause hepatitis or hepatic necrosis	Prostate carcinoma (with simultaneous leuprolide)

(table continued on next page)

TABLE 1 (continued)

Drug	Classification	Route(s) of Administration	Elimination
Goserelin Acetate [Zoladex]	LHRH[4] agonist	Subcutaneous	Renal and metabolic
Leuprolide Acetate [Lupron Injection, Lupron Depot]	LHRH[4] agonist	Subcutaneous (Lupron Injection), intramuscular (Lupron Depot)	Metabolic
Hydroxyprogesterone Caproate [Prodrox]	Progestin	Intramuscular	Metabolic
Medroxyprogesterone Acetate [Provera, Depo-Provera]	Progestin	Oral, intramuscular	Metabolic
Megestrol Acetate [Megace]	Progestin	Oral	Metabolic
Aminoglutethimide [Cytadren]	Aromatase inhibitor	Oral	Metabolic and renal
Mitotane (o, p′-DDD) [Lysodren]	Adrenocortical suppressant	Oral	Metabolic
BIOLOGICAL RESPONSE MODIFIERS			
Aldesleukin (Interleukin-2, IL-2) [Proleukin]	Recombinant lymphokine	Intravenous	Metabolic and renal
Interferon Alfa-2a [Roferon A] Interferon Alfa-2b [Intron A]	Blocks transition from G_0 to the proliferative state	Subcutaneous, intramuscular, intravenous, intravesical, intraperitoneal, intralesional	Metabolic
BCG, Live; BCG Vaccine [TheraCys; TICE BCG]	Immunostimulant	Intravesical	Voiding of bladder contents
Isotretinoin [Accutane]	Vitamin A analogue	Oral	Metabolic

Major Toxicity[2]		
Acute	**Delayed**	**Indications**
Transient increases in bone pain; hot flashes	Impotence; gynecomastia; lower urinary tract disorders	Breast and prostate carcinomas
Transient increase in bone pain; hot flashes	Gynecomastia; impotence; amenorrhea; testicular atrophy	Breast and prostate carcinomas
Local pain	Fluid retention (mild); hypercalcemia, cholestatic jaundice; weight gain	Endometrial carcinoma
Local pain (injectable)	Fluid retention (mild); hypercalcemia; weight gain	Breast, prostate, and endometrial carcinomas
None	Fluid retention (mild); hypercalcemia; weight gain	Breast, endometrial, and renal cell carcinomas; cancer-associated cachexia
Lethargy; ataxia; skin rash; orthostatic dizziness; fever; nausea	Masculinization; hypothyroidism (rare); bone marrow depression	Breast carcinoma
Nausea and vomiting; diarrhea	Neurologic toxicity (mental depression, visual disturbances); dermatitis	Adrenocortical carcinoma
Fever; capillary leak syndrome (edema, hypotension, arrhythmia, angina, myocardial ischemia or infarction, dyspnea or pulmonary congestion, gastrointestinal bleeding or infarction, renal insufficiency, and/or mental status changes); nausea and vomiting; diarrhea; pruritus; chills; pain; erythema; rash; fatigue, weakness, and/or malaise	Neuropsychiatric disorders; oliguria/anuria; hypothyroidism; liver dysfunction; anemia; thrombocytopenia; leukopenia; stomatitis; anorexia; infections (including sepsis, secondary to impaired neutrophil function)	Metastatic renal cell carcinoma; metastatic malignant melanoma (with or without lymphokine-activated killer cells or tumor-infiltrating lymphocytes)
Fever; mild nausea and vomiting; constitutional symptoms; headaches; myalgia; arthralgia; fatigue	Bone marrow depression; wasting syndrome; liver enzyme elevations; minor cognitive impairment with decreased ability to concentrate	Hairy cell and chronic myelogenous leukemias; non-Hodgkin's and cutaneous T-cell lymphomas; Kaposi's sarcoma; renal cell cancer; melanoma; carcinoid syndrome; multiple myeloma; bladder (intravesical) and ovarian (intraperitoneal) cancers; basal cell carcinoma (intralesional)
None	Dysuria; frequent urination; hematuria; cystitis; urinary tract infection; "flu-like" syndrome; localized or systemic BCG infection	Primary and relapsed carcinoma in situ of the urinary bladder (with or without papillary tumors)
None	Dry skin and mucous membranes; cheilitis; corneal opacities; elevated serum lipids and cholesterol; elevated liver enzymes	Basal cell carcinomas; cutaneous T-cell lymphomas

(table continued on next page)

TABLE 1 (continued)

Drug	Classification	Route(s) of Administration	Elimination
Levamisole [Ergamisol]	Immunostimulant	Oral	Metabolic and renal
Octreotide Acetate [Sandostatin]	Somatostatin analogue	Subcutaneous, intravenous	Renal, biliary, and metabolic

plete inclusion in this table. In these instances, some of the regimens used most frequently are listed as representative examples. Because the ideal drug treatment protocol has not been clearly defined for most cancers, preferred drugs or combinations of drugs are likely to change as clinical trials identify more effective regimens. New developments in clinical cancer chemotherapy are being evaluated regularly by leading medical oncologists, and some of the preferences listed in Table 2 are likely to become obsolete with time. For many less responsive tumors and for most patients with recurrent metastatic disease, the best therapy available at present is entry into appropriate clinical trials (McCabe and Friedman, 1989; Karjalainen and Palva, 1989; Stiller, 1989).

Combination Chemotherapy

In general, combinations of drugs have proven superior to single agents (see Table 2); circumvention of drug resistance may be an important reason. As discussed earlier, selection of de novo resistant cell lines from a heterogeneous tumor population can result in drug resistance. In addition, many antineoplastic agents are mutagenic and may directly produce a drug-resistant line. Multiple drug resistance also may develop. However, when combination chemotherapy using two or more noncross-resistant drugs is employed, therapeutic failure due to emergence of drug resistance is less likely.

Another major reason for the greater success of combination chemotherapy is that each drug can provide a maximal tumor cell kill within the range of toxicity tolerated by the host. If the drugs have minimal overlapping toxicities, optimal antitumor doses of each agent can be given. Thus, the total tumor cytoreduction will be much greater with an effective drug combination than with any single agent (Riggs, 1986 C; DeVita, 1989; Haskell, 1990 A; Chabner, 1990).

Although some effective drug combinations have been designed entirely on the basis of biochemical or cytokinetic principles, most successful combination chemotherapy regimens used clinically have been derived empirically. The following guidelines are usually employed when choosing drugs for combination chemotherapy. (1) Drugs that are active against the tumor when used alone should be selected. If available, drugs that produce some fraction of complete responses are preferred to those that produce only partial responses. (2) The drugs included should have different mechanisms of action to minimize the possibility of drug resistance. (3) Drugs selected should have minimally overlapping toxicities to allow the administration of full or nearly full doses of each active agent to result in a greater tumor cell kill. (4) The individual drugs should be optimally scheduled and the combination given at consistent intervals. Usually, the interval selected between cycles is the narrowest possible to allow recovery of the most sensitive normal target tissue, which usually is the bone marrow (Pratt and Ruddon, 1979; Perry, 1986; DeVita, 1989; Rosove and Schwartz, 1990).

An excellent example of the principles discussed above is the MOPP regimen used to treat advanced Hodgkin's disease and other cancers. The drugs and dosage schedules employed in this combination are: mechlorethamine [Mustargen] 6 mg/M^2 intravenously on days one and eight; vincristine [Oncovin] 1.4 mg/M^2 intravenously on days one and eight; procarbazine [Matulane] 100 mg/M^2 orally on days one to fourteen; and prednisone 40 mg/M^2 orally on days one to fourteen (cycles one and four only). The cycle is repeated every four weeks for a minimum of six cycles or as many cycles as needed for complete remission, plus two additional cycles to consolidate the remission (DeVita et al, 1980; for reviews see Hellman et al, 1989; Haskell and Parker, 1990).

When used alone, each of the drugs in the MOPP regimen is active in Hodgkin's disease but produces complete remissions in only a small percentage of patients. The individual drugs have different mechanisms: Mechlorethamine is an alkylating agent that cross-links DNA; vincristine is an M phase specific mitotic inhibitor that disrupts microtubules; procarbazine is a monofunctional alkylator that inhibits DNA and RNA synthesis; and prednisone is lympholytic after binding to the glucocorticoid receptor. Although the dose-limiting toxicities of both mechlorethamine and procarbazine are bone marrow depression and therefore overlap, vincristine (dose-limiting

Major Toxicity[2]		
Acute	**Delayed**	**Indications**
Nausea; vomiting; diarrhea; altered sense of taste or smell	Dermatitis; stomatitis; leukopenia; alopecia; fatigue; fever; infections; arthralgia; myalgia; dizziness; headache; ataxia; blurred vision; confusion; seizures; tardive dyskinesia; anxiety; insomnia; mental depression; somnolence; agranulocytosis (sometimes fatal) at doses higher than those used in adjuvant therapy (all above toxicities are rare)	Adjuvant therapy of Stage III (Dukes Stage C) colon cancer (combined with fluorouracil)
Nausea; diarrhea; abdominal pain	Steatorrhea	Control of symptoms in carcinoid tumors and vasoactive intestinal peptide-secreting adenomas; management of diarrhea induced by fluorouracil plus leucovorin

1 *See the evaluations in the following four chapters and Pratt and Ruddon, 1979, pp 64–272,* Med Lett Drugs Ther, *1993; Carter et al, 1981, pp 53–126; Frei, 1985; Chabner, 1993; Krakoff, 1991; Lane, 1985; Riggs and Bennett, 1991 A, 1991 B; Haskell, 1990 B; Chabner and Collins, 1990, pp 59-490; Black and Livingston, 1990 A and B; Holland et al, 1993.*

2 *Usual dose-limiting toxicity is italicized.*

3 *Individual hormone preparations listed are the ones most commonly employed in cancer chemotherapy.*

4 *Luteinizing hormone-releasing hormone.*

neurotoxicity) and prednisone do not depress the bone marrow. Thus, the criteria of individually active drugs, different mechanisms of action, and nonoverlapping toxicities to allow maximally tolerated doses of each drug are essentially satisfied in the MOPP regimen. Furthermore, the scheduling of cycles four weeks apart accommodates the recovery time for bone marrow. Approximately 80% of patients achieve complete remission, and more than 50% remain free of disease for more than ten years and are considered cured. Other data suggest that alternating cycles of treatment with MOPP and ABVD (see Table 2) may further increase the cure rate (relative to MOPP alone) for patients with stage IV Hodgkin's disease (Bonadonna and Santoro, 1982). However, whether alternating the two regimens improves cure rates compared with ABVD alone has not been established.

Combination chemotherapy has significantly prolonged survival, with some probable cures, in acute lymphocytic leukemia, certain non-Hodgkin's lymphomas, and germ cell tumors (see Table 2). It should be noted that bone marrow-sparing agents (eg, vincristine, bleomycin, cisplatin, asparaginase, prednisone) are included in each of these regimens.

In other cancers, particularly those that show good responses to a number of individual drugs, combination chemotherapy has clearly been superior to single-agent chemotherapy and now is employed routinely. Examples include small cell carcinoma of the lung, acute myelogenous leukemia, and breast carcinoma. In contrast, for many cancers that are only marginally sensitive to presently available drugs (eg, colorectal and renal carcinomas, melanoma), drug combinations have not significantly improved survival over single agents and may cause greater toxicity. Thus, combination chemotherapy for these malignancies is best administered in the context of an appropriate randomized comparative clinical trial. (See Table 2 and the references for more detailed information on specific combination regimens for the various tumor types.)

Adjuvant Chemotherapy

For many solid tumors, cures can be achieved with surgery or radiation therapy alone if the cancer is localized at the time of treatment. However, a high percentage of patients with apparently localized disease harbor undetectable metastases (micrometastases). Eventual relapse is likely in these patients, and cure of late, macrometastatic disease with chemotherapy is rare. As a result, adjuvant systemic chemotherapy is being employed; systemic cytotoxic therapy is initiated immediately after local surgery and/or radiation therapy despite the absence of clinically evident systemic disease to eradicate the micrometastases presumed to be present (Klastersky, 1986; Salmon, 1987). Chemotherapy is presumed to be most effective immediately after cytoreductive surgery when the total micrometastatic body burden is smallest. This has been demonstrated in a number of animal model systems (Martin, 1981).

Clinically, adjuvant chemotherapy is now well accepted for a number of cancers, particularly pediatric cancers (eg, Wilms' tumor, rhabdomyosarcoma, Ewing's sarcoma), osteogenic sarcoma, and breast carcinoma (depending on stage of disease and other prognostic factors). In most of these tumors, adjuvant chemotherapy has increased the duration of survival and/or disease-free survival. However, there is disagreement about the use of adjuvant therapy in the earliest

TABLE 2.
CLINICAL RESPONSES TO CHEMOTHERAPY

Type of Cancer[1]	Drugs or Regimens Currently Preferred	Alternative or Secondary Drugs or Regimens	Other Drugs or Regimens With Reported Activity
RESPONSIVE CANCERS (PROLONGED SURVIVAL AND SOME CURES)			
Acute lymphocytic leukemia	*Induction:* Vincristine + prednisone ± (doxorubicin or daunorubicin) ± asparaginase *Prophylaxis of CNS disease:* Intrathecal methotrexate and/or cranial irradiation; high-dose systemic methotrexate (with leucovorin) ± cytarabine *Postremission therapy:* Methotrexate + mercaptopurine ± vincristine ± prednisone *Relapsed or refractory disease:* Bone marrow transplantation (allogeneic or autologous)	Cyclophosphamide, methotrexate, cytarabine, etoposide, teniposide	Cytarabine + mitoxantrone; cytarabine + idarubicin; cytarabine + amsacrine[2]; mercaptopurine, thioguanine, vindesine[2], ifosfamide + mesna, interferon alfa-2
Acute myelogenous leukemia	*Induction:* (Daunorubicin, idarubicin, or mitoxantrone) + cytarabine *Postremission therapy:* Cytarabine-based regimens (using various dosages) ± etoposide or an anthracycline *Relapsed disease or after a second remission:* Bone marrow transplantation (allogeneic or autologous)	Daunorubicin + cytarabine + (thioguanine or etoposide); doxorubicin + cytarabine + thioguanine	Azacitidine[2], amsacrine[2], teniposide, ifosfamide + mesna, cyclophosphamide, diaziquone[2], aldesleukin
Anal carcinoma	Fluorouracil + mitomycin + radiation therapy		
Breast carcinoma Adjuvant therapy of early-stage disease for women at higher risk of recurrence based on analyses of tumor markers, nodal status, and other prognostic indicators	*Premenopausal:* Cyclophosphamide + methotrexate + fluorouracil (CMF) or cyclophosphamide + doxorubicin + fluorouracil (CAF); if receptor-positive, tamoxifen ± ovarian ablation is added *Postmenopausal:* Tamoxifen (± CMF or CAF) if receptor-positive; CMF or CAF (± tamoxifen) if receptor-negative	CMF + biochemical modulation with leucovorin; CMF + prednisone (CMFP) ± vincristine (CMFVP)	

(table continued on next page)

TABLE 2 (continued)

Type of Cancer[1]	Drugs or Regimens Currently Preferred	Alternative or Secondary Drugs or Regimens	Other Drugs or Regimens With Reported Activity
Advanced disease (therapy rarely curative)	*Endocrine therapy (for receptor-positive tumors):* Tamoxifen followed by a progestin or diethylstilbestrol or fluoxymesterone or aminoglutethimide for postmenopausal women; ovarian ablation or tamoxifen for premenopausal women	Progestins (medroxyprogesterone acetate, megestrol acetate), LHRH agonists (leuprolide, goserelin, buserelin[2])	Androgens, estrogens, corticosteroids, aminoglutethimide (plus replacement hydrocortisone)
	Chemotherapy (for receptor-negative tumors): CMF, CMFP, CMFVP *or* CAF ± methotrexate (CAMF)	Doxorubicin + cyclophosphamide (AC) *or* doxorubicin + vincristine (AV) *or* regimen composed of other active drugs not used in primary therapy *or* sequential monotherapy with active drugs not used in primary therapy	Methotrexate, doxorubicin, melphalan, vinblastine, thiotepa, mitomycin, vindesine[2], leuprolide, mitoxantrone, etoposide, ifosfamide + mesna, cisplatin, carboplatin, fluorouracil + leucovorin, paclitaxel (formerly taxol)
Burkitt's lymphoma	Cyclophosphamide + vincristine + methotrexate (with leucovorin if high dose) ± high-dose cytarabine + intrathecal therapy with methotrexate + cytarabine	Carmustine, ifosfamide + mesna, doxorubicin	Cytarabine, high-dose cyclophosphamide
Embryonal rhabdomyosarcoma	Vincristine + dactinomycin + cyclophosphamide (VAC) *or* cyclophosphamide + doxorubicin + vincristine (CAV)	(VAC or CAV) ± cisplatin ± etoposide	Thiotepa, methotrexate, dacarbazine, ifosfamide + mesna
Ewing's sarcoma	Cyclophosphamide (or ifosfamide + mesna) + doxorubicin + vincristine (CAV)	Dactinomycin *or* CAV + etoposide *or* VAC + doxorubicin	Methotrexate (high dose with leucovorin rescue), fluorouracil
Gestational trophoblastic tumors			
Low risk	Methotrexate ± leucovorin, dactinomycin	Vinblastine, chlorambucil, etoposide	Hydroxyurea, doxorubicin, cisplatin
High risk	Methotrexate + dactinomycin + chlorambucil *or* methotrexate + dactinomycin + cyclophosphamide + hydroxyurea + vincristine + doxorubicin (CHAMOCA)	Methotrexate + dactinomycin + cyclophosphamide *or* cisplatin + vinblastine + bleomycin (PVB) *or* etoposide + methotrexate/leucovorin + dactinomycin + cyclophosphamide + doxorubicin *or* cisplatin + etoposide + bleomycin (PEB)	Etoposide
Hairy cell leukemia	Interferon alfa-2, pentostatin, cladribine	Chlorambucil	Melphalan

(table continued on next page)

TABLE 2 (continued)

Type of Cancer[1]	Drugs or Regimens Currently Preferred	Alternative or Secondary Drugs or Regimens	Other Drugs or Regimens With Reported Activity
Hodgkin's disease (advanced stages)	Mechlorethamine + vincristine + procarbazine + prednisone (MOPP) *or* doxorubicin + bleomycin + vinblastine + dacarbazine (ABVD) *or* MOPP/ABVD "hybrid" regimen	MOPP alternating with ABVD *or* carmustine + vinblastine + cyclophosphamide + procarbazine + prednisone (BCVPP) *or* chlorambucil + (vincristine or vinblastine) + procarbazine + prednisone (LOPP or ChlVPP) *Relapsed or refractory disease:* myeloablative high-dose chemotherapy (eg, cyclophosphamide + carmustine + etoposide) and bone marrow transplantation	Lomustine, thiotepa, etoposide, altretamine, teniposide, streptozocin, interferon alfa-2, cytarabine, ifosfamide + mesna
Non-Hodgkin's lymphomas Intermediate-grade and aggressive (high-grade) types (eg, diffuse large cell lymphoma)	Various combination regimens, eg: Cyclophosphamide + doxorubicin + vincristine + prednisone (CHOP) ± high-dose methotrexate with leucovorin rescue (M-CHOP) *or* CHOP + etoposide *or* prednisone + methotrexate/leucovorin + doxorubicin + cyclophosphamide + etoposide + cytarabine + vincristine + bleomycin (ProMACE-CytaBOM) *or* bleomycin + doxorubicin + cyclophosphamide + methotrexate with leucovorin rescue + dexamethasone (M-BACOD) *or* bleomycin + doxorubicin + cyclophosphamide + vincristine + prednisone (BACOP) ± high-dose methotrexate with leucovorin rescue (M-BACOP) *or* cyclophosphamide + vincristine + methotrexate (high dose with leucovorin rescue) + cytarabine (COMLA) *or* prednisone + methotrexate with leucovorin rescue + doxorubicin + cyclophosphamide + etoposide + mechlorethamine + vincristine + procarbazine + prednisone (ProMACE-MOPP) *or* bleomycin + doxorubicin + cyclophosphamide + vincristine + prednisone + procarbazine (COP-BLAM)	Combination of active agents not previously utilized (eg, dexamethasone + cytarabine + cisplatin *or* etoposide + methylprednisolone + high-dose cytarabine + cisplatin *or* ifosfamide/mesna + mitoxantrone + etoposide) *Relapsed or refractory disease:* Myeloablative high-dose chemotherapy (eg, cyclophosphamide + carmustine + etoposide or high-dose cyclophosphamide and total body irradiation) and bone marrow transplantation	Mechlorethamine, chlorambucil, vinblastine, procarbazine, carmustine, lomustine, cytarabine, altretamine, etoposide, cisplatin, teniposide, ifosfamide + mesna

(table continued on next page)

TABLE 2 (continued)

Type of Cancer[1]	Drugs or Regimens Currently Preferred	Alternative or Secondary Drugs or Regimens	Other Drugs or Regimens With Reported Activity
Osteogenic sarcoma	*Adjuvant therapy:* Doxorubicin + cisplatin + methotrexate (standard dose or high dose with leucovorin) ± bleomycin ± cyclophosphamide ± dactinomycin ± vincristine	Combination regimens, including doxorubicin and cisplatin, not used for primary treatment	Melphalan, mitomycin, bleomycin, ifosfamide + mesna, etoposide
Small cell carcinoma of lung	Various combination regimens, eg: Etoposide + cisplatin (PE) ± doxorubicin ± cyclophosphamide *or* cyclophosphamide + doxorubicin ± vincristine (CAV) ± etoposide (CAVE or CAE) ± cisplatin (CAVEP or CAEP) *or* PE alternated with CAV *or* cisplatin + vincristine + doxorubicin + etoposide (CODE) *or* cyclophosphamide + lomustine + methotrexate ± vincristine	Combination regimens not used for primary treatment, eg: ifosfamide + mesna + carboplatin + etoposide (ICE); daily oral etoposide	Procarbazine, carboplatin, teniposide, ifosfamide + mesna, altretamine, epirubicin[2], nimustine[2], vindesine[2], paclitaxel (formerly taxol)
Testicular cancer (nonseminomatous germ cell tumors)	Cisplatin + etoposide (PE) ± bleomycin (PEB) *or* cisplatin + vinblastine + bleomycin (PVB)	Carboplatin + etoposide ± bleomycin (CEB) *or* vinblastine + dactinomycin + bleomycin + cisplatin + cyclophosphamide (VAB-VI) *or* cisplatin + ifosfamide/mesna + [vinblastine (VIP) or etoposide (PIE)]; high-dose myeloablative chemotherapy (eg, carboplatin + etoposide) with autologous bone marrow transplantation as salvage therapy for recurrent disease	Doxorubicin, plicamycin, methotrexate, carboplatin
Wilms' tumor	Dactinomycin + vincristine ± doxorubicin (± cyclophosphamide for tumors with unfavorable histology)	Cisplatin, etoposide	Ifosfamide + mesna
MODERATELY RESPONSIVE CANCERS (PALLIATION AND PROBABLE PROLONGATION OF LIFE)			
Adrenocortical carcinoma	Mitotane, cisplatin	Etoposide, suramin[2], *or* fluorouracil + doxorubicin + cisplatin	Cyclophosphamide, fluorouracil, doxorubicin, aminoglutethimide
Bladder (also renal pelvis and ureters) transitional cell carcinoma	*Local therapy for superficial tumors:* Intravesical instillation of BCG *Systemic therapy for invasive tumors:* Cisplatin + methotrexate + vinblastine (CMV) ± doxorubicin (M-VAC)	*Local therapy for high-risk superficial tumors:* Intravesical instillation of thiotepa, doxorubicin, mitomycin, or interferon alfa-2 *Systemic therapy for invasive or metastatic tumors:* Cisplatin + doxorubicin (CA) ± cyclophosphamide (CISCA or CAP) *or* other drugs not used for primary treatment	Cyclophosphamide, fluorouracil, mitomycin, interferon alfa-2, fluorouracil + leucovorin, carboplatin

(table continued on next page)

TABLE 2 (continued)

Type of Cancer[1]	Drugs or Regimens Currently Preferred	Alternative or Secondary Drugs or Regimens	Other Drugs or Regimens With Reported Activity
Cervical carcinoma	Cisplatin + bleomycin ± methotrexate *or* bleomycin + mitomycin + vincristine ± cisplatin *or* cisplatin + bleomycin + ifosfamide + mesna	Interferon alfa-2, etoposide + ifosfamide + mesna + cisplatin	Methotrexate, fluorouracil, vincristine, vinblastine, cyclophosphamide, doxorubicin, altretamine, ifosfamide + mesna
Chronic lymphocytic leukemia	Chlorambucil ± prednisone	Fludarabine phosphate, cladribine, cyclophosphamide *or* cyclophosphamide + vincristine + prednisone (COP) ± doxorubicin (CHOP)	Doxorubicin, pentostatin
Chronic myelogenous leukemia	*Chronic phase:* Busulfan, hydroxyurea, interferon alfa-2, high-dose myeloablative therapy with cyclophosphamide and (busulfan or total body irradiation) and with allogeneic bone marrow transplantation (most often curative) *Blast crisis* *Myeloblastic:* Same regimens as for acute myelogenous leukemia (see above) *Lymphoblastic:* Vincristine + prednisone ± daunorubicin	Daunorubicin + high-dose cytarabine	Mercaptopurine, thioguanine, melphalan, cytarabine
Colon carcinoma (Stage III or Dukes Stage C)	Adjuvant therapy with levamisole + fluorouracil	Fluorouracil + leucovorin	
Endometrial carcinoma	Progestins (eg, megestrol, hydroxyprogesterone, medroxyprogesterone) *or* doxorubicin	Doxorubicin ± cisplatin ± (cyclophosphamide or ifosfamide + mesna) ± megestrol *or* cyclophosphamide + bleomycin + cisplatin	Fluorouracil, tamoxifen, melphalan, carboplatin, bleomycin, altretamine
Gastric carcinoma (advanced)	Fluorouracil *or* fluorouracil + doxorubicin (FA) ± methotrexate (FAMTX) *or* fluorouracil + leucovorin	Fluorouracil + doxorubicin + mitomycin (FAM) *or* etoposide + fluorouracil + cisplatin (EFP) *or* etoposide + cisplatin ± doxorubicin (EAP) *or* etoposide + leucovorin + fluorouracil (ELF) *or* fluorouracil + epirubicin[2] + carmustine (FEB)	Semustine[2], tegafur[2]
Glioblastoma and anaplastic astrocytoma	Carmustine *or* lomustine	Procarbazine, cisplatin *or* procarbazine + lomustine + vincristine (PCV)	Semustine[2], etoposide, vincristine, cyclophosphamide, mechlorethamine, carboplatin

(table continued on next page)

TABLE 2 (continued)

Type of Cancer[1]	Drugs or Regimens Currently Preferred	Alternative or Secondary Drugs or Regimens	Other Drugs or Regimens With Reported Activity
Head and neck squamous cell carcinoma (radiation therapy is added to chemotherapy for organ preservation in patients with laryngeal tumors)	Cisplatin + fluorouracil ± leucovorin *or* cisplatin + bleomycin ± vincristine	Vincristine + bleomycin + mitomycin *or* cisplatin + bleomycin + (methotrexate or vinblastine) *or* carboplatin + fluorouracil *or* cyclophosphamide + vincristine + methotrexate + fluorouracil + bleomycin	Fluorouracil, cyclophosphamide, doxorubicin, vinblastine, mitomycin, mitoguazone[2]
Islet cell carcinoma	Streptozocin ± fluorouracil ± doxorubicin	Doxorubicin, dacarbazine, interferon alfa-2, leuprolide	Octreotide
Kaposi's sarcoma (AIDS-related)	Etoposide, interferon alfa-2, vinblastine (systemic or intralesional)	Bleomycin + vincristine + doxorubicin	Cyclophosphamide, vincristine
Medulloblastoma	Vincristine + carmustine ± mechlorethamine ± methotrexate *or* vincristine + cisplatin ± cyclophosphamide *or* lomustine + vincristine + prednisone + methotrexate	Mechlorethamine + vincristine + procarbazine + prednisone (MOPP) *or* lomustine + vincristine + cisplatin *or* cisplatin + etoposide	Carboplatin
Multiple myeloma	Melphalan + prednisone ± vincristine ± cyclophosphamide ± carmustine *or* vincristine + doxorubicin + dexamethasone (VAD)	Doxorubicin *or* etoposide + dexamethasone + cytarabine + cisplatin *or* teniposide + dexamethasone + cyclophosphamide; for high-risk patients, high-dose myeloablative chemotherapy with bone marrow transplantation; interferon alfa-2 (for maintenance)	Dexamethasone, chlorambucil, interferon alfa-2 (for induction), cisplatin, etoposide, teniposide, cytarabine
Neuroblastoma, advanced disease	Cyclophosphamide + vincristine + dacarbazine ± doxorubicin *or* doxorubicin + cyclophosphamide ± cisplatin ± teniposide	Doxorubicin (if not used in primary regimen) *or* cisplatin + cyclophosphamide; for metastatic or recurrent disease, high-dose myeloablative chemotherapy (eg, using melphalan) with autologous bone marrow transplantation	Daunorubicin, vinblastine, prednisone, etoposide, mechlorethamine, dacarbazine, idarubicin
Non-Hodgkin's lymphomas Indolent types (eg, most nodular lymphomas)	Cyclophosphamide + vincristine + prednisone (CVP) *or* chlorambucil ± prednisone *or* cyclophosphamide	Doxorubicin + bleomycin + prednisone (ABP) *or* fludarabine phosphate *or* (chlorambucil or cyclophosphamide) + etoposide	Mechlorethamine, vinblastine, procarbazine, carmustine, lomustine, altretamine, etoposide, interferon alfa-2, cladribine
Ovarian carcinoma	Cyclophosphamide + (cisplatin or carboplatin) ± doxorubicin	Doxorubicin or cisplatin or carboplatin or altretamine depending on primary treatment; paclitaxel (formerly taxol) ± cisplatin; *salvage therapy for recurrent or residual disease:* intraperitoneal chemotherapy with cisplatin ± (etoposide or fluorouracil) *or* chromic phosphate P 32	Chlorambucil, thiotepa, progestins, ifosfamide + mesna, fluorouracil, leuprolide

(table continued on next page)

TABLE 2 (continued)

Type of Cancer[1]	Drugs or Regimens Currently Preferred	Alternative or Secondary Drugs or Regimens	Other Drugs or Regimens With Reported Activity
Advanced prostatic carcinoma	An estrogen *or* leuprolide ± flutamide *or* goserelin ± flutamide	*Hormone refractory relapsed tumors:* Doxorubicin *or* cyclophosphamide *or* cisplatin *or* estramustine	Fluorouracil, ethinyl estradiol, mitoxantrone, methotrexate, megestrol, aminoglutethimide + hydrocortisone, cyproterone acetate[2], ketoconazole
Rectal adenocarcinoma (adjuvant therapy of Stages II and III [Duke's B and C])	Fluorouracil ± leucovorin + pelvic radiation therapy ± semustine[2] ± vincristine		
Soft tissue sarcoma (adult)	Doxorubicin ± dacarbazine ± (cyclophosphamide or ifosfamide + mesna)	Other combinations under investigation	Doxorubicin, methotrexate, vincristine, cisplatin, ifosfamide + mesna
Thyroid carcinoma	Doxorubicin ± cisplatin	Doxorubicin + vincristine + bleomycin ± melphalan	Cisplatin, mitoxantrone
PARTIALLY TO MINIMALLY RESPONSIVE CANCERS (POSSIBLE PALLIATION; MINIMAL TO NO INCREASE IN SURVIVAL)			
Bronchogenic carcinoma (non-small cell)	Various regimens, eg: Cyclophosphamide + doxorubicin ± cisplatin (CAP) *or* (vinblastine or vindesine[2]) + cisplatin ± mitomycin (MVP) *or* cisplatin + etoposide	Methotrexate + doxorubicin + cyclophosphamide + lomustine (MACC) *or* cisplatin + fluorouracil + leucovorin *or* fluorouracil + doxorubicin + mitomycin; doxorubicin; cyclophosphamide; cisplatin, paclitaxel (formerly taxol)	Methotrexate, mitomycin, lomustine, vindesine[2], etoposide, fluorouracil, carboplatin, paclitaxel (formerly taxol)
Metastatic colorectal carcinoma	Fluorouracil + leucovorin ± methotrexate (4 to 24 hours before fluorouracil), intra-arterial floxuridine (hepatic metastases)	Mitomycin *or* semustine[2] *or* fluorouracil + interferon alfa-2 ± leucovorin	Carmustine, lomustine, tegafur[2], methotrexate, interferon alfa-2, *N*-phosphonoacetyl-*L*-aspartate[2]
Esophageal carcinoma	Various regimens, eg: Cisplatin + fluorouracil *or* cisplatin + methotrexate *or* cisplatin + vindesine[2] + bleomycin	Cisplatin + doxorubicin + fluorouracil *or* cisplatin + vindesine[2] + mitoguazone[2]	Bleomycin, mitomycin, vindesine[2], methotrexate, mitoguazone[2], etoposide, interferon alfa-2
Hepatocellular carcinoma	Fluorouracil, doxorubicin	Intra-arterial floxuridine	Mitomycin, methotrexate
Melanoma (metastatic)	Dacarbazine, aldesleukin ± LAK[2] or TIL[2] cells	Nitrosourea (eg, carmustine, lomustine, semustine[2]) *or* cisplatin + dacarbazine ± vinblastine or vindesine[2] *or* bleomycin + vincristine + lomustine + dacarbazine (BOLD)	Interferon alfa-2 ± dacarbazine (alone or in various combination regimens), dactinomycin, tamoxifen + dacarbazine (alone or in various combination regimens)
Pancreatic carcinoma	Fluorouracil + doxorubicin + mitomycin (FAM) *or* streptozocin + mitomycin + fluorouracil (SMF)	Fluorouracil + leucovorin *or* various single agents and combinations under study, eg: altretamine + mitomycin + fluorouracil *or* fluorouracil + cyclophosphamide + methotrexate + vincristine + mitomycin *or* fluorouracil + doxorubicin + cisplatin (FAP)	Leuprolide, semustine[2], ifosfamide + mesna

(table continued on next page)

TABLE 2 (continued)

Type of Cancer[1]	Drugs or Regimens Currently Preferred	Alternative or Secondary Drugs or Regimens	Other Drugs or Regimens With Reported Activity
Renal cell carcinoma	Aldesleukin ± LAK[2] cells, interferon alfa-2	Vinblastine, lomustine, floxuridine	Progestins

[1] For many types of cancer listed, treatment routinely includes surgery and/or radiation therapy in addition to chemotherapy. The reader should consult other references for detailed recommendations on the treatment of the various individual cancers as well as for specific dosage schedules of the currently preferred drug regimens.

[2] Investigational drug

stages of some of these cancers (eg, those with node-negative breast cancer identified as good-risk patients by various prognostic indicators) (Pritchard, 1989). For some other tumors (eg, Stage III [or Duke's stage C] colon cancer), unequivocal data establishing a positive effect of adjuvant chemotherapy on survival have been obtained only recently (Moertel et al, 1990). Furthermore, in other stages of the same (eg, Stage II [or Duke's stage B] colon cancer) or closely related tumors (eg, stage II rectal carcinoma), a sufficient benefit from adjuvant chemotherapy to justify its acceptance as standard treatment has not yet been demonstrated conclusively (Mayer et al, 1989; Mayer, 1990). In still other instances (eg, stage III rectal cancer), postoperative radiation therapy must be combined with adjuvant chemotherapy to increase recurrence-free survival maximally. Major problems in evaluating the effectiveness of adjuvant chemotherapy regimens have been the long follow-up time and large number of patients required for reliable statistical analysis of minor effects. In the absence of conclusive evidence that adjuvant therapy improves the outcome, the risks and benefits of all treatment strategies should be discussed with the patient, and enrollment in a clinical trial of adjuvant chemotherapy should be offered as one option.

Selection of appropriate drugs for adjuvant chemotherapy is based primarily on their effectiveness against advanced cancer. In general, adjuvant chemotherapy has been more successful against chemosensitive (eg, breast carcinoma) than chemoinsensitive (eg, non-small cell lung carcinoma) cancers. Combinations of drugs usually are more effective than single agents, and high-dose, intermittent courses of therapy are preferred. This presents another problem, however. Since a significant number of patients may remain disease-free with surgery or radiotherapy alone, the added risk of drug toxicity (and, in some cases, the induction of secondary malignancies, such as leukemia) must be weighed carefully against the potential benefit. This latter point emphasizes the importance of identifying high-risk recurrence groups who should receive adjuvant chemotherapy (Pratt and Ruddon, 1979; Martin, 1981; DeVita, 1989; Klastersky, 1986; Salmon, 1987).

Investigators also are evaluating induction chemotherapy before definitive surgery or radiotherapy. This approach, which has been referred to as neoadjuvant chemotherapy, has several potential advantages (Frei et al, 1987). As with classic adjuvant therapy, there may be an increased effect on micrometastatic disease. Early treatment limits development of de novo drug resistance, and a higher tumor growth fraction may be exposed to the drugs. Induction chemotherapy provides an in vivo assay system for assessment of response (thereby facilitating evaluation of chemotherapeutic efficacy), identifies patients who might benefit from adjuvant chemotherapy, and offers an opportunity for histopathologic analysis of tumor response. If effective, a decrease in local/regional tumor size may permit improved local/regional control by surgery or radiotherapy, may increase the number of resectable lesions, and may permit a decrease in the extent of local treatment. In addition, induction chemotherapy is administered prior to any alteration of tumor vascularity by surgery or radiation therapy and is generally better tolerated than adjuvant chemotherapy.

SHARED TOXICITIES

Because of the lack of readily exploitable biochemical differences between cancer and normal cells, the cytotoxic nature of most antineoplastic drugs, and the necessity for optimum dosing to produce the best response, most anticancer drugs have low therapeutic indices and produce cytotoxic effects in normal cells. The major acute and delayed toxicities for each of the various drugs are listed in Table 1 and are discussed in the evaluations in the following four chapters. A number of adverse effects are shared among antineoplastic drugs with diverse chemical structures and intracellular targets (Perry, 1986; DeVita et al, 1989; Chabner and Collins, 1990). These are discussed below.

Myelosuppression: Bone marrow suppression is most significant in terms of morbidity and mortality caused by antineoplastic drugs and is the usual dose-limiting toxicity. Hormones, vincristine, bleomycin, asparaginase, and cisplatin have other major dose-limiting toxicities, which makes them desirable components of combination chemotherapy regimens.

Generally, leukopenia is more severe than thrombocytopenia, and anemia is less common. This is because the half-lives (and, thus, the doubling times of precursor marrow cells) of granulocytes (six hours) and platelets (five to seven days) are considerably shorter than that of red blood cells (about 120 days) and, therefore, they are more susceptible to the cytotoxicity of the drugs. Different types of agents produce different patterns of myelosuppression. Phase-specific agents that act only on proliferating cells (eg, methotrexate, vinblastine, antipurines, antipyrimidines) usually produce a rapid granulocytopenia with a rapid recovery. In contrast, certain cycle nonspecific agents cause more prolonged bone marrow depression characterized by slow recovery and cumulative effects. Busulfan, mitomycin, and, in particular, the chloroethylnitrosoureas (carmustine, lomustine, semustine [investigational]) can cause severe thrombocytopenia three to five weeks after drug administration. Other agents (eg, phase nonspecific but with a preference for proliferating cells) usually show an intermediate pattern. The effect on the platelet count may be more or less pronounced than the effect on the granulocyte count, and the kinetics to maximum depression (nadir) may differ. For example, cyclophosphamide and etoposide primarily affect granulocytes and produce thrombocytopenia less often; the opposite is seen with plicamycin. Bone marrow depression is delayed with the nitrosoureas, with the nadir for thrombocytopenia (28 days) appearing approximately one week before the nadir for granulocytopenia (35 days).

The myelosuppression produced by biological agents, such as interferon alfa-2, follows a different pattern. Myelosuppression has a rapid onset and is rapidly reversible (within 24 hours of dose modification or discontinuation of therapy). This appears to be related to retention of mature blood elements in the bone marrow rather than to cytotoxicity among bone marrow stem cells.

Although the severity of bone marrow depression varies among the antineoplastic drugs, it also depends on dose and patient factors, including age, nutritional status, marrow reserve, and prior radiation or chemotherapy (Hoagland, 1982; Perry, 1986; Rosove and Schwartz, 1990).

Careful monitoring of blood counts during and after therapy is essential in patients receiving myelosuppressive drugs. Dosage reductions are often necessary when the white blood cell and platelet counts fail to return to adequate levels before the next course of therapy. The major consequences of granulocytopenia and thrombocytopenia are infection and bleeding, respectively. Supportive measures, including antibiotics, platelet transfusions, and protected environments, may be required (Hoagland, 1982; Deisseroth and Wallerstein, 1989 A; Pizzo and Myers, 1989; Ho, 1990; Young, 1990). The development of allogeneic and autologous bone marrow transplantation (Storb, 1989; Champlin, 1990; Blume, 1990) has allowed administration of dose-intensified chemotherapy regimens without compromising the eventual recovery of bone marrow function. In investigational studies, hematopoietic colony-stimulating factors (see index entry Growth Factors, Hematopoietic) have been administered to patients being treated with myelosuppressive drugs (either with or without bone marrow transplantation). These factors have reduced the duration and, to a lesser extent, the severity of chemotherapy-induced neutropenia (Moore, 1988; Deisseroth and Wallerstein, 1989 B; Groopman, 1990; DiPersio and Golde, 1990; Golde and Glaspy, 1990).

Cytotoxicity to Other Proliferating Cells: Other proliferating normal tissues that are most susceptible to the cytotoxic effects of the antineoplastic drugs are the gastrointestinal and germinal epithelium, hair follicles, and lymphoid organs.

Gastrointestinal mucositis, most commonly stomatitis, can occur with a number of drugs. Severe mucositis with possible ulceration is observed most commonly with methotrexate, the fluorinated pyrimidines (eg, fluorouracil), dactinomycin, doxorubicin, bleomycin, and vinblastine, and it may be dose limiting (Dreizen et al, 1986; Sonis, 1989). Stomatitis occurs more frequently in young patients (age 1 to 20) than in older individuals, and it can result from direct effects of chemotherapeutic drugs on proliferating epithelial cells or as a secondary effect of immunosuppression caused by bone marrow toxicity. Oral evaluation and intervention to reduce potential sources of infection before therapy is begun, combined with preventive measures during drug treatment, can reduce the incidence of mucositis. A number of drugs cause partial or complete hair loss. In particular, cyclophosphamide and doxorubicin cause severe alopecia (Joss et al, 1988; Seipp, 1989). Several approaches, including scalp hypothermia and scalp tourniquets, have been used in attempts to reduce the hair loss. A variety of antineoplastic drugs, particularly the alkylating agents, depress spermatogenesis and can cause sterility and premature menopause (Gradishar and Schilsky, 1989; Schilsky and Erlichman, 1990).

Most antineoplastic drugs suppress cellular and humoral immunity (Pizzo and Myers, 1989). Immunosuppression often does not persist for long periods after treatment is discontinued and is less of a problem when intermittent scheduling is employed. However, cell-mediated immunity appears to be an important defense mechanism against the tumor and the immunocompromised patient is more susceptible to infection.

Immediate Side Effects: Most antineoplastic drugs have acute and delayed effects that can be both frequent and severe (Craig and Powell, 1987; Gralla, 1989). Among the immediate side effects, nausea and vomiting are caused by most antineoplastic agents. Mechlorethamine, cisplatin, streptozocin, and dacarbazine cause vomiting, often severe, in essentially all patients. The sensory and stimulatory inputs underlying chemotherapy-induced vomiting are complex and in part mediated through the chemoreceptor trigger zone in the brain. For this reason, combinations of antiemetics (eg, phenothiazines, butyrophenones, metoclopramide [Reglan], dronabinol [Marinol], dexamethasone, lorazepam [Ativan]) are utilized to provide the most effective control. See index entry Cancer, Chemotherapy, Vomiting Associated With.

Local tissue necrosis will occur in most instances of drug extravasation, and thus great care should be taken to avoid this preventable toxicity. Doxorubicin, daunorubicin, dactinomycin, mechlorethamine, plicamycin, streptozocin, vincristine, vinblastine, and mitomycin are local irritants and must be administered intravenously with care to avoid extravasation (Hubbard et al, 1989; Hubbard and Jenkins, 1990).

Organ-Specific Toxicity: Important toxicities to individual organs and the antineoplastic drugs most frequently implicated are as follows:

Skin—Bleomycin (very common and includes hyperpigmentation, induration, erythema, vesicles, bullae), busulfan (hyperpigmentation), and fluorouracil (palmar-plantar erythrodysesthesia when given by infusion; dermatitis).

Lung—Bleomycin (usual dose-limiting toxicity; most often pneumonitis, but fatal pulmonary fibrosis can occur), busulfan, cyclophosphamide, chloroethylnitrosoureas and most other alkylating agents (pulmonary fibrosis), mitomycin (pneumonitis, fibrosis), and methotrexate (pneumonitis).

Heart—Doxorubicin and daunorubicin (cumulative toxicity limits total dose to 550 mg/M^2 and to 400 mg/M^2 in patients with prior thoracic irradiation; ranges from transient EKG changes to cardiomyopathy with irreversible congestive heart failure) and high-dose cyclophosphamide (severe and sometimes fatal congestive heart failure).

Liver—Mercaptopurine, thioguanine, and sex steroids (cholestatic jaundice), asparaginase (fatty metamorphosis), nitrosoureas (hepatitis), and methotrexate (fibrosis and cirrhosis with prolonged use).

Pancreas—Asparaginase (hyperglycemia, hemorrhagic pancreatitis) and streptozocin (hyperglycemia).

Bladder—Cyclophosphamide and ifosfamide (sterile hemorrhagic cystitis; concomitant administration of mesna prevents or reduces this effect).

Kidney—Cisplatin (usual dose-limiting toxicity; acute renal tubular necrosis), streptozocin (usual dose-limiting toxicity; ranges from proteinuria to renal tubular atrophy), chloroethylnitrosoureas and mitomycin (delayed-onset nephrotoxicity that can progress to renal failure), high-dose methotrexate (renal tubular necrosis), and, indirectly, many cytotoxic drugs (hyperuricemic nephropathy due to large purine breakdown from tumor subsequent to cell killing; allopurinol often is used to counteract this response).

Blood Coagulation—Plicamycin (hemorrhagic diathesis) and asparaginase (decreased clotting factors, reduced fibrinolytic activity).

Nervous System—Vincristine (usual dose-limiting toxicity; peripheral neuropathy ranging from decreased Achilles tendon reflex to areflexia; constipation due to autonomic dysfunction; and ptosis and diplopia due to cranial nerve palsies), asparaginase (cerebral dysfunction ranging from lethargy and confusion to severe depression and coma), fluorinated pyrimidines (cerebellar ataxia), procarbazine (altered consciousness, peripheral neuropathy), cytarabine (cerebellar syndrome and hearing loss), cisplatin (ototoxicity, peripheral neuropathy), intrathecal methotrexate (acute meningeal irritation, progressive meningoencephalopathy), and prednisone (manic psychosis or depression, altered sleep patterns).

Hypersensitivity Reactions: Hypersensitivity reactions may be common and severe. Type I reactions characterized by urticaria, angioedema, and anaphylaxis are most commonly observed with asparaginase (1% mortality) followed by cisplatin and intravenous melphalan. Bleomycin-induced hyperpyrexia is quite common in lymphoma patients. Hypersensitivity reactions have been reported infrequently for methotrexate, doxorubicin, daunorubicin, cyclophosphamide, cytarabine, oral melphalan, procarbazine, and etoposide.

Mutagenicity, Teratogenicity, and Carcinogenicity: Many commonly employed antineoplastic drugs are mutagenic as well as teratogenic, and some, including procarbazine and the alkylating agents, are carcinogenic in animals. The frequency of secondary malignancies, particularly acute leukemia, is increased in patients treated for Hodgkin's disease, non-Hodgkin's lymphomas, multiple myeloma, ovarian cancer, and possibly some other cancers (Kaldor et al, 1990 A and B; Zarrabi, 1990; Schilsky and Erlichman, 1990). The risk of secondary malignancies, which may not appear for many years after chemotherapy, must be considered in weighing benefits versus risks for any new therapy. This is particularly true for adjuvant chemotherapy, in which improved survival must be balanced against the side effects of the drugs, and for treatment of pediatric neoplasms, in which high cure rates and prolonged survival provide ample time for development of secondary malignancies. When possible, combination regimens that are less likely to produce secondary malignancies should be selected from among regimens with comparable curative potential.

Cited References

Drugs of choice for cancer chemotherapy. *Med Lett Drugs Ther* 35:43-50, 1993.

Arrick BA, Nathan CF: Glutathione metabolism as a determinant of therapeutic efficacy: A review. *Cancer Res* 44:4224-4232, 1984.

Bishop JM: The molecular genetics of cancer. *Science* 235:305-311, 1987

Black DJ, Livingston RB: Antineoplastic drugs in 1990: A review (part I). *Drugs* 39:489-501, 1990 A.

Black DJ, Livingston RB: Antineoplastic drugs in 1990: A review (part II). *Drugs* 39:653-673, 1990 B.

Blume KG: Marrow transplantation, in Williams WJ, et al (eds): *Hematology*, ed 4. New York, McGraw-Hill, 1990, 1674-1685.

Bonadonna G, Santoro A: ABVD chemotherapy in treatment of Hodgkin's disease. *Cancer Treat Rev* 9:21-35, 1982.

Carter SK, et al: *Chemotherapy of Cancer,* ed 2. New York, John Wiley & Sons, 1981.

Chabner BA: Clinical strategies for cancer treatment: The role of drugs, in Chabner BA, Collins JM (eds): *Cancer Chemotherapy: Principles and Practice.* Philadelphia, JB Lippincott, 1990, 1-15.

Chabner BA: Articancer drugs, in DeVita VT Jr, et al (eds): *Cancer: Principles & Practice of Oncology*, ed 4. Philadelphia, JB Lippincott, 1993, 325-417.

Chabner BA, Collins JM (eds): *Cancer Chemotherapy: Principles and Practice.* Philadelphia, JB Lippincott, 1990.

Champlin RE: Bone marrow transplantation, in Haskell CM (ed): *Cancer Treatment*, ed 3. Philadelphia, WB Saunders, 1990, 918-930.

Collins JM: Pharmacokinetics and clinical monitoring, in Chabner BA, Collins JM (eds): *Cancer Chemotherapy: Principles and Practice.* Philadelphia, JB Lippincott, 1990, 16-31.

Craig JB, Powell BL: Review: The management of nausea and vomiting in clinical oncology. *Am J Med Sci* 293:34-44, 1987.

Croce CM: Chromosome translocations and human cancer. *Cancer Res* 46:6019–6023, 1986.

Dalton WS, et al: Drug-resistance in multiple myeloma and non-Hodgkin's lymphoma: Detection of P-glycoprotein and potential circumvention by addition of verapamil to chemotherapy. *J Clin Oncol* 7:415-424, 1989.

Deisseroth A, Wallerstein R Jr: Use of blood and blood products, in DeVita VT Jr, et al (eds): *Cancer: Principles & Practice of Oncology*, ed 3. Philadelphia, JB Lippincott, 1989 A, 2045-2059.

Deisseroth A, Wallerstein R Jr: Use of hematopoietic growth factors, in DeVita VT Jr, et al (eds): *Cancer: Principles & Practice of Oncology*, ed 3. Philadelphia, JB Lippincott, 1989 B, 2060-2063.

Deuchars KL, Ling V: P-glycoprotein and multidrug resistance in cancer chemotherapy. *Semin Oncol* 16:156-165, 1989.

DeVita VT Jr: Principles of chemotherapy, in DeVita VT Jr, et al (eds): *Cancer: Principles & Practice of Oncology*, ed 3. Philadelphia, JB Lippincott, 1989, 276-300.

DeVita VT Jr, et al: Curability of advanced Hodgkin's disease with chemotherapy: Long-term follow-up of MOPP-treated patients at the National Cancer Institute. *Ann Intern Med* 92:587-595, 1980.

DeVita VT Jr, et al (eds): Adverse effects of treatment, in *Cancer: Principles & Practice of Oncology*, ed 3. Philadelphia, JB Lippincott, 1989, 2135-2190.

DiPersio JF, Golde DW: Hematopoietic growth factors, in Haskell CM (ed): *Cancer Treatment*, ed 3. Philadelphia, WB Saunders, 1990, 931-940.

Dreizen S, et al: Quantitative analysis of the oral complications of antileukemia chemotherapy. *Oral Surg Oral Med Oral Pathol* 62:650-653, 1986.

Druker BJ, et al: Oncogenes, growth factors, and signal transduction. *N Engl J Med* 321:1383-1390, 1989.

Einhorn LH: Testicular cancer as model for curable neoplasm: Richard and Hinda Rosenthal Foundation Award Lecture. *Cancer Res* 41:3275-3280, 1981.

Frei E III: Curative cancer chemotherapy. *Cancer Res* 45:6523-6537, 1985.

Frei E III, et al: The concept of neoadjuvant chemotherapy, in Salmon SE (ed): *Adjuvant Therapy of Cancer V*. Orlando, Grune & Stratton, 1987, 67-78.

Fry RJM: Principles of carcinogenesis: Physical, in DeVita VT Jr, et al (eds): *Cancer: Principles & Practice of Oncology*, ed 3. Philadelphia, JB Lippincott, 1989, 136-148.

Gazdar AF, et al: Correlation of in vitro drug-sensitivity testing results with response to chemotherapy and survival in extensive-stage small cell lung cancer: A prospective clinical trial. *J Natl Cancer Inst* 82:117-123, 1990.

Golde DW, Glaspy J: Therapeutic use of granulocyte and monocyte colony-stimulating factors, in Williams WJ, et al (eds): *Hematology*, ed 4. New York, McGraw-Hill, 1990, 273-278.

Goldie JH, Coldman AJ: Mathematical model for relating the drug sensitivity of tumors to their spontaneous mutation rate. *Cancer Treat Rep* 63:1727-1733, 1979.

Gradishar WJ, Schilsky RL: Ovarian function following radiation and chemotherapy for cancer. *Semin Oncol* 16:425-436, 1989.

Gralla RJ: Nausea and vomiting, in DeVita VT Jr, et al (eds): *Cancer: Principles & Practice of Oncology*, ed 3. Philadelphia, JB Lippincott, 1989, 2137-2143.

Groopman JE: Status of colony-stimulating factors in cancer and AIDS. *Semin Oncol* 17 (suppl 1):31-37, 1990.

Haskell CM: Principles and practice of cancer chemotherapy, in Haskell CM (ed): *Cancer Treatment*, ed 3. Philadelphia, WB Saunders, 1990 A, 21-43.

Haskell CM: Drugs used in cancer chemotherapy, in Haskell CM (ed): *Cancer Treatment*, ed 3. Philadelphia, WB Saunders, 1990 B, 44-101.

Haskell CM, Parker RG: Hodgkin's disease, in Haskell CM (ed): *Cancer Treatment*, ed 3. Philadelphia, WB Saunders, 1990, 655-681.

Hellman S, et al: Hodgkin's disease, in DeVita VT Jr, et al (eds): *Cancer: Principles & Practice of Oncology*, ed 3. Philadelphia, JB Lippincott, 1989, 1696-1740.

Heppner GH, Miller BE: Therapeutic implications of tumor heterogeneity. *Semin Oncol* 16:91-105, 1989.

Ho WG: Transfusion and apheresis of blood cells, in Haskell CM (ed): *Cancer Treatment*, ed 3. Philadelphia, WB Saunders, 1990, 862-865.

Hoagland HC: Hematologic complications of cancer chemotherapy. *Semin Oncol* 9:95-102, 1982.

Holland JF, et al (eds): *Cancer Medicine*, ed 3. Philadelphia, Lea & Febiger, 1993, 698-948.

Howley PM: Principles of carcinogenesis: Viral, in DeVita VT Jr, et al (eds): *Cancer: Principles & Practice of Oncology*, ed 3. Philadelphia, JB Lippincott, 1989, 149-166.

Hubbard SM, Jenkins JF: Chemotherapy administration: Practical guidelines, in Chabner BA, Collins JM (eds): *Cancer Chemotherapy: Principles and Practice*. Philadelphia, JB Lippincott, 1990, 449-464.

Hubbard SM, et al: Administration of cancer treatments: Practical guide for physicians and oncology nurses, in DeVita VT Jr, et al (eds): *Cancer: Principles & Practice of Oncology*, ed 3. Philadelphia, JB Lippincott, 1989, 2369-2402.

Jordan VC, et al: Hormone receptor assays: Clinical usefulness in the management of carcinoma of the breast. *Crit Rev Clin Lab Sci* 26:97-152, 1988.

Joss RA, et al: Fighting alopecia in cancer chemotherapy. *Recent Results Cancer Res* 108:117-126, 1988.

Kaldor JM, et al: Leukemia following chemotherapy for ovarian cancer. *N Engl J Med* 322:1-6, 1990 A.

Kaldor JM, et al: Leukemia following Hodgkin's disease. *N Engl J Med* 322:7-13, 1990 B.

Karjalainen S, Palva I: Do treatment protocols improve end results? A study of survival of patients with multiple myeloma in Finland. *BMJ* 299:1069-1072, 1989.

Killion JJ, Fidler IJ: The biology of tumor metastasis. *Semin Oncol* 16:106-115, 1989.

Klastersky J: Adjuvant chemotherapy, in Moossa AR, et al (eds): *Comprehensive Textbook of Oncology*. Baltimore, Williams & Wilkins, 1986, 239-243.

Krakoff IH: Cancer chemotherapeutic and biologic agents. *CA Cancer J Clin* 41:264-278, 1991.

Kramer RA, et al: Role of the glutathione redox cycle in acquired and de novo multidrug resistance. *Science* 241:694-697, 1988.

Lane M: Chemotherapy of cancer, in del Regato JA, et al (eds): *Cancer: Diagnosis, Treatment, and Prognosis*. St. Louis, CV Mosby, 1985, 93-118.

Liu LF: DNA topoisomerase poisons as antitumor drugs. *Annu Rev Biochem* 58:351-375, 1989.

Loehrer PJ Sr, et al: Testicular cancer: The quest continues. *J Natl Cancer Inst* 80:1373-1382, 1988.

Lokich JJ: *Cancer Chemotherapy by Infusion*, ed 2. Chicago, Precept Press, 1990.

Markman M: Intracavitary chemotherapy for malignant disease confined to body cavities. *West J Med* 142:364-368, 1985.

Markman M, et al: Intraperitoneal therapy in the management of ovarian carcinoma. *Yale J Biol Med* 62:393-403, 1989.

Martin DS: Scientific basis for adjuvant chemotherapy. *Cancer Treat Rev* 8:169-189, 1981.

Mayer RJ: Does adjuvant therapy work in colon cancer? *N Engl J Med* 322:399-401, 1990.

Mayer RJ, et al: Status of adjuvant therapy for colorectal cancer. *J Natl Cancer Inst* 81:1359-1363, 1989.

McCabe M, Friedman MA: Impact of third-party reimbursement on cancer clinical investigation: A consensus statement coordinated by the National Cancer Institute, letters. *J Natl Cancer Inst* 81:1585-1586, 1989.

Merkel DE, McGuire WL: Ploidy, proliferative activity and prognosis: DNA flow cytometry of solid tumors. *Cancer* 65:1194-1205, 1990.

Moertel CG, et al: Levamisole and fluorouracil for adjuvant therapy of resected colon carcinoma. *N Engl J Med* 322:352-358, 1990.

Moore MAS: The use of hematopoietic growth and differentiation factors for bone marrow stimulation, in DeVita VT Jr, et al (eds): *Important Advances in Oncology 1988*. Philadelphia, JB Lippincott, 1988, 31-54.

Moscow JA, Cowan KH: Multidrug resistance. *J Natl Cancer Inst* 80:14-20, 1988.

Nowell PC: Chromosomal and molecular clues to tumor progression. *Semin Oncol* 16:116-127, 1989.

O'Connell MJ: Is portal-vein fluorouracil hepatic infusion effective colon cancer surgical adjuvant therapy? editorial. *J Clin Oncol* 8:1454-1456, 1990.

Park M, Vande Woude GF: Principles of molecular cell biology of cancer: Oncogenes, in DeVita VT Jr, et al (eds): *Cancer: Principles & Practice of Oncology*, ed 3. Philadelphia, JB Lippincott, 1989, 45-66.

Perry MC: Complications of chemotherapy, in Moossa AR, et al (eds): *Comprehensive Textbook of Oncology*. Baltimore, Williams & Wilkins, 1986, 244-256.

Pierce GB, Speers WC: Tumors as caricatures of the process of tissue renewal: Prospects for therapy by directing differentiation. *Cancer Res* 48:1996-2004, 1988.

Pitot HC: Principles of carcinogenesis: Chemical, in DeVita VT Jr, et al (eds): *Cancer: Principles & Practice of Oncology*, ed 3. Philadelphia, JB Lippincott, 1989, 116-135.

Pizzo PA, Myers J: Infections in the cancer patient, in DeVita VT Jr, et al (eds): *Cancer: Principles & Practice of Oncology*, ed 3. Philadelphia, JB Lippincott, 1989, 2088-2134.

Pratt WB, Ruddon RW: *The Anticancer Drugs.* New York, Oxford University Press, 1979.

Pritchard KI: Systemic adjuvant therapy for node-negative breast cancer: Proven or premature? *Ann Intern Med* 111:1-4, 1989.

Riggs CE Jr, Bennett JP: Principles of cancer chemotherapy, in Moossa AR, et al (eds): *Comprehensive Textbook of Oncology,* ed 2. Baltimore, Williams & Wilkins, 1991 A, vol 1, 527-536.

Riggs CE Jr, Bennett JP: Clinical pharmacology of individual antineoplastic agents, in Moossa AR, et al (eds): *Comprehensive Textbook of Oncology,* ed 2. Baltimore, Williams & Wilkins, 1991 B, vol 1, 537-564.

Riggs CE Jr, Bennett JP: Combination chemotherapy, in Moossa AR, et al (eds): *Comprehensive Textbook of Oncology,* ed 2. Baltimore, Williams & Wilkins, 1991 C, 565-568.

Roberts AB, Sporn MB: Principles of molecular cell biology of cancer: Growth factors related to transformation, in DeVita VT Jr, et al (eds): *Cancer: Principles & Practice of Oncology*, ed 3. Philadelphia, JB Lippincott, 1989, 67-80.

Rosove MH, Schwartz GE: Hematologic complications of cancer and its treatment, in Haskell CM (ed): *Cancer Treatment*, ed 3. Philadelphia, WB Saunders, 1990, 850-861.

Ross WE, et al: Altered function of DNA topoisomerases as a basis for antineoplastic drug action, in DeVita VT Jr, et al (eds): *Important Advances in Oncology 1988*. Philadelphia, JB Lippincott, 1988, 65-82.

Rowley JD: Principles of molecular cell biology of cancer: Chromosomal abnormalities, in DeVita VT Jr, et al (eds): *Cancer: Principles & Practice of Oncology*, ed 3. Philadelphia, JB Lippincott, 1989, 81-97.

Rowley JD: Recurring chromosome abnormalities in leukemia and lymphoma. *Semin Hematol* 27:122-136, 1990.

Sager R: Tumor suppressor genes: The puzzle and the promise. *Science* 246:1406-1412, 1989.

Salmon SE (ed): *Adjuvant Therapy of Cancer V.* Orlando, Grune & Stratton, 1987.

Schilsky RL, Erlichman C: Infertility and carcinogenesis: Late complications of chemotherapy, in Chabner BA, Collins JM (eds): *Cancer Chemotherapy: Principles and Practice*. Philadelphia, JB Lippincott, 1990, 32-58.

Seemayer TA, Cavenee WK: Biology of disease: Molecular mechanisms of oncogenesis. *Lab Invest* 60:585-599, 1989.

Seipp CA: Hair loss, in DeVita VT Jr, et al (eds): *Cancer: Principles & Practice of Oncology*, ed 3. Philadelphia, JB Lippincott, 1989, 2135-2136.

Silverberg E, et al: Cancer statistics, 1990. *CA* 40:9-26, 1990.

Skipper HE, et al: Experimental evaluation of potential anticancer agents, XIII: On the criteria and kinetics associated with "curability" of experimental leukemia. *Cancer Chemother Rep* 35:1-111, 1964.

Skuse GR, Rowley PT: Tumor suppressor genes and inherited predisposition to malignancy. *Semin Oncol* 16:128-137, 1989.

Sonis ST: Oral complications of cancer therapy, in DeVita VT Jr, et al (eds): *Cancer: Principles & Practice of Oncology*, ed 3. Philadelphia, JB Lippincott, 1989, 2144-2152.

Stiller CA: Survival of patients with cancer: Those included in clinical trials do better. *BMJ* 299:1058-1059, 1989.

Storb R: Bone marrow transplantation, in DeVita VT Jr, et al (eds): *Cancer: Principles & Practice of Oncology*, ed 3. Philadelphia, JB Lippincott, 1989, 2474-2480.

Tannock IF: Principles of cell proliferation: Cell kinetics, in DeVita VT Jr, et al (eds): *Cancer: Principles & Practice of Oncology*, ed 3. Philadelphia, JB Lippincott, 1989, 3-13.

Vadlamudi S, Goldin A: Influence of mitotic cycle inhibitors on antileukemic activity of cytosine arabinoside (NSC-63878) in mice bearing leukemia L1210. *Cancer Chemother Rep* 55:547-555, 1971.

van der Bliek AM, Borst P: Multidrug resistance. *Adv Cancer Res* 52:165-203, 1989.

Von Hoff DD: He's not going to talk about in vitro predictive assays again, is he? Commentary. *J Natl Cancer Inst* 82:96-101, 1990.

Von Hoff DD, et al: Selection of cancer chemotherapy for a patient by an in vitro assay versus a clinician. *J Natl Cancer Inst* 82:110-116, 1990.

Weinberg RA: Oncogenes, antioncogenes, and the molecular bases of multistep carcinogenesis. *Cancer Res* 49:3713-3721, 1989.

Weinstein IB: The origins of human cancer: Molecular mechanisms of carcinogenesis and their implications for cancer prevention and treatment: Twenty-seventh G. H. A. Clowes Memorial Award Lecture. *Cancer Res* 48:4135-4143, 1988.

Williams SD, et al: Disseminated testicular cancer: Current chemotherapy strategies. *Semin Oncol* 16(suppl 6):105-109, 1989.

Young LS: Infection in cancer patients, in Haskell CM (ed): *Cancer Treatment,* ed 3. Philadelphia, WB Saunders, 1990, 831-840.

Zarrabi MH: Association of non-Hodgkin's lymphoma and second neoplasms. *Semin Oncol* 17:120-132, 1990.

Other Selected References

Calabresi P, Schein PS (eds): *Medical Oncology*, ed 2. New York, McGraw-Hill, 1993.

Carter SK, et al (eds): *Principles of Cancer Treatment.* New York, McGraw-Hill, 1982.

del Regato JA, et al: *Ackerman and del Regato's Cancer: Diagnosis, Treatment, and Prognosis.* St. Louis, CV Mosby, 1985.

DeVita VT Jr, et al (eds): *Cancer: Principles & Practice of Oncology,* ed 4. Philadelphia, JB Lippincott, 1993.

Dorr RT, Fritz WL: *Cancer Chemotherapy Handbook.* New York, Elsevier, 1980.

Haskell CM (ed): *Cancer Treatment*, ed 3. Philadelphia, WB Saunders, 1990.

Hellmann K, Carter SK (eds): *Fundamentals of Cancer Chemotherapy.* New York, McGraw-Hill, 1987.

Holland JF, et al (eds): *Cancer Medicine*, ed 3. Philadelphia, Lea & Febiger, 1993.

Moossa AR, et al (eds): *Comprehensive Textbook of Oncology.* Baltimore, Williams, & Wilkins, 1986.

Ponder BAJ, Waring MJ (eds): *The Science of Cancer Treatment.* Dordrecht, Kluwer Academic Publishers, 1990.

Tannock IF, Hill RP: *The Basic Science of Oncology*, ed 2. New York, McGraw-Hill, 1992.

Antineoplastic Agents: DNA Damaging Drugs

88

NITROGEN MUSTARDS

Uroprotective Agent

AZIRIDINES

ALKYL SULFONATES

NITROSOUREAS

PLATINUM COMPLEXES

NONCLASSICAL ALKYLATING AGENTS

SYSTEMIC RADIOISOTOPES

Most drugs that damage DNA directly are thought to exert their cytocidal effects by modifying cellular DNA covalently through monoadducts and/or cross-links. The major types of clinically useful DNA cross-linking agents are the nitrogen mustards, chlorambucil, cyclophosphamide, ifosfamide, mechlorethamine, and melphalan; the aziridine, thiotepa; the alkyl sulfonate, busulfan; the nitrosoureas, carmustine and lomustine; and the platinum complexes, cisplatin and carboplatin. Other drugs that covalently modify and damage intracellular DNA without introducing cross-links methylate or otherwise bind to DNA. These include the methyl hydrazine derivative, procarbazine; the triazenes, dacarbazine and altretamine; and the nitrosourea, streptozocin. Internally administered radioisotopes, which damage DNA by introducing strand breaks, also are included in this chapter. Finally, a uroprotective agent (mesna) that has no antitumor effects of its own but is used to prevent or reduce one of the major adverse reactions produced by two of the nitrogen mustards (cyclophosphamide and ifosfamide) is discussed.

The alkylating and cross-linking agents are cell cycle phase nonspecific in that they kill both resting and dividing cells, although most of these drugs are more active against proliferating cells. This may result from enzymatic activities in cells capable of repairing damaged DNA. The more rapidly cells proliferate, the less time is available for repair before replication and mitosis of damaged DNA lead to cell death. Some DNA-damaging drugs also are quantitatively more cytocidal to cells in particular cycle phases (eg, nitrosoureas kill a higher fraction of cells in G_1 or G_2 than in S phase).

Most of these drugs produce positively charged (eg, carbonium ion) intermediates that are short-lived, highly reactive, and readily form covalent bonds with a number of nucleophilic (electron-rich) cellular substances, such as phosphate, amino, sulfhydryl, hydroxyl, carboxyl, and imidazole groups. A particularly important reaction of the nitrogen mustards is alkylation of the 7-nitrogen of guanine in DNA; this can lead to chain scission, depurination, miscoding, and, in the case of these bifunctional alkylating agents, cross-linking between two DNA strands to prevent replication. Although other reactions occur, the alkylation and cross-linking of DNA may be most destructive to the cell.

Most adverse reactions to the alkylating and cross-linking agents also are related to the drugs' cytotoxic effects. The normal tissues most affected are those with a rapid growth rate: the bone marrow, gastrointestinal and germinal epithelia, and hair follicles. Bone marrow depression is the usual dose-limiting toxicity. Nausea and vomiting also are associated with most of these agents, particularly after intravenous administration.

Although all DNA damaging agents possess somewhat similar cytotoxic, mutagenic, and carcinogenic potential, they vary greatly in pharmacokinetic properties, lipid solubility, chemical reactivity, and membrane transport properties and are not uniformly cross-resistant. For example, cyclophosphamide and the nitrosoureas do not show cross resistance in the treatment of lymphomas. Thus, a consideration of the individual agents is necessary in order to understand their unique properties and optimal clinical usage.

NITROGEN MUSTARDS

The common structural feature of the nitrogen mustards is the bis(2-chloroethyl)amine moiety. Covalent bond formation to DNA or other cellular nucleophiles requires an initial cyclization reaction in which chlorine is lost and a positively charged cyclic aziridinium ion is generated. This highly reactive intermediate has a strong affinity for reaction at the N^7 position of guanine in DNA; however, many other sites (eg, phosphoryl oxygens of the sugar/phosphate DNA backbone) also are alkylated. Cyclization of the second chloroethyl moiety followed by reaction with an adjacent guanine on the opposite strand can lead to formation of DNA interstrand cross-links. Cross-links also are formed between DNA and various nuclear proteins, but most available evidence suggests that these lesions contribute little to the antitumor efficacy of nitrogen mustards (for reviews, see Colvin, 1993; Berger, 1993).

Mechlorethamine, the first DNA damaging drug to be developed, was the earliest nonhormonal approach to chemotherapy of cancer. This somewhat more selective analogue of the sulfur mustard gas used in trench warfare during World War I was found to be beneficial in the therapy of lymphomas in the mid-1940s (Rhoads, 1946). However, it has a very low therapeutic index because of its high reactivity. The addition of electron-withdrawing groups to the central nitrogen in the bis(2-chloroethyl)amine structure (phenyl rings in chlorambucil and melphalan and the heterocyclic oxazaphosphorine structure in cyclophosphamide and ifosfamide) reduced the reaction rate and thus markedly improved the selectivity and therapeutic indices of these drugs. However, there are some indications for which regimens that include mechlorethamine are still preferred by some clinicians (see the evaluation).

Chlorambucil and melphalan alkylate and cross-link DNA directly, whereas cyclophosphamide and ifosfamide require metabolic activation to convert from unreactive molecules to active alkylating and cross-linking species. Another advantage resulting from the reduced chemical reactivity (relative to that of mechlorethamine) is the usefulness of cyclophosphamide, chlorambucil, and melphalan when given orally. The four analogues of mechlorethamine are used much more frequently and in a wider range of solid and hematologic malignancies than the parent drug. However, each nitrogen mustard compound has a unique spectrum of activity, and thus the agents in this group are not necessarily interchangeable.

Resistance to nitrogen mustards has been studied extensively in vivo and in cell culture and is known to occur by multiple mechanisms (for reviews, see Morrow and Cowan, 1993; Colvin, 1993). Among these are decreased cell uptake by active transport (mechlorethamine, melphalan), increased cellular content of glutathione or other nonprotein sulfhydryl compounds (all nitrogen mustards), increased activity of glutathione transferases (all nitrogen mustards), increased detoxification by elevated aldehyde dehydrogenase activity (cyclophosphamide and ifosfamide), and increased repair of monoadducts and DNA interstrand cross-links (all nitrogen mustards). Since selection of resistant cell lines in vitro with a single agent often activates more than one of these mechanisms, it is likely that clinical resistance to these drugs in patients who become refractory to nitrogen mustard therapy also involves multiple mechanisms.

CHLORAMBUCIL
[Leukeran]

$$(ClCH_2CH_2)_2N-C_6H_4-CH_2CH_2CH_2COOH$$

ACTIONS AND USES. This aromatic derivative of mechlorethamine is the slowest acting, least toxic nitrogen mustard in clinical use. It is cell cycle nonspecific and has a marked lympholytic effect.

Chlorambucil is used frequently in the treatment of chronic lymphocytic leukemia (Deisseroth et al, 1993; Rai and Rabinowe, 1993). Daily, biweekly, and monthly dosing regimens, with and without prednisone, have been used. More advanced stages of the disease usually are treated with combination regimens, but reports of interim results from a large clinical trial suggest that patients in stage B respond as well to chlorambucil alone as to cyclophosphamide plus vincristine and prednisone (French Cooperative Group on Chronic Lymphocytic Leukemia, 1990 A). However, in patients with a good prognosis (stage A), survival of those treated with chlorambucil was not significantly different from that of untreated patients (French Cooperative Group on Chronic Lymphocytic Leukemia, 1990 B).

Chlorambucil has shown some efficacy in the treatment of Hodgkin's disease, non-Hodgkin's lymphomas, multiple myeloma, polycythemia vera, Langerhans cell histiocytosis (also termed histiocytosis X or Abt-Letterer-Siwe disease), and primary (Waldenstrom's) macroglobulinemia. Chlorambucil currently is preferred therapy only for indolent (low grade) non-Hodgkin's lymphomas (with or without prednisone) and Waldenstrom's macroglobulinemia. In addition, data suggest that both the ChlVPP regimen, which substitutes chlorambucil for mechlorethamine and vinblastine for vincristine in the MOPP regimen (ie, combined with procarbazine and prednisone) (Selby et al, 1990), and the LOPP regimen, which only substitutes chlorambucil for mechlorethamine (Hancock et al, 1991), are as effective as MOPP therapy for Hodgkin's disease and are associated with much less acute toxicity. Complete remissions of comparable duration are induced in equivalent percentages of patients treated with MOPP, LOPP, or ChlVPP. However, the risk for delayed toxicities (eg, leukemogenesis) is equivalent for all three regimens; this risk is thought to be reduced with other regimens used for Hodgkin's disease (eg, ABVD). More effective or less toxic therapeutic regimens are used more frequently than chlorambucil (alone or in combination) for the other diseases.

This agent also has activity against carcinoma of the ovary, testicular cancer, hairy cell leukemia, and choriocarcinoma, but regimens that do not include chlorambucil are currently preferred for these neoplasms. In addition, this drug has been used to treat vasculitis as a complication of rheumatoid arthritis, autoimmune hemolytic anemias associated with cold agglutinins, other immune or autoimmune disorders, and dermatomyositis and polymyositis (see index entry Chlorambucil). Since alkylating agents are carcinogenic (see below) and other effective immunosuppressants are available, use of chlorambucil in these settings has declined.

ADVERSE REACTIONS AND PRECAUTIONS. Hematologic toxicity is most prominent. Myelosuppression is usually moderate, gradual, and reversible. Leukopenia develops after the third week of treatment and continues for up to ten days after the last dose. Subsequently, the leukocyte count usually returns to normal rapidly. The dosage should be decreased if leukocyte or platelet counts fall below normal values, and the drug should be discontinued if depression of blood counts is severe.

Chlorambucil-related gastrointestinal, dermatologic, pulmonary, or hepatic toxicity is seldom encountered with usual therapeutic doses. Seizures have occurred in both children and adults but are rare. Azoospermia in adult males, sterility in prepubertal and pubertal males, and amenorrhea have been reported. This drug is classified in FDA Pregnancy Category D. An increased incidence of secondary acute myelogenous leukemia has been associated with long-term use of chlorambucil.

In addition to blood counts, serum uric acid levels should be monitored frequently to detect hyperuricemia that could lead to renal failure. This is particularly necessary during initial treatment of lymphoma patients with bulky disease.

PHARMACOKINETICS. Chlorambucil is well absorbed after oral administration. The plasma half-life of unmetabolized drug is about 1.5 hours. Chlorambucil is metabolized rapidly to phenylacetic acid mustard, which retains alkylating and cross-linking activity and has a plasma half-life of about 2.5 hours. Renal excretion of other potentially active metabolites is the major route of elimination; $<1\%$ is excreted in the urine as unchanged drug or phenylacetic acid mustard.

DOSAGE AND PREPARATIONS.

Oral: For chronic lymphocytic leukemia and Hodgkin's or non-Hodgkin's lymphomas, 3 to 6 mg/M^2 daily (or 0.1 to 0.2 mg/kg/day) as a single dose or in divided doses. Dosage adjustments are based on blood count.

An alternative schedule for the treatment of chronic lymphocytic leukemia is 15 to 20 mg/M^2 given as a single dose; the dose is repeated every two weeks and increased by 4 mg/M^2 until leukocytosis is controlled or toxicity is observed. A pulsed, high-dose schedule (16 mg/M^2 for five consecutive days each month for one to two years) also has been useful in some advanced low-grade non-Hodgkin's lymphomas (eg, follicular small cleaved-cell lymphoma).

Leukeran (Burroughs Wellcome). Tablets 2 mg.

CYCLOPHOSPHAMIDE

[Cytoxan, Neosar]

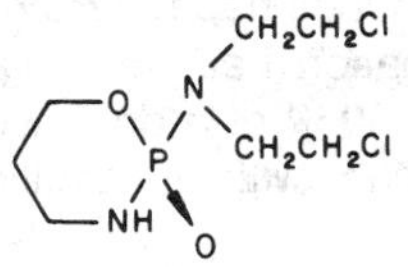

ACTIONS. Cyclophosphamide is the most widely used alkylating agent and can be administered orally or intravenously (for reviews see Colvin, 1993; Berger, 1993). This cyclic oxazaphosphorine derivative of mechlorethamine is cell cycle phase nonspecific. Cyclophosphamide itself does not have alkylating activity and is not a vesicant, but is a prodrug that must be metabolically activated in the liver by the microsomal cytochrome P450 mixed-function oxidase system (Patel, 1990; Moore, 1991) before it can alkylate cellular constituents. It is currently believed that phosphoramide mustard and nor-nitrogen mustard, potent alkylating and DNA cross-linking agents, are the active cytotoxic metabolites.

USES. Cyclophosphamide is used in the treatment of both hematologic and solid cancers. When given intravenously in large doses as a single agent, it has produced cures in some patients with African Burkitt's lymphoma. In combination with other antineoplastic agents, it is used frequently in the treatment of non-Hodgkin's lymphomas (both indolent and aggressive histologic types), multiple myeloma, breast and small cell lung carcinomas, and pediatric solid tumors, such as embryonal rhabdomyosarcoma, Ewing's sarcoma, and neuroblastoma (see index entry Cancer: Clinical Responses to Chemotherapy). It is used in chronic lymphocytic leukemia and ovarian cancers and shows activity in acute lymphocytic leukemia, Hodgkin's disease, choriocarcinoma, and endometrial, cervical, and prostatic cancer. Combination regimens that include cyclophosphamide have sometimes been used to treat soft tissue sarcomas and testicular, bladder, head and neck, and non-small cell lung carcinomas. However, other regimens that do not include cyclophosphamide presently are preferred for all of these neoplasms except perhaps non-small cell lung carcinoma.

High-dose regimens of cyclophosphamide alone or in combination with other agents (eg, busulfan or thiotepa plus carmustine) also have been used to treat various hematologic and solid malignancies in conjunction with autologous or allogeneic bone marrow or peripheral blood stem cell rescue (bone marrow transplantation) to prevent death from the unavoidable myelosuppression that accompanies the intensified treatment schemes (Peters, 1993; O'Reilly and Papadopoulos, 1993; Santos, 1993). A chemically activated analogue of cyclophosphamide, perphosphamide [Pergamid], which does not require enzymatic hydroxylation before it reacts with and cross-links DNA, has been used investigationally for *ex vivo* purging of malignant cells from autologous bone marrow to reduce the rate of tumor recurrence after transplantation. At present, this drug is available only through a Treatment IND from the National Cancer Institute.

Cyclophosphamide has a marked immunosuppressive action and has been used in rheumatoid arthritis, nephrotic syndrome in children, Wegener's granulomatosis, and other immune disorders. Several neurologic diseases thought to have an autoimmune etiology (eg, multiple sclerosis, myasthenia gravis, dermatomyositis/polymyositis) also can be treated with cyclophosphamide when patients do not respond to less toxic drugs. It is also administered before organ or allogeneic bone marrow transplantation for nonmalignant diseases to produce immunosuppression. (See also index entry Cyclophosphamide, Uses.)

DRUG INTERACTIONS. Since this drug is activated in the liver, its metabolism can be affected by drugs that induce (eg, phenobarbital) or inhibit (eg, allopurinol) enzymes of the mixed-function oxidase system. In addition, cyclophosphamide can induce the microsomal enzymes responsible for its own metabolism. Although the half-life of cyclophosphamide may be altered by these enzymatic effects, such interactions do not appear to be clinically relevant since the drug's antitumor activity and therapeutic index do not change.

Recent data suggest that cyclophosphamide may increase the leukopenia and thrombocytopenia caused by carboplatin at any given exposure to the latter (ie, area under the plasma concentration of carboplatin versus time curve) (Reyno et al, 1993). However, the nature and mechanism of this interaction are not understood, and it may reflect only additive myelotoxicity.

ADVERSE REACTIONS AND PRECAUTIONS. A variety of toxic effects have been observed (Fraiser et al, 1991). Nausea and vomiting are common, particularly after intravenous doses >500 mg/M^2. The peak emetogenic response occurs 12 to 18 hours after administration and presumably is caused by direct stimulation of the chemoreceptor trigger zone by the drug or one of its metabolites. This reaction is easily managed with antiemetic therapy (see index entry Vomiting, Treatment).

FD and C Yellow No. 5 (tartrazine), formerly used in tablets, may have caused allergic-type reactions, including bronchospasm, in susceptible individuals. This was removed from the formulation in 1991.

The usual dose-limiting toxicity is bone marrow depression. The major effect is on leukocytes, and thrombocytopenia is less severe than with other alkylating agents. The nadir of leukopenia usually occurs within one to two weeks after the start of administration, and recovery usually takes about ten days after the last dose. Blood counts must be monitored and the dosage reduced as necessary. In some of the high-dose chemotherapy protocols that include cyclophosphamide, results of recent studies demonstrate that recombinant human hematopoietic colony-stimulating factors (with or without bone marrow transplantation) can lessen the severity and/or duration of myelosuppression (see index entry Hematopoietic Hormones).

More than 50% of patients receiving intensive or prolonged therapy with cyclophosphamide experience alopecia, which is usually reversible. Hair loss usually begins within two weeks of initiation of therapy and is most severe after one to two months.

A relatively common and potentially dose-limiting toxic effect of high-dose cyclophosphamide is sterile hemorrhagic cystitis, which can result from a high concentration of active metabolites (eg, acrolein) in the bladder (deVries and Freiha, 1990; Fraiser et al, 1991). However, in the absence of mesna, this reaction occurs less frequently with standard doses of cyclophosphamide than with usual doses of ifosfamide (see the evaluation on Ifosfamide). The incidence of hemorrhagic cystitis can be reduced by ample fluid intake and frequent voiding. Systemic administration of acetylcysteine or mesna also reduces toxicity. Bladder fibrosis and carcinoma have been reported after long-term use of cyclophosphamide.

Other common toxic effects of cyclophosphamide are amenorrhea and azoospermia. Liver dysfunction, hyperpigmentation, oral ulceration, interstitial pneumonitis, and/or irreversible pulmonary fibrosis are less common effects. Decreased renal clearance of water, which may lead to hyponatremia, occurs only with doses ≥60 mg/kg.

Pulmonary toxicity is believed to be caused by metabolites of cyclophosphamide (eg, acrolein, activated alkylating moieties) generated by mixed-function oxidases present in the lung (Patel, 1990). Hyperoxygenation of lung tissue appears to potentiate or increase the incidence of pulmonary toxicity. *Pneumocystis carinii* pneumonia has been reported in patients receiving daily doses of cyclophosphamide and prednisone (Sen et al, 1991).

Cardiac damage (primarily congestive heart failure; less frequently, acute myopericarditis) has been observed with the large doses of cyclophosphamide used in preparative regimens for bone marrow transplantation (Fraiser et al, 1991). Deaths from this adverse reaction have occurred with doses of 60 mg/kg daily for four days or with single doses of 100 mg/kg. For this reason, the largest dose used for bone marrow ablation in preparation for transplantation is now 50 mg/kg each day for four days. The cardiotoxic effects of doxorubicin or radiation therapy also may be potentiated by subsequent therapy with large doses of cyclophosphamide. Secondary malignancies (most often, acute myelocytic leukemia) also have been reported.

This drug is classified in FDA Pregnancy Category C.

PHARMACOKINETICS. Cyclophosphamide is well absorbed orally, and peak plasma levels appear about one hour after oral use (Moore, 1991). It is also administered intravenously. This drug is metabolized in the liver to the cytotoxic metabolite, 4-hydroxycyclophosphamide, which is in equilibrium with the acyclic tautomer, aldophosphamide. Although the major fraction of these metabolites is oxidized further to inactive products, some aldophosphamide is converted to phosphoramide mustard, which alkylates DNA, and to acrolein (a toxic metabolite with no known therapeutic benefit). The nonpolar 4-hydroxycyclophosphamide is thought to deliver the reactive, but poorly diffusible, phosphoramide mustard into the cell.

Approximately 20% of the parent drug and up to 67% of some metabolites present in plasma are bound to proteins (Moore, 1991). The calculated volume of distribution for cyclophosphamide is nearly equal to total body water, which suggests that the drug penetrates most cells and tissues to the same degree. Total body clearance of cyclophosphamide is approximately 5.4 L/hour, primarily by hepatic metabolism. The clearance rate is increased in children and in patients receiving drugs that induce hepatic microsomal enzymes. Estimates of the elimination half-life range from five to eight hours. Approximately 60% of a dose is excreted as inactive metabolites in the urine, with an additional 10% as parent drug.

Although hepatic insufficiency reduces the rates of metabolic activation and clearance of cyclophosphamide, there is no evidence of increased toxicity or decreased efficacy

(Moore, 1991). The total exposure to active metabolites may not change because the unmetabolized drug is cleared very slowly. Similarly, renal impairment does not appear to affect the toxicity or effectiveness of cyclophosphamide, perhaps because the major portion of metabolites excreted in the urine is inactive. Thus, dosage adjustments appear to be unnecessary for patients with reduced liver or kidney function.

DOSAGE AND PREPARATIONS.

Intravenous: For patients with no hematologic deficiency, 500 mg to 1.5 g/M^2 is administered at approximately two- to four-week intervals. The dose is reduced, usually by one-third to one-half, in heavily pretreated patients with reduced bone marrow reserves. Other dosage schedules are frequently used.

Generic. Powder (crystalline) 100, 200, and 500 mg and 1 g.

Cytoxan (Bristol-Myers Oncology). Powder (crystalline, lyophilized) 100, 200, and 500 mg and 1 and 2 g; the lyophilized form contains 75, 150, 375, 750, or 1,500 mg of mannitol, respectively.

Neosar (Adria), ***Generic***. Powder (crystalline, lyophilized) 100, 200, and 500 mg and 1 and 2 g; the lyophilized form contains 82, 164, 410, or 820 mg or 1.64 g of sodium bicarbonate, respectively.

Use of benzyl alcohol-preserved diluents should be avoided.

Oral: When cyclophosphamide is given daily, the dose must be individualized. Doses of 60 to 120 mg/M^2 (or 1 to 5 mg/kg/day) are used. Titration may be required after careful assessment of myelosuppression. Cyclophosphamide is best tolerated when given during or after meals.

Cytoxan (Bristol-Myers Squibb). Tablets 25 and 50 mg.

IFOSFAMIDE

[Ifex]

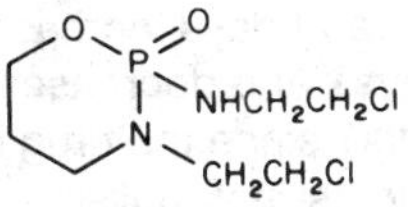

ACTIONS. Ifosfamide is a structural analogue of cyclophosphamide. It differs in that one of the two chloroethyl moieties covalently linked to a central nitrogen, which is characteristic of the nitrogen mustards, is carried by a ring nitrogen. Like cyclophosphamide, activation by hepatic microsomal enzymes is required for conversion of ifosfamide to a cytotoxic metabolite (Dechant et al, 1991; Berger, 1993; Colvin, 1993). The initial metabolic product is subsequently converted to isophosphoramide (alternatively, ifosfamide) mustard, which can alkylate and cross-link cellular DNA. Because ifosfamide is activated at a slower rate than cyclophosphamide, it must be used in larger doses and alternate metabolic pathways (eg, leading to production of chloroacetaldehyde) are of greater importance. The differences in metabolism of these two analogues may explain the marked differences in toxicity (see below).

USES. Ifosfamide combined with cisplatin and either etoposide or vinblastine is an effective salvage regimen for patients with recurrent or refractory disseminated testicular germ cell tumors (Dechant et al, 1991; Motzer et al, 1992; Einhorn et al, 1993). These regimens induce prolonged complete remissions in about 25% of such patients with nonseminomatous tumors; an additional 15% also require surgical resection. Cisplatin plus ifosfamide-based combinations also produce complete responses in >85% of patients with advanced bulky seminoma. Clinical trials are in progress to compare the efficacy of these regimens with that of cisplatin plus bleomycin plus vinblastine or etoposide, the current standard first-line therapy for disseminated testicular cancer.

Results of clinical studies also have demonstrated the activity of ifosfamide against a variety of other malignancies (Dechant et al, 1991; *Semin Oncol*, 1992 A). Ifosfamide plus doxorubicin and dacarbazine produces the highest response rates among combination regimens currently used in patients with advanced soft tissue sarcomas (Antman, 1992). Ifosfamide also is the most active single drug used as salvage therapy for patients with sarcomas unresponsive to other doxorubicin-based regimens. Based on the results of nonrandomized studies and promising response rates to ifosfamide monotherapy in patients previously treated with regimens that include cyclophosphamide, current clinical trials are comparing these two drugs when combined with doxorubicin, vincristine, and radiation for first-line therapy of Ewing's sarcoma (Dechant et al, 1991; Antman, 1992).

Data from clinical trials also support the use of ifosfamide (usually in combination regimens) as alternative or second-line therapy for recurrent or refractory advanced cervical, endometrial, or small cell lung carcinomas or intermediate to high grade non-Hodgkin's lymphoma (Dechant et al, 1991; *Semin Oncol*, 1992 A). (See index entry Cancer: Clinical Responses to Chemotherapy for specific combination regimens used.) In addition, responses to ifosfamide have been reported in patients with advanced, recurrent, or refractory acute lymphocytic and myeloid leukemias; breast, ovarian, and pancreatic carcinomas; osteosarcoma; and Hodgkin's disease. However, at present this drug is reserved for third-line therapy in patients with these malignancies.

The high incidence of urothelial toxicity observed in patients treated with ifosfamide (see below) requires concurrent administration of a prophylactic agent to prevent hemorrhagic cystitis (Dechant et al, 1991; Goren, 1992). Mesna (see the evaluation below) is the uroprotective agent most often employed.

ADVERSE REACTIONS AND PRECAUTIONS. The dose-limiting toxicities of ifosfamide as a single agent are myelosuppression (leukopenia and milder and less frequent thrombocytopenia) and urothelial reactions when a uroprotective drug (eg, mesna) is not used (Dechant et al, 1991). In combination regimens, myelosuppression can be severe. The incidence of hematopoietic toxicity is both dose- and schedule-dependent; fractionated doses cause myelosuppression less frequently than large bolus doses. Nadir white cell counts are observed one to two weeks after therapy begins, and recovery usually occurs three to four weeks after the final dose. Ifosfamide generally is considered less myelosuppressive than cyclophosphamide, although no studies comparing the toxicity of the two analogues in an identical combination regimen have been reported.

Urotoxicity in patients treated with ifosfamide is most often manifested as hemorrhagic cystitis, but dysuria, frequent urination, and other symptoms of bladder irritation also may be noted. Severe bladder toxicity occurs in 20% to 40% of patients treated with ifosfamide without mesna; macrohematuria is observed in <5% of those treated with both drugs (Dechant et al, 1991; Dorr, 1991; Goren, 1992). Accordingly, current recommendations for prophylaxis combine use of ifosfamide with mesna plus adequate hydration.

Ifosfamide can cause nephrotoxicity that may be either acute and reversible or chronic and progressive (Dechant et al, 1991; Skinner et al, 1993). Severe chronic renal damage is rare in adults and more frequent but variable in children (estimates range, 1.4% to 30%). The incidence is greater in patients who were treated with cisplatin previously (cumulative doses >300 mg/M^2), had pre-existing renal impairment, are receiving other nephrotoxic drugs, or have renal tumors. Although products of ifosfamide metabolism are thought to be responsible for both renal and bladder toxicities, concurrent administration of mesna does not appear to prevent the effects on the kidney. The most frequent initial response is damage to the proximal tubules resulting in Fanconi's syndrome; children <5 years of age appear to be most susceptible (Skinner et al, 1992). Hypophosphatemic rickets and growth impairment may result if therapy is not terminated before the glomeruli and distal tubules are irreversibly damaged.

Other commonly observed adverse reactions include alopecia, nausea and vomiting, and central nervous system toxicity (somnolence, confusion, hallucinations, and, rarely, coma). Although an oral preparation is not available in the United States, reports from European investigators suggest that the incidence of encephalopathy is greater with oral than with intravenous administration and also increases with advanced patient age, poorer performance status, and renal or hepatic dysfunction (Dechant et al, 1991). Dose fractionation or continuous infusion over three to five days appears to reduce the frequency of this adverse reaction. Although the biologic mechanism is not understood, the incidence of ifosfamide-induced neurotoxicity in children appears to be related to the previous cumulative dosage of cisplatin (Pratt et al, 1990). Attempts to predict the development of neurotoxicity in adults or children based on results of laboratory measurements and other parameters have been unsuccessful (Watkin et al, 1989).

Reversible liver dysfunction (increased liver enzymes and/or bilirubin) has been noted after treatment with ifosfamide.

Arrhythmias were reported in 5 of 33 patients treated with 6.5 to 10 g/M^2/course, but four of these had previously received cardiotoxic anthracyclines (Kandylis et al, 1989). Data from a retrospective study suggest that larger doses (10 to 18 g/M^2) used in combination regimens prior to autologous bone marrow transplantation are associated with congestive heart failure that usually is reversible after therapy is completed (Quezado et al, 1993). However, all of the patients in this study who required admission to an intensive care unit for treatment of congestive heart failure had received doxorubicin previously.

Ifosfamide should be used cautiously in patients with impaired renal function or compromised bone marrow reserve (eg, leukopenia, granulocytopenia, extensive bone marrow metastases, prior radiation therapy or combination chemotherapy). Blood cell counts (most notably neutrophils and platelets) should be monitored closely during therapy. Urine also must be inspected frequently for evidence of microscopic hematuria.

Ifosfamide is carcinogenic in rats; mutagenic in bacterial and mammalian cells; and embryotoxic and teratogenic in mice, rats, and rabbits (FDA Pregnancy Category D).

PHARMACOKINETICS. Although an oral preparation of ifosfamide is not available in the United States, data from pharmacokinetic studies indicate that oral doses are well absorbed (bioavailability nearly 100%) (Dechant et al, 1991). Peak plasma concentrations are achieved within one hour after an oral dose. The volume of distribution (Vd) at steady state is nearly equal to total body water when the drug is infused intravenously but is somewhat smaller when it is administered orally. The plasma concentration at steady state varies over an approximately two-fold range at doses of either 1 or 2 g/M^2/day by continuous infusion. This reflects variability in the Vd rather than differences in the rate of clearance. Data from studies on small numbers of patients suggest that the Vd may be larger in older and/or obese patients.

Studies that accurately measured ifosfamide and its metabolites indicated that there was no evidence for saturation of clearance at larger doses (for review, see Dechant et al, 1991). Mean values that were independent of dose or route of administration were calculated for the drug's terminal half-life (5.6 hours) and total clearance rate (3.6 L/hour) by combining data from several studies. In contrast, fractionating the total dose over several days increases the clearance rate (by 76% over five days) and decreases the terminal half-life (by 36% over five days) since the drug increases expression of enzymes involved in its metabolism.

As with cyclophosphamide, hepatic microsomal enzymes hydroxylate the ring to generate 4-hydroxy-ifosfamide. This initial metabolite is in tautomeric equilibrium with aldoifosfamide, which spontaneously eliminates acrolein to generate isofosforamide mustard, the active alkylating and cross-linking form. A second metabolic route for ifosfamide involves oxidation and subsequent dechloroethylation. This generates chloroacetaldehyde, which then reacts further to produce S-carboxymethylcysteine or thiodiacetic acid. Because the rate of ring hydroxylation is slower for ifosfamide than for cyclophosphamide, a larger fraction of the ifosfamide dose is metabolized by the alternate route and more chloroacetaldehyde is generated. This, together with the larger doses of ifosfamide required for equivalent DNA cross-linking and therapeutic efficacy, may explain the differences in adverse reactions of the two drugs. In addition, oral administration of ifosfamide produces larger amounts of dechloroethylated metabolites in the urine of patients than intravenous infusion and this may contribute to the greater incidence of severe encephalopathy after oral doses.

DOSAGE AND PREPARATIONS. The dry powder is reconstituted with sterile water for injection or bacteriostatic water for injection to a concentration of 50 mg/ml. Reconstituted solutions are chemically stable for one week at 30° C or three weeks at 5° C. For infusion, solutions may be diluted further in 5% dextrose injection, 0.9% sodium chloride injection, lactated Ringer's injection, or sterile water injection.

Intravenous: For testicular carcinoma, 1.2 g/M^2 per day for five consecutive days, administered as a slow infusion over at least 30 minutes. Alternative schedules (1.5 to 1.8 g/M^2 per day for five days or 2 to 2.5 g/M^2 for four days) have been tolerated in clinical studies. In Phase I trials, the total dose of ifosfamide in a single course was increased to 18 g/M^2, but dose-limiting renal toxicity and significant myelosuppression occurred above 16 g/M^2/course (Elias et al, 1990). Treatment is repeated every three weeks or after recovery from myelosuppression (WBC ≥4,000/microliter; platelets ≥100,000/microliter). To prevent hemorrhagic cystitis, at least 2 L of oral or intravenous fluid should be given daily for hydration, and mesna (at 20% of the ifosfamide dose) should be given with and four and eight hours after each dose of ifosfamide.

Ifex (Bristol-Myers Oncology). Ifex is only available in combination packages with the uroprotective agent, mesna. Powder in 1 and 3 g containers (with 200- and 400-mg ampul of mesna, respectively) and in ten 1-g containers (with ten 1-g containers of mesna).

MECHLORETHAMINE HYDROCHLORIDE

[Mustargen]

$$\begin{matrix} ClCH_2CH_2 \\ \quad\diagdown \\ \quad\quad {}^{+}NHCH_3 \quad Cl^- \\ \quad\diagup \\ ClCH_2CH_2 \end{matrix}$$

ACTIONS AND USES. Mechlorethamine was the first alkylating agent used clinically. The major indication for this bifunctional alkylating agent is in Hodgkin's disease as part of the MOPP regimen (see index entry Cancer: Clinical Responses to Chemotherapy) (DeVita et al, 1993; Takvorian and Canellos, 1993). However, the high incidence of secondary leukemia and other toxicities associated with this regimen has resulted in an increase in the use of alternative combinations (eg, doxorubicin, bleomycin, vinblastine, and dacarbazine [ABVD]) to treat Hodgkin's lymphoma. Some clinicians prefer variants of MOPP in which chlorambucil replaces mechlorethamine (see the evaluation on Chlorambucil). Other oncologists prefer alternating cycles of MOPP and ABVD (or ABV) for Hodgkin's disease. Currently, data from comparative studies are inadequate to establish consensus on the best combination regimen for these patients.

The MOPP regimen also is active in intermediate and aggressive non-Hodgkin's lymphomas (Freedman and Nadler, 1993; Longo et al, 1993). However, it is used infrequently in these patients and is usually restricted to postinduction therapy after remission is induced by ProMACE (prednisone, methotrexate/leucovorin, doxorubicin, cyclophosphamide, and etoposide).

Mechlorethamine may be useful in chronic myelocytic and lymphocytic leukemias, polycythemia vera, and cutaneous T cell lymphomas (mycosis fungoides and Sézary syndrome). Topical mechlorethamine has been effective in patients with plaque-stage cutaneous T cell lymphomas.

ADVERSE REACTIONS AND PRECAUTIONS. The most common immediate adverse reactions are nausea and vomiting, which are direct central nervous system effects. Vomiting may be severe, but usually stops within eight hours; nausea may persist for 24 hours. These reactions usually can be controlled by premedication with a sedative and an antiemetic. Anorexia, weakness, phlebitis, and diarrhea also may occur.

The usual and most serious dose-limiting toxic effect is bone marrow depression. The nadir of granulocytopenia and thrombocytopenia usually occurs within 7 to 21 days after drug administration. Hematologic recovery is usually adequate after four weeks, and rebound hyperplasia may be present from the fifth to seventh week. In contrast to cyclophosphamide, myelosuppression caused by mechlorethamine may be cumulative.

Other toxic effects are maculopapular skin eruptions, alopecia, hearing loss and tinnitus, vertigo, jaundice, menstrual irregularities, impaired spermatogenesis, and total germinal aplasia. Hyperuricemia may develop, particularly in lymphoma patients. Adequate fluid intake should be instituted prior to drug treatment to prevent uric acid nephropathy, or allopurinol should be given. Various chromosomal abnormalities have been reported after mechlorethamine therapy; this drug is teratogenic, mutagenic, and carcinogenic (FDA Pregnancy Category D).

Mechlorethamine is a potent vesicant. Thrombosis and thrombophlebitis may result from direct contact of the drug with the intima of the injected vein. Extravasation into subcutaneous tissue can cause severe, brawny induration and slough may result. If extravasation occurs, the area should be infiltrated with sterile isotonic sodium thiosulfate solution (1/6 molar), and an ice compress should be applied intermittently for 6 to 12 hours. Local corticosteroid injections are of questionable benefit.

Allergic hypersensitivity reactions are common after topical application and often require desensitization.

PHARMACOKINETICS. Mechlorethamine is highly reactive chemically and is hydrolyzed rapidly after intravenous injection; 90% disappears from blood in a few minutes. The drug penetrates cells through an active transport mechanism shared with the physiologic amine, choline. Excretion is via the urine, where approximately 50% appears in metabolized form in 24 hours. Less than 0.01% of unchanged drug is recovered in the urine.

DOSAGE AND PREPARATIONS. Because this agent has a pronounced vesicant action, it is usually injected into the tubing of a freely flowing intravenous infusion. The compound undergoes rapid chemical transformation and decomposes on standing; thus, it must be prepared immediately before administration. The use of surgical gloves is advised during preparation.

Intravenous: For disseminated Hodgkin's disease and other lymphomas, 6 mg/M^2 on days one and eight as a component of the MOPP regimen; the course is repeated every 28 days. (See the section on Combination Chemotherapy in the chapter, Principles of Cancer Chemotherapy.)

Topical: The solution is prepared by dissolving 10 mg mechlorethamine in 50 to 60 ml of sterile water. More dilute preparations are often necessary.

Mustargen (Merck). Powder (crystalline) 10 mg with sodium chloride q.s. 100 mg.

MELPHALAN
[Alkeran]

MELPHALAN HYDROCHLORIDE
[Alkeran for Injection]

ACTIONS. This phenylalanine derivative of nitrogen mustard is cell cycle nonspecific. Like chlorambucil, melphalan contains an aromatic ring. The electron-withdrawing effect of the ring moiety decreases the rate of reactivity of the drug and, therefore, allows time for absorption and distribution after oral administration before alkylation occurs.

USES. Melphalan usually is given orally and is an agent of choice (with and without prednisone) in the treatment of multiple myeloma (Anderson, 1993; Salmon and Cassady, 1993). Because bioavailability of the oral dosage form is inconsistent, an intravenous preparation has been developed for use in patients for whom oral therapy is not appropriate. Although 50% to 60% of patients with multiple myeloma have responded to oral melphalan plus prednisone, it is rarely curative; in a number of studies, median survival ranged from 19 to 39 months.

A meta-analysis of results from 18 randomized trials on patients with multiple myeloma that compared melphalan plus prednisone to regimens that included multiple cytotoxic drugs found no difference in two-year survival rates (Gregory et al, 1992). Melphalan also was a component of most of the combinations used in these patients. Retrospective subgroup analysis suggested that melphalan plus prednisone may be preferable for patients with a more favorable prognosis, while those with a poorer prognosis may survive longer when treated with multidrug cytotoxic regimens. However, more definitive evaluation of prognostic factors and prospective randomized trials in each subgroup are needed before treatment decisions can be based on these results.

High-dose myeloablative regimens using melphalan (alone or combined with other drugs) also have been investigated in patients with multiple myeloma (Cunningham et al, 1994 A, 1994 B) and other malignancies (Crump et al, 1993; Srivastava et al, 1993). In these and similar studies, treatment usually included infusion of bone marrow or peripheral blood stem cells to restore hematopoietic function. Although responses to the high-dose therapy were observed, no data are available from trials comparing duration of survival after high-dose regimens with survival after more conventional doses. Thus, the benefits of myeloablative regimens using melphalan have not been definitively established.

Melphalan also has been used for palliation of unresectable epithelial carcinoma of the ovary, but cisplatin-based combination regimens that do not include melphalan are more effective and currently are preferred (see index entry Cancer: Clinical Responses to Chemotherapy). Ovarian carcinoma (stage II or poorly differentiated stage I) has responded to adjuvant therapy with this agent (Young et al, 1993). Nevertheless, disease-free survival rates are similar after adjuvant therapy with either melphalan or intraperitoneal chromic phosphate P 32, and data are inadequate to establish a definitive role for melphalan in these patients.

In early trials, melphalan was shown to be active in breast carcinoma, and it was studied extensively as a single agent for adjuvant therapy of patients with stage II breast tumors. However, data from subsequent comparative trials demonstrated that combination regimens not including melphalan are more effective (Early Breast Cancer Trialists' Collaborative Group, 1992; Harris et al, 1992); at present, these are preferred to melphalan (see index entry Cancer: Clinical Responses to Chemotherapy).

Melphalan has been used for isolated limb perfusion of extremities affected by malignant melanoma, both at normal body temperatures and under hyperthermic conditions (Hafström and Mattsson, 1993). Although data from several studies suggest that this therapy as an adjunct to surgery improves local control of recurrent or in-transit melanomas, there are no data from well-designed randomized trials that show that duration of survival is improved after isolated limb perfusion with melphalan.

This drug also has been used as part of a combination regimen for second-line therapy of metastatic thyroid carcinoma. In addition, results of older clinical trials demonstrated beneficial effects of melphalan in patients with testicular seminoma, prostate carcinoma, chronic myeloid leukemia, and sarcomas of bone and soft tissues. However, newer, more effective regimens are available for each of these malignancies, and melphalan is no longer used for any of them.

ADVERSE REACTIONS. Melphalan produces dose-limiting bone marrow depression that results in leukopenia, thrombocytopenia, and anemia. Bolus oral doses are followed by gradual declines in the leukocyte and platelet counts; nadirs occur 28 to 35 days after therapy is initiated and recovery is observed two to three weeks after therapy is terminated. Blood counts must be monitored and the dosage reduced as necessary. Alternatively, supportive therapy with hematopoietic growth factors may be considered to hasten recovery from myelotoxicity (see the chapter on Hematopoietic Growth Factors).

Nausea and vomiting have occurred after large doses of melphalan.

In several trials in which large total cumulative doses were administered for one to two years, the risk for developing secondary acute myelogenous leukemia was increased in women successfully treated for ovarian cancer with this drug. There also have been rare reports of pulmonary infiltrates and fibrosis associated with prolonged melphalan therapy.

Although its safety during pregnancy has not been evaluated, this drug is potentially teratogenic and should not be used during this period unless absolutely necessary (FDA Pregnancy Category D). Melphalan is a known carcinogen in rodents.

PHARMACOKINETICS. Absorption is variable after oral administration and may be less than half that after intravenous administration in some patients. Plasma levels can be measured to assure adequate bioavailability. However, assays for melphalan are not widely available and may be inaccurate if samples are not stored and processed properly. Therefore, plasma levels are not monitored routinely; instead, most treatment protocols that include melphalan advise performing blood cell counts midcycle to ensure adequate absorption of drug. Between 20% and 50% is excreted in the stool, which suggests that incomplete gastrointestinal absorption contributes significantly to the poor bioavailability of oral doses. The time between ingestion of oral doses and the appearance of detectable drug levels in the plasma can vary from minutes to as long as six hours.

Melphalan is rapidly distributed throughout the circulation after intravenous injection (half-life, ~10 minutes). The volume of distribution at steady state is approximately 0.5 L/kg. Mean values for peak plasma concentrations after intravenous doses of 10 or 20 mg/M^2 were 1.2 ± 0.4 and 2.8 ± 1.9 ng/ml, respectively. From 60% to 90% of the circulating drug is bound to plasma proteins, with 30% bound irreversibly. The plasma elimination phase half-life of parent drug appears to vary somewhat depending on age (shorter in children than in adults) and the patient's hydration status (faster elimination with hyperhydration) (Lind and Ardiet, 1993). The half-life was approximately 50 to 60 minutes in adults and 37 to 43 minutes in children. Most of an administered dose is chemically altered by rapid hydrolysis, and hydrolysis products and metabolites persist in the body.

Estimates of the total body clearance of melphalan are approximately 7 to 9 ml/min/kg. Melphalan enters cells by an amino acid transport system. Less than 15% is excreted by the kidneys in the unchanged form. However, the drug should be used cautiously in patients with severe renal insufficiency, and dosage adjustments must be considered.

DOSAGE AND PREPARATIONS.

MELPHALAN:

Oral: 6 to 8 mg/M^2 for four consecutive days every six weeks. The dosage is usually adjusted to produce a mild leukopenia (total leukocyte count, 3,000 to 3,500/microliter) for optimal results.

Alkeran (Burroughs Wellcome). Tablets 2 mg.

MELPHALAN HYDROCHLORIDE:

Intravenous: For patients with multiple myeloma, 16 mg/M^2 infused over 15 to 20 minutes is administered once every two weeks for six weeks; the same dose is then administered once every four weeks. See the manufacturer's literature for guidelines on dose reduction based on leukocyte and platelet counts.

Alkeran for Injection (Burroughs Wellcome). Powder (lyophilized) equivalent to 50 mg base plus povidone 20 mg in single-use containers. Supplied with sterile diluent containing 0.2 g sodium citrate, 6 ml propylene glycol, 0.52 ml 96% ethanol, and water for injection to a total of 10 ml. After reconstitution to an initial concentration of 5 mg/ml, the dose to be administered is diluted further with 0.9% sodium chloride injection to a final concentration no greater than 0.45 mg/ml. The time between reconstitution/dilution and administration must be minimized because of the drug's instability in solution.

Uroprotective Agent

Mesna is a synthetic sulfhydryl compound used as a uroprotective agent during chemotherapy with ifosfamide (see evaluation on Ifosfamide). Hemorrhagic cystitis is a relatively frequent adverse effect of therapy with either of the oxazaphosphorine nitrogen mustards, ifosfamide and cyclophosphamide (Dechant et al, 1991; Dorr, 1991; Goren, 1992). Although mesna is not a DNA damaging agent and has no antitumor effects of its own, it is evaluated here in proximity to the alkylating agents with which it is used.

MESNA (Sodium 2-mercaptoethanesulfonate)
[Mesnex]

$$Na^+ \left[HS-CH_2-CH_2-SO_3\right]^-$$

ACTIONS. After intravenous or oral administration of mesna, the sulfhydryl compound is oxidized rapidly to a disulfide (dimesna), the sole class of mesna metabolites in mammals. Entry of dimesna and mesna into cells other than those in the renal tubules is inhibited because of their hydrophilicity. Since dimesna is not reactive, it does not affect the active hepatic metabolites of ifosfamide present in the circulation before they can be taken up by tumor cells. Circulating dimesna is rapidly cleared by the kidney, where it is reduced back to mesna and excreted into the urine. Like many other sulfhydryl compounds, mesna reacts with the acrolein and 4-hydroxylated metabolites generated from the oxazaphosphorines. The result of this reaction is detoxification of the metabolites thought to be responsible for hemorrhagic cystitis and hematuria (Dechant et al, 1991; Dorr, 1991). Since mesna and dimesna are found primarily extracellularly, detoxification of active metabolites in tumor cells probably does not occur. Most available evidence suggests that the use of mesna does not interfere with the intracellular cytotoxic effects and antitumor efficacy of oxazaphosphorines or other drugs.

USES. Mesna is used for prophylaxis to prevent hemorrhagic cystitis in patients being treated with ifosfamide.

Although the incidence of hemorrhagic cystitis is lower in patients treated with cyclophosphamide than with ifosfamide, use of mesna with cyclophosphamide also has been studied (Dorr, 1991; Goren, 1992). Mesna has been compared with intravenous hyperhydration (Shepherd et al, 1991) and hyperhydration plus mesna has been compared with hyperhydration plus continuous bladder irrigation (Vose et al, 1993) for uroprotection in patients receiving high-dose cyclophosphamide as part of a preparative regimen for myeloablation in conjunction with bone marrow transplantation. Results of these randomized trials suggest that the alternative therapies are equally effective as prophylaxis for severe hemorrhagic cystitis in bone marrow transplant patients. However, the incidence of urinary tract infections appears to be lower and discomfort significantly less with mesna plus hyperhydration than with continuous bladder irrigation plus hyperhydration (Vose et al, 1993).

ADVERSE REACTIONS AND PRECAUTIONS. In both animal studies and clinical trials, mesna produced very few acute or chronic toxic effects. In humans, controlled studies comparing ifosfamide plus mesna to ifosfamide with standard hydration or use of diuretics indicated that vomiting, diarrhea, and nausea were the sole side effects that could be attributed to the use of mesna. As might be expected from a sulfhydryl compound, even intravenous administration is accompanied by a bad taste in the mouth. At doses ten times the recommended amount, headache, fatigue, nausea, diarrhea, and limb pain occur frequently, and hypotension and allergic reactions sometimes develop.

Although mesna significantly reduces the incidence of hemorrhagic cystitis in patients being treated with ifosfamide, it has no effect on the nephrotoxicity or the other adverse reactions to ifosfamide, and prophylaxis is not successful in all patients; up to 6% of patients treated with both drugs have developed hematuria.

No studies evaluating carcinogenesis by mesna have appeared in the literature, but this drug is not mutagenic in a variety of in vitro assays. Mesna also is not fetotoxic or teratogenic in rats or rabbits. It is classified in FDA Pregnancy Category B.

PHARMACOKINETICS. Clearance of both mesna and dimesna from plasma is rapid, with half-lives of 15 to 30 minutes for the former and about 70 minutes for the latter. Clearance studies with radioisotope-labeled mesna measured in whole blood yielded a longer half-life (about four hours), possibly due to sequestration in red cells as mixed disulfides with glutathione or other endogenous sulfhydryls. Mixed disulfides of mesna with cysteine also have been detected and are thought to be responsible for the increased excretion of cysteine in patients given mesna. Between 50% and 60% of a dose is excreted into the urine over 24 hours, with the majority eliminated within four hours. Since urotoxic metabolites of ifosfamide continue to be excreted well after most of the mesna has been eliminated, the prophylactic agent is given both at the same time as and after administration of ifosfamide.

The volume of distribution for mesna (0.3 L/kg in rats and 0.65 L/kg in humans) suggests that this agent does not enter cells but is restricted to the circulating and extracellular fluid compartments. About 10% of a dose is bound to plasma proteins by both mixed disulfides and electrostatic interactions.

Although no dosage form of mesna specifically prepared for oral administration is available at present in the United States, this drug is well absorbed from the gastrointestinal tract after this route. Because of the short half-life of mesna, multiple doses must be given after each dose of ifosfamide or cyclophosphamide; therefore, the oral route may be more convenient than intravenous administration, particularly in outpatients. Mesna's disagreeable taste is a disadvantage, but various flavored diluents can be used to improve palatability. Mesna concentrations do not change appreciably for at least 24 hours after dilution in juices, syrups, or other beverages, with the exception of milk (Goren, 1992). Furthermore, the drug's therapeutic activity is retained since the oxidized form (dimesna) also is well absorbed after ingestion and is reduced to the free sulfhydryl in the kidney before excretion in the urine.

The bioavailability of free thiol in the urine after oral administration is 50% to 70% of that after intravenous administration (Goren, 1992). Therefore, some investigators recommend doubling the usual intravenous dose when mesna is given orally. In addition, at least one hour is required for absorption and excretion to produce adequate uroprotective concentrations. Data from a number of studies suggest that the oral and intravenous routes are equivalent in efficacy and safety (Goren, 1992).

DOSAGE AND PREPARATIONS. Prior to administration, mesna should be diluted to a final concentration of 20 mg/ml with 5% dextrose injection, 5% dextrose in 0.9% saline injection, 0.9% saline injection, or lactated Ringer's injection. Although the diluted solutions are stable for 24 hours at 25 °C, it is recommended that they be refrigerated and used within six hours. Mesna is not compatible with cisplatin.

Intravenous: For prevention of hemorrhagic cystitis in patients being treated with ifosfamide, 720 mg/M^2 (or 60% of the daily dose of ifosfamide, w/w) given as bolus injections in three equal fractions at the same time as and four and eight hours after administration of ifosfamide. For adequate protection from ifosfamide urotoxicity, mesna must be administered on each day of ifosfamide treatment, with modifications of mesna dosage in proportion to changes in the amounts of ifosfamide given. The amount remaining after each dose is given should not be used for subsequent administrations, since exposure of mesna to oxygen may generate sulfoxides that are probably inactive.

Mesnex (Bristol-Myers Oncology). Solution (aqueous, sterile) 100 mg/ml in 2, 4, and 10 ml single-dose containers.

AZIRIDINES

Based on the hypothesis that aziridinium intermediates are involved in the chemical reaction mechanisms by which nitrogen mustards alkylate and cross-link DNA, a number of chemically stable aziridine compounds have been synthesized and tested for antitumor efficacy. Drugs that contain three aziridine rings (ie, trifunctional alkylators) include triethylenephosphoramide (tepa), triethylenethiophosphoramide (thiotepa), triethylenemelamine, and trenimon (Colvin, 1993; Berger, 1993). Only thiotepa is still used for chemotherapy of human cancer in the United States. A bifunctional (diaziridine) drug, diaziquone, is under investigation, primarily for use in the treatment of brain tumors. The antibiotic mitomycin also has a single aziridine ring. For evaluation, see index entry on this drug.

THIOTEPA

ACTIONS AND USES. Thiotepa is a cell cycle nonspecific trifunctional alkylating agent. This drug has been employed in the palliative management of carcinoma of the breast and ovary, although more effective agents are available and are preferred (see index entry Cancer: Clinical Responses to Chemotherapy). Thiotepa has limited usefulness in Hodgkin's and non-Hodgkin's lymphomas. Intracavitary instillation may control pleural or peritoneal effusions. Intravesical instillation of thiotepa in superficial papillary carcinomas of the urinary bladder has some efficacy in reducing the incidence of recurrent tumors after transurethral resection or other endoscopic approaches to local control (Whitmore and Yagoda, 1989; Newling, 1990). Intrathecal thiotepa also has been utilized in carcinomatous meningitis.

Use of high-dose thiotepa (alone or in combination with other agents) followed by bone marrow transplantation is being investigated (Antman et al, 1990; Bitran et al, 1990). Data from a Phase I trial suggest that administration of sargramostim without bone marrow or peripheral blood stem cell support is insufficient to overcome the severe thrombocytopenia that occurs after larger doses of thiotepa (O'Dwyer et al, 1992).

ADVERSE REACTIONS AND PRECAUTIONS. The toxic effect on the bone marrow is dose-limiting in the absence of stem cell support; initial effects may not become evident for 5 to 30 days (median, 15 days). As with other alkylating agents, the white blood cell and platelet counts are reliable guides. The larger doses of thiotepa used for bone marrow ablation in preparation for bone marrow transplantation are associated with mucositis and dermatologic and dose-limiting neurologic toxicities.

Thiotepa may produce nausea, anorexia, and headache, but the incidence is less than with mechlorethamine. Amenorrhea and impaired spermatogenesis also have been observed. Thiotepa is teratogenic and, therefore, is contraindicated during the first trimester of pregnancy. The drug is also mutagenic and carcinogenic.

PHARMACOKINETICS. Thiotepa is unstable in acid and poorly absorbed from the gastrointestinal tract. It is not a vesicant and can be administered by direct intravenous injection and by intracavitary or intravesical administration. The pharmacokinetics of thiotepa is dose-dependent (O'Dwyer et al, 1991). With smaller doses ($\leq$55 mg/M^2), thiotepa is cleared at approximately twice the rate observed with larger doses ($\sim$350 ml/min/M^2). The area under the plasma concentration versus time curve is a nonlinear function of thiotepa dose, with the greatest increases occurring at the larger dosages, but the volume of distribution at steady-state remains relatively constant (60 to 70 L/M^2). The drug's elimination half-life varies from 50 to $>$200 minutes but also is independent of dose. Saturation of the rate at which thiotepa undergoes enzymatic oxidative desulfuration to triethylenephosphoramide (tepa) may partially explain the drug's dose-dependent pharmacokinetic behavior. The area under the tepa concentration versus time curve was several-fold larger than that of thiotepa but remained constant at all doses. The half-life for elimination of tepa has ranged from 3 to 21 hours.

Thiotepa crosses the blood-brain barrier. Approximately 85% is excreted in the urine in 24 hours, primarily as metabolites. Patients with renal failure may require reduced doses, but this has not been studied adequately and guidelines for dose reductions have not been established.

DOSAGE AND PREPARATIONS. Dosage must be individualized. The clinical response to thiotepa may be slow, and too frequent administration can cause bone marrow depression.

Intravenous: 0.3 to 0.4 mg/kg at one- to four-week intervals or 50 to 65 mg/M^2 every four weeks, depending on prior treatment status.

Intravesical: For bladder instillation, 30 to 60 mg in 30 to 60 ml of distilled water is instilled into the bladder by catheter and retained for two hours. The patient may be repositioned every 15 minutes for maximum contact. Treatment is repeated at one- to four-week intervals.

Intrathecal (investigational): 1 to 10 mg/M^2 has been given in a concentration of 1 mg/ml in sterile water for injection. An empiric total dose of 10 mg is currently recommended by the manufacturer.

Thiotepa (Immunex). Powder (sterile) 15 mg.

DIAZIQUONE (Aziridinylbenzoquinone, AZQ) (Investigational drug)

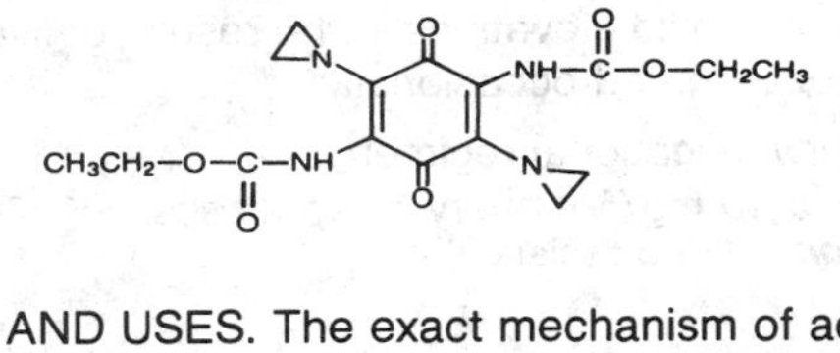

ACTIONS AND USES. The exact mechanism of action is unknown, but the chemical structure suggests that diaziquone may have alkylating and cross-linking activities. Experiments with purified DNA showed that reduction of the quinone moiety (either enzymatic or electrochemical) markedly enhances DNA alkylating and cross-linking activities (Lusthof et al, 1989). This suggests that diaziquone may have enhanced activity against hypoxic tumor cells. The drug may be activated via reduction by NADPH-dependent enzymes at a faster rate in hypoxic tumor cells than in well-oxygenated normal cells. Alternatively, these enzymes may be induced and present in larger amounts in a hypoxic environment, resulting in a net increase in the rate of drug activation. Selective toxicity of alkylating agents for hypoxic cells through this mechanism, which has been demonstrated for other drugs such as mitomycin (see index entry Mitomycin, As Antineoplastic Agent), has been termed bioreductive alkylation (Sartorelli, 1988). Exposure of cultured astrocytoma cells to diaziquone also results in mitochondrial toxicity.

In preclinical studies, diaziquone was reported to exert some action on rodent and human tumors. It was specifically designed to be a highly lipophilic drug able to penetrate the central nervous system; hence, it was used in clinical trials in patients with brain tumors (Kornblith and Walker, 1988; Levin et al, 1993; Prados and Wilson, 1993). In a randomized Phase III trial comparing diaziquone to carmustine in adults who had received surgery and radiation therapy for anaplastic gliomas, no significant difference in survival and time to tumor progression was observed between the two drugs (Schold et al, 1993). However, acute gastrointestinal and chronic pulmonary toxicities were more common in those treated with carmustine.

Diaziquone (administered by intravenous infusion) also has reduced the cerebrospinal fluid blast count in children with leukemic involvement of the central nervous system (Ettinger et al, 1988). However, bone marrow remission in response to this treatment did not occur in any of these patients. High rates of complete and partial response have been reported in patients with meningeal leukemia and other refractory meningeal malignancies who received intrathecal diaziquone therapy (Berg et al, 1992).

In clinical trials of diaziquone in advanced or recurrent solid tumors (eg, endometrial and gastric carcinomas), response rates were disappointing; this may have resulted from its administration as a single slow injection (Slayton et al, 1988; Pugh et al, 1989), given the drug's short half-life in plasma. Diaziquone's activity against primary brain tumors and cerebrospinal fluid blasts in acute leukemia suggests that the drug is retained somewhat longer in the central nervous system. This also may be a consequence of the drug's lipophilicity.

ADVERSE REACTIONS. Myelosuppression is the dose-limiting toxicity. Leukopenia and thrombocytopenia occur with about equal frequency and severity. Anorexia, diarrhea, weight loss, and mild elevations in the results of liver function tests have been noted occasionally.

DOSAGE (investigational regimen).

Intravenous: 40 mg/M^2 every three weeks.

Diaziquone (US Bioscience).

ALKYL SULFONATES

Linear molecules with terminal methylsulfonates separated by methylene chains of varying lengths are capable of alkylating DNA and other cellular molecules (Colvin, 1993; Berger, 1993). These molecules react directly with cellular nucleophiles in a bimolecular (SN-2) reaction that does not involve a reactive intermediate such as the aziridinium moiety postulated for nitrogen mustards. Since the alkyl sulfonates are less reactive than the aziridinium species generated from nitrogen mustards, they are more likely to react with intracellular sulfhydryls than with less nucleophilic nitrogen moieties. Because there are two methylsulfonate groups in each of these compounds, DNA cross-linking is at least theoretically possible and has been reported for busulfan, the analogue with four methylenes separating the terminal methylsulfonates. The preponderance of evidence implicates this as the major mechanism responsible for the cytotoxicity of busulfan. Although alkyl bis-(methylsulfonates) with chains of two to eight methylenes have some antitumor efficacy, busulfan has maximal activity and is the only one of these drugs used clinically at present.

BUSULFAN

[Myleran]

$$CH_3SO_2O(CH_2)_4OSO_2CH_3$$

ACTIONS AND USES. The cytotoxic action of this cell cycle nonspecific bifunctional alkylating agent primarily affects granulocytes and, to some extent, platelets. Busulfan is frequently used in the palliative treatment of chronic myelogenous leukemia (Deisseroth et al, 1993; Silver, 1993); however, some hematologists prefer to use hydroxyurea for this indication because adverse reactions occur less frequently and are milder. Busulfan also may be useful in the myeloproliferative syndromes, polycythemia vera and myelofibrosis with myeloid metaplasia. High-dose regimens of busulfan (with or without cyclophosphamide and sometimes other drugs) are being used as myeloablative treatment in preparation for allogeneic or autologous bone marrow transplantation (O'Reilly and Papadopoulos, 1993; Peters, 1993). The combination of cyclophosphamide and busulfan has been used before transplants for acute and chronic myeloid leukemias, multiple myeloma, lymphoma, and nonmalignant diseases such as aplastic anemia (Santos, 1993).

ADVERSE REACTIONS AND PRECAUTIONS. Toxic effects primarily affect the hematopoietic system, and leukopenia is usually dose limiting. The reduction in white blood cell count begins after about ten days of therapy and continues for two weeks after discontinuation of the drug. Busulfan can cause bone marrow hypoplasia, and peripheral leukopenia and thrombocytopenia may be prolonged (months). Thrombocytopenia may persist after leukocyte counts have returned to normal. The most likely cause of pancytopenia is failure to reduce or discontinue dosage as the blood counts decrease. Therefore, blood cell counts should be measured frequently. Busulfan should be employed with extreme caution in patients with a compromised marrow reserve (eg, because of prior radiation therapy or cytotoxic chemotherapy), unless bone marrow transplantation is planned as part of an overall management strategy.

Hyperpigmentation may develop during prolonged therapy and may be part of an Addison-like syndrome manifested by asthenia, hypotension, nausea, vomiting, and weight loss. Usually there is no objective evidence of adrenal hypofunction. Large doses of busulfan used in preparation for bone marrow transplantation can cause veno-occlusive disease of the liver (Morgan et al, 1991). Individual variability in this drug's pharmacokinetics results in differing exposures (ie, areas under the plasma concentration versus time curve) after identical doses are administered. Data suggest that the risk of this life-threatening complication may be greatest in those patients with the greatest exposure to busulfan. In addition, seizures have been reported in up to 7.5% of children receiving high-dose busulfan without simultaneous prophylaxis with antiepileptic agents (Vassal et al, 1990; Murphy et al, 1992).

Delayed effects, such as cataracts, ovarian fibrosis, amenorrhea, testicular atrophy, aspermia, and gynecomastia, may occur. Esophageal varices and portal hypertension have been associated with the combination of busulfan and thioguanine. A rare and potentially fatal complication is the "busulfan lung" syndrome manifested by persistent cough and progressive dyspnea caused by intra-alveolar exudation of fibrin with subsequent organization. This may not become clinically evident until one to ten years after treatment is begun and usually results in fibrosis and death. Despite the fact that the pathophysiology of this syndrome begins shortly after busulfan treatment, the damage may progress quite slowly. Large doses of corticosteroids may be beneficial, but their use remains controversial.

Serum uric acid levels should be monitored frequently; hyperuricemia, which may result in nephropathy and acute renal failure, can be treated by hydration, alkalization of the urine, and administration of allopurinol.

This drug is classified in FDA Pregnancy Category D.

PHARMACOKINETICS. Busulfan is well absorbed after oral administration. The mean half-life is 140 minutes; 10% to 50% is excreted within 24 hours as metabolites, primarily methanesulfonic acid.

The pharmacokinetics of high-dose busulfan appears to depend on age; the volume of distribution is larger and clearance is more rapid in young children (Vassal et al, 1992; Yeager et al, 1992; Regazzi et al, 1993). As a result, tissue and tumor exposure to the drug (as measured by the area under the plasma concentration versus time curve) in children between 3 and 15 years is approximately 50% that of adults receiving the same dose (by weight) and, in children <3 years, is only 25% that of adults. In children <3 years with lysosomal storage diseases, elimination half-lives were more prolonged, volumes of distribution were larger, and clearance was more rapid than in children of the same age with acute leukemia, immune deficiencies, or other diseases (Vassal et al, 1993).

DOSAGE AND PREPARATIONS.

Oral: For chronic intermittent therapy of chronic myelogenous leukemia, 2 to 5 mg/M^2 daily (or a total of 4 to 8 mg daily) until the white blood cell count decreases to 10,000/microliter; treatment is discontinued until the white blood cell count increases to 50,000/microliter and then is resumed as before. For chronic continuous therapy, 2 to 6 mg/M^2 daily until the white blood cell count decreases to 10,000 to 20,000/microliter; the dose then is reduced as necessary (usually to 2 mg daily) to maintain the white blood cells at this level.

In bone marrow ablative regimens as preparation for transplantation, *adults*, 1 mg/kg every six hours for four days or 600 to 640 mg/M^2 over four days (Vassal et al, 1992; Yeager et al, 1992). *Children,* the dose should be based on body surface area rather than weight to compensate for the more rapid clearance and larger volume of distribution.

Myleran (Burroughs Wellcome). Tablets 2 mg.

NITROSOUREAS

The nitrosoureas most frequently used to treat cancer are the chloroethyl derivatives, carmustine, lomustine, and semustine (investigational) (Berger, 1993; Colvin, 1993). These nitrosoureas are unstable and decompose to alkylating and carbamoylating intermediates in aqueous media. Alkylation at specific sites in DNA can be followed by DNA cross-linking. Although a number of cellular constituents can be alkylated and carbamoylation of the ϵ-amino group of lysines in proteins is common, it appears that DNA cross-linking is the lethal effect of the chloroethylnitrosoureas.

Resistance of human tumor cells to chloroethylnitrosoureas has been studied extensively in vitro and differs markedly from resistance to nitrogen mustards and other DNA cross-linking drugs (Pegg and Byers, 1992). There is much evidence to support the hypothesis that cross-link formation occurs by an initial chloroethylation at the O^6 position of guanine in DNA, followed by cyclization to N^1 and loss of the chlorine. The cross-link is an ethyl (ie, two-carbon) bridge from N^1 of guanine to the cytosine directly across the DNA double helix and forms after opening of the ring at the O^6 to ethyl group bond. Resistance to these drugs involves a repair protein capable of directly removing alkyl groups from the O^6 position of guanine before the cyclization step and cross-link formation can be completed. In contrast, repair of nitrogen mustard cross-links is thought to be a multistep process (the excision-repair pathway) in which the damaged nucleotides plus a variable number of neighboring nucleotides are excised from one strand, after which the gap is filled and ligated by appropriate enzymes.

These differences in DNA repair mechanisms implicated in drug resistance are thought to account for the absence of cross-resistance between the chloroethylnitrosoureas and the nitrogen mustards. Since the protein involved in repair of chloroethylnitrosourea-induced lesions is not a catalyst and is not capable of regeneration, cells have a limited capacity to repair this type of DNA damage. Thus, a number of combination protocols are now under investigation using pretreatment (eg, with the O^6 methylating agent streptozocin or the investigational agent O^6-benzylguanine) to deplete repair capacity and sensitize the tumor to subsequent treatment with a chloroethylnitrosourea (Micetich et al, 1992; Panella et al, 1992).

Carmustine is the least stable of the nitrosoureas; it must be dissolved immediately before use and administered by intravenous infusion. Lomustine and semustine are administered orally and are absorbed rapidly from the gastrointestinal tract. There is considerable nonenzymatic decomposition as well as metabolism for all three of these drugs, and the parent compounds disappear quickly from plasma. Some of the metabolites of lomustine and semustine retain alkylating and cross-linking activity, and many (both active and inactive) have longer half-lives in plasma due to protein binding and enterohepatic recirculation. Nearly all of an administered dose is eliminated by urinary excretion of metabolites and chemical decomposition products.

In contrast to many other antineoplastic drugs, the nitrosoureas are quite lipid soluble and cross the blood-brain barrier. Thus, they have been used to treat central nervous system malignancies.

Delayed, dose-dependent, and cumulative depression of the hematopoietic system is the major adverse reaction. Bone marrow suppression is more pronounced than with the nitrogen mustard alkylating agents. Maximal depression of platelets and leukocytes occurs after three to five and four to six weeks of therapy, respectively, and usually lasts for one to two weeks. In some patients, a second late nadir in the blood cell count may follow an apparent recovery. Severe nausea and vomiting also may be encountered.

Streptozocin, a glycosylated methylnitrosourea, differs from the chloroethylnitrosoureas in a number of its properties, including the absence of a chloroethyl moiety and thus its inability to cross-link DNA. In particular, the sugar moiety facilitates the uptake of this drug by pancreatic islet cells. Bone marrow toxicity is significantly less than with other nitrosoureas used clinically (see the evaluation).

CARMUSTINE (BCNU)
[BiCNU]

$$ClCH_2CH_2N(NO)-C(=O)-NHCH_2CH_2Cl$$

ACTIONS AND USES. Carmustine (bischloroethyl nitrosourea) alkylates and cross-links DNA. This drug also alkylates RNA and proteins, cross-links proteins to DNA, and carbamoylates amino acids, primarily the ϵ-amino group in lysine residues, in proteins. Carbamoylation of membrane constituents results in direct damage to the plasma membrane of normal and malignant cells. The drug's cytocidal efficacy appears to correlate most closely with its ability to cause persistent cross-links in DNA. Carmustine is cell cycle phase nonspecific, although cells in S phase are least affected.

Since carmustine is highly lipid soluble with a relative lack of ionization at physiologic pH, it readily crosses the blood-brain barrier and frequently is used to treat malignant tumors of the central nervous system (Prados and Wilson, 1993; Kramer and Packer, 1992; Lesser and Grossman, 1993; Levin et al, 1993). This drug also is active in multiple myeloma (in combination with prednisone), Hodgkin's disease, and non-Hodgkin's lymphomas. In lymphomas, it is used as secondary therapy in combination with other drugs when patients relapse or do not respond to primary therapy. Carmustine also has been used in melanoma, gastric and colorectal adenocarcinoma, and hepatoma. A topical solution has been employed to treat cutaneous T cell lymphomas.

Recently, carmustine has been used (alone or, more often, combined with other DNA alkylating drugs) for various solid tumors (eg, breast, lung) in high-dose myeloablative regimens followed by autologous bone marrow and/or peripheral blood stem cell rescue. Data suggest that such regimens produce objective (complete and/or partial) responses in a larger percentage of patients than standard doses. However, data are not yet available to compare the duration of survival after high-dose therapy with that after standard doses.

ADVERSE REACTIONS AND PRECAUTIONS. Bone marrow suppression is the usual dose-limiting toxicity. Onset is delayed, with platelet nadirs occurring four to five weeks and leukocyte nadirs five to six weeks after therapy begins. Thrombocytopenia is usually more severe than leukopenia, but both may be dose limiting. Complete blood counts should be performed frequently for at least six weeks after each dose. Carmustine should not be given more often than every six weeks. Since the effect on the bone marrow is cumulative, dosage adjustments must be made on the basis of blood counts obtained after the prior dose.

Nausea and vomiting are noted frequently and are dose related. They occur within two hours and usually last four to six hours. Prior administration of antiemetics may control vomiting (see index entry Vomiting, Drug-induced). Dose-related pulmonary toxicity has been observed often; the frequency is related to the total cumulative dose of carmustine. Symptoms include cough, dyspnea, or acute respiratory distress; deaths have been reported. Pulmonary function tests should be performed before therapy is begun and at regular intervals during treatment. Pulmonary fibrosis has been reported as long as 17 years after children and young adolescents received cumulative doses of 700 mg to 1.8 g/M^2 in combination with cranial irradiation for brain tumors. (O'Driscoll et al, 1990). Delayed-onset nephrotoxicity, including renal failure, also has been reported with the nitrosoureas. Large doses have produced reversible hepatotoxicity in a small percentage of patients; this is manifested by increased transaminase, alkaline phosphatase, and bilirubin levels. There have been isolated reports of optic neuritis. The nitrosoureas are mutagenic, teratogenic, and carcinogenic. Accidental skin contact with the reconstituted drug has caused transient hyperpigmentation.

This drug is classified in FDA Pregnancy Category D.

PHARMACOKINETICS. Because of its chemical instability, only intravenous preparations of carmustine are available. Tissue uptake, chemical decomposition, and metabolism occur rapidly; the elimination half-life of parent drug from serum is approximately 15 minutes. Metabolites and decomposition products are excreted primarily by the kidney. The drug readily enters the cerebrospinal fluid.

DOSAGE AND PREPARATIONS. Carmustine is dissolved in 3 ml of the sterile diluent supplied (ethanol), after which 27 ml of sterile water for injection is added aseptically. The resulting solution contains carmustine 3.3 mg/ml and may be diluted further with sodium chloride injection or 5% dextrose for injection.

Intravenous: As a single agent in previously untreated patients, 200 mg/M^2 is infused over a one- to two-hour period every six weeks. (More rapid infusion may produce intense pain and burning at the injection site.) This may be given as a single dose or 100 mg/M^2 may be given on two successive days. The dose should be reduced when carmustine is used with other myelosuppressive agents or in patients with impaired bone marrow function. Subsequent dosage is determined by the hematologic response to the preceding dose. The course should not be repeated until circulating blood elements have returned to acceptable levels (platelet count $>$100,000/microliter; leukocyte count $>$4,000/microliter), usually within six weeks.

Intra-arterial (carotid): Available data suggest that the efficacy of carmustine is increased in primary brain tumors when this drug is administered into the carotid artery. However, toxicity affecting the retina and normal brain tissue (presumably due to direct damage to cell membranes) severely limits the usefulness of this route.

Topical: Concentrations of 0.5 to 3 mg/ml in an aqueous solution with 30% alcohol have been used topically to treat plaque stage cutaneous T cell lymphoma.

BiCNU (Bristol-Myers Oncology). Powder (lyophilized) 100 mg with 3 ml of sterile diluent (anhydrous ethyl alcohol).

LOMUSTINE (CCNU)
[CeeNU]

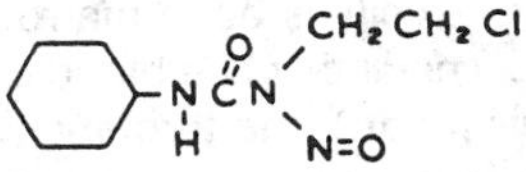

ACTIONS AND USES. This cyclohexylchloroethyl nitrosourea acts as an alkylating and DNA cross-linking agent but, like other nitrosoureas, it also inhibits several key enzymatic processes by protein carbamoylation. Like carmustine, lomustine produces interstrand cross-links in DNA and also has carbamoylating activity. The drug is cell cycle phase nonspecific but has the same selectivity for cells in G_1 or G_2 as carmustine.

Because of its high lipid solubility and relative lack of ionization at physiologic pH, lomustine readily crosses the blood-brain barrier and often is used to treat malignant tumors of the central nervous system (Kramer and Packer, 1992; Lesser and Grossman, 1993; Prados and Wilson, 1993; Levin et al, 1993). Lomustine also has been employed in combination regimens in small cell lung cancer (see index entry Cancer: Clinical Responses to Chemotherapy). Activity has been reported in melanoma, Hodgkin's and non-Hodgkin's lymphomas, and breast, non-small cell lung, and colorectal carcinomas.

ADVERSE REACTIONS AND PRECAUTIONS. The most serious toxic effect is bone marrow suppression, which is delayed, dose related, dose limiting, and cumulative. Thrombocytopenia develops about four weeks and leukopenia about six weeks after a dose of lomustine; both persist for one to two weeks. Complete blood counts should be performed weekly for at least six weeks after each dose. Lomustine should not be given more often than every six weeks. Since the effect on the bone marrow is cumulative, dosage adjustments must be made on the basis of blood counts obtained after the prior dose.

Gastrointestinal disturbances (nausea and vomiting) occur two to six hours after administration and last less than 24 hours. Vomiting can be severe, but prior administration of antiemetics can decrease the frequency and duration (see index entry Vomiting, Drug-induced). Other reactions include stomatitis, alopecia, anemia, and hepatotoxicity manifested by transient, reversible elevation of liver function tests. Neurologic reactions, such as disorientation, lethargy, ataxia, and dysarthria, have been noted but their relationship to medication is unclear. Delayed-onset nephrotoxicity, including renal failure, has been reported with the nitrosoureas.

These drugs are teratogenic, mutagenic, and carcinogenic. This drug is classified in FDA Pregnancy Category D.

PHARMACOKINETICS. Lomustine is rapidly absorbed after oral administration. Parent drug disappears rapidly from plasma. The plasma half-life of metabolites is 16 to 48 hours; 50% of the metabolized drug is excreted in the urine during the first 12 hours. Cerebrospinal fluid levels are 50% of plasma levels.

DOSAGE AND PREPARATIONS.

Oral: *Adults and children,* 130 mg/M^2 as a single dose every six weeks. In patients with impaired bone marrow function, the dose should be reduced to 100 mg/M^2 every six weeks. The dose also must be reduced when lomustine is used with other myelosuppressive drugs. Blood counts should be monitored weekly, and the dose should not be repeated before six weeks; circulating blood elements should return to acceptable levels (platelet count >100,000/microliter; leukocyte count >4,000/microliter). Lomustine should be taken on an empty stomach, and alcohol should be avoided on the day of ingestion.

CeeNU (Bristol-Myers Oncology). Capsules 10, 40, and 100 mg and dose pack containing two 100-mg, 40-mg, and 10-mg capsules each (stable for at least two years when stored at room temperature in tightly closed containers).

NIMUSTINE HYDROCHLORIDE (ACNU) (Investigational drug)

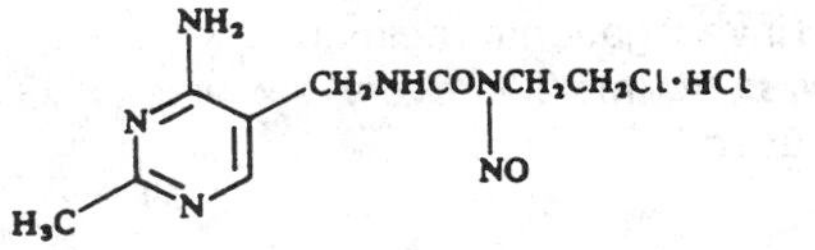

This chloroethylnitrosourea is more water soluble than the other drugs in this class. It has both alkylating and carbamoylating activities and is thought to exert its antitumor effects primarily through the formation of DNA interstrand cross-links.

Nimustine is active when combined with irradiation in the treatment of primary and recurrent malignant gliomas. It has modest efficacy against small-cell lung cancer, Hodgkin's disease, and chronic myelocytic leukemia. This drug has been administered by both the intravenous and intra-arterial routes. When injected intra-arterially, it is reported to cause less retinal and orbital toxicity than carmustine given by the same route. In addition, this route is associated with fewer myelosuppressive effects than intravenous infusion.

Results of early clinical studies determined that the maximal tolerated dose of nimustine was 100 mg/M^2 when administered by intravenous infusion. Cumulative and delayed myelosuppression was the dose-limiting toxicity, and six- to eight-week intervals were required between successive treatments. Other adverse reactions included nausea and vomiting, generalized fatigue, and elevations of serum transaminases.

DOSAGE (investigational regimen).

Intravenous, Intra-arterial: 100 mg/M^2 at six- to eight-week intervals (depending on leukocyte and platelet counts) to a maximum of 300 to 600 mg.

PCNU (Investigational drug)

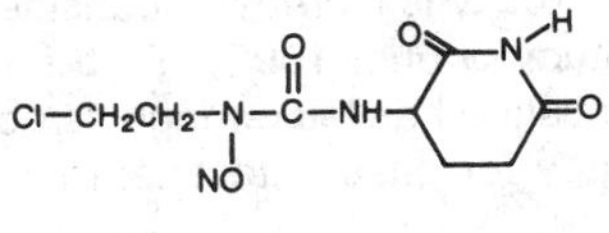

This nitrosourea analogue has high lipid solubility and alkylating activity and low carbamoylating activity. Its primary mechanism of action is DNA cross-linking. Preclinical studies suggest that PCNU has some activity in rodent and human tumors. In clinical trials, PCNU has had modest efficacy against intracerebral tumors when given by intracarotid artery or intravenous infusion. However, data from one randomized trial comparing PCNU with carmustine suggest that the two drugs are equally effective when combined with radiation therapy to increase the median duration of survival and the median time to tumor progression in patients with high-grade gliomas (Dinapoli et al, 1993).

Although leukopenia and thrombocytopenia were more pronounced in the patients receiving PCNU, those treated with carmustine experienced more nausea, vomiting, and other gastrointestinal reactions. Thus, the investigators concluded that PCNU offers no therapeutic advantage over carmustine as therapy for malignant gliomas.

Myelosuppression is dose limiting (less prolonged than with other nitrosoureas). Renal, pulmonary, and hepatic toxicities are rare. Moderate to severe nausea occurs frequently.

DOSAGE (investigational regimen).
Intravenous: 90 mg/M2 every six weeks. Glass syringes should be used.

SEMUSTINE (Methyl-CCNU) (Investigational drug)

CH_3 CH_2CH_2Cl O N C N H N=O

ACTIONS. Semustine (methylcyclohexyl N-[2-chloroethyl] nitrosourea) acts as an alkylating and DNA cross-linking agent. Like other nitrosoureas, semustine may also inhibit several key enzymatic processes as a consequence of its carbamoylating activity. This drug is cell cycle nonspecific.

USES. Therapeutic responses have been observed in patients with brain tumors; gastric, colorectal, and pancreatic adenocarcinomas; Hodgkin's disease; non-Hodgkin's lymphomas; and malignant melanoma. For malignant gliomas, reviews of clinical trials concluded that semustine has no significant therapeutic advantage over carmustine or lomustine when used either alone or in combination with radiation therapy (Kornblith and Walker, 1988; Kramer and Packer, 1992; Lesser and Grossman, 1993).

Although the response rates of gastrointestinal malignancies (eg, stomach, colon, pancreas) to semustine alone are low, one of the more effective regimens for adjuvant treatment of stage II or III rectal cancer combined semustine with fluorouracil (with or without vincristine) and high-dose pelvic irradiation (Fisher et al, 1988; Krook et al, 1991). However, data from a randomized comparative trial suggest that semustine contributes little to the overall efficacy of this multimodality approach and toxicity is increased considerably (Gastrointestinal Tumor Study Group, 1992). Furthermore, data demonstrate that semustine has leukemogenic activity when used as adjuvant therapy for gastrointestinal malignancies (Boice et al, 1983). Thus, most oncologists believe that it is no longer appropriate to include semustine in either experimental or standard multimodality regimens for adjuvant therapy of rectal carcinoma (Steele, 1991).

ADVERSE REACTIONS AND PRECAUTIONS. Nausea and vomiting occur four to six hours after administration and last six to eight hours. Vomiting can be severe; prior administration of antiemetics decreases the frequency and duration.

The dose-limiting toxicity is bone marrow suppression with delayed leukopenia (nadir of white blood cell count occurs six weeks after administration) and thrombocytopenia (nadir occurs after about four weeks). This myelosuppression is cumulative. Anemia is less apparent. Blood counts must be performed frequently for at least six weeks following each dose. Subsequent doses should not be given for at least six weeks, and adjustments must be made on the basis of the nadir from the previous dose. Secondary leukemias occur more frequently in patients treated with semustine than in those given other chloroethylnitrosoureas.

Delayed nephrotoxicity, including renal failure, has been reported frequently, particularly in children. Nephrotoxicity appears to be related to the total cumulative dose. In one study, renal damage occurred in five of six children receiving total doses >1.5 g/M2 (Harmon et al, 1979). Approximately 25% of adults receiving doses in excess of 1.4 g/M2 developed renal abnormalities. Individuals who received a lower total dose were unaffected (Micetich et al, 1981). Renal function must be monitored continually. If results of renal function tests (eg, BUN, creatinine clearance, serum creatinine) are abnormal, semustine should be discontinued. This drug should not be administered with other nephrotoxic drugs.

Other adverse effects include alopecia, pulmonary fibrosis (with prolonged use), and abnormal liver function tests. The drug is teratogenic, mutagenic, and carcinogenic.

PHARMACOKINETICS. Semustine is rapidly absorbed from the gastrointestinal tract following oral administration, and the parent drug rapidly disappears from plasma. The plasma half-lives of metabolites and decomposition products are long (eg, chloroethyl moiety, 36 hours; methylcyclohexyl moiety, 72 hours), but these fragments may be covalently bound to circulating proteins. The adducts are probably eliminated by further metabolism followed by renal excretion. Like other chloroethylnitrosoureas, semustine readily crosses the blood-brain barrier.

DOSAGE (investigational regimen).
Oral: 200 mg/M2 as a single dose every six weeks.

STREPTOZOCIN
[Zanosar]

CH_2OH O HO HO NH OH C NO O N CH_3

ACTIONS. Streptozocin is an antibiotic originally derived from *Streptomyces achromogenes*. Although it is a nitrosourea, the glucose moiety and the absence of a chloroethyl group confer properties that make this drug quite different from the chloroethylnitrosoureas. It has alkylating (methylating) activity but cannot cross-link DNA and also inhibits precursor incorporation into DNA. It lacks the carbamoylating activity of the other nitrosoureas because of a rapid internal cyclization reaction of the glycosyl isocyanate generated from streptozocin. Streptozocin is phase nonspecific. This drug also has direct effects on pancreatic islet beta cells that produce a form of diabetes in many animal species that resembles hyperglycemic, nonketotic diabetes mellitus in humans. This action appears to result from streptozocin-induced reduction in nicotinamide adenine dinucleotide levels in the beta cells.

USES. Streptozocin is taken up selectively by pancreatic islet cells and is cytotoxic to malignant islet cell tumors. Thus, its principal therapeutic use has been in metastatic islet cell tumors (including insulin-secreting and noninsulin-secreting beta cell and nonbeta cell) and gastrinomas (Norton et al, 1993; Vinik et al, 1993). Significant tumor regression (35% response rate) and a return to a normoglycemic state have occurred. Combination regimens containing streptozocin have been studied; a regimen consisting of streptozocin plus fluorouracil was superior to single-agent therapy for advanced islet-cell carcinoma (Moertel et al, 1980). The drug also is effective in patients with malignant carcinoid tumors; those of small bowel origin are most responsive. It may be of some value in combination regimens for advanced pancreatic carcinoma (Brennan et al, 1993; Douglass et al, 1993) and in secondary regimens for Hodgkin's disease. Streptozocin is either inactive or has equivocal status in other cancers.

ADVERSE REACTIONS AND PRECAUTIONS. Renal dysfunction is the major dose-limiting toxicity and occurred in 28% to 73% of patients in various clinical trials. The drug is toxic to both renal tubules and glomeruli. Symptoms include renal tubular acidosis (eg, glycosuria, aminoaciduria, acetonuria), proteinuria, anuria, hyperphosphatemia, and azotemia. Nephrotoxicity can occur with a single dose; however, it is more common with repeated doses, is dose-related, cumulative, and develops in most patients receiving prolonged treatment. The toxicity can be severe or fatal. Serial urinalysis, blood urea nitrogen, plasma creatinine, serum electrolytes, and creatinine clearance should be determined before therapy and at least weekly during and for four weeks after treatment. Mild proteinuria is one of the earliest signs that may indicate further deterioration of renal function and, when detected, should be quantitated with a 24-hour urine collection. If significant renal toxicity develops, the dose should be reduced or the drug discontinued. Mild abnormalities are often reversible on discontinuation of drug, but damage will be irreversible if treatment is continued. Patients with pre-existing renal dysfunction should not receive streptozocin unless the potential therapeutic benefit clearly outweighs the risk of further nephrotoxicity. Streptozocin should not be used with other nephrotoxic drugs. Urinary output should be maintained during and after treatment to ensure maximum dilution of the drug while it is passing through the kidney. Nephrogenic diabetes insipidus has been observed in two patients, one of whom responded to indomethacin.

The other major adverse effects of streptozocin are severe nausea and vomiting; diarrhea has been reported in some patients. Vomiting occurs in almost all patients one to four hours after administration; it can be protracted and occasionally necessitates discontinuation of therapy. Phenothiazine antiemetics do not alleviate symptoms. Some newer antiemetics (eg, ondansetron) may be effective (see index entry Vomiting, Treatment).

Hematologic toxicity is encountered only rarely, which makes this drug potentially useful for combination regimens. When it occurs, mild reduction of the hematocrit is most common. Fatal leukopenia and thrombocytopenia have been reported very rarely. Glucose intolerance develops rarely, is mild to moderate in severity, and is generally reversible. Patients receiving streptozocin for insulinomas should be monitored for hypoglycemia, which may result from release of insulin from drug-induced tumor cell kill. Abnormal liver function tests are common, and hepatotoxicity occasionally is severe. Streptozocin may cause a burning sensation on administration. Miscellaneous untoward effects include fever and eosinophilia.

This drug is classified in FDA Pregnancy Category C. Streptozocin is mutagenic in vitro and is carcinogenic after parenteral administration to some rodent species. The drug also impairs fertility in both male and female rats. Because of the possibility of serious toxicity in infants, nursing should be discontinued by mothers being treated with streptozocin.

PHARMACOKINETICS. Streptozocin is not active orally. After a single intravenous dose, it is rapidly cleared from plasma and parent drug is undetectable after three hours. The initial half-life of parent drug is 5 to 15 minutes, and the terminal half-life is 35 to 40 minutes. Metabolites are detected in plasma for up to 24 hours. Approximately 80% to 90% of the dose is metabolized in the liver. At least three major metabolites are generated, none of which has been clearly identified. The pharmacokinetics of streptozocin given by continuous infusion has been studied in a limited number of patients (Clamon et al, 1986). Mean steady state levels (0.7 to 0.9 mcg/ml) were achieved six hours after the start of infusion) (500 mg/M^2/day). The drug concentrates in certain tissues; the liver and kidneys contain the highest levels and the pancreas lesser amounts. Streptozocin enters the cerebrospinal fluid. Parent drug and metabolites are eliminated by the kidney; 20% to 30% of a dose is recovered in urine within four hours and almost 60% within 24 hours. Approximately 10% of an excreted dose at 24 hours is parent drug; less than 1% is recovered in feces.

DOSAGE AND PREPARATIONS.

Intravenous: For patients with islet cell tumors, the dose and schedule used most often is 500 mg/M^2/day for five consecutive days every four to six weeks. Therapy is continued until a maximal response or dose-limiting toxicity is observed; dose escalation on this schedule is not recommended. In an older regimen that is presently utilized less often, initial single weekly doses of 1 g/M^2 are given for two weeks, with gradual increases in dose up to a maximum of 1.5 g/M^2 in patients who do not respond to and/or experience significant toxicity from the previous course of treatment. Dosage reduction or discontinuation of treatment may be required in patients with renal insufficiency.

Zanosar (Upjohn). Powder (sterile) 1 g. (Refrigerate at 2° to 8° C and protect from light.)

PLATINUM COMPLEXES

As a consequence of their polarizability, the orbitals for outer-shell electrons in platinum form bonds between platinum and its ligands in inorganic coordination complexes, such as cisplatin, that are more covalent than ionic in character. Two features of platinum complexes that result from this chemical property are their spatial configurations and their ability to undergo displacement reactions (for reviews, see Colvin, 1993; Reed, 1993). Complexes of the Pt (II) oxidation state have chemical bonds to four ligands arranged in a square about the central platinum atom (square planar geometry). This allows for *cis-trans* isomerism in the square-planar complexes of cisplatin. Only the *cis* isomer, which carries both chlorides on the same side of the square, is a useful antitumor drug. Although complexes of the Pt (IV) oxidation state, which have six ligands arranged in octahedral geometry around the central platinum, have some antitumor effects (eg, tetraplatin), none are used outside of clinical trials at this time.

The displacement reactions of platinum coordination complexes are functionally analogous to the nucleophilic substitution reactions of alkylating agents. All platinum complexes used in cancer chemotherapy are bifunctional (ie, there are two ligands capable of displacement reactions) and thus can cross-link intracellular molecules. Most cross-links that occur after cisplatin treatment are thought to result from successive reactions in which water molecules displace the chloride ions and then are themselves displaced by amine groups or other intracellular nucleophiles. Some investigators believe that direct reaction without aquation can occur to a limited extent. The N^7 positions of guanine and adenine are the sites in DNA with greatest reactivity for platinum complexes. Second-generation antineoplastic platinum complexes have organic constituents as part of the ligands bound to platinum, either as carboxylates in place of the chloride ions (eg, carboplatin) or as organic amines in place of the ammonia molecules (eg, iproplatin). These were developed in a search for platinum complexes that might retain the antitumor efficacy of cisplatin but cause less nephrotoxicity or acute gastrointestinal toxicity. At present, carboplatin is the only second-generation antineoplastic platinum compound available for clinical use in the United States.

CISPLATIN (CPDD)

[Platinol]

H_3N ---- NH_3
Pt
Cl ---- Cl

ACTIONS. Cisplatin is a heavy metal coordination complex containing a central atom of platinum in the Pt (II) oxidation state surrounded by two chloride atoms and two ammonia molecules in the cis position. Its serendipitous discovery followed an observation that an electric current delivered to bacterial cultures via platinum electrodes led to inhibition of bacterial growth. Subsequent investigation showed that inorganic coordination complexes formed from the metal electrodes and present in solution were responsible for the cytocidal effects and that a continuous electric current was not needed. The cytocidal properties of cisplatin are somewhat similar to those of bifunctional alkylating agents; it damages DNA and is apparently cell cycle nonspecific. However, one consequence of cisplatin at concentrations that are cytocidal in vitro is an arrest in G_2 phase followed much later by cell death (Sorenson et al, 1990).

Cisplatin reacts with RNA more extensively than with DNA and with protein less extensively than with DNA. Most of the data on its mechanism of cytotoxicity support the hypothesis that DNA damage is the principal target responsible for the antitumor efficacy of cisplatin. Several classes of lesions present in DNA from human tumor cells treated with cisplatin can be detected at clinically relevant concentrations. These include monoadducts, intra- and interstrand cross-links, and DNA-protein cross-links (for reviews, see Colvin, 1993; Reed, 1993). Intrastrand cross-links at adjacent purines (d[GpG] or d[ApG]) account for about 90% of the platinum covalently bound to DNA from cisplatin-treated cells; interstrand cross-links are less than 1% of bound platinum. However, the relative contribution of each lesion to overall cisplatin cytotoxicity remains unclear. It is also not yet fully understood why cisplatin is an effective antitumor drug at relatively low concentrations, but its *trans* isomer produces little cytotoxicity and has no antitumor activity despite equivalent ability to produce interstrand DNA cross-links. Some investigators have hypothesized that the markedly reduced activity of *trans* platinum in generating intrastrand cross-links (compared with the activity of cisplatin) may relate to the differences in antitumor efficacy of the two isomers.

Resistance to cisplatin has been studied in both human tumor cell lines and in animal tumor models (Scanlon et al, 1989). Reduced intracellular accumulation of drug (presumably by altered transmembrane transport) is one mechanism that has been identified in cells selected in culture for resistance to cisplatin cytotoxicity (Gately and Howell, 1993). Increased inactivation of cisplatin by elevated concentrations of sulfhydryl compounds (glutathione and/or metallothionein) is a second mechanism of cisplatin resistance and may prove to be amenable to biochemical modulation with investigational agents such as buthionine sulfoximine (an inhibitor of glutathione synthesis). The third mechanism of cisplatin resistance is an increase in repair of cisplatin-induced DNA damage, and cells with this type of resistance also may be cross-resistant to nitrogen mustards or other classical alkylating agents. In addition, some cells resistant through increased DNA repair show cross-resistance to certain antimetabolites (fluorouracil and methotrexate). Data suggest that increased expression of DNA repair genes in ovarian tumor tissue harvested before therapy with cisplatin is associated with clinical resistance to the drug (Dabholkar et al, 1992, 1994). Nevertheless, the relative contributions of these three mechanisms to cisplatin resistance in cancer patients have not been established definitively.

USES. Cisplatin is the most active single drug against testicular tumors. Effective combinations for patients with disseminated seminomatous and nonseminomatous testicular cancer include cisplatin, bleomycin, and vinblastine (PVB) and bleomycin, etoposide, and cisplatin (PEB or $PVP_{16}B$) (*Semin Oncol*, 1992 B; Richie, 1993; Einhorn et al, 1993). Long-term survival and cures occur in more than 70% of patients.

In advanced ovarian carcinoma, the combination of cisplatin and cyclophosphamide is one of the standard regimens of choice for initial treatment. Meta-analyses of data from randomized comparative trials suggest that the response rate is greater and the median duration of disease-free survival is longer after therapy with cisplatin-based combination regimens than with cisplatin alone or combinations without cisplatin (Advanced Ovarian Cancer Trialists Group, 1991; Ovarian Cancer Meta-Analysis Project, 1991). However, a statistically significant difference has not been demonstrated for the overall duration of survival, possibly because patients who relapse after initial therapy with either cisplatin alone or nonplatinum-based regimens often receive salvage therapy with a cisplatin-based drug combination (McGuire, 1993; Thigpen et al, 1993). Evidence from meta-analyses also suggests that adding doxorubicin to a cyclophosphamide/cisplatin regimen increases response rates in patients with advanced ovarian carcinoma (Ovarian Cancer Meta-Analysis Project, 1991; Fanning et al, 1992). It is unclear, however, if the improved response rates are a direct result of adding doxorubicin to this regimen or simply reflect an increase in the total dose intensity when all three drugs are administered. Preliminary data from a randomized trial comparing cisplatin plus cyclophosphamide with cisplatin plus paclitaxel for women with ovarian cancer suggest that response rates are better and the risk of recurrence is reduced with the latter regimen (McGuire, 1994). More definitive data are needed to determine which of these regimens has the greatest benefit for survival of women with ovarian cancer.

Cisplatin also is administered by the intraperitoneal route in patients with advanced ovarian cancer who have an incomplete response to initial systemic therapy (Howell et al, 1991; Markman et al, 1993 A). After intraperitoneal instillation, drug concentration in the peritoneal cavity is approximately 15- to 20-fold higher than in the plasma. This approach to regional therapy appears to benefit some women with small-volume residual ovarian tumors that remain after initial treatment with cisplatin-based regimens. The efficacy of intraperitoneal cisplatin is being assessed in a randomized trial currently in progress.

Cisplatin also is a component of combination regimens used as preferred therapy for carcinomas of the bladder, cervix, lung (small cell and non-small cell), thyroid, and esophagus and for head and neck tumors, osteogenic sarcoma, neuroblastoma, and medulloblastoma (see index entry Cancer: Clinical Responses to Chemotherapy). Alternative and second-line therapeutic regimens for patients with advanced gastric carcinoma, multiple myeloma, melanoma, intermediate- and high-grade non-Hodgkin's lymphomas, high-risk trophoblastic tumors, and glioblastoma also include cisplatin. The drug is reported to be active (alone or in combination) against basal and squamous cell skin cancer, uterine and other soft tissue sarcomas, poorly differentiated carcinomas or adenocarcinomas of unknown primary sites, inoperable alpha-fetoprotein positive hepatoma, and breast carcinoma. However, data to evaluate the efficacy of cisplatin in this last group of cancers are limited.

The intra-arterial and intravesicular routes have been employed (the former for head and neck cancer or malignant melanoma and the latter for bladder tumors), but these approaches to regional chemotherapy cannot yet be considered routine practice.

ADVERSE REACTIONS AND PRECAUTIONS. The most frequent and serious toxicity produced by cisplatin when it is given as a single dose per treatment cycle in the absence of adequate hydration and diuresis is impaired renal function due to a direct toxic effect on renal tubules (Reed, 1993; Colvin, 1993). This is manifested by elevations in BUN, creatinine, and serum uric acid levels and/or decreased creatinine clearance. Nephrotoxicity is usually first noted during the second week of therapy after the initial dose and is dose related and cumulative. Adequate hydration of the patient prior to administration of cisplatin, often with concurrent administration of a diuretic, is the most important and effective measure for decreasing the incidence of drug-induced nephrotoxicity (Cornelison and Reed, 1993). Dose fractionation, slow intravenous infusion, and dilution of the dose in hypertonic saline also have been employed. Although concurrent administration of sodium thiosulfate has been tested as a means of protecting the kidney (Goel et al, 1989; Reichman et al, 1991), there is a concern that thiosulfate may inactivate cisplatin and thus also reduce its effects on the tumor. Other nephrotoxic drugs (eg, aminoglycosides) should be avoided in patients receiving cisplatin.

Other major dose-related manifestations of toxicity are myelosuppression, nausea and vomiting, ototoxicity, and neurotoxicity. Myelosuppression occurs in 25% to 30% of patients treated with cisplatin but usually is milder than with most other myelosuppressive drugs. As a result, cisplatin often is used in combination regimens with other myelotoxic drugs. Myelosuppression caused by cisplatin is most pronounced when doses exceed 50 mg/M^2. The nadirs in circulating platelet and leukocyte counts occur between days 18 and 23 (range, 7.5 to 45), and most patients recover by day 39 (range, 13 to 62). Cumulative anemia, with decreases in hemoglobin levels of more than 2 g Hb/dL, parallels the occurrence of leukopenia and thrombocytopenia.

Nausea and vomiting occur in almost all patients treated with cisplatin and are occasionally so severe that the drug must be discontinued. These reactions usually begin within one to four hours after treatment and last up to 24 hours. Nausea and anorexia may persist for one to two weeks after treatment in some patients. Large intravenous doses of metoclopramide given 30 minutes before cisplatin and every two to three hours thereafter alleviate vomiting in most patients;

however, intravenous ondansetron has replaced metoclopramide for this indication since it appears to be at least equally effective and adverse reactions are milder and less frequent. Administration of lorazepam or large doses of dexamethasone with ondansetron or metoclopramide may be effective in nonresponsive patients (see index entry Vomiting, Treatment, for Antineoplastic Agent-Induced).

Ototoxicity, manifested by tinnitus and/or hearing loss in the high frequency range (4,000 to 8,000 Hz), has been observed in at least 31% of patients treated with a single dose of 50 mg/M^2 of cisplatin. Ototoxic effects may be more severe in children. In addition, ototoxicity occurs at much lower cumulative doses when cisplatin is given after cranial irradiation for brain tumors; however, data suggest that radiation therapy does not potentiate ototoxicity if cisplatin is given prior to cranial irradiation (Kretschmar et al, 1990). Hearing loss may be unilateral or bilateral and tends to become more severe with repeated doses. The ability to hear normal conversational tones may be decreased occasionally. The manufacturer recommends that audiometry be performed prior to and during cisplatin therapy. However, many oncologists rely on clinical rather than audiometric evaluation of hearing and discontinue the drug or reduce the dosage only if significant loss of hearing occurs in the speech frequency range (but not in the high-frequency range).

Neurotoxicity, usually characterized by peripheral neuropathies, may be irreversible in some patients. Loss of taste, visual disturbances, and seizures also have been reported. Although neurotoxicity is not dose limiting with single conventional doses (see below), it may be dose-limiting when cisplatin is diluted in hypertonic saline and given in doses of 40 mg/M^2/day for five consecutive days or in single doses of 200 mg/M^2. In addition, cumulative neuropathy frequently limits the number of cycles of combination regimens containing cisplatin that can be administered.

A randomized trial suggested that Org 2766, a neurotrophic peptide analogue of a segment of adrenocorticotrophic hormone (ACTH[4-9]), may prevent or attenuate cisplatin-induced neuropathy without reducing antitumor efficacy (van der Hoop et al, 1990). However, this protective effect of Org 2766 on cisplatin-induced neuropathy was not confirmed in a more recent and larger double-blind randomized study (Neijt et al, 1994). Amifostine (ethiofos, WR-2721), an investigational organic thiophosphate protective agent, also has been given to reduce the incidence of neuropathy and decrease the ototoxic and nephrotoxic effects in patients treated with cisplatin (Schuchter and Glick, 1993). Since higher concentrations of amifostine accumulate in normal cells and tissues than in tumors, the protection provided may not reduce the antitumor efficacy of cisplatin. However, data are unavailable to determine if the clinical efficacy of cisplatin remains the same with and without amifostine; therefore, use of this protective agent should be restricted to randomized clinical trials.

Decreased levels of serum calcium, magnesium, potassium, and sodium have been observed in patients receiving cisplatin. The decline in calcium and potassium concentrations may be related to the intravenous infusion of large volumes of fluid; in contrast, effects on magnesium and sodium levels are thought to result from loss of these ions in the kidney. In many cases, decreased levels of electrolytes may persist for several weeks and are caused by inappropriate electrolyte excretion resulting from renal tubular damage. Postural hypotension is common in these patients and may be alleviated by use of salt tablets.

In a small percentage of patients previously treated with cisplatin, anaphylactoid reactions (facial edema, wheezing, tachycardia, and hypotension) have been observed within a few minutes after readministration. During the last decade, several physicians have reported that plasma concentrations of antiepileptic drugs decrease to subtherapeutic levels in patients also receiving combination regimens containing cisplatin.

Cisplatin is mutagenic in bacteria and cultured animal cells and teratogenic and embryotoxic in mice. Use of cisplatin in pregnant women should be avoided except when less toxic drugs are not available or the tumor is refractory to other therapy. This drug is classified in FDA Pregnancy Category D. Because of the potential for serious harm to infants, nursing should be discontinued by mothers being treated with cisplatin.

This drug has been reported to be a complete carcinogen and a tumor initiator in animal model systems (for review, see Greene, 1992). It also enhances the conversion of mouse skin tumors from a benign to a malignant phenotype (Hennings et al, 1990). Although data are not available to demonstrate conclusively that cisplatin is a carcinogen in humans, other DNA-damaging drugs with comparable mutagenic potency have been shown to be carcinogenic. There have been several reports of secondary myelodysplasias or acute nonlymphocytic leukemia in patients treated with drug combinations that included cisplatin (for review, see Greene, 1992). However, other known or suspected carcinogens also were used, which precluded identification of a single causative agent.

PHARMACOKINETICS. Cisplatin is administered intravenously. The plasma elimination curve determined by measurement of total platinum is biphasic with half-lives of 25 to 49 minutes and 58 to 73 hours, respectively. More than 90% of the drug present during the second phase is bound irreversibly and covalently to plasma proteins and thus is inactive and nontoxic. The kinetics of ultrafilterable (ie, unbound) platinum also is biphasic; however, the elimination phase half-life of parent drug is only approximately two hours. The major route for clearance of ultrafilterable cisplatin is by covalent reaction with plasma proteins. In contrast, bound platinum is eliminated through protein catabolism followed by renal excretion of platinum adducts with amino acids or small peptides. Up to 30% of the total platinum administered is excreted in the urine during the first 24 hours, but only 25% to 45% is recovered from urine after five days. Very little drug is found in feces. Significant tissue binding occurs, particularly in the liver, kidney, intestine, and skin, and bound platinum persists in the body for prolonged periods. Little cisplatin appears to enter the cerebrospinal fluid but therapeutically adequate amounts penetrate into brain tumor tissue.

DOSAGE AND PREPARATIONS.
Intravenous: When given as a single agent, 60 to 120 mg/M² once every three to four weeks.

When combined with vinblastine or etoposide and bleomycin for testicular cancer, 20 mg/M² daily for five days (days one to five) every three weeks for four courses.

When combined with cyclophosphamide with or without doxorubicin for advanced ovarian carcinoma, 50 to 100 mg/M² once every three weeks for six to eight cycles.

Hydration with 1 to 2 L of 5% dextrose in 0.45% or 0.9% saline infused for several hours prior to and for several hours after cisplatin therapy is recommended. Adequate hydration and urinary output must be maintained during the following 24 hours. However, the drug should not be added directly to 5% dextrose solutions because it decomposes. Mannitol is often administered concomitantly to ensure adequate diuresis. Concurrent therapy with furosemide is no longer recommended unless the patient has clinical fluid overload. Solutions also should not be given through aluminum needles or intravenous sets with parts containing aluminum since chemical reaction of cisplatin with aluminum causes the drug to precipitate and decreases its potency.

Renal function and blood cell counts should be monitored carefully during therapy. The manufacturer also recommends that patients being treated with cisplatin be tested periodically by audiometric analysis.

Platinol (Bristol-Myers Oncology). Powder (lyophilized) 10 and 50 mg; solution 1 mg/ml in 50 and 100 ml containers (***Platinol-AQ***).

CARBOPLATIN (JM-8, CBDCA)
[Paraplatin]

ACTIONS. Of the many cisplatin analogues developed and studied over the past decade, carboplatin is the first to be approved for use outside of clinical trials. It is a platinum (II) coordination complex that differs structurally and chemically from cisplatin in that a dicarboxycyclobutane moiety replaces the two chloride ion ligands present in the earlier drug. Like cisplatin, carboplatin reacts with DNA to generate both interstrand and intrastrand cross-links. Since carboplatin differs only in the composition of the leaving groups, the resulting DNA adducts are structurally identical to those generated by cisplatin. These adducts are probably responsible for the drug's cytocidal effects. Replacement of the carboxylato ligands of carboplatin by water molecules occurs at a slower rate than does aquation at the chloride ligands of cisplatin. Since these reactions produce the active cross-linking species from each drug, the kinetic difference may account for their relative potencies. When used as monotherapy, carboplatin is usually given in doses four times higher than cisplatin. In cells, DNA cross-links appear more slowly after carboplatin than after cisplatin. Carboplatin is not cell cycle specific.

USES. The spectrum of activity of carboplatin is generally similar to that of cisplatin. The major advantage for the newer analogue is its differing profile of toxicity.

Carboplatin is indicated for initial therapy of advanced epithelial ovarian cancer in combination with other chemotherapeutic drugs (usually cyclophosphamide with or without doxorubicin). Results of randomized comparative trials demonstrate that clinical and pathologic response rates and median durations of overall and progression-free survival are comparable for patients receiving regimens with equipotent doses of carboplatin or cisplatin (Conte et al, 1991; Alberts et al, 1992; Swenerton et al, 1992). Data from additional trials established the equivalence of carboplatin and cisplatin monotherapy in equipotent doses for women with advanced ovarian carcinoma (for reviews, see Rozencweig et al, 1990; McGuire and Rowinsky, 1991; Ozols and Young, 1991; McGuire, 1993). The reduced nephrotoxicity, neurotoxicity, and emetogenicity of carboplatin compared with cisplatin may improve the therapeutic index of the carboplatin-based regimen. On the other hand, there is greater overlap in the toxicity profiles of cyclophosphamide and carboplatin, since the latter causes more severe hematologic toxicity (most notably thrombocytopenia) than cisplatin. Consequently, it may be necessary to reduce dosages in later courses more frequently for women receiving carboplatin than for those treated with cisplatin. This could result in delivery of smaller cumulative doses and a lower dose intensity of the platinum agent, thus reducing response rates and durations of survival. Thus, disagreement persists among oncologists on the choice between regimens that include carboplatin or cisplatin for first-line therapy of advanced ovarian carcinoma.

Carboplatin (alone or in combination regimens) also is indicated as salvage therapy for women with recurrent ovarian carcinoma, including those who previously responded to cisplatin-based regimens (Thigpen et al, 1993). However, women whose malignancies progressed during or within six months of initial therapy that included cisplatin are considered to have platinum-resistant tumors and are unlikely to respond to carboplatin. The use of carboplatin combined with cisplatin to increase the magnitude and/or the intensity of the platinum dose administered to women with advanced ovarian carcinoma is being investigated (Dittrich et al, 1993; Waterhouse et al, 1993). Other trials are exploring the use of intraperitoneal carboplatin compared with intraperitoneal cisplatin in women with minimal residual ovarian carcinoma (Pfeiffer et al, 1990; Speyer et al, 1990; Markman et al, 1993 A, 1993 B). Finally, the use of high-dose carboplatin followed by supportive therapy with hematopoietic growth factors to ameliorate drug-induced myelotoxicity also is being investigated (Reed et al, 1993). At present, data are inadequate to allow definitive evaluation of the therapeutic benefits of combining platinum agents, intraperitoneal carboplatin, or high-dose carboplatin for advanced ovarian carcinoma.

Carboplatin (alone or in combination regimens) also is active in patients with squamous cell head and neck tumors (Tobias, 1992; Vokes et al, 1993), small cell lung cancer (Gatzemeier et al, 1991, 1992), and nonseminomatous testicular germ cell tumors (*Semin Oncol*, 1992 B; Richie, 1993; Einhorn et al, 1993). Despite significant rates of objective response to carboplatin, data from randomized comparative trials suggest that cisplatin is more effective in combination chemotherapy for germ cell (Bajorin et al, 1993) and head and neck tumors (Forastiere et al, 1992). No data are available from randomized trials comparing carboplatin to cisplatin in patients with small cell lung cancer. Therefore, use of carboplatin for these indications outside of clinical trials should be restricted to second-line therapy.

Additional uncontrolled studies have provided evidence that carboplatin (alone or in combination) may induce objective responses in some patients with the following advanced or metastatic malignancies: testicular seminoma; non-small cell lung cancer; endometrial, cervical, bladder, and breast carcinoma; soft tissue sarcoma; recurrent glioma and medulloblastoma; acute leukemia; and various pediatric solid tumors. However, data are inadequate to support the use of carboplatin outside of clinical trials for any of these indications, with the possible exception of alternative therapy for breast, bladder, and endometrial carcinomas, glioma and medulloblastoma, and non-small cell lung cancer.

ADVERSE REACTIONS AND PRECAUTIONS. In contrast to cisplatin, renal impairment is minimal and infrequent and hearing loss or neuropathy is rare with usual doses of carboplatin. Myelosuppression is the dose-limiting toxicity and necessitates close hematologic monitoring and the ready availability of supportive therapy. Thrombocytopenia is the predominant hematologic effect (platelet count of $<10^5$/microliter in 37% of patients receiving 400 mg/M^2), with platelet nadirs occurring between two and three weeks and recovery by the fourth week after treatment. Leukopenia and anemia have been observed less frequently and are less severe than the effect on thrombocytes. Nevertheless, data indicate that the incidence of carboplatin-induced thrombocytopenia and leukopenia may approach 100% as the area under the plasma concentration versus time curve (AUC) for carboplatin increases (Jodrell et al, 1992). At any given value for AUC, however, thrombocytopenia is more frequent than leukopenia. Myelotoxicity also is more frequent in patients with poorer performance status, the elderly, and in those with renal dysfunction or a prior history of cytotoxic chemotherapy. The myelotoxicity of any given carboplatin AUC also is increased by concurrent administration of cyclophosphamide (Reyno et al, 1993). Carboplatin-induced myelosuppression may be cumulative, although there are few studies on the toxic effects of repeated courses.

Nausea and vomiting occur frequently but are usually delayed until 6 to 12 hours after treatment and usually disappear within 24 hours. Standard antiemetic regimens control these gastrointestinal reactions (see index entry Vomiting, Drug-induced). Comparative trials have shown that carboplatin causes less intense and less frequent nausea or vomiting than cisplatin in patients not receiving antiemetics. Alopecia is mild and infrequent after a single dose of carboplatin alone, but both the incidence and severity increase after three courses or in combination chemotherapy. Other less frequent side effects include abnormal liver function tests (elevated bilirubin, AST, or alkaline phosphatase levels), hypersensitivity, stomatitis, mucositis, and a "flu-like" syndrome. Sudden onset of cortical blindness was reported in two patients with impaired renal function who received high-dose carboplatin therapy (O'Brien et al, 1992).

Since carboplatin is less nephrotoxic than cisplatin, extensive hydration is not required prior to treatment. However, hydration is necessary for patients with impaired renal function and those receiving high doses, since reductions in creatinine clearance ranging from 36% to 61% of pretreatment values occurred in all patients treated with $\geq$800 mg/M^2 who were not adequately hydrated (Cornelison and Reed, 1993).

Concurrent administration of aminoglycosides with carboplatin can increase the frequency of renal impairment (and ototoxicity). Aluminum can react with carboplatin, resulting in precipitation and decreased potency. Thus, aluminum needles or intravenous sets with parts containing aluminum should not be used.

Carboplatin is mutagenic, probably carcinogenic, embryotoxic, and teratogenic. It is classified in FDA Pregnancy Category D.

PHARMACOKINETICS. In studies estimating the pharmacokinetic parameters of carboplatin in patients, intravenous doses ranged from 11 mg/M^2 to 2.4 g/M^2 and dosage durations ranged from bolus administration to four-day infusions (for review, see van der Vijgh, 1991). The pharmacokinetics of this drug appears to be linear over the entire range of doses. Many studies have determined total and ultrafilterable (ie, nonprotein bound) platinum concentrations in plasma and urine as a function of time after drug administration; a smaller number also have measured unmodified carboplatin in these fluids. In patients with normal renal function, the distribution phase ($t_{1/2\alpha}$=23 min) is followed by an initial elimination phase ($t_{1/2\beta}$=120 min) that represents renal clearance of ultrafilterable platinum and a terminal elimination phase ($t_{1/2}$=5.8 days) that reflects slow breakdown of proteins to which platinum is irreversibly and covalently bound. As with cisplatin, protein-bound carboplatin is inactive and nontoxic. The half-lives for the first two phases are longer in patients with reduced rates of creatinine clearance.

The distribution and elimination-phase half-lives for ultrafilterable carboplatin are significantly longer than those for ultrafilterable cisplatin, probably because the elimination of carboplatin occurs almost exclusively by glomerular filtration while cisplatin is cleared by rapid reaction with plasma proteins. The terminal elimination-phase half-lives of protein adducts for the two drugs are identical; however, significantly less protein binding occurs with carboplatin than with cisplatin. This, together with the absence of tubular secretion, may account for the reduced incidence of nephrotoxicity in patients treated with carboplatin compared with cisplatin.

About 65% of a carboplatin dose is excreted in the first 12 hours and 6% is excreted over the next 12 hours. The remainder probably is tissue- and protein-bound platinum that is eliminated slowly after proteolysis. Almost all of the platinum present in the urine after 24 hours is unmodified carboplatin, which indicates that little, if any, metabolism occurs. Tissue distribution is similar to that of cisplatin, with the highest levels found in the liver, kidney, skin, and tumors.

Response rates to carboplatin and the incidence of myelotoxicity appear to be directly proportional to the area under the plasma concentration versus time curve (AUC) (Jodrell et al, 1992). Since clearance of carboplatin occurs solely by glomerular filtration, the AUC can easily be estimated from the dose and the glomerular filtration rate (GFR). Individualized doses based on a target AUC of 5 to 6 mg/ml x min can be calculated for adults from the formula: Dose (mg) = AUC (mg/ml x min) x (GFR [ml/min] + 25) (Calvert et al, 1989). For children, who have less tissue mass and plasma protein available to react covalently with carboplatin, a modified formula for estimating optimal individualized doses of carboplatin is: Dose = AUC x (GFR + [0.36 x body weight (kg)]) (Newell et al, 1993). Patients with a poor performance status, those who received previous myelotoxic chemotherapy (Jodrell et al, 1992), or those receiving cyclophosphamide concurrently (Reyno et al, 1993) should receive a dose targeted to achieve a smaller AUC.

DOSAGE AND PREPARATIONS. The crystalline drug is reconstituted immediately before use with sterile water for injection, 5% dextrose for injection, or 0.9% saline for injection to a concentration of 10 mg/ml. It can be further diluted to as low as 0.5 mg/ml with 5% dextrose injection or 0.9% saline injection. Solutions are stable for eight hours at room temperature.

Intravenous: When used alone in patients with recurrent ovarian carcinoma, 360 mg/M^2 infused over at least 15 minutes is the standard regimen. Subsequent doses can be given after four weeks or when the platelet count is $\geq 10^5$ and the neutrophil count is $\geq$2,000. As first-line therapy for ovarian carcinoma, 300 mg/M^2 combined with cyclophosphamide 600 mg/M^2 is infused on day 1 every four weeks for six cycles. Subsequent cycles should be delayed until platelet and neutrophil counts recover to the levels indicated above. Dose reductions are recommended for patients with impaired renal function or with previous bone marrow toxicity. Alternatively, doses can be individualized based on a target AUC and the patient's GFR from the equations given in the section on Pharmacokinetics. Other dosages and schedules have been used in clinical studies employing combination regimens for treatment of other solid tumors (see the references cited in the section on Uses).

Paraplatin (Bristol-Myers Oncology). Powder 50, 150, or 450 mg (store at room temperature; protect from light).

NONCLASSICAL ALKYLATING AGENTS

These drugs differ from other alkylating agents used clinically in that they are monofunctional and thus are unable to cross-link cellular macromolecules. Among their common properties are a requirement for metabolic activation to intermediates with antitumor efficacy and the presence in their chemical structures of N-methyl groups that, after metabolism, can covalently modify cellular DNA. Included in this group are the methyl hydrazine derivative, procarbazine; the linear triazene, dacarbazine; and the N-methylated cyclic triazene derivative, altretamine. The precise mechanisms by which each of these drugs kills tumor cells are not completely understood. Nevertheless, procarbazine is used in combination chemotherapy for Hodgkin's disease and also is used (although less frequently) for non-Hodgkin's lymphomas (in both instances, as a component of the MOPP regimen). Dacarbazine also has been beneficial in the chemotherapy of lymphomas as a component of the ABVD regimen and in melanoma and soft tissue sarcoma, and altretamine is useful as second-line therapy for women with persistent or recurrent ovarian carcinoma.

PROCARBAZINE HYDROCHLORIDE

[Matulane]

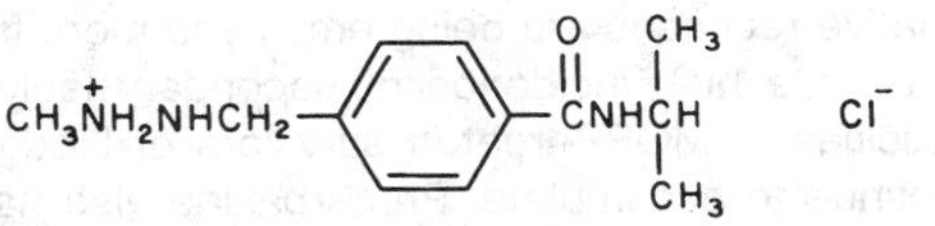

$$CH_3\overset{+}{N}H_2NHCH_2-C_6H_4-\overset{O}{\overset{\|}{C}}NH\underset{CH_3}{\underset{|}{\overset{CH_3}{\overset{|}{C}}}}H \quad Cl^-$$

ACTIONS. Procarbazine was synthesized as part of a program to develop novel inhibitors of monoamine oxidase. It was too cytotoxic in animal models to be useful for that purpose but was found to have promising antitumor activity.

The mechanism of action of this methylhydrazine derivative is uncertain; however, conversion to active metabolites appears to be necessary (for reviews, see Averbuch, 1993; Chabner, 1993). Most studies employing cell culture systems to study the action of procarbazine rely on hepatic microsomes or intact hepatocytes to convert the prodrug to active alkylating intermediates. However, since multiple pathways of metabolism and chemical decomposition can convert procarbazine to a wide variety of reactive species, it has not been determined which of these pathways and products are most germane to its antitumor efficacy. Procarbazine's antitumor efficacy is known to be markedly reduced when it is administered intravenously rather than orally. This may suggest that excretion and/or metabolic inactivation in other organs competes with activation by the liver and that first-pass hepatic metabolism may increase the percentage of drug activated.

The inhibition of DNA, RNA, and subsequent protein synthesis occurs in cells treated with procarbazine. This drug also causes extensive DNA damage, principally as single-strand breaks. The methylation and/or alkylation of nucleic acids, followed by loss (depurination) of the modified bases and cleavage of phosphodiester bonds, are probable steps leading to strand breaks and may contribute significantly to the drug's cytocidal effects. Aberrant transmethylation of purine bases and transfer RNA also has been observed. Autooxidation of procarbazine to hydrogen peroxide and hydroxy radicals produces effects resembling those of ionizing radiation, but these oxidation products do not appear to be the critical cytotoxic intermediates. Procarbazine is cell cycle nonspecific.

Although resistance to this drug develops readily in vitro, the mechanisms involved have not been determined. It is known that there is little or no cross-resistance between procarbazine and the classical alkylating agents (eg, nitrogen mustards); this supports their combined use in regimens such as MOPP. None of the mechanisms that are common in cells resistant to classical alkylating agents (eg, increased glutathione concentrations or glutathione transferase activity, decreased drug uptake) have been reported in procarbazine-resistant cells. Metabolites of procarbazine alkylate the O^6 position of guanines in DNA; thus, the cellular level of the repair enzyme, O^6-alkylguanine-DNA-alkyltransferase, may be a determining factor in tumor cell sensitivity to this drug.

USES. The primary use of procarbazine is in advanced Hodgkin's disease in combination with mechlorethamine, vincristine, and prednisone (MOPP regimen) (DeVita et al, 1993; Takvorian and Canellos, 1993). This regimen produces a high percentage of long-term disease-free survivors (see index entry Cancer: Clinical Responses to Chemotherapy). However, alternative regimens are being employed more frequently, for reports of a high incidence of secondary leukemia and other toxicities in MOPP-treated survivors of Hodgkin's disease continue to accumulate. Procarbazine also has activity in primary and metastatic brain tumors, both as a single agent for recurrent tumors (Rodriguez et al, 1989) and in combination regimens (eg, with lomustine, vincristine [PCV], ± methotrexate) for adjuvant chemotherapy (Kramer and Packer, 1992; Lesser and Grossman, 1993; Prados and Wilson, 1993; Levin et al, 1993). In patients with brain tumors, procarbazine is often combined with cranial irradiation as part of a multimodality approach. Other tumors that have responded to procarbazine (most often in combination with other drugs) include melanoma, small cell lung carcinoma, and non-Hodgkin's lymphomas. However, its use for these malignancies is uncommon outside of clinical trials, and procarbazine usually is reserved for third-line therapies.

ADVERSE REACTIONS AND PRECAUTIONS. Bone marrow depression and gastrointestinal disturbances are the primary toxic manifestations. Leukopenia and thrombocytopenia are usually dose limiting and may be delayed for several weeks after the start of treatment. Like other hydrazine derivatives, procarbazine also may cause hemolysis in individuals deficient in glucose-6-phosphate dehydrogenase activity. Nausea and vomiting occur frequently and may be dose limiting, but tolerance usually develops with continued administration. Gradual escalation of the dose during the first days of treatment may reduce the severity or incidence of gastrointestinal discomfort. Stomatitis, dysphagia, and diarrhea are less common.

Neurologic reactions (eg, lethargy, drowsiness, depression, peripheral neuropathy with paresthesia, nystagmus, ataxia) have been noted in 10% to 20% of patients. These effects may be a result of the drug's inhibitory effects on monoamine oxidase and/or its ability to deplete pyridoxal phosphate. Other untoward effects include myalgia, arthralgia, orthostatic hypotension, dermatitis, pruritus, hyperpigmentation, azoospermia, anovulation, and alopecia. The drug is immunosuppressive and is a potent mutagen. It is teratogenic and carcinogenic in animals (FDA Pregnancy Category D). There have been many reports concerning secondary malignancies in patients successfully treated for various cancers with procarbazine-containing combination regimens (Kaldor et al, 1990; Schilsky and Erlichman, 1990; Zarrabi, 1990). Since many of these regimens also include a nitrogen mustard (eg, mechlorethamine in MOPP), it is difficult to separate the leukemogenic effects of procarbazine from those of the classical alkylating agents with which it is combined.

DRUG INTERACTIONS. The effects of central nervous system depressants (eg, barbiturates, phenothiazines, opioids) may be enhanced. This appears to be due to a procarbazine-induced decrease in cytochrome P450 levels, which decreases the metabolism of these drugs. Procarbazine's hypnotic effect may be additive with that of other drugs. A disulfiram-like reaction may occur when alcohol is ingested concomitantly. Since procarbazine inhibits monoamine oxidase, sympathomimetics, tricyclic antidepressants, and beverages or foods with a high tyramine content (aged cheeses, bananas, caviar, liver, red wine, sausages, yogurt) should be avoided.

PHARMACOKINETICS. Procarbazine is rapidly and completely absorbed following oral administration. The drug initially concentrates in the liver, kidney, intestine, and skin and readily crosses the blood-brain barrier. The plasma half-life of parent drug is approximately 10 minutes. It is rapidly converted, primarily in liver microsomes and also in erythrocytes, to azoprocarbazine, which is metabolized further to active and inactive metabolites (for reviews, see Averbuch, 1993; Chabner, 1993). Approximately 45% to 70% of a dose is excreted in the urine during the first 24 hours as metabolites, particularly the inactive N-isopropylterephthalamic acid derivative. About 30% of the N-methyl group appears in respiratory CO_2.

DOSAGE AND PREPARATIONS.

Oral: Initially, 100 mg/M^2 is given daily; the dose is increased over a one-week period to 150 to 200 mg/M^2. This amount is administered for three weeks and then reduced to 100 mg/M^2 daily until toxicity develops. The dose should be decreased in patients with hepatic, renal, or bone marrow dysfunction.

As a component of the MOPP regimen, 100 mg/M^2 is given daily for 14 days every four weeks.

Matulane (Roche). Capsules equivalent to 50 mg of the base.

DACARBAZINE

[DTIC-Dome]

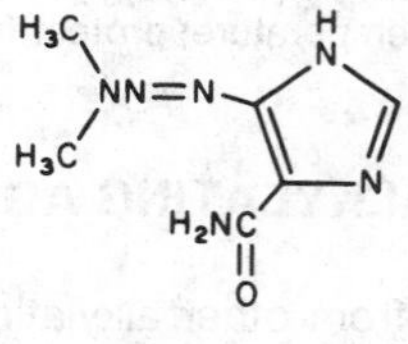

ACTIONS. Dacarbazine, a linear triazene, was originally developed to be an antimetabolite, acting as an inhibitor of purine synthesis, and to interact with sulfhydryl groups in proteins. However, after metabolic activation in the liver, it demonstrated alkylating activity, which is now believed to be the most important action (Averbuch, 1993; Chabner, 1993). This drug inhibits RNA and protein synthesis more markedly than DNA synthesis. In vitro studies on dacarbazine's mechanism of action are complicated by the light-catalyzed decomposition of this drug to products that are themselves capable of causing DNA damage and inhibiting macromolecular synthesis. However, DNA is damaged in human cells treated with the drug in the absence of light (Lönn and Lõhn, 1987). It is cell cycle nonspecific. Resistance to dacarbazine has not been studied adequately.

USES. Dacarbazine is used in the palliative treatment of metastatic melanoma, but the overall response rate is only about 20% when it is given alone for this chemoinsensitive cancer. Dacarbazine more commonly is a component of several multidrug regimens used in the treatment of melanoma, most often with one of the nitrosoureas, a vinca alkaloid, cisplatin, and/or bleomycin (Kirkwood and Agarwala, 1993). It also is a component of the ABVD regimen, which is an alternative to MOPP in the treatment of advanced Hodgkin's disease (see index entry Cancer: Clinical Responses to Chemotherapy) (DeVita et al, 1993; Takvorian and Canellos, 1993) and is a component of combination regimens used to treat soft tissue sarcomas and neuroblastoma. Dacarbazine is active in islet cell cancer and in primary brain tumors.

ADVERSE REACTIONS. Myelosuppression is usually dose limiting and primarily affects leukocytes and platelets. This effect is somewhat delayed compared with classic nitrogen mustards. Leukopenia generally is reported after 10 days of therapy and thrombocytopenia after 10 to 15 days, but both effects may be delayed until two to four weeks after the last dose.

Nausea and vomiting usually occur within one to three hours after administration, and vomiting can last for up to 12 hours. These effects occur in about 90% of patients and may be severe. Some newer antiemetics (eg, ondansetron) can be used successfully to manage this adverse reaction (see index entry Vomiting, Treatment). Rarely, intractable nausea and vomiting have necessitated discontinuance of therapy. Most patients develop tolerance, and these symptoms subside after one to two days of treatment.

An "influenza-like" syndrome consisting of fever, myalgia, and malaise has been described with dacarbazine. Other untoward effects are pain at the infusion site, facial flushing, paresthesia, alopecia, and elevation of hepatic enzyme levels. Hepatic necrosis has been reported. Dacarbazine is teratogenic and carcinogenic in animals. This drug is classified in FDA Pregnancy Category C. Anaphylaxis occurs rarely.

PHARMACOKINETICS. Since oral absorption is incomplete and highly variable, dacarbazine is administered only intravenously. It is metabolized in the liver first by N-demethylation to a monomethyl form and then to amino imidazole carboxamide (AIC) and diazomethane. The active carbonium ion is formed from diazomethane. Dacarbazine has a biphasic plasma decay with half-lives of 19 minutes and five hours. It is rapidly excreted by renal tubular secretion. About 40% of a dose is eliminated unchanged within six hours; the major metabolite in urine is AIC.

DOSAGE AND PREPARATIONS.

Intravenous: 250 mg/M²/day for five days every three to four weeks has been used for solid tumors.

For Hodgkin's disease, as part of the ABVD combination, 375 mg/M²/day is given on days 1 and 15 and the course is repeated every four weeks.

Generic. Powder (sterile) 100, 200, and 500 mg.

DTIC-Dome (Miles). Powder (sterile) 100 and 200 mg.

ALTRETAMINE (Hexamethylmelamine)

[Hexalen]

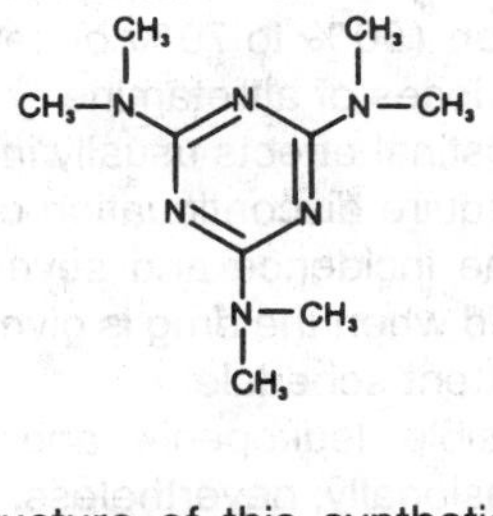

ACTIONS. The structure of this synthetic agent resembles that of triethylenemelamine, an aziridine alkylating and cross-linking agent; however, the precise mechanism of action of altretamine is unknown. It is sequentially demethylated in a series of reactions catalyzed by cytochrome P450 that yield metabolites with alkylating activity (Ames, 1991; Hansen and Hughes, 1991). Although metabolic activation is required for its antitumor effects, altretamine is not consistently cross-resistant with the classical alkylating agents (Averbuch, 1993; Chabner, 1993). This drug inhibits the incorporation of precursors into DNA and RNA in vitro.

USES. Altretamine is used alone as second-line therapy for palliation of persistent or recurrent ovarian cancer in patients whose tumors are resistant to platinum complex- or alkylating agent-based regimens (Ozols and Young, 1991; Thigpen et al, 1993). Data from randomized trials are inadequate to compare the efficacy of altretamine with that of other options (eg, paclitaxel [Taxol], ifosfamide) as salvage therapy for platinum-resistant ovarian cancer. In addition, no randomized studies have compared altretamine alone with combination regimens in these patients. In a clinical trial in women with platinum-refractory ovarian cancer, subgroup analysis suggests that altretamine may be useful for women who relapse within six months of initial chemotherapy but not for those whose tumor progresses or who did not respond to initial treatment (Vergote et al, 1992). Some oncologists believe that women in the former group have tumors that are potentially sensitive to platinum complexes, while those in the latter group may not respond adequately to altretamine either (Muggia and Norris, 1992). Thus, the precise role of altretamine in salvage therapy for recurrent or persistent ovarian carcinoma has not been defined completely.

Altretamine also is a component of several drug combinations (eg, with cyclophosphamide, doxorubicin, and cisplatin [H-CAP]) investigated as first-line therapy for advanced ovarian carcinoma (Ozols and Young, 1991; McGuire, 1993). However, conflicting data have been reported from several small randomized trials that compared response rates and duration of survival in women with ovarian cancer who received regimens that did and did not include altretamine.

Thus, most oncologists currently reserve the use of altretamine for second-line or, more often, subsequent therapy.

Data from uncontrolled studies suggest that this drug also may be active in advanced small cell and non-small cell lung, cervical, endometrial, and breast carcinomas and in refractory lymphomas (Averbuch, 1993; Chabner, 1993). However, data are insufficient to support use of altretamine in patients with these malignancies other than in clinical trials.

ADVERSE REACTIONS AND PRECAUTIONS. Nausea and vomiting are common (50% to 70% of patients) and may be severe when large doses of altretamine are administered daily. These gastrointestinal effects usually increase with subsequent doses and require discontinuation of therapy after two to three weeks. The incidence and severity of nausea and vomiting are reduced when the drug is given in moderate doses using an intermittent schedule.

Moderate, reversible leukopenia and thrombocytopenia have occurred occasionally; nevertheless, this drug is a good candidate for inclusion in combination regimens, since myelosuppression is less frequent and less severe than with most other oncologic drugs.

With repeated courses, peripheral neuropathy has been reported; two cases were irreversible. Other adverse neurologic reactions include numbness, paresthesia, depression, confusion, drowsiness, and hallucinations.

The overlap between altretamine and cisplatin in causing gastrointestinal and neurologic toxicities has raised concern about their use in combination (Muggia and Norris, 1992). However, there are no data thus far to demonstrate that synergy between these drugs produces or increases the incidence of such reactions.

Altretamine is weakly mutagenic in bacteria; however, its ability to induce tumors in mammals has not been investigated. This drug is embryotoxic in rats and rabbits, but has not been studied in pregnant women (FDA Pregnancy Category C). Continuous administration of high-dose altretamine impaired fertility in male rats.

Monoamine oxidase inhibitors should not be given with altretamine since the combination may cause severe orthostatic hypotension.

PHARMACOKINETICS. Altretamine is absorbed following oral administration. It undergoes rapid and extensive first-pass metabolism in the liver. Metabolites are excreted in urine, and 62% of a dose is recovered within 24 hours. The elimination-phase half-life of parent drug in plasma ranges from 4.7 to 10.2 hours.

DOSAGE.

Oral: 260 mg/M^2 daily in a single or in divided doses for 14 to 21 days. In combination regimens, 150 mg/M^2 daily is given for 14 days every four weeks.

Hexalen (U.S. Bioscience). Capsules 50 mg.

SYSTEMIC RADIOISOTOPES

Two radioisotopes, ^{32}P (as sodium phosphate) and ^{89}Sr (as strontium chloride), are now available for systemic treatment of the bone pain of osseous metastases. ^{32}P sodium phosphate also is used to treat polycythemia vera and, occasionally, chronic myelogenous leukemia. The ^{32}P radioisotope has a short half-life (14.2 days) and exerts its effects on biological tissues by emission of β particles (1.7 MeV maximum energy), which penetrate soft tissues to an average depth of 8 to 9 mm. The ^{89}Sr radioisotope has a longer half-life (50.6 days) and emits β particles that are slightly less energetic (1.46 MeV maximum energy) but also penetrate soft tissues to an average depth of approximately 8 mm (*Semin Oncol*, 1993). The maximum β particle ranges in bone for both radioisotopes is approximately 3 mm because of the increased density of bone compared with soft tissues. The emitted radiation from either radioisotope is then thought to cause direct DNA damage as well as to generate activated oxygen and hydroxyl species (radicals) from molecular oxygen and water inside cells that are capable of damaging DNA and other cellular macromolecules.

Instillation of radioisotopic gold-198 was used in the past (intrapleurally for malignant effusions [Pass, 1993] and intraperitoneally for ovarian cancer [Young et al, 1993]), but this isotope is no longer available. ^{32}P as chromic phosphate is still used for these purposes.

In addition to ^{32}P and ^{89}Sr, a radioisotope of iodine (^{131}I) is used for the treatment of thyroid carcinoma (Norton et al, 1993).

Finally, radioisotopes conjugated to monoclonal antibodies directed at tumor-associated antigens are under intensive investigation as a means of targeting delivery of ionizing radiation to tumors after systemic administration. However, thus far, the sole radiolabeled monoclonal antibody generally available in the United States for systemic administration to patients (indium^{111}-satumomab pendetide) is used only for imaging tumors and not for therapy. For discussion of these investigational agents and other therapeutic applications of monoclonal antibodies, see index entry Monoclonal Antibodies, In Cancer.

SODIUM PHOSPHATE P 32

ACTIONS AND USES. Sodium phosphate P 32 is a preparation of the β-emitting radioactive isotope used principally to treat the proliferative phase of polycythemia vera (Athens, 1993) and essential thrombocythemia (Bithell, 1993). When administered orally or intravenously, the isotope is taken up by tissues with high phosphate turnover, including neoplastic and bone marrow cells as well as normal bone. It inhibits proliferation of bone marrow cells and thus reduces the erythrocyte count, packed red blood cell volume, and hypervolemia associated with polycythemia vera. Following an appropriate dose, a latent period of one to three months is succeeded by a smooth progression into complete hematologic remission lasting six months to several years. A second dose of sodium phosphate P 32 may be required within the initial six months for satisfactory remission, and phlebotomies often are performed to maintain the hematocrit at normal levels during the induction period.

Sodium phosphate P 32 also is used as palliative therapy to reduce or relieve pain caused by skeletal metastases from a variety of tumors. In a review of data from 28 clinical trials (Silberstein, 1993), approximately 80% of patients reported some improvement in symptoms. However, there appears to be no dose-response relationship between the activity of administered ^{32}P and the percentage of patients who experience some degree of pain reduction. The therapeutic efficacy of sodium phosphate P 32 for this use probably depends on the quantity of ^{32}P deposited in bone at the site of metastases, which may vary considerably among patients given identical doses.

This isotope may be useful for palliative treatment in the early phase of chronic myelogenous leukemia and has been used to treat some patients with chronic lymphocytic leukemia. Other therapies have largely replaced these uses of the radioisotope.

ADVERSE REACTIONS AND PRECAUTIONS. Although usual doses rarely cause radiation sickness, dosage should be individualized to ensure minimal radiation exposure to the patient and laboratory personnel. Excessive amounts can cause leukopenia, thrombocytopenia, and anemia. Periodic blood cell counts should be performed. This agent is contraindicated when the leukocyte count is approximately 4,500/microliter or the platelet count less than 100,000/microliter. There is evidence that sodium phosphate P 32 is leukemogenic in patients with polycythemia vera, but the incidence appears to be lower than with chlorambucil. Presently, the benefits of sodium phosphate P 32 appear to outweigh the risks of acute leukemia, particularly in patients over age 40 with polycythemia vera, but further studies are required. When used for palliation of bone pain in patients with skeletal metastases, leukemogenesis is not a significant concern since the life expectancy of these patients rarely exceeds two years (Silberstein, 1993).

This agent is classified in FDA Pregnancy Category C.

Treatment with sodium phosphate P 32 is restricted to physicians licensed by the Nuclear Regulatory Commission.

DOSAGE AND PREPARATIONS.

Oral: For polycythemia vera, initially, 6 millicuries.

Intravenous: For polycythemia vera or essential thrombocythemia, 2.3 millicuries/M^2, depending on the initial erythrocyte, leukocyte, and platelet counts and the patient's body surface area. Phlebotomy or plateletpheresis may be performed adjunctively.

For palliation of pain in patients with skeletal metastases, 4 to 10 millicuries has been administered as a single dose, and up to 24 millicuries has been given in divided doses over a period of three to four weeks (Silberstein, 1993).

Sodium Phosphate P32 (Mallinckrodt). Solution 0.67 millicuries/ml in 10 ml containers (5 millicuries radioactivity/container).

CHROMIC PHOSPHATE P 32

[Phosphocol P 32]

USES. The intraperitoneal instillation of chromic phosphate P 32 is employed as adjuvant therapy for early stage ovarian cancer (Young et al, 1993; McGuire, 1993). In addition, clinical trials have evaluated the efficacy of intraperitoneal chromic phosphate P 32 as consolidation therapy after negative "second-look laparotomy" in women treated for advanced ovarian carcinoma. Data from two studies suggest that consolidation therapy has no effect on the rate of relapse or duration of survival (Peters et al, 1992; Vergote et al, 1993), while, in a third study, it was concluded that the risk of recurrence was reduced and survival improved (Rogers et al, 1993). This drug also has been given by intracavitary instillation for malignant pleural effusions and by interstitial injection for prostatic and ovarian carcinomas.

ADVERSE REACTIONS AND PRECAUTIONS. Acute toxicity resulting from the intraperitoneal instillation of chromic phosphate P 32 at standard dosages is limited to mild abdominal discomfort caused by the volume of fluid infused. The most common late complication of intraperitoneal radioisotope administration is small bowel obstruction and stenosis (Spanos et al, 1992). Treatment with chromic phosphate P 32 is restricted to physicians licensed by the Nuclear Regulatory Commission.

DOSAGE AND PREPARATIONS.

Intraperitoneal: For ovarian cancer, 7 to 15 millicuries (diluted with 1,000 ml of sterile saline). Prior to instillation, careful assessment of peritoneal distribution is necessary; technetium 99m sulfur colloid is injected into the peritoneal cavity and scanning of the patient is performed prior to administration.

Phosphocol P 32 (Mallinckrodt). Suspension 10 or 15 millicuries in 10 ml containers (5 millicuries radioactivity/container).

STRONTIUM CHLORIDE Sr 89

[Metastron]

ACTIONS AND USES. Because of its electrochemical similarity to ionized calcium, the divalent strontium cation is incorporated into the hydroxyapatite crystal lattice of bone. The ^{89}Sr radioisotopic form of this element emits β particles, which are toxic to cells adjacent to the sites at which it is retained. There is preferential uptake and retention of strontium cations at sites of active osteogenesis. This may result in a ratio of ≥ 3 to 1 for the radiation dose absorbed by osteoblastic skeletal metastases to that absorbed by normal bone and marrow in adults (*Semin Oncol*, 1993). In addition, strontium cations incorporated into bone hydroxyapatite adjacent to the tumor may be retained for 100 days or more, which is approximately twice the half-life (50.6 days) for radioactive decay of ^{89}Sr. Data from a controlled study with nonradioactive strontium chloride demonstrate that the palliative effects of this drug require the use of the ^{89}Sr radioisotope.

Strontium chloride Sr 89 is indicated as palliative therapy to relieve bone pain in patients with painful osteoblastic skeletal metastases. The greatest amount of experience is in patients with metastatic prostate or breast cancer (*Semin Oncol*, 1993; Robinson, 1993; Porter et al, 1993), approximately 80% of whom experience gradual relief of pain after systemic therapy. A decrease in pain usually begins one to two weeks after administration of a single dose, and the effect lasts 10 to 12 weeks. Therapy can be repeated as often as every 10 weeks, and some patients have been treated up to 10 times (Robinson, 1993). There is no evidence that ^{89}Sr affects patient survival. However, data from two trials suggest that it delays the appearance of new sites of bone pain in patients with prostate cancer and thus may slow the progression of metastatic disease in bone (Porter et al, 1993; Quilty et al, 1994).

Responses have been less frequent in the small number of patients with other primary cancers (eg, lung, 29% response rate) who have received this therapy, but further study is needed in larger groups of patients for a more definitive evaluation of the response rates of skeletal metastases from tumors other than breast and prostate cancer. Patients with metastases limited to soft tissues do not benefit from administration of strontium chloride Sr 89.

ADVERSE REACTIONS AND PRECAUTIONS. Strontium chloride Sr 89 appears to be less likely to cause severe hematopoietic toxicity than sodium phosphate P 32 (Robinson, 1993). However, no comparative studies have been completed. The difference in myelotoxicity probably is due to the relatively high ratio of the ^{89}Sr dose retained by metastatic tumor compared with that retained in marrow. In addition, the kinetics of its biodistribution between normal and metastatic bone and its longer half-life also may reduce its myelotoxicity compared with that of sodium phosphate P 32. The platelet count may drop by 20% to 30% five to six weeks after therapy, but usually returns to pretreatment levels. Leukocyte counts generally do not decline in patients not receiving concurrent external beam radiation therapy. However, more severe myelosuppressive effects occur in patients who previously have received radiation therapy or chemotherapy or in those with extensive metastases to the marrow. Rapid bolus injection may be accompanied by a mild flushing sensation, but this can be prevented by infusing the dose over 60 to 120 seconds. Approximately 10% of patients whose metastatic lesions are responding to ^{89}Sr may experience an initial intensification of bone pain ("flare") 1 to 14 days after treatment begins, and it lasts up to two weeks.

Strontium chloride Sr 89 should not be used in patients with seriously compromised bone marrow reserves as a result of previous chemotherapy or radiation therapy. Peripheral blood cell counts should be monitored at least once every other week.

Although data are inadequate to evaluate the mutagenicity of this drug or its effects on fertility, it is carcinogenic and teratogenic in rats. Women of childbearing age should avoid becoming pregnant while being treated with this agent (FDA Pregnancy Category D), and nursing should be discontinued before treatment, since strontium chloride Sr 89 probably is excreted into human milk as an analogue of calcium. No data are available on the safety of this drug in children under 18 years.

Treatment with strontium chloride Sr 89 is restricted to physicians licensed by the Nuclear Regulatory Commission.

PHARMACOKINETICS. Strontium chloride Sr 89 is rapidly cleared from the circulation but is retained selectively at sites of active osteogenesis. This agent is eliminated from normal bone within 14 days, but more than 50% of an injected dose is retained significantly longer in metastatic bone lesions. Urinary excretion is greatest during the first two days after infusion and accounts for approximately two-thirds of total body clearance in patients with skeletal metastases. Fecal elimination, which accounts for the remaining one-third in these patients, is reduced. Urinary clearance is greater in individuals without bone lesions.

DOSAGE AND PREPARATIONS.

Intravenous: For palliation of pain in patients with skeletal metastases, 148 MBq (4 mCi) administered by slow intravenous injection (over one to two minutes). Alternatively, a dose of 1.5 to 2.2 MBq/kg (40 to 60 μCi/kg) may be used. See the manufacturer's literature for information on radioactive decay factors to be used in adjusting the dosage based on time elapsed since calibration of the radioactive concentration.

Metastron (Medi-Physics/Amersham Healthcare). Solution 37 MBq/ml (1 mCi/ml) in 10 ml vials containing 148 MBq (4 mCi) at a pH of 4.0 to 7.5. The specific activity is 2.96 to 6.17 MBq/mg of strontium chloride (80 to 167 μCi/mg) at calibration, and the concentration of strontium chloride is 10.9 to 22.6 mg/ml. This product must be stored in the original transportation container (shielded with 3 mm thickness lead walls) at room temperature (59° to 77° F).

Cited References

Recent advances in ifosfamide therapy. *Semin Oncol* 19(suppl 12):1-74, 1992 A.

Testicular cancer. *Semin Oncol* 19:117-215, (April) 1992 B.

Palliation of pain in bony metastases. *Semin Oncol* 20(suppl 2):1-49, 1993.

Advanced Ovarian Cancer Trialists Group: Chemotherapy in advanced ovarian cancer: An overview of randomised clinical trials. *BMJ* 303:884-893, 1991.

Alberts DS, et al: Improved therapeutic index of carboplatin plus cyclophosphamide versus cisplatin plus cyclophosphamide: Final report by the Southwest Oncology Group of a Phase III randomized trial in stages III and IV ovarian cancer. *J Clin Oncol* 10:706-717, 1992.

Ames MM: Hexamethylmelamine: Pharmacology and mechanism of action. *Cancer Treat Rev* 18(suppl A):3-14, 1991.

Anderson K: Plasma cell tumors, in Holland JF, et al (eds): *Cancer Medicine*, ed 3. Philadelphia, Lea & Febiger, 1993, 2075-2092.

Antman KH: Chemotherapy of advanced sarcomas of bone and soft tissue. *Semin Oncol* 19:13-22, (Dec) 1992.

Antman K, et al: High-dose thiotepa alone and in combination regimens with bone marrow support. *Semin Oncol* 17:33-38, 1990.

Athens JW: Polycythemia vera, in Lee GR, et al (eds): *Wintrobe's Clinical Hematology*, ed 9. Philadelphia, Lea & Febiger, 1993, 1999-2017.

Averbuch SD: Dacarbazine, procarbazine, hexamethylmelamine, in Holland JF, et al (eds): *Cancer Medicine*, ed 3. Philadelphia, Lea & Febiger, 1993, 755-764.

Bajorin DF, et al: Randomized trial of etoposide and cisplatin versus etoposide and carboplatin in patients with good-risk germ cell tumors: A multiinstitutional study. *J Clin Oncol* 11:598-606, 1993.

Berg SL, et al: Phase I/II trial and pharmacokinetics of intrathecal diaziquone in refractory meningeal malignancies. *J Clin Oncol* 10:143-148, 1992.

Berger NA: Alkylating agents, in DeVita VT Jr, et al (eds): *Cancer: Principles & Practice of Oncology*, ed 4. Philadelphia, JB Lippincott, 1993, 400-409.

Bithell TC: Thrombocytosis, in Lee GR, et al (eds): *Wintrobe's Clinical Hematology*, ed 9. Philadelphia, Lea & Febiger, 1993, 1390-1396.

Bitran JD, et al: High-dose combination chemotherapy with thiotepa and autologous hematopoietic stem cell reinfusion in the treatment of patients with relapsed refractory lymphomas. *Semin Oncol* 17:39-42, 1990.

Boice JD Jr, et al: Leukemia and preleukemia after adjuvant treatment of gastrointestinal cancer with semustine (methyl-CCNU). *N Engl J Med* 309:1079-1084, 1983.

Brennan MF, et al: Cancer of the pancreas, in DeVita VT Jr, et al (eds): *Cancer: Principles & Practice of Oncology*, ed 4. Philadelphia, JB Lippincott, 1993, 849-882.

Calvert AH, et al: Carboplatin dosage: Prospective evaluation of a simple formula based on renal function. *J Clin Oncol* 7:1748-1756, 1989.

Chabner BA: Miscellaneous agents, in DeVita VT Jr, et al (eds): *Cancer: Principles & Practice of Oncology*, ed 4. Philadelphia, JB Lippincott, 1993, 385-389.

Clamon G, et al: Pharmacokinetic studies of streptozotocin (STZ) by continuous infusion (CI). *Proc Am Assoc Cancer Res* 27:(abstract 673) 170, 1986.

Colvin M: Alkylating agents and platinum antitumor compounds, in Holland JF, et al (eds): *Cancer Medicine*, ed 3. Philadelphia, Lea & Febiger, 1993, 733-754.

Conte PF, et al: Carboplatin, doxorubicin, and cyclophosphamide versus cisplatin, doxorubicin, and cyclophosphamide: A randomized trial in stage III-IV epithelial ovarian carcinoma. *J Clin Oncol* 9:658-663, 1991.

Cornelison TL, Reed E: Nephrotoxicity and hydration management for cisplatin, carboplatin, and ormaplatin. *Gynecol Oncol* 50:147-158, 1993.

Crump M, et al: High-dose etoposide and melphalan, and autologous bone marrow transplantation for patients with advanced Hodgkin's disease: Importance of disease status at transplant. *J Clin Oncol* 11:704-711, 1993.

Cunningham D, et al: High-dose melphalan and autologous bone marrow transplantation as consolidation in previously untreated myeloma. *J Clin Oncol* 12:759-763, 1994 A.

Cunningham D, et al: High-dose melphalan for multiple myeloma: Long-term follow-up data. *J Clin Oncol* 12:764-768, 1994 B.

Dabholkar M, et al: ERCC1 and ERCC2 expression in malignant tissues from ovarian cancer patients. *J Natl Cancer Inst* 84:1512-1517, 1992.

Dabholkar M, et al: Messenger RNA levels of XPAC and ERCC1 in ovarian cancer tissue correlate with response to platinum-based chemotherapy. *J Clin Invest* 94:703-708, 1994.

Dechant KL, et al: Ifosfamide/mesna: A review of its antineoplastic activity, pharmacokinetic properties and therapeutic efficacy in cancer. *Drugs* 42:428-467, 1991.

Deisseroth AB, et al: Chronic leukemias, in DeVita VT Jr, et al (eds): *Cancer: Principles & Practice of Oncology*, ed 4. Philadelphia, JB Lippincott, 1993, 1965-1983.

DeVita VT Jr, et al: Hodgkin's disease, in DeVita VT Jr, et al (eds): *Cancer: Principles & Practice of Oncology*, ed 4. Philadelphia, JB Lippincott, 1993, 1819-1858.

deVries CR, Freiha FS: Hemorrhagic cystitis: A review. *J Urol* 143:1-9, 1990.

Dinapoli RP, et al: Phase III comparative evaluation of PCNU and carmustine combined with radiation therapy for high-grade glioma. *J Clin Oncol* 11:1316-1321, 1993.

Dittrich C, et al: In vitro and in vivo evaluation of the combination of cisplatin and its analogue carboplatin for platinum dose intensification in ovarian carcinoma. *Cancer* 71:3082-3090, 1993.

Dorr RT: Chemoprotectants for cancer chemotherapy. *Semin Oncol* 18(suppl 2):48-58, 1991.

Douglass HO Jr, et al: Neoplasms of the exocrine pancreas, in Holland JF, et al (eds): *Cancer Medicine*, ed 3. Philadelphia, Lea & Febiger, 1993, 1466-1484.

Early Breast Cancer Trialists' Collaborative Group: Systemic treatment of early breast cancer by hormonal, cytotoxic, or immune therapy: 133 randomised trials involving 31,000 recurrences and 24,000 deaths among 75,000 women. *Lancet* 339:1-15, 71-85, 1992.

Einhorn LH, et al: Cancer of the testis, in DeVita VT Jr, et al (eds): *Cancer: Principles & Practice of Oncology*, ed 4. Philadelphia, JB Lippincott, 1993, 1126-1151.

Elias AD, et al: High-dose ifosfamide with mesna uroprotection: A Phase I study. *J Clin Oncol* 8:170-178, 1990.

Ettinger LJ, et al: A Phase II study of diaziquone in childhood leukemia: A report from the children's cancer study group. *Am J Pediatr Hematol Oncol* 10:18-22, 1988.

Fanning J, et al: Meta-analysis of cisplatin, doxorubicin, and cyclophosphamide versus cisplatin and cyclophosphamide chemotherapy of ovarian carcinoma. *Obstet Gynecol* 80:954-960, 1992.

Fisher B, et al: Postoperative adjuvant chemotherapy or radiation therapy for rectal cancer: Results from NSABP protocol R-01. *J Natl Cancer Inst* 80:21-29, 1988.

Forastiere AA, et al: Randomized comparison of cisplatin plus fluorouracil and carboplatin plus fluorouracil versus methotrexate in advanced squamous-cell carcinoma of the head and neck: A Southwest Oncology Group study. *J Clin Oncol* 10:1245-1251, 1992.

Fraiser LH, et al: Cyclophosphamide toxicity: Characterising and avoiding the problem. *Drugs* 42:781-795, 1991.

Freedman AS, Nadler LM: Non-Hodgkin's lymphomas, in Holland JF, et al (eds): *Cancer Medicine*, ed 3. Philadelphia, Lea & Febiger, 1993, 2028-2068.

French Cooperative Group on Chronic Lymphocytic Leukemia: A randomized clinical trial of chlorambucil versus COP in stage B chronic lymphocytic leukemia. *Blood* 75:1422-1425, 1990 A.

French Cooperative Group on Chronic Lymphocytic Leukemia: Effects of chlorambucil and therapeutic decision in initial forms of chronic lymphocytic leukemia (stage A): Results of a randomized clinical trial on 612 patients. *Blood* 75:1414-1421, 1990 B.

Gastrointestinal Tumor Study Group: Radiation therapy and fluorouracil with or without semustine for the treatment of patients with surgical adjuvant adenocarcinoma of the rectum. *J Clin Oncol* 10:549-557, 1992.

Gately DP, Howell SB: Cellular accumulation of the anticancer agent cisplatin: A review. *Br J Cancer* 67:1171-1176, 1993.

Gatzemeier U, et al: Carboplatin in small cell lung cancer. *Semin Oncol* 18(suppl 2):8-16, 1991.

Gatzemeier U, et al: Combination chemotherapy with carboplatin, etoposide, and vincristine as first-line treatment in small-cell lung cancer. *J Clin Oncol* 10:818-823, 1992.

Goel R, et al: Effect of sodium thiosulfate on the pharmacokinetics and toxicity of cisplatin. *J Natl Cancer Inst* 81:1552-1560, 1989.

Goren MP: Oral mesna: A review. *Semin Oncol* 19(suppl 12):65-72, 1992.

Greene MH: Is cisplatin a human carcinogen? *J Natl Cancer Inst* 84:306-312, 1992.

Gregory WM, et al: Combination chemotherapy versus melphalan and prednisolone in the treatment of multiple myeloma: An overview of published trials. *J Clin Oncol* 10:334-342, 1992.

Hafström L, Mattsson J: Regional chemotherapy for malignant melanoma. *Cancer Treat Rev* 19:17-28, 1993.

Hancock BW, et al: British National Lymphoma Investigation randomised study of MOPP (mustine, Oncovin, procarbazine, prednisolone) against LOPP (Leukeran substituted for mustine) in advanced Hodgkin's disease—long term results. *Br J Cancer* 63:579-582, 1991.

Hansen LA, Hughes TE: Altretamine. *DICP* 25:146-152, 1991.

Harris JR, et al: Breast cancer (third of three parts). *N Engl J Med* 327:473-480, 1992.

Harmon WE, et al: Chronic renal failure in children treated with methyl CCNU. *N Engl J Med* 300:1200-1203, 1979.

Hennings H, et al: Enhanced malignant conversion of benign mouse skin tumors by cisplatin. *J Natl Cancer Inst* 82:836-840, 1990.

Howell SB, et al: Intraperitoneal cisplatin-based chemotherapy for ovarian carcinoma. *Semin Oncol* 18(suppl 3):5-10, 1991.

Jodrell DI, et al: Relationships between carboplatin exposure and tumor response and toxicity in patients with ovarian cancer. *J Clin Oncol* 10:520-528, 1992.

Kaldor JM, et al: Leukemia following Hodgkin's disease. *N Engl J Med* 322:7-13, 1990.

Kandylis K, et al: Ifosfamide cardiotoxicity in humans. *Cancer Chemother Pharmacol* 24:395-396, 1989.

Kirkwood JM, Agarwala SS: Systemic cytotoxic and biologic therapy of melanoma, in: *PPO Updates*. Philadelphia, JB Lippincott, (Aug) 1993, vol 7.

Kornblith PL, Walker M: Chemotherapy for malignant gliomas. *J Neurosurg* 68:1-17, 1988.

Kramer ED, Packer RJ: Chemotherapy of malignant brain tumors in children. *Clin Neuropharmacol* 15:163-185, 1992.

Kretschmar CS, et al: Ototoxicity of preradiation cisplatin for children with central nervous system tumors. *J Clin Oncol* 8:1191-1198, 1990.

Krook JE, et al: Effective surgical adjuvant therapy for high-risk rectal carcinoma. *N Engl J Med* 324:709-715, 1991.

Lesser GJ, Grossman SA: The chemotherapy of adult primary brain tumors. *Cancer Treat Rev* 19:261-281, 1993.

Levin VA, et al: Neoplasms of the central nervous system, in DeVita VT Jr, et al (eds): *Cancer: Principles & Practice of Oncology*, ed 4. Philadelphia, JB Lippincott, 1993, 1679-1737.

Lind MJ, Ardiet C: Pharmacokinetics of alkylating agents. *Cancer Surv* 17:157-188, 1993.

Longo DL, et al: Lymphocytic lymphomas, in DeVita VT Jr, et al (eds): *Cancer: Principles & Practice of Oncology*, ed 4. Philadelphia, JB Lippincott, 1993, 1859-1927.

Lönn U and Lõhn S: Prevention of dacarbazine damage of human neoplastic cell DNA by aphidicolin. *Cancer Res* 47:26-30, 1987.

Lusthof KJ, et al: DNA alkylation and formation of DNA interstrand cross-links by potential antitumour 2,5-bis(1-aziridinyl)-1,4-benzoquinones. *Chem Biol Interact* 70:249-262, 1989.

Markman M, et al: Intraperitoneal chemotherapy in the management of ovarian cancer. *Cancer* 71:1565-1570, 1993 A.

Markman M, et al: Evidence supporting the superiority of intraperitoneal cisplatin compared to intraperitoneal carboplatin for salvage therapy of small-volume residual ovarian cancer. *Gynecol Oncol* 50:100-104, 1993 B.

McGuire WP: Primary treatment of epithelial ovarian malignancies. *Cancer Suppl* 71:1541-1550, 1993.

McGuire WP: Paclitaxel in the treatment of ovarian cancer, in: *ASCO Educational Book, 30th Annual Meeting, May 14-17, 1994, Dallas, Texas*. Chicago, American Society of Clinical Oncology, 1994.

McGuire WP, Rowinsky EK: Old drugs revisited, new drugs, and experimental approaches in ovarian cancer therapy. *Semin Oncol* 18:255-269, (June) 1991.

Micetich KC, et al: Nephrotoxicity of semustine (methyl-CCNU) in patients with malignant melanoma receiving adjuvant chemotherapy. *Am J Med* 71:967-972, 1981.

Micetich KC, et al: Phase I study of streptozocin- and carmustine-sequenced administration in patients with advanced cancer. *J Natl Cancer Inst* 84:256-260, 1992.

Moertel CG, et al: Streptozocin alone compared with streptozocin plus fluorouracil in treatment of advanced islet-cell carcinoma. *N Engl J Med* 303:1189-1194, 1980.

Moore MJ: Clinical pharmacokinetics of cyclophosphamide. *Clin Pharmacokinet* 20:194-208, 1991.

Morgan M, et al: The toxicity of busulphan and cyclophosphamide as the preparative regimen for bone marrow transplantation. *Br J Haematol* 77:529-534, 1991.

Morrow CS, Cowan KH: Mechanisms of antineoplastic drug resistance, in DeVita VT Jr, et al (eds): *Cancer: Principles & Practice of Oncology*, ed 4. Philadelphia, JB Lippincott, 1993, 340-348.

Motzer RJ, et al: Ifosfamide-based chemotherapy for patients with resistant germ cell tumors: The Memorial Sloan-Kettering Cancer Center Experience. *Semin Oncol* 19(suppl 12):8-12, 1992.

Muggia F, Norris K Jr: Hexamethylmelamine in platinum-resistant ovarian cancer: How active? Editorial. *Gynecol Oncol* 47:279-281, 1992.

Murphy CP, et al: Generalized seizures secondary to high-dose busulfan therapy. *Ann Pharmacother* 26:30-31, 1992.

Neijt J, et al: A double-blind randomised study with ORG-2766, an ACTH(4-9) analog, to prevent cisplatin neuropathy. *Proc ASCO* 13:261, 1994.

Newell DR, et al: Carboplatin pharmacokinetics in children: The development of a pediatric dosing formula. *J Clin Oncol* 11:2314-2323, 1993.

Newling D: Intravesical therapy in the management of superficial transitional cell carcinoma of the bladder: The experience of the EORTC GU group. *Br J Cancer* 61:497-499, 1990.

Norton JA, et al: Cancer of the endocrine system, in DeVita VT Jr, et al (eds): *Cancer: Principles & Practice of Oncology*, ed 4. Philadelphia, JB Lippincott, 1993, 1333-1435.

O'Brien MER, et al: Blindness associated with high-dose carboplatin. *Lancet* 339:558, 1992.

O'Driscoll BR, et al: Active lung fibrosis up to 17 years after chemotherapy with carmustine (BCNU) in childhood. *N Engl J Med* 323:378-382, 1990.

O'Dwyer PJ, et al: Phase I/pharmacokinetic reevaluation of thioTEPA. *Cancer Res* 51:3171-3176, 1991.

O'Dwyer P, et al: Phase I trial of thiotepa in combination with recombinant human granulocyte-macrophage colony-stimulating factor. *J Clin Oncol* 10:1352-1358, 1992.

O'Reilly RJ, Papadopoulos EB: Allogeneic transplantation, in Holland JF, et al (eds): *Cancer Medicine*, ed 3. Philadelphia, Lea & Febiger, 1993, 998-1016.

Ovarian Cancer Meta-Analysis Project: Cyclophosphamide plus cisplatin versus cyclophosphamide, doxorubicin, and cisplatin chemotherapy of ovarian carcinoma: A meta-analysis. *J Clin Oncol* 9:1668-1674, 1991.

Ozols RF, Young RC: Chemotherapy of ovarian cancer. *Semin Oncol* 18:222-232, (June) 1991.

Panella TJ, et al: Modulation of O^6-alkylguanine-DNA alkyltransferase-mediated carmustine resistance using streptozotocin: A Phase I trial. *Cancer Res* 52:2456-2459, 1992.

Pass HI: Treatment of malignant pleural and pericardial effusions, in DeVita VT Jr, et al (eds): *Cancer: Principles & Practice of Oncology*, ed 4. Philadelphia, JB Lippincott, 1993, 2246-2255.

Patel JM: Metabolism and pulmonary toxicity of cyclophosphamide. *Pharmacol Ther* 47:137-146, 1990.

Pegg AE, Byers TL: Repair of DNA containing O^6-alkylguanine. *FASEB J* 6:2302-2310, 1992.

Peters WP: Autologous bone marrow transplantation, in Holland JF, et al (eds): *Cancer Medicine*, ed 3. Philadelphia, Lea & Febiger, 1993, 983-997.

Peters WA III, et al: Intraperitoneal P-32 is not an effective consolidation therapy after a negative second-look laparotomy for epithelial carcinoma of the ovary. *Gynecol Oncol* 47:146-149, 1992.

Pfeiffer P, et al: Intraperitoneal carboplatin in the treatment of minimal residual ovarian cancer. *Gynecol Oncol* 36:306-311, 1990.

Porter AT, et al: Results of a randomized Phase-III trial to evaluate the efficacy of strontium-89 adjuvant to local field external beam irradiation in the management of endocrine resistant metastatic prostate cancer. *Int J Radiat Oncol Biol Phys* 25:805-813, 1993.

Prados MD, Wilson CB: Neoplasms of the central nervous system, in Holland JF, et al (eds): *Cancer Medicine*, ed 3. Philadelphia, Lea & Febiger, 1993, 1080-1119.

Pratt CB, et al: Ifosfamide neurotoxicity is related to previous cisplatin treatment for pediatric solid tumors. *J Clin Oncol* 8:1399-1401, 1990.

Pugh RP, et al: Phase II study of diaziquone in untreated advanced gastric carcinoma: A Southwest Oncology Study Group. *Am J Clin Oncol* 12:11-13, 1989.

Quezado ZMN, et al: High-dose ifosfamide is associated with severe, reversible cardiac dysfunction. *Ann Intern Med* 118:31-36, 1993.

Quilty PM, et al: A comparison of the palliative effects of strontium-89 and external beam radiotherapy in metastatic prostate cancer. *Radiother Oncol* 31:33-40, 1994.

Rai KR, Rabinowe SN: Chronic lymphocytic leukemia, in Holland JF, et al (eds): *Cancer Medicine*, ed 3. Philadelphia, Lea & Febiger, 1993, 1971-1988.

Reed E: Platinum analogs, in DeVita VT Jr, et al (eds): *Cancer: Principles & Practice of Oncology*, ed 4. Philadelphia, JB Lippincott, 1993, 390-400.

Reed E, et al: High-dose carboplatin and recombinant granulocyte-macrophage colony-stimulating factor in advanced-stage recurrent ovarian cancer. *J Clin Oncol* 11:2118-2126, 1993.

Regazzi MB, et al: Disposition of high-dose busulfan in pediatric patients undergoing bone marrow transplantation. *Clin Pharmacol Ther* 53:45-52, 1993.

Reichman B, et al: Phase II trial of high-dose cisplatin with sodium thiosulfate nephroprotection in patients with advanced carcinoma of the uterine cervix previously untreated with chemotherapy. *Gynecol Oncol* 43:159-163, 1991.

Reyno LM, et al: Impact of cyclophosphamide on relationships between carboplatin exposure and response or toxicity when used in the treatment of advanced ovarian cancer. *J Clin Oncol* 11:1156-1164, 1993.

Rhoads CP: Nitrogen mustards in the treatment of neoplastic disease. *JAMA* 131:656-659, 1946.

Richie JP: Detection and treatment of testicular cancer. *CA Cancer J Clin* 43:151-175, 1993.

Robinson RG: Strontium-89—Precursor targeted therapy for pain relief of blastic metastatic disease. *Cancer* 72:3433-3435, 1993.

Rodriguez LA, et al: Reevaluation of procarbazine for the treatment of recurrent malignant central nervous system tumors. *Cancer* 64:2420-2423, 1989.

Rogers L, et al: ^{32}P following negative second-look laparotomy for epithelial ovarian cancer. *Gynecol Oncol* 50:141-146, 1993.

Rozencweig M, et al: Randomized trials of carboplatin versus cisplatin in advanced ovarian cancer, in Bunn PA, et al (eds): *Carboplatin: Current Perspectives and Future Directions.* Philadelphia, Saunders, 1990, 175-186.

Salmon SE, Cassady JR: Plasma cell neoplasms, in DeVita VT Jr, et al (eds): *Cancer: Principles & Practice of Oncology,* ed 4. Philadelphia, JB Lippincott, 1993, 1984-2025.

Santos GW: The development of busulfan/cyclophosphamide preparative regimens. *Semin Oncol* 20 (suppl 4):12-16, 1993.

Sartorelli AC: Therapeutic attack of hypoxic cells of solid tumors: Presidential address. *Cancer Res* 48:775-778, 1988.

Scanlon KJ, et al: Molecular basis of cisplatin resistance in human carcinomas: Model systems and patients. *Anticancer Res* 9:1301-1312, 1989.

Schilsky RL, Erlichman C: Infertility and carcinogenesis: Late complications of chemotherapy, in Chabner BA, Collins JM (eds): *Cancer Chemotherapy: Principles and Practice.* Philadelphia, JB Lippincott, 1990, 32-58.

Schold SC Jr, et al: Randomized comparison of diaziquone and carmustine in the treatment of adults with anaplastic glioma. *J Clin Oncol* 11:77-83, 1993.

Schuchter LM, Glick JH: The current status of WR-2721 (amifostine): A chemotherapy and radiation therapy protector, in DeVita VT Jr, et al (eds): *Biologic Therapy of Cancer Updates.* Philadelphia, JB Lippincott, 1993, vol 3.

Selby P, et al: ChlVPP combination chemotherapy for Hodgkin's disease: Long term results. *Br J Cancer* 62:279-285, 1990.

Sen RP, et al: Pulmonary complications of combination therapy with cyclophosphamide and prednisone. *Chest* 99:143-146, 1991.

Shepherd JD, et al: Mesna versus hyperhydration for the prevention of cyclophosphamide-induced hemorrhagic cystitis in bone marrow transplantation. *J Clin Oncol* 9:2016-2020, 1991.

Silberstein EB: The treatment of painful osseous metastases with phosphorus-32-labeled phosphates. *Semin Oncol* 20 (suppl 2):10-21, 1993.

Silver RT: Chronic myeloid leukemia, in Holland JF, et al (eds): *Cancer Medicine,* ed 3. Philadelphia, Lea & Febiger, 1993, 1934-1942.

Skinner R, et al: The influence of age on nephrotoxicity following chemotherapy in children. *Br J Cancer* 66 (suppl 18):S30-S35, 1992.

Skinner R, et al: Ifosfamide, mesna, and nephrotoxicity in children. *J Clin Oncol* 11:173-190, 1993.

Slayton RE, et al: A Phase II clinical trial of diaziquone in the treatment of patients with recurrent endometrial carcinoma. *Am J Clin Oncol* 11:612-613, 1988.

Sorenson CM, et al: Analysis of events associated with cell cycle arrest at G_2 phase and cell death induced by cisplatin. *J Natl Cancer Inst* 82:749-755, 1990.

Spanos WJ Jr, et al: Complications in the use of intra-abdominal ^{32}P for ovarian carcinoma. *Gynecol Oncol* 45:243-247, 1992.

Speyer JL, et al: Intraperitoneal carboplatin: Favorable results in women with minimal residual ovarian cancer after cisplatin therapy. *J Clin Oncol* 8:1335-1341, 1990.

Srivastava A, et al: Busulphan and melphalan prior to autologous bone marrow transplantation. *Bone Marrow Transplant* 12:323-329, 1993.

Steele G Jr: Combined-modality therapy for rectal carcinoma: The time has come, editorial. *N Engl J Med* 324:764-766, 1991.

Swenerton K, et al: Cisplatin-cyclophosphamide versus carboplatin-cyclophosphamide in advanced ovarian cancer: A randomized Phase III study of the National Cancer Institute of Canada Clinical Trials Group. *J Clin Oncol* 10:718-726, 1992.

Takvorian T, Canellos G: Hodgkin's disease, in Holland JF, et al (eds): *Cancer Medicine,* ed 3. Philadelphia, Lea & Febiger, 1993, 1998-2027.

Thigpen JT, et al: Second-line chemotherapy for recurrent carcinoma of the ovary. *Cancer* 71:1559-1564, 1993.

Tobias JS: Current role of chemotherapy in head and neck cancer. *Drugs* 43:333-345, 1992.

van der Hoop RG, et al: Prevention of cisplatin neurotoxicity with an ACTH (4-9) analogue in patients with ovarian cancer. *N Engl J Med* 322:89-94, 1990.

van der Vijgh WJF: Clinical pharmacokinetics of carboplatin. *Clin Pharmacokinet* 21:242-261, 1991.

Vassal G, et al: Dose-dependent neurotoxicity of high-dose busulfan in children: A clinical and pharmacological study. *Cancer Res* 50:6203-6207, 1990.

Vassal G, et al: Is 600 mg/m^2 the appropriate dosage of busulfan in children undergoing bone marrow transplantation? *Blood* 79:2475-2479, 1992.

Vassal G, et al: Busulfan disposition below the age of three: Alteration in children with lysosomal storage disease. *Blood* 82:1030-1034, 1993.

Vergote I, et al: Hexamethylmelamine as second-line therapy in platin-resistant ovarian cancer. *Gynecol Oncol* 47:282-286, 1992.

Vergote IB, et al: Intraperitoneal radioactive phosphorus therapy in ovarian carcinoma. *Cancer* 71:2250-2260, 1993.

Vinik AI, et al: Neoplasms of the gastroenteropancreatic endocrine system, in Holland JF, et al (eds): *Cancer Medicine,* ed 3. Philadelphia, Lea & Febiger, 1993, 1180-1209.

Vokes EE, et al: Head and neck cancer. *N Engl J Med* 328:184-194, 1993.

Vose JM, et al: Mesna compared with continuous bladder irrigation as uroprotection during high-dose chemotherapy and transplantation: A randomized trial. *J Clin Oncol* 11:1306-1310, 1993.

Waterhouse DM, et al: Combined carboplatin and cisplatin: Limited prospects for dose intensification. *Cancer* 71:4060-4066, 1993.

Watkin SW, et al: Ifosfamide encephalopathy: A reappraisal. *Eur J Cancer Clin Oncol* 25:1303-1310, 1989.

Whitmore WF, Yagoda A: Chemotherapy in the management of bladder tumors. *Drugs* 38:301-312, 1989.

Yeager AM, et al: Optimization of busulfan dosage in children undergoing bone marrow transplantation: A pharmacokinetic study of dose escalation. *Blood* 80:2425-2428, 1992.

Young RC, et al: Cancer of the ovary, in DeVita VT Jr, et al (eds): *Cancer: Principles & Practice of Oncology,* ed 4. Philadelphia, JB Lippincott, 1993, 1226-1263.

Zarrabi MH: Association of non-Hodgkin's lymphoma and second neoplasms. *Semin Oncol* 17:120-132, 1990.

Other Selected References

Calabresi P, et al (eds): *Medical Oncology,* ed 2. New York, Macmillan, 1993.

del Regato JA, et al: *Ackerman and del Regato's Cancer: Diagnosis, Treatment, and Prognosis.* St Louis, CV Mosby, 1985.

DeVita VT Jr, et al (eds): *Cancer: Principles and Practice of Oncology,* ed 4. Philadelphia, JB Lippincott, 1993.

Haskell CM (eds): *Cancer Treatment*, ed 3. Philadelphia, WB Saunders, 1990.

Hellmann K, Carter SK (eds): *Fundamentals of Cancer Chemotherapy*. New York, McGraw-Hill, 1987.

Holland JF, et al (eds): *Cancer Medicine*, ed 3. Philadelphia, Lea & Febiger, 1993.

Tannock IF, Hill RP (eds): *The Basic Science of Oncology*, ed 2. New York, Pergamon Press, 1992.

Antineoplastic Agents: Antimetabolites 89

FOLIC ACID ANALOGUES

PYRIMIDINE ANALOGUES

PURINE ANALOGUES

RIBONUCLEOTIDE REDUCTASE INHIBITORS

INVESTIGATIONAL ANTIMETABOLITES WITH NOVEL TARGETS

Antimetabolites are chemically similar to naturally occurring metabolites, but they differ enough to interfere with normal metabolic pathways. Most antimetabolites used in cancer chemotherapy interfere with important enzymatic reactions in the synthesis of nucleic acids, purines, pyrimidines, and their precursors (Allegra, 1990; Chabner, 1990; Grem, 1990; McCormack and Johns, 1990; Donehower, 1990). Some also may be incorporated into nucleic acids in place of the corresponding normal nucleotides, which alter important cellular functions. These antimetabolites include folic acid analogues, purine and pyrimidine analogues, and ribonucleotide reductase inhibitors. In the last decade, several other enzymes and biochemical pathways in addition to purine, pyrimidine, and nucleic acid biosynthesis have been identified as potentially useful targets for the rational design of cancer chemotherapeutic drugs. For several of these agents, some activity against human cancer has been demonstrated in Phase I or II trials. However, since clinical testing is incomplete, these drugs remain investigational and are available only through ongoing clinical trials.

Folic acid, pyrimidine, and purine analogues and ribonucleotide reductase inhibitors act primarily during the DNA synthesizing phase of the cell cycle (S phase). Some act exclusively in S phase (eg, cytarabine) and others (eg, methotrexate, mercaptopurine) affect cells in both S phase and in G_1. Some drugs in the latter group have self-limiting cytocidal effects since they kill cells only in S phase and prevent entry of G_1 cells into S phase without causing death of these G_1 cells. The fluorinated pyrimidines appear to be exceptions; although they act preferentially on cycling cells, they are not phase specific.

FOLIC ACID ANALOGUES

Folic acid analogues (also referred to as antifolates) used in cancer chemotherapy act by inhibiting the enzyme, dihydrofolate reductase, which converts dihydrofolate (FH_2) to tetrahydrofolate (FH_4) (Allegra, 1990; Schweitzer et al, 1990; Bertino, 1990 A). FH_2 is inactive as a cofactor for any of the folate-dependent one-carbon transfer reactions in cells. Conversion of FH_4 to FH_2 is catalyzed only by thymidylate synthase, the enzyme that converts deoxyuridylate to thymidylate. Since thymidylate is used only for DNA synthesis, antifolates are selectively toxic to proliferating cells, in which they cause accumulation of FH_2 and depletion of FH_4 coenzymes. The latter are required for synthesis of purines, methionine, and glycine, as well as for synthesis of thymidylate. Thus, DNA, RNA, and protein synthesis are inhibited in cells treated with antifolates. In addition, other metabolites of FH_2 (such as formyl-FH_2) may inhibit folate-dependent enzymes and contribute to the toxic effects of antifolates.

Refractoriness to subsequent therapy with antifolates has been reported in patients whose tumors had responded initially. Acquired resistance to methotrexate, the folic acid analogue used most often, has been studied extensively using cell culture systems (Allegra, 1990; Schweitzer et al, 1990; Bertino, 1990 A). Observed mechanisms include reduced intracellular accumulation via active transport catalyzed by the folate transport protein; decreased conversion to polyglutamates (catalyzed by the enzyme, folylpolyglutamyl synthetase) leading to decreased intracellular retention of the drug as well as to less complete inhibition of some folate-dependent enzymes; decreased affinity of FH_2 reductase for drug (but not for substrate) as a result of mutations that change the amino acid sequence; and increased amounts of FH_2 reductase (often as a result of gene amplification, a process resulting in multiple copies of the gene for this enzyme) to levels greater than the drug concentration in the resistant cells. Like other examples of drug resistance in human tumors, the relative contributions of these mechanisms to clinical resistance is unknown. Some of the newer antifolates (eg, trimetrexate) may prove useful in overcoming certain forms of methotrexate resistance.

METHOTREXATE

METHOTREXATE SODIUM

[Folex]

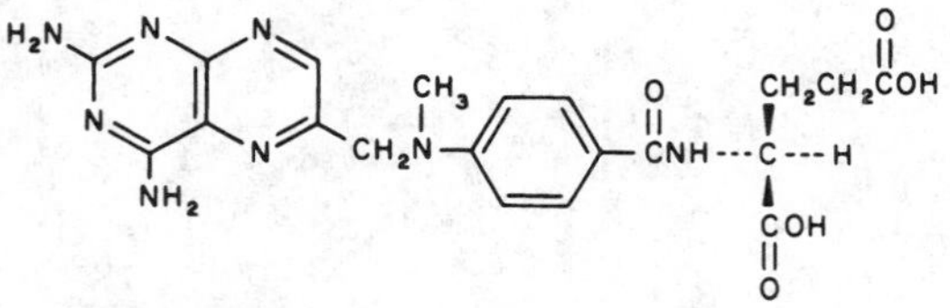

ACTIONS. Methotrexate is the 4-amino, N^{10}-methyl analogue of folic acid. It has a very high affinity for the substrate binding site of mammalian reductase. In addition to the partial depletion of FH_4 coenzymes discussed above, methotrexate polyglutamates, FH_2 polyglutamates, and 10-formyl-FH_2 polyglutamates accumulate after treatment with methotrexate and directly inhibit thymidylate synthase and several enzymes of de novo purine biosynthesis. Thus, multiple mechanisms contribute to the cytocidal effects of methotrexate. This agent is cell cycle specific for the S phase, but it is self-limiting because of other effects on RNA and protein synthesis that slow the entry of G_1 cells into the S phase.

The blockade of dihydrofolate reductase can be bypassed clinically by use of leucovorin calcium (also referred to as folinic acid or citrovorum factor) (Ackland and Schilsky, 1987). This "rescue" agent allows for recovery of normal tissue (which may transport folates into cells at lower extracellular concentrations than some tumors) and thus permits use of larger doses of methotrexate (see Chapter 1 of this Section, Principles of Cancer Chemotherapy). This approach is particularly useful in adjuvant therapy for osteogenic sarcoma. For other tumors (eg, breast, colon, lung), high-dose methotrexate with leucovorin rescue has not provided a therapeutic advantage over standard-dose methotrexate. In some instances (eg, head and neck tumors) and with certain dosages and schedules, data suggest that leucovorin rescue may reduce the antitumor efficacy of methotrexate (Browman et al, 1990). Results of other studies suggest that there are therapeutic benefits from the high-dose/rescue approach in squamous cell carcinoma of the head and neck (Bertino, 1990 B). In addition, thymidine, which restores intracellular pools of thymidine triphosphate, and carboxypeptidase G_2, an enzyme that hydrolyzes and inactivates methotrexate, have been used as rescue measures in clinical trials. However, these approaches are less well established than leucovorin rescue.

USES. Methotrexate, either alone or in combination regimens depending on the patient's risk factors, has been very effective in women with choriocarcinoma and related trophoblastic tumors. Cures have been reported in most individuals treated with low doses of methotrexate plus leucovorin (Bagshawe et al, 1989).

Although methotrexate induces complete remissions in acute lymphocytic leukemia of childhood, it is of more value for maintenance therapy and is an agent of choice in combination with mercaptopurine. Furthermore, intrathecal methotrexate and cranial irradiation are administered routinely to patients with acute lymphocytic leukemia to prevent meningeal metastases.

Methotrexate is a component of combination regimens used to treat non-Hodgkin's and Burkitt's lymphomas and breast, lung, bladder, cervical, gastric, and ovarian carcinomas (see index entry Cancer: Clinical Response to Chemotherapeutic Drugs). High-dose methotrexate plus leucovorin rescue (with or without other drugs) is used to treat osteogenic sarcoma, some non-Hodgkin's lymphomas, and (by some physicians) head and neck tumors.

Methotrexate is a primary agent in the treatment of cutaneous T cell lymphomas and medulloblastoma. It has shown activity as a single agent against testicular cancer; bladder, lung, colorectal, esophageal, hepatocellular, and cervical carcinomas; soft tissue sarcomas; and embryonal rhabdomyosarcoma. For some of these neoplasms (testicular, colorectal, and hepatocellular cancers; soft tissue sarcomas and rhabdomyosarcoma), more effective regimens are available and are used much more frequently than methotrexate. For uses of methotrexate in non-neoplastic diseases, see index entry Methotrexate.

ADVERSE REACTIONS AND PRECAUTIONS. Toxicity to proliferating tissues most often involves the gastrointestinal tract, bone marrow, and oral mucosa. Stomatitis is common and is an indication for interruption of therapy, as is diarrhea. Hemorrhagic enteritis and intestinal perforation can occur if therapy is continued after diarrhea develops.

Myelosuppression (leukopenia, thrombocytopenia, and/or anemia) is the usual dose-limiting toxicity. Following a bolus dose or short-term infusion, the nadir usually appears between 5 and 14 days, and recovery is rapid. More prolonged and severe toxicity has been observed in patients receiving higher doses and in those with poorer performance status or compromised bone marrow, liver, or renal function. The myelosuppressive effects often result in impaired immune responses and increase the risk of infection. Leucovorin may be used to rescue the bone marrow from the myelosuppressive effects of methotrexate if it is given within 42 hours after administration of methotrexate. It is only partially effective when given later.

Since methotrexate is excreted principally by the kidneys, its use in patients with impaired renal function may increase toxicity. Therefore, renal function should be monitored before and during therapy. Use of methotrexate may be contraindicated in patients with severely impaired renal function because of the difficulty in selecting a safe and effective dose for these patients. In addition, large doses have been associated with direct toxicity to the kidney, presumably due to precipitation of the drug or its 7-hydroxy metabolite in the renal tubules. Adequate hydration and alkalinization of the urine (using sodium bicarbonate or acetazolamide) enhance excretion of methotrexate and its metabolite.

Hepatic dysfunction has been observed after short- and long-term use. Acute reversible elevations in hepatic enzyme levels are often seen with high-dose therapy. Prolonged use may lead to fibrosis and occasionally cirrhosis. Liver function should be monitored, but may not provide an adequate indication of the development of hepatic fibrosis. Although not recommended, liver biopsy and histology is the only accurate measure of developing fibrosis.

Alopecia and dermatitis have been reported, and osteoporosis is observed occasionally in children on long-term maintenance therapy. An acute reversible pneumonitis of unknown etiology may develop, especially with intermittent therapy. It is characterized by fever, cough, shortness of breath, peripheral eosinophilia, and patchy pulmonary infiltrates. Acute hypersensitivity (eg, urticaria, wheezing, hypotension) has occurred rarely. Central nervous system toxicity has been observed when methotrexate was given intrathecally, usually when central nervous system irradiation therapy also was administered.

This drug has been reported to be an abortifacient and should not be used during the first trimester of pregnancy. Because of the theoretical possibility of mutagenic effects in humans, the manufacturers recommend that a period of time (one ovulatory cycle in women and three months for men) should elapse between the end of therapy and conception. Methotrexate is classified in FDA Pregnancy Category D.

DRUG INTERACTIONS. Vinca alkaloids, daunorubicin, and cytarabine increase the cellular uptake of methotrexate, while penicillin, hydroxyurea, mercaptopurine, neomycin, kanamycin, corticosteroids, bleomycin, and asparaginase decrease cellular uptake.

Methotrexate may be displaced from plasma albumin by sulfonamides, salicylates, tetracyclines, chloramphenicol, and phenytoin. The resulting increase in the free concentration of methotrexate may potentiate the drug's toxicity. In addition, salicylates and probenecid may compete with methotrexate for renal tubular secretion. Caution should be used if these drugs are given concomitantly, since the reduced rate of excretion may result in elevated plasma levels of methotrexate and more frequent or more severe adverse reactions.

Although vincristine interferes with efflux of methotrexate from cells, the therapeutic effect is not enhanced. Asparaginase may attenuate methotrexate toxicity to the host but not in leukemic lymphoblasts by inhibiting protein synthesis and thus blocking cell entry into S phase. The use of methotrexate followed in 24 hours by asparaginase reportedly can improve antileukemic efficacy in patients with acute lymphocytic leukemia. A synergistic effect has been reported when methotrexate was administered before fluorouracil. Accumulation of intracellular phosphoribosylpyrophosphate as a result of methotrexate therapy increases the formation of fluorouracil nucleotides, which increases cell kill. However, administration of fluorouracil before methotrexate can decrease the efficacy of the latter by inhibiting thymidylate synthase and the conversion of FH_4 to FH_2.

PHARMACOKINETICS. Methotrexate can be given orally, and conventional doses (eg, less than 25 mg/M^2) are readily absorbed; absorption by a saturable active transport system is erratic at higher doses. Peak plasma concentrations are attained in one to four hours. The drug most often is administered intravenously and sometimes is given intramuscularly. The peak plasma concentration is reached within one-half to two hours after intramuscular injection. The initial plasma half-life is two to four hours after parenteral administration; the elimination half-life is 8 to 15 hours after high-dose parenteral use and 3 to 10 hours after oral use.

Drug concentration and duration of cell exposure are critical determinants of cytotoxicity. One-half of the drug is loosely bound to plasma proteins; 50% to 90% is excreted unchanged in the urine within 24 hours by glomerular filtration and active tubular secretion. Dose modifications are required in patients with renal insufficiency, and monitoring of plasma levels is indicated.

Methotrexate enters and exits cells by carrier-mediated active transport systems shared by the physiologic reduced folates. Intracellular storage is in the form of polyglutamate conjugates, which may be important determinants of the duration and site of drug action. The drug accumulates in the liver and kidney. The terminal elimination of methotrexate is very slow, for it persists in the liver and kidney for weeks.

Methotrexate does not enter the cerebrospinal fluid in therapeutic concentrations (except with large intravenous doses, ie, more than 500 mg/M^2), and intrathecal administration is necessary to treat meningeal leukemia and lymphoma. Pleural effusions and ascites may act as drug depots and require evacuation prior to methotrexate administration.

DOSAGE AND PREPARATIONS.
Oral: 2.5 to 5 mg daily.

METHOTREXATE:
Methotrexate (Lederle). Tablets 2.5 mg.

Intramuscular, Intravenous: 25 mg/M^2 once or twice weekly. Dose modifications are based on toxicity. When used with cyclophosphamide and fluorouracil in breast carcinoma, 40 mg/M^2 intravenously on days one and eight every 28 days.
Intravenous (high-dose): 12 to 15 g/M^2 with leucovorin rescue in weeks 4, 5, 6, 7, 11, 12, 15, 16, 29, 30, 44, and 45 after surgery.
Intrathecal: Doses are based on age rather than body surface area, since cerebrospinal fluid volume depends on age. *Children younger than 1 year,* 6 mg; *1 to 2 years,* 8 mg; *2 to 3 years,* 10 mg. *Children older than 3 years and adults,* 12 mg. Doses are administered every two to five days until the cerebrospinal fluid cell count returns to normal. Elliott's B solution is the preferred diluent for intrathecal administration because of its superior buffering capacity; however, it is not commercially available. Preservative-free sodium chloride 0.9% and lactated Ringer's solution are appropriate alternatives.

METHOTREXATE SODIUM:
(Strengths expressed in terms of the base.)
Methotrexate (Lederle). Solution (for injection) 2.5 mg/ml in 2 ml containers and 25 mg/ml in 2, 4, 8, and 10 ml containers; solution (for injection, preservative-free) 25 mg/ml in 2, 4, 8, and 10 ml containers ***(Methotrexate LPF)***; powder (cryodesiccated) 20, 50, 100, and 250 mg and 1 g.
Folex PFS (Adria). Solution 25 mg/ml in 2, 4, 8, and 10 ml containers.

TRIMETREXATE (TMQ) (Investigational drug)

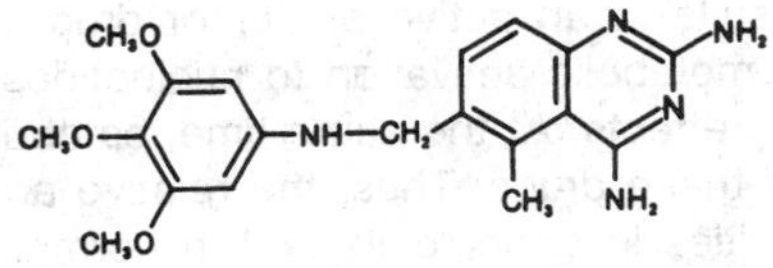

ACTIONS. Trimetrexate is a competitive inhibitor of dihydrofolate reductase. It is a nonclassical antifolate that enters cells by passive diffusion and does not undergo intracellular polyglutamylation because it lacks the terminal benzoylglutamate structure present in the folates and methotrexate. As a result of these structural and biochemical differences, trimetrexate retains activity against cells resistant to methotrexate because of decreased transport or reduced polyglutamation. Trimetrexate can inhibit the incorporation of deoxyuridine, uridine, and thymidine into DNA.

USES. Oncolytic activity against murine and human cell lines and against primary cultures of human tumors has been demonstrated. It is anticipated that trimetrexate may have a wider spectrum of activity than methotrexate, and the incidence of acquired drug resistance may be reduced. Phase II trials in previously treated patients with recurrent gastric, urothelial, lung, and other tumors have demonstrated that trimetrexate has moderate activity when used alone. Clinical trials of combination regimens that include this antifolate are in progress.

For the investigational use of trimetrexate in the treatment of pneumocystis pneumonia, see index entry Trimetrexate.

ADVERSE REACTIONS. Myelosuppression is the dose limiting toxicity, with thrombocytopenia in excess of neutropenia. Administration of leucovorin can reduce the myelosuppressive effects of trimetrexate. Anemia also occurs; the frequency is related to the dose administered. Other adverse reactions to trimetrexate include hepatotoxicity, nausea and vomiting, and mucositis. Arrhythmias have been reported infrequently. Acute maculopapular rashes and hyperpigmentation were reported during Phase I trials.

PHARMACOKINETICS. The terminal plasma half-life of trimetrexate is approximately 12 hours. However, there is considerable variation in the elimination of trimetrexate at a given dose level. It is eliminated primarily by nonrenal clearance. The mechanisms include biotransformation and elimination in the liver.

DOSAGE (investigational regimen).
Intravenous: 8 to 12 mg/M^2 daily for five days, repeated every 14 to 21 days, with dose reductions based on renal function and hematologic toxicity.

Trimetrexate (Parke-Davis).

PYRIMIDINE ANALOGUES

The pyrimidine analogues used in cancer chemotherapy are either nucleosides or bases that have small but therapeutically significant structural differences from the endogenous compounds, cytosine, uridine, and thymidine. For some (eg, cytarabine), the structural change is limited to the sugar ring of the nucleoside; for others (eg, fluorouracil, azacitidine), a single substitution (a fluorine for a hydrogen or a nitrogen for a carbon) results in an active antitumor drug. All of these drugs require metabolic activation to nucleotides in order to exert cytotoxic effects. At the same time, catabolism can inactivate all of these drugs. Thus, the relative activating and catabolic activities in tumor cells and in normal tissues are major determinants of the efficacy and adverse reactions of the pyrimidine analogues.

CYTARABINE (Cytosine Arabinoside)
[Cytosar-U, Tarabine PFS]

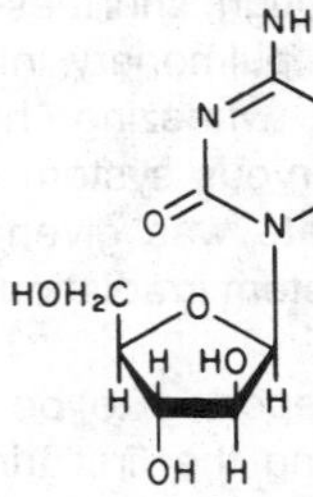

ACTIONS. This synthetic nucleoside differs from the normal nucleosides, cytidine and deoxycytidine, in that the sugar moiety is arabinose rather than ribose or deoxyribose (Chabner, 1990). Cytarabine enters cells by an energy-dependent nucleoside active transport system. It is then converted sequentially by deoxycytidine kinase, dCMP kinase, nucleoside diphosphate kinase, and other nucleotide kinases to the triphosphate derivative, arabinofuranosylcytosine triphosphate (ara-CTP), which is the active metabolite. Ara-CTP may interfere with DNA synthesis by inhibiting DNA polymerase α and is also incorporated into DNA, causing additional defects by chain termination. Incorporation into RNA also has been reported. Incorporation of ara-CTP into DNA appears to be the more important mechanism for the drug's cytocidal effects. The effects are exerted during the S phase. Under certain conditions, cytarabine can also block progression of cells from G_1 into S phase. Because it is a cell cycle-specific drug, the duration of exposure to cytarabine and the amount of activated drug (ara-CTP) retained after the extracellular concentration falls are critical determinants of response to treatment. Since it has a short half-life in vivo, cytarabine is often administered as a continuous infusion.

USES. The primary indication for cytarabine is for induction of remission in adults and children with acute myelogenous leukemia in combination with doxorubicin or daunorubicin (with or without thioguanine) (Wiernik, 1989; Donohue and Charlton, 1989; Chabner, 1990; Buechner and Hiddemann, 1990). Alternative combination regimens employ cytarabine with mitoxantrone or amsacrine. It also is used in combination regimens in the blast crisis phase of chronic myelogenous leukemia, as secondary treatment of acute lymphocytic leukemia, and for some non-Hodgkin's lymphomas. The drug can be administered intrathecally for prophylaxis and treatment of meningeal leukemia. However, focal involvement of the central nervous system may not respond to intrathecal cytarabine and should probably be treated with radiation therapy. Cytarabine has little activity when used alone to treat most solid tumors, possibly because intracellular activation to ara-CTP is inadequate.

Resistance to cytarabine may result from impaired cellular uptake, decreased activation secondary to decreased kinase activity, or enhanced catabolism from increased cytidine deaminase activity. The ratio between deoxycytidine kinase (activating) and cytidine deaminase (degrading) activities is often cited as a major determinant of cellular sensitivity to cytarabine. More recent data suggest that drug transport may play a greater role than drug metabolism. High-dose cytarabine has been effective in overcoming some forms of drug resistance. Recently, low-dose cytarabine has been employed for myelodysplastic syndromes (Doll and List, 1989; Lichtman and Brennan, 1990) and for acute nonlymphocytic leukemia (Tilly et al, 1990). It is not clear whether the predominant effect is cytotoxicity or differentiation in these disorders. Cytarabine also has antiviral activity, but excessive host toxicity precludes its use for viral infections (see index entry Cytarabine, As Antiviral Agent).

ADVERSE REACTIONS AND PRECAUTIONS. The major dose-limiting toxic effect of cytarabine is bone marrow depression, which is dependent on the dose and schedule. It is characterized by leukopenia, thrombocytopenia, reticulocytopenia, anemia, and megaloblastosis. The leukopenia is characterized primarily by granulocyte depression, and circulating lymphocytes are only minimally affected. The white blood cell depression has a biphasic course following continuous infusion for five days or bolus injections of 50 to 600 mg/M^2. There is an initial decrease in the first 24 hours with the nadir occurring on days seven to nine, followed by a brief increase that peaks around the twelfth day. Subsequently, a second and deeper fall reaches a nadir between days 15 to 24, with a rapid rise to above baseline in the next ten days. Platelet depression is noticeable at five days with the nadir occurring between days 12 to 15. Thereafter, a rapid rise to above baseline occurs in the next ten days. Frequent blood counts and bone marrow examinations are required. Leukocyte and platelet counts should be performed daily during induction therapy.

Nausea, vomiting, and diarrhea occur frequently, particularly after rapid intravenous infusion. Stomatitis, thrombophlebitis, hepatic dysfunction, fever, and, rarely, anaphylaxis also have been reported. Acute pancreatitis has occurred during cytarabine therapy in patients who have had prior treatment with asparaginase. Hyperuricemia secondary to rapid lysis of neoplastic cells may occur. Cytarabine is a potent immunosuppressant. It has been shown to be teratogenic in animals. Because cytarabine is metabolized primarily in the liver, caution is necessary when giving this drug to patients with impaired hepatic function; these patients may require a reduction in dosage.

Side effects of high-dose cytarabine regimens (in addition to those seen after standard doses) include reversible corneal toxicity, hemorrhagic conjunctivitis, conjunctival pain, and photophobia (modified with steroid eyedrops); gastrointestinal and pulmonary dysfunction; cerebral and cerebellar dysfunction; and peripheral neuropathy. Risk factors for neurotoxic reactions with high-dose cytarabine therapy include age over 49 years, cumulative dose greater than 48 g/M^2, and concurrent or previous leukemia affecting the central nervous system. Results of recent retrospective studies suggest that renal insufficiency is also a risk factor for neurotoxicity after high-dose cytarabine regimens (Damon et al, 1989) and that fatal pulmonary failure (adult respiratory distress syndrome, noncardiogenic pulmonary edema) may be attributable to this type of regimen (Andersson et al, 1990). Intrathecal cytarabine also may cause central nervous system toxicity. Reversible effects on liver function (cholestatic jaundice and elevations of hepatic enzyme levels in serum) often are observed in patients treated with high-dose cytarabine.

This drug is classified in FDA Pregnancy Category D.

DRUG INTERACTIONS. Because cytarabine inhibits DNA synthesis (for both replication and repair of DNA), there is synergism between this drug and other antineoplastic agents (Chabner, 1990). With some antimetabolites (eg, thioguanine), the synergism is schedule-dependent; cytarabine given 12 hours before thioguanine maximizes thioguanine incorporation into DNA, possibly by partial synchronization of tumor cells after the initial treatment. Other antimetabolites potentiate the effects of cytarabine, either by decreasing deoxycytidine triphosphate pools (eg, hydroxyurea) or by increasing the metabolism of cytarabine to ara-CTP (eg, methotrexate). Inhibition of DNA repair after cytarabine treatment may be responsible for its ability to potentiate the antitumor effects of DNA alkylating and cross-linking agents such as cyclophosphamide or cisplatin.

PHARMACOKINETICS. Cytarabine is rapidly deaminated to uracil arabinoside (an inactive metabolite) in the gastrointestinal tract and on its first pass through the liver. Less than 20% of a dose is absorbed as active, unchanged drug after oral administration; thus, it is given intravenously. The drug also is deaminated rapidly after infusion, primarily in the liver, plasma, and granulocytes, and disappears from the blood in two phases, an initial fast phase with a half-life of 10 minutes and a second phase of approximately one to three hours. Cytarabine concentrations during this second phase are therapeutically adequate only in high-dose regimens. Eighty percent of an intravenous dose is excreted in the urine in 24 hours, 90% as uracil arabinoside and less than 10% as unchanged drug. A carrier-mediated mechanism is responsible for cellular uptake.

Cerebrospinal fluid levels approach 40% of the plasma concentration after a two-hour intravenous infusion. After intrathecal administration, the cerebrospinal fluid concentration follows first-order kinetics with a half-life of about two hours. Because of the low levels of deaminase in the cerebrospinal fluid, little conversion to uracil arabinoside occurs there.

With high-dose cytarabine regimens, peak plasma levels are approximately 100 times those observed with conventional doses. Continuous intravenous infusion of cytarabine in amounts up to 2 g/M^2 per day achieves steady-state plasma levels that are proportional to dose. The deamination reaction is saturated when larger amounts are infused, which leads to unpredictably high concentrations and the risk of severe toxicity.

DOSAGE AND PREPARATIONS. For induction therapy, patients should be hospitalized in a facility with adequate laboratory and supportive resources. In many treatment protocols, cytarabine is used in combination with other cytotoxic drugs. ***Intravenous:*** For continuous intravenous infusion, 100 to 200 mg/M^2/24 hours. Generally, five- to seven-day infusions are given with an anthracycline and thioguanine. If there is no response, the course is repeated; if remission does not occur after the second course, another therapeutic regimen should be substituted. Alternatively, 20 mg/M2/day is given by continuous infusion for 7 to 21 days.

Intravenous (high-dose): 2 to 3 g/M2 infused over a one- to two-hour period every 12 hours for a total of 12 doses. Diluents containing benzyl alcohol should not be used when high-dose regimens of cytarabine are administered.

Subcutaneous: For maintenance therapy in acute leukemia, 50 mg/M2 weekly.

Subcutaneous (low-dose): 10 mg/M2 two times daily for 21 days.

Intrathecal: 5 to 75 mg/M2 in 10 ml of saline given from once every four days to once a day for four days. The most frequently used dose is 30 mg/M2 every four days until cerebrospinal fluid cytology is normal, followed by one additional treatment. Diluents containing benzyl alcohol should not be used for intrathecal administration.

Generic. Powder 100 and 500 mg in 10 and 15 ml containers with diluent.

Cytosar-U (Upjohn). Powder (sterile, cryodesiccated) 100 and 500 mg and 1 and 2 g containers. Store at 15° to 30° C. Supplied with diluent containing benzyl alcohol 0.945%, W/V.

Tarabine PFS (Adria). Solution (for injection, preservative-free) 20 mg/ml in sterile isotonic saline in 5 and 50 ml containers.

FLUOROURACIL (5-FU)

[Adrucil]

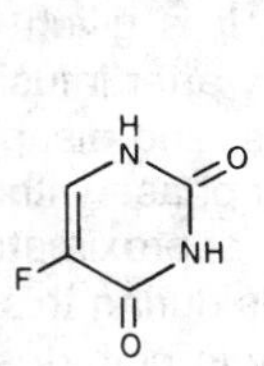

ACTIONS. This fluorinated pyrimidine was developed as a potential antineoplastic agent because of the observation that certain tumor cells incorporate uracil into DNA (after its conversion to thymidine) more effectively than do nontumor cells. Fluorouracil is converted in vivo to the deoxynucleotide, 5-fluoro-2′-deoxyuridine 5′-monophosphate (FdUMP), which is one of the active metabolites (Grem, 1990). In animal tumor models, conversion of fluorouracil to FdUMP correlates well with tumor sensitivity, but this relationship has not been clearly established in human cancer. FdUMP (in the presence of a reduced folate cofactor) inhibits thymidylate synthetase, which catalyzes methylation of deoxyuridylic acid (dUMP) to thymidylic acid (dTMP), and thereby prevents DNA synthesis. Although inhibition of thymidylate synthetase is generally accepted as the primary action, fluorouracil also is converted to the ribonucleotide, fluorouridine monophosphate (FUMP), which is readily incorporated into RNA and inhibits RNA processing and function (Diasio and Harris, 1989; Grem, 1990). A final mechanism is incorporation into DNA after conversion of FdUMP to a triphosphate by intracellular nucleoside monophosphate kinases. DNA with fluorouracil in place of thymine may be less stable than native DNA. The relative contributions of these three mechanisms to overall cytotoxicity after fluorouracil treatment is unclear and may vary among different cells and tissues or depend on extracellular or metabolic conditions.

Fluorouracil is more toxic to proliferating than to nonproliferating cells, but there is no clear-cut cell cycle phase specificity. Resistance to fluorouracil could result from deletion of enzymes required for its activation or from an increase in thymidylate synthetase activity. Other cellular determinants of sensitivity to fluorouracil include the concentrations of cosubstrates required for activation of the drug (eg, donors of ribose-1-phosphate and deoxyribose-1-phosphate or phosphoribosyl-1-pyrophosphate); the stability of the ternary complex formed between thymidylate synthase, FdUMP, and the reduced folate cofactor; the concentration of competing normal substrates for both thymidylate synthase and for RNA and DNA synthesis; the ability to circumvent inhibitory effects of the drug through the "salvage" pathways; and the activities of pathways that degrade fluoropyrimidine nucleosides and nucleotides (Grem, 1990).

USES. Fluorouracil is only useful in solid tumors. It is employed extensively in the palliative treatment of disseminated colorectal and breast carcinomas; when given alone, response rates are only about 20% and 30%, respectively. When given as a component of the CMF or CAF regimens (see index entry Cancer: Clinical Response to Chemotherapeutic Drugs), fluorouracil is used frequently for adjuvant chemotherapy of breast cancer (Henderson et al, 1989; Bonadonna, 1989; Hutchins et al, 1990). Fluorouracil combined with the immunomodulator, levamisole (see index entry Levamisole, In Cancer), is now the preferred regimen for adjuvant chemotherapy of stage III (or Dukes' stage C) colon cancer (Laurie et al, 1989; National Institutes of Health, 1990; Hamilton et al, 1990 A; Moertel et al, 1990). Its use with semustine and high-dose pelvic irradiation is the most effective postsurgical treatment for stage II and III rectal cancer (National Institutes of Health, 1990; Mayer et al, 1989).

This drug also is a component of the FAM and FAMTX combinations used in the palliative treatment of gastric adenocarcinoma (see index entry Cancer: Clinical Response to Chemotherapeutic Drugs). Other responsive tumors are carcinomas of the ovary (eg, Hexa-CAF regimen), bladder, uterine cervix, endometrium, prostate, head and neck, pancreas, and esophagus and hepatoma. Fluorouracil has been used to treat lung carcinoma; malignant melanoma; and malignant pleural, peritoneal, or pericardial effusions. However, regimens that do not include fluorouracil are preferred at present for these indications.

Fluorouracil is used topically in the treatment of multiple actinic keratoses and superficial basal cell carcinomas (see index entry Fluorouracil, In Dermatologic Disorders) and by subconjunctival administration to treat severe ocular inflammation refractory to corticosteroids (see index entry Fluorouracil, In Ocular Inflammation).

ADVERSE REACTIONS AND PRECAUTIONS. The major adverse reactions to fluorouracil result from its effects on rapidly proliferating cells in normal host tissues and affect the gastrointestinal and hematopoietic systems. Anorexia, nausea, and vomiting are common. Stomatitis, esophagopharyngitis, and diarrhea are indications for interruption of therapy because severe ulceration of the oropharynx and bowel may develop. Gastrointestinal toxicity is usually dose limiting when the drug is given by intravenous infusion. There are data suggesting that the severity of gastrointestinal toxicity may be decreased by a circadian-patterned, variable rate infusion, which may increase the maximally tolerated dose by nearly 50% (von Roemeling and Hrushesky, 1989).

Leukopenia is the usual dose-limiting toxicity after bolus intravenous administration. The nadir of the white blood cell count commonly occurs between days 9 and 14 after the first dose, but rarely can be as late as 20 days. Thrombocytopenia is much less prominent and may be observed between days 7 and 17. Monitoring of blood counts is necessary.

Other adverse effects are alopecia, dermatitis, and hyperpigmentation. Acute and chronic conjunctivitis have been seen. Reversible cerebellar ataxia occurs in 1% of patients, is probably dose related, and may occur at any time during therapy (usually after several months). Cerebellar signs may persist for several weeks after discontinuing the drug. Myocardial ischemia and chest pain have developed occasionally (Grem, 1990). Activation of coagulation (increased fibrinopeptide A levels and decreased protein C activity) has been reported in patients treated with fluorouracil alone or in combination with cisplatin (Kuzel et al, 1990). Intraperitoneal administration of fluorouracil for refractory ovarian carcinoma is often associated with chemical peritonitis resulting in abdominal pain. This drug is teratogenic in animals and may be carcinogenic.

Recent clinical observations suggest that the dose of fluorouracil need not be decreased in patients with impaired hepatic function. However, no studies have been published comparing fluorouracil pharmacokinetics in patients with normal liver function and in those with hepatic insufficiency. Fluorouracil should be used with caution in patients with poor nutritional status.

The use of intravenous infusions daily for four or five days markedly decreases hematologic toxicity. However, results of clinical studies do not indicate whether rapid injections or infusions are a superior treatment method. Prolonged infusions (more than two weeks) and, less frequently, bolus administration of fluorouracil have been associated with a hand-foot syndrome (palmar-plantar erythrodysesthesia) associated with pain, erythema, and desquamation.

This drug is classified in FDA Pregnancy Category D.

DRUG INTERACTIONS. Several drug combinations with fluorouracil that either attempt to enhance its efficacy (by modulating intracellular biochemical responses) or to reduce its toxicity to normal host tissues are currently in various stages of clinical trials. Of these, leucovorin with fluorouracil (primarily for metastatic or recurrent colorectal cancer) has received the most attention, and at least nine Phase III trials have been conducted (Einhorn, 1989). In this regimen, leucovorin is used to maximize inhibition of thymidylate synthase by increasing the concentration of the reduced folate cofactor needed for formation of the ternary complex with FdUMP and thymidylate synthase. In three trials using weekly administration of fluorouracil combined with high-dose leucovorin, significant increases in response rates were observed. However, there was no improvement in survival, and the incidence of severe diarrhea was markedly increased with this combination. Results of three of the other six trials, which used five-day courses of fluorouracil with or without leucovorin (repeated every four weeks), indicated that response rates were moderately improved without an increase in the incidence of severe diarrhea. In two of these trials, there were modest increases in the duration of survival in response to the combination. Trials of this regimen in other tumors, including gastric, breast, and head and neck tumors, also have been conducted, but Phase III testing has not been completed (Kerr, 1989).

Other strategies to potentiate the efficacy of fluorouracil include pretreatment with methotrexate (which increases formation of fluorouracil ribonucleotides and thus incorporation into RNA); coadministration with nucleoside transport inhibitors such as dipyridamole (to decrease salvage of thymidine); modulation of pharmacokinetics, catabolism, and incorporation into RNA by pharmacologic doses of thymidine; and putatively synergistic combinations with inhibitors of de novo pyrimidine biosynthesis such as N-(phosphonoacetyl)-L-aspartate (PALA), purines, cisplatin, interferon alfa-2, or ionizing radiation (Grem, 1990). Thus far, none of these combinations have been proven clinically superior to fluorouracil alone in adequate randomized, controlled clinical trials. However, newer doses and schedules for the combination of PALA with fluorouracil appear to yield enhanced response rates (see the evaluation on N-(phosphonoacetyl)-L-aspartate).

Attempts to reduce fluorouracil toxicity to host tissues include combination with allopurinol (a metabolite of which, oxypurinol, indirectly blocks fluorouracil activation in normal tissues), thymidine, purines, interferon alfa-2, hematopoietic growth factors, and uridine rescue (Grem, 1990). Clinical trials are in progress.

PHARMACOKINETICS. Because of erratic absorption and bioavailability, fluorouracil is not administered orally (an oral preparation is available in Europe) (Diasio and Harris, 1989; Grem, 1990). It is usually given intravenously. Most available evidence suggests that continuous infusion yields higher response rates than bolus administration. This drug also has been administered intra-arterially for direct delivery to the tumor (eg, hepatic artery for liver metastases) and by direct injection into effusions in body cavities (eg, intraperitoneally in ovarian cancer). The plasma half-life after intravenous administration is 8 to 20 minutes, and no unchanged drug is detectable after three hours. Intracellular drug levels persist much longer.

Fluorouracil is metabolized extensively in the liver; 60% to 80% is excreted as respiratory carbon dioxide in 8 to 12 hours and 15% is eliminated unchanged in urine within six hours. About 90% of a dose is excreted in the urine within the first hour. The drug enters effusions and the cerebrospinal fluid. Assays for fluorouracil in plasma are available but are not used routinely in clinical practice.

DOSAGE AND PREPARATIONS.

Intravenous: Various regimens have been used. In one, a loading dose of 400 to 500 mg/M^2 (12 mg/kg) is given once daily for four successive days (maximum single daily dose, 800 mg); if no toxicity is observed, this is followed by 200 to 250 mg/M^2 (6 mg/kg) on days 6, 8, 10, and 12. Some investigators repeat the loading dose regimen every four to five weeks. The manufacturers recommend that the dose be reduced by 50% in poor-risk patients or those with inadequate nutrition.

With continuous infusion, 750 mg to 1.1 g/M^2 is administered daily for five days if toxicity is acceptable and the course is repeated every three to four weeks. Dosage adjustments must be made if hematologic or gastrointestinal side effects develop.

Intra-arterial (Hepatic): 750 mg to 1.1 g/M^2/day for 14 to 21 days by continuous infusion.

Intraperitoneal: A 5 mM solution is instilled for 32 to 120 hours.

Adrucil (Adria), ***Generic.*** Solution 50 mg/ml in 10, 50, and 100 ml containers.

FLOXURIDINE
[FUDR]

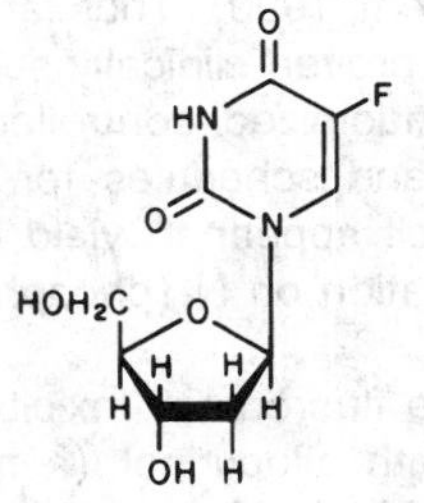

ACTIONS AND USES. Rationale for the use of floxuridine, the deoxyriboside derivative of fluorouracil, is based on its distinctive metabolism, which depends on the mode and rate of administration. Following intravenous or rapid intra-arterial injection, floxuridine is rapidly metabolized to fluorouracil and has the same efficacy and adverse effects. However, when floxuridine is given by slow, continuous, intra-arterial infusion, it is converted by thymidine kinase to the active agent, floxuridine monophosphate (FdUMP), which inhibits thymidylate synthase and thus blocks DNA synthesis. With this method of administration, the dose can be reduced because floxuridine is pharmacologically more active than with bolus injection. Floxuridine administered by slow intra-arterial infusion has less effect on RNA than intravenous fluorouracil.

Although intra-arterial floxuridine has been used for palliation in certain malignancies (eg, carcinoma of the rectum, colon, and gastrointestinal tract), it does not appear to offer any advantages over intravenous fluorouracil. Furthermore, no controlled study has shown superior results with intra-arterial administration, which is both more hazardous and more expensive than intravenous fluorouracil. The sole exception is the use of floxuridine to treat hepatic metastases of gastrointestinal adenocarcinomas by infusion into the hepatic artery. This approach to regional therapy appears to improve the response in the liver metastases but not in the primary tumors. When administered into the hepatic artery, the drug is metabolized immediately by the liver, with 95% removed on the first pass.

ADVERSE REACTIONS AND PRECAUTIONS. Local adverse reactions (eg, mucositis, localized erythema) are more prominent than systemic reactions after intra-arterial injection. Severe, possibly fatal sclerosing cholangitis and/or hepatitis has been observed after hepatic artery infusion, and this method should be used cautiously in patients with hepatic dysfunction.

Systemic reactions are similar to those seen with fluorouracil. The most common are nausea, vomiting, diarrhea, stomatitis, and enteritis. Other adverse effects include anorexia, cramps, duodenal ulcer, gastritis, glossitis, pharyngitis, and dermatologic reactions (alopecia, dermatitis, pruritus, rash, ulceration). Anemia and leukopenia also occur. Elevated alkaline phosphatase, serum transaminase, serum bilirubin, and lactic dehydrogenase values have been noted. Acute and delayed central nervous system toxicity is manifested by ataxia, blurred vision, depression, nystagmus, vertigo, and lethargy. Complications of regional arterial infusion (eg, arterial aneurysm; ischemia and thrombosis; bleeding, leaking, and infection at the catheter site; thrombophlebitis) may occur.

Because of its toxicity and low therapeutic index, floxuridine should be given under the supervision of a physician experienced in both cancer chemotherapy and the intra-hepatic artery infusion technique. Ambulatory patients should be hospitalized for installation of the arterial catheter and attachment to the infusion pump during the first course of treatment, and they should be informed about possible toxic manifestations. White blood cell and platelet counts should be performed regularly.

As with fluorouracil, floxuridine should be discontinued immediately when any of the following signs and symptoms appear: stomatitis, esophagopharyngitis, gastrointestinal ulceration and bleeding, diarrhea (five or more loose stools daily), intractable vomiting, leukocyte count less than 3,500/microliter or a rapidly decreasing count, thrombocytopenia with a platelet count less than 100,000/microliter, or hemorrhage from any site. Use of floxuridine is hazardous in patients with poor nutritional status or bone marrow depression, and it should be avoided in pregnant women, particularly during the first trimester, because of its potential teratogenicity.

DOSAGE AND PREPARATIONS.

Intra-arterial: The specialized nature of this technique requires the combined skills of a surgeon and oncologist. *Adults,* with the patient under general anesthesia, the catheter is inserted into the artery supplying the tumor and sutured to the vessel wall. An infusion pump is used to administer 5 to 20 mg/M^2/24 hr continuously for 14 to 21 days. Infusion is continued until a local toxic reaction (eg, cutaneous erythema, mucositis) or systemic toxicity is noted. The infusion is stopped until the reaction subsides; additional courses then are given for as long as the response continues. Newer regimens rely on the use of implantable infusion pumps (eg, Infusaid), which are now routinely employed for intra-hepatic artery infusions. The most frequently used regimen utilizes a dose of 0.3 mg/kg/day for 14 days, followed by a 14-day drug-free interval. Adequate courses of therapy have varied from one month to several years.

FUDR (Roche), ***Generic***. Powder (sterile) 500 mg.

AZACITIDINE (5-Azacytidine; Ladakamycin) (Investigational drug)

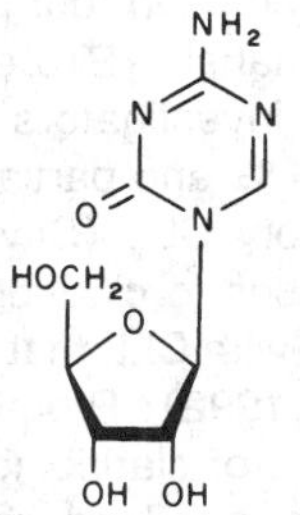

ACTIONS AND USES. This antimetabolite, an analogue of cytidine, is rapidly phosphorylated and incorporated into both RNA and DNA. The substituted pyrimidine ring is chemically unstable and decomposes both before and after its incorporation. The major cytotoxic action of azacitidine appears to be mediated through faulty RNA processing and function after incorporation and decomposition (Chabner, 1990). By disrupting the translation of nucleic acid sequences into protein, protein synthesis is inhibited. Moreover, azacitidine affects de novo pyrimidine synthesis by inhibiting orotidylic acid decarboxylase and also inhibits DNA methylation. It is cell cycle specific for the S phase.

The major indication for azacitidine is acute myelogenous leukemia refractory to conventional therapy. This drug has not shown significant clinical activity against solid tumors.

ADVERSE REACTIONS AND PRECAUTIONS. Dose-limiting toxicity is usually hematologic and is manifested by leukopenia, thrombocytopenia, and anemia. Nausea and vomiting are common and may be severe and prolonged. Symptoms are ameliorated by prolonged or continuous infusion. Antiemetics appear to be most helpful if taken 24 to 48 hours before therapy is begun. Other toxic effects are diarrhea, neuromuscular disturbances, fever, hepatotoxicity, hypotension, and skin rash. Azacitidine has mutagenic and teratogenic effects, decreases male fertility, and is immunosuppressive in various rodent species.

PHARMACOKINETICS. Azacitidine is well absorbed after subcutaneous administration, and the volume of distribution is approximately equal to total body water. There is little or no binding to plasma proteins. Less than 2% of the dose remains as unchanged drug 30 minutes after bolus intravenous administration, but the half-life for metabolites is about 3.5 hours. The parent drug enters cells by means of facilitated nucleoside transport system. Azacitidine is metabolized rapidly, initially by deamination; 70% to 90% of a dose is recovered in urine within 24 hours.

DOSAGE (investigational regimen).

Intravenous: 150 to 400 mg/M^2 daily given by intravenous bolus or by continuous infusion for five days. Preparations must be formulated every three to four hours because the drug is unstable in aqueous solutions.

TEGAFUR (Ftorafur) (Investigational drug)

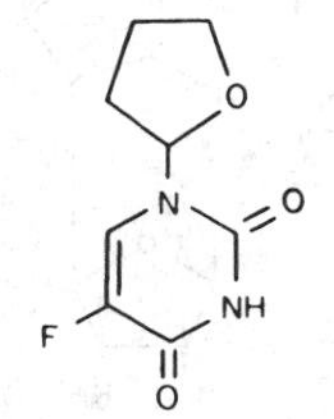

ACTIONS. This furan nucleoside prodrug appears to be converted slowly to fluorouracil in vivo by two different pathways (Grem, 1990). Thus, it probably acts as an inhibitor of thymidylate synthase and is incorporated into nucleic acids.

USES. The clinical and experimental antitumor activity of tegafur is similar to that of fluorouracil; greatest activity is seen in gastric, colorectal, and breast carcinoma. The drug appears to offer no therapeutic advantages over fluorouracil but has a number of toxicologic disadvantages.

ADVERSE REACTIONS AND PRECAUTIONS. The dose-limiting toxicity of tegafur is different from that of fluorouracil. The drug is minimally myelosuppressive. However, it produces considerable diarrhea, cramps, vomiting, and mucositis, which is most often dose limiting. Also, it is more neurotoxic than fluorouracil. Common manifestations are altered mental status and cerebellar ataxia. These differences in spectrums of toxicities can probably be explained by the slow release of fluorouracil from tegafur, which mimics infusion of fluorouracil.

PHARMACOKINETICS. Tegafur is reliably absorbed after oral administration but is more frequently given by the intravenous route in this country. The parent compound has a prolonged plasma half-life of 6 to 16 hours and is eliminated by conversion to hydroxylated metabolites. Tegafur readily penetrates into the central nervous system.

DOSAGE (investigational regimen).

Intravenous: 1.5 to 2.25 g/M^2 daily for five days or 4 g/M^2/week.

PURINE ANALOGUES

Those purine analogues that have long-established roles in cancer chemotherapy (mercaptopurine and thioguanine) are used as free bases and require metabolic activation to nucleotides for cytotoxic efficacy. The activated analogues of these purines have multiple effects on cells, which are mediated through allosteric regulatory sites on enzymes of de novo purine biosynthesis as well as by incorporation into nucleic acids. The more recently developed drugs (cladribine, fludarabine phosphate, and pentostatin) and the investigational agent, tiazofurin, are used either as nucleosides or as nucleotides with actions that markedly differ from those of mercaptopurine and thioguanine.

CLADRIBINE (2-Chlorodeoxyadenosine, CldA)
[Leustatin]

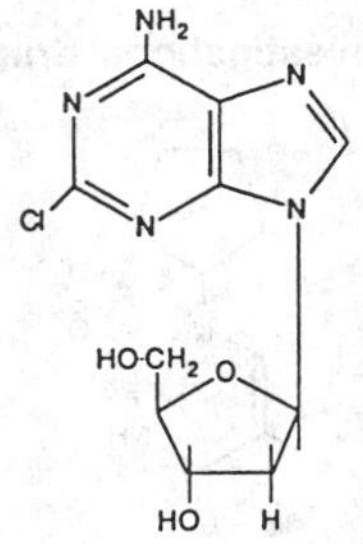

ACTIONS. This analogue of deoxyadenosine was developed as an attempt to mimic metabolic responses to inhibitors of adenosine deaminase (Riscoe et al, 1989). Deficiency of this purine salvage enzyme is the primary genetic defect in some patients with severe combined immunodeficiency. The presence of elevated levels of deoxyadenosine triphosphate in lymphocytes as a result of adenosine deaminase deficiency is thought to impair their function; lymphoid cells appear to be particularly sensitive to this toxic effect. However, the mechanism of action of cladribine has not been determined definitively. This drug is phosphorylated by deoxycytidine kinase and accumulates as a triphosphate that can be incorporated into DNA. In addition, nicotinamide adenine dinucleotide is depleted and adenosine triphosphate levels decrease in cells treated with cladribine. Unlike many other adenosine and deoxyadenosine analogues, it is not inactivated by adenosine deaminase and does not inhibit this enzyme. Low nanomolar concentrations are cytocidal to both proliferating and quiescent cells (Seto et al, 1985).

USES. Cladribine is indicated as therapy for hairy cell leukemia (HCL). Allopurinol usually is administered concomitantly to prevent tumor lysis syndrome (hyperuricemia). In an initial study, 11 of 12 patients with HCL who were given a single course of therapy (0.1 mg/kg/day for seven days by continuous intravenous infusion) had complete remissions (median duration, 15.5 months) (Piro et al, 1990). Subsequently, three single-center studies in larger groups of patients confirmed the promising results reported in this pilot study. Complete remissions occurred in 36 of 46 patients with HCL who received one course of cladribine (4 mg/M^2/day for seven days by continuous infusion) (Estey et al, 1992). Partial remissions were observed in an additional five patients. Similarly, approximately 80% of 86 patients with HCL who were followed for at least six months obtained complete remissions in response to cladribine (0.1 mg/kg/day for seven days by continuous infusion), and partial remissions occurred in most of the remaining 20% (Saven and Piro, 1992). The final study used the identical treatment regimen, and complete remissions were observed in 16 of 20 evaluable patients and partial remissions in the remaining four (Tallman et al, 1992).

The effects of cladribine on survival of patients with HCL cannot be assessed at present, since the duration of patient follow-up has not been sufficient and randomized, placebo-controlled trials have not been performed. Nevertheless, cladribine is considered by many clinicians to be the therapy of choice for patients with symptomatic HCL, whether or not they have been treated previously with other therapies (Beutler, 1992).

Responses to cladribine also have been reported in patients with other malignancies. In a pilot study in patients with previously treated chronic lymphocytic leukemia (CLL), partial responses were observed in four patients and clinical improvement in an additional six (Piro et al, 1988). In a larger group of patients, these investigators reported that complete remissions occurred in 4% and partial remissions in 40% of 90 patients with refractory CLL (Saven et al, 1991). Complete and partial responses to cladribine also have been observed in a few patients with CLL that was resistant to fludarabine (Juliusson et al, 1992). Promising results also were reported in single studies of cladribine in patients with previously treated low-grade non-Hodgkin's lymphomas (eight complete and nine partial responses in 40 evaluable patients) (Kay et al, 1992), therapy-resistant cutaneous T-cell lymphoma (three complete and four partial responses in 15 evaluable patients) (Saven et al, 1992), and relapsed acute myeloid leukemia (eight complete and two partial responses in 17 patients) (Santana et al, 1992).

Current recommendations suggest that use of cladribine as therapy for CLL, low-grade non-Hodgkin's lymphomas, or cutaneous T-cell lymphoma be reserved for those patients whose malignancies are resistant to other therapies (Beutler, 1992). Comparative studies are needed to evaluate the role of cladribine as first-line therapy for these tumors and to optimize its use in combination regimens.

ADVERSE REACTIONS. The most serious adverse reaction to continuous intravenous infusion of cladribine at the dosage recommended for patients with HCL (0.1 mg/kg or 4 mg/M^2 daily for seven days) is bone marrow suppression and its consequences. Serious bleeding episodes as a result of thrombocytopenia did not occur in any of the patients treated with this regimen, but several received prophylactic platelet transfusions to lessen thrombocytopenia. No clinically significant nausea, vomiting, or hair loss occurred at these doses. Patients who received larger doses ($>$0.26 mg/kg/day for 10 to 14 days as part of preparative regimens prior to bone marrow transplantation) experienced neurologic complications (paraparesis/quadraparesis; progressive irreversible motor weakness) and renal dysfunction that, in some patients, required hemodialysis (Beutler, 1992).

Febrile episodes were observed in more than 70% of patients treated with cladribine for HCL. In most cases, the onset of fever occurred between days five and seven of treatment and was not usually due to infection. Although myelosuppression and infection are the most common adverse reactions in patients treated with cladribine for other malignancies, fever occurs less frequently in these patients than in those treated for HCL.

Little information is available regarding the use of cladribine in patients with impaired liver or kidney function. In view of the renal toxicity observed in bone marrow transplant recipients who received the highest doses of this drug, it should be used with caution in patients with baseline renal impairment.

Cladribine is classified in FDA Pregnancy Category D.

PHARMACOKINETICS. The pharmacokinetics of cladribine have been studied in 12 patients who received intravenous infusions of 0.14 mg/kg for 2 and 24 hours (Liliemark and Juliusson, 1991). Analysis of the decline in plasma concentrations after the two-hour infusions using a two-compartment model yielded half-lives of 35 ± 12 minutes for the initial (distribution) phase and 6.7 ± 2.5 hours for the terminal (elimination) phase. The peak concentration of cladribine achieved with the two-hour infusions was 198 ± 87 nmol/L, and the steady-state concentration during the 24-hour infusions was 22.5 ± 11 nmol/L. The areas under the time versus concentration curves for the 2- and 24-hour infusions were nearly identical (552 ± 258 and 588 ± 185 nmol/L/hour, respectively). The mean volume of distribution at steady state was 9.2 ± 5.4 L/kg.

The bioavailability and pharmacokinetics of cladribine have also been investigated after subcutaneous and oral administration (Liliemark et al, 1992). Bioavailability after oral administration was 34% ± 22% in an acid-resistant capsule and 48% ± 8% in an oral solution in phosphate-buffered saline. In contrast, the bioavailability after subcutaneous injection was 102% ± 28%. However, no studies have compared these routes of administration with infusion to assess clinical responses to cladribine.

DOSAGE AND PREPARATIONS. The maximum tolerated single dose has not been determined in *adults* with hematologic disease. In *children* with acute leukemia, 8.9 mg/M^2/day as a continuous infusion was reported to be the maximally tolerated dose (Santana et al, 1991).

Intravenous: For HCL in *adults*, a single course of 0.1 mg/kg or 4 mg/M^2 daily for seven days by continuous infusion. Data are insufficient to determine if a second course of this regimen is necessary or useful; however, if relapse occurs after remission is induced by cladribine, a second course may be given.

For patients with CLL, low-grade non-Hodgkin's lymphoma, or cutaneous T-cell lymphoma resistant to other therapies, the same dose as for HCL may be administered for one week each month until a maximal response is achieved or until persistent thrombocytopenia occurs.

Leustatin (Ortho Biotech). Solution (for injection, preservative-free) 1 mg/ml in 0.9% sodium chloride in 20 ml vials containing 10 ml of solution. Store refrigerated at 2° to 8° C. If solution becomes frozen, thaw at room temperature or in refrigerator; do not heat or microwave. Redissolve any precipitated ingredients by shaking and do not refreeze.

FLUDARABINE PHOSPHATE (2 Fluoro-ara-AMP)

[Fludara]

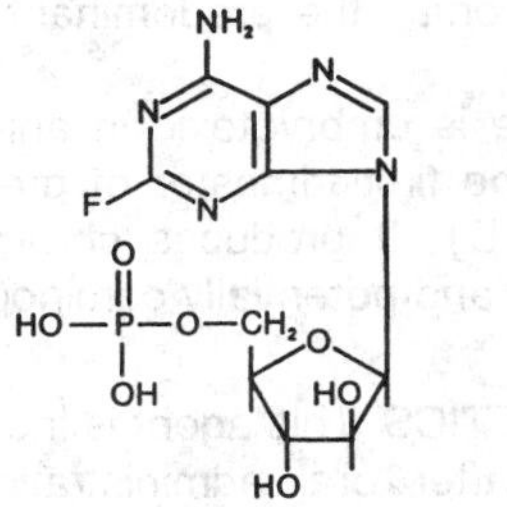

ACTIONS. Fludarabine phosphate is the 2-fluoro, 5′-phosphate derivative of 9-β-D-arabinofuranosyladenine (Ara-A) (Leyland-Jones et al, 1990). Unlike Ara-A, it is resistant to deamination by adenosine deaminase. The phosphate is used because the nucleoside is poorly soluble. Its metabolite, 2-fluoro-ara-ATP, is generated intracellularly (after rapid hydrolysis of the phosphate in the circulation and carrier-mediated transport of fludarabine) in a sequence of reactions that begins with the step catalyzed by deoxycytidine kinase (Chun et al, 1991). The active metabolite competes with deoxyadenosine triphosphate for incorporation into DNA and terminates DNA strand elongation when it is incorporated (Plunkett et al, 1990). It also inhibits ribonucleotide reductase.

USES. Fludarabine phosphate is indicated for patients with refractory B cell chronic lymphocytic leukemia (CLL). Standard regimens for B cell CLL most often combine an alkylating agent with a corticosteroid. In uncontrolled studies in patients with CLL who had not responded to, or whose disease had progressed during treatment with, such regimens, overall objective response rates after use of fludarabine phosphate ranged from 32% to 57% (13% complete responses) (Keating et al, 1989; Keating, 1990; Chun et al, 1991). In an additional uncontrolled study, the total response rate in previously untreated patients with CLL was 79% (Keating et al, 1991). This included complete remissions in 33%, clinically complete remissions (with nodular residual disease) in 39%, and partial remissions in 6% of the patients. Finally, a study of fludarabine phosphate combined with prednisone in patients with CLL reported complete responses in 12%, nodular complete responses in 30%, and partial responses in 18% of the patients (Robertson et al, 1992). No data have been published regarding the effect of fludarabine phosphate therapy on survival of patients with CLL or comparing fludarabine phosphate to other therapies for CLL in randomized, controlled trials.

Data from uncontrolled Phase II studies suggest that fludarabine phosphate also may have significant activity in low-grade (indolent) non-Hodgkin's lymphoma (Hochster and Cassileth, 1990; Hochster et al, 1992; Redman et al, 1992). Limited data suggest fludarabine phosphate also may be useful in patients with hairy cell (Kantarjian et al, 1991 A; Kraut and Chun, 1991) or prolymphocytic (Kantarjian et al, 1991 B) leukemia. This drug does not appear to be useful in treating patients with most common solid tumors (Chun et al, 1991).

ADVERSE REACTIONS AND PRECAUTIONS. At the lower doses currently used for CLL, myelosuppression is dose limiting; leukopenia is most pronounced. Mild neurotoxic effects (eg, lethargy, drowsiness) are common. Nausea and vomiting, stomatitis, renal insufficiency, pulmonary dysfunction, and tumor lysis syndrome also have been noted. With large doses (used for acute leukemia in some early trials but not used presently for CLL), more severe neurotoxicity was observed and was associated with demyelination of nerves.

Fludarabine phosphate is classified in FDA Pregnancy Category D.

PHARMACOKINETICS. Fludarabine phosphate is metabolized rapidly to 2-fluoro-ara-A. The metabolite has a triexponential decay curve with half-lives of 5.42 minutes, 1.4 hours, and 10.2 hours. Total body clearance appears to be related to creatinine clearance.

DOSAGE AND PREPARATIONS.

Intravenous: For chronic lymphocytic leukemia, 25 to 30 mg/M^2/day as a 30-minute infusion administered for five days every four weeks. The manufacturer recommends that three additional cycles of fludarabine phosphate therapy be given to CLL patients after a maximal response is achieved and that the drug then should be discontinued.

In studies in patients with non-Hodgkin's lymphoma and other lymphoid malignancies, 18 to 30 mg/M^2 was administered daily (as a 30-minute infusion) for five days every four weeks.

Fludara (Berlex). Powder (lyophilized) 50 mg, with 50 mg mannitol and sodium hydroxide to adjust pH to 7.7, in 6 ml vials. Reconstitute by dissolving in 2 ml of sterile water for injection. For infusion, this solution may be diluted further in 100 to 125 ml of 5% dextrose injection or 0.9% sodium chloride. The reconstituted product must be used within eight hours.

MERCAPTOPURINE
[Purinethol]

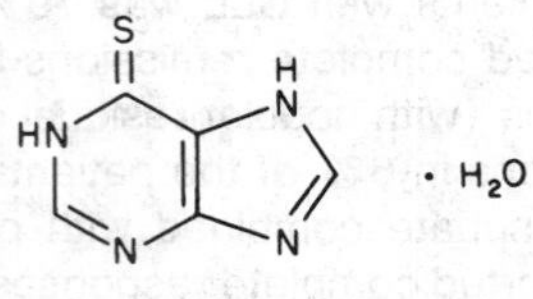

S
HN H
N
N N
· H_2O

ACTIONS. Mercaptopurine, the 6-thio analogue of hypoxanthine, is a prodrug that must be converted to 6-mercaptopurine-ribose-phosphate (6-MPRP) intracellularly by hypoxanthine-guanine phosphoribosyl transferase (HGPRT) (Riscoe et al, 1989; McCormack and Johns, 1990). This has been termed lethal synthesis. 6-MPRP interferes with purine biosynthesis both by feedback inhibition of the first step (phosphoribosylpyrophosphate amidotransferase) in purine biosynthesis and by blocking the conversion of inosinic acid to adenylic acid or guanylic acid. Triphosphorylated nucleotide metabolites are incorporated into DNA, and this may also contribute to the cytotoxic effects of the drug. A small fraction of the mercaptopurine ribonucleotides present in cells also may be converted to thioguanine ribonucleotides and then used for RNA synthesis. However, this mechanism appears to contribute little to the antitumor efficacy of mercaptopurine. Metabolites of the drug also may inhibit RNA synthesis.

Mercaptopurine is cell cycle specific for the S phase but is self-limiting. Biochemical resistance can result from absence of the activating enzyme (HGPRT) or by increased concentration of a degrading enzyme, a membrane-bound alkaline phosphatase. Patients resistant to mercaptopurine are almost always cross-resistant to thioguanine.

USES. When used alone, mercaptopurine induces complete remission in approximately 25% of children and 10% of adults with acute lymphocytic leukemia. However, much better results are obtained with combination regimens (see index entry Cancer: Clinical Response to Chemotherapeutic Drugs). The major role of mercaptopurine in acute lymphocytic leukemia is in maintenance therapy, most often in combination with methotrexate (Wiernik, 1989; Donohue and Charlton, 1989). When administered after a prednisone/vincristine-induced remission, the incidence of prolonged complete bone marrow remissions approaches 80% in children.

Mercaptopurine is marginally effective in acute myelogenous leukemia in adults; complete remissions of short duration occur in less than 20% of patients. It is not a primary drug to induce remission in this type of leukemia. Although mercaptopurine is employed as maintenance therapy for this disease, thioguanine is used more frequently. In the early phase of chronic myelogenous leukemia, mercaptopurine controls the disease in 30% to 50% of adults. It is used as a second-line drug for chronic myelocytic leukemia, particularly in the acute blastic phase.

This drug also is administered as an immunosuppressant in the treatment of inflammatory bowel disease, although a related drug, azathioprine, is preferred (see index entry Mercaptopurine, In Inflammatory Bowel Disease).

ADVERSE REACTIONS AND PRECAUTIONS. The usual dose-limiting toxicity of mercaptopurine is bone marrow depression, including leukopenia, thrombocytopenia, and anemia. It is usually gradual in onset and may persist for several days after cessation of administration. Myelosuppression can be delayed and leukocyte counts should be performed weekly; mercaptopurine should be discontinued if an abnormal reduction occurs. The leukocyte count is used to establish a maintenance dose.

Anorexia, nausea, and vomiting occur in about 30% of adult patients and are usually mild. Gastrointestinal toxicity occurs less frequently in children treated with mercaptopurine. Oral and gastrointestinal ulcerations are much less common than with methotrexate and fluorouracil. Hepatic dysfunction has been observed in a number of adults treated with mercaptopurine; it is less common in children. Cholestatic jaundice is most prominent but is usually reversible on cessation of therapy. Large doses of the drug can cause hepatic necrosis. Smaller doses are recommended in patients with impaired hepatic or renal function to avoid accumulation. Use of mercaptopurine with other hepatotoxic agents should be avoided if possible. Close monitoring of liver function indices is mandatory when mercaptopurine is administered with other hepatotoxic agents.

Since mercaptopurine is metabolized by xanthine oxidase to 6-thiouric acid, the dose should be reduced to one-quarter to one-third of the usual amount if allopurinol, a xanthine oxidase inhibitor, is used concomitantly for hyperuricemia. In the presence of allopurinol, 6-thioxanthine, an intermediate oxidation product, becomes the predominant metabolite eliminated.

Mercaptopurine is embryotoxic in animals and should be avoided during the first trimester of pregnancy (FDA Pregnancy Category D). It produces chromosomal aberrations and is mutagenic and potentially carcinogenic and teratogenic.

PHARMACOKINETICS. This agent is incompletely and erratically absorbed after oral administration. Despite its low

(<20%) and variable bioavailability, mercaptopurine usually is administered orally for maintenance therapy in acute lymphoblastic leukemia. A parenteral formulation is available from the National Cancer Institute for investigational use. Peak plasma concentrations are attained in two hours; after eight hours, no drug is detectable. Mercaptopurine and its active nucleotide are metabolized extensively to a number of inactive products in the liver; 50% of the drug and its metabolites are excreted in the urine in 24 hours. Mercaptopurine is about 30% bound (loosely) to plasma proteins. Although it is widely distributed in body tissues, only a small percentage enters the cerebrospinal fluid after usual doses.

DOSAGE AND PREPARATIONS. The dosage varies from patient to patient, and titration is necessary to obtain maximum effectiveness with acceptable toxicity. The following dosages are frequently employed; modifications may be necessary when mercaptopurine is combined with other cytotoxic drugs. ***Oral:*** For induction of remission, *adults and children over 5 years,* 75 to 100 mg/M^2 daily. If improvement does not occur and leukocytes are not depressed within four weeks, the dose may be increased cautiously to a maximum of 200 mg/M^2 daily. The total daily dose may be given at one time and is calculated to the closest multiple of 25 mg. Alternatively, 500 to 700 mg/M^2/day is given for five days in combination with other drugs.

For maintenance therapy in *children* with acute lymphocytic leukemia in remission, 50 mg/M^2 daily as a single dose, usually in combination with other drugs (most frequently with methotrexate). Administration may be continued for a prolonged period.

Therapy should be discontinued at the first sign of a profound or rapid reduction in the leukocyte or platelet count; it may be reinstituted at one-half the previous dosage after toxic manifestations disappear.

Purinethol (Burroughs Wellcome). Tablets 50 mg.

PENTOSTATIN (2′ Deoxycoformycin)
[Nipent]

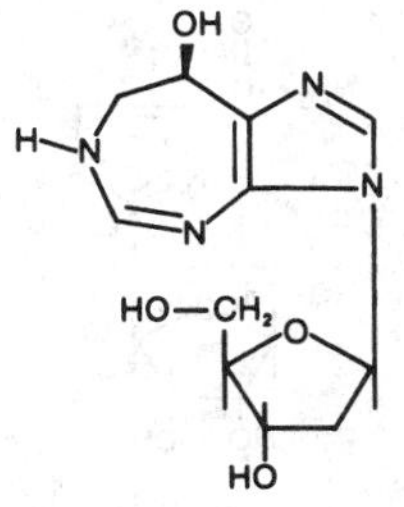

ACTIONS. Pentostatin is a potent inhibitor of adenosine deaminase that binds tightly to the enzyme (McCormack and Johns, 1990). Inhibition of adenosine deaminase leads to an accumulation of deoxyadenosine triphosphate (dATP), which then inhibits ribonucleotide reductase, resulting in decreased DNA synthesis and cell proliferation. Lymphoid cells are particularly sensitive to the cytocidal effects of this drug.

USES. Pentostatin is indicated as therapy for hairy cell leukemia in adults whose disease is refractory to treatment with interferon alfa-2a or 2b (defined as progression after three months of treatment or no response after six months of treatment). Cumulative data from a number of studies demonstrated very high rates of complete (58%) and overall (86%, complete plus partial) responses to pentostatin (Ho et al, 1989; Kraut et al, 1989; Blick et al, 1990; Dutcher et al, 1990; Cassileth et al, 1991). The duration of response ranged from 1.3 to 35 months, with medians of 7.7 and 15.2 months in the two largest studies.

Data from several small Phase II studies suggest that pentostatin also may be active as therapy for various B cell malignancies (eg, chronic lymphocytic leukemia) (Dearden and Catovsky, 1990; Ho et al, 1990), multiple myeloma (Grever et al, 1990), and cutaneous T-cell lymphoma and some T-cell leukemias (Dearden et al, 1991; Cummings et al, 1991). However, more definitive data are needed to determine the role of pentostatin in treating these malignancies.

ADVERSE REACTIONS AND PRECAUTIONS. Pentostatin toxicity has included myelosuppression (lymphopenia may be pronounced), conjunctivitis, and panserositis. Central nervous system side effects are common and range from lethargy to coma. Renal toxicity includes hyperuricemia; pulmonary toxicity has also developed. Immune suppression with reactivation of herpes zoster infection is common.

Pentostatin is classified in FDA Pregnancy Category D.

DOSAGE AND PREPARATIONS.
Intravenous: For hairy cell leukemia, 4 mg/M^2 every two weeks by bolus injection or as a 20- to 30-minute infusion after dilution in a larger volume (25 to 50 ml) with 5% dextrose injection or 0.9% sodium chloride injection. The manufacturer recommends that patients be hydrated with 500 to 1,000 ml of 5% dextrose in 0.5 normal saline before, with an additional 500 ml given after, administration of pentostatin. For patients whose disease responds to pentostatin without accompanying major toxicity, therapy should continue until a complete response is achieved. Some clinicians recommend an additional two doses following the attainment of a complete response. If a complete or partial response is not observed after six months of treatment, pentostatin should be discontinued. In patients who achieve only a partial response, pentostatin should be discontinued after one year.

Nipent (Parke-Davis). Powder (lyophilized) 10 mg in single-use vials. Store refrigerated at 2° to 8° C. Reconstitute by dissolving in 5 ml of sterile water for injection. The reconstituted solution may be stored at room temperature and ambient light but should be used within eight hours.

THIOGUANINE
[Tabloid brand Thioguanine]

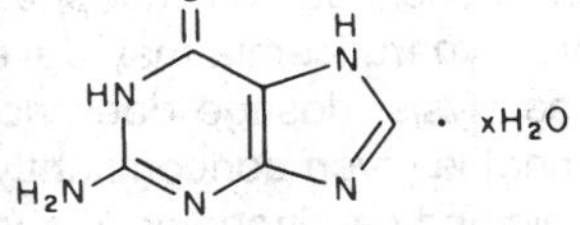

ACTIONS. Thioguanine, the 6-thio analogue of guanine, is a prodrug that is converted to 6-thioguanine-ribose-phosphate

(6-TGRP), an active metabolite, by the same pathway used by mercaptopurine (Riscoe et al, 1989; McCormack and Johns, 1990). 6-TGRP is a feedback inhibitor of the initial (amidotransferase) step in purine biosynthesis. This metabolite also blocks the conversions of inosinic acid to guanylic acid (GMP) and of GMP to GDP. Thioguanine also is converted to the deoxynucleoside triphosphate, which can be incorporated into tumor cell DNA. Although some investigators believe that this is the major mechanism of cytotoxicity, the relative importance of the various sites of action has not been determined. DNA strand breaks and DNA-protein cross-links accumulate in cells treated with thioguanine. Other mechanisms with uncertain relevance to this drug's antitumor efficacy are incorporation of thioguanine ribonucleotides into RNA, inhibition of messenger RNA biosynthesis, and reduced guanosine diphospho sugar levels resulting in deficient cell surface glycoprotein synthesis. The latter effect may be involved in the reported ability of the parent thiopurine to induce differentiation in human leukemic cells (Ishiguro et al, 1984). Thioguanine is cell cycle specific for the S phase. Tumor cells resistant to mercaptopurine usually exhibit cross resistance to thioguanine.

USES. Use of thioguanine is essentially confined to patients with acute leukemias (Wiernik, 1989; Donohue and Charlton, 1989). The combination of thioguanine and cytarabine induces complete responses in approximately 50% of adults with acute myelogenous leukemia. The rate is usually higher when cytarabine is combined with an anthracycline. Thioguanine is often employed as a third drug in these regimens, as well as in combination regimens for maintenance of remission. This drug also is active in the blast crisis of chronic myelogenous leukemia and in both induction and maintenance therapy for acute lymphocytic leukemia.

ADVERSE REACTIONS AND PRECAUTIONS. The usual dose-limiting toxicity of thioguanine is bone marrow depression resulting in leukopenia, thrombocytopenia, and anemia. Hemoglobin levels and white blood cell and platelet counts should be determined weekly or more frequently during remission induction therapy for acute leukemia. Thioguanine should be discontinued if leukocyte or platelet counts decrease suddenly. Therapy may be reinstituted when the cell counts return to normal levels.

Occasionally, nausea, vomiting, anorexia, and stomatitis may develop, especially if large doses are used. Gastrointestinal side effects are usually less severe with thioguanine than with mercaptopurine. Hepatic dysfunction, usually cholestatic jaundice, may occur although less often than with mercaptopurine. Lower doses may be required in patients with impaired hepatic or renal function. The combination of thioguanine with busulfan has been associated with esophageal varices and portal hypertension. Hyperuricemia may develop as a consequence of tumor cell lysis; dosage does not require adjustment when allopurinol is given concomitantly. Thioguanine is potentially mutagenic and carcinogenic. It should not be given during the first trimester of pregnancy because of its potential teratogenic effects (FDA Pregnancy Category D). It is also immunosuppressive.

PHARMACOKINETICS. Thioguanine is incompletely absorbed when given orally, averaging about 30% of an administered dose. Food intake reduces absorption. The elimination half-life of the parent drug is 1.5 hours, but peak plasma levels of metabolites are reached in six to eight hours. Between 24% and 46% is excreted in the urine as metabolites within 24 hours. A parenteral preparation is available for investigational use from the National Cancer Institute. This drug is cleared rapidly from plasma after intravenous administration; more than 80% of a dose is excreted within 24 hours. Although thioguanine crosses the blood-brain barrier in animals after use of large doses, very little enters the cerebrospinal fluid of humans after usual clinical doses are employed.

Thioguanine and its active metabolites are extensively inactivated in the liver, primarily by methylation; 6-methylthioguanine is a major metabolite. Thioguanine is not extensively deaminated, and only a small amount is converted to thiouric acid by xanthine oxidase. Thus, the dose of thioguanine does not require reduction in the presence of allopurinol.

DOSAGE AND PREPARATIONS. The dosage varies from patient to patient, and titration is necessary to obtain maximum effectiveness with acceptable toxicity. The following dosages are frequently employed.

Oral: *Adults and children,* 75 mg/M^2 daily. If there is no response after four weeks, the amount may be increased cautiously to 90 to 100 mg/M^2 daily. The total daily dose may be given at one time and is usually calculated to the closest multiple of 20 mg. If no clinical or laboratory evidence of improvement is observed, another class of drugs should be substituted.

For induction of remission in acute myelogenous leukemia, in combination with daunorubicin and cytarabine, *adults and children,* 100 mg/M^2 every 12 hours on days one through seven.

Tabloid brand Thioguanine (Burroughs Wellcome). Tablets 40 mg.

TIAZOFURIN (Riboxamide, TCAR) (Investigational drug)

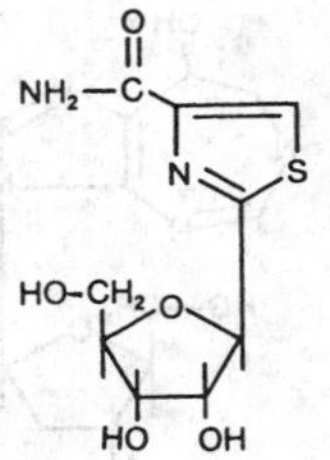

NH_2—C(=O)— [thiazole ring: N, S] ; HO–CH_2 [ribofuranose ring, O] ; HO OH

ACTIONS AND USES. Tiazofurin is converted to an analogue of nicotinamide adenine dinucleotide by a two-step sequence of enzymatic reactions (McCormack and Johns, 1990). This metabolite, thiazole-4-carboxamide adenine dinucleotide (TAD), is a powerful noncompetitive inhibitor of inosine monophosphate dehydrogenase, a critical enzyme in the production of guanine nucleotides. Observations of elevated levels of this enzyme in leukemic cells relative to normal leukocytes led to development of enzyme inhibitors, such as tiazofurin, as potential anticancer and antiviral drugs. Tiazofurin is cytocidal to cultured human and rodent tumor cells at much lower concentrations than are needed for equivalent toxicity to normal human leukocytes. Since TAD can be inactivated by a phosphodiesterase, the balance between synthesis and degradation of this active metabolite contributes to cellular drug sensitivity. Although an animal model of lung cancer was very sensitive to tiazofurin, results of clinical trials in a variety of solid human tumors have been disappointing. However, effects in patients with leukemia have been more promising. Of 13 patients treated with tiazofurin, five achieved complete remissions and three achieved partial remissions in a Phase II trial (Tricot et al, 1989).

ADVERSE REACTIONS AND PRECAUTIONS. The most common adverse reactions include neurotoxicity (most often headache or lethargy, but hemiparesis, weakness of the upper extremities, cortical blindness, seizures, and coma have been reported), nausea and vomiting, and muscle pain. Mild, transient myelosuppression (leukopenia and thrombocytopenia) also occurred but was not dose-limiting. Pleuropericarditis, conjunctivitis, desquamation of the hands and feet, and abnormalities in liver function also were observed in patients treated with tiazofurin. Hyperuricemia, a consequence of the drug's inhibition of inosine monophosphate dehydrogenase, may result in renal damage. Allopurinol is used to prevent this toxic effect and to reduce salvage of guanine (thus potentiating tiazofurin's cytocidal efficacy) by inhibiting hypoxanthine-guanine phosphoribosyl transferase through elevated plasma levels of hypoxanthine.

PHARMACOKINETICS. Tiazofurin is eliminated by the kidney in a biphasic pattern. The half-lives of the two phases are approximately 15 minutes for the first and four to eight hours for the terminal phase. Up to 90% of the drug is recovered in the urine.

DOSAGE (investigational regimen).

Intravenous: 1.65 g/M^2/day for five days every three weeks. In an alternative regimen, the dose was individualized after 2.2 g/M^2 was given initially to reduce concentrations of guanosine triphosphate in bone marrow and peripheral blood mononuclear cells to <20% of control levels (Tricot et al, 1989).

Tiazofurin (Parke-Davis).

RIBONUCLEOTIDE REDUCTASE INHIBITORS

Ribonucleotides, which are substrates for RNA synthesis but cannot be incorporated into DNA, are converted to deoxyribonucleotides as the diphosphates in a reaction catalyzed by the enzyme ribonucleotide reductase. The sole role of deoxyribonucleotides in cells is for DNA synthesis (replication and repair). Thus, inhibition of this enzyme is toxic in a somewhat selective manner to rapidly proliferating cells (Donehower, 1990). Ribonucleotide reductase inhibitors are S phase specific but are also self-limiting, for cells not already in the DNA synthetic phase are unable to progress much beyond initiation of replication. Since RNA and protein metabolism continue despite the inhibition of DNA synthesis, cells treated with these drugs undergo "unbalanced growth," which may contribute to the cytocidal and antineoplastic effects of these enzyme inhibitors.

HYDROXYUREA

[Hydrea]

$$\begin{matrix} NH_2 \\ | \\ C{=}O \\ | \\ NHOH \end{matrix}$$

ACTIONS. Hydroxyurea blocks DNA synthesis by inhibiting ribonucleoside diphosphate reductase (Donehower, 1990). Deoxyribonucleotide pools are depleted in cells treated with hydroxyurea; this leads to an accumulation of cells in very early S phase. The drug enters cells by passive diffusion and interacts with the enzyme's nonheme iron cofactor. Cytotoxicity from hydroxyurea in culture systems can be partially blocked by addition of ferrous iron and can be enhanced by simultaneous treatment with iron chelating agents. These observations have not yet resulted in clinically useful modulation of drug activity. Resistance to hydroxyurea has been observed, usually as a result of increased levels of ribonucleotide reductase in the resistant cells. Increased expression and translation, as well as gene amplification, may contribute to the increased enzyme activity.

USES. Hydroxyurea is most commonly employed in the palliative treatment of chronic myelogenous leukemia (CML), in which it prolongs the chronic phase of the disease and delays blastic transformation (Fialkow and Singer, 1989; Lichtman and Brennan, 1990; Donehower, 1990). Many physicians now consider hydroxyurea the preferred therapy for CML in order to avoid the increased risk of toxic reactions associated with busulfan. This drug also is used to treat some patients with other myeloproliferative diseases, such as polycythemia vera and the hypereosinophilic syndrome; in patients with the latter disease who are refractory to corticosteroids, hydroxyurea is the drug of choice.

Although responses to treatment with hydroxyurea have been reported in patients with some solid tumors (eg, melanoma; head and neck tumors; prostate, renal, and bladder carcinomas), this drug is seldom used for solid tumors, either alone or in combination chemotherapy. When used with radiation therapy, hydroxyurea can provide local control of primary squamous cell carcinoma of the head and neck. Hydroxyurea is also being investigated for use as a radiation sensitizer (eg, in cervical cancer), both as a result of its synchronizing effects (in S phase, a radiation-sensitive phase of the cell cycle) and of its indirect ability to inhibit repair of radiation-induced DNA damage by preventing synthesis of deoxyribonucleotides.

ADVERSE REACTIONS AND PRECAUTIONS. Myelosuppression (leukopenia, thrombocytopenia, anemia, megaloblastosis) is most prominent and is dose-limiting, but recovery is usually rapid when hydroxyurea is discontinued. The nadir in thrombocyte counts usually is delayed by seven to ten days after leukocyte counts begin to rise. Anorexia, nausea, and vomiting occur frequently but are seldom dose-limiting. Stomatitis is rare unless hydroxyurea is used with irradiation. Dermatologic reactions in patients taking hydroxyurea for prolonged periods (maculopapular rash, pruritus, alopecia) are mild and reversible. Less common are central nervous system disturbances (headache, dizziness, disorientation, hallucinations, convulsions). Impairment of renal function with hyperuricemia, uric acid calculi, and elevated BUN levels has been reported.

Blood, bone marrow, renal, and hepatic function should be evaluated prior to and at weekly intervals during therapy. Hydroxyurea should be discontinued if the white blood cell count falls below 2,500/microliter or the platelet count below 100,000/microliter. Administration may be resumed when blood counts return to satisfactory levels. Anemia can be corrected by blood transfusions without discontinuing therapy. Because hydroxyurea is excreted primarily by the kidneys, it must be used with caution in patients with impaired renal function. Since this drug has caused teratogenic effects in experimental animals, it should not be used in women of childbearing age.

PHARMACOKINETICS. Hydroxyurea is readily absorbed from the gastrointestinal tract after oral administration. Peak plasma levels are reached in about one hour; within 24 hours, the plasma concentration is essentially zero. The drug is eliminated primarily by the kidneys. However, recovery of drug in the urine varies widely (range, 10% to 95%).

DOSAGE AND PREPARATIONS.

Oral: 1 g/M^2 daily. Titration is often required. The dose should be decreased in patients with impaired marrow or renal function.

Hydrea (Immunex). Capsules 500 mg.

CARACEMIDE (Investigational drug)

$$CH_3{-}\overset{O}{\overset{\|}{C}}{-}N{-}\overset{O}{\overset{\|}{C}}{-}NH{-}CH_3$$
$$\quad | \\ O{-}\underset{O}{\underset{\|}{C}}{-}NH{-}CH_3$$

ACTIONS. Caracemide inhibits DNA, RNA, and protein synthesis. Its chemical name is N-acetyl-N(methylcarbamoyloxy)-N^1-methylurea. In vitro activity has been demonstrated against ribonucleotide reductase.

USES. Preclinical trials have demonstrated activity against both rodent and human tumors.

ADVERSE REACTIONS. The dose-limiting toxicity of caracemide appears to be central nervous system dysfunction, including agitation, cognitive deficits, depression, lethargy, confusion, and dementia. Electroencephalographic abnormalities appear to correlate with neurobehavioral changes. Mild nausea and vomiting have occurred. Myelosuppression has been observed.

DOSAGE (investigational regimen).

Intravenous: 650 mg/M^2 daily for five days (by continuous infusion) repeated every 21 days.

Caracemide (Marion Merrell Dow).

INVESTIGATIONAL ANTIMETABOLITES WITH NOVEL TARGETS

BUTHIONINE SULFOXIMINE (BSO) (Investigational drug)

$$CH_3(CH_2)_3\overset{O}{\overset{\|}{S}}\underset{NH}{\underset{\|}{}}CH_2CH_2\underset{NH_2}{\underset{|}{CH}}COOH$$

Buthionine sulfoximine is an inhibitor of the enzyme γ-glutamylcysteine synthetase, which catalyzes the initial step in de novo synthesis of glutathione (Leyland-Jones et al, 1990). Glutathione is thought to be involved in intracellular detoxification of and resistance to several DNA alkylating and cross-linking drugs, including melphalan and other nitrogen mustards (Arrick and Nathan, 1984; Kramer et al, 1988). Although it has no antitumor activity when administered alone, studies in cell culture systems and animal tumor models demonstrated that pretreatment with buthionine sulfoximine can potentiate the cytocidal efficacy of some DNA-damaging drugs. Data also suggest that tumor cells are sensitized to melphalan by buthionine sulfoximine to a greater extent than are normal cells.

A Phase I trial is in progress using buthionine sulfoximine for pretreatment followed by its combination with melphalan in patients with advanced refractory cancer. A preliminary report (Hamilton et al, 1990 B) indicated that glutathione levels in peripheral blood mononuclear cells declined after treatment with buthionine sulfoximine and returned to control levels within two days after drug administration ceased. In preclinical toxicology studies, species differences were observed in responses to very high doses of this drug (8 to 9.6 g/kg/day in ten or six fractional doses). In dogs, convulsions, emesis, diarrhea, and hyperactivity occurred. In mice, mild myelosuppression was the only adverse reaction. No toxic reactions to buthionine sulfoximine pretreatment were noted in patients given 1.5 g/M^2 every 12 hours for three days. However, severe neutropenia and/or thrombocytopenia and moderate to severe nausea and vomiting occurred when the same patients received a single dose of melphalan (15 mg/M^2) one hour after the next-to-last dose in a second three-day course of buthionine sulfoximine. Comparative trials of melphalan (and other DNA-damaging antitumor drugs) with and without buthionine sulfoximine are needed to determine whether increased toxicity and/or enhanced antitumor effects occur with the combination.

Polyamine Synthesis Inhibitors

Polyamines (putrescine, spermidine, and spermine) are involved in cell growth and division, and inhibition of their synthesis retards neoplastic growth (Sunkara et al, 1987). In addition, polyamines are known to bind to nucleic acids and may alter their structure or function as a consequence of these interactions (Marton and Morris, 1987). Thus, depletion of cellular polyamines after treatment with inhibitors of their synthesis may alter the efficacy of other antitumor drugs that bind to DNA (Porter and Jänne, 1987).

EFLORNITHINE HYDROCHLORIDE (Difluoromethylornithine, DFMO) (Investigational indication)

[Ornidyl]

$$H_2NCH_2CH_2CH_2-\underset{NH_2}{\overset{CHF_2}{C}}-COOH \cdot HCl \cdot H_2O$$

ACTIONS AND USES. Eflornithine irreversibly inhibits ornithine decarboxylase and thus inhibits polyamine biosynthesis in mammalian cells (Bey et al, 1987; Sunkara et al, 1987; Porter and Jänne, 1987).

In vitro studies utilizing rodent and human tumor cell lines have demonstrated cytostatic activity, and in vitro tests and studies in mice have demonstrated that this drug has activity against human cancer cell lines. To date, eflornithine has not been effective alone in clinical trials (Schechter et al, 1987). It appears, however, that it can potentiate the antitumor effects of nitrosoureas and interferon, as well as increase uptake of mitoguazone into cells.

For the use of eflornithine in the treatment of African trypanosomiasis and pneumocystis pneumonia, see index entry Eflornithine.

ADVERSE REACTIONS AND PRECAUTIONS. Myelosuppression is typically the dose-limiting side effect; thrombocytopenia may be pronounced. Nausea and vomiting are not significant. Anorexia and fatigue occur frequently. Diarrhea is common and often requires dose modification. Reversible ototoxicity has been observed.

PHARMACOKINETICS. Eflornithine has a plasma half-life of three to four hours after an oral dose.

DOSAGE (investigational regimen).

Oral: 2.25 g/M^2 daily in divided doses every six hours.

Ornidyl (Marion Merrell Dow).

MITOGUAZONE (Methylglyoxal Bis[guanylhydrazone], MGBG) (Investigational drug)

$$HN=C(NH_2)NHN=CHCMe=NNHC(NH_2)=NH$$

ACTIONS AND USES. Mitoguazone inhibits the synthesis of spermidine from putrescine by blocking S-adenosylmethionine decarboxylase (Pegg and Williams-Ashman, 1987). Spermidine reverses most of the toxic effects of mitoguazone.

Therapeutic responses have been observed in acute myelocytic leukemia and non-Hodgkin's lymphomas. The drug also has demonstrated activity in solid tumors. Attempts to increase the antitumor efficacy of mitoguazone by increasing its uptake through eflornithine pretreatment resulted in increased toxicity to normal tissues.

ADVERSE REACTIONS AND PRECAUTIONS. Side effects include mucositis, cutaneous lesions, phlebitis, ulceration after extravasation, alopecia, nausea and vomiting, delayed hypoglycemia, peripheral neuropathy, vasculitis, and hypotension after rapid infusion. Fatigue, malaise, and anorexia occur frequently.

PHARMACOKINETICS. There is a biphasic drug elimination. An initial rapid half-life is followed by prolonged terminal elimination. The compound is not extensively metabolized. Approximately 60% of an intravenous dose is excreted primarily as unchanged drug in the urine; less than 20% appears in the feces.

DOSAGE (investigational regimen).

Intravenous: 500 to 700 mg/M^2 every week.

Pyrimidine Synthesis Inhibitors

Compounds that inhibit enzymes in the de novo pathway for biosynthesis of pyrimidines are in various stages of development. Since these are not nucleosides and cannot be converted to nucleotides, they are not incorporated into nucleic acids as are the pyrimidine analogues discussed above. Treatment with these drugs leads to depletion of pyrimidine nucleotide and deoxynucleotide pools; consequently, both DNA and RNA synthesis are inhibited.

N-(PHOSPHONOACETYL)-L-ASPARTATE (PALA) (Investigational drug)

$$HO_2CCH_2\underset{CO_2H}{CH}NHCOCH_2PO_3H_2$$

ACTIONS AND USES. PALA inhibits aspartate carbamoyltransferase, the second enzyme in de novo pyrimidine biosynthesis (Grem et al, 1988; Leyland-Jones et al, 1990). In addition to depletion of pyrimidine nucleotide pools, deoxyguanosine triphosphate levels decline in response to this drug. Its effects on cultured cells and animal tumor models can be reversed by exogenous uridine.

Although PALA lacks significant antitumor activity when administered as a single agent, it is being investigated for use with other antimetabolites whose effects can be enhanced by the biochemical alterations induced in cells treated with PALA. PALA and fluorouracil have received the most attention for exploiting these potentially useful drug interactions. By inhibiting synthesis of endogenous pyrimidine nucleotides, both activation of fluorouracil and incorporation of the activated fluoropyrimidine into nucleic acids are enhanced. Results of more recent Phase II trials have suggested that the response to the combination may be improved compared with the response to fluorouracil alone. However, in many of the earlier trials, inappropriately reduced (and possibly inadequate) doses of fluorouracil were used in the patients given the combination to maximize the dose of PALA. Use of a lower dose of PALA and a larger dose of fluorouracil seems to improve response rates (Ardalan et al, 1988; O'Dwyer et al,

1990). The strategy of increasing activation and incorporation also applies to the combination of PALA with cytarabine. However, studies of these drugs combined with thymidine (to support continued DNA synthesis and incorporation of cytarabine triphosphate despite the inhibitory effects of PALA on de novo pyrimidine biosynthesis) have not progressed beyond Phase I studies.

ADVERSE REACTIONS. The dose-limiting toxicities for PALA when given alone were dermatitis, diarrhea, and mucositis; mild nausea and vomiting and infrequent myelosuppression also were reported. No adverse effects on renal or hepatic function were observed, but neurotoxicity (paresthesias or seizures) occurred rarely. Diarrhea and mucositis were also dose limiting in most of the trials that combined fluorouracil with PALA. The combination of PALA, cytarabine, and thymidine caused marrow aplasia in four of seven patients.

PHARMACOKINETICS. After intravenous administration, plasma decay curves are biphasic, with an initial half-life of 60 to 100 minutes and a terminal half-life of 5 to 13 hours. There is little or no metabolism of PALA, and elimination is predominantly via the kidneys. Between 65% and 85% of an administered dose appears as unchanged drug in the urine. The drug accumulates in bone but not in other tissues.

DOSAGE (investigational regimen).

Intravenous: 1.5 g/M^2 daily for five days every three weeks or 3.75 to 4.5 g/M^2 weekly or 2.5 g/M^2 for two days every two weeks given as a bolus or as a 30- to 60-minute infusion. In trials with fluorouracil (2.6 g/M^2 as a 24-hour infusion once weekly), the dose of PALA was 250 mg/M^2 given as a 15-minute infusion 24 hours before administration of fluorouracil.

PALA (U.S. Bioscience, Wyeth-Ayerst).

BREQUINAR SODIUM (DUP 785) (Investigational drug)

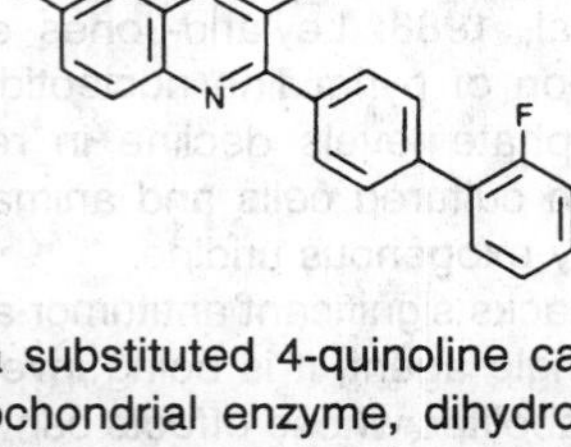

Brequinar is a substituted 4-quinoline carboxylic acid that inhibits the mitochondrial enzyme, dihydroorotic acid dehydrogenase, which is required for de novo pyrimidine biosynthesis (Chen et al, 1986). It has had broad activity against animal and human tumor cell lines and human tumor xenografts. Its activity is reversed by exogenous uridine. Thus far, only Phase I studies in humans have been completed (Bork et al, 1989). Both weekly and biweekly schedules were evaluated for toxicity, and the recommended doses for Phase II trials were 1.5 to 2 g/M^2 weekly or 500 to 750 mg/M^2 biweekly. Thrombocytopenia was the dose-limiting toxicity, but stomatitis/mucositis occurred frequently and dermatologic toxicity was also reported. All adverse reactions were reversible. Elimination of brequinar from the plasma occurred with a median terminal half-life of about 10 hours.

Brequinar Sodium (FMC Corporation).

Cited References

Ackland SP, Schilsky RL: High-dose methotrexate: A critical reappraisal. *J Clin Oncol* 5:2017-2031, 1987.

Allegra CJ: Antifolates, in Chabner BA, Collins JM (eds): *Cancer Chemotherapy: Principles and Practice*. Philadelphia, JB Lippincott, 1990, 110-153.

Andersson BS, et al: Fatal pulmonary failure complicating high-dose cytosine arabinoside therapy in acute leukemia. *Cancer* 65:1079-1084, 1990.

Ardalan B, et al: A randomized Phase I and II study of short-term infusion of high-dose fluorouracil with or without N-(phosphonacetyl)-L-aspartic acid in patients with advanced pancreatic and colorectal cancers. *J Clin Oncol* 6:1053-1058, 1988.

Arrick BA, Nathan CF: Glutathione metabolism as a determinant of therapeutic efficacy: A review. *Cancer Res* 44:4224-4232, 1984.

Bagshawe KD, et al: The role of low-dose methotrexate and folinic acid in gestational trophoblastic tumours (GTT). *Br J Obstet Gynaecol* 96:795-802, 1989.

Bertino JR: Folate antagonists: Toward improving the therapeutic index and development of new analogs. *J Clin Pharmacol* 30:291-295, 1990 A.

Bertino JR: Leucovorin rescue revisited. *J Clin Oncol* 8:193-195, 1990 B.

Beutler E: Cladribine (2-chlorodeoxyadenosine). *Lancet* 340:952-956, 1992.

Bey P, et al: Inhibition of basic amino acid decarboxylases involved in polyamine biosynthesis, in McCann PP, et al (eds): *Inhibition of Polyamine Metabolism: Biological Significance and Basis for New Therapies*. Orlando, Academic Press, 1987, 1-32.

Blick M, et al: Durable complete remissions after 2′-deoxycoformycin treatment in patients with hairy cell leukemia resistant to interferon alpha. *Am J Hematol* 33:205-209, 1990.

Bonadonna G: Conceptual and practical advances in the management of breast cancer. *J Clin Oncol* 7:1380-1397, 1989.

Bork E, et al: A Phase I clinical and pharmacokinetic study of brequinar sodium, DUP 785 (BSC 368390), using a weekly and a biweekly schedule. *Eur J Cancer Clin Oncol* 25:1403-1411, 1989.

Browman GP, et al: Modulation of the antitumor effect of methotrexate by low-dose leucovorin in squamous cell head and neck cancer: A randomized placebo-controlled clinical trial. *J Clin Oncol* 8:203-208, 1990.

Buechner T, Hiddemann W: Treatment strategies in acute myeloid leukemia (AML): A. First-line chemotherapy. *Blut* 60:61-67, 1990.

Cassileth PA, et al: Pentostatin induces durable remissions in hairy cell leukemia. *J Clin Oncol* 9:243-246, 1991.

Chabner BA: Cytidine analogues, in Chabner BA, Collins JM (eds): *Cancer Chemotherapy: Principles and Practice.* Philadelphia, JB Lippincott, 1990, 154-179.

Chen S-F, et al: Mechanism of action of the novel anticancer agent 6-fluoro-2-(2′-fluoro-1,1′-biphenyl-4-yl)-3-methyl-4-quinolinecarboxylic acid sodium salt (NSC 368390): Inhibition of *de novo* pyrimidine nucleotide biosynthesis. *Cancer Res* 46:5014-5019, 1986.

Chun HG, et al: Fludarabine phosphate: A synthetic purine antimetabolite with significant activity against lymphoid malignancies. *J Clin Oncol* 9:175-188, 1991.

Cummings FJ, et al: Phase II trial of pentostatin in refractory lymphomas and cutaneous T-cell disease. *J Clin Oncol* 9:565-571, 1991.

Damon LE, et al: The association between high-dose cytarabine neurotoxicity and renal insufficiency. *J Clin Oncol* 7:1563-1568, 1989.

Dearden C, Catovsky D: Deoxycoformycin in the treatment of mature B-cell malignancies, editorial. *Br J Cancer* 62:4-5, 1990.

Dearden C, et al: Deoxycoformycin in the treatment of mature T-cell leukaemias. *Br J Cancer* 64:903-906, 1991.

Diasio RB, Harris BE: Clinical pharmacology of 5-fluorouracil. *Clin Pharmacokinet* 16:215-237, 1989.

Doll DC, List AF: Myelodysplastic syndromes. *West J Med* 151:161-167, 1989.

Donehower RC: Hydroxyurea, in Chabner BA, Collins JM (eds): *Cancer Chemotherapy: Principles and Practice.* Philadelphia, JB Lippincott, 1990, 225-233.

Donohue SM, Charlton CPJ: Drug treatment of acute leukaemia: Current status. *Drugs* 37:926-938, 1989.

Dutcher JP, et al: Successful treatment of hairy cell leukemia with 2'-deoxycoformin after failure of interferons alpha or beta. *Am J Clin Oncol* 13:290-293, 1990.

Einhorn LH: Improvements in fluorouracil chemotherapy? editorial. *J Clin Oncol* 7:1377-1379, 1989.

Estey EH, et al: Treatment of hairy cell leukemia with 2-chlorodeoxyadenosine (2-CdA). *Blood* 79:882-887, 1992.

Fialkow PJ, Singer JW: Chronic leukemias, in DeVita VT Jr, et al (eds): *Cancer: Principles & Practice of Oncology*, ed 3. Philadelphia, JB Lippincott, 1989, 1836-1852.

Grem JL: Fluorinated pyrimidines, in Chabner BA, Collins JM (eds): *Cancer Chemotherapy: Principles and Practice.* Philadelphia, JB Lippincott, 1990, 180-224.

Grem JL, et al: Biochemistry and clinical activity of *N*-(phosphonacetyl)-L-aspartate: A review. *Cancer Res* 48:4441-4454, 1988.

Grever MR, et al: Phase II investigation of pentostatin in multiple myeloma: A Southwest Oncology Group study. *J Natl Cancer Inst* 82:1778-1779, 1990.

Hamilton JM, et al: 5-Fluorouracil plus levamisole: Effective adjuvant treatment for colon cancer, in DeVita VT Jr, et al (eds): *Important Advances in Oncology 1990*. Philadelphia, JB Lippincott, 1990 A, 115-130.

Hamilton T, et al: Phase I trial of buthionine sulfoximine (BSO) plus melphalan (L-PAM) in patients with advanced cancer. *Proc Am Soc Clin Oncol* 9:73, 1990 B.

Henderson IC, et al: Cancer of the breast, in DeVita VT Jr, et al (eds): *Cancer: Principles & Practice of Oncology*, ed 3. Philadelphia, JB Lippincott, 1989, 1197-1268.

Ho AD, et al: Response to pentostatin in hairy-cell leukemia refractory to interferon-alpha. *J Clin Oncol* 7:1533-1538, 1989.

Ho AD, et al: Pentostatin in refractory chronic lymphocytic leukemia: A Phase II trial of the European Organization for Research and Treatment of Cancer. *J Natl Cancer Inst* 82:1416-1420, 1990.

Hochster H, Cassileth P: Fludarabine phosphate therapy of non-Hodgkin's lymphoma. *Semin Oncol* 17(suppl 8):63-65, 1990.

Hochster HS, et al: Activity of fludarabine in previously treated non-Hodgkin's low-grade lymphoma: Results of an Eastern Cooperative Oncology Group study. *J Clin Oncol* 10:28-32, 1992.

Hutchins L, et al: Breast cancer. *Dis Mon* 35:63-125, 1990.

Ishiguro K, et al: Characterization of the metabolic forms of 6-thioguanine responsible for cytotoxicity and induction of differentiation of HL-60 promyelocytic leukemia cells. *J Cell Physiol* 121:383-390, 1984.

Juliusson G, et al: Response to 2-chlorodeoxyadenosine in patients with B-cell chronic lymphocytic leukemia resistant to fludarabine. *N Engl J Med* 327:1056-1061, 1992.

Kantarjian HM, et al: Fludarabine therapy in hairy cell leukemia. *Cancer* 67:1291-1293, 1991 A.

Kantarjian HM, et al: Efficacy of fludarabine, a new adenine nucleoside analogue, in patients with prolymphocytic leukemia and the prolymphocytoid variant of chronic lymphocytic leukemia. *Am J Med* 90:223-228, 1991 B.

Kay AC, et al: 2-Chlorodeoxyadenosine treatment of low-grade lymphomas. *J Clin Oncol* 10:371-377, 1992.

Keating MJ: Fludarabine phosphate in the treatment of chronic lymphocytic leukemia. *Semin Oncol* 17(suppl 8):49-62, 1990.

Keating MJ, et al: Fludarabine: A new agent with major activity against chronic lymphocytic leukemia. *Blood* 74:19-25, 1989.

Keating MJ, et al: Fludarabine: A new agent with marked cytoreductive activity in untreated chronic lymphocytic leukemia. *J Clin Oncol* 9:44-49, 1991.

Kerr DJ: 5-Fluorouracil and folinic acid: Interesting biochemistry or effective treatment? *Br J Cancer* 60:807-808, 1989.

Kramer RA, et al: Role of the glutathione redox cycle in acquired and de novo multidrug resistance. *Science* 241:694-697, 1988.

Kraut EH, Chun HG: Fludarabine phosphate in refractory hairy cell leukemia. *Am J Hematol* 37:59-60, 1991.

Kraut EH, et al: Pentostatin in the treatment of advanced hairy cell leukemia. *J Clin Oncol* 7:168-172, 1989.

Kuzel T, et al: Thrombogenicity of intravenous 5-fluorouracil alone or in combination with cisplatin. *Cancer* 65:885-889, 1990.

Laurie JA, et al: Surgical adjuvant therapy of large-bowel carcinoma: An evaluation of levamisole and the combination of levamisole and fluorouracil. *J Clin Oncol* 7:1447-1456, 1989.

Leyland-Jones B, et al: Investigational new agents, in Chabner BA, Collins JM (eds): *Cancer Chemotherapy: Principles and Practice*. Philadelphia, JB Lippincott, 1990, 491-530.

Lichtman MA: Chronic myelogenous leukemia and related disorders, in Williams WJ, et al (eds): *Hematology,* ed 4. New York, McGraw-Hill, 1990, 202-222.

Lichtman MA, Brennan JK: Preleukemia and oligoblastic leukemia (myelodysplastic disorders), in Williams WJ, et al (eds): *Hematology*, ed 4. New York, McGraw-Hill, 1990, 175-187.

Liliemark J, Juliusson G: On the pharmacokinetics of 2-chloro-2'-deoxyadenosine in humans. *Cancer Res* 51:5570-5572, 1991.

Liliemark J, et al: On the bioavailability of oral and subcutaneous 2-chloro-2'-deoxyadenosine in humans: Alternative routes of administration. *J Clin Oncol* 10:1514-1518, 1992.

Marton LJ, Morris DR: Molecular and cellular functions of the polyamines, in McCann PP, et al (eds): *Inhibition of Polyamine Metabolism: Biological Significance and Basis for New Therapies.* Orlando, Academic Press, 1987, 79-106.

Mayer RJ, et al: Status of adjuvant therapy for colorectal cancer, commentary. *J Natl Cancer Inst* 81:1359-1364, 1989.

McCormack JJ, Johns DG: Purine and purine nucleoside antimetabolites, in Chabner BA, Collins JM (eds): *Cancer Chemotherapy: Principles and Practice*. Philadelphia, JB Lippincott, 1990, 234-252.

Moertel CG, et al: Levamisole and fluorouracil for adjuvant therapy of resected colon carcinoma. *N Engl J Med* 322:352-358, 1990.

National Institutes of Health: *NIH Consensus Development Conference: Adjuvant Therapy for Patients With Colon and Rectal Cancer*. April, 1990.

O'Dwyer PJ, et al: Phase II study of biochemical modulation of fluorouracil by low-dose PALA in patients with colorectal cancer. *J Clin Oncol* 8:1497-1503, 1990.

Pegg AE, Williams-Ashman HG: Pharmacologic interference with enzymes of polyamine biosynthesis and of 5'-methylthioadenosine metabolism, in McCann PP, et al (eds): *Inhibition of Polyamine Metabolism: Biological Significance and Basis for New Therapies*. Orlando, Academic Press, 1987, 33-48.

Piro LD, et al: 2-chlorodeoxyadenosine: An effective new agent for the treatment of chronic lymphocytic leukemia. *Blood* 3:1069-1073, 1988.

Piro LD, et al: Lasting remissions in hairy-cell leukemia induced by a single infusion of 2-chlorodeoxyadenosine. *N Engl J Med* 322:1117-1121, 1990.

Plunkett W, et al: Metabolism and action of fludarabine phosphate. *Semin Oncol* 17(suppl 8):3-17, 1990.

Porter CW, Jänne J: Modulation of antineoplastic drug action by inhibitors of polyamine biosynthesis, in McCann PP, et al (eds): *Inhibition of Polyamine Metabolism: Biological Significance and Basis for New Therapies*. Orlando, Academic Press, 1987, 203-248.

Redman JR, et al: Phase II trial of fludarabine phosphate in lymphoma: An effective new agent in low-grade lymphoma. *J Clin Oncol* 10:790-794, 1992.

Riscoe MK, et al: Purine metabolism as a target for leukemia chemotherapy. *Blood Rev* 3:162-173, 1989.

Robertson LE, et al: Response assessment in chronic lymphocytic leukemia after fludarabine plus prednisone: Clinical, pathologic, immunophenotypic, and molecular analysis. *Blood* 80:29-36, 1992.

Santana VM, et al: A Phase I clinical trial of 2-chlorodeoxyadenosine in pediatric patients with acute leukemia. *J Clin Oncol* 9:416-422, 1991.

Santana VM, et al: 2-Chlorodeoxyadenosine produces a high rate of complete hematologic remission in relapsed acute myeloid leukemia. *J Clin Oncol* 10:364-370, 1992.

Saven A, Piro LD: Treatment of hairy cell leukemia. *Blood* 79:1111-1120, 1992.

Saven A, et al: 2-Chlorodeoxyadenosine treatment of refractory chronic lymphocytic leukemia. *Leuk Lymphoma* (suppl): 133-138, 1991.

Saven A, et al: 2-Chlorodeoxyadenosine: An active agent in the treatment of cutaneous T-cell lymphoma. *Blood* 80:587-592, 1992.

Schechter PJ, et al (eds): Clinical aspects of inhibition of ornithine decarboxylase with emphasis on therapeutic trials of eflornithine (DFMO) in cancer and protozoan diseases, in McCann PP, et al (eds): *Inhibition of Polyamine Metabolism: Biological Significance and Basis for New Therapies*. Orlando, Academic Press, 1987, 345-364.

Schweitzer BI, et al: Dihydrofolate reductase as a therapeutic target. *FASEB J* 4:2441-2452, 1990.

Seto S, et al: Mechanism of deoxyadenosine and 2-chlorodeoxyadenosine toxicity to nondividing human lymphocytes. *J Clin Invest* 75:377-383, 1985.

Sunkara PS, et al: Inhibitors of polyamine biosynthesis: Cellular and *in vivo* effects on tumor proliferation, in McCann PP, et al (eds): *Inhibition of Polyamine Metabolism: Biological Significance and Basis for New Therapies*. Orlando, Academic Press, 1987, 121-138.

Tallman MS, et al: A single cycle of 2-chlorodeoxyadenosine results in complete remission in the majority of patients with hairy cell leukemia. *Blood* 80:2203-2209, 1992.

Tilly H, et al: Low-dose cytarabine versus intensive chemotherapy in the treatment of acute nonlymphocytic leukemia in the elderly. *J Clin Oncol* 8:272-279, 1990.

Tricot GJ, et al: Biochemically directed therapy of leukemia with tiazofurin: A selective blocker of inosine 5'-phosphate dehydrogenase activity. *Cancer Res* 49:3696-3701, 1989.

von Roemeling R, Hrushesky WJM: Circadian patterning of continuous floxuridine infusion reduces toxicity and allows higher dose intensity in patients with widespread cancer. *J Clin Oncol* 7:1710-1719, 1989.

Wiernik PH: Acute leukemias, in DeVita VT Jr, et al (eds): *Cancer: Principles & Practice of Oncology*, ed 3. Philadelphia, JB Lippincott, 1989, 1809-1835.

Other Selected References

Calabresi P, et al (eds): *Medical Oncology*. New York, Macmillan, 1985.

del Regato JA, et al: *Ackerman and del Regato's Cancer: Diagnosis, Treatment, and Prognosis*. St Louis, CV Mosby, 1985.

DeVita VT Jr, et al (eds): *Cancer: Principles and Practice of Oncology*, ed 3. Philadelphia, JB Lippincott, 1989.

Haskell CM (eds): *Cancer Treatment*, ed 3. Philadelphia, WB Saunders, 1990.

Hellmann K, Carter SK (eds): *Fundamentals of Cancer Chemotherapy*. New York, McGraw-Hill, 1987.

Holland JF, Frei E III (eds): *Cancer Medicine*, ed 2. Philadelphia, Lea & Febiger, 1982.

Tannock IF, Hill RP (eds): *The Basic Science of Oncology*. New York, Pergamon Press, 1987.

Antineoplastic Agents: Antibiotics, Alkaloids, and Enzymes

90

ANTIBIOTICS AND THEIR SYNTHETIC DERIVATIVES

Like other antibiotics, most of these drugs are produced by microbial fermentation. The clinically useful antitumor antibiotics consist of the anthracyclines (daunorubicin, doxorubicin), dactinomycin, plicamycin (mithramycin), mitomycin, and bleomycin. These drugs either bind reversibly to or react with cellular DNA to exert their cytotoxic effects (Myers and Chabner, 1990; Verweij et al, 1990). The anthracyclines and dactinomycin are intercalating agents; however, the anthracyclines also may have several additional cytotoxic mechanisms (see below). Several synthetic intercalating agents were designed in an attempt to reduce the adverse effects of anthracyclines while retaining their broad antitumor efficacy. Although mitoxantrone does not fully achieve this goal, it is the only synthetic intercalator that is generally available at present. Plicamycin also binds DNA noncovalently but is not an intercalating agent. Mitomycin covalently cross-links DNA, and bleomycin causes DNA strand scission. Because antitumor antibiotics are poorly absorbed by the gastrointestinal tract, they are usually administered intravenously.

Anthracyclines

The anthracycline antibiotics, daunorubicin and doxorubicin, are isolated from strains of *Streptomyces peucetius* and are the most broadly active of the natural products used in cancer chemotherapy (Myers and Chabner, 1990). Only the DNA alkylating and cross-linking agents have a wider spectrum of antitumor activity. These drugs are toxic to cells through several mechanisms, and it is not yet known definitively which are primarily responsible for the drugs' clinical efficacy and which are primarily responsible for their adverse effects. The antitumor activity of anthracyclines has very little schedule dependence; responses to continuous infusions, weekly doses, or single monthly boluses are almost equivalent. In contrast, some of the toxic effects of these drugs are related to the schedule used for their administration.

The clinical usefulness of doxorubicin and, to a lesser extent, that of daunorubicin is limited, to some degree, by the cumulative cardiotoxicity they may cause. New anthracyclines (aclarubicin, epirubicin, esorubicin, idarubicin, and menogaril) were developed in attempts to improve the therapeutic indices of daunorubicin and doxorubicin, as well as to increase efficacy against resistant tumor cells. Idarubicin is the first of these agents to become available (for treatment of acute myelogenous leukemia). Epirubicin appears to be the most promising of the remaining investigational anthracyclines.

ACTIONS. Anthracyclines enter cells by passive diffusion of the uncharged drug molecules. Protonation of the daunosamine sugar reduces its ability to cross cell membranes and is affected by both intracellular and extracellular pH. Thus, a low intracellular pH increases drug retention, but the increased acidity of extracellular fluid in solid tumors may hamper drug entry. Retention of these drugs in cells also is affected by an energy-dependent membrane glycoprotein efflux pump (see below). There are a number of mechanisms by which anthracyclines can cause cytotoxicity. Drug entry into cells may not be required for the cytotoxic effect to occur: for example, doxorubicin was covalently bound to agarose beads larger than individual tumor cells and some of the drug's cytocidal effects were retained (Tritton and Yee, 1982). The precise mechanism by which doxorubicin acts at the cell surface is not completely understood, but it may contribute to the total efficacy of the drug.

It is now well established that anthracyclines intercalate between adjacent base pairs in DNA, as well as bind to DNA and other nuclear sites by additional noncovalent modes (Myers and Chabner, 1990). The presence of anthracyclines in the nucleus freezes the enzyme DNA topoisomerase II in its strand cleavage and rejoining cycle, resulting in protein-associated DNA strand breaks in treated cells (Ross et al, 1988; Liu, 1989). There is evidence to suggest that topoisomerase II-mediated DNA damage is a major mechanism contributing to the antitumor effects of anthracyclines. However, nonenzymatic chemical reactions of the quinone moieties also occur under physiologic conditions (Myers and Chabner, 1990). A one-electron reduction followed by several additional steps generates hydrogen peroxide, which then can react further with free ferric ion or with ferric ion/anthracycline complexes to yield activated oxygen species capable of both DNA-strand breakage and oxidative membrane damage. These reactions are thought to be responsible for the cardiotoxicity of daunorubicin and doxorubicin, but may also contribute to their antitumor efficacy. A two-electron reduction is the initial step in a chemical reaction sequence that is thought to result in drug inactivation but that also may contribute to cytotoxicity.

Resistance to anthracyclines occurs readily in vivo and in vitro by several mechanisms. These drugs are substrates for the gp170 glycoprotein drug efflux transporter found at elevated levels in the membranes of multidrug-resistant cells (van der Bliek and Borst, 1989; Deuchars and Ling, 1989). Resistance to anthracyclines mediated by decreased drug accumulation thus can occur without prior exposure to a member of this drug class. A second mechanism of resistance to anthracyclines results from reduced DNA topoisomerase II activity (Ross et al, 1988; Liu, 1989). Since other drugs (eg, epipodophyllotoxins, amsacrine) also interact with topoisomerase II, this mechanism of resistance can be acquired without prior exposure to an anthracycline. A third mechanism of resistance involves elevated levels of glutathione or glutathione peroxidase, leading to increased scavenging and detoxification of hydrogen peroxide and activated oxygen species generated by reduction of the anthracycline quinones (Kramer et al, 1988; Lee et al, 1989). Finally, the absolute levels of reduced nicotinamide adenine dinucleotide phosphate (NADPH) and the ratio between concentrations of the reduced and oxidized (NADP+) forms of this coenzyme indirectly may affect anthracycline sensitivity. NADPH is a cosubstrate for glutathione reductase, and reduced glutathione may be used to inactivate anthracyclines. Alternatively, other enzymes (eg, cytochrome P450 reductase) use NADPH as a cosubstrate in reactions that may activate anthracyclines.

DAUNORUBICIN HYDROCHLORIDE
[Cerubidine]

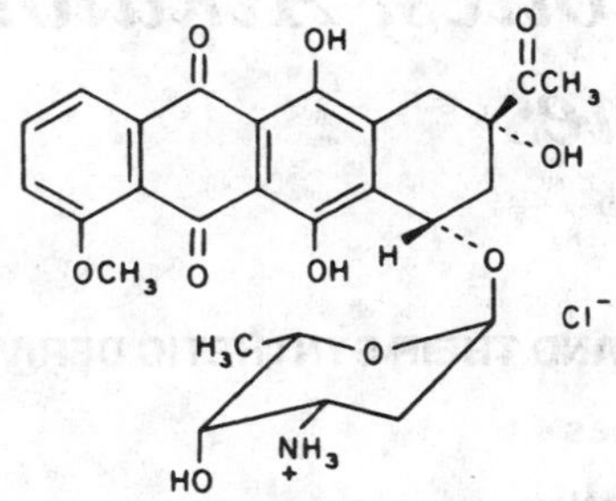

USES. The major indications for daunorubicin, in combination with other active drugs, are acute myelogenous and lymphocytic leukemias (see index entry Cancer: Clinical Response to Chemotherapeutic Drugs). The combination of cytarabine and daunorubicin (with or without thioguanine) is the treatment of choice for induction of remission in acute myelogenous leukemias. Complete response rates exceeding 60% are observed routinely with the combination of cytarabine and daunorubicin (Champlin and Gale, 1987; Donohue and Charlton, 1989; Wiernik, 1989; Lichtman and Henderson, 1990). Daunorubicin is often combined with vincristine and prednisone (with or without asparaginase) to induce remission in acute lymphocytic leukemia (Donohue and Charlton, 1989; Champlin and Gale, 1989; Wiernik, 1989; Mauer, 1990). In children with low- or standard-risk acute lymphocytic leukemia, addition of daunorubicin to vincristine and prednisolone prolongs the duration but does not increase the frequency of induction of complete remissions. The preferred regimen for inducing remission in children with high-risk acute lymphocytic leukemia has not been determined. In adults with this hematologic malignancy, the addition of daunorubicin may increase remission rates slightly above those seen in patients treated with only vincristine and prednisone. Daunorubicin also is active in neuroblastoma.

ADVERSE REACTIONS AND PRECAUTIONS. Myelosuppression is the usual dose-limiting toxicity. Leukopenia is usually more significant than thrombocytopenia, but severe aplasia may develop. The nadir for leukopenia generally occurs between 10 and 14 days, and recovery is gradual over the next one or two weeks. Monitoring of blood counts is essential.

Nausea and vomiting are usually mild but can be severe. Stomatitis also occurs; it typically begins as a burning sensation with erythema of the oral mucosa leading to ulceration in two or three days. Mucositis occurs much less frequently with daunorubicin than with doxorubicin and is less common than myelosuppression. Alopecia develops in about 80% of patients; it often has a sudden onset after three to four weeks of therapy but is usually reversible. Febrile reactions also may occur occasionally.

Cardiotoxicity is the major delayed adverse effect of daunorubicin, although this drug is less cardiotoxic than doxorubicin. An acute syndrome characterized by transient, reversible changes in the electrocardiogram (eg, tachycardia, extrasystoles, ST-T wave alterations) may occur hours to days after a dose and is not related to the total dose. A cumulative, dose-dependent cardiomyopathy also may develop and sometimes leads to congestive heart failure that may not respond to treatment. Cardiotoxicity may be mediated by free radical formation after one-electron reduction of the quinone moiety, and may occur one to six months after treatment is discontinued.

The risk of congestive heart failure is minimal when the total cumulative dose is less than 700 mg/M^2 (900 mg to 1 g/M^2 is the maximum recommended dose) (Myers and Chabner, 1990). Many oncologists recommend that the total dose of daunorubicin be limited to 500 mg/M^2 when radiation therapy to the mediastinum was administered previously and that the total dose also be reduced in children. In addition, the dosage should be modified if previous or concomitant cardiotoxic drug therapy is employed. Daunorubicin should be used with great caution in patients with significant heart disease (ie, recent myocardial infarction, history of congestive heart failure, significant arrhythmia).

Various factors have contributed to continuing use of these drugs despite their potential adverse effects on the heart. One of these is improved monitoring techniques, such as echocardiography, cardiac catheterization, and radionuclide cardiography, to detect cardiotoxicity at an early stage. A second is the identification of risk factors (discussed above) that are associated with increased susceptibility to anthracycline-induced cardiotoxicity and that necessitate reduction of the maximal allowable cumulative dose. Several other approaches are under investigation for reducing the cardiotoxicity of daunorubicin and the other anthracyclines (Myers and Chabner, 1990). Based on the involvement of ferric ion/anthracycline complexes in the biochemical mechanism thought to be responsible for the cardiotoxicity, ICRF-187 (ADR 529), an iron chelator, has been used in clinical trials with combination regimens containing doxorubicin (Speyer et al, 1988). Less impairment of cardiac function occurred in the patients given both drugs, and no loss in antitumor response was observed. Although the effects of daunorubicin alone have not been compared with those of the combination of ICRF-187 and daunorubicin, concurrent use of the iron chelator also may improve the therapeutic index of this anthracycline.

Severe local tissue necrosis and sloughing may develop if extravasation occurs. Thus, daunorubicin should never be administered by subcutaneous or intramuscular injection. Daunorubicin causes transient red discoloration of the urine that is of no clinical significance. The drug is mutagenic, carcinogenic, and teratogenic (FDA Pregnancy Category D).

Dosage reductions may be necessary in patients with impaired hepatic function, since hepatic metabolism and biliary excretion are the major routes of daunorubicin elimination. However, despite some reports of prolonged half-lives for this drug in patients with hepatic impairment, there are no conclusive data demonstrating that toxicity is increased with standard doses. Thus, current recommendations are to reduce the dosage only for patients with severe hepatic dysfunction.

PHARMACOKINETICS. Daunorubicin is poorly absorbed orally. Plasma clearance is biphasic after intravenous administration with a first half-life of 45 minutes, indicating distribution and uptake by tissues, and an elimination half-life of 24 to 55 hours. The drug is metabolized rapidly in the liver and is distributed to the tissues as unchanged drug, a major active metabolite (daunorubicinol), and other metabolites. Conversion of daunorubicin to daunorubicinol occurs at a faster rate and to a greater extent than does the corresponding metabolic transformation of doxorubicin. Daunorubicinol has a much longer plasma half-life than the parent drug; within several hours after administration of a single dose of daunorubicin, it is the major fraction of drug remaining in plasma. Approximately 70% of the drug and its metabolites present in plasma are bound to circulating proteins. Known routes of elimination can only account for about 65% of an administered dose; the remainder is bound to and slowly released from DNA and protein in the tissues. About 40% of the drug is eliminated by biliary excretion of daunorubicinol and other metabolites (a demethylated product, glucuronide and sulfate conjugates, and small amounts of aglycones). Another 25% is eliminated by urinary excretion, primarily of daunorubicinol. Daunorubicin and its metabolites do not enter cerebrospinal fluid to an appreciable extent.

DOSAGE AND PREPARATIONS.

Intravenous: 30 to 60 mg/M^2 daily for three days, repeated at three- to six-week intervals. The drug is administered through a running intravenous line.

Cerubidine (Wyeth-Ayerst). Powder (sterile, lyophilized) equivalent to 20 mg of base with mannitol 100 mg.

DOXORUBICIN HYDROCHLORIDE
[Adriamycin RDF, Adriamycin PFS]

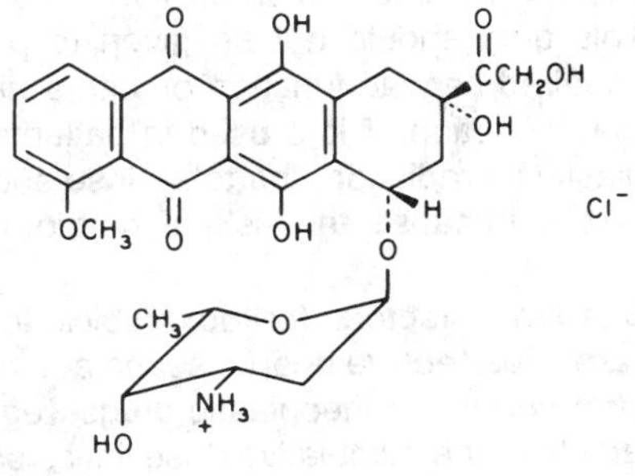

USES. Doxorubicin is one of the most effective antineoplastic agents and has been useful, most often in combination regimens, predominantly against solid tumors (Myers and Chabner, 1990). Doxorubicin is a component of some of the most effective therapies for Hodgkin's disease and non-Hodgkin's lymphoma; sarcomas (Ewing's, osteogenic, rhabdomyosarcoma, soft tissue); neuroblastoma; Wilms' tumor; carcinomas of the breast, lung, stomach, pancreas, bladder, ovary, and thyroid; and hepatoma (see index entry Cancer: Clinical Response to Chemotherapeutic Drugs). Although daunorubicin is usually preferred to induce remission in patients with acute leukemias, doxorubicin is active against both acute lymphocytic and acute myelogenous leukemias. Doxorubicin, alone or with other drugs, is used for secondary therapy in patients with prostatic or endometrial carcinoma. This drug also has marginal activity against carcinoma of the cervix, testes, and head and neck.

ADVERSE REACTIONS AND PRECAUTIONS. Toxicity affects the hematopoietic, cardiac, dermatologic, and gastrointestinal systems. Leukopenia is the usual dose-limiting toxicity, with the nadir occurring 10 to 15 days after initial administration. Blood counts usually return to normal levels approximately 21 days after administration. Thrombocytopenia and anemia follow a similar pattern but are of smaller magnitude. Blood counts must be monitored carefully.

Both acute and cumulative dose-dependent cardiotoxicity may occur. Acute effects may develop within a few minutes after a single intravenous dose (most often after large doses) and may persist for two weeks. They consist of electrocardiographic changes, such as sinus tachycardia, voltage reduction, flattening of the T-wave, depression of the ST segment, and arrhythmias. Such changes are usually transient and reversible, although occasionally they can be fatal. Withdrawal of doxorubicin therapy should take into consideration the patient's overall status.

The second type of cardiotoxicity that may occur is a delayed, cumulative, dose-dependent cardiomyopathy, most often seen during or up to several weeks after completion of treatment. However, congestive heart failure has been reported to occur more than six years after cessation of doxorubicin treatment (Goorin et al, 1990). Doxorubicin must be discontinued when congestive heart failure secondary to diffuse cardiomyopathy develops. Patients should be monitored (see below) for early signs of cardiotoxicity to reduce the morbidity and mortality associated with this adverse reaction. The total dose should not exceed 550 mg/M^2, since the risk of congestive heart failure increases markedly with higher cumulative doses. This drug should not be given to patients with significantly impaired cardiac function or with a history of recent myocardial infarction. If it is used in patients who have received mediastinal irradiation, the total dose should not exceed 400 mg/M^2, because the risk of cardiotoxicity is increased.

Other reported risk factors for doxorubicin-induced cardiomyopathy are hypertensive heart disease and concomitant administration of certain antineoplastic drugs (eg, high-dose cyclophosphamide). The cumulative dose limit also should be reduced for children, who are somewhat more susceptible to doxorubicin-induced cardiomyopathy than adults. Cardiotoxicity is mediated by free radical formation subsequent to one-electron reduction of the quinone moiety. Continuous infusion or weekly administration appears to be less cardiotoxic. This seems to result from the fact that cardiotoxicity is a function of peak plasma levels of doxorubicin, while antitumor efficacy relates more to total drug exposure (area under the curve).

Several other strategies have been investigated for reducing the incidence of cardiomyopathy in patients treated with doxorubicin (Myers and Chabner, 1990). Close monitoring of patients with improved physiologic tests of cardiac function (eg, echocardiography, cardiac catheterization, radionuclide cardiography) can lead to earlier detection and cessation of drug treatment before irreversible toxicity and congestive heart failure occur. Reducing the maximal cumulative dose administered to patients at increased risk of cardiotoxicity (those with hypertension, pre-existing cardiac disease, or previous cardiac irradiation) also has helped decrease the incidence of this adverse reaction. Since ferric ion complexes of doxorubicin have been implicated in the biochemical mechanism responsible for cardiotoxicity, the iron chelating agent, ICRF-187 (ADR-529), has been studied as a cardioprotective agent in a randomized controlled clinical trial in breast cancer patients treated with the CAF combination regimen (cyclophosphamide, doxorubicin, and fluorouracil) (Speyer et al, 1988). The antitumor efficacy of the combination regimen was not altered by the addition of the iron chelating agent and the cardiotoxic effects were reduced. Many of the patients given ICRF-187 were able to tolerate cumulative doses of doxorubicin larger than 600 mg/M^2. However, additional confirmatory trials of doxorubicin with and without ICRF-187 are needed. One other strategy that is in the early stages of clinical investigation involves targeted delivery of doxorubicin to tumors by encapsulating the drug in liposomes, in some instances with antibodies to tumor-associated antigens on their surfaces. The therapeutic potential of such liposomes remains to be determined.

Alopecia occurs in about 80% of patients, and regrowth of hair is usually complete two to five months after cessation of therapy. Doxorubicin also may cause a recurrence of radiation-induced skin reactions and exacerbates tissue changes due to irradiation in mucous membranes and the liver.

Nausea and vomiting are common and usually moderate; diarrhea occurs occasionally. Mucositis (eg, stomatitis, esophagitis) may be severe with ulceration. The incidence and severity of mucositis after bolus administration of doxorubicin are similar to those of myelosuppression; with weekly administration or continuous infusion, mucositis can become dose limiting. In contrast, daunorubicin causes mucositis much less frequently. Fever, chills, and urticaria have been observed, and anaphylaxis may occur.

The urine may become red after administration of doxorubicin, but the discoloration is transient, is due to the presence of drug in the urine, and is of no clinical significance.

Erythematous streaking and/or hives along the vein proximal to the site of injection may be observed. Extravasation causes severe tissue necrosis and sloughing; thus, great care in administration is needed. Doxorubicin should not be given by subcutaneous or intramuscular injection.

Doxorubicin and related compounds are mutagenic, carcinogenic, and teratogenic in animals.

Dosage reductions may be necessary in patients with impaired hepatic function. However, some experts believe that the evidence on which this suggestion is based is inconclusive.

PHARMACOKINETICS. Doxorubicin is poorly absorbed orally and is administered intravenously. Injection is followed by an initial rapid plasma clearance and significant tissue binding. Approximately 75% of the drug present in plasma is bound to circulating proteins. The plasma decay curve of unaltered doxorubicin is triphasic with half-lives of 10 minutes, one to three hours, and 30 to 50 hours. Hepatic metabolism is less rapid than for daunorubicin, but several metabolites exist in plasma; the major metabolite is doxorubicinol. Slow release from tissue binding sites prolongs the duration of drug and metabolites in plasma. As a result of this slow release, cytotoxic concentrations are maintained in the plasma for nearly a week after bolus administration of doxorubicin. Drug concentrations achieved in cerebrospinal fluid are inadequate for therapeutic efficacy. After seven days, 40% to 50% of a dose is eliminated in bile, 50% as unchanged drug and 23% as active metabolite (doxorubicinol), as well as inactive sulfate and glucuronide conjugates and inactive aglycones. Only 5% to 10% is excreted in the urine.

DOSAGE AND PREPARATIONS.

Intravenous: 60 to 75 mg/M^2 given as a single dose every three weeks; alternatively, 10 to 30 mg/M^2 repeated every week. Continuous infusion over 96 hours also has been used. The drug is administered slowly by direct intravenous administration into the side arm of a freely running intravenous line. If daunorubicin has been given previously, the weekly schedule employing smaller doses should be used or the total cumulative dose of anthracyclines should not exceed 500 mg/M^2.

Doxorubicin Hydrochloride (Cetus). Powder (lyophilized) 10, 20, and 50 mg containers; solution 2 mg/ml in 5, 10, and 25 ml containers.

Adriamycin RDF (Adria). Powder (cryodesiccated) 10, 20, 50, and 150 mg containers; solution 2 mg/ml (preservative-free) in 5, 10, 25, and 100 ml containers ***(Adriamycin PFS)***.

IDARUBICIN HYDROCHLORIDE (4-Demethoxydaunorubicin)
[Idamycin]

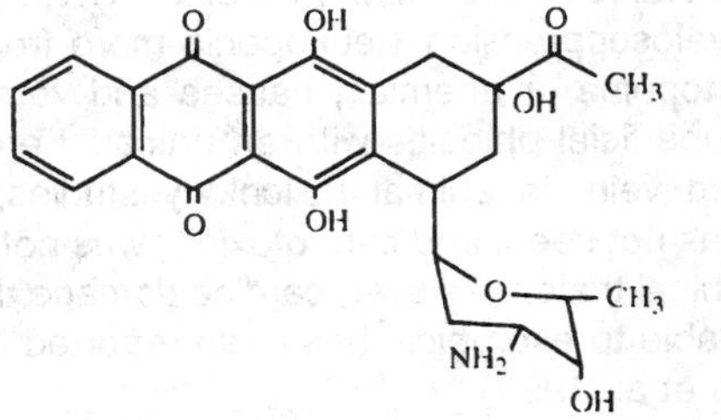

ACTIONS AND USES. Idarubicin is an anthracycline analogue that differs from daunorubicin by the absence of a methoxyl substituent at the 4 position of the anthraquinone ring system. It probably acts at the same intracellular targets as doxorubicin and daunorubicin. In some cell culture systems, idarubicin and its metabolite, idarubicinol, are significantly more potent inducers of protein-associated DNA strand breaks and cytocidal agents than other anthracyclines and their analogous metabolites (Kuffel et al, 1990).

Idarubicin in combination with cytarabine is indicated for the treatment of acute myelogenous leukemia in adults. High response rates (>80% complete remissions) were also obtained when idarubicin was combined with etoposide for the treatment of acute myelogenous leukemia or with cytarabine, vincristine, and prednisone for acute lymphocytic leukemia (Carella et al, 1990). Results of comparative trials of idarubicin and daunorubicin, each combined with cytarabine for the treatment of acute myelogenous leukemia in adults, suggest that the frequency of complete remission is higher in the group treated with idarubicin (Carella et al, 1990). Survival time also may be slightly longer in those given idarubicin. In a randomized trial comparing oral idarubicin with intravenous doxorubicin as single agents in the treatment of advanced breast cancer, response rate in the patients given doxorubicin was more than twofold higher (Lopez et al, 1989). However, those in the group treated with doxorubicin did not survive longer, and toxicity was more severe.

ADVERSE REACTIONS AND PRECAUTIONS. The myelosuppressive effects of idarubicin appear to be equivalent to those of doxorubicin (Lopez et al, 1989). This drug also can cause both acute and chronic cardiotoxicity, although data suggest that therapeutic doses of idarubicin are less cardiotoxic than comparably effective doses of daunorubicin or doxorubicin (Carella et al, 1990). Other toxic effects include reversible alopecia, nausea, vomiting, mucositis, diarrhea, fever, chills, skin rash, and elevated serum levels of liver enzymes or bilirubin. The manufacturer recommends that dose reductions be considered for patients with elevated serum levels of bilirubin or creatinine. As with other anthracyclines, idarubicin can impart a transient red color to the urine, but this is of no clinical significance. Extravasation of the drug can cause severe local tissue necrosis and should be avoided.

Idarubicin is embryotoxic and teratogenic in rats and embryotoxic (but not teratogenic) in rabbits. No data are available on the effects of idarubicin in pregnant women or on human fertility in males or females. This drug is classified in FDA Pregnancy Category D.

PHARMACOKINETICS. Idarubicin is one of the few anthracyclines that can be administered orally. Its bioavailability is approximately 30% by this route. The unchanged drug disappears from the circulation and has a mean half-life of about 20 hours; its major metabolite, idarubicinol, is retained much longer (mean half-life, >45 hours). No aglycone metabolite has been detected in the circulation. Since idarubicinol is cytotoxic and has such a long half-life, it probably contributes significantly to the antitumor effects of the parent drug. Idarubicin has a very large volume of distribution, which suggests that tissue binding is extensive. The major fraction of idarubicin is cleared (as idarubicinol) by biliary excretion, with a small amount eliminated by the kidneys.

DOSAGE.

Intravenous: For induction of remission in acute leukemia, 10 to 12 mg/M^2 daily for three to five days. Alternatively, in patients with solid tumors, 10 to 15 mg/M^2 once every three weeks.

Oral (investigational): 45 mg/M^2 once every three weeks or 25 to 30 mg/M^2 daily for three days, with intervals depending on recovery from myelosuppression.

Idamycin (Adria). Powder (lyophilized) 5 and 10 mg single-dose containers with 50 and 100 mg of lactose, respectively.

EPIRUBICIN HYDROCHLORIDE (4′-Epidoxorubicin) (Investigational drug)

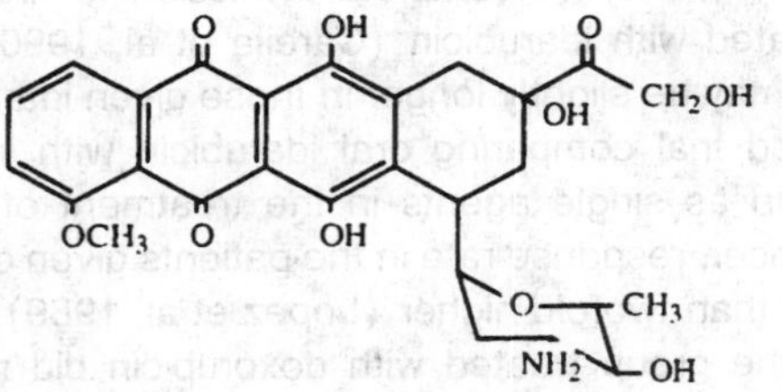

ACTIONS AND USES. Epirubicin is an epimer (stereoisomer) of doxorubicin that differs from the parent compound only in the stereochemistry at the 4′ position of the daunosamine sugar. Its actions are probably the same as those of doxorubicin, with induction of DNA strand breaks by an effect on topoisomerase II, by generation of free radicals, or both. Resistance to epirubicin mediated by the gp-170 cell surface glycoprotein efflux pump has been observed. However, it is not yet known if alterations in topoisomerase II activity can result in resistance to epirubicin.

Clinical trials have demonstrated that epirubicin has some efficacy in patients with advanced and metastatic breast cancer and in non-small cell lung cancer. Several trials have compared epirubicin with doxorubicin as single agents (Jain et al, 1985) or in combination with cyclophosphamide and fluorouracil (French Epirubicin Study Group, 1988; Italian Multicentre Breast Study With Epirubicin, 1988) in patients with advanced breast cancer. Data from these studies suggest that response rates and median survival times in patients treated with epirubicin are about the same as or slightly less than those in patients given doxorubicin in equivalent weight-based doses. However, the incidence of congestive heart failure was slightly lower in those treated with epirubicin. Data also suggest that when administered in equally myelosuppressive doses, the response rate in patients with advanced breast cancer may be slightly higher with epirubicin than with doxorubicin.

ADVERSE REACTIONS. Toxic effects associated with epirubicin therapy include reversible myelosuppression (leukopenia and thrombocytopenia most often dose-limiting), alopecia, and gastrointestinal effects (nausea, vomiting, and mucositis/stomatitis). There is disagreement among investigators regarding the potency of this drug's cardiotoxic effects: Some investigators indicate that it is as cardiotoxic as doxorubicin, while others believe that epirubicin is less cardiotoxic. Randomized comparative trials are needed to resolve this disagreement.

PHARMACOKINETICS. Epirubicin is not absorbed when administered orally. The unchanged drug is cleared from the circulation (half-life, approximately 18 hours). Two major metabolites are present in plasma, 13-epirubicinol and a glucuronide conjugate; these also are cleared and have half-lives of 21 and 12 hours, respectively. The parent compound, as well as the two major metabolites, are excreted in the urine.

DOSAGE (investigational regimen).

Intravenous: 100 to 120 mg/M^2 every three weeks.

ESORUBICIN HYDROCHLORIDE (4′-Deoxydoxorubicin, 4′-DxDx) (Investigational drug)

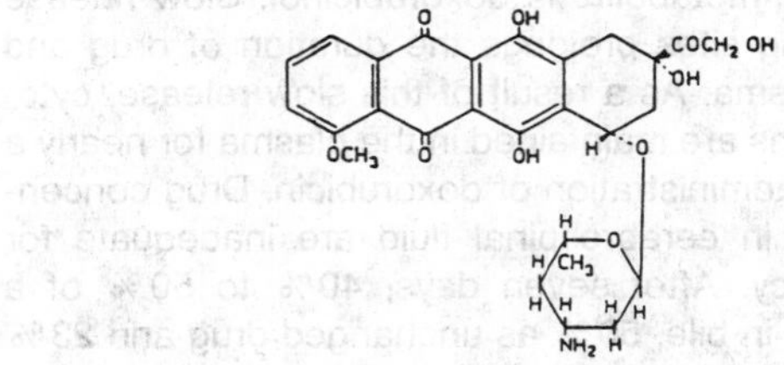

ACTIONS. Esorubicin, a derivative of doxorubicin, differs from the parent compound only in the reduction of the 4′ position on the glycosamine moiety. Its postulated mechanism of action is the same as that for other anthracycline compounds, but esorubicin causes greater stabilization of the DNA helix against heat denaturation and is a more potent inhibitor of DNA synthesis. In vitro and in animal models, the antitumor activity of esorubicin can equal that of doxorubicin at approximately one-half the molar concentration.

USES. Esorubicin is expected to have a spectrum of activity similar to that of doxorubicin. In animal models, esorubicin was not totally cross resistant with doxorubicin. However, it is anticipated that this derivative may be significantly less active against tumors previously exposed to the parent compound. In Phase II clinical trials, esorubicin induced objective responses (complete or partial remissions) in colorectal and breast carcinoma and in multiple myeloma. No randomized trials comparing esorubicin with doxorubicin have been published, but, thus far, response rates to esorubicin have been equivalent to those reported for doxorubicin.

ADVERSE REACTIONS AND PRECAUTIONS. Side effects include myelosuppression (leukopenia more frequently than thrombocytopenia or anemia), nausea and vomiting, alopecia, and superficial phlebitis with an urticarial eruption along the injected vein. In animal toxicology studies, myocardial damage was not seen, and cardiotoxicity was not observed in Phase I clinical trials. However, cardiac damage that is probably attributable to esorubicin has been reported in a Phase II trial (Muss et al, 1990).

PHARMACOKINETICS. Esorubicin can be administered orally or intravenously. The plasma decay curve after intravenous use is multiphasic with half-lives of four to six minutes and 66 hours. The aglycone metabolite is detected only for the first hour, and the largest degradation product is deoxydoxorubicinol. Excretion is primarily through the biliary system.

DOSAGE (investigational regimen).

Intravenous, Oral: 30 to 40 mg/M^2 every three weeks.

MENOGARIL (7-OMEN) (Investigational drug)

[Tomosar]

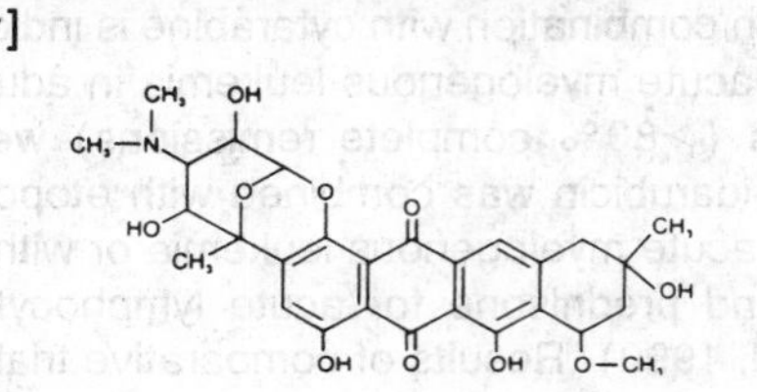

ACTIONS AND USES. Menogaril is a semisynthetic derivative of the anthracycline antibiotic, nogalamycin. Analogues of nogalamycin differ from other anthracyclines by the attachment of a sugar to the D ring rather than to the A ring. Menogaril appears to differ substantially from doxorubicin in its mechanism of action; it binds only weakly to DNA and does not inhibit RNA polymerase activity. In contrast to doxorubicin, intracellular menogaril is concentrated in the cytoplasm rather than in the nucleus.

It is anticipated that menogaril will have a spectrum of activity similar to that of doxorubicin. However, preclinical studies suggest that menogaril is six times less potent. Menogaril has moderate activity against breast tumors, and combination regimens for mammary cancer that include this drug are undergoing clinical trial. Response rates with its administration alone in patients with melanoma; myeloma; colon, lung, prostatic, and renal carcinomas; or metastatic sarcoma have been disappointing. Randomized trials comparing menogaril with doxorubicin have not been published.

ADVERSE REACTIONS AND PRECAUTIONS. Menogaril has produced leukopenia, anemia, local cutaneous reactions, diarrhea, nausea, vomiting, alopecia, fatigue, paresthesias, and inflammation of previously irradiated sites ("radiation recall"). A relative platelet-sparing effect has been observed. Menogaril is cardiotoxic in rabbits, although less so than doxorubicin. Extravasation of the drug from the infusion site can cause ulceration of the skin. Hepatic, renal, and pulmonary toxic effects have occurred in animals.

PHARMACOKINETICS. Menogaril can be administered orally or intravenously. Orally, menogaril has a bioavailability of approximately 35%. As with other anthracycline derivatives, plasma clearance is biphasic, with half-lives of <12 minutes and 7.5 to 15 hours. Excretion through the biliary system and in the urine accounts for $<20\%$ of an administered dose.

DOSAGE (investigational regimens).

Intravenous: 200 mg/M^2 every three to four weeks.

Oral: 150 mg/M^2/day for three days every four weeks or 225 mg/M^2 once weekly.

Tomosar (Upjohn).

RAZOXANE (ICRF-159, ICRF-187, ADR 529) (Investigational drug)

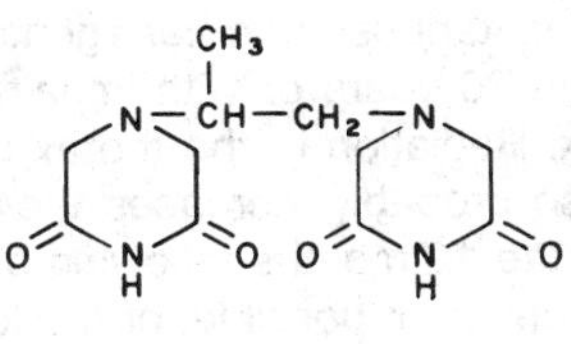

ACTIONS AND USES. This bis-dioxopiperazine compound has a single chiral center and can be prepared as a racemic mixture (razoxane or ICRF-159) or as a single pure stereoisomer. ICRF-187 (ADR 529) is the + enantiomer, which is approximately five times more soluble than the racemate, razoxane. Early in vitro studies with razoxane as a single agent indicated that this drug inhibits cell proliferation and blocks cell cycle progression in the G_2 or M phases of the cell cycle. The precise mechanism of action for razoxane when it is used alone remains to be determined, but it may be related to the drug's ability to chelate ferric ion and other metal cations. DNA synthesis is inhibited in cells treated with razoxane. Significant activity has been reported in leukemia and non-Hodgkin's lymphomas. Although razoxane is obviously not an anthracycline, it is included here because current interest focuses on the ability of ICRF-187, the more soluble pure enantiomer, to attenuate anthracycline cardiotoxicity as a result of its iron-chelating activity (Herman et al, 1988; Speyer et al, 1988).

This bicyclic compound is relatively nonpolar and enters cells by passive diffusion. Hydrolysis and ring-opening of the two piperazines inside cells generates a bidentate chelating agent similar to edetate (ethylenediaminetetraacetic acid). Considerable evidence supports the hypothesis that interactions between activated oxygen species (generated from one-electron reduction of the anthracycline quinone) and a doxorubicin/ferric ion complex results in lipid peroxidation of membranes in cardiac tissue and is responsible for the cardiotoxicity produced by anthracyclines (Myers and Chabner, 1990). Chelation of iron by the hydrolysis product of ICRF-187 attenuates this toxic effect of anthracyclines in beagles (Herman et al, 1988) and in women with advanced breast cancer (Speyer et al, 1988). Neither the antitumor efficacy of doxorubicin nor any of its noncardiac toxic effects were reduced by pretreatment of breast tumor patients with ICRF-187.

ADVERSE REACTIONS AND PRECAUTIONS. Leukopenia is the principal toxic effect of razoxane and ICRF-187 when either is used alone. Nausea and vomiting are common and usually mild. Alopecia, dermatitis, and a "flu-like" syndrome have been reported. The drug is immunosuppressive, radiosensitizing, and teratogenic. When used as a cardioprotective agent in combination regimens with anthracyclines, ICRF-187 increased myelosuppressive effects slightly but did not increase the frequency or severity of other adverse reactions and had no additional toxic effects of its own.

PHARMACOKINETICS. Bioavailability of oral razoxane is erratic because of its poor solubility. The pure enantiomer, ICRF-187, is sufficiently soluble for intravenous administration. The plasma half-life is approximately 3.5 hours. The drug is extensively metabolized (or subject to nonenzymatic hydrolysis) and appears to be excreted by the kidneys and biliary system (with possible significant enterohepatic recirculation).

DOSAGE (investigational regimens).

Oral: 3 g/M^2 of razoxane in divided doses every six hours for one day/week for six weeks.

Intravenous: For use of ICRF-187 as a cardioprotective agent, 1g/M^2 as a 15-minute infusion 30 minutes before doxorubicin administration. For use as a single agent, 1 g/M^2/day for three days every three weeks, with dose reductions based on recovery from hematopoietic toxicity.

Razoxane (ICI Pharma).

Other Antibiotics

In addition to the anthracyclines, a number of clinically useful antitumor antibiotics have been isolated from the fermentation products of various species of *Streptomyces*. Other than their similar derivations, these drugs have little in common with regard to chemical structures or mechanisms of action. However, they all bind to and affect cellular DNA as their common target. The bleomycins are glycopeptides that bind ferrous ion, intercalate between adjacent base pairs in DNA, and then generate activated oxygen species that cause DNA strand breaks. Dactinomycin also binds to DNA by intercalation, but its primary action is inhibition of RNA transcription rather than DNA damage. Mitomycin can generate cross-links between strands of DNA after activation by intracellular reductases. Plicamycin binds to DNA on the outside of the helix rather than by intercalation, and it inhibits replication and transcription by altering DNA conformation. In addition to these, several newer antibiotics are under investigation as potential antineoplastic drugs, including one (didemnin B) isolated from a marine organism.

BLEOMYCIN SULFATE

[Blenoxane]

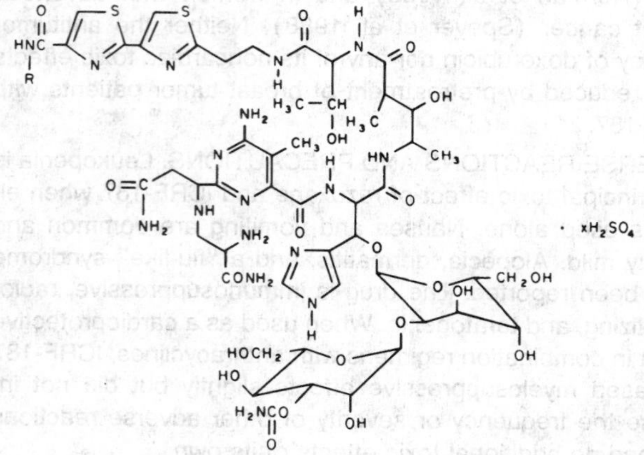

$\cdot\ xH_2SO_4$

(Main Component: Bleomycin A_2, in which R is $(CH_3)_2S^+CH_2CH_2CH_2—$)

ACTIONS. The bleomycins are a family of complex glycopeptides extracted from a strain of *Streptomyces verticillus*. The bleomycin used clinically is a mixture consisting predominantly of bleomycin A_2 and B_2. A bleomycin-ferrous iron-molecular oxygen ternary complex intercalates between DNA base pairs, which causes the double helix to unwind and relaxes supercoiling in circular DNA (Chabner, 1990 A). The bleomycin-ferrous iron complex also catalyzes reduction of molecular oxygen to superoxide or hydroxyl radicals causing DNA strand breaks and inhibition of DNA synthesis. There is some evidence that resistance to bleomycin is mediated by an enhanced capacity for repair of drug-induced DNA damage.

Bleomycin appears to exhibit some degree of cell cycle phase specificity. It is most active during G_2 phase but also has some activity in late G_1, early S, and M phases.

USES. Bleomycin is useful in the treatment of testicular cancer and malignant lymphomas. It is active against squamous cell carcinomas of the head and neck region (eg, buccal mucosa, tongue, tonsil, pharynx, larynx), uterine cervix, penis, and esophagus. This antibiotic has been administered intravesically to treat recurrent superficial bladder tumors and intralesionally to treat warts (see index entry Bleomycin, In Warts). Bleomycin also has been used to treat osteosarcoma, some soft tissue sarcomas, and melanoma. Intrapleural and intraperitoneal instillation of bleomycin has controlled malignant effusions resulting from breast, lung, or ovarian tumors.

Because it lacks significant myelosuppressive activity, bleomycin has been used extensively with other drugs (see index entry Cancer: Clinical Response to Chemotherapeutic Drugs and the discussion on Combination Chemotherapy in Chapter 1 of this Section). The combination of bleomycin, cisplatin, and either vinblastine or etoposide is very effective in disseminated seminomatous and nonseminomatous testicular cancer and produces a high percentage of long-term disease-free survivors who are probably cured of disease (Loehrer et al, 1988; Williams et al, 1989 A). These regimens also are active against malignant germ cell tumors of the ovary (Williams et al, 1989 B; Gershenson et al, 1990). In Hodgkin's disease, bleomycin has been added to the MOPP regimen; the combination of doxorubicin, bleomycin, vinblastine, and dacarbazine (ABVD) is an effective alternative to MOPP (Hellman et al, 1989; Haskell and Parker, 1990). The ABVD regimen is especially preferred in young males, since it causes fewer gonadal complications and results in sterility less often than does the MOPP regimen. Complete responses with long-term disease-free survival also have been observed in many patients with non-Hodgkin's lymphoma who received one of several regimens containing bleomycin (eg, BACOP) (Gaynor and Fisher, 1989; Sarna and Kagan, 1990). The combination of bleomycin, mitomycin, and vincristine is active in the treatment of metastatic carcinoma of the cervix, but there are few complete responses (<30%) and remissions are of short duration (Hoskins et al, 1989).

ADVERSE REACTIONS AND PRECAUTIONS. The usual dose-limiting effect of bleomycin is pulmonary toxicity, which occurs in approximately 10% of patients treated with total doses >450 mg and in 3% to 5% of those given <450 mg. The incidence and severity also are related to the patient's age and the concomitant use of other agents (Comis, 1990). Patients older than 70 years or with impaired renal function are at greater risk. Radiation to the thorax or high-dose oxygen inhalation also probably increases the risk. Patients requiring surgery in the 12 months following bleomycin therapy should breathe room air, if possible, or the lowest concentration of supplemental oxygen that will yield adequate saturation. Doses of bleomycin should be reduced in patients with impaired renal function. Although signs and symptoms of pulmonary toxicity may revert to normal in many patients within two years after bleomycin treatment, the pulmonary fibrosis can be irreversible and fatal. As many as 10% of those treated after thoracic irradiation may succumb to this adverse reaction.

The development of pulmonary toxicity is usually delayed and may occur four to ten weeks after initiation of therapy. The radiographic appearance is typical of interstitial pneumonitis that may progress to pulmonary fibrosis. Rales, rhonchi, and, occasionally, pleural friction rubs usually precede radiographic changes. The lesions are found most frequently in the lower lobes and subpleural areas and consist of a fibrinous exudate, atypical proliferation of alveolar cells, hyaline membranes, interstitial and intra-alveolar fibrosis, and squamous metaplasia of the distal air spaces. Pulmonary function tests are not necessarily predictive. The most sensitive method for early detection of pulmonary toxicity may be serial determination of carbon monoxide diffusion capacity, and the drug should be discontinued if the value falls below 30% to 35% of the pretreatment level. The drug also should be discontinued if other clinical signs of pulmonary dysfunction appear (eg, fine rales or rhonchi, dyspnea, dry cough). Data reported in a retrospective study suggest that the risk of pulmonary toxicity may be less with 72-hour continuous infusions than with weekly bolus administration (Jensen et al, 1990). However, a prospective randomized trial is needed to confirm this possibility.

The incidence of hypersensitivity reactions ranging from chills and fever (usually occurring four to six hours after administration) to anaphylaxis is high (20% to 60% of patients). Severe reactions are most common in lymphoma patients, and test doses are recommended. Mucocutaneous changes (eg, alopecia; hyperpigmentation; pruritic erythema; hyperkeratosis; desquamation of hands, feet, and pressure areas; edema; mucositis) also occur frequently. Nausea and vomiting occur in 15% to 30% of patients. Delayed and reversible alopecia also may result from bleomycin treatment. Neither clinically significant myelosuppression nor immunosuppression has been reported.

The safety of bleomycin during pregnancy or lactation is unknown. However, the drug is teratogenic when administered to pregnant mice.

PHARMACOKINETICS. Bleomycin is inactive orally. When administered parenterally, it is distributed rapidly throughout the body. The highest concentrations appear in the skin, lung, kidney, peritoneum, and lymph nodes. Bleomycin does not enter the cerebrospinal fluid. The drug is inactivated by an aminohydrolase present in most tissues. The highest levels of this activity are found in liver and kidney, followed by bone marrow and lymph nodes. Activity is very low in the lung and skin, the tissues at highest risk for bleomycin toxicity. The plasma elimination terminal phase half-life is about two to four hours; 45% to 70% is recovered in urine within 24 hours as active drug. Drug clearance is decreased and the plasma half-life is prolonged in patients with impaired renal function; dosage modifications are required for those with creatinine clearance below 35 ml/min.

DOSAGE AND PREPARATIONS. A unit of activity is defined based on the preparation's antimicrobial activity and ranges between 1.5 and 2 units/mg (dry weight). For intramuscular or subcutaneous use, the contents of the ampul are dissolved in 1 to 5 ml of sterile water for injection, sodium chloride injection, or 5% dextrose injection. For intravenous use, the contents of the ampul are dissolved in 5 ml or more of sodium chloride injection or 5% dextrose injection and administered slowly over ten minutes.

Intramuscular, Intravenous, Subcutaneous: For squamous cell carcinomas, lymphomas, and testicular carcinoma, 10 to 20 units/M^2 once or twice weekly (to a total dose of 300 to 400 units). Because anaphylactic reactions may occur, patients with lymphomas should receive 2 units or less as the initial dose. If no acute reaction is observed, the regular dosage schedule may be used. For continuous infusion, 15 units/M^2/day for four or five days.

Intracavitary: After thoracostomy tube drainage, 15 to 120 units diluted in 50 to 100 ml of normal saline or 5% dextrose injection is administered into the pleural space. The most common regimen consists of 60 units administered in 50 ml of 5% dextrose injection. Intraperitoneal instillation of 60 to 120 units in 100 ml of normal saline is also utilized. In all instances, the drug solutions are removed after 24 hours.

Blenoxane (Bristol-Myers). Powder (sterile) 15 units.

DACTINOMYCIN (Actinomycin D)

[Cosmegen]

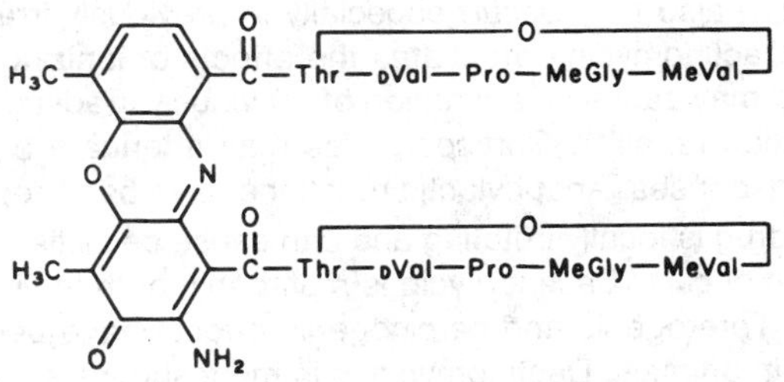

ACTIONS. This antitumor antibiotic, derived from *Streptomyces parvullus*, binds avidly to DNA by intercalation of the planar phenoxazine ring system between adjacent base pairs with the circular polypeptides in the minor groove of the double helix (Verweij et al, 1990). The drug has highest affinity for the sequence dGpdC, but it also binds to other sequences. The major consequence of the drug's binding to DNA is inhibition of RNA synthesis (transcription), with chain elongation more sensitive than initiation, termination, or release. As a result of impaired mRNA production, protein synthesis also declines after dactinomycin therapy. Dactinomycin also causes single-strand DNA breaks. This drug is cell cycle nonspecific. In vitro, acquired resistance to dactinomycin involves the gp-170 drug efflux membrane pump (multidrug resistance); the role of this mechanism in resistance to dactinomycin clinically is not known.

USES. Dactinomycin is effective in gestational choriocarcinoma; regimens combining dactinomycin and methotrexate (with or without other drugs) are standard therapy for those with high-risk tumors (Hoskins et al, 1989; Berkowitz and Goldstein, 1990). Effective therapy of Wilms' tumor requires multiple treatment modalities, including surgery, radiation therapy, and combination chemotherapy with dactinomycin and vincristine. Dactinomycin also is active in testicular tumors, neuroblastoma, endometrial and ovarian carcinomas, embryonal rhabdomyosarcoma, Ewing's sarcoma, osteosarcoma, and other sarcomas. In nearly all of these cancers, dactinomycin is used in combination with other drugs (see index entry Cancer: Clinical Response to Chemotherapeutic Drugs).

ADVERSE REACTIONS AND PRECAUTIONS. The usual dose-limiting toxicity is bone marrow depression, usually leukopenia and thrombocytopenia; anemia (including rare instances of aplastic anemia) also can develop. The nadir usually occurs between one to two weeks after a course of therapy. Thrombocytopenia is often seen first; leukopenia may be dose limiting. Blood counts should be monitored carefully. Dactinomycin should be given cautiously to those with renal or liver disease or impaired bone marrow function.

Anorexia, nausea, and vomiting usually occur within a few hours after administration and may be ameliorated by antiemetics (eg, phenothiazines) given prior to therapy. Abdominal pain and diarrhea may occur. Stomatitis, cheilitis, glossitis, and proctitis are common and may be dose limiting. Oral and gastrointestinal ulcerations may develop.

Dermatologic reactions include alopecia and acneiform eruption. Cutaneous erythema, desquamation, and hyperpigmentation also may occur, especially in previously irradiated areas. Dactinomycin potentiates the effects of ionizing radiation and may cause inflammation of previously irradiated sites ("radiation recall"). Corticosteroids may attenuate or block these responses. Anaphylactic reactions have been reported.

This drug is locally irritating and can cause cellulitis if extravasation occurs. Dactinomycin is mutagenic both in vitro and in vivo. Teratogenic and carcinogenic effects have been observed in animals. Dactinomycin is immunosuppressive.

This drug is classified in FDA Pregnancy Category C.

PHARMACOKINETICS. Dactinomycin is poorly absorbed orally and is administered intravenously. The drug is cleared rapidly from plasma by tissue uptake and DNA binding. It does not enter the cerebrospinal fluid. Dactinomycin has long tissue (47 hours) and plasma (36 hours) half-lives due to slow release from tissue stores. It is metabolized minimally, and about 30% of a dose is excreted in bile and urine over seven days.

DOSAGE AND PREPARATIONS.

Intravenous: The usual dose is 0.4 to 0.6 mg/M^2 daily for a maximum of five days. In both adults and children, a second course may be administered after four to six weeks have elapsed, provided all signs of toxicity have disappeared. Dactinomycin is administered through a running intravenous infusion.

Isolation Perfusion Technique: The dosage schedule and technique vary; the manufacturer's literature should be consulted for details. In general, the following doses are suggested: 0.15 to 0.2 mg/M^2 for lower extremity or pelvis; 0.1 to 0.15 mg/M^2 for upper extremity. After bone marrow function has recovered (three to four weeks), the course is repeated.

Cosmegen (Merck Sharp & Dohme). Powder (lyophilized) 0.5 mg with mannitol 20 mg.

MITOMYCIN

[Mutamycin]

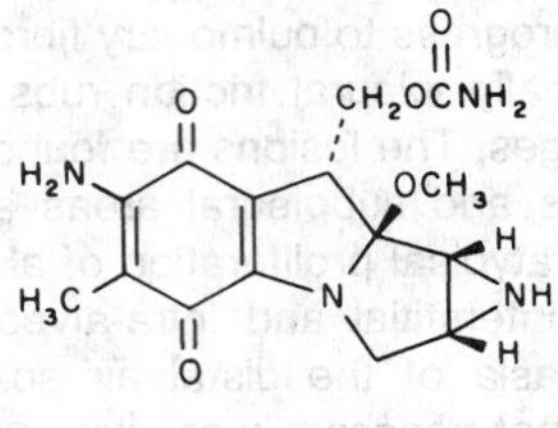

ACTIONS. Mitomycin is isolated from *Streptomyces caespitosus*. After activation by chemical reduction or by intracellular reductases, the drug functions as a mono- and bifunctional alkylating and DNA cross-linking agent (Verweij et al, 1990). Increased rates of reductive activation in hypoxic, relative to well-oxygenated, cells confer some preferential activity for mitomycin against hypoxic solid tumor cells (Sartorelli, 1988). Chemical decomposition in a mildly acidic pH environment also may contribute to drug activation. Cytotoxicity is probably due to the inhibition of DNA synthesis that results from cross-linking of DNA, although only 10% of the drug-DNA adducts are cross-links. Monofunctional alkylation accounts for the remaining 90% of the drug covalently bound to DNA. At high concentrations, RNA and protein synthesis also are inhibited. Mitomycin also can participate in free radical reactions. It is cell cycle nonspecific but appears to be most active in the late G_1 and early S phases. Decreased drug activation, increased inactivation by conjugation to glutathione, and increased DNA repair have been implicated in mitomycin resistance induced in cultured cell lines (Dorr, 1988). Mitomycin also has induced multidrug resistance in one cell line.

USES. Mitomycin is used in the palliative treatment of various solid tumors. It is part of the FAM regimen used in gastric carcinoma (see index entry Cancer: Clinical Response to Chemotherapeutic Drugs). Other indications are non-small cell lung, cervical, colorectal, breast, bladder, pancreatic, prostatic, and esophageal carcinomas. In addition to its systemic use in combination regimens for these tumors, mitomycin has been used as a single agent given by intrahepatic infusion for hepatic metastases from colorectal carcinoma and by intravesical instillation for carcinoma in situ of the bladder. Mitomycin also has been combined with fluorouracil and radiation therapy for carcinoma of the anal canal. Compared to traditional surgical approaches, combined chemoradiotherapy improves survival and enhances the quality of life by preserving organ function (Vokes and Weichselbaum, 1990). Solutions of mitomycin also have been used as ophthalmic drops for treatment of primary and recurrent pterygium (Singh et al, 1988; Hayasaka et al, 1989).

ADVERSE REACTIONS AND PRECAUTIONS. The most significant toxic effect is dose-limiting myelosuppression, which is delayed and appears to be dose- and schedule-dependent. After a single dose of 20 mg/M^2, the average time to nadir is three and one-half weeks for leukopenia and four weeks for thrombocytopenia. Leukopenia persists for one to two weeks and thrombocytopenia for two to three weeks. The blood count recovers in about 75% of patients within eight weeks but does not return to within normal limits in the remaining 25%. With total doses >50 mg, thrombocytopenia is more frequent than leukopenia or anemia. There also is a cumulative effect and more profound and prolonged myelosuppression is noted in subsequent courses.

Other adverse reactions include nausea, vomiting, anorexia, and stomatitis. Severe alopecia and skin rashes occur infrequently. The reported incidence of mild hair loss in patients treated with mitomycin (alone or in combination with mitoxantrone) varies from about 18% to almost 100%. When administered by intravesical instillation, multiple treatments can cause cystitis and eczematous eruptions.

Renal toxicity, in the form of glomerular sclerosis, has been observed after several months of therapy. It does not appear to be dose related and is manifested by increased levels of BUN and serum creatinine and often severe hypertension. Abnormal liver function tests also have been reported, and large doses of mitomycin can cause lethal veno-occlusive liver disease. Severe pulmonary toxicity (interstitial pneumonitis) also may occur. Other rare manifestations of toxicity include fever, drowsiness, and diarrhea.

Cardiomyopathy has been reported in patients treated initially with doxorubicin and subsequently with mitomycin. The length of the interval between the final dose of doxorubicin and the onset of congestive heart failure after mitomycin administration suggests that mitomycin may have enhanced subclinical cardiac damage that resulted from the administration of doxorubicin. Cardiotoxicity has not been reported in patients treated with mitomycin who did not receive other cardiotoxic drugs.

With multiple courses of mitomycin, a thrombotic microangiopathy resembling the hemolytic uremic syndrome has been observed. The mechanism responsible for this reaction is unknown, and no consistently effective treatment has been identified. Immunoperfusion (column pheresis) through immobilized staphylococcal protein A may be used in an attempt to remove circulating immune complexes. However, recovery from hemolytic uremic syndrome has not been consistent or long-lasting in immunoperfused patients.

Extravasation causes severe cellulitis and ulceration, sometimes necessitating plastic surgery.

Mitomycin is teratogenic and carcinogenic in animals.

PHARMACOKINETICS. Absorption of mitomycin after oral administration is erratic; therefore, it is given intravenously for systemic chemotherapy. The drug is cleared rapidly from plasma after intravenous administration (distribution half-life, 2 to 10 minutes and a β half-life of 50 to 60 minutes). The agent is widely distributed throughout body tissues, except the central nervous system, and is metabolized rapidly, primarily in the liver. However, hepatic or renal dysfunction does not appear to alter mitomycin clearance, and thus does not require dose modifications. From 1% to 20% of a dose is excreted unchanged in the urine. Urinary excretion increases with increasing dose, however, due to saturation of metabolic pathways.

DOSAGE AND PREPARATIONS.

Intravenous: 10 to 20 mg/M^2 as a bolus every six to eight weeks administered through a running intravenous line. Because of cumulative myelosuppression, patients must be reevaluated after each course. Subsequent doses are adjusted on the basis of the nadir of myelosuppression from the previous dose and should not be administered until the leukocyte count has returned to 4,000/mm^3 and the platelet count to 100,000/mm^3. Doses greater than 20 mg/M^2 are more toxic but not more effective. The dose must be reduced when this drug is used with other myelosuppressive agents.

Mutamycin (Bristol-Myers Squibb). Powder 5, 20, and 40 mg with 10, 40, and 80 mg of mannitol, respectively.

PLICAMYCIN (Mithramycin)
[Mithracin]

For chemical formula, see index entry Plicamycin, In Hypercalcemia.

ACTIONS. This chromomycin antibiotic is produced by *Streptomyces plicatus*. It binds tightly to DNA by nonintercalative modes to inhibit nucleic acid synthesis. RNA synthesis is more severely affected than DNA synthesis. It is cell cycle nonspecific with some S phase selectivity. Plicamycin also affects calcium metabolism, probably by suppressing osteoclastic bone resorption.

USES. The only indication for plicamycin is embryonal cell carcinoma of the testes. Since it exhibits considerable toxicity and other effective drugs (eg, cisplatin, bleomycin, vinblastine) are available, plicamycin is now a secondary drug for testicular cancer. Lower doses of plicamycin have been effective in severe hypercalcemia unresponsive to conventional therapy (see index entry Plicamycin, In Hypercalcemia).

ADVERSE REACTIONS AND PRECAUTIONS. The most important toxic effect associated with plicamycin is a dose-related bleeding syndrome that usually begins with an episode of epistaxis. Severe coagulation defects resulting in hemorrhagic diathesis and even death due to uncontrolled gastrointestinal hemorrhage have been reported. This syndrome is manifested by thrombocytopenia, prolonged prothrombin time, and depressed clotting factors II, V, VII, and X. The drug should be administered only to hospitalized patients and those who can be observed carefully with frequent monitoring of platelet count and prothrombin time during and after therapy. Leukopenia occurs less frequently.

Most patients experience anorexia, nausea, and vomiting, which may begin one to two hours after initiation of therapy and persist for 12 to 24 hours. The prior use of antiemetics may be helpful. Diarrhea and stomatitis occur occasionally. Other adverse effects are fever, facial flushing, acneiform rashes, drowsiness, lethargy, malaise, headache, and depression.

Abnormal results of liver and renal function tests have been observed, and the serum calcium level is often decreased. Before each dose, the lactic dehydrogenase and blood urea nitrogen levels, prothrombin time, and platelet count must be monitored. Plicamycin is contraindicated in patients with coagulation disorders or thrombocytopenia. It should be used with extreme caution in those with impaired liver and kidney function.

Plicamycin is classified in FDA Pregnancy Category X.

PHARMACOKINETICS. Plicamycin has minimal activity after oral administration and is usually given by intravenous infusion. It is excreted rapidly in the urine (25% within two hours and 40% after 15 hours). Cerebrospinal fluid levels are comparable to those in the blood at four to six hours.

DOSAGE AND PREPARATIONS.

Intravenous: The manufacturer's recommended dose is 0.025 to 0.03 mg/kg/day for 8 to 10 days. An alternative schedule is 0.05 mg/kg (or 1.75 mg/M^2) every two days for three to eight doses every four weeks. This schedule is less toxic than daily administration. The dose is diluted in 1,000 ml of 5% dextrose in water or normal saline and infused over four to six hours. Extravasation can cause local irritation and cellulitis.

For the dosage used in hypercalcemia, see index entry Plicamycin, In Hypercalcemia.

Mithracin (Miles). Powder (cryodesiccated) 2.5 mg with mannitol 100 mg and sufficient disodium phosphate to adjust to pH 7.

DIDEMNIN B (DID-B) (Investigational drug)

ACTIONS AND USES. Didemnin B is a novel cyclic peptide antibiotic extracted from the sea squirt, *Trididemnum*. Cells exposed to didemnin B are killed throughout the cell cycle. Inhibition of progression from G_1 to S phase has been noted. Protein synthesis is affected more than DNA or RNA synthesis. However, the exact mechanism of action is unknown.

Didemnin B has antineoplastic, immunosuppressive, and antiviral properties. In preclinical studies, didemnin B was shown to have activity against rodent and human tumors.

ADVERSE REACTIONS. In Phase I trials, the dose-limiting toxicity was nausea and vomiting. Hepatic dysfunction, diarrhea, anorexia, fatigue, malaise, and phlebitis also may occur. Hypersensitivity reactions (probably related to the vehicle, polyoxyethylated castor oil) have been observed. Myelosuppression has not been reported.

DOSAGE (investigational regimen).

Intravenous: 3.47 mg/M^2 every 28 days.

ECHINOMYCIN (Investigational drug)

ACTIONS AND USES. Echinomycin is a cyclic peptide that is one of a family of quinoxaline antibiotics originally isolated from *Streptomyces echinatus*. Antitumor activity appears to result from intercalation into double-stranded DNA. Because the drug has two quinoxaline rings and each can bind to DNA, echinomycin is a bifunctional intercalator.

Preclinical trials have demonstrated activity against rodent and human tumors. Some responses were observed in previously treated women with metastatic or recurrent cervical carcinoma who were given 1.5 mg/M^2 once every four weeks. Phase II trials using weekly administration and larger doses are in progress.

ADVERSE REACTIONS. The dose-limiting toxicity appears to be severe and often protracted nausea and vomiting. Transient hepatic enzyme elevations occur. Allergic reactions including rash, hypotension, bronchospasm, and flushing have been reported. Prerenal azotemia, phlebitis, fever, anorexia, diarrhea, and mild thrombocytopenia also are seen.

DOSAGE (investigational regimen).

Intravenous: 1.2 mg/M^2 infused over a 30-minute period once weekly.

DEOXYSPERGUALIN (Investigational drug)

ACTIONS AND USES. Deoxyspergualin is a synthetic derivative of the antibiotic, spergualin, isolated from culture broths of *Bacillus laterosporus*. This guanidino compound is structurally related to the polyamine, spermine. The drug's mechanism of action is not yet known but may involve metabolic activation to an aldehyde catalyzed by an amine oxidase (Leyland-Jones et al, 1990). Macromolecular synthesis declines in cells exposed to deoxyspergualin; inhibition of DNA synthesis occurs first (about one hour after drug exposure), followed later by inhibition of RNA and protein synthesis. Deoxyspergualin also has a wide range of stimulant and suppressive effects on the immune system, some of which may be related to its antineoplastic activity.

In preclinical studies, the drug was active against leukemia cell lines but was not consistently active against solid tumor lines in various animal tumor models and human tumor xenografts. Schedule dependence was observed: in vivo efficacy was greater when the drug was given as a continuous infusion rather than by bolus administration. Therefore, current clinical trials are evaluating the usefulness of five-day infusions of deoxyspergualin for antitumor therapy. This drug also has immunosuppressant activity through a mechanism that is not mediated by T cells.

PHARMACOKINETICS. Clearance of deoxyspergualin from the circulation appears to follow a biexponential decay curve, with half-lives for the two phases of about 10 minutes and about 70 minutes. The route of elimination is unknown.

ADVERSE REACTIONS. Hypotension is dose limiting and occurs when >2 g/M^2/day is administered. Other adverse reactions include myelosuppression (thrombocytopenia, leukopenia, and anemia), gastrointestinal effects (nausea, vomiting, and diarrhea), and paresthesias. Gastrointestinal bleeding and epithelial ulceration have occurred in some patients.

DOSAGE (investigational regimen).

Intravenous: 1.5 g/M^2/day by continuous infusion for five days.

Deoxyspergualin (Bristol-Myers Squibb).

Synthetic Intercalators and Topoisomerase Inhibitors

Because of the serious cumulative cardiotoxicity caused by the anthracycline antibiotics, a variety of analogues was synthesized in attempts to reduce their ability to cause this adverse reaction yet retain their broad spectrum and potent activity as antitumor agents. In addition to semisynthetic derivatives that retained the anthracycline aglycone ring structure (eg, epirubicin, esorubicin, idarubicin), several other planar polycyclic ring systems have been synthesized and evaluated for antineoplastic activity. It was recognized that the planar ring systems were capable of binding to DNA by intercalation between adjacent base pairs and that such binding contributed to the antitumor effects of the anthracyclines. Among the synthetic intercalators, the anthracenedione compound, mitoxantrone, is the first to become generally available for cancer treatment. An aminoacridine, amsacrine, is used in a variety of investigational combination regimens for leukemias and some lymphomas. A third group of synthetic intercalators, the anthrapyrazoles, is represented by the investigational drug, piroxantrone. Once the role of topoisomerase II had been identified as a target for antitumor drug actions, most of the synthetic intercalators were shown to inhibit this enzyme and to generate protein-linked DNA strand breaks as a consequence. Two newer investigational agents, amonafide and merbarone, whose structures are not derived from those of the anthracyclines, also appear to interact with topoisomerase.

MITOXANTRONE HYDROCHLORIDE (Dihydroxyanthracenedione, DHAQ)

[Novantrone]

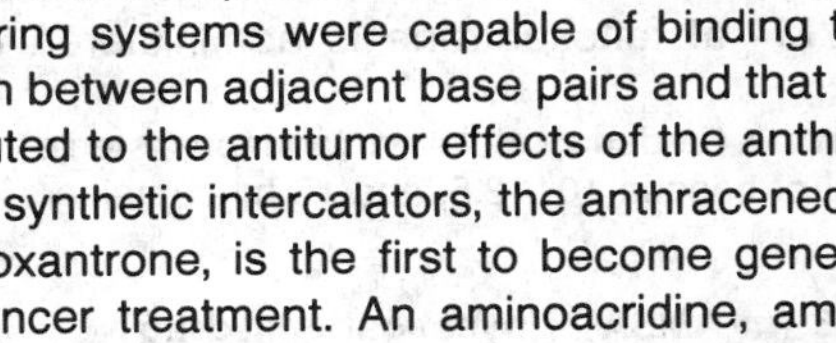

OH O $NHCH_2CH_2NHCH_2CH_2OH$

· 2HCl

OH O $NHCH_2CH_2NHCH_2CH_2OH$

ACTIONS. Mitoxantrone is a substituted aminoalkylanthracenedione originally synthesized as a structural analogue of doxorubicin. Although the mechanism of action is not definitively understood, mitoxantrone is known to inhibit both RNA and DNA synthesis in cell culture systems (Shenkenberg and Von Hoff, 1986). Mitoxantrone intercalates into double-stranded DNA in vitro, but this binding mode does not appear to be responsible for its antitumor efficacy. A second electrostatic mode of DNA binding is thought to be involved in the generation of DNA strand breaks in cells treated with mitoxantrone.

The drug also causes DNA-protein cross-links and protein-associated DNA strand breaks. The latter appear to be mediated by binding to and inhibition of topoisomerase II. In cell culture systems, cross-resistance has been demonstrated between mitoxantrone and the anthracyclines, as well as between mitoxantrone and the vinca alkaloids. Thus, both the gp-170 mediated drug efflux and altered topoisomerase activity forms of multidrug resistance can contribute to loss of cellular sensitivity to mitoxantrone. Mitoxantrone has been reported to be less active in generating oxygen, peroxide, and hydroxyl radicals than other antineoplastic quinones (eg, the anthracyclines). Its effects do not seem to be cell cycle specific; however, the concentrations required to produce cytotoxicity are significantly higher in nonproliferating cells than in proliferating cells. Cell kinetic studies have demonstrated that the drug blocks progression in the G_2 phase.

USES. Mitoxantrone is used in a variety of combination regimens for initial therapy of acute myelogenous leukemia in adults. In a recent randomized trial, mitoxantrone plus cytarabine was compared with daunorubicin plus cytarabine (at equitoxic dose levels) for induction of remission in previously untreated adults with acute myelogenous leukemia. The frequency of complete remissions after a single course was higher with the mitoxantrone/cytarabine combination (Arlin et al, 1990); however, these observations require confirmation by additional randomized trials. The combination of mitoxantrone with high-dose cytarabine also was shown to be active in adults with advanced acute lymphocytic leukemia who had not responded to previous chemotherapy (Kantarjian et al, 1990).

In addition, mitoxantrone currently is being investigated for use in other malignancies and has produced some objective responses when administered as a single agent in patients with advanced or metastatic breast cancer and refractory malignant lymphoma (primarily non-Hodgkin's). Worldwide, mitoxantrone has been used more extensively for treatment of breast cancer than for acute leukemia. In trials comparing mitoxantrone with doxorubicin (both as single agents and in combination with cyclophosphamide and fluorouracil) in patients with advanced breast cancer, mitoxantrone produced slightly lower response rates, similar survival time, and less nonhematologic toxicity (Bennett et al, 1988; Henderson et al, 1989). The high-dose cytarabine/mitoxantrone regimen is also under investigation as salvage therapy for refractory non-Hodgkin's lymphoma.

ADVERSE REACTIONS AND PRECAUTIONS. The repeated daily doses of mitoxantrone used in induction therapy for leukemias almost invariably cause profound myelosuppression. Hematologic toxicity following single bolus doses is manifested primarily as granulocytopenia; the nadir occurs in one to two weeks and recovery is usually noted by the third week but may be delayed as long as four to six weeks. Although mild anemia has been observed in patients treated repeatedly with mitoxantrone, acute effects on erythrocyte levels were not found. Thrombocytopenia occurs in most patients given mitoxantrone as induction therapy for acute leukemia.

Other toxic effects seen frequently include nausea, vomiting, mucositis, fever, and alopecia. Transient blue-green coloration of the urine may result during the first 24 hours after administration, and blue discoloration of the sclera or skin also has been reported. Hepatic and renal toxicity has been observed infrequently. Cardiovascular reactions (arrhythmias, decreased left ventricular ejection fraction sometimes leading to congestive heart failure) also may occur. Their frequency and severity were similar in each arm of a study comparing mitoxantrone plus cytarabine with daunorubicin plus cytarabine for initial treatment of acute myelogenous leukemia in adults (Arlin et al, 1990). When mitoxantrone was given in multiple intermittent doses to patients with solid tumors, the probability of developing congestive heart failure was related to the cumulative dose and to prior treatment with doxorubicin. The probability increased above 5% at cumulative doses >160 mg/M² for patients who did not receive prior doxorubicin therapy and at doses >100 mg/M² for previously treated patients.

The vesicant actions of mitoxantrone are considerably less severe than those of many other antineoplastic drugs (eg, nitrosoureas, anthracyclines, vinca alkaloids). However, tissue necrosis following extravasation of mitoxantrone has been reported rarely.

Mitoxantrone is mutagenic in bacterial systems and can cause chromosomal aberrations, DNA damage, and sister chromatid exchanges in mammalian cells and in animals. The drug was fetotoxic in rats and rabbits but is not teratogenic in rabbits. It is classified in FDA Pregnancy Category D.

PHARMACOKINETICS. Mitoxantrone is rapidly and extensively distributed after intravenous administration to humans. Plasma decay curves appear to be triphasic. An initial rapid phase with a half-life of about 4 to 11 minutes is followed by an intermediate phase with a half-life of 0.3 to 3.1 hours (Ehninger et al, 1990). The long and variable terminal phase (half-life of nine hours to nine days) probably reflects release of the drug from tissue binding sites. The large volume of distribution and high concentrations of drug that can be measured in extracts of autopsy tissue also suggest that mitoxantrone is extensively bound in tissue. Most of the drug present in plasma is bound to protein regardless of the concentration and despite the presence of other drugs known to bind extensively to proteins (eg, phenytoin, doxorubicin, methotrexate, prednisone, aspirin).

Mitoxantrone is excreted by both the biliary and renal routes. Up to 25% of a dose can be recovered in the feces over five days after treatment; only 6% to 11% of the dose is recovered in the urine during the same period, 65% of which is unchanged drug. The remainder consists of two inactive metabolites and their glucuronide conjugates. Mitoxantrone is metabolized in the liver and generates primarily mono- and dicarboxylic acid derivatives. It may be eliminated more slowly in patients with impaired liver function.

No pharmacokinetic data have been reported in patients receiving multiple daily doses.

DOSAGE AND PREPARATIONS. The concentrated solution should be diluted to at least 50 ml with 0.9% sodium chloride injection or 5% dextrose injection. The diluted solution should be introduced slowly into the tubing of a freely flowing intravenous infusion of 0.9% sodium chloride injection or 5% dextrose injection over not less than three minutes. Mitoxantrone should not be administered in the same infusion as heparin, since precipitation may occur. Mitoxantrone should be stored at 15° to 30° C and should not be frozen.

Intravenous: For induction therapy in adult acute myelogenous leukemia, 12 mg/M² daily on days one to three, with cytarabine given as a continuous infusion over 24 hours on days one to seven. If a complete remission does not occur, additional courses may be given after myelosuppression or other severe toxicity reverses; mitoxantrone is administered for two days and cytarabine for five days. Consolidation therapy, when applied, employs the same dose and schedule as the subsequent courses of induction at six weeks and ten weeks after the final induction course.

When mitoxantrone is given alone for treatment of advanced breast cancer, 12 to 14 mg/M² once every three weeks. When it is used with cyclophosphamide and fluorouracil, 10 mg/M² of mitoxantrone is administered once every three weeks.

Novantrone (Lederle). Solution (aqueous, sterile) equivalent to 2 mg/ml of base in 10, 12.5, and 15 ml containers.

AMSACRINE (m-AMSA) (Investigational drug)
[Amsidyl]

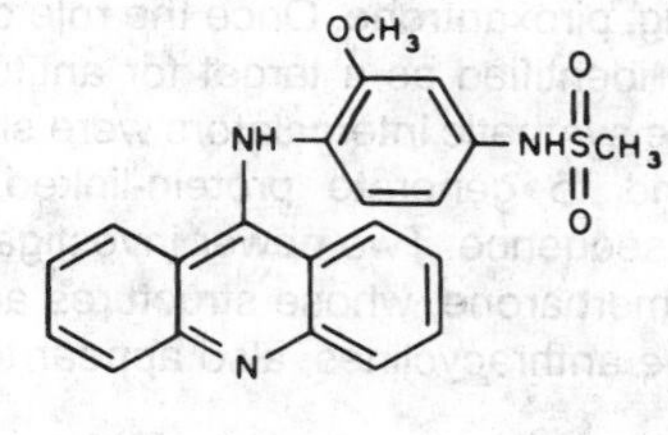

ACTIONS. Amsacrine is a synthetic aminoacridine that exerts its cytotoxic effect by intercalating DNA and inhibiting DNA synthesis. The drug is probably cell cycle nonspecific, but cells in G_2 and S phases are more sensitive. Although the mechanism of action of amsacrine is not known definitively, the drug does form a ternary complex with DNA and the enzyme, topoisomerase II, which results in inhibition of the enzyme's strand-rejoining reaction (Ross et al, 1988; Liu, 1989). Consequently, protein-linked strand breaks are introduced into cellular DNA, and the function of topoisomerase in DNA replication, repair, and transcription is impaired. In vitro, resistance to amsacrine can follow one of several patterns, and may include contributions from the gp-170 mediated drug efflux pump and alterations in either the quantity or the sensitivity to drug inhibition of topoisomerase II (Tan et al, 1989; Finlay et al, 1990).

USES. The primary use of this drug is for induction of remission in acute leukemia in adults who have relapsed or failed to respond to first-line drugs. Amsacrine has induced complete remissions in 10% to 20% of patients with acute myelogenous leukemia unresponsive to cytarabine and anthracyclines. However, remission durations have been short. Amsacrine also has modest activity in acute lymphocytic leukemia and non-Hodgkin's lymphoma.

ADVERSE REACTIONS AND PRECAUTIONS. Leukopenia develops in almost all patients and is the usual dose-limiting toxicity. Nadirs occur around day 12 and recovery occurs between days 25 and 28. Amsacrine can cause serious ventricular arrhythmias with increased QT intervals on the electrocardiogram and polymorphic ventricular tachycardia (torsades de pointes). In patients who receive both amsacrine and anthracyclines, the cardiotoxic effects produced by these drugs may be additive. Other reported adverse reactions include mild nausea and vomiting, mucositis, seizures, and local tissue irritation.

PHARMACOKINETICS. The terminal half-life after intravenous administration ranges from 7 to 17.4 hours. Amsacrine is metabolized in the liver and excreted via the bile. Patients with hepatic dysfunction require dosage adjustments.

DOSAGE (investigational regimen).
Intravenous: For induction of remission in acute leukemia, 120 to 200 mg/M^2 daily for five days.

Amsacrine (Bristol-Myers Squibb), ***Amsidyl*** (Parke-Davis).

AMONAFIDE (5-Aminomitonafide, nafidimide, BIDA) (Investigational drug)

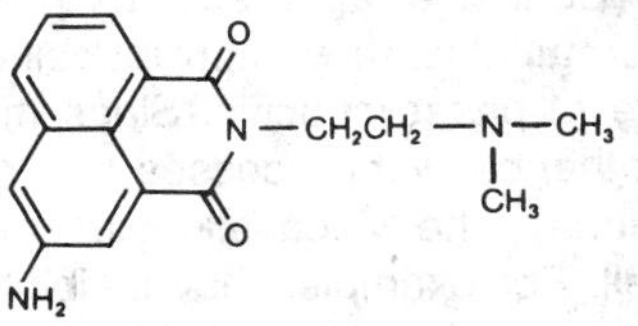

ACTIONS AND USES. Amonafide is a synthetic intercalating agent whose structure is derived from naphthalene-1,8-dicarboxylic acid (Leyland-Jones et al, 1990). Concentrations of the drug needed to inhibit DNA replication are lower than those needed to block RNA synthesis. Protein-linked DNA strand breaks can be detected in cultured cells treated with amonafide, but it is unclear if these result from the drug's interaction with topoisomerase I, topoisomerase II, or both (Andersson et al, 1987).

Preclinical studies demonstrated that amonafide has promising activity against a variety of animal tumor models, human tumor cell lines, and xenografts. Data suggest that amonafide might not be fully cross-resistant with all other topoisomerase inhibitors (eg, amsacrine). Phase II trials to identify the spectrum of clinical activity for amonafide are in progress.

ADVERSE REACTIONS. Reversible myelosuppression was the dose-limiting toxicity for amonafide in Phase I trials (Legha et al, 1987). The severity was quite variable, but blood cell counts returned to near normal three to four weeks after treatment in all patients. Bolus administration caused chest pain, flushing, and shortness of breath in most patients, but these symptoms were not observed with longer infusions. Other adverse reactions included mild nausea and vomiting, phlebitis, alopecia, malaise, fatigue, anorexia, and, rarely, allergic reactions.

PHARMACOKINETICS. After intravenous administration, amonafide is cleared by metabolism, followed by urinary excretion. The plasma concentration curve follows a triexponential decay, with mean half-lives of 12 to 17 minutes, 150 minutes, and 11 to 16 hours in humans. At least five different metabolites have been detected, including an N-acetyl derivative. This suggests that acetylator phenotype may affect clearance rates. Very little unchanged drug can be detected in the urine, and some of the drug or its metabolites may appear in the cerebrospinal fluid.

DOSAGE (investigational regimens).
Intravenous: 300 to 400 mg/M^2/day for five days every three to four weeks, with dose reductions in subsequent cycles based on nadir blood counts. Alternative schedules include 690 to 800 mg/M^2 given as a 30- to 60-minute infusion on day 1 only or 1.6 g/M^2 as a 24-hour continuous infusion every 21 days.

MERBARONE (Investigational drug)

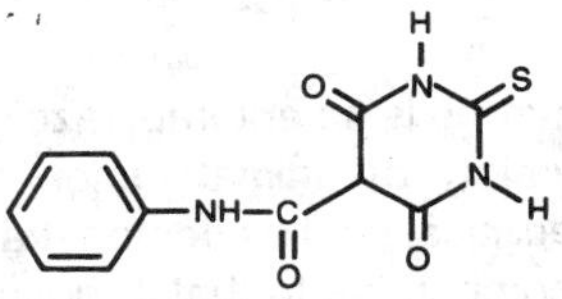

ACTIONS. This aniline amide of thiobarbituric acid has activity against a broad spectrum of animal tumors (Leyland-Jones et al, 1990). The mechanism of action has not yet been established, but cells treated with merbarone accumulate protein-linked DNA strand breaks as a result of the drug's inhibition of topoisomerase II. Merbarone is cross-resistant with amsacrine and other topoisomerase inhibitors but not with vincristine in cells expressing high levels of the drug efflux pump (gp-170). Merbarone inhibits DNA synthesis, and cell cycle progression appears to be blocked in late S phase. Preclinical studies of this drug in animal tumor models showed that it was most active when given on consecutive days. Phase II trials are underway.

ADVERSE REACTIONS. The dose-limiting toxicity for merbarone (administered as a continuous infusion for five days) was reversible renal dysfunction (interstitial nephritis or renal tubular injury). Hypouricemia (as a result of the drug or its metabolites inhibiting tubular reabsorption, through their inhibition of xanthine oxidase, or both) was observed in all patients. Phlebitis occurred when the drug was infused into a peripheral vein but not when it was given through a large central venous catheter. Other adverse responses include nausea and vomiting, diarrhea, and sporadic instances of myelosuppression.

PHARMACOKINETICS. Plasma levels of merbarone decline following a biexponential decay curve, with half-lives of about one hour and 12.5 to 14.2 hours for the two phases. Clearance rates do not appear to be dose- or schedule-dependent. Less than 30% of the drug is cleared by renal excretion, and nearly all of that fraction is present in the urine as metabolites. The major routes of metabolism involve hydroxylation (of the aniline ring) and desulfuration of the thiobarbiturate moiety. Plasma concentrations of the metabolites are maintained at much lower levels than those of merbarone, suggesting that the biotransformation products are excreted much more rapidly than the parent drug.

DOSAGE (investigational regimen).

Intravenous: 1.5 g/M^2/day by continuous 24-hour infusion for five days.

PIROXANTRONE HYDROCHLORIDE (PIX) (Investigational drug)

CH_2CH_2—NH—CH_2CH_2—OH
OH N—N
1.7 HCl
OH O NH—$(CH_2)_3$—NH_2

ACTIONS. Piroxantrone is an anthrapyrazole with curative activity against a variety of animal tumor models (Leyland-Jones, 1990). Preclinical studies demonstrated that the activity of this drug is comparable to that of doxorubicin and that it is more potent than mitoxantrone and amsacrine in some systems. This, together with the fact that it has considerably less potent cardiotoxic effects than the anthracyclines, resulted in clinical investigation of piroxantrone as an antitumor drug. Phase II trials have begun.

Piroxantrone has a high affinity for intercalative binding with DNA and inhibits DNA synthesis at low concentrations and RNA synthesis at higher levels. The inhibition appears to result from binding to the template rather than directly to DNA polymerase. Protein-linked DNA strand breaks accumulate in cells treated with piroxantrone, suggesting that the drug inhibits topoisomerase II. However, concentrations required for strand-break production are tenfold higher than those needed for cytocidal effects, which suggests that other mechanisms may be more important for cytotoxicity.

ADVERSE REACTIONS. Myelosuppression (possibly cumulative) is the dose-limiting toxicity for piroxantrone, with neutropenia more common than thrombocytopenia. Other reactions include nausea, vomiting, mucositis, alopecia, and local effects (phlebitis, erythema, pain, burning, and pruritus) at the site of infusion.

PHARMACOKINETICS. Clearance of the drug in humans follows a biexponential decay curve, with mean half-lives of about 3 and 20 minutes. The drug is unstable in plasma, but its metabolism in patients has not yet been determined.

ALKALOIDS AND THEIR DERIVATIVES

Alkaloids are nitrogenous bases, most often isolated from plants, which usually are protonated and thus carry positive charge at physiologic pH. Many alkaloids have been identified in extracts of folk remedies and medicinal herbs. The periwinkle (*Catharanthus roseus*; formerly named *Vinca rosea*) is a plant whose medicinal properties had been described in various cultures from different parts of the world. The vinca alkaloids, vincristine and vinblastine, were fractionated from extracts of this plant, identified, and shown to have potent antineoplastic activity more than 30 years ago. An extensive screening program sponsored by the National Cancer Institute and the United States Department of Agriculture resulted in identification of other alkaloids with antitumor properties. Podophyllotoxin, isolated from the mayapple or mandrake plant, was one such compound; its excessive toxicity led to the development of semisynthetic analogues, the epipodophyllotoxins, etoposide and teniposide. A number of other plant alkaloids are in various stages of investigation for development as new antineoplastic drugs.

Vinca Alkaloids

Vinca alkaloids are mitotic inhibitors that act by complexing with tubulin, the protein component of microtubules and the mitotic spindle (Bender et al, 1990). By interfering with the assembly of microtubules, they interrupt cell division in metaphase. They are M phase specific. Since microtubules also are involved in other cellular processes (eg, axonal transport, secretory functions), the vinca alkaloids may affect these functions as well. For example, they inhibit the secretion of some hormones (eg, glucose-induced insulin release, TSH-mediated thyroid hormone secretions) and proteins.

Although vincristine and vinblastine have similar chemical structures and mechanisms of action, there are important differences in antitumor activity and dose-limiting toxicities. Also, patients who become resistant to one often respond to the other, which probably reflects differences in dosage rather than a true absence of cross-resistance.

Because the gastrointestinal absorption of vincristine and vinblastine is unpredictable, these drugs are given intravenously. They are highly irritating to tissue, however, and special precautions must be taken to avoid extravasation. Although the pharmacokinetics of the vinca alkaloids have not been delineated clearly, both drugs show triphasic elimination, primarily by biliary excretion and metabolism. Very little (3% to 8%) of either drug is recovered in the urine. The presently available pharmacologic data fail to explain the important clinical differences between vincristine and vinblastine.

Resistance to the vinca alkaloids may result from mutations in the tubulin protein, which affects drug binding; by decreased uptake; or by increased capacity for drug efflux. This latter phenomenon may account for concomitant resistance to anthracyclines and dactinomycin (ie, multiple drug resistance) and is associated with increased expression of the membrane glycoprotein (gp-170) drug efflux pump (Deuchars and Ling, 1989; van der Bliek and Borst, 1989).

A related compound, vindesine, was first isolated as a metabolite of vinblastine but is now produced as a semisynthetic derivative of vinblastine. It is an investigational agent in the United States but is marketed in many European and other countries.

VINBLASTINE SULFATE
[Velban, Velsar]

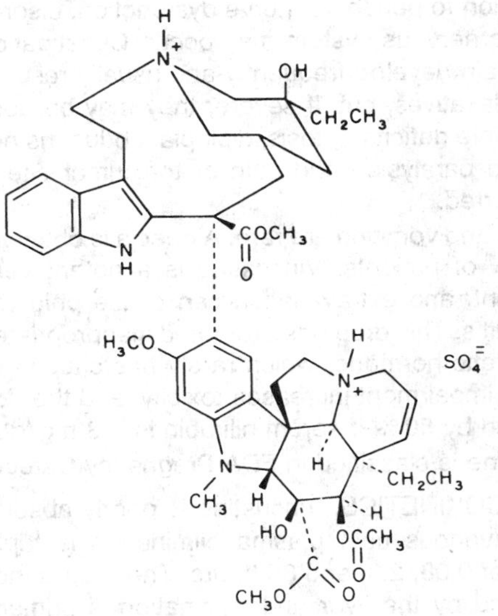

ACTIONS. Vinblastine is the sulfate salt of a dimeric alkaloid derived from the periwinkle plant, *Catharanthus*. It binds to tubulin and prevents the assembly of the microtubular components of the mitotic spindle, leading to metaphase arrest (Bender et al, 1990).

USES. Vinblastine, in combination with cisplatin and bleomycin, is a preferred regimen in disseminated nonseminomatous testicular cancer (Loehrer et al, 1988; Williams et al, 1989 A). Most patients treated with this regimen achieve long-term disease-free survival. This drug also is a component of the ABVD regimen, an effective alternative to MOPP, in the treatment of advanced Hodgkin's disease (see index entry Cancer: Clinical Response to Chemotherapeutic Drugs) (Hellman et al, 1989; Haskell and Parker, 1990). Vinblastine is active (either alone or with other drugs) in non-Hodgkin's lymphomas; choriocarcinoma; breast, bladder, cervical, non-small cell lung, and renal carcinomas; neuroblastoma; head and neck cancer; melanoma; cutaneous T-cell lymphomas; Kaposi's sarcoma (systemic or intralesional); and Langerhans cell histiocytosis (also called histiocytosis X or Abt-Letterer-Siwe disease).

ADVERSE REACTIONS AND PRECAUTIONS. Dose-limiting leukopenia is the most common toxic effect of vinblastine, with the nadir occurring within five to ten days; recovery is observed within 7 to 14 days. With larger doses, the white blood cell count may not return to normal levels for three weeks. Thrombocytopenia occurs less frequently and anemia is uncommon.

Neurotoxic effects have been reported in 5% to 20% of patients and include paresthesias, loss of deep tendon reflexes, peripheral neuritis, mental depression, headache, and convulsions. Neurotoxicity is much less common than with vincristine at the usual clinical doses of vinblastine.

Nausea and vomiting are common but usually can be controlled by antiemetic agents. Other gastrointestinal effects are stomatitis, glossitis, constipation, and adynamic ileus. Raynaud's phenomenon has recently been reported with use of vinblastine and/or bleomycin in testicular cancer.

Alopecia is reversible. Extravasation can cause phlebitis and severe cellulitis. Local injection of hyaluronidase and application of moderate heat have been suggested to help disperse the drug, minimize discomfort, and possibly avoid cellulitis when extravasation occurs. However, treatment regimens for extravasation of vinca alkaloids have not been evaluated in controlled clinical trials or animal studies.

Caution is necessary when vinblastine is used during pregnancy because animal studies suggest that teratogenic effects may occur (FDA Pregnancy Category D).

PHARMACOKINETICS. Vinblastine is poorly absorbed when given orally. After intravenous administration, there is a triphasic plasma clearance (first half-life, 0.06 hours; second half-life, 1.6 hours; third half-life, 25 hours). Approximately 80% of the drug is bound to plasma proteins. Vinblastine is excreted primarily in bile; 30% is excreted in stool as metabolites over the first three days, and 21% is excreted in the urine.

DOSAGE AND PREPARATIONS. Vinblastine is usually given as a bolus once every seven days, but it also has been administered as a five-day continuous infusion. However, there are no data to suggest that antitumor activity is enhanced by continuous infusion rather than bolus administration. Dosage is based on body surface area and weekly white blood cell counts and should be decreased in the presence of liver disease (at least a 50% reduction if the serum bilirubin is >3 mg/dL). *Vinblastine should never be given intrathecally, since this route will cause fatal neurotoxicity.*

Intravenous: Initially, 3.7 mg/M^2 for *adults* and 2.5 mg/M^2 for *children,* repeated once weekly. Subsequent doses may be increased progressively if the preceding dose did not reduce leukocyte counts below 3,000/mm^3. Doses of 18.5 mg/M^2 for *adults* and 12.5 mg/M^2 for *children* should not be exceeded. If given as a continuous infusion, 1 to 2 mg/M^2/day for five days. In combination with cisplatin and bleomycin for testicular cancer, 0.3 to 0.4 mg/kg is given once every three weeks for four courses.

Velban (Lilly), ***Velsar*** (Adria), ***Generic.*** Powder (lyophilized, sterile) 10 mg.

VINCRISTINE SULFATE
[Oncovin, Vincasar PFS]

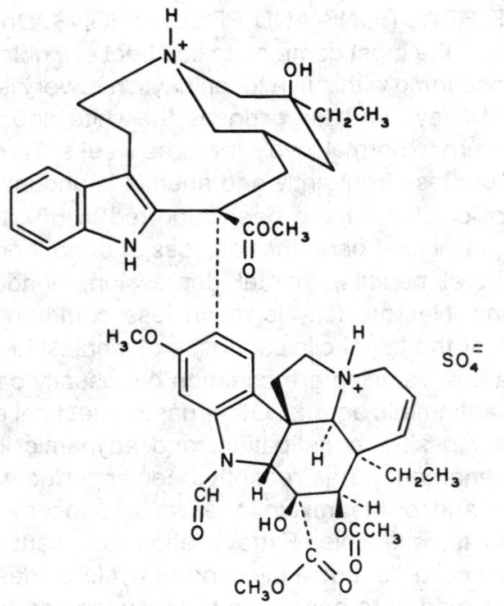

ACTIONS. Vincristine is the sulfate salt of a dimeric alkaloid extracted from the periwinkle plant. It is M phase specific and blocks mitosis with metaphase arrest by binding to tubulin and inhibiting the assembly of microtubules (Bender et al, 1990).

USES. Vincristine is active in a number of neoplastic diseases, including leukemias, lymphomas, sarcomas, and some carcinomas. Because it lacks dose-limiting myelosuppressive activity (see below), this drug is used extensively in combination regimens (see index entry Cancer: Clinical Response to Chemotherapeutic Drugs and the section on Combination Chemotherapy in Chapter 1 of this Section).

When vincristine is combined with prednisone, complete remissions are induced in up to 90% of children with acute lymphocytic leukemia (Poplack et al, 1989; Donohue and Charlton, 1989; Mauer, 1990). The further addition of asparaginase or daunorubicin prolongs disease-free remissions. Similar regimens that include vincristine are used to treat acute lymphocytic leukemia in adults. Vincristine also is very effective in combination regimens used to treat malignant lymphomas, including Hodgkin's, non-Hodgkin's, and Burkitt's lymphomas. For example, the combination of mechlorethamine, vincristine, procarbazine, and prednisone (MOPP) is one of the preferred regimens for treating advanced Hodgkin's disease and a high percentage of patients are cured (Hellman et al, 1989; Haskell and Parker, 1990). Combination regimens containing vincristine also are among the treatments of choice in Ewing's sarcoma, neuroblastoma, embryonal rhabdomyosarcoma, Wilms' tumor, soft tissue sarcomas, and small-cell lung carcinoma (see index entry Cancer: Clinical Response to Chemotherapeutic Drugs). Vincristine also is active in acute myelogenous leukemia, chronic lymphocytic leukemia, multiple myeloma, and breast and cervical carcinomas.

ADVERSE REACTIONS. In contrast to vinblastine, vincristine does not produce serious bone marrow depression, which makes it particularly useful in combination with myelosuppressive agents. Leukopenia may develop but there is no effect on red blood cells or platelets.

Neurologic toxicity, particularly peripheral neuropathy, is usually dose limiting and is caused by vincristine binding to tubulin in neurotubules. Because of its marked neurotoxic effects, *vincristine should never be injected intrathecally.* The drug is almost invariably fatal when given by this route. Mild sensory neuropathy is common after intravenous administration but does not require discontinuance of therapy. Sensory changes and mild paresthesias, followed by loss of the Achilles tendon reflex, are usually the first signs of peripheral neuropathy. More serious manifestations include severe paresthesias (occasional), loss of deep tendon reflexes, ataxia, foot drop, slapping gait, and muscle wasting. The primary muscle groups involved are the dorsiflexors of the hands and wrists and the extensors of the feet.

In addition to peripheral nerve dysfunction, disorders of the autonomic nervous system may occur. Constipation and abdominal pain develop frequently and usually respond to enemas and laxatives, but, if severe, they may be dose limiting. Cranial nerve deficits (ptosis, diplopia, abducens nerve palsy, vocal cord paralysis) and pain at the tumor site also have been reported.

Nausea and vomiting are rare. Alopecia is observed in more than 20% of patients. Vincristine is a potent vesicant and local irritant, and extravasation can cause phlebitis and severe cellulitis. This drug has promoted inappropriate secretion of antidiuretic hormone, which rarely has caused hyponatremia. Liver impairment increases toxicity, and the dose should be reduced by 50% if serum bilirubin is >3 mg/dL.

Vincristine is classified in FDA Pregnancy Category D.

PHARMACOKINETICS. Vincristine is poorly absorbed orally. After intravenous use, plasma elimination is triphasic with half-lives of 0.08, 2.3, and 85 hours. The drug is incompletely metabolized by the liver and elimination is primarily via the bile; approximately 70% of a dose is excreted in the feces and about 12% is eliminated in the urine. Obstruction of liver outflow may require careful adjustment of dosage. Vincristine does not penetrate the central nervous system.

DOSAGE AND PREPARATIONS.

Intravenous: *Adults,* 1.4 mg/M^2 once weekly. *Children older than 1 year,* 2 mg/M^2 once weekly. *Children less than 10 kg or with body surface area less than 1 M^2,* 0.05 mg/kg once weekly to avoid excessive neurotoxicity. The therapeutic effect does not appear to be dose related, and toxic reactions increase significantly without increased benefit with larger doses. The drug is administered through a running intravenous line or is injected with care to prevent extravasation. The dose should be reduced in patients with liver disease (at least a 50% reduction if the serum bilirubin concentration is >3 mg/dL). Concurrent radiation to the liver can affect vincristine's metabolism. *Vincristine should not be given intrathecally since this causes fatal ascending paralysis.*

Oncovin (Lilly), ***Generic.*** Solution 1 mg/ml in 1, 2, and 5 ml containers.

Vincasar PFS (Adria). Solution 1 mg/ml in 1 and 2 ml containers.

VINDESINE SULFATE (Investigational drug)
[Eldisine]

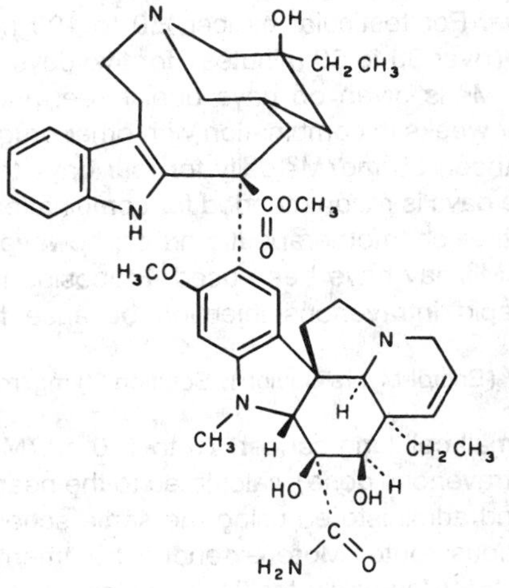

ACTIONS AND USES. This semisynthetic derivative of vinblastine produces mitotic arrest by disrupting the assembly of microtubules.

Vindesine has been active in a variety of cancers, including acute lymphoblastic leukemia, Hodgkin's and non-Hodgkin's lymphomas, breast and esophageal carcinoma, malignant melanoma, and non-small cell lung cancer.

ADVERSE REACTIONS AND PRECAUTIONS. Like vinblastine, the usual dose-limiting toxicity of vindesine is reversible myelosuppression, with neutropenia predominating over thrombocytopenia. Neurotoxicity is usually less severe than that caused by vincristine but may be dose limiting. *Intrathecal injection of vindesine causes death from ascending paralysis.* Neurotoxic reactions occur significantly less frequently with vindesine than with vincristine but are more common than with vinblastine. Paresthesias, muscle weakness, and loss of deep tendon reflexes occur frequently. Cumulative neurotoxicity precludes the use of vindesine with other vinca alkaloids. Gastrointestinal symptoms include nausea, vomiting, and diarrhea. Alopecia ranges from mild to total hair loss. Dermatitis, stomatitis, fever, and myalgias are less common. Vindesine is a tissue irritant.

PHARMACOKINETICS. Vindesine appears to resemble other vinca alkaloids in its pharmacokinetic and pharmacologic behavior. Elimination from the blood is triphasic after intravenous administration; the mean half-lives are approximately 0.05, 1.6, and 20 hours. The major route of excretion has not been determined in humans, but less than 15% of an administered dose can be recovered from the urine.

DOSAGE (investigational regimens). Each 5-mg ampul is reconstituted with 5 ml of the diluent provided. When refrigerated, the solution is stable for four weeks.

Intravenous: Administration is by slow push into the tubing of a free-flowing intravenous line. The most common dose employed is 3 to 4 mg/M^2 every week. Continuous infusions of 1.2 mg/M^2/day for five days or 2 mg/M^2/day for two days have also been used.

Eldisine (Lilly).

Epipodophyllotoxins

Podophyllotoxin is an alkaloid that was extracted and purified from the mayapple or mandrake plant and was shown to have significant antitumor activity in a variety of preclinical screening systems using cultured human and animal cell lines (Bender et al, 1990). Studies in animal tumor models demonstrated that the level of systemic toxicity was unacceptable, and this led to the development of semisynthetic derivatives that might have improved therapeutic indices. Etoposide and teniposide are two such analogues, collectively termed epipodophyllotoxins.

The site at which podophyllotoxin binds to tubulin is different from that of the vinca alkaloids. Podophyllotoxin's major effect on cells is to prevent microtubule assembly and thus block cells in mitosis. It was first assumed that the epipodophyllotoxins had actions similar to those of the parent alkaloid. It is now known that both etoposide and teniposide form ternary complexes with topoisomerase II and its substrate DNA, inhibit the strand-rejoining reaction of the enzyme's catalytic cycle, and introduce protein-linked strand breaks in the DNA of treated cells. In contrast to podophyllotoxin and the vinca alkaloids, which cause cells to accumulate in the mitotic phase of the cell cycle by inhibiting microtubule assembly, etoposide and teniposide arrest cells in either late S or early G_2 phase and neither bind to tubulin nor affect microtubule assembly.

ETOPOSIDE (VP-16)
[VePesid]

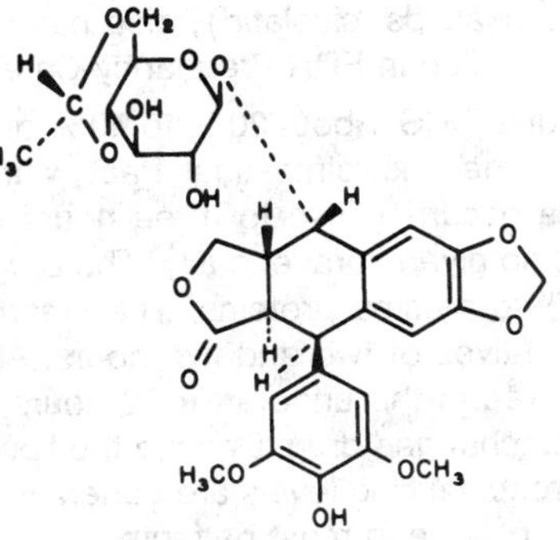

ACTIONS AND USES. Currently, the antineoplastic efficacy of etoposide is believed to result from its action as an inhibitor of DNA topoisomerase II (Bender et al, 1990; Henwood and Brogden, 1990). In addition to the protein-linked DNA damage etoposide causes, the drug also inhibits DNA and RNA synthesis and nucleoside transport in treated cells. Resistance to etoposide can occur by gp-170 mediated drug efflux (Deuchars and Ling, 1989; van der Bliek and Borst, 1989), in which there is cross-resistance to vinca alkaloids as well as to anthracyclines, or by alterations in topoisomerase II activity (Ross et al, 1988; Liu, 1989), in which there is cross-resistance to amsacrine and the anthracyclines but not to vinca alkaloids. A third mechanism of resistance to etoposide involves increased DNA repair activity and is associated with cross-resistance to irradiation in a human tumor cell line (Hill and Bellamy, 1984).

Etoposide exhibits considerable activity in small cell lung carcinoma (average response rate, 40%) and is a component of combination regimens used in this disease (Minna et al, 1989; Carney et al, 1990). It is active in advanced testicular cancer and is a preferred agent in combination with bleomycin and cisplatin (Loehrer et al, 1988; Williams et al, 1989 A). Etoposide also is active in choriocarcinoma, acute lymphocytic and myelogenous leukemias, Hodgkin's and non-Hodgkin's lymphomas, gastric carcinoma, gliomas, Kaposi's sarcoma in AIDS patients, and childhood solid tumors and exhibits some activity in acute myelogenous leukemia, non-small cell lung cancer, ovarian carcinoma, and breast cancer. High-dose etoposide also appears promising in cytoablative combination regimens followed by either autologous or allogeneic bone marrow transplantation (Stadtmauer et al, 1989).

ADVERSE REACTIONS AND PRECAUTIONS. Hematologic toxicity, predominantly leukopenia, is most frequently dose limiting. White blood cell count nadirs occur between 8 and 14 days, and recovery occurs by days 16 to 21. Nausea and vomiting are usually mild. Hypotension can occur following intravenous push injection, and this drug should be given only by intravenous infusion over 30 to 60 minutes. Anaphylactoid hypersensitivity reactions occur rarely. Alopecia is relatively common but is mild and reversible. Fever, chills, and palpitations have been reported. Mucositis is rare after standard doses but is often dose-limiting in the ablative regimens used before bone marrow transplantation. Peripheral neuropathy, which may be cumulative with that caused by other neurotoxins (eg, vinca alkaloids, cisplatin), also has been observed. This drug is classified in FDA Pregnancy Category D.

PHARMACOKINETICS. About 20% to 80% of an oral dose is absorbed from the gastrointestinal tract, with peak plasma concentrations occurring two to three hours after ingestion. Etoposide is also given intravenously. The drug is extensively bound (94%) to plasma proteins. The plasma decay is biphasic with half-lives of two and five hours. About 45% of a dose is recovered in the urine after 72 hours, approximately two-thirds as unchanged drug. Despite the lipophilicity of etoposide, cerebrospinal fluid levels are generally less than 10% of those in the plasma in most patients.

The dose of etoposide should be reduced in patients with severe renal dysfunction. However, there is disagreement regarding the necessity for reducing the dose in patients with obstructive jaundice and normal renal function. Results of some investigations have shown that total systemic clearance is similar in patients with jaundice and in controls with adequate hepatic function (Hande et al, 1990). The investigators believe that no dose reduction is needed in patients in whom serum levels of bilirubin become elevated when etoposide is administered. Other investigators focus on the cumulative exposure to unbound etoposide (ie, area-under-the-curve for free drug); the value is higher in patients with impaired hepatic function, and this suggests that reduced doses may be advisable in these patients (Stewart et al, 1990).

DOSAGE AND PREPARATIONS.

Intravenous: For testicular cancer, 50 to 100 mg/M^2 is infused daily (over 30 to 60 minutes) for five days. Alternatively, 100 mg/M^2 is given on days one, three, and five every three to four weeks in combination with other drugs. For small cell lung cancer, 35 mg/M^2 daily for four days to 50 mg/M^2 daily for five days is recommended for combinations of etoposide with other chemotherapeutic drugs; however, doses up to 100 mg/M^2/day have been used. Etoposide must not be given by rapid intravenous injection because hypotension may occur.

VePesid (Bristol-Myers Squibb). Solution 20 mg/ml in 5 ml containers.

Oral: For small cell lung cancer, 70 to 100 mg/M^2 (ie, about twice the intravenous dose) calculated to the nearest multiple of 50 mg and administered using the same schedules as for the intravenous route. More extended treatment schedules (eg, 50 mg/M^2/day orally for 21 days) are under investigation to determine if they increase survival and/or response rates. Intrapleural administration to patients with malignant pleural effusions also is under investigation.

VePesid (Bristol-Myers Squibb). Capsules 50 mg.

TENIPOSIDE (VM-26)

[Vumon]

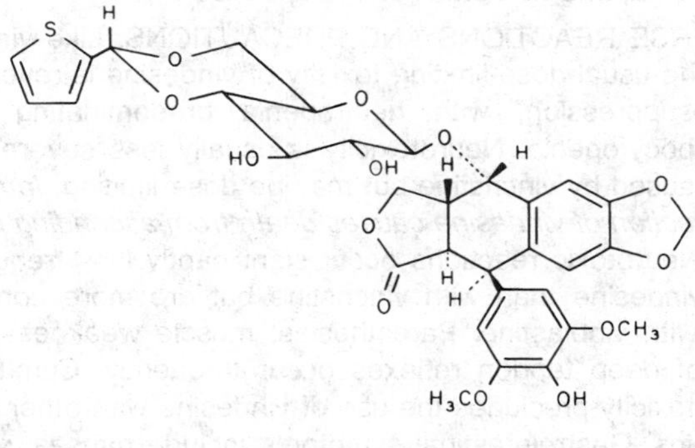

ACTIONS. Teniposide is a semisynthetic epipodophyllotoxin that inhibits DNA topoisomerase II (Bender et al, 1990). It is five to ten times more potent than etoposide in producing protein-linked DNA strand breaks in treated cells. DNA synthesis declines after exposure to teniposide. Teniposide is usually cross-resistant with etoposide and has the same patterns of cross-resistance with anthracyclines, vinca alkaloids, amsacrine, and irradiation.

USES. Teniposide is indicated as a component of combination regimens to induce remission in children with acute lymphoblastic leukemia whose malignancies are no longer responding to standard therapies (refractory ALL). Responses to teniposide also have been reported in patients with previously untreated ALL, Hodgkin's and non-Hodgkin's lymphomas, neuroblastoma, acute myeloid leukemia, multiple myeloma, and small cell lung cancer. However, data are insufficient to permit definitive evaluation of teniposide's efficacy in malignant diseases other than refractory ALL in children.

ADVERSE REACTIONS. Myelosuppression is the dose-limiting toxicity. Mild to moderate nausea and vomiting and alopecia are the other most common toxic reactions to teniposide. Hypotension has occurred after rapid intravenous injection. Anaphylactic reactions have been reported, and chemical phlebitis is not uncommon.

PHARMACOKINETICS. Teniposide is extensively bound to serum proteins (>99%). Plasma clearance is biphasic, with a terminal half-life of 8 to 24 hours in different studies (Bender et al, 1990). The drug is extensively metabolized. Approximately 10% to 20% of a dose appears in the urine as unchanged drug and an additional 30% to 35% as metabolites. Preliminary data suggest that the oral bioavailability of teniposide is about 30% to 35% of an ingested dose. The precise contributions of hepatic and renal clearance to the plasma decay curve have not been determined.

DOSAGE AND PREPARATIONS. The concentrate should be diluted to a final concentration of 0.1, 0.2, 0.4, or 1 mg/ml with either 5% dextrose injection or 0.9% sodium chloride injection. Final concentrations of 0.1, 0.2, or 0.4 mg/ml should be infused within 24 hours of preparation, while those of 1 mg/ml must be infused within four hours to reduce the possibility of precipitation.

Intravenous: *Children with refractory ALL*, 165 mg/M^2 (combined with intravenous cytarabine 300 mg/M^2) twice weekly for eight or nine doses. Alternatively, teniposide 250 mg/M^2 and intravenous vincristine 1.5 mg/M^2 may be given once weekly for four to eight weeks with oral prednisone 40 mg/M^2 given once daily for 28 days. The dose of teniposide is infused over 30 to 60 minutes.

Vumon (Bristol-Myers Squibb). Solution (concentrate) 10 mg/ml in single-use containers. Undiluted solutions should be stored at 2° to 8° C and diluted solutions at room temperature.

Other Alkaloids

Continued screening efforts have identified additional plant alkaloids with potential antineoplastic activity. Of these, paclitaxel (formerly taxol) is the first to become generally available for treatment of a human malignancy (advanced ovarian carcinoma). Other newer alkaloids are investigational and are not available except through sponsored clinical trials.

PACLITAXEL

[Taxol]

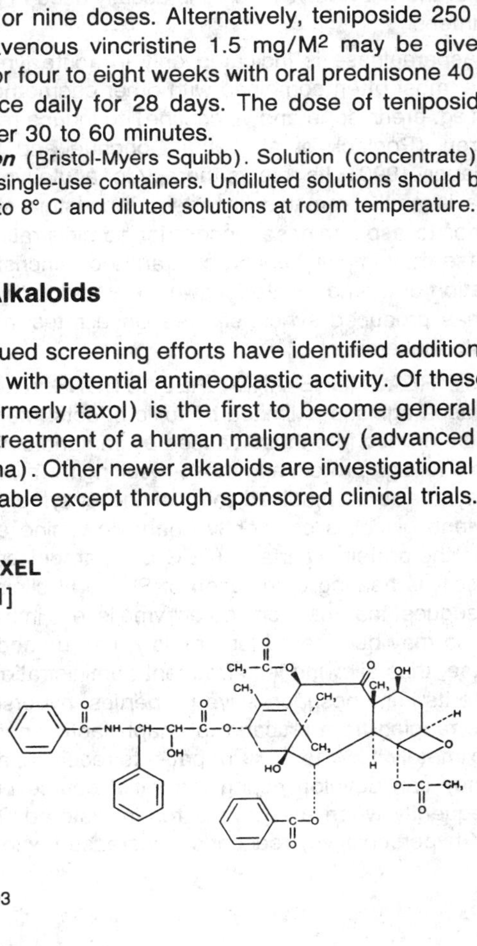

ACTIONS. Paclitaxel is a novel plant diterpene isolated from the stem bark of the western yew, *Taxus brevifolia*. It stabilizes cytoplasmic microtubules as a consequence of binding to polymerized tubulin (Rowinsky et al, 1990). As a result of the drug's inhibitory effects on microtubule depolymerization, cell cycle progression is arrested in late G_2 phase or in mitosis. Its effects on microtubules are in contrast to those of vinca alkaloids, which bind to soluble tubulin dimers and block microtubule polymerization.

Paclitaxel also inhibits other microtubule-dependent cellular processes such as motility and secretion. Studies with paclitaxel-resistant cells have shown that either enhanced drug efflux (mediated by the glycoprotein membrane pump, gp-170) or a mutated tubulin with reduced affinity for paclitaxel can be responsible for the loss of drug sensitivity.

USES. Paclitaxel is indicated as therapy for advanced ovarian carcinoma in women whose tumors have not responded to first-line or subsequent therapy. Results from Phase II studies in women with refractory ovarian cancer demonstrated response rates of 20% to 36% (McGuire et al, 1989; Thigpen et al, 1990; Einzig et al, 1992). Despite these results and the recent approval of this drug by the FDA, a number of questions remain to be answered in order to optimize its use in ovarian cancer. A randomized study currently is comparing the efficacy of paclitaxel plus cisplatin with that of cyclophosphamide plus cisplatin in previously untreated women with stage III or IV ovarian carcinoma. A second study is randomizing similar patients to treatment with paclitaxel alone, cisplatin alone, or both drugs. Finally, a randomized study comparing three doses of paclitaxel (135, 175, and 250 mg/M^2) in women with cisplatin-refractory advanced ovarian carcinoma also is ongoing; women receiving the highest dose are being further randomized to receive one of two doses of G-CSF (filgrastim) to stimulate recovery of neutrophil counts.

Administration of paclitaxel also has been reported to yield significant response rates in patients with a variety of other tumors, including breast cancer, non-small cell lung cancer, and metastatic melanoma. However, data are insufficient to permit definitive evaluation of this drug's efficacy as therapy for malignancies other than refractory ovarian cancer.

ADVERSE REACTIONS. Peripheral neuropathy appears to be the dose-limiting toxicity. Neutropenia is common, although of brief duration. Alopecia, fatigue, mild nausea, rash, and pruritus have been observed. Hypersensitivity reactions (probably related to the vehicle, polyoxyethylated castor oil [Cremophor EL]) may occur, and premedication should be employed.

PHARMACOKINETICS. The plasma disappearance curve is biphasic, with half-lives of 16 to 20 minutes and 6.5 to 8.5 hours. The drug is metabolized; only 5% of the administered dose is excreted unchanged. Significant binding to plasma proteins occurs.

DOSAGE AND PREPARATIONS. The concentrate should be diluted (in 0.9% sodium chloride injection, 5% dextrose injection, 5% dextrose and 0.9% sodium chloride injection, or 5% dextrose in Ringer's injection) to a final concentration of 0.3 to 1.2 mg/ml and infused within 27 hours of dilution.

Intravenous: *Women with refractory ovarian carcinoma*, although adequate dose-finding trials have not been completed, the manufacturer recommends administration of 135 mg/M^2 as a 24-hour infusion once every three weeks. All patients should receive oral dexamethasone 20 mg 12 and 6 hours before treatment, intravenous diphenhydramine 50 mg 30 to 60 minutes before treatment, and intravenous cimetidine or ranitidine 300 or 50 mg, respectively, 30 to 60 minutes before treatment to reduce the possibility of severe hypersensitivity reactions to the Cremophor EL vehicle used to dissolve paclitaxel. Courses of paclitaxel should not be repeated until the patient's neutrophil count is at least 1,500 cells/mm^3 and the platelet count is at least 100,000 cells/mm^3. The dose of paclitaxel should be reduced by 20% for subsequent courses in patients who experienced severe neutropenia (neutrophil count <500 cells/mm^3 for a week or longer) or severe peripheral neuropathy.

Taxol (Bristol-Myers Squibb). Solution 6 mg/ml with 527 mg of Cremophor EL and 49.7% (by volume) of dehydrated alcohol in single-use containers. Undiluted solutions should be stored at 2° to 8° C and diluted solutions at room temperature (approximately 25° C) for no more than 27 hours.

HOMOHARRINGTONINE (Investigational drug)

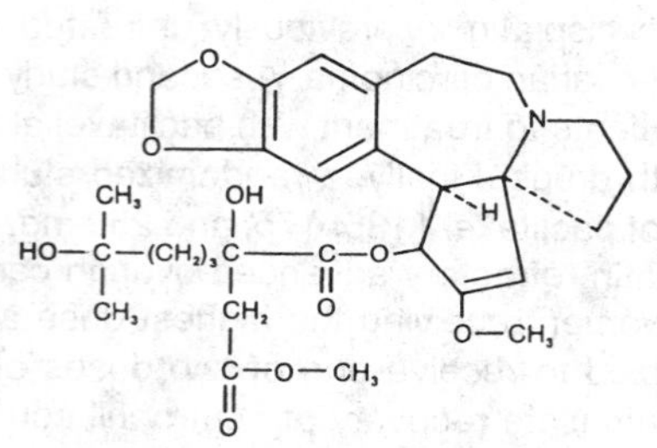

ACTIONS AND USES. Homoharringtonine and its congener, harringtonine, are cephalotoxine alkaloids derived from evergreen trees in China. Homoharringtonine inhibits protein synthesis and thus the synthesis of DNA and RNA. There also is evidence that the drug can induce differentiation in some tumor cell lines with loss of proliferative activity.

Preclinical studies suggest that homoharringtonine has some activity in rodent and human tumors. Responses in acute myelocytic leukemia have been observed in preliminary clinical trials.

ADVERSE REACTIONS AND PRECAUTIONS. Bolus injections have been associated with severe, sometimes irreversible hypotension. Other significant side effects include arrhythmias (ameliorated by prolonged infusion), myelosuppression, fluid retention, hyperglycemia, diarrhea, nausea, alopecia, neuralgias, and mucositis.

PHARMACOKINETICS. Homoharringtonine has a biphasic terminal plasma half-life of 14.4 hours.

DOSAGE (investigational regimen).

Intravenous: 3.25 to 4 mg/M^2 by continuous infusion daily for five days every four weeks.

ENZYME PREPARATIONS

ASPARAGINASE

[Elspar]

ACTIONS. Asparaginase is an enzyme derived from cultures of either *Escherichia coli* or *Erwinia carotovora*. (Elspar is derived from *E. coli*. The *Erwinia* asparaginase is an investigational preparation available through a sponsored clinical trial for patients who have experienced sensitivity reactions to the *E. coli* enzyme.) It catalyzes the hydrolysis of the amino acid, asparagine, to aspartic acid and ammonia, thus depleting the amount of asparagine available to tumor cells. Unlike normal cells, certain leukemic cells appear to lack asparagine synthetase and cannot convert aspartic acid to asparagine (Chabner, 1990 B). Thus, they depend on an exogenous source. The asparagine-depleting action interferes with the synthesis of protein and subsequently DNA and RNA in tumor cells. Asparaginase probably is cell cycle-specific for the postmitotic G_1 phase.

Asparaginase was originally considered to be an antitumor agent that exploited a unique biochemical difference between normal and neoplastic cells. However, it is now known that many normal tissues are sensitive to asparaginase and various toxic effects can result. In addition, human leukemic cells can quickly become resistant due to the emergence of strains that either induce asparagine synthetase or produce a mutated form of the enzyme. This drug is usually used in combination regimens.

USES. Asparaginase is indicated only in acute lymphocytic leukemia, most often combined with other chemotherapeutic agents (eg, prednisone and vincristine) to induce remissions in children (Poplack et al, 1989; Donohue and Charlton, 1989; Mauer, 1990). Its role as therapy for acute lymphocytic leukemia in adults remains uncertain. Vincristine should be given prior to asparaginase since prior administration of asparaginase may impair hepatic clearance of vincristine. The combination of methotrexate followed in 24 hours by asparaginase has produced synergistic response rates in patients with acute leukemia.

ADVERSE REACTIONS AND PRECAUTIONS. The usefulness of asparaginase is limited by toxic effects. Major toxicities can be divided into those caused by immunologic sensitization to a foreign protein and those resulting from decreased protein synthesis. A modified form of the enzyme, in which polyethylene glycol is covalently bound to amino acid side chains on the protein's surface (PEG-L-asparaginase or pegaspargase), is nearing completion of Phase III clinical trials. Studies suggest that the modified enzyme is less immunogenic and also may be cleared less rapidly than unmodified asparaginase, thus allowing less frequent administration.

Despite its immunosuppressive properties, hypersensitivity reactions ranging from urticaria to anaphylactic shock occur in approximately 10% to 15% of patients receiving asparaginase. They can develop during the initial course but occur more frequently when the drug is readministered. The incidence of hypersensitivity reactions is increased when the interval between doses is seven days or longer. Allergic reactions are not completely predictable on the basis of an intradermal skin test. Physicians should be aware of the potential for anaphylactic shock, and appropriate supportive measures should be readily available. Intravenous epinephrine usually terminates hypersensitivity reactions. Since there is no apparent cross reactivity between the *Escherichia coli* and *Erwinia carotovora* enzymes, patients sensitized to the *E. coli* enzyme may be treated with the *Erwinia* enzyme.

Neurotoxic reactions are observed primarily in adults. Approximately 25% of patients exhibit a decreased level of consciousness ranging from confusion to coma. Seizures or focal neurologic signs are rare. Although blood ammonia levels are increased, this does not appear to correlate with central nervous system toxicity, which is currently believed to be caused by decreased levels of asparagine and glutamine or inhibition of protein synthesis in the brain.

Inhibition of protein synthesis also may cause hypoalbuminemia resulting in peripheral edema or decreased circulating insulin resulting in hyperglycemia. In addition, decreased protein synthesis causes hypofibrinogenemia and decreases other clotting factors, particularly V, VII, VIII, and IX. However, severe bleeding is uncommon. Paradoxically, thrombosis may occur due to depletion of factors required for fibrinolysis. Reduction of circulating platelets also has occurred.

Pancreatitis has been observed in less than 15% of patients but may progress to severe hemorrhagic pancreatitis. Hepatotoxicity, with abnormal results of liver function tests, occurs in 50% to 75% of patients, and fatty metamorphosis of the liver has been observed. Azotemia, usually prerenal, occurs frequently. Acute renal shutdown and fatal renal insufficiency have been reported during treatment. Fatal hyperthermia also has been observed.

Approximately two-thirds of patients receiving asparaginase experience immediate side effects including nausea, vomiting, chills, and fever.

Myelosuppression is rare and usually not severe, although marked leukopenia has been reported.

Asparaginase is classified in FDA Pregnancy Category C.

PHARMACOKINETICS. Asparaginase is administered either intravenously or intramuscularly; peak blood levels are 50% lower after intramuscular injection. Plasma concentrations are proportional to the dose. The plasma half-life ranges from 14 to 22 hours and varies among preparations and individuals but is usually stable in a single individual. In patients who develop hypersensitivity to the enzyme, the half-life is shortened. This is probably due to a binding antibody that causes more rapid plasma clearance.

Little of the drug is distributed out of the vascular compartment, because of its large molecular size and highly ionized state in the body. Eventually, concentrations in lymph fluid approach 25% of those in the plasma. Very little drug is found in bile, urine, and cerebrospinal fluid. The inactivation of asparaginase is presumed to be due to serum proteases and the immune and reticuloendothelial systems.

DOSAGE AND PREPARATIONS. When administered intravenously, asparaginase should be injected into the tubing of a running infusion of sodium chloride injection or 5% dextrose in water over a period of at least 30 minutes. Because allergic reactions may occur, an intradermal skin test should be performed prior to initial administration and when the drug is readministered after a week or more has elapsed between courses. However, negative results do not preclude the possibility of an allergic reaction.

Intravenous: *Children,* when used following therapy with prednisone and vincristine, 1,000 IU/kg/day for 10 successive days beginning on day 22 of the treatment cycle. The administration of asparaginase with or immediately before a course of vincristine and prednisone may increase toxicity.

Intramuscular: *Adults and children,* in a combination induction regimen with prednisone and vincristine, 6,000 IU/M^2 on days 4, 7, 10, 13, 16, 19, 22, 25, and 28.

Elspar (Merck Sharp & Dohme). Lyophilized plug or powder containing 10,000 IU with 80 mg of mannitol in 10 ml containers. For reconstitution *(intravenous)*, 5 ml of sterile water for injection or sodium chloride injection is added. The solution may be used within an eight-hour period following reconstitution if it remains clear. For reconstitution *(intramuscular)*, 2 ml of sodium chloride injection is added. The solution should be used within an eight-hour period and only if clear.

Cited References

Andersson BS, et al: *In vitro* toxicity and DNA cleaving capacity of benzisoquinolinedione (nafidimide; NSC 308847) in human leukemia. *Cancer Res* 47:1040-1044, 1987.

Arlin Z, et al: Randomized multicenter trial of cytosine arabinoside with mitoxantrone or daunorubicin in previously untreated adult patients with acute nonlymphocytic leukemia (ANLL). *Leukemia* 4:177-183, 1990.

Bender RA, et al: Plant alkaloids, in Chabner BA, Collins JM (eds): *Cancer Chemotherapy: Principles and Practice.* Philadelphia, JB Lippincott, 1990, 253-275.

Bennett JM, et al: A randomized multicenter trial comparing mitoxantrone, cyclophosphamide, and fluorouracil with doxorubicin, cyclophosphamide, and fluorouracil in the therapy of metastatic breast carcinoma. *J Clin Oncol* 6:1611-1620, 1988.

Berkowitz RS, Goldstein DP: Gestational trophoblastic neoplasia, in Haskell CM (ed): *Cancer Treatment*, ed 3. Philadelphia, WB Saunders, 1990, 366-372.

Carella AM, et al: Idarubicin in the treatment of acute leukemias: An overview of preclinical and clinical studies. *Haematologica* 75:159-169, 1990.

Carney DN, et al: Single-agent oral etoposide for elderly small cell lung cancer patients. *Semin Oncol* 17(suppl 2):49-53, 1990.

Chabner BA: Bleomycin, in Chabner BA, Collins JM (eds): *Cancer Chemotherapy: Principles and Practice.* Philadelphia, JB Lippincott, 1990 A, 341-355.

Chabner BA: Enzyme therapy: L-asparaginase, in Chabner BA, Collins JM (eds): *Cancer Chemotherapy: Principles and Practice.* Philadelphia, JB Lippincott, 1990 B, 397-407.

Champlin R, Gale RP: Acute myelogenous leukemia: Recent advances in therapy. *Blood* 69:1551-1562, 1987.

Champlin R, Gale RP: Acute lymphoblastic leukemia: Recent advances in biology and therapy. *Blood* 73:2051-2066, 1989.

Comis RL: Detecting bleomycin pulmonary toxicity: A continued conundrum, editorial. *J Clin Oncol* 8:765-767, 1990.

Deuchars KL, Ling V: P-glycoprotein and multidrug resistance in cancer chemotherapy. *Semin Oncol* 16:156-165, 1989.

Donohue SM, Charlton CPJ: Drug treatment of acute leukaemia: Current status. *Drugs* 37:926-938, 1989.

Dorr RT: New findings in the pharmacokinetic, metabolic, and drug-resistance aspects of mitomycin C. *Semin Oncol* 15(suppl 4):32-41, 1988.

Ehninger G, et al: Pharmacokinetics and metabolism of mitoxantrone: A review. *Clin Pharmacokinet* 18:365-380, 1990.

Einzig AI, et al: Phase II study and long-term follow-up of patients treated with taxol for advanced ovarian adenocarcinoma. *J Clin Oncol* 10:1748-1753, 1992.

Finlay GJ, et al: Multiple patterns of resistance of human leukemia cell sublines to amsacrine analogues. *J Natl Cancer Inst* 82:662-667, 1990.

French Epirubicin Study Group: A prospective randomized Phase III trial comparing combination chemotherapy with cyclophosphamide, fluorouracil, and either doxorubicin or epirubicin. *J Clin Oncol* 6:679-688, 1988.

Gaynor ER, Fisher RI: Recent advances in the management of non-Hodgkin's lymphomas. *Dis Mon* 35:597-652, 1989.

Gershenson DM, et al: Treatment of malignant germ cell tumors of the ovary with bleomycin, etoposide, and cisplatin. *J Clin Oncol* 8:715-720, 1990.

Goorin AM, et al: Initial congestive heart failure, six to ten years after doxorubicin chemotherapy for childhood cancer. *J Pediatr* 116:144-147, 1990.

Hande KR, et al: Etoposide kinetics in patients with obstructive jaundice. *J Clin Oncol* 8:1101-1107, 1990.

Haskell CM, Parker RG: Hodgkin's disease, in Haskell CM (ed): *Cancer Treatment*, ed 3. Philadelphia, WB Saunders, 1990, 655-681.

Hayasaka S, et al: Postoperative instillation of mitomycin C in the treatment of recurrent pterygium. *Ophthalmic Surg* 20:580-583, 1989.

Hellman S, et al: Hodgkin's disease, in DeVita VT Jr, et al (eds): *Cancer: Principles & Practice of Oncology*, ed 3. Philadelphia, JB Lippincott, 1989, 1696-1740.

Henderson IC, et al: Randomized clinical trial comparing mitoxantrone with doxorubicin in previously treated patients with metastatic breast cancer. *J Clin Oncol* 7:560-571, 1989.

Henwood JM, Brogden RN: Etoposide: A review of its pharmacodynamic and pharmacokinetic property and therapeutic potential in combination chemotherapy of cancer. *Drugs* 39:438-490, 1990.

Herman EH, et al: Effect of pretreatment with ICRF-187 on the total cumulative dose of doxorubicin tolerated by beagle dogs. *Cancer Res* 48:6918-6925, 1988.

Hill BT, Bellamy AS: Establishment of an etoposide-resistant human epithelial tumour cell line *in vitro*: Characterization of patterns of cross-resistance and drug sensitivities. *Int J Cancer* 33:599-608, 1984.

Hoskins WJ, et al: Gynecologic tumors, in DeVita VT Jr, et al (eds): *Cancer: Principles & Practice of Oncology*, ed 3. Philadelphia, JB Lippincott, 1989, 1099-1161.

Italian Multicentre Breast Study With Epirubicin: Phase III randomized study of fluorouracil, epirubicin, and cyclophosphamide *v* fluorouracil, doxorubicin, and cyclophosphamide in advanced breast cancer: An Italian multicentre trial. *J Clin Oncol* 6:976-982, 1988.

Jain KK, et al: A prospective randomized comparison of epirubicin and doxorubicin in patients with advanced breast cancer. *J Clin Oncol* 3:818-826, 1985.

Jensen JL, et al: The effect of corticosteroid administration on bleomycin lung toxicity. *Cancer* 65:1291-1297, 1990.

Kantarjian HM, et al: Mitoxantrone and high-dose cytosine arabinoside for the treatment of refractory acute lymphocytic leukemia. *Cancer* 65:5-8, 1990.

Kramer RA, et al: Role of the glutathione redox cycle in acquired and de novo multidrug resistance. *Science* 241:694-697, 1988.

Kuffel MJ, et al: Characterization of cytotoxicity and DNA damage of idarubicin (ID), idarubicinol (IDOL) and related anthracyclines and their alcohol metabolites following incubation with human leukemia cells. *Proc Am Assoc Cancer Res* 31:399, 1990.

Lee FYF, et al: Changes in cellular glutathione content during adriamycin treatment in human ovarian cancer: A possible indicator of chemosensitivity. *Br J Cancer* 60:291-298, 1989.

Legha SS, et al: Phase I clinical investigation of benzisoquinolinedione. *Cancer Treat Rep* 71:1165-1169, 1987.

Leyland-Jones B, et al: Investigational new agents, in Chabner BA, Collins JM (eds): *Cancer Chemotherapy: Principles and Practice*. Philadelphia, JB Lippincott, 1990, 491-530.

Lichtman MA, Henderson ES: Acute myelogenous leukemia, in Williams WJ, et al (eds): Hematology, ed 4. New York, McGraw-Hill, 1990, 251-272.

Liu LF: DNA topoisomerase poisons as antitumor drugs. *Annu Rev Biochem* 58:351-375, 1989.

Loehrer PJ, et al: Testicular cancer: The quest continues. *J Natl Cancer Inst* 80:1373-1382, 1988.

Lopez M, et al: A prospective randomized trial of doxorubicin versus idarubicin in the treatment of advanced breast cancer. *Cancer* 64:2431-2436, 1989.

Mauer AM: Acute lymphocytic leukemia, in Williams WJ, et al (eds): *Hematology*, ed 4. New York, McGraw-Hill, 1990, 994-1005.

McGuire WP, et al: Taxol: A unique antineoplastic agent with significant activity in advanced ovarian epithelial neoplasms. *Ann Intern Med* 111:273-279, 1989.

Minna JD, et al: Cancer of the lung, in DeVita VT Jr, et al (eds): *Cancer: Principles & Practice of Oncology*, ed 3. Philadelphia, JB Lippincott, 1989, 591-705.

Muss HB, et al: Esorubicin (4'-deoxydoxorubicin, NSC 267469) in advanced breast cancer. *Am J Clin Oncol* 13:233-237, 1990.

Myers CE Jr, Chabner BA: Anthracyclines, in Chabner BA, Collins JM (eds): *Cancer Chemotherapy: Principles and Practice*. Philadelphia, JB Lippincott, 1990, 356-381.

Poplack DG, et al: Leukemias and lymphomas of childhood, in DeVita VT Jr, et al (eds): *Cancer: Principles & Practice of Oncology*, ed 3. Philadelphia, JB Lippincott, 1989, 1671-1695.

Ross WE, et al: Altered function of DNA topoisomerases as a basis for antineoplastic drug action, in DeVita VT Jr, et al (eds): *Important Advances in Oncology 1988*. Philadelphia, JB Lippincott, 1988, 65-82.

Rowinsky EK, et al: Taxol: A novel investigational antimicrotubule agent. *J Natl Cancer Inst* 82:1247-1259, 1990.

Sarna GP, Kagan AR: Non-Hodgkin's lymphomas, in Haskell CM (ed): *Cancer Treatment*, ed 3. Philadelphia, WB Saunders, 1990, 682-717.

Sartorelli AC: Therapeutic attack of hypoxic cells of solid tumors: Presidential address. *Cancer Res* 48:775-778, 1988.

Shenkenberg TD, Von Hoff DD: Mitoxantrone: New anticancer drug with significant clinical activity. *Ann Intern Med* 105:67-81, 1986.

Singh G, et al: Mitomycin eye drops as treatment for pterygium. *Ophthalmology* 95:813-821, 1988.

Speyer JL, et al: Protective effect of the bispiperazinedione ICRF-187 against doxorubicin-induced cardiac toxicity in women with advanced breast cancer. *N Engl J Med* 319:745-752, 1988.

Stadtmauer EA, et al: Etoposide in leukemia, lymphoma and bone marrow transplantation. *Leukemia Res* 13:639-650, 1989.

Stewart CF, et al: Changes in the clearance of total and unbound etoposide in patients with liver dysfunction. *J Clin Oncol* 8:1874-1879, 1990.

Tan KB, et al: Nonproductive rearrangement of DNA topoisomerase I and II genes: Correlation with resistance to topoisomerase inhibitors. *J Natl Cancer Inst* 81:1732-1735, 1989.

Thigpen T, et al: Phase II trial of taxol as second-line therapy for ovarian carcinoma: A gynecologic oncology group study. *Proc ASCO* 9:156, 1990.

Tritton TR, Yee G: The anticancer agent adriamycin can be actively cytotoxic without entering cells. *Science* 217:248-250, 1982.

van der Bliek AM, Borst P: Multidrug resistance. *Adv Cancer Res* 52:165-203, 1989.

Verweij J, et al: Antitumor antibiotics, in Chabner BA, Collins JM (eds): *Cancer Chemotherapy: Principles and Practice*. Philadelphia, JB Lippincott, 1990, 382-396.

Vokes EE, Weichselbaum RR: Concomitant chemoradiotherapy: Rationale and clinical experience in patients with solid tumors. *J Clin Oncol* 8:911-934, 1990.

Wiernik PH: Acute leukemias, in DeVita VT Jr, et al (eds): *Cancer: Principles & Practice of Oncology*, ed 3. Philadelphia, JB Lippincott, 1989, 1809-1835.

Williams SD, et al: Disseminated testicular cancer: Current chemotherapy strategies. *Semin Oncol* 16 (suppl 6):105-109, 1989 A.

Williams SD, et al: Cisplatin, vinblastine, and bleomycin in advanced and recurrent ovarian germ-cell tumors. *Ann Intern Med* 111:22-27, 1989 B.

Other Selected References

Calabresi P, et al (eds): *Medical Oncology*. New York, Macmillan, 1985.

del Regato JA, et al: *Ackerman and del Regato's Cancer: Diagnosis, Treatment, and Prognosis*. St Louis, CV Mosby, 1985.

DeVita VT Jr, et al (eds): *Cancer: Principles & Practice of Oncology*, ed 3. Philadelphia, JB Lippincott, 1989.

Haskell CM (eds): *Cancer Treatment*, ed 3. Philadelphia, WB Saunders, 1990.

Hellmann K, Carter SK (eds): *Fundamentals of Cancer Chemotherapy*. New York, McGraw-Hill, 1987.

Holland JF, Frei E III (eds): *Cancer Medicine*, ed 2. Philadelphia, Lea & Febiger, 1982.

Tannock IF, Hill RP (eds): *The Basic Science of Oncology*. New York, Pergamon Press, 1987.

New Evaluation 90

PEGASPARGASE
[Oncaspar]

ACTIONS. Pegaspargase is a chemically modified preparation of the enzyme, L-asparaginase, that is isolated from *Escherichia coli.* The partially purified enzyme is covalently attached through succinate linkages to units of monomethoxypolyethyleneglycol (PEG) that have a molecular weight of 5,000 daltons each (Capizzi and Holcenberg, 1993). The substrate affinity and other enzyme kinetic parameters are similar for hydrolysis of asparagine to aspartic acid and ammonia by native asparaginase and its PEG-modified derivative. Depletion of asparagine from the circulation inhibits cellular protein synthesis and thus is toxic to tumor cells (primarily those of lymphoid origin) that lack adequate intracellular levels of asparagine synthetase (Keating et al, 1993; Capizzi, 1993). As with the native enzyme, most normal cells are less affected because they either constitutively express asparagine synthetase or induce this enzyme in the absence of asparagine. The attached PEG monomers decrease the immunogenicity of pegaspargase and reduce its cross-reactivity with antibodies to native asparaginase (Weiss, 1992).

USES. Pegaspargase is indicated as a component of combination regimens used to induce and/or consolidate remission in patients with acute lymphoblastic leukemia (ALL) (Keating et al, 1993; Capizzi, 1993; Capizzi and Holcenberg, 1993). For this indication, pegaspargase (or native asparaginase) usually is combined with one or more of the following: vincristine, an anthracycline (doxorubicin or daunorubicin), prednisone, cytarabine, or methotrexate (see index entry Leukemia, Clinical Response to Chemotherapy). Data from the manufacturer's product information indicate that approximately 50% of 42 patients with acute leukemia who experienced a second or subsequent relapse (93% of whom had ALL) and had previous hypersensitivity to asparaginase responded to reinduction with regimens that included pegaspargase (36% complete and 14% partial remissions). These rates were not significantly different from those reported for otherwise similar but nonhypersensitive patients treated with regimens that included native asparaginase (Capizzi and Holcenberg, 1993).

Only one published study has compared pegaspargase directly with native asparaginase (both drugs combined with vincristine and prednisone) as induction chemotherapy for children with ALL in a second relapse (Kurtzberg et al, 1993). Thirty-five patients without previous hypersensitivity to asparaginase were randomly assigned to one of the two regimens, and 39 patients with previous hypersensitivity were assigned to the regimen with pegaspargase. No significant differences were observed in the rates of overall response (55% to 61%) in the three groups. However, the number of patients randomized to receive asparaginase or pegaspargase may not have been large enough to provide adequate statistical power for a definitive conclusion. Similarly, in a study cited in the manufacturer's product information, 20 patients were randomized to receive either drug; there was no significant difference in the rates of response or complete remission, but the statistical power of this study also may be insufficient.

Other potential indications for pegaspargase that have been studied include its use alone in relapsed patients with ALL who had previously been treated with asparaginase (22% response rate after a single dose of pegaspargase) (Kurtzberg, 1992) and in combination regimens as maintenance therapy for patients with ALL in remission (see the manufacturer's product information). It also has been investigated as consolidation therapy after bone marrow transplantation for patients with ALL experiencing a second or subsequent remission (Graham et al, 1993). Data are insufficient to evaluate the efficacy of pegaspargase for any of these uses.

ADVERSE REACTIONS, PRECAUTIONS, AND CONTRAINDICATIONS. Covalent modification with PEG reduces but does not eliminate the immunogenicity of asparaginase. Data in the manufacturer's product information indicate that, during clinical trials, hypersensitivity reactions to intramuscular injection of pegaspargase occurred in 30% of patients previously hypersensitive to asparaginase and in 11% of nonhypersensitive patients. With intravenous administration, hypersensitivity reactions occurred in 60% of those with and in 12% of those without hypersensitivity to asparaginase. Symptoms included rash, erythema, edema (generalized or localized to the lip), induration, pain, tenderness, swelling, fever, chills, arthralgia, urticaria, dyspnea, or bronchospasm. Because anaphylaxis may occur occasionally, epinephrine, oxygen, intravenous steroids, and antihistamines should be available for immediate use if necessary. Pegaspargase also may be an irritant, and appropriate measures should be used to avoid inhalation or contact (eg, by wearing gloves).

Other adverse reactions occurred more often in adults than in children. These included hepatotoxicity (eg, increased serum levels of hepatic enzymes, increased bilirubin concentration, jaundice, ascites, hypoalbuminemia) and coagulopathies (eg, hypofibrinogenemia, prolonged prothrombin or partial thromboplastin times, decreased antithrombin III levels). However, most of these reactions observed in clinical trials of pegaspargase were not clinically significant, and the abnormalities in liver function usually reversed upon discontinuation of therapy. Coagulopathies may increase the risk of bleeding, especially in patients using other drugs with anticoagulant effects (eg, aspirin, nonsteroidal anti-inflammatory agents). Thrombosis occurred in 4%, hyperglycemia requiring insulin therapy in 3%, and pancreatitis in 1% of 174 patients included in these studies. Serum amylase and blood glucose should be monitored during therapy, and measurements of fibrinogen levels and/or prothrombin or partial thromboplastin times also may be indicated. Renal, gastrointestinal, cardiovascular, neurologic, and other adverse reactions also have occurred rarely in patients treated with pegaspargase for hematologic malignancies (see the manufacturer's product information).

Pegaspargase is contraindicated in patients with pancreatitis or a history of pancreatitis, in those who have had significant hemorrhagic events after therapy with asparaginase, and in those who have had serious allergic reactions to this drug.

Although pegaspargase is not mutagenic in vitro (as determined by the Ames assay using *Salmonella typhimurium*), data on its potential carcinogenicity in animals or humans are not available. Its effects on fertility and reproduction and on fetal toxicity also have not been studied (FDA Pregnancy Category C). It is unknown whether pegaspargase is excreted in human milk; however, its administration to a lactating woman probably would deplete the milk of asparagine.

PHARMACOKINETICS. The plasma half-life of pegaspargase appears to be independent of dose, age, sex, body surface area, renal or hepatic function, diagnosis, or extent of disease. The apparent volume of distribution is approximately equal to the plasma volume. In previously untreated patients with ALL, the plasma half-life of pegaspargase was 5.7 days (Asselin et al, 1993). This was significantly longer than the half-lives of native asparaginase from either *E. coli* (1.2 days) or *Erwinia* (0.65 days). As a result, plasma asparagine concentrations are suppressed for much longer after a single dose of pegaspargase than after a single dose of native asparaginase (Capizzi, 1993). A mathematical model has been developed that estimates plasma asparagine concentrations based on the kinetic properties of the enzyme, a monoexponential function for its clearance from plasma, and an input function for entry of asparagine into the circulation. The model predicts that doses producing peak plasma levels of enzyme activity of 2 IU/ml would deplete plasma asparagine for approximately six days with asparaginase and for approximately one month with pegaspargase (Capizzi and Holcenberg, 1993).

Data from a multicenter study indicate that a significant number of previously treated patients without hypersensitivity to asparaginase have high titers of antibodies to the native enzyme (Kurtzberg et al, 1993). The half-life of native asparaginase is shorter in these patients than in those without such "silent" antibodies and they are less likely to respond to asparaginase therapy. Although the half-life of pegaspargase is shorter in patients who are hypersensitive to asparaginase than in those who are not hypersensitive (1.8 versus 5.7 days) (Asselin et al, 1993), the former appears to be cleared less rapidly than the native enzyme in patients with high titers of the silent antibodies (Kurtzberg et al, 1993). Thus, pegaspargase may remain clinically useful in those patients whose resistance to asparaginase results from faster clearance. Additional preliminary data suggest that asparagine may be depleted more effectively in some patients with a history of hypersensitivity to native asparaginase when pegaspargase is administered every week rather than every other week (Kurtzberg et al, 1994).

DOSAGE AND PREPARATIONS. The enzymatic activity of pegaspargase is expressed in International Units (IU) defined as the amount of enzyme that generates 1 μmol of ammonia per minute from L-asparagine at pH 7.3 and 37° C. The specific activity of pegaspargase preparations is at least 85 IU/mg of protein.

Intravenous, Intramuscular: As a component of combination regimens for acute lymphoblastic leukemia (ALL), *adults,* 2,500 IU/M^2 every 14 days. In patients with a history of hypersensitivity to asparaginase, the frequency may be increased to every seven days. *Children,* the manufacturer's recommended doses are as follows: *body surface area* $\geq$*0.6* M^2, 2,500 IU every 14 days; *body surface area* $<$*0.6* M^2, 82.5 IU/kg every 14 days.

The intramuscular route is preferred by many clinicians because the incidence of severe allergic reactions, hepatotoxicity, coagulopathy, renal toxicity, and gastrointestinal disorders is lower than with the intravenous route. No more than 2 ml should be injected at a single intramuscular site; doses that require larger volumes should be administered by injection at multiple sites. Intravenous doses should be diluted in 100 ml of sodium chloride for injection or 5% dextrose for injection and infused over one to two hours through a line that is already running.

Oncaspar (Rhone-Poulenc Rorer). Solution (injection) 750 IU/ml in phosphate-buffered saline (pH 7.3) in 5 ml single-use containers. Store refrigerated at 36° to 46° F (2° to 8° C). The enzymatic activity of pegaspargase is destroyed by freezing. Excessive agitation should be avoided.

Cited References

Asselin BL, et al: Comparative pharmacokinetic studies of three asparaginase preparations. *J Clin Oncol* 11:1780-1786, 1993.

Capizzi RL: Asparaginase revisited. *Leukemia Lymphoma* 10 (suppl):147-150, 1993.

Capizzi RL, Holcenberg JS: Asparaginase, in Holland JF, et al (eds): *Cancer Medicine*, ed 3. Philadelphia, Lea & Febiger, 1993, 796-805.

Graham ML, et al: Feasibility of consolidation therapy with PEG-L-asparaginase after bone marrow transplant for acute lymphoblastic leukemia in second or subsequent remission. *Proc Am Soc Clin Oncol* 12:324, 1993.

Keating MJ, et al: L-asparaginase and PEG asparaginase—Past, present, and future. *Leukemia Lymphoma* 10(suppl):153-157, 1993.

Kurtzberg J: International multicenter study of PEG-L-asparaginase for reinduction therapy for children with acute lymphoblastic leukemia. *Blood* 80(suppl 1):206a, 1992.

Kurtzberg J, et al: PEG-L-asparaginase (PEGasp) vs native *E. coli* asparaginase (asp) for reinduction of relapsed acute lymphoblastic leukemia (ALL): POG #8866 Phase II trial. *Proc Am Soc Clin Oncol* 12:325, 1993.

Kurtzberg J, et al: PEG-L-asparaginase (PEG-ASP) pharmacology in pediatric patients with acute lymphoblastic leukemia (ALL). *Proc Am Soc Clin Oncol* 13:144, 1994.

Weiss RB: Hypersensitivity reactions. *Semin Oncol* 19:458-477, 1992.

Antineoplastic Agents: Hormonal Agents

91

INTRODUCTION

CORTICOSTEROIDS AND ADRENOCORTICAL SUPPRESSANT

ESTROGENS AND ANTIESTROGENS

ANDROGENS AND ANTIANDROGENS

GONADOTROPIN RELEASING HORMONE ANALOGUES

PROGESTINS

INHIBITORS OF STEROID BIOSYNTHESIS OR ACTIVATION

Hormone-sensitive tumors may be hormone-dependent, hormone-responsive, or both. A hormone-dependent tumor regresses on removal or alteration of the hormonal stimulus (for reviews, see Hamm and Allegra, 1991 A, 1991 B; Kennedy, 1993; Sutherland and Mobbs, 1992). This may be accomplished by ablative surgery, as in oophorectomy for the initial treatment of premenopausal women with estrogen receptor-positive advanced breast cancer (Fisher et al, 1993; Harris et al, 1993) and in orchiectomy for men with advanced prostate cancer (Trump and Robertson, 1993; Hanks et al, 1993).

Hormonal stimulation of hormone-dependent tumors also may be prevented with drugs. Tamoxifen, an antiestrogen, and aminoglutethimide, an inhibitor of aromatase-catalyzed estrogen synthesis as well as of adrenal corticosteroid synthesis, prevent estrogen stimulation of breast cancer cells. At present, tamoxifen is used frequently in the treatment of pre- and postmenopausal women with estrogen receptor-positive advanced breast cancer. It also is employed as adjuvant therapy in many women with early-stage breast cancer. Flutamide, an antiandrogen, is used in the treatment of prostate cancer, primarily for metastatic disease and in combination with leuprolide or goserelin (luteinizing hormone-releasing hormone [LHRH] agonists). Synthetic LHRH agonists initially stimulate the release of follicle-stimulating hormone (FSH) and luteinizing hormone (LH); however, further release of LH and FSH is inhibited after 10 to 14 days of continuous treatment. This action results in a decrease of testicular and ovarian steroidogenesis.

Hormone-responsive tumors may regress when pharmacologic amounts of hormones are administered. In patients with carcinomas of the breast, prostate, and endometrium, the tumors most likely to respond to pharmacologic doses of sex steroids are those that have the capacity to respond to other hormonal manipulations (ie, have sex steroid receptors, have responded to another hormonal treatment). Myeloma, lymphomas, and certain leukemias may respond to pharmacologic doses of glucocorticoid agonists. Hormonal substances that inhibit the growth of certain human tumors include estrogens, progestins, androgens, and glucocorticoids. Each of these classes of steroids has been used in advanced breast carcinoma. Estrogens can be used as initial therapy in advanced prostatic carcinoma; these agents exert their effects primarily by inhibiting secretion of LH and FSH. Progestins are drugs of choice in advanced endometrial carcinoma and have activity in carcinomas of the breast, ovary, and prostate.

In pharmacologic doses, the antitumor effects of all three classes of sex steroids are cytostatic, and therapy with these agents is rarely curative. In contrast, glucocorticoids are lympholytic and are important constituents of drug combinations that may be curative in patients with certain leukemias or lymphomas. Examples include the MOPP regimen for Hodgkin's disease, the CHOP and BACOP regimens for large cell lymphomas, and remission-inducing regimens for acute lymphocytic leukemia (see index entry Cancer: Clinical Responses to Chemotherapy). Glucocorticoids also are important constituents of combination regimens used to lengthen the duration of survival of patients with multiple myeloma.

The precise mechanisms of action of the steroid hormones are not completely understood. In some cancers (eg, breast, lymphoid, probably endometrial), the effectiveness of therapy depends on the presence of specific steroid receptor proteins in the cytoplasm or nucleus of tumor cells and, in most cases, binding of the hormone to the receptor appears to be required. The hormone/receptor complexes then alter the spectrum of genes and their encoded proteins being expressed in the target cells. In some instances (eg, the lympholytic effects of glucocorticoids), the end result of altered gene expression in response to hormone therapy is the induction of apoptosis (programmed cell death). The absence or loss of specific hormone receptor proteins can be correlated with a lack of antineoplastic effects. For example, estrogen receptor-negative breast tumors usually do not respond to hormonal therapy (see the discussion on Antineoplastic Drug Selection in Chapter 1 of this Section). See the Section, Endocrine Drugs, for a comprehensive discussion of steroid hormones.

Corticosteroids and Adrenocortical Suppressant

Two classes of corticosteroids are synthesized in the adrenal cortex, glucocorticoids and mineralocorticoids. Of these, only glucocorticoids are used in cancer chemotherapy, in which their cytotoxicity to lymphoid cells is exploited. Cortisol (the principal endogenous glucocorticoid) and cortisone (the first synthetic glucocorticoid, which is readily converted to cortisol in vivo) seldom are used in the therapy of malignant diseases. The synthetic glucocorticoids used in cancer chemotherapy (prednisone, prednisolone, methylprednisolone, dexamethasone) are more potent glucocorticoid agonists, have reduced mineralocorticoid activity, and are metabolized less rapidly than cortisol. Although it is not a hormone or hormone analogue, the adrenocortical suppressant, mitotane, is discussed in this chapter since it is toxic to cells of the adrenal cortex in a highly selective manner. Because of its selectivity, mitotane is used only to treat tumors of the adrenal cortex.

SYNTHETIC GLUCOCORTICOIDS

For individual chemical formulas, see index entry Adrenal Corticosteroids, Chemistry.

ACTIONS. The precise mode of action of the adrenal corticosteroids (glucocorticoids) is unknown, but they must bind to specific cytoplasmic receptor proteins in tumor cells to exert their antitumor effect (Distelhorst, 1989; Jusko, 1990; Cidlowski and Schwartzman, 1993). Many cells are targets for the adrenal corticosteroids, and physiologic effects vary widely. In lymphoid tissues, glucocorticoids induce cell death. This effect does not depend on proliferation of the lymphoid cells and is accompanied by activation of intracellular endonucleases and by fragmentation of nuclear DNA (apoptosis). Inhibition of glucose transport and lipid biosynthesis are among the many other biochemical alterations that glucocorticoids induce in lymphoid cells that may contribute to their lympholytic effects. These drugs interfere with lymphoid proliferation and cause dissolution of lymphocytes and regression of lymphatic tissue. A decrease in utilization of energy due to glucose deprivation also may contribute to their effects.

USES. Because of their cytotoxic effect on lymphoid tissues, the major indications for adrenal corticosteroids are acute and chronic lymphocytic leukemia (Keating et al, 1993; Deisseroth et al, 1993; Schiffer, 1993; Rai and Rabinowe, 1993), Hodgkin's disease (DeVita et al, 1993; Takvorian and Canellos, 1993; DeVita and Hubbard, 1993), non-Hodgkin's lymphomas (Longo et al, 1993; Freedman and Nadler, 1993), and multiple myeloma (Alexanian et al, 1992). Adrenal corticosteroids are not myelosuppressive and usually are given in combination with other chemotherapeutic agents (see index entry Cancer: Clinical Responses to Chemotherapy.) However, significant response rates have been reported in patients with multiple myeloma given dexamethasone as a single agent (Friedenberg et al, 1991; Alexanian et al, 1992). In addition, synthetic glucocorticoids are used infrequently as palliative therapy in some patients with advanced breast or prostate cancer.

Adrenal corticosteroids may be given to treat certain complications of cancer. They may be useful in combination with other drugs to reverse severe hypercalcemia in women with metastatic breast cancer. However, in patients with most other malignancies, hypercalcemia does not respond adequately to glucocorticoids and more effective therapies are not available (see index entry Hypercalcemia, Treatment). Glucocorticoids are employed to reduce brain edema in critical areas (eg, superior mediastinum, brain, spinal cord) in patients with intracranial metastases. Synthetic glucocorticoids also are useful to reduce lymphocytic infiltration of solid tumors and metastases (eg, in lung, liver) and thus relieve some symptoms. The corticosteroids also may produce temporary symptomatic improvement in critically ill patients by suppressing fever, sweating, and pain and by restoring appetite, lost weight and strength (if protein intake is adequate), and a sense of well-being. However, some clinicians hesitate to administer glucocorticoids for these temporary benefits, since their use is accompanied by an increased risk of immunosuppression and susceptibility to infection as well as other complications.

Response should be assessed after one week of therapy, and the drug should be discontinued if symptoms have not decreased (Needham et al, 1992; Twycross, 1992) or no longer respond to corticosteroids. If the duration of therapy or the dosage has been sufficient to suppress the hypothalamic-pituitary-adrenal axis (usually longer than one month, but as soon as one week with large doses), the amount must be tapered to avoid the risks associated with abrupt withdrawal (see index entries Adrenal Corticosteroids, Adverse Reactions; Adrenal Corticosteroids, Withdrawal from Therapy).

Corticosteroids also are used to reduce the nausea and vomiting resulting from cytotoxic chemotherapy (see index entry Vomiting, Treatment).

ADVERSE REACTIONS AND PRECAUTIONS. Long-term therapy can cause cushingoid features with accumulation of fat on the trunk and face. Metabolic effects include sodium retention, which may result in edema, heart failure, and hypertension; potassium loss, which may produce muscle weakness; and decreased glucose tolerance, which may result in glycosuria and overt diabetes mellitus. Loss of skin collagen can result in thinning of the skin, petechiae, ecchymoses, and cutaneous striae. Proximal myopathy, osteoporosis, osteonecrosis, and vertebral compression fractures occur frequently and, during long-term therapy, may produce significant morbidity. Peptic ulcerations may develop. Retardation or interruption of growth has been observed in children. Euphoria is common, and some patients may develop psychoses. Other possible effects on the central nervous system include increased appetite and insomnia. The acute tumor lysis syndrome (hyperkalemia, hyperuricemia, hyperphosphatemia, hypocalcemia, lactic acidosis, and acute renal insufficiency) can occur, although it is rare in patients treated with glucocorticoids alone.

Caution should be exercised in patients receiving long-term steroid therapy, since they are more susceptible to severe infections. Sudden withdrawal of medication or development of stress may result in acute adrenocortical insufficiency; to avoid this problem, the dosage must be tapered gradually when long-term therapy is discontinued (see index entry Adrenal Corticosteroids, Withdrawal from Therapy). To diminish the complications of corticosteroid therapy, an attempt should be made to minimize the dosage and duration of treatment.

For a more detailed discussion, see index entry Adrenal Corticosteroids, Adverse Reactions.

PHARMACOKINETICS. See index entry Glucocorticoids: Properties and Routes of Administration (Table).

DOSAGE AND PREPARATIONS. For comparative information on equivalent dosages of individual adrenal corticosteroids, see index entry Glucocorticoids: Relative Potencies (Table).

PREDNISONE:

Oral: 10 to 100 mg daily.

In combination with vincristine (with or without daunorubicin or asparaginase) to induce remission in acute lymphocytic leukemia, 40 mg/M^2 daily in divided doses for four to six weeks.

As a component of the MOPP regimen in advanced Hodgkin's disease, 40 mg/M^2 daily on days 1 through 14 (cycles one and four only).

As a component of the CVP regimen in indolent non-Hodgkin's lymphomas (ie, histologies associated with a favorable prognosis), 100 mg/M^2 daily on days 1 through 5 every four weeks. As a component of the CHOP regimen in aggressive non-Hodgkin's lymphomas (ie, histologies associated with an unfavorable prognosis), 100 mg/M^2 daily on days 1 through 5 every three weeks.

In combination with melphalan to induce remission in patients with multiple myeloma, 40 mg/M^2 daily on days 1 through 4, repeated every four weeks.

DEXAMETHASONE, DEXAMETHASONE SODIUM PHOSPHATE:

Oral, Intramuscular, Intravenous: To reduce cerebral edema in patients with primary or metastatic brain tumors, initially 10 mg is given intravenously and then 4 mg is injected intramuscularly or intravenously or given orally every six hours until symptoms subside. Some response is usually seen after 12 to 24 hours; signs and symptoms of cerebral edema gradually disappear over 48 to 72 hours. Dosage can be reduced after two to four days, and the drug is either continued through the course of radiation therapy or is gradually discontinued over five to seven days. For maintenance therapy, 2 mg either orally or parenterally is administered two or three times daily to reduce intracranial pressure in patients with recurrent or inoperable brain tumors. Patients who are deteriorating because of continued tumor growth and who are not responding to lower doses have been made comfortable temporarily with doses as high as 64 mg/day or more for short courses of therapy followed by rapid tapering. For patients with spinal cord compression, an initial intravenous bolus of 100 mg is followed by doses of 24 mg every six hours for three days; the amount then is tapered gradually over the following 11 days. The dose can be increased again if neurologic symptoms return during tapering.

For aggressive non-Hodgkin's lymphomas, in combination with other drugs (eg, the M-BACOD and m-BACOD regimens), 6 $mg/M^2/day$ orally on days 1 through 5, repeated every 21 days.

For patients with advanced refractory multiple myeloma, 40 mg orally on days 1 through 4, 9 through 12, and 17 through 20 in combination with vincristine and doxorubicin (the VAD regimen), repeated every 28 days.

PREDNISOLONE:

Oral: 10 to 100 mg daily; used interchangeably with prednisone in equivalent dosages.

PREDNISOLONE SODIUM PHOSPHATE:

Oral, Intramuscular, Intravenous: To reduce cerebral edema in patients with intracranial tumors, can be used interchangeably with dexamethasone but requires doses six- to sevenfold higher.

METHYLPREDNISOLONE, METHYLPREDNISOLONE ACETATE, METHYLPREDNISOLONE SODIUM SUCCINATE:

Oral, Intramuscular, Intravenous: Can be used interchangeably with dexamethasone (at doses fivefold higher) to treat cerebral edema in patients with intracranial tumors.

For preparations, see index entry Adrenal Corticosteroids, Preparations, Systemic.

MITOTANE

[Lysodren]

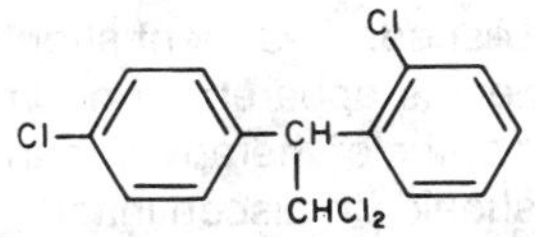

ACTIONS. Chemically, mitotane (*o,p'*-DDD) is similar to the insecticides, DDD and DDT. In toxicology studies in dogs, mitotane produced necrosis and atrophy of the adrenal cortex, particularly the zona fasciculata and zona reticularis. Although it is selectively toxic to adrenal cortical cells, the precise mechanism of action is unknown.

USES. Mitotane is indicated in the palliative treatment of both functional and nonfunctional inoperable carcinoma of the adrenal cortex. The tumor mass is reduced significantly in 34% to 54% of patients with functional tumors, and the mean duration of response is about ten months. Clinical responses occur less frequently in patients with anaplastic, nonfunctional adrenal tumors. Mitotane also is used as adjuvant chemotherapy after surgical resection of adrenocortical carcinoma, but its effects are palliative and transient; it has no significant effect on survival (Luton et al, 1990; Vassilopoulou-Sellin et al, 1993).

Mitotane rapidly decreases the level of corticosteroids and their metabolites in blood and urine. This response is useful for adjusting the dose and monitoring the course of hyperadrenocorticism (Cushing's syndrome) due to adrenal tumor or hyperplasia.

ADVERSE REACTIONS AND PRECAUTIONS. Gastrointestinal disturbances (anorexia, nausea, vomiting, and diarrhea) occur in 80% of patients and are usually dose limiting. About 40% of patients experience central nervous system side effects (lethargy and somnolence, 25%; dizziness or vertigo, 15%). About 15% of patients develop dermatitis. Less frequent adverse effects are visual disturbances (eg, blurred vision, diplopia, lens opacities, retinopathy), albuminuria, hemorrhagic cystitis, flushing, hyperpyrexia, orthostatic hypotension, and hypertension. Hypersensitivity to mitotane has been reported and is a contraindication to use.

This drug is classified in FDA Pregnancy Category C.

PHARMACOKINETICS. Approximately 40% of an oral dose is absorbed from the gastrointestinal tract; the remaining 60% is recovered unchanged in feces. Daily doses of 5 to 15 g produce blood concentrations of 10 to 90 mcg/ml of unchanged drug and 30 to 50 mcg/ml of a metabolite. Plasma concentrations of mitotane are measurable for six to nine weeks after discontinuation of therapy. Although the drug is found in all tissues, fat is the primary site of storage. Approximately 25% of an oral or parenteral dose can be recovered in urine as a water-soluble metabolite.

DOSAGE AND PREPARATIONS.
Oral: Initially, 2 to 6 g is given in three or four divided doses daily. The dose is increased gradually to the maximum tolerated amount, which may vary from 2 to 16 g but is usually 7 to 10 g daily. If adverse reactions occur, the dose is reduced until the maximal tolerated amount is determined. Therapy should be supervised by a physician familiar with the use of mitotane, and patients may be hospitalized until a maintenance dose is established. Treatment should be continued as long as clinical benefit is apparent. If no improvement is observed after three months of therapy with the maximal tolerated dose, the drug should be discontinued.

Lysodren (Bristol-Myers). Tablets 500 mg.

Estrogens and Antiestrogens

Estrogens (and androgens) administered in supraphysiologic amounts were the first agents available to treat cancer. Nonsteroidal synthetic estrogen agonists currently are used more frequently than the naturally occurring molecules or other steroidal estrogens. However, all of these agents are used much less often than tamoxifen, a nonsteroidal drug that is an estrogen receptor antagonist in breast tissue but a partial agonist in some other tissues (Jordan, 1993; Sutherland and Mobbs, 1992).

The mechanisms responsible for the therapeutic effects of, and tumor growth inhibition by, estrogen agonists are not well understood. In males with prostate cancer, high concentrations of circulating estrogens act on normal feedback regulatory mechanisms through suppression of gonadotropin release to decrease production of androgens required to support growth of the tumor. In both prostate and breast cancer, some of the synthetic nonsteroidal estrogens may have direct cytotoxic actions on tumor cells that may or may not be mediated by hormone receptors. Other possibilities include effects of estrogens on chromosomes or on mitosis, stimulation of growth inhibitors such as transforming growth factor-β or mammostatin, and receptor down-regulation (or inhibition of resynthesis of receptor molecules) in response to the high agonist concentration.

Estrogen antagonists prevent stimulation of the growth of hormone-dependent tumor cells by endogenous estrogen as a consequence of competitive binding to the receptor. It is far from clear, however, whether this is the only action of tamoxifen that is responsible for its therapeutic efficacy (Glauber and Kiang, 1992; Jordan et al, 1992; Jordan, 1993).

At present, tamoxifen is the only antiestrogen available for treatment of breast cancer other than in sponsored clinical trials. Several others (eg, toremifene, trioxifene, droloxifene) are being studied in Phase II or III trials. Because tamoxifen and other triphenylethylene antiestrogens are partial agonists in some tissues other than breast, efforts to develop pure antagonists that are more selective in their antitumor effects than tamoxifen continue (Jordan et al, 1992; Jordan, 1993).

ESTROGENS

USES. Estrogens have been used in the palliative management of estrogen receptor-positive metastatic breast carcinoma in postmenopausal women. Although the antiestrogen, tamoxifen, is now the primary therapy for these patients, estrogens may induce regression in those who relapse after initially responding to tamoxifen.

Estrogen induces objective tumor responses in 50% to 60% of patients with estrogen receptor-positive breast tumors. Positive responses are confined primarily to metastatic disease in soft tissues, lung, and bone and generally last about 12 to 14 months. Tumor regression may not be apparent for several weeks, and therapy may have to be continued for 8 to 12 weeks before effectiveness can be evaluated. If the response is favorable, therapy should be continued until there is evidence of disease progression. Occasionally, the tumor may again regress when estrogen subsequently is withdrawn.

Estrogens also have been used in the palliative treatment of advanced carcinoma of the prostate. However, their use as initial therapy for this indication has declined in recent years because of the increased risk of cardiovascular disease in men receiving estrogens and the availability of LHRH agonists. In randomized trials, the length of survival for patients with advanced prostatic cancer was similar for patients who received estrogens, LHRH agonists, or had undergone orchiectomy as primary endocrine therapy (Trump and Robertson, 1993; Hanks et al, 1993). A palliative effect in disseminated prostatic carcinoma can be produced in about 75% of patients by each of these therapeutic options. Successful treatment is manifested almost immediately by reduced bone pain and decreased levels of prostate-specific antigen (PSA) and acid phosphatase. High-dose intravenous diethylstilbestrol diphosphate or oral diethylstilbestrol also have been reported to relieve bone pain and produce objective signs of response in patients with advanced or metastatic prostate cancer that has become refractory to other hormonal therapies.

Of the estrogens available, oral diethylstilbestrol is used most frequently for patients with breast or prostate carcinoma; chlorotrianisene is employed least often.

ADVERSE REACTIONS AND PRECAUTIONS. When estrogens are used to treat breast carcinoma, adverse effects include edema, nausea, anorexia, altered libido, breast swelling and tenderness, abdominal cramps, diarrhea, dizziness, irritability, and urinary incontinence. Fluid retention may be severe, especially in patients with cardiovascular disease. Pigmentation of the nipples, areola, and axilla occurs frequently.

Occasionally, bone pain and the neoplastic process are exacerbated at the onset of estrogen therapy for breast cancer. Hypercalcemia is a potentially fatal complication, and appropriate treatment must be instituted. However, hypercalcemia may indicate the likelihood of a favorable antitumor response later and, unless the tumor is progressing rapidly by objective measures, treatment may be continued.

Since the liver inactivates estrogens, toxic effects tend to be more severe in the presence of hepatic damage. Rarely, cholestatic jaundice may occur.

Urinary incontinence when coughing or straining (stress incontinence) is a frequent complaint of older women receiving estrogen therapy. Postmenopausal patients should be warned that uterine bleeding often occurs with prolonged high-dose estrogen therapy or on withdrawal of estrogen. Vaginal carcinoma has been reported rarely in the offspring of women who received diethylstilbestrol during pregnancy.

When estrogens are used for prostatic carcinoma, gynecomastia and impotence are expected adverse effects. Fluid retention may be hazardous and should be treated appropriately. Diethylstilbestrol diphosphate (a nonsteroidal estrogen agonist) can cause pruritus and burning pain in the anogenital region or at metastatic sites during or after rapid administration. These effects may be ameliorated by slowing the rate of intravenous infusion and administering antihistamines or sedatives simultaneously. The risk of cardiovascular complications (eg, myocardial infarction, cerebrovascular accidents, deep vein thrombosis, pulmonary embolism) is 10% to 20% with a dose of 3 mg/day of diethylstilbestrol and increases with larger doses (5 mg/day) (Trump and Robertson, 1993; Hanks et al, 1993). Hypophosphatemia secondary to renal excretion may occur.

DOSAGE AND PREPARATIONS. Diethylstilbestrol is the estrogen agonist used most frequently in patients with breast or prostate cancer.

CHLOROTRIANISENE:

Oral: For prostatic carcinoma, 12 to 25 mg daily.

CONJUGATED ESTROGENS:

Oral: For breast carcinoma, 10 mg three times daily; for prostatic carcinoma, 3.75 to 7.5 mg daily.

DIETHYLSTILBESTROL (DES):

Oral: For breast carcinoma, 1 to 5 mg three times daily; for prostatic carcinoma, 1 to 3 mg daily.

DIETHYLSTILBESTROL DIPHOSPHATE:

Intravenous: For prostatic carcinoma, 500 mg dissolved in 300 ml of saline or 5% dextrose on the first day; 1 g in 300 ml of saline or dextrose is then given daily for five days or more, depending on the response of the patient. The infusion should be administered slowly (20 to 30 drops/min) during the first 10 to 15 minutes and then the rate of flow adjusted so that the entire amount is given within one hour. Following the first intensive course of therapy, 250 to 500 mg may be administered in a similar manner once or twice weekly, or oral maintenance therapy may be instituted.

Oral: For prostatic carcinoma, 50 mg three times daily, increased to 200 mg or more if necessary.

ESTERIFIED ESTROGENS:

Oral: For breast carcinoma, 10 mg three times daily; for prostatic carcinoma, 1.25 mg or more three times daily.

ESTRONE:

Intramuscular: For prostatic carcinoma, 2 to 4 mg two or three times weekly.

ETHINYL ESTRADIOL:

Oral: For breast carcinoma, 0.5 to 1 mg three times daily; for prostatic carcinoma, 0.15 to 3 mg daily.

POLYESTRADIOL PHOSPHATE:

Intramuscular (deep): For prostatic carcinoma, initially, 40 mg every two to four weeks or less frequently. If the response is not satisfactory, up to 80 mg may be given.

For preparations, see index entry Estrogens, Preparations.

ESTRAMUSTINE PHOSPHATE SODIUM

[Emcyt]

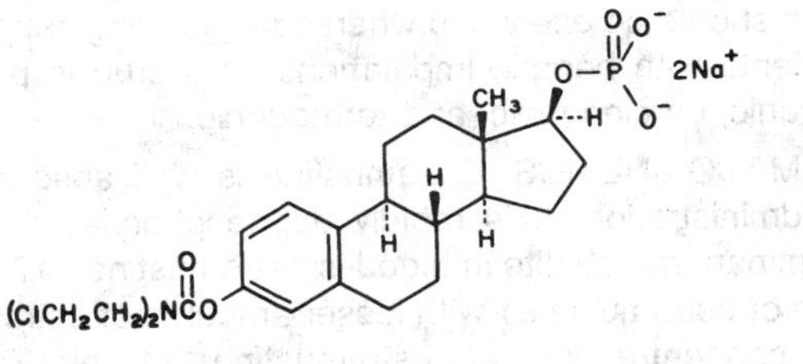

ACTIONS. Estramustine phosphate is composed of nor-nitrogen mustard covalently linked to estradiol. The drug is concentrated in the prostate through the action of an "estramustine binding protein" distinct from known steroid receptors. Although the mechanism by which this protein transports estramustine is not fully understood, its presence in prostatic cells is probably related to the drug's efficacy for prostatic tumors. Estramustine has a dual mode of action: the intact molecule acts as an antimitotic agent by promoting microtubule disassembly and, after hydrolysis of the carbamate ester bridge, the released estrogen exerts an antigonadotropin effect (Tew and Stearns, 1989). It also has weak estrogenic properties and causes little or no bone marrow depression with usual therapeutic doses.

USES. Estramustine is indicated for the palliative management of patients with advanced prostatic carcinoma. A wide range of response rates has been reported; however, the criteria for determination of response often have been poorly defined and, in some studies, may have included maintenance of stable disease. Estramustine's effectiveness appears to be similar to that of estrogen alone. The rates generally are higher (approximately 80%) (Benson and Gill, 1986) in previously untreated patients than in those who had received other hormonal therapy (approximately ≤35%), although a higher rate was reported in those studies that included stable disease as a response to therapy. Durations of responses also are variable (3 to 36 months). Since some patients who have become refractory to estrogen therapy respond to estramustine, its major indication appears to be in this group (Murphy et al 1986; Benson and Gill, 1986). Recent data suggest that the combination of estramustine and vinblastine (a vinca alkaloid that also interferes with microtubule assembly) is useful in patients with prostate cancer refractory to other hormonal therapy (Hudes et al, 1992; Seidman et al, 1992).

Clinical trials also have demonstrated that patients with breast tumors, melanoma, or renal cell carcinoma respond to estramustine (Tew and Stearns, 1989); however, the drug rarely is used for these indications at present.

ADVERSE REACTIONS AND PRECAUTIONS. The adverse effects associated with estramustine are primarily due to the estrogenic component. Gynecomastia is most common. Fluid retention is relatively common, and the drug should be used with caution in patients with cardiovascular disease. An increased risk of stroke is associated with estrogen therapy, particularly when large doses are employed. Hypercalcemia, although uncommon, is serious. Minor gastrointestinal disturbances (nausea, diarrhea) occasionally are observed. Altered liver function tests (eg, LDH, AST) are common, and caution should be exercised when administering estramustine to patients with hepatic impairment. This drug is potentially mutagenic, carcinogenic, and teratogenic.

PHARMACOKINETICS. Estramustine is well absorbed after oral administration. It is rapidly dephosphorylated, and the predominant metabolite in blood is estromustine (17-keto analogue of estramustine) with lesser amounts of estramustine. Peak concentrations of estramustine (1 mcg/ml) are reached two to three hours following a dose of 7.5 mg/kg. Elimination from plasma appears to be multiphasic; the half-life of the terminal phase is about 20 hours. In addition to estromustine and estramustine, estrone and estradiol are biotransformation products of estramustine phosphate. Excretion via the biliary route appears most likely.

DOSAGE AND PREPARATIONS.

Oral: Doses range from 1 to 10 capsules daily (usually 6 to 8) in three or four divided doses. Although responses (eg, decreased bone pain) have occurred after two weeks, patients should be treated for 30 to 90 days before therapy is evaluated. Treatment should be continued until evidence of disease progression is observed.

Emcyt (Kabi Pharmacia). Capsules equivalent to 140 mg estramustine phosphate. (Refrigerate; protect from light.)

TAMOXIFEN CITRATE

[Nolvadex]

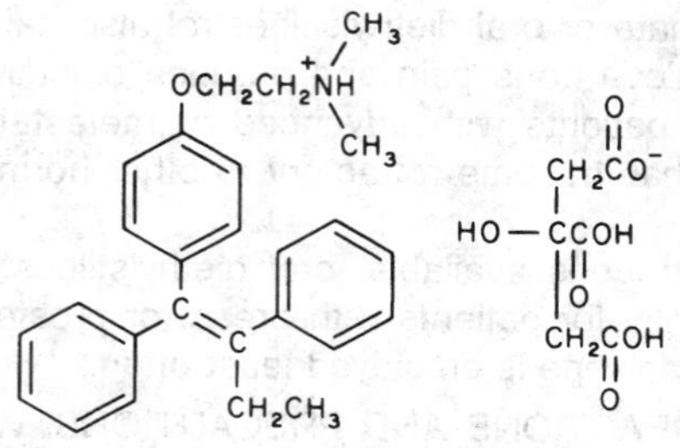

ACTIONS. Tamoxifen is a nonsteroidal antiestrogenic agent. The antiestrogenic effects appear to be at least partly related to the drug's ability to compete with estradiol for binding to estrogen receptors (eg, in breast cancer cells) (Jensen and DeSombre, 1993; Jordan, 1993). Tamoxifen forms a stable complex with the estrogen receptor in the nucleus of receptor-positive cells, but the tamoxifen-receptor complex does not induce expression of all estrogen-responsive genes. Furthermore, estrogen receptor content is depleted in the presence of this drug. Recent data suggest that tamoxifen also may inhibit replication by additional mechanisms, including decreasing transforming growth factor-α and increasing transforming growth factor-β expression.

USES. Tamoxifen is the most widely used endocrine therapy for palliation of metastatic breast cancer in women with indolent tumors that are positive for estrogen and/or progesterone receptors (Fisher et al, 1993; Harris et al, 1993). Tamoxifen is the therapy of first choice for this indication in postmenopausal women and is an alternative that appears to produce response rates comparable to oophorectomy in premenopausal women (Sunderland and Osborne, 1991). Nevertheless, tamoxifen does not induce a complete medical oophorectomy, and responses to surgical oophorectomy have been observed in some premenopausal women whose breast tumors did not respond or relapsed after tamoxifen therapy. Patients with rapidly growing tumors (most often receptor-negative) or with visceral involvement are usually treated with combination chemotherapy, with tamoxifen reserved for later use if the tumor is receptor-positive (see index entry Cancer: Clinical Responses to Chemotherapy).

Approximately 30% of women with advanced breast cancer whose receptor status is unknown will benefit from tamoxifen; in contrast, fewer than 10% of women with receptor-negative tumors will benefit. Overall response rates in postmenopausal women with advanced estrogen receptor-positive breast cancer average about 60%; the durations range from 4 to more than 40 months (median, 14 to 16 months). Soft tissue and osseous lesions respond better than visceral disease. Previous hormonal therapy with or without previous cytotoxic treatment does not preclude a response to tamoxifen. In postmenopausal women with receptor-positive tumors that progress after an initial response to tamoxifen, aminoglutethimide or a progestin (megestrol acetate or medroxyprogesterone acetate) is most commonly chosen for subsequent therapy. However, estrogen therapy also may be useful for these women, and withdrawal of tamoxifen has been beneficial occasionally. Premenopausal patients whose tumors respond to tamoxifen initially but then progress are somewhat more likely to respond to ovarian ablation (using surgery, radiation, or LHRH agonists) as subsequent therapy than those whose tumors had been refractory to the antiestrogen.

Tamoxifen also is indicated as adjuvant therapy for early-stage breast cancer to reduce the rates of local or distant recurrence and to increase survival in specific patient subpopulations (Early Breast Cancer Trialists' Collaborative Group, 1992; National Institutes of Health Consensus Development Panel, 1992; Harris et al, 1992; Council on Scientific Affairs, 1993; Fisher et al, 1993; Harris et al, 1993). Current recommendations for management of these patients are based on a meta-analysis of 133 randomized clinical trials that included a total of 75,000 women (Early Breast Cancer Trialists' Collaborative Group, 1992) and on a consensus development conference sponsored by the U.S. National Cancer Institute in 1990 (*J Natl Cancer Inst Monographs*, 1992).

Although data are not yet available from the randomized, controlled trials presently in progress (eg, the National Surgical Adjuvant Breast Project trial B-21), most clinicians currently believe that adjuvant therapy with tamoxifen usually is not indicated in women with axillary node-negative tumors ≤1cm in diameter. In postmenopausal women with estrogen receptor-positive tumors >1 cm in diameter, tamoxifen monotherapy usually is the recommended adjuvant therapy for most patients with axillary node-negative and for some with node-positive tumors. A combination chemotherapy regimen (see index entry Cancer: Clinical Responses to Chemotherapy) may be indicated for those at highest risk of recurrence. Postmenopausal women with receptor-negative tumors may be given a combination regimen of cytotoxic drugs as adjuvant therapy, although some may benefit from the addition of tamoxifen (chemohormonal therapy). Similarly, most clinicians recommend a combination of cytotoxic agents as adjuvant therapy for early-stage breast cancer in premenopausal women with a significant risk of recurrence. Some women with receptor-positive tumors may be given tamoxifen after completion of the chemotherapy course (in rare instances with ovarian ablation). Some data suggest that ovarian ablation may be an acceptable or even superior alternative to adjuvant therapy with multidrug regimens of cytotoxic agents in premenopausal women with receptor-positive tumors and some nodal involvement (stage II breast carcinoma) (Scottish Cancer Trials Breast Group and ICRF Breast Unit, 1993).

Estimates of the risk of recurrence after primary therapy are based on prognostic indicators such as tumor size, number of positive axillary nodes, histologic subtype, nuclear grade, and hormone receptor status. Assays of the tumor cell proliferative rate (most often by the fraction of cells in S phase or the degree of aneuploidy) also may provide prognostic information. A number of additional tumor markers are under clinical investigation (Fisher et al, 1993; Harris et al, 1993).

Many questions about optimal adjuvant therapy for early-stage breast cancer are unanswered. Data are insufficient to determine if chemotherapy followed by tamoxifen is more effective than tamoxifen alone for preventing tumor recurrence or death in women with node-negative, receptor-positive tumors or in those with node-positive, receptor-positive tumors. It also is unknown if tamoxifen is useful in women with node-negative, receptor-negative tumors. Finally, the optimal duration of adjuvant therapy with tamoxifen remains to be determined (two, three, or five years or longer). Physicians are urged to enroll patients with early-stage breast cancer in one of the ongoing clinical trials designed to address these questions. The recommendations summarized above can serve to guide the choice of therapy for patients (and their physicians) who either choose not to participate or are ineligible for a clinical trial.

Tamoxifen also is being studied for chemoprevention of breast cancer (Powles et al, 1990; Rutqvist et al, 1991; Nayfield et al, 1991). Data from several adjuvant therapy trials indicate that tamoxifen reduces the occurrence of second (contralateral) primary breast tumors in postmenopausal women. A large-scale primary prevention trial is underway in the United States, and additional trials are planned or in progress in Italy, the United Kingdom, and Australia. The American trial is enrolling women older than 60 years and those women between 35 and 59 years whose risk of developing breast cancer (based on factors such as history of breast tumors in first-degree relatives, previous breast biopsies, age at menarche, age at first birth) is equal to that of a 60-year-old woman. Women enrolled in this trial are randomized to receive tamoxifen (20 mg/day for five years) or placebo. The effects of tamoxifen on the incidence of breast cancer, osteoporosis and bone fractures, and myocardial infarction will be studied in a total of 16,000 women. Because the benefits of such therapy remain unproven and many years must elapse before the results of these studies will become available, this use of tamoxifen is not recommended at present outside of the trial.

Tamoxifen also is used as first-line therapy for metastatic breast cancer in males because these rare tumors usually are positive for estrogen receptors. Response rates to tamoxifen in males are similar to those produced by orchiectomy (approximately 50% overall and 70% in those with receptor-positive tumors).

Randomized trials of adjuvant therapy for breast cancer in males have not been conducted because this disease occurs very infrequently. However, data from an uncontrolled series of 39 men with node-positive stage II or III breast tumors suggest that adjuvant therapy with tamoxifen increases overall and disease-free survival compared with historical controls (Ribeiro and Swindell, 1992).

The efficacy of tamoxifen also has been studied in patients with metastatic tumors other than breast cancer. Results of several studies suggest that this drug can increase objective response rates to dacarbazine (with or without other cytotoxic drugs) in patients with metastatic melanoma (McClay et al, 1992; Cocconi et al, 1992 A). In one study, the enhanced response to chemotherapy in patients also given tamoxifen was observed in females but not in males (Cocconi et al, 1992 A). Other investigators have not observed a significant interaction between tamoxifen and dacarbazine-based combination chemotherapy regimens (Buzaid et al, 1991). Additional clinical trials addressing this issue are in progress.

Responses to tamoxifen also have been observed in some patients with advanced ovarian carcinoma that did not respond to first-line combination chemotherapy (Hatch et al, 1991), in a small percentage of patients with metastatic renal cell carcinoma (Stahl et al, 1992; Papac and Keohane, 1993), and in some patients with desmoid tumors (Wilcken and Tattersall, 1991). However, data are inadequate to support the use of tamoxifen for these indications outside of controlled clinical trials. No responses were reported in patients with advanced hepatocellular carcinoma (Engstrom et al, 1990).

ADVERSE REACTIONS AND PRECAUTIONS. Adverse effects of tamoxifen occur less frequently and are significantly milder than with androgens or estrogens. In early trials of tamoxifen therapy for advanced breast cancer, no life-threatening adverse reactions were reported in more than 1,000 patients, and less than 3% were unable to tolerate the drug. Those who temporarily withdrew from therapy or required dosage reduction because of side effects often were able to tolerate reduced dosage or resume therapy.

In the more recent trials of tamoxifen as adjuvant therapy for early-stage breast cancer, similar percentages of patients (3% to 5%) from both treated and placebo-control groups withdrew from the studies because of adverse reactions. The most common reactions were nausea or vomiting and hot flashes, which occurred in 10% to 20% of patients in each study arm. Vaginal bleeding or discharge, menstrual irregularities, and rash were reported less frequently.

Similar adverse effects were reported by women enrolled in a randomized, controlled, double-blind study of the symptoms associated with tamoxifen therapy in postmenopausal women with node-negative breast cancer. This study used a detailed questionnaire to elicit comprehensive responses regarding hot flashes, gynecologic symptoms, fatigue, joint pain, gastrointestinal distress, depression, and headache (Love et al, 1991 A). Significantly more women in the tamoxifen arm than in the control arm reported severe hot flashes or other vasomotor symptoms. These adverse reactions occurred in most women, but their severity gradually decreased over several months. Nausea occurred in many women during the first several weeks of tamoxifen therapy but disappeared thereafter. Approximately 20% of women in the tamoxifen arm reported gynecologic complaints (significant vaginal discharge, pruritus, increased vaginal dryness) at six months. Although depression was reported more frequently among those receiving tamoxifen, headache occurred less often than in control subjects. Overall, 48% of the women in the tamoxifen arm and 21% of those in the control arm reported one or more persistent major side effects.

Increased tumor and bone pain, hypercalcemia, and local disease flare-up have occurred shortly after the start of tamoxifen therapy in a few patients with advanced disease. These usually resolve after a brief period in spite of continued therapy and appear to be predictive of a good response. Thromboembolic events also have been reported infrequently, but no direct causal relationship has been established between tamoxifen administration and their occurrence. They are most common when tamoxifen is combined with cytotoxic chemotherapy and may even be fatal.

Abnormal results of liver function tests have been reported rarely.

In animals, tamoxifen is carcinogenic and interferes with reproductive function. There is no conclusive evidence that this drug is carcinogenic in humans; however, in several studies, an increase in the incidence of endometrial cancer was reported in women given tamoxifen for one, two, or five years as adjuvant therapy for breast cancer (for review, see Wolf and Jordan, 1992). In some of these studies, the incidence of endometrial carcinoma was correlated with the duration of tamoxifen administration. Although the first report was from a trial using twice the presently recommended dose of tamoxifen (ie, 40 mg/day) (Fornander et al, 1989), other studies that reported an increased risk of endometrial cancer used the current standard dose of 20 mg/day. Furthermore, there are numerous reports of endometriosis, endocervical and endometrial polyps, and increased proliferation in the uterine mucosa in association with tamoxifen therapy (for review, see Wolf and Jordan, 1992). It should be noted that the increased risk of endometrial carcinoma is comparable to that reported for postmenopausal women using estrogen replacement therapy without progestins.

Unpublished data from a randomized, placebo-controlled trial in Sweden using tamoxifen 40 mg/day as adjuvant therapy in women with resected breast cancer and published data from a similar trial in the United States using tamoxifen 20 mg/day recently were incorporated into the labeling for this drug (Fisher et al, 1994). After seven to nine years' follow-up, results of both studies indicate that secondary uterine cancer occurred more frequently in the patients given tamoxifen for two to five years (in the Swedish study, 23 of 1,372 in the tamoxifen arm versus 4 of 1,357 controls; in the U.S. study, 15 of 1,419 women in the tamoxifen arm versus 2 of 1,424 controls). Most of the tumors were endometrial carcinoma, but the incidence of less common malignancies (eg, mixed müllerian tumors, uterine sarcomas) also may have increased. Although most of the secondary tumors were diagnosed at early stages and were generally considered curable, fatalities from uterine cancer have occurred after treatment with tamoxifen for breast cancer. Although data from a retrospective study had suggested that endometrial carcinomas that develop after tamoxifen therapy may be more aggressive or of higher grade than in untreated women (Magriples et al, 1993), the results of both randomized trials do not support this conclusion (Fornander et al, 1993; Fisher et al, 1994). In addition, it should be stressed that the quantitative benefit from adjuvant therapy with tamoxifen (ie, delayed or reduced recurrence of breast cancer) far outweighs the risk of endometrial and other uterine cancers. Women who receive tamoxifen as adjuvant hormonal therapy should be instructed to have regular gynecologic examinations and should promptly inform their physicians of any menstrual irregularities, abnormal vaginal bleeding, change in vaginal discharge, or pelvic pain or pressure.

Some premenopausal women developed ovarian cysts or enlargement of uterine fibroids after treatment with tamoxifen.

Induction of ovarian steroidogenesis and elevation of serum estrogen and estradiol concentrations during the follicular phase of the menstrual cycle also have occurred (for review, see Wolf and Jordan, 1992). These effects are not accompanied by major changes in the circulating levels of follicle stimulating hormone or luteinizing hormone. Premenopausal women continue to menstruate while taking tamoxifen and thus can become pregnant. They should be counseled regarding the use of barrier contraceptives to avoid pregnancy. The manufacturer recommends that pregnant women not take tamoxifen, since this drug may cause birth defects, fetal deaths, spontaneous abortions, vaginal bleeding in pregnant women, or a diethylstilbestrol-like syndrome in the daughters of women treated with tamoxifen during pregnancy. This drug is classified in FDA Pregnancy Category D.

A few cases of retinal and corneal damage occurred following use of very large doses in Phase I studies (120 to 160 mg twice daily for more than 17 months). This is equivalent to 20 to 30 years of therapy at recommended dosage levels. In a prospective study in patients receiving tamoxifen 20 mg/day for up to three years, the incidence of retinopathy and/or keratopathy was 6.3% (Pavlidis et al, 1992). Most of these ocular effects were reversible on drug withdrawal.

DRUG INTERACTIONS. In some women taking the coumarin anticoagulant, warfarin, at the same time as tamoxifen, an increase in prothrombin time has been noted and occasionally has resulted in life-threatening bleeding episodes. This interaction presumably results from displacement of warfarin from protein binding sites by tamoxifen and requires close monitoring of prothrombin times (with anticoagulant dose reductions when necessary).

CARDIOVASCULAR AND METABOLIC EFFECTS. In randomized placebo-controlled, double-blind studies of hemostatic changes in women receiving tamoxifen as adjuvant therapy (Love et al, 1992 A) or for chemoprevention (Jones et al, 1992), decreases in the plasma concentrations of fibrinogen and, in postmenopausal women, much smaller declines in antithrombin III concentrations were reported. Platelet counts also decreased in the adjuvant therapy trial. In addition, retrospective analyses of the data from the Scottish Adjuvant Tamoxifen Trial and the Stockholm Breast Cancer Study Group demonstrated that the incidence of fatal myocardial infarction and of hospital admissions for cardiac disease were significantly reduced by long-term tamoxifen therapy (McDonald et al, 1991; Rutqvist and Mattsson, 1993).

The effects of long-term therapy with tamoxifen on blood lipids and other cardiovascular risk factors also have been studied in postmenopausal women with early-stage breast cancer (Love et al, 1991 B; Dewar et al, 1992). Reductions were observed in the concentrations of total and low-density lipoprotein cholesterol in patients treated with tamoxifen. In one of these studies (Love et al, 1991 B), a greater cholesterol-lowering effect occurred in women with the highest baseline levels of total cholesterol. These investigators also reported increased levels of apolipoprotein A-1 and decreased levels of apolipoprotein B among tamoxifen recipients; other cardiovascular risk factors did not appear to change. The magnitude of the decrease in cholesterol levels appeared sufficient to contribute to a reduction in the incidence of fatal myocardial infarction reported earlier (McDonald et al, 1991). However, periodic monitoring of plasma triglycerides and cholesterol may be advisable in patients with pre-existing hyperlipidemias because lipid levels have been reported to increase infrequently in these women.

Despite the antiestrogenic effects of tamoxifen and the role of estrogen in maintenance of bone density in women, tamoxifen therapy does not appear to cause osteoporosis. In fact, clinical studies suggest that the drug may protect women from bone mineral loss, possibly because of its estrogen agonist actions on bone. Bone mineral density (measured by photon absorptiometry) and biochemical measures of bone metabolism were monitored in a randomized, placebo-controlled, double-blind trial of tamoxifen therapy in postmenopausal women with early-stage breast cancer (Love et al, 1992 B). Although the mean mineral density of the lumbar spine decreased by approximately 1% per year among women in the placebo arm of this trial, it increased by 0.61% per year in those taking tamoxifen. In addition, serum osteocalcin and alkaline phosphatase concentrations decreased significantly in the women given tamoxifen; no difference was observed between the two groups in serum concentrations of parathyroid hormone or 1,25-dihydroxyvitamin D. Results of a second study confirmed that serum concentrations of alkaline phosphatase decreased in women taking tamoxifen, and bone histomorphometry (by image analysis of bone biopsy specimens) documented the fact that the rate of bone remodeling decreased in those taking the antiestrogen (Wright et al, 1993). Data from these studies are insufficient to determine if the decrease in the loss of bone mineral in postmenopausal women receiving tamoxifen will be associated with reductions in the incidence of fractures.

PHARMACOKINETICS. Data on the pharmacokinetics of tamoxifen were established, in part, by radioisotope studies in women. Peak plasma levels occur at four to seven hours after a single dose, and only 20% to 30% is present as parent drug. There is an initial half-life of 7 to 14 hours with a second phase of four to seven days. With prolonged administration, three to four weeks are required to attain steady state plasma levels. Radiolabeled tracer studies reveal that tamoxifen is excreted slowly in the feces, and only a small amount is detectable in the urine. N-demethylation followed by deamination is the principal route of metabolism. Most of a single dose is eliminated as conjugates of the deaminated metabolite; less than 30% is excreted in hydroxylated or unchanged form. Tamoxifen apparently undergoes enterohepatic circulation.

DOSAGE AND PREPARATIONS.

Oral: For advanced breast carcinoma, 20 mg daily in a single or in two divided doses. If there is no response to this dose in two to three months, the amount may be increased to 20 mg twice daily. However, few patients who did not respond to the lower dose benefit from larger doses; an alternative form of endocrine therapy (aminoglutethimide, a progestin, or an estrogen) or cytotoxic chemotherapy might be considered for nonresponsive patients.

For adjuvant therapy, 20 mg in a single or in two divided doses has been given for two to five years or longer in various clinical trials. The optimal duration of adjuvant therapy has not been established.

Nolvadex (ZENECA). Tablets equivalent to 10 mg of the base. (Protect from heat and light.)

Androgens and Antiandrogens

Although the mechanisms responsible for the efficacy of androgens as therapy for breast cancer are not completely understood, they appear to be mediated by the estrogen receptor; a requirement for aromatization of the exogenous androgens to estrogens has not been excluded (Bruchovsky, 1993). The actions of androgens on breast cancer probably are not analogous to those of estrogens on prostate cancer (ie, suppression of gonadotropin production and thus blockade of gonadal steroidogenesis), since androgens are active in postmenopausal as well as premenopausal women. Potential indirect actions of androgens in patients with breast cancer include inhibition of growth factor production or activity, stimulation of growth inhibitor production or activity, and induction of differentiation in malignant stem cells. Because of their virilizing effects and because other effective therapies with more acceptable side effects are available, the use of androgens for breast cancer is declining (Bruchovsky, 1993; Fisher et al, 1993).

Antiandrogens, or androgen receptor antagonists, block hormonal stimulation of prostate tumor growth in a manner analogous to the effects of tamoxifen on breast cancer cells. At this time, flutamide is the sole antiandrogen generally available for treatment of prostatic carcinoma outside of clinical trials; other antiandrogens (eg, cyproterone acetate, nilutamide, casodex) are in various stages of development. Flutamide is used most often in combination with a gonadotropin-releasing hormone agonist (eg, leuprolide, goserelin).

Newer approaches to blocking the stimulatory effects of androgens on prostate tumor growth include administration of inhibitors of steroid hydroxylation, such as ketoconazole, and inhibitors of 5α reductase (the enzyme that converts testosterone to dihydrotestosterone), such as finasteride. Treatment with ketoconazole acutely reduces plasma testosterone levels by preventing its biosynthesis, while finasteride prevents the conversion of testosterone to dihydrotestosterone in prostate cells.

ANDROGENS

For individual chemical formulas, see index entry Anabolic Steroids (Table).

USES. Androgens have been used in the palliative management of estrogen receptor-positive, disseminated breast carcinoma in postmenopausal women, although the antiestrogen, tamoxifen, is now the primary therapy for these patients. Response rates to androgens are lower than with other forms of hormonal therapy (eg, one-half of that observed with diethylstilbestrol). Thus, androgens are rarely used. Patients with advanced breast cancer who do not respond to tamoxifen rarely if ever respond to androgens.

In women with hormone-dependent metastatic breast cancer, remissions induced by androgens generally last 12 to 14 months. Soft tissue metastases are most responsive, followed by osseous lesions; metastases to viscera are least responsive. As with estrogens, several weeks may elapse before a beneficial action is evident (see the preceding evaluation on Estrogens).

The prototype parenteral androgen preparations, testosterone propionate and enanthate, although as effective as other androgens, are now rarely used because of their marked virilizing effect. Fluoxymesterone is less virilizing than testosterone and is the most commonly employed androgen for women with advanced breast cancer. Testolactone is relatively inert hormonally, produces less masculinization, and induces remission slightly less often than other androgens.

ADVERSE REACTIONS AND PRECAUTIONS. Adverse effects include fluid retention, hypercalcemia, masculinization (clitoral enlargement, hirsutism, deepening of the voice, increased libido, acne), and alopecia. Erythrocythemia is common, and this side effect of androgens has been exploited in the treatment of some anemias. Cholestatic jaundice has been noted with oral therapy, and hepatocellular neoplasms rarely have been associated with long-term therapy. Rarely, exacerbation of the malignant process may occur.

Androgens are contraindicated in patients with serious cardiac, hepatic, or renal disease or hypercalcemia and in women known or suspected of being pregnant or in nursing mothers. If hypercalcemia develops, the androgen should be discontinued immediately and appropriate corrective measures instituted (eg, hydration, diuretics, adrenal corticosteroids, oral phosphate therapy, plicamycin). Androgens also are contraindicated in males with breast cancer or with known or suspected prostatic carcinoma.

DOSAGE AND PREPARATIONS.

FLUOXYMESTERONE:

Oral: 10 to 40 mg daily in divided doses for at least two to three months. In responding patients, therapy may be continued until the tumor progresses if toxicity is acceptable.

METHYLTESTOSTERONE:

Oral: 200 mg in divided doses.

Buccal: 100 mg daily in divided doses.

TESTOLACTONE:

Oral: 250 mg four times daily.

TESTOSTERONE ENANTHATE, TESTOSTERONE PROPIONATE:

Intramuscular: 100 mg three times weekly.

For androgen preparations, see index entry Androgens.

FLUTAMIDE

[Eulexin]

CF_3

$CH_3CHCONH$ — NO_2

CH_3

ACTIONS. Flutamide, an acetanilid nonsteroidal androgen antagonist, is devoid of androgen agonist or any hormonal activity other than its antiandrogen effects (Bruchovsky, 1993; Brogden and Chrisp, 1991). Its antagonist actions are primarily mediated by the hydroxylated metabolite, 2-hydroxyflutamide. This metabolite appears to have some specificity for binding to androgen receptors of the seminal vesicles and ventral prostate without activating expression of genes regulated by the receptors. In target tissues, it inhibits the uptake of testosterone and/or binding of dihydrotestosterone to the nuclear androgen receptor. It does not, however, inhibit conversion of testosterone to dihydrotestosterone.

When flutamide is administered alone, the absence of antigonadotropic activity present in other antiandrogens (eg, cyproterone acetate), plus the antiandrogen effects that block negative feedback by testosterone in the hypothalamus result in increased circulating levels of testosterone, estradiol, and luteinizing hormone (LH). When used with an LH-releasing hormone (LHRH) agonist such as leuprolide or goserelin (see evaluations) or in castrated men, complete androgen blockade is achieved and the compensatory increases are prevented (Crawford, 1989). In surgically or pharmacologically castrated patients, flutamide blocks the growth-stimulating effects of adrenal androgens (about 9% of total androgens in intact males) on prostate cancer cells due to its receptor antagonist effects. This is the primary rationale for the use of combined androgen blockade in the hormonal treatment of prostate carcinoma.

USES. Flutamide is most frequently used in combination with an LHRH agonist such as leuprolide or goserelin (ie, combined or maximal androgen blockade) as therapy for metastatic prostate carcinoma (stage D_2). However, there is disagreement about the benefits of combined androgen blockade compared with those of other therapies (eg, surgical or pharmacologic castration alone) for this disease.

In one of the first completed trials, flutamide plus leuprolide was reported to significantly increase progression-free survival and median length of survival (compared with leuprolide alone) in previously untreated patients (Crawford et al, 1989). Simultaneous treatment with the two drugs clearly decreased the incidence and severity of disease flare-up seen in the early stage of leuprolide monotherapy, an adverse effect resulting from initial stimulation of gonadotropin release and testosterone production by the LHRH agonist. To achieve maximal androgen blockade, it is important that flutamide therapy precede the start of LHRH agonist administration and that simultaneous administration of the two drugs then be continued. However, other clinicians argue that LHRH agonist monotherapy may not increase overall and progression-free survival to the same degree as surgical castration (for review, see Trump and Robertson, 1993; Bruchovsky, 1993; Hanks et al, 1993). Initial studies comparing orchiectomy with combined androgen blockade did not demonstrate any difference in overall or progression-free survival (Denis and Mettlin, 1990). Thus, many clinicians found it difficult to justify the expense of long-term therapy with an LHRH agonist and flutamide and suggested that this therapeutic approach be reserved for patients who choose not to undergo orchiectomy. A more recent evaluation of the data from this study, with longer patient follow-up, showed that progression-free survival and overall survival were significantly increased (from 85 to 133 weeks and from 27.1 to 34.4 months, respectively) in the group given goserelin acetate plus flutamide compared with those given bilateral orchiectomy (Denis et al, 1993).

Results of most studies have demonstrated modest but definite advantage for the use of flutamide with an LHRH agonist when compared with monotherapy with the LHRH agonist. Some urologists hypothesized that this may result solely from flutamide's ability to prevent disease flare-up and stimulation of tumor growth during the first one or two weeks after the start of therapy with the LHRH agonist. Data from clinical trials suggest that responses to combined androgen blockade are usually of short duration in patients with extensive bone or soft tissue metastases and poor performance status (Hanks et al, 1993). In those with only minimal bone metastases and with good performance status, survival appears to be enhanced after use of combined androgen blockade. For the large majority of patients who fall between these two extremes and who choose not to undergo orchiectomy, some urologists recommend the use of flutamide with an LHRH agonist during the initial one to two weeks of therapy, followed by treatment with the LHRH agonist alone. Others believe that combined androgen blockade should be continued for all patients who refuse orchiectomy.

In a subset of men in whom prostate cancer progressed during combined androgen blockade therapy, symptoms improved and serum levels of prostate-specific antigen decreased significantly when the antiandrogen was withdrawn (Kelley and Scher, 1993; Scher and Kelley, 1993; Dupont et al, 1993). This "withdrawal response" did not occur in patients who had not responded upon addition of flutamide to previous hormonal therapy when the tumor progressed and in whom the flutamide was withdrawn. These observations suggest that flutamide withdrawal may be a useful strategy to try before more toxic therapies are employed for managing patients whose condition progresses after an initial response to flutamide plus surgical or pharmacologic castration.

Data from uncontrolled studies suggest that treatment with flutamide alone can produce objective signs of response and subjective improvement (decreased bone pain) in some patients with either previously untreated or refractory advanced prostate carcinoma. Not surprisingly, response rates are higher in patients not previously treated with other hormonal therapies. Response rates for flutamide and diethylstilbestrol are nearly equivalent when these drugs are used alone for advanced prostate cancer. However, only preliminary results on survival and disease progression have been reported from randomized, double-blind, controlled trials comparing the effects of surgical castration plus flutamide with orchiectomy alone. Thus far, results of these studies suggest that survival and the mean time to treatment failure may be increased after total androgen ablation (at the expense of a modest increase in adverse reactions) when compared with surgical castration alone. Meta-analysis of the data from seven randomized trials comparing orchiectomy plus the investigational antiandrogen, nilutamide, with orchiectomy plus placebo showed statistically significant increases in the response rate and the duration of responses for the combined treatment (Hucher et al, 1993). There also was a trend toward increased survival in the group given orchiectomy plus nilutamide, but the increased duration was not statistically significant.

ADVERSE REACTIONS AND PRECAUTIONS. In noncastrated men treated with flutamide alone, the major side effects are gynecomastia (incidence, between 34% and 100% in various studies) and gastrointestinal discomfort (nausea, vomiting, diarrhea). When used in surgically castrated patients or with an LHRH agonist, gynecomastia occurs much less frequently (incidence, about 9%).

When flutamide is used alone in noncastrated men, the incidence of impotence and loss of libido are reduced by >80% compared with other hormonal therapies for prostate cancer (eg, diethylstilbestrol, estramustine phosphate, surgical castration). Impaired potency and decreased libido occur frequently (incidence, 30% to 35%) in men treated with flutamide and leuprolide. The other frequent side effect reported with the drug combination is hot flashes, although the incidence is comparable to that in men treated with leuprolide alone. In trials comparing leuprolide alone with leuprolide plus flutamide (Crawford et al, 1989), mild diarrhea was the only adverse reaction that occurred significantly more often in the group treated with both drugs.

Elevations in results of liver function tests (alanine aminotransferase and bilirubin) that reverse when treatment is discontinued have been reported in up to 33% of patients; some cases of severe toxic hepatitis (with several fatalities) also have been noted (Wysowski et al, 1993). Thus, periodic monitoring of liver function may be advisable and physicians should warn patients to report promptly any nausea, vomiting, fatigue, jaundice, or other signs and symptoms of liver damage that occur during therapy with flutamide.

Adverse reactions observed rarely include hemolytic and macrocytic anemias, methemoglobinemia, photosensitivity reactions, and discoloration of the urine.

Although flutamide is not mutagenic in vitro (even in the presence of liver microsomes), daily doses 3- to 17-fold higher than those recommended in humans were administered to rats for one year and produced testicular interstitial cell adenomas. In human males, flutamide reduces sperm counts. It does not interfere with the estrous cycle of female rats or with mating behavior of male or female rats even at doses 15 times higher than those used in humans. Conception rates were decreased at doses only five times higher than those used clinically. When flutamide was given to pregnant rats or rabbits, survival of the offspring was decreased. Developmental abnormalities and feminization of male offspring also were observed at higher doses. Flutamide is classified in FDA Pregnancy Category D.

PHARMACOKINETICS. Flutamide is rapidly and almost completely absorbed after oral administration. The major fraction of an absorbed dose is converted to the active metabolite, 2-hydroxyflutamide, during its first pass through the liver. After a single oral dose (250 mg), maximum concentrations of unchanged drug (10 to 20 mcg/L) are achieved within one hour; maximal concentrations of 2-hydroxyflutamide are much higher (about 1.3 mg/L) and peak somewhat later (about two hours). Both flutamide and its principal active metabolite are bound extensively (about 95% at steady state) to plasma proteins. In male rats, the prostate is the only tissue in which flutamide or its metabolites accumulate.

The elimination half-life for 2-hydroxyflutamide is about six hours after a dose of 250 mg but is extended to more than nine hours with a dose of 500 mg. Less than 4% of the dose remains as unchanged flutamide one hour after administration, and by eight hours no unmetabolized drug can be detected. At least ten metabolites are present but not all have been identified. After conversion of the major fraction to the 2-hydroxy metabolite, glucuronide formation is the next step in its elimination. Almost one-half of the dose is recovered in urine within 72 hours, with an additional 4% present in feces. The major metabolite present in urine is 2-amino-5-nitro-4-(trifluoromethyl)phenol.

After multiple doses (250 mg every eight hours) in normal geriatric volunteers, steady-state plasma levels of both flutamide (24 to 78 ng/ml) and 2-hydroxyflutamide (1,500 to 2,300 ng/ml) are achieved after the fourth dose. Since plasma concentrations of testosterone in surgically or pharmacologically castrated males are approximately 1 nmol/L, even trough concentrations of 2-hydroxyflutamide are 5,000 to 10,000 times higher than the dihydrotestosterone level. This ensures continuous occupancy of all prostatic androgen receptors by the antagonist.

DOSAGE AND PREPARATIONS.

Oral: For patients with metastatic prostate carcinoma receiving an LHRH agonist simultaneously, 250 mg three times daily at eight-hour intervals. The same schedule for a total dose of 750 mg/day is used in castrated males being treated with flutamide alone.

Eulexin (Schering). Capsules 125 mg.

Gonadotropin Releasing Hormone Analogues

Pulsatile secretion of gonadotropin releasing hormone (LHRH, luteinizing hormone-releasing hormone) from the hypothalamus stimulates the pituitary gland to release the gonadotropins, luteinizing hormone (LH) and follicle stimulating hormone (FSH). Testicular biosynthesis of androgens in males and ovarian synthesis of estrogens in females are regulated by LH and by the combination of LH and FSH, respectively. Continuous (as opposed to pulsatile) administration of LHRH or one of its agonist analogues results in down-regulation of LHRH receptors in the pituitary and thus blocks LH and FSH secretion and gonadal steroidogenesis (Conn and Crowley, 1991; Schally et al, 1993).

Two synthetic analogues of LHRH (leuprolide and goserelin) currently are available, and others (buserelin and triptorelin) are in various stages of development. (Nafarelin, another LHRH analogue, is available for the treatment of endometriosis and precocious puberty but has not been studied as an agent for hormonal therapy of prostate or breast cancer.) These analogues share structural features that increase their potencies as agonists and half-lives in vivo relative to the natural hormone. They also have identical mechanisms of action and nearly identical uses and adverse reactions. The

LHRH agonists provide an alternative to surgery (orchiectomy or oophorectomy) and are preferred to exogenous estrogens for steroid hormone-dependent prostatic tumors. Advantages to their use include reduced morbidity, patient preference (when compared with surgical castration), and fewer and milder side effects (when compared with estrogens).

LEUPROLIDE ACETATE
[Lupron Injection, Lupron Depot]

pyro Glu—His—Trp—Ser—Tyr—D—Leu—
Leu—Arg—Pro—NHEt • CH_3COOH

GOSERELIN ACETATE
[Zoladex]

pyro Glu—His—Trp—Ser—Tyr—D—Ser (tert Butyl)—
Leu—Arg—Pro—Azgly • CH_3COOH

BUSERELIN ACETATE (Investigational drug)

pyro Glu—His—Trp—Ser—Tyr—D—Ser (tert Butyl)—
Leu—Arg—Pro—ethylamide • CH_3COOH

ACTIONS. Leuprolide acetate, a nonapeptide; goserelin acetate, a decapeptide; and buserelin acetate, an investigational nonapeptide, are synthetic analogues of LHRH, a decapeptide, and have greater potency than the natural hormone. In these and other potent agonists, a D-amino acid is substituted in the sixth position. In leuprolide and buserelin, the N-terminus is modified by substitution of an ethylamide moiety for glycine; in goserelin, an azaglycine moiety is substituted.

LHRH agonists act as potent inhibitors of gonadotropin secretion when therapeutic doses are given continuously (Chrisp and Sorkin, 1991; Chrisp and Goa, 1991). Initial doses increase LH and FSH, resulting in transient increases in testosterone and dihydrotestosterone in males and estrone and estradiol in premenopausal females. Prolonged administration suppresses LH and FSH secretion and thus decreases testosterone to castration levels in males and reduces estrogens to postmenopausal levels in premenopausal females. The decreases are observed two to four weeks after initiation of treatment. Castration levels of testosterone persist for up to five years with continued therapy. In addition to the effects mediated by inhibition of gonadotropin secretion, data from animal studies suggest that LHRH agonists may directly inhibit testicular steroidogenesis by interfering with 17-hydroxylase and 17,20-desmolase activity. When the analogue is discontinued, gonadotropin and sex steroid levels usually return to normal gradually, but occasionally the levels remain low.

LHRH agonists do not affect adrenal androgen production or alter serum prolactin or cortisol levels.

USES. LHRH agonists are indicated for the palliative treatment of advanced prostatic carcinoma when orchiectomy is unacceptable to the patient.

As with castration or administration of diethylstilbestrol (DES) or other estrogen agonists, complete responses to LHRH agonists are rare in patients with stage D_2 prostatic carcinoma. Results of comparative studies suggest that the suppression of plasma testosterone levels (to <1 ng/ml), the rates and durations of responses (25% to 35% partial responses; stabilized disease in about 50%, with median durations of 10 to 18 months), and the median survival of these patients (24 to 30 months) are similar for all three forms of treatment (Chrisp and Sorkin, 1991; Chrisp and Goa, 1991; Schally et al, 1993; Trump and Robertson, 1993; Hanks et al, 1993). Relief of bone pain and urinary symptoms occurs in 60% to 80% of patients, while plasma levels of prostate-specific antigen are significantly decreased in 80% to 90%.

Although orchiectomy, DES, and LHRH agonists do not differ in efficacy as therapies for advanced prostate cancer, there are differences in patient preference, convenience, onset of response, safety, and cost (Chrisp and Sorkin, 1991; Chrisp and Goa, 1991; Schally et al, 1993; Trump and Robertson, 1993; Hanks et al, 1993).

Orchiectomy and LHRH agonist therapy cause fewer long-term adverse responses or morbidities than DES and other estrogen agonists. The risk of cardiovascular toxicity or thromboembolism is unacceptably high with doses of estrogen equivalent to DES >3 mg/day. Moreover, DES (but not orchiectomy or LHRH agonists) appears to cause painful gynecomastia in a larger percentage of patients than either of the other two therapies. Although it is widely assumed that therapy with LHRH agonists is the most costly, the limited data available suggest that the difference in cost between these agents and orchiectomy is modest (Rutqvist and Wilking, 1992). Since their endocrine effects are comparable, they impair potency and decrease libido to the same degree.

While orchiectomy may be most convenient since no further treatment is required after the surgical procedure, many men consider it the least preferred therapy for psychological reasons. Furthermore, castration may be associated with surgical complications such as wound infection or thrombosis, although the frequency of these adverse events is low.

The dosage form of leuprolide used in early clinical trials required daily subcutaneous injection, making it the least convenient of the therapies. However, with the depot forms of leuprolide and goserelin now available, the frequency of administration is reduced to once monthly without loss of efficacy. Because of initial stimulation of testosterone production by LHRH agonists, their onset of action (ie, the time required to reduce plasma concentrations of testosterone to <1 ng/ml) is delayed 7 to 10 days compared with the immediate effects of castration or estrogen therapy. This drawback can be overcome by concomitant administration of the androgen antagonist, flutamide, during the first two weeks of therapy with an LHRH agonist. (See the evaluation on this drug.)

LHRH agonists also are used as an alternative to oophorectomy in premenopausal women with advanced breast cancer (Chrisp and Goa, 1991; Schally et al, 1993; Fisher et al, 1993; Harris et al, 1993). These drugs reduce serum estrogen concentrations to levels found in postmenopausal women. Despite the initial increase in ovarian steroidogenesis that precedes down-regulation of LHRH receptors, the phenomenon of "tumor flare-up" is less well studied in women with advanced breast cancer than in men with advanced prostatic carcinoma. Data from clinical trials on women with metastatic disease indicate that overall response rates to LHRH agonists range from 30% to 50%, which compares favorably with response rates to oophorectomy. Response rates are highest among patients whose tumors are positive for estrogen and/or progesterone receptors. However, data from randomized clinical trials are not available yet to directly compare LHRH agonists with oophorectomy, to determine if the combination of tamoxifen with an LHRH agonist is superior to either drug alone, or to compare LHRH agonist therapy with cytotoxic chemotherapy.

In a few studies, responses to therapy with an LHRH agonist have been observed in postmenopausal women with advanced breast cancer (Schally et al, 1993). The mechanism is not fully understood but has been attributed to one of two possible actions. In the first, high levels of circulating LH and FSH in postmenopausal women stimulate ovarian secretion of androgens that are aromatized to estrogens in adipose tissue and then support the growth of estrogen receptor-positive breast tumors. Because LHRH agonists decrease secretion of LH and FSH, they decrease ovarian secretion of androgens and block tumor growth. In the second proposed mechanism, the LHRH analogue may directly inhibit breast tumor cells. Reports that receptors for LHRH agonists can be detected in breast cancer cell lines and fresh tumor specimens support this hypothesis; however, in clinical trials, responses to LHRH agonists have been observed in postmenopausal women with receptor-positive or indeterminate tumors but not in those with receptor-negative tumors; this suggests that the first proposed mechanism may be more likely (Saphner et al, 1993).

A few patients with other tumors have been treated with LHRH agonists (Schally et al, 1993). Promising rates of response to therapy with leuprolide, goserelin, or other analogues have been observed in several uncontrolled studies on patients with advanced epithelial ovarian tumors. Fewer patients with advanced endometrial carcinoma have been studied, but the response rates reported thus far suggest that further clinical trials are warranted. Clinical investigations on use of LHRH agonists in patients with pancreatic and colorectal cancer also are beginning. However, the clinical role of these drugs in any tumors other than advanced prostatic and breast carcinomas cannot be determined until randomized, controlled studies are performed.

For uses of LHRH agonists in non-neoplastic endocrine disorders, see index entries Buserelin, Goserelin, Leuprolide, Nafarelin, and Triptorelin.

ADVERSE REACTIONS. Initial stimulation of gonadotropin release and sex steroid production may cause disease flare-up during the first weeks of therapy with an LHRH agonist in patients with advanced prostatic carcinoma. Between 3% to 10% of patients complain of increased bone pain and urinary tract disorders, but these usually decline with continued treatment. Concomitant use of an antiandrogen (eg, flutamide) with leuprolide or goserelin to achieve combined androgen blockade may prevent or attenuate disease flare-up (Crawford, 1989; Schulze and Senge, 1990). However, pretreatment with the antiandrogen for several days may be more effective than simultaneously initiating therapy to prevent tumor flare-up at the start of LHRH agonist administration (Schulze and Senge, 1990). A few patients, primarily those with pre-existing urinary obstruction, may have a transient elevation in BUN levels. Exacerbations of signs and symptoms are of concern in patients with vertebral metastases and/or urinary obstruction because this may lead to neurologic problems or increased obstruction.

Hot flashes are the most common adverse response to LHRH agonist therapy for advanced prostate cancer (incidence, 56% to 59%), but these may decrease in frequency and severity over time. They also may respond to low doses of clonidine or alpha-adrenergic blocking agents. Hot flashes also occur frequently in response to LHRH agonist therapy in premenopausal women with advanced breast cancer. Gynecomastia, nausea and vomiting, edema, and thrombophlebitis are reported infrequently in male patients. As with DES, impotence and loss of libido occur frequently. Patients receiving DES experienced gynecomastia, nausea and vomiting, edema, and thromboembolism more frequently than those receiving LHRH agonists; however, hot flashes are reported more often in those treated with leuprolide or goserelin.

See also the evaluation on Flutamide.

PRECAUTIONS. Prostate cancer patients with metastatic vertebral lesions, large tumor volumes, and/or urinary tract obstruction should be monitored during the first few weeks of therapy. These patients may be unable to tolerate the worsening of symptoms that may occur during this period due to the initial increase in circulating testosterone levels. Although not specified in the package labeling approved by the FDA for these drugs, some physicians recommend that LHRH agonists be used only in combination with an antiandrogen in these patients to avoid exposing them to the risk of disease flare-up.

Serum levels of testosterone and prostatic acid phosphatase have been measured in many of the clinical trials evaluating the efficacy of LHRH agonists but need not be monitored routinely in patients receiving these drugs in clinical practice. Castration levels of testosterone usually are reached in two to four weeks, and acid phosphatase levels decrease to values near baseline by the fourth week. Measurements of prostate-specific antigen (PSA) levels in the serum may be the most useful method to monitor response to therapy and recurrence or progression of prostate cancer (Kelly et al, 1993; Armbruster, 1993; Gerber, 1993). In patients who respond to therapy, PSA values may continue to decline for up to six months after therapy begins, whereas significant increases in PSA levels usually predict tumor recurrence or progression.

Leuprolide and goserelin are classified in FDA Pregnancy Category X.

PHARMACOKINETICS. The plasma half-life of leuprolide is about three hours and that of goserelin is between four and five hours (Chrisp and Sorkin, 1991; Chrisp and Goa, 1991). In contrast, the half-life of naturally occurring LHRH is only 30 minutes, undoubtedly because of its greater susceptibility to peptidase activity. None of the LHRH agonists are active when given orally because they are hydrolyzed by peptidases in the gastrointestinal tract. Bioavailability after subcutaneous injection of the preparation used daily (ie, dosage forms other than the depot preparations) is comparable to that with intravenous administration.

No data are available regarding metabolism of leuprolide or goserelin in humans. Based on data from animal model systems, it is likely that these agents are cleaved by proteolysis to smaller peptides that are excreted principally in the urine. The volume of distribution of leuprolide at steady state is between 30 and 40 L (Chrisp and Sorkin, 1991) and that of goserelin (approximately 13.7 L) is slightly in excess of the extracellular fluid volume (Chrisp and Goa, 1991). This difference probably is at least partly responsible for the twofold difference in the recommended dosages of these drugs (see Dosage and Preparations below). The total body clearance of each drug is 8 to 9 L/hr.

With the depot preparation of leuprolide, peak serum concentrations of 13.1 and 47.4 mcg/L are achieved within three hours after subcutaneous injection of 3.75 and 7.5 mg, respectively, of leuprolide incorporated into lactic acid/glycolic acid copolymeric microcapsules (Chrisp and Sorkin, 1991). Therapeutic effects are maintained by uniform daily release of 2.8% of the total administered dose from a single monthly injection of this formulation.

An initial peak in the serum concentration of goserelin (between 0.2 and 2 mcg/L) occurs two to eight hours after administration of the depot preparation containing 3.6 mg of the drug (Chrisp and Goa, 1991). A second peak (between 2 and 3 mcg/L) is observed 14 to 15 days later. The polymeric matrix releases goserelin at a continuous mean rate of 120 mcg/day (3.3% per day) over a 28-day period.

DOSAGE AND PREPARATIONS.

LEUPROLIDE:

Subcutaneous: *Adults*, 1 mg as a single daily injection.

Lupron Injection (TAP). Solution 5 mg/ml in 2.8 ml containers.

Intramuscular: A depot preparation containing 7.5 mg of leuprolide acetate in a biodegradable copolymer of lactic and glycolic acids is injected once monthly as a suspension of lyophilized microspheres reconstituted in 1 ml of sterile diluent.

Lupron Depot (TAP). Single-dose vials containing 7.5 mg of leuprolide acetate in 66.2 mg of copolymer (plus 1.3 mg gelatin and 13.2 mg D-mannitol). Supplied with sterile diluent (carboxymethylcellulose sodium, D-mannitol, acetic acid, and polysorbate 80 in water for injection).

GOSERELIN:

Subcutaneous: A depot preparation is injected into the upper abdominal wall for continuous release over 28 days. Use of a local anesthetic before injection of goserelin is optional.

Zoladex (ZENECA). Single-use disposable syringes prefilled with goserelin acetate equivalent to 3.6 mg of the acid in 13.3 to 14.3 mg of lactic acid/glycolic acid copolymer matrix. (Store at room temperature below 25° C.)

Progestins

ACTIONS. Several hypotheses have been proposed to account for the antitumor effects of progestins (Swain and Lippman, 1990). Among the possibilities are endocrinologic effects (suppression of sex steroid biosynthesis in the adrenal glands; decreased expression of estrogen receptors in tumor cells), direct cytotoxic actions, and regulatory effects on the production of autocrine growth factors or their receptors in tumor cells. However, which of these alternatives is most likely to be responsible for clinical responses to these drugs has not been established. The response to progestins depends on the presence of functionally competent progesterone receptors in the tumor cells (McCarty and McCarty, 1993). See index entry Progesterone, Physiology, for a more complete discussion of responses to natural and synthetic progestins.

USES. Progestins are the hormones of choice for the palliative management of disseminated endometrial carcinoma (Hoskins et al, 1993; Creasman, 1993). Response rates range from 15% to >30%; well-differentiated tumors respond more frequently. Treatment is continued until the disease recurs. Administration of progestins as adjuvant therapy for low-risk, early-stage endometrial cancer does not appear to increase survival or delay disease progression.

In several single-case reports and a few older studies in limited numbers of patients, those with renal cell carcinoma also responded to progestin therapy. Medroxyprogesterone acetate and megestrol acetate are the progestins used most frequently for renal cell carcinoma at present; hydroxyprogesterone caproate should be equally effective. However, recent reviews suggest that when the stricter criteria presently used to define objective responses are employed, the overall response rate to progestin therapy for renal cell carcinoma is <5% (Richie, 1993; Linehan et al, 1993).

Progestins have shown activity as second-line therapy for advanced breast cancer and have some activity in prostate and (rarely) ovarian cancers. Megestrol acetate is the progestin used most frequently as therapy for metastatic breast cancer in the United States; medroxyprogesterone acetate is used most often in Europe. A review of data compiled from 16 clinical trials showed that the overall response rate to megestrol acetate in patients with advanced breast cancer was 26% (Schacter et al, 1990). Almost all women included in these trials were postmenopausal and had received previous treatment. However, limited data suggest that progestins also may be effective for breast cancer in premenopausal women and in males. Response rates were highest (43%) in women whose tumors were positive for both estrogen and progesterone receptors.

In four randomized comparative trials, megestrol acetate was almost as effective as tamoxifen as first-line therapy for advanced breast cancer (30% response rate versus 35% for tamoxifen with little to no difference in times to disease progression or median survival). At present, however, most patients with advanced breast cancer are treated initially with tamoxifen since it is better tolerated. On tumor progression, a progestin is one of several options for second-, third- or fourth-line hormonal therapy. Data suggest that patients whose recurrent breast tumors progressed after initially responding to tamoxifen are unlikely to respond if a progestin is added (Paterson et al, 1990). In contrast, some patients whose tumors progressed after an initial response to progestin therapy did respond to the addition of tamoxifen. Nevertheless, efficacy does not appear to be enhanced by the combined use of tamoxifen with a progestin.

Megestrol acetate also appears to be equal to the aromatase inhibitor, aminoglutethimide, in its effects on survival and in producing objective responses in women with breast cancer who were treated previously with tamoxifen.

Although response rates in women with breast cancer are not consistently improved with doses of tamoxifen >20 mg/day, data from European investigators indicate that high-dose therapy with medroxyprogesterone acetate yields better results than the standard-dose regimen of either drug. Based on the European data, several trials were initiated to evaluate high-dose megestrol acetate in patients with advanced breast cancer (Abrams et al, 1990). Data from one of these studies suggest that, in women receiving megestrol acetate after previous treatment with tamoxifen either for metastatic disease or as adjuvant therapy, the objective response rate, duration of response, and duration of survival were greater with a dose of 800 mg/day than with the standard dose of 160 mg/day (Muss et al, 1990). In contrast, results from a three-arm trial that randomized women with stage IV breast cancer to receive megestrol acetate 160 or 800 mg or 1.6 g daily revealed a dose-dependent increase in side effects and decrease in quality of life at the two higher doses (Kornblith et al, 1993). These investigators concluded that unless subsequent analysis demonstrates a significant improvement in the duration of survival with the higher doses, women with advanced breast cancer should continue to receive the standard megestrol acetate dose of 160 mg/day.

The use of progestins in patients with advanced prostate cancer is based on the ability of these agents to suppress gonadotropin production and inhibit conversion of testosterone to dihydrotestosterone and on their antiandrogenic effects (Trump and Robertson, 1993; Hanks et al, 1993). Progestins are usually reserved for second-line endocrine therapy in patients whose tumors progress after castration or therapy with an LHRH agonist. Significant palliation of symptoms occurs in only 10% to 20% of these patients, and progestin therapy rarely remains effective for more than a brief period.

Epithelial ovarian tumors also have been treated with progestins; overall response rates in clinical trials ranged from 5% to 15% (Young et al, 1993; Berek et al, 1993). Thus, the use of progestins should be limited to individuals who have not responded to standard chemotherapy regimens and are not candidates for aggressive salvage chemotherapy or clinical trials.

Mifepristone (RU486), a progesterone receptor antagonist (or antiprogestin), has been studied as therapy for unresectable meningioma (Grunberg et al, 1991) and for advanced breast cancer in previously treated patients (Horwitz, 1992). Although some responses have been observed, more extensive clinical trials are needed to evaluate the efficacy and safety of this drug for these indications (Spitz and Bardin, 1993).

There is considerable interest in the use of megestrol acetate as therapy for cancer-associated anorexia and cachexia (Loprinzi et al, 1990, 1993; Tchekmedyian et al, 1992; Schmoll et al, 1991). Results of several randomized, placebo-controlled clinical trials employing both standard and high-dose regimens indicate that megestrol acetate decreases nausea, improves appetite, increases food intake, and stimulates weight gain in severely debilitated patients with breast cancer or other tumors. Several of these trials restricted enrollment to patients with hormone-insensitive tumors to avoid confounding effects of the therapy on appetite and weight gain with direct tumor-suppressing responses.

In a recent study, a positive antianorexic dose-response effect for megestrol acetate in dosages ranging from 160 mg to 1.28 g/day was observed (Loprinzi et al, 1993). However, 160 mg/day has been recommended as a reasonable initial dose, with subsequent escalation of the amount as needed. This recommendation was based primarily on the cost and inconvenience of larger doses because, until recently, megestrol was marketed only in 20- and 40-mg tablets in the United States. However, a more concentrated preparation of megestrol acetate [Megace Oral Suspension] is now available that allows more convenient and less costly therapy at the higher dosages.

Two randomized, placebo-controlled trials in patients with AIDs-related cachexia demonstrated that lean muscle mass increased significantly in those given megestrol acetate while those in the placebo group lost weight. In one of these studies, there was a dose-dependent increase in the magnitude of weight gain in those receiving megestrol acetate 100, 400, and 800 mg/day. Based on these data, it may be reasonable to begin therapy in cancer patients with cachexia at a dose of 400 to 800 mg/day for several weeks and, after initial weight gain is achieved, to reduce the daily dose for maintenance therapy. Nevertheless, most clinicians continue to prefer initiating therapy at 160 mg/day and increasing the dose as needed in order to avoid too rapid weight gain at the start of therapy.

In a randomized, double-blind, placebo-controlled trial in anorexic patients with advanced malignancies, medroxyprogesterone acetate 100 mg orally three times daily for six weeks increased appetite but did not stimulate weight gain, suggesting the need for additional studies using higher dosages (Downer et al, 1993).

See index entry Progestins, Uses, for discussion of progestins as therapy for non-malignant endocrine disorders.

ADVERSE REACTIONS AND PRECAUTIONS. Adverse reactions with standard-dose regimens are rare and are usually minimal. Fluid retention and pain at the site of injection may occur. Hypercalcemia develops occasionally if there are osseous metastases.

In women treated with standard-dose regimens of megestrol acetate for breast cancer, the most common side effects were nonfluid weight gain (23% of patients) and vaginal bleeding (2% of patients). Stimulation of appetite and undesired weight gain can be a significant problem for women with breast cancer who are overweight at the start of progestin therapy. The amount of weight gained and the incidence of edema were greater in those given high-dose regimens. It also is advisable to warn postmenopausal breast cancer patients that a withdrawal menses frequently occurs one to three weeks after progestin therapy is discontinued. The frequency of all other adverse events was 1% or less (Schacter et al, 1990). An asymptomatic but dramatic decrease in serum cortisol concentration occurs in patients receiving megestrol acetate (Loprinzi et al, 1992).

Weight gain also occurs in most patients taking medroxyprogesterone acetate. Other adverse reactions to standard doses of this progestin in cancer patients include edema, fatigue, sweating, vaginal discharge, and amenorrhea. Gluteal abscesses, tremors, leg cramps, and moon-shaped facies were observed in those receiving large doses of medroxyprogesterone acetate intramuscularly in combination regimens.

See index entry Progestins, Adverse Reactions, Precautions for a more detailed discussion of toxic effects of these drugs.

PHARMACOKINETICS. In the United States, medroxyprogesterone acetate usually is injected intramuscularly when used to treat neoplastic diseases. Oral administration of larger doses has been studied by a number of European investigators. This drug is metabolized extensively by hydroxylation and glucuronidation in the liver. Between 35% and 40% of a dose is eliminated by urinary excretion of metabolites (<1% is recovered as intact drug) and about 8% is eliminated in the feces. The biologic half-life of the drug is 14 to 15 hours.

A greater quantity of megestrol acetate is absorbed and more is bioavailable after oral administration than with medroxyprogesterone acetate. Peak plasma levels occur two to three hours after a single oral dose. Estimates of the elimination-phase half-life range from 15 to more than 30 hours. Renal excretion accounts for 60% to 80% of an administered dose, and fecal elimination accounts for the remainder. About 12% of the amount found in urine is present as unmetabolized parent compound. Hydroxylation in the liver appears to be the major route of metabolism for megestrol.

DOSAGE AND PREPARATIONS.

HYDROXYPROGESTERONE CAPROATE:

Intramuscular: For advanced endometrial carcinoma, 1 g one to seven times weekly.

MEDROXYPROGESTERONE ACETATE:

Intramuscular: For advanced endometrial or renal cancer, initially, 400 mg to 1 g weekly; for maintenance, 400 mg monthly. In high-dose regimens used by European investigators for advanced breast cancer, 1 to 1.5 g has been given daily.

MEGESTROL ACETATE:

Oral: For breast carcinoma (standard regimen), 160 mg/day in a single or in four divided doses. For advanced breast cancer (high-dose regimens), 800 mg or 1.6 g daily. For endometrial carcinoma, 40 to 320 mg daily in divided doses. To stimulate appetite and promote weight gain, 800 mg to 1.6 g/day has been employed in clinical trials, but most investigators recommend an initial dose of 160 to 320 mg/day. To avoid the necessity of swallowing large numbers of tablets, the new concentrated dosage form [Megace Oral Suspension] is most convenient for high-dose regimens.

For progestin preparations, see index entry Progestins.

Inhibitors of Steroid Biosynthesis or Activation

The rate-limiting step of estrogen biosynthesis involves loss of a methyl group at C-19 and aromatization of the A ring in the steroid nucleus to convert androstenedione to estrone (Santen, 1993; Höffken, 1993; Johannessen and Lønning, 1992). No other endogenous steroid hormones are synthesized via this reaction. Inhibition of aromatase, the enzyme catalyzing this conversion, is highly specific as a means of reducing estrogen biosynthesis, and aromatase inhibition is a rational strategy for treatment of estrogen-dependent tumors. Aromatase inhibitors also have been studied in patients with advanced prostate cancer (Johannessen and Lønning, 1992).

Aminoglutethimide, the only aromatase inhibitor generally available at this time, inactivates the cytochrome P450 prosthetic group of the enzyme complex. However, this drug also inhibits enzymes required for adrenal corticosteroid biosynthesis. Newer aromatase inhibitors (eg, 4-hydroxyandrostenedione [formestane], CGS 16949A [fadrozole], CGS 20267 [letrozole], pyridoglutethimide [rogletimide]) bind to the substrate site within the aromatase catalytic center, and thus they compete with endogenous substrate. These investigational agents, which are in Phase I and II of clinical trials in the United States, are being developed in an attempt to achieve aromatase inhibition without requiring concomitant administration of corticosteroids. Formestane is marketed in the United Kingdom as a second-line hormonal agent for advanced breast cancer.

Inhibitors of androgen biosynthesis or activation are being tested for the treatment of prostate cancer. Ketoconazole, a drug initially developed for antifungal chemotherapy (see index entry Ketoconazole, Uses), inhibits several cytochrome P450-dependent steroid hydroxylases in the testis, ovary, adrenal gland, and other tissues. It rapidly (but only temporarily) reduces plasma testosterone concentrations to castration levels and is active as therapy for advanced prostate cancer.

Finasteride is an inhibitor of 5α reductase, the enzyme that activates testosterone in prostatic cells by catalyzing its conversion to dihydrotestosterone (Gormley, 1991; Sudduth and Koronkowski, 1993). This drug was developed as therapy for benign prostatic hypertrophy (see index entry Finasteride, In Prostatic Hyperplasia) but currently is under investigation for both chemoprevention and treatment of prostate cancer. Initial data in men with advanced prostatic carcinoma suggest that finasteride is, at best, minimally active in these patients (Presti et al, 1992).

AMINOGLUTETHIMIDE

[Cytadren]

O, HN, CH_2CH_3, O, NH_2

ACTIONS. Aminoglutethimide inhibits the enzymatic conversion of cholesterol to Δ^5-pregnenolone, the first step in adrenal corticosteroid biosynthesis, thereby reducing the synthesis of glucocorticoids, mineralocorticoids, and other steroids. In addition, it inhibits the aromatase enzyme that converts androstenedione to estrone and estradiol in extra-adrenal tissues. Because the adrenal gland is the principal source of estrogens in postmenopausal and oophorectomized women, this dual inhibitory action lowers plasma estrogen levels to the same extent as surgical adrenalectomy (Santen, 1993).

USES. Aminoglutethimide plus replacement doses of hydrocortisone (to prevent reflex ACTH hypersecretion from overcoming adrenal inhibition and to prevent addisonian crisis) is as effective as surgical adrenalectomy for second- or third-line therapy in postmenopausal women with estrogen receptor-positive advanced breast carcinoma (Santen, 1993; Höffken, 1993; Johannessen and Lønning, 1992). Thus, "medical adrenalectomy" appears to be a preferred alternative to surgical adrenalectomy and its associated high morbidity and occasional mortality. Overall response rates are approximately 50% in women with estrogen receptor-positive tumors. Durations of response average 30 months in complete responders and 14 months in partial responders. Responses occur primarily in soft tissue (47%) and bone (35%) metastases.

In a randomized crossover trial comparing tamoxifen with aminoglutethimide plus hydrocortisone, response rates and durations were approximately the same. Because of its lower potential for toxicity and greater experience with its use, tamoxifen should be considered the drug of choice in postmenopausal women with estrogen receptor-positive advanced breast cancer, but aminoglutethimide plus hydrocortisone is one of the alternatives for patients who do not respond or relapse with tamoxifen. Objective responses to aminoglutethimide plus hydrocortisone are observed in approximately 50% of patients who relapse after initially responding to tamoxifen but in only 25% of nonresponders (Santen, 1993). Nevertheless, because of the greater severity of side effects associated with aminoglutethimide, progestins are preferred by most clinicians as second-line therapy for advanced breast cancer except in those patients with severe bone pain or lytic metastases. Some patients who relapse after response to progestins may benefit from therapy with aminoglutethimide plus hydrocortisone.

In premenopausal women, aminoglutethimide should only be used after surgical oophorectomy. Enhanced ovarian steroidogenesis in response to the compensatory increase in LH secretion and increased production of new aromatase enzyme molecules in response to increased FSH secretion make the intact ovary resistant to the effects of aromatase inhibition.

In dose-response studies in patients with advanced breast cancer, differences in the rates of objective response to dosages of aminoglutethimide between 250 mg and 1 g/day (Santen, 1993; Johannessen and Lønning, 1992) were not significant; however, the number of patients studied was relatively small. Some of the drug's side effects (eg, those resulting from its CNS sedative properties) occurred less frequently at the smaller doses, but others (eg, morbilliform rash) were equally common with smaller or larger doses.

Some investigators have tried to achieve more specific inhibition of aromatase by using smaller doses of aminoglutethimide to obviate the need for use of hydrocortisone to replace endogenous adrenal glucocorticoid (Santen, 1993). The rates of objective response to aminoglutethimide 250 mg/day without hydrocortisone were lower than expected, and suppression of estrogen biosynthesis at that dose was more complete with than without hydrocortisone. However, in a randomized trial that increased the dose of aminoglutethimide to 500 mg daily, hydrocortisone did not affect the rate or duration of objective responses (Cocconi et al, 1992 B).

Aminoglutethimide plus hydrocortisone also has been investigated in patients with other advanced tumors that were either hormone dependent or contained aromatase activity (Johannessen and Lønning, 1992). Partial responses and disease stabilization were observed in some patients with relapsed endometrial carcinoma or metastatic melanoma; however, data are insufficient to evaluate the benefits of aminoglutethimide therapy for tumors other than advanced breast cancer. Infrequent objective and subjective responses to therapy have been observed in heavily pretreated patients with advanced prostate cancer. The responses may have resulted from the hydrocortisone rather than from aminoglutethimide. Hydrocortisone does suppress plasma androgen levels, while aminoglutethimide had no such effect in castrated males.

Aminoglutethimide also suppresses adrenal function in some patients with Cushing's syndrome (see index entry Aminoglutethimide, Uses, Adrenal Dysfunction).

ADVERSE REACTIONS AND PRECAUTIONS. Aminoglutethimide causes acute soporific side effects; 40% of patients experience lethargy and 10% have ataxia. Tolerance usually develops to these adverse effects after four to six weeks, presumably due to induction of drug metabolizing enzymes. Morbilliform rash and nausea and anorexia also are common side effects, but they usually disappear after one to two weeks of therapy. Orthostatic hypotension characterized by dizziness and weakness occurs in about 10% of patients, and mineralocorticoid supplements may be required. Headache, tachycardia, myalgia, fever, vomiting, and pruritus have been reported. Masculinization and hirsutism can occur in women and precocious sexual development in boys. Goiters with mild hypothyroidism have been observed with long-term use because the drug blocks iodination of tyrosine. Hematologic abnormalities (eg, leukopenia, thrombocytopenia, pancytopenia, agranulocytosis) and elevations in liver enzymes (eg, AST, alkaline phosphatase) have been reported. Since aminoglutethimide accelerates the metabolism of dexamethasone, the latter should not be used in glucocorticoid replacement therapy.

This drug is a teratogen in animals. It is classified in FDA Pregnancy Category D.

PHARMACOKINETICS. Aminoglutethimide is absorbed by the gastrointestinal tract after oral administration. Between 20% and 25% is bound to plasma proteins. At the initial drug exposure, the plasma half-life is 13 hours; after one to two weeks of drug administration, the half-life decreases to seven hours due to induction of drug metabolizing enzymes (Santen, 1993; Johannesson and Lønning, 1992). Four metabolites have been identified, of which aceto-aminoglutethimide is most prominent. After oral administration, 50% of a dose is excreted in the urine unchanged and 20% to 50% is excreted as aceto-aminoglutethimide.

DOSAGE AND PREPARATIONS.

Oral: For breast carcinoma, the most commonly employed regimen is 250 mg twice daily for two weeks, increased to 250 mg four times daily thereafter. This schedule reduces soporific symptoms and compensates for increased rate of drug metabolism. Hydrocortisone is given concomitantly in large doses (60 mg at bedtime, 20 mg in the morning and at 5 PM for a total of 100 mg daily) for the initial two weeks to reduce the severity of rash; thereafter, the dose is reduced to 40 mg daily (20 mg at bedtime, 10 mg in the morning, and 10 mg at 5 PM). Alternatively, aminoglutethimide 125 mg and hydrocortisone 20 mg are administered twice daily for two weeks, after which the aminoglutethimide dosage is increased to 250 mg twice daily.

Cytadren (CIBA). Tablets 250 mg. (Protect from light.)

KETOCONAZOLE
[Nizoral]

For chemical formula, see index entry Ketoconazole, Uses.

ACTIONS. Ketoconazole inhibits a variety of cytochrome P450-dependent enzymes that catalyze steroid hydroxylation reactions (Sonino, 1987). This drug was developed as an antifungal agent (see index entry Ketoconazole, Uses). Higher concentrations of ketoconazole are required to inhibit steroid hydroxylation in mammalian cells than those that inhibit cholesterol biosynthesis in fungi; nevertheless, adequate dosages block androgen production in the testis, ovary, adrenal gland, and other tissues. Treatment with large doses of ketoconazole decreases the plasma concentration of testosterone within two hours and reduces it to levels observed in orchiectomized men within one to two days. In contrast, other pharmacologic approaches (eg, LHRH agonists, progestins, estrogens) may require up to two weeks. Continued therapy with ketoconazole can maintain castration levels of testosterone for up to six months, but, after the initial period of therapy, a gradual reflex increase in LH and FSH concentrations tends to override the effect of ketoconazole on testosterone production. Thus, ketoconazole is less effective than orchiectomy or an LHRH analogue for long-term treatment.

USES. Ketoconazole has been used as palliative therapy in patients with advanced prostate cancer (Lowe and Bamberger, 1990; Percy, 1992). Although data from randomized controlled trials are not available, results of uncontrolled studies suggest that relief of pain and other symptoms usually occurs one to three days after therapy is initiated. However, ketoconazole is not recommended for use as first-line therapy because plasma testosterone concentrations are not suppressed for longer than six months. Lack of compliance with the dosing regimen as a result of gastrointestinal upset, lethargy, and/or hepatic dysfunction also can contribute to the drug's limited efficacy.

At present, the major indications for ketoconazole in advanced prostate cancer appear to be when the patient's condition requires a prompt therapeutic response, when orchiectomy and/or estrogens are contraindicated, and as initial empirical therapy while establishing the diagnosis of metastatic prostate cancer or waiting for the patient to undergo orchiectomy (Lowe and Bamberger, 1990). This drug may be particularly useful for acute reduction of plasma testosterone levels in those with metastatic prostate cancer and disseminated intravascular coagulation or acute paraparesis/paraplegia. A few patients have been treated with ketoconazole at the start of therapy with an LHRH agonist to prevent the disease flare-up that accompanies the initial rise in testosterone production; however, no data are available to compare ketoconazole to antiandrogens (eg, flutamide) for this purpose.

ADVERSE REACTIONS. The side effects of ketoconazole in patients with advanced prostate cancer rarely are life-threatening and usually cease when therapy is discontinued. These include mild gynecomastia, transient elevations in serum levels of aspartate aminotransferase, lethargy, hypertension, and mild symptoms of Addison's disease (Percy, 1992). The latter usually can be controlled by administering a glucocorticoid concomitantly. Gastrointestinal intolerance (nausea, vomiting, anorexia) can be severe and cause some patients to withdraw from further therapy. Histamine$_2$ receptor antagonists (eg, cimetidine) must not be given concomitantly, since they prevent absorption of ketoconazole.

For more detailed discussion of adverse reactions, precautions, and drug interactions, see index entry Ketoconazole.

PHARMACOKINETICS. See index entry Ketoconazole, Uses.

DOSAGE AND PREPARATIONS.

Oral: For metastatic carcinoma of the prostate, 400 mg every eight hours for up to six months.

Nizoral (Janssen). Tablets 200 mg.

Cited References

Consensus development conference on the treatment of early-stage breast cancer. *J Natl Cancer Inst Monographs* 11:1-187, 1992.

Abrams JS, et al: Current status of high-dose progestins in breast cancer. *Semin Oncol* 17 (suppl 9):68-72, 1990.

Alexanian R, et al: Primary dexamethasone treatment of multiple myeloma. *Blood* 80:887-890, 1992.

Armbruster DA: Prostate-specific antigen: Biochemistry, analytical methods, and clinical application. *Clin Chem* 39:181-185, 1993.

Benson RC Jr, Gill GM: Estramustine phosphate compared with diethylstilbestrol: Randomized, double-blind, crossover trial for stage D prostate cancer. *Am J Clin Oncol* 9:341-351, 1986.

Berek JS, et al: Ovarian cancer, in Holland JF, et al (eds): *Cancer Medicine*, ed 3. Philadelphia, Lea & Febiger, 1993, vol 2, 1659-1690.

Brogden RN, Chrisp P: Flutamide: A review of its pharmacodynamic and pharmacokinetic properties, and therapeutic use in advanced prostatic cancer. *Drugs Aging* 1:104-115, 1991.

Bruchovsky N: Androgens and antiandrogens, in Holland JF, et al (eds): *Cancer Medicine*, ed 3. Philadelphia, Lea & Febiger, 1993, vol 1, 884-896.

Buzaid AC, et al: High-dose cisplatin with dacarbazine and tamoxifen in the treatment of metastatic melanoma. *Cancer* 68:1238-1241, 1991.

Chrisp P, Goa KL: Goserelin: A review of its pharmacodynamic and pharmacokinetic properties, and clinical use in sex hormone-related conditions. *Drugs* 41:254-288, 1991.

Chrisp P, Sorkin EM: Leuprorelin: A review of its pharmacology and therapeutic use in prostatic disorders. *Drugs Aging* 1:487-509, 1991.

Cidlowski JA, Schwartzman RA: Corticosteroids, in Holland JF, et al (eds): *Cancer Medicine*, ed 3. Philadelphia, Lea & Febiger, 1993, vol 1, 845-857.

Cocconi G, et al: Treatment of metastatic malignant melanoma with dacarbazine plus tamoxifen. *N Engl J Med* 327:516-523, 1992 A.

Cocconi G, et al: Low-dose aminoglutethimide with and without hydrocortisone replacement as a first-line endocrine treatment in advanced breast cancer: A prospective randomized trial of the Italian Oncology Group for Clinical Research. *J Clin Oncol* 10:984-989, 1992 B.

Conn PM, Crowley WF Jr: Gonadotropin-releasing hormone and its analogues. *N Engl J Med* 324:93-103, 1991.

Council on Scientific Affairs: Report of the Council on Scientific Affairs: Management of patients with node-negative breast cancer. *Arch Intern Med* 153:58-67, 1993.

Crawford ED: Combined androgen blockade. *Urology* 34 (suppl):22-26, 1989.

Crawford ED, et al: Controlled trial of leuprolide with and without flutamide in prostatic carcinoma. *N Engl J Med* 321:419-424, 1989.

Creasman WT: Adenocarcinoma of the uterine corpus, in Holland JF, et al (eds): *Cancer Medicine*, ed 3. Philadelphia, Lea & Febiger, 1993, vol 2, 1647-1655.

Deisseroth AB, et al: Chronic leukemias, in DeVita VT Jr, et al (eds): *Cancer: Principles & Practice of Oncology*, ed 4. Philadelphia, JB Lippincott, 1993, vol 2, 1965-1983.

Denis L, Mettlin C: Conclusions from the workshop. *Cancer* 66 (suppl):1086-1089, 1990.

Denis LJ, et al: Goserelin acetate and flutamide versus bilateral orchiectomy: A Phase III EORTC trial (30853). *Urology* 42:119-129, (Aug) 1993.

DeVita VT Jr, Hubbard SM: Hodgkin's disease. *N Engl J Med* 328:560-565, 1993.

DeVita VT Jr, et al: Hodgkin's disease, in DeVita VT Jr, et al (eds): *Cancer: Principles & Practice of Oncology*, ed 4. Philadelphia, JB Lippincott, 1993, vol 2, 1819-1858.

Dewar JA, et al: Long term effects of tamoxifen on blood lipid values in breast cancer. *BMJ* 305:225-226, 1992.

Distelhorst CW: Recent insight into the structure and function of the glucocorticoid receptor. *J Lab Clin Med* 113:404-412, 1989.

Downer S, et al: A double-blind placebo controlled trial of medroxyprogesterone acetate (MPA) in cancer cachexia. *Br J Cancer* 67:1102-1105, 1993.

Dupont A, et al: Response to flutamide withdrawal in advanced prostate cancer in progression under combination therapy. *J Urol* 150:908-913, 1993.

Early Breast Cancer Trialists' Collaborative Group: Systemic treatment of early breast cancer by hormonal, cytotoxic, or immune therapy: 133 randomised trials involving 31,000 recurrences and 24,000 deaths among 75,000 women. *Lancet* 339:1-15, 71-85, 1992.

Engstrom PF, et al: A Phase II trial of tamoxifen in hepatocellular carcinoma. *Cancer* 65:2641-2643, 1990.

Fisher B, et al: Neoplasms of the breast, in Holland JF, et al (eds): *Cancer Medicine*, ed 3. Philadelphia, Lea & Febiger, 1993, vol 2, 1706-1774.

Fisher B, et al: Endometrial cancer in tamoxifen-treated breast cancer patients: Findings from the National Surgical Adjuvant Breast and Bowel Project (NSABP) B-14. *J Natl Cancer Inst* 86:527-537, 1994.

Fornander T, et al: Adjuvant tamoxifen in early breast cancer: Occurrence of new primary cancers. *Lancet* 1:117-120, 1989.

Fornander T, et al: Descriptive clinicopathologic study of 17 patients with endometrial cancer during or after adjuvant tamoxifen in early breast cancer. *J Natl Cancer Inst* 85:1850-1855, 1993.

Freedman AS, Nadler LM: Non-Hodgkin's lymphomas, in Holland JF, et al (eds): *Cancer Medicine*, ed 3. Philadelphia, Lea & Febiger, 1993, vol 2, 2028-2068.

Friedenberg WR, et al: High-dose dexamethasone for refractory or relapsing multiple myeloma. *Am J Hematol* 36:171-175, 1991.

Gerber GS: Prostate specific antigen. *PPO Updates* 7, (Oct) 1993.

Glauber JG, Kiang DT: The changing role of hormonal therapy in advanced breast cancer. *Semin Oncol* 19:308-316, 1992.

Gormley GJ: Role of 5α-reductase inhibitors in the treatment of advanced prostatic carcinoma. *Urol Clin North Am* 18:93-98, 1991.

Grunberg SM, et al: Treatment of unresectable meningiomas with the antiprogesterone agent mifepristone. *J Neurosurg* 74:861-866, 1991.

Hamm JT, Allegra JC: Hormonal therapy, in Moossa AR, et al (eds): *Comprehensive Textbook of Oncology*, ed 2. Baltimore, Williams & Wilkins, 1991 A, vol 1, 567-600.

Hamm JT, Allegra JC: Hormonal therapy for cancer, in Wittes RE (ed): *Manual of Oncologic Therapeutics 1991/1992*. Philadelphia, JB Lippincott, 1991 B, 122-126.

Hanks GE, et al: Cancer of the prostate, in DeVita VT Jr, et al (eds): *Cancer: Principles & Practice of Oncology*, ed 4. Philadelphia, JB Lippincott, 1993, vol 1, 1073-1113.

Harris JR, et al: Breast cancer (third of three parts). *N Engl J Med* 327:473-480, 1992.

Harris JR, et al: Cancer of the breast, in DeVita VT Jr, et al (eds): *Cancer: Principles & Practice of Oncology*, ed 4. Philadelphia, JB Lippincott, 1993, vol 1, 1264-1332.

Hatch KD, et al: Responsiveness of patients with advanced ovarian carcinoma to tamoxifen: A gynecologic oncology group study of second-line therapy in 105 patients. *Cancer* 68:269-271, 1991.

Höffken K: Experience with aromatase inhibitors in the treatment of advanced breast cancer. *Cancer Treat Rev* 19 (suppl B): 37-44, 1993.

Horwitz KB: The molecular biology of RU486: Is there a role for antiprogestins in the treatment of breast cancer? *Endocr Rev* 13:146-163, (May) 1992.

Hoskins WJ, et al: Gynecologic tumors, in DeVita VT Jr, et al (eds): *Cancer: Principles & Practice of Oncology*, ed 4. Philadelphia, JB Lippincott, 1993, 1152-1225.

Hucher M, et al: Anandron (nilutamide) combined with orchiectomy in stage D prostate cancer patients. *Cancer* 72 (12 suppl):3886-3887, 1993.

Hudes GR, et al: Phase II study of estramustine and vinblastine, two microtubule inhibitors, in hormone-refractory prostate cancer. *J Clin Oncol* 10:1754-1761, 1992.

Jensen EV, DeSombre ER: Steroid hormone binding and hormone receptors, in Holland JF, et al (eds): *Cancer Medicine*, ed 3. Philadelphia, Lea & Febiger, 1993, vol 1, 815-823.

Johannessen DC, Lønning PE: Aromatase inhibitors in malignant diseases of aging. *Drugs Aging* 2:530-545, 1992.

Jones AL, et al: Haemostatic changes and thromboembolic risk during tamoxifen therapy in normal women. *Br J Cancer* 66:744-747, 1992.

Jordan VC: Estrogens and antiestrogens, in Holland JF, et al (eds): *Cancer Medicine*, ed 3. Philadelphia, Lea & Febiger, 1993, vol 1, 857-865.

Jordan VC, et al: Hormonal strategies for breast cancer: A new focus on the estrogen receptor as a therapeutic target. *Semin Oncol* 19:299-307, 1992.

Jusko WJ: Corticosteroid pharmacodynamics: Models for a broad array of receptor-mediated pharmacologic effects. *J Clin Pharmacol* 30:303-310, 1990.

Keating MJ, et al: Acute leukemia, in DeVita VT Jr, et al (eds): *Cancer: Principles & Practice of Oncology*, ed 4. Philadelphia, JB Lippincott, 1993, vol 2, 1938-1964.

Kelly WK, Scher HI: Prostate specific antigen decline after antiandrogen withdrawal: The flutamide withdrawal syndrome. *J Urol* 149:607-609, 1993.

Kelly WK, et al: Prostate-specific antigen as a measure of disease outcome in metastatic hormone-refractory prostate cancer. *J Clin Oncol* 11:607-615, 1993.

Kennedy BJ: Hormone physiology and endocrine ablation, in Holland JF, et al (eds): *Cancer Medicine*, ed 3. Philadelphia, Lea & Febiger, 1993, vol 1, 823-827.

Kornblith AB, et al: Effect of megestrol acetate on quality of life in a dose-response trial in women with advanced breast cancer. *J Clin Oncol* 11:2081-2089, 1993.

Linehan WM, et al: Cancer of the kidney and ureter, in DeVita VT Jr, et al (eds): *Cancer: Principles & Practice of Oncology*, ed 4. Philadelphia, JB Lippincott, 1993, vol 1, 1023-1051.

Longo DL, et al: Lymphocytic lymphomas, in DeVita VT Jr, et al (eds): *Cancer: Principles & Practice of Oncology*, ed 4. Philadelphia, JB Lippincott, 1993, vol 2, 1859-1927.

Loprinzi CL, et al: Controlled trial of megestrol acetate for the treatment of cancer anorexia and cachexia. *J Natl Cancer Inst* 82:1127-1132, 1990.

Loprinzi CL, et al: Effect of megestrol acetate on the human pituitary-adrenal axis. *Mayo Clin Proc* 67:1160-1162, 1992.

Loprinzi CL, et al: Phase III evaluation of four doses of megestrol acetate as therapy for patients with cancer anorexia and/or cachexia. *J Clin Oncol* 11:762-767, 1993.

Love RR, et al: Symptoms associated with tamoxifen treatment in postmenopausal women. *Arch Intern Med* 151:1842-1847, 1991 A.

Love RR, et al: Effects of tamoxifen on cardiovascular risk factors in postmenopausal women. *Ann Intern Med* 115:860-864, 1991 B.

Love RR, et al: Antithrombin III level, fibrinogen level, and platelet count changes with adjuvant tamoxifen therapy. *Arch Intern Med* 152:317-320, 1992 A.

Love RR, et al: Effects of tamoxifen on bone mineral density in postmenopausal women with breast cancer. *N Engl J Med* 326:852-856, 1992 B.

Lowe FC, Bamberger MH: Indications for use of ketoconazole in management of metastatic prostate cancer. *Urology* 36:541-545, 1990.

Luton J-P, et al: Clinical features of adrenocortical carcinoma, prognostic factors, and the effect of mitotane therapy. *N Engl J Med* 322:1195-1201, 1990.

Magriples U, et al: High-grade endometrial carcinoma in tamoxifen-treated breast cancer patients. *J Clin Oncol* 11:485-490, 1993.

McCarty KS Jr, McCarty KS Sr: Progestins, in Holland JF, et al (eds): *Cancer Medicine*, ed 3. Philadelphia, Lea & Febiger, 1993, vol 1, 877-884.

McClay EF, et al: Effective combination chemo/hormonal therapy for malignant melanoma: Experience with three consecutive trials. *Int J Cancer* 50:553-556, 1992.

McDonald CC, et al: Fatal myocardial infarction in the Scottish adjuvant tamoxifen trial. *BMJ* 303:435-437, 1991.

Murphy GP, et al: Results of another trial of chemotherapy with and without hormones in patients with newly diagnosed metastatic prostate cancer. *Urology* 28:36-46, 1986.

Muss HB, et al: High- versus standard-dose megestrol acetate in women with advanced breast cancer: A Phase III trial of the Piedmont Oncology Association. *J Clin Oncol* 8:1797-1805, 1990.

National Institutes of Health Consensus Development Panel: Consensus statement: Treatment of early-stage breast cancer. *J Natl Cancer Inst Monographs* 11:1-5, 1992.

Nayfield SG, et al: Potential role of tamoxifen in prevention of breast cancer. *J Natl Cancer Inst* 83:1450-1459, 1991.

Needham PR, et al: Steroids in advanced cancer: Survey of current practice. *BMJ* 305:999, 1992.

Papac RJ, Keohane MF: Hormonal therapy for metastatic renal cell carcinoma combined androgen and provera followed by high dose tamoxifen. *Eur J Cancer* 29A:997-999, 1993.

Paterson AHG, et al: Comparison of antiestrogen and progestogen therapy for initial treatment and consequences of their combination for second-line treatment of recurrent breast cancer. *Semin Oncol* 17 (suppl 9):52-62, 1990.

Pavlidis NA, et al: Clear evidence that long-term, low-dose tamoxifen treatment can induce ocular toxicity: A prospective study of 63 patients. *Cancer* 69:2961-2964, 1992.

Percy LA: Ketoconazole in advanced prostate cancer. *Ann Pharmacother* 26:1527-1529, 1992.

Powles TJ, et al: Prevention of breast cancer with tamoxifen: An update on the Royal Marsden Hospital pilot programme. *Eur J Cancer* 26:680-684, 1990.

Presti JC Jr, et al: Multicenter, randomized, double-blind, placebo controlled study to investigate the effect of finasteride (MK-906) on stage D prostate cancer. *J Urol* 148:1201-1204, 1992.

Rai KR, Rabinowe SN: Chronic lymphocytic leukemia, in Holland JF, et al (eds): *Cancer Medicine*, ed 3. Philadelphia, Lea & Febiger, 1993, vol 2, 1971-1988.

Ribeiro G, Swindell R: Adjuvant tamoxifen for male breast cancer (MBC). *Br J Cancer* 65:252-254, 1992.

Richie JP: Renal cell carcinoma, in Holland JF, et al (eds): *Cancer Medicine*, ed 3. Philadelphia, Lea & Febiger, 1993, vol 2, 1529-1538.

Rutqvist LE, Mattson A: Cardiac and thromboembolic morbidity among postmenopausal women with early-stage breast cancer in a randomized trial of adjuvant tamoxifen. *J Natl Cancer Inst* 85:1398-1406, 1993.

Rutqvist LE, Wilking N: Analogues of LHRH versus orchidectomy: Comparison of economic costs for castration in advanced prostate cancer. *Br J Cancer* 65:927-929, 1992.

Rutqvist LE, et al: Contralateral primary tumors in breast cancer patients in a randomized trial of adjuvant tamoxifen therapy. *J Natl Cancer Inst* 83:1299-1306, 1991.

Santen RJ: Clinical use of aromatase inhibitors in breast carcinoma, in Holland JF, et al (eds): *Cancer Medicine*, ed 3. Philadelphia, Lea & Febiger, 1993, vol 1, 865-877.

Saphner T, et al: Phase II study of goserelin for patients with postmenopausal metastatic breast cancer. *J Clin Oncol* 11:1529-1535, 1993.

Schacter LP, et al: Overview of hormonal therapy in advanced breast cancer. *Semin Oncol* 17 (suppl 9):38-46, 1990.

Schally AV, et al: Hypothalamic and other peptide hormones, in Holland JF, et al (eds): *Cancer Medicine*, ed 3. Philadelphia, Lea & Febiger, 1993, vol 1, 827-840.

Scher HI, Kelly WK: Flutamide withdrawal syndrome: Its impact on clinical trials in hormone-refractory prostate cancer. *J Clin Oncol* 11:1566-1572, 1993.

Schiffer CA: Acute myeloid leukemia in adults, in Holland JF, et al (eds): *Cancer Medicine*, ed 3. Philadelphia, Lea & Febiger, 1993, vol 2, 1907-1933.

Schmoll E, et al: Megestrol acetate in cancer cachexia. *Semin Oncol* 18 (suppl 2):32-34, 1991.

Schulze H, Senge T: Influence of different types of antiandrogens on luteinizing hormone-releasing hormone analogue-induced testosterone surge in patients with metastatic carcinoma of the prostate. *J Urol* 144:934-941, 1990.

Scottish Cancer Trials Breast Group and ICRF Breast Unit, Guy's Hospital, London: Adjuvant ovarian ablation versus CMF chemotherapy in premenopausal women with pathological stage II breast carcinoma: The Scottish trial. *Lancet* 341:1293-1298, 1993.

Seidman AD, et al: Estramustine and vinblastine: Use of prostate specific antigen as a clinical trial end point for hormone refractory prostatic cancer. *J Urol* 147:931-934, 1992.

Sonino N: The use of ketoconazole as an inhibitor of steroid production. *N Engl J Med* 317:812-818, 1987.

Spitz IM, Bardin CW: Mifepristone (RU 486)—A modulator of progestin and glucocorticoid action. *N Engl J Med* 329:404-412, 1993.

Stahl M, et al: A Phase II study of high dose tamoxifen in progressive, metastatic renal cell carcinoma. *Ann Oncol* 3:167-168, 1992.

Sudduth SL, Koronkowski MJ: Finasteride: The first 5α-reductase inhibitor. *Pharmacotherapy* 13:309-329, 1993.

Sunderland MC, Osborne CK: Tamoxifen in premenopausal patients with metastatic breast cancer: A review. *J Clin Oncol* 9:1283-1297, 1991.

Sutherland DJ, Mobbs BG: Hormones and cancer, in Tannock IF, Hill RP (eds): *The Basic Science of Oncology*, ed 2. New York, McGraw-Hill, 1992, 207-231.

Swain SM, Lippman ME: Endocrine therapies of cancer, in Chabner BA, Collins JM (eds): *Cancer Chemotherapy: Principles and Practice*. Philadelphia, JB Lippincott, 1990, 59-109.

Takvorian T, Canellos G: Hodgkin's disease, in Holland JF, et al (eds): *Cancer Medicine*, ed 3. Philadelphia, Lea & Febiger, 1993, vol 2, 1998-2027.

Tchekmedyian NS, et al: Megestrol acetate in cancer anorexia and weight loss. *Cancer* 69:1268-1274, 1992.

Tew KD, Stearns ME: Estramustine: A nitrogen mustard/steroid with antimicrotubule activity. *Pharmacol Ther* 43:299-319, 1989.

Trump DL, Robertson CN: Neoplasms of the prostate, in Holland JF, et al (eds): *Cancer Medicine*, ed 3. Philadelphia, Lea & Febiger, 1993, vol 2, 1562-1586.

Twycross R: Corticosteroids in advanced cancer: If they are not working stop them. *BMJ* 305:969-970, 1992.

Vassilopoulou-Sellin R, et al: Impact of adjuvant mitotane on the clinical course of patients with adrenocortical cancer. *Cancer* 71:3119-3123, 1993.

Wilcken N, Tattersall MHN: Endocrine therapy for desmoid tumors. *Cancer* 68:1384-1388, 1991.

Wolf DM, Jordan VC: Gynecologic complications associated with long-term adjuvant tamoxifen therapy for breast cancer. *Gynecol Oncol* 45:118-128, 1992.

Wright CDP, et al: Effect of long term tamoxifen treatment on bone turnover in women with breast cancer. *BMJ* 306:429-430, 1993.

Wysowski DK, et al: Fatal and nonfatal hepatotoxicity associated with flutamide. *Ann Intern Med* 118:860-864, 1993.

Young RC, et al: Cancer of the ovary, in DeVita VT Jr, et al (eds): *Cancer: Principles & Practice of Oncology*, ed 4. Philadelphia, JB Lippincott, 1993, vol 1, 1226-1263.

Other Selected References

Calabresi P, et al (eds): *Medical Oncology*, ed 2. New York, McGraw-Hill, 1993.

del Regato JA, et al: *Ackerman and del Regato's Cancer: Diagnosis, Treatment, and Prognosis*. St Louis, CV Mosby, 1985.

DeVita VT Jr, et al (eds): *Cancer: Principles & Practice of Oncology*, ed 4. Philadelphia, JB Lippincott, 1993.

Haskell CM (eds): *Cancer Treatment*, ed 3. Philadelphia, WB Saunders, 1990.

Hellmann K, Carter SK (eds): *Fundamentals of Cancer Chemotherapy*. New York, McGraw-Hill, 1987.

Holland JF, et al (eds): *Cancer Medicine*, ed 3. Philadelphia, Lea & Febiger, 1993.

Tannock IF, Hill RP (eds): *The Basic Science of Oncology*, ed 2. New York, McGraw-Hill, 1992.

Antineoplastic Agents: Biological Response Modifiers

92

MACROMOLECULES

- **Interferons**
  - **Interferon alpha**
  - **Interferon beta**
  - **Interferon gamma**
- **Other Cytokines**
  - **Aldesleukin (Interleukin 2, IL-2)**
  - **Interleukin 1 (IL-1)**
  - **Tumor Necrosis Factor**
- **Nonspecific Immune Stimulants**
  - **BCG**
- **Monoclonal Antibodies**

SMALL-MOLECULE BIOMODULATORS

- **Immunomodulator**
  - **Levamisole Hydrochloride**
- **Inducers of Differentiation**
  - **Retinoids**
  - **Polar/Planar Compounds**
- **Miscellaneous Biomodulators**
  - **Octreotide Acetate**
  - **Suramin Sodium**

Biological response modifiers exert their antitumor effects through mediation of host responses (Miller and Tannock, 1992; Rosenberg, 1993; Holland et al, 1993; Mitchell, 1993). They act by one or more of the following mechanisms: augmenting and/or restoring antitumor effector mechanisms, promoting differentiation and/or interfering with transformation, altering gene expression in tumor cells, inhibiting signal transduction from cell surface receptors to the interior of tumor cells, preventing growth of new blood vessels or otherwise interfering with the blood supply of tumors, modifying tumor cell responses to other therapies, direct antiproliferative activity on the tumor cell, or improving the ability of the host to tolerate damage caused by cytotoxic cancer therapy. Those agents used primarily for supportive therapy rather than for their antitumor effects (eg, hematopoietic growth factors) are discussed elsewhere (see index entry Hematopoietic Hormones).

Biological response modifiers and biotherapeutic techniques include nonspecific immunomodulating agents (eg, Bacillus Calmette-Guerin [BCG], levamisole); interferons and interferon inducers; lymphokines and cytokines (eg, aldesleukin [interleukin 2], tumor necrosis factor [TNF]); monoclonal antibodies; vaccines; effector cells; plasmapheresis; and transplantation. Biological response modifiers can be macromolecular (almost invariably proteins; eg, interferons, interleukins, TNF, monoclonal antibodies) or small- to intermediate-sized monomeric molecules (eg, retinoids, levamisole, N-methylformamide, hexamethylene-*bis*-acetamide). Combinations of biological response modifiers or their combination with cytocidal drugs also are being studied; combined therapy is more likely to decrease morbidity and mortality associated with malignant disease than the modifiers given alone (Mulé and Rosenberg, 1991; *Semin Oncol*, 1992; Sznol and Longo, 1993).

In contrast to cytotoxic agents that are selected solely on the basis of their direct antitumor activity, many biological agents also must be evaluated for their activity on host effector cells, which makes screening of these compounds more difficult. In addition, cytotoxic drugs are tested at the maximum tolerated dose, while biological response modifiers may be optimally therapeutic at high, low, or intermediate dosages. To assess a biological reagent adequately both in vitro and in vivo, tests for biologic activity on each relevant effector cell and evaluation of antitumor activity in appropriate tumor models must be performed.

MACROMOLECULES

Interferons

Interferon refers to a family of more than 20 glycoproteins that are defined biologically by their ability to inhibit viral replication (Rosenberg, 1993; Borden, 1993; Borden et al, 1993; Dorr, 1993). These polypeptides were the first group of lymphokines/cytokines identified, and they were the first genetically engineered anticancer agents. Initially, three classes of human interferons, designated HuIFN-α (leukocyte), HuIFN-β (fibroblast), and HuIFN-γ (T lymphocyte), were defined (Kurzrock et al, 1991 A; Baron et al, 1991; Itri, 1992). A fourth class, designated interferon-ω, now has been characterized; it is related to the trophoblastic interferons identified in domestic ruminants. (For discussion of these agents in other chapters, see index entry Interferons.)

Interferons are 143 to 166 amino acids in length with molecular weights of 17,000 to 25,000 daltons. Approximately 20 nonallelic genes that control the production of alpha interferons have been identified; in contrast, only single genes coding for beta and gamma interferon have been discovered. Approximately 30% of the amino acid sequences of alpha and beta interferon are shared and these interferons generally have been thought to interact with the same high-affinity cell surface receptor. However, the alpha and beta interferon receptors may have some distinguishing features, including some components that may be specific for certain alpha interferon subtypes and/or beta interferon. The number of high-affinity interferon receptor molecules present on the surface of responsive cells is relatively small (<2,000 per cell). The amino acid composition of gamma interferon, produced by lymphocytes following antigenic or mitogenic stimulation, differs significantly from that of the other interferons, and it binds to a distinctly different receptor.

Interferons are species specific and receptor dependent. They have pleiotropic biological activities that include antiviral, immunomodulatory, and antiproliferative effects (Kurzrock et al, 1991 A; Baron et al, 1991; Borden, 1993; Borden et al, 1993; Dorr, 1993). Interferons can promote cell differentiation, induce phenotypic reversion, inhibit autocrine growth regulation, and mediate regulation of oncogene expression. Among the biochemical responses that have been identified following interferon treatment are induction of an oligoadenylate synthetase (2′, 5′ synthetase), protein kinase, phosphodiesterase, and indolamine dioxygenase, as well as other changes in gene expression.

The results of clinical trials utilizing alpha (alfa), beta, and gamma interferon preparations demonstrate that the interferons have activity against a variety of hematologic and solid malignancies (DeVita et al, 1991; Itri, 1992; Volz and Kirkpatrick, 1992; Wadler, 1992 A). The compounds were administered by the subcutaneous, intramuscular, intravenous, intravesical, intralesional, and intraperitoneal routes, and various schedules and dosages were used.

INTERFERON ALFA-2a
[Roferon A]

INTERFERON ALFA-2b
[Intron A]

ACTIONS. Interferons alfa-2a and alfa-2b are produced by recombinant DNA technology. They differ only by a single amino acid at position 23 in the amino acid sequence (alfa-2a, lysine; alfa-2b, arginine). In contrast to these homogeneous polypeptides, interferon alfa-n1 [Wellferon] and interferon alfa-n3 [Alferon N] are purified mixtures of naturally occurring interferon alpha subtypes. These preparations are isolated from human lymphoblastoid cells (alfa-n1) or pooled human leukocytes (alfa-n3) that have been induced to produce interferon by infection with Sendai virus. There are differing proportions of the interferon alpha subtypes in the two mixtures. Interferon alfa-n1 is available in Canada but not in the United States, while interferon alfa-n3 has been licensed for marketing in the United States only for the treatment of recurrent or refractory external genital warts (condylomata acuminatum; see index entry Interferon Alfa-n3, In Warts). Nevertheless, no data are available that demonstrate differences in the actions of the four interferon alfa preparations.

The precise mode of action responsible for the antineoplastic effects of interferon alfa is unknown; however, it seems likely that induced expression of some genes and repressed expression of others mediate cellular responses to interferon (Kurzrock et al, 1991 A; Borden, 1993; Dorr, 1993). Interferons inhibit cellular proliferation. They block the transition of some cells from a quiescent (G_0) to the proliferating state. Although the molecular mechanisms involved in the antiproliferative response at the cellular level have not yet been fully elucidated, it is likely that at least part of this response may be mediated by inhibitors of DNA, RNA, and protein synthesis. Interferons also promote differentiation of some malignant cells. In addition, pleiotropic effects on immune effector cells such as T and B lymphocytes, macrophages, polymorphonuclear leukocytes, natural killer (NK) cells, killer lymphocytes, and lymphokine-activated killer cells have been observed.

The immunomodulating properties of interferons have been theorized to play a role in control of tumor proliferation (Borden, 1993; Dorr, 1993; Gutterman, 1994). The binding of interferons to high-affinity cell surface receptors is necessary for their action. The mechanism(s) for transducing signals derived from binding of interferon alfa to its receptor into the cell interior are not fully understood (Kurzrock et al, 1991 A; Borden, 1993; Dorr, 1993). However, it appears that receptor-ligand interaction leads to phosphorylation of specific tyrosine residues in three cytoplasmic subunits of a multimeric protein, termed the interferon-stimulated gene factor 3 (ISGF-3) (Sen and Lengyel, 1992; Pellegrini and Schindler, 1993). The phosphorylated subunits translocate to the cell nucleus and assemble with a fourth protein into an activated ISGF-3 complex. ISGF-3 then induces specific gene transcription by binding with high affinity to DNA at interferon-alfa dependent response elements in the promoter regions of these genes.

Treatment results in induction of many cellular enzymes: those most thoroughly studied include a protein kinase that is activated by double-stranded RNA and that may have tumor suppressor activity, a 2′, 5′-oligoadenylate synthetase, a guanosine triphosphate cyclohydrolase (guanylate cyclase), a pyrimidine nucleoside phosphorylase, a tRNA synthetase, and an indolamine-2, 3-dioxygenase (IDO) (Borden, 1993). IDO degrades tryptophan to kynurenine; induction of this enzyme activity and the resulting depletion of tryptophan may contribute to a decrease in protein synthesis and inhibition of growth in response to interferon treatment. Effects on the cell surface may also be important; the net cell charge becomes negative, and the density of membrane tumor-associated antigens and major histocompatibility antigens may increase, partly due to an increase in the expression of these proteins.

USES. In vitro biologic studies suggest that interferons alfa-2a, alfa-2b, alfa-n1, and alfa-n3 are probably of comparable efficacy, although some differences in relative effectiveness are possible. There are no data from randomized, comparative studies that demonstrate that their efficacy differs for any indication. Nevertheless, in the United States, patients with malignant diseases are treated almost exclusively with one of the recombinant interferons (alfa-2a or alfa-2b).

Hematologic Malignancies: Interferons alfa-2a and alfa-2b are given alone for various hematologic malignancies, including hairy cell and chronic myelogenous leukemias, advanced multiple myeloma, and advanced nodular (indolent) non-Hodgkin's and cutaneous T-cell lymphomas (Baron et al, 1991; DeVita et al, 1991; Itri, 1992; Borden, 1993; Dorr, 1993; Gutterman, 1994).

From 80% to 90% of patients with hairy cell leukemia respond to interferon alfa-2 as initial therapy. Responses include rapid disappearance of hairy cells from the peripheral circulation and their more gradual disappearance from the bone marrow, normalization of peripheral blood counts, and reduced need for transfusions. However, complete remissions are infrequent and one-third to one-half of patients relapse (median time to progression, six months to two years after therapy is discontinued) (Golomb and Vardiman, 1993; Dorr, 1993; Jaiyesimi et al, 1993). Thus, interferon alfa-2 is not considered curative for hairy cell leukemia. Randomized trials are in progress to compare the efficacy of newer agents for this disease (see index entries Cladribine, Pentostatin) with that of interferon alfa-2.

The optimal dose and duration of therapy for hairy cell leukemia have not been determined definitively (Golomb and Vardiman, 1993; Jaiyesimi et al, 1993). Significantly fewer patients treated with 200,000 units/M^2/day respond than those given 2 million units/M^2/day. In some studies, no significant differences were observed in the degree or duration of responses between patients given interferon alfa-2 for 12 or for 18 months. Other investigators reported that maintenance therapy can extend the median duration of response to five years.

Interferon alfa-2 also produces hematologic remissions in more than 70% of patients with early chronic myelogenous leukemia (CML) that is positive for the Philadelphia chromosome (Ph+) (Deisseroth et al, 1993; Silver, 1993; Dorr, 1993). Fewer patients (40%) also have a complete or partial cytogenetic response (ie, disappearance of Ph+ cells), and the duration of remissions in these patients generally is significantly longer than in those who have no cytogenetic response. Data also suggest that interferon alfa-2 may increase the duration of survival (Kantarjian et al, 1993; Ozer et al, 1993). Nevertheless, almost all patients with a complete cytogenetic response to interferon alfa-2 have a few residual Ph+ cells (one in 10^5 to 1 in 10^6) that can be detected only by use of the polymerase chain reaction assay. Thus far, only one randomized trial has compared interferon alfa-2 with conventional cytotoxic chemotherapy in patients with Ph+ CML (The Italian Cooperative Study Group on Chronic Myeloid Leukemia, 1994). The rate of cytogenetic responses (30% vs 5%), the median time to progression (>72 vs 45 months), and the median duration of survival (72 vs 52 months) were significantly greater in those receiving interferon alfa-2 than in those treated with busulfan or hydroxyurea. For optimal response, patients with CML require larger doses (5 million units/M^2/day) than those used for patients with hairy cell leukemia. In addition, response rates are higher when therapy is given daily, and maintenance therapy appears to sustain hematologic and cytogenetic remissions (Borden, 1993; Kantarjian et al, 1993; Dorr, 1993).

Chemotherapy with melphalan plus prednisone or a more intensive combination regimen (see index entry Cancer: Clinical Responses to Chemotherapy [Table]) is the treatment of choice to induce remission in patients with multiple myeloma. Although the addition of interferon alfa-2 to one of these regimens does not increase the percentage of newly diagnosed patients who enter remission (Cooper et al, 1993), maintenance therapy with interferon alone (3 million units/M^2 three times weekly) reduces the rate of relapse and extends the duration of remissions (Camba and Durie, 1992; Dorr, 1993; Lokhorst and Dekker, 1993; Dunbar and Nienhuis, 1993). Maintenance therapy with interferon also may extend survival in patients with complete or near-complete responses to induction therapy. When combined with cytotoxic drugs, interferon alfa-2 also has limited activity in inducing remission in patients who have relapsed or are refractory to initial therapy for myeloma.

Patients with certain advanced-stage indolent non-Hodgkin's lymphomas (NHL) (primarily follicular or nodular lymphomas) frequently respond to interferon alfa-2 (Gaynor and Fisher, 1991; Oken, 1992; Longo et al, 1993). However, less than one-quarter of the remissions are complete, and their median duration is only eight months. The optimal dose, schedule, and duration of therapy are not known. Dosages used in clinical trials have varied from 1 million units daily for one month to 50 million units/M^2 three times weekly for eight weeks. Although response rates were higher with the largest doses, toxicity necessitated dose reductions in almost all patients who received these amounts.

When combined with doxorubicin-based cytotoxic chemotherapy, interferon alfa-2 extended the duration of complete remissions and prolonged the time to treatment failure of patients with clinically aggressive low- or intermediate-grade NHL when compared with the same combination regimen without interferon (Smalley et al, 1992). Although the high rate of objective responses (approximately 30% complete responses and 86% overall) was identical in both arms of this randomized comparative trial, data from a subsequent study suggest that inclusion of interferon alfa-2 in the regimen may increase the percentage of patients who respond and survive for at least three years (Solal-Celigny et al, 1993). In contrast to its efficacy in patients with indolent NHL, fewer than 20% of patients with high-grade NHL respond to interferon alfa-2.

This drug also is active in patients with cutaneous T-cell lymphomas (ie, mycosis fungoides, Sézary syndrome) (Bunn and Hoppe, 1993; Dorr, 1993). Response rates are approximately 50% for previously treated patients with advanced disease and about 90% for newly diagnosed patients with early-stage disease. However, randomized trials are needed to determine the optimal dose and schedule for interferon alfa-2, to compare its efficacy with that of other therapies in previously untreated patients, and to compare the efficacy of interferon plus cytotoxic chemotherapy with that of each therapy used alone.

Interferon alfa-2 also has been investigated in patients with chronic lymphocytic leukemia and myeloproliferative disorders (including polycythemia vera and essential thrombocytosis) (Schiffer, 1991; Dorr, 1993; Borden, 1993). Because the numbers of patients included in these studies have been small, data are insufficient to determine definitively the role of interferon alfa-2 in these diseases. More extensive randomized clinical trials are justified.

Solid Tumors (systemic therapy): Kaposi's sarcoma, malignant melanoma, metastatic renal cell carcinoma, and endocrine pancreatic and midgut carcinoid tumors are among the solid tumors that respond to systemic therapy with interferon alfa-2 (Borden, 1993; Dorr, 1993; Gutterman, 1994). About 30% of patients with AIDS-related Kaposi's sarcoma respond to interferon alfa-2 ≥20 million units/M^2/day; the response appears to correlate with the absence of prior opportunistic infections or systemic lymphoma-like symptoms and with higher CD4-positive cell counts (Mitsuyasu, 1991; Kaplan and Volberding, 1993, Karp et al, 1993). Data suggest that interferon alfa-2 combined with zidovudine is synergistic, but the maximal interferon dose must be reduced to 15 million units/day. Although interferon alfa-2 has been administered intralesionally in some studies, the intramuscular, subcutaneous, or intravenous route is usually used in patients with asymptomatic but rapidly progressing Kaposi's sarcoma.

Response rates to single-agent therapy with interferon alfa-2 have ranged from 15% to more than 20% in melanoma patients with distant metastases (Kirkwood, 1991; Morton et al, 1993; Balch et al, 1993). These results are comparable to those obtained with cytotoxic drugs used either as single agents or in combination regimens. It is unclear if the maximally tolerated dose of interferon alfa-2 is more effective than intermediate doses in these patients. Response rates were generally higher with daily or alternate-day administration than with interrupted or intermittent schedules. Response rates also varied inversely with tumor size.

Regimens that combine interferon alfa-2 with cytotoxic drugs (eg, dacarbazine) or interleukin 2 (IL-2) in various schedules and dosages also are being tested in patients with advanced melanoma. Preliminary results have been promising for some combinations and dosages (Falkson et al, 1991; Garbe et al, 1992; Keilholz et al, 1993). However, comparison of the data from two studies suggests that the sequential combination of interferon alfa-2 with IL-2 and cisplatin (Khayat et al, 1993) may be more consistently effective than IL-2 plus interferon without any cytotoxic chemotherapy (Sparano et al, 1993). Ongoing studies are evaluating the use of interferon alfa-2 as adjuvant therapy for early-stage melanoma. Although preliminary analysis of data from a randomized trial suggests that adjuvant therapy with interferon alfa-2 prolongs the relapse-free interval and a trend toward increased survival has been observed (Kirkwood et al, 1993), confirmatory studies are needed to support this use of interferon outside of clinical trials.

Approximately one-fourth of patients with metastatic renal cell carcinoma respond to therapy with interferon alfa-2 administered daily at maximally tolerated doses (Richie, 1993; Linehan et al, 1993); however, the median duration of response is less than one year. The median duration of survival also was less than one year in 159 patients who participated in three clinical trials of interferon alfa-2 in renal cell carcinoma (Minasian et al, 1993). The combination of interferon alfa-2 with IL-2 also is being studied intensively as therapy for this malignancy (Figlin et al, 1991, 1992; Atzpodien et al, 1991; Vogelzang et al, 1993).

Interferon alfa-2 is active as therapy for malignant carcinoid tumors and other malignant endocrine tumors of the gastroenteropancreatic system (Vinik et al, 1993; Norton et al, 1993). In 40% to 50% of patients with carcinoid syndrome, symptoms such as flushing, diarrhea, and excretion of serotonin metabolites are reduced by therapy with interferon alfa-2; the duration of response has varied considerably in different studies (median, 40 weeks to 34 months). There also is considerable variation in the objective response rate (from zero to 20%). Relief of symptoms and reduction of peptide hormone secretion (median duration in 75% to 80% of patients, nine months) are the principal responses to interferon alfa-2 as therapy for pancreatic endocrine tumors. Fewer than 30% of patients have measurable decreases in tumor size.

Solid Tumors (regional therapy): The early stages of several solid tumors, including bladder, cervical, ovarian, and basal cell carcinomas, respond to regional therapy with interferon alfa-2 (Wadler, 1992 A; Borden, 1993; Dorr, 1993). Intravesical instillation of interferon alfa-2 is effective in patients with papillary or in situ transitional cell carcinoma of the bladder (Glashan, 1990; Lamm et al, 1992 A). Complete responses, with durations lasting six months to more than two years, were reported in 25% of those with papillary tumors and in nearly 50% of those with in situ tumors. Nevertheless, BCG is preferred at present as first-line intravesical immunotherapy in these patients because more data on its safety and efficacy are available from clinical trials.

Although most women with cervical intraepithelial neoplasia (CIN) are managed surgically, the involvement of human papilloma virus in the etiology of this disease prompted investigation of interferon therapy in these patients. Data pooled from several studies show that approximately 50% of women in stages I to III respond completely to topical application of interferon alfa-2, and 43% respond completely to intralesional or perilesional injections (Bornstein et al, 1993). Optimal dosages and schedules for this therapy have not been determined definitively. In addition, some studies suggest that complete responses may occur in a larger percentage of women with CIN after systemic therapy with interferon beta than after local therapy with interferon alfa-2. Therefore, randomized comparative trials are needed. Data are insufficient to support the routine use of interferon alfa-2 as therapy for invasive carcinoma outside of clinical trials.

Patients with basal or squamous cell carcinoma of the skin also have responded to intralesional injection of interferon alfa-2 (Kurzrock et al, 1991 B). However, the number of patients who have received this therapy is relatively small, and some experts believe that data are insufficient to support the routine intralesional injection of interferon alfa-2 in these tumors (Preston and Stern, 1992). At present, its use for this indication should probably be limited to patients for whom surgical excision is contraindicated.

Intraperitoneal injection of interferon alfa-2 has been used in women with minimal residual or recurrent ovarian cancer (Bookman and Bast, 1991; Runowicz, 1992). The rates of complete response have been approximately 30% for interferon alfa-2 used alone and approximately 40% for combined therapy with cisplatin (Berek et al, 1993). This drug has only limited activity when administered systemically in patients with ovarian cancer, particularly those with large tumor burdens.

Modulating Responses to Cytotoxic Drugs: Interferon alfa-2 has been used to modulate tumor cell responses to cytotoxic chemotherapy (Wadler and Schwartz, 1992; Sznol and Longo, 1993). Results of several Phase II trials have demonstrated that the combination of fluorouracil and interferon alfa-2 is promising in metastatic colon cancer (Wadler, 1992 B). This combination appears to be more effective at inhibiting tumor cell thymidylate biosynthesis than fluorouracil alone and it also may increase serum levels and/or reduce the clearance of the antimetabolite. Phase III trials comparing the combination to fluorouracil plus leucovorin and to fluorouracil alone are in progress. Preliminary data suggest that these regimens are equally effective.

This and other combinations of cytotoxic drugs with interferon alfa-2 are being studied in patients with metastatic renal or transitional cell carcinomas, multiple myeloma, metastatic melanoma, ovarian or esophageal cancer, malignant glioma, and several other malignancies (Wadler, 1992 A, 1992 B; Wadler and Schwartz, 1992; Wadler et al, 1993; Sznol and Longo, 1993). At present, data are insufficient to support the routine use of interferon alfa-2 in combination with cytotoxic drugs outside of clinical trials.

Other Uses: In addition to its antitumor actions, interferon alfa-2 appears to be effective in life-threatening pulmonary hemangiomas in infants, a benign proliferative disease (Ezekowitz et al, 1992).

For use of interferon alfa-2 in patients with viral and other nonmalignant diseases, see index entry Interferons, Uses.

ADVERSE REACTIONS. An influenza-like syndrome that includes fever, chills, myalgias, fatigue, headache, and weakness occurs in most patients soon after therapy is initiated. The initial intensity of these symptoms varies greatly among patients but the reactions usually lessen or disappear with continued administration. Anorexia, weight loss, lethargy, and a decreased ability to concentrate are observed in some patients, most commonly after prolonged therapy or large doses. Gastrointestinal side effects are less common and include nausea, vomiting, altered taste, and diarrhea. Cardiovascular effects (eg, hypotension, hypertension, arrhythmias, ischemic heart disease; after prolonged treatment with large doses, reversible congestive cardiomyopathy) have been reported rarely (Sonnenblick and Rosin, 1991). When large doses are not appropriately reduced, neurologic effects can be pronounced and include headaches, mood alterations, dizziness, lightheadedness, peripheral neuropathy, and seizures (uncommon). Local inflammation, urticaria, stomatitis, and deep vein thrombophlebitis are occasional complications. Increased eyelash growth has been noted. Interferons can enhance radiation toxicity.

Rarely, pulmonary infiltrates, pneumonitis, and pneumonia (including several fatalities) have been reported in patients receiving interferon alfa-2. Although the etiology of these adverse reactions is unknown, patients who develop fever, cough, dyspnea or other respiratory symptoms should have a chest x-ray taken. If there is evidence of pulmonary infiltrates or impairment of pulmonary function, it may be appropriate to discontinue interferon therapy.

Myelosuppression can occur but rarely is dose limiting. Mild granulocytopenia is the most frequently observed hematologic effect, although anemia can occur with chronic therapy. The myelosuppression usually is reversible within 24 to 48 hours after dosage adjustment or discontinuation of therapy. The mechanism of myelosuppression appears to be related to retention of mature cells in the bone marrow. Bone marrow hypoplasia and aplasia have been reported in <2% of patients receiving interferon alfa-2 for chronic myelogenous leukemia (Talpaz et al, 1992).

Transient elevation of hepatic enzymes is seen frequently. Interferon alfa-2 also may increase plasma concentrations of theophylline by reducing the activity of hepatic enzymes responsible for its metabolism (Israel et al, 1993). Rarely, metabolic and renal toxic effects occur.

Adverse reactions after administration of interferon alfa-2a and alfa-2b generally are dose related and reversible. Patients may develop antibodies against the recombinant interferon preparation. Interferon alfa-2a may be more antigenic than interferon alfa-2b; both the frequency of antibody responses and the antibody titer in responding patients are greater with the alfa-2a form (Grander et al, 1990; Antonelli et al, 1991; von Wussow et al, 1992). Antibodies induced by one interferon alfa-2 preparation usually cross-react with the other recombinant protein but not with purified endogenous interferon alpha. The clinical significance of neutralizing antibodies to interferon alfa-2 is unknown, for not all patients who develop such antibodies become resistant to the therapeutic effects of the drug.

Although no causal relationship has been established, autoimmune disorders were reported in 19% of patients with malignant carcinoid tumors treated with interferon alfa-2 or natural interferon (Rönnblom et al, 1991). Their incidence appeared to correlate with the presence of autoantibodies in these patients. Interferon alfa-2 therapy was reported to have either induced or exacerbated psoriasis in three patients with carcinoid syndrome and in one with renal cell carcinoma (Funk et al, 1991).

Very few women have received interferon alfa-2 therapy for malignant diseases during pregnancy and no randomized trials have been performed in these patients. However, two women with hairy cell leukemia and two with chronic myelogenous leukemia who received interferon alfa-2 during pregnancy had normal deliveries followed by normal growth and development of the infants (Baer et al, 1992). Both forms of recombinant interferon are classified in FDA Pregnancy Category C.

PHARMACOKINETICS. Interferon alfa-2 is filtered by the glomeruli and undergoes rapid proteolysis within the kidney; the parent compound does not appear in the urine and only negligible amounts are reabsorbed into the systemic circulation. Intravenous administration produces transiently high serum concentrations, but disappearance of the drug from the plasma compartment is rapid compared with intramuscular injection. Estimates of its volume of distribution vary between 20% and 60% of body weight (Wills, 1990). Penetration into the cerebrospinal fluid is poor. Peak serum concentrations after intramuscular injection are achieved within six to eight hours and are only 10% of those attained when equivalent doses are given intravenously. However, therapeutically adequate serum concentrations are maintained after intramuscular or subcutaneous administration due to gradual absorption of approximately 80% of the administered dose from the injected site. Oral administration of interferon alfa-2 is ineffective since the drug would be digested by proteolytic enzymes in the digestive tract.

DOSAGE AND PREPARATIONS. Interferons can be administered intramuscularly, subcutaneously, intravesically, intralesionally, or intraperitoneally. Local administration usually results in higher concentrations of interferon alfa-2 in the tumor than can be achieved with systemic administration. Intravenous administration is not recommended because of the more rapid rate of clearance when this route is used. Dosage depends on the preparation and route of administration. For convenience, the subcutaneous route was utilized in most clinical studies. The optimal dose and schedule differ for each tumor type. See the manufacturers' product information and/or the reviews cited in the section on Uses for specific recommendations.

Preparations should be stored between 2° and 8° C before and after reconstitution.

INTERFERON ALFA-2a:

Roferon A (Recombinant Interferon Alfa-2a) (Roche). Solution 3 and 36 million IU/vial in 1 ml containers, 9 million IU/vial in 0.9 ml containers, and 18 million IU/vial in 3 ml containers; powder (lyophilized) 18 million IU/vial; reconstitute with diluent (3 ml aqueous saline solution containing human serum albumin and phenol). The manufacturer's package insert specifies that the 9 and 36 million IU containers be used only in patients with AIDS-associated Kaposi's sarcoma.

INTERFERON ALFA-2b:

Intron A (Recombinant Interferon Alfa-2b) (Schering). Solution 10 million IU/vial in 2 ml containers and 25 million IU/vial in 5 ml containers; powder 3, 5, 10, 18, 25, and 50 million IU/vial. Reconstitute with diluent (bacteriostatic water) using 1 ml for 3, 5, and 50 million IU; 1 or 2 ml for 10 million IU; 3 ml for 18 million IU; and 5 ml for 25 million IU. The manufacturer's package insert specifies that the 10 and 25 million IU/vial strengths of Intron A solution not be used for patients with Kaposi's sarcoma and that the 50 million IU/vial strength of Intron A powder be used only for patients with Kaposi's sarcoma.

INTERFERON BETA-1b

[Betaseron]

Interferon beta differs from interferon alfa in amino acid structure (see discussion on Interferons and the evaluation on Interferon Alfa). At least three preparations of interferon beta have been investigated. These include purified natural (endogenous) beta interferon, recombinant interferon beta from transfected Chinese hamster ovary cells, and a recombinant mutant protein produced in transfected bacterial cells [Betaseron]. The bacterially derived recombinant protein differs from the others in several ways: a serine replaces a cysteine at position 17 in the amino acid sequence, the N-terminal methionine of natural interferon beta is absent, and this preparation lacks the glycosylation found on interferons produced in mammalian cells. Consequently, some of the properties of bacterially derived interferon beta may differ from those of the mammalian-derived proteins. The cysteine-to-serine substitution eliminates disulfide bridging at position 17 that is thought to result in reduced activity of other bacterially expressed recombinant preparations compared with endogenous interferon beta (Borden et al, 1993). This substitution also confers increased stability.

Interferon beta binds to the same class of receptors as the natural and recombinant alfa interferons. Available data suggest that the affinity of the bacterially derived recombinant interferon beta for this receptor is five- to tenfold greater than that of any of the alfa interferons. Some other features also may distinguish receptors for interferon beta from those that bind alfa interferons.

Interferon beta has a greater antiproliferative effect in vitro than interferon alfa for some cell lines. Phase II clinical trials are currently in progress with interferon beta. Thus far, response rates to interferon beta in patients with hairy cell leukemia or renal cell carcinoma have been slightly below those for interferon alfa-2. Interferon beta also is being studied in patients with AIDS-related Kaposi's sarcoma, recurrent glioma and other malignant brain tumors, and, in combination with fluorouracil, in patients with colorectal carcinoma. Intravesical instillation (for patients with superficial bladder cancer) and intraperitoneal injection (for patients with recurrent ovarian cancer) of interferon beta also are being investigated. At present, data are insufficient to support use of interferon beta outside of sponsored clinical trials for any malignant disease.

For use of interferon beta in multiple sclerosis and other nonmalignant diseases, and for more complete information on adverse reactions, dosage, and preparations, see index entries Interferons and Interferon Beta.

The spectrum of toxicity in patients with malignant diseases is similar to that observed with interferon alfa preparations. However, several reports suggest that the toxic effects associated with interferon beta may be less severe or frequent than with interferon alfa-2.

INTERFERON BETA-1B:

Betaseron (Berlex). NOTE: A new reference standard was adopted in 1993 for measurement of the specific activity of interferon beta preparations (The IFNB Multiple Sclerosis Study Group, 1993). As a result, units of activity used in clinical trials whose results were published prior to 1993 are not equivalent to the units of activity on the current packaging of Betaseron. Doses given as 9 or 45 million IU relative to the previous reference standard (native interferon beta, prepared by the National Institutes of Health) are equal to 1.6 and 8 million IU, respectively, relative to the recombinant interferon beta reference standard adopted by the World Health Organization. Thus, doses measured in the older units must be multiplied by the conversion factor 0.1778 before measurement using the new units.

INTERFERON GAMMA-1a
[Immuneron]

INTERFERON GAMMA-1b
[Actimmune]

Interferon gamma shares some of the antiproliferative, antiviral, and immunomodulating effects of interferons alfa and beta (see discussion on Interferons and the evaluations on Interferon Alfa and Beta). However, it has some unique biological properties. Interferon gamma recognizes a distinct cell surface receptor, has more potent antiviral and antiproliferative effects in certain cell lines, and induces a select set of polypeptides. A more effective enhancement of both major histocompatibility complex (MHC) class I and II antigens is seen with interferon gamma at equivalent doses. Some leukemic cell lines undergo terminal differentiation after exposure to interferon gamma. Production of interferon gamma in response to treatment with some cytokines (eg, interleukin 2, interleukin 12) or in most models of cellular immunotherapy is required for antitumor efficacy. In addition, interferon gamma has macrophage-activating effects (eg, stimulation of peroxidase generation) and augments Fc receptor expression and antibody-dependent cellular cytotoxicity.

Interferon gamma-1b is indicated to reduce the frequency and severity of infections in patients with chronic granulomatous disease. For discussion of this and other uses of interferon gamma as an immunomodulator and as therapy for nonmalignant diseases, see index entries Interferon Gamma-1b and Interferons, Actions and Uses. Interferon gamma-1a is not available in the United States at present outside of sponsored clinical trials.

Clinical trials of interferon gamma in patients with neoplastic diseases are currently in progress. Responses have been reported in patients with chronic myelogenous leukemia, metastatic renal cell carcinoma, ovarian carcinoma, advanced cutaneous T-cell lymphoma, and metastatic melanoma. However, a randomized clinical trial of interferon gamma as adjuvant therapy in patients with cutaneous melanoma who were at high risk for recurrence after surgical excision of stage I or II lesions was terminated when an interim analysis found increased rates of relapse or death and shorter median times to relapse among those receiving this agent than among the controls who were followed by observation only (Meyskens et al, 1990). A few patients have responded to this cytokine after it was injected intrapleurally for malignant pleural mesothelioma or intra- or perilesionally for basal cell carcinoma or cervical intraepithelial neoplasia.

In vitro studies suggest that the combination of interferon gamma plus alfa or beta interferons may be synergistic. Initial clinical trials of interferon alfa-2 plus interferon gamma have been conducted in patients with renal cell carcinoma, chronic myelogenous leukemia, non-small cell lung cancer, and metastatic melanoma. Additional trials are studying responses to the combination of interferon gamma with tumor necrosis factor, aldesleukin (interleukin 2), a monoclonal antibody preparation, or fluorouracil in patients with various malignancies.

At present, data are insufficient to support the use of interferon gamma (either alone or in combination with other drugs) for any malignancy other than in sponsored clinical trials.

Toxicity in patients treated with interferon gamma for malignant diseases is similar to that observed with other interferon preparations.

INTERFERON GAMMA-1a:
Immuneron (recombinant interferon gamma-1a) (Biogen).
INTERFERON GAMMA-1b:
Actimmune (recombinant interferon gamma-1b) (Genentech).
For preparations, see index entry Interferon gamma-1b, In Chronic Granulomatous Disease.

Other Cytokines

ALDESLEUKIN (Interleukin 2, IL-2)
[Proleukin]

ACTIONS. Endogenous interleukin 2 (IL-2) is a glycoprotein containing 133 amino acids, and its molecular size is estimated to be 14 to 16 kilodaltons on the basis of its electrophoretic mobility. The calculated molecular weight of the amino acid portion is 15.4 kilodaltons, based on the primary structure inferred from the nucleotide sequence of the cloned human gene (Lotze, 1991; Whittington and Faulds, 1993; Bradley and Grimm, 1993; Rosenberg, 1993). Variability in the extent of O-linked glycosylation at position 3 in the amino acid sequence results in heterogeneity in the size and charge of IL-2 molecules. The endogenous cytokine is produced and secreted by T-cells activated by antigen binding and stimulated by IL-1. Among its biological actions, IL-2 stimulates the proliferation of activated T-cells, activates the cellular cytotoxicity of T-cells and natural killer (NK) cells and tumor cell lysis by monocytes, acts as a cofactor for the growth and differentiation of B-cells, is a chemotactic factor for T-cells and thus participates in inflammatory responses, and induces the expression and release of other cytokines (eg, interferon gamma, tumor necrosis factor) by responsive cells.

IL-2 acts through a trimolecular receptor complex found on the surface of NK and T- and B-cells (Lotze, 1991; Whittington and Faulds, 1993; Bradley and Grimm, 1993; Rosenberg, 1993; Smith, 1993). This high-affinity form of the IL-2 receptor consists of a 55-kilodalton α chain, a 75-kilodalton β chain, and a 64-kilodalton γ chain. Monomers of the α chain bind IL-2 with reduced affinity and cannot transduce signals from binding of this cytokine to the cell's interior. In contrast, heterodimers formed from the β and γ chains have an intermediate affinity for IL-2 and can transduce signals to activate and/or stimulate lymphocytes upon binding of the cytokine. The γ chain also is a component of the receptors for other cytokines including IL-4, IL-7, and IL-13.

The antitumor activity of IL-2 is thought to result from its ability to stimulate cell-mediated immunity leading to tumor cell lysis, since IL-2 has no direct antiproliferative or cytotoxic effect on cancer cells. The ability of this cytokine to stimulate lymphocyte proliferation is the basis of its use for in vitro expansion of lymphokine-activated killer (LAK) or tumor-infiltrating lymphocyte (TIL, also called tumor-derived activated cells or TDAC) cell populations (Topalian and Rosenberg, 1991; Yang and Rosenberg, 1991). The expanded pools of LAK or TIL cells are reinfused (with additional IL-2) as adoptive cellular immunotherapy for certain solid tumors (see Uses) (Rosenberg, 1991 A, 1991 B).

Aldesleukin is a recombinant DNA preparation of IL-2 produced in *Escherichia coli*. It differs from endogenous IL-2 by the lack of post-translational glycosylation that occurs in mammalian but not bacterial cells, by the absence of the N-terminal alanine residue in the cytokine's amino acid sequence, and by substitution of a serine for the cysteine moiety at position 125 of the sequence. The cysteine residues at positions 58 and 105 are retained in all active IL-2 preparations, since the disulfide bond between these moieties appears to be required for full biological activity. Despite its structural differences from endogenous IL-2, aldesleukin retains all the biological activities of the native cytokine that have been tested in vitro. Other recombinant human IL-2 preparations (eg, teceleukin) are in various phases of clinical trials but are not yet approved for marketing in the United States.

USES. ***Renal Cell Carcinoma:*** Aldesleukin is indicated as therapy for metastatic renal cell carcinoma (Linehan et al, 1993). The clinical trials reviewed by the FDA before approval of aldesleukin included highly selected hospitalized patients with metastatic or unresectable renal carcinoma, approximately 85% of whom had undergone nephrectomy prior to aldesleukin therapy. A 15-minute infusion of 7.2×10^5 IU/kg was administered every eight hours for up to five days (to a maximum of 14 doses), followed by nine days without therapy and then a second cycle of administration three times daily for up to five days (to a maximum of 14 additional doses). A second course of two cycles was given to patients who responded or whose disease stabilized after the first course.

Since doses frequently were withheld (rather than reduced) to allow recovery from toxicity, the patients in these trials received a median of 20 of the 28 scheduled doses in the first course. Tumors regressed completely in 4% and partially in an additional 11% of the patients. The response rate was highest (18%) among those with the most favorable performance status (asymptomatic patients; Eastern Cooperative Oncology Group [ECOG] performance status 0). In contrast, 9% of patients who were symptomatic but ambulatory (ECOG status, 1) experienced partial remissions, and none of the patients with ECOG performance status ≥ 2 responded. The median duration was 23.2 months for all responses and 18.8 months for partial responses. In these trials, adoptive immunotherapy with LAK cells was not utilized.

Additional studies in patients with renal cell carcinoma investigated alternative routes, dosages, and schedules for administration of aldesleukin. In several trials, 18×10^6 IU/M^2/day was infused continuously for five days, followed by six days without therapy and then by a second 4½-day cycle at the same daily dose (Negrier et al, 1989; von der Maase et al, 1991; Palmer et al, 1992). Patients were scheduled to receive two identical courses of aldesleukin as induction therapy followed by up to four five-day cycles at the same daily dose as maintenance therapy. Response rates to aldesleukin monotherapy using this dose and schedule without LAK cells were comparable to those observed in patients given short infusions every eight hours (5% complete and 11% partial remissions).

The use of aldesleukin as outpatient therapy for metastatic or inoperable renal carcinoma also has been studied. Intravenous boluses of 10×10^6 IU/M^2 infused over 5 to 10 minutes three times weekly caused toxicity that required dose modification after the fourth dose in 73% of patients and resulted in an overall response rate of only 12% (one complete and four partial remissions among 41 patients) (Bukowski et al, 1990). A smaller study evaluated a lower-dose subcutaneous regimen (Sleijfer et al, 1992). Two complete (8%) and four partial (15%) remissions were observed in 26 patients given aldesleukin 18×10^6 IU once a day for five days each week over a six-week period; the disease was stabilized in an additional 50% of the patients. Although results with these alternative regimens are comparable to those achieved with high-dose intravenous boluses or continuous infusions, randomized comparative trials are now in progress and must be completed to determine the optimal dose, schedule, and route of administration for aldesleukin.

Regimens combining aldesleukin with LAK cell infusions generally use a five-day priming period of high-dose aldesleukin administered as three daily boluses of 7.2×10^5 IU/kg each (Rosenberg et al, 1985, 1987) or by continuous infusion of 18×10^6 IU/M^2/day (West et al, 1987). This is followed by leukapheresis on four or more days during the rest period to harvest cytotoxic lymphocytes. The cells are activated by three to four days of culture in the presence of aldesleukin and then infused on three or four days during a second five-day cycle of aldesleukin given at the same dose.

In a randomized trial in patients with renal carcinoma, the intravenous bolus and continuous infusion high-dose regimens of aldesleukin plus LAK cells appeared to be comparable in efficacy and toxicity (Weiss et al, 1992). A second study used a different recombinant IL-2 preparation to compare two continuous infusion regimens (Thompson et al, 1992). These investigators found that reducing the dosage from 18×10^6 to 6×10^6 IU/day and extending the duration of administration from five to ten days during the second (maintenance) cycle reduced the toxicity of this therapy with no loss of efficacy. Furthermore, data from an uncontrolled trial suggest that a low-dose regimen of IL-2 (3×10^4 IU/kg every eight hours during both the priming and maintenance cycles) combined with LAK-cell infusions extends survival of both responding and nonresponding patients beyond that projected based on analysis of their risk factors (Schoof et al, 1993). At present, however, there are no convincing data that LAK cell infusions increase the response rates, prolong the durations of response, or increase the progression-free or overall survival of patients with renal cell carcinoma treated with aldesleukin (Palmer et al, 1992; Rosenberg et al, 1993; Linehan et al, 1993). Studies are in progress to determine if TIL cells, generated by IL-2 stimulation in vitro of lymphocytes isolated from disaggregated tumor specimens, are more effective than

LAK cells in patients receiving aldesleukin therapy for this malignancy.

Malignant Melanoma: Aldesleukin also is active as therapy for malignant melanoma in patients with disseminated metastases (stage IV) (Balch et al, 1993; Morton et al, 1993). In a number of clinical trials, 10% to 25% of patients responded to one of the high-dose regimens used in advanced renal carcinoma. Data are not available from randomized studies comparing the efficacy of different dosages, routes, or schedules in melanoma patients. However, response rates appear to be somewhat higher in the studies that employed bolus administration than in those using continuous infusion. Although most responses were partial and of short duration, remissions were complete and long-lasting in some patients.

Additional uncontrolled studies in patients with melanoma have combined aldesleukin with cytotoxic agents (dacarbazine, cisplatin, or cyclophosphamide) or with other biological response modifiers (interferon alfa-2). Some trials used dosages of aldesleukin that were smaller than the bolus and continuous infusion regimens considered standard for renal carcinoma; the data indicated that response rates were comparable and toxicity was reduced (Mitchell, 1992). Data from randomized trials are needed to compare aldesleukin used alone with aldesleukin (low- or high-dose) combined with other drugs as therapy for metastatic melanoma.

The LAK cell regimens that have been used as therapy for metastatic melanoma are identical to those in patients with renal carcinoma. In one randomized trial, investigators reported that there was a trend toward increased survival for melanoma patients receiving LAK cell infusions combined with aldesleukin (Rosenberg et al, 1993). However, data from most single-arm studies suggest that there is no advantage to the combination compared with aldesleukin monotherapy (Balch et al, 1993; Morton et al, 1993). Response rates of 20% to 50% have been reported in pilot studies in which patients with disseminated malignant melanoma received TIL cell infusions combined with high-dose aldesleukin administered either by intravenous bolus or continuous infusion (Rosenberg et al, 1988; Dillman et al, 1991). Clinical trials are in progress to determine if aldesleukin combined with TIL cell infusions is more effective therapy for metastatic melanoma than aldesleukin alone or with LAK cells.

Miscellaneous Malignancies: Aldesleukin (with or without LAK cells) also has been evaluated in patients with a variety of other advanced, metastatic, or recurrent malignancies refractory to therapy with cytotoxic drug regimens (Lotze and Rosenberg, 1991; Rosenberg, 1991 A, 1991 B; Whittington and Faulds, 1993; Bradley and Grimm, 1993; Rosenberg, 1993). Among these are colorectal, bladder, lung, ovarian, breast, and head and neck carcinomas; primary and metastatic brain tumors; leukemias; and lymphomas. In addition, aldesleukin and other IL-2 preparations have been administered (by intrapleural or intraperitoneal infusion) following bone marrow transplantation and have been evaluated in a few patients as therapy for malignant pleural effusions or ascites. Although responses have been observed in a few patients, data are insufficient to support the routine use of aldesleukin outside of clinical trials as therapy for malignancies other than metastatic renal cell carcinoma or malignant melanoma.

Combination Regimens: Aldesleukin also has been studied in combination regimens that utilized either simultaneous or sequential administration of this cytokine with cytotoxic drugs or with other biologic response modifiers (Rosenberg et al, 1989 A; Dillman et al, 1993). Examples include its use with dacarbazine (Flaherty et al, 1990; Stoter et al, 1991), cisplatin (Demchak et al, 1991), both drugs (Flaherty et al, 1993), or in a low-dose regimen with low-dose cyclophosphamide (Mitchell et al, 1988; Mitchell, 1992) in patients with metastatic melanoma. A regimen that combines aldesleukin with fluorouracil and cisplatin has been investigated in patients with non-small cell lung cancer and head and neck tumors (Valone et al, 1991).

In single-arm uncontrolled trials, aldesleukin (or other IL-2 preparations) has shown activity when combined with interferon alfa-2 as therapy for patients with advanced melanoma (Rosenberg et al, 1989 B; Garbe et al, 1992; Keilholz et al, 1993) and renal cell carcinoma (Rosenberg et al, 1989 B; Figlin et al, 1991, 1992; Atzpodien et al, 1991; Vogelzang et al, 1993). Results from subsequent randomized trials have not demonstrated that the combination is clearly superior in efficacy to either cytokine used alone (Sparano et al, 1993; Atkins et al, 1993). In addition, a within-subject comparison of IL-2 with and without interferon-alfa failed to detect any difference in clinical or immunologic effects (Schiller et al, 1993). In contrast, preliminary data from a trial in 39 patients suggest that there may be synergy when cisplatin followed by interleukin 2 is combined with interferon alfa-2 (Khayat et al, 1993). Sequential chemoimmunotherapy using these two cytokines and a three-drug regimen (carmustine, cisplatin, and dacarbazine) also is being evaluated as therapy for metastatic melanoma (Richards et al, 1992). Additional clinical trials have studied aldesleukin in combination with tumor necrosis factor (Yang et al, 1991), interferon gamma (Redman et al, 1990), the pineal hormone melatonin (Lissoni et al, 1992, 1993), and flavone acetic acid (O'Reilly et al, 1993). Data are insufficient to support use of any of these regimens outside of clinical trial protocols.

ADVERSE REACTIONS AND DRUG INTERACTIONS. The toxicities observed in patients treated with high-dose regimens of aldesleukin have been reviewed (Margolin et al, 1989; Siegel and Puri, 1991; Vial and Descotes, 1992; Whittington and Faulds, 1993). Although many adverse reactions can be serious and life-threatening and often may require support in an intensive care unit, most resolve when therapy is discontinued. In addition, their frequency and severity are dose-related; the severe complications of the vascular leak syndrome (see below) associated with high doses of aldesleukin occur much less frequently in patients receiving intermediate doses by continuous infusion. Furthermore, the low-dose regimens used in some clinical trials (see Uses) have been administered to outpatients.

The most common adverse reaction to high-dose therapy with aldesleukin is a vascular leak syndrome that results in fluid retention, peripheral and pulmonary edema, pleural effusions, and significant weight gain. In the most serious cases, this can be accompanied by severe hypotension, oliguria or anuria, and respiratory failure. Vasopressors (eg, dopamine, phenylephrine) often must be administered to treat the severe hypotension. Because some vasopressors can exacerbate arrhythmia that may accompany aldesleukin therapy (see following paragraph), the more arrhythmogenic agents should not be used. Fluid administration to correct the hypovolemia often is not advisable because it may exacerbate the edema as a result of increased vascular permeability.

Other cardiovascular disorders that have been observed include arrhythmias, cardiac ischemia, myocarditis, hypocontractility, angina, and (rarely) myocardial infarction. Thus, patients with an abnormal thallium stress test or stress electrocardiogram (as well as those with abnormal pulmonary, renal, or hepatic function tests) should not receive aldesleukin.

Reduced renal perfusion as a result of hypotension combined with decreased myocardial contractility usually causes azotemia and decreased sodium excretion and increases plasma renin activity and serum creatinine levels. Pulmonary edema caused by the vascular leak syndrome produces respiratory distress in approximately 20% of patients receiving high-dose therapy with aldesleukin and requires intubation and mechanical ventilation in 5% to 10%. Some patients also develop reversible bronchospasm during aldesleukin therapy.

Mild to severe influenza-like symptoms (eg, fever, chills, malaise, nasal congestion) also are common. Acetaminophen or indomethacin often are used prophylactically to prevent aldesleukin-induced fever. However, renal function must be monitored closely in patients receiving indomethacin (or other nonsteroidal anti-inflammatory drugs) with aldesleukin, since they may cause additive or synergistic nephrotoxicity. Meperidine also is administered to control the chills that occur in nearly all patients receiving high-dose aldesleukin.

Gastrointestinal reactions that develop in most patients during aldesleukin therapy include nausea, vomiting, and diarrhea. These usually respond to standard antiemetic and antidiarrheal therapy. Anorexia and stomatitis also are common, and bowel hemorrhage, infarction, or perforation may occur occasionally. Histamine (H_2) receptor antagonists (eg, ranitidine, cimetidine) may be used prophylactically to control gastric acid secretion in patients receiving aldesleukin. However, these drugs as well as the nonsteroidal anti-inflammatory agents used to reduce fever may affect the response to therapy (Mertens et al, 1992). Reversible hepatotoxicity (cholestasis that elevates circulating levels of bilirubin) occurs in most patients. Acute pancreatitis has been reported in a few instances.

Hypothyroidism developed in 22% of patients after aldesleukin therapy (with or without interferon alfa-2) in two prospective studies (Schwartzentruber et al, 1991; Kruit et al, 1993). Although some investigators have suggested that thyroid toxicity appears to correlate with tumor response, no such correlation was reported in these studies. In the more recent trial, the incidence of thyroid dysfunction was dependent on the cumulative dose of IL-2 and duration of therapy (Kruit et al, 1993). Thyroid toxicity in patients receiving aldesleukin (or other immunotherapies) may be mediated by an autoimmune process. It also appears to be biphasic, since hypothyroidism follows a short period of hyperthyroidism in many patients (Kruit et al, 1993).

Pruritus and erythema are common in patients receiving IL-2 preparations (Wolkenstein et al, 1993). Most cases are mild and are easily controlled with hydroxyzine or diphenhydramine. However, generalized erythroderma with desquamation, severe urticaria, necrotic lesions, or blisters can occur. These more severe reactions also generally resolve when cytokine therapy is discontinued. Subcutaneous injection of aldesleukin may produce an indurated erythematous wheal at the injection site that may become intensely pruritic and persist for weeks. Local or diffuse vitiligo may occur occasionally during or after aldesleukin therapy.

Neurologic toxicities associated with aldesleukin therapy include confusion, disorientation, lethargy, somnolence, and combative behavior. Occasionally patients may become psychotic or comatose or experience hallucinations or seizures. Aldesleukin therapy should be withheld in those who develop moderate to severe lethargy, confusion, or somnolence to avoid the risk of coma.

Hematologic responses to aldesleukin therapy include an initial lymphocytopenia (probably resulting from margination), followed by rebound lymphocytosis one to two days after therapy is discontinued. Anemia and eosinophilia occur frequently, thrombocytopenia less often, and granulocytopenia only occasionally. The severity of anemia requires red blood cell transfusions in more than half of patients treated with high-dose regimens. Eosinophilia results from IL-2-stimulated production of IL-5 and occurs in nearly all patients (MacDonald et al, 1990; Pisani et al, 1991). However, this response usually does not require intervention or specific therapy. Platelet counts fall below 2×10^4/microliter in approximately 20% of those treated with aldesleukin.

The incidence of bacterial infections was between 10% and 30% in studies in which high-dose bolus aldesleukin therapy was employed (Siegel and Puri, 1991). When it was given by continuous infusion without cytotoxic chemotherapy, the infection rate was <10% (Dillman et al, 1993), and it was substantially lower in patients treated with low subcutaneous doses (Schomburg et al, 1992). The increased susceptibility to bacteremia, most often with staphylococcal species, may result from reversible defects in neutrophil chemotaxis and F_c receptor expression caused by IL-2. Risk factors for sepsis include the presence of vascular access catheters, open wounds, or biliary obstruction. Prophylactic antibiotic therapy may be recommended for some patients with indwelling central vascular catheters who are receiving high-dose bolus aldesleukin. Data from a retrospective review of 519 patients suggest that the incidence of infections declined over the three-year study period (Pockaj et al, 1993). Furthermore, infections resolved in almost all patients; only two deaths (0.2%) caused by sepsis were reported.

There are no data evaluating carcinogenesis, mutagenesis, or impairment of fertility in humans or animals receiving aldesleukin. Its effects on the fetus or on pregnant women or animals also have not been studied, and it is not known if the drug is excreted in human milk. Aldesleukin is classified in FDA Pregnancy Category C. Several studies have demonstrated that this drug can be administered safely to children with refractory malignancies (Chien and Hsieh, 1990; Ribeiro et al, 1993).

PHARMACOKINETICS. Based on studies in animals, approximately 70% of an intravenous bolus is sequestered on first pass through the liver, kidneys, and lungs where it distributes throughout the extravascular, extracellular space. The distribution and elimination half-lives of aldesleukin in cancer patients are 13 and 85 minutes, respectively (Konrad et al, 1990). These measurements are comparable to those reported for other recombinant IL-2 preparations and for the endogenous cytokine (Lotze and Rosenberg, 1991; Bocci, 1991). Based on its rapid rate of disappearance from plasma, aldesleukin usually is administered either as three daily boluses or by continuous infusion.

Steady-state plasma levels of aldesleukin are directly proportional to the dose and are achieved within the first one to two hours of a continuous intravenous infusion (Konrad et al, 1990). Serum concentrations approximately 2% of those obtained shortly after an intravenous bolus are maintained for eight hours after subcutaneous or intramuscular injection. Based on measurements of the area under the plasma concentration versus time curves, an estimated 30% of an intramuscular dose appears in the circulation. Data are not available to estimate the bioavailability of aldesleukin after subcutaneous injection.

Aldesleukin is cleared primarily in the kidney by glomerular filtration and peritubular extraction. The mean rate of clearance in patients with advanced malignancies reported in the manufacturer's labeling information is approximately 270 ml/min; however, other investigators have reported a rate of approximately 120 ml/min (Konrad et al, 1990). More than 80% of the aldesleukin cleared by the kidney is metabolized to amino acids in the peritubular cells. The ability of patients with rising serum creatinine concentrations to maintain clearance of aldesleukin is attributed to the dual mechanisms for its removal by the kidney.

DOSAGE AND PREPARATIONS. The activity of aldesleukin (and other IL-2 preparations) is measured in International Units (IU) by comparison to a reference standard adopted by the World Health Organization's National Institute of Biological Standards and Controls. Before establishment of this reference standard, the manufacturers of recombinant IL-2 preparations defined their own units (Cetus Units, Roche Units) and many clinical studies were published with dosages specified only in these units. One Cetus Unit equals 6 IU; one Roche Unit equals approximately 3 IU.

Intravenous, Subcutaneous: For metastatic renal carcinoma or malignant melanoma, aldesleukin is given by intravenous bolus, continuous infusion, or subcutaneous injection. When lymphokine-activated killer cells are used, they are harvested after an initial (priming) cycle of therapy, expanded in vitro, and infused during a subsequent cycle. See the manufacturer's product information, the section on Uses, and the clinical studies cited therein for specific dosages and schedules of administration.

Bacteriostatic water for injection and 0.9% sodium chloride for injection are incompatible with parenteral solutions of aldesleukin and should not be used for reconstitution or dilution. Doses administered as a bolus are infused over 15 minutes, after diluting the reconstituted solution in 50 ml of 5% dextrose injection. When given by continuous infusion, aldesleukin should be diluted to a final concentration of 85,000 to 1 million IU/ml (5 to 60 mcg/ml) in 5% dextrose injection containing human serum albumin to achieve a final concentration of 0.1%. Reconstituted aldesleukin is administered by subcutaneous injection without further dilution. Reconstituted or diluted solutions are stable for at least 48 hours at temperatures from 2° to 25° C. Diluted solutions for continuous infusion (with 0.1% human serum albumin) are stable in the environment of an infusion pump maintained at 32° C for up to six days.

Proleukin (Cetus Oncology). Cake (lyophilized) 22 million IU (1.3 mg) per vial. When reconstituted with 1.2 ml sterile water for injection, each ml contains 18 million IU aldesleukin with mannitol 50 mg and sodium dodecyl sulfate 0.18 mg, buffered with approximately 0.17 mg monobasic and 0.89 mg dibasic sodium phosphate to a pH of 7.5 (range, 7.2 to 7.8). Store refrigerated at 2° to 8° C.

INTERLEUKIN 1 (IL-1) (Investigational drug)

ACTIONS AND USES. Two structurally related forms of interleukin 1 (IL-1) have been identified, IL-1α and IL-1β, each encoded by a distinct gene (Neta and Oppenheim, 1992; Dinarello and Wolff, 1993; Bradley and Grimm, 1993). The two share approximately 27% amino acid sequence homology, and each is synthesized as a precursor with a molecular weight of 31 kilodaltons, cleaved by proteolysis, and glycosylated to yield the biologically active form with a molecular weight of 17 kilodaltons. Glycosylation is apparently not required for biological activity since recombinant IL-1 expressed in *E. coli*, which is not glycosylated, is biologically active. IL-1α is primarily a membrane-bound molecule, while IL-1β is secreted by unknown mechanisms. The human genes for both IL-1α and IL-1β have been cloned, and recombinant preparations of these cytokines are being studied in clinical trials.

Two cell surface receptors capable of binding both forms of IL-1 have been identified, although they are not simultaneously expressed in the same cells (Neta and Oppenheim, 1992; Dinarello and Wolff, 1993). The first is present on T-cells (among others) and transduces signals upon binding of IL-1 by protein phosphorylation on serine and/or threonine residues. The second is found on B-cells (and others), but has not been demonstrated to transduce signals into the cell from ligand binding. An endogenous protein homologous to IL-1α and IL-1β also has been identified (IL-1 Receptor Antagonist, IL-1Ra) that binds to both receptors with affinity equal to both IL-1 species and acts as an antagonist.

The two forms of IL-1 mediate a variety of immune responses and induce the proliferation and maturation of progenitor cells from various hematopoietic lineages (Neta and Oppenheim, 1992; Dinarello and Wolff, 1993; Bradley and Grimm, 1993). These effects probably result from production of colony stimulating factors and other cytokines, as well as induced expression of their receptors, upon binding of IL-1 to responsive cells. The two IL-1 species also have direct antiproliferative activities against certain human tumor cell lines and in animal tumor models.

In addition to their potential use for stimulating hematopoietic recovery from cytotoxic chemotherapy (Crown et al, 1991; Smith et al, 1992 A, 1993), clinical trials of recombinant IL-1α and IL-1β are evaluating their efficacy in tumor immunotherapy (Neta and Oppenheim, 1992). Preliminary data from a Phase II trial in patients with malignant melanoma indicate that there is no response in those with visceral metastases but that the response rate is 13% in those with metastases at other sites.

ADVERSE REACTIONS. Influenza-like symptoms, including chills, fever, nausea and vomiting, fatigue, headache, myalgia, arthralgia, and somnolence, have been the most frequent adverse reactions to IL-1. Although the severe vascular leak syndrome seen in patients receiving high-dose aldesleukin therapy has not been observed, hypotension is the dose-limiting toxicity for most patients in clinical trials of IL-1. Those receiving doses >0.3 mcg/kg require treatment with intravenous vasopressors to maintain blood pressure at levels adequate for tissue perfusion. Increased concentrations of triglycerides, cortisol, C-reactive protein, and thyroid stimulating hormone and decreased concentrations of cholesterol, testosterone, and protein C also have been observed in patients receiving IL-1.

DOSAGE.

Intravenous: The maximum tolerated dose of IL-1α or IL-1β is 0.3 mcg/kg administered as a 15-minute infusion once daily for seven days (Smith et al, 1992 A; Neta and Oppenheim, 1992).

Interleukin-1α (Dainippon Pharmaceuticals).
Interleukin-1β (Immunex).

TUMOR NECROSIS FACTOR (Investigational drug)

ACTIONS. Tumor necrosis factor (TNF-α) is a protein (also known as cachectin) primarily produced by macrophages conditioned by BCG or other immunostimulating agents and triggered by endotoxin (ie, lipopolysaccharide [LPS]) (Spriggs, 1991; Economou, 1993). Other cell types also produce TNF-α in response to various stimuli. A closely related cytotoxic protein, lymphotoxin, is 35% identical and 50% homologous in amino acid sequence with TNF-α, acts at the same receptor, and often is referred to as TNF-β. The monomer polypeptide of TNF-α has a molecular weight of 17 kilodaltons. In solution, it exists primarily as a trimer, and the affinity of cell surface receptors for the trimer is almost 1,000 times greater than for the monomer.

TNF-α mediates a broad range of biological processes, including septic shock, inflammatory responses, and the cachexia accompanying neoplastic diseases and chronic infections (Spriggs, 1991; Economou, 1993). Interest in its potential use in cancer therapy originated with the observation that it can induce hemorrhagic necrosis in many experimental tumor systems. The gene for TNF-α has been cloned and expressed in bacteria to provide quantities of the purified cytokine that are adequate for conducting clinical trials. Although the gene for TNF-β also has been cloned and expressed, clinical trials of this product have not yet begun.

The mechanism of action of TNF-α as an antitumor agent is not well understood. At cell surfaces, it binds to receptors whose molecular structure was determined by cloning of the receptor gene (Spriggs, 1991; Economou, 1993). There may be at least two receptors for TNF-α, each of which may differ in ligand affinity, cell type, size, and glycosylation. Receptors of 55 to 60 and 75 to 80 kilodaltons, to which trimers of TNF-α bind, have been studied most extensively. The mechanism(s) by which TNF receptors transduce signals from ligand binding into the cell interior are not known. TNF-α directly inhibits the proliferation of many cultured malignant cell lines; it is much less inhibitory to the growth of normal (nontransformed) cells. In some cases, however, TNF-α has stimulated tumor cell growth in vitro and may be acting as an autocrine or paracrine growth factor. The density of TNF receptors on the surface of tumor or normal cells and their ligand affinity bear no relationship to the cells' sensitivity to this direct antiproliferative effect.

A second factor contributing to its antitumor effects is the pronounced sensitivity of endothelial cells in the newly formed vasculature of growing tumors between 5 and 6 mm in diameter to direct toxicity from TNF-α. The consequences of this interaction are hemorrhagic necrosis and thrombosis in the central regions of the tumor, although a rim of malignant cells usually remains viable. Finally, TNF-α also may augment some immune responses to tumor cells. The relative contributions of these mechanisms to the antitumor actions of TNF-α are not clearly delineated.

USES. A number of Phase I and II clinical trials of TNF-α have been completed in patients with various malignancies (Alexander and Rosenberg, 1991; Budd et al, 1991; Feldman et al, 1992; Fraker and Alexander, 1993). In some studies, this protein has demonstrated little to no antitumor activity when administered systemically as a single agent even at maximally tolerated doses. In other studies, regional administration was employed. Hepatic artery infusion produced objective responses in 14% of patients with liver metastases but did not increase the maximally tolerated dose above that utilized for intravenous infusion (Mavligit et al, 1992). Tumors regressed partially or completely after intralesional injections in nearly 45% of patients, but the usefulness of this route was limited by the short duration of responses and the lack of effects on noninjected lesions (Bartsch et al, 1989; Kahn et al, 1989). In addition, systemic toxicity limited the total dose and thus the number of lesions that could be treated at one time (Kahn et al, 1989).

The most promising approaches to future therapy with TNF-α may be in combination with other cytokines (eg, interleukin 2, interferon gamma) (Alexander and Rosenberg, 1991; Mulé and Rosenberg, 1991) or in isolated limb perfusion for melanoma or sarcoma when combined with interferon gamma and melphalan (Lienard et al, 1992; Fraker and Alexander, 1993). However, additional trials are needed to evaluate the efficacy of these therapeutic strategies more fully. The TNF-α gene also is being used in gene therapy trials.

ADVERSE REACTIONS. Reactions to TNF-α include rigor, fever, nausea and vomiting, headache, inflammation at the injection site, hypotension, peripheral vasoconstriction, hypertension, rhinorrhea, and chest discomfort (Economou, 1993). It also causes transient decreases in circulating lymphocyte and platelet counts and striking reductions in serum iron concentrations. In normal subjects given TNF-α systemically, subclinical evidence of disseminated intravascular coagulation is apparent (van Hinsbergh et al, 1990; van der Poll et al, 1990). Hemorrhagic gastritis was reported as the dose-limiting toxicity in a Phase I study in which TNF-α was infused intravenously for 15 minutes daily for five days (Krigel et al, 1991). However, in most other studies, severe hypotension was dose limiting. Acute pulmonary toxicity also may occur occasionally.

Tumor Necrosis Factor-α (Genentech, Cetus Oncology).

Nonspecific Immune Stimulants

BCG LIVE (Intravesical)
[TheraCys]

BCG VACCINE
[TICE BCG]

ACTIONS AND USES. Two BCG preparations currently are available for use in patients with superficial bladder tumors. BCG live (intravesical) [TheraCys] is a lyophilized suspension of an attenuated strain of *Mycobacterium bovis* (Bacillus of Calmette and Guerin). BCG vaccine [TICE BCG] is an attenuated live culture preparation of the TICE strain of the same organism and is also lyophilized. Both act as nonspecific immunostimulants when instilled intravesically in the treatment of primary and relapsed carcinoma-in-situ of the urinary bladder (with or without associated papillary tumors) (Hersh and Taylor, 1991; Herr, 1991 A; Bast and Morton, 1993). The resulting inflammatory and immune responses then act by unknown mechanisms to cause regression of superficial tumor lesions in the bladder mucosa (Groves, 1993).

Patients with recurrent papillary tumors of any grade, grade III papillary tumors (stage Ta grade III), carcinoma in situ (stage Tis), or tumors invading the lamina propria (stage T1) are appropriate candidates for intravesical BCG therapy (Fair et al, 1993; Macfarlane et al, 1993). Adjuvant therapy is unnecessary after transurethral resection (TUR) of single, isolated low-grade papillary tumors (stage Ta grades I or II) because recurrences occur infrequently and an effective resection precludes progression. However, patients with recurrent stage Ta tumors should receive adjuvant therapy even if the grade remains I or II. BCG appears to be equally effective in preventing recurrences after resection of stage Ta (recurrent or grade >II), stage Tis, or stage T1 tumors (Klimberg et al, 1991; Eure et al, 1992). The rate of recurrence after TUR has been reduced to less than 50% of that in control subjects. Some patients with endoscopically unresectable lesions also have had remissions after therapy with intravesical BCG.

Data suggest that intravesical BCG is more effective than cytotoxic chemotherapy (eg, intravesical thiotepa, doxorubicin, or mitomycin) as adjuvant therapy after TUR (Lamm et al, 1992 A; Fair et al, 1993; Macfarlane et al, 1993). Pooled data from six Phase II trials indicated that the median duration for remissions induced by BCG in patients with stage Tis lesions is at least four years (DeJager et al, 1991). There were no differences in response rates (75%) or the duration of remissions between those with Tis lesions who received intravesical BCG as primary therapy and those who were treated after not responding to intravesical therapy with cytotoxic drugs. Of 61 patients followed for ≥10 years after TUR and BCG, 31% remained free of tumor and progression and 28% had superficial recurrences but no progression of stage or grade (Herr et al, 1992). These data suggest that long-term survival after TUR plus BCG compares favorably with that after radical cystectomy. However, in other studies the tumor progressed in >80% of patients with recurrent stage T1 lesions three months after BCG therapy (Herr, 1991 B). Cystectomy rather than simple resection with or without additional BCG should be considered for these patients.

Although BCG vaccine [TICE BCG] is indicated for immunization against tuberculosis (see index entry BCG Vaccine, As Immunizing Agent), BCG live (intravesical) [TheraCys] is not intended for use to prevent tuberculosis. In addition, neither preparation is indicated as a vaccine for the prevention of any form of cancer. For use of BCG preparations as an immunostimulant in nonmalignant disorders, see index entry BCG Vaccine, As Immunostimulant.

ADVERSE REACTIONS AND PRECAUTIONS. When instilled intravesically, local reactions are the most frequent side effects of BCG (Lamm et al, 1992 B). These include dysuria, frequent urination, hematuria, cystitis, and urinary tract infection. Most occur two to four hours after the third instillation in a course of therapy and persist for one to three days. Incontinence, cramps and pain, and decreased bladder capacity develop much less frequently. Systemic reactions (fever, malaise, chills, anemia, nausea and vomiting, anorexia) occur in <5% of patients. Granulomatous prostatitis, pneumonitis, or hepatitis as a result of systemic infection with BCG each occur in <1% and BCG sepsis occurs in approximately 0.4% of patients. Arthritis and arthralgia have been reported in 0.5% and rash in 0.3%.

Patients being treated with immunosuppressive drugs or those with impaired immune function should not receive intravesical BCG because the risk of systemic infection is increased. Patients with fever of unknown cause or with infection of the urinary tract or at other sites also should not receive these preparations. Careful monitoring of urinary status and of symptoms associated with systemic BCG infection is necessary during BCG therapy. If systemic BCG infection occurs, the organism responds to therapy with the standard antimycobacterial drugs used for management of patients with tuberculosis.

DRUG INTERACTION. Investigational data suggest that the efficacy of intravesical BCG therapy may require attachment of the BCG organisms to fibronectin during fibrin clot formation at sites of urothelial disruption. Data from a retrospective analysis suggested that the response rate may be lower among patients receiving concomitant therapy with inhibitors of fibrin clot formation (48%) than among those not receiving these medications (67%) (Hudson et al, 1990). Furthermore, 35% of those treated with fibrin clot inhibitors during intravesical BCG therapy had recurrent superficial tumors; in contrast, only 8% of those not treated developed these tumors.

DOSAGE AND PREPARATIONS.

Intravesical: Treatment for carcinoma-in-situ of the urinary bladder should begin 7 to 14 days after biopsy or transurethral resection. For induction therapy with BCG live (intravesical) [TheraCys], suspensions from three vials are instilled once weekly for six weeks. Lyophilized BCG from each vial is reconstituted in 1 ml of the diluent supplied and then added to 50 ml of sterile, preservative-free saline (for a total of 53 ml). For induction therapy with BCG vaccine [TICE BCG], a single ampule suspended in 50 ml of sterile, preservative-free saline is instilled once weekly for six weeks. If the clinical circumstances warrant and if remission has not been induced, a second course of BCG vaccine may be given.

The bladder is either voided by the patient or is drained through a urethral catheter immediately before BCG is administered. The dose of suspended BCG is then instilled slowly by gravity. The catheter is removed, and the manufacturers' product information suggests that the patient be instructed to lie in the prone and supine positions and on each side for 15 minutes each (ie, total of 60 minutes). The suspension should be retained for an additional 60 minutes (or as close to that as possible) with the patient allowed to be upright or lying down. However, some urologists believe that the initial hour in the prone and supine positions is unnecessary and that patients may be ambulatory but should retain the bladder contents for as close as possible to two hours after instillation.

After completion of the induction course, maintenance therapy should be given at 3, 6, 12, 18, and 24 months if BCG live (intravesical) [TheraCys] is being used or monthly for at least 6 to 12 months if BCG vaccine [TICE BCG] is being used.

BCG LIVE (INTRAVESICAL):

TheraCys (Connaught/Merieux). Single-use vial containing 27 mg (dry weight) BCG and 5% (w/v) monosodium glutamate, with diluent (0.85% sodium chloride, 0.025% Tween 80, 0.06% sodium dihydrogen phosphate, and 0.25% disodium hydrogen phosphate). The reconstituted preparation from each vial contains $3.4 \pm 3 \times 10^8$ colony-forming units of BCG. Store refrigerated between 2° and 8° C and protected from direct light. The preparation should be used within two hours after reconstitution.

BCG VACCINE:

TICE BCG (Organon). Single-use 2 ml ampule containing 1 to 8 $\times 10^8$ colony-forming units of BCG (equivalent to approximately 50 mg, wet weight), as lyophilized powder, without preservative. Store refrigerated between 2° and 8° C and protected from direct light. The suspension should be administered within two hours after reconstitution.

Monoclonal Antibodies

Monoclonal antibodies have been produced against a variety of tumor-associated antigens (Bast et al, 1993; Goldenberg, 1993). These reagents are homogenous and each recognizes a single antigenic determinant. Their specificity makes them ideal tools for detecting the qualitative and quantitative differences in the antigenic composition of normal and malignant cells. Monoclonal antibodies are being studied as therapeutic agents and for tumor visualization in patients with cancer. They also are of interest for purging autologous bone marrow from residual tumor cells before reinfusion in bone marrow transplantation.

The first monoclonal antibody-derived product licensed for clinical use in cancer patients, indium^{111}-satumomab pendetide [OncoScint CR/OV Kit] (Cytogen), is used to visualize extrahepatic metastases in patients with colorectal or ovarian tumors. It consists of a murine monoclonal antibody (MAb B72.3) directed against a tumor-associated glycoprotein antigen (TAG-72) covalently conjugated to a chelating agent that binds the gamma-emitting indium^{111} radioisotope that is added immediately prior to use. Tumors are visualized by immunoscintigraphy after intravenous infusion of the radiolabeled antibody. The sensitivity and specificity of this technique for detecting extrahepatic metastases from colorectal (Doerr et al, 1991; Collier et al, 1992) and ovarian (Surwit et al, 1993) carcinomas compare favorably with the results of computed tomography. Hepatic metastases cannot be detected because the radioisotope accumulates nonspecifically in the liver. This radiolabeled antibody should not be used for the initial detection, screening, or diagnosis of colorectal or ovarian carcinomas.

No monoclonal antibodies are available at present for therapeutic uses other than in clinical trials in patients with malignancies. Initial clinical studies tested the safety and efficacy of unconjugated ("naked") murine monoclonal antibodies against various tumor-associated antigens. Results of such trials suggest that these antibodies can be administered safely and that tumor binding can be achieved (LoBuglio and Saleh, 1992; Distasio and Cheung, 1992; Goldenberg, 1993; Bast et al, 1993). Direct inhibition of growth, complement-dependent tumor cell lysis, and antibody-dependent, cell-mediated cytotoxicity are among the mechanisms that may contribute to the antitumor effects of unconjugated monoclonal antibodies. Complete responses may occur in hematologic malignancies, but they are observed only occasionally (most notably B-cell lymphomas treated with anti-idiotypic antibodies) after therapy with "naked" murine monoclonals. Factors that may limit the efficacy of monoclonal serotherapy include quantitatively inadequate levels, heterogeneity, and/or modulation of antigen expression by tumor cells; inadequate and/or uneven delivery of antibody to tumor cells; the presence of circulating shed antigen molecules; saturation or inadequate recruitment of appropriate host effector cell populations; and the human antibody response to mouse monoclonals.

The adverse reactions that have developed after administration of monoclonal antibodies include anaphylactic reactions, chills, diaphoresis, diarrhea, dyspnea, fever, flushing, headache, hypertension, hypotension, myelosuppression, nausea and vomiting, pain, rash, serum sickness, and urticaria.

Current investigational studies are directed at increasing the antitumor efficacy of monoclonal antibodies by covalent conjugation to cytotoxic moieties that are selectively delivered to tumor cells by the affinity of antibodies to antigen. Radioimmunotherapy is a strategy for selectively delivering cytocidal quantities of radionuclides to tumors (Kuzel and Duda, 1992; Abrams et al, 1993; Bast et al, 1993). It has the theoretical advantage of emitting ionizing radiation after a radiolabeled antibody binds to tumor cells expressing the targeted antigen; the radiation also can be lethal to neighboring tumor cells not expressing that antigen.

Conjugating antibodies to toxins (eg, ricin, arbrin, diphtheria toxin, *Pseudomonas* endotoxin) or ribosome-inactivating proteins (eg, bryodin, saporin, gelonin) is a second strategy employed to increase the antitumor efficacy of monoclonal antibodies (Cobb and LeMaistre, 1992; Byers and Baldwin, 1992; Vitetta et al, 1993; Pai and Pastan, 1993; Grossbard and Nadler, 1994). After selectively binding to the cell-surface target antigen, these conjugates are internalized and the toxin is released by cleavage of the covalent bond that joins it to the antibody. A theoretical advantage of this approach is the small number of toxin molecules required to enter a single tumor cell to kill that cell.

A third approach being investigated utilizes antibody-drug conjugates (Reisfeld et al, 1991; Biddle and Foon, 1993; Bast et al, 1993). This strategy relies on administration of molecules that consist of conventional chemotherapeutic agents (eg, vinca alkaloids, anthracyclines, antifolates) covalently bound to a spacer molecule (eg, dextran, albumin) that is also bound to the antibody. The drug molecules are released inside (or adjacent to) tumor cells that express the target antigen by cleavage of the labile bond that held them on the spacer.

Clinical trials to evaluate the safety and efficacy of conjugated monoclonals are in progress or have been completed. Although some improvements over the results with "naked" antibodies have been observed, no therapeutic monoclonal-based products have completed all three clinical trial phases and none is available yet for use outside of clinical trial protocols. Some factors that have limited the utility of unconjugated monoclonals are equally applicable to conjugated antibodies. For example, the human anti-mouse response also can neutralize radiolabeled antibodies, immunotoxins, or drug-antibody conjugates. Additional research seeks to develop human monoclonal antibodies as well as to modify mouse antibodies ("humanize" them). By limiting or eliminating the human anti-mouse response, the effectiveness of repeated administration will be facilitated and interaction of the monoclonal antibodies with host cellular immune responses may be enhanced.

SMALL-MOLECULE BIOMODULATORS

This diverse group of useful drugs and investigational agents has little in common other than the fact that cytocidal activity is not required in their mechanisms of action. Some (eg, levamisole) may act as immunomodulators in vivo, although at some concentrations they may be cytocidal in vitro. Others (eg, retinoids, N-methylformamide, hexamethylene-*bis*-acetamide) induce differentiation of tumor cells. These agents usually inhibit proliferation of cultured tumor cells without causing cell death. Suramin, an investigational trypanosomicide that is being studied for use in metastatic hormone-refractory prostate cancer, appears to act by blocking the binding of certain growth factors (GF) (eg, platelet-derived GF, epidermal GF, basic fibroblast GF, transforming GF-β) to their glycosaminoglycan cell surface receptors. Finally, the somatostatin analogue, octreotide, has no direct antitumor action; however, it is very useful in controlling life-threatening symptoms caused by hormone-secreting tumors of the gastrointestinal tract.

Various other approaches to the biological therapy of cancer are in the early stages of laboratory and/or clinical investigation. For example, drugs that can inhibit the development of new vasculature and thus prevent the growth of solid tumors (antiangiogenic agents) have been identified (Folkman, 1993). Oligonucleotides complementary to specific genes or messenger RNA molecules (antisense oligonucleotides) that block expression of their protein products as a consequence of their sequence-specific binding also are being studied as potential therapeutic agents (Crooke, 1993; Calabretta et al, 1993; Stein, 1993 A).

Immunomodulator

LEVAMISOLE HYDROCHLORIDE

[Ergamisol]

For chemical formula, see index entry Levamisole, As Immunostimulant.

ACTIONS. Levamisole is the levorotatory isomer of tetramisole. In addition to its established role as an anthelmintic drug, levamisole is a weak immunostimulant. Results of in vitro and in vivo studies suggest that this drug acts to improve depressed immune function rather than to enhance immune responses to greater than baseline levels (Van Wauwe and Janssen, 1991; Stevenson et al, 1991; Amery and Bruynseels, 1992). Cellular immune functions that are enhanced by levamisole include monocyte chemotaxis and phagocytosis, natural-killer cell activity, delayed-type hypersensitivity, and lymphocyte proliferative responses to antigens or mitogens. However, there is no clear relationship between these immunologic effects and clinical responses to the drug in patients with cancer.

The molecular mechanism(s) and target cell(s) through which levamisole improves depressed immune function also are poorly understood (see index entry Levamisole, As Immunostimulant). Evidence of monocyte activation, including increased production of neopterin and soluble IL-2 receptor molecules and enhanced expression of cell surface markers of monocyte activation, has been reported in cancer patients receiving levamisole (Janik et al, 1993). These responses occurred only after administration of at least three doses of ≥ 5 mg/kg every other day. However, it is unknown if these are direct responses to levamisole or one of its metabolites or are indirect effects mediated by cytokines whose production may be induced by levamisole.

The synergy observed when levamisole is combined with fluorouracil as adjuvant therapy for stage III colon adenocarcinoma also is not understood. No cytotoxicity occurred when cultured human colon tumor cells were treated with levamisole alone at concentrations achievable clinically (Grem and Allegra, 1989). Furthermore, levamisole enhanced cytotoxic responses to fluorouracil only at concentrations that far exceeded the clinically achievable serum concentration of the immunomodulator.

USES. Levamisole combined with fluorouracil is the currently recommended regimen for adjuvant chemotherapy of stage III (Duke's stage C) colon cancer (Laurie et al, 1989; National Institutes of Health, 1990; Hamilton et al, 1990; Moertel et al, 1990). This regimen has decreased the risk of recurrence at a median follow-up time of three years by 41% and the death rate by 33% compared with controls given no treatment after surgical excision of their tumors (Moertel et al, 1990). A subsequent analysis after a median of five years follow-up showed that recurrence rates were reduced by 39% and cancer-related deaths by 32% (Moertel et al, 1992). When used alone after surgery, levamisole had no effect on duration of survival but caused a small decline in the rate of tumor recurrence, and adjuvant therapy with fluorouracil alone has had only marginal effects on survival and recurrence. Data are insufficient to evaluate the effects of the combination regimen for adjuvant therapy of stage II (Duke's stage B) colon cancer. Patients with stage I tumors should not receive adjuvant therapy after surgery, since they are at very low risk for recurrence.

Conflicting data were reported from two randomized studies of levamisole alone for adjuvant therapy of malignant melanoma. In a Canadian trial with a median duration of 8.5 years follow-up, patients receiving levamisole 2.5 mg/kg on two consecutive days each week for three years had a longer duration of survival and fewer recurrences than patients who received no therapy (Quirt et al, 1991). The second trial was placebo-controlled, utilized a lower dose intensity of 150 mg (not adjusted for weight of the patient) for three consecutive days every two weeks for up to two years, and had a mean follow-up of 10.5 years (Spitler, 1991). No effect on the duration of survival or rate of tumor recurrence was observed. These data highlight the need for additional trials to determine the effect of dose on responses to adjuvant therapy with levamisole for malignant melanoma.

The efficacy of levamisole (alone or with other agents) as primary or adjuvant therapy also has been investigated in patients with other solid or hematologic malignancies (Stevenson et al, 1991; Schiller and Witt, 1992). These include breast, lung, bladder, ovarian, and head and neck carcinomas, acute myeloid and lymphocytic leukemias, lymphoma, and myeloma. Although responses have been observed in a few patients with some of these malignancies, at present the only established role for levamisole in cancer therapy is its use with fluorouracil as adjuvant therapy for stage III colon cancer.

ADVERSE REACTIONS AND PRECAUTIONS. The maximum tolerated dose of levamisole alone in patients with advanced malignancies or resected melanoma was 5 mg/kg administered every other day for 12 days (Janik et al, 1993). Adverse reactions included myalgia, arthralgia, fatigue, fever, chills, rash, nausea, vomiting, anorexia, and CNS effects (headache, lightheadedness, anxiety, depression, difficulty in concentrating, and insomnia). The frequency and severity of adverse reactions depended on the dose. A syndrome of fever, chills, diffuse erythema, moderate to severe headache, and severe nausea and vomiting that caused dehydration occurred in four of ten patients after four or five doses of 10 mg/kg and was the dose-limiting toxicity.

The most frequent toxic reactions to the combination of levamisole with fluorouracil are similar to those of fluorouracil alone and include nausea, vomiting, stomatitis, diarrhea, dermatitis, and leukopenia (Moertel et al, 1990). Adverse effects observed less often include thrombocytopenia, anemia, fatigue or fever, altered sense of taste or smell, arthralgia, dizziness, headache, and abnormal tearing. With the doses and schedules recommended for adjuvant therapy, the severity of toxic effects resulted in discontinuation of treatment in 14% of patients. Adverse responses in control patients given the same dose of levamisole alone were mild and infrequent and included nausea, dermatitis, and leukopenia. These patients also did not experience the mild and reversible laboratory test abnormalities consistent with hepatotoxicity that were observed in those given levamisole plus fluorouracil (Moertel et al, 1993). Levamisole has been associated with agranulocytosis (sometimes fatal), but most often at doses larger than those used with fluorouracil for adjuvant therapy of colon cancer.

A syndrome resembling encephalopathy associated with cerebral demyelination has been reported rarely in individuals treated with levamisole. This includes a few patients receiving this agent in combination with fluorouracil as adjuvant therapy for colon carcinoma (Hook et al, 1992; Kimmel and Schutt, 1993). Symptoms are quite varied and may include confusion, speech disturbances, muscle weakness, lethargy, and paresthesia. If any acute neurologic symptom occurs, immediate discontinuation of adjuvant therapy should be considered.

PHARMACOKINETICS. Levamisole is active after oral administration. Peak plasma concentrations are attained 1.5 to 2 hours after a single oral dose of 50 mg. The drug is extensively metabolized by the liver, and the metabolites are excreted in the urine. Hydroxylation and glucuronidation are among the pathways of levamisole biotransformation. Approximately 70% of an administered dose can be recovered in the urine after three days (<5% as unchanged drug). The plasma half-life of unchanged drug is three to four hours but is 16 hours for metabolites of levamisole.

DOSAGE AND PREPARATIONS.

Oral: For adjuvant therapy of stage III colon cancer, in combination with fluorouracil, 50 mg given every eight hours for three days, with the course repeated every two weeks. Treatment should begin 7 to 30 days after surgery and should continue for one year. Fluorouracil therapy (450 mg/M^2/day by rapid intravenous push for five days during the first week and weekly thereafter) should begin with the second course of levamisole if administration is begun before day 20 after surgery. If therapy begins later, fluorouracil should be given with the first course of levamisole. The manufacturer recommends that the dose of fluorouracil be reduced based on leukocyte counts and that administration of both drugs be deferred if the white cell counts remain <2,500/mm³ for more than 10 days or if platelet counts are <100,000/mm³. (See also the manufacturer's package insert.)

Ergamisol (Janssen). Tablets 59 mg (equivalent to 50 mg levamisole base).

Inducers of Differentiation

The traditional view that cancer results from unregulated cell proliferation recently has been supplemented by convincing evidence that arrested cell differentiation contributes significantly to the malignant phenotype (Fingert et al, 1993; Young and Warrell, 1993). This concept has led to the development of novel therapies for neoplastic diseases; the goal is to induce differentiation in malignant cells so that they cease unregulated proliferation and either carry out the normal differentiated functions of the tissues from which they originated or die (apoptosis or programmed cell death). The two classes of differentiating agents furthest along in clinical trials are the retinoids and the polar/planar compounds; other molecular classes include certain vitamins (eg, calcitriol), fatty acids (eg, butyrate), phorbol esters, and analogues of endogenous cyclic nucleotides or modulators of their metabolism. In addition, several conventional cytotoxic agents (eg, cytarabine, azacitidine, methotrexate, tiazofurin, anthracyclines) and interferons can, under some conditions, cause selected malignant cell lines to differentiate. The degree to which this effect contributes to the therapeutic efficacy of these agents is unknown at present.

RETINOIDS. This class of molecules includes naturally occurring metabolites and semisynthetic analogues of vitamin A (retinol). The principal dietary sources include certain vegetables and animal tissues, which contain carotenoids and retinyl esters, respectively (see index entry Vitamin A). All-*trans* retinoic acid is an endogenous metabolite generated after absorption of dietary retinoids, while 13-*cis* retinoic acid can be produced in vivo by light-catalyzed or enzymatic isomerization of the all-*trans* isomer.

Retinoids are essential for biochemical reactions that mediate vision and also function to regulate growth, embryologic morphogenesis, epithelial cell differentiation, and immune function (Smith et al, 1992 B; Young and Warrell, 1993). All-*trans* retinoic acid can substitute for vitamin A in all of its functions except that in vision; the 13-*cis* isomer also may be unable to function in regulating normal embryologic morphogenesis. Distinct cytoplasmic binding proteins specific for retinol and for retinoic acid are thought to mediate their entry into cells, intracellular metabolism, and translocation to the nucleus. Physiologic functions of retinoids other than vision may be mediated through their interactions with specific nuclear receptors that alter gene expression in target cells in response to ligand binding. These receptors are in the steroid/thyroid hormone receptor superfamily.

Many retinoids induce differentiation of malignant cells in vitro and in vivo (Smith et al, 1992 B; Young and Warrell, 1993). One possible clinical application of this effect is to reverse or prevent progression of early neoplastic changes. In addition, isotretinoin (a preparation of 13-*cis* retinoic acid) and tretinoin (a preparation of all-*trans* retinoic acid) are used in pharmacologic doses as therapy for certain malignancies.

ISOTRETINOIN (13-*cis*-retinoic acid)

[Accutane]

For chemical formula, see index entry Isotretinoin, In Acne.

ACTIONS. Small amounts of 13-*cis*-retinoic acid are produced in humans from endogenous all-*trans* retinoic acid by light- and/or enzyme-catalyzed isomerization (Smith et al, 1992 B; Young and Warrell, 1993). This retinoid interacts with the same cellular retinoic acid-binding proteins as the all-*trans* isomer; however, the affinity of nuclear receptors for 13-*cis* retinoic acid is fivefold less than that for all-*trans* retinoic acid. Agonist actions at the retinoic acid receptor are mediated by alteration(s) of gene expression resulting from activation of the receptor as a transcription factor.

In pharmacologic doses, isotretinoin induces the differentiation of responsive malignant cells by acting either directly as an agonist at the retinoic acid receptor or, more likely, via isomerization to all-*trans* retinoic acid (Smith et al, 1992 B; Young and Warrell, 1993). Tumor cells derived from squamous epithelium appear to be most sensitive to this effect of the drug. In addition, clinically achievable plasma concentrations of isotretinoin may inhibit the proliferation of tumor cells (without inducing differentiation), may induce paracrine responses that result in differentiation and/or arrest of growth of tumor cells, and may induce programmed cell death (apoptosis) (Smith et al, 1992 B). The contribution of each mechanism to the clinical responses to isotretinoin is not well defined. Additional data from preclinical studies suggest that isotretinoin may sensitize tumor cells to other differentiating agents, resulting in synergy (Smith et al, 1992 B; Young and Warrell, 1993).

USES. Isotretinoin is being investigated as therapy for various malignancies, for chemoprevention of cancer, and for reversal of early premalignant lesions (Smith et al, 1992 B; Young and Warrell, 1993). Topical therapy has induced partial or complete regression of most lesions in patients with basal cell carcinoma of the skin. Although there are no data from randomized controlled trials, patients in uncontrolled studies have received oral isotretinoin as monotherapy for advanced squamous or basal cell skin cancer or squamous cell carcinoma of the head and neck; modest activity has been demonstrated. However, the doses required for these responses usually were associated with significant acute and chronic toxicities. Limited activity of oral isotretinoin as a single agent also has been observed in patients with other solid tumors, acute myelogenous leukemia, or myelodysplastic syndromes.

Although a few instances in which patients with refractory acute promyelocytic leukemia (APL) entered remission after therapy with isotretinoin have been documented (for review, see Lippman et al, 1987), concentrations at least tenfold higher than those of tretinoin are needed to show activity against fresh human APL cells in vitro (Chomienne et al, 1990); in addition, a more recent study reported that isotretinoin lacked clinical activity in patients with APL (Runde et al, 1992).

Results from uncontrolled Phase II studies suggest that the combination of isotretinoin plus interferon alfa-2 may be beneficial in some squamous cell cancers. Seven complete and 12 partial responses were observed in 28 patients (68% overall response rate) who received oral isotretinoin and subcutaneous interferon alfa-2 for advanced squamous cell skin cancer (Lippman et al, 1992 A). The median duration of responses was >5 months. In a similar study, 16 of 32 previously untreated patients with locally advanced squamous cell carcinoma of the cervix who received the same combination regimen experienced regression of their tumors (4 complete and 12 partial responses) (Lippman et al, 1992 B, 1993 A). The median duration of responses was three months. However, these results require confirmation in more extensive Phase III trials, since no responses to isotretinoin plus interferon alfa-2 were observed in a group of women with advanced squamous cell carcinoma of the cervix who had received multiple cycles of previous cytotoxic chemotherapy (Alberts et al, 1993). Data from small pilot trials in patients with advanced, refractory, or recurrent tumors suggest that it is unlikely that this combination will have significant clinical activity against squamous cell cancers of the lung or head and neck (Rinaldi et al, 1993; Voravud et al, 1993; Arnold et al, 1994; Roth et al, 1994) or metastatic melanoma (Dhingra et al, 1993).

Positive results have been reported from clinical trials of isotretinoin for chemoprevention of cancer. A randomized, placebo-controlled trial demonstrated that isotretinoin (1 to 2 mg/kg/day administered orally for three months) reversed leukoplakia (a premalignant lesion) in the oral cavity (Hong et al, 1986). However, toxicity precluded continued administration of the drug and there was a high rate of relapse after therapy was withdrawn. In another randomized trial in patients with oral leukoplakia, isotretinoin 1.5 mg/kg/day was administered for three months as induction therapy, followed by maintenance therapy with low-dose isotretinoin (0.5 mg/kg/day) or beta carotene (30 mg/day) for an additional nine months (Lippman et al, 1993 B). Isotretinoin was more effective than beta carotene in preventing clinical progression of oral premalignant lesions. In addition, the rate of relapse was lower than in the earlier study that did not use maintenance therapy.

High-dose oral therapy with this retinoid (50 to 100 mg/M^2/day for 12 months) prevented second primary tumors after local therapy for squamous cell carcinoma of the head and neck (Hong et al, 1990). The therapy did not prevent recurrences of the original tumor, however, and toxicity resulted in discontinuation of therapy or noncompliance in 33% of the patients. Second primary tumors within the upper aerodigestive tract also occurred less frequently in the patients treated with isotretinoin (for one year) after a median follow-up time of 54.5 months (Benner et al, 1994). In contrast to these results, no benefit was observed in a randomized placebo-controlled trial of isotretinoin 10 mg daily for three years to prevent recurrence of basal cell carcinoma in patients previously treated for two or more lesions (Tangrea et al, 1992).

ADVERSE REACTIONS AND PRECAUTIONS. Isotretinoin is teratogenic and should not be given to women who are pregnant or who may become pregnant while undergoing treatment (Smith et al, 1992 B) (FDA Pregnancy Category X). Major human fetal abnormalities resulting from administration of isotretinoin have been documented. Female patients must use reliable contraceptive methods for one month before beginning therapy, during therapy, and for one month following discontinuation of therapy. (See the manufacturer's package insert for more detailed information on the fetal toxicity of isotretinoin.)

Most adverse reactions with isotretinoin occur less often than with tretinoin (Smith et al, 1992 B). Most notably, headache and other CNS reactions are observed in approximately 80% of patients after systemic therapy with tretinoin but in only 10% of those receiving isotretinoin.

Cheilitis is the most frequent adverse reaction with isotretinoin at the dosages used in most clinical trials. It occurs slightly more often than with tretinoin at comparable doses (Smith et al, 1992 B). Dry skin and mucous membranes also are common. Exfoliation and increased susceptibility to sunburn may occur. Data suggest that the use of oral alpha-tocopherol (vitamin E, 800 mg once daily) may ameliorate the mucocutaneous and other reactions caused by isotretinoin (Besa et al, 1990).

Conjunctivitis is less common than the cutaneous effects. Corneal opacities also have been reported. Decreased night vision, occasionally of sudden onset, has occurred rarely in patients being treated with isotretinoin but is reversible.

Inflammatory bowel disease has been reported in patients with no prior history of intestinal disorders. Nonspecific gastrointestinal and musculoskeletal disorders are common. Pseudotumor cerebri has developed. Skeletal hyperostosis has been reported, particularly in patients receiving high-dose, long-term therapy with isotretinoin.

Laboratory abnormalities include altered serum lipids with elevated plasma triglyceride levels and a mild to moderate decrease in high density lipoprotein levels. Cholesterol may be minimally elevated during treatment. These lipid abnormalities are reversible with cessation of therapy. Mild myelosuppression may develop but is uncommon. Transient increases in liver enzymes are noted.

Toxic effects were milder and less frequent with the lower doses of isotretinoin (0.5 mg/kg/day for nine months) used to maintain remissions of oral leukoplakia that had been induced with a dose of 1.5 mg/kg/day for three months (Lippman et al, 1993 B). An intermediate dose of isotretinoin (1 mg/kg/day) given with interferon alfa-2 to patients with squamous cell carcinoma of the skin or cervix produced a similar spectrum of reactions at a slightly lower frequency than with the higher dose of isotretinoin (Lippman et al, 1992 A, 1992 B, 1993 A). Dose reductions were required in 18 of 32 patients with skin cancer but in none of 32 patients with cervical cancer. Interestingly, use of very small doses (10 mg/day) for three years also was associated with a significant incidence of mild mucocutaneous and other minor adverse reactions in a chemoprevention trial in patients with previously treated basal cell carcinoma (Tangrea et al, 1992).

Patients sensitive to parabens should not receive isotretinoin, for they are used as preservatives in the formulation. See also index entry Isotretinoin, In Acne.

PHARMACOKINETICS. See index entry Isotretinoin, In Acne.

DOSAGE AND PREPARATIONS.

Oral: In studies on isotretinoin as treatment for hematologic or solid malignancies, 1 to 3 mg/kg/day has been given in a single or in two divided doses. In chemoprevention studies, 50 or 100 mg/M²/day (approximately 1 to 2 mg/kg/day) was administered. The dose was reduced to 0.5 mg/kg/day in one study to maintain remissions of oral leukoplakia induced by three months of therapy at the higher dose.

Accutane (Roche). Capsules 10, 20, and 40 mg.

TRETINOIN (all-*trans* retinoic acid) (Investigational Route)
[Vesanoid]

For chemical formula, see index entry Tretinoin, In Acne.

ACTIONS. Studies using cultured human and animal tumor cells, in vivo animal tumor models, and cells isolated from patients with malignancies who were included in clinical trials suggest several possible mechanisms that may contribute to the antitumor effects of tretinoin. These include direct induction of differentiation, inhibition of tumor cell growth (without differentiation), paracrine responses that result in either inhibition of growth or induction of differentiation, and induction of programmed cell death (apoptosis) (Parkinson et al, 1992; Smith et al, 1992 B). Paracrine responses to tretinoin may result from this drug's ability to increase expression of some members of the transforming growth factor-β family in some cell types. The relative contributions of these mechanisms to the overall clinical responses seen in patients treated with tretinoin are not clearly understood. Additional studies suggest that tretinoin may enhance cellular responses to other differentiating agents, resulting in synergism in some combinations (Smith et al, 1992 B; Parkinson et al, 1992).

USES. Results of clinical trials in patients with acute promyelocytic leukemia (APL) demonstrated that oral tretinoin induces complete remission in >80% of patients (Castaigne et al, 1990; Chen et al, 1991; Warrell et al, 1991; Frankel et al, 1994). APL is an uncommon form of acute myeloid leukemia ($\simeq$10% of AML cases) characterized by the t[15,17] chromosomal translocation, a unique promyelocytic morphology, evidence of disseminated intravascular coagulation at diagnosis, and more frequent complete remissions after chemotherapy than in those with other subtypes of acute myeloid leukemia (Parkinson et al, 1992; Smith et al, 1992 B; Warrell et al, 1993). The break point on chromosome 17 in the above translocation occurs in the gene for one of the retinoic acid receptors (RAR-α), which probably relates to the efficacy of tretinoin for this malignancy.

Clinical trials of tretinoin for APL enrolled previously untreated patients, a few who did not respond to conventional cytotoxic chemotherapy, and some in their first to third relapse after response(s). Most patients in each subgroup achieved complete remissions. Randomized trials to compare tretinoin as induction therapy for APL with combination chemotherapy employing cytotoxic drugs (daunorubicin plus cytarabine) are currently in progress. A randomized trial that compared tretinoin plus cytotoxic chemotherapy to chemotherapy alone demonstrated a significant improvement in event-free survival among newly diagnosed patients treated with tretinoin and chemotherapy (Fenaux et al, 1993).

The optimal dose and duration of tretinoin administration have not been defined. However, with doses of 25 mg/M²/day, rates of complete remission of APL were comparable to those obtained with the more commonly used dose of 45 mg/M²/day (Castaigne et al, 1993). Induction of remission often required one to two months of therapy. The persistence of the t[15,17] translocation in mature myelocytes from patients who responded suggests that tretinoin induced the differentiation of the malignant promyelocytes. However, the durations of responses were short, averaging approximately four months. Preliminary data suggest that tretinoin followed by cytotoxic chemotherapy may extend the duration of remissions in patients with APL (Fenaux et al, 1992, 1993; Warrell et al, 1993; Frankel et al, 1994). Randomized comparative trials are needed to identify optimally effective maintenance therapies.

Clinical trials of tretinoin in patients with other hematologic or solid malignancies or with myelodysplastic syndromes have been completed or are in progress. This drug is unlikely to be of significant usefulness as a single agent for treatment of myelodysplastic syndromes (Aul et al, 1993; Kurzrock et al, 1993; Ohno et al, 1993) or solid tumors (Smith et al, 1992 B; Young and Warrell, 1993). At present, it appears that tretinoin probably will be used in combination regimens with other differentiating agents in these patients.

ADVERSE REACTIONS. The most common reactions after systemic administration of tretinoin in dermatologic disorders were those associated with the hypervitaminosis A syndrome. They included cheilitis, headache, lethargy or fatigue, xerosis or inflammation, anorexia, dry mucous membranes, nausea and vomiting, visual disturbances, pruritus, and epistaxis (Smith et al, 1992 B; Young and Warrell, 1993; Warrell et al, 1993). The frequency of CNS reactions was dose related; only 4% of patients who received 30 mg/day, but 50% of those given 70 to 100 mg/day, experienced headaches. The mucocutaneous effects were made tolerable with the use of emollients.

In a Phase I trial of tretinoin in children, 60 mg/M²/day was the maximally tolerated dose and pseudotumor cerebri was the dose-limiting toxicity, with severe headaches and vomiting the major clinical manifestations (Smith et al, 1992 C). Other reactions in pediatric cancer patients were similar to those in adults. However, adults with solid tumors appear to tolerate doses up to 150 mg/M²/day; dermatologic effects (erythema with desquamation and paronychia) are dose limiting (Lee et al, 1993).

Metabolic effects of tretinoin include hypertriglyceridemia and hypercholesterolemia. Increased serum concentrations of bilirubin and liver enzymes (transaminases and alkaline phosphatase) are evidence of transient hepatotoxicity.

Induction therapy with tretinoin causes a life-threatening "retinoic acid syndrome" in ≃25% of patients with APL (Frankel et al, 1992; Parkinson et al, 1992; Warrell et al, 1993). Symptoms include fever, respiratory distress, weight gain, lower extremity edema, pleural/pericardial effusions, and episodic hypotension. This syndrome was lethal in three of nine patients in whom it occurred, and infiltration of the pulmonary interstitium with maturing myeloid cells was apparent on autopsy in two of these patients. Administration of large doses of corticosteroids appeared to relieve symptoms and prevent mortality if given early in the course of the syndrome. Thus far, the "retinoic acid syndrome" has not been reported in patients with malignancies other than APL.

Leukocytosis has occurred in up to 40% of patients receiving tretinoin for APL (Young and Warrell, 1993; Warrell et al, 1993). This response appears to be unrelated to the "retinoic acid syndrome" and may indicate tretinoin-induced maturation of malignant promyelocytes. No additional therapy is needed for leukocytosis if there are no other signs of leukostasis. Despite the leukocytosis, tretinoin-induced remission usually improves the disseminated intravascular coagulation seen in many patients with APL.

Very high levels of histamine (to approximately 100 times the normal concentration) and a marked increase in the basophil count was reported in one patient treated with tretinoin for APL (Koike et al, 1992). Shock and severe gastric and duodenal ulceration resulted from the excess histamine. Therapy was discontinued after the patient entered hematologic remission, and the ulcers gradually healed.

Systemically administered tretinoin is a potent teratogen in animals. It should not be administered to pregnant women (Smith et al, 1992 B; Young and Warrell, 1993). A pregnancy test should be performed before it is used for therapy in women of childbearing age. The topical preparation of tretinoin is classified in FDA Pregnancy Category B (see index entry Tretinoin, In Acne). The oral preparation has not been classified yet.

PHARMACOKINETICS. The bioavailability and absorption of tretinoin from the gastrointestinal tract appears to be highly variable and unpredictable. A twofold increase in dose elevated plasma levels from 1.2-fold to >10-fold in a study that used within-subject comparisons (Adamson et al, 1993). Peak plasma levels (347 ± 266 ng/ml) were achieved one to two hours after a single oral dose of 45 mg/M^2 (Muindi et al, 1992 A). In comparison, circulating plasma levels of endogenous retinoic acid in untreated subjects are approximately 1 to 2 ng/ml (Young and Warrell, 1993). Circulating tretinoin is bound extensively to plasma proteins, primarily albumin, after systemic administration of pharmacologic amounts. It appears to enter cells by simple passive diffusion.

The disappearance of tretinoin from plasma follows a monoexponential decay curve, with a clearance half-life of 0.8 ± 0.1 hours in adults (Muindi et al, 1992 A). A similar half-life of approximately 45 minutes was reported in children (Smith et al, 1992 C). Only one metabolite (4-oxo-tretinoin) was detected in plasma, and the glucuronide conjugate of this metabolite was found in urine (Muindi et al, 1992 A). After an initial dose, the metabolite accounted for <10% of the drug in plasma and, with its conjugate, for <1% of the total dose administered.

Peak plasma levels and the area under the concentration-time curve (AUC) are decreased significantly with continued oral administration of tretinoin (45 mg/M^2 daily in two divided doses) (Muindi et al, 1992 A, 1992 B). This is accompanied by a tenfold increase in the urinary excretion of the 4-oxo-tretinoin glucuronide conjugate. Increased metabolism of the drug may result from induction of a cytochrome P450-like enzyme system. This may contribute to the brief duration of remissions and the resistance of relapsed patients to further therapy with tretinoin. Data suggest that ketoconazole (200 mg to 1.2 g administered as a single oral dose one hour before ingestion of tretinoin) can significantly attenuate the decline in AUC that occurs after several weeks of daily treatment with tretinoin (Rigas et al, 1993). However, further clinical studies are needed to determine if this combination can result in clinical responses to tretinoin in patients with relapsed and/or resistant APL.

Promyelocytes isolated from some patients who relapsed after a response remained at least partially sensitive to in vitro induction of differentiation by tretinoin (Muindi et al, 1992 B). However, more recent data showed that higher concentrations of tretinoin were required to induce differentiation in APL cells isolated from patients who relapsed after treatment with tretinoin than had been effective with cells isolated from the same patients before treatment began (Delva et al, 1993). These investigators also demonstrated that the expression of a cytoplasmic retinoic acid binding protein (CRABP-II) was increased in the resistant cells. Binding of tretinoin to this protein in cells may facilitate presentation of the retinoid to catabolic enzymes (eg, cytochrome P450) (see Warrell, 1993, for review). Thus, increased metabolic degradation of and resistance to tretinoin may be mediated by induction of CRABP-II expression rather than by induction of one or more isozymes of P450 itself. This mechanism may be more important in contributing to resistance if systemic therapy induces CRABP-II expression not only in tumor cells but in many tissues and thus increases the drug's metabolic elimination and reduces the achievable blood concentrations as therapy continues.

DOSAGE (Investigational regimen).

Oral: For acute promyelocytic leukemia, 45 mg/M^2/day in two divided doses for up to three months or until complete remission is achieved.

Vesanoid (Roche Dermatologics).

POLAR/PLANAR COMPOUNDS. The observation that dimethylsulfoxide, a polar organic solvent, could induce differentiation in cultured murine erythroleukemic cells stimulated studies of other chemically similar molecules as potential therapies for neoplastic diseases (Marks and Rifkind, 1991; Young and Warrell, 1993). Some polar/planar differentiating agents (eg, hexamethylene-*bis*-acetamide) include two polar regions in their molecular structure linked by a lipophilic spacer. This amphipathic structure is thought to allow noncovalent interaction of the polar/planar compounds with constituents of the cell membrane, possibly resulting in biochemical activation (or inactivation) of signal-transducing components of cell surface receptors. Other differentiating agents (eg, N-methylformamide) are thought to alter cell membrane structure and influence its function because of their properties as polar organic solvents. Although other polar/planar molecules have been studied in cell culture systems, hexamethylene-*bis*-acetamide and N-methylformamide have progressed furthest in clinical trials.

HEXAMETHYLENE-*BIS*-ACETAMIDE (HMBA) (Investigational drug)
[Hexabid]

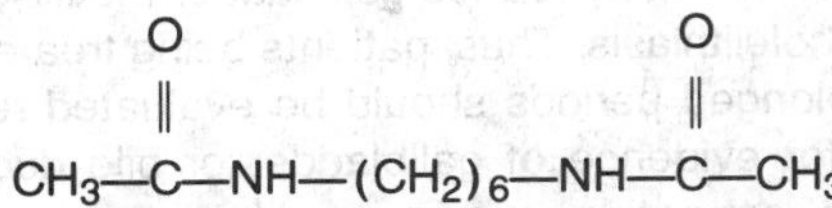

ACTIONS AND USES. Hexamethylene-*bis*-acetamide is a polar/planar molecule that induces differentiation in cultured tumor cells (Marks and Rifkind, 1991; Young and Warrell, 1993). In vitro studies have shown that prolonged exposure to this agent is required to commit cells to differentiation. It is thought that alterations in membrane fluidity and structure due to physicochemical interactions of drug molecules with membrane lipids may activate membrane-associated enzymes that are involved in signal transduction pathways; these enzymes then may influence gene expression and cellular differentiation.

In Phase I and II trials, hexamethylene-*bis*-acetamide has been infused continuously for five or ten days (Young and Warrell, 1993). No responses to therapy were observed in patients treated for five days. One patient with non-small cell lung cancer receiving ten-day infusions every 28 days achieved a partial remission that was sustained through >17 courses of therapy administered over >28 months (Young et al, 1988). Transient regressions of cutaneous metastases were observed in four other patients with solid tumors. Of 28 patients with myelodysplastic syndrome or acute myelogenous leukemia who received ten-day infusions for two or more cycles in a Phase II trial, three achieved complete remissions and six achieved partial remissions (Andreeff et al, 1992). The median duration of complete response was 6.8 months, whereas it was only 3.7 months for partial responses. None of 13 patients who received only one cycle responded to therapy.

ADVERSE REACTIONS. In Phase I trials, this drug produced metabolic acidosis, neurotoxicity, thrombocytopenia, renal dysfunction, nausea, vomiting, mucositis, and elevation of hepatic transaminases in the serum. The dose-limiting toxicities caused by ten-day infusions of hexamethylene-*bis*-acetamide were thrombocytopenia with hemorrhage and CNS dysfunction (disorientation and confusion) (Young et al, 1988). Although the maximally tolerated dose was 28 g/M^2/day, 24 g/M^2/day was recommended for use in Phase II trials because of the frequency of severe toxicity at the higher dose. The reactions observed in a Phase I trial in which this drug was administered by nasogastric tube every four hours for five days were identical to those in patients receiving the drug intravenously (Ward et al, 1991). The maximally tolerated dose by the nasogastric route was 30 g/M^2/day.

PHARMACOKINETICS. Hexamethylene-*bis*-acetamide is metabolized by deacetylation followed by oxidative deamination. Its bioavailability after oral administration by nasogastric tube is nearly 100% (Ward et al, 1991). Clearance of the drug follows a monoexponential decay curve with a half-life of two to four hours. Both the parent compound (20% to 45%) and metabolites (18% to 34%) are excreted in the urine. The steady-state plasma level is approximately 0.9 mM in patients given ten-day infusions at the dose recommended in Phase II studies (Young et al, 1988; Andreeff et al, 1992). Pharmacokinetic parameters following nasogastric administration were identical to those after infusion (Ward et al, 1991).

Hexabid (Roberts).

N-METHYLFORMAMIDE (N-MF) (Investigational drug)

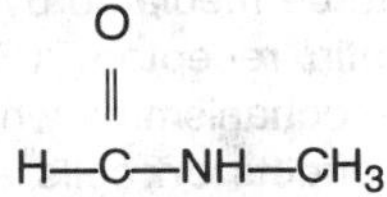

ACTIONS AND USES. N-methylformamide is a polar/planar compound that induces differentiation of specific cells in vitro (Marks and Rifkind, 1991; Young and Warrell, 1993). Both murine virus-infected erythroleukemia cells and human promyelocytic leukemia cells (HL-60) differentiate in the presence of N-methylformamide. It is thought that polar compounds act by changing membrane structure so as to activate receptor-regulated enzymes, which then alter expression of the genes that regulate cellular differentiation.

Preclinical studies suggest that N-methylformamide has some activity in certain rodent and human tumors. Phase II clinical trials in patients with advanced solid tumors, including colon, renal, head and neck, cervical, and ovarian carcinomas, have been completed. Little to no efficacy was observed in these trials (McGuire et al, 1990 A, 1990 B).

ADVERSE REACTIONS AND PRECAUTIONS. Anorexia, nausea, and vomiting are common side effects. Reversible hepatotoxicity has been observed. A syndrome consisting of pain, lethargy, anorexia, and declining performance status occurs in 30% to 40% of patients (McGuire et al, 1990 A, 1990 B). Oral administration of slightly lower doses was tolerated better than the intravenous doses used in the first Phase II trials.

DOSAGE (investigational regimens).

Intravenous: 800 mg/M^2/day for five days every four weeks. Glass syringes or glass containers should be used.

Oral: 600 mg/M^2 has been given three times weekly for four weeks every six weeks.

Miscellaneous Biomodulators

OCTREOTIDE ACETATE
[Sandostatin]

For chemical formula, see index entry Octreotide, In Diarrhea.

ACTIONS. Octreotide, a synthetic octapeptide analogue of the hormone, somatostatin, shares with somatostatin the tetrapeptide sequence required for agonist activity (phe-trp-lys-thr). However, because of the inclusion of two D-amino acids and a modified threonine in octreotide, this drug is much more resistant to degradation by serum peptidases and thus has a longer half-life than somatostatin (Evers et al, 1991; Schally et al, 1993).

The pharmacologic actions of octreotide are similar to those of the natural hormone, namely, it inhibits secretion of serotonin, growth hormone, and a wide variety of gastroenteropancreatic peptides. The latter group includes gastrin, vasoactive intestinal peptide (VIP), insulin, glucagon, secretin, motilin, and pancreatic polypeptide. In animals, octreotide is more potent than the natural hormone in inhibiting secretion of growth hormone, glucagon, and insulin. In humans, it is more potent and more selective than somatostatin in suppressing growth hormone secretion; effects on insulin release are less pronounced. The effects of octreotide on susceptible target tissues appear to be mediated by its agonist activity at cell-surface somatostatin receptors (Schally et al, 1993). Further details of the mechanism by which somatostatin and octreotide exert their effects on cells are obscure, but it is known that somatostatin is internalized after binding to its receptor. Subsequent effects may result from inhibition of adenylate cyclase and decreased accumulation of cAMP or by reduced influx of calcium ions.

USES. Octreotide is indicated for control of symptoms in patients with metastatic carcinoid tumors or VIP-secreting adenomas (VIPomas). Carcinoid tumors, which secrete several peptide hormones and serotonin, are most often found in the small intestine and can metastasize to the liver. Carcinoid syndrome, which occurs only after liver metastasis, is accompanied by flushing, diarrhea, wheezing, and bronchoconstriction. In one study, octreotide reversed the diarrhea or flushing in 22 of 25 patients with metastatic carcinoid tumors (Kvols et al, 1986). Convenient biochemical markers for successful therapy in these patients included decreases in the urinary excretion of 5-hydroxyindole acetic acid and in plasma levels of serotonin.

A frequent symptom of VIPomas, which are rare neuroendocrine tumors of non-beta pancreatic islet cells, is a profuse watery diarrhea. Fluid and electrolyte support of these patients can be reduced and electrolyte imbalances such as hypokalemia can be reversed after octreotide administration. A decrease in plasma VIP levels indicates that the patient is responding to therapy. Octreotide also has been used for management of symptoms produced by hormone-secreting pituitary adenomas, gastrinomas, glucagonomas, and insulinomas. It appears to reduce secretion of thyroid stimulating hormone (TSH) by pituitary adenomas that produce TSH (Chanson et al, 1993 A). Partial shrinkage of the tumors occurred in about one-third of patients.

Octreotide therapy has been accompanied by partial tumor regression in a small percentage of patients with carcinoid tumors. However, data are insufficient to determine if these remissions result directly from the drug. Although data from an uncontrolled study suggest that octreotide may improve the survival rate in patients with neuroendocrine tumors (Saltz et al, 1993), little to no antitumor efficacy was observed in a Phase II trial of this drug in patients with pancreatic, colon, or gastric adenocarcinoma (Klijn et al, 1990). In contrast, other analogues of somatostatin appear to have greater potential than octreotide as direct antitumor agents (Evers et al, 1991; Schally et al, 1993).

ADVERSE REACTIONS AND PRECAUTIONS. Octreotide has not caused any major adverse effects that necessitate discontinuation of therapy. The side effects reported include nausea, diarrhea, loose stools, pain at the site of injection, abdominal pain or discomfort, and vomiting. Each of these occurred in less than 10% of nearly 500 patients.

Because of its hormonal effects, octreotide may cause fat malabsorption and may reduce gallbladder motility, ultimately producing cholelithiasis. Thus, patients being treated with this drug for prolonged periods should be evaluated regularly by ultrasound for evidence of gallbladder or bile duct obstructions. Since octreotide suppresses hormone secretion in many tissues, it can alter the homeostatic balance in circulating levels of insulin, glucagon, and growth hormone, resulting in either hyperglycemia or hypoglycemia. Glucose intolerance also may develop. Reductions in the dose of insulin for insulin-dependent diabetics may be needed. In addition, a progressive decline in thyroid hormone levels resulting in hypothyroidism has been reported in one patient.

Octreotide has not been reported to be mutagenic in animals, but results of long-term carcinogenicity studies have not been reported. Doses as high as 1 mg/kg/day did not reduce fertility in rats. Octreotide is not embryotoxic and is classified in FDA Pregnancy Category B.

PHARMACOKINETICS. Octreotide is absorbed rapidly and completely from the site of subcutaneous injection. After a single dose of 100 mcg, peak plasma levels (5.5 ng/ml) were achieved about 25 minutes after injection. There was a proportional relationship between dose and peak plasma levels after subcutaneous or intravenous injections of up to 400 mcg and after three injections of 200 mcg each at eight-hour intervals. Octreotide is rapidly distributed from the plasma compartment, with a half-life of approximately 12 minutes. About 65% in plasma is bound, mostly to lipoproteins but some to albumin. It is cleared from the plasma with an apparent half-life of 1.5 hours (Chanson et al, 1993 B). In contrast, endogenous somatostatin has a half-life of one to three minutes. The volume of distribution of octreotide ranges from 18 to 30 L. About 32% of a dose is excreted unchanged in the urine. In dialysis patients, clearance is reduced to about one-half that in patients with normal renal function, and doses should be adjusted accordingly. It is not known if hepatic dysfunction affects octreotide clearance.

DOSAGE AND PREPARATIONS.

Subcutaneous: For metastatic carcinoid tumors, 100 to 600 mcg is given daily in two to four divided doses (mean daily dose, 300 mcg) for the first two weeks of therapy. Dose adjustments should be made as needed to control symptoms. In some carcinoid patients, as much as 1.5 mg/day was necessary, but this is rare. For VIPomas, daily doses of 200 to 300 mcg in two to four equal injections are recommended for the first two weeks. Again, dose adjustments should be made as necessary to control symptoms, but amounts exceeding 450 mcg/day usually are not needed.

Sandostatin (Sandoz). Solution (sterile, for injection) 0.05, 0.1, or 0.5 mg (as the acetate salt) in 1 ml single-use containers and 0.2 and 1 mg/ml in 5 ml multidose containers. The containers may be kept at room temperature for up to 14 days if they are protected from light, but should be stored at 2° to 8° C if kept for longer periods.

SURAMIN SODIUM (Investigational Drug)
[Fourneau 309]

For chemical formula, see index entry Suramin, In African Trypanosomiasis.

ACTIONS. Suramin is a symmetrical polysulfonated naphthyl urea that has been used for the treatment of African trypanosomiasis and onchocerciasis (see index entry Suramin). Data from in vitro studies showed that suramin inhibits reverse transcriptase and suggested that it may protect uninfected T-cells from HIV-1 infection and cytopathic effects (Voogd et al, 1993; Scher and Kelly, 1993; Stein, 1993 B). These and similar observations led to its evaluation in the treatment of HIV-associated neoplastic diseases.

Additional studies in cell culture systems demonstrated that suramin binds avidly to various heparin-binding growth factors (GF) and thus inhibits their binding and the activation of specific cell-surface receptors (Voogd et al, 1993; Scher and Kelly, 1993; Stein, 1993 B). Among these are platelet-derived GF, basic fibroblast GF, transforming GF-β, and insulin-like GF-I. These actions of suramin, which are thought to derive from the multiple negative charges of the drug's sulfate moieties that are ionized at physiologic pH, inhibit the proliferation of cultured human tumor cells from a variety of tumor types. Other effects of suramin on tumor cells and some normal tissues include induction of differentiation and inhibition of mitochondrial function, biosynthesis of adrenal steroids, protein kinase C activity, glycolysis, synthesis and accumulation of glycosaminoglycans, ATP-dependent ion transport across membranes, and cell motility. The latter action may influence the metastatic potential of responsive tumor cells. The contribution made by each of these cellular and biochemical effects to suramin's clinical efficacy as an antineoplastic agent is unknown. It is probable that more than one mechanism is responsible for suramin's antitumor effects and that the relative contributions of its actions vary with tissue type (Stein, 1993 B).

USES. Noncomparative, uncontrolled clinical trials have suggested that suramin is an effective palliative therapy for hormone-refractory metastatic prostate cancer (Myers et al, 1992; Eisenberger et al, 1993). Quantifiable reductions in tumor mass were observed in 12 of 29 patients (41.4%) with measurable disease who were included in these two trials. In addition, the circulating levels of prostate-specific antigen (PSA) decreased by ≥75% in 30 of 69 patients (43.5%), including those with metastatic tumor limited to bone. Data from one of these studies demonstrated that the one-year survival rate was nearly 85% in patients who responded to suramin therapy with a decline in PSA levels of this magnitude but was only 20% in less responsive patients (Myers et al, 1992). Furthermore, more than 50% of the responding patients remain alive at 3.5 years of follow-up (Stein, 1993 B). These results are particularly encouraging in view of the generally poor prognosis (average survival time, 30 weeks) and poor response rate to standard chemotherapy (7%) in patients with metastatic hormone-refractory prostate cancer. Nevertheless, randomized trials are needed for a definitive evaluation of the effect of suramin on survival and comparison with the effects of standard therapies in patients with this malignancy.

Isolated responses to suramin also were reported from early Phase II trials in patients with adrenocortical carcinoma or follicular lymphoma (Stein, 1993 B). In contrast, no responses were observed in trials of suramin in renal cell carcinoma (La Rocca et al, 1991; Motzer et al, 1992) or cisplatin-resistant ovarian cancer (Stein, 1993 B).

ADVERSE REACTIONS. Potentially life-threatening coagulopathies (increased thrombin and partial thromboplastin times), a severe demyelinating sensorimotor polyneuropathy (a Guillain-Barré-like syndrome), vortex keratopathy, and adrenal insufficiency occurred in early trials of suramin in cancer patients (Voogd et al, 1993; Scher and Kelly, 1993; Stein, 1993 B). Retrospective analysis suggested an association between these reactions and plasma suramin concentrations ≥350 mcg/ml. In subsequent Phase II trials in patients with metastatic prostate cancer, plasma drug concentrations were carefully monitored and maintained below 300 mcg/ml. As a result, the number of patients who experienced severe neurotoxicity or severe coagulopathy was reduced to slightly more than 10%, and reactions were mild in 80% of patients (Myers et al, 1992; Eisenberger et al, 1993). The use of hydrocortisone as replacement therapy for all patients included in these trials prevented the problems associated with adrenal insufficiency, and clinically significant vortex keratopathy did not occur.

Other adverse reactions encountered in these trials included anemia, lymphocytopenia, thrombocytopenia, renal (decreased creatinine clearance) and hepatic (increased bilirubin concentrations and transaminase levels) dysfunction, hyperglycemia, rash, fatigue, fever, nausea, and infection. Severe lymphocytopenia and anemia each occurred in almost 40% of patients, while severe renal toxicity was reported in 16% (Myers et al, 1992). The remaining severe reactions occurred in ≤11% of patients.

Hypophosphatemia was observed in all 15 patients included in a Phase I trial of suramin (Rago et al, 1994). The mean serum phosphate concentration declined from 4 to 3 mg/dL over 42 days of therapy. Reversible mitochondrial myopathy was detected by electron microscopy of a biopsy specimen from one patient.

For discussion of adverse reactions in patients treated with suramin for nonmalignant diseases, see index entries Suramin, As Anthelmintic and In African Trypanosomiasis.

PHARMACOKINETICS. Suramin is bound extensively to plasma proteins, and ≤0.3% is present in the circulation as free drug. Clearance is predominantly via the kidney but at a very slow rate (approximately 0.4 ml/min). After a course of intravenous therapy in which 200 mg was given by bolus on day 1, followed by injection of 1 g on days 3, 7, 14, 21, 28, and 35, the elimination phase half-life was estimated to be 44 to 54 days (Collins et al, 1986). However, subsequent measurements based on the plasma decay curves after completion of a continuous infusion regimen resulted in a shorter elimination phase half-life of 28.2 ± 5 hours as well as a distribution half-life of 22.3 ± 2.7 hours (Scher et al, 1992). Analysis of the data from this study using a two-compartment model also yielded volumes of 4.5 ± 6.7 L/M² and 10.6 ± 1.4 L/M², respectively for the central and peripheral compartments.

Although there is very little interpatient variation in the rate of clearance for single doses, there is considerable variability between patients in the plasma level attained during the first one to three weeks of continuous infusions (Stein, 1993 B). This appears to result from variance in the rate of drug movement from the central to the peripheral (tissue and organ) compartments, coupled with a constant but slow rate of clearance from only the central compartment.

DOSAGE (Investigational Regimens). Various strategies have been used in clinical trials to maximize the safety and efficacy of suramin as therapy for metastatic prostate cancer. These are required because of the complex and variable pharmacokinetic behavior of this drug, the need to maintain plasma levels <350 mcg/ml to prevent severe neurotoxicity and other adverse reactions, and the apparent lack of clinical response to therapy with plasma levels <200 mcg/ml. In spite of these efforts, the optimal dosage regimen has not been determined.

The initial clinical trial in patients with metastatic prostate cancer used a now-obsolete schedule for continuous intravenous infusion of 350 mg/M²/day for the first week (Myers et al, 1992). Plasma drug levels were measured, and therapy was discontinued when they reached 280 to 300 mcg/ml. For those whose plasma concentrations remained below the target level, the dose rate was adjusted each week based on a nomogram and the result of weekly monitoring. Subsequent studies developed individualized dosing protocols based on monitoring of plasma drug concentrations, estimation of patient-specific pharmacokinetic parameters using a Bayesian algorithm, and a strategy of adaptive control with feedback (Cooper et al, 1992; Scher et al, 1992; Jodrell et al, 1994).

Five regimens for rapid loading doses and two regimens for weekly maintenance doses have been compared (van Rijswijk et al, 1992). The data obtained in this study suggested that continuous infusion of 600 mg/M²/day for three to four days may be the safest and most rapid of the loading doses evaluated to achieve plasma concentrations >200 mcg/ml. In addition, weekly six-hour infusion of individualized doses using Bayesian modeling of patient-specific pharmacokinetics appeared to be optimal for maintenance therapy. However, this study used a target plasma concentration of only 150 mcg/ml during the maintenance phase.

Cited References

Cytokines as modulators of cytotoxic drugs in experimental and clinical hematology and oncology. *Semin Oncol* 19(suppl 4):1-102, 1992.

Abrams PG, et al: Imaging and therapy of cancer with specifically targeted radionuclides, in Mitchell MS (ed): *Biological Approaches to Cancer Treatment: Biomodulation.* New York, McGraw-Hill, 1993, 277-301.

Adamson PC, et al: Variability in the oral bioavailability of all-*trans*-retinoic acid. *J Natl Cancer Inst* 85:993-996, 1993.

Alberts DS, et al: Phase II trial of 13-*cis*-retinoic acid (13-cRA) plus interferon-a2A (IFN) for advanced, heavily treated squamous cell carcinoma of the cervix (SCCC), abstract 852. *Proc ASCO* 12:266, (March) 1993.

Alexander RB, Rosenberg SA: Tumor necrosis factor: Clinical applications, in DeVita VT Jr, et al (eds): *Biologic Therapy of Cancer.* Philadelphia, JB Lippincott, 1991, 378-392.

Amery WKP, Bruynseels JPJM: Levamisole, the story and the lessons. *Int J Immunopharmacol* 14:481-486, 1992.

Andreeff M, et al: Hexamethylene bisacetamide in myelodysplastic syndrome and acute myelogenous leukemia: A Phase II clinical trial with a differentiation-inducing agent. *Blood* 80:2604-2609, 1992.

Antonelli G, et al: Neutralizing antibodies to interferon-alpha: Relative frequency in patients treated with different interferon preparations. *J Infect Dis* 163:882-885, 1991.

Arnold A, et al: Phase II trial of 13-*cis*-retinoic acid plus interferon α in non–small-cell lung cancer. *J Natl Cancer Inst* 86:306-309, 1994.

Atkins MB, et al: Randomized Phase II trial of high-dose interleukin-2 either alone or in combination with interferon alfa-2b in advanced renal cell carcinoma. *J Clin Oncol* 11:661-670, 1993.

Atzpodien J, et al: Alpha-interferon and interleukin-2 in renal cell carcinoma: Studies in nonhospitalized patients. *Semin Oncol* 18 (suppl 7):108-112, 1991.

Aul CA, et al: All-*trans* retinoic acid in patients with myelodysplastic syndromes: Results of a pilot study. *Blood* 82:2967-2974, 1993.

Baer MR, et al: Interferon-α therapy during pregnancy in chronic myelogenous leukaemia and hairy cell leukaemia. *Br J Haematol* 81:167-169, 1992.

Balch CM, et al: Cutaneous melanoma, in DeVita VT Jr, et al (eds): *Cancer: Principles & Practice of Oncology,* ed 4. Philadelphia, JB Lippincott, 1993, 1612-1661.

Baron S, et al: The interferons: Mechanisms of action and clinical applications. *JAMA* 266:1375-1383, 1991.

Bartsch HH, et al: Intralesional application of recombinant human tumor necrosis factor alpha induces local tumor regression in patients with advanced malignancies. *Eur J Cancer Clin Oncol* 25:287-291, 1989.

Bast RC Jr, Morton DL: Immunostimulants, in Holland JF, et al (eds): *Cancer Medicine*, ed 3. Philadelphia, Lea & Febiger, 1993, vol 1, 905-913.

Bast RC Jr, et al: Monoclonal serotherapy, in Holland JF, et al (eds): *Cancer Medicine*, ed 3. Philadelphia, Lea & Febiger, 1993, vol 1, 968-982.

Benner SE, et al: Prevention of second primary tumors with isotretinoin in patients with squamous cell carcinoma of the head and neck: Long-term follow-up. *J Natl Cancer Inst* 86:140-141, 1994.

Berek JS, et al: Ovarian cancer, in Holland JF, et al (eds): *Cancer Medicine*, ed 3. Philadelphia, Lea & Febiger, 1993, vol 2, 1659-1690.

Besa EC, et al: Treatment with 13-*cis*-retinoic acid in transfusion-dependent patients with myelodysplastic syndrome and decreased toxicity with addition of alpha-tocopherol. *Am J Med* 89:739-747, 1990.

Biddle WC, Foon KA: Monoclonal antibodies in therapy, alone or conjugated with drugs, in Mitchell MS (ed): *Biological Approaches to Cancer Treatment: Biomodulation.* New York, McGraw-Hill, 1993, 209-251.

Bocci V: Interleukins: Clinical pharmacokinetics and practical implications. *Clin Pharmacokinet* 21:274-284, 1991.

Bookman MA, Bast RC Jr: The immunobiology and immunotherapy of ovarian cancer. *Semin Oncol* 18:270-291, 1991.

Borden EC: Interferons, in Holland JF, et al (eds): *Cancer Medicine*, ed 3. Philadelphia, Lea & Febiger, 1993, vol 1, 927-936.

Borden EC, et al: Antitumor effects of interferons: Mechanisms and therapeutic activity, in Mitchell MS (ed): *Biological Approaches to Cancer Treatment: Biomodulation.* New York, McGraw-Hill, 1993, 440-476.

Bornstein J, et al: Treatment of cervical intraepithelial neoplasia and invasive squamous cell carcinoma by interferon. *Obstet Gynecol Surv* 48:251-260, 1993.

Bradley EC, Grimm E: Interleukins, in Holland JF, et al (eds): *Cancer Medicine*, ed 3. Philadelphia, Lea & Febiger, 1993, vol 1, 941-948.

Budd GT, et al: A Southwest Oncology Group Phase II trial of recombinant tumor necrosis factor in metastatic breast cancer. *Cancer* 68:1694-1695, 1991.

Bukowski RM, et al: Phase II trial of high-dose intermittent interleukin-2 in metastatic renal cell carcinoma: A Southwest Oncology Group study. *J Natl Cancer Inst* 82:143-146, 1990.

Bunn PA Jr, Hoppe RT: Cutaneous lymphomas, in DeVita VT Jr, et al (eds): *Cancer: Principles & Practice of Oncology*, ed 4. Philadelphia, JB Lippincott, 1993, 1928-1937.

Byers VS, Baldwin RW: Targeted kill: From umbrellas to monoclonal antibodies. *J Clin Immunol* 12:391-405, 1992.

Calabretta B, et al: Prospects for gene-directed therapy with antisense oligodeoxynucleotides. *Cancer Treatment Rev* 19:169-179, 1993.

Camba L, Durie BGM: Multiple myeloma: New treatment options. *Drugs* 44:170-181, 1992.

Castaigne S, et al: All-trans retinoic acid as a differentiation therapy for acute promyelocytic leukemia: I. Clinical results. *Blood* 76:1704-1709, 1990.

Castaigne S, et al: Effectiveness and pharmacokinetics of low-dose all-*trans* retinoic acid (25 mg/m^2) in acute promyelocytic leukemia. *Blood* 82:3560-3563, 1993.

Chanson P, et al: Octreotide therapy for thyroid-stimulating hormone–secreting pituitary adenomas: A follow-up of 52 patients. *Ann Intern Med* 119:236-240, 1993 A.

Chanson P, et al: Clinical pharmacokinetics of octreotide: Therapeutic applications in patients with pituitary tumours. *Clin Pharmacokinet* 25:375-391, 1993 B.

Chen Z-X, et al: A clinical and experimental study on all-*trans* retinoic acid-treated acute promyelocytic leukemia patients. *Blood* 78:1413-1419, 1991.

Chien C-H, Hsieh K-H: Interleukin-2 immunotherapy in children. *Pediatrics* 86:937-943, 1990.

Chomienne C, et al: All-trans retinoic acid in acute promyelocytic leukemias: II. In vitro studies: Structure-function relationship. *Blood* 76:1710-1717, 1990.

Cobb PW, LeMaistre CF: Therapeutic use of immunotoxins. *Semin Hematol* 29 (suppl 2):6-13, 1992.

Collier BD, et al: Immunoscintigraphy performed with In-111-labeled CYT-103 in the management of colorectal cancer: Comparison with CT. *Radiology* 185:179-186, 1992.

Collins JM, et al: Clinical pharmacokinetics of suramin in patients with HTLV-III/LAV infection. *J Clin Pharmacol* 26:22-26, 1986.

Cooper MR, et al: Adaptive control with feedback strategies for suramin dosing. *Clin Pharmacol Ther* 52:11-23, 1992.

Cooper MR, et al: A randomized clinical trial comparing melphalan/prednisone with or without interferon alfa-2b in newly diagnosed patients with multiple myeloma: A cancer and leukemia group B study. *J Clin Oncol* 11:155-160, 1993.

Crooke ST: Progress toward oligonucleotide therapeutics: Pharmacodynamic properties. *FASEB J* 7:533-539, 1993.

Crown J, et al: A Phase I trial of recombinant human interleukin-1β alone and in combination with myelosuppressive doses of 5-fluorouracil in patients with gastrointestinal cancer. *Blood* 78:1420-1427, 1991.

Deisseroth AB, et al: Chronic leukemias, in DeVita VT Jr, et al (eds): *Cancer: Principles & Practice of Oncology*, ed 4. Philadelphia, JB Lippincott, 1993, 1965-1983.

DeJager R, et al: Long-term complete remission in bladder carcinoma in situ with intravesical tice bacillus Calmette Guerin: Overview analysis of six Phase II clinical trials. *Urology* 38:507-513, 1991.

Delva L, et al: Resistance to all-*trans* retinoic acid (ATRA) therapy in relapsing acute promyelocytic leukemia: Study of in vitro ATRA sensitivity and cellular retinoic acid binding protein levels in leukemic cells. *Blood* 82:2175-2181, 1993.

Demchak PA, et al: Interleukin-2 and high-dose cisplatin in patients with metastatic melanoma: A pilot study. *J Clin Oncol* 9:1821-1830, 1991.

DeVita VT Jr, et al: Interferons: Clinical applications, in DeVita VT Jr, et al (eds): *Biologic Therapy of Cancer*. Philadelphia, JB Lippincott, 1991, 275-353.

Dhingra K, et al: Phase II study of alpha-interferon and 13-cis-retinoic acid in metastatic melanoma. *Invest New Drugs* 11:39-43, (Feb) 1993.

Dillman RO, et al: Continuous interleukin-2 and tumor-infiltrating lymphocytes as treatment of advanced melanoma: A national biotherapy study group trial. *Cancer* 68:1-8, 1991.

Dillman RO, et al: Inpatient continuous-infusion interleukin-2 in 788 patients with cancer. *Cancer* 71:2358-2370, 1993.

Dinarello CA, Wolff SM: The role of interleukin-1 in disease. *N Engl J Med* 328:106-113, 1993.

Distasio JA, Cheung N-KV: Current therapies using monoclonal antibodies: II. Malignant disease. *Compr Ther* 18:40-44, (April) 1992.

Doerr RJ, et al: Radiolabeled antibody imaging in the management of colorectal cancer: Results of a multicenter clinical study. *Ann Surg* 214:118-124, 1991.

Dorr RT: Interferon-α in malignant and viral diseases: A review. *Drugs* 45:177-211, 1993.

Dunbar CE, Nienhuis AW: Multiple myeloma: New approaches to therapy. *JAMA* 269:2412-2416, 1993.

Economou JS: Tumor necrosis factor, in Holland JF, et al (eds): *Cancer Medicine,* ed 3. Philadelphia, Lea & Febiger, 1993, vol 1, 937-940.

Eisenberger MA, et al: Suramin, an active drug for prostate cancer: Interim observations in a Phase I trial. *J Natl Cancer Inst* 85:611-621, 1993.

Eure GR, et al: Bacillus Calmette-Guerin therapy for high risk stage T1 superficial bladder cancer. *J Urol* 147:376-379, 1992.

Evers BM, et al: Somatostatin and analogues in the treatment of cancer: A review. *Ann Surg* 213:190-198, 1991.

Ezekowitz RAB, et al: Interferon alfa-2a therapy for life-threatening hemangiomas of infancy. *N Engl J Med* 326:1456-1463, 1992.

Fair WR, et al: Cancer of the bladder, in DeVita VT Jr, et al (eds): *Cancer: Principles & Practice of Oncology,* ed 4. Philadelphia, JB Lippincott, 1993, 1052-1072.

Falkson CI, et al: Improved results with the addition of interferon alfa-2b to dacarbazine in the treatment of patients with metastatic malignant melanoma. *J Clin Oncol* 9:1403-1408, 1991.

Feldman ER, et al: Phase II trial of recombinant tumor necrosis factor in disseminated malignant melanoma. *Am J Clin Oncol* 15:256-259, 1992.

Fenaux P, et al: All-transretinoic acid followed by intensive chemotherapy gives a high complete remission rate and may prolong remissions in newly diagnosed acute promyelocytic leukemia: A pilot study on 26 cases. *Blood* 80:2176-2181, 1992.

Fenaux P, et al: Effect of all transretinoic acid in newly diagnosed promyelocytic leukemia: Results of a multicenter randomized trial. *Blood* 82:3241-3249, 1993.

Figlin RA, et al: The role of interferon and interleukin-2 in the immunotherapeutic approach to renal cell carcinoma. *Semin Oncol* 18:102-107, 1991.

Figlin RA, et al: Concomitant administration of recombinant human interleukin-2 and recombinant interferon alfa-2A: An active outpatient regimen in metastatic renal cell carcinoma. *J Clin Oncol* 10:414-421, 1992.

Fingert HJ, et al: Cell proliferation and differentiation, in Holland JF, et al (eds): *Cancer Medicine*, ed 3. Philadelphia, Lea & Febiger, 1993, vol 1, 1-14.

Flaherty LE, et al: A Phase I-II study of dacarbazine in combination with outpatient interleukin-2 in metastatic malignant melanoma. *Cancer* 65:2471-2477, 1990.

Flaherty LE, et al: A Phase II study of dacarbazine and cisplatin in combination with outpatient administered interleukin-2 in metastatic malignant melanoma. *Cancer* 71:3520-3525, 1993.

Folkman J: Tumor angiogenesis, in Holland JF, et al (eds): *Cancer Medicine*, ed 3. Philadelphia, Lea & Febiger, 1993, vol 1, 153-170.

Fraker DL, Alexander HR: The use of tumor necrosis factor in isolated limb perfusions for melanoma and sarcoma, in: *Principles & Practice of Oncology Updates*. Philadelphia, JB Lippincott, (May) 1993, vol 7, 1-10.

Frankel SR, et al: The 'retinoic acid syndrome' in acute promyelocytic leukemia. *Ann Intern Med* 117:292-296, 1992.

Frankel SR, et al: All-*trans* retinoic acid for acute promyelocytic leukemia: Results of the New York study. *Ann Intern Med* 120:278-286, 1994.

Funk J, et al: Psoriasis induced by interferon-α. *Br J Dermatol* 125:463-465, 1991.

Garbe C, et al: Combined treatment of metastatic melanoma with interferons and cytotoxic drugs. *Semin Oncol* 19 (suppl 4):63-69, 1992.

Gaynor ER, Fisher RI: Clinical trials of α-interferon in the treatment of non-Hodgkin's lymphoma. *Semin Oncol* 18 (suppl 7):12-17, 1991.

Glashan RW: A randomized controlled study of intravesical α-2b-interferon in carcinoma in situ of the bladder. *J Urol* 144:658-661, 1990.

Goldenberg DM: Monoclonal antibodies in cancer detection and therapy. *Am J Med* 94:297-312, 1993.

Golomb HM, Vardiman J: Hairy cell leukemia, in Holland JF, et al (eds): *Cancer Medicine*, ed 3. Philadelphia, Lea & Febiger, 1993, vol 2, 1989-1997.

Grander D, et al: Interferon-induced enhancement of 2′,5′-oligoadenylate synthetase in mid-gut carcinoid tumours. *Lancet* 336:337-340, 1990.

Grem JL, Allegra CJ: Toxicity of levamisole and 5-fluorouracil in human colon carcinoma cells. *J Natl Cancer Inst* 81:1413-1417, 1989.

Grossbard ML, Nadler LM: Immunotoxin therapy of lymphoid neoplasms. *Semin Hematol* 31:88-97, 1994.

Groves MJ: Pharmaceutical characterization of *Mycobacterium bovis* bacillus Calmette-Guérin (BCG) vaccine used for the treatment of superficial bladder cancer. *J Pharm Sci* 82:555-562, 1993.

Gutterman JU: Cytokine therapeutics: Lessons from interferon α. *Proc Natl Acad Sci USA* 91:1198-1205, 1994.

Hamilton JM, et al: 5-Fluorouracil plus levamisole: Effective adjuvant treatment for colon cancer, in DeVita VT Jr, et al (eds): *Important Advances In Oncology 1990*. Philadelphia, JB Lippincott, 1990, 115-130.

Herr HW: Instillation therapy for bladder cancer, in DeVita VT Jr, et al (eds): *Biologic Therapy of Cancer*. Philadelphia, JB Lippincott, 1991 A, 643-650.

Herr HW: Progression of stage T1 bladder tumors after intravesical bacillus Calmette-Guerin. *J Urol* 145:40-44, 1991 B.

Herr HW, et al: Bacillus Calmette-Guerin therapy for superficial bladder cancer: A 10-year followup. *J Urol* 147:1020-1023, 1992.

Hersh EM, Taylor CW: Immunotherapy by active immunization: Use of nonspecific stimulants and immunomodulators, in DeVita VT Jr, et al (eds): *Biologic Therapy of Cancer*. Philadelphia, JB Lippincott, 1991, 613-626.

Holland JF, et al: Principles of biotherapeutics, in Holland JF, et al (eds): *Cancer Medicine*, ed 3. Philadelphia, Lea & Febiger, 1993, vol 1, 905-982.

Hong WK, et al: 13-*cis*-retinoic acid in the treatment of oral leukoplakia. *N Engl J Med* 315:1501-1505, 1986.

Hong WK, et al: Prevention of second primary tumors with isotretinoin in squamous-cell carcinoma of the head and neck. *N Engl J Med* 323:795-801, 1990.

Hook CC, et al: Multifocal inflammatory leukoencephalopathy with 5-fluorouracil and levamisole. *Ann Neurol* 31:262-267, 1992.

Hudson MA, et al: Adverse impact of fibrin clot inhibitors on intravesical bacillus Calmette-Guerin therapy for superficial bladder tumors. *J Urol* 144:1362-1364, 1990.

The IFNB Multiple Sclerosis Study Group: Interferon beta-1b is effective in relapsing-remitting multiple sclerosis: I. Clinical results of a multicenter, randomized, double-blind, placebo-controlled trial. *Neurology* 43:655-661, 1993.

Israel BC, et al: Effects of interferon-α monotherapy on hepatic drug metabolism in cancer patients. *Br J Clin Pharmacol* 36:229-235, 1993.

The Italian Cooperative Study Group on Chronic Myeloid Leukemia: Interferon alfa-2a as compared with conventional chemotherapy for the treatment of chronic myeloid leukemia. *N Engl J Med* 330:820-825, 1994.

Itri LM: The interferons. *Cancer* 70 (suppl):940-945, 1992.

Jaiyesimi IA, et al: Advances in therapy for hairy call leukemia: A review. *Cancer* 72:5-16, 1993.

Janik J, et al: Dose-related immunologic effects of levamisole in patients with cancer. *J Clin Oncol* 11:125-135, 1993.

Jodrell DI, et al: Suramin: Development of a population pharmacokinetic model and its use with intermittent short infusions to control plasma drug concentration in patients with prostate cancer. *J Clin Oncol* 12:166-175, 1994.

Kahn JO, et al: Intralesional recombinant tumor necrosis factor-α for AIDS-associated Kaposi's sarcoma: A randomized, double-blind trial. *J Acquired Immune Deficiency Syndromes* 2:217-223, 1989.

Kantarjian HM, et al: Chronic myelogenous leukemia: A concise update. *Blood* 82:691-703, 1993.

Kaplan LD, Volberding PA: Neoplasms in acquired immunodeficiency syndrome, in Holland JF, et al (eds): *Cancer Medicine*, ed 3. Philadelphia, Lea & Febiger, 1993, vol 2, 2105-2120.

Karp JE, et al: Cancer in AIDs, in DeVita VT Jr, et al (eds): *Cancer: Principles & Practice of Oncology*, ed 4. Philadelphia, JB Lippincott, 1993, 2093-2110.

Keilholz U, et al: Interferon-α and interleukin-2 in the treatment of metastatic melanoma: Comparison of two Phase II trials. *Cancer* 72:607-614, 1993.

Khayat D, et al: Sequential chemoimmunotherapy with cisplatin, interleukin-2, and interferon alfa-2a for metastatic melanoma. *J Clin Oncol* 11:2173-2180, 1993.

Kimmel DW, Schutt AJ: Multifocal leukoencephalopathy: Occurrence during 5-fluorouracil and levamisole therapy and resolution after discontinuation of chemotherapy. *Mayo Clin Proc* 68:363-365, 1993.

Kirkwood JM: Studies of interferons in the therapy of melanoma. *Semin Oncol* 18 (suppl 7):83-90, 1991.

Kirkwood J, et al: A randomized controlled trial of high-dose IFN alfa-2b for high-risk melanoma, abstract 1331. *Proc ASCO* 12:390, (March) 1993.

Klijn JGM, et al: Treatment of patients with metastatic pancreatic and gastrointestinal tumours with the somatostatin analogue Sandostatin: A Phase II study including endocrine effects. *Br J Cancer* 62:627-630, 1990.

Klimberg IW, et al: Intravesical bacillus Calmette-Guerin for patients with high-risk superficial bladder cancer. *Urology* 37:180-184, (Feb) 1991.

Koike T, et al: Brief report: Severe symptoms of hyperhistaminemia after the treatment of acute promyelocytic leukemia with tretinoin (all-*trans*-retinoic acid). *N Engl J Med* 327:385-387, 1992.

Konrad MW, et al: Pharmacokinetics of recombinant interleukin 2 in humans. *Cancer Res* 50:2009-2017, 1990.

Krigel RL, et al: Hemorrhagic gastritis as a new dose-limiting toxicity of recombinant tumor necrosis factor. *J Natl Cancer Inst* 83:129-131, 1991.

Kruit WHJ, et al: Interleukin-2-induced thyroid dysfunction is correlated with treatment duration but not with tumor response. *J Clin Oncol* 11:921-924, 1993.

Kurzrock R, et al: Interferons—α, β, γ: Basic principles and preclinical studies, in DeVita VT Jr, et al (eds): *Biologic Therapy of Cancer*. Philadelphia, JB Lippincott, 1991 A, 247-274.

Kurzrock R, et al: Other tumors, in DeVita VT Jr, et al (eds): *Biologic Therapy of Cancer*. Philadelphia, JB Lippincott, 1991 B, 334-346.

Kurzrock R, et al: All-*trans* retinoic acid: Tolerance and biologic effects in myelodysplastic syndrome. *J Clin Oncol* 11:1489-1495, 1993.

Kuzel TM, Duda RB: The current status of radiolabeled monoclonal antibodies for the diagnosis and treatment of human malignancies. *Compr Ther* 18:16-20, (June) 1992.

Kvols LK, et al: Treatment of the malignant carcinoid syndrome: Evaluation of a long-acting somatostatin analogue. *N Engl J Med* 315:663-666, 1986.

Lamm DL, et al: Current perspectives on diagnosis and treatment of superficial bladder cancer. *Urology* 39:301-308, (April) 1992 A.

Lamm DL, et al: Incidence and treatment of complications of bacillus Calmette-Guerin intravesical therapy in superficial bladder cancer. *J Urol* 147:596-600, 1992 B.

La Rocca RV, et al: A pilot study of suramin in the treatment of metastatic renal call carcinoma. *Cancer* 67:1509-1513, 1991.

Laurie JA, et al: Surgical adjuvant therapy of large-bowel carcinoma: An evaluation of levamisole and the combination of levamisole and fluorouracil. *J Clin Oncol* 7:1447-1456, 1989.

Lee JS, et al: Phase I evaluation of all-*trans*-retinoic acid in adults with solid tumors. *J Clin Oncol* 11:959-966, 1993.

Lienard D, et al: High-dose recombinant tumor necrosis factor alpha in combination with interferon gamma and melphalan in isolation perfusion of the limbs for melanoma and sarcoma. *J Clin Oncol* 10:52-60, 1992.

Linehan WM, et al: Cancer of the kidney and ureter, in DeVita VT Jr, et al (eds): *Cancer: Principals & Practice of Oncology,* ed 4. Philadelphia, JB Lippincott, 1993, 1023-1057.

Lippman SM, et al: Retinoids as preventive and therapeutic anticancer agents, parts I and II. *Cancer Treat Rep* 71:391-405, 493-515, 1987.

Lippman SM, et al: 13-*cis*-retinoic acid and interferon α-2a: Effective combination therapy for advanced squamous cell carcinoma of the skin. *J Natl Cancer Inst* 84:235-241, 1992 A.

Lippman SM, et al: 13-*cis*-retinoic acid plus interferon α-2a: Highly active systemic therapy for squamous cell carcinoma of the cervix. *J Natl Cancer Inst* 84:241-245, 1992 B.

Lippman SM, et al: 13-*cis*-retinoic acid plus interferon-α2a in locally advanced squamous cell carcinoma of the cervix. *J Natl Cancer Inst* 85:499-500, 1993 A.

Lippman SM, et al: Comparison of low-dose isotretinoin with beta carotene to prevent oral carcinogenesis. *N Engl J Med* 328:15-20, 1993 B.

Lissoni P, et al: Biological and clinical results of a neuroimmunotherapy with interleukin-2 and the pineal hormone melatonin as a first line treatment in advanced non-small cell lung cancer. *Br J Cancer* 66:155-158, 1992.

Lissoni P, et al: Immunotherapy with subcutaneous low-dose interleukin-2 and the pineal indole melatonin as a new effective therapy in advanced cancers of the digestive tract. *Br J Cancer* 67:1404-1407, 1993.

LoBuglio AF, Saleh MN: Advances in monoclonal antibody therapy of cancer. *Am J Med Sci* 304:214-224, 1992.

Lokhorst HM, Dekker AW: Tumor review: Advances in the treatment of multiple myeloma. *Cancer Treat Rev* 19:113-128, 1993.

Longo DL, et al: Lymphocytic lymphomas, in DeVita VT Jr, et al (eds): *Cancer: Principles & Practice of Oncology*, ed 4. Philadelphia, JB Lippincott, 1993, 1859-1927.

Lotze MT: Interleukin-2: Basic principles, in DeVita VT Jr, et al (eds): *Biologic Therapy of Cancer.* Philadelphia, JB Lippincott, 1991, 123-141.

Lotze MT, Rosenberg SA: Interleukin-2: Clinical applications, in DeVita VT Jr, et al (eds): *Biologic Therapy of Cancer*. Philadelphia, JB Lippincott, 1991, 159-177.

MacDonald D, et al: Interleukin-2 treatment associated eosinophilia is mediated by interleukin-5 production. *Br J Haematol* 76:168-173, 1990.

Macfarlane MT, et al: Neoplasms of the bladder, in Holland JF, et al (eds): *Cancer Medicine*, ed 3. Philadelphia, Lea & Febiger, 1993, vol 2, 1546-1559.

Margolin KA, et al: Interleukin-2 and lymphokine-activated killer cell therapy of solid tumors: Analysis of toxicity and management guidelines. *J Clin Oncol* 7:486-498, 1989.

Marks PA, Rifkind RA: Differentiating factors, in DeVita VT Jr, et al (eds): *Biologic Therapy of Cancer.* Philadelphia, JB Lippincott, 1991, 754-762.

Mavligit GM, et al: Regional biologic therapy: Hepatic arterial infusion of recombinant human tumor necrosis factor in patients with liver metastases. *Cancer* 69:557-561, 1992.

McGuire WP III, et al: Phase II study of N-methylformamide (N-MF) (NCS 3051) in patients with advanced epithelial ovarian cancer: A Gynecologic Oncology Group study. *Invest New Drugs* 8:191-194, 1990 A.

McGuire WP III, et al: Phase II study of N-methylformamide (N-MF) (NSC 3051) in patients with advanced squamous cancer of the cervix: A Gynecologic Oncology Group study. *Invest New Drugs* 8:195-197, 1990 B.

Mertens WC, et al: Effect of indomethacin plus ranitidine in advanced melanoma patients on high-dose interleukin-2. *Lancet* 340:397-398, 1992.

Meyskens FL Jr, et al: Recombinant human interferon γ: Adverse effects in high-risk stage I and II cutaneous malignant melanoma, correspondence. *J Natl Cancer Inst* 82:1071, 1990.

Miller RG, Tannock IF: Immunology and immunotherapy of cancer, in Tannock IF, Hill RP (eds): *The Basic Science of Oncology*, ed 2. New York, McGraw-Hill, 1992, 232-255.

Minasian LM, et al: Interferon alfa-2a in advanced renal cell carcinoma: Treatment results and survival in 159 patients with long-term follow-up. *J Clin Oncol* 11:1368-1375, 1993.

Mitchell MS: Chemotherapy in combination with biomodulation: A 5-year experience with cyclophosphamide and interleukin-2. *Semin Oncol* 19 (suppl 4):80-87, 1992.

Mitchell MS (ed): *Biological Approaches to Cancer Treatment: Biomodulation*. New York, McGraw-Hill, 1993.

Mitchell MS, et al: Effectiveness and tolerability of low-dose cyclophosphamide and low-dose intravenous interleukin-2 disseminated melanoma. *J Clin Oncol* 6:409-424, 1988.

Mitsuyasu RT: Interferon alpha in the treatment of AIDS-related Kaposi's sarcoma. *Br J Haematol* 79 (suppl 1):69-73, 1991.

Moertel CG, et al: Levamisole and fluorouracil for adjuvant therapy of resected colon carcinoma. *N Engl J Med* 322:352-358, 1990.

Moertel C, et al: The intergroup study of fluorouracil (5-FU) plus levamisole (LEV) and levamisole alone as adjuvant therapy for stage C colon cancer: A final report, abstract 457. *Proc ASCO* 11:161, (March) 1992.

Moertel CG, et al: Hepatic toxicity associated with fluorouracil plus levamisole adjuvant therapy. *J Clin Oncol* 11:2386-2390, 1993.

Morton DL, et al: Malignant melanoma, in Holland JF, et al (eds): *Cancer Medicine*, ed 3. Philadelphia, Lea & Febiger, 1993, vol 2, 1793-1824.

Motzer RJ, et al: Phase II trial of suramin in patients with advanced renal cell carcinoma: Treatment results, pharmacokinetics, and tumor growth factor expression. *Cancer Res* 52:5775-5779, 1992.

Muindi JRF, et al: Clinical pharmacology of oral all-*trans* retinoic acid in patients with acute promyelocytic leukemia. *Cancer Res* 52:2138-2142, 1992 A.

Muindi J, et al: Continuous treatment with all-*trans* retinoic acid causes a progressive reduction in plasma drug concentrations: Implications for relapse and retinoid 'resistance' in patients with acute promyelocytic leukemia. *Blood* 70:299-303, 1992 B.

Mulé JJ, Rosenberg SA: Combination cytokine therapy: Experimental and clinical trials, in DeVita VT Jr, et al (eds): *Biologic Therapy of Cancer*. Philadelphia, JB Lippincott, 1991, 393-416.

Myers C, et al: Suramin: A novel growth factor antagonist with activity in hormone-refractory metastatic prostate cancer. *J Clin Oncol* 10:881-889, 1992.

National Institutes of Health: *NIH Consensus Development Conference: Adjuvant Therapy for Patients With Colon and Rectal Cancer.* April, 1990.

Negrier S, et al: Interleukin-2 with or without LAK cells in metastatic renal cell carcinoma: A report of a European multicentre study. *Eur J Cancer Clin Oncol* 25 (suppl 3):S21-S28, 1989.

Neta R, Oppenheim JJ: IL-1: Can we exploit Jekyll and subjugate Hyde? in DeVita VT Jr, et al (eds): *Biologic Therapy of Cancer Updates*. Philadelphia, JB Lippincott, (Oct) 1992, vol 2, 1-11.

Norton JA, et al: Cancer of the endocrine system, in DeVita VT Jr, et al (eds): *Cancer: Principles & Practice of Oncology*, ed 4. Philadelphia, JB Lippincott, 1993, 1333-1435.

Ohno R, et al: Treatment of myelodysplastic syndromes with all-trans retinoic acid: Leukemia Study Group of the Ministry of Health and Welfare. *Blood* 81:1152-1154, 1993.

Oken MM: New agents for the treatment of multiple myeloma and non-Hodgkin lymphoma. *Cancer* 70:946-948, 1992.

O'Reilly SM, et al: Flavone acetic acid (FAA) with recombinant interleukin-2 (rIL-2) in advanced malignant melanoma: I. Clinical and vascular studies. *Br J Cancer* 67:1342-1345, 1993.

Ozer H, et al: Prolonged subcutaneous administration of recombinant α2b interferon in patients with previously untreated Philadelphia chromosome-positive chronic-phase chronic myelogenous leukemia: Effect on remission duration and survival: Cancer and Leukemia Group B Study 8583. *Blood* 82:2975-2984, 1993.

Pai LH, Pastan I: Immunotoxin therapy for cancer. *JAMA* 269:78-81, 1993.

Palmer PA, et al: Continuous infusion of recombinant interleukin-2 with or without autologous lymphokine activated killer cells for the treatment of advanced renal cell carcinoma. *Eur J Cancer* 28A:1038-1044, 1992.

Parkinson DR, et al: Trans-retinoic acid and related differentiation agents. *Semin Oncol* 19:734-741, 1992.

Pellegrini S, Schindler C: Early events in signalling by interferons. *Trends Biochem Sci* 18:338-342, 1993.

Pisani CVH, et al: Administration of interleukin-2 (IL-2) results in increased plasma concentrations of IL-5 and eosinophilia in patients with cancer. *Blood* 78:1538-1544, 1991.

Preston DS, Stern RS: Nonmelanoma cancers of the skin. *N Engl J Med* 327:1649-1662, 1992.

Pockaj BA, et al: Infectious complications associated with interleukin-2 administration: A retrospective review of 935 treatment courses. *J Clin Oncol* 11:136-147, 1993.

Quirt IC, et al: Improved survival in patients with poor-prognosis malignant melanoma treated with adjuvant levamisole: A Phase III study by the National Cancer Institute of Canada Clinical Trials Group. *J Clin Oncol* 9:729-735, 1991.

Rago RP, et al: Suramin-induced weakness from hypophosphatemia and mitochondrial myopathy: Association of suramin with mitochondrial toxicity in humans. *Cancer* 73:1954-1959, 1994.

Redman BG, et al: A Phase I trial of recombinant interleukin-2 combined with recombinant interferon-gamma in patients with cancer. *J Clin Oncol* 8:1269-1276, 1990.

Reisfeld RA, et al: Antibody-drug conjugates for cancer therapy: Promises and problems. *Immunol Allergy Clin North Am* 11:341-358, (May) 1991.

Ribeiro RC, et al: Continuous infusion of interleukin-2 in children with refractory malignancies. *Cancer* 72:623-628, 1993.

Richards JM, et al: Sequential chemoimmunotherapy in the treatment of metastatic melanoma. *J Clin Oncol* 10:1338-1343, 1992.

Richie JP: Renal cell carcinoma, in Holland JF, et al (eds): *Cancer Medicine*, ed 3. Philadelphia, Lea & Febiger, 1993, vol 2, 1529-1538.

Rigas JR, et al: Constitutive variability in the pharmacokinetics of the natural retinoid, all-*trans*-retinoic acid, and its modulation by ketoconazole. *J Natl Cancer Inst* 85:1921-1926, 1993.

Rinaldi DA, et al: Phase II study of 13-cis-retinoic acid and interferon-alpha 2a in patients with advanced squamous cell lung cancer. *Anticancer Drugs* 4:33-36, (Feb) 1993.

Rönnblom LE, et al: Autoimmunity after alpha-interferon therapy for malignant carcinoid tumors. *Ann Intern Med* 115:178-183, 1991.

Rosenberg SA: Adoptive cellular therapy: Clinical applications, in DeVita VT Jr, et al (eds): *Biologic Therapy of Cancer*. Philadelphia, JB Lippincott, 1991 A, 214-236.

Rosenberg SA: Adoptive cellular therapy in patients with advanced cancer: An update, in DeVita VT Jr, et al (eds): *Biologic Therapy of Cancer Updates*. Philadelphia, JB Lippincott, (May/June) 1991 B, vol 1, 1-15.

Rosenberg SA: Principles and applications of biologic therapy, in DeVita VT Jr, et al (eds): *Cancer: Principles & Practice of Oncology*, ed 4. Philadelphia, JB Lippincott, 1993, 293-324.

Rosenberg SA, et al: Observations on the systemic administration of autologous lymphokine-activated killer cells and recombinant interleukin-2 to patients with metastatic cancer. *N Engl J Med* 313:1485-1492, 1985.

Rosenberg SA, et al: A progress report on the treatment of 157 patients with advanced cancer using lymphokine-activated killer cells and interleukin-2 or high-dose interleukin-2 alone. *N Engl J Med* 316:889-897, 1987.

Rosenberg SA, et al: Use of tumor-infiltrating lymphocytes and interleukin-2 in the immunotherapy of patients with metastatic melanoma: A preliminary report. *N Engl J Med* 319:1676-1680, 1988.

Rosenberg SA, et al: Experience with the use of high-dose interleukin-2 in the treatment of 652 cancer patients. *Ann Surg* 210:474-485, 1989 A.

Rosenberg SA, et al: Combination therapy with interleukin-2 and alpha-interferon for the treatment of patients with advanced cancer. *J Clin Oncol* 7:1863-1874, 1989 B.

Rosenberg SA, et al: Prospective randomized trial of high-dose interleukin-2 alone or in conjunction with lymphokine-activated killer cells for the treatment of patients with advanced cancer. *J Natl Cancer Inst* 85:622-632, 1993.

Roth AD, et al: 13-cis-retinoic acid plus interferon-alpha: A Phase II clinical study in squamous cell carcinoma of the lung and the head and neck. *Oncology* 51:84-86, 1994.

Runde V, et al: Retinoic acid in the treatment of acute promyelocytic leukemia: Inefficacy of the 13-cis isomer and induction of complete remission by the all-trans isomer complicated by thromboembolic events. *Ann Hematol* 64:270-272, (June) 1992.

Runowicz CD: Advances in the screening and treatment of ovarian cancer. *CA Cancer J Clin* 42:327-349, (Nov/Dec) 1992.

Saltz L, et al: Octreotide as an antineoplastic agent in the treatment of functional and nonfunctional neuroendocrine tumors. *Cancer* 72:244-248, 1993.

Schally AV, et al: Hypothalamic and other peptide hormones, in Holland JF, et al (eds): *Cancer Medicine*, ed 3. Philadelphia, Lea & Febiger, 1993, vol 1, 827-840.

Scher HI, Kelly WK: Suramin: Defining the role in the clinic, in: *PPO Updates*. Philadelphia, JB Lippincott, (Sept) 1993, vol 7, 1-16.

Scher HI, et al: Use of adaptive control with feedback to individualize suramin dosing. *Cancer Res* 52:64-70, 1992.

Schiffer CA: Interferon studies in the treatment of patients with leukemia. *Semin Oncol* 18 (suppl 7):1-6, 1991.

Schiller JH, Witt PL: Levamisole: Clinical and biological effects, in DeVita VT Jr, et al (eds): *Biologic Therapy of Cancer Updates*. Philadelphia, JB Lippincott, 1992, vol 2, 1-14.

Schiller JH, et al: A direct comparison of immunological and clinical effects of interleukin 2 with and without interferon-α in humans. *Cancer Res* 53:1286-1292, 1993.

Schomburg AG, et al: Cytokines and infection in cancer patients, letter. *Lancet* 339:1061, 1992.

Schoof DD, et al: Survival characteristics of metastatic renal cell carcinoma patients treated with lymphokine-activated killer cells plus interleukin-2. *Urology* 41:534-539, (June) 1993.

Schwartzentruber DJ, et al: Thyroid dysfunction associated with immunotherapy for patients with cancer. *Cancer* 68:2384-2390, 1991.

Sen GC, Lengyel P: The interferon system: A bird's eye view of its biochemistry. *J Biol Chem* 267:5017-5020, 1992.

Siegel JP, Puri RK: Interleukin-2 toxicity. *J Clin Oncol* 9:694-704, 1991.

Silver RT: Chronic myeloid leukemia, in Holland JF, et al (eds): *Cancer Medicine*, ed 3. Philadelphia, Lea & Febiger, 1993, vol 2, 1934-1942.

Sleijfer DTh, et al: Phase II study of subcutaneous interleukin-2 in unselected patients with advanced renal cell cancer on an outpatient basis. *J Clin Oncol* 10:1119-1123, 1992.

Smalley RV, et al: Interferon alfa combined with cytotoxic chemotherapy for patients with non-Hodgkin's lymphoma. *N Engl J Med* 327:1336-1341, 1992.

Smith KA: Lowest dose interleukin-2 immunotherapy. *Blood* 81:1414-1423, 1993.

Smith JW II, et al: The toxic and hematologic effects of interleukin-1 alpha administered in a Phase I trial to patients with advanced malignancies. *J Clin Oncol* 10:1141-1152, 1992 A.

Smith MA, et al: Retinoids in cancer therapy. *J Clin Oncol* 10:839-864, 1992 B.

Smith MA, et al: Phase I and pharmacokinetic evaluation of all-*trans*-retinoic acid in pediatric patients with cancer. *J Clin Oncol* 10:1666-1673, 1992 C.

Smith JW II, et al: The effects of treatment with interleukin-1α on platelet recovery after high-dose carboplatin. *N Engl J Med* 328:756-761, 1993.

Solal-Celigny P, et al: Recombinant interferon alfa-2b combined with a regimen containing doxorubicin in patients with advanced follicular lymphoma. *N Engl J Med* 329:1608-1614, 1993.

Sonnenblick M, Rosin A: Cardiotoxicity of interferon: A review of 44 cases. *Chest* 99:557-561, 1991.

Sparano JA, et al: Randomized Phase III trial of treatment with high-dose interleukin-2 either alone or in combination with interferon alfa-2a in patients with advanced melanoma. *J Clin Oncol* 11:1969-1977, 1993.

Spitler LE: A randomized trial of levamisole versus placebo as adjuvant therapy in malignant melanoma. *J Clin Oncol* 9:736-740, 1991.

Spriggs DR: Tumor necrosis factor: Basic principles and preclinical studies, in DeVita VT Jr, et al (eds): *Biologic Therapy of Cancer*. Philadelphia, JB Lippincott, 1991, 354-377.

Stein CA: Antisense inhibition of gene expression, in DeVita VT Jr, et al (eds): *Cancer: Principles & Practice of Oncology*, ed 4. Philadelphia, JB Lippincott, 1993 A, 2646-2655.

Stein CA: Suramin: A novel antineoplastic agent with multiple potential mechanisms of action. *Cancer Res* 53:2239-2248, 1993 B.

Stevenson HC, et al: Levamisole: Known effects on the immune system, clinical results, and future applications to the treatment of cancer. *J Clin Oncol* 9:2052-2066, 1991.

Stoter G, et al: Sequential administration of recombinant human interleukin-2 and dacarbazine in metastatic melanoma: A multicenter Phase II study. *J Clin Oncol* 9:1687-1691, 1991.

Surwit EA, et al: Clinical assessment of ^{111}In-CYT-103 immunoscintigraphy in ovarian cancer. *Gynecol Oncol* 48:285-292, 1993.

Sznol M, Longo DL: Chemotherapy drug interactions with biological agents. *Semin Oncol* 20:80-93, (Feb) 1993.

Talpaz M, et al : Bone marrow hypoplasia and aplasia complicating interferon therapy for chronic myelogenous leukemia. *Cancer* 69:410-412, 1992.

Tangrea JA, et al: Long-term therapy with low-dose isotretinoin for prevention of basal cell carcinoma: A multicenter clinical trial. *J Natl Cancer Inst* 84:328-332, 1992.

Thompson JA, et al: Prolonged continuous intravenous infusion interleukin-2 and lymphokine-activated killer-cell therapy for metastatic renal cell carcinoma. *J Clin Oncol* 10:960-968, 1992.

Topalian SL, Rosenberg SA: Adoptive cellular therapy: Basic principles, in DeVita VT Jr, et al (eds): *Biologic Therapy of Cancer*. Philadelphia, JB Lippincott, 1991, 178-196.

Valone FH, et al: Interleukin-2, cisplatin, and 5-fluorouracil for patients with non-small cell lung and head/neck carcinomas. *J Immunother* 10:207-213, 1991.

van der Poll T, et al: Activation of coagulation after administration of tumor necrosis factor to normal subjects. *N Engl J Med* 322:1622-1627, 1990.

van Hinsbergh VVM, et al: Progress of fibrinolysis during tumor necrosis factor infusions in humans: Concomitant increase in tissue-type plasminogen activator, plasminogen activator inhibitor type-1, and fibrin(ogen) degradation products. *Blood* 76:2284-2289, 1990.

van Rijswijk REN, et al: Suramin: Rapid loading and weekly maintenance regimens for cancer patients. *J Clin Oncol* 10:1788-1794, 1992.

Van Wauwe J, Janssen PAJ: On the biochemical mode of action of levamisole: An update. *Int J Immunopharmacol* 13:3-9, 1991.

Vial T, Descotes J: Clinical toxicity of interleukin-2. *Drug Safety* 7:417-433, 1992.

Vinik AI, et al: Neoplasms of the gastroenteropancreatic endocrine system, in Holland JF, et al (eds): *Cancer Medicine*, ed 3. Philadelphia, Lea & Febiger, 1993, vol 1, 1180-1209.

Vitetta ES, et al: Immunotoxin therapy, in DeVita VT Jr, et al (eds): *Cancer: Principles & Practice of Oncology*, ed 4. Philadelphia, JB Lippincott, 1993, 2624-2636.

Vogelzang NJ, et al: Subcutaneous interleukin-2 plus interferon alfa-2a in metastatic renal cancer: An outpatient multicenter trial. *J Clin Oncol* 11:1809-1816, 1993.

Volz MA, Kirkpatrick CH: Interferons 1992: How much of the promise has been realised? *Drugs* 43:285-294, 1992.

von der Maase H, et al: Recombinant interleukin-2 in metastatic renal cell carcinoma—A European multicentre Phase II study. *Eur J Cancer* 27:1583-1589, 1991.

von Wussow P, et al: RIFN-α2A is more immunogenic than RIFN-α2b in patients with CML. *J Interferon Res* 12(suppl 1):S72, 1992.

Voogd TE, et al: Recent research on the biological activity of suramin. *Pharmacol Rev* 45:177-203, 1993.

Voravud N, et al: Phase II trial of 13-cis-retinoic acid plus interferon-alpha in recurrent head and neck cancer. *Invest New Drugs* 11:57-60, (Feb) 1993.

Wadler S: The role of interferons in the treatment of solid tumors. *Cancer* 70:949-958, 1992 A.

Wadler S: Antineoplastic activity of the combination of 5-fluorouracil and interferon: Preclinical and clinical results. *Semin Oncol* 19(suppl 4):38-40, 1992 B.

Wadler S, Schwartz EL: Principles in the biomodulation of cytotoxic drugs by interferons. *Semin Oncol* 19(suppl 3):45-48, 1992.

Wadler S, et al: Treatment of carcinoma of the esophagus with 5-fluorouracil and recombinant alfa-2a-interferon. *Cancer* 71:1726-1730, 1993.

Ward FT, et al: A Phase I bioavailability and pharmacokinetic study of hexamethylene bisacetamide (NSC 95580) administered via nasogastric tube. *Cancer Res* 51:1803-1810, 1991.

Warrell RP Jr: Retinoid resistance in acute promyelocytic leukemia: New mechanisms, strategies, and implications, editorial. *Blood* 82:1949-1953, 1993.

Warrell RP Jr, et al: Differentiation therapy of acute promyelocytic leukemia with tretinoin (all-*trans*-retinoic acid). *N Engl J Med* 324:1385-1393, 1991.

Warrell RP Jr, et al: Acute promyelocytic leukemia. *N Engl J Med* 329:177-189, 1993.

Weiss GR, et al: A randomized Phase II trial of continuous infusion interleukin-2 or bolus injection interleukin-2 plus lymphokine-activated killer cells for advanced renal cell carcinoma. *J Clin Oncol* 10:275-281, 1992.

West WH, et al: Constant-infusion recombinant interleukin-2 in adoptive immunotherapy of advanced cancer. *N Engl J Med* 316:898-905, 1987.

Whittington R, Faulds D: Interleukin-2: A review of its pharmacological properties and therapeutic use in patients with cancer. *Drugs* 46:446-514, 1993.

Wills RJ: Clinical pharmacokinetics of interferons. *Clin Pharmacokinet* 19:390-399, 1990.

Wolkenstein P, et al: Cutaneous side effects associated with interleukin 2 administration for metastatic melanoma. *J Am Acad Dermatol* 28:66-70, 1993.

Yang JC, Rosenberg SA: Adoptive cellular therapy: Preclinical studies, in DeVita VT Jr, et al (eds): *Biologic Therapy of Cancer*. Philadelphia, JB Lippincott, 1991, 197-213.

Yang SC, et al: Clinical and immunomodulatory effects of combination immunotherapy with low-dose interleukin 2 and tumor necrosis factor α in patients with advanced non-small cell lung cancer: A Phase I trial. *Cancer Res* 51:3669-3676, 1991.

Young CW, Warrell RP Jr: Differentiating agents, in DeVita VT Jr, et al (eds): *Cancer: Principles & Practice of Oncology*, ed 4. Philadelphia, JB Lippincott, 1993, 2636-2646.

Young CW, et al: Phase I trial and clinical pharmacological evaluation of hexamethylene bisacetamide administration by ten-day continuous intravenous infusion at twenty-eight-day intervals. *Cancer Res* 48:7304-7309, 1988.

Other Selected References

Calabresi P, et al (eds): *Medical Oncology*, ed 2. New York, McGraw-Hill, 1993.

del Regato JA, et al: *Ackerman and del Regato's Cancer: Diagnosis, Treatment, and Prognosis*. St Louis, CV Mosby, 1985.

DeVita VT Jr, et al (eds): *Biologic Therapy of Cancer*. Philadelphia, JB Lippincott, 1991.

DeVita VT Jr, et al (eds): *Cancer: Principles & Practice of Oncology*, ed 4. Philadelphia, JB Lippincott, 1993.

Haskell CM (eds): *Cancer Treatment*, ed 3. Philadelphia, WB Saunders, 1990.

Hellmann K, Carter SK (eds): *Fundamentals of Cancer Chemotherapy*. New York, McGraw-Hill, 1987.

Holland JF, et al (eds): *Cancer Medicine*, ed 3. Philadelphia, Lea & Febiger, 1993.

Tannock IF, Hill RP (eds): *The Basic Science of Oncology*, ed 2. New York, McGraw-Hill, 1992.

Drugs Used for Glaucoma

The glaucomas are characterized by progressive physical changes in the optic disc (deepening and enlargement of the cup) and a loss of nerve fiber substance (Hurvitz et al, 1991; Hoskins and Kass, 1989). They generally are divided into open-angle and angle-closure types based on the appearance of the anterior chamber angle as determined by gonioscopy and are further subdivided into primary and secondary forms. The primary glaucomas are precipitated by intrinsic ocular pathologic changes, and the secondary forms are associated with other eye or systemic diseases.

All forms of glaucoma result from interference with aqueous outflow. Aqueous humor is secreted by the ciliary epithelium and transported into the posterior chamber from which it passes through the pupil into the anterior chamber. The aqueous humor leaves the eye by two routes: About 80% of the total outflow passes through the trabecular meshwork in the anterior chamber angle, enters Schlemm's canal, and then appears in the venous system. The remaining 20% flows through the uveoscleral pathway to the ciliary body and into the suprachoroidal space and then is drained to the venous circulation in the ciliary body, choroid, and sclera. Intraocular pressure is determined by the balance between the rate of aqueous humor produced by the ciliary body, the resistance to aqueous outflow at the angle of the anterior chamber, and the level of episcleral venous pressure.

The likelihood of development of glaucoma increases almost exponentially with escalating intraocular pressure ($\geq$20 mm Hg). However, not all patients with ocular hypertension develop the disease because modest elevations of intraocular pressure sometimes can be tolerated without injury to the optic nerve; conversely, some patients with glaucoma have an intraocular pressure in the normal range (15 $\pm$ 2.5 mm Hg) (Shiose, 1990). Other risk factors for glaucoma include heredity, black race (Tielsch et al, 1991), diabetes mellitus, high myopia, systemic vascular disease, and advancing age.

In the United States, 5 to 10 million people are estimated to have an elevated intraocular pressure. At least 2 million have glaucoma, although 50% are unaware of its presence. An estimated 80,000 Americans are blind as a result of the disease (Hurvitz et al, 1991).

PRINCIPLES OF THERAPY

Treatment of glaucoma depends on the type of glaucoma and the presence of underlying conditions. The primary goal is to prevent damage to the ganglion cells and optic nerve fibers and loss of visual field. Other goals include prevention of damage to aqueous humor outflow channels and relief of ocular symptoms.

Drugs reduce intraocular pressure by increasing outflow of aqueous humor (miotics and epinephrine), by decreasing aqueous production (beta-adrenergic blocking drugs, alpha-adrenergic agonists, and carbonic anhydrase inhibitors), or by transiently reducing the volume of intraocular fluids (osmotic agents). Laser or conventional surgery also is performed to reduce intraocular pressure.

PRIMARY OPEN-ANGLE (CHRONIC SIMPLE) GLAUCOMA. Primary open-angle glaucoma is the most prevalent form and is one of the major causes of blindness in the United States (Kanski, 1989). It is most common in individuals over age 40, especially blacks. This form is characterized by an open angle, glaucomatous cupping, and loss of visual field. As many as one-third of these patients have an intraocular pressure >22 mm Hg on a single measurement. The elevated intraocular pressure is usually due to obstruction of aqueous outflow through the trabecular meshwork-Schlemm's canal system. The pathologic process may involve a decrease in the number or activity of the trabecular cells.

Primary open-angle glaucoma is a chronic, slowly progressing, multifactorial disorder that usually is asymptomatic until extensive, irreversible loss of visual field has occurred. Drug therapy is the primary treatment and is usually initiated with a topical beta blocker, a miotic, or epinephrine. Drug selection often depends largely on how well the patient tolerates side effects (Begg and Cottle, 1988). If the first topical drug fails to reduce pressure sufficiently and noncompliance has been ruled out as a cause of treatment failure, substitution of another drug is recommended before proceeding to combined therapy. Laser trabeculoplasty or filtering surgery is usually reserved for patients whose intraocular pressure has not been lowered sufficiently to prevent further optic nerve damage and visual field loss despite maximally tolerated therapy with a topical beta blocker, miotic, epinephrine, and, possibly, an orally administered carbonic anhydrase inhibitor. When evaluating pressure-lowering effectiveness, the intraocular pressure should be measured at different times of day, since variations of as much as 10 mm Hg or more may occur over a 24-hour period. In addition, the condition of the optic nerve and status of the visual field must be determined regularly (twice a year or more frequently when indicated) to ensure that there is no further progressive ocular damage from insufficient pressure-lowering, intermittent noncompliance, or other causes.

Special consideration should be given to treatment of open-angle glaucoma in patients with cataracts. A beta blocker or dipivefrin is usually preferred for topical therapy because miotics may further impair vision, and the long-acting miotics may exacerbate cataracts and increase the risk of complications during or after cataract surgery. In addition, prolonged use of miotics (particularly the long-acting agents) may lead to permanent miosis and thus interfere with evaluation of the optic disc and macula (Hoskins and Kass, 1989).

OCULAR HYPERTENSION. Individuals with an intraocular pressure ≥21 mm Hg, a normal visual field and optic disc, an open angle, and no other ocular or systemic disorders that contribute to elevated ocular pressure have ocular hypertension, and the possibility that they have glaucoma must be considered. The risk of developing visual field loss in these individuals ranges from 0.5% to 1% per year. They require periodic examination, including tonometry, perimetry, and optic disc assessment, but therapy is needed only in those judged to be at high risk of developing primary open-angle glaucoma.

NORMAL-TENSION GLAUCOMA. This disease resembles primary open-angle glaucoma except that the intraocular pressure usually is within or below the normal range (18 to 19 mm Hg) and is sometimes accompanied by wide diurnal and postural fluctuation. Patients with the stable form of normal-tension glaucoma do not require treatment, but underlying disorders (eg, anemia, arrhythmia, congestive heart failure) should be treated to prevent ischemia of the optic nerve. In patients with the progressive form of the disease, drug therapy, argon laser trabeculoplasty, or filtering surgery is often performed to reduce the intraocular pressure to a level at which no further optic damage occurs (ie, <12 mm Hg) (Reiss et al, 1991).

PRIMARY ANGLE-CLOSURE GLAUCOMA. This disease affects approximately one in 1,000 individuals over age 40 and is especially prevalent in women (female:male ratio of 4:1 in Caucasians and Eskimos). Affected eyes are characterized by a relatively anterior location of the iris-lens diaphragm, a shallow anterior chamber, and a narrow entrance to the chamber angle. When pupillary block is present, passage of aqueous humor from the posterior chamber to the anterior chamber is restricted. The pressure differential created is adequate to push the peripheral iris far enough forward to come into contact with the trabecular meshwork; this leads to restriction of outflow in proportion to the extent of angle closure and a corresponding elevation of intraocular pressure. When approximately two-thirds of the angle is occluded, intraocular pressure rises substantially, producing extensive peripheral anterior synechiae and damaged outflow channels.

Many cases of acute angle-closure glaucoma are precipitated by pupillary dilation in predisposed individuals as a result of emotional upset, low level of illumination, or ingestion of drugs that dilate the pupil (eg, antianxiety agents, bronchodilators, vasoconstrictors, appetite suppressants, antiparkinsonism agents, cold preparations, antispasmodics). An acute attack of primary angle-closure glaucoma with pupillary block is often accompanied by pain, blurred vision, and redness; nausea, vomiting, sweating, and bradycardia also may occur.

Laser iridotomy or conventional iridectomy is the definitive treatment for primary angle-closure glaucoma. The intraocular pressure should be lowered medically prior to these procedures. A combination of two or more of the following agents are often employed: An osmotic agent, a carbonic anhydrase inhibitor, a topical beta blocker, and an alpha-adrenergic ago-

DRUGS USED TO TREAT CHRONIC GLAUCOMAS

Drug	Dosage	Comments
BETA BLOCKERS		
Timolol Maleate [Timoptic]	*Topical:* Initially, one drop of the 0.25% solution is instilled in the conjunctival sac twice daily. If a satisfactory response is not obtained, dosage may be increased to one drop of the 0.5% solution twice daily.	Beta blockers are useful for initial and maintenance therapy. They cause fewer local side effects than miotics and thus are better tolerated in patients with active accommodation or cataracts. Systemic reactions are not uncommon.
Betaxolol Hydrochloride [Betoptic, Betoptic S]	*Topical:* Initially, one drop of a 0.5% solution or 0.25% suspension is instilled twice daily.	
Levobunolol Hydrochloride [Betagan]	*Topical:* Initially, one drop of a 0.25% or 0.5% solution is instilled once or twice daily.	
Metipranolol Hydrochloride [OptiPranolol]	*Topical:* Initially, one drop of 0.3% solution is instilled twice daily.	
PARASYMPATHOMIMETIC MIOTICS		
Pilocarpine Hydrochloride (Solution) [Adsorbocarpine, Akarpine, Isopto Carpine, Pilocar, Generic] Pilocarpine Nitrate [Pilagan]	*Topical:* Initially, one drop of a 0.25%, 0.5%, 1%, or 2% solution is instilled in the conjunctival sac every four to eight hours. The concentration and frequency of administration may be adjusted later as needed. For maintenance, drops are usually instilled four times daily (range, three to six times daily). Concentrations of 4% or 6% may be necessary, especially in patients with heavily pigmented irides or advanced glaucoma. Stronger concentrations may have a longer duration of action but cause side effects more frequently.	Pilocarpine is useful for initial and maintenance therapy. It should be given in a dosage adequate to maintain intraocular pressure at the level necessary to prevent further damage to the optic nerve and progressive loss of visual field. Allergic reactions or systemic side effects are rare. This miotic may be poorly tolerated by patients with active accommodation or cataracts.
Pilocarpine (Ocular Insert) [Ocusert Pilo-20, Pilo-40 Systems]	*Topical:* The unit is placed in the upper or lower cul-de-sac at bedtime and should be replaced every seven days.	
Pilocarpine (Gel) [Pilopine HS Gel]	*Topical:* One-eighth inch of 4% ointment is applied to the lower conjunctival cul-de-sac once daily at bedtime. More frequent application may be required in some patients.	
Carbachol [Isopto Carbachol]	*Topical:* Initially, one drop of a 0.75% to 3% solution is instilled in the conjunctival sac every eight hours.	Carbachol is most commonly used when resistance or intolerance to pilocarpine has developed.
ANTICHOLINESTERASE MIOTICS		
Demecarium Bromide [Humorsol]	*Topical:* Initially, one drop of a 0.125% or 0.25% solution is instilled in the conjunctival sac every 12 to 48 hours.	Because of their cataractogenic potential and other adverse effects, these strong miotics should be used in the lowest effective dosage and should generally be reserved for patients refractory to weaker miotics and other antiglaucoma drugs. These agents should not be used in patients with phakitis.
Echothiophate Iodide [Phospholine Iodide]	*Topical:* Initially, one drop of a 0.03% to 0.125% solution is instilled in the conjunctival sac every 12 to 48 hours. A stronger concentration (0.25%) may be required in highly pigmented eyes.	
Isoflurophate [Floropryl]	*Topical:* Initially, a one-quarter inch strip of 0.025% ointment is applied every 8 to 72 hours.	

(table continued on next page)

TABLE (continued)

Drug	Dosage	Comments
EPINEPHRINE AND ANALOGUES		
Epinephrine Hydrochloride [Epifrin, Glaucon] Epinephrine Bitartrate [Epitrate] Epinephryl Borate [Epinal, Eppy/N]	*Topical:* One drop of a 0.25% to 2% solution is instilled in the conjunctival sac, usually once or twice daily. The stronger concentration may be required in patients with dark irides.	Epinephrine is useful for initial and maintenance therapy, especially in patients who cannot tolerate the accommodative spasm and miosis induced by miotics. Local irritation is common and systemic reactions may occur. The effect of epinephrine may not be additive when a nonselective beta blocker (timolol, levobunolol, metipranolol) is given concomitantly.
Dipivefrin Hydrochloride [Propine]	*Topical:* In primary open-angle glaucoma and other chronic glaucomas, one drop of 0.1% solution is instilled in the conjunctival sac every 12 hours.	Dipivefrin has fewer side effects than epinephrine.
CARBONIC ANHYDRASE INHIBITORS		
Acetazolamide [AK-Zol, Dazamide, Diamox, Generic]	*Oral: Adults,* 62.5 to 250 mg (tablets) two to four times daily or 500 mg (capsules) once or twice daily. *Children,* 10 to 15 mg/kg daily in divided doses.	Carbonic anhydrase inhibitors are useful in patients refractory to short-acting miotics, beta blockers, and epinephrine. Many patients cannot tolerate these drugs for prolonged therapy because of side effects. The prolonged-release preparation of acetazolamide given once daily is better tolerated by some patients.
Dichlorphenamide [Daranide]	*Oral: Adults,* 50 to 200 mg every six to eight hours.	
Methazolamide [Neptazane]	*Oral: Adults,* 25 to 50 mg two or three times daily.	
ALPHA-ADRENERGIC AGONIST		
Apraclonidine Hydrochloride [Iopidine]	*Topical:* One drop of 1% solution is instilled one hour before laser surgery and a second drop is instilled immediately after surgery.	Apraclonidine is used primarily to control intraocular pressure in patients undergoing argon laser trabeculoplasty.

nist. After laser iridotomy, residual glaucoma is treated in stepwise fashion with drug therapy, laser trabeculoplasty, and filtering surgery, as required.

SECONDARY GLAUCOMAS. The secondary glaucomas are associated with various ocular or systemic diseases, trauma, or the use of certain drugs and may be either open-angle or closed-angle (synechial). They are less common than the primary forms and are usually detected upon diagnosis or during treatment of the patient's other illnesses. The primary goal of treatment is to control the underlying disorder if possible. Drugs employed in primary open-angle glaucoma are useful in most cases of noninflammatory secondary glaucoma. In glaucoma associated with inflammation, miotics should be avoided because they may worsen the inflammation and increase synechia formation. Mydriatics, cycloplegics, and corticosteroids are useful to treat the iritis; beta blockers, carbonic anhydrase inhibitors, and dipivefrin are used to reduce the intraocular pressure. See index entry Glaucoma, Secondary.

CONGENITAL GLAUCOMA. Although this form of glaucoma is present at birth (Kanski, 1989), symptoms are not apparent in about 50% of affected infants but develop during the first year of life. In about 40% of cases, the intraocular pressure is elevated in the fetus, and the infant is born with ocular enlargement. Both eyes are affected in 75% of the infants, but the severity of the disorder in each eye frequently varies. Congenital glaucoma is treated surgically. Drug therapy to lower intraocular pressure may be used preoperatively to obtain optimal conditions for surgery and postoperatively to treat residual glaucoma.

BETA-ADRENERGIC BLOCKING DRUGS

Beta-adrenergic receptors have been identified in ocular tissue, primarily in the iris, ciliary body, and trabecular meshwork. Beta-blocking drugs combine reversibly with these receptors to block the response to sympathetic nerve stimulation or circulating catecholamines. The various beta-blocking drugs differ in their affinity for cardiac ($beta_1$) and noncardiac ($beta_2$) receptors, and some have local anesthetic and partial agonist activity (see index entry Beta-Adrenergic Blocking Agents).

Beta-blocking agents lower intraocular pressure, presumably by decreasing the production of aqueous humor. Although the precise mechanism of action is unknown, these agents may act by antagonizing the effect of circulating catecholamines on $beta_2$ receptors in the ciliary epithelium. Because $beta_1$ selectivity is not absolute and/or because mixed populations of $beta_1$ and $beta_2$ receptors are present in the ciliary epithelium, the intraocular pressure is reduced by both selective ($beta_1$) and nonselective ($beta_{1,2}$) agents. Either topical or systemic administration is effective; the topical route is usually preferred because the incidence of systemic side effects is lower. Oral therapy may be very useful when there are additional indications for a beta-blocking drug (eg, systemic hypertension, angina pectoris).

Four beta-blocking drugs are currently available for topical ophthalmic use. Timolol, levobunolol, and metipranolol are nonselective, while betaxolol is relatively selective for the $beta_1$ receptor. All four drugs reduce intraocular pressure for at least 12 hours; the ocular hypotensive effect of levobunolol, timolol, and metipranolol may persist for 24 hours or more.

Drug Evaluations

TIMOLOL MALEATE

[Timoptic]

For chemical formula, see index entry Beta-Adrenergic Blocking Agents.

USES. This nonselective beta blocker is useful in treating primary open-angle glaucoma, chronic glaucoma in aphakia, and secondary glaucoma due to obstruction of aqueous flow induced by alpha chymotrypsin, sodium hyaluronate, or laser procedures. When instilled prior to laser capsulotomy, timolol may reduce the incidence and severity of pressure increases (Migliori et al, 1987). Timolol also may be useful in the emergency treatment of acute angle-closure glaucoma when given with systemic ocular hypotensive drugs and pilocarpine and in some childhood glaucomas.

Timolol appears to be as effective as pilocarpine or epinephrine in lowering intraocular pressure in open-angle glaucoma and is often better tolerated (Moss et al, 1978). The beta-adrenergic blockers have replaced pilocarpine as the usual drug selected for initial and maintenance therapy. Timolol is of particular benefit in young individuals with active accommodation and in older patients with lens opacities who cannot tolerate miotics. Its effect on intraocular pressure is additive with that of miotics and carbonic anhydrase inhibitors (Berson and Epstein, 1981; Dailey et al, 1982; Kass et al, 1982).

ADVERSE REACTIONS, PRECAUTIONS, AND INTERACTIONS. Timolol may cause mild ocular irritation, conjunctival hyperemia, ocular pain, headache, decreased corneal sensitivity, transitory dry-eye syndrome, local hypersensitivity reactions, superficial punctate keratitis, blepharoptosis, and blurring of central vision (sometimes associated with a reversible myopia). Refractive changes due to withdrawal of miotics given concomitantly may have been responsible for some reports of blurred vision.

An abrupt rise in intraocular pressure may occur when timolol replaces other antiglaucoma medication, and the pressure should be checked shortly after the previous drug is discontinued. When used alone, timolol does not dilate the pupil; however, the mydriatic effect of epinephrine is enhanced when this drug is used with timolol; therefore, combined therapy may be dangerous in patients with narrow filtration angles. Aqueous suppression therapy has occasionally been associated with development of hypotony and ciliochoroidal detachment after filtering surgery (Vela and Campbell, 1985).

Timolol is absorbed into the systemic circulation and may produce side effects related to blockade of cardiac and noncardiac beta receptors. Gentle eyelid closure for a few minutes reduces the likelihood of systemic reactions and increases ocular contact time, and there may be added benefit from digital pressure at the inner canthus to block lacrimal drainage (Passo et al, 1984; Zimmerman et al, 1984).

Timolol significantly reduces forced expiratory volume in patients with chronic obstructive airway disease and may precipitate bronchospasm (Schoene et al, 1981). Like other nonselective beta blockers, timolol should not be used in patients with a history of asthma or chronic airway disease. Rarely, this drug has induced vasomotor rhinitis. Both the cardiac and pulmonary side effects of timolol may be additive with those of the anticholinesterase miotics.

Cardiac sympathetic tone and inotropy are reduced by timolol even when plasma levels are low or undetectable (Leier et al, 1986). The effects of timolol are additive with those of other beta-blocking drugs, and patients who are also receiving a systemically administered beta blocker should be observed carefully. Timolol also may have additive effects with calcium channel blocking agents. Bradycardia has been associated with the concurrent use of timolol eyedrops and oral quinidine. If the patient is being treated by another physician for a cardiac disorder, this physician should be consulted prior to instituting therapy.

Bradycardia is the most common systemic side effect of timolol and blood pressure also may be decreased; therefore, the pulse rate and blood pressure should be monitored. Congestive heart failure, syncope, heart block, atrial fibrillation with a slow ventricular rate, and myocardial infarction have been reported rarely. Timolol should be used cautiously in patients with uncontrolled congestive heart failure or AV conduction disturbances. Sudden death has occurred occasionally shortly after timolol therapy was instituted, but a cause-and-effect relationship was not established in all cases (Van Buskirk, 1980).

Timolol occasionally has increased the frequency of hypoglycemic episodes and masked the symptoms of hypoglycemia in diabetic patients receiving insulin. Rarely it has caused hyperkalemia.

Central nervous system effects are similar to those reported with systemically administered beta blockers and include fatigue, lethargy, depression, anxiety, psychic dissociation, confusion, and hallucinations (McMahon et al, 1979; Van Buskirk, 1980). Timolol also may cause sexual dysfunction (impotence, decreased libido). It has occasionally aggravated symptoms of myasthenia gravis and caused arthropathy.

Anorexia, nausea, and dyspepsia have been reported. Reversible nail pigmentation has occurred rarely.

Although indomethacin may attenuate the antihypertensive effect of oral beta blockers, it does not antagonize the ocular hypotensive action of timolol (Goldberg et al, 1985).

Very high blood levels of timolol occur in infants after ocular administration, and this may lead to episodes of apnea and other complications (Passo et al, 1984). Timolol is excreted in breast milk and should be used cautiously in nursing mothers. Its safety in pregnancy has not been determined (FDA Pregnancy Category C).

DOSAGE AND PREPARATIONS.

Topical: For primary open-angle glaucoma and other chronic glaucomas, see Table.

Timoptic (Merck Sharp & Dohme). Solution (sterile, aqueous) 0.25% and 0.5% with benzalkonium chloride 0.01% in 2.5, 5, 10, and 15 ml containers ***(Ocumeter)***; solution 0.25% and 0.5% (preservative-free) in 0.45 ml containers ***(Ocudose)***.

BETAXOLOL HYDROCHLORIDE

[Betoptic]

For chemical formula, see index entry Beta-Adrenergic Blocking Agents.

USES. Betaxolol is a selective $beta_1$ adrenergic blocking agent (Buckley et al, 1990). In placebo-controlled studies, administration of betaxolol 0.25% twice daily reduced intraocular pressure in patients with primary open-angle glaucoma or ocular hypertension by 13% to 27% compared with 2% to 13% in placebo recipients.

In comparative trials lasting four weeks to six months, betaxolol 0.5% or timolol 0.25% reduced the intraocular pressure to the same degree (26% to 37%) in patients with primary open-angle glaucoma or ocular hypertension (Buckley et al, 1990). However, when the effectiveness of therapeutically equivalent concentrations of betaxolol and timolol (0.25% or 0.5%) was compared, the decrease in intraocular pressure was more pronounced with timolol (Allen et al, 1986). In these studies, betaxolol was administered in the form of the racemate and timolol was instilled as a pure solution of the active *l*-isomer; thus, the true efficacy of the *l*-isomer of betaxolol is still unclear.

After two weeks of treatment with dipivefrin 0.1% administered twice daily, addition of betaxolol 0.5% twice daily further reduced the intraocular pressure in patients with open-angle glaucoma or ocular hypertension (Allen and Epstein, 1986). Incremental reduction also was observed when betaxolol 0.5% twice daily was used with oral acetazolamide. The combination of betaxolol and epinephrine also produced synergic effects.

A suspension formulation of betaxolol appears to be more effective than the solution (Weinreb et al, 1990). In a double-blind, three-month trial of 352 patients with primary open-angle glaucoma, a 0.25% suspension reduced intraocular pressure as effectively as the 0.5% solution. Ocular discomfort after topical instillation also was significantly reduced with use of the suspension.

Also see the evaluation on Timolol Maleate.

ADVERSE REACTIONS AND PRECAUTIONS. Betaxolol may cause more local irritation than timolol. Although it is safer than a nonselective beta blocker, $beta_1$ selectivity is not absolute and bronchospasm has occurred occasionally in patients with asthma or chronic obstructive lung disease (Dunn et al, 1986; Weinreb et al, 1988). Bradycardia, syncope, and sinus arrest have occurred rarely. For other adverse effects of topical beta blockers, see the evaluation on Timolol Maleate.

This drug is classified in FDA Pregnancy Category C.

DOSAGE AND PREPARATIONS.

Topical: For primary open-angle glaucoma and other chronic glaucomas, see Table.

Betoptic (Alcon). Solution (sterile, aqueous) 0.5% (as base) with benzalkonium chloride 0.01% in 2.5, 5, 10, and 15 ml containers; suspension (aqueous) 0.25% in 5 and 10 ml containers (***Betoptic S***).

LEVOBUNOLOL HYDROCHLORIDE

[Betagan]

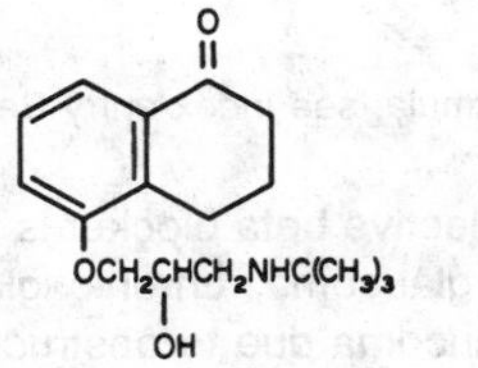

USES. Levobunolol, the active *l*-isomer of bunolol, is a potent nonselective ($beta_1$ and $beta_2$) beta-adrenergic blocking agent that is structurally similar to timolol and propranolol (Gonzalez and Clissold, 1987). It has no intrinsic sympathomimetic or membrane-stabilizing properties.

Levobunolol is effective in patients with primary open-angle glaucoma and ocular hypertension. It also may decrease the incidence and severity of the increase in intraocular pressure that occurs soon after cataract extraction (West et al, 1988) and prevents an elevation in pressure following posterior capsulotomy (Silverstone et al, 1988).

In a double-blind, placebo-controlled, single-dose study involving 48 patients with ocular hypertension, levobunolol 0.3% to 2% produced dose-related reductions in intraocular pressure of 30% to 40%. Concentrations of 0.3% and 0.6% reduced intraocular pressure for up to four hours and the 1% concentration was effective for up to 12 hours. Single daily doses of levobunolol 0.25%, 0.5%, or 1% may be as effective and safe as twice-daily instillation of lower concentrations (Wandel et al, 1986; Silverstone et al, 1991).

The efficacy of levobunolol 0.5% to 1% in reducing intraocular pressure in patients with glaucoma is similar to that of timolol 0.5%, befunolol 0.25% to 0.5% (not available in the United States), or metipranolol 0.6% (Gonzalez and Clissold, 1987; Levobunolol Study Group, 1989). In double-blind crossover studies, levobunolol was slightly more potent than betaxolol in normal subjects and in patients with ocular hypertension (Long et al, 1988; Gaul et al, 1989).

When used with dipivefrin in patients with open-angle glaucoma, the efficacy of levobunolol was comparable to that of timolol (Allen et al, 1988). A combination of levobunolol and pilocarpine maintained a reduction of intraocular pressure in patients with open-angle glaucoma or ocular hypertension who were only marginally responsive to a topical beta-adrenergic blocking drug alone (David et al, 1987).

ADVERSE REACTIONS AND PRECAUTIONS. Topical instillation of levobunolol 0.25% to 1% was generally well tolerated in studies lasting up to four years (Gonzalez and Clissold, 1987). The most significant adverse reactions were blepharitis, conjunctivitis, decreased visual acuity, superficial punctate keratitis, redness, itching, and burning. Systemic effects on hemodynamic parameters were minor. However, subjects with cardiovascular or bronchospastic disease were generally excluded from most studies and hence the true systemic effects of topical administration of levobunolol have not been established. For adverse systemic effects of topical beta blockers, see the evaluation on Timolol Maleate.

This drug is classified in FDA Pregnancy Category C.

DOSAGE AND PREPARATIONS.

Topical: For primary open-angle glaucoma and other chronic glaucomas, see Table.

Betagan (Allergan). Solution (sterile) 0.25% and 0.5% with benzalkonium chloride 0.004% and edetate disodium in 2, 5, 10, and 15 ml containers.

METIPRANOLOL HYDROCHLORIDE

[OptiPranolol]

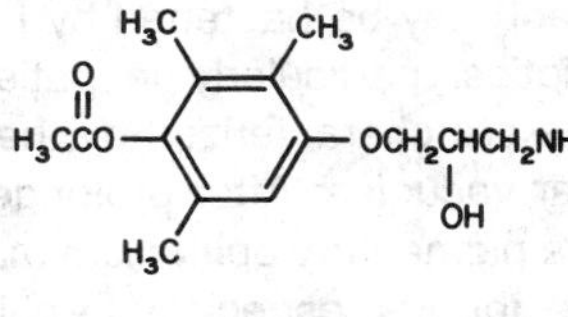

USES. This nonselective ($beta_1$ and $beta_2$) beta-adrenergic blocking agent has no intrinsic sympathomimetic or membrane-stabilizing properties.

In healthy subjects and in patients with ocular hypertension and open-angle glaucoma, metipranolol 0.1% to 0.6% reduced intraocular pressure by 25% to 34% (Battershill and Sorkin, 1988). Peak effects appeared two hours following instillation, and the reduction in intraocular pressure persisted for 24 hours. Tolerance did not develop for up to 12 months (Battershill and Sorkin, 1988). In comparative single-dose studies in patients with chronic open-angle glaucoma, the ability of metipranolol 0.6% to reduce intraocular pressure was comparable to that of timolol 0.5%, levobunolol 0.5% to 1%, and befunolol 0.25% to 0.5% (not available in the United States).

In combination therapy, metipranolol 0.1% and pilocarpine 2% produced a greater reduction in intraocular pressure in patients with open-angle glaucoma than either agent alone. In a six-month multicenter study involving 143 patients, a combination of pilocarpine 2% and metipranolol 0.1% four times daily stabilized intraocular pressure in up to 95% of patients who were inadequately controlled by previous antiglaucoma medication. In a 10-day double-blind study, metipranolol 0.6% reduced the reactive elevation of intraocular pressure after cataract extraction.

ADVERSE REACTIONS AND PRECAUTIONS. Ocular instillation of metipranolol 0.1% to 0.6% is generally well tolerated and no significant changes have been observed in visual acuity, visual field, pupil diameter, corneal sensitivity, Schirmer tear-test values, and in results of biomicroscopic and ophthalmoscopic examination (Battershill and Sorken, 1988). The most frequent side effect is an initial stinging or burning sensation, which may be of longer duration than that produced by comparable doses of timolol and levobunolol. Mild hyperemia of the lid and conjunctiva were observed following treatment with metipranolol 0.6%. However, in 15 patients with glaucoma (26 eyes being treated), metipranolol 0.6% and 0.3% caused granulomatous anterior uveitis, which is characterized by keratic precipitates, flare, and cells in the anterior chamber (Akingbehin and Villada, 1991). Following the discontinuation of metipranolol, all patients recovered with no evidence of ocular inflammation even when other antiglaucoma therapy, including other ophthalmic topical beta-blocking agents, was substituted. In view of these findings, multidose preparations of metipranolol 0.6%, 0.3%, and 0.1% have been withdrawn from the market in the United Kingdom and only the single-dose disposable form is still available.

Because of its systemic effects, metipranolol should be avoided in patients with bronchospastic disease, bradycardia, or congestive heart failure.

Metipranolol is classified in FDA Pregnancy Category C.

DOSAGE AND PREPARATIONS.

Topical: For chronic open-angle glaucoma or ocular hypertension, see Table.

OptiPranolol (Bausch & Lomb). Solution (sterile, isotonic, aqueous) 0.3% with benzalkonium chloride 0.004% in 5 and 10 ml containers.

MIOTICS

ACTIONS AND USES. The miotics are cholinergic drugs that stimulate parasympathetic effector cells directly (parasympathomimetic agents) or indirectly by inhibiting cholinesterase (anticholinesterase agents). Topical instillation of these drugs causes constriction of the pupil and contraction of the ciliary muscle.

In chronic open-angle glaucoma, a miotic has long been the principal and initial drug used, but beta blockers are now usually preferred for initial therapy. Miotics lower intraocular pressure in open-angle glaucoma by reducing outflow resistance, thereby increasing outflow of aqueous humor. This reduction in outflow resistance probably occurs because contraction of the ciliary muscle produces traction on the scleral spur and enhances porosity within the trabecular meshwork. Increased aqueous outflow is the desired effect; miosis and spasm of accommodation are side effects that may interfere with vision and cause discomfort.

In contrast, the beneficial effect of miotics in angle-closure glaucoma results not from ciliary body contraction but from constriction of the pupil, which pulls the peripheral iris away from the trabecular meshwork. Rarely, miotics (particularly strong miotics) may close rather than open the angle and worsen angle closure. This paradoxical effect results from increased pupillary block induced by miosis and/or forward movement of the lens associated with ciliary muscle contraction.

Although miotics are beneficial in many forms of noninflammatory secondary glaucoma, they are not as effective when obstruction of the outflow channels is due to particulate matter (eg, lens cortex or macrophages with lens material in phacolytic glaucoma; zonular fragments in alpha-chymotrypsin-induced glaucoma; viscous material in sodium hyaluronate-induced glaucoma; inflammatory cells in iridocyclitis; tumor cells; red blood cells). Miotics should be avoided when iritis is present because they may aggravate the inflammatory process. Moreover, iridolenticular adhesions (posterior synechiae) may result from inflammation and are particularly undesirable in the presence of a small pupil.

Parasympathomimetic Miotics: The parasympathomimetic agent, pilocarpine, has long been the preferred miotic for therapy in primary open-angle glaucoma and many other chronic glaucomas. It often controls intraocular pressure when used alone. Pilocarpine should be given in a dosage adequate to maintain the intraocular pressure at the level required to prevent further damage to the optic disc and progressive loss of visual field. Variations in pressure at different times of day should be taken into consideration. Stronger concentrations may be required in patients with dark irides, because topical miotics are less effective in heavily pigmented eyes. In addition to the eyedrop preparation, pilocarpine is available in a long-acting gel formulation [Pilopine HS Gel] and a timed-release system [Ocusert].

In patients over age 50 who do not have cataracts, pilocarpine is better tolerated than other miotics available in the United States. Carbachol is sometimes substituted when resistance or intolerance develops to pilocarpine or when a slightly longer acting drug is needed.

Pilocarpine is also the miotic usually given (in low concentrations) for emergency treatment of acute angle-closure glaucoma. It generally should not be administered for long periods to avoid or postpone laser iridectomy, especially if the pressure remains elevated, because many patients experience a recurrence of acute angle closure despite miotic therapy and others may develop chronic angle closure with formation of peripheral anterior synechiae. Pilocarpine is also used for long-term therapy after laser or conventional surgery if the intraocular pressure remains elevated or if a patent iridotomy does not relieve the angle closure.

Anticholinesterase Miotics: Demecarium [Humorsol] and the organophosphorus compounds, isoflurophate [Floropryl] and echothiophate [Phospholine], are long-acting, potent cholinesterase inhibitors employed in the treatment of chronic open-angle glaucoma. Because of their cataractogenic properties and the rare precipitation of retinal detachment, these drugs should be reserved for patients refractory to short-acting miotics, epinephrine, beta-blocking drugs, and, possibly, carbonic anhydrase inhibitors. Filtering surgery or laser trabeculoplasty may be preferred to long-acting miotics, especially if the lens is present. In the absence of the lens, strong miotics can be used to treat chronic glaucoma in aphakic patients when there is no sign of an imminent retinal detachment. Anticholinesterase miotics should not be administered for two weeks prior to surgery. They may be used after surgery if continued drug therapy is required and weaker miotics are inadequate.

The short-acting anticholinesterase drug, physostigmine (eserine), is not well tolerated and is seldom used today for prolonged therapy.

ADVERSE REACTIONS AND PRECAUTIONS. Miotics cause a variety of untoward reactions as a result of their local effects on ocular structures. Accommodative myopia can be troublesome in younger patients, and pupillary constriction may interfere with vision, particularly in patients with central lens opacities. Presbyopic patients may need a change in eyeglass prescription if a miotic is discontinued because the "pinhole" effect of a small pupil (which compensates for presbyopia) is no longer present.

Most patients taking miotics have poor vision in dim light, making night driving hazardous. Other common local effects include twitching of the eyelids, browache, headache, ocular pain, ciliary and conjunctival congestion, and lacrimation. Localized allergy, manifested by conjunctivitis and contact dermatitis, may develop. This complication was more prevalent when physostigmine solutions were used. Long-term therapy with the strong miotics may cause conjunctival thickening and obstruction of the nasolacrimal canals.

Cataract development may be hastened by treatment with anticholinesterase miotics, particularly in patients over 60 years. These cataracts are characterized by the appearance of anterior subcapsular vacuoles. After prolonged treatment, rounded nodules of the pigmentary epithelium may develop at the pupillary margin of the iris, especially in children. These nodules may enlarge sufficiently to interfere with vision and rarely may rupture or break free into the aqueous. They generally disappear when the drug is discontinued, and their incidence may be reduced if one drop of phenylephrine 2.5% or epinephrine 0.5% to 1% is instilled simultaneously.

Pupillary block, local vascular congestion, and occasional forward movement of the lens induced by the strong miotics may cause a sudden or, more often, an insidious closure of the angle and an increase in intraocular pressure even in eyes with only moderately narrow angles. Patients with swollen lenses due to advanced cataracts may be particularly at risk.

Strong miotics should be discontinued two weeks prior to surgery in angle-closure glaucoma, in open-angle glaucoma with an excessively narrow angle, and in secondary glaucomas with angle closure. Occasionally, parasympathomimetic miotics have similarly aggravated angle closure in predisposed eyes. Rarely, if miotics are administered after surgery for angle closure, the anterior chamber may become very shallow and the intraocular pressure may rise due to development of malignant (ciliary block) glaucoma.

When there is an active inflammatory process (eg, in glaucoma secondary to anterior uveitis), miotics usually are of little therapeutic value and predispose to the development of posterior synechiae. Long-acting miotics increase the frequency of hemorrhage during ocular surgery, aggravate postoperative inflammation, and promote formation of posterior synechiae. If possible, these agents should be discontinued at least two weeks prior to ocular surgery.

Following prolonged (months to years) use of miotics, particularly the cholinesterase inhibitors, miosis may persist when the drug is discontinued. This complication may be caused by fibrosis of the sphincter muscle, by loss of tone of the dilator muscle, or occasionally by the formation of dense posterior synechiae.

Retinal detachment, an occasional complication of miotic therapy in predisposed individuals, may result from drug-induced spasm of accommodation, which causes the lens and vitreous to move forward and create a retinal tear. It may occur from one hour to several weeks after beginning miotic therapy (Beasley and Fraunfelder, 1979). Miotics should be used with caution in patients at high risk of retinal detachment (eg, aphakic or myopic patients, those with retinovitreal pathology or previous retinal detachment in the opposite eye).

Topical miotics, particularly echothiophate and demecarium, occasionally cause systemic effects. Such reactions are very rare following routine administration of pilocarpine, carbachol, or the rapidly hydrolyzed anticholinesterase, isoflurophate, but have been seen with excessive treatment. Symptoms of systemic anticholinesterase toxicity include muscle weakness, hypersalivation, sweating, nausea, vomiting, abdominal pain, urinary incontinence, diarrhea, bradycardia, severe hypotension, and bronchospasm. These agents should be used with caution in patients with bronchial asthma, bradycardia, or hypotension. An increase in blood pressure, due to a nicotinic effect on sympathetic ganglia, may occur rarely.

Toxic doses of anticholinesterase drugs can cause central nervous system (CNS) effects (ataxia, confusion, seizures, coma) and muscular paralysis. Death can result from respiratory failure. Patients who have undergone lacrimal surgery with placement of lacrimal drainage tubes are at increased risk because of enhanced drug absorption.

The most common symptoms of systemic toxicity in children are abdominal cramps and diarrhea; mild rhinorrhea, lacrimation, and upper respiratory congestion also may be observed. Children with Down's syndrome may be particularly prone to develop CNS disturbances from anticholinesterase miotics.

Severe toxic reactions are treated with intravenous atropine; pralidoxime [Protopam] may be used concomitantly when required.

DRUG INTERACTIONS. Plasma cholinesterase levels are depressed significantly during topical therapy with anticholinesterase miotics, and prolonged apnea and cardiovascular collapse may develop if succinylcholine is given to patients using these drugs. These strong miotics should be discontinued, if possible, two to four weeks prior to administration of succinylcholine, and the anesthesiologist should be informed that the patient has been receiving an anticholinesterase drug. The hydrolysis of procaine also is decreased by topical anticholinesterase agents.

Because of possible adverse additive effects, anticholinesterase miotics should be administered cautiously to patients with myasthenia gravis who are receiving systemic anticholinesterase therapy. Similarly, caution should be exercised in the use of a systemic anticholinesterase drug for myasthenia gravis when the patient is already receiving topical therapy with a strong miotic. An adverse interaction between organophosphate miotics and organophosphate insecticides is possible, and these miotics are considered hazardous in farm workers exposed to insecticides. The cardiac and pulmonary side effects of these drugs may be additive with those of the beta blockers.

Drug Evaluations

PARASYMPATHOMIMETIC MIOTICS

PILOCARPINE HYDROCHLORIDE

[Adsorbocarpine, Akarpine, Isopto Carpine, Pilocar]

PILOCARPINE NITRATE

[Pilagan]

ACTIONS AND USES. Pilocarpine is the miotic of choice for therapy in primary open-angle glaucoma and many other chronic glaucomas and in the emergency treatment of acute angle-closure glaucoma. This agent penetrates the eye well. After topical instillation, miosis begins in 15 to 30 minutes and lasts four to eight hours. The maximal reduction of intraocular pressure occurs in two to four hours, which correlates with the maximal decrease in outflow resistance. Pilocarpine does not appear to have a clinically important effect on aqueous production.

In patients with Adie's (tonic pupil) syndrome, a weak concentration of pilocarpine (0.125%) is useful for demonstrating denervation supersensitivity and possibly for long-term treatment.

ADVERSE REACTIONS AND PRECAUTIONS. Pilocarpine generally is tolerated better than other miotics. Nevertheless, stinging and local irritation may occur and ciliary spasm and miosis may be troublesome initially. Allergic reactions and systemic effects are uncommon. (See also the preceding section on Adverse Reactions and Precautions.)

Pilocarpine is classified in FDA Pregnancy Category C.

DOSAGE AND PREPARATIONS.
Topical: For long-term administration in primary open-angle glaucoma and other chronic glaucomas, see Table.

In primary acute angle-closure glaucoma, initially, drops (usually the 1% or 2% solution) are instilled frequently (eg, every 15 minutes for four doses, then hourly for several doses). Occasionally, pilocarpine is unsuccessful in opening the angle, particularly when the pressure is high enough to impede circulation to the sphincter muscle. The unaffected eye may be treated every six to eight hours to avoid a bilateral attack.

For preoperative preparation before laser iridotomy, surgical iridectomy, or filtration surgery, the 2% solution is instilled two or three times during the hour before surgery. Laser iridotomy is facilitated by a taut iris, and the iris is reposited more easily after surgical iridectomy if the sphincter muscle is contracted.

In congenital glaucoma, a constricted iris protects the lens during surgery; therefore, some surgeons apply one drop of a 2% solution to the affected eye every six hours for 24 hours before surgery.

All preparations are available as ophthalmic solutions.

PILOCARPINE HYDROCHLORIDE:

Generic. Solution 0.5%, 1%, 2%, 3%, 4%, 5%, 6%, and 8%.

Adsorbocarpine (Alcon). Solution (sterile) 1%, 2%, and 4% with benzalkonium chloride 0.004% and edetate disodium 0.1% in 15 ml containers.

Akarpine (Akorn). Solution (aqueous) 1%, 2%, and 4% with benzalkonium chloride 0.01% and edetate disodium 0.01% in 15 ml containers.

Isopto Carpine (Alcon). Solution (sterile) 0.25%, 0.5%, 1%, 2%, 3%, 4%, 5%, 6%, 8%, and 10% with benzalkonium chloride 0.01% in 15 and 30 ml containers.

Pilocar (Iolab). Solution (sterile) 0.5%, 1%, 2%, 3%, 4%, and 6% with benzalkonium chloride and edetate disodium in 1 and 15 ml containers.

Pilocarpine Steri-Units (Alcon). Solution (sterile) 1%, 2%, 4%, and 8% in 2 ml presterilized containers (preservative free).

Additional Trademarks.

Ocu-Carpine (Ocumed), ***Pilokair*** (Texas).

PILOCARPINE NITRATE:

Pilagan (Allergan). Solution (sterile) 1%, 2%, and 4% with chlorobutanol 0.5% and polyvinyl alcohol in 15 ml containers.

PILOCARPINE OCULAR INSERT

[Ocusert Pilo-20/Pilo-40 Systems]

ACTIONS AND USES. The Ocusert pilocarpine system is a drug delivery unit consisting of two outer membranes with a central reservoir of pilocarpine. It is used in patients with chronic open-angle glaucoma who are responsive to pilocarpine. When placed in the upper or lower cul-de-sac, pilocarpine gradually diffuses across the two outer polymeric layers that serve as rate-controlling membranes. The unit is available in two strengths, Pilo-20 and -40, which correspond in effectiveness roughly to 0.5% or 1% and 2% or 3% pilocarpine. Patients who are inadequately controlled with the Pilo-40 unit may require concomitant use of other antiglaucoma drugs. The Ocusert system is more expensive than eyedrops, but it may provide better diurnal control of intraocular pressure and improve compliance in unreliable patients. In younger patients, miosis and spasm of accommodation are less severe than with use of the eyedrops; however, because these symptoms can be troublesome during the first few hours after insertion of a new unit (caused by rapid drug release when the unit becomes wet), the device should be inserted at bedtime or it may be soaked in a glass of water for one hour before placement in the cul-de-sac.

Although the Ocusert system is labeled for replacement every seven days, the duration of action and rate of release of pilocarpine may vary among patients.

ADVERSE REACTIONS AND PRECAUTIONS. Conjunctival irritation may be noted, particularly during initial use. Rarely, sudden leakage of pilocarpine has produced marked miosis and decreased vision associated with a further fall in intraocular pressure. Rarely, the Ocusert may migrate onto the cornea, obstructing vision and causing pain. Some patients, particularly those with loose lids, have difficulty retaining the Ocusert and may lose it without noting the loss. Since the unit may fall out at night, the patient should be instructed to make sure that it is in place every morning.

DOSAGE AND PREPARATIONS.
Topical: See Table.

Ocusert Pilo-20 Ocular Therapeutic System (20 mcg/hour for one week), ***Ocusert Pilo-40 Ocular Therapeutic System*** (40 mcg/hour for one week) (Alza). Ophthalmic prolonged-release systems (sterile) in packages of eight units.

PILOCARPINE GEL

[Pilopine HS Gel]

This long-acting preparation contains pilocarpine hydrochloride in an aqueous gel. It is applied before bedtime to treat chronic open-angle glaucoma. After one application, intraocular pressure is lowered for 18 to 24 hours.

ADVERSE REACTIONS AND PRECAUTIONS. Pilocarpine gel often causes irritation, blurred vision, and transient superficial punctate keratitis. Some patients are bothered by their eyelids sticking together in the morning.

DOSAGE AND PREPARATIONS.
Topical: See Table.

Pilopine HS Gel (Alcon). Gel (sterile) containing pilocarpine hydrochloride 4% with benzalkonium chloride 0.008% in 5 g containers.

CARBACHOL

[Isopto Carbachol]

$$H_2N\overset{O}{\overset{\|}{C}}OCH_2CH_2\overset{+}{N}(CH_3)_3 \quad Cl^-$$

ACTIONS AND USES. Carbachol is sometimes used in primary open-angle and other chronic glaucomas, usually to replace pilocarpine when resistance or intolerance to the latter has developed or when a slightly longer acting drug is needed. However, replacing pilocarpine with carbachol only rarely improves long-term control of intraocular pressure (Reichert et al, 1988).

Carbachol does not penetrate the eye as well as pilocarpine and is usually prepared with a wetting agent to enhance corneal penetration.

ADVERSE REACTIONS AND PRECAUTIONS. Carbachol may cause more accommodative spasm and headache than pilocarpine and produces slight conjunctival hyperemia. Resistance has been reported to develop suddenly. Other local and systemic adverse reactions occur rarely (see the section on Adverse Reactions and Precautions in the Introduction).

DOSAGE AND PREPARATIONS.

Topical: For primary open-angle glaucoma and other chronic glaucomas, see Table.

All preparations are available as ophthalmic solutions.

Isopto Carbachol (Alcon). Solution (sterile) 0.75%, 1.5%, 2.25%, and 3% with benzalkonium chloride 0.005% in 15 and 30 ml containers.

Intracameral: See index entry Miotics, In Ocular Surgery.

ANTICHOLINESTERASE MIOTICS

DEMECARIUM BROMIDE
[Humorsol]

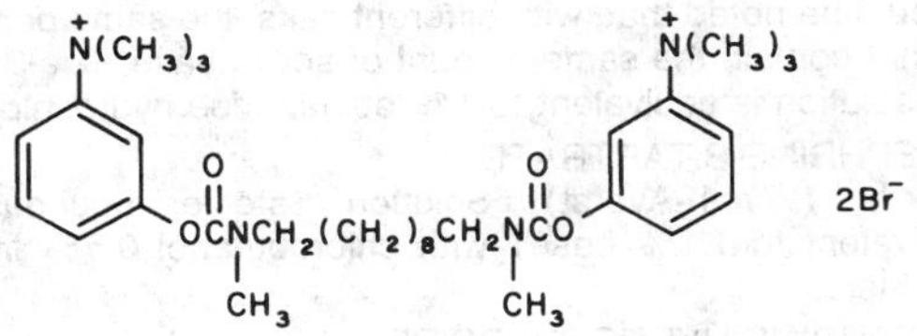

ECHOTHIOPHATE IODIDE
[Phospholine Iodide]

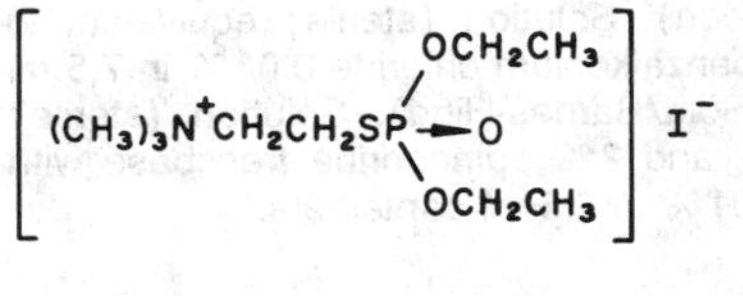

ISOFLUROPHATE (DFP)
[Floropryl]

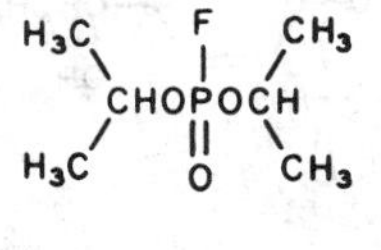

ACTIONS AND USES. These potent, long-acting miotics are used to treat primary open-angle glaucoma and other chronic glaucomas when short-acting miotics and other agents are inadequate. They are used most frequently to treat glaucoma in aphakic patients. Maximal reduction of intraocular pressure occurs within 24 hours after a single instillation, and residual effects may persist for days. When instilled once daily for a number of days, the effect is cumulative; the maximal reduction in pressure is attained after several days of therapy.

In addition to their use in glaucoma, the strong miotics have been employed to diagnose and treat accommodative esotropia. By inducing accommodation peripherally, they decrease accommodative effort and thereby reduce accommodative convergence. The lowest effective concentration should be employed.

ADVERSE REACTIONS AND PRECAUTIONS. The development of cataracts after long-term administration has limited the usefulness of these agents in glaucoma therapy. Although cataract formation has not been observed in children or young adults, the usefulness of these agents in young patients with strabismus must be balanced against the possible risk that they will hasten the development of cataracts later in life. These drugs should not be used in patients with phakitis. (See also the section on Adverse Reactions and Precautions in the Introduction.)

DOSAGE AND PREPARATIONS. For primary open-angle glaucoma and other chronic glaucomas, see Table. These strong miotics should be applied topically in the lowest effective dosage.

DEMECARIUM BROMIDE:

Humorsol (Merck Sharp & Dohme). Solution (sterile, aqueous) 0.125% and 0.25% with benzalkonium chloride 0.02% in 5 ml containers.

ECHOTHIOPHATE IODIDE:

Phospholine Iodide (Wyeth-Ayerst). Powder (lyophilized) 1.5, 3, 6.25, and 12.5 mg with 5 ml of diluent containing mannitol 1.2%, boric acid 0.06%, exsiccated sodium phosphate 0.026%, and chlorobutanol 0.5% to make 0.03%, 0.06%, 0.125%, and 0.25% solution, respectively.

ISOFLUROPHATE:

Floropryl (Merck Sharp & Dohme). Ointment (sterile) 0.025% in polyethylene-mineral oil gel in 3.5 g containers.

ADRENERGIC AGONISTS

The dilator muscle of the iris contains mainly alpha-adrenergic receptors, and activation of these receptors causes pupillary dilation. Although the sphincter and ciliary muscles are largely under parasympathetic control, adrenergic receptors have also been described in these tissues, primarily beta receptors in the ciliary muscle and both alpha and beta receptors in the sphincter muscle of the iris. The data are conflicting regarding the mechanisms involved in adrenergic control of aqueous humor dynamics. Current evidence suggests that both aqueous formation and outflow facility are modulated primarily by beta-adrenergic mechanisms: Activation of $beta_2$ receptors in the outflow channels increases outflow facility (Allen and Epstein, 1986), an action that may involve stimulation of prostaglandin synthesis and hence increase uveoscleral outflow (Camras et al, 1985). Activation of beta receptors in the ciliary processes causes a slight, transient, clinically unimportant increase in aqueous production, while blockade of these receptors decreases production (Schenker et al, 1981).

Epinephrine and Analogues

EPINEPHRINE BITARTRATE
[Epitrate]

EPINEPHRINE HYDROCHLORIDE
[Epifrin, Glaucon]

EPINEPHRYL BORATE
[Epinal, Eppy/N]

For chemical formula, see index entry Epinephrine, In Asthma.

ACTIONS AND USES. Epinephrine acts on both alpha- and beta-adrenergic receptors. When instilled in eyes with primary open-angle glaucoma, it reduces intraocular pressure for 12 to 24 hours or, rarely, longer. Its pressure-lowering effect is currently thought to be due largely to an increase in aqueous outflow facility, primarily uveoscleral outflow. Brief constriction of the conjunctival vessels is followed by a more prolonged vasodilation. Transient mydriasis may occur in some patients.

Epinephrine is used to treat primary open-angle glaucoma and other chronic glaucomas. It may be administered alone for initial treatment, especially when beta blockers are ineffective or not tolerated. Epinephrine also is used to supplement miotics and/or carbonic anhydrase inhibitors.

ADVERSE REACTIONS AND PRECAUTIONS. Epinephrine produces browache, headache, blurred vision, ocular irritation, and lacrimation in some patients. Epinephryl borate may cause less local discomfort than the hydrochloride and especially the bitartrate salts. Repeated use of epinephrine may cause reactive hyperemia, allergic conjunctivitis, and contact dermatitis; discontinuation of the medication may be required in 20% or more of patients. Corneal edema has been reported very rarely after long-term administration.

Of particular importance in aphakic eyes is the possibility of inducing cystoid macular edema. This complication has been reported in 10% to 20% of aphakic patients during long-term therapy. Fortunately, the maculopathy is usually reversible if epinephrine is discontinued when visual acuity first begins to decrease. Many ophthalmologists prefer not to use epinephrine in aphakic eyes unless the glaucoma is sufficiently severe to justify the risk. When needed, it may be used if vision and macular status are monitored.

Topical epinephrine can cause pupillary dilation, even when used with miotics. It is contraindicated before iridectomy in angle-closure glaucoma because it may precipitate an acute attack. When instilled without miotics in patients with open-angle glaucoma, epinephrine rarely may cause a temporary elevation of intraocular pressure upon initial administration. This phenomenon may be associated with release of pigment particles from the iris into the aqueous humor. With long-term administration, adrenochrome deposits may appear in the bulbar or palpebral conjunctiva, in the lacrimal canaliculi, in roughened or edematous areas of the cornea, or in soft contact lenses.

Supersensitivity, manifested by mydriasis and lid retraction, has been reported after long-term topical therapy. Prolonged use rarely contributes to the development of benign ocular mucous membrane pemphigoid.

The ocular hypotensive effect of epinephrine is partially inhibited by oral indomethacin (Camras et al, 1985).

Systemic reactions to topical epinephrine include tachycardia, premature ventricular contractions, hypertension, headache, sweating, tremors, blanching, and disorientation. In several instances, systemic effects occurred when the drug was applied after conjunctival permeability was increased by tonometry or administration of local anesthetics.

Epinephrine should be used with care in patients with arrhythmias, hypertension, hyperthyroidism, recent myocardial infarction, or arteriosclerotic heart disease. It may cause ventricular premature contractions, tachycardia, and fibrillation in patients undergoing general anesthesia with halothane, cyclopropane, or other agents that sensitize the heart to catecholamines. Increased cardiovascular toxicity may also occur in patients receiving topical epinephrine who are taking systemic monoamine oxidase inhibitors, tricyclic antidepressants, or sympathomimetic drugs.

Epinephrine is classified in FDA Pregnancy Category C.

DOSAGE AND PREPARATIONS. Discolored solutions should be discarded.

Topical: For primary open-angle glaucoma and other chronic glaucomas, see Table.

All preparations are available for ophthalmic use.

It should be noted that, with different salts, the same percentage may not contain the same amount of active base. The 2% bitartrate solution is equivalent to 1% epinephrine hydrochloride.

EPINEPHRINE BITARTRATE:

Epitrate (Wyeth-Ayerst). Solution (sterile, aqueous) 2% (equivalent to 1.1% base) with chlorobutanol 0.5% in 7.5 ml containers.

EPINEPHRINE HYDROCHLORIDE:

Epifrin (Allergan). Solution (sterile) equivalent to 0.25%, 0.5%, 1%, and 2% free base with benzalkonium chloride 0.01% in 15 ml containers.

Glaucon (Alcon). Solution (sterile) equivalent to 1% or 2% base with benzalkonium chloride 0.01% in 10 ml containers.

EPINEPHRYL BORATE:

Epinal (Alcon). Solution (sterile) equivalent to 0.5% or 1% base with benzalkonium chloride 0.01% in 7.5 ml containers.

Eppy/N (Sola/Barnes-Hind). Solution (sterile) equivalent to 0.5%, 1%, and 2% epinephrine free base with benzalkonium chloride 0.01% in 7.5 ml containers.

DIPIVEFRIN HYDROCHLORIDE (Dipivalyl Epinephrine)
[Propine]

$(CH_3)_3CCO$ (O) – ring – $CHCH_2NHCH_3$ (OH)
$(CH_3)_3CCO$ (O)

ACTIONS AND USES. Dipivefrin is a lipophilic analogue of epinephrine that is formed by the addition of two pivalic acid side chains to the parent compound. It is converted to epinephrine by esterases in the ocular tissues. Because of its lipophilic properties, dipivefrin penetrates the corneal epithelium more readily than epinephrine and reduces intraocular pressure at a lower concentration. The onset of action occurs in 30 minutes, and the maximal reduction in pressure is attained in one hour.

Dipivefrin 0.1% is an effective ocular hypotensive agent in patients with open-angle glaucoma. Its effect on intraocular pressure is slightly less than that of 2% epinephrine hydrochloride, but its mydriatic effect is comparable (Kass et al, 1979; Kohn et al, 1979).

ADVERSE REACTIONS. Dipivefrin produces less burning and irritation than epinephrine and may cause fewer allergic reactions. Allergic or follicular conjunctivitis may occur during long-term therapy (Theodore and Leibowitz, 1979). As with epinephrine, cystoid macular edema has been reported. Because a lower concentration is required for corneal penetration, systemic side effects may be reduced.

For other potential adverse effects, see the previous evaluation.

Dipivefrin is classified in FDA Pregnancy Category B.

DOSAGE AND PREPARATIONS.

Topical: For primary open-angle glaucoma and other chronic glaucomas, see Table.

Propine (Allergan). Solution (sterile) 0.1% with benzalkonium chloride 0.004% in 5, 10, and 15 ml containers.

EPINEPHRINE BITARTRATE AND PILOCARPINE HYDROCHLORIDE

Mixtures containing pilocarpine and epinephrine are used to treat open-angle glaucoma when both drugs are required and one of the available combinations is effective in controlling intraocular pressure. Use of a combination product may improve compliance and avoids the inconvenience of waiting between instillation of two separate drop preparations; however, an excessive dose of epinephrine may be administered.

Preparations are available as ophthalmic solutions.

E-Pilo-1, E-Pilo-2, E-Pilo-3, E-Pilo-4, and ***E-Pilo-6*** (Iolab). Solution (sterile) containing epinephrine bitartrate 1% (equivalent to 0.55% base) and pilocarpine hydrochloride 1%, 2%, 3%, 4%, or 6% with benzalkonium chloride and edetate disodium in 10 ml containers.

P1E1, P2E1, P3E1, P4E1, and ***P6E1*** (Alcon). Solution (sterile) containing epinephrine bitartrate 1% (equivalent to 0.5% base) and pilocarpine hydrochloride 1%, 2%, 3%, 4%, or 6% with edetate disodium and benzalkonium chloride 0.01% in 15 ml containers.

Alpha-Adrenergic Agonist

APRACLONIDINE HYDROCHLORIDE

[Iopidine]

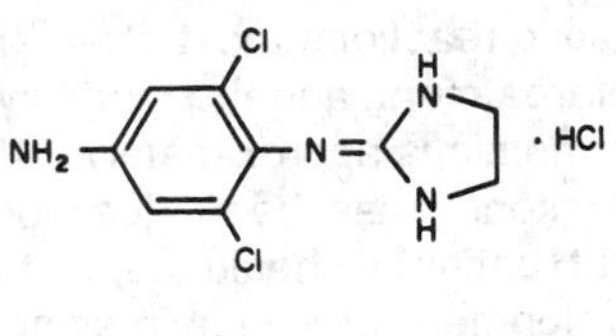

NH_2 · Cl · Cl · N= · H · N · H · HCl

ACTIONS AND USES. This selective alpha$_2$-agonist is chemically related to clonidine, a centrally acting antihypertensive drug. Topical forms of both drugs lower intraocular pressure by decreasing the production of aqueous humor; however, clonidine has caused pronounced decreases in pulse rate and blood pressure (Kitazawa et al, 1989 A, 1989 B). Apraclonidine is used to prevent elevation of intraocular pressure following argon laser trabeculoplasty, iridotomy and capsulotomy, and cataract surgery.

In two double-blind studies (Hurvitz et al, 1991), patients with severe open-angle glaucoma received either placebo or apraclonidine one hour before and immediately after argon laser trabeculoplasty. The mean intraocular pressure increased slightly during the first three hours after the procedure in the placebo-treated eyes, but fell in the apraclonidine-treated eyes. Large intraocular pressure spikes ≥10 mm Hg over baseline were observed in 18.4% of placebo-treated eyes compared with 2.5% of those treated with apraclonidine. The effectiveness of apraclonidine 1% in preventing a postoperative increase in intraocular pressure is significantly greater than that of timolol 0.5%, pilocarpine 4%, dipivefrin 0.1%, and acetazolamide 250 mg (Robin, 1989). Similarly, apraclonidine prevented elevation of the intraocular pressure in patients with angle-closure glaucoma who had laser iridotomy and capsulotomy (Robin et al, 1987 A, 1987 B; Brown et al, 1988; Hurvitz et al, 1991). In separate studies, neither pilocarpine nor beta-adrenergic blocking agents (eg, timolol) were as efficacious as apraclonidine in patients who had these two procedures (Hurvitz et al, 1991).

Apraclonidine also has been tested for control of postoperative intraocular pressure in patients undergoing extracapsular cataract extraction (Wiles et al, 1991). The pressure increased in all patients after cataract surgery, but none who received apraclonidine 1% before surgery had a postoperative intraocular pressure >24 mm Hg two to five hours after surgery (average preoperative level, 14.4 mm Hg). In contrast, 45% and 44% of patients treated postoperatively with apraclonidine or artificial tears, respectively, had intraocular pressure ≥30 mm Hg in the early postoperative period (mean preoperative level, 14.9 to 15.7 mm Hg).

ADVERSE REACTIONS AND PRECAUTIONS. Conjunctival blanching, mydriasis, and lid retraction (all alpha-adrenergic side effects) were noted frequently in volunteers with normal eyes (Robin, 1988). In patients, mydriasis may not occur because of prior miotic therapy. Local irritation and, rarely, allergic reactions have been reported.

Rare systemic reactions include taste disturbances, bradycardia, vasovagal episodes, and central nervous system and gastrointestinal disturbances.

The most common systemic side effect of apraclonidine is a sensation of dry mouth or nose, which occurs more frequently in patients treated with the 1% than the 0.25% or 0.125% concentration.

Apraclonidine is classified in FDA Pregnancy Category C.

DOSAGE AND PREPARATIONS.

Topical: See Table.

Iopidine (Alcon). Solution (sterile) 1% in 0.1 ml dispensers packaged in pairs (one for pre- and one for post-treatment use).

CARBONIC ANHYDRASE INHIBITORS

ACETAZOLAMIDE
[AK-Zol, Dazamide, Diamox]

ACETAZOLAMIDE SODIUM
[Diamox]

DICHLORPHENAMIDE
[Daranide]

METHAZOLAMIDE
[Neptazane]

ACTIONS AND USES. The carbonic anhydrase inhibitors are given orally to reduce intraocular pressure. These drugs were originally introduced as diuretics, but their effect on intraocular pressure does not depend on diuresis. They reduce aqueous production by blocking ocular carbonic anhydrase in the ciliary epithelium and thus lower pressure. Systemic acidosis enhances the ocular hypotensive effect. When maximal doses are given, carbonic anhydrase inhibitors reduce aqueous flow by about 40%. Acetazolamide may have a more consistent pressure-lowering effect than methazolamide (Lichter et al, 1989).

The major use of carbonic anhydrase inhibitors is for long-term treatment of primary open-angle glaucoma and other chronic glaucomas refractory to parasympathomimetic miotics, beta blockers, and epinephrine. Although these drugs are generally given orally, the sodium salt of acetazolamide also can be given intravenously or intramuscularly.

Carbonic anhydrase inhibitors are used with osmotic agents, miotics, and topical beta blockers for the emergency treatment of acute angle-closure glaucoma. By reducing aqueous formation, carbonic anhydrase inhibitors decrease intraocular pressure, usually resulting in pupillary miosis and opening of the anterior chamber angle. These agents should be used only for *short-term* treatment prior to iridectomy because the lowered pressure may mask the fact that the angle is still partly closed. Peripheral anterior synechiae may then develop and cause permanent closure of the angle.

Carbonic anhydrase inhibitors also are used in other acute glaucomas (eg, glaucomatocyclitic crisis syndrome; glaucoma induced by sodium hyaluronate or laser procedures; glaucoma secondary to anterior uveitis or trauma) and in the preoperative treatment of congenital glaucoma.

For discussion of topical carbonic anhydrase inhibitors, see the section on Investigational Agents.

ADVERSE REACTIONS, PRECAUTIONS, AND INTERACTIONS. Transient myopia has been reported and may result from changes in lens hydration or forward movement of the lens. Carbonic anhydrase inhibitors commonly cause malaise, weight loss, fatigue, headache, weakness, nervousness, loss of libido, impotence, paresthesias, and, in infants, failure to thrive (Hurvitz et al, 1991). Lethargy and depression are common and often unrecognized until the drug is discontinued and the patient notices a sudden improvement in emotional state. Many patients cannot tolerate these agents for prolonged periods because of this malaise syndrome. Confusion, ataxia, tremor, and tinnitus have been observed rarely.

Carbonic anhydrase inhibitors frequently cause gastric distress, anorexia, nausea, vomiting, and diarrhea. Constipation also has been reported. Taking the medication with meals, lowering the dosage, supplementation with sodium bicarbonate, or substitution of one carbonic anhydrase inhibitor for another also may alleviate some side effects. Patients under 40 years of age tolerate these drugs better than older patients. Acetazolamide in prolonged-release capsule form may be better tolerated than the tablet form.

Diuresis may be troublesome initially but often subsides during continued therapy. The serum potassium level may fall during the first few weeks of treatment but usually returns to a near normal level unless a potassium-wasting diuretic (thiazide, loop diuretic) is taken concurrently. The hypokalemia is not associated with a clinically significant reduction in total body potassium; however, serum potassium levels should be monitored in patients taking another potassium-wasting diuretic.

Renal colic, hematuria, and oliguria or anuria may occur during prolonged therapy and are usually evidence of ureteral calculus formation. The renal stones may be precipitated by the reduced urinary excretion of citrate and/or magnesium, which decreases the solubility of calcium. Because of more extensive renal excretion, nephrolithiasis may occur more frequently with acetazolamide than with methazolamide. Carbonic anhydrase inhibitors reduce the glomerular filtration rate in patients with diabetic nephropathy (Skott et al, 1987).

The carbonic anhydrase inhibitors reduce uric acid excretion and increase the blood uric acid level. The hyperuricemia is usually asymptomatic but rarely has led to an exacerbation of gout. Other untoward effects include rash (due to sulfonamide sensitivity) and, rarely, drug fever, hirsutism, thrombocytopenia, leukopenia, agranulocytosis, and aplastic anemia. Adverse hemopoietic reactions most often appear within the first six months of treatment, and the mortality in patients who develop aplastic anemia is approximately 50%. The value of routine blood monitoring has been questioned (Mogk and Cyrlin, 1988), but patients should be instructed to report promptly the development of systemic symptoms such as a persistent sore throat, fever, fatigue, pallor, easy bruising, epistaxis, purpura, or jaundice (Fraunfelder et al, 1985).

Since carbonic anhydrase inhibitors may have teratogenic effects, these drugs should be avoided during early pregnancy. Negligible amounts of acetazolamide are excreted in breast milk.

Carbonic anhydrase inhibitors should be used cautiously in patients with obstructive pulmonary disease because they may precipitate acute respiratory failure. Rarely, these drugs have caused severe hyperchloremic acidosis in diabetic patients. Because they increase blood ammonia levels, carbonic anhydrase inhibitors should be avoided in patients with advanced liver disease.

Postoperative use of carbonic anhydrase inhibitors may adversely affect the outcome of filtering operations by reducing the size of the resultant drainage bleb and delaying reformation of the anterior chamber; therefore, these drugs are generally avoided after surgery. However, carbonic anhydrase inhibitors are used to slow aqueous humor flow and promote healing of fistulas with excessive leak. They also have been recommended when the filtration bleb shows signs of being compacted into a dense subconjunctival capsule. Aqueous suppression therapy has occasionally been associated with development of hypotony and ciliochoroidal detachment after filtration surgery (Vela and Campbell, 1985).

PHARMACOKINETICS. Carbonic anhydrase inhibitors are widely distributed throughout the body, with the highest concentrations present in tissues containing high concentrations of carbonic anhydrase, especially erythrocytes and the renal cortex. The drugs also enter the aqueous humor.

Different brands of acetazolamide may vary in bioavailability, and significant lot-to-lot variation has been found in some products. For this reason, bioequivalence requirements have been proposed for all carbonic anhydrase inhibitors. Therapeutic plasma levels of acetazolamide range from 4 to 10 mcg/ml. Acetazolamide is 93% protein bound. It is not metabolized, and 70% of an administered dose is recovered in the urine within 24 hours. The half-life is five hours. The nonsteroidal anti-inflammatory drug, diflunisal, competes with acetazolamide for plasma protein binding sites, thereby increasing both the therapeutic and toxic effects of the carbonic anhydrase inhibitor (Yablonski et al, 1988).

Methazolamide is well absorbed. It is only 55% protein bound and diffuses into tissues more readily than acetazolamide. Only 25% of a dose is excreted unchanged in the urine, but there is no information about metabolites.

Dichlorphenamide appears to be well absorbed, and maximal effects are observed two to four hours after administration. Its pharmacokinetic properties have not been studied extensively.

The absorption of carbonic anhydrase inhibitors does not appear to be reduced by food, and some ophthalmologists recommend taking them with food to decrease gastric irritation.

DOSAGE AND PREPARATIONS.

ACETAZOLAMIDE:

Oral: For primary open-angle glaucoma and other chronic glaucomas, see Table.

Generic. Tablets 125 and 250 mg.
AK-Zol (Akorn), ***Dazamide*** (Major). Tablets 250 mg.
Diamox (Storz). Capsules (prolonged-release) 500 mg; tablets 125 and 250 mg.

ACETAZOLAMIDE SODIUM:

Intravenous, Intramuscular: *Adults,* initially, 500 mg; the dose may be repeated, if necessary, in two to four hours. *Infants and children,* 5 to 10 mg/kg every six hours.

Diamox (Storz), ***Generic.*** Powder 500 mg (should be reconstituted with at least 5 ml of sterile water for injection).

DICHLORPHENAMIDE:

Oral: For primary open-angle glaucoma and other chronic glaucomas, see Table.

Daranide (Merck Sharp & Dohme). Tablets 50 mg.

METHAZOLAMIDE:

Oral: For primary open-angle glaucoma and other chronic glaucomas, see Table.

Neptazane (Storz). Tablets 25 and 50 mg.

OSMOTIC AGENTS

Hypertonic solutions of glycerin [Osmōglyn], isosorbide [Ismotic], urea [Ureaphil], or mannitol [Osmitrol] are used for the short-term reduction of intraocular pressure and vitreous volume. By increasing blood osmolarity, these agents induce the withdrawal of fluid from the eyeball by an osmotic effect. They also may decrease aqueous production by an effect on hypothalamic osmoreceptors. Osmotic agents cause an immediate, marked fall in intraocular pressure and reduction of vitreous volume and are generally effective even in patients who do not respond to miotics and carbonic anhydrase inhibitors.

In acute angle-closure glaucoma, osmotic agents are used to reduce intraocular pressure rapidly prior to iridectomy and to help reduce corneal edema. When the pressure elevation is pronounced, the iris sphincter becomes ischemic and may not respond to miotics unless pressure is reduced initially with an osmotic agent. Osmotic agents also may aid in opening the angle by reducing the volume of the posterior segment of the eye and temporarily reducing pressure behind the iris. If the miotic is then effective in opening the angle, the pressure may remain normal even after the osmotic effect has worn off.

In chronic glaucomas, osmotic agents are used only for pre- and postoperative treatment. They also are used pre- and postoperatively in congenital glaucoma, retinal detachment surgery, routine cataract extraction, and keratoplasty, and they may be of temporary benefit in some secondary glaucomas. Since their action depends on an intact blood-aqueous barrier, osmotic agents may be less effective in inflammatory secondary glaucomas and after iridectomy.

Mannitol and urea are given intravenously; they are equally effective in reducing intraocular pressure and vitreous volume, but mannitol is more convenient to administer and less toxic. Orally administered glycerin and isosorbide are not as rapidly effective as the intravenous agents but often are preferred because of their safety and convenience. Ethanol also has an osmotic action and may be given orally to reduce intraocular pressure in an emergency.

See the evaluations for adverse reactions and precautions.

Drug Evaluations

GLYCERIN

[Osmoglyn]

CH_2OH
$CHOH$
CH_2OH

USES. Oral glycerin is used to reduce intraocular pressure and vitreous volume prior to various ocular surgical procedures, such as cataract surgery and iridectomy, and for short-term treatment of some secondary glaucomas. Glycerin is probably safer than the intravenously administered agents, urea and mannitol, but it has a slower onset of action. A maximal reduction in intraocular pressure and vitreous volume occurs about one hour after administration, with a return to the pretreatment level in about five hours. Because it is rapidly metabolized, glycerin produces little diuresis, and routine urinary bladder catheterization for surgery is not required.

ADVERSE REACTIONS AND PRECAUTIONS. Headache, nausea, and vomiting are the most common untoward effects. Diarrhea occurs occasionally. Glycerin may cause hyperglycemia and glycosuria and should be used cautiously in diabetic patients. Confusion and amnesia may occur in older patients, but frank hyperosmolar nonketotic coma is a rare complication. Pulmonary edema has occurred rarely. The systemic effects of dehydration that occur with use of the intravenous osmotic agents are less likely with glycerin.

Glycerin is classified in FDA Pregnancy Category C.

DOSAGE AND PREPARATIONS.

Oral: *Adults and children,* 1 to 1.5 g/kg, given as a 50% or 75% solution. The drug may be administered more than once daily, if necessary. Lemon juice or instant coffee may be added to unflavored preparations. Palatability is also enhanced by pouring the solution over crushed ice and drinking through a straw, but patients should not be permitted to drink additional water.

Available generically in bulk form (unflavored) and may be diluted.

Osmoglyn (Alcon). Solution (oral) 50% (0.6 g/ml) in 220 ml containers.

ISOSORBIDE

[Ismotic]

Isosorbide is an oral osmotic agent used to reduce intraocular pressure and vitreous volume prior to ocular surgical procedures and for short-term treatment of some secondary glaucomas. It apparently has the same onset and duration of action as glycerin.

Untoward effects also are similar, although isosorbide does not adversely affect blood glucose levels and is preferred in diabetic patients. It also may cause less nausea and vomiting. Isosorbide produces a more significant diuresis than glycerin, and catheterization may be necessary. It also may cause diarrhea.

This drug is classified in FDA Pregnancy Category B.

DOSAGE AND PREPARATIONS.

Oral: *Adults,* initially, 1.5 g/kg. The drug may be given up to four times daily, if indicated. It may be poured over cracked ice to increase palatability.

Note: Isosorbide should not be confused with isosorbide dinitrate, an antianginal drug.

Ismotic (Alcon). Solution (oral) 45% (0.45 g/ml) in 220 ml containers.

MANNITOL

[Osmitrol]

CH_2OH
$HOCH$
$HOCH$
$HCOH$
$HCOH$
CH_2OH

ACTIONS AND USES. Mannitol is given intravenously to reduce intraocular pressure and vitreous volume prior to ocular surgical procedures and for short-term treatment of some secondary glaucomas. A maximal reduction in intraocular pressure occurs in 30 to 60 minutes and lasts six to eight hours.

If an intravenous osmotic agent is indicated, mannitol is generally preferred to urea because it is more convenient and less toxic. Impaired renal function is not a contraindication to its use, and it does not cause tissue necrosis if extravasation occurs. Mannitol may be less likely than urea to penetrate ocular fluids in the presence of inflammation and, in this situation, it would be more effective than urea.

ADVERSE REACTIONS AND PRECAUTIONS. Headache, nausea, vomiting, dehydration, and massive diuresis are common untoward effects of mannitol. Urinary bladder catheterization should be considered in patients who are undergoing surgery. Chills, dizziness, and chest pain also have been reported. The drug occasionally has caused agitation, disorientation, convulsions, and anaphylactoid reactions. Cardiovascular status should be evaluated before using mannitol. Because of the large amount of fluid required, an acute increase in intravascular volume with subsequent overload may result in pulmonary edema or intracranial hemorrhage. Fatalities have been reported.

Mannitol is classified in FDA Pregnancy Category C.

DOSAGE AND PREPARATIONS.

Intravenous: *Adults and children,* 0.5 to 2 g/kg as a 20% solution is infused over a period of 30 to 60 minutes. Administration may be discontinued when the desired effect has been obtained, even if the full dose has not been given. A total dose of 1 g/kg is usually sufficient, and smaller doses are sometimes effective.

Note: Mannitol should not be confused with mannitol hexanitrate, an antianginal drug.

Generic. Solution 5%, 10%, 15%, 20%, and 25%.

Osmitrol (Baxter Healthcare). Solution 5% in 1,000 ml containers, 10% in 500 and 1,000 ml containers, 15% in 500 ml containers, and 20% in 250 and 500 ml containers.

UREA FOR INJECTION
[Ureaphil]

Urea is used less commonly than other osmotic agents. Because the eye is permeable to urea, a rebound elevation in intraocular pressure and vitreous volume may occur after the ocular hypotensive effect has terminated (about 8 to 12 hours after administration), but this is not usually a significant clinical problem.

The systemic toxicity of urea is similar to that of mannitol. Urea is irritating to the tissues; it causes pain at the site of infusion and necrosis may result if extravasation occurs. Superficial and deep thrombosis may develop if urea is infused into the veins of the lower extremities. This agent should not be used in patients with severely impaired renal or hepatic function. Cardiovascular status should be evaluated before administering urea.

Urea is classified in FDA Pregnancy Category C.

Urea is often reconstituted with invert sugar solution. Invert sugar contains fructose, which can cause severe reactions (hypoglycemia, nausea, vomiting, tremors, coma, and convulsions) in patients with hereditary fructose intolerance (aldolase deficiency).

DOSAGE AND PREPARATIONS. The solution should be prepared just prior to use.

Intravenous: *Adults,* 0.5 to 2 g/kg of a 30% solution is administered at a rate of 60 drops/min. The usual dose is 1 g/kg. *Children,* 0.5 to 1.5 g/kg of a 30% solution is infused over a 30-minute period.

Ureaphil (Abbott). Powder (lyophilized, for injection) 40 g.

INVESTIGATIONAL AGENTS

Topical Carbonic Anhydrase Inhibitors

Adverse reactions associated with oral carbonic anhydrase inhibitors have led to their withdrawal in more than 50% of patients; thus, development of topical preparations that would be effective in lower doses and cause fewer reactions is desirable.

The investigational topical carbonic anhydrase inhibitors, MK-417 (sezolamide), MK-927, and MK-507, are based on modifications of an ethoxzolamide-like structure. MK-417 is the slightly more potent S-enantiomer of the racemic compound, MK-927. MK-507, the most recently synthesized compound, is specific for carbonic anhydrase isoenzyme II, the isoenzyme present in ciliary processes. The concentrations needed to inhibit isolated human carbonic anhydrase isoenzyme II are 0.2 nM, 0.5 nM, 1.2 nM, and 3.4 nM for MK-507, MK-417, MK-927, and acetazolamide, respectively (Lippa et al, 1991 B). In several clinical trials, these topical agents reduced ocular hypertension with minimal side effects.

MK-927, MK-417: In a single-dose study in patients with primary open-angle glaucoma, one drop of MK-927 1% or 2% reduced intraocular pressure by approximately 20% for six and eight hours, respectively (Higginbotham et al, 1990; Pfeiffer et al, 1990). A similar reduction in intraocular pressure with MK-927 2% was observed in patients with ocular hypertension (Serle et al, 1990). Multiple dosing and long-term treatment did not alter the efficacy (Lippa et al, 1991 A).

In a double-blind, randomized, placebo-controlled trial of patients with ocular hypertension or open-angle glaucoma, MK-417 1.8% reduced intraocular pressure by 20%, with the peak effect occurring two hours after instillation of the drops (Bron et al, 1991). MK-417 1.8% was slightly more effective than MK-927 2% in the four to ten hours after administration; however, transient ocular discomfort (burning, blurred vision, tearing, itching) occurred more frequently with MK-417 than with MK-927. Because of the short duration of activity of these compounds, topical application three times daily (MK-417 1.8% or MK-927 2%) as monotherapy is recommended.

MK-507: This agent lowered intraocular pressure in normal individuals and in patients with primary open-angle glaucoma or ocular hypertension (Lippa et al, 1991 B). The efficacy of MK-507 and MK-417 did not differ significantly in a comparative study, but more patients experienced transient stinging or burning with MK-417 instilled every eight hours than with MK-507 every eight hours or MK-507 every 12 hours. Common systemic adverse effects for both compounds were bitter taste and headache.

As with MK-927 and MK-417, instillation of drops three times daily is recommended for MK-507 2%.

Prostaglandins

The prostaglandins, a group of naturally occurring compounds derived from the conversion of arachidonic acid through the cyclooxygenase pathway, are potent coronary, systemic, and pulmonary vasodilators and inhibitors of platelet aggregation. In the eye, prostaglandins (PGFs), especially $PGF_{2\alpha}$, decrease intraocular pressure, probably through their action on uveoscleral drainage. Invasive perfusion studies in the eyes of monkeys showed that single doses of $PGF_{2\alpha}$ 4 mcg increased uveoscleral outflow by 60%, and twice-daily topical therapy for several days increased it two- to fourfold (Hurvitz et al, 1991).

Two forms of $PGF_{2\alpha}$, the tromethamine salt and the isopropyl ester (IE) derivative, have been tested in human eyes. The latter is much more potent, has better corneal penetration, and produces milder adverse effects (Camras et al, 1989; Kerstetter et al, 1988). One instillation of $PGF_{2\alpha}$-IE 1.12 mcg lowered the intraocular pressure by 20% in healthy individuals, with the peak effect noted eight hours after treatment (Kerstetter et al, 1988). In patients with ocular hypertension or open-angle glaucoma, the intraocular pressure was consistently reduced by 20% to 25% throughout an eight-day treatment period during which $PGF_{2\alpha}$-IE 0.5 mcg was instilled twice daily (Camras et al, 1989). There were no adverse effects on the pupillary diameter or visual acuity, but many patients experienced conjunctival hyperemia, ocular irritation, and a foreign body sensation.

$PGF_{2\alpha}$ is a very potent ocular hypotensive agent and may be a pharmacologic alternative to laser therapy or full-thickness filtering procedures for patients with low-tension glaucoma who have optic nerve and field vision loss.

LASER TRABECULOPLASTY

In addition to the use of medical therapy for lowering of intraocular pressure in various forms of glaucoma, the obstruction of aqueous outflow at the trabecular meshwork can be lessened by the use of a laser. Argon laser trabeculoplasty plays an important role in the treatment of severe primary open-angle glaucoma, pigmentary and exfoliation glaucoma, and normal-tension glaucoma, especially in patients refractory to medical therapy (Reiss et al, 1991). It also has been suggested that this procedure could be used in early primary open-angle glaucoma and hence can be regarded as an alternative treatment (The Glaucoma Laser Trial Research Group, 1990). In large studies of patients with primary open-angle glaucoma, argon laser trabeculoplasty reduced the intraocular pressure by one-third in 70% to 97% of patients during follow-up periods of five months to two years. Similar success rates were observed in patients with pigmentary and exfoliation glaucoma.

In general, older patients are more responsive to argon laser trabeculoplasty than younger patients. Since primary open-angle glaucoma is usually a bilateral disease, a good response in one eye usually signifies that the second eye will also do well. The greatest absolute reduction in pressure occurs in those with the highest initial pressures. The average reduction obtained in primary open-angle glaucoma is usually 30% or less.

A transient elevation of pressure was routinely observed in at least 25% of patients several hours after treatment (Reiss et al, 1991). The increase ranged from several mm Hg to >20 mm Hg. Although the duration of elevation in pressure is brief in most patients, the effect may be permanent. In addition, loss of central vision may occur. However, the post-treatment pressure spike usually can be alleviated by apraclonidine. In a prospective randomized, double-blind study in patients with open-angle glaucoma, pretreatment with apraclonidine 1% decreased the elevation of intraocular pressure to >10 mm Hg in laser-treated eyes (Robin et al, 1987 A, 1987 B). In addition, only 21% of those in the apraclonidine-treated group had any elevation of intraocular pressure as compared with 59% in the placebo group.

The formation of peripheral anterior synechiae also has been reported in more than 20% of the patients following argon laser trabeculoplasty (Reiss et al, 1991). The incidence was higher when this procedure was the initial treatment (The Glaucoma Laser Trial Research Group, 1990). Even though peripheral anterior synechiae, which usually extend just to the scleral spur, may be of no clinical significance, treatment at the anterior aspects of the trabecular meshwork may minimize their formation.

Other adverse effects of argon laser trabeculoplasty include transient uveitis, hyphema, corneal sequelae, and syncope. In addition, this procedure may lessen the chances of success of conventional filtration surgery, possibly because of the formation of encapsulated blebs (incidence, 28%) (Reiss et al, 1991).

Thus, argon laser trabeculoplasty may not be a curative measure in patients with glaucoma. However, it does control intraocular pressure for extended periods in many patients and, in some, it may delay the need for filtering surgery. The procedure can be useful for most patients with primary open-angle glaucoma, exfoliation syndrome glaucoma, pigmentary glaucoma, and angle-closure glaucoma who have been successfully treated with laser iridectomy but have a residual uncontrolled increase in intraocular pressure. It is considered to be less effective in normal-tension and aphakic/pseudophakic glaucoma.

Cited References

Akingbehin T, Villada JR: Metipranolol-associated granulomatous anterior uveitis. *Br J Ophthalmol* 75:519-523, 1991.

Allen RC, Epstein DL: Additive effect of betaxolol and epinephrine in primary open angle glaucoma. *Arch Ophthalmol* 104:1178-1184, 1986.

Allen RC, et al: A double-masked comparison of betaxolol vs timolol in the treatment of open-angle glaucoma. *Am J Ophthalmol* 101:535-541, 1986.

Allen RC, et al: Combination of levobunolol and dipivefrin for treatment of glaucoma. *Arch Ophthalmol* 106:904-907, 1988.

Battershill PE, Sorkin EM: Ocular metipranolol: A preliminary review of its pharmacodynamic and pharmacokinetic properties, and therapeutic efficacy in glaucoma and ocular hypertension. *Drugs* 36:601-615, 1988.

Beasley H, Fraunfelder FT: Retinal detachments and topical ocular miotics. *Ophthalmology* 86:95-98, 1979.

Begg LS, Cottle RW: Epidemiologic approach to open-angle glaucoma: 1. Control of intraocular pressure. Report of the Canadian Ocular Adverse Drug Reaction Registry Program. *Can J Ophthalmol* 23:273-278, 1988.

Berson FG, Epstein DL: Separate and combined effects of timolol maleate and acetazolamide in open-angle glaucoma. *Am J Ophthalmol* 92:788-791, 1981.

Bron A, et al: Multiple-dose efficacy comparison of the two topical carbonic anhydrase inhibitors sezolamide and MK-927. *Arch Ophthalmol* 109:50-53, 1991.

Brown RH, et al: ALO 2145 reduces the intraocular pressure elevation after anterior segment laser surgery. *Ophthalmology* 95:378-384, 1988.

Buckley MM-T, et al: Ocular betaxolol: A review of its pharmacological properties, and therapeutic efficacy in glaucoma and ocular hypertension. *Drugs* 40:75-90, 1990.

Camras CB, et al: Inhibition of epinephrine-induced reduction of intraocular pressure by systemic indomethacin in humans. *Am J Ophthalmol* 100:169-175, 1985.

Camras CB, et al: Maintained reduction of intraocular pressure by prostaglandin F2α-1-isopropylester applied in multiple doses in ocular hypertensive and glaucoma patients. *Ophthalmology* 96:1329-1337, 1989.

Dailey RA, et al: Effects of timolol maleate and acetazolamide on rate of aqueous formation in normal human subjects. *Am J Ophthalmol* 93:232-237, 1982.

David R, et al: Treatment of elevated intraocular pressure with concurrent levobunolol and pilocarpine. *Can J Ophthalmol* 22:208-211, 1987.

Dunn TL, et al: Effect of topical ophthalmic instillation of timolol and betaxolol on lung function in asthmatic subjects. *Am Rev Respir Dis* 133:264-268, 1986.

Fraunfelder FT, et al: Hematologic reactions to carbonic anhydrase inhibitors. *Am J Ophthalmol* 100:79-81, 1985.

Gaul GR, et al: Comparison of a noncardioselective β-adrenoceptor blocker and a cardioselective blocker in reducing aqueous flow in humans. *Arch Ophthalmol* 107:1308-1311, 1989.

The Glaucoma Laser Trial Research Group: The glaucoma laser trial (GLT): 2. Results of argon laser trabeculoplasty versus topical medicines. *Ophthalmology* 97:1403-1413, 1990.

Goldberg HS, et al: Effect of topical indomethacin and timolol maleate on intraocular pressure in normal subjects. *Am J Ophthalmol* 99:576-578, 1985.

Gonzalez JP, Clissold SP: Ocular levobunolol: Review of its pharmacodynamic and pharmacokinetic properties, and therapeutic efficacy. *Drugs* 34:648-661, 1987.

Higginbotham EJ, et al: MK-927: A topical carbonic anhydrase inhibitor: Dose response and duration of action. *Arch Ophthalmol* 108:65-68, 1990.

Hoskins HD, Kass M: *Becker-Shaffer's Diagnosis and Therapy of the Glaucomas*, ed 6. St. Louis, Mo, CV Mosby, 1989, 2-9.

Hurvitz LM, et al: New developments in the drug treatment of glaucoma. *Drugs* 41:514-532, 1991.

Kanski JJ: *Clinical Ophthalmology: A Systemic Approach,* ed 2. Boston, Mass, Butterworths, 1989.

Kass MA, et al: Dipivefrin and epinephrine treatment of elevated intraocular pressure: Comparative study. *Arch Ophthalmol* 97:1865-1866, 1979.

Kass MA, et al: Timolol and acetazolamide: Study of concurrent administration. *Arch Ophthalmol* 100:941-942, 1982.

Kerstetter JR, et al: Prostaglandin $F_{2\alpha}$-1-isopropyl ester lowers intraocular pressure without decreasing aqueous humor flow. *Am J Ophthalmol* 105:30-34, 1988.

Kitazawa Y, et al: The prevention of an acute rise in intraocular pressure following Q-switched Nd:YAG laser iridotomy with clonidine. *Graefe's Arch Clin Exp Ophthalmol* 227:13-16, 1989 A.

Kitazawa Y, et al: Use of apraclonidine to reduce acute intraocular pressure rise following Q-switched Nd:YAG laser iridotomy. *Ophthalmol Surg* 20:49-52, 1989 B.

Kohn AN, et al: Clinical comparison of dipivalyl epinephrine and epinephrine in treatment of glaucoma. *Am J Ophthalmol* 87:196-201, 1979.

Leier CV, et al: Cardiovascular effects of ophthalmic timolol. *Ann Intern Med* 104:197-199, 1986.

Levobunolol Study Group: Levobunolol: Four-year study of efficacy and safety in glaucoma treatment. *Ophthalmology* 96:642-645, 1989.

Lichter PR, et al: Intraocular pressure effects of carbonic anhydrase inhibitors in primary open-angle glaucoma. *Am J Ophthalmol* 107:11-17, 1989.

Lippa EA, et al: Multiple-dose, dose-response relationship for the topical carbonic anhydrase inhibitor MK-927. *Arch Ophthalmol* 109:46-49, 1991 A.

Lippa EA, et al: MK-507 versus sezolamide: Comparative efficacy of two topically active carbonic anhydrase inhibitors. *Ophthalmology* 98:308-313, 1991 B.

Long DA, et al: Levobunolol and betaxolol: Double-masked controlled comparison of efficacy and safety in patients with elevated intraocular pressure. *Ophthalmology* 95:735-741, 1988.

McMahon CD, et al: Adverse effects experienced by patients taking timolol. *Am J Ophthalmol* 88:736-738, 1979.

Migliori ME, et al: Intraocular pressure changes after neodymium-YAG laser capsulotomy in eyes pretreated with timolol. *Arch Ophthalmol* 105:473-475, 1987.

Mogk LG, Cyrlin MN: Blood dyscrasias and carbonic anhydrase inhibitors. *Ophthalmology* 95:768-771, 1988.

Moss AP, et al: Comparison of effects of timolol and epinephrine on intraocular pressure. *Am J Ophthalmol* 86:489-495, 1978.

Passo MS, et al: Plasma timolol in glaucoma patients. *Ophthalmology* 91:1361-1363, 1984.

Pfeiffer N, et al: A single dose of the topical carbonic anhydrase inhibitor MK-927 decreases IOP in patients. *Br J Ophthalmol* 74:405-408, 1990.

Reichert RW, et al: Intraocular pressure response to replacing pilocarpine with carbachol, letter. *Am J Ophthalmol* 106:747-748, 1988.

Reiss GR, et al: Laser trabeculoplasty. *Surv Ophthalmol* 35:407-428, 1991.

Robin AL: Short-term effects of unilateral 1% apraclonidine therapy. *Arch Ophthalmol* 106:912-915, 1988.

Robin AL: The role of apraclonidine hydrochloride in laser therapy for glaucoma. *Trans Am Ophthalmol Soc* 97:729-761, 1989.

Robin AL, et al: Effects of ALO 2145 on intraocular pressure following argon laser trabeculoplasty. *Arch Ophthalmol* 105:646-650, 1987 A.

Robin AL, et al: Effects of topical ALO 2145 (*p*-aminoclonidine hydrochloride) on acute intraocular pressure rise after argon laser iridotomy. *Arch Ophthalmol* 105:1208-1211, 1987 B.

Schenker HI, et al: Fluorophotometric study of epinephrine and timolol in human subjects. *Arch Ophthalmol* 99:1212-1216, 1981.

Schoene RB, et al: Timolol-induced bronchospasm in asthmatic bronchitis. *JAMA* 245:1460-1461, 1981.

Serle JB, et al: MK-927: A topical carbonic anhydrase inhibitor: Dose response and reproducibility. *Arch Ophthalmol* 108:838-841, 1990.

Shiose Y: Intraocular pressure: New perspectives. *Surv Ophthalmol* 34:413-435, 1990.

Silverstone DE, et al: Prophylactic treatment of intraocular pressure elevations after neodymium: YAG laser posterior capsulotomies and extracapsular cataract extractions with levobunolol. *Ophthalmology* 95:713-718, 1988.

Silverstone D, et al: Evaluation of once-daily levobunolol 0.25% and timolol 0.25% therapy for increased intraocular pressure. *Am J Ophthalmol* 112:56-60, 1991.

Skott P, et al: Effect of carbonic anhydrase inhibitors on glomerular filtration rate in diabetic nephropathy. *Br Med J* 294:549, 1987.

Theodore J, Leibowitz HM: External ocular toxicity of dipivalyl epinephrine. *Am J Ophthalmol* 88:1013-1016, 1979.

Tielsch JM, et al: Racial variations in the prevalence of primary open-angle glaucoma: The Baltimore Eye Survey. *JAMA* 266:369-374, 1991.

Van Buskirk EM: Adverse reactions from timolol administration. *Ophthalmology* 87:447-450, 1980.

Vela MA, Campbell DG: Hypotony and ciliochoroidal detachment following pharmacologic aqueous suppressant therapy in previously filtered patients. *Ophthalmology* 92:50-57, 1985.

Wandel T, et al: Glaucoma treatment with once-daily levobunolol. *Am J Ophthalmol* 101:298-304, 1986.

Weinreb RN, et al: Long-term betaxolol therapy in glaucoma patients with pulmonary disease. *Am J Ophthalmol* 106:162-167, 1988.

Weinreb RN, et al: A double-masked three-month comparison between 0.25% betaxolol suspension and 0.5% betaxolol ophthalmic solution. *Am J Ophthalmol* 110:189-192, 1990.

West DR, et al: Comparative efficacy of the β-blockers for prevention of increased intraocular pressure after cataract extraction. *Am J Ophthalmol* 106:168-173, 1988.

Wiles SB, et al: Control of intraocular pressure with apraclonidine hydrochloride after cataract extraction. *Am J Ophthalmol* 111:184-188, 1991.

Yablonski ME, et al: Enhancement of ocular hypotensive effect of acetazolamide by diflunisal. *Am J Ophthalmol* 106:332-336, 1988.

Zimmerman TJ, et al: Improving therapeutic index of topically applied ocular drugs. *Arch Ophthalmol* 102:551-553, 1984.

Mydriatics, Cycloplegics, Local Anesthetics, and Intraocular Miotics

94

MYDRIATICS AND CYCLOPLEGICS

The eye is served by both the parasympathetic and sympathetic autonomic nervous systems. The parasympathetic fibers innervate the ciliary body and iris sphincter and the sympathetic fibers innervate the dilator muscles of the iris and the ciliary muscles. Parasympathetic stimulation constricts the longitudinal muscles of the ciliary body (accommodation) and the iris sphincter (miosis). Sympathetic stimulation constricts the dilator muscle of the iris, resulting in pupillary dilation (mydriasis).

Anticholinergic drugs are applied topically to the eye to produce cycloplegia (paralysis of accommodation of ciliary muscles) and mydriasis. They are used primarily as an aid in refraction, internal examination of the eye, and other diagnostic procedures; to produce mydriasis and cycloplegia before, during, and after intraocular surgery; and to treat anterior uveitis and some secondary glaucomas. The anticholinergic drugs available commercially as ophthalmic preparations include atropine, scopolamine (hyoscine), homatropine, cyclopentolate, and tropicamide.

Adrenergic agents produce mydriasis without cycloplegia. Phenylephrine and epinephrine act directly on the adrenergic receptors, whereas cocaine has an indirect action. Cocaine prevents neuronal reuptake of the neurotransmitter, thereby increasing its concentration at the neuronal synapse.

Phenylephrine, the most commonly administered topical adrenergic drug, is useful for diagnostic purposes, ocular surgery, and as an adjunct in the treatment of anterior uveitis to prevent formation of posterior synechiae (adhesions). Epinephrine dilates the pupil when a dilute solution is instilled into the anterior chamber during ophthalmic surgery. It does not produce significant mydriasis when applied topically unless the corneal epithelium is disturbed. Since adrenergic and anticholinergic drugs act by different mechanisms, wider mydriasis can be obtained by using a combination of both agents.

Uses

DIAGNOSIS. Refraction: Both the cycloplegic and mydriatic actions of anticholinergic drugs are useful in estimating errors of refraction. Cycloplegia prevents accommodation during refraction and reveals latent refractive errors (eg, in hyperopia); mydriasis facilitates retinoscopic estimation of the refractive error. Highly pigmented eyes are relatively resistant to topical cycloplegics, and more frequent instillation or use of a stronger solution may be required.

Atropine is the most potent mydriatic-cycloplegic drug in clinical use. It has a slow onset and a very long duration of action; in adults, residual cycloplegia may persist for six days or more and mydriasis for two or three weeks. Because of its prolonged action, atropine is not used for refraction in adults, but it is useful for children up to 5 or 6 years of age, especially when esotropia is present (Hiatt and Jerkins, 1983). Scopolamine has a cycloplegic effect almost equal to that of atropine. Although its duration of action is somewhat shorter (approximately three days), it is still too long for refraction in adults.

The shorter acting cycloplegics, particularly cyclopentolate and tropicamide, are used for refraction in adults, older children, and sometimes in young children. Homatropine is also used occasionally for refraction in children. It is longer acting than cyclopentolate or tropicamide; residual cycloplegia may persist for 36 to 48 hours. Cyclopentolate induces maximal cycloplegia in 25 to 75 minutes with complete recovery in 6 to 24 hours. It is preferred to atropine by some ophthalmologists for refraction in children over 2 to 3 years of age, including those with convergent strabismus. Tropicamide is a weaker cycloplegic, but its potency and duration of action are sufficient for refraction in adults. Examination must be performed within 20 to 35 minutes or it may be necessary to instill an additional drop. However, one drop of cyclopentolate given with the initial drop of tropicamide extends the period of cycloplegia to 60 to 70 minutes. Complete recovery of accommodation occurs two to six hours after administration. Mydriasis, especially of blue irides, may persist for 24 to 36 hours with cyclopentolate and rarely with tropicamide.

For dosage of drugs used for refraction, see Table 1.

Funduscopic Examination: Adrenergic and short-acting anticholinergic drugs are used to dilate the pupil for examination of the intraocular structures. Tropicamide (1%) produces adequate pupillary dilation in most adults within 15 minutes, which makes it useful for routine funduscopic screening (Steinmann et al, 1987). Phenylephrine produces mydriasis without cycloplegia, thus avoiding the inconvenience of residual blurring of vision.

Because of the reflex contraction of the iris sphincter caused by exposure to the light from an ophthalmoscope, an anticholinergic agent must be used with an adrenergic drug when wide mydriasis is needed. Phenylephrine 2.5% may be combined with tropicamide 0.5% or 1% or cyclopentolate 0.5% in a single solution or separately. The combination eliminates the need for multiple instillations and usually produces adequate mydriasis in patients with dark irides (whose pupils may be difficult to dilate). The effect of mydriatics is enhanced by prior instillation of a local anesthetic (Apt and Henrick, 1980; Sinclair et al, 1980). Closing the eye after instillation also enhances absorption and produces more rapid mydriasis.

In patients with open-angle glaucoma, prolonged miotic therapy may lead to fibrotic changes in the sphincter muscle and loss of tone of the dilator muscle. Combined use of phenylephrine and tropicamide may be necessary to produce mydriasis in these patients. The pupils of diabetic patients also respond poorly to topical anticholinergics, but a tropicamide/phenylephrine combination produces satisfactory mydriasis (Huber et al, 1985).

After ocular examination, the alpha-adrenergic blocking agents, dapiprazole [Rev-Eyes] (Allinson et al, 1990) or the investigational agent, moxisylyte (thymoxamine) (Relf et al, 1988; Wright et al, 1990), can be used to constrict the pupil without affecting intraocular pressure, outflow of aqueous humor, ciliary muscle, or anterior chamber depth. Dapiprazole 0.03% and moxisylyte 0.1% safely and effectively reverse phenylephrine-induced mydriasis. Both agents are more effective in light irides, possibly because of pigmentary binding in dark irides (Wright et al, 1990). Pilocarpine also reverses mydriasis induced by phenylephrine (Saheb et al, 1982); however, it may increase pupillary block by constricting the iris sphincter and it may precipitate angle closure.

For dosages of drugs used for ophthalmoscopy, see Table 2.

TABLE 1.
AGENTS USED FOR REFRACTION

Drug	Dosage (Topical)
Atropine Sulfate	*Children:* One drop of 0.125% solution (in infants less than 1 year), 0.25% solution (in children 1 to 5 years and in all children with blue irides), 0.5% solution or ointment (in children over 5 years), or 1% solution or ointment (in children with dark irides) is applied three times daily for three days prior to refraction and once on the morning of refraction. (If ointment is used, it should not be applied for several hours prior to refraction because it will impair the transparency of the cornea and alter the regularity of its refraction.) Administration should be discontinued if systemic effects occur.
Cyclopentolate Hydrochloride	*Adults:* One drop of 1% solution (or 2% in patients with dark irides) is instilled once, or one drop of 0.5% solution is instilled and repeated in five minutes.
	Children: One drop of 1% solution is instilled and repeated in ten minutes. *Infants under 1 year:* 0.5% solution should be used.
Homatropine Hydrobromide	*Children:* One drop of 2% or 5% solution is instilled and may be repeated if necessary in 5 to 10 minutes.
Scopolamine Hydrobromide	*Children:* One drop of 0.25% solution is instilled twice daily for two days prior to refraction.
Tropicamide	*Adults:* Two drops of 1% solution are instilled and repeated in five minutes.

TABLE 2.
AGENTS USED FOR OPHTHALMOSCOPY

Drug	Dosage (Topical)
Cyclopentolate Hydrochloride	One drop of 0.5% solution, repeated in five minutes if necessary. For *preterm infants,* a 0.2% solution should be used. For wider mydriasis in *older children and adults,* one drop of a solution containing 0.5% cyclopentolate and 2.5% phenylephrine.
Cyclopentolate Hydrochloride and Phenylephrine Hydrochloride	One drop of solution containing 0.2% cyclopentolate and 1% phenylephrine, repeated in five minutes if necessary (may be used safely in *preterm infants).*
Tropicamide	One drop of 0.5% or 1% solution, repeated in five minutes if necessary. For wider mydriasis, one drop of a solution containing 0.5% tropicamide and 2.5% phenylephrine. For examination of patients with primary open-angle glaucoma who are being treated with miotics or for diabetics, a solution containing equal parts of 0.5% tropicamide and 10% phenylephrine may be used.
Phenylephrine Hydrochloride	One drop of 2.5% solution, repeated in five minutes if necessary.

Provocative Test for Angle-Closure Glaucoma: Angle-closure glaucoma can be detected by instillation of a short-acting mydriatic such as tropicamide or phenylephrine (Hoskins and Kass, 1989). Results are considered positive if the pressure increases by 8 mm Hg within one hour and the angle is gonioscopically closed at the time of the elevation.

Horner's Syndrome: Horner's syndrome is characterized by total or partial interruption of sympathetic innervation to the eye; this causes a moderate degree of ptosis, miosis, and anhidrosis. Unilateral Horner's syndrome can be diagnosed by bilateral instillation of cocaine eyedrops, which dilates the pupil in the unaffected eye but not in the affected one.

Once the presence of Horner's syndrome is confirmed, the lesion usually can be localized by instilling hydroxyamphetamine 1% 48 hours later to allow cocaine to dissipate (Cremer et al, 1990). The denervated pupil should dilate if the lesion is preganglionic but not if it is postganglionic. The production of hydroxyamphetamine [Paredrine] was discontinued in 1989 (Burde and Thompson, 1991), but this drug may be obtained from the manufacturer on a compassionate-use basis.

INTRAOCULAR SURGERY. Mydriatic eyedrops are instilled prior to some ocular surgical procedures, particularly cataract extraction, retinal detachment operations, and vitreous surgery. Full mydriasis allows direct visualization to ensure adequate capsulotomy, phacoemulsification, and aspiration of lens material. Phenylephrine may produce sufficient mydriasis for intracapsular cataract extraction. For procedures requiring maximal mydriasis (eg, extracapsular cataract extraction, vitreous surgery), phenylephrine may be given with an anticholinergic drug (Barraquer and Barraquer, 1985). Short-acting mydriatics are preferred for implantation of a posterior chamber intraocular lens.

Manipulation of the iris during surgery is believed to release prostaglandins that have a constrictor effect on the iris sphincter. Since this action is independent of the cholinergic and adrenergic receptors, miosis will occur even in the presence of anticholinergic or adrenergic drugs. Prostaglandin synthetase inhibitors (topical flurbiprofen [Ocufen], suprofen [Profenal], or topical indomethacin [investigational preparation]) have been given prior to surgery to prevent or reduce surgically induced miosis (Keates and McGowan, 1984; Keulen-De Vos et al, 1983).

Another possible local mediator is the neuropeptide, Substance P, which is found in various small-diameter nerve fibers, including the iris sphincter innervation (Caprioli et al, 1985). Miosis induced by surgical trauma may be mediated by the action of Substance P on the iris sphincter muscle, an effect that cannot be prevented by cholinergic blockade. Adrenergic drugs counteract the miosis by acting on the dilator muscle of the iris (Barraquer and Barraquer, 1985).

Epinephrine hydrochloride may be administered intracamerally in a very dilute solution to produce mydriasis during surgery. Since the commercial 1:1,000 solution contains sodium bisulfite as a preservative and most preservatives are highly toxic to the corneal endothelium, the commercial preparation should be diluted with a solution appropriate for intraocular use. Endothelial damage can be prevented if the commercial epinephrine solution is diluted to a concentration not exceeding 1:5,000. Phenylephrine, which is a pure alpha agonist, has been suggested for use when halogenated anesthetics are employed (Barraquer and Barraquer, 1985).

The pupil is dilated daily after some ocular surgical procedures to prevent formation of posterior synechiae. Atropine, scopolamine, or a shorter-acting anticholinergic agent may be instilled one to several times daily until slit-lamp examination shows minimal iritis. An alpha-adrenergic agonist, such as phenylephrine, may be given as well. In addition to their use for postoperative iritis, cycloplegics are useful to prevent or treat a shallow or flat anterior chamber after filtering surgery.

Strong mydriatics and cycloplegics are *not* instilled after extracapsular cataract surgery with placement of a posterior chamber intraocular lens, because mydriasis may cause the iris to become trapped behind the lens. Intraocular miotics, such as acetylcholine [Miochol] or carbachol [Miostat], are used at the end of this procedure. Short-acting mydriatic agents have been employed with some success to reposition dislocated intraocular lens implants, especially the iris-clip type.

ANTERIOR UVEITIS. Uveitis is an inflammation of the uveal tract and its adjacent structures; anterior uveitis encompasses inflammation of the iris and anterior part of the ciliary body. The primary symptoms of acute anterior uveitis are photophobia, pain, redness, decreased vision, and lacrimation. Topical corticosteroids are the mainstay in the treatment of anterior uveitis (see index entry Adrenal Corticosteroids, Uses, Ocular Disorders); antibiotics are given when ocular infection is present. Cycloplegics are used adjunctively to relieve pain by relaxing the ciliary muscles and to prevent iris-lens adhesions by dilating the pupil and reducing abnormal vascular permeability. Atropine and scopolamine are often preferred because the duration of action of shorter-acting agents is further reduced in the inflamed eye and because the latter drugs are more expensive. The cycloplegic may be supplemented with phenylephrine for maximal mydriasis. Shorter acting anticholinergics (eg, homatropine, cyclopentolate) are used when inflammation is mild and may be preferred when the intraocular pressure is elevated. The shorter-acting agents also may be employed in acute iritis to keep the iris in motion and prevent it from becoming sealed by synechiae in a mydriatic position.

SECONDARY GLAUCOMAS. ***Glaucoma Associated with Intraocular Inflammation:*** In acute anterior uveitis, increased permeability of the nonpigmented epithelium of the ciliary body and blood vessels of the iris leads to an outpouring of protein and inflammatory cells into the anterior chamber. The exudates may obstruct the trabecular meshwork and increase resistance to outflow of aqueous humor. If the inflammation persists, permanent obstruction may develop due to adhesions that seal the iris to the angle structures (peripheral anterior synechiae). These may occur with or without pupillary block (Hoskins and Kass, 1989).

Treatment of anterior uveitis with topical corticosteroids and cycloplegics may prevent these complications. A topical beta blocker and/or epinephrine and systemic antiglaucoma drugs (a carbonic anhydrase inhibitor and, for short-term therapy, an osmotic agent) may be used to reduce elevated intraocular pressure. (See index entry Glaucoma.) Miotics should be avoided in the presence of active inflammation, but may be helpful later if glaucoma persists after uveitis has subsided; they may be useful as long as the anterior chamber angle is open. It is important to rule out steroid therapy as a cause of the glaucoma.

Pupillary block is another potential complication of chronic or recurrent anterior uveitis. Contact between the inflamed iris and the anterior surface of the lens allows the formation of adhesions that seal the iris to the lens. These posterior synechiae prevent passage of aqueous humor from the posterior to the anterior chamber through the pupil (pupillary block). As a result, the iris bulges forward (iris bombé) closing the anterior chamber angle and causing the intraocular pressure to rise. Pupillary block also may occur in the absence of the lens (aphakia) when posterior synechiae seal the iris to the bulging vitreous face or lens capsule. Predisposing causes are an occluded iridectomy or iridotomy and wound leak.

Dilation of the pupil reduces contact between the iris and the lens or the vitreous face and may prevent formation of posterior synechiae or aid in breaking them once they have formed. Intensive mydriatic-cycloplegic therapy with atropine or scopolamine and phenylephrine may be required, along with topical corticosteroids (if inflammation is active) and antiglaucoma therapy (see the chapter, Drugs Used for Glaucoma). By reducing vitreous volume, an osmotic agent may be particularly helpful to break pupillary block in eyes with angle closure. Subconjunctival injection of 0.1 ml of a mixture containing equal proportions of cocaine 4%, atropine 1%, and epinephrine 1:1,000 has been used rarely to break resistant synechiae in aphakia; the blood pressure should be monitored when this combination is used because it will rise alarmingly in an occasional patient. If medical treatment fails to relieve pupillary block, surgery should be performed.

Malignant (Ciliary Block) Glaucoma: In malignant glaucoma, a rare complication of ocular surgery, forward displacement of the lens, ciliary processes, and iris flattens the anterior chamber and closes its angle. Blockage of aqueous flow past the ciliary process (ciliary block), increased vitreous pressure, and an abnormal laxity in the zonules are believed to be the causative factors.

Mydriatic-cycloplegic therapy with atropine (or scopolamine) and phenylephrine may promote re-formation of the anterior chamber and opening of the angle, presumably by increasing tension on the zonules and by relieving ciliary block. A beta-adrenergic blocking agent or carbonic anhydrase inhibitor can be administered to reduce pressure from within the vitreous. If drug therapy is successful, the systemic drugs and phenylephrine may be discontinued but, in many cases, the cycloplegic must be administered indefinitely. Surgery may be necessary in unresponsive patients. Medical therapy is rarely effective in aphakic malignant (ciliovitreal block) glaucoma; laser or surgical disruption of the anterior hyaloid may be the treatment of choice.

Lens Subluxation: Although mydriatic-cycloplegic drugs have been used to treat acute glaucoma associated with anterior dislocation of the lens, pupillary dilation in the presence of a dislocated lens in the posterior chamber may promote anterior migration of the loose lens.

MISCELLANEOUS USES. Cycloplegic drugs have been used to discourage accommodation in other ocular disorders. In patients with severe functional spasm of accommodation, atropine is sometimes applied daily for three or four weeks to provide a period of accommodative rest.

Because of evidence that close work may contribute to the progression of myopia, there has been some interest in the use of atropine to retard its progression (Brodstein et al, 1984). The efficacy of chronic cycloplegia for treating myopia remains highly controversial and the potential adverse effects of long-term therapy are of concern.

In suppression amblyopia when occlusion therapy is unsuccessful or not feasible, atropine has been employed to blur vision in the normal eye, thus forcing fixation with the amblyopic eye. Atropine is most effective if the fixing eye is significantly hyperopic because cycloplegia impairs both near and distance vision in hyperopes, while it primarily blurs near vision in myopes and emmetropes.

Atropine has been used occasionally in accommodative esotropia to prevent convergence by paralyzing accommodation. This form of therapy is not consistently effective because the blurred vision induced by the cycloplegic may increase accommodative effort and thereby increase the degree of esotropia, especially initially or as the effect of the drug wears off.

Adverse Reactions and Precautions

LOCAL REACTIONS. Both anticholinergic and adrenergic mydriatics can precipitate an attack of acute angle-closure glaucoma in eyes with anatomically narrow angles (Fraunfelder, 1989). An abrupt elevation of intraocular pressure occurs when the pupil is mid-dilated, because this position maximizes iris-lens contact and blocks the forward movement of aqueous through the pupil (pupillary block). The increased pressure behind the iris causes it to bow forward, obstructing outflow through the anterior chamber angle. An attack of closed-angle glaucoma also can be precipitated by crowding of the peripheral iris into the chamber angle in patients with plateau-type irides. Angle closure sometimes reverses spontaneously, but therapy often is required to break the block. Long-acting mydriatics (atropine or scopolamine) should not be used preoperatively in eyes predisposed to angle closure, and shorter-acting mydriatics should be used cautiously, if at all.

Topical anticholinergic drugs increase intraocular pressure to some degree in 25% to 30% of eyes with open-angle glaucoma (Shaw and Lewis, 1986) and occasionally in normal eyes. The rise in pressure is self-limited and is not caused by closure of the angle. It appears to be due to increased resistance to aqueous outflow associated with loss of ciliary muscle tone or to blocking of the trabecular meshwork by pigment liberated from the iris.

When treating anterior uveitis, posterior synechiae may form if mydriatic drugs (particularly the long-acting agents) are applied for prolonged periods without moving the pupil. Periodic brief discontinuation of the mydriatic may prevent this complication.

Patients with keratoconus and Down's syndrome are particularly sensitive to the mydriatic effect of anticholinergic drugs. Atropine and scopolamine should be used cautiously in these individuals.

Anticholinergic drugs cause blurred vision, glare, and photophobia. Atropine may cause contact dermatitis of the lids and allergic conjunctivitis. Allergic reactions are less common with the other anticholinergic agents.

Adrenergic drugs may cause browache, headache, blurred vision, hypersensitivity reactions, pain, and lacrimation. Pigment granules in the anterior chamber may be observed with slit lamp biomicroscopy several minutes after instillation. They disappear within 12 to 24 hours and occur with decreasing frequency when the drug is administered repeatedly. These granules are apparently released from the iris and are derived from degenerated cells in the iris pigment epithelium that rupture when the dilator muscle contracts. They occur most commonly in older patients with dark irides and in those with pigment dispersion syndrome and exfoliation syndrome. If the angle of the anterior chamber is open, the effect is transient and usually requires no treatment unless the optic nerve is vulnerable to pressure damage.

SYSTEMIC REACTIONS. Systemic reactions may occur after instillation of anticholinergic or adrenergic drugs, particularly in children and elderly patients. These drugs should be instilled in the lowest effective concentration and no more often than needed to obtain the desired response. Systemic absorption can be reduced and corneal contact time prolonged by gentle eyelid closure for five minutes after instillation (which reduces the action of the nasolacrimal pump) and pressure at the inner canthus (which minimizes drainage into the nose and throat) (Zimmerman et al, 1984). Excess solution should be blotted with a tissue.

Symptoms of anticholinergic toxicity include dryness of the mouth and skin, flushing, fever, rash, thirst, tachycardia, irritability, dizziness, depression, weeping, hyperactivity, ataxia, confusion, somnolence, hallucinations, delirium, and, rarely, seizures, coma, and death. Systemic reactions are most common after instillation of atropine, scopolamine, or cyclopentolate 2% [Cyclogyl]. Cyclopentolate and scopolamine in particular have caused transient, acute psychosis. Children with fair complexions or brain damage may be especially susceptible.

Some cases of delirium after cataract surgery may be caused by anticholinergic toxicity (Summers and Reich, 1979). Atropine eyedrops have been associated with the development of arrhythmias (atrial fibrillation, supraventricular tachycardias) in elderly hypertensive patients undergoing glaucoma surgery (Merli et al, 1986). Bladder atony and urinary retention may be a problem, especially in elderly men with prostatic hypertrophy. Cyclopentolate 0.5% affects gastrointestinal function in preterm infants, but a 0.25% solution does not (Isenberg et al, 1985).

For ophthalmoscopy, one drop of a dilute solution of a combination of phenylephrine and tropicamide or cyclopentolate provides adequate mydriasis and reduces the risk of systemic toxicity from multiple applications and/or higher concentrations (Apt and Henrick, 1980; Sinclair et al, 1980). Physostigmine salicylate is an effective antidote for anticholinergic toxicity (see index entry Physostigmine, In Anticholinergic Toxicity).

Tachycardia, hypertension, ventricular arrhythmias, anginal pain, myocardial infarction, cardiac arrest, subarachnoid hemorrhage, hyperhidrosis, blanching, tremors, agitation, and confusion may occur following ocular instillation of adrenergic drugs. These systemic reactions are most common when a strong concentration (phenylephrine 10%) is instilled repeatedly (Fraunfelder, 1989). Neonates, elderly patients, adults with orthostatic hypotension, and patients given systemic atropine are particularly at risk. For neonates, elderly patients, and those with known cardiovascular disease, the 2.5% solution of phenylephrine is safer than the 10% solution but is still too concentrated for low-weight (less than 1,600 g) neonates. The risk of systemic toxicity in neonates and infants can be reduced by decreasing the drop volume (Lynch et al, 1987). A solution containing cyclopentolate 0.2% and phenylephrine 1% [Cyclomydril] appears to be safe and effective for mydriasis in premature infants (Isenberg et al, 1984).

The sulfites present in many mydriatic solutions can cause severe bronchospasm and occasionally anaphylactic reactions in sensitive patients (Onorato, 1985). Asthmatic patients are particularly likely to manifest sensitivity to these compounds.

Drug Evaluations

ANTICHOLINERGIC AGENTS

ATROPINE SULFATE

[Atropair, Atropine-Care, Atropisol, Isopto Atropine, Ocu-Tropine]

ACTIONS AND USES. Atropine is a potent, long-acting mydriatic and cycloplegic. Its effect on accommodation may last six days or longer and mydriasis may persist for two or three weeks. Atropine is used for pre- and postoperative mydriasis, in anterior uveitis, and in some secondary glaucomas. It may be used for refraction in children up to age 5 or 6 years and is the most potent cycloplegic for use in children with convergent strabismus (Hiatt and Jerkins, 1983). Because of its long duration of action, atropine is not useful for refraction in adults.

ADVERSE REACTIONS AND PRECAUTIONS. Acute angle-closure glaucoma may occur if atropine is instilled in eyes with anatomically narrow angles. This agent also may increase intraocular pressure in eyes with open-angle glaucoma and in some normal eyes. Systemic reactions may occur, particularly in children and elderly patients. Contact dermatitis and allergic conjunctivitis are not uncommon. See also the section on Adverse Reactions and Precautions in the Introduction.

Atropine is classified in FDA Pregnancy Category C.

DOSAGE AND PREPARATIONS.

Topical: For preoperative mydriasis, one drop of a 1% solution, often supplemented with one drop of phenylephrine, is instilled prior to surgery. Some surgeons prefer to instill drops for several days prior to surgery as well.

In anterior segment inflammation, the concentration and frequency of administration are determined by the severity of inflammation and the pupillary response. Atropine may be supplemented with phenylephrine for maximal mydriasis.

For anterior uveitis or postoperative mydriasis, one drop of a 1% to 2% solution instilled once daily is often adequate, but more frequent use (maximum, three times daily) may be required in the presence of severe inflammation. A 0.5% solution or ointment applied one to three times daily is often adequate in children. When slit-lamp examination reveals minimal inflammation, a less potent agent, such as homatropine, may be substituted.

To break posterior synechiae, drops may be instilled more frequently, eg, one drop of a 2% solution (alternately with phenylephrine 10%) every five to ten minutes for five applications of each. The risk of toxicity from each drug is increased with increasing dosage.

For malignant (ciliary block) glaucoma, initially, one drop of a 1% or 2% solution and one drop of phenylephrine 10% three or four times daily. For maintenance, one drop of a 1% or 2% solution daily or every other day.

For refraction in *children,* see Table 1.

All preparations available in topical ophthalmic forms.

Atropair (Texas). Solution (sterile) 1% in 2 and 15 ml containers; ointment (sterile) 1% in 3.75 g containers.

Atropine-Care (Akorn). Solution (sterile) 1% with benzalkonium chloride 0.01% in 2, 5, and 15 ml containers.

Atropine Sulfate (Allergan). Solution (sterile) 1% with chlorobutanol 0.5% in 15 ml containers; ointment (sterile) 0.5% and 1% (***S.O.P.***) with chlorobutanol 0.5% in 3.5 g containers.

Atropine Sulfate Steri-Unit (Alcon). Solution (sterile) 1% and 2% (preservative free) in 2 ml containers.

Atropisol (Iolab). Solution (sterile) 0.5%, 1%, and 2% with benzalkonium chloride in 1 ml containers and 1% with benzalkonium chloride and edetate disodium in 5 and 15 ml containers.

Isopto Atropine (Alcon). Solution (sterile) 0.5%, 1%, and 3% with benzalkonium chloride 0.01% in 5 and 15 (1% concentration only) ml containers.

Ocu-Tropine (Ocumed). Solution (sterile) 1% in 15 ml containers; ointment (sterile) 1% in 3.5 g containers.

Ophthalmic forms also marketed by other manufacturers under generic name: Solution 1% and 2%; ointment 0.5% and 1%.

CYCLOPENTOLATE HYDROCHLORIDE

[AK-Pentolate, Cyclogyl, Ocu-Pentolate, Pentolair]

ACTIONS AND USES. Cyclopentolate is an effective mydriatic and cycloplegic with a rapid onset and relatively short duration of action. Cycloplegia is maximal 25 to 75 minutes after instillation, and recovery of accommodation is complete in 6 to 24 hours. This drug is used as an aid in refraction, for ophthalmoscopy, and for preoperative mydriasis. The mydriatic effect may be greater than that of other cycloplegic drugs and is enhanced by phenylephrine. One drop of a solution containing 0.5% cyclopentolate and 2.5% phenylephrine is usually adequate for ophthalmoscopy; maximal effects occur 60 minutes after instillation.

ADVERSE REACTIONS AND PRECAUTIONS. Cyclopentolate has caused systemic reactions in both children and adults. Mild reactions of short duration are common. Severe central nervous system disturbances, manifested by ataxia, hallucinations, and seizures, have occurred rarely in children. Vomiting, abdominal distention, and adynamic ileus developed in a pair of premature twins following instillation of six drops of the 1% solution. One of the twins subsequently died from necrotizing enterocolitis. Even the 0.5% solution affects gastric function in premature infants (Isenberg et al, 1985) and full-term neonates (Hermansen and Sullivan, 1985). Acute angle closure may occur if cyclopentolate is instilled in eyes with anatomically narrow angles. See also the section on Adverse Reactions and Precautions in the Introduction.

Cyclopentolate is classified in FDA Pregnancy Category C.

DOSAGE AND PREPARATIONS.
Topical: For refraction, see Table 1. For ophthalmoscopy, see Table 2.

All preparations available as topical ophthalmic solutions.

AK-Pentolate (Akorn). Solution (sterile) 0.5% and 1% with edetate disodium 0.01% and benzalkonium chloride 0.01% in 2 (1% concentration only) and 15 ml containers.

Cyclogyl (Alcon). Solution (sterile) 0.5%, 1%, and 2% with edetate disodium and benzalkonium chloride 0.01% in 2, 5, and 15 ml containers.

Ocu-Pentolate (Ocumed), ***Pentolair*** (Texas). Solution (sterile) 1% in 2, 5, and 15 ml containers.

Ophthalmic forms also marketed by other manufacturers under generic name: Solution 1%.

CYCLOPENTOLATE HYDROCHLORIDE AND PHENYLEPHRINE HYDROCHLORIDE
[Cyclomydril]

This combination is used to produce wide mydriasis for ophthalmoscopy and for preoperative mydriasis. It may be the mydriatic of choice in premature neonates (Isenberg et al, 1984).

See the individual evaluations on Cyclopentolate Hydrochloride and on Phenylephrine Hydrochloride and the section on Adverse Reactions and Precautions in the Introduction.

DOSAGE AND PREPARATIONS.
Topical: For ophthalmoscopy, see Table 2.

Cyclomydril (Alcon). Solution (sterile) containing cyclopentolate hydrochloride 0.2% and phenylephrine hydrochloride 1% with benzalkonium chloride 0.01% and edetate disodium in 2 and 5 ml containers.

HOMATROPINE HYDROBROMIDE
[AK-Homatropine, Isopto Homatropine]

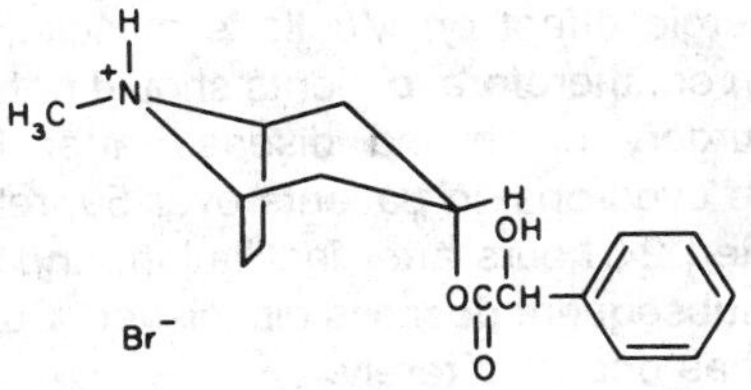

H
H_3C—$\overset{+}{N}$
H
OH
OCCH
O
Br^-

Homatropine is a mydriatic and cycloplegic used for refraction and for treatment of anterior uveitis. Repeated instillation of the 2% solution at ten-minute intervals produces maximal cycloplegia in 60 minutes. Effects may persist for 36 to 48 hours.

For adverse effects, see the section on Adverse Reactions and Precautions in the Introduction. Homatropine is classified in FDA Pregnancy Category C.

DOSAGE AND PREPARATIONS.
Topical: For refraction, see Table 1. For mild anterior uveitis, one drop of a 2% or 5% solution is instilled two or three times daily. When homatropine is used for continuing therapy after administration of atropine or scopolamine, the drops may be instilled initially one or more times daily, followed by twice daily administration.

All preparations available as topical ophthalmic solutions.

AK-Homatropine (Akorn). Solution 5% with benzalkonium chloride 0.01%, hydroxyethylcellulose, and edetate disodium in 15 ml containers.

Homatropine Hydrobromide (Iolab). Solution (sterile) 2% and 5% with benzalkonium chloride in 1 ml containers.

Isopto Homatropine (Alcon). Solution (sterile) 2% and 5% with benzalkonium chloride 0.01% (2% concentration) or 0.005% (5% concentration) in 5 and 15 ml containers.

Homatropine Hydrobromide Steri-Unit (Alcon). Solution 5% (preservative-free) in 2 ml containers.

Drug also marketed by other manufacturers under generic name: Solution 2% and 5%.

SCOPOLAMINE HYDROBROMIDE
[Isopto Hyoscine]

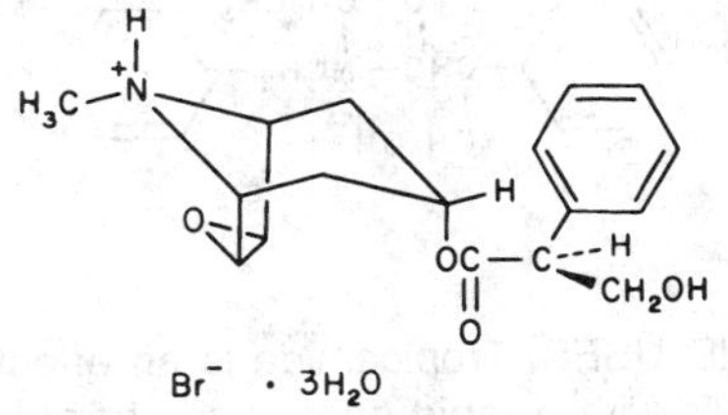

H
H_3C—$\overset{+}{N}$
O
H
OC—C---H
O CH_2OH
$Br^- \cdot 3H_2O$

ACTIONS AND USES. Scopolamine is a potent mydriatic and cycloplegic. In the concentrations used clinically, it has a shorter duration of action than atropine; cycloplegia may persist for three days. Scopolamine rarely causes local allergic reactions and is useful in patients who are allergic to atropine. It is administered occasionally for refraction in children but is employed most commonly for postoperative mydriasis, in anterior uveitis, and in some secondary glaucomas.

ADVERSE REACTIONS AND PRECAUTIONS. Scopolamine can cause acute angle-closure glaucoma if instilled in eyes with anatomically narrow angles. It also may increase intraocular pressure in eyes with open-angle glaucoma. Acute psychotic reactions may occur, particularly in children and elderly patients (see the section on Adverse Reactions and Precautions in the Introduction). Scopolamine may cause drowsiness.

DOSAGE AND PREPARATIONS.

Topical: In anterior segment inflammation, the concentration and frequency of administration are determined by the severity of inflammation and pupillary response. Scopolamine may be supplemented with phenylephrine for maximal mydriasis.

For postoperative mydriasis, one drop of a 0.25% solution instilled once daily is often adequate.

For anterior uveitis, one drop of a 0.25% solution is instilled once daily or more frequently in severe inflammation. When slit-lamp examination reveals minimal inflammation, a less potent agent, such as homatropine, may be substituted.

To break posterior synechiae, one drop of solution is instilled more frequently and may be alternated with phenylephrine 10% to enhance the mydriatic effect. The risk of toxicity from each drug is increased with increasing dosage.

For malignant (ciliary block) glaucoma, initially, one drop of a 0.25% solution and one drop of phenylephrine 10% three or four times daily or more often if required. For maintenance, one drop of a 0.25% or 0.3% solution once daily.

For refraction in children, see Table 1.

All preparations available in topical ophthalmic forms.

Isopto Hyoscine (Alcon). Solution (sterile) 0.25% with benzalkonium chloride 0.01% in 5 and 15 ml containers.

Available Mixture.

Murocoll-2 (Bausch & Lomb). Solution (sterile) containing scopolamine 0.3% and phenylephrine 10% with benzalkonium chloride 0.01% in 5 ml containers.

TROPICAMIDE

[Mydriacyl, Mydriafair, Ocu-Tropic, Tropicacyl]

ACTIONS AND USES. Tropicamide is an effective mydriatic and cycloplegic with a rapid onset and short duration of action. It is used as an aid in refraction, for ophthalmoscopy and retinal photography, for preoperative mydriasis, and occasionally in provocative testing for acute angle-closure glaucoma. Maximal cycloplegia occurs within 20 to 35 minutes after two drops of the 1% solution are instilled five minutes apart. The duration of action is very brief and complete recovery of accommodation occurs in two to six hours. A preparation containing 0.5% tropicamide and 2.5% phenylephrine produces maximal pupillary dilation within 45 minutes.

ADVERSE REACTIONS AND PRECAUTIONS. Because of its short duration of action, tropicamide rarely causes systemic reactions. For adverse effects of anticholinergic drugs, see the section on Adverse Reactions and Precautions in the Introduction.

DOSAGE AND PREPARATIONS.

Topical: For refraction, see Table 1. For ophthalmoscopy and retinal photography, see Table 2.

All preparations available as topical ophthalmic solutions.

Mydriacyl (Alcon). Solution (sterile) 0.5% and 1% with benzalkonium chloride 0.01% and edetate disodium in 3 (1% concentration only) and 15 ml containers.

Mydriafair (Texas). Solution (sterile) 0.5% and 1% in 2 and 15 ml containers.

Ocu-Tropic (Ocumed). Solution (sterile) 0.5% in 15 ml containers.

Tropicacyl (Akorn). Solution (sterile) 0.5% and 1% with benzalkonium chloride 0.1% in 2 and 15 (0.5% concentration) ml containers.

Drug also marketed under generic name: Solution 0.5% and 1%.

ADRENERGIC AGENT

PHENYLEPHRINE HYDROCHLORIDE

[AK-Dilate, Dilatair, Mydfrin, Neo-Synephrine, Ocu-Phrin]

ACTIONS AND USES. Phenylephrine is an alpha-adrenergic agonist. It is used to produce mydriasis without cycloplegia for examination of the intraocular structures; to facilitate ocular surgery; as an adjunct in the treatment of anterior uveitis, postoperative inflammation, and some secondary glaucomas; and occasionally for provocative testing for acute angle-closure glaucoma. It is often given with an anticholinergic drug to achieve wider mydriasis.

After ocular instillation of a 10% solution, maximal mydriasis is obtained in 60 to 90 minutes and recovery occurs in about six hours. Maximal plasma concentrations are achieved within 20 to 30 minutes after instillation of a 2.5% solution regardless of the vehicle (aqueous or viscous) employed (Kumar et al, 1986). For preoperative mydriasis, a 2.5% solution is as effective as a 10% solution when instilled every 15 minutes for 90 minutes, but the 10% solution is more effective (particularly in highly pigmented eyes) when drops are applied three times in conjunction with cyclopentolate (Duffin et al, 1983). A solution containing 2.5% phenylephrine and 0.5% tropicamide or cyclopentolate is useful for ophthalmoscopy (Apt and Henrick, 1980).

ADVERSE REACTIONS, PRECAUTIONS, AND INTERACTIONS. Local adverse reactions include transient pain, release of pigment granules from the iris with a transitory increase in intraocular pressure, and occlusion of structurally narrow angles resulting in angle-closure glaucoma. Because of the adrenergic effect on Mueller's muscle, lid retraction may be observed; therefore, patients should not be evaluated for ptosis surgery or thyroid disease after instillation of phenylephrine eyedrops. In patients over 50, rebound miosis has been noted 24 hours after instillation, and the mydriatic response to subsequent doses is diminished. Subconjunctival hemorrhage has occurred rarely.

Phenylephrine occasionally may cause systemic reactions (eg, tachycardia, hypertension and reflex bradycardia, angina, ventricular arrhythmias, myocardial infarction, cardiac failure, cardiac arrest, subarachnoid hemorrhage), particularly when a strong concentration is instilled repeatedly. Although the incidence of severe hypertensive responses to 10% phenylephrine eyedrops may be low (Brown et al, 1980), a pronounced increase in blood pressure can occur in neonates and elderly patients. Severe nausea and vomiting resulting in dehydration, hyperviscosity, venous thrombosis, and pulmonary embolism were reported in a diabetic patient who received the 10% solution.

Adverse cardiovascular effects usually can be avoided by use of the 2.5% solution (Meyer and Fraunfelder, 1980). The 10% solution should be used cautiously, if at all, in patients with hypertension and/or coronary artery disease and should be avoided in neonates and elderly patients. Even the 2.5% solution can markedly increase the blood pressure in preterm infants and patients with idiopathic orthostatic hypotension. Patients at high risk for adverse cardiovascular effects should be monitored for 20 to 30 minutes following instillation of phenylephrine eyedrops (Kumar et al, 1986).

Monoamine oxidase inhibitors and tricyclic antidepressants may increase the pressor response to phenylephrine. There is one report of an adverse cardiovascular reaction to phenylephrine eyedrops that was attributed to an interaction with propranolol; however, in a controlled study on hypertensive patients, beta blockade did not enhance the pressor effect of phenylephrine (Myers, 1984).

Phenylephrine is classified in FDA Pregnancy Category C.

See also the section on Adverse Reactions and Precautions in the Introduction.

DOSAGE AND PREPARATIONS. Phenylephrine solutions are unstable and should not be exposed to light, heat, or air.

Topical: For ophthalmoscopy, see Table 2. For preoperative mydriasis, one drop of a 2.5% solution every 15 minutes for two to four doses, or one drop of a 10% solution instilled one to two hours prior to surgery.

For postoperative mydriasis after iridectomy, one drop of a 10% solution is instilled once or twice daily. Atropine should be substituted if inflammation is severe. After cyclodialysis, one drop of a 10% solution is instilled once daily for three days in conjunction with miotics.

For use of phenylephrine to supplement atropine or scopolamine, see the evaluations on these drugs.

All preparations available as topical ophthalmic solutions.

AK-Dilate (Akorn). Solution (sterile) 2.5% and 10% with edetate disodium and benzalkonium chloride 0.01% in 2 (10% concentration) and 15 (2.5% concentration) ml containers.

Dilatair (Texas). Solution (sterile) 2.5% in 2 and 15 ml containers.

Mydfrin (Alcon). Solution (sterile) 2.5% with edetate disodium and benzalkonium chloride 0.01% in 3 and 5 ml containers.

Neo-Synephrine (Sanofi Winthrop). Solution (sterile) 2.5% with benzalkonium chloride 0.014% in 15 ml containers; 10% (viscous, nonviscous) with benzalkonium chloride 0.01% in 5 ml containers.

Ocu-Phrin (Ocumed). Solution (sterile) 0.12% in 15 ml containers and 2.5% and 10% in 5 ml containers.

Phenylephrine Hydrochloride (Iolab). Solution (sterile) 2.5% and 10% with thimerosal 0.01% in 1 and 15 (2.5% concentration only) ml containers.

Drug also marketed by other manufacturers under generic name: Solution 2.5% and 10%.

PROSTAGLANDIN INHIBITORS

FLURBIPROFEN SODIUM

[Ocufen]

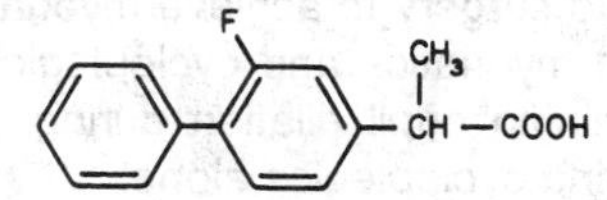

ACTIONS AND USES. This nonsteroidal anti-inflammatory drug is applied topically to prevent miosis during ophthalmic surgery. It is a more potent inhibitor of prostaglandin biosynthesis than ibuprofen, indomethacin, or aspirin. In patients undergoing extracapsular cataract extraction, the effect of one drop of flurbiprofen 0.03% instilled every 30 minutes into the operative eye beginning two hours before surgery is additive to that of mydriatic agents (eg, phenylephrine, cyclopentolate, epinephrine) used concomitantly; moreover, the combination was more effective in maintaining pupillary dilation than the mydriatic alone (Drews and Katsev, 1989; Gimbel, 1989; Keates and McGowan, 1984; Heinrichs and Leith, 1990).

ADVERSE REACTIONS AND PRECAUTIONS. Transient burning and stinging are the most common side effects of flurbiprofen. This drug does not elevate intraocular pressure in individuals who respond to corticosteroids, but it may delay wound healing and interfere with the clotting mechanism. Flurbiprofen can be absorbed into the systemic circulation and generally should be avoided in pregnant women (FDA Pregnancy Category C).

DOSAGE AND PREPARATIONS.

Topical: One drop is instilled every 30 minutes beginning two hours before surgery (total dose, four drops).

Ocufen (Allergan). Solution (sterile) 0.03% in 2.5 ml containers.

SUPROFEN

[Profenal]

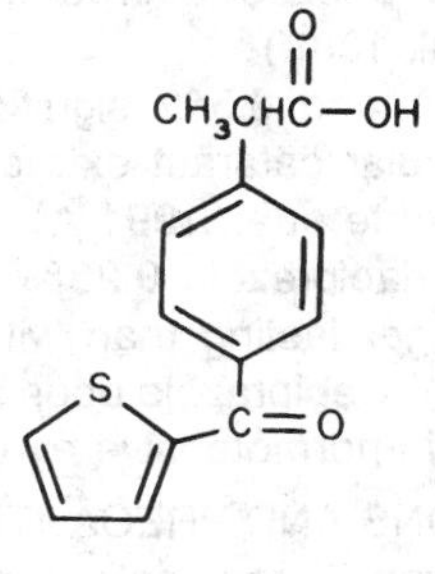

USES. Suprofen is a peripheral analgesic that has a potent inhibitory action on prostaglandin biosynthesis. This nonsteroidal anti-inflammatory drug is applied topically to prevent miosis during ophthalmic surgery.

In a double-blind, multicenter study, two drops of suprofen 1% were instilled into the operative eye one day prior to hospitalization in patients undergoing intracapsular or extracapsular cataract surgery with or without implantation of an intraocular lens (Stark et al, 1986). Two drops of suprofen were then instilled into the operative eye hourly for three hours prior to surgery. Phenylephrine, tropicamide, homatropine, or atropine sulfate also were instilled in selected groups of patients prior to surgery to achieve mydriasis. Suprofen, in combination with mydriatics and cycloplegics, was more effective in maintaining pupil dilation during cataract surgery than mydriatics and cycloplegics alone.

ADVERSE REACTIONS AND PRECAUTIONS. Suprofen may cause transient burning and stinging, itching, and redness. Photophobia, ocular pain, allergic reactions, chemosis, iritis, and punctate epithelial staining occur rarely. When administered with nonsteroidal anti-inflammatory drugs, suprofen may increase the bleeding time due to interference with thrombocyte aggregation. There have been reports that the bleeding tendency of ocular tissues increases during surgery.

Suprofen is classified in FDA Pregnancy Category C.

DOSAGE AND PREPARATIONS.

Topical: Two drops are applied three, two, and one hours prior to surgery. Two drops also may be applied every four hours during waking hours on the day prior to surgery.

Profenal (Alcon). Solution (sterile) 1% in 2.5 ml containers.

ALPHA-ADRENERGIC BLOCKING AGENTS

DAPIPRAZOLE HYDROCHLORIDE

[Rev-Eyes]

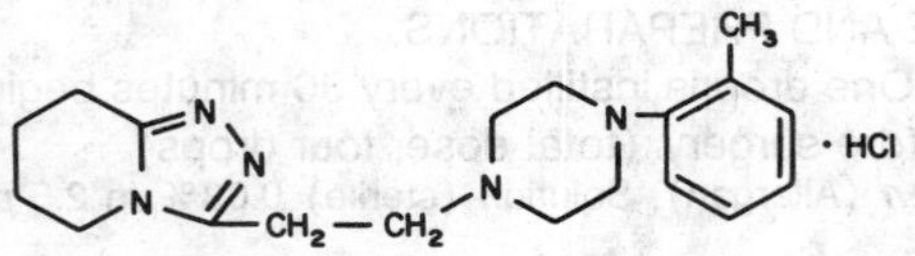

ACTIONS AND USES. Dapiprazole, an alpha-adrenergic blocking agent that acts on the dilator muscle of the iris, produces miosis and is used to reverse mydriasis produced by phenylephrine and, to a lesser degree, tropicamide (Allinson et al, 1990; Lodi et al, 1988).

Dapiprazole 0.25% and 0.5% significantly reverses mydriasis after extracellular cataract extraction with intraocular lens implantation (Ponte et al, 1991 A). The reversal of mydriasis produced by dapiprazole 0.25% has a slower onset but the effect is longer lasting than with acetylcholine 1% (Ponte et al, 1991 B). Dapiprazole does not significantly alter intraocular pressure in normotensive eyes.

ADVERSE REACTIONS AND PRECAUTIONS. The most frequent adverse reaction is conjunctival injection, which lasts 20 minutes in more than 80% of patients. Burning on instillation occurs in approximately 50% of patients. In addition, ptosis, lid erythema or edema, chemosis, itching, punctate keratitis, corneal edema, browache, photophobia, and headache have been reported. Rarely, dryness of the eyes, tearing, and blurring of vision also occur.

Dapiprazole is classified in FDA Pregnancy Category B.

DOSAGE AND PREPARATIONS.

Topical: To reverse mydriasis after ophthalmic examination, two drops applied to the conjunctiva of each eye, followed in five minutes by an additional two drops in each eye.

Rev-Eyes (Storz/Lederle). Powder (lyophilized) 25 mg with 5 ml of diluent to make a 0.5% solution.

MOXISYLYTE HYDROCHLORIDE (Thymoxamine Hydrochloride) (Investigational drug)

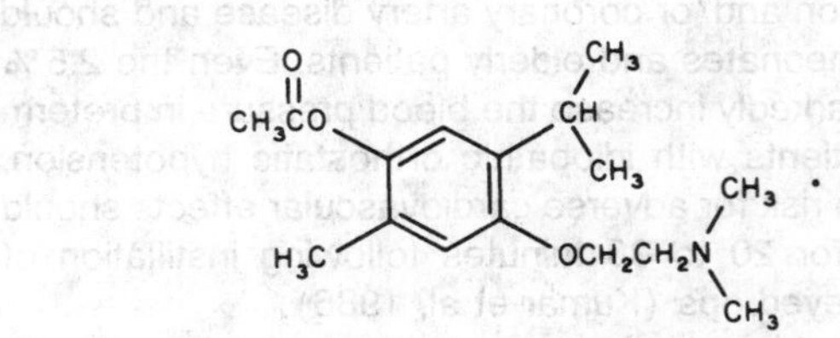

ACTIONS. This alpha-adrenergic blocking agent constricts the pupil by blocking alpha receptors in the dilator muscle of the iris, thereby permitting parasympathetic dominance via the sphincter muscle. Since moxisylyte has no effect on the ciliary muscle, it induces miosis without causing shallowing of the anterior chamber as may occur with cholinergic drugs (Saheb et al, 1980; Susanna et al, 1978).

USES. When applied topically, moxisylyte induces a rapid and sustained reversal of phenylephrine-induced mydriasis. It appears to be safer than pilocarpine for this purpose in eyes with narrow angles (Relf et al, 1988; Saheb et al, 1982). Moxisylyte also may be useful in glaucoma therapy (see index entry Glaucoma) and in the differential diagnosis and treatment of lid retraction (Dixon et al, 1979).

ADVERSE REACTIONS. The 0.5% concentration may cause ocular irritation. Marked chemosis and ptosis have occurred with stronger concentrations.

DOSAGE AND PREPARATIONS.

Topical: For reversing phenylephrine-induced mydriasis, one drop induces significant miosis, which may persist for 24 hours.

Moxisylyte Hydrochloride (Iolab).

LOCAL ANESTHETICS

Agents Used for Surface Anesthesia

COCAINE HYDROCHLORIDE

PROPARACAINE HYDROCHLORIDE

[Ak-Taine, Alcaine, Kainair, Ocu-Caine, Ophthaine, Ophthetic]

TETRACAINE HYDROCHLORIDE
[Pontocaine]

ACTIONS AND USES. These agents are applied topically to the eye to anesthetize the conjunctiva and cornea. Surface anesthesia alone provides sufficient analgesia for superficial procedures, such as tonometry, gonioscopy, removal of superficial foreign bodies and sutures, conjunctival and corneal scrapings, and lacrimal canalicular manipulation. Topical anesthetics also may be used as adjuncts to locally injected anesthetics for operations on deeper structures.

Topical anesthetics produce adequate corneal anesthesia within one minute after instillation. The duration of anesthesia (which may be increased by repeated application) is approximately 15 minutes with proparacaine 0.5% or tetracaine 0.5%. Cocaine 4% may have a slightly shorter duration of action (Jordan and Baum, 1980), but its vasoconstrictor effect is useful for conjunctival surgery. It also may loosen the corneal epithelium more readily than other anesthetics, thus facilitating debridement or total removal of the surface epithelium.

ADVERSE REACTIONS AND PRECAUTIONS. Topical anesthetics cause transient irregularities in the surface of the corneal epithelium that may interfere with visualization of the intraocular structures. Because protective eyelid reflexes are suppressed, the corneal epithelium may become dry. Repeated administration may retard healing and cause pitting and sloughing of the corneal epithelium with formation of a yellow-white ring in the corneal stroma around the original area of disease (Burns et al, 1977). Cocaine may be more toxic in this respect than other topical anesthetics, but all of these agents can cause severe keratitis and visual loss.

The patient should be warned not to touch the eye after instillation. Topical anesthetics should not be used repeatedly except under close medical supervision, and they should never be given to the patient for self-medication. Long-term unsupervised use has caused corneal scarring and permanent loss of vision.

Proparacaine causes less local discomfort than the other topical anesthetics, although this varies with the proprietary product. Allergic reactions have been reported most frequently with tetracaine. Allergy to the preservative also may occur occasionally.

Cocaine dilates the pupil and has precipitated acute angle closure in predisposed eyes.

The amount of anesthetic absorbed after topical application to the eye is usually not sufficient to cause systemic reactions, but excessive doses can cause central nervous system disturbances.

DOSAGE AND PREPARATIONS. See Table 3.

TABLE 3.
AGENTS USED FOR SURFACE ANESTHESIA

Drug	Dosage (Topical)	Ophthalmic Preparation
Cocaine Hydrochloride, U.S.P.	One or two drops of 0.5% to 2% solution instilled before procedure.	No pharmaceutical dosage form available; compounding necessary for prescription.
Proparacaine Hydrochloride	One or two drops of 0.5% solution instilled before procedure. For deeper anesthesia, more frequent instillation required.	*Generic.* Solution 0.5% in 2 and 15 ml containers. *Ak-Taine* (Akorn). Solution (sterile) 0.5% with benzalkonium chloride in 2 and 15 ml containers. *Alcaine* (Alcon). Solution (sterile) 0.5% with glycerin, sodium hydroxide and/or hydrochloric acid, and benzalkonium chloride in 15 ml containers. *Kainair* (Texas), *Ocu-Caine* (Ocumed). Solution (sterile) 0.5% in 2 and 15 ml containers. *Ophthaine* (Apothecon). Solution (sterile) 0.5% with glycerin, chlorobutanol, and benzalkonium chloride in 15 ml containers. *Ophthetic* (Allergan). Solution (sterile) 0.5% with glycerin, sodium chloride, and benzalkonium chloride in 15 ml containers.
Tetracaine Hydrochloride	One or two drops of 0.5% solution instilled before procedure. For deeper anesthesia, two to four instillations required. Alternatively, one-half to one inch of ointment is applied to the lower conjunctival fornix.	*Generic.* Solution 0.5% in 1, 2, and 15 ml containers. *Pontocaine* (Sanofi Winthrop). Solution 0.5% with chlorobutanol 0.4% in 15 and 60 ml containers; ointment 3.5 g with white petrolatum and light mineral oil in 3.75 g containers. *Tetracaine Steri-Units* (Alcon). Solution (sterile) 0.5% in 2 ml containers (preservative free).

Agents Used For Local Injection

BUPIVACAINE HYDROCHLORIDE
[Marcaine, Sensorcaine]

ETIDOCAINE HYDROCHLORIDE
[Duranest]

LIDOCAINE HYDROCHLORIDE
[Xylocaine]

MEPIVACAINE HYDROCHLORIDE
[Carbocaine, Polocaine]

PROCAINE HYDROCHLORIDE
[Novocain]

ACTIONS AND USES. These agents are injected locally adjacent to the muscle cone (retrobulbar or peribulbar injection) or in the region of the facial nerve (facial nerve akinesia) to reduce pain and to prevent eye and lid movements during surgery. Epinephrine may be added to the solution to reduce systemic absorption and thereby prolong the action and decrease the toxicity of the anesthetic, but it is usually not required when slowly absorbed agents, such as mepivacaine and bupivacaine, are employed. Hyaluronidase [Wydase] enhances diffusion of the anesthetic into the tissues.

Procaine, lidocaine, and mepivacaine also are used to block nerve endings in the immediate area of surgery (infiltration anesthesia) for procedures such as minor lid operations. Subconjunctival infiltration anesthesia is sometimes employed prior to intraocular surgery or some operations on the surface of the eye (eg, pterygium).

Because it is metabolized rapidly, procaine has a short duration of action and is relatively safe. Lidocaine diffuses more readily than procaine and is more potent, longer acting, and more toxic on a milligram-for-milligram basis. Mepivacaine is similar to lidocaine in potency and toxicity, but it may have a longer action. Bupivacaine is the most potent of these anesthetics, and strict adherence to the safe dosage range is essential. Bupivacaine has a slow onset of action but the duration of akinesia and analgesia is prolonged. Etidocaine is long-acting.

Combinations of locally injected anesthetics (eg, lidocaine and bupivacaine) are employed in an attempt to produce both a rapid onset and a long duration of analgesia and akinesia. The toxic effects of combined local anesthetics are additive.

ADVERSE REACTIONS AND PRECAUTIONS. Allergic reactions are less common with the amide group of local anesthetics (lidocaine, mepivacaine, bupivacaine, etidocaine) than with the ester group (procaine). Transient pain may follow the injection of bupivacaine. Occlusion of the central retinal artery has occurred following retrobulbar injection of anesthetics. Another adverse consequence of retrobulbar injection is the inadvertent penetration of the globe or the optic nerve.

Locally injected anesthetics can cause seizures, respiratory and cardiac arrest, and other severe systemic reactions if excessive amounts are absorbed or if the anesthetic is inadvertently given intravenously (see index entry Anesthetics, Local). Respiratory arrest, often unaccompanied by central nervous system or cardiovascular symptoms, has occurred as a complication of retrobulbar injection (Smith, 1981; Wittpenn et al, 1986) and appears to be caused by inadvertent subarachnoid injection (Ahn and Stanley, 1987; Chang et al, 1984). Systemic reactions (eg, tachycardia, hypertension) also may occur if sufficient quantities of epinephrine are absorbed; however, the blood catecholamine levels produced by fear or pain can exceed those produced by the anesthetic solution.

Buffering the anesthetic with sodium bicarbonate can hasten the onset of action (Zahl et al, 1990) and reduce the pain associated with injection (Christoph et al, 1988).

DOSAGE AND PREPARATIONS. See Table 4.

INTRAOCULAR MIOTICS

ACETYLCHOLINE CHLORIDE
[Miochol]

ACTIONS AND USES. Acetylcholine is the neurohumoral transmitter at numerous sites in the nervous system, including the neuroeffector junction of the iris sphincter muscle. When applied topically to the eye, acetylcholine is of no therapeutic value because of poor corneal penetration and rapid hydrolysis by acetylcholinesterase. However, it produces prompt, pronounced miosis when introduced into the anterior chamber and is useful during surgical procedures on the anterior segment of the eye when a deep anterior chamber and lens protection are required.

Acetylcholine is commonly used during cataract surgery to produce miosis after implantation of an intraocular lens. It may attenuate the early postoperative increase in intraocular pressure (Hollands et al, 1987 A).

During peripheral iridectomy, acetylcholine may be introduced into the anterior chamber to permit excision of only peripheral iris tissue and to aid in repositing of the iris. It also is used during penetrating keratoplasty to facilitate suturing of the graft by protecting the lens and preventing iris incarceration.

Acetylcholine has a shorter duration of action than other miotics, which is an advantage during ocular surgery, because prolonged miosis can cause severe postoperative pain or predispose to pupillary block. If miosis is desired postoperatively, a longer acting miotic (ie, carbachol, physostigmine, pilocarpine) must be instilled.

ADVERSE REACTIONS AND PRECAUTIONS. Because it is rapidly inactivated, acetylcholine seldom produces adverse effects. Systemic reactions (hypotension, bradycardia, flushing, sweating, and dyspnea) occur rarely. The bradycardia should be treated with intravenous atropine. Bronchospasm has been reported following intraocular administration of ace-

**TABLE 4.
AGENTS USED FOR LOCAL INJECTION**

Drug	Dosage* Facial Nerve Akinesia†	Dosage* Retrobulbar Block‡	Dosage* Infiltration Anesthesia	Preparations§
Procaine Hydrochloride	4 to 10 ml of 1% to 2% solution	2 to 4 ml of 1% to 2% solution	0.25% to 0.5% solution	*Generic.* Solution 1% and 2% (with and without epinephrine). *Novocain* (Sanofi Winthrop). Solution 1% and 2%.
Lidocaine Hydrochloride	4 to 10 ml of 1% to 2% solution	2 to 4 ml of 2% or 4% solution	0.5% solution	*Xylocaine Hydrochloride* (Astra), *Generic.* Solution 0.5%, 1%, 1.5%, and 2% (with and without epinephrine 1:200,000) and 4% (without epinephrine).
Mepivacaine Hydrochloride	4 to 10 ml of 2% solution	2 to 4 ml of 2% solution	1% solution	*Generic.* Solution 1% and 2%. *Carbocaine.* (Sanofi Winthrop), *Polocaine* (Astra). Solution 1%, 1.5%, and 2%.
Bupivacaine Hydrochloride	5 to 10 ml of 0.5% solution or 5 to 7 ml of 0.75% solution	2 to 4 ml of 0.75% solution	—	*Generic.* Solution 0.5% and 0.75%. *Marcaine* (Sanofi Winthrop), *Sensorcaine* (Astra). Solution 0.5% and 0.75% (with and without epinephrine bitartrate 1:200,000). Solutions without epinephrine may be autoclaved.
Etidocaine Hydrochloride	5 ml of 1% solution	2 to 4 ml of 1% solution	—	*Duranest* (Astra). Solution 1% (with and without epinephrine). Solutions without epinephrine may be reautoclaved.

**Hyaluronidase may be added to increase diffusion of the anesthetic.*

†Solution is injected in region of terminal branches of facial nerve or around the proximal trunk of the nerve.

‡Solution is injected inside the muscle cone behind the globe. Low pressure may be applied to the eye intermittently for three to five minutes after the injection. Some ophthalmologists combine two different anesthetics for retrobulbar block (eg, 2 ml lidocaine and 2 ml bupivacaine).

§For complete product information, see index entry Anesthetics, Local.

tylcholine to a patient who was taking a beta blocker (Rasch et al, 1983).

No local toxic effects produced by acetylcholine itself have been reported; however, the hypertonic solution may cause transient lens opacities. Serious ocular complications (corneal edema, intraocular inflammation, opacity of the anterior lens capsule, retinal toxicity, and optic atrophy) have occurred when acetylcholine was gas sterilized, because the ethylene oxide used in the process may enter through or around the rubber stopper of the two-compartment vial and react chemically with the water and/or chloride ion in the pharmaceutical product. Ethylene glycol and/or ethylene chlorhydrin may form, and both are highly toxic to the eye.

DOSAGE AND PREPARATIONS.

Intracameral: 0.5 to 2 ml of a freshly prepared 1:100 solution is instilled into the anterior chamber.

Miochol (Iolab). Two-compartment vial containing lyophilized acetylcholine chloride 20 mg and mannitol 60 mg in the lower compartment and sterile water 2 ml in the upper compartment in 2 ml containers.

CARBACHOL

[Miostat]

For chemical formula, see index entry Carbachol, In Glaucoma.

ACTIONS AND USES. This parasympathomimetic agent may be preferred to acetylcholine during ocular surgery when more prolonged miosis is desired. In contrast to the transient effect of acetylcholine, the miosis induced by carbachol is still evident 15 hours after intracameral injection. Carbachol and acetylcholine are equally effective in producing prompt, complete miosis after cataract extraction. Carbachol reduces the intraocular pressure for 24 to 48 hours postoperatively (Hollands et al, 1987 B; Linn et al, 1989). This drug is stable in solution and may be the agent of choice for achieving intrasurgical miosis and preventing an intraocular pressure rise after cataract surgery (Ruiz et al, 1989).

ADVERSE REACTIONS AND PRECAUTIONS. Corneal edema may occur if excessive amounts of carbachol are introduced into the anterior chamber or if the drug is used in patients with an already compromised endothelium (eg, Fuchs' dystrophy, corneal transplants, cataract surgery that requires unusual manipulation) (Fraunfelder, 1989).

DOSAGE AND PREPARATIONS.

Intracameral: 0.4 to 0.5 ml of a 0.01% solution is instilled into the anterior chamber.

Miostat (Alcon). Solution (sterile, for intraocular use) 0.01% in 1.5 ml containers.

Cited References

Ahn JC, Stanley JA: Subarachnoid injection as a complication of retrobulbar anesthesia. *Am J Ophthalmol* 103:225-230, 1987.

Allinson RW, et al: Reversal of mydriasis by dapiprazole. *Ann Ophthalmol* 22:131-138, 1990.

Apt L, Henrick A: Pupillary dilatation with single eyedrop mydriatic combinations. *Am J Ophthalmol* 89:553-559, 1980.

Barraquer RI, Barraquer J: Intraoperative mydriasis and miosis, in Sears ML, Tarkkanen A (eds): *Surgical Pharmacology of the Eye.* New York, Raven Press, 1985, 271-288.

Brodstein RS, et al: Treatment of myopia with atropine and bifocals: Long-term prospective study. *Ophthalmology* 91:1373-1379, 1984.

Brown MM, et al: Lack of side effects from topically administered 10% phenylephrine eyedrops: Controlled study. *Arch Ophthalmol* 98:487-489, 1980.

Burde RM, Thompson HS: Hydroxyamphetamine: A good drug lost? *Am J Ophthalmol* 111:100-102, 1991.

Burns RP, et al: Chronic toxicity of local anesthetics on cornea, in Leopold IH, Burns RP (eds): *Symposium on Ocular Therapy.* New York, John Wiley & Sons, 1977, vol 10, 31-44.

Caprioli J, et al: Pupillary response to trauma, in Sears M, Tarkkanen A (eds): *Surgical Pharmacology of the Eye.* New York, Raven Press, 1985, 257-267.

Chang JL, et al: Brain stem anesthesia following retrobulbar block. *Anesthesiology* 61:789-790, 1984.

Christoph RA, et al: Pain reduction in local anesthetic administration through pH buffering. *Ann Emerg Med* 17:117-120, 1988.

Cremer SA, et al: Hydroxyamphetamine mydriasis in Horner's syndrome. *Am J Ophthalmol* 110:71-76, 1990.

Dixon RS, et al: Use of thymoxamine in eyelid retraction. *Arch Ophthalmol* 97:2147-2150, 1979.

Drews RC, Katsev DA: Ocufen and pupillary dilation during cataract surgery. *J Cataract Refract Surg* 15:445-448, 1989.

Duffin RM, et al: 2.5% v 10% phenylephrine in maintaining mydriasis during cataract surgery. *Arch Ophthalmol* 101:1903-1906, 1983.

Fraunfelder FT: *Drug-Induced Ocular Side Effects and Drug Interactions*, ed 3. Philadelphia, Lea & Febiger, 1989.

Gimbel HV: Effect of treatment with topical nonsteroidal anti-inflammatory drugs with and without intraoperative epinephrine on the maintenance of mydriasis during cataract surgery. *Ophthalmology* 96:585-588, 1989.

Heinrichs DA, Leith AB: Effect of flurbiprofen on the maintenance of pupillary dilation during cataract surgery. *Can J Ophthalmol* 25:239-242, 1990.

Hermansen MC, Sullivan LS: Feeding intolerance following ophthalmologic examination. *Am J Dis Child* 139:367-368, 1985.

Hiatt RL, Jerkins G: Comparison of atropine and tropicamide in esotropia. *Ann Ophthalmol* 15:341-343, 1983.

Hollands RH, et al: Effect of acetylcholine on early postoperative intraocular pressure. *Am J Ophthalmol* 103:749-753, 1987 A.

Hollands RH, et al: Effect of intracameral carbachol on intraocular pressure after cataract extraction. *Am J Ophthalmol* 104:225-228, 1987 B.

Hoskins HD, Kass MA: *Becker-Shaffer's Diagnosis and Therapy of the Glaucomas,* ed 6. St Louis, CV Mosby, 1989.

Huber MJE, et al: Mydriatic drugs for diabetic patients. *Br J Ophthalmol* 69:425-427, 1985.

Isenberg S, et al: Comparison of mydriatic eyedrops in low-weight infants. *Ophthalmology* 91:278-279, 1984.

Isenberg SJ, et al: Effects of cyclopentolate eyedrops on gastric secretory function in preterm infants. *Ophthalmology* 92:698-700, 1985.

Jordan A, Baum J: Basic tear flow: Does it exist? *Ophthalmology* 87:920-930, 1980.

Keates RH, McGowan KA: Clinical trial of flurbiprofen to maintain pupillary dilation during cataract surgery. *Ann Ophthalmol* 16:919-921, 1984.

Keulen-De Vos HCJ, et al: Effect of indomethacin in preventing surgically induced miosis. *Br J Ophthalmol* 67:94-96, 1983.

Kumar V, et al: Aqueous vs viscous phenylephrine: I. Systemic absorption and cardiovascular effects. *Arch Ophthalmol* 104:1189-1191, 1986.

Linn DK, et al: Effect of intracameral carbachol on intraocular pressure after cataract extraction. *Am J Ophthalmol* 107:133-136, 1989.

Lodi M, et al: Reversal of tropicamide and phenylephrine mydriasis in ten patients with narrow iridocorneal angle (I-II according to Shaffer): Comparison of dapiprazole with thymoxamine. *Acta XXV Concilium Ophthalmologicum* 25:2425-2427, 1988.

Lynch MG, et al: Reduction of phenylephrine drop size in infants achieves equal dilation with decreased systemic absorption. *Arch Ophthalmol* 105:1364-1365, 1987.

Merli GJ, et al: Cardiac dysrhythmias associated with ophthalmic atropine. *Arch Intern Med* 146:45-47, 1986.

Meyer SM, Fraunfelder FT: Phenylephrine hydrochloride. *Ophthalmology* 87:1177-1180, 1980.

Myers MG: Beta adrenoceptor antagonism and pressor response to phenylephrine. *Clin Pharmacol Ther* 36:57-63, 1984.

Onorato DJ: Ophthalmic medications that contain sulfites, letter. *Arch Ophthalmol* 103:1274-1276, 1985.

Ponte F, et al: Intraocular dapiprazole for the reversal of mydriasis after extracapsular cataract extraction with intraocular lens implantation: Part I, dose-response correlation. *J Cataract Refract Surg* 17:780-784, 1991 A.

Ponte F, et al: Intraocular dapiprazole for the reversal of mydriasis after extracapsular cataract extraction with intraocular lens implantation: Part II, comparison with acetylcholine. *J Cataract Refract Surg* 17:785-789, 1991 B.

Rasch D, et al: Bronchospasm following intraocular injection of acetylcholine in patient taking metoprolol. *Anesthesiology* 59:583-585, 1983.

Relf SJ, et al: Thymoxamine reverses phenylephrine-induced mydriasis. *Am J Ophthalmol* 106:251-255, 1988.

Ruiz RS, et al: Effects of carbachol and acetylcholine on intraocular pressure after cataract extraction. *Am J Ophthalmol* 107:7-10, 1989.

Saheb NE, et al: Effect of thymoxamine and pilocarpine on depth of anterior chamber. *Can J Ophthalmol* 15:170-171, 1980.

Saheb NE, et al: Thymoxamine versus pilocarpine in reversal of phenylephrine-induced mydriasis. *Can J Ophthalmol* 17:266-267, 1982.

Shaw BR, Lewis RA: Intraocular pressure elevation after pupillary dilation in open angle glaucoma. *Arch Ophthalmol* 104:1185-1188, 1986.

Sinclair SH, et al: Mydriatic solution for outpatient indirect ophthalmoscopy. *Arch Ophthalmol* 98:1572-1574, 1980.

Smith JL: Retrobulbar Marcaine can cause respiratory arrest. *J Clin Neuroophthalmol* 1:171-172, 1981.

Stark WJ, et al: Reduction of pupillary constriction during cataract surgery using suprofen. *Arch Ophthalmol* 104:364-366, 1986.

Steinmann WC, et al: Pupillary dilation with tropicamide 1% for funduscopic screening: Study of duration of action. *Ann Intern Med* 107:181-184, 1987.

Summers WK, Reich TC: Delirium after cataract surgery: Review and two cases. *Am J Psychiatry* 136(4A):386-391, 1979.

Susanna R, et al: Effects of thymoxamine on anterior chamber depth in human eyes. *Can J Ophthalmol* 13:250-251, 1978.

Wittpenn JR, et al: Respiratory arrest following retrobulbar anesthesia. *Ophthalmol* 93:867-870, 1986.

Wright MM, et al: Time course of thymoxamine reversal of phenylephrine-induced mydriasis. *Arch Ophthalmol* 108:1729-1732, 1990.

Zahl K, et al: pH-adjusted bupivacaine and hyaluronidase for peribulbar block. *Anesthesiology* 72:230-232, 1990.

Zimmerman TJ, et al: Improving the therapeutic index of topically applied ocular drugs. *Arch Ophthalmol* 102:551-553, 1984.

Ophthalmic Anti-inflammatory Agents, Decongestants, and Antiallergy Agents

ANTI-INFLAMMATORY AGENTS

Three groups of anti-inflammatory agents are used in ocular diseases: adrenal corticosteroids, nonsteroidal anti-inflammatory agents, and immunosuppressive drugs. Corticosteroids have been the primary agents of choice and are most often used topically or subconjunctivally; however, serious side effects may accompany their use and some patients may not respond to therapy. As understanding of the immune system and of the role of prostaglandins in inflammation improves, nonsteroidal agents are increasingly being employed for mild inflammatory conditions such as uveitis and episcleritis. Immunosuppressive drugs are now being used for severe ocular disorders (eg, Behcet's syndrome, Wegener's granulomatosis). Most are administered systemically.

ADRENAL CORTICOSTEROIDS

ACTIONS AND USES. Adrenal corticosteroids are used to control ocular inflammation, reduce scarring, and prevent visual loss. Steroid therapy is useful in ocular allergic disorders (eg, vernal conjunctivitis, contact dermatitis of the lids and conjunctiva, allergic blepharitis), Thygeson's superficial punctate keratopathy, uveal tract inflammation (iritis, iridocyclitis, posterior uveitis), episcleritis, scleritis, temporal arteritis, orbital inflammation associated with Graves' disease, chalazia, and congenital hemangiomas.

Corticosteroids also are useful to prevent corneal graft rejection and control postoperative iridocyclitis, but the benefits of their prophylactic use must be weighed against potential adverse effects (ie, delayed wound healing, increased susceptibility to infection, masking of postoperative infection). Steroids do not significantly reduce the incidence of uveitis or choroidal detachment following retinal detachment surgery, and they do not prevent the increase in intraocular pressure frequently associated with laser trabeculoplasty.

Use of steroids in ocular infections requires concomitant antimicrobial therapy that is effective against the specific causative organism; if used alone, these drugs may weaken ocular defense mechanisms and worsen the course of infectious disease. An exception is their local use in chronic herpes zoster ophthalmicus. Herpes simplex stromal keratitis and uveitis may be treated cautiously with steroids, but an antiviral agent must be used concomitantly to prevent reactivation of the epithelial infection.

ROUTES OF ADMINISTRATION. Topical therapy usually controls inflammation of the lids, conjunctiva, cornea, or anterior sclera. Ophthalmologists also inject solutions or suspensions of corticosteroids by the subconjunctival route to supplement topical therapy in resistant inflammation. For a very prolonged action, the repository form of methylprednisolone or triamcinolone acetonide may be used. Intralesional injection of these long-acting steroids has resolved chalazia, congenital hemangiomas of the lids, and cutaneous palpebral sarcoid dermatitis.

Anterior uveitis sometimes is controlled by steroids applied topically or injected subconjunctivally, but systemic therapy also may be needed. Inflammatory disorders of the posterior segment of the globe (eg, posterior uveitis, scleritis) may require both systemic and periocular (posterior subconjunctival or retrobulbar) administration.

Dexamethasone, dexamethasone sodium phosphate, fluorometholone, fluorometholone acetate (investigational), medrysone, prednisolone acetate, and prednisolone sodium phosphate are available as drops or ointment for topical application. Ophthalmic preparations of hydrocortisone and its acetate ester are available only in fixed-dose combinations. Medrysone, hydrocortisone, and low concentrations of prednisolone (0.125%) and fluorometholone (0.1%) have mild anti-inflammatory activity and are useful for treating superficial inflammatory conditions. Dexamethasone and its esters and stronger concentrations of prednisolone and fluorometholone and their esters readily penetrate the cornea and are preferred for treatment of corneal inflammatory disorders and anterior uveitis.

Many steroid preparations are available only as suspensions, which may be packaged in opaque bottles. Their liquid phases contain the corticosteroid at saturation concentrations, but their particulate phases tend to settle with gravity. Therefore, unequal doses may be administered if the bottle is not shaken sufficiently before use.

ADVERSE REACTIONS AND PRECAUTIONS. Topically applied corticosteroids may cause stinging and burning. Although the severe adverse reactions associated with systemic therapy occur only rarely, corticosteroid eyedrops are absorbed in amounts sufficient to cause partial adrenal suppression in adults and, occasionally, Cushing's syndrome in young children.

Corticosteroids lower resistance to fungal, bacterial, and some viral infections and, by reducing inflammation, they can mask the warning symptoms of pain and hyperemia. The concomitant use of an antibiotic and the presence of a corneal abrasion may increase susceptibility to fungal infections. If steroids are used to treat stromal herpes simplex of the cornea or herpetic uveitis, an antiviral drug should be given concomitantly to prevent reactivation of the epithelial infection.

Corticosteroids should not be used without prior slit-lamp examination of the cornea for evidence of herpes simplex involvement, and long-term use requires periodic re-examination. Corticosteroids should be given in the lowest effective concentration, and long-term use should be avoided when possible. Exacerbation of active but controlled inflammation may occur if the corticosteroid is discontinued abruptly; therefore, when therapy is to be withdrawn, the interval between applications should be lengthened gradually.

Repeated local administration of corticosteroids may increase intraocular pressure. This response has been attributed to a reduction in the facility of outflow of aqueous humor through the trabecular meshwork. The elevation in pressure is not accompanied by pain and is reversible upon discontinuation of the drug; if undetected, it may damage the optic nerve.

The ocular hypertensive response to prolonged administration of topical corticosteroids is variable and may be genetically determined. In the general population, an insignificant pressure elevation occurs in about 65% of individuals. Marked elevations occur frequently in patients with primary open-angle glaucoma and their relatives, myopes, diabetics, and males with connective tissue disorders. The magnitude of the pressure elevation also depends on the drug used, the concentration, frequency of administration, and duration of treatment. Dexamethasone and its esters and prednisolone and its esters produce the greatest pressure elevations (Mindel et al, 1979). The pressure elevation produced by fluorometholone 0.1% is one-half that caused by dexamethasone 0.1% but is four times that caused by medrysone 1% (Mindel et al, 1980). A clinically important increase in pressure is rare with medrysone, hydrocortisone 0.5%, or dilute concentrations of more potent steroids, eg, 0.01% dexamethasone (Podos and Becker, 1972). Increased intraocular pressure is less common with systemic therapy.

Intraocular pressure should be measured before initiation of long-term topical therapy and then every two months or more frequently in patients predisposed to a steroid-induced pressure elevation. Particular caution should be observed when using repository corticosteroids in predisposed individuals because their effects may persist for months and the residual steroid may have to be removed surgically in order to reduce intraocular pressure.

Posterior subcapsular cataracts have developed during long-term corticosteroid therapy. This complication was first noted in patients receiving large systemic doses but also has been associated with topical use. Early lens changes may regress when steroids are discontinued but, if the opacities are more distinct, regression is uncommon and the cataracts may progress. Intraocular inflammation also may cause cataracts, and it is difficult to distinguish those caused by disease from those promoted by therapy.

Corticosteroids may delay wound healing. After cataract surgery, this may result in wound dehiscence and the development of a filtering bleb.

Topical corticosteroid preparations should be used sparingly in any conditions that cause thinning of the cornea, for perforation may occur.

Retrobulbar injection of repository steroids has rarely caused atrophy of orbital rim fat and delayed hypersensitivity reactions.

Products containing sulfites as preservatives may cause bronchospasm in asthmatic patients.

PREPARATIONS.

DEXAMETHASONE:

Generic. Suspension 0.1% in 5 ml containers.

Maxidex Suspension (Alcon). Suspension (sterile) 0.1% with benzalkonium chloride 0.01% in 5 and 15 ml containers.

DEXAMETHASONE SODIUM PHOSPHATE:

Generic. Ointment 0.05% in 3.75 g containers; solution 0.1% in 5 and 15 ml containers.

Ak-Dex (Akorn), ***Dexair*** (Bausch & Lomb), ***Ocu-Dex*** (Ocumed). Ointment (sterile) 0.05% in 3.5 g containers; solution (sterile) 0.1% in 5 ml containers.

Decadron Phosphate (Merck Sharp & Dohme). Ointment (sterile) 0.05% in 3.5 g containers; solution (sterile) 0.1% with sodium bisulfite 0.1%, phenylethanol 0.25%, and benzalkonium chloride 0.02% in 5 ml containers.

Maxidex Ointment (Alcon). Ointment (sterile) 0.05% (dexamethasone phosphate equivalent) in 3.5 g containers.

FLUOROMETHOLONE:

Fluor-Op (Iolab). Suspension (sterile) 0.1% in 3, 5, 10, and 15 ml containers.

FML (Allergan). Suspension (sterile) 0.1% or 0.25% ***(Forte)*** with polyvinyl alcohol 1.4%, benzalkonium chloride, and edetate disodium in 1 (0.1% only), 2 (0.25% only), 5, 10, and 15 ml containers; ointment (sterile) 0.1% with phenylmercuric acetate, petrolatum, mineral oil, and lanolin alcohol in 3.5 g containers.

MEDRYSONE:

HMS (Allergan). Suspension (sterile) 1% with polyvinyl alcohol 1.4%, benzalkonium chloride, and edetate disodium in 5 and 10 ml containers.

PREDNISOLONE ACETATE:

Generic. Suspension 1% in 5, 10, and 15 ml containers.

AK-Tate (Akorn). Suspension (aqueous, sterile) 1% with benzalkonium chloride and edetate disodium in 5, 10, and 15 ml containers.

Econopred, Econopred Plus (Alcon). Suspension (sterile) 0.125% (***Econopred***) or 1% (***Econopred Plus***) with benzalkonium chloride 0.01% in 5 and 10 ml containers.

Ocu-Pred-A (Ocumed), ***Predair-A*** (Bausch & Lomb). Suspension (sterile) 1% in 5 and 10 ml containers.

Pred Mild, Pred Forte (Allergan). Suspension (sterile) 0.12% (***Mild***) or 1% (***Forte***) with benzalkonium chloride in 5 and 10 ml (***Mild***) and 1, 5, 10, and 15 ml (***Forte***) containers.

PREDNISOLONE SODIUM PHOSPHATE:

Generic. Solution 0.125% and 1% in 5 and 15 ml containers.

Ak-Pred (Akorn). Suspension (aqueous, sterile) 0.125% or 1% (equivalent to 0.1% or 0.8% base) with benzalkonium chloride 0.01% in 5 ml containers.

Inflamase (Iolab). Solution (sterile) 0.125% (***Mild***) and 1% (***Forte***) (equivalent to 0.1% or 0.8% base) with benzalkonium chloride in 5 and 10 ml (***Mild***) and 3, 5, 10, and 15 ml (***Forte***) containers.

Metreton (Schering). Solution (sterile) 0.5% (prednisolone phosphate equivalent) with edetate disodium and benzalkonium chloride in 5 ml containers.

Ocu-Pred (Ocumed). Solution (sterile) 0.125% and 1% (***Forte***) in 5 and 15 ml containers.

Predair (Bausch & Lomb). Solution (sterile) 0.125% in 5 ml containers and 1% (***Forte***) in 5 ml containers.

STEROID-ANTIBACTERIAL MIXTURES

Mixtures containing a fixed-dose combination of a corticosteroid and one or more antibacterial agents are used to treat conditions in which both may be required, eg, marginal keratitis secondary to staphylococcal infection, allergic conjunctivitis with chronic bacterial conjunctivitis, blepharoconjunctivitis, phlyctenular keratoconjunctivitis, selected cases of postoperative inflammation. The antibacterial agents used in these mixtures include chloramphenicol, gentamicin, neomycin, and polymyxin B. Preparations containing neomycin should not be used for prolonged periods (eg, more than seven days) because they may produce toxic allergic reactions in the corneal or conjunctival epithelium. In addition, none of these mixtures should be used to treat conjunctivitis or blepharitis of unknown origin. Corticosteroids reduce resistance to infection and may have an adverse effect if the invading organism is resistant to the antibiotic. See index entry Eye Infection.

PREPARATIONS.

CHLORAMPHENICOL AND STEROID:

Chloromycetin Hydrocortisone Ophthalmic (Parke-Davis). Powder (sterile) containing chloramphenicol 12.5 mg and hydrocortisone acetate 25 mg (preservative free) with 5 ml sterile water for suspension.

CHLORAMPHENICOL, POLYMYXIN B, AND STEROID:

Ophthocort (Parke-Davis). Ointment (sterile) containing chloramphenicol 1%, polymyxin B sulfate 10,000 units/g, and hydrocortisone acetate 0.5% (preservative free) in 3.5 g containers.

GENTAMICIN AND STEROID:

Pred-G (Allergan). Ointment (sterile) containing gentamicin 0.3% and prednisolone acetate 0.6% with chlorobutanol 0.5% in 3.5 g containers (***S.O.P***); suspension (sterile) containing gentamicin 0.3% and prednisolone acetate 1% with polyvinyl alcohol 1.4% and benzalkonium chloride 0.005% in 2, 5, and 10 ml containers.

NEOMYCIN AND STEROID:

AK-Neo-Cort (Akorn), ***Ortho Drops*** (Vortech). Suspension (aqueous, sterile) containing neomycin sulfate 0.5% (equivalent to 0.35% base) and hydrocortisone acetate 1.5% with chlorobutanol 0.5% in 5 ml containers.

NeoDecadron Ophthalmic (Merck Sharp & Dohme). Ointment (sterile) containing neomycin sulfate 0.5% (equivalent to 0.35% base) and dexamethasone sodium phosphate 0.05% (equivalent to dexamethasone phosphate 0.05%) in 3.5 g containers; solution (sterile) containing neomycin sulfate 0.5% (equivalent to 0.35% base) and dexamethasone sodium phosphate (equivalent to dexamethasone phosphate 0.1%) with benzalkonium chloride 0.02% and sodium bisulfite 0.1% in 5 ml containers.

NEOMYCIN, POLYMYXIN B, AND STEROID:

AK-Trol (Akorn), ***Dexacidin*** (Iolab), ***Dexasporin*** (Bausch & Lomb). Ointment (sterile) containing neomycin sulfate 0.5%, polymyxin B sulfate 10,000 units, and dexamethasone 0.1% with white petrolatum and mineral oil in 3.5 g containers; suspension (sterile) containing neomycin sulfate 0.5%, polymyxin B sulfate 10,000 units/ml, and dexamethasone 0.1% with benzalkonium chloride in 5 ml containers.

Maxitrol (Alcon). Ointment (sterile) containing neomycin sulfate 0.5% (equivalent to 0.35% base), polymyxin B sulfate 10,000 units/g, and dexamethasone 0.1% with methylparaben 0.05% and propylparaben 0.01% in 3.5 g containers; suspension (sterile) containing neomycin sulfate 0.5% (equivalent to 0.35% base), polymyxin B sulfate 10,000 units/ml, and dexamethasone 0.1% with benzalkonium chloride 0.004% in 5 ml containers.

Poly-Pred Ophthalmic (Allergan). Suspension (sterile) containing neomycin sulfate 0.5% (equivalent to 0.35% base), polymyxin B sulfate 10,000 units/ml, and prednisolone acetate 0.5% with thimerosal 0.001% in 5 and 10 ml containers.

Cortisporin (Burroughs Wellcome), ***Triple-Gen*** (Goldline). Suspension (sterile) containing neomycin sulfate 0.5%, polymyxin B sulfate 10,000 units/ml, and hydrocortisone 1% with benzalkonium chloride 0.01% or thimerosal 0.001% (***Cortisporin***) in 7.5 ml containers.

NEOMYCIN, POLYMYXIN B, BACITRACIN, AND STEROID:

Cortisporin Ophthalmic (Burroughs Wellcome). Ointment (sterile) containing neomycin sulfate 0.5% (equivalent to 0.35% base), polymyxin B sulfate 10,000 units/g, bacitracin zinc 400 units/g, and hydrocortisone 1% in 3.75 g containers.

SULFACETAMIDE SODIUM AND STEROID:

AK-Cide (Akorn). Ointment (sterile) containing sulfacetamide sodium 10% and prednisolone acetate 0.5% in 3.5 g containers; suspension (sterile) containing sulfacetamide sodium 10% and prednisolone acetate 0.5% with benzalkonium chloride 0.01% in 5 and 15 ml containers.

Blephamide (Allergan). Suspension (sterile) containing sulfacetamide sodium 10% and prednisolone acetate 0.2% with benzalkonium chloride in 2.5, 5, and 10 ml containers (***Liquifilm***); ointment (sterile) containing sulfacetamide sodium 10% and prednisolone acetate 0.2% with phenylmercuric acetate 0.0008% in 3.5 g containers (***S.O.P.***).

Cetapred (Alcon). Ointment (sterile) containing sulfacetamide sodium 10% and prednisolone acetate 0.25% with methylparaben 0.05% and propylparaben 0.01% in 3.5 g containers; suspension (sterile) containing sulfacetamide sodium 10% and prednisolone acetate 0.25% with methylparaben 0.05%, propylparaben 0.01%, and benzalkonium chloride 0.025% in 5 and 15 ml containers (***Isopto Cetapred***).

FML-S (Allergan). Suspension (sterile) containing sulfacetamide sodium 10% and fluorometholone 0.1% with polyvinyl alcohol 1.4%, benzalkonium chloride, edetate disodium, and povidone in 5 and 10 ml containers.

Metimyd (Schering). Ointment (sterile) containing sulfacetamide sodium 10% and prednisolone acetate 0.5% with methylparaben 0.05% and propylparaben 0.01% in 3.5 g containers; suspension (sterile) containing sulfacetamide sodium 10% and prednisolone acetate 0.5% with phenylethyl alcohol 0.5% and benzalkonium chloride 0.025% in 5 ml containers.

Optimyd (Schering). Solution (sterile) containing sulfacetamide sodium 10% and prednisolone sodium phosphate 0.5% (equivalent to prednisolone phosphate 0.5%) with benzalkonium chloride 0.025% and phenylethyl alcohol 0.5% in 5 ml containers.

Predsulfair (Texas). Ointment (sterile) containing sulfacetamide sodium 10% and prednisolone acetate 0.5% with white petrolatum, mineral oil, and parabens in 3.5 g containers; suspension (sterile) containing sulfacetamide sodium 10% and prednisolone acetate 0.5% with hydroxypropyl methylcellulose, sodium thiosulfate, and benzalkonium chloride 0.01% in 3.5 g and 5 and 15 ml containers.

Sulphrin (Bausch & Lomb). Ointment (sterile) containing sulfacetamide sodium 10% and prednisolone acetate 0.5% in 3.5 g containers; suspension (sterile) containing sulfacetamide sodium 10% and prednisolone acetate 0.5% with methylparaben 0.05% and propylparaben 0.01% in 5 and 15 ml containers.

Sulpred (Bausch & Lomb). Suspension (sterile) containing sulfacetamide sodium 10% and prednisolone acetate 0.2% with bezalkonium chloride 0.01% in 5 and 10 ml containers.

Vasocidin (Iolab). Ointment (sterile) containing sulfacetamide sodium 10% and prednisolone acetate 0.5% in 3.5 g containers; solution (sterile) containing sulfacetamide sodium 10% and prednisolone sodium phosphate 0.25% (equivalent to prednisolone 0.2%) with thimerosal 0.01% in 5 and 10 ml containers.

NONSTEROIDAL ANTI-INFLAMMATORY DRUGS

There has been increasing interest in the role of prostaglandins in ocular inflammation and in the effect of agents that inhibit their synthesis or release. Aspirin and indomethacin [Indocin], which inhibit prostaglandin synthesis, have been given systemically to treat uveitis, episcleritis, and postsurgical cystoid macular edema, but reports on their efficacy conflict. Aspirin may be useful as an adjunct in the treatment of vernal conjunctivitis. Systemically administered phenylbutazone [Azolid, Butazolidin] has been reported to be effective in some patients with scleritis, episcleritis, and mild anterior uveitis.

Flurbiprofen [Ocufen] and suprofen [Profenal] have been used to prevent surgically induced miosis. Two drops of suprofen 1% applied four times daily significantly reduced ocular signs, papillae, and mucus strands in patients with giant papillary conjunctivitis associated with the use of contact lenses (Wood et al, 1988). Diclofenac sodium [Voltaren] eye drops can be used to treat inflammation after cataract surgery.

An indomethacin eye drop preparation (not available commercially) also has been used to treat surgical miosis and for prophylaxis of angiographic aphakic or pseudophakic cystoid macular edema associated with cataract or retinal detachment surgery, but it does not appear to improve long-term prognosis (Jampol, 1982, 1985; Kraff et al, 1982; Miyake et al, 1983; Yannuzzi et al, 1981). Indomethacin eyedrops are not effective for the treatment of *established* cystoid macular edema (Jampol, 1985). Postoperative complications following argon laser trabeculoplasty are not decreased by preoperative treatment with topical indomethacin (Pappas et al, 1985).

Several other nonsteroidal anti-inflammatory drugs are being investigated for topical treatment of ocular inflammatory disorders. Ketorolac tromethamine eyedrops were reported to improve visual acuity in patients with established cystoid macular edema (Flach et al, 1987, 1990). Oxyphenbutazone eyedrops have been used abroad in the management of postoperative ocular inflammation, superficial eye injuries, and episcleritis. Ibuprofen has been studied for its effect on ocular inflammation in laboratory animals, and limited data suggest that it may be useful clinically.

For preparations, see index entries on these drugs.

IMMUNOSUPPRESSIVE AGENTS

Sight-threatening, corticosteroid-resistant ocular diseases can require the use of immunosuppressive agents (see Table). Although many of these drugs were originally developed to treat malignant neoplasms, they are increasingly being recognized as the agents of choice for a number of severe ocular inflammatory diseases (Hemady et al, 1991). For example, cyclosporine reduces inflammation and improves visual acuity in selected patients with refractory posterior uveitis (Nussenblatt et al, 1983). It also has improved corneal graft survival in high-risk patients (Hill, 1989). Cyclosporine eyedrops improve symptoms of severe vernal keratoconjunctivitis, but the disease usually recurs when treatment is discontinued (Ben Ezra et al, 1986).

Fluorouracil, given in small doses by the subconjunctival route after filtering surgery, improves the surgical outcome of eyes with an initially poor prognosis (Ruderman et al, 1987). It has caused severe corneal epithelial defects and wound leaks (Knapp et al, 1987), but a reduction in dosage appears to decrease the incidence of these adverse reactions (Weinreb, 1987).

When administered in properly adjusted doses by physicians familiar with their pharmacodynamics, these potentially toxic agents appear to produce fewer adverse effects than corticosteroids.

Some commonly used immunosuppressive agents that have been useful in severe ocular diseases are listed in the Table. Most of these agents are administered orally; the development of topical preparations (eg, cyclosporine [Pesko, 1990]) will enhance their usefulness.

DECONGESTANTS AND ANTIALLERGY AGENTS

In addition to their mydriatic and antiglaucoma actions (see the chapter, Drugs Used for Glaucoma), the adrenergic drugs discussed below are occasionally used to produce vasoconstriction and relieve symptoms of allergic reactions and hyperemia of the conjunctiva.

IMMUNOSUPPRESSIVE DRUGS FOR IMMUNE AND INFLAMMATORY OCULAR DISEASES

Immunosuppressive Agent	Dosage	Possible Ocular Indications	Adverse Reactions
Azathioprine [Imuran]	*Oral:* 1-2.5 mg/kg/day in a single or divided doses.	Peripheral uveitis, Behcet's syndrome, ocular inflammation associated with juvenile rheumatoid arthritis, cicatricial pemphigoid	Minimal complications; however, bone marrow suppression and leukopenia may occur.
Bromocriptine [Parlodel]	*Oral:* 2.5 mg three or four times daily.	Iridocyclitis, Behcet's syndrome, thyroid ophthalmopathy	Early adverse effects include nausea, vomiting, and orthostatic hypotension.
Chlorambucil [Leukeran]	*Oral:* Initially, 0.1 mg/kg/day; maximal dose, 18 mg/day.	Behcet's syndrome, sympathetic ophthalmia, ocular inflammation associated with juvenile rheumatoid arthritis	Interference with spermatogenesis; irreversible azoospermia occurs in some. Moderate but rapid myelosuppression necessitates monitoring.
Colchicine	*Oral:* 0.5-0.6 mg two or three times daily.	Behcet's syndrome	Gastrointestinal upset is common. Hemorrhagic gastroenteritis, nephrotoxicity, vascular damage, muscular depression, and ascending paralysis of the central nervous system also occur.
Cyclophosphamide [Cytoxan, Neosar]	*Oral, Intravenous:* 1-2 mg/kg/day.	Wegener's granulomatosis, necrotizing scleritis associated with rheumatoid arthritis or relapsing polychrondritis, cicatricial pemphigoid	Reversible alopecia and anemia with relative thrombocytopenia, sterile hemorrhagic cystitis, dry eyes, increased ocular pressure, and transient blurring of vision occur.
Cyclosporine [Sandimmune]	*Oral:* 5-7 mg/kg/day.	Behcet's syndrome, birdshot retinochoroiditis, sarcoidosis, pars planitis, Vogt-Koyanagi-Harada syndrome, sympathetic ophthalmia, idiopathic vitritis	Nephrotoxicity is the most serious reaction. Paresthesias, temperature hypersensitivity, nausea, and vomiting are common.
Dapsone	*Oral:* Initially, 25 mg twice daily for one week, then increased to 50 mg twice daily.	Cicatricial pemphigoid, relapsing polychondritis	Hemolytic anemia is most common. Infectious mononucleosis-like syndrome, methemoglobinemia, gastrointestinal upset, blurred vision, reversible peripheral neuropathy, and psychosis also may occur.
Fluorouracil [Adrucil]	*Subconjunctival injection:* 5 mg.	Inflammatory glaucoma, filtering surgery for uncontrolled glaucoma	Gastrointestinal and hematopoietic reactions, anorexia, nausea, and vomiting are common. Stomatitis, diarrhea, and alopecia occur less frequently. Pruritus and irritation are common after topical application.

(table continued on next page)

Immunosuppressive Agent	Dosage	Possible Ocular Indications	Adverse Reactions
Methotrexate [Folex, Mexate]	*Oral, Intravenous, Intramuscular:* 10-25 mg divided over 36-48 hours and administered every one to four weeks.	Cyclitis, sympathetic ophthalmia, ocular inflammation associated with juvenile rheumatoid arthritis, cicatricial pemphigoid	Hepatic fibrosis and cirrhosis, ulcerative stomatitis, and diarrhea are common; bone marrow suppression and other side effects are relatively uncommon.

NAPHAZOLINE HYDROCHLORIDE

OXYMETAZOLINE

PHENYLEPHRINE HYDROCHLORIDE

TETRAHYDROZOLINE HYDROCHLORIDE

ACTIONS AND USES. These topically applied adrenergic drugs constrict dilated conjunctival vessels and are widely used by the public to whiten the eye. The FDA Advisory Review Panel on OTC Ophthalmic Drug Products has found the following concentrations to be safe and effective for relief of redness of the eye due to minor irritations: phenylephrine 0.08% to 0.2%, naphazoline 0.01% to 0.03%, and tetrahydrozoline 0.01% to 0.05% (*Federal Register*, 1980, 1988).

ADVERSE REACTIONS AND PRECAUTIONS. In the concentrations present in decongestant products, adrenergic drugs rarely cause serious untoward effects. However, prolonged or indiscriminate use should be avoided, since this could lead to neglect of symptoms of serious eye disease.

Ocular stinging and burning and reactive hyperemia may occur with excessive use. Mydriasis develops occasionally, particularly in patients with light irides, in those who wear contact lenses, or in those with corneal abrasions. Mydriasis may precipitate an attack of acute angle-closure glaucoma in predisposed eyes.

For local and systemic adverse effects of stronger concentrations of adrenergic drugs, see index entries Mydriatics; Cycloplegics.

Naphazoline and tetrahydrozoline are more stable in solution than phenylephrine; the activity of phenylephrine is greatly reduced by oxidation.

DOSAGE AND PREPARATIONS.

Topical: One or two drops instilled up to four times daily.

All preparations available in topical ophthalmic form.

NAPHAZOLINE HYDROCHLORIDE:

Generic. Solution 0.01% and 0.25%.

AK-Con (Akorn). Solution (sterile) 0.1% with benzalkonium chloride 0.01% and edetate disodium 0.01% in 15 ml containers.

Albalon (Allergan). Solution (sterile) 0.1% with benzalkonium chloride and edetate disodium in 5 and 15 ml containers.

Allerest (Fisons), ***Clear Eyes*** (Ross). Solution (sterile) 0.012% with edetate disodium 0.1% and benzalkonium chloride 0.01% in 15 and 30 ml containers (nonprescription).

Allergy Drops (Bausch & Lomb). Solution (sterile) 0.012% with edetate disodium 0.1% and benzalkonium chloride 0.01% in 15 ml containers (nonprescription).

Comfort Eye Drops (Sola/Barnes-Hind). Solution 0.03% with benzalkonium chloride 0.005% and edetate disodium 0.02% in 15 ml containers (nonprescription).

Degest 2 (Sola/Barnes-Hind). Solution (sterile) 0.012% with benzalkonium chloride 0.0067% and edetate disodium 0.02% in 15 ml containers (nonprescription).

Muro's Opcon (Bausch & Lomb). Solution (sterile) 0.1% with benzalkonium chloride 0.01% in 15 ml containers.

Nafazair (Bausch & Lomb). Solution (sterile) 0.1% with benzalkonium chloride 0.01% and edetate disodium in 15 ml containers.

Naphcon (Alcon). Solution 0.012% (nonprescription) or 0.1% (***Naphcon Forte***) with benzalkonium chloride 0.01% in 15 ml containers.

Ocu-Zoline (Ocumed). Solution (sterile) 0.1% in 15 ml containers.

VasoClear (Iolab). Solution (sterile) 0.02% in Lipiden polymeric system with benzalkonium chloride 0.01% in 15 ml containers (nonprescription).

Vasocon Regular (Iolab). Solution (sterile) 0.1% with benzalkonium chloride in 15 ml containers.

OXYMETAZOLINE:

OcuClear (Schering), ***Visine L.W.*** (Pfizer). Solution (sterile) 0.025% with benzalkonium chloride 0.01% in 15 and 30 ml containers.

PHENYLEPHRINE HYDROCHLORIDE:

Generic. Solution (sterile) 0.12% (nonprescription).

AK-Nefrin (Akorn). Solution (sterile) 0.12% with benzalkonium chloride 0.01% in 15 ml containers (nonprescription).

Isopto Frin (Alcon). Solution (sterile) 0.12% with benzalkonium chloride 0.01% and hydroxypropyl methylcellulose in 15 ml containers (nonprescription).

Ocugestrin (Texas), ***Ocu-Phrin*** (Ocumed). Solution (sterile) 0.12% in 15 ml containers (nonprescription).

Prefrin (Allergan). Solution (sterile) 0.12% with benzalkonium chloride 0.004% in 20 ml containers (nonprescription).

Relief (Allergan). Solution (sterile) 0.12% with edetate disodium in 30 single-use containers (nonprescription).

TETRAHYDROZOLINE HYDROCHLORIDE:

Generic. Solution (sterile) 0.05% (nonprescription).

Collyrium Fresh Eye Drops (Wyeth-Ayerst). Solution 0.05% with benzalkonium chloride 0.01% and edetate disodium 0.1% in 15 ml containers (nonprescription).

Eye Drops (Bausch & Lomb). Solution (sterile) 0.05% in 15 ml containers (nonprescription).

Eye-Zine (Ocumed). Solution (sterile) 0.05% in 15 ml containers (nonprescription).

Murine Plus (Ross). Solution (sterile) 0.05% with edetate disodium 0.1% and benzalkonium chloride 0.01% in 15 and 30 ml containers (nonprescription).

Optigene 3 (Pfeiffer). Solution (sterile) 0.05% with edetate disodium 0.1% and benzalkonium chloride 0.01% in 15 ml containers (nonprescription).

Soothe (Alcon). Solution (sterile) 0.05% with benzalkonium chloride 0.004% and edetate disodium 0.1% in 15 ml containers (nonprescription).

Visine (Pfizer). Solution (sterile) 0.05% with edetate disodium 0.1% and benzalkonium chloride 0.01% in 15, 22.5, and 30 ml containers (***Visine***) and polyethylene glycol 1% in 15 and 30 ml containers (***Visine Extra***) (nonprescription).

ANTIHISTAMINES WITH DECONGESTANTS

Antihistamines block the H_1 receptor sites and are used to treat acute allergic reactions of the eyelids and conjunctiva that are caused by release of histamine in the affected area. Decongestants are included in the formulation to produce an additive effect.

ACTIONS AND USES. Products containing an antihistamine and decongestant are promoted for the treatment of allergic conjunctivitis. In studies using a histamine model of ocular allergy, pretreatment with a topical antihistamine-decongestant combination prevented redness and pruritus induced by application of histamine to the eye.

The antihistamines used in ophthalmic solutions include antazoline, pheniramine, and pyrilamine. A highly specific H_1 antagonist, levocabastine, is being investigated for topical ophthalmic therapy. H_2 receptors are also present in ocular tissue and may play a role in ocular allergy (Abelson and Udell, 1981).

ADVERSE REACTIONS AND PRECAUTIONS. Antihistamines can cause eczematous contact dermatitis following topical use. Individuals sensitized to one antihistamine may exhibit cross sensitivity to other antihistamines or related agents. These agents may dilate the pupil and, in patients predisposed to angle-closure glaucoma, could precipitate an acute attack.

All preparations available in topical ophthalmic form.

AK-Con-A (Akorn), ***Muro's Opcon-A*** (Bausch & Lomb), ***Naphcon-A*** (Alcon). Solution (sterile) containing pheniramine maleate 0.3% and naphazoline hydrochloride 0.025% with benzalkonium chloride 0.01% and edetate disodium in 15 ml containers.

Albalon-A (Allergan). Solution (sterile) containing antazoline phosphate 0.5% and naphazoline hydrochloride 0.05% with benzalkonium chloride 0.004% and edetate disodium in 5 and 15 ml containers.

Prefrin-A (Allergan). Solution (sterile) containing pyrilamine maleate 0.1% and phenylephrine hydrochloride 0.12% with benzalkonium chloride 0.01% in 15 ml containers.

Vasocon-A (Iolab). Solution (sterile) containing antazoline phosphate 0.5% and naphazoline hydrochloride 0.05% with benzalkonium chloride 0.01% in 15 ml containers.

Cited References

Ophthalmic drug products for over-the-counter human use; establishment of a monograph, proposed rulemaking. *Federal Register* 45:30002-30050, 1980.

Ophthalmic drug products for over-the-counter human use; final monograph; final rule. *Federal Register* 53:7076-7098, 1988.

Abelson MB, Udell IJ: H_2-receptors in human ocular surface. *Arch Ophthalmol* 99:302-304, 1981.

Ben Ezra D, et al: Cyclosporine eyedrops for treatment of severe vernal keratoconjunctivitis. *Am J Ophthalmol* 101:278-282, 1986.

Flach AJ, et al: Effectiveness of ketorolac tromethamine 0.5% ophthalmic solution for chronic aphakic and pseudophakic cystoid macular edema. *Am J Ophthalmol* 103:479-486, 1987.

Flach AJ, et al: Prophylaxis of aphakic cystoid macular edema without corticosteroids: A paired-comparison, placebo-controlled double-masked study. *Ophthalmology* 97:1253-1258, 1990.

Hemady R, et al: Immunosuppressive drugs in immune and inflammatory ocular disease. *Surv Ophthalmol* 35:369-385, 1991.

Hill JC: Use of cyclosporine in high-risk keratoplasty. *Am J Ophthalmol* 107:506-510, 1989.

Jampol LM: Pharmacologic therapy of aphakic cystoid macular edema. *Ophthalmology* 80:891-897, 1982.

Jampol LM: Pharmacologic therapy of aphakic and pseudophakic cystoid macular edema. *Ophthalmology* 92:807-810, 1985.

Knapp A, et al: Serious corneal complications of glaucoma filtering surgery with postoperative 5-fluorouracil. *Am J Ophthalmol* 103:183-187, 1987.

Kraff MC, et al: Prophylaxis of pseudophakic cystoid macular edema with topical indomethacin. *Ophthalmology* 89:885-890, 1982.

Mindel JS, et al: Similarity of intraocular pressure response to difference corticosteroid esters when compliance is controlled. *Ophthalmology* 86:99-107, 1979.

Mindel JS, et al: Comparative ocular pressure elevation by medrysone, fluorometholone, and dexamethasone phosphate. *Arch Ophthalmol* 98:1577-1578, 1980.

Miyake K, et al: Incidence of cystoid macular edema after retinal detachment surgery and use of topical indomethacin. *Am J Ophthalmol* 95:451-456, 1983.

Nussenblatt RB, et al: Cyclosporin A therapy in treatment of intraocular inflammatory disease resistant to systemic corticosteroids and cytotoxic agents. *Am J Ophthalmol* 96:275-282, 1983.

Pappas HR, et al: Topical indomethacin therapy before argon laser trabeculoplasty. *Am J Ophthalmol* 99:571-575, 1985.

Pesko LJ: Cyclosporine eyedrops. *Am Druggist* 60, (Oct) 1990.

Podos SM, Becker B: Intraocular pressure effects of diluted and new topical corticosteroids, in Leopold IH (ed): *Symposium on Ocular Therapy.* St Louis, CV Mosby, 1972, vol 5, 90-95.

Ruderman JM, et al: Randomized study of 5-fluorouracil and filtration surgery. *Am J Ophthalmol* 104:218-224, 1987.

Weinreb RN: Adjusting the dose of 5-fluorouracil after filtration surgery to minimize side effects. *Ophthalmology* 94:564-570, 1987.

Wood TS, et al: Suprofen treatment of contact lens-associated giant papillary conjunctivitis. *Ophthalmology* 95:822-826, 1988.

Yannuzzi LA, et al: Incidence of aphakic cystoid macular edema with use of topical indomethacin. *Ophthalmology* 88:947-954, 1981.

Miscellaneous Ophthalmic Preparations

96

AGENT FOR BLEPHAROSPASM AND STRABISMUS

AGENTS USED FOR DRY-EYE SYNDROMES

CORNEAL DEHYDRATING AGENTS

DYES

ENZYMES

VISCOELASTIC AGENTS

CHELATING AGENTS

IRRIGATING SOLUTIONS

ASTRINGENTS

AGENT FOR BLEPHAROSPASM AND STRABISMUS

In blepharospasm and strabismus, dysfunction of the extraocular skeletal muscles interferes with vision (Jankovic and Brin, 1991).

Blepharospasm is a form of focal dystonia manifested by intermittent or sustained closure of the eyelids caused by involuntary contractions of the orbicularis oculi muscle. Symptoms range from increased blinking to functional blindness due to persistent, involuntary closure of the eyelids. Symptomatic relief may be achieved temporarily in about one third of patients by administration of clonazepam [Klonopin], lorazepam [Ativan], baclofen [Lioresal], and trihexyphenidyl [Artane].

Although relief of symptoms of blepharospasm also can be obtained in most patients by surgical procedures such as orbicularis myectomy, facial-nerve sectioning, and brow lift, exposure keratitis, local sensory impairment, lower-lid ectropion, ptosis, and eyelid necrosis are possible complications. Blepharospasm also may recur within months after surgery. Alternatively, injections of botulinum toxin type A into the orbicularis muscles has produced moderate to marked symptomatic and functional improvement in 70% to 90% of patients; relief from spasm begins two to five days after injection and may be maintained for an average of three to four months (American Academy of Ophthalmology, 1989; Jankovic and Brin, 1991; Taylor et al, 1991).

Strabismus (squint, heterotropia) is an anomaly of binocular vision in which the visual axis of one eye fails to pass through the point of regard. This condition usually is a developmental defect that occurs during early childhood, but it also may be caused by trauma or disease. Injection of botulinum toxin type A into the extraocular muscle has been used as an alternative to conventional incisional surgery. At least 60% of patients experience satisfactory relief (American Academy of Ophthalmology, 1989; Scott et al, 1990).

BOTULINUM TOXIN TYPE A
[Oculinum]

ACTIONS. Botulinum toxin is produced by *Clostridium botulinum* as six antigenically distinct forms; at present, only type A is available for clinical use. Botulinum toxin type A blocks neuromuscular transmission at cholinergic junctions by binding irreversibly to presynaptic sites and preventing release of ace tylcholine from the motor nerve terminals. The toxin thus denervates the muscle and produces a temporary paralysis that persists until new fibrils develop (in several weeks to months).

USES. Botulinum toxin type A is injected locally as an alternative to surgery for the treatment of extraocular muscle disorders. In patients with essential blepharospasm (Jankovic and Brin, 1991; Taylor et al, 1991), involuntary blinking is relieved. Functional improvement is seen within a few days after injection and is maximal in seven to ten days. The duration of relief from symptoms varies widely (6 to 48 weeks) (Taylor et al, 1991); for sustained efficacy, the injections must be repeated every three to four months. Up to 98% of patients with blepharospasm benefit from the initial injections, although between 10% to 15% require larger than usual doses. A small number of patients who appear to have essential blepharospasm manifested by apraxia of eyelid opening or an inability to voluntarily elevate the levator palpebrae superioris do not respond to botulinum toxin, even though marked paralysis of the orbicularis oculi is observed after treatment.

Injection of botulinum toxin is effective in patients with strabismus; this agent is especially useful when the angles are under 50 prism diopters, when residual strabismus occurs two to eight weeks after surgery, when treatment of the antagonist muscle in paralytic strabismus is required, and when surgery is inappropriate (eg, in active thyroid ophthalmopathy or inflamed or prephthisical eyes). Paralysis of an ocular rotary muscle for several weeks produced by botulinum toxin improves ocular alignment permanently. After an average of 26 months, about 60% of children maintain an alignment correction within 10 prism diopters of the ortho position (Scott et al, 1990). Better results are obtained in those with esotropia (60%) than exotropia (45%) regardless of the outcome of previous surgery. Success rates are higher when botulinum toxin is injected into the medial recti muscles for esotropia.

Botulinum toxin has been used in conjunction with surgery to relieve medial rectus contracture and regain eye alignment in patients with recent sixth cranial nerve paralysis (Fitzsimmons et al, 1988). It also has been injected into the orbicularis oculi muscle to relieve spastic lower eyelid entropion (Carruthers, 1985). In patients with corneal disease, it has been injected into the levator palpebrae superioris muscle to induce a temporary protective ptosis (Kirkness et al, 1988).

In addition to its use in disorders of the extraocular muscles, botulinum toxin has been employed to treat focal dystonias such as spasmodic torticollis (see index entry Dystonias, Focal).

ADVERSE REACTIONS AND PRECAUTIONS. Dry eye and exposure keratitis are the most common side effects of locally injected botulinum toxin type A. They are caused by a combination of decreased blink frequency and decreased lid excursion during blinking. Transient ptosis, the second most common side effect, is caused by spread of the toxin to the levator palpebrae superioris muscle. Deep or misplaced injections can cause transient diplopia (Patrinely et al, 1988). Lagophthalmos, ectropion, and entropion have been reported when the drug was injected into the lower lid. Local side effects are dose related.

Systemic side effects have not occurred, although electrophysiologic studies revealed that large doses produced subclinical effects on neuromuscular transmission in distant muscles (Lange et al, 1987). Antibodies have been detected only after administration of large doses.

Botulinum toxin type A is classified in FDA Pregnancy Category C.

DOSAGE AND PREPARATIONS. For reconstitution, see manufacturer's literature.

Intramuscular: *Adults,* for blepharospasm, initially 1.25 to 2.5 units (0.05 to 0.1 ml at each site) is injected into the medial and lateral pretarsal orbicularis oculi of the upper lid and the lateral pretarsal orbicularis oculi of the lower lid. Injections can be repeated indefinitely every three months. Dosage may be increased up to 5 units at subsequent sessions.

Adults and children, for strabismus, 0.05 to 0.15 ml per muscle (maximum recommended dose for a single injection in any one muscle, 25 units). Lower doses are employed for small deviations and larger doses for large deviations. For vertical muscles and horizontal strabismus of less than 20 prism diopters, initially 1.25 to 2.5 units in any one muscle; for horizontal strabismus of 20 to 50 prism diopters, initially 2.5 to 5 units in any one muscle. For sixth cranial nerve palsy persisting for one month or longer, 1.25 to 2.5 units in the medial rectus muscle.

Patients should be re-examined 7 to 14 days after each dose. Those requiring subsequent injections should receive an amount comparable to the initial dose if paralysis was adequate; if paralysis was incomplete, dosage may be increased up to twice the previous amount. Subsequent injections should not be given until the effect of the previous dose has dissipated.

Oculinum (Allergan). Powder (lyophilized, sterile) 100 units with human albumin 0.5 mg and sodium chloride 0.9 mg (preservative free).

AGENTS USED FOR DRY-EYE SYNDROMES

About 95% of the aqueous component of tears is produced by the primary lacrimal gland. Deficiency in secretion of aqueous tears, as in keratoconjunctivitis sicca, may be caused by atrophy and fibrosis or inflammation of the lacrimal gland. Dry-eye syndromes also can be caused by damage or destruction of the lacrimal tissues or blockage of the secretion ducts. The most common symptoms are irritation, a foreign body sensation, presence of stringy mucus, and transient blurring of vision. Although there is no cure for dry-eye syndromes, a number of demulcents and emollients are available; these solutions relieve symptoms by replacing tear fluids.

DEMULCENTS

ACTIONS AND USES. Ocular demulcents (artificial tears) are used to prevent corneal damage and alleviate symptoms in patients with keratoconjunctivitis sicca, neuroparalytic keratitis, exposure keratopathy, and other dry-eye syndromes. They also are used in normal eyes for temporary relief of discomfort and dryness caused by exposure to irritants, wind, or sun. These preparations contain water-soluble polymers (usually cellulose esters or polyvinyl alcohol) that act as a substitute for natural tears. More recently developed artificial tears contain long-chain polymeric systems that adsorb to the cornea, rendering it more wettable. These preparations have a relatively long duration of action (Lemp, 1987).

The comfort of an artificial tear preparation is influenced by various factors, including pH, tonicity, and preservative, and the choice of the best preparation for an individual patient is usually determined by trial and error (Laibson, 1980).

Formulations containing higher concentrations of cellulose esters are more viscous than those containing polyvinyl alcohol, but retention times are comparable. Preparations reported to be mucomimetic (eg, Adsorbotear, Celluvisc, Tears Naturale II) may be retained longer and have been suggested for use in mucus-deficient dry-eye conditions, such as ocular pemphigoid (Lemp et al, 1975). Patients with keratoconjunctivitis sicca may prefer a hypotonic solution [eg, HypoTears] to help balance the elevated tear film osmolarity that occurs in this disorder (Gilbard and Kenyon, 1985). The effect of hypotonic solutions on the tear film osmolarity is brief. A dilute 0.1% solution of sodium hyaluronate also has been used as a tear substitute. Unit-dose, preservative-free preparations (eg, Refresh) are useful for patients whose symptoms are worsened by preservatives (Lemp, 1987). Other available preservative-free solutions include Celluvisc, Cellufresh, HypoTears PF, and Tears Naturale Free. These solutions are recommended for patients who need to apply artificial tears more frequently than four times a day.

Patients who require frequent administration of artificial tear solutions may benefit from Lacrisert. This prolonged-release ocular insert consists of a water-soluble hydroxypropylcellulose pellet that is placed in the lower conjunctival cul-de-sac once or twice daily. The most common problems associated with Lacrisert are blurred vision and inadvertent loss of the insert (Lamberts, 1983).

In addition to their use in artificial tear preparations, cellulose esters and polyvinyl alcohol are employed as vehicles for ophthalmic drugs and as lubricants to moisten hard contact lenses and to protect the cornea during gonioscopy. A product [Enuclene] containing the detergent, tyloxapol, is used to lubricate artificial eyes.

ADVERSE REACTIONS AND PRECAUTIONS. Ophthalmic demulcents are nonirritating to ocular tissue and can be used for prolonged periods without damaging the eye. Solutions containing preservatives can cause irritation and superficial punctate keratitis if they are used more than four times daily. Viscous preparations may cause discomfort if excess solution is allowed to dry on the lids (see also *Federal Register*, 1980, 1988).

DOSAGE AND PREPARATIONS.

Topical: Artificial tears must be used regularly and as often as necessary to keep the conjunctiva moist. In patients with dry-eye syndrome, it may be necessary to apply preservative-free drops as often as every 15 minutes during warm dry weather. Occlusion of the lacrimal puncta by cauterization or insertion of punctum plugs may help to preserve existing lacrimal secretion and prolong the retention of artificial tears.

All preparations available in ophthalmic form (nonprescription).

ARTIFICIAL TEARS.

CARBOXYMETHYLCELLULOSE:

Cellufresh (Allergan). Solution (sterile) 0.5% in 30 single-use containers (preservative free).

Celluvisc (Allergan). Solution (sterile) 1% in 30 single-use containers (preservative free).

HYDROXYETHYLCELLULOSE:

Comfort Tears (Sola/Barnes-Hind). Solution (sterile) with benzalkonium chloride 0.005% and edetate disodium 0.02% in 15 ml containers.

TearGard (Medtech). Solution (sterile) with lecithin 0.05% and edetate disodium 0.1% in 15 ml containers.

HYDROXYPROPYLCELLULOSE (Sterile Ocular Insert):

Lacrisert (Merck Sharp & Dohme). Water-soluble insert containing hydroxypropylcellulose 5 mg in packages containing 60 units.

HYDROXYPROPYLMETHYLCELLULOSE:

Isopto Alkaline (Alcon). Solution (sterile) 1% with benzalkonium chloride 0.01% in 15 ml containers.

Isopto Plain (Alcon). Solution 0.5% with benzalkonium chloride 0.01% in 15 ml containers.

Isopto Tears (Alcon). Solution (sterile) 0.5% with benzalkonium chloride 0.01% in 15 and 30 ml containers.

Just Tears (Blairex). Solution (sterile) with benzalkonium chloride 0.01%, edetate disodium 0.025%, sodium chloride, and boric acid in 15 ml containers.

Lacril (Allergan). Solution 0.5% with gelatin A 0.01% and chlorobutanol 0.5% in 15 ml containers.

Lubrifair (Bausch & Lomb). Solution (sterile) with dextran in 15 ml containers.

Moisture Drops (Bausch & Lomb). Solution (sterile) 0.5% and dextran 40 with benzalkonium chloride 0.01% in 15 and 30 ml containers.

Tearisol (Iolab). Solution (sterile) 0.5% with benzalkonium chloride 0.01% and edetate disodium 0.01% in 15 ml containers.

Tears Renewed (Akorn). Solution (sterile) with dextran 70, benzalkonium chloride 0.01%, and edetate disodium 0.05% in 15 ml containers.

Ultra-Tears (Alcon). Solution (sterile) 1% with benzalkonium chloride 0.01% in 15 ml containers.

METHYLCELLULOSE:

Murocel (Bausch & Lomb). Solution (sterile) 1% with propylparaben 0.01% and methylparaben in 15 ml containers.

POLYVINYL ALCOHOL:

Akwa Tears (Akorn). Solution (sterile) with 0.01% benzalkonium chloride and edetate disodium in 15 ml containers.

Liquifilm Tears (Allergan). Solution (sterile) 1.4% with chlorobutanol 0.5% in 15 and 30 ml containers.

Liquifilm Forte (Allergan). Solution (sterile) 3% with thimerosal 0.002% and edetate disodium in 15 and 30 ml containers.

Refresh (Allergan). Solution (sterile) 1.4% with povidone 0.6% in 0.3 ml unit doses (preservative free).

Tears Plus (Allergan). Solution 1.4% with povidone 0.6% and chlorobutanol 0.5% in 15 and 30 ml containers.

OTHER POLYMERIC SYSTEMS.

Adsorbotear (Alcon). Solution (sterile) containing water-soluble polymers, povidone 1.67%, hydroxyethylcellulose, thimerosal 0.004%, and edetate disodium 0.1% in 15 ml containers.

HypoTears (Iolab). Solution (sterile, hypotonic) containing ***Lipiden*** polymeric system with benzalkonium chloride 0.01% and edetate disodium 0.03% (tonicity adjusted with nonionic agents) in 15 and 30 ml containers.

HypoTears PF (Iolab). Solution (hypotonic) containing polyvinyl alcohol in ***Lipiden*** polymeric system (polyethylene glycol 400, dextrose, edetate disodium, and purified water) in 30 0.6-ml single-use containers (preservative free).

Tears Naturale II (Alcon). Solution containing ***Duasorb*** water-soluble polymers, polyquad 0.001%, and sodium borate in 15 and 30 ml containers.

Tears Naturale Free (Alcon). Solution containing ***Duasorb*** polymeric system (dextran 70 and hydroxypropyl methylcellulose 2910) and sodium borate in 24 0.6-ml single-use containers (preservative free).

ARTIFICIAL EYE LUBRICANT.

Enuclene (Alcon). Solution (sterile) containing tyloxapol 0.25% and benzalkonium chloride 0.02% in 15 ml containers.

GONIOSCOPY LUBRICANTS.

Gonioscopic Prism Solution (Alcon). Solution (sterile) containing hydroxyethylcellulose with thimerosal 0.004% and edetate disodium 0.1% in 15 ml containers.

Gonak (Akorn), ***Goniosol*** (Iolab). Solution (sterile) containing hydroxypropylmethylcellulose 2.5% with benzalkonium chloride 0.01% and edetate disodium in 15 ml containers.

EMOLLIENTS

ACTIONS AND USES. Emollients are sterile, bland ointments that usually contain petrolatum, mineral oil, and lanolin derivatives. They form an occlusive film on the surface of the eye and are used to lubricate and protect the eye from drying during and after surgery, exposure to wind or sun, or foreign body removal. Emollients are useful to protect the cornea of patients with dry-eye syndromes, particularly as nighttime medication. They also are used as vehicles for ophthalmic drugs.

ADVERSE REACTIONS AND PRECAUTIONS. Emollients cause temporary blurring of vision. Although oleaginous vehicles are toxic to the interior of the eye, no adverse effects have been reported when emollients were used immediately after ocular surgery or in the presence of corneal abrasions or corneal ulcers (*Federal Register*, 1980, 1988).

DOSAGE AND PREPARATIONS.

Topical: One-fourth inch of ointment is applied to the inside of the lower lid.

All preparations available in topical ophthalmic form (nonprescription).

Akwa Tears (Akorn). Ointment (sterile) with white petrolatum, mineral oil, and lanolin in 3.5 g containers (preservative free).

Duolube (Bausch & Lomb). Ointment (sterile) containing white petrolatum and mineral oil in 3.5 g containers.

Duratears (Alcon). Ointment (sterile) with white petrolatum, anhydrous liquid lanolin, and mineral oil in 3.5 g containers.

HypoTears (Iolab). Ointment (sterile) with white petrolatum and light mineral oil in 3.5 g containers.

Lacri-Lube NP (Allergan). Ointment (sterile) with white petrolatum 57.3%, mineral oil 42.5%, and lanolin alcohol in 0.7 g-unit dose.

Lacri-Lube S.O.P. (Allergan). Ointment (sterile) with white petrolatum 56.8%, mineral oil 42.5%, lanolin alcohols, and chlorobutanol 0.5% in 3.5 and 7 g containers and 0.7 g unit dose.

Refresh PM (Allergan). Ointment (sterile) with white petrolatum 56.8%, mineral oil 41.5%, and lanolin alcohol (and) sodium chloride in 3.5 g containers.

INVESTIGATIONAL AGENTS

Tretinoin: Because vitamin A plays an important role in epithelial growth and differentiation, tretinoin ophthalmic ointment [Lacramore] is being investigated for the treatment of various *severe, refractory* dry-eye disorders. In an uncontrolled study in patients with keratoconjunctivitis sicca, Stevens-Johnson syndrome, inactive ocular pemphigoid, or dry-eye syndromes induced by drugs, surgery, or radiation, tretinoin relieved symptoms, improved visual acuity, decreased the use of artificial tear preparations, increased tear production in some patients, and reversed squamous metaplasia as evidenced by impression cytology (Tseng et al, 1985). In a controlled trial, tretinoin was ineffective in improving signs and symptoms of keratoconjunctivitis sicca but reversed ocular surface keratinization associated with conjunctival cicatricial diseases (Soong et al, 1988). Tretinoin also has been studied for use as an adjunct to systemic vitamin A therapy in children with retinal lesions caused by vitamin A deficiency (Sommer, 1983).

The most common adverse effects reported with tretinoin are local irritation, erythema, and photophobia. A more serious complication, corneal calcification, occurred in two patients (Avisar et al, 1988).

Fibronectin: Fibronectin is a glycoprotein present in plasma and on cell surfaces that plays an important role in wound healing and hemostasis. Acting as an adhesive protein, fibronectin facilitates uptake of intravascular debris by the reticuloendothelial system (Pussell et al, 1985). Limited data suggest that fibronectin eyedrops may be useful for treatment of severe corneal epithelial defects refractory to conventional therapy (Phan et al, 1987).

Aprotinin: The tear fluid of patients with severe, resistant corneal lesions shows high proteolytic activity. Preliminary studies suggest that epithelial healing may be improved following topical therapy with the serine proteinase inhibitor, aprotinin, sometimes combined with fibronectin (Salonen et al, 1987).

Acetylcysteine: Acetylcysteine eyedrops may alleviate symptoms in patients with filamentary keratitis that is usually secondary to severe keratoconjunctivitis sicca. The usefulness of this approach is limited because the solution is irritating, expensive, and malodorous (Lemp, 1987).

Bromhexine: Another mucolytic drug, bromhexine [Bisolvon], has been reported to alter the mucous phase of keratoconjunctivitis sicca when given orally. The efficacy of topical therapy is currently being studied (Norn, 1985).

Epidermal Growth Factor (EGF): In laboratory studies, this growth-regulating protein, which is produced by genetic engineering techniques, promoted corneal wound healing. Its potential clinical applications include treatment of corneal ulcers and promotion of corneal healing in recurrent erosion syndromes and other surgical procedures.

CORNEAL DEHYDRATING AGENTS

Corneal edema is caused by impaired epithelial function as a result of disease or injury (eg, implantation of poorly designed intraocular lens). Anhydrous glycerin and hypertonic sodium chloride are used to treat these conditions.

ANHYDROUS GLYCERIN

[Ophthalgan]

HYPERTONIC SODIUM CHLORIDE

[Adsorbonac, AK-NaCl, Muro-128]

ACTIONS AND USES. These hypertonic agents are applied topically to reduce corneal epithelial edema. They act by rendering the precorneal tear film hypertonic, thereby extracting water from the corneal epithelium. Hypertonic agents are effective in the short-term treatment of epithelial edema to clear the cornea, improve visual acuity, and enhance the view for optical examination through the cornea. Topical osmotherapy extracts only a small volume of stromal fluid and does not reduce stromal edema. Hypertonic agents also do not improve visual acuity if scarring or edema of the epithelium or stroma has occurred (Dohlman, 1983).

Glycerin is used prior to ophthalmoscopy or gonioscopy when the cornea is too edematous to permit diagnosis. It is very effective as a dehydrating agent, but instillation is painful and long-term therapy is not used.

Hypertonic sodium chloride is used for prolonged treatment of epithelial edema associated with cataract extraction, trauma, or recurrent corneal erosions. When treating corneal edema of long duration, best results may be obtained when the patient is also fitted with a hydrophilic soft contact lens (Gasset and Kaufman, 1971). The lens usually relieves pain and occasionally improves visual acuity.

ADVERSE REACTIONS AND PRECAUTIONS. Topical osmotic agents may cause transient stinging and burning. Glycerin causes more local discomfort than sodium chloride. Anhydrous glycerin is classified in FDA Pregnancy Category C.

DOSAGE AND PREPARATIONS.

ANHYDROUS GLYCERIN:

Topical: To facilitate diagnosis, one to three drops are instilled prior to the examination. A topical anesthetic should be instilled before glycerin is applied.

Ophthalgan (Wyeth-Ayerst). Solution (ophthalmic, sterile) with chlorobutanol 0.55% in 7.5 ml containers.

HYPERTONIC SODIUM CHLORIDE:

Topical: For treatment of corneal edema, one or two drops of the solution are instilled every three or four hours or as needed and the ointment may be applied at bedtime. In patients with bullous keratopathy, topical hyperosmotic agents should be avoided if the eye is painful. After pain has subsided, one or two drops of the 5% solution are instilled as needed to reduce epithelial edema. (The solution is used with a hydrophilic soft contact lens; the ointment is not appropriate.) The frequency of administration may be reduced or the drug discontinued if edema subsides.

All preparations available in topical ophthalmic form.

Adsorbonac (Alcon). Solution (sterile) 2% and 5% with thimerosal 0.004% and edetate disodium 0.1% in 15 ml containers (nonprescription).

Ak-NaCl (Akorn). Ointment (sterile) 5% in 3.5 g containers (nonprescription); solution (sterile) 5% with hydroxypropylmethylcellulose, propylene glycol, methylparaben, and propylparaben in 15 ml containers.

Muro-128 (Bausch & Lomb). Ointment (sterile) 5% in 3.5 g containers; solution (sterile) 2% and 5% with methylparaben 0.023% and propylparaben 0.01% in 15 (2% concentration only) and 30 ml containers (nonprescription).

DYES

The dyes, fluorescein and rose bengal, are used topically as diagnostic tools to detect corneal and conjunctival epithelial defects. Fluorescein also can be injected intravenously for evaluation of retinal function.

FLUORESCEIN SODIUM

ACTIONS AND USES. Fluorescein is an indicator dye that appears yellow-green in normal tear film and bright green in a more alkaline medium, such as the aqueous humor. Fluorescence is activated by blue and ultraviolet light.

Fluorescein is applied topically to detect corneal epithelial defects by staining the exposed stroma where the epithelium is absent. Because it makes the tear fluid visible, this dye is used to fit hard contact lenses and to delineate the margins of the applanated area in applanation tonometry. Since the intensity of green fluorescence increases when the dye is in contact with aqueous humor, fluorescein is useful for locating the site of a wound leak (eg, in patients with a flat or shallow anterior chamber after eye surgery). It also is instilled in the eye to test lacrimal patency; if drainage is normal, the dye will appear in the nasal secretions.

The usual fluorescein products should not be used to fit soft contact lenses because the lens will absorb the dye. Fluorexon [Fluoresoft] is available for use with soft contact lenses having a water content of less than 60%. This solution can be removed by repeated rinsing with physiologic saline.

Fluorescein is given intravenously as an aid in retinal angiography. It is used to evaluate diabetic retinopathy and to detect occlusion or obliteration of retinal vessels, vascular malformations, retinal or subretinal neovascularization, changes in vascular permeability, ocular tumors, reticular degeneration of the retinal pigment epithelium, and abnormalities of the iris vasculature (iris angiography). Intravenous administration or multiple topical applications may be used to study aqueous humor flow rate. Measurement of the arm-to-retina circulation time is employed for diagnosis of carotid artery occlusion.

ADVERSE REACTIONS AND PRECAUTIONS. Preservatives with positive charges are inactivated by the negatively charged fluorescein molecule. Contaminated fluorescein solutions have been a source of ocular infections, particularly by *Pseudomonas* organisms. Sterile, single-dose containers and individually packaged filter-paper strips impregnated with fluorescein are safer than multiple-dose containers.

Nausea and vomiting occur occasionally when fluorescein is given intravenously. Pruritus, urticaria, paresthesias, dizziness, and syncope also have been reported. Acute pulmonary edema, acute myocardial infarction, and cardiac arrest are uncommon complications of intravenous fluorescein. Topical preparations of fluorescein are classified in FDA Pregnancy Category C.

DOSAGE AND PREPARATIONS.

Topical: To detect epithelial defects, a fluorescein strip moistened with ophthalmic irrigating solution is used to touch the inferior palpebral conjunctiva, or one drop of a 0.5% to 2% solution is placed in the conjunctival sac. To provide contrast between the lesion and surrounding areas, excess dye may be removed by use of an irrigating solution.

To fit hard contact lenses, with the contact lens in place, a fluorescein strip moistened with ophthalmic irrigating solution is lightly touched to the inferior conjunctiva. The patient should be instructed to blink several times to circulate the dye. Under blue light, areas that lack fluorescein-stained tears appear black, indicating that the contact lens is touching the cornea at those points. Areas with fluorescein pooling indicate vaulting of the lens and askew fit.

In applanation tonometry, following topical anesthesia, one drop of a 0.25% solution or a fluorescein strip moistened with ophthalmic irrigating solution is applied to the conjunctiva immediately before tonometry. Combination products containing benoxinate or proparacaine and fluorescein may be used for simultaneous staining and local anesthesia, but the use of the fluorescein strip is preferable. Tetracaine generally should be avoided because it may reduce the intensity of fluorescence.

To test lacrimal patency, one drop of a 2% solution is instilled in the conjunctival sac. The patient should be instructed to blink at least four times after the dye is instilled. After six minutes, nasal secretions are examined under blue light; the presence of traces of the dye indicates that the nasolacrimal drainage system is open. In a modification of this procedure (Hecht, 1978), one drop of the 2% solution is instilled three times at 15-minute intervals. One minute after instillation of the third drop, the patient is instructed to place his head downward at a 45° angle to prevent posterior loss of the dye and to avoid sniffing back the fluid. The nasal secretions are then examined after 10 minutes.

To test for aqueous leak following ocular surgery or trauma, a moistened fluorescein strip is used to detect the wound. Gentle pressure on the globe may be applied to determine the site of the leak but is usually not necessary or desirable.

All preparations available in ophthalmic forms.

Generic. Solution 2% in 1, 2, and 15 ml containers.

Fluorescein Sodium Steri-Units (Alcon). Solution (sterile) 2% with phenylmercuric nitrate 0.04% in 2 ml containers.

Fluorets (Akorn). Sterile applicators impregnated with fluorescein sodium 1 mg/strip in boxes containing 100 individual strips.

Fluor-I-Strip (Wyeth-Ayerst). Sterile applicators impregnated with fluorescein sodium 9 mg/strip (lint free) with chlorobutanol 0.5% in individual envelopes in boxes containing 200 envelopes.

Fluor-I-Strip A.T. (Wyeth-Ayerst). Sterile applicators impregnated with fluorescein sodium 1 mg/strip (lint free) with chlorobutanol 0.5% in boxes containing 100 envelopes (2 strips/envelope).

Ful-Glo (Sola/Barnes-Hind). Sterile applicators impregnated with fluorescein sodium 0.6 mg/strip in boxes containing 300 individual strips.

Available Mixtures.

Fluoracaine (Akorn). Solution (sterile) containing fluorescein sodium 0.25% and proparacaine hydrochloride 0.5% with thimerosal 0.01% in 5 ml containers.

Fluress (Sola/Barnes-Hind). Solution (sterile) containing fluorescein sodium 0.25% and benoxinate hydrochloride 0.4% with chlorobutanol 1% in 5 ml containers.

Product Used for Fitting Soft Contact Lenses with Water Content <60%:

FLUOREXON:

Fluoresoft (Holles Laboratories). Solution (sterile, without preservatives) 0.35% in 0.5 ml containers.

Intravenous: *Adults,* 500 mg (10 ml of a 5% solution or 5 ml of a 10% solution) is injected rapidly into an arm vein. Some investigators believe that better visualization can be attained with 3 ml of a 25% solution (750 mg). The dye should appear in the central retinal artery in 9 to 15 seconds.

Ak-Fluor (Akorn). Solution (sterile) 25% in 2 ml containers and 10% in 5 ml containers.

Fluorescite (Alcon). Solution (sterile) 10% in 5 ml containers, 10% in 5 ml syringe containers, and 25% in 2 ml containers.

Funduscein (Iolab). Solution 10% in 5 ml containers and 25% in 3 ml containers.

ROSE BENGAL

Rose bengal is a vital stain that does not stain the precorneal tear film but has a particular affinity for devitalized corneal and conjunctival epithelium. When viewed under the slitlamp, the stain consists of rose-colored dots. Rose bengal is used to determine the extent of epithelial damage in various conjunctival or corneal disorders. It is particularly useful for diagnosis of keratoconjunctivitis sicca (Laibson, 1980; Lamberts, 1983) and for the fine differentiation of the margin of corneal ulcers caused by herpes simplex virus.

Although rose bengal is more irritating to the eye than fluorescein, a local anesthetic is generally not necessary if small amounts are used. Rose bengal discolors the lids and surrounding facial area for several days when the undiluted 1% solution is applied in the form of eyedrops.

DOSAGE AND PREPARATIONS.

Topical: Ocular irritation and staining of the lids and surrounding facial area can be minimized by placing a drop of the 1% solution on the stick end of a cotton-tipped applicator, which permits application of about one-fourth of a normal drop. Alternatively, the 1% solution may be diluted and then instilled in drop form or ophthalmic strips impregnated with rose bengal may be used.

Rose Bengal (Akorn). Solution (ophthalmic, sterile) 1% with thimerosal 0.01% in 5 ml containers.

Rose Bengal Ophthalmic Strips (Sola/Barnes-Hind). Sterile strips impregnated with 1.3 mg in packages containing 100 strips.

ENZYMES

The enzymes, chymotrypsin and hyaluronidase, are employed as adjuncts in ophthalmic surgical procedures. Chymotrypsin is used to dissolve the zonules of the lens (zonulysis) during intracapsular cataract surgery. Hyaluronidase facilitates the penetration of anesthetics during surgery.

CHYMOTRYPSIN

[Catarase, Zolyse]

ACTIONS AND USES. During intracapsular cataract extraction, the proteolytic enzyme, chymotrypsin, is introduced behind the iris into the posterior chamber, where it dissolves the zonular fibers within two to four minutes. It reduces the risk of capsule rupture and of traction-induced retinal detachment, especially in young adults, high myopes, and patients with intumescent cataract or prior retinal detachment (Barraquer and Barraquer, 1985). Chymotrypsin also can be used to aid in removal of residual cortical and capsular material of the lens following pars plana lensectomy. This enzyme is used less commonly today than in the past because of the increasing employment of extracapsular surgery.

ADVERSE REACTIONS AND PRECAUTIONS. A transient increase in intraocular pressure is a common untoward effect of chymotrypsin; if the pressure is very high, ocular pain and corneal edema may occur. Enzyme-induced increase in intraocular pressure may persist for a week. The cause is unknown but may involve the accumulation of zonular fragments in the trabecular meshwork or a toxic effect on the trabecular meshwork and ciliary body. Administration of chymotrypsin also has been associated with wound leak and shallowing of the anterior chamber. These complications apparently result from the enzyme-induced glaucoma; the incidence can be reduced by use of multiple corneoscleral sutures and postoperative administration of a topical beta blocker and a systemic carbonic anhydrase inhibitor.

Chymotrypsin is extremely toxic to the retina and should not be allowed to penetrate into the vitreous. In patients with fluid vitreous, enzymatic zonulysis can result in loss of the lens posteriorly and, possibly, entry of chymotrypsin into the vitreous body. Uveitis also has been observed. Systemic reactions have not been reported.

DOSAGE AND PREPARATIONS. Alcohol, disinfectants, and blood may inactivate the enzyme.

Injection: 0.2 to 0.5 ml of a freshly prepared 1:5,000 to 1:10,000 solution is injected slowly behind the iris into the posterior chamber. The chamber then may be irrigated with 2 ml of the diluent or a balanced salt solution. A second application of chymotrypsin may be required if the zonules are resistant.

Catarase (Iolab). Two-compartment vial containing lyophilized chymotrypsin 150 (1:10,000) or 300 (1:5,000) units in the lower compartment and sodium chloride injection 2 ml in the upper compartment.

Zolyse (Alcon). Powder (lyophilized, for solution) 750 units with 9 ml of diluent.

HYALURONIDASE

[Wydase]

ACTIONS AND USES. Hyaluronidase hydrolyzes hyaluronic acid, a polysaccharide found in interstitial spaces of tissues where it blocks invasive substances. This enzyme is used during ophthalmic surgical procedures to enhance diffusion of locally injected anesthetics by increasing tissue permeability. When it is added to the injection solution, the time required for induction of complete akinesia is reduced and anesthesia is enhanced (Thomson, 1988). Hyaluronidase may increase the rate of absorption of the anesthetic and thus reduce its duration of action, but this problem can usually be avoided if epinephrine is added to the injection solution.

ADVERSE REACTIONS AND PRECAUTIONS. Adverse reactions are rare. Local irritation and allergic reactions have been reported.

Hyaluronidase is classified in FDA Pregnancy Category C.

DOSAGE AND PREPARATIONS. 150 units are added to each 10 ml of anesthetic solution.

Wydase (Wyeth-Ayerst). Powder (lyophilized) 150 and 1,500 units with lactose and thimerosal; solution (stabilized) 150 units/ml with edetate disodium and thimerosal in sterile sodium chloride injection in 1 and 10 ml containers.

VISCOELASTIC AGENTS

Viscoelastic agents are used as aids in cataract surgery, lens implantation, filtering operations for glaucoma, and keratoplasty (Liesegang, 1990). They deepen the anterior chamber and protect the corneal endothelium during these procedures.

SODIUM HYALURONATE

[AMO Vitrax, Amvisc, Healon]

ACTIONS AND USES. Sodium hyaluronate is the sodium salt of hyaluronic acid. A highly purified fraction of this naturally occurring polymer is available as a 1% or 3% transparent, noninflammatory, viscoelastic solution for use as an aid in ophthalmic surgery.

Cataract Surgery-Intraocular Lens Implant: When placed in the anterior chamber prior to lens extraction, sodium hyaluronate reduces endothelial cell loss and prevents flattening of the anterior chamber during surgery (Barraquer, 1985; Pape and Balazs, 1980). Sodium hyaluronate is particularly useful to protect the corneal endothelium during primary or secondary implantation of an intraocular lens (Miller and Stegmann, 1981, 1982; Polack et al, 1981).

Filtering Operations for Glaucoma: In conjunction with trabeculectomy, injection of sodium hyaluronate into the anterior chamber and subconjunctival space may deepen the anterior chamber and promote formation of a superior filtration bleb. Postoperatively, it dissolves in newly formed aqueous and is eliminated slowly from the anterior chamber (Barraquer, 1985; Pape and Balazs, 1980).

Keratoplasty: Sodium hyaluronate is useful in corneal grafting procedures to protect the corneal endothelium of the graft and to facilitate graft suturing. It may aid in hemostasis (Barraquer, 1985; Pape and Balazs, 1980; Polack et al, 1981). It also is useful in dissecting iridocorneal adhesions.

Retinal Detachment Surgery: During vitrectomy procedures, sodium hyaluronate may be injected into the vitreous cavity to facilitate treatment of giant retinal tears and to assist in dissolution of fibrovascular membranes associated with proliferative diabetic retinopathy. However, it appears to offer no particular advantage over other methods in patients with proliferative vitreoretinopathy (Gerke et al, 1985; Vatne and Syrdalen, 1986).

ADVERSE REACTIONS AND PRECAUTIONS. The intraocular pressure should be monitored carefully during the first 24 to 48 hours after use of sodium hyaluronate in anterior segment surgery (Pape, 1980). If a significant elevation in pressure occurs, a carbonic anhydrase inhibitor and/or a topical beta blocker should be given until the intracameral sodium hyaluronate is diluted by newly formed aqueous (Pape and Balazs, 1980). Alternatively, a carbonic anhydrase inhibitor or beta blocker may be given prophylactically immediately after surgery (Lewin and Insler, 1985). Replacement of sodium hyaluronate by balanced salt solution or physiologic saline at the end of the operation may minimize the increase in pressure (Miller and Stegmann, 1981; Pape, 1980).

When used as an adjunct in retinal detachment surgery, sodium hyaluronate can pass through retinal tears and prevent reattachment (Vatne and Syrdalen, 1986).

Rarely, iritis, hypopyon, corneal edema, and corneal opacities have been reported postoperatively. Their relationship to sodium hyaluronate has not been established. Small intraocular foreign bodies have been observed after injection of sodium hyaluronate. These foreign bodies, which in most cases could be removed successfully, were found to originate in the rubber membrane sealing the ampule.

DOSAGE AND PREPARATIONS. Whenever feasible, sodium hyaluronate should be removed at the end of any surgical procedure.

Intracameral: For cataract surgery-intraocular lens implant, a sufficient amount is introduced slowly and carefully into the anterior chamber (using a cannula or needle) before or after delivery of the lens. Injection prior to lens delivery is preferred to protect the corneal endothelium during surgery. Additional amounts may be added to replace any that is lost during surgery. Sodium hyaluronate also may be used to coat intraocular lenses and surgical instruments.

For glaucoma surgery, in conjunction with trabeculectomy, a sufficient amount of sodium hyaluronate is injected slowly and carefully through a corneal paracentesis to reform the anterior chamber. Additional amounts may be injected to permit the preparation to extrude into the subconjunctival filtration site through and around the sutured outer scleral flap.

For corneal transplant surgery, after removal of the corneal button, the anterior chamber is filled with sodium hyaluronate; the donor graft is then placed on top of the preparation and sutured in place.

AMO Vitrax (Allergan). Solution 30 mg/ml with sodium chloride 3.2 mg, potassium chloride 0.75 mg, calcium chloride 0.48 mg, magnesium chloride 0.3 mg, sodium acetate 3.9 mg, and sodium citrate 1.7 mg in 0.5 ml containers.

Amvisc (Iolab). Solution (sterile, ophthalmic) 10 mg/ml in 0.25, 0.5, 0.8, and 4 ml containers; and 16 mg/ml in 0.25, 0.5, and 8 ml containers (***Amvisc Plus***).

Healon (Pharmacia). Solution (sterile, ophthalmic) 10 mg/ml with sodium chloride 8.5 mg, disodium hydrogen phosphate dihydrate 0.28 mg, and sodium dihydrogen phosphate 0.04 mg in 0.4, 0.75, and 2 ml containers.

SODIUM CHONDROITIN SULFATE/SODIUM HYALURONATE
[Viscoat]

ACTIONS AND USES. Sodium chondroitin sulfate is a naturally occurring polymer found in relatively high concentrations in the cornea. It is claimed to provide more protection for the corneal endothelium than sodium hyaluronate but is less viscous. The combination of the two polymers is used as an aid in cataract surgery and intraocular lens implantation to maintain the anterior chamber and reduce endothelial cell loss.

ADVERSE REACTIONS AND PRECAUTIONS. The postoperative rise in intraocular pressure induced by this combination is comparable to that caused by sodium hyaluronate alone (Barron et al, 1985). The original formulation caused calcific band keratopathy, identified as calcium-phosphate precipitates, which responded to edetate disodium chelation therapy (Ullman et al, 1986). The product was subsequently reformulated with a reduced concentration of phosphate buffer to reduce the risk of corneal deposits. Sodium chondroitin sulfate has anticoagulant properties, but there have been no reports of impaired ocular hemostasis (Pandolfi and Hedner, 1984).

DOSAGE AND PREPARATIONS.

Intracameral: 0.5 ml is introduced into the anterior chamber using a needle or cannula.

Viscoat (Alcon). Each milliliter of solution (sterile, ophthalmic) contains sodium chondroitin sulfate 40 mg, sodium hyaluronate 30 mg, sodium dihydrogen phosphate hydrate 0.45 mg, disodium hydrogen phosphate, and sodium chloride 4.3 mg in 0.5 ml containers.

HYDROXYPROPYLMETHYLCELLULOSE
[Occucoat]

ACTIONS AND USES. Hydroxypropylmethylcellulose is a space occupying, tissue protective substance that is used as an aid in surgical procedures involving the anterior segment, including cataract extraction, intraocular lens implantation, and corneal transplant surgery. This agent maintains a deep chamber during anterior segment surgery, thereby facilitating surgical manipulation with less trauma to the corneal endothelium and other ocular tissue. The viscoelasticity of hydroxypropylmethylcellulose enables the vitreous face to be pushed back and prevents the formation of a flat chamber postoperatively.

ADVERSE REACTIONS. Hydroxypropylmethylcellulose is well tolerated after injection into the eye. A transient increase in intraocular pressure postoperatively has been reported in a few patients; thus, this agent should be removed from the anterior chamber at the end of surgery. Appropriate glaucoma therapy should be initiated if postoperative intraocular pressure rises above accepted values (see the chapter, Drugs Used for Glaucoma).

DOSAGE AND PREPARATIONS.

Intracameral: For cataract extract and intraocular lens implantation, hydroxypropylmethylcellulose should be carefully introduced into the anterior chamber using a 20-gauge or larger cannula prior to or following delivery of the crystalline lens. The intraocular lens and tips of surgical instruments also may be coated with hydroxypropylmethylcellulose prior to implantation.

Occucoat (Storz). Solution (sterile, nonpyrogenic) 20 mg/ml dissolved in a physiologic balanced salt solution containing sodium chloride 0.49%, potassium chloride 0.075%, calcium chloride 0.048%, magnesium chloride 0.03%, sodium acetate 0.39%, and sodium citrate 0.17% in a single-use glass syringe with a Luer tip and cannula.

CHELATING AGENTS

Chelating agents are used to remove corneal calcium or iron deposits that impair vision or cause pain. These agents are applied topically in ocular siderosis, band keratopathy, and chronic uveitis.

DEFEROXAMINE MESYLATE

[Desferal]

For chemical formula, see index entry Deferoxamine, In Iron Poisoning.

ACTIONS AND USES. This chelating agent may be applied locally to the eye to treat ocular siderosis involving the cornea. It is applied topically to remove superficial iron deposits and injected subconjunctivally to remove deposits in the stroma or iris.

ADVERSE REACTIONS. Hyperemia and allergic reactions have been reported after local use.

DOSAGE AND PREPARATIONS.

Topical: A 10% solution of deferoxamine in 1% methylcellulose is applied four times daily for several weeks, or a 5% concentration in an ointment base is used.

Subconjunctival: 0.5 ml of a 10% solution is injected twice weekly for eight to ten weeks.

Desferal (CIBA). Powder (lyophilized, sterile) 500 mg.

EDETATE DISODIUM (EDTA)

[Chealamide, Disotate, Endrate]

```
          O                          O
          ||                         ||
Na⁺ ⁻OCCH₂                    CH₂CO⁻ Na⁺
           \                 /
      O     NCH₂CH₂N       O
      ||   /         \     ||
   HOCCH₂             CH₂COH
```

ACTIONS AND USES. This chelating agent is applied topically to remove corneal calcium deposits that impair vision or cause pain. It dissolves calcium deposits of endogenous origin (eg, band keratopathy and other calcific corneal deposits associated with chronic uveitis, advanced interstitial keratitis, hypercalcemia).

Edetate disodium extracts calcium from the conjunctiva, corneal epithelium, and anterior layers of the stroma but does not affect deposits in the deep stroma. The removal of superficial calcium deposits should improve vision unless scarring and vascularization have occurred or vision is reduced by coexistent posterior segment diseases; however, calcium deposits of endogenous origin tend to recur. Edetate disodium does not penetrate the corneal epithelium. Unless the deposit extends to the surface, the epithelium must be removed completely during treatment using a cotton-tip applicator.

ADVERSE REACTIONS AND PRECAUTIONS. Edetate disodium is well tolerated when applied topically. Transient stinging and chemosis may occur. The stronger concentration (1.85%) may cause stromal edema.

DOSAGE AND PREPARATIONS.

Topical: For removal of calcium deposits from the anterior layers of the stroma, a local anesthetic should be instilled before the procedure; cocaine is often preferred because it facilitates epithelial removal. The corneal epithelium then is removed completely and the denuded area is irrigated with edetate disodium (0.35% to 1.85% solution) for 15 to 20 minutes. The solution is applied as a corneal bath, by continuous irrigation, or by application of a pledget soaked in the solution to the cornea. After the procedure, the eye should be irrigated with sodium chloride injection or a balanced salt solution.

For emergency treatment of calcium hydroxide burns, the eye should first be flushed with water as quickly as possible and then irrigated with a 0.35% to 1.85% solution of edetate disodium for 15 minutes.

For emergency treatment of zinc chloride injury, after flushing with water, the eye may be irrigated with a 1.7% solution for 15 minutes. Treatment may be ineffective if not begun within two minutes after injury.

No ophthalmic preparation is available. The intravenous solution must be diluted to the desired concentration with isotonic sodium chloride injection (usually one part edetate sodium to three parts sodium chloride).

Chealamide (Vortech), ***Disotate*** (Forest), ***Endrate*** (Abbott), ***Generic.*** Solution (injection) 150 mg/ml in 20 ml containers.

IRRIGATING SOLUTIONS

External and internal irrigating solutions are used to cleanse the eye tissues. Internal irrigating solutions also are used to supply nutrients to the anterior segment, particularly the corneal endothelium.

Internal Irrigating Solutions: These preparations are administered during ocular surgery to irrigate the anterior chamber, extraocular muscles, or lacrimal system; to wash out lens fragments during cataract surgery; to irrigate the eye during vitrectomy; and to moisten the cornea. Irrigating solutions differ in their ability to preserve corneal endothelial structure and function.

In corneal perfusion studies, glutathione-bicarbonate-Ringer's solution [BSS Plus], which is chemically similar to aqueous humor, was more effective than lactated Ringer's solution in maintaining corneal thickness and endothelial structure (Edelhauser and MacRae, 1985). In patients undergoing pars plana vitrectomy, BSS Plus caused less corneal swelling than lactated Ringer's on the first day after surgery, but, by the seventh postoperative day, there was no significant difference between the two solutions (Benson et al, 1981). Endothelial cell loss, measured six months after cataract surgery, was greater in eyes irrigated with BSS (which lacks bicarbonate, dextrose, and glutathione) compared to those irrigated with BSS Plus (Kline et al, 1983). However, no significant difference was observed in another study (Rosenfeld et al, 1986).

Results of a multi-institutional evaluation of intraocular irrigating solutions showed that BSS Plus may be appropriate for surgical procedures with a duration exceeding one hour or those in which viscoelastic agents are not used, in patients younger than 50 years, and in patients with diabetes mellitus or evidence of pre-existing corneal endothelial compromise in the affected eye (Closson et al, 1990).

BSS (Alcon), ***Iocare Balance Salt Solution*** (Iolab). Solution (sterile) containing sodium chloride 0.64%, potassium chloride 0.075%, calcium chloride 0.048%, magnesium chloride 0.03%, sodium acetate 0.39%, sodium citrate 0.17%, and sodium hydroxide and/or hydrochloric acid in 15, 30, 250 (***BSS*** only), and 500 ml containers.

BSS Plus (Alcon). Two-container preparation: (Part I, 500 ml) Solution (sterile) containing sodium chloride 7.44 mg, potassium chloride 0.395 mg, dried sodium phosphate 0.433 mg, sodium bicarbonate 2.19 mg, and sodium hydroxide and/or hydrochloric acid to be reconstituted with (Part II, 20 ml) solution (sterile) containing calcium chloride dihydrate 3.85 mg, magnesium chloride hexahydrate 5 mg, dextrose 23 mg, and glutathione disulfide 4.6 mg/ml.

External Irrigating Solutions: These solutions are used for flushing the eye to remove foreign bodies, air pollutants, chemicals, and gases and for irrigation after diagnostic and surgical procedures. The boric acid present in some preparations may form an insoluble complex with the polyvinyl alcohol contained in some contact lens wetting solutions.

All preparations available in topical ophthalmic forms (nonprescription).

AK-Rinse (Akorn). Solution (sterile) containing sodium chloride 0.49%, potassium chloride 0.075%, calcium chloride 0.048%, magnesium chloride 0.03%, sodium acetate 0.39%, sodium citrate 0.17%, and benzalkonium chloride 0.013% in 30 and 118 ml containers.

Blinx (Sola/Barnes-Hind). Solution (sterile) containing sodium and potassium chloride, sodium phosphate, benzalkonium chloride 0.005%, and edetate disodium 0.02% in 120 ml containers.

Collyrium Fresh Eyes (Wyeth-Ayerst). Solution containing boric acid, sodium borate, and thimerosal 0.002% in 180 ml containers.

Dacriose (Iolab). Solution (sterile) containing sodium chloride, potassium chloride, sodium phosphate, sodium hydroxide, benzalkonium chloride, and edetate disodium in 15, 30, and 120 ml containers.

Eye-Stream (Alcon). Each milliliter contains a balanced salt solution of sodium chloride 0.49%, potassium chloride 0.075%, calcium chloride 0.48%, magnesium chloride 0.03%, sodium acetate 0.39%, sodium citrate 0.17%, sodium hydroxide and/or hydrochloric acid, purified water, and benzalkonium chloride 0.013% in 30 and 120 ml containers.

Murine Regular Formula (Ross). Solution (sterile) containing sodium chloride, potassium chloride, sodium phosphate, and glycerine with benzalkonium chloride 0.01% and edetate disodium 0.05% in 45 ml containers.

ASTRINGENTS

ZINC SULFATE

Zinc sulfate has mild astringent properties when applied topically to the eye. In the concentration used in ophthalmic products, it may act by clearing mucus from the surface of the eye. The FDA Advisory Review Panel on OTC Ophthalmic Drug Products has found the 0.25% solution (which is usually marketed in combination with a decongestant) to be safe and effective for temporary relief of discomfort caused by minor eye irritation (*Federal Register*, 1980, 1988).

Zinc sulfate may cause transient stinging or burning. Other adverse effects have not been reported.

DOSAGE AND PREPARATIONS.

Topical: One or two drops of a 0.25% solution are instilled into the affected eye(s) up to four times daily.

All preparations available in topical ophthalmic forms (nonprescription).

Optised (Rugby). Solution (sterile) 0.25% with phenylephrine 0.12% in 15 ml containers.

Phenylzin (Iolab). Solution (sterile) 0.25% with phenylephrine 0.12%, benzalkonium chloride, and edetate disodium in 15 ml containers.

Visine-A.C. (Pfizer). Solution (sterile, isotonic) 0.25% with tetrahydrozoline hydrochloride 0.05% and benzalkonium chloride 0.01% in 15 and 30 ml containers.

Zincfrin (Alcon). Solution (sterile) 0.25% with phenylephrine hydrochloride 0.12% and benzalkonium chloride 0.01% in 15 ml containers.

Cited References

Ophthalmic drug products for over-the-counter human use; establishment of a monograph, proposed rulemaking. *Federal Register* 45:30002-30050, 1980.

Ophthalmic drug products for over-the-counter human use; final monograph; final rule. *Federal Register* 53:7076-7098, 1988.

American Academy of Ophthalmology: Botulinum toxin therapy of eye muscle disorders. *Ophthalmology* 96(part 2):37-40, 1989.

Avisar R, et al: Corneal calcification in dry eye disorders associated with retinoic acid therapy, letter. *Am J Ophthalmol* 106:753-755, 1988.

Barraquer J: Viscous solutions in anterior segment surgery, in Sears M, Tarkkanen A (eds): *Surgical Pharmacology of the Eye.* New York, Raven Press, 1985, 391-407.

Barraquer RI, Barraquer J: Useful enzymes, in Sears M, Tarkkanen A (eds): *Surgical Pharmacology of the Eye.* New York, Raven Press, 1985, 321-360.

Barron BA, et al: Comparison of effects of Viscoat and Healon on postoperative intraocular pressure. *Am J Ophthalmol* 100:377-384, 1985.

Benson WE, et al: Intraocular irrigating solutions for pars plana vitrectomy: Prospective, randomized, double-blind study. *Arch Ophthalmol* 99:1013-1015, 1981.

Carruthers JDA: Ophthalmologic use of botulinum A exotoxin. *Can J Ophthalmol* 20:135-141, 1985.

Closson RG, et al: Multi-institutional drug-use evaluation of intraocular irrigating solutions. *Am J Hosp Pharm* 47:2255-2259, 1990.

Dohlman CH: Physiology of the cornea: Corneal edema, in Smolin G, Throft RA (eds): *The Cornea: Scientific Foundations and Clinical Practice.* Boston, Little Brown, 1983, 3-17.

Edelhauser HF, MacRae SM: Irritating and viscous solutions, in Sears M, Tarkkanen A (eds): *Surgical Pharmacology of the Eye.* New York, Raven Press, 1985, 363-388.

Fitzsimmons R, et al: Treatment of sixth nerve palsy in adults with combined botulinum toxin chemodenervation and surgery. *Ophthalmology* 95:1535-1542, 1988.

Gasset AR, Kaufman HE: Bandage lenses in treatment of bullous keratopathy. *Am J Ophthalmol* 72:376-380, 1971.

Gerke E, et al: Use of hyaluronic acid in complicated retinal detachments, in Sears M, Tarkkanen A (eds): *Surgical Pharmacology of the Eye.* New York, Raven Press, 1985, 411-415.

Gilbard JP, Kenyon KR: Tear diluents in treatment of keratoconjunctivitis sicca. *Ophthalmology* 92:646-650, 1985.

Hecht SD: Evaluation of the lacrimal drainage system. *Ophthalmology* 85:1250-1258, 1978.

Jankovic J, Brin MF: Therapeutic uses of botulinum toxin. *N Engl J Med* 324:1186-1194, 1991.

Kirkness CM, et al: Botulinum toxin A-induced protective ptosis in corneal disease. *Ophthalmology* 95:473-480, 1988.

Kline OR Jr, et al: Effect of BSS Plus on the corneal endothelium with intraocular lens implantation. *J Toxicol Clin Ocular Toxicol* 2:243-247, 1983.

Laibson PR: Diagnosis and treatment of keratoconjunctivitis sicca, in: *Symposium on Medical and Surgical Disease of the Cornea.* St Louis, Mo, CV Mosby, 1980, 36-47.

Lamberts DW: Keratoconjunctivitis sicca, in Smolin G, Throft RA (eds): *The Cornea: Scientific Foundations and Clinical Practice.* Boston, Little Brown, 1983, 293-309.

Lange DJ, et al: Distant effects of local injection of botulinum toxin. *Muscle Nerve* 10:552-555, 1987.

Lemp MA: Recent developments in dry eye management. *Ophthalmology* 94:1299-1304, 1987.

Lemp MA, et al: Effect of tear substitutes on tear film break-up time. *Invest Ophthalmol* 14:255-258, 1975.

Lewin R, Insler MS: Effect of prophylactic acetazolamide on intraocular pressure rise associated with Healon-aided intraocular lens surgery. *Ann Ophthalmol* 17:315-318, 1985.

Liesegang TJ: Viscoelastic substances in ophthalmology. *Surv Ophthalmol* 34:268-293, 1990.

Miller D, Stegmann R: Use of sodium hyaluronate in human IOL implantation. *Ann Ophthalmol* 13:811-815, 1981.

Miller D, Stegmann R: Secondary intraocular lens implantation using sodium hyaluronate. *Ann Ophthalmol* 14:621-623, 1982.

Norn MS: Keratoconjunctivitis sicca, in Fraunfelder FT, Roy FH (eds): *Current Ocular Therapy 2.* Philadelphia, WB Saunders, 1985, 322-324.

Pandolfi M, Hedner U: Effect of sodium hyaluronate and sodium chondroitin sulfate on coagulation system in vitro. *Ophthalmology* 91:864-866, 1984.

Pape LG: Intracapsular and extracapsular technique of lens implantation with Healon. *Ann Intraoc Implant Soc J* 6:342-343, 1980.

Pape LG, Balazs EA: Use of sodium hyaluronate (Healon) in human anterior segment surgery. *Ophthalmology* 87:699-705, 1980.

Patrinely JR, et al: Local side effects of botulinum toxin injections. *Adv Neurol* 49:493-500, 1988.

Phan T-MM, et al: Topical fibronectin in treatment of persistent corneal epithelial defects and trophic ulcers. *Am J Ophthalmol* 104:494-501, 1987.

Polack FM, et al: Sodium hyaluronate (Healon) in keratoplasty and IOL implantation. *Ophthalmology* 88:425-431, 1981.

Pussell BA, et al: Human fibronectin metabolism. *J Clin Invest* 76:143-148, 1985.

Rosenfeld SI, et al: Comparison of intraocular irrigating solutions in pars plana vitrectomy. *Ophthalmology* 93:109-115, 1986.

Salonen E-M, et al: Plasmin in tear fluid of patients with corneal ulcers: Basis for new therapy. *Acta Ophthalmol* 65:3-12, 1987.

Scott AB, et al: Botulinum treatment of childhood strabismus. *Ophthalmology* 97:1434-1438, 1990.

Sommer A: Treatment of corneal xerophthalmia with topical retinoic acid. *Am J Ophthalmol* 95:349-352, 1983.

Soong HK, et al: Topical retinoid therapy for squamous metaplasia of various ocular surface disorders: Multicenter, placebo-controlled double-masked trial. *Ophthalmology* 95:1442-1446, 1988.

Taylor JDN, et al: Treatment of blepharospasm and hemifacial spasm with botulinum A toxin: A Canadian multicentre study. *Can J Ophthalmol* 26:133-138, 1991.

Thomson I: Addition of hyaluronidase to lignocaine with adrenaline for retrobulbar anaesthesia in the surgery of senile cataract. *Br J Ophthalmol* 72:700-702, 1988.

Tseng SCG, et al: Topical retinoid treatment for various dry-eye disorders. *Ophthalmology* 92:717-727, 1985.

Ullman S, et al: Corneal opacities secondary to Viscoat. *J Cataract Refract Surg* 12:489-492, 1986.

Vatne HO, Syrdalen P: Use of sodium hyaluronate (Healon) in treatment of complicated cases of retinal detachment. *Acta Ophthalmol* 64:169-172, 1986.

Vitamins and some minerals are essential for normal metabolism. Vitamins are organic compounds that are required in minute amounts to maintain good health and often act as cofactors to a number of metabolic enzymes. Trace elements are inorganic compounds required for growth and maintenance of tissues and bones.

Food is the best source of vitamins and minerals, and healthy persons consuming an adequate balanced diet will not benefit from additional vitamins. However, individuals on low-calorie diets (less than 1,200 calories/day) often do not ingest adequate vitamins and may require a supplement. Purified or synthetic products are available individually or in various combinations. Products intended for prophylactic use should be distinguished from those preparations suitable only for therapeutic purposes.

Although there are few valid indications for vitamin or mineral supplements, nearly 50% of adults in the United States are thought to take such preparations. The danger of toxic effects from excessive amounts of vitamin A or D and all minerals, particularly in infants and children, should be considered (Reuter and Hellriegel, 1983; Lewis, 1980; Marshall, 1983). Massive-dose therapy usually is justified only in patients who cannot utilize nutrients properly, in those with certain diseases, or in those with inborn errors of metabolism that respond to pharmacologic doses of vitamins (see the evaluations).

Vegetarian diets utilizing multiple food sources can provide essential nutrients if milk products or eggs are added to supply vitamin B_{12}. Inadequate vitamin intake is not a problem for individuals consuming lactovegetarian diets (which include milk or milk products) or lacto-ovovegetarian diets (which include dairy products and eggs) (Council on Scientific Affairs, 1987). As these diets become more restrictive, the risk of nutritional inadequacies increases greatly, especially deficiencies of protein, vitamin B_{12}, calcium, vitamin D, and riboflavin.

The toxic substances known as vitamin B_{15} (pangamic acid) and vitamin B_{17} (laetrile) are neither nutrients nor vitamins. Laetrile contains 6% cyanide by weight and has caused chronic cyanide poisoning and death (Herbert, 1980; Moertel et al, 1982). Pangamic acid or pangamate may be mutagenic (Herbert, 1979). Neither substance has any established nutritional or other usefulness (Herbert, 1988).

TABLE 1.
RECOMMENDED DAILY DIETARY ALLOWANCES, 1989*

Category	Age (years) or Condition	Weight (kg)	Weight (lb)	Height (cm)	Height (in)	Protein (g)	Fat-Soluble Vitamins: Vitamin A (mcg RE)[1]	Vitamin D (mcg)[2]	Vitamin E (mg α-TE)[3]	Vitamin K (mcg)
Infants	0.0-0.5	6	13	60	24	13	375	7.5	3	3
	0.5-1.0	9	20	71	28	14	375	10	4	10
Children	1-3	13	29	90	35	16	400	10	6	15
	4-6	20	44	112	44	24	500	10	7	20
	7-10	28	62	132	52	28	700	10	7	30
Males	11-14	45	99	157	62	45	1,000	10	10	45
	15-18	66	145	176	69	59	1,000	10	10	65
	19-24	72	160	177	70	58	1,000	10	10	70
	25-50	79	174	176	70	63	1,000	5	10	80
	51+	77	170	173	68	63	1,000	5	10	80
Females	11-14	46	101	157	62	46	800	10	8	45
	15-18	55	120	163	64	44	800	10	8	55
	19-24	58	128	164	65	46	800	10	8	60
	25-50	63	138	163	64	50	800	5	8	65
	51+	65	143	160	63	50	800	5	8	65
Pregnant	1st 6 months					60	800	10	10	65
Lactating	2nd 6 months					65	1,300	10	12	65
						62	1,200	10	11	65

Food and Nutrition Board, National Academy of Sciences-National Research Council, 1989.

[1] *Retinol equivalents. 1 retinol equivalent = 1 mcg retinol or 6 mcg B-carotene.*

[2] *As cholecalciferol. 10 cholecalciferol = 400* IU of vitamin D.

[3] *α-Tocopherol equivalents. 1 mg d-α tocopherol = 1 α*-TE.

[4] *1* NE *(niacin equivalent) is equal to 1 mg of niacin or 60 mg of dietary tryptophan.*

Allowances

The Recommended Dietary Allowances (RDA) for vitamins and minerals established by the Food and Nutrition Board of the National Academy of Sciences-National Research Council provide authoritative information to assist the physician in evaluating the formulas of multivitamin preparations (see also the section on Multivitamin Preparations With or Without Minerals).

The RDA (see Table 1) are "The levels of intake of essential nutrients considered, in the judgment of the Committee on Dietary Allowances of the Food and Nutrition Board on the basis of available scientific knowledge, to be adequate to meet the known nutritional needs of practically all healthy persons" (*Recommended Dietary Allowances*, 1989). They are set approximately two standard deviations above the mean requirement, thereby encompassing the needs of 97% of the population. RDA were not established for pantothenic acid and biotin because adequate data are lacking and deficiency due to dietary lack has never been reported in the United States. However, the RDA Committee did establish ranges of Estimated Safe and Adequate Daily Dietary Intakes for these vitamins (Table 2).

RDA should not be confused with the United States Recommended Daily Allowances (U.S. RDA), which is the largest amount of each nutrient recommended for any age group as determined by the National Academy of Sciences/National Research Council in 1968 (see Table 3). The U.S. RDA is used by the Food and Drug Administration for labeling purposes. The RDA is used throughout this chapter for comparison, except in the section on Multivitamin Preparations With or Without Minerals, in which the U.S. RDA is used. The FDA has authority to regulate the vitamin and mineral content of supplements only for use in children under 12 years and in pregnant or lactating women. However, the labels provide information on the proportion of established allowances that are supplied by a product and permit the consumer to judge the appropriateness of the product (see the section on Multivitamin Preparations With or Without Minerals for discussion of recommended composition).

Prophylactic Uses of Vitamins

Requirements of Infants: Full-term infants breast fed by well-nourished mothers generally receive adequate amounts

Water-Soluble Vitamins							Minerals						
Vitamin C (mg)	Thiamin (mg)	Riboflavin (mg)	Niacin (mg NE)[4]	Vitamin B_6 (mg)	Folate (mcg)	Vitamin B_{12} (mcg)	Calcium (mg)	Phosphorus (mg)	Magnesium (mg)	Iron (mg)	Zinc (mg)	Iodine (mcg)	Selenium (mcg)
30	0.3	0.4	5	0.3	25	0.3	400	300	40	6	5	40	10
35	0.4	0.5	6	0.6	35	0.5	600	500	60	10	5	50	15
40	0.7	0.8	9	1.0	50	0.7	800	800	80	10	10	70	20
45	0.9	1.1	12	1.1	75	1.0	800	800	120	10	10	90	20
45	1.0	1.2	13	1.4	100	1.4	800	800	170	10	10	120	30
50	1.3	1.5	17	1.7	150	2.0	1,200	1,200	270	12	15	150	40
60	1.5	1.8	20	2.0	200	2.0	1,200	1,200	400	12	15	150	50
60	1.5	1.7	19	2.0	200	2.0	1,200	1,200	350	10	15	150	70
60	1.5	1.7	19	2.0	200	2.0	800	800	350	10	15	150	70
60	1.2	1.4	15	2.0	200	2.0	800	800	350	10	15	150	70
50	1.1	1.3	15	1.4	150	2.0	1,200	1,200	280	15	12	150	45
60	1.1	1.3	15	1.5	180	2.0	1,200	1,200	300	15	12	150	50
60	1.1	1.3	15	1.6	180	2.0	1,200	1,200	280	15	12	150	55
60	1.1	1.3	15	1.6	180	2.0	800	800	280	15	12	150	55
60	1.0	1.2	13	1.6	180	2.0	800	800	280	10	12	150	55
70	1.5	1.6	17	2.2	400	2.2	1,200	1,200	320	30	15	175	65
95	1.6	1.8	20	2.1	280	2.6	1,200	1,200	355	15	19	200	75
90	1.6	1.7	20	2.1	260	2.6	1,200	1,200	340	15	16	200	75

of vitamins and minerals, except vitamins K and D. Vitamin K deficiency has been reported during the first week of life before the intestinal flora become established. Human milk contains low quantities of vitamin K. Therefore, newborns should be given 0.5 to 1 mg of vitamin K_1 (phytonadione) intramuscularly or intravenously immediately after birth to prevent hemorrhage and loss of vitamin K-dependent coagulation factors. Low-birth-weight infants may require a second injection at about 1 week of age.

The quantity of vitamin D in breast milk may be insufficient for some infants, especially those protected from sunlight or nursed by malnourished mothers, to maintain adequate

TABLE 2. ESTIMATED SAFE AND ADEQUATE DAILY DIETARY INTAKE OF SELECTED VITAMINS*

		Vitamins		Trace Elements†				
Category	Age (years)	Biotin (mcg)	Pantothenic Acid (mg)	Copper (mg)	Manganese (mg)	Fluoride (mg)	Chromium (mcg)	Molybdenum (mcg)
Infants	0-0.5	10	2	0.4-0.6	0.3-0.6	0.1-0.5	10-40	15-30
	0.5-1	15	3	0.6-0.7	0.6-1.0	0.2-1.0	20-60	20-40
Children and adolescents	1-3	20	3	0.7-1.0	1.0-1.5	0.5-1.5	20-80	25-50
	4-6	25	3-4	1.0-1.5	1.5-2.0	1.0-2.5	30-120	30-75
	7-10	30	4-5	1.0-2.0	2.0-3.0	1.5-2.5	50-200	50-150
	11+	30-100	4-7	1.5-2.5	2.0-5.0	1.5-2.5	50-200	75-250
Adults		30-100	4-7	1.5-3.0	2.0-5.0	1.5-4.0	50-200	75-250

**Food and Nutrition Board, National Academy of Sciences-National Research Council, 1989.*

†The upper levels for the trace elements given in this table should not be exceeded.

25(OH)-D concentrations and reduced bone mineralization may result (Tsang, 1983). A daily supplement of 200 to 300 IU is recommended for breast-fed infants who are not exposed to sunlight.

Supplemental administration of vitamin A or E is rarely indicated. The rationale for adding vitamin A to most supplements containing vitamin D is historical; both vitamins are contained in cod liver oil. Supplemental doses of water-solu-

TABLE 3.
U.S. RDA FOR DIETARY SUPPLEMENTS[1]

	Units of Measurement	Infants (birth-1 yr)	Children (1-4 yrs)	Adults and Children Over 4 yrs	Pregnant and Lactating Women
VITAMINS					
A	RE[2] (IU)	450 (1,500)	750 (2,500)	1,500 (5,000)	2,400 (8,000)
D	mcg[3] (IU)	10 (400)	10 (400)	10 (400)	10 (400)
E	mg[4] (IU)	3.3 (5)	6.7 (10)	20 (30)	20 (30)
C	mg	35	40	60	60
Thiamin	mg	0.5	0.7	1.5	1.7
Riboflavin	mg	0.6	0.8	1.7	2.0
Niacin	mg	8.0	9.0	20	20
B_6	mg	0.4	0.7	2.0	2.5
B_{12}	mcg	2.0	3.0	6.0	8.0
Folic Acid	mg	0.1	0.2	0.4	0.8
Biotin	mg	0.5	0.15	0.3	0.3
Pantothenic Acid	mg	3.0	5.0	10	10
MINERALS					
Calcium	mg	600	800	1,000	1,300
Iron	mg	15	10	18	18
Phosphorus	mg	500	800	1,000	1,300
Iodine	mcg	45	70	150	150
Magnesium	mg	70	200	400	450
Zinc	mg	5	8	15	15
Copper	mg	0.6	1	2	2

[1] These values usually represent the highest allowance for any age group within the broad category and are the amounts judged necessary to maintain health.
[2] RE = Retinol Equivalents (1 RE = 3.3 IU vitamin A)
[3] As cholecalciferol (10 mcg cholecalciferol = 400 IU vitamin D)
[4] As d-alpha tocopherol (1 mg d-alpha tocopherol = 1.5 IU vitamin E)

ble vitamins also are rarely indicated. Infants fed a strict vegan diet may require daily vitamin B_{12} supplementation in doses similar to those recommended for infants receiving commercial formula (ie, 0.15 mcg/100 kcal) (Committee on Nutrition, American Academy of Pediatrics, 1976). Formula-fed infants should receive supplemental amounts of ascorbic acid if less than 25 mg of this vitamin is ingested daily.

Iron deficiency seldom occurs before age 4 to 6 months and usually can be managed by adding iron-fortified cereal to the diet. Iron supplements may be necessary if the infant receives an inadequate quantity from iron-fortified foods.

Fluoride supplementation for infants should take the infant's age and nutritional source into account. Breast-fed infants should receive fluoride supplements (0.25 mg/day) shortly after birth. For formula-fed infants, the dose depends upon the type of formula used. Powdered and concentrated formulas are mixed with water from the local water supply; therefore, dosage recommendations are based on the concentration of fluoride in the local water (see Table 4). Ready-to-use formulas are required by federal law to be manufactured using water with low fluoride levels; therefore, infants receiving these products should receive the same dose of fluoride as breast-fed infants (ie, 0.25 mg/day).

Commercial infant formulas sold in the United States must contain vitamins and minerals in quantities established by the Infant Formula Act of 1980. Healthy infants fed proprietary formulas usually do not require supplementation during the first six months. Supplementation may be required during the second six months of life if the amount of formula ingested is inadequate.

Preterm infants should receive vitamin and mineral supplementation during the first weeks of life. The dosage should supply the equivalent of the RDA for term infants and also should contain vitamin E and folic acid. The prescription of iron should be delayed until after the first weeks.

When parenteral preparations of vitamin E are necessary, only those approved for marketing by the FDA should be utilized.

Requirements of Children: Normal children usually receive adequate amounts of vitamins and minerals from their diet and do not require supplementation. An important exception is fluoride, which should be supplemented when there are insufficient quantities in the local water supply. Children and adolescents from deprived families, those who are neglected or abused, or those with poor eating habits are considered to be at high risk for vitamin and mineral deficiency and should receive supplementation as shown in Table 5.

Requirements of Pregnant and Lactating Women: The routine prescription of multivitamin and mineral supplements for pregnant and lactating women is common but often unnecessary. A well-balanced diet designed to meet their needs minimizes the need for supplementation. However, there are some exceptions (see Table 5).

During pregnancy and for two to three months postpartum, the requirements for iron exceed the level normally available from dietary intake; 15 mg of supplemental iron daily is recommended. Therapeutic doses of iron should be considered for women at risk of developing iron deficiency anemia (ie, packed cell volume less than 30%, hemoglobin less than 11 mg/dl). Iron should be administered orally whenever feasible; if the patient is unable to ingest sufficient iron due to side effects or is likely to be noncompliant, parenteral administration may be necessary.

Supplementation with folic acid is recommended for pregnant women. The RDA is 400 mcg daily and, although this amount is larger than most pregnant women need, it is intended to meet the requirements of women with low body folate stores, low dietary intake of folate, and multiple or twin pregnancies. Lactating women also may benefit from folic acid supplements. The allowance for folate during lactation is 260 to 280 mcg daily.

A small number of women have very low hepatic reserves of vitamin A. Therefore, an additional intake of a maximum of 200 mcg is recommended during the third trimester (Olson, 1987).

Those who cannot tolerate milk may require calcium supplementation. See index entry Calcium for additional information. There are a few special conditions in which other vitamins and minerals should be prescribed to supplement the diet of pregnant and lactating women.

Requirements of Vegetarians: Patients who consume a vegan-vegetarian diet may require riboflavin, vitamin B_{12}, and vitamin D. Lacto-ovo vegetarians, who consume some animal foods, may need only iron supplements to maintain a normal dietary intake of the essential vitamins and minerals.

Requirements of Individuals on Weight Reduction Diets: Even a well-planned weight reduction diet may provide an inadequate supply of vitamins, especially when the energy intake is limited to 800 to 1,000 kcal/day. In these individuals, a supplemental multivitamin preparation may be advisable. Periodic monitoring of individuals on very low energy diets is recommended.

Requirements of Elderly Individuals: It has not been determined whether elderly persons consuming an adequate diet have higher requirements for vitamins or minerals than other healthy adults. Since some elderly individuals do not eat an adequate diet, especially those living alone, some physicians recommend a multiple vitamin and mineral supplement. However, adding just the U.S. RDA amount of vitamin A as a

TABLE 4.
SUPPLEMENTAL FLUORIDE DOSE (MG FLUORIDE ION/DAY) BASED ON FLUORIDE CONCENTRATION IN DRINKING WATER*

	Concentration of Fluoride in Water (ppm)		
Age (years)	**<0.3**	**0.3-0.7**	**>0.7**
Birth to 2	0.25	0	0
2 to 3	0.50	0.25	0
3 to 13	1.00	0.50	0

* *Adapted from Accepted Dental Therapeutics, 1984*

TABLE 5.
GUIDELINES FOR VITAMIN AND MINERAL SUPPLEMENTATION IN HEALTHY INFANTS AND CHILDREN AND PREGNANT OR LACTATING WOMEN*

		Vitamins			Minerals	
	Multivitamins/Minerals	**D**	**E**	**Folate**	**Iron**	**Fluoride[1]**
PRETERM INFANT[2]						
Breast-fed	+	+	0[3]	0	+	0
Formula-fed	+	+	0[3]	0	+[4]	0
TERM INFANT						
Breast-fed	–	0	–	–	0[4]	+
Formula-fed	–	–	–	–	–	+
OLDER INFANT (6 mos)						
Normal	–	–	–	–	0[4]	+
High-risk[5]	+	–	–	–	0	+
CHILD						
Normal	–	–	–	–	–	+
High-risk	+	–	–	–	–	+
PREGNANT AND LACTATING WOMEN	+		–	+	+	+/–

+: Supplement usually indicated
0: Supplement sometimes indicated
–: Supplement not usually indicated

[1] *Fluoride supplements should be started shortly after birth in term infants and continued throughout life. The dose depends upon the concentration in the water supply. Ready-to-use formulas are manufactured with water low in fluoride.*

[2] *Multivitamin supplement (plus added folate) is usually needed primarily when the calorie intake is <300 kcal/day or when the infant weighs <2.5 kg. Vitamin D should be supplemented in breast-fed infants until at least age 6 months. Iron should be started at age 2 months.*

[3] *Vitamin E should be in a preparation that is well absorbed by preterm infants. Breast-fed preterm infants are less susceptible to vitamin E deficiency.*

[4] *Iron supplements are usually unwarranted before age 4 to 6 months. After age 6 months, iron should be supplemented either by adding iron-fortified cereal to the diet (preferred) or by prescribing an iron supplement.*

[5] *Multivitamin and mineral preparations (with iron) are preferred to the use of iron alone.*

* *Adapted from Committee on Nutrition, American Academy of Pediatrics, 1980.*

supplement to their regular diet has been associated with abnormal liver enzyme blood concentrations. Housebound elderly persons may benefit from routine supplementation with vitamin D 400 IU daily (Suter and Russell, 1987).

Therapeutic Uses of Vitamins

Alcoholism: The diet of alcoholic individuals often is poor, which may result in multiple vitamin deficiencies, especially the water-soluble vitamins (thiamine, folate, pyridoxine, riboflavin, and ascorbic acid). Thiamine deficiency can lead to Wernicke's encephalopathy, a medical emergency requiring immediate thiamine administration. This deficiency occurs because an inadequate amount of the vitamin is consumed, alcohol interferes with the active transport mechanism of thiamine in the gastrointestinal tract, and alcohol may inhibit the biotransformation of thiamine to its active form, thiamine pyrophosphate. A deficiency of folic acid in alcoholics results from a poor diet, impaired enterohepatic circulation leading to poor reutilization of the vitamin, and actual destruction of folate by a product of alcohol catabolism. Pyridoxine deficiency is caused by increased metabolism of an active analogue. Acetaldehyde, a major metabolite of alcohol, competes for the same plasma protein binding sites with pyridoxal phosphate, causing an increased concentration of free pyridoxal phosphate, which is then susceptible to hydrolysis by phosphatases. Ascorbic acid and riboflavin deficiencies occur because of decreased intake and increased elimination.

A patient with alcoholism should receive a single therapeutic dose of B-complex vitamins parenterally during withdrawal and detoxification to prevent vitamin deficiency disease, including Wernicke's encephalopathy (Council on Scientific Affairs, 1987).

See also index entry Alcoholism.

Requirements of Patients on Hemodialysis: Hemodialysis removes circulating coenzymatic compounds derived from folate, pyridoxine, and ascorbic acid; therefore, compensatory amounts (100% to 300% of the RDA) of these vitamins should be prescribed. The requirements for other vitamins, with the possible exception of vitamin E, apparently are not increased.

Parenteral Administration: Vitamins and minerals should be administered parenterally only in certain special circumstances (see the discussion on Therapeutic Multivitamin Preparations and Table 6). They should not be combined with other intravenous medications unless admixture is specified in the labeling. Compatibility data are available in most hospital pharmacies and should be consulted.

FAT-SOLUBLE VITAMINS

The fat-soluble vitamins (A, D, E, and K) are absorbed by complex processes that parallel the absorption of fat. Thus, any condition that causes malabsorption of fat (eg, bile acid deficiency, pancreatic insufficiency, obstructive jaundice, celiac disease, tropical sprue, regional enteritis) may result in deficiency of one or all of these vitamins. Fat-soluble vitamins affect permeability or transport in various cell membranes and act as oxidation-reduction agents, coenzymes, or enzyme inhibitors. Vitamin A has some, and vitamin D has extensive, hormonal activity. Fat-soluble vitamins are stored principally in the liver and are excreted in the feces. Since these vitamins are metabolized very slowly, doses relatively close to the RDA may produce toxic effects.

Drug Evaluations

VITAMIN A (Retinol)

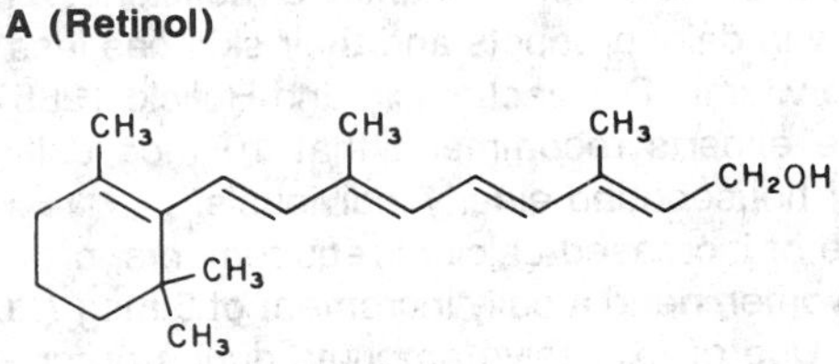

Vitamin A is essential for growth and bone development in children, for vision (particularly in dim light), for integrity of mucosal and epithelial surfaces, and for reproduction. For use of vitamin A derivatives in dermatologic disorders, see index entry Retinoids.

SOURCES. Vitamin A includes several active compounds including beta-carotene, alpha-carotene, retinol, and various carotenoids. Retinol is the major naturally occurring form. Precursor carotenoid pigments, especially beta-carotene, may be obtained from green and yellow vegetables, but only about one-sixth is converted to vitamin A in man. Preformed vitamin A (retinols) is acquired from animal sources (eggs, dairy products, and liver) and fish liver oils. Dietary fat is necessary for effective absorption of carotene, and proteins stimulate absorption of retinols. Sufficient vitamin A to satisfy requirements for several months is stored in the liver of well-nourished people. Protein and possibly zinc may be required to mobilize hepatic reserves.

Human milk supplies sufficient vitamin A for infants unless the maternal diet is grossly inadequate, in which case enough vitamin A should be given during the first six months after birth to provide a daily total of 420 retinol equivalents (1,400 IU). Healthy children and adults consuming a well-balanced diet do not require supplementation.

HYPOVITAMINOSIS A. Vitamin A deficiency occurs most commonly when the dietary intake is inadequate in preschool children, when intestinal absorption is impaired (eg, cystic fibrosis, steatorrhea, biliary obstruction), when the ability to store or transport vitamin A is impaired (eg, hepatic cirrhosis, abetalipoproteinemia), when metabolic requirements are increased (eg, in growing infants, pregnant and lactating women), or when hyperthyroidism is present.

The initial manifestation of hypovitaminosis A is night blindness (nyctalopia), which may progress to xerophthalmia and keratomalacia with corneal perforation and, eventually, blindness, particularly in young children. Hyperkeratosis of the skin and metaplasia of mucous membranes, which impair local defenses against infection, also may occur. Acute hypovitaminosis A is extremely rare in the United States; however, in less developed countries it causes an estimated 250,000 cases of blindness in children annually (Olson, 1987).

HYPERVITAMINOSIS A. Toxicity of vitamin A usually results from ingestion of more than 210 to 900 retinol equivalents/kg/day for several months to years. However, liver damage has resulted from ingestion of as little as the adult RDA for years by a child and as little as five times the RDA for seven to ten years by an adult (Herbert, 1982). Acute intoxication has followed the ingestion of a single dose of 450,000 retinol equivalents (1,500,000 IU) in adults and 90,000 retinol equivalents (300,000 IU) in infants. In adults, the symptoms of acute intoxication include dizziness, nausea, vomiting, and erythema with eventual desquamation that persists for several weeks; in infants, the symptoms include transient hydrocephalus and vomiting.

Chronic hypervitaminosis A in infants and children produces pseudotumor cerebri, tinnitus, bulging fontanelles, increased cerebrospinal fluid pressure, bone pain, lethargy, pruritus, exfoliative dermatitis, angular stomatitis, hyperostosis, metaphyseal cupping, and paronychia. Diplopia and papilledema occur; in long-standing cases, optic atrophy and blindness may result. Common symptoms in adults are vomiting, skin changes, irritability, headache, hypomenorrhea, and weakness. Psychiatric symptoms also may be observed, and such patients rarely have been placed in psychiatric hospitals with a diagnosis of severe depression or schizophrenia. Hepatic dysfunction, often associated with hepatosplenomegaly, may occur and marked hypercalcemia and ascites have been reported. In children and adults, chronic hypervitaminosis A may cause dryness of the skin and mucous membranes, alopecia, anorexia, brittle nails, myalgia, ostealgia, arthralgia, abdominal pain, splenomegaly, and hypoplastic anemia with leukopenia. Most symptoms disappear when the vitamin is discontinued, but growth retardation caused by premature epiphyseal closure may occur in children. Water-soluble vitamin A preparations are absorbed more readily than oily formulations. Doses of an oily emulsion must be approximately six times higher than those of a water-miscible preparation to cause the same degree of toxicity (Silverman et al, 1987).

TERATOGENICITY. Overdosage of vitamin A in animals has produced malformations of the central nervous system, eye, palate, and urogenital tract. The maximal nonteratogenic dose is somewhat species dependent, ranging from 40,000 retinol equivalents/kg in rats to 750 retinol equivalents/kg in mice. The relative sensitivity of humans is unknown (*Federal Register*, 1983). Because of possible teratogenic effects on the human fetus, doses exceeding the RDA should not be administered during pregnancy (FDA Pregnancy Category X). Isotretinoin-like deformities have been reported in infants of mothers who ingested as little as 25,000 IU of vitamin A daily just before and through the first months of pregnancy (Public Affairs Committee, Teratology Society, 1987).

DOSAGE AND PREPARATIONS.

THERAPEUTIC:

Doses exceeding 7,500 retinol equivalents (25,000 IU) daily should not be prescribed unless the deficiency is severe. The safety of doses exceeding 1,800 retinol equivalents (6,000 IU) daily during pregnancy and lactation has not been established. Oral administration is preferred; the intramuscular route may be used for short-term therapy when absorption is grossly impaired, ocular symptoms are prominent, or oral administration is not feasible.

Intramuscular: In severe deficiency, *adults and children over 8 years,* 15,000 to 30,000 retinol equivalents (50,000 to 100,000 IU) daily for three days, followed by 15,000 retinol equivalents (50,000 IU) daily for two weeks; *1 to 8 years,* 1,500 to 4,500 retinol equivalents (5,000 to 15,000 IU) daily for ten days; *infants,* 1,500 to 3,000 retinol equivalents (5,000 to 10,000 IU) daily for ten days.

Aquasol A (Armour). Solution 50,000 IU/ml in 2 ml containers.

Oral: In deficiency, *adults and children over 8 years,* 1,500 to 3,000 retinol equivalents (5,000 to 10,000 IU) daily for one to two weeks. In severe deficiency, 30,000 retinol equivalents (100,000 IU) daily for three days, followed by 15,000 retinol equivalents (50,000 IU) daily for two weeks, then 3,000 to 6,000 retinol equivalents (10,000 to 20,000 IU) daily for another two months.

Generic. Capsules 10,000, 25,000 (nonprescription), and 50,000 IU; tablets 10,000 (nonprescription) and 50,000 IU.

Available Trademark.

Aquasol A (Armour) (water-dispersible).

DIETARY SUPPLEMENTATION OR PROPHYLAXIS:

The dosage should not exceed the RDA after evaluation of the patient's diet. The diet should be corrected or the dose adjusted on the basis of the RDA. No single-entity preparations are available; see the section on Multivitamin Preparations With or Without Minerals.

VITAMIN D

For chemical formula, see index entry Vitamin D, In Hypocalcemia.

Vitamin D is the generic designation for several sterols and their metabolites that have antirachitic properties. Ergocalciferol (vitamin D_2), derived from yeast and fungal ergosterol, is the usual active ingredient supplied commercially. Irradiation of the provitamin, 7-dehydrocholesterol, in the skin or irradiation of food produces cholecalciferol (vitamin D_3).

METABOLISM AND FUNCTIONS. Vitamin D is stored mainly in the liver but also in adipose tissue and muscle and is excreted slowly. The vitamin is stable and is well absorbed from the gastrointestinal tract. Following absorption, it is hydroxylated in the liver to form 25-hydroxy-vitamin D (25-(OH)D_3 or calcifediol). Further hydroxylation occurs in the kidney in response to the need for calcium and phosphorus, and 1,25-dihydroxy-vitamin D (1,25-$(OH)_2D_3$ or calcitriol) is produced. In conjunction with calcitonin and parathyroid hormone, calcitriol regulates calcium and phosphorus metabolism in the intestine, bone, and possibly kidney; it facilitates the intestinal absorption of calcium and may initiate phosphorus transport, thus increasing serum calcium and phosphorus levels to allow normal mineralization of the skeleton. Paradoxically, vitamin D also mobilizes calcium from bone to maintain proper plasma levels of calcium. It may suppress parathyroid hormone secretion, thus preventing phosphaturia, and may have a direct action on the proximal tubules to promote phosphorus retention.

REQUIREMENTS. Although vitamin D is essential, the daily requirement in adults is very small and may be obtained by adequate exposure to sunlight or in the diet. Products containing more than 10 mcg (400 IU) should be used only when deficiency is documented. Members of dark-skinned races inhabiting northern climates have a slightly higher requirement for vitamin D because melanin interferes with absorption.

There is increasing evidence that the elderly have an increased risk of developing vitamin D deficiency. Their diet often is low in dairy products and their skin has less capacity to produce vitamin D (MacLaughlin and Holick, 1985). Therefore, some experts recommend that 10 mcg daily be prescribed for housebound elderly individuals.

Because of increased calcium requirements, pregnant and lactating women need a daily increment of 5 mcg (200 IU) of vitamin D. Use of excessive amounts during pregnancy may produce hy-percalcemia, which is potentially teratogenic; supravalvular aortic stenosis, vascular injury, and suppression of parathyroid function may occur in the neonate.

Premature infants and those who are breast-fed or fed unfortified formulas should receive enough supplemental vitamin D to provide a daily intake of 5 to 7.5 mcg. Infants and children receiving adequate amounts of vitamin D-fortified food require no supplementation; in fact, use of a supplement can result in overdosage.

Vitamin D is classified in FDA Pregnancy Category C.

HYPOVITAMINOSIS D. Primary nutritional deficiency of vitamin D is rare in the United States. An absolute or relative deficiency may occur secondary to malabsorption syndromes, in individuals not exposed to the sun, or in patients with metabolic disorders. Deficiency causes hypocalcemia and hypophosphatemia, which stimulates parathyroid hormone secretion to restore plasma calcium levels at the expense of bone. This causes rickets in infants and children and osteomalacia in adults. When produced by dietary deficiency, these conditions respond rapidly to adequate doses of vitamin D, but treatment of other disorders may depend upon blood levels of calcium, phosphate, and parathyroid hormone, as well as the degree of derangement of vitamin D metabolism. For discussion of the therapeutic uses of vitamin D, see index entry Vitamin D, In Hypocalcemia.

In all deficiency states, the dose of vitamin D should be reduced to the RDA after symptoms are relieved and before normal biochemical levels are achieved or bone healing is complete. When bone healing has occurred, the requirement may decrease suddenly and, since the action of vitamin D may persist long after administration is discontinued, hypercalcemia and renal damage may result.

Administration of vitamin D to treat lupus vulgaris is obsolete, and its topical use for other dermatoses is not justified.

HYPERVITAMINOSIS D. Vitamin D is very toxic in large doses. In infants and children, the margin of safety between prophylactic or therapeutic and toxic doses is narrow. Hypercalcemia may develop in hypersensitive infants at doses very close to 10 mcg. In addition, large amounts may be ingested inadvertently by children who consume a great variety of foods fortified with vitamin D.

Prolonged hypervitaminosis D in infants causes mental and physical retardation, elfin facies, renal failure, and death. Symptoms of toxicity may occur with doses greater than 25 mcg (1,000 IU) daily, and retardation of linear growth has been reported after daily doses of 45 mcg (1,800 IU) (Beeson et al, 1979). Amounts exceeding 1.25 mg (50,000 IU) daily produce hypercalcemia in normal adults and children. Initial manifestations of toxicity are associated with symptoms of hypercalcemia (eg, weakness, anorexia, vomiting, diarrhea, polydipsia, polyuria, mental changes). Proteinuria may indicate renal impairment, and prolonged hypercalcemia may result in soft tissue calcifications (calcinosis universalis). Prolonged use of massive doses ultimately results in irreversible renal failure and death.

Vitamin D intoxication usually is reversible after administration is discontinued unless renal impairment is severe. Some patients also require a low-calcium diet, glucocorticoids, and other measures to reduce plasma calcium levels to normal.

DOSAGE AND PREPARATIONS. Dosage for vitamin D is preferably expressed in terms of cholecalciferol (10 mcg of cholecalciferol equals 400 IU).

PROPHYLACTIC:

Oral: *Premature or breast-fed infants when maternal milk is inadequate or infants given unfortified formulas,* 5 to 7.5 mcg (200 to 300 IU) daily. *Infants abnormally susceptible to rickets* (eg, malabsorption syndrome, born to mothers with vitamin D deficiency), up to 750 mcg (30,000 IU) daily for a short period. In *adults,* based on dietary intake and exposure to sunlight, supplementation may be needed during pregnancy and lactation and in the elderly to assure a daily intake of 10 mcg. If larger doses are used for prolonged periods, blood calcium levels and 24-hour urine specimens should be monitored frequently. Blood calcium levels should be maintained at 9 to 10 mg/dL.

Generic. Capsules and tablets 400 and 1,000 IU (nonprescription) and 25,000 and 50,000 IU.

THERAPEUTIC:

See index entry Vitamin D.

VITAMIN E (Tocopherol)

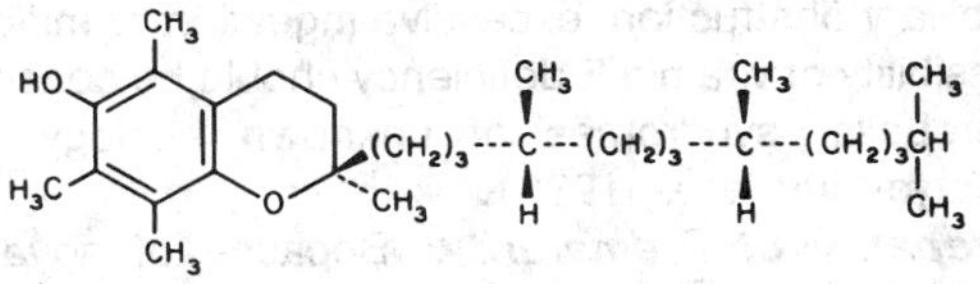

Vitamin E refers to a group of fat-soluble substances occurring in plants. Alpha-tocopherol is the most active form; soybean products contain gamma-tocopherol, which is less potent but contributes somewhat to vitamin E intake. When only the amount of alpha-tocopherol is reported on the labeling, total milligrams of alpha-tocopherol equivalents may be calculated by increasing the value in milligrams by 20% to account for other tocopherols present in a mixed diet.

FUNCTIONS. Vitamin E is considered to be an essential nutrient, but its biochemical functions are not completely understood; 50% to 80% is absorbed and transported by lipoprotein in essentially the same manner as fats. It is stored in adipose tissue and is thought to stabilize the lipid portions of cell membranes. Vitamin E protects polyunsaturated fatty acids (PUFA) from oxidation. Other functions attributed to vitamin E are enhancement of vitamin A utilization, inhibition of prostaglandin production, and stimulation of an essential cofactor in steroid metabolism. It also helps maintain the normal neurologic structure and function. A number of other substances that occur naturally in foods (eg, selenium, sulfur, amino acids, coenzyme Q) can function as partial substitutes for vitamin E in certain metabolic reactions.

REQUIREMENTS. Surveys indicate that adequate amounts of vitamin E are supplied by the usual diet, that human requirements are small, and that the RDA exceeds the actual needs of normal persons. The requirement for vitamin E increases as the intake of PUFA increases. However, foods that supply PUFA (vegetable oils, shortenings, and margarine) also are good sources of vitamin E. Nevertheless, consumption of excessive amounts of PUFA (more than 20 g/day over normal dietary intake) may warrant supplementation with vitamin E, particularly if the PUFA intake is discontinued abruptly, thus producing a relative deficiency of the vitamin.

Vitamin E requirements may be increased in people exposed to high-oxygen environments or in those taking therapeutic doses of iron or large doses of thyroid hormone. Skin lesions, hematologic changes, and edema have developed in premature infants receiving formulas high in PUFA and low in vitamin E; the deficiency of vitamin E may be aggravated by the large iron supplements given these infants. Recovery followed administration of 25 to 50 mg of alpha-tocopherol equivalent (37.5 to 75 IU) daily or reduction of the iron supplements and quantity of PUFA.

USES. ***Deficiency States:*** Vitamin E therapy should be restricted to deficiency states demonstrable by low serum vitamin E levels and/or increased fragility of red cells to hydrogen peroxide. These may occur in premature low birth weight infants and in patients who have malabsorption syndromes with steatorrhea (eg, celiac disease, tropical sprue, gastrointestinal resections) and other conditions characterized by prolonged malabsorption of fats (eg, cystic fibrosis, hepatic cirrhosis, biliary obstruction, excessive ingestion of mineral oil). The possibility of vitamin E deficiency should be considered in spinocerebellar syndromes of unknown etiology (Muller, 1986; Satya-Murti et al, 1986).

Retinopathy of Prematurity: Because of advances in neonatal intensive care, more premature infants of extremely low birth weight are surviving. In infants weighing less than 1,500 g and of less than 31 weeks gestational age at birth, the risk of retinopathy of prematurity (ROP) remains high. In an effort to reduce its incidence and severity, large oral doses of vitamin E (100 mg/kg/day) have been given to premature infants beginning within hours after birth with administration continued until the eyes mature or for as long as active neovascularization continues. The role of vitamin E in this condition remains controversial. One double-blind study indicated that vitamin E does not prevent ROP but does reduce its severity (Hittner et al, 1981). However, a second controlled double-blind study reported that vitamin E neither prevents ROP nor reduces the severity. Further, infants receiving vitamin E developed grades three and four intraventricular hemorrhages more frequently than those receiving placebo (Phelps et al, 1987). Additional studies are required to resolve this question.

Unsubstantiated Uses: There is no evidence to support the efficacy of vitamin E in the numerous conditions for which it is popularly used. Large doses do not protect against arteriosclerosis, cancer, pulmonary damage from air pollution, or deterioration from aging, and vitamin E is ineffective in inflammatory skin disorders, habitual abortion, heart disease, menopausal syndrome, infertility, peptic ulcer, burns, and porphyria.

ADVERSE REACTIONS AND PRECAUTIONS. In anemic children, the hematologic response to parenteral iron is suppressed by large doses of alpha-tocopherol. Excessive use of vitamin E may deplete vitamin A stores and inhibit the absorption or action of vitamin K, although adverse effects (eg, increased hypoprothrombinemic response to oral anticoagulants) occur only rarely when 200 to 270 mg daily is taken for prolonged periods. However, the long-term use of doses as low as 270 to 540 mg daily has been reported to produce nausea, muscular weakness, fatigue, headache, and blurred vision in a few patients, and very large doses (1.3 to 8 g daily) have been reported to cause gastrointestinal upset, decreased gonadal function, and creatinuria (Hayes and Hegsted, 1973). Symptoms disappeared within a few weeks when excessive doses were discontinued. An intravenous vitamin E preparation (no longer marketed) caused hepatic, renal, pulmonary, and hematopoietic toxicity when used in premature infants to prevent ROP.

DOSAGE AND PREPARATIONS.

Oral: For deficiency in *adults and children,* four to five times the RDA. Commercial formulas for infant feeding that are high in polyunsaturated fats should contain at least 3.3 mg/L (5 IU/L). For low-birth-weight or premature infants, the formula should contain 4.7 mg/L (7 IU/L); the Committee on Nutrition of the American Academy of Pediatrics (1980) has recommended an additional oral supplement of 3.3 mg (5 IU) of water-miscible alpha-tocopherol.

Generic. Capsules 100, 200, 400, 600, and 1,000 IU (nonprescription); tablets 100, 200, 400, and 1,000 IU (nonprescription); tablets (chewable) 100 and 200 IU (nonprescription).

Aquasol E (Armour). Capsules (tocopheryl acetate) 100 and 400 IU; drops 50 IU/ml (both forms nonprescription).

E-ferol (Forest). Capsules (tocopheryl succinate) 200 and 400 IU (nonprescription).

Eprolin (Lilly). Capsules (tocopheryl acetate) 100 IU (nonprescription).

VITAMIN K

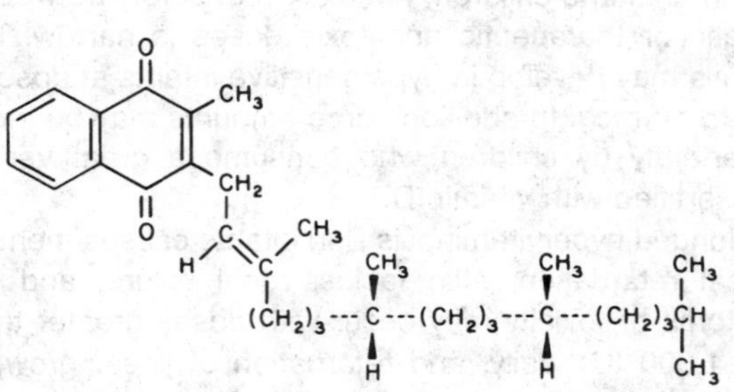

In normal individuals, synthesis of vitamin K by intestinal mucosa provides about one-half the estimated daily requirement; the remainder is supplied by the average diet.

Hypoprothrombinemia due to vitamin K deficiency may be secondary to malabsorption of fats, prolonged hyperalimentation, or inhibition of intestinal bacterial biosynthesis (eg, long-term administration of antibiotics). Relative deficiency also may result from an imbalance of fat-soluble vitamins following excessive doses of one or all of the other fat-soluble vitamins (A, D, E). Newborn infants, especially those who are premature, have low concentrations of vitamin K-dependent clotting factors that decrease for a few days after birth. Small doses (0.5 to 1 mg) of phytonadione (vitamin K_1) administered either intramuscularly or intravenously immediately after birth are advocated for all newborn infants. This dose may be repeated after one week if required.

Oral liquid nutritional products containing vitamin K can be purchased at health food stores, and patients who require oral anticoagulants should be warned that these products may interfere with the hypoprothrombinemic response.

Vitamin K is classified in FDA Pregnancy Category C.

For a detailed discussion on the therapeutic and prophylactic uses of vitamin K, see index entry Vitamin K.

WATER-SOLUBLE VITAMINS

The water-soluble vitamins include ascorbic acid and the B-complex vitamins, biotin, folic acid (folate), niacin (nicotinic acid), pantothenic acid, pyridoxine (B_6), riboflavin (B_2), thiamine (B_1), and cyanocobalamin (B_{12}). Since cyanocobalamin and folic acid are used principally to treat deficiency anemias (see index entry Anemia, Megaloblastic), they are discussed only briefly in this chapter.

Water-soluble vitamins are structurally diverse and act as coenzymes or as oxidation inhibitors. Metabolism is rapid, any excess is excreted in the urine, and, except for niacin and pyridoxine, overdosage seldom causes toxic effects in individuals with normal renal function.

Drug Evaluations

ASCORBIC ACID

ASCORBATE CALCIUM

ASCORBATE SODIUM

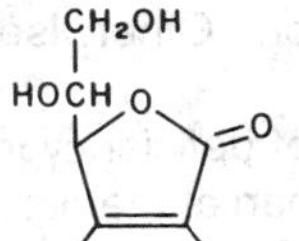

Ascorbic acid (vitamin C) acts as a coenzyme and, under certain conditions, as a reducing agent and antioxidant. It directly or indirectly supplies electrons to enzymes that require reduced metal ions and acts as a cofactor for prolyl and lysyl hydroxylases in the biosynthesis of collagen (Levine, 1986).

REQUIREMENTS. Like other primates, man lacks the microsomal enzyme necessary to convert L-gulonolactone to ascorbic acid; therefore, vitamin C must be supplied exogenously. Intake of 60 to 75 mg of vitamin C daily produces a serum ascorbate concentration of approximately 0.75 mg/dl (7.5 mg/L) and a total body pool of approximately 900 to 1,700 mg in the average healthy adult male. Requirements are increased during pregnancy and lactation, as reflected in the RDA (see Table 1). Environmental stresses (eg, extremes in temperature, surgery, thermal burns, trauma) also increase the daily requirement by 300% to 500%. Cigarette smokers are estimated to require as much as 50% more ascorbic acid to maintain serum concentrations within the normal range; however, these amounts are still within the RDA (Sauberlich, 1984). Women taking oral contraceptives also have decreased serum ascorbate concentrations, but the clinical relevance of this is unknown.

SOURCES. Vitamin C is present in relatively high concentrations in citrus fruits, tomatoes, potatoes, and leafy vegetables.

HYPOVITAMINOSIS C. Clinical scurvy occurs after three to five months in those ingesting an ascorbic acid-free diet and is relatively rare in the United States. In adults, scurvy is most common in elderly or chronically ill individuals, alcoholics, and dietary cultists. Infants fed diets deficient in ascorbic acid are also susceptible.

Pathology is manifest in most body tissues, especially those of mesodermal origin (ie, collagen, growing bones, teeth, blood vessels), and symptoms are associated with plasma vitamin C concentrations less than 2 mg/L, leukocyte concentration less than 2 mcg/10^8, and a body pool of less than 300 mg (Olson and Hodges, 1987). Defective ground substance is formed and development of scar tissue is delayed. Capillary fragility combined with defective calcification of cartilage causes subperiosteal hemorrhages and, eventually, bone resorption, abnormal bone development, and defective development of teeth in growing children. Ecchymoses appear and hemorrhages into muscles and joints may occur. A normocytic or macrocytic anemia, which is multifactorial in origin, is common. Rarely, megaloblastic anemia is observed (only associated with deficiency of both ascorbic and folic acids). If untreated, hypotension, convulsions, coma, and death occur.

USES. Ascorbic acid is indicated to prevent and treat scurvy. It also is used to treat a number of syndromes not associated with deficiency. However, efficacy in most of the purported uses is unfounded, unproven, or unsubstantiated. Vitamin C does not affect the incidence of colds, although it may attenuate the severity and duration of the symptoms slightly. There is good evidence that pharmacologic doses of ascorbic acid have no beneficial effect in patients with advanced cancer (Moertel et al, 1985).

Other conditions treated with megadoses of vitamin C that have been studied and found to be unaffected include atherosclerosis, healing of wounds, and schizophrenia.

There are various diseases for which vitamin C has been promoted, but further research is required. Among these are asthma, pressure sores, male infertility due to nonspecific spermagglutination, osteogenesis imperfecta, and adjunctive therapy in opioid withdrawal (Ovesen, 1984).

ADVERSE REACTIONS. The incidence of adverse reactions from even megadoses of vitamin C is low. Doses exceeding 1 g/day may cause diarrhea due to direct irritation of the intestinal mucosa that increases peristalsis. The irritant action also may cause nonspecific urethritis with dysuria and clear watery discharge primarily limited to the distal urethra (Fong, 1981). Chronic ingestion of very large doses may lead to vitamin C dependency, in which the abrupt change from large to moderate but normally adequate levels may provoke rebound scurvy. This complication can be avoided by reducing the vitamin C intake gradually. Metastatic oxalosis may occur with chronic ingestion or parenteral administration of very large doses (Olson and Hodges, 1987).

Ascorbic acid increases iron absorption and, thus, large doses may be dangerous in patients with heterogenous or homozygous hemochromatosis, thalassemia, or sideroblastic anemia. Mild hemolysis has been reported in patients with G6PD deficiency receiving large doses of vitamin C; in one patient, acute hemolysis resulted in disseminated intravascular coagulation, acute renal failure, and death (Campbell et al, 1975). Megadoses of ascorbic acid also may produce sickle cell crisis by converting oxidized SS hemoglobin to reduced SS hemoglobin. In megadoses, parenteral ascorbic acid has caused severe renal damage as well as metastatic oxalosis with cardiac arrhythmias (Balcke et al, 1984; Schwartz et al, 1984).

Ascorbic acid is classified in FDA Pregnancy Category C.

INTERACTIONS. In doses of 1 g/day, ascorbic acid has been reported to increase ethinyl estradiol plasma levels. This interaction may cause breakthrough bleeding and contraceptive failure when women taking oral contraceptives containing ethinyl estradiol abruptly discontinue ascorbic acid (Morris et al, 1981).

INTERFERENCE WITH LABORATORY TEST RESULTS. Large doses of ascorbic acid can affect results of the enzyme test for glycosuria used by many diabetics to regulate the dosage of hypoglycemic drugs. The Testape test is falsely negative, and the Clinitest is falsely positive. Megadoses also can cause false-positive results when Benedict's solution is used as a test for glycosuria. Tests for occult blood in the stool may be falsely negative in patients with carcinoma of the colon.

DOSAGE AND PREPARATIONS. For prophylaxis or correction of deficiency, vitamin C may be given as fresh or frozen orange juice (contains approximately 0.5 mg of ascorbic acid/ml). Crystalline ascorbic acid is a suitable alternative; oral administration is preferred, but the vitamin also may be injected intramuscularly or intravenously in patients receiving total parenteral nutrition.

PROPHYLACTIC:

Oral, Intramuscular: *Infants,* for the first six months of life, 30 mg daily; *premature infants* may require a larger dose. *Older infants, children, and adults,* at least 60 to 120 ml of orange juice or other source of vitamin C or 40 to 60 mg of crystalline ascorbic acid daily. During pregnancy 70 mg daily and during lactation 90 to 95 mg daily of ascorbic acid is recommended. During periods of increased requirement (eg, infections, trauma), 150 mg daily.

THERAPEUTIC:

Oral, Intramuscular, Intravenous: *Adults and children,* the diet should be corrected by ingesting at least 60 to 120 ml of orange juice or other source of vitamin C daily. For treatment of scurvy, 100 mg three times daily for one week, followed by 100 mg daily for several weeks until tissue saturation is normal. For severe burns, 200 to 500 mg daily until healing has occurred or grafting operations are completed.

ASCORBIC ACID:

Generic. Capsules (prolonged-release) 500 mg; solution (injection) 250 mg/ml in 2 and 30 ml containers and 500 mg/ml in 50 and 100 ml containers; syrup 20, 50, and 100 mg/ml; tablets 50, 100, 250, and 500 mg and 1 g; tablets (chewable) 100, 250, and 500 mg; tablets (prolonged-release) 500 mg and 1 and 1.5 g (all oral forms and sizes nonprescription).

Cecon (Abbott). Drops 100 mg/ml (nonprescription).

Cevalin (Lilly). Solution (intramuscular) 100 mg/ml in 10 ml containers and 500 mg/ml in 1 ml containers.

Cevi Bid (Geriatric). Capsules (prolonged-release) 500 mg (nonprescription).

Ce-Vi-Sol (Mead Johnson). Drops (pediatric) 35 mg/0.6 ml (alcohol 5%, nonprescription).

ASCORBATE CALCIUM:

Generic. Tablets 500, 610, and 1,111 mg (nonprescription).

ASCORBATE SODIUM:

Generic. Solution (injection) 250 mg/ml in 10 and 30 ml containers and 500 mg/ml in 30 and 50 ml containers.

Cenolate (Abbott). Solution (injection) equivalent to ascorbic acid 500 mg/ml in 1 and 2 ml containers.

BIOTIN

This member of the B-complex group of vitamins is a coenzyme essential for fatty acid and carbohydrate metabolism and other carboxylation reactions and is synthesized by intestinal bacteria. Persons with multiple carboxylase deficiency, an inborn error of biotin-dependent enzyme systems, respond to 10 mg of biotin given once or twice daily (Nyhan, 1980). Deficiency can be produced by prolonged ingestion of large amounts of raw egg white, which contains the inactivating protein, avidin. Biotin deficiency also may occur during long-term parenteral nutrition. Otherwise, biotin deficiency has never been reported.

In adults, symptoms of deficiency include alopecia, anorexia, mental depression, partial memory loss, and dermatitis. In young infants, deficiency causes seborrheic dermatitis, and the Committee on Nutrition of the American Academy of Pediatrics (1980) recommends that formulas contain 15 mcg/1,000 kcal. Because the amounts produced by intestinal microorganisms may meet most needs, no firm RDA has been determined. (See Table 2).

FOLIC ACID

Folate is the generic term for several compounds having folic acid activity. Adequate varied diets provide sufficient amounts for normal individuals. Chronic alcoholics are susceptible to folate deficiency; 40% to 87% of alcoholics admitted to municipal hospitals have low serum folate concentrations (Wagner, 1984).

Amounts present in human or cow's milk are adequate to fulfill infant requirements. Supplementation may be needed in low-birth-weight infants, those who are breast-fed by mothers with folic acid deficiency, infants who do not receive solid foods until quite late, or those with infections or prolonged diarrhea. During pregnancy and lactation, folic acid requirements are markedly increased and deficiency will adversely affect the infant. See Table 1.

In patients with megaloblastic anemia, the diagnosis of vitamin B_{12} deficiency should be excluded before therapeutic doses of folic acid are prescribed. Patients with pernicious anemia who receive more than 400 mcg of folic acid daily and who are inadequately treated with vitamin B_{12} may show reversion of hematologic parameters to normal, while neurologic damage due to vitamin B_{12} deficiency progresses.

Doses of folic acid exceeding the RDA should not be included in multivitamin preparations; if therapeutic amounts are necessary, folic acid should be given separately.

For a more detailed discussion of folic acid, see index entry Anemia, Megaloblastic.

PREPARATIONS.

Generic. Tablets 0.4, 0.8 (nonprescription), and 1 mg; solution (injection) 5 and 10 mg/ml in 10 ml containers.

Folvite (Lederle). Tablets 1 mg; solution (injection) 5 mg/ml in 10 ml containers.

NIACIN (Nicotinic Acid)

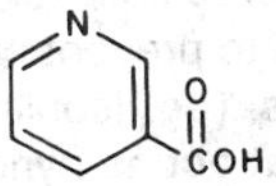

NIACINAMIDE (Nicotinamide)

FUNCTIONS. Niacin, including niacinamide and tryptophan, is converted to physiologically active diphosphopyridine nucleotide (DPN or NAD) and triphosphopyridine nucleotide (TPN or NADP). As coenzymes of numerous dehydrogenases, these nucleotides are functional groups of electron transfer agents active in cellular respiration, glycolysis, and lipid synthesis.

SOURCES AND METABOLISM. Chief dietary sources of niacin are proteins of animal origin, yeast, and green vegetables. Bound forms, which are unavailable for conversion to nucleotides, are present in many foods, especially cereals. The conversion of dietary tryptophan to NAD and NADP requires thiamine, riboflavin, and pyridoxine; approximately 60 mg of precursor tryptophan is equivalent to 1 mg of niacin. Thus, the dietary requirement for niacin is influenced by the protein content of the diet. Larger amounts are needed during periods of increased metabolism (eg, pregnancy, lactation, prolonged infection, hyperthyroidism, burns).

DEFICIENCY. Primary dietary deficiency is rare in the United States except in areas where corn (which is low in tryptophan) is the main constituent of the diet. Secondary deficiency may occur in those with malabsorption syndromes, in alcoholics, or in dietary cultists.

Deficiency causes pellagra, which is characterized by erythematous lesions on areas of the skin exposed to sun, friction, or pressure. As lesions become chronic, pigmentation and hyperkeratinization occur. Diarrhea and abdominal pain are prominent. Other symptoms include mental depression or apathy, headache, insomnia, atrophy of sebaceous glands and hair follicles, inflammation and atrophy of mucous membranes, angular stomatitis, sialorrhea, and glossitis. As pellagra progresses, psychoses (eg, hallucinations, disorientation) often occur. The condition may be complicated by thiamine deficiency with associated peripheral neuritis. The macrocytic anemia that sometimes accompanies pellagra probably is related to concomitant folic acid deficiency. Therefore, patients treated for pellagra also should receive small doses of all B-complex vitamins and consume a well-balanced diet with adequate protein to provide tryptophan.

Pellagra may be associated with isoniazid therapy (competitive inhibition of niacin incorporation into NAD), carcinoid syndrome (deviation of precursor tryptophan for conversion by tumor to serotonin), Hartnup disease (a genetic disorder characterized by impaired absorption of tryptophan), or hepatic cirrhosis (decreased hepatic dehydrogenases leading to decreased niacin activity).

OTHER USES. The vasodilating effect of niacin is of doubtful therapeutic value (see index entry Niacin). The large doses used in psychiatric disorders lack any beneficial effect (Petrie and Ban, 1985). Niacin (but not niacinamide) reduces blood lipid levels (see index entry Niacin).

ADVERSE REACTIONS. Therapeutic doses of niacin may cause pruritus, flushing, headache, paresthesias, nausea, and other symptoms of gastrointestinal irritation. Large doses may activate peptic ulcer, impair glucose tolerance, or produce liver damage and hyperuricemia. These reactions are usually reversible when therapy is discontinued. Rarely, anaphylaxis has been reported following intravenous administration.

Niacin is classified in FDA Pregnancy Category C.

DOSAGE AND PREPARATIONS.

Oral (preferred): For pellagra, *adults,* initially, 300 to 500 mg niacinamide daily in divided doses; *children,* initially, 100 to 300 mg daily in divided doses. For maintenance, a preparation containing RDA amounts of niacinamide, thiamine, riboflavin, and pyridoxine should be given daily. Associated anemia may require the use of iron, folic acid, or vitamin B_{12}. For less severe deficiency, 50 to 100 mg daily.

As dietary supplement, 5 to 20 mg daily.

Intravenous (preferred parenteral route): For pellagra, initially, 25 to 100 mg niacinamide every two or three hours to a maximum of 1 g/day. The vitamin must be given very slowly at a concentration of no more than 10 mg/ml or it may be diluted in 500 ml of 0.9% sodium chloride injection and given at a rate of 2 mg/min. The oral route should be substituted and ingestion of a well-balanced diet should begin as soon as possible.

Intramuscular: For pellagra, *adults and children,* 50 to 100 mg niacinamide daily in five or more divided doses.

NIACIN:
Generic, Nicotinic Acid. Capsules (prolonged-release) 125, 250, 400, and 500 mg; tablets 25, 50, 100, 250, and 500 mg (nonprescription); solution (injection, sodium salt) 100 mg/ml in 30 ml containers.
Nicobid (Rorer). Capsules (prolonged-release) 125, 250, and 500 mg (nonprescription).
Nicolar (Rorer). Tablets 500 mg.
Nico-400 (Jones). Capsules (prolonged-release) 400 mg (nonprescription).
Nicotinex (Fleming). Elixir 50 mg/5 ml (alcohol 14%) (nonprescription).

NIACINAMIDE (Nicotinamide):
Generic. Tablets 50, 100, and 500 mg (nonprescription); solution (injection) 100 mg/ml in 30 ml containers.

PANTOTHENIC ACID

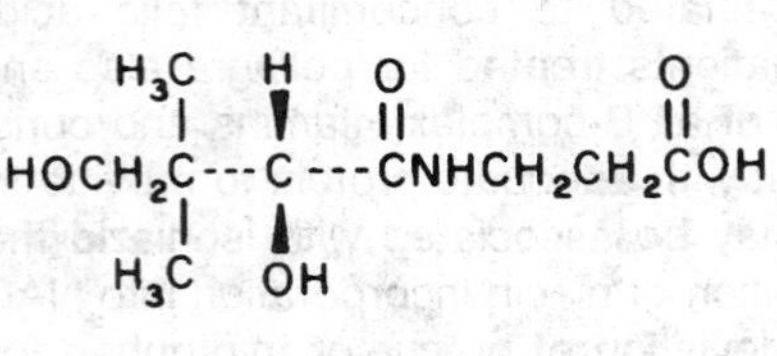

```
      H3C   H    O            O
       |    ▼    ||           ||
HOCH2C---C---CNHCH2CH2COH
       |    ▲
      H3C   OH
```

As a precursor of coenzyme A, pantothenic acid is essential in the intermediary metabolism of fats, carbohydrates, and proteins and in the synthesis of steroids, porphyrins, acetylcholine, and other substances. The RDA has not been established, but a daily intake of 4 to 7 mg is recommended for adults and 3 to 4 mg for children. A balanced diet containing 2,500 calories supplies about 10 mg. Pantothenic acid is considered suitable for inclusion in multivitamin preparations in amounts of 5 to 20 mg.

Spontaneous clinical deficiency has not been observed, presumably because pantothenic acid is present in almost all plant and animal tissues and also is produced by intestinal bacteria. Body needs may be met by absorption of pantothenate synthesized by intestinal flora. Deficiency is unlikely except in association with other B-vitamin deficiencies (eg, pellagra, beriberi, alcoholism), and there is no indication for use of this vitamin alone.

Large doses are ineffective in the prevention or treatment of graying hair, adynamic ileus, diabetic neuropathy, or psychiatric states.

Pantothenic acid is largely nontoxic, although large doses reportedly cause liver disease in rats.

Generic. Tablets 100, 200, 250, and 500 mg (nonprescription).

PYRIDOXINE HYDROCHLORIDE (Vitamin B_6)

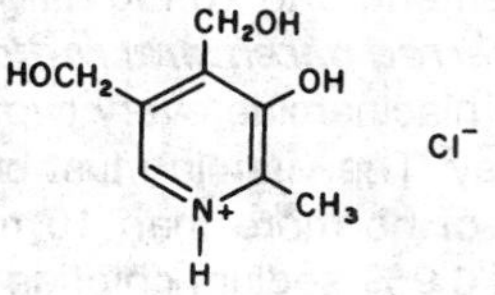

```
            CH2OH
HOCH2             OH
                        Cl⁻
            N+    CH3
            |
            H
```

The vitamin B_6 group is composed of three compounds (pyridoxine, pyridoxal, pyridoxamine) that are metabolically and functionally interrelated. These compounds are converted to pyridoxal phosphate and, to a lesser extent, pyridoxamine phosphate, which function principally in protein and amino acid metabolism (eg, as coenzymes for decarboxylations or transaminations).

REQUIREMENTS. The requirement for pyridoxine appears to parallel protein intake (approximately 0.02 mg/g of protein compound). Most balanced diets provide adequate amounts, but home-prepared artificial formulas for infants should be fortified with pyridoxine. Intake must be increased during pregnancy and lactation and in some women taking oral contraceptives.

DEFICIENCY. Dietary deficiency is rare except in combination with other vitamin B-complex deficiencies (eg, in alcoholism, malabsorption syndromes). However, inadequate utilization of pyridoxine due to inborn errors of metabolism has been implicated in pyridoxine-dependent seizures, pyridoxine-responsive anemia, homocystinuria, xanthinuric aciduria, and cystathioninuria. Pyridoxine-dependent seizures should be considered in all infants with intractable convulsions. The proposed biochemical pathology is decreased affinity of the enzyme, glutamic acid decarboxylase, which converts glutamic acid to GABA, for pyridoxal phosphate. Thus, larger than usual amounts of pyridoxine are required to overcome the depressed enzyme binding and maintain normal GABA, an inhibitory neurotransmitter, in the central nervous system.

USES. Pyridoxine-responsive anemia (usually sideroblastic) is uncommon and may occur in patients without deficiency. It cannot be induced in normal persons either by deficiency in the diet or administration of pyridoxine antagonists. Therefore, a genetic defect is presumed to be the cause (see also index entry Anemia, Sideroblastic).

Pyridoxine is indicated to prevent or treat peripheral neuritis caused by certain drugs (eg, isoniazid, cycloserine, hydralazine, penicillamine) that act as pyridoxine antagonists and/or increase its excretion in the urine. Pyridoxine may be given prophylactically in doses 300% to 500% higher than the RDA during therapy with pyridoxine antagonists.

Patients with homocystinuria, xanthinuric aciduria, and cystathioninuria require large doses of pyridoxine to overcome inborn errors of metabolism.

This agent has been reported to improve symptoms, such as cheilosis, seborrheic dermatitis, glossitis, and stomatitis, that do not respond to thiamine, riboflavin, and niacin and to relieve the symptoms associated with premenstrual tension (see index entry Premenstrual Tension).

ADVERSE REACTIONS. Pyridoxine can cause sensory neuropathy or neuropathic syndromes when given in doses exceeding 50 mg to 2 g daily over prolonged periods (Schaumburg et al, 1983; Dalton and Dalton, 1987). The initial findings are unstable gait and numb feet, followed by numbness and awkwardness of the hands and perioral numbness. Pinprick and temperature sensations are less affected. Symptoms gradually resolve over a period of months once the intake of pyridoxine is stopped.

Pyridoxine is classified in FDA Pregnancy Category A.

DRUG INTERACTIONS. Pyridoxine supplements should not be given to patients receiving levodopa, because the action of the latter is antagonized. However, this vitamin may be used concurrently with a preparation containing both carbidopa and levodopa.

DOSAGE AND PREPARATIONS.

Oral (preferred), Intramuscular, Intravenous: In pyridoxine dependency syndromes, *infants,* 2 to 15 mg daily; *adults and children,* 10 to 250 mg daily. For drug-induced peripheral neuritis, *adults and children,* 50 to 200 mg daily. For prophylaxis in patients taking drugs that affect pyridoxine disposition, 25 to 50 mg daily. For deficiency, *adults and children,* 5 to 25 mg daily for three weeks, followed by 1.5 to 2.5 mg daily in a multivitamin preparation for maintenance. During pregnancy and lactation, same dose as for deficiency.

Generic. Solution (injection) 100 mg/ml in 1, 10, and 30 ml containers; tablets 10, 25, 50, 100, 250, and 500 mg (nonprescription).

Hexa-Betalin (Lilly). Solution (injection) 100 mg/ml in 10 ml containers; tablets 25 and 50 mg (nonprescription).

RIBOFLAVIN (Vitamin B_2)

FUNCTIONS AND REQUIREMENTS. Riboflavin functions as the coenzyme for flavin adenine dinucleotide (FAD) and flavin mononucleotide (FMN), which primarily influence hydrogen transport in oxidative enzyme systems (eg, cytochrome C reductase, succinic dehydrogenase, xanthine oxidase).

This vitamin is readily absorbed from the intestine and is distributed to all tissues, but little is stored. A well-balanced diet provides adequate amounts for normal individuals. A minimum of 1.2 mg/day is recommended for persons with low caloric intake. Requirements parallel carbohydrate intake and are increased during pregnancy, lactation, and possibly in women taking oral contraceptives. The requirement also is reported to be increased by prolonged administration of phenothiazines or heterocyclic antidepressants.

DEFICIENCY. Ariboflavinosis is characterized by cheilosis, angular stomatitis, glossitis, seborrheic dermatitis of the nose and scrotum, and corneal vascularization (injection and proliferation of capillaries in the limbic plexus). Ocular symptoms include pruritus, burning, blepharospasm, photophobia, and visual impairment. The lesions of the skin and mucous membranes also are noted in other B-complex deficiencies.

Riboflavin deficiency seldom occurs alone; it often is associated with pellagra and other vitamin B-complex deficiency states (eg, alcoholism, malabsorption syndromes). Therefore, ariboflavinosis should be treated with multivitamin B preparations.

There is no acceptable evidence that riboflavin has any effect other than in the treatment or prevention of its deficiency state. No toxic effects have been reported clinically.

DOSAGE AND PREPARATIONS.

Oral: For deficiency, 5 to 25 mg daily, preferably in a preparation containing the other B-complex vitamins.

Generic. Tablets 5, 10, 25, 50, and 100 mg (nonprescription).

THIAMINE HYDROCHLORIDE (Vitamin B_1)

Following the conversion to thiamine pyrophosphate, the active form of thiamine hydrochloride, this vitamin acts as a coenzyme in the decarboxylation of α-keto acids and is essential for carbohydrate metabolism. Additionally, thiamine may help modulate neurotransmitter activity, although further studies are required to verify this role and its relative importance. Requirements parallel caloric intake, particularly of carbohydrate, and are increased during pregnancy and lactation.

DEFICIENCY. Mild deficiency may occur even with apparently adequate diets, especially when energy needs are increased (eg, in hyperthyroidism, during heavy manual labor). Elderly persons should maintain an intake of 1 mg/day, for impaired utilization of thiamine has been reported in this age group.

Severe deficiency (beriberi) is relatively rare. It is most common in alcoholics, in pregnant women receiving inadequate diets, or in patients with malabsorption syndromes, prolonged diarrhea, or hepatic diseases causing defective utilization of thiamine. Beriberi has two principal forms: (1) chronic dry beriberi characterized mainly by polyneuropathy, and (2) acute wet beriberi, in which edema and serous effusions predominate.

Chronic dry beriberi occurs most often in adults and usually is associated with malabsorption or multiple vitamin deficiencies. It also may occur during long-term dialysis or parenteral feeding. In chronic alcoholism with associated malnutrition, Wernicke's encephalopathy may develop. The characteristic symptoms (ophthalmoplegia, ataxia, polyneuropathy, mental deterioration) often are accompanied by Korsakoff syndrome (amnestic confabulatory psychosis). This condition is considered a medical emergency and immediate parenteral administration of thiamine is necessary to limit permanent damage of the central nervous system.

Wet beriberi is endemic in areas where polished, unenriched rice forms a large part of the diet. In adults, it may progress from anorexia, muscle weakness, and personality changes to severe circulatory disturbances with edema and high-output heart failure. Severe deficiency in infants may cause death within 24 hours after the onset of symptoms (anorexia, vomiting, convulsions, cyanosis) unless intensive treatment is begun immediately.

A small number of case reports document the existence of thiamine dependency in genetically predisposed individuals. The symptoms include severe anemia, diabetes, and deafness, all of which improve following the administration of large doses (100 mg daily) of thiamine (Mandel et al, 1984).

Several patients with branched-chain ketoaciduria (maple syrup urine disease) have been reported to respond favorably to large doses of thiamine. This disorder is caused by impairment of branched-chain α-ketoacid dehydrogenase, resulting in the accumulation of α-ketoacids in the bloodstream. Patients with residual enzyme activity in mononuclear blood cells exceeding 5% are more likely to respond than those with less enzyme activity. In addition to dietary restriction of branched-chain amino acids, a trial with large doses of thiamine (10 to 20 mg/kg/day in infants and 150 mg/day in older patients) should be undertaken (Fernhoff et al, 1985).

Oral administration corrects most uncomplicated deficiencies, but the parenteral route may be utilized in severe, acute situations. In all individuals, the absorptive capacity is limited; the maximum individual oral dose absorbed probably is 5 mg.

ADVERSE REACTIONS. Thiamine produces no toxic effects when given orally and the excess is excreted rapidly in the urine. Anaphylactoid reactions, a few of which were fatal, have occurred rarely after intravenous administration of large amounts in sensitive patients.

Thiamine is classified in FDA Pregnancy Category A.

DOSAGE AND PREPARATIONS.

Oral, Intramuscular, Intravenous: For deficiency, 5 to 10 mg three times daily. Larger parenteral doses have been recommended in severe cases, but no satisfactory evidence exists to show that an increased response occurs with doses larger than 30 mg daily. After signs of deficiency have been corrected, the dose should be no greater than the RDA as supplied by correction of the diet, if possible, or by a daily supplement. Unless evidence indicates that the deficiency is clearly one of thiamine alone or a therapeutic test is being employed, administration of a vitamin B-complex preparation is preferred until a well-balanced diet is restored.

Generic. Tablets 10, 25, 50, 100, 250, and 500 mg (nonprescription); elixir 2.25 mg/5 ml (nonprescription); solution (injection) 100 mg/ml in 1, 2, 10, and 30 ml containers.

Available Trademark.

Betalin S (Lilly).

Similar Preparation.

Thiamine Mononitrate, U.S.P. Used in some multivitamin preparations.

VITAMIN B_{12} (Cyanocobalamin)

For chemical formula, see index entry Cyanocobalamin, In Deficiency Anemias.

Vitamin B_{12} is a generic term for several cobalt-containing compounds. As a component of various coenzymes, it is important in the synthesis of nucleic acid and of myelin, thereby influencing cell maturation and maintenance of the integrity of neuronal tissue. Animal products are the primary food sources, and dietary deficiencies are rare except in strict vegetarians. Since milk is a relatively good source of vitamin B_{12}, supplementation is unnecessary in infants unless artificial formulas lacking this vitamin are used.

The average U.S. diet supplies an estimated 5 to 15 mcg daily, but there is a large variation among individuals. The absorption of vitamin B_{12} requires sufficient intrinsic factor and calcium ions. The ileum contains receptor sites that bind to intrinsic factor, promoting the absorption of vitamin B_{12}. The intrinsic factor is destroyed during passage through the intestinal mucosa, and vitamin B_{12} is transferred to transcobalamin II (Herbert, 1987). Intrinsic factor deficiency causes pernicious anemia, which may be associated with demyelination of the spinal cord, as may occur with any form of vitamin B_{12} deficiency. Prompt parenteral administration of vitamin B_{12} prevents progression of neurologic damage. Oral dietary supplements are inadequate to treat this disorder, except in very large doses, and should be reserved for patients in whom pernicious anemia has been ruled out.

Supplemental amounts of vitamin B_{12} may be necessary during pregnancy and lactation in vegetarians. A daily intake of 0.15 mcg/100 kcal for all infants receiving commercial formulas is now required. Vitamin B_{12} should be included in B-complex preparations that also contain folic acid.

Also see index entry Cyanocobalamin, In Deficiency Anemias.

MINERALS

Many mineral elements function as essential constituents of enzymes, regulate a variety of physiologic functions (eg, maintenance of osmotic pressure, oxygen transport, muscle contraction, central nervous system integrity), and are required for growth and maintenance of tissues and bones. Some elements (calcium, phosphorus, sodium, potassium, magnesium, sulfur, and chloride) are present in relatively large amounts, while others appear only in trace quantities. Trace elements recognized as essential in man are cobalt (as vitamin B_{12}), copper, fluorine, iodine, iron, zinc, chromium, selenium, manganese, and molybdenum. Because of their effects in experimental animals, nickel, tin, silicon, and arsenic also are considered essential.

Unless absorption is impaired, severe mineral deficiency is uncommon in the United States, since most minerals (except zinc) are widely distributed in foods. However, iron deficiency is relatively common in infants, children up to age 4, and women of childbearing age. Marginal zinc deficiencies also occur frequently in vegetarians. A balanced, varied diet supplies adequate amounts of most trace elements, and dietary supplements containing minerals should be used only when there is evidence of deficiency or when demands are known to be increased (eg, during pregnancy and lactation).

Trace element deficiencies may develop during prolonged total parenteral nutrition (TPN) (see index entry Nutrition, Parenteral). Minerals should be given routinely when the need for supplementation is anticipated (eg, patients with Crohn's disease, ileal bypass surgery or other resections, malabsorption syndromes). In patients with renal disease or biliary tract obstruction, caution is necessary to avoid excessive dosage.

Minerals Present in Relatively Large Amounts

Calcium: This element is present in the body in greater amounts than any other mineral. Its metabolism, functions, and uses are discussed elsewhere; see index entry Calcium Metabolism.

Vitamin D is required for efficient absorption of calcium. Dietary requirements are increased in growing children, during pregnancy and lactation, and in postmenopausal women. Infants fed artificial formulas require supplementation. Intake of calcium also should be increased when high-protein and/or high-phosphorus diets are consumed. Various investigators have suggested an intake of approximately 1.2 g/day of calcium for alcoholics, patients with malabsorption syndromes, and those receiving corticosteroids, isoniazid, tetracycline, or aluminum-containing antacids.

Magnesium: Magnesium activates many enzyme systems (alkaline phosphatase, enolases, leucine aminopeptidase) and is an essential cofactor in oxidative phosphorylation, thermoregulation, muscular contractility, and nerve excitability. Deficiency is uncommon in normal individuals eating a varied diet, but the requirement for magnesium parallels the amount of protein, calcium, and phosphorus ingested.

Hypomagnesemia increases neuronal excitability and neuromuscular transmission; severe deficiency may result in tetany and convulsions. Hypomagnesemia has been observed in alcoholics; in patients with kwashiorkor, infantile tetany, diabetes, malabsorption syndromes, hyper- or hypoparathyroidism, and renal diseases; during diuretic therapy; in burn patients treated with daily saline baths; in patients receiving total parenteral nutrition without adequate magnesium supplements; in patients receiving cisplatin [Platinol]; and postoperatively.

Hypermagnesemia produces peripheral vasodilation and loss of tendon reflexes; it has a curare-like effect at the myoneural junction and blocks release of catecholamine from the adrenal glands. Respiratory failure and cardiac arrest occur after very large doses.

For a more detailed discussion of magnesium imbalances, see index entry Magnesium Imbalances.

Phosphorus: This mineral is necessary for utilization of many B-complex vitamins. It is present in bones and teeth in amounts nearly equal to those of calcium, is a prominent component of all body tissues, and is very important as a buffer in body fluids. Lipids, proteins, carbohydrates, and various enzymes involved in energy transfer contain phosphorus.

A varied diet supplies sufficient phosphorus. The calcium:phosphorus ratio also is important. If an appropriate amount of vitamin D is ingested, diets supplying excess phosphorus in relation to calcium are tolerated. Deficiency does not occur in adults unless there is prolonged excessive use of alcohol or nonabsorbable antacids, prolonged vomiting, liver disease, or, less commonly, hyperparathyroidism.

For further discussion of the therapeutic use of phosphorus, see index entry Calcium Metabolism.

Potassium: The differential concentration of potassium (the principal cation of intracellular fluid) and sodium (the principal cation of extracellular fluid) across the cell wall regulates the excitability of the cell, nerve impulse conduction, and body fluid balance and volume.

Although dietary deficiency is rare in individuals consuming an adequate diet, hypokalemia may occur in children whose diet lacks protein. The most common cause of hypokalemia is diuretic therapy, especially when thiazides or a loop diuretic are given. Other causes of hypokalemia include prolonged diarrhea, particularly in infants; hyperaldosteronism; inappropriate or inadequate parenteral fluid therapy; and long-term use of adrenal corticosteroids or laxatives. The most serious consequences of hypokalemia are cardiac arrhythmias and neuromuscular disorders.

Hyperkalemia most commonly is caused by impaired renal excretion of potassium, which may occur in patients with adrenocortical insufficiency, acute renal failure, or terminal chronic renal failure; inappropriate vitamin K supplementation; or use of aldosterone antagonists. Severe arrhythmias and conduction defects are the most serious sequelae. Other manifestations include weakness and paresthesias.

For the therapeutic uses of potassium, see index entries Diuretics; Potassium Chloride.

Sodium: Sodium helps to maintain fluid balance and volume. Its concentration in body fluids is under homeostatic control. Imbalances occur only when these mechanisms fail or losses are greater than the compensatory abilities of adaptive mechanisms. Sodium often is added during the processing of food. Most individuals consume more sodium than necessary. Dietary restriction often is recommended in patients with congestive heart failure, hepatic cirrhosis, and hypertension. Intake of less than usual amounts of sodium starting in childhood and continuing throughout adult life may aid in preventing hypertension in susceptible individuals. However, dietary restriction of sodium in healthy women during pregnancy is not recommended.

Hyponatremia is encountered rarely in normal individuals but may occur after prolonged diarrhea or vomiting, particularly in infants; in renal disorders, cystic fibrosis, or adrenocortical insufficiency; or with use of thiazide diuretics. Excessive sweating may cause pronounced sodium loss, and replacement therapy should include both water and sodium chloride.

Chloride: Chloride is the most important anion in the maintenance of electrolyte balance. Hypochloremic metabolic alkalosis may develop following prolonged vomiting or excessive use of diuretics. Excessive loss may accompany excessive loss of sodium and, when sodium intake is curtailed, substitution of another source of chloride may be necessary. If potassium chloride is used, the possibility of hyperkalemia and its associated dangers should be considered.

Sulfur: Several essential amino acids, thiamine, and biotin contain sulfur. Although this mineral is known to be essential for man, its precise function other than as an atom in the above essential molecules is not known and no daily requirements have been established.

Trace Elements

Chromium: Trivalent chromium plays a role in a cofactor complex for insulin and thus is involved in normal glucose utilization. The organic form of chromium exists in a dinicotino-glutathionine complex in natural foods and appears to be absorbed better than the inorganic form.

Deficiency has been reported in a few patients receiving total parenteral nutrition for five months to three years. These patients had peripheral neuropathy and/or encephalopathy that was alleviated by administration of chromium 150 mcg daily. Symptoms included a diabetes-like condition with impaired utilization of glucose. Other patients with similar symptoms of glucose intolerance also had protein-calorie malnutrition.

Marginal levels of chromium have been associated with decreased glucose utilization during pregnancy and in the elderly. In these patients, administration of the metal improved glucose tolerance. However, the clinical significance of these findings requires further clarification. Supplemental amounts of chromium do not have a hypoglycemic effect in normal individuals. Excessive chromium is toxic.

Cobalt: Cobalt is a component of vitamin B_{12}; it has no other known function in human nutrition. The daily requirement is easily obtained from a balanced, varied diet.

Cobalt salts have been used with dubious success to treat certain types of anemias refractory to other therapy; they appear to act via selective toxicity. In massive doses (ie, 20 to 30 mg daily), cobalt can produce polycythemia, thyroid hyperplasia, and cardiomyopathy.

Copper: Copper is absorbed in the proximal portion of the small intestine and then transported to the liver bound loosely to albumin and other proteins. In the liver, copper is incorporated into ceruloplasmin, its major blood carrier protein. Copper is an essential component of a number of proteins (eg, erythrocuprein, hepatocuprein) and enzymes (eg, lysyl hydroxylase, dopamine beta-hydroxylase). This mineral is thought to act as a catalyst in the storage and release of iron to form hemoglobin. It is believed to be essential for connective tissue formation, hematopoiesis, and central nervous system function.

Most unprocessed foods are excellent sources of copper and deficiency was thought to be rare. However, a typical American diet may supply only one-half the RDA for copper (Patterson et al, 1984). Copper deficiency has also been reported in malnourished children with anemia and neutropenia. Hypocupremia has been observed in adults with sickle cell anemia who received large doses of zinc for several months. In addition, the administration of zinc in doses slightly in excess of the RDA reduces the absorption of copper and increases its fecal excretion (Festa et al, 1985). Competitive inhibition of copper by iron and certain sugars has been demonstrated in experimental animals and possibly in a premature infant receiving an iron-fortified formula. Copper supplements should be given during prolonged parenteral or enteral nutrition.

Hypocupremia unrelated to nutritional factors may result from reduced or defective formation of ceruloplasmin; this occurs in newborn infants (especially premature infants). In Menkes' syndrome (kinky hair disease), an inherited disease, there is abnormal copper transport by intestinal cells. Although hypocupremia has been observed in patients with protein-calorie malnutrition, tropical sprue, celiac disease, and nephrotic syndrome, it is thought to be secondary to disturbances of protein metabolism with loss of copper-protein complexes.

Elevated serum levels of copper occur in various diseases and are produced by some drugs (eg, estrogens, thyroid, corticotropin), but associated abnormalities are rare. Acute toxicity has occurred following the oral ingestion of as little as 10 to 15 mg of inorganic copper and may be manifested by nausea and vomiting, epigastric pain, diarrhea, malaise, and, in more severe poisoning, acute hemolysis and renal tubular disorders. For the treatment of hypercupremia, see index entry Penicillamine, in Metal Poisoning.

Fluoride: Fluoride is incorporated into teeth and decreases the incidence of dental caries, especially in children. There is evidence that it also aids in retention of calcium in bones. However, evidence regarding fluoride supplementation as a means of preventing or alleviating bone diseases, such as osteoporosis, remains controversial. (See index entry Calcium Metabolism.)

Fluoridation of the water supply (optimum concentration, 0.7 to 1.2 ppm) is the most efficient and economical method of assuring adequate intake. The prevalence of dental caries has decreased 30% to 60% in the past 20 years, principally because of the widespread fluoridation of drinking water and the use of dentifrices containing fluoride (Glass, 1986). For maximal anticariogenic effects, fluoride should be ingested daily from birth throughout life. Dietary supplements should be used only when water supplies contain less than 0.7 ppm, and the dose should be adjusted according to the amount of fluoride in the water (see Table 3). Approximately one-half the daily dose is recommended when drinking water contains between 0.3 and 0.7 ppm fluoride. Use of fluoride should be reviewed if the family moves or when the fluoride content of the water changes. In trace quantities, fluoride is a nutrient; in large quantities, it is a poison.

Chronic toxicity (fluorosis) usually results from prolonged exposure to insecticides or industrial dusts or from prolonged daily ingestion of water containing more than 4 ppm. Mottled enamel (dental fluorosis) may occur if teeth are developing, and osteomalacia and osteosclerosis may be induced in older people. Considerable mottling of teeth and bone disorders occur when more than 8 ppm are present in the water supply or with combined intake from water and fluoride supplements. Except for orthopedic and supportive measures, there is no treatment for fluorosis; therefore, all efforts should be directed at prevention.

Claims that persons residing in areas where water supplies are fluoridated have experienced a higher incidence of cancer have been refuted by the National Cancer Institute (*J Am Diet Assoc*, 1977) and others (Clemmesen, 1983).

Iodine: Iodine is an integral part of the thyroid hormones, tetraiodothyronine (thyroxine) and triiodothyronine. Deficiency results in compensatory hyperplasia and hypertrophy of the thyroid gland (endemic goiter). Endemic goiter occurs in areas where the soil is deficient in iodine and was common before the iodization of table salt. It no longer appears to be a problem in the United States, where recent nutrition surveys suggest that iodine intake exceeds requirements. Iodate in bread and use of iodophores as antiseptics by the dairy industry are the main sources of iodide in most diets. Iodized table salt is another economical and efficient source of iodine. Seafoods are a reliable food source.

Amounts of 100 to 300 mcg daily are desirable and up to 1 mg daily may be consumed safely. Requirements for iodine are increased in growing children and in pregnant or lactating women. However, the prolonged ingestion of large amounts of iodides during pregnancy may result in neonatal thyroid enlargement, hypothyroidism, or cretinism.

Manifestations of acute iodine intoxication are related to the organ systems that incorporate iodine (eg, thyroid gland, salivary apparatus, eye) and include edema, fever, and conjunctivitis. Laryngeal edema resulting in airway obstruction is potentially fatal. Local reactions in the gastrointestinal tract include abdominal pain, vomiting, and diarrhea (sometimes bloody), which may lead to dehydration and shock.

Chronic iodine poisoning (iodism) is more common. There is considerable individual variation in sensitivity to iodine, and 6 mg or more daily may inhibit thyroid activity and lead to development of hypothyroidism. Hypersensitivity reactions include rash and dermatoses (which appear to be dose related), nausea, edema of the face and eyes, headache, cough, and gastric irritation.

For therapeutic use of iodine, see index entry Iodides.

Iron: Ionic iron is an essential component of a number of enzymes necessary for energy transfer and also is present in compounds required for oxygen transport and utilization. On the average, 10% of inorganic and food iron is absorbed when given orally; increased absorption occurs in iron-deficient individuals. Absorption of nonheme iron also is increased by concomitant use of ascorbic acid. Iron from meat (heme iron) is absorbed an average of five times better than that from vegetables (primarily nonheme iron).

Requirements are increased in infants and young children, adolescents, and menstruating, pregnant, and lactating women. They are greatest during infancy and, because of the low iron content of milk, formulas should supply 10 to 15 mg of iron daily during the first year of life. Pregnant women cannot obtain sufficient iron from a normal diet unless large amounts of meat are consumed or iron pots are used for cooking. This deficit can be corrected only by supplementation (usually 30 mg of elemental iron daily). Supplements should be continued for two to three months after parturition to increase iron stores depleted during pregnancy.

Tannins, phosphates, and antacids bind iron in relatively insoluble complexes and thus decrease its absorption; inorganic iron in food also is often bound in these poorly absorbed insoluble complexes.

Bleeding associated with gastrointestinal disease (eg, hemorrhoids, peptic ulcer, ulcerative colitis, neoplasms) frequently produces iron deficiency, and malabsorption of iron may occur in those with tropical sprue or celiac disease, gastrectomy, prolonged diarrhea, or achlorhydria. Deficiency may increase the absorption of other elements, which may lead to chronic lead, cobalt, and manganese poisoning. Copper deficiency decreases iron mobilization and, if uncorrected, causes anemia even in the presence of abundant iron stores, which cannot be adequately utilized. After iron stores in ferritin and hemosiderin are depleted, hemoglobin production is reduced and anemia results. See index entry Anemia, Iron Deficiency.

Excess iron is stored in the liver, kidneys, heart, and other organs, and iron overload can be hazardous, particularly in patients with certain diseases (eg, primary and secondary hemochromatosis, porphyria cutanea tarda). Acute iron poisoning is most common in children under 5 years. Iron-containing medications should be labeled as hazardous, kept out of the reach of children, and packaged in childproof containers. For treatment of iron poisoning, see index entry Metal Antagonists.

Manganese: This element is concentrated in cell mitochondria, mostly in the pituitary gland, liver, pancreas, kidney, and bone. It influences the synthesis of mucopolysaccharides, stimulates hepatic synthesis of cholesterol and fatty acids, and is a cofactor in many enzymes, including arginase and alkaline phosphatase in the liver. Manganese is abundant in many foods. Deficiency is unknown clinically, but a daily intake of 2 to 5 mg is thought to be safe and adequate for adults. Manganese should be supplemented during long-term total parenteral nutrition.

Chronic manganese intoxication by inhalation is an occupational hazard in mining and industrial areas, although manganese released into the atmosphere from its many industrial uses has not been a general hazard. In cases of exposure, the onset of parkinsonian symptoms is subtle and may progress unless the exposure ends quickly. Levodopa may relieve rigidity or dystonia.

Molybdenum: This element is an essential constituent of many enzymes. It is well absorbed and is present in the bones, liver, and kidneys. Deficiency is rare. Ingestion of 0.15 to 0.5 mg/day for adults has been estimated to be safe and adequate, and this apparently is provided by the usual diet.

Intake of 10 to 15 mg of molybdenum daily has been associated with a gout-like syndrome, and a moderate excess of 0.54 mg/daily may be associated with significant urinary loss of copper. Therefore, ingestion of amounts in excess of normal dietary intake is not recommended.

Selenium: Glutathione peroxidase, a selenium-dependent enzyme present in most tissues, has peroxidase-destroying capabilities, which explains much of the biological activity of selenium. There appears to be a close relationship between vitamin E and selenium.

Evidence that selenium is an essential trace element in man is provided by a study of Keshan disease (a fatal cardiomyopathy of children and young women) in China. The incidence of this disease is high in children living in areas where selenium levels in the staple food are low. Large-scale selenium supplementation in children has practically abolished Keshan disease. A similar cardiomyopathy has been found in a few patients after long-term parenteral feeding and may be due, at least partially, to selenium deficiency. However, more information is needed before definite requirements are known.

It is assumed that the dietary intake of selenium is adequate, since dietary deficiency has not been encountered in this country. Tolerance in humans has not been determined, but 0.05 to 0.2 mg/day appears to be safe for adults. Its use for either life extension or the prevention of cancer or ischemic heart disease is not supported by currently available data. Selenium is toxic in massive quantities and may cause alopecia, loss of nails, fatigue, nausea, vomiting, and sour-milk breath (Jensen et al, 1984).

Zinc: Zinc is a cofactor for over 100 enzymes and is important in nucleic acid metabolism and protein synthesis. It is necessary for growth, sexual maturation and function (primarily in males), appetite and taste acuity, and wound healing.

The absorption of zinc is a saturable process involving an active transport mechanism facilitated by low-molecular-weight ligands of pancreatic origin. About 20% to 30% of orally administered zinc is absorbed, primarily in the duodenum and proximal small intestine. The percentage absorbed depends upon a number of factors, including the source of the element. Zinc from animals generally is better absorbed than that from plant sources, probably due to the presence of phytates and fiber in plants that bind to zinc in the intestine, rendering it unavailable. Phosphates, iron, copper, lead, cadmium, and calcium also inhibit zinc absorption. Absorption is enhanced by pregnancy, corticosteroids, endotoxin, and leukocyte endogenous mediator (Jeejeebhoy, 1984).

Zinc is distributed throughout the body. The highest concentrations appear in the choroid of the eye, spermatozoa, hair, nails, prostate, and bone. In the plasma, most zinc is protein bound, predominately to albumin, alpha 2-macroglobulin, and transferrin. Human breast milk contains about 3 mg/L immediately after delivery, but the concentration tends to decrease over time.

The major route of excretion is intestinal, with fecal loss accounting for approximately two-thirds of the normal dietary intake. Only about 2% of the daily intake is excreted in the urine. Patients with diarrhea or drainage from a stoma or fistula can lose a large amount of zinc that must be replaced.

Zinc deficiency may be due to inadequate dietary intake (eg, debilitated or elderly patients, alcoholics with cirrhosis and poor diets), decreased absorption (eg, malabsorption syndrome, cystic fibrosis), increased excretion (eg, sickle cell disease, major burns, draining fistulas), or an inherited defect in metabolism (ie, acrodermatitis enteropathica). Evidence of marginal to mild deficiency has been found among some groups of children, but severe deficiency in this country probably occurs only secondary to malabsorption syndromes. It has been suggested that maternal zinc deficiency during pregnancy may have teratogenic effects, since malformation and behavioral disturbances occur in animal offspring.

Cutaneous manifestations of deficiency resembling acrodermatitis enteropathica have been reported following long-term parenteral nutrition. Patients on total parenteral nutrition should receive zinc supplements after about one month of therapy. When enterally administered defined formula diets are the sole source of nutrients, 100% of the RDA for zinc should be given.

Symptoms of deficiency include disturbances in taste and smell, anorexia, and suboptimal growth in children. More severe deficiency results in delayed bone maturation, hepatosplenomegaly, hypogonadism, testicular hypofunction, and decreased growth or dwarfism. Other manifestations are alopecia, rashes, multiple cutaneous lesions, glossitis, stomatitis, blepharitis, and paronychia.

Gonadal dysfunction and impotence in patients with renal disease can sometimes be corrected partially by administering zinc. During dialysis, zinc chloride may be added to the dialysate in sufficient quantities (400 mcg/L) to maintain the plasma concentrations between 100 and 150 mg/dl.

Evidence suggesting that zinc may promote healing of wounds or chronic ulcers is controversial; accelerated healing following zinc administration probably occurs only in those with deficiency. However, many hospitalized and elderly individuals are marginally deficient. Therefore, zinc supplementation may be worthwhile for patients experiencing delay in wound healing (Prasad, 1985).

Zinc is notable for its relatively large margin of safety. Doses required to treat zinc deficiency (ie, elemental zinc 1 mg/kg/day) cause essentially no adverse reactions. However, ingestion of excessive doses for prolonged periods is not recommended. High concentrations alter the immune response by inhibiting neutrophil migration and accumulation. Excessive intake also may induce copper and iron deficiency by interfering with their absorption and utilization and may cause nausea, vomiting, headache, chills, fever, malaise, and abdominal pain (*Med Lett Drugs Ther*, 1978).

Miscellaneous Elements: Deficiencies of elements such as nickel, tin, silicon, and vanadium have been produced in animals under rigid experimental conditions, but their importance in human nutrition is unknown.

MULTIVITAMIN PREPARATIONS WITH OR WITHOUT MINERALS

Clinically apparent vitamin deficiencies are uncommon in the United States, and subclinical deficiencies are difficult to detect. Excessive use of one or more vitamins may cause relative deficiencies of other essential micronutrients, and large doses of all minerals, fat-soluble vitamins, and some water-soluble vitamins are toxic. Also, multivitamin preparations used by adequately nourished individuals may grossly exceed nutrient needs and represent unnecessary expense.

When needed, properly formulated multivitamin preparations are useful, since clinical vitamin deficiencies are frequently multiple. Such preparations should contain only those ingredients essential for human nutrition in amounts proportional to the U.S. RDA. Additional components, such as liver, yeast, and wheat germ, do not confer any special advantage over the pure chemical ingredients, and inclusion of agents that have no proved value (eg, choline, methionine, lecithin, bioflavonoids, inositol) is unwarranted (Herbert, 1988). The amount of vitamin D in the preparation should not exceed the

U.S. RDA (10 mcg, 400 IU) because of the dangers of hypervitaminosis D. Quantities of folic acid should not exceed the U.S. RDA. Although excessive amounts produce a satisfactory hematologic response in pernicious anemia, they do not prevent progression of the neurologic symptoms of this disorder and, in fact, may mask these symptoms, rendering diagnosis difficult.

Caution is necessary when selecting multivitamin preparations because many manufacturers use the same general trademark for several preparations having very different formulas. Additionally, some manufacturers make drastic changes in product formulation while maintaining the same trademark. Until multivitamin preparations are brought into greater conformity with current nutritional knowledge, the physician should make an effort to prescribe only those having a rational quantitative basis. There seems to be little logic in a formulation containing less than 50% of the U.S. RDA for some vitamins and more than 500% of the U.S. RDA for others (particularly the interrelated B vitamins). Dosage should take into account the contribution of the patient's diet, especially vitamins A and D and all minerals.

Supplemental Multivitamin Preparations (With or Without Minerals)

Prophylactic multivitamin preparations may reasonably contain 50% to 150% of the U.S. RDA (except that vitamin D should not exceed the U.S. RDA) and should be chosen to fit the needs of the individual. These preparations may be useful during periods of increased requirements (eg, pregnancy, lactation), during relatively brief illnesses that impair absorption of nutrients, and in patients who are not eating properly. They should be discontinued after recovery or when correction of the diet has been assured. Preparations containing 150% of the U.S. RDA may be useful to supplement therapeutic, but nutritionally inadequate, diets (eg, in allergy) or when food intake is reduced drastically (eg, in rapid weight reduction programs, during prolonged illness). During pregnancy and lactation, supplemental preparations should contain folic acid and iron, for these nutrients probably cannot be supplied adequately by the diet.

Supplemental amounts of a particular vitamin are sometimes contraindicated. For example, vitamin D supplements

TABLE 6.
SUGGESTED COMPOSITION FOR INTRAVENOUS MULTIVITAMIN FORMULATIONS

Vitamin[1]	Units of Measurement	Infants/Children (<11 years)	Adults
A	RE[2] (IU)	690 (2,300)	990 (3,300)
D	mcg[3] (IU)	10 (400)	5 (200)
E	mg[4] (IU)	4.7 (7)	6.7 (10)
K_1 (Phytonadione)	mg	0.2	—
Ascorbic Acid	mg	80	100
Folacin	mg	0.14	0.4
Niacin	mg	17	40
Riboflavin	mg	1.4	3.6
Thiamin	mg	1.2	3.0
B_6 (Pyridoxine)	mg	1.0	4.0
B_{12} (Cyanocobalamin)	mcg	1.0	5.0
Pantothenic Acid	mg	5.0	15.0
Biotin	mcg	20.0	60.0

1 May be provided in appropriate salt or ester form in equivalent potency
2 RE = Retinol Equivalents (1 RE = 3.33 IU vitamin A)
3 As cholecalciferol (10 mcg cholecalciferol = 400 IU vitamin D)
4 As d-α tocopherol (1 mg d-α tocopherol = 1.5 IU vitamin E)

should be avoided in individuals, especially infants and children, who have adequate exposure to sunlight or a normal diet. Pyridoxine may interfere with the effectiveness of levodopa in the treatment of parkinsonism and, therefore, amounts exceeding the U.S. RDA should be avoided in these patients.

The individual preparations are not listed because the formulations are often changed by the manufacturers, frequently without notice, while the tradenames are unaltered.

Therapeutic Multivitamin Preparations (With or Without Minerals)

Therapeutic multivitamin preparations should be labeled as such and prescribed only to treat deficiency states and for supportive therapy in pathologic conditions that markedly increase nutritional requirements (eg, alcoholism, postoperative cachexia). *They should not be used as dietary supplements,* and medical supervision is important when such amounts are administered.

Multivitamin preparations for therapeutic use may contain as much as five times the U.S. RDA. If the required dose for a vitamin exceeds 500% of the U.S. RDA, that vitamin should be given separately. Therapeutic multivitamin preparations should not contain more than the U.S. RDA of vitamin D. In addition, the intake of vitamin A must be limited in order to avoid hypervitaminosis A.

Multivitamin preparations for parenteral administration are essential during long-term total parenteral nutrition (TPN) or to treat conditions in which oral intake or absorption of vitamins is inadequate. Guidelines for formulations of intravenously administered vitamins were established by an Expert Panel of the Nutrition Advisory Group, AMA Department of Foods and Nutrition in December 1975 (see Table 6). It was recommended that a pediatric formulation be prepared for infants and children to age 10 and an adult formulation be prepared for those age 11 and older.

The vitamin preparations used during TPN should be incorporated into daily intravenous feedings and include the fat-soluble vitamins. All essential minerals should also be included during long-term TPN. When parenteral administration of vitamins is necessary in other conditions, intramuscular injection is usually preferred. For intramuscular use, the same formulation shown in Table 6 for water-soluble vitamins only is recommended; when the fat-soluble vitamins are also needed, they should be given separately as single entities in an appropriate form for intramuscular administration. The fat-soluble vitamins are not indicated for routine use except in patients with specific deficiencies.

Cited References

Fluoride compounds, in: *Accepted Dental Therapeutics,* ed 40. Chicago, American Dental Association, 1984, 395-420.

National nutrition consortium endorses fluoridation. *J Am Diet Assoc* 10:354, 1977.

Recommended Dietary Allowances, ed 10. Washington, DC, National Academy of Sciences, 1989.

Vitamin A; proposed affirmation of Gras status as direct human food ingredient. *Federal Register* 48:1745-1758, (Jan 14) 1983.

Zinc. *Med Lett Drugs Ther* 20:57-59, 1978.

Balcke P, et al: Ascorbic acid aggravates secondary hyperoxemia in patients on chronic hemodialysis. *Ann Intern Med* 101:344-345, 1984.

Beeson PB, et al (eds): Diseases of nutrition, in: *Textbook of Medicine,* ed 15. Philadelphia, WB Saunders, 1979, 1670-1691.

Campbell GD Jr, et al: Ascorbic acid-induced hemolysis in G-6-PD deficiency. *Ann Intern Med* 82:810, 1975.

Clemmesen J: Alleged association between artificial fluoridation of water supplies and cancer: Review. *Bull WHO* 61:871-883, 1983.

Committee on Nutrition, American Academy of Pediatrics: Commentary on breast-feeding and infant formulas, including proposed standards for formulas. *Pediatrics* 57:278-285, 1976.

Committee on Nutrition, American Academy of Pediatrics: Vitamin and mineral supplementation in normal children in the United States. *Pediatrics* 66:1015-1021, 1980.

Council on Scientific Affairs, AMA: Vitamin preparations as dietary supplements and as therapeutic agents. *JAMA* 257:1929-1936, 1987.

Dalton K, Dalton MJT: Characteristics of pyridoxine overdose neuropathy syndrome. *Acta Neurol Scand* 76:8-11, 1987.

Fernhoff PM, et al: Thiamine response in maple syrup urine disease. *Pediatr Res* 19:1011-1016, 1985.

Festa MD, et al: Effect of zinc intake on copper excretion and retention in man. *Am J Clin Nutr* 41:285-292, 1985.

Fong T: Problems associated with megadose vitamin C therapy, letter. *West J Med* 134:264, 1981.

Glass RL: Fluoride dentifrices: Basis for the decline in caries prevalence. *J R Soc Med* 79(suppl 14):16-17, 1986

Hayes KC, Hegsted DM: Toxicity of vitamins, in: *Toxicants Occurring Naturally in Foods,* ed 2. Washington, DC, National Academy of Sciences, 1973, 235-253.

Herbert V: Pangamic acid ("vitamin B_{15}"). *Am J Clin Nutr* 32:1534-1540, 1979.

Herbert V: The vitamin craze. *Arch Intern Med* 140:173-176, 1980.

Herbert V: Toxicity of 25,000 IU vitamin A supplements in "health" food users. *Am J Clin Nutr* 36:185-186, 1982.

Herbert V: Recommended dietary intakes (RDI) of vitamin B-12 in humans. *Am J Clin Nutr* 45:671-678, 1987.

Herbert V: Pseudovitamins, in Shils ME, Young VR (eds): *Modern Nutrition in Health and Disease,* ed 7. Philadelphia, Lea & Febiger, 1988.

Hittner HM, et al: Retrolental fibroplasia: Efficacy of vitamin E in double-blind clinical study of preterm infants. *N Engl J Med* 305:1365-1371, 1981.

Jeejeebhoy KN: Zinc and chromium in parenteral nutrition. *Bull NY Acad Med* 60:118-124, 1984.

Jensen R, et al: Selenium intoxication: New York. *Morbid Mortal Week Rep* 33:157-158, 1984.

Levine M: New concepts in the biology and biochemistry of ascorbic acid. *N Engl J Med* 314:892-902, 1986.

Lewis JG: Adverse reactions to vitamins. *Adverse Drug React Bull* 82:296-299, (June) 1980.

MacLaughlin S, Holick MF: Aging decreases the capacity of human skin to produce vitamin D. *J Clin Invest* 76:1536-1538, 1985.

Mandel H, et al: Thiamine-dependent beriberi in the "thiamine-responsive anemia syndrome." *N Engl J Med* 311:836-836, 1984.

Marshall CW: *Vitamins and Minerals: Help or Harm?* Philadelphia, Stickley, 1983.

Moertel CG, et al: Clinical trial of amygdalin (Laetrile) in treatment of human cancer. *N Engl J Med* 306:201-206, 1982.

Moertel CG, et al: High-dose vitamin C versus placebo in treatment of patients with advanced cancer who have had no prior chemotherapy. *N Engl J Med* 312:137-141, 1985.

Morris JC, et al: Interaction of ethinyloestradiol with ascorbic acid in man, letter. *Br Med J* 283:503, 1981.

Muller DPR: Vitamin E: Its role in neurologic function. *Postgrad Med J* 62:107-112, 1986.

Nyhan WL: Understanding inherited metabolic disease: Treatment. *Clin Symp* 32:30-31, 1980.

Olson JA: Recommended dietary intakes (RDI) of vitamin A in humans. *Am J Clin Nutr* 45:704-716, 1987.

Olson JA, Hodges RE: Recommended dietary intakes (RDI) of vitamin C in humans. *Am J Clin Nutr* 45:693-703, 1987.

Ovesen L: Vitamin therapy in absence of obvious deficiency: What is the evidence? *Drugs* 27:148-170, 1984.

Patterson KY, et al: Zinc, copper, and manganese intake and balance for adults consuming self-selected diets. *Am J Clin Nutr* 40:1397-1403, 1984.

Petrie WM, Ban TA: Vitamins in psychiatry: Do they have a role? *Drugs* 30:58-65, 1985.

Phelps DL, et al: Tocopherol efficacy and safety for preventing retinopathy of prematurity: Randomized, controlled, double-masked trial. *Pediatrics* 79:489-500, 1987.

Prasad AS: Clinical, endocrinological and biochemical effects of zinc deficiency. *Clin Endocrinol Metab* 14:567-589, 1985.

Public Affairs Committee, Teratology Society: Position paper by the Teratology Society: Vitamin A during pregnancy, editorial. *Teratology* 35:267-268, 1987.

Reuter H, Hellriegel KP: Vitamins, in Dukes MNG (eds): *Side Effects of Drugs Annual 7.* Amsterdam, Excerpta Medica, 1983, 370-373.

Satya-Murti S, et al: Spectrum of neurologic disorders from vitamin E deficiency. *Neurology* 36:917-921, 1986.

Sauberlich HE: Ascorbic acid, in: *Nutrition Reviews' Present Knowledge in Nutrition,* ed 5. Washington, DC, The Nutrition Foundation, 1984, 260-272.

Schaumberg H, et al: Sensory neuropathy from pyridoxine abuse: New megavitamin syndrome. *N Engl J Med* 309:445-448, 1983.

Schwartz RD, et al: Hyperoxaluria and renal insufficiency due to ascorbic acid administration during total parenteral nutrition. *Ann Intern Med* 100:530-531, 1984.

Silverman AK, et al: Hypervitaminosis A syndrome: Paradigm of retinoid side effects. *J Am Acad Dermatol* 16:1027-1039, 1987.

Suter PM, Russell RM: Vitamin requirements of the elderly. *Am J Clin Nutr* 45:501-512, 1987.

Tsang RC: Quandary of vitamin D in newborn infant. *Lancet* 1:1370-1372, 1983.

Wagner C: Folic acid, in: *Nutrition Reviews' Present Knowledge in Nutrition,* ed 5. Washington, DC, The Nutrition Foundation, 1984, 332-346.

Other Selected References

Bieri JG, et al: Medical uses of vitamin E. *N Engl J Med* 308:1063-1071, 1983.

Committee on Nutrition, American Academy of Pediatrics: *Pediatric Nutrition Handbook,* ed 2. Elk Grove Village, IL, American Academy of Pediatrics, 1985.

DeLuca HF: Vitamin D endocrinology. *Ann Intern Med* 85:367-377, 1976.

Herbert V: *Nutrition Cultism: Facts and Fictions.* Philadelphia, Stickley, 1981.

Herbert V, Barrett S: *Vitamins and "Health" Foods: The Great American Hustle.* Philadelphia, Stickley, 1981.

James MB, et al: Hypervitaminosis A: Case report. *Pediatrics* 69:112-115,1982.

Memon AS: Role of vitamin C in causation and outcome of cancer. *Res Staff Physician* 30:63-71, 1984.

Schneider HA, et al (eds): *Nutritional Support of Medical Practice,* ed 2. Philadelphia, Harper & Row, 1983.

Shils ME, Young VR (eds): *Modern Nutrition in Health and Disease,* ed 7. Philadelphia, Lea & Febiger, 1988.

Ulmer DD: Trace elements. *N Engl J Med* 297:318-321, 1977.

Parenteral and Enteral Nutrition

98

Nutritional support provided by central or peripheral parenteral nutrition or enteral tube feeding is indicated in patients who are unable to ingest or absorb enough nutrients to maintain or restore healthy nutritional status. It is undertaken in order to provide sufficient nutriture to preserve lean body mass, enhance wound healing, maintain immunocompetence, and decrease postoperative complications associated with malnutrition. Guiding principles motivating the use of nutritional support include the concepts that there is no disease process whose treatment benefits from starvation, malnutrition, or fasting; that progressive malnutrition results in wasting of vital organ protein, functional impairment, and increasing morbidity and mortality; and that nutritional support is best used in the prevention of malnutrition (ASPEN Board of Directors, 1986; Grant, 1992).

Patients with either chronic malnutrition or conditions predisposing to acute malnutrition respond to nutritional support. The latter include comatose, incapacitated, incompetent, or dysphagic patients and those with severe diarrhea, intractable vomiting, severe persistent hyperemesis gravidarum, intestinal obstruction, renal or hepatic failure, extensive burns, trauma, severe prolonged infection, systemic inflammatory response syndrome (SIRS; often referred to as multiple systems organ failure [MSOF]), or other causes of persistent hypermetabolic status. Nutritional support also benefits patients with intestinal mucosal damage caused by starvation, AIDS, chemotherapy accompanying bone marrow transplantation, acute symptomatic inflammatory bowel disease, acute enteritis induced by chemotherapy or radiation, severe acute necrotizing pancreatitis, enterocutaneous fistulas, massive bowel resection, and short-gut syndrome. Nonvolitional feeding may be required when mechanical problems exist (dysphagia, head or neck surgery) and during the perioperative and postoperative periods, especially in severely malnourished patients and those with inflammatory bowel disease or enteroenteric, enterocutaneous, or perianal fistulas (Sitzmann et al, 1989; Kotler et al, 1990; Pillar and Perry, 1990; Singer et al, 1991; The Veterans Affairs Total Parenteral Nutrition Cooperative Study Group, 1991; Grant, 1992).

When a patient's overall physical and medical condition (subjective global assessment) suggests the presence of malnutrition, a comprehensive assessment of nutrition should be undertaken (Grant, 1992). Such an assessment should include the evaluation of data obtained from a thorough history and physical examination. In addition, serum albumin or prealbumin or plasma transthyretin or transferrin concentrations can be measured to estimate protein status crudely, and triceps and subscapular skinfold thicknesses can be measured to estimate fat stores. Immunologic competence may be evaluated with a skin test for delayed hypersensitivity or other simple indicators.

Assessment of nutritional status in premature infants, neonates, and infants with low body weight for age requires careful selection of diagnostic tests. Poor nutritional status in these infants is indicated by failure to thrive, delayed growth, plasma transferrin concentrations <1.5 g/L, or plasma transthyretin concentrations <80 mg/L (Polberger et al, 1990 A). The nutritional status of older children and adolescents is best estimated by comparison of body size and, if possible, growth rates with norms for both incremental and absolute growth (Wetzel, 1946, 1948; Roche and Himes, 1980; National Center for Health Statistics, 1987).

PARENTERAL NUTRITION

Parenteral nutrition delivers fluids and nutrients directly into the circulation by cannulation of high flow blood vessels. The use of parenteral nutrition is indicated only in patients who are unable to adequately ingest, digest, or absorb nutrients via the alimentary tract. However, parenteral nutrition offers no advantage over enteral feeding when the gastrointestinal tract is functioning properly (The Veterans Affairs Total Parenteral Nutrition Cooperative Study Group, 1991; Campos and Meguid, 1992), and generally it is not indicated in patients expected to regain adequate gastrointestinal function within one to two weeks of the onset of illness. Emergency surgery should not be delayed by catheterization for administration of parenteral nutrition (ASPEN Board of Directors, 1986).

Withholding parenteral nutrition from patients with extremely poor prognoses has become a predominately legal issue, and appropriate counsel should be consulted.

Total Parenteral Nutrition (TPN)

Parenteral nutrition delivered via central venous infusion (total parenteral nutrition, TPN) is indicated in patients with serious gastrointestinal disease, in home-care patients with inadequate gastrointestinal function, when enteral feeding is contraindicated or inadequate, or pre- and postoperatively in debilitated patients when repletion is desirable to improve surgical risk. As adjunctive therapy, TPN can enhance drug-induced intestinal healing in most patients with Crohn's disease (Cravo et al, 1991; Sitrin, 1992).

TPN is administered to hospitalized patients and also may be given at home by trained patients or family members. Home TPN is less expensive than similar therapy in a hospital and is safe provided the patient is in a reasonably stable condition and the home situation is conducive to this technique. A home TPN program may be indicated for individuals with persistent gastrointestinal hypomotility or obstruction, massive bowel resection, short-gut syndrome, severe radiation enteritis and other malabsorption states, low-output fistulas or stomas located in the upper intestine, carcinoid tumors, advanced cystic fibrosis, chronic pancreatitis, intractable sprue, chronic ulcerative colitis, hyperemesis gravidarum, and AIDS-associated enteropathy and for bone marrow transplant recipients (ASPEN Board of Directors, 1987 A; Singer et al, 1991; Allen and Van Way, 1992). Home TPN may reduce dependence on steroids in patients with Crohn's disease (Sitrin, 1992). It also may be employed for up to three months when rest for the gastrointestinal tract is necessary temporarily.

At home, TPN often is administered cyclically rather than continuously, with nutrients being delivered nocturnally and venous access maintained during the day by a heparin or saline lock (Matuchansky et al, 1992). Cyclical TPN maintains metabolic status as effectively as continuous TPN and delivers the required amounts of energy, amino acids, electrolytes, minerals, trace elements, and vitamins. However, cyclical TPN may result in greater urine calcium excretion compared with continuous TPN (Wood et al, 1985). Most important, home TPN often permits patients to maintain normal activities, and, if cyclical, may encourage supplemental oral intake during the day.

Complications of home TPN include fluid or electrolyte imbalances, glucose intolerance, septicemia, thrombosis, and catheter displacement (Herfindal et al, 1992; Matuchansky et al, 1992). Standards for home TPN have been developed (Pillar and Perry, 1990; American Society for Parenteral and Enteral Nutrition, 1992; Grant, 1992).

Peripheral Parenteral Nutrition (PPN)

Parenteral nutrition delivered via peripheral veins (peripheral parenteral nutrition, PPN) may be used to supply nutrients for a limited time (7 to 10 days) when oral or enteral intake is insufficient; central venous infusion is not feasible, advisable, or definitely necessary; and access to a peripheral vein of sufficient patency to pass large volumes of hypertonic fluid is possible (Fairfull-Smith and Freeman, 1993). PPN also may be useful during the transition period of readaptation to enteral feeding. It is generally safer and simpler than central TPN and is most often employed in hospitalized patients.

A solution containing a final concentration of 2.5% to 4.25% amino acids, dextrose, and maintenance doses of electrolytes, vitamins, and trace elements is commonly used. In adults, up to 40% to 60% of the calories (less in children) may be supplied by concomitantly administered lipid emulsions of low osmolality, which decrease the osmolar insult of the mixture entering the vein and reduce the potential for phlebitis to develop. In addition, small amounts of potassium, magnesium, calcium, phosphate, chloride, and acetate are needed to facilitate anabolism and maintain normal plasma composition. Some clinicians prefer to add only routine electrolytes and administer other minerals separately as needed to correct any developing abnormalities in plasma concentrations.

The major complications associated with PPN are thrombophlebitis, infiltration due to dislodgement of the catheter, embolism, and infection (Jeejeebhoy, 1983). The use of long silastic cannulas inserted into an arm vein and directed into a central vein (peripherally inserted central [PIC] lines) has greatly reduced the incidence of such complications. Intravenous sites should be changed routinely to prevent peripheral vein phlebitis.

Preparation and Administration of TPN Solutions

Preparation of TPN Solutions: To reduce bacterial contamination, TPN solutions are prepared aseptically under a laminar air flow hood or using a computerized admixture system, refrigerated, and administered within 24 to 48 hours in a hospital setting. Home TPN solutions that do not contain perishable vitamins or lipids can be premixed under aseptic conditions and refrigerated for up to one month. Darkened or cloudy solutions and those that show signs of destabilization should be discarded.

The usual TPN solution, which contains more than 10% dextrose, must be infused into a central vein with a high blood flow for rapid dilution. Appropriate TPN solutions for fluid-restricted patients must be maximally concentrated to prevent excess water loading. Algorithms allowing full parenteral nutrition support in a limited volume have been developed (Driscoll and Blackburn, 1990).

Preparation of Total Nutrient Admixtures: Traditional TPN solutions are prepared by mixing hypertonic dextrose, most commonly a 50% or 70% concentration, with a 5.5% to 15% amino acid solution and appropriate amounts of electrolytes, trace elements, and vitamins. Substituting lipids for some of the dextrose decreases the risk of glucose intolerance and pulmonary dysfunction in susceptible patients (Driscoll, 1990).

Total nutrient admixtures (TNA, three-in-one admixtures) contain carbohydrates, amino acids, and lipids in a single bag and can be formulated to meet individual needs. Their physical stability is maintained by the negative surface charge of fat droplets; high concentrations of electrolytes (especially divalent cations such as calcium and magnesium) neutralize this surface charge, causing the emulsion to aggregate (Go and Grant, 1987; Grimble and Silk, 1987; Driscoll, 1990). The lipid contents of selected TNA containing moderate amounts of electrolytes have remained stable without aggregating for at least four weeks when stored at 4° C (Tannuri et al, 1992). Unstable admixtures have light yellow or amber oil globules or a ring at the liquid/air interface that clings to the interior wall of the container, flocculation, or visible "creaming" of the emulsion; such admixtures should be discarded.

Compared with solutions without fat, TNA are associated with increased rates of mechanical complications (eg, catheter obstruction) resulting from spontaneous microparticulation (Jacobson and Glaumann, 1988). Extraction of container plasticizers by lipid is not a problem because plasticizer-free ethylene vinyl acetate and polyester CR3 bags are available for TNA. Lipid emulsions by themselves are excellent media for bacterial and fungal growth, but when used as TNA are as resistant to microorganisms as TPN solutions without fat (Fuksa et al, 1987, Driscoll, 1990).

Adding Drugs to TPN Solutions. The infusion of nutrients should not be interrupted to administer intravenous medications. The few medications that are compatible with nutrient solutions may be added to decrease fluid requirements for drug dilution, reduce the need for ancillary injection sites, reduce the possibility of line contamination, and decrease staff time required for drug administration. Drugs that can be admixed with nutrient solutions, providing that strict admixing guidelines are followed, include those that are physically and chemically compatible for at least 24 hours and can be infused continuously (eg, insulin, heparin, albumin, cimetidine, ranitidine, metoclopramide, hydrocortisone and methylprednisolone sodium succinates, cytarabine) (Reed et al, 1979; Niemiec and Vanderveen, 1984; Garabedian-Ruffalo and Ruffalo, 1986; Perry et al, 1987; LaFrance and Miyagawa, 1991). Drugs that cannot be admixed under any conditions include those with suboptimal therapeutic indices when administered by continuous infusion, drugs that require dosage titration to patient response, and drugs that are incompatible. Adding drugs directly to the nutrient solution via Y-site injection into the flowing solution increases the risk of infection and should be avoided.

Little is known about the physical and chemical stability of drugs added to TPN solutions that contain lipids. Although most drugs should not be added to TPN solutions, stability has been demonstrated for ampicillin, cefamandole, cefazolin, cefoxitin, cephapirin, cimetidine, clindamycin, dopamine, erythromycin lactobionate, famotidine, furosemide, isoproterenol, lidocaine, ranitidine, ticarcillin, and tobramycin (Shea and Souney, 1990; LaFrance and Miyagawa, 1991).

Important interactions can follow the introduction of a drug into the circulation of a patient receiving TPN. For example, increases in plasma free fatty acid concentrations resulting from infusion of lipid emulsions can cause displacement of drugs that are highly bound to plasma proteins (eg, clofibrate, morphine, phenytoin, salicylate, valproate).

Administration of TPN Solutions. Infusion of TPN solutions over 24 hours minimizes the risk of contamination and encourages more efficient use of infused fatty acids by the liver (Driscoll, 1990). In contrast, some authorities advocate an administration time of 12 to 18 hours for patients who are stable on long-term continuous TPN in order to prevent the hepatic enzyme abnormalities and fatty infiltration and steatosis that have occasionally been associated with continuous TPN. This administration schedule also allows increased mobility and activity (Matuchansky et al, 1992).

For detailed instructions on catheter placement and management and on nutrient delivery, see Beam et al, 1990; Flowers et al, 1991; Warner, 1991; Grant, 1992; and Van Way and Allen, 1992.

Monitoring of TPN: Bedside examinations and determinations of serum and urine chemistries should be performed initially and at frequent intervals for several days after initiating TPN (Brown and Begley, 1991). Serum electrolyte and blood urea nitrogen or creatinine concentrations should be measured two or three times weekly or more often if the patient is metabolically unstable. If initial values are within a reasonable range, liver function studies and measurement of serum albumin, calcium, phosphorus, and magnesium concentrations may be performed once or twice weekly. If initial values indicate the presence of hypokalemia, hypomagnesemia, and/or hypophosphatemia, the appropriate elements should be measured daily to detect any marked fall in their concentration. Additions or deletions to TPN solutions should be made as necessary to correct any electrolyte or fluid imbalance.

The efficacy of nutritional support is determined most simply by weight measurements assessed in relation to possible edema formation and, in stable patients, to visceral protein status. The body weight of malnourished patients should be

TABLE 1.
FORMULAS FOR CALCULATING ENERGY AND PROTEIN REQUIREMENTS OF ADULTS NOURISHED BY TPN

Basal Energy Expenditure (BEE) in Healthy Adults:

(1[1]) Males: $BEE_{kcal} = 66.5 + 13.8\ (BW_{kg}) + 5\,(Height_{cm}) - 6.75\,(Age_{yr})$

Females: $BEE_{kcal} = 655.1 + 9.6\ (BW_{kg}) + 1.85\,(Height_{cm}) - 4.7\,(Age_{yr})$

Daily Energy Expenditure (DEE) in Healthy Adults:

$DEE_{kcal} = 1.25\ BEE_{kcal}$

Daily Energy Expenditure (DEE) in Disease:

(1) $DEE_{kcal} = (BEE_{kcal})$ (Sum of Adjustment Factors)

Clinical Condition:	Adjustment Factor:
Malnutrition (chronic, severe)	0.70
Chronic renal failure (nondialyzed)	1.00
Surgery (elective, uncomplicated)	1.00
Infections (mild)	1.00
Maintenance hemodialysis	1.00
Ventilator support	1.10
Bed rest	1.15
Peritonitis	1.15
Soft tissue trauma	1.15
Fractures (appendicular)	1.20 - 1.25
Infections (moderate)	1.20 - 1.40
Head trauma	1.30 - 1.50
Sepsis (moderate)	1.30
Surgery (abdominal)	1.50
Trauma (severe)	1.50
Infections (severe)	1.40 - 1.60
Active cancer	1.60
Sepsis (severe)	1.60
Hyperthyroidism (untreated))	2.00

(2) Burn Patients (BSAB = percent of body surface area burned):

(a[2]) $DEE_{kcal} = (BEE_{kcal}) + [\,(X)\ (BSAB)/100]$

(b[3]) $DEE_{kcal} = (BEE_{kcal})\ (AF^4)\ (IF^5)$

(c[6]) $DEE_{kcal} = 24\ (2.338\ (BEE_{kcal}) - 1.338e^{(-0.0286)\ (BSAB)})$

(d[7]) $DEE_{kcal} = 10.5\ (BSAB) + 0.023\ (CI^8) + 0.84\ (BEE_{kcal}) + 114\ (BT^9) - 4.5\ (PBD^{10}) - 4343$

Daily Protein Requirements of Thermally Injured Patients:

(1[6]) First week post-burn:

$Protein_g = 7.8\ (UUN^{11}{}_g) + 1.2\ (BSAB)\ (BSA^{12}) + 25\ g$

Second week post-burn:

$Protein_g = 7.8\ (UUN_g) + 0.6\ (BSAB)\ (BSA) + 25\ g$

(2[13]) $Protein_g = (0.04167)\ (DEE_{kcal})$

1 Decrease by 25% in those over 65 (Driscoll and Bistrian, 1992).

2 For age < 1 year, X = 1,500 kcal; 1 to 3 years, X = 2,500 kcal; 4 to 59 years, X = 4,000 kcal; ≥ 60 years, X = 6,500 kcal.

3 Long, 1979.

4 Activity factor: AF = 1.2 if patient is confined to bed; AF = 1.3 otherwise.

5 Injury factor: IF = 1.0 if BSAB = 0.01; IF = 2.0 if BSAB = 1.00.

6 Becker and Pruitt, 1991.

7 Allard et al, 1990.

8 Caloric intake for past 24 hours.

9 Body temperature (°C).

10 Number of days post-burn.

11 Daily urinary urea nitrogen excretion (g).

12 Body surface area (M^2); $BSA_{M^2} = [\,(BW_{kg}{}^{0.425})\ (Height_{cm}{}^{0.725})\ (71.84)\,]/10{,}000$

13 Buerk, 1992.

measured daily. Weight gain of more than 0.5 kg in 24 hours reflects undesirable fluid retention. If overhydration occurs, it may be treated by restricting sodium or fluid intake. Clinical observation of changes in the rate of wound healing, the patient's sense of well-being and strength, and serum concentrations of transferrin, pre-albumin, and retinol-binding proteins also are useful indicators of effectiveness.

Nutritional Requirements Provided by TPN

Energy: The daily caloric requirements of individuals may be estimated initially by calculating basal energy expenditure (BEE) using the Harris-Benedict equation (see Table 1). Adjustments can then be made to account for increased caloric needs during disease. However, use of the Harris-Benedict equation may overestimate BEE and does not take into account large individual variability (Brandi et al, 1992). When possible, many clinicians prefer to estimate daily energy requirements of individual patients by the use of indirect calorimetry (McClave and Snider, 1992). After the initiation of TPN using solutions formulated on the basis of either of these methods, periodic nutritional assessments should be performed and further adjustments made as warranted.

Protein: Total protein requirements of healthy adults generally average 1 g/kg/day (Driscoll and Bistrian, 1992). During metabolic stress, this requirement increases. For example, patients on maintenance hemodialysis or peritoneal dialysis should receive 1.1 to 1.5 g/kg/day (Vehe et al, 1991), and those with hypermetabolism should receive 1.5 to 2.5 g/kg/day (Grant, 1992). In contrast, those with nephrotic syndrome, acute renal failure, or diabetic nephropathy should receive 0.55 to 0.8 g/kg/day initially, gradually increasing to 1.5 g/kg (Brouhard and LaGrone, 1990; Kaysen, 1992). Nitrogen balance should be maintained in burn patients during recovery (Table 1).

Electrolytes and Minerals: Adults without abnormal electrolyte loss or retention and with normal renal function

TABLE 2.
ELECTROLYTES, MINERALS, AND TRACE ELEMENTS: RECOMMENDED DAILY INTRAVENOUS INTAKE DURING TPN[1,2,3]

Nutrient	Preterm Infants	Term Infants	Children [maximum/day]		Adults
	mg/kg/day			mg/day	
Calcium	60-90	60-90	20-40	400	200
Chloride	70-105	40-120	70	1,400	2,000
Magnesium	4.3-7.2	4.3-7.2	2-4	80	120
Phosphorus	47-70	47-70	15-30	500	1,000
Potassium	78-120	55-120	80	1,600	800
Sodium	70-105	35-100	45	900	700
	mcg/kg/day				
Chromium	0.05-0.2	0.2	0.2	5	0.3
Copper[4]	20	20	20	300	20
Iodine[5]	1	1	1	70	12
Manganese[4,6]	1	1	1	50	10
Molybdenum[7]	0.25	0.25	0.25	5	3
Selenium[8]	1.5-2	2	2	30	1.2
Zinc	400	250 (<3 mo) 100 (>3 mo)	50	5,000	50-80[9]

[1] *Adapted from Szwanek et al, 1987; Cochran et al, 1988; Fleming, 1989; National Research Council, 1989; Koo and Tsang, 1991; Moukarzel et al, 1992 A; Tsang et al, 1993.*

[2] *Patients should be monitored for signs and symptoms of deficiency or excess of each component and appropriate changes made to assure optimum level of intake. When parenteral nutrition is only supplemental or is limited to one or two weeks, only zinc should be added to the infusate.*

[3] *The contamination levels of trace elements in intravenous fluids vary markedly. The values in this table refer to total intake that is present in the fluids as contaminants plus the additives. For molybdenum and manganese, dilution of the manufacturer's product may be necessary for pediatric use.*

[4] *Not routinely administered to those with significant liver impairment, including children with TPN cholestasis.*

[5] *Iodine may not be necessary in patients taking some food orally or when dermal preparations of povidone-iodine are being used (Moukarzel et al, 1992 A).*

[6] *Even though manganese is recommended for infants and children, there is no convincing evidence that it is essential for adult patients on TPN.*

[7] *Molybdenum supplements are recommended only with long-term TPN.*

[8] *Because selenium is excreted primarily via the kidneys, lower dosage should be given to patients with impaired renal function.*

[9] *Add zinc 40 mg/day for those in acute catabolic state. Add 12 mg/L of small bowel fluid lost and 17 mg/L of stool or ileostomy effluent lost, because a positive nitrogen balance is facilitated by a positive zinc balance (Shils and White, 1984).*

require approximately 80 to 120 mEq of sodium and 60 to 100 mEq of potassium daily. However, requirements vary with the clinical condition (see also index entries Electrolytes; Sodium; Potassium). Sodium and potassium are generally added to TPN solutions as mixtures of chloride or acetate salts to achieve a proper ratio of anions to cations and to provide an acidifying or alkalizing effect as necessary. Acetate salts are especially useful because they are oxidized by the liver to bicarbonate.

Phosphorus requirements are increased when glycolytic activity is increased, urinary losses are high (eg, persistent acidosis, proximal renal tubular defect), and during repletion of body mass. Approximately 1 g (30 mmol) of phosphorus is required daily for maintenance, but larger amounts are often needed when initiating TPN in malnourished patients to maintain the serum phosphate concentration >2.5 mg/dL. Because insulin stimulates cellular uptake of phosphate, phosphorus requirements are proportional to carbohydrate and nitrogen intake; two to three times more phosphorus may be needed when employing more concentrated solutions of dextrose or amino acids. For each 500 ml of 50% dextrose in water infused, 400 mg of phosphorus is recommended.

Hypomagnesemia will develop unless 120 mg (10 mEq) of magnesium is provided daily. Some commercial solutions provide only 120 mg/L. Usually a total of 400 to 600 mg daily is adequate, but more may be needed in the presence of extensive gastrointestinal fluid loss, alcoholism, or renal tubular damage or with long-term use of diuretics or amphotericin B; these conditions increase urinary magnesium excretion. Magnesium status should be monitored by measuring the plasma concentration and 24-hour urinary excretion.

The average adult on TPN requires 200 mg (10 mEq) of elemental calcium daily, which should be supplied as calcium gluceptate or gluconate. Calcium chloride should never be used in TPN; it will form potentially lethal insoluble calcium phosphate precipitates. Hypoalbuminemia, which is common among patients on TPN, may artificially suppress measurements of plasma total calcium concentration; measurements may be corrected as follows: measured plasma total calcium concentration (mg/dL) − plasma albumin concentration (g/dL) + 4 mg/dL = adjusted plasma total calcium concentration. Alternatively, plasma ionized calcium concentration, which is not affected by hypoalbuminemia, may be measured. Calcium status may be maintained by limiting the amount of calcium supplied so that the 24-hour urinary calcium excretion is <4 mg/kg.

Essential Trace Elements: The need for trace elements varies among patients depending on age, clinical and metabolic status, and the need to replace any gastrointestinal losses. When prolonged TPN is anticipated, these minerals should be provided from the beginning in order to prevent deficiencies, especially in malnourished patients (see Table 2).

Zinc, copper, chromium, selenium, and molybdenum are essential during long-term TPN. Iodine also may be needed, but exact amounts have not been determined. There is no convincing evidence that manganese is required by adults on TPN. For salts of trace elements that are available for addition to TPN solutions, see Table 3.

Iron supplementation during TPN remains controversial but is probably required by preterm infants on long-term TPN (Tsang et al, 1993). When iron is indicated, iron dextran complex is compatible with TPN solutions.

Vitamins: All vitamins may be depleted in malnourished patients, especially those with prolonged malabsorption. Requirements may be increased during severe trauma, major surgery, and serious illness. A parenteral multivitamin preparation that provides sufficient amounts of fat- and water-soluble vitamins (see Table 4) should be added to the intravenous solution daily (see also index entry Vitamins).

Care should be taken to avoid overdosage of vitamins A and D because of potential toxicity. Vitamin A overdose also may impair the utilization of vitamin E. On the other hand, vitamin A is adsorbed rapidly onto both plastic and glass and may be destroyed on exposure to light. Vitamin K (1 mg) can be added to TPN solutions daily. It may be necessary to administer vitamin K subcutaneously to adults (5 to 10 mg once weekly).

Deaths attributed to thiamine deficiency, manifested as a refractory lactic acidosis, have been reported in patients receiving TPN who did not receive multivitamin supplements (*MMWR,* 1989).

Fat: Essential fatty acid deficiency may develop during prolonged lipid-free TPN. Intravenous fat emulsions [Intralipid, Liposyn II, Liposyn III] contain linoleic, oleic, palmitic, linolenic, and stearic acids, and prevent or correct essential fatty acid deficiencies when infused in amounts that provide 3% to 5% of the total caloric input as linoleic acid (approximately 500 ml of a 10% fat emulsion two or three times weekly).

These isotonic emulsions can be infused peripherally as a major source (30% to 50%) of non-nitrogen calories, and patients receiving a significant proportion of nonprotein calories as fatty acids can achieve positive nitrogen balance. However, overzealous administration of lipids may overwhelm physiologic clearance mechanisms and cause hypertriglyceridemia and impair the function of the reticuloendothelial and immune systems (McCrae et al, 1993). If more than 2,800 calories are needed, more dextrose can be infused through a central venous catheter.

Medium-chain triglycerides (MCT) contain medium-chain fatty acids that are not stored or incorporated into lipoproteins but instead rapidly enter mitochondria and are oxidized to acetyl CoA, hydroxybutyrate, and acetoacetate (Weissman et al, 1988). Although MCT are mildly ketogenic and increase resting energy expenditure (without increasing body temperature), they are a useful noncarbohydrate source of dietary energy, especially in those with glucose intolerance (Mascioli et al, 1991). Nitrogen balance has been improved by the addition of MCT to the TPN regimen of patients with a wide variety of conditions (Dennison et al, 1988; Hatton et al, 1990). Intravenous administration of pure MCT causes dyspnea, vomiting, and back pain; use of mixtures containing equal amounts of MCT and long-chain triglycerides eliminates adverse effects and decreases serum total cholesterol concentrations in adults and neonates (Crowe et al, 1985; Lima

TABLE 3.
TRACE METALS FOR TPN

Preparation	Chromium mcg/ml	Copper mcg/ml	Iodine mcg/ml	Manganese mg/ml	Molybdenum mcg/ml	Selenium mcg/ml	Zinc mg/ml
Chromium Chloride (Abbott, McGuff)	4						
Chromic Chloride (Fujisawa)	4 or 20						
Chroma-Pak (SoloPak Pharmaceuticals)	4 or 20						
Copper Chloride (Abbott)		400					
Cupric Sulfate (Loch, Fujisawa)		400 or 2000					
Iodopen (Fujisawa)			100				
Manganese Chloride (Abbott)				0.1			
Manganese Sulfate (Fujisawa)				0.1			
Ammonium Molydate (American Regent)					25		
Molypen (Fujisawa)					25		
Selenium (American Regent, McGuff)						40	
Sele-Pak (SoloPak Pharmaceuticals)						40	
Selepen (Fujisawa)						40	
Zinc Chloride; Zinc Sulfate (Various)							1;5
Zinca-Pak (SoloPak Pharmaceuticals)							1;5
Pedtrace-4 (Fujisawa)	0.85	100		0.025			0.5
Multiple Trace Element Neonatal (American Regent)	0.85	100		0.025			1.5
Neotrace-4 (Fujisawa)	0.85	100		0.025			1.5
PedTE-PAK-4 (SoloPak Pharmaceuticals)	1	100		0.025			1
P.T.E.-4 (Fujisawa)	1	100		0.025			1
Multiple Trace Element Pediatric (American Regent)	1	100		0.03			0.5
Trace Metals Additive on 0.9% NaCl (Abbott)	2	200		0.16			0.8
M.T.E.-4 (Fujisawa)	4	400		0.1			1
MulTE-PAK-4 (SoloPak Pharmaceuticals)	4	400		0.1			1
Multiple Trace Element (American Regent)	4	400		0.1			1
Multiple Trace Element Concentrated (American Regent)	10	1000		0.5			5

(table continued on next page)

TABLE 3 (continued)

Preparation	Chromium mcg/ml	Copper mcg/ml	Iodine mcg/ml	Manganese mg/ml	Molybdenum mcg/ml	Selenium mcg/ml	Zinc mg/ml
ConTE-PAK-4 (SoloPak Pharmaceuticals)	10	1000		0.5			5
M.T.E.-4 Concentrated (Fujisawa)	10	1000		0.5			5
P.T.E.-5 (Fujisawa)	1	100		0.025		15	1
M.T.E.-5 (Fujisawa)	4	400		0.1		20	1
MulTE-PAK-5 (SoloPak Pharmaceuticals)	4	400		0.1		20	1
Multiple Trace Element with Selenium (American Regent)	4	400		0.1		20	1
M.T.E.-5 Concentrated (Fujisawa)	10	1000		0.5		60	5
Multiple Trace Element with Selenium Concentrated (American Regent)	10	1000		0.5		60	5
M.T.E.-6 (Fujisawa)	4	400	25	0.1		20	1
M.T.E.-6 Concentrated (Fujisawa)	10	1000	75	0.5		60	5
M.T.E.-7 (Fujisawa)	4	400	25	0.1	25	20	1
Tracelyte[1] (Fujisawa)	0.6	60		0.015			0.15
Tracelyte with Double Electrolytes[1] (Fujisawa)	0.3	30		0.0075			0.075
Tracelyte-II[2] (Fujisawa)	0.6	60		0.015			0.15
Tracelyte-II with Double Electrolytes[2] (Fujisawa)	0.3	30		0.0075			0.075

[1] Contains acetate 122 mg/ml, calcium 10 mg/ml, chloride 60 mg/ml, gluconate 0.25 mEq/ml, magnesium 9.6 mg/ml, potassium 80 mg/ml, sodium 30 mg/ml; 7.57 mOsm/ml.

[2] Contains acetate 89 mg/ml, calcium 9 mg/ml, chloride 62 mg/ml, magnesium 6 mg/ml, potassium 40 mg/ml, sodium 40 mg/ml; 6.2 mOsm/ml.

et al, 1988; Hatton et al, 1990; Ball, 1991). Unfortunately, intravenous lipid emulsions containing MCT are not yet commercially available in the United States.

Carbohydrate: The amount of dextrose given initially is 800 to 1,000 kcal/day or 250 to 300 g/day, usually as a 25% solution delivered at 40 to 50 ml/hr. The dose gradually is increased by 500 to 1,000 kcal every one to two days until energy needs are satisfied. An initial dose of 500 to 700 kcal/day or 150 to 200 g/day is appropriate for malnourished individuals, known or suspected diabetic patients, and elderly patients. Optimal rates of glucose oxidation usually can be obtained by limiting dextrose infusion to 5 to 7 mg/kg/min in adults or 15 to 20 mg/kg/min in neonates.

Blood glucose concentrations should be determined until glucose tolerance is demonstrated (usually in two to three days as endogenous insulin production increases). However, steady-state plasma glucose concentrations between 150 and 220 mg/dL are acceptable in ill patients in order to avoid hypoglycemia. Fractional urine glucose concentrations are not dependable and should only be relied on when the blood glucose concentration cannot be measured (eg, in premature infants and neonates). If the concentration remains highly elevated, the rate of infusion may be decreased or glucose may be replaced with lipids. Glucose tolerance should be monitored when there is any increase in the amount of carbohydrate administered.

The carbohydrate infusion rate should be reduced in severely malnourished patients to avoid triggering oversecretion of insulin, producing "refeeding syndrome" (ie, shift of potassium, phosphate, and magnesium ions into their intercellular compartments); interstitial fluid retention; pulmonary edema; cardiovascular overload; and nutritional cardiomyopathy. In addition, excessive infusion of dextrose or of total calories increases carbon dioxide production and oxygen consumption, which can complicate weaning of hypermetabolic patients from respirators or precipitate respiratory distress in patients with pulmonary abnormalities (Askanazi et al, 1980; Talpers et al, 1992). Reduction in total calories by substitution of intravenous fat emulsion for a part of the energy normally supplied as glucose is recommended for patients with respiratory quotients >1.

Other Components: In most patients requiring TPN, the serum albumin concentration is low as a result of hepatic disease, nephropathy, enteropathy, and cytokine-mediated reduction in albumin synthesis and increases in albumin catabolism and leakage into interstitial spaces (the stress response). Initial volume resuscitation further decreases the serum albumin concentration by dilution. During TPN, the serum albumin concentration will increase gradually over a number of weeks as adequate amino acids and calories are given, provided there are no persisting underlying pathologic conditions that impair the synthesis of albumin or increase its catabolism. Consequently, the routine administration of albumin for the sole purpose of increasing serum albumin is unnecessary and should be avoided (Blackburn and Driscoll, 1992; Subcommittee of the Victorian Drug Usage Advisory Committee, 1992). Infusion of albumin can result in an increase in colloid oncotic pressure that can trigger oliguria, hypervolemia, and hypocalcemia (Nearman and Herman, 1991).

Glutamine provides nitrogen and carbon skeletons for many biosynthetic pathways; plays a role in the regulation of hepatic glycogen synthesis and the modulation of muscle protein turnover; enhances recovery from critical illness and injury; acts as an energy source for intestinal mucosal cells, pancreatic cells, stimulated lymphocytes, and macrophages; and is required for phagocytosis and secretion of interleukin-1 by macrophages and for lymphocyte replication (Souba et al, 1990; Wallace and Keast, 1992). Animal studies have demonstrated that TPN solutions enriched in glutamine enhance intestinal mucosal growth and help maintain intestinal structure, integrity, and immune function during illness (Alverdy, 1990); reduce gastrointestinal toxicity after chemotherapy; prevent pancreatic atrophy; and attenuate hepatic steatosis.

Plasma glutamine concentrations decline and skeletal muscle glutamine release is increased in humans after major surgery (Parry-Billings et al, 1992); in contrast, parenteral glutamine (12 or 20 g daily) reduces postoperative skeletal muscle proteolysis (Hammarqvist et al, 1989; Stehle et al, 1989). After bone marrow transplantation, glutamine 0.57 g/kg daily improved nitrogen balance, reduced the incidence of infection and microbial colonization, and shortened hospital stay (Ziegler et al, 1992). Even in healthy subjects, parenteral glutamine (0.57 g/kg with adequate calories and protein 1.5 g/kg daily) increased nitrogen retention and had no adverse clinical or biochemical effects (Lowe et al, 1990; Ziegler et al, 1990). These findings suggest that glutamine may be a conditionally essential nutrient during severe illness (although it may be contraindicated in patients with malignancies that utilize glutamine for fuel [Fischer and Chance, 1990] and those with elevated serum ammonia or urea concentrations). However, this amino acid currently is not included in any commercially available TPN solutions because of its instability during long-term storage. However, glutamine is stable in solution for up to six weeks at 4° C. Glutamine dipeptide analogues (L-alanyl-L-glutamine; glycyl-L-glutamine) are under study (Klimberg, 1991; Tamada et al, 1992).

Arginine also may be conditionally essential during recovery from malnutrition or trauma because it functions as an essential component of polyamine and nucleic acid synthesis. Supplemental arginine enhances immune function in trauma, starvation, burns, and infection by stimulating T-lymphocyte proliferation and activation (Daly et al, 1988; Barbul, 1990). It also promotes nitrogen retention and wound healing and stimulates secretion of growth hormone, prolactin, insulin, and glucagon (Daly et al, 1988).

Carnitine is required for the transport of long-chain fatty acids into mitochondria, and may stimulate the oxidation of MCT (although MCT transport into mitochondria is independent of carnitine). Carnitine is manufactured in the liver and kidney from the essential amino acids, lysine and methionine, a process requiring vitamin C, vitamin B_6, niacin, and iron. Lack of substrates or cofactors may limit carnitine synthesis in malnutrition. Hemodialysis reduces plasma free and total carnitine concentrations; however, although postdialysis injections of levocarnitine increase plasma carnitine concentrations, they have no effect on functional indices of carnitine status (Golper et al, 1990).

Taurine is a component of bile acids and is involved in the regulation of cardiac rhythm and maintenance of membrane integrity. Hepatic synthesis of taurine from cysteine or methionine may be impaired in those with liver disease. TPN solutions lacking taurine are associated with deficiencies in bile acid conjugation that result in intracellular and intracanalicular cholestasis with varying degrees of portal fibrosis, bile duct proliferation and inflammation, biliary cirrhosis, and bile plugging (Howard and Thompson, 1992).

TPN in Pediatric Patients

The indications for TPN in pediatric patients are similar to those in adults. In addition, certain congenital anomalies prevent the use of the gastrointestinal tract; these include gastroschisis, omphalocele, tracheoesophageal fistula, intestinal atresia, meconium ileus, neonatal necrotizing enterocolitis, and the enterocolitis associated with Hirschsprung's disease. TPN provides nutritional support until surgical correction of the anomaly allows enteral feeding to be resumed (Warner, 1991). Additional indications for use of TPN include short-bowel syndrome following massive intestinal resection, intractable diarrhea of infancy, necrotizing enterocolitis in premature infants, and very low birth weight (<1,200 g).

Premature infants require 110 to 120 kcal/kg/day (American Academy of Pediatrics Committee on Nutrition, 1985; Heird et al, 1992). Most of these infants tolerate a daily parenteral intake of dextrose 5 g/kg and lipids 1 g/kg; however, most will require additional energy (Heird et al, 1992). Controlled infusion of insulin can allow administration of up to 30 g/kg of dextrose daily (Collins et al, 1991), and 20% lipid emulsions given at infusion rates of up to 0.15 g/kg/hr are often tolerated to total daily intakes of 3 to 4 g/kg (Gilbertson et al, 1991).

Daily caloric needs reflect both age and body weight: Infants <1 year require 100 to 110 kcal/kg; 1 to 3 years, 100 kcal/kg; 4 to 6 years, 90 kcal/kg; 7 to 10 years, 70 kcal/kg; and adolescents, 45 to 60 kcal/kg (National Research Council, 1989). Children with extensive burns require 2,200 kcal/M^2 of body surface area burned (Carvajal, 1993).

Generally, 2.5 to 3 g/kg/day of parenteral amino acids promotes nitrogen retention in premature neonates and infants (Heird et al, 1992). Protein requirements slowly decrease to 1.5 to 2 g/kg/day by adolescence. Burned children should receive 20% to 25% of their calories as amino acids.

The nutritional status of premature infants can be dramatically improved by the concurrent administration of albumin (0.5 to 1 g/day) to increase the serum albumin concentration to 3 g/dL (Kanarek et al, 1992).

Taurine is a β-amino acid that is considered essential for the normal development of the brain and retina. Because the immature kidney has limited ability to upregulate tubular taurine reabsorption, taurine deficiency during the first weeks of life may result in abnormal electroretinograms and auditory brain stem-evoked responses (Zelikovic et al, 1990). TPN solutions for infants (especially low-birth-weight infants) should provide taurine 8 to 12 g/kg daily (Rassin et al, 1990; Thornton and Griffin, 1991).

Plasma concentrations of carnitine, which is required for the transport and metabolism of fatty acids, are reduced in children receiving prolonged TPN with carnitine-free solutions (Christensen et al, 1989; Moukarzel et al, 1992 B). Similarly, premature infants and full-term neonates are unable to synthesize adequate amounts of carnitine, but lipid utilization is normalized during levocarnitine supplementation (2 to 16 mg/kg daily) (Helms et al, 1986, 1990; Rubaltelli et al, 1987; Smith et al, 1988; Olson et al, 1989; Melegh, 1990). Genetic defects in carnitine metabolism (decreased synthesis or increased renal excretion) or excessive elimination of carnitine secondary to long-term renal dialysis, hepatic cirrhosis, Fanconi's syndrome, and valproate toxicity responds to supplemental levocarnitine (Siliprandi et al, 1989) (see index entry Carnitine Deficiency Disorders).

Endogenous carnitine is almost entirely the L-isomer, while D-carnitine is produced synthetically. All of the effects attributed to carnitine result from use of levocarnitine. In contrast, D-carnitine inhibits carnitine acetyltransferase and palmitate oxidation, and its use has resulted in myasthenia and failure to protect against levocarnitine-responsive doxorubicin cardiotoxicity. Administration of D-carnitine depletes L-carnitine reserves and can produce cardiomyopathies. In addition, use of D-carnitine can exacerbate L-carnitine deficiency. The use of DL-carnitine is contraindicated in any condition requiring levocarnitine.

Providing enough calcium for neonates is difficult because of the solubility limitations of calcium and phosphorus in TPN solutions. However, because L-cysteine hydrochloride decreases solution pH, calcium 1 g/L and phosphate 2 g/L (phosphorus 600 mg/L) are compatible in a solution containing 1% TrophAmine or Aminosyn-PF, 10% dextrose, and L-cysteine hydrochloride at 40 mg of L-cysteine per g of protein plus additives (Pelegano et al, 1988). When used to treat early neonatal hypocalcemia, 18 mg/kg of calcium should be administered as a bolus infusion of calcium gluconate 10%; this solution should be infused over 10 minutes to minimize potential decreases in blood pH and plasma phosphorus concentrations (Venkataraman et al, 1991).

For daily electrolyte requirements, see Table 2; for daily vitamin requirements, see Table 4.

TABLE 4.
VITAMINS:
RECOMMENDED DAILY INTRAVENOUS INTAKE DURING TPN[1,2]

Nutrient	Preterm[3] Infants (per kg/day)	Term Infants (per day)	Children (per day)	Adults (per day)
Vitamin A (mcg)	500	700	700	3300
Vitamin D (mcg)	4	10	10	5
Vitamin E (mg)	2.8	7	7	10
Vitamin K (mcg)	80	200	200	50-80
Vitamin C (mg)	25	80	80	100
Thiamine (mg)	0.35	1.2	1.2	3
Riboflavin (mg)	0.15	1.4	1.4	3.6
Vitamin B_6 (mg)	0.18	1	1.0	4
Niacin (mg)	6.8	17	17	40
Folate (mcg)	56	140	140	400
Vitamin B_{12} (mcg)	0.3	1	1	5
Biotin (mcg)	6	20	20	60
Pantothenic Acid (mg)	2	5	5	15

[1] Adapted from American Medical Association, 1979; Levy et al, 1992; Tsang et al, 1993.

[2] Patients should be monitored for signs and symptoms of deficiency or excess of each component and appropriate changes made to assure optimum level of intake.

[3] Maximum intake not to exceed recommendations for term infants.

Intradialytic (Perdialytic) and Intraperitoneal Parenteral Nutrition

Malnutrition is common among long-term hemodialysis patients (Cano et al, 1990). If serum transthyretin concentrations fall below 300 mg/L, intravenous infusion of lipids (16 kcal/kg) and protein (0.5 g/kg) in 16 ml of infusate per kg three times weekly during four hours of filtration-controlled hemodialysis (intradialytic or perdialytic parenteral nutrition) can increase appetite; body weight; arm muscle circumference; and serum concentrations of transthyretin, albumin, and HDL-cholesterol.

Continuous ambulatory peritoneal dialysis (CAPD) may preserve renal function more effectively than center-based hemodialysis (Nolph, 1992). However, CAPD is associated with metabolic abnormalities resulting from glucose absorption from the dialysate, protein and amino acid losses into the dialysate, poor appetite, and recurrent peritonitis. Protein-energy malnutrition with hypoalbuminemia, muscle wasting, and loss of subcutaneous fat is common. However, manipulation of concentration gradients can be used to transfer nutrients from the dialysis solution to the circulation.

Providing lipids, amino acids, and glucose via intraperitoneal dialysis solutions (intraperitoneal nutrition [IPN]) may improve nutritional status, but additional parenteral or enteral feeding may be required to satisfy all nutrient needs. Complete nutriture via IPN is possible only rarely. Alternating dextrose-based and amino acid-based solutions (see Table 5) should be most effective. In addition, peritoneal permeability and nutrient transfer are increased by alkalization of dialysate solutions and the addition of hypertonic dextrose, lipids, and a number of drugs and hormones (see Table 6). IPN may be a useful adjunctive nutritional therapy for individuals with end-stage renal failure, pediatric patients with limited venous access, and patients for whom fluid restriction is required (Wolk, 1992). However, additional validation of the effectiveness of IPN is required.

TABLE 5. AMINO ACID FORMULAS TO ALTERNATE WITH STANDARD DIALYSIS FORMULAS DURING INTRAPERITONEAL NUTRITION*

Nutrient	High Amino Acid	Low Amino Acid
Amino Acids (g/L)	25	10
Acetate (g/L)	2	0
Lactate (g/L)	0	3
Calcium (mg/L)	180	120
Chloride (g/L)	3.6	3.8
Magnesium (mg/L)	36	36
Potassium (mg/L)	0	0
Sodium (mg/L)	2.3	3
Osmolarity (mOsm/L)	460	364

**Adapted from Wolk, 1992.*

Adverse Reactions and Precautions

The major complications of TPN are catheter-related sepsis, metabolic abnormalities, and mechanical problems related to the catheter and infusion apparatus (Flowers et al, 1991; Grant, 1992). The cause of a low-grade fever during TPN should be investigated immediately. Blood for bacterial and fungal cultures should be obtained by venipuncture and from the TPN line using strict aseptic technique, and a search for systemic infectious foci should be undertaken (Vanhuynegem et al, 1985). If the number of colonies grown from the TPN line sample in 24 hours exceeds five times the number grown from the peripheral blood sample, catheter sepsis is indicated (Mosca et al, 1987). Rarely, the solution may be contaminated. If the temperature remains elevated for 24 hours, especially in association with rigor, and no other explanation can be found, the catheter may be empirically incriminated as a source of infection.

TABLE 6. DRUGS AND HORMONES THAT INCREASE PERITONEAL ABSORPTION OF NUTRIENTS

Albumin	Indomethacin
Arachidonic acid	Insulin
Bradykinin	Methylprednisolone
Cholecystokinin	Nitroprusside
Deferoxamine	Phentolamine
Diazoxide	Procaine hydrochloride
Dioctyl sodium sulfosuccinate	Prostaglandin A_1
Dipyridamole	Prostaglandin E_1
Dopamine	Prostaglandin E_2
Edetate calcium disodium	Protamine
Ethacrynic acid	Salicylate
Furosemide	Secretin
Glucagon	Serotonin
Histamine	Streptokinase
Hydralazine	Tolazoline

Recurrent catheter tip sepsis can cause right atrial and superior vena caval thrombi and fungal or bacterial endocarditis, resulting in congestive heart failure (Naidoo et al, 1992). Patients with suspected subclavian vein thrombosis, suggested by neck or arm swelling with venous distension, should be examined by two-dimensional echocardiography for the presence of right atrial thrombi before the catheter is removed. A temporary catheter should be removed unless the thrombus is very large and attempted removal could result in embolic shower. Unless they are grossly infected, centrally placed catheters may be exchanged using guidewires.

The tip of the removed catheter should be cultured and appropriate antibiotic therapy initiated if defervescence does not occur rapidly. Alternatively, a permanent subcutaneous catheter may be left in place and an appropriate antibiotic given in an attempt to salvage the catheter. Prompt administration of antibiotics and thrombolytic agents often is effective; however, tunnel infections and infections caused by *Staphylococcus aureus*, *Pseudomonas*, or fungi warrant prompt catheter removal. Unresponsive thrombi, those occluding the tricuspid valve orifice, and those associated with antibiotic-resistant organisms should be removed surgically. Treatment of catheter-related sepsis with a local antibiotic-lock has resolved sepsis without necessitating catheter removal in >90% of a series of cases (Matuchansky et al, 1992).

Septicemia and multiple organ sepsis occur frequently in stressed patients (Martindale and Andrassy, 1991; Ryan et al, 1992). Disuse of the gastrointestinal tract, especially when combined with physical stress, causes villous atrophy and loss of mucosal epithelial function and integrity. Reduced mucosal IgA secretion into the lumen, microfloral overgrowth, and loss of mucosal barrier function may contribute to enhanced extraluminal relocation of indigenous intestinal microflora (bacterial translocation) and secondary sepsis (Alverdy, 1990; Bragg et al, 1991). These complications cannot be prevented by selective decontamination of the digestive tract using nonabsorbable, aerobic bacteria-specific antibiotics (Hammond et al, 1992); however, their incidence can be reduced by limiting the use of TPN to situations in which enteral feeding is impossible or by combining TPN with partial enteral feeding.

Excessive infusion of dextrose may cause hyperglycemia, glycosuria, osmotic diuresis, steatosis, and an elevated respiratory quotient. The rate of dextrose infusion must be decreased if hyperglycemia (plasma glucose concentration >220 mg/dL) persists.

If TPN must be stopped suddenly, 5% dextrose should be infused peripherally for one to two hours to prevent hypoglycemia. Accidental or emergency cessation of TPN during anesthesia may cause hypoglycemia, which may be unrecognized and result in irreversible brain damage or death.

Hyperammonemia occasionally has been associated with infusion of amino acid solutions lacking arginine. The mechanism is uncertain, but the condition appears to occur less frequently with amino acid solutions that contain arginine.

Liver disease in premature infants receiving long-term parenteral nutrition has been attributed to many factors, including essential fatty acid deficiency; however, this complication also has occurred in infants receiving Intralipid. The use of taurine-free TPN solutions may be one cause (Howard and Thompson, 1992).

Adults with inflammatory bowel disease, short-gut syndrome, or radiation enteritis often develop cholestasis, bile duct proliferation, extensive hepatic fatty infiltration and fibrosis, and focal hepatic necrosis when TPN is used for over one year (Freund, 1991). In some cases, these reversible abnormalities are caused by excessive amounts of carbohydrates, lipids, or protein (Freund, 1991; Messing et al, 1992).

Bone disease is a common complication of long-term TPN, although its etiology has not been determined (see reviews by Hurley and McMahon, 1990; Koo, 1992). In adults, TPN-related bone disease may be associated with back pain, periarticular bone pain, and fractures. In infants, signs include osteopenia, fractures, and rickets. Symptoms may appear after only two to four months of TPN.

In adults, TPN may result in significant calciuresis and negative calcium balance and, paradoxically, negative phosphorus balance despite decreased urinary phosphorus excretion. Maintenance of calcium and phosphorus balance may not be possible in all adults who receive the amounts of calcium and phosphorus typically provided by commonly used TPN solutions and many may require mineral supplementation. Similarly, many TPN solutions given to infants are deficient in calcium, phosphorus, and vitamin D and predispose to hypophosphatemia, decreased urinary phosphorus excretion, hypercalciuria, osteopenia, and spontaneous fractures (Adams and Rowe, 1992).

Many other factors can contribute to increases in urinary mineral losses, including excessive infusion of fluid, sodium, chloride, magnesium, calcium, phosphorus, vitamin D, and amino acids. Non-nutritional factors (especially long-term use of loop diuretics, amphotericin, and chemotherapeutic agents [eg, cisplatin]) also increase urinary excretion of minerals. In addition, cyclic TPN (infusion time <24 hours daily) loads the circulation more quickly and results in greater rates of urinary excretion of minerals.

Contamination of TPN nutrients with aluminum may result in aluminum toxicity and osteomalacia or rickets. Infants on TPN are exposed to amounts of aluminum (20 to 40 mcg/kg) that may surpass their ability to excrete this mineral. Such levels have triggered symptomatic bone pain in adults. However, osteopenia in small TPN-nourished preterm infants improved when they were given additional minerals known to be contaminated with aluminum (Koo and Tsang, 1991).

Drug Evaluations

AMINO ACID SOLUTIONS

[Aminosyn, Aminosyn II, FreAmine III, Novamine, ProcalAmine, Travasol]

COMPOSITION AND USES. These solutions contain a mixture of essential and nonessential crystalline amino acids with or without electrolytes or dextrose. One preparation [ProcalAmine] contains glycerol 3%. Amino acid solutions are indicated for intravenous administration when there is interference with ingestion, digestion, or absorption of protein for long periods or when parenteral supplementation of oral protein intake is required.

ADVERSE REACTIONS AND PRECAUTIONS. Mild thrombophlebitis has occurred occasionally during peripheral infusion of amino acid solutions. This is more common when solution osmolality exceeds 600 mOsm/L. Flushing, fever, and nausea also have been reported. Because amino acids increase the blood urea nitrogen level, they should be given cautiously in restricted amounts and with adequate amounts of nonprotein calories to patients with impaired renal function.

In patients with chronic or acute liver disease, hepatic coma may be precipitated because of accumulation of nitrogenous substances in the blood. For this reason, standard amino acid solutions should be used cautiously (ie, at low total amino acid concentrations) in patients with cirrhosis, severe viral hepatitis, and major involvement of the liver by cancer. Specially formulated amino acid solutions for patients with chronic encephalopathy are available (see the evaluation on Amino Acid Solutions: Hepatic Formulas).

Amino acid solutions containing significant amounts of sodium should be used cautiously in patients who must restrict sodium intake, and those containing significant amounts of potassium, phosphorus, and magnesium generally should be avoided in patients with renal failure who are not on dialysis.

DOSAGE. The dosage must be individualized.

PREPARATIONS. See Tables 7, 8, 9, and 10.

AMINO ACID SOLUTIONS: RENAL FAILURE FORMULAS

[Aminess, Aminosyn-RF, NephrAmine, RenAmin]

COMPOSITION AND USES. Renal failure formulas contain essential amino acids (EAA) plus histidine or EAA plus nonessential amino acids (NEAA) [Aminosyn RF, RenAmin]. They are formulated to be mixed with hypertonic dextrose solution (final concentration of dextrose as high as 48%). When mixed with appropriate vitamins, minerals, and electrolytes, these formulas provide about 1,200 calories in 750 to 800 ml.

The goal of parenteral nutrition in the treatment of acute renal failure is to reduce the workload on the kidneys and the biochemical consequences of renal failure. EAA plus histidine may improve survival, renal function, and nitrogen and mineral balances, although this is controversial. This approach requires a ratio of EAA to total amino acids >0.65 and a ratio of branched chain amino acids (BCAA) to EAA of >0.5 (Proietti et al, 1983). A sensible approach is to use EAA plus histidine in early renal failure before dialysis is necessary; as renal function deteriorates, both EAA and NEAA balances become negative and both EAA and NEAA are required. TPN with EAA plus NEAA is most beneficial in severely malnourished patients undergoing daily dialysis (Li, 1991).

ADVERSE REACTIONS AND PRECAUTIONS. Administration of excessive amounts of renal failure formulas without arginine occasionally has been associated with hyperammonemia leading to central nervous system disorders and coma; the role of arginine in this reaction is unclear. For further information on adverse reactions and precautions, see the evaluation on Amino Acid Solutions.

DOSAGE. Renal failure formulas that are prepared with 70% dextrose are infused into a central vein because of their high osmolality. The dosage must be individualized.

PREPARATIONS. See Table 11.

AMINO ACID SOLUTIONS: HEPATIC FORMULA

[HepatAmine]

COMPOSITION. HepatAmine contains reduced quantities of aromatic amino acids (phenylalanine, tyrosine, and tryptophan) and methionine and increased quantities of arginine and the BCAA (see Table 11).

USES. The use of amino acid solutions that are low in aromatic amino acid (AAA) content to treat hepatic encephalopathy is based on the neurotransmitter amino acid hypothesis, which presumes that hepatic encephalopathy is caused, at least in part, by elevated plasma concentrations of AAA that result from decreased clearance of AAA by the cirrhotic liver (Mullen and Weber, 1991). Increased transport of AAA into the central nervous system causes overproduction of the false neurotransmitters, octopamine and tyramine, and the putative neurotransmitter, serotonin, in the central nervous system. These false neurotransmitters then replace the true neurotransmitters, dopamine and norepinephrine, and excitatory neurotransmission is impaired (Lockwood, 1992). BCAA competes with AAA for entry into the central nervous system and, following their infusion by TPN, are believed to reduce abnormal production of false neurotransmitters and resolve the encephalopathy.

In several studies, patients with latent subclinical or chronic hepatic encephalopathy who were given 60% of their daily amino acid requirement as BCAA exhibited greater improvements in psychomotor function and alertness compared with those receiving standard amino acid formulas (Horst et al, 1984; Marchesini et al, 1990). In a controlled, multicenter study of patients with acute hepatic encephalopathy, HepatAmine was more effective in improving hepatic encephalopathy, normalizing plasma amino acid patterns, providing nutritional support, and improving survival than treatment with neomycin and glucose (no protein was provided) (Cerra et al, 1985).

A meta-analysis concluded that BCAA enrichment improves survival in acute hepatic encephalopathy, even in patients resistant to standard therapy (Naylor et al, 1989). HepatAmine has been recommended for individuals in whom standard amino acid solutions produce encephalopathy (Pillar and Perry, 1990).

For adverse reactions and precautions, see the evaluation on Amino Acid Solutions.

DOSAGE. The dosage must be individualized; most patients will improve when given 80 g amino acids daily.

PREPARATIONS. See Table 11.

AMINO ACID SOLUTIONS: BRANCHED CHAIN AMINO ACID-ENRICHED STRESS FORMULAS

[Aminosyn-HBC, BranchAmin, FreAmine HBC]

COMPOSITION. Aminosyn-HBC and FreAmine HBC contain high concentrations of branched chain amino acids (BCAA) (leucine, isoleucine, and valine); standard quantities of phenylalanine, tryptophan, and methionine; and relatively low quantities of glycine. BranchAmin contains only the BCAA, isoleucine, leucine, and valine, and must be added to a standard amino acid formula.

USES. Patients with sepsis, trauma, or thermal injury often become hypermetabolic, tripling muscle and visceral protein catabolism to supply alanine for hepatic gluconeogenesis. During metabolic stress, skeletal muscle preserves intracellular protein by preferentially oxidizing available BCAA; 80% of the oxidation of BCAA occurs in muscle. When used as part of a balanced nutrition regimen in critically ill patients, BCAA-enriched TPN improves nitrogen balance, preserves visceral proteins, normalizes plasma amino acid concentrations (and by decreasing the ratio of aromatic amino acids to BCAA, protects against metabolic and hepatic encephalopathy), and

TABLE 7.
BALANCED AMINO ACID SOLUTIONS FOR PARENTERAL NUTRITION

	Aminosyn (Abbott)						Aminosyn II (Abbott)	
AMINO ACID CONCENTRATION	**3.5%**	**5%**	**7%**	**8.5%**	**10%**	**10% (pH 6.0)**	**3.5%**	**5%**
NORMALIZED AMINO ACID CONTENT (mg/100 ml)								
Essential (% Nitrogen)								
Isoleucine (10.7)	252	360	510	620	720	720	231	330
Leucine (10.7)	329	470	660	810	940	940	350	500
Lysine (19.2)	252	360	510	624	720	720	368	525
Methionine (9.4)	140	200	280	340	400	400	60	86
Phenylalanine (8.5)	154	220	310	380	440	440	104	149
Threonine (11.8)	182	260	370	460	520	520	140	200
Tryptophan (13.7)	56	80	120	150	160	160	70	100
Valine (12.0)	280	400	560	680	800	800	175	250
TOTAL EAA	1645	2350	3320	4064	4700	4700	1498	2140
Nonessential (% Nitrogen)								
Alanine (15.7)	448	640	900	1100	1280	1280	348	497
Arginine (32.2)	343	490	690	850	980	980	356	509
Histidine (27.1)*	105	150	210	260	300	300	105	150
Proline (12.2)	300	430	610	750	860	860	253	361
Serine (13.3)	147	210	300	370	420	420	186	265
Tyrosine (7.7)*	31	44	44	44	44	44	95	135
Glycine (18.9)	448	640	900	1100	1280	1280	175	250
Glutamic Acid	—	—	—	—	—	—	258	369
Aspartic Acid	—	—	—	—	—	—	245	350
Cysteine (11.6)	—	—	—	—	—	—	—	—
TOTAL NEAA	1822	2604	3654	4474	5164	5164	2021	2886
ELECTROLYTES (mEq/L)								
Sodium	7	—	—	—	—	—	16.3	19.3
Potassium	—	5.4	5.4	5.4	5.4	2.7	—	—
Magnesium	—	—	—	—	—	—	—	—
Chloride	—	—	—	35	—	—	—	—
Acetate	46	86	105	90	148	111	25.2	35.9
Phosphate (mMol/L)	—	—	—	—	—	—	—	—
EAA/TAA%	47	47	48	48	48	48	43	43
BCAA/EAA%	52	52	52	52	52	52	50	50
BCAA/TAA%	25	25	25	25	25	25	21	21
Nitrogen (g/100 ml)	0.55	0.79	1.1	1.34	1.57	1.57	0.54	0.77
Osmolarity (mOsm/L)	357	500	700	850	1000	993	308	438
Supplied in (ml)	1000	500 1000	500	500 1000	500 1000	500 1000	1000	500 1000

* *Histidine and tyrosine are generally considered essential amino acids in infants and patients with renal failure.*

promotes immune function (Cerra et al, 1987; Okada et al, 1988; Skeie et al, 1990).

Patients who are most likely to respond favorably to BCAA-enriched TPN have an elevated oxygen consumption index, increased total urinary nitrogen excretion, hyperglycemia, hypoalbuminemia (<2.5 mg/dL), and depressed serum transferrin concentration (Brown et al, 1990; Mattox and Teasley-Strausburg, 1992). Although decreased mortality has yet to be demonstrated, BCAA-enriched TPN may be indicated in patients with sepsis; renal, pulmonary, or liver dysfunction; multiple organ failure; or impaired immunocompetence (Söreide et al, 1991; Mattox and Teasley-Strausburg, 1992).

For adverse reactions and precautions, see the evaluation on Amino Acid Solutions.

DOSAGE. The dosage must be individualized.

PREPARATIONS. See Table 11.

AMINO ACID SOLUTION: PEDIATRIC FORMULAS

[Aminosyn-PF, TrophAmine]

COMPOSITION AND USES. These mixtures of essential and

Aminosyn II (Abbott)				FreAmine III (McGaw)		Novamine (Clintec)		Travasol (Clintec)		
7%	8.5%	10%	15%	8.5%	10%	11.4%	15%	5.5%	8.5%	10%
462	561	660	990	590	690	570	749	263	406	600
700	850	1000	1500	770	910	790	1040	340	526	730
735	893	1050	1575	620	730	900	1180	318	492	580
120	146	172	258	450	530	570	749	318	492	400
209	253	298	447	480	560	790	1040	340	526	560
280	340	400	600	340	400	570	749	230	356	420
140	170	200	300	130	150	190	250	99	152	180
350	425	500	750	560	660	730	960	252	390	580
2996	3638	4280	6420	3350	4630	5110	6717	2160	3340	4050
695	844	993	1490	600	710	1650	2170	1140	1760	2070
713	865	1018	1527	810	950	1120	1470	570	880	1150
210	255	300	450	240	280	680	894	241	372	480
505	614	722	1083	950	1120	680	894	230	356	680
371	450	530	795	500	590	450	592	—	—	500
189	230	270	405	—	—	30	39	22	34	40
350	425	500	750	1190	1400	790	1040	1140	1760	1030
517	627	738	1107	—	—	570	749	—	—	—
490	595	700	1050	—	—	330	434	—	—	—
—	—	—	—	<20	<24	—	—	—	—	—
4040	4675	5771	8657	4290	5050	5400	8282	3343	5162	5950
31.3	33.3	45.3	62.7	10	10	—	—	—	—	—
—	—	—	—	—	—	—	—	—	—	—
—	—	—	—	—	—	—	—	—	—	—
—	—	—	—	<3	<3	—	—	22	34	40
50.3	61.1	71.8	107.6	72	89	114	151	43	67	87
—	—		—	10	10	—	—	—	—	—
43	44	43	43	48	48	49	45	39	39	41
50	50	50	50	49	49	41	41	40	40	47
21	22	21	21	23	23	20	18	16	16	19
1.07	1.3	1.53	2.3	1.3	1.53	1.8	2.37	0.925	1.43	1.65
612	742	873	1300	810	950	1057	1388	569	880	898
500	500	500	2000	500	500	500	500	500	500	200
	1000	1000		1000	1000	1000	1000	1000	1000	500
								2000	2000	1000
										2000

nonessential amino acids, taurine, and tyrosine are formulated specifically for use in infants and young children. Because certain enzymes are poorly developed in neonates, cysteine, taurine, tyrosine, and histidine may be essential amino acids in these infants. TrophAmine produces plasma amino acid concentrations similar to those found in breast-fed infants and induces weight gain and positive nitrogen balance more efficiently than standard adult formulas (Heird et al, 1987, 1988).

Premature and newborn infants are particularly at risk for hepatobiliary complications associated with TPN. The incidence of cholestatic liver disease increases with younger gestational age, lower birth weight, and increasing duration of TPN therapy (Warner, 1991). A growing body of evidence indicates that taurine is an essential amino acid for premature infants and neonates and that the incidence of TPN-associated cholestasis can be reduced by using solutions containing taurine [Aminosyn PF 7% (50 mg/dL), Trophamine 6% (15 mg/dL)] (Howard and Thompson, 1992) (see also discussion on TPN in Pediatric Patients).

For adverse reactions and precautions, see the evaluation on Amino Acid Solutions.

TABLE 8.
BALANCED AMINO ACID SOLUTIONS WITH ELECTROLYTES FOR PARENTERAL NUTRITION

	Aminosyn (Abbott)			Aminosyn II (Abbott)				FreAmine III (McGaw)		ProcalAmine (McGaw)	Travasol (Clintec)		
AMINO ACID CONCENTRATION	**3.5%**	**7%**	**8.5%**	**3.5%**	**7%**	**8.5%**	**10%**	**3%**	**8.5%**	**3%**	**3.5%**	**5.5%**	**8.5%**
NORMALIZED AMINO ACID CONTENT (mg/100 ml)													
Essential (% Nitrogen)													
Isoleucine (10.7)	252	510	620	231	462	561	660	210	590	210	168	263	406
Leucine (10.7)	329	660	810	350	700	850	1000	270	770	270	217	340	526
Lysine (19.2)	252	510	624	368	735	893	1050	220	620	220	203	318	492
Methionine (9.4)	140	280	340	60	120	146	172	160	450	160	203	318	492
Phenylalanine (8.5)	154	310	380	104	209	253	298	170	480	170	217	340	526
Threonine (11.8)	182	370	460	140	280	340	400	120	340	120	147	230	356
Tryptophan (13.7)	56	120	150	70	140	170	200	46	130	46	63	99	152
Valine (12.0)	280	560	680	175	350	425	500	200	560	200	161	252	390
TOTAL EAA	1645	3320	4064	1498	2996	3638	4280	1396	3940	1396	1379	2160	3340
Nonessential (% Nitrogen)													
Alanine (15.7)	448	900	1100	348	695	844	993	210	600	210	728	1140	1760
Arginine (32.2)	343	690	850	356	713	865	1018	290	810	290	364	570	880
Histidine (27.1)*	105	210	260	105	210	255	300	85	240	85	154	241	372
Proline (12.2)	300	610	750	253	505	614	722	340	950	340	147	230	356
Serine (13.3)	147	300	370	186	371	450	530	180	500	180	—	—	—
Tyrosine (7.7)*	31	44	44	95	189	230	270	—	—	—	14	22	34
Glycine (18.9)	448	900	1100	175	350	425	500	420	1190	420	728	1140	1760
Glutamic Acid	—	—	—	258	517	627	738	—	—	—	—	—	—
Aspartic Acid	—	—	—	245	490	595	700	—	—	—	—	—	—
Cysteine (11.6)	—	—	—	—	—	—	—	<20.	<20	<20	—	—	—
TOTAL NEAA	1822	3654	4474	2021	4040	4905	5771	1525	4310	1525	2135	3343	5162
ELECTROLYTES (mEq/L)†													
Sodium	47	70	70	36	76	80	87	35	60	35	25	70	70
Potassium	13	66	66	13	66	66	66	24.5	60	24	15	60	60
Magnesium	3	10	10	3	10	10	10	5	10	5	5	10	10
Chloride	40	96	98	37	86	86	86	41	60	41	25	70	70
Acetate	58	124	142	25	50	61	72	44	125	47	52	102	141
Phosphate (mMol/L)	3.5	30	30	3.5	30	30	30	3.5	20	3.5	7.5	30	30
EAA/TAA%	47	48	48	43	43	43	43	47	48	47	39	39	39
BCAA/EAA%	52	52	52	50	50	50	50	49	49	49	40	40	40
BCAA/TAA%	25	25	25	21	21	21	21	23	23	23	16	16	16
Nitrogen (g/100 ml)	0.55	1.1	1.34	0.54	1.07	1.3	1.53	0.46	1.3	0.46	0.59	0.925	1.43
Osmolarity (mOsm/L)	477	1013	1160	425	869	999	1130	405	1045	735	450	850	1160
Supplied in (ml)	1000	500	500	1000	500	500	1000	1000	500	1000	500	500	500
									1000		1000	1000	1000
												2000	2000

** Histidine and tyrosine are generally considered essential amino acids in infants and patients with renal failure.*
† To determine the electrolyte concentrations in a 500 ml bottle, divide the mEq/L values by 2.

DOSAGE. The dosage must be individualized.

PREPARATIONS. See Table 11.

FAT EMULSIONS

[Intralipid, Liposyn II, Liposyn III]

USES. Intravenous fat emulsions are used to prevent or correct essential fatty acid deficiency and to provide calories in high-density form on a regular basis during prolonged TPN, especially in patients with insulin resistance. They also are used in patients with chronic obstructive pulmonary disease to lower the respiratory quotient and decrease arterial CO_2 concentrations. Lipids can be administered parenterally or orally to prevent essential fatty acid deficiency. Because they are isotonic with plasma, these preparations are suitable for peripheral infusion. Fat emulsions may be used to supplement calories, and the need to administer hypertonic (>5%) dex-

TABLE 9.
BALANCED AMINO ACID SOLUTIONS WITH DEXTROSE FOR PARENTERAL NUTRITION

	Aminosyn II (Abbott)						Travasol (Clintec)				
AMINO ACID CONCENTRATION	**3.5%**	**3.5%**	**4.25%**	**4.25%**	**4.25%**	**5%**	**2.75%**	**2.75%**	**4.25%**	**4.25%**	**4.25%**
DEXTROSE CONCENTRATION	5%	25%	10%	20%	25%	25%	5%	10%	5%	10%	25%
NORMALIZED AMINO ACID CONTENT (mg/100 ml)											
Essential (% Nitrogen)											
Isoleucine (10.7)	231	231	280	280	280	330	132	132	203	203	203
Leucine (10.7)	350	350	425	425	425	500	170	170	263	263	263
Lysine (19.2)	368	368	446	446	446	525	159	159	246	246	246
Methionine (9.4)	60	60	73	73	73	86	159	159	246	246	246
Phenylalanine (8.5)	104	104	126	126	126	149	170	170	263	263	263
Threonine (11.8)	140	140	170	170	170	200	115	115	178	178	178
Tryptophan (13.7)	70	70	85	85	85	100	50	50	76	76	76
Valine (12.0)	175	175	212	212	212	250	126	126	195	195	195
TOTAL EAA	1498	1498	1817	1817	1817	2140	1081	1081	1470	1470	1470
Nonessential (% Nitrogen)											
Alanine (15.7)	348	348	422	422	422	496	570	570	880	880	880
Arginine (32.2)	356	356	432	432	432	509	285	285	440	440	440
Histidine (27.1)*	105	105	128	128	128	150	120	120	186	186	186
Proline (12.2)	252	252	307	307	307	361	115	115	178	178	178
Serine (13.3)	186	186	225	225	225	265	—	—	—	—	—
Tyrosine (7.7)*	94	94	115	115	115	135	11	11	17	17	17
Glycine (18.9)	175	175	212	212	212	250	570	570	880	880	880
Glutamic Acid	258	258	314	314	314	369	—	—	—	—	—
Aspartic Acid	245	245	298	298	298	350	—	—	—	—	—
Cysteine (11.6)	—	—	—	—	—	—	—	—	—	—	—
TOTAL NEAA	2021	2021	2453	2453	2453	2885	1671	1671	2581	2581	2581
ELECTROLYTES (mEq/L)											
Sodium	18	18	19	19	19	22.2	—	—	—	—	—
Potassium	—	—	—	—	—	—	—	—	—	—	—
Magnesium	—	—	—	—	—	—	—	—	—	—	—
Chloride	—	—	—	—	—	—	11	11	17	17	17
Acetate	25.2	25.2	30.6	30.6	30.6	35.9	21	21	34	34	34
Phosphate (mMol/L)	—	—	—	—	—	—	—	—	—	—	—
EAA/TAA%	43	43	43	43	43	43	39	39	36	36	36
BCAA/EAA%	50	50	50	50	50	50	40	40	45	45	45
BCAA/TAA%	21	21	21	21	21	21	16	16	16	16	16
Nitrogen (g/100 ml)	0.54	0.54	0.65	0.65	0.65	0.77	0.46	0.46	0.7	0.7	0.7
Osmolarity (mOsm/L)	585	1515	894	1295	1536	1539	535	790	690	945	1700
Supplied in (ml)	—[1]	—[2]	—[1]	—[1]	—[3]	—[4]	—[2]	—[2]	—[2]	—[2]	—[2]

** Histidine and tyrosine are generally considered essential amino acids in infants and patients with renal failure.*

[1] 1000 ml with 1000 ml dextrose.

[2] 500 ml with 500 ml dextrose.

[3] 750 and 1000 ml with 750 and 1000 ml dextrose.

[4] 500, 750, and 1000 ml with 500, 750, and 1000 ml dextrose.

trose via a central vein catheter may be avoided. This may be especially beneficial in patients who require partial parenteral nutritional support and can tolerate limited enteral feeding (Jeejeebhoy, 1991).

Fatty acids are the major fuel oxidized during malnutrition, trauma, and serious infection. The commercially available lipid emulsions are comparable to carbohydrate in promoting energy and nitrogen balance in a variety of conditions (Bruder et al, 1991; Gilbertson et al, 1991; Jarnberg, 1991; Jeejeebhoy, 1991). Weight gain, healing of fistulas, and increased serum protein concentrations have been observed in adults receiving fat emulsions providing up to 83% of nonprotein calories during long-term TPN.

Intravenous fat emulsions should supply 3% to 5% of total caloric intake when used to prevent essential fatty acid deficiency and 4% to 10% when used to correct existing defi-

TABLE 10.
BALANCED AMINO ACID SOLUTIONS WITH DEXTROSE AND ELECTROLYTES FOR PARENTERAL NUTRITION

	Aminosyn II M (Abbott)	
AMINO ACID CONCENTRATION	**3.5%**	**4.25%**
DEXTROSE CONCENTRATION	5%	10%
NORMALIZED AMINO ACID CONTENT (mg/100 ml)		
Essential (% Nitrogen)		
Isoleucine (10.7)	231	280
Leucine (10.7)	350	425
Lysine (19.2)	368	446
Methionine (9.4)	60	73
Phenylalanine (8.5)	104	126
Threonine (11.8)	140	170
Tryptophan (13.7)	70	85
Valine (12.0)	175	212
TOTAL EAA	1498	1817
Nonessential (% Nitrogen)		
Alanine (15.7)	348	422
Arginine (32.2)	356	432
Histidine (27.1)*	105	128
Proline (12.2)	252	307
Serine (13.3)	186	225
Tyrosine (7.7)*	94	115
Glycine (18.9)	175	212
Glutamic Acid	258	314
Aspartic Acid	245	298
Cysteine (11.6)	—	—
TOTAL NEAA	2021	2453
ELECTROLYTES (mEq/L)		
Sodium	41	43.7
Potassium	13	13
Magnesium	3	3
Chloride	36.5	36.5
Acetate	25.1	30.5
Phosphate (mMol/L)	3.5	3.5
EAA/TAA%	43	43
BCAA/EAA%	50	50
BCAA/TAA%	21	21
Nitrogen (g/100 ml)	0.535	0.65
Osmolarity (mOsm/L)	616	919
Supplied in (ml)	—1	—2

** Histidine and tyrosine are generally considered essential amino acids in infants and patients with renal failure.*
1 500 and 1000 ml with 500 and 1000 ml dextrose.
2 500 ml with 500 ml dextrose.

ciency. When used as a source of calories, they should comprise no more than 60% of the total caloric intake in adults and no more than 40% in children; the remainder should be supplied by dextrose and a source of amino acids.

The particle size (0.1 to 0.5 microns), clearance, and elimination of available lipid emulsions are similar to those of chylomicrons.

ADVERSE REACTIONS AND PRECAUTIONS. Currently available fat emulsions rarely cause severe adverse reactions in adults at daily doses of lipids up to 4 g/kg and in children and infants at daily doses up to 2 g/kg.

Hyperlipidemia may occur if these preparations are infused too rapidly, given to patients with impaired fat metabolism, or administered with an excessive amount of dextrose. Small increases (5 to 25 mg/dL) in plasma total and LDL-cholesterol concentrations may accompany the use of fat emulsions given daily for more than seven days (Messing et al, 1990; Nichoalds et al, 1991).

Persistent hypertriglyceridemia, increased prostaglandin, prostacyclin, and thromboxane concentrations, and impairment of immune and reticuloendothelial systems function also have been associated with rapid infusion (Bedrick, 1988).

Long-term TPN often is associated with formation of biliary sludge. Bile stasis (decreased gallbladder emptying) results from decreased food-stimulated intestinal secretion of hormones. Infusion of fat emulsions increases biliary cholesterol and phospholipid concentrations and the cholesterol saturation index and may predispose to cholelithiasis if continued for prolonged periods (Rubin et al, 1992).

Long-term (>30 days) TPN with fat emulsions containing polyunsaturated fatty acids may increase tumor necrosis factor synthesis and secretion, inhibit neutrophil chemotaxis and migration, impair complement synthesis, and stimulate synthesis of inflammatory prostaglandins (Argilés et al, 1992; Gogos et al, 1992; Standiford and Strieter, 1992). In addition, Kupffer cells may proliferate and a brown pigment may be deposited throughout the reticuloendothelial system; however, these effects do not appear to be clinically significant.

Newborn infants, particularly those who are premature, small, or acutely ill, may metabolize intravenous fat emulsions slowly (Dahlström et al, 1988; Jensen and Jensen, 1992 A, 1992 B). In particular, the high lecithin content of 10% emulsions can exceed the ability of lecithin cholesteryl acyltransferase, resulting in hypercholesterolemia. Because free fatty acids compete with bilirubin for albumin binding sites, intravenous fats may increase the risk of kernicterus in infants with hyperbilirubinemia and may interfere with estimation of serum bilirubin concentration. Deaths have been reported following too rapid infusion in preterm infants; however, these were related to overinfusion without proper administration controls.

Thrombophlebitis, vomiting, pain in the chest or back, hypersensitivity reactions, hepatomegaly, thrombocytopenia, anemia, transient abnormalities in liver function tests, and decreased pulmonary diffusing capacity have been reported rarely. The "overloading syndrome" (focal seizures, edema, fever, leukocytosis, thrombocytopenia, splenomegaly, and shock) associated with use of the previously available cotton seed oil emulsions also is rare following infusion of currently available preparations. However, caution is advised when administering fat emulsions to patients with severe liver disease, anemia, blood coagulation disorders, or allergy to egg yolks.

Baseline and periodic liver function tests, determination of plasma lipid concentrations, hemogram, blood coagulation tests, and platelet counts should be performed periodically during long-term therapy. Infusion rates must be adjusted to maintain plasma triglyceride concentrations below 100 mg/dL in infants and below 400 mg/dL in adults. The lipemia must clear between daily infusions (Brans et al, 1988). These preparations should be discontinued if a significant abnormality is attributable to fat infusion.

DOSAGE. Intravenous fat emulsions may be infused via a peripheral or central vein. A total of 500 ml of a 20% emulsion provides 1,000 kcal; the same volume of a 10% emulsion provides 550 kcal. A 20% fat emulsion is useful when volume restriction is necessary. Compatibility should be verified before admixing with other solutions, drugs, or vitamins. Three-in-one systems, in which fats, amino acids, and dextrose are admixed in one container, are available. Fat emulsions should always be examined for signs of destabilization (such as oil droplets) prior to and after admixture and prior to and during administration. The contents of any partly used bottle must be discarded. Bottles should be stored in the refrigerator until immediately prior to use; if accidentally frozen, the bottle must be discarded.

Intravenous: *Adults,* the manufacturers recommend that the initial infusion rate should not exceed 1 ml/min (10% oil emulsion) or 0.5 ml/min (20% oil emulsion) for 15 minutes. If no adverse effects occur (fever, chills, pain in chest or back), the rate may be increased to provide a maximum of 500 ml over six hours (10%) or eight hours (20%). No more than 500 ml of the 20% preparations should be given on the first day of therapy. On the following day, the dosage may be increased to 1 g of fat/kg of body weight daily infused over 20 to 24 hours.

In *children,* the initial infusion rate is 0.1 ml/min (10%) or 0.05 ml/min (20%) for 15 minutes; if tolerated, the rate then may be increased to provide 1 g of fat/kg in four hours. The amount of fat should not routinely exceed 3 g/kg/day. Even smaller doses should be used in patients with infection, compromised pulmonary function, and/or hyperbilirubinemia.

In *newborn infants,* intravenous fat emulsions should be infused at a constant rate over 20 to 24 hours with a maximal daily dose calculated to provide 2 to 4 g of fat/kg and no more than 0.15 g/kg hourly (Gilbertson et al, 1991). Lipemic response should be monitored.

PREPARATIONS. See Table 12.

ENTERAL NUTRITION

Enteral nutrition (EN) is indicated for patients with at least partially patent and functioning alimentary tracts who cannot or will not ingest adequate amounts of food and for those with digestive disorders whose small intestines can absorb adequate amounts of nutrients. EN is preferred to TPN whenever possible; it is more physiologic, cost-effective, and convenient than TPN and is less prone to complications (Alverdy et al, 1985; ASPEN Board of Directors, 1987 B; Moore et al, 1992). In addition, exposure of the intestinal tract to intraluminal nutrients is required to maintain intestinal mass, integrity, absorptive functions, and hormone secretion (Alverdy et al, 1988).

EN may comprise part of the total daily diet for those who can ingest and absorb some nutrients, or it may comprise the total intake for those unable to ingest anything. Patients with otherwise adequate intestinal function require EN when they are unable to ingest food orally for more than five days due to such conditions as severe dysphagia, major full-thickness burns, massive small bowel resection, cystic fibrosis, congenital anomalies of the digestive tract, head or neck cancer, Guil-

TABLE 11.
PARENTERAL AMINO ACID SOLUTIONS FOR SPECIFIC SITUATIONS

AMINO ACID CONCENTRATION	Aminess (Clintec) 5.2%	Renal Failure Formulations Aminosyn-RF (Abbott) 5.2%	NephrAmine (McGaw) 5.4%	RenAmin (Clintec) 6.5%
NORMALIZED AMINO ACID CONTENT (mg/100 ml)				
Essential (% Nitrogen)				
Isoleucine (10.7)	525	462	560	500
Leucine (10.7)	825	726	880	600
Lysine (19.2)	600	535	640	450
Methionine (9.4)	825	726	880	500
Phenylalanine (8.5)	825	726	880	490
Threonine (11.8)	375	330	400	380
Tryptophan (13.7)	188	165	200	160
Valine (12.0)	600	528	640	820
TOTAL EAA	5,175†	4,627†	5,330†	4,320†
Nonessential (% Nitrogen)				
Alanine (15.7)	—	—	—	560
Arginine (32.2)	—	600	—	630
Histidine (27.1)†	412†	429†	250†	420†
Proline (12.2)	—	—	—	350
Serine (13.3)	—	—	—	300
Taurine	—	—	—	—
Tyrosine (7.7)†	—	—	—	40†
Glycine (18.9)	—	—	—	300
Glutamic Acid	—	—	—	—
Aspartic Acid	—	—	—	—
Cysteine (11.6)	—	—	<20	—
TOTAL NEAA	0†	600†	<20†	2,140†
ELECTROLYTES (mEq/L)				
Sodium	—	—	5	—
Potassium	—	5.4	—	—
Magnesium	—	—	—	—
Chloride	—	—	<3	31
Acetate	50	105	44	60
Phosphate (mMol/L)	—	—	—	—
EAA/TAA%	100	89	100	66
BCAA/EAA%	38	37	39	44
BCAA/TAA%	38	33	39	30
Nitrogen (g/100 ml)	0.66	0.79	0.65	1
Osmolarity (mOsm/L)	416	475	435	600
Supplied in (ml)	400	300	250	250 500

** Some authorities use BranchAmin for the treatment of hepatic disorders. For formulation, see under High Branched-Chain Formulations.*
† Histidine and tyrosine are considered essential amino acids in infants and in patients with renal failure. This is reflected in the total EAA, total NEAA, and ratios.

lain-Barré syndrome, and low-output enterocutaneous fistulas (Ramsey et al, 1992; Roubenoff et al, 1992; Vanderhoof, 1992; Wright, 1992; Goodwin and Byers, 1993). EN stimulates growth and weight gain in very-low-birth-weight infants (Shulman and Kanarek, 1993) and is beneficial in helping adults meet the increased nutritional needs associated with major trauma, radiation therapy, mild chemotherapy, hepatic failure, severe renal dysfunction, superior mesenteric artery syndrome, and prolonged underfeeding (Moore and Moore, 1991; Anderson et al, 1992; Johnson et al, 1993; Milner et al, 1993; Mowatt-Larssen and Brown, 1993). When begun within 12 hours postoperatively, EN is superior to standard TPN therapy in improving nitrogen balance and constitutive protein synthesis and in reducing septic morbidity, synthesis of acute-phase proteins, plasma glucagon concentration, and urinary catecholamine excretion following surgery (Enzi et al, 1990;

High Branched-Chain Formulations			Hepatic Formulation*	Pediatric Formulations			
Aminosyn-HBC (Abbott) 7%	BranchAmin (Clintec) 4%	FreAmine HBC (McGaw) 6.9%	HepatAmine (McGaw) 8%	Aminosyn-PF (Abbott) 7%	Aminosyn-PF (Abbott) 10%	TrophAmine (McGaw) 6%	TrophAmine (McGaw) 10%
789	1,380	760	900	534	760	490	820
1,576	1,380	1,370	1,100	831	1,200	840	1,400
265		410	610	475	677	490	820
206		250	100	125	180	200	340
228		320	100	300	427	290	480
272		200	450	360	512	250	420
88		90	66	125	180	120	200
789	1,240	880	840	452	673	470	780
4,213	4,000	3,992	4,166	3,422†	4,921†	3,440†	5,980†
660	—	400	770	490	698	320	540
507	—	580	600	861	1,227	730	1,200
154	—	160	240	220†	312†	290†	480†
448	—	630	800	570	812	410	680
221	—	330	500	347	495	230	380
—	—	—	—	50	70	15	25
33	—	—	—	44†	44†	140	240†
660	—	330	900	270	385	220	360
—	—	—	—	576	820	300	500
—	—	—	—	370	527	190	320
—	—	<20	<20	—	—	<20	<16
2,650	—	2,450	3,810	3,534†	5,034†	2,415	5,021†
7	—	10	10	3.4	3.4	5	5
—	—	—	—	—	—	—	—
—	—	—	—	—	—	—	—
—	—	<3	<3	—	—	<3	<3
72	—	57	62	33	46	56	97
—	—	—	10	—	—	—	—
61	100	62	52	49	49	49	54
75	100	75	68	53	54	52	50
46	100	47	36	26	26	26	27
1.12	0.443	0.97	1.2	1.07	1.52	0.93	1.55
665	316	620	785	586	829	525	875
500	500	750	500	250	1,000		500
1,000				500		500	

Meguid et al, 1990 A, 1990 B; Moore and Moore, 1991; Baskin, 1992; Campos and Meguid, 1992; Deitch, 1992; Moore et al, 1992). It is as effective in achieving long-term remission in acute nonulcerative inflammatory bowel disease as primary therapy with drugs or TPN (Teahon et al, 1990, 1991; Cravo et al, 1991; Lochs et al, 1991; Kushner, 1992; Sitrin, 1992; González-Huix et al, 1993 A) and is safe and nutritionally effective during episodes of ulcerative colitis (González-Huix et al, 1993 B).

EN is contraindicated in patients with (1) severe malabsorption with uncontrollable diarrhea; (2) total bowel obstruction; (3) severe intestinal hypomotility; (4) persistent uncontrolled vomiting; (5) high-output enteric fistulas; (6) severe acute pancreatitis; (7) shock; and (8) a tendency to aspirate (especially in the presence of serious pulmonary disease, although appropriate tube placement and adherence to aspiration precautions in persons at risk for aspiration can limit this complication) (ASPEN Board of Directors, 1987 B).

Enteral formulas differ in digestibility, caloric density, palatability, osmolality, viscosity, composition, and expense. Some products contain minimally altered foods and others contain processed food derivatives or synthetic nutrients. Prepara-

TABLE 12. COMPOSITION OF FAT EMULSIONS FOR PARENTERAL NUTRITION[1]

Preparation	Fatty Acids					Calories per ml
	Linoleic	Oleic	Palmitic	Linolenic	Stearic	
Intralipid (Clintec)						
10%[2]	50%	26%	10%	9%	3.5%	1.1
20%[3]	50%	26%	10%	9%	3.5%	2
Liposyn II (Abbott)						
10%[4]	65.8%	17.7%	8.8%	4.2%	3.4%	1.1
20%[5]	65.8%	17.7%	8.8%	4.2%	3.4%	2
Liposyn III (Abbott)						
10%[2]	54.5%	22.4%	10.5%	8.3%	4.2%	1.1
20%[3]	54.5%	22.4%	10.5%	8.3%	4.2%	2

[1] *All preparations contain purified egg phospholipid (1.2%) as an emulsifier and glycerol (2.25% or 2.5%) to make the final emulsion isotonic.*

[2] *10% soybean oil.*

[3] *20% soybean oil.*

[4] *5% soybean oil and 5% safflower oil.*

[5] *10% soybean oil and 10% safflower oil.*

tions containing intact proteins generally are more palatable than those made from hydrolyzed protein or crystalline amino acids and should be used for oral EN when tolerated, although proteins hydrolyzed to dipeptides and tripeptides may be absorbed more efficiently by some patients.

Patients receiving EN frequently are given medications concurrently, often through the feeding tube. The administration of drugs may accompany either intermittent feeding or continuous infusion. Limited data are available on the compatibility of drugs with enteral formulas. It is usually assumed that drug absorption, distribution, metabolism, and excretion are not affected by the components of the formula; however, this assumption is not always warranted and subtherapeutic or toxic effects can occur. Direct admixing of drugs in formulas may change the chemical or physical characteristics of the drugs or the formulas. These changes can range from an increase in viscosity to phase separation, resulting in altered drug dissolution, poor formula flow characteristics, tube obstruction, nausea, abdominal cramping, or diarrhea. In addition, effects on bioavailability of drugs given through tubes placed in different parts of the digestive tract must be considered.

Some drugs are known to be incompatible with administration through enteral feeding tubes (brompheniramine, cephalexin, chlorpromazine, cimetidine, guaifenesin, ketoconazole, mandelamine, pseudoephedrine, sucralfate; the combination products, Dimetapp and Mylanta; all enteric-coated tablets; all prolonged-release capsules). A number of other drugs exhibit decreased bioavailability when added to enteral feeding solutions (captopril, carbamazepine, dicumarol, digoxin, hydralazine, hydrochlorothiazide, isoniazid, methyldopa, metoprolol, phenacetin, phenytoin, procainamide, propranolol, rifampin, tetracycline, theophylline). As a general rule, medications other than H_2 blockers or paregoric should not be added to EN formulas (Enteral Nutrition Council, 1987).

Detailed instructions on choice of delivery method; access points; placement of standard nasogastric, nasojejunal, percutaneous endoscopic gastrostomy, and percutaneous endoscopic jejunostomy tubes; and prevention of reflux are available (Mobarhan and Barch, 1989; Shike et al, 1989; Byrd, 1990; Forlaw et al, 1990; DeLegge and Kirby, 1991; Baskin, 1992; Drickamer and Cooney, 1993; Fuchs, 1993; Marian, 1993). Manuals and workbooks for patients receiving EN also are available (Shronts, 1983; Piepmeyer et al, 1988; Ross Laboratories, 1988 A, 1988 B; Clintec Nutrition, 1992).

Components of Enteral Formulas

Several criteria can guide the selection of appropriate enteral formulas, depending on a patient's specific nutritional and metabolic requirements. The most important are nutrient composition, caloric distribution, caloric density, protein source and content, route of administration, and cost. If more than one formula satisfies these criteria for an individual patient, somewhat less important criteria can be considered, such as osmolality, complexity, fat content, fat source, fiber content, lactose content, protein source, form (powder or ready-to-use), and whether clinical trials have demonstrated effectiveness (DeChicco and Matarese, 1992).

For the specific quantitative energy and protein requirements of patients on EN, see discussions on Nutritional Requirements Provided by TPN and TPN in Pediatric Patients. For the requirements for vitamins and minerals not specifically discussed below, see index entry Vitamins: Recommended Daily Allowances.

Carbohydrates: These constitute the main source of calories in most enteral formulations. Carbohydrates are available as dextrose, sucrose, lactose, hydrolyzed corn starch, starch, and glucose oligosaccharides. Dextrose, sucrose, and lactose contribute to high osmolality and are slightly more likely to produce osmotic diarrhea than the more complex forms. The absorptive and digestive capacity of the mucosa also should be considered when selecting a source of carbohydrates. Complex carbohydrates (eg, dextrins, starch) require a larger segment of functional gastrointestinal tract for absorption than simple sugars. Glucose transport can become saturated when jejunal length is limited; partial replacement of glucose polymers with sucrose allows distinct fructose transporters to increase carbohydrate absorption (Silk and Grimble, 1992). However, fructose absorption is slow and incomplete, and significant fructose intake can cause abdominal distension, cramps, diarrhea, hypertriglyceridemia, hyperuricemia, and hypertension. Glucose oligosaccharides (eg, hydrolyzed corn starch) have low osmolality but are readily hydrolyzed to simple sugars, are easily absorbed even in patients with moderate gastrointestinal dysfunction, and produce plasma glucose and insulin responses indistinguishable from those produced by simple glucose.

Lactose intolerance is common in many adolescents and adults, particularly blacks, Orientals, Mexicans, American Indians, and Jews, and can be associated with diseases of malabsorption (eg, celiac disease, tropical sprue, regional enteritis), short bowel syndrome, and recovery from illness or surgery. Thus, formulations containing lactose should be avoided in individuals with genetic or secondary lactase deficiency. Patients with severe malabsorption secondary to disease or resection also may have deficiency of other disaccharidases and large amounts of sucrose should be avoided. Formulas containing hydrolyzed corn starch or other glucose oligosaccharides have lower osmolality and are preferred. These carbohydrates can be mixed with small amounts of sucrose or fructose to increase palatability.

The carbohydrate content of enteral formulations must be considered when treating diabetic patients. Administration of a formula with lower carbohydrate content or adjustment of insulin or oral hypoglycemic dosage may be required.

Amino Acids: These are available as intact proteins (eg, pureed meat), protein isolates (eg, casein isolated from milk, soy isolates), hydrolyzed proteins, small peptides, and free amino acids.

In general, the absorption of dipeptides and tripeptides is greater than that of free amino acids in healthy humans because these molecules are absorbed by a distinct intestinal peptide transport system with greater capacity than the transport system for free amino acids (Silk and Grimble, 1992). Disease (eg, malabsorption, pancreatitis) has less effect on impairment of absorption of dipeptides and tripeptides than free amino acids (Adibi and Allen, 1970; Milla et al, 1983; Vazquez et al, 1985; Zaloga, 1993). In addition, peptide-based diets cause less nausea, vomiting, and diarrhea in severely ill patients and have a greater trophic effect on the intestinal mucosa. However, commercially available "peptide-based" formulas are composed largely of peptides containing five or more amino acids (Andrassy, 1991); the absorption of the amino acids in these peptides requires luminal pancreatic enzyme proteolysis. Consequently, in the presence of adequate pancreatic function and 50 cm or more of functioning small intestine, whole proteins can be utilized as efficiently as protein hydrolysates or "small" peptides (Rees et al, 1992). In pancreatic disease, brush border hydrolysis of large peptides and intact proteins becomes rate limiting and amino acid absorption may decrease. Those with severely impaired small bowel or pancreatic function require free amino acids or dipeptides and tripeptides (Zaloga, 1993). Those with an inherited inability to absorb certain amino acids (eg, cystinuria, Hartnup disease) may require dipeptide- and tripeptide-based elemental formulas (Grimble and Silk, 1990; Mowatt-Larssen et al, 1992). Nevertheless, an advantage of hydrolysates, small peptides, and free amino acids is their greater solubility compared with whole proteins, which allows delivery of more amino acids in less volume. This may be advantageous in hypermetabolic or elderly patients, who often require increased amounts of protein but have limited ability to tolerate large volumes of fluid (Feller et al, 1990).

Selection of a formula that provides sufficient total nitrogen as protein or amino acids is essential for all patients. However, low-protein formulations [Amin-Aid, Suplena, Travasorb Renal] are indicated for patients with severe renal failure who should not receive more than 0.3 g/kg daily (Talbot, 1990). In contrast, dialysis patients require 1 to 1.2 g/kg daily to maintain nitrogen balance (Lindsay et al, 1994). Formulas enriched with branched-chain amino acids [Hepatic-Aid II, NutriHep] may be useful for adults and children with impending or actual encephalopathy secondary to hepatic insufficiency or portacaval shunts (Talbot, 1990; Chin et al, 1992). Preparations containing increased amounts of protein or amino acids (supplying 2 to 2.5 g/kg daily) [Impact, Replete, Perative, Promote, Traum-Aid HBC, TraumaCal, Stresstein] are indicated when the nitrogen requirement is increased, as in those with malnutrition, decubitus ulcers, trauma, burns, sepsis, or other causes of hypermetabolism; for wound healing following surgery; and during initial treatment of chronic pulmonary disease (Talbot, 1990; Breslow et al, 1993; Beal and Cerra, 1994). The efficient utilization of amino acids for tissue synthesis depends on adequate intake of calories, vitamins, and minerals.

Small amounts of levocarnitine are added to a number of enteral formulas. Although urinary carnitine excretion is elevated during recovery from trauma or surgery, signs of carnitine deficiency are rare (Rebouche, 1992; Wennberg et al, 1992). Endogenous synthesis of L-carnitine can satisfy requirements in virtually all patients without genetic carnitine deficiency, but those with carnitine-sensitive cardiomyopathies, hemodialysis patients, and those taking valproate or anthracycline antineoplastic agents may benefit from formulas fortified with carnitine (Po, 1990; Rose et al, 1992; Tanphaichitr and Leelahagul, 1993; Leibovitz and Mueller, 1993). See also the discussion on TPN in Pediatric Patients.

Glutamine may be a conditionally essential nutrient during critical illness (Souba, 1993; see also discussion in Central Venous Nutrition, Other Components). The amount of protein-bound glutamine present in whole protein or peptide-based enteral formulas depends on the protein source and amount used and is not affected by the method of processing. The estimated glutamine content of commercially available enteral formulas is given in Table 13.

Choline is required for the biosynthesis of phosphatidylcholine, lysophosphatidylcholine, choline plasmalogen, sphingomyelin, and acetylcholine and is a source of labile methyl groups. Choline deficiency in infants may result in memory impairment later in life; choline deficiency in adults causes liver dysfunction (elevated serum ALT activity, inability to secrete VLDL, and accumulation of 1,2-diacylglycerol) and leads to hepatic stenosis and predisposition to hepatocarcinoma (Buchman et al, 1992; Zeisel, 1992). Adults on nutri-

TABLE 13.
ESTIMATED GLUTAMINE CONTENT OF ENTERAL FORMULAS[1]

Preparations	Manufacturer	Glutamine g/1,000 kcal
Entrition HN	Clintec Nutrition	3.84 - 5.49
Nutren 1.0		3.47 - 5.11
Nutren 1.5		3.47 - 5.11
Nutren 2.0		3.47 - 5.11
Peptamen		3.00 - 3.80
Replete		5.43 - 7.99
Deliver 2.0	Mead Johnson Nutritionals	3.26 - 4.80
Isocal		2.80 - 3.91
Linisorb Liquid		3.69 - 5.43
Respalor		4.34 - 6.39
Sustacal		5.35 - 7.33
Sustacal HC		3.53 - 5.20
Sustacal with Fiber		3.79 - 5.27
Traumacal		4.80 - 7.07
Ultracal		3.61 - 5.32
Fiberlan	Elan Pharma	3.62 - 5.32
Isolan		3.27 - 4.82
Nitrolan		4.20 - 6.19
Ultralan		3.49 - 4.99
Ensure	Ross Laboratories	3.07 - 4.36
Ensure HN		3.65 - 5.21
Ensure Plus		3.19 - 4.54
Ensure Plus HN		3.63 - 5.19
Ensure with Fiber		3.15 - 4.46
Glucerna		3.63 - 5.34
Jevity		3.63 - 5.35
Osmolite		3.07 - 4.36
Osmolite HN		3.65 - 5.20
Pulmocare		3.62 - 5.33
TwoCal HN		3.64 - 5.35
Fibersource	Sandoz Nutrition	3.11 - 4.58
Fibersource HN		3.83 - 5.64
Impact		3.79 - 5.58
Isosource		3.11 - 4.58
Isosource HN		3.83 - 5.64
Resource		3.07 - 4.36
Resource Plus		3.19 - 4.54
Vivonex T.E.N.		4.90
Attain	Sherwood Medical	3.47 - 5.11
Comply		3.47 - 5.11
Magnacal		3.04 - 4.48
Profiber		3.47 - 5.11

[1] *Adapted from Swails et al, 1992.*

tion support require at least 800 mg of choline daily, and elderly patients often benefit from >2 g/day (Zeisel, 1992).

The rationale for selecting specific enteral formulas for stressed patients or those with renal, hepatic, or pulmonary disease parallels the rationale for selecting similar TPN formulas and is equally controversial. See the evaluations on Amino Acid Solutions: Renal Failure Formulas; Amino Acid Solutions: Branched Chain Amino Acid-Enriched Stress Formulas; and Amino Acid Solutions: Hepatic Formula for further discussion.

Fat: The amount of fat in enteral formulas varies considerably. Many commercial formulas contain a high percentage of their total calories as polyunsaturated fatty acids, but some have a very low total fat content. Fat sources included most commonly are canola oil and corn oil, which contain medium-chain triglycerides (MCT), and soy oil and safflower oil, which contain predominantly long-chain triglycerides (LCT). All LCT are absorbed efficiently by patients with normal digestive and absorptive capabilities, although unsaturated LCT are better absorbed than saturated LCT.

Inclusion of oils containing MCT in enteral formulations is common. MCT are absorbed better than LCT (1) when the intestinal endothelium is damaged and fat absorption is inhibited (as in resection of the small intestine, celiac disease, Whipple's disease, Crohn's disease, enteritis, and gluten enteropathy); (2) when transport of fat from epithelial cells into the lymphatic system is impaired or lymphatic flow is obstructed (as in chylomicron deficiency, intestinal lymphangiectasia, chyluria, chylous ascites, and chylothorax); and (3) when the secretion of conjugated bile salts or pancreatic enzymes is decreased (as in biliary atresia, obstructive jaundice, primary biliary cirrhosis, pancreatitis, pancreatectomy, and cystic fibrosis). However, MCT do not provide essential fatty acids, provide only 8.3 kcal/g, and their use in large amounts can lead to ketosis. MCT should be used with caution in patients with diabetes or advanced cirrhosis.

Low-fat formulations are useful for the patient with maldigestion with malabsorption of fat (as in acute pancreatitis) (Pisters and Ranson, 1992). To prevent fatty acid deficiency, especially during long-term use, some source of linoleic acid is present in all low-fat formulations. In *adults,* the amount of total essential fatty acids should approximate 3% to 5% of total calories ingested.

If malabsorption is severe, a low-fat formulation is recommended initially with LCT or MCT added gradually as tolerated. In patients with cirrhosis or portacaval shunts, excessive intake of fatty acids of any chain length may act synergistically with ammonia and other toxins to exacerbate or cause hepatic encephalopathy. Patients with pulmonary dysfunction may benefit from a high-fat preparation (eg, NutriVent, Pulmocare), because metabolism of lipids generates less CO_2 than does oxidative glycolysis. Unfortunately, immune suppression, diarrhea, and delayed gastric emptying are common adverse reactions to high-fat formulas and often require their discontinuation.

Many of the conditions requiring EN are characterized by overproduction of cytokines and eicosanoids (Hardin, 1993; Lowry, 1993; Meydani and Dinarello, 1993; Shronts, 1993). Oral administration of omega-3 polyunsaturated fatty acids (ω-3 PUFA) has been shown to reduce production of these biologic response mediators in several clinical conditions, including ulcerative colitis (Ross, 1993), and during postoperative recovery (Daly et al, 1992; Alexander, 1993). However, substantial reduction in immune system responsiveness may impair normal healing and disease resistance. In addition, ω-3 PUFA reduce antioxidant status and may themselves contribute to free radical production and accelerated lipid peroxidation.

Residue: The amount of residue in the formulation largely determines fecal bulk. Some residue is produced from intestinal cell sloughing or bacteria even when no food is ingested orally. Patients with chronic partial bowel obstruction should consume low-residue preparations.

Dietary Fiber: Fiber is a natural component of most foods. Its primary physiologic function is to regulate bowel function. Commercially available liquid diets have traditionally been low in fiber and residue, but soy fiber, guar, and oat fiber have been incorporated into enteral formulas. Soy fiber is rich in insoluble cellulose (16.4% of total fiber) and insoluble noncellulose saccharides (arabinose, 17.5% of total fiber; xylose, 6.1%; and galactose, 32.5%) and contains a substantial proportion of uronic acids (pectins, 13.5% of total fiber) (Elia, 1989); guar consists entirely of soluble polysaccharides. These saccharides and polysaccharides are extensively fermented by human cecal anaerobic microflora, generating the short-chain fatty acids (SCFA), acetate, propionate, and butyrate, and contribute little to fecal bulk. Acetate and propionate are absorbed by the colon and stimulate the resorption of water by solvent drag and of sodium by a sodium-hydrogen cotransporter. The process of microbial fermentation enriches the microflora, and increased stool weight results from increased fecal bacterial mass. These properties of dietary fiber and its fermentation products reduce the incidence of diarrhea in humans during EN (Liebl et al, 1990). The fermentation waste product, butyrate, is metabolized directly by colonocytes and stimulates crypt proliferation; this function may be critical to maintain large bowel integrity (Shronts, 1988). Whether added dietary fiber is beneficial in those with impaired bowel function remains to be demonstrated (Scheppach and Bartram, 1993).

Soy polysaccharide inhibits calcium and magnesium absorption in a dose-dependent fashion (Taper et al, 1988), but the amounts of fiber added to EN formulas do not significantly affect mineral balance.

Purines: The small intestine lacks a pathway of de novo purine biosynthesis, and purine-free diets are immunosuppressive (Seidman et al, 1991). In contrast, exogenous nucleotides promote T-lymphocyte maturation and cytokine secretion, increase natural killer cell activity, and enhance small intestinal growth and resistance to bacterial infections. A formula that combines added arginine, nucleotides, and ω-3 fatty acids [Impact] has stimulated lymphocyte proliferative responses in patients with persistent sepsis and after abdominal surgery (Cerra et al, 1991) and has decreased postoperative complications and length of hospital stay (Daly et al, 1992).

Flavoring: Flavored oral preparations are preferred by most patients, and the medical staff should be aware of the taste characteristics of these formulations. Oral formulations are best tolerated when served at temperatures consistent with the patient's preference. Flavorings also can be added to some enteral formulas via available flavor packets. Diets given by tube should be unflavored, particularly when used in infants.

Fluid and Electrolytes: Fluid must be available to satisfy water requirements, especially for patients who are completely dependent on these formulations or those who have impaired renal concentrating ability. To prevent dehydration, sufficient intake of fluid is needed to replace insensible water loss, sweat, a reasonable amount of urine, and gastrointestinal losses. Standard EN formulas (1 kcal/ml) contain approximately 80% to 85% water. Additional electrolytes may be required in patients with some salt-losing nephropathies, diarrhea, fistulas, burns, or other conditions in which there is excessive electrolyte loss.

Vitamins and Minerals: A minimum volume of any EN formula must be ingested to satisfy 100% of all micronutrient requirements (see Table 15). Some formulas provide inadequate amounts of minerals, particularly zinc, potassium, and magnesium, for patients with pronounced gastrointestinal losses, and these must be supplemented if enteral formulas are the sole source of nutrition for prolonged periods. Manufacturers now are adding a variety of trace elements to the formulations. To avoid hypoprothrombinemia, vitamin K also should be a component if administration is prolonged. However, patients receiving oral anticoagulants should be monitored because the dietary vitamin K content of some preparations can interfere with anticoagulation.

Nutrient Delivery

Oral Feeding: Nutritionally complete, liquified food and defined formulas are indicated for patients with no special nutritional requirements and those with mild to moderate impairment of absorptive surface area or digestive enzyme function who are capable of digesting intact protein, long-chain fats, or complex branched-chain polysaccharides. If oral ingestion is feasible and gastrointestinal tract function is adequate, enteral formulas can be given to increase nutrient intake in patients with trauma, malignancies, cachexia, or protein-calorie malnutrition.

Tube Feeding: Tube feedings using nasogastric, nasoduodenal, nasojejunal, esophagostomy, gastrostomy, or jejunostomy tubes may be necessary for infants, patients with mechanical chewing or swallowing problems, comatose patients, and those with partially impaired gastrointestinal function or anorexia. Because of the irritation caused by the nasal tube and its lack of cosmetic appeal to the patient and public in long-term feeding situations, ostomy tubes are often used. The percutaneous placement of a small-bore tube into the stomach (percutaneous endoscopic gastrostomy) or jejunum (percutaneous endoscopic jejunostomy) under local anesthesia and endoscopic control are gaining wide popularity for patients who require long-term feeding.

Commercial formulations, especially when delivered via pump, must pass through small-bore (8F) tubes. Finely suspended preparations are required when tube feeding is necessary. Food blended in ordinary kitchen equipment is not suitable because the larger particles may clog small-bore tubes. In addition, the risk of bacterial contamination is greater when home-blending is used.

The amount and rate of administration should be individualized, based on the patient's condition, the specific formula administered, and the method of administration. Hyperosmolar formulations should be started at full-strength but initial infusion rates of 15 to 25 ml/hr are preferable. Incremental increases of up to 25 ml/hr each 8- to 24-hour period are generally tolerated and will allow the patient to achieve estimated nutrient needs within three days of initiation of EN feedings (ASPEN, 1993). However, adjustment can be a lengthy process during which the patient is not receiving the daily nutritional requirements, and TPN may need to be continued during the transition to EN feedings (Epps, 1988). Other clinicians feel that this conservative regimen offers no benefit compared with full feeding with isotonic formulations beginning on the first day (Zarling et al, 1986; Pesola et al, 1990; Koruda, 1991).

To provide optimal nutritional support for the patient in transition from parenteral to enteral support, the feeding regimen should allow for adaptive increases in digestive enzymes and digestive surface area within the gut by progressing with small increases in the volume of full-strength formula delivered (Braunschweig et al, 1988).

For slow-drip feeding into the small intestine, use of an automated infusion pump is recommended; absorption and tolerance are improved and the incidence of adverse reactions is reduced by slow constant feeding over many hours rather than repeated bolus feedings that are typical with gastric administration. This method of administration prevents the dumping syndrome, which occurs when hyperosmolar solutions are introduced rapidly into the small intestine. Jejunal feeding should be initiated with slow infusion of full-strength formulas and gradually increasing the infusion rate ('Gottschlich et al, 1988).

Adverse Reactions and Precautions

Overall, 10% of patients receiving EN through a nasogastric tube experience some type of complication (Cataldi-Betcher et al, 1983). Gastrointestinal disturbances (eg, diarrhea, inadequate gastric emptying, vomiting, gastrointestinal bleeding) are the most common complications. About 25% to 50% of patients experiencing gastrointestinal complications require TPN, at least temporarily. Administration of a mucilaginous hydrophilic colloid bulk laxative (7 g/L of liquid formula), cholestyramine (4 g/L), bismuth subsalicylate (20 mg/L), or kaolin (200 g/L) plus pectin (300 mg/L) can reduce nonspecific diarrhea without additional complications or discontinuation of EN, although these medications may clog small-bore feeding tubes (Frank and Green, 1979; Koruda, 1991).

Concomitant administration of oral electrolyte solutions and certain medications through the EN feeding tube often causes gastrointestinal disturbances (Edes et al, 1990; Koruda, 1991; Eisenberg, 1993). Hyperosmolar electrolyte solutions and medications can be diluted with water, mixed with EN solutions to reduce osmolarity, or given parenterally. Many drugs commonly given in elixir form during EN feedings contain sorbitol (Table 14) in amounts sufficient to cause diarrhea, and these elixirs should be discontinued if diarrhea occurs. Many antibiotics affect the colonic microflora and can cause diarrhea; their use may necessitate concomitant administration of antidiarrheal medications (see above).

TABLE 14.
ORAL MEDICATIONS CONTAINING SORBITOL[1]

Acetaminophen elixir [Tylenol]
Aluminum hydroxide gels [generic]
Amantadine hydrochloride solution [Symmetrel]
Aminocaproic acid syrup [Amicar]
Calcium carbonate suspension [generic]
Carbamazepine suspension [Tegretol]
Chloral hydrate syrup [generic]
Chlorpromazine hydrochloride solution [Chlorpromazine Hydrochloride Intensol]
Cimetidine solution [Tagamet]
Co-trimoxazole suspension [generic]
Diazepam solution [generic]
Digoxin elixir [generic]
Diphenoxylate hydrochloride [generic]
Ferrous sulfate solution [Fer-in-sol]
Furosemide solution [generic; Lasix]
Guaifenesin syrup [generic[2]]
Hydroxyzine solution [generic]
Ibuprofen suspension [generic[2]]
Isoniazid syrup [generic]
Lithium citrate syrup [generic]
Methadone hydrochloride solution [generic]
Metoclopramide syrup [generic]
Molindone concentrate [Moban]
Morphine sulfate solution [generic]
Oxybutynin syrup [Ditropan]
Perphenazine solution [Trilafon]
Pseudoephedrine syrup [Actifed; Sudafed]
Pyridostigmine bromide syrup [Mestinon]
Ranitidine syrup [Zantac]
Tetracycline hydrochloride suspension [Sumycin]
Theophylline solution [generic]
Valproate sodium syrup [Depakene]
Vitamin E solution [Aquasol]

1 Adapted from Lutomski et al, 1993.
2 Sorbitol-free: Dilantin-125 (phenobarbital elixir), Pedia-Profen (ibuprofen suspension), Robitussin (guaifenesin syrup)

The most serious and most frequent mechanical complication of tube feeding is aspiration pneumonitis, although pleural effusion, empyema, pneumomediastinum, bronchopleural fistula, and hydropneumothorax can occur (Cabré and Gassull, 1993). Patients should be kept in a semisitting position (head of the bed elevated 30°) during feeding and for one hour thereafter. The loss of gag reflex, hiccuping, a tendency to vomit, or a history of pulmonary aspiration of gastric contents is a contraindication to bolus feeding through a nasopharyngeal tube, and even feeding by slow drip should be undertaken with great caution. In high-risk patients receiving slow-drip feeding, the tube should be inserted into the duodenum or jejunum with simultaneous nasogastric decompression. Otherwise, intravenous feeding should be instituted. When tube feeding is used cautiously, aspiration secondary to tracheobronchial passage of feeding tubes occurs in less than 1% of patients.

Metabolic complications secondary to EN feeding can be minimized by close monitoring of the serum pH, osmolarity, and electrolyte and glucose concentrations every two to three days initially until the optimum dose and rate of administration is attained. The monitoring interval then can be extended gradually to once or twice weekly. Hyperglycemia progressing to nonketotic coma can result from administration of excessive carbohydrate and protein. Caution is required in patients prone to hyperglycemia (eg, those with pancreatitis or diabetes mellitus; those taking glucocorticoids, adrenergic drugs, or potent diuretics). Large amounts of carbohydrates with inadequate phosphate also can cause significant hypophosphatemia in three to seven days. If necessary, phosphate supplements should be given intravenously because administration through the tube may cause diarrhea.

The electrolyte content of enteral preparations should be reviewed carefully. Patients with excessive intestinal loss of fluid and electrolytes (eg, fistula, diarrhea) may require oral or intravenous administration of additional sodium, potassium, and trace elements.

Occasionally, malnourished patients develop congestive heart failure during nonvolitional refeeding. In some cases, this has been attributed to excessive fluid and nutrient loading, which may be inadvertent but also may result from intentional efforts to compensate for presumed absorptive inefficiencies. Malnourished patients absorb nutrients only slightly less efficiently than well-nourished individuals, and careful monitoring of fluid, calorie, and sodium infusion rates is required during continuous EN to avoid the cardiovascular complications associated with overfeeding (Casper et al, 1990; Benya et al, 1991).

Contaminated enteral products may cause diarrhea, nausea, vomiting, chills, and fever. Contamination of enteral solutions occurs primarily during the preparation process. After dry or liquid preparations are mixed or diluted with water, respectively, they serve as excellent culture media and should be refrigerated promptly and used within 24 to 48 hours. Unopened dry preparations can be kept at room temperatures below 95° F (see the manufacturers' literature).

Four variables that significantly affect microbial growth in enteral solutions after preparation are initial microbial inoculation, solution hang time, the pH of the solution, and the presence of a preservative (Sami et al, 1988). Except for unopened liquid formulas, enteral formulas and containers generally are not sterile, and precautions must be taken to minimize additional microbial contamination. However, use of vacuum-packed, prefilled enteral formulas has reduced the likelihood of contamination and bacterial growth.

It is essential to compound the product as soon as possible before use, refrigerate the final product until it is to be administered, and minimize hang time at room temperature. It may be advantageous to provide eight-hour containers so that a minimal amount of final product is exposed to room temperature at a time. With pre-packaged products in closed systems, hang time for up to 24 to 36 hours is acceptable (Epps, 1988).

Freezing enteral products should be avoided. Freezing may damage packaging and allow contamination. Thawing after freezing may result in prolonged warming and spoilage (Enteral Nutrition Council, 1988).

Manufacturers' instructions should be consulted for specific recommendations concerning individual products.

Available Formulations

POLYMERIC FORMULAS. These preparations contain intact protein, complex carbohydrates, and fats of high molecular weight for patients with normal gastrointestinal function. The source of protein is generally casein, soy protein, pureed meats, or egg albumin. A few formulas containing lactose as a source of carbohydrate are generally used as oral supplements. Fats provide approximately 20% to 45% of the total calories and usually improve the palatability of polymeric formulas. Depending on the type of enteral formula, 1 to 2 L/day are required to provide 100% of all vitamin and mineral requirements (Mobarhan and Trumbore, 1991). (See Table 15.)

Polymeric formulations also are indicated for patients with an obstruction below the small bowel and for those with mild to moderate impairment of the absorptive surface area or digestive enzyme activities who are capable of digesting intact proteins, long-chain fats, and complex branched-chain polysaccharides. Patients with obstruction can be fed via tube if food enters the digestive tract beyond the site of obstruction. Many polymeric formulas are flavored and are accepted by patients when taken orally. Polymeric diets designed for tube feeding usually are isotonic, but those intended as oral supplements often are hypertonic.

A complex diet (the Shriners' burn diet) supplemented with arginine (5 g/1,000 kcal), histidine (1 g/1,000 kcal), cysteine (1 g/1,000 kcal), and ω-3 fatty acids (6 g/1,000 kcal) markedly reduces the incidence of bacteremia, wound infection, and pneumonia and decreases length of hospital stay in patients with extensive third-degree burns (Alexander and Gottschlich, 1990).

ELEMENTAL DIETS. These formulas provide essential nutrients in a readily assimilated form, require little or no active digestion of the dietary components, decrease gastric secretions and reduce stool bulk, and often have minimal residue (Table 15). They flow easily through a small-bore tube directly into the stomach, duodenum, or jejunum. Many are composed of chemically isolated food derivatives that may not require digestion and may be well absorbed in the jejunum and upper ileum. The degree of absorption depends on the efficacy of the absorption processes and the amount of normal absorptive surface present.

Elemental diets are indicated only when luminal hydrolysis or absorption is impaired (eg, in patients with inflammatory bowel disease, severe exocrine pancreatic enzyme deficiency, AIDS, cystic fibrosis, or short bowel syndrome; after surgery or radiation therapy to the gastrointestinal tract; in patients who have had no enteral stimulation for prolonged periods and who probably have mucosal atrophy). They should be used as adjuncts to or instead of TPN when EN can provide adequate calories.

Elemental diets are more effective than polymeric formulas in a number of conditions. Spontaneous closure of lower alimentary tract fistulas has occurred with the use of elemental diets. Pancreatitis complicated by alcoholism or gallstones when oral feeding is not feasible may respond well to elemental diets administered through a tube with the tip in the small bowel (ideally, past the ligament of Treitz). In patients with chronic pancreatic insufficiency, steatorrhea has been reduced by elemental diets that replace a portion of the LCT with MCT. However, patients with pancreatic disorders also may have diabetes mellitus, and the additional glucose load imposed by the generally greater carbohydrate content of elemental diets may require adjustment of the dose of hypoglycemic drug. Peptide-based elemental formulas (eg, Peptamen) contain less carbohydrate and may be preferable in patients with diabetes mellitus who require a pre-digested formula.

Elemental diets also may be more effective than polymeric formulas in achieving remission in patients with nonulcerative inflammatory bowel disease (Lochs et al, 1991; Raouf et al, 1991; Kushner, 1992; Sitrin, 1992; Sutton, 1992); the addition of glutamine may increase their effectiveness (Giaffer et al, 1990). The duration of remission depends on the disease site and is greater in more proximal sites (Teahon et al, 1990). In children with Crohn's disease, elemental diets (eg, Neocate One+) reverse growth failure and malnutrition; often induce and maintain remission, even in steroid-dependent individuals; reduce the required doses of immunosuppressive medications; control diarrhea; and enhance healing after surgery (Seidman et al, 1991).

Malabsorption and short bowel syndrome respond well to elemental diets administered as a slow drip over many hours following initial use of TPN. This stimulates luminal absorption and reverses the intestinal mucosal atrophy induced by prolonged TPN. Elemental diets also are useful for individuals with galactosemia, lactase deficiency, allergy to milk protein, and glycogen storage disease and for diagnosing food allergy.

Commercial elemental diets are formulated for adults but can be used in infants and children if the rate of administration is reduced and the patient is observed closely and monitored carefully to prevent hyperosmolar dehydration. In addition, the rate of gastric emptying can be increased and the incidence of gastric reflux and vomiting decreased in children by using whey-based elemental diets (Fried et al, 1992). However, these formulas require supplementation in order to satisfy the nutritional requirements of infants and children. For infants and children on long-term feeding without oral supplements, a formula containing a source of essential fatty acids with linolenic acid and linoleic acid is advisable.

See Table 15.

MODULAR FORMULAS. Modular formulas are used as supplements or as base formulas to which specified components are added as needed (Table 16). They are not intended to be the sole source of nutrients and, depending on which formula is used, must be compounded with sources of carbohydrate, protein, fat, minerals, and vitamins or used with ordinary foods to provide complete nutrition. Familiarity with the composition of these products before prescription is essential, since they may provide some nutrients in excess of requirements for certain patients.

FORMULAS FOR NORMAL INFANTS. These formulas may be used to provide nutrients for normal full-term bottle-fed infants or as a supplement for breast-fed infants (Table 17). They have been formulated to provide nutrients in proportions similar to those present in human breast milk and to support growth and development as effectively as human breast milk; formulas are available as ready-to-feed preparations or as concentrated liquid or powder for dilution with water. Standard infant formulas are nutritionally complete and meet or exceed FDA guidelines (Table 17), although, contrary to common belief, their composition is not standardized.

All standard infant formulas contain a minimum of 0.15 mg of iron/100 kcal; those providing less than 1 mg of iron/100 kcal may not provide sufficient iron for low-birth-weight infants. If the formula contains insufficient iron, supplemental amounts should be given. The American Academy of Pediatrics recommends at least 1 mg iron/100 kcal of formula (American Academy of Pediatrics Committee on Nutrition, 1989). Use of supplemental amounts of iron should be initiated immediately when iron deficiency is suspected (Oski, 1993); developmental deficits caused by iron deficiency may be reversible through 18 months of age (Idjradinata and Pollitt, 1993).

Lactose is the carbohydrate found in human breast milk and its presence in infant formulas enhances the absorption of calcium, magnesium, and zinc; helps establish normal colonic microflora; and can be used to synthesize brain glycolipids. Lactose-free formulas given during episodes of gastroenteritis with diarrhea may accelerate recovery (Chandra et al, 1989), although whether they are more effective than lactose-containing formulas is controversial (Brown et al, 1994). Infants who have galactosemia (a rare inherited disorder occurring in 1 to 4 of 100,000 births) should not be fed formulas containing lactose.

Human breast milk contains at least 50 fatty acids of chain length 10 or greater (Jensen et al, 1992). On average, palmitic acid comprises 22% of the total fatty acid content of human milk, stearic acid 8%, oleic acid 31%, linoleic acid 11%, linolenic acid 1%, eicosapentaenoic acid 0.2%, and docosahexaenoic acid 0.25%. It has been recommended that infant formulas provide 12% to 20% of their total fatty acids as linoleic acid (500 to 700 mg/kg/day) and 1.6% to 4% as the sum of all ω-3 fatty acids (70 to 150 mg/kg/day), with the latter equally divided between linolenic acid and the sum of eicosapentaenoic and docosahexaenoic acids (Jensen and Jensen, 1992 A). Docosahexaenoic acid improves visual function in infants, and arachidonic acid may be needed for improved growth (Carlson et al, 1993 A, 1993 B). Infant formulas with lipid composition resembling that of human milk (eg, Good Start) may be preferable (Williams, 1993; Cockburn, 1994).

FORMULAS FOR PRETERM INFANTS. Premature birth interrupts growth and overall nutrient accretion, resulting in poorer body stores of fat, minerals, trace metals, and some vitamins. Preterm infants fed standard infant formulas or nonfortified, banked human breast milk often are growth-retarded and have moderate motor impairment at 9 and 18 months of age (Lucas et al, 1989 A, 1989 B, 1990). Formulas designed specially for preterm infants increase linear growth, weight gain, and motor function (Lucas et al, 1990, 1992), and they should be fed to infants born before 36 weeks of gestational age and to all those weighing <1.5 kg at birth (Table 17). The efficiency of fat and total energy utilization is greater when preterm infants receive continuous enteral infusions than when they receive intermittent bolus feedings (Grant and Denne, 1991; Harrison and Peat, 1992).

Inadequate intake of several key nutrients may limit growth in preterm infants. Daily calcium and phosphorus intakes over 100 mg/100 kcal and 50 mg/100 kcal, respectively, markedly accelerate bone mineral accretion and increase body length in preterm infants compared with standard infant formulas (Horsman et al, 1989; Lucas et al, 1992; Bishop et al, 1993; Chan, 1993). Low-phosphorus formula feeding also has been associated with sodium deficiency (Manz et al, 1992). Preterm infants weighing <1.5 kg who ingest 2.9 g of protein/100 kcal (160% the minimum required by law) gain weight significantly faster (American Academy of Pediatrics Committee on Nutrition, 1985; Polberger et al, 1990 B). Increasing protein intake to 3.2 g/100 kcal significantly improved scores on the Neonatal Behavior Assessment Scale (Bhatia et al, 1991). Detailed guidelines for enteral feeding of preterm infants have been provided by Lucas (1993).

Medium-chain fatty acids (MCT) are substituted for up to one-half of the LCT in several formulas. However, when formulas low or high in MCT content were fed to infants weighing <1.8 kg on a presumably equal gross energy basis, no improvements in energy digestibility, metabolism, expenditure, or storage; nitrogen absorption or retention; calcium, phosphorus, or magnesium absorption or retention; or weight gain occurred (Whyte et al, 1986; Sulkers et al, 1992 A, 1992 B). The lack of positive effect of replacing LCT with MCT may result from the adherence of substantial amounts of MCT to feeding tubes (Mehta et al, 1991). In addition, the absorption of MCT and LCT is similar in preterm infants (Hamosh et al, 1991). It is doubtful that amounts of MCT exceeding 10% to 15% of total fatty acids will be beneficial in the absence of malabsorption (Jensen and Jensen, 1992 B).

FORMULA INTOLERANCE. Intolerance or sensitivity to formulas develops in as many as one in five infants. Immunologic, metabolic, pharmacologic, toxic, and idiosyncratic reactions occur; symptoms range from crying to anaphylaxis and involve the gastrointestinal, respiratory, dermatologic, or central nervous systems. Sleep disturbances also may be attributable to formula intolerance. The increased natural perme-

TABLE 15.
ELEMENTAL AND POLYMERIC DIETS FOR ENTERAL FEEDING

Preparations	kcal/ml	mOsm/kg	Per 1,000 kcal Protein (g)	Fat (g)	CHO[1] (g)	Sodium (mg)	Potassium (mg)	Calcium (mg)
LACTOSE-CONTAINING FORMULAS								
Milk-Based Formulas								
Lonalac Powder (Mead Johnson Nutritionals)	1.01	360	53	55	74	40	2000	1760
Meritene Powder (Sandoz Nutrition)	1.06	690	65	32	113.2	1020	2640	2075
Compleat Regular Liquid (Sandoz Nutrition)	1.07	450	40	40	120	1200	1300	630
Sustacal Powder (Mead Johnson Nutritionals)	1.08	950	72	2.4	166	1110	3300	2000
Sustagen Powder (Mead Johnson Nutritionals)	1.86	1130	62	9	169	560	1820	1820
LACTOSE-FREE FORMULAS								
Protein Source: Amino Acids								
Tolerex Liquid (Sandoz Nutrition)	1	550	21	1.5	230	468	1173	556
Vivonex T.E.N. Liquid (Sandoz Nutrition)	1	630	38	2.8	210	460	780	500
Vivonex Plus (Sandoz Nutrition)	1	650	45	7.0	189	611	1060	556
Protein Source: Amino Acids and Enzymatically Hydrolyzed Proteins								
Accupep HPF Liquid (Sherwood)	1	490	40	10	189	680	1150	625
Peptamen Liquid (Clintec Nutrition)	1	270	40	39	127	500	1250	800
Peptamen Oral (Clintec Nutrition)	2	380	40	39	127	500	1252	800
Peptamen VHP Diet (Clintec Nutrition)	1	300	63	39	104	560	1500	800
Reabilan Liquid (Elan Pharma)	1	350	31.5	38.9	131.5	699	1251	499
Travasorb STD Powder (Clintec Nutrition)	1	560	30	13.5	190	921	1170	—
Vital High Nitrogen Powder (Ross)	1	500	41.7	10.8	185	566	1400	667
Criticare HN Liquid (Mead Johnson Nutritionals)	1.06	650	36	5	200	600	1240	500
Isosource Liquid (Sandoz Nutrition)	1.2	360	36	34	140	1000	1400	560
Isosource HN Liquid (Sandoz Nutrition)	1.2	330	44	34	130	890	1400	560
Protein Source: Enzymatically Hydrolyzed Proteins								
Half-Strength Entrition Liquid (Clintec Nutrition)	0.5	120	35	35	136	700	2000	500
Pre-Attain Liquid (Sherwood)	0.5	150	40	40	120	680	1150	—
Introlan (Elan Pharma)	0.53	150	35.8	34.9	134.8	597	997	594
Introlite Liquid (Ross)	0.53	220	41.9	34.7	133	1755	2963	1430

[1] *Carbohydrate*

Per 1,000 kcal						Volume to Supply 1,000 kcal (ml)	kcal to Supply 100% of USRDA for Vitamins	Volume to Supply 100% of USRDA (ml)	Comment
Phosphorus (mg)	Magnesium (mg)	Zinc (mg)	Copper (mg)	Chromium (mcg)	Selenium (mcg)				
1560	141	—	—	—	—	990	—	—	Low sodium.
1820	360	13.6	1.82	—	0	945	1100	1040	Gluten-free.
1130	250	14.4	1.25	94	62.5	943	1600	1500	Contains dietary fiber 4.2 g/ 1000 ml.
1720	460	17.2	2.4	—	—	930	910	830	
1360	230	11.3	1.1	—	—	540	1770	950	
556	222	8.3	1.11	28	83	1000	1800	1800	Cholesterol-free.
500	200	10	1	17	50	1000	2000	2000	Cholesterol-free.
556	222	12.5	1.11	—	55.6	1000	—	—	Cholesterol-free.
625	250	15	1.50	—	—	1000	1600	1600	Contains MCT. For GI conditions.
700	400	14	1.40	40	40	1000	1500	1500	Gluten-free; cholesterol-free. Contains MCT.
700	400	14	1.4	40	40	1500	1500	1500	Cholesterol-free. Contains MCT.
700	300	24	2	—	50	1000	1500	1500	Cholesterol-free. Contains MCT.
499	251	10	1.60	62	50.7	1000	2250	2250	Contains MCT.
500						1000	2000	2000	Gluten-free. Contains MCT.
667	267	15	1.4	67	47	1000	1500	1500	Contains MCT.
500	200	10	1	—	—	940	2000	1890	Cholesterol-free.
560	220	14	1.1	83	83.3	833	1800	1500	Gluten-free. Contains canola oil, MCT.
560	220	14	1.1	83	83.3	833	1800	1500	Gluten-free. Contains canola oil, MCT.
500	200	7.5	1	—	—	2000	2000	4000	
625	500	30	3	—	—	2000	800	2560	
594	239	9	1.20	—	—	1887	1060	2000	Contains MCT.
1430	574	32.3	2.87	143.4	100	1887	700	1321	

(table continued on next page)

TABLE 15 (continued)

Preparations	kcal/ml	mOsm/kg	Per 1,000 kcal Protein (g)	Fat (g)	CHO (g)	Sodium (mg)	Potassium (mg)	Calcium (mg)
Citrotein Powder (Sandoz Nutrition)	0.67	490	62	2.4	183	1000	824	1590
Citrisource (Sandoz Nutrition)	0.76	700	49	0	200	306	83	750
Precision Isotonic Powder (Sandoz Nutrition)	0.96	300	30	31	150	800	821	670
Attain Liquid (Sherwood)	1	300	40	35	135	805	1600	960
Entrition HN Liquid (Clintec Nutrition)	1	300	44	41	114	920	1579	770
Impact Liquid (Sandoz Nutrition)	1	375	56	28	130	1070	1270	800
Impact with Fiber (Sandoz Nutrition)	1	375	56	28	140	1070	1270	800
Lipisorb Powder (Mead Johnson Nutritionals)	1	320	35	48	115	740	1250	700
Nutren 1.0 Liquid (Clintec Nutrition)	1	300	40	38	127	500	1250	700
Nutren 1.0 with Fiber (Clintec Nutrition)	1	300	40	38	127	500	1250	700
Pediasure Liquid (Ross)	1	310	30	50	110	380	1310	970
Portagen Powder (Mead Johnson Nutritionals)	1	350	35	48	115	550	1250	940
Profiber Liquid (Sherwood)	1	330	40	35	147	800	1500	80
Replete Liquid-Flavored (Clintec Nutrition)	1	350	62.5	34	112.8	500	1550	800
Replete Liquid-Unflavored (Clintec Nutrition)	1	290	62.5	34	113	500	1560	1000
Replete with Fiber (Clintec Nutrition)	1	290	62.5	34	113	500	1560	1000
Sustacal Liquid (Mead Johnson Nutritionals)	1	650	61	23	140	930	2000	1010
Travasorb MCT Powder (Clintec Nutrition)	1	312	49.3	33	122.8	350	1000	—
Vitaneed Liquid (Sherwood)	1	300	40	40	128	630	1250	667
Ensure Liquid (Ross)	1.06	470	35.2	35.2	137.2	800	1480	500
Ensure HN Liquid (Ross)	1.06	470	42	33.6	133.6	760	1480	715
Isocal Liquid (Mead Johnson Nutritionals)	1.06	270	32.1	41.5	128	500	1240	600
Isocal HN Liquid (Mead Johnson Nutritionals)	1.06	270	41.5	42.4	116.9	877	1509	791

Per 1,000 kcal						Volume to Supply 1,000 kcal (ml)	kcal to Supply 100% of USRDA for Vitamins	Volume to Supply 100% of USRDA (ml)	Comment
Phosphorus (mg)	**Magnesium (mg)**	**Zinc (mg)**	**Copper (mg)**	**Chromium (mcg)**	**Selenium (mcg)**				
1590	630	23.5	3.1	—	0	1490	730	1100	Cholesterol-free.
890	278	21	1.4	—	0	1320	1890	1890	Cholesterol-free.
670	270	10	1.3	100	67	1040	1500	1560	Gluten-free; cholesterol-free; purine-free.
800	320	24	1.60	100	100	1000	1250	1250	Gluten-free. Contains MCT.
770	308	11.6	1.54	—	—	1000	1300	1300	Contains structured lipids, menhaden oil, arginine, purines, and dietary fiber 10 g/1000 ml.
800	267	15.3	1.70	100	100	1000	1500	1500	Contains structured lipids, menhaden oil, arginine, purines.
800	270	15.3	1.67	100	100	1000	1500	1500	
700	200	10	1	—	—	1000	2000	2000	Contains MCT.
700	340	14	1.40	40	40	1000	1500	1500	Gluten-free; cholesterol-free. Contains MCT.
700	340	14	1.40	40	40	1000	1500	1500	Gluten-free; cholesterol-free. Contains MCT.
800	200	12	1	30	23	1000	1000	1000	Gluten-free. Contains MCT.
700	200	9.4	1.56	—	—	1000	3800	3800	Contains MCT.
800	320	24	1.60	150	100	1000	1250	1250	Contains dietary fiber 12 g/1000 kcal.
720	400	14	1.40	—	0	1000	1500	1500	Gluten-free; cholesterol-free.
1000	400	24	2	140	100	1000	1000	1000	Cholesterol free. Contains MCT.
1000	400	24	2	140	100	1000	1000	1000	Cholesterol free. Contains MCT.
930	380	13.9	2	—	—	1000	1080	1060	
—	—	—	—	—	—	—	—	—	Gluten-free. Contains MCT.
667	267	20	1.50	—	—	1000	1500	1500	Contains dietary fiber 8 g/1000 kcal
500	200	11.3	1	50	35	943	2000	1887	
715	286	16.1	1.51	72	50	943	1400	1321	
500	200	10	1.04	50	50	943	2003	1890	Contains MCT.
792	321	16	1.60	79	56	943	1251	1180	Contains MCT.

(table continued on next page)

TABLE 15 (continued)

Preparations	kcal/ml	mOsm/kg	Per 1,000 kcal Protein (g)	Fat (g)	CHO (g)	Sodium (mg)	Potassium (mg)	Calcium (mg)
Jevity Liquid (Ross)	1.06	300	42	33.9	143.1	877	1480	860
Nutrilan Liquid (Elan Pharma)	1.06	450	35.8	34.9	134.8	597	997	594
Isolan Liquid (Elan Pharma)	1.06	300	37.7	33.9	135.8	651	1103	754
Osmolite Liquid (Ross)	1.06	300	35.2	35.5	137.2	600	960	500
Osmolite HN Liquid (Ross)	1.06	300	42	33.9	133	877	1480	715
Resource Crystals (Sandoz Nutrition)	1.06	450	35.2	35.2	137.2	800	1480	500
Resource Liquid (Sandoz Nutrition)	1.06	430	35.2	35.2	137.2	840	1520	500
Sustacal Basic (Mead Johnson Nutritionals)	1.06	500	35	33	140	800	1520	500
Sustacal with Fiber Liquid (Mead Johnson Nutritionals)	1.06	480	43.4	33	133	679	1311	802
Ultracal Liquid (Mead Johnson Nutritionals)	1.06	310	41.5	42.5	116	880	1519	802
Compleat Modified Liquid (Sandoz Nutrition)	1.07	300	40.2	34.6	130.9	938	1310	625
Ensure Liquid with Fiber (Ross)	1.1	480	36.2	33.8	147.3	769	1538	654
Fibersource Liquid (Sandoz Nutrition)	1.2	390	35.8	34.2	141.6	940	1500	558
Fibersource HN Liquid (Sandoz Nutrition)	1.2	390	44.1	34.2	133.3	940	1500	558
Isotein HN Liquid (Sandoz Nutrition)	1.2	300	56.6	28.3	133.3	524	905	476
Fiberlan Liquid (Elan Pharma)	1.2	310	41.7	33.3	133.3	767	1300	667
Nitrolan Liquid (Elan Pharma)	1.24	310	48.4	32.2	129	556	944	645
Reabilan HN Liquid (Elan Pharma)	1.33	490	43.7	39.1	118.9	752	1249	339
Comply Liquid (Sherwood)	1.5	410	40	40	120	734	1234	667
Crucial (Clintec Nutrition)	1.5	490	63	45	90	780	1250	670
Ensure Plus Liquid (Ross)	1.5	690	36.6	35.5	133.2	704	1296	470
Ensure Plus HN Liquid (Ross)	1.5	650	41.7	33.2	133.2	786	1213	705

Per 1,000 kcal						Volume to Supply 1,000 kcal (ml)	kcal to Supply 100% of USRDA for Vitamins	Volume to Supply 100% of USRDA (ml)	Comment
Phosphorus (mg)	**Magnesium (mg)**	**Zinc (mg)**	**Copper (mg)**	**Chromium (mcg)**	**Selenium (mcg)**				
716	286	16.1	1.44	72	50	943	1400	1321	Contains MCT; dietary fiber 13.6 g/1000 kcal; taurine 0.108 g/1000 kcal; L-carnitine 0.108 g/1000 kcal.
594	239	9	1.20	—	—	943	1680	1585	Contains MCT.
754	302	11.3	1.51	113.2	113.2	943	1325	1250	Contains MCT.
500	200	11.5	1	50	35	943	2000	1887	Contains MCT; taurine 0.075 g/1000 kcal; L-carnitine 0.075 g/1000 kcal.
715	286	16.1	1.43	72	50	943	1400	1321	Contains taurine 0.108 g/1000 kcal; L-carnitine 0.108 g/1000 kcal.
500	200	15.1	1.04	—	0	943	2014	1900	
500	200	15.1	1.04	—	0	943	2003	1890	Gluten-free.
500	200	10	1	50	50	943	2000	1890	
670	270	13.1	1.31	—	—	943	1500	1420	Contains dietary fiber.
802	321	16	1.6	80	56	943	1251	1180	Contains MCT, dietary fiber.
813	252	14.4	1.25	93.5	62.5	935	1605	1500	Gluten-free. Contains dietary fiber 4.2 g/1000 ml.
654	262	14.7	1.31	66	46	909	1530	1391	Gluten-free; low cholesterol. Contains dietary fiber 13.1 g/1000 kcal.
558	225	14.2	1.11	83.3	83.3	833	1800	1500	Contains dietary fiber 8.3 g/1000 kcal; MCT.
558	225	14.2	1.11	83.3	83.3	833	1800	1500	Contains dietary fiber 5.7 g/1000 kcal; MCT.
476	192	7.1	0.95	70.8	71.4	833	2124	1770	Contains MCT.
667	267	10	1.33	100	100	833	1500	1250	Contains MCT; dietary fiber 11.7 g/1000 kcal.
645	—	9.7	1.29	96.8	96.8	806	1550	1250	Contains MCT.
376	—	10	1	62.2	50.2	752	2500	1875	Contains MCT.
667	267	20	1.34	—	—	667	1500	1000	
670	270	24	2	—	67	667	—	—	Cholesterol-free. Contains MCT.
470	189	10.6	0.96	47	33	667	2130	1420	
705	282	15.9	1.42	71	50	667	1421	947	Contains taurine 0.106 g/1000 kcal; L-carnitine 0.106 g/1000 kcal.

(table continued on next page)

TABLE 15 (continued)

Preparations	kcal/ml	mOsm/kg	Per 1,000 kcal Protein (g)	Fat (g)	CHO (g)	Sodium (mg)	Potassium (mg)	Calcium (mg)
Ultralan Liquid (Elan Pharma)	1.5	610	40	33.3	134.7	690	1170	667
Nutren 1.5 Liquid (Clintec Nutrition)	1.5	410	40	45	113.3	500	1251	690
Resource Plus Liquid (Sandoz Nutrition)	1.5	600	36.7	35.4	133.4	845	1380	470
Sustacal Plus (Mead Johnson Nutritionals)	1.5	670	40.1	38.2	125	559	974	559
Deliver 2.0 (Mead Johnson Nutritionals)	2	640	37.5	51	100	400	845	500
Magnacal Liquid (Sherwood)	2	590	35	40	125	500	625	500
Nutren 2.0 Liquid (Clintec Nutrition)	2	710	40	53	98	500	1250	700
Two Cal Liquid (Ross)	2	690	41.7	45.3	108.2	653	1228	526
SPECIALIZED FORMULAS								
Renal Failure Formulas								
Travasorb Renal Powder (Clintec Nutrition)	1.35	590	17	13.1	200.4	0	0	0
Amin-Aid Instant Powder (McGaw)	2	700	10	23.6	187	176	0	0
Nepro Liquid (Ross)	2	635	34.9	47.8	107.6	415	528	686
Suplena Liquid (Ross)	2	600	14.9	47.8	127.6	392	558	693
Hepatic Encephalopathy Formulas								
Generaid Plus Powder (Scientific Hospital Supplies)	1	333	24.2	42	136	152	103	686
Hepatic-Aid II (McGaw)	1	560	37.5	31	143	293	0	0
NutriHep Liquid (Clintec Nutrition)	1.5	690	26.7	14	193	213.3	880	667
Trauma/Stress Formulas								
Alitra Q (Ross)	1	—	53	15.5	165	1000	1200	750
Traum-Aid HBC Powder (McGaw)	1	675	56	12.4	166	533	1136	—
Stresstein Powder (Sandoz Nutrition)	1.2	910	58.4	23.4	141.7	541	916	417
Perative (Ross)	1.3	—	50	27.7	136	833	1370	690
TraumaCal Liquid (Mead Johnson Nutritionals)	1.5	560	55	46	95	790	930	500

Per 1,000 kcal						Volume to Supply 1,000 kcal (ml)	kcal to Supply 100% of USRDA for Vitamins	Volume to Supply 100% of USRDA (ml)	Comment
Phosphorus (mg)	**Magnesium (mg)**	**Zinc (mg)**	**Copper (mg)**	**Chromium (mcg)**	**Selenium (mcg)**				
667	267	10	1.34	80	80	667	1500	1000	Contains MCT.
690	330	13	1.33	40	40	667	1500	1000	Gluten-free; cholesterol-free. Contains MCT.
470	211	16	1.07	—	0	667	2100	1140	Gluten-free.
559	224	11.1	1.12	56	39	670	1800	1180	
510	200	10	1	50.5	50.5	500	2000	1000	Contains MCT.
500	200	15	1	—	—	500	2000	1000	
700	340	14	1.40	40	40	500	1500	750	Gluten-free; cholesterol-free. Contains MCT.
526	211	11.9	1.1	53	37	500	1900	950	Gluten-free.
0	0	0	0	0	0	741	—	—	Contains MCT; only water-soluble vitamins.
0	0	0	0	0	0	500	0	0	Cholesterol-free; vitamin-free; mineral-free.
343	105	11.8	1.05	—	51	500	1900	950	Contains taurine 0.080 g/1000 kcal; L-carnitine 0.131 g/1000 kcal.
364	105	11.8	1.05	—	38	500	1886	943	Contains taurine 0.080 g/1000 kcal; L-carnitine 0.080 g/1000 kcal.
517	95	5.9	0.60	17.8	17.8	1000	—	—	For children >1 year old and adults with hepatic disorders.
0	0	0	0	0	0	1000	0	0	(70%) branched-chain amino acids, (2%) aromatic amino acids. Cholesterol-free; mineral-free; vitamin-free.
670	270	10	1.33	—	0	667	—	—	
750	270	20	1.33	71	50	1000	—	—	Contains glutamine 14 g/1000 kcal; arginine 3 g/1000 kcal.
400	—	—	—	—	—	1000	3000	3000	
417	167	6.3	0.83	50	50	833	2400	2000	Contains MCT.
690	270	15.9	1.40	70	50	777	1500	1154	
500	132	9.9	1	—	—	670	3000	2000	Contains MCT.

(table continued on next page)

TABLE 15 (continued)

Preparations	kcal/ml	mOsm/kg	Per 1,000 kcal					
			Protein (g)	Fat (g)	CHO (g)	Sodium (mg)	Potassium (mg)	Calcium (mg)
Miscellaneous Formulas								
Glucerna Liquid (Ross)	1	375	41.8	55.7	93.7	928	1561	704
Immun-Aid (McGaw)	1	460	80	22	120	580	1060	500
Advera (Ross)	1.28	680	47	17.5	16.4	800	2000	700
NutriVent Liquid (Clinic Nutrition)	1.5	450	45	67	63	500	1493	800
Pulmocare Liquid (Ross)	1.5	520	41.7	61.4	70.4	873	1155	704
Respalor (Mead Johnson Nutritionals)	1.52	580	50	47	97	830	970	460
OptiHealth Gain (Metagenics)	1.54	380	38	2	205	600	700	700

ability of the intestinal mucosa of young infants may enhance absorption of large protein molecules, including intact food antigens. Intact proteins from any source, including soy and milk casein, are equally antigenic. In contrast, protein hydrolysates are much less antigenic. Whey hydrolysates appear to be less antigenic than standard soy or cow's milk-based formulas (Chandra et al, 1989; Merritt et al, 1990) and promote growth rates and bone mineralization equal to those of breast-fed infants (Mimouni et al, 1993). The protein efficiency ratio and biological value of whey proteins are 20% and 25% greater, respectively, than those of casein. However, a moderate ratio of whey to casein (35:65) may result in the most efficient absorption of nitrogen, fat, calcium, phosphorus, magnesium, and zinc (Cooke et al, 1992).

Infants demonstrating allergy to milk protein, milk-induced steatorrhea, or glycogen storage disease should be fed formulas that do not contain intact milk proteins (see Table 18). Appropriate formulas for such infants contain extensively hydrolyzed casein (Wahn et al, 1992). Intolerance to galactose (galactosemia) or lactose (lactase deficiency) can be avoided by substituting sucrose, maltose, dextrose, dextrins, or corn syrup solids (Büller and Grand, 1990; Sinden and Sutphen, 1991). Sucrose intolerance (sucrose deficiency) can be avoided by substituting glucose polymers.

SPECIALIZED FORMULAS FOR SPECIFIC DISEASES IN INFANTS AND CHILDREN. Special nutritional formulations are available for use in infants and children with specific diseases.

Phenylketonuria: In phenylketonuria (PKU), phenylalanine hydroxylase deficiency results in hyperphenylalaninemia (>4 mg/dL), mental retardation, seizures, ataxia, and behavior problems. Patients with classical PKU (plasma phenylalanine concentration >20 mg/dL) are most severely affected. Atypical PKU (plasma phenylalanine concentration 10 to 20 mg/dL) and benign PKU (plasma phenylalanine concentration 4 to 10 mg/dL) also occur and are of decreasing severity. Women with plasma phenylalanine concentration >6 mg/dL during pregnancy usually give birth to low-birth-weight babies with a wide variety of congenital anomalies, including microcephaly and congenital heart disease (Medical Research Council Working Party on Phenylketonuria, 1993).

Successful therapy at all ages requires limiting dietary phenylalanine intake to maintain the plasma phenylalanine concentration between 2 and 10 mg/dL. This can be managed by providing the following amounts of phenylalanine daily: 0 to 3 months, 40 to 70 mg/kg; 4 to 6 months, 30 to 50 mg/kg; 7 to 9 months, 25 to 40 mg/kg; 10 to 12 months, 20 to 40 mg/kg; 1 to 3 years, 15 to 40 mg/kg; 4 to 6 years, 10 to 35 mg/kg; over 6 years, 10 to 30 mg/kg. Infants should be fed low-phenylalanine formulas, and older children should be fed a phenylalanine-free enteral formula, supplemented by foods providing phenylalanine in order to support physical and mental development. Other low-protein foods should be added, as required, to provide calories. Frequent monitoring of plasma phenylalanine and tyrosine concentrations and of urinary phenylalanine and tyrosine excretion is essential, with dietary adjustment as necessary. In addition, deficiencies in carnitine, zinc, selenium, and copper have been reported in children treated with diets modified for amino acid composition (Acos-

Per 1,000 kcal						Volume to Supply 1,000 kcal (ml)	kcal to Supply 100% of USRDA for Vitamins	Volume to Supply 100% of USRDA (ml)	Comment
Phosphorus (mg)	Magnesium (mg)	Zinc (mg)	Copper (mg)	Chromium (mcg)	Selenium (mcg)				
704	282	15.9	1.50	71	50	1000	1422	1422	For abnormal glucose tolerance. Gluten-free. Contains dietary fiber 14.4 g/1000 kcal; taurine 0.106 g/1000 kcal; L-carnitine 0.141 g/1000 kcal.
500	200	30	2	—	100	1000	—	—	For immunocompromised patients. 60% branched-chain amino acids. Contains MCT.
700	282	12.5	2	71	50	780	1515	1183	For immunocompromised patients. Contains MCT. Lactose-free. Gluten-free.
800	400	14	1.41	46	40	660	1420	1420	For impaired pulmonary function and CO_2 retention.
704	282	15.9	1.41	71	50	667	1420	947	For impaired pulmonary function and CO_2 retention.
460	186	9.2	0.83	46	33	660	1420	1420	For impaired pulmonary function and CO_2 retention.
433	433	80	0.8	33.3	40	650	—	—	For immunocompromised patients. Contains MCT. Lactose-free. Gluten-free.

ta et al, 1982; McCabe and McCabe, 1986; Acosta et al, 1987) and may occur despite trace mineral supplementation (McCabe and McCabe, 1986).

Available Formulations:
Lofenalac (Mead Johnson Nutritionals), ***Phenex-1, Phenex-2*** (Ross), ***PKU 1, PKU 2*** (Mead Johnson Nutritionals). See the manufacturers' literature for product composition.

Maple Syrup Urine Disease: Maple syrup urine disease (MSUD; branched-chain ketoaciduria) is one of nine inherited disorders in the metabolism of the branched-chain amino acids (BCAA), leucine, isoleucine, and valine. Deficiency in α-ketoacid dehydrogenase results in elevated concentrations of the BCAA and their ketoacids in plasma, spinal fluid, and urine. Irritability, poor feeding, lethargy, absent Moro and rooting reflexes, irregular jerky respirations, elevated plasma BCAA concentrations, and detectable plasma alloisoleucine concentration first appear shortly after birth; loss of tendon reflexes, alternating periods of hypertonicity and hypotonicity, seizures, coma, and apnea follow in rapid succession, with death often occurring within three weeks. The typical odor from which the disease derives its name is apparent by the end of the first week of life. Affected infants may survive but usually suffer severe mental retardation and other signs of irreversible central nervous system damage.

Three categories of MSUD have been identified: classic MSUD with <2% normal α-ketoacid dehydrogenase activity; intermediate MSUD with 2% to 20% normal α-ketoacid dehydrogenase activity; and intermittent MSUD, in which symptoms may be triggered by infections, immunizations, trauma, surgery, or consumption of a large amount of protein.

Treatment must be initiated as soon as MSUD is diagnosed, and consists of providing sufficient amounts of BCAA to allow tissue repair and normal growth without exceeding requirements (Table 19). Solid foods other than meat and milk products can be introduced at usual ages. By 1 year of age, BCAA can be supplied by a low-protein diet (American Academy of Pediatrics Committee on Nutrition, 1976). Thiamine (5 to 20 mg/kg daily) may enhance the activity of mutant α-ketoacid dehydrogenase in MSUD (Danner and Elsas, 1989).

Available Formulations:
Ketonex-1, Ketonex-2 (Ross), ***MSUD Diet Powder, MSUD 1, MSUD 2*** (Mead Johnson Nutritionals). See the manufacturers' literature for product composition.

Hereditary Tyrosinemia: In hereditary tyrosinemia, tyrosine metabolism is impaired as a result of fumarylacetoacetase deficiency, causing accumulation of tyrosine and succinylacetone in blood and urine (Lindblad et al, 1977). Para-OH-phenylpyruvate dioxygenase deficiency and hypermethioninemia also occur secondary to severe liver damage. Clinical symptoms include vomiting, diarrhea, failure to thrive, abdominal distension, hepatomegaly, splenomegaly, ascites, edema, hemorrhage, bilateral cataracts, nystagmus, keratitis, hyperactivity, mental retardation, microcephaly, and corneal erosions (Kretchmer and Etzwiler, 1958). Vitamin D-resistant rickets, hyperphosphaturia, and hypophosphatemia caused by progressive renal tubular dysfunction are common. Hereditary tyrosinemia must be distinguished from transient neonatal tyrosinemia (benign tyrosinemia) resulting from im-

TABLE 16.
MODULAR FORMULA DIETS FOR ENTERAL FEEDING

Preparations	kcal/ml	kcal/g	Per 100 kcal Protein g	Fat g	CHO[1] g	Sodium mg	Potassium mg	Chloride mg	Calcium mg	Phosphorus mg
GLUCOSE POLYMERS										
Polycose Liquid (Ross)	2	—	0	0	25	35	3	70	10	1.5
Polycose Powder (Ross)	—	3.8	0	0	24.7	28.9	2.6	58.7	7.9	1.3
Moducal Powder (Mead Johnson (Nutritionals)	—	3.8	0	0	25	18.4	2.6	39	0	0
Sumacal Powder (Sherwood)	—	3.8	0	0	25	26.3	10.3	55.3	5.3	8.2
PROTEIN SUPPLEMENTS										
Gevral Protein Powder (Lederle)	—	3.7	16.4	0.5	7.4	52.4	13.6	0	0	0
Elementra Powder (Clintec Nutrition)	—	3.8	20.9	1.4	0.5	10.4	400	12	240	120
ProMod Powder (Ross)	—	4.3	17.9	2.1	2.4	53.6	235.7	0	142.9	107.1
Propac (Sherwood)	—	4	18.8	2	1.5	56.3	125	57.9	87.5	75
LIPID SUPPLEMENTS										
Corn Oil:										
Lipomul Liquid (Roberts)	6	—	0	11.1	0	15	0	0	0	0
Safflower Oil:										
Microlipid Emulsion (Sherwood)	4.5	—	0	11.1	0	0	0	0	0	0
Medium Chain Triglycerides from Coconut Oil:										
MCT Oil (Mead Johnson Nutritionals)	7.7	—	0	12.2	0	0	0	0	0	0
CARBOHYDRATE/LIPID SUPPLEMENT										
Pro-Phree (Ross)	—	5.2	0	5.96	11.5	48	168	67	144	101
DIETARY FIBER SUPPLEMENTS										
Fibrad Powder (Ross)	—	0.55	0	0	0.78[2]	1.5	1.5	0	0	0

[1] *Carbohydrate*
[2] *Dietary fiber*

maturity of the digestive system; the presence of succinylacetone in blood and urine is diagnostic.

The goal of dietary management is to provide strictly controlled amounts of phenylalanine and tyrosine; when hypermethioninemia exists, sulfur-containing amino acids also must be limited. Plasma tyrosine concentration should be maintained between 0.9 and 2.7 mg/dL and plasma methionine concentrations between 0.7 and 1.3 mg/dL (Elsas and Acosta, 1988). These goals have been attained with a diet containing 0.009% L-tyrosine and 0.08% L-phenylalanine (Scriver et al, 1967).

Available Formulations:
Tyrex-2, Tyromex-1 (Ross), ***TYR 1, TYR 2, Low Phe/Tyr Diet Powder*** (Mead Johnson Nutritionals). See the manufacturers' literature for product composition.

Homocysteinemia: Homocysteinemia results from cystathionine β-synthase deficiency or from defective remethylation of homocysteine to methionine (secondary to impaired metabolism of N^5-methyltetrahydrofolate or methylcobalamin). In either case, plasma homocysteine concentration is elevated. Patients with cystathionine β-synthase deficiency have ectopia lentis, fine hair, malar flush, and thromboembolic episodes early in life; they later develop skeletal abnormalities such as scoliosis, long extremities, or arachnodactyly. Mental deficits occur in some patients. Those with a homocysteine remethylation defect have clinical signs ranging from megaloblastic anemia and muscle weakness to psychoneuroses and varying degrees of developmental delay, movement disorders, and spinal cord or retinal degeneration.

The goals of treatment are to maintain nearly normal plasma methionine and cystine concentrations; eliminate homocystine excretion in urine; reduce plasma homocysteine concentration; and maintain normal growth and development. Some patients respond to supplementation with pyridoxine, dipyridamole, folate, cobalamin, or betaine. Unresponsive patients must be provided a low-methionine diet, restricted to amounts sufficient for normal growth, and supplemented with milk or solid foods. Daily dietary requirements for methionine are: 0 to 6 months, 20 to 50 mg/kg; 6 to 12 months, 15 to 40 mg/kg; 1 to 15 years, 10 to 30 mg/kg; over 15 years, 5 to 10 mg/kg. Daily dietary requirements for cystine are: 0 to 6 months, 200 to 300 mg/kg; 6 to 12 months, 200 to 250 mg/kg; 1 to 15 years, 150 to 200 mg/kg; over 15 years, 100 to 150 mg/kg.

Available Formulations:
HOM 1, HOM 2, Low Methionine Diet Powder (Mead Johnson Nutritionals), ***Hominex-1, Hominex-2*** (Ross). See the manufacturers' literature for product composition.

Galactosemia: The most prevalent of three recessively inherited disorders resulting in galactosemia results from deficiency of galactose-1-phosphate uridyltransferase (Segal, 1989). Galactokinase deficiency and uridine diphosphate-4-epimerase deficiency also result in galactose in blood and urine. Most patients with galactose-1-phosphate uridyltransferase deficiency can metabolize only a small fraction of galactose to carbon dioxide (Segal et al, 1965; Segal and Cuatrecasas, 1968). Treatment consists of dietary restriction of galactose intake. In addition, medications containing galactose should be avoided.

Urea Cycle Disorders: Deficiencies of carbamyl phosphate synthetase (CPS), ornithine transcarbamylase (OTC), argininosuccinic acid synthetase (AS), argininosuccinase (AL), arginase (AR), and N-acetylglutamate synthetase (NAS) impair the synthesis of urea and cause the accumulation of systemic ammonium. Therapy is directed primarily toward reducing the need for ureagenesis by limiting protein intake to the minimum required for adequate growth (about 2 g/kg daily.) In addition, the activity of alternative excretory routes for ammonia can be stimulated. For example, argininosuccinate and citrulline metabolism can be stimulated by arginine supplementation (400 to 700 mg/kg daily) and the effectiveness of phenylacetylglutamine as an ammonia sink can be increased by supplementation with sodium phenylbutyrate (600 mg/kg daily) or sodium phenylacetate (500 mg/kg daily).

In arginase deficiency, the *de novo* synthesis of arginine should be minimized. Dietary therapy should be based on a low-protein diet; supplementation with sodium phenylbutyrate will divert nitrogen to phenylacetylglutamine synthesis.

In CPS and OTC deficiencies, supplementation with L-citrulline (170 mg/kg daily) must accompany other therapy. Similarly, patients with AS or AL deficiencies require supplemental arginine (400 to 600 mg/kg daily).

Available Formulations:
Cyclinex-1, Cyclinex-2 (Ross), ***UCD 1, UCD 2*** (Mead Johnson Nutritionals). See the manufacturers' literature for product composition.

Organic Acidemias: Inherited disorders of amino acid and fatty acid oxidation are characterized by the accumulation of nonamino organic acids in the urine. Such disorders include isovaleric acidemia, 3-methylcrotonylglycinemia, combined carboxylase deficiency (defective biotinidase or holocarboxylase synthetase), hydroxymethylglutaric acidemia, propionic acidemia, methylmalonic acidemia (defective methylmalonyl-CoA mutase or adenosyl-B_{12}), β-ketothiolase deficiency, glutaric acidemia Types I and II, 5-oxoprolinemia, and deficiencies of various acyl-CoA dehydrogenases. Symptomatic infants will be hyperammonemic, acidemic, ketotic, or hypoglycemic; older children may have Reye's syndrome-like symptoms, episodes of hypoketotic hypoglycemia, a progressive dystonic movement disorder, or the combination of alopecia, ataxia, and seborrheic rash. Each acidemia also causes specific symptoms reflecting the exact enzymatic error.

Treatment usually emphasizes dietary restriction of the substrates of the defective enzyme present in order to minimize the production of toxic organic acids. For example, in isovaleric acidemia, leucine intake is restricted; in propionic or methylmalonic acidemias, ingestion of threonine, valine, methionine, and isoleucine is limited; and in glutaric acidemia, lysine and tryptophan are avoided (Table 20). In addition, carnitine supplementation (>100 mg/kg daily) may be necessary to prevent the secondary carnitine deficiency that commonly accompanies organic acidemias (Chalmers et al, 1984).

Available Formulations: (Methylmalonic Aciduria, Propionic Acidemia) ***OS 1, OS 2, Protein-Free Diet Powder*** (Mead Johnson Nutritionals), ***Pro-Phree Powder, Propimex-1, Propimex-2*** (Ross). **(Glutaric Aciduria)** ***Glutarex-1, Glutarex-2***

TABLE 17.
FORMULA DIETS FOR NORMAL INFANTS

Nutrients	Human Breast Milk[1]	FDA (1985)[2]	Enfamil[3]	Enfamil with Iron[3]	Enfamil Premature[3]
kcal/ml					
Calories	0.68 - 0.78		0.676	0.676	0.676
g/100 kcal					
Protein	1.1 - 1.7	1.8 - 4.5	2.2	2.2	3
Fat	4.8 - 5.9	3.3 - 6	5.6	5.6	5.1
Carbohydrate	9.5 - 10.2		10.3	10.3	11.1
mg/100 kcal					
Linoleic Acid	540	300	910	910	1060
Linolenic Acid	100		95	95	95
Cholesterol	20		trace	trace	trace
Choline	12.5	7	15.6	15.6	12
Inositol	14.9	4	4.7	4.7	17
L-Carnitine	0.95		2.5	2.5	2.5
Taurine	5.6		5.9	5.9	5.9
Histidine	34		43	43	
Isoleucine	85		134	134	
Leucine	154		230	230	
Lysine	100		153	153	
Tryptophan	31		33	33	
Phenylalanine	63		86	86	
Threonine	76		116	116	
Valine	96		136	136	
Methionine	29		43	43	
Cystine	27		26	26	
Calcium	35 - 42	60[6]	78	78	165
Chloride	49 - 67	55 - 150	63	63	85
Iron	0.03 - 0.05	0.15 - 3	0.47	1.88	0.25
Magnesium	4.5 - 5.3	6	7.8	7.8	6.8
Phosphorus	16 - 22	30[6]	53	53	83
Potassium	67 - 80	80 - 200	108	108	103
Sodium	19 - 31	20 - 60	27	27	39
Zinc	0.14 - 0.2	0.5	0.78	0.78	1.5
mcg/100 kcal					
Copper	30 - 40	60	94	94	125
Iodine	9.6 - 21	5 - 75	6	6	25
Manganese	0.05 - 0.11	5	15.6	15.6	6.3
Selenium					
per 100 kcal					
Vitamin A (RE[7])	64 - 122	75 - 225	93	93	210
Vitamin D (mcg[8])	0.06 - 0.10	1 - 2.5	1.58	1.58	6.8
Vitamin E (TE[9])	0.17 - 0.47	0.5[10]	1.3	1.3	6.3
Vitamin K (mcg)	0.27 - 0.31	4	8	8	8
Vitamin C (mg)	4 - 6	8	8.1	8.1	20
mcg/100 kcal					
Thiamine	24 - 34	40	78	78	200
Riboflavin	44 - 54	60	150	150	300
Niacin	178 - 238	250	1250	1250	4000
Folic Acid	6.6 - 7.4	4	15.6	15.6	35
Pantothenic Acid	220 - 280	300	470	470	1200

Enfamil Premature with Iron[3]	Gerber[3]	Similac[4]	Similac with Iron[4]	Similac Special Care with Iron[4]	SMA with Iron[5]
0.676	0.676	0.676	0.676	0.806	0.676
3	2.2	2.14	2.14	2.71	2.2
5.1	5.4	5.4	5.4	5.43	5.3
11.1	10.7	10.7	10.7	10.6	10.6
1060	880	1300	1300	700	500
95	95		245	115	
trace	trace		1.6	3.1	4.9
12	16	16	16	10	15
17	4.7	4.7	4.7	5.5	4.7
2.5	2.1		1.6	5.8	5.5
5.9	5.9		6.7	6.7	5.9
	56		44	53	54
	116		104	143	124
			202	267	221
	168		153	214	175
	30		27	31	36
	97		104	89	93
	93		92	158	119
	138		116	147	133
	54		60	67	55
	19		18	43	42
165	75	73	73	180	63
85	70	64	64	81	56
1.88	1.8	0.22	1.8	1.8	1.8
6.8	6	6	6	12	7
83	58	56	56	90	42
103	108	105	105	129	83
39	30	27	27	43	22
1.5	0.75	0.75	0.75	1.5	0.8
125	90	90	90	250	70
25	8	9	9	6	9
6.3	5	5	5	12	22
	2.8		2.2	1.8	1.8
210	90	90	90	90	90
6.8	1.5	1.5	1.5	3.75	1.5
6.3	1.3	3	2	4.0	1.4
8	8	8	8	12	8
20	9	9	9	37	8.5
200	100	100	100	250	100
300	150	150	150	620	150
4000	1050	1050	1050	5000	750
35	15	15	15	37	7.5
1200	450	450	450	1900	315

(table continued on next page)

TABLE 17 (continued)

Nutrients	Human Breast Milk[1]	FDA (1985)[2]	Enfamil[3]	Enfamil with Iron[3]	Enfamil Premature[3]
mcg/100 kcal					
Biotin	0.4 - 0.8	1.5	2.3	2.3	4
Vitamin B_6	11.6 - 45.4	35	63	63	150
Vitamin B_{12}	0.07 - 0.1	0.15	0.23	0.23	0.25
% of total protein					
Protein:					
Casein	30		40	40	40
Whey protein	70		60	60	60
% of total fatty acids					
Lipids:					
Polyunsaturated	14.2		19	19	
Monounsaturated	41.6		38	38	
Saturated	44.2		40	40	
Source:					
Coconut Oil			20	20	
MCT[11]			—[12]	—[12]	—[12]
Palm Oil			45	45	
High Oleic Safflower Oil			15	15	
Soy Oil			20	20	
% of total carbohydrates					
Carbohydrates:					
Source:					
Lactose	100		100	100	100
Soy Sugars					
mOsm/kg					
Osmolality	300		360	360	310
mOsm/L					
Osmolarity	255		320	320	270
mOsm/100 kcal					
Renal Solute Load[13]	11.1		20.0	20.0	26.0

Enfamil Premature with Iron[3]	Gerber[3]	Similac[4]	Similac with Iron[4]	Similac Special Care with Iron[4]	SMA with Iron[5]
4	4.4	4.4	4.4	37	2.2
150	60	60	60	250	62.5
0.25	0.25	0.25	0.25	0.55	0.2
40	82	82	82	40	40
60	18	18	18	60	60
	19	37.3	37.3	37.3	14.5
	38	17.7	17.7	17.7	41.2
	40	45	45	45	44.2
		40	40	40	40
—[12]					
		60	60	60	60
100	100	100	100	100	100
310	320	300	300	300	300
270	290	270	270	270	270
26	20	14.3	14.3	14.3	13.5

1 *Tsang and Nichols, 1988; Institute of Medicine, 1991.*

2 *Infant Formula Act of 1980 (Public Law 96-359); Food and Drug Administration, 1985.*

3 *Mead Johnson Nutritionals.*

4 *Ross.*

5 *Wyeth-Ayerst.*

6 *Calcium to phosphorus ratio between 1.1 and 2.0.*

7 *Retinol equivalents (μg retinol).*

8 *Cholecalciferol.*

9 *Tocopherol equivalents (mg d-α-tocopherol).*

10 *At least 0.7 TE per g of linoleic acid.*

11 *Saturated medium chain triglycerides.*

12 *Contains MCT as 40% of total triglycerides.*

13 *Renal Solute Load (mOsm/100 kcal) =*

$4 * (Protein_{g/100\ kcal}) + (Na_{mEq/100\ kcal}) + (K_{mEq/100\ kcal}) + (Cl_{mEq/100\ kcal})$ *(Ziegler and Ryu, 1976).*

TABLE 18.
HYPOALLERGENIC FORMULA DIETS FOR INFANTS AND CHILDREN[1]

Nutrients	Alimentum[2]	Gerber Soy Liquid[3]	Good Start[4]	Isomil[2]	Isomil SF[2]
kcal/ml					
Calories	0.676	0.676	0.670	0.676	0.676
g/100 kcal					
Protein	2.75	3.0	2.4	2.45	2.66
Fat	5.54	5.3	5.1	5.46	5.46
Carbohydrate	10.2	10.0	11.0	10.3	10.1
mg/100 kcal					
Linoleic Acid	1600	860	850	1300	1300
Linolenic Acid	54	86	100	245	245
Cholesterol	1.5	0	10	0	0
Choline	8	8	12	8	8
Inositol	5	5	18	5	5
L-Carnitine	1.6	1.88	1.6	1.7	1.6
Taurine	6.7	5.9	8	6.7	6.7
Histidine	71	69	57	62	62
Isoleucine	148	138	130	115	115
Leucine	243	230	245	213	213
Lysine	237	180	221	153	153
Tryptophan	38	36	53	28	28
Phenylalanine	121	147	78	133	133
Threonine	129	96	169	100	100
Valine	195	138	142	111	111
Methionine	74	54	53	59	59
Cystine	44	27	11	30	30
Calcium	105	94	64	105	105
Chloride	80	88	59	62	62
Iron	1.8	1.8	1.5	1.8	1.8
Magnesium	7.5	7.5	6.7	7.5	7.5
Phosphorus	75	74	36	75	75
Potassium	118	115	98	108	108
Sodium	44	47	24	44	44
Zinc	0.75	0.75	0.75	0.75	0.75
mcg/100 kcal					
Copper	75	75	80	75	75
Iodine	15	15	8	15	15
Manganese	30	30	7	30	30
Selenium	2.8	2.8	0.18	2.1	2.1
per 100 kcal					
Vitamin A (RE[7])	90	90	90	90	90
Vitamin D (mcg[8])	1.3	1.5	1.5	1.5	1.5
Vitamin E (TE[9])	2.0	2.0	1.2	2.0	2.0
Vitamin K (mcg)	15	15	8.2	15	15
Vitamin C (mg)	9	9	8	9	9
mcg/100 kcal					
Thiamine	60	60	60	60	60
Riboflavin	90	90	135	90	90
Niacin	1350	1350	750	1350	1350
Folic Acid	15	15	9	15	15
Pantothenic Acid	750	750	450	750	750
Biotin	4.5	4.5	2.2	4.5	4.5
Vitamin B_6	60	60	75	60	60
Vitamin B_{12}	0.45	0.45	0.22	0.45	0.45

Lactofree[3]	Nursoy[3]	PediaSure[2]	PediaSure with Fiber[2,6]	RCF[2]	Soyalac[5]	I-Soyalac[5]
0.676	0.676	1	1	0.41	0.69	0.69
2.2	2.7	3	3	4.95	3.1	3.1
5.5	5.3	5	5	8.91	5.5	5.5
10.4	10.2	11	11	0	10	10
900	500	1072	1072	2170	2810	2810
95	53	100	100			
trace	2.3	2.1	2.1		0	0
12	13	30	30	13	12	12
17	4.1	8	8	8	10	10
2	1.2	1.7	1.7			
6	5.6	7.2	7.2		6.2	6.2
56	72	72	72		81	81
116	140	144	144		142	150
210	233	288	288		240	240
168	156	228	228		188	188
30	39	39	39		28	30
97	141	144	144		152	163
93	109	144	144		120	112
138	135	171	171		140	140
54	68	84	84		66	72
19	37	27	27			
82	90	97	97	173	94	102
67	56	101	101	103	65	78
1.8	1.8	1.4	1.4	0.37	1.9	1.9
8	10	20	20	12.4	12	11
55	63	80	80	124	55	63
110	105	131	131	180	117	117
30	30	38	38	73	44	42
1	0.8	1.2	1.2	1.24	0.78	0.78
75	70	100	100	124	78	117
15	9	9.7	9.7	25	7.8	7.8
15	30	250	250	50	90	30
2.8	1	2.3	2.3	3.5		
90	90	77	77	170	93	93
1.5	1.5	1.3	1.3	2.5	1.55	1.58
1.3	1.4	1.5	1.5	3.1	2.3	2.3
8	15	3.8	3.8	25	7.8	7.8
12	8.3	10	10	13.6	12	12
80	100	270	270	100	78	94
90	150	210	210	150	94	94
1000	750	1700	1700	2230	1250	1250
16	7.5	37	37	25	15.6	15.6
500	450	1000	1000	1240	469	469
3	5.5	32	32	7.5	9.4	7.8
60	63	260	260	100	70	86
0.3	0.3	0.6	0.6	0.75	0.31	0.31

(table continued on next page)

TABLE 18 (continued)

Nutrients	Alimentum[2]	Gerber Soy Liquid[3]	Good Start[4]	Isomil[2]	Isomil SF[2]
% of total protein					
Protein:					
Soy Protein		100		100	100
Casein	100[10]				
Whey Protein			100		
% of total fatty acids					
Lipids:					
Polyunsaturated	38	19	22.2	38.6	38.5
Monounsaturated	8	38	33.2	17.1	17.3
Saturated	54	40	44.6	44.3	44.2
Source:					
Coconut Oil			21	40	40
MCT[11]	50				
Palm Oil			47		
High Oleic Safflower Oil	40		6		
Soy Oil	10	100	26	60	60
% of total carbohydrates					
Carbohydrates:					
Source:					
Corn Syrup				60	
Glucose Polymers			30		100
Lactose			70		
Soy Sugars		100			
Sucrose	70			40	
Tapioca Dextrin					
Tapioca Starch	30				
mOsm/kg					
Osmolality	370	230	264	240	180
mOsm/L					
Osmolarity	330	210	238	220	160
mOsm/100 kcal					
Renal Solute Load[13]	18.2	27	14.8	16.2	17.1

Lactofree[3]	Nursoy[3]	PediaSure[2]	PediaSure with Fiber[2,6]	RCF[2]	Soyalac[5]	I-Soyalac[5]
	100			100	100	100
82		82	82			
18		18	18			
19	14.5	27.7	27.7	20	60	60
38	41.2	44.7	44.7	40	16.4	16.4
40	44.2	27.6	27.6	40	23.6	23.6
				40		
		20	20			
		50	50			
		30	30	60	100	100
100					100	100
		70	70			
	100[12]	30	30			
200	240	310	345	200	240	270
180	220	260		182	215	241
20	17.1	19.8	19.8	19	19.1	19.4

[1] *For infants and children with galactosemia, colic, sensitivity or allergy to corn or cow's milk, lactase deficiency, lactose intolerance, or sucrose intolerance, and for those desired to be on vegetarian diets.*

[2] *Ross.*

[3] *Mead Johnson Nutritionals.*

[4] *Carnation Nutritionals.*

[5] *Not intended for those under 1 year of age.*

[6] *Nutricia.*

[7] *Retinol equivalents (μg retinol).*

[8] *Cholecalciferol.*

[9] *Tocopherol equivalents (mg d-α-tocopherol).*

[10] *Supplemented with amino acids.*

[11] *Includes saturated medium chain fatty acids 55%.*

[12] *Nursoy liquid; Nursoy powder provides carbohydrates as sucrose (25%) and corn syrup solids (75%).*

[13] *Renal Solute Load (mOsm/100 kcal) =*

$$4 * (Protein_{g/100\ kcal}) + (Na_{mEq/100\ kcal}) + (K_{mEq/100\ kcal}) + (Cl_{mEq/100\ kcal})$$ *(Ziegler and Ryu, 1976).*

TABLE 19.
DAILY NUTRIENT REQUIREMENTS IN MAPLE SYRUP URINE DISEASE (MSUD)[1]

Nutrient	Unit	0-2 Months	2-5 Months	6-12 Months	1-2 Years	2-3 Years	3-4 Years	4-6 Years	6-8 Years	>8 Years
Carbohydrate	g	15/kg	14/kg	13/kg	138	156	175	200	250	275
Protein	g	2.2/kg	2.0/kg	1.8/kg	25	25	30	30	35	40
Fat	g	4.7/kg	4.3/kg	3.9/kg	43	49	55	62	78	86
Leucine	mg		76-150/kg				750-1,000			
Isoleucine	mg		79-110/kg				500-750			
Valine	mg	65-105/kg		50-80/kg			400-600			

[1] *American Academy of Pediatrics Committee on Nutrition, 1976.*

TABLE 20.
DAILY NUTRIENT REQUIREMENTS IN ORGANIC ACIDEMIAS[1]

	0-6 months	6-12 months	1-4 years	4-7 years	7-11 years	11-15 years	15-19 years
PROPIONIC OR METHYLMALONIC ACIDEMIA							
mg/kg							
Isoleucine	30-90	30-90	20-85	20-80	20-30	20-30	10-30
Methionine	20-50	15-40	10-30	10-20	10-20	10-20	5-10
Valine	40-95	30-60	30-85	30-50	25-30	20-30	15-30
ISOVALERIC ACIDEMIA							
mg/kg							
Leucine	60-100	40-75	40-70	35-65	30-60	30-50	15-40

[1] *Adapted from Elsas and Acosta, 1988.*

(Ross). See the manufacturers' literature for product composition.

Histidinemia: Histidase deficiency results in plasma histidine concentrations in excess of 4.5 mg/dL (Levy et al, 1974). Whether histidinemia is clinically significant is controversial; however, histidinemia may predispose individuals to central nervous system disorders during perinatal hypoxia (Scriver and Levy, 1983). For the majority of asymptomatic cases, treatment is not indicated. When intervention is desired, the goal is to provide 20 to 35 mg/kg of histidine daily (Snyderman et al, 1979).

Available Formulations:
HIST 1, HIST 2 (Mead Johnson Nutritionals). See the manufacturer's literature for product composition.

Hyperlysinemia: Familial hyperlysinemia may be accompanied by plasma lysine concentrations in excess of 10 mg/dL. Although hyperlysinemia may be clinically inconsequential, some practitioners advocate strict control of lysine intake in affected infants until the process of brain myelination is complete (at about 2 years) (Gregory et al, 1989).

Available Formulations:
LYS 1, LYS 2 (Mead Johnson Nutritionals). See the manufacturer's literature for product composition.

Gluten Enteropathy (Celiac Disease): This chronic intestinal malabsorption disorder is caused by intolerance to gluten and is characterized by a flat jejunal mucosa. Clinical and/or histologic improvement is noted following withdrawal of dietary gluten. A gluten-sensitive jejunopathy similar to that found in celiac disease is observed in many patients with dermatitis herpetiformis; thus, the jejunopathy and dermatitis are considered components of the same disease complex. (Also see index entry Dermatitis Herpetiformis).

Available Formulations:
Nutramigen, ProSobee (Mead Johnson Nutritionals). See the manufacturer's literature for product composition.

Miscellaneous Disorders: In addition to the above, specialized formulas are available for infants and children with the following disorders. See the manufacturers' literature for product composition.

Idiopathic Hypercalcemia: *Calcilo XD, Similac PM 60/40* (Ross), ***Special Formula S-44*** (Wyeth-Ayerst).

Leucine-Sensitive Hypoglycemia: *Special Formula S-14* (Wyeth-Ayerst).

Disaccharidase Deficiency: *Mono- and Disaccharide-Free Diet Powder* (Mead Johnson Nutritionals).

Severe Malabsorption Disorders (intractable diarrhea, short gut syndrome, steatorrhea, cystic fibrosis, severe protein-calorie malnutrition, recovery from surgery, intestinal resection, fat intolerance, fat malabsorption): *Isomil DF, ProViMin* (Ross), ***Portagen, Pregestimil*** (Mead Johnson Nutritionals).

Cited References

Deaths associated with thiamine-deficient total parenteral nutrition. *MMWR* 38:43-46, 1989.

Mastering the Technique of Tube Feeding at Home: By Nasogastric, Nasoduodenal, or Nasojejunal Tube. Columbus, Ohio, Ross Laboratories, 1988 A.

Mastering the Technique of Tube Feeding at Home: By Gastrostomy or Jejunostomy. Columbus, Ohio, Ross Laboratories, 1988 B.

Nutrition Support Dietetics: Core Curriculum, ed 2. Rockville, Md, ASPEN, 1993.

Your Guide to Home Tube Feeding. Deerfield, Ill, Clintec Nutrition, 1992.

Acosta PB, et al: Zinc status and growth of children undergoing treatment for phenylketonuria. *J Inherit Metab Dis* 5:107-110, 1982.

Acosta PB, et al: Trace element status of PKU children ingesting an elemental diet. *J Parenter Enter Nutr* 11:287-292, 1987.

Adams ND, Rowe JC: Nephrocalcinosis. *Clin Perinatol* 19:179-195, (March) 1992.

Adibi SA, Allen ER: Impaired jejunal absorption rates of essential amino acids induced by either dietary caloric or protein deprivation in man. *Gastroenterology* 59:404-411, 1970.

Alexander JW: Immunoenhancement via enteral nutrition. *Arch Surg* 128:1242-1245, 1993.

Alexander JW, Gottschlich MM: Nutritional immunomodulation in burn patients. *Crit Care Med* 18:S149-S153, 1990.

Allard JP, et al: Validation of a new formula for calculating the energy requirements of burn patients. *J Parenter Enter Nutr* 14:115-118, 1990.

Allen JR, Van Way CW III: Home nutritional support, in Van Way CW III (ed): *Handbook of Surgical Nutrition.* Philadelphia, JB Lippincott, 1992, 132-144.

Alverdy JC: Effects of glutamine-supplemented diets on immunology of the gut. *J Parenter Enter Nutr* 14(suppl):109S-113S, 1990.

Alverdy J, et al: Effect of parenteral nutrition on gastrointestinal immunity: Importance of enteral stimulation. *Ann Surg* 202:681-684, 1985.

Alverdy JC, et al: Total parenteral nutrition promotes bacterial translocation from the gut. *Surgery* 104:185-190, 1988.

American Academy of Pediatrics Committee on Nutrition: Special diets for infants with inborn errors of amino acid metabolism. *Pediatrics* 57:786, 1976.

American Academy of Pediatrics Committee on Nutrition: Nutritional needs of low-birth-weight infants. *Pediatrics* 75:479-490, 1985.

American Academy of Pediatrics Committee on Nutrition: Iron-fortified infant formulas. *Pediatrics* 84:1114-1115, 1989.

American Medical Association, Department of Foods and Nutrition: Multivitamin preparations for parenteral use: A statement by the Nutrition Advisory Group, 1975. *J Parenter Enter Nutr* 3:258, 1979.

American Society for Parenteral and Enteral Nutrition: Standards for home nutrition support. *Nutr Clin Pract* 7:65-69, (April) 1992.

Anderson JD, et al: Enteral feeding in the critically injured patient. *Nutr Clin Pract* 7:117-122, 1992.

Andrassy RJ: Free amino acids and peptides—The pros and cons, in: *Nutritional Support Strategies for the Catabolic Patient: Proceedings From a Symposium Held at the 1990 American Dietetic Association Meeting.* Norwich, NY, Norwich Eaton Pharmaceuticals, 1991, 21-28.

Argilés JM, et al: The role of cytokines in muscle wasting: Its relation with cancer cachexia. *Med Res Rev* 12:637-652, 1992.

Askanazi J, et al: Respiratory changes induced by large glucose loads of total parenteral nutrition. *JAMA* 243:1444-1447, 1980.

ASPEN Board of Directors: Guidelines for use of total parenteral nutrition in the hospitalized adult patient. *J Parenter Enter Nutr* 10:441-445, 1986.

ASPEN Board of Directors: Guidelines for use of home total parenteral nutrition. *J Parenter Enter Nutr* 11:342-344, 1987 A.

ASPEN Board of Directors: Guidelines for the use of enteral nutrition in the adult patient. *J Parenter Enter Nutr* 11:435-439, 1987 B.

Ball MJ: Hematological and biochemical effects of parenteral nutrition with medium-chain triglycerides: Comparison with long-chain triglycerides. *Am J Clin Nutr* 53:916-922, 1991.

Barbul A: Arginine and immune function. *Nutr* 6(suppl):53-58, 1990.

Baskin W: Advances in enteral nutrition techniques. *Am J Gastroenterol* 87:1547-1553, 1992.

Beal AL, Cerra FB: Multiple organ failure syndrome in the 1990s. Systemic inflammatory response and organ dysfunction. *JAMA* 271:226-233, 1994.

Beam TR, et al: Preventing central venous catheter-related complications: A roundtable discussion. *Infect Surg* 1-13, (Oct) 1990.

Becker WK, Pruitt BA Jr: Parenteral nutrition in the thermally injured patient. *Compr Ther* 17:47-53, 1991.

Bedrick AD: Metabolic tolerance of parenteral lipid in neonates: Better late than never, editorial. *Am J Dis Child* 142:135-136, 1988.

Benya R, et al: Protein and carbohydrate absorptive efficiency of chronically malnourished and well-nourished patients during enteral feeding initiation. *J Am Coll Nutr* 10:50-56, 1991.

Bhatia J, et al: Effect of protein/energy ratio on growth and behavior of premature infants: Preliminary findings. *J Pediatr* 119:103-110, 1991.

Bishop NJ, et al: Increased bone mineral content of preterm infants fed with a nutrient enriched formula after discharge from hospital. *Arch Dis Child* 68:573-578, 1993.

Blackburn GL, Driscoll DF: Time to abandon routine albumin supplementation, editorial. *Crit Care Med* 20:157-158, 1992.

Bragg LE, et al: Influence of nutrient delivery on gut structure and function. *Nutrition* 7:237-243, (July/Aug) 1991.

Brandi LS, et al: Energy expenditure and gas exchange measurements in postoperative patients: Thermodilution versus indirect calorimetry. *Crit Care Med* 20:1273-1284, 1992.

Brans YW, et al: Tolerance of fat emulsions in very-low-birth-weight neonates. *Am J Dis Child* 142:145-152, 1988.

Braunschweig CL, et al: Rationale and guidelines for parenteral and enteral transition feeding of the 3 to 30 kg child. *J Am Diet Assoc* 88:479-482, 1988.

Breslow RA, et al: The importance of dietary protein in healing pressure ulcers. *J Am Geriatr Soc* 41:357-362, 1993.

Brouhard BH, LaGrone L: Effect of dietary protein restriction on functional renal reserve in diabetic nephropathy. *Am J Med* 89:427-431, (Oct) 1990.

Brown SJ, Begley JP: Biochemical monitoring of total parenteral nutrition. *Pharm J* 247:40-45, 1991.

Brown RO, et al: Comparison of modified amino acids and standard amino acids in parenteral nutrition support of thermally injured patients. *Crit Care Med* 18:1096-1101, 1990.

Brown KH, et al: Use of nonhuman milks in the dietary management of young children with acute diarrhea: A meta-analysis of clinical trials. *Pediatrics* 93:17-27, 1994.

Bruder N, et al: Evolution of energy expenditure and nitrogen excretion in severe head-injured patients. *Crit Care Med* 19:43-48, 1991.

Buchman AL, et al: Lecithin increases plasma free choline and decreases hepatic steatosis in long-term total parenteral nutrition patients. *Gastroenterology* 102:1363-1370, 1992.

Buerk C: Nutrition in thermal injuries, in Van Way CW III (ed): *Handbook of Surgical Nutrition.* Philadelphia, JB Lippincott, 1992, 197-206.

Büller HA, Grand RJ: Lactose intolerance. *Annu Rev Med* 41:141-148, 1990.

Byrd TM: Enteral nutrition therapy. *Resident Staff Physician* 36:47-50, (Sept) 1990.

Cabré E, Gassull MA: Complications of enteral feeding. *Nutrition* 8:1-9, 1993.

Campos AC, Meguid MM: A critical appraisal of the usefulness of perioperative nutritional support. *Am J Clin Nutr* 55:117-130, 1992.

Cano N, et al: Perdialytic parenteral nutrition with lipids and amino acids in malnourished hemodialysis patients. *Am J Clin Nutr* 52:726-730, 1990.

Carlson SE, et al: Arachidonic acid status correlates with first year growth in preterm infants. *PNAS* 90:1073-1077, 1993 A.

Carlson SE, et al: Visual acuity development in healthy preterm infants: Effect of marine oil supplementation. *Am J Clin Nutr* 58:35-42, 1993 B.

Carvajal HF: Energy and protein metabolism in the pediatric burn patient, in Suskind RM, Lewinter-Suskind L (eds): *Textbook of Pediatric Nutrition,* ed 2. New York, Raven Press, 1993, 217-223.

Casper K, et al: Overfeeding: Cardiovascular and metabolic response during continuous formula infusion in adult humans. *Am J Clin Nutr* 52:602-609, 1990.

Cataldi-Betcher EL, et al: Complications occurring during enteral nutrition support: Prospective study. *J Parenter Enter Nutr* 7:546-552, 1983.

Cerra FB, et al: Disease-specific amino acid infusion (F080) in hepatic encephalopathy: Prospective, randomized, double-blind, controlled trial. *J Parenter Enter Nutr* 9:288-295, 1985.

Cerra FB, et al: Effect of stress level, amino acid formula, and nitrogen dose on nitrogen retention in traumatic and septic stress. *Ann Surg* 205:282-287, 1987.

Cerra FB, et al: Improvement in immune function in ICU patients by enteral nutrition supplemented with arginine, RNA, and menhaden oil is independent of nitrogen balance. *Nutrition* 7:193-199, (May/June) 1991.

Chalmers RA, et al: L-carnitine insufficiency in disorders of organic acid metabolism: Response to L-carnitine by patients with methylmalonic acidemia and 3-hydroxy-3-methyl-glutaric acidemia. *J Inherit Metab Dis* 7 (suppl 2):109-110, 1984.

Chan GM: Growth and bone mineral status of discharged very low birth weight infants fed different formulas of human milk. *J Pediatr* 123:439-443, 1993.

Chandra RK, et al: Effect of feeding whey hydrolysate, soy and conventional cow milk formulas on incidence of atopic disease in high risk infants. *Ann Allergy* 63:102-106, (Aug) 1989.

Chin SE, et al: Nutritional support in children with end-stage liver disease: A randomized crossover trial of a branched-chain amino acid supplement. *Am J Clin Nutr* 56:158-163, 1992.

Christensen ML, et al: Plasma carnitine concentration and lipid metabolism in infants receiving parenteral nutrition. *J Pediatr* 115:794-798, 1989.

Cochran EB, et al: Parenteral nutrition in pediatric patients. *Clin Pharm* 7:351-366, 1988.

Cockburn F: Neonatal brain and dietary lipids. *Arch Dis Child* 70:F1-F2, 1994.

Collins JW Jr, et al: A controlled trial of insulin infusion and parenteral nutrition in extremely low birth weight infants with glucose intolerance. *J Pediatr* 118:921-927, 1991.

Cooke RJ, et al: Effects of type of dietary protein on acid-base status, protein nutritional status, plasma levels of amino acids, and nutrient balance in the very low birth weight infant. *J Pediatr* 121:444-451, 1992.

Cravo M, et al: Nutritional support in Crohn's disease: Which route? *Am J Gastroenterol* 86:317-321, (March) 1991.

Crowe PJ, et al: A new intravenous emulsion containing medium-chain triglyceride: Studies of its metabolic effects in the perioperative period compared with a conventional long-chain triglyceride emulsion. *J Parenter Enter Nutr* 9:720-724, 1985.

Dahlström KA, et al: Lipid tolerance in children receiving long-term parenteral nutrition: A biochemical and immunologic study. *J Pediatr* 113:985-990, 1988.

Daly JM, et al: Immune and metabolic effects of arginine in the surgical patient. *Ann Surg* 208:512-522, 1988.

Daly JM, et al: Enteral nutrition with supplemental arginine, RNA, and omega-3 fatty acids in patients after operation: Immunologic, metabolic, and clinical outcome. *Surgery* 112:56-67, 1992.

Danner DJ, Elsas LJ: Disorders of branched chain amino acid and keto acid metabolism, in Scriver CR, et al (eds): *Metabolic Basis of Inherited Disease*, ed 6. New York, McGraw Hill, 1989, 671-692.

DeChicco RS, Matarese LE: Selection of nutrition support regimens. *Nutr Clin Pract* 7:239-245, 1992.

Deitch EA: Multiple organ failure: Pathophysiology and potential future therapy. *Ann Surg* 216:117-134, 1992.

DeLegge MH, Kirby DK: Enteral nutrition overview part I, enteral access devices. *Pract Gastroenterol* 15 (No. 10):21-27, 1991.

Dennison AR, et al: Total parenteral nutrition using conventional and medium chain triglycerides: Effect on liver function tests, complement, and nitrogen balance. *J Parenter Enter Nutr* 12:15-19, 1988.

Drickamer MA, Cooney LM Jr: A geriatrician's guide to enteral feeding. *J Am Geriatr Soc* 41:672-679, 1993.

Driscoll DF: Clinical issues regarding the use of total nutrient admixtures. *DICP* 24:296-303,1990.

Driscoll DF, Bistrian BR: Special considerations required for the formulation and administration of total parenteral nutrition therapy in the elderly patient. *Drugs Aging* 2:395-405, 1992.

Driscoll DF, Blackburn GL: Total parenteral nutrition 1990: A review of its current status in hospitalised patients, and the need for patient-specific feeding. *Drugs* 40:346-363, 1990.

Edes TE, et al: Diarrhea in tube-fed patients: Feeding formula not necessarily the cause. *Am J Med* 88:91-93, (Feb) 1990.

Eisenberg PG: Causes of diarrhea in tube-fed patients: A comprehensive approach to diagnosis and management. *Nutr Clin Pract* 8:119-123, 1993.

Elia M: Artificial enteral nutrition: Patient profiles and the use of fiber, in Cummings JH (ed): *The Role of Dietary Fiber in Enteral Nutrition*. Abbott Park, Ill: Abbott International, 1989, 85-92.

Elsas LJ, Acosta PB: Nutrition support of inherited metabolic diseases, in Shils ME, Young VR (eds): *Modern Nutrition in Health and Disease,* ed 7. Philadelphia, Lea & Febiger, 1988, 1337-1379.

Enteral Nutrition Council: *Position Paper on Medication/Enteral Formula Interactions*. Atlanta, Enteral Nutrition Council, 1987.

Enteral Nutrition Council: *Position Paper on Freezing/Thawing Enteral Nutrition Products*. Atlanta, Enteral Nutrition Council, 1988.

Enzi G, et al: Metabolic and hormonal effects of early nutritional supplementation after surgery in burn patients. *Crit Care Med* 18:719-721, 1990.

Epps DR: Enteral nutrition: Overview. *J Pharm Pract* 1:109-120, 1988.

Fairfull-Smith RJ, Freeman JB: Peripheral parenteral nutrition, in Deitel M (ed): *Nutrition in Clinical Surgery*. Baltimore, Williams and Wilkins, 1993, 143-149.

Feller AG, et al: Effects of three liquid diets on nutrition-sensitive plasma proteins of tube-fed elderly men. *J Am Geriatr Soc* 38:663-668, 1990.

Fischer JE, Chance WT: Total parenteral nutrition, glutamine, and tumor growth. *J Parenter Enter Nutr* 14 (suppl):86S-89S, 1990.

Fleming CR: Trace element metabolism in adult patients requiring total parenteral nutrition. *Am J Clin Nutr* 49:573-579, 1989.

Flowers JF, et al: Catheter-related complications of total parenteral nutrition, in Fischer JE (ed): *Total Parenteral Nutrition*, ed 2. Boston, Little Brown, 1991, 25-45.

Food and Drug Administration: Nutrient requirements for infant formulas. *Federal Register* 50:45106-45108, (Oct) 1985.

Forlaw L, et al: Enteral delivery systems, in Rombeau JL, Caldwell MD (eds): *Enteral and Tube Feeding*, ed 2. Philadelphia, WB Saunders, 1990, 174-191.

Frank HA, Green LC: Successful use of a bulk laxative to control the diarrhea of tube feeding. *Scand J Plast Reconstr Surg* 13:193-194, 1979.

Freund HR: Abnormalities of liver function and hepatic damage associated with total parenteral nutrition. *Nutrition* 7:1-6, 1991.

Fried MD, et al: Decrease in gastric emptying time and episodes of regurgitation in children with spastic quadriplegia fed a whey-based formula. *J Pediatr* 120:569-572, 1992.

Fuchs GJ III: Enteral support of the hospitalized child, in Suskind RM, Lewinter-Suskind L (eds): *Textbook of Pediatric Nutrition*, ed 2. New York, Raven Press, 1993, 239-246.

Fuksa M, et al: Growth of microorganisms in 3-in-1 TPN admixtures. *Nutr Support Services* 7:22-24, (Dec) 1987.

Garabedian-Ruffalo SM, Ruffalo RL: Drug and nutrient interactions. *Am Fam Physician* 165-174, (Feb) 1986.

Giaffer MH, et al: Controlled trial of polymeric versus elemental diet in treatment of active Crohn's disease. *Lancet* 335:816-819, 1990.

Gilbertson N, et al: Introduction of intravenous lipid administration on the first day of life in the very low birth weight neonate. *J Pediatr* 119:615-623, 1991.

Go J, Grant DJW: Total nutrient admixtures, part 2. *Nutr Support Serv* 7:11-21, (Dec) 1987.

Gogos CA, et al: Tumor necrosis factor production by human mononuclear cells during total parenteral nutrition containing long-chain triglycerides. *Nutrition* 8:26-29, 1992.

Golper TA, et al: Multicenter trial of L-carnitine in maintenance hemodialysis patients: I. Carnitine concentrations and lipid effects. *Kidney Int* 38:904-911, 1990.

González-Huix F, et al: Polymeric enteral diets as primary treatment of active Crohn's disease: A prospective steroid controlled trial. *Gut* 34:778-782, 1993 A.

González-Huix F, et al: Enteral *versus* parenteral nutrition as adjunct therapy in acute ulcerative colitis. *Am J Gastroenterol* 88:227-232, 1993 B.

Goodwin WJ, Byers PM: Nutritional management of the head and neck cancer patient. *Med Clin North Am* 77:597-610, 1993.

'Gottschlich MM, et al: Diarrhea in tube fed burn patients. *JPEN* 12:338-345, 1988.

Grant JP: *Handbook of Total Parenteral Nutrition*, ed 2. Philadelphia, Harcourt Brace Jovanovich, 1992.

Grant J, Denne SC: Effect of intermittent versus continuous enteral feeding on energy expenditure in premature infants. *J Pediatr* 118:928-932, 1991.

Greene HL, et al: Guidelines for the use of vitamins, trace elements, calcium, magnesium, and phosphorus in infants and children receiving total parenteral nutrition: Report of the Subcommittee on Pediatric Parenteral Nutrient Requirements from the Committee on Clinical Practice Issues of the American Society for Clinical Nutrition. *Am J Clin Nutr* 48:1324-1342, 1988.

Gregory JW, et al: Dietary treatment of hyperlysinaemia. *Arch Dis Child* 64:716-720, 1989.

Grimble GK, Silk DBA: Administration of fat emulsions with nutritional mixtures from the three-liter delivery system: TPN, efficacy and safety. *Nutr Support Serv* 10:14-16, (Oct) 1987.

Grimble GK, Silk DBA: The nitrogen source of elemental diets—An unresolved issue? *Nutr Clin Pract* 227-230, (Dec) 1990.

Hammarqvist F, et al: Addition of glutamine to total parenteral nutrition after elective abdominal surgery spares free glutamine in muscle, counteracts the fall in muscle protein synthesis, and improves nitrogen balance. *Ann Surg* 209:455-461, 1989.

Hammond JMJ, et al: Double-blind study of selective decontamination of the digestive tract in intensive care. *Lancet* 340:5-9, 1992.

Hamosh M, et al: Fat absorption in premature infants: Medium-chain triglycerides and long-chain triglycerides are absorbed from formula at similar rates. *J Pediatr Gastroenterol Nutr* 13:143-149, 1991.

Hardin TC: Cytokine mediators of malnutrition: Clinical implications. *Nutr Clin Pract* 8:55-59, 1993.

Harrison VC, Peat GM: Feeding intervals and fat absorption in preterm babies. *S Afr Med J* 81:160-161, 1992.

Hatton J, et al: Safety and efficacy of a lipid emulsion containing medium-chain triglycerides. *Clin Pharm* 9:366-371, 1990.

Heird WC, et al: Amino acid mixture designed to maintain normal plasma amino acid patterns in infants and children requiring parenteral nutrition. *Pediatrics* 80:401-408, 1987.

Heird WC, et al: Pediatric parenteral amino acid mixture in low birth weight infants. *Pediatrics* 81:41-50, 1988.

Heird WC, et al: Practical aspects of achieving positive energy balance in low birth weight infants. *J Pediatr* 120:S120-S128, 1992.

Helms RA, et al: Enhanced lipid utilization in infants receiving oral L-carnitine during long-term parenteral nutrition. *J Pediatr* 109:984-988, 1986.

Helms RA, et al: Effect of intravenous L-carnitine on growth parameters and fat metabolism during parenteral nutrition in neonates. *J Parenter Enter Nutr* 14:448-453, 1990.

Herfindal ET, et al: Complications of home parenteral nutrition. *Clin Pharm* 11:543-548, 1992.

Horsman A, et al: Bone mineral accretion rate and calcium intake in preterm infants. *Arch Dis Child* 64:910-918, 1989.

Horst D, et al: Comparison of dietary protein with an oral, branched chain-enriched amino acid supplement in chronic portal-systemic encephalopathy: A randomized controlled trial. *Hepatology* 4:279-287, 1984.

Howard D, Thompson DF: Taurine: An essential amino acid to prevent cholestasis in neonates? *Ann Pharmacother* 26:1390-1392, 1992.

Hurley DL, McMahon MM: Long-term parenteral nutrition and metabolic bone disease. *Endocrinol Metab Clin North Am* 19:113-131, (March) 1990.

Idjradinata P, Pollitt E: Reversal of developmental delays in iron-deficient anaemic infants treated with iron. *Lancet* 341:1-4, 1993.

Institute of Medicine: *Nutrition During Lactation.* Washington, DC, National Academy Press, 1991.

Jacobson S, Glaumann H: Utilization and metabolic effects of the all-in-one total nutrient admixture compared to conventional TPN postoperatively. *Nutr Support Serv* 8:25-29, (Jan) 1988.

Jarnberg P-O: Liposyn versus Intralipid: A comparative study of two lipid emulsions in critically ill patients receiving total parenteral nutrition. *Curr Ther Res* 50:38-44, 1991.

Jeejeebhoy KN (ed): *Total Parenteral Nutrition in the Hospital and at Home.* CRC Press, Boca Raton, FL, 1983, 82.

Jeejeebhoy KN: Lipid emulsions, in Fischer JE (ed): *Total Parenteral Nutrition,* ed 2. Boston, Little Brown, 1991, 403-421.

Jensen GL, Jensen RG: Specialty lipids for infant nutrition: II. Concerns, new developments, and future applications. *J Pediatr Gastroenterol Nutr* 15:382-394, 1992 A.

Jensen RG, Jensen GL: Specialty lipids for infant nutrition: I. Milks and formulas. *J Pediatr Gastroenterol Nutr* 15:232-245, 1992 B.

Jensen RG, et al: Lipids in human milk and infant formulas. *Annu Rev Nutr* 12:417-441, 1992.

Johnson LE, et al: Oral nutritional supplement use in elderly nursing home patients. *J Am Geriatr Soc* 41:947-952, 1993.

Kanarek KS, et al: Concurrent administration of albumin with total parenteral nutrition in sick newborn infants. *J Parenter Enter Nutr* 16:49-53, 1992.

Kaysen GA: Nutritional management of nephrotic syndrome. *J Renal Nutr* 2:50-58, (April) 1992.

Klimberg VS: Glutamine: A key factor in establishing and maintaining intestinal health, in Andrassy R (ed): *Nutritional Support Strategies for the Catabolic Patient: Proceedings From a Symposium Held at the 1990 American Dietetic Association Meeting.* Norwich, NY, Norwich Eaton Pharmaceuticals, 1991, 39-47.

Koo WWK: Parenteral nutrition-related bone disease. *J Parenter Enter Nutr* 16:386-394, 1992.

Koo WWK, Tsang RC: Mineral requirements of low-birth-weight infants. *J Am Coll Nutr* 10:474-486, 1991.

Koruda MJ: Controlling diarrhea in tube-fed patient. *Support Line* 13(1):10-14, 1991.

Kotler DP, et al: Effect of home total parenteral nutrition on body composition in patients with acquired immunodeficiency syndrome. *J Parenter Enter Nutr* 14:454-458, 1990.

Kretchmer N, Etzwiler DD: Disorders associated with the metabolism of phenylalanine and tyrosine. *Pediatrics* 21:454, 1958.

Kushner RF: Should enteral nutrition be considered as primary therapy in acute Crohn's disease? *Nutr Rev* 50:166-178, (June) 1992.

LaFrance RJ, Miyagawa CI: Pharmaceutical considerations in total parenteral nutrition, in Fischer JE (ed): *Total Parenteral Nutrition*, ed 2. Boston, Little Brown, 1991, 57-97.

Leibovitz B, Mueller J: Carnitine. *J Optimal Nutr* 2:90-109, 1993.

Levy HL, et al: Routine newborn screening for histidinemia: Clinical and biochemical results. *N Engl J Med* 291:1214, 1974.

Levy R, et al: Thiamine, riboflavin, folate, and vitamin B_{12} status of low birth weight infants receiving parenteral and enteral nutrition. *J Parenter Enter Nutr* 16:241-247, 1992.

Li S: Acute renal failure, in Fischer JE (ed): *Total Parenteral Nutrition,* ed 2. Boston, Little Brown, 1991, 191-202.

Liebl BH, et al: Dietary fiber and long-term large bowel response in enterally nourished nonambulatory profoundly retarded youth. *JPEN* 14:371-375, 1990.

Lima LAM, et al: Neonatal parenteral nutrition with a fat emulsion containing medium chain triglycerides. *Acta Paediatr Scand* 77:332-339, 1988.

Lindblad B, et al: On the enzymic defects in hereditary tyrosinemia. *PNAS* 74:4641-4645, 1977.

Lindsay RM, et al: Adequacy of hemodialysis and nutrition—Important determinants of morbidity and mortality. *Kidney Intern* 45(suppl 44):S85-S91, 1994.

Lochs H, et al: Comparison of enteral nutrition and drug treatment in active Crohn's disease: Results of the European Cooperative Crohn's Disease Study IV. *Gastroenterology* 101:881-888, 1991.

Lockwood AH: *Hepatic Encephalopathy.* Boston, Butterworth-Heinemann, 1992.

Long CL: Energy expenditure of major burns. *J Trauma* 19:904, 1979.

Lowe DK, et al: Safety of glutamine-enriched parenteral nutrient solutions in humans. *Am J Clin Nutr* 52:1101-1106, 1990.

Lowry SF: Cytokine mediators of immunity and inflammation. *Arch Surg* 128:1235-1241, 1993.

Lucas A: Enteral nutrition, in Tsang RC, et al (eds): *Nutritional Needs of the Preterm Infant: Scientific Basis and Practical Guidelines.* Baltimore, Williams and Wilkins, 1993, 209-223.

Lucas A, et al: High alkaline phosphatase activity and growth in preterm neonates. *Arch Dis Child* 64:902-909, 1989 A.

Lucas A, et al: Early diet in preterm babies and developmental status in infancy. *Arch Dis Child* 64:1570-1578, 1989 B.

Lucas A, et al: Early diet in preterm babies and developmental status at 18 months. *Lancet* 335:1477-1481, 1990.

Lucas A, et al: Randomised trial of nutrition for preterm infants after discharge. *Arch Dis Child* 67:324-327, 1992.

Lutomski DM, et al: Sorbitol content of selected oral liquids. *Ann Pharmacother* 27:269-274, 1993.

Manz F, et al: Low renal net acid excretion, high calciuria and biochemical signs of sodium deficiency in low-birth-weight infants fed a new low-phosphorus formula. *Acta Paediatr* 81:969-973, 1992.

Marchesini G, et al: Long-term oral branched-chain amino acid treatment in chronic hepatic encephalopathy. *J Hepatol* 11:92-101, 1990.

Marian M: Pediatric nutrition support. *Nutr Clin Pract* 8:199-209, 1993.

Martindale RG, Andrassy RJ: Elemental nutrition overview, in Andrassy R (ed): *Nutritional Support Strategies for the Catabolic Patient: Proceedings From a Symposium Held at the 1990 American Dietetic Association Meeting.* Norwich, NY, Norwich Eaton Pharmaceuticals, 1991, 2-13.

Mascioli EA, et al: Thermogenesis from intravenous medium-chain triglycerides. *J Parenter Enter Nutr* 15:27-31, 1991.

Mattox TW, Teasley-Strausburg KM: Brief communication: Clinical experience with high branched-chain parenteral nutrition. *J Am Coll Nutr* 11:25-28, 1992.

Matuchansky C, et al: Cyclical parenteral nutrition. *Lancet* 340:588-592, 1992.

McCabe ER, McCabe L: Issues in the dietary management of phenylketonuria: Breast-feeding and trace-metal nutriture. *Ann NY Acad Sci* 477:215, 1986.

McClave SA, Snider HL: Use of indirect calorimetry in clinical nutrition. *Nutr Clin Pract* 7:207-221, 1992.

McCrae JD, et al: Parenteral nutrition: Hospital to home. *J Am Diet Assoc* 93:664-670, 1993.

Medical Research Council Working Party on Phenylketonuria: Recommendations on the dietary management of phenylketonuria. *Arch Dis Child* 68:426-427, 1993.

Meguid MM, et al: Nutritional support in surgical practice: Part I. *Am J Surg* 159:345-358, 1990 A.

Meguid MM, et al: Nutritional support in surgical practice: Part II. *Am J Surg* 159:427-443, 1990 B.

Mehta NR, et al: Adherence of medium-chain fatty acids to feeding tubes of premature infants fed formula fortified with medium-chain triglyceride. *J Pediatr Gastroenterol Nutr* 13:267-269, 1991.

Melegh B: Carnitine supplementation in the premature. *Biol Neonate* 58(suppl 1):93-106, 1990.

Merritt RJ, et al: Whey protein hydrolysate formula for infants with gastrointestinal intolerance to cow milk and soy protein in infant formulas. *J Pediatr Gastroenterol Nutr* 11:78-82, 1990.

Messing B, et al: Effect of fat-emulsion phospholipids on serum lipoprotein profile during 1 mo of cyclic total parenteral nutrition. *Am J Clin Nutr* 52:1094-1100, 1990.

Messing B, et al: Chronic cholestasis and macronutrient excess in patients treated with prolonged parenteral nutrition. *Nutrition* 8:30-36, 1992.

Meydani SN, Dinarello CA: Influence of dietary fatty acids on cytokine production and its clinical implications. *Nutr Clin Pract* 8:65-72, 1993.

Milla PJ, et al: Small intestinal absorption of amino acids and a dipeptide in pancreatic insufficiency. *Gut* 24:818-824, 1983.

Milner EA, et al: Superior mesenteric artery syndrome in a burn patient. *Nutr Clin Pract* 8:264-266, 1993.

Mimouni F, et al: Bone mineralization in the first year of life in infants fed human milk, cow-milk formula, or soy-based formula. *J Pediatr* 122:348-354, 1993.

Mobarhan S, Barch DH: Nutritional management of patients with deglutition disorders, transfer dysphagia and esophageal carcinoma. *Dis Esophagus* 2:15-22, 1989.

Mobarhan S, Trumbore LS: Enteral tube feeding: A clinical perspective on recent advances. *Nutr Rev* 49:129-138, 1991.

Moore EE, Moore FA: Immediate enteral nutrition following multisystem trauma: A decade perspective. *J Am Coll Nutr* 10:633-648, 1991.

Moore FA, et al; Early enteral feeding, compared with parenteral, reduces postoperative septic complications: The results of a meta-analysis. *Ann Surg* 216:172-183, 1992.

Mosca R, et al: The benefits of isolator cultures in the management of suspected catheter sepsis. *Surgery* 102:718-723, 1987.

Moukarzel AA, et al: Iodine supplementation in children receiving long-term parenteral nutrition. *J Pediatr* 121:252-254, 1992 A.

Moukarzel AA, et al: Carnitine status of children receiving long-term total parenteral nutrition: A longitudinal prospective study. *J Pediatr* 120:759-762, 1992 B.

Mowatt-Larssen CA, Brown RO: Specialized nutritional support in respiratory disease. *Clin Pharm* 12:276-292, 1993.

Mowatt-Larssen CA, et al: Comparison of tolerance and nutritional outcome between a peptide and a standard enteral formula in critically ill, hypoalbuminemic patients. *J Parenter Enter Nutr* 16:20-24, 1992.

Mullen KD, Weber FL Jr: Role of nutrition in hepatic encephalopathy. *Semin Liver Dis* 11:292-304, 1991.

Naidoo DP, et al: Cardiovascular complications of parenteral nutrition. *Postgrad Med J* 68:629-633, 1992.

National Center for Health Statistics: *NCHS* Percentiles. Genentech, 1987.

National Research Council: *Recommended Dietary Allowances*, ed 10. Washington, DC, National Academy Press, 1989.

Naylor CD, et al: Parenteral nutrition with branched-chain amino acids in hepatic encephalopathy: A meta-analysis. *Gastroenterology* 97:1033-1042, 1989.

Nearman HS, Herman ML: Toxic effects of colloids in the intensive care unit. *Crit Care Med* 71:713-722, 1991.

Nichoalds GE, et al: Lipid and lipoprotein levels in adults receiving Liposyn II. *Nutrition* 7:329-332, 1991.

Niemiec PW Jr, Vanderveen TW: Compatibility considerations in parenteral nutrient solutions. *Am J Hosp Pharm* 41:893-911, 1984.

Nolph KD: What's new in peritoneal dialysis—An overview. *Kidney Int* 42(suppl 38):S-148-S-152, 1992.

Okada A, et al: Branched-chain amino acids metabolic support in surgical patients: A randomized, controlled trial in patients with sub-total or total gastrectomy in 16 Japanese institutions. *J Parenter Enter Nutr* 12:332-337, 1988.

Olson AL, et al: Low carnitine intake and altered lipid metabolism in infants. *Am J Clin Nutr* 49:624-628, 1989.

Oski FA: Iron deficiency in infancy and childhood. *N Engl J Med* 329:190-193, 1993.

Parry-Billings M, et al: Effects of major and minor surgery on plasma glutamine and cytokine levels. *Arch Surg* 127:1237-1240, 1992.

Pelegano JF, et al: Calcium/phosphorus ratio of 1.7:1 in parenteral nutrition (PN) promotes efficient Ca and P retention in preterm infants, abstract. *Pediatr Res* 23:490A, 1988.

Perry M, et al: Stability of penicillins in total parenteral nutrient solution. *Am J Hosp Pharm* 44:1625-1628, 1987.

Pesola GR, et al: Hypertonic nasogastric tube feedings: Do they cause diarrhea? *Crit Care Med* 18:1378-1382, 1990.

Piepmeyer J, et al: *Tube Feeding at Home: A Manual of Instruction for Home Tube-Feeding Care.* Evansville, Ind, Bristol-Myers, 1988.

Pillar B, Perry S: *Evaluating Total Parenteral Nutrition: Final Report and Core Statement of the Technology Assessment and Practice Guidelines Forum.* Washington, DC, Dept of Health and Human Services, 1990.

Pisters PW, Ranson JH: Nutritional support for acute pancreatitis. *Surg Gynecol Obstet* 175:275-284, 1992.

Po ALW: Carnitine: A scientifically exciting molecule. *Pharm J* 388-389, (Sept) 1990.

Polberger SKT, et al: Amino acid concentrations in plasma and urine in very low birth weight infants fed protein-unenriched or human milk protein-enriched human milk. *Pediatrics* 86:909-915, 1990 A.

Polberger SKT, et al: Eleven plasma proteins as indicators of protein nutritional status in very low birth weight infants. *Pediatrics* 86:916-921, 1990 B.

Proietti R, et al: Nutrition in acute renal failure. *Resuscitation* 10:159-166, 1983.

Ramsey BW, et al: Nutritional assessment and management in cystic fibrosis: A consensus report. *Am J Clin Nutr* 55:108-116, 1992.

Rassin DK, et al: Taurine and cholesterol supplementation in the term infant: Responses of growth and metabolism. *J Parenter Enter Nutr* 14:392-397, 1990.

Raouf AH, et al: Enteral feeding as sole treatment for Crohn's disease: Controlled trial of whole protein υ amino acid based feed and a case study of dietary challenge. *Gut* 32:702-707, 1991.

Rebouche CJ: Carnitine function and requirements during the life cycle. *FASEB J* 6:3379-3386, 1992.

Reed MD, et al: Antibiotic compatibility and stability in a parenteral nutrition solution. *Chemotherapy* 25:336-345, 1979.

Rees RGP, et al: Do patients with moderately impaired gastrointestinal function requiring enteral nutrition need a predigested nitrogen source? A prospective crossover controlled clinical trial. *Gut* 33:877-881, 1992.

Roche AF, Himes JH: Incremental growth charts. *Am J Clin Nutr* 33:2041-2052, 1980.

Rose SJ, et al: Carnitine deficiency associated with long-term pivampicillin treatment: The effect of a replacement therapy regime. *Postgrad Med J* 68:932-934, 1992.

Ross E: The role of marine fish oils in the treatment of ulcerative colitis. *Nutr Rev* 51:47-49, 1993.

Roubenoff RA, et al: Hypermetabolism and hypercatabolism in Guillain-Barré syndrome. *JPEN* 16:464-472, 1992.

Rubaltelli FF, et al: Carnitine and the premature. *Biol Neonate* 52 (suppl 1):65-77, 1987.

Rubin M, et al: Effect of lipid infusion on bile composition and lithogenicity in patients without cholesterol gall stones. *Gut* 33:1400-1403, 1992.

Ryan CM, et al: Increased gut permeability early after burns correlates with the extent of burn injury. *Crit Care Med* 20:1508-1512, 1992.

Sami H, et al: New technique in enteral nutrition: Sterile and modular system allowing ambulatory nutritional support. *Nutrition* 4:289-292, 1988.

Scheppach WM, Bartram H-P: Experimental evidence for and clinical implications of fiber and artificial enteral nutrition. *Nutrition* 9:399-405, 1993.

Scriver CR, Levy HL: Histidinemia Part I: Reconciling retrospective and prospective findings. *J Inherit Metab Dis* 6:51-53, 1983.

Scriver CR, et al: Hereditary tyrosinemia and tyrosyluria in a French Canadian geographic isolate. *Am J Dis Child* 113:41-46, 1967.

Segal S: Disorders of galactose metabolism, in: Scriver CR, et al (eds): *Metabolic Basis of Inherited Disease,* ed 6. New York, McGraw-Hill Information Services, 1989, 453-480.

Segal S, Cuatrecasas P: The oxidation of 14C galactose by patients with congenital galactosemia. *Am J Med* 44:340-347, 1968.

Segal S, et al: The metabolism of galactose by patients with congenital galactosemia. *Am J Med* 38:62-70, 1965.

Seidman E, et al: Nutritional issues in pediatric inflammatory bowel disease. *J Pediatr Gastroenterol Nutr* 12:424-438, 1991.

Shea BF, Souney PF: Stability of famotidine in a 3-in-1 total nutrient admixture. *DICP Ann Pharmacother* 24:232-235, 1990.

Shike M, et al: Skin-level gastrostomies and jejunostomies for long-term enteral feeding. *J Parenter Enter Nutr* 13:648-650, 1989.

Shils ME, White PL: Introduction to trace element conference. *Bull NY Acad Med* 60:115-117, 1984.

Shronts EP: *The Patient's Guide to Tube Feeding at Home.* Minneapolis, Clinical Products Division, Sandoz Nutrition Corporation, 1983.

Shronts EP: Enteral formulas update. *Nutr Support Serv* 4:16, (April) 1988.

Shronts EP: Basic concepts of immunology and its application to clinical nutrition. *Nutr Clin Pract* 8:177-183, 1993.

Shulman DI, Kanarek K: Gastrin, motilin, insulin, and insulin-like growth factor-I concentrations in very-low-birth-weight infants receiving enteral or parenteral nutrition. *JPEN* 17:130-133, 1993.

Siliprandi N, et al: Carnitine: Metabolism and clinical chemistry. *Clin Chimica Acta* 183:3-12, 1989.

Silk DBA, Grimble GK: Relevance of physiology of nutrient absorption to formulation of enteral diets. *Nutrition* 8:1-12, 1992.

Sinden AA, Sutphen JL: Dietary treatment of lactose intolerance in infants and children. *J Am Diet Assoc* 91:1567-1571, 1991.

Singer P, et al: Risks and benefits of home parenteral nutrition in the acquired immunodeficiency syndrome. *J Parenter Enter Nutr* 15:75-79, 1991.

Sitrin MD: Nutrition support in inflammatory bowel disease. *Nutr Clin Pract* 7:53-60, (April) 1992.

Sitzmann JV, et al: Statement on guidelines for total parenteral nutrition. *Digest Dis Sci* 34:489-496, 1989.

Skeie B, et al: Branch-chain amino acids: Their metabolism and clinical utility. *Crit Care Med* 18:549-571, 1990.

Smith RB, et al: Plasma carnitine alterations in premature infants receiving various nutritional regimes. *J Parenter Enter Nutr* 12:37-42, 1988.

Snyderman SE, et al: The nutritional therapy of histidinemia. *J Pediatr* 95:712-715, 1979.

Söreide E, et al: Branched-chain amino acid in chronic renal failure patients: Respiratory and sleep effects. *Kidney Int* 40:539-543, 1991.

Souba WW: Glutamine and cancer. *Ann Surg* 218:715-728, 1993.

Souba WW, et al: Gut glutamine metabolism. *J Parenter Enter Nutr* 14 (suppl):45S-50S, 1990.

Standiford TJ, Strieter RM: TNF and IL-1 in sepsis: Good cytokines gone bad, editorial. *J Lab Clin Med* 179-180, (Aug) 1992.

Stehle P, et al: Effect of parenteral glutamine peptide supplements on muscle glutamine loss and nitrogen balance after major surgery. *Lancet* 1:231-233, 1989.

Subcommittee of the Victorian Drug Usage Advisory Committee: Human albumin solutions: Consensus statements for use in selected clinical situations. *Med J Aust* 157:340-343, 1992.

Sulkers EJ, et al: Comparison of two preterm formulas with or without addition of medium-chain triglycerides (MCTs), I: Effects on nitrogen and fat balance and body composition changes. *J Pediatr Gastroenterol Nutr* 15:34-41, 1992 A.

Sulkers EJ, et al: Comparison of two preterm formulas with or without addition of medium-chain triglycerides (MCTs), II: Effects on mineral balance. *J Pediatr Gastroenterol Nutr* 15:42-47, 1992 B.

Sutton MM: Nutritional needs of children with inflammatory bowel disease. *Compr Ther* 18:21-25, (Oct) 1992.

Swails WS, et al: Glutamine content of whole proteins: Implications for enteral formulas. *Nutr Clin Pract* 7:77-80, (April) 1992.

Szwanek M, et al: Trace elements and parenteral nutrition. *Nutr Support Services* 7:8-14, (Aug) 1987.

Talbot JM: *Guidelines for the Scientific Review of Enteral Food Products for Special Medical Purposes.* Washington, DC, Center for

Food Safety and Applied Nutrition, Department of Health and Human Services, 1990.

Talpers SS, et al: Nutritionally associated increased carbon dioxide production: Excess total calories vs high proportion of carbohydrate calories. *Chest* 102:551-555, 1992.

Tamada H, et al: The dipeptide alanyl-glutamine prevents intestinal mucosal atrophy in parenterally fed rats. *J Parenter Enter Nutr* 16:110-116, 1992.

Tannuri U, et al: Long-term stability of lipid emulsions with parenteral nutrition solutions. *Nutrition* 8:98-100, 1992.

Tanphaichitr V, Leelahagul P: Carnitine metabolism and human carnitine deficiency. *Nutrition* 9:246-254, 1993.

Taper LJ, et al: Mineral retention in young men consuming soy-fiber-augmented liquid-formula diets. *Am J Clin Nutr* 48:305-311, 1988.

Teahon K, et al: Ten years' experience with an elemental diet in the management of Crohn's disease. *Gut* 31:1133-1137, 1990.

Teahon K, et al: The effect of elemental diet on intestinal permeability and inflammation in Crohn's disease. *Gastroenterology* 101:84-89, 1991.

Thornton L, Griffin E: Evaluation of a taurine containing amino acid solution in parenteral nutrition. *Arch Dis Child* 66:21-25, 1991.

Tsang RC, Nichols BL: *Nutrition During Infancy.* Philadelphia, Hanley and Belfus, 1988.

Tsang RC, et al (eds): *Nutritional Needs of the Preterm Infant: Scientific Basis and Practical Guidelines.* Pauling, NY, Caduceus Medical Publishers, 1993.

Van Way CW III, Allen JA: Intravenous nutrition, in Van Way CW III (ed): *Handbook of Surgical Nutrition.* Philadelphia, JB Lippincott, 1992, 73-92.

Vanderhoof JA: Short bowel syndrome: Smoothing the road to recovery. *Contemp Pediatr* 9:19-34, (Oct) 1992.

Vanhuynegem L, et al: Detection of central venous catheter-associated sepsis. *Eur J Clin Microbiol* 4:46-48, 1985.

Vazquez JA, et al: Effect of starvation on amino acid and peptide transport and hydrolysis in humans. *Am J Physiol* 249:G563-G566, 1985.

Vehe KL, et al: The efficacy of nutrition support in infected patients with chronic renal failure. *Pharmacotherapy* 11:303-307, 1991.

Venkataraman PS, et al: Effect of intravenous calcium infusions on serum chemistries in neonates. *J Pediatr Gastroenterol Nutr* 13:134-138, 1991.

The Veterans Affairs Total Parenteral Nutrition Cooperative Study Group: Perioperative total parenteral nutrition in surgical patients. *N Engl J Med* 325:525-532, 1991.

Wahn U, et al: Comparison of the residual allergenic activity of six different hydrolyzed protein formulas. *J Pediatr* 121:S80-S84, 1992.

Wallace C, Keast D: Glutamine and macrophage function. *Metabolism* 41:1016-1020, 1992.

Warner BW: Parenteral nutrition in the pediatric patient, in Fischer JE (ed): *Total Parenteral Nutrition,* ed 2. Boston, Little Brown, 1991, 299-322.

Weissman C, et al: Intravenous infusion of a medium-chain triglyceride-enriched lipid emulsion. *Crit Care Med* 16:1183-1190, 1988.

Wennberg A, et al: Prevalence of carnitine depletion in critically ill patients with undernutrition. *Metabolism* 41:165-171, (Feb) 1992.

Wetzel NC: The baby grid: An application of the grid technique to growth and development in infants. *J Pediatr* 29:439-454, 1946.

Wetzel NC: Grid for evaluating physical fitness in terms of physique (body build), developmental level and basal metabolism, in: *A Guide to Individual Progress From Infancy to Maturity.* Cleveland, Ohio, NEA Service Inc, 1948.

Whyte RK, et al: Energy balance in low birth weight infants fed formula of high or low medium-chain triglyceride content. *J Pediatr* 108:964-971, 1986.

Williams AF: Human milk and the preterm baby: Mothers should breast feed. *BMJ* 306:1628-1629, 1993.

Wolk R: Intraperitoneal nutrition. *Hosp Pharm* 27:893-905, 1992.

Wood RJ, et al: Calciuretic effect of cyclic versus continuous total parenteral nutrition. *Am J Clin Nutr* 41:614-619, 1985.

Wright JK Jr: Short gut syndrome—Options for management. *Compr Ther* 18 (No. 8):5-8, 1992.

Zaloga GP: Studies comparing intact protein, peptide and amino acid formulas, in: *Uses of Elemental Diets in Clinical Nutrition.* Boca Raton, Fla, CRC Press, 1993, 201-217.

Zarling EJ, et al: Effect of enteral formula infusion rate, osmolality, and chemical composition upon clinical tolerance and carbohydrate absorption in normal subjects. *J Parenter Enter Nutr* 10:588-590, 1986.

Zeisel SH: Choline: An important nutrient in brain development, liver function and carcinogenesis. *J Am Coll Nutr* 11:473-481, 1992.

Zelikovic I, et al: Taurine depletion in very low birth weight infants receiving prolonged total parenteral nutrition: Role of renal immaturity. *J Pediatr* 116:301-306, 1990.

Ziegler EE, Ryu JE: Renal solute load and diet in growing premature infants. *J Pediatr* 89:609-611, 1976.

Ziegler TR, et al: Safety and metabolic effects of L-glutamine administration in humans. *J Parenter Enter Nutr* 14 (suppl):137S-146S, 1990.

Ziegler TR, et al: Clinical and metabolic efficacy of glutamine-supplemented parenteral nutrition after bone marrow transplantation: A randomized, double-blind, controlled study. *Ann Intern Med* 116:821-828, 1992.

Blood, Blood Components, and Plasma Expanders

99

Blood is transfused most often to provide temporary support during treatment of an underlying condition. However, a blood transfusion is potentially hazardous and should not be given unless the risk/benefit ratio is clearly favorable. Viral infections, particularly hepatitis and, rarely, human immunodeficiency virus (HIV) and other retroviruses, may be transmitted (Barker and Dodd, 1989; Barbara and Contreras, 1990). In addition, there is some evidence that transfusion has an immunosuppressive effect, and this may increase susceptibility to infection and may enhance metastasis or recurrence of malignancies (Blumberg and Heal, 1989; Brunson and Alexander, 1990; Contreras and Mollison, 1990; Liewald et al, 1990). However, other retrospective studies found no increase in the rates of metastasis or recurrence in patients given perioperative blood transfusions (Weiden et al, 1987; Moriguchi et al, 1990). Randomized clinical trials are needed to resolve this disparity in findings. Although transmission of HIV and other similar infectious agents by transfusion is relatively rare, immunosuppression can occur with as little as one transfusion (Perkins, 1988; Petricciani and Epstein, 1988). This effect may be beneficial in patients undergoing kidney or heart transplantation, even in those given cyclosporine for immunosuppression (Ross and Yap, 1990).

Whole blood is obtained from a donor and collected into a bag containing an acidified anticoagulant preservative solution (usually CPD/adenine-saline). Blood components are usually produced from single units of whole blood by differential centrifugation. Some components (eg, platelets, plasma) also are obtained through apheresis procedures. Further processing by filtration, fractionation, and freeze-thawing is used to prepare some plasma derivatives. Utilization of a closed system of presterilized, interconnected bags or sterile connection devices reduces bacterial contamination to a minimum but does not affect infectious agents present in the donor's blood. The availability and proper use of component preparations have minimized some risks and markedly reduced the need for whole blood transfusions. The required component (eg, red blood cells, platelets, fresh frozen plasma) usually can be administered without burdening the circulation; exposure to donor alloantibodies, potentially harmful cations, and metabolites is reduced; and utilization of each unit of blood is maximized, since components not needed by one patient are available for other recipients. Quality control measures ensure that blood components meet minimal acceptable standards (eg, for number and survival of red blood cells).

Plasma derivatives (eg, albumin, factor VIII, factor IX complex, gamma globulins, plasma protein fraction) are prepared from large pools of plasma and are sterilized by filtration. Some derivatives are solvent-, heat-, and/or detergent-treated to eliminate or at least minimize the potential for transmission of infectious agents; others undergo immunoaffinity chromatography (monoclonal antibody purification) to accomplish this goal. Most recently, recombinant DNA technology has produced some plasma derivatives (eg, factor VIII) that are free of infectious agents. Plasma derivatives, unlike blood components, can be assayed and standardized for potency.

For a detailed discussion of donor selection, transfusion procedures, and current accepted standards, see publications on blood banking, such as *Standards for Blood Banks and Transfusion Services* (Holland, 1991), *Clinical Practice of Transfusion Medicine* (Petz and Swisher, 1989), and *The Technical Manual* (Walker et al, 1990).

When acute bleeding occurs, attempts should be made to maintain (1) blood volume at ≥90% of normal; (2) hemoglobin level of at least 7 g/dL and hematocrit of 0.21 to allow adequate oxygen transport to tissues (however, rigorous clinical trials to establish these thresholds have not been performed, and individual clinical situations should be considered in applying guidelines [National Institutes of Health, 1988]; eg, patients with impaired cardiovascular or pulmonary status may require higher levels to achieve adequate oxygenation); (3) total serum protein level of at least 60% of normal; (4) plasma coagulation factors above 35% of normal, except factor VIII at 50% of normal; and (5) platelets above 50,000/microliter. To achieve these levels, the following is suggested: When blood loss is 25% or less of total volume, a crystalloid solution (eg, balanced electrolyte solution) without red blood cell replacement usually is adequate. With further blood loss, nonprotein plasma volume expanders may be preferred and red blood cells may be required. When blood loss exceeds 50%, red blood cells are administered with crystalloid and/or colloid solutions. If available, whole blood may be given in place of this combination. Massive transfusion (the replacement of the total blood volume in less than 24 hours) may result in dilutional thrombocytopenia and, less often, reduction of some plasma coagulation factors (Rudolph and Boyd, 1990). Platelet concentrates and fresh frozen plasma then may be necessary, but, to avoid the risk of transfusion-transmitted diseases, they usually are administered only when microvascular hemorrhage, thrombocytopenia, or significant prolongation of prothrombin or partial thromboplastin times are demonstrated.

AUTOLOGOUS TRANSFUSION. Autologous blood can be collected prior to surgery, stored, and later administered to the individual who donated it. Other techniques for collecting and administering autologous blood are termed autotransfusions and include phlebotomy with hemodilution during surgery (acute normovolemic hemodilution) with intra- or postoperative retransfusion (Stehling, 1989; National Blood Resource Education Program Expert Panel, 1990), intraoperative blood salvage and retransfusion, postoperative collection of shed blood, or salvage and reinfusion of blood from closed spaces following trauma or surgery. In most elective surgical procedures, prior collection of blood is preferred. In some instances (eg, cardiopulmonary bypass procedures) acute normovolemic hemodilution may improve small vessel perfusion and tissue oxygenation by decreasing blood viscosity. Perioperative blood salvage is usually contraindicated when the operative field may be contaminated with bacteria and when tumor resections are performed.

The advantages of autologous transfusion of any type are avoidance of immunologic mismatch and disease transmission and conservation of available blood resources. With most forms of autotransfusion, anticoagulants must be added; shed blood collected postoperatively is usually defibrinated and does not require further anticoagulation. For perioperative salvage, the blood is often specially filtered or red blood cells are saline-washed before reinfusion.

Major disadvantages of autotransfusion include the risk of reinfusing contaminants, dilutional coagulopathy, and the undesired reinfusion of anticoagulant. In addition, hemolyzed red blood cells that either remain or are generated after washing can result in hemoglobinuria and rarely may cause mild renal insufficiency.

Autologous transfusion is preferred whenever possible for anyone undergoing an elective surgical procedure that may require replacement of 1 to 4 units of blood (National Blood Resource Education Program Expert Panel, 1990; Perkins, 1990). The number of units recommended for deposit before surgery depends on the elective procedure and individual patient characteristics but most often should equal the number of units of homologous blood that would be required for cross-match in preparation for surgery on an identical patient. Collection should start at least two weeks prior to surgery and may continue up to 72 hours before the procedure is to begin. When the need for larger volumes is anticipated, the availability of anticoagulant/preservative solutions allows collection and storage of autologous blood to begin as much as five to six weeks before surgery. For some individuals (eg, cardiac and vascular surgery patients), the benefits of use of autologous blood must be weighed against the risk of delaying surgery until sufficient stores are collected. The decision to transfuse should not be influenced by the availability of autologous blood, since unnecessary blood administration can produce circulatory overload and may result in serious or potentially fatal complications through clerical errors or ex vivo hemolysis. Patients undergoing procedures that are unlikely to require transfusions during or after surgery should not be encouraged to deposit autologous blood (Silvergleid, 1991).

Although higher levels are required for homologous blood donors, patients with hemoglobin concentrations ≥11 g/dL (hematocrit ≥0.33) are candidates for preoperative donation. Standards defining minimal waiting periods between successive homologous blood donations do not apply to patients storing autologous blood for use during or after elective surgery. Individuals usually excluded from homologous blood donation (eg, pediatric patients, the elderly, patients with a history of hepatitis or cancer, those weighing <49.5 kg) should not automatically be excluded from presurgical deposit of autologous blood if it is likely that transfusion will be required. However, those who would not be suitable donors because of their underlying medical problem (eg, unstable angina, severe aortic stenosis) should receive homologous blood if needed. Patients with possible bacteremia are not eligible for autologous blood collection, since bacteria can proliferate during the storage or transport of blood. There is disagreement about the advisability of collecting autologous blood from pregnant women in preparation for delivery (Kruskall, 1990; Sayers, 1990). Current recommendations suggest limiting collection to those women who are most likely to need transfusions (eg, those with placenta previa or placenta accreta, those delivering twins or triplets, those with bleeding disorders, those planning a cesarean section coupled with hysterectomy).

Therapeutic doses of oral iron (see index entry Iron Compounds, In Deficiency Anemia) usually should be prescribed during and after autologous blood collection, since increased hematopoiesis induced by repeated phlebotomy (sometimes as frequently as every three days) may deplete iron stores. The use of epoetin alfa [Epogen, Procrit] to increase the amount of autologous blood that can be collected before surgery is under investigation (Goodnough et al, 1989) (see index entry Epoetin Alfa, In Anemia). However, questions have been raised about the need for and benefits of this use of epoetin (Mintz et al, 1990). Thus far, it appears that epoetin therapy will benefit only those patients who must store four or more units of autologous blood in the three weeks before surgery.

Many experts believe that blood collected for autologous use should be tested for evidence of transfusion-transmitted diseases in the same manner employed for donated blood intended for homologous use. However, others maintain that fewer tests are necessary for autologous blood donations, and the FDA requires that only tests for antibodies to hepatitis B surface antigen (HbSAg) and HIV–1 and a serologic test for syphilis be performed on such units (Silvergleid, 1991). If positive test results for exposure to HIV or hepatitis viruses are confirmed, the blood or its products may be released by the collecting facility for autologous use if the patient's physician submits a signed and dated written order, the hospital agrees to accept such units into its inventory, and the units are labeled to indicate their potential hazard. Additional data on outcome after transfusion are needed to resolve current controversies and standardize hospital and blood bank policies on release of contaminated units of blood donated for autologous use (Silvergleid, 1991). FDA regulations prohibit shipment of such units across state lines.

Some authorities maintain that unused autologous blood with sufficient hemoglobin concentrations that meets all other criteria for protection of blood recipients can be added to supplies for homologous transfusion (Popovsky and Kruskall, 1989). This requires the autologous donor's consent and release of the stored blood by the donor's physician. Other experts disagree because of the higher frequency of abnormal laboratory test results in autologous blood than in homologous blood (Starkey et al, 1989; Grossman and Grindon, 1989). Also, there is some concern that patients donating blood for their own (autologous) use may be less frank than homologous donors in response to questions regarding exposure to viral illnesses through behaviors that place them at risk of infection.

DIRECTED DONATIONS. This term refers to blood donated for the use of single, specified patients by individuals recruited by the patient or his/her family. These donors are most often family members or friends who seek to reduce the perceived risk of disease transmission accompanying transfusion of homologous blood.

Much controversy exists within the blood banking community regarding the advisability of directed donor programs. Arguments against widespread employment of this practice (Page, 1989; Collins and Churchill, 1989) include (1) decreased safety of the donated blood (since most directed donors are first-time donors and thus the rate of abnormal laboratory test results is higher, and because directed donors are often under real or perceived pressure to donate, which may lead to concealment of exposure history); (2) concern about the possibility of reduced donations to the general blood supply (since potential donors may refrain from donating to save their blood for possible need by relatives or friends); (3) increased complexity of blood banking procedures (leading to increased costs and a greater possibility of clerical errors that result in transfusion of mismatched blood and adverse reactions); (4) the introduction of a two-tiered system for providing blood (directed donations for those with large families or many friends and anonymous donors for all others); and (5) the loss of donor anonymity and confidentiality (particularly important if the donated blood is not used because of positive test results for exposure to pathogenic viruses).

Those who support directed donation of blood to patients who request it (Yalon and Perkins, 1989; Goldfinger, 1989) argue that directed-donor blood is as safe as anonymous-donor blood since units that produce abnormal test results are not made available for transfusion; these programs have little or no documented impact on the general blood supply; and these programs help to reduce or limit the number of donors to which a multiply transfused patient is exposed (thus possibly decreasing alloimmunization). Furthermore, proponents argue that the benefits of decreased anxiety and resistance to blood transfusion in patients who request directed donations exceed the disadvantages listed above. The increased cost of providing directed donor blood to patients is usually passed on in the form of a surcharge. Despite the fact that autologous blood clearly is safer than directed-donor blood, some data suggest that suitable candidates for autologous blood donation may choose not to participate in such programs if directed-donor blood is available (Chambers et al, 1990).

There are certain medical conditions for which blood or blood components obtained from a specified donor are indicated and may be the treatment of choice; these are not considered directed donations. Examples include maternal platelets given to a neonate with alloimmune thrombocytopenia; blood from a living kidney or bone marrow donor given to the transplant recipient; platelets from close relatives given to patients refractory to best-match platelets; and red blood cells from family members with compatible rare red blood cell types. Directed donations are contraindicated from the prospective father to the prospective mother of a potential future child, from a marrow donor to the marrow recipient before the transplant is performed, and when donor suitability and compatibility have not been thoroughly tested.

A recent report from the Pediatric Hemotherapy Committee, American Association of Blood Banks, recommends that mothers should not provide blood components containing plasma to their children and that maternal red blood cells and platelets should be washed before transfusion into neonates with alloimmune thrombocytopenia (Strauss et al, 1990). Furthermore, fathers and paternal relatives should not provide blood products containing cells to their infant children unless a major crossmatch is carried out through at least the antiglobulin phase. Adherence to these recommendations avoids immunologically mediated transfusion reactions. In addition, to prevent graft-versus-host disease, all blood components obtained from parents, children, or siblings (ie, first degree relatives) must be irradiated to at least 15 Gy before they are transfused into neonates (Anderson and Weinstein, 1990). The Committee also agreed that programs designed to limit the number of donors to which pediatric patients who require multiple transfusions are exposed provide benefits that justify their expense and the logistical problems; however, no data were provided to support this recommendation.

APHERESIS. Techniques employing centrifugation, filtration, or spinning membrane filtration may be used to separate the various components of blood. The desired component is retained and the remaining fractions are returned to the donor. Apheresis allows the harvesting of large quantities of non-red cell blood products from donors and has the advantage of reducing the number of donors to whom a patient is exposed. This technique also can be used therapeutically to remove cells or soluble molecules that might contribute to pathologic conditions if allowed to remain in the circulation. Examples include leukemic blast cells, antigen-antibody complexes, autoantibodies, myeloma proteins, and platelets from patients with symptomatic thrombocytosis.

Two types of apheresis are used: (1) With *cytapheresis*, one or more cellular elements are withdrawn and the plasma and remaining cellular elements are returned to the donor. Leukapheresis and plateletpheresis represent types of cytapheresis. Plateletpheresis separates platelets from donor blood, with plasma and red blood cells returned to the donor. With continuous or intermittent flow centrifugation, the equivalent of six or more units of platelets is obtained from one donor in a typical single session. Platelets obtained by apheresis must be administered within 24 hours if an open system procedure is used because of the risk of bacterial contamination. In a closed system procedure, the platelets may be stored for five days.

(2) With *plasmapheresis*, plasma is removed from the cellular constituents, which are returned to the donor. It is performed on healthy donors to provide plasma for further fractionation in the preparation of plasma derivatives (eg, cryoprecipitate, factor VIII and other clotting factor concentrates, immune globulins). Therapeutic plasmapheresis (also referred to as plasma exchange) is the treatment of choice for patients with thrombotic thrombocytopenic purpura (TTP), Guillain-Barré syndrome, Goodpasture's syndrome, and other disorders. It is also used rarely to remove some ingested poisons when dialysis cannot be performed. Plasma is used as the sole replacement solution only in therapy for TTP. It is usually replaced with a combination of albumin and saline (volume for volume) for other indications; occasionally, other plasma expanders have been used. It is not necessary to add electrolytes or globulins to the replacement solution. (See also the discussion on Plasma Exchange.)

EXCHANGE TRANSFUSIONS. Exchange transfusions of whole blood are used to treat hemolytic disease of the newborn and other neonatal disorders, some red blood cell disorders, and various other diseases. Automated red blood cell exchanges have replaced manual exchange transfusion in many nonpediatric patients.

Red blood cell exchanges using a cell separator have been effective in sickle cell anemia during crises and also have been used prior to surgery. Operative mortality may be reduced when sickle cells are replaced with normal red blood cells; red blood cell transfusion alone may not be as effective as exchange transfusions. However, no well-controlled studies have addressed the requirements for and efficacy of exchange transfusion before surgery for sickle cell patients. Cell separators also have been used rarely to separate young red blood cells (neocytes) from older ones in donor blood. Neocytes survive longer after transfusion and have been used in the treatment of thalassemias to reduce the frequency of transfusion and thereby diminish the iron load. Because the efficacy of this therapy has not been documented by results of controlled trials, the procedure is still considered experimental. Currently, exchange transfusion is being used to reduce the level of parasitemia in patients with severe malaria.

WHOLE BLOOD OR RED BLOOD CELL TRANSFUSION. During storage of blood, changes in red blood cell metabolism and hemoglobin structure and function occur that reduce the survival time of transfused red blood cells and decrease hemoglobin function (Mollison et al, 1987; Beutler, 1989). Current standards require that at least 70% of erythrocytes be circulating 24 hours after transfusion.

Whole blood may be preferred by some physicians when there is acute loss of more than 25% of blood volume, as in surgical or medical catastrophes, but appropriate components can be used instead. Because most blood suppliers keep little whole blood in inventory, it may not be readily available.

When the sole aim of transfusion is to increase oxygen-carrying capacity, red blood cells should be used. Transfusion of red blood cells with a hematocrit of 70% to 80% reduces the danger of hypervolemia and associated congestive heart failure and is preferred in patients with cardiac disease and chronic anemia. (Red blood cells to which adenine-saline [AS] has been added have a hematocrit of 55% to 65% [*American Red Cross*, revised, 1989].)

During dire emergencies, group O red blood cells should be used if non-ABO group-specific transfusion is necessary because group O cells can be given to persons of any blood group and removal of the plasma reduces the amount of donor anti-A and/or anti-B alloantibodies present. The presence of these antibodies may lead to destruction of the recipient's own red blood cells. However, the risk of transmitting infectious organisms is not reduced by concentrating the red blood cells.

To reduce the risk of febrile, nonhemolytic transfusion reactions, blood banks can now use filtration to prepare red blood cells that are depleted of various other cellular components (eg, platelets, leukocytes) to a greater extent than could be achieved previously by centrifugation techniques. When the preparative technique does not utilize a closed, self-contained, sterile multiple-bag system or a sterile connection device, the product's shelf-life is 24 hours. Leukocyte-poor red blood cells can be stored for up to 42 days if they are prepared using closed multiple-bag systems with in-line filters and adenine-saline additive solutions (Davey et al, 1989). Requirements for crossmatching and the method of administration of leukocyte-poor red blood cells are the same as for whole blood or red blood cells. As an alternative, in-line filters that remove more than 99% of contaminating leukocytes are available for bedside use during transfusion of red blood cells.

Frozen red blood cells are prepared in some blood centers. The high cost of preparation and storage, the time required to thaw and wash the cells (to remove cryoprotective agent) before they can be transfused, and the short post-thaw shelf-life (24 hours) limit their routine use. At present, the principal use for frozen red blood cells is to maintain inventories of rare blood types (ie, those with uncommon antigens). The risk of bacterial contamination during preparation, thawing, and washing also is somewhat greater than for red blood cells or whole blood unless sterile connection devices are used. Furthermore, the risk of transfusion-transmitted infection is not eliminated.

After thawing and washing (deglycerolizing), frozen red blood cells contain very little plasma protein and cellular debris from leukocytes or platelets, thus minimizing alloimmunization to HLA and leukocyte- or platelet-specific antigens and the incidence of febrile nonhemolytic transfusion reactions. Suitably filtered red blood cells may be superior for this purpose because then filters can remove a higher percentage of white blood cells. Thawed, deglycerolized red blood cells should be reserved for patients who continue to experience reactions to saline-washed or leukocyte-poor red blood cells, for those with IgA deficiency, or for those who have had anaphylactoid transfusion reactions. Results from one retrospective analysis of 23 patients with paroxysmal nocturnal hemoglobinuria who were observed over a 38-year period suggest that the risk of hemolysis is not increased in such patients who receive blood group-specific, unwashed red blood cells rather than saline-washed or thawed deglycerolized red blood cells (Brecher and Taswell, 1989). This conclusion needs confirmation in prospective randomized trials.

Hemolytic disease in newborn infants caused by maternal antibodies against common antigens can be treated with frozen red blood cells obtained from the mother during early pregnancy. If necessary, the blood can be collected after delivery and washed to remove plasma proteins prior to transfusion. Autologous frozen red blood cells may be accumulated to meet anticipated needs in selected persons. However, logistics and cost limit their use for routine autologous blood transfusion. A recent retrospective analysis showed that almost 80% of individuals for whom autologous frozen red blood cells were stored without a specific anticipated use did not receive the stored blood during a mean follow-up period of eight years (DePalma et al, 1990). In contrast, 50% of those who donated blood for storage of autologous frozen red blood cells prior to elective surgery received some of the stored units.

Frozen red blood cells were once preferred for patients scheduled to undergo organ transplantation, but most data now indicate that survival of renal transplants is decreased when only frozen red blood cells are employed. Prior transfusion of whole blood from living, related kidney donors enhances renal homograft survival but has been replaced, for the most part, by immunosuppression with cyclosporine. In contrast, prior transfusion appears to have a deleterious effect in patients with aplastic anemia who undergo bone marrow transplantation.

PLATELET TRANSFUSION. Platelets are prepared by differential centrifugation of random units of never-refrigerated whole blood (within eight hours after phlebotomy) and suspended in 50 to 70 ml of the original plasma. Platelets from one unit of blood (one random-donor platelet concentrate) should increase the platelet count of a 70-kg adult by at least 5,000/microliter (measured one hour after transfusion). The usual adult dose necessary to achieve hemostasis is one unit for each 10 kg of body weight or six to eight such concentrates in a typical 70-kg individual (Snyder, 1989; Tomasulo and Petz, 1989). The equivalent of six or more units of platelets can be obtained at one time from a single donor by plateletpheresis (single-donor platelets).

Platelet transfusions are indicated when severe acute thrombocytopenia is associated with active or imminent bleeding, especially that resulting from decreased platelet production. However, there are no convincing data to support the establishment of a uniform, unvarying threshold for platelet counts that must be maintained to prevent hemorrhage in all patients. The platelet count at which spontaneous bleeding occurs will vary with the cause of the thrombocytopenia and the degree to which impairment of platelet function exists. Thrombocytopenia may be caused by decreased production or increased destruction of platelets, and dilutional thrombocytopenia can develop following massive transfusion of stored blood. Serious spontaneous bleeding usually does not occur unless the platelet count is less than 20,000/microliter or even lower if platelet function is not impaired by disease or drugs. Patients with leukemia and other malignancies who are receiving intensive chemotherapy often are given prophylactic platelet transfusions when the platelet count falls to 10,000 to 20,000/microliter. Some authorities recommend that prophylactic platelet transfusions in the absence of clinically significant bleeding be limited to patients with platelet counts below 5,000/microliter (Slichter, 1990). Certain complicating clinical factors (eg, fever and sepsis, administration of platelet-inhibitory drugs, gastrointestinal ulceration, coagulopathies) increase the risk of hemorrhage in patients undergoing myelosuppressive chemotherapy for malignant diseases, and thus prophylactic platelet transfusions to maintain counts above 20,000/microliter may be justified (Murphy, 1990). Furthermore, patients with acute leukemia and blast counts greater than 100,000/microliter are at risk for cerebral and pulmonary leukostasis, and their platelet counts should be maintained above 40,000 to 50,000/microliter (Heyman and Schiffer, 1990). During major surgery and the postoperative period, the platelet count should be maintained between 50,000 and 100,000/microliter in these high-risk patients.

Patients with aplastic anemia and some other conditions characterized by prolonged suppression of bone marrow function who have low (less than 20,000/microliter) but stable platelet counts may not require maintenance platelet transfusions unless hemorrhage occurs. Prophylactic platelet transfusions should be avoided because these patients often develop alloantibodies that decrease the effectiveness of subsequent transfusions.

Platelet transfusions are less likely to be effective in conditions associated with increased platelet destruction (eg, sepsis, fever). They are not recommended when platelet destruction is caused by systemic consumption (disseminated intravascular coagulation [DIC] before the consumptive process is controlled) or an antibody (idiopathic thrombocytopenic purpura [ITP]) except when life-threatening hemorrhage occurs. Platelet transfusion is contraindicated in patients with TTP. Patients with splenomegaly may require large doses of platelets because of splenic sequestration.

More complete discussions of criteria and indications for platelet transfusions are available (National Institutes of Health, 1987; Murphy, 1988, 1990).

Prolonged preservation by freezing with a cryoprotective agent has been accomplished but remains investigational at present because of technical difficulties and expense. Cryopreserved platelets obtained during remissions from patients with hematologic malignancies have been used to combat hemorrhage during subsequent relapse. Cryopreservation may be particularly important if HLA-matched single-donor platelets obtained by plateletpheresis are not available because of an uncommon HLA phenotype.

Refractoriness to repeated administration of random-donor platelets is not uncommon. This usually is caused by antibodies directed against histocompatibility antigens (HLA) or, less frequently, against platelet-specific antigens. For this reason, some authorities have advocated that prophylactic platelet transfusions not be given to nonbleeding patients. Patients refractory to pooled or single-donor random platelets may sometimes benefit from platelets collected from siblings or other family members. This approach may delay the need to substitute HLA-matched platelets but should not be employed in patients who may later receive bone marrow from a family member. Other strategies to reduce the development of refractoriness in patients who require multiple platelet transfusions include the use of leukocyte-depleted concentrates, administration of immunosuppressive drugs to transfusion recipients, and ultraviolet irradiation of the concentrates to inactivate donor antigen-presenting cells (Snyder, 1989; Slichter, 1990; Heyman and Schiffer, 1990). The impact of these measures on the development of refractoriness in patients who receive a number of platelet transfusions is as yet unclear.

HLA-matched platelets collected from single donors by plateletpheresis can increase the platelet increment and survival time after alloimmunization has developed (McFarland et al, 1989). Transfusion of platelets from the "preferred" donor (sometimes an HLA-matched sibling) can provide long-term support, but the use of siblings as donors is contraindicated when marrow transplantation from that sibling or another family member is contemplated. Many centers have developed lists of HLA-typed donors for rapid matching to thrombocytopenic patients who are refractory to random-donor platelets. Platelet compatibility testing (crossmatching) also is available in many laboratories and has been recommended to provide platelets to alloimmunized patients.

Although platelet concentrates usually contain few erythrocytes, they may contain large amounts of plasma and substantial numbers of leukocytes, and determination of ABO compatibility is desirable but usually not practical. Data from recent randomized trials suggest that the use of ABO-mismatched platelets results in lower platelet increments and may contribute to the development of platelet refractoriness (Lee and Schiffer, 1989; Carr et al, 1990). Platelets do not contain the Rh antigen, but the red blood cells present can cause sensitization, and infusion of platelets from an Rh-positive donor into an Rh-negative recipient could result in Rh sensitization. Therefore, Rh-negative female children and women of childbearing age may be given $Rh_0(D)$ immune globulin immediately after receiving platelets from an Rh-positive donor unless there is no likelihood of a future pregnancy.

GRANULOCYTE TRANSFUSION. Severe thrombocytopenia and leukopenia caused by marrow hypoplasia frequently result from aggressive cancer chemotherapy, but platelet transfusion has decreased mortality from thrombocytopenic hemorrhage in these patients. As a result, infections, particularly those caused by gram-negative bacteria and fungi, rather than hemorrhage are now the leading cause of death in patients with bone marrow failure.

The incidence of infection increases as the granulocyte count falls below 1,000/microliter and becomes severe when it falls below 250/microliter. Newer, more effective antibiotics developed during the last decade have contributed to a marked improvement in the management of infection in neutropenic patients (see index entry Fever, Treatment). In addition, effective combination chemotherapy protocols that minimize the degree of neutropenia induced are available for most neoplastic diseases. Nevertheless, many patients treated with myelosuppressive drugs remain at serious risk for infection until marrow function returns. Results of recent studies showed that recombinant preparations of myeloid growth factors (G-CSF and GM-CSF) can reduce the duration of neutropenia in such patients (see index entry Hematopoietic

Hormones). Two such preparations are now available for clinical use (see index entries G-CSF, GM-CSF, Filgrastim, and Sargramostim). In some patients who remain febrile despite appropriate antibiotic therapy for at least 48 hours, granulocyte transfusion has had some efficacy in combating bacterial infections (Dutcher, 1989; Nusbacher, 1990). In contrast, prophylactic transfusion of granulocytes to neutropenic patients with no evidence of infection does not appear to reduce the incidence of infections, although bacterial septicemia may develop less frequently.

The yield of granulocytes that can be obtained from a single donor is limited by the low number of granulocytes in the circulation and the difficulty of separating phagocytic cells from lymphocytes and red blood cells. The addition of hydroxyethyl starch (a sedimenting agent) to the blood during leukapheresis and pretreatment of donors with glucocorticoids (to increase blood granulocyte counts) can increase the yield of phagocytic cells. These techniques usually are combined and yield 1.5 to 3.0×10^{10} granulocytes per leukapheresis procedure. The minimal dose recommended for granulocyte transfusions, 1×10^{10} cells, is only about 10% of the normal daily production, but this appears to provide enough white blood cells to overcome infection in responsive patients.

Data from clinical trials have demonstrated that granulocyte transfusions improve survival of neutropenic patients with documented gram-negative sepsis (McCullough, 1989). However, data are insufficient to evaluate the effects of granulocyte transfusion on survival in neutropenic patients with pneumonia, urinary tract infections, cellulitis or abscess, or fungal infections. Mixed results have been reported in clinical trials on newborn infants. In some reports, the survival rate of neutropenic neonates with sepsis may be improved in response to granulocyte transfusions (see McCullough, 1989, for review). The infants who are likely to benefit most from this procedure are those with >75% immature granulocytes in their peripheral blood and those with antibiotic-resistant gram-negative sepsis. Granulocyte transfusion also may be useful to support bone marrow transplantation, particularly in patients infected with antibiotic-resistant bacteria or fungi (Strauss, 1987; Petz, 1989). Finally, in some congenital diseases associated with impaired granulocyte function (eg, chronic granulomatous disease), granulocyte transfusions appear to be beneficial in patients with severe infections who did not respond to antibiotics (McCullough, 1989).

Since granulocyte preparations also contain red blood cells, ABO compatibility should be assured. HLA-compatible granulocytes may be required in alloimmunized patients. Febrile reactions are very common, and respiratory distress may develop in some individuals.

PLASMA TRANSFUSION. Plasma, the cell-free portion of anti-coagulated blood, constitutes approximately 60% of blood volume and contains the blood proteins, electrolytes, coagulation factors, and other elements, including immunoglobulins. When a unit of whole blood is converted to red blood cells, plasma is removed. Plasma also can be obtained by plasmapheresis. The plasma can be fractionated into plasma derivatives (eg, albumin, plasma protein fraction) or used as a source of procoagulants. Fresh plasma and thawed fresh frozen plasma may be used as a source of all the coagulation factors. Supernatant plasma remaining after removal of cryoprecipitate, platelets, or both is useful to replace the stable clotting factors (II, VII, IX, X, XI, XII).

Plasma is employed primarily in the management of bleeding associated with liver disease and the dilutional coagulopathy caused by massive blood transfusion that results from clotting factor deficiency as documented by measurement of prothrombin or partial thromboplastin times. Because the activity of labile clotting factors (V and VIII) stored in plasma decreases during storage, fresh frozen single-donor plasma generally is preferred to correct deficiencies of factor V; factor VIII deficiency preferably is treated by replacement with factor VIII concentrates (see index entry Hemostatics). Although plasma is useful to treat minor bleeding episodes in factor IX deficiency, as well as in multiple coagulation factor deficiencies, large volumes usually are required to achieve hemostatic levels of these factors.

Plasma may be useful adjunctively to control bleeding associated with oral anticoagulant (ie, warfarin) therapy, particularly prior to emergency surgery. Plasma also has been used to maintain circulating blood volume but is not currently recommended for this use (except possibly in burn patients with infection) because of the risk of disease transmission and the availability of safer alternatives for plasma volume expansion (Swisher and Petz, 1989). Other inappropriate uses of fresh frozen plasma and other plasma products include empiric treatment or prophylaxis of bleeding before or after procedures such as coronary bypass surgery; nutritional supplementation for patients with wasting diseases; treatment of chronic hypoproteinemia; and administration to improve healing, control infection, or replace vaguely defined "factors." Fresh frozen plasma also should not be used to reconstitute a unit of whole blood by addition to a unit of red blood cells. Whole blood should be administered when indicated to minimize exposure to multiple donors (National Institutes of Health Consensus Conference, 1985; Swisher and Petz, 1989).

Single-donor or fresh frozen plasma carries approximately the same risk of transmitting disease as a single unit of whole blood because it does not undergo viral inactivation or reduction procedures. However, there may be less risk of cell-associated viruses (eg, HTLV-I or -II, CMV), and there is less risk of graft-versus-host disease with plasma than with whole blood. If it is not obtained from an AB donor, the plasma contains anti-A (found in group O and group B blood) and/or anti-B alloagglutinins (found in group O and group A blood).

PLASMA EXCHANGE. When large volumes of plasma are replaced by normal plasma or other proteins and an equal volume of fluid, the process is known as plasma exchange. During this process, plasma is separated from the cellular elements, which are then returned to the patient.

Plasma sometimes is employed as the replacement fluid in plasma exchange (therapeutic plasmapheresis), either as the sole exchange fluid or with electrolyte solutions, usually saline. Plasma has been used in conjunction with therapeutic plasma exchange for TTP, for infants with protein-losing enteropathy, and for selected patients with other immune deficiencies (National Institutes of Health Consensus Conference, 1985; Savage et al, 1988). Plasma exchange with plasma replacement is now preferred therapy for TTP. However, because of the potential for disease transmission, plasma generally is not used for other indications of plasma exchange. Instead, albumin or plasma protein fraction plus crystalloid solutions is effective, and there is no risk of disease transmission.

Some autoimmune diseases can be treated by plasma exchange. Examples include myasthenia gravis, acute Guillain-Barré syndrome, chronic inflammatory demyelinating polyneuropathy, and Goodpasture's syndrome (Shumak and Nusbacher, 1989). Since it is difficult to remove only immune globulins, the entire plasma portion of blood is replaced. If only 1 or 2 L is exchanged, the substitute fluid may be crystalloid (eg, saline, electrolyte solutions), albumin, or other colloid solutions. The therapeutic benefits of plasma exchange also have been demonstrated in some uncommon disorders, such as hyperviscosity syndrome and posttransfusion purpura, and in factor VIII-deficient patients with factor VIII antibodies. Plasma exchange is an investigational therapy for some other diseases (eg, warm antibody hemolytic anemia, ITP, hemolytic disease due to anti-Rh) in which adequate clinical trials have not yet been completed or in which a specific abnormal molecule responsible for the pathogenesis and removed by plasma exchange has not yet been demonstrated (Shumak and Nusbacher, 1989).

PLASMA VOLUME EXPANDERS. If temporary maintenance of near-normal blood volume is the sole therapeutic objective, plasma volume expanders should be used instead of whole blood, and crystalloid solutions can be used if the estimated volume deficit is small. Plasma should not be administered for this purpose. Albumin [Albuminar, Albutein, Buminate, Plasbumin] and plasma protein fraction (PPF) [Plasmanate, Plasma Plex, Plasmatein, Protenate] are processed from human plasma and may be indicated in the emergency treatment of shock. These preparations are sterile-filtered and heated for ten hours at 60° C, which eliminates the risk of hepatitis and HIV infection.

Plasma expanders (eg, dextran 70 [Macrodex], dextran 75 [Gentran 75], hetastarch [Hespan], pentastarch [Pentaspan]) support the circulation in hypovolemic states (eg, cardiogenic shock, respiratory distress syndrome). They can be given to restore blood volume after hemorrhage while typing and crossmatching of blood is being performed, to correct the oligemia of burn shock, or to maintain colloid osmotic pressure temporarily in emergencies or during certain types of cardiovascular surgery. They are not substitutes for blood components in the treatment of anemia or hypoproteinemia. Dextran 40 [Gentran-40, Rheomacrodex, 10% LMD] may be used as an adjunct in the treatment of shock, but the effects are of shorter duration than those of higher molecular weight dextran.

Dextrans and, to a lesser extent, hetastarch have been associated with histamine release and major anaphylactoid reactions (Ljungström et al, 1988). Most of the allergic reactions have been mild, but anaphylaxis and death have been reported. Dextran 1 [Promit] can be used as a hapten inhibitor to block anaphylaxis mediated by dextran-reactive antibodies. Dextrans also have been associated with increased bleeding tendencies secondary to interference with platelet function and increased fibrinolysis and renal failure. Because of these hazards, the use of dextran solutions has declined.

Most physicians now believe that moderate hypovolemia and hemoconcentration can be treated by temporary replacement with a balanced electrolyte solution (in amounts three or four times the estimated blood loss). Sodium chloride and lactated Ringer's solutions also can be used, but the effects of all crystalloid solutions last only two hours or less. (See index entry Hydration, Abnormal States.)

HEMOGLOBIN SUBSTITUTES. Perfluorochemicals: Studies in animals have demonstrated that perfluorochemicals transport oxygen and remove carbon dioxide, thus suggesting that these compounds be investigated as hemoglobin substitutes. They are effective only when oxygenated (eg, when high concentrations of oxygen are inhaled by patients with severely depleted hemoglobin), and they do not provide platelets or coagulation factors. Pure fluorocarbons are immiscible with blood; hence, they must be used as stabilized aqueous emulsions.

Fluosol, a 20% emulsion of perfluorodecalin and perfluorotri-*n*-propylamine, has been used investigationally in Japan as a red blood cell substitute and has been used experimentally in patients who refused blood transfusion for religious reasons (Faithfull, 1988; Vercellotti and Hammerschmidt, 1988). However, because of lack of evidence of efficacy (Gould et al, 1986), the potential for pulmonary toxicity from prolonged breathing of air with a high oxygen concentration (required for adequate oxygenation of tissues), and insufficient data on the safety of the emulsifier used in these preparations, perfluorochemicals are not approved in the United States for use in humans as a substitute for red blood cells (Kahn et al, 1985). Adverse pulmonary reactions to perfluorochemical infusions, possibly mediated by activation of the complement cascade, also have been noted in a number of patients.

Presently, the sole indication for use of Fluosol in this country is for intracoronary infusion during percutaneous transluminal coronary angioplasty (PTCA) to prevent myocardial ischemia in patients at high risk of ischemic complications during the procedure (Jaffe et al, 1988; Cowley et al, 1990; Kent et al, 1990). Fluosol and other perfluorochemical preparations also are being investigated for use as an oxygen-carrying supplement for regional perfusion of various tissues, in treatment of evolving myocardial infarction, preoperative treatment of anemia in surgical patients, as therapy for sickle cell crisis, and to increase tissue oxygenation in solid tumors prior to radiation or chemotherapy (Faithfull, 1988; Vercellotti and Hammerschmidt, 1988). However, data are insufficient to establish the efficacy and safety of administering perfluorochemicals in any condition other than during PTCA.

Hemoglobin Solutions: Hemoglobin solutions are prepared either by hemolyzing red blood cells and using membrane ultrafiltration to remove all of the contaminating stroma, which is nephrotoxic, or by recombinant DNA technology. Hemoglobin solutions are stable, may be stored for up to 18 months, and do not require crossmatching. However, they have a short intravascular half-life and problems with toxicity have not been satisfactorily resolved. Chemical modifications of the purified hemoglobin have been employed to alter the clearance rate and the ability of the hemoglobin to deliver oxygen at the usual partial pressures found in the tissues (Keipert et al, 1989; Gould et al, 1990). Conjugation of hemoglobin to polymeric molecules, covalent attachment of pyridoxal in the 2,3-diphosphoglycerate binding site, and cross-linking of the hemoglobin tetramer with bis-pyridoxal tetraphosphate are among the modifications being studied. Although these solutions of modified hemoglobin have not yet proved clinically acceptable as red blood cell substitutes, they are being investigated intensively (Chang and Geyer, 1988; Moss et al, 1988; Lowe, 1988 A).

Cryoprecipitate and Coagulation Factor Concentrates: See index entry Hemostatics.

Adverse Reactions and Precautions

Viral Hepatitis: This is the most common serious adverse reaction associated with transfusion therapy and may occur after the use of any blood, blood component, or blood derivative preparation (eg, whole blood, red blood cell concentrates, plasma, platelets, granulocytes) or after the use of some plasma derivatives (eg, cryoprecipitated antihemophilic factor, antihemophilic and prothrombin complex concentrates). Since hepatitis viruses cannot be eliminated totally from these preparations, components prepared from the blood of volunteer (as opposed to paid) donors should be used whenever possible and all blood *must* be screened by tests for hepatitis B surface antigen (HBsAg), a specific marker for hepatitis B virus. However, there are no data demonstrating that coagulation factor concentrates processed from pooled plasma obtained from unpaid donors are less likely to transmit viral hepatitis than concentrates derived from paid blood donors. Testing of donor blood or plasma for HBsAg is required by the FDA, the American Red Cross (ARC), the American Association of Blood Banks (AABB), and the Council of Community Blood Centers (CCBC). A repeatedly reactive test for HBsAg or a history of hepatitis precludes donation.

The exclusion of HBsAg-positive donors has markedly reduced the incidence of post-transfusion hepatitis caused by hepatitis B virus. As a result, this virus now causes only 10% or less of post-transfusion hepatitis. The remaining 90% probably is caused primarily by agent(s) designated non-A, non-B (now usually referred to as hepatitis C). A test kit for detection of antibodies to the hepatitis C virus was licensed by the FDA in May 1990, and testing of donated blood for antibodies to this virus is now required by the FDA, AABB, ARC, and CCBC. Blood that repeatedly tests positive for antibodies to hepatitis C virus, the infectious agent apparently responsible for 70% to 90% of non-A, non-B hepatitis, is not used. Type A (infectious) hepatitis rarely is transmitted by blood transfusion. Other viruses (eg, cytomegalovirus, Epstein-Barr virus) can be transmitted by transfusion and also may cause a type of hepatitis.

Indirect testing for non-A, non-B hepatitis was required by the ARC, AABB, and CCBC prior to licensing of the test for antibodies to the hepatitis C virus. Since no direct test was available for routine use, surrogate tests were used. Serum alanine aminotransferase (ALT) activity was measured, and the presence of antibody to hepatitis B core antigen was determined. The test for antibody to hepatitis B core antigen had the added benefit of identifying the relatively few donors who harbored the hepatitis B virus but tested negative for HBsAg. Blood that tested positive for the antibody or that had a serum ALT level above a laboratory-specific cut-off level was not used for transfusion.

The precise incidence of post-transfusion hepatitis is not known, because the true incidence can be determined only if blood recipients are followed prospectively and concentrations of serum aminotransferases are measured periodically at close intervals. Such studies have not been completed; however, two large-scale prospective studies conducted in the 1970s (ie, before introduction of the surrogate tests for non-A, non-B hepatitis and the direct test for antibodies to the hepatitis C virus) indicated that 5% to 10% of patients receiving multiple transfusions of volunteer donor blood developed hepatitis (estimated risk, 2%/unit transfused). Most cases were subclinical and anicteric, but even icteric cases were not necessarily reported to the institution that provided the blood. Despite the apparently benign course of the acute phase of anicteric hepatitis, it predisposes to chronic liver disease in more than 50% of patients and to a carrier state. The current risk, while unknown, is undoubtedly much smaller than that suggested by these older studies.

In general, although type B hepatitis tends to be more severe in the acute phase, hepatitis C more frequently progresses to chronic liver disease. Liver biopsy specimens from patients with hepatitis C frequently show histologic findings consistent with chronic active hepatitis.

Acquired Immunodeficiency Syndrome (AIDS): Retrovirus transmission is the most recently discovered infectious complication of blood transfusion. AIDS is caused by the human immunodeficiency virus (HIV), formerly called human T-lymphotropic virus type III (HTLV-III). Infected persons are capable of transmitting HIV during the period in which they remain asymptomatic as well as in the symptomatic stages of the disease.

HIV is transmitted by infected persons to their sexual partners, by infected persons sharing equipment used to administer intravenous drugs of abuse, and from infected mothers to their fetuses and newborn infants. Although uncommon, HIV also can be transmitted by transfusion of contaminated blood and blood products. In 1983, blood banks initiated programs to restrict donation of blood from persons in high-risk groups (eg, homosexual men, bisexual men and their female partners, intravenous drug abusers). Detection and exclusion of any donors with HIV antibodies have markedly reduced the transmission of HIV through blood transfusion since the introduction of tests for this purpose in 1985 (Cumming et al, 1989; Barker and Dodd, 1989; Menitove, 1990). The sensitivity of current test procedures to detect individuals who have been exposed to HIV is well in excess of 99%. The false-negative test results (estimated at between 1 in 30,000 and 1 in 153,000 units collected) are attributed mainly to individuals who donate during the time between exposure and seroconversion. Increased use of autologous transfusion also is valuable to reduce the risk of HIV infection, hepatitis, and all transfusion-transmitted diseases in patients not requiring repeated blood replacement.

Other Infectious Diseases: Many infections can be transmitted by blood transfusion, including cytomegalovirus, Epstein-Barr virus, syphilis, toxoplasmosis, filariasis, human parvovirus, human herpes virus type 6, HTLV-I and -II, malaria, Chagas' disease, babesiosis, Lyme disease, *Yersinia enterocolitica* bacteremia, and brucellosis. Cytomegalovirus and Epstein-Barr infection are usually asymptomatic and self-limited, but associated fever and hepatosplenomegaly may be hazardous in pregnant women, immunodeficient or immunosuppressed patients, and premature infants. Blood products from seronegative donors or that are processed to deplete white cells and thus reduce the risk of cytomegalovirus transmission are recommended for these patients (Hillyer et al, 1990).

HTLV-I, the first pathogenic human retrovirus identified, causes adult human T-cell leukemia and myelopathy in about 3% to 5% of infected individuals two to three decades after infection. The virus also causes a degenerative neuropathy that can occur several years after the infection. Testing of donors for antibody to HTLV-I was instituted late in 1988.

There has been a recent increase in the number of reported cases of probable transfusion-related sepsis and fatal endotoxin shock attributed to contamination with *Y. enterocolitica* (Tipple et al, 1990; *MMWR*, 1991). This organism grows at the storage temperature used for banked red blood cells after a delay of 10 to 20 days. Sufficient endotoxin is produced by the 25th day of refrigerated storage to cause acute severe illness and death, especially in elderly recipients. Measures being considered to reduce or prevent *Y. enterocolitica* contamination of transfused blood include screening donors for recent gastrointestinal illness, reducing the shelf life of red blood cells, and testing units older than 24 days for endotoxin or bacteria.

Hypersensitivity Reactions: Donor blood causes allergic responses in 1% to 3% of recipients (Holland, 1989 B). Urticarial rashes and generalized pruritus are mild and transitory, but severe bronchospasm and angioedema occur occasionally and cause death rarely. Mild urticarial reactions that are not accompanied by any other signs or symptoms do not require termination of the transfusion or discarding of the blood product (Holland, 1989 B). These are most often managed by administration of an antihistamine and slowing or temporarily discontinuing the flow of the blood product. The normal rate of transfusion usually can be resumed after 15 to 30 minutes once the urticaria are no longer visible. More severe hypersensitivity reactions are much less common and require termination of the transfusion and possibly administration of epinephrine. Since anaphylaxis can often result in severe hypotension, it is important to use normal saline solution to maintain patency of the intravenous line through which the transfusion was being administered. (For treatment, see index entry Shock, Anaphylactic.) Patients who lack IgA may become sensitized and experience anaphylactic reactions mediated by their anti-IgA with subsequent transfusions. These patients require blood products from IgA-deficient donors or thoroughly saline-washed or thawed, deglycerolized red cells. However, anti-IgA antibodies do not account for all anaphylactic transfusion reactions.

Febrile Reactions: Fever may exceed 39.4 to 40° C (103 to 104° F) and usually occurs within 15 to 60 minutes after transfusion is begun, although it may develop two hours or more after completion of transfusion. It frequently is accompanied by chills, headache, and malaise. When fever develops, the transfusion should be interrupted (with patency of the intravenous line maintained) and the cause investigated, since increased temperature may be an early manifestation of a more serious problem, especially hemolytic transfusion reaction or the presence of endotoxin due to bacterial contamination (Holland, 1989). However, most febrile reactions are of unknown cause or are attributable to leukoagglutinins, antibodies directed against HLA, or other antigens located on granulocytes and platelets. These reactions almost always respond to standard antipyretic therapy (see index entry Analgesic-Antipyretics and Nonsteroidal Anti-inflammatory Agents). After two febrile, nonhemolytic reactions, administration of leukocyte-poor preparations (saline-washed red blood cells; red blood cells filtered to remove leukocytes; or, as a last choice, thawed, deglycerolized red blood cells) is indicated.

Delayed febrile reactions that are not accompanied by hemolysis and are not the result of infection may be an early indication of transfusion-associated graft-versus-host disease (GVHD). This is a rare, often fatal, consequence of susceptible immunocompromised recipients receiving donor lymphocytes in whole blood, red blood cells, fresh plasma, or platelets. Directed blood donations from first-degree relatives also may cause GVHD in immunologically normal patients. Gamma irradiation of blood components for patients at risk is the preferred approach for prevention. The use of leukocyte-poor products (washed, filtered, or thawed and deglycerolized red blood cells) may minimize the incidence of GVHD. Ongoing studies are investigating the use of ultraviolet irradiation of platelet concentrates (Deeg, 1989), which also may prevent GVHD in patients treated with platelet transfusions.

Hemolysis: This potentially fatal complication results from the administration of incompatible blood and usually is caused by clerical error (eg, mislabeling of specimens, misidentification of recipients). Only rarely does it result from technical errors in blood typing and crossmatching. The transfusion of as little as 5 to 20 ml of ABO- and other antigen-incompatible blood may cause flushing, nausea, hypotension, tachycardia, restlessness, dyspnea, chills, fever, headache, substernal and/or flank pain, and vomiting (Holland, 1989). Hemoglobinemia and hemoglobinuria occur and often are followed by oliguria and acute renal failure. Hemorrhagic diathesis with thrombocytopenia and spontaneous bleeding may be observed and is caused by disseminated intravascular coagulation (DIC). Its severity is generally proportional to the dose of incompatible erythrocytes. Hypotension and unexpected surgical bleeding may be the only findings in an anesthetized patient. Extreme caution is required in treating DIC while the cause of the incompatibility is being ascertained (see index entry Disseminated Intravascular Coagulation). Rarely, shock and death occur shortly after transfusion of ABO-incompatible red blood cells is initiated.

If a hemolytic reaction is suspected, the transfusion must be stopped immediately. Prompt intravenous administration of fluids (0.9% saline solution) and furosemide [Lasix] or possibly a suitable osmotic diuretic (eg, mannitol) may prevent acute renal failure. The transfusion service should be consulted immediately and supplied with both clotted and anticoagulated samples of the patient's blood together with all containers and attachments used; other fluids infused through the same tubing either during or immediately prior to the transfusion should be identified.

Some experts advocate the administration of dopamine [Dopastat, Intropin] to patients in shock caused by a hemolytic transfusion reaction. Although small doses of this drug can increase arterial blood pressure, cardiac output, and renal perfusion, careful monitoring of urine production, hemodynamic parameters, and electrocardiogram are required (Holland, 1989) (see index entry Dopamine, In Shock). The use of heparin to prevent DIC in patients experiencing hemolytic transfusion reactions is controversial, since this agent may exacerbate the bleeding that led to the initial transfusion. However, because of the severity of the hemolytic reaction, the benefits of heparin may outweigh the risks of further bleeding in patients who have received >200 ml of incompatible blood (Goldfinger, 1977). In some cases, rapidly instituted renal dialysis may be lifesaving.

Acute hemolysis in the absence of red blood cell incompatibility can result from inadvertent freezing (without cryoprotective agents), heating (to temperatures >50° C), or contact of red blood cells with hypertonic or hypotonic solutions or certain drugs. This type of hemolysis most often results in asymptomatic hemoglobinuria and occasionally causes renal insufficiency but rarely can lead to DIC. The remaining transfused product should be tested for the presence of free hemoglobin, and immune-mediated hemolysis must be ruled out. Only normal saline (0.9% sodium chloride solution) should be used in conjunction with whole blood or red blood cells unless there is clearcut evidence that another intravenous solution does not cause hemolysis, coagulation, or agglutination.

Delayed hemolytic transfusion reactions sometimes are observed in patients who do not have serologically detectable antibodies at the time of transfusion but who later develop an increased antibody titer anamnestically. Since the hallmark of the delayed transfusion reaction is a transiently positive direct antiglobulin test, this type of reaction may mimic autoimmune hemolytic anemia. With the exception of fever and developing anemia, most delayed reactions are benign and do not produce symptoms. However, occasionally they are severe and can be life-threatening in individuals who received multiple transfusions. Treatment is similar to that employed for a severe acute hemolytic reaction.

Reactions from Contaminated Products: Administration of whole blood, blood components, or plasma contaminated by bacteria or bacterial endotoxins is a rare cause of catastrophic transfusion reactions. Despite storage of most blood components at refrigerator temperature, a potential for bacterial growth exists. Endotoxin shock caused by transfusion of red blood cells contaminated with *Yersinia* is an example of this problem (Tipple et al, 1990; *MMWR*, 1991). A severe reaction, manifested by nausea and vomiting, chills, fever, profound shock with marked cutaneous erythema (red shock), coma, convulsions, DIC, and, frequently, death, may occur after the injection of the first 50 to 100 ml of a product contaminated by gram-negative bacilli. Treatment must be prompt and aggressive and includes immediate termination of the transfusion, management of shock, and administration of a broad spectrum antibiotic followed by use of the most specific antibiotic for the organism once it has been identified and sensitivity tests have been performed. Bacterial contamination is rare in the United States even for platelet concentrates, which are kept at room temperature. However, even proper preparation and storage cannot prevent it entirely at present, and it should be considered when fever accompanies a transfusion. No medicinal agents should be added to blood or blood components intended for transfusion in an attempt to prevent bacterial contamination.

Hypervolemia: Hypervolemia, possibly resulting in congestive heart failure, can be a serious consequence of transfusions with whole blood, plasma, or plasma substitutes, particularly in the elderly, the very young, and patients with pulmonary or cardiac disease (Holland, 1989). However, this acute transfusion reaction can occur in any patient when the flow rate is excessively rapid. The use of red blood cells greatly reduces but does not eliminate this hazard. Hematocrit determinations are commonly employed as guides for transfusion therapy but do not detect hypervolemia. In patients who have secondary congestive heart failure and one or more of the risk factors listed above for hypervolemia, the rate should be significantly slower than the usual 200 ml/hour. Monitoring of central venous or pulmonary wedge pressure is useful to detect volume overexpansion. When serious hypervolemia and congestive heart failure occur, prompt intravenous administration of a suitable diuretic (eg, furosemide) and/or phlebotomy may be indicated.

Adult Respiratory Distress Syndrome (ARDS): ARDS (noncardiogenic pulmonary edema) occurs very infrequently (Holland, 1989). It should be suspected in patients with respiratory distress or evidence of poor oxygenation in whom problems secondary to hypervolemia are not likely. The transfusion should be discontinued immediately and some experts advocate administration of the diuretic, furosemide. The use of oxygen (by mask or endotracheal tube, if in place), corticosteroids, and epinephrine also may be considered.

The cause of this syndrome is not known. It has been associated with microaggregate debris in patients who received massive transfusions. Other possible contributing factors include humoral mediators liberated during storage from disintegrating cellular components, anti-HLA antibodies, or leukoagglutinins in donor plasma. A strong association exists between sepsis and the development of ARDS. It is most severe in patients receiving plasma or whole blood and less severe in recipients of platelets and red blood cells. It also may occur in recipients of granulocyte transfusions if leukoagglutinins are present.

Immunization: The recipient of transfusions may become immunized to one or a combination of red blood cell, white blood cell, platelet, and plasma protein antigens. This is more common in patients who have received multiple transfusions or have been pregnant. Although symptoms do not necessarily develop, when subsequent transfusions become necessary in these immunized individuals, it may be increasingly difficult to obtain compatible blood products that do not show clinically significant anti-red blood cell antibody reactivity in crossmatching tests. Providing blood products for these patients is thus significantly more difficult and potentially more hazardous than for patients in the general population.

Immunization to antigens found on platelet membranes can mediate destruction of transfused platelets and thus be responsible for refractoriness after administration of multiple units of random-donor platelets. There is evidence to suggest that white cell-associated HLA antigens rather than platelet-associated antigens are required for the initial sensitizing event. The effectiveness of leukocyte filters in reducing this sensitization is being studied and appears promising (vanMarwijk Kooy et al, 1991; Schiffer, 1991). The use of ultraviolet irradiation to functionally inactivate residual white cells in platelet concentrates and other blood products and thus prevent alloimmunization also is under investigation (Deeg, 1989).

Post-transfusion purpura with severe thrombocytopenia is a very rare consequence of transfusion in women immunized to platelet antigens during pregnancy or in men or women who have previously received transfusions. Corticosteroid treatment, plasma exchange, and high doses of intravenous immune globulin are among the therapeutic strategies used to manage this delayed but often life-threatening transfusion reaction. Immunization to a platelet antigen in the neonate can result in neonatal alloimmune thrombocytopenia, which requires platelet transfusions from donors who lack this antigen. The donor is usually the mother, and the platelets must be washed before administration to the neonate. An autoimmune thrombocytopenia also can occur in neonates whose mothers have ITP. This disease, which is refractory to platelet transfusions, often may be prevented by administration of corticosteroids to the mother during pregnancy; administration of corticosteroids to the infant also may be required.

Miscellaneous Adverse Effects: Massive transfusion (defined by some as administration of more than 10 units of whole blood or red blood cells or replacement of more than one blood volume within 24 hours) may cause coagulopathy due to a combination of dilution and consumption of platelets and clotting factors (Rudolph and Boyd, 1990). Data from several studies show that clinically significant bleeding does not occur until after transfusion of at least one blood volume, although slower clotting times (PT, APTT, and TT), reduced concentrations of clotting factors, and decreased platelet counts can be detected earlier (Reed et al, 1986; Ciavarella et al, 1987; Murray et al, 1988). Stored units of red blood cells are deficient in platelets and clotting factors. Most patients who continue to bleed after massive transfusion can be managed by infusion of platelets. Prophylactic administration of platelet concentrates should be reserved for those patients whose platelet counts fall below 50×10^9/L with massive transfusion (Ciavarella et al, 1987). Fresh frozen plasma or cryoprecipitate should be administered when fibrinogen levels fall below 0.8 g/L or when clotting times (PT or APTT) are $\geq$1.8 times control values despite adequate fibrinogen levels, which suggest deficiency of factors V or VIII:C.

Rapid administration of citrate during massive transfusions may sometimes produce muscle tremors, circulatory depression, and electrocardiographic changes consistent with hypocalcemia if citrate metabolism is impaired. Up to 1 g of calcium (as calcium chloride) may be administered intravenously to neutralize the citrate load if the hypocalcemia is associated with hypothermia or hepatic or cardiac dysfunction or if the rate of blood infusion is >100 ml/min (Rudolph and Boyd, 1990). Calcium replacement is not advocated routinely in massive transfusion because excessive calcium may be administered and possibly cause ventricular arrhythmias. Thus, all patients who require administration of calcium chloride must be monitored closely.

Other chemical alterations that may occur rarely after massive transfusion of stored blood include acidosis and hyperkalemia. Long-term storage of red blood cells results in release of intracellular potassium, which can increase the serum potassium level after massive transfusion. Nevertheless, hypokalemia is observed more frequently in massively transfused patients, probably because of reabsorption of potassium by the transfused red blood cells and as a consequence of alkalosis from metabolism of citrate to bicarbonate. The rare cases of acidosis in patients receiving massive transfusions probably result from inadequate perfusion and shock; alkalosis is observed more frequently, but it is rarely of clinical consequence. In contrast, rapid transfusion of large amounts of refrigerated and unwarmed blood can have hypothermic effects on the heart and may cause arrhythmias.

Hemosiderosis develops after repeated transfusions (ie, >100 units) in patients with some chronic anemias (eg, thalassemia major; aplastic anemia; less frequently, sickle cell anemia). Hemosiderosis appears to be less common in other patients receiving chronic transfusion therapy. In patients with thalassemia or sideroblastic anemias, iron overload may be life-threatening as a result of organ damage associated with secondary hemochromatosis (eg, arrhythmias, congestive heart failure, cirrhosis, diabetes). Iron-chelating agents have been employed to forestall this process. Iron excretion may be increased if deferoxamine [Desferal] is given by slow intravenous infusion or by continuous subcutaneous infusion over a 12-hour period several times each week. Automated delivery systems for continuous administration of deferoxamine are available.

Drug Evaluations

BLOOD AND BLOOD COMPONENTS

CPD WHOLE BLOOD

CP2D WHOLE BLOOD

CPDA-1 WHOLE BLOOD

WHOLE BLOOD

Whole blood is drawn from a screened and selected donor under aseptic conditions and flows into blood bags containing premeasured amounts of anticoagulant-preservative solutions; ABO and Rh groups are identified. The content (eg, hemoglobin level, number of viable erythrocytes) of a unit of blood varies according to the donor. Citrate ion (usually as a citrate-phosphate-dextrose-adenine mixture [CPDA-1] or citrate-phosphate-dextrose mixture [CPD or CP2D]) is used as the anticoagulant. Following compatibility testing, blood is administered through a recipient set with a 170- to 210-micron mesh filter.

Whole blood is stored between 1° and 6° C, except during shipment when the temperature may vary from 1° to 10° C. Limits on storage times (shelf-lives) for whole blood and red blood cells are set to establish that, even at the maximum storage time, at least 70% of the transfused cells are intact and viable in the recipient's circulation 24 hours after the transfusion. These limits depend on the composition of the anticoagulant-preservative solution used. The expiration date is not later than 21 days after collection if a CPD or CP2D formulation is used and 35 days if CPDA-1 is used. Red blood cells can be stored in adenine-saline solution for 42 days. Units on which the hermetic seal is broken are outdated within 24 hours if they are stored between 1° and 6° C but must be used within 6 hours if they are kept at 20° to 24° C.

Transfusion orders that specifically request fresh whole blood less than 24 hours old cannot be justified except possibly for children under 2 years who are undergoing cardiopulmonary bypass (Manno et al, 1991). In all other circumstances, components (eg, platelets or clotting factor concentrates) should be administered with the stored whole blood (or red blood cells plus fluids) when necessary.

Only 4% of red blood cell-containing transfusions are in the form of whole blood. The routine use of whole blood is wasteful and may produce hypervolemia in some patients. Whole blood transfusion should be reserved for patients with massive bleeding (>25% of the blood volume). However, it is often not necessary even when >25% of the original blood volume has been lost, since the need for oxygen-carrying capacity and volume expansion often can be met by administration of red blood cells plus 0.9% saline solution. Conventional cell-free resuscitation fluids cannot restore circulating red blood cell volume and do not provide sufficient oxygen following severe hemorrhage. (See also the Introduction.)

After 24 hours of storage at 1° to 6° C, blood contains few functioning platelets or granulocytes but retains viable lymphocytes. Coagulation factors V and VIII decrease to about 50% of normal after five to seven days, but factor IX is stable. Massive blood transfusions of stored blood may produce significant dilutional thrombocytopenia.

DOSAGE AND PREPARATIONS.

Intravenous: One unit (450 ± 45 ml with 63 ml of CPD, CP2D, or CPDA-1), repeated as needed. Units must be administered through a standard 170- to 210-micron filter. Other medications should not be added.

Available through hospital blood banks and community blood centers.

MODIFIED WHOLE BLOOD

Whole blood can be modified by removing one or more of its components and is prepared in a closed system of integrally attached containers in order to maintain its full shelf-life. Plasma is removed from a fresh unit of whole blood, platelets are separated by differential centrifugation, and/or antihemophilic factor is removed by cryoprecipitation. The remaining platelet- and/or factor VIII-poor plasma then is reintroduced into the original container and mixed with the red blood cells. Units from which cryoprecipitate has been removed should not be used to treat labile factor coagulation deficiencies. Otherwise, side effects, hazards, dosage, storage, and dating period are the same as for whole blood. This product is rarely given and its use is not encouraged. Leukocytes can be removed by filtration to reduce the incidence of febrile nonhemolytic transfusion reaction (see the evaluation, Red Blood Cells Leukocytes Removed).

RED BLOOD CELLS IN CPD OR CP2D

RED BLOOD CELLS IN CPDA-1

Human red blood cells are prepared by removing most of the plasma from whole blood at any time during the dating period; the ABO and Rh groups are identified, and the hematocrit of the final product usually ranges from 70% to 80%.

Characteristics of this product may vary with the donor, the process used, and the duration of storage of the whole blood before red blood cell extraction. The characteristics of red blood cells contained in a unit may not be apparent from the label, but the product may contain platelet or leukocyte debris and products of red blood cell metabolism, and hematocrit levels may vary.

Liquid red blood cells should be stored at 1° to 6° C. The expiration date for red blood cells in CPD or CPDA diluents is the same as that of the whole blood from which it was derived or 24 hours after the hermetic seal is broken.

Red blood cells provide the same hemoglobin content and oxygen-carrying capacity as the whole blood from which they were derived in approximately 50% of the volume. This is the product of choice when an increased red blood cell mass is required (except in patients with massive hemorrhage who also require volume replacement and who may require coagulation factor replacement). In neonates, red blood cells less than seven days old may be preferable to whole blood to prevent hypervolemia, hyperkalemia, and hyperammonemia.

Red blood cells may be mixed with 50 to 100 ml of 0.9% sodium chloride injection to increase the flow rate but should not be mixed with other solutions.

For adverse reactions and precautions, see the Introduction.

DOSAGE AND PREPARATIONS.

Intravenous: One unit usually elevates the venous hematocrit level by approximately 3% in a 70-kg recipient; 50 to 100 ml of 0.9% sodium chloride injection may be added to a unit of red blood cells through a standard Y-administration set.

Available through hospital blood banks and community blood centers.

RED BLOOD CELLS IN ADENINE-SALINE

Most of the plasma and possibly platelet and/or leukocyte fractions from whole blood, collected in CPD or CP2D anticoagulant, are removed, and an additive solution is mixed with the red blood cells to provide a product with a hematocrit of 55% to 65%. This probably is the most widely available product containing red blood cells. Typical additive solutions are dextrose and adenine in 0.9% sodium chloride injection with mannitol (AS-1 or AS-5; the former contains more dextrose and mannitol and slightly less adenine) or without mannitol but with more citrate and phosphate, an intermediate amount of dextrose, and a greater amount of adenine (AS-3). Red blood cells collected in CPD anticoagulant that are then concentrated and placed in adenine-saline solution can be stored for 42 days. These products are labeled to identify the anticoagulant and additive solution. They have approximately the same flow rate as whole blood and no further dilution is required.

The actions, indications, and contraindications are the same as for Red Blood Cells in CPD or CPDA-1. Furthermore, because of the dilution with saline, large amounts of these products should not be used in patients at risk of circulatory overload.

DOSAGE AND PREPARATIONS. The dosage is the same as for Red Blood Cells in CPD or CPDA-1.

AS-1:
Adsol (Fenwal/Baxter).
AS-3:
Neutricel (Cutter).
AS-5:
Optisol (Terumo).

RED BLOOD CELLS LEUKOCYTES REMOVED

About 1% of transfusions are associated with nonhemolytic febrile reactions following transfusion of red blood cells or whole blood. These reactions may result from alloimmunization to antigens associated with white blood cells, platelets, plasma proteins, and other nonerythrocyte elements. More than 80% of patients who develop febrile reactions after a single transfusion do not react to a subsequent transfusion (Holland, 1989). Therefore, most patients do not require leukocyte-poor preparations after a single transfusion has caused a febrile reaction. However, febrile reactions are common in patients who receive multiple transfusions (particularly those with diseases such as leukemia or aplastic anemia) and immunosuppressed or immunodeficient individuals. If febrile reactions occur, these patients should receive preparations from which leukocytes have been removed.

Leukocyte-poor (ie, $<5 \times 10^8$ leukocytes/unit) or buffy coat-poor red blood cells can be prepared simply by removing the sedimented buffy coat after centrifugation of whole blood. Removal of leukocytes is more efficient from blood stored for more than 10 days. Preparations from which at least 70% of the original white cells are removed (with retention of at least 80% of the original red blood cells) are usually adequate for uncomplicated situations. However, in persons with high titers of leukoagglutinins or HLA antibodies, further removal of white blood cell and platelet debris may be necessary. Several techniques involving filtration (in the blood bank prior to issue of the unit or at the bedside at the time of transfusion), inverted centrifugation, or sedimentation are available (Walker et al, 1990); filtration is preferred.

DOSAGE AND PREPARATIONS. Same as for Red Blood Cells in CPD or CPDA-1.

RED BLOOD CELLS SALINE-WASHED

Significant amounts of leukocytes, platelets, plasma, microaggregates, and cell-derived debris are removed by washing, especially when automated blood cell processors are used. However, currently available filters remove a larger percentage of white cells than washing and are less labor intensive. The red blood cells are washed with normal saline within 24 hours before transfusion, but products vary according to the shelf-age before washing. The more efficient batch washing process removes approximately 90% of leukocytes and almost all plasma but also results in the loss of about 20% of erythrocytes. Although the risk of leukocyte contamination is slightly greater than with thawed, deglycerolized red blood cells, these preparations can be used in most alloimmunized patients with recurrent nonhemolytic febrile transfusion reactions. Red blood cells washed with saline five or more times also may be used to reduce the incidence of urticarial and anaphylactic transfusion reactions in IgA-deficient patients with anti-IgA antibodies.

DOSAGE AND PREPARATIONS. Same as for Red Blood Cells in CPD or CPDA-1.

RED BLOOD CELLS FROZEN

A unit of red blood cells less than six days old is frozen rapidly after addition of a cryoprotective agent, usually glycerol, and stored at -65° C or colder. One of two methods (using high or low glycerol concentrations) is used at most blood banks in the United States. The expiration date is ten years, but units have demonstrated adequate in vivo recovery after storage for more than ten years. Transfusion must be preceded by thawing and deglycerolizing to replace the cryoprotectant with saline. Thawed red blood cells are outdated in 24 hours. These preparations contain about 2% of the original leukocytes and almost no measurable plasma protein or platelets. The newer filtration methods are more efficient at removing leukocytes. The method used to deglycerolize frozen red blood cells must be compatible with the procedure used for freezing. If glycerol has not been removed sufficiently, intravascular hemolysis may result.

Although processing is expensive and time consuming, this type of preparation is particularly useful for storing erythrocytes of rare phenotypes and for autologous blood donation in special circumstances (eg, anticipated needs during pregnancy, elective surgery, or neonatal exchange transfusions). (See the Introduction.)

Thawed, deglycerolized red blood cells are the most desirable choice for patients with rare phenotypes when supplies of liquid refrigerated red blood cells are inadequate and for patients with confirmed severe febrile or allergic transfusion reactions who continue to experience reactions to saline-washed or leukocyte-poor red blood cells.

DOSAGE AND PREPARATIONS. Same as for Red Blood Cells in CPD or CPDA-1.

PLASMA FRESH FROZEN

This preparation is the liquid portion of a single unit of citrated (CPD, CPDA-1) whole blood that has been separated from the cells and frozen within eight hours of donation. It may be stored at -18° C or lower for up to one year after the date of collection. Storage at temperatures below -30° C is now preferred since this allows retention of about 90% of factor VIII activity (Calhoun, 1989; Walker et al, 1990). The unit is thawed in a water bath at 37° C (with gentle agitation to facilitate thawing), and it must be administered within six hours if used for labile coagulation factors and within 24 hours if used for replacement of stable clotting factors or for any other indication. The product usually contains 70% or more of the coagulation factors present in fresh plasma.

USES. Fresh frozen plasma may be used to replace coagulation factor II, VII, IX, X, or XI deficiencies and is the agent of choice to replace coagulation factor V deficiency. Although fresh frozen plasma also contains factor VIII, antihemophilic factor preparations (cryoprecipitate and concentrates) are preferred for deficiency of this factor (see index entry Hemostatics). Plasma should not be employed routinely to treat hemophilia; it is reserved for patients with acute blood loss who have a documented coagulation factor deficiency. Cryoprecipitated factor VIII preparations also are preferred to treat hypofibrinogenemia or, experimentally, fibronectin deficiency. Plasma may be used prior to surgery in patients with severe liver disease and multiple clotting factor deficiencies and for the rapid reversal of warfarin overdose.

Plasma from donors known to be deficient in IgA is indicated for the treatment and prophylaxis of immunoglobulin deficiencies when class-specific anti-IgA antibodies are present, and it may provide the only source of IgA-free IgG and IgM currently available. These patients may have anaphylactic reactions to transfusion of IgA-containing materials, including albumin and immune globulin. For most other patients who require replacement therapy for immune globulin deficiencies, intramuscular or intravenous (IVIG) preparations of immune globulin are preferred to the use of fresh frozen plasma, since these preparations carry less risk for transmission of viral and other infectious diseases and for hypervolemia (see index entries Immune Globulin and Immune Globulin Intravenous). Fresh frozen plasma may be indicated for the treatment of infants with secondary immunodeficiency associated with severe protein-losing enteropathy if IVIG is not available.

When plasma exchange is used to treat thrombotic thrombocytopenic purpura (TTP), the replacement fluid of choice is fresh frozen plasma. In some cases, equivalent therapeutic benefits can be obtained by plasma transfusion without exchange in patients with TTP if a sufficient amount of plasma can be infused without causing hypervolemia (and potentially congestive heart failure). When bleeding is caused by coumarin anticoagulants, fresh frozen plasma is indicated for rapid hemostasis (eg, prior to emergency surgery). Plasma can be used in antithrombin III deficiency, particularly before surgery or in patients who require heparin for the treatment of thrombosis. Also, the use of plasma for its oncotic properties in burn patients with infection appears to be promising. However, albumin provides equivalent oncotic effects and is free of risk for transmission of HIV or hepatitis.

ADVERSE REACTIONS AND PRECAUTIONS. Plasma may cause circulatory overload and carries a risk of disease transmission since viruses are not inactivated or reduced prior to administration. It should not be used when blood volume can be adequately and more safely replaced by crystalloids or colloids (eg, albumin, plasma protein fraction).

Other possible adverse reactions to plasma include urticaria, acute lung syndrome, and anaphylaxis.

DOSAGE AND PREPARATIONS.

Intravenous: Dosage is determined by clinical response and, when possible, by laboratory assays of appropriate coagulation factors. ABO compatibility is required, but crossmatching is not necessary.

PLASMA

Plasma (also referred to as single-donor plasma) is the liquid portion of a single unit of citrated (CPD, CPDA-1) whole blood separated up to five days after the dating period (21 days [CPD] or 35 days [CPDA-1]). Plasma also may be obtained by plasmapheresis. It may be stored at 1° to 6° C for no more than 26 days (CPD) or 40 days (CPDA-1) after collection of the whole blood. This product contains variable amounts of stable coagulation factors depending on the duration of storage, but labile clotting factors and platelets decrease during the first few days of blood storage and are not present in the plasma prepared from stored blood. It also contains significant quantities of cellular debris, adenine, citrate, sodium, potassium, and other ions, which may increase the metabolic burden in a bleeding patient with hepatic or renal disease. It has all the disadvantages of fresh frozen plasma and no compensating advantages.

Plasma may be used to treat mild deficiencies of stable clotting factors (eg, II, VII, IX, X, XI, XIII). It may be of value to counteract warfarin overdose in patients who are bleeding or require emergency surgery. This product should not be used as a plasma volume expander because of the risk of disease transmission.

DOSAGE AND PREPARATIONS.

Intravenous: Dosage is determined by clinical response and, when possible, by laboratory assays of appropriate coagulation factors. ABO compatibility is necessary, but crossmatching is not required.

PLATELETS

Platelets (one of the primary products obtained from routine processing of whole blood into red blood cells) are prepared by centrifugation of citrated (CPD or CPDA-1) whole blood at 20° to 24° C within eight hours after collection. An average unit of random-donor platelets obtained from whole blood contains more than 5.5 X 10^{10} platelets suspended in approximately 50 ml of the original plasma. Single-donor platelets may be obtained by automated apheresis techniques. The dating period of random-donor platelets prepared using sterile closed systems is up to five days (depending on the plastic container used after collection) when stored at 20° to 24° C. Platelets preserved at room temperature must be gently and continuously agitated.

Ordinarily, ABO-identical platelets are used but, when unavailable, platelets from non-ABO-identical donors may be administered if not grossly contaminated with red blood cells. However, large volumes of the suspending incompatible plasma should not be given to children. If necessary, some of the incompatible plasma may be removed just prior to administration. Rh-negative platelets should be used in Rh-negative females before and during the childbearing period to prevent Rh alloimmunization by contaminating red blood cells. If it is necessary to give a platelet transfusion to an Rh-negative woman from an Rh-positive donor, Rh_o(D) immune globulin should be administered to prevent sensitization (for dosage, see index entry Rh_o(D) Immune Globulin).

For indications, see the Introduction.

DOSAGE AND PREPARATIONS.

Intravenous: Units must be administered through an approved 170- to 210-micron filter *(microaggregate filters must not be used)*. Adults, initially, 1 unit/10 kg; the appropriate number of units (usually 6 to 8) is pooled immediately prior to infusion. In patients without platelet (HLA) antibodies, splenomegaly, sepsis, or disseminated intravascular coagulation, this dose should increase the platelet count by approximately 35,000 to 50,000/microliter in a 70-kg person (measured one hour after transfusion). In patients with splenomegaly, an initial dose of 1.5 to 2 units/10 kg may be helpful. See also the section on Platelet Transfusion in the Introduction.

GRANULOCYTES

Granulocyte transfusion became practical only after technology for obtaining granulocytes by continuous or intermittent flow centrifugation or by filtration (leukapheresis) was developed. Steroids may be given to the donor, and a sedimenting agent (eg, hydroxyethyl starch) may be used to increase the harvest of granulocytes. With mechanical leukapheresis, a single donor can provide at least 1 X 10^{10} granulocytes in two to three hours. Although this is only about 10% of the normal daily granulocyte production, it may be sufficient to combat infection in the recipient. ABO compatibility is necessary since most granulocyte concentrations contain red blood cells. If the patient is immunized against HLA antigens, it also may be advisable to provide granulocyte transfusions only from HLA-matched donors.

USES. Granulocyte transfusions are used infrequently because antibiotics usually control most infections and obviate the need for this component. Granulocytes may be transfused to treat sepsis if (1) the patient's granulocyte count is less than 500/microliter, and (2) fever persists for 72 hours despite appropriate antibiotic therapy. However, results of clinical trials thus far have indicated that granulocyte transfusions are only useful to treat gram-negative sepsis (McCullough, 1989). Granulocytes should be administered for at least four consecutive days in conjunction with appropriate antibiotics. Daily (or twice daily) therapy is usually necessary until the patient's absolute granulocyte count exceeds 500/microliter or the sepsis resolves. Additionally, there should be a reasonable likelihood of recovery and significant improvement after recovery from the infection. Granulocytes should not be given to patients with widespread malignant disease that is unresponsive to chemotherapy. If recovery of bone marrow function is unlikely, granulocyte transfusion will not alter the course of the disease and may cause additional problems (eg, pulmonary toxicity) because of sensitization to the infused granulocytes. The prophylactic use of granulocyte transfusions is not recommended. However, HLA-matched granulocytes have been beneficial in some patients recovering from bone marrow transplants. (It is necessary to irradiate all blood products given to bone marrow recipients to prevent transfusion-associated graft-versus-host disease.)

Results of in vitro tests suggest that granulocytes from normal donors may retain some phagocytic and microbicidal functions for as long as 24 hours. However, 30% to 50% of the chemotactic response is lost after 24 hours at refrigerator temperatures and approximately 30% is lost after storage for 24 hours at room temperature. Granulocytes should be used within six hours after collection to assure maximum benefit.

ADVERSE REACTIONS AND PRECAUTIONS. Fever and chills often follow granulocyte transfusion and can be ameliorated by an antipyretic. The more severe transfusion reactions, hypotension and respiratory distress, occur much less frequently (after about 1% of transfusions; in comparison, the mild to moderate reactions are observed in 25% to 50% of recipients).

Pulmonary reactions (eg, respiratory insufficiency) may result from sequestration of granulocytes in the pulmonary capillaries. The reaction may be particularly severe in those with pulmonary infections or congestive heart failure. Severe pulmonary reactions have been attributed to amphotericin B given with granulocyte transfusions. Although this observation has not been confirmed, it is advisable not to administer granulocytes and amphotericin B simultaneously.

The risk of transmitting viral or other infectious diseases always accompanies granulocyte (or any other) transfusions. However, transmission of cytomegalovirus is of particular concern in bone marrow transplant recipients who are given granulocyte transfusions; therefore, granulocyte transfusion donors should be seronegative if both the marrow donor and recipient are seronegative. Graft-versus-host disease is another possible adverse reaction, since granulocyte concentrates contain viable lymphocytes; this can be prevented by irradiation of the component before transfusion.

DOSAGE AND PREPARATIONS.
Intravenous: A minimum of 1 X 10^{10} granulocytes is administered slowly once daily on at least four consecutive days. Two transfusions per day may be advisable if the concentrates contain no more than the minimal number of granulocytes. Some physicians recommend that the duration of each course of therapy be at least seven days. The optimum duration of an infusion has not been determined, but one suggested regimen is administration over a two-hour period via standard blood administration sets. Micropore filters should *not* be used.

ALBUMIN (HUMAN)
[Albuminar, Albutein, Buminate, Plasbumin]

This sterile plasma protein preparation is obtained by fractionating plasma in a series of controlled precipitations with cold ethanol. The plasma must be nonreactive for hepatitis B surface antigen (HBsAg) and anti-HIV-I. Plasma obtained from whole blood donations is tested for antibody to HTLV-I and hepatitis B core antigen. However, most plasma for fractionation is obtained from paid plasmapheresis donors, and the latter two tests are not performed routinely because the fractionation process eliminates the risk of transmission. Human albumin contains no coagulation factors or blood group antibodies. Heating for ten hours at 60° C removes the hazard of undetected HIV and viral hepatitis. Albumin preparations contain caprylate and acetyltryptophanate as stabilizers. Unopened preparations can be stored for up to three years at temperatures not exceeding 37° C and up to five years at temperatures between 2° and 8° C. All albumin preparations should be used within four hours after the container has been opened. Unused portions should be discarded.

USES. Albumin 25 g is equivalent osmotically to about 500 ml of plasma. This preparation is used to restore the colloidal osmotic pressure of plasma in hypovolemic states (eg, burns, hemorrhage, surgical procedures, during plasma exchange). The advantages and disadvantages of using albumin or other colloid solutions rather than crystalloid solutions for resuscitation of hypovolemic patients remain controversial. Some experts assert that use of crystalloid solutions may be associated with a greater risk of pulmonary edema because plasma proteins are diluted and thus plasma oncotic pressure is reduced. Others maintain that albumin is readily distributed out of the vasculature into the interstitium (even when capillary permeability remains unaltered) and thus also can result in retention of tissue water.

Albumin binds bilirubin and has been used adjunctively during exchange transfusion to treat hyperbilirubinemia, most frequently that associated with hemolytic disease in the newborn; however, newer treatment methods are preferred. Albumin has been given to patients with acute nephrosis, ascites, and protein-losing enteropathy, but most authorities consider these uses to be of temporary benefit at best. Other uses of albumin include maintenance of colloid osmotic pressure for priming of cardiopulmonary bypass pumps when marked hemodilution is employed and in adult respiratory distress syndrome (if capillary permeability in the lung has not increased significantly). Albumin should not be used to treat malnutrition, chronic nephrosis, or chronic hepatic cirrhosis and also should not be used in media for resuspension of red blood cells before transfusion.

The 5% solution is preferred for most indications. The 25% preparation is hyperoncotic and should be used cautiously because it can cause hypervolemia unless it is diluted appropriately.

ADVERSE REACTIONS AND PRECAUTIONS. Since albumin is a constituent of human blood, it usually can be given with relative safety, although chills, fever, urticaria, and variable effects on blood pressure, pulse, and respiration have been noted. This preparation does not interfere with normal coagulation mechanisms or promote clotting. Albumin preparations contain 130 to 160 mEq/L of sodium, and this should be considered when salt intake must be restricted. Patients with heart failure should be given albumin cautiously. Because patients with low cardiac reserve or severe anemia and those not deficient in albumin are more likely to develop hypervolemia and congestive heart failure, they should not receive large amounts of albumin.

Albumin should not be administered if the solution is turbid or contains sediment.

Albumin preparations are classified in FDA Pregnancy Category C.

DOSAGE AND PREPARATIONS.
Intravenous: Dosage should be determined by monitoring the pulmonary artery, wedge, or central venous pressure during administration to avoid hypervolemia. No more than 250 g/48 hours should be given. When more than this is necessary, plasma should be substituted.

The 5% solution is given undiluted, usually at a rate of 2 to 4 ml/min. The 25% solution can be administered undiluted or it can be diluted with sterile, nonpyrogenic sodium chloride injection or 5% dextrose injection. (In the presence of edema, the undiluted 25% concentrate should be used, but 5% dextrose injection may be employed if dilution is necessary.)

Albumin 25% must be administered slowly (1 ml/min), especially to patients with low cardiac reserve, to prevent rapid expansion of plasma volume and possible pulmonary edema. For shock caused by diminished plasma volume, it may be given as rapidly as desired, preferably diluted (an approximately isotonic solution can be prepared by diluting each 20 ml of 25% solution to a volume of 100 ml).

For shock, *adults and older children,* 25 g initially, repeated in 15 to 30 minutes if necessary. Whole blood may be required if the patient is hemorrhaging.

For burns, the extent of the burn determines the amount and duration of administration. The dose should be sufficient to restore plasma volume and to decrease hemoconcentration. Initially, 500 ml of 5% solution or 100 ml of 25% solution has been used in addition to electrolyte solutions. For nonemergency treatment of *children,* 6.25 to 12.5 g.

Generic. Solution 5% in 250 ml containers and 25% in 10 and 50 ml containers.

Albuminar-5, Albuminar-25 (Armour), ***Albutein 5% and 25%*** (Alpha Therapeutic), ***Buminate 5%, 25%*** (Baxter), ***Plasbumin-5, Plasbumin-25*** (Miles). Solution (aqueous) 5% in 50 ml containers (***Albuminar-5, Plasbumin-5***), 250 and 500 ml containers with intravenous administration sets (***Albuminar-5, Albutein 5%, Buminate 5%, Plasbumin-5***), and 1,000 ml containers (***Albuminar-5***); solution (aqueous) 25% in 20, 50, and 100 ml containers (***Albuminar-25, Albutein 25%, Buminate 25%, Plasbumin-25***). The 50 and 100 ml containers are supplied with intravenous administration sets.

Use of 4% and 20% solutions is permitted by the Code of Federal Regulations. The 20% concentration is produced by some manufacturers in the United States for export; it is not generally available in this country.

PLASMA PROTEIN FRACTION (HUMAN)

[Plasmanate, Plasma Plex, Plasmatein, Protenate]

Plasma protein fraction (PPF) (human) is a 5% solution of stabilized human plasma proteins (at least 83% albumin, no more than 17% globulin, and no more than 1% of total protein as gamma globulin), which contains 130 to 160 mEq/L of sodium. The material is prepared from large pools of normal human plasma, which is nonreactive for hepatitis B surface antigen (HBsAg) and antibody to HIV-I, by fractionation involving a series of controlled precipitations with cold ethanol. Plasma obtained from whole blood donations is tested for antibodies to HTLV-I and hepatitis B core antigen. However, most plasma for fractionation is obtained from paid plasmapheresis donors and tests for these two antibodies are not done routinely since the fractionation process eliminates the risk of transmission. Products are heated at 60° C for 10 hours to minimize the risk of transmitting viral diseases.

PPF has been used to treat hypovolemic shock, but albumin may be preferable for expanding plasma volume because it is less likely to cause hypotension and is a more purified preparation. PPF also has been used for the initial treatment of shock in infants and small children with dehydration, hemoconcentration, and electrolyte deficiency caused by diarrhea. Albumin products are not recommended in the treatment of chronic hypoproteinemia (eg, nephrotic syndrome, cirrhosis), because they are not effective in these disorders. PPF does not provide labile clotting factors and should not be given to correct coagulation defects.

ADVERSE REACTIONS AND PRECAUTIONS. Chills, fever, urticaria, nausea, and vomiting have occurred. Serious hypotension was reported in surgical patients undergoing extracorporeal circulation following transfusion of earlier preparations of PPF. Contamination of some of these lots with prekallikrein activator (PKA) was implicated as the cause of bradykinin-induced peripheral vasodilation. This usually could have been avoided by slowing the rate of infusion to less than 10 ml/minute. PKA levels have been reduced in all preparations and hypotension has been rare since this change was made. Nevertheless, PPF probably should not be given when rapid intravenous infusion is necessary.

All patients should be observed carefully for signs of hypervolemia (eg, pulmonary edema) or cardiac failure. Administration of large quantities to patients with impaired renal function has caused electrolyte imbalances resulting in metabolic alkalosis.

Solutions should not be mixed with or administered through the same sets as other intravenous fluids. Administration is contraindicated if the preparation is turbid or a precipitate forms.

PPF is classified in FDA Pregnancy Category C.

DOSAGE AND PREPARATIONS.

Intravenous: The following amounts serve as guides; the total amount administered must be adjusted to meet the needs of each patient. *Adults,* for hypoproteinemia, 1 to 1.5 L of solution containing 50 to 75 g of protein infused at a rate of 5 to 8 ml/min, repeated as necessary. *Infants and young children,* for dehydration, 33 ml/kg infused at a rate of 5 to 10 ml/min.

Plasmanate (Miles), ***Plasma Plex*** (Armour), ***Generic.*** Solution 5% in 50 ml containers and in 250 and 500 ml containers with intravenous administration set.

Plasmatein (Alpha Therapeutic), ***Protenate*** (Baxter). Solution 5% in 250 and 500 ml containers with intravenous administration set.

PLASMA EXPANDERS

DEXTRAN 40

[Gentran-40, Rheomacrodex, 10% LMD]

DEXTRAN 70

[Macrodex, Gentran-70]

DEXTRAN 75

Dextran is a water-soluble glucose polymer biosynthesized by *Leuconostoc mesenteroides* from sucrose. The native dextrans consist of glucose molecules joined by alpha-glucosidic linkages with a molecular weight of seven to ten million daltons. Dextran is hydrolyzed and fractionated to produce preparations with average molecular weights of 40, 70, and 75 kilodaltons.

USES. Because they tend to remain in the intravascular space, the high-molecular-weight preparations may be used as plasma volume expanders. They also may be used to correct the oligemia of burn shock or to maintain colloidal osmotic pressure temporarily during certain types of cardiovascular surgery.

Dextran 40 is used as a priming fluid (alone or as an additive) for pump-oxygenators during extracorporeal circulation and as an adjunct in the treatment of shock or impending shock. More recently, dextran 40 has been administered to prevent venous thrombosis and thromboembolism (see index entry Dextran, As Antiplatelet Drug). Use of dextran 40 also has been studied as therapy for intermittent claudication in patients with occlusive peripheral artery disease (Ernst et al, 1990). Data from a double-blind trial suggest that both the maximal and pain-free distances that the treated patients were able to walk were increased.

ADVERSE REACTIONS. Hypersensitivity reactions (rash, pruritus, nasal congestion, dyspnea, chest tightness, and mild hypotension) are the most common untoward effects. The incidence is very low and reactions generally are mild. Both dextran 40 and dextran 70 have produced urticaria, angioedema, bronchospasm, and anaphylactic reactions. Patients also may develop nausea, vomiting, and, occasionally, acute hypotension. Histamine release and major anaphylactoid reactions have been reported.

Discontinuation of therapy usually relieves the milder reactions. More serious adverse effects may require rapid plasma volume expansion with an agent other than dextran and immediate subcutaneous administration of 1:1,000 epinephrine 0.5 ml, followed if necessary by intravenous injection of 0.25 to 0.5 ml of a 1:10,000 solution. Antihistamines, steroids, and other supportive measures also may be required to counteract shock and hypotension. (For treatment of anaphylaxis, see also index entry Shock, Anaphylactic.) Equipment for emergency resuscitation should be readily available. Because death from anaphylactic reactions has occurred after intravenous administration of as little as 10 ml of dextran 70 solution, blood pressure should be monitored and the patient observed closely during at least the first 30 minutes of infusion of any dextran preparation.

The incidence and severity of anaphylactic reactions can be markedly reduced by the administration of dextran 1 [Promit], a hapten inhibitor of dextran reactive antibodies with a molecular weight of 1,000, one to two minutes prior to the use of dextran 40, 70, or 75 (Ljungström et al, 1988). Dextran 1 is given intravenously in the following amounts: *adults*, 20 ml (150 mg/ml); *children*, 0.3 ml/kg. It should not be diluted or mixed with high-molecular-weight dextran preparations.

Increased bleeding time caused by interference with platelet function occurs in many patients receiving dextran, especially when the higher molecular weight products are used and the dose exceeds 1 to 1.5 L. This reaction may not appear for six to nine hours following infusion, and bleeding may occur, especially if there is a pre-existing coagulation defect. Dextran also can reduce serum levels of fibrinogen and factors V, VIII, and IX.

All of the dextrans are degraded enzymatically to glucose; the average rate of metabolism is 70 to 90 mg/kg daily. In patients with adequate urine flow, dextran has little effect on urine viscosity. However, when urine flow is diminished, dextran markedly increases urine viscosity and specific gravity and possibly causes subsequent acute tubular failure.

EFFECTS ON LABORATORY TESTS, PRECAUTIONS, AND CONTRAINDICATIONS. Currently available dextran solutions induce minimal rouleaux formation and do not interfere with blood typing and crossmatching when these tests are carried out by saline agglutination and indirect antiglobulin methods. However, difficulties may be encountered, especially with dextran 70 and 75, when proteolytic enzyme techniques are used to crossmatch blood.

Dextran is contraindicated in patients with known hypersensitivity, severe congestive heart failure, renal failure, hypervolemic conditions, or severe bleeding disorders. It should be used with caution in patients with chronic liver disease or impaired renal function or in those likely to develop pulmonary edema or congestive heart failure.

Dextran is classified in FDA Pregnancy Category C.

DOSAGE AND PREPARATIONS. Dextran may precipitate from solution on storage. It can be redissolved by heating in a water bath for a short time at the minimal temperature required to effect solution.

DEXTRAN 40:

Intravenous: *Adults and children,* for shock, the first 10 ml/kg of 10% solution may be infused as rapidly as necessary to effect improvement; the remainder of the dose is given more slowly. Monitoring of the pulmonary artery, wedge, or central venous pressure is strongly recommended as a guide to dosage. The total dosage during the first 24 hours should not exceed 20 ml/kg. If therapy is continued for more than 24 hours, the total daily dose should not exceed 10 ml/kg. Therapy should not be continued for more than five days.

Dextran 40 (McGaw), ***Gentran-40*** (Baxter), ***Rheomacrodex*** (Kabi Pharmacia), ***10% LMD*** (Abbott). Solution 10% in 0.9% sodium chloride solution or 5% dextrose in 500 ml containers.

DEXTRAN 70, DEXTRAN 75:

Intravenous: *Adults*, in an emergency, 500 ml of 6% solution may be infused at a rate of 20 to 40 ml/min. *Children*, the best guide to dosage is the body weight or surface area of the patient. The total dosage should not exceed 20 ml/kg during the first 24 hours.

Dextran 70 (McGaw), ***Gentran-70*** (Baxter). Solution 6% in 0.9% sodium chloride solution in 500 ml containers.

Dextran 75 (Abbott). Solution 6% in 0.9% sodium chloride solution or 5% dextrose solution in 500 ml containers.

Macrodex (Kabi Pharmacia). Solution 6% in 0.9% sodium chloride solution or 5% dextrose in water in 500 ml containers.

HETASTARCH

[Hespan]

ACTIONS. Hetastarch (hydroxyethyl starch, HES) is a colloid derived from waxy maize starch. The molecular weight of at least 80% of the polymer units ranges from 10,000 to 3,000,000 daltons. The weight of the average-sized molecule is 70,000 daltons, but the distribution is skewed with a preponderance of large molecules.

A 6% solution of hetastarch has approximately the same osmotic properties as 5% albumin at physiologic concentration. The pH is approximately 5.5 (range, 4.5 to 7.0) and the osmolality is approximately 310 mOsmol/L. Following intravenous infusion of hetastarch, the plasma volume is expanded slightly in excess of the actual volume given. This effect gradually disappears 18 to 24 hours after infusion; 40% of a dose is eliminated within 24 hours. About 64% of the dose is eliminated within eight days, and approximately 90% in 42 days; the average half-life is 17 days. The remaining 10% is eliminated slowly over a prolonged period. Additional doses have additive effects. The small molecules (<50,000 daltons) are removed from the circulation by glomerular filtration. Large molecules are degraded in the plasma by amylase to a size that can be eliminated by the kidneys. A small residue of glucose is produced by the degradation process. The largest molecules are stored temporarily in the reticuloendothelial cells of various body tissues, principally the liver and spleen. These larger molecules also are degraded by amylase.

USES. Hetastarch is used to expand plasma volume in the treatment of hypovolemia, shock, or impending shock caused by hemorrhage, burns, surgery, sepsis, or other trauma.

The choice of crystalloid versus colloid solutions for treatment of hypovolemic shock remains unresolved. An advantage of colloid solutions is maintenance of hemodynamic parameters with smaller volumes of infused fluids and without reduction of colloid oncotic pressure. However, resuscitation with crystalloid solutions is much less costly. Advocates of each premise assert that their approach is associated with less risk of pulmonary edema and dysfunction. In randomized clinical trials comparing crystalloids with colloids, results were conflicting; the conclusions drawn may relate to differences in fluid replacement protocols and in choice of endpoints. However, recent data suggest that in patients undergoing coronary artery bypass grafts or valve surgery, the reduced fluid volumes of hetastarch solutions required may improve hemodynamic performance and shorten intensive care stays more than when normal saline solution is used (Ley et al, 1990). Few studies have compared the use of different colloids for plasma volume expansion. For the most part, 6% hetastarch appears to provide hemodynamic effects comparable to those of 5% albumin and other colloidal plasma volume expanders.

Hemodilution with other preparations of hydroxyethyl starch has been studied as therapy for peripheral artery occlusive disease (Ernst et al, 1987; Kiesewetter et al, 1990). Data from randomized, double-blind trials show that hemodilution improves exercise tolerance in these patients.

Hetastarch also is useful as a sedimenting agent in the preparation of granulocytes by leukapheresis (continuous and intermittent flow cytapheresis). In these healthy donors, the main concern is the delayed excretion of hetastarch.

ADVERSE REACTIONS AND PRECAUTIONS. Nausea, vomiting, mild febrile reactions, chills, pruritus, and urticaria have occurred. Rarely, anaphylactoid reactions have been reported (incidence, less than 0.1% according to the manufacturer's literature). Larger doses decrease the hematocrit, dilute plasma proteins and coagulation factors, have a mild direct effect in reducing factor VIII levels, and interfere with platelet function. Thus, hetastarch is contraindicated in patients with severe bleeding disorders.

As with all plasma fluid expanders, hypervolemia is a potential danger. Because hetastarch is excreted relatively slowly, primarily by the kidneys, slow dissipation of plasma expansion occurs in patients with impaired renal function. Accordingly, this agent is contraindicated in patients with severe congestive heart failure and renal failure with oliguria or anuria not due to plasma volume depletion.

No teratogenic effects were demonstrated during studies in mice, but extrapolation of animal data to humans may not be appropriate, and the risk/benefit potential must be considered carefully before this drug is used in pregnant women (FDA Pregnancy Category C). Similarly, no data are available on the use of hetastarch in children.

DOSAGE AND PREPARATIONS.

Intravenous Infusion: *Adults,* for plasma volume expansion, total dosage and rate of infusion depend on the amount of blood or plasma fluid lost and the resultant hemoconcentration. The usual amount administered is 500 to 1,000 ml. The total dosage does not usually exceed 1,500 ml or approximately 20 ml/kg for the typical 70-kg patient, but doses of 3 to 4 L have been given in severe hypovolemia (eg, trauma) with monitoring for dilutional coagulopathy. Hetastarch should not be administered repeatedly over several days.

In acute hemorrhagic shock, the total dose of 20 ml/kg may be given over a one-hour period; in burn or septic shock, the rate is usually slower.

For leukapheresis in continuous flow centrifugation (CFC) procedures, 250 to 700 ml is typically infused at a constant fixed ratio to venous whole blood, usually 1:8. Multiple CFC procedures of up to two per week to a total of seven to ten have been reported to be safe and effective. Adequate data are not available to establish the safety of more frequent or a greater number of procedures.

Hespan (DuPont-Merck). Solution 6% in 0.9% sodium chloride solution in 500 ml containers.

PENTASTARCH

[Pentaspan]

ACTIONS. Pentastarch is a colloid derived almost entirely from amylopectin. This low-molecular-weight hydroxyethyl starch is more rapidly degraded by circulating amylase than the chemically similar hetastarch. The molecular weight of the polymer units is between 10,000 and 2 million daltons. The weight of the average-size molecule is 63,000 daltons, but the distribution is skewed toward the larger molecules.

A 10% solution of pentastarch has approximately the same oncotic properties as albumin 5%. The pH is approximately 5.0 and the osmolality is about 326 mOsmol/L. Following intravenous infusion of pentastarch, the plasma volume is expanded approximately 1.5 times the actual volume given. This effect dissipates after 12 to 18 hours; 70% of a dose is eliminated within 24 hours, and about 80% to 90% of a dose is eliminated within one week. The remaining fraction is presumed to undergo slower elimination. The average half-life is 1.7 days. The small molecules (<50,000 daltons) are rapidly eliminated by glomerular filtration. The larger molecules are degraded in the plasma by amylase to a size that can be filtered by the kidneys. A modest residue of glucose results from this process. The largest molecules are stored temporarily within the reticuloedothelial cells of various body tissues, principally the liver and spleen, until they are degraded by amylase and eliminated in the urine.

USES. Pentastarch is used as an adjunct in leukapheresis to improve the harvesting and increase the yield of leukocytes by centrifugal means. It also is being tested clinically to expand plasma volume in the treatment of patients with hypovolemia caused by shock from severe sepsis and systemic hypoperfusion (Rackow et al, 1989). Preliminary results suggest that it is equivalent to albumin for fluid resuscitation.

ADVERSE REACTIONS AND PRECAUTIONS. Hypersensitivity reactions of wheezing and urticaria have been reported with pentastarch; however, these effects are readily reversible upon discontinuation of infusion. Administration of an antihistamine facilitates reversal. Larger doses decrease the hematocrit level, dilute plasma proteins and coagulation factors, and interfere with platelet function. Thus, pentastarch is contraindicated in patients with severe bleeding disorders.

As with all plasma expanders, hypervolemia is a potential danger. Because pentastarch is excreted relatively slowly, primarily by the kidneys, elimination is delayed in patients with impaired renal function. Therefore, the agent is contraindicated in patients with severe congestive heart failure and renal failure with oliguria and anuria not due to hypovolemia.

Pentastarch has been shown to be embryocidal in rabbits and mice when given in amounts five times larger than the human dose; therefore, this agent should be used during pregnancy only if the potential benefits justify the potential risk to the fetus (FDA Pregnancy Category C). No data are available on the use of pentastarch in children or in breast-feeding women.

DOSAGE AND PREPARATIONS.

Intravenous Infusion: *Adults,* for leukapheresis in continuous flow centrifugation (CFC) procedures, pentastarch 250 to 700 ml, to which citrate anticoagulant has been added, is administered by aseptic addition to the input line of the centrifugation apparatus in a ratio of 1:8 to 1:13 to venous whole blood. The bottle containing pentastarch and citrate should be thoroughly agitated to assure effective anticoagulation of blood as it flows through the leukapheresis machine. For systemic hypoperfusion or impending shock due to severe sepsis (investigational use), 250 ml has been administered every 15 minutes until either the wedge pressure is ≥15 mmHg or a maximum of 2 L has been given.

Pentaspan (DuPont-Merck). Solution 10% in 0.9% sodium chloride injection in 500 ml containers.

HEMOGLOBIN SUBSTITUTE

INTRAVASCULAR PERFLUOROCHEMICAL EMULSION

[Fluosol]

ACTIONS AND USES. Fluosol is a stable aqueous emulsion of perfluorodecalin (14%, w/v) and perfluorotri-n-propylamine (6%, w/v) combined with various emulsifiers, nonionic surfactants, electrolytes, and dextrose. Oxygenation of Fluosol by bubbling 95% O_2/5% CO_2 for at least 15 minutes yields an oxygen partial pressure higher than 600 mmHg and an oxygen content of >6 vol%. In contrast, bubble oxygenation of electrolyte solutions such as Ringer's lactate results in oxygen partial pressures of approximately 450 mmHg and an oxygen content <2 vol%.

Fluosol is indicated for intracoronary infusion to prevent ischemia during percutaneous transluminal coronary angioplasty (PTCA) in patients at high risk of ischemic complications. Balloon inflation during this procedure, which occludes the coronary artery, adversely affects myocardial function in the ischemic region. With balloon inflation times of 45 seconds or more, reduced contractility in the affected myocardial segments may decrease left ventricular ejection fraction. In many angioplasty procedures, inflation times of 90 to 120 seconds are not uncommon. Patients with decreased left ventricular function, a large area of myocardium in jeopardy, low baseline ejection fraction (<45%), recent myocardial infarction, or unstable or refractory angina requiring hospitalization are at particularly high risk of ischemic complications during angioplasty procedures.

Early clinical trials investigating transcatheter infusions of Fluosol during PTCA provided evidence that the oxygenated perfluorochemical emulsion delayed the onset and shortened the duration of angina (Anderson et al, 1985) and prevented left ventricular wall motion abnormalities (Cleman et al, 1986). Subsequent studies showed that distal coronary infusion of Fluosol also attenuated the decline in left ventricular ejection fraction that accompanies balloon inflations without infusion (Jaffe et al, 1988). These observations, made in patients with stable angina, single-vessel coronary artery disease, and normal baseline left ventricular function, were extended to patients with unstable angina or higher risk lesions (Cowley et al, 1990). Fluosol perfusion also reduced myocardial ischemia and maintained left ventricular systolic function in patients who were at higher risk. However, recent data suggest that Fluosol infusion during PTCA has no effect on left ventricular diastolic dysfunction during balloon inflation (Bell et al, 1990). Global diastolic dysfunction may be an earlier and more sensitive index of myocardial ischemia than decline in systolic function.

ADVERSE REACTIONS AND PRECAUTIONS. Use of Fluosol during PTCA has not been shown to reduce the incidence of adverse reactions that result from factors other than ischemia distal to the inflated balloon. These risks include coronary arterial dissection with occlusion, coronary artery spasm and vasospastic angina, myocardial infarction, distal intraluminal thrombus, arrhythmias, and ventricular fibrillation requiring cardioversion. Consequently, only individuals experienced in the use of PTCA should perform this procedure and institutional policy regarding emergency coronary artery bypass graft surgery should be followed.

Only angioplasty catheters with a central lumen of sufficient diameter to permit Fluosol infusion at adequate flow rates should be used. Proper positioning of the balloon catheter must be verified before starting the transcatheter infusion of Fluosol. During the PTCA procedure the patient must be continuously monitored by electrocardiography and other available measures to detect signs of ischemia.

In some patients, ischemia (angina and elevation of the ST segment on electrocardiograms, transient elevations of pulmonary artery wedge pressure) may occur during PTCA despite the Fluosol infusion. This may develop if the inflated balloon occludes a branch artery that is not perfused with Fluosol. In other patients, an ST segment elevation artifact may occur. Fluosol infusion into the *unoccluded* coronary artery of dogs resulted in ST segment elevations but did not decrease ejection fractions (Schaer et al, 1989). These observations suggest that ST segment elevations during Fluosol infusion occur by a mechanism other than myocardial ischemia.

Other potential adverse responses to Fluosol infusion during PTCA include ventricular tachycardia, ventricular fibrillation, bradycardia, chest discomfort, dyspnea, hypotension, increased respiratory rate, and coughing. In clinical trials, the incidence of one or more of these adverse reactions was only 0.7% when Fluosol had been warmed to 37° C. However, arrhythmias were observed in 1.4% of patients when Fluosol was infused at ambient temperature. Thus, this perfluorochemical should be warmed to 37° C before administration.

Mild hypersensitivity reactions (eg, mild pruritus, mild chills, urticaria, nausea, vomiting, mild back pain) were observed in about 1.2% of the patients during clinical trials. Therefore, it is recommended that a test dose of 0.5 ml be administered intravenously and that the patient be observed for at least ten minutes before the transcatheter infusion is started. Patients who react to the test dose can be given an intravenous antihistamine and/or corticosteroid to control the hypersensitivity and alternative therapeutic procedures (angioplasty without perfusion or bypass graft surgery) should be employed.

Transcatheter infusion of Fluosol is contraindicated in patients who have additional stenoses downstream from the lesion. It is also recommended that Fluosol be given no more than once in a six-month period because of concern, based on animal studies, that frequent doses may cause toxic reactions.

Centrifugation of blood samples from patients who received large volumes of Fluosol yields three separated phases: a perfluorochemical phase at the bottom, red blood cells in the middle, and the plasma phase at the top. Estimation of the volume percent for the bottom layer yields the fluorocrit, a measure of the perfluorochemical concentration in the blood. Results of laboratory tests (radioimmunoassays, spectrophotometry-based assays) may be altered by high fluorocrits. Transcatheter infusion during PTCA does not usually produce high fluorocrit values and often may not yield a measurable third (perfluorochemical) phase after centrifugation. However, the ability of perfluorochemicals to dissolve and retain lipid-soluble anesthetics may extend the latter's duration of action during PTCA procedures.

Clinical and animal studies using perfluorochemical emulsions for transfusions reveal some additional adverse effects (Lowe, 1988 B; Vercellotti and Hammerschmidt, 1988). These include morphologic alterations (appearance of foamy vesicles) and reduced clearance by cells of the reticuloendothelial system, interference with immune system function, and prolonged coagulation times and other hematologic disturbances. Some of these responses were attributed to impurities in the perfluorochemicals or to the surfactants used to prepare the emulsion; others were thought to result from the high concentrations of oxygen required when Fluosol is used for transfusions. Nevertheless, it seems unlikely that the amounts of Fluosol infused during PTCA would cause similar adverse responses.

In animal studies, Fluosol infusion (at about three times the human dose) into either male or female rats prior to mating had no effect on fertility, fetal development, or growth of the offspring. No mutagenic effects could be demonstrated by in vitro assays. Fluosol is classified in FDA Pregnancy Category B, although no adequate and well-controlled studies have been carried out in pregnant women. Neither are any data available on the possible effects of Fluosol on either the mother or the neonate when this preparation is used during labor and delivery. The perfluorodecalin component of Fluosol has been detected in breast milk one day after intravenous infusion, although no perfluorotri-n-propylamine was found. Thus, nursing mothers should not breast feed after administration of Fluosol.

PHARMACOKINETICS. Perfluorochemicals are eliminated primarily by expiration through the lungs. Both perfluorodecalin and perfluorotri-n-propylamine are taken up by reticuloendothelial cells in the liver, spleen, and bone marrow. Despite their lipophilicity, perfluorochemicals were not detected in brain tissue and there is no evidence to suggest that perfluorochemicals are metabolized in vivo.

The half-lives of perfluorochemicals in blood and tissues varies with the dose administered. In early studies in which Fluosol was used for transfusions in a dose of 10 to 20 ml/kg, the circulatory half-life was about eight hours; about 4% to 6% was retained in the liver and 1% to 2% was retained in the spleen four days after transfusion. Trace amounts remained for as long as 80 days. At the doses used for PTCA (3 to 5 ml/kg), half-lives and tissue retention have not yet been determined.

The other major components of the emulsion are cleared by different mechanisms from those involved in perfluorochemical clearance. The poloxamer 188 surfactant is eliminated by renal clearance and is not metabolized. The egg-yolk phospholipids are metabolized as dietary nutrients. Glycerin is metabolized to carbon dioxide and glycogen or is used for synthesis and storage of fats.

DOSAGE AND PREPARATIONS. Fluosol is supplied as 400 ml of frozen emulsion in 500-ml bags, together with 30 ml of a sodium bicarbonate/potassium chloride solution (solution 1) and 70 ml of a dextrose/electrolyte solution (solution 2). The latter two solutions are stored at room temperature and mixed with the thawed perfluorochemical emulsion immediately before use. The reconstituted emulsion should be warmed to 37° C and oxygenated to >600 mmHg partial pressure of O_2 by bubbling 95% O_2/5% CO_2 for at least 15 minutes. Use of 100% O_2 may alter the pH of the emulsion and therefore should be avoided.

Intracoronary: The emulsion should be loaded into an angiographic power injector with a warming jacket and administered during inflation at a rate of 60 to 90 ml/min through the central lumen of the angioplasty balloon catheter, depending on the size of the distal vessel. However, if the catheter design prohibits a flow rate of 60 ml/min, infusion at a rate of 40 to 60 ml/min may be used. The reduced flow rate was tolerated in clinical trials and allowed balloon inflation times up to five minutes. If the clinician judges that a satisfactory clinical result cannot be obtained with the guidewire in place, it may be withdrawn. Unused emulsion should be discarded. Total infusion volumes greater than 500 ml have not been administered. Fluosol should not be filtered before administration, since the stability of emulsion may be adversely affected.

Fluosol (Alpha Therapeutic). Single-use kits with 400 ml of emulsion in a flexible plastic bag, two glass vials containing 30 ml of solution 1 and 70 ml of solution 2, and disposable accessories for aseptic oxygenation of the reconstituted emulsion. The emulsion should be stored between −5° and −30° C, and the other solutions and accessories should be stored as liquids between 1° and 30° C.

Cited References

Circular of Information for the Use of Human Blood and Blood Components, pamphlet. American Red Cross, revised, 1989.

Update: *Yersinia enterocolitica* bacteremia and endotoxin shock associated with red blood cell transfusions—United States, 1991. *MMWR* 40:176-178, 1991.

Anderson KC, Weinstein HJ: Transfusion-associated graft-versus-host disease. *N Engl J Med* 323:315-321, 1990.

Anderson HV, et al: Distal coronary artery perfusion during percutaneous transluminal coronary angioplasty. *Am Heart J* 110:720-726, 1985.

Barbara JAJ, Contreras M: Infectious complications of blood transfusion: Viruses. *Br Med J* 300:450-453, 1990.

Barker LF, Dodd RY: Viral hepatitis, acquired immunodeficiency syndrome, and other infections transmitted by transfusion, in Petz LD, Swisher SN (eds): *Clinical Practice of Transfusion Medicine,* ed 2. New York, Churchill Livingstone, 1989, 667-712.

Bell MR, et al: Does intracoronary infusion of Fluosol-DA 20% prevent left ventricular diastolic dysfunction during coronary balloon angioplasty? *J Am Coll Cardiol* 16:959-966, 1990.

Beutler E: Erythrocyte metabolism and its relation to the liquid preservation of blood, in Petz LD, Swisher SN (eds): *Clinical Practice of Transfusion Medicine,* ed 2. New York, Churchill Livingstone, 1989, 271-296.

Blumberg N, Heal JM: Transfusion and host defenses against cancer recurrence and infection. *Transfusion* 29:236-245, 1989.

Brecher ME, Taswell HF: Paroxysmal nocturnal hemoglobinuria and the transfusion of washed red cells: A myth revisited. *Transfusion* 29:681-685, 1989.

Brunson ME, Alexander JW: Mechanisms of transfusion-induced immunosuppression. *Transfusion* 30:651-658, 1990.

Calhoun L: Blood product preparation and administration, in Petz LD, Swisher SN (eds): *Clinical Practice of Transfusion Medicine,* ed 2. New York, Churchill Livingstone, 1989, 239-270.

Carr R, et al: Transfusion of ABO-mismatched platelets leads to early platelet refractoriness. *Br J Haematol* 75:408-413, 1990.

Chambers LA, et al: Directed-donor programs may adversely affect autologous donor participation. *Transfusion* 30:246-248, 1990.

Chang TMS, Geyer RP (eds): *Blood Substitutes.* New York, Marcel Dekker, 1988.

Ciavarella D, et al: Clotting factor levels and the risk of diffuse microvascular bleeding in the massively transfused patient. *Br J Haematol* 67:365-368, 1987.

Cleman M, et al: Prevention of ischemia during percutaneous transluminal coronary angioplasty by transcatheter infusion of oxygenated Fluosol DA 20%. *Circulation* 74:555-562, 1986.

Collins ML, Churchill LR: The case against directed donations. *Transfus Sci* 10:139-145, 1989.

Contreras M, Mollison PL: Immunological complications of transfusion. *Br Med J* 300:173-176, 1990.

Cowley J, et al: Perfluorochemical perfusion during coronary angioplasty in unstable and high-risk patients. *Circulation* 81 (suppl IV):IV-27-IV-34, 1990.

Cumming PD, et al: Exposure of patients to human immunodeficiency virus through the transfusion of blood components that test antibody-negative. *N Engl J Med* 321:941-946, 1989.

Davey RJ, et al: Preparation of white cell-depleted red cells for 42-day storage using an integral in-line filter. *Transfusion* 29:496-499, 1989.

Deeg HJ: Transfusions with a tan: Prevention of allosensitization by ultraviolet irradiation. *Transfusion* 29:450-455, 1989.

DePalma L, et al: Utilization patterns of frozen autologous red blood cells: Experience in a referral center and a community hospital. *Arch Pathol Lab Med* 114:516-518, 1990.

Dutcher JP: The potential benefit of granulocyte transfusion therapy. *Cancer Invest* 7:457-462, 1989.

Ernst E, et al: Placebo-controlled, double-blind study of haemodilution in peripheral arterial disease. *Lancet* 1:1449-1451, 1987.

Ernst E, et al: A double-blind trial of Dextran-haemodilution *vs.* placebo in claudicants. *J Intern Med* 227:19-24, 1990.

Faithfull NS: Potential applications of perfluorochemical emulsions in medicine and research, in Lowe KC (ed): *Blood Substitutes: Preparation, Physiology and Medical Applications.* Chichester, England, Ellis Horwood, 1988, 130-148.

Goldfinger D: Acute hemolytic transfusion reactions: A fresh look at pathogenesis and considerations regarding therapy. *Transfusion* 17:85-98, (March-April) 1977.

Goldfinger D: Directed blood donations: Pro. *Transfusion* 29:70-74, 1989.

Goodnough LT, et al: Increased preoperative collection of autologous blood with recombinant human erythropoietin therapy. *N Engl J Med* 321:1163-1168, 1989.

Gould SA, et al: Fluosol-DA as a red-cell substitute in acute anemia. *N Engl J Med* 314:1653-1656, 1986.

Gould SA, et al: The efficacy of polymerized pyridoxylated hemoglobin solution as an O_2 carrier. *Ann Surg* 211:394-398, 1990.

Grossman BJ, Grindon AJ: Autologous blood: A greater risk for the homologous recipient. *Transfus Sci* 10:125-130, 1989.

Heyman MR, Schiffer CA: Platelet transfusion therapy for the cancer patient. *Semin Oncol* 17:198-209, 1990.

Hillyer CD, et al: The risk of cytomegalovirus infection in solid organ and bone marrow transplant recipients: Transfusion of blood products. *Transfusion* 30:659-666, 1990.

Holland PV: The diagnosis and management of transfusion reactions and other adverse effects of transfusion, in Petz LD, Swisher SN (eds): *Clinical Practice of Transfusion Medicine,* ed 2. New York, Churchill Livingstone, 1989, 713-736.

Holland PV (ed): *Standards for Blood Banks and Transfusion Services,* ed 14. Arlington, Va, American Association of Blood Banks, 1991.

Jaffe CC, et al: Preservation of left ventricular ejection fraction during percutaneous transluminal coronary angioplasty by distal transcatheter coronary perfusion of oxygenated Fluosol DA 20%. *Am Heart J* 115:1156-1164, 1988.

Kahn RA, et al: Alternate sources and substitutes for therapeutic blood components. *Blood* 66:1-12, 1985.

Keipert PE, et al: Functional properties of a new crosslinked hemoglobin designed for use as a red cell substitute. *Transfusion* 29:768-773, 1989.

Kent KM, et al: Reduction of myocardial ischemia during percutaneous transluminal coronary angioplasty with oxygenated Fluosol. *Am J Cardiol* 66:279-284, 1990.

Kiesewetter H, et al: Haemodilution with medium molecular weight hydroxyethyl starch in patients with peripheral arterial occlusive disease stage IIb. *J Intern Med* 227:107-114, 1990.

Kruskall MS: Controversies in transfusion medicine: The safety and utility of autologous donations by pregnant patients: Pro. *Transfusion* 30:168-171, 1990.

Lee EJ, Schiffer CA: ABO compatibility can influence the results of platelet transfusion: Results of a randomized trial. *Transfusion* 29:384-389, 1989.

Ley SJ, et al: Crystalloid versus colloid fluid therapy after cardiac surgery. *Heart Lung* 19:31-40, 1990.

Liewald F, et al: Influence of blood transfusions on tumor recurrence and survival rate in colorectal carcinoma. *Eur J Cancer* 26:327-335, 1990.

Ljungström KG, et al: Hapten inhibition and dextran anaphylaxis. *Anaesthesia* 43:729-732, 1988.

Lowe KC (ed): *Blood Substitutes: Preparation, Physiology and Medical Applications*. Chichester, England, Ellis Horwood, 1988 A.

Lowe KC: Biological assessment of perfluorochemical emulsions, in Lowe KC (ed): *Blood Substitutes: Preparation, Physiology and Medical Applications.* Chichester, England, Ellis Horwood, 1988 B, 149-172.

Manno CS, et al: Comparison of the hemostatic effects of fresh whole blood, stored whole blood, and components after open heart surgery in children. *Blood* 77:930-936, 1991.

McCullough J: Granulocyte transfusion, in Petz LD, Swisher SN (eds): *Clinical Practice of Transfusion Medicine*, ed 2. New York, Churchill Livingstone, 1989, 469-484.

McFarland JG, et al: Factors influencing the transfusion response to HLA-selected apheresis donor platelets in patients refractory to random platelet concentrates. *Br J Haematol* 73:380-386, 1989.

Menitove JE: Current risk of transfusion-associated human immunodeficiency virus infection. *Arch Pathol Lab Med* 114:330-334, 1990.

Mintz PD, et al: Erythropoietin and preoperative blood donation, correspondence. *N Engl J Med* 322:1157-1158, 1990.

Mollison PL, et al: *Blood Transfusion in Clinical Medicine,* ed 8. Palo Alto, Calif, Blackwell Scientific, 1987, 134-141.

Moriguchi S, et al: Lack of relationship between perioperative blood transfusion and survival time after curative resection for gastric cancer. *Cancer* 66:2331-2335, 1990.

Moss GS, et al: Results of the first clinical trial with a polymerized hemoglobin solution. Clinical Congress, American College of Surgeons, October 23, 1988.

Murphy S: Guidelines for platelet transfusion. *JAMA* 259:2453-2454, 1988.

Murphy S: Preservation and clinical use of platelets, in Williams WJ, et al (eds): *Hematology*, ed 4. New York, McGraw-Hill, 1990, 1654-1659.

Murray DJ, et al: Coagulation changes during packed red cell replacement of major blood loss. *Anesthesiology* 63:839-845, 1988.

National Blood Resource Education Program Expert Panel: The use of autologous blood. *JAMA* 263:414-417, 1990.

National Institutes of Health Consensus Conference: Fresh-frozen plasma: Indications and risks. *JAMA* 253:551-553, 1985.

National Institutes of Health: National consensus conference on platelet transfusion therapy. *JAMA* 257:1777-1780, 1987.

National Institutes of Health: Perioperative red blood cell transfusion. *JAMA* 260:2700-2703, 1988.

Nusbacher J: Preservation and clinical use of leukocytes, in Williams WJ, et al (eds): *Hematology*, ed 4. New York, McGraw-Hill, 1990, 1647-1653.

Page PL: Controversies in transfusion medicine: Directed blood donations: Con. *Transfusion* 29:65-70, 1989.

Perkins HA: Transfusion-induced immunologic unresponsiveness. *Transfus Med Rev* 2:196-203, 1988.

Perkins HA: Autologous transfusions. *Adv Intern Med* 35:221-233, 1990.

Petricciani JC, Epstein JS: Effects of the AIDS epidemic on the safety of the nation's blood supply. *Public Health Rep* 103:236-241, 1988.

Petz LD: Bone marrow transplantation, in Petz LD, Swisher SN (eds): *Clinical Practice of Transfusion Medicine*, ed 2. New York, Churchill Livingstone, 1989, 485-510.

Petz LD, Swisher SN (eds): *Clinical Practice of Transfusion Medicine*, ed 2. New York, Churchill Livingstone, 1989.

Popovsky MA, Kruskall MS: Safety of autologous blood for homologous transfusion. *Transfus Sci* 10:117-123, 1989.

Rackow EC, et al: Effects of pentastarch and albumin infusion on cardiorespiratory function and coagulation in patients with severe sepsis and systemic hypoperfusion. *Crit Care Med* 17:394-398, 1989.

Reed RL II, et al: Prophylactic platelet administration during massive transfusion: A prospective, randomized, double-blind clinical study. *Ann Surg* 203:40-48, 1986.

Ross WB, Yap PL: Blood transfusion and organ transplantation. *Blood Rev* 4:252-258, 1990.

Rudolph R, Boyd CR: Massive transfusion: Complications and their management. *South Med J* 83:1065-1070, 1990.

Savage COS, et al: Therapeutic applications of plasma exchange. *Br J Hosp Med* 40:272-279, 1988.

Sayers MH: Controversies in transfusion medicine: Autologous blood donation in pregnancy: Con. *Transfusion* 30:172-174, 1990.

Schaer GL, et al: Dissociation of ST segment elevation and regional wall motion with open-artery, intracoronary Fluosol. *Am Heart J* 118:679-685, 1989.

Schiffer CA: Prevention of alloimmunization against platelets, editorial. *Blood* 77:1-4, 1991.

Shumak K, Nusbacher J: Therapeutic apheresis, in Petz LD, Swisher SN (eds): *Clinical Practice of Transfusion Medicine*, ed 2. New York, Churchill Livingstone, 1989, 635-648.

Silvergleid AJ: Preoperative autologous donation: What have we learned? Editorial. *Transfusion* 31:99-101, 1991.

Slichter SJ: Platelet transfusion therapy. *Hematol Oncol Clin North Am* 4:291-311, 1990.

Snyder EL (ed): *Blood Transfusion Therapy: A Physician's Handbook,* ed 3. Washington, DC, American Association of Blood Banks, 1989 A.

Snyder EL: Clinical use of white cell-poor blood components, editorial. *Transfusion* 29:568-571, 1989 B.

Starky JM, et al: Markers for transfusion-transmitted disease in different groups of blood donors. *JAMA* 262:3452-3454, 1989.

Stehling L: Acute normovolemic hemodilution during surgery. *Transfus Sci* 10:101-106, 1989.

Strauss RG: Granulocyte transfusions: Uses, abuses and indications, in Kolins J, McCarthy LJ (eds): *Contemporary Transfusion Practice.* Arlington, Va, American Association of Blood Banks, 1987.

Strauss RG, et al: Directed and limited-exposure blood donations for infants and children. *Transfusion* 30:68-72, 1990.

Swisher SN, Petz LD: Plasma products and blood substitutes, in Petz LD, Swisher SN (eds): *Clinical Practice of Transfusion Medicine,* ed 2. New York, Churchill Livingstone, 1989, 649-666.

Tipple MA, et al: Sepsis associated with transfusion of red cells contaminated with *Yersinia enterocolitica*. *Transfusion* 30:207-213, 1990.

Tomasulo PA, Petz LD: Platelet transfusions, in Petz LD, Swisher SN (eds): *Clinical Practice of Transfusion Medicine*, ed 2. New York, Churchill Livingstone, 1989, 427-468.

van Marwijk Kooy M, et al: Use of leukocyte-depleted platelet concentrates for the prevention of refractoriness and primary HLA alloimmunization: A prospective, randomized trial. *Blood* 77:201-205, 1991.

Vercellotti GM, Hammerschmidt DE: Human studies involving perfluorochemical emulsions, in Lowe KC (ed): *Blood Substitutes: Preparation, Physiology and Medical Applications.* Chichester, England, Ellis Horwood, 1988, 173-183.

Walker R, et al: *The Technical Manual*, ed 10. Arlington, Va, American Association of Blood Banks, 1990.

Weiden PL, et al: Perioperative blood tranfusion does not increase the risk of colorectal cancer recurrence. *Cancer* 60:870-874, 1987.

Yalon V, Perkins HA: The arguments for directed donations. *Transfus Sci* 10:131-137, 1989.

Drugs Affecting Calcium Metabolism 100

Calcium is the most abundant mineral in the body. Its metabolic role has priority over structural function, and maintenance of calcium ion homeostasis will occur, if necessary, at the expense of bone. Calcium homeostasis is determined by the amount of calcium ingested in the diet, the net amount of dietary calcium absorbed into the blood stream by the gut (total amount absorbed minus the amount excreted in feces), the net uptake and release of calcium by bone, and the amounts reabsorbed by the kidney and excreted in the urine (Charles, 1992; Forman and Lorenzo, 1991).

The amount of calcium absorbed is related to the quantity ingested; average net absorption is 15% to 20%, which is equivalent to the amount excreted in the urine in 24 hours by an adult, although as much as 50% may be absorbed when calcium intake is low. The small intestine is the main site of calcium absorption, although the entire bowel probably is capable of this function. The duodenum has the greatest active absorption capacity per unit length, but the majority of calcium is absorbed in the jejunum because of its greater total length.

Intestinal absorption of calcium is regulated primarily by the active metabolite of vitamin D_3, 1,25-dihydroxycholecalciferol (1,25-$(OH)_2D_3$). Vitamin D_3 is available from dietary sources and from the skin, where it is formed from 7-dehydrocholesterol by ultraviolet irradiation. Vitamin D_3 is converted in the liver and circulated in the blood as the less active form, 25-OHD_3, which is then converted to 1,25-$(OH)_2D_3$ in the kidney.

The absorption of calcium may be enhanced indirectly by hormones (eg, parathyroid hormone [PTH], growth hormone) that stimulate renal conversion of 25-OHD_3 to 1,25-$(OH)_2D_3$. Likewise, calcium absorption may be suppressed indirectly when renal conversion of 1,25-$(OH)_2D_3$ is inhibited (eg, excess of thyroid hormones and possibly calcitonin). Glucocorticoids may directly impair intestinal absorption of calcium. Absorbed calcium and phosphorus participate in the regulation of more complete calcium absorption through the effects of serum calcium on PTH secretion and of phosphate and PTH on the renal production of 1,25-$(OH)_2D_3$. Calcium is continuously lost into the intestinal lumen because of the secretion of digestive juice. Part of the calcium in the digestive juice is reabsorbed and the rest is excreted in the feces.

Calcium absorption declines with age; this is probably more pronounced in women than in men and may be caused by dietary vitamin D deficiency and a fall in endogenous production of vitamin D due to decline in the dermal production of 17-dehydrocholesterol and reduced exposure to the sun in the elderly. In addition, impairment of renal function with age reduces renal 1,25-$(OH)_2D_3$ production.

Almost all endogenous calcium is present in skeletal tissue (>98%) as part of the hydroxyapatite crystal that provides the structural integrity of the bones; 1% is in soft tissue and only 0.1% is in body fluids where it may be ionized, protein bound, or complexed with various ions (eg, phosphate, carbonate, citrate, sulfate). The ionized calcium in extracellular

TABLE 1.
DIRECT ACTIONS AND INDICATIONS FOR DRUGS USED TO TREAT DISORDERS OF CALCIUM METABOLISM

Drug	Actions: Calcium Excretion	Calcium Intestinal Absorption	Bone Formation	Bone Resorption	Indications for Use
Adrenal Corticosteroids	+	−	−		Certain types of hypercalcemia
Calcitonin	+		+ ?	−	Paget's disease, hypercalcemic states associated with high bone mineral loss, postmenopausal osteoporosis
Calcium Preparations		+			Hypocalcemia, osteoporosis
Estrogens				−	Postmenopausal osteoporosis
Etidronate			−*	−	Paget's disease, heterotopic ossification due to spinal cord injury or total hip replacement; hypercalcemia due to malignancy (parenteral)
Fluoride			+		Osteoporosis (investigational)
Furosemide	+				Hypercalcemia
Gallium nitrate			+ ?	−	Cancer-related hypercalcemia
Pamidronate			− ?	−	Cancer-related hypercalcemia
Phosphates	−		+	−	Hypophosphatemic rickets or osteomalacia, hypercalciuria, hypercalcemia
Plicamycin (mithramycin)				−	Severe hypercalcemia associated with carcinoma, Paget's disease
Thiazides	−				Hypercalciuria with renal calculi
Vitamin D Preparations		+	+		Vitamin D deficiency, hypoparathyroidism, osteomalacia, rickets

− *decreases*
+ *increases*
* *Not associated with cyclical etidronate in treatment of osteoporosis.*

fluid and serum is in constant equilibrium with the small fraction of skeletal calcium (4 to 6 g) that is available for rapid exchange. Only unbound, ionized calcium is physiologically active and is essential for maintenance of heart rhythm and myocardial contraction, functioning of nerves and muscles, blood coagulation, and other physiologic reactions.

The concentration of total calcium in serum is maintained within a narrow range (8.6 to 10.5 mg/dL). The normal ionized calcium levels are 4.4 to 5.4 mg/dL and are in equilibrium with the rest of the calcium, being mainly bound to albumin (0.8 mg calcium/g albumin). Acidosis increases and alkalosis decreases the fraction of calcium that is ionized. The serum calcium concentration usually is controlled by a negative feedback mechanism involving ionized serum calcium and PTH. A *fall* in ionized serum calcium stimulates secretion of PTH, which, in turn, promotes the renal tubular reabsorption of calcium, decreases the renal reabsorption of phosphate, and, if the decrement is large, increases osteoclastic mobilization of calcium from bone. In addition, PTH enhances the renal synthesis of 1,25-$(OH)_2D_3$; the latter is probably necessary for osteoclast formation. Synthesis of 1,25-$(OH)_2D_3$ also is stimulated by a decrease in the serum concentration of inorganic phosphate caused by the effects of PTH on renal phosphate excretion. A *rise* in the level of ionized serum calcium inhibits the release of PTH and, secondarily, the renal production of 1,25-$(OH)_2D_3$. In addition, calcium acts directly on the renal tubule to inhibit synthesis of 1,25-$(OH)_2D_3$. The effects are opposite those noted above.

Calcitonin is a calcium-regulating hormone that is secreted by the parafollicular cells of the thyroid. Its major actions are to inhibit bone resorption and renal tubular reabsorption of calcium, thus promoting the reduction in serum calcium. Although secretion of calcitonin is stimulated by increasing serum calcium levels, this hormone appears to have little, if any, effect on normal calcium homeostasis. In infants and children, enhanced secretion of calcitonin after feeding may modulate the tendency toward postabsorptive hypercalcemia.

Several adjustments in calcium metabolism occur during pregnancy. Increased secretion of PTH helps to balance the tendency toward lower maternal serum calcium concentration caused by expansion of extracellular fluid volume and the active transport of calcium from mother to fetus. Bone turnover in the mother is increased during the third trimester because of increased demand of mineralization of the fetal skeleton. The concentration of calcium in the fetus is high relative to that in the mother until parturition. The neonatal serum calcium level drops on delivery and becomes normal about two days after delivery (Pitkin, 1985). Since much more calcium is lost through the milk to the breast-feeding infant, bone turnover continues to be increased in lactating women (Cole et al, 1987).

The mechanism of action of certain drugs used in disorders of calcium metabolism and the indications for their use appear in Table 1.

HYPERCALCEMIA

DIAGNOSIS. Most patients with mild hypercalcemia are asymptomatic and usually are identified by routine blood chemistry screening. Diagnostic studies most often identify asymptomatic primary hyperparathyroidism as the etiology of mild hypercalcemia (Lafferty, 1991). The hyperparathyroidism usually (~80% of the time) is caused by a single adenoma, but it may be due to hyperplasia of all parathyroid glands or, in <1% of patients, a parathyroid carcinoma (see reviews by Parisien et al, 1990; Bilezikian, 1991; Melton, 1991; Salti et al, 1992). Guidelines for management of patients with asymptomatic primary hyperparathyroidism are available (Potts, 1990; Consensus Development Conference Panel, 1991; Bilezikian, 1991).

Less common disorders of hypercalcemia that must be considered and evaluated include sarcoidosis and other granulomatous diseases (eg, tuberculosis, fungal infections, berylliosis, leprosy), hypervitaminosis D, hyperthyroidism, milk-alkali syndrome, and thiazide therapy (Pont, 1989). Thiazides usually are associated with hypercalcemia only in patients with subclinical or overt hyperparathyroidism or other disorders associated with increased bone turnover. Hypercalcemia also can occur with renal osteodystrophy, particularly in dialysis patients. Less commonly, hypercalcemia may be associated with hypervitaminosis A, hyperthyroidism in children, acute adrenocortical insufficiency and abrupt cessation of glucocorticoid therapy, pheochromocytoma, AIDS (generally in those with AIDS-associated lymphoma), and immobilization. A familial syndrome of idiopathic hypercalcemia, an autosomal dominant disorder also known as familial hypocalciuric hypercalcemia, must be considered in the differential diagnosis as well (Kristiansen, 1992). (This disorder also has been termed familial benign hypercalcemia since not all patients are hypocalciuric.)

When symptoms occur as a result of mild hypercalcemia, they frequently include polyuria, nausea and vomiting, constipation, and neuropsychiatric disturbances. As severity increases, hypercalcemia also may affect the kidneys (eg, renal vasoconstriction, nephrocalcinosis, decreased concentrating ability), central nervous system (eg, depression, lethargy, confusion, weakness), gastrointestinal tract (eg, anorexia, peptic ulcer, pancreatitis), and cardiovascular system (eg, arrhythmias, ECG changes, hypertension). Abnormal deposition of calcium also may occur (eg, cornea, myocardium, kidney, conjunctiva, other soft tissues).

Life-threatening hypercalcemia is most often caused by neoplasms. Breast and non-small cell lung carcinomas are most commonly associated with cancer-related hypercalcemia, but this condition also occurs with a variety of other malignancies, whether or not bone metastases are present (Warrell, 1993; Pritchard and Burch, 1993). Certain tumors synthesize and secrete substances that stimulate bone resorption focally (in areas of skeletal metastasis) or systemically (in the absence of bone metastases). Although these substances may include "osteoclast-activating factors," prostaglandins of the E series, and transforming growth factors (Mundy, 1989, 1991), the parathyroid hormone-related peptide (PTHrP) is now believed to be the most common cancer-related hypercalcemic substance produced by solid tumors (Martin, 1990; Burtis et al, 1990; Kao et al, 1990; Grill et al, 1991; Warrell, 1993). Elevated levels of PTHrP are present in the serum of most patients with humoral hypercalcemia of malignancy. Furthermore, local production of PTHrP at sites of bone metastases has been demonstrated using immunohistochemistry (Southby et al, 1990; Powell et al, 1991). Thus, the classic mechanistic distinction between humoral and local osteolytic etiologies for hypercalcemia of malignancy appears to be invalid. PTH itself is suppressed in hypercalcemia caused by malignancy. Dysregulated production of 1,25-$(OH)_2D_3$, the active metabolite of vitamin D, is thought to be a major mechanism of hypercalcemia in patients with Hodgkin's disease or non-Hodgkin's lymphomas (Seymour and Gagel, 1993) and in granulomatous diseases (Pont, 1989).

THERAPY. The primary objective of treatment is to establish control of the underlying disease (Bilezikian, 1992). Conservative therapy such as hydration may be adequate in asymptomatic patients with mild hypercalcemia, but more aggressive intervention almost always is indicated when total serum calcium exceeds 12 mg/dL. Levels >15 mg/dL require immediate intensive treatment. There is no consistent correlation between the total serum calcium concentration and the severity of symptoms; some symptoms (eg, mental changes) may occur in older individuals with mild hypercalcemia. In patients with symptomatic hypercalcemia caused by hyperparathyroidism, surgical removal of the adenoma or of all but one-half of one gland in the case of parathyroid hyperplasia is commonly utilized (Bilezikian, 1991, 1992; Salti et al, 1992).

The drugs used to treat hypercalcemia reduce serum calcium levels (1) by increasing the renal excretion of calcium (isotonic saline with or without loop diuretics), (2) by inhibiting bone resorption (plicamycin [Mithracin]; calcitonin [Calcimar, Cibacalcin, Miacalcin]; phosphates; corticosteroids; intravenous bisphosphonates such as etidronate [Didronel] and pamidronate [Aredia]; and gallium nitrate [Ganite]), (3) by reducing gastrointestinal absorption of calcium (phosphates, corticosteroids, cellulose phosphate), or (4) by promoting calcium uptake by bone and other tissues (phosphates). Therapy depends on the etiology and severity of hypercalcemia, the status of renal function, and the response to prior therapy (Bilezikian, 1992). Blood calcium levels should be measured frequently so that treatment can be modified as needed. The treatment of hypercalcemia of malignancy has been reviewed (Bilezikian, 1992; Warrell, 1993; Nussbaum, 1993; Hall and Burns Schaiff, 1993).

Symptomatic patients usually are dehydrated because of reduced fluid intake, vomiting, and polyuria; therefore, *hydration* with isotonic saline is the first step in treatment. Recommended regimens include 2.5 to 4 L daily (Bilezikian, 1992) or 300 to 500 ml/hr for the first three to four hours (Warrell, 1993). The fluid deficit may be as much as 5 to 10 L, and more aggressive measures to increase hydration may be necessary to compensate for ongoing losses. Both the volume and the rate of administration must be adjusted based on the severity of hypercalcemia, the extent of dehydration, and the capacity of the patient's renal and circulatory systems to handle the increased plasma volume. The diet may include moderate amounts of calcium-containing foods. The value of further restriction of calcium consumption (other than elimination of dietary supplements) is doubtful. Other electrolyte deficits (eg, potassium, magnesium) also should be corrected. Ambulation is encouraged to reduce bone resorption resulting from immobility. The saline infusion may be continued (when volume overload is not a problem) to increase sodium excretion and maintain volume expansion, since both factors enhance a calcium diuresis.

Only after expansion of plasma volume has been accomplished may a loop diuretic (furosemide [Lasix] or ethacrynic acid [Edecrin]) be given (with monitoring to prevent electrolyte imbalance and hypovolemia) in therapeutic doses (eg, furosemide 10 to 20 mg intravenously at 6- to 12-hour intervals) as needed to prevent volume overload. (Thiazides should not be used for this purpose because they increase the tubular reabsorption of calcium.) Care should be taken not to overuse diuresis in these patients, for this may worsen hypercalcemia. "Standing orders" for diuretic therapy are inappropriate because of the risk of worsening dehydration. Some patients may tolerate the necessary amount of fluid without requiring a diuretic. It should be noted that these measures do not reduce the excessive mobilization of calcium from bone, and they rarely are adequate to correct symptomatic hypercalcemia completely.

Patients with severe renal insufficiency or life-threatening hypercalcemia (generally, serum calcium concentration >18 mg/dL) may require *hemodialysis or peritoneal dialysis* (using calcium-free or low-calcium dialysis fluids) to remove large amounts of calcium. Other methods to promote calciuresis are obsolete. Infusions of sodium sulfate or citrate may increase calciuresis, but they have no significant advantage over sodium chloride and may precipitate acute renal failure due to the affinity of ionized calcium for the sulfate and citrate anions.

Calcitonin may be useful in many forms of acute, severe hypercalcemia and is generally devoid of serious side effects. This drug both inhibits bone resorption due to osteoclast activity and increases excretion of calcium. With the exception of intravenous phosphate, calcitonin has the most rapid onset of action among the drugs used for therapy of hypercalcemia. Transient reductions (1 to 3 mg/dL) in the serum calcium concentration frequently can be achieved rapidly. However, the concentrations often rebound once the nadir is achieved after the first 24 to 48 hours of therapy, despite continued administration of calcitonin. Loss of efficacy may be due to an escape phenomenon secondary to the down-regulation of calcitonin receptors or to other as yet unidentified factors. Responsiveness may be maintained or possibly enhanced in some patients by providing a drug-free interval (eg, administration five days out of seven) or by administering glucocorticoids (eg, prednisone 30 mg/day) concomitantly. Lack of effectiveness may reflect inadequate doses.

Glucocorticoids may be effective in hypercalcemia associated with sarcoidosis or other granulomatous diseases and hypervitaminosis D (Adams, 1989), but they are not useful for hypercalcemia associated with hyperparathyroidism. This specificity probably is a consequence of their actions to reduce serum concentrations of 1,25-$(OH)_2D_3$ to values within or below the normal range. Glucocorticoids also may reduce serum calcium concentrations in patients with hypercalcemia associated with hematologic tumors (eg, lymphoma, multiple myeloma). This probably results from their antitumor effects on malignant lymphoid cells rather than from direct hypocalcemic effects (Bilezikian, 1992; Warrell 1993). However, most hypercalcemic patients with solid tumors do not respond to glucocorticoid therapy (Bilezikian, 1992), and their routine use in these patients is not recommended (Warrell, 1993). Since the prolonged use of moderate doses of glucocorticoids may produce serious adverse effects, these drugs should be administered only for short periods when other therapy is inadequate.

Plicamycin (mithramycin), a cytotoxic agent, kills osteoclasts and thus reduces elevated serum calcium concentrations. This drug usually is not administered for initial therapy but may be particularly useful in recurrent or resistant hypercalcemia associated with advanced neoplastic disease. Serum calcium concentrations begin to decline by 12 hours after this drug's administration in most responsive patients and usually reach a nadir in 48 to 72 hours (Bilezikian, 1992). Although a single dose may achieve normocalcemia in some patients, administration can be repeated at intervals of 24 to 48 hours when necessary. After successful therapy, normocalcemia may last from several days to weeks.

Plicamycin may cause hemorrhagic complications due to platelet deficiency. Because this effect is dose related and is cumulative, the usefulness of this drug is limited when it is given with many forms of primary antineoplastic chemotherapy. However, transient or permanent renal impairment is rare except when prolonged therapy is required. The serum calcium level must be measured frequently during therapy, and the patient should be monitored for hematologic and renal complications before administering the next dose. Caution is advised when using plicamycin in patients with hypokalemia. When combined with hypercalcemia, hypokalemia may increase cardiac automaticity and predispose to ventricular fibrillation. Although the hypocalcemic effect of plicamycin may be delayed for 24 to 48 hours, serum potassium falls after the first hour and remains low (Avioli, 1982). The use of plicamycin has declined recently as agents with equal efficacy but reduced toxicity (eg, bisphosphonates, gallium nitrate) have become available.

The *bisphosphonates* are analogues of pyrophosphate that resist enzymatic degradation by phosphatases because the labile phosphorus-oxygen-phosphorus bond system present in the latter is replaced by a more stable phosphorus-carbon-phosphorus moiety (Bilezikian, 1992; Warrell, 1993). The bisphosphonates inhibit osteoclast function by binding avidly to hydroxyapatite in bone resulting in its decreased susceptibility to resorptive activity. They also decrease the viability of osteoclasts. Etidronate and pamidronate are the only bisphosphonates available in the United States at present; clodronate and alendronate are available in some European countries.

Intravenous *etidronate* is effective and safe for the treatment of mild to moderate hypercalcemia due to malignancy. However, its use should be limited to patients with serum creatinine <5 mg/dL, and it should be infused slowly over a period of two to four hours. Etidronate should only be administered after the patient has been rehydrated with intravenous saline and adequate urinary output has been established. Recommended doses will significantly reduce albumin-adjusted calcium levels in 25% to 40% of patients (Singer et al, 1991; Warrell et al, 1991; Gucalp et al, 1992). The usual regimen is 5 to 7.5 mg/kg infused once daily for three to five days. The calcium concentration begins to decline within 24 to 48 hours in responding patients, and reaches a nadir within four to seven days. If serum calcium levels fall to near or within the normal range before three days of therapy are completed, the drug should be withdrawn (Shane, 1993).

The duration of normocalcemia varies after discontinuing the drug in responsive patients and depends on the individual's rate of bone resorption. Although some investigators have used oral etidronate for maintenance in an attempt to prevent recurrent hypercalcemia after an initial response, there are no convincing data to demonstrate the efficacy of this approach (Bilezikian, 1992). In addition, long-term administration of etidronate can cause osteomalacia, although this may be of minor importance in patients with widely disseminated metastases who have a poor long-term prognosis.

Pamidronate, a newer bisphosphonate, has become the therapy of choice for many patients with moderate to severe hypercalcemia of malignancy. As with etidronate, adequate hydration and urine output must be established before administration of pamidronate is begun. In addition, its safety has not been established in patients with renal impairment (serum creatinine >5 mg/dL).

The response to pamidronate is relatively independent of tumor type. However, tumors that elaborate PTHrP (eg, squamous carcinomas) may be less responsive (Beex et al, 1989; Thiébaud et al, 1990 A; Fitton and McTavish, 1991). Diminished efficacy has been noted after repeated administration of pamidronate for treatment of hypercalcemic relapses (Thiébaud et al, 1990 A).

The usual dosage is 60 to 90 mg given as a single 24-hour continuous intravenous infusion. The rate of response to single infusions of pamidronate 30 to 90 mg may be dose related (Nussbaum et al, 1993). Many investigators have shortened the duration of infusion to as little as two to four hours without loss of efficacy (Coleman and Rubens, 1989; Dodwell et al, 1990; Millward et al, 1990; Sawyer et al, 1990), but the occurrence of complications at the site of infusion (eg, erythema, irritation, phlebitis) may increase slightly with shorter infusions, particularly if doses >60 mg are given in <4 hours. Although regimens employing multiple infusions (eg, 30 to 60 mg daily for three days) are effective (Shane, 1993), there is little advantage in administering more than one large infusion to patients with hypercalcemia of malignancy (Yates et al, 1987; Morton et al, 1988 A; Ralston et al, 1988; Body et al, 1989; Dodwell et al, 1990). Single intravenous infusions of pamidronate 30 or 60 mg have resulted in more rapid onset of hypocalcemic action, greater reduction in serum calcium concentration by day 6, and more prolonged normocalcemic remission than three consecutive daily intravenous infusions of etidronate (7.5 mg/kg/day) (Ralston et al, 1989 A; Ritch et al, 1990; Gucalp et al, 1992).

Pamidronate is approximately 100 times more potent than etidronate in inhibiting bone resorption (Fleisch, 1991). Approximately twice as many patients achieved normocalcemia with either 30 or 60 mg of pamidronate than with etidronate. Pamidronate also has been more effective than either plicamycin or prednisolone plus calcitonin (Ralston et al, 1985; Thuerlimann et al, 1989). Enhanced effectiveness has been achieved when a single infusion of pamidronate (45 to 60 mg) was combined with calcitonin suppositories (900 units/day for three days) (Thiébaud et al, 1990 B). A randomized trial comparing pamidronate with gallium nitrate in patients with hypercalcemia of malignancy is ongoing.

Pamidronate and other bisphosphonates also may have important applications in the treatment of skeletal metastases. Intravenous pamidronate monotherapy (30 to 60 mg once weekly or biweekly or 60 to 90 mg once monthly) reduces urinary calcium and hydroxyproline excretion in patients with osteolytic bone metastases accompanying advanced breast cancer (Coleman et al, 1988; Morton et al, 1988 B; Thiébaud et al, 1991). In a number of studies, reduction of bone pain and (possibly) reduced incidence of new pathologic fractures and hypercalcemia have been reported in such patients and in those with skeletal metastases from prostate cancer (van Holten-Verzantvoort et al, 1987; Coleman et al, 1988; Morton et al, 1988 B; Pelger et al, 1989; Lipton, 1990; Thiébaud et al, 1991). Evidence of bone healing and stabilization of previously progressive osteolytic bone lesions also were observed in some of the patients.

Clodronate was one of the first bisphosphonates to be used as therapy for the hypercalcemia of malignancy, but it is available at present only in Europe (Bilezikian, 1992). It has been administered in doses of 4 to 6 mg/kg as single infusions of two to nine hours' duration and as multiple daily infusions of two to five hours' duration for three to five days. Oral dosage forms of clodronate also are used by some European physicians to maintain normocalcemia after responses to intravenous therapy. Data from a randomized trial on patients receiving melphalan and prednisolone for multiple myeloma suggest that oral clodronate also may delay the progression of osteolytic bone lesions, reduce the degree of hypercalcemia and hypercalciuria, and decrease bone pain (Lahtinen et al, 1992).

Gallium nitrate is another potent inhibitor of bone resorption with demonstrated efficacy as therapy for the hypercalcemia of malignancy. This drug binds to hydroxyapatite in bone and reduces its solubility without directly altering osteoclast function or viability (Todd and Fitton, 1991; Bilezikian, 1992; Warrell, 1993). Studies in rodents suggest that this drug also may stimulate bone formation (Bockman et al, 1986). Gallium nitrate should not be used in patients receiving other nephrotoxic drugs (eg, aminoglycosides, cisplatin) or in those with renal insufficiency (serum creatinine >2.5 mg/dL), since the incidence of nephrotoxicity may be increased. As with the bisphosphonates, adequate hydration with normal saline and urine output must be established before initiating therapy. A urinary volume of 2 L/day should be maintained during treatment.

Results of early studies demonstrated that serum calcium levels were reduced to a greater degree and normocalcemia was achieved more frequently with doses of 200 mg/M^2/day than with half that amount. Currently, treatment is begun with the larger dose for up to five days, but the infusion is discontinued if normocalcemia is achieved before day five.

In a randomized double-blind trial, gallium nitrate (200 mg/M^2/day for five days by continuous intravenous infusion) was more effective than salmon calcitonin (8 IU/kg by intramuscular injection every six hours for five days) in normalizing serum calcium concentrations (75% versus 31% of patients) and in sustaining the effect (six days versus one day) (Warrell et al, 1988). Although calcitonin reduced serum calcium concentration more rapidly than gallium nitrate in responding patients, the brief duration of responses to calcitonin necessitated treatment with other hypocalcemic agents or cytotoxic drugs when hypercalcemia recurred. Furthermore, gallium nitrate was effective regardless of tumor type or the presence or absence of skeletal metastases, while calcitonin was relatively ineffective in patients with epidermoid tumors. There was no significant difference in the incidence of renal insufficiency among patients in the two groups.

A second randomized double-blind trial compared gallium nitrate with etidronate for therapy of acute hypercalcemia of malignancy (Warrell et al, 1991). Patients in the gallium nitrate arm received the same regimen as in the previous trial; those in the etidronate arm were given four-hour intravenous infusions of 7.5 mg/kg daily for five days. Gallium nitrate was more effective than etidronate in achieving normocalcemia (82% vs 43% of patients). In addition, the median duration of response to gallium nitrate (eight days) was greater than to etidronate (three days). Normocalcemia was achieved after five to six days with both drugs. However, a larger percentage (27%) of the patients in the etidronate arm required additional therapy with hypocalcemic drugs (eg, plicamycin) during the poststudy period compared with those in the gallium nitrate arm (9%). Furthermore, significantly larger volumes of intravenous fluids were administered (to help reduce persistent hypercalcemia) during the five days following completion of the study with etidronate than with gallium nitrate. There also was no significant difference in the incidence of renal insufficiency among patients in these two groups.

A randomized trial comparing gallium nitrate with pamidronate as therapy for hypercalcemia of malignancy is in progress. Data from separate single-arm studies suggest that the rapidity of response to the two drugs may be equivalent, but more patients may respond to gallium nitrate than to pamidronate.

Gallium nitrate appears to control hypercalcemia associated with excess PTH secretion (ie, parathyroid carcinoma) or production of PTH-like peptides by epidermoid tumors. This drug has not been compared with plicamycin in controlled trials, but theoretically it may be preferable to that agent due to the lack of myelosuppressive activity and maintenance of skeletal integrity.

Data from a recent randomized pilot study suggest that gallium nitrate also may be useful for patients with skeletal metastases (Warrell et al, 1993). Patients with multiple myeloma who were stabilized on cytotoxic chemotherapy and also received adjuvant treatment with low-dose gallium nitrate had increased skeletal calcium content; decreased bone pain; and preservation of height, which is indicative of the absence of vertebral fractures. The dosage of gallium nitrate used in this six-month study was 30 mg/M^2/day for two weeks followed by a two-week drug-free interval, and then 100 mg/M^2/day for five days every other month.

Elevated serum calcium levels also have been reduced by *phosphate*, which promotes the deposition of calcium in bone and soft tissues. However, phosphate should not be administered until the serum phosphorus level and renal function have been determined. Serum calcium and phosphate levels should be monitored closely to avoid hypocalcemia and even mild hyperphosphatemia. Phosphate may be used in the presence of hypophosphatemia (<3.5 mg/dL) but is contraindicated in the presence of hyperphosphatemia. Adequate hydration must be maintained during treatment.

Intravenous administration is discouraged because of the possibility of death caused by hypocalcemia as a consequence of deposition of calcium and phosphate in the lungs, kidneys, and other soft tissue. Most authorities consider the use of intravenous phosphate for hypercalcemia to be obsolete. The oral route is least hazardous and, if renal function is normal, can be used daily for prolonged periods without loss of effectiveness. However, fatalities have occurred in hypercalcemic patients with parathyroid adenomas who were treated with oral phosphates and in whom the serum phosphorus level only slightly exceeded the normal range (Vernava et al, 1987). Phosphate may be given rectally when oral administration is not feasible; phosphate enemas also will alleviate the constipation that frequently is present in hypercalcemic patients.

Measures that reduce the gastrointestinal absorption of calcium are important in treating hypercalcemia associated with the milk-alkali syndrome, sarcoidosis, hypervitaminosis D, and idiopathic hypercalcemia. Although reduction of calcium intake alone may be effective, especially in the milk-alkali syndrome, low calcium diets have no place in the management of patients with cancer-related hypercalcemia. The next measure to be employed depends on the disease state and its severity.

HYPOCALCEMIA

Symptomatic hypocalcemia occurs when serum levels of ionized calcium fall below 2.5 to 3 mg/dL (0.6 to 0.75 mmol/L). It primarily affects the central and peripheral nervous systems and muscular function. In infants and young children, seizures are the most common manifestation. In older children and adults, the most frequent disorder is tetany, with spasms of involuntary contraction in the hands and feet. Hypocalcemia results primarily from a deficiency of PTH or vitamin D (or its active metabolites). Hypocalcemia with hyperphosphatemia may be due to PTH deficiency, resistance to PTH (pseudohypoparathyroidism), or advanced renal insufficiency. Hypocalcemia with hyperphosphatemia also may occur when there is a large influx of phosphate into the circulation, as in leukemia or lymphoma when chemotherapy induces rapid tissue lysis; after large amounts of phosphate are administered; or when phosphate enemas are used in children.

Hypocalcemia with hypophosphatemia usually indicates deficiency or altered metabolism of vitamin D or a malabsorption syndrome. Prolonged administration of antiepileptic agents (eg, phenytoin [Dilantin], phenobarbital), rifampin [Rifadin, Rimactane], glutethimide, and probably other enzyme-inducing drugs also may induce hypocalcemia and hypophosphatemia secondary to increased metabolism of vitamin D. Marked hypocalcemia with hypophosphatemia may occur during the acute phase of hemorrhagic pancreatitis and may be secondary to extraskeletal deposition of calcium. The low serum calcium level encountered occasionally in conditions associated with hypomagnesemia is believed to be secondary to a decrease in the release of PTH and/or impaired tissue responsiveness to PTH (most commonly seen in acute alcoholism). Replenishment of magnesium stores usually corrects this condition.

In severe alcoholism, hypocalcemia is frequently secondary to inadequate intake of calcium, magnesium, and vitamin D; transient malabsorption; and excessive urinary excretion of calcium and magnesium. Osteoblastic metastases (eg, prostate and occasionally breast) rarely cause hypocalcemia.

In most chronic hypocalcemic disorders (except those associated with primary hypoparathyroidism and hypomagnesemia), there is a compensatory increase in the secretion of PTH (secondary hyperparathyroidism), which mobilizes mineral from bone. As a result, the serum calcium level may be raised toward normal at the expense of bone, and there may be evidence of excessive PTH.

Several clinical conditions also lead to disturbances in the calcium balance (Forman and Lorenzo, 1991). Hypocalcemia may develop during massive transfusions when citrated blood is administered to the patient. The degree of hypocalcemia is dependent on the rate of infusion of citrate-treated blood, how quickly peripheral stores of calcium are mobilized in response to the lowering of ionic calcium, and the rate of citrate clearance by the liver and the kidneys. Patients with underlying hepatic and renal diseases have a higher baseline level of lactate and citrate and are at greater risk for developing hypocalcemia. In general, a transfusion rate >90 ml/hr greatly increases the risk of development of hypocalcemia.

In patients undergoing liver transplantation, the inability of the liver to metabolize citrate products increases risks for hypocalcemia during the surgical and postsurgical period.

Hypocalcemia is common in critically ill patients, especially those with sepsis and/or renal, cardiac, or pulmonary failure following surgery or in burn patients, because of lowering of serum protein and albumin levels, the presence of acid-base abnormalities, and the need for citrated blood products (Zaloga, 1992). Hypocalcemia is associated with increased mortality in patients in intensive care units (Burchard et al, 1990).

THERAPY. Regardless of etiology, treatment is necessary to prevent complications (eg, convulsions, tetany, laryngospasm, respiratory and other muscle spasms). The initial treatment of severe symptomatic hypocalcemia is intravenous infusion of a source of rapidly available calcium ion, such as 10% calcium gluconate (see Table 2). For maintenance, a calcium salt is given orally. The calcium content of available oral calcium salts ranges from 9% (calcium gluconate) to 40% (calcium carbonate).

Calcitriol [Calcijex, Rocaltrol] is indicated for hypocalcemia and bone disease caused by defective conversion of vitamin D to 1,25-$(OH)_2D_3$, as in patients undergoing renal dialysis and in those with postsurgical or idiopathic hypoparathyroidism or pseudohypoparathyroidism (Chan et al, 1985). Parathyroid hormone injection (synthetic 1-34 PTH) [Parathar] is no longer used therapeutically, but it is still employed to distinguish pseudohypoparathyroidism from idiopathic and postsurgical hypoparathyroidism (Elsworth-Howard test).

If functional or actual vitamin D deficiency exists, the vitamin or its active metabolites should be administered after acute hypocalcemic symptoms have been controlled. When the deficiency is severe, the increase in serum calcium concentration after treatment may be delayed, and additional oral and/or intravenous calcium may be required to ameliorate symptoms. Vitamin D itself also can be employed to increase the serum calcium level in hypoparathyroidism; this is often accompanied by a reciprocal decline in serum phosphate levels.

OSTEOMALACIA AND RICKETS

Deficiency of vitamin D, calcium, or phosphorus may result in rickets or osteomalacia. Rickets is a disorder of impaired mineralization of the bone matrix, or osteoid, in growing bone; it involves the epiphyses and newly formed trabecular and cortical bone. In children with rickets, epiphyseal changes are dominant; delayed bone development, skeletal deformity, growth retardation, and muscle weakness are the principal manifestations. Mineralization of the bone matrix also is defective in osteomalacia; however, in contrast to rickets, this disorder occurs after cessation of growth. Backache, diffuse bone pain, muscle weakness, bowing of the legs, fractures of the long bones, kyphosis (particularly when associated with osteoporosis), and waddling gait are clinical features of osteomalacia.

Osteomalacia and rickets are produced by an imbalance in the metabolism of calcium or phosphate (Glorieux, 1991).

Hypocalcemia is caused by dietary calcium deficiency, primary and secondary vitamin D deficiency (due to fat malabsorption or renal failure), and pseudodeficiency of vitamin D. Two known forms of vitamin D-pseudodeficiency rickets (vitamin D-dependent rickets Type I and Type II) are inherited as autosomal recessive traits. Type I is due to impaired activity of renal 1α-hydroxylase and hence an inadequate synthesis of 1,25-$(OH)_2D_3$. Type II is caused by point mutations affecting the structure and function of the receptor of 1,25-$(OH)_2D_3$.

Hypophosphatemia results from decreased intake (eg, in premature infants), decreased absorption due to vitamin D deficiency, or renal wasting of inorganic phosphate (eg, in tumor-induced rickets or osteomalacia, Fanconi's syndrome). There are various forms of hereditary hypophosphatemia. The most common is X-linked hypophosphatemic rickets, which is expressed by decreased phosphate levels, elevated serum alkaline phosphatase activity, and inappropriately normal serum levels of 1,25-$(OH)_2D_3$.

Osteomalacia also may result from increased metabolism of vitamin D caused by the prolonged administration of antiepileptic drugs (Hahn, 1980). Inadequate diet combined with limited exposure to sunlight may contribute to the osteomalacia commonly seen in elderly, bedridden patients and in institutionalized individuals of all ages.

THERAPY. Most of the acquired forms of rickets or osteomalacia can be controlled by measures to increase the uptake of vitamin D, calcium, or phosphate or by excision of tumor.

In patients with Type I vitamin D-pseudodeficiency rickets, lifelong administration of calcitriol is required. In Type II vitamin D-dependent rickets, large amounts of a calcium supplement appear to be effective but intravenous administration often is required. In hereditary hypophosphatemia with hypercalciuria, phosphate supplementation alone may promote mineralization. In X-linked hypophosphatemic rickets, combined use of phosphate and calcitriol increases intestinal absorption of phosphate, reverses hyperparathyroidism, and improves symptoms of osteomalacia (Petersen et al, 1992; Verge et al, 1991). However, nephrocalcinosis may be induced with this combination therapy and ultimately may impair renal function.

Selected patients with renal hypophosphatemic rickets due to renal wastage of phosphate may benefit from the addition of hydrochlorothiazide and amiloride [Moduretic] to the calcitriol/phosphate regimen. The renal threshold for phosphate is raised and the serum phosphate concentration is increased; therefore, smaller doses of supplemental phosphate are required, thus avoiding the diarrhea that often accompanies use of this mineral (Alon and Chan, 1985).

RENAL OSTEODYSTROPHY

Osteodystrophy often accompanies end-stage renal disease and has been attributed to hormonal and metabolic responses to loss of functioning nephrons and to accumulation of uremic toxins (McCarthy and Kumar, 1990). In many patients, renal osteodystrophy is manifested by some degree of osteomalacia, osteitis fibrosa, and osteosclerosis, while in others only osteitis fibrosa or osteomalacia may be present.

Renal osteodystrophy also is often accompanied by osteoporosis, which may progress despite treatment. Hyperphosphatemia and elevated serum alkaline phosphatase levels are common in these patients, but the serum calcium level may be low, normal, or high depending on the stage of the disease. Phosphate retention, secondary hyperparathyroidism, impaired vitamin D metabolism, calcium malabsorption, and chronic acidosis are important in the pathogenesis of renal osteodystrophy. 1,25-$(OH)_2D_3$ may act as a hormone to inhibit PTH production directly; therefore, reduced renal production of 1,25-$(OH)_2D_3$ in renal failure may remove the inhibition of PTH secretion (Sherwood, 1987). Alternatively, a decrease in the number of 1,25-$(OH)_2D_3$ receptors or binding to receptors in parathyroid tissue may be instrumental in causing an increase in PTH secretion in renal failure (Korkor, 1987).

Osteitis fibrosa is caused by severe secondary hyperparathyroidism. PTH secretion is increased because of the fall in the serum calcium level, which occurs in response to phosphate retention, decreased levels of 1,25-$(OH)_2D_3$, and decreased intestinal calcium absorption. The increase in PTH activity helps to restore homeostasis by decreasing renal phosphate reabsorption and increasing renal calcium retention; however, prolonged parathyroid stimulation eventually may cause hyperparathyroid bone disease with or without hypercalcemia. Hypercalcemia may appear or persist after renal transplantation due to persistent hyperplasia of the parathyroid glands (sometimes requiring surgery) despite the removal of factors that cause resistance to PTH stimulation (Hahn, 1985).

Osteomalacia may be caused by a decrease in the renal production of 1,25-$(OH)_2D_3$, and, as a result, intestinal absorption of calcium may be impaired. However, most cases of osteomalacia and many cases of low-turnover bone disease are associated with excessive deposits of aluminum, especially in long-term dialysis patients (McCarthy and Kumar, 1990; Malluche and Faugere, 1990). Aluminum is deposited at the bone-osteoid interface and within the bony trabeculae in approximately 50% of patients with chronic renal failure. Aluminum is present in the normal daily diet, and the intestinal tract is an effective barrier to its absorption. The small amount that is absorbed is rapidly excreted by the normal kidney. However, in those with renal insufficiency, the total aluminum level in the body will increase and accumulate primarily in bone, brain, and liver. Its excessive deposition in these patients is augmented by the ingestion of aluminum-containing antacids used as oral phosphate binders and by the transfer from dialysate water that is contaminated with a high level of aluminum during dialysis.

The high levels of aluminum found in the brain tissue of deceased uremic patients are thought to be one cause of dialysis encephalopathy (Andress et al, 1987), which may be either sporadic or endemic. Sporadic encephalopathy is believed to be caused by aluminum toxicity due to the prolonged use of phosphate binders containing aluminum during therapy. Endemic encephalopathy may be due to insufficient water intake. Osteodystrophy also has been observed in patients with severe hepatic disease who had received aluminum antacids for long periods and in whom biliary excretion of aluminum presumably was inadequate (Williams et al, 1986).

Removal of aluminum from the dialysate water and substitution of phosphate binders containing calcium have significantly decreased the occurrence of osteomalacia in renal failure patients requiring dialysis (Sherrard et al, 1993). The incidence of osteodystrophy in patients with hepatic disease and encephalopathy that are caused by aluminum toxicity also should decrease.

Aplastic bone lesion is caused by low turnover without an increase in osteoid area (Malluche and Faugere, 1990). It occurs in the presence or absence of aluminum toxicity. Because of improvements in histologic techniques, aplastic bone lesion now is observed more frequently in patients undergoing dialysis, especially peritoneal dialysis (Sherrard et al, 1993). Usually patients with aplastic bone lesion are asymptomatic, and the lesion may merely be the response of bone to aggressive parathyroid control (Sherrard et al, 1993). In the absence of aluminum, this lesion may not be particularly dysfunctional.

THERAPY. An understanding of the pathophysiology of renal osteodystrophy provides a rational approach to therapy.

Maintenance of normal serum phosphate is important in managing secondary hyperparathyroidism and in preventing soft tissue calcification in patients with advanced renal failure and in those receiving dialysis. In early renal failure, secondary hyperparathyroidism may be avoided by progressively reducing phosphate absorption in proportion to the decrease in glomerular filtration rate. This may be accomplished in part through dietary measures, including restriction of protein intake. Administration of phosphate-binding antacids usually is required to control hyperphosphatemia when the glomerular filtration rate is 25% to 30% of normal. To reduce the risk of aluminum toxicity, aluminum-containing phosphate-binding gels generally should be avoided (Committee on Nutrition, 1986). Calcium carbonate, which forms insoluble complexes with dietary phosphates, is preferable and often can maintain adequate serum phosphate levels in those undergoing dialysis, although hypercalcemia can occur (Norris and Coburn, 1985). Daily doses should be proportional to the amount of phosphate in meals and may range between 4 and 14 g (Goodman et al, 1993). The dose should be adjusted to maintain serum phosphate levels between 4 and 5 mg/dL; further depletion may induce or worsen osteomalacia.

Some patients require combined therapy with aluminum hydroxide and calcium carbonate for adequate maintenance of serum phosphate levels. Other forms of calcium, particularly calcium acetate, also have been used in patients with renal osteodystrophy (Mai et al, 1989). Calcium also may be administered by high-calcium dialysis.

Despite the above measures, secondary hyperparathyroidism often develops in dialysis patients. Thus, the administration of calcitriol [Calcijex, Rocaltrol], calcifediol [Calderol], or large doses of vitamin D also may be required to increase serum calcium levels, decrease PTH secretion, and improve radiologic and histologic signs of osteitis fibrosa with or without osteomalacia. Many clinicians favor the use of calcitriol (oral dose, 0.25 to 1.25 mcg/day) for patients with symptomatic renal osteodystrophy; however, this compound frequently induces hypercalcemia, especially in patients receiving calcium carbonate, and it may worsen hyperphosphatemia. Intravenous administration of calcitriol may be more effective in suppressing secondary hyperparathyroidism independent of its effect on serum calcium (Slatopolsky et al, 1984). Intermittent (or pulse) oral therapy also has been used (Fukagawa et al, 1990). Similar results have been reported in patients treated orally with an investigational vitamin D_3 analogue, alfacalcidol, which is converted in the liver to form calcitriol. An analogue of calcitriol, 22-oxacalcitriol, suppresses PTH secretion and has virtually no effect on the calcium level (Brown et al, 1989; Finch et al, 1993); this compound is undergoing clinical trials for treatment of secondary hyperparathyroidism.

Osteomalacia due to aluminum toxicity frequently is unresponsive to vitamin D preparations. The chelating agent, deferoxamine [Desferal], has been effective in removing aluminum during hemodialysis (Coburn and Henry, 1984; Felsenfeld et al, 1989).

OSTEOPOROSIS

Primary Osteoporosis

PATHOGENESIS. Bone mass increases during childhood and adolescence, peaks in the third or early in the fourth decade of life, and declines progressively thereafter. Bone loss results from excessive activity of osteoclasts, decreased activity of osteoblasts, or both. Slow, age-related bone loss occurs in all individuals and is characterized by gradual thinning of trabeculae due to the decline in osteoblast function. This process may be hastened when bone remodeling is activated by secondary hyperparathyroidism, which develops in response to reduced calcium absorption and impaired renal hydroxylation of 25-OHD_3.

Osteoporosis is a "disease characterized by low bone mass, microarchitectural deterioration of bone tissue leading to enhanced bone fragility, and a consequent increase in fracture risk" (*Am J Med*, 1993). The magnitude of peak bone mass and the rate and duration of postmenopausal and age-associated bone loss determine the likelihood of developing osteoporosis. Although a large number of factors influence the bone mass of elderly women, results of a cross-sectional analysis indicate that the most important are age, weight, muscle strength, and estrogen use (Bauer et al, 1993). Osteoporotic fractures can occur in any bone but mainly affect the spine (vertebral crush fractures), hip, and distal radius (Colles' fracture).

Patients with age-related (senile, Type 2) osteoporosis have lost significant amounts of cortical as well as trabecular bone. Typically, hip and multiple wedge fractures of the vertebrae occur in these patients, usually after age 70. In contrast, women with postmenopausal (Type 1) osteoporosis tend to be younger and have lost predominantly trabecular bone. Thirty to forty percent of women over age 60 experience vertebral crush fractures; fractures of the distal radius also are typical in this group. Some patients with osteoporosis (eg, very elderly, institutionalized) also may develop osteomalacia, which contributes to structural weakness and pain. However, osteomalacia is rare in patients with vertebral compression fractures.

In women, bone loss, particularly from the vertebrae, may occur prior to menopause because of the gradual decline in estrogen production (Johnston et al, 1985). After menopause, bone turnover increases and the rate of cancellous bone loss is much greater than that of cortical bone. Rapid postmenopausal bone loss is mediated by osteoclasts. Estrogen withdrawal causes an increase in the formation or activation of osteoclasts, probably mediated by increased generation of local factors (eg, interleukin 1, interleukin 6, prostaglandin E_2) that influence osteoclast formation from precursor cells. Estrogen also may exert a direct but modest anabolic effect through receptors on osteoblasts. Thus, its withdrawal causes increased bone resorption coupled with inadequate bone formation. Persistent bone loss is associated with thinning of trabeculae and perforation of trabecular plates that causes loss of template for further bone formation.

At greatest risk for osteoporosis are postmenopausal Caucasian and Asian women who are thin (<58 kg) and have a small body frame and a positive family history. Other risk factors for osteoporosis include inadequate peak bone mass, chronic calcium deficiency, inactivity or immobilization, smoking, nulliparity, and early menopause. Estrogen deficiency or amenorrhea (eg, due to hyperprolactinemia, excessive exercise, or anorexia nervosa) in premenopausal women also may be associated with osteoporosis. However, osteoporosis may occur in the absence of any of these risk factors. Osteoporosis and fractures are less common in black postmenopausal women, in whom the incidence of hip fractures is approximately one-third that of Caucasian women. In elderly Caucasian men, the incidence of vertebral fractures is one-third and hip fractures one-half that of Caucasian women. Younger Caucasian males may be afflicted with a rare idiopathic osteoporotic disorder (Jackson and Kleerekoper, 1990).

DIAGNOSIS. Measurement of bone mass in vivo (single and double photon beam absorptiometry, quantitative computed tomography, dual energy radiographic absorptiometry) may detect osteoporosis before symptoms become severe. Measurement of bone mineral density (BMD) currently is the only method that accurately predicts fracture risk. Generally, individuals who develop osteoporotic fractures have lower bone mass than those of similar age who do not experience fractures, although there is overlap between the two groups (Hui et al, 1989; Ross et al, 1991; Cummings et al, 1993). The relative risk of fracture increases approximately twofold for every standard deviation decrease in bone mass from that of healthy young adults. Depending on the site, this is equivalent to the risk associated with a 13-(hip) to 17-(vertebrae) year increase in age (Melton et al, 1993). BMD measurement at one site predicts fracture risk at all susceptible sites; however, measurement at a specific site (eg, proximal femur) most accurately predicts fracture risk at that site (eg, hip). Some patients who have normal bone mass at menopause may have sufficient bone loss within two to three years to greatly increase fracture risk. Standards are being developed on the use of biochemical markers to help identify patients at risk for osteoporosis and those with high bone turnover (Christiansen et al, 1987; Hansen et al, 1991; Uebelhart et al, 1991; Delmas, 1993). Results of recent studies indicate that common allelic variants in the gene encoding the vitamin D receptor are major determinants of bone mass and hence of the risk of fracture (Morrison et al, 1994).

Dual energy radiographic absorptiometry is probably the method of choice to measure spine, hip, and total body bone mass. It has a precision of about 1% and is the least expensive, safest, and most readily available technique. Although it is a valuable research tool, there is controversy regarding the use of bone densitometry for a particular clinical situation (Health and Public Policy Committee, 1987; Bellantoni and Blackman, 1988; Eastell and Riggs, 1988; Riis and Christiansen, 1988; Mazess et al, 1989). Most of the controversy concerns the use of BMD measurements as a widespread screening tool in perimenopausal women. A task force of the National Osteoporosis Foundation concluded that measurement of bone density is appropriate if a treatment decision depends on assessment of fracture risk (Johnston et al, 1989). Such indications include (1) measurement of bone mass in order to make decisions about hormone replacement therapy; some postmenopausal women who are treated with conventional doses of estrogen continue to lose bone at an accelerated rate. BMD measurement can be used to determine secondary bone loss, adjust the estrogen dose, and enhance compliance in this group. (2) Diagnosis of spinal osteoporosis in individuals with vertebral abnormalities identified by roentgenography in order to make decisions about further evaluation and therapy. (3) Diagnosis of low bone mass in patients receiving prolonged glucocorticoid therapy in order to adjust dosage. (4) Diagnosis of low bone mass in patients with asymptomatic primary hyperparathyroidism in order to identify those at risk of severe skeletal disease who may be candidates for surgery. Routine radiography is inadequate in these situations.

THERAPY. The prevention and treatment of osteoporosis primarily involves the use of antiresorptive agents (eg, calcium, vitamin D, estrogen, calcitonin, bisphosphonates); treatment of established disease also may involve the use of agents that stimulate bone formation (eg, fluoride, PTH). For reviews, see Riggs and Melton, 1992; Lindsay, 1993; and *Am J Med*, 1993.

Calcium and Vitamin D Preparations: A large number of studies on the relationship between calcium intake and bone mass, bone loss, or bone fragility have been conducted (Dawson-Hughes et al, 1990; Reid et al, 1993; Heaney, 1993 A, 1993 B). In virtually all trials in which the total calcium intake was controlled (range, 900 mg to 1.75 g per day) and that excluded women within the first five years after menopause, adequate calcium intake slowed or stopped bone loss, at least in the short term (Heaney, 1993 A). The majority of studies on calcium supplementation also demonstrate a beneficial effect on bone mass in adolescents (Sentipal et al, 1991; Lloyd et al, 1993) as well as in other pre- and postmenopausal women. In one large controlled trial on ambulatory institutionalized elderly women, supplemental calcium (1.2 g) with modest amounts of vitamin D (800 IU) reduced the incidence of hip and other nonvertebral fractures (Chapuy et al, 1992). These results indicate that calcium and vitamin D supplements can favorably affect steady-state calcium balance.

Patients with inadequate dietary calcium should receive oral calcium supplements. Postmenopausal women given estrogen replacement therapy should receive a total of 1 g of calcium daily, and those not taking estrogen should receive 1.5 g daily (National Institutes of Health Consensus Conference, 1984). Regular weight-bearing exercise should be encouraged whether or not replacement therapy is prescribed. Small doses of vitamin D (400 to 800 IU) also may be indicated if there is a deficiency of the vitamin and lack of exposure to sunlight. The latter may be a problem during winter months, particularly in northern states, or at any time of year with chronic use of sunscreens (Matsuoka et al, 1988). Also, vitamin D may not be synthesized in the elderly as effectively as in younger people (Morley et al, 1988).

Several trials have been conducted on the use of calcitriol in women with osteoporosis, with conflicting results. In two of the more recent trials, calcitriol 0.5 mcg plus calcium 1.2 g or calcitriol alone (mean dose 0.62 mcg) increased spine density and reduced the rate of new vertebral compression fractures in women with postmenopausal osteoporosis (Gallagher and Goldgar, 1990; Tilyard et al, 1992). However, most physicians do not routinely prescribe calcitriol to prevent or treat osteoporosis because of the risk of hypercalcemia and hypercalciuria and the need for frequent monitoring of serum and urinary calcium. Calcitriol may be indicated in patients who cannot adequately hydroxylate the parent compound.

Estrogen: Estrogen replacement is the therapy of choice to prevent postmenopausal osteoporosis. Nevertheless, estrogen replacement is underutilized because of physician uncertainty about patient selection and duration of treatment and the reluctance of patients to accept the side effects and risks associated with long-term treatment.

Women who have undergone oophorectomy and hysterectomy in the pre- or perimenopausal period are prime candidates for prophylactic therapy because (1) there is a relationship between early loss of ovarian function and subsequent osteoporosis, (2) estrogen prevents bone loss in this group, (3) symptoms of estrogen deficiency (eg, senile vaginitis, vasomotor disturbances) are likely to develop, and (4) these patients are not at risk of endometrial carcinoma. Since bone loss is most rapid during the first few years after oophorectomy, therapy should be initiated promptly. In addition, young individuals with amenorrhea caused by intense physical activity or anorexia should be considered for estrogen therapy. Postmenopausal oophorectomy is not associated with rapid loss of bone.

In patients with natural menopause, indications for replacement therapy are less clear-cut, particularly when there are no symptoms of estrogen deficiency. However, estrogen replacement therapy is probably indicated in women with early natural menopause or a strong family history of osteoporosis. The patient's age, race, body build, and muscle mass also can be considered in assessing the potential benefits of prophylactic therapy.

A woman's decision to use estrogen replacement therapy should be based on consideration of potential beneficial effects of estrogen on menopausal symptoms, quality of life, osteoporosis, and cardiovascular disease versus the side effects and reported risks associated with estrogen use, specifically the increased risk of endometrial and possibly breast cancer. Recent data regarding the latter are reassuring (Henrich, 1992). Bone mass measurement provides the most accurate assessment of the risk of osteoporosis at menopause; use of biochemical markers may aid in the identification of individuals who are experiencing rapid bone loss (see discussion under Diagnosis). *Unless it is contraindicated, patients with low bone mass or evidence of rapid bone loss should be offered estrogen replacement at menopause.*

Results of several controlled trials have shown that estrogen replacement slows or eliminates bone loss in the early postmenopausal period and reduces the risk of subsequent fractures (Hammond et al, 1979; Hutchinson et al, 1979; Paganini-Hill et al, 1981; Lindsay, 1988). *Estrogen is most effective when given before significant bone loss has occurred.* Prospective studies have demonstrated that estrogen replacement decreases the incidence of vertebral fractures by 60% and the rate of all nontraumatic fractures by 50%, especially those involving the spine, forearm, and rib (Weiss et al, 1980; Kiel et al, 1987; Lufkin et al, 1992). There is less protection from fractures of the proximal femur, humerus, and tibia in treated patients (Kiel et al, 1987; Lindsay et al, 1984; Ettinger et al, 1985).

The minimum effective daily dose for prevention of bone loss is 0.625 mg of conjugated estrogens, 1 to 2 mg of estradiol, or equivalent doses of other orally active estrogens (National Institutes of Health Consensus Conference, 1984). The same dose of estrogen is employed to treat established osteoporosis.

Transdermal administration of estrogen (estradiol 0.05 mg to 0.1 mg) also prevents postmenopausal bone loss (Adami et al, 1989; Ribot et al, 1990; Stevenson et al, 1990) and decreases the vertebral fracture rate in postmenopausal women with established osteoporosis (Lufkin et al, 1992). Transdermal application of 0.05 mg appears to be equivalent to 0.625 mg of conjugated estrogens orally (see Balfour and McTavish, 1992).

Significant bone loss appears to be prevented as long as estrogen is administered (Ettinger et al, 1985; Al-Azzawi et al, 1987). However, when estrogen is discontinued, bone mineral density declines at a rate similar to that just after menopause. Results of a recent cross sectional study on bone density in postmenopausal women suggest that at least seven years of estrogen therapy is necessary for a persistent long-term effect (Felson et al, 1993). Even this duration of prophylactic therapy may have little residual effect on bone density among women 75 years and older, who have the highest risk of fracture.

The use of estrogen for prevention of osteoporosis in older women is more controversial. Women can respond to estrogen more than 10 years after the menopause, and it is likely that those with low bone mass, height loss, and other risk factors will benefit. Estrogen therapy also may stabilize skeletal mass in those with established osteoporosis (Lindsay and Tohme, 1990). *All postmenopausal women with vertebral crush fractures should be considered for estrogen therapy unless there is a specific contraindication.*

There is some evidence that a combination of estrogen and progestin further increases bone mass (Nachtigall et al, 1979; Upton, 1982; Christiansen et al, 1981, Johnansen et al, 1990), but the combination may provide less cardiovascular protection than estrogen alone. Most women experience monthly bleeding during sequential therapy, which many consider unacceptable. In order to avoid the persistence of menses, an increasing number of patients are selecting continuous rather than intermittent prophylaxis. Doses of 2.5 to 5 mg/day of medroxyprogesterone given continuously with estrogen can protect the endometrium from hyperplasia without producing regular menses, but irregular bleeding often occurs in these patients during the first several months.

For further information on the risks and benefits of postmenopausal hormone replacement therapy, see the chapter on Drugs Used for Gynecologic Indications.

Calcitonin: Current data suggest that either parenteral or intranasal (investigational) administration of salmon calcitonin [Calcimar, Miacalcin] stabilizes bone mass at multiple skeletal sites; this effect appears to be greatest in individuals with high bone turnover, which is consistent with calcitonin's ability to inhibit bone resorption (Wallach et al, 1977; Gennari et al, 1985; Mazzuoli et al, 1986; Reginster et al, 1987; Civitelli et al, 1988; MacIntyre et al, 1988; Overgaard et al, 1989). Results of other studies indicate that administration of calcitonin for one to two years prevents vertebral and hip fractures, although resistance to therapy or tachyphylaxis may occur in some patients after 6 to 12 months of continuous use (Kanis et al, 1992; Rico et al, 1992; Overgaard et al, 1992). Trials are ongoing to determine the duration of protection from fractures. Additional data are required to determine (1) the specific effects of calcitonin, especially in the estrogen-dependent phase of bone loss (recent data indicate that intranasal administration of 200 to 250 IU is ineffective in reducing bone loss immediately after menopause), (2) optimal dosage, and (3) roles of intermittent and combination regimens.

Despite the inconvenience of parenteral administration, calcitonin may be useful for older osteoporotic patients or those with high bone turnover and in those in whom estrogen is contraindicated. Long-term investigations to study the potential benefit of calcitonin in the treatment of osteoporosis are in progress. Results of studies reveal that a significant decrease in bone loss occurs with the more convenient nasal spray forms of calcitonin (Reginster et al, 1987; Overgaard et al, 1989).

In addition to its effect on bone structure, calcitonin (100 units daily) appears to have an analgesic effect that may occur earlier than biochemical indices of effects on bone disease. The mechanism of this action may be related to endorphins; a dose-dependent increase in circulating β-endorphin is observed after calcitonin is administered intravenously. A direct effect of calcitonin on the central nervous system also is possible; analgesia is produced by intracerebral or epidural administration. Calcitonin has been found in the pituitary and cerebrospinal fluid, and calcitonin-binding sites have been observed in brain areas involved in pain perception (Gennari and Agnusdei, 1988). The salmon form of calcitonin appears to be more effective than the human form for analgesia. Progressive pain relief has been observed in Paget's disease of bone, in osteoporotic patients with recent vertebral collapses, and in bone pain associated with malignancy, in which calcitonin was more effective than indomethacin.

Bisphosphonates: Bisphosphonates such as etidronate [Didronel] and pamidronate [Aredia] are potent inhibitors of bone resorption. Because the dosage of etidronate that inhibits bone resorption also impairs the mineralization of newly synthesized bone matrix, long-term continuous use is not feasible. Double-blind, placebo-controlled studies have demonstrated the apparent effectiveness of cyclical etidronate regimens for postmenopausal osteoporosis. Patients receiving etidronate cyclically (400 mg daily, 2 weeks on and 13 weeks off) with calcium supplementation for three years had increased vertebral bone mass and a decreased rate of vertebral fracture rate after the first year compared with placebo controls (Storm et al, 1990). The gain in vertebral bone mass was approximately 5%, which is similar to results obtained with estrogen and calcitonin.

In a multicenter, randomized, placebo-controlled study, patients treated with etidronate (400 mg daily, 2 weeks on and 10 weeks off) and calcium supplementation with or without phosphate (2 g daily) also had increased vertebral bone mass and decreased vertebral fractures at two years compared with controls treated with placebo or phosphate alone. The greatest decrease in fractures occurred in a subgroup with the lowest bone density. Bone density in the hip and wrist did not improve (Watts et al, 1990).

In a continuation of this study that included a third year of blinded treatment followed by an open-label phase in the fourth year, the gains in spinal bone mass achieved at two years persisted and increased slightly during the third year, and proximal femur bone density increased over the initial three-year period (Harris et al, 1993). During the open-label phase, bone mass was maintained and low fracture rates were observed. Although there was only a trend toward reduction in the overall incidence of fracture, post-hoc analysis revealed a significant reduction in vertebral fracture rates in patients at higher risk; this subgroup was comprised of women who at baseline had three or more vertebral fractures and spinal BMD below the 50th percentile for the study population as a whole. Further prospective study is required to determine the role of cyclical etidronate administration in the treatment of women at lower risk for recurrent vertebral fracture and in the prevention of nonvertebral fractures (Marcus, 1993). Until additional data become available, cyclical etidronate therapy is an additional treatment option for osteoporosis to be employed for a limited time period.

Various studies have demonstrated the effects of pamidronate. Multiple intravenous doses of pamidronate (15 to 30 mg/day for eight consecutive days) have produced positive calcium balances in patients with osteoporosis (Goldstein et al, 1989). After six months of additional treatment with 1 mg/kg once monthly, calcium balance remained positive and lumbar BMD was increased significantly. Administration of 30 mg/day for five consecutive days every two months for two years given with oral sodium fluoride (75 mg/day) and elemental calcium (1.5 g/day) increased lumbar spinal and distal and proximal forearm BMD in osteoporotic women (Devogelaer et al, 1990). One year of treatment with oral pamidronate 150 mg/day improved calcium balance and increased bone density that was sustained during three years of follow-up.

A regimen known as ADFR (activate-depress-free-repeat) or "coherence therapy" has been suggested for treatment of osteoporosis. Initially, bone resorption is stimulated by phosphate, then etidronate is given to depress resorption. Theoretically, bone formation occurs during an extended drug-free period. The cycle is then repeated (Anderson et al, 1984; Hodsman, 1989). In general, however, data are limited, and beneficial effects have not been supported by experimental results.

Other Antiresorptive Agents: *Thiazide Diuretics.* Thiazide diuretics produce a sustained reduction in urinary calcium excretion. Results of several cross-sectional and case control studies (for review see LaCroix, 1991) and longitudinal follow-up of one male cohort (Wasnich et al, 1990) indicate that use of thiazide diuretics in patients with hypertension is associated with higher bone density at several skeletal sites including the hip (Lindsay et al, 1987). The association between thiazide use and reduction in fracture risk is more tenuous. Although results of several case control and one prospective cohort study indicate that thiazide use is associated with reduced rates of hip fracture (Ray et al, 1989; LaCroix et al, 1990; Felson et al, 1991), several other studies have found no protective effect on risk for hip fracture and one found an increased risk (Heidrich et al, 1991).

Although low doses of thiazides generally are well tolerated by elderly hypertensive patients, it remains to be determined whether these drugs can be used safely in elderly normotensive patients. In particular, their use may be associated with orthostatic hypotension that may increase falls. Thus, results from randomized prospective trials of sufficient length are required before thiazides can be considered for routine use in the treatment of involutional osteoporosis. However, they are commonly employed in prophylaxis of glucocorticoid-induced osteoporosis because hypercalciuria is common in these patients. Bone loss associated with idiopathic hypercalciuria also may be reversed by thiazides. The combination of hydrochlorothiazide and amiloride [Moduretic] may be most effective in reducing hypercalciuria and is less likely to cause hypokalemia (see index entry Thiazides, Uses).

Anabolic Steroids. These agents may slow bone loss and increase bone mass (Chesnut, 1981), but side effects, including masculinization and adverse effects on serum lipids, are a problem in postmenopausal women. No studies comparing the effectiveness of anabolic steroids with that of an estrogen/progestin regimen are available. Anabolic steroids may be appropriate for osteoporotic men, but there are no controlled studies to support their efficacy in these patients.

Agents Stimulating Bone Formation: *Fluoride.* Fluoride stimulates osteoblasts to synthesize and secrete osteoid matrix. Bone mass and skeletal density are increased by increasing the width of existing trabeculae. Results of some population surveys have suggested that the incidence of osteoporosis may be reduced in areas with a high fluoride content in the drinking water; however, other studies suggest that the incidence of hip fractures is increased in women who reside in such areas. Thus, further information is required to establish the relationship between the fluoride content of water and susceptibility to osteoporosis (Melton, 1990).

Results of two prospective, randomized, double-blind placebo-controlled NIH-sponsored trials on sodium fluoride therapy in postmenopausal osteoporosis (Riggs et al, 1990; Kleerekoper et al, 1991) indicated that a daily dose of 75 mg did not reduce the occurrence of vertebral compression fractures despite an annual average increase of 8% to 10% in spinal bone mass. In addition, the risk of peripheral fractures may be increased. The results of these trials are in accord with a smaller study on 23 patients that used a similar dose (80 mg daily) (Dambacher et al, 1986). Large doses of fluoride may be associated with formation of brittle bone and an increased fracture rate. In addition, a significant number of patients experience gastric irritation, arthralgia, and pain in the lower extremities that may be associated with incomplete fractures at the site of pain. Fluoride may accumulate and its use is contraindicated in patients with renal insufficiency.

In contrast, in another study, survival analysis indicated that the probability of new vertebral crush fracture was reduced in patients treated with sodium fluoride, calcium, and vitamin D. However, the effect was only temporary after 6 to 18 months of therapy, and no difference was noted between treated and untreated patients after 18 to 24 months (Mamelle et al, 1988). In an uncontrolled trial on patients with osteoporosis, intermittent therapy with a slow-release sodium fluoride preparation and continuous calcium citrate supplementation resulted in increased vertebral density, improved bone morphology, and decreased vertebral fractures. The fluoride concentration was maintained within a therapeutic but nontoxic range, and side effects were tolerable; no effect on hip fractures was observed (Pak et al, 1989).

Interim results were reported recently from a placebo-controlled, randomized trial using slow-release fluoride plus calcium citrate in patients (n=99) with postmenopausal osteoporosis (Pak et al, 1994). Treatment consisted of slow-release sodium fluoride 25 mg twice daily in repeated 14-month cycles (12 months on treatment followed by 2 months off treatment) or placebo. Both groups took calcium citrate (400 mg elemental calcium twice daily) continuously. A total of 48 fluoride recipients and 51 placebo recipients completed a mean 2.44 and 2.14 cycles/patient, respectively. In fluoride recipients, the mean lumbar (L2 to L4) bone mineral content increased by 4% to 6% in each cycle and the mean femoral neck bone density increased by 4.1% and 2.1% during the first two cycles; radial bone density did not change. Bone mass was unchanged in the placebo group. Fluoride recipients also had a lower individual new vertebral fracture rate (0.057/patient cycle compared with 0.204/patient cycle), a higher fracture-free rate (83.3% compared with 64.7%), and a lower group fracture rate. Side effects previously reported with use of higher fluoride doses (ie, microfractures, hip fracture, anemia) did not occur. These results indicate that intermittent slow-release sodium fluoride plus continuous calcium citrate inhibits new vertebral fractures and is safe to use. The study is ongoing to determine if the effect is sustained. Based on current information, fluoride treatment should be restricted to clinical trials until the optimal dose and schedule are determined.

Parathyroid Hormone. Although high concentrations of PTH directly stimulate bone resorption, low doses, particularly when given intermittently, may exert anabolic effects. The short-term subcutaneous administration of low doses of the amino terminal fragment (1-34) of synthetic human PTH increases bone accretion, and long-term therapy appears to increase cancellous bone in the axial skeleton (spine or ilium) with no significant change in forearm cortical bone (Reeve et al, 1980; Slovik et al, 1986). In one trial, the increase in vertebral bone density reached a plateau at 12 months and then began to decrease (Neer et al, 1990). It has not been determined whether the increase in bone mass is sustained and is sufficient to reduce fracture risk.

In summary, no currently available drug restores the 30% to 40% loss of bone mass that occurs in symptomatic osteoporosis. Most of the agents studied inhibit bone resorption and have less effect on bone formation. Thus, they are of greater use in prophylaxis and stabilization than in restoration of bone mass. Agents that increase bone formation (sodium fluoride, possibly calcitonin) do not necessarily prevent fractures. Until a more potent stimulant of bone formation becomes available, efforts should continue to develop precise methods of identifying susceptible individuals (eg, by bone mass measurement) and detecting osteoporosis in its early stages. The benefits of estrogen in peri- and postmenopausal women should be emphasized.

Secondary Osteoporosis

Prolonged therapy with glucocorticoids is the most common cause of secondary osteoporosis. Other drugs that may be associated with its development include GnRH agonists, lithium, antiepileptic drugs (eg, phenytoin, carbamazepine, phenobarbital), thyroid hormones, methotrexate, and heparin. Osteoporosis also may be secondary to chronic liver and kidney disease, alcoholism, primary hyperparathyroidism, idiopathic hypercalciuria, Cushing's syndrome, hypogonadism, hyperthyroidism, insulin-dependent diabetes, gastrectomy or malabsorption, systemic mastocytosis, lymphoproliferative disorders, blood dyscrasias, rheumatoid arthritis, and ankylosing spondylitis.

GLUCOCORTICOID-INDUCED OSTEOPOROSIS. Patients who receive large doses of glucocorticoids may experience rapid loss of bone, and vertebral compression fractures can occur within weeks to months after initiation of therapy. The rate of bone loss is dose-dependent but is greatest in the first year and is reduced during the second and third years (Adachi et al, 1993). Patients treated chronically or who have received a large cumulative dose ($\geq$5 g prednisone equivalent) are at increased risk; significant osteopenia has been observed in those treated chronically with prednisone in doses as low as 7.5 to 10 mg daily (Hahn, 1980). Risk also is increased in those younger than 15 years or older than 50 years and in postmenopausal females. Other general risk factors for osteoporosis also increase susceptibility. Bone loss is diffuse and affects both the cortical and axial skeleton; however, bone loss is most rapid and significant in areas of the skeleton containing the greatest proportion of trabecular bone. Pharmacologic effects of glucocorticoids that contribute to osteoporosis include suppression of bone formation (osteoblast function), inhibition of intestinal calcium absorption leading to secondary hyperparathyroidism, hypogonadism, and increased renal calcium excretion.

Therapy: Sufficient data are not available to formulate definitive recommendations for prevention and treatment of glucocorticoid-induced osteoporosis. Vitamin D deficiency augments the adverse effects of glucocorticoids and its status (ie, serum 25-hydroxyvitamin D concentration) should be assessed. Patients with low serum concentrations of 25-hydroxyvitamin D should be considered deficient and should receive small supplemental doses of vitamin D, calcifediol, or calcitriol.

Measurement of 24-hour urinary calcium excretion is helpful in assessing calcium balance and susceptibility to secondary hyperparathyroidism. In most patients treated with glucocorticoids, serum osteocalcin concentrations are low and may be useful in assessing inhibition of osteoblast activity.

General preventive guidelines include use of the lowest possible dose of glucocorticoid (alternate-day therapy typically does not prevent osteoporosis). Gonadal hormones should be replaced in postmenopausal women or in women with corticosteroid-induced amenorrhea and in hypogonadal men. Other measures include a regular program of weight-bearing physical activity, cessation of smoking, avoidance of excessive alcohol intake, and adequate calcium intake (Hahn, 1993).

Pharmacologic doses of vitamin D preparations have been used to treat or prevent glucocorticoid-induced bone loss, although the results of most previous studies have not supported their efficacy or study designs were flawed (see Luckert and Raisz, 1990). However, results of a randomized, placebo-controlled trial indicate that prophylactic daily use of calcitriol (mean dose 0.6 mcg) and calcium (1 g) for one year prevented corticosteroid-induced bone loss in the lumbar spine but not at the femoral neck or distal radius (Sambrook et al, 1993). The protective effect was increased by the addition of salmon calcitonin 400 IU given intranasally.

Use of large doses of vitamin D in patients who have normal serum concentrations of 25-hydroxyvitamin D can be hazardous. Hypercalciuria and hypercalcemia frequently develop. Furthermore, initiation of vitamin D and calcium therapy may aggravate steroid-induced hypercalciuria and/or cause hypercalcemia. Thus, most clinicians reserve pharmacologic vitamin D therapy for patients with low bone mass or clinical osteoporosis who will receive close follow-up care (Luckert and Raisz, 1990; Adachi et al, 1993). Nevertheless, vitamin D intake should be adequate, and this can be assured in most patients with a daily supplement of 400 to 800 U or alternatively with calcitriol 0.5 to 1 mcg.

Hypercalciuria (24-hour calcium excretion >4 mg/kg) can be reduced with a thiazide diuretic (eg, 25 mg hydrochlorothiazide twice daily). Adjunctive use of a potassium-sparing diuretic also is recommended so that steroid-induced potassium loss is not aggravated. Because thiazide diuretics also tend to exacerbate hypercalcemia in glucocorticoid-treated patients, some clinicians may choose to use either calcitriol or thiazides, but not both together. Serum calcium should be monitored and, if thiazides are used, the dose adjusted to maintain the daily urinary calcium loss within 2.5 to 3.5 mg/kg. In any event, therapy with a vitamin D metabolite or pharmacologic doses of vitamin D requires careful follow-up to monitor for hypercalcemia and hypercalciuria and to make appropriate adjustments in dosage.

Treatment of established glucocorticoid-induced osteopenia follows the general measures for prophylaxis. Some patients may benefit from therapy with calcitonin or bisphosphonates (see Meunier, 1993). In one study, intermittent therapy with etidronate for six months prevented vertebral bone loss in postmenopausal women with temporal arteritis who were treated with prednisone (Mulder and Shelder, 1992). Therapy with pamidronate also has been reported to cause a short-term increase and stabilization of axial and appendicular bone density in patients treated with glucocorticoids. Anabolic steroids may be beneficial in those who continue to experience vertebral crush fractures or marked bone loss.

For further information on clinical presentation, assessment, prevention, and treatment guidelines for glucocorticoid-induced osteoporosis, see Adachi et al, 1993; Hahn, 1993.

PAGET'S DISEASE OF BONE

Paget's disease of bone (osteitis deformans) is a chronic focal disorder that occurs primarily in individuals over age 40 (for review, see Bone and Kleerekoper, 1992). This disease is characterized by greatly increased size and activity of osteoclasts in association with increased bone resorption, formation of structurally abnormal replacement bone, and increased vascularity in the affected regions. It can occur in any bone but most often affects the femur, pelvis, and spine; the skull, humerus, and tibia also are affected frequently. Lesions may be lytic and/or sclerotic, resulting in pain, deformity (eg, thickening of the skull), fractures, and a variety of functional abnormalities involving structures (eg, spinal or cranial nerves) that are associated with affected skeletal sites. The pathogenesis is not established, but the disease may be a late consequence of a paramyxoviral infection (Kaplan, 1992).

The rate of progression, degree of disability, and extent of involvement vary. Patients with mild disease are often asymptomatic, and pagetic lesions may be localized. In about 25% of patients, the disease is associated with moderate to severe bone pain, and osteoarthritic changes in joints adjacent to affected areas are common. Rarely, high-output congestive heart failure develops when extensive skeletal involvement is associated with greatly increased blood flow to bone. Perhaps 1% of patients develop osteogenic sarcoma or fibrosarcoma, which usually is fatal within two years.

The serum calcium level is normal in ambulatory patients with Paget's disease but may be elevated and associated with hypercalciuria if the patient is immobilized. When active disease involves a significant proportion of the skeleton, the increased bone turnover is reflected by elevated serum alkaline phosphatase and urinary hydroxyproline levels.

THERAPY. Asymptomatic patients with small areas of bone involvement are usually not treated. Mild pain often can be managed with analgesics and anti-inflammatory agents. In symptomatic patients with more extensive skeletal involvement, agents that inhibit excessive bone turnover (ie, calcitonin, bisphosphonates) are employed to relieve symptoms and perhaps retard progression of the disease. Of the calcitonins, the salmon preparation [Calcimar, Miacalcin] has a longer duration of action and greater potency; human calcitonin [Cibacalcin] also is available. Of the bisphosphonates, clinical experience is greatest with etidronate; pamidronate also has been used. Calcitonin and bisphosphonates have not been compared in controlled clinical trials.

Serum alkaline phosphatase and the urinary concentration of hydroxyproline and pyridinoline cross-links usually decrease and bone pain is relieved during calcitonin or etidronate therapy; calcitonin provides more rapid pain relief. Neurologic symptoms may be alleviated and functional capacity may increase; improved bone histology and radiologic evidence of regression of abnormalities also may occur. Calcitonin is generally well tolerated, and it has been suggested that its administration to asymptomatic patients might delay complications, such as fractures, bone deformities, and premature deafness.

A problem with use of salmon calcitonin is the development of antibodies in 40% to 70% of patients; however, their formation is not always associated with resistance (Grauer et al, 1990). The risk of diminishing effectiveness as a result of antibody formation or hypersensitivity reaction is less with human calcitonin than with nonhuman forms of the hormone. Nevertheless, the effectiveness of human calcitonin also may diminish over time in some patients.

The dose and duration of treatment with etidronate are limited by the propensity of large doses (10 to 20 mg/kg/day) to interfere with mineralization of newly formed bone. The effect is time- and dose-dependent but also may occur with lower therapeutic doses (5 mg/kg/day). Since the mineralization defect can result in fractures, patients with lytic lesions of long bones should be monitored radiographically and biochemically to permit termination of therapy in unresponsive individuals.

In young patients, active disease should be treated with calcitonin administered three times per week or etidronate 20 mg/kg/day for one month with follow-up to detect relapse. Patients with bone pain unrelieved by analgesics and anti-inflammatory agents may be treated weekly with calcitonin or etidronate 5 mg/kg/day orally for six months. Calcitonin administered daily until the lesion is healed is the treatment of choice for patients with lytic lesions in the long bones, since these may be accelerated during therapy with etidronate. Patients with early hearing loss or other neurologic complications should be treated immediately with daily administration of calcitonin and/or etidronate 4.3 mg/kg/day intravenously for seven days. Calcitonin also often is used three months prior to, and six months after, corrective orthopedic surgery in pagetic patients. Salmon calcitonin nasal spray (investigational) appears to produce results similar to the injectable form.

Pamidronate disodium also appears to be effective in Paget's disease, and it has induced remission in some patients who are resistant to etidronate (Delmas et al, 1987). Various dosage schedules have been employed. Normalization of urinary excretion of hydroxyproline and of serum alkaline phosphatase activity occurred within one year in those receiving intravenous pamidronate 15, 30, or 45 mg infused over two to six hours at six-week intervals (Stone et al, 1990). Daily infusions of 20 to 60 mg for 2 to 10 days normalized urinary hydroxyproline excretion within 5 to 10 days (Papapoulos et al, 1987; Fenton et al, 1991). Infusions of 30 mg once weekly reduced serum alkaline phosphatase activity in six weeks (Gallacher et al, 1988; Gray et al, 1990). A single 60-mg infusion normalized urinary hydroxyproline excretion within two weeks and serum alkaline phosphatase activity within three months; these effects were sustained for more than 12 months without further treatment (Thiébaud et al, 1988). Successful treatment was accompanied by reduced bone pain and repair of osteolytic bone lesions with no signs of defective mineralization. Guidelines on the use of pamidronate in the treatment of Paget's disease are available (Siris, 1994).

The rapid inhibition of bone resorption and delayed effect on osteoblastic activity suggest that pamidronate inhibits osteoclasts rapidly but does not interfere with ongoing cycles of bone formation (Fitton and McTavish, 1991). However, one case of transient, asymptomatic early mineralization defects after cumulative dosages of 180 to 260 mg has been reported (Adamson et al, 1993). The dissociation of the antiresorptive effects of pamidronate from antianabolic activity has led to the suggestion that pamidronate be discontinued when urinary hydroxyproline excretion is normalized, regardless of the serum alkaline phosphatase status (Harinck et al, 1987).

Limited data are available comparing the relative effectiveness of intravenous pamidronate with other agents in Paget's disease of bone. Other bisphosphonates under investigation for treatment of Paget's disease include tiludronate (Reginster et al, 1993; Audran et al, 1989) and alendronate (O'Doherty et al, 1990, 1992).

Gallium nitrate also has been used successfully in several patients with advanced Paget's disease (Siris et al, 1992). Although large intravenous doses have been administered (Matkovic et al, 1990), most investigators have given small doses by the subcutaneous route (see the evaluation on Gallium Nitrate).

Plicamycin is sometimes employed to treat symptomatic patients unresponsive to other agents. It is also useful when a rapid response is desired, as in spinal cord compression. However, toxicity and the need for intravenous administration limit this drug's usefulness.

NEPHROLITHIASIS

For a discussion of the pathogenesis and management of nephrolithiasis, see index entry Urolithiasis.

Drug Evaluations

ADRENAL CORTICOSTEROIDS

Glucocorticoids reduce the intestinal absorption of calcium by antagonizing the action of vitamin D and by reducing serum concentrations of 1,25-$(OH)_2D_3$ in sarcoidosis and in some patients with lymphoma. They are effective in hypercalcemia due to hypervitaminosis D, sarcoidosis, and adrenocortical insufficiency. Because of additional direct or indirect effects on bone resorption, they also are useful in some patients with hypercalcemia due to myeloma, leukemia, and lymphoma and in some patients with solid (particularly breast) tumors. Large doses may be necessary initially. The onset of action varies, but improvement may occur within 24 to 72 hours. Smaller doses of glucocorticoids administered with calcitonin may lower serum calcium levels safely and effectively, but this action has not been observed consistently.

The adverse effects of prolonged glucocorticoid therapy are an important consideration (see index entry Adrenal Corticosteroids, Adverse Reactions).

DOSAGE AND PREPARATIONS.

Intravenous, Intramuscular: *Adults,* for severe hypercalcemia, parenteral preparations are preferred (hydrocortisone sodium succinate 100 to 500 mg daily in three or four divided doses or prednisolone sodium phosphate 20 to 100 mg daily); these drugs may be given intramuscularly, intravenously, or, preferably, by intravenous infusion.

Oral: *Adults,* initially, 40 to 80 mg of prednisone or the equivalent daily until the serum calcium level is controlled. Dosage then is reduced gradually; final dosage is determined by the results of serum calcium determinations.

See index entry Adrenal Corticosteroids, Preparations, Systemic for listings of preparations.

CALCITONIN (HUMAN)

[Cibacalcin]

ACTIONS AND USES. This synthetic polypeptide contains the exact sequence of amino acids found in natural human calcitonin. Human calcitonin has the same actions and uses in Paget's disease of bone and other disorders as salmon calcitonin (see below); however, it may be less potent.

ADVERSE REACTIONS. Adverse effects are similar to those observed with salmon calcitonin with the exception of antibody formation. Because this preparation is chemically identical to the naturally occurring hormone, antibody formation is much less common. Patients who have developed resistance to salmon calcitonin may respond to this preparation, and long-term effectiveness can be anticipated. Allergic reactions may occur rarely. No contraindications to human calcitonin have been identified.

This drug is classified in FDA Pregnancy Category C.

DOSAGE AND PREPARATIONS.

Subcutaneous: For Paget's disease of bone, *adults,* initially 0.5 mg daily. In patients troubled by nausea and flushing, treatment should begin with 0.25 mg, which can be increased in a stepwise fashion at intervals of one to two weeks until a dose of 0.5 mg/day is achieved. If the patient responds favorably, the maintenance dosage may be reduced to 0.5 mg two or three times per week or 0.25 mg daily. Patients with severe disease may require up to 0.5 mg twice daily. Treatment generally is continued for six months.

Cibacalcin (CIBA). Double-chambered syringe containing 0.5 mg calcitonin plus 20 mg mannitol in sterile, lyophilized form in one chamber and 30 mg mannitol in 1 ml water for injection in the other chamber.

CALCITONIN (SALMON)

[Calcimar, Miacalcin]

ACTIONS AND USES. This synthetic polypeptide derived from salmon differs from the human form at 16 of the 32 amino acid sites. Salmon calcitonin reduces bone resorption and thereby controls symptoms, prevents complications, and possibly halts progression of Paget's disease of bone. It is indicated primarily in symptomatic patients with moderate to severe involvement and is the drug of choice for rapid relief of pain. In almost all patients, calcitonin reduces (but seldom to normal) increased levels of serum alkaline phosphatase and urinary hydroxyproline, and it often relieves bone pain. Neurologic defects caused by compression of the spinal cord, spinal nerves, or cranial nerves may be relieved and functional capacity increased. Calcitonin does not reverse hearing loss but may prevent its progression. If cardiac output is elevated because of increased blood flow to bone, calcitonin may relieve the congestive symptoms. There is radiologic evidence that abnormalities in some affected bones regress in a few patients, but it is not yet known whether long-term calcitonin therapy will prevent bony overgrowth and deformities and improve skeletal structure.

After about one year of calcitonin therapy, a partial loss of effectiveness has been noted in approximately 20% of patients with Paget's disease who initially responded well. The biochemical parameters (serum alkaline phosphatase and urinary hydroxyproline) may continue to improve despite the loss of corresponding symptomatic relief. In some cases, loss of response is probably related to high titers of neutralizing antibodies to salmon calcitonin. However, low antibody titers occur in up to two-thirds of patients, most of whom do not become resistant to the drug. Substitution of human calcitonin is effective in most patients in whom reduced response is attributable to high titers of antibodies to salmon calcitonin.

Salmon and human calcitonin also have been used to treat hypercalcemic states associated with high rates of bone mineral loss, such as hyperparathyroidism, immobilization (particularly in association with Paget's disease), and malignancies. Calcitonin is useful for acute control of mild to moderate hypercalcemia of malignancy and in emergencies because it usually produces a rapid but slight hypocalcemic effect. Effectiveness in these patients may decrease after several days of therapy; institution of a drug-free interval or the addition of corticosteroids to the regimen may restore responsiveness.

Calcitonin has been used as an adjunct to chemotherapy and anabolic steroids in the treatment of bone metastases from breast or prostate carcinoma or multiple myeloma. However, data are inadequate to establish the efficacy of calcitonin for this indication.

Calcitonin also may be used to treat postmenopausal osteoporosis, especially in elderly patients, those with symptomatic vertebral crush fractures, those in whom estrogen is contraindicated, or those with high bone turnover (see the section on Osteoporosis). Calcitonin is the treatment of choice in young males with idiopathic osteoporosis and also may be useful in the treatment of glucocorticoid-induced osteopenia.

ADVERSE REACTIONS. Calcitonin is generally well tolerated, but rash, nausea, vomiting, diarrhea, facial flushing, and malaise may occur. The gastrointestinal and skin reactions usually diminish with continued therapy. A transient, marked increase in sodium and water excretion has been noted during initial therapy and probably is related to both a direct renal effect and to improved circulatory dynamics. Soreness and inflammation at the site of injection may occur. This drug is classified in FDA Pregnancy Category C.

DOSAGE AND PREPARATIONS.

Subcutaneous, Intramuscular (subcutaneous generally preferred): For Paget's disease of bone, *adults with early hearing loss or other neurologic complications*, 100 IU twice daily for seven days followed by 50 to 100 IU three times per week for one month or until a satisfactory clinical or biochemical response is obtained; *adults with active disease,* 50 to 100 IU is given for a duration similar to that above; *adults with bone pain unrelieved by analgesics and anti-inflammatory agents*, 50 to 100 IU daily for six months; *adults with lytic lesions in long bones*, 100 IU twice daily until the lesions are healed.

For hypercalcemia, the manufacturers recommend an initial dose of 4 IU/kg every 12 hours. If the response is unsatisfactory after one or two days, the dose may be increased to 8 IU/kg every 12 hours. If the response is still unsatisfactory after two more days, a maximum of 8 IU/kg may be administered every six hours. Some clinicians prefer to initiate therapy with the larger dose and most frequent schedule of administration (8 IU/kg every six hours for two days) to achieve the maximal hypocalcemic effect rapidly, since the duration of responsiveness to calcitonin is usually quite limited. The dose and schedule can then be decreased to 4 IU/kg every 12 hours in patients who continue to respond. Others prefer to use a fixed dose of 50 to 100 IU every 12 hours throughout therapy because of the nausea caused by higher doses in some patients.

For postmenopausal osteoporosis, doses range from 50 IU three times/week to 100 IU daily.

Calcimar (Rhone-Poulenc Rorer). Solution (sterile) 200 IU/ml in 2 ml containers.

TABLE 2. CALCIUM PREPARATIONS

Generic Name	Amount of Elemental Calcium	Dosage	Preparations	Elemental Calcium Present in Preparation	Indications Comments
ORAL PREPARATIONS					
Calcium carbonate	40%	*Oral: Adults,* 1 to 2 g (equivalent to 400 to 800 mg elemental calcium) three times daily with meals.	Generic. Tablets 500 (chewable), 600, 650 mg, 1.25 and 1.5 g (plain, chewable)	200, 240, 260, 500, and 600 mg	Nonprescription. Calcium carbonate is probably the most commonly used calcium preparation for mild hypocalcemia, osteomalacia, rickets, osteoporosis, and renal osteodystrophy. It is converted in the stomach to soluble calcium salts by interaction with hydrochloric acid. In patients with achlorhydria, absorption is impaired in the fasting state.
			Caltrate 600 (Lederle). Tablets 1.5 g	600 mg	
			Equilet (Mission). Tablets (chewable) 500 mg	200 mg	
			OS-Cal 500 (SmithKline Beecham). Tablets (plain, chewable) 1.25 g	500 mg	
			Titralac (3M). Tablets (plain, chewable) 420 mg	168 mg	
			Titralac Extra Strength (3M). Tablets (chewable) 750 mg	300 mg	
			Tums (SmithKline Beecham). Tablets (chewable) 500 and 750 mg (Tums E-X)	200 and 300 mg	
Calcium citrate	21.2%	*Oral:* 950 mg to 1.9 g (equivalent to 200 to 400 mg elemental calcium) three or four times daily.	Citracal 950 (Mission). Tablets 950 mg	200 mg	Nonprescription. More soluble and is absorbed more effectively than calcium carbonate in fasting normal (Nicar and Pak, 1985) and achlorhydric individuals. The incidence of achlorhydria increases with age and thus may affect postmenopausal women and elderly men who are at risk for osteoporosis. A preliminary report suggested that urinary calcium oxalate crystal and kidney stone formation may be decreased when this preparation is used for calcium supplementation (Harvey et al, 1985).
			Citracal 1500D (Mission). Tablets 1.5 g with 200 USP units vitamin D	381 mg	
			Citracal Liquitab (Mission). Effervescent tablets 2.376 g	500 mg	

(table continued on next page)

TABLE 2 (continued)

Generic Name	Amount of Elemental Calcium	Dosage	Preparations	Elemental Calcium Present in Preparation	Indications Comments
Calcium glubionate	6.5%	*Oral: Adults,* 15 g daily in divided doses; *children,* 500 mg/kg daily in divided doses.	Neo-Calglucon (Sandoz). Syrup 1.8 g/5 ml	23.8 mg/ml	Nonprescription. May cause diarrhea. Probably obsolete.
Calcium lactate	13%	*Oral:* See manufacturers' literature for dosage recommendation.	Generic. Tablets 325 and 650 mg	42.2 and 84.5 mg	Nonprescription. May be used to treat mild hypocalcemia and for maintenance therapy. However, use is impractical because of the large number of tablets needed to achieve a therapeutic effect. Probably obsolete.
PARENTERAL PREPARATIONS					
Calcium chloride	27.2%	*Intravenous: Adults,* 5 to 10 ml of a 10% solution infused slowly.	Generic. Solution 10% in 10 ml containers	27.2 mg/ml	Effective in severe hypocalcemia, but other salts usually preferred because calcium chloride is more irritating to the veins and subcutaneous tissue and care must be taken to avoid extravasation. Should never be administered intramuscularly. Rarely given orally because this salt irritates the gastrointestinal tract. Probably obsolete.
Calcium gluceptate	8.2%	*Intravenous: Adults,* 5 to 20 ml. *Newborn infants,* to prevent hypocalcemia during exchange transfusion, 0.5 ml after every 100 ml of blood exchanged. *Intramuscular:* 2 to 5 ml in gluteal region or, in *infants,* in the lateral thigh.	Generic. Solution 220 mg/ml in 1, 5, 50, and 100 ml containers	18 mg/ml	Effective for severe hypocalcemia when given intravenously. Also given intramuscularly to infants and other patients in whom intravenous administration is not feasible. This salt is well tolerated, although mild local reactions may occur. Transient tingling sensation and metallic taste may be noted after intravenous injection.
Calcium gluconate	9%	*Intravenous: Adults,* initially, 20 ml of a 10% solution injected slowly over 10 minutes, followed by slow infusion of 1 mg elemental calcium/kg/hr. *Infants,* 2 ml/kg of 10% solution.	Generic. Solution 10% in 10, 50, 100, and 200 ml containers	9 mg/ml	Intravenous administration is treatment of choice in severe hypoglycemia. Not irritating to the veins but has been reported to cause skin necrosis and sloughing in infants. Intramuscular route should not be used because it is irritating, painful, and may cause abscess formation.

Miacalcin (Sandoz). Solution (sterile) 200 IU/ml in 2 ml containers.

CALCIUM PREPARATIONS

For information on specific calcium compounds, see Table 2.

Hypercalcemia may occur during long-term therapy with any calcium preparation, particularly in patients also receiving a vitamin D preparation.

Intravenous calcium should be administered cautiously to patients taking digitalis because calcium enhances the effect of this glycoside and may precipitate arrhythmias. If intravenous administration is necessary in these patients because of severe hypocalcemia (ie, tetany), the infusion should be given very slowly.

All calcium preparations are classified in FDA Pregnancy Category C.

ESTROGENS

Estrogens are used in postmenopausal women (natural or surgical menopause) for prophylaxis of osteoporosis or to prevent progression of established disease. Although any estrogen may be used, oral preparations of conjugated estrogens are most widely prescribed in the United States. Transdermal application is an alternative route.

DOSAGE AND PREPARATIONS.

Oral: For prophylaxis of osteoporosis in postmenopausal women, 0.625 mg conjugated estrogens or the equivalent daily for 25 days each month. A progestin may be added during the last 10 to 13 days of medication or used continuously with estrogen, especially in women with an intact uterus, to prevent endometrial hyperplasia and carcinoma. Alternatively, estrogen may be administered daily (continuous) with a progestin added daily (continuous) or for 14 consecutive days each calendar month (cyclical). (See also index entry Estrogens, Uses, Osteoporosis.)

CONJUGATED ESTROGENS:

Premarin (Wyeth-Ayerst). Tablets 0.3, 0.625, 0.9, 1.25, and 2.5 mg.

For other estrogen preparations, see index entry Estrogens, Preparations.

Transdermal: See index entry Estradiol, Uses, Gynecologic Disorders.

ESTRADIOL:

Estraderm (CIBA). Transdermal system 0.05 and 0.1 mg.

ETIDRONATE DISODIUM

[Didronel, Didronel I.V. Infusion]

$$Na^{+}\,{}^{-}O-\underset{\underset{O}{\|}}{\overset{\overset{OH}{|}}{P}}-\underset{\underset{CH_3}{|}}{\overset{\overset{OH}{|}}{C}}-\underset{\underset{O}{\|}}{\overset{\overset{OH}{|}}{P}}-O^{-}\,Na^{+}$$

ACTIONS AND USES. This bisphosphonate compound slows osteoclastic activity and the coupled response of osteoblastic activity. It is used to treat symptomatic patients with Paget's disease of bone. The oral route of administration for this drug is more convenient than the parenteral route required with calcitonin.

Like calcitonin, etidronate lowers serum alkaline phosphatase and urinary hydroxyproline levels, reduces cardiac output by decreasing bone vascularity, and may improve bone histology and reduce bone pain. One to three months of therapy may elapse before biochemical improvement occurs (60% of patients show symptomatic improvement). However, reduction in urinary hydroxyproline occurs earlier. Maximal effects are achieved within six months, and bone turnover may be reduced to one-half the pretreatment rate. Elevated osteoclast counts decrease, and resorption surfaces are reduced (Johnston et al, 1980).

The greatest effectiveness and longest remissions are achieved in patients with moderate disease. Although biochemical remission may persist for 18 months or more after a single course of therapy, the serum alkaline phosphatase and urinary hydroxyproline levels may increase when the drug is discontinued. When relapse occurs, subsequent courses should be given *intermittently* because the safety of long-term continuous therapy, which may lead to significant osteomalacia, has not been established. The use of etidronate to treat Paget's disease has been reviewed (Altman, 1985).

Results of two randomized, placebo-controlled, double-blind prospective trials in women with postmenopausal osteoporosis and vertebral fractures indicate that cyclical administration of etidronate for two to three years (400 mg daily for two weeks, followed by a 10- to 13-week drug-free interval) increases the bone mineral density of the spine and decreases the rate of new vertebral fractures (Storm et al, 1990; Watts et al, 1990). However, after three years, the decreased fracture rate may be restricted to patients at highest risk for recurrent fractures; others may experience a relative increase in new fractures after this period (Harris et al, 1993). Further study is required to determine the role of long-term, cyclical administration of etidronate, particularly in patients who are at lower risk for recurrent fractures.

The intravenous preparation of etidronate is used to reduce hypercalcemia associated with malignancy by reducing bone resorption, which results in lowering of serum calcium (see the section on Hypercalcemia). Saline and diuretics are given concurrently.

Etidronate also is given to prevent and treat heterotopic ossification due to spinal cord injury and total hip replacement.

ADVERSE REACTIONS AND PRECAUTIONS. Etidronate is usually well tolerated, but nausea and diarrhea have been reported, particularly in patients receiving oral doses of 10 to 20 mg/kg/day. These effects are often alleviated by dividing the total daily dose. The serum phosphate level may increase when this dosage is given, presumably because of increased renal reabsorption, but therapy should not be discontinued. This elevation usually does not occur when 5 mg/kg/day is employed. Elevated serum phosphate levels generally return to normal two to four weeks after therapy ceases. Patients with impaired renal function (reduced glomerular filtration rates) should receive smaller doses and should be monitored closely.

The most serious adverse effect of etidronate is inhibition of bone mineralization. Accumulation of unmineralized osteoid is common in patients receiving large doses (10 to 20 mg/kg daily) for prolonged periods but also may occur when lower doses (5 mg/kg/day) are given for long periods. New episodes of incapacitating bone pain and fractures have occurred during a six-month period of treatment with doses of 10 to 20 mg/kg daily (Canfield et al, 1977). Although unusual, fractures also have been reported with doses as low as 5 mg/kg daily (Boyce et al, 1984). Bone pain alone occurs in up to 10% of patients receiving 5 mg/kg daily.

This drug is classified in FDA Pregnancy Category C.

PHARMACOKINETICS. Approximately 1% of an oral dose of 5 mg/kg/day is absorbed; the amount is increased to about 2.5% at 10 mg/kg/day and to 6% at 20 mg/kg/day. The rest is excreted unchanged in the feces. Approximately 50% of the absorbed dose is chemisorbed to bone; the rest is excreted unchanged in the urine.

DOSAGE AND PREPARATIONS.

Oral: *Adults,* for Paget's disease, etidronate should be given as a single daily dose with water. Eating should be avoided for two hours before and after taking the medication. Initially, 5 mg/kg is given daily for no longer than six months. Larger doses should be reserved for use when there is a need for rapid suppression of increased bone turnover or prompt reduction of elevated cardiac output. When more than 10 mg/kg daily is given (maximum, 20 mg/kg), the treatment period should not exceed three months. Increased or recurrent bone pain and/or pain at previously asymptomatic sites has been reported. If therapy is continued, pain may resolve in some patients but persist in others. If fractures occur, the drug should be withheld until signs of callus formation are evident. Serum alkaline phosphatase and/or urinary hydroxyproline levels should be monitored during and after therapy. Treatment may be initiated again after a drug-free period of at least three months if there is biochemical, symptomatic, or other evidence of active disease.

For heterotopic ossification due to spinal cord injury, 20 mg/kg daily is given for two weeks, followed by 10 mg/kg daily for ten weeks (total treatment period, 12 weeks). For heterotopic ossification following total hip replacement, 20 mg/kg is given daily for one month before and three months after surgery (four months total).

For osteoporosis, 400 mg for two weeks followed by a 10- to 13-week drug-free interval; calcium 1.5 g should be given daily during the drug-free interval. Cyclic administration may continue for up to three years.

Didronel (Procter & Gamble). Tablets 200 and 400 mg.

Intravenous: *Adults,* for hypercalcemia due to malignancy, initially, 7.5 mg/kg, diluted in at least 250 ml of sterile isotonic sodium chloride injection, is infused daily over a period of *at least four hours* for three to five consecutive days. If the hypercalcemia recurs, another course of therapy may be given, but there should be at least a seven-day interval between courses. The dose and manner of retreatment are the same as for initial treatment.

For patients with Paget's disease who have early hearing loss or other neurologic complications, 4.3 mg/kg/day intravenously for seven days.

Didronel I.V. Infusion (MGI Pharma). Solution 50 mg/ml in 6 ml containers.

FUROSEMIDE

[Lasix]

For chemical formula, see index entry Furosemide, As Diuretic.

ACTIONS AND USES. Furosemide reduces the serum calcium concentration by increasing urinary calcium excretion. This diuretic blocks active sodium chloride transport in the thick ascending limb of Henle's loop. Since the calcium ion is handled like the sodium ion in this segment of the nephron, a parallel increase in calcium excretion occurs due to blocked resorption of calcium. However, large intravenous doses (100 mg every two hours) are required to achieve direct calciuretic and hypocalcemic effects. This is not a convenient method of treatment and is associated with significant side effects (eg, ototoxicity, dehydration). Thus, the major role of furosemide in therapy for hypercalcemia is as a diuretic administered in small doses to prevent fluid overload during aggressive saline hydration.

For treatment of hypercalcemia, it is important to restore normal blood volume by hydration, which will increase urine calcium excretion by 100 to 300 mg per day. Furosemide may be given intravenously in conjunction with isotonic sodium chloride to reduce the serum calcium level rapidly in the emergency treatment of hypercalcemia. The saline solution should be administered before the diuretic to ensure adequate expansion of the extracellular fluid volume. Aggressive hydration therapy may decrease serum calcium by 4 mg/dL or more within 24 hours. During diuresis, urinary loss of water and electrolytes (including sodium, potassium, and magnesium) should be measured carefully and replaced. If these measures are not followed, severe fluid and electrolyte disturbances may occur. In addition, volume contraction may increase reabsorption of calcium in the proximal tubule and reduce the therapeutic response.

ADVERSE REACTIONS AND PRECAUTIONS. See index entry Furosemide, As Diuretic.

DOSAGE AND PREPARATIONS.

Intravenous: Large doses should be given at a rate not exceeding 4 mg/min to avoid ototoxic reactions. Maintenance of extracellular fluid volume to avoid hypovolemia and exacerbation of hypercalcemia is essential. *Adults,* for severe hypercalcemia, a bolus infusion of 40 to 160 mg after infusion of isotonic sodium chloride. The diuretic response should be assessed before subsequent doses are given. It is essential that fluid status be carefully monitored to avoid dehydration and exacerbation of the hypercalcemic condition. In general, "standing orders" for administration of furosemide in these patients are not advisable. Smaller doses may be given every two to four hours in less severely affected patients. *Children,* 25 to 50 mg every four hours.

Lasix (Hoechst), ***Generic***. Solution 10 mg/ml in 2, 4, and 10 ml containers.

GALLIUM NITRATE
[Ganite]

ACTIONS. This hydrated nitrate salt of the group IIIa element gallium exerts a hypocalcemic effect by inhibiting bone resorption; bone formation may increase as well. In animal studies, no cytotoxic effects on bone cells were observed. In rats, gallium nitrate localizes in metabolically active regions of the bone such as the growth plate and endosteal and periosteal surfaces of cortical bone. Urinary calcium and hydroxyproline excretion are reduced in patients with bone metastases and hypercalcemia. The drug increases calcium and osteocalcin content of bone and enhances incorporation of hydroxyproline into new bone collagen, which suggests that it has a stimulatory effect on bone protein formation. Myelosuppression has not been observed.

USES. Gallium nitrate is indicated for the treatment of cancer-related hypercalcemia that has not responded to hydration. It is equally effective in patients with epidermoid and nonepidermoid malignancies, unlike calcitonin and etidronate, which are relatively ineffective in patients with the former. The drug is being investigated for use (primarily by subcutaneous injection) in the treatment of Paget's disease of bone, for skeletal metastases, and for osteoporosis.

ADVERSE REACTIONS AND PRECAUTIONS. When administered according to the regimen below, gallium nitrate may be nephrotoxic. Thus, it should be given only after the patient has been adequately hydrated with intravenous fluids. Careful monitoring of urine output and renal function is important. Gallium nitrate should not be used in patients with severe renal impairment (serum creatinine ≥ 2.5 mg/dL) or those who are otherwise at risk for nephrotoxicity (Warrell et al, 1988). Hypophosphatemia (asymptomatic) and mild respiratory alkalosis occur commonly after treatment with this drug. Mild hypochromic microcytic anemia has been reported in several patients in whom the subcutaneous route was used for extended periods.

This drug is classified in FDA Pregnancy Category C.

PHARMACOKINETICS. Gallium nitrate has an initial plasma half-life of one hour and, upon prolonged intravenous administration, a plasma half-life of 72 to 115 hours. Continuous infusion of 200 mg/M^2/day achieves plasma steady-state levels of 1 to 1.5 mg/L within 48 hours (Warrell et al, 1986; Todd and Fitton, 1991). The mean volume of distribution at steady-state and plasma clearance are 1.27 L/kg and 0.04 L/hour/kg, respectively. The drug is excreted mainly in the urine.

DOSAGE AND PREPARATIONS.

Intravenous: For hypercalcemia, after the patient has been hydrated adequately with intravenous fluids, 200 mg/M^2 is diluted with one liter of 5% dextrose or 0.9% sodium chloride and administered by continuous infusion over 24 hours daily for five days. In patients with mild hypercalcemia or few symptoms, 100 mg/M^2/day for five days may be adequate. If the serum calcium concentration decreases to the normal range in less than five days, treatment should be discontinued.

Subcutaneous: For palliation of skeletal metastases and for therapy of Paget's disease of bone, 20 mg/M^2 (or a fixed dose of 30 mg in adults) once daily for 14 days. In patients with skeletal metastases, the initial two weeks of therapy is followed by a two-week drug-free interval, and this cycle can be repeated monthly. Patients who do not respond after three cycles are unlikely to respond to further administration of gallium nitrate. For patients with Paget's disease, the first two weeks of therapy are followed by a drug-free interval of two to four weeks, and this cycle can be repeated over the following 6 to 12 months.

Ganite (Fujisawa). Solution (for injection) containing gallium nitrate (anhydrous) 25 mg and sodium citrate dihydrate 28.75 mg/ml in 20 ml containers. When gallium nitrate is added to 0.9% sodium chloride or 5% dextrose, the solution is stable for at least 48 hours at room temperature and for seven days if refrigerated.

PAMIDRONATE DISODIUM
[Aredia]

ACTIONS. This amino-substituted bisphosphonate analogue of pyrophosphate rapidly chemisorbs to calcium on the surface of hydroxyapatite crystals, preferentially in areas of high bone turnover, thereby reducing the solubility of the mineralized matrix and rendering it more resistant to osteoclastic resorption (Kellihan and Mangino, 1992). In addition, the attachment of osteoclast precursors to the mineralized matrix is impaired when previously bound pamidronate is released in high local concentrations from the matrix surface during the early phase of resorption; transformation of precursors into mature, functioning osteoclasts and dissolution of bone matrix are then inhibited (Boonekamp et al, 1987; Lowik et al, 1988; Ralston et al, 1988).

Concentrations of pamidronate that inhibit bone resorption have little effect on osteoblastic activity or on the mineralization of newly formed bone; half-maximal inhibition of mineralization requires doses 50 times larger than those required for half-maximal inhibition of resorption (Reitsma et al, 1980). These properties result in inhibited bone resorption, reduced release of minerals into the circulation, and decreased serum mineral concentrations when pamidronate is administered in therapeutic doses.

USES. Pamidronate disodium, in conjunction with adequate hydration (resulting in urine output of at least 2 L/day), is the therapy of choice in the treatment of moderate or severe hypercalcemia associated with malignancy with or without bone metastases.

The safety and efficacy of pamidronate in the treatment of hypercalcemia associated with conditions that are not tumor-related have not been established. Single intravenous infusions of pamidronate (30 mg) reduced plasma calcium concentrations in patients with mild primary hyperparathyroidism, but clinical status was unaffected (Schmidli et al, 1990). In a small number of patients, hypercalcemia secondary to immobilization has been reported to respond well to intravenous pamidronate (10 to 45 mg) (Gallacher et al, 1990). Multiple intravenous infusions of 20 to 30 mg did not retard the radiographic progression of periarticular bone lesions associated with rheumatoid arthritis (Ralston et al, 1989 B; Tan et al, 1989).

Pamidronate also may be effective in the treatment of a variety of other conditions characterized by pathologic bone loss, such as Paget's disease and osteoporosis. (See the discussion on these disorders in the Introduction.)

The safety and effectiveness of pamidronate in children have not been established.

ADVERSE REACTIONS. Intravenous doses of up to 90 mg/day are generally well tolerated. Transient fever, leukopenia, and lymphopenia occurred within the first 72 hours after drug administration in up to 50% of patients in clinical trials (Fitton and McTavish, 1991; Fleisch, 1991). Fatigue, swelling and pain at the site of injection, nausea, and anorexia are common in patients receiving 90 mg of pamidronate but uncommon in those receiving 60 mg. At least 15% of patients treated with pamidronate for hypercalcemia of malignancy experience fluid overload, hypertension, abdominal pain, constipation, and bone pain. Other adverse reactions include malaise, rash, thrombophlebitis, and granulocytopenia. Focal osteomalacia also has occurred.

Asymptomatic hypophosphatemia (8%), hypokalemia (18%), hypomagnesemia (12%), and hypocalcemia (12%) have been reported in patients receiving doses of 90 mg; the incidence of these reactions is much lower when 60 mg is used. More severe hypophosphatemia may occur and require supplemental phosphate therapy.

Several patients with symptomatic hypercalcemia of malignancy and renal impairment have been treated successfully with intravenous pamidronate without further deterioration in renal function (Yap et al, 1990). However, large intravenous doses have been associated with reversible degenerative nephropathies (focal tubular fibrosis, tubulointerstitial nephritis) in rats and dogs.

PRECAUTIONS. Serum calcium, sodium, potassium, phosphate, magnesium, and creatinine concentrations must be monitored closely during pamidronate treatment. Patients with pre-existing anemia, leukopenia, or thrombocytopenia should be monitored carefully during the first two weeks following treatment.

Patients should be hydrated adequately throughout treatment, but overhydration should be avoided. Renal function should be evaluated periodically. When the serum creatinine concentration exceeds 5 mg/dL, the benefit-to-risk ratio should be considered carefully.

Pamidronate is classified in FDA Pregnancy Category C.

This drug should not be used in patients who are hypersensitive to bisphosphonates.

DRUG INTERACTIONS. *Pamidronate must not be mixed with infusion solutions containing calcium.*

PHARMACOKINETICS. In cancer patients, 45% to 53% of an intravenous dose of 60 mg infused over 24 hours is rapidly adsorbed to bone, preferentially in areas of high turnover, and the remainder is excreted unchanged in the urine within 72 hours (Fitton and McTavish, 1991). Three groups of patients with skeletal metastases were given infusions of pamidronate 60 mg for 1, 4, or 24 hours (Leyvraz et al, 1992). The median body retention at 24 hours did not vary significantly with the rate of infusion and was 60% to 70% of the dose in all three groups. The percentage retained varied approximately threefold within each group. Most of the variance was attributable to a direct correlation between the number of skeletal metastases and body retention of pamidronate, although differences in patients' creatinine clearance rates also appeared to contribute to the variance. Estimates of pharmacokinetic parameters in the group given one-hour infusions included a mean half-life for the distribution phase of 0.8 ± 0.3 hours, a mean area under the plasma concentration x time curve of 22.0 ± 8.8 μmol/L x hours, and a mean maximal plasma concentration of 9.7 μmol/L. The half-life for the elimination phase could not be estimated because plasma concentrations fell below the limit of detection in most patients between 5 and 24 hours after the one-hour infusion. The rate of release of bound pamidronate from bone is slow and depends on the rate of local bone turnover; this also makes it difficult to estimate the half-life for the elimination phase.

DOSAGE AND PREPARATIONS. *Pamidronate must not be mixed with infusion solutions containing calcium.* The powder is diluted in 1,000 ml of sterile isotonic sodium chloride injection for infusion.

Intravenous: For moderate hypercalcemia associated with malignancy, *adults,* initially, 60 to 90 mg infused over 2 to 24 hours, depending on patient response. If hypercalcemia recurs, treatment may be repeated, but seven days or more should elapse between doses.

For symptomatic bone metastases, *adults,* 30 to 60 mg biweekly or 60 to 90 mg monthly over 1 to 24 hours, depending on patient response.

For Paget's disease of bone, *adults,* initially, 60 mg infused over 1 to 24 hours, depending on patient response. Treatment may be repeated after three to six months, if necessary.

Aredia (Ciba). Powder (lyophilized, sterile) 30 mg.

PHOSPHATE SALTS

Phosphates are used for the long-term treatment of patients with hypophosphatemic rickets or osteomalacia. They also have been administered to treat hypercalcemia, but this use is not encouraged because of the risks, including fatalities, that can result from precipitation of calcium phosphate in the soft tissues.

Intravenous administration of phosphates is no longer justified. Hypocalcemia, hypotension and shock, myocardial infarction, tetany, and acute renal failure have occurred, and deaths have been reported. Deposition of calcium phosphate in the kidney, heart, lungs, and blood vessels also may be fatal.

Although oral administration is less hazardous, deaths have been reported when phosphate was administered by this route for hypercalcemia (Vernava et al, 1987) (see also the discussion on Hypercalcemia in the Introduction). If oral phosphate is administered for hypercalcemia, careful monitoring of serum electrolyte levels and renal function is necessary. Hypocalcemia and even mild hyperphosphatemia must be avoided.

Phosphates should not be administered to patients with impaired renal function or hyperphosphatemia. They also should not be given to patients with alkaline urine due to urinary tract infections because increased calcium and phosphate concentrations in the alkaline urine increase the risk of calcium phosphate stones. Phosphate should be given as the potassium rather than the sodium salt because the latter causes volume expansion and inhibits phosphate reabsorption, thus negating the therapeutic effect.

These products are classified in FDA Pregnancy Category C.

DOSAGE AND PREPARATIONS.

Oral: *Adults,* 1 to 2 g of phosphorus daily in divided doses. The sodium-free preparations (K-Phos Original, Neutra-Phos K) should be used in patients on sodium-restricted diets. Following remission, the dose should be reduced to maintain a normal serum calcium concentration.

K-Phos M.F. (Beach). Each tablet contains potassium acid phosphate 155 mg and sodium acid phosphate 350 mg.

K-Phos Neutral (Beach). Each tablet contains phosphorus 250 mg, sodium 298 mg, and potassium 45 mg.

K-Phos No. 2 (Beach). Each tablet contains potassium acid phosphate 305 mg and sodium acid phosphate 700 mg.

K-Phos Original (Sodium Free) (Beach). Each tablet contains potassium acid phosphate 500 mg.

Neutra-Phos (Baker Norton). Each 75 ml of solution (after reconstitution) or packet contains phosphorus 250 mg, sodium 164 mg, and potassium 278 mg (both forms nonprescription).

Neutra-Phos K (Baker Norton). Each 75 ml of solution (after reconstitution) or packet contains phosphorus 250 mg and potassium 556 mg (sodium-free) (both forms nonprescription).

PLICAMYCIN (Mithramycin)

[Mithracin]

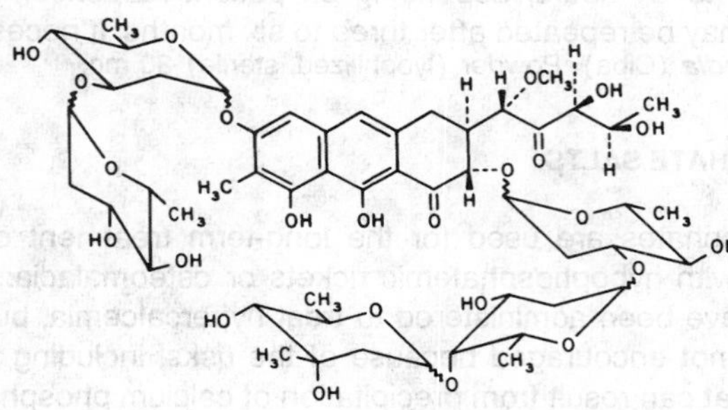

ACTIONS AND USES. Plicamycin is a cytotoxic antibiotic formerly used to treat testicular neoplasms; newer combination regimens have, for the most part, replaced it for this indication. It decreases serum calcium levels in both hypercalcemic and normocalcemic individuals, probably by a direct toxic effect on osteoclasts in bone. Plicamycin presently is used only to treat severe hypercalcemia associated with carcinoma (with or without bony metastases) and is one of the more effective agents for this purpose. In some patients, a single infusion reduces serum calcium levels within 24 to 48 hours without serious toxic effects; in others, a satisfactory response may require several infusions. The duration of action may be only a few days but occasionally persists for longer periods. Because newer agents with comparable efficacy but reduced toxicity have become available in the last several years (eg, pamidronate, gallium nitrate), plicamycin has been replaced as first-line therapy for acute management of patients with cancer-related hypercalcemia.

Plicamycin has been used in Paget's disease of bone, but calcitonin and etidronate are less toxic. Occasionally, plicamycin is used in patients with severe disease who are unresponsive to other therapy.

ADVERSE REACTIONS AND PRECAUTIONS. In addition to anorexia, nausea, and vomiting, plicamycin can produce severe thrombocytopenia and abnormalities in multiple clotting factors that may progress to a hemorrhagic diathesis. The gastrointestinal distress can be minimized by using a slow infusion rate. Abnormal results of hepatic and renal function tests also have been reported. With the exception of nausea and vomiting, adverse reactions are infrequent after single doses of 25 mcg/kg or when multiple doses are separated by intervals of several days. They occur more frequently if the interval between doses is shorter or if more than three to four doses must be given (Bilezikian, 1992). Although lower doses are used for hypercalcemia than for neoplasms, the same precautions and contraindications apply (see index entry Plicamycin, As Antineoplastic Agent). It also is important to monitor serum calcium and potassium levels closely when treating hypercalcemic patients. Plicamycin generally should not be used in patients with renal or hepatic disease, bone marrow depression, thrombocytopathy, coagulation disorders, or increased susceptibility to bleeding from other causes.

Plicamycin is classified in FDA Pregnancy Category X.

DOSAGE AND PREPARATIONS.

Intravenous: 10 to 50 mcg/kg (25 mcg/kg in most patients with normal kidney function; 10 to 20 mcg/kg in patients with impaired renal function) is added to 5% dextrose in water or isotonic saline and infused over 30 minutes. Prolonged infusions over several hours are unnecessary and may cause protracted vomiting. Appropriate prophylactic antiemetic therapy should be given. If serum calcium levels are not reduced after 48 hours, 25 mcg/kg may be given every other day for two to four doses. Additional courses may be administered if hypercalcemia is not controlled, but this increases potential toxicity. Alternatively, one to three doses may be given weekly, depending on the patient's response. The drug should be discontinued after three infusions or sooner when a favorable effect has been achieved.

Mithracin (Miles). Powder (cryodesiccated) 2.5 mg with mannitol 100 mg and sufficient disodium phosphate to adjust to pH 7.

THIAZIDES

Although most diuretics that promote renal sodium loss also increase renal calcium loss, the thiazide diuretics reduce urinary calcium excretion. The mechanism is not completely understood but appears to involve enhanced calcium reabsorption in the distal tubule.

Thiazides (in conjunction with a low-sodium diet) have been recommended as adjuncts to calcium and vitamin D in hypoparathyroidism, but their efficacy in this condition must be confirmed. It is unlikely that the thiazides alone will be effective in patients with severe hypoparathyroidism (eg, serum calcium <7.5 mg/dL) because urinary calcium excretion is already minimal in such patients.

Because thiazides reduce urinary calcium excretion temporarily, it has been suggested that selection of a thiazide when a diuretic is needed may help prevent bone loss in older individuals. However, thiazides are not suggested as a treatment per se for osteoporosis except as an adjunct during prolonged glucocorticoid therapy to minimize urinary calcium excretion and prevent the development of secondary osteoporosis (see the section on Osteoporosis).

The adverse effects of prolonged thiazide therapy are discussed elsewhere; see index entry Thiazides, Uses, Diuresis.

DOSAGE AND PREPARATIONS. See index entry Thiazides, Uses, Diuresis.

VITAMIN D PREPARATIONS

The vitamin D requirement of the body is fulfilled by ingestion of vitamin D_2 (ergocalciferol) or D_3 (cholecalciferol) or by ultraviolet irradiation of 7-dehydrocholesterol to vitamin D_3 in the skin. Vitamin D_3 (or D_2) is hydroxylated at C-25 in the liver to produce 25-OHD_3 (or D_2), which is the major metabolite circulating in the plasma. This compound is available commercially as calcifediol [Calderol]. The metabolite is further hydroxylated in the kidney to 1,25-$(OH)_2D_3$ (or D_2), the most active metabolite in initiating intestinal transport of calcium and phosphate and mobilization of mineral from bone. 1,25$(OH)_2D_3$ is available commercially as calcitriol [Calcijex, Rocaltrol]. An analogue of this metabolite, alfacalcidol (1-α-OHD_3), is used in Europe, Canada, and Japan to treat renal osteodystrophy and is under investigation in this country. Alfacalcidol is converted in the liver to calcitriol. Another metabolite of vitamin D, 24,25-$(OH)_2D_3$, is formed in the kidney and bone, but its metabolic actions are uncertain.

In general, the onset of action of vitamin D is slow and the duration of action is long. The metabolites act more rapidly (a calcemic response may be obtained with calcitriol in one or two days) and have shorter biological half-lives.

VITAMIN D_2 (Ergocalciferol)
[Calciferol, Drisdol]

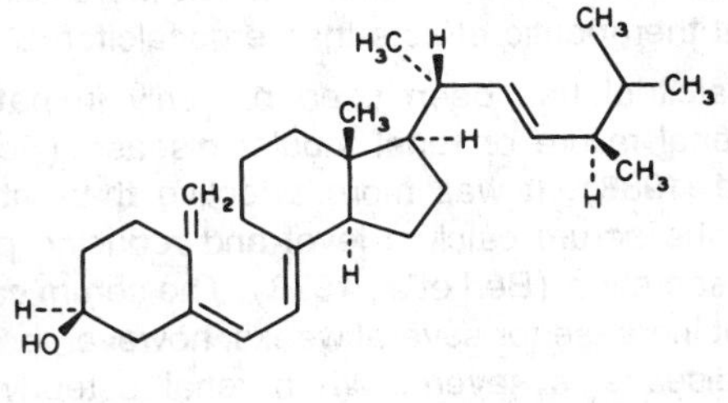

ACTIONS AND USES. Vitamin D is used in hypoparathyroidism, vitamin D deficiency states (eg, simple and conditioned deficiencies, genetic vitamin D-dependent rickets, malabsorption, impaired renal or hepatic metabolism), and as an adjunct in osteomalacia associated with hypophosphatemia and renal tubular disorders. In parathyroid hormone deficiency, large doses of vitamin D increase serum calcium levels and there may be a moderate reciprocal decrease in serum phosphorus levels. Large doses may be associated with phosphaturia, increased mobilization of mineral from bone, and increased intestinal absorption of calcium, phosphate, and magnesium; these effects account for the elevation of serum calcium concentrations.

Rickets and osteomalacia caused by dietary deficiency of vitamin D and inadequate exposure to sunlight respond rapidly to physiologic doses of vitamin D, but much larger doses are required to treat vitamin D-dependent and resistant rickets. In malabsorption disorders, effective treatment of the primary cause usually cures associated osteomalacia or rickets, but if the underlying condition does not respond to therapy, life-long administration of large doses of vitamin D and calcium may be necessary. In hypophosphatemic states (vitamin D-resistant or familial hypophosphatemic rickets) and renal tubular disorders, large doses of vitamin D may be needed, but correction of hypophosphatemia or acidosis is of primary importance.

The low serum levels of 25-OHD_3 observed in patients receiving long-term phenytoin, phenobarbital, rifampin, or glutethimide therapy have been attributed to drug-induced stimulation of hepatic microsomal enzymes, which is presumed to accelerate the metabolism of vitamin D_3 to inactive metabolites. For this reason, prophylactic doses of vitamin D may be desirable during prolonged therapy with these drugs. Pharmacologic doses are indicated when overt bone disease is associated with impaired hepatic or renal metabolism of vitamin D.

The lag between initiation of vitamin D therapy and onset of effectiveness is 10 to 14 days or longer, depending on the preparation used. The onset of action of ergocalciferol is somewhat slower than that of dihydrotachysterol and the duration of effect is more prolonged.

The dose of vitamin D should be based on measurement of the serum calcium concentration (in the early treatment period, weekly; with chronic treatment, about every three months). Urinary calcium excreted per day should be used as a guide, since this parameter often increases before the serum calcium concentration. Determination of the serum alkaline phosphatase level also may be helpful in monitoring the therapeutic response. It usually is elevated in patients with untreated rickets or osteomalacia and rises transiently during the first weeks to months of therapy ("alkaline phosphatase flare") before returning toward normal as skeletal healing continues. The dose of vitamin D should be reduced when the serum alkaline phosphatase level stops rising after the "flare."

ADVERSE REACTIONS AND PRECAUTIONS. Vitamin D is potent and potentially harmful. Hypercalcemia produced by overdosage can cause gastrointestinal and central nervous system disturbances and soft tissue calcification. Renal complications may be severe, and death may result. If hypercalcemia persists, the possibility of renal damage continues long after the drug is discontinued. Adverse effects occasionally result from increased sensitivity in patients not receiving excessive doses.

Vitamin D should be given cautiously to patients receiving digitalis because hypercalcemia may precipitate arrhythmias.

This drug is classified in FDA Pregnancy Category C. (See also index entry Vitamin D.)

DOSAGE AND PREPARATIONS.

Oral: For hypoparathyroidism, *adults,* initially, 50,000 to 200,000 IU daily as soon as acute tetany is controlled with an intravenous calcium preparation. The maintenance dose is usually 25,000 to 100,000 IU daily. *Children,* 10,000 to 25,000 IU daily.

For osteomalacia and rickets caused by dietary deficiency of vitamin D, *adults,* initially, 1,000 to 2,000 IU daily; for maintenance, 400 IU daily. *Children,* initially, 1,000 to 4,000 IU daily; for maintenance, 400 IU daily.

For genetic vitamin D-dependent rickets, *children,* 5,000 to 50,000 IU daily.

For familial hypophosphatemia or other forms due to renal phosphate wasting (vitamin D-resistant rickets), *children,* 25,000 to 100,000 IU daily in conjunction with a high phosphate intake and calcium supplements. *Adults,* 50,000 to 200,000 IU daily in conjunction with a high phosphate intake.

For osteomalacia in malabsorption syndromes, *adults,* 10,000 to 50,000 IU daily. *Children,* 10,000 to 25,000 IU daily. For osteomalacia in hepatobiliary disease, *adults,* 10,000 to 40,000 IU daily. *Children,* 10,000 to 25,000 IU daily. For osteomalacia associated with anticonvulsant therapy, *adults and children,* 1,000 IU daily.

For renal osteodystrophy (now rarely used in chronic renal failure), *adults,* 20,000 to 50,000 IU daily.

VITAMIN D_2 (ERGOCALCIFEROL):
Available generically under name Vitamin D (capsules 25,000 and 50,000 IU).

Calciferol (Schwarz). Liquid 8,000 IU/ml (nonprescription); tablets 50,000 IU.

Drisdol (Sanofi Winthrop). Capsules 50,000 IU; liquid 8,000 IU/ml (nonprescription).

DIHYDROTACHYSTEROL (DHT)

[DHT, Hytakerol]

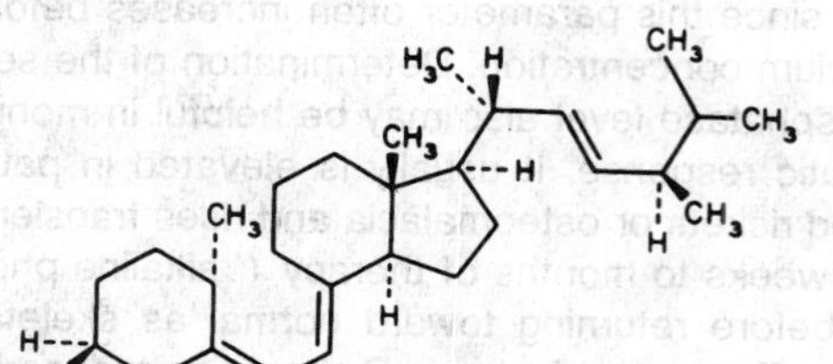

This form of vitamin D is hydroxylated in the liver but does not require renal activation. It acts somewhat more rapidly than the D_2 and D_3 forms. In comparison to ergocalciferol, the phosphate diuresis produced by dihydrotachysterol is almost as great, the intestinal absorption of calcium is less (on a molar basis), and the serum calcium concentration rises more rapidly. Because its duration of action is shorter, the hazards of hypercalcemia are fewer with dihydrotachysterol than with ergocalciferol. (For adverse reactions and precautions, see index entry Vitamin D.)

Dihydrotachysterol has only weak antirachitic activity (about 1/450 that of vitamin D).

This drug is classified in FDA Pregnancy Category C.

DOSAGE AND PREPARATIONS.

Oral: For hypoparathyroidism, *adults,* initially, 0.75 to 2.5 mg daily; specific dosage is determined by frequent monitoring of serum calcium levels. For maintenance, 0.25 to 1.75 mg weekly has been given, but larger doses may be required in some patients.

For prevention of renal osteodystrophy, *adults,* initially, 0.1 to 0.25 mg daily. *Children,* initially, 0.01 mg daily. For patients on long-term hemodialysis, *adults,* initially, 0.25 to 0.375 mg daily. Some patients may require doses as large as 1 mg daily.

DHT (Roxane). Tablets 0.125, 0.2, and 0.4 mg; solution 0.2 mg/ml in 30 ml containers.

Hytakerol (Sanofi Winthrop). Capsules 0.125 mg; solution (in oil) 0.25 mg/ml in 15 ml containers.

CALCITRIOL

[Calcijex, Rocaltrol]

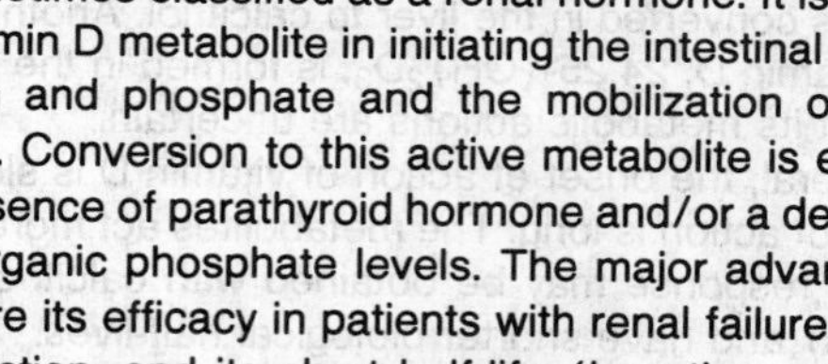

ACTIONS. Calcitriol is the synthetic preparation of 1,25-$(OH)_2D_3$. The endogenous product is produced in the kidney and is sometimes classified as a renal hormone. It is the most active vitamin D metabolite in initiating the intestinal transport of calcium and phosphate and the mobilization of mineral from bone. Conversion to this active metabolite is enhanced by the presence of parathyroid hormone and/or a decrease in serum inorganic phosphate levels. The major advantages of calcitriol are its efficacy in patients with renal failure, its rapid onset of action, and its short half-life (less than one day in contrast to three to four weeks for vitamin D), which makes toxic reactions easier to manage. On the other hand, the extreme potency and rapid onset of action of calcitriol necessitate caution in determining dosage because toxicity can occur very rapidly. Moreover, calcitriol is much more expensive for equivalent therapeutic effects than ergocalciferol.

USES. Calcitriol has been used primarily in patients with chronic renal failure or renal tubular disease (Feinfeld and Sherwood, 1988). It was more effective than vitamin D in elevating the serum calcium level and reducing parathyroid hormone secretion (Berl et al, 1978). The serum calcium level may not increase for several weeks, however, particularly if skeletal disease is severe. When renal osteodystrophy is present, calcitriol often relieves bone pain, permits increased physical activity, and may improve bone histology.

Calcitriol is effective in the treatment of hypoparathyroidism following thyroidectomy or parathyroid surgery. Idiopathic hypoparathyroidism also responds to calcitriol. Larger doses may be required during episodes of malabsorption and diarrhea. Calcitriol also is the preferred treatment for pseudoparathyroidism.

Calcitriol is used in various forms of rickets and osteomalacia and is the preferred treatment for Type I vitamin D-dependent rickets. Phosphate may be added to the regimen when hypophosphatemia also is present (eg, X-linked hypophosphatemic rickets).

ADVERSE REACTIONS. Calcitriol stimulates intestinal absorption of both calcium and phosphate, which are utilized in remineralization of the skeleton initially. A decrease in serum alkaline phosphatase serves as a warning of an impending increase in serum calcium. Metastatic calcification, decreased renal function, and increased serum phosphate concentrations are possible consequences. These complications may be avoided by decreasing the dose of calcitriol when the serum alkaline phosphatase concentration declines, by administering phosphate-binding agents to combat hyperphosphatemia, and by monitoring serum calcium and phosphate levels. (See the section on Renal Osteodystrophy.) To avoid soft tissue calcifications, the product of serum calcium and phosphate (Ca × P) should not be allowed to exceed 70. For other adverse reactions and precautions, see the evaluation on Vitamin D.

Calcitriol is classified in FDA Pregnancy Category C.

DOSAGE AND PREPARATIONS.

Oral: Initially, 0.25 mcg/day. If the response is not adequate, the dosage may be increased by 0.25 mcg/day at two- to four-week intervals for hypoparathyroid patients and at four- to eight-week intervals for dialysis patients, although some physicians suggest increasing dosage on a more rapid schedule. Serum calcium concentrations should be measured at least twice weekly, and the drug should be discontinued if hypercalcemia occurs. Treatment may be reinstituted when the serum calcium concentration is normal. Patients with normal or only slightly reduced serum calcium levels may respond to 0.25 mcg every other day. Most patients undergoing hemodialysis require 0.5 or 1 mcg/day. Most *adults and children 6 years and older* with hypoparathyroidism have responded to 0.5 to 2 mcg daily. Hypoparathyroid *children 1 to 5 years* are usually given 0.25 to 0.75 mcg daily.

Rocaltrol (Roche). Capsules 0.25 and 0.5 mcg.

Intravenous: *Adults,* initially, 0.5 mcg infused rapidly three times weekly or about every other day for dialysis patients. If the response is not adequate, the dosage may be increased by 0.25 to 0.5 mcg at two- to four-week intervals. If hypercalcemia occurs, the drug should be discontinued until the serum calcium concentration returns to normal. Treatment may be reinstituted at a dosage lower than the amount that induced hypercalcemia. Most patients require 0.5 to 3 mcg three times weekly.

Calcijex (Abbott). Solution (isotonic) 1 and 2 mcg/ml in 1 ml containers.

CALCIFEDIOL
[Calderol]

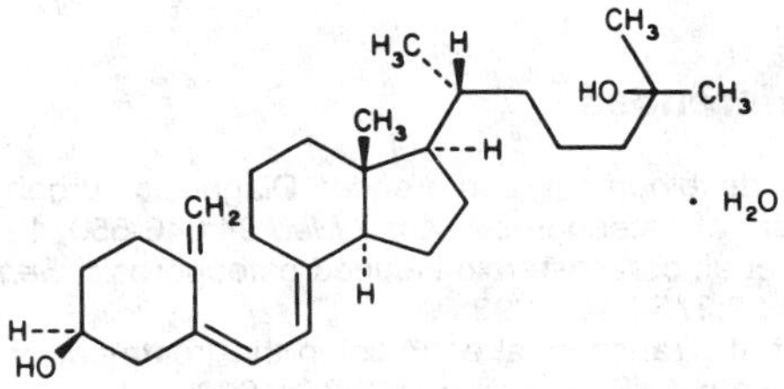

ACTIONS AND USES. Calcifediol is the synthetic preparation of 25-OHD_3. The endogenous product is formed in the liver from hydroxylation of vitamin D_3 and is the major form of vitamin D circulating in the blood. Levels of 25-OHD_3 can be monitored readily. Calcifediol is useful therapeutically because it is converted to the potent metabolite, 1,25-$(OH)_2D_3$ (calcitriol), and has some intrinsic activity. It is used in metabolic bone diseases associated with chronic renal failure in patients undergoing dialysis. This agent increases serum calcium and may decrease alkaline phosphatase and parathyroid hormone levels. Bone resorption, signs of hyperparathyroid bone disease, and mineralization defects are reduced.

Because vitamin D metabolites other than 1,25-$(OH)_2D_3$ may have direct effects on bone, calcifediol, the common precursor, may be more advantageous than calcitriol in patients with osteomalacia and in children with renal osteodystrophy or hypoparathyroidism who have not achieved full bone growth. In such cases, a mixture of calcifediol and calcitriol may be used. Calcifediol is the preferred agent for treatment of osteomalacia associated with gastrointestinal disease. It is used investigationally in osteomalacia secondary to hepatic disease when endogenous production of 25-OHD_3 is impaired.

ADVERSE REACTIONS AND PRECAUTIONS. As with all vitamin D metabolites, excessive doses of calcifediol can result in hypercalcemia and possibly hypercalciuria. Serum calcium should be monitored at least weekly during dosage adjustment, and the drug should be discontinued if hypercalcemia develops.

There are no well-controlled studies on use of calcifediol in pregnant women, but teratogenic effects were observed in experimental animals. Calcifediol is classified in FDA Pregnancy Category C.

For other adverse reactions and precautions, see the evaluation on Vitamin D_2 (ergocalciferol).

PHARMACOKINETICS. Calcifediol is rapidly absorbed and a peak serum concentration is attained in four to eight hours. It is transported bound to protein and has a half-life of about 16 days.

DOSAGE AND PREPARATIONS.

Oral: Dosage must be individualized and adequate intake of calcium assured. In patients with chronic renal failure on dialysis, initially, 50 mcg daily or 100 mcg on alternate days. Dosage may be increased at four-week intervals if a satisfactory response is not obtained. Serum calcium should be measured at least weekly during dosage adjustment. Most patients respond to doses of 50 to 100 mcg daily or 100 to 200 mcg on alternate days.

Calderol (Organon). Capsules 20 and 50 mcg.

Cited References

Consensus development conference: Diagnosis, prophylaxis, and treatment of osteoporosis. *Am J Med* 94:646-650, 1993.

Adachi JD, et al: corticosteroid-induced osteoporosis. *Semin Arthritis Rheum* 22:375-384, 1993.

Adami S, et al: Transdermal estradiol in the treatment of postmenopausal women. *Bone Miner* 7:79-86, 1989.

Adams JS: Vitamin D metabolite-mediated hypercalcemia. *Endocrinol Metab Clin North Am* 18:765-778, 1989.

Adamson BB, et al: Mineralization defects with pamidronate therapy for Paget's disease. *Lancet* 342:1459-1460, 1993.

Al-Azzawi F, et al: Long term effect of oestrogen replacement therapy on bone mass as measured by dual photon absorptiometry. *BMJ* 294:1261-1262, 1987.

Alon U, Chan JCM: Effects of hydrochlorothiazide and amiloride in renal hypophosphatemic rickets. *Pediatrics* 75:754-763, 1985.

Altman RD: Long-term follow-up therapy with intermittent etidronate disodium in Paget's disease of bone. *Am J Med* 79:583-590, 1985.

Anderson C, et al: Preliminary observations of a form of coherence therapy for osteoporosis. *Calcif Tissue Int* 36:341-343, 1984.

Andress DL, et al: Osteomalacia and aplastic bone disease in aluminum related osteodystrophy. *J Clin Endocrinol Metab* 65:11-16, 1987.

Audran M, et al: Treatment of Paget's disease of bone with (4-chlorophenyl) thiomethylene bisphosphonate. *Clin Rheumatol* 8:1-9, 1989.

Avioli LV: Calcitonin therapy for bone disease and hypercalcemia, editorial. *Arch Intern Med* 142:2076-2078, 1982.

Balfour JA, McTavish D: Transdermal estradiol: A review of its pharmacological profile, and therapeutic potential in the prevention of postmenopausal osteoporosis. *Drugs Aging* 2:487-507, 1992.

Bauer DC, et al: Factors associated with appendicular bone mass in older women. *Ann Intern Med* 118:657-665, 1993.

Beex L, et al: Pamidronate and hypercalcaemia of malignancy, letters. *Lancet* 2:617-618, 1989.

Bellantoni MF, Blackman MR: Osteoporosis: Diagnostic screening and its place in current care. *Geriatrics* 43:63-70, 1988.

Berl T, et al: 1,25 dihydroxycholecalciferol effects in chronic dialysis: Double-blind controlled study. *Ann Intern Med* 88:774-780, 1978.

Bilezikian JP: Primary hyperparathyroidism, in Bardin CW (ed): *Current Therapy in Endocrinology and Metabolism*, ed 4. Philadelphia, BC Decker, 1991, 448-452.

Bilezikian JP: Management of acute hypercalcemia. *N Engl J Med* 326:1196-1203, 1992.

Bockman RS, et al: Gallium increases bone calcium and crystallite perfection of hydroxyapatite. *Calcif Tissue Int* 39:376-381, (Dec) 1986.

Body JJ, et al: Aminohydroxypropylidene bisphosphonate (APD) treatment for tumor-associated hypercalcemia: A randomized comparison between a 3-day treatment and single 24-hour infusions. *J Bone Miner Res* 4:923-928, 1989.

Bone HG, Kleerekoper M: Paget's disease of bone. *J Clin Endocrinol Metab* 75:1179-1182, 1992.

Boonekamp PM, et al: Enhancement of the inhibitory action of APD on the transformation of osteoclast precursors into resorbing cells after dimethylation of the amino group. *Bone Miner* 2:29-42, 1987.

Boyce BF, et al: Focal osteomalacia due to low-dose bisphosphonate therapy in Paget's disease. *Lancet* 1:821-824, 1984.

Brown AJ, et al: The noncalcemic analogue of vitamin D, 22-oxacalcitriol, suppresses parathyroid hormone synthesis and secretion. *J Clin Invest* 84:728-732, 1989.

Burchard KW, et al: Ionized calcium, parathormone, and mortality in critically ill surgical patients. *Ann Surg* 212:543-549, 1990.

Burtis WJ, et al: Immunochemical characterization of circulating parathyroid hormone-related protein in patients with humoral hypercalcemia of cancer. *N Engl J Med* 322:1106-1112, 1990.

Canfield R, et al: Diphosphonate therapy of Paget's disease of bone. *J Clin Endocrinol Metab* 44:96-106, 1977.

Chan JCM, et al: Calcium and phosphate metabolism in children with idiopathic hypoparathyroidism or pseudohypoparathyroidism: Effects of 1,25-dihydroxyvitamin D_3. *J Pediatr* 106:421-426, 1985.

Chapuy MC, et al: Vitamin D_3 and calcium to prevent hip fractures in elderly women. *N Engl J Med* 327:1637-1642, 1992.

Charles P: Calcium absorption and calcium bioavailability. *J Intern Med* 231:161-168, 1992.

Chesnut CH III: Treatment of postmenopausal osteoporosis: Some current concepts. *Scott Med J* 26:72-80, 1981.

Christiansen C, et al: Bone mass in postmenopausal women after withdrawal of oestrogen/gestagen replacement therapy. *Lancet* 1:459-461, 1981.

Christiansen C, et al: Prediction of rapid bone loss in postmenopausal women. *Lancet* 1:1105-1108, 1987.

Civitelli R, et al: Bone turnover in postmenopausal osteoporosis: Effect of calcitonin treatment. *J Clin Invest* 82:1268-1274, 1988.

Coburn JW, Henry DA: Renal osteodystrophy. *Adv Intern Med* 387-424, 1984.

Cole DEC, et al: Changing osteocalcin concentrations during pregnancy and lactation: Implications for maternal mineral metabolism. *J Clin Endocrinol Metab* 65:290-294, 1987.

Coleman RE, Rubens RD: APD for the treatment of hypercalcaemia of malignancy (HOM): A comparison of different doses and schedules of administration. *Br J Cancer* 60:448, 1989.

Coleman RE, et al: Treatment of bone metastases from breast cancer with (3-amino-1-hydroxypropylidene)-1,1-bisphosphonate (APD). *Br J Cancer* 58:621-625, 1988.

Committee on Nutrition: Aluminum toxicity in infants and children. *Pediatrics* 78:1150-1154, 1986.

Consensus Development Conference Panel: Diagnosis and management of asymptomatic primary hyperparathyroidism: Consensus Development Conference Statement. *Ann Intern Med* 114:593-597, 1991.

Cummings SR, et al: Bone density at various sites for prediction of hip fractures. *Lancet* 341:72-75, 1993.

Dambacher MA, et al: Long term fluoride therapy of postmenopausal osteoporosis. *Bone* 7:199-205, 1986.

Dawson-Hughes B, et al: A controlled trial of the effect of calcium supplementation on bone density in postmenopausal women. *N Engl J Med* 323:878-883, 1990.

Delmas PD: Markers of bone formation and resorption, in Favus MJ (ed): *Primer on the Metabolic Bone Diseases and Disorders of Mineral Metabolism*. New York, Raven Press, 1993, 108-112.

Delmas PD, et al: Beneficial effects of aminohexane diphosphonate in patients with Paget's disease of bone resistant to sodium etidronate. *Am J Med* 83:276-282, 1987.

Devogelaer JP, et al: A randomized, controlled trial of APD (disodium pamidronate) given intravenously with and without sodium fluoride in involutional osteoporosis, abstract, in Overgaard K, Christiansen C (eds): *Third International Symposium on Osteoporosis*. Denmark, (Oct 14-18) 1990, 157.

Dodwell D, et al: Treatment of tumour-induced hypercalcaemia (TIH) with pamidronate (APD): Effect of infusion rate and scheduling. *Br J Cancer* 62:483, 1990.

Eastell R, Riggs BL: Diagnostic evaluation of osteoporosis. *Endocrinol Metabol Clin North Am* 17:547-571, 1988.

Ettinger B, et al: Long-term estrogen replacement therapy prevents bone loss and fractures. *Ann Intern Med* 102:319-324, 1985.

Feinfeld DA, Sherwood LM: Parathyroid hormone and 1,25$(OH)_2D_3$ in chronic renal failure. *Kidney Int* 33:1049-1058, 1988.

Felsenfeld AJ, et al: Desferrioxamine therapy in hemodialysis patients with aluminum-associated bone disease. *Kidney Int* 35:1371-1378, 1989.

Felson DT, et al: Thiazide diuretics and the risk of hip fracture: Results from the Framingham Study. *JAMA* 265:370-373, 1991.

Felson DT, et al: The effect of postmenopausal estrogen therapy on bone density in elderly women. *N Engl J Med* 329:1141-1146, 1993.

Fenton AJ, et al: Intravenous aminobisphosphonate in Paget's disease: Clinical, biochemical, histomorphometric and radiological responses. *Clin Endocrinol* 34:197-204, 1991.

Finch JL, et al: Differential effects of 1,25-$(OH)_2D_3$ and 22-oxacalcitriol on phosphate and calcium metabolism. *Kidney Int* 43:561-566, 1993.

Fitton A, McTavish D: Pamidronate: A review of its pharmacological properties and therapeutic efficacy in resorptive bone disease. *Drugs* 41:289-318, 1991.

Fleisch H: Bisphosphonates: Pharmacology and use in the treatment of tumour-induced hypercalcaemic and metastatic bone disease. *Drugs* 42:919-944, 1991.

Forman DT, Lorenzo L: Ionized calcium: Its significance and clinical usefulness. *Ann Clin Lab Sci* 21:297-304, 1991.

Fukagawa M, et al: Suppression of parathyroid gland hyperplasia by 1,25$(OH)_2D_3$ pulse therapy. *N Engl J Med* 315:421-422, 1990.

Gallacher SJ, et al: A study of the effects of aminohydroxypropylidene diphosphonate (APD) on the alleviation of symptoms in Paget's disease of bone. *Scott Med J* 33:252, 1988.

Gallacher SJ, et al: Immobilization-related hypercalcaemia—A possible novel mechanism and response to pamidronate. *Postgrad Med J* 66:918-922, 1990.

Gallagher JC, Goldgar D: Treatment of postmenopausal osteoporosis with high doses of synthetic calcitriol: A randomized controlled study. *Ann Intern Med* 113:649-655, 1990.

Gennari C, Agnusdei D: Calcitonin in bone pain management. *Curr Ther Res* 44:712-722, 1988.

Gennari C, et al: Comparative effects on bone mineral content of calcium and calcium plus salmon calcitonin given in two different regimens in postmenopausal osteoporosis. *Curr Ther Res* 38:455-464, 1985.

Glorieux FH: Rickets, the continuing challenge, editorial. *N Engl J Med* 325:1875-1877, 1991.

Goldstein AJ, et al: Treatment of osteoporosis with aminohydroxypropylidene diphosphonate (APD). *Bone* 10:475, 1989.

Goodman WG, et al: Renal osteodystrophy in adults and children, in Favus MJ, et al (eds): *Primer on the Metabolic Bone Diseases and Disorders of Mineral Metabolism*, ed 2. New York, Raven Press, 1993, 304-323.

Grauer A, et al: In vitro detection of neutralizing antibodies after treatment of Paget's disease of bone with nasal salmon calcitonin. *J Bone Miner Res* 5:387-391, 1990.

Gray RES, et al: Treatment of Paget's disease of bone with intravenous pamidronate, abstract, *Br J Rheumatol* 29(suppl 2):138, 1990.

Grill V, et al: Parathyroid hormone-related protein: Elevated levels in both humoral hypercalcemia of malignancy and hypercalcemia complicating metastatic breast cancer. *J Clin Endocrinol* 73:1309-1315, 1991.

Gucalp R, et al: Comparative study of pamidronate disodium and etidronate disodium in the treatment of cancer-related hypercalcemia. *J Clin Oncol* 10:134-142, 1992.

Hahn TJ: Drug-induced disorders of vitamin D and mineral metabolism. *Clin Endocrinol Metab* 9:107-129, 1980.

Hahn TJ: Parathyroid hormone, calcitonin, vitamin D, mineral and bone: Metabolism and disorders, in Mazzaferri EL (ed): *Endocrinology*, ed 3. New Hyde Park, NY, Medical Examination Pub. Co., Inc., 1985, 458-575.

Hahn TJ: Steroid and drug-induced osteopenia, in Favus MJ (ed): *Primer on the Metabolic Bone Diseases and Disorders of Mineral Metabolism*. New York, Raven Press, 1993, 250-255.

Hall TG, Burns Schaiff RA: Update on the medical treatment of hypercalcemia of malignancy. *Clin Pharm* 12:117-125, 1993.

Hammond CB, et al: Effects of long-term estrogen therapy: I. Metabolic effects. *Am J Obstet Gynecol* 133:525-536, 1979.

Hansen MA, et al: Role of peak bone mass and bone loss in postmenopausal osteoporosis: Twelve year study. *BMJ* 303:961-964, 1991.

Harinck HIJ, et al: Paget's disease of bone: Early and late responses to three different modes of treatment with aminohydroxypropylidene bisphosphonate (APD). *BMJ* 295:1301-1305, 1987.

Harris ST, et al: Four-year study of intermittent cyclic etidronate treatment of postmenopausal osteoporosis: Three years of blinded therapy followed by one year of open therapy. *Am J Med* 95:557-567, 1993.

Harvey JA, et al: Calcium citrate: Reduced propensity for crystallization of calcium oxalate in urine resulting from induced hypercalciuria of calcium supplementation. *J Clin Endocrinol Metab* 61:1223-1225, 1985.

Health and Public Policy Committee: Bone mineral densitometry. *Ann Intern Med* 107:932-936, 1987.

Heaney RP: Thinking straight about calcium, editorial. *N Engl J Med* 328:503-505, 1993 A.

Heaney RP: Nutritional factors in osteoporosis. *Annu Rev Nutr* 13:287-316, 1993 B.

Heidrich FE, et al: Diuretic drug use and the risk for hip fracture. *Ann Intern Med* 115:1-6, 1991.

Henrich JB: The postmenopausal estrogen/breast cancer controversy. *JAMA* 268:1900-1902, 1992.

Hodsman AB: Effects of cyclical therapy for osteoporosis using an oral regimen of inorganic phosphate and sodium etidronate: Clinical and bone histomorphometric study. *Bone Miner* 5:201-212, 1989.

Hui SL, et al: Baseline measurements of bone mass predicts fracture in white women. *Ann Intern Med* 111:362-367, 1989.

Hutchinson TA, et al: Postmenopausal oestrogens protect against fractures of hip and distal radius: Case-control study. *Lancet* 2:705-709, 1979.

Jackson JA, Kleerekoper M: Osteoporosis in men: Diagnosis, pathophysiology, and prevention. *Medicine* 69:137-149, 1990.

Johansen JS, et al: Time-dependent variations in bone turnover parameters during 2 months' cyclic treatment with different doses of combined estrogen and progestogen in postmenopausal women. *Metabolism* 11:1122-1126, 1990.

Johnston CC Jr, et al: Use of etidronate (EHDP) in Paget's disease of bone. *Arthritis Rheum* 23:1172-1176, 1980.

Johnston CC Jr, et al: Early menopausal changes in bone mass and sex steroids. *J Clin Endocrinol Metab* 61:905-911, 1985.

Johnston CC Jr, et al: Clinical indications for bone mass measurements: A report from the Scientific Advisory Board of the National Osteoporosis Foundation. *J Bone Miner Res* 4(suppl 2):1-28, 1989.

Kanis JA, et al: Evidence for efficacy of drugs affecting bone metabolism in preventing hip fracture. *BMJ* 305:1124-1128, 1992.

Kao PC, et al: Parathyroid hormone-related peptide in plasma of patients with hypercalcemia and malignant lesions. *Mayo Clin Proc* 65:1399-1407, 1990.

Kaplan F: Paget's disease of bone: Exploring the questions. *Calcif Tissue Int* 51:1-3, 1992.

Kellihan MJ, Mangino PD: Pamidronate. *Ann Pharmacother* 26:1262-1269, 1992.

Kiel DP, et al: Hip fracture and the use of estrogens in postmenopausal women: The Framingham Study. *N Engl J Med* 317:1169-1174, 1987.

Kleerekoper M, et al: A randomized trial of sodium fluoride as a treatment for post-menopausal osteoporosis. *Osteop Int* 1:115-162, 1991.

Korkor AB: Reduced binding of [^{3}H] 1,25-dihydroxyvitamin D_3 in parathyroid glands of patients with renal failure. *N Engl J Med* 316:1573-1577, 1987.

Kristiansen JH: Familial hypocalciuric hypercalcaemia. *Dan Med Bull* 39(4):321-334, 1992.

LaCroix AZ: Thiazide diuretic agents and prevention of hip fracture. *Compr Ther* 17:30-39, (Aug) 1991.

LaCroix AZ, et al: Thiazide diuretic agents and the incidence of hip fracture. *N Engl J Med* 322:286-290, 1990.

Lafferty FW: Differential diagnosis of hypercalcemia. *J Bone Miner Res* 6(suppl 2):S51-S59, 1991.

Lahtinen R, et al: Randomised, placebo-controlled multicentre trial of clodronate in multiple myeloma. *Lancet* 340:1049-1052, 1992.

Leyvraz S, et al: Pharmacokinetics of pamidronate in patients with bone metastases. *J Natl Cancer Inst* 84:788-792, 1992.

Lindsay R: Sex steroids in the pathogenesis and prevention of osteoporosis, in Riggs BL (ed): *Osteoporosis: Etiology, Diagnosis and Management.* New York, Raven Press, 1988, 333-358.

Lindsay R: Prevention and treatment of osteoporosis. *Lancet* 341:801-805, 1993.

Lindsay R, Tohme J: Estrogen treatment of patients with established postmenopausal osteoporosis. *Obstet Gynecol* 76:1-6, 1990.

Lindsay R, et al: Minimum effective dose of estrogen for prevention of postmenopausal bone loss. *Obstet Gynecol* 63:759-763, 1984.

Lindsay R, et al: Increased axial bone mass in women with hypertension: Role of thiazide therapy. *J Bone Miner Res* 2 (suppl 2):S29, 1987.

Lipton A: Pamidronate disodium—a dose-seeking study in patients with prostate cancer, in: *Current Perspectives in the Management of Bone-Related Complications of Malignancy*. Banff, Canada, (Nov 15-16) 1990, 15.

Lloyd T, et al: Calcium supplementation and bone mineral density in adolescent girls. *JAMA* 270:841-844, 1993.

Lowik CWGM, et al: Migration and phenotypic transformation of osteoclast precursors into mature osteoclasts: The effect of a bisphosphonate. *J Bone Miner Res* 3:185-192, 1988.

Luckert BP, Raisz LG: Glucocorticoid-induced osteoporosis: Pathogenesis and management. *Ann Intern Med* 112:352-364, 1990.

Lufkin EG, et al: Treatment of postmenopausal osteoporosis with transdermal estrogen. *Ann Intern Med* 117:1-9, 1992.

MacIntyre I, et al: Calcitonin for prevention of postmenopausal bone loss. *Lancet* 1:900-902, 1988.

Mai ML, et al: Calcium acetate, an effective phosphorous binder in patients with renal failure. *Kidney Int* 36:690-695, 1989.

Malluche HH, Faugere M-C: Effects of 1,25 $(OH)_2D_3$ administration on bone in patients with renal failure. *Kidney Int* 38 (suppl 29): S-48-S-53, 1990.

Mamelle N, et al: Risk benefit ratio of sodium fluoride treatment in primary vertebral osteoporosis. *Lancet* 2:361-365, 1988.

Marcus R: Cyclic etidronate: Has the rose lost its bloom? Editorial. *Am J Med* 95:555-556, 1993.

Martin TJ: Properties of parathyroid hormone-related protein and its role in malignant hypercalcaemia. *Q J Med* 76:771-786, 1990.

Matkovic V, et al: Use of gallium to treat Paget's disease of bone: A pilot study. *Lancet* 335:72-75, 1990.

Matsuoka LY, et al: Chronic sunscreen use decreases circulating concentrations of 25-hydroxyvitamin D: Preliminary study. *Arch Dermatol* 124:1802-1804, 1988.

Mazess RB, et al: Monitoring skeletal response to estrogen. *Am J Obstet Gynecol* 161:843-848, 1989.

Mazzuoli GE, et al: Effects of salmon calcitonin in postmenopausal osteoporosis: Controlled double-blind clinical study. *Calcif Tissue Int* 38:3-8, 1986.

McCarthy JT, Kumar R: Renal osteodystrophy. *Endocrinol Metab Clin North Am* 19:65-93, 1990.

Melton LJ: Fluoride in the prevention of osteoporosis and fractures. *J Bone Miner Res* 5 (suppl 1):S163-S167, 1990.

Melton LJ III: Epidemiology of primary hyperparathyroidism. *J Bone Miner Res* 6 (suppl 2):S25-S30, 1991.

Melton LJ III, et al: Long-term fracture prediction by bone mineral assessed at different skeletal sites. *J Bone Miner Res* 8:1227-1233, 1993.

Meunier PJ: Is steroid-induced osteoporosis preventable? Editorial. *N Engl J Med* 328:1781-1782, 1993.

Millward MJ, et al: Comparison of 1-hour vs 2-hour infusions of disodium pamidronate (APD) in breast cancer with bone metastases. *Br J Cancer* 62:521, 1990.

Morley JE, et al: UCLA geriatric grand rounds: Osteoporosis. *J Am Geriatr Soc* 36:845-859, 1988.

Morrison NA, et al: Prediction of bone density from vitamin D receptor alleles, letter. *Nature* 367:284-287, 1994.

Morton AR, et al: Single dose versus daily intravenous aminohydroxypropylidene bisphosphonate (APD) for the hypercalcaemia of malignancy. *BMJ* 296:811-814, 1988 A.

Morton AR, et al: Sclerosis of lytic bone metastases after disodium aminohydroxypropylidene bisphosphonate (APD) in patients with breast carcinoma. *BMJ* 297:772-773, 1988 B.

Mulder H, Shelder HA: Effect of cyclical etidronate regimen on prophylaxis of bone loss of glucocorticoid therapy in postmenopausal women. *Bone Miner* 17 (suppl 1):168, 1992.

Mundy GR: Hypercalcemic factors other than parathyroid hormone-related protein. *Endocrinol Metab Clin North Am* 18:795-806, 1989.

Mundy GR: Ectopic production of calciotropic peptides. *Endocrinol Metab Clin North Am* 20:473-487, 1991.

Nachtigall LE, et al: Estrogen replacement therapy: I. 10-year prospective study in relationship to osteoporosis. *Obstet Gynecol* 53:277-281, 1979.

National Institutes of Health Consensus Conference: Osteoporosis. *JAMA* 252:799-802, 1984.

Neer R, et al: Treatment of postmenopausal osteoporosis with daily parathyroid hormone plus calcitriol, in Christiansen C, Overgaard K (eds): *Osteoporosis 1990*. Copenhagen, Denmark, Osteopress ApS, 1990, 1314-1317.

Nicar MJ, Pak CYC: Calcium bioavailability from calcium carbonate and calcium citrate. *J Clin Endocrinol Metab* 61:391-393, 1985.

Norris KC, Coburn JW: Rocaltrol (calcitriol): Guidelines for management. *Dialysis Transplant* Suppl 1-8, (July) 1985.

Nussbaum SR: Pathophysiology and management of severe hypercalcemia. *Endocrinol Metab Clin North Am* 22:343-362, 1993.

Nussbaum SR, et al: Single-dose intravenous therapy with pamidronate for the treatment of hypercalcemia of malignancy: Comparison of 30-, 60-, and 90-mg dosages. *Am J Med* 95:297-304, 1993.

O'Doherty DP, et al: Intravenous aminohydroxybutylidene bisphosphonate in the treatment of Paget's disease of bone. *J Bone Miner Res* 5:483-491, 1990.

O'Doherty DP, et al: Effects of five daily 1 h infusions of alendronate in Paget's disease of bone. *J Bone Miner Res* 7:81-87, 1992.

Overgaard K, et al: Nasal calcitonin for treatment of established osteoporosis. *Clin Endocrinol* 30:435-442, 1989.

Overgaard K, et al: Effect of salcatonin given intranasally on bone mass and fracture rates in established osteoporosis: A dose-response study. *BMJ* 305:556-561, 1992.

Paganini-Hill A, et al: Menopausal estrogen therapy and hip fractures. *Ann Intern Med* 95:28-31, 1981.

Pak CYC, et al: Safe and effective treatment of osteoporosis with intermittent slow release sodium fluoride: Augmentation of vertebral bone mass and inhibition of fractures: *J Clin Endocrinol Metab* 68:150, 1989.

Pak CYC, et al: Slow-release sodium fluoride in the management of postmenopausal osteoporosis: A randomized controlled trial. *Ann Intern Med* 120:625-632, 1994.

Papapoulos SE, et al: Serum osteocalcin in Paget's disease of bone: Basal concentrations and response to bisphosphonate treatment. *J Clin Endocrinol* 55:89-94, (July) 1987.

Parisien M, et al: Bone disease in primary hyperparathyroidism. *Endocrinol Metab Clin North Am* 19:19-34, 1990.

Pelger RCM, et al: Short-term metabolic effects of pamidronate in patients with prostatic carcinoma and bone metastases. *Lancet* 2:865, 1989.

Petersen DJ, et al: X-linked hypophosphatemic rickets: A study (with literature review) of linear growth response to calcitriol and phosphate therapy. *J Bone Miner Res* 7:583-597, 1992.

Pitkin RM: Calcium metabolism in pregnancy and perinatal period: Review. *Am J Obstet Gynecol* 151:99-109, 1985.

Pont A: Unusual causes of hypercalcemia. *Endocrinol Metab Clin North Am* 18:753-764, 1989.

Potts JT Jr: Management of asymptomatic hyperparathyroidism. *J Clin Endocrinol Metab* 70:1489-1493, 1990.

Powell GJ, et al: Localization of parathyroid hormone-related protein in breast cancer metastases: Increased incidence in bone compared with other sites. *Cancer Res* 51:3059-3061, 1991.

Pritchard DJ, Burch PA: Orthopedic complications, in Holland JF, et al (eds): *Cancer Medicine*, ed 3. Philadelphia, Lea & Febiger, 1993, 2290-2293.

Ralston SH, et al: Comparison of aminohydroxypropylidene diphosphonate, mithramycin, and corticosteroids/calcitonin in treatment of cancer-associated hypercalcaemia. *Lancet* 2:907-910, 1985.

Ralston SH, et al: Clinical experience with aminohydroxypropylidene bisphosphonate (APD) in the management of cancer-associated hypercalcaemia. *Q J Med* 69:825-834, 1988.

Ralston SH, et al: Comparison of three intravenous bisphosphonates in cancer-associated hypercalcaemia. *Lancet* 2:1180-1182, 1989 A.

Ralston SH, et al: Clinical, biochemical, and radiographic effects of aminohydroxypropylidene bisphosphonate treatment in rheumatoid arthritis. *Ann Rheum Dis* 48:396-399, 1989 B.

Ray WA, et al: Long-term use of thiazide diuretics and risk of hip fracture. *Lancet* 1:687-690, 1989.

Reeve J, et al: Anabolic effect of human parathyroid hormone fragment on trabecular bone in involutional osteoporosis: A multicentre trial. *BMJ* 280:1340-1344, 1980.

Reginster JY, et al: One-year controlled randomised trial of prevention of early postmenopausal bone loss by intranasal calcitonin. *Lancet* 2:1481-1483, 1987.

Reginster JY, et al: Paget's disease of bone treated with a five day course of oral tiludronate. *Ann Rheum Dis* 52:54-57, 1993.

Reid IR, et al: Effect of calcium supplementation on bone loss in postmenopausal women. *N Engl J Med* 328:460-464, 1993.

Reitsma PH, et al: Kinetic studies of bone and mineral metabolism during treatment with (3-amino-1-hydroxypropylidene)-1,1-bisphosphonate (APD) in rats. *Calcif Tissue Int* 32:145-157, 1980.

Ribot C, et al: Preventive effects of transdermal administration of 17β-estradiol on postmenopausal bone loss: A 2-year prospective study. *Obstet Gynecol* 75(suppl):42S-46S, 1990.

Rico H, et al: Salmon calcitonin reduces vertebral fracture rate in postmenopausal crush fracture syndrome. *Bone Miner* 16:131-138, 1992.

Riggs BL, Melton LJ III: The prevention and treatment of osteoporosis. *N Engl J Med* 327:620-627, 1992.

Riggs BL, et al: Effect of fluoride treatment on the fracture rate in postmenopausal women with osteoporosis. *N Engl J Med* 322:802-809, 1990.

Riis BJ, Christiansen C: Measurement of spinal or peripheral bone mass to estimate early postmenopausal bone loss? *Am J Med* 84:646-653, 1988.

Ritch P, et al: Pamidronate (APD) and etidronate disodium (EHDP) in hypercalcaemia of malignancy—Preliminary report of a comparative multicentre trial, in Rubens RD (ed): *The Management of Bone Metastases and Hypercalcaemia by Osteoclast Inhibition.* Toronto, Canada, Hogrefe & Huber, 1990, 47-49.

Ross PD, et al: Pre-existing fractures and bone mass predict vertebral fracture incidence in women. *Ann Intern Med* 114:919-923, 1991.

Salti GI, et al: Continuing evolution in the operative management of primary hyperparathyroidism. *Arch Surg* 127:831-837, 1992.

Sambrook P, et al: Prevention of corticosteroid osteoporosis: A comparison of calcium, calcitriol, and calcitonin. *N Engl J Med* 328:1747-1752, 1993.

Sawyer N, et al: Fast (4-h) or slow (24-h) infusions of pamidronate disodium (aminohydroxypropylidene diphosphonate) (APD) as single shot treatment of hypercalcaemia. *Bone Miner* 9:121-128, 1990.

Schmidli RS, et al: Aminopropylidine diphosphonate (APD) in mild primary hyperparathyroidism: Effect on clinical status. *Clin Endocrinol* 32:293-300, 1990.

Sentipal JM, et al: Influence of calcium intake and growth indexes on vertebral bone mineral density in young females. *Am J Clin Nutr* 54:425-428, 1991.

Seymour JF, Gagel RF: Calcitriol: The major humoral mediator of hypercalcemia in Hodgkin's disease and non-Hodgkin's lymphomas. *Blood* 82:1383-1394, 1993.

Shane E: Management of hypercalcemia, in Favus MJ, et al (eds): *Primer on the Metabolic Bone Diseases and Disorders of Mineral Metabolism*, ed 2. New York, Raven Press, 1993, 185-187.

Sherrard DJ, et al: The spectrum of bone disease in end-stage renal failure—An evolving disorder. *Kidney Int* 43:436-442, 1993.

Sherwood LM: Vitamin D, parathyroid hormone, and renal failure, editorial. *N Engl J Med* 316:1601-1603, 1987.

Singer FR, et al: Treatment of hypercalcemia of malignancy with intravenous etidronate: A controlled, multicenter study. *Arch Intern Med* 151:471-476, 1991.

Siris ES: Perspectives: A practical guide to the use of pamidronate in the treatment of Paget's disease. *J Bone Miner Res* 9:303-304, 1994.

Siris E, et al: Cyclical treatment of advanced Paget's disease with gallium nitrate: A 12-week dose finding study, abstract 816. *J Bone Miner Res* 7(suppl 1):S296, 1992.

Slatopolsky E, et al: Marked suppression of secondary hyperparathyroidism by intravenous administration of 1,25-dihydroxy-cholecalciferol in uremic patients. *J Clin Invest* 74:2136-2143, 1984.

Slovik DM, et al: Restoration of spinal bone in osteoporotic men by treatment with human parathyroid hormone (1-34) and 1,25-dihydroxyvitamin D. *J Bone Miner Res* 1:377-381, 1986.

Southby J, et al: Immunohistochemical localization of parathyroid hormone-related protein in human breast cancer. *Cancer Res* 50:7710-7716, 1990.

Stevenson JC, et al: Effects of transdermal versus oral hormone replacement therapy on bone density in spine and proximal femur in postmenopausal women. *Lancet* 335:265-269, 1990.

Stone MD, et al: Treatment of Paget's disease with intermittent low-dose infusions of disodium pamidronate (APD). *J Bone Miner Res* 5:1231-1235, 1990.

Storm T, et al: Effect of intermittent cyclical etidronate therapy on bone mass and fracture rate in women with postmenopausal osteoporosis. *N Engl J Med* 322:1265-1271, 1990.

Tan PLJ, et al: Preliminary report: Effects of aminobisphosphonate infusion on biochemical indices of bone metabolism in rheumatoid arthritis. *Br J Rheumatol* 28:325-328, 1989.

Thiébaud D, et al: Dose-response in the treatment of hypercalcemia of malignancy by a single infusion of the bisphosphonate AHPrBP. *J Clin Oncol* 5:762-768, 1988.

Thiébaud D, et al: Response to retreatment of malignant hypercalcemia with the bisphosphonate AHPrBP (APD): Respective role of kidney and bone. *J Bone Miner Res* 5:221-226, 1990 A.

Thiébaud D, et al: Fast and effective treatment of malignant hypercalcemia: Combination of suppositories of calcitonin and a single infusion of 3-amino 1-hydroxypropylidene-1-bisphosphonate. *Arch Intern Med* 150:2125-2128, 1990 B.

Thiébaud D, et al: Treatment of bone metastases from breast cancer and myeloma with pamidronate. *Eur J Cancer* 27:37-41, 1991.

Thuerlimann B, et al: Mithramycin and APD in symptomatic tumour-related hypercalcaemia—A comparative randomised trial, in Burckhardt P (ed): *Disodium Pamidronate (APD) in the Treatment of Malignancy-Related Disorders.* Toronto, Canada, Hans Huber Publishers, 1989, 81-84.

Tilyard MW, et al: Treatment of postmenopausal osteoporosis with calcitriol or calcium. *N Engl J Med* 326:357-362, 1992.

Todd PA, Fitton A: Gallium nitrate: A review of its pharmacological properties and therapeutic potential in cancer-related hypercalcaemia. *Drugs* 42:261-273, 1991.

Uebelhart D, et al: Effect of menopause and hormone replacement therapy on the urinary excretion of pyridinium crosslinks. *J Clin Endocrinol Metab* 72:367-373, 1991.

Upton GV: Perimenopause: Physiologic correlates and clinical management. *J Reprod Med* 27:1-28, 1982.

van Holten-Verzantvoort ATh, et al: Reduced morbidity from skeletal metastases in breast cancer patients during long-term bisphosphonate (APD) treatment. *Lancet* 2:983-985, 1987.

Verge CF, et al: Effects of therapy in X-linked hypophosphatemic rickets. *N Engl J Med* 325:1843-1848, 1991.

Vernava AM III, et al: Lethal hyperparathyroid crisis: Hazards of phosphate administration. *Surgery* 102:941-948, 1987.

Wallach S, et al: Effect of salmon calcitonin on skeletal mass in osteoporosis. *Curr Ther Res* 22:556-572, 1977.

Warrell RP Jr: Metabolic emergencies, in DeVita VT Jr, et al (eds): *Cancer: Principles & Practice of Oncology*, ed 4. Philadelphia, JB Lippincott, 1993, 2128-2141.

Warrell RP Jr, et al: Gallium nitrate for acute treatment of cancer-related hypercalcemia: Clinicopharmacological and dose response analysis. *Cancer Res* 46:4208-4212, 1986.

Warrell RP, et al: Gallium nitrate for acute treatment of cancer-related hypercalcemia. *Ann Intern Med* 108:669-674, 1988.

Warrell RP Jr, et al: A randomized double-blind study of gallium nitrate compared with etidronate for acute control of cancer-related hypercalcemia. *J Clin Oncol* 9:1467-1475, 1991.

Warrell RP Jr, et al: Low-dose gallium nitrate for prevention of osteolysis in myeloma: Results of a pilot randomized study. *J Clin Oncol* 11:2443-2450, 1993.

Wasnich R, et al: Effect of thiazide on rates of bone mineral loss: A longitudinal study. *BMJ* 301:1303-1305, 1990.

Watts ND, et al: Intermittent cyclical etidronate treatment of postmenopausal osteoporosis. *N Engl J Med* 323:73-79, 1990.

Weiss NS, et al: Decreased risk of fractures of the hip and lower forearm with postmenopausal use of estrogen. *N Engl J Med* 303:1195-1198, 1980.

Williams JW, et al: Biliary excretion of aluminum in aluminum osteodystrophy with liver disease. *Ann Intern Med* 104:782-785, 1986.

Yap AS, et al: Use of aminohydroxypropylidene bisphosphonate (AHPrBP, 'APD') for the treatment of hypercalcemia in patients with renal impairment. *Clin Nephrol* 34:225-229, 1990.

Yates AJP, et al: A comparison of single and multiple intravenous infusions of 3-amino-1-hydroxypropylidene-1,1-bisphosphonate (APD) in the treatment of hypercalcemia of malignancy. *Aust N Z J Med* 17:387-391, 1987.

Zaloga GP: Hypocalcemia in critically ill patients. *Crit Care Med* 20:251-262, (Feb) 1992.

Hematinic Agents

Hematinic agents are used to treat anemia, which is defined as a condition in which the concentration of hemoglobin in the blood falls below normal. It results from one or more of a great variety of underlying disorders (Erslev, 1990; Bunn, 1991); therefore, the physician should identify and, if possible, correct the specific underlying cause (Lindenbaum, 1992). It has become increasingly common for physicians either to fail to recognize anemia or to approach its treatment in an empiric manner without adequate attention to differential diagnosis and specific therapy (Welborn and Meyers, 1991; Brown, 1991).

Nutritional anemias are characterized by impaired erythropoiesis that is caused by lack of one or more nutrients required for red blood cell production. The impairment may be quantitative, resulting in hypoproliferative anemia, or qualitative, resulting in a maturation abnormality with ineffective erythropoiesis and short-lived red cells (eg, megaloblastic anemias). Iron deficiency is by far the most common nutritional anemia, followed by folate deficiency and vitamin B_{12} deficiency (Beutler, 1988; Bridges and Bunn, 1991; Babior and Bunn, 1991). Other "nutritional anemias" (eg, pyridoxine-responsive anemia) develop infrequently and probably are not strictly a consequence of nutritional deficiencies. Differential diagnosis is made more complicated by the occurrence of multiple deficiencies in the same patient. For instance, iron deficiency often coexists with folate deficiency, particularly during pregnancy and in alcoholism.

Nutritional anemias result from decreased dietary intake, increased loss (eg, blood loss causing iron deficiency), inadequate absorption, poor utilization, increased nutrient requirements, or a combination of factors. In many instances, nutritional anemias may provide the principal clue to an unsuspected serious underlying illness. Of these, the most important is unrecognized gastrointestinal bleeding due to occult colon carcinoma in the iron-deficient adult.

Each patient with anemia must be evaluated carefully and thoroughly before treatment is undertaken, both to establish the underlying cause of the anemia and to ensure appropriate and safe treatment (Beutler, 1988; Erslev, 1990; Lindenbaum, 1992). It is a common misconception that the hemoglobin level or hematocrit normally declines in elderly individuals. Reduced values for these parameters in older patients should lead to suspicions of anemia at the same thresholds as in middle-aged or young adults (Babitz and Freedman, 1988; Stander, 1989). In addition to a careful history and physical examination, basic studies in all anemic patients should include examination of the blood smear, red blood cell indices (mean corpuscular volume, mean corpuscular hemoglobin), a reticulocyte count, and an evaluation of the white blood cells and platelets for abnormalities in other cell lines. Based on the results of these initial tests, further studies should be selected to provide a pathophysiologic classification and a specific etiologic diagnosis of the anemia. In particular, laboratory evaluation of the patient with nutritional anemia should permit identification of both the specific nutrient that is deficient and the cause of that deficiency (eg, blood loss as the cause of iron deficiency). The goals are to correct the nutrient deficiency to treat the anemia and to correct the underlying disorder to prevent recurrence of the anemia or other consequences of the underlying disease.

IRON DEFICIENCY ANEMIA

Iron Distribution: Iron is distributed throughout the body, where it is found primarily in the form of heme or stored as hemosiderin or ferritin iron. The hemoglobin contained in circulating red blood cells is the largest repository of iron in the body. Iron is stored in hepatocytes and in reticuloendothelial cells in the spleen, liver, and bone marrow bound to ferritin and hemosiderin (Dallman, 1989; Brock, 1989). Other iron compartments (in decreasing size) include myoglobin, a labile pool (interstitial and intracellular fluids), tissue iron (cytochromes and other enzymes), and the plasma transport pool. Together, these compartments comprise approximately 6% of total body iron, with the smallest (the plasma transport pool) being the most kinetically active (Fairbanks and Beutler, 1990 A).

Iron balance is maintained by mechanisms operative within the duodenal mucosa, with homeostasis controlled primarily by regulation of the rate of iron absorption within the duodenum and proximal jejunum. Stored iron is rigidly conserved, with only small amounts lost through desquamation of epithelium from the skin and gastrointestinal mucosa. In normal adults, these losses average approximately 1 mg/day for 70-kg males and 0.8 mg/day for 55-kg females (Harju, 1989). Additional amounts are lost as blood from the gastrointestinal tract and, in premenopausal women, as menstrual blood. However, there is no regulated excretory mechanism for iron.

Regulation of iron balance is achieved primarily through alterations in intestinal absorption. During periods of relative abundance of iron stores, the rate of absorption is minimal (5% to 10% of dietary intake for the typical Western diet). However, when iron requirements are increased due to growth, blood loss, pregnancy, or iron deficiency, the rate of absorption is increased to 25% of the amount ingested. Absorption occurs principally in the proximal small intestine, with the absorptive capacity of the gut decreasing progressively from the duodenum to the ileum. Some of the iron that enters mucosal cells is transported into the circulation, but the major portion is retained as ferritin, then lost as cells are shed into the lumen and excreted. Absorbed iron is transported through the circulation attached to the iron binding and transport protein, transferrin. It is taken up by developing erythroid cells in the bone marrow and is incorporated into heme. Iron that is not utilized in red blood cell production or other replication is transferred into reticuloendothelial and parenchymal storage sites, from which it later can be mobilized to meet the requirements for erythropoiesis. A portion of the iron derived from breakdown of senescent red blood cells is incorporated into reticuloendothelial storage pools, but the majority is reutilized immediately for erythropoiesis.

Iron Deficiency: Iron deficiency occurs when homeostasis is disrupted because of decreased iron intake, growth, or increased iron losses resulting from blood loss (Fairbanks and Beutler, 1990 B; Kushner, 1992). Its severity varies, in overlapping degrees, from iron depletion (reduced storage pools but normal blood iron and hemoglobin levels) through iron deficiency without anemia (normal hemoglobin levels but reduced storage pools and serum levels of iron) to iron deficiency anemia. Dietary iron deficiency is uncommon when iron requirements are low because of the abundance of iron in dietary sources. Intake is inadequate during periods of increased iron requirement (eg, in children during periods of rapid growth, during pregnancy). Rarely, iron absorption may be decreased because of intestinal disease associated with severe malabsorption or because of the rapid transit of luminal iron past the absorptive surface of the duodenum following partial or total gastrectomy. In all other circumstances, iron deficiency *must* be presumed to have resulted from blood loss. In residents of and recent immigrants from less developed countries, the most common cause of iron deficiency may be infection with hookworm (uncinariasis). In developed nations, menstruation is the usual cause of negative iron balance in young women, while drug-induced gastrointestinal blood loss (eg, from salicylates) is relatively common in both men and women.

The single most important point regarding diagnosis of iron deficiency in men and postmenopausal women is that iron deficiency should be presumed to result from pathologic blood loss unless proven otherwise (Lutcher, 1992; Kushner, 1992). Bleeding caused by unsuspected gastrointestinal tract cancer is the cause of iron deficiency in at least 2% of iron-deficient adults; this percentage increases significantly when menstruating women are excluded.

Although empiric trials of iron therapy may be appropriate in populations at low risk for occult blood loss (eg, growing children, menstruating or pregnant women), specific diagnosis of iron deficiency is essential in men or postmenopausal women for the reasons stated above. Furthermore, because anemia may occur in individuals with iron overload, specific diagnosis of iron deficiency prior to initiation of therapy becomes even more important (Herbert, 1987). The diagnosis of iron deficiency anemia requires demonstration of both a restricted supply of iron to the bone marrow and depletion of iron storage depots. Hypochromia and microcytosis are common in iron deficiency, but they are not invariably present, particularly early in the development of the disorder. Furthermore, although these red blood cell changes are typically found in iron deficiency, they may occur in any disorder in which the rate of hemoglobin synthesis is restricted by hemoglobinopathy (eg, thalassemia trait), defective pyrrole synthesis (eg, sideroblastic anemia), or limited iron supply to the red blood cell precursors in noniron-deficient individuals (eg, anemia associated with severe inflammation and neoplasm, often called the anemia of chronic disease). In children, hypochromic microcytic anemia also may result from lead poisoning, which must be distinguished from iron deficiency and treated promptly to prevent central nervous system damage.

The expense and discomfort associated with bone marrow examination preclude routine use of the most direct and definitive test, absence of stainable iron from the bone marrow, in the routine diagnosis of iron deficiency. Iron supply to the bone marrow is more easily estimated by determining the percentage of the total iron binding capacity (TIBC, a measure of circulating transferrin) that is saturated with iron. The triad of a low serum iron concentration (in a sample obtained from a fasting patient), an elevated TIBC, and a saturation less than 15% is diagnostic of iron deficiency. Determining only serum iron concentrations can be misleading. For example, patients with inflammatory or neoplastic disease may have low serum iron despite the presence of adequate iron stores, although the TIBC usually also is low in these patients. Furthermore, because patients with iron deficiency also may have inflammation or neoplasia, even the results of measurement of serum iron, TIBC, and percent of saturation may not be diagnostic. Some authorities recommend relying on the absolute magnitude of the unsaturated iron binding capacity (>54 micromole/L) as a guide for diagnosis of iron deficiency (Beutler, 1988). Others believe that examination of bone marrow aspirates is required in severely ill patients with inflammation, neoplasia, or liver disease.

The concentration of ferritin in the serum correlates closely with body iron storage levels in healthy individuals. A serum ferritin concentration less than 10 mcg/L is characteristic of iron deficiency anemia, while values between 10 and 20 mcg/L suggest this diagnosis (Fairbanks and Beutler, 1990 B). However, inflammatory and neoplastic disease can elevate the serum ferritin level into the low-normal range even in iron-deficient individuals and extensive cell damage or turnover (eg, after surgery, in some types of liver disease) also can cause elevated serum ferritin levels even in the presence of iron deficiency. Furthermore, the threshold serum ferritin level indicating iron deficiency is elevated and unpredictable in long-term hemodialysis patients. For these reasons, a normal serum ferritin concentration cannot absolutely exclude a diagnosis of iron deficiency. Nevertheless, in the elderly, the serum ferritin level probably is the most reliable laboratory measurement other than examination of bone marrow for establishing the diagnosis of iron deficiency anemia (Guyatt et al, 1990). A less readily available assay that some experts believe may be useful when diagnosis is difficult is the free erythrocyte protoporphyrin concentration (FEP), which is increased in iron-deficient patients (Fairbanks and Beutler, 1990 B). However, other conditions (eg, some hemolytic anemias, sideroblastic anemias, the anemias of chronic disease) also can be accompanied by increased FEP. Therefore, FEP may be useful primarily to screen large populations (eg, school children) for iron deficiency.

Iron Compounds

In adults and in most children and infants, prevention of iron deficiency is best accomplished by dietary means including, when necessary, iron-fortified foods. In one double-blind, randomized, placebo-controlled trial, 6-month-old infants from low-income minority families who had low or low-normal hemoglobin levels were fed an iron-fortified formula with or without additional oral iron (3 or 6 mg/kg/day of ferrous sulfate drops administered before meals); the mild anemia was not corrected more rapidly by supplementation with oral iron (Irigoyen et al, 1991). Although the prevalence of anemia among children from low-income families continues to decline because of government-sponsored nutrition programs (Yip et al, 1987), these children still have a threefold greater risk of iron deficiency than those in families with higher incomes (Yip, 1989). See the chapter on Vitamins and Minerals for recommended allowances.

Prophylactic use of oral iron preparations should be restricted to those individuals at especially high risk for development of iron deficiency anemia (ie, pregnant and lactating women, low-birth-weight or preterm infants, infants fed unsupplemented formulas). Others who may be appropriate candidates for iron prophylaxis are rapidly growing children who consume food low in available iron (eg, meatless diets) and adults with known chronic blood loss, such as menorrhagia or hereditary hemorrhagic telangiectasia. Iron prophylaxis should be avoided under other circumstances because there is a risk of iron overload with resultant tissue damage (Herbert, 1987; Fairbanks and Baldus, 1990), because occult gastrointestinal neoplasms may be masked, and because iron overdose is a common cause of poisoning in children.

Therapeutic doses of iron are used only to treat iron deficiency anemia. Oral administration of iron salts is the treatment of choice in patients who are not iron intolerant. Since ferrous salts (sulfate, fumarate, and gluconate) are the most bioavailable forms of iron, they should be selected in preference to any form of ferric salts.

Formulations and Dosage: Ferrous sulfate is the standard preparation of oral iron. Patients who do not respond to ferrous sulfate are unlikely to respond to any oral iron preparation, and therefore the use of more expensive preparations is rarely justified. Side effects of oral iron preparations are directly related to their bioavailability, since they result from the presence of ionized iron within the proximal gastrointestinal tract. Therefore, when equivalent doses of ionic elemental iron are administered as different salts, equivalent side effects usually will occur.

Some preparations contain iron salts in a prolonged-release or enteric-coated form. These are intended to reduce side effects by delaying dissolution and release of ionized iron until the medication has passed from the stomach into the proximal duodenum. The effectiveness of such preparations varies from one formulation to another, since the iron may be released distal to the site of maximal absorption. The selection of a particular formulation should be based on published bioavailability data (Cook et al, 1982; Delorme et al, 1990). Data from a pilot study suggest that incorporation of ferrous sulfate into a gastric delivery system that results in retention and slow dissolution of the dose in the stomach may yield a higher rate of iron absorption with a lower incidence of gastrointestinal side effects than with the conventional dosage form (Cook et al, 1990).

The iron content in various preparations varies greatly, and thus dosage should be calculated in terms of elemental iron. Hydrated 300-mg ferrous sulfate tablets contain approximately 60 mg of elemental iron (325-mg tablets contain 65 mg of elemental iron). In general, for oral iron replacement in deficient adults, most hematologists and manufacturers recommend a dose of 50 to 60 mg of elemental iron (eg, one ferrous sulfate tablet) three times daily, administered on an empty stomach to prevent interference with absorption by food. With this regimen, anemia will be corrected rapidly if the patient does not have continuing blood loss (ie, two weeks for recovery to 50% of normal and six to eight weeks for recovery to normal). Iron replacement therapy must be continued for a total of about six months despite the reversal of anemia, since iron stores will not be restored until after this time. However, some experts favor a more conservative approach and recommend doses of 30 to 60 mg of elemental iron daily taken with food to retard absorption and reduce gastrointestinal disturbances (Crosby, 1986; Lutcher, 1992). This regimen also generally will correct anemia rapidly, since iron is absorbed at a maximal rate during periods of frank iron deficiency. As with the regimen utilizing higher doses, iron therapy must be continued for at least four months after the anemia is corrected in order to replenish iron stores. However, it may take somewhat longer to replenish these stores fully because the rate of iron absorption falls dramatically as the degree of iron deficiency diminishes. In patients who have continuing blood loss, maintenance iron therapy may be necessary indefinitely. Dosage recommendations for correction of iron deficiency in children range from 3 to 6 mg/kg/day.

Carbonyl iron is a microspherical form of elemental (as opposed to ionized) iron that is produced by controlled heating of vaporized iron pentacarbonyl. Since the particle size is about one-tenth that of other forms, the bioavailability of carbonyl iron is somewhat improved relative to that of other elemental iron preparations. Studies in anemic women showed that carbonyl iron could correct iron deficiency anemia, but the prevalence of gastrointestinal side effects was similar to that in patients given ferrous sulfate (Gordeuk et al, 1986). In menstruating blood donors, supplementation with carbonyl iron replaced the iron lost by donation and reduced the rate of deferral from repeat donation compared with women receiving a placebo (Gordeuk et al, 1990). However, in randomized double-blind trials comparing carbonyl iron 600 mg with ferrous sulfate 300 mg (equivalent to 60 mg elemental iron) and with placebo (each given three times daily for one week to premenopausal women who were repeat blood donors), carbonyl iron prevented the reduction in iron stores found in placebo-treated individuals but not to the degree observed with ferrous sulfate (Gordeuk et al, 1987 A). Furthermore, the incidence of gastrointestinal side effects was similar in the two groups receiving iron preparations. Results of a three-week trial comparing identical regimens of carbonyl iron and ferrous sulfate in anemic menstruating women showed that nearly identical durations of therapy are required to replenish iron stores with both regimens (Gordeuk, 1987 B). Thus, carbonyl iron does not appear to have any major therapeutic advantage over other iron preparations.

Many factors affect the rate of absorption of the dose of iron (Harju, 1989; Dallman, 1989; Fairbanks and Beutler, 1990 A; Bridges and Bunn, 1991). Some iron preparations do not dissolve in the stomach or duodenum. This can be documented by measuring the serum iron level in a fasting patient and then repeating this measurement two to three hours after ingestion of a single dose of iron. When iron is being absorbed, the serum level will increase by approximately 100 mcg/dL. A variety of substances in food (phytates, oxalates, or phosphates) and medications bind iron or cause it to be oxidized to an insoluble form within the intestinal lumen, which reduces bioavailability and diminishes absorption markedly. Certain vegetables may decrease absorption by 60% or more. Iron absorption also is reduced by some antacids, tetracyclines, and tea. Pancreatic juice also inhibits iron absorption.

Ascorbic acid and other reducing agents are thought by some to enhance absorption by facilitating conversion of ferric to ferrous iron. However, addition of ascorbic acid to ferrous sulfate did not improve the rate at which iron stores were replenished in anemic patients following gastrointestinal surgery compared with patients treated only with ferrous sulfate (Harju, 1989). Furthermore, ascorbic acid also may increase the incidence of reactions to oral iron. Consequently, monotherapy with ferrous sulfate is preferred in the treatment of uncomplicated iron deficiency. Ascorbic acid does aid iron absorption in patients with achlorhydria.

In patients who are not actively bleeding, the hemoglobin concentration should increase by approximately 0.1 g/dL/day within two weeks after starting oral iron therapy. An increase in the reticulocyte count may be a better indicator of response to iron replacement therapy, since the response occurs even in patients who continue to bleed actively. When anemia is severe, there is sometimes a brief erythropoietic burst with a rapid but fleeting initial rise in hemoglobin, after which the patient responds at the same rate as those less severely affected.

Lack of response to oral iron therapy most commonly results from the patient's failure to take the prescribed dose, either because of side effects of iron (or fear of side effects) or because of inadequate understanding of the need for the medication. Another frequent cause of treatment failure is incorrect diagnosis. Less commonly, the response to oral iron is blunted or even nullified by continued blood loss, which should be suspected when there is a brisk reticulocytosis without an increase in hemoglobin concentration during iron therapy. Finally, a small proportion of patients do not respond either because of rapid transit of the administered dose past the absorptive surface (eg, in postgastrectomy patients) or because of frank iron malabsorption (eg, in patients with sprue). Those in whom transit is rapid usually will respond when iron salts are given separately from food as an elixir or suspension.

Parenteral iron (iron dextran injection [InFeD]) acts similarly to oral iron in correcting iron deficiency. However, since serious and even fatal reactions can occur after administration of parenteral iron, its use should be reserved for those with a confirmed diagnosis of iron deficiency anemia who do not respond adequately to oral iron (eg, those with continued blood loss), those who require immediate replacement of their iron deficit, those who are unable to take oral iron because of severe side effects that cannot be controlled conservatively, or those who adamantly refuse oral iron despite counseling regarding the risks of parenteral treatment (Kumpf and Holland, 1990). Because of possible adverse reactions to transfusion, some experts recommend parenteral iron for the correction of anemia caused by blood loss in patients who require surgery or in prepartum patients who would otherwise require red blood cell transfusions. (See also index entry Transfusion Therapy, Adverse Reactions, Precautions.)

Generally, malabsorption of iron, postgastrectomy states, and apparent intolerance for oral iron are not valid indications for parenteral iron therapy. As noted above, iron malabsorption severe enough to preclude oral iron therapy is rare, and patients with transit-related iron malabsorption after gastrectomy usually respond to liquid iron preparations. Patients who cannot tolerate oral iron usually can be managed successfully by reducing the dose, by administering the entire dose at bedtime, or by administering iron with meals. These measures decrease side effects at the expense of bioavailability, but a sufficient amount of iron usually can be absorbed to correct the anemia.

For information on combination products containing iron, see the section on Mixtures.

Pharmacokinetics: Peak plasma levels are achieved about two hours after an oral dose of ferrous sulfate (Harju, 1989). Measurement of the serum iron concentration in a blood sample obtained two to three hours after ingestion of a single dose of iron can confirm or exclude the occurrence of iron malabsorption. Both the peak levels and the amount of iron absorbed are approximately in linear relation to the dose ingested. Nevertheless, absorption after a single dose is higher than after the same amount given as two divided doses. The half-life of iron after peak plasma levels are achieved is about six hours.

Adverse Reactions and Precautions: Iron compounds are contraindicated in patients with primary or secondary iron overload, including hereditary hemochromatosis, thalassemia major, and transfusion hemosiderosis (Fairbanks and Baldus, 1990). Secondary siderosis also may occur if iron is given to patients with chronic inflammation, chronic renal failure, or hemolytic anemia (unless intravascular hemolysis is associated with urinary iron losses). Secondary iron overload is a particular risk in patients with refractory anemias (especially sideroblastic anemias) erroneously diagnosed as iron deficiency. It also may occur in patients treated with excessive amounts of parenteral iron and in patients given *both* oral and parenteral iron. Those receiving blood transfusions regularly should not receive iron because each milliliter of transfused packed red blood cells contains approximately 1 mg of iron. Prolonged iron therapy should be reserved for patients with continuing blood loss or menorrhagia or for women with repeated pregnancies.

Paroxysmal nocturnal hemoglobinuria is a disease in which red blood cells are abnormally sensitive to complement. This causes intravascular hemolysis and iron deficiency secondary to urinary iron losses, which are manifested as hemoglobinuria and hemosiderinuria. Treatment of such patients with large doses of iron may induce a brisk reticulocytosis resulting in a dangerous hemolytic crisis. This complication may be prevented by using very small oral doses of iron to avoid a rapid erythropoietic response or by administering blood transfusions prior to iron therapy to suppress endogenous production of complement-sensitive erythrocytes.

Oral iron therapy is always preferred to parenteral iron. Use of parenteral iron bypasses the intestinal mechanisms that regulate iron absorption, thus increasing the risk of secondary siderosis. Parenteral iron is associated with a variety of toxic and uncomfortable reactions, including phlebitis, urticaria, fever, regional lymphadenopathy, and arthralgias. Dangerous and even fatal anaphylaxis has occurred after administration of parenteral iron dextran, even in patients with no prior exposure to this drug. These life-threatening reactions can occur with any route of parenteral administration (see above).

There is no rationale for simultaneous oral and parenteral iron therapy, because the principal indications for parenteral iron are failure of oral iron therapy or presence of a pre-existing condition that precludes successful oral administration.

Oral iron only rarely causes overload, except when it is administered chronically to patients with abnormally increased iron absorption (eg, those with hemolytic anemia, hemochromatosis, refractory sideroblastic anemias). Heterozygotes for hemochromatosis may comprise up to 10% of the population. Iron should be reserved for patients with demonstrated iron deficiency or a well-documented requirement for supplemental iron.

The major side effects of oral iron are gastrointestinal disturbances. Nausea and vomiting are dose related and generally can be controlled by changing the quantity or timing of the iron dose or by substituting another dosage form. Constipation and occasionally diarrhea are not dose related, but rarely are they so severe that treatment cannot be continued. In a very small number of individuals, successful therapy with oral iron (sulfate or gluconate) was followed by rapid, but transient, declines in platelet counts (Soff and Levin, 1988).

Intolerance for oral iron is strongly influenced by a well-recognized "conditioning" effect that occurs when the patient is cautioned to expect some gastrointestinal distress. In these individuals, some gastrointestinal disturbances would occur even if a placebo were administered. Reassurance and symptomatic treatment are often sufficient to control side effects, especially since these tend to subside spontaneously with continued oral iron therapy. When reassurance alone is insufficient, decreasing the total daily dose, giving part or all of the dose at bedtime, or giving each dose with meals will usually control symptoms. Substitution of ferrous gluconate for ferrous sulfate is sometimes effective in patients with severe gastrointestinal side effects. Each ferrous gluconate tablet contains 30 to 50 mg of elemental iron, thus slightly reducing the concentration of ionized iron within the stomach after each dose. Any of these measures that result in a decreased effective daily dose may require that treatment be continued longer than four to six months to ensure adequate replacement of iron stores.

In general, infants and children tolerate oral iron preparations better than adults. Pregnant women are especially susceptible to gastrointestinal side effects, but there is no absolute intolerance for oral iron. In those pregnant patients in whom iron produces uncomfortable effects that do not subside with continued administration, appropriate timing of administration or adjustment in dose usually is successful.

Iron salts are very dangerous for young children. The tablets resemble small candies, and children can easily ingest enough to produce toxic and even lethal effects. Reversible staining of teeth also may occur in children. All iron preparations should be labeled as potentially hazardous and kept securely away from children.

Drug Evaluations

ORAL IRON PREPARATIONS

The usual therapeutic doses cited in this section reflect manufacturers' recommendations and the traditionally prescribed regimens. One tablet of an iron salt three times daily on an empty stomach is the usual prescribed dose. Some authorities prefer smaller doses, especially if gastrointestinal side effects are a problem. Patients can be successfully treated with as little as 30 mg of elemental iron daily (Crosby, 1986). Larger doses do not appreciably enhance the rate of correction of the hemoglobin deficit in iron-deficient patients, although some patients may require a longer total period of treatment for complete replacement of depleted iron stores.

FERROUS SULFATE

[Feosol, Fer-In-Sol, Mol-Iron, Slow Fe]

ACTIONS AND USES. Iron is required for hemoglobin synthesis and red blood cell production (see the Introduction). It is also incorporated into myoglobin and serves as a cofactor for several essential enzymes.

Oral ferrous sulfate is the agent of choice for prophylaxis and treatment of uncomplicated iron deficiency anemia. Enteric-coated and prolonged-release preparations are more expensive than plain tablets. Although it is claimed that the former decrease gastrointestinal side effects, the iron may not be adequately solubilized until after the preparation has passed the area of greatest absorptive capacity in the proximal small intestine, thus diminishing the effective bioavailability of the preparation. Prolonged-release forms of iron should be used only if adverse reactions cannot be managed by reducing the dosage of standard forms or there are specific objective data showing adequate bioavailability of the preparation.

ADVERSE REACTIONS, PRECAUTIONS, AND DRUG INTERACTIONS. Except for constipation and the occasional occurrence of diarrhea, gastrointestinal side effects are dose related (Fairbanks and Beutler, 1990 B; Lutcher, 1992). These include nausea, bloating, anorexia, or pyrosis. In about 10% of patients, these effects are severe enough to be intolerable. Although ferrous sulfate is best absorbed when taken on an empty stomach, side effects can be minimized in most patients by decreasing the daily dose, giving part or all of the dose at bedtime, or administering the dose with meals. However, some grain products and tea can severely impair iron absorption; thus, oral iron should never be taken with tea or with meals containing grains. Alternatively, the dose can be reduced to as little as 30 mg of elemental iron daily (Crosby, 1986), and all or part of the dose can be taken at bedtime. Such measures will adequately control side effects in most patients.

Ferrous sulfate, like virtually all iron salts, can aggravate pre-existing gastrointestinal disorders such as acid peptic disease, ulcerative colitis, and regional enteritis. This usually can be avoided by reducing the dose of iron. Furthermore, prolonged-release preparations may cause bowel obstruction in patients with bowel strictures, since these forms of iron are sometimes contained in a wax matrix that is delivered intact into the distal intestine.

Administration of ferrous sulfate or ferrous gluconate with ciprofloxacin [Cipro] was reported to reduce the bioavailability of the fluoroquinolone antibiotic (Polk et al, 1989; Kara et al, 1991). Both the peak plasma level and the area under the concentration-time curve were markedly reduced. Therefore, patients taking ciprofloxacin should avoid products containing iron salts. Absorption of tetracyclines also is reduced because of ferrous ion chelation (Campbell and Hasinoff, 1991); two to three hours should elapse between oral administration of iron salts and tetracyclines. Other drugs with decreased bioavailability as a result of concurrent ingestion of iron preparations include penicillamine, methyldopa, levodopa, and carbidopa.

Severe acute iron poisoning is rare in adults, but it does occur in children who accidentally ingest iron preparations intended for adults. As little as 400 mg of elemental iron has caused fatalities in children. Death results from acute circulatory failure and shock, massive gastrointestinal hemorrhage due to coagulation necrosis of the gastric mucosa, and acute massive hepatic necrosis. See index entry Iron Compounds, Poisoning, for information on the management of acute iron toxicity.

DOSAGE AND PREPARATIONS.

Therapeutic:

The manufacturers' recommended doses are given. Before deciding on the dose for a particular patient, see the discussion under Formulations and Dosage in the Introduction.

Oral: *Adults,* initially 30 to 60 mg of elemental iron daily, increased in 30- to 60-mg increments to 180 mg of elemental iron daily in three divided doses. *Children 6 to 12 years,* 24 to 120 mg (3 mg/kg) of elemental iron daily in three or four divided doses, as the syrup or elixir; *2 to 5 years,* 15 to 45 mg (3 mg/kg) of elemental iron daily in three or four divided doses, as the syrup or elixir; *6 months to 2 years,* up to 6 mg/kg of elemental iron daily in three or four divided doses, as the syrup or elixir; *infants under 6 months,* a quantity of pediatric preparation sufficient to provide 10 to 25 mg of elemental iron daily in three or four divided doses.

Prophylactic (supplemental):

Oral: *Women of childbearing age, adolescents, and children,* approximately 20 mg of elemental iron daily; *pregnant and lactating women,* 30 to 60 mg of elemental iron daily. *Men and postmenopausal women* should not receive routine supplemental iron, for this may mask chronic iron (blood) loss and thus delay diagnosis of occult gastrointestinal neoplasia. If there is a well-documented increased risk of iron deficiency, such as frequent blood donation in a closely monitored patient, supplemental iron may be given. *Low-birth-weight infants and infants with low iron stores,* initially, 2 mg/kg of elemental iron daily, decreased gradually to approximately 1 mg/kg daily; *normal infants,* 10 to 15 mg elemental iron daily, including any supplemental iron contained in the formula fed to the infant.

Generic. Capsules (plain, prolonged-release) 150 and 250 mg (30 and 50 mg elemental iron, respectively); drops 75 mg (15 mg elemental iron)/0.6 ml and 125 mg (25 mg elemental iron)/ml; elixir 220 mg (44 mg elemental iron)/5 ml; solution 300 mg/5 ml (60 mg elemental iron); tablets (plain, enteric-coated) 300 and 325 mg (60 and 65 mg elemental iron, respectively); tablets (prolonged-release) 250 and 325 mg (50 and 65 mg elemental iron, respectively) (all forms nonprescription).

Feosol (SmithKline Beecham). Capsules (exsiccated, prolonged-release) 159 mg (50 mg elemental iron); elixir 220 mg (44 mg elemental iron)/5 ml (alcohol 5%); tablets (exsiccated) 200 mg (65 mg elemental iron) (all forms nonprescription).

Fer-In-Sol (Mead Johnson). Capsules (exsiccated) 190 mg (60 mg elemental iron); drops 75 mg (15 mg elemental iron)/0.6 ml (alcohol 0.02%); syrup 90 mg (18 mg elemental iron)/5 ml (alcohol 5%) (all forms nonprescription).

Mol-Iron (Schering-Plough). Tablets 195 mg (39 mg elemental iron) (nonprescription).

Slow Fe (CIBA). Tablets (exsiccated, prolonged-release) 160 mg (50 mg elemental iron) (nonprescription).

FERROUS FUMARATE

[Femiron, Feostat, Fumerin, Hemocyte, Ircon]

FERROUS GLUCONATE

[Fergon, Ferralet, Simron]

ACTIONS AND USES. These compounds are pharmacologically similar to ferrous sulfate for the treatment of uncomplicated iron deficiency anemia. They are claimed to be less irritating to the gastrointestinal tract than ferrous sulfate by virtue of a slower rate of dissolution (ferrous fumarate) or a lower concentration of elemental iron per tablet (ferrous gluconate). Because of reduced solubility, these preparations should not be used in achlorhydric patients.

ADVERSE REACTIONS. Gastrointestinal side effects are comparable to those of ferrous sulfate when similar amounts of elemental iron are present in a bioavailable (soluble) form in the proximal gastrointestinal tract. Overdosage may be fatal to children, and these preparations should be considered as dangerous as ferrous sulfate.

DOSAGE AND PREPARATIONS. The manufacturers' recommended doses are given. Before deciding on the dose for a particular patient, see the discussion under Formulations and Dosage in the Introduction.

FERROUS FUMARATE:

Therapeutic:

Oral: *Adults,* 100 to 400 mg (approximately 33 to 133 mg of elemental iron) daily in one to four doses; *children 6 to 12 years,* 100 to 300 mg (33 to 100 mg of elemental iron) daily in one to four doses as the suspension; *1 to 5 years,* initially, a quantity of pediatric suspension sufficient to provide 15 mg of elemental iron (12 drops or one-half teaspoonful of the suspension), increased gradually to a maximum of 45 mg of elemental iron daily, if necessary, in three or four divided doses; *infants,* 10 to 20 mg of elemental iron daily (5 to 16 drops) divided into two to four doses.

Prophylactic:

Same as for ferrous sulfate.

Generic. Capsules 300 mg (99 mg elemental iron); tablets 300 and 325 mg (prolonged-release) (99 and 106 mg elemental iron, respectively) (both forms nonprescription).

Femiron (Menley & James). Tablets 60 mg (20 mg elemental iron) (nonprescription).

Feostat (Forest). Drops 45 mg (15 mg elemental iron)/0.6 ml; suspension 100 mg (33 mg elemental iron)/5 ml; tablets (chewable) 100 mg (33 mg elemental iron) (all forms nonprescription).

Fumerin (Laser). Tablets 195 mg (64 mg elemental iron) (nonprescription).

Hemocyte (U.S. Pharmaceutical Corp.). Tablets 324 mg (106 mg elemental iron) (nonprescription).

Ircon (Kenwood). Tablets 200 mg (66 mg elemental iron) (nonprescription).

FERROUS GLUCONATE:

Therapeutic:

Oral: *Adults,* 320 to 640 mg (38 to 77 mg of elemental iron) three times daily; *children,* 100 to 300 mg (12 to 36 mg of elemental iron) three times daily; *infants,* initially, 120 mg (30 drops of elixir equivalent to 15 mg of elemental iron), increased gradually if needed to 300 mg (36 mg of elemental iron) daily.

Prophylactic:

Same as for ferrous sulfate.

Generic. Tablets 300 and 325 mg (34 and 38 mg elemental iron, respectively) (nonprescription).

Fergon (Winthrop Consumer Products), ***Ferralet*** (Mission). Tablets 320 mg (37 mg elemental iron) (nonprescription).

Simron (SmithKline Beecham). Capsules 86 mg (10 mg elemental iron) (nonprescription).

POLYSACCHARIDE-IRON COMPLEX

[Niferex, Nu-Iron]

ACTIONS AND USES. This preparation contains ferric iron (as ferrihydrite) complexed to carbohydrate (Berg et al, 1984; Bereman and Berg, 1989). The iron is present in the core of spherical particles with diameters ranging from 3 to 10 nanometers. These particles carry a negative charge at pH >4.6 and a positive charge at pH <4.0; they are neutral between pH 4.0 and 4.6. Polysaccharide-iron complex is soluble when charged but insoluble within the narrow pH range at which it remains neutral. No data have been published comparing the bioavailability of iron from polysaccharide-iron complex with that from ferrous salts. Unpublished studies (sponsored by the manufacturer) in a small number of subjects suggest that oral absorption of iron from this complex is comparable to that from ferrous sulfate.

Results of uncontrolled trials of polysaccharide-iron complex in anemic geriatric patients (Sanders, 1968) showed that clinical responses (rise in hemoglobin and hematocrit) occurred after 28 days of treatment in 15 of 19 patients given doses equal to 200 mg of elemental iron per day. In randomized trials in anemic premature infants (Newton et al, 1980), which compared oral polysaccharide-iron complex (6 mg elemental iron/kg/day) with oral ferrous succinate (5 mg elemental iron/kg/day) and with intramuscular iron dextran (100 mg elemental iron/day), no differences were observed in the ability of these preparations to correct the early anemia of prematurity. In a double-blind randomized trial (using unspecified doses of iron), oral polysaccharide-iron complex was reported to be comparable to oral ferrous fumarate in correcting iron deficiency anemia in patients aged 13 to 73 years (Piccinini and Ricciotti, 1982). Although these studies suggest that polysaccharide-iron complex is effective for iron deficiency, each study has at least one defect in experimental design (lack of controls; unequal or unspecified doses of iron). Because of these flaws and the lack of published comparative bioavailability studies in an adequate number of subjects, ferrous salts are preferred for iron deficiency anemia.

ADVERSE REACTIONS. Mild gastrointestinal disturbances are the most common adverse effects. Although this complex appears to be less toxic on a weight basis and better tolerated than the ferrous salts, this reflects the smaller quantity of ionic iron reaching the gastric and intestinal mucosa. Equal amounts of ionic iron from polysaccharide-iron complex and the ferrous salts are probably equally toxic. The rationale for use of this preparation to reduce adverse reactions in iron-intolerant patients is that little, if any, free (ie, uncomplexed) ionic iron is present in the gastrointestinal tract when polysaccharide-iron complex is ingested and that comparable fractions of oral doses are absorbed for equimolar amounts of elemental iron as the complex and as a ferrous salt. The latter hypothesis requires confirmation in adequate, well-controlled published studies. The danger of severe iron poisoning still exists, particularly in children. Like other iron preparations, polysaccharide-iron complex may aggravate gastrointestinal disease.

DOSAGE AND PREPARATIONS. The manufacturers' recommended doses are given. Before determining the dose for a particular patient, see the discussion under Formulations and Dosage in the Introduction.

Oral: *Adults,* to correct iron deficiency anemia, 150 to 300 mg of elemental iron per day in single or divided doses; *children 6 to 12 years,* 50 to 100 mg of elemental iron per day; *2 to 6 years,* 50 mg of elemental iron per day. *Infants,* for prophylaxis, 25 mg of elemental iron per day. See also the Introduction to this section.

Strengths are expressed in terms of elemental iron.

Niferex (Central). Capsules 150 mg ***[Niferex-150]***; elixir 100 mg/5 ml (alcohol 10%); tablets 50 mg (all forms nonprescription).

Nu-Iron (Mayrand). Capsules 150 mg; elixir 100 mg/5 ml (alcohol 10%) (both forms nonprescription).

PARENTERAL IRON PREPARATION

IRON DEXTRAN INJECTION

[InFeD]

USES. Iron dextran injection is indicated for use *only* in patients with a confirmed diagnosis of iron deficiency anemia in whom one or more of the following circumstances exist: (a) oral iron therapy has clearly failed; (b) the rate of continuing blood loss exceeds the rate at which iron can be absorbed from oral ferrous sulfate; (c) immediate replacement is necessary and it is desirable to avoid transfusion (eg, late pregnancy, prior to emergency surgery, use in individuals with religious objections to transfusion); (d) pre-existing gastrointestinal disease, such as ulcerative colitis, has been or may be seriously exacerbated by oral iron therapy; (e) the patient has severe iron deficiency anemia and is incapable of compliance; or (f) an infant will not receive any iron supplementation at home (Kumpf and Holland, 1990). (However, parenteral iron may be dangerous in infants, especially newborns.)

Bioavailability of iron from iron dextran complex depends on the actions of phagocytic cells of the reticuloendothelial system. A small proportion of injected iron dextran may remain biologically unavailable regardless of the route of administration for several months after injection. This amount is usually small after intravenous injection but may be substantial after intramuscular injection. This unavailable complexed iron is stainable and may provide falsely positive evidence of bone marrow iron stores, thus masking recurrence of iron deficiency in patients with relatively rapid blood loss who are treated with iron dextran injection.

ADVERSE REACTIONS AND PRECAUTIONS. Serious and even life-threatening toxic reactions may occur following administration of iron dextran injection. These include anaphylaxis (even in patients never previously exposed to iron dextran injection), circulatory collapse with shock, and cardiac arrest. Less serious effects include urticaria, phlebitis, arthralgias and myalgias, regional lymphadenopathy, fever, nausea, vomiting, and headache.

Despite common misconceptions to the contrary, anaphylactic reactions can occur after either intramuscular or intravenous injection; the overall incidence is $<1\%$. Because intravenous injection permits the rate of infusion to be controlled, anaphylaxis may be detected before the full dose is given and the infusion terminated more readily than with intramuscular injection. Emergency resuscitative equipment, epinephrine, and other appropriate drugs should be readily available whenever iron dextran injection is administered. It is recommended that a small test dose of 0.1 ml (5 mg) be administered before each course of therapy to detect sensitivity to iron dextran. Since fatal reactions have occurred after administration of as little as 0.01 ml (0.5 mg), patients should be continuously monitored even during the test dose.

Because of the unpredictable absorption of intramuscular iron dextran, the greater risk of uncontrolled anaphylaxis, and the problem of irritation at the site of intramuscular injection, most clinicians recommend that the drug not be given intramuscularly. When this route is employed, a Z-track technique deep in the muscle should be utilized to avoid irritation and discoloration to the skin. Even with this technique, skin discoloration is a common complication of intramuscular injection, but this usually resolves after one to two months or, rarely, within one to two years. Although the relationship to iron injection has not been clearly established, sarcomas have been reported to develop in animals at sites of intramuscular iron dextran injection.

There are reports of abnormalities in the offspring of non-anemic animals given large single doses (125 mg/kg) of iron dextran during early pregnancy. Therefore, the drug should not be used during early pregnancy unless there are compelling reasons to do so (FDA Pregnancy Category C). Intravenous infusion of iron dextran appears to be safe as therapy for anemia in late pregnancy (final one to two months).

Parenteral and oral iron preparations should not be administered concomitantly.

DOSAGE AND PREPARATIONS. Dosages are expressed in terms of elemental iron. Iron dextran injection is available in a concentration of 50 mg of elemental iron per ml. The total dose of iron required to correct the anemia (restore the circulating hemoglobin mass) and to replenish iron stores is individualized and is calculated by one of a number of formulas or tables. The following is an example of such a formula:

$$0.66 \times \text{body weight (kg)} \times (100 - [\frac{\text{patient's Hb} \times 100}{14.8}]) =$$

total milligrams of iron required

This formula calculates the total amount of elemental iron (in milligrams) necessary to restore the circulating hemoglobin mass and replenish iron stores.

The following alternative formula may be somewhat easier to remember and calculates only the deficit in circulating hemoglobin iron (ie, the amount of iron required to correct the anemia):

$$\text{body weight (kg)} \times 70 \text{ ml/kg} \times [0.45 - \frac{\text{patient's Hct}}{100}] =$$

circulating hemoglobin iron deficit in milligrams

An additional 5 to 10 mg/kg should be added to replenish iron stores.

An adult who is not actively bleeding should receive no more than 1.5 to 2 g of iron as iron dextran injection per course of treatment. Unless there is well-documented further iron loss (generally in the form of bleeding), the calculated total deficit plus 5 to 10 mg/kg should not be exceeded. If the patient fails to show an expected erythropoietic response, either the diagnosis of iron deficiency is incorrect or the patient has another complicating disorder that blunts the erythropoietic response to iron.

Intravenous: *Adults and children,* (undiluted) an initial test dose of one or two drops, followed in about 15 minutes by an additional test dose of 0.5 ml (25 mg). If no reaction is evident, a total of 100 mg (2 ml) of undiluted drug may be given daily at a rate not exceeding 50 mg (1 ml)/min. These doses may be repeated on consecutive days until the total calculated dose has been given. When larger doses are needed, most authorities believe that infusion of the total calculated amount as a single dose is the safest method of administering iron dextran injection to an adult (Lutcher, 1992). *Adults and children,* (diluted) after dilution to a concentration of 250 mg iron/ml in 0.9% sodium chloride injection or 5% dextrose in water, a test dose of a few milliliters should be infused slowly. After 10 to 15 minutes, the diluted solution may be administered at a rate of 1 L in four to six hours. In elderly or severely anemic patients, the large volume may cause circulatory overload and pulmonary edema unless a loop diuretic (eg, furosemide) is given concomitantly. In patients in whom volume is of particular concern, the diluted total dose may be infused in two or three sessions rather than at one time.

It is emphasized that iron dextran injection can cause severe or fatal anaphylactic reactions. All patients *must* be observed constantly during the first 30 to 60 minutes of infusion and at very frequent intervals thereafter until the infusion is completed. Emergency drugs and resuscitative equipment should be readily available during infusion.

Intramuscular (deep): This route of administration is not recommended. See the manufacturer's literature for dosage information. Experiments using iron dextran injection labeled with a radioisotope indicate that approximately 30% of the injected dose remains at the site of intramuscular injection for more than 30 days.

Generic. Solution 50 mg/ml of elemental iron in 2 ml (intravenous) and 10 ml (intramuscular) containers.

InFeD (Schein). Solution equivalent to 50 mg/ml of elemental iron in 2 ml (intramuscular, intravenous) and 10 ml (intramuscular) containers.

MEGALOBLASTIC ANEMIAS (FOLATE AND VITAMIN B_{12} DEFICIENCIES)

Folic acid is required for the synthesis of purine nucleotides for DNA biosynthesis, as well as for metabolism of some amino acids. In addition, a folate cofactor is essential for conversion of deoxyuridylate to thymidylate (Babior, 1990 A). Vitamin B_{12} and other cobalamins act as cofactors in conversion of homocysteine to methionine and of methylmalonyl coenzyme-A to succinyl coenzyme-A. The folates and cobalamins are interrelated through the participation of N^5-methyltetrahydrofolate as a methyl donor in the conversion of homocysteine to methionine. Therefore, deficiency of one or both of these vitamins will result in a nuclear maturation abnormality within the cell (Babior, 1990 B; Babior and Bunn, 1991; Allen, 1992). In the bone marrow, the effect of this maturation defect is the production of abnormal hematopoietic elements and ineffective hematopoiesis, causing a decrease in the number of circulating blood elements in all cell lineages. These disorders, referred to as megaloblastic anemias, are characterized by vigorous proliferation of bone marrow cells with striking cellular gigantism. It is emphasized, however, that they would more properly be called megaloblastic *pancytopenias* rather than anemias, since the effects are trilinear and are not restricted to erythroid cells. The large cells that are produced are characteristic of macrocytic anemia. However, the diagnosis of megaloblastic anemia must be confirmed by bone marrow examination, because other conditions (eg, thyroid deficiency) also can cause macrocytic anemia.

The defective hematopoietic cells produced in these disorders may be destroyed prematurely within the bone marrow, which results in ineffective erythropoiesis (defined as intramedullary hemolysis). Those cells that do reach the circulation also are subject to shortened survival, and an element of peripheral hemolysis contributes to the anemia in megaloblastic anemias.

Other rapidly proliferating cells are affected similarly to hematopoietic elements of the bone marrow, including the mucosal cells lining the gastrointestinal tract. Thus, glossitis, gastritis, and small intestinal mucosal atrophy with malabsorption may accompany the megaloblastic anemias.

Folic acid deficiency is much more common than vitamin B_{12} deficiency, because folate stores are depleted within four months during periods of decreased dietary intake, whereas reserves of vitamin B_{12} may last for several years (Babior and Bunn, 1991; Allen, 1992). Maximal vitamin B_{12} absorption occurs in the distal ileum, whereas maximal folate absorption occurs in the upper third of the small intestine. Absorption of both vitamins requires an intact small bowel.

Megaloblastic anemias may result from deficiency of folate, vitamin B_{12}, or both. In addition, conditions such as malabsorption (eg, tropical sprue, celiac disease, blind loop syndrome, ileal resection); impaired utilization; competition for the vitamins by intestinal parasites (eg, intestinal bacteria or, more rarely, fish tapeworm competing for vitamin B_{12}); or increased losses in association with other diseases, chronic infection, or drugs may produce or exacerbate anemia. Prolonged exposure to nitrous oxide also can chemically inactivate vitamin B_{12} and lead to a megaloblastic state that may be fatal if left untreated. An acute megaloblastic reaction to nitrous oxide anesthesia is unusual, however, and probably occurs only in patients with underlying deficiencies of folate or cobalamin. Conditions that increase requirements for one or both of these vitamins, such as hemolysis or pregnancy, may aggravate existing anemias or produce relative deficiencies of the vitamins and thus cause anemia. Several primary disorders of nuclear maturation affecting bone marrow cells (eg, certain myelodysplastic syndromes) also cause megaloblastoid anemia, but they do not respond to either folate or vitamin B_{12}.

Pernicious anemia is a specific form of vitamin B_{12} deficiency in which the vitamin is malabsorbed because of a lack of gastric intrinsic factor, a protein that binds the vitamin to enable it to be absorbed (Babior and Bunn, 1991; Allen, 1992; Karnad and Krozser-Hamati, 1992). The intrinsic factor deficiency usually results from chronic gastritis with damage to gastric parietal cells and loss of capacity to produce intrinsic factor. Deficiency of intrinsic factor in the absence of gastritis may be hereditary.

Diagnosis: The hematologic findings in both folate and vitamin B_{12} deficiency are identical, and large doses of folate may overcome the megaloblastosis of vitamin B_{12} deficiency. Nevertheless, these vitamins are *not* interchangeable therapeutic agents, and it is essential to make a specific diagnosis in each patient (Babior and Bunn, 1991; Allen, 1992; Cooper, 1992). This is particularly important in pernicious anemia and other forms of cobalamin deficiency, because although the anemia responds to large doses of folic acid, without appropriate vitamin B_{12} therapy the neurologic damage progresses unabated and gradually becomes irreversible.

Initial diagnostic studies should include a complete blood count, red cell indices, blood smear, and reticulocyte count. The presence of macro-ovalocytes and hypersegmented polymorphonuclear leukocytes is strong evidence of megaloblastosis, which can be confirmed by examination of a bone marrow sample. Serum levels of isoenzymes 1 and 2 of lactate dehydrogenase (LDH-1 and LDH-2) often are increased approximately in proportion to the severity of the anemia. However, some patients with megaloblastic anemia have normal or only moderately increased LDH levels. In contrast to other types of anemia, serum from patients with megaloblastic anemia usually contains higher levels of LDH-1 than LDH-2. Several other serum enzymes (lysozyme, malic dehydrogenase, 6-phosphogluconate dehydrogenase, and thymidine kinase) as well as serum erythropoietin levels also are elevated in these patients.

Assays of serum vitamin B_{12}, serum folate, and red blood cell folate usually permit a diagnosis of the specific vitamin deficiency, although the assays are somewhat difficult to perform and may yield equivocal or misleading results (Dawson et al, 1987). Pernicious anemia can be present with only a minimal reduction in the serum cobalamin level and without anemia or macrocytosis (Carmel, 1990; Herbert, 1990 A; Stabler et al, 1990; Fine and Soria, 1991). Concurrent deficiencies of iron and vitamin B_{12} frequently are responsible for the absence of macrocytosis. Determinations of serum levels of methylmalonic acid and total homocysteine are very useful follow-up tests to diagnose and distinguish between cobalamin and folate deficiencies (Stabler et al, 1990; Beck, 1991; Allen, 1992). Homocysteine concentrations are elevated in both cobalamin and folate deficiency, while methylmalonic acid concentrations are elevated only in the former.

A Schilling test both with and without intrinsic factor helps to determine the mechanism of vitamin B_{12} deficiency and usually confirms a diagnosis of pernicious anemia. However, a normal Schilling test does not exclude vitamin B_{12} deficiency. A food Schilling test may be necessary, since malabsorption of vitamin B_{12} contained in food (often due to an inability to release protein-bound cobalamin) sometimes occurs in patients showing no malabsorption of free B_{12} (Carmel, 1990; Herbert, 1990 B). Patients with pernicious anemia frequently also have antibodies to either parietal cells or to intrinsic factor detectable in serum. In addition, it is important to remember that patients may have coexisting folate and B_{12} deficiency, especially since severe deficiency of either vitamin can cause malabsorption that may diminish absorption of the other.

Therapy: In most instances, treatment can be delayed until a specific diagnosis is made. However, immediate therapy may be necessary in patients with thrombocytopenia associated with bleeding, with granulocytopenia associated with infection, with severe anemia associated with circulatory compromise or heart failure, or with severe neurologic damage.

Prior to initiating treatment in such patients, a serum sample should be obtained and frozen for later vitamin assays. Both vitamin B_{12} 1,000 mcg and folic acid 5 mg then should be given intramuscularly, followed by daily oral administration of folic acid 1 mg and parenteral vitamin B_{12} 1,000 mcg for one week. If intramuscular injection is contraindicated because of a low platelet count, the drugs may be infused. In nearly all other circumstances, the intravenous route is inadvisable because it causes more rapid excretion of vitamin B_{12} and thus reduces the portion of the dose that is retained.

It is also important to remember that severely ill, malnourished patients, especially those with overwhelming infection who are hospitalized in critical care units, may be folate deficient despite normal serum folate levels. These patients may develop life-threatening granulocytopenia and/or thrombocytopenia unless they are given folic acid supplementation, and they are appropriate candidates for empiric folic acid replacement therapy.

Transfusions are seldom needed to correct the anemia associated with deficiencies of folate or vitamin B_{12}. Furthermore, the anemia is usually well tolerated because it develops so slowly; thus, extensive compensatory processes can occur concurrently. When transfusions are required, volume overload is a major risk, because the circulatory adjustments to anemia, which may include an expanded plasma volume, put considerable stress on the heart. This risk may be minimized by exchange transfusion, performing exchanges in 50-ml increments with a three-way stopcock and a 50-ml syringe.

The response to treatment with vitamin replacement therapy requires two or three weeks to reach 50% and six to eight weeks for cell counts to be restored to normal. The megaloblastic cells present at the initiation of therapy are destroyed and a new generation of normal cells is produced from vitamin-replenished precursors that are responding to high levels of erythropoietin.

Patients with pernicious anemia may have other medical problems that require attention in addition to the megaloblastic anemia. These include neurologic disorders, such as peripheral neuropathy, dementia, and combined system disease, which may respond to replacement therapy if the disorder has been of moderate duration (Beck, 1991); other autoimmune phenomena, such as Hashimoto's thyroiditis; late-onset immunoglobulin deficiency; and a somewhat higher risk of gastric carcinoma, which occurs in many patients despite adequate replacement therapy (Talley et al, 1989). Because of the risk of gastric cancer, some authorities recommend that patients with pernicious anemia be evaluated for occult gastric cancer at regular intervals. Iron deficiency also frequently accompanies pernicious anemia (Carmel et al, 1987; Atrah and Davidson, 1988).

Vitamin B_{12} Compounds

Vitamin B_{12} Metabolism: Vitamin B_{12} is the common name for cyanocobalamin, one of several cobalt-containing compounds called cobalamins. These molecules consist of a macrocyclic tetrapyrrole group, known as a corrin, covalently linked to a dimethylbenzimidazolyl nucleotide. The coordinated cobalt ligand is held in the center of the corrin ring system. The cobalamins are produced by microorganisms that are ingested by animals, and the only sources of vitamin B_{12} compounds for humans are fish, meat, and, to a small extent, dairy products. Strict vegans may become deficient in vitamin B_{12}, although such a deficiency may take many years to develop.

A typical diet will supply 5 to 30 mcg of the vitamin daily in a protein-bound form that can be absorbed with intrinsic factor after normal digestion. Of this amount, 1 to 5 mcg is absorbed. Vitamin B_{12} is bound to intrinsic factor as it traverses the gastrointestinal tract, and the complex is absorbed in the distal ileum in the presence of calcium. Once absorbed, the vitamin is transported through the circulation bound to specific transport proteins called transcobalamins. A small additional amount of vitamin B_{12} can be absorbed by simple diffusion, but this is negligible unless huge doses of the vitamin are ingested.

Two cofactors, adenosylcobalamin and methylcobalamin, are synthesized in vivo from hydroxocobalamin. Most plasma cobalamin in humans is in the form of methylcobalamin. Adenosylcobalamin is the cofactor required for conversion of methylmalonyl coenzyme A (from propionate catabolism) to succinyl coenzyme A. Thus, cobalamin deficiency is accompanied by increased serum levels of methylmalonic acid. Serum levels of homocysteine also are elevated in vitamin B_{12}-deficient patients, because methylcobalamin is the methyl donor required for conversion of homocysteine to methionine. (Urinary excretion of these metabolites also has been reported to increase in cobalamin deficiency, but this has been studied in relatively few patients.) Methylcobalamin is then regenerated by transfer of the methyl moiety from N^5-methyltetrahydrofolate. In cobalamin-deficient cells, folate accumulates as N^5-methyltetrahydrofolate; this metabolite cannot be used as a substrate or cofactor for other biosynthetic reactions. Large doses of folate can correct the hematologic abnormalities (but not the neurologic deficits) that accompany vitamin B_{12} deficiency by bypassing this reaction and providing the methylene tetrahydrofolate needed for thymidylate synthesis.

Cobalamin Deficiency: Cobalamin deficiency is a continuous and progressive series of stages from the clinically silent condition of negative nutrient balance through nutrient depletion leading to biochemical deficits, and finally results in clinical deficiency and frank anemia (Herbert, 1990 A, 1990 B; Stabler et al, 1990). It has been reported that the earliest stage, negative balance, can be detected by a decline in saturated transcobalamin II holoenzyme levels and that vitamin B_{12} depletion occurs after serum cobalamin levels fall below 200 picomol/L even though other findings (deoxyuridine suppression, hypersegmented neutrophils, RBC folate levels) remain normal (Herbert 1990 A, 1990 B). In contrast, other investigators emphasize the imprecision of the assay method for determination of saturated transcobalamin II holoenzyme (Griffiths, 1991) and question the hypothesis that reduced serum levels are predictive of a negative balance for cobalamin (Stabler et al, 1991). Furthermore, 5% to 10% of cobalamin-depleted patients (some with severe life-threatening deficiency) have normal serum B_{12} levels (Lindenbaum et al, 1988, 1990), and some patients with serum B_{12} levels below 200 picomol/L may not be cobalamin-depleted. In the former viewpoint (Herbert 1990 A, 1990 B), the earliest deficits that may result from cobalamin deficiency are an abnormal deoxyuridine suppression test and/or hypersegmented granulocyte nuclei and neutropenia. Clinical symptoms, macro-ovalocytosis, and reduced hemoglobin levels occur only in the final stages.

In pernicious anemia, vitamin B_{12} cannot be adequately absorbed due to the lack of gastric intrinsic factor. Because of the magnitude of stores of the enzyme-bound vitamin in the liver, it takes 2 to 12 years for frank deficiency to develop once the patient develops intrinsic factor deficiency. In pernicious anemia patients, it has been estimated that the total deficit of vitamin B_{12} is approximately 4 to 5 mg. Patients with dietary deficiency of vitamin B_{12} take much longer to develop clinical deficiency syndromes because of the still intact enterohepatic recirculation of the vitamin.

Rarely, congenital transcobalamin II deficiency has been reported to cause vitamin B_{12} deficiency in infants. In these patients, prompt injection of vitamin B_{12} 1,000 mcg twice weekly can prevent the early impairment of mental development (Hall, 1992).

Diminished vitamin B_{12} absorption occurs after total gastric resection (due to loss of the capacity to produce gastric intrinsic factor). If prophylactic therapy is not begun or is interrupted, vitamin B_{12} deficiency occurs in an average of five to six years. Reduced absorption also frequently accompanies partial gastric resection or severe malabsorption disorder, such as tropical sprue, celiac disease, or regional enteritis. Cobalamin therapy may be necessary in these patients. Renal transplant and dialysis patients apparently maintain normal serum levels of the vitamin.

Formulations and Uses: Hydroxocobalamin is identical in hematopoietic activity to the antianemia factor in purified liver extract. Cyanocobalamin, the stable pharmaceutical form of the vitamin, is equally active once it loses its cyanide adduct. Vitamin B_{12} preparations have no demonstrated role in the treatment of any nonhematologic disorder, although they have been used for many years to "treat" a variety of ailments and as a general tonic.

Hydroxocobalamin is somewhat more tightly protein bound than cyanocobalamin, and at least theoretically its rate of loss from the body may be slightly less. However, this is of no clinical significance, and both forms of the vitamin are equally effective in the treatment of megaloblastic anemias due to vitamin B_{12} deficiency. Some patients develop antibodies to the complex of hydroxocobalamin and transcobalamin II, but there is no evidence that these antibodies interfere with the action of hydroxocobalamin. Cyanocobalamin is more widely available and less costly than hydroxocobalamin and thus is preferred by many physicians for general clinical use.

Cyanocobalamin is rapidly and completely absorbed from intramuscular and subcutaneous injection sites. Between 50% and 98% of a large injected dose is excreted unchanged in the urine. Even more rapid renal clearance occurs following intravenous administration; thus, there is little likelihood that much of the injected dose will go into hepatic storage sites.

To avoid the discomfort, inconvenience, and cost of monthly injections of cyanocobalamin, some physicians advocate the use of large oral doses to treat patients with pernicious anemia; this is based on data indicating an adequate therapeutic response with long-term oral administration of 1,000 mcg/day (Lederle, 1991). However, other authorities stress problems with patient compliance, the need for close patient monitoring during the first few months of therapy, and data that suggest that 50% of those with pernicious anemia prefer monthly injections (Hathcock and Troendle, 1991).

Preparations are marketed that contain both vitamin B_{12} and intrinsic factor, the rationale being to provide an orally absorbable form of the vitamin for patients with pernicious anemia so that they will not require parenteral administration. However, these preparations are not reliably absorbed, they frequently induce allergic sensitization that renders them ineffective, and they are not absorbed in the presence of diseases of the small intestine. Therefore, there is no justification for their use in clinical practice.

Although liver extracts contain active vitamin B_{12}, they can cause serious sensitization and have been outmoded by purified cobalamins. They should not be used.

Gastric atrophy in patients with pernicious anemia often responds to glucocorticoids, and secretion of intrinsic factor may be resumed by the regenerated mucosa as long as steroid therapy is continued. However, treatment of pernicious anemia with steroids is not recommended.

Administration: For patients with pernicious anemia or intestinal malabsorption causing vitamin B_{12} deficiency, crystalline hydroxocobalamin or cyanocobalamin should be given by intramuscular or subcutaneous injection. Oral administration of vitamin B_{12} compounds at standard dosages should be reserved *only* for patients with nutritional deficiency with normal absorption of the vitamin demonstrated by a Schilling test without intrinsic factor. Massive oral doses of at least 1,000 mcg daily may permit sufficient absorption by mass action to be used for maintenance therapy for patients with pernicious anemia in remission (Lederle, 1991).

The hematologic response to parenteral administration of hydroxocobalamin or cyanocobalamin is usually dramatic. Typically, the bone marrow converts from megaloblastic to normoblastic erythroid hyperplasia within six to eight hours after administration of an intramuscular dose, and a brisk reticulocytosis follows five to eight days thereafter. Psychiatric problems associated with pernicious anemia may respond within 24 hours, but neurologic problems respond more slowly because their correction requires regeneration of myelin damaged by vitamin B_{12} deficiency (Herbert, 1987; Beck, 1991). The neuropsychiatric consequences of vitamin B_{12} deficiency are not always preceded by frank anemia. Anemia and macrocytosis can be absent in nearly 30% of patients with cobalamin-responsive neuropsychiatric disorders (Herbert, 1987, 1990 B; Lindenbaum et al, 1988; Stabler et al 1990). However, most of these patients will be neutropenic.

For the patient with pernicious anemia, maintenance therapy with vitamin B_{12} compounds must continue for life to pre-

vent the development of irreversible neurologic damage. The same is true for vitamin B_{12} deficiency resulting from any other irreversible defect in absorption of the vitamin. After discontinuation of vitamin B_{12} therapy, the time to relapse is at least 18 months and as long as 12 years (Lindenbaum et al, 1990). If the neurologic problems resulting from vitamin B_{12} deficiency are permitted to progress untreated for even relatively short times, they may become permanent. Failure of these to reverse after 12 to 18 months of vitamin B_{12} therapy is an indication that the neurologic injury is irreversible.

Drug Evaluations

CYANOCOBALAMIN

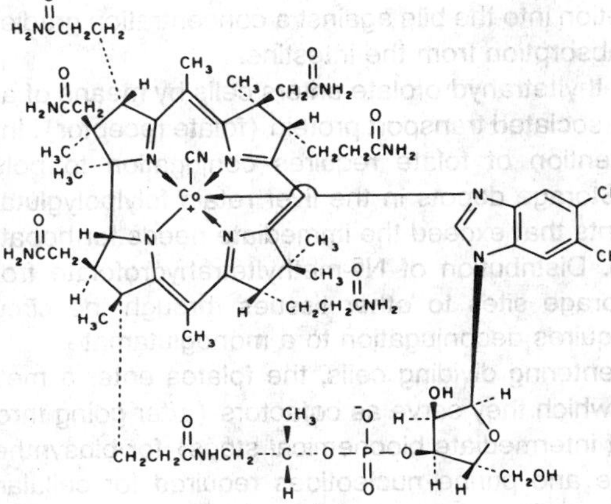

HYDROXOCOBALAMIN

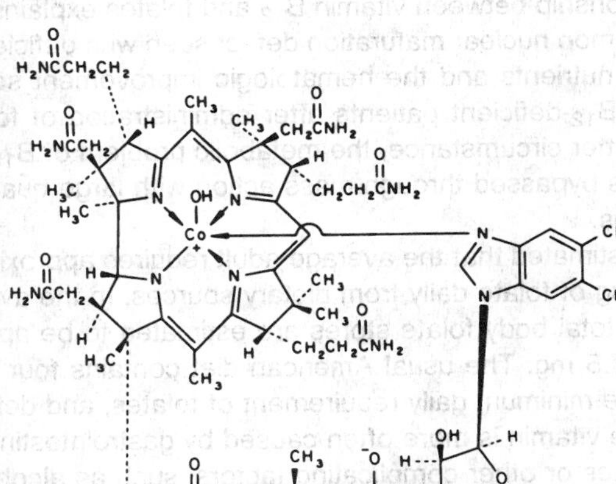

ACTIONS AND USES. The primary uses for these preparations are to treat documented deficiencies of vitamin B_{12} and to saturate vitamin B_{12} binding sites in performance of the Schilling test for pernicious anemia or malabsorption. In addition, they are used occasionally in patients suspected of having pernicious anemia while awaiting results of serum assays for vitamin B_{12}, particularly in critically ill patients who require immediate treatment. Oral forms of vitamin B_{12} are appropriate for use as supplements in vegetarians, particularly strict vegans who exclude all animal and fish products from their diet. Massive oral doses also have been suggested for maintenance of remission in patients with pernicious anemia. A vitamin B_{12}-fortified cereal may be prescribed for patients who object to taking medications on religious grounds.

Hydroxocobalamin has a somewhat longer duration of action than cyanocobalamin due to increased protein binding. It is the preferred therapeutic choice in patients with inborn errors of cobalamin metabolism. In spite of the occasional development of antibodies to the transcobalamin II/hydroxocobalamin complex, the choice between hydroxocobalamin and cyanocobalamin in all other patients most often is determined by cost and/or availability, since these antibodies do not appear to affect therapeutic responses. When parenteral doses in excess of 30 mcg per day are administered, there is no increase in the hematopoietic response, although vitamin stores may be replenished slightly more quickly. In general, most of the excess dose is excreted in the urine. Cyanocobalamin should only rarely be administered intravenously because most of the drug is excreted unchanged in the urine.

ADVERSE REACTIONS. Benzyl alcohol preservatives can cause a fatal "gasping syndrome" in premature infants. Injections are essentially painless and produce no local inflammation or adverse reactions except in patients with thrombocytopenia. Cyanocobalamin and hydroxocobalamin are classified in FDA Pregnancy Category C.

DRUG INTERACTIONS. A variety of drugs can diminish intestinal absorption of vitamin B_{12} preparations. These include aminoglycoside antibiotics, colchicine, certain antiepileptic drugs, prolonged-release potassium supplements, and aminosalicylic acid, as well as chronic ethanol ingestion. Most of these interactions have little or no clinical significance, since (except for chronic alcoholics) patients being treated with these drugs rarely become cobalamin deficient.

DOSAGE AND PREPARATIONS.

Intramuscular, Subcutaneous (deep): The following regimen is usually recommended: For treatment of uncomplicated pernicious anemia or vitamin B_{12} malabsorption, *adults,* 100 mcg daily for five to ten days, followed by 100 to 200 mcg monthly until remission is complete. Alternatively, 100 mcg daily may be given for one week, followed by 100 mcg every other day for two weeks, then 100 mcg every three to four days until remission is complete. With either regimen, remission should be maintained with a monthly 100-mcg dose.

Some experts recommend that injections of 1,000 mcg (rather than 100 mcg) be given initially and for maintenance in spite of the fact that a greater amount of the administered drug is lost by excretion with the larger doses. In their view, a larger absolute amount of cobalamin is retained by the body than when the smaller dose is given, which allows more rapid repletion with fewer injections overall. Furthermore, the larger doses do not increase toxicity and are only slightly more costly.

For serious complications requiring immediate therapy, both vitamin B_{12} 1,000 mcg and folic acid 5 mg are given intramuscularly, followed by daily administration of oral folic acid 1 mg and parenteral vitamin B_{12} 1,000 mcg for one week.

Children, a total of 1,000 to 5,000 mcg is given. Some clinicians prefer to divide this into doses of 30 to 50 mcg per day for two or more weeks. Others use larger doses (eg, 100 mcg) in order to reduce the total number of injections. Thereafter, 100 mcg every four weeks will maintain remission. *Infants,* for congenital transcobalamin deficiency, 1,000 mcg twice weekly.

In all patients with abnormal B_{12} absorption, therapy must be lifelong to maintain remission.

Intramuscular: For a therapeutic trial to establish diagnosis of vitamin B_{12} deficiency, 1 mcg/day for ten days plus a diet low in folic acid and vitamin B_{12}. However, with the availability of serum assays for B_{12}, methylmalonic acid, and homocysteine, therapeutic trials are no longer necessary. The flushing dose to saturate binding sites for the Schilling test is 1,000 mcg.

CYANOCOBALAMIN:

Generic. Solution 30 mcg/ml in 30 ml containers and 100 and 1,000 mcg/ml in 1, 10, and 30 ml containers. Also available in Tubex.

Available Trademarks.

Crysti-12 (Hauck), ***Rubesol-1000*** (Central), ***Rubramin PC*** (Apothecon).

HYDROXOCOBALAMIN:

Generic. Solution 100 mcg/ml in 30 ml containers and 1,000 mcg/ml in 10 and 30 ml containers (intramuscular use only).

Oral: (therapeutic) For maintenance of remission in pernicious anemia, *adults and children*, 1,000 mcg once daily (see Lederle, 1991; Hathcock and Troendle, 1991; not all authorities consider oral maintenance therapy acceptable, because monthly documentation that vitamin B_{12} concentrations remain above 250 pg/ml is required).

CYANOCOBALAMIN:

Generic. Tablets 25, 50, 100, 200, 250, 500, and 1,000 mcg (nonprescription).

Oral: (dietary supplements) For dietary vitamin B_{12} supplementation to prevent vitamin B_{12} deficiency, *adults and children,* 6 mcg daily (in vegans); *infants up to 1 year,* 2 to 3 mcg daily.

For oral dietary supplements, multivitamin preparations may be appropriate, but this usage is controversial. Single-entity oral vitamin B_{12} preparations also are available.

LIVER INJECTION

The crude soluble vitamin B_{12} activity contained in liver can be obtained in purified, generic form, either as a vitamin mixture for injection or as a single-entity preparation. There is no indication for use of these preparations, since cyanocobalamin crystalline injection is superior in all respects. Allergic reactions can occur.

Liver injection should not be used, and therefore no dosage information is provided.

Folates

Intracellular folate derivatives exist primarily in conjugated forms with multiple glutamic acid residues, most commonly in the heptaglutamate form (Babior, 1990 A). Although present in nearly all foods, they are readily destroyed by heat and may be lost from foods during processing or prolonged cooking. Absorption of folates from dietary sources requires enzymatic action of conjugase (gamma glutamyl transpeptidase) to remove the multiple glutamate residues leaving the monoglutamate form (folates with longer glutamate chains cannot be absorbed efficiently in the proximal small intestine). A carrier-mediated active transport mechanism drives folate monoglutamate into the epithelial cells of the proximal jejunum. The absorbed folates are reduced if necessary and then converted to N^5-methyltetrahydrofolate in the intestinal cells before being transported into the blood stream. Folate recirculates by secretion into the bile against a concentration gradient and then reabsorption from the intestine.

N^5-methyltetrahydrofolate enters cells by means of a membrane-associated transport protein (folate receptor). Intracellular retention of folate requires conjugation to polyglutamates. Storage depots in the liver retain folylpolyglutamates in amounts that exceed the immediate needs for hepatic metabolism. Distribution of N^5-methyltetrahydrofolate from hepatic storage sites to other tissues through the circulation again requires deconjugation to a monoglutamate.

After entering dividing cells, the folates enter a metabolic cycle in which they serve as cofactors (after going through a series of intermediate biochemical steps) for biosynthesis of thymidine and purine nucleotides required for cellular DNA synthesis. A vitamin B_{12}-dependent enzyme, N^5-methyltetrahydrofolate-homocysteine methyltransferase, "regenerates" free (ie, unmethylated) tetrahydrofolic acid that can then reenter the metabolic pathway for purine biosynthesis. This interrelationship between vitamin B_{12} and folates explains both the common nuclear maturation defect seen with deficiencies of both nutrients and the hematologic improvement seen in vitamin B_{12}-deficient patients after administration of folates. In the latter circumstance, the metabolic problem of B_{12} deficiency is bypassed through mass action with large quantities of folates.

It is estimated that the average adult requires approximately 50 mcg of folate daily from dietary sources. In the average person, total body folate stores are estimated to be approximately 7.5 mg. The usual American diet contains four to six times the minimum daily requirement of folates, and deficiency of the vitamin is more often caused by gastrointestinal abnormalities or other complicating factors, such as alcoholism or increased folate requirements, than by dietary deficiency. Alcoholics may have inadequate dietary folate intake if they are also malnourished.

Pregnant and lactating women, premature infants, children on synthetic diets, critically ill patients (especially those with severe infection), patients with chronic hemolytic anemia, hemodialysis patients, or those with chronic diseases (eg, renal failure, inflammation, neoplasia) also may have deficiency caused by increased folate requirements or inadequate intake.

Dietary folate deficiency is best treated by dietary measures rather than supplemental medications. Adequate correction can usually be achieved by adding one uncooked fruit or vegetable or glass of fruit juice each day. During pregnancy and lactation, folate requirements are especially high and may be difficult to meet through diet alone. Therefore, vitamin preparations containing supplemental folic acid are usually indicated prenatally.

The sodium salt of folic acid may be given by intramuscular, intravenous, or deep subcutaneous injection. Parenteral administration has no advantage over the oral route, but it may be preferred when this drug is a constituent of total parenteral nutrition solutions. It is also preferred in critically ill patients or patients with gastrointestinal disease that may limit or prevent absorption of the vitamin.

Indications: Folate-deficient patients with megaloblastic anemia usually respond quickly to folic acid; normalization of the bone marrow morphology occurs very rapidly and a brisk reticulocytosis begins two to five days after initiating treatment (Babior and Bunn, 1991; Allen, 1992; Cooper, 1992).

Folic acid is indicated in the treatment of infantile megaloblastosis, the megaloblastic anemias occurring during pregnancy, and in celiac disease or tropical sprue. It also is indicated in situations in which brisk erythropoiesis and rapid turnover of red blood cells (hemolytic disease) may cause relative folate deficiency, especially in patients with myeloid metaplasia or in children with thalassemia major or intermedia. There is evidence suggesting that daily oral doses of 100 mcg of folic acid in the month before contemplated pregnancy and during pregnancy may significantly reduce the frequency of neural tube defects. Recommendations issued before more definitive data became available suggested that pregnant women or those contemplating pregnancy take daily folate supplements of 50 to 100 mcg (depending on amounts of folate in their usual diets) (Herbert, 1990 C). More recent guidelines recommend a dose of 400 mcg/day (*MMWR,* 1992).

A daily prophylactic dose of folate should be given routinely during pregnancy and lactation, since dietary intake often cannot meet demands. In pregnant women taking antiepileptic drugs, administration of up to 1 mg daily did not adversely affect seizure control (Hillesmaa et al, 1983). Since folate storage in the fetus occurs primarily during the latter part of gestation, premature infants are likely to be born with smaller stores and are therefore more prone to develop folate deficiency.

Hospitalized critically ill patients, especially those maintained on unsupplemented intravenous fluids, may develop subtle folate deficiency that can cause granulocytopenia or decreases in other circulating elements when marrow demands are increased (eg, during episodes of infection). Inclusion of folates in the parenteral fluids is essential in such patients.

Some authorities believe that folate deficiency can result in several neurologic or psychiatric disorders, manifested by a variety of complaints. However, the use of folic acid in patients with such complaints in the absence of documented reduced serum folate levels has not been proved effective. In addition, vitamin B_{12} deficiency should always be excluded in such patients.

Patients with pernicious anemia or other vitamin B_{12} deficiency anemias will respond with correction of the hematologic abnormalities when given large doses of folic acid. One mg of folic acid per day may be enough to produce such a response (Crosby, 1986). However, folates do *not* prevent the development or progression of the neurologic symptoms of vitamin B_{12} deficiency or reverse such symptoms once they develop. Therefore, indiscriminate prophylactic use of folates should be avoided to prevent masking of vitamin B_{12} deficiency; before folate is given, serum and red blood cell folate concentrations as well as serum vitamin B_{12} concentrations should be measured to confirm the deficiency.

Several drugs can induce folate deficiency. Antiepileptic drugs may block absorption of folates, and some antimalarial drugs interfere with dihydrofolate reductase, thus interfering with both metabolic activation of the vitamin and its transport into the cell. Some data suggest that folate requirements also may be increased by long-term use of some contraceptives, analgesics, steroids, or doses of sulfasalazine exceeding 2 g/day.

Leucovorin calcium (folinic acid) is a metabolically reduced form of folate (in the tetrahydrofolate form) that does not require the enzymatic action of dihydrofolate reductase for its activation. It is used principally to "rescue" patients treated for neoplastic disease with the folate antagonist (dihydrofolate reductase inhibitor), methotrexate, and also is effective in patients treated with other dihydrofolate reductase inhibitors, such as trimethoprim. Leucovorin also is used to modulate the antitumor effects of fluorouracil used in the treatment of metastatic colon cancer.

Drug Evaluations

FOLIC ACID
[Folvite]

FOLATE SODIUM
[Folvite Solution]

These synthetic unreduced folates are indicated specifically for the treatment of folate deficiency. They are *not* appropriate, may be dangerous, and should never be used as the sole treatment of pernicious anemia or other vitamin B_{12} deficiency states for the reasons cited above. There also is no evidence to support the use of folates to treat various psychiatric and neurologic disorders, for which they have been advocated, in the absence of evidence of reduced levels of serum and red blood cell folate and without excluding vitamin B_{12} deficiency.

Some patients with small bowel disease are unable to break down the nonabsorbable polyglutamate forms of folate found in foodstuffs. However, the vast majority of such patients will be able to absorb folic acid, because it is presented to the gut in much higher concentrations than naturally occurring folates.

Patients with a life-threatening illness caused by severe megaloblastic anemia with circulatory compromise, severe thrombocytopenia, or severe granulocytopenia may require initiation of treatment before a specific diagnosis can be established. These patients should have serum and whole blood samples frozen for later assay of folate and vitamin B_{12} levels, after which they should be treated empirically with both folic acid and vitamin B_{12}.

Oral doses exceeding 100 mcg daily should be avoided unless vitamin B_{12} deficiency has been excluded or is already being treated, or unless the patient's condition is complicated by infection, uremia, arthritis, ulcerative colitis, liver disease, or another inflammatory or myelosuppressive disorder. Doses larger than 5 mg daily are never indicated, because the excess amount is excreted in the urine and no further increase in hematopoiesis occurs.

There is no known direct toxicity of folic acid in humans, although oral doses of 350 mcg or more may interfere with absorption of zinc (Herbert, 1990 C). However, the seizure threshold of patients taking antiepileptic drugs (eg, phenytoin) may be lowered significantly when megadoses of folic acid are given concomitantly; therefore, these patients should not receive doses in excess of 1 mg and preferably not more than 300 mcg.

DOSAGE AND PREPARATIONS.

Therapeutic:

Intramuscular, Intravenous, Subcutaneous: *Adults and children,* 0.5 to 1 mg daily for most deficiencies. When symptoms subside and blood tests become normal, a maintenance dose of 0.25 to 0.5 mg daily should be given orally if possible. Patients with severe megaloblastic anemia requiring immediate therapy should receive folic acid 5 mg with vitamin B_{12} 1,000 mcg parenterally, followed by folic acid 1 mg and vitamin B_{12} 1,000 mcg daily for one week.

Oral: The manufacturers' recommended oral replacement dose for *adults and children* is 0.25 to 1 mg daily. In most adults with uncomplicated folic acid deficiency, as little as 0.1 mg daily will be efficacious without risk of masking vitamin B_{12} deficiency (Crosby, 1986).

Prophylactic:

Oral: *Adults and children,* during periods of high demand, such as hemolysis or infection, 0.5 to 1 mg daily. *During pregnancy and lactation*, 0.8 mg daily. For all prophylactic indications after vitamin B_{12} deficiency has been excluded or is already being treated, 1 mg daily is a reasonable dose. *Low-birth-weight infants and those fed goat's milk formulas,* 0.05 mg daily.

FOLIC ACID:

Generic. Tablets 0.1, 0.4, 0.8 (nonprescription), and 1 mg.

Folvite (Lederle). Tablets 1 mg.

FOLATE SODIUM:

Generic. Solution (for injection) equivalent to folic acid 5 and 10 mg/ml in 10 ml containers.

Folvite Solution (Lederle). Solution (for injection) equivalent to folic acid 5 mg/ml in 10 ml containers.

LEUCOVORIN CALCIUM (Folinic Acid)

[Wellcovorin]

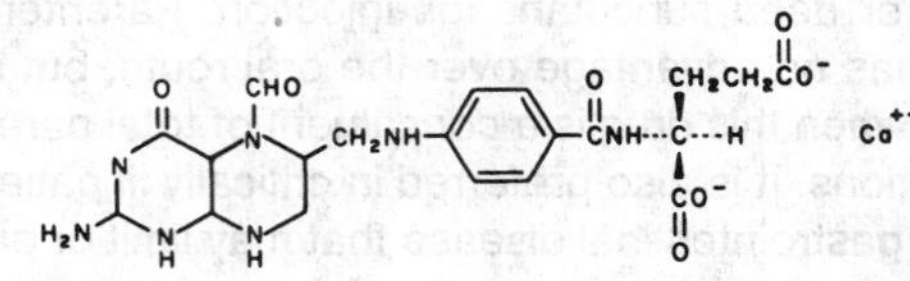

ACTIONS. Leucovorin calcium is a metabolically active form of tetrahydrofolate, also known as N^5-formyltetrahydrofolic acid or citrovorum factor. It is functionally identical to folic acid, except that it is already in reduced form and does not require the action of dihydrofolate reductase. It is converted to N^5-methyltetrahydrofolic acid 20 to 30 minutes after administration of an oral dose. Its plasma peak occurs in 1.5 to 2 hours, and therapeutic plasma levels are maintained for three to six hours. It is excreted almost completely in the urine.

USES. This drug can be used interchangeably with folic acid for the treatment of folate deficiency. However, because it is much more expensive than folic acid, its use should be reserved for those situations in which there is a specific requirement to bypass the dihydrofolate reductase step. The most important of these are for "leucovorin rescue" of patients given large doses of antifols (especially methotrexate) and to modulate responses to fluorouracil. It also may be useful in patients who are receiving other folate antagonists.

The preservatives present in some leucovorin preparations occasionally produce allergic reactions. This drug is classified in FDA Pregnancy Category C.

DOSAGE AND PREPARATIONS.

Oral, Intramuscular, Intravenous: *Adults and children,* no more than 1 mg daily for the treatment of folate deficiency. Doses for use in "rescue" protocols must be individualized according to the antifol used, its dose, and its serum levels and pharmacokinetics.

Generic. Powder for injection (cryodesiccated, preservative-free) 50, 100, and 350 mg; solution (injection) 5 mg/ml in 5 ml containers; tablets 5, 15, and 25 mg.

Wellcovorin (Burroughs Wellcome). Powder (for injection) 50 and 100 mg (preservative-free); tablets 5 and 25 mg.

SIDEROBLASTIC ANEMIAS

Sideroblastic anemias are virtually never simple deficiency anemias, although some patients respond to administration of vitamin B_6 (pyridoxine). These disorders have several features in common, including ineffective erythropoiesis (apparently resulting from abnormal cytoplasmic maturation, thus distinguishing them from megaloblastic anemias) and an extraordinary accumulation of iron (in hemosiderin) within the mitochondria of erythroblasts in a ring form around the nucleus (Beutler, 1990; Bridges and Bunn, 1991; Kushner, 1992).

The mitochondria are the site of porphyrin biosynthesis and insertion of iron into the porphyrin ring to form heme. The abnormal accumulation of iron in the mitochondria is presumably the result of some defect in heme synthesis, either during synthesis of the porphyrin ring itself or during incorporation of iron into the ring (Bottomley and Muller-Eberhard, 1988). Sideroblastic anemia rarely may occur as a congenital abnormality (eg, as a result of delta-aminolevulinic acid [ALA] synthetase, uroporphyrinogen decarboxylase, heme synthetase, or coproporphyrin oxygenase deficiency) and may respond to long-term administration of pyridoxine. Pyridoxal phosphate, which is enzymatically synthesized from pyridoxine in vivo, is a required cofactor for ALA synthetase and for the conversion of serine to glycine. The latter reaction is also important for erythropoiesis, since it generates the specific folate cofactor needed for thymidylate biosynthesis. It is unclear, however, why pharmacologic doses of pyridoxine are effective in some types of sideroblastic anemia.

Sideroblastic anemia also may occur as an acquired disorder, either as a consequence of alcoholism (often accompanied by megaloblastic anemia due to folate deficiency) or as an idiopathic disorder. In the latter circumstance, some patients have evidence of disordered nuclear maturation as well as of disordered maturation of other cellular elements of the bone marrow. These are now classified as myelodysplastic syndromes (or dysmyelopoietic syndromes) and, in many patients, will progress to acute leukemia. An analysis of the prognostic factors that are predictive of leukemic conversion showed that elevated percentages of myeloblasts in the bone marrow correlated positively, while increased numbers of ringed sideroblasts correlated negatively with leukemic transformation (Vandermolen et al, 1988). Patients who do not develop neoplasia often become transfusion-dependent and suffer from the effects of iron overload (Cazzola et al, 1988).

In alcoholic patients, the ringed sideroblasts may develop as the result of a relative intracellular deficiency of pyridoxal phosphate, perhaps because the phosphorylation step fails to take place. Some of these individuals will respond to administration of pyridoxine 50 to 200 mg daily. However, the sideroblastic changes usually reverse spontaneously within 7 to 12 days, and there is little evidence that they are caused by a pyridoxine deficiency state (Lindenbaum, 1987). Since alcoholic patients frequently have coexistent folate deficiency, they also should be given folic acid. This will often correct both the megaloblastosis and sideroblastosis.

Patients with idiopathic sideroblastic anemias *not* associated with other marrow abnormalities sometimes respond to pyridoxine (50 to 200 mg/day), although the response tends to be transient. However, those with myelodysplasia only infrequently respond to pyridoxine (Cazzola et al, 1988; Vandermolen et al, 1988).

Improvements in several hematologic parameters after infusion of heme arginate have been reported in a small number of patients with either acquired myelodysplasia (Volin et al, 1988) or hereditary sideroblastic anemia that did not respond to pyridoxine (Volin, 1989). However, other investigators have reported that there was no improvement in erythropoiesis in response to heme arginate therapy for primary acquired sideroblastic anemia (Houston et al, 1992).

Finally, several drugs can interfere with porphyrin synthesis or pyridoxine metabolism and cause sideroblastic anemia. Isoniazid, pyrazinamide, cycloserine, and chloramphenicol are examples of agents that can cause sideroblastosis, which can be prevented by administration of pyridoxine 50 mg daily. Although lead intoxication is often included among the causes of sideroblastic anemia (Beutler, 1990), some investigators report that ring sideroblasts in iron-stained marrow aspirates are absent from patients with lead intoxication (Bottomley and Muller-Eberhard, 1988).

MIXTURES

Deficiency anemias must be diagnosed accurately and specifically before therapy is initiated. Once a diagnosis is established, the most appropriate treatment is usually administration of the specific nutrient that is deficient. This is the proper approach except when multiple deficiencies are present.

Except in nutritional anemias resulting from very poor diets or malnutrition in which a multiple vitamin supplement is appropriate, the use of mixtures of hematinics is strongly discouraged. Combination therapy is indicated only when it can be demonstrated clearly that one type of deficiency anemia is superimposed on another. Even in this circumstance, the use of specific replacement therapy is preferred. Avoidance of mixtures is better therapy and, in some situations, may be mandatory. For example, combined iron and vitamin B_{12} deficiencies mandate two different preferred routes of administration, and use of a mixture in this situation would be totally inappropriate.

Mixtures also often add needlessly to the cost of replacement therapy. For instance, iron preparations containing ascorbate are substantially more expensive than generic ferrous sulfate tablets. Even though ascorbate will enhance iron absorption, in clinical practice it is almost never necessary to add that additional absorptive "boost." In addition, many of the commercially available mixtures are irrational combinations of multiple hematinic agents, such as iron plus vitamin B_{12}, folate, pyridoxine, and ascorbate. Trace metals, such as copper, often are also included and are of no value in these preparations except for the rare patient with documented copper deficiency anemia. Furthermore, there are data demonstrating that ascorbate, thiamine, and copper interact to convert vitamin B_{12} to analogues that may interfere with absorption or retention of vitamin B_{12} (Kondo et al, 1982).

Because these preparations have no justifiable use in the treatment of nutritional deficiency anemias, a partial listing is provided for identification only. Patients who require multiple vitamin or vitamin and mineral supplementation may be appropriately treated with nutritional supplements not designed to treat anemia, and these are described elsewhere; see index entry Vitamins, Multivitamin Preparations.

Caltrate 600 Plus Iron & Vitamin D (Lederle). Each tablet contains ferrous fumarate 54 mg (equivalent to elemental iron 18 mg), calcium carbonate 1.5 g, and vitamin D 125 IU (nonprescription).

Cevi-Fer (Geriatric). Each capsule (prolonged-release) contains ferrous fumarate 60 mg (equivalent to elemental iron 20 mg), ascorbic acid 300 mg, and folic acid 1 mg.

Chromagen Capsules (Savage). Each capsule contains ferrous fumarate 200 mg (equivalent to elemental iron 66 mg), cyanocobalamin 10 mcg, ascorbic acid 250 mg, and desiccated stomach substance 100 mg.

Ferancee (Johnson & Johnson/Merck Consumer). Each tablet (chewable) contains ferrous fumarate 209 mg (equivalent to elemental iron 67 mg) and vitamin C 150 mg (ascorbic acid 59 mg and sodium ascorbate 136 mg) (nonprescription).

Fero-Folic-500 (Abbott). Each tablet (prolonged-release) contains ferrous sulfate 525 mg (equivalent to elemental iron 105 mg), folic acid 0.8 mg, and sodium ascorbate 500 mg.

Fero-Grad-500 (Abbott). Each tablet (prolonged-release iron) contains ferrous sulfate 525 mg (equivalent to elemental iron 105 mg) and sodium ascorbate 500 mg (nonprescription).

Ferro-Sequels (Lederle). Each capsule (prolonged-release) contains ferrous fumarate 150 mg (equivalent to elemental iron 50 mg) and docusate sodium 100 mg (nonprescription).

Iberet (Abbott). Each tablet (prolonged-release iron) or 20 ml of liquid contains ferrous sulfate 525 mg (equivalent to elemental iron 105 mg), cyanocobalamin 25 mcg, sodium ascorbate 150 mg (tablet) or ascorbic acid 150 mg (liquid), thiamine mononitrate 6 mg, riboflavin 6 mg, niacinamide 30 mg, pyridoxine hydrochloride 5 mg, and calcium pantothenate 10 mg (alcohol 1% [liquid]) (both forms nonprescription).

Iberet-500 (Abbott). Each tablet (prolonged-release) or 20 ml of liquid contains same formulation as ***Iberet*** except sodium ascorbate 500 mg (tablet) or ascorbic acid 500 mg (liquid) (both forms nonprescription).

Iberet-Folic-500 (Abbott). Each tablet (prolonged-release) contains same formulation as ***Iberet-500*** plus folic acid 0.8 mg.

Ircon-FA (Kenwood). Each tablet contains ferrous fumarate 250 mg (equivalent to elemental iron 82 mg) and folic acid 0.8 mg (nonprescription).

Iromin-G (Mission). Each tablet contains ferrous gluconate 260 mg (equivalent to 30 mg elemental iron), vitamin B_{12} (crystalline or resin) 2 mcg, ascorbic acid 100 mg, thiamine mononitrate 5 mg, riboflavin 2 mg, pyridoxine hydrochloride 25 mg, niacinamide 10 mg, folic acid 0.8 mg, calcium pantothenate 1 mg, vitamin A acetate 4,000 IU, vitamin D_2 400 IU, calcium carbonate 70 mg (calcium 50 mg), calcium gluconate 100 mg, and calcium lactate 100 mg (nonprescription).

Niferex-150 Forte (Central). Each capsule contains polysaccharide-iron complex 150 mg, vitamin B_{12} 25 mcg, and folic acid 1 mg; each 5 ml of elixir contains polysaccharide-iron complex 100 mg, vitamin B_{12} 25 mcg, and folic acid 1 mg (alcohol 10%).

Nu-Iron Plus (Mayrand). Each 5 ml of elixir contains polysaccharide-iron complex 100 mg, vitamin B_{12} 25 mcg, and folic acid 1 mg (alcohol 10%).

Simron Plus (SmithKline Beecham). Each capsule contains ferrous gluconate 86 mg (equivalent to elemental iron 10 mg), cyanocobalamin 3.3 mcg, sodium ascorbate 50 mg, pyridoxine hydrochloride 1 mg, and folic acid 0.1 mg (nonprescription).

Stuartinic (Johnson & Johnson/Merck Consumer). Each tablet contains ferrous fumarate 300 mg (equivalent to elemental iron 100 mg), ascorbic acid and sodium ascorbate 500 mg, cyanocobalamin 25 mcg, thiamine mononitrate 4.9 mg, riboflavin 6 mg, pyridoxine hydrochloride 0.8 mg, niacinamide 20 mg, and calcium pantothenate 9.2 mg (nonprescription).

Tabron (Parke-Davis). Each tablet contains ferrous fumarate 304.2 mg (equivalent to 100 mg elemental iron), ascorbic acid 500 mg, cyanocobalamin 25 mcg, folic acid 1 mg, thiamine mononitrate 6 mg, riboflavin 6 mg, pyridoxine hydrochloride 5 mg, niacinamide 30 mg, calcium pantothenate 10 mg, vitamin E 30 IU, and docusate sodium 50 mg.

Theragran Hematinic (Apothecon). Each tablet contains ferrous fumarate equivalent to elemental iron 66.7 mg, cyanocobalamin 50 mcg, folic acid 0.33 mg, sodium ascorbate 100 mg, thiamine mononitrate 3.3 mg, riboflavin 3.3 mg, niacinamide 33.3 mg, pyridoxine hydrochloride 3.3 mg, vitamin A acetate 0.42 mg (1,400 IU), ergocalciferol 3.5 mg (140 IU), vitamin E 5 mg (5 IU), calcium pantothenate 11.7 mg, copper sulfate 0.67 mg, and magnesium carbonate 41.7 mg.

TriHEMIC 600 (Lederle). Each tablet contains ferrous fumarate 350 mg (equivalent to elemental iron 115 mg), cyanocobalamin 25 mcg, intrinsic factor concentrate 75 mg, folic acid 1 mg, ascorbic acid 600 mg, vitamin E 30 IU, and docusate sodium 50 mg.

Trinsicon (Whitby). Each capsule contains ferrous fumarate equivalent to elemental iron 110 mg, vitamin B_{12} (activity equivalent) 15 mcg, liver-stomach concentrate (containing intrinsic factor) 240 mg, folic acid 0.5 mg, and ascorbic acid 75 mg.

Vitron-C (Fisons). Each tablet (chewable) contains ferrous fumarate 200 mg (equivalent to elemental iron 66 mg) and ascorbic acid 125 mg (nonprescription).

Cited References

Recommendations for the use of folic acid to reduce the number of cases of spina bifida and other neural tube defects. *MMWR* 41 (No. RR-14):1-7, 1992.

Allen RH: Megaloblastic anemias, in Wyngaarden JB, et al (eds): *Cecil Textbook of Medicine*, ed 19. Philadelphia, WB Saunders, 1992, 846-854.

Atrah HI, Davidson RJL: Iron deficiency in pernicious anaemia: A neglected diagnosis. *Postgrad Med J* 64:110-111, 1988.

Babior BM: Metabolic aspects of folic acid and cobalamin, in Williams WJ, et al (eds): *Hematology.* New York, McGraw-HIll, 1990 A, 339-355.

Babior BM: The megaloblastic anemias, in Williams WJ, et al (eds): *Hematology.* New York, McGraw-Hill, 1990 B, 453-481.

Babior BM, Bunn HF: Megaloblastic anemias, in Wilson JD, et al (eds): *Harrison's Principles of Internal Medicine*, ed 12. New York, McGraw-Hill, 1991, 1523-1529.

Babitz LE, Freedman ML: Anemia in the aged. *Compr Ther* 14:55-64, (June) 1988.

Beck WS: Neuropsychiatric consequences of cobalamin deficiency. *Adv Intern Med* 36:33-56, 1991.

Bereman RD, Berg KA: Structure, size and solution chemistry of a polysaccharide iron complex (Niferex). *Inorg Chim Acta* 155:183-189, 1989.

Berg KA, et al: Identification of ferrihydrite in polysaccharide iron complex by Mossbauer spectroscopy and x-ray diffraction. *J Inorg Biochem* 22:125-135, 1984.

Beutler E: The common anemias. *JAMA* 259:2433-2437, 1988.

Beutler E: Hereditary and secondary acquired sideroblastic anemias, in Williams WJ, et al (eds): *Hematology.* New York, McGraw-Hill, 1990, 554-557.

Bottomley SS, Muller-Eberhard U: Pathophysiology of heme synthesis. *Semin Hematol* 25:282-302, 1988.

Bridges KR, Bunn HF: Anemias with disturbed iron metabolism, in *Harrison's Principles of Internal Medicine*, ed 12. New York, McGraw Hill, 1991, 1518-1523.

Brock JH: The biology of iron, in de Sousa M, Brock JH (eds): *Iron in Immunity, Cancer and Inflammation.* Chichester, England, John Wiley & Sons, 1989, 35-53.

Brown RG: Determining the cause of anemia: General approach, with emphasis on microcytic hypochromic anemias. *Postgrad Med* 89:161-170, (May) 1991.

Bunn HF: Pathophysiology of the anemias, in Wilson JD, et al (eds): *Harrison's Principles of Internal Medicine*, ed 12. New York, McGraw-Hill, 1991, 1514-1518.

Campbell NRC, Hasinoff BB: Iron supplements: A common cause of drug interactions. *Br J Clin Pharmacol* 31:251-255, 1991.

Carmel R: Subtle and atypical cobalamin deficiency states. *Am J Hematol* 34:108-114, 1990.

Carmel R, et al: Iron deficiency occurs frequently in patients with pernicious anemia. *JAMA* 257:1081-1083, 1987.

Cazzola M, et al: Natural history of idiopathic refractory sideroblastic anemia. *Blood* 71:305-312, 1988.

Cook JD, et al: Absorption of controlled-release iron. *Clin Pharmacol Ther* 32:531-539, 1982.

Cook JD, et al: Gastric delivery system for iron supplementation. *Lancet* 335:1136-1139, 1990.

Cooper BA: Pernicious anemia and other megaloblastic anemias, in Rakel RE (ed): *1992: Conn's Current Therapy*. Philadelphia, WB Saunders, 1992, 306-308.

Crosby WH: Overtreating the deficiency anemias. *Arch Intern Med* 146:779, 1986.

Dallman PR: Review of iron metabolism, in Filer LJ Jr (ed): *Dietary Iron: Birth to Two Years*. New York, Raven Press, 1989, 1-17.

Dawson DW, et al: Laboratory diagnosis of megaloblastic anemia: Current methods assessed by external quality assurance trials. *J Clin Pathol* 40:393-397, 1987.

Delorme MA, et al: Prescribing and dispensing practices for oral iron tablets: A Canadian experience. *DICP* 24:874-877, 1990.

Erslev AJ: Clinical manifestations and classification of erythrocyte disorders, in Williams WJ, et al (eds): *Hematology*. New York, McGraw-Hill, 1990, 423-429.

Fairbanks VF, Baldus WP: Iron overload, in Williams WJ, et al (eds): *Hematology*, ed 4. New York, McGraw-Hill, 1990, 752-758.

Fairbanks VF, Beutler E: Iron metabolism, in Williams WJ, et al (eds): *Hematology*. New York, McGraw-Hill, 1990 A, 329-339.

Fairbanks VF, Beutler E: Iron deficiency, in Williams WJ, et al (eds): *Hematology*. New York, McGraw-Hill, 1990 B, 482-505.

Fine EJ, Soria ED: Myths about vitamin B_{12} deficiency. *South Med J* 84:1475-1481, 1991.

Gordeuk VR, et al: Carbonyl iron therapy for iron deficiency anemia. *Blood* 67:745-752, 1986.

Gordeuk VR, et al: Carbonyl iron for short-term supplementation in female blood donors. *Transfusion* 27:80-85, 1987 A.

Gordeuk VR, et al: High-dose carbonyl iron for iron deficiency anemia: A randomized double-blind trial. *Am J Clin Nutr* 46:1029-1034, 1987 B.

Gordeuk VR, et al: Prevention of iron deficiency with carbonyl iron in female blood donors. *Transfusion* 30:239-245, 1990.

Griffiths A: Diagnosis of cobalamin deficiency, correspondence. *Blood* 77:1853, 1991.

Guyatt GH, et al: Diagnosis of iron-deficiency anemia in the elderly. *Am J Med* 88:205-209, 1990.

Hall CA: The neurologic aspects of transcobalamin II deficiency. *Br J Haematol* 80:117-120, 1992.

Harju E: Clinical pharmacokinetics of iron preparations. *Clin Pharmacokinet* 17:68-89, 1989.

Hathcock JN, Troendle GH: Oral cobalamin for treatment of pernicious anemia? Editorial. *JAMA* 265:96-97, 1991.

Herbert V: The Herman Award Lecture. Nutrition science as a continually unfolding story: The folate and vitamin B_{12} paradigm. *Am J Clin Nutr* 46:387-402, 1987.

Herbert V: Vitamin B_{12}, in Brown ML (ed): *Present Knowledge in Nutrition*, ed 6. Washington, DC, International Life Sciences Institute/Nutrition Foundation, 1990 A, 170-178.

Herbert V: Low holotranscobalamin II is the earliest serum marker for subnormal vitamin B_{12} (cobalamin) malabsorption in patients with AIDS. *Am J Hematol* 34:132-139, 1990 B.

Herbert V: Development of human folate deficiency, in Picciano MF, et al (eds): *Folic Acid Metabolism in Health and Disease*. New York, Wiley-Liss, 1990 C, 195-210.

Hillesmaa V, et al: Serum folate concentrations during pregnancy in women with epilepsy: Relation to antiepileptic drug concentrations, numbers of seizures, and fetal outcome. *BMJ* 287:577-579, 1983.

Houston T, et al: Treatment of primary acquired sideroblastic anaemia with haem arginate, correspondence. *Br J Haematol* 80:263-264, 1992.

Irigoyen M, et al: Randomized, placebo-controlled trial of iron supplementation in infants with low hemoglobin levels fed iron-fortified formula. *Pediatrics* 88:320-326, 1991.

Kara M, et al: Clinical and chemical interactions between iron preparations and ciprofloxacin. *Br J Clin Pharmacol* 31:257-261, 1991.

Karnad AB, Krozser-Hamati A: Pernicious anemia: Early identification to prevent permanent sequelae. *Postgrad Med* 91:231-237, (Feb) 1992.

Kondo H, et al: Presence and formation of cobalamin analogues in multivitamin-mineral pills. *J Clin Invest* 70:889-989, 1982.

Kumpf VJ, Holland EG: Parenteral iron dextran therapy. *DICP* 24:162-166, 1990.

Kushner JP: Hypochromic anemias, in Wyngaarden JB, et al (eds): *Cecil Textbook of Medicine*, ed 19. Philadelphia, WB Saunders, 1992, 839-846.

Lederle FA: Oral cobalamin for pernicious anemia: Medicine's best kept secret? *JAMA* 265:94-95, 1991.

Lindenbaum J: Hematologic complications of alcohol abuse. *Semin Liver Dis* 7:169-181, 1987.

Lindenbaum J: An approach to the anemias, in Wyngaarden JB, et al (eds): *Cecil Textbook of Medicine*, ed 19. Philadelphia, WB Saunders, 1992, 822-831.

Lindenbaum J, et al: Neuropsychiatric disorders caused by cobalamin deficiency in the absence of anemia or macrocytosis. *N Engl J Med* 318:1720-1728, 1988.

Lindenbaum J, et al: Diagnosis of cobalamin deficiency: II. Relative sensitivities of serum cobalamin, methylmalonic acid, and total homocysteine concentrations. *Am J Hematol* 34:99-107, 1990.

Lutcher CL: Iron deficiency, in Rakel RE (ed): *1992: Conn's Current Therapy*. Philadelphia, WB Saunders, 1992, 295-297.

Newton RW, et al: Prophylaxis of iron-deficiency anaemia of prematurity: Oral and intramuscular iron in preterm infants. *Clin Trials J* 17:106-111, 1980.

Piccinini L, Ricciotti M: Therapeutic effectiveness of an iron-polysaccharide complex in comparison with iron fumarate in the treatment of iron deficiency anaemias. *Panminerva Med* 24:213-220, 1982.

Polk RE, et al: Effect of ferrous sulfate and multivitamins with zinc on absorption of ciprofloxacin in normal volunteers. *Antimicrob Agents Chemother* 33:1841-1844, 1989.

Sanders JF: Clinical response to iron-polysaccharide complex in geriatric patients with iron-deficiency anemia. *Mich Med* 67:726-727, 1968.

Soff GA, Levin J: Thrombocytopenia associated with repletion of iron in iron-deficiency anemia. *Am J Med Sci* 295:35-39, 1988.

Stabler SP, et al: Clinical spectrum and diagnosis of cobalamin deficiency. *Blood* 76:871-881, 1990.

Stabler SP, et al: Diagnosis of cobalamin deficiency: Response, correspondence. *Blood* 77:1854, 1991.

Stander PE: Anemia in the elderly: Symptoms, causes, and therapies. *Postgrad Med* 85:85-96, (Feb) 1989.

Talley NJ, et al: Risk for colorectal adenocarcinoma in pernicious anemia. *Ann Intern Med* 111:738-742, 1989.

Vandermolen L, et al: Ringed sideroblasts in primary myelodysplasia. *Arch Intern Med* 148:653-656, 1988.

Volin L: Haem arginate treatment for hereditary sideroblastic anaemia. *Eur J Haematol* 42:60-66, 1989.

Volin L, et al: Heme arginate treatment for myelodysplastic syndromes. *Leuk Res* 12:423-431, 1988.

Welborn JL, Meyers FJ: A three-point approach to anemia. *Postgrad Med* 89:179-186, (Feb) 1991.

Yip R: Iron nutritional status defined, in Filer LJ Jr (ed): *Dietary Iron: Birth to Two Years*. New York, Raven Press, 1989, 19-36.

Yip R, et al: Declining prevalence of anemia among low-income children in the United States. *JAMA* 258:1619-1623, 1987.

Drugs Used in Obesity

OBESITY

Excess adiposity, the most common form of nutrient imbalance in developed countries, occurs when more energy from foodstuffs is stored than is used for metabolism and physical activities. Social, scientific, and philosophical views on overweight and obesity are changing based on new data available on the etiology, pathogenesis, associated morbidity and mortality, and management of this complex disorder (Bray, 1988 Gray,1988 A, 1988 B; Bray, 1989 B).

CLINICAL CLASSIFICATIONS. Although the terms overweight and obesity frequently are used interchangeably, they are not necessarily synonymous. *Overweight* is an increase in body weight above some arbitrary standard defined in relation to height and is not necessarily due to an increase in total body fat. For example, it can occur in athletes as a result of increased muscle mass or in women primarily as a result of fluid retention caused by estrogen-containing oral contraceptives. *Obesity* is a condition of increased adipose tissue mass. The percentage of fat in nonobese young men and women is 15% to 18% and 22% to 30%, respectively, and tends to increase with age in both sexes. Increased lean body mass also is present in obese individuals; however, about 75% of the excess weight consists of fat (Gray and Bauer, 1991).

Obesity can be classified by age of onset (ie, childhood-onset, adult-onset), the character and distribution of adipose tissue, the degree of obesity, and its etiology. During the first year of life, both nonobese and obese infants store fat by increasing the size of fat cells present at birth. After the first year of life, fat cells remain large in obese children (*hypertrophic obesity*) but decrease in volume in nonobese children. Fat cells multiply through the developing years of childhood but the increase in number normally stops in adolescence. However, the number of fat cells continues to increase (*hypercellular obesity*), even into adult life, in individuals destined to become severely overweight. Moderately overweight individuals characteristically have hypertrophic obesity; those who are severely obese usually have a combination of hypercellular and hypertrophic obesity (Hirsch et al, 1989). Hypercellular obesity is a poor prognostic sign; the number of fat cells appears to be irreversible, and body weight in these individuals tends to remain significantly above the ideal even after some success in weight reduction.

Etiologic classification of obesity reflects its multifactorial nature. Differential diagnosis must take into account all of the following genetic and/or environmental causes: complex polygenic and the relatively rare single-gene dysmorphic obesities, dietary practices, use of certain drugs (eg, phenelzine, tricyclic antidepressants, methysergide, lithium, adrenal corticosteroids [Bernstein, 1987]), lack of physical activity, age, psychological and neuroendocrine disorders (eg, hypothyroidism, hyperadrenalism, hyperinsulinemia, hypogonadism), and socioeconomic factors. Algorithms are available to facilitate treatment-oriented diagnosis (Bray, 1989 B).

CLINICAL MEASUREMENT. Relative weight, body mass index, and fat distribution are the three major indices currently available for diagnosing obesity and monitoring therapeutic interventions.

Relative weight is the actual body weight divided by an arbitrary "desirable" standard weight based on height. For many years the accepted desirable-weight standards have been those published by the Metropolitan Life Insurance Company. However, these standards have been criticized because they are based on actuarial data that do not relate relative body weight to health status while alive (Knapp, 1983; Harrison, 1985).

The U.S. Department of Health and Human Services has published an alternative table of suggested "healthy" weight ranges (Table 1). Individuals whose weight falls outside these ranges are either underweight or overweight. This table does not distinguish between men and women, but it does recognize that good health is not inconsistent with some additional weight gain after maturity (Andres et al, 1985; Rissanen et al, 1989; Tuomilehto, 1991). Although some criticism has focused on the upper limits within each weight range, the ranges have been calculated to correspond to what have become accepted as healthy ranges of Body Mass Index (19 to 25 kg/M^2 for adults up to age 34; 21 to 27 kg/M^2 for adults older than age 34) (see Jéquier, 1987; Bray and Gray, 1988 A; Bray, 1989 B; Committee on Diet and Health, 1989; Gray, 1989).

The *Body Mass Index* (BMI) is now recommended as the measure of choice for interpreting body weight in adults (National Institutes of Health Consensus Development Panel, 1985). This indicator is expressed as weight/height^2 (kg/M^2) obtained from subjects wearing neither clothes nor shoes (see Figure 1) and correlates well with body fat estimated by measuring total body water, total body potassium, or body water displacement (Revicki and Israel, 1986; Heitmann, 1990; Gray and Fujioka, 1991; Knowler et al, 1991). However, the average BMI tends to increase from childhood to maturity (see Figures 2 and 3), which decreases its usefulness in assessing individuals under 18 years (Jonides, 1990). For suggested systems for classifying body weight according to BMI, see Figures 1 and 4 (Frankel, 1986; Gray, 1989; Bray, 1991 A).

TABLE 1.
SUGGESTED WEIGHTS FOR ADULTS[1]

Height[2]		Weight (lb)[3]	
Ft	In	19-34 Years	35 Years and Older
5	0	97-128	108-138
5	1	101-132	111-143
5	2	104-137	115-148
5	3	107-141	119-152
5	4	111-146	122-157
5	5	114-150	126-162
5	6	118-155	130-167
5	7	121-160	134-172
5	8	125-164	138-178
5	9	129-169	142-183
5	10	132-174	146-188
5	11	136-179	151-194
6	0	140-184	155-199
6	1	144-189	159-205
6	2	148-195	164-210
6	3	152-200	168-216
6	4	156-205	173-222
6	5	160-211	177-228
6	6	164-216	182-234

[1] *From* Nutrition and Your Health: Dietary Guidelines for Americans, *ed 3, 1990. U.S. Dept. of Health and Human Services.*

[2] *Without shoes.*

[3] *Without clothing.*

NOMOGRAM FOR BODY MASS INDEX

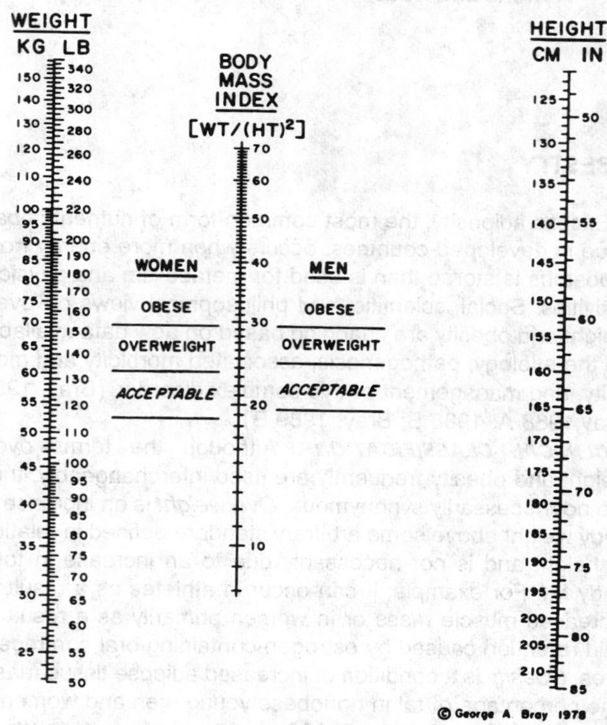

Figure 1. Nomogram for determining body mass index (BMI). Place a straight edge between the column for weight and the column for height and read the BMI from the point where this straight edge crosses the BMI line. (Bray, 1978. Reprinted with permission.)

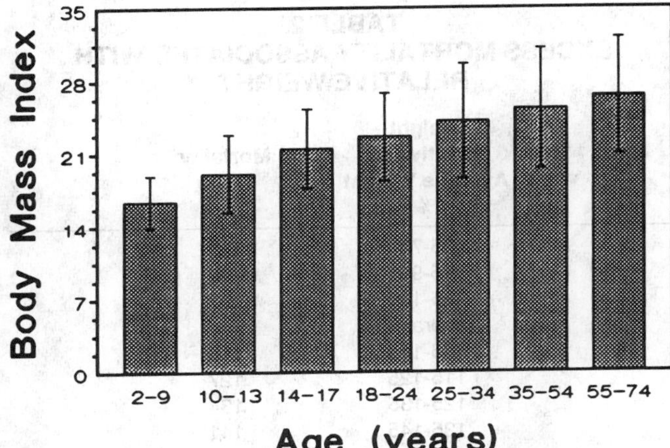

Figure 2. Body mass index (BMI) for females aged 2-74 years, grouped by related ages (mean ± SD). Adapted from Najjar and Rowland, 1987, based on NHANES II data (all races, U.S., 1976-1980).

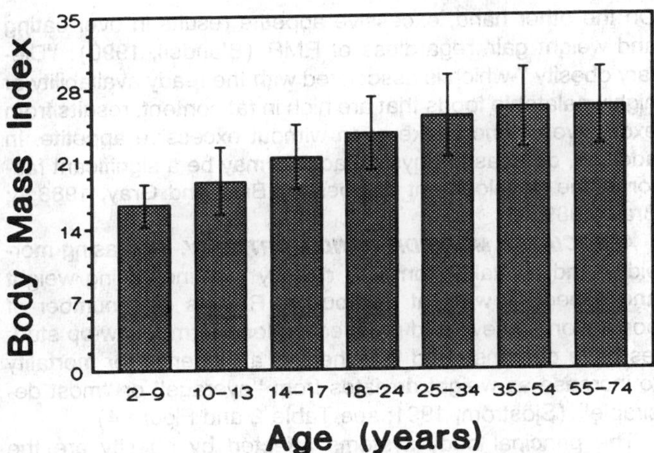

Figure 3. Body mass index (BMI) for males aged 2-74 years, grouped by related ages (mean ± SD). Adapted from Najjar and Rowland, 1987, based on NHANES II data (all races, U.S., 1976-1980).

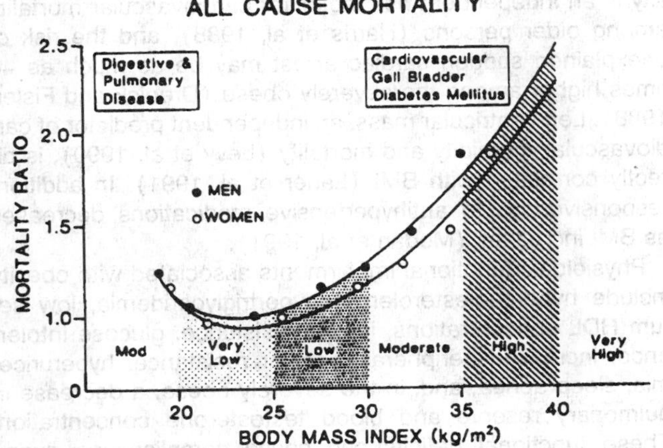

Figure 4. Mortality ratios for men and women at different levels of body mass index. From Gray, 1989. Reprinted with permission.

Fat distribution or localization measurements may employ determination of skinfold thicknesses at one or several sites (eg, subscapular skinfold, sum of triceps and subscapular thickness), measurement of abdominal to gluteal circumference ratio (AGR), or waist to hip circumference ratio (WHR). The latter is measured as the circumference of the waist at its narrowest level and the circumference of the hips at the level of greatest protuberance of the gluteal muscles. A nomogram for the determination of the AGR or WHR is shown in Figure 5. Because BMI and indices of body fat distribution may not account for age-related differences in body composition (Hammer et al, 1991), skinfold measurements (Figure 6) are often recommended for assessment of children and adolescents (Jonides, 1990; Sangi and Mueller, 1991).

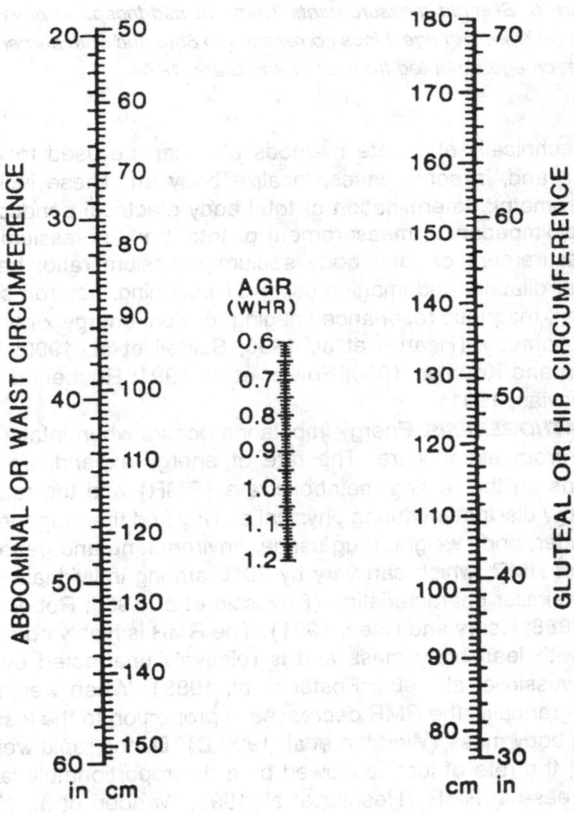

Figure 5. Nomogram for determining abdominal (waist) to gluteal (hips) ratio. Place a straight edge between the column for waist circumference and the column for hip circumference and read the ratio from the point where this straight edge crosses the AGR (WHR) line. The waist or abdominal circumference is the smallest circumference below the rib cage and above the umbilicus, and the hips or gluteal circumference is taken as the largest circumference at the posterior extension of the buttocks. From Bray, 1989 B. Reprinted with permission.

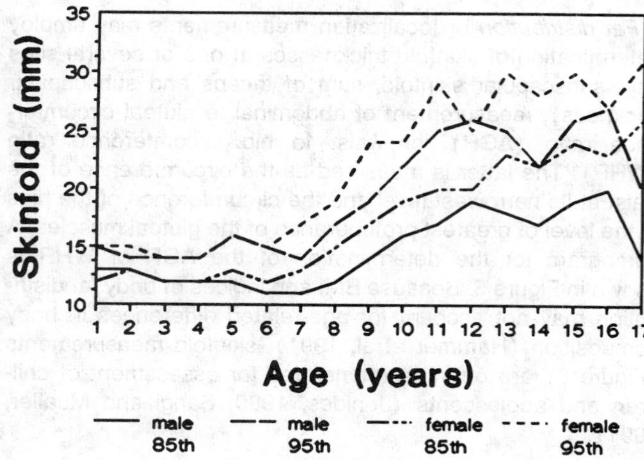

Figure 6. Skinfold measurements (mm) at mid-triceps in boys and girls 1-17 years of age. Lines correspond to 85th and 95th percentiles for each age. Adapted from Garn and Clark, 1976.

TABLE 2. EXCESS MORTALITY ASSOCIATED WITH RELATIVE WEIGHT

Weight Relative to Average Weight (%)	Mortality Ratio (%)
65-75	105
75-95	93
95-105 (average)	95
105-115	110
115-125	127
125-135	134
135-145	141
145-155	211
155-165	277

From Abraham et al, 1983. Reprinted with permission.

Technically elaborate methods also can be used to estimate and, in some cases, localize body fat. These include hydrometry; determination of total body electrical conductivity; bioimpedance; measurement of total body potassium-40; measurement of total body sodium:potassium ratio; heavy water dilution; and imaging using CT scanning, neutron scattering, magnetic resonance imaging, or dual-energy x-ray absorptiometry (Haarbo et al, 1990; Seidell et al, 1990; Van Loan and Koehler, 1990; Fowler et al, 1991; Roubenoff and Kehayias, 1991).

PATHOGENESIS. Energy imbalance occurs when intake differs from expenditure. The rate of energy expenditure depends on the resting metabolic rate (RMR) and the rate of energy dissipation during physical activity and thermogenesis. Gender, body weight, drug usage, environment, and genetics affect RMR, which can vary by 20% among individuals with very similar characteristics (Ravussin et al, 1988; Roberts et al, 1988; Henry and Rees, 1991). The RMR is highly correlated with lean body mass and is relatively unaffected by fat (Ravussin et al, 1986; Foster et al, 1988). When weight is lost gradually, the RMR decreases in proportion to the loss of lean body mass (Wadden et al, 1990 B). During rapid weight loss, the rate of loss is slowed by a disproportionately large decrease in RMR (Heshka et al, 1990; Wadden et al, 1990 B). Because adults tend to increase fat and lean body mass in an approximately 3:1 ratio, RMR increases during weight gain.

Individuals with an RMR below average for their lean body mass will tend to be obese (Elliot et al, 1989; Griffiths et al, 1990; Howard et al, 1991). In affected individuals, a "thrifty gene" may enhance energy efficiency and promote fat accumulation (Neel, 1962). A genetic predisposition to obesity may increase the difficulty of maintaining an appropriate body weight; obesity is more common among adults who were either obese at 6 months of age (Charney et al, 1976) or weighed over 3,500 g (7.7 lb) at birth (Seidman et al, 1991). On the other hand, excessive appetite results in over-eating and weight gain regardless of RMR (Blundell, 1990). "Dietary obesity," which is associated with the ready availability of highly palatable foods that are high in fat content, results from excessive caloric intake even without excessive appetite. In addition, decreased physical activity may be a significant factor in the development of obesity (Bray and Gray, 1988 A; Bray, 1989 A).

ASSOCIATED MORBIDITY AND MORTALITY. Increasing morbidity and mortality correlate directly with increasing weight and especially with fat distribution. Results of a number of population surveys and prospective long-term follow-up studies have demonstrated that there is a tendency for mortality to increase as weight deviates from "average" or "most desirable" (Sjöström, 1991; see Table 2 and Figure 4).

The principal body systems affected by obesity are the cardiovascular, pulmonary, endocrine-metabolic, gastrointestinal, reproductive, and central nervous systems (National Institutes of Health Consensus Development Panel, 1985; Kissebah et al, 1989; Pi-Sunyer, 1991 A; Terry, et al 1991). Obesity is an independent risk factor for cardiovascular mortality among older persons (Harris et al, 1988), and the risk of unexplained sudden cardiac arrest may be as much as 40 times higher among the severely obese (Drenick and Fisler, 1988). Left ventricular mass, an independent predictor of cardiovascular morbidity and mortality (Levy et al, 1990), is directly correlated with BMI (Lauer et al, 1991). In addition, responsiveness to antihypertensive medications decreases as BMI increases (Modan et al, 1991).

Physiologic functional impairments associated with obesity include hypercholesterolemia, hypertriglyceridemia, low serum HDL concentrations, insulin resistance, glucose intolerance, increased peripheral vascular resistance, hyperuricemia, sleep apnea, and, in the severely obese, a decrease in pulmonary reserve and blood testosterone concentration. These functional deficits can cause complications during anesthesia, surgery, and childbirth and can affect development of hypertension, coronary artery disease, stroke, noninsulin-dependent diabetes mellitus, lithogenic bile gallbladder disease, and early menarche. Individuals with BMI >30 secrete smaller amounts of growth hormone in response to growth hormone releasing factor (Argenio et al, 1991), potentiating the tendency to partition dietary nutrients into adipose tissue instead of muscle (Rutherford et al, 1991). Development of cancer is less strongly correlated with obesity but the prevalence of colorectal and prostate cancer in men and cancer of the endometrium, gallbladder, cervix, ovary, and breast in women may be increased. The excess weight also can aggravate arthritic signs and symptoms as well as other musculoskeletal syndromes. Psychologically, obesity is associated with a higher incidence of negative self-image and depression (Tsai et al, 1988). In contrast, moderate weight loss (10% to 20% of initial weight) can improve glycemic control in individuals with noninsulin dependent diabetes mellitus, reduce hypertension, and decrease total serum cholesterol concentration (Blackburn and Kanders, 1987; Wood et al, 1988; Hypertension Prevention Trial Research Group, 1990; Wing et al, 1991).

Obesity can substantially affect drug disposition and pharmacologic response (see index entry Obesity, Effect on Response to Drugs). For example, increased adipose tissue pool increases both the half-life and the volume of distribution of benzodiazepines, resulting in a slower onset of drug effect and a prolonged residual effect upon discontinuation. Although obesity appears to have little effect on protein binding of drugs, free fatty acids, whose plasma concentrations are increased in obesity, can displace a number of drugs from their binding proteins (eg, morphine, phenytoin, clofibrate, valproate, salicylate). Obesity stimulates the hepatic clearance of ibuprofen, prednisolone, acetaminophen, lorazepam, and oxazepam and the renal clearance of procainamide, vancomycin, gentamicin, tobramycin, and amikacin. In contrast, the volume of distribution and clearance rate of methylprednisolone are decreased and its plasma half-life is extended in obese individuals.

The regional distribution of body fat appears to be as important as total body fat in predicting risks from obesity (see Figure 7) (Bouchard et al, 1990; Sosenko et al, 1990; Kannel et al, 1991; Kaye et al, 1991). The ratio of abdominal to gluteal fat is independently correlated with the occurrence of hypertension, diabetes, hypercholesterolemia, hypertriglyceridemia, low serum HDL concentrations, glucose intolerance, hyperinsulinemia, stroke, endometrial cancer, and premature mortality (Micciolo et al, 1991; Pi-Sunyer, 1991 A; Schapira et al, 1991; Terry et al, 1991).

There is evidence that repeated weight loss/gain cycles ("weight cycling") may carry risks out of proportion to actual weight. Subjects with highly variable body weights participating in the Framingham Heart Study had a significantly increased risk of cardiovascular morbidity and mortality, regardless of weight status (Lissner et al, 1991).

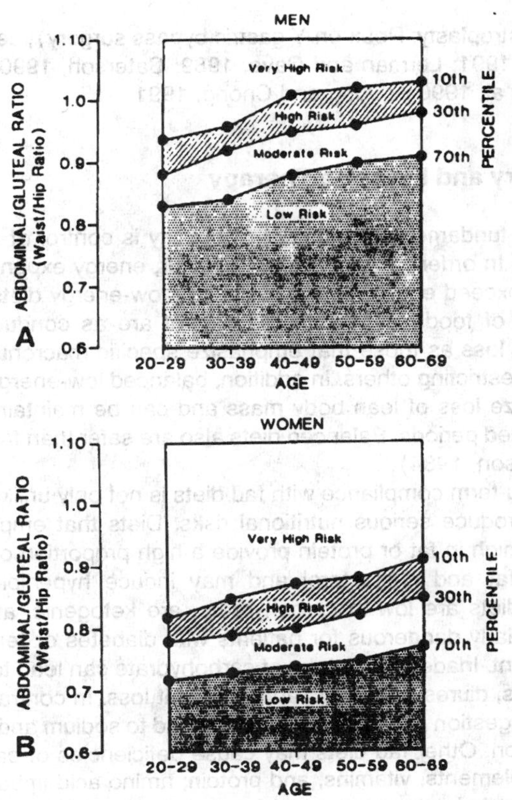

Figure 7. Percentiles for fat distribution. The percentiles for the ratio of abdominal circumference to gluteal circumference (ratio of waist to hips) are depicted for men (A) and women (B) by age groups. The relative risk for these percentiles is indicated based on the available information. From Bray, 1989 B. Reprinted with permission.

MANAGEMENT OF OBESITY

For most patients, dietary control and normalization, exercise, and behavioral therapy form the basis for weight management (Council on Scientific Affairs, 1988; Malcolm et al, 1988; Bray and Gray, 1988 A; Weintraub and Bray, 1989; Rees, 1990) and are most effective when incorporated into a structured, supervised program (Perri et al, 1988). Because weight management is a long-term endeavor, patients benefit from at least one year of active support and guidance (Rees, 1990) and may require lifelong treatment (Goodrick and Foreyt, 1991).

Occasionally, *adjunctive* use of anorexiants will help patients who respond unsatisfactorily, who have a high rate of recidivism when adhering to an otherwise adequate and comprehensive management program, or who are no longer losing weight. Anorexiants should be used no longer than required to achieve the desired changes in behavior, diet, physical activity, and body weight and should not be used alone when a comprehensive management program is terminated.

For discussion of more radical treatment of obesity (eg, very-low-calorie diet regimens, liposuction, external abdominal constriction, mandibular fixation, lipectomy, vertical banded gastroplasty, Roux-en-Y gastric bypass surgery), see Kral, 1989, 1991; Lerman and Cave, 1989; Caterson, 1990; Wadden et al, 1990 A; Jung and Chong, 1991.

Dietary and Exercise Therapy

The fundamental treatment of obesity is control of energy intake. In order for weight loss to occur, energy expenditures must exceed energy intake. Balanced low-energy diets composed of foods familiar to the patient are as conducive to weight loss as those that emphasize specific macronutrients while restricting others. In addition, balanced low-energy diets minimize loss of lean body mass and can be maintained for extended periods. Balanced diets also are safer than fad diets (Atkinson, 1984).

Long-term compliance with fad diets is not only unlikely but may produce serious nutritional risks. Diets that emphasize foods high in fat or protein provide a high proportion of saturated fat and cholesterol and may induce hyperlipidemia. Such diets are low in carbohydrate, are ketogenic, and are particularly dangerous for patients with diabetes or renal impairment. Inadequate intake of carbohydrate can lead to sodium loss, diuresis, and an "apparent" fat loss. In contrast, excess ingestion of carbohydrates can lead to sodium and water retention. Other fad diets may cause deficiencies of calcium, trace elements, vitamins, and protein; amino acid imbalance; and hypokalemia or other electrolyte imbalance. It is especially important that the growth and development of children and adolescents not be compromised by enforced or voluntary dietary restrictions.

A nutritionally balanced low-energy diet (1,000 to 1,200 kcal/day) provides a conventional distribution of the macronutrients, ie, carbohydrates (≥50% of total energy intake), protein (20% to 25%), and fat (<30%). Very-low-calorie diets (VLCD) provide 400 to 800 kcal/day and may accelerate initial weight loss. However, >35% of calories consumed must be from high-quality protein in order to avoid muscle wasting, loss of organ tissue protein, and cardiac dysfunction (Stunkard, 1987; Doherty et al, 1991). When energy intake falls below 1,000 kcal/day, it also becomes very difficult to obtain the required amounts of other nutrients (eg, iron, calcium, magnesium, pyridoxine, zinc, copper) without marked alterations in food choices. Therefore, vitamin and mineral supplementation is usually necessary under these circumstances and supervision by a physician experienced in weight reduction techniques is recommended (Council on Scientific Affairs, 1988; Atkinson, 1989; Wadden et al, 1990 A). Unfortunately, one-third to one-half of the weight lost during adherence to these strict diets is typically regained within one year (Amatruda et al, 1988).

The determination of the desired daily dietary energy deficit has traditionally been based on the caloric equivalence of fatty tissue (approximately 3,500 kcal/lb). Thus, a daily deficit of 500 kcal could result in an average weight loss of about 1 lb a week, although individual variability in energy efficiency strongly influences the actual amount of weight lost. Because weight loss in excess of 1% of body weight per week is inconsistent with good health, daily dietary energy deficits should not exceed 1,000 kcal for most people.

A diet designed to support management of body weight should provide all necessary nutrients, be palatable, and be readily available from the viewpoints of economics and convenience. The intake of foods containing natural fiber (eg, fresh fruits, vegetables, whole grains) should be increased, and the intake of foods containing fats and refined carbohydrates (eg, sugar, white flour) should be reduced. A nutritional management team can provide education, guidance, and emotional support to patients while they are learning to control their dietary intake. Nutrition management materials (eg, on weight loss, diabetes, hyperlipidemia) are available from the departments of dietetics associated with large clinics or medical schools, and the food and drug industry supplies numerous pamphlets that can assist physicians in the education of their patients.

Increased energy expenditure through increased physical activity facilitates achievement of an energy deficit of 500 to 1,000 kcal/day without having to reduce energy intake below 1,200 to 1,500 kcal/day. However, exercise alone is a relatively inefficient way to incur an energy deficit; walking or jogging for an hour expends only about 300 and 600 kcal, respectively. Nevertheless, 30 minutes of brisk walking per day for one year can theoretically result in an additional loss of 10 pounds (Jung and Chong, 1991). A regular, moderate exercise program in conjunction with dietary control may increase the rate of weight loss and the ability to maintain reduced weight (Perri et al, 1988; Wing et al, 1988). Exercise also increases cardiorespiratory fitness, reduces some cardiovascular disease risk factors, and promotes a sense of well-being (Segal and Pi-Sunyer, 1989; Pi-Sunyer, 1991 B). In addition, it may help conserve lean body mass during weight loss (Hill et al, 1987) and increase peripheral insulin sensitivity regardless of body weight (Lampman and Schteingart, 1991).

After one or two weeks on a successful diet and exercise program, a gradual reduction in the rate of weight loss will occur because of decreased metabolic and energy needs as a result of lower weight. Muscle mass also may increase. Many patients then require renewed encouragement to continue a program of dietary modification and exercise.

Behavioral Therapy

Behavioral change is a prerequisite for successful management of obesity. Three strategic components of behavioral therapy are used to effect desirable changes in lifestyle that promote and maintain weight loss and avoid behaviors that promote weight gain (Stunkard, 1987; Brownell and Kramer, 1989). *Self-monitoring* is necessary initially to determine which behaviors are problematic and to provide criteria and standards for monitoring and evaluation. *Stimulus control* attempts to eliminate or minimize those cues that patients associate with eating. Such cues may be visual, time and place oriented, or habitual eating routines. *Reinforcement* techniques reward weight loss through pleasures other than eating and improve the patient's self-image. In addition, realistic body weight goals should be set on the basis of rational assessment of the individual. Table 1 and Figure 1 can assist in the determination of an appropriate final target weight for a given height and desirable (and attainable) BMI.

Intensive behavior modification programs incorporate balanced low-calorie diets, structured exercise regimens, incentive systems, and training in techniques such as relapse prevention and are most effective when conducted by behavioral psychologists. When followed for one to five years, such programs result in high compliance; low recidivism; long-term weight loss as great as that obtained by mandibular fixation, VLCD, or gastrointestinal surgery; and better maintenance of reduced body weight (Björvell and Rossner, 1985, 1990; Stunkard, 1987; Kraemer et al, 1989; Wing, 1991). For some individuals, self-help groups (Take Off Pounds Sensibly [TOPS], Overeaters Anonymous, Weight Watchers) can provide considerable help in achieving desirable modifications of behavior and reaching and maintaining desired weight goals, although such programs typically have high attrition rates. Reliance on self-management alone may result in cyclic compliance and potentially harmful weight cycling (Goodrick and Foreyt, 1991).

Anorexiant (Appetite Suppressant) Therapy

RECOMMENDATIONS FOR USE. Drug use as a primary therapy to promote weight loss is not recommended. All anorexiants have side effects, encourage reliance on drugs, and do not change behaviors that may have contributed to the development of obesity. Anorexiant therapy should be reserved for *adults* and used *only* as an adjunct to a combination of caloric restriction, exercise, and behavior modification when an acceptable management program utilizing these measures has been inadequate. The limited usefulness of these agents should be weighed against the risks inherent in their use.

Anorexiants reduce hunger and food intake to various degrees, depending on dose and individual response (Silverstone, 1987). When they are effective, the average total amount of weight loss ascribed to anorexiants compared with placebo in a *comprehensive program* is modest (an additional 0.25 to 0.5 lb/week); over time, this can result in significant weight loss. In a comprehensive program, if significant weight loss is not achieved within four to six weeks after dosage adjustments or at maximum tolerated dose levels, drug therapy should be discontinued.

The optimal duration of treatment with anorexiants has not been established (Bray, 1991 B). Some clinicians prefer diet therapy initially, followed by short-term use of anorexiants only when weight loss has reached a plateau. When weight goals are achieved after 12 to 24 weeks of anorexiant therapy, it may be preferable to then use these drugs intermittently (with the exception of fenfluramine), timing drug administration during times of stress or anticipated recidivism (eg, holidays). Others advocate more prolonged use of anorexiants to prevent recidivism even when further weight loss does not occur (Bray and Gray, 1988 B; Weintraub and Bray, 1989; Bray, 1991 B).

Fenfluramine [Pondimin], the investigational drug dexfenfluramine [Adifax, Isomeride], diethylpropion [Tenuate, Tepanil], and phentermine resin [Ionamin] have induced and, more important, have maintained significant weight losses when used for 24 to 52 weeks without producing adverse effects, tolerance, or dependence (Sullivan and Comai, 1978; Bray, 1984; Weintraub et al, 1984; Guy-Grand et al, 1989). Abrupt discontinuation of treatment after long-term administration of therapeutic doses or short-term use of large doses (especially Schedule II anorexiants and fenfluramine) is sometimes followed by temporary fatigue, marked lethargy, paranoid psychosis (after large doses or abuse), and mental depression that may be severe.

Drugs should not be prescribed for the treatment of obesity in *growing children*, including *adolescents*. Although data are conflicting, growth impairment has been reported with use of fenfluramine and mazindol.

PRESCRIPTION DRUG SELECTION. The amphetamines (amphetamine, dextroamphetamine [Dexedrine], methamphetamine [Desoxyn], and phenmetrazine [Preludin]) were the first drugs prescribed widely for appetite suppression. These agents, as well as mixtures that combine more than one amphetamine (eg, Biphetamine, Obetrol), are no more effective than other available agents; they are no longer recommended for the treatment of obesity because the risk of dependence is great. All are classified as Schedule II controlled substance drugs. The FDA Center for Drug Evaluation and Review has concluded that the amphetamines have no advantage over other safer anorexiants (*Federal Register*, 1979), and a few states and Canada have prohibited their use for weight control (Richard and Lasagna, 1988).

Benzphetamine [Didrex], diethylpropion, fenfluramine, mazindol [Mazanor, Sanorex], phendimetrazine [Adipost, Bontril PDM, Melfiat, Plegine, Prelu-2, Statobex], phentermine hydrochloride [Adipex-P, Fastin], and phentermine resin are available only by prescription. Benzphetamine and phendimetrazine are Schedule III controlled-substance drugs; the remainder are Schedule IV agents. Despite some differences in pharmacologic actions and untoward effects, all induce about the same degree of weight loss.

All prescription anorexiant drugs in Schedules III and IV have only one approved indication: short-term adjunctive treatment of obesity. None are used in the treatment of attention deficit hyperactivity disorder or narcolepsy.

Actions and Uses: Most prescription anorexiants are beta-phenylethylamine derivatives of amphetamine that are presumed to act centrally to increase sympathetic activity by stimulating the release of the catecholamine neurotransmitters, norepinephrine and dopamine. Satiety and decreased food intake are associated with increased sympathetic activity and decreased parasympathetic activity (Bray, 1989 A). These drugs also may elevate blood pressure.

All amphetamine derivatives are central nervous system stimulants. Their potency, degree of stimulation, and abuse potential vary. However, even those in Schedule III are of low abuse potential.

Mazindol also is capable of producing central nervous system stimulation, but this effect is observed only at doses approaching the toxic level. This drug is structurally related to the tricyclic antidepressants, which also block the neuronal uptake of norepinephrine and serotonin.

In contrast to amphetamine derivatives, serotonin appears to reduce food intake (Angel et al, 1988; Bray, 1989 A; Leibowitz, 1990). Obese adults given 8 mg/kg/day of oral 5-hydroxytryptophan, a serotonin precursor, for five weeks decreased their daily carbohydrate and total food intakes by 21% and 22%, respectively, and lost three times more weight than when given a placebo (Ceci et al, 1989).

Fenfluramine and dexfenfluramine stimulate the release of serotonin at synapses and inhibit its reuptake by afferent neurons (Garattini et al, 1989). In addition to reducing carbohydrate intake and inducing initial weight loss in adults, dexfenfluramine has maintained reduced body weight for more than one year in chronically obese patients (Guy-Grand et al, 1989; Turner, 1990). Its use also has resulted in additional weight loss following cessation of a VLCD (Finer et al, 1989). Because most of the anorexiant activity of fenfluramine (a combination of d- and l-isomers) is attributed to dexfenfluramine (the d-isomer), effective doses of dexfenfluramine may be only one-half those required with fenfluramine (*Lancet*, 1991).

The antidepressants, fluoxetine [Prozac], fluvoxamine, and sertraline, also inhibit serotonin reuptake (see index entries Fluoxetine; Fluvoxamine). Unlike the tricyclic antidepressants, which tend to promote weight gain, they may facilitate sustained weight loss in some patients (Abell et al, 1986; Leibowitz, 1990; Marcus et al, 1990; Fuller et al, 1991). However, many patients regain the weight previously lost while still on drug therapy.

Satietin has been isolated from human plasma and identified as an alpha$_1$-glycoprotein with a molecular weight of 64 kilodaltons. It has anorectic activity, although its mechanism of action appears to differ from that of serotoninergic agents and has not been established (Knoll, 1988). Further studies are needed in this promising area of research before satietin and related derivatives can be used clinically.

The gastrointestinal hormone, cholecystokinin (CCK), may mediate satiety in humans. Parenteral administration of CCK results in reduced food intake and less time spent eating, but whether these behavioral responses reflect satiety or mild aversive effects is controversial (Peikin, 1989; Stricker and Verbalis, 1990; Uvnäs-Moberg, 1990). CCK also may contribute to satiety in humans by inhibiting gastric emptying and prolonging the postprandial duration of gastric distention (Moran and McHugh, 1982; Robinson et al, 1988).

Investigational sympathomimetic (thermogenic) drugs stimulate norepinephrine release and increase RMR in addition to inhibiting appetite. Beta-adrenergic agonists such as ephedrine selectively stimulate the hydrolysis of fatty acids and increase RMR in a dose-dependent fashion, possibly by stimulating T_4 deiodination (Silva and Larsen, 1983; Reeds and Mersmann, 1991). However, doses of ephedrine that are sufficient to cause weight loss also often cause acute elevations in blood pressure and tremors. The beneficial effects of low doses of ephedrine may be potentiated by aspirin and caffeine (Dulloo and Miller, 1989). Long-term controlled clinical trials of such drugs or drug combinations are required before their utility in obesity therapy can be assessed.

Other agents being investigated for their involvement in the homeostatic regulation of body weight in adults include agonists to CCK, corticotropin-releasing hormone, bombesin, neurotensin, and growth hormone; antagonists to opioid peptides, galanin, and neuropeptide Y; stimulators of beta$_3$-adrenergic receptors; and inhibitors of glucocorticoid and aldosterone receptors (Blundell, 1991). Because multiple mechanisms apparently are involved in the regulation of food intake, effective weight management in the future may utilize combinations of agents in conjunction with nonpharmacologic therapies (Bray, 1991 C).

Adverse Reactions: Anorexiants that are directly or indirectly related structurally to amphetamine produce central nervous system stimulation and can cause widely differing side effects depending on whether they affect adrenergic or serotoninergic receptors. Manifestations include nervousness, irritability, insomnia, decreased sense of fatigue, increased alertness and ability to focus one's thoughts, and euphoria. As the stimulant actions decline, fatigue and depression occur. The central nervous system effects may be severe enough to require discontinuing drug therapy.

Sympathetic nervous system effects include dryness of the mouth, blurred vision and mydriasis, dizziness and lightheadedness, tachycardia and other arrhythmias, hypertension, nausea, constipation, and sweating. These effects are less common with mazindol.

Sedation rather than central nervous system stimulation occurs with use of fenfluramine. Severe vomiting, diarrhea with abdominal pain, and constipation also have been reported.

For additional adverse effects, see the evaluations. For discussion of the dependence potential of these drugs, see the section on Dependence below.

Acute Overdosage (Poisoning): Acute overdosage accentuates the usual pharmacologic effects of excitement, agitation, hypertension, tachycardia and other arrhythmias, mydriasis, tremor, hyperreflexia, tachypnea, fever, headache, confusion, aggressiveness, and toxic psychoses characterized by panic, auditory and visual hallucinations, and paranoid delusions. In severe cases, overdosage may cause hyperpyrexia, rhabdomyolysis, chest pain, hypotension, acute circulatory failure, convulsions, and coma; fatalities have been reported. Gastrointestinal symptoms include nausea, vomiting, diarrhea, and abdominal cramps. Fenfluramine poisoning appears to have some specific characteristics, including rotary nystagmus and continuous tremor of the lower jaw. Either pronounced drowsiness or agitation may occur.

Management of acute amphetamine intoxication is largely symptomatic. A quiet environment and supportive care is desirable, and sedation is useful. Gastric lavage or induced vomiting may be indicated. Urinary acidifying agents facilitate excretion of some beta-phenylethylamines. Haloperidol [Haldol] may be of value in blocking severe central nervous agitation.

Dependence: Susceptible patients may develop physical dependence with use of anorexiant agents, although this is less likely with fenfluramine (Rowland and Carlton, 1986). Accordingly, amphetamine, dextroamphetamine, methamphetamine, phenmetrazine, and mixtures containing amphetamine compounds are classified as Schedule II drugs under the Controlled Substances Act. Because of the risk of dependence, Schedule II drugs have no place in the treatment of obesity. Benzphetamine and phendimetrazine are classified as Schedule III drugs and diethylpropion, fenfluramine, mazindol, and phentermine as Schedule IV drugs. See also the index entry Prescription Practices.

Withdrawal of amphetamines or other anorexiants from abusers may unmask symptoms of chronic fatigue (mental depression, asthenia, tremors, and gastrointestinal disturbances), which may be followed by drowsiness and prolonged sleep or lethargy. Sudden withdrawal of fenfluramine may cause severe depression whether or not the patient has a history of depression.

Pregnancy: Although suggested weight gains for obese women during pregnancy are lower than those for the nonobese, dietary restriction and weight reduction efforts are not recommended (Institute of Medicine, 1990). Anorexiants are contraindicated in pregnant and lactating women.

Precautions: Before prescribing any anorexiant, the patient's medical history must be ascertained to determine whether there is any tendency to abuse drugs, including alcohol. Anorexiants should not be given to such patients.

Anorexiant therapy should be supervised closely by a physician, and the amount of drug prescribed should be limited to that sufficient for a two-week period. It is advisable to schedule office visits for these intervals, and anorexiants should be given at subsequent consultations only if the patient continues to comply with the management program and is not experiencing symptoms of psychological disturbance. When tolerance to an anorectic effect develops, the drug should be discontinued.

Because of their stimulant effects on the cardiovascular system, anorexiants with adrenergic activity should not be prescribed for individuals with ischemic heart disease, hypertension, hyperthyroidism, or advanced arteriosclerosis (see the evaluations). Fenfluramine or fluoxetine are suitable alternatives for such patients.

Interactions: Most anorexiants theoretically release norepinephrine and/or dopamine from adrenergic neurons and also inhibit uptake of some hypotensive drugs (eg, guanethidine, guanadrel) into the adrenergic neuron. However, interference with the action of antihypertensive drugs probably is clinically unimportant with usual doses of anorexiants. Nevertheless, blood pressure should be monitored weekly for the first four to six weeks of therapy.

The risk of developing arrhythmias or cardiac arrest is increased when anorexiants are given with thyroid hormones, potassium-losing diuretics, laxatives, or phenylpropanolamine (Riddell, 1982; Griffin et al, 1988). Since anorexiants can precipitate a hypertensive crisis when used with monoamine oxidase inhibitors, they should not be given within 14 days after administration of any of these agents.

The half-lives and durations of action of amphetamine derivatives are increased by agents that alkalize the urine (eg, acetazolamide, sodium bicarbonate) and are decreased by those that acidify the urine.

Pharmacokinetics: A peak blood concentration is attained one to two hours after oral administration of all prescription anorexiants except phentermine, which peaks at four to eight hours. Only fragmentary data on volumes of distribution, clearance, and metabolic disposition are available. The half-lives of Schedule III and IV drugs range from 8 to 20 hours. If desirable, a prolonged-release formulation of diethylpropion is available for once-a-day administration. With the exception of fenfluramine, these drugs are excreted unchanged in acid urine; the amounts vary from 20% to 75% (Bray and Gray, 1988 B). Fenfluramine is metabolized in the liver to norfenfluramine, which has a plasma half-life twice that of fenfluramine; these compounds are excreted in the urine as 3-trifluoromethylhippuric acid. Benzphetamine is metabolized to amphetamine and methamphetamine.

NONPRESCRIPTION DRUGS. The FDA considers two OTC drugs to be safe and effective as aids in weight reduction. The first, phenylpropanolamine, has few central nervous system stimulant properties in normal individuals but may cause sympathomimetic effects on the cardiovascular system and other adverse effects, particularly when it is used for prolonged periods in amounts exceeding the approved dose of 75 mg/day. It should not be used indiscriminately. Benzocaine, the other drug used in proprietary preparations, has no particular merit as an anorexiant and its usefulness in a weight reduction program is questionable. Its appetite suppressant effect theoretically results from numbness of the oral cavity and gastrointestinal mucosa that modifies taste sensitivity and thus discourages snacking.

MISCELLANEOUS DRUGS. Many OTC fad diets and drugs have been misused as anorexiants; the latter include thyroid hormones, digitalis, diuretics, and chorionic gonadotropin (O'Donnell, 1988). Use of any of these agents as an aid to weight reduction is unjustified.

Thyroid extract and levothyroxine (T_4) are ineffective in overweight euthyroid patients when doses within the range of usual hormone replacement therapy are given. Larger doses may increase the metabolic rate up to 30% and produce a negative energy balance but have potentially dangerous effects on protein catabolism and cardiac function, including cardiomegaly and tachyarrhythmias, and may contribute to the development of osteoporosis. Self-medication with phenylpropanolamine may be especially dangerous in patients taking thyroid hormones. Because rapid weight loss is a variant of the nonthyroidal illness or starvation syndromes, it is accompanied by decreased serum T_3 concentrations, reduced RMR, and increasing difficulty in losing more weight. In obese subjects, restoration of RMR by ingestion of liothyronine requires doses that result in hypertriiodothyroninemia and may trigger clinical hyperthyroidism (Welle and Campbell, 1986).

Digitalis may induce anorexia but this usually is a sign of toxicity. Diuretics are of no use in decreasing adipose tissue mass in normally hydrated persons, although they may cause transient fluid loss and, therefore, deceptive weight loss. In numerous studies, human chorionic gonadotropin had no greater effect on weight reduction than placebo injections (Bosch et al, 1990). The Food and Drug Administration now requires that the labeling for thyroid, digitalis, or related drugs warn against use of these agents in the treatment of obesity.

Oral bulk-producing agents have been used to promote satiety and inhibit carbohydrate and lipid absorption. Water-soluble agents (agar; carboxymethylcellulose; carrageenan; glucomannan; kelp; methylcellulose; pectin; psyllium; polycarbophil; tragacanth; and guar, karaya and xanthan gums) may be effective, but rapid hydration and swelling after ingestion have caused esophageal obstruction, choking, and death (Di Lorenzo et al, 1988; Caterson, 1990; *Federal Register*, 1990), and these agents are no longer classified as OTC products (*Federal Register*, 1991).

Many other substances have been used as ingredients of nonprescription diet aids, including alcohols, oils, vitamins, minerals, herbal extracts, tissue concentrates, purified nutrients, and microbial fermentation byproducts. Inclusion of these substances in nonprescription weight loss products is now prohibited by the FDA because of the complete absence of data that any of them are effective (*Federal Register*, 1991).

Drug Evaluations

Schedule IV Drugs

DIETHYLPROPION HYDROCHLORIDE

[Tenuate, Tepanil]

Diethylpropion is comparable to other anorexiants in suppressing the appetite. Although mild restlessness, dryness of the mouth, and constipation are common, the overall incidence of central nervous system side effects (nervousness, excitability, euphoria, and insomnia) is considerably lower than with other anorexiants. Psychic and physical dependence may occur, but the incidence is low despite common worldwide use. In one study, administration of diethylpropion for 25 weeks did not produce tolerance or dependence (Sullivan and Comai, 1978).

Diethylpropion is considered to be one of the safest of the anorexiant drugs for patients with mild to moderate hypertension even when myocardial ischemia is present. No adverse cardiovascular effects have been reported to date in patients with angina pectoris or hypertension, but use of this drug in patients with severe cardiovascular disease or marked hypertension generally is inadvisable. Diethylpropion may increase convulsions in some individuals with epilepsy.

The safety and efficacy of diethylpropion during pregnancy and lactation have not been established; however, it does cross the placenta and may affect the fetus. Therefore, this anorexiant should not be given to women who are or are likely to become pregnant (FDA Pregnancy Category B).

DOSAGE AND PREPARATIONS.

Oral: *Adults,* 25 mg three times daily one hour before meals. An additional 25 mg may be taken in the evening if needed to overcome night hunger. Alternatively, one prolonged-release tablet may be taken once daily in midmorning.

Tenuate (Marion Merrell Dow), ***Tepanil*** (3M Pharmaceuticals), ***Generic***. Tablets 25 mg; tablets (prolonged-release) 75 mg (***Tenuate Dospan, Tepanil Ten-Tab***).

FENFLURAMINE HYDROCHLORIDE

[Pondimin]

ACTIONS AND USES. This agent, a substituted phenethylamine, has little sympathomimetic activity and differs from other available anorexiants in that it usually depresses rather than stimulates the central nervous system at therapeutic doses. Therefore, fenfluramine is useful in nervous or tense patients or when central nervous system stimulant effects are undesirable. This drug principally stimulates the release of serotonin and blocks its reuptake; therefore, its neurochemical action differs from that of sympathomimetic drugs. Its primary action is to reduce the feeling of hunger.

Fenfluramine is comparable to other anorexiants in its ability to suppress the appetite. When given for six months, it has induced loss of approximately 9 to 10 kg more than was lost with placebos. In some studies, the weight loss has been maintained for six months or more after drug therapy was discontinued; in other studies, regain of lost weight was common and rapid. This drug may be beneficial when taken before the evening meal by patients who snack excessively in the evening. Also, when taken late in the day, its sedative effects are less disruptive for patients who must remain alert during the day.

Fenfluramine improves glucose tolerance in some patients, probably by increasing glucose uptake in muscle. However, it should not be used to treat glucose intolerance, even though it is considered the anorexiant of choice for patients with non-insulin-dependent diabetes mellitus (NIDDM) who do not have depression (see index entry Fenfluramine, Interaction with Sulfonylureas). At therapeutic dose levels, fenfluramine has been used safely in patients with hypertension. At toxic dose levels or in sensitive patients, an increase in blood pressure could occur.

ADVERSE REACTIONS AND PRECAUTIONS. Fenfluramine is well tolerated, although dry mouth, a symptom common with most anorexiants, can be aggravating. Drowsiness occurs frequently. Occasionally, severe vomiting, diarrhea with abdominal pain, and constipation have occurred during use of this drug. Dizziness, headache, sleep disturbances, vivid dreams, urinary frequency, impotence, and loss of libido also may occur rarely. Paradoxically, libido may increase with prolonged use. Several cases of reversible pulmonary hypertension have been reported.

Fenfluramine appears to be mildly hallucinogenic in some individuals and rarely may cause physical dependence. Sudden withdrawal after prolonged use can cause depression, which may be severe; reinstitution of therapy followed by gradual reduction of the dose appears to be satisfactory for such patients. Because of the tendency to induce depression upon withdrawal, this drug should not be used intermittently. Fenfluramine should not be given to patients who are being or have been treated for major depression or migraine headaches or who are receiving other central nervous system depressants. The side effects in an individual patient are unpredictable.

Overdosage produces amphetamine-like symptoms and some specific characteristics (rotary nystagmus, continuous tremor of the lower jaw). Convulsions, coma, and a few deaths have been reported. Ventricular extrasystoles culminating in irreversible ventricular fibrillation have been fatal in several patients. Standard supportive measures are effective in most cases of overdosage; forced diuresis with acidification of the urine and/or large doses of diazepam may be helpful in severe cases.

An interaction between halothane and fenfluramine has been reported; it is suggested that fenfluramine be discontinued gradually one week prior to elective surgery (Bennett and Eltringham, 1977).

The safety and efficacy of fenfluramine during pregnancy and lactation have not been established; therefore, this anorexiant should not be given to women who are or are likely to become pregnant (FDA Pregnancy Category C).

DOSAGE AND PREPARATIONS.

Oral: *Adults,* initially, 20 mg three times daily one hour before meals. Dosage may be increased to 40 mg three times daily one hour before meals (maximum, 120 mg/day). The drug must not be discontinued abruptly; dosage should be decreased gradually to prevent withdrawal reactions. Initiating therapy with lower doses, ie, 10 to 20 mg taken prior to bedtime for several days, may minimize adverse reactions.

Pondimin (Robins). Tablets 20 mg.

MAZINDOL

[Mazanor, Sanorex]

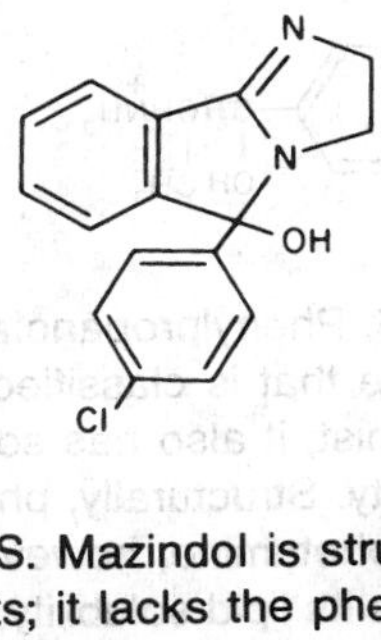

ACTIONS AND USES. Mazindol is structurally related to tricyclic antidepressants; it lacks the phenethylamine structure of other anorexiant agents. It appears to act principally by blocking the neuronal reuptake of norepinephrine and synaptically released dopamine.

Mazindol is comparable to other anorexiants in suppressing the appetite.

ADVERSE REACTIONS AND PRECAUTIONS. Mazindol does not appear to produce euphoria; therefore, its abuse potential is low. Otherwise, the stimulant effects are similar to those of the amphetamines, but the incidence is very much lower and reactions are less severe. However, the incidence of central nervous system stimulation (eg, insomnia, dizziness, agitation) is greater with mazindol than diethylpropion, particularly during the first two weeks of treatment.

Psychological and physical dependence have not been reported during several decades of use, but the possibility of their occurrence remains.

Although the only cardiovascular action attributed to mazindol is an increase of 10 beats/minute in the orthostatic heart rate, use of this drug in patients with severe cardiovascular disease, including marked hypertension, is inadvisable. There is some evidence that mazindol may be safe in patients with stable atherosclerotic heart disease or mild to moderate hypertension. Control of diabetes mellitus or rheumatic diseases does not appear to be affected adversely by this drug. However, it may cause hyperinsulinemia, which reduces the effectiveness of both long-term glycemic control and appetite suppression.

Mazindol is a tricyclic compound and can potentiate the effects of catecholamines. Therefore, extreme care is needed during concomitant use of pressor amines.

The safety and efficacy of mazindol during pregnancy and lactation have not been established; therefore, this drug should not be given to women who are or are likely to become pregnant.

DOSAGE AND PREPARATIONS.

Oral: *Adults,* 1 to 2 mg daily one hour before the midday meal.

Mazanor (Wyeth-Ayerst). Tablets 1 mg.

Sanorex (Sandoz). Tablets 1 and 2 mg.

PHENTERMINE HYDROCHLORIDE

[Adipex-P, Fastin, Obermine]

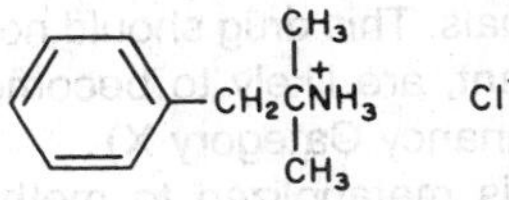

PHENTERMINE RESIN

[Ionamin]

Phentermine is available as the hydrochloride salt and as a complex of the base with an ion exchange resin. It is comparable to other anorexiants in suppressing the appetite.

The incidence and severity of central nervous system stimulation are less than with dextroamphetamine, but the incidence of insomnia is higher than with diethylpropion and is unacceptable to some patients. Although insomnia is rare when phentermine resin is given, both forms may increase blood pressure, produce tachycardia, and commonly cause dryness of the mouth. Therefore, phentermine is not advocated for patients with hypertension and cardiovascular disease. Because euphoria is rare, the abuse potential is low.

The safety and efficacy of phentermine during pregnancy and lactation have not been established; therefore, this drug should not be given to women who are or are likely to become pregnant.

DOSAGE AND PREPARATIONS.

PHENTERMINE HYDROCHLORIDE:

Oral: *Adults,* 8 mg three times daily one-half hour before meals or 15 to 37.5 mg once daily two hours after breakfast. Administration during the evening should be avoided to decrease the likelihood of insomnia.

Generic. Capsules 15, 18.75, 30, and 37.5 mg; tablets 8, 18.75, 30, and 37.5 mg.

Adipex-P (Gate). Tablets 37.5 mg (equivalent to 30 mg of base).

Fastin (SmithKline Beecham), ***Obermine*** (Forest). Capsules 30 mg (equivalent to 24 mg of base).

PHENTERMINE RESIN:

Oral: *Adults,* 15 to 30 mg before breakfast or 10 to 14 hours before bedtime.

Generic. Capsules 30 mg.

Ionamin (Fisons). Capsules 15 and 30 mg.

Schedule III Drugs

BENZPHETAMINE HYDROCHLORIDE

[Didrex]

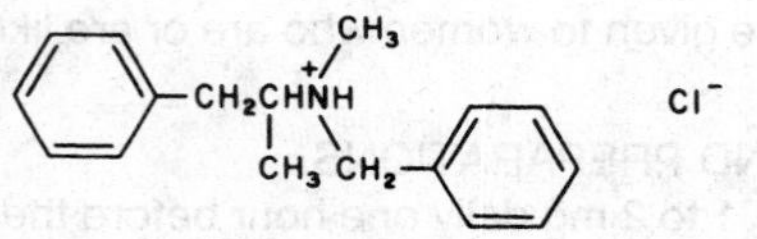

Benzphetamine is comparable to dextroamphetamine in suppressing the appetite and causes similar, but fewer, untoward effects. Psychotic episodes are rare when recommended doses are used.

Benzphetamine is a secondary agent for use in obesity because it may produce euphoria and, rarely, dependence in susceptible individuals. This drug should not be given to women who are pregnant, are likely to become pregnant, or are nursing (FDA Pregnancy Category X).

Benzphetamine is metabolized to methamphetamine and will therefore result in a positive finding of methamphetamine in urine drug testing.

DOSAGE AND PREPARATIONS. Dosage should be individualized according to patient response.

Oral: *Adults,* 25 to 50 mg daily. Preferably, a single dose is given in midmorning or midafternoon depending on the patient's eating habits.

Didrex (Upjohn). Tablets 25 and 50 mg (contain tartrazine).

PHENDIMETRAZINE TARTRATE

[Adipost, Bontril PDM, Melfiat-105, Plegine, Prelu-2, Statobex]

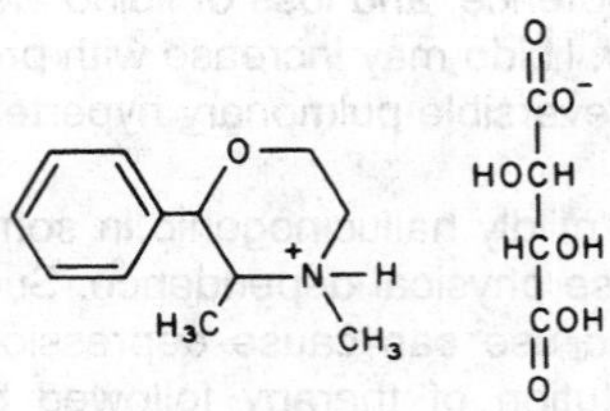

Phendimetrazine is comparable to other anorexiants in its ability to suppress the appetite and stimulate the central nervous system. This drug is a secondary agent for use in obesity because it produces euphoria with the potential for abuse and because the degree of central nervous stimulation is unacceptable to some patients.

Cardiovascular effects occur infrequently. Phendimetrazine should be used with caution in patients with even mild hypertension and is contraindicated in those with moderate or severe hypertension. It also should not be given to patients with other cardiovascular disorders, hyperthyroidism, or glaucoma.

Glossitis, stomatitis, abdominal cramps, headache, and dysuria are noted occasionally. Phendimetrazine may decrease the hypotensive effect of guanethidine and may alter insulin requirements in diabetics.

The safety and efficacy of phendimetrazine during pregnancy and lactation have not been established; therefore, this anorexiant should not be given to women who are or are likely to become pregnant.

DOSAGE AND PREPARATIONS.

Oral: *Adults,* 35 mg (range, 17.5 to 70 mg) two or three times daily one hour before meals. Alternatively, one prolonged-release capsule (105 mg) taken in the morning.

Generic. Capsules 35 and 105 mg; capsules (prolongedrelease) 105 mg; tablets (plain, prolonged-release) 35 mg.

Adipost (Ascher), ***Melfiat-105*** (Solvay), ***Prelu-2*** (Boehringer Ingelheim). Capsules (prolonged-release) 105 mg.

Bontril PDM (Carnrick). Tablets 35 mg; capsules (prolonged-release) 105 mg (***Bontril***).

Plegine (Wyeth-Ayerst), ***Statobex*** (Lemmon). Tablets 35 mg.

Nonprescription Drug

PHENYLPROPANOLAMINE HYDROCHLORIDE

[Acutrim, Dexatrim]

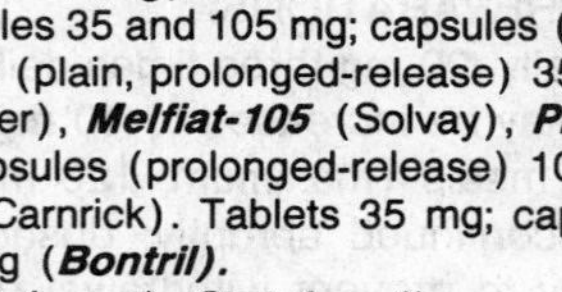

ACTIONS AND USES. Phenylpropanolamine is a beta-phenylethylamine derivative that is classified primarily as a direct alpha-adrenergic agonist; it also has some indirect catecholamine-releasing activity. Structurally, phenylpropanolamine is closely related to amphetamine; however, the presence of a hydroxyl group impairs its lipid solubility and probably its central nervous system penetration. Thus, in clinically recommended doses, it has few significant central nervous system stimulant effects and it does not produce dependence.

Phenylpropanolamine has been used widely for 40 years as an OTC topical and systemic nasal decongestant and systemically as an appetite suppressant. When used adjunctively in a comprehensive management program that includes diet, exercise, and behavioral modification, it has increased the rate of weight loss by about 0.25 to 0.5 lb weekly more than placebo for up to 16 weeks in controlled clinical trials; this rate of weight loss is comparable to that achieved with use of currently available prescription anorexiants (Lasagna, 1988).

ADVERSE REACTIONS AND PRECAUTIONS. Phenylpropanolamine was judged to be well tolerated in an evaluation of nearly 50 placebo-controlled trials (Winick, 1991). Side effects (confusion, headache, nervousness, tachycardia, palpitations, sleeplessness) occur at a low rate, are of mild to moderate severity, and usually are of brief duration.

Phenylpropanolamine is not addictive in recommended doses; therefore, it is not an effective drug of abuse (Morgan et al, 1989). Nevertheless, during the past two decades concerns have arisen about its safety. Phenylpropanolamine is a widely available OTC drug, is inappropriately regarded and/or sold as an "amphetamine-like" stimulant among the drug abuse population, and is often confused with illegal combination and/or look-alike drugs when serious adverse drug reactions are reported. When used in excessive doses, phenylpropanolamine may produce altered perception or mild psychosis.

Although a statistically significant but clinically unimportant pressor effect was observed during short-term administration in 881 healthy subjects (Blackburn et al, 1989), no changes were observed in 26 stable hypertensive patients taking 25 mg five times daily (Kroenke et al, 1989). Clinically significant central nervous system stimulation and hypertension are rare at recommended doses and usually occur only in sensitive patients (idiosyncratic reaction) or, most commonly, in patients with relevant associated illnesses (eg, autonomic dystonia, orthostatic hypotension). The current warning label states that individuals being treated for high blood pressure, depression, heart disease, diabetes, or thyroid disease should take this medication only under the supervision of a physician. In the peer-reviewed literature, the most common concern expressed about the safety of phenylpropanolamine is that 75 mg of the immediate-release (*not* prolonged-release) product, ie, three times the recommended dose of 25 mg, may increase the potential for the development of a hypertensive adverse reaction, and serious toxicity (eg, intracranial hemorrhage, severe hypertension) may occur in a few of these patients.

These concerns have prompted the FDA and investigators to re-evaluate this agent's efficacy and safety (Pentel, 1984; Morgan and Kagan, 1985; Liebson et al, 1987; Lasagna, 1988; Miller, 1989). Although some controversy remains about the safety of higher than recommended doses for prolonged periods, all investigators support the concept that the safe OTC use of phenylpropanolamine is especially dependent on following the warning and dose instructions on the label.

No birth defects have been attributed to phenylpropanolamine in large retrospective and prospective studies. Nevertheless, because weight loss is not recommended during pregnancy, the drug is not recommended for pregnant or lactating women.

Although a considerable potential for drug interactions with phenylpropanolamine exists, well-documented serious drug interactions are uncommon. Cardiovascular complications may occur when patients given thyroid hormones also use phenylpropanolamine. To avoid the possibility of a hypertensive episode, the drug should not be used in patients who are taking monoamine oxidase inhibitors.

PHARMACOKINETICS. Phenylpropanolamine is well absorbed orally, and the peak blood concentration is attained within one to two hours. The half-life ranges from 2.7 to 3.4 hours. The drug is principally excreted unchanged; the major route of excretion is renal. Since phenylpropanolamine is a weak base, elimination is enhanced in acid urine.

DOSAGE AND PREPARATIONS.

Oral: *Adults,* 25 mg of the immediate-release product two or three times daily one hour before meals (maximum, 75 mg/day). Alternatively, a prolonged-release preparation (75 mg) is taken once daily in the morning.

Acutrim (CIBA). Tablets (prolonged-release) 75 mg (nonprescription).

Dexatrim (Thompson). Tablets 25 and 75 mg; capsules (prolonged-release) 50 and 75 mg (both forms nonprescription).

Cited References

Amphetamines: Drugs for human use; drug efficacy study implementation. *Federal Register* 44:41552-41571, (July 17) 1979.

Dexfenfluramine, editorial. *Lancet* 337:1315-1316, 1991.

Warning statements required for over-the-counter drugs containing water-soluble gums as active ingredients. *Federal Register* 55:45782-45785, (Oct 30) 1990.

Weight control drug products for over-the-counter human use; certain active ingredients; final rule. *Federal Register* 56:37792-37799, (Aug 8) 1991.

Abell CA, et al: Placebo controlled double-blind trial of fluvoxamine maleate in the obese. *J Psychosom Res* 30:143-146, 1986.

Abraham S, et al: Overweight and obese adults in the United States. *Vital and Health Statistics.* DHHS Publ No (PHS) 83-1680, National Health Survey Series 11, 230:1-28, 1983.

Amatruda JM, et al: The safety and efficacy of a controlled low-energy ('very-low calorie') diet in the treatment of non-insulin-dependent diabetes and obesity. *Arch Intern Med* 148:873-877, 1988.

Andres R, et al: Impact of age on weight goals. *Ann Intern Med* 103:1030-1033, 1985.

Angel I, et al: Anorectic activities of serotonin uptake inhibitors: Correlation with their potencies at inhibiting serotonin uptake in vivo and ^{3}H-mazindol and binding in vitro. *Life Sci* 43:651-658, 1988.

Argenio GF, et al: Blunted growth hormone (GH) responsiveness to GH-releasing hormone in obese patients: Influence of prolonged administration of the serotonergic drug fenfluramine. *Metabolism* 40:724-727, 1991.

Atkinson RL: Effects of fad diets for weight reduction, in: *Malnutrition: Determinants and Consequences.* New York, Alan R. Liss, 1984, 405-413.

Atkinson RL: Low and very low calorie diets. *Med Clin North Am* 73:203-215, 1989.

Bennett JA, Eltringham RJ: Possible dangers of anaesthesia in patients receiving fenfluramine: Results of animal studies following case of human cardiac arrest. *Anaesthesia* 32:8-13, 1977.

Bernstein JG: Induction of obesity by psychotropic drugs. *Ann NY Acad Sci* 499:203-215, 1987.

Björvell H, Rössner S: Long term treatment of severe obesity: Four year follow up of results of combined behavioural modification programme. *Br Med J* 291:379-382, 1985.

Björvell H, Rössner S: A ten year follow-up of weight change in severely obese subjects treated in a behavioural modification-like program. *Int J Obes* 14:88, 1990.

Blackburn GL, Kanders BS: Medical evaluation and treatment of the obese patient with cardiovascular disease. *Am J Cardiol* 60:55G-58G, 1987.

Blackburn GL, et al: Determinants of the pressor effect of phenylpropanolamine in healthy subjects. *JAMA* 261:3267-3272, 1989.

Blundell JE: Appetite disturbance and the problems of overweight. *Drugs* 39 (suppl 3):1-19, 1990.

Blundell J: Pharmacological approaches to appetite suppression. *Trends Pharmacol Sci* 12:147-157, 1991.

Bosch B, et al: Human chorionic gonadotrophin and weight loss: A double-blind, placebo-controlled trial. *S Afr Med J* 77:185-189, 1990.

Bouchard C, et al: Basic and clinical aspects of regional fat distribution. *Am J Clin Nutr* 52:946-950, 1990.

Bray GA: Definitions, measurements and classifications of the syndromes of obesity. *Int J Obes* 2:99-113, 1978.

Bray GA: Treating obesity with drugs. *Drug Ther* 14:93-100, (July) 1984.

Bray GA: Nutrient balance and obesity: Approach to control of food intake in humans. *Med Clin North Am* 73:29-45, 1989 A.

Bray GA: Classification and evaluation of the obesities. *Med Clin North Am* 73:161-184, 1989 B.

Bray GA: Pathophysiology of obesity, in: *Gastrointestinal Surgery for Severe Obesity.* Bethesda, Md, National Institutes of Health, 1991 A, addendum.

Bray GA: Barriers to the treatment of obesity. *Ann Intern Med* 115:152-153, 1991 B.

Bray GA: Treatment for obesity: A nutrient balance/nutrient partition approach. *Nutr Rev* 49:33-45, (Feb) 1991 C.

Bray GA, Gray DS: Obesity: Part I. Pathogenesis. *West J Med* 149:429-441, 1988 A.

Bray GA, Gray DS: Obesity: Part II. Treatment. *West J Med* 149:555-571, 1988 B.

Brownell KD, Kramer FM: Behavioral management of obesity. *Med Clin North Am* 73:185-201, 1989.

Caterson ID: Management strategies for weight control: Eating, exercise and behaviour. *Drugs* 39 (suppl 3):20-32, 1990.

Ceci F, et al: The effects of oral 5-hydroxytryptophan administration on feeding behavior in obese adult female subjects. *J Neural Transm* 76:109-117, 1989.

Charney E, et al: Childhood antecedents of adult obesity: Do chubby infants become obese adults? *N Engl J Med* 295:6-9, 1976.

Committee on Diet and Health: *Diet and Health: Implications for Reducing Chronic Disease Risk.* Washington, DC, National Academy Press, 1989.

Council on Scientific Affairs: Treatment of obesity in adults. *JAMA* 260:2547-2551, 1988.

Di Lorenzo C, et al: Pectin delays gastric emptying and increases satiety in obese subjects. *Gastroenterology* 95:1211-1215, 1988.

Doherty JU, et al: Long-term evaluation of cardiac function in obese patients treated with a very-low-calorie diet: A controlled clinical study of patients without underlying cardiac disease. *Am J Clin Nutr* 53:854-858, 1991.

Drenick EJ, Fisler JS: Sudden cardiac arrest in morbidly obese surgical patients unexplained after autopsy. *Am J Surg* 155:720-726, 1988.

Dulloo AG, Miller DS: Ephedrine, caffeine and aspirin: "Over-the-counter" drugs that interact to stimulate thermogenesis in the obese. *Nutrition* 5:7-9, 1989.

Elliott DL, et al: Sustained depression of the resting metabolic rate after massive weight loss. *Am J Clin Nutr* 49:93-96, 1989.

Finer N, et al: Prolonged use of a very low calorie diet (Cambridge diet) in massively obese patients attending an obesity clinic: Safety, efficacy and additional benefit from dexfenfluramine. *Int J Obes* 12 (suppl 2):91-93, 1989.

Foster GD, et al: Resting energy expenditure, body composition, and excess weight in the obese. *Metabolism* 37:467-472, 1988.

Fowler PA, et al: Total and subcutaneous adipose tissue in women: The measurement of distribution and accurate prediction of quantity by using magnetic resonance imaging. *Am J Clin Nutr* 54:18-25, 1991.

Frankel HM: Determination of body mass index, letter. *JAMA* 255:1292, 1986.

Fuller RW, et al: Fluoxetine, a selective inhibitor of serotonin uptake. *Med Res Rev* 11:17-34, 1991.

Garattini S, et al: Reduction of food intake by manipulation of central serotonin: Current experimental results. *Br J Psychiatry* 155 (suppl 8):41-51, 1989.

Garn SM, Clark DC: Trends in fatness and the origins of obesity. *Pediatrics* 57:443-456, 1976.

Goodrick GK, Foreyt JP: Why treatments for obesity don't last. *J Am Diet Assoc* 91:1243-1247, 1991.

Gray DS: Diagnosis and prevalence of obesity. *Med Clin North Am* 73:1-13, 1989.

Gray DS, Bauer M: The relationship between body fat mass and fat-free mass. *J Am Coll Nutr* 10:63-68, 1991.

Gray DS, Fujioka K: Use of relative weight and body mass index for the determination of adiposity. *J Clin Epidemiol* 44:545-550, 1991.

Griffin JP, et al: *A Manual of Adverse Drug Interactions,* ed 4. London, Wright, 1988.

Griffiths M, et al: Metabolic rate and physical development in children at risk of obesity. *Lancet* 336:76-78, 1990.

Guy-Grand B, et al: International trial of long-term dexfenfluramine in obesity. *Lancet* 2:1142-1144, 1989.

Haarbo J, et al: Body composition by dual-energy X-ray absorptiometry (DEXA). *J Bone Miner Res* 5 (suppl 2):S180, 1990.

Hammer LD, et al: Impact of pubertal development on body fat distribution among white, Hispanic, and Asian female adolescents. *J Pediatr* 118:975-980, 1991.

Harris T, et al: Body mass index and mortality among nonsmoking older persons: The Framingham Heart Study. *JAMA* 259:1520-1524, 1988.

Harrison GG: Height-weight tables. *Ann Intern Med* 103:989-994, 1985.

Heitmann BL: Evaluation of body fat estimated from body mass index, skinfolds and impedance: A comparative study. *Eur J Clin Nutr* 44:831-837, 1990.

Henry CJK, Rees DG: New predictive equations for the estimation of basal metabolic rate in tropical peoples. *Eur J Clin Nutr* 45:177-185, 1991.

Heshka S, et al: Weight loss and change in resting metabolic rate. *Am J Clin Nutr* 52:981-986, 1990.

Hill JO, et al: Effects of exercise and food restriction on body composition and metabolic rate in obese women. *Am J Clin Nutr* 46:622-630, 1987.

Hirsch J, et al: The fat cell. *Med Clin North Am* 73:83-96, 1989.

Howard BV, et al: Studies of the etiology of obesity in Pima Indians. *Am J Clin Nutr* 53:1577S-1585S, 1991.

Hypertension Prevention Trial Research Group: The hypertension prevention trial: Three-year effects of dietary changes on blood pressure. *Arch Intern Med* 150:153-162, 1990.

Institute of Medicine: *Nutrition During Pregnancy.* Washington, DC, National Academy Press, 1990.

Jéquier E: Energy, obesity, and body weight standards. *Am J Clin Nutr* 45:1035-1047, 1987.

Jonides LK: Childhood obesity: An update. *J Pediatr Health Care* 4:244-251, 1990.

Jung RT, Chong P: The management of obesity. *Clin Endocrinol* 35:11-20, 1991.

Kannel WB, et al: Regional obesity and risk of cardiovascular disease: The Framingham study. *J Clin Epidemiol* 44:183-190, 1991.

Kaye SA, et al: Increased incidence of diabetes mellitus in relation to abdominal adiposity in older women. *J Clin Epidemiol* 44:329-334, 1991.

Kissebah AH, et al: Health risks of obesity. *Med Clin North Am* 73:111-138, 1989.

Knapp TR: A methodological critique of the 'ideal weight' concept. *JAMA* 250:506-510, 1983.

Knoll J: Endogenous anorectic agents—satietins. *Ann Rev Pharmacol Toxicol* 28:247-268, 1988.

Knowler WC, et al: Obesity in the Pima Indians: Its magnitude and relationship with diabetes. *Am J Clin Nutr* 53:1543S-1551S, 1991.

Kraemer FM, et al: Long-term follow-up of behavioral treatment for obesity: Patterns of weight regain among men and women. *Int J Obes* 13:123-136, 1989.

Kral JG: Surgical treatment of obesity. *Med Clin North Am* 73:251-264, 1989.

Kral JG: Overview of surgical techniques for treating obesity, in: *Gastrointestinal Surgery for Severe Obesity.* Bethesda, Md, National Institutes of Health, 1991, 63-69.

Kroenke K, et al: Safety of phenylpropanolamine in patients with stable hypertension. *Ann Intern Med* 111:1043-1044, 1989.

Lampman RM, Schteingart DE: Effects of exercise training on glucose control, lipid metabolism, and insulin sensitivity in hypertriglyceridemia and non-insulin dependent diabetes mellitus. *Med Sci Sports Exercise* 23:703-712, 1991.

Lasagna L: *Phenylpropanolamine: A Review.* New York, John Wiley & Sons, 1988.

Lauer MS, et al: The impact of obesity on left ventricular mass and geometry: The Framingham Heart Study. *JAMA* 266:231-236, 1991.

Leibowitz SF: The role of serotonin in eating disorders. *Drugs* 39(suppl 3):33-48, 1990.

Lerman RH, Cave DR: Medical and surgical management of obesity. *Adv Intern Med* 34:127-164, 1989.

Levy D, et al: Prognostic implications of echocardiographically determined left ventricular mass in the Framingham Heart Study. *N Engl J Med* 322:1561-1566, 1990.

Liebson I, et al: Phenylpropanolamine: Effects on subjective and cardiovascular variables at recommended over-the-counter dose levels. *J Clin Pharmacol* 27:685-693, 1987.

Lissner L, et al: Variability of body weight and health outcomes in the Framingham population. *N Engl J Med* 324:1839-1844, 1991.

Malcolm R, et al: Update on the management of obesity. *South Med J* 81:632-639, 1988.

Marcus MD, et al: A double-blind, placebo-controlled trial of fluoxetine plus behavior modification in the treatment of obese binge-eaters and non-binge-eaters. *Am J Psychiatry* 147:876-881, 1990.

Micciolo R, et al: The association of body fat location with haemodynamic and metabolic status in men and women aged 21-60 years. *J Clin Epidemiol* 44:591-608, 1991.

Miller LG: Phenylpropanolamine: A controversy unresolved, editorial. *J Clin Psychopharmacol* 9:1-3, 1989.

Modan M, et al: Obesity, glucose intolerance, hyperinsulinemia, and response to antihypertensive drugs. *Hypertension* 17:565-573, 1991.

Moran TH, McHugh PR: Cholecystokinin suppresses food intake by inhibiting gastric emptying. *Am Physiol Soc* R491-R497, 1982.

Morgan JP, Kagan DV (eds): Phenylpropanolamine: Risks, benefits, and controversies, in: *Clinical Pharmacology and Therapeutics.* New York, Praeger, 1985.

Morgan JP, et al: Subjective profile of phenylpropanolamine: Absence of stimulant or euphorigenic effects at recommended dose levels. *J Clin Psychopharmacol* 9:33-38, 1989.

Najjar MF, Rowland M: Anthropometric reference data and prevalence of overweight, United States, 1976-1980, in National Center for Health Statistics: *Vital and Health Statistics.* DHHS Pub No (PHS) 87-1688. Washington DC, Public Health Service, 1987.

National Institutes of Health Consensus Development Panel: Health implications of obesity. *Ann Intern Med* 103:1073-1077, 1985.

Neel JV: Diabetes mellitus: A "thrifty" phenotype rendered detrimental by "progress"? *Am J Human Genet* 14:353-362, 1962.

O'Donnell JT: Nutrition fraud: Vitamins and obesity: Pharmacists' responsibilities. *J Pharm Pract* 1:131-149, (Oct) 1988.

Peikin SR: Role of cholecystokinin in the control of food intake. *Gastroenterol Clin North Am* 18:757-775, 1989.

Pentel P: Toxicity of over-the-counter stimulants. *JAMA* 252:1898-1903, 1984.

Perri MG, et al: Effects of four maintenance programs on the long-term management of obesity. *J Consult Clin Psychol* 56:529-534, 1988.

Pi-Sunyer FX: Health implications of obesity. *Am J Clin Nutr* 53:1595S-1603S, 1991 A.

Pi-Sunyer FX: Obesity: Determinants and therapeutic initiatives. *Nutrition* 7:292-294, (July/Aug) 1991 B.

Ravussin E, et al: Determinants of 24-hour energy expenditure in man: Methods and results using a respiratory chamber. *J Clin Invest* 78:1568-1578, 1986.

Ravussin E, et al: Reduced rate of energy expenditure as a risk factor for body-weight gain. *N Engl J Med* 318:467-472, 1988.

Reeds PJ, Mersmann HJ: Protein and energy requirements of animals treated with β-adrenergic agonists: A discussion. *J Anim Sci* 69:1532-1550, 1991.

Rees JM: Management of obesity in adolescence. *Med Clin North Am* 74:1275-1292, 1990.

Revicki DA, Israel RG: Relationship between body mass indices and measures of body adiposity. *Am J Public Health* 76:992-994, 1986.

Richard BW, Lasagna L: Anorectic drugs: Drug policy making at the state level. *J Clin Pharmacol* 28:395-400, 1988.

Riddell RH: *Pathology of Drug-Induced and Toxic Diseases.* New York, Churchill Livingstone, 1982.

Rissanen A, et al: Weight and mortality in Finnish men. *J Clin Epidemiol* 42:781-789, 1989.

Roberts SB, et al: Energy expenditure and intake in infants born to lean and overweight mothers. *N Engl J Med* 318:461-466, 1988.

Robinson PH, et al: Gastric control of food intake. *J Psychosom Res* 32:593-606, 1988.

Roubenoff R, Kehayias JJ: The meaning and measurement of lean body mass. *Nutr Rev* 49:163-175, (June) 1991.

Rowland NE, Carlton J: Neurobiology for an anorectic drug: Fenfluramine. *Prog Neurobiol* 27:16-62, 1986.

Rutherford OM, et al: Changes in skeletal muscle and body composition after discontinuation of growth hormone treatment in growth hormone deficient young adults. *Clin Endocrinol* 34:469-475, 1991.

Sangi H, Mueller WH: Which measure of body fat distribution is best for epidemiologic research among adolescents? *Am J Epidemiol* 133:870-883, 1991.

Schapira DV, et al: Upper-body fat distribution and endometrial cancer risk. *JAMA* 266:1808-1811, 1991.

Segal KR, Pi-Sunyer FX: Exercise and obesity. *Med Clin North Am* 73:217-236, 1989.

Seidell JC, et al: Visceral fat accumulation in men is positively associated with insulin, glucose, and C-peptide levels, but negatively with testosterone levels. *Metabolism* 39:897-901, 1990.

Seidman DS, et al: A longitudinal study of birth weight and being overweight in late adolescence. *Am J Dis Child* 145:782-785, 1991.

Silva JE, Larsen PR: Adrenergic activation of triiodothyronine production in brown adipose tissue. *Nature* 305:712-713, 1983.

Silverstone T: Appetite-suppressant drugs in the management of obesity: The current view. *Int J Obesity* 11(suppl 3):135-139, 1987.

Sjöström L: Morbidity and mortality of obese subjects, in: *Gastrointestinal Surgery for Severe Obesity.* Bethesda, Md, National Institutes of Health, 1991, addendum.

Sosenko JM, et al: The relation between the plasma lipoprotein pattern and the waist/hip ratio in non-diabetic individuals. *J Clin Epidemiol* 43:1149-1156, 1990.

Stricker EM, Verbalis JG: Control of appetite and satiety: Insights from biologic and behavioral studies. *Nutr Rev* 48:49-56, (Feb) 1990.

Stunkard AJ: Conservative treatments for obesity. *Am J Clin Nutr* 45:1142-1154, 1987.

Sullivan AC, Comai K: Pharmacological treatment of obesity. *Int J Obes* 2:167, 1978.

Terry RB, et al: Contributions of regional adipose tissue depots to plasma lipoprotein concentrations in overweight men and women: Possible protective effects of thigh fat. *Metabolism* 40:733-740, 1991.

Tsai SP, et al: Obesity and morbidity prevalence in a working population. *J Occup Med* 30:589-591, 1988.

Tuomilehto J: Body mass index and prognosis in elderly hypertensive patients: A report from the European Working Party on High Blood Pressure in the Elderly. *Am J Med* 90 (suppl 3A):3A-34S-3A-41S, 1991.

Turner P: Dexfenfluramine: Its place in weight control. *Drugs* 39 (suppl 3):53-62, 1990.

Uvnäs-Moberg K: Endocrinologic control of food intake. *Nutr Rev* 48:57-63, (Feb) 1990.

Van Loan MD, Koehler LS: Use of total-body electrical conductivity for the assessment of body composition in middle-aged and elderly individuals. *Am J Clin Nutr* 51:548-552, 1990.

Wadden TA, et al: Responsible and irresponsible use of very-low-calorie diets in the treatment of obesity. *JAMA* 263:83-85, 1990 A.

Wadden TA, et al: Long-term effects of dieting on resting metabolic rate in obese outpatients. *JAMA* 264:707-711, 1990 B.

Weintraub M, Bray GA: Drug treatment of obesity. *Med Clin North Am* 73:237-249, 1989.

Weintraub M, et al: Double-blind clinical trial in weight control: Use of fenfluramine and phentermine alone and in combination. *Arch Intern Med* 144:1143-1148, 1984.

Welle SL, Campbell RG: Decrease in resting metabolic rate during rapid weight loss is reversed by low dose thyroid hormone treatment. *Metabolism* 35:289-291, 1986.

Wing RR: Behavioral treatment of severe obesity, in: *Gastrointestinal Surgery for Severe Obesity.* Bethesda, Md, National Institutes of Health, 1991, 49-62.

Wing RR, et al: Exercise in a behavioural weight control programme for obese patients with type 2 (non-insulin-dependent) diabetes. *Diabetologia* 31:902-909, 1988.

Wing RR, et al: Effects of a very-low-calorie diet on long-term glycemic control in obese type 2 diabetic subjects. *Arch Intern Med* 151:1334-1340, 1991.

Winick C: Phenylpropanolamine: Toward resolution of a controversy, editorial. *J Clin Psychopharmacol* 11:79-81, (April) 1991.

Wood PD, et al: Changes in plasma lipids and lipoproteins in overweight men during weight loss through dieting as compared with exercise. *N Engl J Med* 319:1173-1179, 1988.

Treatment of Disorders of Cholesterol and Lipoprotein Metabolism

103

The risk of developing atherosclerotic plaque with subsequent myocardial infarction is increased in most individuals with disorders of lipid metabolism and transport. Impaired hepatic or peripheral lipid metabolism or excessive ingestion of cholesterogenic dietary substances can result in a variety of dyslipidemias associated with increased risk of coronary heart disease (CHD). These include elevated serum concentrations of total cholesterol, low density lipoprotein-associated cholesterol (LDL-cholesterol), very low density lipoprotein-associated cholesterol (VLDL-cholesterol), lipoprotein (a) (Lp[a]), or triglyceride-rich chylomicrons and their remnants, and low serum concentrations of high density lipoprotein-associated cholesterol (HDL-cholesterol). Factors that interact with disorders of lipid metabolism and transport to further increase the risk of CHD include poorly controlled hypertension, cigarette smoking, sedentary habits, diabetes mellitus, obesity, left ventricular hypertrophy, male sex, female sex postmenopause, chronic renal failure, hyperhomocysteinemia, low antioxidant reserve potential, and a family history of CHD, cerebrovascular, or peripheral vascular disease before age 55 (Hopkins and Williams, 1981; Pathobiological Determinants of Atherosclerosis in Youth Research Group, 1990; Clinical Experience Network, 1991; Assmann and Schulte, 1992; Genest et al, 1992; Kang et al, 1992; Manson et al, 1992; Markussis et al, 1992; Neaton and Wentworth, 1992; Stampfer et al, 1992; Ross, 1993).

The primary goal of intervention in dyslipidemias is to retard the development of atherosclerotic disease by reducing the contributions of circulating factors to disease progression. Aggressive intervention can cause some atherosclerotic plaques to regress and may reduce the incidence or severity of CHD in patients with familial hypercholesterolemia or established CHD, including recipients of coronary artery bypass surgery

TABLE 1.
CLASSIFICATION AND PROPERTIES OF LIPOPROTEINS

Lipoprotein Class	Major Lipids	Apolipoproteins	Density (g/ml)
Chylomicrons	Dietary triglycerides and cholesteryl esters	A-I, A-II, A-IV B-48 C-I, C-II, C-III E	<0.95
Chylomicron remnants	Dietary cholesteryl esters and triglycerides	B-48 E	<1.006
VLDL	Endogenous triglycerides and cholesteryl esters	B-100 C-I, C-II, C-III E	<1.006
IDL, VLDL remnants	Cholesteryl esters and triglycerides	B-100 E	1.006 to 1.019
LDL	Cholesteryl esters	B-100	1.019 to 1.063
HDL_2	Cholesteryl esters Phospholipids	A-I, A-II, A-IV C-I, C-II, C-III DE	1.063 to 1.125
HDL_3	Cholesteryl esters Phospholipids	A-I, A-II, A-IV C-I, C-II, C-III D E	1.125 to 1.210
Lp (a)	Cholesteryl esters	(a) B-100	1.055 to 1.088

and angioplasty (Lipid Research Clinics Program, 1984; Anderson et al, 1987; Holme, 1990; Ornish et al, 1990; Reis et al, 1991; Rifkind and Rossouw, 1991; Blankenhorn et al, 1992; Gould et al, 1992; Shah and Amin, 1992; Alva et al, 1993; Blankenhorn et al, 1993 A; Brown et al, 1993; Vos et al, 1993).

In general, each 1% reduction in serum total cholesterol concentration, 1.5% reduction in serum LDL-cholesterol concentration, or 1 mg/dL increase in serum HDL-cholesterol concentration reduces the risk of myocardial infarction in high-risk hypercholesterolemic men and women by approximately 2% to 3% (Lipid Research Clinics Program, 1984; Frick et al, 1987; Gordon et al, 1989; Stampfer et al, 1991; Buring et al, 1992; Manson et al, 1992). In addition, each 1-unit decrease in the ratio of serum total to HDL-cholesterol concentrations may cut the risk of myocardial infarction in men by half (Stampfer et al, 1991). It has been estimated that reducing serum total cholesterol concentration from 300 to 200 mg/dL may increase life expectancy by up to three years and may delay symptomatic CHD by up to five years (Grover et al, 1992). However, concerns have been raised that spontaneous or drug-induced decreases in serum total cholesterol concentrations to below 140 mg/dL may be associated with increased risk of noncardiovascular death (Frank et al, 1992; Harris et al, 1992; Lindberg et al, 1992).

Conditions favoring atherosclerotic plaque formation (atherogenesis) usually reflect abnormal metabolism of circulating lipoproteins (Ginsberg, 1990; Galton and Krone, 1991; Gotto, 1991 A; Frishman, 1992). The selection of appropriate treatment options requires accurate characterization of the lipoprotein disorders present.

LIPOPROTEINS AND APOLIPOPROTEINS

Dietary and endogenous fatty acids and cholesterol are transported after incorporation into lipoprotein particles (Dietschy, 1990; Gotto, 1991 A; Grundy, 1991 A). Lipoproteins consist of an inner core of nonpolar cholesteryl esters and triglycerides surrounded by a surface coat of apoproteins, phospholipids, and nonesterified cholesterol (Table 1). Apoproteins combine with phospholipids in lipoproteins to provide a soluble complex for transporting lipids (Table 2) (Gotto, 1991 A). They also serve as binding ligands or recognition sites for cell surface lipoprotein receptors and as cofactors to several enzymes involved in lipoprotein metabolism. Disturbances of lipoprotein metabolism often result from alterations of apoprotein metabolism (Young, 1990).

The lipoproteins involved in lipid transport are dynamic and metabolically interrelated. They are separated by density and electrophoretic migration into five major classes (Table 1): (1) *chylomicrons,* the largest lipoproteins, consisting of 90% triglycerides derived from absorbed dietary fatty acids and about 5% cholesterol by weight; (2) *very low density lipoproteins* (VLDL, prebeta lipoproteins), consisting of 60% triglycerides synthesized from endogenous free fatty acids (FFA) and glycerol and 10% to 15% cholesterol; (3) *intermediate density lipoproteins* (IDL), intermediates in the conversion of VLDL to LDL consisting of roughly equal proportions of cho-

TABLE 2.
CLASSIFICATION, PROPERTIES, AND FUNCTIONS OF APOLIPOPROTEINS

Apolipoprotein Class	Tissue Expression	Functions
Apo (a)	Liver	Structural component of Lp (a); ligand for plasminogen receptors
Apo A-I	Liver, Intestine	Structural component of HDL; activator of LCAT
Apo A-II	Liver	Structural component of HDL; activator of hepatic lipase
Apo A-IV	Liver, Intestine	Activator of LCAT
Apo B-48	Intestine	Structural component of chylomicrons; essential for chylomicron secretion; undetectable in fasting plasma
Apo B-100	Liver	Structural component of VLDL and LDL; essential for VLDL secretion; ligand for LDL receptors
Apo C-I	Liver, Intestine	Inhibitor of premature clearance of triglyceride-rich lipoproteins and activator of LCAT
Apo C-II	Liver, Intestine	Inhibitor of premature clearance of triglyceride-rich lipoproteins and activator of LPL
Apo C-III	Liver, Intestine	Inhibitor of premature clearance of triglyceride-rich lipoproteins and inhibitor of LPL
Apo D	Liver, Intestine, Kidney	Stimulator of CETP
Apo E	Liver, Macrophages	Ligand for LDL receptors; ligand for chylomicron remnant receptors

lesterol and triglycerides; (4) *low density lipoproteins* (LDL, beta lipoproteins), consisting of almost 50% cholesterol and <10% triglycerides and carrying 60% to 75% of the total circulating cholesterol; and (5) *high density lipoproteins* (HDL, alpha lipoproteins), consisting of about 20% to 30% cholesterol and <5% triglyceride. An additional lipoprotein, lipoprotein (a) (Lp[a]), is very similar to LDL but carries a molecule of apo (a) linked to apo B-100. Serum concentrations of the major lipoproteins are affected by a number of factors, including diet, age, sexual maturation, and race (Berenson et al, 1991).

LIPOPROTEIN METABOLISM

Monoglycerides and FFA released from ingested fats are re-esterified into triglycerides in enterocytes and are combined with several apoproteins (apo B-48, apo A-I, and apo A-IV) to form chylomicrons. These lipoproteins are secreted into lymph and pass into plasma where they receive apo C-I, apo C-II, and apo C-III from HDL. Chylomicrons bind to the luminal surface of the capillary endothelium in adipose tissue and muscle. Apo C-II is required to activate lipoprotein lipase (LPL) on the endothelial cell surface, which then hydrolyzes the triglyceride core of the chylomicron, releasing FFA and monoglycerides. Once released, FFA are bound to albumin and are taken up by adipose tissue, muscle, or the liver. As its triglyceride core is depleted, the chylomicron shrinks and transfers triglycerides, apo A-I, and apo A-IV to circulating HDL particles in exchange for apo E and cholesteryl esters. The exchange of triglyceride for cholesteryl ester is facilitated by plasma cholesteryl ester transfer protein (CETP). The resulting chylomicron remnant is cleared rapidly from plasma by the liver via an apo E receptor-mediated process. LPL may combine with a chylomicron remnant after dissociation from the endothelial surface to facilitate remnant removal. The plasma half-life of chylomicrons and most of their remnants is four to five minutes; however, smaller chylomicron remnants may persist for much longer. Triglyceride-rich chylomicrons may not be atherogenic; in contrast, cholesterol-rich chylomicron remnants can pass through the endothelium and become sequestered within periendothelial monocytes and macrophages and are highly atherogenic.

The endogenous lipid transport pathway originates in the liver, where triglycerides and cholesterol are either synthesized de novo or recycled (via VLDL, IDL, and LDL; see below). The rate of hepatic cholesterol synthesis is regulated by 3-hydroxy-3-methylglutaryl Coenzyme A (HMG-CoA) reductase, which catalyzes the conversion of HMG-CoA to mevalonate (Goldstein and Brown, 1990). HMG-CoA reductase activity is regulated by negative feedback from oxysterols generated by cytochrome P450 oxidation of intracellular cholesterol.

Triglycerides, apo B-100, apo C-I, apo C-II, apo C-III, apo E, and cholesterol are incorporated into nascent VLDL whenever synthesis of fatty acids and triglycerides is stimulated (eg, diabetes, obesity, insulin resistance). VLDL synthesis is altered by ingestion of alcohol and by changes in caloric intake, cholesterol intake, dietary fat intake, body weight, stress, exercise, hormones, and HMG-CoA reductase activity.

Mature VLDL also interact with endothelial LPL and circulating CETP and HDL. As triglyceride is removed, the size of the VLDL particle decreases, its density increases, and an IDL particle is formed. About 25% to 75% of IDL is cleared rapidly by the liver via hepatic LDL receptors that recognize both apo E and apo B-100; the rate of IDL clearance is proportional to the number of hepatic LDL receptors. IDL particles remaining in circulation undergo further lipolysis by LPL and hepatic triglyceride lipase (HL), as well as continued exchange of triglycerides for cholesteryl esters. As a result, most triglycerides are removed, all apoproteins except apo B-100 are lost, and LDL are formed. Inadequate LPL activity, apo CII deficiency, or apo C-III excess can result in hypertriglyceridemia and low LDL-cholesterol concentration or LDL particles that are abnormally high in triglyceride content and particularly susceptible to peroxidation and involvement in atherogenesis (Malmendier et al, 1991; Regnström et al, 1992; Karpe et al, 1993).

LDL delivers cholesterol to extrahepatic cells and to the liver, where most LDL is catabolized. In normal individuals, about two-thirds of the LDL in plasma bind via apo B-100 to high affinity LDL receptors, whose number is regulated by the intracellular free cholesterol concentration. Following binding, receptor-ligand complexes invaginate and internalize LDL by endocytosis, lysosomal hydrolases degrade apoproteins to amino acids, and acid cholesterol ester hydrolase liberates free cholesterol. Within hepatocytes, free cholesterol is either converted to oxysterols by cytochrome P450, esterified for storage by acyl CoA:cholesterol acyl transferase (ACAT), converted to bile acids and excreted into the intestine, secreted into the bile as nonesterified cholesterol, or incorporated into nascent VLDL. Some of the cholesterol is reabsorbed from the intestine and incorporated into chylomicrons; a small portion is excreted in the feces. Some LDL is catabolized by the liver via nonreceptor-mediated mechanisms.

LDL particles can become highly atherogenic after surface oxidation in the subendothelial space of the peripheral vasculature (Steinberg, 1993). This process is dramatically accelerated by the presence of pro-oxidants. Aldehydes formed by the oxidation of surface phospholipids bind to apo B-100 through acetylation reactions and trigger LDL binding to "scavenger" receptors on macrophages of the reticuloendothelial system. Binding and internalization of modified LDL and storage of cholesteryl esters are not subject to feedback inhibition and continue until these cells accumulate excessive amounts of lipid and become foam cells typical of atherosclerotic lesions. Oxidized LDL also are toxic to endothelial cells and trigger secretion of platelet activation factors; activated platelets in turn secrete platelet-derived growth factor (PDGF), which stimulates smooth muscle cell proliferation, tissue hyperplasia, and progression and expansion of atherosclerotic lesions.

HDL metabolism is complex and not completely understood (see review by Silverman et al, 1993). Nascent HDL particles are synthesized in the liver and intestine and contain phospholipid, free cholesterol, and either apo A-I (LpA-I) or apo A-I and apo A-II (LpA-I/A-II). Some nascent HDL particles also carry apo E. As nascent HDL enters the blood, apo A-I activates plasma lecithin-cholesterol acyltransferase (LCAT), which converts lecithin and cholesterol on the HDL surface to lysolecithin and cholesteryl ester. Lysolecithin is transferred to serum albumin, and cholesteryl esters migrate toward the HDL particle's center. As cholesteryl esters accumulate within HDL, the particle becomes spherical and is termed either HDL_{3a} or HDL_{3b}, depending on its size and cholesteryl ester content. Most HDL in humans circulates as $HDL_{3(a+b)}$. Continued uptake and esterification of free cholesterol obtained from the outer surfaces of other lipoproteins and from peripheral cells, possibly via an apo A-I receptor-mediated process, further expand the particle; eventually it becomes a cholesterol-enriched HDL_{2a} particle. Although most HDL_{2a} lack apo E, cholesterol-rich HDL_{2a} carrying apo E are directly catabolized by hepatocytes via apo E receptor-mediated endocytosis. CETP transport cholesteryl esters from HDL_{2a} that lack apo E to chylomicrons and VLDL particles in exchange for triglycerides, apoproteins, and phospholipids; cholesterol-rich HDL_{2a} become cholesterol-depleted, triglyceride-rich HDL_{2b}.

Apo A-II on triglyceride-rich HDL_{2b} activate HL, which hydrolyses HDL_{2b} triglyceride and regenerates smaller, denser, triglyceride-depleted HDL_{3c}. HL also has substantial phospholipase activity, resulting in removal of surface lipids from HDL_{2b} and facilitating its conversion to HDL_3. In addition, some apo A-I is lost in the conversion of HDL_2 to HDL_3 as particle surface area decreases.

Variability in serum HDL-cholesterol concentration usually reflects changes in the amount of HDL_2 present. Genetic LCAT or apo A-I deficiency results in failure of HDL to capture and esterify cholesterol, and serum HDL-cholesterol concentration is reduced. In genetic CETP deficiency, cholesteryl esters and triglycerides are not exchanged, HDL_{2a} particles become abnormally large, HDL_{2a} clearance is inhibited, and serum HDL_{2a}-cholesterol (and therefore total HDL-cholesterol) concentration remains high. Conversely, in genetic CETP elevation, exchange of cholesteryl esters and triglycerides and conversion of HDL_2 to HDL_3 are accelerated, and serum HDL concentration is decreased. In LPL deficiency, triglyceride hydrolysis in chylomicrons and VLDL is slowed, fewer FFA are released, triglyceride/cholesteryl ester exchange is increased, HDL_{2b} formation and subsequent clearance by HL are accelerated, and serum HDL-cholesterol concentration is decreased. In HL deficiency, large triglyceride-rich HDL_{2b} particles are not metabolized and accumulate in serum. In contrast, high HL activity accelerates regeneration of HDL_{3c}, and serum HDL_{2b}-cholesterol (and therefore total HDL-cholesterol) concentration decreases. Hypertriglyceridemia stimulates both CETP and HL activities and accelerates the conversion of HDL_{2a} to HDL_{2b} and HDL_3; this mechanism probably results in the inverse relationship typically found between fasting triglyceride and HDL-cholesterol concentrations.

Experimental and epidemiologic evidence suggests that HDL may inhibit atherogenesis. In addition to participation in reverse cholesterol transport, HDL facilitates lipoprotein metabolism, inhibits LDL oxidation, stimulates prostacyclin secretion (reducing platelet aggregability), promotes fibrinolysis, and inhibits platelet activation and oxidized LDL aggregation and binding to "scavenger" receptors (Badimon et al, 1992).

The functions of Lp(a) are unknown; it may transport cholesterol to sites of tissue injury for cell membrane synthesis. Plasminogen-like domains of apo(a) bind to fibrin at sites of vascular injury, allowing Lp(a) to traverse the endothelium, become oxidized, and contribute to foam cell formation. Lp(a) also may suppress local fibrinolysis, although in vivo studies have not confirmed this hypothesis (Hajjar et al,

TABLE 3.
PRIMARY LIPOPROTEIN DISORDERS

Lipid Disorder	Lipoprotein Profile	Clinical Manifestations
HYPERCHOLESTEROLEMIA		
Familial heterozygous	↑↑ serum LDL-cholesterol	Tendon xanthomas (finger extensors and Achilles) occur in one-third of patients. Strongly associated with premature atherosclerosis and family history of hypercholesterolemia.
Familial homozygous Familial defective Apolipoprotein B-100	↑↑↑ serum LDL-cholesterol	All of the above signs are exaggerated and a cutaneous planar xanthoma is usually evident. Aortic stenosis may develop as a result of cholesterol deposition in the aortic valve. Premature catastrophic CHD is common.
Polygenic	↑ serum LDL-cholesterol	Xanthomas are absent. This disorder often is associated with obesity and/or excess intake of saturated fat and cholesterol in the diet. Premature coronary atherosclerosis often is present.
HYPERTRIGLYCERIDEMIA		
Familial Hypertriglyceridemia	↑ plasma triglycerides ↓ serum HDL-cholesterol	Usually asymptomatic. Difficult to distinguish from major secondary hypertriglyceridemias (see Table 4). Concentration of VLDL is increased by alcohol ingestion, obesity, and excess carbohydrate and saturated fat intake. Glucose intolerance and elevated uric acid concentrations may be present. Family often includes individuals with lesser degrees of hypertriglyceridemias.
FAMILIAL COMBINED HYPERLIPIDEMIA		Xanthomas do not occur. Family history of elevation of LDL, VLDL, or both is common. Premature coronary atherosclerosis is common. Recurrent pancreatitis is occasionally present.
With isolated hypercholesterolemia	↑ serum LDL-cholesterol borderline plasma triglycerides ↓ serum HDL-cholesterol	
With isolated hypertriglyceridemia	↑ plasma triglycerides borderline serum LDL-cholesterol ↓ serum HDL-cholesterol	
Hypercholesterolemia plus hypertriglyceridemia	↑ serum LDL-cholesterol and ↑ plasma triglycerides ↓ serum HDL-cholesterol	
FASTING HYPERCHYLOMICRONEMIA	Marked fasting chylomicronemia ↑↑↑ plasma triglycerides	Usually recurrent abdominal pain, pancreatitis, and hepatosplenomegaly are present. Eruptive xanthomas and lipemia retinalis are common.

(table continued on next page)

TABLE 3 (continued)

Lipid Disorder	Lipoprotein Profile	Clinical Manifestations
FAMILIAL DYSBETALIPOPROTEINEMIA	Mild fasting chylomicronemia ↑ serum IDL-, VLDL-, and β-VLDL-cholesterol	Palmar/planar xanthomas are practically pathognomonic; tuberoeruptive xanthomas on elbows, knees, buttocks and tendon are common. The disorder is markedly exaggerated by hypothyroidism, alcohol ingestion, estrogen deficiency, diabetes, and obesity. Uric acid concentrations often are elevated. Premature coronary and peripheral vascular disease are common.
FAMILIAL MIXED HYPERTRIGLYCERIDEMIA	Mild fasting chylomicronemia ↑ ↑ ↑ plasma triglycerides ↓ serum HDL-cholesterol	Eruptive xanthomas, recurrent abdominal pain, and pancreatitis may be present unless the elevated triglyceride level and fasting chylomicronemia are controlled. Glucose intolerance and hyperuricemia may be present.
HYPOALPHALIPOPROTEINEMIA	↓ serum HDL-cholesterol	Asymptomatic. Many patients have a secondary cause for this disorder (see Table 4). Increased risk of premature CHD.
HYPERALPHALIPOPROTEINEMIA	↑ ↑ serum HDL-cholesterol	Extremely rare CETP deficiency. CHD very rare.
HYPOBETALIPOPROTEINEMIA	↓ serum total, LDL-, VLDL-, and HDL-cholesterol	Not uncommon. Marked attenuation of postprandial hypertriglyceridemia. Reduced incidence of CHD and exceptional longevity.
ABETALIPOPROTEINEMIA	Absence of VLDL- and LDL-cholesterol	Extremely rare. Malabsorption of fat and fat-soluble vitamins, neurologic lesions, and erythrocyte abnormalities.
DIABETIC DYSLIPIDEMIA		Insulin-dependent or noninsulin-dependent diabetes mellitus present. Premature atherosclerosis and CHD common.
Severe hypertriglyceridemia	↑ ↑ ↑ plasma triglycerides ↓ serum LDL- and HDL-cholesterol	
Moderate hypertriglyceridemia	↑ plasma triglycerides ↑ ↑ serum LDL-cholesterol ↓ serum HDL-cholesterol	

1989; Miles et al, 1989; Harpel and Borth, 1992; Glueck et al, 1993).

Lp(a) is atherogenic (Seidel et al, 1992). Patients with renal failure and heterozygous familial hypercholesterolemia or poorly controlled diabetes mellitus tend to have elevated serum Lp(a) concentrations (Seed et al, 1990; Kapelrud et al, 1991; Haffner et al, 1992), and those with the highest concentrations are most at risk for CHD (Labeur et al, 1992). In contrast, serum Lp(a) concentration and CHD risk are reduced in patients with hepatic cirrhosis (Feely et al, 1992). Elevated serum Lp(a) concentrations also are correlated with increased risk of early extracoronary atherosclerotic plaque formation (Cambillau et al, 1992), peripheral vascular disease (Tyrrell et al, 1992), stenosis after coronary artery bypass surgery (Hoff et al, 1988), and restenosis after percutaneous transluminal coronary angioplasty (Hearn et al, 1992).

Serum Lp(a) concentration in adults ranges from undetectable to >100 mg/dL and is relatively constant in any given individual (Albers et al, 1990). The serum concentration of Lp(a) is inversely correlated with the number of allele duplications coding for a repeated portion of apo(a) in an individual; the size polymorphism of apo(a) accounts for 40% to 70% of the interindividual variability in serum Lp(a) concentrations. Although the hepatic LDL receptor plays a minor role in Lp(a) clearance, drugs that increase the expression of those receptors do not affect serum Lp(a) concentrations.

TABLE 4.
MAJOR CAUSES OF SECONDARY LIPIDEMIC ABNORMALITIES

Elevated Triglycerides	Elevated LDL-cholesterol	Reduced HDL-cholesterol
Excess dietary saturated fat Excess dietary carbohydrate Excess alcohol ingestion Bulimia Cushing's disease Hypothyroidism Obesity Diabetes mellitus (poorly controlled) Uremia Nephrotic syndrome Pregnancy Glycogen storage disease Systemic lupus erythematosus LCAT deficiency Drugs: isotretinoin, thiazide diuretics[1], furosemide, beta blockers[2], oral contraceptives[3], estrogens, corticosteroids, cimetidine, phenothiazines	Excess dietary saturated fat Excess dietary cholesterol Obesity Hypothyroidism Nephrotic syndrome Anorexia nervosa Pregnancy Acute intermittent porphyria Anxiety Extrahepatic biliary obstruction Growth hormone deficiency Hepatoma Insulin-like growth factor-I (IGF-I) deficiency Infantile hypercalcemia Primary biliary cirrhosis Sexual ateliotic dwarfism Werner's syndrome Dysglobulinemias, multiple myeloma, monoclonal gammopathy, Drugs: isotretinoin, thiazide diuretics, cyclosporine, amiodarone, retinoids, androgens, mitotane, corticosteroids, progestin[3], beta blockers	Excess dietary carbohydrate Elevated triglycerides Obesity Cigarette smoking Lack of exercise Diabetes mellitus (poorly controlled) Drugs: beta blockers[2], anabolic steroids, androgens, progestins, retinoids, phenothiazines, probucol

[1] *Not all patients on thiazide diuretics will exhibit hypertriglyceridemia. Patients should be monitored and, if required, other diuretics can be considered for substitution. Calcium channel blockers, angiotensin-converting enzyme inhibitors, and alpha blockers do not possess this action.*

[2] *Not all patients on beta blockers will develop hypertriglyceridemia or reduced HDL-cholesterol. Patients should be monitored and, if required, beta blockers with intrinsic sympathomimetic activity (eg, pindolol) can be considered for substitution.*

[3] *Progestin-only formulations or progestin-estradiol combinations containing desogestrel or low-dose norethindrone have little effect on plasma triglyceride or serum cholesterol concentrations (Godsland et al, 1990).*

PRIMARY AND SECONDARY LIPOPROTEIN DISORDERS

The major lipoprotein disorders (dyslipidemias) are classified on the basis of the lipid abnormality present, the family history and pedigree, and the clinical manifestations. These disorders are broadly regarded as primary or secondary. Primary dyslipidemias are genetically determined (Table 3); secondary dyslipidemias are associated with certain diseases, diets, and drug therapy (Table 4) (Henkin et al, 1992). Dyslipidemia may result from malfunction in any of the metabolic steps involved in the synthesis, transport, interconversion, or catabolism of lipoproteins.

Abnormalities in lipoprotein metabolism are classified clinically on the basis of plasma triglyceride concentrations and serum concentrations of chylomicrons, VLDL-cholesterol, remnant particles, LDL-cholesterol, and HDL-cholesterol. High concentrations of total or LDL-cholesterol (hypercholesterolemia) or triglycerides (hypertriglyceridemia) are considered to be clinically significant and are termed hyperlipidemias. Hypercholesterolemia often is accompanied by elevated serum Lp(a) concentrations. Fasting chylomicronemia (which is rare) or a low serum concentration of HDL-cholesterol (which is common) also are considered to be of clinical significance. Hypercholesterolemia and hypertriglyceridemia occur both independently and together. Hypoalphalipoproteinemia ("low HDL-cholesterolemia") frequently occurs in association with hypertriglyceridemia.

HYPERCHOLESTEROLEMIA. Definitions of desirable (<200 mg/dL), borderline (200 to 239 mg/dL), and high (≥240 mg/dL) serum total cholesterol concentrations refer to concentration ranges associated with baseline, increasing, and more than doubled risks of death from cardiovascular disease and do not differ for men and women (Expert Panel, 1993). The "high" classification corresponds approximately to the 75th percentile for the US adult population and the borderline classification to about the 45th percentile. Because LDL-cholesterol may be the principal atherogenic component of circulating lipids, ranges of serum LDL-cholesterol concentrations also are classified as desirable <130 mg/dL), borderline high risk (130 to 159 mg/dL), and high risk (≥160 mg/dL). These classifications have been endorsed by the American

Diabetes Association for individuals with either insulin-dependent diabetes mellitus (IDDM) or noninsulin-dependent diabetes mellitus (NIDDM) (American Diabetes Association, 1993).

Hypercholesterolemia is redefined in the presence of multiple risk factors or when secondary prevention of CHD is the goal (Expert Panel, 1993). Patients with existing CHD or other atherosclerotic diseases are at substantially increased risk for adverse clinical events when serum LDL-cholesterol concentrations exceed 130 mg/dL; in these patients, serum LDL-cholesterol concentrations <100 mg/dL are now considered desirable (Expert Panel, 1993).

Familial hypercholesterolemia is an autosomal dominant disorder characterized by elevated serum LDL-cholesterol and apoprotein B-100 concentrations but relatively normal plasma triglyceride and serum VLDL concentrations. This disorder is caused by decreased numbers of high-affinity hepatic LDL receptors or by defective receptors with either reduced affinity for LDL or aberrant structures that permit binding but prevent internalization of LDL (Harada-Shiba et al, 1992). Heterozygotes have approximately one-half the number of normal receptors, and homozygotes have no or few functional LDL receptors. Reduction in LDL clearance causes LDL particles to accumulate in the circulation and increases their rate of deposition in the artery wall.

The degree of hypercholesterolemia is inversely proportional to the extent of the receptor defect or deficiency. Tendinous xanthomas, especially in the Achilles tendon, occur in both homozygotes and heterozygotes; planar lesions often are evident in homozygotes. In untreated homozygous patients, CHD is almost inevitable before age 20; in male heterozygotes, the probability of CHD is at least 50% by age 50. Therefore, early detection is important. Approximately 90% of individuals with serum total cholesterol concentrations >360 mg/dL and plasma triglyceride concentrations <250 mg/dL have familial hypercholesterolemia (Williams et al, 1992). Because about one-half of first-degree family members of a patient with familial hypercholesterolemia also will be affected, blood relatives should be screened.

Polygenic hypercholesterolemia occurs in patients with elevated serum LDL-cholesterol concentrations for whom it is not possible to establish a monogenic cause. Such patients usually have milder hypercholesterolemia and fewer clinical signs than those with familial hypercholesterolemia.

HYPERTRIGLYCERIDEMIA. Fasting plasma triglyceride concentrations are now classified as follows: normal (<200 mg/dL), borderline-high (200 to 400 mg/dL), high (400 to 1000 mg/dL), and very high (>1000 mg/dL) (Expert Panel, 1993).

Hypertriglyceridemia >1000 mg/dL is often independently associated with recurrent acute pancreatitis and CHD. Individuals at very high risk should be evaluated to determine if high serum LDL-cholesterol concentration, serum HDL-cholesterol concentration <45 mg/dL, or a positive family history of premature CHD is present. Patients at increased risk for the development of CHD should be further evaluated to determine whether hypertriglyceridemia is familial or secondary. An aggressive management program may be indicated (Expert Panel, 1993; NIH Consensus Development Panel on Triglyceride, High-Density Lipoprotein, and Coronary Heart Disease, 1993). Individuals with plasma triglyceride concentrations <1000 mg/dL but with desirable serum LDL-cholesterol concentrations and HDL-cholesterol concentrations >45 mg/dL and no family history of premature CHD generally are not considered to be at increased risk of developing CHD; only modification of diet or elimination or treatment of secondary causes may be required to reduce fasting plasma triglyceride concentrations to the desirable range.

Familial hypertriglyceridemia is characterized by hypertriglyceridemia and hypoalphalipoproteinemia. About one-half of those at genetic risk exhibit elevated plasma triglyceride concentrations by age 25. The risk of premature CHD is much lower than in those with familial or polygenic hypercholesterolemia or familial combined hyperlipidemia; there usually are no prior external signs. Many patients have carbohydrate intolerance with an excessive insulin response to a glucose or sucrose load, and more than 40% have hyperuricemia. Secondary causes (Table 4) can lead to more pronounced hypertriglyceridemia with fasting hyperchylomicronemia.

FAMILIAL COMBINED HYPERLIPIDEMIA. This common lipid disorder is characterized by overproduction of apo B-100-containing lipoproteins and moderate elevations of serum LDL-cholesterol and plasma triglyceride concentrations. A family history of hyperlipidemia (either similar or different type) is common. Premature CHD, recurrent pancreatitis, corneal arcus, and xanthelasma may be present, but xanthomas usually do not occur. Some patients also may have LPL deficiency and delayed catabolism of triglycerides.

FASTING HYPERCHYLOMICRONEMIA. This form of hypertriglyceridemia is characterized by massive fasting chylomicronemia present even with normal dietary fat intake (Chait and Brunzell, 1991). It can be caused by deficiency of either LPL or the required chylomicron surface cofactor for LPL, apo C-II (Fojo and Brewer, 1992). Insulin deficiency is a relatively common cause of LPL deficiency and secondary hyperchylomicronemia (Schwartz et al, 1992). In either case, chylomicrons are not cleared from the circulation and plasma triglyceride concentration can be markedly elevated (>2000 mg/dL); serum total and VLDL-cholesterol concentrations are increased but serum LDL-cholesterol concentrations are low.

Patients with this disorder can become symptomatic before age 10 (occasionally within the first year of life); lipemia retinalis, colic, recurrent abdominal pain, eruptive xanthomas, and hepatosplenomegaly often develop in early childhood. Adults also may experience pain (pancreatitis) that mimics acute abdominal crises and often is accompanied by fever, leukocytosis, anorexia, and vomiting. Acute hemorrhagic pancreatitis is the most severe, and often fatal, complication of this disorder. However, premature CHD is not associated with this form of lipidemia. An aggressive dietary management program (including a low fat diet with ω-3 fatty acid supplementation) is required to control the disorder; drug therapy is less helpful, but gemfibrozil or niacin may be indicated in selected patients.

FAMILIAL DYSBETALIPOPROTEINEMIA. Homozygous inheritance of substitution of abnormal apo E_2 for normal apo E_3 or

E_4 or genetic apo E deficiency produces a partial block in the clearance of chylomicron and VLDL remnants (β-VLDL) (Mahley et al, 1991). The hepatic uptake of VLDL and chylomicron remnants is impaired because LDL and chylomicron remnant receptors do not recognize the E_2 isoform of apo E, and remnants accumulate in blood and tissues. Circulating lipoprotein concentrations usually are not elevated. However, in the presence of a second defect, such as apo B receptor deficiency or VLDL overproduction, serum total cholesterol and plasma triglyceride concentrations are markedly elevated and VLDL migrates as β-VLDL on electrophoresis. Definitive diagnosis requires a complete lipid evaluation.

Symptoms may appear by early adulthood, especially in males. Palmar/planar xanthomas and tuberoeruptive lesions on the elbows, knees, or buttocks are characteristic. Accelerated and premature coronary and peripheral vascular disease frequently occur, even in the absence of markedly elevated cholesterol or triglyceride concentrations (Sentí et al, 1992). Glucose intolerance and hyperuricemia are observed in about 40% of patients and may reflect the common association of abdominal obesity with hypertriglyceridemia.

FAMILIAL MIXED HYPERTRIGLYCERIDEMIA. This disorder is characterized by accumulation of VLDL and fasting chylomicrons in the circulation, probably caused by a combination of increased VLDL synthesis and varying degrees of defective VLDL catabolism. This disorder can be markedly exaggerated by secondary causes of hypertriglyceridemia. Serum total cholesterol concentrations may be elevated if hypertriglyceridemia is severe. The disorder may be genetically heterogeneous. Patients with the familial disorder usually do not develop hyperlipidemia until after age 20. This disorder is exacerbated by obesity and often is accompanied by glucose intolerance and hyperuricemia, particularly in patients with abdominal obesity. An association between familial mixed hypertriglyceridemia and premature CHD has not been established unequivocally, but plasma triglyceride concentrations should be reduced to decrease the likelihood of eruptive xanthomas, pancreatitis, and abdominal pain.

HYPOALPHALIPOPROTEINEMIA. The only clinically significant lipid disorder in this class is a low serum concentration of HDL-cholesterol (<35 mg/dL), which has been established definitively as an independent risk factor for CHD. Most commonly (but not consistently), low serum HDL-cholesterol concentration occurs in association with hypertriglyceridemia, with virtually all HDL present as HDL_3; the CETP-regulated exchanges of cholesteryl esters and triglycerides between HDL and other lipoprotein particles may account for this reciprocal relationship. Treatment of the hypertriglyceridemia will often improve low serum HDL-cholesterol concentration.

A number of distinct genetic disorders (eg, LCAT deficiency [fish eye disease], LCAT absence, accelerated apo A-I clearance [Tangier disease], reduced apo A-I production, defective apo A-I) have been described in patients with very low numbers of circulating HDL particles. Most but not all are associated with premature CHD. Hypoalphalipoproteinemia also has been correlated with obesity, lack of exercise, cigarette smoking, and drug therapy (see Table 4).

No specific diet or drug therapy is yet available for reliably increasing isolated low serum HDL-cholesterol concentration. Elimination of secondary causes of hypoalphalipoproteinemia is most beneficial. Aerobic training may help. No drug therapy should be prescribed unless hypoalphalipoproteinemia is accompanied by other lipoprotein abnormalities (against which therapy should be primarily targeted) or CHD; in the latter case, low-dose niacin may be effective (Kreisberg, 1993).

HYPERALPHALIPOPROTEINEMIA. Individuals with serum HDL-cholesterol concentrations >150 mg/dL may have familial hyperalphalipoproteinemia, a generally benign disorder of uncertain genetic etiology (serum HDL-cholesterol concentrations >150 mg/dL have been associated with CETP deficiency in a few patients). However, the prevalence of these genetic defects in adults is $<10^{-8}$. Individuals with serum HDL-cholesterol concentrations between 100 and 150 mg/dL have nongenetic hyperalphalipoproteinemia secondary to treatment with ranitidine, estrogen replacement therapy, biliary cirrhosis, marathon running, or alcoholism (Weitzman and Vladutiu, 1992).

FAMILIAL DEFECTIVE APOLIPOPROTEIN B-100. A single amino acid substitution in apo B-100 reduces the ability of the associated LDL particle to bind to the hepatic LDL receptor, resulting in delay of LDL clearance and accumulation of excess cholesteryl ester within LDL (Defesche et al, 1993). Abnormally large LDL of subnormal density accumulate in serum, and the serum LDL-cholesterol concentration often exceeds 250 mg/dL. The resulting dyslipidemia and its consequences are clinically indistinguishable from severe familial hypercholesterolemia. Therapeutic intervention is similar.

HYPOBETALIPOPROTEINEMIA. Familial hypobetalipoproteinemia is an autosomal dominant disorder resulting in synthesis of abnormal apo B-100 and serum total cholesterol concentration <100 mg/dL and serum LDL-cholesterol concentration <80 mg/dL. There usually are no clinical sequelae; the incidence of CHD is reduced and longevity is prolonged.

ABETALIPOPROTEINEMIA. A number of genetic defects in apo B synthesis or release can severely diminish ability to secrete chylomicrons and VLDL (Farese et al, 1992; Rader and Brewer, 1993). In the complete absence of apo B (abetalipoproteinemia), absorption of dietary fat is severely impaired, and neuroretinal degeneration resulting from essential fatty acid and fat-soluble vitamin deficiencies occurs. Selective deficiency of functional apo B-48 restricts the ability to secrete chylomicrons (chylomicron retention disease); similarly, isolated apo B-100 deficiency (normotriglyceridemic abetalipoproteinemia) prevents VLDL secretion. Increased fecal sterol losses from intestinal malabsorption and failure to produce LDL for hepatic binding and uptake result in two- to sixfold stimulation of HMG-CoA reductase and hepatic cholesterogenesis.

DYSLIPIDEMIA ASSOCIATED WITH DIABETES MELLITUS. Both insulin-dependent and non-insulin dependent diabetes mellitus (IDDM and NIDDM, respectively) are associated with increased risks of myocardial infarction, angina, and sudden death. In patients with either hypoinsulinemia or peripheral insulin resistance, LPL and HL are inhibited and hepatic triglyceride synthesis and lipolysis are slowed. Hyperinsulinemia stimulates CETP activity; transfer of cholesteryl esters from HDL to VLDL and LDL is abnormally accelerated and the serum concentration of small, dense, cholesterol-enriched LDL increases. Consequently, hypertriglyceridemia, hypercholesterolemia, hypoalphalipoproteinemia, atherosclerosis, and CAD are common among patients with poorly controlled diabetes, but diabetics with good glycemic control may have elevated serum HDL-cholesterol concentrations (Modan et al, 1991; Bierman, 1992; Laws and Reaven, 1992; Russell, 1992). In addition, plasma Lp(a) concentration is greater in uncontrolled IDDM and NIDDM than in nondiabetic patients, but it is not increased in patients with good glycemic control (Haffner et al, 1992; Ramirez et al, 1992).

Biochemical and functional changes induced by diabetes that contribute to atherogenesis include basement membrane thickening, diminished vasodilator response to stimulation, increased fibronectin and decreased elastin content of arterial media, and glycosylation of laminin and collagen (Schwartz et al, 1992). Macrophage phagocytosis of extracellular lipid is impaired and lesion regression is retarded. Nonenzymatic glycosylation of proteins may link hyperglycemia and the cardiovascular complications of diabetes mellitus. Glycosylation of apo B on LDL enhances LDL oxidative modification and accumulation in macrophages via the scavenger receptor pathway and slows LDL clearance by decreasing LDL recognition by the hepatic apo B/E receptor. Lipoprotein binding to collagen within arterial intima is prolonged after collagen glycosylation, and the susceptibility of bound lipoprotein to oxidation is increased. In addition, endothelial resistance to thrombus formation may be reduced by increases in plasma von Willebrand factor, t-PA antigen, fibrinogen, and plasminogen activator-inhibitor concentrations; increased endothelial cell procoagulant activity; increased platelet activation, adhesiveness, and aggregability; and decreased fibrinolytic activity, platelet survival, and plasmin degradation of glycosylated fibrin (Schwartz et al, 1992).

In obese patients with NIDDM, weight reduction attenuates hypertriglyceridemia and increases serum HDL-cholesterol concentration. In nonobese patients with NIDDM, isocaloric replacement of monounsaturated dietary fat for carbohydrate improves hypertriglyceridemia and slightly increases serum HDL-cholesterol concentration (Garg et al, 1992). Control with insulin or oral hypoglycemic agents improves the lipoprotein profile (Elkeles, 1991; Merrin and Elkeles, 1991). When necessary, pharmacologic intervention should focus on alleviating hypertriglyceridemia, reducing serum LDL-cholesterol concentration, and, if possible, increasing serum HDL-cholesterol concentration.

HYPOCHOLESTEROLEMIA. Serum total cholesterol concentrations <160 mg/dL may result from chronic illness or other conditions stimulating cytokine activation, untreated or iatrogenic hyperthyroidism, progressive AIDS, or familial hypobetalipoproteinemia or from increased frequency of expression of the apo E_2 phenotype (Snyder et al, 1993).

Compared with those who have serum total cholesterol concentrations between 160 and 199 mg/dL, middle-aged men and women with concentrations below 160 mg/dL (about 6% of the total population) have a 20% to 30% increase in the age-adjusted rate of cancer deaths (especially cancers of the lung and liver) and a 40% increase in noncardiovascular, noncancer deaths: increases of 35% in deaths from trauma (especially suicide and violent accidents), 15% in deaths from respiratory disease (especially chronic obstructive pulmonary disease, possibly from production of cholesterol-deficient surfactant), 50% in deaths from digestive system diseases (especially hepatic cirrhosis), and 70% in deaths from other causes (Hulley et al, 1992; Jacobs et al, 1992; Kritchevsky and Kritchevsky, 1992). Furthermore, rates of death from lung cancer, noncancer respiratory disease, and digestive disease decrease continuously in men and women as serum total cholesterol concentration increases, and rates of death from nonatherosclerotic cardiovascular disease increase in women as serum total cholesterol concentration decreases (Jacobs et al, 1992). In addition, the risk of intracranial hemorrhage is doubled (Neaton et al, 1992), possibly following degenerative change in intracerebral arterioles through increased fragility of media muscle cells resulting from reduced cell membrane cholesterol content. Serum total cholesterol concentrations <160 mg/dL in elderly men and women also are associated with a doubling of the prevalence of diabetes and of lower plasma concentrations of hemoglobin, albumin, and factor VII, suggesting that hypocholesterolemia may be a consequence of impaired hepatic synthetic functions (Manolio et al, 1993). Moreover, the threefold increase in the incidence of clinical depression reported among elderly men with serum total cholesterol concentrations <160 mg/dL (Morgan et al, 1993) may cause undernutrition or alcohol dependence that in turn result in hypocholesterolemia (Glueck et al, 1993).

Meta-analysis of primary prevention trials confirmed that rates of deaths from cancer and trauma were significantly higher among men who received pharmacologic agents to decrease their serum cholesterol concentration (Muldoon et al, 1990; Jacobs et al, 1992). The magnitude of the increase in noncardiovascular deaths is similar to the magnitude of the decrease in CHD mortality, and total mortality is not reduced. In contrast, meta-analysis of secondary prevention trials has found decreases in both cardiovascular and noncardiovascular deaths (Jacobs et al, 1992). It is not known whether the apparent increase in noncardiovascular deaths in primary prevention reflects epidemiologic confounding, effects of low serum cholesterol concentration per se, effects of rapid rates of change in serum cholesterol concentration during active therapy, or effects of unsuspected factors. However, a low-fat ("cholesterol-lowering") diet has been reported to reduce depression and hostility (Weidner et al, 1992). These uncertainties notwithstanding, reduction of serum total cholesterol concentration to <140 mg/dL may be accompanied by unidentified harmful effects (Jacobs and Blackburn, 1993).

GUIDELINES FOR IDENTIFYING AND EVALUATING LIPIDEMIC ABNORMALITIES

ADULTS. Recommendations of the National Cholesterol Education Program of the National Heart, Blood, and Lung Institute of the National Institutes of Health for the detection of covert dyslipidemias in adults have recently been revised (Table 5; Expert Panel, 1993). The system for classifying individuals by serum total cholesterol concentration is unchanged from previous recommendations, and dietary and life-style modification remain the cornerstones of efforts to reduce serum total cholesterol concentrations. However, a greater appreciation for the limitations and hazards of lifetime pharmacologic treatment for more than 20% of the adult population has refocused attention on individuals at high risk for the development of atherosclerotic cardiovascular disease, CHD, and myocardial infarction.

It is now recommended that universal screening to identify individuals with hypercholesterolemia begin at age 20 years or older and be repeated at least once every five years. Screening should include measurement of serum total and HDL-cholesterol concentrations. Further clinical evaluation and more detailed lipoprotein analysis are recommended if serum total cholesterol concentration is >240 mg/dL or serum HDL-cholesterol concentration is <35 mg/dL. In addition, a serum total cholesterol concentration >200 mg/dL in the presence of two or more other risk factors for CHD is now considered sufficient to warrant further analysis. Risk factors to be considered with the results of laboratory analyses now include hypertension, cigarette smoking, diabetes mellitus, chronic renal failure, the nephrotic syndrome, age 45 years or older in men and 55 years or older in women, premature menopause, and a family history of myocardial infarction or sudden CHD death before 55 years in first-degree male relatives or before 65 years in first-degree female relatives. Although they probably do not directly potentiate CHD risk, obesity and sedentary life habits should be considered indicators of the likely presence of one or more risk factors. In a new emphasis on positive preventive measures, it is now recommended that a serum HDL-cholesterol concentration ≥60 mg/dL be treated as a "negative risk factor" able to negate one CHD risk factor.

Further clinical evaluation, when indicated, should include a complete history and physical examination and should attempt to identify any possible causes of secondary hypercholesterolemia. Lipoprotein analysis should include measurement of fasting plasma triglyceride concentration, which will allow calculation of serum LDL-cholesterol concentration.

Clinical classification is then based on serum LDL-cholesterol concentration and the presence of other risk factors. Individuals without evidence of CHD and with serum LDL-cholesterol concentration <130 mg/dL ("desirable") are at low risk for CHD and can be re-evaluated in five years. Those with serum LDL-cholesterol concentrations between 130 and 159 mg/dL ("borderline-high-risk") and fewer than two other CHD risk factors should be given instruction in dietary therapy and the benefits of physical activity and then re-evaluated in one year. Patients with borderline high-risk serum LDL-cholesterol concentrations and two or more other CHD risk factors and those with serum LDL-cholesterol concentrations ≥160 mg/dL ("high-risk") should be enrolled in a program of dietary and life habits therapy. A combination of dietary, life habits, and pharmacologic therapies can be considered if serum LDL-cholesterol concentration is >220 mg/dL.

A nonfasting blood sample is adequate for determination of serum total and HDL-cholesterol concentration. However, 12-hour fasting samples are required for accurate measurement of triglyceride concentrations and calculation of LDL-cholesterol concentrations. It has been suggested that determination of plasma apo A-I or apo B concentrations may better facilitate identification of patients at increased risk of CHD and may be more reliable than serum cholesterol concentrations measured in blood sampled in the nonfasting state or when fasting status is uncertain (Dennison et al, 1990; Deslypere, 1991; Kwiterovich et al, 1992 A; Levinson and Wagner, 1992; Zunić et al, 1992). However, lack of standardization currently prevents routine clinical use of apo A-I and apo B measurements.

Because measurements of serum cholesterol concentrations are affected by a number of sources of variability, misdiagnosis from a single sample can occur in as many as 40% of patients (Frishman et al, 1992; Weissfeld and Holloway, 1992). A minimum of two samples obtained on different days is required; if the difference in serum total cholesterol concentration between the two measurements is >30 mg/dL, a third sample is necessary and the two measurements differing by <30 mg/dL should be averaged (Expert Panel, 1993). When sampled, patients should be in their usual state of health; major surgery, trauma or burns, prolonged fasting, recent weight change, pregnancy, a change in diet, and serious illness can transiently affect serum cholesterol concentrations. To minimize the effects of posture on measurements, venipuncture should be performed on patients after at least five minutes in a sitting position. Serum is preferable for laboratory analyses of lipoprotein concentrations. The clinical laboratory utilized must participate in a reliable standardization program and should have its lipid assays standardized through one of the National Network Laboratories of the Centers for Disease Control and Prevention.

ELDERLY PATIENTS. The major cause of death in persons over 60 years is atherosclerotic CHD. Although some data suggest that the relative risk of CHD associated with hypercholesterolemia may decrease with advancing years (Jacobsen et al, 1992), the attributable risk (the percentage of cases of CHD attributed to hypercholesterolemia after correcting for the presence of other risk factors) increases with age (Denke and Grundy, 1990; Shipley et al, 1991; Castelli et al, 1992; Manolio et al, 1992).

Aging is associated with increased serum LDL-cholesterol concentrations resulting from a decrease in the number of hepatic LDL receptors and therefore in the fractional catabolism of LDL particles (Ericsson et al, 1991). Concurrently, serum HDL-cholesterol concentration declines in postmenopausal women not receiving estrogen replacement therapy. Low serum HDL-cholesterol concentrations coupled with high LDL-cholesterol concentrations increase CHD risk even in those over 75 years (Zimetbaum et al, 1992; Castelli et al, 1992; Mangion and Roy, 1993). Serum HDL-cholesterol concentration may be the most important single predictor of CHD and carotid atherosclerosis in the elderly (Nikkilä and Heikkinen, 1990; O'Leary et al, 1992).

Because the absolute number of CHD events occurring in persons with serum total cholesterol concentrations in the

TABLE 5.
GUIDELINES FOR IDENTIFYING AND EVALUATING LIPOPROTEIN DISORDERS IN ADULTS[1]

Serum Concentration (mg/dL)	Status	Recommended Follow-up
INITIAL CLASSIFICATION AND RECOMMENDED FOLLOW-UP BASED ON TOTAL SERUM CHOLESTEROL CONCENTRATION		
<200	Desirable	Repeat in five years.
200 to 240	Borderline high risk	For those *without* definite CHD[2] or two other CHD risk factors,[3] supply dietary information and recheck annually.
		For those *with* definite CHD *or* two other CHD risk factors, perform lipoprotein analysis; further management based on serum LDL-cholesterol concentration.
>240	High risk	Perform lipoprotein analysis; further management based on serum LDL-cholesterol concentration.
INITIAL CLASSIFICATION AND RECOMMENDED FOLLOW-UP BASED ON SERUM HDL-CHOLESTEROL CONCENTRATION		
>35	Desirable	Repeat in five years.
<35	Increased risk	Perform lipoprotein analysis; further management based on serum LDL-cholesterol and fasting plasma triglyceride concentrations.
CLASSIFICATION AND TREATMENT DECISIONS BASED ON SERUM LDL-CHOLESTEROL CONCENTRATION		
<130	Desirable	Repeat in five years.
130 to 160	Borderline high risk	For those *without* definite CHD or two other CHD risk factors, supply dietary information, advise to exercise, and recheck annually.
		For those *without* definite CHD but *with* two other CHD risk factors, initiate dietary changes to reduce serum LDL-cholesterol concentration to <130 mg/dL.
		For those *with* definite CHD, initiate dietary changes followed by drug treatment if needed to reduce serum LDL-cholesterol concentration to <100 mg/dL.[4]
161 to 220	High risk	For those *without* definite CHD or two other CHD risk factors, initiate dietary changes to reduce serum LDL-cholesterol concentration to <160 mg/dL.
		For those *without* definite CHD but *with* two other CHD risk factors, initiate dietary changes followed by drug treatment if needed to reduce serum LDL-cholesterol concentration to <130 mg/dL.
		For those *with* definite CHD, initiate dietary changes followed by drug treatment if needed to reduce serum LDL-cholesterol concentration to <100 mg/dL.
>220	High risk	Initiate dietary and lifestyle changes followed by drug treatment if needed to reduce serum LDL-cholesterol concentration to <190 mg/dL.
CLASSIFICATION AND TREATMENT DECISIONS BASED ON FASTING PLASMA TRIGLYCERIDE CONCENTRATION		
<200	Normal	Repeat in five years.
200 to 400	Borderline high risk	For those *without* definite CHD or two other CHD risk factors, supply dietary information, advise to exercise, and recheck annually.
400 to 1,000	High risk	For those *without* definite CHD or two other CHD risk factors, initiate dietary changes, advise to exercise, and recheck annually.
		For those *with* definite CHD or two other CHD risk factors, initiate dietary and lifestyle changes and drug treatment to reduce fasting plasma triglyceride concentration to <400 mg/dL.
>1,000	Very high risk	Initiate dietary and lifestyle changes and drug treatment to reduce fasting plasma triglyceride concentration to <1,000 mg/dL.

[1] *See text for discussion.*

[2] *CHD = coronary heart disease.*

[3] *Risk factors: male sex, diabetes mellitus, hypertension, smoking, family history of premature CHD, definite cerebrovascular or peripheral vascular disease, serum HDL-cholesterol concentration <35 mg/dL, severe obesity, left ventricular hypertrophy, a positive exercise test for cardiovascular disease, postmenopausal status.*

[4] *Drug treatment for hypercholesterolemia may not be advisable in those over age 60 with congestive heart failure, stroke, cancer, chronic obstructive lung disease, dementia, debilitating arthritis, or other reasons for a poor prognosis for an extended lifetime (Denke and Grundy, 1990).*

highest quartile increases with increasing age and because serum total and LDL-cholesterol concentrations are correlated with potentially modifiable factors (obesity, glucose intolerance, sedentary life-style, renal impairment, medication use) in the elderly, reducing serum cholesterol concentrations should benefit the elderly (Kafonek and Kwiterovich, 1990; Aronow, 1992; Ettinger et al, 1992; Kannel and Vokonas, 1992). The presence of either asymptomatic or overt CHD in elderly patients may warrant attempts to reduce serum LDL-cholesterol concentrations to <100 mg/dL and increase serum HDL-cholesterol concentrations to >35 mg/dL (Expert Panel, 1993). However, aggressive hypocholesterolemic regimens are not appropriate in patients of very advanced age who have very low cardiac ejection fraction, chronic congestive heart failure, stroke, metastatic cancer, chronic obstructive lung disease, deterioration of mental function, debilitating arthritis, or other reasons for a poor prognosis for an extended lifetime (Denke and Grundy, 1990; Hazzard, 1992; Expert Panel, 1993).

WOMEN. Atherosclerotic disease is an important cause of morbidity and mortality among women, who tend to develop CHD an average of 10 years later than men (Kuhn and Rackley, 1993). In general, premenopausal women are at very low risk for CHD; even severe genetic forms of hypercholesterolemia usually do not produce CHD before menopause unless other risk factors are present. However, exercise-induced amenorrhea increases serum total and LDL-cholesterol concentrations (Friday et al, 1993).

High concentrations of LDL-cholesterol and triglycerides and low (<35 mg/dL) concentrations of HDL-cholesterol are independent risk factors for CHD in women after age 65 (The Bezafibrate Infarction Prevention [BIP] Study Group, 1992; Kannel and Vokonas, 1992; Stensvold et al, 1993). Aggressive lipid-lowering may slow atherosclerotic progression in women who survive myocardial infarction (Buchwald et al, 1992; Rifici and Khachadurian, 1992).

LDL receptor activity is reduced after menopause (Arca et al, 1994). In contrast, estrogen increases hepatic LDL-receptor expression (Angelin et al, 1992) and biliary excretion of cholesterol (Everson et al, 1991). Estrogen replacement therapy is widely recommended for postmenopausal women and appears to be able to improve postmenopausal lipoprotein metabolism, reduce coronary artery narrowing, and decrease the risk of CHD (Jensen, 1992; Kuhn and Rackley, 1993; Nabulsi et al, 1993; Psaty et al, 1993).

INFANTS. Serum total cholesterol concentration ranges between 50 and 100 mg/dL at birth and is approximately equally distributed among LDL and HDL (Innis and Hamilton, 1992). Serum LDL-cholesterol concentration doubles during the first week of life and is independent of diet. Human breast milk contains much more cholesterol than do most infant formulas, and exclusive breast feeding after the first week of life is associated with significantly higher serum total cholesterol concentrations in infants. This difference does not persist after weaning, which suggests that, when fed to neonates, infant formulas may be cholesterol-deficient compared with human milk (Jooste et al, 1991; Kallio et al, 1992). Substitution of linolenic acid for linoleic acid in infant formulas has decreased serum total and LDL-cholesterol concentrations and increased serum HDL-cholesterol concentrations (Hayes et al, 1992; Van Biervliet et al, 1992).

Serum lipoprotein concentrations in most infants appear to bear very little relationship to adult concentrations (Hamosh, 1988; Kallio et al, 1993), but infants with a strong familial tendency to develop CHD may have thickening of the internal elastic lamina of the coronary arteries (Kaprio et al, 1993). In addition, low growth rates in utero or during infancy are associated with increased adult mortality from CHD (Barker et al, 1993). Fat-restricted diets (<20% of total calories as fats) often are deficient in essential nutrients required for proper growth and development (Sigman-Grant et al, 1993); such diets are inappropriate in infants (Lifshitz, 1992).

CHILDREN. The development of atherosclerosis is a lifelong process that begins in childhood; children aged 8 to 16 years with serum total cholesterol concentrations >300 mg/dL have increased evidence of subendothelial cholesterol deposits and early plaque formation (Celermajer et al, 1992). The extent and severity of aortic and coronary arterial lesions in young men and women without clinical CHD are proportional to serum total, VLDL-, and LDL-cholesterol concentrations (Pathobiological Determinants of Atherosclerosis in Youth Research Group, 1990). In addition, hypercholesterolemic adults and those with documented CHD are likely to have hypercholesterolemic children (Berenson et al, 1991; Benuck et al, 1992). Therefore, the American Academy of Pediatrics (AAP) and the NCEP advocate selective testing of serum cholesterol concentrations of children over 2 years with a family history of premature CHD or a parent with hypercholesterolemia; or who have hypertension, obesity, sedentary life-style, diabetes, or nephrotic syndrome; use tobacco, alcohol, oral contraceptives, or anticonvulsants; or had low birth weight (<2.5 kg) (National Institutes of Health, 1991; Committee on Nutrition, American Academy of Pediatrics, 1992; NCEP Expert Panel on Blood Cholesterol Levels in Children and Adolescents, 1992).

Screening based on selected risk factors may fail to identify many hypercholesterolemic children and adolescents even if applied comprehensively. However, the AAP and NCEP have identified the following as significant drawbacks to universal childhood screening: the spontaneous transient decrease in serum cholesterol concentration that often occurs during adolescence; the potential for the results of universal screening to label many children as "patients with a disease;" the potential for overuse of lipid-lowering medications during childhood and adolescence; and concerns that dietary or drug therapy to reduce serum cholesterol concentration might adversely affect growth and development.

The AAP has endorsed the diagnostic categories established by the NCEP for the interpretation of serum total and LDL-cholesterol concentrations in those under 20 years: acceptable (<170 mg/dL and <110 mg/dL), borderline (170 to 199 mg/dL and 110 to 129 mg/dL), and high (≥200 mg/dL and ≥130 mg/dL) (National Institutes of Health, 1991; NCEP Expert Panel on Blood Cholesterol Levels in Children and Adolescents, 1992). However, given the uncertainty of an unrepeated measurement, the actual range of borderline serum total cholesterol concentrations is 155 to 215 mg/dL, if diagnosis is based on a single measurement (Gillman et al, 1992).

Despite advocacy of a classification system based on childhood serum total or LDL-cholesterol concentrations, treatment recommendations for hypercholesterolemic children are conservative and concentrate on universally beneficial dietary and lifestyle adjustments. These recommendations generally reflect concern over the potential for overmedication of children and uncertainties associated with potential long-term adverse effects of lipid-lowering drugs in children and adolescents. They also acknowledge the limited ability of childhood cholesterol concentration to predict adult hypercholesterolemia (Newman et al, 1990 A; Berenson et al, 1991; Bao et al, 1993; Gidding, 1993; Guo et al, 1993). For example, in two long-term studies (the Beaver County and Bogalusa Heart studies), only 50% of preadolescent children with serum total or LDL-cholesterol concentrations above the 75th percentile remained in this category 12 or 16 years later (Berenson et al, 1991; Stuhldreher et al, 1991; Webber et al, 1991). In another 12-year study, only 57% of girls and 30% of boys 8 to 18 years old with serum total cholesterol concentrations above the 90th percentile for children had serum total cholesterol concentrations below the 75th percentile for adults when 20 to 30 years old (Lauer and Clarke, 1990). In addition, in the Bogalusa Heart Study only 45% of preadolescent and young adolescent children with serum HDL-cholesterol concentrations in the lowest quartile remained in that quartile 12 years later (Berenson et al, 1991). It has been estimated that fewer than half of those with childhood hypercholesterolemia are likely to be hypercholesterolemic as adults, even without explicit intervention (Lauer and Clarke, 1990; Newman et al, 1990 A), and that only 7% to 15% of hypercholesterolemic boys and 5% to 8% of hypercholesterolemic girls will manifest CHD before age 65 (Newman et al, 1990 A; Holtzman, 1991). Nevertheless, a considerable percentage of children with high serum total cholesterol concentrations will have high concentrations as adults; decisions regarding early intervention should rely on clinical expertise and judgment concerning the relative risks and benefits in each case.

Despite the limited diagnostic value of childhood hypercholesterolemia itself, children and adolescents with elevated serum cholesterol concentrations often have the "deadly quartet" (elevated blood pressure, obesity, hypercholesterolemia, and impaired glucose tolerance) (Berenson et al, 1991), and those affected will benefit from aggressive treatment of all four disorders. Overweight children can reduce their serum total and LDL-cholesterol concentrations and increase their serum HDL-cholesterol concentrations by restricting dietary energy and fat intakes and by increasing their physical activity level (Nicklas et al, 1991; Endo et al, 1992). However, children >2 years should maintain dietary fat intakes of no less than 30% and no more than 40% of total daily calories, with saturated fat intake providing no more than 10% (Committee on Nutrition, American Academy of Pediatrics, 1992). Not starting or discontinuing tobacco use also is highly beneficial. The adoption of healthy life-styles by children and adolescents (and their parents) is safe and effective if undertaken prudently.

The impact of drug-induced lipid-lowering in children and adolescents on the development of CHD is unknown. Bile acid sequestering agents are the only lipid-lowering drugs currently recommended for use in selected children with very high serum total or LDL-cholesterol concentrations (National Institutes of Health, 1991; NCEP Expert Panel on Blood Cholesterol Levels in Children and Adolescents, 1992). These agents, in combination with dietary adjustments and increased exercise, have reduced serum total cholesterol concentrations in children with initial serum total cholesterol concentrations >500 mg/dL (Kwiterovich, 1990). However, long-term compliance often is poor.

MONITORING HYPERCHOLESTEROLEMIA. Evaluations should be performed at five-year intervals in adults not at risk and more often in those at risk and during therapeutic intervention. Although the primary goal of therapy is to reduce serum LDL-cholesterol concentration, the serum total cholesterol concentration tends to parallel serum LDL-cholesterol concentration and is more convenient and less expensive to obtain. Therefore, it may be used to monitor response to treatment. For most patients, a serum total cholesterol concentration of 240 mg/dL corresponds to a serum LDL-cholesterol concentration of about 160 mg/dL, and a serum total cholesterol concentration of 200 mg/dL corresponds to a serum LDL-cholesterol concentration of about 130 mg/dL. Once a serum total cholesterol concentration suggests that a therapeutic goal has been attained, the serum LDL-cholesterol concentration should be measured to confirm that the LDL-cholesterol target also has been reached.

In hypertriglyceridemic patients or patients losing weight, it is advisable to continue to measure serum LDL-cholesterol concentration because significant increases in serum HDL-cholesterol concentration may mask decreases in serum LDL-cholesterol concentration if only serum total cholesterol concentration is measured.

Comparisons of cholesterol, triglyceride, lipoprotein, or apoprotein concentrations over time must acknowledge the intra-individual variability caused by day length, diet, life-style, menstrual cyclicity, concurrent drug therapy, postural effects, level of acute mental stress, specimen handling, and, perhaps most important, analytic uncertainty (Tangney et al, 1991; Karpanou et al, 1992; Kritchevsky, 1992; Miller et al, 1992). Estimates of these variabilities define the limits that must be exceeded in order for change to be detected with confidence in an individual when testing the effects of therapy. For serum total cholesterol concentration, a subsequent determination must differ from a previous measurement by at least 13%; for LDL-cholesterol by 20%; for HDL-cholesterol by 15%; for HDL_2-cholesterol by 40%; for triglycerides by 35%; for apo A by 25%; and for apo B by 35% (Bookstein et al, 1990; Irwig et al, 1991; Gallagher et al, 1992; Ortolá et al, 1992; Smith et al, 1993).

MANAGEMENT

DIETARY MANAGEMENT. Responses to therapeutic diets (Table 6) differ among patients, and the variations in response are determined by both environmental and genetic

TABLE 6.
NONDRUG MANAGEMENT OF LIPOPROTEIN DISORDERS

Lipid Disorder	Dietary and Life-style Measures
General Population[1]	All adults should adopt a prudent diet that restricts the intake of saturated plus *trans*-fatty acids to <10% of total calories and polyunsaturated fatty acids to no more than 10% of total calories, while providing 10% to 15% of total calories as monounsaturated fatty acids. Dietary cholesterol intake should be restricted to less than 300 mg daily. Proteins should provide 10% to 20% of total calories and complex carbohydrates 50% to 60%. Total dietary fiber intake of at least 20 g daily should be maintained; 30 g would be preferable. It is important to minimize or eliminate all causes of secondary hypercholesterolemia and hypertriglyceridemia.
Hypercholesterolemia Familial heterozygous Familial homozygous Polygenic	The response to the prudent diet recommended for the general population should be evaluated for six weeks. Only a small percentage of hypercholesterolemic individuals will have large decreases in serum LDL-cholesterol concentration while adhering to this diet. If serum LDL-cholesterol concentration target is not achieved, more stringent restriction of saturated plus *trans*-fatty acids (to no more than 7% of total daily caloric intake) and cholesterol (no more than 200 mg daily) should be initiated and its impact on serum LDL-cholesterol concentration evaluated after four to six weeks. Compliance with this more restrictive diet typically is poor, and drug therapy usually is indicated for patients with familial hypercholesterolemia.
Hypertriglyceridemia Familial hypertriglyceridemia Familial combined hyperlipidemia Familial dysbetalipoproteinemia	When hypertriglyceridemia is present, the patient must (1) minimize or eliminate alcohol intake; (2) reduce fat intake to below 30% of total daily calories and substitute polyunsaturated and monounsaturated fatty acids and dietary fiber for saturated fatty acids as often as possible; (3) reduce intake of simple sugars; (4) achieve and maintain ideal body weight; and (5) increase exercise. Plasma triglyceride concentrations above 500 mg/dL may require drug therapy in addition to dietary management.
Fasting Hyperchylomicronemia	Restrict dietary fat intake to no more than 25 g, and replace a portion with medium-chain triglycerides whose absorption bypasses the chylomicron pathway. Protein intake should exceed 20% of total calories, permitting a lower intake of carbohydrates. Alcohol must be avoided. Restriction of dietary cholesterol intake and weight reduction when indicated also are important for overall risk reduction.
Familial Mixed Hypertriglyceridemia	Restrict dietary fat intake to no more than 25 g, and replace a portion with medium-chain triglycerides whose absorption bypasses the chylomicron pathway. Protein intake should exceed 20% of total calories. Alcohol must be avoided. Restriction of dietary cholesterol intake and weight reduction also are important for overall risk reduction. Plasma triglyceride concentrations above 500 mg/dL may require drug therapy in addition to dietary management.
Hypoalphalipoproteinemia	Adherence to the prudent diet recommended for the general population and, when indicated, achieving and maintaining ideal body weight, adhering to a regular program of moderate exercise, and normalization of triglyceridemia will increase serum HDL-cholesterol concentration. Smoking should be eliminated. The use of anabolic steroids, progestational agents, and beta blockers without intrinsic sympathomimetic activity depresses serum HDL-cholesterol concentration and should be avoided if possible.

[1] *The fat and cholesterol contents of the diets of children <2 years old should not be restricted.*

variables. Strong patient motivation and physician support are prerequisites if prolonged dietary modification is to succeed, and it is usually necessary to be specific about foods to be avoided. An appropriate dietary pattern must be established that can be maintained throughout life rather than as a temporary treatment. Understanding of and adherence to a diet may require several months of adjustment with frequent follow-up, instruction, and encouragement by the physician. The use of team-based Continuous Quality Improvement techniques may be effective (Headrick et al, 1992). General guidance in the development of lipid-lowering diets is available to the physician (Greene and Feldman, 1991; Ulbricht and Southgate, 1991; Expert Panel, 1993).

Serum LDL-cholesterol concentration should be measured after 4 and 12 weeks of dietary, weight reduction, and exercise therapy. If the target goal for serum LDL-cholesterol concentration has been achieved, reinforcement of lifetime adherence to these life-style changes should be given. If the target has not been achieved, additional dietary restrictions may be initiated in compliant patients. Even if the goal is not achieved in 12 weeks, healthier life habits should be encouraged while consideration is given to pharmacologic therapy.

In a minority of patients, life-style modification will not adequately decrease high serum LDL-cholesterol concentrations. These patients will not achieve cholesterol-lowering goals despite a high degree of compliance and may be candidates for drug therapy. Unfortunately, it is not possible to determine the inherent responsiveness of an individual other than after a trial of dietary, exercise, and life-style modification.

Cholesterol: Epidemiologic data have been used to support the suggestion that each 100 mg decrease in daily dietary cholesterol intake reduces serum total cholesterol concentration an average of 2 to 10 mg/dL, thereby reducing CHD risk by an average of 9% to 15% (Hegsted and Ausman, 1988; Stamler and Shekelle, 1988; Grundy, 1991 B; Sonnenberg et al, 1992). However, results from prospective studies indicate that serum total cholesterol concentration decreases the least in response to decreased cholesterol intake when the initial intake is large because a change in dietary cholesterol intake can exert only a relatively small influence on hepatic cholesterol concentration and LDL receptor activity in the presence of excess dietary cholesterol (Hopkins, 1992). In addition, it has been speculated that only about 25% to 35% of hypercholesterolemic individuals may be sensitive to dietary cholesterol intake ("high responders") (McNamara, 1990; Gotto, 1991 B). Serum total cholesterol concentrations tend to change much less in response to changes in dietary cholesterol intake among "average" responders, and successful dietary therapy often requires dramatic reductions in daily cholesterol intake. Among responders, responses to decreased cholesterol intakes are usually proportional to initial serum LDL-cholesterol concentrations.

Individual differences in cholesterol absorption efficiency also may affect responsiveness to dietary cholesterol intake, although perhaps less than the effects of level of intake (Enig, 1993). In contrast, inherent differences in the sensitivity of HMG-CoA reductase to regulation by intracellular cholesterol concentration may influence the response to dietary cholesterol (Jones et al, 1993). Hyporesponsive individuals also may excrete excessive amounts of cholesterol in bile, in effect diverting cholesterol of dietary origin away from inclusion in new VLDL (Gotto, 1991 B). Responsiveness to dietary cholesterol also may be influenced by the apo E genotype (Mäntärri et al, 1991) and body adiposity (Goff et al, 1993).

Some clinicians dismiss dietary cholesterol as an important cause of elevated serum cholesterol concentrations (Krummel et al, 1992; Enig, 1993). Others assert that despite limited quantitative effects on circulating cholesterol, dietary cholesterol is an independent risk factor for CHD (Shekelle and Stamler, 1989), although the findings of the Framingham Heart Study do not support this conclusion (Posner et al, 1991). Responsiveness to dietary cholesterol has not been considered in recommendations concerning dietary cholesterol intake. Because the small percentage of patients who will respond dramatically to dietary therapy cannot be identified except by observing their response to dietary change and, except in rare disease conditions, adults do not require dietary cholesterol for health, dietary therapy that includes reduction in cholesterol and saturated fat intakes is always the first hypocholesterolemic option for reducing serum cholesterol concentrations in adults (see Table 6).

Saturated Fatty Acids: The short chain saturated fatty acids (SFA), caproic, caprylic, and capric acids, do not affect serum cholesterol concentrations. The long-chain SFA, stearic acid, a major component of animal fats, also appears to have little effect on serum cholesterol concentration, possibly because of rapid conversion in vivo to oleic acid (Denke and Grundy, 1991). In contrast, lauric, myristic, and palmitic acids, SFA found primarily in animal fats and coconut, palm, and palm kernel oils, are markedly hypercholesterolemic (Dupont et al, 1991; Cobb et al, 1992; Denke and Grundy, 1992).

Reduction of dietary fat intake to 30% of total caloric intake does not decrease serum total or LDL-cholesterol concentrations unless the reduction includes decreased intake of SFA (Barr et al, 1992). In addition, high and low responders to dietary SFA intake appear to exist and responsiveness increases with advancing age (Cobb and Risch, 1993). Among responders, each reduction in SFA intake equal to 1% of total calories is associated with a 2- to 3-mg/dL decrease in serum total cholesterol concentration and a 3% to 5% decrease in CHD risk (Graves et al, 1990; Burke et al, 1991; Grundy, 1991 B), with the greatest effects observed in those with the highest baseline serum total cholesterol concentrations (Denke and Frantz, 1993). Clearly, it is important to limit SFA intake to no more than 10% of total daily calories in any regimen attempting to reduce serum cholesterol concentrations.

ω-6 Polyunsaturated Fatty Acids: The predominant ω-6 polyunsaturated fatty acid (PUFA) is α-linoleic acid. It is synthesized in plants but not animals, and is usually ingested as corn, safflower, soybean, and sunflower oils or as walnuts. Replacement of dietary SFA with PUFA increases LDL receptor activity and decreases serum LDL-cholesterol concentration (Mensink and Katan, 1992). In addition, high α-linoleic acid intake may reduce blood pressure and protect against arrhythmias and CHD (Grundy, 1991 B). However, studies in humans have demonstrated that consumption of >10% of total calories as α-linoleic acid decreases serum HDL-cholesterol concentration; this effect is greatest in women (Cobb et al, 1992) and may predispose to the formation of cholesterol gallstones. Because α-linoleic acid is highly susceptible to peroxidation, large amounts in the diet (>20% of total calories) may increase endothelial exposure to oxidatively modified LDL (Parthasarathy et al, 1990; Berry et al, 1991). In addition, there may be positive correlations between α-linoleic acid intake and the incidence of breast, colon, and prostate cancers, although direct evidence for these relationships is lacking (Dolecek, 1992). Therefore, dietary PUFA should not exceed 10% of total daily caloric intake.

Cis-*Monounsaturated Fatty Acids:* Oleic acid is the major monounsaturated fatty acid (MUFA) synthesized by both plants and animals. Olive oil, canola oil, certain forms of sunflower and safflower oils, peanuts, almonds, hazelnuts, and walnuts are rich sources. Substitution of MUFA-containing foods for foods high in SFA decreases serum LDL-cholesterol concentration, while maintaining serum HDL-cholesterol concentration and reducing the risk of myocardial infarction as effectively as substitution with foods high in PUFA (Dreon et al, 1990; Grundy and Denke, 1990; Trevisan et al, 1990; Wardlaw and Snook, 1990; Berry et al, 1991, 1992; Fraser et al, 1992 A). The beneficial effects of MUFA are similar to those of PUFA (Mensink and Katan, 1989; Mata et al, 1992).

Some evidence suggests that oleic acid as olive oil is not prone to oxidation and therefore could be mildly antiatherogenic (Grundy, 1991 B). However, data from the Cholesterol Lowering Atherosclerosis Study suggest that increasing MUFA intake to >7% of total calories may increase the risk of development of new atherosclerotic lesions in the coronary arteries (Blankenhorn et al, 1990). Nevertheless, oleic acid has been consumed in large quantities as olive oil for centuries with no evidence that it is harmful. In contrast to findings for SFA and PUFA, there is no evidence that MUFA increase cancer risk (Prentice and Sheppard, 1990). Patients unable to comply with therapeutic dietary recommendations (usually because of palatability problems) may be able to substitute oleic acid-containing foods for foods high in SFA.

Trans-*Monounsaturated Fatty Acids:* The most common *trans*-monounsaturated fatty acid (*trans*-MUFA) is elaidic acid, the *trans*-isomer of oleic acid. The *trans* double bond, in contrast to the *cis* bond, promotes rigidity and packing of fatty acid molecules and raises their melting points; fats rich in *trans*-MUFA usually are solids at room temperature. During the partial hydrogenation of polyunsaturated vegetable oils to produce margarines and shortenings, some *trans*-PUFA are generated.

Trans fatty acids typically provide about 3% to 10% of daily caloric intake in the United States (Enig et al, 1990; Dupont et al, 1991). Oils high in *trans*-MUFA raise serum LDL-cholesterol and plasma triglyceride and Lp (a) concentrations and also decrease serum HDL-cholesterol concentration (Mensink et al, 1992; Nestle et al, 1992; Troisi et al, 1992; Siguel and Lerman, 1993) and may increase the risk for CHD (Willett et al, 1993). Lipids containing *trans*-PUFA facilitate platelet aggregation in response to thrombin. It may be prudent to consider SFA, *trans*-MUFA, and *trans*-PUFA together and limit the sum of their intakes to 10% of total daily calories (Grundy, 1991 B).

Carbohydrates: The influence of dietary carbohydrates (monosaccharides, disaccharides, and polysaccharides or starches) on lipid metabolism is not fully understood. Long-term consumption of diets high in simple sugars and low in fat is associated with slightly higher plasma triglyceride and lower serum LDL- and HDL-cholesterol concentrations compared with lower carbohydrate, higher fat intakes (West et al, 1990). Experimental replacement of SFA with sugars or simply adding fructose to the existing diet has similar effects (Mensink and Katan, 1992; Hollenbeck, 1993). In the Framingham Heart Study, increasing daily carbohydrate intake by 100 g (presumably at least in part at the cost of fat intake) appeared to reduce serum total cholesterol concentration by 22 mg/dL (Sonnenberg et al, 1992). Acutely increasing dietary carbohydrate intake increases VLDL production and may accelerate apo A-I clearance from plasma (Abbott et al, 1990; Brinton et al, 1991). The significance of these metabolic responses to dietary carbohydrate is not yet established.

Soluble Dietary Fiber: Soluble fibers (eg, pectins in citrus fruits, mucilages [water-soluble hemicelluloses] in psyllium seeds, gums in oat products and beans) have a modest effect in lowering serum cholesterol concentrations. Insoluble dietary fibers (eg, cellulose and lignin in wheat bran; most hemicelluloses) do not affect serum cholesterol concentrations (see review by Kritchevsky, 1991). The degrees to which soluble fibers reduce serum cholesterol concentrations are proportional to their pectin or β-glucan contents (Davidson et al, 1991). In general, dietary fiber is recommended as a part of a prudent dietary lifestyle rather than as a dietary factor possessing pharmacologic properties.

The hypocholesterolemic action of soluble fibers is ascribed to one or more mechanisms that include binding of bile acids, cholesterol, and/or fatty acids in the gut to diminish their absorption. Soluble fibers also provide fermentation substrate for colonic bacteria, which produce short-chain fatty acids that are absorbed and may inhibit hepatic synthesis of cholesterol. The LDL-cholesterol-lowering action of soluble fiber ranges from 3% to 5% and may be attenuated by dietary SFA (Kritchevsky, 1991; Leadbetter et al, 1991; Anderson et al, 1992 A; Clevidence et al, 1992; Jenkins et al, 1993 B). Long-term safety and efficacy in reducing the incidence of coronary events remain unproven. Most soluble dietary fiber is well tolerated; complaints are usually limited to gaseous distention, flatulence, and the sensation of uncomfortable fullness due to increased stool bulk.

Psyllium decreases serum LDL-cholesterol concentrations by stimulating bile acid synthesis (Everson et al, 1992), is well tolerated, and has no effect on blood pressure, weight, serum HDL-cholesterol concentration, or plasma triglyceride, glucose, iron, or zinc concentrations. Although the soluble fiber content of the diet can be raised by judicious selection of foods, use of psyllium or other soluble fiber products may provide a reasonably useful adjunct to dietary therapy in the treatment of mild to moderate elevated serum LDL-cholesterol concentration. Adding psyllium-enriched cereal to a low fat diet also may contribute to cholesterol-lowering (Anderson et al, 1992 B; Sprecher et al, 1993). Psyllium (2.5 to 5 g twice daily) has safely decreased serum total cholesterol concentration when added to fat-restricted diets of preadolescent children (Glassman et al, 1990).

The consumption of oat bran as a dietary constituent or as a supplement in daily amounts of 3 to 150 g has lowered serum total and LDL-cholesterol concentrations by 3% or more (see reviews by Grant, 1991; Ripsin et al, 1992). Serum

HDL-cholesterol concentrations usually are not affected. Oat bran is significantly more effective than wheat bran or rice bran on an equal-weight basis (Anderson and Siesel, 1990; Kestin et al, 1990; Jenkins et al, 1993 A). Oat bran cereal may be as effective as supplemental oat bran (Anderson et al, 1990).

Alcohol: Moderate alcohol consumption (one or two glasses of wine or beer per day) appeared to increase serum HDL-cholesterol concentration and decrease CHD risk among the participants in the Framingham Heart Study (Castelli, 1990). In the Multiple Risk Factor Intervention Trial, each increment of average weekly alcohol consumption of seven "drinks" increased serum HDL-cholesterol concentration about 5% and reduced CHD risk 6% in men (Suh et al, 1992). Alcohol ingestion may increase serum HDL-cholesterol concentration by increasing apo A-I synthesis and inhibiting CETP (Amarasuriya et al, 1992; Hirano et al, 1992). Alternatively, wine may contain powerful antioxidants (Frankel et al, 1993). However, the adverse effects of chronic alcohol consumption (hypertriglyceridemia, high blood pressure, stroke, cancer, liver disease, pancreatitis, alcoholism and its consequences) prevent advocacy of this method of cardioprotection, although modest intake should not precipitate adverse cardiovascular events.

Coffee: Boiled coffee contains a factor that raises serum LDL-cholesterol concentration that is not found in filtered coffee (Zock et al, 1990; Ahola et al, 1991; van Dusseldorp et al, 1991). Neither filtered regular nor filtered decaffeinated coffee consumption up to four cups a day affect serum lipid concentrations (Rosmarin et al, 1990; van Dusseldorp et al, 1990; Bak and Grobbee, 1991; Fried et al, 1992; Jossa et al, 1993), although more than five cups daily may increase serum LDL-cholesterol concentration by 10 to 20 mg/dL through unknown mechanisms (Fried et al, 1992). However, even more than 10 cups of filtered coffee daily failed to increase the risk of myocardial infarction (Grobbee et al, 1990; Fraser et al, 1992 A; Myers and Basinski, 1992; Klatsky et al, 1993). Brewed tea (one to two cups daily) has no effect on cholesterolemia (Kark et al, 1985). The possible lipidemic effects of "instant" coffees and teas have not been examined.

Dietary Proteins: Atherosclerosis and CHD are more prevalent in populations consuming larger amounts of animal protein. Substituting soybean protein for animal protein has reduced serum total cholesterol concentrations an average of 20% to 30% in hypercholesterolemic patients and 8% to 12% in normocholesterolemic subjects (Carroll, 1992). In rabbits, dietary casein is associated with a decrease in receptor-mediated LDL catabolism whose magnitude corresponds to that of a subsequent increase in serum LDL-cholesterol concentration. This effect appears to result from actions of the essential amino acids, particularly lysine, but other amino acids may contribute to the effect; a mixture of amino acids corresponding to soy protein is less hypercholesterolemic than a mixture of amino acids corresponding to casein.

Fish Oil Supplements (ω-3 Fatty Acids): Extensive epidemiologic evidence has demonstrated an association between the consumption of fish, sea mammals, or their oils; reduced circulating lipid and lipoprotein concentrations; and decreased cardiovascular mortality. Data from clinical trials suggest that enrichment of the diet with ω-3 FA-rich foods, substitution of ω-3 FA for other dietary fats, or supplementation with ω-3 FA can decrease fasting plasma triglyceride concentrations, frequently by over 50%, in patients with severe hypertriglyceridemia or familial hyperchylomicronemia (Richter et al, 1992; see also reviews by Harris et al, 1988 A; Kromhout, 1989; Connor and Connor, 1990; Kinsella et al, 1990; Knapp, 1990).

Docosahexaenoic acid (DHA) and α-linolenic acid must be obtained from exogenous sources; eicosapentaenoic acid (EPA) can be synthesized from α-linolenic acid by elongation and desaturation, although conversion is inefficient and slow (Singer, 1992). The ω-3 FA are completely absorbed within six hours of ingestion, incorporated into chylomicrons, and transported into hepatocytes where they may be preferentially oxidized (Nordøy et al, 1991). EPA and DHA are equally effective in inhibiting phosphatidate hydrolase activity (and therefore hepatic triglyceride and VLDL synthesis) (Coniglio, 1992). EPA and DHA also reduce the extent and duration of postprandial accumulation of VLDL and chylomicrons in familial mixed hypertriglyceridemia and markedly reduce fasting hypertriglyceridemia in IDDM and NIDDM (Malasanos and Stacpoole, 1991).

EPA and DHA have opposite effects on hepatic LDL receptors (EPA: downregulation; DHA: upregulation) and serum LDL-cholesterol concentration (EPA: increase; DHA: decrease) (Childs et al, 1990; Franceschini et al, 1991 A). DHA also may decrease serum cholesterol concentration by increasing biliary excretion of cholesterol (Smit et al, 1991). Whether fish oil supplements increase or decrease serum total and LDL-cholesterol concentrations may reflect their ratio of EPA to DHA.

EPA and DHA appear to be incorporated into atherosclerotic plaques in humans, where they may compete with arachidonic acid (ω-6 FA) for both the cyclooxygenase and lipoxygenase enzymes (see the review by Kinsella et al, 1990). The lipoxygenase pathway catalyzes the formation of leukotrienes; substitution of ω-3 FA for ω-6 FA results in the formation of relatively more mildly atherogenic leukotriene B_5 than strongly atherogenic leukotriene B_4 (Mori et al, 1992). In addition, synthesis of interleukin-1β (IL-1β), IL-2, IL-6, and tumor necrosis factor is inhibited by ω-3 FA, and lymphocyte proliferation in response to a mitogenic stimulus is reduced (Meydani et al, 1991). Although there is no direct evidence that ω-3 FA are involved in the regression or reversibility of human atherosclerosis, treatment of patients undergoing percutaneous transluminal coronary angioplasty with ω-3 FA has resulted in dose-dependent decreases in the incidence of restenosis (defined as a loss of at least 50% of coronary luminal diameter) (Gapinski et al, 1993; Goodnight, 1993). The likelihood of restenosis was inversely related to the level of ω-3 FA consumption.

The antithrombogenic effects of the ω-3 FA may be more clinically significant than their antiatherogenic actions (Hart Hansen et al, 1990: Nordøy, 1991). It has been reported that ω-3 FA increase the endothelial-dependent relaxation of coronary arteries in response to bradykinin, serotonin, adenosine diphosphate, and thrombin; reduce the vasospastic response to catecholamines; decrease thromboplastin synthesis in endothelial cells; and stimulate endogenous fibrinolysis (Nordøy, 1991). However, ω-3 FA may inhibit fibrinolysis in hypercholesterolemic patients by stimulating plasma plasminogen activator inhibitor activity (Hornstra, 1991).

No differences have been noted in the responses to ω-3 FA whether present in crude fish oil, highly purified fish oil, or fish. Responses to equivalent doses of EPA and DHA from different sources of either the triglyceride or ethyl ester forms have been similar (Harris et al, 1988 B; Nordøy et al, 1991). However, ethyl esters of ω-3 FA are incompletely absorbed when taken in large doses, and their effects can be sporadic (Lawson and Hughes, 1988; Schectman et al, 1989). Ingestion of ethyl esters with meals may increase their absorption (Nordøy et al, 1991).

EPA and DHA are substantially more effective than α-linolenic acid (Singer, 1992). Optimal levels of consumption have not been established. A rather low dietary intake over a lifetime may afford effective prophylaxis from cardiovascular events. A total of 3 to 4 g/day of (EPA + DHA) may exert maximal triglyceride-lowering effects (Childs et al, 1990; Harris et al, 1990; Schmidt et al, 1990). Ethyl esters of ω-3 FA are less effective (Nenseter et al, 1992). Dietary α-linolenic acid is not biologically equivalent to EPA or DHA from fish oil.

Concerns about daily consumption of over 2 g (EPA + DHA) have included increased bleeding, increased peroxidation of cell membranes and lipids, carcinogenesis, deterioration of glycemic control in diabetic patients, and poor absorption of vitamin D (Connor and Connor, 1990; Malasanos and Stacpoole, 1991). However, more than 150 studies have not revealed toxicity in healthy or hyperlipidemic adults at daily doses of up to 7 g. In addition, ω-3 FA attenuate the tumorigenic response to high intakes of linoleic acid (Cave, 1991).

Fish oils can provide a significant amount of supplemental calories. Their beneficial effects are obliterated when they are simply added to diets high in saturated or *trans*-fatty acids, cholesterol, or alcohol (Drevon, 1992).

Between 1% and 2% of maternal caloric intake as ω-3 FA stimulates normal intrauterine growth and development; this suggests that purified EPA and DHA might be both safe and necessary to consume during pregnancy. Similarly, human milk normally contains 9 to 25 mg ω-3 FA/g total fats, depending on maternal dietary intake (Sanders et al, 1978). Little is known concerning the effects of ω-3 FA on children.

Antioxidants: Recent research findings have suggested that nutrients with antioxidant properties can reduce the susceptibility of LDL to oxidation (see review by Harris, 1992). Vitamins C and E and β-carotene inhibit chemical and cell-mediated oxidation of LDL-borne lipids, and ascorbic acid also protects the vitamin E and β-carotene incorporated into LDL during VLDL synthesis (eg, vitamin E and β-carotene) (Frei, 1991; Jialal and Grundy, 1991; Rifici and Khachadurian, 1993).

Vitamin E is a powerful antioxidant; lipid oxidation is delayed until LDL particles are depleted of vitamin E (Niki et al, 1991). Plasma α-tocopherol concentration, LDL α-tocopherol content, and LDL resistance to oxidation are proportional to α-tocopherol intake (Dieber-Rotheneder et al, 1991; Jialal and Grundy, 1992), and plasma α-tocopherol concentration and CHD severity may be inversely related (Gey et al, 1991). Long-term vitamin E intakes >20 mg/day (women) or 60 mg/day (men) were associated with decreased risk for CHD in the Nurses' Health Study (Stampfer et al, 1993) and the Health Professionals Follow-up Study (Rimm et al, 1993). In addition, 300 mg of vitamin E (α-tocopherol) daily reduced free radical-mediated myocardial dysfunction after coronary artery bypass grafting (Yau et al, 1990), and 1.2 g daily reduced the incidence of restenosis after percutaneous transluminal coronary angioplasty by 30% compared to placebo (DeMaio et al, 1992).

Similarly, when taken in large doses, β-carotene also accumulates in lipoproteins and, in the Physicians' Health Study, 50 mg every other day reduced the incidence of major secondary coronary events by 44% compared with placebo (Gaziano et al, 1990). Selenium also inhibits lipid peroxidation by scavenging free radicals. It has been suggested that low serum selenium concentration may be an independent risk factor for the progression of atherosclerosis (Salonen et al, 1991). Increased intakes of the antioxidant bioflavonoids, quercetin, kaempferol, myricetin, apigenin, and luteolin, is associated with a reduced incidence of myocardial infarction and decreased mortality from CHG (Hertog et al, 1993). If proven effective, antioxidants can join the armamentarium available for the prevention of atherosclerosis, CHD, and ischemic peripheral and cerebrovascular disease.

Pro-Oxidants: Transition metals are extremely effective promoters of free radical reactions and lipid peroxidation. Copper is especially efficient in catalyzing lipoprotein peroxidation directly and also facilitates the conversion of xanthine dehydrogenase to xanthine oxidase, which increases the reduction of O_2 to superoxide (O_2^-). Serum copper concentration is positively correlated with serum malondialdehyde concentration, an index of plasma lipid peroxidation. High serum copper concentration may be an independent risk factor for accelerated atherogenesis (Salonen et al, 1991).

Vitamin D: Pathologic calcification of the arterial wall is an underlying feature of atherosclerosis. Excessive vitamin D intake is a well-documented cause of dystrophic cardiovascular calcification. Vitamin D has been implicated as a hypercholesterolemic agent in infantile hypercalcemia, vitamin D poisoning, and in adults with atherosclerosis (see review by Moon et al, 1992). Although the relationship between vitamin D intake and the incidence of CHD has not been thoroughly investigated, vitamin D intake generally should not exceed the RDA of 400 IU.

EXERCISE. Physical activity can reduce the risk of developing CHD and slow the progression of existing CHD (Fletcher et al, 1992; Fletcher, 1993). These benefits are mediated by substantial decreases in plasma triglyceride concentration, slight increases in serum HDL-cholesterol concentration, and weight reduction. The diameters of stenotic lesions also may decrease (Hambrecht et al, 1993). The effects appear to be related to exercise intensity, duration, and frequency and accrue to both males and females from childhood through at least 90 years of age (Nieman et al, 1990; Reaven et al,

1990; Fraser et al, 1992 B; DuRant et al, 1993; Taylor and Ward, 1993). Brisk walking appears to be as effective as jogging on an equal-distance basis (Tucker and Friedman, 1990; Superko, 1991). However, it is uncertain whether weight lifting is lipid-lowering (Kohl et al, 1992; Boyden et al, 1993). Regular vigorous aerobic exercise has repeatedly been shown to increase serum HDL-cholesterol concentrations in children and adolescents (Rowland, 1985; Epstein et al, 1989). Exercise may increase serum HDL-cholesterol concentration by reducing CETP activity (Seip et al, 1993).

WEIGHT REDUCTION. Obesity is clearly associated with a significant increase in the incidence of myocardial infarction, even among those who are otherwise at low risk (Fraser et al, 1992 B). Obese people have higher plasma triglyceride and serum total cholesterol concentrations and lower serum HDL-cholesterol concentrations than nonobese individuals of the same age at all ages (Denke et al, 1993). In a group of young men aged 18 and 19 years who were followed for ten years, every unit-increase in body mass index (BMI) (1 kg/M^2) was associated with an increase in serum total cholesterol concentration of 8 mg/dL and a decrease in serum HDL-cholesterol concentration of 1 mg/dL (Berns et al, 1989). Fractional catabolic rates of HDL are proportional to BMI and increasing central adiposity (Terry et al, 1992).

On average, for every 1-kg decrease in body weight, serum total cholesterol concentration decreases 2 to 3 mg/dL and serum LDL-cholesterol and fasting plasma triglyceride concentrations decrease 1 to 3 mg/dL (Dattilo and Kris-Etherton, 1992; Kasim et al, 1993). Decreases in fasting plasma triglyceride concentration are even greater in renal transplant recipients following weight reduction. Changes in serum HDL-cholesterol concentration during active weight loss have been variable. Transient increases in serum LDL-cholesterol concentrations during massive weight loss may represent the effects of stored cholesterol being released from mobilized adipose tissues. Despite changes in other circulating lipid fractions, serum Lp(a) concentrations are not affected by BMI, weight loss, or diet in general.

DRUG THERAPY. *Drugs usually are indicated for adults only when lifestyle modifications including dietary modifications, weight reduction when necessary, an exercise program, and elimination or minimization of the causes of concurrent secondary lipidemic abnormalities are unsuccessful in attaining desired target serum LDL- and HDL-cholesterol and plasma triglyceride concentration goals. In some patients, increased risk of atherosclerotic (eg, transient ischemic attacks, intermittent claudication, myocardial infarction, stroke) or other complications (eg, pancreatitis, abdominal pain, xanthomas) justifies their use. Dietary regulation must continue during drug therapy because effects are additive and pharmacologic therapy may be ineffective without dietary modification.*

Following initiation of drug treatment, serum total, LDL-, and HDL-cholesterol concentrations should be determined at 8- to 12-week intervals until they become stable and at gradually longer intervals thereafter. In most instances, dosage should be modified or another drug substituted or added if serum cholesterol concentrations are not reduced significantly after an adequate trial (usually three to six months) that includes evaluation of patient compliance. Drug therapy must be continuous and lifelong in those with lipoprotein disorders; circulating cholesterol concentrations usually return to pretreatment levels within a few weeks if treatment is discontinued. Therefore, decisions to initiate drug therapy must be made only after careful assessment that includes consideration of potential side effects of long-term medication. In addition, the patient must be monitored indefinitely at regular intervals to assess the effectiveness of therapy and because dosage adjustments are required if diet or body weight changes, if concomitant medications are used, if adverse reactions occur, and as patients age.

The serum LDL-cholesterol concentrations that justify initiation of drug therapy and setting of target goals depend on whether the clinical objective is primary or secondary prevention (Expert Panel, 1993), and the severity of hypercholesterolemia is an important factor in clinical decision-making. In general, in the absence of two or more other risk factors, drug therapy should be considered in men $\geq$45 years and women $\geq$55 years if the serum LDL-cholesterol concentration is $>$190 mg/dL, with the goal of reducing this to $<$160 mg/dL; when two or more other risk factors are present, drug therapy should be considered if the serum LDL-cholesterol concentration is $>$160 mg/dL, with the goal of reducing this to $<$130 mg/dL. These guidelines also are recommended for primary prevention in patients with diabetes.

For younger people, drug therapy for serum LDL-cholesterol concentrations $>$220 mg/dL generally is appropriate, whereas prescription of drugs may be delayed when serum LDL-cholesterol concentrations range between 190 and 220 mg/dL if no other risk factors are present. However, pharmacologic therapy may be indicated in young adults when serum LDL-cholesterol concentrations are $>$190 mg/dL and they have a family history of CHD or a genetic hypercholesterolemia.

Most patients with CHD should be treated to reduce the serum LDL-cholesterol concentration to $<$100 mg/dL. Whether to initiate drug therapy for patients with CHD whose serum LDL-cholesterol concentration is between 100 and 129 mg/dL after dietary, weight reduction, and exercise therapy depends on a variety of factors and must be left to the judgment of the physician. If drug therapy is initiated and the goal of therapy is not attained after three months with a single drug, consideration can be given to adding a second agent. However, similar clinical judgment is required in deciding whether to raise the dose of a drug or to add a second drug when the serum LDL-cholesterol concentration decreases but remains $>$100 mg/dL. If the serum LDL-cholesterol concentration is consistently below target levels, the dose of drug should be decreased to establish the minimum amount required to maintain the desired target.

At the time of hospitalization for an acute coronary event, consideration can be given to initiating drug therapy at discharge if the serum LDL-cholesterol concentration is $>$130 mg/dL. Serum LDL-cholesterol concentrations often are decreased in the first weeks following a coronary event, and a serum LDL-cholesterol concentration $>$130 mg/dL at discharge typically will be even higher later when the patient has not only recovered from the acute event but has re-established normal life-style habits. On the other hand, patients may be particularly receptive to risk factor management after sustaining a coronary event.

Patients with serum LDL-cholesterol concentrations <130 mg/dL at discharge initially can be managed with intensive dietary therapy alone; however, if the concentration increases to >130 mg/dL after three months, drug therapy may be necessary. If the concentration remains between 100 and 130 mg/dL, the decision to use drugs will depend on physician judgment.

Some patients with CHD may not be candidates for cholesterol-lowering drug therapy because of very advanced age, poor cardiac prognosis (eg, chronic congestive heart failure), or coexisting medical conditions that severely impair quality of life or life expectancy. Primary prevention trials in middle-aged men using drug therapy reveal that at least two years are required before a reduction in risk for CHD becomes manifest; therefore, before pharmacologic therapy is begun in older persons, a good prognosis for several years of healthy life seems to be essential.

Hormone changes during the second and third trimesters of pregnancy increase serum total and LDL-cholesterol and plasma triglyceride concentrations by approximately 35% (Hegele, 1991). The use of drugs that decrease serum cholesterol concentrations during pregnancy is contraindicated because the effects on the fetus caused by interference with maternal or fetal cholesterol metabolism have not been established. However, gestational pancreatitis triggered by chylomicronemic crisis in women with severe gestational hypertriglyceridemia is dangerous for mother and fetus. Susceptible women typically are hypertriglyceridemic when not pregnant and are likely to have had a previous episode of chylomicronemic pancreatitis when not pregnant. Early diagnosis of hypertriglyceridemia during the first trimester followed by monitoring to determine the onset of severe hypertriglyceridemia can alert the clinician to the possibility of a hyperlipidemic abdominal crisis. Careful dietary management (severe fat restrictions with concurrent ω-3 fatty acids), or, if necessary, total parenteral nutrition often is successful.

Whether hypolipidemic drugs are excreted in breast milk and the possible consequences of such excretion are unknown.

Little information is available concerning the treatment of children with lipid-lowering drugs. The benefits of treating children with less than severe hypercholesterolemia or hypertriglyceridemia are not clear, and treatment before the completion of puberty is controversial.

Available Drugs: No single drug is consistently effective in all types of lipoprotein disorders, and the long-term safety of some agents has not been established. Drugs currently approved by the FDA for treatment of lipoprotein disorders are cholestyramine resin [Questran, Questran Light], colestipol [Colestid], clofibrate [Atromid-S], fenofibrate [Lipidil], gemfibrozil [Lopid], niacin (nicotinic acid) [Niacor, Nicolar], lovastatin [Mevacor], pravastatin [Pravachol], simvastatin [Zocor], fluvastatin [Lescol], and probucol [Lorelco].

Several agents used in the past are no longer recommended. The poorly absorbed aminoglycoside antibiotic neomycin, given in a daily dose of 500 mg orally (maximum, 2 g/day), was an alternative to the bile-acid sequestrants but was used infrequently because it impairs cholesterol absorption from the gut. Serum LDL-cholesterol concentration decreases 12% to 25%, but HDL-cholesterol concentration also decreases by up to 16% (Kesäniemi and Miettinen, 1991). Approximately 3% of a dose is absorbed; in patients with impaired renal function, blood concentrations may accumulate to nephrotoxic and ototoxic levels. Therefore, neomycin is no longer recommended for use in lipid disorders.

Dextrothyroxine [Choloxin] lowers serum LDL-cholesterol concentration, but doses that result in clinical hyperthyroidism are required (Bantle et al, 1984). In the Coronary Drug Project, dextrothyroxine increased the incidence of all-cause mortality in patients with one or more previous episodes of myocardial infarction (Coronary Drug Project Research Group, 1972). Because agents with more favorable risk/benefit profiles are available, dextrothyroxine should not be used to treat lipid disorders.

Chelation therapy has been advocated by some physicians to treat atherosclerosis, but it has not been shown to be effective (DATTA, 1983; Scott, 1988) and potential side effects may be harmful. Thus, chelating agents have no place in the treatment of atherosclerosis with or without hyperlipidemia.

The investigational drug, acipimox, is a pyrazine *N*-oxide derivative of niacin that is a potent inhibitor of mobilization of free fatty acids in adipose tissue (Fucella et al, 1980). Acipimox also may decelerate VLDL synthesis to decrease the triglyceride content of LDL particles and their density and increase the efficiency of their interaction with the LDL receptor (Franceschini et al, 1991 B; Griffin et al, 1992). It also decreases blood viscosity and the cholesterol saturation of bile (potentially reducing the risk of gallstone formation) in patients with familial combined hyperlipidemia (Montefusco et al, 1988; Ericsson et al, 1990). The lipid-lowering effects of doses of 250 mg taken three times daily after meals in patients with hypercholesterolemia and hypertriglyceridemia are similar to those produced by clofibrate (2 g/d) (Stuyt et al, 1985; Crepaldi et al, 1988; Barlow et al, 1990). Acipimox is less likely to produce glucose intolerance than niacin.

The use of low doses (0.625 or 1.25 mg daily) of oral conjugated estrogens in postmenopausal women accelerates LDL catabolism and produces large, triglyceride-rich VLDL (Walsh et al, 1991). Serum total and LDL-cholesterol concentrations decrease, serum HDL_2-cholesterol concentration increases, and fasting plasma triglyceride concentrations usually increase (Campos et al, 1990; Miller et al, 1991; Walsh et al, 1991). Despite this mixed response, the prevalence of coronary artery stenosis confirmed by angiography in postmenopausal women may be reduced (Hong et al, 1992). Combining estradiol continuously with cyproterone or sequentially with levonorgestrel, medroxyprogesterone, or desogestrel also has reduced serum total and LDL-cholesterol concentrations in postmenopausal women (Haarbo et al, 1991). However, serum HDL-cholesterol and apo A-I concentrations were elevated only during periods of estradiol monotherapy. Postmenopausal women with mildly elevated serum LDL-cholesterol concentrations but without hypertriglyceridemia may benefit from low-dose oral estrogen replacement therapy. Estrogens are contraindicated in men because they are feminizing, increase the incidence of thromboembolism and myocardial infarction, and may increase CHD and cancer mortality (Coronary Drug Project Research Group, 1973).

Drug Selection: The drugs used to treat lipoprotein disorders can be grouped either on the basis of common mechanisms of action or on common effects on plasma lipids.

Bile acid sequestering resins (cholestyramine and colestipol) interfere with the absorption of cholesterol-derived bile acids from the gut, resulting in a reduction in hepatic cholesterol content and an increase in hepatic uptake of circulating LDL. The resins are considered interchangeable, are used exclusively for their hypocholesterolemic effect, and have traditionally been considered the drugs of choice in lipoprotein disorders in which serum LDL-cholesterol concentration cannot be adequately decreased by diet alone. They may aggravate hypertriglyceridemia, resulting in pancreatitis. Bile acid sequestering resins are not used together.

The fibric acid derivatives (clofibrate, gemfibrozil, fenofibrate, bezafibrate, ciprofibrate) produce somewhat variable decreases in serum total or LDL-cholesterol concentrations but are very effective in controlling hypertriglyceridemia. Bezafibrate and ciprofibrate are investigational drugs in the United States but are widely used in Europe. Bezafibrate, ciprofibrate, and fenofibrate are more effective than clofibrate or gemfibrozil in reducing serum LDL-cholesterol concentrations. Fibric acid derivatives are especially useful in disorders characterized by hypertriglyceridemia and in familial dysbetalipoproteinemia (Frick et al, 1987). When combined with bile acid sequestering resins or niacin, fenofibrate or bezafibrate have additive effects in decreasing serum LDL-cholesterol and plasma triglyceride concentrations and in increasing serum HDL-cholesterol concentrations. In some early studies on clofibrate, an appreciable number of serious adverse reactions occurred; its use is now limited to patients with familial dysbetalipoproteinemia who do not respond to gemfibrozil (Coronary Drug Project Research Group, 1975).

The effects of pharmacologic doses of niacin (as nicotinic acid) on VLDL and HDL are similar to those of the fibric acid derivatives; however, decreases in serum LDL-cholesterol concentration generally are larger with niacin. Side effects are frequent, bothersome, and reduce compliance; when facial flushing is the major complaint, encouragement by the physician during the early phases of treatment may significantly improve compliance and allow tolerance to develop. Although impaired liver function, glucose intolerance, and gout occur infrequently, these reactions can be serious. Niacin has a long-term record of efficacy and relative safety as an alternative to bile acid sequestrants and is the drug of choice when the goal of therapy is to normalize elevated serum LDL-cholesterol, VLDL, and triglyceride concentrations (except in diabetes mellitus, where niacin may exacerbate glucose intolerance). It frequently is combined with cholestyramine or colestipol because actions on serum LDL-cholesterol concentration are complementary. However, timed-release formulations of niacin can be hepatotoxic and cannot be recommended.

The HMG-CoA reductase inhibitors (fluvastatin, lovastatin, pravastatin, and simvastatin) directly inhibit cholesterogenesis and accelerate LDL clearance. They are more potent in reducing serum total and LDL-cholesterol concentrations than other available drugs and are generally well tolerated. These drugs are preferred alternatives in hypercholesterolemia when niacin or bile acid sequestrants are inadequate or not tolerated and are initial drugs of choice in patients with primary hypercholesterolemia. Combining HMG-CoA reductase inhibitors with bile acid sequestering resins or niacin enhances the effects on cholesterol metabolism.

Probucol [Lorelco] is unrelated chemically to all other drugs that affect serum lipids. It reduces serum total and LDL-cholesterol concentrations moderately; however, it can markedly reduce serum HDL-cholesterol concentration (Chiesa et al, 1993). Concerns about its potential for lengthening the electrocardiographic QT interval and long persistence in tissues limit its use. Nevertheless, probucol possesses an antioxidant action that interferes with the oxidative modification of LDL, an action that is apparently antiatherogenic in animals, and it may retard restenosis after percutaneous transluminal coronary angioplasty (Setsuda et al, 1993). The combination of probucol plus bile acid sequestering resins produces additive effects on serum LDL-cholesterol concentrations and the serum HDL-concentration lowering effect of probucol is attenuated.

Most therapeutic failures in the pharmacologic treatment of disorders of cholesterol and lipoprotein metabolism result from poor compliance. However, even in compliant patients, dyslipidemias may persist and require alternative forms of therapy. One approach is to use selected combinations of drugs that act by different mechanisms in these patients. For further information on drug combinations, see the evaluations.

TREATMENT OF SPECIFIC LIPOPROTEIN DISORDERS. Table 7 summarizes drug therapy for the major lipoprotein disorders.

Familial Hypercholesterolemia: Bile acid sequestrants (cholestyramine, colestipol) and HMG-CoA reductase inhibitors are the agents of choice to treat heterozygous patients. If the response to monotherapy is inadequate, these drugs may be combined.

The familial homozygous form of hypercholesterolemia is the most malignant; myocardial infarction is common before age 10, and untreated patients seldom live beyond early adulthood. Because these patients either have no or defective LDL receptors, little or no response can be expected from therapy designed to increase LDL receptor activity. Referral to a lipid specialist is recommended, although treatment is rarely successful; LDL apheresis or liver transplantation may be indicated. Some success has been reported with a combination of diet, cholestyramine, and niacin or HMG-CoA reductase inhibitors in patients with defective receptors.

Polygenic Hypercholesterolemia/Secondary Hypercholesterolemia: In most individuals, elevated serum LDL-cholesterol concentrations are caused by subtle aberrations of many genes whose detrimental effects are elicited by environmental cofactors (eg, high intake of dietary cholesterol or

TABLE 7.
DRUG SELECTION FOR LIPIDEMIC ABNORMALITIES

Lipid Disorder	Preferred Therapies[1]	Alternative Therapies
Hypercholesterolemia		
Familial heterozygous	HMG-CoA reductase inhibitor Bile acid sequestering resin HMG-CoA reductase inhibitor + bile acid sequestering resin	Niacin Niacin + bile acid sequestering resin
Familial homozygous[2]	HMG-CoA reductase inhibitor + bile acid sequestering resin	Specialist referral for LDL apheresis
Polygenic	HMG-CoA reductase inhibitor Bile acid sequestering resin HMG-CoA reductase inhibitor + bile acid sequestering resin Niacin	Probucol + bile acid sequestering resin
Familial Hypertriglyceridemia	Niacin	Gemfibrozil[3] or fenofibrate
Familial Combined Hyperlipidemia		
Isolated hypercholesterolemia	Bile acid sequestering resin Niacin Niacin + bile acid sequestering resin	HMG-CoA reductase inhibitor HMG-CoA reductase inhibitor + bile acid sequestering resin
Isolated hypertriglyceridemia	Niacin	Gemfibrozil or fenofibrate
Hypercholesterolemia plus hypertriglyceridemia	Niacin HMG-CoA reductase inhibitor	Gemfibrozil or fenofibrate
Fasting Hyperchylomicronemia	Special dietary therapy (see text)	
Familial Dysbetalipoproteinemia	Gemfibrozil or fenofibrate Niacin	HMG-CoA reductase inhibitor Estrogen in postmenopausal women
Familial Mixed Hypertriglyceridemia	Gemfibrozil or fenofibrate	
Isolated Hypoalphalipoproteinemia	No specific drug therapy[4]	
Diabetic Dyslipidemia		
Severe hypertriglyceridemia	Gemfibrozil or fenofibrate	
Moderate hypertriglyceridemia	Gemfibrozil or fenofibrate	HMG-CoA reductase inhibitor

1 Combination drug regimens should not be employed unless indicated.
2 Drug therapy is ineffective in homozygous receptor-negative familial hypercholesterolemia.
3 Other fibric acid derivatives (eg, bezafibrate) are being investigated; however, sufficient data are not yet available to document their effectiveness in decreasing mortality and morbidity in cardiovascular disease.
4 When niacin, gemfibrozil, or lovastatin, dietary therapy, and exercise are used to treat elevated triglyceride and/or LDL-cholesterol concentrations, serum HDL-cholesterol concentration will often rise; serum HDL-cholesterol concentration is not affected by bile acid sequestrants and often are depressed by probucol.

fat, excessive calories). Dietary modification, increased exercise, and elimination or treatment of other risk factors (see Table 6) usually are effective to some degree. If the response is inadequate, drug therapy of this disorder is identical to that described for the heterozygous form of familial hypercholesterolemia.

Familial Hypertriglyceridemia/Secondary Hypertriglyceridemia: Plasma triglyceride concentrations are elevated and symptoms are similar in these disorders; differential diagnosis will be difficult unless a secondary cause of hypertriglyceridemia is obvious or relatively complete family data are available. Individuals with borderline hypertriglyceridemia

(250 to 500 mg/dL) without elevated serum LDL-cholesterol concentrations may require only modification of diet and/or elimination of secondary causes. More severe hypertriglyceridemia may respond to diet therapy and niacin or gemfibrozil. Bile acid sequestrants are contraindicated.

Familial Combined Hyperlipidemia: The decision to add drug therapy to the treatment regimen will depend on the severity of the disorder and the response to diet, exercise, and elimination of secondary causes of hypertriglyceridemia. If drug therapy is indicated, drug selection is based on the type and degree of hyperlipidemia. Relatively isolated elevation of serum LDL-cholesterol concentration can be managed by the dietary and drug treatment recommended for familial heterozygous or polygenic hypercholesterolemia. Relatively isolated hypertriglyceridemia can be managed the same as familial hypertriglyceridemia. When both hypercholesterolemia and hypertriglyceridemia are present, drug therapy should be initiated with niacin or an HMG-CoA reductase inhibitor. The latter should not be added to niacin because of the increased risk of myopathy. Gemfibrozil or niacin may be combined with a bile acid sequestrant in combined hyperlipidemia (Hunninghake et al, 1990) unless hypertriglyceridemia is severe.

Fasting Hyperchylomicronemia: Restriction of dietary fat (25 g/day or less) markedly decreases plasma triglyceride concentrations, resolves eruptive xanthomas, and relieves abdominal pain, although moderate lipemia may persist. A fat-free diet may be required initially when the disorder is very severe. At least 1% of total calories should consist of linoleic acid to meet essential fatty acid requirements, and fat-soluble vitamins should be prescribed if they are not provided in the diet. The addition of medium-chain triglycerides, which are transported directly to the liver without chylomicron formation, increases palatability and dietary compliance. To supply adequate calories, complex carbohydrate should be substituted for fat; however, a protein intake of greater than the normal 15% to 20% of calories minimizes reliance on excessive amounts of carbohydrate and may improve dietary compliance. Alcohol consumption should be avoided to prevent abdominal pain and acute pancreatitis. Dietary cholesterol restriction and weight reduction without fat restriction are of little value in this disorder and none of the currently available drugs is consistently effective.

Familial Dysbetalipoproteinemia: Dietary restriction and exercise to achieve ideal body weight, followed by adherence to a low-cholesterol, low-saturated fat diet, frequently is the only therapy needed. In some patients, restriction of alcohol consumption and intake of simple sugars also may be required. If this does not normalize lipid concentrations, administration of gemfibrozil, niacin, or an HMG-CoA reductase inhibitor usually reduces serum lipid concentrations to normal ranges and causes regression of xanthomas. Estrogen therapy may be very useful in women with this disorder. Cholestyramine and colestipol are not useful in this type of hyperlipoproteinemia and may even worsen it.

Familial Mixed Hypertriglyceridemia: In addition to pronounced hypertriglyceridemia, fasting chylomicronemia is present. This pattern may occur in some patients with familial hypertriglyceridemia who have an exacerbation of their disorder due to secondary causes, especially diabetes, alcohol excess, or estrogen therapy. Administration of gemfibrozil to reduce the triglyceride level and limitation of daily fat intake to no more than 25 g to eliminate the fasting chylomicronemia are required.

Dyslipidemia Associated with Diabetes Mellitus: Fibric acid derivatives, especially gemfibrozil, are the preferred lipid-lowering agents in diabetic patients with severe hypertriglyceridemia and mild hypercholesterolemia in the absence of both impaired creatinine clearance and microalbuminuria >1 g/day (Durrington, 1991; Merrin and Elkeles, 1991; Lahdenperä et al, 1993; Vinik et al, 1993). Fibric acid derivatives markedly reduce plasma triglyceride concentrations; serum VLDL- and LDL-cholesterol concentrations decrease slightly and serum HDL-cholesterol concentrations often increase (Onuma et al, 1992). However, HMG-CoA reductase inhibitors are the treatment of choice in diabetic patients with hypercholesterolemia and established cardiovascular disease and only moderate hypertriglyceridemia (Durrington, 1991; Zambon et al, 1992). Glycemic control is not affected by either gemfibrozil or HMG-CoA reductase inhibitors. Niacin also can decrease serum total cholesterol concentration in diabetic patients but can interfere with glycemic control (Garg and Grundy, 1990).

Bile acid sequestrants are not indicated in diabetic hyperlipidemia because they tend to increase the plasma triglyceride concentration. Probucol, despite its antiatherogenic antioxidant properties, is not recommended because serum HDL-cholesterol concentrations tend to decrease further with its use. Although fish oils appear to dramatically decrease plasma triglyceride concentrations and increase serum HDL-cholesterol concentration in diabetes, they may worsen glycemic control.

Elevated Serum Lp(a) Concentration: Niacin (3 g/day) has been reported to reduce elevated serum Lp(a) concentrations, but this high dose is often accompanied by adverse reactions. Intravenous administration of tissue plasminogen activator has temporarily reduced serum Lp(a) concentrations in patients with unstable angina (Hegele et al, 1992). Acetylcysteine (1.2 to 4 g/day) may have a limited capacity to inhibit hepatic Lp(a) production by preventing disulfide linkage between apo(a) and apo B-100 when serum Lp(a) concentration exceeds 40 mg/dL (Kroon et al, 1991). Danazol (600 mg/day) markedly reduces serum Lp(a) concentrations but also reduces serum HDL-cholesterol and increases LDL-cholesterol concentrations (Crook et al, 1992).

Dyslipidemias Associated with Other Endocrine Diseases: Serum total and LDL-cholesterol concentrations and fasting plasma triglyceride concentrations are positively correlated with serum thyroid stimulating hormone (TSH) concentrations and inversely related to serum free T_3 concentration in patients with serum TSH concentration >5 microunits/ml. Serum HDL-cholesterol concentrations may be increased or decreased (Caron et al, 1990). In overtly hypothyroid patients without primary hypercholesterolemia, normalization of serum TSH concentration with levothyroxine also normalizes serum LDL-cholesterol concentration within eight weeks (Arem and Patsch, 1990). However, levothyroxine has no effect on Lp(a) (Klausen et al, 1992).

Spontaneous hyperthyroidism or mild overuse of levothyroxine replacement therapy result in substantially lower than average serum total and LDL-cholesterol concentrations. Serum HDL-cholesterol and plasma triglyceride concentrations are usually unaffected.

Growth hormone and insulin-like growth factor-I (IGF-I) deficiencies have been linked to elevated serum total cholesterol concentration. Serum IGF-I and apo B concentrations have been reported to be inversely correlated in humans (Ostlund et al, 1991). However, growth hormone replacement or augmentation therapy has little effect on lipoprotein metabolism.

Drug Evaluations

BILE ACID SEQUESTERING RESINS

CHOLESTYRAMINE RESIN

[Questran]

COLESTIPOL HYDROCHLORIDE

[Colestid]

ACTIONS. Cholestyramine and colestipol are chloride salts of indigestible basic anion exchange resins. They reversibly bind bile acids in the small intestine. Interruption of the enterohepatic circulation of bile acids increases their fecal excretion and stimulates bile acid synthesis from cholesterol. In response, expression of hepatic LDL receptors is upregulated, LDL clearance and apolipoprotein B catabolism are accelerated, and serum LDL-cholesterol concentration decreases. However, HMG-CoA reductase and phosphatidic acid phosphatase activities also are increased and the rates of hepatic VLDL synthesis and secretion may be doubled, resulting in significantly increased plasma VLDL-triglyceride concentration. The extent of stimulation of bile acid synthesis is apparently sufficient to normalize secretion of biliary bile acid, phospholipid, and cholesterol and the cholesterol saturation of bile, and there is no increased risk of gallstone formation (Carrella et al, 1991; Einarsson et al, 1991).

USES. Cholestyramine and colestipol are the drugs of choice for familial and polygenic hypercholesterolemia to reduce the risks of atherosclerotic coronary artery disease and myocardial infarction. When used as adjuncts to dietary control, they reduce serum LDL-cholesterol concentration an average of an additional 20% to 30% in a dose-dependent manner (Lipid Research Clinics Program, 1984 A; Brensike et al, 1984). The maximum effect on serum total and LDL-cholesterol concentrations is apparent within 28 days if the usual therapeutic dose is well tolerated; however, it may be more appropriate to increase the dose gradually (adding 4 or 5 g/day every three to four weeks) to minimize side effects and improve compliance. Beneficial effects have been maintained for more than 13 years of continued use (The Lipid Research Clinics Investigators, 1992). In the usual dosage range, bile acid sequestering resins may aggravate familial dysbetalipoproteinemia or hypertriglyceridemia.

Colestipol is more effective than gemfibrozil in lowering serum LDL-cholesterol concentrations but is less effective in lowering plasma triglyceride concentrations. The combination of niacin and cholestyramine has reduced LDL-cholesterol concentrations more than maximal doses of either agent alone (eg, 40% to 60%). Similar decreases have followed combinations of either resin and an HMG-CoA reductase inhibitor.

Use of cholestyramine 24 g/day by asymptomatic hypercholesterolemic middle-aged men on moderate cholesterol-lowering diets was associated with significantly decreased rates of cardiovascular disease-related death, nonfatal myocardial infarction, new-onset angina, intermittent claudication, and need for coronary bypass surgery (Lipid Research Clinics Program, 1984; Probstfield and Rifkind, 1991). Beneficial effects were most apparent in individuals with the highest baseline serum cholesterol concentrations. However, six years after completion of this trial there were no differences in the incidence of cardiovascular disease-related death or nonfatal myocardial infarction in treated and untreated individuals (The Lipid Research Clinics Investigators, 1992). Colestipol 15 g/day lowered serum cholesterol concentrations, significantly reduced the incidence of cardiovascular disease-related death, and stabilized atherosclerotic lesions in similar populations of patients (Kuo et al, 1979).

Patients with hypercholesterolemia and a history of coronary artery disease given either cholestyramine (16 or 24 g/day) or colestipol (15 g/day) in addition to dietary therapy for up to seven years had decreased progression of coronary artery narrowing, increased frequency of lesion regression, and decreased frequency of fatal and nonfatal myocardial infarction, stroke, angina, coronary artery bypass surgery, and angioplasty (Brensike et al, 1984; Ast and Frishman, 1990).

The use of cholestyramine or colestipol by children decreased serum LDL-cholesterol concentrations when compliance was good, and there was no evidence of major side effects or changes in growth rates (West et al, 1980; Koletzko et al, 1992; Liacouras et al, 1993). However, adverse effects limit compliance in children (Liacouras et al, 1993), and the effects of life-long use of these agents beginning in childhood have not been determined.

ADVERSE REACTIONS AND PRECAUTIONS. Cholestyramine and colestipol are among the safest drugs currently available to treat isolated hypercholesterolemia; cholestyramine has been no more toxic than placebo with up to 13 years of use (The Lipid Research Clinics Investigators, 1992). These drugs are not absorbed from the gastrointestinal tract and have no significant systemic toxic effects. The most frequent untoward effects are bloating, flatulence, mild nausea, and constipation; they usually subside with continued therapy or are minimized by increasing the dose gradually. Constipation can be prevented in most patients by large fluid intake, dietary fiber (bran or psyllium), or regular use of a stool softener. Other adverse reactions include epigastric distress and diarrhea. Bile acid sequestering agents should be avoided in patients with pre-existing bowel disease or intractable constipation.

The increase in the synthesis of triglyceride-rich VLDL during cholestyramine use is nearly double the accompanying increase in VLDL catabolism; as a result, serum triglyceride concentrations are increased (Angelin et al, 1990). Bile acid sequestering resins should not be used alone when plasma triglyceride concentration exceeds 300 mg/dL (Ast and Frishman, 1990).

Bile acid sequestering resins directly interfere with intestinal absorption of dietary magnesium, iron, and zinc and indirectly decrease calcium absorption by inhibiting vitamin D absorption. Hyperchloremia and increased urinary excretion of calcium may result from the absorption of chloride released from large doses of the resin. Large doses of cholestyramine or colestipol may interfere with the absorption of folic acid and vitamins A, E, and K. Recommended doses taken with meals retain full efficacy (Sirtori et al, 1991).

Appropriate studies in the elderly have not been conducted. However, these patients may be increasingly prone to gastrointestinal side effects and the consequences of age-related impairment of renal function.

DRUG INTERACTIONS. Bile acid sequestering resins may bind to and decrease the absorption of other drugs given concomitantly (particularly fibric acid derivatives, thiazides, levothyroxine, acetaminophen, methotrexate, piroxicam, chenodiol, ursodiol, digitoxin, propanolol, penicillin G, hydrocortisone, iron compounds, phenylbutazone, tetracycline, vancomycin, barbiturates, cyclosporine, and warfarin). These drugs should be given at least one hour before or four hours after the resin.

PHARMACOKINETICS. Less than 0.05% of an oral dose of cholestyramine is absorbed. Exchange with chloride ions of the resin increases chloremia and acidifies urine. Only about 10% of available binding sites retain bile acids during intestinal transit (Luner and Amidon, 1992). Total serum cholesterol concentration decreases within 48 hours of initiation of therapy and returns to baseline within four weeks after discontinuation of therapy.

DOSAGE AND PREPARATIONS.

CHOLESTYRAMINE RESIN:

Oral: *Adults,* initially, 4 g one or two times daily for the first week as tolerance permits, increased to 8 g twice daily the second week, and to 12 g twice daily thereafter. Dosage should be reduced temporarily if symptoms such as bloating or constipation are troublesome. Although the dosage in *children over 6 years* has not been definitively established, the usual dose is 4 to 8 g twice daily with meals; often 8 to 12 g/day is adequate. *Children under 6 years,* dosage has not been established.

The powder should never be swallowed dry because of the hazard of esophageal irritation or blockage. It should be mixed with 120 to 180 ml of water, fruit juice, soup, or pulpy fruit. A three-day supply can be premixed. An aspartame-containing formulation, Questran Light, may be more palatable and may increase compliance without loss of lipid-lowering effect. A tablet formulation designed to be swallowed intact (investigational) also may alleviate palatability problems (Kwiterovich et al, 1992 B).

Questran (Bristol Myers Squibb). Powder in packets (9 g) and cans (378 g) providing 4 g of anhydrous cholestyramine resin/9 g of powder; powder (for oral suspension) in packets (5 g) and cans (210 g) providing 4 g of anhydrous cholestyramine resin and 17 mg phenylalanine as aspartame/5 g of powder (***Questran Light***).

COLESTIPOL HYDROCHLORIDE:

Oral: *Adults,* 10 to 20 g daily (maximum, 30 g/day); 5 g daily may be adequate when baseline serum LDL-cholesterol concentration is <160 mg/dL (Superko et al, 1992). Colestipol can be mixed with 120 to 180 ml of suitable liquid and taken in two to four divided doses with meals. This drug should be given at least one hour before or four hours after other drugs. It appears to be safe and effective in *children*, but this has not been definitively established; 10 to 15 g daily divided into two doses (mixed with liquids at the morning and evening meals) has been used in children with familial hypercholesterolemia.

Colestid (Upjohn). Granules (unflavored) in 5-g packets and 300- and 500-g containers; granules (flavored for oral suspension) in 7.5-g packets and 450-g containers. Each packet or level scoopful provides 5 g.

FIBRIC ACID DERIVATIVES

CLOFIBRATE

[Atromid-S]

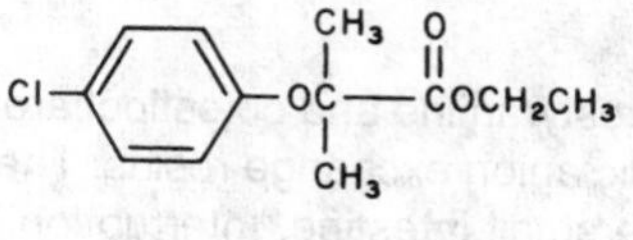

CH_3 O
Cl– –OC– COCH$_2$CH$_3$
CH_3

FENOFIBRATE

[Lipidil]

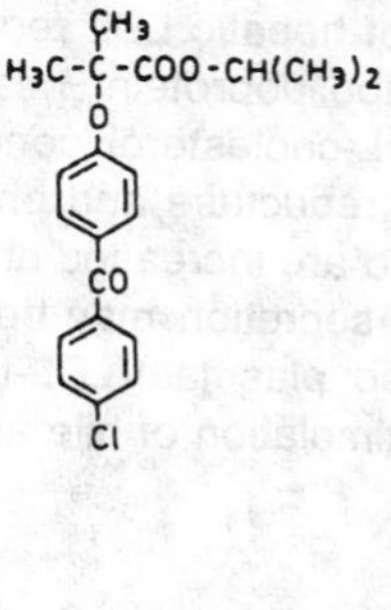

CH_3
H_3C-C-COO-CH$(CH_3)_2$
O
CO
Cl

GEMFIBROZIL
[Lopid]

BEZAFIBRATE (Investigational drug)

ACTIONS. The fibric acid derivatives reduce serum VLDL and plasma triglyceride concentrations by stimulating lipoprotein lipase (LPL) activity and the hydrolysis of triglycerides in plasma (Balfour et al, 1990; Schwandt, 1991; Shepherd, 1993). As LPL activity increases, reduced availability of triglycerides for exchange with cholesterol esters increases serum HDL_{2a}- and total HDL-cholesterol concentrations (Caslake et al, 1993; Silverman et al, 1993), although this effect may be apparent only when plasma triglyceride concentrations fall below 75 mg/dL (Rubins and Robins, 1992). The changes in serum HDL-cholesterol and plasma triglyceride concentrations do not appear to be related. Fibric acid derivatives also reduce the incorporation of long-chain fatty acids into triglycerides, inhibiting VLDL synthesis and secretion (Kesäniemi and Grundy, 1984). Apo A-I synthesis and serum HDL-cholesterol concentration (especially HDL_2) increase (Resta and Capurso, 1991). Fibric acid derivatives also may mildly inhibit HMG-CoA reductase, upregulating LDL receptor activity and decreasing serum LDL-cholesterol concentration (Shepherd, 1993). In contrast, serum LDL concentrations may increase in patients with isolated hypertriglyceridemia or familial combined hyperlipidemia as conversion of VLDL to LDL is accelerated.

Gemfibrozil may inhibit plasminogen activator inhibitor type I (Avellone et al, 1992; Fujii and Sobel, 1992) and decrease circulating concentrations of fibrinogen, fibrinopeptide A, t-PA, plasminogen, and factor VII (Avellone et al, 1992). Fenofibrate decreases platelet and erythrocyte aggregability and inhibits platelet-derived, growth factor-induced proliferation of arterial smooth muscle cells (Balfour et al, 1990). Bezafibrate also decreases plasma fibrinogen concentration and platelet aggregability (Pazzucconi et al, 1992).

USES. Gemfibrozil is especially useful in lipoprotein disorders characterized by elevated serum VLDL and IDL-cholesterol and plasma triglyceride concentrations. It decreases circulating concentrations of all lipoproteins, especially those rich in triglycerides, and is a drug of choice for patients with familial dysbetalipoproteinemia, familial combined hyperlipidemia, familial mixed hypertriglyceridemia, or diabetic hypertriglyceridemia (plasma triglyceride concentration >500 mg/dL) with serum LDL-cholesterol concentration ≤240 mg/dL (Vinik et al, 1993).

In a primary prevention trial, gemfibrozil reduced the risk of cardiovascular disease, particularly Q-wave myocardial infarction, by approximately 2% for each 1% decrease in serum LDL-cholesterol concentration and 3% for every 1% increase in serum HDL-cholesterol concentration (Mänttäri et al, 1990). In patients with the "lipid triad" (elevated ratio of serum LDL-cholesterol concentration to serum HDL-cholesterol concentration and plasma triglyceride concentration >500 mg/dL) but without established CHD, gemfibrozil reduced the incidence of primary cardiac events by 70% (Miettinen, 1991). In a secondary prevention trial, gemfibrozil reduced the rate of progression of arterial wall lesions (Belcaro et al, 1992). However, in the Helsinki secondary prevention study, gemfibrozil treatment was associated with an increase in the incidence of cardiac events. The effects of gemfibrozil and cholestyramine on serum LDL- and HDL-cholesterol concentrations are additive (Ödman et al, 1991).

Clofibrate may decrease serum LDL-cholesterol and plasma triglyceride concentrations, especially in familial dysbetalipoproteinemia; xanthomas regress and peripheral vascular disease improves. However, long-term use of clofibrate is associated with an increase in the incidence of peripheral vascular disease, intermittent claudication, pulmonary embolism, thrombophlebitis, angina pectoris, increased heart size, arrhythmias, cholelithiasis, decreased libido, and breast tenderness (Coronary Drug Project Research Group, 1975). Furthermore, a large primary prevention trial conducted in Europe confirmed that clofibrate can cause excessive mortality from noncardiac causes (Oliver et al, 1984). Because of the risks, most clinicians avoid clofibrate entirely or restrict its use to patients with familial dysbetalipoproteinemia who do not respond to gemfibrozil, niacin, or HMG-CoA reductase inhibitors.

In double-blind trials, fenofibrate (100 mg three times daily) or bezafibrate (400 to 600 mg daily) given with modified-fat diets for one to six months reduced serum LDL-cholesterol concentrations by an additional 5% to 37% and plasma triglyceride concentrations by 13% to 67% and increased serum HDL-cholesterol concentrations by 10% to 34% in hypercholesterolemic patients with mild hypertriglyceridemia when compared with the effects achieved with diet therapy and placebo (see reviews by Monk and Todd, 1987; Balfour et al, 1990). In open-label trials, similar effects were maintained with use of fenofibrate for up to seven years and bezafibrate for up to 4.5 years (Olsson et al, 1985). Fenofibrate (200 to 400 mg/day) has stimulated regression of narrowing of coronary arteries (Hahmann et al, 1991). Fenofibrate and bezafibrate have reduced plasma triglyceride concentrations by more than 80% compared with placebo in patients with severe hypertriglyceridemia, but serum LDL-cholesterol concentrations have increased by as much as 100% in some patients (Goldberg et al, 1989); the largest increases occurred with bezafibrate. The drug-induced increases may not be detrimental in patients with severe hypertriglyceridemia because their baseline serum LDL-cholesterol concentrations often are abnormally low.

Fenofibrate (100 mg three or four times daily) and bezafibrate (200 mg three or four times daily) have comparable effects on lipidemia, and both are somewhat superior to clofibrate (Monk and Todd, 1987; Balfour et al, 1990). There is no advantage to administration of bezafibrate 200 mg three times daily compared with 400 mg once daily, and a prolonged-release formulation (400 mg daily) is no more effective than a standard preparation containing 400 mg given once daily (Bimmermann et al, 1991).

Bezafibrate may be more effective than gemfibrozil in lowering serum LDL-cholesterol concentrations but is less effective in raising serum HDL-cholesterol concentrations (Kremer et al, 1989). Fenofibrate has decreased plasma triglyceride concentrations more than either simvastatin or probucol, and bezafibrate has had a greater effect than probucol (Moreno and González, 1989). In contrast, simvastatin was more effective than fenofibrate in reducing serum LDL-cholesterol concentrations (Bard et al, 1992). Fenofibrate or bezafibrate plus bile acid sequestering resins or niacin have additive effects in decreasing serum LDL-cholesterol and plasma triglyceride concentrations and in increasing serum HDL-cholesterol concentrations.

Fenofibrate and bezafibrate retain their effectiveness in either IDDM or NIDDM accompanied by elevated serum cholesterol and plasma triglyceride concentrations and do not adversely affect glycemic control (Karhapää et al, 1992), and they can be used to reduce hypertriglyceridemia in adults with pancreatitis (Zimetbaum et al, 1991). Bezafibrate has been safe and effective in the treatment of hypertriglyceridemia and low serum HDL-cholesterol concentration in patients with chronic renal insufficiency and in those on renal dialysis.

ADVERSE REACTIONS. Use of clofibrate increases the risk of cholelithiasis, cholecystitis requiring surgery, peripheral vascular disease, intermittent claudication, pulmonary embolism, thrombophlebitis, angina pectoris, arrhythmias, elevated plasma urea nitrogen, and depressed hematocrit.

Gemfibrozil, bezafibrate, and fenofibrate are quite well tolerated. Gastrointestinal disturbances (nausea, vomiting, diarrhea, dyspepsia, and flatulence) occur in about 10% of patients but are usually transient and disappear with continued therapy. Less frequently, anemia, weight gain, decreased libido, headache, impotence, breast tenderness, leukopenia, hypokalemia, rash, drowsiness, and alopecia areata have been noted.

Potentially serious effects on skeletal and cardiac muscle are infrequent during gemfibrozil monotherapy. Serum creatinine phosphokinase (CPK) activity may increase, and frank myositis with asthenia, myalgia, and malaise may develop. Patients with the nephrotic syndrome and those with low serum albumin concentrations are at particularly high risk for these side effects. Elevated serum CPK activity may persist after other serum enzyme activities have returned to normal and the patient has become asymptomatic.

Fenofibrate and bezafibrate may reduce plasma fibrinogen concentrations (Branchi et al, 1993).

Reversible elevations in serum ALT and AST activities have been noted, especially with clofibrate.

Doses five to eight times higher than those used in humans have increased the incidence of malignant hepatic tumors in rodents. Clofibrate may tend to increase the incidence of hepatobiliary and rectal tumors in humans (Oliver et al, 1984).

PRECAUTIONS. Patients receiving long-term therapy must be supervised closely. Fibric acid derivatives should be used with caution and in reduced doses in those with impaired renal or hepatic function, since delayed detoxification and excretion make the duration of action unpredictable. Serum ALT and AST activities should be determined periodically in all patients receiving clofibrate.

These drugs increase biliary cholesterol saturation, which may promote gallstone formation; therefore, they are contraindicated in patients with pre-existing gallbladder disease. Gemfibrozil may increase plasma fibrinogen concentration (Stringer et al, 1990).

Fibric acid derivatives may cross the placenta and may be excreted in milk; their use is contraindicated during pregnancy and lactation. No information is available concerning the safety or effectiveness of these drugs in children or the elderly.

DRUG INTERACTIONS. Fibric acid derivatives potentiate the action of coumarin anticoagulants. The dose of anticoagulants must be reduced by at least one-half for most patients, and prothrombin times should be determined frequently, especially during initiation of therapy.

Gemfibrozil and clofibrate may displace sulfonylureas from plasma protein binding sites and precipitate severe hypoglycemia (Ahmad, 1991 A). Probenecid may decrease binding of clofibrate to plasma proteins and accelerate clofibrate clearance.

The absorption of fibric acid derivatives is reduced by bile acid sequestrants; administration of drugs in these two classes should be separated by at least two hours (Forland et al, 1990).

The incidence of skeletal muscle myopathy is about 3% to 5% when gemfibrozil is administered with lovastatin. In contrast, the risk of clinical myopathy may be lower during combination therapy with gemfibrozil and pravastatin (Wiklund, 1993).

PHARMACOKINETICS. Absorption of clofibrate in oral doses of up to 2 g daily is complete and is followed by rapid gastrointestinal and hepatic de-esterification to an active metabolite, chlorophenoxyisobutyric acid (CPIB). Peak plasma concentrations of CPIB are usually attained in three to six hours. The mean plasma elimination half-life of CPIB is 15 hours. Plasma protein binding decreases as the dose increases and is associated with increased plasma clearance of CPIB. Approximately 10% to 20% of CPIB is recovered in the urine unchanged; 40% to 70% is excreted as a glucuronide ester. Peak effect is obtained after three weeks of use, and pretreatment serum VLDL concentrations recur within three weeks after discontinuation of the drug.

Gemfibrozil is completely absorbed. Peak plasma and tissue concentrations and maximum tissue contents are attained in one to two hours. Plasma concentrations are proportional to the dose, and there is no evidence of accumulation with twice daily administration. Gemfibrozil is 95% bound to serum albumin. The plasma elimination half-life is 1.5 hours; 70% of a dose is excreted unchanged, primarily in the urine.

About 30% of a dose of fenofibrate is absorbed; absorption increases twofold when the drug is taken with food. Fenofibrate is hydrolyzed to fenofibric acid during absorption, and peak plasma fenofibric acid concentrations occur four to six hours after ingestion. Plasma concentration reaches a steady state after five days. Over 99% of circulating fenofibric acid is bound to plasma proteins. Maximum tissue concentrations are reached after eight hours. About 30% of a dose is excreted in the urine as fenofibryl glucuronide. The plasma elimination half-life of fenofibric acid is 20 to 27 hours.

Bezafibrate is absorbed virtually completely. Peak plasma concentrations occur two hours after a single dose of 300 mg. Circulating bezafibrate is 94% to 96% bound to plasma proteins. About 40% of a dose is excreted unchanged in the urine; an additional 22% is excreted as glucuronides and 20% as other metabolites. The mean plasma elimination half-life is about two hours.

DOSAGE AND PREPARATIONS.

CLOFIBRATE:

Oral: *Adults,* 500 mg two to four times daily.
Atromid-S (Wyeth-Ayerst), ***Generic***. Capsules 500 mg.

FENOFIBRATE:

Oral: *Adults,* 100 mg once daily.
Lipidil (Fournier). Tablets 100 mg.

GEMFIBROZIL:

Oral: *Adults,* 600 mg once or twice daily (one-half hour before breakfast and dinner). Doses of 600 mg to 1.2 g/day are equally effective in postmenopausal women and middle-aged men (Koskinen et al, 1992).
Lopid (Parke-Davis). Capsules 300 mg; tablets 600 mg.

HMG-CoA REDUCTASE INHIBITORS

FLUVASTATIN SODIUM
[Lescol]

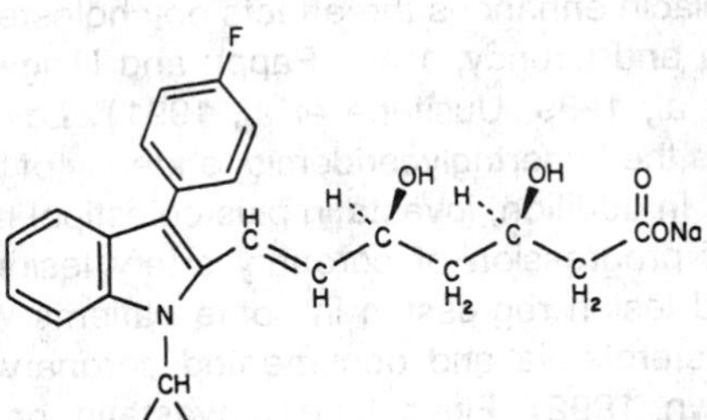

LOVASTATIN
[Mevacor]

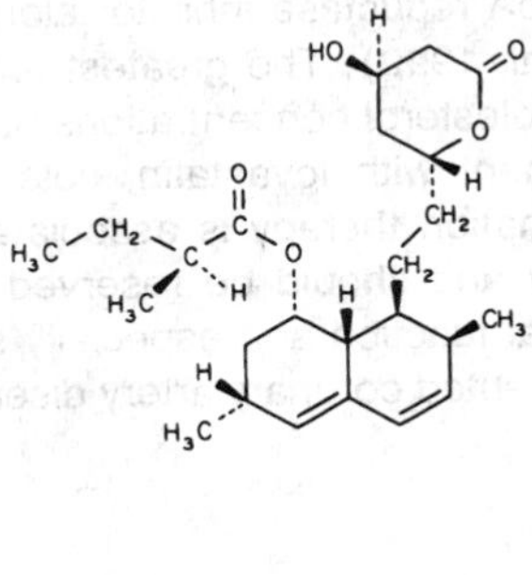

PRAVASTATIN SODIUM
[Pravachol]

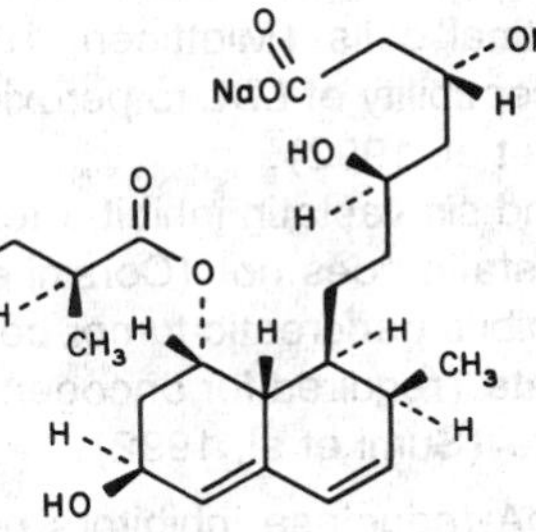

SIMVASTATIN
[Zocor]

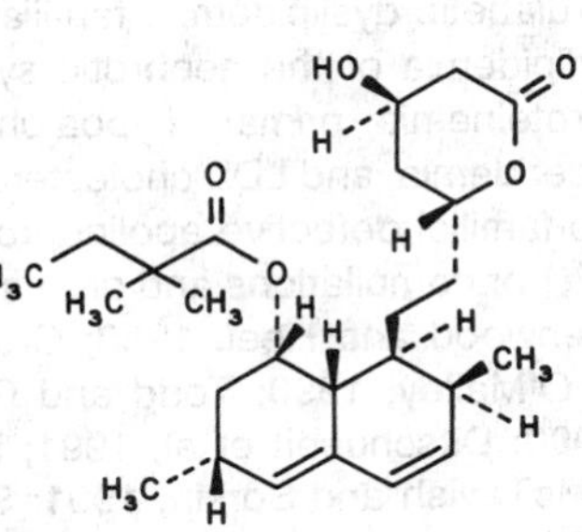

ACTIONS. The drugs in this class of oral lipid-lowering agents directly inhibit cholesterol synthesis. Pravastatin is the sodium salt of pravastatin β-hydroxyacid, fluvastatin is the sodium salt of fluvastatin dihydroxyacid, and lovastatin and simvastatin are inactive tricyclic lactone prodrugs. These drugs undergo extensive carrier-mediated first-pass extraction by the liver, where the lactones are activated by hydroxylation to open β-hydroxyacids; the β-hydroxyacids and fluvastatin dihydroxyacid are potent inhibitors of hepatic HMG-CoA reductase (Hoeg and Brewer, 1987; Grundy, 1988).

Inhibition of cholesterol synthesis stimulates up-regulation of high-affinity cell surface receptors for LDL; as hepatic uptake of LDL increases, serum total and LDL-cholesterol concentrations decrease. In addition, hepatic synthesis of apolipoprotein B and VLDL is inhibited by HMG-CoA reductase inhibitors, especially fluvastatin (Jokubaitis et al, 1993; Levy et al, 1993). Ultimately, the number of LDL particles in the circulation is reduced as a new steady-state is attained (Vega et al, 1990; Levy et al, 1993). However, lipoprotein(a) concentrations and whole-body cholesterol metabolism are unchanged (O'Connor et al, 1992; Goldberg et al, 1990 A).

Through mechanisms that are poorly understood, increases in serum HDL-cholesterol concentrations frequently accompany decreases in serum LDL-cholesterol concentrations, although the correlation between changes in these two lipoprotein complexes is unknown (Alessandri et al, 1992; Kaeser et al, 1992; Levy et al, 1993). Simvastatin has been shown to increase the HDL_{2b} subfraction (Johannson et al, 1991; Neuman et al, 1991).

HMG-CoA reductase inhibitors significantly inhibit the absorption of dietary cholesterol (Vanhanen et al, 1992), possibly by reducing acyl coenzyme A:cholesterol acyltransferase activity in intestinal cells (Miettinen, 1991). They also decrease the susceptibility of LDL to peroxidation (Aviram et al, 1992; Hoffman et al, 1992).

Fluvastatin and simvastatin inhibit arterial myocyte proliferation, but pravastatin does not (Corsini et al, 1993).

Lovastatin inhibits pancreatic tumor cell synthesis of farnesyl pyrophosphate (required for oncogene activation) and reduces tumor size (Sumi et al, 1992).

USES. HMG-CoA reductase inhibitors produce dose-related decreases in serum concentrations of total, LDL-, and VLDL-cholesterol; apolipoprotein B; and triglycerides in the following disorders: heterozygous familial and polygenic (nonfamilial) primary hypercholesterolemias, familial combined hyperlipidemia, diabetic dyslipidemia, familial dysbetalipoproteinemia, hyperlipidemia of the nephrotic syndrome, primary hypoalphalipoproteinemia, primary hypoalphalipoproteinemia with hypertriglyceridemia, and LDL-cholesterol concentrations in heterozygous familial defective apolipoprotein B-100 dyslipoproteinemia. (For compilations and discussions of individual trials, see Henwood and Heel, 1988; Grundy et al, 1990; Illingworth and O'Malley, 1990; Todd and Goa, 1990; Vega and Grundy, 1990; Ditschuneit et al, 1991; Mauro and MacDonald, 1991; McTavish and Sorkin, 1991; Stuyt et al, 1991; Chrisp et al, 1992; Hunninghake, 1992; Illingworth et al, 1992 A; Jungnickel et al, 1992; Miccoli et al, 1992; Shear et al, 1992; Torri et al, 1992; Jokubaitis et al, 1993; Levy et al, 1993; Mauro, 1993.) Because their primary action depends on the presence of functioning LDL receptors to decrease serum total and LDL-cholesterol concentrations, HMG-CoA reductase inhibitors are much less effective in homozygous receptor-defective familial hypercholesterolemia (Brown and Goldstein, 1986) and are ineffective in homozygous receptor-negative familial hypercholesterolemia (Uauy et al, 1988; Levy et al, 1993).

Beneficial effects on serum total and LDL-cholesterol concentrations have been sustained during three to five years of continued treatment with lovastatin, pravastatin, and simvastatin, but initial decreases in VLDL-cholesterol, triglyceride, and apolipoprotein B concentrations have diminished after one to three years (Lintott et al, 1991; Nakandakare et al, 1991; Simons et al, 1992 A). Long-term experience with fluvastatin has been limited to one year; initial therapeutic effects were not diminished at that time. Lovastatin, pravastatin, and simvastatin have been safe and effective in the treatment of hypercholesterolemic patients with renal disease, diabetic nephropathy, elevated blood pressure, or coronary heart disease; after renal or cardiac transplantation; and during continuous ambulatory peritoneal dialysis (Kuo et al, 1989; Kannel et al, 1990; Kasiske et al, 1990 A, 1990 B; Barbir et al, 1991; Bazzato et al, 1991; Wanner et al, 1991; Ballantyne et al, 1992; Biesenbach and Zazgornik, 1992; Yoshimura et al, 1992; Lal, 1993; Arca et al, 1994). The few available data suggest that the efficacy and safety of HMG-CoA reductase inhibitors in women and elderly men are comparable to their effects in younger male patients (D'Agostino et al, 1992; Lintott and Scott, 1992; Bradford et al, 1993; Arca et al, 1994).

Lovastatin, pravastatin, and simvastatin consistently have been more effective than gemfibrozil, probucol, neomycin, cholestyramine, or colestipol in reducing serum total and LDL-cholesterol concentrations and increasing serum HDL-cholesterol concentrations in hypercholesterolemias. They also blunt the tendency of bile acid sequestrants to increase plasma triglyceride concentration. In contrast, gemfibrozil has been more effective than lovastatin, pravastatin, or simvastatin in reducing hypertriglyceridemia and in increasing serum HDL-cholesterol concentration in individuals with isolated hypoalphalipoproteinemia (Hunninghake, 1992; Muggeo et al, 1992) and in heart transplant recipients (Peters et al, 1993). The comparative efficacy of fluvastatin has not been examined.

Results of trials comparing the HMG-CoA reductase inhibitors in the treatment of primary hypercholesterolemia have shown that lovastatin and pravastatin (20 to 80 mg/day) are comparable (Richter et al, 1991 A; Vanhanen and Miettinen, 1992). On a milligram-for-milligram basis, low doses of simvastatin (2.5 to 10 mg/day) are twice as effective as lovastatin in decreasing serum total and LDL-cholesterol, apolipoprotein B, and triglyceride concentrations (Malini et al, 1991; The European Study Group, 1992; Farmer et al, 1992; Illingworth et al, 1992 B; Volpe et al, 1992). Similarly, low doses of simvastatin are one to one and a half times as effective as equal doses of pravastatin (The Simvastatin Pravastatin Study Group, 1993). With larger doses of simvastatin (eg, 20 mg twice daily), there are few differences in the effects of the HMG-CoA reductase inhibitors on lipid metabolism (Pan et al, 1990 A; Ditschuneit et al, 1991).

Combining lovastatin with colestipol, cholestyramine, neomycin, or niacin enhances the effects on cholesterol metabolism (Vega and Grundy, 1987; Pappu and Illingworth, 1989; Witztum et al, 1989; Uusitupa et al, 1991). Lovastatin also counteracts the hypertriglyceridemic tendency of bile acid sequestrants. In addition, lovastatin plus colestipol has reduced the rate of progression of coronary artery lesions and has accelerated lesion regression in some patients with primary hypercholesterolemia and documented coronary artery disease (Brown, 1992). Fluvastatin, pravastatin, or simvastatin plus cholestyramine or colestipol has reduced serum lipid concentrations to a greater extent than any HMG-CoA reductase inhibitor alone (Hoogerbrugge et al, 1990; Pan et al, 1990 B; Kostis et al, 1992; Simons et al, 1992 B; Levy et al, 1993). However, the combination of probucol and pravastatin or lovastatin did not improve the response over that observed with the HMG-CoA reductase inhibitor alone (Witztum et al, 1989; Kostis et al, 1992). The greatest reductions in serum total and LDL-cholesterol concentrations have occurred after combined treatment with lovastatin, colestipol, and niacin. However, combination therapy is associated with increased risk of myopathy and should be reserved for patients who have normal renal function and especially severe lipoprotein disorders, documented coronary artery disease, or resistance to monotherapy.

Preliminary evidence suggests that these drugs also may reduce biliary cholesterol excretion, accelerate gallstone dissolution, and decrease the incidence of cholesterol gallstones (Mazzella et al, 1992; Smit et al, 1992).

HMG-CoA reductase inhibitors should be employed as adjuncts to dietary management, exercise, and, when appropriate, weight reduction to reduce elevated total and LDL-cholesterol concentrations in patients with hypercholesterolemia. However, strict compliance with a low-fat diet may allow a reduction in the dosage of drug required to achieve a therapeutic goal (Cobb et al, 1991; Smith et al, 1993).

Small groups of hypercholesterolemic children have been successfully and safely treated with simvastatin 10 to 40 mg/day (Ducobu et al, 1992) or lovastatin 20 mg/day (Sinzinger et al, 1992) for relatively short periods. However, the safety and effectiveness of these agents in children under 18 years have not been established, and their use in this population is not recommended.

ADVERSE REACTIONS. HMG-CoA reductase inhibitors are generally well tolerated for at least five years and cause fewer adverse reactions than bile sequestering resins (Boccuzzi et al, 1993; Nakandakare et al, 1991; Lovastatin Study Groups I Through IV, 1993; McGovern and Mellies, 1993). This conclusion appears valid for patients up to 83 years old (Antonicelli et al, 1990; Ruiz et al, 1991; D'Agostino et al, 1992). The adverse reactions observed with fluvastatin, lovastatin, pravastatin, and simvastatin are similar.

Rhabdomyolysis with myalgia, with or without acute renal failure secondary to myoglobinuria, has occurred in fewer than 0.2% of patients receiving HMG-CoA reductase inhibitor monotherapy (Bradford et al, 1991). The incidence increases to 1% to 2% when lovastatin is administered with niacin, to 3% to 5% when it is combined with gemfibrozil, and may reach 30% in immunosuppressed patients receiving cyclosporine. Myopathy has been reported in some patients receiving lovastatin and erythromycin (Spach et al, 1991). However, combining pravastatin with these agents is less risky. Patients unable to tolerate gemfibrozil may be switched to HMG-CoA reductase inhibitor therapy without an adverse effect (Ojala et al, 1990). Lovastatin alone may increase the risk of exertional myopathy (Reust et al, 1991).

Reversible elevation of serum AST and ALT concentrations occurs in 1% to 2% of patients receiving these drugs. The increases may be gradual or abrupt and often are asymptomatic and transient. Rarely, lovastatin has been associated with jaundice or other signs or symptoms, including hypersensitivity (McQueen, 1990). If the serum AST or ALT concentration exceeds three times normal at successive determinations, HMG-CoA reductase inhibitor therapy should be discontinued. There is some evidence to suggest that alcoholic patients may be more prone to this adverse reaction.

Minor gastrointestinal disturbances include constipation, diarrhea, flatulence, nausea, and dyspepsia; their incidence ranges from 2% to 6% and is similar to the response to placebo. Intestinal cell growth and turnover are apparently not affected (Gebhard et al, 1991). Blurred vision, dysgeusia, headache, and rash have been noted infrequently. A few patients have developed a lupus erythematosus-like syndrome during lovastatin therapy (Ahmad, 1991 B). Although several small studies have suggested that lovastatin and simvastatin (but not pravastatin) may disturb sleep patterns (Newman et al, 1990 B; Scott et al, 1991; Vgontzas et al, 1991) and impair ability to concentrate (Roth et al, 1992), such effects have not been observed in large placebo-controlled trials (Bradford et al, 1991).

Anemia, thrombocytopenia, leukopenia, and transient asymptomatic eosinophilia have been reported. Blood fibrinogen concentrations may increase during treatment with HMG-CoA reductase inhibitors (Beigel et al, 1991). However, this has not been a consistent finding, and other investigators have observed either a slight decrease or no change (McDowell et al, 1991; Sandset et al, 1991; Illingworth et al, 1992).

Initial concerns that treatment with HMG-CoA reductase inhibitors may interfere with cholesterol-dependent steroid hormone synthesis have not been substantiated. In three studies, 24 weeks of treatment with pravastatin or one year of simvastatin therapy did not alter testosterone, sex hormone binding globulin, androstenedione, dehydroepiandrosterone sulfate, estradiol, 17α-hydroxyprogesterone, follicle-stimulating hormone, or luteinizing hormone concentrations in males or premenopausal or postmenopausal females with heterozygous familial hypercholesterolemia (Jay et al, 1991; Azzarito et al, 1992; Honjo et al, 1992). Similarly, 14 weeks of simvastatin therapy did not affect sperm number, concentration, motility, velocity, or vitality or the frequency of abnormalities (Purvis et al, 1992). Neither pravastatin nor simvastatin has affected the synthesis or secretion of cortisol, ACTH, renin, or vitamin D_3 (unhydroxylated cholecalciferol) (Mol et al, 1989; Ide et al, 1990; Dobs et al, 1991; Jay et al, 1991; Prihoda et al, 1991; Azzarito et al, 1992).

Adverse ophthalmologic findings in dogs given very high doses of HMG-CoA reductase inhibitors resulted in a recommendation that ocular slit-lamp examinations be performed periodically in patients taking lovastatin. However, no statistically or clinically significant adverse ophthalmologic effects have been reported in humans during up to five years of therapy with lovastatin or pravastatin; visual acuity was higher in lovastatin recipients than in those receiving placebo (Newman et al, 1990 B; Laties et al, 1991). Subsequently, the Food and Drug Administration eliminated the recommendation for periodic eye examinations of patients treated with lovastatin.

In rodents, the incidence of hepatocellular carcinoma and adenoma, malignant lymphoma, lung adenoma, thyroid follicular adenoma, and adenoma of the Harderian glands in the eye increased in those given very high daily doses of HMG-CoA reductase inhibitors for one to two years. No evidence of mutagenicity has been observed, and no predisposition to human cancers has been associated with HMG-CoA reductase inhibitor use.

PRECAUTIONS. Before initiating drug therapy, the importance of dietary modification should be stressed. Care should be taken to exclude secondary causes of dyslipidemia, including poorly controlled diabetes mellitus, hypothyroidism, nephrotic syndrome, dysproteinemias, obstructive liver disease, alcoholism, and treatment with amiodarone, progestins, anabolic steroids, isotretinoin, corticosteroids, cyclosporine, or thiazide diuretics (O'Leary et al, 1987; Durrington, 1990; Glazer, 1991; Henkin et al, 1992).

Because of the potential effects of HMG-CoA reductase inhibitors on the liver and muscle (see Adverse Reactions), serum AST and ALT concentrations should be determined prior to initiation of therapy, every six weeks for the first three months of therapy, every eight weeks for the remainder of the first year, and then semiannually. If the concentration of either enzyme increases, more frequent monitoring is required. If the increase is progressive or persistently exceeds three times the upper limit of normal, therapy should be discontinued. A liver biopsy should be considered if the elevation persists after discontinuation of therapy.

HMG-CoA reductase inhibitors should be used with caution in patients who consume substantial quantities of alcohol or have a history of liver disease, which can increase plasma half-lives (Smith et al, 1993). Active liver disease or unexplained elevations in serum transaminase concentrations are contraindications to their use.

HMG-CoA reductase inhibitor therapy should be discontinued if myopathy, defined as muscle aching or weakness with increases in serum creatine phosphokinase concentrations exceeding 10 times the upper limit of normal, is diagnosed or suspected. Therapy also should be temporarily withheld from any patient experiencing an acute or serious condition predisposing to the development of renal failure secondary to rhabdomyolysis (eg, sepsis; hypotension; major surgery; trauma; severe metabolic, endocrine, or electrolyte disorders; uncontrolled epilepsy).

Patients with cholestasis should not be given HMG-CoA reductase inhibitors; impaired drug excretion may elevate serum drug concentrations, inducing myopathy.

DRUG INTERACTIONS. The risk of myopathy and life-threatening rhabdomyolysis increases when lovastatin is combined with immunosuppressive agents, gemfibrozil, niacin, or erythromycin (Pierce et al, 1990; Spach et al, 1991). Cyclosporine may increase peripheral tissue exposure to HMG-CoA reductase inhibitors by inducing cholestasis and inhibiting drug excretion via bile (Smith et al, 1991).

Hypoprothrombinemia, prolonged prothrombin time, and bleeding have occurred in a few patients stabilized on warfarin and then treated with lovastatin (Ahmad, 1990). In contrast, fluvastatin, pravastatin, or simvastatin has not affected prothrombin time in warfarin-treated patients (Feely and O'Connor, 1991). Simvastatin (but not fluvastatin, lovastatin, or pravastatin) inhibits the clearance of digoxin. Propranolol may slightly increase first-pass hepatic extraction of HMG-CoA reductase inhibitors, but the clinical significance of this effect is limited (Pan et al, 1991 A; Smith et al, 1993).

Cholestyramine decreases the absorption of fluvastatin (Smith et al, 1993) or pravastatin (Pan et al, 1990 B) when these agents are taken together. Aspirin, niacin, gemfibrozil, and probucol have no effect on absorption of pravastatin (Pan, 1991).

Caution should be exercised if HMG-CoA reductase inhibitors are administered to patients receiving drugs that may decrease the secretion or activity of endogenous steroid hormones (eg, ketoconazole, spironolactone, cimetidine). Patients who develop clinical evidence of endocrine dysfunction should be re-evaluated.

HMG-CoA reductase inhibitors have no effect on the microsomal oxidizing enzyme systems responsible for the metabolism of many drugs. No drug interactions have occurred with angiotensin-converting enzyme inhibitors, antihypertensive agents, nitroglycerin, calcium-channel blocking agents, diuretics, insulin, oral hypoglycemic agents, and nonsteroidal anti-inflammatory agents (Goldberg et al, 1990 B; Johnson et al, 1990; Garg, 1992; Ikeda et al, 1992; Pool et al, 1992; Jokubaitis et al, 1993; Levy et al, 1993).

PREGNANCY AND LACTATION. The safety of HMG-CoA reductase inhibitors in pregnant women has not been established; cholesterol and its metabolites are essential for proper fetal development and the effect of reducing maternal cholesterol synthesis on the human fetus is unknown. However, very high doses of lovastatin have produced malformations in rat and mouse fetuses, and lovastatin and simvastatin are known to cross the placenta. These drugs should be administered to women of childbearing potential only when they are unlikely to conceive and have been informed of the potential hazards (FDA Pregnancy Category X). If a woman conceives while taking one of these agents, therapy should be discontinued and the potential for fetal harm emphasized.

It is not known whether fluvastatin, lovastatin, or simvastatin is excreted in human milk. Because a small fraction of pravastatin is excreted by the lactating breast (Pan, 1991) and inhibition of cholesterol synthesis in infants may be dangerous, all HMG-CoA reductase inhibitors are contraindicated during lactation.

PHARMACOKINETICS. HMG-CoA reductase inhibitors are only partially absorbed and undergo extensive first-pass extraction in the liver; less than 5% of an oral dose of these drugs reaches the systemic circulation (Pan et al, 1990 A; Tse et al, 1992; Mauro, 1993). Peak plasma concentrations are achieved within two to four hours after ingestion of lovastatin and simvastatin and 0.7 to 1.5 hours after ingestion of fluvastatin or pravastatin. With once-daily administration, steady-state serum concentrations of active metabolites are attained after two to three days. Although serum concentrations of active metabolites are highly variable and correlate poorly with therapeutic efficacy, they correlate directly with the incidence and severity of adverse reactions.

Lovastatin and simvastatin β-hydroxyacids are, respectively, 75 and 200 times more lipophilic than pravastatin and appear to penetrate nonhepatic cells much more readily (Roth et al, 1991; Serajuddin et al, 1991). In addition, lovastatin and simvastatin cross the blood-brain and placental barriers, but fluvastatin and pravastatin do not (Botti et al, 1991; Terasaki et al, 1991; Guillot et al, 1993). The poor lipophilicity of fluvastatin and pravastatin may contribute to their limited penetration into nonhepatic cells (Jokubaitis et al, 1993).

These drugs are primarily excreted in bile; 60%, 70%, 83%, and 95% of the dose of simvastatin, pravastatin, lovastatin, and fluvastatin, respectively, appear in the feces. Both lovastatin and simvastatin and their β-hydroxyacid metabolites are highly bound ($>$95%) to human plasma proteins;

only 50% of circulating pravastatin is protein bound. The major end products of metabolism of these drugs are the 3α-hydroxyisomer of pravastatin and the 6′-hydroxyacid derivatives of simvastatin and lovastatin (Henwood and Heel, 1988; Singhvi et al, 1990; Everett et al, 1991; Tse et al, 1992; Mauro, 1993; Smith et al, 1993).

DOSAGE AND PREPARATIONS. Dosage should be individualized on the basis of pretreatment serum total and LDL-cholesterol concentrations, the goal of therapy, and the patient's response. Serum total and LDL-cholesterol concentrations should be monitored periodically, and any dosage adjustments should be made at intervals of four weeks or more. The dosage for patients with renal insufficiency should be increased gradually and in small increments.

FLUVASTATIN:

Oral: *Adults,* initially, 20 mg daily at bedtime; for maintenance, the range is 20 to a maximum of 40 mg once daily at bedtime or in two divided doses. Fluvastatin may be taken without regard to meals, but it should be taken at least four hours after bile acid sequestering resins.

Lescol (Sandoz). Capsules 20 and 40 mg.

LOVASTATIN:

Oral: *Adults,* initially, 10 mg (serum total cholesterol concentration <240 mg/dL) or 20 mg (serum total cholesterol concentration >240 mg/dL) once daily in the evening (Lovastatin Study Groups I Through IV, 1993). High-fiber diets may impede drug absorption and should precede drug administration by several hours (Richter et al, 1991 B). The recommended range is 20 to a maximum of 80 mg/day in single or divided doses. Divided doses may be more effective (Bradford et al, 1991). In *elderly patients,* the maximum therapeutic effect may be obtained with doses ≤40 mg/day (D'Agostino et al, 1992).

Mevacor (Merck). Tablets 10, 20, and 40 mg.

PRAVASTATIN:

Oral: *Adults,* initially, 10 or 20 mg once daily at bedtime; for maintenance, the range is 10 to a maximum of 40 mg once daily at bedtime. There are no important differences in effects between divided and once-daily doses, but this drug is most effective when taken in the evening (Hunninghake et al, 1990; Pan et al, 1991 B). In *elderly patients,* initially, 10 mg/day at bedtime; the maximum therapeutic effect may be obtained with doses of ≤20 mg/day (Bo et al, 1991). Pravastatin may be taken without regard to meals, but it should be taken one hour before or four hours after bile acid sequestering resins.

Pravachol (Bristol-Myers Squibb). Tablets 10 and 20 mg.

SIMVASTATIN:

Oral: *Adults,* initially, 5 or 10 mg once daily in the evening (Saito et al, 1991); for maintenance, the range is 5 to a maximum of 40 mg/day. In *elderly patients,* the maximum therapeutic effect may be obtained with doses of ≤20 mg/day (Antonicelli et al, 1990; Bach et al, 1990; Walker et al, 1990).

Zocor (Merck). Tablets 5, 10, 20, and 40 mg.

OTHER AGENTS

NIACIN (Nicotinic Acid)

[Niacor, Nicolar, Nico-400]

For chemical formula, see index entry Niacin, As Vitamin.

ACTIONS. Niacin (as nicotinic acid) decreases hepatic VLDL synthesis and secretion. As a result, plasma triglyceride and serum VLDL and LDL-cholesterol concentrations decrease. Niacin also stimulates the synthesis and secretion of nascent HDL and apo A-I, which often increase serum HDL_3 concentration. Serum HDL_2 concentration also may rise. In familial dysbetalipoproteinemia, serum lipid concentrations may be reduced to normal.

Niacinamide has no lipid-lowering properties (Parsons, 1960).

USES. Niacin in doses of 1.2 g/day or greater is quite effective in lowering elevated serum LDL-cholesterol and plasma triglyceride concentrations and may be useful in all types of lipoprotein disorders except familial hyperchylomicronemia (Figge et al, 1988; Alderman et al, 1989; Henkin et al, 1991; Expert Panel, 1993). Niacin may significantly increase serum HDL concentrations in hypoalphalipoproteinemia (Vega and Grundy, 1994). When given with other hypolipidemic drugs, smaller doses may be adequate and the drug may be better tolerated.

Niacin (3 g/day for six years) reduced serum total cholesterol and plasma triglyceride concentrations, the incidence of nonfatal myocardial infarction, and total and cardiovascular mortality in the Coronary Drug Project trial of secondary prevention of cardiovascular disease in men with previous myocardial infarction (Coronary Drug Project Research Group, 1975; Canner et al, 1986). However, niacin may have prevented only milder nonfatal myocardial events (Berge and Canner, 1991).

Large doses of niacin (3 to 12 g daily) plus colestipol (30 g daily) given in addition to stringent dietary restriction to patients following coronary bypass surgery (Cholesterol-Lowering Atherosclerosis Study) reduced serum total and LDL-cholesterol concentrations, increased serum HDL-cholesterol concentrations, and decreased atheroma formation and progression for up to four years (Blankenhorn et al, 1993 B; Cashin-Hemphill et al, 1990). Similarly, niacin (2.5 to 4.5 g daily) and colestipol (30 g daily) were superior to colestipol alone in a 32-month study of men with documented coronary arterial atherosclerosis (Familial Atherosclerosis Treatment Study); the incidence of myocardial infarction or need for revascularization also were reduced by combination drug treatment (Brown et al, 1990).

Niacin has reduced serum total, LDL-, and VLDL-cholesterol concentrations in cardiac transplant recipients, although serum HDL-cholesterol concentrations were not changed (Henkin et al, 1991).

Doses of 2 g/day or less, used to minimize the incidence and severity of adverse reactions, do not always decrease serum total or LDL-cholesterol or plasma triglyceride concentrations (Alderman et al, 1989; Henkin et al, 1991). However, even 1 g/day may be sufficient to increase serum HDL-cholesterol concentrations.

Prolonged-release forms of niacin have been developed in attempts to improve patient compliance by limiting adverse reactions. However, in one study, compliance decreased when prolonged-release niacin 3 g/day was given (Knopp et al, 1985). Among the compliant, reductions in serum LDL-cholesterol and plasma triglyceride concentrations were only 62% and 30% as large, respectively, as those achieved with standard niacin formulations. In addition, serum total HDL- and HDL_2-cholesterol concentrations were not affected by prolonged-release niacin compared with 26% and 36% increases, respectively, with standard niacin. In contrast, a wax matrix-based prolonged-release formulation produced effects on total and LDL-cholesterol concentrations resembling those produced by similar doses of standard niacin and compliance was comparable (Keenan et al, 1991 A). The beneficial effects of this preparation may be more pronounced in patients older than 50 years (Keenan et al, 1991 B).

A generic niacin compound, inositol hexaniacinate [Nicinol], has been developed in an effort to reduce the adverse effects of oral niacin. This compound is de-esterified in the liver, gradually releasing nicotinic acid into the circulation. Inositol hexaniacinate is as effective as niacin in reducing serum total cholesterol and fasting plasma triglyceride concentrations, and few of the adverse reactions that occur with conventional niacin therapy have been reported (El-Enein et al, 1983).

ADVERSE REACTIONS AND PRECAUTIONS. Niacin often produces potentially troublesome side effects, but 2 g/day or less is usually well tolerated. Flushing (mediated through prostaglandin release) occurs initially in almost all patients and persists in 10% to 15%. This effect often can be ameliorated by concomitant use of aspirin 325 mg taken 30 minutes before niacin or by use of a prolonged-release formulation; however, an increase in gastrointestinal side effects may necessitate cessation of therapy with the latter preparation. Other common untoward effects are pruritus, dry skin with scaling, and gastrointestinal irritation (eg, nausea, gastritis, vomiting, flatulence, diarrhea). Gastrointestinal symptoms may subside with continued therapy. Use of small initial doses that are increased gradually reduces the severity of these reactions in most patients.

More serious reactions are activation of peptic ulcer, impaired glucose tolerance, hyperuricemia, and liver dysfunction, including cholestatic jaundice and chronic active hepatitis. These effects are usually reversible when the drug is discontinued. However, irreversible chronic hepatitis has been reported in a few patients, especially with daily doses exceeding 3 g. Many patients with lipoprotein disorders have pre-existing hyperglycemia and hyperuricemia that may be aggravated by niacin. Allopurinol can be used to minimize the hyperuricemia. Atrial arrhythmias and blurred vision due to toxic amblyopia have been reported rarely.

Liver function tests should be performed periodically in all patients receiving niacin, and the drug should be discontinued if any liver enzymes are elevated significantly. Hepatotoxicity is more likely to occur with prolonged-release preparations (Henkin et al, 1990; Rader et al, 1992). Niacin should not be given to patients with hepatic disease, peptic ulcer, gouty arthritis, or after renal transplantation. Niacin should be avoided in patients with glucose intolerance or in those treated with oral hypoglycemic agents because of the risk of inducing hyperglycemia. However, niacin can be very useful for patients already receiving insulin. Prolonged-release preparations may cause clotting factor deficiency and coagulopathy (Dearing et al, 1992).

This drug is classified in FDA Pregnancy Category C. The safety and effectiveness of niacin in the treatment of lipid disorders in pregnant or lactating women or in children have not been established; in children, initial efficacy often is accompanied by adverse effects that require discontinuation of therapy (Colletti et al, 1993).

DRUG INTERACTIONS. Niacin may potentiate the vasodilating effects of antihypertensive drugs. If lipid-lowering doses of niacin are administered with lovastatin, myopathy may result.

PHARMACOKINETICS. Niacin is absorbed rapidly; peak concentrations are achieved in about 45 minutes. It disappears rapidly from the blood and is concentrated mainly in the liver but also appears in adipose tissue and the kidneys. Niacin has a high hepatic extraction ratio and plasma clearance may be reduced in the elderly and in patients with hepatic impairment. Renal clearance depends on the plasma concentration and may be decreased when the therapeutic concentration is high.

A greater percentage of ingested niacin from prolonged-release formulations is metabolized to nicotinuric acid, resulting in very low bioavailability and a greater likelihood of hepatotoxicity (Neuvonen et al, 1991).

DOSAGE AND PREPARATIONS.

Oral: *Adults,* initially, 100 mg three times daily, increased gradually over six to eight weeks to 1.5 to 3 g given in three or four divided doses with or after meals. Doses exceeding 4 g daily are not recommended (Havel, 1990).

NIACIN:

Available generically and under the name Nicotinic Acid: Capsules (prolonged-release) 125, 250, and 400 mg; tablets 25, 50, 100, 250 (nonprescription), and 500 mg.

Niacor (Upsher-Smith). Tablets 500 mg.

Nicolar (Rorer). Tablets 500 mg.

Nico-400 (Jones). Capsules (prolonged-release) 400 mg (nonprescription).

PROBUCOL

[Lorelco]

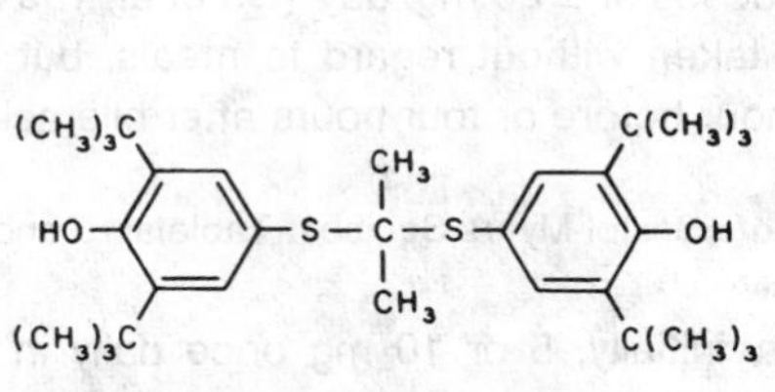

ACTIONS. Probucol, a lipophilic *bis*-phenol, decreases serum LDL-cholesterol concentrations by enhancing hepatic LDL uptake through a receptor-independent pathway and by increasing fecal bile acid excretion. It does not reduce serum triglyceride concentrations appreciably in most patients.

Serum HDL-cholesterol concentrations often decrease during probucol treatment. Although the synthesis of apo A-I may be inhibited (Berg et al, 1991), the primary mechanism that reduces serum HDL-cholesterol concentrations may be accelerated by hepatic removal of cholesterol esters from cholesterol-rich HDL ("reverse cholesterol transport"). Hepatic uptake of radiolabeled cholesterol esters from HDL is increased in probucol-treated rats with no loss of net mass transport of cholesterol into the liver despite a decrease in serum HDL-cholesterol concentrations (Richard et al, 1992). Probucol also stimulates apo E synthesis, and the fraction of HDL_{2a} cleared via the hepatic apo E receptor-mediated pathway is increased (McPherson and Marcel, 1991). CETP activity also is stimulated, triglyceride-cholesterol ester exchange between VLDL and HDL particles is increased, and cholesterol clearance via hepatic uptake of relatively cholesterol-rich VLDL remnants is accelerated (McPherson and Marcel, 1991). Accelerated clearance of HDL-cholesterol without compensatory increase in HDL synthesis would result in decreased serum HDL-cholesterol concentrations despite increased efficiency of the cholesterol efflux pathways (Zimetbaum et al, 1990).

Probucol inhibits oxidative modification of LDL particles, reducing their atherogenicity (Steinberg et al, 1989; Masana et al, 1991). The antioxidant actions of probucol may be more important than its lipid-lowering effects in preventing cardiovascular disease.

USES. Probucol is effective primarily in familial and polygenic hypercholesterolemia. Compared with diet therapy alone, diet therapy plus probucol has reduced serum LDL-cholesterol concentrations by 10% to 15% with no attenuation of effect for up to nine years (McCaughan, 1981). This effect may be even greater in those over 65 years (Morisaki et al, 1990). However, probucol also lowers serum HDL-cholesterol concentrations. Because a low serum HDL-cholesterol concentration may be a risk factor for atherogenesis, the usefulness of probucol monotherapy may be limited.

The combination of probucol plus colestipol or cholestyramine produces additive effects on serum LDL-cholesterol concentrations, while the serum HDL-cholesterol concentration-lowering effect of probucol tends to be ameliorated (Kuo et al, 1986; Sommariva et al, 1986). In contrast, probucol has not increased the effectiveness of lovastatin or pravastatin (Witztum et al, 1989; Kostis et al, 1992).

ADVERSE REACTIONS AND PRECAUTIONS. The most common adverse reactions are mild gastrointestinal disturbances (diarrhea, flatulence, abdominal pain, and nausea), which are usually transient. Less common reactions include excessive or fetid perspiration, angioedema, headache, dizziness, paresthesias, and eosinophilia. Transient elevations of serum transaminases, alkaline phosphatase, creatine phosphokinase, bilirubin, uric acid, blood urea nitrogen, and blood glucose levels have occurred rarely.

Administration of probucol to rhesus monkeys and dogs fed high-cholesterol, high-fat diets produced cardiotoxic effects, especially arrhythmias, in some of these animals. Prolongation of the QT interval may occur in humans and rarely can cause life-threatening arrhythmias. Probucol is not advocated for patients with arrhythmias.

Although probucol crosses the human placenta, clinical experience does not indicate an adverse effect on the fetus (FDA Pregnancy Category B). Nevertheless, it should not be used in pregnant women, and women of childbearing age should exercise strict birth control both during and for six months after therapy is discontinued, since the drug remains in adipose tissue for about six months after termination of administration. It is not known whether probucol is excreted in human milk, but lactating mothers should not receive this drug.

Probucol does not appear to increase the incidence of biliary tract disease (cholecystectomy, cholelithiasis, cholecystitis) (Zimetbaum et al, 1990).

DRUG INTERACTIONS. Probucol may potentiate the action of agents known to prolong the QT conduction interval.

No interactions have been reported to date between probucol and insulin, oral hypoglycemic agents, or anticoagulants.

Diarrhea results from stimulation of bile acid secretion and can be reduced by the concurrent administration of a bile acid sequestering agent.

PHARMACOKINETICS. Bioavailability is limited to less than 10%, but peak blood concentrations are higher when probucol is administered with meals because the drug is incorporated into and transported with chylomicrons. Probucol is carried in plasma as a constituent of VLDL, LDL, and HDL. Blood concentrations increase gradually for three or four months with continued oral administration and remain relatively constant thereafter. There is no correlation between blood concentrations and the hypocholesterolemic action.

With prolonged treatment, this fat-soluble agent accumulates slowly in fatty tissues. The major pathway of excretion is through the biliary system into the feces; renal clearance is negligible.

DOSAGE AND PREPARATIONS.

Oral: *Adults,* usually 250 or 500 mg with the morning and evening meal. Once-daily administration after dinner may be as effective in lowering serum LDL-cholesterol as twice-daily dosing and more effective than once-daily dosing after breakfast, with smaller reduction in serum HDL-cholesterol concentration (Fujimura et al, 1992).

The safety and efficacy of probucol in *children* have not been established.

Lorelco (Marion Merrell Dow). Tablets 250 and 500 mg.

Cited References

National Cholesterol Education Program: Report of the Expert Panel on Blood Cholesterol Levels in Children and Adolescents. Bethesda, Md, National Institutes of Health, 1991.

Abbott WGH, et al: Effect of a high-carbohydrate, low-saturated-fat diet on apolipoprotein B and triglyceride metabolism in Pima indians. *J Clin Invest* 86:642-650, 1990.

Ahmad S: Lovastatin: Warfarin interaction. *Arch Intern Med* 150:2047, 1990.

Ahmad S: Gemfibrozil: Interaction with glyburide. *Clin Alert* 5, 1991 A.

Ahmad S: Lovastatin-induced lupus erythematosus. *Arch Intern Med* 151:1667-1668, 1991 B.

Ahola I, et al: The hypercholesterolaemic factor in boiled coffee is retained by a paper filter. *J Intern Med* 230:293-297, 1991.

Albers JJ, et al: The unique lipoprotein(a): Properties and immunochemical measurement. *Clin Chem* 36:2019-2026, 1990.

Alderman JD, et al: Effect of a modified, well-tolerated niacin regimen on serum total cholesterol, high density lipoprotein cholesterol and the cholesterol to high density lipoprotein ratio. *Am J Cardiol* 64:725-729, 1989.

Alessandri C, et al: Effect of simvastatin treatment of high-density lipoprotein cholesterol. *Curr Ther Res* 52:98-105, 1992.

Alva F, et al: Structural and dynamic changes in the elastic arteries due to arterial hypertension and hypercholesterolemia. *Clin Cardiol* 16:614-618, 1993.

Amarasuriya RN, et al: Ethanol stimulates apolipoprotein A-I secretion by human hepatocytes: Implications for a mechanism for atherosclerosis protection. *Metabolism* 41:827-832, 1992.

American Diabetes Association: Detection and management of lipid disorders in diabetes. *Diabetes Care* 16:828-834, 1993.

Anderson JW, Siesel AE: Hypocholesterolemic effects of oat products, in Furda I, Brine CJ (eds): *New Developments in Dietary Fiber.* New York, Plenum Press, 1990, 17.

Anderson KM, et al: Cholesterol and mortality: 30 years of follow-up from the Framingham Study. *JAMA* 257:2176-2180, 1987.

Anderson JW, et al: Oat-bran cereal lowers serum total and LDL cholesterol in hypercholesterolemic men. *Am J Clin Nutr* 52:495-499, 1990.

Anderson JW, et al: Prospective, randomized, controlled comparison of the effects of low-fat and low-fat plus high-fiber diets on serum lipid concentrations. *Am J Clin Nutr* 56:887-894, 1992 A.

Anderson JW, et al: Cholesterol-lowering effects of psyllium-enriched cereal as an adjunct to a prudent diet in the treatment of mild to moderate hypercholesterolemia. *Am J Clin Nutr* 56:93-98, 1992 B.

Angelin B, et al: Increased turnover of very low density lipoprotein triglyceride during treatment with cholestyramine in familial hypercholesterolaemia. *J Intern Med* 227:201-206, 1990.

Angelin B, et al: Hepatic cholesterol metabolism in estrogen-treated men. *Gastroenterology* 103:1657-1663, 1992.

Antonicelli R, et al: Simvastatin in the treatment of hypercholesterolemia in elderly patients. *Clin Ther* 12:165-171, 1990.

Arca M, et al: Hypercholesterolemia in postmenopausal women. *JAMA* 271:453-459, 1994.

Arem R, Patsch W: Lipoprotein and apolipoprotein levels in subclinical hypothyroidism: Effect of levothyroxine therapy. *Arch Intern Med* 150:2097-2100, 1990.

Aronow WS: Is hyperlipidemia a risk factor for atherosclerosis in the elderly? *Cardiovasc Rev Rep* 10-13, (Jan) 1992.

Assmann G, Schulte H: Relation of high-density lipoprotein cholesterol and triglycerides to incidence of atherosclerotic coronary artery disease (the PROCAM experience). *Am J Cardiol* 70:733-737, 1992.

Ast M, Frishman WH: Bile acid sequestrants. *J Clin Pharmacol* 30:99-106, 1990.

Avellone G, et al: Effect of gemfibrozil treatment on fibrinolysis system in patients with hypertriglyceridemia. *Curr Ther Res* 52:338-348, 1992.

Aviram M, et al: Lovastatin inhibits low-density lipoprotein oxidation and alters its fluidity and uptake by macrophages: In vitro and in vivo studies. *Metabolism* 41:229-235, 1992.

Azzarito C, et al: Long-term therapy with high-dose simvastatin does not affect adrenocortical and gonadal hormones in hypercholesterolemic patients. *Metabolism* 41:148-153, 1992.

Bach LA, et al: The use of simvastatin, an HMG CoA reductase inhibitor, in older patients with hypercholesterolemia and atherosclerosis. *J Am Geriatr Soc* 38:10-14, 1990.

Badimon JJ, et al: Role of high density lipoproteins in the regression of atherosclerosis. *Circulation* 86(suppl III):III-86-III-94, 1992.

Bak AAA, Grobbee DE: Caffeine, blood pressure, and serum lipids. *Am J Clin Nutr* 53:971-975, 1991.

Balfour JA, et al: Fenofibrate: A review of its pharmacodynamic and pharmacokinetic properties and therapeutic use in dyslipidaemia. *Drugs* 40:260-290, 1990.

Ballantyne CM, et al: Hyperlipidemia after heart transplantation: Report of a 6-year experience, with treatment recommendations. *J Am Coll Cardiol* 19:1315-1321, 1992.

Bantle JP, et al: Comparison of effectiveness of thyrotropin-suppressive doses of D- and L-thyroxine in treatment of hypercholesterolemia. *Am J Med* 77:475-481, 1984.

Bao W, et al: Tracking of serum apolipoproteins A-I and B in children and young adults: The Bogalusa Heart Study. *J Clin Epidemiol* 46:609-616, 1993.

Barbir M, et al: Low-dose simvastatin for the treatment of hypercholesterolaemia in recipients of cardiac transplantation. *Int J Cardiol* 33:241-246, 1991.

Bard JM, et al: A multicenter comparison of the effects of simvastatin and fenofibrate therapy in severe primary hypercholesterolemia, with particular emphasis on lipoproteins defined by their apolipoprotein composition. *Metabolism* 41:498-503, 1992.

Barker DJP, et al: Fetal nutrition and cardiovascular disease in adult life. *Lancet* 341:938-941, 1993.

Barlow CW, et al: Safety, tolerability and efficacy of acipimox in type II hyperlipidaemia. *S Afr Med J* 77:504-505, 1990.

Barr SL, et al: Reducing total dietary fat without reducing saturated fatty acids does not significantly lower total plasma cholesterol concentrations in normal males. *Am J Clin Nutr* 55:675-681, 1992.

Bazzato G, et al: Treatment of nephrotic syndrome hyperlipidemia with simvastatin. *Curr Ther Res* 50:744-752, 1991.

Beigel Y, et al: Lovastatin therapy in heterozygous familial hypercholesterolaemic patients: Effect on blood rheology and fibrinogen levels. *J Intern Med* 230:23-27, 1991.

Belcaro C, et al: Four-year follow-up of the progression of arterial wall changes associated with gemfibrozil therapy of hyperlipidemia. *Adv Ther* 9:52-61, 1992.

Benuck I, et al: Usefulness of parental serum total cholesterol levels in identifying children with hypercholesterolemia. *Am J Cardiol* 69:713-717, 1992.

Berenson GS, et al: *Cardiovascular Risk in Early Life: The Bogalusa Heart Study.* Kalamazoo, Mich, Upjohn, 1991.

Berg A, et al: Clinical and therapeutic use of probucol. *Eur J Clin Pharmacol* 40(suppl 1):S81-S84, 1991.

Berge KG, Canner PL: Coronary Drug Project: Experience with niacin. *Eur J Clin Pharmacol* 40(suppl 1):S49-S51, 1991.

Berns MAM, et al: Increase in body fatness as a major determinant of changes in serum total cholesterol and high density lipoprotein cholesterol in young men over a 10-year period. *Am J Epidemiol* 130:1109-1122, 1989.

Berry EM, et al: Effects of diets rich in monounsaturated fatty acids on plasma lipoproteins—the Jerusalem Nutrition Study: High MUFAs vs high PUFAs. *Am J Clin Nutr* 53:899-907, 1991.

Berry EM, et al: Effects of diets rich in monounsaturated fatty acids on plasma lipoproteins—the Jerusalem Nutrition Study: II monounsaturated fatty acids vs carbohydrates. *Am J Clin Nutr* 56:394-403, 1992.

The Bezafibrate Infarction Prevention (BIP) Study Group, Israel: Lipids and lipoproteins in symptomatic coronary heart disease: Distribution, intercorrelations, and significance for risk classification in 6,700 men and 1,500 women. *Circulation* 86:839-848, 1992.

Bierman EL: Atherogenesis in diabetes. *Arterioscler Thromb* 12:647-656, 1992.

Biesenbach G, Zazgornik J: Lovastatin in the treatment of hypercholesterolemia in nephrotic syndrome due to diabetic nephropathy state IV-V. *Clin Nephrol* 37:274-279, 1992.

Bimmermann A, et al: Effective therapeutic measures for reducing lipoprotein (A) in patients with dyslipidemia: Lipoprotein (A) reduction with sustained-release bezafibrate. *Curr Ther Res* 49:635-643, 1991.

Blankenhorn DH, et al: The influence of diet on the appearance of new lesions in human coronary arteries. *JAMA* 263:1646-1652, 1990.

Blankenhorn DH, et al: Evaluation of colestipol/niacin therapy with computer-derived coronary end point measures: A comparison of different measures of treatment effect. *Circulation* 86:1701-1709, 1992.

Blankenhorn DH, et al: Coronary angiographic changes with lovastatin therapy: The Monitored Atherosclerosis Regression Study (MARS). *Ann Intern Med* 119:969-976, 1993 A.

Blankenhorn DH, et al: Beneficial effects of colestipol-niacin therapy on the common carotid artery: Two- and four-year reduction of intima-media thickness measured by ultrasound. *Circulation* 88:20-28, 1993 B.

Bo M, et al: One-year experience in the treatment of elderly hypercholesterolemic patients with pravastatin. *Curr Ther Res* 50:151-158, 1991.

Boccuzzi SJ, et al: Long term experience with simvastatin. *Drug Invest* 5:135-140, 1993.

Bookstein L, et al: Day-to-day variability of serum cholesterol, triglyceride, and high-density lipoprotein cholesterol levels: Impact on the assessment of risk according to the National Cholesterol Education Program guidelines. *Arch Intern Med* 150:1653-1657, 1990.

Botti RE, et al: Concentrations of pravastatin and lovastatin in cerebrospinal fluid in healthy subjects. *Clin Neuropharmacol* 14:256-261, 1991.

Boyden TW, et al: Resistance exercise training is associated with decreases in serum low-density lipoprotein cholesterol levels in premenopausal women. *Arch Intern Med* 153:97-100, 1993.

Bradford RH, et al: Expanded clinical evaluation of lovastatin (EXCEL) study results: I. Efficacy in modifying plasma lipoproteins and adverse event profile in 8245 patients with moderate hypercholesterolemia. *Arch Intern Med* 151:43-49, 1991.

Bradford RH, et al: Efficacy and tolerability of lovastatin in 3390 women with moderate hypercholesterolemia. *Ann Intern Med* 118:850-855, 1993.

Branchi A, et al: Effect of three fibrate derivatives and of two HMG-CoA reductase inhibitors on plasma fibrinogen level in patients with primary hypercholesterolemia. *Thromb Haemost* 70:241-243, 1993.

Brensike JF, et al: Effects of therapy with cholestyramine on progression of coronary arteriosclerosis: Results of the NHLBI type II coronary intervention study. *Circulation* 69:313-324, 1984.

Brinton EA, et al: Increased apo-I and apo-II fractional catabolic rate in patients with low high density lipoprotein-cholesterol levels with or without hypertriglyceridemia. *J Clin Invest* 87:536-544, 1991.

Brown BG: Effect of lovastatin or niacin combined with colestipol and regression of coronary atherosclerosis. *Eur Heart J* 13 (suppl B):17-20, 1992.

Brown MS, Goldstein JL: A receptor-mediated pathway for cholesterol homeostasis. *Science* 232:34-47, 1986.

Brown G, et al: Regression of coronary artery disease as a result of intensive lipid-lowering therapy in men with high levels of apolipoprotein B. *N Engl J Med* 323:1289-1298, 1990.

Brown BG, et al: Lipid lowering and plaque regression: New insights into prevention of plaque disruption and clinical events in coronary disease. *Circulation* 87:1781-1791, 1993.

Buchwald H, et al: Women in the POSCH trial: Effects of aggressive cholesterol modification in women with coronary heart disease. *Ann Surg* 216:389-397, 1992.

Buring JE, et al: Decreased HDL_2 and HDL_3 cholesterol, apo A-1 and apo A-II, and increased risk of myocardial infarction. *Circulation* 85:22-29, 1992.

Burke GL, et al: Trends in serum cholesterol levels from 1980 to 1987: The Minnesota Heart Survey. *N Engl J Med* 324:941-946, 1991.

Cambillau M, et al: Serum Lp(a) as a discriminant marker of early atherosclerotic plaque at three extracoronary sites in hypercholesterolemic men. *Arterioscler Thromb* 12:1346-1352, 1992.

Campos H, et al: Differences in apolipoproteins and low-density lipoprotein subfractions in postmenopausal women on and off estrogen therapy: Results from the Framingham Offspring Study. *Metabolism* 30:1033-1038, 1990.

Canner PL, et al: Fifteen year mortality in Coronary Drug Project patients: Long-term benefit with niacin. *J Am Coll Cardiol* 8:1245-1255, 1986.

Caron P, et al: Decreased HDL cholesterol in subclinical hypothyroidism: The effect of L-thyroxine therapy. *Clin Endocrinol* 33:519-523, 1990.

Carrella M, et al: Effect of cholestyramine treatment on biliary lipid secretion rates in normolipidaemic men. *J Intern Med* 229:241-246, 1991.

Carroll KK: Dietary protein, cholesterolemia and atherosclerosis. *Can Med Assoc J* 147:900, 1992.

Cashin-Hemphill L, et al: Beneficial effects of colestipol-niacin on coronary atherosclerosis: A 4-year follow-up. *JAMA* 264:3013-3017, 1990.

Caslake MJ, et al: Fenofibrate and LDL metabolic heterogeneity in hypercholesterolemia. *Arterioscler Thromb* 13:702-711, 1993.

Castelli WP: Diet, smoking, and alcohol: Influence on coronary heart disease risk. *Am J Kidney Dis* 16 (suppl 1):41-46, 1990.

Castelli WP, et al: Lipids and risk of coronary heart disease: The Framingham Study. *Ann Epidemiol* 2:23-28, 1992.

Cave WT Jr: Dietary n-3 (ω-3) polyunsaturated fatty acid effects on animal tumorigenesis. *FASEB J* 5:2160-2166, 1991.

Celermajer DS, et al: Non-invasive detection of endothelial dysfunction in children and adults at risk of atherosclerosis. *Lancet* 340:1111-1115, 1992.

Chait A, Brunzell JD: Chylomicronemia syndrome. *Adv Intern Med* 37:249-273, 1991.

Chiesa G, et al: Mechanisms of high-density lipoprotein reduction after probucol treatment: Changes in plasma cholesterol esterification/transfer and lipase activities. *Metabolism* 42:229-235, 1993.

Childs MT, et al: Divergent lipoprotein responses to fish oils with various ratios of eicosapentaenoic acid and docosahexaenoic acid. *Am J Clin Nutr* 52:632-639, 1990.

Chrisp P, et al: Simvastatin: A pharmacoeconomic evaluation of its cost-effectiveness in hypercholesterolaemia and prevention of coronary heart disease. *Pharmacoeconomics* 1:124-145, 1992.

Clevidence BA, et al: Plasma lipid and lipoprotein concentrations of men consuming a low-fat, high-fiber diet. *Am J Clin Nutr* 55:689-694, 1992.

Clinical Experience Network: Low high-density lipoprotein cholesterol and other coronary heart disease risk factors in patients with total cholesterol levels greater than 5.17 mmol/L (200 mg/dL) in family practice: A report from CEN. *J Am Board Fam Pract* 4:285-297, 1991.

Cobb MM, Risch N: Low-density lipoprotein cholesterol responsiveness to diet in normolipidemic subjects. *Metabolism* 42:7-13, 1993.

Cobb MM, et al: Lovastatin efficacy in reducing low-density lipoprotein cholesterol levels on high- vs low-fat diets. *JAMA* 265:997-1001, 1991.

Cobb MM, et al: Influence of dietary fat, apolipoprotein E phenotype, and sex on plasma lipoprotein levels. *Circulation* 86:849-857, 1992.

Colletti RB, et al: Niacin treatment of hypercholesterolemia in children. *Pediatrics* 92:78-82, 1993.

Committee on Nutrition, American Academy of Pediatrics: Statement on cholesterol. *Pediatrics* 90:469-473, 1992.

Coniglio JG: How does fish oil lower plasma triglycerides? *Nutr Rev* 195-206, 1992.

Connor WE, Connor SL: Diet, atherosclerosis and fish oil. *Adv Intern Med* 35:139-172, 1990.

Coronary Drug Project Research Group: The Coronary Drug Project: Findings leading to further modifications of its protocol with respect to dextrothyroxine. *JAMA* 220:996-1008, 1972.

Coronary Drug Project Research Group: The Coronary Drug Project: Findings leading to discontinuation of the 2.5-mg/day estrogen group. *JAMA* 226:652-657, 1973.

Coronary Drug Project Research Group: Clofibrate and niacin in coronary heart disease. *JAMA* 231:360-381, 1975.

Corsini A, et al: Relationship between mevalonate pathway and arterial myocyte proliferation: In vitro studies with inhibitors of HMG-CoA reductase. *Atherosclerosis* 101:117-125, 1993.

Crepaldi G, et al: Plasma lipid lowering activity of acipimox in patients with type II and type IV hyperlipoproteinemia: Results of a multicenter trial. *Atherosclerosis* 70:115-121, 1988.

Crook D, et al: Lipoprotein Lp(a) levels are reduced by danazol, an anabolic steroid. *Atherosclerosis* 92:41-47, 1992.

D'Agostino RB, et al: Efficacy and tolerability of lovastatin in hypercholesterolemic women. *Clin Ther* 14:390-395, 1992.

DATTA (Diagnostic and Therapeutic Technology Assessment): Chelation therapy. *JAMA* 250:672, 1983.

Dattilo AM, Kris-Etherton PM: Effects of weight reduction on blood lipids and lipoproteins: A meta-analysis. *Am J Clin Nutr* 56:320-328, 1992.

Davidson MH, et al: The hypocholesterolemic effects of β-glucan in oatmeal and oat bran: A dose-controlled study. *JAMA* 265:1833-1839, 1991.

Dearing BD, et al: Niacin-induced clotting factor synthesis deficiency with coagulopathy. *Arch Intern Med* 152:861-863, 1992.

Defesche JC, et al: Familial defective apolipoprotein B-100 is clinically indistinguishable from familial hypercholesterolemia. *Arch Intern Med* 153:2349-2356, 1993.

DeMaio SJ, et al: Vitamin E supplementation, plasma lipids and incidence of restenosis after percutaneous transluminal coronary angioplasty (PTCA). *J Am Coll Nutr* 11:68-73, 1992.

Denke MA, Frantz ID Jr: Response to a cholesterol-lowering diet: Efficacy is greater in hypercholesterolemic subjects even after adjustment for regression to the mean. *Am J Med* 94:626-631, 1993.

Denke MA, Grundy SM: Hypercholesterolemia in elderly persons: Resolving the treatment dilemma. *Ann Intern Med* 112:780-792, 1990.

Denke MA, Grundy SM: Effects of fats high in stearic acid on lipid and lipoprotein concentrations in men. *Am J Clin Nutr* 54:1036-1040, 1991.

Denke MA, Grundy SM: Comparison of effects of lauric acid and palmitic acid on plasma lipids and lipoproteins. *Am J Clin Nutr* 56:895-898, 1992.

Denke MA, et al: Excess body weight: An underrecognized contributor to high blood cholesterol levels in white American men. *Arch Intern Med* 153:1093-1103, 1993.

Dennison BA, et al: Measurement of apolipoprotein B as a screening test for identifying children with elevated levels of low-density lipoprotein cholesterol. *J Pediatr* 117:358-363, 1990.

Deslypere JP: Apolipoproteins and coronary heart disease, in Rosseneu M, et al (eds): *Apolipoproteins in Lipid Disorders: Risk Assessment and Monitoring.* New York, Springer-Verlag Wein, 1991, 27-40.

Dieber-Rotheneder M, et al: Effect of oral supplementation with D-α-tocopherol on the vitamin E content of human low density lipoproteins and resistance to oxidation. *J Lipid Res* 32:1325-1332, 1991.

Dietschy JM: LDL cholesterol: Its regulation and manipulation. *Hosp Pract* 67-78, (June) 1990.

Ditschuneit HH, et al: Comparison of different HMG-CoA reductase inhibitors. *Eur J Clin Pharmacol* 40(suppl 1):S27-S32, 1991.

Dobs AS, et al: Effects of pravastatin, a new HMG-CoA reductase inhibitor, on vitamin D synthesis in man. *Metabolism* 40:524-528, 1991.

Dolecek TA: Epidemiological evidence of relationships between dietary polyunsaturated fatty acids and mortality in the Multiple Risk Factor Intervention Trial. *PSEBM* 200:177-182, 1992.

Dreon DM, et al: The effects of polyunsaturated fat vs monounsaturated fat on plasma lipoproteins. *JAMA* 263:2462-2466, 1990.

Drevon CA: Marine oils and their effects. *Nutr Rev* 50:38-45, 1992.

Ducobu J, et al: Simvastatin use in children, letter. *Lancet* 339:1488, 1992.

Dupont J, et al: Saturated and hydrogenated fats in food in relation to health. *J Am Coll Nutr* 10:577-592, 1991.

DuRant RH, et al: Association among serum lipid and lipoprotein concentrations and physical activity, physical fitness, and body composition in young children. *J Pediatr* 123:185-192, 1993.

Durrington PN: Secondary hyperlipidaemia. *Br Med Bull* 46:1005-1024, 1990.

Durrington PN: Specific lipid lowering therapy in the management of diabetes. *Postgrad Med J* 67:947-952, 1991.

Einarsson K, et al: Bile acid sequestrants: Mechanisms of action on bile acid and cholesterol metabolism. *Eur J Clin Pharmacol* 40(suppl 1):S53-S58, 1991.

El-Enein AMA, et al: The role of nicotinic acid and inositol hexanicotinate as anticholesterolemic and antilipidemic agents. *Nutr Rep Intern* 28:899-911, 1983.

Elkeles RS: Lipids in non-insulin dependent diabetes: A case for treatment? *Royal Soc Med* 84:393-394, 1991.

Endo H, et al: Beneficial effects of dietary intervention on serum lipid and apolipoprotein levels in obese children. *Am J Dis Child* 146:303-305, 1992.

Enig MG: Diet, serum cholesterol, and coronary heart disease, in Mann GV (ed): *Coronary Heart Disease: The Dietary Sense and Nonsense.* London, Janice Publishing, 1993, 36-60.

Enig MG, et al: Isomeric *trans* fatty acids in the U.S. diet. *J Am Coll Nutr* 9:471-486, 1990.

Epstein LH, et al: The effect of weight control on lipid changes in obese children. *Am J Dis Child* 143:454-457, 1989.

Ericsson ES, et al: Biliary lipids in familial combined hyperlipidaemia: Effects of acipimox therapy. *Eur J Clin Invest* 20:261-265, 1990.

Ericsson S, et al: Influence of age on the metabolism of plasma low density lipoproteins in healthy males. *J Clin Invest* 87:591-596, 1991.

Ettinger WH, et al: Lipoprotein lipids in older people: Results from the Cardiovascular Health Study. *Circulation* 86:858-869, 1992.

The European Study Group: Efficacy and tolerability of simvastatin and pravastatin in patients with primary hypercholesterolemia (multicountry comparative study). *Am J Cardiol* 70:1281-1286, 1992.

Everett DW, et al: Biotransformation of pravastatin sodium in humans. *Drug Metab Dispos* 19:740-748, 1991.

Everson GT, et al: Mechanisms of gallstone formation in women: Effects of exogenous estrogen (Premarin) and dietary cholesterol on hepatic lipid metabolism. *J Clin Invest* 87:237-246, 1991.

Everson GT, et al: Effects of psyllium hydrophilic mucilloid on LDL-cholesterol and bile acid synthesis in hypercholesterolemic men. *J Lipid Res* 33:1183-1192, 1992.

Expert Panel: National Cholesterol Education Program: *Second Report of the Expert Panel on Detection, Evaluation, and Treatment of High Blood Cholesterol in Adults (Adult Treatment Panel II).* Washington, DC, National Cholesterol Education Program, 1993.

Farese RV Jr, et al: Apolipoprotein B gene mutations affecting cholesterol levels. *J Intern Med* 231:643-652, 1992.

Farmer JA, et al: Comparative effects of simvastatin and lovastatin in patients with hypercholesterolemia. *Clin Ther* 14:708-717, 1992.

Feely J, O'Connor P: Effects of HMG CoA reductase inhibitors on warfarin binding. *Drug Invest* 3:315-316, 1991.

Feely J, et al: Lipoprotein(a) in cirrhosis. *BMJ* 304:545-546, 1992.

Figge HL, et al: Nicotinic acid: Review of its clinical use in the treatment of lipid disorders. *Pharmacotherapy* 8:287-294, 1988.

Fletcher GF: The value of exercise in preventing coronary atherosclerotic heart disease. *Heart Dis Stroke* 2:183-187, (May/June) 1993.

Fletcher GF, et al: Statement on exercise: Benefits and recommendations for physical activity programs for all Americans: A statement for health professionals by the Committee on Exercise and Cardiac Rehabilitation of the Council on Clinical Cardiology, American Heart Association. *Circulation* 86:340-344, 1992.

Fojo SS, Brewer HB: Hypertriglyceridaemia due to genetic defects in lipoprotein lipase and apolipoprotein C-II. *J Intern Med* 231:669-677, 1992.

Forland SC, et al: Apparent reduced absorption of gemfibrozil when given with colestipol. *J Clin Pharmacol* 30:29-32, 1990.

Franceschini G, et al: ω-3 fatty acids selectively raise high-density lipoprotein 2 levels in healthy volunteers. *Metabolism* 40:1283-1286, 1991 A.

Franceschini G, et al: Increased affinity of LDL for their receptors after acipimox treatment in hypertriglyceridemia. *Eur J Clin Pharmacol* 40(suppl 1):S45-S48, 1991 B.

Frank JW, et al: Will lowering population levels of serum cholesterol affect total mortality? Expectations from the Honolulu Heart Program. *J Clin Epidemiol* 45:333-346, 1992.

Frankel EN, et al: Inhibition of oxidation of human low-density lipoprotein by phenolic substances in red wine. *Lancet* 341:454-457, 1993.

Fraser GE, et al: A possible protective effect of nut consumption on risk of coronary heart disease: The Adventist Health Study. *Arch Intern Med* 152:1416-1424, 1992 A.

Fraser GE, et al: Effects of traditional coronary risk factors on rates of incident coronary events in a low-risk population: The Adventist Health Study. *Circulation* 86:406-413, 1992 B.

Frei B: Ascorbic acid protects lipids in human plasma and low-density lipoprotein against oxidative damage. *Am J Clin Nutr* 54:1113S-1118S, 1991.

Frick MH, et al: Helsinki Heart Study: Primary-prevention trial with gemfibrozil in middle-aged men with dyslipidemia; Safety of treatment, changes in risk factors, and incidence of coronary heart disease. *N Engl J Med* 317:1237-1245, 1987.

Friday KE, et al: Elevated plasma low-density lipoprotein and high-density lipoprotein cholesterol levels in amenorrheic athletes: Effects of endogenous hormone status and nutrient intake. *J Clin Endocrinol Metab* 77:1605-1609, 1993.

Fried RE, et al: The effect of filtered-coffee consumption on plasma lipid levels: Results of a randomized clinical trial. *JAMA* 267:811-815, 1992.

Frishman WH (ed): *Medical Management of Lipid Disorders: Focus on Prevention of Coronary Artery Disease.* Mount Kisco, NY, Futura Publishing, 1992.

Frishman WH, et al: Serum lipids and lipoproteins in advanced age: Intraindividual changes. *Ann Epidemiol* 2:43-50, 1992.

Fuccella LM, et al: Inhibition of lipolysis by nicotinic acid and by acipimox. *Clin Pharmacol Ther* 28:790-795, 1980.

Fujii S, Sobel BE: Direct effects of gemfibrozil on the fibrinolytic system: Diminution of synthesis of plasminogen activator inhibitor type 1. *Circulation* 85:1888-1893, 1992.

Fujimura A, et al: Time-dependent change in the effect of probucol in subjects with elevated cholesterol. *Eur J Clin Pharmacol* 43:299-301, 1992.

Gallagher SK, et al: Short- and long-term variability of selected indices related to nutritional status: II. Vitamins, lipids, and protein indices. *Clin Chem* 38:1449-1453, 1992.

Galton DJ, Krone W: *Hyperlipidemia In Practice*. London, Gower Medical Publishing, 1991.

Gapinski JP, et al: Preventing restenosis with fish oils following coronary angioplasty. *Arch Intern Med* 153:1595-1601, 1993.

Garg A: Lipid-lowering therapy and macrovascular disease in diabetes mellitus. *Diabetes* 41 (suppl 2):111-115, 1992.

Garg A, Grundy SM: Nicotinic acid as therapy for dyslipidemia in non-insulin-dependent diabetes mellitus. *JAMA* 264:723-726, 1990.

Garg A, Grundy SM: Nicotinic acid as therapy for dyslipidemia in non-insulin-dependent diabetes mellitus. *JAMA* 264:723-726, 1990.

Garg A, et al: Effect of high carbohydrate intake hyperglycemia, islet function, and plasma lipoproteins in NIDDM. *Diabetes Care* 15:1572-1580, 1992.

Gaziano JM, et al: Beta carotene therapy for chronic stable angina. *Circulation* 82 (suppl III):III-201, 1990.

Gebhard RL, et al: Effect of 3-hydroxy-3-methylglutaryl coenzyme A reductase inhibition on human gut mucosa. *Lipids* 26:492-494, 1991.

Genest JJ Jr, et al: Familial lipoprotein disorders in patients with premature coronary artery disease. *Circulation* 85:2025-2033, 1992.

Gey KF, et al: Inverse correlation between plasma vitamin E and mortality from ischemic heart disease in cross-cultural epidemiology. *Am J Clin Nutr* 53:326S-334S, 1991.

Gidding SS: The rationale for lowering serum cholesterol levels in American children. *Am J Dis Child* 147:386-392, 1993.

Gillman MW, et al: Impact of within-person variability on identifying children with hypercholesterolemia: Framingham Children's Study. *J Pediatr* 121:342-347, 1992.

Ginsberg HN: Lipoprotein physiology and its relationship to atherogenesis. *Endocrinol Metab Clin North Am* 19:211-228, 1990.

Glassman M, et al: Treatment of type IIa hyperlipidemia in childhood by a simplified American Heart Association diet and fiber supplementation. *Am J Dis Child* 144:973-976, 1990.

Glazer G: Atherogenic effects of anabolic steroids on serum lipid levels: A literature review. *Arch Intern Med* 151:1925-1933, 1991.

Glueck CJ, et al: Relationships between lipoprotein(a), lipids, apolipoproteins, basal and stimulated fibrinolytic regulators, and D-dimer. *Metabolism* 42:236-246, 1993.

Godsland IF, et al: The effects of different formulations of oral contraceptive agents on lipid and carbohydrate metabolism. *N Engl J Med* 323:1375-1381, 1990.

Goff DC Jr, et al: Does body fatness modify the effect of dietary cholesterol on serum cholesterol? Results from the Chicago Western Electric Study. *Am J Epidemiol* 137:171-177, 1993.

Goldberg AC, et al: Fenofibrate for the treatment of type IV and V hyperlipoproteinemias: A double-blind, placebo-controlled multicenter US study. *Clin Ther* 11:69-83, 1989.

Goldberg IJ, et al: Lack of effect of lovastatin therapy on the parameters of whole-body cholesterol metabolism. *J Clin Invest* 86:801-808, 1990 A.

Goldberg R, et al: Comparison of the effects of lovastatin and gemfibrozil on lipids and glucose control in non-insulin-dependent diabetes mellitus. *Am J Cardiol* 66:16B-21B, 1990 B.

Goldstein JL, Brown MS: Regulation of the mevalonate pathway. *Nature* 343:425-430, 1990.

Goodnight SH: The effects of n-3 fatty acids on atherosclerosis and the vascular response to injury. *Arch Pathol Lab Med* 117:102-106, 1993.

Gordon DJ, et al: High-density lipoprotein cholesterol and cardiovascular disease: Four prospective American studies. *Circulation* 79:8-15, 1989.

Gotto AM Jr: *The Role of Lipids in Coronary Heart Disease*. Kalamazoo, Mich, Upjohn, 1991 A.

Gotto AM: Cholesterol intake and serum cholesterol level. *N Engl J Med* 324:912-913, 1991 B.

Gould KL, et al: Improved stenosis geometry by quantitative coronary arteriography after vigorous risk factor modification. *Am J Cardiol* 69:845-853, 1992.

Grant KI: Oat bran: Panacea or placebo? *S Afr Med J* 80:421-422, 1991.

Graves KI, et al: Trends in serum cholesterol levels and dietary intake in a metropolitan area between 1980-82 and 1985-87: The Minnesota Heart Survey, abstract. *Circulation* 82 (suppl 3) III-347, 1990.

Greene JM, Feldman EB: Physician's office guide to a lipid-lowering diet. *J Am Coll Nutr* 10:443-452, 1991.

Griffin BA, et al: Effects of cholestyramine and acipimox on subfractions of plasma low density lipoprotein: Studies in normolipidaemic and hypercholesterolemic subjects. *Eur J Clin Invest* 22:383-390, 1992.

Grobbee DE, et al: Coffee, caffeine, and cardiovascular disease in men. *N Engl J Med* 323:1026-1032, 1990.

Grover SA, et al: The benefits of treating hyperlipidemia to prevent coronary heart disease: Estimating changes in life expectancy and morbidity. *JAMA* 267:816-822, 1992.

Grundy SM: HMG-CoA reductase inhibitors for treatment of hypercholesterolemia. *N Engl J Med* 319:24-32, 1988.

Grundy SM: Multifactorial etiology of hypercholesterolemia: Implications for prevention of coronary heart disease. *Arterioscler Thromb* 11:1619-1635, 1991 A.

Grundy SM: *Evaluation of Publicly Available Scientific Evidence Regarding Certain Nutrient-Disease Relationships: 9. Lipids and Cardiovascular Disease.* Bethesda, Md, Life Sciences Research Office, Federation of American Societies For Experimental Biology, 1991 B.

Grundy SM, Denke MA: Dietary influences on serum lipids and lipoproteins. *J Lipid Res* 31:1149-1172, 1990.

Grundy SM, et al: Use of 3-hydroxy-3-methylglutaryl coenzyme A reductase inhibitors in various forms of dyslipidemia. *Am J Cardiol* 66:31B-38B, 1990.

Guillot F, et al: Comparison of fluvastatin and lovastatin blood-brain barrier transfer using in vitro and in vivo methods. *J Cardiovasc Pharmacol* 21:339-346, 1993.

Guo S, et al: Serial analysis of plasma lipids and lipoproteins from individuals 9-21 y of age. *Am J Clin Nutr* 58:61-67, 1993.

Haarbo J, et al: Serum lipids, lipoproteins, and apolipoproteins during postmenopausal estrogen replacement therapy combined with either 19-nortestosterone derivatives or 17-hydroxyprogesterone derivatives. *Am J Med* 90:584-589, 1991.

Haffner SM, et al: Lp(a) concentrations in NIDDM. *Diabetes* 41:1267-1272, 1992.

Hahmann HW, et al: Progression and regression of minor coronary arterial narrowings by quantitative angiography after fenofibrate therapy. *Am J Cardiol* 67:957-961, 1991.

Hajjar KA, et al: Lipoprotein (a) modulation of endothelial cell surface fibrinolysis and its potential role in atherosclerosis. *Nature* 339:303-305, 1989.

Hambrecht R, et al: Various intensities of leisure time physical activity in patients with coronary artery disease: Effects on cardiorespiratory fitness and progression of coronary atherosclerotic lesions. *J Am Coll Cardiol* 22:468-477, 1993.

Hamosh M: Does infant nutrition affect adiposity and cholesterol levels in the adult? *J Pediatr Gastroenterol Nutr* 7:10-16, 1988.

Harada-Shiba M, et al: Siblings with normal LDL receptor activity and severe hypercholesterolemia. *Arterioscler Thromb* 12:1071-1078, 1992.

Harpel PC, Borth W: Identification of mechanisms that may modulate the role of lipoprotein (a) in thrombosis and atherogenesis. *Ann Epidemiol* 2:413-417, 1992.

Harris WS: The prevention of atherosclerosis with antioxidants. *Clin Cardiol* 15:636-640, 1992.

Harris WS, et al: Effects of a low saturated fat, low cholesterol fish oil supplement in hypertriglyceridemic patients: Placebo-controlled trial. *Ann Intern Med* 109:465-470, 1988 A.

Harris WS, et al: ω-3 fatty acids in hypertriglyceridemic patients: Triglycerides vs methyl esters. *Am J Clin Nutr* 48:992-997, 1988 B.

Harris WS, et al: Fish oils in hypertriglyceridemia: A dose-response study. *Am J Clin Nutr* 51:399-406, 1990.

Harris T, et al: The low cholesterol-mortality association in a national cohort. *J Clin Epidemiol* 45:595-601, 1992.

Hart Hansen JP, et al: Atherosclerosis in native Greenlanders: An ultrasonographic investigation. *Arctic Med Res* 49:151-156, 1990.

Havel RJ: Experience with individual lipid-lowering drugs: Nicotinic acid. *Cardiovasc Rev Rep* 76-77, (June) 1990.

Hayes KC, et al: Modulation of infant formula fat profile alters the low-density lipoprotein/high-density lipoprotein ratio and plasma fatty acid distribution relative to those with breast-feeding. *J Pediatr* 120:S109-S116, 1992.

Hazzard WR: Dyslipoproteinemia in the elderly: Should it be treated? *Clin Geriatr Med* 8:89-102, 1992.

Headrick LA, et al: Efforts to improve compliance with the National Cholesterol Education Program guidelines: Results of a randomized controlled trial. *Arch Intern Med* 152:2490-2496, 1992.

Hearn JA, et al: Usefulness of serum lipoprotein (a) as a predictor of restenosis after percutaneous transluminal coronary angioplasty. *Am J Cardiol* 69:736-739, 1992.

Hegele RA: Hyperlipidemia in pregnancy. *Can Med Assoc J* 145:1596, 1991.

Hegele RA, et al: Acute reduction of lipoprotein (a) by tissue-type plasminogen activator. *Circulation* 85:2034-2038, 1992.

Hegsted DM, Ausman LM: Diet, alcohol and coronary heart disease in men. *J Nutr* 118:1184-1189, 1988.

Henkin Y, et al: Rechallenge with crystalline niacin after drug-induced hepatitis from sustained-release niacin. *JAMA* 264:241-243, 1990.

Henkin Y, et al: Niacin revisited: Clinical observations on an important but underutilized drug. *Am J Med* 91:239-246, 1991.

Henkin Y, et al: Secondary dyslipidemia: Inadvertent effects of drugs in clinical practice. *JAMA* 267:961-968, 1992.

Henwood JM, Heel RC: Lovastatin: A preliminary review of its pharmacodynamic properties and therapeutic use in hyperlipidaemia. *Drugs* 36:429-454, 1988.

Hertog MGL, et al: Dietary antioxidant flavonoids and risk of coronary heart disease: The Zutphen Elderly Study. *Lancet* 342:1007-1011, 1993.

Hirano K-i, et al: Polydisperse low-density lipoproteins in hyperalphalipoproteinemic chronic alcohol drinkers in association with marked reduction of cholesteryl ester transfer protein activity. *Metabolism* 41:1313-1318, 1992.

Hoeg JM, Brewer HB Jr: 3-hydroxy-3-methylglutaryl-coenzyme A reductase inhibitors in treatment of hypercholesterolemia. *JAMA* 258:3532-3536, 1987.

Hoff HF, et al: Serum Lp (a) level as a predictor of vein graft stenosis after coronary artery bypass surgery in patients. *Circulation* 77:1238-1244, 1988.

Hoffman R, et al: Hypolipidemic drugs reduce lipoprotein susceptibility to undergo lipid peroxidation: In vitro and ex vivo studies. *Atherosclerosis* 93:105-113, 1992.

Hollenbeck CB: Dietary fructose effects on lipoprotein metabolism and risk for coronary artery disease. *Am J Clin Nutr* 58 (suppl):800S-809S, 1993.

Holme I: An analysis of randomized trials evaluating the effect of cholesterol reduction on total mortality and coronary heart disease incidence. *Circulation* 82:1916-1924, 1990.

Holtzman NA: The great god cholesterol, commentary. *Pediatrics* 87:943-945, 1991.

Hong MK, et al: Effects of estrogen replacement therapy on serum lipid values and angiographically defined coronary artery disease in postmenopausal women. *Am J Cardiol* 69:176-178, 1992.

Honjo H, et al: Menopause and hyperlipidemia: Pravastatin lowers lipid levels without decreasing endogenous estrogens. *Clin Ther* 14:699-707, 1992.

Hoogerbrugge N, et al: The efficacy and safety of pravastatin, compared to and in combination with bile acid binding resins, in familial hypercholesterolaemia. *J Intern Med* 228:261-266, 1990.

Hopkins PN: Effects of dietary cholesterol on serum cholesterol: A meta-analysis and review. *Am J Clin Nutr* 55:1060-1070, 1992.

Hopkins PN, Williams RR: A survey of 246 suggested coronary risk factors. *Atherosclerosis* 40:1-52, 1981.

Hornstra G: Effect of dietary marine lipids on (anti-) thrombotic mechanisms, in Herman AG (ed): *Antithrombotics.* Netherlands, Kluwer Academic, 1991, 233-249.

Hulley SB, et al: Health policy on blood cholesterol: Time to change directions, editorial. *Circulation* 86:1026-1029, 1992.

Hunninghake DB: HMG CoA reductase inhibitors. *Curr Opin Lipidol* 3:22-28, 1992.

Hunninghake DB, et al: Efficacy and safety of pravastatin in patients with primary hypercholesterolemia: II. Once-daily versus twice-daily dosing. *Atherosclerosis* 85:219-227, 1990.

Ide H, et al: Effects of simvastatin, an HMG-CoA reductase inhibitor, on plasma lipids and steroid hormones. *Clin Ther* 12:410-420, 1990.

Ikeda T, et al: Comparison of the effects of small doses of probucol and pravastatin on serum lipids and apolipoproteins in nonobese, non-insulin-dependent diabetes mellitus patients with hypercholesterolemia. *Curr Ther Res* 51:593, 1992.

Illingworth DR, O'Malley JP: The hypolipidemic effects of lovastatin and clofibrate alone and in combination in patients with type III hyperlipoproteinemia. *Metabolism* 39:403-409, 1990.

Illingworth DR, et al: Hypocholesterolaemic effects of lovastatin in familial defective apolipoprotein B-100. *Lancet* 339:598-600, 1992 A.

Illingworth DR, et al: Comparative hypolipidemic effects of lovastatin and simvastatin in patients with heterozygous familial hypercholesterolemia. *Atherosclerosis* 96:53-64, 1992 B.

Innis SM, Hamilton JJ: Effects of developmental changes and early nutrition on cholesterol metabolism in infancy: A review. *J Am Coll Nutr* 11:63S-68S, 1992.

Irwig L, et al: Estimating an individual's true cholesterol level and response to intervention. *JAMA* 266:1678-1685, 1991.

Jacobs DR Jr, Blackburn H: Models of effects of low blood cholesterol on the public health: Implications for practice and policy, editorial. *Circulation* 87:1033-1036, 1993.

Jacobs D, et al: Report of the conference on low blood cholesterol: Mortality associations. *Circulation* 86:1046-1060, 1992.

Jacobsen SJ, et al: Cholesterol and coronary artery disease: Age as an effect modifier. *J Clin Epidemiol* 45:1053-1059, 1992.

Jay RH, et al: Effects of pravastatin and cholestyramine on gonadal and adrenal steroid production in familial hypercholesterolaemia. *Br J Clin Pharmacol* 32:417-422, 1991.

Jenkins DJA, et al: The apolipoprotein E gene and the serum low-density cholesterol response to dietary fiber. *Metabolism* 42:585-593, 1993 A.

Jenkins DJA, et al: Effect on blood lipids of very high intakes of fiber in diets low in saturated fat and cholesterol. *N Engl J Med* 329:21-26, 1993 B.

Jensen J: Lipid and lipoprotein profiles in postmenopausal women: Effects of combined hormone replacement therapy. *Dan Med Bull* 39:64-80, (Feb) 1992.

Jialal I, Grundy SM: Preservation of the endogenous antioxidants in low density lipoprotein by ascorbate but not probucol during oxidative modification. *J Clin Invest* 87:597-601, 1991.

Jialal I, Grundy SM: Effect of dietary supplementation with alphatocopherol on the oxidative modification of low density lipoprotein. *J Lipid Res* 33:899-906, 1992.

Johansson J, et al: Plasma high density lipoprotein particle size alteration by simvastatin treatment in patients with hypercholesterolaemia. *Atherosclerosis* 91:175-184, 1991.

Johnson BF, et al: Effects of lovastatin in diabetic patients treated with chlorpropamide. *Clin Pharmacol Ther* 48:467-472, 1990.

Jokubaitis LA, et al: Clinical experience with fluvastatin, the first synthetic HMG-CoA reductase inhibitor, in Catapano AL (ed): *Drugs Affecting Lipid Metabolism*. Netherlands, Kluwer Academic Publishers, 1993, 269-276.

Jones PJH, et al: Response of cholesterol synthesis to cholesterol feeding in men with different apolipoprotein E genotypes. *Metabolism* 42:1065-1071, 1993.

Jooste PL, et al: Effect of breast feeding on the plasma cholesterol and growth of infants. *J Pediatr Gastroenterol Nutr* 13:139-142, 1991.

Jossa F, et al: Coffee and serum lipids: Findings from the Olivetti Heart Study. *Ann Epidemiol* 3:250-255, 1993.

Jungnickel PW, et al: Pravastatin: A new drug for the treatment of hypercholesterolemia. *Clin Pharm* 11:677-689, 1992.

Kaeser P, et al: Compositional changes in serum lipoproteins during simvastatin therapy in type II hyperlipoproteinemia. *Curr Ther Res* 51:848-858, 1992.

Kafonek SD, Kwiterovich PO: Treatment of hypercholesterolemia in the elderly. *Ann Intern Med* 112:723-725, 1990.

Kallio MJT, et al: Exclusive breast-feeding and weaning: Effect on serum cholesterol and lipoprotein concentrations in infants during the first year of life. *Pediatrics* 89:663-666, 1992.

Kallio MJT, et al: Tracking of serum cholesterol and lipoprotein levels from the first year of life. *Pediatrics* 91:949-954, 1993.

Kang Soo-Sang, et al: Hyperhomcyst(e)inemia as a risk factor for occlusive vascular disease. *Annu Rev Nutr* 12:279-298, 1992.

Kannel WB, Vokonas PS: Demographics of the prevalence, incidence, and management of coronary heart disease in the elderly and in women. *Ann Epidemiol* 2:5-14, 1992.

Kannel WB, et al: Efficacy and tolerability of lovastatin in a six-month study: Analysis by gender, age and hypertensive status. *Am J Cardiol* 66:1B-10B, 1990.

Kapelrud H, et al: Serum Lp(a) lipoprotein concentrations in insulin dependent diabetic patients with microalbuminuria. *BMJ* 303:675-678, 1991.

Kaprio J, et al: Intimal thickening of the coronary arteries in infants in relation to family history of coronary artery disease. *Circulation* 87:1960-1968, 1993.

Karhapää P, et al: Effects of bezafibrate on insulin sensitivity and glucose tolerance in subjects with combined hyperlipidemia. *Clin Pharmacol Ther* 52:620-626, 1992.

Kark JD, et al: Coffee, tea, and plasma cholesterol: The Jerusalem Lipid Research Clinic Prevalence Study. *BMJ* 291:699-704, 1985.

Karpanou EA, et al: Disparate serum lipid changes between normotensive and hypertensive women during the menstrual cycle. *Am J Cardiol* 70:111-113, 1992.

Karpe F, et al: Metabolism of triglyceride-rich lipoproteins during alimentary lipemia. *J Clin Invest* 91:748-758, 1993.

Kasim SE, et al: Dietary and anthropometric determinants of plasma lipoproteins during a long-term low-fat diet in healthy women. *Am J Clin Nutr* 57:146-153, 1993.

Kasiske BL, et al: The effects of lovastatin in hyperlipidemic patients with the nephrotic syndrome. *Am J Kidney Dis* 15:8-15, 1990 A.

Kasiske BL, et al: Lovastatin treatment of hypercholesterolemia in renal transplant recipients. *Transplantation* 49:95-100, 1990 B.

Keenan JM, et al: Niacin revisited: A randomized, controlled trial of wax-matrix sustained-release niacin in hypercholesterolemia. *Arch Intern Med* 151:1424-1432, 1991 A.

Keenan JM, et al: Treatment of hypercholesterolemia: Comparison of younger versus older patients using wax-matrix sustained-release niacin. *J Am Geriatr Soc* 40:12-18, 1991 B.

Kesäniemi YA, Grundy SM: Influence of gemfibrozil and clofibrate on metabolism of cholesterol and plasma triglycerides in man. *JAMA* 251:2241-2246, 1984.

Kesäniemi YA, Miettinen TA: Inhibition of cholesterol absorption by neomycin, benzodiazepine derivatives and ketoconazole. *Eur J Clin Pharmacol* 40(suppl 1):S65-S67, 1991.

Kestin M, et al: Comparative effects of three cereal brans on plasma lipids, blood pressure, and glucose metabolism in mildly hypercholesterolemic men. *Am J Clin Nutr* 52:661-666, 1990.

Kinsella JE, et al: Dietary n-3 polyunsaturated fatty acids and amelioration of cardiovascular disease: Possible mechanisms. *Am J Clin Nutr* 52:1-28, 1990.

Klatsky AL, et al: Coffee, tea, and mortality. *Ann Epidemiol* 3:375-381, 1993.

Klausen IC, et al: Treatment of hypothyroidism reduces low-density lipoproteins but not lipoprotein(a). *Metabolism* 41:911-914, 1992.

Knapp HR: Polyunsaturates, endogenous eicosanoids, and cardiovascular disease. *J Am Coll Nutr* 9:344-351, 1990.

Knopp RH, et al: Contrasting effects of unmodified and time-release forms of niacin on lipoproteins in hyperlipidemic subjects: Clues to mechanism of action of niacin. *Metabolism* 34:642-650, 1985.

Kohl HW III, et al: Musculoskeletal strength and serum lipid levels in men and women. *Med Sci Sports Exerc* 24:1080-1087, 1992.

Koletzko B, et al: Treatment of hypercholesterolemia in children and adolescents. *Acta Paediatr* 81:682-685, 1992.

Koskinen P, et al: Gemfibrozil also corrects dyslipidemia in postmenopausal women and smokers. *Arch Intern Med* 152:90-96, 1992.

Kostis JB, et al: The use of pravastatin alone and in combination with colestipol or probucol in the treatment of primary hypercholesterolemia. *Curr Ther Res* 51:487-494, 1992.

Kreisberg RA: Low high-density lipoprotein cholesterol: What does it mean, what can we do about it, and what should we do about it? Editorial. *Am J Med* 94:1-6, 1993.

Kremer P, et al: Therapeutic effects of bezafibrate and gemfibrozil in hyperlipoproteinaemia type IIa and IIb. *Curr Med Res Opin* 11:293-303, 1989.

Kritchevsky D: *Evaluation of Publicly Available Scientific Evidence Regarding Certain Nutrient-Disease Relationships: 6. Dietary Fiber and Cardiovascular Disease*. Bethesda, Md, Life Sciences Research Office, Federation of American Societies for Experimental Biology, 1991.

Kritchevsky D: Variation in plasma cholesterol levels. *Nutr Today* 21-23, (Sept/Oct) 1992.

Kritchevsky SB, Kritchevsky D: Serum cholesterol and cancer risk: An epidemiologic perspective. *Annu Rev Nutr* 12:391-416, 1992.

Kromhout D: n-3 fatty acids and coronary heart disease: Epidemiology from Eskimos to Western populations. *J Int Med* 225(suppl 1):47-51, 1989.

Kroon AA, et al: N-acetylcysteine and serum concentrations of lipoprotein(a). *J Intern Med* 230:519-526, 1991.

Krummel DA, et al: Prediction of plasma lipids in a cross-sectional sample of young women. *J Am Diet Assoc* 92:942-948, 1992.

Kuhn FE, Rackley CE: Coronary artery disease in women: Risk factors, evaluation, treatment, and prevention. *Arch Intern Med* 153:2626-2636, 1993.

Kuo PT, et al: Use of combined diet and colestipol in long-term (7-7½ years) treatment of patients with type II hyperlipoproteinemia. *Circulation* 59:199-211, 1979.

Kuo PT, et al: Effects of combined probucol-colestipol treatment for familial hypercholesterolemia and coronary artery disease. *Am J Cardiol* 57:43H-48H, 1986.

Kuo PC, et al: Lovastatin therapy for hypercholesterolemia in cardiac transplant recipients. *Am J Cardiol* 64:631-635, 1989.

Kwiterovich PO Jr: Diagnosis and management of familial dyslipoproteinemia in children and adolescents. *Pediatr Clin North Am* 37:1489-1523, 1990.

Kwiterovich PO Jr, et al: Comparison of the plasma levels of apolipoproteins B and A-1, and other risk factors in men and women with premature coronary artery disease. *Am J Cardiol* 69:1015-1021, 1992 A.

Kwiterovich PO Jr, et al: Treatment of patients with elevated plasma levels of low-density lipoproteins with a cholestyramine tablet compared with cholestyramine powder. *Curr Ther Res* 52:330-337, 1992 B.

Labeur C, et al: Plasma lipoprotein(a) values and severity of coronary artery disease in a large population of patients undergoing coronary angiography. *Clin Chem* 38:2261-2266, 1992.

Lahdenperä S, et al: Effects of gemfibrozil on low-density lipoprotein particle size, density distribution, and composition in patients with type II diabetes. *Diabetes Care* 16:584-592, 1993.

Lal SM: Hyperlipidemia in continuous ambulatory peritoneal dialysis patients. *ASAIO J* 39:87-88, 1993.

Laties AM, et al: Expanded Clinical Evaluation of Lovastatin (EXCEL) study results II: Assessment of the human lens after 48 weeks of treatment with lovastatin. *Am J Cardiol* 67:447-453, 1991.

Lauer RM, Clarke WR: Use of cholesterol measurements in childhood for the prediction of adult hypercholesterolemia: The Muscatine Study. *JAMA* 264:3034-3038, 1990.

Laws A, Reaven GM: Evidence for an independent relationship between insulin resistance and fasting plasma HDL-cholesterol, triglyceride and insulin concentrations. *J Intern Med* 231:25-30, 1992.

Lawson LD, Hughes BG: Human absorption of fish oil fatty acids as triacylglycerols, free acids, or ethyl esters. *Biochem Biophys Res Commun* 152:328-335, 1988.

Leadbetter J, et al: Effects of increasing quantities of oat bran in hypercholesterolemic people. *Am J Clin Nutr* 54:841-845, 1991.

Levinson SS, Wagner SG: Measurement of apolipoprotein B-containing lipoproteins for routine clinical laboratory use in cardiovascular disease. *Arch Pathol Lab Med* 116:1350-1354, 1992.

Levy RI, et al: A quarter century of drug treatment of dyslipoproteinemias, with a focus on the new HMG-CoA reductase inhibitor fluvastatin. *Circulation* 87(suppl 4):III45-III53, 1993.

Liacouras CA, et al: Use of cholestyramine in the treatment of children with familial combined hyperlipidemia. *J Pediatr* 122:477-482, 1993.

Lifshitz F: Children on adult diets: Is it harmful? Is it healthful? *J Am Coll Nutr* 11:84S-90S, 1992.

Lindberg G, et al: Low serum cholesterol concentration and short term mortality from injuries in men and women. *BMJ* 305:277-279, 1992.

Lintott CJ, Scott RS: HMG-CoA reductase inhibitor use in the aged: A review of clinical experience. *Drugs Aging* 2:518-529, 1992.

Lintott CJ, et al: Treatment of primary hypercholesterolaemia with simvastatin: New Zealand multicentre evaluation. *Med J Aust* 155:433-436, 1991.

The Lipid Research Clinics Investigators: The Lipid Research Clinics Coronary Primary Prevention Trial: Results of 6 years of post-trial follow-up. *Arch Intern Med* 152:1399-1410, 1992.

Lipid Research Clinics Program: The Lipid Research Clinics Coronary Primary Prevention Trial results: I. Reduction in incidence of coronary heart disease. II. The relationship of reduction in incidence of coronary heart disease to cholesterol lowering. *JAMA* 251:351-364, 365-374, 1984.

Lovastatin Study Groups I Through IV: Lovastatin 5-year safety and efficacy study. *Arch Intern Med* 153:1079-1087, 1993.

Luner PE, Amidon GL: Equilibrium and kinetic factors influencing bile sequestrant efficacy. *Pharm Res* 9:670-676, 1992.

Mahley RW, et al: Genetic defects in lipoprotein metabolism: Elevation of atherogenic lipoproteins caused by impaired catabolism. *JAMA* 265:78-83, 1991.

Malasanos TH, Stacpoole PW: Biological effects of ω-3 fatty acids in diabetes mellitus. *Diabetes Care* 14:1160-1179, 1991.

Malini PL, et al: Simvastatin versus pravastatin: Efficacy and tolerability in patients with primary hypercholesterolemia. *Clin Ther* 13:500-510, 1991.

Malmendier CL, et al; Apolipoprotein C-II and C-III metabolism in a kindred of familial hypobetalipoproteinemia. *Metabolism* 40:45-50, 1991.

Mangion DM, Roy SS: Serum lipids and coronary heart disease in British elderly. *Postgrad Med J* 69:609-614, 1993.

Manolio TA, et al: Cholesterol and heart disease in older persons and women: Review of an NHLBI workshop. *Ann Epidemiol* 2:161-176, 1992.

Manolio TA, et al: Epidemiology of low cholesterol levels in older adults: The Cardiovascular Health Study. *Circulation* 87:728-737, 1993.

Manson JE, et al: The primary prevention of myocardial infarction. *N Engl J Med* 326:1406-1416, 1992.

Mänttäri M, et al: Reduction in Q wave myocardial infarctions with gemfibrozil in the Helsinki Heart Study. *Am Heart J* 119:991-995, 1990.

Mänttäri M, et al: Apolipoprotein E polymorphism influences the serum cholesterol response to dietary intervention. *Metabolism* 40:217-221, 1991.

Markussis V, et al: Detection of premature atherosclerosis by high-resolution ultrasonography in symptom-free hypopituitary adults. *Lancet* 340:1188-1192, 1992.

Masana I, et al: Effectiveness of probucol in reducing plasma low-density lipoprotein cholesterol oxidation in hypercholesterolemia. *Am J Cardiol* 68:863-867, 1991.

Mata P, et al: Effects of long-term monounsaturated- vs polyunsaturated-enriched diets on lipoproteins in healthy men and women. *Am J Clin Nutr* 55:846-850, 1992.

Mauro VF: Clinical pharmacokinetics and practical applications of simvastatin. *Clin Pharmacokinet* 24:195-202, 1993.

Mauro VF, MacDonald JL: Simvastatin: A review of its pharmacology and clinical use. *DICP* 25:257-264, 1991.

Mazzella G, et al: Effect of simvastatin, ursodeoxycholic acid and simvastatin plus ursodeoxycholic acid on biliary lipid secretion and cholic acid kinetics in nonfamilial hypercholesterolemia. *Hepatology* 15:1072-1078, 1992.

McCaughan D: The long-term effects of probucol on serum lipid levels. *Arch Intern Med* 141:1428-1432, 1981.

McDowell IFW, et al: Simvastatin in severe hypercholesterolaemia: A placebo controlled trial. *Br J Clin Pharmacol* 31:340-343, 1991.

McGovern ME, Mellies MJ: Long-term experience with pravastatin in clinical research trials. *Clin Ther* 15:57-64, 1993.

McNamara DJ: Relationship between blood and dietary cholesterol in Pearson AM, Dutson TR (eds): *Meat and Health.* London, Elsevier, 1990, vol 6 of Advances in Meat Research, 63-87.

McPherson R, Marcel Y: Role of cholesteryl ester transfer protein in reverse cholesterol transport. *Clin Cardiol* 1:31-34, 1991.

McQueen MJ: Cholestatic jaundice associated with lovastatin (Mevacor) therapy. *Can Med Assoc J* 142:841-842, 1990.

McTavish D, Sorkin EM: Pravastatin: A review of its pharmacological properties and therapeutic potential in hypercholesterolaemia. *Drugs* 42:65-89, 1991.

Mensink R, Katan MB: Effect of a diet enriched with monounsaturated or polyunsaturated fatty acids on levels of low-density and high-density lipoprotein cholesterol in healthy women and men. *N Engl J Med* 321:436-441, 1989.

Mensink RP, Katan MB: Effect of dietary fatty acids on serum lipids and lipoproteins: A meta-analysis of 27 trials. *Arterioscler Thromb* 12:911-919, 1992.

Mensink RP, et al: Effect of dietary *cis* and *trans* fatty acids on serum lipoprotein[a] levels in humans. *J Lipid Res* 33:1493-1501, 1992.

Merrin PK, Elkeles RS: Treatment of diabetes: The effect on serum lipids and lipoproteins. *Postgrad Med J* 67:931-937, 1991.

Meydani SN, et al: Oral (*n*-3) fatty acid supplementation suppresses cytokine production and lymphocyte proliferation: Comparison between young and older women. *J Nutr* 121:547-555, 1991.

Miccoli R, et al: Simvastatin for lowering cholesterol levels in non-insulin-dependent diabetes mellitus and in primary hypercholesterolemia. *Curr Ther Res* 51:66-74, 1992.

Miettinen TA: Inhibition of cholesterol absorption by HMG-CoA reductase inhibitor. *Eur J Clin Pharmacol* 40 (suppl 1):S19-S21, 1991.

Miles LA, et al: A potential basis for the thrombotic risks associated with lipoprotein (*a*). *Nature* 339:301-303, 1989.

Miller VT, et al: Effects of conjugated equine estrogen with and without three different progestogens on lipoproteins, high-density lipoprotein subfractions, and apolipoprotein A-I. *Obstet Gynecol* 77:235-240, 1991.

Miller M, et al: Normal variation of plasma lipoproteins: Postural effects on plasma concentrations of lipids, lipoproteins, and apolipoproteins. *Clin Chem* 38:569-574, 1992.

Modan M, et al: Hyperinsulinemia, sex, and risk of atherosclerotic cardiovascular disease. *Circulation* 84:1165-1175, 1991.

Mol MJTM, et al: Effects of inhibition of cholesterol synthesis by simvastatin of the production of adrenocortical steroid hormones and ACTH. *Clin Endocrinol* 31:679-689, 1989.

Monk JP, Todd PA: Bezafibrate: Review of its pharmacodynamic and pharmacokinetic properties, and therapeutic use in hyperlipidaemia. *Drugs* 33:539-576, 1987.

Montefusco S, et al: Blood and plasma viscosity after acipimox treatment in hypertriglyceridemic patients. *Int J Clin Pharmacol Ther Toxicol* 26:492-494, 1988.

Moon J, et al: Hypothesis: Etiology of atherosclerosis and osteoporosis: Are imbalances in the calciferol endocrine system implicated? *J Am Coll Nutr* 11:567-583, 1992.

Moreno JP, González G: Comparative study of bezafibrate and probucol in hyperlipidaemia. *Curr Med Res Opin* 11:523-532, 1989.

Morgan RE, et al: Plasma cholesterol and depressive symptoms in older men. *Lancet* 341:75-79, 1993.

Mori TA, et al: Plasma lipid levels and platelet and neutrophil function in patients with vascular disease following fish oil and olive oil supplementation. *Metabolism* 41:1059-1067, 1992.

Morisaki N, et al: Effects of long-term treatment with probucol on serum lipoproteins in cases of familial hypercholesterolemia in the elderly. *J Am Geriatr Soc* 38:15-18, 1990.

Muggeo M, et al: Long term treatment with pravastatin, simvastatin and gemfibrozil in patients with primary hypercholesterolemia: A controlled study. *Drug Invest* 4:376-385, 1992.

Muldoon MF, et al: Lowering cholesterol concentrations and mortality: A quantitative review of primary prevention trials. *BMJ* 301:309-314, 1990.

Myers MG, Basinski A: Coffee and coronary heart disease. *Arch Intern Med* 152:1767-1772, 1992.

Nabulsi AA, et al: Association of hormone-replacement therapy with various cardiovascular risk factors in postmenopausal women. *N Engl J Med* 328:1069-1075, 1993.

Nakandakare E, et al: Long term treatment of hypercholesterolaemia with simvastatin. *Drug Invest* 3:34-38, 1991.

NCEP Expert Panel on Blood Cholesterol Levels in Children and Adolescents: National Cholesterol Education Program (NCEP): Highlights of the report of the Expert Panel on Blood Cholesterol Levels in Children and Adolescents. *Pediatrics* 89:495-501, 1992.

Neaton JD, Wentworth D: Serum cholesterol, blood pressure, cigarette smoking, and death from coronary heart disease: Overall findings and differences by age for 316,099 white men. *Arch Intern Med* 152:56-64, 1992.

Neaton JD, et al: Serum cholesterol level and mortality findings for men screened in the Multiple Risk Factor Intervention Trial. *Arch Intern Med* 152:1490-1500, 1992.

Nenseter MS, et al: Effect of dietary supplementation with n-3 polyunsaturated fatty acids on physical properties and metabolism of low density lipoprotein in humans. *Arterioscler Thromb* 12:369-379, 1992.

Nestle M, et al: Plasma lipoprotein lipid and Lp (a) changes with substitution of elaidic acid for oleic acid in the diet. *J Lipid Res* 33:1029-1036, 1992.

Neuman MP, et al: Significant increase of high-density lipoprotein$_2$-cholesterol under prolonged simvastatin treatment. *Atherosclerosis* 91:S11-S19, 1991.

Neuvonen PJ, et al: The bioavailability of sustained release nicotinic acid formulations. *Br J Clin Pharmacol* 32:473-476, 1991.

Newman TB, et al: The case against childhood cholesterol screening. *JAMA* 264:3039-3043, 1990 A.

Newman TJ, et al: Safety of pravastatin in long-term clinical trials conducted in the United States. *J Drug Dev* 3 (suppl 1):275-281, 1990 B.

Nicklas TA, et al: Dietary studies in children: Cardiovascular disease prevention: The Bogalusa Heart Study. *Compr Ther* 17:8-15, 1991.

Nieman DC, et al: Reducing-diet and exercise-training effects on serum lipids and lipoproteins in mildly obese women. *Am J Clin Nutr* 52:640-645, 1990.

NIH Consensus Development Panel on Triglyceride, High-Density Lipoprotein, and Coronary Heart Disease: Triglyceride, high-density lipoprotein, and coronary heart disease. *JAMA* 269:505-510, 1993.

Niki E, et al: Membrane damage due to lipid oxidation. *Am J Clin Nutr* 53:201S-205S, 1991.

Nikkilä M, Heikkinen J: Serum cholesterol, high-density lipoprotein cholesterol and five-year survival in elderly people. *Age Aging* 19:403-408, 1990.

Nordøy A: Is there a rational use for n-3 fatty acids (fish oils) in clinical medicine? *Drugs* 42:331-342, 1991.

Nordøy A, et al: Absorption of the n-3 eicosapentaenoic and docosahexanoic acids as ethyl esters and triglycerides by humans. *Am J Clin Nutr* 53:1185-1190, 1991.

O'Connor P, et al: Effects of HMG Co-A reductase inhibitors on lipids and lipoprotein (a) in hypercholesterolaemia. *Drug Invest* 4:227-231, 1992.

Ödman B, et al: Gemfibrozil in familial combined hyperlipidaemia: Effect of added low-dose cholestyramine on plasma and biliary lipids. *Eur J Clin Invest* 21:344-349, 1991.

Ojala J-P, et al: Switch from gemfibrozil to lovastatin (mevinolin) therapy in patients with primary hypercholesterolaemia: A multicentre study. *Drug Invest* 2 (suppl 2):40-47, 1990.

O'Leary TJ, et al: Changes in serum lipoproteins and high-density lipoprotein composition during isotretinoin therapy. *Clin Invest Med* 10:355-360, 1987.

O'Leary DH, et al: Cholesterol and carotid atherosclerosis in older persons: The Framingham Study. *Ann Epidemiol* 2:147-153, 1992.

Oliver MF, et al: WHO cooperative trial of primary prevention of ischaemic heart disease with clofibrate to lower serum cholesterol: Final mortality follow-up: Report of committee of principal investigators. *Lancet* 2:600-604, 1984.

Olsson AG, et al: Effect of bezafibrate during 4.5 years of treatment of hyperlipoproteinaemia. *Atherosclerosis* 55:195-203, 1985.

Onuma T, et al: Effects of bezafibrate on abnormal lipoprotein metabolism and glucose tolerance in patients with non-insulin-dependent diabetes mellitus. *Curr Ther Res* 51:439-447, 1992.

Ornish D, et al: Can lifestyle changes reverse coronary heart disease? The Lifestyle Heart Trial. *Lancet* 336:129-133, 1990.

Ortolá J, et al: Biological variation data applied to the selection of serum lipid ratios used as risk markers of coronary heart disease. *Clin Chem* 38:56-59, 1992.

Ostlund RE Jr, et al: Insulin-like growth factor and apolipoprotein B, letter. *JAMA* 266:1937, 1991.

Pan HY: Clinical pharmacology of pravastatin, a selective inhibitor of HMG-CoA reductase. *Eur J Clin Pharmacol* 40 (suppl 1):S15-S18, 1991.

Pan HY, et al: Comparative pharmacokinetics and pharmacodynamics of pravastatin and lovastatin. *J Clin Pharmacol* 30:1128-1135, 1990 A.

Pan HY, et al: Pharmacokinetics and pharmacodynamics of pravastatin alone and with cholestyramine in hypercholesterolemia. *Clin Pharmacol Ther* 48:201-207, 1990 B.

Pan HY, et al: Pharmacokinetic interaction between propranolol and the HMG-CoA reductase inhibitors pravastatin and lovastatin. *Br J Clin Pharmacol* 31:665-670, 1991 A.

Pan HY, et al: Comparative efficacy of once-daily versus twice-daily pravastatin in primary hypercholesterolemia. *Clin Ther* 13:368-372, 1991 B.

Pappu AS, Illingworth DR: Contrasting effects of lovastatin and cholestyramine on low-density lipoprotein cholesterol and 24-hour urinary mevalonate excretion in patients with heterozygous familial hypercholesterolemia. *J Lab Clin Med* 114:554-562, 1989.

Parsons WB Jr: The effect of nicotinic acid on serum lipids. *Am J Clin Nutr* 8:471-479, 1960.

Parthasarathy S, et al: Low density lipoprotein rich in oleic acid is protected against oxidative modifications: Implications for dietary prevention of atherosclerosis. *Proc Natl Acad Sci USA* 87:3894-3898, 1990.

Pathobiological Determinants of Atherosclerosis in Youth Research Group: Relationship of atherosclerosis in young men to serum lipoprotein cholesterol concentrations and smoking: A preliminary report from the Pathobiological Determinants of Atherosclerosis in Youth (PDAY) Research Group. *JAMA* 264:3018-3024, 1990.

Pazzucconi F, et al: Bezafibrate lowers plasma lipids, fibrinogen and platelet aggregability in hypertriglyceridaemia. *Eur J Clin Pharmacol* 43:219-223, 1992.

Peters JR, et al: Treatment of hyperlipidemia in heart transplant recipients with gemfibrozil ± lovastatin. *Am J Cardiol* 71:1485-1488, 1993.

Pierce LR, et al: Myopathy and rhabdomyolysis associated with lovastatin-gemfibrozil combination therapy. *JAMA* 264:71-75, 1990.

Pool JL, et al: Lovastatin and coadministered antihypertensive/cardiovascular agents. *Hypertension* 19:242-248, 1992.

Posner BM, et al: Dietary lipid predictors of coronary heart disease in men: The Framingham Study. *Arch Intern Med* 151:1181-1187, 1991.

Prentice RL, Sheppard L: Dietary fat and cancer: Consistency of the epidemiologic data, and disease prevention that may follow from a practical reduction in fat consumption. *Cancer Causes Control* 1:81-97, 1990.

Prihoda JS, et al: The influence of simvastatin on adrenal corticosteroid production and urinary mevalonate during adrenocorticotropin stimulation in patients with heterozygous familial hypercholesterolemia. *J Clin Endocrinol Metab* 72:567-574, 1991.

Probstfield JL, Rifkind BM: The Lipid Research Clinics Coronary Primary Prevention Trial: Design, results, and implications. *Eur J Clin Pharmacol* 40 (suppl 1):S69-S75, 1991.

Psaty BM, et al: A review of the association of estrogens and progestins with cardiovascular disease in postmenopausal women. *Arch Intern Med* 153:1421-1427, 1993.

Purvis K, et al: Short-term effects of treatment with simvastatin on testicular function in patients with heterozygous familial hypercholesterolaemia. *Eur J Clin Pharmacol* 42:61-64, 1992.

Rader DJ, Brewer HB Jr: Abetalipoproteinemia: New insights into lipoprotein assembly and vitamin E metabolism from a rare genetic disease. *JAMA* 270:865-869, 1993.

Rader JI, et al: Hepatic toxicity of unmodified and time-release preparations of niacin. *Am J Med* 92:77-81, 1992.

Ramirez LC, et al: Lipoprotein (a) levels in diabetes mellitus: Relationship to metabolic control. *Ann Intern Med* 117:42-47, 1992.

Reaven PD, et al: Leisure time exercise and lipid and lipoprotein levels in an older population. *J Am Geriatr Soc* 38:847-854, 1990.

Regnström J, et al: Susceptibility to low-density lipoprotein oxidation and coronary atherosclerosis in man. *Lancet* 339:1183-1186, 1992.

Reis GJ, et al: Effects of serum lipid levels on restenosis after coronary angioplasty. *Am J Cardiol* 68:1431-1435, 1991.

Resta F, Capurso A: Modifications in serum lipids and apolipoproteins induced by gemfibrozil. *Curr Ther Res* 50:144-149, 1991.

Reust CS, et al: Lovastatin use and muscle damage in healthy volunteers undergoing eccentric muscle exercise. *West J Med* 154:198-200, 1991.

Richard BM, et al: Transport of HDL cholesterol esters to the liver is not diminished by probucol treatment in rats. *Arterioscler Thromb* 12:862-869, 1992.

Richter WO, et al: Comparative effects of two HMG-CoA reductase inhibitors (lovastatin and pravastatin) on serum lipids and lipoproteins. *Int J Tissue React* 13:107-110, 1991 A.

Richter W, et al: Interaction between fibre and lovastatin, letter. *Lancet* 338:706, 1991 B.

Richter WO, et al: Treatment of primary chylomicronemia due to familial hypertriglyceridemia by ω-3 fatty acids. *Metabolism* 41:1100-1105, 1992.

Rifici VA, Khachadurian AK: The inhibition of low-density lipoprotein oxidation by 17-β estradiol. *Metabolism* 41:1110-1114, 1992.

Rifici VA, Khachadurian AK: Dietary supplementation with vitamins C and E inhibits in vitro oxidation of lipoproteins. *J Am Coll Nutr* 12:631-637, 1993.

Rifkind BM, Rossouw JE: The case for secondary prevention of CHD, in Stein O, et al (eds): *Atherosclerosis IX: Proceedings of the Ninth International Symposium on Atherosclerosis, Rosemont-Chicago, Illinois, October 6-11, 1991.* Tel Aviv, Israel, R&L Creative Communications, 1991, 395-400.

Rimm EB, et al: Vitamin E consumption and the risk of coronary heart disease in men. *N Engl J Med* 328:1450-1456, 1993.

Ripsin CM, et al: Oat products and lipid lowering: A meta-analysis. *JAMA* 267:3317-3325, 1992.

Rosmarin PC, et al: Coffee consumption and serum lipids: A randomized, crossover clinical trial. *Am J Med* 88:349-356, 1990.

Ross R: The pathogenesis of atherosclerosis: A perspective for the 1990's. *Nature* 362:801-809, 1993.

Roth BD, et al: Relationship between tissue selectivity and lipophilicity for inhibitors of HMG-CoA reductase. *J Med Chem* 34:463-466, 1991.

Roth T, et al: Comparative effects of pravastatin and lovastatin on nighttime sleep and daytime performance. *Clin Cardiol* 15:426-432, 1992.

Rowland TW: Exercise and atherosclerosis in children and adolescents. *Cardiovasc Rev Rep* 6:851-857, 1985.

Rubins HB, Robins SJ: Effect of reduction of plasma triglycerides with gemfibrozil on high-density-lipoprotein-cholesterol concentrations. *J Intern Med* 231:421-426, 1992.

Ruiz M-J, et al: Simvastatin in the treatment of type II hyperlipoproteinemia in the elderly: A two-year experience. *Curr Ther Res* 50:731-739, 1991.

Russell JC: Insulin resistance and atherosclerosis. *Can Med Assoc J* 146:951, 1992.

Saito Y, et al: Comparison between morning and evening doses of simvastatin in hyperlipidemic subjects: A double-blind comparative study. *Arteriosclerosis Thromb* 11:816-826, 1991.

Salonen JT, et al: Interactions of serum copper, selenium, and low density lipoprotein cholesterol in atherogenesis. *BMJ* 302:756-760, 1991.

Sanders TAB, et al: Studies of vegans: The fatty acid composition of plasma choline phosphoglycerides, erythrocytes, adipose tissue, and breast milk, and some indicators of susceptibility to ischemic heart disease in vegans and omnivore controls. *Am J Clin Nutr* 31:805-813, 1978.

Sandset PM, et al: Treatment with hydroxymethylglutaryl-coenzyme A reductase inhibitors in hypercholesterolemia induces changes in the components of the extrinsic coagulation system. *Arteriosclerosis Thromb* 11:138-145, 1991.

Schectman G, et al: Can the hypotriglyceridemic effect of fish oil concentrate be sustained? *Ann Intern Med* 110:346-352, 1989.

Schmidt EB, et al: Dose-response studies on the effect of n-3 polyunsaturated fatty acids on lipids and haemostasis. *Thromb Haemost* 63:1-5, 1990.

Schwandt P: Fibrates and triglyceride metabolism. *Eur J Clin Pharmacol* 40 (suppl 1):S41-S43, 1991.

Schwartz CJ, et al: Pathogenesis of the atherosclerotic lesion: Implications for diabetes mellitus. *Diabetes Care* 15:1156-1167, 1992.

Scott J: Chelation therapy-evolution or devolution of a nostrum? *NZ Med J* 101:109-110, 1988.

Scott RS, et al: Simvastatin and side effects. *NZ Med J* 104:493-495, 1991.

Seed M, et al: Relation of serum lipoprotein(a) concentration and apolipoprotein(a) phenotype to coronary heart disease in patients with familial hypercholesterolemia. *N Engl J Med* 322:1494-1499, 1990.

Seidel D, et al: Lipoprotein(a) in internal medicine, in Stein O, et al (eds): *Atherosclerosis IX. Proceedings of the Ninth International Symposium on Atherosclerosis, Rosemont-Chicago, Illinois, October 6-11, 1991.* Tel Aviv, Israel, R&L Creative Communications, 1992.

Seip RL, et al: Exercise training decreases plasma cholesteryl ester transfer protein. *Arterioscler Thromb* 13:1359-1367, 1993.

Sentí M, et al: Lipoprotein profile in men with peripheral vascular disease: Role of intermediate density lipoproteins and apoprotein E phenotypes. *Circulation* 85:30-36, 1992.

Serajuddin ATM, et al: Relative lipophilicities, solubilities, and structure-pharmacological considerations of 3-hydroxy-3-methylglutaryl-coenzyme A (HMG-CoA) reductase inhibitors pravastatin, lovastatin, mevastatin, and simvastatin. *J Pharm Sci* 80:830-834, 1991.

Setsuda M, et al: Probucol therapy in the prevention of restenosis after successful percutaneous transluminal coronary angioplasty. *Clin Ther* 15:374-382, 1993.

Shah PK, Amin J: Low high density lipoprotein level is associated with increased restenosis rate after coronary angioplasty. *Circulation* 85:1279-1285, 1992.

Shear CL, et al: Expanded clinical evaluation of lovastatin (EXCEL) study results: Effect of patient characteristics on lovastatin-induced changes in plasma concentrations of lipids and lipoproteins. *Circulation* 85:1293-1303, 1992.

Shekelle RB, Stamler J: Dietary cholesterol and ischaemic heart disease. *Lancet* 1:1177-1179, 1989.

Shepherd J: Mechanism of action of fibrates. *Postgrad Med J* 69(suppl 1):S34-S41, 1993.

Shipley MJ, et al: Does plasma cholesterol concentration predict mortality from coronary heart disease in elderly people? 18 year follow up in Whitehall study. *BMJ* 303:89-92, 1991.

Sigman-Grant M, et al: Dietary approaches for reducing fat intake of preschool-age children. *Pediatrics* 91:955-960, 1993.

Siguel EN, Lerman RH: Trans-fatty acid patterns in patients with angiographically documented coronary artery disease. *Am J Cardiol* 71:916-920, 1993.

Silverman DI, et al: High-density lipoprotein subfractions. *Am J Med* 94:636-645, 1993.

Simons LA, et al: Treatment of primary hypercholesterolaemia with pravastatin: Efficacy and safety over three years. *Med J Aust* 157:584-589, 1992 A.

Simons LA, et al: Successful management of primary hypercholesterolaemia with simvastatin and low-dose colestipol. *Med J Aust* 157:455-459, 1992 B.

The Simvastatin Pravastatin Study Group: Comparison of the efficacy, safety and tolerability of simvastatin and pravastatin for hypercholesterolemia. *Am J Cardiol* 71:1408-1414, 1993.

Singer P: α-linolenic acid vs. long-chain n-3 fatty acids in hypertension and hyperlipidemia. *Nutrition* 8:133-135, (March/April) 1992.

Singhvi SM, et al: Disposition of pravastatin sodium, a tissue-selective HMG-CoA reductase inhibitor, in healthy subjects. *Br J Clin Pharmacol* 29:239-243, 1990.

Sinzinger H, et al: Treatment of hypercholesterolaemia in children, letter. *Lancet* 340:548-549, 1992.

Sirtori M, et al: Efficacy of cholestyramine does not vary when taken before or during meals. *Atherosclerosis* 88:249-252, 1991.

Smit MJ, et al: Dietary fish oil-induced changes in intrahepatic cholesterol transport and bile acid synthesis in rats. *J Clin Invest* 88:943-951, 1991.

Smit JWA, et al: Successful dissolution of cholesterol gallstone during treatment with pravastatin. *Gastroenterology* 103:1068-1070, 1992.

Smith PF, et al: HMG-CoA reductase inhibitor-induced myopathy in the rat: Cyclosporine A interaction and mechanism studies. *J Pharmacol Exp Ther* 257:1225-1235, 1991.

Smith HT, et al: Pharmacokinetics of fluvastatin and specific drug interactions. *Am J Hypertens* 6:375S-382S, 1993.

Snyder SM, et al: Relationship of apolipoprotein E phenotypes to hypocholesterolemia. *Am J Med* 95:480-488, 1993.

Sommariva D, et al: Probucol and cholestyramine combination in the treatment of severe hypercholesterolemia. *Int J Clin Pharmacol Ther Toxicol* 24:505-510, 1986.

Sonnenberg LM, et al: Dietary predictors of serum cholesterol in men: The Framingham cohort population. *J Clin Epidemiol* 45:413-418, 1992.

Spach DH, et al: Rhabdomyolysis associated with lovastatin and erythromycin use. *West J Med* 154:213-215, 1991.

Sprecher DL, et al: Efficacy of psyllium in reducing serum cholesterol levels in hypercholesterolemic patients on high- or low-fat diets. *Ann Intern Med* 119:545-554, 1993.

Stamler J, Shekelle R: Dietary cholesterol and human coronary heart disease: The epidemiologic evidence. *Arch Pathol Lab Med* 112:1032-1040, 1988.

Stampfer MJ, et al: A prospective study of cholesterol, apolipoproteins, and the risk of myocardial infarction. *N Engl J Med* 325:373-381, 1991.

Stampfer MJ, et al: A prospective study of plasma homocyst(e)ine and risk of myocardial infarction in US physicians. *JAMA* 268:877-881, 1992.

Stampfer MJ, et al: Vitamin E consumption and the risk of coronary disease in women. *N Engl J Med* 328:1444-1449, 1993.

Steinberg D: Modified forms of low-density lipoprotein and atherosclerosis. *J Intern Med* 233:227-232, 1993.

Steinberg D, et al: Beyond cholesterol: Modifications of low-density lipoprotein that increase its atherogenicity. *N Engl J Med* 320:915-924, 1989.

Stensvold I, et al: Non-fasting serum triglyceride concentration and mortality from coronary heart disease and any cause in middle aged Norwegian women. *BMJ* 307:1318-1322, 1993.

Stringer MD, et al: Gemfibrozil in hyperlipidaemic patients with peripheral arterial disease: Some undiscovered actions. *Curr Med Res Opin* 12:207-214, 1990.

Stuhldreher WL, et al: Cholesterol screening in childhood: Sixteen-year Beaver County Lipid Study experience. *J Pediatr* 119:551-556, 1991.

Stuyt PMJ, et al: A comparative study of the effects of acipimox and clofibrate in type III and type IV hyperlipoproteinemia. *Atherosclerosis* 55:51-62, 1985.

Stuyt PMJ, et al: Long-term effects of simvastatin in familial dysbetalipoproteinaemia. *J Intern Med* 230:151-155, 1991.

Suh I, et al: Alcohol use and mortality from coronary heart disease: The role of high-density lipoprotein cholesterol. *Ann Intern Med* 116:881-887, 1992.

Sumi S, et al: Inhibition of pancreatic adenocarcinoma cell growth by lovastatin. *Gastroenterology* 103:982-989, 1992.

Superko HR: Exercise training, serum lipids, and lipoprotein particles: Is there a change threshold? *Med Sci Sports Exerc* 23:677-685, 1991.

Superko HR, et al: Effectiveness of low-dose colestipol therapy in patients with moderate hypercholesterolemia. *Am J Cardiol* 70:135-140, 1992.

Tangney C, et al: Impact of menstrual periodicity on serum lipid levels and estimates of dietary intakes. *J Am Coll Nutr* 10:107-113, 1991.

Taylor PA, Ward A: Women, high-density lipoprotein cholesterol, and exercise. *Arch Intern Med* 153:1178-1184, 1993.

Terasaki T, et al: Restricted transport of pravastatin sodium through the blood-brain barrier, in: *Ninth International Symposium on Atherosclerosis.* Rosemont, Ill, International Atherosclerosis Society, 1991, 192.

Terry RB, et al: High-density apolipoprotein A-I and A-II kinetics in relation to regional adiposity. *Metabolism* 41:1386-1392, 1992.

Todd PA, Goa KL: Simvastatin: A review of its pharmacological properties and therapeutic potential in hypercholesterolaemia. *Drugs* 40:583-607, 1990.

Torri, et al: Long-term effects of low-dose simvastatin in hypercholesterolemic type 2 diabetic patients. *Curr Ther Res* 51:28-36, 1992.

Trevisan M, et al: Consumption of olive oil, butter, and vegetable oils and coronary heart disease risk factors. *JAMA* 263:688-692, 1990.

Troisi R, et al: *Trans*-fatty acid intake in relation to serum lipid concentrations in adult men. *Am J Clin Nutr* 56:1019-1024, 1992.

Tse FL, et al: Pharmacokinetics of fluvastatin after single and multiple doses in normal volunteers. *J Clin Pharmacol* 32:630-638, 1992.

Tucker LA, Friedman GM: Walking and serum cholesterol in adults. *Am J Public Health* 80:1111-1113, 1990.

Tyrrell J, et al: Lipoprotein [Lp (a)] and peripheral vascular disease. *J Intern Med* 232:349-352, 1992.

Uauy R, et al: Lovastatin therapy in receptor-negative homozygous familial hypercholesterolemia: Lack of effect on low-density lipoprotein concentrations or turnover. *J Pediatr* 113:387-392, 1988.

Ulbricht TLV, Southgate DAT: Coronary heart disease: Seven dietary factors. *Lancet* 338:985-992, 1991.

Uusitupa M, et al: Combination therapy with lovastatin and guar gum versus lovastatin and cholestyramine in treatment of hypercholesterolemia. *J Cardiovasc Pharmacol* 18:496-503, 1991.

Van Biervliet J-P, et al: Serum cholesterol, cholesteryl ester, and high-density lipoprotein development in newborn infants: Response to formulas supplemented with cholesterol and γ-linolenic acid. *J Pediatr* 120:S101-S108, 1992.

van Dusseldorp M, et al: Effect of decaffeinated versus regular coffee on serum lipoproteins: A 12-week double-blind trial. *Am J Epidemiol* 132:33-40, 1990.

van Dusseldorp M, et al: Cholesterol-raising factor from boiled coffee does not pass a paper filter. *Arterioscler Thromb* 11:586-593, 1991.

Vanhanen H, Miettinen TA: Pravastatin and lovastatin similarly reduce serum cholesterol and its precursor levels in familial hypercholesterolaemia. *Eur J Clin Pharmacol* 42:127-130, 1992.

Vanhanen H, et al: Pravastatin lowers serum cholesterol, cholesterol-precursor sterols, fecal steroids, and cholesterol absorption in man. *Metabolism* 41:588-595, 1992.

Vega GL, Grundy SM: Treatment of primary moderate hypercholesterolemia with lovastatin (mevinolin) and colestipol. *JAMA* 257:33-38, 1987.

Vega GL, Grundy SM: Management of primary mixed hyperlipidemia with lovastatin. *Arch Intern Med* 150:1313-1319, 1990.

Vega GL, Grundy SM: Lipoprotein responses to treatment with lovastatin, gemfibrozil, and nicotinic acid in normolipidemic patients with hypoalphalipoproteinemia. *Arch Intern Med* 154:73-82, 1994.

Vega GL, et al: Pravastatin therapy in primary moderate hypercholesterolaemia: Changes in metabolism of apolipoprotein B-containing lipoproteins. *J Intern Med* 227:81-94, 1990.

Vgontzas AN, et al: Effects of lovastatin and pravastatin on sleep efficiency and sleep stages. *Clin Pharmacol Ther* 50:730-737, 1991.

Vinik AI, et al: Effects of gemfibrozil on triglyceride levels in patients with NIDDM. *Diabetes Care* 16:37-44, 1993.

Volpe R, et al: The efficacy and safety of pravastatin and simvastatin in patients with primary hypercholesterolemia. *Curr Ther Res* 51:422-430, 1992.

Vos J, et al: Retardation and arrest of progression or regression of coronary artery disease: A review. *Prog Cardiovasc Dis* 35:435-454, (May/June) 1993.

Walker JF, et al: Efficacy and tolerability of simvastatin (epistatin) in the elderly. *Drug Invest* 2(suppl 2):53-56, 1990.

Walsh BW, et al: Effects of postmenopausal estrogen replacement on the concentrations and metabolism of plasma lipoproteins. *N Engl J Med* 325:1196-1204, 1991.

Wanner C, et al: Effects of HMG-CoA reductase inhibitors in hypercholesterolemic patients on hemodialysis. *Kidney Int* 39:754-760, 1991.

Wardlaw GM, Snook JT: Effect of diets high in butter, corn oil, or high oleic acid sunflower oil on serum lipids and apolipoproteins in men. *Am J Clin Nutr* 51:815-821, 1990.

Webber LS, et al: Tracking of serum lipids and lipoproteins from childhood to adulthood: The Bogalusa Heart Study. *Am J Epidemiol* 133:884-899, 1991.

Weidner G, et al: Improvements in hostility and depression in relation to dietary change and cholesterol lowering: The Family Heart Study. *Ann Intern Med* 117:820-823, 1992.

Weissfeld JL, Holloway JJ: Precision of blood cholesterol measurement and high blood cholesterol case-finding and treatment. *J Clin Epidemiol* 9:971-984, 1992.

Weitzman JB, Vladutiu AO: Very high values of serum high-density lipoprotein cholesterol. *Arch Pathol Lab Med* 116:831-836, 1992.

West R, et al: Long-term follow up of children with familial hypercholesterolemia treated with cholestyramine. *Lancet* 2:873-875, 1980.

West CE, et al: Boys from populations with high-carbohydrate intake have higher fasting triglyceride levels than boys from populations with high-fat intake. *Am J Epidemiol* 131:271-282, 1990.

Wiklund U: Pravastatin and gemfibrozil alone and in combination for the treatment of hypercholesterolemia. *Am J Med* 94:13-20, 1993.

Willett WC, et al: Intake of *trans* fatty acids and risk of coronary heart disease among women. *Lancet* 341:581-585, 1993.

Williams RR, et al: Prevention of familial cardiovascular disease by screening for family history and lipids in youths. *Clin Chem* 38:1555-1560, 1992.

Witztum JL, et al: Intensive combination drug therapy of familial hypercholesterolemia with lovastatin, probucol, and colestipol hydrochloride. *Circulation* 79:16-28, 1989.

Yau T, et al: Vitamin E improved myocardial protection. *Circulation* 82(suppl III):III-146, 1990.

Yoshimura N, et al: The effects of pravastatin on hyperlipidemia in renal transplant recipients. *Transplantation* 53:94-99, 1992.

Young SG: Recent progress in understanding apolipoprotein B. *Circulation* 82:1574-1594, 1990.

Zambon S, et al: Long-term treatment with simvastatin in hypercholesterolemic non-insulin-dependent diabetic patients. *Curr Ther Res* 52:221-229, 1992.

Zimetbaum P, et al: Probucol: Pharmacology and clinical application. *J Clin Pharmacol* 30:3-9, 1990.

Zimetbaum P, et al: Effects of gemfibrozil and other fibric acid derivatives on blood lipids and lipoproteins. *J Clin Pharmacol* 31:25-37, 1991.

Zimetbaum P, et al: Plasma lipids and lipoproteins and the incidence of cardiovascular disease in the very elderly: The Bronx Aging Study. *Arterioscler Thromb* 12:416-423, 1992.

Zock PL, et al: Effect of a lipid-rich fraction from boiled coffee on serum cholesterol. *Lancet* 335:1235-1237, 1990.

Zunić G, et al: Reference values for apolipoproteins A-1 and B in healthy subjects, by age. *Clin Chem* 38:566-569, 1992.

Therapy for Inborn Errors of Metabolism

104

There are approximately 3,000 inborn errors of metabolism, and relatively few drugs have been found to be useful in these conditions. In some instances, dietary restriction remains the basis of therapy. Recently, with the advent of orphan drug programs and advances in biotechnology some new therapeutic agents have been approved for certain inherited metabolic disorders and others are being investigated. Information on these rare diseases and their therapy, as well as a brief discussion of metabolic errors, appears in this chapter.

Inborn errors of metabolism are biochemical disorders caused by genetically determined defects in protein molecules. This definition encompasses not only enzymes but proteins involved in transport processes in the serum or across cell membranes, regulatory proteins, structural proteins, and virtually any protein product of the gene. Geneticists refer to the clinical manifestations of a disease as phenotypes. Phenotypes of inborn errors are quite variable; some are essentially benign but others may be fulminant and fatal (Valle and Mitchell, 1988).

The most effective management for many of these metabolic disorders continues to be prevention, ie, patient education, genetic testing, and prenatal diagnosis (Valle, 1987). Recent advances in molecular genetics have resulted in the development of tests for prenatal, perinatal, and presymptomatic diagnosis and for detection of carriers of many inherited conditions (Crawfurd, 1988; Smith et al, 1989; Ostrer and Hetmancik, 1988). Most states have mandatory screening programs for newborn infants to detect certain metabolic disorders. However, there are no federal guidelines for these programs. In all 50 states and the District of Columbia, screening is available for phenylketonuria (PKU) and congenital hypothyroidism (Stevens et al, 1988). In most instances, early detection allows for therapeutic intervention.

Accurate diagnosis and an understanding of the pathophysiology of the metabolic disease are essential to management. A monogenic disease begins with a mutant gene that manufactures abnormal messenger RNA, which in turn leads to the production of a dysfunctional protein. The protein abnormality results in some biochemical or metabolic imbalance. If the protein functions as an enzyme, the abnormality can cause (1) an excess of toxic precursors, (2) an excess of toxic metabolites, or (3) a deficiency of essential metabolites. Cell and organ function are disrupted to produce the characteristic clinical phenotype.

The Metabolic Information Network (MIN) was developed recently to provide physicians and researchers with selected information on patients with specified disorders, including the names and geographic locations of physicians and researchers studying these disorders. At present the database includes information on biotin defects, galactosemias, glycogen storage diseases, hereditary tyrosine disorders, homocystinurias, hyperphenylalaninemias, maple syrup urine diseases, mucopolysaccharidoses, organic acidurias, and urea cycle disorders. The information is provided by physicians, neonatal screening laboratories, reference laboratories, or by patients or their parents. Confidentiality is assured, and cases are screened to avoid duplication. Presently the data collected are from North America; however, the program may be expanded to other areas of the world. Further information can be obtained from the Metabolic Information Network, P.O. Box 670847, Dallas, TX 75367 (800/945-2188).

Therapy for many of these conditions is discussed in other chapters. Some of the disorders associated with amino acid metabolism are managed through dietary restriction and administration of vitamins (eg, biotin, cyanocobalamin, pyridoxine). Errors in purine metabolism that result in hyperuricemia are treated with allopurinol. Orphan products discussed elsewhere are alpha$_1$-antitrypsin and alpha$_1$-proteinase inhibitor for pulmonary emphysema and tiopronin for the prevention of cystine nephrolithiasis (see index entries).

Alpha-Galactosidase Deficiency (Fabry's Disease)

Fabry's disease is an inborn error of glycosphingolipid metabolism with an incidence of 1:40,000 births. It is an X-linked recessive trait most commonly manifested in hemizygous males. Heterozygous females may exhibit an attenuated form or, rarely, the full syndrome. The molecular defect in Fabry's disease is the inability to cleave the terminal galactose from globotriosylceramide and other glycosphingolipids with terminal α-galactosyl moieties and results in the accumulation of these glycosphingolipid substrates throughout the body.

Clinical manifestations are varied. Angiokeratomas appear in childhood and increase in size and number with age; they usually are distributed in a "bathing suit pattern" and do not blanch with pressure. Sweating is decreased, and facial hair may be sparse. Ocular lesions may appear in all areas of the eye, but they are most prevalent in the cornea, conjunctiva, and retina. Most heterozygotes have corneal opacities. Patients usually experience episodes of acroparesthesia. These burning pains in the hands and feet occur during the first 10 to 20 years of life; they may last from a few minutes to several days or may persist for weeks. The pain may be associated with fever and there may be joint involvement suggesting rheumatic fever. Acute abdominal or flank pain may mimic appendicitis.

Renal function gradually deteriorates with age and results in renal failure. Cardiovascular manifestations include angina, myocardial infarction, cardiomegaly, congestive heart failure, and stroke. Death usually results from uremia or cardiovascular disease (Nyhan and Sakati, 1987 A).

There is no effective therapy to manage the excruciatingly painful episodes associated with this disease. Opioid analgesics have been only partially effective, and nonsteroidal anti-inflammatory drugs are without value. Phenytoin [Dilantin] or carbamazepine [Tegretol] has provided symptomatic relief in some patients. Chronic hemodialysis and renal transplantation have been employed to manage renal failure. Plasmapheresis has reduced levels of glycosphingolipid substrates in the plasma, but the effectiveness of chronic plasmapheresis has not been established (Desnick and Bishop, 1989).

Characterization of alpha-galactosidase samples purified from human spleen and serum show that, although the enzymes are the same protein, they are glycosylated differently. The serum form is high in sialic acid residues and remains in the circulation longer; the splenic form is cleared rapidly by the liver. Subsequent studies in patients have shown that the toxic substrate levels could be reduced to normal utilizing enzyme replacement. However, not enough enzyme can be produced using classic enzyme purification techniques (Desnick, 1988). Alpha-galactosidases derived from various sources are currently investigational orphan products sponsored independently by David Calhoun, Ph.D., Robert Desnick, M.D., Ph.D., and the Genzyme Corporation (Coppola et al, 1989).

Nephropathic Cystinosis

This genetic disorder is characterized by cystine storage within the lysosomes. Three forms are recognized: nephropathic, intermediate, and benign. The primary clinical features of the nephropathic phenotype are nephropathy progressing to renal failure, glycosuria, phosphaturia, generalized aminoaciduria, acidosis, rickets, growth retardation, retinopathy, refractile corneal bodies, cystine crystals in bone marrow and other tissues, increased intracellular cystine, and a defective ATP-dependent lysosomal efflux system (Nyhan and Sakati, 1987 C).

Although infants with nephropathic cystinosis appear normal at birth, polyuria and polydipsia occur during the first year of life. Urinalysis reveals the classic elements of Fanconi's syndrome. A pathognomonic crystalline keratopathy and "salt and pepper" retinopathy are present. The children are fair-complexioned, have marked photophobia, and fail to thrive. Life-threatening episodes of dehydration and/or sodium and potassium depletion occur during the early years. Fluid, salt, and phosphate replacement is required, usually with Shohl's solution [Bicitra] (1 mEq of sodium/ml) or Polycitra (1 mEq each of sodium and potassium/ml). The average dose is 45 to 60 ml/day.

Patients develop progressive glomerular dysfunction at age 6 to 8. During this phase, the requirements for salt and water replacement may decrease. Renal rickets is managed by phosphate replacement or 10,000 to 15,000 IU/day of vitamin D or equivalent 1,25-dihydroxycholecalciferol. Carnitine deficiency due to Fanconi's syndrome can be treated with levocarnitine 100 mg/kg/day given orally in divided doses every six hours. Hypothyroidism also may occur in some patients and responds well to standard doses of levothyroxine (Gahl et al, 1989). By the time the children are 10 years old, the end-stage renal disease must be managed by chronic hemodialysis or renal transplantation. Growth is not enhanced after the transplant, and visual problems seem to progress (Gahl et al, 1986). Cystine does not reaccumulate in parenchyma of the transplanted kidney because the defect leading to cystine storage is located intracellularly within the lysosomes. In cystinosis, the genetic defect is presumed to be in the carrier protein for cystine in the lysosomal membrane.

Therapy with cysteamine (mercaptamine) enhances cystine depletion (Thoene et al, 1976). Cysteamine eye drops 10 mM were effective in removing corneal crystals in children under 2 years (Kaiser-Kupfer et al, 1987). For systemic therapy, the average oral dose is 51.3 mg/kg/day (as free base) given every six hours. Results of a multicenter study begun in 1978 indicate that cysteamine enhances growth and preserves kidney function (Gahl et al, 1988). This preparation has been designated as an orphan product and is sponsored by Jess G. Thoene. In the past there have been problems in obtaining an adequate supply of this compound. The Generic Pharmaceutical Association Institute of Orphan Drugs has been instrumental in finding a source of cysteamine, and currently a grant from a consortium of companies (Warner-Lambert, Biocraft, and Mylan) provides funding for its manufacture and distribution. Another difficulty associated with cysteamine therapy is the unpleasant odor and taste that make it unpalatable to patients.

Efforts are continuing to develop a more acceptable, effective agent. A phosphorothioester of cysteamine, phosphocysteamine, not only smells and tastes better but is more stable at room temperature and is less toxic. Early reports showed cystine depletion to be similar to that produced with cysteamine (Thoene and Lemons, 1980). Results of a multicenter study indicate that, when taken orally, cysteamine and phosphocysteamine can be regarded as equivalent and should be equally effective for the treatment of cystinosis (Smolin et al, 1988). Phosphocysteamine has been designated as an orphan product; it is sponsored by Medea Research Laboratories and is being tested in collaborative studies in the United States.

Glucocerebrosidase (Beta-Glucosidase) Deficiency (Gaucher's Disease Type 1)

This non-neuropathic form of Gaucher's disease is the most common lysosomal storage disease. Although the incidence is lower in the general population, 1:600 to 1:2,500 Ashkenazi Jews may be affected. Nearly one-third of the cases of this so-called adult-type disease are diagnosed in the first decade of life. Splenomegaly and thrombocytopenia secondary to hypersplenism are the usual clinical manifestations (Kolodny, 1988). Bone is affected in most patients; manifestations range from bone pain to aseptic necrosis of the femoral head. Fractures of the vertebrae and long bones may occur secondary to erosion. Many patients have symptoms of pulmonary involvement.

Gaucher cells (enlarged lipid-containing histiocytes) are present in the bone marrow. Diagnosis is established by assaying glucosylceramide-beta-D-glucosidase in leukocytes or cultured fibroblasts. Because splenectomy performed for persistent thrombocytopenia may hasten the pace of lipid deposition in liver and bones, it has been suggested that this procedure be postponed or avoided if possible. Partial splenectomy is being explored as an alternative. Bone marrow transplantation and enzyme replacement therapy have been carried out in a few patients. In initial trials, purified human enzyme cleared rapidly from the circulation but was taken up by hepatocytes and was unable to hydrolyze glucocerebroside in the hepatic macrophages (Kupffer cells).

A modified placenta-derived preparation of glucocerebrosidase, alglucerase [Ceredase], is targeted to the specific mannose lectin on the lysosomes of the macrophages where the glucocerebroside is stored. Patients who received the modified enzyme improved clinically as evidenced by increased hemoglobin concentration and platelet counts and decreased serum acid phosphatase activity and plasma glucocerebroside levels. Splenic and hepatic volume decreased and there were early signs of skeletal response (Barton et al, 1991).

Alglucerase is now being used for long-term enzyme replacement therapy for Gaucher's disease type 1. The manufacturer has estimated the cost of therapy would be between $20,000 and $60,000 per year, but in a 50-kg patient with severe disease the amount could be as high as $550,000. The recommended initial dose of 60 units/kg every two weeks may be inadequate in some patients; in contrast, a total of 30 units/kg monthly given in divided doses every other day or three times a week was effective in eight children. Optimum dosage should be established on an individual basis (Beutler, 1991). Once response is achieved, dosage may be reduced; however, lifelong replacement is required.

A recombinant glucocerebrosidase (beta-glucosidase) is being developed by Genzyme Corporation for replacement therapy in all three types of Gaucher's disease.

Another approach to therapy is the use of a specific inhibitor of glucocerebroside synthesis. Results of studies in mice indicate that subcutaneous injections of levcycloserine significantly reduce cerebrosides and have only negligible effects on other glycosphingolipids, gangliosides, sulfatides, or sphingomyelins. This drug currently is under investigation as an orphan drug product (Lev and Sundaram, 1987).

Somatic gene therapy for Gaucher's disease also is being explored (Barranger and Ginns, 1989; Beaudet, 1987; Goldblatt, 1988; Cournoyer and Caskey, 1990).

Drug Evaluation

ALGLUCERASE
[Ceredase]

ACTIONS AND USES. Alglucerase catalyzes the hydrolysis of glucocerebroside and thus prevents this lipid from accumulating in tissue macrophages resulting in the appearance of Gaucher cells in the liver, spleen, bone marrow, lung, kidney, and intestine. These cells are responsible for the anemia, thrombocytopenia, hepatosplenomegaly, osteonecrosis, and osteopenia with secondary fractures observed in this disease. Alglucerase is used to replace glucocerebrosidase in patients with Gaucher's disease type 1 who have any of the above symptoms.

ADVERSE REACTIONS AND PRECAUTIONS. Pain and swelling at the site of injection have been reported. A few patients have experienced low-grade fever, chills, abdominal discomfort, nausea, or vomiting. None of the reactions required medical intervention. Antibodies were detected in one patient, but no diminution in clinical response was seen with continuation of therapy. Therapy with alglucerase should be directed by physicians knowledgeable in the management of Gaucher's disease.

Caution is advised when treating nursing mothers, for the possibility of excretion of alglucerase in human milk is unknown. This drug is classified in FDA Pregnancy Category C.

DOSAGE AND PREPARATIONS.

Intravenous: Dosage should be individualized. The recommended initial dose is up to 60 units/kg diluted to a total volume of 100 ml and infused over one to two hours. The usual frequency of infusion is once every two weeks, but this should be determined by patient response and disease severity. It may be possible to lower the dosage progressively at three- to six-month intervals.

Ceredase (Genzyme). Solution (injection) 80 units/ml in 5 ml containers.

Adenosine Deaminase Deficiency (Severe Combined Immunodeficiency Disease [SCID])

This disease occurs about once in one million births and is usually fatal in early childhood if untreated. Patients may be diagnosed at any age. The failure of the immune system to develop is thought to result from sensitivity of lymphocytes or their precursors to the adenosine deaminase (ADA) substrates, adenosine and 2′-deoxyadenosine. A significant amount of 2′-deoxyadenosine triphosphate (dATP) accumulates in red cells. Expansion of the dATP pool is toxic to lymphocytes and is thought to be responsible for profound T-cell depletion. The clinical picture is a triad of persistent diarrhea, progressive pulmonary disease, and extensive candidiasis. Skeletal abnormalities also may be present (Nyhan and Sakati, 1987 B).

Transplantation of HLA-matched bone marrow is potentially curative, but HLA-identical donors are not available in the majority of cases; transplantation of HLA-haploidentical marrow carries a greater risk of graft-versus-host disease and is less successful in restoring immune function. In recent years, partial exchange transfusion with irradiated erythrocytes has been used to provide exogenous ADA activity, but success has been limited. Injection of purified ADA is impractical because of its very short circulating life and the potential for immunogenicity. The conjugation of monomethoxypolyethylene glycol (PEG) to purified bovine adenosine deaminase has little effect on the catalytic activity of ADA but does block attack by proteases and antibodies and greatly slows clearance by renal or reticuloendothelial mechanisms. In animal studies, this modification also diminished the immunogenicity of ADA.

Evaluation of the clinical response to pegademase bovine has been challenging because of the small number of patients available for study, their varied clinical and therapeutic histories, and the fact that the period of clinical observation will be short relative to the lifelong therapy needed. An orphan NDA application for pegademase bovine [Adagen] was approved by the FDA in 1990.

Pegademase bovine was given to ADA-deficient patients once weekly by intramuscular injection. This treatment has been safe, is well tolerated, and is effective in maintaining levels of plasma ADA adequate to correct the deficiency. Pegademase bovine appears to be more effective than monthly transfusion of irradiated erythrocytes, and it avoids the risks of virus transmission, iron overload, and sensitization to erythrocyte antigens.

Gene replacement therapy for SCID associated with adenosine deaminase deficiency is underway. Gene Therapy, Inc. has a collaborative research and development agreement with the National Institutes of Health (clinical studies are being conducted by W. French Anderson, M.D., and R. Michael Blaese, M.D.). At least nine months of therapy with pegademase bovine is required before gene therapy can be instituted. The first patient's T-cell count rose to the normal range at 200 days and adenosine deaminase activity was 20% of normal. She also has developed an isohemagglutin titer. Her lymphocytes are used as vehicles for the ADA gene. A large number of T-cells with normal ADA gene to enhance the partial immune reconstruction are returned to the patient. It is not yet known if these cells can produce a sufficient amount of ADA so that pegademase replacement requirements are reduced (Sharp, 1991). Thus far, patients involved in the gene therapy study have continued to receive full doses of pegademase.

Drug Evaluation

PEGADEMASE BOVINE
[Adagen]

Pegademase bovine, a modified enzyme, provides replacement of adenosine deaminase in patients with severe combined immunodeficiency disease (SCID) who are not suitable candidates for or have not benefitted from bone marrow transplantation. Close medical supervision and appropriate diagnostic tests and therapy for intercurrent illnesses should be maintained.

ADVERSE REACTIONS AND PRECAUTIONS. Pegademase bovine should be used with caution in patients with thrombocytopenia and should not be administered if the platelet count is severely depressed. Headache and pain at the injection site have been reported. Potency may vary between lots of this preparation, and any laboratory or clinical indication of less than optimum potency should be reported immediately to the manufacturer. Concomitant use of pegademase bovine and vidarabine should be avoided.

It is not known if this agent is excreted in human milk, and it should be used with caution in nursing mothers. Pegademase bovine is classified in FDA Pregnancy Category C.

DOSAGE AND ADMINISTRATION. Pegademase bovine should not be diluted or mixed with other drugs. The prescribing physician must be thoroughly familiar with the requirements for monitoring therapy. Plasma ADA activity and red blood cell dATP levels must be measured before the initial series and prior to maintenance injections. The monitoring schedule will change as immune function improves. For more complete information, contact Enzon, Inc. (201/668-1800).

Intramuscular: This agent is administered once or twice weekly. New patients, particularly if severely ill, are treated twice weekly with 30 units/kg, based on ideal body weight (ie, 50th percentile for a normal child of the same age). When the patient is stable and shows evidence of improving immune function, once weekly injections are began. The usual maintenance dose is 20 to 30 units/kg/week (Hershfield, 1992).

Adagen (Enzon) solution (injection) 250 units/ml in 1.5 ml containers.

Carnitine Deficiency Disorders

Levocarnitine (L-carnitine) occurs naturally as an essential cofactor of fatty acid metabolism. It is produced endogenously and can be obtained from dietary sources. Deficiency of levocarnitine affects mitochondrial oxidation of free fatty acids and causes lipids to accumulate in the cytoplasm and acylcoenzyme A (acylCoA) esters to accumulate in the mitochondria, thus producing a toxic effect on the cell. In addition, an energy deficit is created by the inability of free fatty acids to enter the Krebs cycle (Goa and Brogden, 1987).

Primary carnitine deficiencies are due to an inherent defect in the transport of this compound. Deficiencies of carnitine may present either as a "myopathic" form with abnormal muscle lipid storage resulting in progressive weakness, hypotonia, atrophy, and cardiomyopathy, or as a "systemic" form in which carnitine levels in liver, muscle, and plasma are reduced resulting in clinical symptoms similar to those of Reye's syndrome (nausea, vomiting, weakness, hypoglycemia, and coma from metabolic encephalopathy) (Chapoy et al, 1980; Greene et al, 1988). Death may occur as a result of respiratory, cardiac, or hepatic failure. A mixed syndrome with some of the myopathic as well as systemic characteristics also has been described.

Secondary carnitine deficiencies occur in patients with disorders of amino acid metabolism, specifically organic acidemias (propionic, isovaleric, methylmalonic) in which there is an accumulation of short-chain acylCoA within the mitochondria. Severe metabolic acidosis may develop during the neonatal period, and episodic ketoacidosis or developmental retardation occurs later. The addition of levocarnitine to the treatment regimen increases the excretion of the toxic anion and may improve motor skills (Nyhan and Sakati, 1987 D). When children with propionic acidemia or methylmalonic aciduria are given large doses of levocarnitine (200 mg/kg/day), they excrete 60% to 70% of the total carnitine in the form of acylcarnitines. With larger doses, bacterial degradation in the intestine produces trimethylamine. In these instances, intravenous administration may be more beneficial.

Secondary carnitine deficiency also has been reported to play a role in the hyperammonemia of ornithine transcarbamylase deficiency (Ohtani et al, 1988). In disorders such as renal Fanconi's syndrome, there is excessive urinary loss of carnitine. Other factors that may contribute to secondary carnitine deficiency are total parenteral nutrition, changing the source of protein in infant formula from milk-based to soy-based, and deficiency of ascorbic acid and pyridoxine (Roe and Coates, 1989). Patients undergoing repeated hemodialysis may develop secondary deficiencies. Improvement in "post dialysis syndrome" and an increase in the hematocrit level have been noted in patients with reduced carnitine levels who were given levocarnitine orally. Levocarnitine also has been administered intravenously after dialysis or added to the dialysate. The ideal dosage and route of administration have not been determined (Rebouche and Engel, 1983; Goa and Brogden, 1987).

Drug Evaluation

LEVOCARNITINE
[Carnitor, VitaCarn]

ACTIONS AND USES. Levocarnitine is an essential cofactor of fatty acid metabolism and is used as a nutritional supplement for the treatment of primary or secondary carnitine deficiencies (see above). Only the prescription form of levocarnitine is indicated for the treatment of carnitine deficiency. Over-the-counter and health food store products should never be substituted. Substances labeled L-carnitine are not therapeutically equivalent, and the D form of the racemic mixture, D,L-carnitine, can competitively inhibit levocarnitine.

Another possible use of levocarnitine is as a supplement in neonates and debilitated patients on total parenteral nutrition; however, more studies are needed to determine if there is a beneficial effect on fat metabolism. Levocarnitine also may protect patients from the cardiotoxic effects of daunorubicin or doxorubicin and the hepatotoxic effects of valproic acid.

ADVERSE REACTIONS AND PRECAUTIONS. Mild gastrointestinal complaints (nausea, vomiting, diarrhea) have been reported in patients receiving long-term therapy. In patients receiving the liquid preparation, these effects may be minimized by dilution and slow consumption. An unpleasant body odor also has been reported. A reduction in the dosage should eliminate these effects.

Levocarnitine is classified in FDA Pregnancy Category B.

DOSAGE AND PREPARATIONS. The blood chemistry and plasma carnitine concentration should be monitored, and the clinical condition should be evaluated.

Oral: *Adults* (Tablets), 990 mg two or three times a day with meals. (Liquid), initially, 1 g once daily with food. The dosage may be increased gradually as tolerated. The usual dose for a 50-kg patient is 1 g one to three times a day. *Infants and children* (Tablets or Liquid), 50 mg/kg daily with food. The amount may be increased slowly. The usual dosage is 50 to 100 mg/kg daily (maximum, 300 mg/kg/day).

Carnitor (Sigma Tau). Liquid 100 mg/ml; tablets 330 mg.
VitaCarn (McGaw). Liquid 100 mg/ml.

Urea Cycle Disorders

Inborn errors of urea synthesis, which are caused by deficiencies of carbamoyl phosphate synthetase (CPSD), ornithine transcarbamylase (OTCD), argininosuccinic acid synthetase (ASD), and argininosuccinase (ALD), cause nitrogen precursors (amino acids and ammonium ion) to accumulate, and the replacement of arginine, the intermediate product of ureagenesis, is essential. These deficiencies have similar phenotypes. Hyperammonemia produces lethargy, irritability, vomiting, confusion, stupor, and coma associated with increased intracranial pressure (Brusilow and Horwich, 1989). This may lead to brain stem compression and death. Arginine depletion can result in net proteolysis (Brusilow, 1985). A deficiency of the fifth enzyme involved in the cycle, arginase (AD), produces a distinctly different phenotype characterized by spasticity and mental retardation (Smith, 1988).

The classic urea cycle defect usually produces symptoms during the neonatal period, although great heterogeneity exists that results in considerable phenotypic variability. Symptoms may not occur until later in infancy, childhood, or adulthood. Neonates are essentially normal for up to 48 hours

TABLE 1. PROTOCOL FOR MANAGEMENT OF INTERCURRENT HYPERAMMONEMIA

Note: All nitrogen intake should be discontinued. After plasma ammonium levels approach normal, dietary nitrogen can be reintroduced gradually, following which oral medication can be substituted for intravenous therapy.

CARBAMYL PHOSPHATE SYNTHETASE OR ORNITHINE TRANSCARBAMYLASE DEFICIENCY	
Priming infusion, mg/kg over 90 min in 35 ml/kg 10% dextrose	
Sodium benzoate	250
Sodium phenylacetate	250
10% arginine hydrochloride	210 (2 ml/kg)
Sustaining infusion I, mg/kg for *no more than 12 hours**	
Sodium benzoate	250 followed by sustaining infusion II *immediately* after plasma NH decreases
Sodium phenylacetate	250 followed by sustaining infusion II *immediately* after plasma NH decreases
10% arginine hydrochloride	105 (1 ml/kg)
Sustaining infusion II, mg/kg/24 hours*	
Sodium benzoate	250
Sodium phenylacetate	250
10% arginine hydrochloride	210 (2 ml/kg)
Hemodialysis if plasma ammonium level does not decrease within 12 to 24 hours	
ARGININOSUCCINIC ACID SYNTHETASE DEFICIENCY	
Priming infusion, mg/kg over 90 min in 35 ml/kg 10% dextrose	
Sodium benzoate	250
Sodium phenylacetate	250
10% arginine hydrochloride	660 (6 ml/kg)
Sustaining infusion, mg/kg/24 hours	
Sodium benzoate	250
Sodium phenylacetate	250
10% arginine hydrochloride	660 (6 ml/kg)
Hemodialysis if plasma ammonium level does not decrease within 12 to 24 hours	
ARGININOSUCCINASE DEFICIENCY	
Priming infusion, mg/kg over 90 min in 35 ml/kg 10% dextrose	
10% arginine hydrochloride	660 (6 ml/kg)
Sustaining infusion, mg/kg/24 hours	
10% arginine hydrochloride	660 (6 ml/kg)
Hemodialysis if unresponsive to above therapy	

**For patients with partial defects, including females heterozygous for OTCD, sustaining infusion II may be omitted in favor of sustaining infusion I.*

From Brusilow and Horwich, 1989. Reprinted with permission.

TABLE 2. MANAGEMENT OF INBORN ERRORS OF UREAGENESIS

	g/kg/day
CARBAMYL PHOSPHATE SYNTHETASE OR ORNITHINE TRANSCARBAMYLASE DEFICIENCY	
Diet*	
Essential amino acids	0.5-0.7
Protein	0.5-0.7
Caloric supplementation with Mead Johnson # 80056	
Sodium (or calcium) benzoate	0-0.25
Medication	
Sodium phenylacetate	0.30-0.55
Citrulline	0.17
ARGININOSUCCINIC ACID SYNTHETASE DEFICIENCY	
Diet	
Protein	1.25-1.5
Caloric supplementation with Mead Johnson # 80056	
Medication	
Sodium (or calcium) benzoate	0-0.25
Sodium phenylacetate	0.30-0.55
Arginine (free base)	0.40-0.70
ARGININOSUCCINASE DEFICIENCY	
Diet	
Protein	1.25-1.75 g/day
Caloric supplementation with Mead Johnson # 80056	
Medication	
Arginine (free base)	0.40-0.70

** Patients with partial deficiencies, including females heterozygous for OTCD, should receive a diet containing the age-determined minimal daily protein requirement. Essential amino acids are not prescribed.*

From Brusilow and Horwich, 1989. Reprinted with permission.

after birth and then anorexia, lethargy, convulsions, and coma develop. Hyperammonemia occurs in all of these conditions with the occasional exception of arginase deficiency. Other abnormal metabolic findings are increased glutamine and alanine levels in CPSD, OTCD, ASD, and ALD as well as a marked increase in citrulline level in ASD. Urinalysis reveals orotic aciduria in OCTD and ASD and argininosuccinic aciduria in ALD. Organic acidemias should be ruled out. Transient hyperammonemia of the newborn can mimic urea cycle defect, but it usually occurs in preterm infants with respiratory distress; these patients do not have elevated levels of specific amino acids.

The therapeutic rationale is to provide an alternative pathway for nitrogen waste that cannot be excreted by means of the urea cycle and to correct the arginine deficit. Techniques employed in the past (eg, dietary restriction, exchange transfusions, peritoneal dialysis) usually were ineffective in neonatal hyperammonemic crisis (Donn et al, 1979). In one study of 26 children who survived neonatal coma, nitrogen restriction and alternative-pathway therapy resulted in a survival rate of 92% after one year; however, 79% of those affected had at least one developmental disability. IQ scores at 12 months directly correlated with the duration of coma (Msall et al, 1984). The importance of prenatal or early neonatal diagnosis and treatment is stressed.

Hemodialysis is the treatment of choice for hyperammonemic crisis during the neonatal period and for episodes of hyperammonemic coma unresponsive to medical therapy. Suggested therapy for recurrent episodes of acute hyperammonemia appears in Table 1.

Long-term management is initiated with a combination of drug therapy and dietary restriction. A suggested protocol appears in Table 2. Either sodium phenylacetate or sodium phenylbutyrate may be used alone in a dosage of 550 mg/kg/day; the latter drug does not have the repugnant odor of sodium phenylacetate. A preparation containing sodium benzoate and sodium phenylacetate [Ucephan] is available (see evaluation). The recommended dosage of this mixture will provide slightly less sodium phenylacetate than that suggested in Table 2.

Drug Evaluation

SODIUM BENZOATE AND SODIUM PHENYLACETATE
[Ucephan]

ACTIONS AND USES. Sodium benzoate and sodium phenylacetate activate conjugation pathways involved in the acylation of amino acids and elimination of nitrogen. The oral solution is indicated as adjunctive therapy to prevent and treat hyperammonemia associated with the long-term management of urea cycle enzymopathies.

ADVERSE REACTIONS AND PRECAUTIONS. Nausea and vomiting have occurred. Because of structural similarities between benzoate and salicylates, exacerbation of peptic ulcer, mild hyperventilation, and mild respiratory alkalosis may develop. Hypernatremia is possible, especially in patients with diminished renal function.

Although there are no known contraindications, low-birth-weight infants may not be able to metabolize these compounds adequately; therefore, the risk/benefit ratio must be carefully assessed. In vitro studies suggest that benzoate competes for bilirubin binding sites on albumin, and it should be used with caution in those with neonatal hyperbilirubinemia.

This mixture is classified in FDA Pregnancy Category C.

DRUG INTERACTIONS. Some antibiotics (eg, penicillin) may compete with the conjugated products of sodium benzoate and sodium phenylacetate for active secretion by the renal tubules. Probenecid also may inhibit renal transport. Valproic acid should not be administered to hyperammonemic patients.

PHARMACOKINETICS. Pharmacokinetic studies have not been conducted in the primary patient population (neonates, infants, and children). Preliminary studies in three normal adults suggest that peak plasma levels occur within one hour after a single oral dose; 80% to 100% of a dose is excreted by the kidney as the respective conjugated products, hippurate or phenylacetylglutamine, within 24 hours. The major sites for metabolism are the liver and kidney.

DOSAGE AND PREPARATIONS. *This product is for oral use only and must be diluted.*

Oral: 2.5 ml/kg/day (250 mg each of sodium benzoate and sodium phenylacetate) is given in three to six equally divided doses. The total daily dose should not exceed 100 ml (10 g each sodium benzoate and sodium phenylacetate). Each dose should be diluted in 4 to 8 ounces of infant formula or milk and is administered as or with a meal. If given in other beverages, precipitation may occur; therefore, the solution should be inspected before it is administered.

Ucephan (Kendall-McGaw). Solution (oral) containing 10% each of sodium benzoate and sodium phenylacetate in 100 ml containers.

Porphyrias

Porphyrias are a group of metabolic diseases characterized by acquired or genetic derangements in heme biosynthesis resulting in overproduction and build-up of intermediates in the metabolic pathway of heme synthesis (Sekula et al, 1986). They are manifested by neurologic and/or cutaneous dysfunction. The types of porphyria generally may be identified by characteristic enzyme deficiencies and the pattern of porphyrin excretion in urine and feces.

In most susceptible individuals, the disease is latent until clinical expression is precipitated by environmental, metabolic, or chemical factors. Except for porphyria cutanea tarda, onset of all forms usually occurs in infancy, but may be delayed until childhood or early adulthood.

Congenital erythropoietic porphyria (CEP) is very rare. The disease is characterized by photosensitivity that results in severe cutaneous lesions with scarring and hypertrichosis, hemolytic anemia, and erythrodontia. The skin must be protected from sunlight (sunscreens are ineffective) and skin trauma must be avoided. Splenectomy may be helpful in some patients.

Erythropoietic protoporphyria (EPP) is more common than CEP. Most patients have mild to moderate photosensitivity but little or no hemolysis. However, a few patients develop progressive liver damage due to hepatic deposition of protoporphyrin; also, the incidence of cholelithiasis is increased. The skin must be protected from sunlight, and beta carotene 60 to 180 mg/day is given orally to increase tolerance to sunlight. Other therapeutic regimens (high carbohydrate intake, administration of cholestyramine, vitamin E, or hemin) are being studied (Mustajoki et al, 1989).

Acute intermittent porphyria (AIP) occurs in 2 to 10/100,000 population, and there is regional variation. AIP is more prevalent in women and often recurs prior to the onset of menstruation. Precipitating factors (drugs, malnutrition, female sex hormones, infection) induce delta-aminolevulinic acid synthase, the rate-limiting enzyme necessary for hepatic heme biosynthesis. Photosensitivity does not occur. Symptoms of the acute attack may be manifested as neurologic disturbances, and any part of the nervous system may be involved. Abdominal pain, labile hypertension, painful extremities, depression and organic brain syndrome, tachycardia, and paresthesia often occur. Neuropathy may progress to hypothalamic dysfunction, respiratory paralysis, and death. Although patients may recover completely from an acute attack, neurologic deficits may persist. This failure to reverse the deficit may be related to inadequate or delayed treatment (Yeung-Laiwah and McColl, 1987) (see discussion on variegate porphyria).

Hereditary coproporphyria (HCP) is much less common than AIP, and similar but milder neurovisceral symptoms occur during an acute attack. Photosensitivity can develop but usually does not persist after the acute attack.

Variegate porphyria (VP) produces symptoms common to those of the hepatic porphyrias (AIP, HCP) in which there is increased hepatic production and increased urinary excretion of the porphyrin precursors, delta-aminolevulinic acid (ALA) and porphobilinogen (PBG). However, cutaneous disease resembling porphyria cutanea tarda can occur either simultaneously or separately. Variegate porphyria is less prevalent than AIP in the United States but is much more common in Europe and in South African whites.

The same treatment is required as for hepatic porphyrias. Of primary importance is avoidance of precipitating factors. This may be difficult in females whose exacerbations are associated with their menstrual cycles. Hormonal manipulation of menstrual cycles to prevent attacks may precipitate them instead. When an attack occurs, large amounts of carbohydrate (450 to 500 g daily) are given to decrease the excretion of porphyrin precursors by blocking the hepatic induction of delta-aminolevulinic acid synthase. Hemin apparently acts in the same fashion. Supportive treatment of neurologic dysfunctions is also important; this may include administration of phenothiazines and/or propranolol for autonomic symptoms, potent analgesics for pain, antiemetics, and anticonvulsants. Assisted ventilation may be indicated for impaired pulmonary function. Long-term occupational and physical therapy may be needed for established neuropathy.

Porphyria cutanea tarda (PCT) is the most common form of porphyria and usually appears sporadically in middle life or later, more frequently in males than in females. Cutaneous manifestations are prominent with scarring, hirsutism, and pigmented or depigmented areas; disfiguring changes occur in severe untreated disease. Liver disease often is present, and common predisposing factors are excessive alcohol or iron intake and use of estrogens or oral contraceptives. Chlorinated hydrocarbon insecticides and fungicides have been implicated as precipitating factors. PCT is differentiated from the hepatic porphyrias (AIP, HCP, and VP) by the absence of acute neurovisceral symptoms and by normal PBG excretion. In PCT, there is increased excretion of urinary uroporphyrin with a lesser increase in coproporphyrin excretion. The opposite is true in VP and this distinguishes the two diseases, which are treated differently. When iron levels are elevated, phlebotomy is employed.

Therapy for Heme Deficiency: A lyophilized form of hemin hydroxide [Panhematin] has been approved as an orphan drug and has been effective in the treatment of acute porphyric attacks. The therapeutic effect of hemin in acute porphyrias is thought to be due to its capacity to depress the increased activity of delta-aminolevulinic acid synthase (ALA synthase), the rate-limiting enzyme in heme biosynthesis. This preparation has a short shelf life and undergoes rapid degradation after reconstitution. Another approach is to provide heme as an infusion concentrate dissolved and stabilized by L-arginine, ethanol, and propylene glycol. Heme arginate [Normosang], sponsored by Leiras Oy is currently being investigated as an orphan drug in the therapy of porphyrias (Mustajoki et al, 1989).

Drug Evaluation

HEMIN
[Panhematin]

ACTIONS. This iron-containing metalloporphyrin is derived from processed red blood cells (approximately 1.8 g of hemin is obtained from 250 ml of packed red cells). Following intravenous injection in nonicteric patients, fecal urobilinogen increases in amounts roughly proportional to the dose of hemin. This suggests a hepatic pathway as one route of elimination.

USES. Hemin is indicated for the amelioration of recurrent attacks of acute intermittent porphyria temporally related to the menstrual cycle in susceptible women. Pain, hypertension, tachycardia, abnormal mental status, and neurologic signs may be controlled in selected patients with this disorder. Similar response has been reported in patients with other hepatic porphyrias (variegate porphyria and hereditary coproporphyria).

During an acute attack, prompt administration of hemin is essential to prevent progression of porphyria and avoid irreversible neuronal damage (pre-existing neuronal damage is not affected). However, therapy should not be started until alternative therapy (ie, 400 g of dextrose/day) given for one to two days has failed.

Hemin therapy is not curative. After discontinuation of treatment, symptoms generally return, although remission may be prolonged. Some neurologic symptoms have improved weeks to months after therapy was terminated, although little or no response was noted at the time of treatment.

ADVERSE REACTIONS. One case of reversible renal shutdown occurred when an excessive amount (12.2 mg/kg) was administered as a single dose. Phlebitis with or without leukocytosis and pyrexia has occurred after administration of hemin. Coagulopathy with prolonged prothrombin and partial thromboplastin times, thrombocytopenia, mild hypofibrinogenemia, mild elevation of fibrin split products, and a 10% decrease in hematocrit have been reported. Local thrombophlebitis at the site of infusion is common (Simionatto et al, 1988).

Teratogenicity has not been studied (FDA Pregnancy Category C). Effects on nursing mothers and children are not known.

PRECAUTIONS. Diagnosis of acute porphyria should be made by evaluating symptoms and performing a Watson-Schwartz or Hoesch test for urinary porphyrobilinogen before hemin therapy is started.

Hemin for injection should be used only by physicians experienced in the management of porphyrias and in hospitals where the recommended clinical and laboratory diagnostic and monitoring techniques are available. It is contraindicated in patients with known hypersensitivity to the drug and in those with porphyria cutanea tarda.

Since hemin is thought to act by inhibiting delta-aminolevulinic acid synthetase, drugs that increase the activity of this enzyme should be avoided. These include estrogens, barbiturates, and steroids.

Anticoagulant effects have been noted infrequently during clinical studies. These have been linked to the instability of hemin; degradation products have an anticoagulant action (Goetsch and Bissell, 1986). Therefore, concomitant anticoagulant therapy should be avoided.

Reversible renal shutdown may result if recommended dosage levels are exceeded.

MONITORING THERAPY. The efficacy of treatment is demonstrated by decreased urinary concentrations of aminolevulinic acid (ALA) and porphobilinogen (PBG).

DOSAGE AND PREPARATIONS.

Intravenous: A large arm vein or central venous catheter must be used to avoid phlebitis. No drug or chemical agent should be added unless its effect on the chemical and physical stability of hemin has been determined.

For acute attacks of porphyria that do not respond to dextrose, infusion of 1 to 4 mg/kg/day over 10 to 15 minutes for 3 to 14 days may be given. Based on the clinical signs in more severe cases, this dose may be repeated no more often than every 12 hours. No more than 6 mg/kg should be infused in any 24-hour period.

Reconstituted material is not transparent and should be administered through a sterile 0.45-micron or smaller filter to prevent administration of particulate material. For information regarding preparation of solution, stability, and storage, see the manufacturer's literature.

Panhematin (Abbott). Powder (301 mg/container [7 mg/ml] after reconstitution with 43 ml of sterile water for injection). Because Panhematin is unstable and is suitable for only a limited number of patients, it is available only from Abbott Laboratories, Chicago distribution center. Abbott ships the drug on the next available commercial airline flight. To order, call 800/222-6883, Monday through Friday, from 7:00 AM to 4:30 PM Central Time. After business hours, call collect: 708/937-7970.

Wilson's Disease

Wilson's disease is an autosomal, recessively inherited abnormality in copper metabolism characterized by a reduction in the rate of incorporation of copper into ceruloplasmin and a reduction in the biliary excretion of copper. It results in progressive accumulation of copper in the liver. Increases in nonceruloplasmin copper in the plasma cause increased excretion of copper by the kidneys and deposition in other tissues and organs (eg, brain, cornea, kidney, skeletal and heart muscle, bones and joints) (Danks, 1989). Patients usually have symptoms of liver or neurologic disease. Other symptoms and disorders include acute hemolytic crisis, joint pain, kidney stones, renal tubular acidosis, pancreatic disease, cardiomyopathy, and hypoparathyroidism.

Wilson's disease usually occurs in children or young adults, but has been diagnosed in a few patients 30 to 60 years of age. All children with neurologic symptoms (eg, incoordination, involuntary movements, disorders of posture and tone) that develop after age 8 and young patients with chronic or recurrent liver disease should be tested for Wilson's disease. If untreated, this disorder is fatal.

The appearance of copper deposits in the eye (Kayser-Fleischer rings), low serum ceruloplasmin concentration, and elevated urine copper excretion after administration of penicillamine usually confirm diagnosis. In some cases, liver biopsy is necessary.

The current treatment is based on two principles: eliminating stored copper with chelating agents that increase copper excretion in the urine and decreasing intestinal copper absorption by reducing dietary copper intake. Penicillamine is the drug that is most effective for eliminating stored copper. The outcome of treatment usually depends on the amount of damage present before therapy is started. Improvement in neurologic symptoms may occur after several months, but improvement in liver function may require longer. Undesirable side effects occur in 5% to 20% of patients, and in some cases neurologic symptoms may worsen (Tankanow, 1991).

Trientine [Syprine], an orphan drug approved in 1985, is a useful alternative in patients unable to tolerate penicillamine. Toxicity is low, but iron deficiency anemia has occurred. Although the chelating effect and urinary excretion of copper is less than that with penicillamine on a molar basis, results of recent studies indicate that trientine also decreases intestinal copper absorption (Siegemund et al, 1991). Thus, it may be more useful than penicillamine in the therapy of Wilson's disease; more studies are required to assess long-term comparative effectiveness.

Ammonium tetrathiomolybdate is being evaluated as an alternative to penicillamine in the initial treatment of Wilson's disease in patients with neurologic disease. On theoretical grounds this agent should be effective since it is capable of blocking copper absorption from the gastrointestinal tract and forms nontoxic complexes with copper in the blood; this renders copper unavailable for cellular uptake and depletes the toxic pools. A pilot study was conducted in six patients for eight weeks using ammonium tetrathiomolybdate alone for six weeks and in combination with zinc acetate (50 mg three times a day) for two weeks, followed by zinc acetate maintenance therapy. This was the initial therapy employed in five patients; the sixth had been treated with penicillamine previously but was noncompliant. The daily dose of ammonium tetrathiomolybdate, 2 to 3 mg/kg with one-third taken with meals and two-thirds between meals, seemed optimal. Blockade of copper absorption was immediate, but 8 to 29 days of therapy were required to neutralize the nonceruloplasmin copper. Qualitative neurologic ratings improved in two patients, was unchanged in two, and not evaluated in two (one patient because of antiepileptic medication and the other because of prior penicillamine treatment). These initial findings indicate that ammonium tetrathiomolybdate deserves further investigation (Brewer et al, 1991).

Zinc salts block copper absorption by induction of intestinal metallothionein, which preferentially binds to copper to prevent its passage into the blood stream. The bound copper-zinc-metallothionein complex is excreted in the feces (Brewer et al, 1991). Thus, zinc salts may be promising for maintenance therapy for patients with active disease or as initial prophylaxis for asymptomatic individuals (Mayet, 1990). Zinc acetate has been given orphan drug status and is being developed by the Lemmon Company.

Patients should be informed that lifelong therapy for copper overload is imperative. Discontinuation of treatment results in recurrence of severe symptoms within two to three years, sometimes with rapidly fatal outcomes (Danks, 1989).

Drug Evaluations

PENICILLAMINE

[Cuprimine, Depen]

For chemical formula, see index entry Penicillamine, Uses, Metal Poisoning.

ACTIONS AND USES. This chelating agent combines with copper to form soluble complexes that are readily excreted by the kidney. Most patients with Wilson's disease respond to oral penicillamine, often dramatically. However, some neurologic symptoms may worsen during early therapy with this agent. After the accumulation of copper is reduced, patients who receive continued therapy have a normal lifespan. Asymptomatic homozygotes also benefit from penicillamine prophylaxis.

ADVERSE REACTIONS. Approximately 20% of patients develop acute hypersensitivity reactions manifested by morbilliform rash, fever, lymphadenopathy, leukopenia, thrombocytopenia, or a combination of these effects, usually between the first and third week of treatment. Loss of taste, proteinuria, and anorexia occur rarely. Serious adverse reactions are rare and include nephrotic syndrome, thrombocytopenia, and autoimmune disorders (systemic lupus erythematosus, Goodpasture's syndrome, polymyositis, myasthenia gravis, pemphigus). Most of these adverse reactions are reversible upon discontinuation of the drug.

DOSAGE AND PREPARATIONS. Penicillamine should be given in divided doses on an empty stomach before meals and at bedtime. The last dose should be given at least three hours after the evening meal. Urinary excretion of copper should be measured before therapy is initiated and periodically thereafter to ascertain compliance and adequacy of the dosage.

Oral: The usual daily dose is 1 to 2 g, depending on the severity of the disease and the amount of copper excreted in the urine, which should total 0.5 to 1 mg or more every 24 hours. *Children over 10 and adults*, initially, 250 mg is given four times daily. In patients in whom the disease has been stabilized, the total daily dose may be reduced to 750 mg. Administration of penicillamine should be continued during pregnancy but the dosage should be limited to 1 g/day. If cesarean section is contemplated, dosage should be reduced to 250 mg/day during the last six weeks of pregnancy and for two weeks postoperatively. *Infants over 6 months and children under 10* should receive 20 mg/kg rounded to the nearest multiple of 125 mg.

Cuprimine (Merck Sharp & Dohme). Capsules 125 and 250 mg.
Depen (Wallace). Tablets 250 mg.

TRIENTINE HYDROCHLORIDE

[Syprine]

$$H_2N(CH_2)_2NH(CH_2)_2NH(CH_2)_2NH_2 \cdot 2HCl$$

Trientine is a chelating agent employed to remove excess copper in patients with Wilson's disease who cannot tolerate penicillamine.

ADVERSE REACTIONS AND PRECAUTIONS. Iron deficiency anemia has been reported. Since iron and trientine inhibit each other's absorption, administration of these agents should be separated by at least two hours. Contact dermatitis, bronchitis, and asthma have been reported from exposure to the powder present in the capsule. Thus, the skin should be washed following exposure to the capsule contents. Any episodes of fever or skin lesions should be reported to the manufacturer.

Trientine is classified in FDA Pregnancy Category C.

DOSAGE AND PREPARATIONS. Trientine should be given on an empty stomach at least one hour before or two hours after meals and at least one hour apart from any other drug, food, or milk. The capsules should be swallowed whole with water.

Oral: Initiallly, 500 to 750 mg/day for *children* and 750 mg to 1.25 g/day for *adults* in two to four divided doses. The dosage may be increased to a maximum of 1.5 g/day in children under 12 years and to 2 g/day in adults. The daily dosage is increased only if the clinical response is inadequate or the concentration of free copper in the serum remains above 20 mcg/dL.

Syprine (Merck Sharp & Dohme). Capsules 250 mg.

Cited References

Barranger JA, Ginns I: Glucosylceramide lipidoses: Gaucher disease, in Scriver CR, et al (eds): *The Metabolic Basis of Inherited Disease, I*, ed 6. New York, McGraw-Hill, 1989, 1677-1698.

Barton NW, et al: Replacement therapy for inherited enzyme deficiency: Macrophage-targeted glucocerebrosidase for Gaucher's disease. *N Engl J Med* 324:1464-1470, 1991.

Beaudet AL: Gaucher's disease. *N Engl J Med* 316:619-621, 1987.

Beutler E: Gaucher's disease. *N Engl J Med* 325:1354-1360, 1991.

Brewer GJ, et al: Initial therapy of patients with Wilson's disease with tetrathiomolybdate. *Arch Neurol* 48:42-47, 1991.

Brusilow SW: Inborn errors of urea synthesis, in Scriver C, Lloyd J (eds): *Genetic and Metabolic Diseases in Pediatrics.* Stoneham, Mass, Butterworth International Medical Reviews, 1985, vol 5, 140-165.

Brusilow SW, Horwich AL: Urea cycle enzymes, in Scriver CR, et al (eds): *The Metabolic Basis of Inherited Disease, I,* ed 6. New York, McGraw-Hill, 1989, 629-663.

Chapoy PR, et al: Systemic carnitine deficiency: Treatable inherited lipid-storage disease presenting as Reye's syndrome. *N Engl J Med* 303:1389-1394, 1980.

Coppola G, et al: Construction of baculovirus derivatives that overproduce human α-galactosidase A, abstract. *J Cell Biochem* (suppl 13D): 39, (March-April) 1989.

Cournoyer D, Caskey CT: Gene transfer into humans: A first step, editorial. *N Engl J Med* 323:601-602, 1990.

Crawfurd Md'A: Prenatal diagnosis of common genetic disorders. *Br Med J* 297:502-506, 1988.

Danks DM: Wilson's disease (hepatolenticular degeneration), in Scriver CR, et al (eds): *The Metabolic Basis of Inherited Disease, I,* ed 6. New York, McGraw-Hill, 1989, 1416-1421.

Desnick RJ: Proteins as orphan drugs, in: *Transcript of Proceedings: National Conference on Orphan Drugs.* Washington, DC, May 18, 1988, 74-95.

Desnick RJ, Bishop DF: Fabry disease: Alpha-galactosidase deficiency; Schindler disease: Alpha-N-acetylgalactosaminidase deficiency, in Scriver CR, et al (eds): *The Metabolic Basis of Inherited Disease, I,* ed 6. New York, McGraw-Hill, 1989, 1751-1796.

Donn SW, et al: Comparison of exchange transfusion, peritoneal dialysis, and hemodialysis in an anuric newborn infant. *J Pediatr* 95:67-70, 1979.

Gahl WA, et al: Course of nephropathic cystinosis after age 10 years. *J Pediatr* 109:605-608, 1986.

Gahl WA, et al: Cystinosis: Progress in a prototypic disease. *Ann Intern Med* 109:557-569, 1988.

Gahl WA, et al: Lysosomal transport disorders: Cystinosis and sialic acid storage disorders, in Scriver CR, et al (eds): *The Metabolic Basis of Inherited Disease, II,* ed 6. New York, McGraw-Hill, 1989, 2619-2647.

Goa KL, Brogden RN: L-carnitine: Preliminary review of its pharmacokinetics, and its therapeutic use in ischaemic cardiac disease and primary and secondary carnitine deficiencies in relationship to its role in fatty acid metabolism. *Drugs* 34:1-24, 1987.

Goetsch CA, Bissell DM: Instability of hematin used in the treatment of acute hepatic porphyria. *N Engl J Med* 315:235-238, 1986.

Goldblatt J: Type I Gaucher disease. *J Med Genet* 25:415-418, 1988.

Greene C, et al: Inborn errors of metabolism and Reye syndrome: Differential diagnosis. *J Pediatr* 113:156-159, 1988.

Hershfield MS: Personal communication, 1992.

Kaiser-Kupfer MI, et al: Removal of corneal crystals by topical cysteamine in nephropathic cystinosis. *N Engl J Med* 316:775-779, 1987.

Kolodny EH: Gaucher's disease, in Wyngaarden JB, Smith LH (eds): *Textbook of Medicine.* Philadelphia, WB Saunders, 1988, vol 1, 1145-1147.

Lev M, Sundaram KS: Gaucher's disease, letter. *N Engl J Med* 317:572, 1987.

Mayet IY: Low-dose zinc therapy for maintenance treatment of Wilson's Disease. *Clin Pharm* 9:951-953, 1990.

Msall M, et al: Neurologic outcome in children with inborn errors of urea synthesis: Outcome of urea-cycle enzymopathies. *N Engl J Med* 310:1500-1505, 1984.

Mustajoki P, et al: Heme in treatment of porphyrias and hematological disorders. *Semin Hematol* 26:1-9, 1989.

Nyhan WL, Sakati NA: Fabry disease: Alpha-galactosidase A deficiency, in: *Diagnostic Recognition of Genetic Disease.* Philadelphia, Lea & Febiger, 1987 A, 352-357.

Nyhan WL, Sakati NA: Adenosine deaminase deficiency, in: *Diagnostic Recognition of Genetic Disease.* Philadelphia, Lea & Febiger, 1987 B, 19-23.

Nyhan WL, Sakati NA: Cystinosis: Syndrome of Lignac, Fanconi, Debre, and De Toni, in: *Diagnostic Recognition of Genetic Disease.* Philadelphia, Lea & Febiger, 1987 C, 239-245.

Nyhan WL, Sakati NA: Propionic acidemia; Isovaleric acidemia, in: *Diagnostic Recognition of Genetic Disease.* Philadelphia, Lea & Febiger, 1987 D, 36-41, 69-73.

Ohtani Y, et al: Secondary carnitine deficiency in hyperammonemic attacks of ornithine transcarbamylase deficiency. *J Pediatr* 112:409-414, 1988.

Ostrer H, Hejtmancik JF: Prenatal diagnosis and carrier detection of genetic disease by analysis of deoxyribonucleic acid. *J Pediatr* 112:679-687, 1988.

Rebouche CJ, Engel AG: Carnitine metabolism and deficiency syndromes. *Mayo Clin Proc* 58:533-540, 1983.

Roe CR, Coates PM: Acyl-CoA dehydrogenase deficiencies, in Scriver CR, et al (eds): *The Metabolic Basis of Inherited Disease, II,* ed 6. New York, McGraw-Hill, 1989, 889-914.

Sekula SA, et al: The porphyrias. *Am Fam Physician* 33:219-232, (March) 1986.

Sharp D: Gene therapy. *Lancet* 337:1277-1278, 1991.

Siegemund R, et al: Mode of action of triethylenetetramine dihydrochloride on copper metabolism in Wilson's disease. *Acta Neurol Scand* 83:364-366, 1991.

Simionatto CS, et al: Thrombophlebitis and disturbed hemostasis following administration of intravenous hematin in normal volunteers. *Am J Med* 85:538-540, 1988.

Smith LH Jr: Diseases of the urea cycle, in Wyngaarden JB, Smith LH Jr (eds): *Textbook of Medicine,* ed 18. Philadelphia, WB Saunders, 1988, vol 1, 1158-1159.

Smith ML, et al: Diagnosis of cystinosis with use of placenta, letter. *N Engl J Med* 321:397-398, 1989.

Smolin LA, et al: Comparison of the effectiveness of cysteamine and phosphocysteamine in elevating plasma cysteamine concentration and decreasing leukocyte free cystine in nephropathic cystinosis. *Pediatr Res* 23:616-620, 1988.

Stevens MB, et al: State screening for metabolic disorders in newborns. *Am Fam Physician* 37:223-228, (April) 1988.

Tankanow RM: Pathophysiology and treatment of Wilson's disease. *Clin Pharm* 10:839-849, 1991.

Thoene JG, Lemons R: Cystine depletion of cystinotic tissues by phosphocysteamine (WR638). *J Pediatr* 96:1043-1044, 1980.

Thoene JG, et al: Intracellular cystine depletion by aminothiols in vitro and in vivo. *J Clin Invest* 58:180-189, 1976.

Valle D: Genetic disease: Overview of current therapy. *Hosp Pract* 22:167-182, (July) 1987.

Valle DL, Mitchell GA: Inborn errors of metabolism in the molecular age, in Childs B, et al (eds): *Molecular Genetics in Medicine.* New York, Elsevier, 1988, vol 7, 100-129.

Yeung-Laiwah AC, McColl KEL: Management of attacks of acute porphyria. *Drugs* 34:604-616, 1987.

Hematopoietic Growth Factors 105

REGULATION OF HEMATOPOIESIS

Hematopoiesis is a complex and highly regulated process (see Figure) by which multipotential stem cells with maximal capabilities for self-renewal are stimulated to proliferate and differentiate along one of several pathways (Quesenberry, 1990; Golde, 1991; Sachs, 1991). Proliferative capacity declines as maturation progresses. The conventional viewpoint of most investigators is that the first major branch point in hematopoietic differentiation involves commitment to either the lymphoid or myeloid lineages. (Further lymphoid differentiation, which generates the T-cells and B-cells of the immune system, is not discussed in this chapter.) Alternatively, other investigators suggest that the first major branch point is between the T-cells and all other lineages, with subsequent differentiation of B-cells from the myeloid lineage.

Myeloid differentiation produces erythrocytes, granulocytes, platelets, monocytes/macrophages, eosinophils, and basophils and depends on the actions of interacting cytokines: the interleukins (IL) and colony-stimulating factors (CSF). Early progenitor cells (also referred to as committed stem cells) from each of the myeloid lineages respond to multiple cytokines, and most cytokines act on more than one cell lineage and at several stages of differentiation (Quesenberry, 1990; Golde, 1991; Sachs, 1991). Detection and quantitation of progenitor cells in fresh suspensions prepared from blood or bone marrow rely on in vitro or in vivo (mouse spleen) colony formation assays (Caro, 1990; Moore, 1991 A).

Pluripotent progenitor cells represent a very small fraction (<0.1%) of the cells present in bone marrow. They have been characterized by the presence or absence of various cell-surface antigens (most notably CD34) and their ability to repopulate the bone marrow in lethally irradiated experimental animals (Golde, 1991). These progenitor cells can be purified to varying degrees from suspensions of bone marrow cells, peripheral blood cells, or umbilical cord blood cells using automated cell separators, antibody-based T-lymphocyte depletion, counterflow centrifugal elutriation, chemical purging in culture, flow cytometric sorting, or other techniques, alone or in combination (Ciavarella, 1991). A multipotent growth factor stimulates the proliferation of quiescent human hematopoietic stem cells (Bernstein et al, 1991; Carow et al, 1991; Brandt et al, 1992). This glycoprotein has been referred to as stem cell factor (SCF), mast cell growth factor, and *c-kit* ligand (since it appears to be the endogenous agonist for a cell surface receptor that is the product of the *c-kit* proto-oncogene). Under the influence of SCF and other cytokines, including IL-3 (formerly termed multi-CSF), IL-1, IL-4, and IL-6, pluripotent progenitor cells proliferate and partially differentiate to generate early myeloid progenitor cells that are most likely represented by the colony-forming unit-blast or the high proliferative potential colony-forming cell (McNiece et al, 1990; Grosh and Quesenberry, 1992).

Under the influence of the cytokines listed above, together with granulocyte/macrophage-CSF (GM-CSF) and granulocyte-CSF (G-CSF), the early myeloid progenitor cells differentiate further to yield the committed progenitors of the myeloid lineages. The proliferation and terminal maturation of erythroid precursors also require the actions of multiple cytokines (SCF, G-CSF, GM-CSF, IL-3, IL-4, and IL-9) as well as of erythropoietin (Quesenberry, 1990; Erslev, 1990). These cytokines have been characterized as having burst-promoting activity because, in the presence of erythropoietin, they stimulate formation of large colonies of erythroid cells that have a "burst-like" appearance. The progenitor cells that give rise to these colonies are referred to as BFU-E.

In addition to the BFU-E, four other progenitor cells are thought to arise from the early myeloid progenitor cell (CFU-GEMM): granulocyte/macrophage precursors (CFU-GM), megakaryocyte precursors (BFU-Meg), eosinophil precursors (CFU-Eos), and basophil precursors (CFU-Baso) (Grosh and Quesenberry, 1992). The further action of IL-3, GM-CSF, and other cytokines results in differentiation of CFU-GM into progenitors that are committed to the neutrophil (CFU-G [CFU-N in the Figure]) or monocyte/macrophage (CFU-M) cell lineages. Maturation and proliferation of CFU-G to neutrophils are regulated primarily by G-CSF, although IL-3 and GM-CSF enhance the effects of G-CSF (Quesenberry, 1990; Golde, 1990). Proliferation and maturation of monocytes and macrophages from CFU-M require macrophage-CSF (M-CSF; also referred to as CSF-1); IL-3 and GM-CSF participate at several stages of the pathway (Quesenberry, 1990; Golde and Groopman, 1990). Basophil production from CFU-Baso is enhanced by SCF, GM-CSF, IL-3, and IL-4 (Quesenberry, 1990; Galli et al, 1990). Eosinophil growth and differentiation from CFU-Eos depend on actions of multiple factors. IL-5 appears to be selective for eosinophil production, while IL-3 and GM-CSF stimulate neutrophils, monocytes, and eosinophils (Zucker-Franklin, 1990). Finally, production of megakaryocytes and platelets from early progenitors (BFU-Meg and CFU-Meg) requires SCF, GM-CSF, G-CSF, IL-3, IL-6, and IL-11 (and probably IL-1, erythropoietin, and IL-4) (Quesenberry, 1990; Paulus and Aster, 1990). Maturation (but not colony formation) of megakaryocytes and platelets appears to require a plasma-borne protein or proteins, which may be members of the interleukin family (IL-6, IL-7) (Paulus and Aster, 1990; McDonald, 1988).

Information on some of the properties, actions, and sources of many hematopoietic growth factors has been available for some time. Erythropoietin, the first to be identified, was purified from the urine of patients with aplastic anemia more than 15 years ago (Miyake et al, 1977). However, until the advent of recombinant DNA technology, it was not possible to produce any of the hematopoietic growth factors in amounts sufficient for administration to patients. Thus far, genes for many of these glycoproteins have been cloned and expressed in suitable vectors, and the active recombinant hematopoietic factors are available for clinical investigation and, in three cases, for therapeutic administration (Golde and Glaspy, 1990; Kanz et al, 1991; Moore, 1991 B; St. Onge and Jacobson, 1992; Lieschke and Burgess, 1992). The genes for GM-CSF, IL-3, IL-4, IL-5, M-CSF, and the M-CSF receptor (the c-*fms* proto-oncogene) have been localized to the long arm of chromosome 5 and may be coordinately expressed. Deletions in this region have been associated with the "5q minus" myelodysplastic disorder (Nimer and Golde, 1987); however, data are insufficient to establish a causal relationship between this deletion and the myelodysplasia.

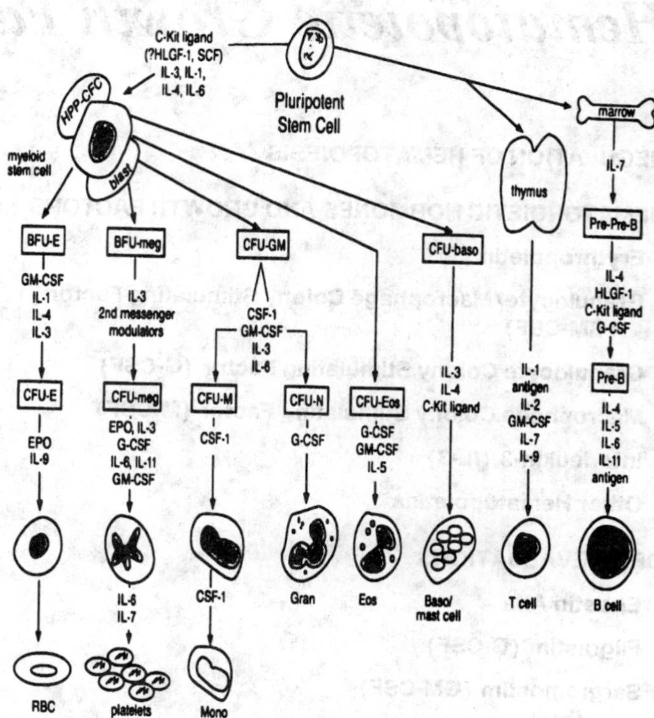

Regulation of hematopoiesis. Reprinted with permission (Grosh and Quesenberry, 1992).

Epoetin alfa [Epogen, Procrit], the first commercially available recombinant hematopoietic factor, is used to treat the anemia of chronic renal failure and zidovudine-induced anemia in HIV-infected patients. It also has been studied for use in several other anemic conditions. Preparations of recombinant GM-CSF (sargramostim) [Leukine, Prokine] and G-CSF (filgrastim) [Neupogen] are used to accelerate marrow engraftment after transplantation and for neutropenia resulting from cancer chemotherapy. Clinical trials on a second recombinant form of GM-CSF (molgramostim [Leucomax]) have been conducted; however, this product is not yet available in the United States. Trials of M-CSF, IL-1, IL-3, and IL-4 in the treatment of various neutropenias, aplasias, myelodysplasias, and infectious diseases have either been completed recently or are ongoing.

HEMATOPOIETIC HORMONES AND GROWTH FACTORS

ERYTHROPOIETIN. In adults, approximately 90% of the hormone, erythropoietin, is produced in the peritubular interstitial cells of the kidney and approximately 10% is produced in the liver (Erslev, 1991; Jelkmann, 1992; Krantz, 1991). Erythropoietin is classified as a hematopoietic mitogen and survival factor. It is responsible for recruiting quiescent BFU-E to progress through the cell cycle and for maintaining their viability and facilitating their differentiation. The latter action may be mediated through erythropoietin-induced expression of genes that are not transcribed (or are transcribed at lower rates) in its absence. For example, erythropoietin activates globin gene transcription (Nijhof et al, 1987) and enhances the enzyme activities required for heme synthesis (Beru and Goldwasser, 1985; Abraham et al, 1989). These actions of erythropoietin are mediated by specific receptors present on the surface of responsive cells (D'Andrea and Zon, 1990). Signal transduction into the cell interior after ligand-receptor binding may be mediated by activation of phospholipases and then of protein kinase C (Mason-Garcia and Beckman, 1991). Adequate stores of iron, folic acid, and vitamin B_{12} are essential for the action of erythropoietin (Van Wyck et al, 1989; Macdougall et al, 1989). Other colony-stimulating factors and interleukins also are necessary for the complete regulatory control of the earliest stages of erythropoiesis (Quesenberry, 1990; Erslev, 1990).

Tissue hypoxia or anemia cause elevated erythropoietin concentrations in individuals with normal kidney function (Jelkmann, 1992). Although serum concentrations of erythropoietin in most patients with anemia of end-stage renal disease (ESRD) or chronic renal failure are within the normal range, the levels are inappropriately low for the degree of anemia in these patients (Ad Hoc Committee for the National Kidney Foundation, 1989; Adamson and Eschbach, 1990). Individuals with renal insufficiency caused by polycystic kidney disease usually have higher concentrations of erythropoietin than other ESRD patients and often are only moderately anemic because erythropoietin is produced by stromal cells in the cyst walls (Eckardt et al, 1989). An elevated erythropoietin concentration also is observed in individuals with certain tumors that produce the hormone inappropriately in the absence of tissue hypoxia.

Before the advent of recombinant DNA technology, supplies of human erythropoietin were inadequate for widespread use in the therapy of anemia. However, both cDNA and genomic clones for the human erythropoietin gene have now been developed. Recombinant human erythropoietin (epoetin) has been expressed in both bacterial and mammalian cells; since glycosylation is required for in vivo activity, only the mammalian cell-derived preparations are therapeutically useful.

The primary amino acid sequence of recombinant erythropoietin is identical to that of the mature endogenous glycoprotein (ie, 165 amino acids after removal of a carboxy-terminal arginine during post-translational processing). Different recombinant preparations vary in the extent of glycosylation and in the degree of branching found in the sugar chains. These differences do not affect erythropoietin activity when measured in bone marrow cultures, but in vivo activity in mice is much greater for tetra-antennary than for biantennary glycoproteins. The increased branching significantly enhances the biological half-life (ie, reduces the rate of clearance) relative to that of less-branched glycoprotein (Takeuchi et al, 1989). The clinical significance of these differences is not known. Desialylation also increases clearance in vivo because of the action of an asialoglycoprotein-binding protein found in the liver (Spivak and Hogans, 1989).

Uses: Erythropoietin therapy reverses the anemia of chronic renal failure and has eliminated the need for blood transfusion in almost all of these patients (Ad Hoc Committee for the National Kidney Foundation, 1989; Adamson and Eschbach, 1990; Erslev, 1991). Use of the recombinant hormone now is standard therapy for the hypoproliferative, generally normocytic anemia of chronic renal failure. It has replaced the use of androgen therapy to stimulate production of endogenous erythropoietin. Although initial clinical trials were limited to anemic hemodialysis patients, it is now clear that erythropoietin therapy also is safe and effective in anemic predialysis patients (Lim et al, 1989; Watson et al, 1990; Erslev, 1991; The US Recombinant Human Erythropoietin Predialysis Study Group, 1991; Jelkmann, 1992). Furthermore, it can be administered subcutaneously to correct anemia in individuals maintained on continuous ambulatory peritoneal dialysis (Lui et al, 1990; Rotellar et al, 1991).

In a small number of patients, as an indirect result of the reduced transfusion dependence, HLA sensitization was decreased; this resulted in shorter waiting times and improved survival rates for renal allografts (Grimm et al, 1990). Other benefits of erythropoietin therapy include improvement in exercise tolerance as a consequence of increasing the oxygen-carrying capacity of the blood (Canadian Erythropoietin Study Group, 1990; Robertson et al, 1990; Metra et al, 1991). Data suggest that brain and cognitive functions also may improve (Marsh et al, 1991; Wolcott, 1991), depression may be reduced (Canadian Erythropoietin Study Group, 1990), and uremic pruritus may be relieved, possibly mediated by a decrease in plasma histamine concentration (De Marchi et al, 1992) with long-term therapy. Thus, it is not surprising that the quality of life of these patients appears to improve once the hematocrit has been restored to within the normal range (Lundin, 1989; Lundin et al, 1990; Evans et al, 1990).

Erythropoietin also is used to treat the severe anemia often seen in patients with AIDS who are taking zidovudine (Fischl et al, 1990; Groopman, 1990; Henry et al, 1992 A). Measurements of serum immunoreactive erythropoietin in anemic individuals infected with the human immunodeficiency virus (HIV) showed levels that were inappropriately low in this population when compared with serum levels in patients with iron deficiency anemia of equivalent severity (Spivak et al, 1989). The increase in erythropoietin associated with a decline in hemoglobin was significantly less in the HIV-infected group than in iron-deficient individuals. Treatment with zidovudine resulted in marked elevation of erythropoietin levels but was accompanied by an apparent worsening of the anemia. Results of a randomized, double-blind, placebo-controlled trial indicated that hematopoiesis improves and transfusion requirements are reduced in response to erythropoietin in those AIDS patients with baseline levels of erythropoietin <500 milliunits/ml (Fischl et al, 1990). In comparison, the range for normal individuals is 10 to 30 milliunits/ml. AIDS patients with anemia whose erythropoietin levels were >500 milliunits/ml did not benefit from the exogenously administered hormone at the dose used in this study (100 units/kg administered intravenously three times weekly). Similar results were reported in a review of four clinical trials that included 297 anemic AIDS patients receiving zidovudine therapy who were randomized to receive either epoetin (100 to 200 units/kg three times weekly subcutaneously or intravenously) or placebo (Henry et al, 1992 A).

Despite the ability of erythropoietin to correct the anemia in AIDS patients receiving zidovudine, the dose of zidovudine must be reduced in most of these individuals because of the neutropenia it produces. Consequently, there is interest in the combined use of erythropoietin with myeloid CSFs (GM-CSF or G-CSF) to allow continued full-dose therapy with zidovudine (Groopman, 1990; Miles et al, 1991). Preliminary data indicate that combined use of the two growth factors does not reduce the response to each of them.

Limited data from a small randomized trial on use of erythropoietin in 15 AIDS patients who are anemic but are not receiving zidovudine suggest that transfusion requirements also may be reduced in these individuals (Henry et al, 1992 B).

The efficacy and safety of erythropoietin therapy has been studied in a variety of other anemias (Erslev, 1991; Jelkmann, 1992). Patients with advanced cancer often are anemic, as a result of either their disease (the anemia of chronic disease) or chemotherapy (Abels et al, 1991; Means and Krantz, 1991; Abels, 1992; Spivak, 1992). Erythropoietin is now also indicated for chemotherapy-associated anemia in patients with nonmyeloid malignancies. Separate, randomized trials have shown that erythropoietin therapy increases the hematocrit and reduces transfusion requirements in anemic patients with a variety of solid tumors, B-cell lymphomas, or multiple myeloma being treated with regimens that do or do not include cisplatin, as well as in those not receiving chemotherapy.

Small randomized controlled (Stein et al, 1991) and uncontrolled (Bowen et al, 1991; van Kamp et al, 1991; Cazzola et al, 1992) trials also have employed erythropoietin to treat refractory anemia in patients with myelodysplastic syndromes (MDS). Increased hemoglobin levels and/or reduced transfusion requirements were noted in small and variable percentages of these patients. The only predictive factor for response to erythropoietin in MDS patients appears to be a low baseline concentration of the endogenous glycoprotein. Thus, some investigators suggest that a trial of erythropoietin is warranted only in MDS patients with endogenous levels of erythropoietin <100 units/ml (Mittelman et al, 1992).

Erythropoietin appears to be quite promising as therapy for infants with anemia of prematurity. In one randomized study in which erythropoietin was compared with transfusion, the degree of reduction in the signs and symptoms of anemia was similar with both therapies, but symptoms recurred and additional transfusion was required in the majority of infants who did not receive erythropoietin (Ohls and Christensen, 1991). Other randomized, placebo-controlled trials demonstrated that transfusion requirements were reduced and erythropoiesis was enhanced in premature infants receiving erythropoietin (Shannon et al, 1991, 1992; Carnielli et al, 1992). An increase in the rate of recovery from postpartum maternal anemia after erythropoietin therapy was reported in a placebo-controlled, randomized trial (Huch et al, 1992).

Other anemias that have responded to erythropoietin therapy in some patients include the anemia associated with rheumatoid arthritis (Means et al, 1989; Pincus et al, 1990) and that secondary to trauma, surgery, or burns in patients with religious objections to transfusion (Pousada et al, 1990; Green and Handley, 1990; Boshkov et al, 1991; Connor and Olsson, 1992). In contrast, the limited data available suggest that anemia in patients with sickle cell disease probably does not respond to erythropoietin administered as a single agent (Goldberg et al, 1990, 1992). Results reported in pilot studies of erythropoietin combined with hydroxyurea in these patients depended on the dosage schedule. When erythropoietin was administered in two intravenous boluses of 1,500 units/kg each one day each week for four weeks plus oral hydroxyurea given daily, the combination did not increase the percentage of fetal hemoglobin-containing reticulocytes or red blood cells more than hydroxyurea alone (Goldberg et al, 1990, 1992). However, combining the two drugs in an alternating schedule of oral hydroxyurea for four days followed by intravenous erythropoietin for three days (with dosage escalating from 1,000 to 3,000 units/kg/day) appeared to enhance fetal hemoglobin production (Rodgers et al, 1993). Further clinical trials are necessary to determine if this response, and the improved erythrocyte rheology that accompanies it, offer significant benefits for patients with sickle cell disease.

Erythropoietin also is useful in nonanemic patients scheduled for elective surgery who plan to donate autologous blood for use if transfusion is necessary. Results from randomized, placebo-controlled trials demonstrate that administration of erythropoietin during three weeks of blood collection (one or two phlebotomies each week) maintained higher hematocrits and yielded significantly larger volumes of red blood cells than in the control groups (Goodnough et al, 1989, 1992; Tasaki et al, 1992). However, the increase in the yield of autologous red blood cells in response to erythropoietin is higher in men and postmenopausal women than in premenopausal women. Data suggest that erythropoiesis may be limited by the rate of absorption of oral iron in premenopausal women (Goodnough et al, 1991) and that intravenous iron supplementation may be needed for these women.

Erythropoietin has been used inappropriately by a few athletes to increase the hematocrit and thus the oxygen-carrying capacity of the blood (Catlin and Hatton, 1991; Smith and Perry, 1992) and thereby enhance endurance and aerobic capacity, particularly in those athletes participating in long-distance events. This goal is similar to that of "blood doping"—transfusion of autologous or homologous red blood cells to increase the hematocrit shortly before competition. The risks associated with these practices include increased blood viscosity due to an elevated hematocrit and dehydration resulting in decreased cardiac output and possible thrombosis (Catlin and Hatton, 1991; Adamson and Vapnek, 1991; Smith and Perry, 1992).

Erythropoietin should not be used routinely for anemia. It is imperative that the cause of the anemia be determined prior to administration of any antianemic drug, including epoetin.

GRANULOCYTE/MACROPHAGE COLONY STIMULATING FACTOR (GM-CSF). In vivo, GM-CSF is produced by various cells, including T-cells, endothelial cells, macrophages, and fibroblasts (Gasson, 1991; Lieschke and Burgess, 1992; Grant and Heel, 1992). The cloned gene for recombinant human GM-CSF has been expressed in bacteria, yeast, and mammalian cells. The endogenous factor is a monomeric glycoprotein with a molecular weight of about 22 kilodaltons. The recombinant preparation derived from bacterial cells is unglycosylated (and thus has a substantially lower molecular weight), while the yeast- and mammalian-derived recombinant proteins are glycosylated, although to varying degrees and patterns. Glycosylation does not seem to be required for either in vitro or in vivo activity, since the recombinant protein from bacteria induces leukocytosis in humans. The extent and pattern of glycosylation may influence pharmacokinetics and in vivo half-life.

GM-CSF stimulates the proliferation, differentiation, and function of a variety of target cells at different stages of hematopoietic maturation (Gasson, 1991; Lieschke and Burgess, 1992; Grant and Heel, 1992). It directly stimulates production of granulocyte and macrophage colonies in vitro and acts with other factors to increase colony formation by BFU-Meg and CFU-Meg, blast cells, and BFU-E. In vivo, GM-CSF enhances production of granulocytes, macrophages, and possibly platelets in humans, other primates, and mice. Thus, the progenitor cells that are targets for GM-CSF include CFU-Blast, CFU-GEMM, CFU-GM, CFU-G, CFU-M, CFU-Eos, CFU-Meg, and BFU-E. In addition to its colony-stimulating effects, GM-CSF acts on mature end-stage cells of several lineages to activate or enhance some of their functions. Among the latter actions of GM-CSF are stimulation of the production of cytokines (tumor necrosis factor, IL-1, and M-CSF) and leukotriene B_4 by appropriate target cells, activation of mature granulocytes and monocytes, enhancement of antibody-dependent and independent cellular cytotoxicity, an increase in macrophage tumorcidal activity, and an increase in the adhesion and inhibition of migration of mature neutrophils. The mature end-stage cells that respond to GM-CSF include granulocytes, monocytes, macrophages, and eosinophils.

Uses: An extensive series of clinical trials have evaluated the response to therapy with GM-CSF in patients with a variety of pathologic conditions (Lieschke and Burgess, 1992; Grant and Heel, 1992). In early Phase I/II trials of GM-CSF in patients with advanced malignancies, there was an initial rapid but transient decline in peripheral blood leukocyte counts, followed by progressive dose-dependent increases in the number of neutrophils, monocytes, and eosinophils. The initial decline appears to result from sequestration of neutrophils in the lung, and baseline levels usually are restored within four hours by re-entry of these sequestered cells into the peripheral circulation.

GM-CSF is used to enhance the rate of engraftment and shorten the duration of neutropenia in patients undergoing bone marrow transplants (Nemunaitis and Singer, 1991; Singer, 1992; Lieschke and Burgess, 1992; Grant and Heel, 1992; St. Onge and Jacobson, 1992). Many Phase II trials that used historical controls and a smaller number of randomized, placebo-controlled studies have evaluated the efficacy and safety of GM-CSF therapy in patients receiving high-dose chemotherapy and autologous bone marrow transplantation (ABMT) for lymphoid malignancies or some solid tumors. Results from these studies indicate that administration of GM-CSF results in more rapid recovery of hematopoiesis (neutrophil and, in some studies, platelet counts), reduced transfusion requirements for red blood cells and platelets, shorter hospital stays, a lower risk of serious infection, and reduced use of antibiotics (Gulati and Bennett, 1992; Advani et al, 1992; Nemunaitis, 1993; and reviews cited above). Data also suggest that the administration of GM-CSF in patients receiving ABMT can reduce the total cost of treatment incurred after marrow infusion (Gulati and Bennett, 1992). It appears that chemical purging of marrow for ABMT (eg, with 4-hydroperoxycyclophosphamide) can decrease the number of infused CFU-GM below levels that are adequate for GM-CSF enhancement of neutrophil recovery (Blazar et al, 1989). GM-CSF therapy did not affect the rate of disease relapse or survival after high-dose chemotherapy and ABMT in any of the randomized trials.

GM-CSF also is used to increase the number of peripheral blood progenitor cells that can be harvested by leukapheresis during recovery from moderate-dose chemotherapy (Lieschke and Burgess, 1992; Grant and Heel, 1992). This probably results from the ability of GM-CSF to mobilize progenitor cells and enhance their transit from the bone marrow into the circulation (Rosenfeld and Nemunaitis, 1992). The harvested progenitor cells are then reinfused after high-dose chemotherapy. Successful engraftment of peripheral blood progenitors used alone has been reported in patients from whom adequate amounts of autologous marrow could not be obtained (Haas et al, 1990) or when marrow was held in reserve (Elias et al, 1992). When infused with autologous marrow, the GM-CSF-stimulated peripheral progenitors result in a more rapid recovery of neutrophil counts (Lieschke and Burgess, 1992; Grant and Heel, 1992).

Recovery after high-dose chemotherapy and allogeneic bone marrow transplant also is more rapid in patients treated with GM-CSF (Singer, 1992; Lieschke and Burgess, 1992; Grant and Heel, 1992). Results from a placebo-controlled, randomized trial in patients receiving marrow from HLA-identical siblings showed that patients given GM-CSF had significantly higher early leukocyte and absolute neutrophil counts and reduced rates of infection (De Witte et al, 1992). The incidence or severity of graft-versus-host disease (GVHD) and transplant-related mortality did not differ between the GM-CSF treated and control groups. However, in an earlier study, the response to GM-CSF after infusion of allogeneic marrow was significantly decreased in patients who received cyclosporine plus methotrexate as prophylaxis for GVHD compared with those given cyclosporine and methylprednisolone (followed by prednisone) for prophylaxis (Nemunaitis et al, 1991 A). Data from a trial of GM-CSF therapy in patients receiving allogeneic marrow from unrelated donors who were compared with historical controls who had not received GM-CSF suggest that the number of days with fever and the incidence of septicemia may be reduced by GM-CSF administration (Nemunaitis et al, 1992). As in the studies with HLA-matched sibling donors, the incidence and severity of GVHD were unaffected, as was the incidence of graft rejection. However, the time after marrow infusion required to reach absolute neutrophil counts >500/mm³ did not appear to be shorter in those treated with GM-CSF.

GM-CSF also is used as therapy for early or late failure of marrow engraftment in patients who receive either autologous or allogeneic marrow (Nemunaitis and Singer, 1991; Singer, 1992; Grant and Heel, 1992). About 50% of the patients experiencing graft failure respond to GM-CSF with an increase in neutrophil counts; no effect on platelet or red blood cell counts was reported in these patients.

Clinical trials investigating the effects of GM-CSF therapy on recovery from neutropenia in patients treated for hematologic malignancies or solid tumors with one of a variety of chemotherapeutic regimens also have been reviewed (Grant and Heel, 1992; St. Onge and Jacobson, 1992). Many of these trials used patients as their own controls by comparing recovery in a chemotherapy cycle without GM-CSF with recovery in a subsequent or previous cycle with GM-CSF. Other studies compared recovery in GM-CSF treated patients with historical controls who received the same chemotherapy regimen. Only one study used a randomized, double-blind, placebo-controlled design (de Vries et al, 1991). In nearly all studies, the duration of chemotherapy-induced neutropenia was significantly shortened by GM-CSF therapy. In some of the studies, the incidence and severity of mucositis and the incidence of stomatitis also were reduced after GM-CSF administration. Little if any effect on platelet counts as a result of GM-CSF administration was observed in most studies, and, in some studies, the ability to deliver subsequent cycles of high-dose chemotherapy on schedule and at full dose was improved as a consequence of treatment with GM-CSF. There was no evidence that GM-CSF stimulated tumor growth or reduced the response to chemotherapy.

Results of several studies in patients with acute myeloid leukemia have suggested that stimulation of the leukemic cells with GM-CSF may increase the fraction of cells in S phase and thus sensitize them to the effects of cytarabine, an S phase-specific cytotoxic drug (Bettelheim et al, 1991; Grant and Heel, 1992). However, in a more recent study, the rates of complete remission and survival were lower in patients given GM-CSF plus cytarabine (and daunorubicin) than in those treated with cytarabine (with or without amsacrine or mitoxantrone) and no GM-CSF (Estey et al, 1992).

A number of clinical trials also have used GM-CSF in the treatment of myelodysplastic syndromes (Lieschke and Burgess, 1992; Grant and Heel, 1992: Greenberg, 1992). GM-CSF increased neutrophil counts in about 80% of the patients, and the counts returned to pretreatment levels when GM-CSF administration was terminated. Monocyte and eosinophil counts also increased in most patients. In contrast, reticulocyte and platelet counts increased in less than 25% of those treated with GM-CSF. Preliminary data have raised concern that GM-CSF may accelerate the transformation to acute leukemia in patients with ≥15% blasts in the bone marrow (ie, those with refractory anemia with excess blasts with or without transformation, those with chronic myelomonocytic leukemia) (Ganser et al, 1989). GM-CSF does not appear to stimulate leukemic transformation in those with subtypes of myelodysplastic syndromes that are associated with better prognoses (refractory anemia and refractory anemia with ringed sideroblasts).

In patients with HIV infection, neutropenia can occur as a toxic response to zidovudine therapy, as a direct consequence of AIDS, or as an adverse reaction to other therapies (eg, ganciclovir for cytomegalovirus-induced retinitis, zidovudine plus interferon alfa for Kaposi's sarcoma) (Groopman, 1990; Lieschke and Burgess, 1992; Grant and Heel, 1992). Results from a series of Phase I/II trials showed that daily administration of GM-CSF to neutropenic AIDS patients increased neutrophil and eosinophil counts in a dose-dependent manner, allowed continued therapy with myelosuppressive antiretroviral drugs (eg, zidovudine, ganciclovir), and did not alter the rate of progression of AIDS. This observation is significant because in vitro studies have suggested that GM-CSF may stimulate the proliferation of HIV in monocytes in the absence of antiretroviral drugs. However, continuation of ganciclovir therapy as a result of GM-CSF's reversal of neutropenia prevented progression of retinitis. Similarly, continuation of zidovudine therapy after correction of neutropenia by GM-CSF (and anemia by erythropoietin) appears to slow HIV proliferation (as determined by p24 antigen levels). GM-CSF also ameliorates neutropenia induced by combination chemotherapy for AIDS-associated non-Hodgkin's lymphoma (Kaplan et al, 1991).

Investigations of the efficacy of GM-CSF therapy for various chronic neutropenic conditions have been reviewed (Lieschke and Burgess, 1992; Grant and Heel, 1992). One randomized, double-blind, placebo-controlled trial confirmed results reported in pilot studies in patients with aplastic anemia who did not respond to immunomodulator therapy and for whom compatible bone marrow donors were unavailable. In these studies, GM-CSF increased neutrophil counts two- to eightfold except in patients with severe aplasia of long duration. This response was maintained only during continued administration of GM-CSF. Monocyte and eosinophil counts and bone marrow cellularity increased as well, but lymphocyte counts increased less often. There was no evidence that GM-CSF therapy had any effect on survival of these patients.

In most patients with chronic neutropenias (idiopathic, congenital, cyclic, or autoimmune neutropenias; Felty's syndrome; glycogen storage disease type 1b) who were treated with GM-CSF in a series of small pilot studies, marked eosinophilia without clinically significant improvement in neutrophil counts was observed (Grant and Heel, 1992). In a few of the patients, severe infection improved after GM-CSF administration despite the minimal effect on neutrophil counts. Several of the studies on patients with congenital or cyclic neutropenia compared the effects of GM-CSF and G-CSF; the latter was reported to be more effective in increasing neutrophil counts (see the discussion on G-CSF). However, in one case study, a patient with cyclic neutropenia was treated with GM-CSF at one-tenth the dosage used by other investigators (Kurzrock et al, 1991 A). This very low dose of GM-CSF abolished the neutropenia and resolved the patient's infections, stomatitis, and malaise. Randomized trials of low-dose GM-CSF in similar patients are necessary.

Results from two small uncontrolled studies of GM-CSF as therapy for drug-induced agranulocytosis conflicted (Nand et al, 1991; Delannoy, 1992). In the first report, two patients appeared to respond to GM-CSF with an increase in the absolute neutrophil count, but only one of five patients treated in the second study showed any benefit from GM-CSF. Controlled trials are necessary to evaluate the efficacy of GM-CSF for this indication.

GRANULOCYTE COLONY STIMULATING FACTOR (G-CSF). This hematopoietic growth factor is more lineage-specific than GM-CSF. The native glycoprotein has a molecular mass of approximately 20 kilodaltons and is produced in vivo by monocytes, macrophages, endothelial cells, and fibroblasts (Demetri and Griffin, 1991; Hollingshead and Goa, 1991; Lieschke and Burgess, 1992). The human gene coding for G-CSF has been cloned and expressed in both bacterial and mammalian cells and has been localized to chromosome 17. The bacterially derived recombinant preparation (with a molecular mass of 18.6 kilodaltons) is not glycosylated but retains biological activity both in vitro and in vivo.

The predominant action of G-CSF in vitro is to stimulate formation of neutrophilic granulocyte colonies; thus, the major progenitor cell target for G-CSF is the CFU-G (Demetri and Griffin, 1991; Hollingshead and Goa, 1991; Lieschke and Burgess, 1992). In addition, it synergizes with IL-3 to stimulate formation of blast, megakaryocyte, and giant macrophage colonies, and it potentiates colony formation in response to GM-CSF. Some malignant cell lines derived from human solid and hematologic tumors show increased proliferation in response to G-CSF, and several myeloid leukemic lines undergo in vitro maturation in its presence. G-CSF also affects the functions of some mature end-stage cells, primarily neutrophils. Among these effects are priming of neutrophils to respond to chemotactic peptides and enhancing neutrophil antibody-dependent cellular cytotoxicity and phagocytosis of granulocytes. G-CSF's major effect in vivo is to increase circulating numbers of neutrophil granulocytes, but small increases are also seen in monocytes.

Uses: Clinical trials with G-CSF in healthy volunteers and in patients with a variety of diseases have been reviewed (Hollingshead and Goa, 1991; Lieschke and Burgess, 1992). A transient decrease in the number of circulating neutrophils and monocytes occurs within the first hour after intravenous or subcutaneous administration of G-CSF. This is usually followed by a sustained, dose-dependent increase in neutrophil count that reaches a plateau after about one week of therapy and returns to baseline levels four to seven days after cessation of G-CSF administration. Small increases in the numbers of monocytes and lymphocytes usually are noted if doses ≥ 10 mcg/kg/day are given; platelet counts may decrease by up to 25% if doses ≥ 30 mcg/kg/day (higher than recommended) are given for two weeks. G-CSF also increases the circulating levels of peripheral blood progenitor cells from all lineages.

Many Phase I/II trials (ie, using historical controls or using patients as their own controls by comparing cycles of chemotherapy with and without G-CSF) and fewer, more recent randomized, controlled Phase III studies of G-CSF in patients receiving myelosuppressive chemotherapy for various malignancies have been reviewed (Hollingshead and Goa, 1991; Lieschke and Burgess, 1992; St. Onge and Jacobson, 1992). Results demonstrate that G-CSF is safe and effective in reducing the duration and severity of neutropenia. Benefits include reductions in the incidence of febrile neutropenia and documented infections, the duration of hospital stays and antibiotic therapy, and the number of patients who require hospitalization or antibiotic therapy. G-CSF also increased the number of patients able to receive subsequent cycles of chemotherapy at full dose and on schedule.

G-CSF reduces neutropenia both in those who have previously received cytotoxic chemotherapy and in those not previously treated and retains its efficacy for at least six cycles of chemotherapy followed by G-CSF therapy. Included in the trials were patients with lung, breast, ovarian, urothelial, and lymphoid malignancies, as well as relapsed or refractory acute leukemia. Despite concerns that G-CSF therapy might stimulate proliferation of leukemic cells and accelerate disease progression, in several trials recovery from chemotherapy-induced neutropenia was enhanced and there was no progression of leukemia.

In studies to determine the efficacy of G-CSF in patients receiving high-dose chemotherapy with autologous or allogeneic bone marrow transplantation (Hollingshead and Goa, 1991; Lieschke and Burgess, 1992), the duration of neutropenia was shortened in those given G-CSF therapy after marrow infusion. No effect on thrombocytopenia was observed. In some of the trials, G-CSF therapy also reduced the number of days with fever, the number of days of antibiotic therapy, and the number of days of hospitalization. Results from two recent reports indicate that G-CSF can increase the yield of peripheral blood progenitor cells that can be harvested by leukapheresis and that autotransplantation of the progenitor cells can increase the rate of myeloid reconstitution after high-dose chemotherapy when infused with (Sheridan et al, 1992) or without (Fukuda et al, 1992) autologous bone marrow cells.

Clinical trials also have evaluated G-CSF therapy in patients with myelodysplastic syndromes (Hollingshead and Goa, 1991; Lieschke and Burgess, 1992; Greenberg, 1992). Increased neutrophil counts were reported in a study of very short-term use (one to two weeks) of G-CSF in 41 patients with myelodysplastic syndromes (Yoshida et al, 1991). Of 18 patients who were treated for six weeks or longer in initial studies of short-term therapy, G-CSF increased absolute neutrophil counts in 16, including 9 of 11 of those with severe neutropenia. In some patients, increases in reticulocyte counts and decreases in transfusion requirements also were observed. Platelet, lymphocyte, monocyte, and eosinophil counts were not affected, and neutrophil counts returned to baseline levels two to four weeks after G-CSF therapy was discontinued. However, in 5 of the 18 patients (4 of whom had refractory anemia with excess blasts in transformation) the myelodysplasia progressed to acute leukemia during G-CSF therapy. Eleven patients were maintained on G-CSF therapy for 6 to 28 months, and 10 continued to respond with persistently elevated neutrophil counts (Negrin et al, 1990). The risk of infection decreased in many of these individuals during the periods when neutrophil counts were $>1,500/mm^3$

and, in some, increases in hematocrits or decreases in transfusion requirements persisted during G-CSF therapy.

G-CSF also has been investigated as therapy for a variety of chronic neutropenic disorders (Hollingshead and Goa, 1991; Lieschke and Burgess, 1992; Boxer et al, 1992). Patients with severe congenital (Kostmann's syndrome) and chronic neutropenias have responded to G-CSF with an increase in neutrophil counts and a decrease in the risk of infection. These improvements were maintained for the duration of therapy in most of the patients. In contrast to the results observed after therapy with GM-CSF, eosinophils do not account for the major portion of the increase in granulocyte counts noted in patients with severe congenital neutropenia who are treated with G-CSF. Small uncontrolled studies in patients with cyclic neutropenia suggest that G-CSF therapy may increase neutrophil levels, shorten the cycle length, and decrease the incidence of fever, infection, and mucositis. Finally, most children with moderate or severe aplastic anemia also respond to G-CSF therapy with an increase in absolute neutrophil counts.

G-CSF therapy also has increased neutrophil counts and improved neutrophil function in patients with AIDS who were being treated with zidovudine (Miles et al, 1991; van der Wouw et al, 1991). The reversal of neutropenia, when combined with erythropoietin therapy for anemia, allowed continued administration of antiretroviral therapy.

Single case reports or uncontrolled studies with fewer than five patients have documented the clinical response to G-CSF therapy in neutropenic patients with hairy cell leukemia, Shwachman's syndrome, and drug-induced neutropenia (Hollingshead and Goa, 1991).

Randomized, placebo-controlled trials of G-CSF therapy in myelodysplastic syndromes, chronic neutropenias, AIDS, and other disorders are needed.

MACROPHAGE COLONY STIMULATING FACTOR (M-CSF). This homodimeric protein (also known as CSF-1) is extensively glycosylated; the degree depends on the source. Consequently, estimates of its molecular mass vary. Human urinary M-CSF has an estimated mass of 45 kilodaltons, while preparations purified from culture media range from 70 to 90 kilodaltons. This hematopoietic growth factor is produced in vivo by many cell types, including monocytes, fibroblasts, and endothelial cells. The primary progenitor cell target for M-CSF is the CFU-M, while monocytes and macrophages are the major end-stage cells responsive to this factor. Among the effects of M-CSF on mature target cells are increased production and secretion of other cytokines (interferon, tumor necrosis factor, IL-1, plasminogen activators) and enhancement of antibody-dependent cellular cytotoxicity against tumor cells.

In early clinical studies with a preparation partially purified from human urine (largely M-CSF), periods of neutropenia associated with chemotherapy for various malignancies were shortened (Motoyoshi et al, 1986). No other myeloid lineages were affected, including (rather surprisingly) the monocyte series. This preparation also has been reported to accelerate recovery of hematopoiesis and improve survival during the initial 120 days after bone marrow transplantation (Masaoka et al, 1990). In contrast, no effect of purified human urinary M-CSF on the rate of hematopoietic recovery following ABMT was observed in another study (Khwaja et al, 1992). However, in a subset of patients who received large inocula ($>2 \times 10^8$) of nucleated marrow cells, M-CSF increased the rate of platelet recovery and reduced the length of hospitalization. In hematologically normal patients with malignant lymphoma, a two-hour infusion of 4 to 16 million units/M^2 enhanced various in vitro and in vivo functions of monocytes (Khwaja et al, 1991). Among these were migration of monocytes into inflammatory "skin windows," priming of the respiratory burst, and phagocytosis and killing of *Candida*; these results suggest that M-CSF may be useful as therapy for severe infection, particularly in immunocompromised patients. A recombinant preparation of human M-CSF has been evaluated (in combination with conventional antifungal therapy) in a Phase I trial in bone marrow transplant patients with invasive fungal infections (Nemunaitis et al, 1991 B). The initial results (resolution of the infection in 6 of 12 evaluable patients) are sufficiently encouraging to warrant a randomized trial of M-CSF in a larger group of similar patients.

The partially purified human urinary preparation of M-CSF also has stimulated neutrophil production in children with chronic neutropenia (Komiyama et al, 1988). Both this response and the response in patients with chemotherapy-induced neutropenia may indirectly be due to the production of endogenous G-CSF rather than to a direct effect of the M-CSF itself. The sole side effect associated with the urinary CSF preparation has been mild fever in about one-third of treated patients. Transient, dose-related thrombocytopenia was reported in the trial of recombinant M-CSF (Nemunaitis et al, 1991 B). It is noteworthy that neither preparation alters the severity of GVHD in recipients of allogeneic bone marrow transplants.

INTERLEUKIN-3 (IL-3). This glycoprotein (also known as multi-CSF) is a hematopoietic cytokine that is produced by activated T-lymphocytes, mast cells, and eosinophils (Frendl, 1992) and has a molecular mass of 24 kilodaltons. The progenitor cell target specificity for IL-3 is even broader than that for GM-CSF and includes early progenitors from all of the myeloid lineages. In addition to its effects when used alone, IL-3 acts synergistically with GM-CSF and other growth factors, such as IL-5, erythropoietin, G-CSF, and M-CSF, to stimulate colony formation in marrow cell cultures. IL-3 supports mast cell growth and may stimulate some T-cell populations. Mature eosinophils and monocytes (but not neutrophils) are functionally activated by IL-3. Administration of IL-3 in vivo enhances production of all myeloid cell lineages (Ganser et al, 1990 A; Lindemann et al, 1991).

Recombinant human IL-3 has been produced by expression of the cloned cDNA in bacteria, yeast, and mammalian cells. Although the preparation from bacterial cells is not glycosylated, it retains biological activity both in vitro and in vivo. Thus far, clinical trials of recombinant IL-3 have focused primarily on hematologic responses, toxicities, and pharmacokinetics and have included cancer patients with normal hematopoiesis as well as patients with bone marrow failure (myelodysplasias, aplastic anemia, or secondary to cancer chemotherapy). The doses administered ranged from 30 to 500 mcg/M^2/day (Ottmann et al, 1990; Ganser et al, 1990 A) and 1,000 mcg/M^2/day (Kurzrock et al, 1991 B). In some studies, patients received daily subcutaneous injections for 15 days (Ottmann et al, 1990; Ganser et al, 1990 A); in others, IL-3 was infused for four hours each day for 28 days (Kurzrock et al, 1991 B). Increased numbers of white blood cells (neutrophils, eosinophils, and basophils), platelets, and reticulocytes were observed in varying percentages of the patients treated with IL-3. Bone marrow cellularity increased in response to IL-3 in most patients with myelodysplastic syndromes (Ganser et al, 1990 B) and in several with aplastic anemia (Ganser et al, 1990 C). After therapy with IL-3, three of six patients with congenital pure red cell aplasia (Diamond-Blackfan anemia) had increased reticulocyte counts and transfusion dependence also was reduced in two (Dunbar et al, 1991).

The most frequently observed adverse effects have been headache, fever, chills, and bone pain, but doses $\leq$500 mcg/M^2/day generally have been well tolerated. The serum half-life after intravenous infusion lengthened as the dose increased (from 19 minutes at 60 mcg/M^2 to 53 minutes at 250 mcg/M^2) (Kurzrock et al, 1991 B). The half-life after subcutaneous injection is considerably longer (>200 minutes) (Lindemann et al, 1991).

Although occasional therapeutic responses (eg, reduced red blood cell or platelet transfusion requirements) to IL-3 were observed in these Phase I/II studies, randomized, controlled trials of IL-3 (administered over longer periods) are needed to evaluate its potential as therapy for bone marrow failure. In a recent study, subcutaneous injection of IL-3 (8 or 16 mcg/kg/day for 14 days) in outpatients who received chemotherapy for relapsed small-cell lung cancer reduced the period of neutropenia to a mean of three days after a second cycle of chemotherapy; this compared with a mean of seven days of neutropenia in the same patients after a previous cycle without IL-3 (Postmus et al, 1992).

Sequential administration of recombinant IL-3 followed by GM-CSF also is being investigated. In a Phase I trial in cancer patients with normal hematopoiesis, the increases in the number of neutrophils and peripheral blood progenitor cells were larger with the combination than with either hematopoietin alone (Ganser et al, 1992). However, the combination was no more effective than IL-3 alone in increasing platelet counts. Results of a subsequent study suggest that the combination of IL-3 followed by GM-CSF (given after a one-day course of standard-dose chemotherapy) may increase the yield of peripheral blood progenitors that could be harvested for reinfusion after high-dose (myeloablative) chemotherapy (Brugger et al, 1992).

Interest in the potential of combination cytokine therapy has resulted in the development of a fusion protein (PIXY321) that is transcribed from a recombinant DNA fragment containing coding sequences of both the IL-3 and GM-CSF genes (Curtis et al, 1991). In vitro, this fusion protein has a higher receptor affinity and stimulates proliferation and colony formation more than either IL-3 or GM-CSF alone or in combination.

OTHER HEMATOPOIETINS. In addition to the hematopoietic growth factors discussed above, SCF, IL-1, IL-4, IL-5, and IL-6 have been produced by recombinant DNA techniques. Clinical trials of these cytokines in cancer patients are now under way, and studies investigating their therapeutic efficacy in various hematologic conditions should begin in the near future. Since IL-1, IL-4, IL-5, and IL-6 act primarily on late progenitors, they are likely to be most useful when combined with factors such as SCF, IL-3, or GM-CSF that stimulate early progenitor cells. The same may be true for G-CSF and M-CSF. Some investigators have suggested that the ultimate therapeutic promise for hematopoietic growth factors, particularly as therapy for aplastic anemia or to stimulate recovery after bone marrow transplantation, may lie in the design of appropriate "cocktails" of these glycoproteins. However, with the exception of IL-3 followed by administration of GM-CSF, there is little or no information available regarding strategies, schedules, or dosage regimens that might provide synergistic responses to such combinations. In addition, there is some concern that the earliest acting cytokines, such as SCF, may deplete stem cells and thus may be less beneficial (or more harmful) than currently anticipated; this question must be resolved by clinical trials.

Drug Evaluations

EPOETIN ALFA
[Epogen, Procrit]

ACTIONS AND USES. Epoetin alfa is the human hormone, erythropoietin, manufactured by recombinant DNA technology. The naturally occurring 165-amino acid glycoprotein has a molecular weight of 30.4 kilodaltons and is produced principally by the kidney. Erythropoietin is both a hematopoietic growth and differentiating factor that acts on erythroid burst-forming units and colony-forming units to promote their maturation and stimulate red blood cell production.

Epoetin is indicated in the treatment of the hypoproliferative, generally normocytic anemia associated with chronic renal failure in both dialyzed and nondialyzed patients (see the Introduction for discussion of the results of clinical trials). Onset of action is within one to two weeks, and desired hematocrits are attained within 8 to 12 weeks, depending on the degree of anemia, the dose employed, and the available iron stores. The increased blood viscosity that results from correction of anemia by epoetin and the hypertension that occasionally accompanies its use (incidence 10% to 20% of patients) do not appear to accelerate the deterioration of renal function in these patients (Lim et al, 1990).

Stimulation of erythropoiesis by epoetin occurs only in the presence of adequate iron stores. Therefore, it is imperative to evaluate iron stores before and during epoetin therapy. All dialysis patients except those with transfusional iron overload will require iron supplementation (Van Wyck, 1989). Transferrin saturation should be at least 20%, and the ferritin concentration should be at least 100 ng/ml.

Erythropoietin deficiency is not the only cause of anemia in patients receiving prolonged hemodialysis; vitamin B_{12} and folate deficiencies, gastrointestinal blood loss, and blood loss during dialysis also can be contributing factors. Aluminum overload may be a contributory factor in anemic patients with renal failure who do not respond adequately to epoetin (Grützmacher et al, 1990; Rosenlöf et al, 1990) or in whom hematopoietic responses to epoetin are delayed (Hollomby et al, 1990). However, aluminum overload does not account for all instances of epoetin-refractory anemia in hemodialysis patients (Adamson et al, 1990). Active inflammatory disease, infection, and malignancies also appear to reduce the response to epoetin (Adamson and Eschbach, 1990; Jelkmann, 1992).

Epoetin also is indicated for the anemia associated with zidovudine therapy in patients with AIDS and that caused by chemotherapy in patients with nonmyeloid malignancies. In randomized, controlled clinical trials, epoetin corrected the anemia resulting from myelosuppressive cancer chemotherapy, as well as the anemia that occurs in some untreated cancer patients. Highly positive results also have been reported from trials of epoetin as therapy for the anemia of prematurity and as an erythropoietic stimulant in candidates for elective surgery who are donating more than four units of autologous blood. Epoetin also is being evaluated as therapy for the anemias that accompany some myelodysplastic syndromes, rheumatoid arthritis, and blood loss in patients with religious objections to transfusion. See the Introduction for discussion of use of epoetin in all of these indications.

Epoetin should not be used to enhance athletic performance by increasing the hematocrit and thus the oxygen-carrying capacity of the blood.

ADVERSE REACTIONS AND PRECAUTIONS. In general, epoetin is well tolerated (Wong et al, 1990). No serious allergic or anaphylactic reactions have been reported. Headache and arthralgias are the most common adverse reactions attributable to this agent. Hypertension is associated with the increase in hematocrit produced by epoetin in patients with chronic renal failure. Blood pressure may rise soon after treatment is begun (rise in diastolic pressure >10 mm) in about one-third of patients. In previously hypertensive patients, episodes of elevated blood pressure may increase in frequency during epoetin therapy; therefore, blood pressure should be well controlled with medication before initiating therapy. About 25% to 30% of dialysis patients will require either a change in antihypertensive medication or an increase in dosage after correction of anemia with epoetin.

The hypertensive effects of epoetin seem to result from multiple factors. These include an increase in red blood cell mass without a proportional increase in plasma volume and an increase in peripheral vascular resistance, possibly due to correction of peripheral vasodilation accompanying the anemia. The latter hemodynamic change has been observed in dialysis patients in whom the hematocrit was increased to normal by transfusions over a three-week period. Since the resting blood pressure does not increase in normal volunteers (Berglund and Ekblom, 1991) or increases only when the hematocrit is elevated above the normal range in patients treated with epoetin for indications other than renal failure (Erslev, 1991), it also seems apparent that this agent has no direct pressor effect.

Because the hemodynamic changes underlying the decrease in blood pressure control may be associated with the increasing hematocrit or its rate of rise, some experts suggest that doses should be adjusted so that the hematocrit rises no more than 4 points in any two-week period. However, an analysis of patients in one study suggested that the severity of anemia at the start of epoetin therapy was the major risk factor contributing to hypertension in anemic patients with chronic renal failure (Buckner et al, 1989). A previous history of hypertension, the rate of rise of hematocrit, and other factors (eg, age, sex, number of years on dialysis, presence or absence of kidneys) did not seem to affect the incidence of hypertension in this study. Thus, other experts suggest that doses of epoetin be reduced when hematocrit values exceed 30% and that this agent be withheld until the blood pressure is reduced if serious hypertension occurs during the acute phase of treatment (Adamson and Eschbach, 1990).

Data suggest that dialyzer efficiency may decrease after anemia is corrected by epoetin therapy (van Geelen, 1991). This may be a result of an increase in blood viscosity. The hypocoagulability of uremic serum usually reverses after epoetin corrects the anemia in these patients. Therefore, it may be necessary to increase the dose of heparin used during dialysis to prevent or minimize clotting in the artificial kidney or the vascular access device (Evans et al, 1990; Wong et al, 1990).

In uncontrolled clinical trials, worsening hypertension may have contributed to a lower seizure threshold and a higher incidence of seizures in dialysis patients during the first 90 days of epoetin therapy; the incidence of seizures was 2.5%. However, the incidence of seizures in patients with end-stage renal disease who are treated with epoetin appears to be similar to that in untreated dialysis patients (Eschbach et al, 1989 A). Blood pressure and premonitory neurologic symptoms must be monitored closely during the early period of therapy. The manufacturer recommends that patients at risk be advised to avoid potentially hazardous activities such as driving or operating heavy machinery during this time.

Hypertension and seizures have not been associated with epoetin therapy in patients with AIDS or cancer. Nevertheless, blood pressure should be controlled before epoetin therapy is initiated in these individuals.

Hyperkalemia is not uncommon in patients with chronic renal failure and has been observed in those treated with epoetin. Most often, hyperkalemia is associated with poor compliance with medication or dietary prescriptions and/or dialysis requirements.

If the patient has a significantly delayed or diminished response to epoetin therapy, an alternative or additional cause of the anemia should be considered (eg, absolute or relative [functional] iron deficiency; underlying infectious, inflammatory, or malignant process; occult blood loss; another underlying hematologic disease [ie, thalassemia, refractory anemia or other myelodysplastic disorder, folic acid or vitamin B_{12}

deficiencies]; hemolysis; aluminum intoxication; osteitis fibrosa cystica).

No evidence of interaction of epoetin with other drugs was observed during clinical trials.

Epoetin has had adverse effects on the offspring of rats who received five times the human dose during pregnancy. This agent has been used successfully to treat anemia in a few pregnant women with chronic renal failure (Yankowitz et al, 1992); however, because no adequate and well-controlled studies have been conducted in pregnant women, epoetin should be used during pregnancy only if the potential benefit justifies the potential risk to the fetus (FDA Pregnancy Category C). It is not known whether epoetin is excreted in human milk. Thus, caution should be exercised when this hormone is administered to nursing women.

PHARMACOKINETICS. This glycoprotein may be degraded in the intestinal tract; therefore, it is administered intravenously or subcutaneously. Epoetin's effect on hematocrit is observed within one to two weeks, and an increase in reticulocytes is observed within seven to ten days after initiating therapy. The mean plasma elimination half-life after a single intravenous dose is between 4 and 12 hours (Macdougall et al, 1991). Epoetin appears to be cleared somewhat more rapidly after multiple doses than after a single dose (McMahon et al, 1990). With equal intravenous and subcutaneous doses, the peak plasma levels following subcutaneous administration are considerably lower, clearance rates are much slower, and plateau plasma levels are maintained for more extended periods than after intravenous administration (Macdougall et al, 1991). It seems probable that these differences result from a slow rate of absorption from the subcutaneous injection site. Bioavailability of epoetin after subcutaneous administration is between 20% and 30%. Because of the more rapid clearance of intravenous doses, biological responses are equivalent or better after subcutaneous administration of an identical dose. In patients with progressive renal failure who began epoetin therapy before they needed hemodialysis, no change in the dose of epoetin required to maintain hematopoiesis was needed at the start of dialysis (Eschbach et al, 1989 B).

DOSAGE AND PREPARATIONS.

Intravenous, Subcutaneous: *Adults and children,* for the anemia of chronic renal failure, the manufacturer recommends initial doses of 50 to 100 units/kg three times weekly. Some experts recommend starting therapy at 50 units/kg three times weekly for all patients. Others suggest an initial dose of 35 units/kg three times weekly, which produces a slower but steady rise in hematocrit (Erslev, 1991). The dose may be administered as an intravenous bolus or subcutaneously. The amount should be adjusted to achieve a targeted hematocrit range of 30% to 33% (maximum, 36%), with no more than a 4-unit increase in any two-week period in patients with renal disease. The dose should be reduced if a more rapid increase in hematocrit occurs.

The amount of epoetin administered should be increased by 25 units/kg if the hematocrit does not increase by 5 to 6 points after eight weeks of therapy when iron stores are adequate and the hematocrit is below the target range. The hematocrit should be measured twice weekly following dose increases. Once the targeted hematocrit is achieved, the maintenance dose must be individualized. If the hematocrit exceeds 36%, treatment may be withheld temporarily until the level decreases to about 33%, and the dose should be reduced by 25 units/kg when therapy is resumed. Information from clinical trials showed that intravenous doses of 75 to 150 units/kg *per week* (25 to 50 units/kg three times weekly) were adequate to maintain a hematocrit of 36% to 38% for up to six months in patients with chronic renal failure not on dialysis. Currently, the subcutaneous route is being used for maintenance therapy in most patients. For those on dialysis, about 10% have required 25 units/kg or less three times weekly and 10% have required more than 200 units/kg three times weekly; the median dose was 75 units/kg three times weekly, and 65% of patients required 100 units/kg or less three times weekly. In the clinical trials, dose adjustments resulted in an overall response rate of 97%.

For anemia in AIDS patients being treated with zidovudine who have serum erythropoietin levels ≤500 milliunits/ml, initially, 100 to 200 units/kg three times weekly for eight weeks given either intravenously or subcutaneously. The patient's hematocrit should be monitored and, if the response to initial therapy is inadequate, the dose, which is given three times weekly, may be increased by 50 to 100 units/kg every four to eight weeks to a maximum of 300 units/kg. Patients who do not respond to therapy at that dose are unlikely to benefit from larger amounts. For those who do respond (with either a decreased transfusion dependence or an increased hematocrit), maintenance doses must be individualized. If the hematocrit exceeds 40%, epoetin administration should be discontinued until the hematocrit declines below 36%. The dose should be reduced by 25% when therapy is resumed and adjusted to maintain the desired hematocrit.

Epogen (Amgen), ***Procrit*** (Ortho Biotech). Solution (sterile) 2,000, 3,000, 4,000, or 10,000 units in 1 ml containers (preservative-free) with water for injection buffered at a pH of 6.9 ± 0.3 and human albumin 2.5 mg/ml. Store at 2° to 8° C. Do not freeze or shake.

FILGRASTIM (G-CSF)

[Neupogen]

ACTIONS. Filgrastim is a recombinant preparation of human G-CSF that is produced by expression of the transfected human gene in bacteria (*Escherichia coli*). This protein contains 175 amino acids and has a molecular mass of 18.8 kilodaltons; it differs from endogenous G-CSF by the addition of an N-terminal methionine and by not being glycosylated. Endogenous G-CSF regulates the production of neutrophils (granulocytes) from progenitor cells in the bone marrow; it has few direct effects on other hematopoietic cell lineages. In addition to stimulating proliferation of neutrophil progenitors, filgrastim induces differentiation and affects some functions of end-stage (ie, differentiated) cells. The latter effects include stimulation of phagocytosis, antibody-dependent cellular cytotoxicity, and chemotactic responses. See the Introduction for a more detailed discussion of responses to G-CSF (filgrastim).

USES. Filgrastim is indicated to shorten the duration of severe neutropenia in patients with nonmyeloid malignancies who are receiving myelosuppressive oncolytic drugs in dosages known to reduce the neutrophil count to <500/mm^3. Results from clinical trials also demonstrate the efficacy and safety of filgrastim in patients receiving autologous or allogeneic bone marrow transplantation. Encouraging responses to filgrastim therapy have been reported in patients with chronic severe or congenital neutropenias. Promising initial results have been observed in separate uncontrolled clinical studies in which filgrastim was used to hasten recovery from chemotherapy-induced myelosuppression in patients with acute leukemia or to increase granulocyte counts in those with some myelodysplastic syndromes; to increase the yield of peripheral blood progenitor cells for transplantation after high-dose myelosuppressive chemotherapy for cancer; and when this agent was given to patients with cyclic neutropenia or aplastic anemia or to those with neutropenia caused by zidovudine therapy for AIDS. See the Introduction for detailed discussions of the results from clinical trials of filgrastim in these diseases.

ADVERSE REACTIONS AND PRECAUTIONS. Mild to moderate medullary bone pain is the only adverse response to filgrastim that was reported consistently in randomized, placebo-controlled trials. Nonopioid analgesics (eg, acetaminophen) controlled the pain in most patients, although a small number required opioid analgesics. The incidence of bone pain was higher in patients who received large intravenous doses (20 to 100 mcg/kg/day) than in those given small subcutaneous doses (3 to 10 mcg/kg/day).

Most of the other adverse effects reported in trials with filgrastim probably are attributable to the underlying cancer or to the larger cumulative doses of antineoplastic drugs being administered. Therefore, anemia or thrombocytopenia may be observed more frequently or may be more severe in patients who receive filgrastim. There are no data on the maximum tolerated dose. The largest intravenous dose given thus far (115 mcg/kg/day administered to six patients) did not produce more toxic effects than smaller doses.

Although the safety and efficacy of filgrastim therapy in pediatric patients have not been determined, the responses in adults and the small number of children studied thus far appear to be similar. Determination of the appropriate dose of filgrastim for use in pediatric cancer patients with chemotherapy-induced neutropenia is ongoing.

This drug is contraindicated in patients with a history of hypersensitivity to proteins produced in *E. coli*.

Responses of myeloid cells in the bone marrow and peripheral circulation to filgrastim include stimulation of cell proliferation, which sensitizes these nonmalignant cells to cytotoxic antineoplastic drugs. Consequently, filgrastim should not be administered until 24 hours after the last dose of chemotherapy in a cycle, and it should be discontinued at least 24 hours before the next cycle is begun. In addition, since growth of tumor cells with myeloid characteristics may be stimulated, patients with these malignancies may not be appropriate candidates for filgrastim therapy. However, several studies demonstrate that progression of acute myeloid leukemia is not accelerated by administration of filgrastim to stimulate neutrophil recovery after induction chemotherapy (see Lieschke and Burgess, 1992 for review).

Leukocytosis (white cell count ≥100,000/mm^3) occurs in about 2% of patients treated with ≥5 mcg/kg/day of filgrastim. Although this response does not appear to be clinically significant, it is best to avoid excessive increases of white blood cell counts; dose reduction or discontinuation of therapy should be considered if excessive leukocytosis does occur. Complete blood and platelet counts should be obtained before the start of filgrastim therapy and should be repeated twice weekly during continued administration.

Less frequent or rare side effects associated with filgrastim therapy include erythema or pain at the site of subcutaneous injection, Sweet's syndrome (acute febrile neutrophilic dermatosis), vasculitis, wheezing, and transient supraventricular arrhythmia.

The safety and efficacy of long-term therapy with filgrastim have not been studied adequately. A small number of patients have been treated for up to three years. Splenomegaly was observed by CT or MRI (both required by the study protocol) in about one third of recipients, but clinical symptoms were reported in only 3% of those receiving long-term therapy with filgrastim.

Filgrastim is not mutagenic for bacteria in vitro, but its carcinogenic potential has not been studied. This drug has no effects on fertility in male or female rats or on gestation of pregnant rats with doses up to 500 mcg/kg. Filgrastim has caused fetal toxicity in rabbits when given in doses two- to tenfold larger than those used in humans. No data are available on the use of filgrastim in pregnant women. This drug is classified in FDA Pregnancy Category C.

PHARMACOKINETICS. Filgrastim can be administered as a bolus subcutaneous injection, a continuous subcutaneous infusion, or a short (20- to 30-minute) intravenous infusion. Absorption and clearance rates are not dose dependent and follow simple first-order pharmacokinetics in adults (Petros, 1992). The clearance rate in adults is about 0.5 to 0.7 ml/min/kg. There is no evidence that the drug accumulates in adults when it is administered as a continuous 24-hour infusion for up to 20 days. The elimination half-life and volume of distribution are about 3.5 hours and 150 ml/kg, respectively, and no differences in these parameters were observed between healthy subjects and cancer patients. The half-life after a single dose and after 14 days of daily intravenous administration remained the same. Half-lives also were similar after intravenous and subcutaneous administration. In children receiving combination chemotherapy for advanced neuroblastoma, the elimination half-life declined from 5.8 to 4.5 hours and the clearance rate decreased from 0.57 to 0.31 ml/min/kg between days 1 and 10 of filgrastim therapy (Stute et al, 1992).

DOSAGE AND PREPARATIONS. Filgrastim should not be diluted in saline solutions. Albumin should be added if filgrastim is diluted (with dextrose in water for injection) to less than 15 mcg/ml.

Intravenous, Subcutaneous: *Adults and children,* as an adjunct to standard-dose chemotherapy, an initial dose of 5 mcg/kg/day is given as a single injection. However, the optimal dose and schedule in pediatric patients have not been determined in clinical trials. The amount of drug administered probably should be based on lean or ideal body weight. If the response is delayed or inadequate, the dose may be increased by 5 mcg/kg/day after five to seven days. Therapy with filgrastim should not be initiated until 24 hours after the final dose of a chemotherapy cycle and should be discontinued 24 hours before the start of the next cycle or within 12 hours before or after radiation therapy. Within a given cycle, filgrastim should be administered daily until the neutrophil count returns to normal levels (ie, >10,000/mm³). In patients receiving intensified regimens of antineoplastic drugs, filgrastim should be continued until two consecutive neutrophil counts are normal. For most chemotherapy regimens, the time to neutrophil count nadir is two to three days earlier in patients treated with filgrastim than in those not given the hematopoietic growth factor.

To promote myeloid engraftment after bone marrow transplantation, 5 to 10 mcg/kg/day is administered by intravenous or subcutaneous injection for up to 21 days (until recovery of neutrophil counts) beginning two to four hours after marrow infusion. Optimal dosage regimens for other indications have not been established in clinical trials.

Neupogen (Amgen). Solution (sterile) 300 and 480 mcg in water for injection with 0.59 mg acetate, 50 mg mannitol, 0.004% Tween 80, and 0.035 mg sodium per ml, buffered at a pH of 4.0 (preservative-free) in 1 and 1.6 ml containers, respectively. Store at 2° to 8° C. Do not freeze or shake.

SARGRAMOSTIM (GM-CSF)

[Leukine]

ACTIONS. Sargramostim is a recombinant preparation of human GM-CSF that is produced by expression of the transfected human gene in yeast (*Saccharomyces cerevisiae*). This protein contains 127 amino acids and differs from endogenous human GM-CSF by substitution of leucine at position 23. Since it is produced in yeast rather than in bacteria, sargramostim is glycosylated. The purified preparation contains three molecular forms with masses of 15.5, 16.8, and 19.5 kilodaltons, which differ from each other in the extent of glycosylation.

Endogenous GM-CSF and sargramostim stimulate the proliferation and differentiation of partially committed hematopoietic progenitor cells to produce end-stage cells of both the granulocyte (neutrophil) and monocyte/macrophage lineages. They also activate some functions of fully differentiated cells, including chemotaxis of granulocytes, monocytes, and macrophages and cytotoxicity of these cell types against bacteria, fungi, protozoa, and tumor cells. Endogenous and recombinant GM-CSF also support the survival in vitro of cells in the granulocyte and monocyte lineages. GM-CSF stimulates the proliferation of erythroid and megakaryocyte progenitors, but it cannot induce differentiation of these cells when used alone. Thus, sargramostim therapy usually does not increase red blood cell or platelet counts. Administration of sargramostim and other GM-CSF preparations stimulates myelopoiesis. See the Introduction for discussion of hematologic responses to GM-CSF.

USES. Sargramostim is indicated to accelerate myeloid repopulation in patients with non-Hodgkin's lymphoma (NHL), acute lymphoblastic leukemia (ALL), or Hodgkin's disease who are undergoing autologous bone marrow transplantation (ABMT) as supportive therapy after high-dose chemotherapy (with or without total body irradiation) that ablates the bone marrow. It also is used to shorten the duration of neutropenia in patients with solid tumors who are undergoing ABMT, to hasten engraftment after allogeneic bone marrow transplant, and to increase the yield of peripheral blood progenitor cells that can be harvested and stored for reinfusion after high-dose chemotherapy.

Sargramostim also is indicated to improve survival in patients who experience graft failure or delayed engraftment after allogeneic or autologous bone marrow transplants. Data from clinical trials support its use to accelerate recovery from neutropenia and reduce the incidence and severity of infections after standard-dose myelosuppressive chemotherapy for a variety of malignancies. In addition, promising results have been reported in patients with some myelodysplastic syndromes, aplastic anemia, or HIV infection or AIDS who are neutropenic as a consequence of either their underlying disease or the antiretroviral or oncolytic drugs they are receiving. Additional investigation is needed to determine if sargramostim therapy will benefit patients with chronic or drug-induced neutropenias or will be useful as adjunctive therapy for myeloid leukemias by sensitizing leukemic cells to S phase-specific cytotoxic drugs. See the Introduction for detailed discussions of results from clinical trials of sargramostim in patients with each of these diseases.

ADVERSE REACTIONS AND PRECAUTIONS. Sargramostim is relatively well tolerated at dosages <16 mcg/kg/day or <500 mcg/M²/day. In placebo-controlled trials using doses below these thresholds in patients undergoing ABMT, the only adverse reactions reported with frequencies increased by >5% were diarrhea (89% versus 82% for controls), asthenia (66% versus 51% for controls), rash (44% versus 38% for controls), and malaise (57% versus 51% for controls); however, these differences were not clinically significant. Mild to severe bone pain was not reported in these trials but was noted in earlier uncontrolled studies and occasionally has been reported during postmarketing surveillance. It usually can be treated with nonopioid analgesics but rarely may require treatment with opioids. All other adverse reactions were attributed to the marrow-ablative chemotherapy or to the underlying malignancy. In uncontrolled Phase I and II studies, the most frequently reported untoward effects were fever, asthenia, headache, chills, and myalgia, which were of mild to moderate severity and were managed successfully with nonopioid analgesics. Dyspnea and rash were reported infrequently.

Some patients respond to the first dose of GM-CSF with a characteristic syndrome that includes transient flushing, tachycardia, hypotension, musculoskeletal pain, dyspnea, nausea and vomiting, and arterial oxygen desaturation (Lieschke and Burgess, 1992). This first-dose reaction is more common after intravenous than subcutaneous administration. Patients who discontinued GM-CSF therapy because of this syndrome are at increased risk for its recurrence when therapy is resumed.

Edema, capillary leak syndrome, and pleural and/or pericardial effusion have been reported after sargramostim administration. In placebo-controlled studies in 156 patients in whom sargramostim 250 mcg/M^2 was infused daily for two hours, the reported incidences of fluid retention (sargramostim versus placebo) were as follows: peripheral edema, 11% versus 7%; pleural effusion, 1% versus 0%; and pericardial effusion, 4% versus 1%. Capillary leak syndrome was not observed in this limited number of patients; based on other uncontrolled studies and isolated reports, its incidence is estimated to be less than 1%.

In uncontrolled studies, transient increases in serum creatinine or bilirubin concentrations or levels of hepatic enzymes were observed in some patients with pre-existing renal or hepatic dysfunction. Reduction of the dose or discontinuation of the drug reversed these effects. In controlled trials, no differences in these parameters were noted between patients treated with sargramostim and those given placebo.

Leukocytosis or thrombocytosis can occur after administration of sargramostim. The eosinophil count should be monitored because high levels are possible. Dose reduction or discontinuation of therapy should be considered if neutrophil counts are $\geq$20,000/mm^3 or platelet counts exceed 500,000/mm^3. Blood cell counts exceeding the normal range returned to baseline levels three to seven days after sargramostim therapy was discontinued. To avoid leukocytosis, a complete blood count (with differential) should be obtained twice weekly during therapy.

Sargramostim is contraindicated in patients with a history of hypersensitivity to yeast-derived proteins. It should not be administered within 24 hours before or after chemotherapy or within 12 hours before or after radiation therapy, since stimulation of normal myeloid cell proliferation by the growth factor can sensitize these cells to cytotoxic therapies.

No data are available on carcinogenesis or mutagenesis, effects on fertility in males or females, or on toxicity to the fetus or mother in humans or animals. Sargramostim is classified in FDA Pregnancy Category C.

No controlled studies have assessed the safety or efficacy of sargramostim in children, but data from clinical trials that included pediatric patients suggest that the response and adverse reactions are similar in adults and children. Data from a study of sargramostim in pediatric patients receiving myelosuppressive chemotherapy suggest that children may tolerate significantly larger doses of this hemopoietin than adults (Furman et al, 1991).

PHARMACOKINETICS. The disappearance of sargramostim from plasma after intravenous administration follows biphasic kinetics (Petros, 1992; Grant and Heel, 1992; Lieschke and Burgess, 1992). The half-life of the distribution phase is 5 to 15 minutes and that of the elimination phase is about 1.5 to 2 hours. When administered subcutaneously, plasma levels are detectable within five minutes, reach peak levels within two hours, and decline with an apparent elimination half-life of approximately three hours. The myelopoietic response is about the same whether sargramostim is given as a continuous intravenous infusion or subcutaneous injection. However, intravenous bolus administration is generally thought to be less effective because serum concentrations decline more rapidly below the minimal level required for biological responses. Neutralizing antibodies have been observed in 2.3% of patients; however, all patients with such antibodies had impaired hematopoiesis before administration of sargramostim. Consequently, the effect of neutralizing antibodies on hematopoietic responses to the drug could not be determined.

DOSAGE AND PREPARATIONS. No more than six hours before use, the lyophilized powder should be dissolved in preservative-free sterile water for injection to a concentration of 500 mcg/ml; the diluent should be directed gently against the wall of the container, and the solution should be swirled without agitation or shaking to avoid foaming. This solution can be further diluted for intravenous infusion with 0.9% sodium chloride for injection. Human albumin (0.1%) should be added if the final concentration of sargramostim is <10 mcg/ml to prevent adsorption of the cytokine to the walls of the infusion system. Any unused portion of the single-dose container should be discarded.

Intravenous, Subcutaneous: *Adults and children,* to accelerate marrow engraftment, 250 mcg/M^2/day for 21 days as a two-hour infusion or subcutaneous injection. Extending the duration of the infusion to six or more hours may ameliorate some of the side effects seen occasionally with this drug. Subcutaneous injection or longer infusion times also will have a greater therapeutic effect because adequate blood concentrations will be maintained for longer periods. Treatment should begin two to four hours after infusion of bone marrow, which should occur at least 24 hours after the last dose of chemotherapy and 12 hours after the last dose of radiation therapy. Treatment with this cytokine should be discontinued if blast cells appear or the malignancy progresses.

As therapy for graft failure or delayed engraftment, 250 mcg/M^2/day is administered for 14 days as a two-hour infusion or subcutaneous injection. If neutrophil counts continue to be inadequate, after seven days without therapy the same dose is administered for a second 14-day cycle. If needed, a dose of 500 mcg/M^2/day may be given after a seven-day period without sargramostim therapy for a third 14-day cycle.

In patients who are neutropenic as a result of myelosuppressive chemotherapy for malignancy, 250 mcg/M^2/day is infused over a period of two hours or injected subcutaneously. Therapy with sargramostim should begin 24 or more hours after the last dose of a chemotherapy cycle and is continued for up to 14 days or until the absolute neutrophil count returns to 10,000/mm^3 following its nadir. When used in patients receiving high-dose chemotherapy, sargramostim therapy should continue until two successive counts are at that level. If the myelopoietic response is inadequate, the dosage may be increased to 500 mcg/M^2/day.

For other indications, dosages that yielded clinically useful responses to sargramostim in clinical trials have generally been in the range of 200 to 300 mcg/M^2/day or 3 to 10 mcg/

kg/day, administered as a two-hour infusion or subcutaneous injection.

Leukine (Immunex). Powder (lyophilized) 250 and 500 mcg in single-use containers with 40 mg mannitol, 10 mg sucrose, and 1.2 mg tromethamine per vial to yield an isotonic solution with a pH of 7.4 ± 0.3 after addition of 1 ml of water for injection. Store at 2° to 8° C. Do not freeze or shake.

Cited References

Abels RI: Use of recombinant human erythropoietin in the treatment of anemia in patients who have cancer. *Semin Oncol* 19 (suppl 8):29-35, 1992.

Abels RI, et al: Recombinant human erythropoietin (r-HuEPO) for the treatment of the anemia of cancer, in Murphy MJ Jr (ed): *Blood Cell Growth Factors: Their Present and Future Use in Hematology and Oncology.* Dayton, Ohio, AlphaMed Press, 1991.

Abraham NG, et al: Erythropoietin controls heme metabolic enzymes in normal human bone marrow culture. *Exp Hematol* 17:908-913, 1989.

Ad Hoc Committee for the National Kidney Foundation: Statement on the clinical use of recombinant erythropoietin in anemia of end-stage renal disease. *Am J Kidney Dis* 14:163-169, (Sept) 1989.

Adamson JW, Eschbach JW: Treatment of the anemia of chronic renal failure with recombinant human erythropoietin. *Annu Rev Med* 41:349-360, 1990.

Adamson JW, Vapnek D: Recombinant erythropoietin to improve athletic performance. *N Engl J Med* 324:698-699, 1991.

Adamson JW, et al: Why do some hemodialysis patients (HDP) need large doses of recombinant erythropoietin (rHuEPO)? abstract. *Kidney Int* 37:235, 1990.

Advani R, et al: Granulocyte-macrophage colony-stimulating factor (GM-CSF) as an adjunct to autologous hemopoietic stem cell transplantation for lymphoma. *Ann Intern Med* 116:183-189, 1992.

Berglund B, Ekblom B: Effect of recombinant human erythropoietin treatment on blood pressure and some haematological parameters in healthy men. *J Intern Med* 229:125-130, 1991.

Bernstein ID, et al: Recombinant human stem cell factor enhances the formation of colonies by CD34+ and CD34+lin− cells, and the generation of colony-forming cell progeny from CD34+lin− cells cultured with interleukin-3, granulocyte colony-stimulating factor, or granulocyte-macrophage colony-stimulating factor. *Blood* 77:2316-2321, 1991.

Beru N, Goldwasser E: The regulation of heme biosynthesis during erythropoietin-induced erythroid differentiation. *J Biol Chem* 260:9251-9257, 1985.

Bettelheim P, et al: Recombinant human granulocyte-macrophage colony-stimulating factor in combination with standard induction chemotherapy in de novo acute myeloid leukemia. *Blood* 77:700-711, 1991.

Blazar BR, et al: In vivo administration of recombinant human granulocyte/macrophage colony-stimulating factor in acute lymphoblastic leukemia patients receiving purged autografts. *Blood* 73:849-857, 1989.

Boshkov LK, et al: Recombinant human erythropoietin for a Jehovah's Witness with anemia of thermal injury. *Am J Hematol* 37:53-54, 1991.

Bowen D, et al: The treatment of anaemia in the myelodysplastic syndromes with recombinant human erythropoietin. *Br J Haematol* 77:419-423, 1991.

Boxer LA, et al: Recombinant human granulocyte-colony-stimulating factor in the treatment of patients with neutropenia. *Clin Immunol Immunopathol* 62:S39-S46, 1992.

Brandt J, et al: Role of c-*kit* ligand in the expansion of human hematopoietic progenitor cells. *Blood* 79:634-641, 1992.

Brugger W, et al: Mobilization of peripheral blood progenitor cells by sequential administration of interleukin-3 and granulocyte-macrophage colony-stimulating factor following polychemotherapy with etoposide, ifosfamide, and cisplatin. *Blood* 79:1193-1200, 1992.

Buckner FS, et al: Correction of the anemia in hemodialysis (HD) patients (PTS) with recombinant human erythropoietin (rHuEpo): Hemodynamic changes and risks for hypertension, abstract. *Kidney Int* 35:190, 1989.

Canadian Erythropoietin Study Group: Association between recombinant human erythropoietin and quality of life and exercise capacity of patients receiving haemodialysis. *BMJ* 300:573-578, 1990.

Caro J: Clonal assays for hemopoietic progenitor cells, in Williams WJ, et al (eds): *Hematology.* New York, McGraw-Hill, 1990, 1695-1698.

Carnielli V, et al: Effect of high doses of human recombinant erythropoietin on the need for blood transfusions in preterm infants. *J Pediatr* 121:98-102, 1992.

Carow CE, et al: Mast cell growth factor (*c-kit* ligand) supports the growth of human multipotential progenitor cells with a high replating potential. *Blood* 78:2216-2221, 1991.

Catlin DH, Hatton CK: Use and abuse of anabolic and other drugs. *Adv Intern Med* 36:399-424, 1991.

Cazzola M, et al: Subcutaneous erythropoietin for treatment of refractory anemia in hematologic disorders: Results of a Phase I/II clinical trial. *Blood* 79:29-37, 1992.

Ciavarella D: Hematopoietic stem cell processing and storage, in Goldstein J (ed): *Biotechnology of Blood.* New York, Butterworth-Heinemann, 1991.

Connor JP, Olsson CA: The use of recombinant human erythropoietin in a Jehovah's Witness requiring major reconstructive surgery. *J Urol* 147:131-132, 1992.

Curtis BM, et al: Enhanced hematopoietic activity of a human granulocyte/macrophage colony-stimulating factor—interleukin 3 fusion protein. *Proc Natl Acad Sci USA* 88:5809-5813, 1991.

D'Andrea AD, Zon LI: Erythropoietin receptor: Subunit structure and activation. *J Clin Invest* 86:681-687, 1990.

Delannoy A: GM-CSF therapy for drug-induced agranulocytosis. *J Intern Med* 231:269-271, 1992.

De Marchi S, et al: Relief of pruritus and decreases in plasma histamine concentrations during erythropoietin therapy in patients with uremia. *N Engl J Med* 326:969-974, 1992.

Demetri GD, Griffin JD: Granulocyte colony-stimulating factor and its receptor. *Blood* 78:2791-2808, 1991.

de Vries EGE, et al: A double-blind placebo-controlled study with granulocyte-macrophage colony-stimulating factor during chemotherapy for ovarian carcinoma. *Cancer Res* 51:116-122, 1991.

De Witte T, et al: Recombinant human granulocyte-macrophage colony-stimulating factor accelerates neutrophil and monocyte recovery after allogeneic T-cell-depleted bone marrow transplantation. *Blood* 79:1359-1365, 1992.

Dunbar CE, et al: Treatment of Diamond-Blackfan anaemia with haematopoietic growth factors, granulocyte-macrophage colony stimulating factor and interleukin 3: Sustained remissions following IL-3. *Br J Haematol* 79:316-321, 1991.

Eckardt KU, et al: Erythropoietin in polycystic kidneys. *J Clin Invest* 84:1160-1166, 1989.

Elias AD, et al: Mobilization of peripheral blood progenitor cells by chemotherapy and granulocyte-macrophage colony-stimulating factor for hematologic support after high-dose intensification for breast cancer. *Blood* 79:3036-3044, 1992.

Erslev AJ: Production of erythrocytes, in Williams WJ, et at (eds): *Hematology.* New York, McGraw-Hill, 1990, 389-398.

Erslev AJ: Erythropoietin. *Drug Ther* 324:1339-1344, 1991.

Eschbach JW, et al: Recombinant human erythropoietin in anemic patients with end-stage renal disease. *Ann Intern Med* 111:992-1000, 1989 A.

Eschbach JW, et al: Treatment of the anemia of progressive renal failure with recombinant human erythropoietin. *N Engl J Med* 321:158-163, 1989 B.

Estey E, et al: Treatment of newly diagnosed acute myelogenous leukemia with granulocyte-macrophage colony-stimulating factor (GM-CSF) before and during continuous-infusion high-dose ara-C+ daunorubicin: Comparison to patients treated without GM-CSF. *Blood* 79:2246-2255, 1992.

Evans RW, et al: The quality of life of hemodialysis recipients treated with recombinant human erythropoietin. *JAMA* 263:825-830, 1990.

Fischl M, et al: Recombinant human erythropoietin for patients with AIDS treated with zidovudine. *N Engl J Med* 322:1488-1493, 1990.

Frendl G: Interleukin 3: From colony-stimulating factor to pluripotent immunoregulatory cytokine. *J Immunopharmacol* 14:421-430, 1992.

Fukuda M, et al: Autotransplantation of peripheral blood stem cells mobilized by chemotherapy and recombinant human granulocyte colony-stimulating factor in childhood neuroblastoma and non-Hodgkin's lymphoma. *Br J Haematol* 80:327-331, 1992.

Furman WL, et al: Therapeutic effects and pharmacokinetics of recombinant human granulocyte-macrophage colony-stimulating factor in childhood cancer patients receiving myelosuppressive chemotherapy. *J Clin Oncol* 9:1022-1028, 1991.

Galli SJ, et al: Morphology, biochemistry, and function of basophils and mast cells, in Williams WJ, et al (eds): *Hematology.* New York, McGraw-Hill, 1990, 840-845.

Ganser A, et al: Recombinant human granulocyte-macrophage colony-stimulating factor in patients with myelodysplastic syndromes: A Phase I/II trial. *Blood* 73:31-37, 1989.

Ganser A, et al: Effects of recombinant human interleukin-3 in patients with normal hematopoiesis and in patients with bone marrow failure. *Blood* 76:666-676, 1990 A.

Ganser A, et al: Effects of recombinant human interleukin-3 in patients with myelodysplastic syndromes. *Blood* 76:455-462, 1990 B.

Ganser A, et al: Effects of recombinant human interleukin-3 in aplastic anemia. *Blood* 76:1287-1992, 1990 C.

Ganser A, et al: Sequential in vivo treatment with two recombinant human hematopoietic growth factors (interleukin-3 and granulocyte-macrophage colony-stimulating factor) as a new therapeutic modality to stimulate hematopoiesis: Results of a Phase I study. *Blood* 79:2583-2591, 1992.

Gasson JC: Molecular physiology of granulocyte-macrophage colony-stimulating factor. *Blood* 77:1131-1145, 1991.

Goldberg MA, et al: Treatment of sickle cell anemia with hydroxyurea and erythropoietin. *N Engl J Med* 323:366-372, 1990.

Goldberg MA, et al: Hydroxyurea and erythropoietin therapy in sickle cell anemia. *Semin Oncol* 19:74-81, 1992.

Golde DW: Production, distribution, and fate of neutrophils, in Williams WJ, et al (eds): *Hematology.* New York, McGraw-Hill, 1990, 795-801.

Golde DW: The stem cell. *Sci Am* 86-93, (Dec) 1991.

Golde DW, Glaspy J: Therapeutic use of granulocyte and monocyte colony-stimulating factors, in Williams WJ, et al (eds): *Hematology.* New York, McGraw-Hill, 1990, 273-278.

Golde DW, Groopman JE: Production, distribution, and fate of monocytes and macrophages, in Williams WJ, et al (eds): *Hematology.* New York, McGraw-Hill, 1990, 874-878.

Goodnough LT, et al: Increased preoperative collection of autologous blood with recombinant human erythropoietin therapy. *N Engl J Med* 321:1163-1168, 1989.

Goodnough LT, et al: Iron-restricted erythropoiesis as a limitation to autologous blood donation in the erythropoietin-stimulated bone marrow. *J Lab Clin Med* 118:289-296, 1991.

Goodnough LT, et al: Preoperative red cell production in patients undergoing aggressive autologous blood phlebotomy with and without erythropoietin therapy. *Transfusion* 32:441-445, 1992.

Grant SM, Heel RC: Recombinant granulocyte-macrophage colony-stimulating factor (rGM-CSF): A review of its pharmacological properties and prospective role in the management of myelosuppression. *Drugs* 43:516-560, 1992.

Green D, Handley E: Erythropoietin for anemia in Jehovah's Witnesses. *Ann Intern Med* 113:720-721, 1990.

Greenberg PL: Treatment of myelodysplastic syndromes with hemopoietic growth factors. *Semin Oncol* 19:106-114, 1992.

Grimm PC, et al: Effects of recombinant human erythropoietin on HLA sensitization and cell mediated immunity. *Kidney Int* 38:12-18, 1990.

Groopman JE: Management of the hematologic complications of human immunodeficiency virus infection. *Rev Infect Dis* 12:931-937, 1990.

Grosh WW, Quesenberry PJ: Recombinant human hematopoietic growth factors in the treatment of cytopenias. *Clin Immunol Immunopathol* 62:S25-S38, 1992.

Grützmacher P, et al: Response to recombinant erythropoietin in aluminium overload and hyperparathyroidism, abstract. *Kidney Int* 37:299, 1990.

Gulati SC, Bennett CL: Granulocyte-macrophage colony-stimulating factor (GM-CSF) as adjunct therapy in relapsed Hodgkin disease. *Ann Intern Med* 116:177-182, 1992.

Haas R, et al: Successful autologous transplantation of blood stem cells mobilized with recombinant human granulocyte-macrophage colony-stimulating factor. *Exp Hematol* 18:94-98, 1990.

Henry DH, et al: Recombinant human erythropoietin in the treatment of anemia associated with human immunodeficiency virus (HIV) infection and zidovudine therapy: Overview of four clinical trials. *Ann Intern Med* 117:739-748, 1992 A.

Henry DH, et al: Recombinant human erythropoietin and the treatment of anemia in patients with AIDS or advanced ARC not receiving ZDV, letter. *J Acquired Immune Deficiency Syndromes* 5:847-852, 1992 B.

Hollingshead LM, Goa KL: Recombinant granulocyte colony-stimulating factor (rG-CSF): A review of its pharmacological properties and prospective role in neutropenic conditions. *Drugs* 42:300-330, 1991.

Hollomby DJ, et al: The role of aluminum (AL) and PTH in erythropoietin (EPO) resistance in hemodialysis patients, abstract. *Kidney Int* 37:301, 1990.

Huch A, et al: Recombinant human erythropoietin in the treatment of postpartum anemia. *Obstet Gynecol* 80:127-131, 1992.

Jelkmann W: Erythropoietin: Structure, control of production, and function. *Physiol Rev* 72:449-489, 1992.

Kanz L, et al: Hemopoietins in clinical oncology. *Am J Clin Oncol* 14(suppl 1):S27-S33, 1991.

Kaplan LD, et al: Clinical and virologic effects of recombinant human granulocyte-macrophage colony-stimulating factor in patients receiving chemotherapy for human immunodeficiency virus-associated non-Hodgkin's lymphoma: Results of a randomized trial. *J Clin Oncol* 9:929-940, 1991.

Khwaja A, et al: *In vivo* effects of macrophage colony-stimulating factor on human monocyte function. *Br J Haematol* 77:25-31, 1991.

Khwaja A, et al: The effect of macrophage colony-stimulating factor on haemopoietic recovery after autologous bone marrow transplantation. *Br J Haematol* 81:288-295, 1992.

Komiyama A, et al: Increases in neutrophil counts by purified human urinary colony-stimulating factor in chronic neutropenia of childhood. *Blood* 71:41-45, 1988.

Krantz SB: Erythropoietin. *Blood* 77:419-434, 1991.

Kurzrock R, et al: Treatment of cyclic neutropenia with very low doses of GM-CSF. *Am J Med* 91:317-318, 1991 A.

Kurzrock R, et al: Phase I study of recombinant human interleukin-3 in patients with bone marrow failure. *J Clin Oncol* 9:1241-1250, 1991 B.

Lieschke GJ, Burgess AW: Granulocyte colony-stimulating factor and-granulocyte—macrophage colony-stimulating factor. *N Engl J Med* 327:28-35, 99-106, 1992.

Lim VS, et al: Recombinant human erythropoietin treatment in predialysis patients: A double-blind placebo-controlled trial. *Ann Intern Med* 110:108-114, 1989.

Lim VS, et al: Effect of recombinant human erythropoietin on renal function in humans. *Kidney Int* 37:131-136, 1990.

Lindemann A, et al: Biologic effects of recombinant human interleukin-3 in vivo. *J Clin Oncol* 9:2120-2127, 1991.

Lui SF, et al: Pharmacokinetics and pharmacodynamics of subcutaneous and intraperitoneal administration of recombinant human erythropoietin in patients on continuous ambulatory peritoneal dialysis. *Clin Nephrol* 33:47-51, 1990.

Lundin AP: Quality of life: Subjective and objective improvements with recombinant human erythropoietin therapy. *Semin Nephrol* 9(suppl 1):22-29, 1989.

Lundin AP, et al: Perspectives on the improvement of quality of life with epoetin alfa therapy. *Pharmacotherapy* 10(2 part 2):22S-26S, 1990.

Macdougall IC, et al: Poor response to treatment of renal anaemia with erythropoietin corrected by iron given intravenously. *BMJ* 299:157-158, 1989.

Macdougall IC, et al: Clinical pharmacokinetics of epoetin (recombinant human erythropoietin). *Clin Pharmacokinet* 20:99-113, 1991.

Marsh JT, et al: rHuEPO treatment improves brain and cognitive function of anemic dialysis patients. *Kidney Int* 39:155-163, 1991.

Masaoka T, et al: Double-blind test of human urinary macrophage colony-stimulating factor for allogeneic and syngeneic bone marrow transplantation: Effectiveness of treatment and 2-year follow-up for relapse of leukaemia. *Br J Haematol* 76:501-505, 1990.

Mason-Garcia M, Beckman BS: Signal transduction in erythropoiesis. *FASEB J* 5:2958-2964, 1991.

McDonald TP: Thrombopoietin: Its biology, purification, and characterization. *Exp Hematol* 16:201-205, 1988.

McMahon FG, et al: Pharmacokinetics and effects of recombinant human erythropoietin after intravenous and subcutaneous injections in healthy volunteers. *Blood* 76:1718-1722, 1990.

McNiece IK, et al: Colony-forming cells with high proliferative potential (HPP-CFC). *Int J Cell Cloning* 8:146-160, 1990.

Means RT Jr, Krantz SB: Erythropoietin in cancer therapy. *Biol Ther Cancer Updates* 1:1-7, (Nov/Dec) 1991.

Means RT Jr, et al: Treatment of the anemia of rheumatoid arthritis with recombinant human erythropoietin: Clinical and in vitro studies. *Arthritis Rheum* 32:638-642, 1989.

Metra M, et al: Improvement in exercise capacity after correction of anemia in patients with end-stage renal failure. *Am J Cardiol* 68:1060-1066, 1991.

Miles SA, et al: Combined therapy with recombinant granulocyte colony-stimulating factor and erythropoietin decreases hematologic toxicity from zidovudine. *Blood* 77:2109-2117, 1991.

Mittelman M, et al: Subcutaneous erythropoietin for treatment of refractory anemia in hematologic disorders. *Blood* 80:841, 1992.

Miyake T, et al: Purification of human erythropoietin. *J Biol Chem* 252:5558-5564, 1977.

Moore MAS: Clinical implications of positive and negative hematopoietic stem cell regulators. *Blood* 78:1-19, 1991 A.

Moore MAS: The clinical use of colony stimulating factors. *Annu Rev Immunol* 9:159-191, 1991 B.

Motoyoshi K, et al: Protective effect of partially purified human urinary colony-stimulating factor on granulocytopenia after antitumor chemotherapy. *Exp Hematol* 14:1069-1075, 1986.

Nand S, et al: Granulocyte-macrophage colony stimulating factor for the treatment of drug induced agranulocytosis. *Am J Hematol* 37:267-269, 1991.

Negrin RS, et al: Maintenance treatment of patients with myelodysplastic syndromes using recombinant human granulocyte colony-stimulating factor. *Blood* 76:36-43, 1990.

Nemunaitis J: Granulocyte-macrophage—colony-stimulating factor: A review from preclinical development to clinical application. *Transfusion* 33:70-83, 1993.

Nemunaitis J, Singer JW: The use of recombinant human granulocyte-macrophage colony stimulating factor in autologous bone marrow transplantation. *Am J Clin Oncol* 14(suppl 1):S15-S18, 1991.

Nemunaitis J, et al: Phase I/II trial of recombinant human granulocyte-macrophage colony-stimulating factor following allogeneic bone marrow transplantation. *Blood* 77:2065-2071, 1991 A.

Nemunaitis J, et al: Phase I trial of recombinant human macrophage colony-stimulating factor in patients with invasive fungal infections. *Blood* 78:907-913, 1991 B.

Nemunaitis J, et al: Phase II trial of recombinant human granulocyte-macrophage colony-stimulating factor in patients undergoing allogeneic bone marrow transplantation from unrelated donors. *Blood* 79:2572-2577, 1992.

Nijhof W, et al: Induction of globin mRNA transcription by erythropoietin in differentiating erythroid precursor cells. *Exp Hematol* 15:779-784, 1987.

Nimer SD, Golde DW: The 5q− abnormality. *Blood* 70:1705-1712, 1987.

Ohls RK, Christensen RD: Recombinant erythropoietin compared with erythrocyte transfusion in the treatment of anemia of prematurity. *J Pediatr* 119:781-788, 1991.

Ottmann OG, et al: Effects of recombinant human interleukin-3 on human hematopoietic progenitor and precursor cells in vivo. *Blood* 76:1494-1502, 1990.

Paulus JS, Aster RH: Production, distribution, life-span, and fate of platelets, in Williams WJ, et al (eds): *Hematology.* New York, McGraw-Hill, 1990, 1251-1260.

Petros WP: Pharmacokinetics and administration of colony-stimulating factors. *Pharmacotherapy* 12(suppl)32S-38S, 1992.

Pincus T, et al: Multicenter study of recombinant human erythropoietin in correction of anemia in rheumatoid arthritis. *Am J Med* 89:161-168, 1990.

Postmus PE, et al: Effects of recombinant human interleukin-3 in patients with relapsed small-cell lung cancer treated with chemotherapy: A dose-finding study. *J Clin Oncol* 10:1131-1140, 1992.

Pousada L, et al: Erythropoietin and anemia of gastrointestinal bleeding in a Jehovah's Witness, letter. *Ann Intern Med* 112:552, 1990.

Quensenberry PJ: Hemopoietic stem cells, progenitor cells, and growth factors, in Williams WJ, et al (eds): *Hematology.* New York, McGraw-Hill, 1990, 129-147.

Robertson HT, et al: Recombinant erythropoietin improves exercise capacity in anemic hemodialysis patients. *Am J Kidney Dis* 15:325-332, 1990.

Rodgers GP, et al: Augmentation by erythropoietin of the fetal-hemoglobin response to hydroxyurea in sickle cell disease. *N Engl J Med* 328:73-80, 1993.

Rosenfeld CS, Nemunaitis J: The role of granulocyte-macrophage colony-stimulating factor—stimulated progenitor cells in oncology. *Semin Hematol* 29(suppl 3):19-26, 1992.

Rosenlöf K, et al: Erythropoietin, aluminum, and anaemia in patients on haemodialysis. *Lancet* 335:247-249, 1990.

Rotellar C, et al: Low-dose subcutaneous erythropoietin in continuous ambulatory peritoneal dialysis. *Am J Hematol* 37:31-33, 1991.

Sachs L: The control of growth and differentiation in normal and leukemic blood cells. *Cancer* 67(suppl):2684-2694, 1991.

Shannon KM, et al: Recombinant human erythropoietin in the anemia of prematurity: Results of a placebo-controlled pilot study. *J Pediatr* 118:949-955, 1991.

Shannon KM, et al: Enhancement of erythropoiesis by recombinant human erythropoietin in low birth weight infants: A pilot study. *J Pediatr* 120:586-592, 1992.

Sheridan WP, et al: Effect of peripheral-blood progenitor cells mobilised by filgrastim (G-CSF) on platelet recovery after high-dose chemotherapy. *Lancet* 339:640-644, 1992.

Singer JW: Role of colony-stimulating factors in bone marrow transplantation. *Semin Oncol* 19(suppl 7):27-31, (June) 1992.

Smith DA, Perry PJ: The efficacy of ergogenic agents in athletic competition Part II: Other performance-enhancing agents. *Ann Pharmacother* 26:653-659, 1992.

Spivak JL: The application of recombinant erythropoietin in anemic patients with cancer. *Semin Oncol* 19(suppl 8):25-28, 1992.

Spivak JL, Hogans BB: The in vivo metabolism of recombinant human erythropoietin in the rat. *Blood* 73:90-99, 1989.

Spivak JL, et al: Serum immunoreactive erythropoietin in HIV-infected patients. *JAMA* 261:3104-3107, 1989.

St. Onge J, Jacobson RJ: The role of hematopoietic growth factors in the treatment of neoplastic diseases. *Semin Hematol* 29(suppl 2):53-63, (July) 1992.

Stein RS, et al: Pharmacologic doses of recombinant human erythropoietin in the treatment of myelodysplastic syndromes. *Blood* 78:1658-1663, 1991.

Stute N, et al: Pharmacokinetics of subcutaneous recombinant human granulocyte colony-stimulating factor in children. *Blood* 79:2849-2854, 1992.

Takeuchi M, et al: Relationship between sugar chain structure and biological activity of recombinant human erythropoietin produced in Chinese hamster ovary cells. *Proc Natl Acad Sci USA* 86:7819-7822, 1989.

Tasaki T, et al: Recombinant human erythropoietin for autologous blood donation: Effects on perioperative red-blood-cell and serum erythropoietin production. *Lancet* 339:773-775, 1992.

The US Recombinant Human Erythropoietin Predialysis Study Group: Double-blind, placebo-controlled study of the therapeutic use of recombinant human erythropoietin for anemia associated with chronic renal failure in predialysis patients. *Am J Kidney Dis* 18:50-59, (July) 1991.

van der Wouw PA, et al: Effects of recombinant human granulocyte colony-stimulating factor on leucopenia in zidovudine-treated patients with AIDS and AIDS related complex, a Phase I/II study. *Br J Haematol* 78:319-324, 1991.

van Geelen JA, et al: Influence of erythropoietin treatment on urea kinetic parameters in hemodialysis patients. *Clin Nephrol* 35:165-170, 1991.

van Kamp H, et al: Effect of subcutaneously administered human recombinant erythropoietin on erythropoiesis in patients with myelodysplasia *Br J Haematol* 78:488-493, 1991.

Van Wyck DB: Iron management during recombinant human erythropoietin therapy. *Am J Kidney Dis* 14:9-13, 1989.

Van Wyck DB, et al: Iron status in patients receiving erythropoietin for dialysis-associated anemia. *Kidney Int* 35:712-716, 1989.

Watson AJ, et al: Treatment of the anemia of chronic renal failure with subcutaneous recombinant human erythropoietin. *Am J Med* 89:432-435, 1990.

Wolcott DL: Erythropoietin treatment effects on cognitive function and quality of life in patients on chronic dialysis, in Nissenson AR (moderator): Recombinant human erythropoietin and renal anemia: Molecular biology, clinical efficacy, and nervous system effects. *Ann Intern Med* 114:410-413, 1991.

Wong KC, et al: The adverse effects of recombinant human erythropoietin therapy. *Adverse Drug React Acute Poisoning Rev* 9:183-206, 1990.

Yankowitz J, et al: Erythropoietin in pregnancies complicated by severe anemia of renal failure. *Obstet Gynecol* 80:485-488, 1992.

Yoshida Y, et al: A Phase II trial of recombinant human granulocyte colony-stimulating factor in the myelodysplastic syndromes. *Br J Haematol* 78:378-384, 1991.

Zucker-Franklin D: Eosinophils: Morphology, production, biochemistry, and function, in Williams WJ, et al (eds): *Hematology*. New York, McGraw-Hill, 1990, 835-839.

Manufacturers

Abbott Laboratories, Pharm. Products Div., One Abbott Park Road, Abbott Park, Illinois 60064 (800/255-5162)

ACME United Corporation, Medical Products Division, 75 Kings Highway Cut Off, Fairfield, Connecticut 06430 (203/332-7330; 800/243-9852)

Adria Laboratories, Inc., P.O. Box 16529, Columbus, Ohio 43216-6529 (614/764-8100)

Alcon Laboratories, Inc., 6201 S. Freeway, P.O. Box 6600, Ft. Worth, Texas 76134 (817/293-0450)

Allen & Hanburys, Division of Glaxo, Inc., Five Moore Drive, Research Triangle Park, North Carolina 27709 (919/248-2100)

Allercreme, Div. of Owen Laboratories, P.O. Box 6600, Ft. Worth, Texas 76115 (817/293-0450)

Allergan, Herbert, Inc., 2525 Dupont Drive, P.O. Box 19534, Irvine, California 92713 (714/752-4500)

Aloe Creme Laboratories, Div. of ALO Science, Inc., 738 Union Avenue, Middlesex, New Jersey 08846 (908/563-0077)

Alpha Therapeutic Corp., 5555 Valley Blvd., Los Angeles, California 90032 (800/421-0008; fax 213/227-9053)

Alza Corporation, 950 Page Mill Road, P.O. Box 10950, Palo Alto, California 94303-0802 (800/634-8977; fax 415/494-5151)

Americal Corp., 950 Flanders Rd., Mystic, Connecticut 06355

American Cyanamid Company, Davis and Geck Div., One Cyanamid Plaza, Wayne, New Jersey 07470 (800/225-5341)

American Red Cross, Blood Services, Plasma Operations 1730 E. Street, Washington, D.C. 20006 (202/639-3261; fax 202/783-3402)

American Optical Corp., Soft Contact Lens Div., 14 Mechanic Street, Southbridge, Massachusetts 01550

Amgen, Inc., 1900 Oak Terrace Lane, Thousand Oaks, California 91320 (805/499-5725)

AMI Medical Electronics, Inc., Subs. Distinctive Devices, Inc., P.O. Box 148, Ronkonkoma, New York 11779

Anaquest, Inc., Subsidiary of BOC Health Care, Inc., 110 Allen Road, P.O. Box 804, Liberty Corner, New Jersey 07938-0804 (800/262-3784)

Antigen Supply House, 9215-H Partlenia Street, Northridge, California 91324

Apothecon, A Bristol-Myers Squibb Company, P.O. Box 4500, Princeton, New Jersey 08543 (800/321-1335)

Apthalmic Division, P.O. Box 6600, Ft. Worth, Texas 76115

Elizabeth Arden, Inc., 55 East 52nd Street, New York, New York 10022

Armour Pharmaceutical Company, Subsidiary of Rhône-Poulenc Rorer, 500 Arcola Road, PO Box 1200, Mail Stop 3B22, Collegeville, Pennsylvania 19426 (215/454-8000)

B.F. Ascher & Company, Inc., P.O. Box 717, Shawnee Mission, Kansas 66201-0717 (913/888-1880)

Astra Pharmaceutical Products, Inc., Div. of AB ASTRA (Sodertalje, Sweden) 50 Otis Street, Westborough, Massachusetts 01581-4428 (800/225-6333; fax 508/366-7406; 508/366-1100)

Atlanta, Inc., 60 Baylis Rd., Melville, New York 11747

Baker Cummins Pharmaceuticals, Div. of IVAX Corporation, 8800 NW 36th Street, Miami, Florida 33178-2404, (305/590-2282; 800/347-4774)

Basel Pharmaceuticals, Division of CIBA-GEIGY Corp, 556 Morris Ave., Summit, New Jersey 07901 (908/277-5000)

Bausch & Lomb Pharmaceuticals, 1400 North Goodman Street, Rochester, New York 14692 (716/338-6000)

Baxter Healthcare Corp., Fenwal Division, 1425 Lake Cook Road, Deerfield, Illinois 60015 (800/766-1077)

Baxter Healthcare Corp., Hyland Division, 550 N. Brand Boulevard, Glendale, California 91203 (818/956-3200; 800/423-2090)

Baxter Healthcare Corp., I.V. Systems Division, 1425 Lake Cook Road, Deerfield, Illinois 60015 (708/940-5000; 800/933-0303)

Bayer AG, 5090 Leverkusen, West Germany

Beach Pharmaceuticals, Div. of Beach Products, Inc., 5220 S. Manhattan Avenue, P.O. Box 13447, Tampa, Florida 33681 (813/839-6565)

Becton Dickinson Consumer Products Division, One Becton Drive, Franklin Lakes, New Jersey 07417 (201/847-7100)

Beiersdorf, Inc., Div. of Beirsdorf AG, BFD Plaza, 360 Martin Luther King Drive, P.O. Box 5529, Norwalk, Connecticut 06856 (203/853-8008)

Berlex Laboratories, 300 Fairfield Road, Wayne, New Jersey 07470

Berna Products, Inc., 4216 Ponce De Leon Blvd., Coral Gables, Florida 33146 (201/694-4100; 800/533-5899; 305/443-2900)

Biocraft Laboratories, Inc., 18-01 River Road, Fair Lawn, New Jersey 07410 (201/703-0400; 800/631-0165)

Biogen, 14 Cambridge Center, Cambridge, Massachusetts 02142, (617/864-8900)

Bionetics Research, Inc., 115 S. Sangamen Street, Chicago, Illinois 60607

Bio Products Ophthalmics, Inc., Post Road West, Westport, Connecticut 06880

Biosearch Medical Products, Inc., 35 Industrial Parkway, P.O. Box 1700, Somerville, New Jersey 08876, (908/722-5000; 800/326-5976)

Biotechnology Research Institute, 1333 A Piccard Dr., Rockville, Maryland 20850

Bird Products Corp., 4371 Latham Street, Suite 202, Riverside, California 92501

Blaine Company, Inc., 1465 Jamike Lane, Erlanger, Kentucky 41018 (606/283-9437; fax 606/283-9460)

Blairex Laboratories, Inc., P.O. Box 15190, Evansville, Indiana 47716 (800/252-4739)

Blair Laboratories, Inc., Affiliate of The Purdue Frederick Company, 100 Connecticut Ave., Norwalk, Connecticut 06856 (203/853-0123)

Bock Pharmacal Company, P.O. Box 8519, St. Louis, Missouri 63126 (314/343-0994)

Boehringer Ingelheim Pharmaceuticals, Inc., 900 Ridgebury Road, P.O. Box 368, Ridgefield, Connecticut 06877 (203/798-9988)

Bolar Pharmaceutical Company, 33 Ralph Avenue, Copiague, New York 11726-0030, (516/842-8383)

Boots Pharmaceuticals, 300 Tri-State International Center, Suite 200, Lincolnshire, Illinois 60069 (708/405-7400; fax 708/405-7505)

Boots PLC, Travenol Laboratories, Inc., 1425 Lake Cook Road, Deerfield, Illinois 60015

Bowman Pharmaceutical, Inc., 119 Schroyer Avenue Northwest, Canton, Ohio 44702

Braintree Laboratories, Inc., P.O. Box 361, 60 Columbian Street, Braintree, Massachusetts 02184 (617/843-2202)

Bristol Meyers Oncology Division, A Bristol Meyers-Squibb Company, P.O. Box 4500, Princeton, New Jersey 08543-4500 (609/921-4000)

Bristol-Myers Squibb, US Pharmaceutical Division, P.O. Box 4500, Princeton, New Jersey 08543-4500 (609/243-6000)

Bristol-Myers Squibb Company, Bristol-Myers Pharmaceutical Research & Development Division, 5 Research Parkway, P.O. Box 5100, Wallingford, Connecticut 06492-7660

Britannia Pharmaceuticals Limited, Hamilton House, 87/89 Bell Street, Reigate, Surrey, Great Britain RH27YZ

Burroughs Wellcome Company, 3030 Cornwallis Road, Research Triangle Park, North Carolina 27709 (800/722-9292)

Carnrick Laboratories, Inc., 65 Horse Hill Road, Cedar Knolls, New Jersey 07927 (201/267-2670)

Carrington Laboratories, Inc., 1300 E. Rochelle Blvd., Irving, Texas 75356-9500 (214/518-1300)

Carter Products, Div. Carter-Wallace Inc., One-Half Acre Road, Cranbury, New Jersey 08512 (609/655-6000)
Central Pharmaceuticals, Inc., 120 East Third Street, PO Box 328, Seymour, Indiana 47274 (812/522-3915)
Century Pharmaceuticals, Inc., 10377 Hague Road, Indianapolis Indiana 46256 (317/849-4210)
Cetus Oncology Corporation, 4560 Horton St., Emeryville, California 94608 (800/238-8779)
Chesebrough-Ponds, U.S.A. Company, Div. of Unilever, 33 Benedict Place, Greenwich, Connecticut 06830 (203/661-2000)
Chiron Ophthalmics, Inc., 9342 Geronimo Rd., Irvine, California 92718-1903 (714/768-4690)
CIBA Consumer Pharmaceuticals, Div. of CIBA-Geigy Corp., Mack Woodbridge II, 581 Main Street, Woodbridge, New Jersey 07095 (908/602-6600)
CIBA-Geigy Corporation, Pharmaceuticals Division, 556 Morris Avenue, Summit, New Jersey 07901 (908/277-5000)
Otis Clapp & Sons, Inc., 143 Albany Street, Cambridge, Massachusetts 02139
Clintec Nutrition Company, Affiliate of Baxter Healthcare Corp., & Nestle SA, 3 Parkway N., Suite 500, Box 760, Deerfield, Illinois 60015 (800/388-0300)
Colgate-Hoyt, Division of Colgate-Palmolive Company, 1 Colgate Way, Canton, Massachusetts 02021 (800/225-3756)
Colgate-Palmolive Company, 300 Park Avenue, New York, New York 10022 (212/310-2000)
Commerce Drug Company, Division of Del Laboratories, Inc., 565 Broad Hollow Road, Farmingdale, New Jersey 11735 (516/293-7070)
Connaught Laboratories, Inc., A Pasteur Merleux Co., Subsidiary of Connaught Laboratories Limited Rt. 611, P.O. Box 187, Swiftwater, Pennsylvania 18370 (717/839-7187)
CooperVision, Inc., 3495 Winton Place, Rochester, NY 14623 (408/434-7000; 800/225-2578)
Curatek Pharmaceuticals, Inc., 1965 Pratt Blvd., Elk Grove Village, Illinois 60007 (708/806-7680)
Cutter Biological, Division of Miles Pharmaceuticals, 400 Morgan Lane, West Haven, Connecticut 06516 (203/937-2000)
Davis & Geck, Division of American Cyanamid, One Cyanamid Plaza, Wayne, New Jersey 07470 (800/225-5341; 201/831-2000)
Degussa Corporation, 65 Challenger Road, Ridgefield Park, New Jersey 07660 (201/641-6100)
DEP Corporation, DEP Consumer Products Division, 2102 E. Via Arado, Rancho Domenguez, California 90220 (213/604-0777)
Dermalab, LTD, 2809 Higgins Road, Elk Grove Village, Illinois 60007 (708/640-0590)
Dermik Laboratories Inc., Division of Rhône-Poulenc Rorer Inc., 500 Arcola Road, P.O. Box 1200, Collegeville, Pennsylvania 19426 (215/454-8000)
Dey Laboratories, Inc., 2751 Napa Valley Corporate Dr., Napa, California 94558 (800/755-5560; fax 707/224-3235)
Dista Products Company, Division of Eli Lilly & Company, Lilly Corporate Center, Box 1407, Indianapolis, Indiana 46285 (317/276-4000)
Dixon & Williams Pharmaceutical Company, Inc., 43 Old Wood Road, Bernardsville, New Jersey 07924 (908/766-3558)
Doak Pharmacal Company, Inc., 67 Sylvester St., Westbury, New York 11590 (516/333-7222)
Dorsey Laboratories, Division of Sandoz Pharmaceutical Corp., Route 10, East Hanover, New Jersey 07936 (201/503-7500)
E. I. DuPont de Nemours & Company, Inc., dba DuPont Pharmaceuticals, P.O. Box 80016, Wilmington, Delaware 19880 (800/441-7515)
DuPont Pharmaceuticals, Barley Mill Plaza, P.O. Box 80026, Wilmington, Delaware 19880-0026 (302/992-4240; fax 302/992-7771)
Elder Pharmaceuticals, Inc., ICN Plaza, 3300 Hyland Avenue, Costa Mesa, California 92626 (800/556-1937)
Enzon, Inc., 40 Kingsbridge Road, Piscataway, New Jersey 08854 (908/980-4500; fax 908/980-5911)
Ethicon, Inc., Div. of Johnson & Johnson, Route 22, P.O. Box 151, Somerville, New Jersey 08876 (201/218-0707)
Ethigen, 6320 Commodore Sloat Drive, Los Angeles, California 90048
Ethitek Pharmaceuticals Company, 7855 Gross Point Road, Unit L, Skokie, Illinois 60077 (708/675-6611)
Farmitalia Carb Erba GmbH, Merzhauser Strasse 112, Postfach 480, 7800 Freiburg, West Germany
Ferndale Laboratories, Inc., 780 West Eight Mile Road, Ferndale, Michigan 48220 (313/548-0900; fax 313/548-0708)
Ferring Laboratories, Inc., 400 Rella Boulevard, Suite 201, Suffern, New York 10901 (800/445-3690)
Fisons Pharmaceuticals, Prescription Product Div., P.O. Box 1766, Rochester, New York 14603 (716/475-9000)
C.B. Fleet Company, Inc., 4615 Murray Place, Lynchburg, Virginia 24506-2235 (804/528-4000)
Fleming & Company, 1600 Fenpark Drive, Fenton, Missouri 63026 (314/343-8200)
Forest Pharmaceuticals, Inc., Subsidiary of Forest Laboratories, 2510 Metro Blvd., St. Louis, Missouri 63043 (314/569-3610)
E. Fougera & Company, Inc., Div. of Altana, Inc., 60 Baylis Road, Melville, New York 11747 (516/454-6996; 800/645-9833)
Fujisawa Pharmaceutical Company, Division of Fujisawa USA, Inc., Three Parkway North, Third Floor, Deerfield, Illinois 60015-2548 (800/888-7704)
Gate Pharmaceuticals, Division of The Lemmon Company, 650 Cathill Road, Sellersville, Pennsylvania 18960 (800/292-4283)
Geigy Pharmaceuticals, Division of Ciba-Geigy Corp., 556 Morris Avenue, Summit, New Jersey 07901 (908/277-5390)
GenDerm Corporation, 600 Knightsbridge Pkwy., Lincolnshire, Illinois 60069 (708/634-7373; 800/533-3376)
Genentech, Inc., 460 Point San Bruno Blvd., San Francisco, California 94080 (415/225-1000)
Genzyme Corporation, 1 Kendall Square, Cambridge, Massachusetts 02139-1562 (800/745-4447; fax 617/252-7600)
Gerber Products Company, 445 State Street, Fremont, Michigan 49412 (616/928-2000)
Geriatric Pharmaceutical Corp., Subsidiary of W.E. Hauck, Inc., 11525 N. Fulton Industrial Blvd., P.O. Box 1065, Alpharetta, Georgia 30201 (404/475-4758)
Gilbert Laboratories, 31 Fairmont Avenue, Chester, New Jersey 07930
Glaxo, Inc., Five Moore Drive, Research Triangle Park, North Carolina 27709 (919/248-2100)
Glenbrook Laboratories, Division of Sterling Drug Inc., 90 Park Avenue, 17th Fl., New York, New York 10016 (212/907-2000)
Glenwood Laboratories, Inc., P.O. Box 518, 83 N. Summit Street, Tenafly, New Jersey 07670 (201/569-0050; 800/542-0772)
Goldline Laboratories, Inc., 1900 W. Commercial Blvd., Ft. Lauderdale, Florida 33309 (305/491-4000; 800/327-4114)
Guardian Laboratories, Div. United Guardian, Inc., 230 Marcus Boulevard, P.O. Box 2500, Smithtown, New York 11787 (800/645-5566)
Gulf Bio-Systems, Inc., 5310 Harvest Hill Road, Dallas, Texas 75230
GynoPharma Laboratories, 50 Division St., Somerville, New Jersey 08876 (908/725-3100; 800/322-4966)
Harber Pharmaceuticals Company, 350 Meadowlands Parkway, Secaucus, New Jersey 07094 (201/343-3700)
Hauck Pharmaceuticals, Division of W.E. Hauck, Inc., 11525 N. Fulton Industrial Blvd., P.O. Box 1065, Alpharetta, Georgia 30201 (404/475-4758; 800/426-4309)
Herald Phamacal, Inc., 6503 Warwick Road, Richmond, Virginia 23225 (804/745-3400)
Herbert Laboratories, Div. of Allergan, Inc. 18600 Von Karman Avenue, Irvine, California 92713 (714/955-6200)
Hermal Pharmaceutical Laboratories, Inc., Affiliate of Hermal-Kurt Hermann, West Germany, 163 Delaware Ave, Delmar, New York 12054 (518/475-2175; 800/437-6251)
Dow B. Hickman, Inc., 10410 Corporate Drive, P.O. Box 2006, Sugar Land, Texas 77487-2006 (713/240-1000; 800/231-3052)
Hoechst-Roussel Pharmaceuticals Inc., Div. of Hoechst Celanese Corp., Route 202-206, P.O. Box 2500 North, Somerville, New Jersey 08876 (800/445-4774; 908/231-2000; fax 908/231-3154)

Hollister-Stier Laboratories, Division of Miles Laboratories, Inc., 3525 N. Regal Street, P.O. Box 3145, Spokane, Washington 99220 (509/489-5656)

Hyland Therapeutics Division, Travenol Laboratories, Inc., P.O. Box 1976, 444 West Glenoaks Blvd., Glendale, California 91202

Hynson Westcott & Dunning, Div. of Becton Dickinson, 250 Schilling Circle, Cockeysville, Maryland 21030 (301/771-0100; 800/638-8663)

Hyrex Pharmaceuticals, 3494 Democrat Road, P.O. Box 18385, Memphis, Tennessee 38118 (901/794-9050; fax: 901/794-9051)

ICN-Elder, 3300 Hyland Avenue, Costa Mesa, California 92626, (714/545-0100)

ICN Pharmaceuticals, Inc., ICN Plaza, 3300 Hyland Ave., Costa Mesa, California 92626 (800/556-1937)

IDEC, Inc., 11099 N. Torrey Pines Rd., #160, LaJolla, California 92037 (619/458-0600)

Immunex Corporation, 51 University Street, Seattle, Washington 98101 (800/334-6273; 206/587-0430; fax: 206/587-0606)

Immuno U.S., Inc. 1200 Parkdale Road, Rochester, MI 48307 (313/652-7872; fax 313/652-0670)

International Ethical Labs, Avenue Americo Miranda, #1021, Repto., Metropolitano, San Juan, Puerto Rico 00921 (809/765-3510; fax 809/767-1110)

Iolab Pharmaceuticals, 500 Iolab Drive, Claremont, California 91711 (714/624-2020; 800/443-6440 fax: 714/399-1425)

Ives Laboratories, Inc., 685 Third Avenue, New York, New York 10017

Jacobus Pharmaceutical Company, Inc., 37 Cleveland Lane, P.O. Box 5290 Princeton, New Jersey 08540 (609/921-7447)

Janssen Pharmaceutica, Inc., 1125 Trenton-Harbourton Road, P.O. Box 200, Titusville New Jersey 08560-0200 (800/253-3682; fax 609/730-3044; 609/730-2000)

The Andrew Jergens Company, 2535 Spring Grove Avenue, Cincinnati, Ohio 45214 (513/421-1400)

Johnson and Johnson, Merck Pharmaceuticals, Camp Hill Road, Ft. Washington, PA 19034 (215/233-7000; fax: 215/233-3307)

Jones Medical Industries, Inc., Western Division, 11604 Liburn Park Drive, P.O. Box 46903, St. Louis, Missouri 63146 (314/432-7557, fax: 432-3785)

Kabi Pharmacia, Inc., 800 Centennial Ave., P.O. Box 1327, Piscataway, New Jersey 08855-1327 (800/526-3610, 908/457-8000, fax: 908/457-8283)

KabiVitrum, Inc., 160 Industrial Drive, Franklin, Ohio 45005 (800/526-5224)

Kay Pharmacal Company, Inc., P.O. Box 50375, 1312 N. Utica Avenue, Tulsa, Oklahoma 74150

Keene Pharmaceuticals, Inc., 333 S. Mockingbird, P.O. Box 7, Keene, Texas 76059 (817/645-8083)

Kenwood Laboratories, Inc., Div. of Bradley Pharmaceuticals, Inc., 383 Route 46 West, Fairfield, New Jersey 07004 (201/882-1505, 800/866-1521, fax: 201/575-5366)

Key Pharmaceuticals, Inc., Div. of Schering-Plough Corp., 2000 Galloping Hill Rd., Kenilworth, New Jersey 07033 (908/298-4000, fax: 908/298-5661)

Knoll Pharmaceutical Company, A unit of BASF K&F Corporation, 30 North Jefferson Road, Whippany, New Jersey 07981 (800/526-0710, 201/887-8300, fax: 201/887-8131)

Lafayette Pharmacal, Inc., P.O. Box 4499, Lafayette, Indiana 47903 (317/447-3129)

Lakeside Pharmaceuticals Division of Merrell Dow Pharmaceuticals, Inc., P.O. Box 429553, Cincinnati, Ohio 45242-9553 (513/948-9110)

The Lannett Company, Inc., 9000 State Road, Philadelphia, Pennsylvania 19136 (215/333-9000, fax: 215/333-9004)

Laser Pharmaceuticals, 2000 N. Main Street, P.O. Box 905, Crown Point, Indiana 46307 (219/769-0110)

Lederle Laboratories, American Cyanamid Company, One Cyanamid Plaza, Wayne, New Jersey 07470 (800/533-3753, 201/831-2000, fax; 831-4097)

Leeming Division, Pfizer, Inc., 100 Jefferson Road, Parsippany, New Jersey 07054

Leeming/Pacquin Division, Division of Pfizer, Inc., 235 E. 42nd Street, New York, New York 10017 (212/573-3131)

Legere Pharmaceuticals, Inc., 7326 East Evans Road, Scottsdale, Arizona 85260 (602/991-4033; fax 602/483-0792)

Lemmon Company, P.O. Box 904, Sellersville, Pennsylvania 18960 (800/545-8800; 215/723-5544; fax 215/721-9669)

Lever Brothers Company, 390 Park Avenue, 19th Floor, New York, New York 10022

Eli Lilly and Company, Lilly Corporate Center, Indianapolis, Indiana 46285 (317/276-2000; fax 317/276-2095)

Lypho-med Fujisawa, Division of Fujisawa USA, Inc., Three Parkway North, Deerfield, Illinois 60015-2548, (708/317-0600; fax 708/317-7296)

Major Pharmaceutical Corp., 8330 Arjons Drive, San Diego, CA 92126 (619/693-6080)

Mallard, Inc., 3021 Wabash Avenue, Detroit, Michigan 48216

Mallinckrodt Medical, Inc., 675 McDonnell Boulevard, P.O. Box 5840, St. Louis, Missouri 63134 (314/895-2000; 800/822-2075; fax 314/895-2136)

Marion Merrell-Dow Laboratories, Inc., 9300 Ward Parkway, P.O. Box 8480, Kansas City, Missouri 64114-0408 (800/522-3656; 800/966-4000; fax: 816/966-3270)

Jeffrey Martin, Inc., 410 Clermont Terrace, Union, New Jersey 07083

Massachusetts Public Health, Biologic Laboratories, 305 South Street, Jamaica Plain, Massachusetts 02130 (617/522-3700)

Mayrand, Inc., 4 Dundas Circle, PO Box 8869, Greensboro, North Carolina 27419 (919/292-5347)

McGaw, Inc., 2525 McGaw Ave., Box 19791, Irvine, California 92713-9791 (714/660-2000; fax: 714/660-2767)

McNeil Pharmaceutical, Welsh & McKean Road, Springhouse, Pennsylvania 19477 (215/628-5000; fax 215/628-8689)

Mead Johnson Laboratories, A Bristol-Myers Squibb Company, 2400 W. Lloyd Expressway, Evansville, Indiana 47721 (800/468-7746; 609/243-6986)

Medchem Products, Inc., 444 Washington Street, Woburn, Massachusetts 01801 (617/938-9328)

Med-Corp, Division of Life Medical Systems, Inc., 5001 Spring Valley Road, Dallas, Texas 75244 (214/385-7214)

Medco Research, Inc., 8733 Beverly Blvd., Suite 404, Los Angeles, California 90048 (213/854-1954)

Medical Market Specialties, P.O. Box 150, Boonton, New Jersey 07005 (201/263-4243)

Medicone Company, 225 Varick Street, New York, New York 10014 (212/924-5166)

Medtech Laboratories, Inc., 3510 N. Lake Creek, P.O. Box 1108, Jackson, Wyoming 83001 (307/733-1680; 800/443-4908)

Medtronic, Inc., 7000 Central Avenue, N.E., Minneapolis, Minnesota 55432 (612/574-4000; 612/574-6072; fax 612/574-4879)

Melville Biologics, New York Blood Center, Inc., 155 Duryea Road, Melville, New York 11747 (516/752-8753)

Mephra AG, 4143 Dormach, Postfast 137, Aesch Basel, Switzerland

Merck Sharp & Dohme, Div. of Merck & Company, Inc., Sumneytown Pike, West Point, Pennsylvania 19486 (215/652-5000)

Merck Sharp & Dohme International, WP38M-2, West Point, Pennsylvania 19486 (215/652-5000)

Michigan Dept. of Health, 3424 N. Logan, P.O. Box 30195, Lansing, Michigan 48909

Miles, Inc., 400 Morgan Lane, West Haven, Connecticut 06516 (800/468-0894; 203/937-2000)

Misemer Pharmaceutical, Inc., 4553 South Campbell, Springfield, Michigan 65810 (417/881-0660)

Mission Pharmacal Company, 1325 E. Durango Street, P.O. Box 1676, San Antonio, Texas 78210 (512/650-3273; fax 512/650-0520)

Montedison Farmaceuttica, Arcos 2626, Buenos Aires, Argentina

H.L. Moore Drug Exchange, 389 John Downey Drive, P.O. Box 1500 New Britain, Connecticut 06050 (203/826-3600)

Muro Pharmaceutical, Inc., 890 East Street, Tewksbury, Massachusetts 01876 (800/225-0974; 508/851-5981)

National Cancer Institute, Division of Cancer Treatment, National Institutes of Health, Bldg. 31, Room 3A49, Bethesda, Maryland 20892

Neutrogena Dermatologics, 5760 W. 96th Street, P.O. Box 45036, Los Angeles, California 90045 (310/642-1150; 800/421-6857; fax 310/337-5557)

Newport Pharmaceutical International, Inc., 897 West 16th, Newport Beach, California 92663 (714/642-7511)

Norcliff Thayer, Inc., 303 South Broadway, Tarrytown, New York 10591

Nordisk-USA, 3202 Tower Oaks Blvd., Suite 100, Rockville, Maryland 20852

Norwich Eaton Pharmaceuticals, Inc., A Procter & Gamble Company, 17 Eaton Avenue, P.O. Box 191, Norwich, New York 13815 (800/448-4878; 607/335-2111; fax 607/335-2098)

Novo Nordisk Pharmaceuticals, 100 Overlook Center, Suite 200, Princeton, New Jersey 08540 (609/987-5800; fax: 609/921-8082)

Oclassen Pharmaceuticals, 100 Pelican Way, San Rafael, California 94901 (800/288-4508; 415/258-4500; fax 415/258-4550)

Ocumed, Inc., 119 Harrison Ave., Roseland, New Jersey 07068 (201/226-2330)

ONY Inc., Baird Research Park, 1576 Sweet Home Road, Amhurst, New York 14221 (716/636-9096)

Optopics Laboratories Corp., P.O. Box 210, Fairton, New Jersey 08320 (800/223-0865; 609/451-9350; fax 609/451-2177)

Oral B Laboratories, Division of Gillette Company, 1 Lagoon Drive, Redwood City, California 94065 (415/598-5000; fax 800/322-1329)

Organon, Inc., 375 Mount Pleasant Avenue, West Orange, New Jersey 07052 (201/325-4500; fax 201/325-4589)

Organon Teknika Corporation, 100 Akzo Ave., Durham, North Carolina 27704 (919/620-2000; 800/682-2666; fax 919/620-2107)

Ortho Diagnostic Systems, Inc., Route 202, P.O. Box 300, Raritan, New Jersey 08869 (800/322-6374)

Ortho Pharmaceutical Corporation, Route 202 South, P.O. Box 300, Raritan, New Jersey 08869-0602 (800/682-6532; 908/218-6000; fax 908/218-1416)

Paddock Laboratories, Inc., 3101 Louisiana Avenue North, Minneapolis, Minnesota 55427 (800/328-5113; 612/546-4676; fax 612/546-4842)

Palisades Pharmaceuticals, Inc., 219 County Rd., Tenafly, New Jersey 07670 (800/237-9083; 201/569-8502; fax 201/569-7416)

Parke-Davis, Div. of Warner-Lambert Company, 201 Tabor Road, Morris Plains, New Jersey 07950 (201/540-2000; fax 201/540-4624)

Pedinol Pharmacal, Inc., 30 Banfi Plaza North, Farmingdale, New York 11735 (516/293-9500; 800/PED-INOL; fax 516/293-7359)

Peninsula Laboratories, 611 Taylor Way, Belmont, California 94002

Pennwalt Corporation, Pharmacraft Division, P.O. Box 1710, 155 Jefferson Road, Rochester, New York 14603

Person & Covey, Inc., 616 Allen Avenue, Glendale, California 91201 (800/423-2341; 818/240-1030; fax 818/547-9821)

The Pfeiffer Company, P.O. Box 100, 43-45 North Washington Ave., Wilkes Barre, Pennsylvania 18773 (717/826-9000; 800/342-6450; fax 717/826-9009)

Pfipharmecs Division, Pfizer, Inc., 235 E. 42nd Street, New York, New York 10017 (212/573-2323)

Pfizer Pharmaceuticals, 235 East 42nd Street, New York, New York 10017 (212/573-2323)

Pharmachemie B.V., Nijverheidsweg 48-50, P.O. Box 552, 2003 RN Harlem, Holland 023-319209

Pharmacia-Chiron Partnership, 4560 Horton Street, Emeryville, California 94608

Pharmacia Inc., Medical Products Group, P.O. Box 1327, 800 Centennial Ave., Piscataway, New Jersey 08855-1327 (800/526-3619; fax 908/457-8283; 201/457-8000)

Pharmacraft Division, Pennwalt Corporation, 755 Jefferson Road, Rochester, New York 14623

Pharmaquest Corporation, 3301 Kerner Boulevard, Suite 200, San Raphael, California 94901

PharmaFair, Inc., 205C Kelsey Lane, Tampa, Florida 33619 (813/972-7705)

Plough, Inc., Div. of Shering-Plough Healthcare Products, 110 Allen Rd., Liberty Bell, New Jersey 07938 (908/604-1995)

Porton Products Limited, 30401 Agoura Road, #102, Agoura Hills, California 91301 (800/727-6737; 818/879-2200)

Poythress & Company, Inc., 16 North 22nd Street, P.O. Box 26946, Richmond, Virginia 23261 (804/644-8591)

Praxis Biologics, 30 Corporate Woods, Suite 300, Rochester, New York 14623 (716/272-7000)

Princeton Pharmaceutical Products, Div. of Bristol-Myers Squibb, P.O. Box 4000, New Brunswick, New Jersey 08543-4000 (609/243-6000)

Procter & Gamble Company, P.O. Box 599, 1137 Reed Hartman Highway, Cincinnati, Ohio 45201 (513/983-1100)

Purdue Frederick Company, 100 Connecticut Ave., Norwalk, Connecticut 06856 (203/853-0123); (800-733-1333) (fax 203/838-1576)

Quad Pharmaceuticals Inc., 6340 LaPas Trail, Indianapolis, Indiana 46268 (317/299-6611)

Recsei Laboratories, 330 South Kellogg, Building M, Goleta, California 93117-3875 (805/964-2912)

Rachelle Laboratories, Inc., P.O. Box 187, Culver, Indiana 46511 (219/842-3305)

Reed & Carnrick, Division of Block Drug Co., Inc., 257 Cornelison Ave., Jersey City, New Jersey 07302-9988 (201/434-4000; fax 201/434-3032)

Reid-Provident Laboratories, Inc., 640 Tenth Street, N.W., Atlanta, Georgia 30318

Reid-Rowell, Inc. (see Solvay Pharmaceuticals)

Research Industries Corporation, Pharmaceutical Div., 6864 South 300 West, Midvale, UT 84047 (801/972-5500; fax 801/562-1122)

Research Medical, Inc., Subsidiary of Research Industries Corporation, 1847 West 2300 South, Salt Lake City, Utah 84119 (801/972-5500)

Revlon Health Care Group, Ethical Products Division, (Armour & USV), 303 South Broadway, Tarrytown, New York 10591

Rhone-Poulenc Rorer Pharmaceutical, 500 Arcola Road, Collegeville, Pennsylvania 19426-0107 (215/454-8000)

Richardson-Vicks, A Procter & Gamble Co., P.O. Box 5516, Cincinnati, Ohio 45201 (800/358-8707)

Roberts Laboratories, 2084 R.D. J25, Austin, Colorado 81410 (303/835-3913)

Roberts Pharmaceutical Corp., Meridian Center III, 6-G Industrial Way West, Eatontown, New Jersey 07724 (908/389-1182; fax 908/389-1014)

A.H. Robins Company, 1407 Cummings Drive, P.O. Box 26609, Richmond, Virginia 23220-6609 (804/257-2000)

Roche Laboratories, Div. of Hoffmann La Roche Inc., 340 Kingsland Street, Nutley, New Jersey 07110-1199 (201/235-5000; 201/235-3843)

Roerig, Division of Pfizer, Inc., 235 East 42nd Street, New York, New York 10017 (212/573-2323)

Ross Laboratories, Div. of Abbott Laboratories, 625 Cleveland Avenue, Columbus, Ohio 43231 (614/624-7677; 800/255-5162)

Rowell Laboratories, Inc., 210 Main Street, West, Baudette, Minnesota 56623

Roxane Laboratories, Inc., 1809 Wilson Road, P.O. Box 16532, Columbus, Ohio 43216 (614/276-4000)

Rugby Laboratories, Inc., 898 Orlando Ave., West Hempstead, New York 11552 (516/536-8565)

Russ Pharmaceuticals, 1211 Sherwood Avenue, Richmond, Virginia 23220 (804/254-4400)

Rydelle Laboratories, Inc., Div. of S.C. Johnson & Son, Inc., 1525 Howe Street, Racine, Wisconsin 53403 (414/631-2000)

Sandoz Pharmaceuticals, 59 Route 10, East Hanover, New Jersey 07963 (201/503-7500; 800/221-3951; fax 201/503-8265)

Sanofi Winthrop Pharmaceuticals, Inc., 90 Park Avenue, New York, New York 10016 (212/907-2000)

Savage Laboratories, Div. of Altana, Inc., 60 Baylis Road, Melville, New York 11747 (800/231-0206; 516/454-9071)

Schering Corp., 2000 Galloping Hill Road, Kenilworth, New Jersey 07033 (908/298-4000)

Schering-Plough Corporation, 110 Allen Road, Liberty Corner, New Jersey 07938 (908/604-1995)

Schmid Products Company, Route 46 West, Little Falls, New Jersey 07424 (201/256-5500)

Schwarz Pharmaceuticals, Kremers Urban Company, P.O. Box 2038, Milwaukee, Wisconsin 53201 (800/558-5114; 414/354-4300)

Scientific Testing, Inc., 783 Jersey Avenue, New Brunswick, New Jersey 08085

Sclavo, Inc., 5 Mansard Court, Wayne, New Jersey 07470 (201/696-8300)

Searle, P.O. Box 5110, Chicago, Illinois 60680-9899 (800/323-1603; 708/470-9710; 708/982-7000)

The Seatrace Company, P.O. Box 363, Gadsden, Alabama 35902 (205/442-5023)

Seres Laboratories, Inc., 3331 Industrial Drive, P.O. Box 470, Santa Rosa, California 95402 (707/526-4526)

Serono Laboratories, Inc., Division of: Ares-Serono Group, 100 Longwater Circle, Norwell, MA 02061 (800/283-8088); (617/982-9000)

Sherwood Laboratories, Inc., 1601 East 361st Street, Willoughby, Ohio 44094

Sigma F and D Division Ltd., Sigma Chemical Company, 3050 Spruce Street, St. Louis, Missouri 63103

Sigma Tau, Inc., 200 Orchard Ridge Drive, Gathersburg, Maryland 20878 (301/948-1041; 800/447-0169)

Smith Laboratories, Inc., 2211 Sanders Road, P.O. Box 3044, Northbrook, Illinois 60062

SmithKline Beecham Pharmaceuticals, Division of SmithKline Beecham Corporation, One Franklin Plaza, P.O. Box 7929, Philadelphia, Pennsylvania 19101 (215/751-4000)

Sola/Barnes-Hind Pharmaceuticals, Inc., A Pilkington Visioncare Co., 810 Kifer Road, Sunnyvale, California 94086-5200, (619/277-9893; 800/538-1680)

Solvay Pharmaceuticals, 901 Sawyer Rd., Marietta, Georgia 30062 (404/578-9000; fax 404/578-5586)

Somerset Pharmaceuticals, Inc., 777 South Harbour Island Boulevard, Suite 800, Tampa, Florida 33602 (813/223-7677)

Spectra Pharmaceuticals Service, Hanover Business Park, 155 Webster Street, Hanover, Massachusetts 02339 (617/871-3991)

Sporocidin Company, Rt. 8 Box 338, Jonesboro, Tennessee 37659

Squibb-Connaught Inc., 330 Alexander Street, Princeton, NJ 08540

Squibb-Mark, Div. E. R. Squibb & Sons, P.O. Box 4500, Princeton, New Jersey 08543-4500

Squibb-Marsam, Div. Bristol-Myers Squibb, P.O. Box 1022, Cherry Hill, New Jersey 08034 (609/424-5600)

Squibb-Novo, Inc., Suite 200, 100 Overlook Center, Princeton, New Jersey 08540-7810 (609/987-5800)

Star Pharmaceuticals, 1990 N.W. 44th Street, Pompano Beach, Florida 33064 (305/971-9704)

Steri-Med, Inc., P.O. Box 459, Lindenhurst, New York 11757

Sterling Winthrop, Inc., Div. of Sterling Drug, Inc. 90 Park Ave., New York, New York 10016 (212/907-2000)

Stiefel Laboratories, Inc., 255 Alhambra Circle, Suite 1000, Coral Gables, Florida 33134-6988 (305/443-3807)

Storz/Lederle Ophthalmic Pharmaceuticals, Div. American Cyamid Co., One Cyanamid Plaza, Wayne, New Jersey 07470 (800/533-3753)

Stuart Pharmaceuticals, Division of ICI Americas, Inc., Concord Pike & Murphy Road, Wilmington, Delaware 19897 (302/886-2231; 800/441-7758)

Summit Pharmaceuticals, CIBA-GEIGY Corp., 556 Morris Ave., Summit, New Jersey 07901 (201/277-5000)

Syntex Laboratories, Division of Syntex Corporation, 3401 Hillview Avenue, P.O. Box 10850, Palo Alto, California 94303 (415/852-1386; 815/855-5050)

Syosset Laboratories, 150 Eileen Way, Syosset, New York 11791 (516/921-6306)

TAG Pharmaceuticals, c/o Lemmon Company, P.O. Box 904, Sellersville, Pennsylvania 18960 (215/723-5544)

TAP Pharmaceuticals, Bannockburn Lake Office Plaza, 2355 Waukegan Rd., Deerfield, Illinois 60015 (800/621-1020)

Terumo Corporation, 2100 Cottontail Lake, Somerset, New Jersey 08873 (800/283-7866); (908/302-4900)

Texas Drug Company, P.O. Box 790771, San Antonio, Texas 78279

Theragenics Corporation, 900 Atlantic Drive NW, Atlanta, Georgia 03019

Thompson Medical Company, Inc., 222 Lakview Avenue, 17th Floor, West Palm Beach, Florida 33401-6112 (407/820-9900)

3M Pharmaceuticals, Div. of 3M Corporation, 3M Center Building 275-3W-01, St. Paul, Minnesota 55144 (612/736-4930; 612/736-4911)

Travenol Laboratories, Inc., One Baxter Parkway, Deerfield, Illinois 60015

Trimen Laboratories, Inc., 80 26th Street, Pittsburgh, Pennsylvania 15222 (412/261-0339)

Triton Bioscience, Inc., 1501 Harbor Bay Parkway, Alameda, California 94501 (415/769-5200)

UAD Laboratories, Inc., 8339 Highway 18 West, P.O. Box 10587, Jackson, Mississippi 39209 (601/372-7773)

UCB Secteur Pharmaceutique, 326 Avenue, Luise, 1050, Brussels, Belgium

Ueno Fine Chemicals Industry, Ltd., 2-31 Koraibashiigashi-Ku, Osaka 541, Japan (06/203-0761)

Ulmer Pharmacal, Div of James Phillips Co., 2440 Fernbrook Lane, Plymouth, Minnesota 55447 (612/559-3333)

Unimed, Inc., 35 Columbia Road, Somerville, New Jersey 08876-3587 (201/526-6894)

The Upjohn Company, 7000 Portage Road, Kalamazoo, Michigan 49001 (616/323-4000)

Upsher-Smith Laboratories, Inc., 14905 23rd Avenue, North, Minneapolis, Minnesota 55447 (612/475-4412)

U.S. Bioscience, One Tower Bridge, 100 Front St., Suite 400, West Conshohocken, Pennsylvania 19428 (215/832-0570)

U.S. Pharmaceutical Corp., 2401C Mellon Court, Decatur, Georgia 30035 (404/987-4745)

U.S. Products, Inc., 16636 N.W. 54th St., Miami Lakes, Florida 33014 (305/620-9540)

USV Laboratories-North America, 500 Virginia Drive, Ft. Washington, Pennsylvania 19034-2707

Vale Chemical Company, Inc., 1202 Liberty Street, Allentown, Pennsylvania 18102

Vestal Laboratories, 5075 Manchester Avenue, St. Louis, Missouri 63110

Vicks Health Care, Div. of Richardson Vicks Inc., One Far Mill Crossing, Shelton, Connecticut 06484 (203/925-7701)

VioBin Corporation, Subsidiary of A.H. Robins Company, 226 W. Livingston Street, Monticello, Illinois 61856

Viratek/ICN Pharmaceuticals, 3300 Hyland Avenue, Costa Mesa, California 92627 (714/540-1866)

Vitaline Formulas, 722 Jefferson Avenue, Ashland, OR 97520 (800/648-4755; fax 503/482-9231)

VLI Corp., 2031 Main Street, Irvine, California 92714

Vortech Pharmaceuticals, Ltd., P.O. Box 189, Dearborn, Michigan 48121 (313/584-4088; 800/521-4686)

Waksman Institute, Rutgers University, New Brunswick, New Jersey 08903

Wallace Laboratories, Div. of Carter-Wallace, Inc., P.O. Box 1001, Half-Acre Road, Cranbury, New Jersey 08512 (609/655-6000)

Warner-Chilcott Laboratories, Div. Park-Davis Group/Warner Lambert Company, 182 Tabor Road, Morris Plains, New Jersey 07950 (201/540-2000; 800/521-8813; fax 201/540-3283)

Warner-Lambert Company, Parke Davis Division, 201 Tabor Road, Morris Plains, New Jersey 07950 (201/540-2000); (fax 201/540-3283)

Webcon Pharmaceuticals Division, Alcon Laboratories, Inc., 6201 South Freeway T4-4, Fort Worth, Texas 76134-2099 (817/293-0450)

West Chemical Products, Inc., 1855 S. Mt. Prospect Road, Des Plaines, Illinois 60618

Westwood Squibb Pharmaceuticals, Inc., Division of Bristol-Myers Squibb, 100 Forest Avenue, Buffalo, New York 14213 (716/887-3400)

Wharton Laboratories, Inc., 500 Arcola Road, Collegeville, PA 19426-2911 (215/454-8000)

Whitehall Laboratories, Div. of American Home Products Corp., 685 Third Avenue, New York, New York 10017-4076 (800/343-0856; 212/878-5500)

Willen Drug Company, 18 N. High Street, Baltimore, Maryland 21202 (301/752-1865)

The J.B. Williams Company, Inc., 750 Walnut Avenue, Cranford, New Jersey 07016

Wyeth-Ayerst Laboratories, Division of American Home Products Corp., 150 Radnor-Chester Rd., Location A-1, St. Davids, Pennsylvania 19087 (215/688-4400; 800/590-5099)

W.F. Young, Inc., 111 Lyman Street, Springfield, Massachusetts 01101 (413/737-0201)

Xoma Corp., 2910 Seventh Street, Berkeley, California 94710 (415/644-1170)

Youngs Drug Products Corporation, 865 Centennial Avenue, Piscataway, New Jersey 08854

ZENECA Pharmaceuticals Group, Division of ICI Americas Inc., Concord Pike and Murphy Road, Wilmington, Delaware 19897 (302/886-3000; 800/822-8215; fax: 302/886-3119)

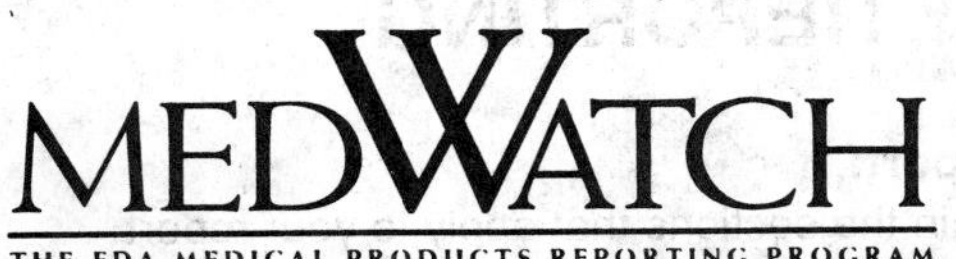

For VOLUNTARY reporting by health professionals of adverse events and product problems

Form Approved: OMB No. 0910-0291 Expires: 12/31/94
See OMB statement on reverse

FDA Use Only (AMA)

Triage unit sequence #

Page ____ of ____

A. Patient information

1. **Patient identifier** In confidence
2. **Age at time of event:** or **Date of birth:**
3. **Sex** ☐ female ☐ male
4. **Weight** ____ lbs or ____ kgs

B. Adverse event or product problem

1. ☐ **Adverse event** and/or ☐ **Product problem** (e.g., defects/malfunctions)
2. **Outcomes attributed to adverse event** (check all that apply)
   - ☐ death ________ (mo/day/yr)
   - ☐ life-threatening
   - ☐ hospitalization – initial or prolonged
   - ☐ disability
   - ☐ congenital anomaly
   - ☐ required intervention to prevent permanent impairment/damage
   - ☐ other: ________
3. **Date of event** (mo/day/yr)
4. **Date of this report** (mo/day/yr)
5. **Describe event or problem**
6. **Relevant tests/laboratory data**, including dates
7. **Other relevant history, including preexisting medical conditions** (e.g., allergies, race, pregnancy, smoking and alcohol use, hepatic/renal dysfunction, etc.)

C. Suspect medication(s)

1. **Name** (give labeled strength & mfr/labeler, if known)
   #1
   #2
2. **Dose, frequency & route used**
   #1
   #2
3. **Therapy dates** (if unknown, give duration) from/to (or best estimate)
   #1
   #2
4. **Diagnosis for use** (indication)
   #1
   #2
5. **Event abated after use stopped or dose reduced**
   #1 ☐ yes ☐ no ☐ doesn't apply
   #2 ☐ yes ☐ no ☐ doesn't apply
6. **Lot #** (if known)
   #1
   #2
7. **Exp. date** (if known)
   #1
   #2
8. **Event reappeared after reintroduction**
   #1 ☐ yes ☐ no ☐ doesn't apply
   #2 ☐ yes ☐ no ☐ doesn't apply
9. **NDC #** (for product problems only)
   – –
10. **Concomitant medical products** and therapy dates (exclude treatment of event)

D. Suspect medical device

1. **Brand name**
2. **Type of device**
3. **Manufacturer name & address**
4. **Operator of device**
   - ☐ health professional
   - ☐ lay user/patient
   - ☐ other: ________
5. **Expiration date** (mo/day/yr)
6. model # ________
   catalog # ________
   serial # ________
   lot # ________
   other #
7. **If implanted, give date** (mo/day/yr)
8. **If explanted, give date** (mo/day/yr)
9. **Device available for evaluation?** (Do not send to FDA)
   ☐ yes ☐ no ☐ returned to manufacturer on ________ (mo/day/yr)
10. **Concomitant medical products** and therapy dates (exclude treatment of event)

E. Reporter (see confidentiality section on back)

1. **Name, address & phone #**
2. **Health professional?** ☐ yes ☐ no
3. **Occupation**
4. **Also reported to**
   - ☐ manufacturer
   - ☐ user facility
   - ☐ distributor
5. **If you do NOT want your identity disclosed to the manufacturer, place an " X " in this box.** ☐

FDA

Mail to: MEDWATCH
5600 Fishers Lane
Rockville, MD 20852-9787

or **FAX to:**
1-800-FDA-0178

FDA Form 3500 (6/93)

Submission of a report does not constitute an admission that medical personnel or the product caused or contributed to the event.

ADVICE ABOUT VOLUNTARY REPORTING

Report experiences with:

- medications (drugs or biologics)
- medical devices (including in-vitro diagnostics)
- special nutritional products (dietary supplements, medical foods, infant formulas)
- other products regulated by FDA

Report SERIOUS adverse events. An event is serious when the patient outcome is:

- death
- life-threatening (real risk of dying)
- hospitalization (initial or prolonged)
- disability (significant, persistent or permanent)
- congenital anomaly
- required intervention to prevent permanent impairment or damage

Report even if:

- you're not certain the product caused the event
- you don't have all the details

Report product problems – quality, performance or safety concerns such as:

- suspected contamination
- questionable stability
- defective components
- poor packaging or labeling

How to report:

- just fill in the sections that apply to your report
- use section C for all products except medical devices
- attach additional blank pages if needed
- use a separate form for each patient
- report either to FDA or the manufacturer (or both)

Important numbers:

- 1-800-FDA-0178 to FAX report
- 1-800-FDA-7737 to report by modem
- 1-800-FDA-1088 for more information or to report quality problems
- 1-800-822-7967 for a VAERS form for vaccines

If your report involves a serious adverse event with a device and it occurred in a facility outside a doctor's office, that facility may be legally required to report to FDA and/or the manufacturer. Please notify the person in that facility who would handle such reporting.

Confidentiality: The patient's identity is held in strict confidence by FDA and protected to the fullest extent of the law. The reporter's identity may be shared with the manufacturer unless requested otherwise. However, FDA will not disclose the reporter's identity in response to a request from the public, pursuant to the Freedom of Information Act.

The public reporting burden for this collection of information has been estimated to average 30 minutes per response, including the time for reviewing instructions, searching existing data sources, gathering and maintaining the data needed, and completing and reviewing the collection of information. Send your comments regarding this burden estimate or any other aspect of this collection of information, including suggestions for reducing this burden to:

Reports Clearance Officer, PHS
Hubert H. Humphrey Building, Room 721-B
200 Independence Avenue, S.W.
Washington, DC 20201
ATTN: PRA

and to:
Office of Management and Budget
Paperwork Reduction Project (0910-0230)
Washington, DC 20503

Please do NOT return this form to either of these addresses.

FDA Form 3500-back

Please Use Address Provided Below – Just Fold In Thirds, Tape and Mail

Department of Health and Human Services
Public Health Service
Food and Drug Administration
Rockville, MD 20857

Official Business
Penalty for Private Use $300

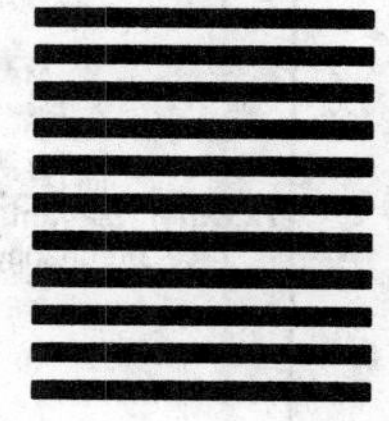
NO POSTAGE
NECESSARY
IF MAILED
IN THE
UNITED STATES
OR APO/FPO

BUSINESS REPLY MAIL

FIRST CLASS MAIL PERMIT NO. 946 ROCKVILLE, MD

POSTAGE WILL BE PAID BY FOOD AND DRUG ADMINISTRATION

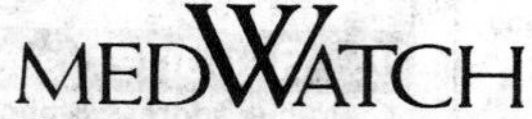
MEDWATCH

The FDA Medical Products Reporting Program
Food and Drug Administration
5600 Fishers Lane
Rockville, MD 20852-9787

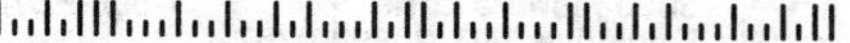